Tintinalli's Emergency Medicine

A Comprehensive Study Guide

NOTICE

Medicine is an ever-changing science. As new research and clinical experience broaden our knowledge, changes in treatment and drug therapy are required. The authors and the publisher of this work have checked with sources believed to be reliable in their efforts to provide information that is complete and generally in accord with the clinical practices accepted at the time of publication. However, in view of the possibility of human error or changes in medical sciences, neither the authors nor the publisher nor any other party who has been involved in the preparation or publication of this work warrants that the information contained herein is in every respect accurate or complete, and they disclaim all responsibility for any errors or omissions or for the results obtained from use of the information contained in this work. Readers are encouraged to confirm the information contained herein with other sources. For example and in particular, readers are advised to check the product information sheet included in the package of each drug they plan to administer to be certain that the information contained in this work is accurate and that changes have not been made in the recommended dose or in the contraindications for administration. This recommendation is of particular importance in connection with new or infrequently used drugs.

Tintinalli's Emergency Medicine

A Comprehensive Study Guide

Eighth Edition

Editor-in-Chief

Judith E. Tintinalli, MD, MS
Professor and Chair Emeritus
Department of Emergency Medicine
Adjunct Professor
Department of Health Policy and Administration
Adjunct Professor
School of Journalism and Mass Communications
University of North Carolina
Chapel Hill, North Carolina

Co-Editors

J. Stephan Stapczynski, MD
Professor, Department of Emergency Medicine
University of Arizona College of Medicine - Phoenix
Phoenix, Arizona

O. John Ma, MD
Professor and Chair
Department of Emergency Medicine
Oregon Health & Science University
Portland, Oregon

Donald M. Yealy, MD
Chair, Department of Emergency Medicine
University of Pittsburgh/University of Pittsburgh Physicians
Senior Medical Director, Health Services Division, UPMC
Professor of Emergency Medicine, Medicine, and Clinical and Translational Sciences
University of Pittsburgh School of Medicine
Pittsburgh, Pennsylvania

Garth D. Meckler, MD, MSHS
Associate Professor and Division Head
Pediatric Emergency Medicine
University of British Columbia/BC Children's Hospital
Vancouver, British Columbia

David M. Cline, MD
Professor and Director of Departmental Research
Department of Emergency Medicine
Wake Forest School of Medicine
Winston-Salem, North Carolina

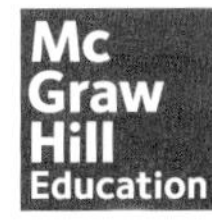

New York Chicago San Francisco Athens London Madrid Mexico City
Milan New Delhi Singapore Sydney Toronto

TINTINALLI'S EMERGENCY MEDICINE: A Comprehensive Study Guide, Eighth edition

1 2 3 4 5 6 7 8 9 0 DOW/DOW 20 19 18 17 16 15

ISBN 978-0-07-179476-3
MHID 0-07-179476-X

This book was set in Minion by Cenveo® Publisher Services
The Editors were Brian Belval and Christie Naglieri
The Production Supervisor was Catherine Saggese.
The Illustration manager was Armen Ovsepyan.
Project Management was provided by Yashmita Hota, Cenveo Publisher Services.
Cover Photo: BKFox, TarpanGroupLLC, used with permission.
RR Donnelley was printer and binder.

This book is printed on acid-free paper.

Library of Congress Cataloging-in-Publication Data

Tintinalli's emergency medicine : a comprehensive study guide/editor-in-chief,
Judith E. Tintinalli ; co-editors, J. Stephan Stapczynski, O. John Ma, Donald M. Yealy,
Garth D. Meckler, David M. Cline.—Eighth edition.
p. ; cm.
Emergency medicine
Includes bibliographical references and index.
ISBN 978-0-07-179476-3 (hardcover : alk. paper)—ISBN 0-07-179476-X
(hardcover : alk. paper)
I. Tintinalli, Judith E., editor. II. Stapczynski, J. Stephan, editor. III. Ma, O. John, editor.
IV. Yealy, Donald M., editor. V. Meckler, Garth D., editor. VI. Cline, David, editor.
VII. Title: Emergency medicine.
[DNLM: 1. Emergency Medicine. 2. Emergencies. WB 105]
RC86.7
616.02′5—dc23

2015030053

To the clinicians, residents, medical students, NPs, PAs, EMTs, and paramedics who provide emergency care around the world.

Judith E. Tintinalli, MD, MS

Co-Editors

Dedicated with love and respect to my father and father-in-law, two veterans from the Greatest Generation, on the 70th anniversary of the end of World War II.

J. Stephan Stapczynski, MD

For my parents: my mother, Simone, for her continued love and support, and in loving memory of my father, Mark.

O. John Ma, MD

I thank: My family, who always believe in me and make this all possible; my partners, who bring excellence to my eyes each day; and those seeking emergency care, trusting that all will be well.

Donald M. Yealy, MD

To the patients, nurses, students, and mentors who teach me every day, and to my family and partner for their love and support.

Garth D. Meckler, MD, MSHS

To my family, mentors, residents, and students who continue to give meaning to this work.

David M. Cline, MD

Contents

About the Video

To access the collection of more than 50 emergency medicine videos, please scan the QR code above or visit www.tintinalliem.com. The password to access videos is **tem8**

Contributors

Benjamin S. Abella, MD, MPhil, FACEP [26]
Department of Emergency Medicine and Center for Resuscitation Science
University of Pennsylvania
Philadelphia, Pennsylvania

Kathleen Adelgais, MD, MPH [137]
Associate Professor, Pediatrics
Pediatric Emergency Medicine
Department of Pediatrics
University of Colorado School of Medicine
Aurora, Colorado

Srikar Adhikari, MD, MS [241]
Associate Professor of Emergency Medicine
University of Arizona
Chief, Emergency Ultrasound Section
University of Arizona Medical Center
Tucson, Arizona

Dewesh Agrawal, MD [120]
Associate Professor of Pediatrics and Emergency Medicine
George Washington University School of Medicine
Director, Pediatric Residency Program
Children's National Medical Center
Washington, DC

William D. Alley, MD [54]
Assistant Professor
Department of Emergent Medicine
Wake Forest Baptist Medical Center
Winston-Salem, North Carolina

Mohammed Al Mogbil, MD [144]
Consultant
Pediatric Emergency Medicine
Department of Emergency Medicine
King Faisal Specialist Hospital and Research Center
Riyadh, Kingdom of Saudi Arabia

Mohammed A. Alsultan, PharmD, PhD [4]
Associate Professor of Emergency Medicine and Critical Care
College of Medicine
King Saud bin Abdulaziz University for Health Sciences (KSA-HS)
Riyadh, Kingdom of Saudi Arabia

Eric Anderson, MD, MBA, FACEP, FAAEM [65,66]
Cleveland Clinic Emergency Department
Faculty Cleveland Clinic Lerner College of Medicine at Case Western Reserve University
Faculty Cleveland Clinic Metro Health Emergency Medicine Residency Program
Cleveland, Ohio

Phillip Andrus, MD, FACEP [172]
Assistant Professor of Emergency Medicine
Mount Sinai School of Medicine
Attending Physician
The Mount Sinai Hospital
New York City, New York

Arash Armin, DO, FACOEP [74]
Associate Clinical Professor
Michigan State University
College of Osteopathic Medicine
Medical Director and Core Faculty
Department of Emergency Medicine
Beaumont Trenton-Southshore Campus
Trenton, Michigan

Kim Askew, MD [91]
Associate Professor
Department of Emergency Medicine
Wake Forest School of Medicine
Winston-Salem, North Carolina

Peter S. Auerbach, MD [114]
Adjunct Assistant Professor of Emergency Medicine
Oregon Health & Science University
Pediatric Emergency Medicine Fellowship Site Director
Randall Children's Hospital at Legacy Emanuel
Portland, Oregon

Caitlin Bailey, MD [218]
Attending Physician, Highland Hospital-Alameda Health System
Oakland, California
Assistant Clinical Professor
UCSF School of Medicine
San Francisco, California

John Bailitz, MD [259]
Emergency Ultrasound Division Director
Cook County Hospital
Associate Professor of Emergency Medicine
Rush University Medical School
Chicago, Illinois

Joseph A. Barbera, MD [9]
Associate Professor of Engineering Management and Systems Engineering
Clinical Associate Professor of Emergency Medicine
The George Washington University
Washington, DC

Ciara J. Barclay-Buchanan, MD [102, 272]
Clinical Assistant Professor
Wayne State University
Associate Program Director, Emergency Medicine Residency Program
Sinai-Grace Hospital/Detroit Medical Center
Tenet Health System
Detroit, Michigan

Kristen Barrio, MD [288]
Geriatric Emergency Medicine Fellow
Clinical Instructor
Department of Emergency Medicine
University of North Carolina
Chapel Hill, North Carolina

Melissa A. Barton, MD [102, 272]
Clinical Assistant Professor
Wayne State University
Program Director, Emergency Medicine Residency Program
Sinai-Grace Hospital/Detroit Medical Center
Tenet Health System
Detroit, Michigan

Craig G. Bates, MD, MS, FACEP [70]
Assistant Professor of Emergency Medicine
Case Western Reserve University School of Medicine
Faculty, Department of Emergency Medicine
MetroHealth Medical Center
Medical Director, Metro Life Flight
Assistant Medical Director, Department of Public Safety at City of Cleveland
Cleveland, Ohio

Brigitte M. Baumann, MD, MSCE [57, 58]
Associate Professor of Emergency Medicine
Head, Division of Clinical Research
Cooper Medical School of Rowan University
Camden, New Jersey

Ashley S. Bean, MD, MA, FACEP, FAAEM [260]
Associate Professor
Department of Emergency Medicine
Adjunct Faculty, Division of Academic Affairs
Office of Global Health
University of Arkansas for Medical Sciences
Little Rock, Arkansas

Ronald W. Beaudreau, DMD, MD [245]
Shanghai United Family Hospital and Clinics
Department of Emergency Medicine
Attending Emergency Physician
Shanghai, People's Republic of China

Solomon Behar, MD [139]
Assistant Professor of Emergency Medicine and Pediatrics
LAC+USC Medical Center and Children's Hospital Los Angeles
Keck School of Medicine, University of Southern California
Los Angeles, California

Rachel R. Bengtzen, MD [274]
Assistant Professor
Department of Emergency Medicine
Department of Family Medicine (Sports Medicine)
Oregon Health & Science University
Portland, Oregon

Edward Bernstein, MD [292]
Professor of Emergency Medicine
Vice Chair for Academic Affairs
Department of Emergency Medicine, Boston University School of Medicine
Professor of Community Health Sciences, Co-Director of the BNI ART Institute
Boston University School of Public Health
Boston, Massachusetts

Judith A. Bernstein, RNC, PhD [292]
Professor of Community Health Sciences, Co-Director of the BNI-ART Institute
Boston University School of Public Health
Professor of Emergency Medicine
Department of Emergency Medicine
Boston University School of Medicine
Boston, Massachusetts

Bart Besinger, MD, FAAEM [79]
Assistant Professor of Clinical Emergency Medicine
Department of Emergency Medicine
Indiana University School of Medicine
Indianapolis, Indiana

Rachna Bhandari, MD, PhD [253]
Resident, University of North Carolina
Chapel Hill, North Carolina

Kevin Biese, MD, MAT [288]
Associate Professor
Department of Emergency Medicine and Department of Internal Medicine, Division of Geriatrics
University of North Carolina
Chapel Hill, North Carolina

Lars Petter Bjoernsen, MD, FACEP [271]
Clinical Assistant Professor, Emergency Medicine
The University of Wisconsin School of Medicine & Public Health
Madison, Wisconsin
Department of Emergency Medicine, St. Olav's Hospital
Trondheim, Norway

Karen J. L. Black, MD, MSc [140]
British Columbia Children's Hospital
Vancouver, British Columbia

Tyler R. Black, BSc, MD, FRCPC [147]
Medical Director
CAPE Unit, BC Children's Hospital
Assistant Clinical Professor, Department of Psychiatry
University of British Columbia
Vancouver, British Columbia

Bentley J. Bobrow, MD, FACEP [26]
Department of Emergency Medicine
Maricopa Medical Center
University of Arizona College of Medicine
Phoenix, Arizona

Andy Boggust, MD [2]
Instructor in Emergency Medicine
College of Medicine
Mayo Clinic
Rochester, Minnesota

Angela Bogle, MD [78]
Assistant Professor
Emergency Medicine
University of Missouri Kansas City School of Medicine
Truman Medical Center, Kansas
Kansas City, Missouri

Gary Bonfante, DO, FACOEP, FACEP [141]
Clinical Professor of Medicine
The Commonwealth Medical College
Scranton, Pennsylvania
Department of Emergency Medicine
Lehigh Valley Health Network
Allentown, Pennsylvania

Michael J. Bono, MD [7]
Vice Chair
Department of Emergency Medicine
Eastern Virginia Medical School
Norfolk, Virginia

Susan Bork, MD [72]
Associate Residency Director
Department of Emergency Medicine
William Beaumont Hospital
Royal Oak, Michigan

Nicole C. Bouchard, MD, FRCPC [200]
Assistant Clinical Professor of Medicine
Assistant Site Director, Adult Emergency Medicine
Director of Medical Toxicology
New York-Presbyterian Hospital
Columbia University
New York City, New York

Edith V. Bowers, MD [252]
Department of Dermatology
University of North Carolina
Chapel Hill, North Carolina

Stephen H. Boyce, MBChB, FRCS(A&E), FIMC, FRCEM, MSc (Sports Medicine), Dip SEM, FFSEM [301]
Consultant in Emergency Medicine, Glasgow Royal Infirmary
Glasgow, Scotland

William J. Brady, MD [18, 248, 249]
Professor of Emergency Medicine & the David A. Harrison Distinguished Educator
Medical Director, Emergency Preparedness and Response
University of Virginia School of Medicine
Operational Medical Director, Albemarle County Fire Rescue
Charlottesville, Virginia

Anne F. Brayer, MD [219]
Professor of Emergency Medicine and Pediatrics
University of Rochester School of Medicine
Rochester, New York

Daniel E. Brooks, MD [192]
Associate Professor
Departments of Internal Medicine and Emergency Medicine,
University of Arizona College of Medicine – Phoenix
Phoenix, Arizona

Kara Luersen Brooks, MD [251]
University of North Carolina
Department of Dermatology
University of North Carolina
Chapel Hill, North Carolina

Eric J. Brown, MD, MS [34]
Staff Physician
Department of Emergency Medicine
St. John Medical Center
Tulsa, Oklahoma

Doug Brown, MD, FRCPC [209]
Emergency Physician
Royal Columbian Hospital
Clinical Instructor
UBC Department of Emergency Medicine
Vancouver, British Columbia

Brian E. Burgess, PT, MD, FACEP, FAAEM [85]
Assistant Professor of Emergency Medicine
Jefferson Medical College
Philadelphia, Pennsylvania
Assistant Residency Director
Emergency Medicine Residency Program
Christiana Care Health System
Wilmington, Delaware

Guillermo Burillo-Putze, MD, PhD [192, 207]
Emergency Department
Hospital Universitario de Canarias and Associated Professor
Department of Pharmacology, Universidad de La Laguna
Tenerife, Spain

Boyd Burns, DO, FACEP, FAAEM [25]
Assistant Professor
Department of Emergency Medicine
University of Oklahoma School of Community Medicine
Tulsa, Oklahoma

John Burton, MD [284]
Chair
Department of Emergency Medicine
Carilion Clinic
Virginia Tech Carilion School of Medicine
Roanoke, Virginia

Alia Busuttil [124]
Queen's School of Medicine
Kingston, Ontario

Donald Byars, MD [84]
Associate Professor
Department of Emergency Medicine
Eastern Virginia Medical School
Norfolk, Virginia

Derya Caglar, MD [121]
Assistant Professor
Department of Pediatrics
University of Washington, School of Medicine
Attending Physician
Division of Emergency Medicine, Seattle Children's Hospital
Seattle, Washington

J. Hayes Calvert, MD [297]
Clinical Affiliate
Wake Forest School of Medicine
Winston-Salem, North Carolina

Peter Cameron, MBBS, MD, FACEM, FIFEM [254]
Professor Emergency and Trauma Centre
The Alfred Hospital
Melbourne, Australia

Donna L. Carden, MD [156]
Professor
Director of Faculty Development
Department of Emergency Medicine
University of Florida College of Medicine
Gainesville, Florida

Jestin N. Carlson, MD [28]
Department of Emergency Medicine Saint Vincent Health System
Erie, Pennsylvania
Department of Emergency Medicine, University of Pittsburgh School of Medicine
Pittsburgh, Pennsylvania

Michele Carney, MD [143]
Assistant Professor, Pediatric Emergency Medicine
Director, Pediatric Emergency Medicine Fellowship
Department of Emergency Medicine
Children's Emergency Services
Ann Arbor, Michigan

David Carr, MD, CCFP, EM [61]
Assistant Director of Risk Management and Faculty Development
University Health Network
Assistant Professor
Department of Family and Community Medicine
Toronto, Ontario

Wallace A. Carter, MD [40, 191, 200, 206]
Program Director, Emergency Medicine Residency
Senior Associate Medical Director, Emergency Medical Services
New York Presbyterian
White Plains, New York
Associate Professor of Emergency Medicine in Medicine
Weill Cornell Medical College
Associate Professor of Clinical Medicine
Columbia University College of Physicians & Surgeons
New York City, New York

Melissa Chan, MD, FRCPC (PEM) [129]
Division of Pediatric Emergency Medicine
Department of Pediatrics
University of Alberta
Edmonton, Alberta

Michael E. Chansky, MD [225]
Chair
Department of Emergency Medicine
Associate Professor of Emergency Medicine and Internal Medicine
Cooper Medical School of Rowan University
Adjunct Associate Professor of Emergency Medicine and Internal Medicine
UMDNJ/Robert Wood Johnson Medical School
Cooper University Hospital
Camden, New Jersey

Betty C. Chen, MD [220]
Acting Instructor, Division of Emergency Medicine, University of Washington School of Medicine
Attending Physician, Harborview Medical Center
Seattle, Washington

Anil Chopra, MD, FRCP, DABEM [61]
Head and Medical Director, Emergency Medicine
University Health Network
Associate Professor, Department of Medicine
Toronto, Ontario

Yvonne C. Chow, MD [270]
Assistant Professor of Emergency Medicine and Internal Medicine
Associate Residency Program Director
Department of Emergency Medicine
Albany Medical College
Albany, New York

Stephen John Cico, MD, MEd, FAAEM, FAAP [215, 232]
Associate Professor of Pediatrics
University of South Dakota Sanford School of Medicine
Attending Physician, Pediatric Emergency Medicine
Sanford USD Medical Center and Sanford Children's Hospital
Sioux Falls, South Dakota

Richard F. Clark, MD [211]
Professor of Emergency Medicine
Director, Division of Medical Toxicology
UCSD School of Medicine
San Diego, California

Michelle S. Clarke, MD, FRCP(C) [148]
Clinical Instructor
Division of Emergency Medicine, Department of Pediatrics, University of British Columbia
Child Protection Service Unit, British Columbia Children's Hospital
Vancouver, British Columbia

Ilene Claudius, MD [115, 138, 142]
Associate Professor
Emergency Medicine
USC, Keck School of Medicine
Los Angeles, California

David M. Cline, MD [15]
Professor and Director of Departmental Research
Department of Emergency Medicine
Wake Forest School of Medicine
Winston-Salem, North Carolina

Wendy C. Coates, MD [42]
Professor of Medicine
UCLA David Geffen School of Medicine
Senior Education Specialist
Harbor-UCLA Emergency Medicine
Torrance, California

Daniel J. Cobaugh, Pharm D, DABAT, FAACT [181]
Vice President
ASHP Research and Education Foundation
Bethesda, Maryland

Joanna S. Cohen, MD [120]
Assistant Professor of Pediatrics and Emergency Medicine
George Washington University School of Medicine
Children's National Medical Center
Washington, DC

Jennifer P. Cohen, MD [185]
Attending Emergency Physician
Mt Graham Regional Medical Center
Safford, Arizona
Attending Toxicologist
Banner-University Medical Center
Tucson, Arizona

Clinton J. Coil, MD, MPH, FACEP [238]
Assistant Clinical Professor of Medicine
Patient Safety Officer
Harbor-UCLA Medical Center
Torrance, California

Margaret Colbourne, MD, FRCP(C) [148]
Clinical Associate Professor
Department of Pediatrics, University of British Columbia
Director, Child Protection Service Unit, British Columbia Children's Hospital
Vancouver, British Columbia

Marc F. Collin, MD [109]
Associate Professor of Pediatrics
Medical Director, Neonatal Intensive Care Unit
MetroHealth Medical Center
Case Western Reserve University
Cleveland, Ohio

Sean P. Collins, MD, MSc [53]
Associate Vice Chair for Research
Department of Emergency Medicine
Vanderbilt University
Nashville, Tennessee

Alessandra Conforto, MD [138, 142]
Assistant Professor of Clinical Emergency Medicine
Keck School of Medicine of USC
University of Southern California
Los Angeles, California

Carmen Coombs, MD, MPH [118]
Assistant Clinical Professor
Division of Emergency Medicine
Seattle Children's Hospital
Seattle, Washington

Joseph Copeland, MD, CCFP-EM, FCFP [125]
Clinical Assistant Professor
Department of Emergency Medicine
University of British Columbia/BC Children's Hospital
Vancouver, British Columbia

Francis L. Counselman, MD, FACEP [89]
Distinguished Professor of Emergency Medicine
Department of Emergency Medicine
Eastern Virginia Medical School
Emergency Physicians of Tidewater
Norfolk, Virginia

Rita K. Cydulka, MD, MS, FACEP [69,70]
Professor, Emergency Medicine
Case Western Reserve University School of Medicine
Faculty, Department of Emergency Medicine
MetroHealth Medical Center
Cleveland, Ohio

Shawn M. D'Andrea, MD, MPH [161]
Instructor of Emergency Medicine
Harvard Medical School
Attending Physician
Brigham and Women's Hospital
Boston, Massachusetts

Kevin W. Dahle, MD [250]
Department of Dermatology
University of North Carolina
Chapel Hill, North Carolina

Dan Danzl, MD, FACEP [29]
Professor and Chair
Department of Emergency Medicine
University of Louisville
Louisville, Kentucky

Richard C. Dart, MD, PhD [212]
Director, Rocky Mountain Poison and Drug Center
Denver Health and Hospital Authority
Denver, Colorado

Moira Davenport, MD [43, 268]
Associate Professor of Emergency Medicine, Associate Emergency Medicine Residency Director
Allegheny General Hospital
Temple University School of Medicine
Pittsburgh, Pennsylvania

Jonathan E. Davis, MD [93]
Program Director
Georgetown University Hospital/Washington Hospital Center Emergency Medicine Residency
Associate Professor
Department of Emergency Medicine
Georgetown University School of Medicine
Washington, DC

Christopher B. Davis [221]
Assistant Professor of Emergency Medicine
University of Colorado School of Medicine
Aurora, Colorado

E. Paul DeKoning, MD, MS [81, 216]
Assistant Residency Director
Assistant Professor of Emergency Medicine
Dartmouth-Hitchcock Medical Center
The Geisel School of Medicine at Dartmouth
Lebanon, New Hampshire

David Della-Giustina, MD, FACEP, FAWM [279, 280]
Associate Professor of Emergency Medicine
Program Director of Emergency Medicine Residency
Chief of Education Section
Department of Emergency Medicine
Yale School of Medicine
New Haven, Connecticut

Nicole M. Delorio, MD [256]
Professor and Co-chief, Education Section, Department of Emergency Medicine
Assistant Dean, Student Affairs, Undergraduate Medical Education
Oregon Health and Science University
Portland, Oregon

H. Scott Derstine, MD [272]
Clinical Assistant Professor, Wayne State University
Assistant Program Director, Emergency Medicine Residency Program
Sinai-Grace Hospital/Detroit Medical Center
Tenet Health System
Detroit, Michigan

Tracy M. DeSelm, MD [289]
Assistant Professor
Department of Emergency Medicine
UNC School of Medicine Academic Advisor
University of North Carolina
Chapel Hill, North Carolina

Alicia Devine, MD [264]
Assistant Professor
Eastern Virginia Medical School
Norfolk, Virginia

John J. Devlin, MD [213]
Emergency Medicine, Naval Medical Center
Emergency Physicians of Tidewater
Virginia Beach, Virginia

Deborah B. Diercks, MD, MSc [49]
Professor and Chair, Department of Emergency Medicine
University of Texas Southwestern Medical Center

Douglas Dillon, MD [36]
Associate Professor Emergency Medicine
University of Utah
Park City, Utah

Jeffrey Ditkoff, MD [72]
Director of Operations
Department of Emergency Medicine
William Beaumont Hospital
Royal Oak, Michigan

Laurie Ann Dixon, MD, MPH [237]
Emergency Medicine
Emergency Physicians Medical Group
St. Joseph Mercy Hospital Ann Arbor/Livingston
Ann Arbor, Michigan

Andrew Dixon, MD, FRCPC [119, 127, 134]
Program Director-Pediatric Emergency Medicine Residency, Assistant Professor Division of Pediatric Emergency Medicine Department of Pediatrics, University of Alberta
Edmonton, Alberta

Quynh H. Doan, MDCM, MHSc, FRCPC [114, 147]
Clinical Assistant Professor
UBC Pediatrics, Division of Pediatric Emergency,
Clinician Scientist Child and Family Research Institute,
University of British Columbia
Vancouver, British Columbia

Gail D'Onofrio, MD, MS [292]
Professor of Emergency Medicine; and Chair, Department of Emergency Medicine
Yale School of Medicine
New Haven, Connecticut

Jeffrey S. Dubin, MD, MBA [279]
Associate Professor of Clinical Emergency Medicine
Vice-Chair, Department of Emergency Medicine
Washington Hospital Center
Washington, DC

James Ducharme, MD, CM, FRCP [35]
Clinical Professor
Department of Medicine
McMaster University
Hamilton, Ontario

Catherine Duffy, MD, FRCS [140]
Belfast Health and Social Care Trust
Musgrave Park Hospital
Belfast, Northern Ireland

Amy Lewis Dunn, DO, MPH [141]
Attending Physician, Department of Emergency Medicine
Section of Pediatric Emergency Medicine
Lehigh Valley Health Network
Allentown, Pennsylvania

Alexander Ebinger, MD [271]
Assistant Professor, Emergency Medicine, University of Colorado School of Medicine
Aurora, Colorado

Paul Enarson, MD, PhD, FRCPC (PEM) [129]
Division of Emergency Medicine, Department of Pediatrics
University of British Columbia
Vancouver, British Columbia

Jennifer L. Englund, MD [200]
Attending Physician, Department of Emergency Medicine
HealthEast Care System
Maplewood, Minnesota
Toxicology Consultant, Minnesota Poison Control System
Minneapolis, Minnesota

Robert Escarza, MD [269]
Associate Clinical Professor
Department of Surgery
University of Illinois College of Medicine at Rockford
Rockford Memorial Hospital
Rockford, Illinois

Brenna M. Farmer, MD [207]
Assistant Professor of Medicine
Attending Physician
Division of Emergency Medicine
Weill-Cornell College of Medicine/New York Presbyterian Hospital
New York City, New York

Ana Felix, MD [165]
Assistant Professor, Adult Neurology
University of North Carolina School of Medicine
Chapel Hill, North Carolina

Ross J. Fleischman, MD [130, 255]
Assistant Professor
Department of Emergency Medicine
Oregon Health & Science University
Portland, Oregon

Heather Miller Fleming, MD [97]
Assistant Professor of Clinical Emergency Medicine and Pediatrics
Assistant Program Director
Indiana University
Indianapolis, Indiana

Ninfa Mehta, MD [90]
Associate Medical Director SUNY Downstate
Ultrasound Fellowship Director SUNY Downstate/Kings County Hospital
Emergency Department
SUNY Downstate Hospital, Kings County Emergency Department
Brooklyn, New York

Timothy J. Fortuna, DO [284]
Assistant Professor
Associate Program Director, Emergency Medicine
Virginia Tech Carilion School of Medicine
Roanoke, Virginia

Sarah Elisabeth Frasure, MD [100]
Department of Emergency Medicine
Brigham and Women's Hospital
Boston, Massachusetts

Stephen Freedman, MDCM, MSc, FAAP, FRCPC [128]
Alberta Children's Hospital Foundation Professor in Child Health and Wellness
Associate Professor of Pediatrics
Department of Pediatrics
Sections of Pediatric Emergency Medicine and Gastroenterology
Alberta Children's Hospital
Alberta Children's Hospital Research Institute
Cumming School of Medicine, University of Calgary
Calgary, Alberta

Loren K. French, MD [263, 265]
Assistant Professor
Emergency Department
Oregon Health & Science University
Portland, Oregon

Adam D. Friedlander, MD [22]
Chief Resident, Combined Residency in Emergency Medicine and Pediatrics
Department of Emergency Medicine
Department of Pediatrics
University of Maryland School of Medicine
Baltimore, Maryland

Phillip A. Friesen, DO [75]
Pediatric Emergency Medicine Fellow, The University of Texas at Austin, Dell Medical School
Austin, Texas

William Frohna, MD [279]
Professor of Clinical Emergency Medicine
Chairman, MedStar Emergency Physicians
Chairman, Department of Emergency Medicine
Washington Hospital Center
Washington, DC

Lynette Froula, MD [219]
Department of Emergency Medicine
University of Rochester Medical Center
Rochester, New York

Theodore J. Gaeta, DO, MPH [14]
Vice-chair and Program Director in Emergency Medicine
New York Methodist Hospital
Associate Professor of Emergency Medicine, in Medicine
Weill Cornell School of Medicine
West Harrison, New York

John P. Gaillard, MD [12, 247]
Assistant Professor
Department of Anesthesiology-Critical Care
Department of Emergency Medicine
Department of Internal Medicine-Pulmonary/Critical Care Wake Forest Baptist Health
Winston-Salem, North Carolina

Sarah Andrus Gaines, MD [173]
Assistant Professor
Department of Emergency Medicine
Brown University
Providence, Rhode Island

Shauna S. Garris, PharmD, BCPP, BCPS [287]
Pharmacy Clinical Specialist, Psychiatry/Neurology
UNC Healthcare
Adjunct Assistant Professor
Division of Practice Advancement and Experiential Education
UNC Eshelman School of Pharmacy
Chapel Hill, North Carolina

Kulleni Gebreyes, MD, MBA [80]
Physician Executive
Washington, DC

Carl A. Germann, MD [283]
Assistant Professor, Tufts University School of Medicine
Maine Medical Center
Portland, Maine

Chris A. Ghaemmaghami, MD [18]
Associate Professor of Emergency Medicine and Medicine
Medical Director & Vice Chair for Academics
Department of Emergency Medicine
Chief Medical Officer and Senior Associate Dean
University of Virginia School of Medicine
University of Virginia Health System
Charlottesville, Virginia

Jaylaine Ghoubrial, MD [25]
OB/GYN
Reading Hospital
West Reading, Pennsylvania

Michael A. Gibbs, MD [36]
Professor, Department of Emergency Medicine
Tufts University School of Medicine
Chief of Emergency Medicine
Department of Emergency Medicine, Maine Medical Center
Portland, Maine

Jeffrey N. Glaspy, MD [274]
Department Chief Emergency Medicine
Aurora West Allis Medical Center
ERMED, SC
Milwaukee, Wisconsin

Casey Glass, MD [16, 50]
Assistant Professor, Department of Emergency Medicine
Director of Community Emergency Ultrasound Programs
Wake Forest School of Medicine
Winston Salem, North Carolina

Jonathan Glauser, MD, MBA, FACEP [295]
Professor, Emergency Medicine
Case Western Reserve University School of Medicine
Faculty MetroHealth Medical Center
Residency Program Emergency Medicine
Cleveland, Ohio

Steven Go, MD [167, 258]
Associate Professor of Emergency Medicine
Department of Emergency Medicine
University of Missouri—Kansas City School of Medicine
Kansas City, Missouri

H. Brian Goldman, MD, FACEP, FCFP [170]
Staff Emergency Physician, Schwartz Reisman Emergency Centre
Mount Sinai Hospital
Assistant Professor, Department of Family and Community Medicine
University of Toronto
Toronto, Ontario

Stephanie Gordy, MD, FACS [263]
Assistant Professor of Surgery
Ben Taub Hospital
Baylor College of Medicine
Michael E. DeBakey Department of Surgery
Houston, Texas

Nikhil Goyal, MD [223]
EM/IM Combined Residency Director
Transitional Year Residency Director
Henry Ford Hospital
Clinical Assistant Professor, Wayne State University
Detroit, Michigan

Charles S. Graffeo, MD, ABEM-UHM [227]
Professor and Assistant Residency Director
Department of Emergency Medicine
Eastern Virginia Medical School
Norfolk, Virginia

Autumn Graham, MD [82]
Associate Program Director
Medstar Georgetown University Hospital/Medstar Washington Hospital Center
Washington, DC

Matthew C. Gratton, MD [78]
Professor and Chair, Emergency Medicine
University of Missouri, Kansas City School of Medicine
Truman Medical Center
Kansas City, Missouri

Matthew C. Gratton, MD [265]
Professor and Chair, Emergency Medicine
University of Missouri, Kansas City School of Medicine
Truman Medical Center
Kansas City, Missouri

Shaun Greene, FACEM [176]
Emergency Physician and Clinical Toxicologist
Austin Health
Melbourne, Australia

Chip Gresham, MD [182, 192, 204]
Director of Education
Department of Emergency Medicine
Middlemore Hospital
Auckland, New Zealand

Thomas Grosheider, MD [296]
Attending Physician
Tuba City Regional Care
Tuba City, Arizona

Joseph M. Grover, MD [248]
Clinical Instructor and EMS Fellow
Department of Emergency Medicine
University of North Carolina
Chapel Hill, North Carolina

Camilo E. Gutiérrez, MD [110, 143]
Assistant Professor of Pediatrics / Pediatric Emergency Medicine
Boston University School of Medicine
Boston Medical Center
Boston, Massachusetts

Peter H. Hackett, MD [221]
Clinical Professor
Department of Emergency Medicine
University of Colorado Denver School of Medicine
Aurora, Colorado
Founder and Director, Institute for Altitude Medicine
Telluride, Colorado

Jeffrey L. Hackman, MD [166]
Assistant Professor
Department of Emergency Medicine
University of Missouri-Kansas City School of Medicine
Truman Medical Center
Kansas City, Missouri

Paul Haller, MD [275, 278]
HealthPartners Medical Group
Assistant Professor
Department of Emergency Medicine
University of Minnesota
Minneapolis, Minnesota

Pinchas Halpern, MD [7]
Associate Professor of Emergency Medicine
Tel Aviv University Faculty of Medicine
Chair, Emergency Department
Tel Aviv Medical Center
Tel Aviv, Israel

Mary Hancock, MD [294]
Attending Physician
Emergency Services Institute
Cleveland Clinic
Cleveland, Ohio

Daniel A. Handel, MD, MPH [173]
Assistant Professor
Department of Emergency Medicine
Oregon Health & Science University
Portland, Oregon

Bophal Sarha Hang, MD [72, 96, 104]
Department of Emergency Medicine
William Beaumont Oakland University, School of Medicine
Rochester, Michigan

Matthew Hansen, MD [113, 188]
Assistant Professor
Department of Emergency Medicine
Oregon Health & Science University
Portland, Oregon

Michael Harrigan, MD, FACEP [165]
Assistant Professor
Department of Emergency Medicine
UNC Chapel Hill School of Medicine
Chapel Hill, North Carolina

Nicholas D. Hartman, MD, MPH [246]
Assistant Professor
Department of Emergency Medicine
Wake Forest School of Medicine
Winston-Salem, North Carolina

William E. Hauda II, MD [110]
Associate Professor of Emergency Medicine
Virginia Commonwealth University School of Medicine—Inova Campus
Assistant Professor of Pediatrics
University of Virginia School of Medicine
Falls Church, Virginia

Heather A. Heaton, MD [98]
Instructor of Emergency Medicine, Mayo Clinic College of Medicine
Department of Emergency Medicine
Mayo Clinic
Rochester, Minnesota

Tarlan Hedayati, MD [259]
Associate Program Director
Emergency Medicine Residency Program
Cook County (Stroger) Hospital
Assistant Professor
Department of Emergency Medicine
Rush University Medical Center
Chicago, Illinois

James Heilman, MD [266]
Assistant Professor
Department of Emergency Medicine
Oregon Health & Science University
Portland, Oregon

C. William Heise, MD [199]
Assistant Professor, University of Arizona College of Medicine—Phoenix Center for Toxicology and Pharmacology Education and Research Department of Medical Toxicology, Banner—University Medical Center
Phoenix, Arizona

Corey R. Heitz, MD [243]
Virginia Tech Carilion School of Medicine, Carilion Clinic Department of Emergency Medicine
Roanoke, Virginia

Robin R. Hemphill, MD [231, 232, 233, 234, 235, 237]
Veterans Health Administration
Chief Patient Safety and Risk Awareness Officer
Director, VA National Center for Patient Safety
Ann Arbor, Michigan

Robert G. Hendrickson, MD [5, 8]
Medical Director, Emergency Management
Associate Professor
Department of Emergency Medicine
Program Director, Fellowship in Medical Toxicology
Oregon Health & Science University
Associate Medical Director, Oregon Poison Center
Portland, Oregon

Melanie Heniff, MD, FACEP, FAAEM, FAAP [97]
Assistant Professor Clinical Emergency Medicine
Indiana University
Indianapolis, Indiana

Stephanie H. Hernandez, MD [198]
Icahn School of Medicine at Mount Sinai
Department of Emergency Medicine
New York City, New York

David Hile, MD [280]
Assistant Professor of Emergency Medicine
Associate Program Director of Emergency Medicine Residency
Department of Emergency Medicine
Yale School of Medicine
New Haven, Connecticut

Jon Mark Hirshon, MD [22]
Associate Professor
Department of Emergency Medicine
University of Maryland School of Medicine
University of Maryland Medical Center
Baltimore, Maryland

Cherri Hobgood, MD, FACEP [300]
Chair and Rolly McGrath Professor
Department of Emergency Medicine
Indiana University School of Medicine
Indianapolis, Indiana

Rachel Holland, PharmD, BCPS [19, 20]
Pharmacist
Emergency Department
Wake Forest Baptist Health
Department of Pharmacy
Winston-Salem, North Carolina

Judd E. Hollander, MD [39, 41, 47, 49]
Associate Dean for Strategic Health Initiatives
Vice Chair, Finance and Healthcare Enterprises
Department of Emergency Medicine
Sidney Kimmel Medical College of Thomas Jefferson University
Philadelphia, Pennsylvania

Maija Holsti, MD, MPH [135]
Associate Professor
Division of Pediatric Emergency Medicine
Department of Pediatrics
University of Utah
Salt Lake City, Utah

Edmond A. Hooker, MD [87]
Assistant Professor and Resident Research Director
Department of Emergency Medicine
University of Cincinnati
Cincinnati, Ohio

Courtney Hopkins-Mann, MD [140]
Medical Director
Children's Emergency Department
Wake Medical Center
University of North Carolina, Chapel Hill
Chapel Hill, North Carolina

B. Zane Horowitz, MD, FACMT [5, 8]
Professor
Department of Emergency Medicine
Oregon Health & Science University
Medical Director, Oregon Poison Center
Portland, Oregon

Kathleen Hosmer, MD, FACEP [51, 242]
Assistant Professor
Department of Emergency Medicine
Wake Forest University School of Medicine
Winston-Salem, North Carolina

David T. Huang, MD, MPH [32]
Associate Professor, Critical Care Medicine, Emergency Medicine, Clinical and Translational Science
Director, Multidisciplinary Acute Care Research Organization (MACRO)
University of Pittsburgh School of Medicine
Pittsburgh, Pennsylvania

J. Stephen Huff, MD [164, 168 , 169]
Associate Professor
Emergency Medicine and Neurology
Department of Emergency Medicine
University of Virginia
Charlottesville, Virginia

Caitlin M. Hughes, PharmD [287]
Assistant Professor
Department of Clinical & Administrative Sciences
Notre Dame of Maryland University School of Pharmacy
Baltimore, Maryland

Oliver L. Hung, MD [190]
Attending Physician
Department of Emergency Medicine
Morristown Memorial Hospital
Morristown, New Jersey

Fredric M. Hustey, MD [295]
Staff Physician, Emergency Services Institute
Cleveland Clinic
Cleveland, Ohio

Alzamani Mohammad Idrose, MBBS, MMed(Emergency), MITM, EMDM [228, 229, 230]
Consultant Emergency Physician
Emergency & Trauma Department
Hospital Kuala Lumpur, Kuala Lumpur, Malaysia

Andy Jagoda, MD [172]
Professor and Chair
Department of Emergency Medicine
Mount Sinai School of Medicine
New York City, New York

Mohammad Jalili, MD [224]
Associate Professor of Emergency Medicine
Tehran University of Medical Sciences
Tehran, Iran

Gary A. Johnson, MD, FACEP [59,60]
Associate Professor and Chair, Department of Emergency Medicine
Upstate Medical University
Syracuse, New York

Alan E. Jones, MD [151]
Professor and Chair of Emergency Medicine, University of Mississippi Medical Center
Jackson, Mississippi

David Jones, MD [261]
Department of Emergency Medicine
Oregon Health and Science University
Portland, Oregon

Elaine B. Josephson, MD [95]
Assistant Professor of Emergency Medicine in Clinical Medicine
Weill Cornell Medical College of Cornell University
Program Director, Emergency Medicine Residency Department of Emergency Medicine
Lincoln Medical and Mental Health Center Bronx
New York City, New York

Turan Kayagil, MD [84]
EVMS Emergency Medicine
Norfolk, Virginia

Gabor D. Kelen, MD, FRCP(C), FACEP, FAAEM [15]
Professor and Chair, Department of Emergency Medicine
Johns Hopkins University
Director, Johns Hopkins Office of Critical Event Preparedness and Response
The Johns Hopkins Institutions
Baltimore, Maryland

Elizabeth W. Kelly, MD [152]
Assistant Professor
Department of Emergency Medicine
Wake Forest University Baptist Medical Center
Winston-Salem, North Carolina

Osama Kentab, MD, FAAP, FACEP [144]
Assistant Professor Emergency Medicine—KSAU
Clinical Assistant Professor of Pediatrics—KSU
Consultant Pediatric Emergency Medicine
Department of Emergency Medicine
King Abdulaziz Medical City
Riyadh, Kingdom of Saudi Arabia

William P. Kerns II, MD, FACEP, FACMT [194]
Professor of Emergency Medicine
Program Director, Medical Toxicology Fellowship
Department of Emergency Medicine
Carolinas Medical Center
Charlotte, North Carolina

Benjamin D. Kessler, MD [181]
Medical Toxicology Fellow
North Shore University Hospital
Manhasset, New York

Janeva Kircher, MD [119]
Pediatric Emergency Medicine Fellow
Department of Peditatrics and Department of Emergency Medicine
University of Alberta
Edmonton, Alberta

Niranjan Kissoon, MD [114]
Associate Head and Professor
Division of Critical Care,
Department of Pediatrics, University of British Columbia
Vice-President, Medical Affairs, BC Children's Hospital
Vancouver, British Columbia

Bryan B. Kitch, MD [160]
Clinical Instructor
Department of Emergency Medicine
Brody School of Medicine at East Carolina University
Greenville, North Carolina

Andy Kitlowski, MD [75]
Emergency Medicine
University of Texas at Austin
Dell Medical School
Austin, Texas

Jeffrey A. Kline, MD [56]
Vice Chair of Research
Department of Emergency Medicine
Professor, Department of Cellular and Integrative Physiology
Indiana University School of Medicine
Indianapolis, Indiana

Nicholas E. Kman, MD, FACEP [73]
Associate Professor
Department of Emergency Medicine
The Ohio State University
Columbus, Ohio

Barry J. Knapp, MD [254]
Residency Program Director
Department of Emergency Medicine
Eastern Virginia Medical School
Norfolk, Virginia

Kevin J. Knoop, MD, MS [213]
Staff Physician
Naval Medical Center, Portsmouth, Virginia
Assistant Professor of Military and Emergency Medicine
Uniformed Services University of the Health Sciences
Bethesda, Maryland

Joshua G. Kornegay, MD [171]
Assistant Professor
Department of Emergency Medicine
Oregon Health & Science University
Portland, Oregon

Nancy S. Kwon, MD, MPA [44]
Associate Chair of Academics and Research
Department of Emergency Medicine
Long Island Jewish Medical Center
Assistant Professor of Emergency Medicine
Hofstra North Shore-LIJ School of Medicine at Hofstra University
Hempstead, New York

Richard Kwun, MD [121]
Attending Physician
Department of Emergency Medicine
Swedish Medical Center
Issaquah, Washington

Jay G. Ladde, MD, FACEP, FAAEM [175]
Associate Program Director, Orlando Health EM Residency
Orlando, Florida
Associate Professor, University of Central Florida College of Medicine
Assistant Professor, University of Florida College of Medicine
Assistant Professor, Florida State University School of Medicine

David S. Lambert, MD [21]
Associate Professor
Department of Emergency Medicine
Associate Medical Director
Hospital of the University of Pennsylvania
PennStar Life Flight Medical Command Physician
Undersea and Hyperbaric Medicine Physician

Richard L. Lammers, MD [45]
Assistant Dean for Simulation
Professor of Emergency Medicine
Western Michigan University Homer Stryker, MD School of Medicine
Kalamazoo, Michigan

Stephanie A. Lareau, MD, FAWM [243]
Assistant Professor Emergency Medicine
Emergency Physician Carilion Clinic
Virginia Tech-Carilion School of Medicine
Roanoke, Virginia
Carilion Franklin Memorial Hospital
Rocky Mount, Virginia

Thomas S. Laughrey, MD [18]
Chief Resident
Department of Emergency Medicine
University of Virginia Health System
Charlottesville, Virginia

Chen-Hsen Lee, MD [92]
Professor
Department of Surgery
Taipei Veterans General Hospital
Institute of Emergency and Critical Care Medicine
National Yang-Ming University
Taipei, Taiwan

Cedric W. Lefebvre, MD [64]
Assistant Professor
Department of Emergency Medicine
Wake Forest School of Medicine
Medical Center Blvd
Winston-Salem, North Carolina

Amy Levine, MD [117]
Associate Professor
Pediatrics and Emergency Medicine
Department of Pediatrics
University of North Carolina at Chapel Hill
Chapel Hill, North Carolina

Michael Levine, MD [180, 184]
Department of Emergency Medicine, Section of Medical Toxicology
University of Southern California.
Los Angeles, California

Rachel Levitan, MD [189]
Emergency Department
Flagstaff Medical Center
Flagstaff, Arizona

Gemma C. Lewis, MD [291]
Emergency Medicine—BayCare Clinics, LLP
Adjunct Assistant Clinical Professor
Department of Medicine
University of Wisconsin
Madison, Wisconsin

Stephen Y. Liang, MD [150]
Instructor of Medicine
Divisions of Emergency Medicine & Infectious Diseases
Washington University School of Medicine
Saint Louis, Missouri

Swee Han Lim, MBBS, FRCS Edin (A&E), FRCP Edin, FAMS [23, 24, 33]
Senior Consultant, Department of Emergency Medicine, Singapore General Hospital
Outram Road, Singapore
Clinical Associate Professor, Yong Loo Lin School of Medicine, National University of Singapore
Adjunct Associate Professor, Duke-NUS Graduate Medical School Singapore

Deborah R. Liu, MD [133]
Faculty, Division of Emergency and Transport Medicine
Children's Hospital Los Angeles
Assistant Professor of Pediatrics
USC Keck School of Medicine
Los Angeles, California

Bruce M. Lo, MD, RDMS [76,89]
Assistant Professor of Department of Emergency Medicine
Eastern Virginia Medical School
Norfolk, Virginia

Maurice F. Loeffel III, MD [269]
Assistant Clinical Professor
Department of Emergency Medicine
Rockford Memorial Hospital
Rockford, Illinois

Heather Long, MD [203]
Director, Medical Toxicology
Albany Medical College
Albany, New York

Annette M. Lopez, MD [10]
Clinical Instructor, Department of Emergency Medicine
Oregon Health & Science University
Portland, Oregon

Frank LoVecchio, DO, MPH, FACEP, ABMT [177, 178, 179, 180, 182, 189, 196, 197, 199, 202, 204, 210]
Vice Chair of Research, Department of Emergency Medicine, Maricopa Medical Center
Banner Poison Drug and Information Center, BUMC-PHX
Professor of Emergency Medicine, Research Scholar, University of Arizona College of Medicine
Phoenix, Arizona

Cary L. Lubkin, MD [225]
Associate Professor of Emergency Medicine and Internal Medicine
Cooper Medical School of Rowan University
Adjunct Associate Professor of Emergency Medicine and Internal Medicine
UMDNJ/Robert Wood Johnson Medical School
Cooper University Hospital
Camden, New Jersey

Robert H. Lutz, MD [302]
Emergency Medicine Physician
United States Army Special Operations Command
Fort Bragg, North Carolina

Michael Lynch, MD [217]
Medical Director, Pittsburgh Poison Center
Assistant Professor, Division of Medical Toxicology, Department of Emergency Medicine
Divisions of Adolescent and Pediatric Emergency Medicine, Department of Pediatrics University of Pittsburgh School of Medicine
Pittsburgh, Pennsylvania

O. John Ma, MD [166, 174, 255, 261, 263]
Professor and Chair
Department of Emergency Medicine
Oregon Health & Science University
Portland, Oregon

Sharon E. Mace, MD, FACEP, FAAP [66]
Director, Observation Unit Emergency Services Institute
Director, Research Emergency Services Institute
Professor, Cleveland Clinic Lerner College of Medicine at Case Western Reserve University
Faculty Cleveland Clinic Metro Health Emergency Medicine Residency Program
Cleveland, Ohio

Anthony G. Macintyre, MD [9]
Associate Professor of Emergency Medicine
George Washington University
Washington, DC

David Magilner, MD, MSPH [152]
Assistant Professor, Pediatric Emergency Medicine
Director, Fellowship in Pediatric Emergency Medicine
Department of Emergency Medicine
Wake Forest University Baptist Medical Center
Winston-Salem, North Carolina

Simon A. Mahler, MD, FAAEM [48, 54, 154]
Assistant Professor
Associate Residency Program Director
Louisiana State University Health Sciences Center-Shreveport
Shreveport, Louisiana

Gerald Maloney, DO, CPPS, FACEP [65, 222]
Assistant Professor of Emergency Medicine
Case Western Reserve University/MetroHealth Medical Center
Cleveland, Ohio

David E. Manthey, MD [50, 68, 94]
Professor of Emergency Medicine
Vice Chair of Education
Wake Forest School of Medicine
Winston-Salem, North Carolina

Elisa Mapelli, MD [123]
Clinical Fellow
Department of Pediatric Emergency Medicine
University of British Columbia
Vancouver, British Columbia

Catherine A. Marco, MD, FACEP [15, 154, 155]
Professor of Emergency Medicine
Department of Emergency Medicine
Wright State University Boonshoft School of Medicine
Dayton, Ohio

Asa M. Margolis, DO, MPH, MS [4]
Senior Resident
Department of Emergency Medicine
Johns Hopkins University School of Medicine
Baltimore, Maryland

Roberta Marino, MD [17]
Emergency Medicine Unit
S. Andrea Hospital
Vercelli, Italy

John P. Marshall, MD [142]
Chair
Department of Emergency Medicine
Maimonides Medical Center
Brooklyn, New York

Erik Mattison, MD [178]
Emergency Physician
Chandler Regional Medical Center
Chandler, Arizona

Henderson D. McGinnis, MD, FACEP [244]
Associate Professor
Department of Emergency Medicine
Wake Forest Baptist Health
Winston-Salem, North Carolina

C. Crawford Mechem, MD, MS, FACEP [1]
Associate Professor
Department of Emergency Medicine
University of Pennsylvania School of Medicine
Philadelphia, Pennsylvania

Garth D. Meckler, MD, MSHS [106, 126, 136, 144]
Associate Professor and Division Head
Pediatric Emergency Medicine
University of British Columbia/BC Children's Hospital
Vancouver, British Columbia

Ninfa Mehta, MD [90]
Associate Medical Director SUNY Downstate
Ultrasound Fellowship Director SUNY Downstate/ Kings County Hospital
Emergency Department
SUNY Downstate Hospital, Kings County Emergency Department
Brooklyn, New York

Sarah A. Mellion, MD [137]
Clinical Instructor
Pediatric Emergency Medicine
Department of Pediatrics
University of Colorado School of Medicine
Aurora, Colorado

Moss Mendelson, MD, FACEP [77]
Associate Professor of Emergency Medicine
Eastern Virginia Medical School
Emergency Physicians of Tidewater
Norfolk, Virginia

Jeffrey S. Menkes, MD, FACEP [267]
Physician Informatics
Department of Hospital Information Systems
St. Francis Hospital and Medical Center
Hartford, Connecticut
Clinical Instructor
Emergency Medicine
University of Connecticut School of Medicine
Farmington, Connecticut

Lisa H. Merck, MD, MPH [257]
Assistant Professor, Emergency Medicine
Assistant Professor, Diagnostic Imaging
Director, Neurological Emergencies Research Program
Department of Emergency Medicine
The Warren Alpert Medical School of Brown University
University Emergency Medicine Foundation
Providence, Rhode Island

John T. Meredith, MD, FACEP [160]
Clinical Assistant Professor
Department of Emergency Medicine
Brody School of Medicine at East Carolina University
Greenville, North Carolina

Nate Mick, MD [111]
Associate Chief, Pediatric Emergency Medicine, Maine Medical Center
Portland, Maine
Department of Emergency Medicine
Associate Professor, Tufts University School of Medicine
Boston, Massachusetts

Megan E. Mickley, MD [143]
Boston Medical Center
Boston, Massachusetts

Chadwick D. Miller, MD, MS [51]
Associate Professor
Wake Forest School of Medicine
Medical Center Boulevard
Winston-Salem, North Carolina

Michael G. Millin, MD, MPH, FACEP [4]
Assistant Professor
Department of Emergency Medicine
Johns Hopkins University School of Medicine
Baltimore, Maryland

Lisa D. Mills, MD [6]
Professor, Department of Emergency Medicine
University of California at Davis School of Medicine
Sacramento, California

Trevor J. Mills, MD, MPH [6]
Professor of Emergency Medicine, Department of Emergency Medicine, University of California, Davis
Chief of Emergency Medicine Services, Northern California Veterans Affairs Health Care System
Sacramento, California

Alicia B. Minns, MD [195]
Assistant Clinical Professor of Medicine
Department of Emergency Medicine
Fellowship Director
Medical Toxicology Fellowship
University of California
San Diego, California

Óscar Miró, MD, PhD [186, 192]
Senior Consultant
Research Coordinador. Emergency Department.
Hospital Clinic
Barcelona, Spain

Joel L. Moll, MD [156]
Assistant Professor
Residency Program Director
Virginia Commonwealth University School of Medicine
Richmond, Virginia

Malcolm E. Molyneux, MD, FRCP [158]
Emeritus Professor of Tropical Medicine
Liverpool School of Tropical Medicine, Liverpool, UK and College of Medicine, University of Malawi
Blantyre, Malawi

Gregory J. Moran, MD [153]
Professor of Clinical Medicine, David Geffen School of Medicine at UCLA
Department of Emergency Medicine and Division of Infectious Diseases
Olive View-UCLA Medical Center
Los Angeles, California

Lisa Moreno-Walton, MD, MSCR [293]
Associate Professor of Clinical Emergency Medicine
Director of Research, Section of Emergency Medicine
Director of Diversity, Section of Emergency Medicine
Assistant Professor of Research, Department of Genetics
Assistant Professor of Medicine—Research
Associate Professor of Surgery
Tulane University School of Medicine
Louisiana State University Health Sciences Center – New Orleans
New Orleans, Louisiana

Donna Moro-Sutherland, MD [140]
Assistant Professor
Department of Emergency Medicine
University of North Carolina at Chapel Hill
Chapel Hill, North Carolina

Dean S. Morrell, MD [250, 251, 252, 253]
Professor
Director of Dermatology Residency Training Program
Director of Pediatric & Adolescent Dermatology
UNC Department of Dermatology
Chapel Hill, North Carolina

Sean W. Mulvaney, MD [302]
Assistant Professor
Department of Military and Emergency Medicine
Uniformed Services University of the Health Sciences
Bethesda, Maryland

Jessie G. Nelson, MD [234]
Associate Professor of Emergency Medicine
Senior Staff Physician, Emergency Medicine
University of Minnesota/Regions Hospital
St. Paul, Minnesota

R. Darrell Nelson, MD, FACEP, FAAEM [282]
Assistant Professor
Director EMS and Disaster Fellowship Program
Department of Emergency Medicine
Wake Forest University Health Sciences
Medical Center Boulevard
Winston-Salem, North Carolina

Anna S. Nelson, MD [166, 261]
Department of Emergency Medicine
Oregon Health & Science University
Portland, Oregon

Lewis S. Nelson, MD [190, 198, 203, 207, 220]
Professor and Vice Chair for Academic Affairs
Ronald O. Perelman Department of Emergency Medicine
New York University School of Medicine
Director, Fellowship in Medical Toxicology
New York City Poison Control Center
New York City, New York

Tom S. Neuman, MD, FACP, FACPM, FUHM [214]
Emeritus Professor of Emergency Medicine
University of California
San Diego, California

H. Bryant Nguyen, MD [32]
Professor of Emergency Medicine
Medicine-Critical Care, and Basic Sciences
Vice-Chair, Medicine Research
Director, Center for Comparative Effectiveness and Outcomes Research
Loma Linda University
Loma Linda, California

Bret A. Nicks, MD, MHA, FACEP [12, 68, 94]
Associate Professor, Emergency Medicine
Associate Dean, Global Health
Wake Forest School of Medicine
Winston-Salem, North Carolina

David D. Nicolaou, MD, MS, FACEP [16]
Clinical Assistant Professor
Department of Emergency Medicine
Michigan State University College of Human Medicine
Attending Physician
Munson Medical Center
Traverse City, Michigan

James T. Niemann, MD [55]
Professor of Medicine
Department of Emergency Medicine
Harbor-UCLA Medical Center
Torrance, California

Mahtab Niroomand, MD [224]
Assistant Professor of Endocrinology
Shahid Beheshti University of Medical Sciences
Tehran, Iran

Flavia Nobay, MD [149]
Associate Professor and Associate Chair for Education
Director, Emergency Medicine Residency Program
Department of Emergency Medicine
University of Rochester Medical Center
School of Medicine and Dentistry
Rochester, New York

Andrew L. Nyce, MD [225]
Assistant Professor of Emergency Medicine
Cooper Medical School of Rowan University
Adjunct Assistant Professor of Emergency Medicine
UMDNJ/Robert Wood Johnson Medical School
Cooper University Hospital
New Brunswick, New Jersey

Mary Claire O'Brien, MD [71]
Associate Professor
Department of Emergency Medicine
Wake Forest University School of Medicine
Winston-Salem, North Carolina

Damilola Ogunnaike-Joseph, MD [140]
Wake Emergency Physicians
Raleigh, North Carolina

Kelly Patrick O'Keefe, MD [281]
Associate Professor, University of South Florida Morsani College of Medicine
Program Director, Emergency Medicine Residency
University of South Florida and Tampa General Hospital
Tampa, Florida

Lila O'Mahony, MD [146]
Departments of Emergency Medicine and Pediatrics
Pediatric Emergency Medicine Fellow,
University of Washington and Seattle Children's Hospital
Seattle, Washington

Susan R. O'Mara, MD, FAAEM [80]
Washington Hospital Center
Department of Emergency Medicine
Washington, DC

Ricardo C. Ong, MD, DiMM [302]
Command Surgeon
1st Special Forces Command (Airborne)
Fort Bragg, North Carolina

Marcus E. H. Ong, MBBS, MPH, FAMS [23, 24]
Associate Professor
Office of Clinical Sciences
Duke-National University of Singapore Graduate Medical School
Senior Consultant and Clinician Scientist
Department of Emergency Medicine
Singapore General Hospital
Outram Road, Singapore

Joseph P. Ornato, MD, FACP, FACC, FACEP [11]
Professor and Chairman
Department of Emergency Medicine
Virginia Commonwealth University
Medical College of Virginia Hospitals
Virginia Commonwealth University
Richmond, Virginia

Raymond J. Orthober, MD [83]
Assistant Professor
Department of Emergency Medicine
School of Medicine
University of Louisville
Louisville, Kentucky

Charissa B. Pacella, MD [162]
Associate Professor, University of Pittsburgh Department of Emergency Medicine
Vice Chair of Operations, UPMC Department of Emergency Medicine
Pittsburgh, Pennsylvania

Michael T. Paddock, DO, MS [208]
Clinical Associate, Section of Emergency Medicine
University of Chicago Medicine
Chicago, Illinois

Amit Pandit, MD [249]
Critical Care Medicine Fellow Memorial Sloan Kettering
New York City, New York

Peter Peacock, MD [88]
Assistant Professor, Emergency Medicine
State University of New York, Downstate
Chief Medical Informatics Officer
Kings County and Woodhull Hospital Centers
Brooklyn, New York

Andre M. Pennardt, MD, FAWM, FACEP, DiMM [302]
Professor of Emergency Medicine & Hospitalist Services
Medical College of Georgia, Georgia Regents University
Augusta, Georgia

Debra G. Perina, MD [226]
Associate Professor
Department of Emergency Medicine
Quality Director, Prehospital Division Director,
EMS Fellowship Director
Department of Emergency Medicine
University of Virginia Hospital
Charlottesville, Virginia

Andrew D. Perron, MD, FACEP, FACSM [164]
Professor and Residency Program Director
Department of Emergency Medicine
Maine Medical Center
Portland, Maine

Jeanmarie Perrone, MD [187]
Professor, Emergency Medicine Director, Division of Medical Toxicology, Department of Emergency Medicine
Perelman School of Medicine, University of Pennsylvania
Philadelphia, Pennsylvania

Roberta Petrino, MD [17]
President Elect of the European Society for Emergency Medicine
Chair Emergency Medicine Unit
S. Andrea Hospital
Vercelli, Italy

Vu D. Phan, MD [67]
Staff Physician
Emergency Department
Aultman Hospital
Canton, Ohio

Michael R. Pinsky, MD, CM, Dr hc [32]
Professor of Critical Care Medicine, Bioengineering, Anesthesiology, Cardiovascular Diseases, and Clinical & Translational Sciences
Vice-Chair, Academic Affairs
Department of Critical Care Medicine
University of Pittsburgh School of Medicine
University of Pittsburgh
Pittsburgh, Pennsylvania

R. Dustin Pippin, PharmD [19]
Pharmacist
Emergency Department
Wake Forest Baptist Health
Department of Pharmacy
Winston-Salem, North Carolina

Anthony F. Pizon, MD [217]
Chief, Medical Toxicology
Department of Emergency Medicine
University of Pittsburgh Medical Center
Pittsburgh, Pennsylvania

Charles V. Pollack, Jr., MA, MD [239]
Professor of Emergency Medicine
Chairman, Department of Emergency Medicine
Pennsylvania Hospital
University of Pennsylvania School of Medicine
Philadelphia, Pennsylvania

Janet Poponick, MD [67]
Assistant Professor
Department of Emergency Medicine
Metro Health Medical Center
Case Western Reserve University
Cleveland, Ohio

Samuel Josiah Prater, MD [107]
Fellow
Pediatric Emergency Medicine
Baylor College of Medicine
Houston, Texas
Texas Children's Hospital
Houston, Texas

Timothy G. Price, MD [83]
Associate Professor
Department of Emergency Medicine
School of Medicine
University of Louisville
Louisville, Kentucky

Louise A. Prince, MD, FACEP [59,60]
Associate Professor, Department of Emergency Medicine
Upstate Medical University
Syracuse, New York

Susan B. Promes, MD [149]
Chairman and Professor
Department of Emergency Medicine
Pennsylvania State University School of Medicine
Hershey, Pennsylvania

Jane M. Prosser, MD [187]
Assistant Professor, Medicine Division of Emergency Medicine, Weill Cornell Medical School
New York City, New York

Katherine M. Prybys, DO [188]
Assistant Professor
Department of Emergency Medicine
University of Maryland School of Medicine
Baltimore, Maryland

Michael A. Puskarich, MD [151]
Assistant Professor of Emergency Medicine
University of Mississippi Medical Center
Jackson, Mississippi

Linda Quan, MD [215]
Professor of Pediatrics
Seattle Children's Hospital
Seattle, Washington

Dan Quan, DO [183, 184, 185, 196, 202]
Associate Professor
Department of Emergency Medicine,
University of Arizona College of Medicine – Phoenix
Phoenix, Arizona

Nadeemuddin Quereshi, MD, FAAP, FCCM [144]
Consultant Pediatric Emergency Medicine
Department of Emergency Medicine
King Faisal Specialist Hospital and Research Centre
Riyadh, Kingdom of Saudi Arabia

James Quinn, MD, MS [44, 50]
Associate Professor of Surgery/Emergency Medicine
Stanford University
Stanford, California

Ralph H. Raasch, PharmD [163]
Associate Professor of Pharmacy (retired)
Division of Practice Advancement and Clinical Education, Eshelman School of Pharmacy
The University of North Carolina at Chapel Hill
Chapel Hill, North Carolina

John C. Ray, MD [231]
Assistant Professor of Emergency Medicine
Department of Emergency Medicine
Medical College of Wisconsin
Milwaukee, Wisconsin

Sarah M. Reid, MD, FRCPC [131]
Assistant Professor, Departments of Pediatrics and Emergency Medicine, University of Ottawa
Children's Hospital of Eastern Ontario
Ottawa, Ontario

Joseph G. Rella, MD [191, 206]
Assistant Professor
Emergency Medicine
Weill Cornell Medical College
New York City, New York

Vito Rocco, MD, FACE [74]
Vice chief
Emergency medicine
St. John hospital Macomb-Oakland
Warren, Michigan

Christopher Ross, MD, FRCPC, FACEP, FAAEM [262]
Associate Professor of Emergency Medicine
Associate Chair of Professional Education
Attending Physician Emergency Medicine
Cook County (Stroger) Hospital
Department of Emergency Medicine
Chicago, Illinois

Richard Rothman, MD, PhD [154, 155]
Professor
Johns Hopkins University, School of Medicine
Baltimore, Maryland

Brian H. Rowe, MD, MSc, CCFP(EM), FCCP [14]
Tier I Canada Research Chair in Evidence-Based Emergency Medicine
Scientific Director, Emergency Strategic Clinical Network
Professor, Department of Emergency Medicine
University of Alberta
Edmonton, Alberta

William Rushton, MD [248]
University of Virginia School of Medicine
Charlottesville, Virginia

William A. Rutala, PhD, MPH [157]
Professor of Medicine
Director, Hospital Epidemiology
Department of Infectious Diseases
University of North Carolina
Chapel Hill, North Carolina

Vikram Sabhaney, BSc, MD, FRCPC [122, 123]
Pediatric Emergency Medicine Fellowship Director, BC Children's Hospital
Clinical Assistant Professor, Department of Pediatrics
University of British Columbia
Vancouver, British Columbia

Justin W. Sales, MD, MPH [132]
Division of Pediatric Emergency Medicine
Director, Prehospital Coordination
Randall Children's Hospital
Portland, Oregon

Annabella Salvador-Kelly, MD, FACEP [44]
Associate Medical Director
Long Island Jewish Medical Center
New Hyde park, New York
Assistant professor
Hofstra-Northshore LIJ School of Medicine
Hempstead, New York

Tracy G. Sanson, MD, FACEP [281]
Associate Clinical Professor
Division of Emergency Medicine
Department of Internal Medicine
University of South Florida
Tampa, Florida

Sally A. Santen, MD, PhD [233, 238]
Assistant Dean, Educational Research & Quality Improvement
Associate Chair, Education, Department of Emergency Medicine
University of Michigan School of Medicine
Ann Arbor, Michigan

John Sarko, MD (Deceased) [62]
Associated Professor, Department of Emergency Medicine
University of Arizona College of Medicine – Phoenix
Maricopa Integrated Health System
Phoenix, Arizona

Adam B. Schlichting, MD, MPH [223]
Fellow, Critical Care Medicine
Departments of Emergency Medicine and Internal Medicine
Henry Ford Hospital
Detroit, Michigan

Sandra M. Schneider, MD, FACEP [181]
Senior Research Director
North Shore Hospital
Manhasset, New York
Professor
Hofstra North Shore LIJ School of Medicine
Hempstead, New York

Aaron Schneir, MD [211]
Professor of Clinical Medicine
Division of Medical Toxicology
Department of Emergency Medicine
University of California San Diego Health System
La Jolla, California

Abigail Schuh, MD [121]
Assistant Professor
Pediatric Emergency Medicine
Medical College of Wisconsin
Milwaukee, Wisconsin

Theresa M. Schwab, MD [262]
Assistant Professor
Department of Emergency Medicine
Advocate Christ Medical Center
University of Illinois at Chicago
Oak Lawn, Illinois

Robert W. Shaffer, MD [233]
Assistant Professor
University of Michigan Medical School
Department of Emergency Medicine
University of Michigan Medical Center
Ann Arbor, Michigan

Manish I. Shah, MD [107]
Assistant Professor
Department of Pediatrics, Section of Emergency Medicine
Baylor College of Medicine
Attending Physician
Emergency Center, Texas Children's Hospital
Houston, Texas

Allan Shefrin, MD, FRCPC [124]
Division of Pediatric Emergency Medicine
Department of Pediatrics
Children's Hospital of Eastern Ontario
Assistant Professor, University of Ottawa
Ottawa, Ontario

Suzanne M. Shepherd, MD, DTM&H [103, 296]
Professor
Education Officer
Chair, COAP Committee
Department of Emergency Medicine
Penn Medicine-Hospital of the University of Pennsylvania
Philadelphia, Pennsylvania

David C. Sheridan, MD [136]
Pediatric Emergency Medicine
Oregon Health & Science University
Portland, Oregon

Sara Haney Shields, PharmD, BCPS [19, 20]
Pharmacy System Manager, Emergency Department & Perioperative Services
Department of Pharmacy
Wake Forest Baptist Medical Center
Winston-Salem, North Carolina

William H. Shoff, MD [103]
Associate Professor
Director of Travel Medicine
Department of Emergency Medicine
Hospital of the University of Pennsylvania
Philadelphia, Pennsylvania

Jonathan E. Siff, MD, MBA, FACEP [303]
Associate Chief Medical Informatics Officer
The MetroHealth System
Associate Professor
Department of Emergency Medicine
Case Western Reserve University School of Medicine
Cleveland, Ohio

Troy Sims, DO [63]
Clinical Assistant Professor
University of Pittsburgh
Pittsburgh, Pennsylvania

Richard Sinert, DO [88,90]
Professor of Emergency Medicine
Vice-Chair In-Charge of Research
State University of New York—Downstate Medical Center
and Kings County Hospital Center
Health and Hospitals Corporation
Brooklyn, New York

Adam J. Singer, MD [39, 41, 47]
Professor and Vice Chairman for Research
Department of Emergency Medicine
Stony Brook University
Stony Brook, New York

Aaron Skolnik, MD [193]
Banner-University Medical Center Phoenix
Assistant Medical Director, Banner Poison & Drug Information Center
Assistant Professor, Department of Emergency Medicine
University of Arizona College of Medicine
Phoenix, Arizona

David E. Slattery, MD, FACEP, FAAEM [239]
Assistant Professor and Research Director
Department of Emergency Medicine
University of Nevada School of Medicine
Las Vegas, Nevada

Benjamin Small, PharmD, BCPS [19]
Pharmacist
Emergency Department
Wake Forest Baptist Health
Department of Pharmacy
Winston-Salem, North Carolina

Michael D. Smith, MD, MBA [30]
Associate Professor, Case Western Reserve University
Attending Physician, MetroHealth Medical Center
Cleveland, Ohio

Lane M. Smith, MD, PhD, FACEP [159]
Assistant Professor
Department of Emergency Medicine
Wake Forest School of Medicine
Winston Salem, North Carolina

Brian K. Snyder, MD [214]
Clinical Professor of Emergency Medicine
Attending, Hyperbaric Medicine Division
University of California, San Diego Health System

Mark Sochor, MD [249]
Associate Professor of Emergency Medicine
Research Director, Emergency Medicine Research Office
Department of Emergency Medicine
Charlottesville, Virginia

Mitchell C. Sokolosky, MD [285]
Associate Professor of Emergency Medicine
Wake Forest Health Sciences Center
Winston-Salem, North Carolina

David M. Somand, MD, FACEP [13]
Clinical Lecturer
Department of Emergency Medicine
University of Michigan
Ann Arbor, Michigan

J. Stephan Stapczynski, MD [62, 240]
Professor, Department of Emergency Medicine
University of Arizona College of Medicine - Phoenix
Phoenix, Arizona

Brandy Stauffer, MD [134]
Pediatric Emergency Medicine Fellow
Department of Pediatrics
Department of Emergency Medicine
University of Alberta
Edmonton, Alberta

Mark T. Steele, MD [273, 274]
Department of Emergency Medicine
University of Missouri—Kansas City
Truman Medical Center
Kansas City, Missouri

Christine R. Stehman, MD [79]
Assistant Professor of Clinical Emergency Medicine
Department of Emergency Medicine
Indiana University School of Medicine
Indianapolis, Indiana

Jennifer A. Stephani, MD [10]
Clinical Instructor, Department of Emergency Medicine
Oregon Health & Science University
Portland, Oregon

Richard J. Stevenson, MBChB, BMSc (Hons), FRCEM, MRCP, MFFLM, DFM, DMedTox [301]
Consultant in Emergency Medicine
Glasgow Royal Infirmary
Glasgow, Scotland

C. Keith Stone, MD, FACEP [3]
Professor and Chair
Department of Emergency Medicine
Texas A&M University, Health Science Center
College of Medicine
Scott & White Healthcare
Temple, Texas

Susan C. Stone, MD, MPH [40]
Associate Professor of Emergency Medicine
Los Angeles County Medical Center
Keck School of Medicine of University of South Carolina
Los Angeles, California

Alan B. Storrow, MD [53]
Associate Professor of Emergency Medicine
Vice Chairman for Research and Academic Affairs
Vanderbilt University
Nashville, Tennessee

Charles E. A. Stringer, MD, MSc [122]
Resident, Emergency Medicine
Department of Emergency Medicine
University of British Columbia
Vancouver, British Columbia

Amy M. Stubbs, MD [273]
Assistant Professor
Department of Emergency Medicine
University of Missouri—Kansas City
Truman Medical Center
Kansas City, Missouri

Gerald W. Surrett, MD, FAWM, DiMM [302]
Group Surgeon
10th Special Forces Group
Fort Carson, Colorado

Carolyn Synovitz, MD, MPH [34]
Clinical Associate Professor
Department of Emergency Medicine
Oklahoma School of Community Medicine
Tulsa, Oklahoma
Jackson County Memorial Hospital
Altus, Oklahoma

Sukhjit S. Takhar, MD [153]
Instructor of Medicine (Emergency Medicine)
Harvard Medical School
Brigham and Women's Hospital
Boston, Massachusetts

Peter Tang, MD, MPH [268]
Director
Hand, Upper Extremity & Microvascular Fellowship
Associate Professor
Drexel University College of Medicine
Allegheny General Hospital
Allegheny Health Network
Pittsburgh, Pennsylvania

Mary E. Tanski, MD [174]
Assistant Professor
Department of Emergency Medicine
Oregon Health & Science University
Portland, Oregon

Wee Siong Teo, MBBS, M Med (Int Med), FRCP (Edin), FACC, FHRS [33]
Senior Consultant
Department of Cardiology
National Heart Centre
Singapore

Stephen R. Thom, MD, PhD [21]
Professor, Emergency medicine
University of Maryland School of Medicine
Baltimore, Maryland

Stephen H. Thomas, MD, MPH [3]
George Kaiser Family Foundation Professor and Chair
Department of Emergency Medicine
University of Oklahoma School of Community Medicine
Tulsa, Oklahoma

Jennifer Thull-Freedman, MD, MSc [128]
Clinical Associate Professor
University of Calgary
Calgary, Alberta

Aleksandr M. Tichter, MD [40]
Assistant Program Director
Emergency Medicine Residency
NewYork-Presbyterian Hospital
Assistant Professor of Clinical Medicine
Columbia University College of Physicians and Surgeons
New York City, New York

Joel S. Tieder, MD, MPH [115]
Assistant Professor
Department of Pediatrics
Division of Hospital Medicine
Seattle Children's Hospital
The University of Washington
Seattle, Washington

Adam Z. Tobias, MD, MPH [290]
Assistant Professor of Emergency Medicine
University of Pittsburgh, School of Medicine
Pittsburgh, Pennsylvania

Christian Tomaszewski, MD, MS, MBA, FACEP, FACMT, FIFEM [195]
Professor of Clinical Emergency Medicine
Medical Director, Department of Emergency Medicine
Attending in Medical Toxicology and Hyperbarics
University of California San Diego Health Sciences
San Diego, California

Richard Tovar, MD, FACEP, FACMT [205]
Medical Toxicology
Clinical Forensic Medicine
Wisconsin Poison Center
Milwaukee, Wisconsin

Dennis T. Uehara, MD, MS, FACEP [269]
Chair, Department of Emergency Medicine
Rockford Memorial Hospital
Clinical Professor of Surgery, University of Illinois
College of Medicine, Rockford
Rockford, Illinois

Adam Vella, MD [145]
Associate Professor of Emergency Medicine
Pediatrics and Medical Education
Icahn School of Medicine at Mount Sinai
New York City, New York

Anantharaman Venkataraman, MBBS, FRCP (Edin), FRCS Ed (A&E), FAMS [23, 24, 33]
Professor and Senior Consultant, Department of Emergency Medicine
Singapore General Hospital
Adjunct Professor, Duke-NUS Graduate Medical School, Singapore
Advisor, International Co-operation
SingHealth Corporate Office
Singapore

Raghu Venugopal, MD, MPH, FRCPC [161]
Assistant Professor of Medicine
University of Toronto
Attending Physician
University Health Network Emergency Department
Toronto, Ontario

Robert J. Vissers, MD [29, 111]
CEO and President, Boulder Community Health, Boulder, CO
Clinical Professor of Emergency Medicine, University of Colorado
Instructor, School of Management, Oregon Health Sciences University,
Portland, Oregon

Richard A. Walker, MD [241]
Associate Professor
Department of Emergency Medicine
University of Nebraska Medical Center
Clinical Director
Department of Emergency Medicine
The Nebraska Medical Center
Omaha, Nebraska

Nikki Waller, MD [106]
Assistant Professor
Assistant Residency Program Director
Department of Emergency Medicine
University of North Carolina School of Medicine
Chapel Hill, North Carolina

Vincent J. Wang, MD, MHA [116]
Associate Professor of Pediatrics
Keck School of Medicine of the University of Southern California
Associate Division Head
Division of Emergency Medicine
Children's Hospital Los Angeles
Los Angeles, California

Henry E. Wang, MD, MS [28]
Department of Emergency Medicine
University of Alabama School of Medicine
Birmingham, Alabama

Kevin R. Ward, MD [13]
Professor
Department of Emergency Medicine
University of Michigan
Michigan Center for Integrative Research in Critical Care (MCIRCC)
Ann Arbor, Michigan

Christopher S. Weaver, MD, MBA [37]
Associate Professor of Emergency Medicine
Indiana University School of Medicine
Indianapolis, Indiana

Lindsay Weaver, MD [300]
Assistant Professor of Clinical Emergency Medicine
Indiana University School of Medicine
Indianapolis, Indiana

David J. Weber, MD, MP [157]
Professor of Medicine
Pediatrics and Epidemiology
Medical Director, Hospital Epidemiology
Department of Infectious Diseases
University of North Carolina
Chapel Hill, North Carolina

Ian S. Wedmore, MD, FACEP, FAWM, DiMM [302]
Program Director, Austere and Wilderness Medicine Fellowship
Department of Emergency Medicine
Madigan Army Medical Center
Tacoma, Washington

Scott G. Weiner, MD, MPH [292]
Associate Professor of Emergency Medicine,
Department of Emergency Medicine, Tufts University School of Medicine and Director of Research, Tufts Medical Center
Boston, Massachusetts

Brian Weiss, MD [103]
University of Pennsylvania
Philadelphia, Pennsylvania

Janna M. Welch, MD [75]
Emergency Medicine
University of Texas at Austin
Dell Medical School
Austin, Texas

Howard A. Werman, MD, FACEP [73]
Professor of Clinical Emergency Medicine
The Ohio State University
Columbus, Ohio

Lori J. Whelan, MD [99]
Assistant Professor & Director of Ultrasound
Assistant Program Director
Assistant Medical Student Director
Department of Emergency Medicine
University of Oklahoma School of Community Medicine
Tulsa, Oklahoma

Julian White, MB, BS, MD, FACTM [212]
Professor and Department Head
Toxinology Department
Women's & Children's Hospital
North Adelaide, Australia

Eric Williams, BSc, MBBS, MSc, DM [236]
Associate Lecturer
Department of Surgery, Radiology, Anesthesia and Intensive Care
The Emergency Medicine Division Faculty of Medical Sciences
University of the West Indies
Mona, Jamaica

Joanne Williams, MD, FAAEM [298]
Adjunct Clinical Professor of Emergency Medicine
Keck School of Medicine of USC
Associate Professor of Emergency Medicine
Charles Drew University of Medicine and Science
Los Angeles, California

Jean Williams-Johnson, BSc, MBBS, MSc, DM [236]
Senior Lecturer/ Emergency Medicine Residency Program Director
Department of Surgery
Faculty of Medical Sciences
The University of the West Indies
Medical Director/Consultant Emergency Physician
The Emergency Medicine Division
The University Hospital of the West Indies
Mona, Jamaica

Michael E. Winters, MD, FACEP, FAAEM [57, 58]
Associate Professor of Emergency Medicine and Medicine
Co-Director, Combined Emergency Medicine, Internal Medicine, Critical Care Program
University of Maryland School of Medicine
Baltimore, Maryland

Michael D. Witting, MD, MS [86]
Associate Professor
Department of Emergency Medicine
University of Maryland School of Medicine
Maryland, Baltimore

David A. Wohl, MD [157]
Associate Professor
Division of Infectious Diseases
The University of North Carolina at Chapel Hill
Chapel Hill, North Carolina

William A. Woods, MD [226]
Program Director Emergency Medicine Residency
Associate Professor, Departments of Emergency Medicine,
Pediatrics, and Mechanical and Aerospace Engineering
Director, Pediatric Emergency Department
University of Virginia Hospital
Charlottesville, Virginia

Daniel J. Worman, MD [167]
Associate Professor
Department of Emergency Medicine
Medical College of Wisconsin
Milwaukee, Wisconsin

David W. Wright, MD, FACEP [257]
Associate Professor, Emergency Medicine
PI, ProTECT III Clinical Trial
Director, Emergency Neurosciences
Department of Emergency Medicine
Emory University School of Medicine
Atlanta, Georgia

Chris Wyatt, MD [31]
Assistant Professor
MetroHealth Medical Center/Case Western Reserve University School of Medicine
Cleveland, Ohio

Santiago Nogue Xarau, MD, PhD [201]
Clinical Toxicology Unit, Emergency Department
Hospital Clinic, Universidad de Barcelona
Barcelona, Spain

Samuel Yang, MD [154, 155]
Associate Professor
Stanford University
Stanford, California

Donald M. Yealy, MD [30, 65]
Chair, Department of Emergency Medicine
University of Pittsburgh / University of Pittsburgh Physicians
Senior Medical Director, Health Services Division, UPMC
Professor of Emergency Medicine, Medicine, and Clinical and Translational Sciences
University of Pittsburgh School of Medicine
Pittsburgh, Pennsylvania

David Hung-Tsang Yen, MD, PhD [92]
Associate Professor
Department of Emergency Medicine
Taipei Veterans General Hospital
Institute of Emergency and Critical Care Medicine
National Yang-Ming University
Taipei, Taiwan

Janet S. Young, MD [100]
Assistant Professor
Department of Emergency Medicine
Virginia Tech- Carilion School of Medicine
Roanoke, Virginia

Esther L. Yue, MD [126]
Pediatric Emergency Medicine Fellow
Department of Emergency Medicine
Division of Pediatric Emergency Medicine
Oregon Health and Science University
Portland, Oregon

Robert J. Zalenski, MD [299]
Brooks F. Bock Professor of Emergency Medicine
Wayne State University
School of Medicine
Director, Center to Advance Palliative-Care Excellence
Detroit, Michigan

Roger Zemek, MD, FRCPC [124]
Associate Professor, Department of Pediatrics,
Children's Hospital of Eastern Ontario, University of Ottawa
Ottawa, Ontario

Christopher M. Ziebell, MD, FACEP [75]
Chairman, Department of Emergency Medicine, University Medical Center Brackenridge
Executive Director, SETON Event Medicine Institute,
Assistant Professor, Dell Medical School
University of Texas
Austin, Texas

Erin Zimny, MD [299]
Clinical Assistant Professor, Wayne State University
Senior Staff Physician, Henry Ford Hospital
Department of Emergency Medicine
Detroit, Michigan

Leslie S. Zun, MD [286]
Professor and Chair
Department of Emergency Medicine
Rosalind Franklin University of Medicine and Science
The Chicago Medical School
North Chicago, Illinois
Chair, Department of Emergency Medicine
Mount Sinai Hospital
Chicago, Illinois

Pharmacy Reviewers

Chapter 17, Fluids and Electrolytes

Christopher B. Adams, PharmD
Emergency Medicine Clinical Pharmacist

Nathan Mah, PharmD
Emergency Medicine Clinical Pharmacy Specialist
Oregon Health and Science University
Portland, Oregon

Chapter 19, Pharmacology of Antiarrhythmics and Antihypertensives

Andrea Julia Miura, PharmD, BCPS
Critical Care and Emergency Medicine Clinical Pharmacist

Nathan Mah, PharmD
Emergency Medicine Clinical Pharmacy Specialist
Oregon Health and Science University
Portland, Oregon

Chapter 109, Resuscitation of Children

Kate M. Kokanovich, PharmD
PGY2 Emergency Medicine Pharmacy Resident
University of Rochester Medical Center
Rochester, New York

Nicole Acquisto, PharmD
Emergency Medicine Clinical Pharmacy Specialist
Assistant Professor, Department of Emergency Medicine
Director, PGY2 Emergency Medicine Pharmacy Residency
University of Rochester Medical Center
Rochester, New York

Chapter 194, Beta-Blockers

Nathan Mah, PharmD
Emergency Medicine Clinical Pharmacy Specialist
Oregon Health and Science University
Portland, Oregon

Chapter 195, Calcium Channel Blockers

Nathan Mah, PharmD
Emergency Medicine Clinical Pharmacy Specialist
Oregon Health and Science University
Portland, Oregon

Chapter 20, Pharmacology of Vasopressors and Inotropes

Cassie A. Barton, PharmD, BCPS
Critical Care Pharmacist

Chapter 25, Resuscitation in Pregnancy

Ceirra N. Treu, PharmD
PGY2 Emergency Medicine Pharmacy Resident
University of Rochester Medical Center
Rochester, New York

Nicole Acquisto, PharmD
Emergency Medicine Clinical Pharmacy Specialist
Assistant Professor, Department of Emergency Medicine
Director, PGY2 Emergency Medicine Pharmacy Residency
University of Rochester Medical Center
Rochester, New York

Chapter 239, Thrombotics and Antithrombotics

Kristan E. Vollman, PharmD
Emergency Medicine Clinical Pharmacy Specialist
Owensboro Health Regional Hospital
Owensboro, Kentucky

Nathan Mah, PharmD
Emergency Medicine Clinical Pharmacy Specialist
Oregon Health and Science University
Portland, Oregon

Chapter 289, Mood and Anxiety Disorders

Nadia Awad, PharmD, BCPS
Clinical Assistant Professor, Emergency Medicine
Ernest Mario School of Pharmacy
Rutgers, The State University of New Jersey
Piscataway, New Jersey
Emergency Medicine Pharmacist
Robert Wood Johnson University Hospital Somerset
Somerville, New Jersey

Nathan Mah, PharmD
Emergency Medicine Clinical Pharmacy Specialist
Oregon Health and Science University
Portland, Oregon

Chapter 290, Psychoses

Mason H. Bucklin, PharmD
Emergency Medicine Pharmacist
Assistant Professor, Department of Clinical Pharmacy
University of Tennessee Medical Center

Nathan Mah, PharmD
Emergency Medicine Clinical Pharmacy Specialist
Oregon Health and Science University
Portland, Oregon

Preface

This 8th edition marks 37 years of continuous publication of a textbook that began in 1978 as a collection of material used to study for the early board examinations in Emergency Medicine. Each edition has expanded in depth and breadth to represent the complexity and expertise needed to practice emergency medicine in today's environment. For past editions, I have been fortunate to have the editorial collaboration of notable emergency educators—Ron Krome, Ernie Ruiz, Gabe Kelen, and Rita Cydulka. This 8th edition is the result of efforts by Steve Stapczynski, John Ma, Donald M. Yealy, Garth Meckler, and David Cline—and a host of dedicated authors.

How do we identify the scope of practice and knowledge that is today's specialty of emergency medicine? Is it through paper books, blogs, social networking, Google, journals, or clinical practice? While e-information is perfectly suited to the multitasking and frequent-attention shifts of the emergency medicine environment. E-information does not communicate what Emergency Medicine IS. E-information provides information about snippets of care, but not about the comprehensive knowledge set that is our specialty.

Both digital and print materials are available as part of the 8th edition. We have designed the 8th edition, like the past editions, to include the content that comprises the specialty of Emergency Medicine. But this edition is part of a much larger e-work, AccessEmergencyMedicine, the McGraw-Hill compendium of emergency medicine education texts. AccessEmergencyMedicine also includes the digital version of the 8th edition, with online searching of text, videos, tables, and illustrations. Accompanying this print edition is a digital set of procedure videos that were designed for both learner and teacher.

We will continue to combine the best educational tools—print and digital—for contemporary emergency medicine practice as the best way to communicate what Emergency Medicine IS.

Judith E. Tintinalli, MD, MS
Editor-in-chief
Chapel Hill, North Carolina

SECTION 1
Prehospital Care

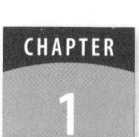

CHAPTER 1 Emergency Medical Services

C. Crawford Mechem

INTRODUCTION

EMS is the extension of emergency medical care into the prehospital setting. The concept of bringing care to the sick or injured dates back to Roman times. However, today's EMS systems have their roots in legislative and clinical developments of the 1960s and 1970s. The 1966 report "Accidental Death and Disability—The Neglected Disease of Modern Society" highlighted the deficiencies of prehospital care for trauma victims, which were attributable to inadequate equipment and provider training. Up until that time, more than half of ambulance services were run by funeral homes because hearses were among the few vehicles able to transport a stretcher. The National Highway Safety Act of 1966 established the Department of Transportation and made it the lead agency responsible for upgrading EMS systems nationwide.[1]

In 1967, J. F. Pantridge began using a physician-staffed mobile coronary care unit in Belfast, Northern Ireland, to extend cardiac care into the prehospital setting. By doing so, he was able to reduce mortality among myocardial infarction patients.[2] Using physicians to staff ambulances never gained popularity in the United States. However, in the late 1960s and 1970s, nonphysician prehospital personnel in the United States began to learn advanced medical skills, including IV placement, administration of medications, cardiac rhythm interpretation, and defibrillation.[3]

The U.S. EMS Systems Act of 1973 set aside large federal grants to develop regional EMS systems across the country. Approximately 300 EMS regions were established and became eligible for federal funding. To receive funding, the Act required that EMS systems address 15 key elements (**Table 1-1**). These elements form the foundation of many EMS systems today.[4]

The 1970s became something of a Golden Age for EMS in the United States. The U.S. Department of Transportation developed curricula for emergency medical technicians, paramedics, and first responders. EMS communications systems were formalized. In 1972, the Federal Communications Commission recommended that 9-1-1 be implemented as the emergency telephone number nationwide. The concept of designated trauma centers within EMS systems was introduced, the idea being that EMS personnel would transport seriously injured patients preferentially to these facilities.

The Omnibus Budget Reconciliation Act of 1981 eliminated direct federal funding for EMS. Instead, federal funds were given to states in the form of block grants. The result was a decrease in overall funding of EMS as well as decreased coordination of EMS systems. EMS systems took on a decidedly local flavor, with great variation between systems within states and across the country. This trend has had long-term consequences for the field.[1]

In 2011, the American Board of Emergency Medicine recognized EMS as its seventh subspecialty. The certification examination is based on the Core Content of EMS Medicine[5] with four major content areas: Clinical Aspects of EMS Medicine, Medical Oversight of EMS, Quality Management and Research, and Special Operations.

EMS SYSTEM OVERVIEW

A review of the 15 elements of EMS systems identified by the EMS Systems Act of 1973 (Table 1-1) provides insight into the current structure of EMS systems and the challenges they face.

MANPOWER

In most urban areas, paid public safety and ambulance personnel provide prehospital medical care. In contrast, suburban, rural, or wilderness EMS systems commonly use volunteers. Regardless of setting, EMS personnel fall into one of four levels of training, or licensure levels, in accordance with the National EMS Scope of Practice Model, set forth by the National Highway Traffic Safety Administration. These are emergency medical responder, emergency medical technician, advanced emergency medical technician, and paramedic. Each type of provider must master a minimum set of psychomotor skills. Emergency medical responders are usually first on the scene of a medical emergency. They are trained to perform CPR, spine immobilization, hemorrhage control, use of an automated external defibrillator, and other basic interventions while awaiting an ambulance. Emergency medical technicians function as part of an ambulance crew and are trained to take care of immediate life threats. Skills include oxygen administration; CPR; hemorrhage control; and patient extrication, immobilization, and transportation. They are also trained to assist patients in using some of their own medications and can administer to patients certain over-the-counter medications under medical oversight. Advanced emergency medical technician training includes additional assessment skills plus IV insertion, use of esophageal-tracheal multi-lumen airway devices, and administration of certain medications. Paramedics have the highest skill level, with greater training and broader scope of practice than advanced emergency medical technicians. Because of their advanced level of training, paramedics function under a designated physician's medical license.[6]

TRAINING

Training includes initial provider training and continuing education. As EMS call volume increases, providers often care for a disproportionate number of patients with minor medical issues. Maintaining proficiency in skills needed to manage critically ill patients may be difficult. Innovative training methods to ensure skills retention must be sought. Use of computerized human patient simulators is one option, both for reviewing skills and learning new ones.

COMMUNICATIONS

The adoption of 9-1-1 as a nationwide emergency number in the United States has greatly facilitated public access to emergency medical care. In many systems, the local answering center or public safety answering point has enhanced equipment that provides the number and location of a caller (enhanced 9-1-1). Widespread use of cellular telephones has prompted the development of enhanced technology to identify and locate these callers as well, in accordance with Federal Communications Commission regulations. Emergency call takers are trained to collect the necessary information, dispatch appropriate resources, and offer first aid or prearrival instructions, while the ambulance is en route. Ambulance personnel should also be able to communicate with the destination hospital. Most EMS personnel operate under standing

TABLE 1-1 Fifteen Key Elements of EMS Systems Defined by U.S. EMS Systems Act of 1973

Manpower
Training
Communications
Transportation
Facilities
Critical-care units
Public safety agencies
Consumer participation
Access to care
Patient transfer
Coordinated patient record keeping
Public information and education
Review and evaluation
Disaster plan
Mutual aid

orders and protocols developed by physicians. However, there are times when providers may require online medical control, talking directly with a physician for direction.[7] Historically, communications represent the weakest link in most disaster responses. It is therefore important that EMS communication systems have built-in redundancy to ensure uninterrupted service.

TRANSPORTATION

Ambulances have evolved from simple transport vehicles into mobile patient care vehicles. Ambulance design must enable EMS personnel to provide airway and ventilatory support while transporting the patient safely. Basic life support ambulances carry equipment appropriate for personnel trained at the emergency medical technician level, such as automated external defibrillators, oxygen, bag-mask ventilation devices, immobilization and splinting devices, and wound dressings. They do not carry medications and cannot transport patients requiring IVs or cardiac monitoring. Advanced life support ambulances are equipped for paramedics or advanced emergency medical technicians with supplies appropriate for their scope of practice, including IV fluids and medications, intubation equipment, cardiac monitors, and pulse oximeters. Ground transportation is appropriate for the majority of patients, especially in urban and suburban areas. However, air transport, generally by helicopter, should be considered for critically ill patients when the ground transport time would be dangerously long or if the terrain is difficult to navigate.[4]

FACILITIES AND CRITICAL-CARE UNITS

Patients are often transported to the closest appropriate hospital. In recent years, the number of specialty hospitals has increased. These include pediatric hospitals, trauma and spinal cord injury centers, burn centers, stroke centers, and centers with advanced cardiac or resuscitation capabilities.[8] Tertiary care centers, often affiliated with medical schools, provide many of these services and may also have a large number of critical-care unit beds. The decision to bypass hospitals to go directly to a specialty center or a hospital with a large critical-care capacity, often at greater distances, is not a simple one. Although specialty hospitals often have more resources, transporting an unstable patient past an ED to get to the specialty hospital is not without risks. Furthermore, bypassing hospitals may have negative financial consequences for those facilities that are bypassed.[1] It is wise to solicit input from the local, regional, or statewide medical community before developing destination policies involving such specialty centers.

Due to increasing hospital inpatient censuses and ED overcrowding, at a given time, even the largest hospitals may not have adequate resources to care for EMS patients. This may result in prolonged offload times of ambulance patients, long wait times for patients to be seen, and ED boarding of admitted patients. Furthermore, some EDs may request that EMS divert patients to other hospitals.[9] Because of these issues, regional EMS systems should develop methods to monitor in real-time available resources of their receiving hospitals. A secure, Internet-based Web site of hospital resources, including ED and inpatient bed availability, is one option.

PUBLIC SAFETY AGENCIES

EMS systems should have strong ties with police and fire departments. Many large U.S. EMS systems are run by municipal fire departments. In addition to providing scene security, public safety agencies can provide first responder services because they are often first on the scene. Fire and police automated external defibrillator programs are common.[10,11] In some locations, these have been shown to improve outcomes for cardiac arrest victims. Finally, EMS personnel often provide medical support to police and fire departments in hazardous circumstances.

CONSUMER PARTICIPATION

Public support, both political and financial, is necessary for a good EMS system. It is therefore important that laypersons contribute to the policy-making process. One way to accomplish this is to encourage representation of the general public on the membership of regional EMS councils. In addition, the public can participate by volunteering for local EMS agencies.

ACCESS TO CARE

Successful EMS systems ensure that all individuals have access to emergency care regardless of ability to pay. Often, the EMS system is a patient's primary point of entry into the healthcare system. There should be no barriers or disincentives preventing timely access. A more difficult problem exists when terrain or low population densities result in longer response times for some citizens, as in rural or wilderness areas of the country. Possible solutions include stationing or predeploying ambulances throughout the area with one central dispatching center. Another option is heavier reliance on air medical services.

PATIENT TRANSFER

Patients are often transferred from one medical facility to another for a higher level of care. Safe transfer is an important concept. Many problems can be avoided if the transferring and receiving facilities develop transfer agreements in advance. The Emergency Medical Treatment and Active Labor Act, passed in 1986, sets forth rules that hospitals participating in the Medicare program must adhere to when considering a patient transfer. Under the Emergency Medical Treatment and Active Labor Act, all patients must receive a medical screening exam and be stabilized before transfer is considered. There must also be explicit acceptance of the transfer by the receiving hospital.[12]

COORDINATED PATIENT RECORD KEEPING

Maintaining good medical records is important to any patient encounter. Prehospital medical records need to be legible, intelligible, and readily accessible to hospital providers. Standardization of EMS medical records among different agencies within a region helps to streamline transfer of information between prehospital and hospital providers. The adoption of electronic charting and cloud-based electronic medical record keeping by many EMS systems is a step toward this goal. Electronic charts can be printed out in the receiving ED or downloaded from a secure Internet Web site. Regardless of the charting system used, EMS systems must comply with the stipulations of the U.S. Health Insurance Portability and Accountability Act of 1996, designed to protect the privacy of patient health information.[13]

PUBLIC INFORMATION AND EDUCATION

EMS systems have a responsibility to train the public on how to access EMS and use it appropriately. As EMS call volumes rise and available resources decline, educating the public to use 9-1-1 only for true emergencies is an appropriate goal. However, given the obstacles that many patients encounter in trying to access office- or hospital-based care, conveying this message is not simple. The public needs to know that EMS will always be there when needed.

Another important message that EMS can convey to the public is the importance of learning CPR, first aid, and basic disaster preparedness. The responses to Hurricanes Katrina, Rita, and Irene and other recent disasters illustrated that, at times, the emergency response infrastructure may be so seriously disrupted that it may take hours, if not days, for help to arrive. A public that is adequately prepared and trained will be in a better position to safely await help.[14]

REVIEW AND EVALUATION

To ensure proper functioning of an EMS system and high-quality patient care, there must be a process for ongoing review and evaluation. This requires input from personnel involved in day-to-day operations and active involvement of a physician medical director. A continuous quality improvement program should be established to assess system performance and formulate improvements.[15] Routine audits of communications, response times, scene times, and patient care records should be performed. Outcome studies of conditions such as cardiac arrest and trauma may be valuable. However, obtaining such outcomes may be problematic. An unforeseen consequence of the Health Insurance Portability and Accountability Act is that hospitals are often resistant to releasing patient information, even to EMS services, for fear of liability. Solutions to this problem are being investigated.

EMS research is invaluable to evaluate prehospital interventions and develop new ones. It is not valid to assume that what works in the hospital will also work in the prehospital setting. Issues such as limited funding, barriers to obtaining patient outcomes, and obtaining informed consent from critically ill patients, or waivers of consent, can make prehospital research daunting. However, these barriers must be overcome if patients are to receive quality care.[16]

DISASTER PLAN

The EMS system is an integral part of disaster preparedness and should be involved in planning along with other agencies and the medical community. The Omnibus Budget Reconciliation Act legislation of 1981 ended direct federal block grants to EMS. Because EMS is often not considered to fall into the category of public safety, emergency preparedness funding for EMS has fallen behind that of police and fire services.[1] Despite this, EMS agencies must maintain a high level of disaster preparedness. This involves having written policies and procedures, stockpiling supplies that may be rapidly depleted in multi-casualty situations, and participating in regional disaster drills with other emergency response agencies and hospitals.[17]

MUTUAL AID

EMS services should develop mutual aid agreements with neighboring jurisdictions so that emergency care is available when local agencies are overwhelmed or unable to respond.[18] Depending on the size and resources of the system, mutual aid may be required frequently or only under dire circumstances. Working out in advance details such as reimbursement, credentialing, liability, and chain of command at incident scenes will streamline the process.

CHALLENGES AND FUTURE TRENDS

The 2006 Institute of Medicine publication *Emergency Medical Services at the Crossroads*[1] detailed many of the challenges facing EMS. These include fragmentation and lack of interoperability between EMS systems, between EMS and other public safety agencies, and between EMS and the rest of the healthcare infrastructure. These limit the efficiency of EMS systems and may have serious consequences in disaster response. In addition, the fallout from the Omnibus Budget Reconciliation Act legislation of 1981 is still being felt. Funding for EMS continues to fall behind other public safety agencies, both for day-to-day operations and for emergency preparedness. Also, restructuring of how Medicare pays for advanced life support and basic life support services jeopardizes reimbursements. Therefore, many EMS agencies must either find other funding sources or cut services. This is occurring at a time when call volumes are rising in many parts of the country, in part due to the aging of the population and limited access to health care.[1]

Although demand for EMS steadily grows, in many parts of the country EMS staffing is not keeping pace. Factors such as low pay, high stress, and limited advancement opportunities cause high turnover rates among providers. As the length of EMS training curricula increases, alternative careers in health care may appear more appealing.[19] Many EMS systems are currently experiencing real or perceived paramedic shortages, prompting them to look at alternative staffing configurations or resource deployment.

As a consequence of funding and staffing constraints amid increasing call volumes, many EMS systems routinely operate at full capacity. As a result, their surge capacity, or ability to accommodate a sudden, large increase in demand for services, is limited. Surge capacity is determined by a system's staffing capabilities, its available resources, and the ability of its organizational structure to react effectively to the increased demand. To enhance surge capacity, EMS systems need funding for additional personnel, vehicles, and stockpiles of supplies that can be readily deployed. They must also participate in frequent training that is realistic and based on those threats they are most likely to encounter.[20-23]

Despite the many challenges EMS faces, the quality of care provided by EMS personnel continues to improve, driven in part by EMS research. Some of the advances involve regionalization of care, resuscitation of cardiac arrest victims, and management of ST-elevation myocardial infarction patients. The quality of cardiac arrest studies has been enhanced by adoption of the **Utstein template** for data reporting. Developed in 1990, the Utstein style presents a systematic and standardized format for reporting cardiac arrest data. This facilitates the comparison of results of studies performed in different EMS systems.[24] The importance of basic life support skills in cardiac arrest and other emergencies is being rediscovered. Basic interventions in some cases can have a greater impact on outcome than advanced life support skills. More widespread use of automated external defibrillators by first responders and the public has the potential to increase rates of resuscitation in cardiac arrest. The emphasis on high-quality, uninterrupted CPR, as set forth by the international 2007 guidelines for CPR and emergency cardiovascular care,[25] is widely reflected in EMS protocols across the United States.[26,27] Automatic chest compression devices and devices that provide instant feedback on the quality of CPR are being introduced in the prehospital setting.[28] Some EMS systems are beginning to induce hypothermia in resuscitated cardiac arrest patients.[29,30] Prehospital use of 12-lead electrocardiograms on patients with chest pain is becoming common.[31-34] Some systems transmit electrocardiograms to receiving EDs. Others activate cardiac catheterization labs directly when an ST-elevation myocardial infarction is identified on electrocardiogram.

EMS is maturing as an important subspecialty of emergency medicine in the United States and abroad. Growing populations and increased urbanization are driving the development of EMS systems worldwide.[35,36] The aftermath of the 2004 Asian tsunami emphasized the need for organized and effective prehospital care in developing countries, as well as for international cooperation among EMS agencies.[37,38] Although EMS systems in some countries are very similar to those in the United States, in other countries, differences in geography, healthcare system design, funding, and political structure present unique challenges and the potential for novel solutions. These developing EMS systems have the advantage of not being encumbered by decades of tradition, so they can take advantage of lessons learned elsewhere. They also present the opportunity for collaboration on international research initiatives that can lead to improved patient outcomes.[39]

REFERENCES

The complete reference list is available online at www.TintinalliEM.com.

CHAPTER 2

Prehospital Equipment

Andy Boggust

INTRODUCTION

To a large extent, early EMS equipment began as hospital equipment that was extrapolated to the field; it was assumed that if something worked in the hospital, then it would work in the field. It soon became apparent that hospital equipment did not always perform under the more rigorous conditions of prehospital care. Over the last 30 years, equipment has evolved specifically for EMS that is better adapted to field use in terms of size, weight, and durability. This equipment is directed at resuscitating and packaging the patient for transport to the hospital and for maintenance of stability during emergency or interfacility transport. As the science of EMS continues to mature, more equipment will be scrutinized for effectiveness.[1] The four basic questions regarding efficacy of EMS equipment are:

1. Does it do the job?
2. Is it safe?
3. Can it be applied to the field environment?
4. Can it be used effectively by prehospital personnel?

The nature of EMS equipment is changing due to the expanded scope of practice by paramedics and the blurring of care levels between basic life support (BLS) and advanced life support (ALS) personnel. Equipment once considered only for ALS care is now being carried on some BLS ambulances (e.g., defibrillators and airway adjuncts). This chapter discusses EMS vehicles; communications; the electronic patient record; personal protective equipment; and specific equipment for stabilization, resuscitation, and treatment.

VEHICLES

The vehicles may be ground ambulances, helicopters, fixed-wing aircraft, or a variety of first-response vehicles (fire engines, police cruisers, or sport utility vehicles). The most common vehicle used is the ground ambulance, categorized into three common varieties:

Type I: A standard truck (e.g., pick-up) chassis with a separate modular box to carry personnel, patient, and equipment

Type II: An enlarged van-type vehicle

Type III: A van chassis with an integrated modular box on the back for medical care and equipment

In types II and III, there is physical access between the driver's and patient care compartments, as opposed to type I, in which these spaces are separate.

Ground vehicles typically have warning devices (lights and siren) as part of their equipment. Unwarranted use of red lights and sirens is dangerous for the EMS crew, the patient onboard (if present), and the general public on the streets.[2] Protocols or guidelines to limit the use of these devices only to times when they are medically indicated are important.

COMMUNICATIONS

The two-way radio is an important piece of equipment carried by prehospital providers. As the arena of wireless communication changes, EMS systems will need to adapt their communications system to best fit their needs. The spectrum of frequencies available for emergency services is limited and shared with other industries that require wireless communications. In the United States, EMS services may use specific frequencies (*channels*) in the very high frequency (around 170 MHz), ultra-high frequency (around 460 MHz), and public safety (around 800 MHz) bands. In an attempt to create more channels for users, the Federal Communications Commission has decreased channel spacing from 25 to 12.5 kHz, and there is a Federal Communications Commission mandate to continue spacing down to 6.25 kHz. Although newer radio equipment can be reprogrammed to allow for the change in channel spacing, older equipment may not function correctly with this spacing.

EMS systems in rural or suburban settings may have no difficulties with local communications; however, as they transport patients into urban settings and attempt to communicate with urban providers, the problems of compatible frequencies and channel congestion may develop. Urban systems may use trunking, in which communications pathways are managed by a central processor between end users, allowing large numbers of users to share a relatively small number of communications frequencies. Trunked systems may be analog, very high frequency/ultra-high frequency digital radio, or 800-MHz digital radio. An 800-MHz digital trunked system is popular because of the advantages of shared equipment between different providers (EMS, police, and fire), enhanced radio coverage, shared or lowered cost, and wide-area communications. The main disadvantage with all trunked systems is the cost necessary to upgrade the current system. In the United States, 800-MHz trunking is slowly being implemented for emergency services providers, largely due to sponsorship by the U.S. Department of Homeland Security, because of improved communications during terrorist incidents and other disasters. Although 800 MHz is a more effective means of communication, the transition to it is slow due to the difficulties with simultaneous upgrading by police, fire, and EMS.

Many urban and suburban EMS providers are choosing cellular/personal communication systems as a means of communication. These systems are abundant in urban settings because they are often inexpensive and easier to use. However, at times, these cellular/personal communication systems are congested, and there are still dead spots, even in urban areas. During many disasters, when landline phones have not worked, cellular systems have also failed to function, so reliance on cell service during major incidents is problematic.[3,4]

ELECTRONIC MEDICAL RECORD

Use of the prehospital electronic medical record has increased substantially over the past 5 years. As usage of these electronic systems increases, research and system quality assurance analysis should become easier because of better data access.[5]

Large systems with enough resources often have their own software specifically written for that system. Smaller EMS systems often use off-the-shelf alternatives. Using one of the latter products may require either modification of a vendor's product or modification of the EMS system workflow to make the software fully functional. Many states are in the process of generating or have already generated a common data set and are collecting statewide data, which are submitted to the state EMS agency. Local and state data systems should be coordinated so they are compatible.

One common difficulty with the prehospital electronic medical record is incompatibility with the hospital electronic medical record. This means that the ambulance record cannot be expeditiously transferred to the hospital database. Long-term solutions need to be devised to ensure that all of these record systems are compatible.

PERSONAL PROTECTIVE EQUIPMENT

Every EMS provider must be protected against exposure to blood and other body fluids from patients. Equipment such as masks, goggles, and gloves for routine use should be carried on every EMS vehicle. On occasion, gowns or sturdy gloves may be needed.[6]

Exposure to hazardous material or biologic or chemical weapons of mass destruction requires more protective equipment. **Minimum personal protective equipment for such exposure should include a high-efficiency particulate air filter mask that filters 99.97% of airborne particles 0.3 μm in diameter (or an acceptable alternative for the purpose, such as an M95 military gas mask), goggles, gloves, and protective clothing.** Protective clothing should be nonabsorbent and puncture resistant (**Figure 2-1**).[7]

Some urban EMS providers wear soft body armor as a standard part of the uniform. Suburban and rural providers can be placed in situations that

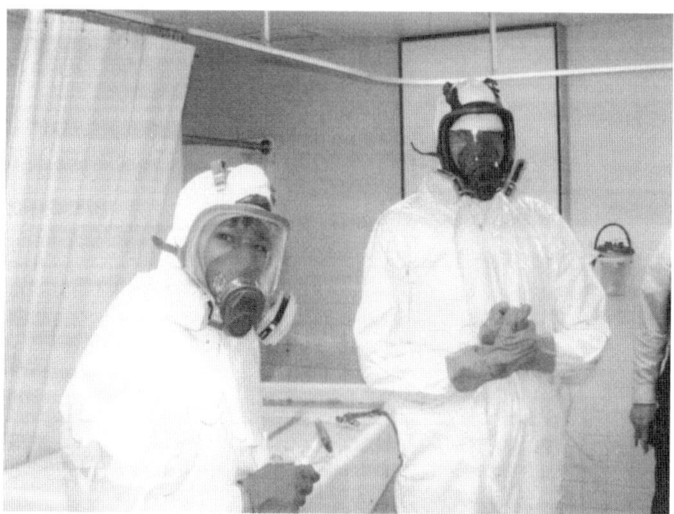

FIGURE 2-1. Personal protective equipment: filtered (high-efficiency particulate air, M95, N95, or chemical-specific) mask, goggles, gloves, and protective clothing.[7]

necessitate similar protection. With advances in soft-armor technology, there are now a variety of styles and levels of protection from which to choose. Although each service must consider such variables as comfort, heat, weight, and cost, for EMS providers, a combination of ballistic/stab protection is optimal.

EQUIPMENT FOR STABILIZATION, RESUSCITATION, AND TREATMENT

This section reviews defibrillators, electrocardiograms, airway and ventilation adjuncts, vascular access devices, spinal immobilization, and extremity immobilization.

DEFIBRILLATORS

Defibrillators have been an essential part of prehospital care since Pantridge showed that defibrillation could be done in the field on the streets of Belfast in 1965. **Early defibrillation is the most important factor in surviving a cardiac arrest.** Because of this, defibrillators have become smaller and less costly to expand their use. Paramedic-staffed ALS services typically carry manual monitor/defibrillators, often with additional functions (e.g., 12-lead electrocardiogram, external cardiac pacing, and synchronized cardioversion). An increasing percentage of BLS services carry automated external defibrillators. These devices are shock advisory defibrillators. Automated external defibrillators analyze the patient's rhythm by computer algorithm, determine if the rhythm meets defibrillation criteria, inform the operator that a shock is advised, charge the capacitor, and deliver a defibrillation when the operator pushes the appropriate button. Automated external defibrillators are designed only to shock ventricular fibrillation and very fast ventricular or supraventricular tachycardias (usually >180 beats/min). Automated external defibrillators have become so easy to use and are so effective that many health and medical organizations are promoting these devices for first-responder public safety personnel and for public-access defibrillation by laypersons.[8-10]

Automated external defibrillators are simple and relatively inexpensive. They often do not have monitor screens that display the patient's rhythm. This actually may be better because a rhythm on the screen may only serve to distract a non-ALS operator. The device should have recording capabilities so that the cardiac arrest can later be reviewed for medical oversight and quality assurance reasons. The medical director should be involved in choosing such devices, training in their use, establishing protocols for their use, and reviewing their use afterward for quality assurance.

A defibrillator used by ALS personnel is typically a different, more sophisticated device, usually with additional functions. Defibrillation is facilitated using hands-off combination monitoring/defibrillation adhesive pads rather than with handheld paddles. Pads give better contact with the skin and decrease skin resistance to allow for a higher success rate of rhythm conversion. It is also safer for the operator who does not have direct contact with the patient when the shock is delivered. The ALS defibrillator has a screen for interpreting rhythms and so is also used for ongoing monitoring of patients' rhythms. It may be used for cardioversion of nonlethal rhythms or pacing bradyasystolic rhythms. Additional critical care patient monitoring can be incorporated into an ALS defibrillator, including noninvasive blood pressure, pulse oximetry, end-tidal partial pressure of carbon dioxide in intubated patients, and other physiologic parameters. ALS personnel can use these machines for closely monitoring very ill patients during emergent calls or interfacility transfers.

Modern defibrillators use biphasic waveforms for shock delivery (as opposed to the traditional monophasic waveform). Monophasic waveforms deliver energy in one direction, from the positive to the negative pole. Biphasic waveforms deliver energy in two phases, one toward the positive pole and one toward the negative pole. Biphasic defibrillators defibrillate and cardiovert at lower energy levels and thus decrease myocardial injury.[11]

Prehospital 12-lead electrocardiograms have become increasingly important in the management of ST-elevation myocardial infarctions (STEMI). Both BLS and ALS ambulance services can perform electrocardiograms in the prehospital setting.[12] Analysis of electrocardiograms provided immediately by the electrocardiograph has demonstrated limited sensitivity for detecting ST-elevation myocardial infarction.[13] However, sensitivity can be increased using serial prehospital electrocardiograms, training paramedics to interpret electrocardiograms, and providing computer-assisted interpretation or remote physician overread of the electrocardiogram.[14,15] Irrespective of the method of interpretation, patients with a prehospital 12-lead electrocardiogram showing ST-elevation myocardial infarction arriving at a hospital with a dedicated percutaneous coronary intervention team in place have reduced door-to-balloon time and reduced mortality when compared with similar patients arriving without a prehospital 12-lead electrocardiogram.[16-18]

AIRWAY AND VENTILATION ADJUNCTS

In a patient with acute respiratory failure or arrest, these devices maintain a patent airway that otherwise would have to be maintained by the paramedic. In addition, some airway adjuncts aid in preventing complications of airway management, such as gastric distention or aspiration (**Figure 2-2**). See chapter 28, Noninvasive Airway Management,

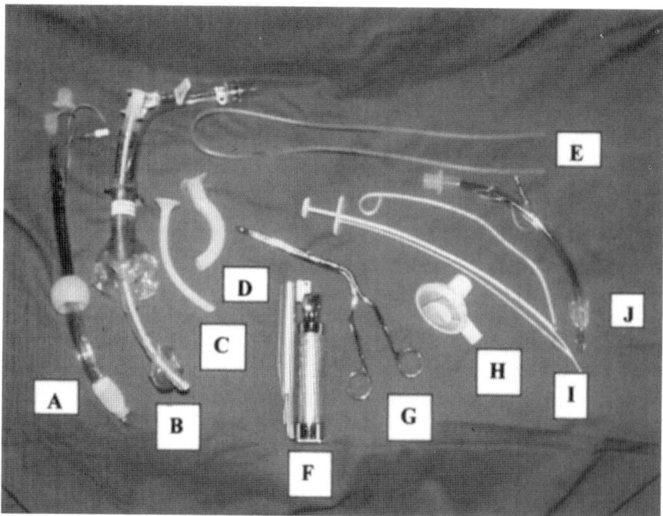

FIGURE 2-2. Airway devices and adjuncts. **A.** Combitube®. **B.** Pharyngeal tracheal lumen airway. **C.** Nasopharyngeal airway. **D.** Oropharyngeal airway. **E.** Tube exchanger. **F.** Laryngoscope. **G.** Magill forceps. **H.** Qualitative expiratory carbon dioxide detector. **I.** Stylets for endotracheal intubation. **J.** Endotracheal tube.

and 29, Intubation and Mechanical Ventilation, for detailed discussions of these topics.

Oral and Nasal Airways The simplest devices for airway management after manual airway maneuvers are the oropharyngeal and nasopharyngeal airways. These basic airway adjuncts usually are paired in the field with a simple bag-valve mask device for ventilation and will work quite well together. Ventilation with the bag-valve mask can be difficult for a single person to both attain a good seal with the mask and compress the bag to produce an adequate tidal volume for the patient. It is probably more effective (especially for first-responder and ambulance personnel who do not perform the skill often) to make this a two-person task (one person to maintain the seal and one person to compress the bag to maintain tidal volume). Along with these adjuncts, effective portable suction devices are available to be carried to the patient's side to help clear the airway.

Supraglottic Airways More advanced airway devices are used if the patient appears to need more prolonged airway management or is at greater risk for aspiration. At the BLS level, these airways include, most commonly, the **pharyngeal tracheal lumen airway (PtL®)**, the **esophagotracheal Combitube** or **King LTS-D airway**, and the **laryngeal mask airway (LMA®)**. Each of these is used in conjunction with a bag-valve mask for ventilation. These devices are great improvements over the esophageal obturator airway and esophageal gastric tube airway, which have unacceptably high complication rates and are no longer recommended for use. Both the PtL® and the Combitube® are for unconscious patients >14 years and >48 inches tall. They improve the airway seal to promote better ventilation than the bag-valve mask with the oral airway and seal the esophagus off with a balloon to prevent aspiration. If either device goes into the trachea, which occurs a small percentage of the time, the device can function equivalently to an endotracheal tube. The Combitube® may be a more reliable device than the PtL® because the large mouth balloon of the PtL® is more easily broken than the more robust Combitube® balloon, and basic emergency medical technicians (EMTs) may find ventilation easier with the Combitube®.[19-22] There are few data on the use of the LMA® for prehospital care. The LMA® provides a seal for ventilation but may not prevent aspiration. One possible advantage of the LMA® is that it may be less expensive than the Combitube® or the PtL®. The PtL® and Combitube® are mostly used by BLS ambulance personnel, but may be used by ALS personnel (or even by hospital personnel) as a fallback rescue device for a patient who has a difficult airway and cannot be intubated with an endotracheal tube (**Table 2-1**).[23-26]

A review of pediatric alternative airway devices in prehospital care discusses the problems encountered in the field with airway management of children.[27] Unlike the PtL® or Combitube®, there are pediatric-sized LMAs® available. It is not clear how useful the LMA® is as a prehospital rescue airway because it is not clear if the LMA® prevents aspiration. Table 2-1 compares the PtL®, Combitube®, LMA®, and King LTS-D® devices.

Endotracheal Intubation Endotracheal intubation is the "gold standard" for airway management in all patients and is especially useful in patients in whom the other airway adjuncts are not satisfactory.[28] The majority of ALS systems use endotracheal intubation as the airway of choice for patients in respiratory failure or with an unprotected airway. Numerous adjuncts to assist with endotracheal intubation can be found in the ED as well as the prehospital setting. However, provider procedural experience is a primary determinant for successful placement. For further discussion, see chapter 29, Intubation and Mechanical Ventilation.

The basic EMT curriculum has an optional module for endotracheal intubation training. Therefore, intubation equipment may be found on some BLS ambulances. Increasing the number of ambulance personnel in need of endotracheal intubation training in an EMS system may cause logistic problems for the medical director. It is sometimes difficult to obtain adequate live intubation opportunities for the personnel in an EMS system to maintain skills. Some studies have shown that basic EMTs do not maintain endotracheal intubation skills and have low rates of successful completion.[29,30] This might suggest that intubation should remain an ALS skill.[31,32]

TABLE 2-1 Comparison of PtL®, Combitube®, LMA®, and King LTS-D®

Device	Use	Comments
PtL®	Adults Adolescents >48 inches tall or age >14 years old	Prevents/minimizes aspiration If inadvertently placed in trachea, will still ventilate Cannot use if gag reflex present Balloon may not be as sturdy as Combitube® balloon
Combitube®	Adults Adolescents >48 inches tall or age >14 years old	Prevents/minimizes aspiration If inadvertently placed in trachea, will still ventilate Cannot use if gag reflex present Sturdy balloon
LMA®	Sizes for adults and children	May not prevent aspiration Can cause respiratory obstruction if incorrectly placed Cannot use if gag reflex present
King LTS-D®	Sizes for adults and children	Prevents/minimizes aspiration If inadvertently placed in trachea, will still ventilate Cannot use if gag reflex present Sturdy balloon Port for gastric decompression tube

Abbreviations: LMA® = laryngeal mask airway; PtL® = pharyngeal tracheal lumen airway.

Rapid-Sequence Intubation Another intubation-related modality that has bearing on the equipment carried on an ambulance is **rapid-sequence intubation**. Critical care transport services have been performing rapid-sequence intubation for more than a decade, and now this same level of care is provided in ALS systems as well. Rapid-sequence intubation raises the level of training, judgment, and psychomotor skills needed by the paramedic but has the advantage of being able to secure more difficult airways. In addition to the usual equipment required for intubation, rapid-sequence intubation requires ALS services to carry the medications needed for sedation and paralysis.[33] The technique increases the need for oversight and vigilance by the medical director. Los Angeles,[34] San Diego,[35] and Orlando[36] have all indicated difficulties with ALS intubation, with or without the assistance of neuromuscular junction blockade/sedation. Intubation, especially rapid-sequence intubation, is a training-intensive modality. Large systems with many paramedics may have difficulties with training type and intensity.[32] Smaller services, such as air medical services, which have a smaller group to train, a smaller span of medical control, and more intubation experience per provider, may be able to attain and maintain the complex skills needed for rapid-sequence intubation.

CONTINUOUS POSITIVE AIRWAY PRESSURE AND BILEVEL POSITIVE AIRWAY PRESSURE

Continuous positive airway pressure (CPAP) maintains a continuous level of positive airway pressure throughout the respiratory cycle. Similarly, bilevel positive airway pressure (BiPAP) delivers CPAP in a preset or measured inspiratory positive airway pressure phase and expiratory positive airway pressure phase. BLS and ALS services become competent in the use of this adjunct with additional training and a broadened understanding of respiratory physiology.[37-39] Use of either modality in the ED and prehospital setting is lifesaving and cost-effective in the treatment of the severely dyspneic patient.[40-42]

VASCULAR ACCESS EQUIPMENT

The equipment used to establish IV access is the same as at the hospital: tourniquets, cleaning agent, IV catheters, IV fluid bags, and IV tubing. ALS ambulances need IV access for fluid resuscitation and for administration of medications. In general, vascular access for medication administration is completed as soon as possible after the patient is assessed and it is determined that pharmacologic intervention is needed. For fluid resuscitation, usually in trauma patients, vascular access usually is started en route to the hospital after the patient is immobilized, unless there is prolonged scene time due to extrication. This is to avoid prolonged scene times that may be detrimental to a trauma patient who may need intervention in the operating room. In any event, the amount of fluid that can be administered during transport is modest and may not be physiologically significant. Some data show that aggressive fluid resuscitation of hypovolemic trauma patients is detrimental, in that it may increase morbidity and mortality by enhancing exsanguination from vascular or organ injury requiring operative intervention.[43,44] The difference between hospital and EMS usage of IV equipment is that the medical director must provide guidelines for when and how to institute vascular access to allow appropriate interventions at the appropriate time. Use of vascular access should be examined in the quality assurance process in an ongoing manner.

Intraosseous access devices are important adjuncts for difficult vascular access. Studies have not conclusively demonstrated the superiority of one device over another. One small study indicated that the EZ-IO® device (Vidacare Corporation, San Antonio, TX) may be superior to the FAST1® device (Pyng Medical Corporation, Richmond, British Columbia, Canada) because of higher insertion success.[45] Guidance is provided in a position paper from the National Association of EMS Physicians (http://www.naemsp.org).[46,47]

Vascular access is also used by some BLS services for fluid resuscitation. Because BLS services are usually more rural and have longer transport times, fluid resuscitation may be more beneficial in rural hypovolemic trauma patients with blunt rather than penetrating trauma.

PREHOSPITAL ULTRASOUND

US is an important diagnostic tool in the practice of emergency medicine. New diagnostic applications for bedside US in the ED are reported in emergency medicine literature almost monthly. Moving US into the prehospital setting would seem like a logical next step. Multiple investigations demonstrate the feasibility of prehospital US in the United States and Europe.[48-51] Some prospective observational data on prehospital US in European EMS systems is available.[52,53] Remember, however, that these systems are often staffed with physician-level providers. Prospective data from paramedic- and nurse-staffed EMS systems is gradually becoming available.[54,55]

SPINAL IMMOBILIZATION

Preservation of the integrity of the spinal column and spinal cord is of paramount importance in the prehospital setting. The first person to assess the patient should immobilize the cervical spine immediately and, if necessary, simultaneously perform a modified jaw thrust to open the airway. Manual stabilization of the neck is not released until the patient has been transferred and securely strapped to a board. Short or long boards, either alone or in combination, are used to immobilize the spine depending on the initial position in which the patient is found by the EMT or first responder.

Carrying boarded patients takes a physical toll on EMTs and paramedics. Evaluation of the boarded patient is more expensive and time consuming in the ED because of the need to clear the cervical spine. A reasonable approach is for the medical director to develop protocols and guidelines for clearance of the spine in the field. A patient with no neck pain, tenderness, or discomfort (neck pain must be defined liberally and include stiffness or "feels funny"); not in the extremes of age (<10 years or >65 years); no altered sensorium (no drugs or alcohol present, no head injury); and no distracting injuries (long-bone fracture, abdominal or chest injury) may be cleared in the field because there is an extraordinarily low probability of neck injury (**Table 2-2**).[56]

TABLE 2-2 Guidelines for Cervical Spine Clearance in the Field
Absence of neck pain, tenderness, or discomfort
Age between 11 and 65 years
No altered sensorium
No intoxication
No distracting injuries

SPINAL BOARDS AND CERVICAL COLLARS

Long or short spinal boards are made from plastic or wood and provide a rigid surface to minimize movement of the cervical, thoracic, or lumbar spine. Straps secure the patient to the board for transport. Some boards are provided with firm rubber blocks on either side of the head with straps to go across the blocks to keep the head steady. Blanket rolls secured to the board with tape are also effective head blocks. A popular and effective variation of the short board is the **Kendrick Extrication Device® (KED®)** (**Figure 2-3**), which consists of slats of rigid material bound together by heavy cloth.

This board immobilizes the cervical spine, wraps partly around the patient, and is then strapped the rest of the way around the thorax and around the thighs for secure immobilization. If necessary, the patient can be lifted by the straps, allowing for easier and safer upward extrication from the vehicle.

Rigid cervical collars are more accurately called cervical extrication devices. Multiple types are used in the field, such as the Philadelphia® collar, the Miami J® collar (**Figure 2-4**), the Stifneck® (Laerdal Medical, Wappingers Falls, NY), and the Nec Loc® (Junkin Safety Appliance Co., Louisville, KY).

The collars come in two asymmetric pieces, which are used and marked for back and front, or as a single piece that is folded into the correct shape. By themselves, collars are not adequate for cervical immobilization but require additional lateral support to avoid movement in that direction. For adequate immobilization, the patient needs to be strapped on the backboard and secured with head blocks and head straps. Once the patient is well secured to the board, the collar does not add a significant amount of stabilization and actually can be removed without compromise of the spine; however, it is often left in place for added protection. Patients with mandible or soft tissue neck injuries probably should not have a collar applied because of the potential for airway compromise, which could be masked by the collar. Newer collars have openings in the front to allow observation of the trachea and jugular veins, but this may not be adequate for observing other neck areas. Soft cervical collars are not adequate or appropriate for prehospital care.

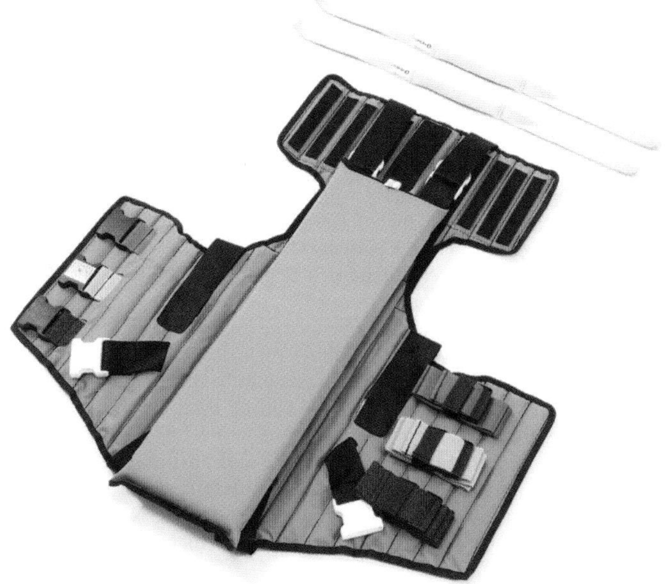

FIGURE 2-3. Kendrick Extrication Device® (KED®) (Armstrong Medical Industries, Lincolnshire, IL). [Reproduced with permission from Armstrong Medical Industries, Inc.]

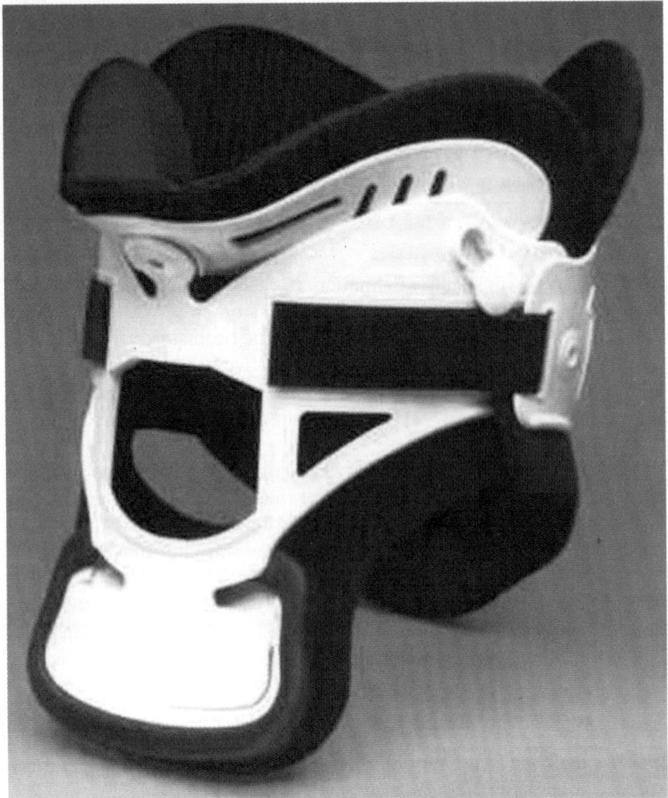

FIGURE 2-4. Miami J® collar. [Reproduced with permission from Ossur Americas, Foot Hill Ranch, CO.]

SEQUENCE OF SPINAL IMMOBILIZATION

Prehospital personnel are taught to have a high index of suspicion for spine trauma. **If the patient is sitting in a car after an accident and is stable from respiratory and circulatory standpoints, a short spine board and rigid cervical collar or Kendrick Extrication Device® are first used to get the patient out of the vehicle safely and onto a long spine board.** If the situation at hand is a critical one because of the patient's condition or the threat of hazards, such as chemicals, fire, or water, the patient can be extricated more rapidly using only the cervical collar. After applying the cervical collar, the patient is carefully rotated out and slid onto the waiting long board.

At a noncritical scene, when the patient is still sitting in the vehicle, one EMT secures the neck with his or her hands and applies the necessary airway maneuvers, while the second EMT applies the rigid cervical collar. The short board is then slid in behind the patient, and the patient is strapped to the short spine board. (Short boards are not used if the patient is not seated in a vehicle.) The first EMT maintains manual stabilization of the neck until the patient is secured to the short board. The patient's head and trunk can then be rotated around as one unit and slid directly onto the long board positioned on the car seat or on the ambulance cot. The patient is then strapped to the long board and then to the cot. A properly boarded patient can be turned on the board or even stood on end if necessary to move the patient to the ambulance. If the patient vomits, for instance, the board can be partly log-rolled up to prevent aspiration.

Because of the difference in relative size and positions of head and body, adults and children need slightly different positioning on a backboard. **An adult needs more padding under the head, whereas a child needs more padding under the body to maintain neutral neck position.**

If a patient is walking at the scene when the paramedical personnel arrive but complains of neck pain, the patient can be boarded from a standing position. If the patient is lying on the ground when the EMTs arrive, the patient can be carefully log-rolled by several attendants onto a long backboard.

Immobilization on a rigid board produces midline cervical pain and tenderness, so examination and radiographs should be performed promptly on arrival.[57] Radiographs can be done without difficulty through short and long boards. In general, patients should not be removed from immobilization until the spine has been cleared clinically and radiographically. Transfer from the hard prehospital board to a padded board at the hospital is desirable if the patient may spend prolonged time immobilized.

FOOTBALL HELMET REMOVAL

The National Athletic Trainer's Association (http://www.nata.org) and the Inter-Association Task Force for the Appropriate Care of the Spine-Injured Athlete have developed guidelines for the prehospital care of athletes with potential spine injury. **These guidelines recommend that the face mask of a football helmet be removed at the earliest opportunity, before transportation and regardless of respiratory status.** However, because a properly fitted football helmet with shoulder pads holds the head in a position of neutral spinal alignment, field removal of these devices is not recommended. It is recommended that the helmet and shoulder pads remain on as the athlete is immobilized and transported on a rigid backboard. Simultaneous removal of the helmet and shoulder pads should be done after clinical assessment and radiographs at the hospital, although radiographs may have to be repeated after equipment removal.[58]

Removal of football shoulder pads and helmet requires several individuals to maintain spinal alignment (**Figure 2-5**). One individual stands at the head of the bed to stabilize the patient's head, neck, and helmet, while others stabilize the spine and body. All straps and laces that secure the pads to the torso and arms are cut, not unbuckled or unsnapped. The laces or straps over the sternum are cut, allowing the right and left anterior portions to be spread open, exposing the chest. The posterior portion of the shoulder pads is kept in place to maintain spinal alignment with the helmet. Another individual cuts the chin strap from below while standing beside the patient's chest. Accessible internal padding should be removed from inside the helmet and any air bladders deflated. The individual standing alongside the patient's chest then reaches up into the helmet to stabilize the head by placing a hand with fingers and thumbs spread alongside the jaw, mastoid region, and occiput.

Two additional individuals stand alongside the patient's chest and place their hands directly on the skin in the thoracic region. On command, the patient is lifted slightly, with all four individuals maintaining spinal alignment. The individual standing at the head of the bed can remove the helmet by a slight forward rotation to slide it off the occiput. Slight traction or anteroposterior motion may be necessary, but care should be taken not to move the head and neck unit. Attempting to assist removal by pulling on the ear holes tightens the helmet in the forehead and occipital regions and does not help. The posterior portion of the shoulder pads is removed, and the patient is lowered. A rigid cervical collar can then be placed.

TRACTION SPLINTS

Pelvic fractures and femoral shaft fractures are potentially life and limb threatening. Field or ED stabilization of pelvic fractures is difficult. Devices, such as the T-POD® (Pyng Medical Corporation), for pelvic fracture immobilization have become available, but their place in prehospital care is unclear.

Fractures of the femur can damage vessels and nerves when bony fragments move. Stabilization in the field is important to minimize blood loss and soft tissue damage. The femoral traction splint is the preferred device for femur fractures.

Several leg traction splint variations are available for use. The two most commonly used types are the Hare® splint (Dynamed, Westbury, Tasmania) and the Sager® splint (Minto Research and Development, Inc., Redding, CA). The underlying technique is the application of traction by a hitch on the ankle against resistance when the splint impinges

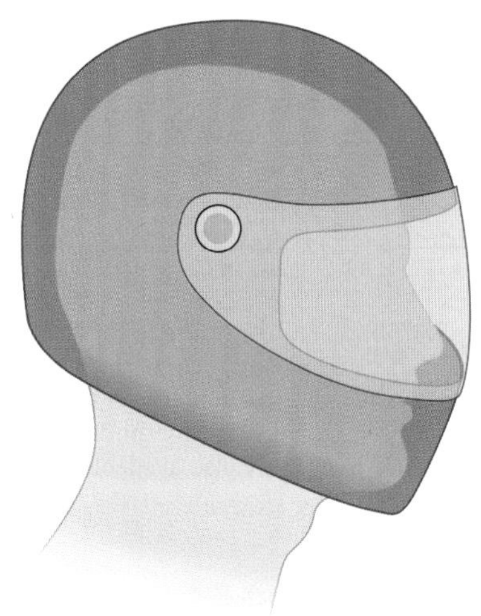

FIGURE 2-5. Helmet removal technique. [Reproduced with permission from American College of Surgeons, Committee on Trauma Brochure, April 1997.]

Helmet Removal

The varying sizes, shapes, and configurations of motorcycle and sports helmets necessitate some understanding of their proper removal from victims of motorcycle crashes. The rescuer who removes a helmet improperly may unintentionally aggravate cervical spine injuries.

The Committee on Trauma believes that physicians who treat the injured should be aware of helmet removal techniques. A gradual increase in the use of helmets is anticipated, because many organizations are urging voluntary wearing of helmets, and some states are reinstating their laws requiring the wearing of helmets.

Types of Helmets

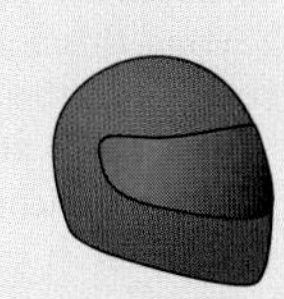

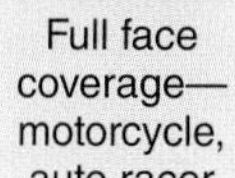

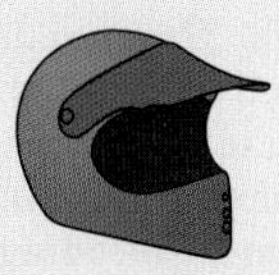

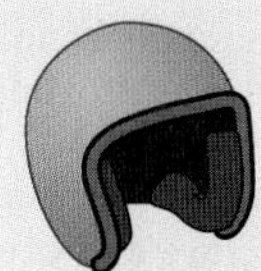

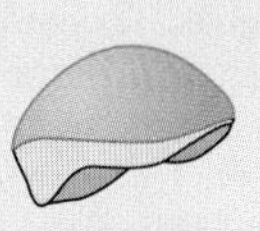

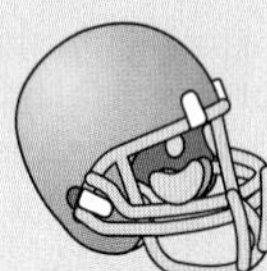

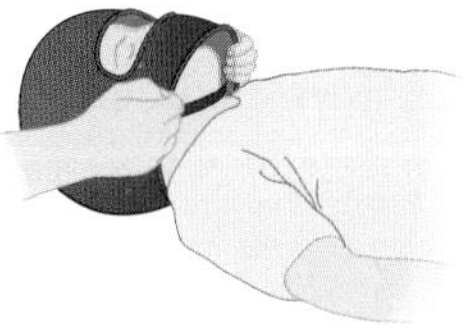

1. One rescuer maintains inline immoblization by placing the hands on each side of the helmet with the fingers on the victim's mandible. This position prevents slippage if the strap is loose.

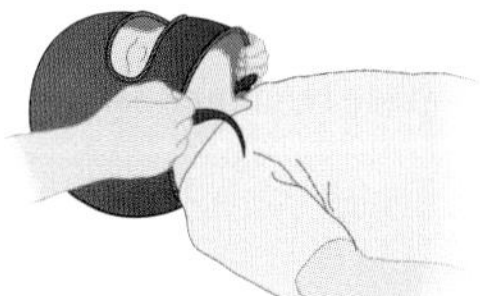

2. A second rescuer cuts or loosens the strap at the D-rings.

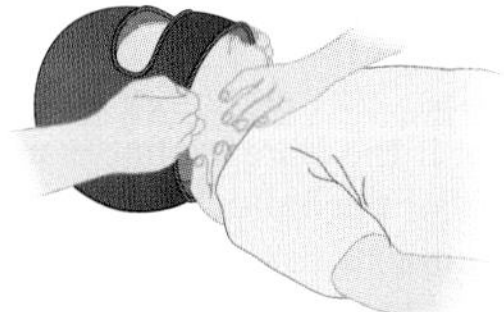

3. The second rescuer places one hand on the mandible at the angle, the thumb on one side, the long and index fingers on the other. With the other hand, pressure is applied from the occipital region. This maneuver transfers the inline immobilization responsibility to the second rescuer.

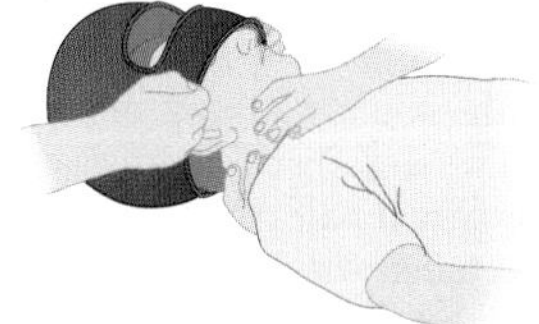

4. The rescuer at the top moves the helmet. Three factors should be kept in mind:

- The helmet is egg shaped and therefore must be expanded laterally to clear the ears.
- If the helmet provides full facial coverage, glasses must be removed first.
- If the helmet provides full facial coverage, the nose may impede removal. To clear the nose, the helmet must be tilted backward and raised over it.

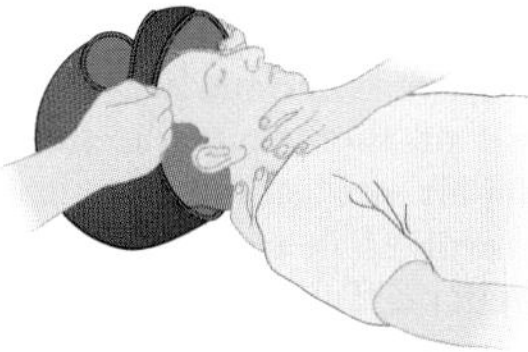

5. Throughout the removal process, the second rescuer maintains inline immobilization from below to prevent unnecessary neck motion.

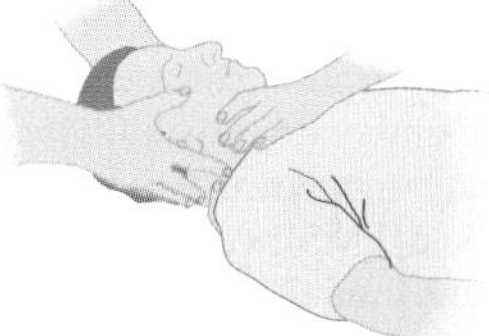

6. After the helmet has been removed, the rescuer at the top replaces the hands on either side of the victim's head with the palms over the ears.

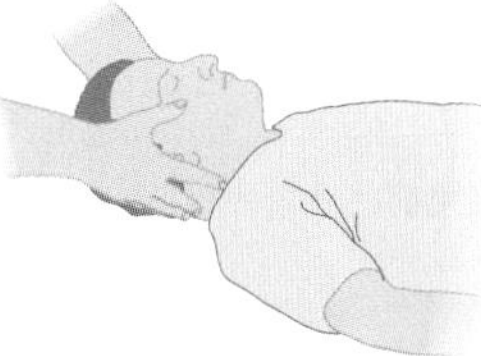

7. Inline immobilization is maintained from above until a backboard is in place and a cervical immobilization device (collar) is applied.

Summary

The helmet must be maneuvered over the nose and ears while the head and neck are held rigid.

- Inline immobilization is first applied from above.
- Inline immobilization is applied from below by a second rescuer with pressure on the jaw and occiput.
- The helmet is removed.
- Inline immobilization is reestablished from above.

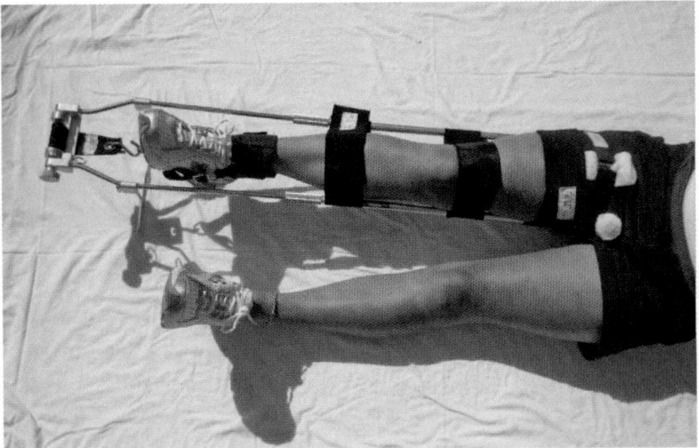

FIGURE 2-6. Hare® traction splint (Dynamed, Westbury, Tasmania). [Courtesy of Jan Smith, RN, MPH, NREMT-P; acknowledgments to Kara Smith and Lucky Bruton, EMT-P.]

proximally on the pelvis. The padded proximal end of the Hare® splint abuts the ischial tuberosity (**Figure 2-6**). The proximal end of the Sager® splint rests against the pubic symphysis (**Figure 2-7**). **These splints cannot be used if a pelvic fracture is suspected because the pressure on the pelvis may further displace a fracture and cause more bleeding. Also, do not apply a traction splint if there is open fracture, hip dislocation, suspicion for neurovascular injury to the extremity, or injury about the knee, as a traction splint may exacerbate neurovascular or knee injury.**

Leg traction splints also may be used for tibial shaft fractures. Traction splints should not be used for fractures near the knee because longitudinal traction may damage neurovascular structures in the popliteal region. Traction splints for the tibia should be reserved for angulated or displaced fractures; otherwise, an air splint or a pillow splint would suffice.

At the scene, clothing should be removed and the extremity assessed for injury and distal neurovascular function. If the Hare® splint is used, the proximal half ring is placed in the crease of the buttocks against the ischial tuberosity. Traction is placed on the ankle with the padded ankle strap by one rescuer while the splint is strapped to the leg. The ankle strap is then attached to a ratcheting mechanism, and traction is tightened. If a Sager® splint is used, the splint is placed on the medial side of the limb up against the groin. The padded ankle hitch is applied, and traction is applied until malalignment is reduced and pain is relieved. Elastic straps are then applied to hold the splint to the leg.

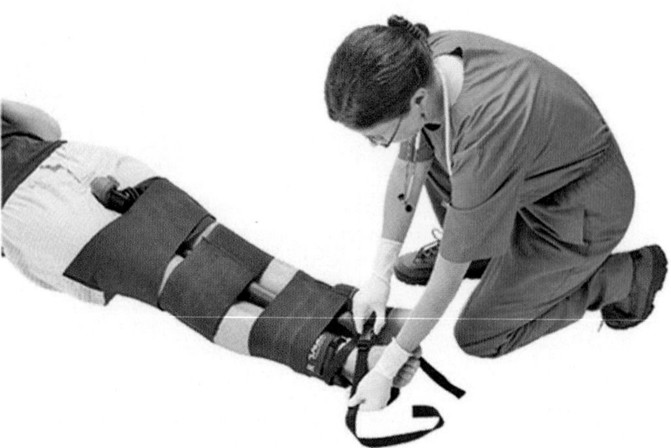

FIGURE 2-7. Sager Emergency Traction Splint; Model S304, Form III Bilateral, Application step 3 "Secure". [Used with permission from: Minto Research & Development, Inc., Redding, CA, USA.]

The Hare® splint can be longer than an ambulance cot when fully extended, and care needs to be taken when closing the rear door of the ambulance. The Sager® splint is shorter than the Hare® splint, and one Sager® splint can be used to splint both legs simultaneously. The Sager® splint is less bulky and therefore takes up less room in an ambulance or a helicopter.

PELVIC STABILIZERS

Unstable pelvic fractures can be immobilized to minimize the risk of bleeding from patient movement and during transport. A sheet wrap, applied around the patient at the level of the trochanter and fastened with a clamp or hemostat, is the simplest stabilization method.[56] Commercial devices, such as the SAM Pelvic Sling®, are also available.

PHARMACEUTICAL SUPPLIES

The basic EMT curriculum has modules that teach EMTs to administer a patient's personal medication in specific circumstances. For example, modules are provided for administering nitroglycerin for chest pain, inhaled β-agonists for bronchospasm, glucagon for hypoglycemia, and epinephrine-preloaded injections for anaphylaxis. Some states have gone beyond this and allow BLS services to stock and provide the medications covered in these modules.

The medications carried by ALS services are more extensive, but prehospital pharmaceutical interventions are limited to the few that make a real difference before or during transport. These include oxygen, glucose, nitroglycerin, inhaled β-agonists, naloxone, parenteral narcotic and nonsteroidal analgesics, benzodiazepines, furosemide, epinephrine, lidocaine, magnesium, amiodarone, adenosine, diltiazem, calcium, and sodium bicarbonate. In the system that provides rapid-sequence intubation, neuromuscular junction–blocking agents (succinylcholine, vecuronium) are also provided.

REFERENCES

The complete reference list is available online at www.TintinalliEM.com.

Air Medical Transport

C. Keith Stone
Stephen H. Thomas

INTRODUCTION

Air medical transport consists of helicopter (or rotor-wing) and airplane (or fixed-wing) transport and is an important component of EMS systems for prehospital care and interfacility transport. These specialized vehicles offer fast speeds, ranging from 100 to 200 miles per hour for helicopters to >500 miles per hour for airplanes. However, planning for appropriate vehicle use involves many other logistic factors in addition to speed. Although many ill and injured patients can be transported safely by ground, air medical transport provides added medical assessment and care capabilities beyond those of the paramedic-staffed ground ambulance. Guidelines for the use of air medical transport exist, but field EMS personnel and physicians involved in transfer decision making should be able to consider situational circumstances to determine the appropriate transportation mode.

With the occasionally important exception of ground transport legs (e.g., from a landing zone to the patient or from an airport to the hospital), air transport modalities are not limited by traffic or road quality. Weather can be an operational limitation, particularly for helicopters. The radius of service differs between helicopters and fixed-wing craft, but, as a general rule, fixed-wing transport is considered when weather conditions are poor or when transport distances exceed 150 to 200 miles.

The complexity of air transport far exceeds the simple act of loading a patient on an airborne vehicle. National organizations such as the Air Medical Physician Association, the Committee on Accreditation of Medical Transport Systems, and the National Association of EMS Physicians have published texts, position statements, and guidelines covering aspects of air medical transport. The Air Medical Physician Association (http://www.ampa.org) *Air Medical Physician Handbook* is a particularly helpful resource for medical issues. The Committee on Accreditation of Medical Transport Systems (http://www.camts.org) accreditation standards address medical, aviation, organizational, and operational issues. The National Association of EMS Physicians (http://www.naemsp.org) has created detailed position statements and guidelines addressing helicopter EMS trauma and nontrauma triage criteria, as well as training of physicians involved as air medical crew or medical directors.

The effectiveness of air medical services is enabled by attention to a myriad of factors that come into play before, during, and after actual patient transport. The transport service should disseminate protocols guiding appropriate triage, and the program's communications personnel (as well as its physician consultants) should be versed and available for rapid decision making as to appropriate vehicle use. Ongoing training of referring agencies should occur to ensure safe and efficient operations during air transport service arrival (e.g., securing of landing zones) and transition of patient care to the flight crew (e.g., loading of patients onto the aircraft). **Rigorous training programs, covering both cognitive and procedural skills, enable flight crews to provide a high level of intratransport care.** In-flight communications capabilities should include the ability of the air medical crew to speak with medical control physicians, as well as arrange for any change of plan (e.g., direct transport to the operating suite) necessitated by patient condition.

HELICOPTER TRANSPORT

AVIATION ISSUES

Individual hospitals, hospital systems, or private for-profit enterprises run most U.S. civilian air transport programs. Because helicopters are expensive (ranging from $750,000 to more than $5 million each) and other aviation needs (e.g., maintenance, pilot training) are also resource intensive, most hospital-based programs lease their helicopters from vendors. The air medical program typically provides and equips communications and medical personnel, whereas the aircraft vendor supplies the helicopters, pilots, and maintenance personnel. Although costs vary depending on geographic region, patient case mix, equipment and aircraft used, and even the methods used for their calculation, annual operating costs for a rotor-wing service typically exceed $2 million.

Safety is an overriding consideration for air transport. Optimization of safety begins well before an actual air transport, with training of the flight crew and of those who interact with them at scenes and hospitals. Training is especially important for scene responses, in which the helicopter may be landing in an unknown area with more nearby obstacles (e.g., wires, trees) than the hospital helipad. Scene setup (depending on the aircraft, an area of up to 100 × 100 ft is required) and demarcation, as well as safety of nearby personnel, must be taught to ground EMS services and others who call for helicopter EMS transport. In addition to providing training for referring agencies, helicopter EMS pilots and medical crew should undergo both initial and recurrent safety training. For added protection, most helicopter EMS programs have followed the lessons of the military experience and adopted injury-prevention maneuvers such as the use of helmets and fire-resistant clothing. As another safety issue, the pilot should be "blinded" to the nature of the call during mission planning; this eliminates the introduction of acuity-related subjectivity as the pilot considers whether the mission should be accepted.

Safety is partially behind the transition of helicopter EMS programs from single-engine helicopters with visual flight rules capability to twin-engine helicopters that can fly under instrument flight rules conditions. The latter aircraft have greater lifting capacity, range, and speed and usually can execute controlled landings in the event of failure of one engine. A visual flight rules aircraft can fly only during good visibility, whereas instrument flight rules aircraft operate safely in poorer conditions; both comply with visibility limitations imposed by the Federal Aviation Administration, but the instrument flight rules helicopter has fewer restrictions. If the pilot unexpectedly encounters bad weather during a flight, an instrument flight rules helicopter (as compared with a visual flight rules aircraft) has a better chance of completing the mission successfully and safely. Due to the complexity of instrument flight rules operations, some programs (especially those with frequent bad weather periods) have elected to use two-pilot instrument flight rules.

Air medical programs operate under rules established by the national aviation authority—in the United States, the Federal Aviation Administration. Additionally, the industry itself has set forth stringent standards under the auspices of the Committee on Accreditation of Medical Transport Systems. On request, the Committee on Accreditation of Medical Transport Systems performs site visits of air medical programs to certify that they comply with strict safety and operational (as well as clinical) standards. As of January 2012, 148 U.S. transport programs were accredited by the Committee on Accreditation of Medical Transport Systems.

AIR MEDICAL CREW

The primary considerations regarding medical members of the flight crew are crew configuration and training. Although there are few absolutes with regard to optimal configuration, initial and recurrent training are at least as important as the credentials of the flight team members.

The air medical team can have multiple compositions: nurse–paramedic, nurse–nurse, nurse–physician, or nurse–respiratory therapist. These differences may be one reason that the literature has failed to answer definitively the seemingly simple question of whether a physician should be on board the helicopter. Studies done outside the United States, where physician staffing is more prevalent, have failed to show outcome improvement associated with physician staffing of helicopter EMS programs.[1,2] Most U.S. programs agree that physicians are not a necessary component of helicopter EMS crews, and individual program staffing configurations generally have remained stable during the ongoing debate on optimal team makeup.

For a number of reasons, it is unlikely that further efforts to define the optimal crew configuration will result in a consensus. The capabilities of most U.S. nonphysician crews represent an *extended scope of practice.* For instance, flight paramedics and/or nurses frequently are credentialed to perform such procedures as neuromuscular blockade–assisted endotracheal intubation and cricothyrotomy. This example of extended practice scope is important, given the importance of prehospital airway considerations and the fact that flight crews represent a highly trained group with particular expertise in this area. Reported success rates for nonphysicians are as high as 94.6% for drug-assisted and 97.7% for rapid sequence intubation–assisted endotracheal intubation and 90.9% for surgical cricothyrotomy.[3] The ability of nonphysicians to perform advanced procedures—and to perform them well—blurs the procedural skills demarcation between physician and nonphysician crew. Physician cognitive contributions are inherently difficult to quantify or associate with patient survival.[1,2]

At this time, the best recommendation with regard to crew configuration is for programs to continue to do what works for them, as the literature does not report the superiority of a particular model. Most U.S. programs perform a variety of scene and interfacility missions for trauma and nontrauma indications, so the nurse–paramedic configuration, combining the complementary skills of prehospital and hospital-based practitioners, is most popular in the United States. Some transport population heterogeneity can be addressed by the accommodation of extra crew members (e.g., neonatal nurses, intra-aortic balloon pump technicians) when logistics allow. Regardless of the background of the air medical crew, initial and recurrent training in both cognitive and procedural skills is necessary to ensure an optimal level of care.

ENVIRONMENTAL FACTORS OF AIR TRANSPORT

Patient care in any transport vehicle differs from that provided while the patient is on a hospital stretcher. Vehicle vibrations, bumpy rides, noise, physiologic stress, ergonomic constraints (**Figure 3-1**), and motion sickness are among the factors that can affect monitoring and interventions.

The impact of most vehicle-related issues in helicopter EMS can be eliminated, or at least reduced. Some solutions are easy (e.g., visual rather

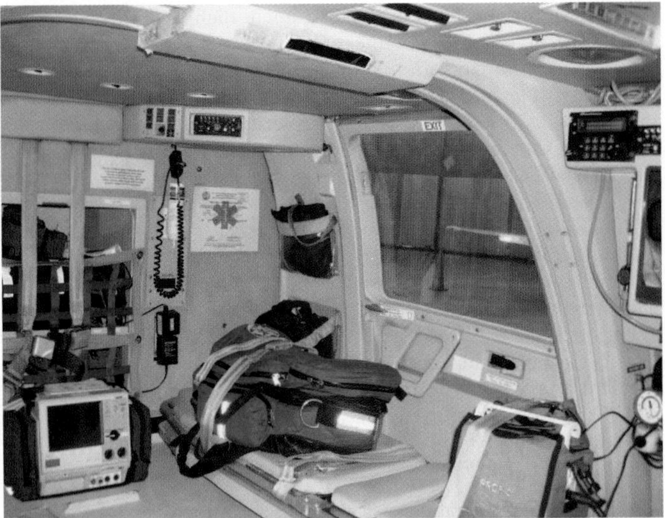

FIGURE 3-1. The patient care compartment in a Dauphin II helicopter.

than aural alarms on ventilators), but flight crews must learn to "work around" other limitations (e.g., perform preflight intubation on patients who appear likely to deteriorate). Some problems will be specific to a service's particular aircraft, mission profile, or crew background. Individual program patient care protocols should take into account the service's equipment and personnel-related capabilities and limitations.

One transport-related issue that cannot be avoided is the question of **altitude and its potential effects on the patient and the crew**. In fact, altitude considerations vary with location—a Denver-based program has concerns that are different from those of a Miami service. Environmental conditions also have an impact on altitude considerations, because aircraft operating under instrument flight rules frequently fly at higher altitudes than those operating under visual flight rules. Of course, fixed-wing transports have more pronounced altitude considerations.

Helicopter (or fixed-wing) altitude and environment have potential effects on patient pathology as well as the crew's ability to monitor and care for the patient. Helicopters generally transport patients at about 1000 to 3500 ft above ground level (not necessarily sea level), although sometimes these altitudes are increased for instrument flight rules flights or for clearing of obstacles or terrain. Therefore, altitude-related problems such as hypoxemia, dehydration, and low temperature tend to be mild or relatively easily to overcome. However, geographic differences are important. Some western U.S. programs fly with supplemental oxygen for the medical crews.

Pressure-related problems related to Boyle's law (the volume of a gas increases when the pressure decreases at a constant temperature) may represent the most important consideration for helicopter-transported patients. For example, even the relatively low transport altitude range for helicopter EMS may affect patients with certain diagnoses (e.g., decompression sickness, cerebral arterial gas embolism) or instrumentation (e.g., tamponading devices for esophageal variceal hemorrhage). Endotracheal intracuff pressures increase an average of 33.9 cm of water at a mean altitude of 2260 ft.[4] This could raise the cuff pressure above the perfusion pressure of the tracheal mucosa, leading to injury. Hand-held commercially available devices can be used to keep cuff pressure within the target range of 20 to 30 cm of water. The devices are held in one hand and connected to the cuff inflation port. An inflation bulb can be used to further inflate the cuff or an air-release button can be used to remove air while the cuff pressure is simultaneously measured by the device.

In some cases, an understanding of altitude issues is important in preventing complications. To minimize aspiration risk, gastric intubation should be performed for unconscious patients transported by air. Alternatively, understanding of the relevant science can be used to prevent overreaction to potential barometric risks. For example, not all patients with small pneumothoraces who do not otherwise require tube thoracostomy require pretransport chest decompression simply because they are to be transported by air.

CLINICAL USE OF HELICOPTERS

While trauma still constitutes the majority of helicopter transports for most programs, as more time-critical treatments develop, **more transports will be arranged for noninjured patients**. There are many schemes (age group, scene/interfacility mission type) for categorization of helicopter EMS transports, but the simplest categorization is into trauma and nontrauma. Logistical issues are important to both categories. Therefore, these are considered first.

LOGISTICS AND HELICOPTER EMS USE

Some logistic prompts for helicopter consideration include **(1) lengthy transport time for ground ambulances to reach the tertiary center, (2) ground vehicle transport time to the local hospital exceeds the time required for helicopter transport to the tertiary center, and (3) for entrapped trauma patients, extrication time is expected to exceed 20 minutes**. In some cases, helicopter EMS is used because local ground EMS personnel lack the expertise to provide the indicated level of intratransport care. Another important consideration is whether a region's ground EMS system can provide transport to the receiving tertiary center while maintaining the ability to cover its base area with appropriate advanced life support care. Questions that can assist healthcare providers in determining the appropriate transport modality for an individual patient are listed in **Table 3-1**.

The ideal helicopter trauma response guideline is appropriate patient selection without overtriage. Various anatomic, physiologic, and mechanism criteria have been tested, without agreement on any detailed protocol. Retrospective utilization review and ongoing education are critical to system evaluation.

HELICOPTER EMS FOR TRAUMA PATIENTS

There is one group of trauma patients—those in **traumatic cardiac arrest**—for whom air medical scene response has shown a very low rate of resuscitation and essentially zero survival.[5] Most helicopter EMS programs have their crews accompany traumatic arrest patients by ground to the nearest facility.

After the initial triage response decision, **the larger issue is whether helicopter EMS actually improves outcome for *any* injured patients.** There is disagreement over this question, but multiple studies have shown improved outcomes.[6-9]

The largest study to demonstrate improved outcomes after traumatic injury related to helicopter transport analyzed 258,827 patients from the National Trauma Data Bank transported by helicopter (16%) or ground EMS (84%). Helicopter transport patients had a 22% decrease in mortality compared to ground transport, regardless of patient age or mechanism of injury.[6] In addition, the study showed that the injury severity scores of patients decreased as the distance of the injury site from the trauma center increased, which demonstrated that the selection criteria used nationwide to use helicopter transport seemed appropriate. Another study of 10,268 trauma patients demonstrated that the 2-week mortality in patients transported by helicopter decreased by 33% compared to ground transport. The subanalysis showed that the reduction

TABLE 3-1 Questions to Aid in Determining Need for Helicopter Transport
Is minimization of time spent out of hospital important?
Is time-sensitive evaluation and treatment involved, and is it available at the referring facility?
Is the patient inaccessible to ground transport?
What are the transport route weather conditions?
Does the weight of the patient preclude air medical transport?
Are aircraft landing facilities available at or near the referring hospital?
Is critical-care life support required that is not available with ground transport?
Would ground transport leave the local area without adequate EMS coverage?
If local ground transport is not an option, are regional ground critical-care transport services available?

was most evident in patients with a Revised Trauma Score (based on the vital signs at the scene) of 3 to 7.[7]

The outcomes of rural trauma patients are thought to be worse than those of urban trauma victims. After controlling for age, gender, and Injury Severity Score, a Utah study[10] of helicopter scene transports from rural and urban trauma scenes found no difference in mortality. This study demonstrated that the helicopter scene transport of rural trauma victims appears to be a mortality equalizer.

A shortcoming of the literature is that studies generally address only the hard endpoint of mortality, with little emphasis on either mechanisms for survival improvement or nonmortality endpoints. Regardless of these shortcomings, the primary issue for trauma helicopter EMS is not whether some patients benefit, but rather how well those patients most likely to benefit from helicopter use can be identified by improved triage criteria. Although definitive criteria are lacking, the National Association of EMS Physicians has published guidelines for clinical situations that are appropriate for air transport (**Table 3-2**).

TABLE 3-2 Air Transport Indications for Scene Trauma

General and mechanism of injury
Trauma score <12
Unstable vital signs
Significant trauma in ages <12 or >55 years and pregnant patients
Multisystem injuries
Ejection from vehicle
Pedestrian or cyclist struck
Death in same passenger compartment
Penetrating trauma of the head, neck, chest, abdomen, or pelvis
Crush injury of the head, chest, or abdomen
Fall from height
Near drowning
Neurologic injuries
Glasgow Coma Scale score <10
Mental status deterioration
Obvious skull fracture
Spinal cord injury
Thoracic injury
Major chest wall injury (e.g., flail chest)
Pneumothorax
Hemothorax
Suspected cardiac injury
Abdominal/pelvic injuries
Significant abdominal pain postinjury
Seatbelt sign or abdominal contusion
Rib fractures below the nipple line
Unstable pelvis
Open pelvic fracture
Pelvic fracture with hypotension
Orthopedic injuries
Amputation of limb (partial or complete)
Finger or thumb amputation when replantation is available
Fracture/dislocation with associated vascular compromise
Limb ischemia
Open long-bone fractures
Two or more long-bone fractures
Thermal injury
Burns of >20% body surface area
Burns of face, head, hands, feet, or genitalia
Inhalation injury
Chemical or electrical burns
Burns associated with other traumatic injuries

HELICOPTER EMS FOR NONTRAUMA PATIENTS

The reason that helicopter EMS trauma literature is (relatively) abundant is that there are ready means for controlling for the differing acuities of air- and ground-transported patients. Unfortunately, there is no such easy methodology for patients with nontrauma diagnoses, and acuity scales for nontrauma patients generally have not been accepted for use in assessing the association between transport mode and outcome.

Some general guidelines are available (**Table 3-3**), and the logistic considerations noted previously in the section "Logistics and Helicopter EMS Use" apply to nontrauma flights. **In most helicopter EMS programs, the largest single nontrauma diagnostic category is cardiac.** Patients in cardiac arrest should be transported to the nearest hospital rather than loaded on an aircraft. Transport for primary or rescue coronary intervention for ST-elevation myocardial infarction is a frequent indication for helicopter use and can be done rapidly and safely.[11,12] Cardiac patients with pacemakers or those who have received thrombolytic therapy can be transported safely and effectively by helicopter EMS.

Another growing indication is the provision of lytic therapy or vascular intervention for ischemic stroke.[13] The American Stroke Association (http://www.strokeassociation.org) Task Force on Development of Stroke

TABLE 3-3 Air Transport Indications for Nontrauma Conditions

Cardiac
Acute coronary syndromes
Cardiogenic shock
Cardiac tamponade
Mechanical cardiac disease (cardiac rupture)
Critically ill medical or surgical patients
Pretransport cardiac arrest
Pretransport respiratory arrest
Mechanical ventricular assist
Continuous vasoactive medications
Risk of airway deterioration
Severe poisoning
Need for hyperbaric oxygen treatment
Emergent dialysis
Unstable GI bleeding
Surgical emergencies (e.g., aortic dissection)
Obstetric
Delivery will require obstetric or neonatal care beyond the capabilities of the referring facility
Active premature labor <34 wk or estimated fetal weight <2000 grams
Acute abdominal emergencies <34 wk or estimated fetal weight <2000 grams
Preeclampsia or eclampsia
Third-trimester hemorrhage
Fetal hydrops
Complicated maternal medical conditions
Predicted severe fetal heart disease
Neurologic
CNS hemorrhage
Spinal cord compression
Status epilepticus
Neonatal
Gestational age <30 wk or fetal weight <2000 grams
Supplemental oxygen exceeding 60%, continuous positive airway pressure, or mechanical ventilation
Extrapulmonary air leak, interstitial emphysema, or pneumothorax
Medical emergencies (e.g., congestive heart failure, disseminated intravascular coagulation)
Surgical emergencies (e.g., diaphragmatic hernia, necrotizing enterocolitis)

Systems[14] identified helicopter EMS as an important part of stroke systems. However, a study of 122 patients transported to a stroke center after receiving recombinant tissue plasminogen activator at the referring hospital demonstrated no benefit in patient outcomes in air-transported patients.[15]

Obstetric transports are a special consideration for air transport because many high-risk patients are best delivered at tertiary care centers. The question for this population is primarily one of safety during transport. In-flight deliveries are a major resuscitation problem for both mother and infant. Experience has provided some reassurance that the use of helicopter EMS to transport high-risk obstetric patients did not result in deliveries in the back of the helicopter, and **neonatal outcomes are not adversely impacted by transport**. Helicopter EMS transport of obstetric patients in an urban area is one solution to the problem of traffic congestion.

FIXED-WING AIR MEDICAL TRANSPORT

Fixed-wing aircraft can serve a wide variety of missions, from urgent to routine, over great distances. Because airplanes land only at airports, they cannot respond to the scene, and fixed-wing transports need ground ambulance connections at both ends of the flight to transport the patient between the hospital and airport. Because of these factors, fixed-wing flights generally take longer to arrange and are uncommonly used for truly emergent patients.

Helicopters are virtually always dedicated as air medical transport vehicles when used by U.S. EMS services, but fixed-wing airplanes used for medical transport may have other roles. When fixed-wing aircraft are used for air medical transport, cabins must be reconfigured. Vendors have developed removable medical equipment modules that can be placed relatively quickly in the aircraft cabin.

On a per-mile basis, fixed-wing transports are less expensive than helicopter EMS transports. However, the optimal transport radius for fixed-wing triage varies with regional and patient-specific considerations. The appropriate aircraft to use for any one mission depends on many factors: distance, the nature of the airport at the patient's pickup point, the condition of the patient, the amount of equipment, and the crew required in transport. A larger plane that can be pressurized can fly above 3000 m (10,000 ft), which means that the aircraft can travel faster, farther, and more comfortably. At these higher altitudes, flight crews must have a deeper understanding of altitude physiology issues. Cabin pressure (i.e., indicated altitude above sea level) should be recorded on medical records because of the importance of pressure issues to physiology, and crew safety training should include measures to take in case of inadvertent cabin depressurization.

All fixed-wing services must comply with civil aviation authority rules for airplanes. The Commission on Accreditation of Medical Transport Systems has developed standards for air medical fixed-wing transport. These standards, which are also a useful primer for more detailed information about fixed-wing air medical transport, deal with aircraft configuration, medical equipment requirements, medical crew configuration and training, and medical director qualifications.

MEDICAL DIRECTION OF AIR MEDICAL SERVICES

Medical direction may be even more important with rotor- and fixed-wing services than with ground services; it is certainly more complicated because it involves most aspects of ground EMS in addition to vehicle-specific and altitude- and acuity-related issues. The medical director should be familiar with the physiology and stress of flight on patients and should oversee the teaching of these and other applicable principles to the air medical crew. Overall, **a flight crew requires more initial and ongoing training than do most ground EMS personnel due to the higher patient acuity and extended practice scope**. Because flight crews are often far from their base of operations and may be out of voice contact, they must be sufficiently trained so that they can act independently when necessary. For nonphysician crew, standing orders or protocols (especially for advanced procedures such as cricothyrotomy) are needed. Periodic review and updating of these protocols, as well as close inspection of every transport record, are among the many responsibilities of the medical director. The Air Medical Physician Association and the National Association of EMS Physicians have published information on the responsibilities and function of the air medical program physician director.

REFERENCES

The complete reference list is available online at www.TintinalliEM.com.

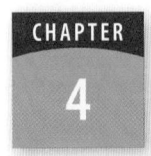

Mass Gatherings

Michael G. Millin

INTRODUCTION

Mass gathering medical care refers to the provision of medical services to organized events or venues with relatively large numbers of people in a defined geographic area. Typically, mass gatherings are considered to be events that have at least 1000 people; however, this does not have to be the case.[1,2] Although the principles of mass gathering medical care traditionally apply to congregations of large numbers of people, these principles also apply to smaller venues with a relatively high concentration of people in a limited space and those where it may not be easy to access the general system of EMS. Therefore, the principles of mass gathering medical care also apply to athletic events with fewer than 1000 people, as well as airplanes, cruise ships, and wilderness environments.

Table 4-1 lists some of the major factors affecting planning for a mass gathering event. Physical barriers may inhibit easy entry and exit from the site. These barriers can make it difficult to get medical resources into, and to get patients out of, the event location. **Reliable communication between medical personnel, event organizers, and outside medical resources is key to a successful medical response.** Environmental factors will also affect the response, especially at extremes of cold, wet weather that can precipitate hypothermia or hot weather that can precipitate dehydration and heat stroke. Finally, event planners should consider possible public health threats of widespread communicable disease and the potential for a terrorist attack with explosive or other devices.

EPIDEMIOLOGY

The need for mass gathering medical care was first described after two spectators collapsed and died during a University of Nebraska football game in 1965.[3] The event organizers were not prepared to manage medical emergencies in the midst of the event, and consequently, when these two patients needed medical care, the organizers were not able to meet the need. Medical directors have become experienced in mass gathering medicine, and case reports are described for sporting events, concerts, expositions, and other large congregations of people.[2]

One of the largest global gatherings, the Islamic Hajj pilgrimage to Mecca, Saudi Arabia (reaching 2.5 million in 2009), has required officials to manage threats to public safety from outbreaks of infectious disease to major traumatic injuries from stampedes. Other notable global mass gatherings include the 2010 World Expo in Shanghai, China,

TABLE 4-1 Factors Affecting Planning for a Mass Gathering Event
Venue entry and exit
Communication
Environment
Potential public health threats

which attracted approximately 70 million visitors, and the FIFA 2010 World Cup in South Africa, during which more than 1 million foreign visitors entered the country.[4] As large-scale global mass gatherings become more common, it is evident that there is a need for a global effort to develop the science of mass gathering medicine. This is exemplified by the mass gathering conference held in collaboration with the Kingdom of Saudi Arabia Ministry of Health in Jeddah, Saudi Arabia, in 2010[4] and the formation of an online registry for mass gathering data collection as developed by the University of British Columbia.[5]

Interestingly, despite the fact that mass gatherings are generally attended by individuals in good health, these events tend to have a higher incidence of illness and injury than that which would be found in the general population.[6] The incidence of usage of medical care at mass gatherings has been reported to range from 4 to 440 patients per 10,000.[2] The wide variance in medical usage rate is a function of the type of event and environmental factors.

COMPONENTS OF A MEDICAL ACTION PLAN

In preparing for a mass gathering event, medical directors should develop an organized approach through the development of a medical action plan.[7]

PHYSICIAN MEDICAL OVERSIGHT

All mass gathering events should have an identified physician medical director who is responsible for developing the medical action plan. The medical director is also responsible for providing medical oversight before and during the event. This person should be board certified in emergency medicine and have a current medical license from the state(s) where the event will be located. The medical director should also have experience in the medical direction of EMS and the provision of medical care at mass gathering events. In the future, it will be desirable for the event medical director to be board certified in EMS. Experience and training in EMS provide an event medical director with skills in field medicine, including creative thinking, the ability to make diagnostic and treatment decisions purely on clinical grounds, and an awareness of operational environments that are very different from a typical ED.

The medical director is responsible for developing plans for indirect medical oversight and ensuring a coordinated system of direct medical oversight. Indirect oversight describes a system of written protocols that provide the medical personnel with a standardized set of directions for the care of a variety of traumatic and medical conditions that may be encountered during the event. **These protocols should always be consistent with local EMS protocols unless the medical director has prior approval from the local jurisdictional EMS medical director to deviate from them.** Direct medical oversight describes a method of direct communication with medical providers during the event to answer questions and provide medical direction in real time during the event. Although direct oversight can be delegated to a team of physicians for an event of long duration, ideally, the medical director should plan to be on site during the event as much as possible.

COMMAND AND CONTROL

In addition to an event medical director, mass gathering plans should have an organized system of command and control. Although many systems exist for the command and control of resources at emergency incidents or mass gatherings, one of the most well-tested and efficient methods is the Incident Command System. It was initially developed as a consequence of poor management of a series of wild-land fires in Southern California in 1970.[8] The system can be used for any type or size of emergency, disaster, or mass gathering, with the purpose of allowing either a single agency or multiple agencies to communicate using common terminology and operating procedures. Further, the ease in putting the system into action allows it to be functional from the time an incident occurs until the requirement for operations no longer exists. In fact, since its original development, the Incident Command System has been adopted by the National Fire Academy and currently provides the structure for the Federal National Incident Management System.[8]

The purpose of establishing a command and control system like the Incident Command System is to define clear lines of reporting and communication among all major functioning components that may coexist during an incident. The organizational structure develops in a modular fashion from the top down and may incorporate five functional divisions.[8] While the Command function is always established, the other divisions, which include Operations, Logistics, Planning, and Finance, form as needed (**Figure 4-1**). The incident commander for a mass gathering event ideally should be someone with experience functioning within an Incident Command System structure. A lead fire official would be well suited as the incident commander, because officers in the fire service typically have extensive experience working within the Incident Command System. However, if the local fire department is not involved with the event, as may be the case in smaller events, command should be managed by someone with EMS experience and ideally should not be a physician. As will be discussed later, the physician's role within the Incident Command System structure should be focused on direct oversight of patient care and not involve the global issues that are the concern of the incident commander. In short, the incident commander must be involved in directing available resources, communicating effectively within the organization, continuously assessing the incident priorities, coordinating activities of outside agencies, and always retaining ultimate responsibility for the incident.

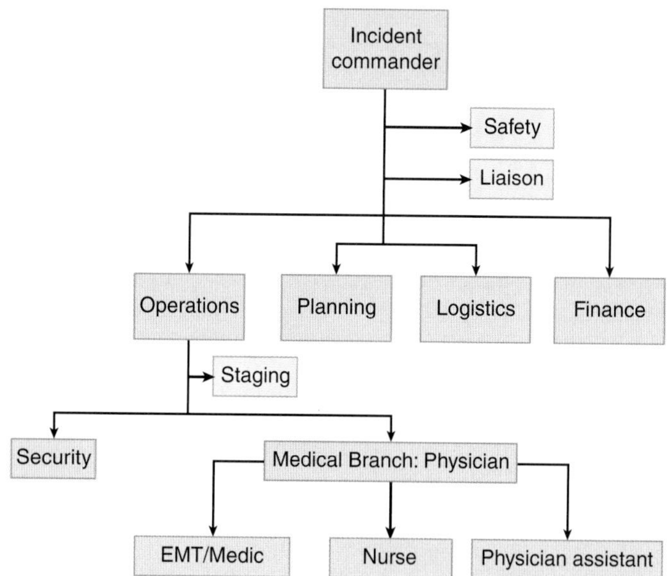

FIGURE 4-1. Incident Command System organizational chart.

Within a typical Incident Command System, the provision of medical care to the public occurs within the Operations Section. Often referred to as the "doers," it is the function of the Operations Section to complete the primary tasks of the mission. The medical branch in Operations should establish a similar modular command framework for organizing the various medical teams, each having at a minimum their own team lead. Members of the medical teams include, but are not limited to, EMTs, paramedics, nurses, physician assistants, and physicians. It is not required that the physician take the lead role of each medical team. In fact, it may be more beneficial to have the individual with EMS or fire service experience in the role of team lead, which ideally may be an EMS physician. Depending on the number of agencies involved, there may be more than one EMS medical director on scene. An agency's medical director should be available for direct medical oversight as needed and should ideally be on site as much as possible. The medical director(s) should function as a commander within the Operations Section and report back to the section head of Operations who ultimately reports to the incident commander. Key to the success of the Incident Command System is that every individual abides by the established hierarchical ranks of command.

Perhaps the most important functional component for ensuring a successful mass gathering event within the Incident Command System structure is the Logistics Section. Logistics personnel are responsible for ensuring that all equipment and supplies are available and in working order when needed. Whereas the Operations personnel are the "doers," the Logistics personnel are the "getters." They "get" the supplies needed by Operations. Because the ability to effectively care for the public at a mass gathering event is highly dependent on having a certain amount of supplies, it cannot be stressed enough that a well-functioning Logistics unit is critical to the success of the event. The event medical director should not have to be responsible for acquiring necessary supplies if Logistics is functioning well.

The Incident Command System also provides a framework for accountability of personnel, which is paramount to maintaining safety during a potentially long and unpredictable event. Within each branch under Operations, there should be a designated safety officer. The sole responsibility of this individual is not to provide care, but instead to maintain a system by which all personnel are accounted for at all times. This may include simply keeping a visual account of personnel, which would only be feasible at a very small event, or implementing a method that uses an identification tag that is kept by the safety officer during the time each individual is operational on scene. Each functional unit safety officer should ultimately report to the command staff safety officer for the event, who reports to the incident commander.

Closely related to the concept of accountability is the notion of force protection. This is a term used by the U.S. military to describe preventive measures taken to mitigate hostile actions against individuals. The number one priority in all events is scene safety. It is well known that if a medical provider becomes sick or injured, the provider will use resources intended for the public and distract other providers from the ability to perform their duties. As such, a sick or injured medical provider has the potential to dramatically disrupt the overall medical mission for the event. While medical personnel are always responsible for assessing and assuring their own safety and those with whom they work, it is imperative to have a well-designed plan for the overall medical care and protection of the medical providers at the event. One of the duties of the event medical director is to be prepared to provide care to the other medical providers should the need arise. In addition, communication with law enforcement personnel will help to ensure the overall protection of the medical providers. Their support should be readily available and have the means to immediately respond to any location should the situation become unsafe. Depending on the type of event, threats could range from those that are readily seen (i.e., crowds at a concert) to those that are hidden (i.e., explosives and other weapons carried by an individual with the goal of using mass gathering events to kill and injure).

RECONNAISSANCE

In the beginning stages of preparation, the medical director and assistants need to assess the site to identify the geographic variants that will affect their ability to provide medical care to the public. Within the Incident Command System structure, this establishes a role for the event medical director in the Planning Section. Most important, the planners will need to determine routes of ingress and egress for the event. Backup plans should also be developed. Planners should determine ideal locations for setting up a base of operations, fixed medical care sites, and staging areas for mobile units. Decisions should take into account the effects of predicted traffic flow, predicted sites of high-volume medical need, natural geographic barriers, and location of receiving medical facilities.

NEGOTIATIONS

The process of developing a medical plan for a mass gathering event requires a cohesive teamwork approach with multiple interest groups. First and foremost, the medical planners should develop a plan that meets the needs of the public and the event planners. This first step may require some negotiations with event planners in determining locations for fixed and mobile medical units, level of care to be provided, and resources provided to the medical units. Negotiations will determine if the medical units will be paid under contractual terms by the event planners or if they will volunteer their services to the event. This negotiation stage should also resolve who will finance the purchase of needed supplies and pay for other needed resources, such as costs of transportation and liability coverage.

Regardless of who pays for supplies, it is important that the medical teams coordinate with the Logistics Section to ensure that equipment and supplies are readily available when needed. Similarly, regardless of who is responsible for acquiring supplies, there is value to the event medical director having ultimate control over the acquisition and maintenance of critical medical supplies, as this will ensure that the medical needs of the public are assured.

Medical planners should also establish communication and agreements with other outside agencies that have a potential need to interact with the medical response team for the event. Medical teams that are formed outside the local jurisdictional EMS system should have an agreement with local EMS that addresses transportation of patients out of the event to local resource hospitals. Transfer and acceptance agreements should be developed with the hospitals. Local law enforcement should be contacted for assistance with traffic flow and security. Events that have the potential to be affected by security issues on a national scale may also require agreements with the U.S. Department of Homeland Security for disaster and security response.

HUMAN RESOURCES, LEVEL OF CARE, AND TRAINING

The event medical director should determine the desired level of care for the event based on the predicted medical need and available resources. Depending on the needs of the event, the desired level of care may range from emergency medical responders to physicians. Once the desired level of care and the predicted patient volume are determined, the medical director will be able to develop a plan for human resource needs. These resources may be acquired through the local EMS system, area hospitals, medical training programs, or other sources such as ski patrols and medical reserve corps.

Medical personnel should be licensed to practice at their level of training in the local jurisdiction. Although the medical personnel should be trained for their established level of care, the medical director may want to have additional training sessions to address specific injuries and medical conditions that are predicted to be encountered by the medical personnel during the event. Regardless, it is important that the providers work within a defined scope of practice as determined by level of training and any operational-specific protocols that may be authorized by local authorities for mass gathering events.

EQUIPMENT

When considering equipment for a mass gathering event, planners and medical directors should take into account the type of event, the weather, and the skill level of the medical staff. Medical units comprised of personnel at the EMT level or lower will need to carry significantly less equipment than units staffed by personnel at the paramedic level or higher. Units with physicians may elect to have on hand supplies to do simple suturing and advanced resuscitation. However, thought should be given to the available time needed to suture a wound in balance to the patient volume and the availability of the fixed standing acute care centers. If available, it may be more advantageous to refer patients needing procedures to acute care hospitals. The appropriate way to manage the need for procedures is dependent on the available resources and the overall mission of the medical care at the event.

Often, a large proportion of time spent planning out supplies is focused on generating a broad list and subsequently obtaining supplies that would be necessary to provide medical care for a critical patient. As discussed earlier, it is important to consider that rapid transport of this patient away from the incident to the controlled environment of an acute care hospital may be more beneficial for the patient and free up the provider to care for other patients who would likely not receive evaluation given the time-consuming nature of the critical patient. In addition, proportionally fewer critical patients are seen at a given event compared with the vast majority who seek aid for minor complaints such as scrapes, blisters, headaches, and sprains. Therefore, more effort should be placed on obtaining supplies in highest demand. As suggested by the number and type of complaints seen, those supplies in highest demand typically include bandages, foam padding for blisters, ice for sprains, fluids for oral rehydration, acetaminophen, and ibuprofen.

In general, the incidence of cardiopulmonary arrest and the need for major resuscitation at mass gathering events is low. However, **medical units should, at the very least, have access to an automated**

external defibrillator. Event-specific protocols should address the use of advanced airway equipment, including the possible use of medications for rapid sequence intubation. Plans for other resuscitation needs should also be addressed prior to the event so that all providers manage these small numbers of cases in a standard format (e.g., fluids for sepsis, postresuscitation care, management of cardiac arrhythmia, status asthmaticus). Although it is rare that there is a need for major resuscitation, there may be value to having supraglottic airways (e.g., KING LT Airway®) and adult intraosseous needles (e.g., EZ-IO®).

In addition to the level of training of the medical staff, equipment needs will be determined by the mobility of the unit. Some events may need mobile medical units that are able to reach patients in difficult locations or easily move through large crowds. Units on foot and other nonmotorized means of travel will be able to carry fewer supplies than those using motorized vehicles such as golf carts. For events using nonmotorized mobile units, it will be important to design a means to bring heavier supplies to a patient should the need arise, such as equipment needed to manage a patient with a high suspicion of spinal cord injury. Units in fixed locations will be able to stock a greater quantity of materials, possibly including cots, shelter, and additional medical supplies.

Although the equipment needs are unique for each event, there are some things that are universal. **Tables 4-2** and **4-3** show suggested items for both mobile and fixed units as well as suggested equipment based on the skill level of medical personnel.

TABLE 4-2 Equipment List for Mobile Units

	Item
Basic (BLS-level EMS provider and above)	Automatic external defibrillator *(May alternatively place in a strategic location in the site venue)*
	Cervical collar *(May strategically place in the site venue a method for transport of a patient requiring in-line spinal immobilization)*
	Airway adjuncts
	Oxygen delivery devices (nasal cannula, nonrebreather mask, bag-valve mask)
	Oxygen and suction *(May be strategically placed in site venue)*
	Bandages (4×4, roller gauze)
	Triangular cravats
	Adhesive bandages
	Nonlatex gloves
	Splints
	Stethoscope
	Sphygmomanometer
	Tape
	Shears
	Flashlight
	Documentation forms
	Hazardous waste bags
	Compact foil space blankets
	Petroleum jelly (used to prevent chaffing by marathon runners)
	Oral fluids for hydration (water, sports drinks)
Advanced (ALS-level EMS provider and above)	Advanced airway equipment including laryngoscope with assorted blades, endotracheal tubes, and cricothyrotomy kit *(May alternatively use a supraglottic airway device)*
	IV access devices and tubing *(May choose to carry an adult intraosseous set)*
	Normal saline in 1-L bags
	Glucometer
	Dextrose for IV administration
	Advanced cardiovascular life support medications: epinephrine, atropine, amiodarone, adenosine
	Aspirin
	Nitroglycerin
	IV diphenhydramine
	Parenteral benzodiazepine
	Multidose inhaler albuterol
	Epinephrine in 1:1000 concentration
	Morphine
	Airway medications: induction agent, paralytic

Abbreviations: ALS = advanced life support; BLS = basic life support.

TABLE 4-3 Equipment List for Fixed Units

	Item
Physician-level care (some of these skills and/or medications may be available for use by EMS providers with authorized operational-specific scope of practice for mass gathering events)	Suture kits with absorbable and nonabsorbable sutures
	Needles and syringes
	Forceps
	Scalpel
	Normal saline for irrigation
	Local anesthetics
	Otoscope
	Analgesics: acetaminophen, ibuprofen, morphine
	Antacids
	Antiemetics
	Prednisone
	Antibiotics: ointment, oral
	Activated charcoal
	Airway management: induction agent, paralytic
Nonmedical equipment	Cots
	Shelter
	Blankets
	Chairs
	Hazardous waste receptacle
	Sharps box

TREATMENT FACILITIES

Medical directors will need to determine if the scope of the event will require fixed treatment facilities or if mobile units will be sufficient. Factors that contribute to this decision are the predicted number of patients expected to seek medical care, length of the event, distance to off-site medical care, and environmental factors. Fixed treatment facilities can be set up in mobile tents or within a permanent structure. Regardless, fixed treatment facilities should be set up in such a way as to be able to withstand the predictable weather conditions that may be encountered during the duration of the event. From a patient care perspective, it is important to have a facility that has environmental control to manage heat-related illness in warm weather and cold-related illness in cold/wet weather. Off-site treatment facilities should be arranged with local hospitals.

TRANSPORTATION

Nonmedical and medical transportation is necessary, taking into account the number, capacity, and staging location for transport units. Nonmedical transportation units move personnel and resources throughout the site. Medical transportation moves patients within the event location and out to area hospitals.

Planners may also need to address nontraditional modes of transportation, such as golf carts, boats, bicycles, horses, snowmobiles, and toboggans. Protocols should also be developed that address the appropriate use of air medical transportation, including location and setup of a safe landing zone.

TABLE 4-4 Public Health Concerns to Be Considered for a Mass Gathering Event

Access to potable water
Proper waste management for human waste
Waste management for nonhuman waste
Proper management of food service to prevent spread of foodborne illness
Proper road/traffic management to prevent traffic-related injuries
Other considerations for injury prevention
Large-scale natural or man-made disaster

PUBLIC HEALTH

Public health concerns during a mass gathering event may be addressed by the event managers or delegated to the local public health authority or the medical director and EMS system. Even if these concerns are not delegated to the medical response team, public health concerns can affect patient care, and therefore the medical director should be aware of these issues. **Table 4-4** lists some potential public health concerns.

ACCESS TO CARE

The event managers and medical director should develop plans to ensure that the public will be able to access emergency care, if needed. These plans should ensure that the locations of fixed treatment facilities are well marked with signs and other visual aids and that there are limited barriers to access these facilities. Fixed treatment facilities should be accessible to all members of the public and comply with guidelines that are in accordance with the Americans with Disabilities Act. Mobile medical personnel should also wear vests or other high-visibility clothing easily identified by the public. Pamphlets or signage can alert the public about methods for accessing emergency care.

COMMUNICATIONS

Successful management of any mass gathering event is contingent upon an effective communication system. To maintain coordination and control, the system must be tailored to the unique needs of the scenario. The design is dictated by a variety of factors, including geography and size of venue, number of participants, budget, and the systems of those with whom providers will be interfacing. Consideration should also be given to environmental factors including temperature extremes, water, and noise. Venues at music concerts and motor sports may require special communication devices to allow for providers to communicate with each other while in the presence of loud background noise.

Modalities can range from simple flag signals to sophisticated radio networks and may include consumer Family Radio Service devices (walkie-talkies), cellular systems, and landline phones. Each has their strengths and weaknesses. Walkie-talkies have a multitude of channel options but are typically limited to a 1- to 2-mile range. Cellular and other phone systems may provide an inexpensive option but are easily overwhelmed by large numbers of users during a crisis. Two-way radios with more power and range than Family Radio Service systems may be analog or digital, using very high frequency, ultra-high frequency, or 800-MHz frequencies. Systems using a repeater antenna allow for communication over greater distances and across rugged terrain. Large-scale, trunked radio systems provide central control of end-user access to selected channels, allowing a greater number of people to function within a limited spectrum. These systems also allow for discrete groups of responders to communicate among themselves without disturbing other groups.

If the communications network is not linked to surrounding resources, a protocol must be in place for making contact and for relaying information as needed. In an urban environment, this may be in the form of an on-site representative from the local EMS system or an identified phone number or frequency designated for the activation of additional resources. In a remote area, one or more people may be tasked with relaying messages via radio or traveling to the nearest telephone or area of cellular service to contact local authorities, or a specific "communications tent" may be organized.

TABLE 4-5 Documentation

Purposes of medical documentation for a mass gathering event
Assist in transfer of care from the event site to off-site medical facilities
Record medical interactions for the purposes of liability control
Establish a means of data capture for continuous quality oversight and research
Essential components of medical documentation for a mass gathering event
Patient's name, contact information, sex, and age
Vital signs
Chief complaint
Focused physical examination
Suspected diagnosis
Medical care rendered
Disposition

DOCUMENTATION

The medical director should develop a system for documentation of patient encounters during the event. This system need not be as extensive as that which would be found in the typical ED setting and, instead, should be focused on the event to address specific components of the patient encounter as outlined in **Table 4-5**. Medical documentation should be easy to complete and not exhaustive, such that it can be quickly completed if large numbers of patients seek medical care at the same time. Medical directors may want to consider a method of electronic documentation. Paper documentation should ideally be on a single sheet that can be used by all providers involved in the patient's care (**Figure 4-2**).

LIABILITY

All members of the medical response team for a mass gathering event should have medical liability coverage. Depending on the restrictions of the carrier, liability coverage may be provided by the policy of one's primary employment or may need to be purchased as additional coverage. The medical director may want to arrange coverage for all members of the medical response team as a group. This should be factored into the cost of providing medical care for the event and should be discussed with planners during the negotiation stage before the event. It is important to note that, if the medical personnel will be reimbursed for services in the form of legal tender or payment in kind (even in the form of a free meal at the event), they may not be protected from liability through Good Samaritan laws, depending on the state. In addition, if the medical providers are advertising their medical services to the public at an event even by setting up an established medical tent, the providers have established a duty to act and are liable to the public to provide care at an established standard. In order to mitigate untoward risk, the medical director should review the laws that pertain to the local area before the event.

CONTINUOUS QUALITY IMPROVEMENT

Unless an event is anticipated to be a one-time occurrence of a short duration, the medical director should establish a method of continuous quality improvement. The continuous quality improvement program should begin with a review of the documentation for patient encounters to identify elements of the system that are performing well and elements that need improvement. The results of continuous quality improvement review should then be used to improve upon the system of delivery of care. The medical director may also consider having regular case reviews with the medical personnel at the event to improve the care being delivered.

COMMERCIAL AIRLINE FLIGHTS

Commercial airline flights represent a special scenario in mass gathering medicine. The steadily rising number of travelers, the increasing

Patient Encounter Form

Event:

DATE & TIME (24hr)
Last Name:
First Name:
Phone #:
Age: ☐ Female ☐ Male ☐ Transgender
DOB*: PHN*:
Family Physician*:

PATIENT CATEGORY
(A=Athlete, E=Event Staff, P=Performer, S=Spectator, U=Unknown)
PARTICIPANT ID
(Race/Bib Number)
TRIAGE ACUITY SCALE**
☐ Black ☐ Red ☐ Yellow ☐ Green ☐ White

PRESENTING COMPLAINT

HISTORY

Past history

Medications

Allergies

Level of Consciousness (AVPU)

R L R L

VITAL SIGNS	#1	#2	#3
Time			
Temp.			
Pulse			
B.P.			
R.R.			
SaO2			
Glucose			
GCS			

PHYSICAL FINDINGS

***DOB, PHN, Family Physician** (Optional)

****Triage/Discharge Acuity Scale Level**
Black/Deceased – obvious non-survivable injury
Red/Emergent – critical, resuscitation, chest pain, collapse
Yellow/Urgent – overdose no ABC compromise, SOB
Green/Minor – assessment required, wound care, prescriptions
White/Dispensary – product requests, customer service

****Level of Training of Care Provider**
PCP, SFA, OFA #, EMR, LPN, RN, NP, MD, Chiro, Physio, etc.

MGM Pt. ID:

RA ID:

CLINICAL IMPRESSION OF CARE PROVIDER
☐ Abrasion ☐ Dental ☐ Hypothermia
☐ Blister ☐ Dislocation ☐ Intoxication
☐ Chest Pain ☐ Dizziness ☐ Laceration
☐ Concussion ☐ Fracture ☐ Sprain/Strain
☐ Contusion ☐ Hyperthermia
☐ Other

MEDICATION or IV GIVEN

Time:	Medication/IV	Provider Name:

TREATMENT & SERVICES PROVIDED
☐ Antacid ☐ Splint/Taping/Tensor
☐ Counselling ☐ Stretching
☐ Ibuprofen ☐ Tylenol
☐ Immobilization ☐ Vaseline
☐ R.I.C.E. ☐ Wound Management
☐ Sling ☐ Other
☐ Other ☐ Other

DISCHARGE ACUITY SCALE**
☐ Black ☐ Red ☐ Yellow ☐ Green ☐ White

FOLLOW-UP
☐ Event Medical Team
☐ ER
☐ Family Physician/Clinic
☐ Other

DISPOSITION
☐ Returned to Event/work
☐ Left Event (private vehicle)
☐ Left Event (taxi)
☐ Left Event (event staff)
☐ Ambulance Transport
☐ Air Evacuation
☐ AMA
☐ Other

DISCHARGE INSTRUCTIONS

ADDITIONAL NOTES

Did the care provided on site prevent a visit to another medical facility (i.e. hospital, clinic, family doctor)? ☐ Yes ☐ No

LEVEL OF TRAINING OF CARE PROVIDER**

LOCATION CARE WAS PROVIDED

DISCHARGE TIME

Name of Attendant (please PRINT)

Signature of Attendant

2011

FIGURE 4-2. Patient encounter form. [Used with permission from the Mass Gathering Medicine On-Line Registry, accessed at http://ubcmgm.ca/registry/.]

mobility of people with chronic illness, and the aging population all contribute to make in-flight medical emergencies more and more common. Yet, the exact incidence is not known because a formal system to report in-flight medical emergencies is not required by the Federal Aviation Administration.[9] However, it is known that cardiac, neurologic, and respiratory emergencies comprise the more serious complaints as defined by a need to divert the aircraft or use ground-based EMS resources.[10-12] GI complaints, such as abdominal pain, nausea, and vomiting, are common yet rarely represent medical emergencies and require little intervention. The combined data suggest that medical emergencies occur at a rate of 20 to 100 per million passengers, with a death rate of 0.1 to 1 per million passengers.[10,13,14]

Factors unique to the airline environment that affect medical care include the lower partial pressure of oxygen, potential exposure to chemical irritants, dry air, virulent airborne particles, and venous stasis. The aircraft cabin is typically pressurized to the equivalent of 5000 to 8000 feet above sea level. For individuals with cardiopulmonary disease, this relative decrease in arterial blood oxygen saturation may compromise cardiovascular reserves, thus precipitating an emergency. For chronic obstructive pulmonary disease and asthma patients, a combination of dry cabin air, respiratory irritants, reduced partial pressure of oxygen, and lack of access to their bronchodilators may trigger respiratory problems. In addition, this setting may aggravate normal health behaviors through alcohol ingestion, dehydration, and the inaccessibility of prescribed medications.

The management and disposition of medical emergencies on commercial airline flights are dependent on available personnel and equipment. Airline crew members receive education in basic first aid and CPR as mandated by the Federal Aviation Administration.[15] In addition, most large commercial flights include passengers with some medical training who are called upon to assist a passenger or crew member in distress. Assuming that care rendered is provided on a volunteer basis, Good Samaritan laws should provide protection from medical malpractice liability.

Onboard medical supplies are limited. The Federal Aviation Administration requires passenger-carrying aircraft weighing more than 7500 pounds maximum capacity with at least one flight attendant to carry an enhanced emergency medical kit in addition to a basic first aid kit, as outlined in **Table 4-6.**[16] Some airlines may choose to supplement these supplies with additional types of medications or equipment. Oxygen supplies are plentiful in the case of cabin depressurization, but there is typically limited availability of supplemental oxygen for sick passengers. In some cases, the pilot may be able to lower the cruising altitude to

Mass Gatherings: Hajj

Mohammed A. Alsultan

The Kingdom of Saudi Arabia is host to the annual event of Hajj (pilgrimage), the largest mass gathering in the world, in the city of Mecca, Saudi Arabia. All Hajj worship activities have to be accomplished in 4 to 5 days; an estimated 4 million pilgrims participated in 2011, 6 million are projected for 2015, and 10 million are projected for 2025. A complex infrastructure is required to handle transportation, accommodation, water, food, sanitation, safety and security, health, and hospitality for the millions of pilgrims who participate in Hajj.

Cultural, socioeconomic, and geographic factors contribute to the complexity of Hajj and require detailed planning. Communication must be provided in multiple languages for pilgrims from 140 countries with vastly different educational backgrounds, cultures, and health literacy, and communication must also accommodate illiterate pilgrims. The city of Mecca sits in a valley just above sea level and lies in a corridor between mountains, so space for population movement is very limited. Hajj is held in the twelfth lunar month and is not synchronized with seasons, so over the years, the weather varies between the extremes of heat in summer and flooding in winter. Most pilgrims are elderly, with considerable variation in health-related behavior, underlying health status, and medical needs. Challenges include visa management, illegal immigrants, illegal pilgrims, and security against terror attacks and for high-profile pilgrims.

Because free health care is provided to all pilgrims, the majority of Saudi Arabia's healthcare resources are redirected to Mecca during Hajj. There are 20 hospitals in Mecca, of which seven are seasonal. One hospital, with 3350 beds, has cardiac catheterization capabilities. During Hajj, there are more than 100 walk-in clinics and emergency centers, which are operated by 20,000 emergency care givers. All of these centers are run mainly by the Ministry of Health, but other governmental institutions (mainly military) participate in healthcare provision, so that coordination between the various centers is challenging.[1] Prehospital care is provided by the Saudi Red Crescent Association with more than 300 ground ambulances, hundreds of homemade wagons, five air ambulances, and many Red Crescent stations. Also, there are hundreds of mini-clinics that come with every international pilgrim group, and while they usually liaise between the hospitals and health centers, they have never been part of strategic health planning.

In 2010, the total number of outpatient visits to hospitals and health centers was 1 million, with an increase of 8.9% from the previous year. The admission rate was 1.1%, with 666 deaths (23.9 deaths/100,000 pilgrims).[2] All healthcare documentation is in English, and treatment records are given to every pilgrim who visits any medical facility. Planning is under way to develop an electronic medical record system that will be integrated with other medical records in or outside of Saudi Arabia.

The Ministry of Health prepares all year for the Hajj. The Ministry conducts several workshops for medical and nonmedical staff on disaster preparedness, triage, and emergency care. During Hajj, public health issues are precisely and completely reported because of the international and intercontinental repercussions in terms of the spread of infectious disease.[3] Regular reports are generated concerning stampedes, motor vehicle crashes, burns, and heatstroke. The Ministry submits a weekly epidemiologic report to the World Health Organization, indicating pilgrim vaccination status before traveling to Mecca (meningococcal meningitis and poliomyelitis if traveling from a polio-endemic country, or yellow fever if traveling from a country at risk of yellow fever) and other recommended health measures (seasonal flu vaccine and health education programs in the pilgrim's country of origin).[3] Different countries have varying vaccination policies and different endemic diseases. Historically, there were many documented outbreaks of plague and cholera during Hajj, involving large numbers of pilgrims, when quarantine was the principal means of control. Today, the speed of air travel means that pilgrims incubating infectious diseases at their time of departure may not manifest illness until after arrival in Mecca, thereby facilitating the spread of disease and even full-blown epidemics.[4] In 2010, the Ministry of Health established 25 health centers at entry points to the Holy Land (Jeddah airport, seaport, and land ports) and provided preventive services to 1.8 million pilgrims at these sites. For example, 435,000 pilgrims were given infectious disease chemoprophylaxis, and 463,000 pilgrims were vaccinated against poliomyelitis.

The Minister of the Interior is the general commander for Hajj. He is the overall leader of the Hajj Higher Committee, which includes the Governor of Mecca province, the Minister of Islamic Affairs, the Minister of Health, the Minister of Municipality, the Minister of Finance, the President of the Saudi Red Crescent Authority, the Minister of Transportation, and other high-ranking government members. This committee acts as the highest command center. Each one of the above members chairs a command center in his field and reports back to the Hajj Higher Committee. For example, the Minister of the Interior heads the military command center, which includes civil defense, traffic police, passport officers, and security police departments, besides chairing the Hajj Higher Committee.

In a disaster situation, the disaster commander is the head of Civil Defense, and the Ministry of Health and Red Crescent teams fall under that command. The Ministry of Health team leader at the scene is responsible for dispatching patients from the scene, and the commander from the Ministry of Health controls patient distribution to all the hospitals. There is a central operational room that serves as headquarters for one representative from each service (e.g., civil defense, traffic, police, Ministry of Health, Red Crescent, municipal affairs). This also serves as the communication center and is fully equipped with radios and telephone landlines.

The Saudi Arabian government is responsible for safety and fire prevention and fire fighting, with more than 40 centers set up during the Hajj period. These centers monitor security, prevent and manage any terrorist acts (e.g., bombing near the holy mosque in 1989), assist in disaster management (76 people were killed when a hotel in Mecca collapsed in a narrow street in 2006), and provide and control travel access to and from the Holy Land borders. The Hajj mass gathering demands an enormous amount of preparation by, and cooperation between, politicians, military staff, media, laboratory scientists, public health officials, emergency physicians, and other Saudi Arabian authorities. Some of the future challenges during the Hajj are the training of pilgrims prior to arrival as part of the visa-issuing process; mega food storing; prohibiting the use of fires inside pilgrim tents; providing special mobile shelters; minimizing air and water pollution; and providing climate control. However, the greatest future challenge is crowd management inside the Holy Mosque during Tawaf, the ritual of circumambulating the Kaaba seven times (Figure 1). The Custodian of the Two Holy Mosques Institute of Hajj Research was established in 1975 to provide support for researchers and scientists in the medical, civil engineering, sociology, cultural, and public health fields to continue to improve all services in the vicinity of the Holy Shrine of Hajj.

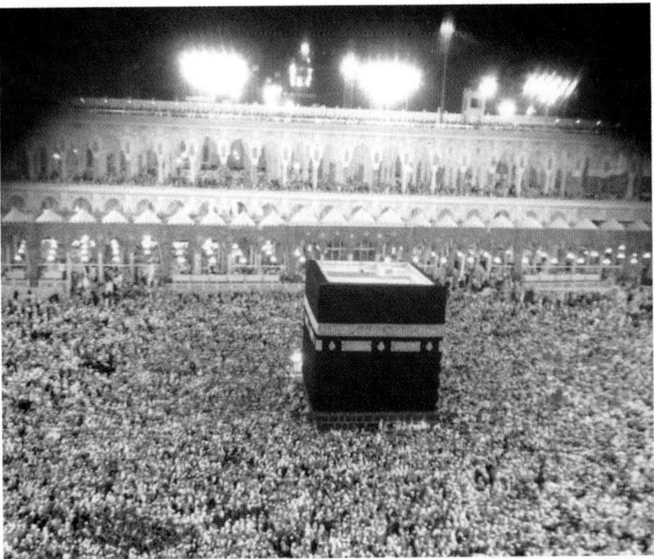

FIGURE 1. Pilgrims during Tawaf, circumambulating the Kaaba. [Photo courtesy of Dr. Mohammed A. Alsultan.]

REFERENCES

1. Al-Anazi A: Hajj 2011: a unique learning experience for final year emergency medical services student. *World J Med Sci* 7: 59, 2012.
2. www.moh.gov.sa (Ministry of Health, Statistical Year Book, 2010.) Accessed on September 5, 2012.
3. http://www.who.int/csr/mass gathering/en/ (World Health Organization: Communicable disease alert and response for mass gatherings.) Accessed on August 3, 2008.
4. Shafi S, Booy R, Haworth E, Rashid H, Memish ZA: Hajj: health lessons for mass gatherings. *J Infect Public Health* 1: 27, 2008. [PMID: 20701842]

TABLE 4-6 Federal Aviation Administration–Mandated Equipment

First Aid Kits	Equipment	Medications
1-inch adhesive bandage	Stethoscope	Acetaminophen
4×4–inch bandage	Sphygmomanometer	Antihistamine
Roller bandage	Gloves	Atropine
Triangular bandage	Syringes	Aspirin
Antiseptic	Needles	Bronchodilator
Ammonia capsules	IV administration set with tubing and venous tourniquet	Dextrose
Splints, arm and leg	Oral airways	Epinephrine, 1:1000 and 1:10,000
Tape	Bag-valve mask	Lidocaine
Scissors	Automated external defibrillator	Nitroglycerin
	CPR masks	Normal saline
		Oxygen

Basic instruction book that explains how to use equipment and medications.

increase the cabin pressure and subsequently increase the level of oxygen. In 2004, the Federal Aviation Administration mandated that all domestic flights carry an automated external defibrillator.[15] Finally, passengers on board may provide their own medicines for use by others during an emergency, providing an inconsistent but possibly valuable resource.

The decision to divert an aircraft for a medical emergency is a balance between medical need, cost, and logistic constraints. Although the final decision to divert is made by the pilot, there are a number of resources available for guidance. Most airlines contract with some form of ground-based online medical support. Usually directed by an emergency physician, these services provide information on resources available at airports in the vicinity and along the route of flight. From a medical perspective, it is necessary to decide if the patient is stable enough to continue to the planned destination or if there is a need for immediate definitive care. The cost of diverting an aircraft, including rebooking of flights and the cost of dumping fuel to meet maximum landing weight, can be quite high, running from $30,000 to $750,000. Logistically, diversion requires finding a landing site that can accommodate the aircraft and has appropriate medical resources nearby. The decision to divert an international flight may be complicated by legal issues, such as landing rights and passenger screening requirements.

The advent of long-haul travel brings to the forefront the issue of global spread of infectious disease. Passengers may travel across the globe between continents while in the prodromal phase of a disease, or they may knowingly travel while ill, making efforts to mask signs and symptoms with medications. It has been reported that risk of infection is greatest on flights longer than 8 hours and among passengers seated within two rows of the infected individual, particularly referring to the transmission of tuberculosis.[17] This is a testament to the well-contained local circulation of cabin air. However, there is the misconception by some that when an infected passenger sneezes, the majority of the passengers of the aircraft will become infected. In reality, cabin air is a mixture of outside air that enters the aircraft engine continuously and recirculated air passing through high-efficiency particulate air filters that remove particles as small as 0.003 μm.[17]

Both the outbreak of severe acute respiratory syndrome in November 2002 and the H1N1 influenza pandemic outbreak of April 2009 demonstrated the urgent need for a rapid, appropriate, and coordinated international response to deal with the spread of pandemics. Consequently, the concept of quarantine is often considered as an option for preventing the spread of disease. Drawing on the most recent experience and analysis of the response efforts to the 2009 H1N1 pandemic, it is evident that airport quarantine inspection is not effective in preventing the spread of influenza virus.[17,18] It has been determined that between the large number of people in the incubation period (thus not showing any symptoms), the low accuracy of the inspection kits used, and the poor cost-effectiveness, quarantine inspection in itself is not effective in preventing the spread of respiratory viruses. However, follow-up information obtained from passengers, follow-up surveys distributed to passengers, and information disseminated on symptoms to be aware of are believed to be important in mitigating the secondary spread of viruses.

TABLE 4-7 Distribution of Common Complaints on Cruise Ships

Complaint	Percentage of Complaints
Shortness of breath	29.1
Injuries	18.2
Neurologic	9.1
Abdominal pain/digestive	8.9
Chest pain	3.3
GU	3.2
Musculoskeletal	3.1
Skin	2.5

CRUISE SHIP MEDICINE

Nearly 10 million people travel on cruise lines each year, the majority of whom are from North America. With an average customer age of 55 years on many ships, the number of people with chronic medical conditions can be quite high.[19] Large vessels carry >2000 passengers and 1000 crew, resulting in a uniquely isolated environment with a high probability of encountering sick patients.[20]

The most common complaints seen in the ship's infirmary are shortness of breath and injuries. Other complaints are outlined in **Table 4-7**. On a typical week-long cruise with 1100 passengers, it is estimated that there will be an average of four potentially life-threatening conditions, with one patient terminating the cruise early as a result.[19] The decision to continue onboard treatment, to transport to a shore-based facility, or to arrange aeromedical evacuation must be made in light of weather forecasts, predicted flight time, and the quality of local resources. This choice is often made in conjunction with online medical support services provided by the cruise line.

WILDERNESS MEDICINE

Mass gathering events that are located within a wilderness environment can present unique challenges to the provision of medical care. Ideally, medical directors for wilderness mass gathering events should be experienced in both wilderness medicine and EMS. The 16-hour National Association of EMS Physicians/Wilderness Medical Society's Wilderness EMS Medical Directors Course provides concrete skills that are beneficial to a medical director for a wilderness mass gathering event. These events can occur in environments with extremes of temperature that medical personnel should be prepared to manage, both for themselves and for the care of patients. Most significantly, mass gatherings in wilderness environments can present challenges in the extrication of patients and may necessitate the use of alternative means of transport such as horses, snowmobiles, and aircraft.

ULTRA-DISTANCE ATHLETIC EVENTS

One of the clinical situations often encountered during exercise, particularly in individuals involved in endurance events such as marathons, triathlons, and ultra-distance athletic races, is the management of fluid and electrolyte repletion, specifically severe and potentially life-threatening hyponatremia. Exercise-associated hyponatremia, first described in the early 1980s, is defined as serum sodium below the normal reference range of the laboratory occurring during or up to 24 hours after prolonged physical activity.[21,22] Both fluid intake in excess of fluid loss and impaired urinary water excretion due to persistent secretion of antidiuretic hormone are important pathologic mechanisms contributing to this rapid, predominately dilutional decrease in serum sodium. Risk factors for developing exercise-associated hyponatremia include a high rate of fluid consumption during and after exercise (often associated with weight gain compared with prerace weight), exercise time longer than 4 hours, female sex, and a low body mass index.[23]

Athletes presenting to first aid tents during ultra-distance events should be evaluated for electrolyte abnormalities.[24] Although a serum sodium level should ideally be checked before administering IV fluids, this may not always be feasible in the mass gathering environment. Therefore, it is critical to be able to identify individuals with signs and symptoms consistent with hyponatremia and to differentiate those with life-threatening presentations. The majority of hyponatremic athletes are asymptomatic or mildly symptomatic, with manifestations such as nausea and vomiting, malaise, lightheadedness, dizziness, headache, and fatigue. Severe, life-threatening manifestations include confusion, seizures, and coma, which may indicate the development of cerebral edema and impending death.

Hyponatremia during athletic events is best managed by preventative means. Oral rehydration using fluids that contain both carbohydrates and sodium, as found in commercial "sports drinks," results in less of a dilutional effect; however, they are still relatively hypotonic compared to plasma. It has also been previously suggested that maintaining a fluid balance during the event by limiting drinking to <500 mL/h will help to prevent hyponatremia. However, given the wide variation in sweat production and renal water excretion between individual athletes, and in the same individual depending on conditions during the race, it is not feasible to develop specific universal guidelines. Overall, recommendations for endurance athletes support the concept of drink according to thirst.[22]

Athletes presenting with the clinical manifestation of mild to moderate hyponatremia should have fluid restriction and observation until the onset of spontaneous diuresis rather than administration of hypertonic saline, since similar symptoms may occur in hypernatremia.[22,25] However, among those with severe symptoms, when it is not feasible to measure serum sodium due to the constraints of the mass gathering event, treatment should be initiated empirically. Recommendations suggest an initial 100 mL bolus of 3% hypertonic saline, which should raise the serum sodium by 2 to 3 mEq/L. The bolus can be followed by an infusion rate of 3% hypertonic saline at 2 to 3 mL/kg/h to establish an increase in the serum sodium concentration of 4 to 5 mmol/L over the first 1 to 2 hours in order to reverse the osmotic gradient.[26] An alternative approach is to administer an additional two boluses of 100 mL of 3% hypertonic saline every 10 minutes until life-threatening symptoms have resolved.[27] Once clinical improvement occurs, the rate of infusion is decreased to follow the guidelines recommend for the safe correction of chronic hyponatremia (maximum increase of 12 mmol/L over 24 hours).[26]

CARDIAC ARRESTS

Although cardiac arrests comprise a small percentage of medical occurrences at mass gathering events, results can be detrimental if planners are not well prepared for this potential need. At the very least, planners should prepare to have an adequate number of automated external defibrillators and make calculated decisions as to where these devices should be placed to minimize response time for all locations within the event. Planners should also consider the placement of ambulances within the event for easy egress and the provision of advance life support care.

MASS CASUALTY

In planning for a mass gathering, the event medical director should be cognizant of and prepared for the potential of a mass casualty incident. Plans should include methods of triage, coordination of the mass casualty with local EMS, and distribution of large numbers of patients as needed to area acute care facilities. Ultimately, the medical teams should function seamlessly in the Incident Command System structure such that patient flow is managed in the same manner regardless of the numbers of patients seen at any point in time and the potential influx of large numbers of patients in the event of a mass casualty situation.

REFERENCES

The complete reference list is available online at www.TintinalliEM.com.

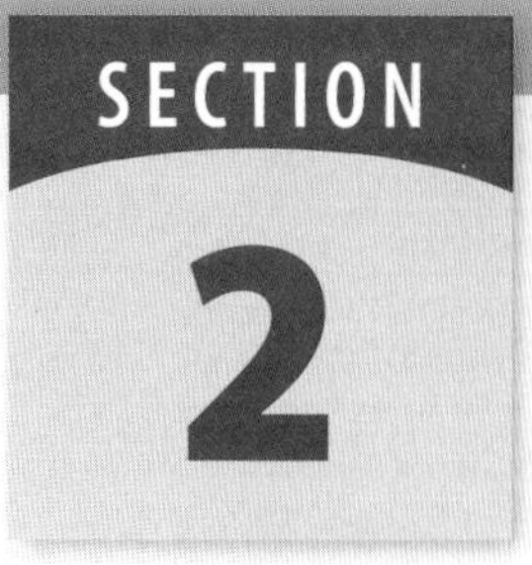

Disaster Management

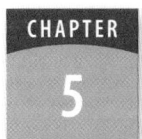

Disaster Preparedness

Robert G. Hendrickson
B. Zane Horowitz

INTRODUCTION

Disasters have claimed millions of lives and cost billions of dollars worldwide in the past few decades. Examples of large-scale disasters include the terrorist attacks of September 11, 2001; the 2004 Pacific Ocean tsunami; the 2010 earthquake in Haiti; the 2011 earthquake and tsunami in Japan; and Superstorm Sandy of 2012. Emergency physicians frequently have extensive responsibilities for community and hospital-level disaster preparedness and response. This chapter discusses the definition of a disaster, disaster preparedness and planning, the hospital emergency operations plan, field disaster response, and the ED disaster response.

DISASTER DEFINITION

The World Health Organization defines a disaster as a sudden ecologic phenomenon of sufficient magnitude to require external assistance. A disaster is an event that overwhelms the resources of the region or location in which it occurs. Furthermore, a hospital disaster may similarly be defined as an event that overwhelms the resources of the receiving hospital. A hospital disaster may be of any size and is not limited to mass casualty incidents. A single patient who ingested an organic phosphorous pesticide may overwhelm the resources of a hospital if that hospital is not prepared to decontaminate external to the ED. A single patient with suspected smallpox or a single influential patient (e.g., world leader or a celebrity) may use so many ED resources that it affects the care of other patients.

Whether an event is a disaster further depends on the time of day, nature of the injuries, type of event, and the amount of preparation time before the arrival of patients. The ED "surge capacity" (ability of the ED to care for more patients than is typical) may be severely limited by hospital overcrowding.

When it appears that the normal procedures of an ED may be interrupted by an event, there must be policies and procedures in place to activate a disaster response, direct the mobilization of personnel and equipment, and permit the rapid triage, assessment, stabilization, and definitive care of victims.

TYPES OF DISASTERS

Disasters are subdivided into several categories (**Table 5-1**). **External disasters occur at locations that are physically separate from the hospital (e.g., transportation accident, industrial accident). An internal disaster is an event that occurs within the confines of the hospital (e.g., bomb scare, laboratory accident involving radiologic agents, power failure).** Disasters can be both internal and external (e.g., earthquake with mass casualties as well as damage to the internal hospital). Further discussions of disasters are provided in the following chapters: chapter 6, Natural Disasters; chapter 8, Chemical Disasters; and chapter 9, Bioterrorism.

DISASTER CHARACTERISTICS

Regardless of the cause, most disasters have common characteristics that are important for disaster preparedness and planning. In an acute disaster, or a disaster with an identifiable time of onset that produces casualties (e.g., explosion, chemical release, fire, earthquake), the event is followed by a large number of minimally injured patients presenting to the nearest hospitals, usually without prehospital triage or evaluation.[1,2] This is typically followed by prehospital transport of the most affected patients to the same hospitals.[3] Initial patients can be expected within minutes, and peak volumes can be expected at 2 to 3 hours after the event.[2,3] The vast majority (~80%) of patients are not transported by prehospital agencies, but instead self-transport by car, van, police vehicle, cabs, foot, or any means available to the nearest ED.[2-4] Even in acute events, ED volumes tend to remain elevated for days to weeks after events.[3] In nonacute events, such as a pandemic of an infectious disease, ED volumes have a slower onset of surge, but ED and hospital volumes remain elevated for extended periods.

Based on previous events, common factors that may hinder ED response are listed in **Table 5-2**. A large amount of federal funding has been supplied to address these issues, but they likely remain as the major common limitations to effective ED disaster response.

DISASTER PREPAREDNESS AND PLANNING

Planning for any type of disaster consists of common elements. A hospital disaster planning group is responsible for generating the hospital's emergency operations plan. Include a diverse membership of hospital employees and decision makers. **Table 5-3** lists some potential members and their roles. The group should meet on a regular basis to assess hazards, develop and update short- and long-term disaster plans, plan exercises and training, and redesign the disaster plan based on evaluations of exercises and real events.

The general components of the disaster plan include hazard vulnerability analysis, compliance with agency requirements, hospital–community coordination, integration with national response assets, and training and disaster drills. Develop specific plans (for radiation, explosions, mass casualties, decontamination) based on an assessment of the potential disasters in the area as well as study of the events that would cause the most disruption to the ED and hospital.

HAZARD VULNERABILITY ANALYSIS

The hospital planning group should address those disasters that are most likely to occur in their community and geographic area. For example, planners on the West Coast of the United States may make earthquake planning a priority and those on the Gulf and Atlantic coasts may prioritize hurricane planning. Give consideration to the proximity of population centers to chemical release threats (military chemical weapons depots, large industrial sites, or transportation hubs).[5] Industrial sites that store large volumes of potentially harmful chemicals are required by Title III of the Superfund Amendments and Reauthorization Act to participate in local emergency planning committees. Industries are required to report spills of potentially harmful chemicals, and the approximate location of these sites may be found at http://toxmap.nlm.nih.gov. Terrorist-related disasters may be prioritized in hospitals that are in proximity to sites that may be significant terrorist targets. Include factors such as proximity to transportation facilities (e.g., ports, airports) as well as locations where large numbers of people collect (e.g., festivals, stadiums, arenas) with the risk assessment.

The hazard vulnerability analysis can prioritize planning efforts because different disasters are characterized by different morbidity and mortality patterns and different challenges to the ED and hospital.

TABLE 5-1 Types of Disasters

Disaster Type	Definition	Examples
Natural disaster	Disaster caused by a naturally occurring event	Earthquakes, tsunamis, tornadoes, hurricanes/typhoons, volcanic eruption, pandemic influenza
Man-made disaster	Nonnatural events that are not purposefully produced	Vehicle crashes (e.g., car, plane, bus), mass casualty events, explosions, fires, industrial accident/chemical release
Terrorist-related disaster	Events that are purposefully produced in an effort to cause terror	Events of September 11, 2001, as well as intentional chemical, biological, radiologic, or toxin releases
Internal disaster	An event that occurs within the hospital	Hazardous materials spill in hospital laboratory, fire or explosion within hospital, power failure
External disaster	An event that occurs external to the hospital	Transportation accident, industrial accident
Acute disaster	Disaster that occurs in a narrow and well-defined time frame	Explosion, industrial release, earthquake
Nonacute disaster	Disaster with no well-defined start point or continuous production of casualties over a broad time frame	Pandemic infectious disease, incremental release of a biological or toxin (e.g., anthrax sent through mail)

TABLE 5-3 Hospital Planning Group

Hospital Planner	Role in Disaster Planning and Response
Public safety	Crowd control, hospital lockdown, and hospital access control
Facilities/engineering	Evaluate structural damage and advise on stability of facilities
Logistics/equipment supply	Provide supplies/equipment; arrange for rapid ordering of additional supplies
Pharmacy	Provide pharmaceuticals, antidotes, and antibiotics; arrange for rapid ordering of additional pharmaceuticals
Transportation	Assist with patient transport
Clinical fields	A wide array of clinical fields should be represented, including representatives from the ED, primary specialties (internal medicine, family medicine, pediatrics), and surgical specialties
Media/public relations	Act as single point of contact for media; liaise between media and clinical areas, emergency operations center, and other hospital resources
Communications officer	Coordinate communication to employees during a disaster through e-mail, Web site, paging groups, phone, or social media
Nonclinical patient care	Housekeeping and food services
Safety officer	Determine and ensure safe practices for employees (e.g., appropriate personal protective equipment for decontamination)
Radiation safety officer	Prepare plan for and respond to radiologic emergencies
Infection control officer	Prepare for and respond to infectious disease emergencies

For example, earthquakes may cause severe traumatic injuries requiring a concentration on surge capacity of the critically ill patient. Rescue operations may last several days. Unique needs, such as dialysis for renal failure for multiple crush injury victims, may need to be considered. Natural disasters often cause large numbers of homeless or displaced persons whose everyday medical needs are exacerbated by limited access to usual health care, as occurred after Hurricane Katrina. Chemical releases may require mass decontamination as well as large numbers of ventilators, oxygen, and specific antidotes that are not typically available in large quantities.

THE JOINT COMMISSION REQUIREMENTS

The Joint Commission requires that member hospitals have a written plan for the timely care of casualties arising from both external and internal disasters, and the hospital must document the training and exercise of these plans.

HOSPITAL–COMMUNITY COORDINATION

Every hospital should integrate its emergency operations plan with those of community disaster management agencies. This is especially important regarding disaster notification and communications, transportation of casualties, and provisions for dispatch of hospital medical teams to a disaster site. Strong relationships with community agencies (e.g., fire department, regional EMS system, local emergency management, or public health agency) are important to ensure a coordinated disaster response. There are a large number of community agencies that have some responsibility for disaster planning and response (**Table 5-4**).

Other organizations that a hospital may interact with during the disaster planning process include the military, local chapters of the American Red Cross, local emergency planning committees, Citizen Corps Councils, and other volunteer agencies, along with state and

TABLE 5-2 Factors That May Hinder ED Response to Disasters

Poor communication between ED and disaster scene
Poor communication within the hospital (e.g., ED to emergency operations center, emergency operations center to patient care areas)
Inability to control volunteer healthcare personnel who are unfamiliar with the ED function and their roles in disaster response
Inability to engage and control convergence of media to the ED
Inability to engage, control, and direct visitors who are searching for loved ones
Inability to control large numbers of patients (i.e., crowd control)
Difficulty maintaining high staffing needs for extended periods

TABLE 5-4 Community Agencies Involved in Disaster Planning

Community Agency	Responsibilities
Federal Bureau of Investigation	Incident command if a federal crime may be involved
FEMA	Incident command in public health disaster
State governor	Authority to declare health emergency; requests federal assistance (e.g., FEMA); responsible for public safety
State health department	Authorized by governor to coordinate disaster response
State emergency management association	State-level equivalent of FEMA
City/county health department	May have jurisdiction for local disasters (variable); may be initial incident command for local health disasters
EMS	Patient triage in field; decontamination in field (if necessary); stabilization and transfer to definitive care facility
Fire service	Overall scene command in an acute disaster; victim rescue and hazard control
Police service	Traffic management and scene security in an acute disaster
Public works	Support equipment and personnel; structural safety expertise
Hazardous materials (HAZMAT) teams	Initial incident command at scene of hazardous materials spill/exposure

Abbreviation: FEMA = Federal Emergency Management Agency.

federal agencies (e.g., National Disaster Medical System, Metropolitan Medical Response System, Centers for Disease Control and Prevention). Medical planning in a community is usually the responsibility of local and state health departments and EMS councils.

INTEGRATION WITH NATIONAL RESPONSE ASSETS

Some of the important federal response resources are listed in **Table 5-5**. During a response, these agencies may play pivotal roles and may interface and coordinate with hospitals and emergency physicians.

TRAINING AND DISASTER DRILLS

Regular training and drills familiarize staff with their disaster roles and responsibilities and identify weaknesses or omissions in the plans that require additions or revisions. Drills can range from full-scale, community-wide simulations, with moulage (use of makeup or theater techniques to represent injuries) victims, to tabletop triage scenarios, mini-drills that test only certain components of the disaster plan (such as call-up of personnel), and tests of communications. The Joint Commission requires two annual drills. The scenarios should reflect incidents that are likely to occur in the community as determined by the hazard vulnerability analysis.

HOSPITAL EMERGENCY OPERATIONS PLAN

The hospital emergency operations plan provides for an organized response of the hospital from the time of notification of a disaster until the situation normalizes (**Table 5-6**).

Functions include activation of the emergency operations plan, establishment of an emergency operations center, assessment of hospital capacity, surge capacity planning, communications, supply and resupply, triage and treatment of casualties, establishment of support areas, and termination of the disaster state to allow for recovery and the return to normal activities.

ACTIVATE THE EMERGENCY OPERATIONS PLAN

Clearly delineate the roles and responsibilities of all employees in the ED and any employees who may respond to the ED in the planning process; those roles must be clearly listed and easily accessed in the event of a disaster. Clarify the reasons for activation of the emergency operations plan. Activation of the emergency operations plan should provide for the immediate mobilization of supplies, equipment, and personnel.

ESTABLISH EMERGENCY OPERATIONS CENTER

The Incident Command System is a standard emergency management system used throughout the United States to provide a flexible command and control structure upon which to organize a response.[6] The Incident Command System is generally used when there is an identifiable single scene for a disaster event, such as the site of a plane crash. By standardizing an organizational structure and using common terminology, the Incident Command System provides a management system that is adaptable to incidents involving a multiagency or multijurisdictional response. At the most basic level, there are five main components to the organizational structure: (1) incident command, (2) operations, (3) planning, (4) logistics, and (5) finance. With this type of organizational infrastructure and the flexibility to expand and collapse as needed, an orderly and efficient response to any incident can theoretically be implemented.

The Hospital Emergency Incident Command System is modeled after the Incident Command System. Upon declaration of a disaster, an emergency operations center within the hospital should be established in a predesignated area. This center should be able to communicate with the ED and triage area and with external authorities (regional EMS, police, fire, public health agencies). Provisions for multiple redundant modes of communication should be made. Other responsibilities of the emergency operations center include opening up additional hospital wards or

TABLE 5-5 Federal Response Resources

Agency	Role
U.S. Public Health Service/Office of Emergency Response; http://www.phe.gov/preparedness/pages/default.aspx	Office within DHHS. Management and coordination of federal health and medical activities related to preparation, response, and recovery from major emergencies or presidentially declared disasters.
Metropolitan Medical Response System For more information: http://www.bt.cdc.gov/planning/CoopAgreementAward/presentations/mmrs-oep10minbriefing-jim11.pdf	Enhance local emergency preparedness systems by promoting coordination between local responders (e.g., police, fire, hazardous materials agencies, EMS, hospitals).
National Disaster Medical System; http://ndms.fhpr.osd.mil/	Asset sharing program between DHHS, Federal Emergency Management Agency, U.S. Department of Defense, U.S. Department of Veterans Affairs, and public/private organizations—developed to provide surge capacity for natural disasters, wartime military casualties, and large-scale bioterrorism events.
DMAT; http://www.phe.gov/Preparedness/responders/ndms/teams/Pages/dmat.aspx	Multidisciplinary teams that deploy in response to federally declared disasters and emergencies to support a local jurisdiction's response. Teams include physicians, nurses, medics, pharmacists, and logisticians.
National Disaster Medical System Response Teams; http://www.phe.gov/Preparedness/responders/ndms/teams/Pages/default.aspx	Specialty teams, based on the DMAT concept, developed to respond to chemical, biological, and radiologic events.
Disaster Mortuary Operational Response Teams; http://www.phe.gov/Preparedness/responders/ndms/teams/Pages/dmort.aspx	Teams that respond to federally declared disasters and emergencies to support a local jurisdiction's ability to process large volumes of deceased patients.
Centers for Disease Control and Prevention http://www.bt.cdc.gov	Centers within DHHS. Lead federal agency in developing and applying disease prevention and control. Advisory agency in bioterrorism response.
CDC Outbreak Response Teams	Teams of CDC epidemiologists to assist with local efforts in investigating potential outbreaks, confirmation of cases and exposures, and environmental clean-up.
Laboratory Response Network; http://www.bt.cdc.gov/lrn/factsheet.asp	Network that links local and state public health laboratories to advanced-capacity laboratories, including military, chemical, veterinarian, agricultural, water, and food testing labs.
National Electronic Disease Surveillance System; http://wwwn.cdc.gov/nndss/script/nedss.aspx	National public health surveillance system.
Health Alert Network; http://emergency.cdc.gov/han/	System that allows for rapid early warning broadcast alerts to health departments for potential emerging infectious diseases or outbreaks.
Strategic National Stockpile; http://www.cdc.gov/phpr/stockpile/stockpile.htm	Two-part system designed to provide local jurisdictions with medications, vaccines, and equipment during a disaster. Prepackaged cache—delivered within 12 h in the U.S. Situation-specific cache—delivered within 36 h in the U.S.
Federal Bureau of Investigation	Lead federal agency for crisis management. Has authority to conduct law enforcement investigations into acts of terrorism.

Abbreviations: CDC = Centers for Disease Control and Prevention; DHHS = Department of Health and Human Services; DMAT = Disaster Medical Assistance Teams.

TABLE 5-6 Components of the Hospital Emergency Operations Plan

Component	Function
Activate emergency operations plan	Notify and mobilize personnel and equipment
Set up emergency operations center	Nerve center for hospital response and communication with outside agencies
Assess hospital capacity	Determine safety of hospital itself; determine capabilities of hospital in all units
Create surge capacity	Determine ways to handle the maximum number of patients
Establish communication systems	Develop multiple and redundant systems, including cellular phones, satellite phones, two-way radios, runners
Provide supplies and equipment	Deliver available supplies to proper areas and plan for resupplying or obtaining other needed materials
Establish support areas	Volunteer, media, and family information centers
Establish decontamination, triage, and treatment areas	Decontamination, triage, resuscitation, acute care, and minor care areas; surgical triage and holding; psychiatric area; morgue
Terminate disaster response and provide for remediation	Return personnel and supplies to normal activity; provide emotional support for caregivers; improve emergency operations plan for future incidents

clinics, obtaining outside assistance, evacuating endangered patients, assigning staff to treatment areas, and terminating the disaster mode of operation.

ASSESS HOSPITAL CAPACITY

Before the hospital can receive casualties, it must be determined if the hospital itself has sustained any structural damage or loss of use as a result of a disaster. These include blocked passageways or inoperable elevators; potential for fire, explosion, or building collapse; failure of utilities; loss of equipment or supplies; contamination of water; and outside access problems. This damage assessment is usually the responsibility of the hospital safety officer or engineer. If the hospital's structural integrity has been compromised, it may be necessary to initiate the evacuation plan to evacuate staff and patients.

Once it is determined that the hospital itself is safe, the hospital should determine how many casualties from the disaster site it can safely manage. This may be limited by available personnel, beds, operating room and intensive care unit capacity, and supplies, as well as by the type of disaster and the availability of other community resources. At the time of disaster notification, it is necessary to know the status of many of the hospital's capabilities: how many beds are available, how much critical supplies and medications are available, how many personnel are on duty, what damage has been done, how many operating rooms are in use, which clinicians are present in the hospital, and so forth.

CREATE SURGE CAPACITY

Surge capacity is the ability to increase hospital bed capacity over normal limits. Intrahospital surge may include doubling patients in rooms, converting an acute care ward to an intensive care level unit, opening previously closed wards, or caring for patients in typically nonclinical locations, such as the cafeteria. Interhospital or regional surge may include discharging hospitalized patients to an external low acuity unit, either mobile or fixed, and altering standards of care (typically a role of the state governor and legislature and only during governor-declared disasters).[7,8] The standards of care should be altered only in the most extreme circumstances, as patient surge has been linked to somewhat worse outcomes for individual patients.[9]

ESTABLISH COMMUNICATIONS SYSTEMS

Establishment of good communications is critical in any disaster or mass casualty situation. Even the best disaster plans fail without well-established communications systems. Unfortunately, experience shows that this essential function is difficult to achieve for a variety of reasons. Many communication modes become inoperative during a disaster. Cellular telephones, in particular, are often overwhelmed in disasters. Disaster planning must include a multi-tiered plan for intrahospital (blackboard, two-way radios, messengers/couriers) and interhospital (citizen band groups, cellular telephones, satellite telephones, two-way radios) communication.

SUPPLIES

During a disaster, necessary supplies and equipment must be ready for immediate distribution to appropriate locations in the hospital. Each hospital will need to estimate the amount of supplies that will be needed in stock over and above their regular hospital supply. Unfortunately, due to "just in time" stocking, most U.S. hospitals do not have a surge of supplies that may be used in a disaster. The Centers for Disease Control and Prevention has arranged a series of medication push-packs throughout the United States that can be delivered to any area of disaster within 12 hours (http://www.bt.cdc.gov/stockpile/index.asp). Once delivered, additional time is necessary to unpack the supplies and deliver the supplies to individual hospitals. The regional/local disaster plan must include a mechanism to unpack the push-packs, determine the hospitals in greatest need of individual items, divide the push-pack contents, and deliver the supplies to the hospital. This logistical issue makes it necessary for most hospitals to rely on their own supplies for a period of at least 96 hours.

ESTABLISH SUPPORT AREAS

Family Information Center During a disaster, families and friends will arrive at the hospital seeking information about victims. This convergence can seriously interfere with efforts of the hospital to respond effectively to the situation. For this reason, predesignate a separate area for family members seeking information. This area may also be used to discharge in-hospital patients and treated disaster victims.

Volunteer Coordination Center In major disasters, anticipate the potential for large numbers of volunteers, including those wishing to donate blood. Although some of these people may have appropriate clinical skills, they are unlikely to be familiar with the hospital functions and could be more hindrance than help. A separate place should be identified to handle these volunteers and, if appropriate, credential and decide how they may best be used. This area should include all equipment and personnel that are required to perform emergency credentialing (if appropriate and necessary).

Media Center Direct members of the media to a room or office of the hospital away from the ED and closely supervised by a hospital administrator or public information officer. Identify a single hospital spokesperson to relay information to the media.

DECONTAMINATION, TRIAGE, AND TREATMENT

Certain areas of the hospital must be designated for specific functions, including decontamination, triage, care of major and minor casualties, presurgical holding and surgical triage, psychiatric care, and morgue facilities. The plan should be quite specific as to the function of these areas, staffing requirements, and basic supplies to be used.

DECONTAMINATION

Perform decontamination in an area that is outside of the clinical care area of the ED.[4] Typically, this area is located external to the ED but may be in internal locations. Use the decontamination facility to remove clothing and cleanse the skin and hair of patients exposed to a chemical or radioisotope (**Table 5-7**).[10] Provide patient coverage and protection from the environment. Make sufficient

TABLE 5-7 Decontamination Guidelines

Decontaminate patients exposed to solids, liquids, vapors, or mists.
Patients exposed only to a fully dispersed gas need to be assessed for pulmonary symptoms and systemic toxicity and do not require decontamination. When uncertain if a substance is a gas or actually a vapor or mist, decontamination should occur.
Hospital personnel should have the **initial ability to decontaminate one patient at a time with a shower or hose system** while setting up a larger tent or a multiple-person decontamination system.
Perform decontamination outside of the ED in a way that prevents patients from entering the ED before decontamination.
Hospital personnel require level C personal protective equipment while performing decontamination. Higher levels of protection are not necessary and should only be used by hospitals that follow stringent training protocols and criteria, and use only personnel who have been specifically trained to use the equipment. **Sufficient equipment for multiple personnel and rotations of personnel in and out of the decontamination zone every 30 min is suggested.**
The first and a very effective method for decontamination is to disrobe, brush off solid dusts or powders, and wash and dry the face. Patient clothing and belongings should be individually bagged and labeled. Watches, earrings, body piercings, jewelry, and contact lenses should be removed. Hearing aids should be wiped with a moistened cloth and may be returned to patients after the decontamination procedure because the need to hear instructions outweighs any risk of wearing the hearing aid.
Warm water is the universal decontamination fluid. Hosing a patient from head to toe (or showering) for 5 min will decontaminate most ambulatory patients.
Patients with adherent materials will need additional scrubbing of hair and affected body parts with soap to remove these; medical assistance will be necessary in some circumstances. An additional check to ensure the removal of all earrings and body piercings should be done.
Young children need assistance and reassurance and should be decontaminated with the aid of a parent or guardian who can hold and reassure the child while medical personnel perform the decontamination.
After the decontamination procedure, provide hospital clothing (cloth or paper gowns) and triage patients to an area to await further assessment. Retriage patients with eye pain after whole-body decontamination for individual irrigation of their eyes with sterile normal saline. Patients with contaminated wounds will likely need additional irrigation of debris in wounds.
Contain runoff water from the decontamination to prevent environmental contamination.
Critical medical devices (infusion pumps, hearing aids, ostomy bags, etc.) may remain with the patient unless a high-risk chemical has been identified. Wash canes and walkers with soap and water or diluted household bleach and return to patients to ensure their mobility.
At least one radiation survey meter (e.g., Geiger-Muller counter) and staff that are trained in its use are necessary for events that potentially involve radioisotopes. Patients may need a radiation survey sweep before and after decontamination, and further decontamination may be needed until levels reach background radiation levels.
Staff involved in the decontamination process and systems need annual training and practice drills. Share an assessment of strengths and weakness learned from each drill with hospital personnel to improve preparedness and performance.

personal protective equipment available for hospital staff assisting with decontamination.

TRIAGE

Restrict patient entry to only one location—the triage area. The primary functions of a disaster triage area are rapid assessment of all incoming casualties or ill patients, patient registration and identification, the assignment of priorities for management, and distribution of patients to appropriate treatment areas in the ED and hospital.

TREATMENT

Patient care in disasters requires alteration of scale and sometimes location of clinical care, but staff should perform the clinical roles that are familiar to them. Several exceptions to this rule may exist (decontamination); however, in general, staff are more efficient at performing typical tasks quickly than learning new tasks in real time.

Organize patient care stations so that clinicians who are familiar with the assessment and treatment of the clinical problems may staff them. One suggested method of organizing patient care stations includes "resuscitation" and "minor treatment" areas.

RESUSCITATION

From the triage location, most, if not all, of the **seriously injured patients will be sent to the resuscitation area** (trauma and cardiac resuscitation, treatment of hypovolemic or septic shock, severe respiratory distress). This is usually physically located in the ED and staffed by emergency physicians.

MINOR TREATMENT AREA

In most disaster situations, the majority of patients are not very seriously injured. **These low-acuity patients can be sent to an "urgent care" area for definitive care**, including splinting of fractures, primary closure of lacerations, tetanus prophylaxis, and observation for delayed symptoms. This minor treatment area can be established in the hospital's outpatient clinics and staffed by the clinic physicians.

PRESURGICAL HOLDING AREA AND SURGICAL TRIAGE

Send trauma patients who are initially stabilized in the ED to the presurgical holding area for preoperative preparation and observation. **The number of operating rooms that can be staffed is the main limiting factor in the provision of definitive care for a large number of severely injured casualties.** The most experienced surgeon available should take the responsibility to prioritize cases and to rapidly assign surgeons to individual cases.

MENTAL HEALTH

In the event of a disaster involving mass casualties, and even property damage with loss of possessions, it is common for patients to present with episodes of anxiety and depression, or exacerbations of their psychiatric disorders.[11] Agitated patients, visitors, or staff can be extremely disruptive to hospital disaster operations. Consider a separate isolated area to receive individuals in need of psychological intervention. Include consideration for assessing patients and hospital staff who are psychologically affected by the disaster. Consider providing a critical stress response team, including social workers and psychiatrists, to provide support and critical stress debriefing.

MORGUE FACILITIES

Disasters can result in a large number of fatalities. Morgue capacities may need to be expanded to other areas of the hospital (medical school anatomy area, auditorium), enhanced by mobilization of local freezer trucks (this must be prearranged during the planning stage), or enhanced by federal assets (Disaster Mortuary Operational Response Teams). Viewing of deceased patients should take place here, not in treatment areas.

TERMINATING DISASTER RESPONSE (RECOVERY)

As soon as appropriate, direct efforts toward returning the hospital to normal operations. Besides restocking and cleaning, give consideration to the emotional stress experienced by both the EMS and hospital staff. In an attempt to reduce the psychological impact of these events on medical responders, a technique known as *critical incident stress debriefing* was introduced in 1993. The critical incident stress debriefing offers immediate emotional support to healthcare workers. Data from previous experiences suggest that such intervention can assist providers in maintaining job performance and satisfaction, resulting in improved patient care.[12] Provide all members who participated in the disaster, not just medical personnel, the opportunity to participate in critical incident stress debriefing.

Carefully record and review deficiencies in a hospital's disaster plan that are revealed during a disaster, and write an after-action report. Take immediate steps to correct these flaws in the plan.

FIELD DISASTER RESPONSE

Elements of field disaster response are field triage and medical care, communications, distribution of casualties, and management of on-site disaster medical teams.

FIELD TRIAGE AND MEDICAL CARE

In the field, rescue personnel often use a simple triage and rapid treatment technique that depends on a rapid assessment of respiratory status, perfusion, hemorrhage control, and mental status. Patients are then triaged to immediate care, delayed care, or dead/dying.[13,14] Subsequently, determining how much and what type of care to administer at the disaster site depends on several factors. If the number of patients is small and there are sufficient prehospital personnel and transportation resources available, on-site medical care can proceed in a fairly normal manner, with rapid stabilization and transportation to nearby hospitals. When extrication will be prolonged, interventions such as fluid resuscitation and pain control should be instituted in the field. On the other hand, early, rapid transportation with a minimum of treatment should be practiced when there is danger to rescuers and casualties from fire, explosion, falling buildings, hazardous materials, and extreme weather conditions.

When patients are likely to have significantly delayed transport from a scene (e.g., number of casualties exceeds transportation capacity or damage to hospital infrastructure), the "Secondary Assessment of Victim Endpoint" triage system may be helpful to identify patients who are most likely to benefit from the care available under austere field conditions.[15] The Secondary Assessment of Victim Endpoint triage system is intended to triage patients into categories that reflect a balance between resource use and probability of survival. Category 1 includes patients who will die regardless of how much care they receive. Category 2 includes patients who will survive whether or not they receive care. Category 3 includes patients who will benefit significantly from austere field interventions.[15]

COMMUNICATION—DISASTER SITE TO HOSPITALS

The local emergency communications or emergency operations center should alert hospitals in the affected area of possible mass/multiple casualty situations or disasters. This report should include the total number of injured, the number of seriously injured (who may need intensive care unit capability), and the number for whom ambulatory treatment is sufficient. Hospitals should report to the local emergency communications center the following information: bed availability, number of casualties received thus far, number of additional casualties that the hospital is prepared to accept, and specific items in short supply.

DISTRIBUTION OF CASUALTIES TO RECEIVING HOSPITALS

Maintain good communication between hospitals and on-site EMS command in order to minimize unequal distribution of victims. **Alert the on-scene incident commander immediately of a potentially overloaded hospital.** In this situation, the less injured and more stable can be sent a further distance to outlying hospitals.

Casualties with special problems, such as major burns, carbon monoxide poisoning, spinal cord injuries, or victims of chemical or biological terrorism, may need to be transferred directly to specialized units, although it may not be possible for these units to accept a large number of ill or injured. For that reason, develop regional plans to allow for the care of specialty patients in nonspecialty hospitals.

MANAGEMENT OF ON-SITE DISASTER MEDICAL TEAMS FROM HOSPITALS

On-site disaster medical teams dispatched from local hospitals may be of value in situations in which victims require prolonged extrication; transportation routes are blocked, preventing easy evacuation to hospitals; or the number of casualties is of such magnitude that they exceed transportation capacities. Dispatch such a team with great caution. Physicians and nurses function optimally in an in-hospital setting. Few, however, are prepared to work under austere field conditions. Such hospital-based teams should probably not come from the ED staff until back-up staff has arrived to care for patients arriving from the disaster site or who are already present. Explicitly describe how such personnel are placed in action in the hospital emergency operations plan and coordinate with state and local agencies through memoranda of understanding.

Carefully map out the resources for such field response teams on a regional basis. At least one institution from each region should maintain an on-site triage team of physicians and nurses. The designated hospital should store disaster triage kits containing essential resuscitation and stabilization equipment for field use.

ED DISASTER RESPONSE

INITIAL RESPONSE

When a call is made to the hospital indicating the occurrence of a disaster or potential mass casualty–producing event, the incident must be verified by the appropriate predesignated official, who then puts the emergency operations plan into effect. In some events, the first sign of a disaster may be patients arriving at the hospital. In this case, contact the regional emergency communications center to notify the regional hospitals of the impending disaster and initiate the emergency operations plan.

This sets a series of activities into motion. The information obtained from the call is given to the charge nurse; the nursing and medical personnel in the ED are notified of the impending arrival of casualties; and the ED's plan for calling additional staff is activated. If hospital telephone communications have been completely disrupted, ED personnel may have to be reached by radio, cellular phone, e-mail, or television announcement. In many disasters, cellular phone and text messaging systems are quickly overwhelmed. Alternatively, a calling station remote from the hospital, such as at the residence of an administrator, physician, or nurse, may be able to handle this extensive calling job without taxing the hospital's phone system.

An initial needs assessment is conducted by the nurse and/or physician in charge, given the information available. They should evaluate the current status of the patients in the ED and make the appropriate disposition decisions. The ED physician or charge nurse becomes the on-site incident commander until the plan-designated incident commander arrives. **Among the decisions to be made are those related to the admission, discharge, or transfer of patients, and decisions about the priority of patient care.** Discharge all nonemergency patients from the ED with responsible individuals.

Based on the initial assessment, the number of patients that the department can receive is determined and communicated to the prehospital disaster communications center. The nurse and the physician in charge then assign staff to those areas in the department to be used during the disaster.

Take all available litters and wheelchairs to the ambulance entrance immediately on announcement of the disaster status. Patients from the disaster site are met at the receiving area by hospital escorts who assist the EMTs in transferring patients to wheelchairs or stretchers.

Place essential equipment, such as endotracheal tubes, IV fluids, cervical collars, splints, and bandages, near the ambulance entrance to permit convenient restocking of the ambulance (when plans call for ambulance restocking from hospitals) and rapid return to the disaster site.

SECURITY

Hospital security diverts nonessential vehicles and ensures a smooth, one-way flow of traffic to the ambulance entrance. Once patients, family, and media arrive, security is also responsible for protecting the treatment areas and inhibiting unplanned entry into the hospital.[4]

TRIAGE

Triage establishes priorities for care and determines the clinical area of treatment. Many seeking help will arrive independent of the EMS system.[3,4] **Triage will need to be performed at the ED entrance even if it was done at the scene.**

Triage category is identified by use of a colored band or trauma/disaster tag that is placed on the patient to document that triage has been done.

The approach to patient evaluation and treatment is quite different when dealing with disaster situations that result in high casualties.[16] To accomplish the most good for the most number of patients, the triage team should evaluate all patients arriving at the ED and classify their condition with regard to severity of injury and need for treatment. Some principles of medical care must be altered to achieve the best overall result. Patient care at triage should be limited to manually opening airways and controlling external hemorrhage.

The most common triage classification in the United States still involves assigning patients to one of four color-coded categories (red, yellow, green, or black), depending on injury severity and prognosis (Table 5-8). In addition to the nature and urgency of the patient's systemic condition, triage decisions should be sensitive to factors affecting prognosis, such as age, general health, and prior physical condition of the patient, as well as the qualifications of the responders and the availability of key supplies and equipment.

Catastrophically injured patients who have a minimal chance for survival despite optimal medical care should be classified as "expectant" ("black": to include patients with burns involving 95% body surface area, and patients in full cardiac arrest or septic shock). Devoting time and resources to patients who are not likely to live jeopardizes other patients who are truly salvageable. The goal with these "expectant" patients should be adequate pain control and the opportunity to be with friends and family.

TRIAGE TEAM

A team consisting of an emergency physician, an ED nurse, and medical records or admitting clerks should receive every patient. In extraordinary situations, several triage teams may be required to handle the casualty load. Acknowledge the physician performing hospital triage as being in command of the triage area (clearly identified by a specially colored vest or other garment) and understanding all triage options.

TABLE 5-8 Triage Categories

Red
First priority
Most urgent
Life-threatening shock or hypoxia is present or imminent, but the patient can likely be stabilized and, if given immediate care, will probably survive.
Yellow
Second priority
Urgent
The injuries have systemic implications or effects, but patients are not yet in life-threatening shock or hypoxia; although systemic decline may ensue, given appropriate care, can likely withstand a 45- to 60-min wait without immediate risk.
Green
Third priority
Nonurgent
Injuries are localized without immediate systemic implications; with a minimum of care, these patients generally are unlikely to deteriorate for several hours, if at all.
Black
Dead
No distinction can be made between clinical and biological death in a mass casualty incident, and any unresponsive patient who has no spontaneous ventilation or circulation is classified as dead. Some place catastrophically injured patients who have a slim chance for survival regardless of care in this triage category.

Assign one member of the triage team (admitting or medical records clerk) the job of recording the victim's name on the disaster tag along with the triage destination within the hospital. If identification of the patient is not available, ethnicity, gender, and approximate age should be noted on the tag. An initial diagnostic impression should also be registered on the tag. This information is entered into a department log or into the electronic medical record, if possible. In some patient tracking systems, a scan of the bar code on the disaster tag may allow for immediate registration by disaster tag number and open an electronic medical record. Additional care can be recorded in the electronic medical record or in a paper disaster chart and kept with the patient at all times and later scanned into the electronic medical record.

ED DISASTER PATIENT CARE

Disaster care concepts often vary from the typical ED routine. Care that is not immediately time sensitive can be provided the next day. For example, wounds may benefit from delayed closure after copious irrigation due to delayed presentations or gross contamination. In the event of prolonged extrication from rubble, assess for delayed signs and symptoms, including cardiac dysrhythmias, hyperkalemia from crush injury, renal failure, and pulmonary blast injury.

Terrorist-related or industrial explosive events may lead to medical conditions or exposure to chemicals that are not familiar to clinicians.[4] Patients may require prolonged observation (e.g., exposure to phosgene or ricin) or unique testing. For infectious exposures, the Centers for Disease Control and Prevention and local/state public health agencies can guide testing, observation time, and treatment. Immediately contact the local public health agency if a biological terrorist agent or a rare and potentially fatal infectious disease is seen or suspected in the ED. In the event of a chemical agent, the Carolinas Poison Center (1-800-222-1222) can provide information and guidance on whether decontamination is necessary, as well as testing, observation time, and antidotal or supportive treatment. Fact sheets on biological, chemical, and radiologic agents are available at http://www.bt.cdc.gov.[4,17]

Use radiographic and laboratory studies sparingly, if at all, in a mass casualty situation, and only if the results of such tests will change treatment. For example, possible closed, nonangulated fractures can be splinted, and radiographs can be safely delayed for 24 to 48 hours. A chest radiograph may be appropriate in those patients complaining of chest pain, dyspnea, or abnormal chest wall motion, or who were potentially exposed to blast waves secondary to bombs. CT imaging may be quicker than plain radiographs in some injuries, and prioritization to CT may be required. Ultrasonography to detect free intraperitoneal fluid, pericardial fluid, and pneumothorax is time- and cost-effective, and has been used in earthquakes to triage operative care.[18]

With the exception of identification of biological and chemical agents, there are few indications for laboratory testing in disaster medicine. If testing will change management, use point-of-care testing to expedite care. For example, obtain a baseline hematocrit and type and crossmatching for blood in cases of hemorrhagic shock. Pulse oximetry monitors may need to be used as spot assessments, rather than continuous bedside monitoring of a single patient. Consider laboratory studies to be accessory and ordered only in specific circumstances (carboxyhemoglobin in cases of smoke inhalation).

In a disaster situation involving many casualties, the blood bank should have up to 50 units of blood available and should have access to volunteer donors who can be rapidly mobilized. Potential donors include friends and family members of patients, as well as mildly injured patients.

Acknowledgments: The authors gratefully acknowledge the contributions of Eric K. Noji, MD, and Gabor D. Kelen, MD, who were the authors of this chapter in the previous edition.

REFERENCES

The complete reference list is available online at www.TintinalliEM.com.

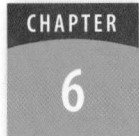

Natural Disasters

Lisa D. Mills
Trevor J. Mills

INTRODUCTION AND EPIDEMIOLOGY

Natural disasters continue to be an unpredictable source of worldwide morbidity and mortality and present unique challenges for practitioners of emergency care. The 2002 to 2011 annual average worldwide mortality rate was 107,000 deaths/year from natural disasters, with an average of 268 million worldwide victims per year during the same time period and an economic cost of $143 billion in 2012.[1] With the increase in rapidly mobilized recovery teams, emergency physicians are at the forefront of patient care following a natural disaster. It is here that we can have the greatest impact in treating survivors and minimizing secondary morbidity and mortality, often in the setting of a significantly impaired healthcare system. Research suggests that the burden of natural disasters is likely to rise in the coming years, due to increasing population density in high-risk areas and risks associated with expanding technology (e.g., fires or earthquakes in larger and taller buildings or critical infrastructure).[2]

Although the mechanics, warning period, and impact vary widely between types of natural disasters, there is a predictable pattern of events that occur and may be used to maximize the subsequent response. Natural disasters result in a combined loss of resources—infrastructure, economic, social, and health. While this may be tempered by pre-event preparedness and infrastructure strength, this combination of resource loss has a synergistic impact on the health of and the delivery of health care to the affected population. Another commonality is the predictable pattern of pathology, seen in the progression from the impact of the event itself, through the acute aftermath, to the immediate postdisaster phase, into the recovery phase (**Table 6-1**). Perhaps most salient for emergency practitioners, relief efforts can be implemented based on data from previous disaster experience, while simultaneously being tailored to the type of disaster (e.g., hurricane, earthquake, tornado, flood, tsunami, or snow) and region affected. Finally, disaster responders should be prepared to face the duty of management of dead bodies, on a scale otherwise only seen in the setting of combat.

LOSS OF RESOURCES

Most natural disasters—whether by water, wind, fire, or snow—cause some disruption of power, communication, and transportation systems. In developed and developing nations, entire cities can be destroyed instantly, overwhelming nearby healthcare facilities and personnel. In such cases, the traditional triage system may not be effective.[3] A Centers for Disease Control and Prevention posthurricane assessment in 2012 determined that most of the resulting public health emergencies were directly due to loss of public health infrastructure and related to clean up and repair activities.[4] Because standard amenities, such as power, running water, and sanitation methods, may be unavailable for extended periods of time, all medical disaster planning must include practical, simple alternatives to technologies that are likely to fail during a disaster.

Lack of communication is a common feature of both the impact and delayed phases of a disaster. Even the most sophisticated equipment may fail due to regionwide outages or loss of electricity for charging devices. In our experience during the active phase of Hurricane Katrina, the only working means of communication within Charity Hospital was a single landline telephone. Difficulty in communication has led to recent innovation with proposals for disaster-specific electronic medical records.[5]

Evidence suggests that the predisaster level of preparedness and resources in a community has a significant impact on its response to a catastrophic event. Analysis of four earthquakes in different regions (developed and developing countries) found that regions with the least preparedness and weakest preexisting medical infrastructure had the highest number of deaths per patients injured.[6] Investment in targeted disaster preparedness efforts before an event occurs, particularly for the most vulnerable populations, is crucial in mitigating the effects of an inevitable disruption in resources during a disaster.[7]

DISEASE BURDEN

Understanding of the likely health emergencies to be encountered in the acute and postdisaster phases is crucial to any emergency response. Although it is widely thought that outbreaks of rare and/or severe disease inevitably follow many types of natural catastrophe, evidence does not support this belief.[8,9] Common medical problems after natural disasters include traumatic injury, infectious disease, exacerbations of chronic medical conditions, and a surge in mental health issues (**Table 6-2**). In addition to the common medical problems previously listed, the handling of bodies has an additional unique impact on the health of the affected population.

TRAUMA

Traumatic injuries frequently occur in the acute phase of a natural disaster, commonly from direct trauma from collapsing structures or flying debris. A second spike in trauma is seen during the recovery/clean-up phase, mainly due to unsafe infrastructure. However, this secondary spike in trauma may also include violent injuries, depending on the level of civil unrest.[10] Although most trauma is minor, management of severe injuries by healthcare professionals can prove especially challenging when resources are lacking, as they often require coordinated surgical care. **This necessitates adequate resources of anesthesia, blood products, surgical equipment and the ability to sterilize it, intensive care capacity, and operating theaters.** When these resources are unavailable, limb amputation, nonunion, and missed injury rates are high, and lack of safe blood products hampers surgical capability.[11,12] Recommendations for adequate surgical capability include mobile blood banks with adequate supply and well-trained staff, at least two units of blood available per operation, adequate supplies of appropriate anesthesia, strict adherence to national or international quality and safety standards, and functioning critical care units.[3,12,13]

INFECTIOUS DISEASE

Infectious diseases are commonly feared and should be anticipated after natural disasters. Although popular media often focuses on the possibility of rare disease epidemics, most postdisaster infections are directly related to the usual pathogens of that region.[9,14] One exception to this was the outbreak of cholera after the 2010 earthquake in Haiti, which is believed to have been brought in by United Nations relief workers.[15] Evidence indicates that the combination of communicable disease and population malnutrition is the major cause of morbidity and mortality in most disasters. Infectious disease predominantly occurs in the extended postevent phase.[16] Infectious disease risks are heightened by certain characteristics common to natural disasters: mass population

TABLE 6-1 Timing of Disease Presentation

Timing of Onset	Presentation						
Acute phase	Trauma	Stress reactions	Drowning	Inhalational injury	Burns		
Immediate postevent phase	Infectious complications of trauma	Exacerbation of chronic disease	Acute stress disorder	Burns	Inhalational injury		
Recovery phase	Trauma	Communicable disease	Infectious complications of trauma	Soft tissue infections	Exacerbation of chronic disease	Vectorborne disease	Posttraumatic stress disorder

TABLE 6-2 Common Disease Patterns

Trauma	Communicable Disease	Chronic Medical Conditions	Infectious Disease	Mental Health
Strains and sprains	Respiratory infections	Hypertension	Soft tissue infections	Stress reactions
Falls	GI infections	Diabetes	Open fractures	Depression
Lacerations		Renal failure	Vectorborne disease	Exacerbation of chronic condition
Burns		Chronic obstructive pulmonary disease	Local diseases	
Fractures				

movement and resettlement; overcrowding; poverty; sanitation and waste issues, including water contamination; absence of shelter, food, and healthcare access; and disruption of public health programs. Respiratory, GI, skin/soft tissue, and vectorborne infectious diseases are most commonly analyzed in disasters.

Respiratory illnesses range from direct aspiration of contaminated water (floods and tsunamis) to airborne droplet transmission to inhalation injuries caused by excess dust or debris. Although most infections are mild, respiratory illness may account for 20% of all natural disaster deaths in children <5 years old.[13] In the acute phase of a flood or tsunami, inhalation of water with polymicrobial contamination may cause aspiration pneumonia.[17] Most respiratory outbreaks, however, emerge several weeks after disaster as disease spreads through shelters and settlement camps. **Both disaster victims and rescue workers are at risk for respiratory illness due to crowded conditions and compromised sanitation.**[18,19] Some respiratory illnesses (pertussis and measles) are preventable with adequate vaccination; thus, knowledge of the predisaster vaccination status of a population and sufficient vaccine stores may prevent severe outbreaks. Tuberculosis presents a special challenge for public health officials. To prevent outbreaks, adequate stores of antimicrobials must be on hand, and strict adherence to surveillance of known infectious cases is essential.[9]

GI illness—primarily diarrheal—is another common feature of postdisaster health care. Approximately 40% of deaths in the acute postevent phase (with 80% of these being children) can be attributed to diarrhea. These diseases are mainly due to issues of water quality and availability, sanitation, and cleaning materials; in one study, the mere presence of soap decreased diarrhea by 27% in a refugee camp.[16] As with respiratory illness, the incidence of GI disease often peaks several weeks after the disaster, and the infections are generally mild. With good health surveillance and attention to typical endemic disease patterns, severe GI illness outbreaks requiring extraordinary public health resources are rare.

Skin and soft tissue infections are seen in a variety of natural disasters. Falling debris from wind, fire, or earthquake can cause traumatic abrasions or lacerations. With a disrupted healthcare system or contaminated water exposure to the wound, the incidence of infection is likely to increase. Although wounds are frequently seen in the acute phase of a disaster, they are also often encountered during the clean-up phase several weeks to months after an event.[20,21] Severe infections are not prevalent; however, organisms such as *Vibrio vulnificus* in water-based disasters and gram-negative bacteria due to soil contamination of wounds in tornadoes and earthquakes have the potential for severe threats to life and limb.[9,22]

Vectorborne illnesses, such as yellow fever, malaria, and dengue fever, generally have a higher incidence during water-based disasters but can occur after any event in a vulnerable population. Although rare, the outbreak can occur up to 8 weeks after disaster.[13] Regions without predisaster populations of vectors or disease are not likely to suddenly acquire such infections; thus, although there was intense media speculation of the perceived risk of malaria, yellow fever, and other vectorborne illnesses after Hurricane Katrina, these illnesses were not seen in the Gulf Coast.[9] In regions where these illnesses are endemic, vector control is key, and initial postdisaster public health efforts should direct resources toward appropriate programs.

TABLE 6-3 Commonly Neglected Disaster Response Medications and Supplies

Antihypertensives
Tetanus prophylaxis
Soap
Analgesics—oral and parenteral
Insulin
Oral hypoglycemics and sulfonylureas
Antibiotics, especially for soft tissue infections
Albuterol and ipratropium inhalers

CHRONIC MEDICAL CONDITIONS

Management of the chronic health conditions of a displaced population is a significant contributor to postdisaster morbidity. Separation from medications or health technology products, removal from the usual sources of care, and disruption of the healthcare infrastructure after a catastrophic event can all contribute to exacerbations of patients' chronic disease. In an analysis of patients presenting to one of the few healthcare facilities available in the 2 months after Hurricane Katrina, 51% of all native patients had at least one preexisting medical condition, and half took at least one regular medication.[20] Other studies have shown that >25% of patients presenting after a variety of natural disasters have chronic medical conditions, and "medication refill" or "chronic medical problem" is frequently among the top five diagnoses made in disaster relief health clinics.[21,23]

Inability to properly control chronic diseases, such as hypertension, diabetes, asthma, or coronary artery disease, may well be the biggest unanticipated health threat to a postdisaster population (Table 6-3).[7] Understanding of the common chronic diseases of a region is essential for health relief efforts. In our experience, well-meaning donations of medications for conditions not normally experienced by our population (e.g., outdated psychiatric medications, older generation antiarrhythmics) went unused. Conversely, we were unable to keep enough antihypertensives or diabetic medications to supply the vast demand.

MENTAL HEALTH

An often-overlooked consequence of natural disasters is the psychological burden inflicted on survivors. Destruction of communities and property, witnessing terrifying and often fatal events, and disruption of normal life for days to years after the disaster can cause severe mental health consequences in survivors. In one study of post–Hurricane Katrina survivors, rates of posttraumatic stress disorder were 10 times the expected population incidence and on par with rates in returning Vietnam War veterans.[24] Psychological disorders may be exacerbated by lack of housing and illness or death of a close family member due to the disaster.[25] Disaster-related physical injury or illness may also contribute to mental health comorbidity. The number of emergency amputations due to the 2004 tsunami in an Indonesian surgical clinic quickly overwhelmed the ability of the healthcare system to provide the necessary psychological counseling for patients.[26] Conversely, mental health conditions, such as major depression, may exacerbate acute or chronic physical ailments due to weakened immune systems, disconnection with the larger community and healthcare systems, or attempts to cope by using drugs or alcohol. Suicide rates may also be elevated years after a significant disaster. Any appropriate healthcare response to disasters must include sufficient resources to deal with the degree and severity of psychological disorders suffered by survivors, including children, first responders, and those who have endured severe trauma or loss.

HANDLING OF BODIES

Any natural disaster with a significant number of casualties requires efficient and sanitary removal and proper burial of dead bodies. Although the fear of disease outbreak from survivor or rescue worker exposure to corpses is prevalent, such exposures are rare. Most initial victims of natural disasters die of traumatic injuries; few are likely to have acute, communicable diseases, although the standard transmission risks of chronic infectious diseases, such as human immunodeficiency virus, tuberculosis, or hepatitis, to body-handling rescue workers are present.[27] Universal precautions for protective coverings, hand washing, disposal bags, and vaccinations should be followed by anyone working with dead bodies; this includes having sufficient refrigerated trucks on standby should morgue capabilities be overwhelmed.

HURRICANES

Hurricanes are among the most destructive natural disasters, particularly in coastal areas. Morbidity in the acute phase may be due to wind forces (collapsing buildings or flying debris) or water (storm surge or rapid flooding). Hurricanes tend to cause more structural damage than floods and therefore can disrupt infrastructure and population resettlement more severely.[28] Hospitals themselves are frequently damaged, but even if structurally intact, they may be affected by loss of power.[29] With catastrophic destruction of a densely populated region, such as in Hurricanes Katrina and Sandy, temporary medical facilities may be needed months after a disaster. **Indeed, hurricanes may be the only natural disaster where more injury and death occur during the recovery period than in the acute phase.**[30]

Most posthurricane illness and injury falls into predictable categories. Studies from eight different hurricanes over the last 15 years all list a handful of patient diagnoses that comprise the vast majority (up to 75%) of visits to healthcare centers: infections (specifically respiratory, GI, and skin); treatment of chronic medical conditions; wounds and lacerations; musculoskeletal injury and trauma; and rashes.[19,20,28-34] In functioning healthcare facilities, ED visits peak several days to weeks after the hurricane as citizens are allowed reentry into the area; there may be an acute, brief influx of several times the normal patient volume or a steady rise in visits over time.[5,20,31]

Initial traumatic injury directly due to hurricanes is relatively uncommon, and simple supplies for minor sprain, strain, and fracture care are recommended. Although surgical units and personnel are an important adjunct, basic supplies and some radiographic capability may provide the best investment of limited resources.[28,30] Unintentional injuries predominate; a post–Hurricane Katrina evaluation of injuries found that only 2% were due to intentional trauma.[18] Causes of traumatic death in the acute period include falling objects, motor vehicle crashes, and electrocution. In the recovery period (weeks to months after the hurricane), clean-up–associated trauma predominates. One study after Hurricane Hugo found that one third of all wounds evaluated in an ED were caused by chainsaw accidents.[32]

As with other disasters, infections are generally mild, reflective of the typical local disease burden, and occur several weeks to months after the hurricane. Scattered outbreaks of mild respiratory and GI illness have been described, with overcrowding in shelters and sanitation issues the main predictors of disease. Unless hurricanes are associated with concomitant prolonged flooding in endemic areas, the risks of waterborne disease are minor. Post–Hurricane Katrina incidence of *V. vulnificus* skin infection was consistent with typical nondisaster rates.[9]

Individuals without transportation or with tenuous connection to community resources are potentially more likely to be negatively impacted by the effects of a severe hurricane. These individuals may not be able to evacuate in advance of a storm and thus suffer greater risks of direct trauma and water- or wind-related morbidity during the initial impact. Effects may persist beyond the acute phase. A study of Hurricane Mitch survivors noted that GI illness and emotional distress were more likely months after the storm in those without access to housing, food, or medical care.[25] Other population concerns often seen in hurricanes include the healthcare burden of relief workers (civilian and military). Recovery efforts often require massive numbers of workers whose living conditions are often on par with storm victims. In one study, relief workers were nearly six times more likely than natives to use nonhospital healthcare facilities, and a spike in respiratory illness was attributed to transmission through a military battalion.[18] Our experience found that although younger than the native population, nearly half of relief workers seeking care had significant comorbidities that further burdened the struggling medical system after Hurricane Katrina.[20] Disaster planning should account for the needs of disenfranchised citizens as well as the expected influx of relief workers, many of whom may have chronic medical conditions.

EARTHQUAKES

Earthquakes are a unique disaster phenomenon in that there is no technology to detect a pending earthquake and thus no opportunity to provide a warning. Due to the lack of warning, supplies and a response plan must be continuously available. As was evidenced by the Haiti experience in January 2010, earthquakes can destroy water, electric, communication, gas, and sewage lines and cause structural instability. With no opportunity to evacuate before an earthquake, there is increased potential for casualties. People are at increased risk for being trapped in rubble or stranded. The first 1 to 14 days of response to an earthquake are dedicated to recovery of the injured. After an earthquake, the majority of fatalities occur within the first 3 hours.[35]

Injuries after earthquakes are the result of falling structures and debris. The most common injuries are fractures and crush injuries.[36,37] One hospital that registered 2892 patients after an earthquake reported that 37% of patients had musculoskeletal injuries. This hospital also reported the frequent occurrence of scalp injuries with large tissue defects.[36] Another hospital that registered 1500 patients in the first 72 hours after an earthquake reported that 78.4% of patients had extremity injuries; 50.4% of injuries were fractures, primarily closed. This same study reported that 37% of injuries required extensive debridement.[12] After the Mansehra earthquake in Pakistan in 2005, the medical equipment that the response teams found most useful was "external fixators that are easily applied."[36]

As with all disaster areas, the most common "illnesses" are the "regular medical needs of the people living in the earthquake zone."[36] In undeveloped regions recovering from large earthquakes, "preventable diseases, such as measles, are on the rise."[37] With proper sanitary and sewage techniques and adequate supplies of potable water, GI disease remains uncommon.

People with compromised mobility, including some geriatric patients, people with paralysis, amputees, people on ventilators, and people in wheelchairs and walkers, will be less likely to evacuate before the disaster and will have increased difficulty extracting themselves from the ruins. These people are more likely to be stranded in debris and to sustain crush injuries (also see chapter 7, "Bomb, Blast, and Crush Injuries") by collapsing buildings. These populations are especially at risk after earthquakes, because there will be no opportunity to evacuate before the disaster. Rescue and health services coordinators should make provisions for larger numbers of patients with increased needs after earthquakes. One study analyzed a metropolitan area in the United States and found that 31.6% of people >65 years old had a disability and 16.6% of people >65 years required assistance to evacuate. Planning for and responding to earthquakes requires an estimate of the number of citizens with special needs.[38]

TORNADOES

The continent of North America sustains more tornadoes than any other location in the world.[39] Nationally, 800 tornadoes are sighted annually. The annual human toll is estimated to be 80 deaths and 1500 injuries.[40] Tornadoes cause focal damage to buildings and lines above ground. It is unusual for entire regions to lose power and communications capacity. It is unusual for multiple hospitals to be disabled by a single tornado.[41,42] As a result, medical infrastructure in developed countries remains functional. Surge capacity may be tested in the immediate aftermath, but the provision of adequate chronic medical care is usually unhampered.

Most commonly, injuries from tornadoes result from being struck by flying debris or being thrown by the force of the tornado. Patients who were thrown or airborne as a result of the tornado sustain more severe injuries than patients who are struck by debris.[43,44] Additional risk factors for hospitalization or death include being struck by broken glass or falling objects, having one's home lifted off of its foundation, collapsed ceiling or floor, or loss of walls of the shelter structure.[44,45] Injuries are commonly multisystem. Fractures and soft tissue trauma are the most common injuries reported.[39,46-48] In one study, most patients (91%) sustained injuries to the extremities. Head, chest, and abdominal injuries were also common, occurring in 45%, 45%, and 27% of patients, respectively.[43] Head injuries are the more common cause of death.[39,47,48] Death from the impact after being thrown by the tornado is thought to most often occur at the scene, rather than en route to or at the hospital.[49-51]

Wound contamination is common among patients who are thrown by the tornado. Polymicrobial contamination is common.[39,46] Gram-negative organisms commonly infect the wounds of those injured by tornadoes.[43] Studies that report low infection rates attribute this to meticulous attention to open wounds.[52]

Where functioning tornado warning systems exist, injury and loss of life are dramatically reduced.[40,53] People in mobile homes or outdoors without cover are more likely to sustain severe and fatal injuries during a tornado.[45,53,54] Deaths are more common in patients who are in mobile homes or in rooms above ground with windows, who are "older," or who have less warning regarding the approaching tornado.[43,44,48,49,55] Use of a tornado shelter is associated with a significant reduction in tornado-associated injuries.[54]

FLOODS AND TSUNAMIS

Water-based natural disasters, such as floods and tsunamis, can be extremely destructive. Although floods can occur from a storm or flowing body of water, tsunamis are formed when a massive force (for example, an underwater earthquake, volcanic eruption, meteorite impact, or landslide) displaces a large amount of water in a rapid period of time. A spring flood of the Yangtze River in China in 1931 caused >3 million deaths, and more recently, deaths from the Indian Ocean tsunami in 2004 approached 300,000. Factors that contribute to the catastrophic nature of these events include the short (if any) warning period to vulnerable populations and their association with other natural events, such as an oceanic earthquake resulting in a tsunami. Key challenges faced by healthcare providers include severe and prolonged incapacitation of physical buildings due to structural damage or persistent standing water; handling and identification of large numbers of dead bodies; and the chronic needs of a large, displaced population in temporary shelter.[26,56,57]

Acute injuries may be caused by sheer force of water, drowning, and trauma from falling objects. A review of flood deaths from 1989 to 2003 found that morbidity and mortality after flood were related not only to direct physical impact but also the socioeconomic conditions of the affected area. Two thirds of fatalities were from drowning, mostly associated with motor vehicles in the acute phase (e.g., when floodwaters are still high); low crossings and bridges were most dangerous. Only 12% of deaths were from trauma, and the vast majority of cases occurred in the initial impact phase of the disaster.[58]

Illnesses from water-based disasters generally occur after the acute phase and are dominated by infectious disease. True epidemics are rare, and respiratory illnesses predominate. These are generally minor and self-limited, although uncommonly severe pulmonary infections or pneumonitis directly related to aspiration of floodwaters (e.g., "tsunami lung") may occur. As long as clean, safe, adequate supplies of potable water are available, acute gastroenteritis and diarrheal illnesses are relatively rare; a Sri Lankan refugee camp after the 2004 tsunami diagnosed GI complaints in <1% of patients.[23] Minor skin trauma is common and has the potential to progress to infected wounds if prolonged exposure to floodwaters and delayed access to care are present.

Certain population groups have been shown to have higher risks of morbidity and mortality after floods and tsunamis. Women had three times the risk of death compared with men after the 2004 tsunami due to heavier clothes impeding escape, risking lives to save their children, lack of swimming ability, and increased dangers in settlement camps.[26] In a comprehensive study of flood deaths, however, men had more than twice the mortality rate of women, which the authors surmised was due to increased risk-taking behavior during the storm (attempting to drive through flooded passages, traveling to unsafe areas in an attempt to retrieve belongings).[58] Public awareness of the rapidity and danger of water, simple swimming instruction, and clear warnings of the dangers of driving during floods may prevent at-risk populations in flood-prone areas from loss of life in future disasters.

BLIZZARDS AND SNOW DISASTERS

A blizzard is a winter storm with wind speeds of 35 miles per hour or higher accompanied by significant falling or blowing snow. The Mid-Atlantic, New England, Midwest, Plains, Rocky Mountain states, and Alaska are affected by blizzards and snow disasters. Above-ground power and communication lines are the primary resources lost during winter storms. Traditionally, these are restored relatively quickly as compared with the duration without resources after other natural disasters.[59]

Generally, ED volumes do not significantly increase after blizzards and snow disasters. However, there is a shift in the presenting complaints.[59-61] Injuries after winter weather disasters most commonly result from slipping on the ice, falling from trees while clearing branches, and injuries from clearing snow. The most common injuries are back injuries and fractures.[62,63] In one study, the incidence of fractures increased until the sixth day after the storm.[64]

Carbon monoxide poisoning increases dramatically during and following winter weather disasters.[60,62,65-68] Most people presenting with carbon monoxide poisoning report using a portable generator.[69] A smaller group reported burning charcoal in the house to generate heat.[65] In one study after a blizzard, the local hyperbarics services were overwhelmed and unable to respond to the sudden surge in carbon monoxide poisonings.[62]

One study documented an increase in the number of myocardial infarctions and angina after a blizzard. This was primarily in association with shoveling snow. The majority of these cases were in people who did not have previously diagnosed coronary artery disease. One fourth of these patients were women.[70]

RELIEF EFFORTS

Of particular importance to the emergency medical practitioner is the experience and effect of postdisaster volunteer relief efforts. Although well meaning, the literature is filled with examples of emergency personnel who ended up burdening rather than assisting a fractured community. Any emergency practitioner who truly wishes to provide meaningful health care to a displaced and disenfranchised patient population should be mindful of the lessons learned from a variety of natural disasters.

Medical relief volunteers are often the first outside help to arrive in the aftermath of a disaster, and although some are well coordinated, many are not. Volunteers are often exuberant, expecting dramatic rescues and emergency interventions. They may be unwilling to provide much-needed routine medical care, unfamiliar with the region or local disease patterns, and unable to fully comprehend the loss of resources.[71] Furthermore, the needs of rescue personnel often strain a fragile infrastructure, with demands on housing, food, health care, and essential resources; one analysis of relief efforts after the 2004 tsunami concluded that "personnel who do not bring essential skills are often a burden—much more should also be done to ensure that the right type of people are sent on relief missions."[26]

Embedding locals familiar with the language, culture, and healthcare patterns of the affected region can significantly enhance the effectiveness of relief efforts and promote cooperation between disparate volunteer groups. Furthermore, appropriate anticipation by relief groups of the true population needs can be crucial: reproductive hygiene kits were distributed to women in a postflood refugee camp after an initial spike in sexual assaults and were widely credited with improving patient morale and health.[26]

The National Disaster Medical System, a government agency responsible for sending highly organized and often experienced teams to disaster areas, recommends the following for disaster response: teams with well-trained and organized support staff; the ability to be self-sufficient for at least 72 hours; clear communication with area hospitals and medical resources; individuals dedicated to transportation issues; a designated coordinator of walk-in volunteers; and professional methods of record keeping, forms, and copy-making capability.[30] Our experience during Hurricane Katrina also suggests that strong, coordinated partnerships between local emergency personnel and formal military medical units have great promise for sophisticated, expanded acute and delayed postdisaster medical relief as well as continuance of medical education and resident training programs in a devastated community.[20]

REFERENCES

The complete reference list is available online at www.TintinalliEM.com.

Bomb, Blast, and Crush Injuries

Michael J. Bono
Pinchas Halpern

BOMB AND BLAST INJURIES

EPIDEMIOLOGY

Blast injuries using conventional weapons have emerged as the terrorist weapon of choice. Terrorist attacks have increased dramatically over the last decade. The National Counterterrorism Center reported more than 14,000 terrorist attacks in 2007, with 44,000 injuries and 22,000 deaths, which was a 20% to 30% increase over 2006.[1] Explosive devices in military conflicts have killed or injured more than 25,000 U.S. and Coalition forces and more than 100,000 Iraqis.[1] Blast injuries are increasing in the civilian setting, particularly suicide bombings, and emergency personnel must be familiar with the management and treatment of blast injuries, ad potential mass casualty incidents.[2-9] The United States is not immune from intentional bombings, with about 36,000 bombing incidents reported from 1983 to 2002 - including explosive, incendiary, premature, and attempted bombings.[6] There were 281 injured in the 2013 Boston Marathon bombing, with most injuries involving the lower extremities and soft tissue.[8] Death, survival, and hospitalization rates vary greatly, depending on the type of explosive, distance from the explosion, and whether the explosion occurred in an open or closed space. Although some victims die immediately at the scene, the majority of injuries suffered by the immediate survivors of bombings are potentially survivable. Blast injuries commonly occur not as isolated incidents, but as part of multiple-casualty incidents of varying sizes. This pattern, combined with the fact that most emergency physicians have never encountered a blast injury victim or a true mass casualty incident, makes the care of often eminently salvageable victims contingent upon appropriate training and skill retention by the individual emergency physician, along with appropriate institutional leadership, planning, and preparation.

Terrorist bombings result in high injury scores for victims as well as higher hospital resource use by victims than by victims of other trauma. Blast victims have increased immediate scene mortality, greater hospital mortality, more frequent need for surgical intervention, longer hospital stays, and greater use of critical care.

PATHOPHYSIOLOGY

An explosion is the instantaneous transformation of a solid or liquid into a gas, releasing tremendous kinetic and heat energy. Detonation of a conventional high explosive generates a blast wave that spreads out from the detonation point and displaces air, water, or anything in its path. The blast wave consists of two parts: a shock wave of high pressure followed closely by a blast wind, which is air mass in motion. The blast wave loses its energy over distance and time.

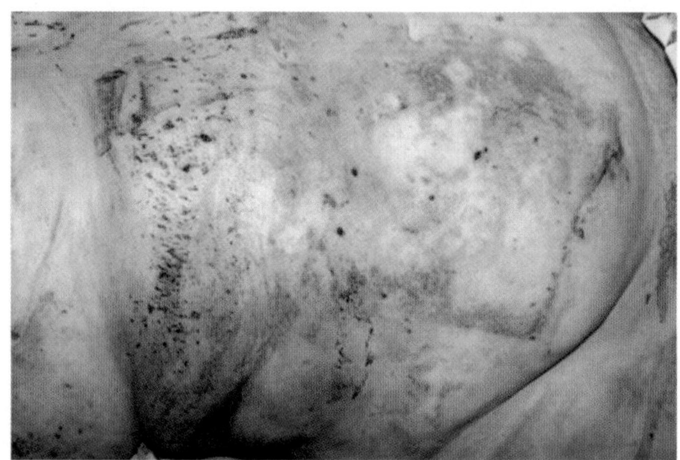

FIGURE 7-1. Secondary blast injury to the chest and abdomen due to flying debris. It is difficult to assess the degree of underlying internal organ injury without imaging and careful clinical follow-up, especially if the patient is unconscious. [Image used with permission of Tel Aviv Medical Center.]

BLAST INJURIES

There are four main types of blast effects. A primary injury is caused by a direct effect of blast wave overpressure on tissue. Primary blast injury mostly (but not exclusively) affects air-filled structures such as the lungs, ears, and GI tract, by the following mechanisms: spalling, shearing, and implosion. Spalling is displacement and fragmentation of a dense medium into a less dense medium.[10] An example is a blast wave causing the lung parenchyma to explode into the alveolar space like a geyser. Shearing, sometimes called inertia, is a stress caused by the blast wave traveling through different tissue densities at different velocities. An example of shearing is the blast wave traveling through the pulmonary vessels and air spaces, resulting in ruptured vascular and bronchial pedicles. Implosion is the opposite of spalling, where the less dense material is displaced into denser material. An example of implosion is the blast wave causing the flexible air spaces to rebound to greater than original size, sometimes causing air embolism from the alveoli into the pulmonary vessels.[10] A secondary blast injury is due to collateral damage from flying objects and shrapnel (**Figures 7-1 and 7-2**). Tertiary blast

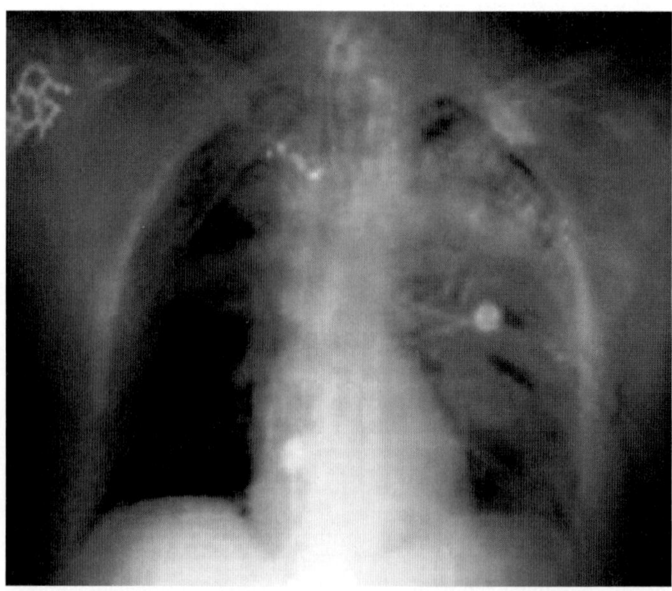

FIGURE 7-2. This young patient came in fully conscious and hemodynamically stable. Multiple externally visible shrapnel wounds required imaging. This x-ray image shows severe lung injury due to shrapnel. She also suffered multiple abdominal injuries, including major liver lacerations and bowel perforations, and required extensive surgery. [Image used with permission of Tel Aviv Medical Center.]

injury results from the victim being propelled through the air and striking stationary objects. A quaternary blast injury is a result of burns, smoke inhalation, or chemical agent release.

FACTORS AFFECTING BLAST INJURY

The effects of a bomb blast are difficult to predict in the individual victim, as well as in the group. However, a number of important principles are known:

Distance of victim from explosion: The intensity of an explosion pressure wave declines with the cubed root of the distance from the explosion. A person 3 m (10 ft) from an explosion experiences eight times more overpressure than a person 6 m (20 ft) away. Proximity of the victim to the explosion is an important factor in a primary blast injury.

Enclosed versus open space: The effects of an explosion in a closed space, like a room, bus, or train, are much greater than in an open space. Injuries are more severe, and mortality is greater.

Surrounding environment: Blast waves are reflected by solid surfaces; thus, a person standing next to a wall may suffer increased primary blast injury.

Quantity of explosive: A greater quantity of explosive produces greater potential for damage at any distance.

Type of explosive: Explosives are commonly classified as either low-order or high-order. Low-order explosives burn rapidly and produce a blast wave of less than 1000 m/s.[11] Black powder is an example of a low-order explosive. High-order explosives detonate when a shock wave passes through them, causing an almost instantaneous transformation of the original explosive material into gases occupying the same volume of space under extremely high pressure. These high-pressure gases expand rapidly, compress the surrounding medium, and produce a supersonic, overpressure blast wave, moving at greater than 4500 m/s, followed closely by a negative pressure wave.

Embedded shrapnel: Many terrorists purposefully embed multiple pieces of metal and plastic in the explosive, maximizing the number and severity of secondary injuries.

CLINICAL FEATURES

The nature of the injury may produce a multiplicity of external signs (**Figure 7-3**), making detection of important internal injuries challenging. Insufficient or suboptimal resources need to be prioritized in a mass casualty incident. High-grade clinical expertise is even more in demand to allow optimal use of resources.[2-9]

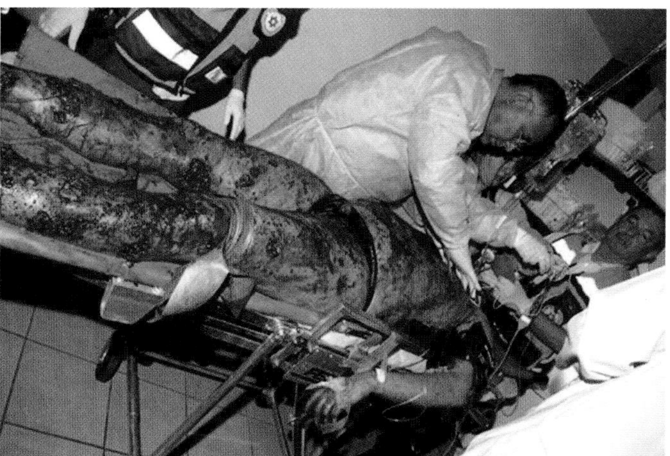

FIGURE 7-3. The severe external injuries often seen with explosive blast may or may not indicate associated severe internal injury. Clinical examination is difficult and requires a high degree of experience and suspicion as well as early use of imaging. [Image used with permission of Tel Aviv Medical Center.]

CARDIOPULMONARY SYSTEM

The lung is very susceptible to primary blast injury. **Pulmonary barotrauma is the most common fatal primary blast injury** and the most common critical injury in people close to the blast center. Pressure differentials across the alveolar–capillary interface can cause disruption, hemorrhage, pulmonary contusion, pneumothorax, hemothorax, pneumomediastinum, and subcutaneous emphysema. Air embolism is another well-recognized consequence of blast lung injury and is probably one of the major factors leading to cardiac dysfunction and immediate death after blast wave exposure, although it is usually difficult to diagnose specifically. The resulting neurologic symptoms caused by air embolism must be differentiated from the direct effects of CNS trauma. Pulmonary fat embolism is a finding of clinical importance in survivors of blast trauma because it can lead to the development of acute respiratory distress syndrome and significantly affects clinical outcomes.

In general, managing blast lung injury is similar to caring for pulmonary contusion and acute respiratory distress syndrome, except that early recognition of the syndrome may be complicated by initially benign symptoms, especially in the context of hectic mass casualty incident situations. Hypoxia is an almost universal finding.[12] Monitoring of respiratory rate and room-air pulse oximetry, as well as serial chest radiographs, may be needed. Fluid administration should ensure tissue perfusion without volume overload. The decision to institute mechanical ventilation must be made carefully because it entails the assignment of what may be scarce critical care unit beds and ventilators and also exposes the patient to the potential complications of pulmonary barotrauma, commonly seen with the friable lungs associated with blast lung syndrome. **Keep tidal volume to 6 to 7 mL/kg ideal body weight to limit the peak inspiratory pressure and to minimize ventilator-induced lung barotrauma.** Often, neuromuscular paralysis and early institution of pressure-limited ventilation (plateau pressures <30 cm H_2O),[13] with the lowest pressures compatible with adequate ventilation, may be the best strategy. Inverse inspiratory-to-expiratory ratio ventilation may be useful. Permissive hypercapnia is acceptable depending on cerebral perfusion pressure or increased intracranial pressure.[13] Aggressive methods of oxygenation, such as extracorporeal membrane oxygenation or intravascular oxygenation, may become necessary within hours of the injury.

There are no definitive guidelines for observation, admission, or discharge of patients with possible blast lung injury. Admit patients requiring complex management to an intensive care unit. In general, asymptomatic patients with normal chest radiographs and normal room-air pulse oximetry may be considered for discharge after 4 to 6 hours of observation as long as there is no clinical deterioration. Survivors of this type of injury typically have no long-term pulmonary complaints, and most have normal physical examinations, chest radiographs, and normal lung function tests.

EARS

The tympanic membrane ruptures at 1 to 8 psi of dynamic overpressure. Dislodgement of ossicles may also occur. Patients with an isolated tympanic membrane perforation and no other immediately identified injuries should have a chest radiograph ordered but do not automatically require an extended period of observation. Conversely, intact tympanic membranes do not imply the absence of serious injury, and the use of the perforation of tympanic membrane as an indicator of primary blast injury missed up to 50% of those suffering a primary blast injury to the lung.[14] Clinical judgment is necessary, and limited observation is reasonable for patients with intact tympanic membranes.

ABDOMEN

Abdominal injuries from explosions may be occult. Reported injury rates are low, but missed injuries may carry significant morbidity due to delayed intestinal perforation and necrosis. A review of the literature on abdominal trauma from primary blast injury reveals an incidence of 1.3% to 33%, and the terminal ileum and cecum were the most commonly injured areas.[15] Serial clinical examinations, serial imaging as needed, and 24- to 48-hour observation are indicated whenever the suspicion arises. **Air is a poor conductor of blast-wave energy; thus,**

patients who were subjected to enough energy to damage abdominal organs probably were situated near the explosive device.

BRAIN INJURY

The conflicts of the Global War on Terror in Iraq and Afghanistan have resulted in over a quarter of a million diagnosed cases of traumatic brain injury.[16] Mild traumatic brain injury has been labeled the "signature injury of the war in Iraq."[1,17-22] The clinical examination may be misleading for penetrating injuries. Shrapnel are low-velocity missiles, often producing small entry wounds in survivors. Small entry wounds may be missed under the hair, and evidence for traumatic brain injury may initially be benign or masked by anesthesia as the patient undergoes treatment for other life-threatening injuries. Neuroimaging is an important early diagnostic tool (**Figure 7-4**).

VASCULAR INJURY

Small entry wounds from shrapnel may mask severe vascular injuries (**Figure 7-5**). Compartment syndrome (see "Crush Injury and the Crush Syndrome," below) may develop and is difficult to diagnose, especially in patients receiving anesthesia. Carefully assess and document pulses and perfusion in affected limbs. **Observe for delayed presentation of compartment syndrome, and measure compartment pressure if any signs or symptoms develop.** Early angiography and intervention are indicated if pulses are lost.

EXTERNAL HEMORRHAGE

Bleeding from wounds is likely to be the most commonly encountered life-threatening finding. Whether venous or arterial, blood loss from multiple wounds (internal and external) may be sufficient to cause hypovolemic shock. Quickly control external bleeding with direct pressure. Military experience has shown that hemorrhage is the most common cause of preventable death in penetrating trauma.[9] Apply tourniquets for extremity hemorrhage whenever blood loss cannot be controlled with direct pressure, or if the resources required to maintain direct pressure are insufficient during either treatment or transportation. Tourniquets have been successfully used for up to 6 hours in battlefield situations.[23] Angiographic vascular occlusion is an attractive treatment option if the time and staff are available. Victims of blast mass casualty incidents may require massive amounts of blood and blood products.[24]

OCULAR INJURIES

Eye injuries from a blast wave may cause shearing damage to the orbit, but ocular injuries are from a combination of primary and secondary processes.[25] Ocular injuries include lid or brow lacerations, conjunctival lacerations, open globe injuries, orbital fractures, retinal detachment, retained intraocular foreign body, lens dislocation, vitreous hemorrhage, retinal tears and retinal detachment.[25] Eye examination is needed for all moderately to severely injured blast victims, and a poor initial visual acuity is not a guarantee of a poor final result.

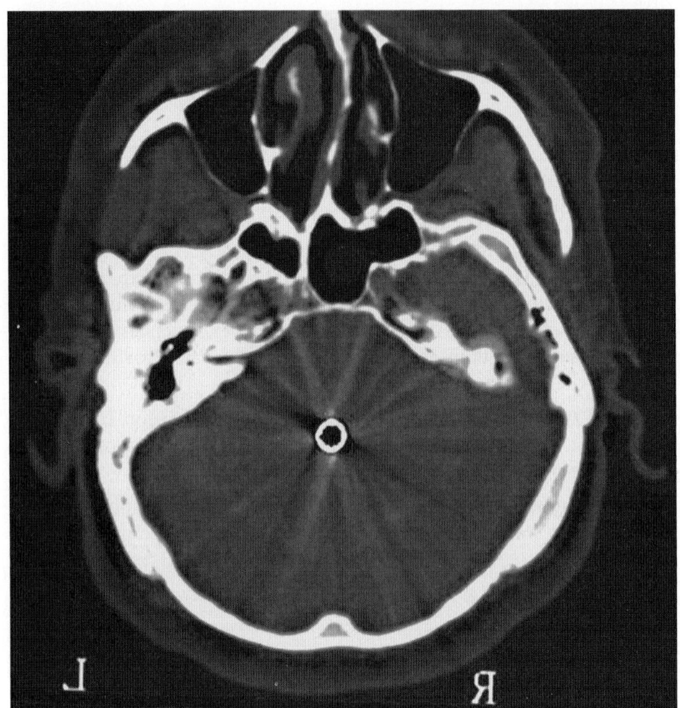

A

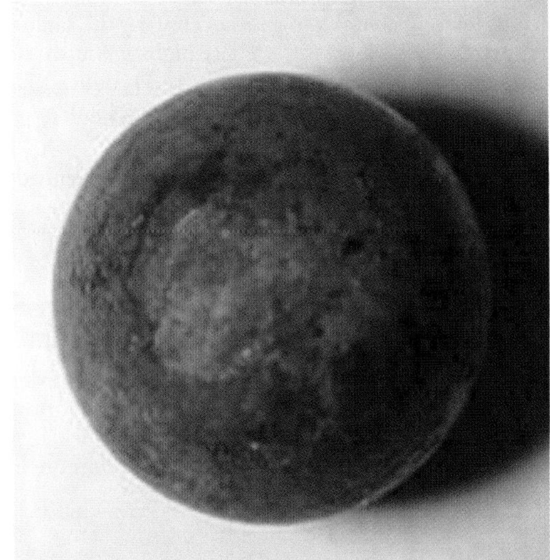

B

FIGURE 7-4. **A.** CT scan image of a 17-year-old female patient injured in a terrorist bomb blast in Israel. This girl walked into the ED unassisted, was triaged "green," but deteriorated after 30 minutes. Fortunately the clinical deterioration was noted, she underwent emergent CT, and then extensive neurosurgical intervention. **B.** A 1-cm metal ball bearing was extracted. Prolonged rehabilitation was later required for residual brain damage. [Image used with permission of Tel Aviv Medical Center.]

DIAGNOSIS

Order diagnostic imaging judiciously in a mass casualty incident. Visualization of a metallic object on a single-plane radiograph is often inadequate for thorough evaluation, but it can direct the treatment team on the need for urgent surgery or for additional imaging. Use the FAST examination liberally. Plain chest radiographs, ultrasonography, and diagnostic peritoneal lavage are the most rapid studies used to evaluate for life-threatening injuries. Order laboratory tests sparingly.

TREATMENT

When blast injuries occur, they tend to be unexpected, occur outside of regular working hours, and often produce moderate to large numbers of simultaneously arriving casualties. Drills and checklists are critical for successful implementation of rarely used protocols. Checklists should be concise, never more than one to two pages, and available in a location known to everyone. Implement the hospital plan for management of mass casualty incidents.

Obtain details about the explosion from patients and rescue teams. **The nature and location of the blast, including size and type of charge, location in open or closed space, structural collapse, associated fire or smoke, and toxic agent release, will be helpful in making informed clinical decisions, especially with regard to disposition of moderately to severely injured casualties.**

Patient triage will be needed when multiple patients arrive. Station an experienced emergency physician or surgeon at the ED entrance to triage

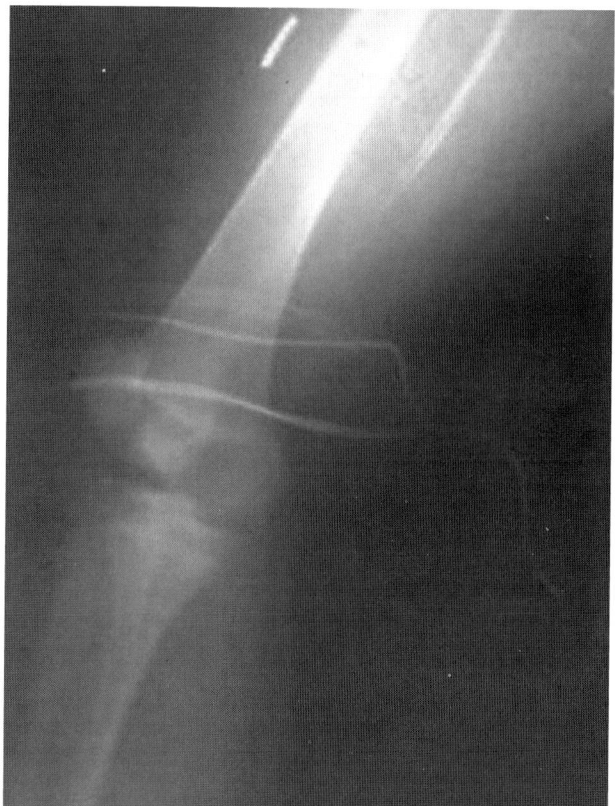

FIGURE 7-5. Vascular injuries may occur with externally minor penetrating injury. This young woman was triaged "green." The significance of a small penetrating injury in her lower limb, one of many throughout her body, was initially misinterpreted, but she lost her pulses after 1 hour and was rushed to angiography and subsequent vascular surgical intervention. [Image used with permission of Tel Aviv Medical Center.]

patients to appropriate, predetermined locations in the ED or elsewhere in the hospital. Patients must be triaged to categories of urgency based on relevant criteria, such as those listed in **Table 7-1**. Many triage methods have been in use in various parts of the world, with varying success and scientific foundation.[2-7]

Apply the basic advanced trauma life support principles of primary and secondary surveys within the logistic limitations that may occur temporarily or permanently. Administer IV fluids and blood products judiciously. Preventing fluid overload is important for lung- and brain-injured patients. Activated factor VII administration or tranexamic acid may be considered in select cases of uncontrollable bleeding.

Copiously irrigate and disinfect wounds urgently, but definitive debridement and closure may wait a few hours. Temporary splinting, traction, and dressings are generally sufficient for initial management of musculoskeletal injuries. Consider prophylactic antibiotics for severely soiled wounds, penetrating abdominal and thoracic wounds, and open fractures, and in patients with diabetes or who are immunocompromised.

TABLE 7-1 Criteria for the Triage in Bomb Injuries

Severely Injured	Lightly Injured
Airway compromise	Minor wounds
Breathing difficulty	Burns, first or second degree
Hemodynamic instability	Isolated trauma to a limb
Altered level of consciousness	Anxiety states
Vascular trauma	Most walking patients
Extensive second- to third-degree burns	

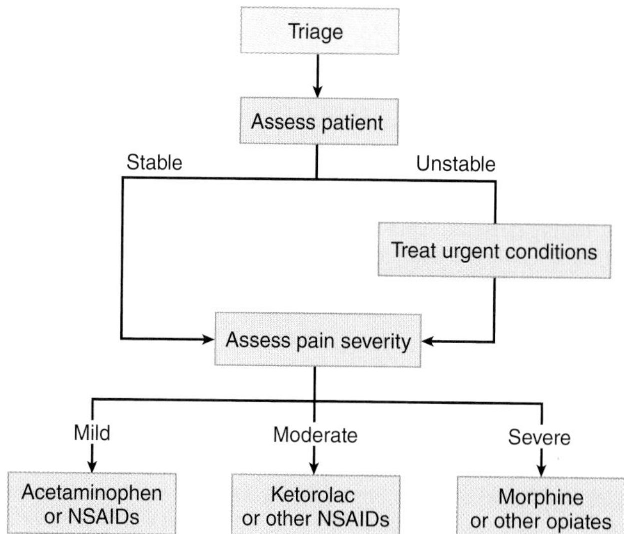

FIGURE 7-6. Algorithm for pain management in blast injury patients in the context of a multiple-casualty incident. NSAID = nonsteroidal anti-inflammatory drug.

Address pain management after life-threatening emergencies have been evaluated. Reserve opiates for patients with severe pain because opiate supplies may become limited (**Figure 7-6**).

Patients exposed to open-space explosions and who have no apparent significant injury, normal vital signs, and an unremarkable physical examination generally can be discharged after a few hours of observation. Asymptomatic patients may be discharged after 4 to 6 hours of observation. Admit all patients with significant burns, suspected air embolism, radiation or chemical contamination, abnormal vital signs, abnormal lung examination findings, clinical or radiographic evidence of pulmonary contusion or pneumothorax, abdominal pain, vomiting, hypoxia, or penetrating injuries to the thorax, abdomen, neck, or head to the hospital.

Patients appropriate for discharge need to be given proper follow-up instructions. Given the austerity of initial care and the propensity to miss injuries in a mass casualty incident, secondary assessments of all casualties should be done before discharge. Because symptoms of pulmonary contusion and intestinal hematoma may take 12 to 48 hours to develop, instruct all discharged patients to return for reevaluation if they develop breathing problems, abdominal pain, or vomiting. Provide relevant follow-up instructions in writing, including audiologic and ear, nose, and throat follow-up, wound care, immunization schedules, medications, psychological support, and social services.

SPECIAL POPULATIONS

PREGNANT WOMEN

Because the fetus is surrounded by amniotic fluid, direct injury to the fetus is uncommon. **Injuries to the placenta, however, are more common.** After life-threatening conditions have been stabilized, admit patients in the second or third trimester of pregnancy who have been exposed to blast injury to the labor and delivery area for continuous fetal monitoring and further testing and evaluation. Pelvic US, fetal nonstress test monitoring, and obstetrics consultation should always be obtained. Consider Rh immune globulin administration if the mother's blood type is Rh negative.

CHILDREN

Children may suffer significant tertiary blast injury because their lighter bodies are more easily hurled by the blast wind. Imaging, such as total-body CT, may be difficult to perform in anxious and frightened children. Children typically require sedation to facilitate imaging.

SPECIAL CONSIDERATIONS

STAFF SAFETY

Issues that may affect staff safety include: (1) possible infiltration of the ED by perpetrators intent on causing second explosions or attacks in the hospital; (2) unexploded explosives inadvertently brought into the ED; (3) transmissible disease in the setting of body fluid exposure or needle sticks during stressful, rapid work; and (4) contamination of victims by chemical, radiologic, and biologic hazards, either accidental or intentionally caused by the perpetrators.

FORENSIC ISSUES

Police and crime scene investigators, as well as counterterrorism and other security services, have legitimate interests in securing forensic and other information. Efforts should be made to accommodate them, but never at the expense of medical care. Prior coordination with all relevant authorities should establish protocols, such as who and how many persons from these agencies are allowed in, when, into which parts of the ED, who controls them, and who is empowered to limit their entry and work. As a rule, however, although a terrorist event is a crime, forensics in the hospital are of minor relevance compared with the actual crime scene. Investigators may wish to interrogate victims with minor injuries regarding the event and obtain shrapnel or clothing from patients for forensic analysis.

INFORMATION MANAGEMENT

Because blast injury is often part of a large event, information becomes a critical component of appropriate management. Such information concerns include: (1) clinical charting and other patient care–centered information, such as imaging; (2) command and control information, such as casualty flow data, resource management data, and interface with other agencies; (3) information provided to relatives; (4) information provided to the media; and (5) information recorded for quality improvement and research. An information center is an indispensable component of such events, providing relief for the relatives and also preventing them from crowding patient care spaces and impeding caregiver workflow.

CRUSH INJURY AND THE CRUSH SYNDROME

A crush injury occurs when a body part is subjected to a high degree of force or pressure, usually after being squeezed between two heavy or immobile objects. **Crush injury that produces ongoing ischemia of a fascial muscle compartment is termed *compartment syndrome*, defined as increased pressure within a confined space that leads to microvascular compromise and ultimately to cell death as a result of oxygen starvation.** Crush syndrome is the systemic manifestation of muscle cell damage resulting from pressure or crushing with or without subsequent compartment syndrome. This chapter discusses crush injury and treatment measures specifically in the context of mass natural disasters. Specific discussion of detailed physiology, compartment anatomy, and compartment pressure measurement is found in chapter 278, "Compartment Syndrome."

EPIDEMIOLOGY

Crush injuries may be seen in two different scenarios: in single-patient situations and in disasters of varying magnitude, like earthquakes or tsunamis. Catastrophes have occurred throughout history, but the recognition of crush syndrome in the twentieth century and the advent of effective treatment for some of the components of the systemic and local injury have made it one of the important aspects of the medical care of natural disaster victims. The increasing number of vehicular and workplace accidents has also led to a rise in the incidence of crush syndrome and in the importance of its timely recognition and treatment. In various reports, the incidence of crush syndrome and subsequent renal failure varies from 1% to 25%, probably resulting from reporting differences, the nature of the disaster, and the timeliness and effectiveness of the rescue efforts and medical care.[26]

Crush injuries are most commonly seen in the extremities, because crush of the trunk or head and neck is quickly lethal. There is a high incidence of associated injuries such as fractures, lacerations, and degloving injury.

PATHOPHYSIOLOGY

Injury to muscles, including crush and ischemia, causes rupture of the sarcolemma and the release of the intracellular contents of the myocytes into the surrounding tissues. Calcium ion is one of the most destructive components released from the myocytes, because calcium stimulates proteolytic enzymes and oxygen free radicals are released. This causes more myocyte destruction, and potassium, phosphate, myoglobin, creatine kinase, and uric acid leak into the bloodstream. Serum haptoglobin binds some of the myoglobin, but its binding capacity is quickly overwhelmed, and myoglobin causes direct kidney injury. Membrane damage to the myocytes and to the systemic capillary endothelium causes vascular volume loss and hypovolemia. Hyperkalemia and hypocalcemia may cause arrhythmias and cardiac arrest. Metabolic acidosis caused by hypovolemia and shock aggravates arrhythmogenicity. **Renal failure is the most serious complication of crush syndrome.** The pathogenesis of renal failure is multifactorial, including systemic hypoperfusion, renal vasoconstriction, nephrotoxicity from myoglobin, and uric acid and phosphate precipitation in the distal tubules. Low urine pH and renal vasoconstriction promote precipitation of nephrotoxins. Myoglobin is indirectly nephrotoxic through the formation of ferrihemate, which produces free hydroxyl radicals and, combined with lipid peroxidation, damages the kidney.[27]

Reperfusion syndrome is a paradoxical phenomenon of exacerbation of cellular dysfunction after restoration of blood flow to previously ischemic tissues. It involves biochemical and cellular changes causing oxidant production and complement activation, which culminates in an inflammatory response, mediated by neutrophils and platelets interacting with the endothelium. The inflammatory response has both local and systemic manifestations.[28] Systemic manifestations include hypotension, vasodilatation, hypovolemia, myocardial depression, hyperkalemia, and acidosis.

Normal muscle compartment pressure is <10 mm Hg. After crush injury, trauma to the microcirculation leads to edema formation, interstitial bleeding, stasis, and obstruction, and the myocytes are no longer able to retain intracellular water. Edema in a closed space causes increased pressure, which further collapses the microcirculation and potentiates the problem.[29] **Pressures >30 mm Hg produce muscle ischemia; irreversible nerve and muscle damage occurs after 4 to 6 hours.**

CLINICAL FEATURES

Obvious external signs of crush injury are usually evident, as is a suggestive history. Lacerations, degloving, deformity, pain, and ischemia may occur in varying degrees.

Compartment syndrome often presents with the five "P's": **pain, paresthesias, passive stretch, pressure, and pulselessness.** Pain is the most common and consistent symptom, described as diffuse and intense; exacerbated with movement, touch, or pressure; and out of proportion to physical examination findings.

Paresthesias are numbness, tingling, or burning sensations in the affected area. Severe pain results when muscles in the affected compartment are stretched.

The affected compartment is very tight to the examiner's touch and sometimes warm, and there are measurable increases in tissue pressure. Pulselessness occurs only in the late stages. Examining for a pulse, or its lack, is the least reliable because compartment syndrome is a disorder of the microvasculature; the major vessels are frequently unaffected.

Crush syndrome is due to the manifestations of muscle toxin release and hypovolemia. Hypovolemic shock may occur, aggravated by hyperkalemic, hypocalcemic, or acidemic cardiotoxicity. Thromboplastin release may cause disseminated intravascular coagulation, which is especially critical in the face of tissue damage, open wounds, or the need for surgery. Renal failure may ensue quickly and is the primary cause of delayed death.[26]

DIAGNOSIS

Testing of the compartment pressure will confirm the diagnosis. A compartment pressure of >30 mm Hg is considered to be a positive test. Measurement is best accomplished with a dedicated device (Stryker STIC; Stryker Co., Kalamazoo, MI) or by inserting a saline-filled needle connected to an intravascular pressure measurement system (arterial or central venous pressure gauges) into each compartment and recording the pressures.[26] See chapter 278 for detailed description of compartment pressure measurement.

Crush syndrome is characterized by protean and rapid metabolic changes. Laboratory tests are crucial to help direct management. Serum creatine kinase levels may not necessarily predict disease severity and risk of renal failure, but they are a useful initial triage and subsequent follow-up tool. Pay close attention to serum potassium, calcium, phosphorus, pH, creatinine, hemoglobin, coagulation indices, and urine pH and electrolytes. A preplanned sequence of laboratory tests every 2 to 4 hours is useful, rather than sporadic checks. Urine collection for total electrolyte excretion and creatinine clearance calculations may be considered.[26]

TREATMENT

Establish two large-bore IV lines and administer normal saline with a 1- to 2-L bolus. Avoid Ringer's lactate and other potassium-containing fluids, because fatal hyperkalemia may occur, even in the absence of renal failure.[26] Initiate IV fluid rate at 1000 mL/h, and then reduce to 500 mL/h after 2 hours. Urine output should be approximately 200 to 300 mL/h (5 to 7 L every 24 hours) for an adult. Monitor serial serum potassium levels. Admit the patient to an intensive care unit setting to monitor fluid administration and electrolyte status.

FASCIOTOMY

In reports of mass casualties from earthquakes, most of the fasciotomy procedures were performed >12 hours after the time of trauma. Reviews of these cases showed high infection rates with increased mortality and amputations and poor long-term outcomes. Fasciotomy creates open wounds, which increases the risk for sepsis, amputation, hemodynamic instability, chronic nerve dysfunction, and death.[26] Most recommendations discourage the use of routine fasciotomy, particularly for crush wounds, and fasciotomy is only indicated for absence of distal pulses, a requirement for debridement of necrotic muscle, compartment pressures >30 mm Hg (measured within 6 hours of injury), and differences between compartmental pressure and diastolic blood pressure of >30 mm Hg.[26] If initial compartment pressures are normal and delayed compartment syndrome develops, fasciotomy may be needed, but infection rates have been reported to be high and prolonged, and profuse local bleeding may develop.

HYPERBARIC OXYGEN THERAPY

Hyperbaric oxygen therapy is a useful adjunct in the treatment of crush injury and compartment syndrome because it supplements oxygen availability to the hypoxic tissues in the early postinjury period.[29] With hyperbaric oxygen therapy at 2 atm, the blood oxygen content (oxygen carried by hemoglobin and plasma) is increased by 125% (by increasing plasma oxygen content), and the oxygen tension in plasma and tissue fluid is increased 10-fold compared to room air breathing.[29] Edema reduction secondary to oxygen-induced vasoconstriction is another beneficial effect of hyperbaric oxygenation. Hyperbaric oxygenation reduces blood flow by 10% to 20%, thereby reducing tissue edema caused by blood flow, but oxygen delivery to the tissues is increased because of higher tissue oxygen tensions.[29] The immediate effects of hyperbaric oxygen therapy are threefold: enhanced oxygen at the tissue level, increased oxygen delivery per unit of blood flow, and edema reduction. Long-term effects may include improved wound repair after fasciotomy, diminished infection rates, and improved outcome of skin grafts.[29]

SPECIAL POPULATIONS

Care of crush injury patients in the setting of mass casualty incidents is radically different than that of the individual victim. Extrication may be delayed, medical treatment during extrication may be unavailable, initial management may occur in makeshift or suboptimal conditions, and medical personnel may have little experience working under such conditions. Transportation to definitive care may be prolonged; critical equipment, such as dialysis machines, may be in short supply; and laboratory, monitoring, and intensive care facilities may be insufficient for the volume demands. Healthcare workers should anticipate these obstacles and develop flexible treatment protocols.

REFERENCES

The complete reference list is available online at www.TintinalliEM.com.

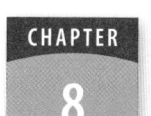

Chemical Disasters

B. Zane Horowitz
Robert G. Hendrickson

INTRODUCTION AND EPIDEMIOLOGY

Although the term "agents of mass destruction" is often used in planning for terrorist events, in reality, few chemicals can be delivered by terrorists in the appropriate fashion to create large numbers of deaths.[1] However, chemical mass casualty events do occur. The setting may involve the release of industrial chemicals, such as the 1984 industrial accident in Bhopal, India, that caused more than 2500 deaths and 200,000 injuries from a methyl isocyanate release,[2] or a natural chemical incident, such as the emission of carbon dioxide in Lake Nyos, Cameroon, that was responsible for 1700 chemical asphyxiant deaths. Chemical terrorism may also occur through acts of willful deployment, as with the sarin release in the Tokyo subway in 1995 in which 12 people died and 5500 sought medical attention.

The emergency physician is most likely to encounter the accidental release of a chemical from a fixed industrial site or transportation accident. In 2005, a freight train collision in Graniteville, South Carolina, caused the release of chlorine gas that resulted in nine deaths and 511 ED visits.[2,3] Environmental contamination, even without injuries, may affect an entire community, including local emergency departments. In 2014, a previously little-known chemical named 4-methylcyclohexane methanol that was used in coal washing leaked into the Elk River in West Virginia, in proximity to the intake area for the water supply for nine counties that served 300,000 people. Although there were no injuries, emergency planners needed to supply clean water to the affected population. Providing risk management advice based on limited data on this chemical and the chemical's strong black licorice odor despite levels below the toxic concentration made it challenging to convince the citizens that the water was safe to use again.[4]

What has been learned from these incidents is that when chemicals are released, the agents create a penumbra effect, in which true chemical emergencies occur in the epicenter and a larger surrounding area of fear and panic arises in individuals with lower, usually nontoxic levels of exposure. **Planning for chemical disasters must take into account both the chemical emergency occurring near the center of any chemical release and the chaos that can ensue through fear of exposure.**[2,3] What makes these events overwhelming for an individual ED is the larger number of victims who are ambulatory, frightened, and make their own way to the hospital, bypassing any scene triage or decontamination.[5] Appropriate planning for management of this large, self-extricated population is paramount to the concept of disaster preparedness for chemical emergencies and perhaps even more important than specific antidotes for rare agents that might be encountered.

PRINCIPLES OF PHYSICS: SOLIDS, LIQUIDS, AND GASES

Solids have a fixed volume and shape and can be bulk solids, powders, dusts, or fumes.[6] Dust particles are visible if they are >100 μm in diameter; particles smaller than this size are imperceptible to the naked eye.[7] Most dust particles settle with time as the result of gravity; however, in a wind-blown environment or an explosion, they can be blown through the air and contaminate mucous membranes or be inhaled. Dust particles between 2.5 and 6.0 μm in diameter deposit in the bronchial mucosa, whereas particles smaller than 2.5 μm can reach the alveoli. Fumes are fine, solid particles created by either combustion or condensation and are smaller than 1 μm in diameter. Chemicals may adhere to fumes or dusts and be deposited in the lungs through inhalation.

Liquids have a fixed volume, but their shape conforms to both gravitation and container shape. They will flow downhill and can accumulate in clothing and shoes. A liquid forced through a small orifice under pressure can be aerosolized into fine liquid droplets (i.e., aerosols). Aerosols, like dust, will settle with gravity over time. A vapor may be a dispersion of a liquid or a volatile solid, like mercury. Vapors and aerosols may penetrate clothing, causing contact injury by soaking the underlying skin or reacting with moisture in mucous membranes.

A gas has a variable shape and volume and will diffuse to fill an enclosed space once released. Many compressed gases are stored as liquids in cylinders and are converted to a gas upon their release. Hazardous risk analysis should take into consideration misuse or theft of these compressed gas cylinders. An endothermic reaction may occur during release of a compressed gas, causing hypothermic skin injury. Gases can be inhaled into the lungs and cause local reaction, systemic toxicity, or, in some cases, delayed reactions deep in the pulmonary tree.

How deeply in the lungs a gas or vapor exerts its effects depends on its degree of water solubility. Highly water-soluble compounds react with water in our mucous membranes and can irritate the eyes and upper airway.[6] Examples of agents with this property includes ammonia and hydrogen chloride. These agents have good warning properties, allowing an awake and ambulatory individual to leave the area of exposure. Low water-soluble compounds may be less irritating, allowing greater duration of exposure and, therefore, greater pulmonary penetration. Phosgene is an example of a low-solubility gas; it has a pleasant smell like new-mown hay and penetrates deep into the alveoli where it slowly is converted to hydrochloric acid.

All liquids at temperatures between their freezing point and their boiling point are in equilibrium between the liquid itself and some amount of gas vaporized into the atmosphere. Below their freezing point, liquids become a solid and pose little risk of vaporization. Above their boiling point, they become a gas, and their vapor pressure equals the atmospheric pressure.[6] The higher the vapor pressure is for a substance, the more likely it is to volatilize into a gas. It is possible to calculate the concentration of a chemical as a vapor knowing its vapor pressure and the atmospheric pressure. This vapor concentration may be used to predict risk of toxicity based on established exposure limit guidelines.

HAZARDOUS MATERIALS EXPOSURE-LIMIT GUIDELINES

Several agencies have created exposure guidelines used for different purposes, of which a few may be useful in assessing health risks during an exposure. The American Conference of Governmental Industrial Hygienists has created threshold limit values for many substances.[8] This value is the maximum allowable airborne concentration of a substance that a worker can be exposed to for an 8-hour workday. Concentrations below this should be regarded as acceptable and safe.[6,8] The American Conference of Governmental Industrial Hygienists has also established a short-term exposure limit for substances to which an individual should not be exposed for >15 minutes.[8] The National Institute for Occupational Safety and Health has established an acute exposure limit called the *immediately dangerous to life or health* limit. This is the maximum environmental air concentration of a substance from which a person without protective equipment could escape within 30 minutes and not sustain irreversible health effects.[6] This applies only to acute health effects and does not take into account chronic health effects or carcinogenicity. The immediately dangerous to life or health level is meant to apply to the work environment and not a chemical accident, where the level of a substance measured in an environment is usually unavailable during an actual disaster and may change over time.

The Environmental Protection Agency created a three-tiered Acute Exposure Guideline Level (AEGL) that is applied to nonoccupational, one-time exposures in the general population.[9] AEGL-1 levels cause discomfort only; AEGL-2 levels cause irreversible, long-lasting effects; and AEGL-3 levels cause serious disease or death. Each level is further rated by time exposure for concentrations of exposure for 10 minutes, 30 minutes, 60 minutes, and 4 and 8 hours.

Exposures at or less than AEGL-1 limits require public health and emergency response agency efforts to educate the public about the minor effects expected to help minimize ED and physician visits. Access to areas with levels higher than AEGL-1 limits should be restricted. **Levels between AEGL-2 and AEGL-3 require accurate and specific information to be given to the public and generally would require people to shelter in place, seal their homes, and perform self-decontamination.**[9] Highly susceptible individuals, such as the elderly, those with lung disease, or the very young, may need priority evacuation and evaluation. Levels anticipated at or greater than AEGL-3 require evacuation, field decontamination, and triage.

SCENE HAZARDOUS MATERIALS RESPONSE

Each year, there are 15,000 to 19,000 hazardous materials (HAZMAT) events in the United States. Planning for chemical exposure events, whether terrorist or accidental, builds on our existing principles of HAZMAT response. Core concepts of planning are listed in **Table 8-1**.

COMMUNITY RISK ASSESSMENT

The Superfund Amendments and Reauthorization Act, also called the Emergency Planning and Community Right-to-Know Act, requires states to create state-level emergency response commissions and communities to form local emergency planning committees to prepare emergency response plans for chemical accidents. Chemical facilities are required to provide local emergency management agencies and local fire departments with annual inventory reports and information about hazardous chemicals. The Environmental Protection Agency maintains a national database containing a Toxics Release Inventory that mandates certain facilities to annually report the quantities of their emissions of toxic chemicals (http://www.epa.gov/tri and http://www.epa.gov/triexplorer/maps.htm). This information includes the chemical name, an estimate of the maximum amount of the hazardous chemical present at the facility at any time during the preceding calendar year, an estimate of the average daily amount of the hazardous chemical present at the facility during the preceding calendar year, a brief description of the manner of storage of the hazardous chemical, and the location within the facility of the hazardous chemical. **Table 8-2** lists the most common chemicals stored in the United States. Appropriate emergency planning would require a laborious review of these databases at each local level and is not often done with any assessment of vulnerability to release. Rather than expect an accurate accounting of local risk, each ED must be knowledgeable in the general principles

TABLE 8-1 Scene HAZMAT Planning Guidelines

Scene HAZMAT Planning Guidelines
Community risk assessment
Recognition of an event
Identification of the substances involved
Isolation and scene control
Decontamination
Stabilization and triage

Abbreviation: HAZMAT = hazardous materials.

TABLE 8-2 Most Common Chemicals Stored in the United States

Most Common Chemicals Stored in the United States
Anhydrous ammonia
Chlorine
Flammable mixtures
Propane
Sulfur dioxide

of HAZMAT decontamination. An awareness of the clinical manifestations of the most common stored chemicals and the availability of just-in-time information sheets can supplement risk assessment in the real world.[10]

RECOGNITION OF AN EVENT

Most chemical releases are recognized early because many chemicals have early warning properties, including a noxious or unusual odor, or cause eye or upper airway irritation. Toxic exposures may produce rapid death at the site of the release. Sometimes, more subtle clues are present, such as large numbers of dead animals in an outdoor environment.

Most HAZMAT events occur in fixed industrial facilities, and many industries have monitors for leaks of chemicals at nontoxic threshold levels that have no warning properties. For example, the semiconductor manufacturing industry has monitoring sensors for many toxic semiconductor gases, such as arsine, and these are triggered at very low levels. However, these agents are gases and pose no risk of secondary contamination.

IDENTIFICATION OF THE SUBSTANCES INVOLVED

The most common agents released in the United States are the pulmonary irritants ammonia and chlorine. There are numerous resources for the identification of which substances are involved in a spill by a transportation accident or industrial site (**Table 8-3**).

Few of these resources will identify the amount, and none will have treatment recommendations. **Although it may be intuitive that an exact identification of a substance is critical to the disaster or HAZMAT process, in reality, it is more important to recognize the clinical syndromic manifestations of the victims.** It is not necessary at the scene to know which organophosphate is involved; it is more important to identify that the symptom complex of a cholinergic crisis is occurring. Similarly, early recognition of the pulmonary irritant effects of a highly water-soluble acid is usually more important than the concentration or the specific chemical identified. Ultimately, identification of the exact agent involved will need to be made. HAZMAT teams have several techniques to identify substances and usually have a standard procedure to enter and evaluate a building where an odor is detected. The treating physician should evaluate all presumptive initial identifications of substances with some caution.[3] **If the symptoms of the patient do not fit the initial chemical identification, then the accuracy of the identification should be called into question.** Experience with chemical events has sometimes revealed that the substance involved must be reidentified during the evolution of the incident, and sometimes, the initial determination of the chemical involved in the release is wrong.

TABLE 8-3 Chemical Identification Aids

Chemical Identification Aids
U.S. Department of Transportation placards with Department of Transportation Emergency Response Guidebook
Container National Fire Protection Association markings (NFPA 704 system)
Chemical Abstracts Service (CAS) number
Material Safety Data Sheets (MSDS)/Safety Data Sheets (SDS)
Bill of lading
Shipping documents
CHEMical TRansportation Emergency Center (CHEMTREC): 1-800-424-9300

ISOLATION AND SCENE CONTROL

Once a suspected chemical release occurs, the EMS response team must establish an incident command system; designation of hot, warm, and cold zones; and an isolation process. The immediate area where the suspected chemicals and victims of exposure are located is designated the hot zone. Only trained personnel in fully encapsulated protective gear should be allowed to enter. **Their primary role is rescue of victims by removing them from further exposure.** There is substantial risk of secondary contamination and, therefore, toxic effects for any rescuer or bystander who enters the hot zone without the proper protective gear.[11]

A surrounding corridor through which each victim is washed off and decontaminated is created outside the hot zone and is designated the warm zone (**Figure 8-1**). Basic treatment, such as opening obstructed airways, may occur simultaneously with decontamination. Once appropriately decontaminated, the patient can be transferred to the cold zone where a lower level of protective equipment is necessary and a very low risk of secondary contamination exists. With less cumbersome protective gear, reevaluation in the cold zone, triage, and initiation of treatment can occur (**Figure 8-2**).

DECONTAMINATION IN THE WARM ZONE

Primary contamination is caused by direct contact with the release. Both people and the environment may suffer primary contamination. Secondary contamination is the inadvertent contamination of rescue personnel through contact with a contaminated patient or environment. **Secondary contamination can be avoided by proper use of personnel protective equipment and adequate decontamination of adherent solids and liquids.** Some rare substances are excreted in sweat and exhaled. Close unprotected contact with wet skin, mouth-to-mouth ventilation, or mouth-to-mask ventilation could be a source of secondary contamination. Equipment can become secondarily contaminated and may be required to be taken out of service until appropriate decontamination is done. This equipment contamination can be something as simple as a stethoscope or as large as a fire truck. Organophosphates can be excreted in sweat and may adhere to leather. Care must be taken with first responders who may not have protective gear; their shoes, belts, and holsters need to be discarded because they cannot be effectively decontaminated and could potentially pose a risk to coworkers or their families at home.

After the victim is removed from the hot zone to the warm zone, the critical management issue is adequate decontamination. The first and most effective method of decontamination is removing clothing, brushing off solid particles, and washing and toweling the face.[11-13] **Water is the universal decontamination agent.** Some guidelines recommend decontamination for nerve agents and vesicants with dilute household bleach, but there is little evidence of superiority over plain water, and bleach is likely to be unavailable in sufficient quantities at the scene. In general, 5 minutes of decontamination with warm water in the warm zone is adequate for most ambulatory patients.[13] Warm water is used to prevent shivering. If the patient has had direct contact with either liquid or vapor, he or she must be hosed off with water, paying critical attention to occult areas where fluids can hide, such as the hair, skin folds, axilla, groin, toes, and eyes. Patients with severe symptoms may require rapid decontamination and simultaneous treatment in the warm zone.

STABILIZATION AND TRIAGE IN THE COLD ZONE

Triage patients in the cold zone. Safety requires the cold zone to be upwind and, if needed, uphill from the hot zone. Once decontaminated, stabilize patients and evaluate for syndromic symptoms and the need for antidotes. **Primary stabilization includes the establishment of airway, applying oxygen, and administering bronchodilators for bronchospasm.** The establishment of IV lines in a disaster or multiple-casualty incidents requires judgment of the need for fluid resuscitation and critical IV medications. Give priority for IV line placement to patients requiring benzodiazepines for stopping seizure activity,

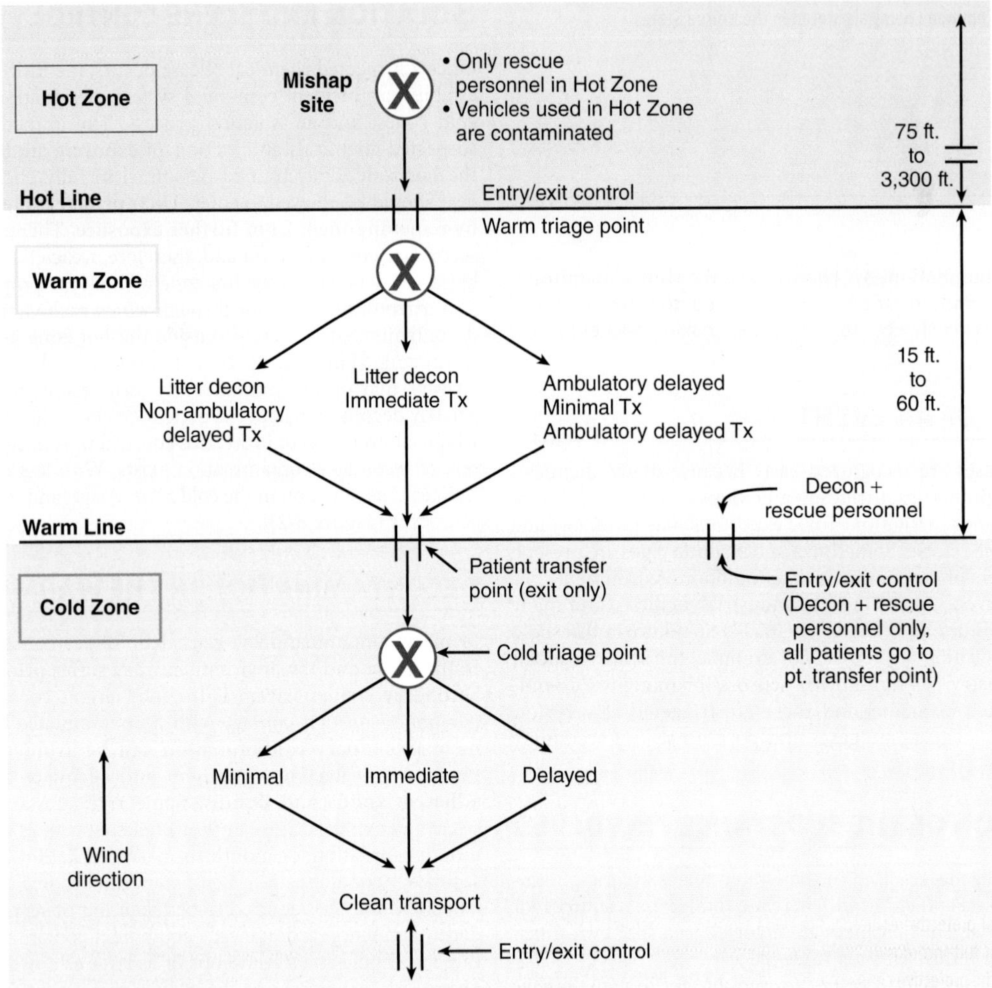

FIGURE 8-1. Control zones of a chemical event. decon = decontamination; pt. = patient; Tx = treatment.

treating cardiac arrhythmias with usual advanced cardiac life support medications, and volume resuscitation for hypotension. Only a few antidotes may truly be beneficial if given early, such as the cyanide antidote, hydroxocobalamin, or atropine for muscarinic effects of organophosphate exposure. The need for additional antidotes in the prehospital phase is unusual unless prolonged on-scene triage is likely to occur.

ED HAZMAT RESPONSE

Despite the best planned and drilled chemical emergency response plan, most individuals will self-rescue and make their way in an uncoordinated fashion to a healthcare facility, so potentially contaminated patients will find their way by private transportation to the ED.[3] In the Tokyo subway release of sarin, 85% of patients who presented to St. Luke's Hospital, the facility closest to the scene, arrived under their own accord.[14-16] Therefore, EDs cannot rely solely on the prehospital system to completely decontaminate and triage every patient. Each facility must consider their physical space and patient flow, create a hospital-based plan for chemical emergencies, and have a policy and training that allow for the identification of chemically exposed patients. There should be an organized plan to perform decontamination and mobilize a system for decontamination of multiple patients, and the plan and equipment must be practiced on a regular basis. Regardless of the specific type of equipment, EDs should have the ability to decontaminate large numbers of patients external to the ED with warm water and proper personal protective equipment. ED decontamination is performed far from the release of the chemical, is not in a warm zone, and does not require fully encapsulated supplied air gear. However, ED decontaminators should wear chemical-resistant covers for all body surfaces (e.g., chemical-resistant gloves, coveralls, and boots) and air-purifying respirator masks with filters that are designed for chemical threats.[11,13]

HIGH-RISK CHEMICALS (TABLE 8-4)

TOXIC INHALANTS

Toxic inhalants tend to interfere with one or more of the four phases of oxygen delivery. Gases that interfere with oxygen uptake by displacement of oxygen from air are **simple asphyxiants**. Interruption of pulmonary diffusion may occur with some of the less soluble irritant agents such as phosgene. Agents that may interrupt oxygen transport include carbon monoxide and the methemoglobin-forming agents. Agents that interfere with oxygen utilization at the cellular level, such as cyanide, azide, and sulfides, produce severe lactic acidosis.

DISPLACEMENT OF OXYGEN FROM AIR: SIMPLE ASPHYXIANTS

Simple asphyxiants create an oxygen-poor environment by displacing oxygen from air. Many inert gases fall into this category, such as carbon dioxide, hydrogen, nitrogen, the noble gases (helium, neon, argon, krypton, xenon, radon), and simple hydrocarbons such as methane, butane, and propane. An occupant confined in a closed unventilated space may die as the concentration of an asphyxiant gas builds up silently.

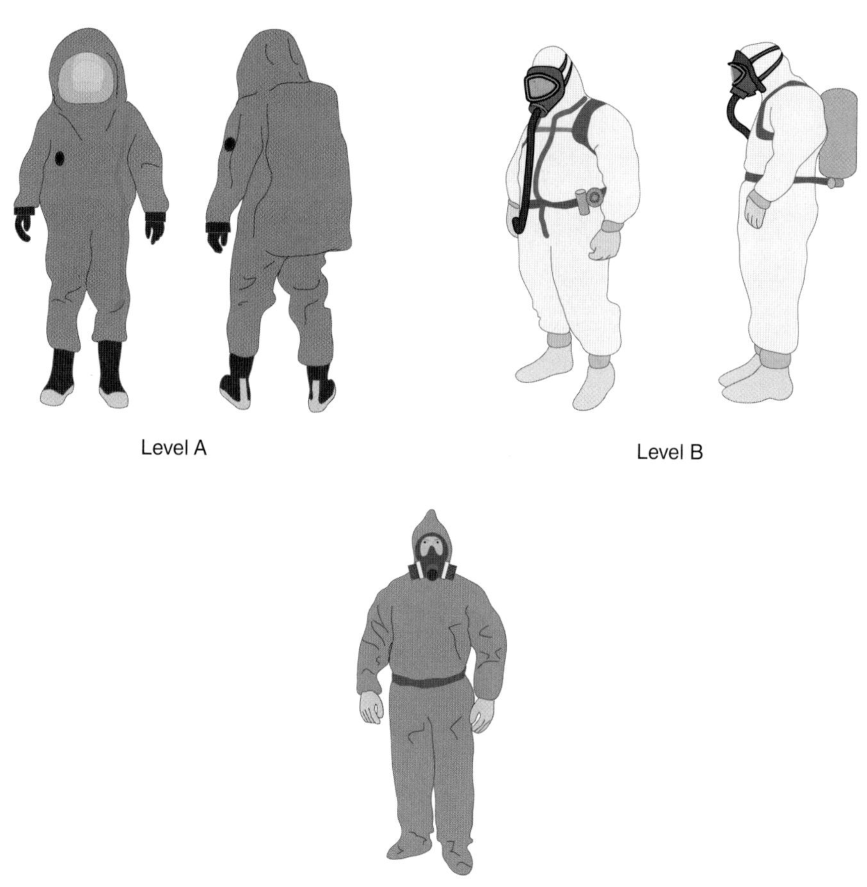

FIGURE 8-2. Personal protective equipment. Level A: Completely encapsulated protection. Requires use of self-contained breathing apparatus (SCBA) inside a chemical-resistant suit sealed at the face. Taped or suit-incorporated gloves and boots make this a completely sealed environment. Level B: Provides either an SCBA or a supplied air respirator and splash protection. The SCBA is worn outside the protective clothing and could expose this equipment to secondary contamination. There may be areas of the skin around the face mask of the SCBA where gas or vapor may penetrate. Level C: Either a gas-mask or air-purifying respirator and skin slash protection. This is the highest level of protection most hospital-based personnel should be trained to use.[12,13] [From U.S. Army Center for Health Promotion and Preventive Medicine Fact Sheet for Acute Exposure Guideline Levels. http://chppm-www.apgea.army.mil.]

TABLE 8-4 High-Risk Chemicals

	Simple Asphyxiants	Irritant Gases or Droplets	Agents that Interrupt Delivery of Oxygen to Tissues	Agents that Interfere with Oxygen Utilization in Mitochondria	Nerve Agents	Incapacitating Agents	Vesicants
Mechanism	Displace oxygen from air	React with H_2O in upper respiratory tract	Alter hemoglobin so it cannot transport O_2; or produce methemoglobin	Bind to cytochrome oxidase	Organophosphates, which bind to acetylcholinesterase	Immobilize victims in a variety of ways	Blistering to eyes, skin, mucous membranes, lungs
Agents	CO, H, N, methane, butane, propane	Ammonia, chloramine, SO_2, HCl, HFl, chlorine, phosgene	CO, methylene chloride, nitrites, benzocaine, phenazopyridine	Cyanide, HS, phosphine, sodium azide, CO	GA, GB (sarin), GD, VX, GF	Mace, narcotic vapors, LSD, BZ	Sulfur mustard, phosgene oxime, lewisite
Treatment	Remove from source, give O_2	Remove from source, give O_2, monitor pulmonary status; for HFl, monitor serum Ca	O_2, methylene blue	Hydroxocobalamin	Identify DUMBELS syndrome; atropine for muscarinic effects; 2-PAM for nicotinic effects, benzodiazepines for seizures; atrovent for wheezing; never give succinylcholine	Individualize for agent	Irrigate with water, supportive care; mustard agents can cause marrow suppression

Abbreviations: BZ = 3-quinuclidinyl benzilate; DUMBELS = defecation, urination, miosis, bradycardia/bronchospasm/bronchorrhea, emesis, lacrimation, and salivation; LSD = lysergic acid diethylamide; 2-PAM = pralidoxime.

For example, deaths have been reported in persons transporting dry ice in the back seat of an automobile with the windows closed. As the solid carbon dioxide sublimes from solid to gas, oxygen concentration drops, and the driver asphyxiates. When the concentration of any of these nonreactive gases increases, the fraction of inspired oxygen (F_{IO_2}) decreases. At an F_{IO_2} of <16%, air hunger, tachypnea, and changes in level of consciousness occur. At F_{IO_2} <10%, loss of consciousness, seizures, or vomiting may occur. Treatment is restoration of a higher F_{IO_2} with supplemental oxygen and correction of the problem that led to the exposure.[17]

IRRITANT AGENTS THAT INTERRUPT PULMONARY DIFFUSION

Irritant agents are classified according to their water solubility as high-, intermediate-, or low-solubility agents. Despite being often referred to as "irritant gases," many of these agents are actually liquid droplets suspended in the air. **Highly water-soluble agents react with water in the upper respiratory tract and produce immediate irritation and discomfort. The most common agent released in chemical events is the highly soluble pulmonary irritant ammonia.** Ammonia, used as an industrial refrigerant, is prototypical of a highly water-soluble vapor. The gas chloramine is created accidentally when bleach and ammonia cleaners are mixed together. Other chemicals with high water solubility include sulfur dioxide and hydrogen chloride. Hydrogen fluoride, in addition to being a highly water-soluble irritant vapor, also reacts with intercellular calcium, causing life-threatening calcium depletion and cardiac dysrhythmias. Because of the immediate discomfort caused by these agents, they have excellent warning properties to those exposed. These agents cause significant eye irritation and edema, burning in the throat, and, at higher concentrations, constriction of the upper airway.[6,17] Treatment is removal from the source, providing supplemental humidified oxygen, and monitoring pulmonary status. Hydrogen fluoride exposure also requires close monitoring of the serum ionized calcium level and administration of supplemental calcium IV.

The only agents classified as intermediate in solubility are chlorine and hydrogen sulfide. Chlorine was the first gas used in chemical warfare in the trenches during the First World War.[17,18] Chlorine is used for chlorinating water in swimming pools and as a disinfectant, making **chlorine releases the second most common hazardous material released. Chlorine reacts with water in the upper airways to produce hydrochloric and hydrochlorous acids.** Symptoms include burning of the conjunctiva, throat, and the bronchial tree. Because of its acrid odor, it has good warning properties. Higher concentrations can produce bronchospasm, lower pulmonary injury, and delayed pulmonary edema.

Phosgene, another chemical warfare agent used extensively in World War I, is prototypical of the minimally soluble agents.[17] At concentrations as low as 25 parts per million, it can be fatal after even brief exposures. It produces only minimal irritation to the eyes and upper airways and, in fact, has a pleasant odor of new-mown hay. However, it slowly hydrolyzes to hydrochloric acid and reacts in the alveoli to cause the delayed onset of severe acute lung injury. Treatment is directed at providing pulmonary monitoring, and the need for intubation and ventilator management is guided by clinical symptoms and radiographic findings of acute lung injury. Noncardiogenic pulmonary edema may require ventilation with positive end-expiratory pressure.

AGENTS THAT INTERRUPT OXYGEN TRANSPORT

Chemicals that react in the body to interrupt the delivery of oxygen do so by altering hemoglobin so that it is no longer capable of binding and transporting oxygen. Examples are carbon monoxide and methylene chloride, which is metabolized to carbon monoxide to generate carboxyhemoglobin. Certain other chemicals, including the nitrites, and some pharmaceuticals, such as benzocaine and phenazopyridine (Pyridium), may cause the iron moiety in hemoglobin to convert from divalent Fe^{2+} to trivalent Fe^{3+}. Hemoglobin with trivalent iron is called *methemoglobin*, and it is incapable of binding and transporting oxygen.[19] Symptoms of either exposure include those consistent with declining oxygenation. Headache, nausea, and fatigue occur at low levels; however, in those with critical fixed coronary artery lesions, angina may occur. Both carboxyhemoglobin and methemoglobin can be measured by co-oximetry on an arterial blood gas analyzer. Pulse co-oximeters are also available that detect both carboxyhemoglobin and methemoglobin and may be used by either prehospital agencies or in hospitals. Both hemoglobinopathies may be treated initially with high concentrations of oxygen. Methemoglobinemia may be treated with methylene blue, which acts as an electron donor and converts trivalent iron back to divalent iron.[19]

AGENTS THAT INTERFERE WITH CELLULAR OXYGEN UTILIZATION (CHEMICAL ASPHYXIANTS)

Chemical asphyxiants are agents that interfere with oxygen utilization at the electron transport chain in the mitochondria. **These agents include cyanide, hydrogen sulfide, phosphine, and sodium azide.**[20,21] Carbon monoxide also interferes with oxygen utilization, in addition to its effect on oxygen delivery. By binding to cytochrome oxidase a_3, these agents disrupt aerobic metabolism and create intracellular acidosis. Cyanogens have been developed for use in chemical warfare, and nitriles used in industry release cyanide.[21,22] Symptoms include headache, alteration of consciousness, seizures, and severe acidosis. Hydroxocobalamin was approved for use in the United States in 2006 for cyanide toxicity and for smoke inhalation and is administered as a 5-gram infusion.[22]

NERVE AGENTS

During World War II, scientists in Germany discovered and manufactured three nerve agents, classified as GA (tabun), GB (sarin), and GD (soman). In 1952, chemists in Great Britain and America manufactured the agents VX and GF.[23,24] Although the preferred terminology for these chemicals is organic phosphorus compounds, they are still referred to as organophosphates in most publications. These agents were chosen as chemical warfare agents over existing insecticides because they had greater CNS activity and higher lethality than many of the organophosphates and carbamates used for insect control.[23-27] With the advent of the Cold War, organophosphate production accelerated, with both the United States and Soviet Union developing large stockpiles of these agents.[24] Occasional accidents occurred, sickening soldiers handling these agents, and one chemical release of VX in Skull Valley, Utah, killed 6000 sheep.[28,29] In the 1980s, Iraq developed an extensive capability to manufacture and weaponize these gases and used both sarin and GF against both its own Kurdish people and the Iranians with whom it was engaged in a prolonged border war.[24] During the Syrian civil war in 2013, nerve agents were confirmed to be used as well, with over 800 civilian casualties.[30,31] Today, not only do many countries have the capability to manufacture these or similar agents, but terrorist groups have used them also. The Aum Shinrikyo cult used sarin in two separate attacks, one in Matsumoto in 1984, which killed seven people, and in a larger release in the Tokyo subway a year later that killed 12 people and sickened 5500 individuals.[14,16]

The organophosphate compounds inhibit several key enzymes by binding to them. They bind to acetylcholinesterase in a two-stage process. The first stage is reversible if the antidote pralidoxime (Protopam) is given.[26] The second stage (aging process) makes the enzyme unavailable to be regenerated by pralidoxime. Acetylcholinesterase breaks down the neurotransmitter acetylcholine. With this enzyme inhibited, acetylcholine remains at its postsynaptic receptor sites, causing excessive cholinergic stimulation. Within the parasympathetic nervous system, there are cholinergic receptors at muscarinic sites, such as tear glands, sweat glands, bronchial secretion glands, and the sinoatrial and atrioventricular nodes of the heart. **Overstimulation of these leads to the "DUMBELS" syndrome, a mnemonic for the following symptom complex: *d*efecation, *u*rination, *m*iosis, *b*radycardia/*b*ronchospasm/*b*ronchorrhea, *e*mesis, *l*acrimation, and *s*alivation.**[6]

The second location within the peripheral nervous system where cholinergic transmission is affected is the neuromuscular junction, or nicotinic receptor. **Excess cholinergic stimulation here causes the progression from muscular fasciculation to profound muscular weakness to complete paralysis in a dose-dependent fashion.** Early in the course, there can also be paradoxical hypertension and tachycardia, but these both subside as the bradycardia from muscarinic receptors predominates in the clinical presentation.

The last location of importance for cholinergic stimulation is the brain, where excessive stimulation produces coma and seizures. Many organophosphates cross the blood–brain barrier freely, and the nerve agents in particular have potent CNS effects.

The treatment strategy for nerve agents must counteract cholinergic excess at all three of these receptor sites. **Atropine counteracts only the muscarinic effects. Pralidoxime counteracts the nicotinic effects. Benzodiazepines treat seizures.**[24,26] The indication for each of these agents varies with the clinical manifestations. For the patient with exposure in low concentrations, such as with vapor releases, only eye findings may develop. Pinpoint pupils, frequently with local pain, may be treated with any of the anticholinergic eye drops, scopolamine, or homatropine. If pulmonary symptoms are isolated to bronchospasm in the reactive airway disease–prone patient, ipratropium bromide (Atrovent) may be adequate. **Administer IV atropine to anyone experiencing hypersalivation, bronchial secretions, or bradycardia.**[25,26] Large doses of IV atropine, sometimes as much as 20 milligrams, may be needed.[26] This has been reported typically in ingestions but could be needed in liquid exposure to the nerve agents. High doses of atropine were not needed in the lower concentration exposures that occurred in the Tokyo subway incident.[14-16] **Titrate atropine administration to clearing of the excess secretions.** Pupil size and heart rate response are poor indicators of adequate atropinization in organophosphate exposure.

Pralidoxime reactivates the enzyme acetylcholinesterase at the neuromuscular junction. It can only reactivate the enzyme if the aging process has not occurred. How rapidly an agent ages varies from agent to agent; VX takes 24 hours, whereas soman takes only 5 to 8 minutes to age and create an irreversible bond.[26] The recommended initial dosage of pralidoxime is 1 to 2 grams IV slowly over 20 to 30 minutes.[24-26] **In a large event with multiple casualties, half this may be given to spread the antidote to the maximal number of patients.** Many patients with neuromuscular weakness will eventually require intubation and mechanical ventilation. Succinylcholine should not be used, if at all possible, because it is metabolized by the same enzymes inhibited by the organophosphates. **The onset of action of succinylcholine will be the same (usually <90 seconds), but the duration of action of this drug will be prolonged to several hours.**[32] Seizures, when they occur, may be refractory and, in combination with diaphragmatic paralysis, will lead to respiratory arrest. Use any of the IV benzodiazepines to treat seizures. Phenytoin and fosphenytoin are not effective for seizure control.

Patients with minor symptoms, such as eye findings only, may be observed for a 6- to 8-hour period and released if no further symptoms occur.[15] Admit any patient who received pralidoxime to an intensive care unit and give either a continuous infusion of pralidoxime at 500 milligrams/h or intermittent bolus dosages of 1 to 2 grams every 6 hours.[14,24]

INCAPACITATING AGENTS

The incapacitating agents are a diverse group of chemicals that immobilize victims.[13] Although riot control agents, such as Mace (Mace Security International, Horsham, PA), are not classically defined in this category, they can be considered incapacitating and are generally nonlethal. Narcotic vapors have also been used, such as the fentanyl derivatives used by Russia when they stormed the Moscow theater in 2002 where terrorists were holding hostages. The potent fentanyl derivatives, carfentanil and remifentanil, may have been mixed with a halothane-like anesthetic agent.[33] Despite the intent of this mixture to immobilize those inside the theater, lack of coordinated rescue efforts and late use of the antidote naloxone led to >100 causalities. 3-Quinuclidinyl benzilate is a long-acting potent anticholinergic agent. The U.S. Army developed it in the 1960s; exact information on how it was used is difficult to substantiate.[24] 3-Quinuclidinyl benzilate causes a severe and prolonged anticholinergic delirium similar to diphenhydramine or atropine. Other agents intended to immobilize victims have been experimented with, such as lysergic acid diethylamide, benzodiazepines, α_2-agonists, vomiting agents, and other exotic agents.

TABLE 8-5 Indications of a Possible Biotoxin Exposure

Occurrence of a disease or syndrome that rarely occurs naturally
Multiple victims of a similar disease with no classic risk factors
Epidemiology suggesting a point source or localized exposure
Possible animal and human morbidity in the same area
High mortality in an otherwise healthy population

VESICANTS

Sulfur mustard was first deployed by Germany in 1917 near Ypres, Belgium, the site of their release of chlorine as a chemical weapon 2 years earlier.[34,35] Vesicant agents were used extensively as military weapons by both sides in World War I and in a variety of regional wars leading up to and during World War II (Ethiopia, Manchuria).[24] The largest number of casualties from sulfur mustard came with the explosion of the Liberty ship *John Harvey*, during World War II in Bari, Italy, where 617 sailors sustained burns from sulfur mustard.[36,37] During the 1980s sulfur mustard was used in the Middle East (Iraq against Iran and the Kurds, Egypt against Yemen); 12 of these patients were transported to Germany, and their therapy was described in detail.[35] A small number of spills have occurred since in the United States at chemical weapons storage facilities.[36] **Vesicants cause damage to eyes, skin, mucous membranes, and potentially the lungs if exposed to high concentrations.** Sulfur mustards [bis(2-chloroethyl) sulfide] make up the most common vesicants used, although the nitrogen mustards were also produced, but never used militarily.[34] Other vesicant agents are phosgene oxime, a solid that liquefies at 35°C (95°F); this agent does not cause blisters but produces severe skin erythema.[24,36] Lewisite, an arsenical compound that smells like geraniums and that was developed in 1918, too late for use in World War I and thus never deployed, is also included in this category.[36] Both lewisite and phosgene oxime produce symptoms on immediate contact.[35-37] Sulfur mustard skin symptoms are delayed in onset for 4 to 8 hours, leading to blistering similar to second-degree burns within 2 to 18 hours of initial exposure.[34] Ocular damage from vapor exposure to all these agents is common, leading to incapacitation of the victims exposed. Corneal vesicle formation and sloughing of epithelium occur. The primary goal of therapy is copious irrigation with water to dilute and remove the chemical, and then monitoring the patient with serial eye examinations, pulmonary monitoring, and careful attention to skin care. The mustard agents may produce a systemic toxicity, with marrow suppression as a delayed component presenting with a falling white blood cell count and increased risk of infection 3 to 5 days after exposure.[35]

BIOTOXINS

The biotoxins differ from biologic agents in that the toxins do not replicate in the body and a sufficient dose needed to cause disease must be delivered. These agents produce unusual symptoms, some with delayed onset. Clues to biotoxin exposure are presented in **Table 8-5**.

With many biotoxins, the lethal dose in 50% of exposed subjects (LD_{50}) is quite low (**Table 8-6**), allowing small amounts to potentially be made into a high-risk weaponized aerosol and dispersed intentionally.[24]

TABLE 8-6 Lethality of Biotoxins

Agent	LD_{50} (micrograms/kg)
Botulinum toxin	0.001
Tetanus toxin	0.002
Staphylococcal enterotoxin B	0.02
Diphtheria toxin	0.10
Ciguatoxin	0.4
Ricin	3.0
Tetrodotoxin	8.0
Saxitoxin	10.0
Trichothecene toxin	1200

Abbreviation: LD_{50} = lethal dose in 50% of exposed subjects.

BOTULINUM TOXIN

Inhalational botulism has been described in humans only after an accidental laboratory exposure. It is estimated that the LD_{50} for inhalation botulism is 1 to 3 nanograms/kg.[24] Three days after performing an autopsy on a lab animal that died of botulism, three technicians developed tightness in the throat, difficulty swallowing, and symptoms characterized as a cold without a fever. They developed ocular paresis, rotatory nystagmus, dilated pupils, dysarthria, ataxia, and generalized weakness. All recovered within 2 weeks with antitoxin treatment.[24] Diagnosis requires the recognition of the clinical presentation, with early subtle cranial nerve palsies, typically presenting with difficulty swallowing, palsies of extraocular muscles, and trouble speaking.[38] **Treatment with antitoxin will prevent progression of the disease but will not reverse paralysis once it occurs. Administer the antitoxin based on clinical suspicion as early as possible; do not wait for the results of laboratory tests.** The heptavalent antitoxin against all subtypes of botulism is available by contacting the Centers for Disease Control and Prevention.[38] Give one vial of antitoxin IV in suspected cases of botulism. Supportive care, including mechanical ventilation, is frequently needed and may be required for 90 days or more in cases presenting with diaphragmatic paralysis before receiving the antitoxin.[38] Antibiotics only have a role in wound botulism and are not indicated in inhalational botulism.

RICIN

Ricin toxin gained notoriety when it was used as the agent to assassinate Bulgarian activist Georgi Markov. At autopsy, a pellet containing ricin was removed from a small wound in the back of his leg. The pellet was fired from a specially designed umbrella into his leg while he waited at a London bus stop.[24] Ricin is a toxin derived from the castor bean, *Ricinus communis*.[39] Ricin is not toxic by ingestion and must either be injected or inhaled as an aerosolized powder to produce disease. Ricin is taken up by cells in many tissues and causes destruction of RNA, leading to cell death. With inhalation exposure, pulmonary symptoms occur after about an 8-hour postexposure delay. Inflammation, exudates, and pulmonary edema occur, producing a necrotizing pneumonitis. After parenteral administration, local pain occurs, followed in a few hours by weakness and flu-like symptoms. Fifteen to 24 hours later, nausea, vomiting, fever, and localized lymphadenopathy proximal to the injection site may occur. After 48 hours, a sepsis-like syndrome occurs with hypotension, leukocytosis, disseminated intravascular coagulation, and multiorgan system failure (involving the liver, kidneys, heart, lungs, and GI hemorrhage). In Georgi Markov's case, death occurred by deterioration to complete atrioventricular dissociation.[24] The differential diagnosis includes other causes of sepsis, but in the setting of an intentional attack, staphylococcal enterotoxin B must also be considered. Diagnosis may be confirmed by an enzyme-linked immunosorbent assay. Contact the Centers for Disease Control and Prevention in any suspicious case. Aggressive supportive care in an intensive care unit is warranted for all cases.

REFERENCES

The complete reference list is available online at www.TintinalliEM.com.

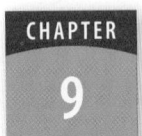

CHAPTER 9 Bioterrorism

Anthony G. Macintyre
Joseph A. Barbera

INTRODUCTION AND EPIDEMIOLOGY

An adequate response to a bioterrorist event of any magnitude requires early recognition and effective coordination of many disparate health and medical entities beyond the ED. Although the emergency physician plays a critical role in these types of events, many other essential functions must be addressed by individuals and organizations representing public health, mental health, law enforcement, emergency management, and others.

A bioterrorist incident is the release, or the threat of a release, of a biologic agent among a civilian population for the purpose of creating fear, illness, and death. Such an occurrence is a low-probability, high-impact incident. For example, in the U.S. anthrax dissemination incident, the U.S. Postal Service was used to deliver letters containing spores of *Bacillus anthracis*. Although the environmental contamination was widespread, only 22 diagnosed cases of anthrax infection occurred: 11 cases of inhalational and 11 cases of cutaneous anthrax. Five patients died as a direct result of the anthrax exposure.[1] Communities on the Eastern Seaboard of the United States were severely affected, with thousands of people receiving prophylaxis for anthrax.[2] Fear then spread across the nation, as concern increased for a wider delivery of anthrax. Much of this national anxiety may have been exacerbated by the perception of an inadequate public health response capability, with the deficiencies demonstrating a critical need to integrate acute care medicine and the public health response.

Biologic agents are classified into two groups: biologically produced toxins and infectious organisms. Biologic toxins usually act as chemical agents in their human impact. The recognition and response requirements for these are very similar to those for chemical incidents. Infectious agents are subdivided into two categories: contagious (propagating person to person) and noncontagious. Contagious agents have additional ramifications, both for protection of the healthcare workforce as well as propagation of the disease beyond the initially exposed population. The contagious agents of greatest concern, such as smallpox, plague (pneumonic), and certain viral hemorrhagic fevers, are person-to-person infectious through airborne or droplet transmission. Suspected biologic agents causing illness should be treated as contagious until demonstrated otherwise.

AGENTS OF CONCERN

Certain characteristics make individual organisms particularly attractive as weapons for generating widespread fear, illness, and death among civilian populations. The Centers for Disease Control and Prevention identified select organisms and the diseases they cause as the priority for focused preparation.[3] Infectious agent selection was based on four general criteria:

1. Potential for public health impact
2. Delivery potential (an estimation of the ease for development and dissemination, including the potential for person-to-person transmission of infection)
3. Public perception (fear) of the agent
4. Special requirements for public health preparedness (diagnostic, logistic, etc.)

The selected agents were then ranked in three categories, based on their overall potential for adverse public health impact (**Table 9-1; Figures 9-1 to 9-3**). **Class A agents have the most severe potential and include viruses and bacteria such as variola major (smallpox), *B. anthracis* (anthrax), and *Yersinia pestis* (plague). Class B agents are considered to have less potential for causing widespread illness and death, and Class C agents are those that, as technology improves, could emerge as future threats.** More common pathogens could be used to cause intentional injury and death, and the intentional etiology of the infections may be apparent only through epidemiologic cohort evaluation. This chapter focuses on Class A agents, but applies also to a range of additional bacteria and viruses that, although not on the Centers for Disease Control and Prevention list, could have a similar human impact if used in a nefarious manner (e.g., hanta virus).

CLINICAL FEATURES: RECOGNITION OF A BIOTERRORISM INCIDENT

Unless the release of an agent is openly announced or the terrorist is caught in the process of delivering the agent, initial indications of attack may be subtle. **Early symptoms of most agents of concern are not**

TABLE 9-1 Infectious Agents of Concern as Defined by the Centers for Disease Control and Prevention

Biologic Agent	Disease Caused	Incubation Period	Signs and Symptoms
Class A agents			
Variola major	Smallpox (Figure 9-1)	7–14 d	Initially fever, severe myalgias, prostration; followed within 2 d by papular rash on the face spreading to extremities (affecting palms and soles) and then to trunk (lesser extent than chickenpox); lesions progress at same rate, becoming vesicular and then pustular with subsequent scab formation
Bacillus anthracis	Cutaneous anthrax (Figure 9-2)	Usually 1 d, up to 2 wk reported	Macule or papule enlarging into eschar with surrounding vesicles and edema; sepsis possible, less common
	GI anthrax	Usually 1–7 d	Abdominal pain, vomiting, GI bleeding progressing to sepsis; mesenteric adenopathy on CT
	Oropharyngeal anthrax	Usually 1–7 d	Sore throat, ulcers on base of tongue, marked unilateral neck swelling
	Inhalational anthrax (Figure 9-3)	Usually <1 wk, 43 d reported at Sverdlovsk[4]	First stage is nonspecific (fever, dyspnea, cough, headache, vomiting, abdominal pain, chest pain); second stage (dyspnea, diaphoresis, shock); hemorrhagic mediastinitis with widened mediastinum on x-ray
Yersinia pestis	Bubonic plague	2–8 d	Initially fever, chills, painful swollen lymph node(s); node progresses to bubo (sometimes suppurative)
	Pneumonic plague	2–3 d	Fever, chills, cough, dyspnea, nausea, vomiting, abdominal pain; clinical condition consistent with gram-negative sepsis
	Primary septicemic plague	2–8 d	The clinical condition is consistent with gram-negative sepsis, disseminated intravascular coagulation (secondary septicemic plague may occur after bubo formation)
Clostridium botulinum	Foodborne botulism	1–5 d	GI symptoms followed by symmetric cranial neuropathies, blurred vision, progressing to descending paralysis
	Inhalational botulism*	12–72 h	Symmetric cranial nerve palsies followed by descending paralysis
Francisella tularensis	Tularemia	1–21 d	Depends on route of exposure: all usually involve abrupt nonspecific febrile illness; inhalation exposure progressing to pleuropneumonitis; cutaneous exposure developing glandular or ulceroglandular lesions; ingestion developing oropharyngeal lesions/tonsillitis
Filoviruses and arenaviruses (Ebola virus)	Viral hemorrhagic fevers	2 d–3 wk, depending on virus	Initial nonspecific febrile illness, sometimes with rash; progresses to bloody vomiting, diarrhea, shock
Class B agents			
Coxiella burnetii	Q fever	2–3 wk	Fever, myalgias, headache, 30% develop pneumonia, rarely lethal (2%)
Brucella spp.	Brucellosis	2–4 wk	Fever, myalgias, back pain; CNS infections and endocarditis possible
Burkholderia mallei	Glanders	10–14 d	Local infection: ulcers, suppurative; pneumonia, pulmonic abscesses, sepsis possible
Burkholderia pseudomallei	Melioidosis	2 d to years reported	Local infection: nodule; pneumonia, pulmonic abscesses, sepsis
Alpha viruses (Venezuelan equine encephalitis, Eastern equine encephalitis, Western equine encephalitis)	Encephalitis	Variable	Fever, headache, aseptic meningitis, encephalitis, focal paralysis, seizures
Rickettsia prowazekii	Typhus fever	7–14 d	Fever, headache, rash
Toxins (ricin, *Staphylococcus*, enterotoxin B)	Toxic syndromes	—	—
Chlamydia psittaci	Psittacosis	6–19 d	Fever, headache, dry cough, pneumonia, endocarditis
Food safety threats (*Salmonella* spp., *Escherichia coli* 0157:H7)	—	—	—
Water safety threats (*Vibrio cholera*, *Cryptosporidium parvum*)	—	—	—
Class C threats			
Emerging threat agents (Nipah virus, hantavirus)	—	—	—

*Inhalational botulism may not be preceded by GI symptoms. Inhalational and foodborne botulisms are caused by botulinum toxin, not the bacteria itself.

Note: Incubation periods should be interpreted with some caution. Data in some instances are limited and in others may be based on natural outbreaks. Intentional releases or engineered organisms could cause variations in expected disease parameters.

readily distinguished from more common, less threatening illnesses. Fever, myalgias, and malaise could be the initial presenting symptoms of a victim of bioterrorism (anthrax and others) or of influenza, parainfluenza, or many common illnesses. This is more than a theoretical risk, as demonstrated when some agents of concern have been documented to occur in the nonbioterrorism setting.[5] During the anthrax dissemination incident in 2001, several anthrax-infected postal workers were evaluated by physicians early in their illness. Their relatively nonspecific symptoms were attributed to other causes, and they were discharged home without antibiotic therapy.[6] Two postal workers in this cohort died from inhalational anthrax. The similarity in early symptoms also creates another response issue: once an attack becomes public, patients with any

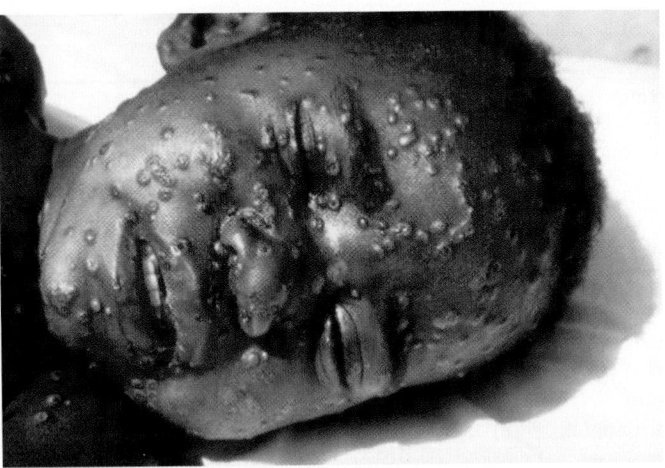

FIGURE 9-1. Smallpox.

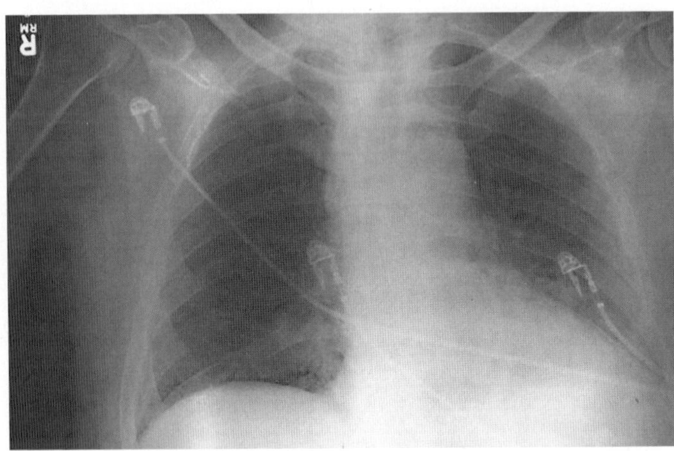

FIGURE 9-3. Chest radiograph with widened mediastinum characteristic of inhalational anthrax.

of those common symptoms or concerns about exposure may seek rapid evaluation in EDs, clinics, or private offices. Extreme patient volume and diagnostic challenge should be anticipated.

The recognition of a biologic attack could occur through several pathways:

1. A patient presents with signs, symptoms, or real-time diagnostic results that obviously indicate a suspect disease process.
2. A patient presents with protean symptoms, but an astute clinician establishes enough criteria (e.g., suspicious historical information, signs, symptoms, short-turnaround laboratory results, public health corroborative information) to designate the patient as a presumptive case until diagnostic confirmation can be accomplished.
3. Patient is evaluated and admitted or released but not suspected as being a victim of bioterrorism. That patient's course then unexpectedly worsens, or diagnostic test results (e.g., blood cultures, immunoassays), even postmortem, subsequently establish a diagnosis.
4. Multiple patients present over a defined period with similar symptoms or historical characteristics, with the cohort pattern raising practitioner suspicions that prompt a report to public health. Further investigation, through environmental and diagnostic testing and/or public health investigation of the cohort, establishes the cause.
5. Public health surveillance systems establish unusual patterns of signs, symptoms, or disease in the community and investigate further to establish the etiology.
6. Sampling technologies (of which there are numerous types related to different jurisdictions and agencies) detect the release of an agent of concern in the community.

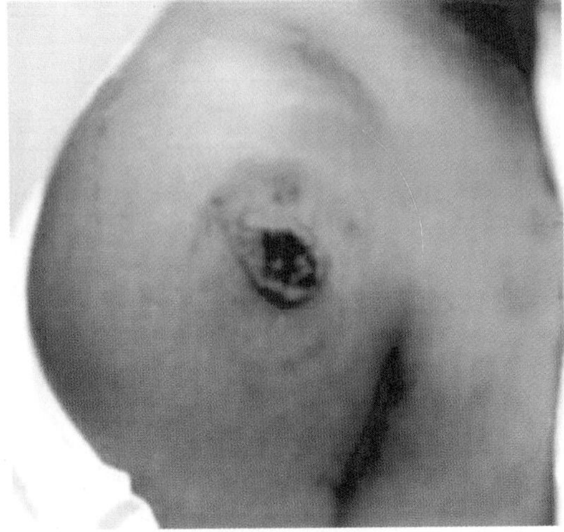

FIGURE 9-2. Ulcer and eschar of cutaneous anthrax.

Based on the few historical cases, the first three scenarios may be the most likely ways in which a bioterrorist event would be detected. Scenario 3 is how the inhalational anthrax index case was initially diagnosed in Florida during the fall of 2001.[7] The initial inhalational anthrax infection in a postal worker was recognized as in scenario 2. Thus, the emergency physician should have an operational knowledge of the biologic agents of concern or understand where to readily access this information. This knowledge should include basic pathologic principles for each agent, modes of dissemination and transmission, disease signs and symptoms, recommended diagnostic testing, recommended treatment (medications, immunizations, or prophylaxis), and infection control practices (Table 9-1 and **Table 9-2**).[8]

DIAGNOSIS

Real-time diagnostic studies to reliably confirm or exclude the presence of potential agents of concern are not available for all Centers for Disease Control and Prevention–designated agents (this actually does not differ from most common infectious processes). In some cases, specialized confirmatory testing by state or federal laboratories may be required (e.g., through the Laboratory Response Network),[10] and methodologies are rapidly evolving. Therefore, clinicians should command sufficient knowledge to initiate available and appropriate test ordering, medical interventions, and reporting when they are **suspicious** of a patient's clinical presentation. The public health authorities with jurisdiction over the involved communities should be consulted early for current diagnostic recommendations and further testing (both patient and environmental).

Be prepared to appropriately respond to notification of a potential disease by another health or medical professional (public health authority, laboratory technician, radiologist, pathologist, or medical examiner). Carefully query the reporting source for pertinent specific information before considering further actions such as those delineated below. Questions to be asked include the methodology of the testing that produced the concern (specimen collection technique and the sensitivity and specificity of the test procedure) and the time until confirmatory test results become available.

Situations that are much more common and pose a great challenge to ED operations are those in which patients present after having been exposed to an unidentified substance (e.g., white powder), with circumstances that raise suspicion for terrorism (e.g., threatening letter, high-profile location, a "very important person"). The source substance may not have been properly evaluated or secured, and any recommended treatment necessarily will involve coordination with outside agencies, especially public health and law enforcement. If no environmental or

TABLE 9-2 Class A Agents: Treatment, Prophylaxis, and Vaccination

Biologic Agent	Vaccination	Prophylaxis	Treatment
Variola major	Vaccinia vaccination: currently not recommended for general public use because of its association with limited numbers of deaths and complications in immunocompromised individuals and those with eczema; useful in preventing disease if given within 4 d of exposure	Vaccinia immune globulin: best given within 2–3 d of exposure; limited supplies are available; consider giving to those exposed who have contraindications to vaccine. Several antivirals are under investigation for postexposure prophylaxis.	Supportive.
Bacillus anthracis	Anthrax vaccination: five-part series vaccination at 0 and 4 wk and then at 6, 12, and 18 mo; annual boosters required; currently not available to the public (offers have been made to the first responder community); efficacy in preventing inhalational anthrax demonstrated in animal models	Ciprofloxacin or doxycycline for 60 d is preferred, but alternatives exist. In addition, amoxicillin and penicillin V potassium for penicillin-susceptible strains; 60-d term established by using latency period for last infection occurring at Sverdlovsk[4]; consider concurrent 3-dose vaccination.* NOTE: 60-d regimen recommended whether vaccinated before event, receiving postexposure vaccination, or no vaccination.[9]	Three-drug IV regimen for presumed or proven meningitis concurrent with illness. Two-drug regimen for illness with meningitis ruled out (see Hendricks et al[9] for specifics). Consider antitoxin administration for systemic anthrax infection (either raxibacumab or anthrax immune globulin).
Yersinia pestis	Killed whole bacilli vaccine no longer available by producers; vaccine had efficacy in preventing bubonic disease but not the pneumonic form	Ciprofloxacin or doxycycline; alternative: chloramphenicol; prophylaxis for 10 d.	Streptomycin or gentamicin preferred choices; alternatives: doxycycline, ciprofloxacin, chloramphenicol.
Clostridium botulinum	Vaccine not available to the public: pentavalent toxoid of C. botulinum toxin types A–E; three-part series with yearly booster	Not applicable.	Antitoxin: requires procurement through local public health agency (state or the Centers for Disease Control and Prevention); antitoxin may preserve remaining neurologic function but does not reverse paralysis; may require prolonged, assisted mechanical ventilation and supportive care.
Francisella tularensis	Live attenuated vaccine was under investigation but now discontinued in United States	Ciprofloxacin or doxycycline for 14 d.	Streptomycin or gentamicin preferred choices; alternatives: doxycycline, ciprofloxacin, chloramphenicol.
Filoviruses (e.g., Ebola virus) and arenaviruses	Not applicable	Not applicable.	Supportive therapy; ribavirin may have applicability in arenaviruses.

*Not approved by the U.S. Food and Drug Administration but potentially available under Emergency Use Authorization.

NOTE: Due to multiple ongoing efforts, some new or adjusted therapies may be available in the near future. Readers are encouraged to check peer-reviewed literature because this is a dynamic field. Specific recommendations exist for some agents and may entail use of therapies traditionally reserved for nonpregnant adults. In some cases, these entail use under Emergency Use Authorization, which is beyond the scope of this chapter.

agent testing was performed, one may attempt to obtain confirmatory studies through the local public health authorities if the substance remains available. Otherwise, the difficult task of stratifying patient exposure risk is necessary, using arguably nonspecific factors such as patient demographics and the specific characteristics of the incident (e.g., white powder found in a local business vs a high-level federal official's office). The public health authorities with jurisdiction over the involved communities should be consulted early in the process, ideally by using a preplanned notification process and decision support tools. When testing has been performed by others, the emergency clinician should request specific information on the testing methodology and judge the reliability of the test procedure. For example, anthrax environmental testing may be performed with a wide range of procedures, including immune-based assays, assays based on polymerase chain reaction, and confirmatory culture testing.[11] Older immune-based assays caused numerous instances of false-positive environmental tests, which were subsequently reported in the media and created serious public concern during and after the 2001 anthrax incident. Clearer understanding of the sensitivity and specificity of these tests could have assisted in interpretation and representation of results.[12]

Methods for potentially detecting a biologic event include the recognition of unusual epidemiologic phenomena such as a high incidence of nonspecific illness, clusters or large numbers of rapidly fatal cases, and steep infection curves identified through public health surveillance systems.[12]

Much effort in the United States has been focused on developing broad-based public health surveillance systems for detection of disease. The surveillance systems currently in use or under development are based on collecting and analyzing public health information and/or patient diagnostic information in specific communities. It is intuitive that this may be further enhanced by the widespread adoption of electronic medical records. Information is sought from many disparate sources, including hospitals, clinics, nursing homes, pharmacies, emergency medical service systems, independent laboratories, medical examiners, and general businesses (e.g., absenteeism rates). Information collected from EDs often is based on symptom complexes (syndromic surveillance). The City of New York Department of Health and Mental Hygiene has operated this type of surveillance system since the late 1990s, which has more recently capitalized on the use of electronic medical records.[13,14]

Air sampling systems to detect inhalation agents have been implemented in some communities and for specific agencies or facilities across the United States. The most well-known is the BioWatch program, which uses strategically placed sensors in specific communities. These sensors operate on the principle of drawing air samples across filters that are subsequently analyzed for some agents of concern.[15,16]

INITIAL RESPONSE TO A BIOTERRORISM INCIDENT

Every receiving facility and ED should have standard operating procedures to manage a bioterrorism threat or actual incident. These should be incorporated into the all-hazards emergency operations plan, with bioterrorism-specific procedures in an attached incident-specific annex. The initial response to a suspected or confirmed bioterrorist event should involve many different hospital departments plus agencies outside the hospital. Initial actions taken by the emergency physician can be pivotal in the success of the hospital performance and the overall community response.

When bioterrorism is confirmed or suspected, critical initial notifications and prompt emergency operations plan activation should include:

1. Activation of processes and procedures (including preplanned surge capacity configuration) as appropriate and as listed in incident-specific annexes to the emergency operations plan
2. Implementation of appropriate infection control procedures (which may extend to how patients are received in the ED), with provision of protective equipment for patients and healthcare workers[17]

TABLE 9-3 Guidelines for Initial Public Health Reporting

1. Diagnosed or suspected agent of concern
2. Whether it is a presumed or confirmed diagnosis (and method for "confirmation")
3. Patient demographics (including occupation)
4. Recent history of travel or participation in special events by the patient(s) (mass gatherings, high-profile events, or at-risk activities)
5. Patient condition
6. Initial testing performed and further diagnostic testing being conducted
7. Treatment being provided
8. Public health assistance required (including environmental and additional patient testing)
9. Preferred method of contacting hospital or treating physicians for follow-up

3. Notification of key departments, including hospital administration, infection control and infectious diseases, security, environmental services, and the hospital laboratory
4. Information flow to all hospital personnel regarding the suspected agent, its characteristics (including potential for person-to-person transmission), and actions to protect the staff
5. Coordination of hospital media messages to external entities (other hospitals, public health, emergency management) to avoid dissemination of conflicting information
6. Notification of the appropriate public health agency, with confirmation that law enforcement was notified by them

Initial information that should be conveyed to the public health department is listed in **Table 9-3**. Ideally, the hospital emergency operations plan fully integrates the hospital into the community response, which is critical for successful bioterrorist incident response.[18]

The local department of health then has the responsibility to notify regional or state public health departments and the Centers for Disease Control and Prevention. With some agents and/or situations, the U.S. Department of Health and Human Services would notify the World Health Organization, because the potential impact could be global and this reporting is mandatory under International Health Regulations administrated by the World Health Organization (the United States is a signatory to International Health Regulations).[19] Public health officials also have the responsibility for notifying local law enforcement and the Federal Bureau of Investigation.

INTEGRATION WITH THE LOCAL HEALTH DEPARTMENT

In any suspected or confirmed case of bioterrorism, the emergency physician can expect to interface with multiple diverse agencies in an ongoing fashion, the most critical of which is the local public health department. In most communities, public health epidemiologists are assigned the task of defining the size and scope of an incident, the at-risk population, and other incident parameters. This type of information becomes critical to acute care clinicians, other medical care providers, and hospitals in the evaluation and treatment of patients and in anticipating medical surge and continuity of operations requirements. Challenges, such as the evaluation of minimally symptomatic individuals or the evaluation of large volumes of patients, can be facilitated by receiving clear and concise information from public health. **The most important assistance public health can provide to all clinicians is in the development of a community-wide patient evaluation and treatment protocol.** Evaluation and treatment protocols provide criteria to stratify individual and population risk for exposure and guide steps for specific evaluation and treatment. The protocol also should include recommended testing, treatment, patient instructions, tracking of at-risk cohorts, and public education.

A single evaluation and treatment protocol provides a uniform method across a community to evaluate patients presenting with possible exposure. This is important not only for individual practitioners but also for the public. During the 2001 anthrax incident, the initial epidemiologic investigation in the Washington metropolitan area used nasal swabs in suspect exposures. This practice was misunderstood by some clinicians and the public as having individual diagnostic utility when, in fact, it was merely an epidemiologic surveillance tool. Anxiety and confusion resulted when individuals received nasal swabbing at some healthcare locations and were (correctly) told it was not useful for diagnosis at other medical facilities. Because no early standardized protocol was developed by the public health system, hospitals implemented their own individual protocols to limit variation between clinicians practicing within individual hospitals. The resultant variability between institutions, however, caused great consternation for patients and, subsequently, for providers.

Critical information that the public health system should also provide includes a clear and concise case definition for the particular agent in question. **A case definition imparts definitive clinical and diagnostic criteria for an individual patient.** Within the case definition, criteria should be supplied that define "presumptive" or "suspect" cases for patients awaiting confirmatory testing. This kind of tool is simple and allows practitioners to officially designate victims as "confirmed" or "presumptive/suspected" for the target illness. Similarly delineated "exposure" categories are helpful in providing criteria for stratifying risk by designating "confirmed" or "presumptive" (suspected) exposure.

INTEGRATION WITH OTHER RESPONSE ASSETS

Requests for assistance or for resources not available within an individual hospital should be coordinated through the hospital administration to other hospitals (through mutual aid mechanisms), the local department of health, and/or the local emergency management agency. From there, requests may be transmitted to the regional, state, or federal levels.[18]

TREATMENT

General treatment principles for victims of bioterrorism should be understood by the practitioner. Specific therapies for individual Class A agents are listed in Table 9-2. From a population perspective, morbidity and mortality are primarily minimized by preventing exposure and providing prophylaxis and immunization as appropriate, and then by treating the infected, symptomatic patients. Treatment may involve specific pharmaceuticals or general supportive care. Depending on the agent involved, prophylaxis or immunization of the hospital staff may be warranted. **Prophylaxis, immunization, or treatment may be indicated even without obvious signs of disease or definitive information about exposure.** This makes the practitioner heavily reliant on the public health sector to stratify patient risk based on exposure and to provide evidence-based prophylaxis and treatment. With specific agents (e.g., anthrax), large community-based efforts have been developed with federal support related to the dispensing of postexposure prophylaxis (i.e., Medical Counter Measures).[20]

MEDICAL SURGE

One of the critical issues in providing treatment to victims of bioterrorism is the development of adequate medical surge.[18] This issue is complicated by current healthcare industry practices that minimize staff, maintain just-in-time inventory, and limit hospital bed capacity. Medical surge capacity is developed by first maximizing individual healthcare facility capacity and capabilities (through an effective emergency operations plan) and then by coordinating regional resources to address and match patient needs to available resources. The development of emergency healthcare coalitions is supported by federal funding through the national Hospital Preparedness Program, in part to achieve this surge requirement through information dissemination and effective mutual aid. State and federal assistance should also be included in planning but not relied upon for at least the first 48 hours.

Federal agencies distinguish medical *surge capacity* from *surge capability*, which similarly can pose challenges.[18] *Medical surge capability* refers to the ability to manage patients requiring unusual or very specialized medical evaluation and care. It is intuitively obvious, for example, that even one patient presenting with signs and symptoms of smallpox would present highly unusual challenges affecting any hospital's continuity of operations.

DISEASE CONTAINMENT

Infection control guidelines for the diagnosed or suspected agent should be put into practice. This is essential to protect clinicians, hospital staff, visitors, and other patients. It is also critical in maintaining the ability of the hospital to continue its regular medical commitment to the community. The Association for Professionals in Infection Control and Epidemiology has published guidelines for hospital infection control in response to a bioterrorist event.[21] Most agents of concern require only standard precautions (gloves, mucous membrane protection when potential for splashing exists, and a gown when the potential exists for soiling), but meticulous attention to detail is required. The more troubling agents are those that are contagious through airborne or droplet transmission. Disease containment for a case of pneumonic plague requires droplet protection and patient isolation. Smallpox requires airborne and contact precautions and, therefore, full patient isolation. If a contagious disease is spreading within the community, procedures must be instituted to screen everyone entering the healthcare facility (e.g., staff, patients, visitors, delivery personnel) for active disease. This screening should ideally take place in an appropriately established "facility" before entering or immediately upon entry into the hospital building.

Isolation of large numbers of infectious patients may be necessary. Current hospital configurations often prohibit large-scale containment of patients in official isolation rooms, but entire wings could be adapted (using fire doors and manipulation of ventilation/air pressure within hospital smoke compartments) to serve as isolation wards. Plans to provide adequate separation from other, noninfected patients, to designate and train specific staff to care for these patients, and to furnish proper personal protective equipment should be developed in the emergency operations plan annex.

Another important initial consideration for ED personnel is whether patient decontamination is indicated. **Decontamination is a consideration only if a patient presents shortly after acute exposure to a substance suspected or confirmed as a biologic agent, in contrast to the presentation of the patient who has already developed symptoms of an infectious disease.** If a realistic concern exists, simply disrobing the patient and showering with soap and warm water should be adequate decontamination, but this must be accomplished in a controlled environment before patient entry into the healthcare facility. Clothing and personal belongings should be secured to assist with the public health and law enforcement investigations. Decontamination agents, such as diluted bleach, should be avoided, due to their potential for harm and the lack of demonstrated clinical or protective efficacy.[22,23]

SUPPLY MANAGEMENT

Just-in-time inventory practices may limit the amount of vaccine, antibiotics, and other pharmaceuticals and supplies available. Vendors for emergency back-up supplies and equipment are commonly shared by multiple institutions, each counting the vendor's back-up cache as their own. Having a community-wide mutual aid system between all the hospitals promotes appropriate sharing of critical supplies, equipment, and staff during an emergency. If prescriptions are being written for antibiotics, the local pharmacies' on-hand supply should be considered (an issue during the anthrax incident in 2001). Writing short-course prescriptions with procedures to provide completion of the medication regimen may be indicated until adequate supplies are available, but this strategy should be implemented on a region-wide basis to not place an individual practitioner's patients at increased risk. Integration of Strategic National Stockpile supplies into a medical community has specific requirements that are available for review through the Centers for Disease Control and Prevention and requires specific planning by the community emergency management and public health agencies.[18]

PATIENT MANAGEMENT

In unusual and very threatening situations such as bioterrorism, addressing the requirements of each patient encountered and maximizing efficiency can markedly facilitate the overall processing of victims. For those patients who are potentially exposed but not physically ill, the patient interaction may require sophisticated explanations as to why the individual is or is not receiving a particular therapy. Preprinted instructions (indicating category of risk stratification and why the patient was placed in that category) can increase efficiency and be helpful for patients being treated and released. These instructions should clearly indicate how the disease is transmitted, measures that prevent spread, and early signs and symptoms of disease with appropriate steps if they should occur. Appropriate follow-up should be established (in a large-scale incident, this may not be with a primary care physician but through a public health venue). It is important to note any change in the epidemiology of the incident (e.g., a new site tests positive for the agent) or if new information becomes available on the etiologic agent itself (e.g., antibiotic resistance patterns). Patients may need to be rapidly re-contacted to change therapy. Proper record keeping and organization of charts based on assigned risk category can assist with this process. Entering all patients into a reliable long-term surveillance database should be a task for the public health agency, but hospitals and EDs could facilitate this process.

For agents of concern that have an available vaccine, such as anthrax and smallpox, in a preincident setting, recommendations are to withhold vaccination for the general public.[23,24] Anthrax vaccination requires a series of five injections followed by yearly updates. A 2003 initiative to vaccinate healthcare workers and willing civilians against smallpox was discontinued after only a minority of the target cohort actually accepted vaccinations. The risk of potential life-threatening side effects, such as generalized vaccinia and potential cardiac sequelae, complicates the recommendations for smallpox vaccination in the absence of known disease.[25]

Therapeutics recommended for some bioterrorism agents are normally not approved for children or for pregnant or lactating women. In many situations, these recommendations are relaxed (e.g., Emergency Use Authorization) when the risk of infection and its consequences exceeds the risks of the medication or vaccine. In addition, some unique treatments (e.g., ciprofloxacin for anthrax prophylaxis in children) have received U.S. Food and Drug Administration approval.

REFERENCES

The complete reference list is available online at www.TintinalliEM.com.

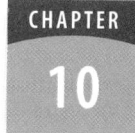

Radiation Injuries

Annette M. Lopez
Jennifer A. Stephani

INTRODUCTION

Radiation exposure may either be accidental or intentional. The year 2015 marked the 70th anniversary of the bombing of Hiroshima and Nagasaki, with nearly 200,000 acute deaths and untold numbers with chronic disability. Accidental exposures can occur during transport, storage, or working with radioactive materials or with errors in dosing radiotherapy. Most civilian incidents involve industrial exposures from sealed radiation sources.[1] The Fukushima Daiichi nuclear disaster resulted in about 1000 disaster-related deaths; however as of this writing, no deaths were related to radiation exposure.[2]

The largest reported accidental exposure took place in Goiania, Brazil in 1987. An "orphaned" cesium-137 radiosource was left in place at an abandoned radiotherapy institute. Individuals looking for scrap metal removed the source and dismantled it. They proceeded to sell it to a junk dealer, who observed the material glowing in the dark. Due to this unique characteristic, he distributed it to family and friends, who quickly became ill with acute radiation syndrome. At the conclusion of this event, there were 112,000 individuals evaluated for exposures, 249 who were contaminated, 20 who required hospital admissions, and four who died.[3,4]

A famous case of malicious intentional exposure involved Alexander Litvinenko, a former KGB agent who had defected to England. In 2006, after a meeting with former co-workers, he suffered a protracted gastrointestinal illness with associated leukopenia. On the day of his death, elevated levels of polonium-210 were identified, confirming his death from radiation exposure. Investigations into his murder revealed that there are had been rehearsals in multiple areas of England leading to contamination.[5] The public health response that followed found that there were 1693 local and international individuals who were potentially exposed during such rehearsals.[6,7]

Radiologic dispersal devices, or "dirty bombs," combine radioactive materials with conventional explosives in attempts to disperse "hot material" over an unsuspecting population. The intended use of these devices is to generate some injuries, but the true goal is to generate massive panic and hysteria, overwhelm local resources, affect the local economy, and lead to prolonged clean-up efforts.[4]

FUNDAMENTALS OF RADIATION PHYSICS

Radiation energy includes the entire electromagnetic spectrum: from low-energy, long-wavelength, and low-frequency *nonionizing radiation*, such as radio waves and microwaves, to high-energy, short-wavelength, and high-frequency forms of *ionizing radiation*. Ionizing radiation has enough energy to remove an electron from an atom and generate charged particles. Sources of ionizing radiation are: alpha particles, beta particles, neutrons, and sole energy waves that include x-rays and gamma rays.[8]

Alpha and beta particles and positrons are charged particles that directly interact with electrons of the atom. Neutrons are not charged, and they lead to expulsion of other particles after interactions with the atomic nuclei, so neutrons indirectly generate charged atoms. Gamma and x-rays are electromagnetic waves that destabilize the atomic nucleus and lead to the expulsion of ionized particles (**Table 10-1**).

ALPHA PARTICLES

Alpha particles have relatively large size (two protons and two neutrons), have limited travel potential, and are unable to penetrate the outer layers of the skin. Thus, alpha particles are easily shielded with a piece of paper. Exposure to alpha particles only leads to pathology in the setting of ingestion, inhalation, or absorption. Detection can be problematic because common Geiger counters do not detect alpha particles without a special attachment.[8]

BETA PARTICLES

Beta particles are much smaller (a single electron) than alpha particles. Small size allows for greater penetration ability. Beta radiation can travel several meters in air, penetrates approximately 8 mm into exposed skin, and can cause serious burns. Beta radiation is a hazard if internally deposited. Most radioisotopes decay by beta radiation followed by gamma emission.[8]

POSITRONS

Positrons are positively charged beta particles that are emitted from the atomic nuclei. They are the antiparticles to the electron, and interactions with electrons lead to the generation of highly energetic photons that requires shielding with lead, steel, or concrete. Positron sources are commonly used in medical procedures such as positron emission tomography scanning.[8]

NEUTRONS

Neutrons are uncharged particles that are capable of generating radiation via alterations of the atomic nuclear proton-to-electron ratio. These particles are capable of traveling large distances and require the use of helium, water, and paraffin as shielding. Neutron exposures are rare and tend to be limited to nuclear fallout, research, industry, and weapons manufacturing.[8]

GAMMA RAYS AND X-RAYS

Gamma rays and high-energy x-rays are able to travel meters in the air and can penetrate centimeters into human tissue. Shielding materials must be very dense, such as concrete or lead. Individuals exposed to high doses of these sources are at high risk of developing acute radiation syndrome.[8]

BIOLOGIC EFFECTS OF IONIZING RADIATION

Ionizing radiation leads to cellular effects at both high and low levels of exposure. At high doses, ionizing radiation causes cell death. At lower doses, it interrupts cellular reproduction through inhibition of mitosis, resulting in cellular injury with delayed onset of effects.[9]

Radiosensitivity refers to the response of cells to radiation injury. Rapidly dividing cells with short life spans are the cells most vulnerable to radiation injury, because they are quickly depleted and new cells are unable to replete the population.[4]

MEASURING RADIATION

There are many ways in which radiation can be measured: dose given, exposure received, absorbed dose, or activity generated. Many conventional units may be used, and confusion can arise between interchanging units. See **Table 10-2** for more information on units of measure.

RADIATION MONITORING EQUIPMENT

Just as there are many radiation units, there are many ways to monitor radiation exposures. Commonly used equipment includes dosimeters and survey meters (**Table 10-3**). In the setting of radiation emergencies, both of these devices should be available to ED staff. Staff should wear dosimeters because of their small size and ability to measure and record an individual's cumulative exposure doses. In contrast, rate meters are survey instruments that record the amount of radiation in an area over a particular time course and are best suited to monitor environmental contamination.

ALLOWED ANNUAL DOSE OF RADIATION

Radiation exposures are an unavoidable hazard of living on our planet. Common sources of unavoidable radiation include cosmic and

TABLE 10-1 Types of Radiation

Type (Symbol)	Charge	Penetration	Shield	Hazard	Source
Alpha	+2	Few centimeters in air	Paper, keratin layer of skin	Internal contamination only; requires special detection devices	Heavy radioisotopes (e.g., plutonium, uranium, radon)
Beta	−1	~8 mm into skin	Clothing	External (skin) and internal contamination	Most radioisotopes decay by beta followed by gamma emission
Positron	+1	~8 mm into skin	Lead, steel or concrete	Interacts with electrons and releases photons of energy	Medical tracers
Neutron	0	Variable	Material with high hydrogen content	Whole-body irradiation	Nuclear power plants, particle accelerators, weapons assembly plants
Gamma and x-rays	0	Several centimeters in tissue	Concrete, lead	Whole-body irradiation	Most radioisotopes decay by beta followed by gamma emission

TABLE 10-2 Radiation Units of Measure

Description	Conventional Units	SI Unit	Conversion
Activity	Curie	Becquerel	1 Bq ~2.7 × 10^{11} Ci
Units of activity describe the amount of radioactivity present.			1 Ci ~3.7 × 10^{10} Bq
Exposure	Roentgen	Coulomb per kilogram	1 R = 2.58 × 10^4 cP/kg
Units of exposure measure the amount of x-ray or gamma radiation that produces a given number of ionizations in air.			
Absorbed dose	rad	Gray	1 rad = 0.01 Gy
Units of absorbed dose can be applied to any type of radiation and reflect the energy imparted to matter.			1 Gy = 100 rad
Dose equivalent	Roentgen equivalents man	Sievert	1 rem = 0.01 Sv
Units that provide a common scale of measure for the different types of radiation.			1 Sv = 100 rem

Abbreviation: SI = International System of Units.

solar rays, naturally occurring elements such as radon and uranium, and even some of the carbon in our bodies. The background radiation dose of individuals living in the United States is approximately 6.2 mSv (620 mrem).[10] The International Commission on Radiological Protection, the National Commission on Radiological Protection and Measurements, and the Health Physics Society have set the annual radiation dose limit for the general public at 1 mSv per year (100 mrem) over natural background radiation. See **Table 10-4** for selected approximate levels of radiation exposure.

LETHAL DOSE OF RADIATION

The $LD_{50/60}$ from exposure to ionizing radiation is defined as the dose of penetrating ionizing radiation that will result in the deaths (lethal dose) of 50% of the exposed population within 60 days without medical treatment. Regarding human survival, the most commonly cited value is an $LD_{50/60}$ of approximately 3.5 to 4.5 Gy (350 to 450 rad).[8] In the setting of supportive medical therapy, including antibiotics, blood products, and reverse isolation, the value is 4.8 to 5.4 Gy (480 to 540 rad). During mass exposures where resources may be limited to basic first aid, the $LD_{50/60}$ falls to approximately 3.4 Gy (340 rad). The use of stem cell transplantation and hematopoietic growth factor administration has theoretically increased the $LD_{50/60}$ to 11 Gy (1100 rad).[11]

TABLE 10-3 Radiation Monitoring Equipment

Equipment Type	Device	Common Type of Measurement	Units Commonly Recorded
Dosimeter	Thermoluminescent dosimeter or film badge	Cumulative dose of beta, x-ray, and gamma	Roentgen equivalents man or sieverts
Dosimeter	Pocket dosimeter	Cumulative exposure to x-ray and gamma	Milliroentgen
Survey meter	Geiger-Müeller tube	Low exposure rates of x-ray, gamma, and beta*	Counts per minute†
Survey meter	Ion chamber	Higher exposure rates of x-ray and gamma	Milliroentgen per hour

*With special instrument probes, alpha radiation can also be detected.

†2500 counts per minute equal approximately 1 mR/h.

TABLE 10-4 Selected Approximate Levels of Radiation Exposure

Natural background radiation	620 mrem/y (U.S. average)
Chest x-ray (effective dose)	10 mrem
Abdominal x-ray	120 mrem
Lumbar spine x-ray	70 mrem
CT head	200 mrem
CT chest	700 mrem
CT abdomen or pelvis	1000 mrem
Jet travel	1 mrem per 1000 miles traveled
Annual radiation dose limit (public)	100 mrem/y*
Occupational exposure limit	5000 mrem/y
Lethal dose in 50% of exposed subjects within 60 d (3.5–4.5 Gy)	350,000–450,000 mrem (350–450 rad†)

*over natural background radiation.

†1 rem (dose equivalent) = 1 rad (absorbed dose or exposure).

CLINICAL EFFECTS OF RADIATION

LOCAL RADIATION INJURY

Most radiation accidents are due to local radiation injury from partial-body exposure. Partial-body irradiation rarely causes systemic manifestations; rather, it leads to a dose-dependent *cutaneous* involvement. Typically, the injury in the first week tends to be asymptomatic, although there may be transient erythema (6 Gy/600 rad), hyperesthesia, and itching. The second week is characterized by the development of erythema that progresses to hair loss (3 Gy/300 rad). The development of skin tenderness, swelling, and pruritus heralds the third week after exposure. Within the fourth week, the wound will develop dry (10 to 15 Gy/1000 to 1500 rad) or wet (15 to 20 Gy/1500 to 2000 rad) desquamation and/or ulceration (>25 Gy/2500 rad).[12]

Skin findings may be indistinguishable from thermal burns. Radiation injuries are hallmarked by episodes of transient erythema and delayed onset of prolonged and severe pain. As long as the exposure is less than 50 Gy (5000 rad), these injuries develop over a much longer time period than thermal burns. When doses exceed 50 Gy, these injuries will progress similarly to thermal burns, and the onset of pain will occur immediately. Surgical intervention such as resection and grafting may be required.

ACUTE RADIATION SYNDROME

Acute Radiation Syndrome occurs after a significant exposure to penetrating ionizing radiation within a 24-hour time period (**Table 10-5**). It

TABLE 10-5 Acute Radiation Syndrome

Approximate Dose	Onset of Prodrome	Duration of Latent Phase	Manifest Illness
>2 Gy (200 rad)	Within 2 d	1–3 wk	Hematopoietic syndrome with pancytopenia, infection, and hemorrhage; survival possible
>6 Gy (600 rad)	Within hours	<1 wk	GI syndrome with dehydration, electrolyte abnormalities, GI bleeding, and fulminant enterocolitis; death likely
>20–30 Gy (2000–3000 rad)	Within minutes	None	Cardiovascular/CNS syndrome with refractory hypotension and circulatory collapse; fatal within 24–72 h

should be expected in cases in which a whole-body gamma dose exceeds of 2 Gy (200 rad). External sources of alpha and beta radiation are unable to penetrate the body, although internal contamination may lead to this syndrome. Neutron sources, although rarely encountered, can also lead to acute radiation syndrome.

Acute radiation syndrome develops in four distinct phases: prodrome, latent phase, manifest-illness, and recovery. The initial **prodrome** involves the transient autonomic nervous system response to the exposure. It is directly related to the dose received. High doses cause acute and severe symptom onset, whereas lower doses may lead to prolonged onset and milder symptoms. Nausea, vomiting, anorexia, and diarrhea may be accompanied by hypotension, pyrexia, diaphoresis, cephalgia, and fatigue.

The prodrome is followed by the **latent phase**, a symptom-free interval whose duration depends on the received dose. Larger doses result in a shorter duration of this phase. Doses less than 4 Gy are associated with a period that may last 1 to 3 weeks, whereas in doses greater than 15 Gy, this phase may only last a few hours.

The **manifest-illness phase** is subdivided into three dose-dependent syndromes that are hallmarked by the affected organ system. The syndromes are not independent of one another, and there is synergy and overlap leading to the clinical manifestations. The final stage is **recovery**.

Hematopoietic Syndrome The hematopoietic system is the first organ system that demonstrates injury when doses exceed 1.5 Gy. The prodromal phase of this subsyndrome occurs within hours to a few days from the exposure, resolves within 48 hours, and is followed by a latent phase that on average lasts 1 to 3 weeks.

Radiation damages the bone marrow stem cells and destroys circulating hematopoietic cells, particularly lymphocytes (**Figure 10-1**). Because of the preferential destruction of lymphocytes, the peripheral lymphocyte count is currently the best marker to grade the extent of the injury. Granulocytes and platelets are also affected. However, being markers of inflammation, their counts rise in the immediate time period following the exposure, and later decline and reach a nadir within 30 days of the injury. Red blood cells are also affected but not to the same extent of the other lines due to the lack of nuclear material. Morbidity and mortality depend on associated pancytopenia, immunosuppression, and hemorrhage. Aggressive medical management with blood products and growth factors may increase survival.

GI Syndrome Doses greater than 6 Gy (>600 rad) cause the GI syndrome. Nausea, vomiting, and diarrhea develop within hours of exposure. This is followed by a short latent phase lasting up to 1 week. The manifest-illness phase is characterized by the recrudescence of severe nausea, vomiting, diarrhea, and abdominal pain. The initial insult leads to the apoptotic death of the GI mucosa, with associated insult to the underlying stem cells responsible for their replenishment. Impaired mucosal integrity causes massive fluid and electrolyte losses and allows the translocation of enteric flora into the bloodstream. Fulminating enterocolitis results.

Cardiovascular and CNS Syndrome The last subsyndromes of the manifest-illness phase are the cardiovascular and CNS syndromes, resulting from doses greater than 20 to 30 Gy (>2000 to 3000 rad). There is immediate hypotension, prostration, nausea, vomiting, and explosive bloody diarrhea. Hypotension is persistent and unresponsive to treatment. CNS symptoms manifest within hours and include seizures, lethargy, disorientation, ataxia, and tremors. The lymphocyte count, the quickest marker available to determine the extent of injury, very quickly falls to near-zero levels. Death from circulatory collapse ensues within 72 hours.

EMERGENCY RESPONSE PLANNING

Emergency response plans should involve multiple community-wide organizations, including hospitals, EDs, public safety, public health, and emergency management officials. Every EMS system should have a prehospital plan for the evacuation of victims from a radiation disaster. Every hospital is required by The Joint Commission to have a written protocol detailing instructions for receiving and treating radiation victims. Hospitals should stage regular disaster drills and train personnel in decontamination procedures, use of personal protective equipment, and radiologic monitoring. Planning templates exist to assist hospitals in developing appropriate radiation emergency response plans.[13,14]

PREHOSPITAL EMERGENCY MEDICAL MANAGEMENT

Emergency responders should rapidly establish incident command in a situation involving radioactive materials. Personal protective equipment and respiratory protection should be used as the situation dictates. Care and transportation of seriously injured victims should not be delayed, even if the patient is contaminated. In medically stable patients, perform radiation monitoring and decontamination at the scene.

ED NOTIFICATION AND PREPARATION

First responders must communicate with hospitals prior to arrival to allow adequate preparation. Provide incident information such as circumstances of the event, number of victims, type of radiologic insult, and identification of radioactive material (if known). Coexisting medical conditions and traumatic injuries need to be reported. Extent of completed patient decontamination should also be relayed. The hospital disaster plan should include steps that need to be initiated by the ED upon notification to prepare for a radiologic event (**Table 10-6**).

The hospital protocol should instruct ED personnel how to contact predetermined local radiation specialists and health physics professionals. These specialists may assist by monitoring radiation doses of personnel,

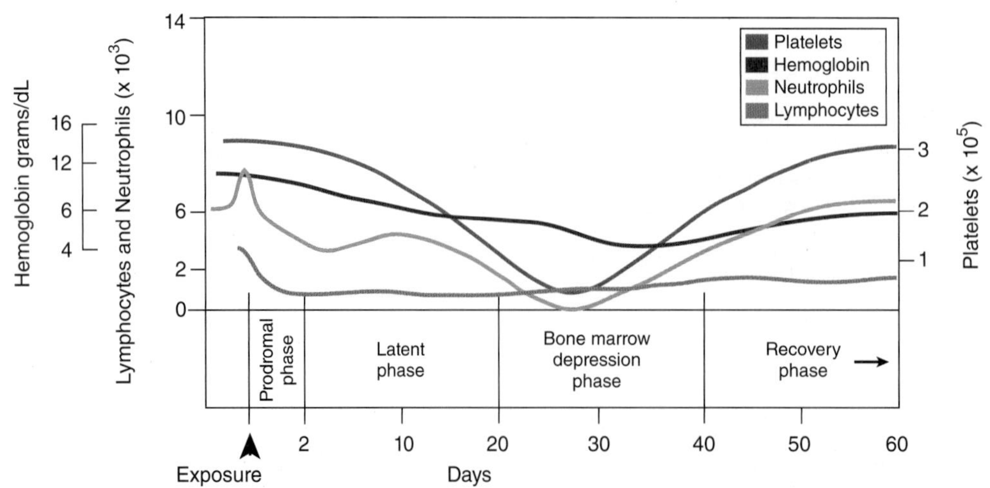

FIGURE 10-1. Typical hematologic course and clinical stages after sublethal (~3 Gy/300 rad) exposure to total-body irradiation.

TABLE 10-6 ED Preparation

Initiate hospital disaster plan.
- Mobilize hospital radiation experts (radiation safety officer, nuclear medicine and radiation oncology experts and staff).
- Request dosimeters for staff and radiation monitoring and survey instruments.

Prepare the ED.
- Establish an ad hoc triage area based on the location designated in the hospital disaster plan.
- Establish a "contaminated" area and "clean" area separated by a buffer zone using ropes, tape, and signs to designate areas.
- Remove contaminated outer garments when leaving contaminated area and have your body surveyed with a radiation meter prior to leaving the area.
- Cover floors with plastic or paper secured with heavy tape.
- Remove pregnant women, nonessential personnel, and nonessential equipment.
- Request extra gloves, other medical supplies, and extra large plastic bags for disposal.

Use standard precautions to protect staff.
- Staff should wear a water-resistant gown, cap, and shoe covers to keep contaminants off skin and clothes.
- Double glove with inner glove taped in place, changing the top pair after handling contaminated items and between patients.
- N95 masks, if available, are recommended, but surgical masks should be adequate.
- Survey hands and clothing at frequent intervals with a radiation meter.
- Dosimeters, if available, should be worn at the collar, under protective clothing.

surveying personnel and areas for contamination, directing contamination control and decontamination efforts, and disposing of contaminated wastes. If radiation monitors are not available, patients should undergo decontamination and then be surveyed for residual contamination when monitoring equipment is available.

TRIAGE PRINCIPLES

When there are multiple victims, field triage protocols will designate patients as minor, delayed, immediate, or deceased depending on physical trauma or burns. Do not alter triage principles based solely on radiation exposure. **Because radioactive contamination is never immediately life-threatening, do not delay treatment of life-threatening injuries for radiologic surveying.** Morbidity and mortality from ionizing radiation injuries increase dramatically in the face of physical trauma, thermal burns, and other significant medical conditions. In a mass-casualty event that could include blast injuries in addition to radiologic insult, resources may be limited and will require a coordinated approach to develop the best management plan.

TREATMENT

Because most radiation injuries are not immediately life-threatening, there is usually time to determine whether the patient was irradiated, externally contaminated, or internally contaminated. Early treatment decisions are based on the signs and symptoms evident in the first 24 to 48 hours and corresponding laboratory test results.[15,16] **Figure 10-2** illustrates the medical treatment prioritization for those exposed to and/or contaminated with radioactivity.

DECONTAMINATION OF EXTERNALLY CONTAMINATED PATIENTS

It is highly unlikely that the radioactivity from a contaminated patient would pose a significant risk to healthcare personnel. However, the goal of decontamination measures is to decrease total exposure of the patient and staff, by minimizing radiation exposure from a source external to the body to a level that is as low as reasonably achievable (**Table 10-7**). This is accomplished by minimizing time of exposure and the quantity of radioactive materials in the area, as well as maximizing distance and shielding from the source.[16,17]

ACUTE RADIATION SYNDROME

Direct treatment of the irradiated patient toward alleviating the symptoms of the prodromal phase. Pain can be managed with acetaminophen and opioids. Because the patient may be at risk for significant GI bleeding if the exposure dose is more than 5 to 6 Gy, avoid using nonsteroidal anti-inflammatory agents.[8] Administer antiemetics for nausea and vomiting. Ondansetron or other 5-hydroxytryptamine-3 antagonists are effective.[18] Use antidiarrheal agents as needed.

Complete laboratory testing as soon as possible. Biologic dosimetry uses laboratory analyses (e.g., rate and nadir of lymphocyte depletion) and clinical signs to estimate absorbed dose. Cytogenetic analysis for chromosomal aberrations (dicentrics) is the gold standard for biodosimetry. Contact the Radiation Emergency Assistance Center/Training Site for assistance with obtaining chromosomal testing.

Perform a targeted history and physical exam. Note time of onset of all symptoms, especially vomiting and diarrhea, which are important in biologic dosimetry. Observe for abnormal vital signs suggestive of acute radiation syndrome, including fever, hypotension, tachycardia, and tachypnea. Monitor for impaired level of consciousness, ataxia, motor or sensory deficits, reflex abnormalities or papilledema, abdominal tenderness, and GI bleeding.

Obtain a baseline CBC with differential and absolute lymphocyte count in the ED and check a CBC every 6 hours for 24–48 hours. Monitor the CBC for progressive declines in lymphocytes as an indicator of total dose. Also obtain a baseline serum amylase and C-reactive protein, because dose-dependent increases are expected after 24 hours in a significant exposure. If vomiting and diarrhea occur in the first 2 to 3 hours (dose estimated to >2 Gy), consider the need for human leukocyte antigen typing in anticipation of pancytopenia requiring further management. This could include administration of blood products, cytokines, colony-stimulating factors, bone marrow cells, or stem cell transplant.[19] The goal is to bridge cytopenic gaps and manage subsequent infections. Patients may require antibiotics, antifungals, and antivirals during their course.

Monitor patients with large exposures who survive the acute phase for severe infectious and metabolic complications. Treat multiorgan failure from a large radiation exposure with standard supportive measures.[20]

LOCAL RADIATION INJURY

Analgesia is important in the early management of cutaneous radiation injury. Cutaneous radiation injury differs from thermal burns in that the cutaneous injury continues to evolve and may not be visible to the naked eye. The primary goal of treatment is interruption of radiation-induced inflammation in the dermis. Perform traditional burn care, including burn dressings, surgical debridement, and grafting, when indicated. Consider applying topical steroids to control local inflammation[16] and giving vitamin A, C, and E supplementation, and pentoxifylline to decrease blood viscosity and increase blood flow.[17] Systemic steroids are not recommended.[20] Although inpatient treatment may not be always be required, close follow-up is essential given the potential for ongoing evolution of cutaneous injury.

INTERNALLY CONTAMINATED PATIENTS

Internal contamination generally does not produce early symptoms but should be considered if persistently high radiation survey readings are notedand with all nose or mouth contamination cases. Obtain a 24-hour urine collection for possible radionuclide identification. Collect other specimens depending on exposure with or without contamination (**Table 10-8**). Consult radiation experts for treatment with cathartics, activated charcoal, gastric lavage, and radionuclide-specific decorporation agents (**Table 10-9**). Duration of therapy is based on dose estimations from radiochemical measurements of urine and fecal samples.

PRENATAL EXPOSURES

Fetal sensitivity to radiation depends on a number of factors, including radiation dose and gestational age. The radiation dose to the fetus may not be the same as the dose to the mother, because the fetus is shielded

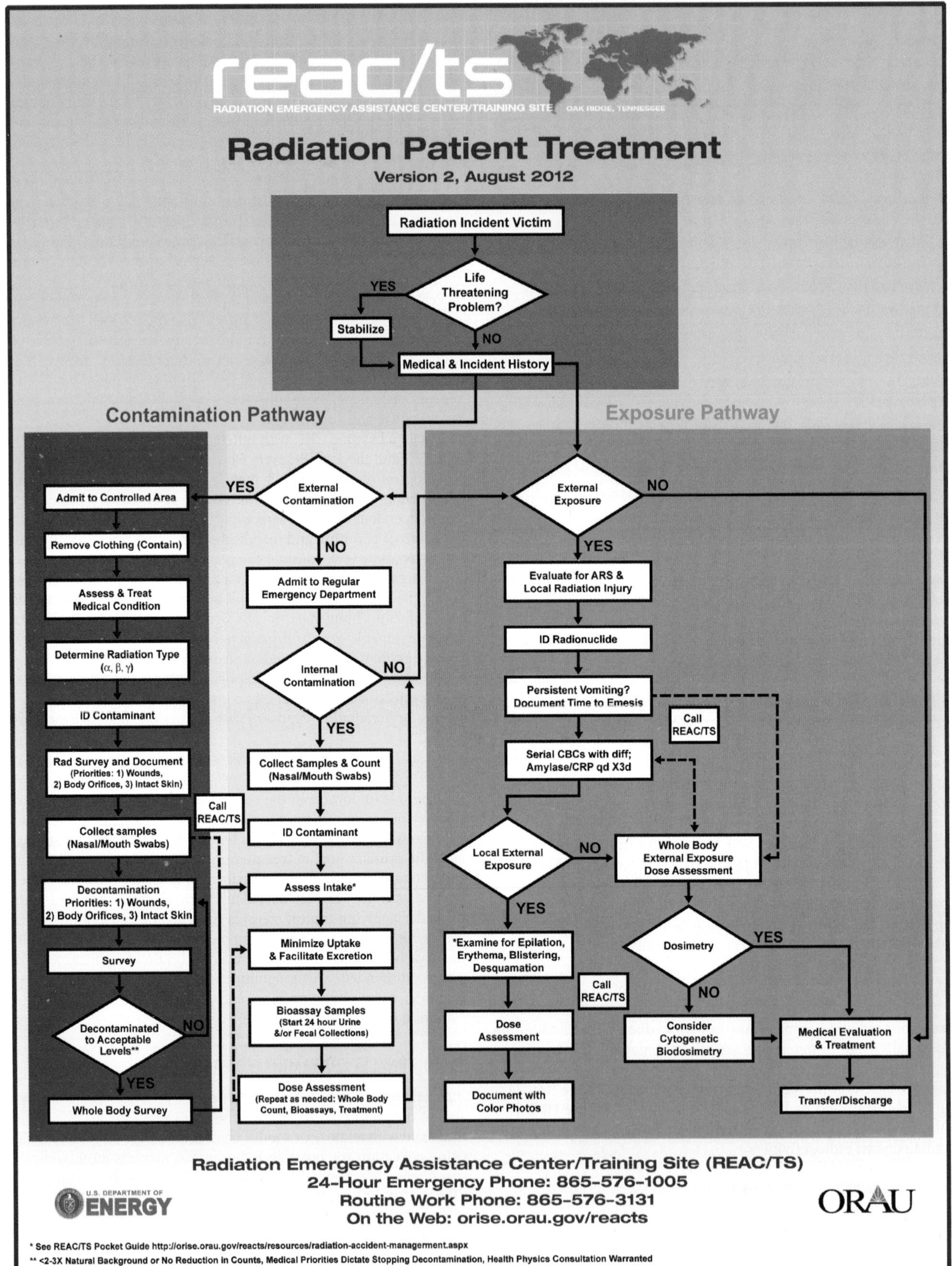

FIGURE 10-2. Medical treatment flow diagram for those exposed to or contaminated with ionizing radiation. [Diagram used with permission of Radiation Emergency Assistance Center/Training Site (REAC/TS), Oak Ridge, TN, under contract number DE-AC05-06OR23100 between the U.S. Department of Energy and Oak Ridge Associated Universities.]

TABLE 10-7 Steps of Patient Decontamination

Assess external contamination.
- Contact radiation safety officer.
- Assess contamination with radiation survey meter (Geiger counter).
- Evaluate for radioactive shrapnel. Easily accessible pieces should be removed with a forceps and placed in a lead container.
- Document contamination pattern on a body diagram.
- Swab each nostril separately to estimate level of internal contamination of the lungs.

Decontaminate whole body.
- Carefully cut and roll clothing away from the face to contain contamination.
- Double bag clothing and label as hazardous waste.
- Wash wounds first with saline or water.
- If facial contamination is present, rinse as appropriate.
- Gently cleanse intact skin and avoid scrubbing.
- Repeat patient scan with radiation survey meter. Repeat washing until radiation is <2 times background. Avoid scrubbing.
- Cover wounds with waterproof dressing.

TABLE 10-9 Internal Contamination Treatment

Radionuclide	Ionizing Radiation	Treatment	Mechanism of Action	Usual Administration
Iodine (I-131)	β, γ	Potassium iodide	Block thyroid uptake	130 milligrams PO for adults
Plutonium (Pu-239)	α	Ca-DTPA or Zn-DTPA	Chelation	1 gram in 250 mL NS or 5% dextrose in water over 60 min
Tritium (H-3)	β	Water	Dilution	Oral: 3–4 L a day for 2 wk
Cesium (Cs-137)	β, γ	Prussian blue	Decrease GI uptake	1 gram in 100–200 mL water three times a day for several days
Uranium (U-235)	α	Bicarbonate	Urine alkalinization	2 ampules in 1 L NS at 125 mL/h

Abbreviations: DTPA = diethylenetriamine pentaacetate; NS = normal saline.

in part by the uterus and surrounding tissues. External exposure of alpha and beta particles is unlikely to reach the fetus, but gamma and x-rays directed toward a pregnant woman's abdomen could harm the fetus. In addition, internal contamination could expose the fetus to higher radiation, because the radioactive material could accumulate in the bladder of the pregnant woman.

The health effects of radiation on the fetus are dependent on the gestational age. Before about 2 weeks of gestation, there is an all-or-none phenomenon, and if the exposure does not result in death of the embryo, no observable effects would be expected. An exposure of greater than 0.1 Gy is expected to be lethal, resulting in resorption of the conceptus. From 2 to 8 weeks, organogenesis occurs. During this time, the embryo is at risk for congenital malformations and growth retardation. In cases of substantial exposures, there is a significant risk of major malformations of the neurologic and motor systems. After 8 weeks of gestation, most organogenesis is complete with the exception of the CNS. Exposures during this period have an increased risk of mental retardation and miscarriage. Throughout gestation, an exposure of less than 0.05 Gy would not be expected to produce an increased risk of noncancer health effects. Consult with radiation medicine physicians regarding fetal dose estimation and risk assessment counseling for the expecting parents.[21] For additional discussion, see chapter 99, Comorbid Disorders in Pregnancy.

TABLE 10-8 Specimens for Medical Assessment

Specimen/Type of Analysis	Reason	Mechanism
Suspected radiation exposure		
Check a CBC every 6 hours for 24–48 hours	Establish baseline and assess lymphocyte depletion as an early predictor of dose.	Venipuncture
Serum amylase and CRP, repeat daily for 3 days	Parotid glands are sensitive to radiation; amylase will rise if exposed to >0.5 Gy.	Venipuncture
Blood: chromosomal analysis (dicentrics)	Gold standard for estimating dose.	Venipuncture. Call REAC/TS for assistance.
Urine: routine urinalysis	Establish baseline kidney function, especially if internal contamination is suspected.	Clean catch
Suspected external contamination		
Swabs of body orifices and samples from dressings/wounds	Assess internal contamination and identify radionuclide.	Use separate saline or water-moistened swabs to wipe the inside of each nostril, ear, and mouth.
Suspected internal contamination		
Urine bioassay: 24-h specimen; repeat for 4 d	Radionuclide identification.	Standard specimen containers
Consider feces bioassay in consult with radiation expert		

CRP = C-reactive protein; REAC/TS = Radiation Emergency Assistance Center/Training Site.

SOURCES OF ASSISTANCE

Two organizations provide medical advice for the treatment of radiation casualties. The Radiation Emergency Assistance Center/Training Site, sponsored by the Department of Energy and managed by the Oak Ridge Institute for Science and Education, provides training programs, consultation assistance, and treatment capabilities, and can dispatch an emergency response team of health professionals to assist at an accident site. After initial treatment and decontamination actions are complete, the Radiation Emergency Assistance Center/Training Site may also accept severely contaminated or irradiated patients for transfer to its facilities for more definitive care.

Radiation Emergency Assistance Center/Training Site (REAC/TS)
Oak Ridge Institute for Science and Education
P.O. Box 117, MS 39, Oak Ridge, TN 37831-0117
865-576-3131 (daytime phone; ask for REAC/TS)
865-576-1005 (24-hour emergency number)

Another organization available for consultation is the Medical Radiobiology Advisory Team, sponsored by the Department of Defense and managed by the Armed Forces Radiobiology Research Institute.

Medical Radiobiology Advisory Team
Armed Forces Radiobiology Research Institute
National Naval Medical Center
8901 Wisconsin Avenue, Building 42
Bethesda, MD 20889-5603
301-295-0316
301-295-0530 (24-hour emergency number)

The US Department of Health & Human Services sponsors the Radiation Emergency Medical Management (REMM) Guidance on Diagnosis & Treatment for Health Care Providers. Information can be found at http://www.remm.nlm.gov.

REFERENCES

The complete reference list is available online at www.TintinalliEM.com.

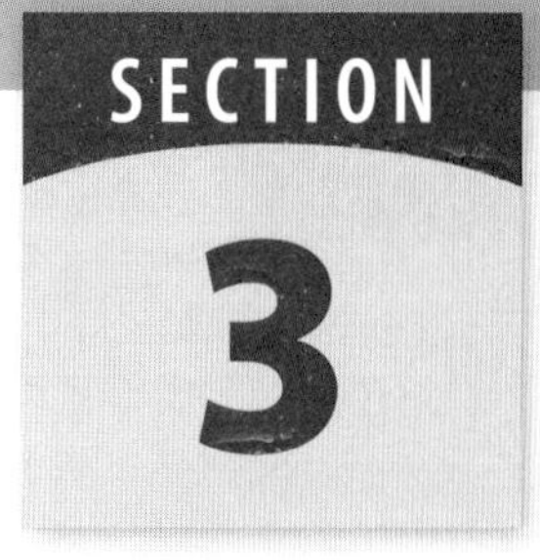

Resuscitation

Chapter 11 Sudden Cardiac Death

Joseph P. Ornato

INTRODUCTION AND EPIDEMIOLOGY

This chapter focuses on the epidemiology and pathophysiology of sudden cardiac death in adults and strategies for prevention and treatment. Discussions of sudden infant death syndrome and cardiac arrest in children are found in chapter 126, Congenital and Acquired Heart Disease, and chapter 127, Syncope, Dysrhythmias, and ECG Interpretation in Children. Chapters 22 and 23 discuss basic and advanced life support, respectively. Chapters 23 and 33 discuss defibrillation and cardioversion, and cardiac pacing, respectively.

Sudden, unexpected out-of-hospital cardiac arrest occurs in approximately 382,800 adult Americans each year.[1] Estimated national survival of EMS-treated cardiac arrest cases is 11.4%, yielding an estimated overall out-of-hospital cardiac arrest survival rate of 6.8% (EMS-treated plus deceased-on-EMS-arrival cases).[1] There is substantial variability in the odds for survival across various geographic locations.[2]

Most episodes of sudden cardiac death occur in the home, although victims who experience cardiac arrest in a public place have a much better chance of survival.[3] The initial recorded cardiac arrest rhythm is more likely to be ventricular fibrillation when cardiac arrest occurs in a public location rather than in the home, likely because patients who experience cardiac arrest in the home are typically older and more likely to have one or more chronic diseases that limit or exclude participation in activities outside the home.[3] Sudden cardiac death is 30% to 80% higher among residents in the lowest compared with the highest socioeconomic quartile.[4] This association is likely due to lifestyle and healthcare disparity issues.

There is a circadian pattern of sudden cardiac death and acute myocardial infarction,[5,6] and both are most likely to occur within the first few hours after awakening from sleep, when there is increased sympathetic stimulation. β-Blockade provides some protection from sudden cardiac death, particularly in patients with known coronary artery disease who have had myocardial infarction and have a low ejection fraction.[7]

There are two peaks in the age-related prevalence of sudden cardiac death: infancy (representing sudden infant death syndrome) and age greater than 45 to 50 years, with 60% in males.[4] There are multiple known factors contributing to the likelihood of sudden cardiac death (**Table 11-1**).

Coronary artery disease (which is often undiagnosed before the event) is the major cause of sudden cardiac death in adults and is present in 80% of cases, followed by cardiomyopathy (10% to 15%) and other miscellaneous conditions (e.g., hereditary channelopathies, valvular disease, congenital anomalies), which account for most of the remaining 5% to 10% of cases.[4]

PATHOPHYSIOLOGY

CORONARY ARTERY DISEASE

Coronary atherosclerosis is present on autopsy in 80% of sudden cardiac death victims.[8] Coronary artery disease is also found in 70% to 80% of cardiac arrest victims who survive and undergo coronary angiography.[9-12] Approximately one third have evidence of acute plaque rupture in areas of long-segment coronary stenosis.[10,11] A documented initial cardiac arrest rhythm of ventricular fibrillation (or shockable rhythm if an automated external defibrillator was applied) suggests that an acute coronary syndrome is the cause, since ventricular fibrillation is noted in the majority of cases in which a coronary occlusion is found on angiography.[9-12] However, ventricular fibrillation is present in only 23% of all cardiac arrests.[13]

SEVERE LEFT VENTRICULAR DYSFUNCTION

Severe left ventricular dysfunction with a reduced ejection fraction is currently the best available predictor of sudden death risk.[4] Patients with an ejection fraction ≤35% are the primary candidates for an implantable cardioverter-defibrillator. However, almost half of sudden deaths occur in individuals with normal left ventricular function.

CARDIOMYOPATHY

Cardiomyopathy with reduced left ventricular function, regardless of cause or presence of decompensated heart failure, is another predictor of sudden cardiac death. Dilated ventricles promote dispersion of ventricular depolarization and/or repolarization, allowing "islands" of ventricular tissue to depolarize and repolarize at different rates. The lack of homogeneity in electrical activation and recovery fosters the development of circus movement reentry, which can initiate and sustain ventricular tachyarrhythmias. Myocardial ischemia and/or infarction can also transiently diminish the homogeneity of left ventricular depolarization and repolarization. Left ventricular hypertrophy (often a result of hypertension and/or valvular heart disease) or conduction disturbances (left or right bundle-branch block or a nonspecific intraventricular conduction disturbance) can create similar functional disturbances.

In-hospital cardiac arrest patients with heart failure are more likely to have ventricular fibrillation as the initial documented cardiac arrest rhythm compared with non–heart failure patients.[14] New York Heart Association functional class II (symptoms with moderate exertion) and III (symptoms with mild exertion) patients are at higher risk of sudden cardiac death than death from pump failure, whereas class IV patients (symptoms at rest) are more likely to die of pump failure than sudden cardiac death.[5,15]

Hypertrophic cardiomyopathy is characterized by unexplained left ventricular hypertrophy associated with nondilated ventricular chambers.[16] The disorder can cluster in families, and the risk of sudden cardiac death increases at a rate of approximately 1% per year.[16] **Hypertrophic cardiomyopathy is the most common cardiovascular cause of sudden cardiac death in young athletes, accounting for one third of such events**, and its presence disqualifies affected individuals from competitive sports.[16] Implantable cardioverter-defibrillator placement is recommended for individuals with prior documented cardiac arrest; ventricular fibrillation; hemodynamically significant or nonsustained ventricular tachycardia; patients with a first-degree relative who has had sudden cardiac death; one or more recent, unexplained episodes of **syncope**; a maximum left ventricular wall thickness ≥30 mm; an abnormal blood pressure response to exercise in the presence of other sudden death risk factors or modifiers; or high-risk children with unexplained syncope, massive left ventricular hypertrophy, or family history of sudden cardiac death.[16]

Arrhythmogenic right ventricular cardiomyopathy is a hereditary form of cardiac muscle disease that is characterized by right-sided heart failure, ventricular arrhythmias of right ventricular origin (i.e., ventricular

TABLE 11-1 Known Factors Contributing to the Likelihood of Sudden Cardiac Death

Cardiovascular pathology
Coronary artery disease
Severe left ventricular dysfunction
Cardiomyopathy
Hypertrophic cardiomyopathy
Arrhythmogenic right ventricular cardiomyopathy
Congenital heart disease, especially coronary artery anomalies
Valvular heart disease
Cardiac pacemaker and conducting system disease
Hereditary channelopathies
Brugada's syndrome
Early repolarization syndrome (ERS)
Long QT syndrome (LQTS)
Short QT syndrome (SQTS)
Catecholaminergic polymorphic ventricular tachycardia (CPVT)
Risk factors and triggers
Long-term risk factor management
Hypertension
Hyperlipidemia
Smoking
Diabetes mellitus
Socioeconomic status
Unstable atherosclerotic plaque
Psychological stress
Physical activity

tachycardia with a left bundle-branch block morphology), syncope, and sudden cardiac death.[17,18] **The electrocardiogram typically shows T-wave inversion in the right precordial leads (V_{1-3}).** Severe right heart failure develops in the majority of cases. Patients suspected of having this disorder should be referred for cardiology evaluation. Implantable cardioverter-defibrillator placement is often the treatment of choice since β-blockers and other antiarrhythmics do not usually prevent symptomatic ventricular arrhythmias in these patients.[17]

CONGENITAL HEART DISEASE

Congenital heart disease occurs in approximately 0.8% of all live births.[19] Because many children with congenital heart disease survive to adulthood as a result of improvements in cardiac surgery, sudden cardiac death is a frequent cause of later morbidity and mortality. Congenital heart defects commonly associated with sudden cardiac death in children and adults are listed in **Table 11-2**.[19]

The most frequent coronary artery anomaly associated with sudden cardiac death is anomalous origin of the left coronary artery from the pulmonary artery syndrome, which results in the left coronary artery traversing between the aorta and main pulmonary artery. This disorder is being diagnosed more frequently in adults by cardiac CT and MRI.[20] Ischemic symptoms, ventricular arrhythmias, and sudden death can be triggered during exercise as a result of increasing venous return, which dilates the main pulmonary artery and compresses the anomalous coronary artery in the space between the aorta and main pulmonary artery. Treatment is surgical correction.

The greatest risk of sudden cardiac death in children and adults with congenital heart disease exists in those with left heart obstructive lesions (e.g., aortic stenosis, aortic coarctation) and cyanotic defects (e.g., Ebstein's anomaly, corrected transposition of the great vessels, tetralogy of Fallot).[19] Most sudden death events in this population occur during exercise, with half of cases resulting from ventricular fibrillation.[19] Nonventricular arrhythmias (e.g., sinus node dysfunction, atrioventricular block, supraventricular tachyarrhythmias) are also common, even after surgical correction.[19]

TABLE 11-2 Congenital Heart Defects Commonly Associated With Sudden Cardiac Death[19]

Coronary artery anomalies (anomalous left coronary artery from the pulmonary artery [ALCAPA] syndrome)
Aortic stenosis
Aortic coarctation
Tetralogy of Fallot
Transposition of the great arteries
Ebstein's anomaly
Single ventricle

VALVULAR HEART DISEASE

Hemodynamically severe aortic stenosis can cause effort-induced dyspnea, myocardial ischemia, and ventricular arrhythmias, which can trigger syncope and sudden cardiac death. The most common causes of aortic stenosis are a congenitally bicuspid aortic valve that typically calcifies and narrows its orifice in mid-adulthood or sclerosis/calcification of a tricuspid aortic valve, which can occur in individuals who are older than 70 or 80 years of age. **A harsh, late-peaking systolic murmur at the upper-right sternal border with radiation to the neck is a typical finding in hemodynamically significant aortic stenosis.**

CARDIAC PACEMAKER AND CONDUCTING SYSTEM DISEASE

Sick sinus syndrome affects the heart's primary pacemaker and can cause intermittent lightheadedness, syncope, or sudden cardiac death. Although it is more common with advancing age, primary electrical failure of the heart can occur in infants and children. The cause is unknown, but pathologic studies reveal histologic degeneration of the sinoatrial node. In addition, the disorder often involves the atrioventricular node and the conduction tissue between the sinoatrial and atrioventricular nodes. Therefore, sick sinus syndrome should be thought of as a diffuse degenerative disease of the heart's electrical generation and conduction system. Idiopathic sclerodegeneration of the AV node and the bundle branches (Lenègre's disease) or invasion of the conduction system by fibrosis or calcification spreading from adjacent cardiac structures (Lev's disease) can lead to bradyasystolic heart block with or without cardiac arrest. In rare cases, a clinical presentation resembling the sick sinus syndrome can occur when the heart's electrical system is affected by systemic disease, vascular compromise, or tumor. Symptomatic bradycardia is treated with pacemaker placement.

HEREDITARY CHANNELOPATHIES

Sudden Arrhythmic Death Syndrome The sudden arrhythmic death syndrome is characterized by sudden cardiac death occurring out of hospital in relatively young adults (mostly men), often during sleep or at rest, usually without any premonitory symptoms (including syncope) and with no anatomic abnormality identified at autopsy.[18,19] Genetic disorders are associated with sudden arrhythmic death syndrome, and many cases can be identified clinically based on their characteristic electrocardiogram patterns.

Ion Channel Disease Cardiovascular and genetic examination of first-degree relatives can identify an inherited form of heart disease known as a "channelopathy" or "ion channel disease" in almost half of cases. Ion channel flux is responsible for the initiation, propagation, and repolarization of the cardiac action potential. Ion channel disease is

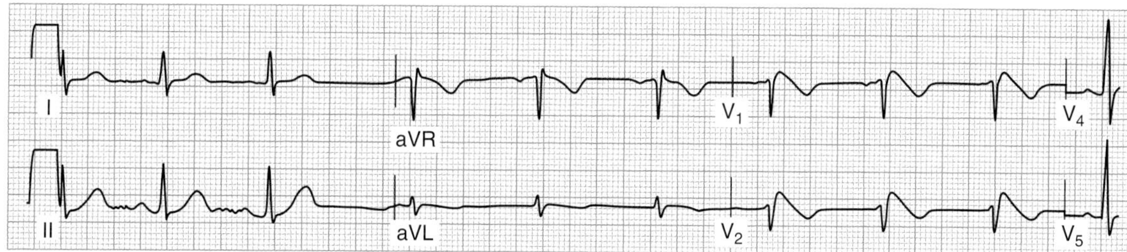

FIGURE 11-1. Brugada's syndrome. Twelve-lead electrocardiogram typical of Brugada's syndrome shows characteristic downsloping ST-segment elevation in leads V_1 and V_2 and QRS morphology resembling a right bundle-branch block.

caused by mutations in the genes that encode the proteins responsible for forming and interacting with the specialized sodium, potassium, and calcium ion channels within the heart.[21] There are many known ion channelopathies, modulated by a variety of causative gene defects that can have variable phenotype penetration in a given family. Genetic testing is used to screen family members for a known mutation. Common subtypes are listed in **Table 11-1**.

Brugada's Syndrome **Brugada's syndrome most commonly affects men and consists of a prominent J-wave with a characteristic downsloping ST-segment elevation in electrocardiogram leads V_{1-3} (Figure 11-1).** This electrocardiogram pattern resembles a right bundle-branch block and is associated with a 40% to 60% incidence of life-threatening ventricular arrhythmias (particularly polymorphic ventricular tachycardia that degenerates into ventricular fibrillation) and sudden cardiac death. The syndrome exhibits an autosomal dominant inheritance that results in total loss of function of the sodium channel or in acceleration of recovery from sodium channel activation.[22] **Brugada's syndrome is common in Southeast Asia (where it is called sudden unexplained nocturnal death syndrome), in the Philippines (*bangungut*, "to rise and moan in sleep"), in Japan (*pokkuri*, "sudden and unexpectedly ceased phenomena"), and in Thailand (*lai tai*, "death during sleep"). It is crucial for emergency physicians to identify this condition from its characteristic electrocardiogram pattern, because the risk of sudden cardiac death is high and can be prevented by internal cardioverter-defibrillator placement.**[23]

Early Repolarization Syndrome **Early repolarization syndrome** is present in 1% to 2% of adults (mostly males) and has long been considered to be a benign variant of normal ventricular repolarization.[24] Its prevalence is higher (10%) in general athletes and reaches as high as 100% in top-performing, endurance-trained individuals.[25] Classic electrocardiogram diagnostic criteria are a prominent, notch-like J wave on the QRS down-slope, followed by upsloping ST-segment elevation (**Figure 11-2**). These changes are seen most prominently in the mid to lateral precordium but can also occur just laterally or inferiorly. There is commonly reciprocal ST-segment depression in aVR. Rapid ventricular pacing or exercise usually normalizes these changes.

There may be similarity or overlap between Brugada's and early repolarization syndromes, but as of this writing, the clinical significance of early repolarization syndrome has not been established.[24] Both syndromes are often familial and more prominent in males, and drugs alter their characteristic electrocardiogram patterns (sodium channel blockers and β-blockers increase, and isoproterenol decreases the ST-segment elevation).[26,27] At this time, cardiology referral might only be warranted in the case of a teenager or young adult with syncope of unknown origin or with a family history of sudden cardiac death at an early age and with an electrocardiogram pattern of early repolarization.

Long QT Syndrome **The long QT syndrome is characterized by prolongation of the corrected QT interval (QT_c), syncope, and sudden death caused by torsade de pointes and ventricular fibrillation.**[21] The QT_c can be calculated by Bazett's equation:

$$QT_c = \frac{QT_m}{\sqrt{R-R}}$$

where QT_c is the corrected QT interval in seconds, QT_m is the measured QT interval in seconds, and R-R is the interval between any two consecutive R waves on the electrocardiogram in seconds. Because the QT interval is heart-rate dependent, the formula "corrects" the measured QT interval to a heart rate of 60 beats/min (at which the R-R interval is 1 second). Because the square root of 1 = 1, the QT_c equals the QT_m at a heart rate of 60 beats/min (at which the normal QT interval limits are 0.35 to 0.44 second).

Prolongation of the QT_c represents dispersion in ventricular repolarization and can be hereditary or acquired (caused by hypokalemia, hypomagnesemia, hypocalcemia, anorexia, ischemia, central nervous system pathology, terfenadine-ketoconazole combinations, or certain antipsychotic or antiarrhythmic drugs).[21,28] Hereditary long QT syndrome can have an autosomal recessive (Jervell and Lange-Neilsen

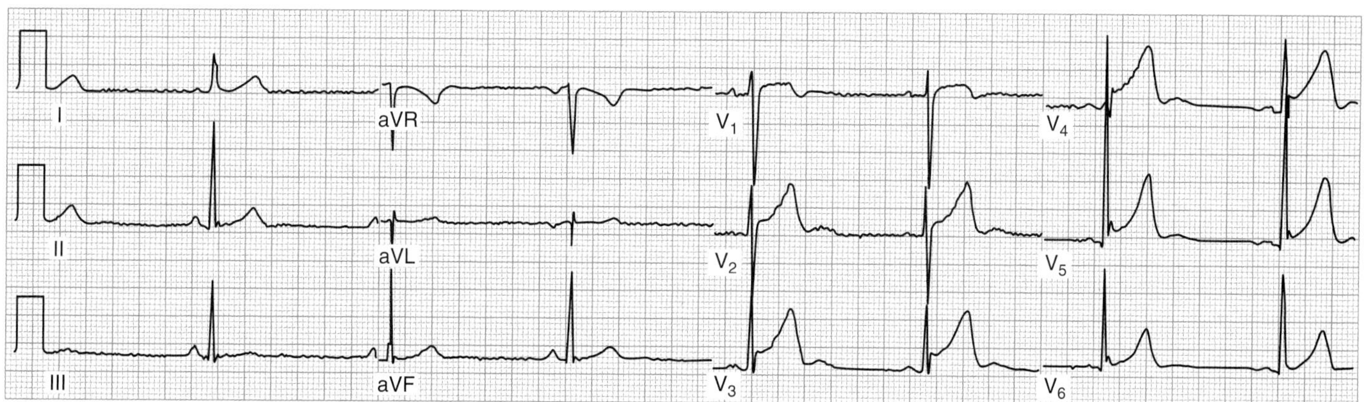

FIGURE 11-2. Early repolarization syndrome. Note in V_5 the prominent notch-like J wave on the QRS downslope, and the upsloping ST-segment.

syndrome with nerve deafness) or dominant (Romano-Ward syndrome without nerve deafness) mode of inheritance.[21] **Management of patients with long QT syndrome involves avoidance of QT-prolonging drugs (an up-to-date list can be found at http://www.azcert.org) and high-intensity sports, as well as cardiology/electrophysiology referral.**[21] A β-blocker is typically prescribed as prophylaxis against sudden cardiac death. Long QT syndrome patients who have syncope, torsade de pointes, or ventricular fibrillation despite β-blocker therapy are candidates for implantable cardioverter-defibrillator placement.[29]

Short QT Syndrome **An abnormally short QT_c (i.e., <0.34 second) can be secondary to hypercalcemia, hyperkalemia, acidosis, systemic inflammatory syndrome, myocardial ischemia, or increased vagal tone or can be inherited in an autosomal dominant genetic pattern.**[30] The genetic variety, dubbed the "short QT syndrome" (SQTS), is associated with atrial arrhythmia, including atrial fibrillation, syncope, polymorphic ventricular tachycardia, ventricular fibrillation, and sudden cardiac death.[30] Early repolarization, especially in the inferolateral leads, is noted in 65% of patients.[31] These individuals should also be referred for cardiology/electrophysiology evaluation and are candidates for cardioverter-defibrillator placement if syncope or life-threatening ventricular arrhythmias are documented.[30]

Catecholaminergic Polymorphic Ventricular Tachycardia Catecholaminergic polymorphic ventricular tachycardia (CPVT) is another genetically determined disorder involving defective myocardial cellular calcium handling. Affected individuals have exercise- and stress-related ventricular tachycardia, syncope, and sudden cardiac death, usually in childhood or early adulthood. Although there are no characteristic abnormalities in the electrocardiogram pattern, a significant number of affected individuals have sinus bradycardia that is not otherwise explainable. Almost half of these individuals carry a diagnosis of epilepsy as the cause of their recurrent syncope before the true cause (i.e., catecholaminergic polymorphic ventricular tachycardia) is identified.[32] β-blockers are the mainstay of prophylaxis, with implantable cardioverter-defibrillator placement as the next step if syncope recurs.[32]

PREVENTION OF SUDDEN CARDIAC DEATH

Unfortunately, the majority of sudden cardiac death victims cannot be identified in advance. Prodromal symptoms in the days to weeks preceding cardiac arrest are common but are usually too nonspecific to be of important predictive value.[33] The most common premonitory symptoms reported by sudden cardiac death survivors or family members of victims are chest discomfort, dyspnea, and "not feeling well."

Various tests have been used to try to "risk stratify" potential sudden cardiac death patients, but none are sensitive or specific enough to be useful. Tests include invasive and noninvasive assessment of left ventricular ejection fraction, coronary angiography, ambulatory electrocardiogram monitoring, exercise testing, detection of ventricular late potentials by using signal averaging, programmed ventricular stimulation of the heart to test the inducibility of ventricular tachyarrhythmias, assessment of heart rate variability, and T-wave alternans (alternating T-wave amplitude from beat to beat on the electrocardiogram, which is only visible with special recording equipment).[34] **The only opportunity for prevention is to recognize signs and symptoms of the syndromes that place a patient at higher risk of sudden cardiac death and to admit or refer such patients for proper evaluation and prophylaxis.**

ANTIARRHYTHMIC DRUG AND DEVICE THERAPY

The Cardiac Arrhythmia Suppression Trial showed that potent class I sodium channel–blocking antiarrhythmic drugs (encainide, flecainide, and moricizine) are proarrhythmic and paradoxically increase the odds of developing sudden cardiac death, as compared with placebo, in patients at relatively low risk for death.[35] The benefits of β-blockade, sotalol, and amiodarone in decreasing mortality from sudden cardiac death pale in comparison with the protective effects of the implantable cardioverter-defibrillator in high-risk patients,[36] including those who have been resuscitated from ventricular fibrillation or cardioverted out of sustained ventricular tachycardia.[37] Although these devices are expensive to insert, their effectiveness over conventional therapy results in a cost of less than $30,000 per year of life saved, which makes them relatively cost-effective for implantation in high-risk individuals.

SUDDEN CARDIAC DEATH RESCUE

The outcome of resuscitation is influenced strongly by the patient's initial cardiac rhythm. In most cases in which the event has been captured during monitoring, the initiating event is either pulseless ventricular tachycardia that degenerates rapidly to ventricular fibrillation or "primary" ventricular fibrillation.[38]

EMS and in-hospital resuscitation systems are the most effective means currently known to rescue patients from sudden cardiac death. Survival from pulseless ventricular tachycardia or ventricular fibrillation is inversely related to the time interval between its onset and termination. Survival is optimal when both CPR and advanced cardiac life support, including defibrillation and drug therapy, are provided early. Community resuscitation strategies should include provision of early CPR, early activation of the EMS system, early defibrillation (including public access defibrillation), early advanced cardiac life support, and regionalized systems of post-resuscitation care.[39,40]

See Chapters 22, 23, and 24 Basic Cardiopulmonary Resuscitation and Defibrillation and Cardioversion, and Advanced Cardiac Life Support, respectively, and Chapter 18, Cardiac Rhythm Disturbances, for detailed discussion of resuscitation pharmacotherapy.

Bystanders who witness the event can improve a victim's chances for survival significantly by alerting the emergency response system promptly. The best survival is attained in EMS systems that can provide early defibrillation to a large percentage of patients. In most cases, this is most cost-effectively accomplished by a tiered response system, in which large numbers of rapid first responders are trained and equipped to provide first aid, CPR, and early defibrillation using an automated external defibrillator. The Public Access Defibrillation randomized clinical trial showed that laypersons trained and equipped to use automated external defibrillators in public places can double survival to hospital discharge compared with that which can be achieved by layperson rescuers who can only perform CPR while awaiting EMS arrival.[41] These results have been confirmed in an analysis of 13,769 out-of-hospital cardiac arrest registry cases.[42]

PULSELESS VENTRICULAR TACHYCARDIA/VENTRICULAR FIBRILLATION

The likelihood of survival is relatively high if the initial rhythm is ventricular tachycardia or ventricular fibrillation (particularly if the ventricular fibrillation is "coarse," the arrest is witnessed, and prompt CPR and defibrillation are provided). If the initial rhythm is not ventricular tachycardia or ventricular fibrillation, survival is typically <5% in most reported series. Asystolic patients whose cardiac arrest is unwitnessed rarely survive to hospital discharge neurologically intact. The only common exceptions are witnessed cardiac arrest patients whose initial asystole is a result of increased vagal tone or other relatively easily correctible factors, such as hypoxia of brief duration.

PULSELESS ELECTRICAL ACTIVITY

Some sudden cardiac death events begin with a bradyarrhythmia or an organized rhythm without a pulse (e.g., pulseless electrical activity). *Bradyasystole* in adults is defined as a ventricular rate <60 beats/min or periods of absent heart rhythm (asystole). Bradyasystolic rhythms other than asystole can be accompanied by a pulse, or there can be no discernible pulse with each QRS (i.e., pulseless electrical activity). Bradyasystole *with* a pulse is often accompanied by a significant decrease in cardiac output, leading to hypotension and/or syncope. Bradycardia *with or without* a pulse occurs frequently during cardiac arrest, either as the initial rhythm, during the course of resuscitation, or after electrical defibrillation. Obviously, asystole occurs eventually in all dying patients. **To ensure that ventricular fibrillation is not masquerading as asystole, rescuers can switch to another lead whenever a "flat line" is recorded on the electrocardiogram during resuscitation or use US if available.**

TABLE 11-3 Common Causes of Bradyasystolic Arrest
Myocardial ischemia or infarction
Sick sinus syndrome
Asphyxiation (including near-drowning)
Hypoxia
Hypercarbia
Stroke
Opiates, β-blockers, calcium channel blockers, adenosine, or parasympathetics

Primary bradyasystole occurs when the heart's electrical system fails to generate and/or propagate an adequate number of ventricular depolarizations per minute to sustain consciousness and other vital functions. Secondary bradyasystole is present when factors external to the heart's electrical system cause it to fail (e.g., hypoxia). Common causes of bradyasystolic arrest are listed in **Table 11-3.**

One of the most baffling mysteries of bradyasystolic cardiac arrest relates to myocardial mechanics. Bradyasystole, unlike ventricular fibrillation, is accompanied by very little myocardial oxygen consumption in animal models. Because of this, myocardial high-energy phosphate stores should decay relatively slowly during bradyasystole. This should theoretically result in a high incidence of return of spontaneous circulation after restoration of a more normal rhythm (e.g., with the early use of electrical pacing). It is unclear why conventional treatment of bradyasystolic cardiac arrest with atropine, epinephrine, or electrical pacemakers rarely results in survival to hospital discharge. Return of spontaneous circulation is infrequent, and long-term neurologically intact survival is rare in bradyasystolic cardiac arrest.

Other factors must play a determining role in the pathophysiology and subsequent outcome of bradyasystolic cardiac arrest. Bradyasystolic arrest is not just a disorder of rhythm generation or propagation; it is a perplexing syndrome characterized by such rhythm disturbances accompanied, in many cases, by profound depression of myocardial and vascular function. Suspected causes include endogenous myocardial depressants (including down-regulation of catecholamine receptors and/or toxic influences of intense sympathetic stimulation), neurogenic influences, postischemic myocardial stunning, and/or free radical injury.

It is important to differentiate pulseless electrical activity from conditions in which the rescuer is unable to detect a pulse, but there is unmistakable evidence that there is adequate blood pressure and cardiac output to maintain vital organ perfusion (e.g., a conscious patient with profound vasoconstriction caused by hypothermia, or "pseudo pulseless electrical activity").[43]

TABLE 11-4 Conditions That Cause Pulseless Electrical Activity
Hypovolemia
Tension pneumothorax
Pericardial tamponade
Pulmonary embolism
Massive myocardial dysfunction due to ischemia or infarction, myocarditis, cardiotoxins, etc.
Drug toxicity (e.g., β-blockers, calcium channel blockers, tricyclic antidepressants)
Profound shock
Hypoxia
Acidosis
Severe hypercarbia
Auto positive end-expiratory pressure
Hypothermia
Hyperkalemia
Pseudo pulseless electrical activity

The underlying physiologic cause of pulseless electrical activity is a marked reduction in cardiac output due to either profound myocardial depression or mechanical factors that reduce venous return or impede the flow of blood through the cardiovascular system. Common conditions that can cause pulseless electrical activity are shown in **Table 11-4**. The management of patients with pulseless electrical activity is directed at identifying and treating the underlying cause or causes.

REFERENCES

The complete reference list is available online at www.TintinalliEM.com.

Approach to Shock

Bret A. Nicks
John Gaillard

EPIDEMIOLOGY

The exact number of cases of shock that present to the ED in the United States is difficult to ascertain due to the insensitivity of clinical parameters, current definitions, and lack of a central database repository. Previous estimates propose that more than 1 million cases of shock are seen in the ED each year in the United States.[1] These estimates are largely based on the assumption that hypotension, defined as a systolic blood pressure <90 mm Hg, is consistent with shock in adults. Using this definition, the incidence of patients with hypotension that present to American EDs is approximately 5.6 million cases per year.[2]

Mortality depends on the inciting event. Septic shock has an estimated mortality of 40% to 60%.[3] Cardiogenic shock has an estimated mortality of 36% to 56%.[4] Approximately 30% to 45% of patients with septic shock and 60% to 90% of patients with cardiogenic shock die within 1 month of presentation.[3,4] With a greater recognition and improved treatment, mortality from neurogenic shock has been reduced significantly. The definition of and treatment approach to shock continue to evolve, but the initial approach to a patient in shock follows similar principles, regardless of the inciting factors or cause.

Patients present to the ED in varying stages of critical illness and shock. These stages are confounded by age, comorbidities, and delays in presentation. A focus on early recognition, rapid diagnosis, and empiric resuscitation is essential. Therapy and patient stabilization may need to occur simultaneously with evaluation.

PATHOPHYSIOLOGY

Shock is a state of circulatory insufficiency that creates an imbalance between tissue oxygen supply (delivery) and oxygen demand (consumption) resulting in end-organ dysfunction. Reduction in effective perfusion may be due to a local or global delivery deficiency or utilization deficiency with suboptimal substrate at the cellular or subcellular level.[5] The mechanisms that can result in shock are frequently divided into four categories: (1) hypovolemic, (2) cardiogenic, (3) distributive, and (4) obstructive.

FACTORS AFFECTING CARDIAC OUTPUT

An understanding of the mechanisms of oxygen delivery and consumption is foundational to the treatment of shock. While the physiology is complex, familiarity with the basic principles, equations, and their interactions is essential (**Tables 12-1 and 12-2**). As noted in the cardiac output (CO) equation, CO is determined by heart rate and stroke volume. Stroke volume is dependent on preload, afterload, and contractility. The mean arterial pressure (MAP) demonstrates the impact that CO has on MAP (which can also be estimated with the formula: 2 × diastolic blood pressure + systolic blood pressure/3). This is important because there is a MAP threshold below which oxygen delivery is decreased. Systemic

TABLE 12-1 Physiologic Equations

Parameter	Equation Specifics
Cardiac output	Cardiac Output = Heart Rate × Stroke Volume $CO = HR \times SV$
Mean arterial pressure	Mean Arterial Pressure = Cardiac Output × Systemic Vascular Resistance $MAP = CO \times SVR$
Oxygen delivery	Oxygen Delivery = Cardiac Output × Arterial Oxygen Content $Do_2 = CO \times [(1.39 \times Hb \times Sao_2) + (Pao_2 \times 0.0031)]$ Do_2 is the amount of O_2 delivered to the tissues per minute. A normal value is 1000 mL O_2 per minute.
Arterial oxygen content	Arterial Oxygen Content = Amount of Oxygen in the Blood $Cao_2 = (1.39 \times Hb \times Sao_2) + (Pao_2 \times 0.0031)$
Oxygen consumption	Oxygen Consumption = Cardiac Output × (Arterial O_2 Content − Venous O_2 Content) $\dot{V}o_2 = CO \times (Cao_2 - Cvo_2)$ Alternative equation: $\dot{V}o_2 = CO \times Hb \times 1.39 \times (Sao_2 - Smvo_2)$ The amount of O_2 consumed by tissues each minute is equal to the difference in O_2 delivered to tissues and the O_2 returning from tissues to the heart. A normal value is about 250 mL O_2 per minute. Note that this formula ignores the small contribution from dissolved oxygen.
Shock index	Shock Index = Heart Rate ÷ Systolic Blood Pressure $SI = HR/SBP$ A normal value is 0.5–0.7. A persistent elevation of the shock index (>1.0) indicates an impaired left ventricular function (as a result of blood loss or cardiac depression) and carries a high mortality rate.

Abbreviations and units: Hb = hemoglobin in grams/dL; HR = heart rate per min; Pao_2 = partial pressure of oxygen in arterial blood in mm Hg; Sao_2 = oxygen saturation expressed as a fraction of 1.0, rather than a percentage; SBP = systolic blood pressure in mm Hg; $Smvo_2$ = mixed venous oxygen saturation expressed as a fraction of 1.0, rather than a percentage; SV = stroke volume in mL; SVR = systemic vascular resistance in mm Hg·min/L.

TABLE 12-2 Abbreviations and Definitions of Hemodynamic Parameters

Cao_2	Arterial oxygen content
CI	Cardiac index (cardiac output/body surface area)
CO	Cardiac output
Cvo_2	Venous oxygen content
CVP	Central venous pressure
Do_2	Systemic oxygen delivery
DBP	Diastolic blood pressure
Hb	Hemoglobin
MAP	Mean arterial pressure
MODS	Multiorgan dysfunction syndrome
$Paco_2$	Partial pressure of arterial carbon dioxide
Pao_2	Partial pressure of arterial oxygen
Sao_2	Arterial oxygen saturation
$Scvo_2$	Central venous oxygen saturation from the superior vena cava
$Smvo_2$ (Svo_2)	Mixed venous oxygen saturation from the pulmonary artery
SBP	Systolic blood pressure
SI	Shock index
SIRS	Systemic inflammatory response syndrome
SVR	Systemic vascular resistance
$\dot{V}o_2$	Systemic oxygen consumption

vascular resistance (SVR) directly impacts MAP, but also impacts afterload and thus CO. The physiologic mechanism of oxygen delivery to peripheral tissues (Do_2) is described in the oxygen delivery equation. Recognize that blood pressure is not represented in this equation. Patients in shock may initially have normal blood pressures (cryptic shock), yet have other objective signs of shock (see "Clinical Features" below). It is from these basic equations that the concept of preload influencing stroke volume, which itself influences CO and Do_2, has become fundamental in shock management.

Tissue oxygenation is predicated on CO being sufficient enough to deliver oxygenated hemoglobin to the tissues. CO is dependent on the interplay of cardiac inotropy (speed and shortening capacity of myocardium), chronotropy (heart contraction rate), and lusitropy (ability to relax and fill heart chambers). Determinants of inotropy include autonomic input from sympathetic activation, parasympathetic inhibition, circulating catecholamines, and short-lived responses to an increase in afterload (Anrep effect) or heart rate (Bowditch effect). Increases in the inotropic state help to maintain stroke volume at high heart rates.[6] Under certain conditions, such as shock states, higher levels of epinephrine will be produced and reinforce adrenergic tone. Epinephrine levels are significantly elevated during induced hemorrhagic shock, but these levels subsequently reduce to almost normal levels after adequate blood pressure is restored.[7] Previous studies have also shown that an acidotic milieu, which is common in shock, further compromises ventricular contractile force and blood pressure.[8] Chronotropy and lusitropy are both influenced by sympathetic input. Norepinephrine interacts with cardiac β_1-receptors, resulting in increased cyclic adenosine monophosphate. This leads to a process of intracellular signaling with an increased chronotropy and sequestration of calcium, leading to myocardial relaxation.[6]

LACTIC ACID

When compensatory mechanisms fail to correct the imbalance between tissue supply and demand, anaerobic metabolism occurs and results in the formation of lactic acid. Lactic acid is rapidly buffered, resulting in the formation of measured serum lactate. Normal venous lactate levels are less than 2.0 mmol/L. Most cases of lactic acidosis are a result of inadequate oxygen delivery, but lactic acidosis occasionally can develop from an excessively high oxygen demand (e.g., status epilepticus). In other cases, lactic acidosis occurs because of impaired tissue oxygen utilization (e.g., septic shock or the postresuscitation phase of cardiac arrest). Elevated lactate is a marker of impaired oxygen delivery or utilization and correlates with short-term prognosis of critically ill patients in the ED.[7]

COMPENSATORY MECHANISMS AND THEIR FAILURE

Shock provokes a myriad of autonomic responses, many of which serve to maintain perfusion pressure to vital organs. Stimulation of the carotid baroreceptor stretch reflex activates the sympathetic nervous system triggering (1) arteriolar vasoconstriction, resulting in redistribution of blood flow from the skin, skeletal muscle, kidneys, and splanchnic viscera; (2) an increase in heart rate and contractility that increases CO; (3) constriction of venous capacitance vessels, which augments venous return; (4) release of the vasoactive hormones epinephrine, norepinephrine, dopamine, and cortisol to increase arteriolar and venous tone; and (5) release of antidiuretic hormone and activation of the renin-angiotensin axis to enhance water and sodium conservation to maintain intravascular volume.[8]

These compensatory mechanisms attempt to maintain Do_2 to the most critical organs (heart and brain), but blood flow to other organs, such as the kidneys and GI tract, may be compromised. The cellular response to decreased Do_2 (adenosine triphosphate depletion) leads to ion-pump dysfunction, influx of sodium, efflux of potassium, and reduction in membrane resting potential. As shock progresses, the loss of cellular integrity and the breakdown in cellular homeostasis result in cellular death. These pathologic events give rise to a cascade of metabolic features including hyperkalemia, hyponatremia, azotemia, hyper- or hypoglycemia, and lactic acidosis.

TABLE 12-3 Clinical Features of Systemic Inflammatory Response Syndrome (SIRS)

Two or more of the following features are required to make a diagnosis of SIRS:
Temperature >38°C (100.4°F) or <36°C (96.8°F)
Heart rate >90 beats/min
Respiratory rate >20 breaths/min (or carbon dioxide tension <32 mm Hg)
WBC count >12.0 × 10^9/L, <4.0 × 10^9/L, or >10% immature forms or bands

In the early phases of shock, these physiologic changes may produce a clinical syndrome called the systemic inflammatory response syndrome or SIRS (**Table 12-3**).

As systemic inflammatory response syndrome progresses, shock ensues, followed by the multiorgan dysfunction syndrome, which is manifested by renal failure, respiratory failure, myocardial depression, liver failure, and then disseminated intravascular coagulation. The fulminant progression from systemic inflammatory response syndrome to multiorgan dysfunction syndrome is determined by the balance of anti-inflammatory and proinflammatory mediators and the level of inadequate tissue perfusion (**Figure 12-1**).

CATEGORIES OF SHOCK

The four categories of shock can be described in terms of their respective physiologic changes and common causes, recognizing that overlap is common (**Table 12-4**). **Hypovolemic shock** occurs when decreased intravascular fluid or decreased blood volume causes decreased preload, stroke volume, and CO. Severe blood loss (hemorrhage) can cause decreased myocardial oxygenation, which decreases contractility and CO. This action may lead to an autonomic increase in the SVR.

TABLE 12-4 Categories of Shock

Type	Hemodynamic Changes	Etiologies
Hypovolemic	Decreased preload, increased SVR, decreased CO	Hemorrhage, capillary leak, GI losses, burns
Cardiogenic	Increased preload, increased afterload, increased SVR, decreased CO	MI, dysrhythmias, heart failure, valvular disease
Obstructive	Decreased preload, increased SVR, decreased CO	PE, pericardial tamponade, tension PTX
Distributive	Decreased preload, increased SVR, mixed CO	Sepsis, neurogenic shock, anaphylaxis

Abbreviations: CO = cardiac output; MI = myocardial infarction; PE = pulmonary embolism; PTX = pneumothorax; SVR = systemic vascular resistance.

Hypovolemic shock can also occur due to volume loss from other etiologies. In **cardiogenic shock**, the left ventricle fails to deliver oxygenated blood to peripheral tissues due to variances in contractility, as well as preload and afterload. Myocardial infarction is the most common cause of cardiogenic shock. Dysrhythmias are another common cause because they can lead to a decreased CO. Bradyarrhythmias result in low CO, and tachyarrhythmias can result in decreased preload and stroke volume. **Obstructive shock** is due to a decrease in venous return or cardiac compliance due to an increased left ventricular outflow obstruction or marked preload decrease. Cardiac tamponade and tension pneumothorax are common causes. In **distributive shock**, there is relative intravascular volume depletion due to marked systemic vasodilatation. This is most commonly seen in septic shock. Compensatory responses to decreased SVR may include increased CO (increased contractility and heart rate) and tachycardia. The concurrent decreased SVR results in a decreased preload and may hinder CO

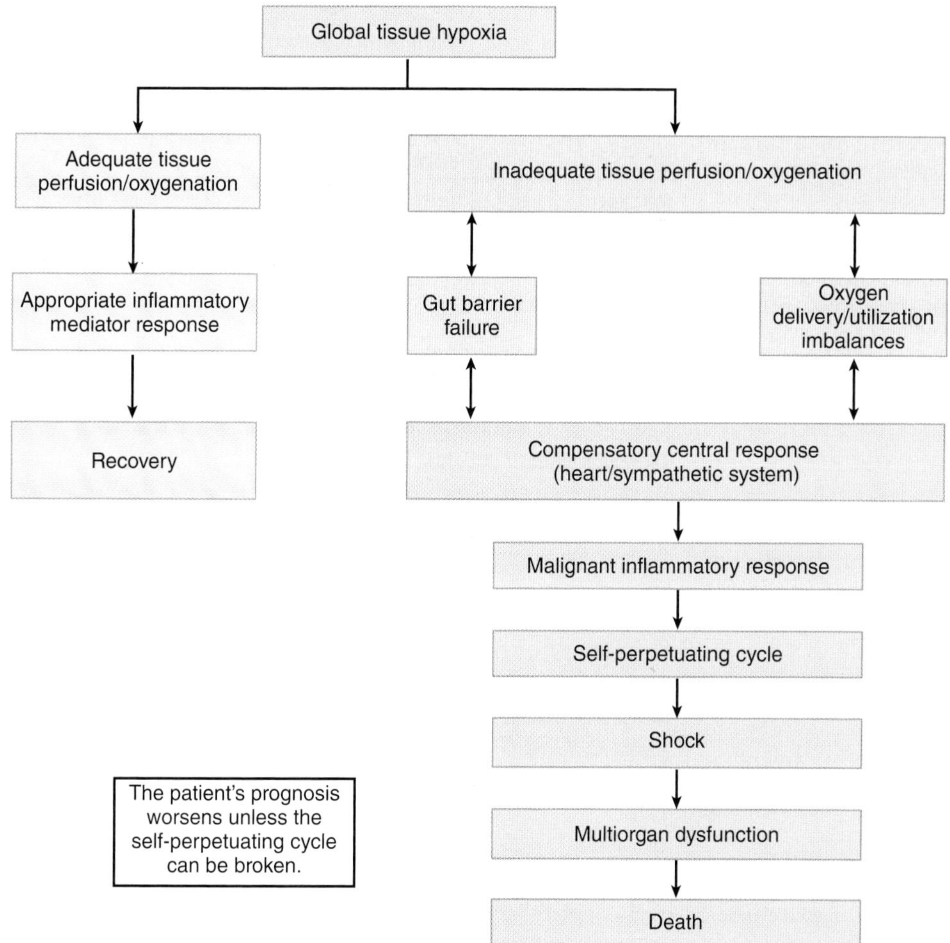

FIGURE 12-1. The pathophysiology of shock, the systemic inflammatory response syndrome, and multiorgan dysfunction.

overall. In sepsis, up to 40% of patients may have a transient cardiomyopathy characterized by decreased contractility and increased mortality.[3,4] Anaphylaxis, adrenal insufficiency and neurogenic shock are additional causes of distributive shock.

CLINICAL FEATURES

HISTORY AND COMORBIDITIES

While the clinical presentation of a patient in shock and the underlying cause may be quite apparent (e.g., acute myocardial infarction, anaphylaxis, or hemorrhage), it may be difficult to obtain a history from patients in shock. Assistance with medical history from EMS, family, or other sources may help determine the cause of shock, especially if the patient has comorbidities. Some patients in shock may have few symptoms other than generalized weakness, lethargy, or altered mental status. If the patient is unresponsive, consider trauma as a primary or secondary complication.

PHYSICAL EXAMINATION

Shock is usually associated with systemic arterial hypotension—systolic blood pressure <90 mm Hg. Blood pressure is the product of flow and resistance (MAP = CO × SVR). Blood pressure may not drop if there is an increase in peripheral vascular resistance in the presence of decreased CO with inadequate tissue hypoperfusion, making blood pressure an insensitive marker for global tissue hypoperfusion. **Shock may occur with a normal blood pressure, and hypotension may occur without shock.** No single vital sign is diagnostic of shock, and blood pressure is particularly insensitive in the presence of peripheral vascular disease, tachycardia with a small pulse pressure, or cardiac dysrhythmias. Composite physical findings are useful in the assessment of shock (**Table 12-5**).

TABLE 12-5 Composite Physical Examination Findings in Shock

Temperature	Hyperthermia or hypothermia may be present. Endogenous hypothermia (hypometabolic shock) must be distinguished from exogenous environmental hypothermia.
Heart rate	Usually elevated; however, paradoxical bradycardia can be seen in shock states due to hypoglycemia, β-blocker use, and preexisting cardiac disease.
Systolic blood pressure	May actually increase slightly when cardiac contractility increases in early shock and then fall as shock advances.
Diastolic blood pressure	Correlates with arteriolar vasoconstriction and may rise early in shock and then fall when cardiovascular compensation fails.
Pulse pressure	Increases early in shock and decreases before systolic pressure begins to drop.
Mean arterial blood pressure	Often low, <65 mm Hg.
CNS	Acute delirium or brain failure, restlessness, disorientation, confusion, and coma secondary to a decrease in cerebral perfusion pressure
Skin/capillary refill	Pallor, pale, dusky, clammy, cyanosis, sweating, altered temperature, and increased capillary refill time of >2–3 s.
Cardiovascular	Neck vein distention or flattening depending on the type of shock. Tachycardia and arrhythmias. An S_3 may result from high-output states. Decreased coronary perfusion pressures can lead to ischemia, decreased ventricular compliance, increased left ventricular diastolic pressure, and pulmonary edema.
Respiratory	Tachypnea, increased minute ventilation, increased dead space, bronchospasm, and hyper- or hypocapnia with progression to respiratory failure.
Splanchnic organs	Ileus, GI bleeding, pancreatitis, acalculous cholecystitis, and mesenteric ischemia can occur due to low flow states.
Renal	Reduced glomerular filtration rate. Renal blood flow redistributes from the renal cortex toward the renal medulla leading to oliguria.
Metabolic	Hyperglycemia, hypoglycemia, and hyperkalemia. As shock progresses, metabolic acidosis occurs with concurrent attempted respiratory compensation.

DIAGNOSIS

LABORATORY EVALUATION

No single laboratory value is sensitive or specific for shock. Laboratory studies are driven by the clinical presentation and the presumptive cause. Common studies are listed in **Table 12-6**. Arterial blood gases are useful to assess acid–base status and ventilation and oxygenation concerns, whereas a venous blood gas is limited to acid–base information. A rise in serum lactate correlates with mortality in many shock states;[7] typically this is due to anaerobic metabolism, but nonhypoxic causes of lactic acidosis due to cellular dysfunction occur in shock states. Serial lactate assessments may be indicated because lactate clearance is associated with improved outcomes in septic shock and may assist with resuscitation.[9] A wide range of laboratory abnormalities may be encountered in shock, but most abnormal values merely point to the particular organ system that is contributing to, or being affected by, the shock state.

TABLE 12-6 Initial Diagnostic Studies to Evaluate a Patient in Shock*

CBC with differential
Electrolytes, glucose, calcium, magnesium, phosphorus
BUN, creatinine
Serum lactate
ECG
Urinalysis
Chest radiograph
Coagulation studies: prothrombin time, PTT, INR
Arterial blood gas (measured pH, carbon dioxide, and oxygen levels)
Hepatic function panel
Cultures: blood, urine, suspicious wounds, quantitative sputum culture
Culture
Cortisol level
Pregnancy test
CT of chest/abdomen/pelvis as indicated history, physical exam

*Ordering of the listed tests should be individualized by patient presentation and history.

IMAGING

Chest X-Ray The portable anteroposterior view chest x-ray is often used in the evaluation of unstable patients to avoid transporting the patient during resuscitation. While limitations exist, evaluation of the heart size, presence of pulmonary edema, free air under the diaphragm, pneumothorax, infiltrates, or effusions may provide useful clinical information.

US Bedside US assessment is an important tool for developing a differential diagnosis, assessing volume status, defining cardiac function, and assisting with procedures. Various US methods are described to determine overall volume status by assessing right-sided filling pressures, including measuring inferior vena cava respiratory variation, end-expiratory vena cava respiratory variation, and other methods. Defining the degree of hypovolemia is inexact.

Bedside cardiac US to assess left ventricular ejection fraction can assist with determining the cause of shock. Emergency physicians trained in focused bedside cardiac US can provide an estimated ejection fraction with high relative correlation to cardiologists.[10]

US may also be used to assess for vascular emergencies. Identifying an abdominal aortic aneurysm on US may lead to further evaluation.

Additional US protocols, such as the Abdominal and Cardiac Evaluation with Sonography in Shock protocol and the Rapid Ultrasound in Shock protocol, have been formulated using many of the aforementioned concepts. The Abdominal and Cardiac Evaluation with Sonography in Shock protocol looks at cardiac function, inferior vena cava dynamics, pulmonary congestion, sliding and consolidation, abdominal free fluid, abdominal aortic aneurysm, and leg venous thrombosis to assist in differential diagnosis generation or narrowing.[11] The Rapid Ultrasound in Shock exam involves a three-part bedside physiologic assessment simplified as the pump (cardiac), the tank (volume status), and the pipes (arterial and venous).[12,13] However, as with any US intervention, operator competency and available resources are essential.

CT Although CT is an accurate and noninvasive approach for detecting internal pathology, patients must travel from the ED to the radiology suite, which may be unadvisable in unstable shock. The potential benefits of CT must be weighed against the associated risks, including concerns about renal function due to hypovolemia and contrast-induced nephropathy. CT scans without IV contrast will add some information to the clinical picture, although not to the degree of a scan with IV contrast.

HEMODYNAMIC MONITORING

Hemodynamic monitoring helps assess the severity of shock and the response to treatment. Monitoring capabilities should initially include pulse oximetry, electrocardiographic monitoring, and noninvasive blood pressure monitoring. In the critical care arena, intra-arterial blood pressure monitoring, end-tidal carbon dioxide monitoring, central venous pressure, and central venous oxygen saturation from the superior vena cava ($Scvo_2$) monitoring are frequently used. When obtaining central access, the average access time, number of attempts, and mechanical complications are reduced when a US-assisted approach is used.[14]

EARLY TREATMENT

Comprehensive and timely ED care can significantly decrease the predicted mortality of critically ill patients in as little as 6 hours of treatment.[15] Application of an algorithmic approach to optimize hemodynamic end points with early goal-directed therapy in the ED reduced mortality by 16% in patients with severe sepsis or septic shock in 2001.[16] That original study, the Surviving Sepsis Campaign that followed,[17] and other algorithmic efforts[18] have changed the approach to sepsis and shock care on a worldwide basis. Two large, multicenter, randomized controlled trials published in 2014 failed to show additional benefits to a rigid algorithmic approach.[19,20] However, we attempt to present below the most beneficial aspects of shock care demonstrated by the medical progress of the last 15 years. **The *ABCDE* tenets of shock resuscitation are establishing *a*irway, controlling the work of *b*reathing, optimizing the *c*irculation, assuring adequate oxygen *d*elivery, and achieving *e*nd points of resuscitation.**[21]

ESTABLISHING THE AIRWAY

Airway control is best obtained through endotracheal intubation. Sedatives used to facilitate intubation may cause arterial vasodilatation, venodilation, or myocardial suppression and may result in hypotension. Positive-pressure ventilation reduces preload and CO. The combination of sedative agents and positive-pressure ventilation will often lead to hemodynamic collapse. To avoid this unwanted situation, initiate volume resuscitation and vasoactive agents before intubation and positive-pressure ventilation.

CONTROLLING THE WORK OF BREATHING

Control of breathing is required when significant tachypnea accompanies shock. Respiratory muscles are significant consumers of oxygen during shock and contribute to lactate production. Mechanical ventilation and sedation allow for adequate oxygenation, improvement of hypercapnia, and assisted, controlled, synchronized ventilation. All of these treatments decrease the work of breathing and improve survival. When starting mechanical ventilation on a patient, it is essential to consider the patient's compensatory minute ventilation prior to intubation to ensure appropriate initial settings are selected. After a patient is placed on mechanical ventilation, obtain an arterial blood gas to evaluate acid–base status, oxygenation, and ventilation. Neuromuscular blocking agents should be considered to further decrease respiratory muscle oxygen consumption and preserve Do_2 to vital organs, especially if patients are severely hypoxemic due to acute respiratory distress syndrome.[22]

OPTIMIZING THE CIRCULATION

Fluids Circulatory or hemodynamic stabilization begins with intravascular access through large-bore peripheral venous lines. The Trendelenburg position does not improve cardiopulmonary performance compared with the supine position. It may worsen pulmonary gas exchange and predispose to aspiration. Passive leg raising above the level of the heart with the patient supine may be effective. If passive leg raising results in an increase in blood pressure or CO, fluid resuscitation is indicated.[23]

Fluid resuscitation should begin with isotonic crystalloid.[24] The amount and rate of infusion are determined by an estimate of the hemodynamic abnormality. Most patients in shock have either an absolute or relative volume deficit. The exception is the patient in cardiogenic shock with pulmonary edema. Administer fluid rapidly (over 5 to 20 minutes), in set quantities of 500 or 1000 mL of normal saline, and reassess the patient after each bolus. Patients with a modest degree of hypovolemia usually require an initial 20 to 30 mL/kg of isotonic crystalloid, as is suggested in the 2012 Surviving Sepsis Campaign Guidelines; however, there are few data to support this uniform recommendation, and fluid volume should be individualized to each patient.[25] More fluids are needed for profound volume deficits. It is common for patients in septic shock to receive 6 L of crystalloid in the first 24 hours of hospital care. For large fluid volumes, consider using lactated ringer's or plasmalyte to avoid hyperchloremic metabolic acidosis.[26,27]

Central venous access may aid in assessing volume status (preload) and monitoring $Scvo_2$. It is also the preferred route for the long-term administration of certain vasopressor therapy. However, there is no need for universal central access in patients with septic shock, and the need for central access should be individually determined.[20]

Vasopressors Vasopressors are used when there has been an inadequate response to volume resuscitation or if there are contraindications to volume infusion.[25] Vasopressors are most effective when the vascular space is "full" and least effective when the vascular space is depleted. Patients with chronic hypertension may be at greater risk of renal injury at lower blood pressures; however, in others, there appears to be no mortality benefit in raising MAP above the 65 to 70 mm Hg range.[28,29]

Vasopressor agents have variable effects on the α-adrenergic, β-adrenergic, vasopressin, and dopaminergic receptors (**Table 12-7**). Although vasopressors improve perfusion pressure in the large vessels, they may decrease capillary blood flow in certain tissue beds, especially the GI tract and peripheral vasculature. If multiple vasopressors are used, they should be simplified as soon as the best therapeutic agent is identified. In addition to a vasopressor, an inotrope may be needed to directly increase CO by increasing contractility and stroke volume.

ASSURING ADEQUATE OXYGEN DELIVERY

Control of oxygen consumption ($\dot{V}o_2$) is important in restoring the balance of oxygen supply and demand to the tissue (oxygen consumption equation). A hyperadrenergic state results from the compensatory response to shock, physiologic stress, pain, and anxiety. Shivering frequently results when a patient is unclothed for examination and then left inadequately covered in a cold resuscitation room. The combination of these variables increases $\dot{V}o_2$. Pain further suppresses myocardial function, further impairing Do_2 and $\dot{V}o_2$. Providing analgesia,

TABLE 12-7 Commonly Used Vasoactive Agents (all vasopressors increase myocardial oxygen demand; most should be titrated to desired effect)

Drug	Dose	Action	Cardiac Contractility	Vasoconstriction	Vasodilation	Cardiac Output
Dobutamine	2.0–20.0 micrograms/kg/min	β_1, some β_2 and α_1 in large dosages	++++	+	++	Increases
Side effects and comments	Inotrope only; Causes tachydysrhythmias, occasional GI distress, hypotension in volume-depleted patients; has less peripheral vasoconstriction than dopamine; can cause fewer arrhythmias than isoproterenol					
Dopamine	0.5–20 micrograms/kg/min	α, β, and dopaminergic	++ at 2.5–5 micrograms/kg/min	++ at 5–20 micrograms/kg/min	+ at 0.5–2.0 micrograms/kg/min	Usually increases
Side effects and comments	Tachydysrhythmias; a cerebral, mesenteric, coronary, and renal vasodilator at low doses; Surviving Sepsis Campaign second line, lot of overlap with α/β/dopaminergic receptors and dose; can be given through a peripheral IV					
Epinephrine	2–10 micrograms/min	α and β	++++ at 0.5–8 micrograms/kg/min	++++ at >8 micrograms/kg/min	+++	Increases
Side effects and comments	Causes tachydysrhythmia, leukocytosis; increases myocardial oxygen consumption; may increase lactate; no real maximum dose					
Isoproterenol	0.01–0.05 micrograms/kg/min	β_1 and some β_2	++++	0	++++	Increases
Side effects and comments	Inotrope; causes tachydysrhythmia, facial flushing, hypotension in hypovolemic patients; increases myocardial oxygen consumption; never use alone in shock					
Norepinephrine	0.5–50 micrograms/min	Primarily α_1, some β_1	++	++++	0	Slightly increases
Side effects and comments	Useful when loss of venous tone predominates; first-line agent for most situations; should be given through a central line					
Phenylephrine	10–200 micrograms/min	Pure α	0	++++	0	Decreases
Side effects and comments	Reflex bradycardia, headache, restlessness, excitability, rarely arrhythmias; can be used on patients in shock with tachycardia or supraventricular arrhythmias; not good comparatively for septic shock					
Vasopressin	0.01–0.04 units/min	Directly stimulates V_1 receptor on smooth muscle	0	++++	0	0
Side effects and comments	Primarily vasoconstriction; usually started at max dose and not titrated					

Note: 0 = no effect; + = mild effect; ++ = moderate effect; +++ = marked effect; ++++ = very marked effect.

muscle relaxation, warm covering, anxiolytics, and even paralytic agents, when appropriate, decreases this inappropriate systemic oxygen consumption.

Once blood pressure is stabilized through optimization of preload and afterload, Do_2 can be assessed and further manipulated. Restore arterial oxygen saturation to ≥91%. In shock states, consider a transfusion of packed red blood cells to maintain hemoglobin ≥7 to 9 grams/dL.[25] If CO can be assessed, it should be increased using volume infusion or inotropic agents in incremental amounts until venous oxygen saturation (mixed venous oxygen saturation [$Smvo_2$] or $Scvo_2$) and lactate are normalized.

Sequential examination of lactate and $Smvo_2$ or $Scvo_2$ is a method to assess adequacy of a patient's resuscitation. Continuous measurement of $Smvo_2$ or $Scvo_2$ can be used in the ED, although recent literature questions the need for this in resuscitation management.[20] A variety of technologic tools may be used to assess tissue perfusion during resuscitation.[30-35] These technologies may be available in some EDs, but it is essentially standard of care in intensive care units. Transfer of the patient to the intensive care unit should not be delayed so that monitoring devices can be placed in the ED.[15,36]

END POINTS OF RESUSCITATION

The goal of resuscitation is to use hemodynamic and physiologic values to guide therapy in order to maximize survival and minimize morbidity. No therapeutic end point is universally effective, and only a few have been tested in prospective trials, with mixed results.[20,28,29] Hypotension at ED presentation is associated with poor outcomes.[37] Noninvasive parameters, such as blood pressure, heart rate, and urine output, may underestimate the degree of remaining hypoperfusion and oxygen debt, so the use of additional physiologic end points may be informative.[20,28,29,37] A goal-directed approach of MAP >65 mm Hg, central venous pressure of 8 to 12 mm Hg, $Scvo_2$ >70%, and urine output >0.5 mL/kg/h during ED resuscitation of septic shock has been shown to decrease mortality, but which of the metrics accounts for the mortality decrease remains in question.[16,19,20,25] Source control, whether with infection, hemorrhage, or other state of shock, is essential in the initial stages of management. If shock or hypotension persists, reassessment at the patient's bedside is essential while considering the important issues in **Table 12-8**.

CONTROVERSIES OF TREATMENT

FLUID THERAPY

Rapid restoration of fluid deficits modulates inflammation and, if the condition progresses to shock, decreases the need for subsequent vasopressor therapy, steroid administration, and invasive monitoring (e.g., pulmonary artery catheterization and arterial line placement).[25,38] Although there is general agreement that volume therapy is an integral component of early resuscitation, there is a lack of consensus for the type of fluid, standards of volume assessment, and end points. **Table 12-9** compares the most commonly used fluid therapies.[39-43]

Colloids are high-molecular-weight solutions that increase plasma oncotic pressure. Colloids can be classified as either natural (albumin) or artificial (starches, dextrans, and gelatins). Due to their higher molecular weight, colloids stay in the intravascular space significantly longer than crystalloids. The intravascular half-life of albumin is 16 hours versus 30 to 60 minutes for normal saline and lactated

TABLE 12-8 Questions to Answer if There Is Persistent Shock or Hypotension

Equipment and monitoring

Is the patient appropriately monitored?

Is there an equipment malfunction, such as dampening of the arterial line or disconnection from the transducer?

Is the IV tubing into which the vasopressors are running connected appropriately?

Are the vasopressor infusion pumps working?

Are the vasopressors mixed adequately and in the correct dose?

Patient assessment

Do mentation and clinical appearance match the degree of hypotension?

Is the patient adequately volume resuscitated?

Does the patient have a pneumothorax after placement of central venous access?

Has the patient been adequately assessed for an occult penetrating injury (a bullet hole or stab wound)?

Is there hidden bleeding from a ruptured spleen, large-vessel aneurysm, or ectopic pregnancy?

Does the patient have adrenal insufficiency? The incidence of adrenal dysfunction can be as high as 30% in this subset of patients.

Is the patient allergic to the medication just given or taken before arrival?

Is there cardiac tamponade in the dialysis patient or cancer patient?

Is there associated acute myocardial infarction, aortic dissection, or pulmonary embolus?

ringer's solution.[24,39-41] Resuscitation with **crystalloids** requires two to four times more volume than colloids.[24,38,39] The outcome advantage between crystalloid and colloids continues to remain unresolved in sepsis, despite multiple studies.[24,38-41] Due to the equivalency and the higher cost of colloids, crystalloids would seem to be a better choice for resuscitation in the ED.

BICARBONATE USE IN SHOCK

Bicarbonate administration shifts the oxygen-hemoglobin dissociation curve to the left, impairs tissue unloading of hemoglobin-bound oxygen, and may worsen intracellular acidosis. However, many clinicians remain uncomfortable withholding bicarbonate if the pH is <7.00. Animal studies of profound acidosis demonstrate decreased ventricular contractility and systolic blood pressure.[7] In settings of a low pH and when evidence of decreased contractility (despite ongoing resuscitative efforts) or development of a dysrhythmia, partially correct the metabolic acidosis, either with sodium bicarbonate boluses or a drip. Recognize the risk of paradoxical intracerebral intracellular acidosis in the process. Consider situations, such as end-stage renal disease and renal tubular acidosis, that cannot reclaim bicarbonate through normal renal processes and whether bicarbonate may be indicated.

TABLE 12-9 Fluid Therapy

Crystalloids	
Normal saline (NS)	Slightly hyperosmolar containing 154 mEq/L of both sodium and chloride. Risk of inducing hyperchloremic metabolic acidosis when given in large amounts due to relatively high chloride concentration.
Lactated ringer's (LR)	Lactate can accept a proton and subsequently be metabolized to carbon dioxide and water by the liver, leading to release of carbon dioxide in the lungs and excretion of water by the kidneys. LR results in a buffering of the acidemia that is advantageous over NS. Theoretical risk of inducing hyperkalemia in patients with renal insufficiency or renal failure due to small potassium content (very small amount).
Colloids	
Albumin	Derived from human plasma. Available in varying strengths from 4% to 25%. Multiple studies have shown that there is no outcome difference whether colloids or crystalloids are used. Colloids cost significantly more than crystalloids. One study actually showed an increase in mortality in trauma patients complicated by head injury.
Hydroxyethyl starch	Synthetic colloid derived from hydrolyzed amylopectin. Hydroxyethyl starch should be avoided in sepsis. Many harmful effects: renal impairment at recommended doses and impairing long-term survival at high doses, coagulopathy and bleeding complications from reduced factor VIII and von Willebrand factor levels, impaired platelet function.

DISPOSITION AND TRANSITION TO THE INTENSIVE CARE UNIT

Early recognition, treatment, and subsequent transfer of critically ill patients to the intensive care unit improves patient outcomes and improves ED throughput.[15,36] Communicate and document all ED resuscitative efforts to the critical care team. Even when resuscitation is systematic and thoughtful, miscommunication can undo the benefits of initial ED treatment. Ideally, before transfer, verbally communicate and document a system-oriented problem list with an assessment and plan, including all procedures and complications. For prolonged or "boarded" ED stays, constantly reassess the critically ill patient and ensure that care plans are continuing. Often, this will entail ordering tests that are not commonly performed on ED patients or ordering subsequent doses of medicines, particularly antibiotics.

PROGNOSIS

Some clinical variables are associated with poor outcome, such as severity of shock, temporal duration, underlying cause, preexisting vital organ dysfunction, and reversibility. Early recognition, intervention, source control, and smooth transitions of care help ensure the most ideal outcomes. While associated morbidity and mortality remain high for patients with shock, integration of protocol-based care pathways, with ongoing refinement in response to new information, may lead to continued reductions over time.[15,20,25,36] Additional outcome predictions related to physiologic scoring systems, ED-based shock interventions, and the balance between invasive and noninvasive or minimally invasive strategies are still being studied.[15,44,45]

REFERENCES

The complete reference list is available online at www.TintinalliEM.com.

Fluid and Blood Resuscitation in Traumatic Shock

David M. Somand
Kevin R. Ward

INTRODUCTION

Circulatory shock has a high mortality. Severe hemorrhage after injury carries a mortality rate of 30% to 40% and is responsible for almost 50% of deaths occurring within 24 hours of injury.[1,2] Septic shock has a mortality of up to 50%.[3] Resuscitation, starting in the prehospital setting and continuing throughout the victim's care in the ED and on into the hospital, has the goal of restoring the necessary level of tissue perfusion and oxygenation for survival while simultaneously limiting further volume loss.

Intravascular volume depletion is a common feature of circulatory shock; crystalloids, colloids, and blood products (packed red blood cells

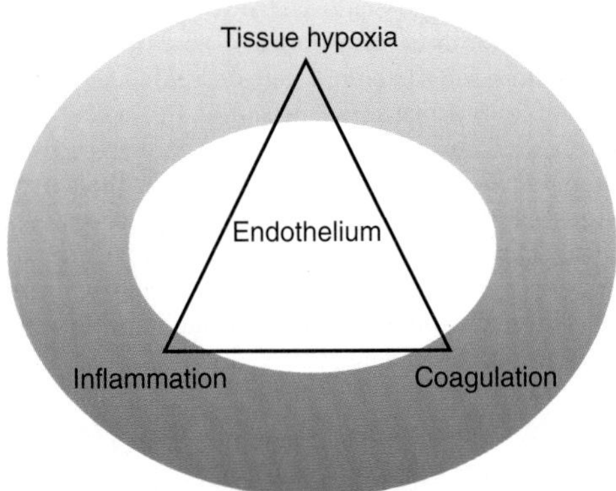

FIGURE 13-1. Endothelium-mediated activation of the triad of hypoxia, inflammation, and coagulation. [©Kevin R. Ward, MD.]

TABLE 13-1 Adult Fluid Spaces

Fluid Compartment	% Body Weight*	% Body Water*	Volume* (70 kg)
Total body water	60	100	42 L
Intracellular	40	67	28 L
Extracellular	20	33	14 L
Interstitial	15	25	10 L
Intravascular	~7–8	~11–13	~5.0–5.5 L
Plasma	~4.0–4.5	~7	~3.0–3.5 L
Red blood cells†	~3.0–3.5	~5	~2.0–2.5 L

*Approximate percentage and amount.

†Percentages do not add up to 100% because fluid contained within intravascular red blood cells is included within the intracellular fluid compartment.

and plasma) are the primary volume expanders to reverse intravascular volume depletion. This chapter focuses on the issues related to fluid and blood resuscitation in traumatic shock, with an emphasis on hemorrhagic shock. Processes that cause loss of plasma fluid and electrolytes (e.g., dehydration, burns, sepsis), often requiring aggressive fluid therapy, are discussed in other chapters (see chapters 150, "Toxic Shock Syndromes," 151, "Sepsis," and 216, "Thermal Burns").

The principal objectives of fluid and blood resuscitation in traumatic shock are: (1) to restore intravascular volume sufficient to maintain oxygen-carrying capacity and tissue perfusion for adequate cellular oxygen delivery, and (2) to prevent or correct derangements in coagulation.

PATHOPHYSIOLOGY

Circulatory shock is a state of impaired oxidative metabolism and homeostasis due to inadequate oxygen delivery to meet metabolic demand, and hypoperfusion leading to inadequate cellular waste removal. Acute shock triggers a complex range of physiologic responses that compensate for intravascular volume loss and maintain perfusion to the most important vascular beds. Shock also produces a global insult to the vascular endothelium that activates the coagulation and inflammatory systems (**Figure 13-1**). When uncorrected, coagulopathy, additional inflammation, and organ system damage result.

While moderate transient hypoperfusion may be well tolerated, prolonged or severe hypoperfusion leads to accumulation of oxygen debt and progressive cellular and organ dysfunction. If rapid and severe, sudden cardiovascular collapse and death may occur.

Coagulopathy observed in trauma victims, termed *trauma-induced coagulopathy*, is ascribed to a combination of factors beginning with loss of coagulation factors from hemorrhage, followed by hemodilution from crystalloid resuscitation, and then exacerbated by acidosis (evidenced by a base deficit) and hypothermia that occur during the course of ongoing hemorrhage and resuscitation.[4] These same principles also apply to other causes of shock.[5] However, acidosis does not, by itself, have a significant effect on coagulation until the pH decreases below 7.0.[6]

The lethal triad of hypothermia, hemodilution, and acidosis can be viewed a partially iatrogenic based on the type of resuscitation provided. The normal total circulating volume of an adult is approximately 7% of ideal body weight or about 5 L for an average 70-kg adult patient divided into about 3 L of plasma and 2 L of red blood cell volume (**Table 13-1**). Understanding this distribution explains how trauma-induced coagulopathy can be iatrogenically produced.

Factors exacerbating trauma-induced coagulopathy, including hyperfibrinolysis and clotting factor and platelet consumption or dysfunction, are related to the degree of injury and hemorrhage.[7] Early trauma-induced coagulopathy is characterized by anticoagulation and hyperfibrinolysis, likely modulated through the protein C pathway. Endothelial damage associated with trauma or sepsis stimulates an increase in thrombomodulin expression on the endothelium that complexes with thrombin and in turn activates protein C (**Figure 13-2**). Complexed thrombin is now no longer available for its usual hemostatic role of cleaving fibrinogen to form fibrin. Subsequent consumption of plasminogen activator inhibitor-1 by activated protein C contributes to hyperfibrinolysis (Figure 13-2).[8]

Thrombomodulin normally found in the endothelium may be viewed as protective because it is able to sequester thrombin and thus allow for generation of adequate levels of protein C to prevent thrombosis caused by low-flow states. However, on a mass systemic level, this appropriate local response may become pathologic, resulting in clotting inhibition.

CLINICAL FEATURES

The clinical appearance of acute traumatic shock is variable and depends on the cause, rate, volume, and duration of volume loss or bleeding; the presence of other acute disorders; the effects of current medications; and the patient's baseline physiologic status.

The hemodynamic response to acute severe hemorrhage-induced hypovolemia traditionally includes tachycardia, hypotension, and signs of poor peripheral perfusion (cool, pale, clammy extremities with weak peripheral pulses and prolonged capillary refill). Arterial and venous vasoconstriction leads to a narrowing of the pulse pressure. Cerebral hypoperfusion causes alterations in mental status. With increasing blood loss, signs and symptoms become more pronounced. Classification of hemorrhage severity as a percentage of blood volume loss based on vital signs is not accurate and should not be used to guide ED resuscitation.[9]

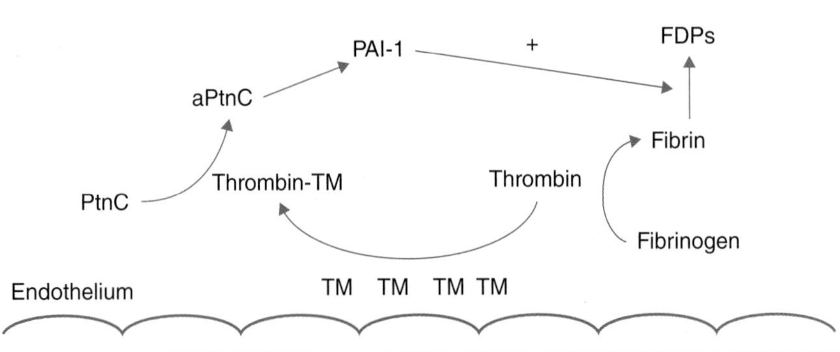

FIGURE 13-2. Endothelial damage results in increased thrombomodulin (TM) expression. TM can complex with thrombin (thrombin-TM complex), leading to activation of the protein C (PtnC to aPntcC) pathway. Modulated through a multistep pathway leading to plasminogen activator inhibitor-1 (PAI-1), fibrinolysis is encouraged, resulting in increased fibrin degradation products (FDPs). In addition, the complexed thrombin is no longer able to perform its usual role in cleaving fibrinogen to fibrin to form clots.

Patients with excellent baseline physiologic status (e.g., young athletes) may have such a robust compensatory response to hemorrhage that they appear stable and do not manifest tachycardia or hypotension, even with large blood volume loss. Signs of peripheral hypoperfusion and subtle mental status alterations may be the only clues that the severity of hemorrhage is greater than predicted based on hemodynamic parameters. Elderly patients may not develop tachycardia due to underlying heart disease or medications such as β-adrenergic blockers. Bradycardia or lack of tachycardia may occur in about 30% of patients with intra-abdominal hemorrhage from increased vagal tone in response to hemoperitoneum. In a pregnant trauma patient, compression of the inferior vena cava by the gravid uterus can decrease central venous return and worsen hypotension and tachycardia in the setting of less severe hemorrhage.

DIAGNOSIS

Vital signs offer little value unless they are in extreme low ranges. Arterial blood pressure does not adequately reflect cardiac output or regional perfusion. Clinical evidence of peripheral hypoperfusion is useful but is not a quantitative measurement. Metabolic information (discussed below), assessment of mechanisms of injury and illness, and appropriate imaging studies offer the best chance for early recognition of severe hemorrhage and for guiding an appropriate response to treatment.

There is a biphasic relationship between oxygen consumption and oxygen delivery (**Figure 13-3**). While this relationship exists for the body as a whole, it also exists for each individual organ system and is largely mediated by the microcirculation. Oxygen debt develops in tissues or organs when oxygen delivery does not meet the metabolic demands and represents the amount of extra oxygen that is needed to metabolize the accumulated products of anaerobic metabolism once perfusion is restored. Oxygen debt is the accumulation of multiple oxygen deficits over time and is a measure of whole-body ischemia. Oxygen debt is the only physiologic measure that has clearly been linked to both mortality and even morbidity in the form of multiple organ failure after shock. The degree of oxygen debt incurred after injury has also been clearly linked to inflammation.[10]

Measurements of lactate and base deficit are in fairly ubiquitous use in trauma centers and EDs and are now even being used as point-of-care testing in the prehospital setting as a triage tool. Using lactate and/or base deficit as a resuscitation trigger and its clearance/normalization as an endpoint is prudent and is associated with improvements in survival. However, elevated lactate and base deficit is a late finding, which is first preceded by increases in oxygen extraction as indicated by a decrease in indicators of oxygen consumption such as mixed or central venous hemoglobin oxygen saturation (Figure 13-2). Furthermore, improvements in oxygen delivery resulting in lactate clearance do not indicate that oxygen extraction is normal.

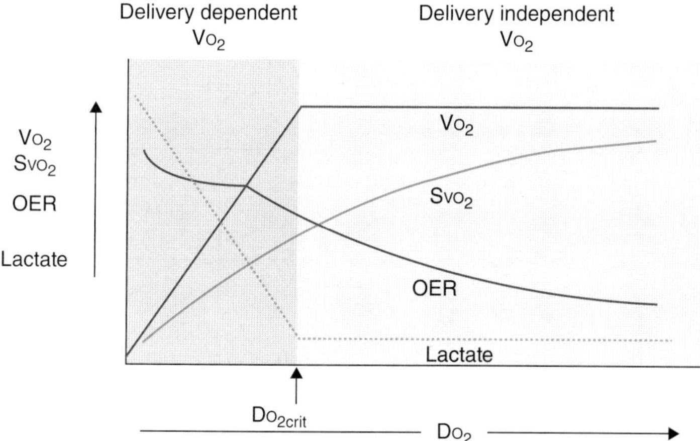

FIGURE 13-3. The biphasic relationship of oxygen delivery (Do_2) and oxygen consumption (Vo_2). As Do_2 decreases, Vo_2 may remain constant due to an increase in the ratio of extracted oxygen (OER) at the tissue level. This is mirrored by a decrease in venous hemoglobin oxygen saturation (Svo_2). However, at some point, OER will not meet the Vo_2 demands of the tissues, resulting in a state of Do_2 dependent Vo_2 whereby aerobic Vo_2 transitions to anaerobic Vo_2. At this point of critical Do_2, oxygen debt begins to accumulate along with metabolic byproducts of anaerobiosis such as lactate. While this relationship exists for the body as a whole, it also exists for each individual organ system and is largely mediated by the microcirculation. [©Kevin R. Ward, MD.]

Although lactate is also a measure of oxygen debt, its resolution during resuscitation does not ensure the important repayment and resolution of oxygen debt. Lactate also suffers from the intermittent and time-dependent nature of its measure and change. To counter these, continuous measures of oxygen consumption surrogates are available in the form of invasive oximetric catheters measuring central venous oxygen saturation ($Scvo_2$) and tissue oxygen saturation (Sto_2) noninvasively from target tissues such as skeletal muscle using near-infrared spectroscopy. Sto_2 measurements with infrared spectroscopy are based on the fact that tissue blood volume is 70% to 80% venous blood with the remaining 10% to 20% a combination of arterial and capillary blood. Thus aggregate measures of hemoglobin oxygenation in the tissue are heavily dominated by the venous blood and thus the postextraction compartment. Although not an exact mirror of $Scvo_2$, ensuring Sto_2 values above 50% appears to be reasonable from both a diagnostic and treatment standpoint to begin and sustain hemostatic resuscitation. A target Sto_2 or $Scvo_2$ between 60% and 70% should be maintained to help ensure resolution of tissue hypoxia.

TREATMENT

Resuscitation begins in the prehospital setting and continues in the ED. The priority for prehospital care is treatment of life-threatening conditions and rapid transport to an appropriate facility. For the hemorrhaging patient, this entails assuring adequate ventilation and oxygenation (including securing an airway if necessary), controlling external bleeding (if present), and protecting the spinal cord (if potentially vulnerable).

In the ED, **restore intravascular volume** to reverse or limit systemic and regional hypoperfusion, **maintain oxygen-carrying capacity** so that tissue oxygen delivery meets demand, and **limit ongoing blood loss** and **prevent the development of coagulopathy**. From the moment resuscitation begins, prevent the development of **hypothermia** by keeping the patient warm and administering warmed IV fluids and blood products.[11] Endogenous hypothermia occurs when heat production from cellular respiration is decreased by hypoperfusion and inadequate tissue oxygen delivery. Major causes of exogenous hypothermia are exposure and the use of below-body-temperature fluid and blood resuscitation. Apply external warming devices early to prevent external heat escape. Warming devices that allow for the rapid warming of infused fluid and blood should be used for all patients in whom large-volume resuscitation is undertaken.[11]

AIRWAY CONTROL, VENTILATION, AND OXYGENATION

If spontaneous ventilation is not adequate, intubate and ventilate to achieve an arterial hemoglobin oxygen saturation of ≥94%. Identify and treat potential respiratory conditions such as pneumothorax, tension pneumothorax, hemothroax, or upper airway obstruction.

VASCULAR ACCESS AND MONITORING

Establish adequate IV access concurrent with airway management. Large-bore (14- to 16-gauge in adults) peripheral lines may be adequate if two or more can be secured. Central venous access may be necessary. Intraosseous lines are suitable for resuscitation.

Institute continuous ECG heart rate monitoring, continuous pulse oximetry, and, if possible, continuous end-tidal carbon dioxide monitoring. Monitor arterial blood pressure, mental status, and peripheral perfusion frequently. Bedside US is useful to identify intraperitoneal bleeding, assess cardiac function and volume status, and assist in central venous cannulation.[12,13]

TABLE 13-3 Isotonic Fluid Composition*							
Fluid	Na^+ (mmol/L)	K^+ (mmol/L)	Ca^{++} (mmol/L)	Mg^{++} (mmol/L)	CL^- (mmol/L)	Buffer (mmol/L)	Osm (mOsm/L)
Normal saline	154	0	0	0	154	None	308
Ringer's lactate	130	4	1.4	0	109	28 lactate	273
Ringer's acetate	130	5	1	1	112	27 acetate	276
Hartmann's	131	5	2	0	111	29 lactate	278
Plasma-Lyte A	140	5	0	1.5	98	27 acetate 23 gluconate	294

*Minor variations may exist between different commercial manufacturers.

HEMOSTATIC-HYPOTENSIVE RESUSCITATION

Hemostatic resuscitation begins in the field. In traumatic shock, the goal is deliberate hypotensive resuscitation, so that intravascular volume expansion is limited and blood pressure is not normalized. Blood pressure goals are systolic blood pressures of 80 to 90 mm Hg (10.7 to 12.0 kPa) in trauma and 90 to 95 mm Hg (12.0 to 12.7 kPa) in head injury. Normalization of blood pressure and the raising of hydrostatic pressure can increase hemorrhage. This is particularly evident in noncompressible hemorrhage where raising blood pressure could potentially "pop the clot" and reestablish active hemorrhage.

Hypotensive resuscitation targets fluid resuscitation only when systolic blood pressure falls below 70 to 80 mm Hg (9.3 to 10.7 kPa) and/or there is evidence of decreasing mental status and, thus cerebral hypoperfusion. This practice has been widely adopted in combat casualty care (see chapter 302, "Military Medicine") and is partially supported by civilian studies.[14] Preliminary results of traumatic injury comparing low versus traditional mean arterial pressure guided resuscitation indicate that a lower mean arterial pressure group sustains less blood loss, requires fewer transfusions, and has improved early and 30-day survival.[15]

Hypotensive resuscitation is problematic for a number of reasons, including the inability to obtain frequent and accurate blood pressures and, in the civilian world, its application to the elderly and those with hypertension or cerebral vascular disease. Hypotensive resuscitation should not be used in patients with myocardial disease, cerebral ischemia, or traumatic brain injury. Obviously there is not an unlimited time span that patients can tolerate hypotensive resuscitation. From a cellular standpoint, patients will at some time incur irreversible damage from prolonged tissue hypoxia if adequate tissue oxygenation is not restored.

ISOTONIC CRYSTALLOID SOLUTIONS

Isotonic crystalloids, normal saline, and lactated Ringer's solution are the most commonly used resuscitation fluids in the United States. Concerns about each fluid are: (1) infusion of large volumes of either normal saline or lactated Ringer's solution can cause increased neutrophil activation, (2) lactated Ringer's solution can increase cytokine release and may increase lactic acidosis when given in large volumes, and (3) normal saline can exacerbate intracellular potassium depletion and cause hyperchloremic acidosis.[16]

Crystalloid solutions are isotonic but hypo-oncotic, because they lack the large protein molecules present in the plasma. Low oncotic pressure results in substantial shifts of crystalloid to the extravascular space corresponding to the relative size of the intravascular and interstitial fluid compartments (**Table 13-2**). This was the physiologic basis for the 3:1 ratio for crystalloid to blood. For every amount of blood lost, three times that amount of isotonic crystalloid is required to restore intravascular volume because, at best, about 30% of the infused fluid stays intravascular. Based on this rule, a loss of 1 L of blood (about 15% to 20% of total circulating blood volume) would require about 3 L of isotonic crystalloid to restore normovolemia, assuming no ongoing blood loss. Bearing this in mind, the recommendations for initial fluid resuscitation have been to administer 2 to 3 L of crystalloid solution in acute hemorrhage and assess the response before initiating blood transfusion. In light of the new data reflecting improved outcomes with plasma-based resuscitation in traumatic hemorrhage, no more than 2 L of crystalloid solution should be administered before giving serious consideration to using blood products, especially if ongoing hemorrhage is expected.

Common modifications of isotonic fluids include use of acetate instead of lactate in Ringer's solution, Hartmann's solution, and Plasma-Lyte (**Table 13-3**). Plasma-Lyte is the shared name for a family of isotonic crystalloid solutions available worldwide, marketed with variation in composition according to regional preferences. Solutions containing lactate or acetate are considered *balanced crystalloids* because they are buffered and have a lower chloride concentration compared to normal saline. There is evidence of low confidence that balanced crystalloids are associated with reduced mortality compared with normal saline when used for fluid resuscitation in sepsis.[17]

TABLE 13-2 Theoretical Volemic Effect of 1 L of Fluid Administration on Fluid Compartments			
	Intracellular (mL)	Interstitial (mL)	Plasma (mL)
5% dextrose in water	660	255	85
Normal saline or Ringer's lactate	−100	825	275
7.5% saline	−2950	2960	990
5% albumin	0	500	500
Whole blood	0	0	1000

COLLOID SOLUTIONS

Colloid solutions contain larger molecular weight particles that have oncotic pressures similar to normal plasma proteins. Therefore, colloids theoretically have several advantages during resuscitation. They would be expected to remain in the intravascular space, replacing plasma proteins lost due to hemorrhage, and more effectively restore circulating blood volume than crystalloid solutions. An argument favoring the use of colloids has been the concern that extravascular shift, or third-spacing, of infused crystalloid solutions has potential adverse effects, including pulmonary interstitial edema with impaired oxygen diffusion and intra-abdominal edema with diminished bowel perfusion. However, pathologic conditions, such as hemorrhagic shock and sepsis, lead to increased vascular permeability that can allow for eventual extravascular leakage of these larger colloid molecules.[18]

The colloids used as resuscitation fluids are a heterogeneous group of agents with widely varying characteristics and effects. These agents have no proven consistent benefit, and there is evidence of harm in some patients with critical illness.[19,20]

Hetastarch is a high-molecular-weight polysaccharide that has no proven benefit in critically ill patients.[21] Currently, for logistical reasons of weight and size, hetastarch is the recommended fluid of choice for the far forward resuscitation of battlefield casualties.[22] It is used as a part of a hypotensive resuscitation strategy with no more than 1000 mL to be given. The administration of 1000 mL of hetastarch is theoretically equal to the administration of 3 L of isotonic crystalloid.

HYPERTONIC SOLUTIONS

Hypertonic saline (7.5% saline) has been proposed as a potential crystalloid alternative that would limit the tissue edema effects that are often of concern with isotonic crystalloid solutions. Hypertonic saline has anti-inflammatory and immunomodulatory effects, with demonstrable decrease in lung and intestinal injury in animal models of hemorrhagic shock.[18] The intravascular shift of fluid from the extravascular space may be potentially beneficial in head trauma patients by limiting cerebral edema, lowering intracranial pressure, and improving cerebral perfusion. The addition of dextran to hypertonic saline was aimed at sustaining the hemodynamic effect of the hypertonic saline. The volume of hypertonic saline solution that can be given during resuscitation is limited due to the potential for hypernatremia. Similar to hetastarch, an approach using smaller volumes (250 mL) of hypertonic saline (7.5%) has also been advocated. Randomized controlled trials have not demonstrated a clinically significant difference in outcome when hypertonic saline was compared with conventional isotonic fluid.[23] However, these studies did not generally incorporate hypotensive resuscitation as a part of the overall strategy, and in the prehospital trail, transport times to trauma centers were short.[24]

PACKED RED BLOOD CELLS

Packed red blood cells (PRBCs) are the most commonly transfused blood product (see chapter 238). Using only PRBCs in the patient with traumatic shock and ongoing bleeding (without plasma and platelets) will do little to promote hemostasis and may not restore tissue oxygenation. If hemorrhage is definitively controlled, do not transfuse if the hemoglobin concentration is > 10 g/dL (> 100 g/L). Consensus recommendations for transfusion are a hemoglobin concentration between 6 and 7 g/dL (60 to 70 g/L) for those without cardiopulmonary, cerebral, or peripheral vascular disease.[25] For a hemoglobin between 6 and 10 g/dL (60 to 100 g/L), use clinical judgement for transfusion.

When possible, typed and cross-matched blood is preferable. However, if time and the patient's clinical status do not permit full cross-matching, type-specific blood is the next option, followed by low-titer O-negative blood. In U.S. blood banks, whole blood is not stocked, and only PRBCs are available (see the chapter 302 for further discussion of whole-blood transfusion).

PRBC transfusion obviously restores lost hemoglobin. Using current preservatives, PRBCs can be stored for up to 45 days, and the average age of a unit of blood administered in the United States is about 21 days. Stored red blood cells can lose deformability, limiting their ability to pass normally through capillary beds or even resulting in capillary plugging. The oxygen dissociation curve is altered by loss of 2,3-diphosphoglycerate in the erythrocytes of stored PRBCs, impeding the off-loading of oxygen at the tissue level.[26] Despite these changes, no consistent harm has been identified with use of "older" stored blood.[27,28]

FRESH FROZEN PLASMA

Fresh frozen plasma (FFP) is plasma obtained after the separation of whole blood from red blood cells and platelets and then frozen within 8 hours. A unit of FFP has a volume of 200 to 250 mL and contains all the coagulation factors present in fresh blood. Kept frozen, FFP can be stored for up to a year after the unit was collected. It takes between 15 and 20 minutes to thaw a unit of FFP in a 37°C water bath, which can limit availability in a massive transfusion situation. However, some major trauma centers and their respective blood banks keep thawed FFP (kept at 1°C to 6°C) available for immediate use. FFP may be kept thawed at this temperature for up to 5 days with little degradation of plasma proteins. FFP ABO compatibility is required, but because there are no red cells in FFP, Rh compatibility is less important, and universal donor FFP is typically AB+ (see chapter 238, "Transfusion Therapy").

PLATELETS

Platelets are collected from whole-blood donations or from single donors using apheresis techniques and can only be stored for up to 5 days. Six units of pooled random-donor platelet concentrate or one apheresis-collected single-donor platelet concentrate in an adult will increase platelet count up to 50,000/mm^3 (50 × 10^9/L).

MASSIVE TRANSFUSION PROTOCOLS

Massive transfusion is generally defined as the requirement for >10 units of PRBCs within the first 24 hours of injury. Massive transfusion is not a substitute for definitive surgical hemostasis but enhances the ability to achieve surgical hemostasis and to limit complications.[29,30] Draw sufficient specimens from the patient early in anticipated massive transfusion because once the patient has received close to one blood volume of transfused products, new blood specimens will contain so much donor blood that cross-matching of subsequent units is difficult. Initially use isotonic solutions to begin resuscitation in predetermined aliquots (250 to 500 mL) while assessing the likelihood of ongoing active hemorrhage and the need for, type, and timing of hemostasis and for hypotensive resuscitation.[31,32] Variables predictive of need for massive transfusion include penetrating mechanism of injury, positive FAST examination, blood pressure <90 mm Hg (< 12.0 kPa), and pulse rate >120 beats/min.[33,34] If hemorrhage is clinically significant and immediate hemostasis is not achievable, transition from crystalloid-based resuscitation to a plasma-based massive transfusion protocol.

An estimated 10% of military trauma patients and 3% to 5% of civilian trauma patients receive massive transfusion.[1] Soldiers receiving high ratios of plasma to PRBC (a plasma:PRBC ratio of about 1:1.4) have significantly improved survival rates than those receiving lower ratios (between 1:1.8 and 1:2.5). Additional evidence supporting this also comes from combat casualty care data suggesting that early administration of fresh whole blood (something not currently practical in civilian trauma) offers survival advantages.[18,35] These survival observations using high plasma-to-PRBC ratios were confirmed by civilian studies, which also appear to indicate less incidence of trauma-induced coagulopathy.[33,36]

High plasma-to-PRBC ratio resuscitation appears to also offer survival benefit independent of coagulopathy, and plasma may enhance cell survival by endothelial repair and reducing vascular permeability. It may also be that plasma is simply a superior fluid for perfusion and tissue oxygenation restoration. In addition, many trauma centers now include early platelet administration in predetermined ratios to plasma and PRBC in their resuscitation protocols based on findings that platelet function can rapidly decrease soon after trauma.[1,34]

Studies routinely using FFP and platelets with PRBCs during massive transfusion have yielded mixed results on reducing mortality.[34,37] The best ratio of PRBCs to platelets to FFP during massive transfusion is controversial.[38] Some experts advocate a 1:1:1 ratio, although lower ratios of platelets and FFP have been used without evidence of inferiority.[39] Likewise, the benefits with adjunctive agents such as calcium chloride, prothrombin complex concentrates, and fibrinogen concentrate included in some protocols are unknown. Tranexamic acid (an antifibrinolytic) is advocated early in the resuscitation process of major trauma victims based on the early fibrinolytic phase of trauma-induced coagulopathy and on clinical studies suggesting improved survival.[40] An institution-specific massive transfusion protocol is recommended to guide the clinician when ordering blood components and to facilitate release from the blood bank (**Figure 13-4**). Tranexamic acid, an antifibrinolytic agent, is not currently a component of massive transfusion protocols in the United States. Its use is discussed in the chapters 254, "Trauma in Adults" and 302, "Military Medicine." If given, it must be administered as soon as possible and within 3 hours of injury. The dose is 1 gram IV bolus in 100 mL normal saline.

Calcium PRBCs and FFP contain citrate that can complex calcium, producing life-threatening hypocalcemia.[41] Most massive transfusion protocols include the administration of calcium and monitoring of ionized calcium. Calcium chloride is preferred over calcium gluconate because a well-perfused liver is required to liberate more free calcium from calcium gluconate. Maintain ionized calcium levels at or above 0.9 mmol/L.[42]

Thromboelastography and Thromboelastometry The blood coagulation system consists of nearly 80 very tightly coupled biochemical reactions. Conventional coagulation testing such as the prothrombin time and activated partial thromboplastin time do not take into account the cellular components of the clot such as red cells and platelets. Because the blood clot itself consists of a complex three-dimensional network of cross-linked fibers made of fibrin, platelets, and red cells entrapped within this mesh, newer viscoelastic tests such as thromboelastography or thromboelastometry are being developed

Massive Transfusion Protocol (MTP) – ADULT

Appropriate initial interventions:
- Intravenous access – 2 large bore IVs and Central Venous Cath
- Labs: T&S, CBC, Plts, INR, PT, PTT, Fibrinogen, Electrolytes. BUN/Creatinine, ionized calcium
- Continual monitoring: VS, U/O, Acid-base status
- Aggressive re-warming
- Prevent/Reverse acidosis
- Correct hypocalcemia: CaGluconate or CaCl
- Target goal ionized calcium 1.2–1.3
- If use CaCl 1 gm, give slowly IV
- Repeat lab testing to evaluate coagulopathy
- Stop crystalloid - avoid dilutional coagulopathy

Other considerations:
- Cell salvage: Anes Tech via front desk
- Heparin reversal: Protamine 1 mg IV/100 U heparin
- Warfarin reversal: Vitamin K 10 mg IV: consider prothromin CC
- Chronic Renal Failure or VW Disease: DDAVP 0.3 microgram/kg IV × 1 dose
- Consider antifibrinolytics:
  - Tranexamic acid 10 mg/kg IV
  - Amicar 5 gm IV bolus then 1 gm/hr IV infusion

Additional help
- Anesthesia: Page

General Guidelines for Lab-based Blood Component Replacement in Adults:

Product	Threshold	Dose
RBCs	No threshold	MD discretion
FFP	INR >1.5	4 units FFP
Platelets	<100,000	One 5-pack Plts
Cryoprecipitate	Fibrinogen <100	Two 5-packs cryoprecipitate

Identify and Manage Bleeding
(Surgery, Angiographic, Embolization, Endoscopy)

↓

Adult: 4U RBCs in <4 hours and ongoing bleeding

↓

Clinical Team Activates MTP & Designates Clinical Contact
Clinical Contact Phones Blood Bank (BB) and:
- Provides name of clinical contact person to BB
- Provides MR#, sex, name, location of patient
- Records name of BB contact, calls if location/contact information changes
- Sends person to pick up the cooler
- Ensures that MTP protocol electronic order is entered

↓

BB prepares MTP pack; transfuse as 1:1:1 ratio
MTP pack: 6U RBCs; 4U FFP; one (1) 5-pack platelets

Hemostasis & resolution of coagulopathy?

No → Clinical contact calls BB for another MTP pack ** MD can adjust pack based on labs PRN → (back to BB prepares MTP pack) → Consider rFVIIa

Consider rFVIIa
- If persistent coagulopathy
- 90 micrograms/kg

No → Repeat labs
- CBC, platelets
- INR/PT, PTT
- Fibrinogen
- ABG (ionized calcium, potassium, lactate, hematocrit)

Yes → Stop MTP
- Notify BB & return any unused blood ASAP
- Resume standard orders
- D/C MTP electronic order

FIGURE 13-4. Massive transfusion protocol (MTP) from the University of Michigan's Level I Trauma Center.

to measure the physical and dynamic characteristics of clotting. Thromboelastography and thromboelastometry can detect trauma-induced coagulopathy and can be used to guide massive transfusion protocols better than traditional prothrombin time and activated partial thromboplastin time assays.[43] However, impact on clinical care is uncertain at this time.[43]

COMPLICATIONS

TRANSFUSION-RELATED ACUTE LUNG INJURY

Acute lung injury is the leading cause of transfusion-related fatalities. It develops within 6 hours of blood transfusion and is felt to be related to an inflammatory reaction.[44] Care is supportive.

TRANSFUSION-ASSOCIATED CIRCULATORY OVERLOAD

Circulatory overload occurs when the recipient's circulatory system is overwhelmed by the rate of transfusion or the volume of products transfused.[45] Clinically, it is characterized by the acute onset of dyspnea, hypertension, tachypnea and tachycardia, and marked elevation in brain natriuretic peptide levels. Care often involves rapid diuresis.

REFERENCES

The complete reference list is available online at www.TintinalliEM.com.

Anaphylaxis, Allergies, and Angioedema

Brian H. Rowe
Theodore J. Gaeta

INTRODUCTION

Anaphylaxis is a serious allergic reaction, with a rapid onset; it may cause death and requires emergent diagnosis and treatment. Consensus clinical criteria have been developed to provide consistency for diagnosis (**Table 14-1**).[1-3]

The terms *anaphylactic* and *anaphylactoid* were previously applied to immunoglobulin E (IgE)-dependent and IgE-independent events, respectively. Because the final pathway in both events is identical, *anaphylaxis* is the term now used to refer to both.[4] Hypersensitivity is an inappropriate immune response to generally harmless antigens, manifesting a continuum from minor to severe manifestations. Anaphylaxis represents the most dramatic and severe form of immediate hypersensitivity.

Foods, medications, insect stings, and allergen immunotherapy injections are the most common provoking factors for anaphylaxis, but any agent capable of producing a sudden degranulation of mast cells or basophils can induce anaphylaxis (**Table 14-2**).[5,6] Latex hypersensitivity is increasing in prevalence in the general population, with a resultant risk for anaphylaxis. In addition, a significant number of anaphylaxis cases

TABLE 14-1 Clinical Criteria for Anaphylaxis

1. Urticaria, generalized itching or flushing, or edema of lips, tongue, uvula, or skin developing over minutes to hours and associated with at least one of the following:
   Respiratory distress or hypoxia
   or
   Hypotension or cardiovascular collapse
   or
   Associated symptoms of organ dysfunction (e.g., hypotonia, syncope, incontinence)
2. Two or more signs or symptoms that occur minutes to hours after allergen exposure:
   Skin and/or mucosal involvement
   Respiratory compromise
   Hypotension or associated symptoms
   Persistent GI cramps or vomiting
3. Consider anaphylaxis when patients are exposed to a known allergen and develop hypotension

have no identified cause, termed idiopathic anaphylaxis.[7] The lifetime individual risk of anaphylaxis is estimated to be 1% to 3%, but the prevalence of anaphylaxis may be increasing.[8] Although allergic reactions are a common cause for ED visits,[9] anaphylaxis is likely underdiagnosed.[10,11]

PATHOPHYSIOLOGY

Anaphylaxis, for the most part, arises from the activation of mast cells and basophils through a mechanism involving crosslinking of IgE and aggregation of the high-affinity receptors for IgE.[6] Upon activation, mast cells and/or basophils quickly release preformed mediators from secretory granules that include histamine, tryptase, carboxypeptidase A, and proteoglycans. Downstream activation of phospholipase A_2, followed by cyclooxygenases and lipoxygenases, produces arachidonic acid metabolites, including prostaglandins, leukotrienes, and platelet-activating factor. The inflammatory cytokine, tumor necrosis factor-α, is released as a preformed mediator and also as a late-phase mediator with other cytokines and chemokines. These mediators are responsible for the pathophysiology of anaphylaxis. Histamine stimulates vasodilation and increases vascular permeability, heart rate, cardiac contraction, and glandular secretion. Prostaglandin D_2 is a bronchoconstrictor, pulmonary and coronary vasoconstrictor, and peripheral vasodilator. Leukotrienes produce bronchoconstriction, increase vascular permeability, and promote airway remodeling. Platelet-activating factor is also a potent bronchoconstrictor and increases vascular permeability. Tumor necrosis factor-α activates neutrophils, recruits other effector cells, and enhances chemokine synthesis. These overlapping and synergistic physiologic effects contribute to the overall pathophysiology of anaphylaxis.[6]

TABLE 14-2 Common Causes for Anaphylaxis, Anaphylactoid, and Allergic Reactions

Drugs	Foods and Additives
β-Lactam antibiotics	Shellfish
Acetylsalicylic acid (ASA)	Soybeans
Trimethoprim-sulfamethoxazole	Nuts (peanuts and tree nuts)
Vancomycin	Wheat
Nonsteroidal anti-inflammatory drugs (NSAIDs)	Milk
Virtually any drug	Eggs
Others	Salicylates
Hymenoptera stings	Seeds
Insect parts	Sulfites
Molds	
Radiographic contrast material	
Vaccines	
Latex	
Blood products	

CLINICAL FEATURES

The classic presentation of anaphylaxis begins with pruritus, cutaneous flushing, and urticaria. These symptoms are followed by a sense of fullness in the throat, anxiety, a sensation of chest tightness, shortness of breath, and lightheadedness. A complaint of a "lump in the throat" and hoarseness heralds life-threatening laryngeal edema in a patient with symptoms of anaphylaxis. These major symptoms may be accompanied by abdominal pain or cramping, nausea, vomiting, diarrhea, bronchospasm, rhinorrhea, conjunctivitis, and/or hypotension. As the cascade progresses, respiratory distress, decreased level of consciousness, and circulatory collapse may ensue. In severe cases, loss of consciousness and cardiorespiratory arrest may result.

Signs and symptoms begin suddenly, often within 60 minutes of exposure, in most patients. In general, the faster the onset of symptoms, the more severe is the reaction—**one half of anaphylactic fatalities occur within the first hour**. After the initial signs and symptoms abate, patients are at a small risk for a recurrence of symptoms caused by a second phase of mediator release, peaking 8 to 11 hours after the initial exposure and manifesting symptoms and signs 3 to 4 hours after the initial clinical manifestations have cleared. The late-phase allergic reaction is primarily mediated by the release of newly generated cysteinyl leukotrienes, the former slow-reacting substance of anaphylaxis. The incidence of this biphasic phenomenon has been reported to vary widely up to 20%, but prospective studies specifically searching for clinically important biphasic events report an incidence of 4% to 5%.[12,13]

DIAGNOSIS

The diagnosis of anaphylaxis is clinical. Consider anaphylaxis when involvement of any two or more body systems is observed, with or without hypotension or airway compromise (**Table 14-3**).[1,14] The diagnosis is easily made if there is a clear history of exposure, such as a bee sting, shortly followed by the multisystem signs and symptoms described above. Unfortunately, diagnosis is not always easy or clear, because symptom onset may be delayed, symptoms may mimic other presentations (e.g., syncope, gastroenteritis, anxiety), or anaphylaxis may be a component of other diseases (e.g., asthma).

The differential diagnosis of anaphylactic reactions is extensive, including vasovagal reactions, myocardial ischemia, arrhythmias, severe acute asthma, seizure, epiglottitis, hereditary angioedema, foreign body airway obstruction, carcinoid, mastocytosis, vocal cord dysfunction, and non–IgE-mediated drug reactions. The most common anaphylaxis imitator is a vasovagal reaction, which is characterized by hypotension, pallor, bradycardia, diaphoresis, and weakness, and sometimes by loss of consciousness.

Laboratory investigations are of minimal utility.[15] Serum histamine levels, elevated for 5 to 30 minutes after reaction, are unhelpful because they are typically normal upon ED presentation. Tryptase is a neutral protease of unknown function in anaphylaxis that is found only in mast

TABLE 14-3 Clinical Manifestations of Anaphylaxis

System	Signs and Symptoms (approximate incidence)
Respiratory	Shortness of breath and/or wheezing (45%–50%)
	Pharyngeal or laryngeal edema (50%–60%)
	Rhinitis (30%–35%)
Cardiovascular	Hypotension (30%–35%)
	Chest pain (4%–5%)
Skin	Urticaria and/or angioedema (60%–90%)
	Flushing (45%–55%)
	Pruritus only (2%–5%)
GI	Nausea, emesis, cramps, or diarrhea (25%–30%)
Neurologic	Headache (5%–8%)
	Seizure (1%–2%)

cell granules and is released with degranulation. Serum tryptase levels are elevated for several hours and have been proposed for later confirmation of a suspected anaphylactic episode, but this test has poor sensitivity; about one third of patients with an acute anaphylaxis episode have a normal serum tryptase level upon ED arrival,[16] and some patients experience severe anaphylaxis without elevated tryptase levels.[17]

TREATMENT

Triage all acute allergic reactions at the highest level of urgency because of the possibility of sudden deterioration.[10] Current treatment recommendations are derived from the clinical experience of experts as professed in consensus statements and guidelines.[15,18-20]

FIRST-LINE THERAPY

Emergency management starts with airway, breathing, and circulation. Assess vital signs and pulse oximetry. Initiate IV access, oxygen administration, and cardiac rhythm monitoring in patients with severe symptoms. The first-line therapies for anaphylaxis (airway protection, oxygen, decontamination, epinephrine, IV crystalloids) have immediate effect during the acute stage.[19-22]

Airway and Oxygenation **In severe anaphylaxis, securing the airway is the first priority.** Examine the mouth, pharynx, and neck for signs and symptoms of angioedema: uvula edema or hydrops, audible stridor, respiratory distress, or hypoxia. If angioedema is producing respiratory distress, intubate early, because delay may result in complete airway obstruction secondary to progression of angioedema. Provide sufficient oxygen to maintain arterial oxygen saturation >90%.

Decontamination If the causative agent can be identified, termination of exposure should be attempted. Gastric lavage is **not recommended** for foodborne allergens and may be associated with complications (i.e., aspiration) and delays in the administration of more effective treatments (e.g., epinephrine). In insect stings, remove any remaining stinging remnants because the stinger continues to inject venom even if it is detached from the insect (see chapter 211, "Bites and Stings").

Epinephrine Epinephrine is a mixed α_1- and β-receptor agent. The α_1-receptor activation reduces mucosal edema and treats hypotension, β1-receptor stimulation increases heart rate and myocardial contractility, and β_2-receptor stimulation provides bronchodilation and limits further mediator release.[15] **Epinephrine is the treatment of choice for anaphylaxis.[15,18,23,24] However, observational studies indicate that it is underused, often dosed suboptimally, and underprescribed upon discharge for potential future self-administration.[9,11]** Most of the reasons proposed to withhold epinephrine are flawed, and the therapeutic benefits of epinephrine exceed the risk when given in appropriate routes and doses.[23]

In patients without signs of cardiovascular compromise or collapse, administer epinephrine IM (**Table 14-4**).[25] Repeat every 5 to 10 minutes

TABLE 14-4 Drug Treatment of Anaphylaxis and Allergic Reactions

Drug	Adult Dose	Pediatric Dose
First-Line Therapy		
Epinephrine	IM: 0.3–0.5 milligram (0.3–0.5 mL of 1:1000 dilution); *or* EpiPen® 0.3 milligram epinephrine (or equivalent preformulated product)	IM: 0.01 milligram/kg (0.01 mL/kg of 1:1000 dilution) *or* EpiPen Junior® 0.15 milligram of epinephrine (or equivalent preformulated product)
	IV bolus: 100 micrograms over 5–10 min; mix 0.1 milligram (0.1 mL of 1:1000 dilution) in 10 mL NS and infuse over 5–10 min	
	IV infusion: start at 1 microgram/min; mix 1 milligram (1 mL of 1:1000 dilution) in 500 mL NS and infuse at 0.5 mL/min; titrate dose as needed	IV infusion: 0.1–0.3 microgram/kg per min; titrate dose as needed; maximum, 1.5 micrograms/kg per min
Oxygen	Titrate to Sao_2 ≥90%	Titrate to Sao_2 ≥90%
IV fluids: NS or LR	1–2 L bolus	10–20 mL/kg bolus
Second-Line Therapy		
H_1 Blockers		
Diphenhydramine	25–50 milligrams every 6 h IV, IM, or PO	1 milligram/kg every 6 h IV, IM, or PO
H_2 Blockers		
Ranitidine	50 milligrams IV over 5 min	0.5 milligram/kg IV over 5 min
Cimetidine	300 milligrams IV	4–8 milligrams/kg IV
Corticosteroids		
Hydrocortisone	250–500 milligrams IV	5–10 milligrams/kg IV (maximum, 500 milligrams)
Methylprednisolone	80–125 milligrams IV	1–2 milligrams/kg IV (maximum, 125 milligrams)
Prednisone	40–60 milligrams/d PO divided twice a day or daily	1–2 milligrams/d PO divided twice a day or daily
	To be used after initial IV dose (for outpatients: 3–5 d; tapering not required)	To be used after initial IV dose (for outpatients: 3–5 d; tapering not required)
Treatment of Bronchospasm, Add:		
Albuterol	Single treatment: 2.5–5.0 milligrams nebulized (0.5–1.0 mL of 0.5% solution)	Single treatment: 1.25–2.5 milligrams nebulized (0.25–0.5 mL of 0.5% solution)
	4–6 puffs from MDI with holding chamber	4–6 puffs from MDI with holding chamber
	Both repeated every 20 min as needed	Both repeated every 20 min as needed
	Continuous nebulization: 5–10 milligrams/h	Continuous nebulization: 3–5 milligrams/h
Ipratropium bromide	Single treatment: 250–500 micrograms nebulized	Single treatment: 125–250 micrograms nebulized
	4–6 puffs from MDI with holding chamber	4–6 puffs from MDI with holding chamber
	Both repeated every 20 min as needed	Both repeated every 20 min as needed
Magnesium sulfate	2 grams IV over 20 min	25–50 milligrams/kg IV over 20 min
Treatment for Patients on β-Blockers with Refractory Hypotension, Add:		
Glucagon	1 milligram IV every 5 min until hypotension resolves, followed by 5–15 micrograms/min infusion	50 micrograms/kg IV every 5 min

Abbreviations: H_1 = histamine-1; H_2 = histamine-2; LR = lactated Ringer's; MDI = metered dose inhaler; NS = normal saline; Sao_2 = arterial oxygen saturation.

according to response or if relapse occurs. Injections into the thigh are more effective at achieving peak blood levels than injections into the deltoid area.[25] IM dosing is recommended because it provides higher, more consistent, and more rapid peak blood epinephrine levels than SC administration.[25,26] For convenience and accurate dosing, many EDs have adopted the use of EpiPen® (0.3 milligram epinephrine for adults; Dey, L.P., Napa, CA) and EpiPen Junior® (0.15 milligram epinephrine for children <30 kg; Dey, L.P.).

Most patients with anaphylaxis need only a single epinephrine dose. Check blood pressure in patients taking β-blockers, because epinephrine use may result in severe hypertension secondary to unopposed α-adrenergic stimulation. Age is not a barrier to epinephrine IM injections in patients with anaphylaxis.

If the patient is refractory to treatment despite repeated doses of epinephrine IM or has signs of cardiovascular compromise or collapse, then institute an epinephrine IV bolus and/or infusion. The initial epinephrine IV bolus is a dilute solution of 100 micrograms (0.1 milligram) IV, given over 5 to 10 minutes.

If the patient is refractory to the initial bolus, institute an epinephrine IV infusion, starting at 1 microgram/min and titrating to effect. There is a higher risk of cardiovascular complications when IV epinephrine is used to treat anaphylaxis.[27] It should be stressed that the initial IV bolus dose is very dilute, is given over 5 to 10 minutes, and should be stopped immediately if arrhythmias or chest pain occur.

IV Crystalloids Hypotension is generally the result of distributive shock and responds to fluid resuscitation.[15] Administer an isotonic crystalloid solution bolus of 1 to 2 L (10 to 20 mL/kg in children) concurrently with epinephrine. There is no evidence that albumin or hypertonic saline should replace crystalloids.[28]

SECOND-LINE THERAPY

The second-line anaphylaxis treatments include corticosteroids, antihistamines, inhaled bronchodilators, vasopressors, and glucagon.[15,18-20] These drugs are used to treat anaphylaxis refractory to the first-line treatments or associated with complications, and also to prevent recurrences.[22]

Corticosteroids Patients with anaphylaxis often receive corticosteroids to prevent protracted and biphasic reactions, although evidence for clinical benefit is scant and primarily derived from acute asthma studies.[18-20,22,29-31] Methylprednisolone, 80 to 125 milligrams IV (2 milligrams/kg in children; up to 125 milligrams), and hydrocortisone, 250 to 500 milligrams IV (5 to 10 milligrams/kg in children; up to 500 milligrams), are equally appropriate. Mineralocorticoid effects of steroids are ranked in declining order. Hydrocortisone and cortisone have the strongest effects, followed by prednisone. Methylprednisolone and dexamethasone have the lowest mineralocorticoid effect and produce less fluid retention than hydrocortisone and cortisone and thus are preferred for the elderly and for those in whom fluid retention would be problematic.

Antihistamines Most patients with anaphylaxis should receive an H_1-antihistamine, such as diphenhydramine, 25 to 50 milligrams IV by slow infusion or via IM injection,[15,18-20,22] although clinical benefit is unproven.[32] In severe cases, especially with circulatory shock, H_2-antihistamines, such as ranitidine or cimetidine, are recommended,[18-20,22] although evidence for benefit is lacking.[33] Cimetidine should not be used for patients who are elderly (side effects), have multiple comorbidities (interference with metabolism of many drugs), have renal or hepatic impairment, or whose anaphylaxis is complicated by β-blocker use (cimetidine prolongs metabolism of β-blockers and may prolong anaphylactic state). After the initial IV dose of steroids and antihistamines, the patient may be switched to oral medication (**Table 14-4**).

Vasopressors In patients with anaphylaxis and shock resistant to initial treatment, including repeated doses of IM epinephrine, oxygen, and intravenous crystalloids, initiate IV epinephrine infusion. If dangerous dysrhythmias or tachycardia result from epinephrine, other agents (e.g., dopamine, dobutamine, epinephrine, norepinephrine, phenylephrine, or vasopressin) may be effective, and superiority from a specific agent has not been demonstrated.[15,18-20] Clinicians should use the agent they feel most comfortable with and titrate according to the clinical response.

AGENTS FOR ALLERGIC BRONCHOSPASM

A β_2 bronchodilator, such as intermittent or continuous nebulized albuterol/salbutamol, should be instituted if wheezing is present. Asthmatics are often more refractory to the treatment of allergic bronchospasm. For severe bronchospasm refractory to inhaled albuterol/salbutamol, inhaled anticholinergics and IV magnesium sulfate can be added (**Table 14-4**).[29,34] Bronchodilators should be used with caution (lower dose and slower rate) in elderly patients. IV aminophylline is not recommended. Leukotriene receptor antagonists are not effective for the treatment of anaphylaxis.

GLUCAGON

Concurrent use of β-blockers is a risk factor for severe prolonged anaphylaxis. For patients taking β-blockers with hypotension refractory to fluids and epinephrine, IV glucagon should be used every 5 minutes until hypotension resolves, followed by an infusion (**Table 14-4**).[15,18-20] The side effects of glucagon include nausea, vomiting, hypokalemia, dizziness, and hyperglycemia.

DISPOSITION AND FOLLOW-UP

With appropriate initial treatment, admission to hospital is rare, only required in about 1% to 4% of acute allergic reactions treated in the ED.[9,13] All unstable patients with anaphylaxis refractory to treatment or in whom airway interventions were required should be admitted to the intensive care unit. Patients who receive epinephrine should be observed in the ED, but the duration of observation necessary is not well established.[12,13] Otherwise healthy patients who remain symptom-free after appropriate treatment following 4 hours of observation can be safely discharged home.

Consider prolonged observation in patients with a past history of severe reaction and those using β-blockers. Although the risk of important biphasic reactions after ED discharge is low,[13] patients who live alone, reside long distances from medical care, have significant comorbidity (including but not limited to asthma), or are elderly should be observed longer before discharge.

Patients with severe allergic reactions or anaphylaxis are usually discharged with prescriptions for antihistamines and corticosteroids for 3 to 5 days. Although prolonged corticosteroid treatment should not be required for most patients, an aggressive longer-term approach (1 to 2 weeks or until symptoms are controlled) appears to reduce the frequency of relapses in patients with idiopathic anaphylaxis.[7]

Discharge instructions should provide recommendations to prevent future episodes (**Table 14-5**).[35] For all allergic reactions, instruct the patient on how to avoid future exposure to the causative agent (if the agent is known). Prescribe an epinephrine autoinjector to patients with serious allergic reactions or anaphylaxis with clear instructions on the use of the autoinjector. If delay in filling a prescription is anticipated, patients can be discharged from the ED with an epinephrine autoinjector (EpiPen®). Reinforce this prescription with documentation in the ED discharge instructions. Because allergic occurrences are unpredictable, prescriptions should include sufficient samples for multiple locations (e.g., home, vehicle, work), and patients should be advised to carry epinephrine with them at all times.

Refer patients with severe or frequent allergic reactions to an allergist for in-depth preventive management and attempts at allergen identification.[36] Offer patients information about this syndrome (e.g., from Web sites), advice on advocacy groups, and education regarding food contamination for food allergies, and encourage wearing of personal identification alerts about this condition (e.g., MedicAlert® bracelets). Because of the potential for severe and prolonged future reactions, patients with anaphylaxis on a β-blocker should be switched to an agent from a different therapeutic class.

ALLERGIES AND ANGIOEDEMA

URTICARIA

Urticaria, or hives, is a cutaneous reaction marked by acute onset of pruritic, erythemic wheals of varying size that generally are described as

TABLE 14-5 Discharge Planning for Patients with Anaphylaxis

Education
Identification of inciting allergen, if possible
Instructions on use of medications and epinephrine autoinjector
Advice about personal identification/allergy alert tag
Prescriptions for current reaction
Antihistamines: Diphenhydramine, 25–50 milligrams PO every 6–8 h for 3–5 d
Corticosteroids: Prednisone, 40–60 milligrams PO daily for 3–5 d
Prevention
Instructions on avoiding future exposure
Prescription for future reactions
Epinephrine autoinjector (at least 2)
Referral to allergist

"fleeting." Erythema multiforme is a more pronounced variation of urticaria, characterized by typical "target" skin lesions. Although these manifestations may accompany many allergic reactions, they also may be nonallergic; many acute urticarial reactions are due to viruses, especially in children, or present as hives persisting or recurring for more than 24 hours. Obtain a detailed history; if an etiologic agent can be identified, future reactions may be avoided, although many acute urticarial reactions are viral in nature.

Treatment of urticarial reactions is generally supportive and symptomatic, with attempts to identify and remove the offending agent. H_1-antihistamines, with or without corticosteroids, are usually sufficient, although epinephrine can be considered in severe or refractory cases. The addition of an H_2-antihistamine, such as ranitidine, may also be useful in more severe, chronic, or unresponsive cases. Cold compresses may be soothing to affected areas. Referral to an allergy specialist is indicated in severe, recurrent, or refractory cases.

ANGIOEDEMA

Angioedema is a similar reaction as urticaria, but with deeper involvement characterized by edema formation in the dermis, generally involving the face and neck, and distal extremities. Angioedema of the tongue, lips, and face has the potential for airway obstruction.[37] Angioedema is caused by a variety of agents, but an angiotensin-converting enzyme inhibitor (ACEI) is a common trigger, with angioedema occurring in 0.1 to 0.7% of patients taking ACEIs.[38,39] The pathophysiology of **ACEI-induced angioedema** is complex, involving both bradykinin and substance P.[38,39]

Management of ACEI-induced angioedema is supportive, with special attention to the airway, which can become occluded rapidly and unpredictably. Allergic reaction drugs, such as epinephrine, antihistamines and corticosteroids, are not beneficial because ACEI-induced angioedema is not mediated by IgE.[38,39] Icartibant, a bradykinin-2 antagonist, is effective agent to reduce swelling and shorten time to complete resolution (**Table 14-6**).[40] C1 esterase inhibitor [human] at a dose of 1000 units IV also appears effective based on a case-series compared to historical controls.[41] Ecallantide, a kallikrein inhibitor, is not effective in ACEI-induced angioedema.[42]

Immediate withdrawal from the ACE inhibitor is indicated, and another antihypertensive should be prescribed, with the important exception that angiotensin II receptor–blocking agents should not be used. Most cases resolve in a few hours to days, so patients with mild swelling and no evidence of airway obstruction should be observed for 12 to 24 hours, and discharged if swelling diminishes. Rebound or recurrent swelling will not occur unless the patient takes an ACE inhibitor again.

Hereditary angioedema is a rare autosomal dominant disorder due to deficiency in C1 esterase inhibitor; either low levels (Type I) or a dysfunctional enzyme (Type II).[43,44] About 25% of cases are due to new mutations.[45] The disorder is characterized by acute edematous reactions involving the upper respiratory, soft tissue of extremities or trunk, or GI tract. Attacks can last from a few hours to 1 to 2 days. Minor trauma often precipitates an acute episode. Typical treatments for allergic reactions, such as epinephrine, corticosteroids, and antihistamines, are ineffective. The best screening test is the C4 level. A C4 level $< 30\%$ of normal suggests hereditary angioedema.

Acute attacks can be shortened by a C1 esterase inhibitor (either human plasma derived or recombinant), by the bradykinin-2 receptor antagonist icatibant, or the kallikrein inhibitor ecallantide (**Table 14-6**).[46,47] Fresh frozen plasma may be used if C1 esterase inhibitor is not available, although the dosing is not standardized, with 2 to 3 units described in most case reports.[48] Prophylaxis of acute attacks is possible with attenuated androgens, such as stanozolol 2 milligrams/d or danazol 200 milligrams/d. Treatment of patients is complex and best done in coordination with the appropriate specialist.

FOOD ALLERGY REACTIONS

Hypersensitivity reactions to ingested foods are generally caused by IgE-coated mast cells lining the GI tract reacting to ingested food proteins

TABLE 14-6 Pharmacologic Treatment of Angioedema in Adults

Agent*	Recommended Adult Dose	Comments
C1 esterase inhibitor [human] (Berinert®)	20 U/kg IV for HAE 1000 U IV for ACEI-induced angioedema	Effective in HAE and ACEI-induced angioedema† Adverse side effects include headache, abdominal pain, nausea, diarrhea, and vomiting
C1 esterase inhibitor [recombinant] (Ruconest®)	50 U/kg IV (max dose 4200 U)	Effective in HAE, but not FDA approved for HAE patients with laryngeal attacks No data for ACEI-induced angioedema Adverse side effects include headache and vertigo
Icatibant (Firazyr®)	30 milligrams SC	Effective in HAE and ACEI-induced angioedema† Bradykin-2 receptor antagonist Single dose highly effective: about 10% require second dose 90% experience mild local reactions: pain ,swelling, erythema
Ecallantide (Kalbitor®)	30 milligrams SC (in three separate 10 milligrams or 1 mL injections)	Effective in HAE, but not ACEI-induced angioedema Kallikrein inhibitor Risk of anaphylaxis in up to 4% May repeat 30 milligram dose within 24 hours if reaction persists Adverse side effects include headache, nausea, fatigue, diarrhea, nasopharyngitis, injection site reactions, and vomiting

Abbreviations: ACEI = angiotensin converting enzyme inhibitor; HAE = hereditary angioedema

*Proprietary names provided to aid in recognition

†Not FDA approved for ACEI-induced angioedema

and, rarely, to additives. Their frequency is rising for unknown reasons and varies based on age (more common in children), country of origin, and definitions and confirmatory tests used.[44] Dairy products, eggs, nuts, and shellfish are the most commonly implicated foods.[49,50]

A detailed dietary history within the 24 hours of allergic symptoms may provide the best clues to food allergy, with particular attention to other allergic history and prior reactions. Diagnosis is often difficult, however, and it may require multiple episodes before an offending agent is identified.[50] Symptoms of food allergy include swelling and itching of the lips, mouth, and pharynx; nausea; abdominal cramps; vomiting; and diarrhea. Cutaneous manifestations, such as angioedema and urticaria, as well as anaphylaxis, can occur. Treatment for mild reactions is supportive, with the administration of antihistamines to lessen symptoms. More severe reactions or anaphylaxis are managed as described above.

ALLERGIC DRUG REACTIONS

Adverse reactions to drugs are a common clinical problem, but true hypersensitivity reactions probably account for less than 10% of these occurrences, with the majority of anaphylaxis from IgE-mediated drug reactions.[51] Most drugs are small organic molecules, generally unable to stimulate an immune response alone. However, when a drug or metabolite becomes protein-bound, either in serum or on cell surfaces, the drug–protein complex can become an allergen and stimulate immune system responses. Thus, the ability of a drug or its metabolites to sensitize the immune system depends on the ability to bind to tissue proteins. Many different drugs and treatments can cause allergic reactions and anaphylaxis.

Penicillin is the drug most commonly implicated in eliciting true allergic reactions and accounts for approximately 90% of all reported allergic drug reactions and about 75% of fatal anaphylactic drug reactions.[52] **Fatal reactions can occur without a prior allergic history; less than 25% of patients who die of penicillin-induced anaphylaxis exhibited allergic reactions during previous treatment with the drug.** Parenteral penicillin administration is more than twice as likely to produce fatal allergic reactions as is oral administration. The cross-reactivity of penicillin allergy with cephalosporins is about 10%, so patients with a previous life-threatening or anaphylactic reaction to penicillin should not be given cephalosporins.

The clinical manifestations of drug allergy vary widely. A generalized reaction similar to immune-complex or serum sickness reactions is very common, especially with trimethoprim-sulfamethoxazole and certain cephalosporins (cefaclor being the most frequent). Sulfa moieties are contained in many drugs, but sulfa allergic reactions upon exposure to the nonantibiotic sulfas are uncommon. See chapter 206, "Antimicrobials" for more discussion of drug allergies.

Serum sickness usually begins in the first or second week after initiation of the drug and can take many weeks to subside after drug withdrawal. Generalized malaise, arthralgias, arthritis, pruritus, urticarial eruptions, fever, adenopathy, and hepatosplenomegaly are common signs and symptoms. Drug fever may occur without other associated clinical findings and may also occur without an immunologic basis. Circulating immune complexes are probably responsible for the lupus-like reactions caused by some drugs.

Other reactions are possible. Cytotoxic reactions include penicillin-induced hemolytic anemia. Skin eruptions include erythema, pruritus, urticaria, angioedema, erythema multiforme, and photosensitivity. Severe reactions, such as those seen in Stevens-Johnson syndrome and toxic epidermal necrolysis, may also occur. Delayed hypersensitivity reactions may manifest as contact dermatitis from drugs applied topically.

Diagnosis is determined by a careful history. Treatment is supportive, with oral or parenteral antihistamines and corticosteroids. Drug cessation is important, but reactions can continue. Referral to an allergy specialist is indicated for severe reactions.

REFERENCES

The complete reference list is available online at www.TintinalliEM.com.

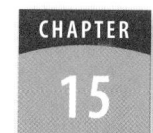

Acid-Base Disorders

Gabor D. Kelen
David D. Nicolaou
David M. Cline

INTRODUCTION

Controversy has existed concerning acid-base physiology and the ideal method to assess acid-base disorders for 130 years.[1] The two most common methods advocated to analyze acid-base disorders are the traditional bicarbonate-centered method[2,3] and the Stewart, or strong ion, method.[4,5] The traditional approach teaches that acid-base homeostasis is maintained by respiratory control of the partial pressure of carbon dioxide (Pco_2) through changes in alveolar ventilation and control of HCO_3^- reabsorption and H^+ excretion by the kidneys. Peter Stewart proposed that acid-base physiology involves the dynamic interaction of body fluids and multiple chemical species including strong ions (primarily Na^+, K^+, Ca^{2+}, Mg^{2+}, and Cl^-) and weak acids, as well as Pco_2 control by the lungs.

Each of these methods has limitations. The traditional bicarbonate-centered model continues to be the most commonly used at the bedside[3] but is criticized for failing to identify acid-base abnormalities that are due to alterations in plasma free water or in complex cases of mixed acid-base disorders.[6,7] The Stewart method is praised for its accuracy in identifying acid-base disorders but is criticized for the difficulty of application at the bedside.[7-11] This chapter does not detail the Stewart method, but we acknowledge its importance and its contribution to underscoring the limitations of the traditional method, which has led to modifications that improve the performance of the traditional method at the bedside.[8] For example, using a correction factor for the albumin level (detailed in this chapter), the traditional method performs as well as the Stewart method for identifying complex acid-base abnormalities in critically ill patients.[8-12]

Many diseases, including those that present an imminent threat to life, produce acid and base (acid-base) disturbances that provide important clues concerning the nature of the underlying illness and suggest immediate therapeutic interventions. Further, ED treatments such as rapid resuscitation of critically ill patients may create unintended acid-base disorders. This chapter describes a practical approach to the clinical evaluation and treatment of acid-base disorders.

PATHOPHYSIOLOGY

MEASUREMENT OF PLASMA ACIDITY

Plasma hydrogen ion concentration ($[H^+]$)* is normally 40 nmol/L, corresponding to a pH of 7.4. Because pH is a logarithmic transformation of $[H^+]$, the relation of $[H^+]$ to pH is not linear for all pH values (**Table 15-1**).

TABLE 15-1 pH and Hydrogen Ion Concentrations

pH	$[H^+]$, nmol/L
6.8	158
6.9	126
7.0	100
7.1	79
7.2	63
7.3	50
7.4	40
7.5	32
7.6	25
7.7	20

*Standard nomenclature is used in this chapter. The presence of brackets, [ ], surrounding an element or molecule implies the term concentration. Without the brackets, the chemical expressions simply refer to the element or molecule.

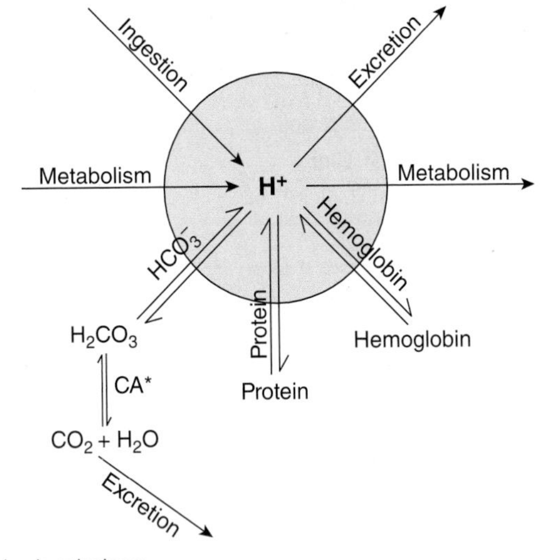

FIGURE 15-1. Schematic representation of hydrogen ion homeostasis.

However, for pH values from 7.20 to 7.50, the relation between $[H^+]$ and pH is nearly linear; pH changes of 0.01 correspond to approximately 1 nmol/L change in $[H^+]$. This linear relation allows for rapid bedside interpretation of blood gas and electrolyte results.

PLASMA ACID-BASE HOMEOSTASIS

Plasma $[H^+]$ is influenced by the rate of endogenous production, the rate of excretion, exogenous addition (e.g., acetylsalicylic acid ingestion), and the buffering capacity of the body. Buffers mitigate the impact of large changes in available hydrogen ion on plasma pH.

Buffer systems that are effective at physiologic pH include hemoglobin, phosphate, proteins, and bicarbonate (**Figure 15-1**). One can consider the $[H^+]$ to be the result of all physiologic buffers acting on the common pool of hydrogen ions.

The familiar Henderson-Hasselbalch equation, shown in Eq. (1),

$$\mathrm{pH} = \mathrm{p}K + \log\frac{[\mathrm{HCO_3^-}]}{[\mathrm{H_2CO_3}]} \qquad (1)$$

specifies the relationship between carbonic acid, bicarbonate, and pH; any two of these determine the value of the third. The clinical use of the Henderson-Hasselbalch equation is limited. However, if all constants are inserted into the Henderson-Hasselbalch equation and the antilogarithm of all its terms is taken, the result is the Kassirer-Bleich equation [Eq. (2)], which is of great clinical utility.

$$[\mathrm{H^+}] = 24 \times \frac{\mathrm{P}\mathrm{CO_2}}{[\mathrm{HCO_3^-}]} \qquad (2)$$

The Kassirer-Bleich equation may be used to estimate the concentration of any component of the bicarbonate buffer system provided the concentrations of the other two components are known. Therefore, it allows clinicians to determine, for example, what the pH must be when the P_{CO_2} and $[HCO_3^-]$ are known.[†] Note that when $[HCO_3^-]$ is normal, the Kassirer-Bleich equation demonstrates that $[H^+]$ = P_{CO_2}, using their respective units of measure.

[†]The "bicarbonate concentration" measured by the clinical laboratory is actually the total CO_2, which is the sum of bicarbonate, dissolved CO_2, and H_2CO_3. H_2CO_3 is the P_{CO_2} multiplied by the solubility coefficient of CO_2 in blood (α), 0.03. Thus, total CO_2 = $[HCO3^-]$ + (0.03) (P_{CO_2}). Most clinicians simply neglect the second term when the P_{CO_2} is normal; when hypercapnia is present, however, the second term measurably contributes to total CO_2.

ACID PRODUCTION AND EXCRETION

The quantity of $[HCO_3^-]$ in relation to carbonic acid buffer in the system is not fixed, but varies according to physiologic need. This flexibility is largely provided by pulmonary exhalation of carbon dioxide (CO_2), which can vary significantly and change rapidly as required by alterations in the underlying acid-base status.

Renal Influence on Acid-Base Balance The kidney regulates HCO_3^- excretion and the formation of new HCO_3^-. The rate of these processes is dependent on the underlying acid-base status. The renal response to pulmonary acid-base disturbances begins within 30 minutes of onset, but requires hours to days to achieve equilibrium.[13] Bicarbonate is filtered into the urine and must be reclaimed to maintain homeostasis. Eighty-five percent of bicarbonate that is filtered is reclaimed by the proximal convoluted tubule in a sodium-dependent process. H^+ is secreted into the tubular lumen, and Na^+ is absorbed from the tubular lumen into the cell. Sodium is then extruded from the tubular cell into the plasma in exchange for K^+ via the Na^+/K^+-ATPase pump. Thus, the H^+ secreted into the tubule combines with the filtered HCO_3^- in the lumen to produce carbonic acid (H_2CO_3), which in turn is converted to CO_2 and H_2O by carbonic anhydrase. The CO_2 diffuses down its concentration gradient into the tubule cell, where cytoplasmic carbonic anhydrase regenerates H_2CO_3, which then dissociates into HCO_3^- and H^+ (creating a supply of H^+ for extrusion). If tubular disease inhibits H^+ extrusion, a proximal renal tubular acidosis results, in which serum $[HCO_3^-]$ decreases to a steady-state level, i.e., reclaimed HCO_3^- effectively equals H^+ extrusion.

The balance (15%) of HCO_3^- reclamation occurs in the distal tubule via a sodium-independent process. Cytoplasmic carbonic anhydrase generates $H_2CO_3^-$, which dissociates. HCO_3^- diffuses into plasma, and H^+ is secreted into the lumen by an H^+-ATPase pump, thereby maintaining cellular electrical neutrality. H^+ is trapped in the lumen by inorganic phosphate or ammonia (NH_4^+). Failure of H^+ secretion is the underlying mechanism of distal renal tubular acidosis.

New HCO_3^- can also be created by the kidney. A sodium-dependent process allows synthesis of HCO_3^- in the distal tubule. Intracellular glutamine generates HCO_3^- and ammonia NH_4^+. The Na^+/K^+ pump moves Na^+ into the lumen, but Na^+ diffuses back across the cell membrane, and NH_4^+ is secreted into the lumen in exchange. The generated HCO_3^- remains in the cell. Formation of HCO_3^- by this process increases during acidosis, but may require 4 to 5 days to reach equilibrium. Drugs that alter uptake or delivery of Na^+ to the distal tubule can significantly alter HCO_3^- synthesis. The process of acid secretion allows the regeneration of HCO_3^- in proportion to the daily production of acid. Urine, especially under conditions of acidosis, can be made almost entirely without HCO_3^-.

FUNDAMENTAL ACID-BASE DISORDERS

Any condition that acts to increase $[H^+]$—whether through endogenous production, decreased buffering capacity, decreased excretion, or exogenous addition—is known as *acidosis*. Similarly, any condition that acts to decrease $[H^+]$ is termed *alkalosis*. The terms *acidemia* and *alkalemia* refer to the net imbalance of $[H^+]$ in the blood. The difference between acidosis and acidemia is not merely semantic, but of great clinical importance. For example, a patient with acidosis and alkalosis of equal magnitude will have a normal pH. A patient with these disturbances thus has neither acidemia nor alkalemia (resulting in the normal pH), but nevertheless has both acidosis and alkalosis. It is important to appreciate that, although acidemia is diagnostic of acidosis and alkalemia of alkalosis, a normal or high pH does not exclude acidosis and a normal or low pH does not exclude alkalosis.

Acid-base disturbances are further classified as respiratory or metabolic. Respiratory acid-base disorders are due to primary changes in P_{CO_2}, and metabolic acid-base disorders reflect primary changes in $[HCO_3^-]$. Compensatory mechanisms are, by definition, not "disorders," but rather normal physiologic responses to acid-base derangements. Terms such as *compensatory respiratory alkalosis* are therefore misleading. The clinician is nonetheless concerned with the adequacy of compensation, because failure of appropriate compensatory response implies the presence of another primary acid-base disturbance.

It is important to note that compensatory mechanisms return the pH toward normal but do not reach baseline.[‡] The fact that compensatory mechanisms cannot reach completion is evident when one considers that complete compensation would necessarily remove the physiologic stimulus driving the compensation.[2]

The "normal" values of pH, P_{CO_2}, and $[HCO_3^-]$ for given laboratory ranges are intended to include 95% of patients without an acid-base disorder. The normal pH range is 7.35 to 7.45, the normal P_{CO_2} range is 35 to 45 mm Hg, and the normal $[HCO_3^-]$ is usually 21 to 28 mEq/L. However, a patient's values may all fall within the "normal range" and still have significant acid-base disturbances. As detailed further below, a patient with metabolic acidosis and a concomitant metabolic alkalosis of nearly approximate magnitude will have a "normal" pH, P_{CO_2}, and $[HCO_3^-]$. In contrast, abnormal values may be appropriate for a given simple acid-base disturbance. For example, in the presence of a metabolic acidosis where $[HCO_3^-] = 15$ and pH = 7.3, an appropriate respiratory compensation should result in a P_{CO_2} of about 30 mm Hg. This P_{CO_2} value is below the "normal" range, but at the expected level of physiologic respiratory compensation for the degree of metabolic acidosis. In this example, the finding of P_{CO_2} in the normal (35 to 45 mm Hg) range actually implies the presence of a respiratory acidosis, because the expected physiologic respiratory response is inadequate.

THE ANION GAP

The principle of electrical neutrality requires that plasma have no net charge. The charge of the predominant plasma cation, Na^+, must therefore be "balanced" by the charge of plasma anions. Although HCO_3^- and Cl^- constitute a significant fraction of plasma anions, the sum of their concentrations does not equal that of sodium. Therefore, there must be other anions present in the serum to maintain electrical neutrality. These anions are primarily serum proteins (albumin, phosphate, sulfate, and organic anions, such as lactate) and the conjugate bases of ketoacids. Because these substances are not commonly measured, they are termed *unmeasured anions*. Unmeasured cations also exist, largely in the form of Ca^{2+} and Mg^{2+}. Because all cations (measured cations [MC] and unmeasured cations [UC]) must equal all anions (measured anions [MA] and unmeasured anions [UA]):

$$MC + UC = MA + UA \quad (3)$$

it follows that:

$$MC - MA = UA - UC = AG \quad (4)$$

Thus, substituting measured ions produces:

$$[Na^+] - ([HCO_3^-] + [Cl^-]) = AG \quad (5)$$

The unmeasured anion concentration is commonly called the *anion gap* (AG), i.e., the difference between the serum $[Na^+]$ and the sum of serum $[Cl^-]$ and $[HCO_3^-]$ equals the concentration of the unmeasured anions. The contribution of $[K^+]$, largely an intracellular ion, is usually neglected (although some hospital laboratories still include the $[K^+]$ as part of the reported AG value). For the purposes of AG determination, correction of serum $[Na^+]$ in the face of hyperglycemia is unnecessary, because this condition similarly dilutes $[Cl^-]$. The normal value of the AG is generally considered to be 12 ± 4 mEq/L, assuming no major deviations in expected concentration of unmeasured anions or cations. Reports have suggested that a normal AG value of 7 ± 4 mEq/L may be more appropriate to electrolyte measurements made with ion-specific electrodes.[14] However, normal range values used by the clinician should reflect institutional practice. As with other acid-base concepts, the accepted "normal" range for the AG is less important than whether it has changed in relation to the patient's steady-state baseline value. Thus, a relative change in the AG, referred to as the *delta gap*, may be more important than the actual AG value. Virtually all AG values above 15 mEq/L can be considered abnormal, even when there are no previous comparison values available.

The AG may change even in the absence of acid-base disturbances. It may rise when (unmeasured) cations decrease, as in severe states of hypomagnesemia, hypokalemia, and hypocalcemia. A reduced, narrow, or even negative AG may result from an increase in the concentration of unmeasured cations, such as lithium; unmeasured positively charged proteins resulting from myeloma and polyclonal gammopathies; or a significant decrease in unmeasured anions, such as albumin and γ-globulin. Albumin is a major component of the AG. Critically ill patients are frequently hypoalbuminemic, which may decrease the AG into the normal range, effectively masking the presence of a wide AG acidosis.[15] The AG should be corrected $[\text{AG-Corr}_{(albumin)}]$[6,8] for an abnormal albumin level to improve the sensitivity of using the AG to identify a metabolic acidosis:[#]

$$\text{AG-Corr}_{(albumin)} = AG + 0.25 \times ([\text{albumin}]_{Reference} - [\text{albumin}]_{measured}) \quad (6)^f$$

A factitiously narrow or even negative AG may result from a number of conditions including measurement artifact. Bromide toxicity yields false elevations of chloride, unless Cl^- specific electrodes are used for detection;[**] triglyceride levels greater than 600 mg/dL falsely elevate chloride levels and lower sodium levels, resulting in an apparently narrow or even negative AG.[16] If these can be excluded, a narrow AG may imply an excess of unmeasured cations such as may occur with hypergammaglobulinemias and myeloma proteins.

Although increases in the AG are traditionally considered in the context of metabolic acidosis, elevation of the AG may be seen with other acid-base disturbances. Metabolic and respiratory alkalosis, for example, may elevate the AG by 2 to 3 mEq/L, due to elevations in lactate (an unmeasured anion) produced by enhancement of glycolysis.[††] Penicillin and carbenicillin, as unmeasured anions, produce elevations in the AG and may be accompanied by a hypokalemic alkalosis.

Elevations of the AG are usually clinically importance in the emergency setting and most commonly associated with metabolic acidosis (**Table 15-2**). Traditional mnemonics for the differential diagnosis of an elevated AG acidosis (MUDPILES, CAT MUDPILES, GOLDMARK, KARMEL, KUPIN, ACE GIFTs) can help the clinician recall elements of the differential diagnosis for this condition. However, these mnemonics leave the dangerous impression that lactic acidosis is a diagnostic endpoint for elevated AG acidosis. It is not. For example, propylene glycol, iron, seizures from isoniazid, carbon monoxide poisoning, and aspirin ingestions, as well as alcoholic ketoacidosis, may produce significant lactic acidosis. We suggest that the differential diagnosis of metabolic acidosis with an elevated AG should emphasize distinctions between endogenous and exogenous unmeasured anion sources and avoid mixing the etiology of lactic acidosis with that of other increased unmeasured anions. Some authors suggest correcting for lactate in patients known to have lactate elevations at baseline;[17,18] if lactate correction is calculated, the delta lactate should be used.

Clinical use of AG values requires an appreciation of their limitations. Although an AG greater than 30 mEq/L is usually caused by lactic acidosis or diabetic ketoacidosis, these conditions may exist even when the AG is normal.[19] Thus, a "normal" AG does not exclude the possibility of the presence of increased concentrations of unmeasured cations. An AG

[‡]The sole exception is in chronic respiratory alkalosis, where bicarbonate levels may decline to a level that nearly normalizes the pH, such that differentiating the actual pH from normal falls within the range of laboratory error.

[#]This correction is generally not of clinical importance in emergency medicine because even a large decrease in albumin will have negligible effect on the anion gap and the delta gap, particularly in patients with severe acidosis.

[f]For SI units (g/L); if the lab reports g/dL, the factor is increased 10-fold, i.e., 2.5 × Δ albumin.

[**]Other techniques cause reactions where bromide is falsely read as chloride.

[††]This form of lactate is not associated with acid production as occurs with states resulting in anaerobic metabolism.

TABLE 15-2 Unmeasured Anions Associated with an Elevated Anion Gap and Metabolic Acidosis

Diagnostic Category	Anion Species	Origin	Diagnostic Adjuncts
Renal failure (uremia)	$[PO_4^{2-}]$, $[SO_4^{2-}]$	Protein metabolism	BUN/creatinine
Ketoacidosis	Ketoacids, lactate	Fatty acid metabolism	Serum/urine ketones
Diabetic	β-Hydroxybutyrate, lactate	Fatty acid metabolism	Specific test now available (older nitroprusside test yields false-negative result for β-hydroxybutyrate)
Alcoholic	Acetoacetate, lactate	Fatty acid metabolism	
Starvation			Consider coexistent dehydration
Lactic acidosis*	Lactate	Metabolism	Lactate level for subtypes
Sepsis	Lactate	Hypoperfusion, anaerobic metabolism	Culture/organism-specific tests
Cardiac arrest	Lactate	Hypoperfusion/reperfusion injury	Consider other acidosis
Liver failure	Lactate	Decreased lactate clearance	Liver function tests
Iron	Lactate	Disruption of cellular metabolism,	Serum iron level
Metformin	Lactate	Inhibition of gluconeogenesis	
Cyanide	Lactate	Mitochondrial dysfunction, histotoxic hypoxia	
Carbon monoxide	Lactate	Hypoxia, anaerobic metabolism	Carbon monoxide level
Thiamine deficiency	Lactate	Aerobic metabolism interrupted, lactate accumulates	Assess peripheral sensory and motor function for neuropathy
Exogenous poisoning*			
Methanol	Formate	Methanol metabolism	Osmolal gap
Ethylene glycol (EG)	Oxalate and organic anions	EG metabolism favors pyruvate conversion to lactate	Osmolal gap Oxalate crystals (urine)
Salicylate	Salicylate	Salicylate, lactate, ketoacids	Concomitant respiratory alkalosis and metabolic acidosis
Isoniazid	Lactate	Anaerobic metabolism, lactate accumulation	

*This is not an exhaustive list; several other causes exist.

increased from baseline but still within the "normal" range may be a clue (delta gap). Direct measurements of lactate, formate (parent of formic acid), ketoacids, methanol, ethylene glycol (parent of oxalic acid and numerous other organic acids), and salicylate should be ordered when the presence of any of these substances is suspected, but the AG is "normal," (when a delta gap exists, or the AG is in the upper range of normal). Measurement of serum osmolarity and subsequent comparison to calculated serum osmolarity are necessary to detect small unmeasured molecules (such as toxic alcohols).[20] Finally, it is important to recognize that several concomitant causes of wide AG–type metabolic acidosis may be present.

A common clinical problem is the diagnosis of mixed acid-base disturbances in the presence of an elevated AG. Simple acid-base disturbances that produce elevated AGs are referred to as wide AG metabolic acidoses. If a wide AG metabolic acidosis is the only disturbance, then the change (elevation from baseline) in value of the AG (the delta gap) should exactly equal the net decrease in the $[HCO_3^-]$. This is a one-to-one relationship. This concept is represented mathematically in Eq. (7).

$$\Delta \text{ increase in AG} = \Delta \text{ decrease in } [HCO_3^-] \qquad (7)$$

If the $[HCO_3^-]$ is lower than the value predicted by the delta AG, then there must be a concomitant hyperchloremic (i.e., normal AG type) metabolic acidosis (**Figure 15-2A**). Similarly, if the $[HCO_3^-]$ is higher than expected based on the delta AG, there must be a concomitant metabolic alkalosis present. Note that acute respiratory conditions (respiratory acidosis or alkalosis) do not affect these determinations, although chronic respiratory conditions may have substantial metabolic compensatory effects. Potential acid-base disturbances related to respiratory status must be further determined, as discussed below (**Figure 15-2A–C**).

PARAMETERS REQUIRED FOR CLINICAL ACID-BASE EVALUATION

When taking a medical history, one should emphasize events that may result in the gain or loss of acid or base, such as vomiting, diarrhea, medications, or ingestions of toxins, and seek evidence of dysfunction of the organs of acid-base homeostasis—the liver, kidneys, and lungs.

Laboratory evaluation requires blood samples for determination of blood gases (pH, P_{CO_2}, and $[HCO_3^-]$), electrolytes ($[Na^+]$, $[K^+]$, $[Cl^-]$, and $[HCO_3^-]$), and other factors that affect the patient's acid-base status (albumin, lactic acid, creatinine, BUN, drug levels of suspected ingestions such as salicylate). Based on current history and physical and past medical history, consider the need for calcium, magnesium, phosphate, serum ketones and glucose, serum osmolality, and urine electrolytes, osmolality, and glucose. Most clinical laboratories measure two of the parameters reported in blood gas results (most commonly the pH and P_{CO_2}) and use the Henderson-Hasselbalch equation to calculate the third ($[HCO_3^-]$).

Blood samples for acid-base evaluation were historically obtained by arterial puncture, but there is increasing evidence that, in many clinical situations, venous or capillary blood may be used instead.[21] Venous P_{CO_2} may be a sensitive screen for hypercarbia (cutoff 45 mm Hg), but the venous and arterial P_{CO_2} values exhibit wide variation and are not interchangeable.[22] With increasing attention to early goal-directed therapy, point-of-care venous lactate levels are useful to screen for hyperlactatemia.[23] Confirming an elevated venous lactate with an arterial sample[24] is not necessary.[22,23]

Inexperienced clinicians frequently resort to arterial blood gas (ABG) determination as a means to determine the pH. However, **the pH per se is often the least important value for diagnosis and management.** When respiratory status is not compromised (which should be presumed only with caution), the pH can be calculated with the aid of the Kassirer-Bleich equation [see Eq. (2)] from the venous $[HCO_3^-]$ alone, as described below.

METABOLIC ACIDOSIS

Metabolic acidosis may result from HCO_3^- loss, administration or ingestion of acid, or endogenous production and accumulation of acid. Loss of HCO_3^- occurs by externalization of intestinal contents (e.g., vomiting, enterocutaneous fistulae) and renal wasting of bicarbonate (e.g., renal tubular acidosis, carbonic anhydrase inhibitor therapy). Administration of acid, unlikely to be seen in the ED, occurs primarily with total parenteral nutrition, whereby patients receive hydrochloric salts of basic amino acids. Endogenous acids accumulate in renal tubular acidosis, ketoacidosis, and lactic acidosis. Acidosis from rapid infusion of normal saline, called dilutional acidosis, has been shown to involve endogenous accumulation from CO_2 hydration.[25]

Unopposed metabolic acidosis results in a decreased serum $[HCO_3^-]$ and an increase in serum $[H^+]$. The increased $[H^+]$ stimulates the respiratory center, resulting in increased minute ventilation. The physiologically based "respiratory compensation" is an attempt to lower the $[H^+]$ by a reduction in P_{CO_2} through increased ventilation. The steady-state relationship between the P_{CO_2} and the $[HCO_3^-]$ is shown in Eq. (8).[12‡‡]

$$P_{CO_2} = (1.5 \times [HCO_3^-] + 8) \pm 2 \qquad (8)$$

‡‡The constants in this equation ($P_{CO_2} = 1.54 \times [HCO_3^-] + 8.36 \pm 2$) have been rounded for ease of use.

While equation (8) expresses the steady-state values after 24 hour of metabolic acidosis, the respiratory response is almost immediate. When $[HCO_3^-]$ is greater than ~8 mEq/L, the relationship between P_{CO_2} and $[HCO_3^-]$ is simpler. With normal respiratory compensation, P_{CO_2} decreases by 1 mm Hg for every 1 mEq/L net decrease in $[HCO_3^-]$. Using these relationships allows the clinician to calculate the expected P_{CO_2} from the measured $[HCO_3^-]$, assuming respiratory compensation is normal. If the expected P_{CO_2} value differs from the measured value in steady-state metabolic acidosis, then respiratory compensation is compromised, and a primary respiratory disorder exists in conjunction with the metabolic acidosis. As an example, if the $[HCO_3^-]$ is 15 mEq/L, the expected P_{CO_2} is ~30 mm Hg. If the actual measured value is higher than expected (e.g., 35 mm Hg), then by definition there is a concomitant respiratory acidosis (Figure 15-2A). If the measured value is lower than expected (e.g., 25 mm Hg), then there is a concomitant respiratory alkalosis. This latter case is not an example of overcompensation, but rather a second, simultaneous primary acid-base disturbance. These are important concepts. The body cannot tolerate metabolic and respiratory mechanisms for acidosis simultaneously, as one cannot buffer or compensate for the other.

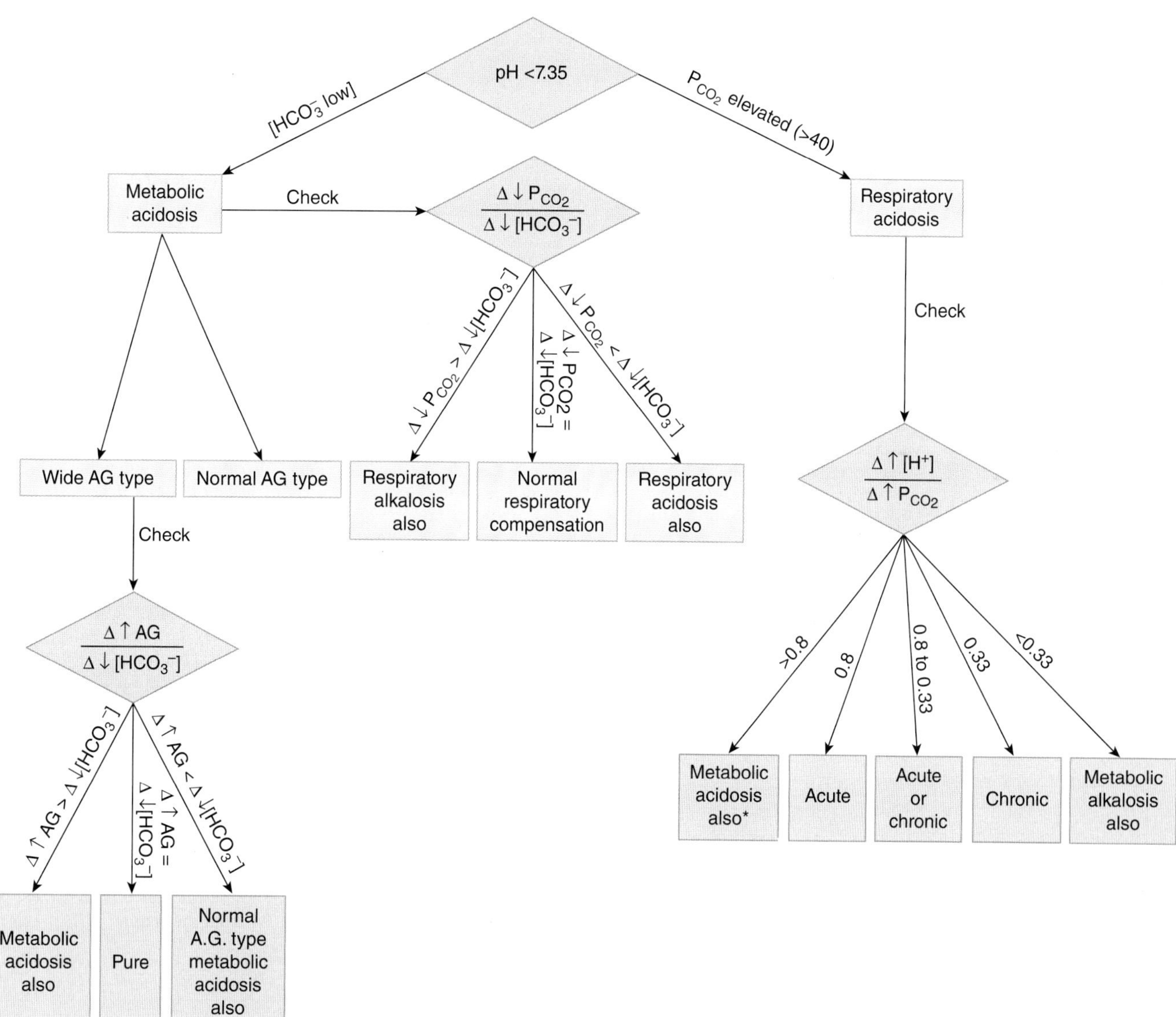

FIGURE 15-2. **A.** Algorithm for determination of type of acidosis and mixed acid-base disturbances when pH indicates acidemia. **B.** (next page) Algorithm for determination of type of alkalosis and mixed acid-base disturbances when pH indicates alkalemia. **C.** (next page) Algorithm to check for acid-base disturbances when pH is within the "normal" range.

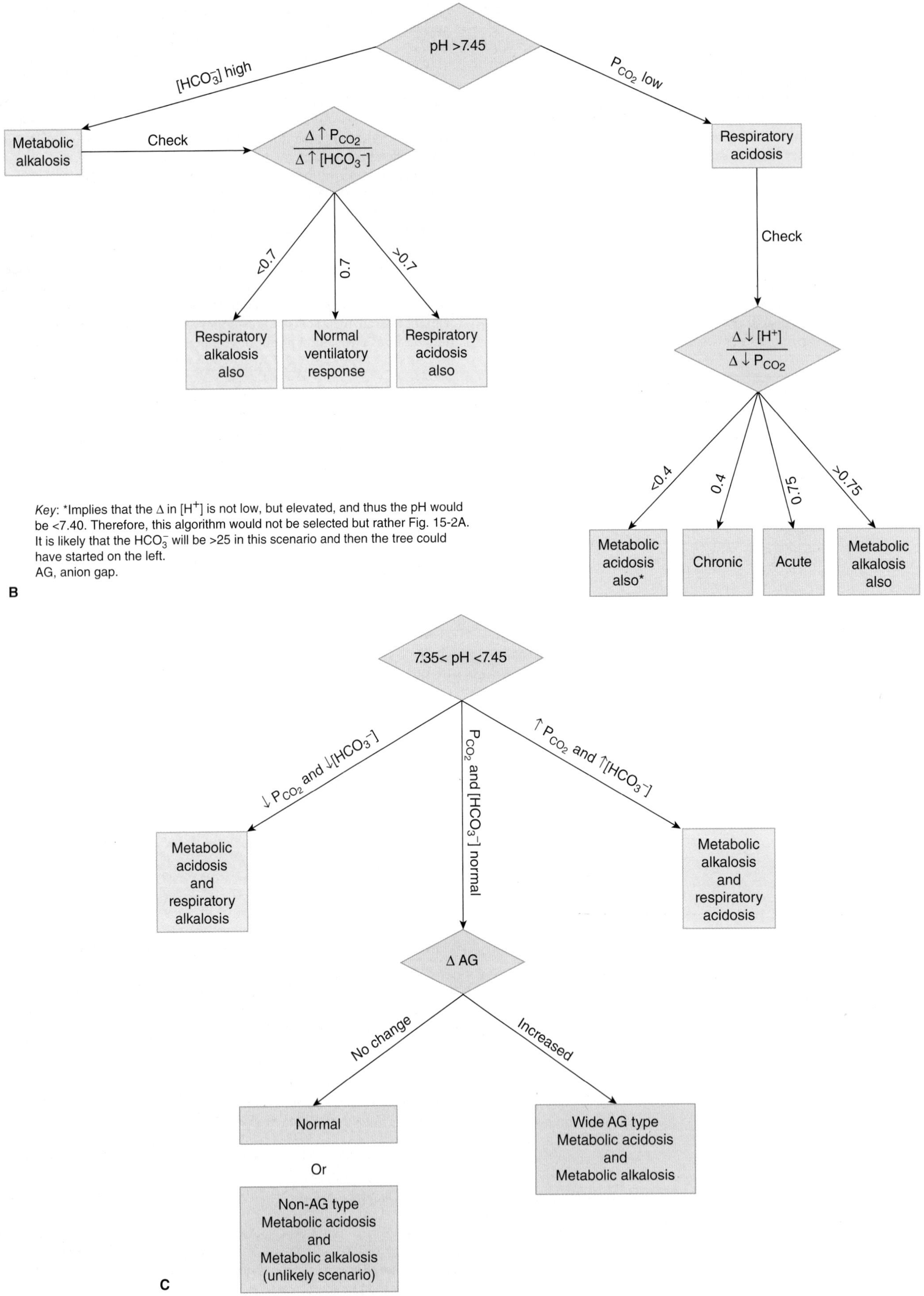

pH >7.45
[HCO3-] high
PCO2 low
Metabolic alkalosis
Check
Δ↑PCO2 / Δ↑[HCO3-]
<0.7
0.7
>0.7
Respiratory alkalosis also
Normal ventilatory response
Respiratory acidosis also
Respiratory acidosis
Check
Δ↓[H+] / Δ↓PCO2
<0.4
0.4
0.75
>0.75
Metabolic acidosis also*
Chronic
Acute
Metabolic alkalosis also
Key: *Implies that the Δ in [H+] is not low, but elevated, and thus the pH would be <7.40. Therefore, this algorithm would not be selected but rather Fig. 15-2A. It is likely that the HCO3- will be >25 in this scenario and then the tree could have started on the left.
AG, anion gap.
B
7.35< pH <7.45
↓PCO2 and ↓[HCO3-]
PCO2 and [HCO3-] normal
↑PCO2 and ↑[HCO3-]
Metabolic acidosis and respiratory alkalosis
Metabolic alkalosis and respiratory acidosis
Δ AG
No change
Increased
Normal
Or
Non-AG type Metabolic acidosis and Metabolic alkalosis (unlikely scenario)
Wide AG type Metabolic acidosis and Metabolic alkalosis
C

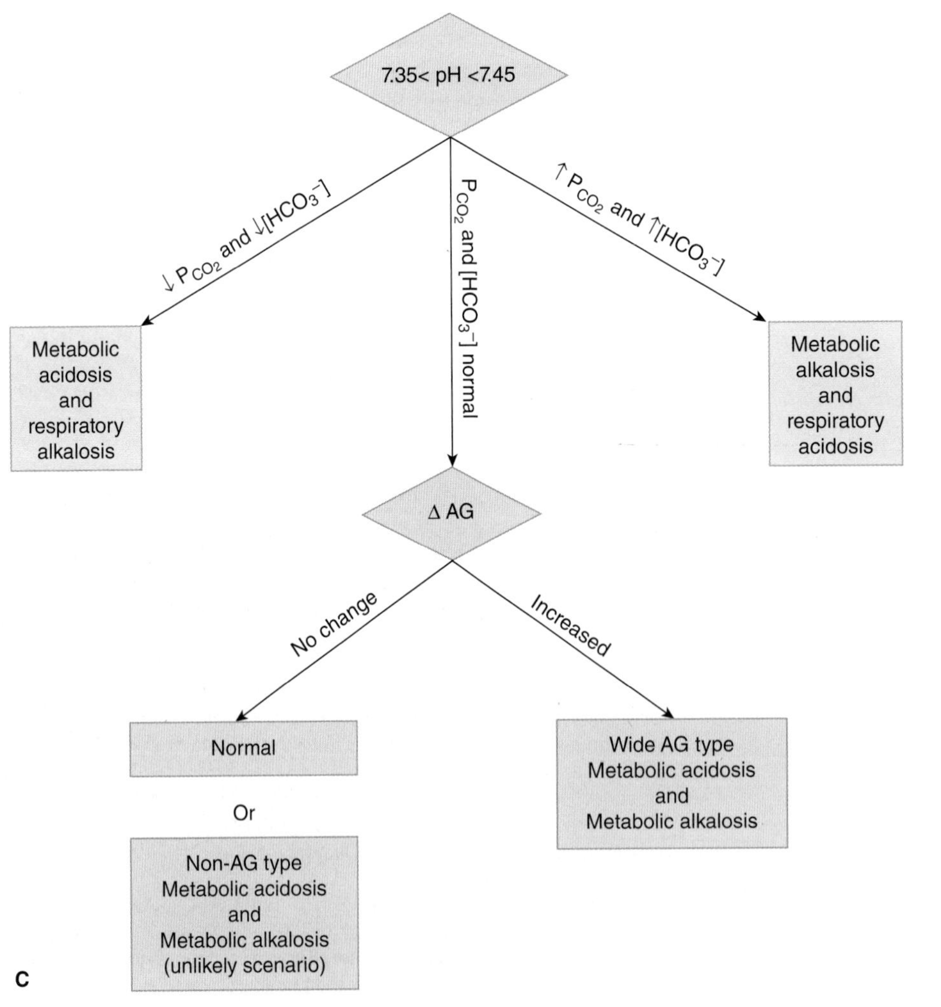

FIGURE 15-2. *(Continued)*

Physiologic studies of otherwise healthy persons with acute metabolic acidosis caused by diarrhea found that the completeness of the respiratory response to metabolic acidosis depends on the duration of the acidosis, the time course of its development, and its severity. When [HCO_3^-] is held constant, steady-state Pco_2 is reached in 11 to 24 hours. When acidosis develops slowly, there is no lag in respiratory compensation. If acidosis develops more quickly, the Pco_2 is often higher than values observed in steady state; the more rapid and severe the acidosis, the larger is the difference between the observed Pco_2 and the predicted steady-state CO_2. The delay in full compensation again indicates the presence of concomitant respiratory acidosis, and the clinician must recognize the contribution of inadequate ventilation to the level of acidosis (e.g., [H^+]). Thus, in the ED setting, the delay in reaching steady state is of passing interest as the labs results signify the reality of the moment. Unfortunately, the ED patient's illness can rarely be assumed to be in steady state.

There are limits to the adequacy of respiratory compensation during metabolic acidosis. Respiratory minute volume actually declines when pH decreases below 7.10. This finding has led clinicians to initiate bicarbonate therapy when pH falls below 7.10. It is particularly important to appreciate any contribution to the acidosis from inadequate respiratory response. Administration of HCO_3^- in the presence of hypoventilation may exacerbate the respiratory acidosis, because the HCO_3^- converts to CO_2 and H_2O.

The development of metabolic acidosis that drives the pH below 7.10 is likely associated with a very high risk of inadequate ventilation response, since there is a limit to respiratory compensation. The lowest Pco_2 level achievable is ~12 mm Hg. This lower limit in obtainable Pco_2 is due to resistance in airflow and increased CO_2 generated by the exertion required for rapid ventilation, both offsetting the ventilator exhalation of CO_2. The superimposition of respiratory acidosis on a patient in such a condition will result in a rapid decline of pH to levels at which organ function drops and pharmacotherapy will fail. Mechanical ventilation usually should be instituted in such situations to ensure the ventilatory rate and volume are sufficient to prevent an increase in Pco_2 at this critical time.

The serum [K^+] level is affected by metabolic acidosis. The movement of H^+ into cells is associated with extrusion of K^+. Changes in [K^+] are more substantial during inorganic acidosis, although elevated serum [K^+] is typically seen in diabetic ketoacidosis. In general, for each 0.10 change in the pH, serum [K^+] will change by approximately 0.5 mEq/L, in an inverse relationship. Whatever the mechanism of the acidosis, it is important to remember that normal values as well as low serum [K^+] likely reflect severe intracellular K^+ depletion. As the acidosis is corrected, serum [K^+] should fall, possibly to levels that may produce clinical symptoms, dysrhythmias, and other adverse outcomes.

CLINICAL FEATURES AND PHYSIOLOGIC CONSEQUENCES OF ACIDOSIS

Symptoms of the primary disorder causing metabolic acidosis dominate the clinical presentation; however, several symptoms are common to various etiologies. Patients may complain of abdominal pain, headache, nausea with or without vomiting, and generalized weakness, and because acidosis stimulates the respiratory center, the patient may complain of dyspnea.

Acidemia has numerous negative physiologic consequences that impair the function of enzymes as well as many different organs through mechanisms not yet well understood. Cardiac contractile function is reduced, likely due to impaired oxidative phosphorylation, intracellular acidosis, and alterations in intracellular calcium concentrations. The threshold for ventricular fibrillation falls as the defibrillation threshold rises. Hepatic and renal perfusion and systemic blood pressure decline, and pulmonary vascular resistance increases. The physiologic effects of catecholamines are attenuated, and when acidosis is sufficiently severe, vascular collapse may result. A catabolic state develops, including a generalized increase in metabolism, resistance to insulin, and inhibition of anaerobic glycolysis. The effect of hypoxia on all organs is aggravated.[26]

CAUSES OF METABOLIC ACIDOSIS

The causes of elevated AG metabolic acidosis are listed in Table 15-2. A comparison with the patient's steady-state AG should be made whenever possible. Measurement and detection of specific anions may be indicated.

Differential Diagnosis of Wide AG Acidosis The differential diagnoses to be considered in emergency practice fall into four broad categories: renal failure (uremia), ketoacidosis (diabetic ketoacidosis, alcoholic ketoacidosis, starvation ketoacidosis), lactic acidosis, and ingestions (methanol, ethylene glycol, salicylates, and many others).

Renal failure should be evident from the serum chemistries. Acidosis seen in initial stages of renal failure may be severe, but tends to be stable, with [HCO_3^-] ~15 mEq/L in cases of chronic renal failure.

Positive serum ketones point to one of the ketoacidoses. In instances of known insulin-dependent diabetes mellitus, diabetic ketoacidosis is likely, although there is usually a component of lactic acidosis. In alcoholics who have recently stopped heavy drinking, alcoholic ketoacidosis should be considered; ketoacids contribute far less to the acidosis in ketoacidosis than lactate. Starvation ketosis will be found in patients with recent oral intake that is inadequate, such as in cases of fasting, dieting, or protracted vomiting, although the magnitude of acid-base disturbance in starvation ketosis should be small. The major ketone present in the serum of a patient with untreated diabetic or alcoholic ketoacidosis may be β-hydroxybutyrate. A specific test is now available. The older nitroprusside test yields a false-negative result for β-hydroxybutyrate. See chapter 223, "Type 1 Diabetes Mellitus for a detailed discussion.

Lactic acidosis occurs whenever lactate production exceeds lactate metabolism and is classified into two types. The first, in which tissue hypoxia is present and lactate production is elevated, is referred to as **type A.** Normal tissue oxygenation and impairment of lactate metabolism define the second, called **type B.** Severe acidosis that is resistant to treatment is seen in various type B lactic acidoses and ingestions. **Lactic acidosis is not a diagnosis, but a syndrome with its own differential diagnosis.** Causes of lactic acidosis include renal failure, shock, sepsis, cardiac arrest, trauma, seizures, tissue ischemia, diabetic ketoacidosis, thiamine deficiency, malignancy (e.g., leukemia), liver dysfunction, genetic disorders (e.g., metabolic diseases), toxins (e.g., methanol), and medications (e.g., metformin, salicylates, iron, isoniazid) (Table 15-2).

Lactate levels should be measured and accounted for in an adjustment of the AG. Ethanol is frequently cited as a cause of wide AG acidosis, but **ethanol should never be considered the etiologic source of any significant metabolic acidosis**; look for other causes. Although ethyl alcohol metabolism may lead indirectly to very mild lactic acidosis, usually due to the same mechanism as alcoholic ketoacidosis, in which lactic acidosis is more substantial, neither the alcohol nor its metabolites directly contribute to the acidosis.

Determination of the osmolal gap will help identify methanol and ethylene glycol from other etiologies. Although methanol is measured in most hospital laboratories, determination of ethylene glycol levels is performed off-site in many institutions. A widened osmolal gap without clear evidence of methanol ingestion may determine the diagnosis long before confirmatory laboratory evidence is available. Calculated adjustments to the osmolal gap may need to be made if ethanol is a co-ingestant (see chapter 185, "Alcohols" for detailed discussion).

Concomitant acid-base disturbance may further assist in determining the etiology. The triple acid-base disturbance of wide AG metabolic acidosis, metabolic alkalosis, and respiratory alkalosis is seen with sepsis (lactic acidosis) and salicylate poisoning. The latter also may be associated with a mild temperature elevation.

The relation of [HCO_3^-] to the AG and the [HCO_3^-] to the expected Pco_2 compensation must be examined in every patient with wide AG acidosis to determine whether other acid-base disturbances, metabolic or respiratory, exist (Figure 15-2A).

Differential Diagnosis of Unchanged (Normal) AG Acidosis The non-AG type of acidosis is often referred to as "normal" AG acidosis.[3] Some texts refer to this as **hyperchloremic metabolic acidosis**, but not all cases of normal AG acidosis are associated with hyperchloremia. If the patient has hyponatremia with a normal AG acidosis, the chloride

TABLE 15-3 Causes of Normal Anion Gap Metabolic Acidosis

With a Tendency to Hyperkalemia	With a Tendency to Hypokalemia
Subsiding diabetic ketoacidosis	Renal tubular acidosis, type I (classical distal acidosis)
Early uremic acidosis	Renal tubular acidosis, type II (proximal acidosis)
Early obstructive uropathy	Acetazolamide
Renal tubular acidosis, type IV	Acute diarrhea with losses of HCO_3^- and K^+
Hypoaldosteronism (Addison's disease)	Ureterosigmoidostomy with increased resorption of [H^+] and [Cl^-] and losses of HCO_3^- and K^+
Infusion or ingestion of HCl, NH_4Cl, lysine-HCl, or arginine-HCl	Obstruction of artificial ileal bladder
Potassium-sparing diuretics	Dilution acidosis (may occur with 0.9% NaCl infusion)

may be in the normal range. Abnormal chloride levels alone usually signify a more serious underlying metabolic disorder, such as metabolic acidosis (elevated chloride) or metabolic alkalosis (low chloride).[27]

Normal AG acidosis results from loss of HCO_3^-, failure to sufficiently excrete H^+, or administration of H^+. Bicarbonate may be lost from the urine or GI tract and is usually accompanied by K^+ loss. However, potassium-sparing diuretics, hypoaldosteronism, urinary tract obstruction, and type IV renal tubular acidosis result in loss of HCO_3^- with retention of K^+ (**Table 15-3**). Acetazolamide exerts its effect through carbonic anhydrase inhibition, inducing a functional renal tubular acidosis.

One should be wary of traditional classification based on [K^+], because serum [K^+] itself is dependent on the actual pH. Thus, in severe acidosis, a normal range [K^+] value may be falsely reassuring. As the acidosis is corrected and acidemia resolves, the [K^+] will concordantly fall.

Because all diuretics may cause a contraction alkalosis, the metabolic acidosis that occurs simultaneously with potassium-sparing diuretics may not be evident, as the two may simply cancel each other out (Figure 15-2C). Because the AG is unchanged, there is no indication that two distinct opposing processes may be occurring. As with wide AG–type acidosis, **the expected P_{CO_2} compensation must be examined in every patient with normal AG acidosis** to determine whether other respiratory acid-base disturbances exist (Figure 15-2A).

TREATMENT

The treatment of acidosis reflects that of the underlying disorder but particularly emphasizes restoration of normal tissue perfusion and oxygenation. The most important step is to determine whether there is a respiratory component to the acidosis (i.e., a primary respiratory acidosis), because the treatment approach differs. If there is inadequate respiratory compensation, the most appropriate treatment will be to first correct the respiratory problem. Address electrolyte disturbances, administer antidotes for toxins as appropriate, and initiate treatment for underlying causes such as sepsis (see chapter 150, "Toxic Shock Syndromes") or diabetic ketoacidosis (see chapter 225, "Diabetic Ketoacidosis").

Buffer Therapy in Acidosis Slow replacement of sodium bicarbonate in patients with sodium bicarbonate loss due to diarrhea or proximal renal tubular acidosis is useful.[28] The adverse effects of acidemia make the concept of buffer therapy teleologically appealing, but its role in instances of cardiac arrest and severe metabolic acidosis is unclear. A small 2013, single-center, randomized controlled trial showed mortality benefit in the treatment of sepsis patients; this study needs confirmation.[29] The traditional therapeutic buffer, sodium bicarbonate, may have negative effects in the treatment of acidosis. Bicarbonate therapy results in the generation of significant quantities of CO_2, which diffuses readily into cells, in particular those of the CNS, which may cause paradoxical worsening of intracellular acidosis. An abrupt CO_2 increase may exceed the ventilatory capacity of a patient already at maximum minute ventilation, thereby producing abrupt and worsening respiratory acidosis. After successful treatment with bicarbonate, "overshoot" alkalosis may result. Bicarbonate therapy imposes an osmotic and sodium load (1000 mEq/L of typical 1 N solution). These concerns suggest that bicarbonate therapy should not be used in the ED treatment of mild to moderate metabolic acidosis.

TABLE 15-4 Potential Indications for Bicarbonate Therapy in Metabolic Acidosis

Indication	Rationale
Severe hypobicarbonatemia (<4 mEq/L)	Insufficient buffer concentrations may lead to extreme increases in acidemia with small increases in acidosis.
Severe acidemia (pH <7.00 to 7.15)* in cases of wide anion gap acidosis, with signs of shock or myocardial irritability that has not responded to supportive measures including adequate ventilation and fluid resuscitation as indicated by the patient's clinical characteristics	Therapy for the underlying cause of acidosis depends on adequate organ perfusion.
Severe hyperchloremic acidemia†	Lost bicarbonate must be regenerated by kidneys and liver, which may require days.

*Presented as a range because recommendations differ among authors; data do not support a specific threshold for treatment.

†No specific threshold indication by pH exists. The presence of serious hemodynamic insufficiency despite supportive care should guide the use of bicarbonate therapy for this indication.

Concerning use of buffer therapy for cardiac arrest, diabetic ketoacidosis, and lactic acidosis, several studies of HCO_3^- use in adult and pediatric cases, including patients with severe acidosis, failed to show any improvement in speed of recovery or decrease in complication rates with buffer therapy.[26,28,30-33] There has been some suggestion of harmful effects, particularly an increased rate of development of cerebral edema in pediatric patients with diabetic ketoacidosis who were treated with bicarbonate. However, it remains unclear whether certain subgroups of patients (for example, those with cardiac or other disease) may benefit from bicarbonate therapy and dialysis.

The goal of bicarbonate and dialysis therapy in lactic acidosis may be to "bridge" the patient physiologically to definitive treatment of the etiology of the acidosis. Bicarbonate therapy may be appropriate for limited indications (**Table 15-4**).[26,28,30-34]

When given, HCO_3^- can be dosed 0.5 mEq/kg for each milliequivalent per liter rise in [HCO_3^-] desired.[26] The goal is to restore adequate buffer capacity ([HCO_3^-] >8 mEq/L) or to achieve clinical improvement in shock or dysrhythmias. Bicarbonate should be given as slowly as the clinical situation permits. Seventy-five milliliters of 8.4% sodium bicarbonate in 500 mL of dextrose 5% in water produces a nearly isotonic solution for infusion. Adequate time should be allowed for the desired effect to be achieved, and close monitoring of acid-base balance, especially in patients with organic acidosis, is critical. Other buffers appeared promising in the treatment of metabolic acidosis during early studies but have failed to provide improvement in clinical outcomes, including carbicarb, and tris-hydroxymethyl amino-methane.

METABOLIC ALKALOSIS

Metabolic alkalosis is typically classified as chloride-sensitive and chloride-insensitive, thus indicating the treatment approach. Metabolic alkalosis results from gain of bicarbonate or loss of acid. The relation of metabolic alkalosis to chloride balance defines pathophysiologic features of the disease and its therapy.

CLINICAL FEATURES AND PHYSIOLOGIC CONSEQUENCES OF ALKALOSIS

Symptoms of the primary disorder causing metabolic alkalosis dominate the clinical presentation; however, several symptoms are common to various etiologies. Patients may complain of generalized weakness, dizziness, myalgia, palpitations, nausea with or without vomiting, paresthesias, and possibly muscle spasm or twitching.

The physiologic effects of alkalemia are substantial. Neurologic abnormalities, especially tetany, neuromuscular instability, and seizures, are common. Reduction in $[H^+]$ results in reductions in ionized calcium, potassium, magnesium, and phosphate levels. Serum proteins, largely polyanionic, buffer H^+; with rapid acid loss, such as that which occurs in respiratory alkalosis, the newly available buffer capacity of those proteins binds calcium and other cations instead. Constriction of arterioles occurs, resulting in reduced coronary and cerebral blood flow. Refractory dysrhythmias may develop.[26] Alkalemia may be of particular concern in patients with chronic obstructive pulmonary disease, because of the shift of the oxygen-hemoglobin dissociation curve to the left, which makes O_2 less available to the tissues. Many patients with chronic obstructive pulmonary disease take diuretics, which lead to a contraction alkalosis. Additionally, the alkalemic environment tends to further depress ventilatory drive.

CAUSES OF METABOLIC ALKALOSIS

Bicarbonate and chloride represent the major serum anions whose concentrations may be readily altered, and their homeostasis is therefore closely intertwined. Conditions that result in chloride loss, such as vomiting (which also causes acid loss), diarrhea, diuretic therapy, and chloride-wasting diseases (e.g., cystic fibrosis and chloride-wasting enteropathy), tend to reduce serum chloride concentration and extracellular volume. The reduction in extracellular volume increases mineralocorticoid activity, which enhances sodium reabsorption and potassium and hydrogen ion secretion in the distal tubule, which in turn enhance bicarbonate generation. The resulting increase in serum $[HCO_3^-]$ eventually exceeds the tubule's maximum ability to reabsorb filtered bicarbonate. The resulting urine is alkaline, and because its anionic content is mostly bicarbonate, it is largely free of chloride (<10 mEq/L). (Nevertheless, the urine chloride may be normal when diuretics are administered.) The result is hypokalemic, hypochloremic alkalosis that responds to normal saline (chloride-responsive alkalosis).

Other diseases that cause metabolic alkalosis are usually associated with normovolemia or hypervolemia and often include hypertension. These diseases usually cause excess mineralocorticoid activity, resulting in the same pathophysiologic cascade described above. However, the excess mineralocorticoid activity is not associated with hypovolemia, so the urine chloride is generally normal or elevated (>10 mEq/L) and the alkalosis cannot be reversed with normal saline. Conditions producing "chloride-unresponsive alkalosis" and hypertension include renal artery stenosis, renin-secreting tumors, adrenal hyperplasia, hyperaldosteronism, Cushing's syndrome, Liddle's syndrome, and exogenous mineralocorticoids (e.g., licorice, fludrocortisone). Chloride-unresponsive alkalosis caused by Bartter's and Gitelman's syndromes is usually associated with normotension.

The compensation for metabolic alkalosis involves reduction in alveolar ventilation, but the exact relation between P_{CO_2} and $[H^+]$ is not well established. Most studies to date have been conducted in dialysis patients or patients with conditions that predispose to alveolar hyperventilation (e.g., sepsis, pneumonia). As a guideline, P_{CO_2} in patients with significant metabolic alkalosis should rise by 0.7 mm Hg for each milliequivalent increase in $[HCO_3^-]$. The P_{CO_2} also rarely rises above 55 mm Hg in compensation for metabolic alkalosis.

TREATMENT

As with all acid-base disorders, therapy of alkalemia emphasizes treatment of the underlying cause with careful supportive care. In the emergency setting, metabolic alkalosis rarely requires active management. Acetazolamide produces significant bicarbonaturia and is effective in the treatment of metabolic alkalosis, but its use requires very careful monitoring of potassium, magnesium, and phosphate concentrations. If alkalosis is severe ($[HCO_3^-]$ >45 mmol/L) and associated with serious signs or symptoms not responsive to supportive care, the use of intravenous hydrochloric acid should be considered. A 0.1 normal solution (100 mmol/L) should be used, infused ideally at 0.1 mmol/kg/h but at no more than 0.2 mmol/kg/h through a central venous catheter. Higher concentrations may degrade the catheter material. An infusion rate of 100 mL/h of 0.1 N solution provides about 10 mmol/h. The dose is calculated using ideal body weight as shown in Eq. (9), with the result in mmol H^+ required.

$$\text{Dose} = (\Delta[HCO_3^-]) * 0.5 \text{ weight, in kg} \qquad (9)$$

RESPIRATORY ACIDOSIS

Respiratory acidosis is defined by alveolar hypoventilation and is diagnosed when the P_{CO_2} is greater than the expected value. Acute respiratory acidosis may have origins in other conditions, such as increased CO_2 production (high-glucose diet) and abnormal gas exchange (e.g., pneumonia). However, the final common path is inadequate ventilation.

Inadequate minute ventilation most frequently results from head trauma, chest trauma, lung disease, or excess sedation. The chronic hypoventilation seen in extremely obese patients is often referred to as the **pickwickian syndrome**. Patients with severe chronic obstructive pulmonary disease have increased dead space and frequently also have decreased minute ventilation.

In general, a rise in the P_{CO_2} stimulates the respiratory center to increase respiratory rate and minute ventilation. However, if the arterial P_{CO_2} chronically exceeds 60 to 70 mm Hg, as may occur in 5% to 10% of patients with severe emphysema, the respiratory acidosis may depress the respiratory center. Under such circumstances, the stimulus for ventilation is provided primarily by hypoxemia acting on chemoreceptors in the carotid and aortic bodies. Giving oxygen could remove the main stimulus to breathe, causing the P_{CO_2} to rise abruptly to extremely dangerous levels. Consequently, when administering oxygen to patients with COPD, careful monitoring for the development of apnea or hypoventilation is required; however, do not withhold oxygen from a patient with severe dyspnea for fear of worsening hypercarbia. Evaluation of ventilation requires attention to several important clinical issues. First, the ventilation that would be expected based on assessment of the respiratory rate and depth should be compared with the actual ventilation of the patient (i.e., P_{CO_2}). A "normal" P_{CO_2} of 40 mm Hg in a tachypneic, dyspneic patient likely reflects significant ventilatory insufficiency. Second, the impact of respiratory acidosis on partial pressure of oxygen in the alveoli (P_{AO_2}) in such a patient may be considerable. The alveolar gas equation suggests that if inspired oxygen concentration and respiratory quotient do not change, increases in P_{CO_2} will result in reductions in P_{AO_2}.

The relation of P_{CO_2} to hydrogen ion concentration in acute respiratory acidosis derived from the Kassirer-Bleich equation shown in Eq. (10):

$$\Delta[H^+] = 0.8\ (\Delta P_{CO_2}) \qquad (10)$$

Each 1-mm Hg increase in P_{CO_2} results in a 1-mmol increase in $[H^+]$. Across the linear portion of the pH-hydrogen ion concentration relationship, each 1-mm Hg increase in P_{CO_2} should theoretically produce a 0.01 decrease in pH. The actual relation between changes in P_{CO_2} (up to values of 90 mm Hg) and changes in $[H^+]$ determined in normal humans is about 8 to 10, as shown in Eq. (10). Thus, a 10-mm Hg increment in P_{CO_2} produces an 8-mmol increase in $[H^+]$, with little change in bicarbonate concentration (usually 1 mEq/L) or urinary acid excretion. If the $[H^+]$ is higher or lower than that suggested by the change in the P_{CO_2}, a mixed disorder is present.

The adaptation to chronic respiratory acidosis is complex. Over time, chronic elevation of P_{CO_2} reduces carotid sinus sensitivity to hypercapnia, and ventilatory drive is then controlled by P_{AO_2}. The acidosis results in significant increases in renal HCO_3^- generation and avid reclamation of filtered HCO_3^-. The relation between $[H^+]$ and $[HCO_3^-]$ in chronic respiratory acidosis at steady state, derived from studies in humans, is shown in Eq. (11).

$$\Delta[H^+] = 0.3 * (\Delta P_{CO_2}) \qquad (11)$$

TABLE 15-5 Evaluation of Acid-Base Status in Respiratory Acidosis

Ratio = $\Delta[H^+]/\Delta P_{CO_2}$				
Ratio < 0.3	Ratio = 0.3	0.3 < Ratio < 0.8	Ratio = 0.8	Ratio > 0.8
Change in hydrogen ion concentration is less than accounted for by chronic change in P_{CO_2}. Metabolic alkalosis is also present.	Change in hydrogen ion concentration matches chronic change in P_{CO_2}. Chronic respiratory acidosis is present.	Change in hydrogen ion concentration is larger than accounted for by chronic change in P_{CO_2}. Chronic respiratory acidosis plus either acute respiratory alkalosis or metabolic acidosis is present; examine pH.	Change in hydrogen ion concentration matches acute change in P_{CO_2}. Acute respiratory acidosis is present.	Change in hydrogen ion concentration is larger than accounted for by acute or chronic change in P_{CO_2}. Metabolic acidosis is also present.

Abbreviation: P_{CO_2} = partial pressure of carbon dioxide.

It is frequently uncertain whether a patient has an acute respiratory acidosis, a chronic respiratory acidosis, or a mixed disorder. Evaluation of the acid-base status in such circumstances does not require "baseline" arterial blood gas values. Instead, the change in $[H^+]$ is compared with the change in P_{CO_2}. If this ratio is 0.3, the patient has a chronic respiratory acidosis; if it is 0.8, the patient has an acute respiratory acidosis. Other ratios suggest a mixed acid-base disturbance, as shown in **Table 15-5**.

TREATMENT

Treatment of respiratory acidosis is designed primarily to improve alveolar ventilation. In general, if the minute ventilation is doubled, the P_{CO_2} will be reduced by 50%. In patients with chronic obstructive pulmonary disease, bronchodilators such as β-agonists, anticholinergics, or systemic sympathomimetic agents, with careful administration of small amounts of oxygen, may substantially improve ventilation. However, ventilatory assistance (intubation or noninvasive ventilatory support) may be required in some patients who do not respond adequately to lesser measures, particularly if the pH falls below 7.25.

In patients with a chronic respiratory acidosis, reduction of the P_{CO_2} should generally proceed slowly. The minute ventilation for a 70-kg person is normally about 6 L/min; in chronic obstructive pulmonary disease patients, it may be less than 4 L/min. It is beyond the scope of this chapter to discuss in detail the approach to management of a patient with chronic obstructive pulmonary disease and severe hypercarbia. If treatment is indicated in the ED, it may be wise to start with a minute ventilation of about 5 L/min and then gradually increase it according to the clinical response and changes in P_{CO_2}.

In patients with a chronic respiratory acidosis, the arterial P_{CO_2} should not be reduced by more than 5.0 mm Hg/h. Rapid correction of a chronic respiratory acidosis can cause sudden development of a severe combined metabolic and respiratory alkalosis, with resulting dysrhythmias. A rapid rise in pH can cause an abrupt fall in ionized calcium levels and hypokalemia. Both may cause dangerous dysrhythmias, seizures, and decreased microvascular blood flow.

RESPIRATORY ALKALOSIS

Respiratory alkalosis is defined by alveolar hyperventilation and exists when P_{CO_2} is less than expected. It is caused by conditions that stimulate respiratory centers, including CNS tumors or stroke, infections, pregnancy, hypoxia, and toxins (e.g., salicylates). Anxiety, pain, and iatrogenic overventilation of patients on mechanical ventilators also cause respiratory alkalosis.

Whatever the etiology, the clinical symptoms of acute respiratory alkalosis are predictable from its physiologic effects. Acute reduction in P_{CO_2} produces a reduction in $[H^+]$, resulting in an increase in negative charge on anionic buffers. The now negatively charged proteins instead bind calcium, and if the effect is sufficiently large, the reduction in ionized calcium produces tetany (e.g., carpopedal spasm) and paresthesias.[26] Hypocapnia also produces substantial reductions in cerebral blood flow and results in reduced tissue oxygen delivery due to a leftward shift in the oxygen-hemoglobin dissociation curve (i.e., increased hemoglobin-oxygen binding).

The theoretical relationship of $[H^+]$ and P_{CO_2} predicted by the Kassirer-Bleich equation is that a 1-mmol decrease in $[H^+]$ results from each 1-mm Hg reduction in P_{CO_2}. The actual observed relationship is very close to the predicted values. Each 1-mm Hg reduction in P_{CO_2} results in a 0.75-mmol reduction in $[H^+]$ (Eq. 12).

$$\Delta[H^+] = 0.75 * (\Delta P_{CO_2}) \qquad (12)$$

Chronic respiratory alkalosis is unique among the acid-base disorders in that its compensation may be complete. Compensatory events include bicarbonaturia and a reduction in acid excretion, requiring 6 to 72 hours to develop fully and at least 1 week to normalize pH. The steady-state relationship between $[H^+]$ and P_{CO_2} in chronic respiratory alkalosis observed in normal human subjects at high altitude is shown in Eq. (13).

$$\Delta[H^+] = 0.4 * (\Delta P_{CO_2}) \qquad (13)$$

TREATMENT

Therapy for acute respiratory alkalosis emphasizes identification and treatment of the underlying cause. The use of "paper-bag" rebreathing in the treatment of respiratory alkalosis should be avoided because it may lead to hypoxia, and patients respond to calm reassurance, which is more effective treatment. Chronic respiratory alkalosis is seen at high altitudes, in particular among mountaineers climbing over 3700 m (12,000 ft), where the partial pressure of O_2 is significantly diminished. Acetazolamide is frequently prescribed to counter the physiologic respiratory effects of such ascents.

CLINICAL APPROACH TO ACID-BASE PROBLEMS AND MIXED ACID-BASE DISTURBANCES

Methodical interpretation of laboratory results followed by correlation with the clinical scenario is necessary to prevent erroneous acid-base evaluation. We present one method that has worked well for the authors; however, the particular method used matters less than the consistency of its application.

1. Look at the pH. If it is decreased, the primary or predominant disturbance is acidosis. If the pH is increased, the predominant disturbance is alkalosis.
2. If the pH indicates acidosis, the primary (or predominant) mechanism can be ascertained by examining the $[HCO_3^-]$ and P_{CO_2} (Figure 15-2A).
   a. If the $[HCO_3^-]$ is low (implying a primary metabolic acidosis), then the AG should be examined and, if possible, compared with a known steady-state value. Correct AG for abnormal albumin level [see Eq. (6), above].
      i. If the AG is increased compared with the known steady-state value or is greater than 15 (or above institutional threshold), then by definition a wide AG metabolic acidosis is present, and the absolute change in the AG should be compared with the

absolute change in the $[HCO_3^-]$ from normal to detect other disturbances.

ii. If the AG is unchanged, then the disturbance is nonwidened or *normal AG* metabolic acidosis, typically with hyperchloremia.

iii. If the change in the AG is equal to the change in the $[HCO_3^-]$ [see Eq. (7) above], then the wide AG acidosis is termed *pure*. If the AG has risen more than the $[HCO_3^-]$ has decreased, then there is also likely to be a concomitant metabolic alkalosis. If the change in the AG is less than the change in the $[HCO_3^-]$, then a normal AG acidosis is also present. (This is a difficult concept, but two separate physiologic mechanisms resulting in increased $[H^+]$ can occur simultaneously.) Next examine whether the ventilatory response is appropriate.

(1) If the decrease in the Pco_2 equals the decrease in the $[HCO_3^-]$, there is appropriate respiratory compensation. Note that the pH will not return to normal.

(2) If the decrease in the Pco_2 is greater than the decrease in the $[HCO_3^-]$, there is a concomitant respiratory alkalosis. Although there are other formulas for this comparison, this is the simplest, as explained earlier in the text.

(3) If the decrease in the Pco_2 is less than the decrease in $[HCO_3^-]$, there is also a concomitant respiratory acidosis.

b. If the Pco_2 is elevated (rather than the $[HCO_3^-]$ being decreased), the primary disturbance is respiratory acidosis (Figure 15-2A). The next step is to determine which type it is by examining the ratio of (i.e., the change in) $[H^+]$ to (the upward change in) Pco_2.

i. If the ratio is 0.8, it is considered acute.

ii. If the ratio is 0.33, it is considered chronic.

iii. If the ratio is between 0.8 and 0.33, it is probably an acute exacerbation of the chronic condition.

iv. If the ratio is greater than 0.8, there must be a metabolic explanation for the excess $[H^+]$.

v. If the ratio is less than 0.33, a metabolic alkalosis must also be present.

3. If the pH is greater than 7.45, the primary or predominant disturbance is alkalosis (Figure 15-2B).

a. It is best to look at the $[HCO_3^-]$ first. If it is elevated, there is a primary metabolic alkalosis. There is an expected ventilatory response, although it is quite varied. The ratio of the change upward in Pco_2 to the change upward in $[HCO_3^-]$ can be examined. If the ratio is much less than 0.7, there is also a respiratory alkalosis (in addition to the metabolic alkalosis). If the ratio is more or less 0.7, this is likely to be a compensatory ventilatory response. If the ratio is well above 0.7, respiratory acidosis is concomitantly present.

b. If the Pco_2 is low, there is a primary respiratory alkalosis, and the ratio of the change in $[H^+]$ to the change in Pco_2 should be examined. Acute respiratory alkalosis has a ratio of about 0.75. If the ratio is well above 0.75, there is probably also a concomitant metabolic alkalosis to explain the greater than expected decline in $[H^+]$. If the ratio is smaller, the condition is chronic or there may also be a metabolic acidosis component.

4. Every arterial blood gas that shows no or minimal pH derangement should still call for examination of the Pco_2, $[HCO_3^-]$, and AG, because there may well be a mixed acid-base disturbance (Figure 15-2C). It is quite possible for the pH, $[HCO_3^-]$, and Pco_2 to be normal and yet have significant acid-base disturbances. The only evident abnormality may be the AG. Take the example of an $[Na^+]$ of 145, $[Cl^-]$ of 97, $[K^+]$ of 4.5, and $[HCO_3^-]$ of 25 and a normal arterial blood gas. All the numbers look reasonably normal. However, the AG is 23, so by definition there must be a wide AG metabolic acidosis. The explanation for the normal numbers is a concomitant metabolic alkalosis.

REFERENCES

The complete reference list is available online at www.TintinalliEM.com.

CHAPTER 16 Blood Gases

Casey Glass

Blood gases provide important clinical information for patients with respiratory disorders, compromised circulation, or abnormal metabolism. In recent years, a number of surrogates for blood gas analysis have entered the daily practice of emergency medicine. Leveraging the benefits of blood gases requires an understanding of the underlying physiology, appropriate use of arterial and venous blood gases, and knowledge of the advantages and limitations of noninvasive monitoring methods. This chapter will be limited to evaluation of oxygen and carbon dioxide levels; for information on carbon monoxide, please refer to chapter 222, "Carbon Monoxide."

RESPIRATORY PHYSIOLOGY

Several factors contribute to overall gas exchange in the lungs. Each breath (*tidal volume*) is composed of functional movement of air in and out of the alveolus and nonfunctional movement of air through bronchioles, bronchi, trachea, and nonperfused areas of lung (*physiologic dead space*). The physiologic dead space is approximately 30% of the tidal volume. The air remaining in the chest at the end of exhalation is referred to as the *functional residual capacity*. Dead space and the functional residual capacity do not contribute to gas exchange. The amount of air inhaled and exhaled in a minute is referred to as *minute ventilation* and is the product of the respiratory rate and tidal volume. Relatively small changes in the functional alveolar space demand large increases in the minute ventilation to maintain the same rate of gas exchange. Either raising the fraction of inspired oxygen (Fio_2) or increasing the surface area or functional residual capacity of the lung can increase total alveolar oxygen (O_2) content. Positive-pressure ventilation increases the functional residual capacity through recruitment of collapsed nonventilated alveolar space.

ESTIMATING OXYGEN DELIVERY TO THE ALVEOLAR SPACE

The Fio_2 is the fraction or percentage of oxygen in the space being measured. At sea level, room air is 21% oxygen (20% is often used for ease of calculation). As Fio_2 increases, the alveolar concentration of oxygen (PAo_2) proportionately increases. Unless the patient is part of a closed system, like a ventilator circuit, the Fio_2 is only estimated. Each liter per minute of O_2 flow delivered via nasal cannula increases the Fio_2 by about 4%. Flow rates >4 L/min through a nasal cannula are poorly tolerated because of upper airway irritation. A simple O_2 mask provides an Fio_2 of 35% to 60% at flows of 10 to 15 L/min. A nonrebreather mask with a reservoir can deliver 95% O_2 at a flow rate of 10 to 12 L/min.

Comparing the measured arterial concentration of oxygen to the expected concentration of oxygen can be useful for determining the nature and severity of respiratory disorders. The approximate arterial oxygen concentration (Pao_2) values that are expected in normal persons who are inhaling various concentrations of O_2 are listed in **Table 16-1**.

The expected Pao_2 for a patient being given supplemental oxygen can be roughly estimated by multiplying the actual delivered percentage of O_2 by 5, the "**Five Times Rule**." Thus, a patient getting 60% O_2 would be

TABLE 16-1 Expected Pao_2 in Patients Inhaling Various Concentrations of Oxygen (mm Hg)

Fraction of inspired oxygen	0.21 (room air)	0.4	0.6	0.8	1.0
~Pao_2*	105†	200	300	400	500

Abbreviation: Pao_2 = partial pressure of arterial oxygen.

*Assuming a patient with normal lung function at sea level and a partial pressure of carbon dioxide (Pco_2) of 40 mm Hg.

†Calculation demonstrates slight overestimation using this technique.

expected to have a Pao_2 of about 60 × 5, or 300 mm Hg. For every 1000 ft (305 m) rise in altitude, barometric pressure drops approximately 25 mm Hg, and the atmospheric partial pressure of oxygen (Po_2) drops about 5 mm Hg. The arterial oxygen estimate would therefore be reduced by the fraction of pressure at elevation compared to sea level. The total alveolar oxygen pressure cannot be greater than atmospheric pressure unless the patient is receiving positive-pressure ventilation. Further discussion of O_2 and ventilation at altitude and depth is found in chapters 221, "High-Altitude Disorders" and 214, "Diving Disorders."

ALVEOLAR GAS EXCHANGE AND SYSTEMIC DELIVERY

Once oxygen or carbon dioxide reaches the alveolus, it moves across the interstitial space to either the red blood cell or alveolar space, respectively. The efficiency of diffusion depends on the distance across the alveolar-capillary membrane (interstitial space), the partial pressure of the gas in the alveolar space, and the solubility of the gas. Both oxygen and carbon dioxide are highly soluble, and carbon dioxide is 20 times more soluble than oxygen. As a result, increases in the distance across the interstitial space (as in pulmonary edema, for example) have greater effect on oxygen diffusion than carbon dioxide (CO_2) diffusion. Gas diffusion requires functioning alveolar space, and conditions that damage the alveolus prevent effective oxygen and carbon dioxide transport. Additionally, the alveolar space must be perfused by the pulmonary circulation. When portions of lung are perfused but not ventilated (as in pneumonia), or ventilated but not perfused (as in pulmonary embolism), there is a *ventilation-perfusion mismatch*. Either scenario may lead to hypoxemia, the first as deoxygenated blood passes through the nonfunctional lung and mixes with oxygenated blood in the left atrium, and the second when too little perfused lung is available for adequate oxygen loading.

The effectiveness of alveolar oxygenation can be estimated either by the alveolar-arterial gradient or the Pao_2/Fio_2 ratio. The alveolar-arterial gradient is the difference between the partial pressure of oxygen in the alveolar space (estimated from Fio_2 at atmospheric pressure) and the measured partial pressure of the gas in an arterial blood gas sample. The alveolar-arterial (A-a) gradient can be estimated by the following simplified formula:

$$P(A\text{-}a)O_2 = 147 - (Paco_2 \times 1.25) - Pao_2$$

A normal gradient for young adults is <15 mm Hg. The gradient increases with age at a rate of approximately 4 to 8 mm Hg per decade or can be estimated with the following formula: age/4 + 4. The Pao_2/Fio_2 ratio correlates with the relative venous shunt across the pulmonary circulation and is calculated as the measured Pao_2 divided by the Fio_2 in decimal form. A healthy person on 40% oxygen would be expected to have a ratio of approximately 600, representing a normal physiologic shunt of approximately 5%. As the shunt increases, the ratio decreases. **Table 16-2** illustrates the fall in the Pao_2/Fio_2 ratio with increasing physiologic shunt in hypothetical patients all receiving oxygen with an Fio_2 of 40%.

TABLE 16-2 Interpretation of Pao_2/Fio_2

Pao_2 (mm Hg)	Fio_2 (mm Hg)	Ratio	QS/QT (%)	Impairment of Oxygenation
240	0.4	600	5	None
120	0.4	300	10	Minimal
100	0.4	250	15	Mild
80	0.4	200	20	Moderate
60	0.4	150	30	Severe*
40	0.4	100	40	Very severe*

Abbreviations: Fio_2 = fraction of inspired oxygen; Pao_2 = partial pressure of arterial oxygen; QS/QT = venous-arterial admixture (shunt).

*Ventilatory support and positive end-expiratory pressure to increase functional residual capacity and reduce the QS/QT to 15% should be considered.

The Pao_2/Fio_2 ratio is the most frequently used parameter for evaluating the severity of lung failure and is included in the current definition for acute lung injury/acute respiratory distress syndrome.[1] The amount of oxygen transported to the body is determined to the greatest extent by the total blood hemoglobin content and cardiac output. Relatively little oxygen is dissolved in the plasma itself. The arterial O_2 content of blood (Cao_2) can be calculated with the following formula (hemoglobin [Hb] in grams/dL, Pao_2 in mm Hg, and arterial oxygen saturation [Sao_2] expressed as a fraction of 1.0):

$$Cao_2 = [Hb \times 1.39 \times Sao_2] + (Pao_2 \times 0.0031)$$

As a result, systemic delivery of oxygen can only be practically modified by either increasing the hemoglobin content or oxygen saturation. Although increasing the hemoglobin by transfusion will increase O_2 content, various qualities of transfused blood limit its benefit to patients, and further discussion is beyond the scope of this chapter (see chapters 13, "Fluid and Blood Resuscitation in Traumatic Shock," and 238, "Transfusion Therapy").

Carbon dioxide is transported by the red blood cell as carbamino compounds bound to hemoglobin and other carbamino-containing proteins, as well as in the form of plasma bicarbonate. Most carbon dioxide (60% to 70%) combines with plasma water to form carbonic acid, which dissociates into bicarbonate and hydrogen ions. This reaction is catalyzed by carbonic anhydrase in the erythrocyte such that the reaction is almost instantaneous. The deoxygenated hemoglobin is a willing receptor for released hydrogen ions. As hemoglobin is oxygenated in the lung, hydrogen ions are released, driving the reaction back toward the production of CO_2.

ARTERIAL BLOOD GAS ANALYSIS

The amount of oxygen and carbon dioxide in the blood can be sampled and reported as the partial pressure of the gas. Blood gas analysis also typically includes a direct measurement of the serum pH and estimates of serum bicarbonate derived from the measured partial pressure of carbon dioxide (Pco_2) and pH (see chapter 15, "Acid-Base Disorders"). Current tests often include other useful information such as direct measurement of lactic acid as lactate, total hemoglobin, and serum electrolytes.

An arterial blood sample is the reference standard for pH, oxygen, carbon dioxide, and lactate content providing a description of the oxygen and CO_2 content of the blood after leaving the pulmonary circulation and before any gas exchange in the peripheral tissues has occurred. In scenarios that require precise determination of these variables, an arterial sample is necessary.

Arterial blood gas samples are sometimes used for evaluation of serum hemoglobin and electrolytes. Blood gas analyzers typically have good concordance with the reference venous sample; however, there may be clinically significant variances when the result falls outside the normal range. Arterial electrolytes and hemoglobin results should be interpreted with caution when the results are significantly abnormal.[2-6]

MIXED VENOUS BLOOD GAS ANALYSIS

Mixed venous blood samples provide a source of information regarding the systemic uptake of oxygen and can be used to calculate cardiac output. The ideal sampling site for a systemic venous sample is at the pulmonary artery because blood from all body sites is equally represented. Sampling blood from the pulmonary artery is limited to situations where the patient has a pulmonary artery catheter placed. More commonly, blood is sampled from the superior vena cava or right atrium after placement of a central venous catheter. Blood from the superior vena cava disproportionally represents cerebral and upper body blood flow but is generally useful for determining systemic oxygen uptake and lactic acid production.

Regular monitoring of the venous O_2 saturation at the superior vena cava ($S_{cv}O_2$) or right atrium ($S_{ra}O_2$) is currently recommended as part of the Surviving Sepsis Campaign.[7,8] Although measurement of the O_2 saturation from a superior vena cava sample is acceptable within the guidelines, this location may not accurately reflect the $S_{ra}O_2$, and neither the $S_{cv}O_2$ nor the $S_{ra}O_2$ may accurately reflect the mixed venous O_2 saturation at the pulmonary artery (S_vO_2) for critically ill patients.[9-13]

PERIPHERAL VENOUS GAS ANALYSIS

Peripheral venous samples are commonly used as the source for gas analysis due to their relative ease of collection and decreased patient discomfort. The substitution of venous blood for an arterial sample is appropriate in particular clinical scenarios as described below.

Peripheral venous blood gases are commonly used to monitor serum pH. When compared to arterial blood gases, the peripheral venous pH correlates very closely such that any differences are not usually clinically significant (+/− 0.05 pH units).[14] Venous Pao_2 values do not correlate with arterial oxygen content and cannot be used for evaluation of oxygenation. Venous CO_2 values trend along with arterial CO_2, although they do vary somewhat (up to +/− 20 mm Hg). Normal venous CO_2 is predictive of normal $Paco_2$; however, the clinical outcomes of substituting venous CO_2 for evaluation of hypercarbia have not been described in the literature.[14-19]

It may be possible to derive a mathematical correction to venous blood gas values that better approximates arterial values. To date, no recognized validated approach has been identified.[20-24]

Peripheral venous estimations of serum lactate production are widely used for patient care; however, most studies describing the clinical utility of serum lactate reference an arterial or mixed venous sample. Peripheral venous lactate measurements correlate with arterial lactate; however, they are not equivalent, and a peripheral venous lactate level may be significantly higher than arterial lactate.[25-27]

NONINVASIVE OXYGEN MONITORING

It is not possible to directly measure the arterial oxygen concentration by noninvasive means. In the clinical context, the arterial oxygen saturation is often as helpful for patient management and treatment decisions. For the last 30 years, the standard bedside tool for estimating arterial oxygen saturation has been the photometric pulse oximeter.

Pulse oximetry measures the relative absorption of oxygenated hemoglobin and deoxygenated hemoglobin and reports the percentage of oxygenated hemoglobin compared to the total. Pulse oximetry is fairly accurate, typically within 2% to 5% of the directly measured value performed at blood gas analysis. Importantly, the discrepancy between peripheral pulse oxygenation results and arterial gas saturation increases with hypoxia and poor circulation. Pulse oxygenation values greater than 92% are highly predictive of arterial saturations greater than 90%.[28] Pulse oxygenation values between 88% and 92% do not necessarily reflect normal arterial saturations and may overestimate arterial oxygen saturation. The pulse oximeter may overestimate saturation when arterial saturations fall below 80% to 90%, and marginally normal values should be interpreted with caution.[29,30] Carbon monoxide also causes hemoglobin to conform to the saturated state and will cause a false elevation in measured saturation (see chapter 222).

Although clinically useful, pulse oximetry does not allow for determination of the partial pressure of oxygen in the arterial blood, which, in combination with total hemoglobin content, is the primary determinant of peripheral oxygen delivery. A basic understanding of the oxygen saturation/dissociation curve is essential for practicing clinicians when using pulse oximetry to guide clinical therapy (**Figure 16-1**). Most notably, arterial oxygen content declines precipitously when the oxygen saturation falls below 92%.

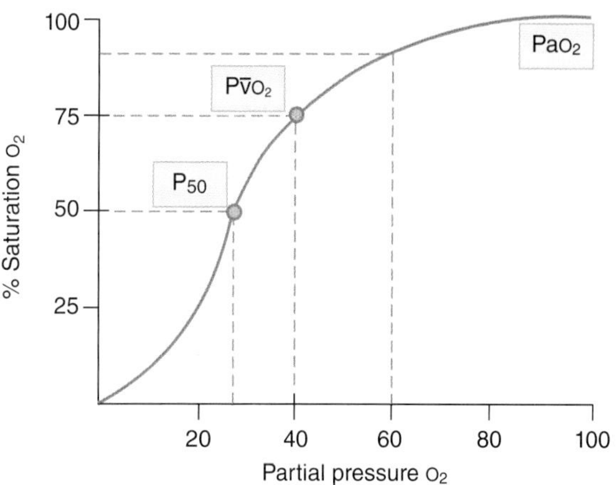

FIGURE 16-1. The oxyhemoglobin dissociation curve. This curve demonstrates the relationship of the partial pressure of oxygen (Po_2) in the plasma to the saturation of hemoglobin molecules with O_2. The P_{50} is the Po_2 at which hemoglobin is 50% saturated and correlates with Po_2 of 27 mm Hg normally. Normal mixed venous blood has an oxygen partial pressure ($Pmvo_2$) of 40 mm Hg and an oxyhemoglobin saturation of 75%. A partial pressure of arterial oxygen (Pao_2) of 60 mm Hg normally results in approximately 90% saturation of hemoglobin.

NONINVASIVE CARBON DIOXIDE MONITORING

The CO_2 content of arterial blood can be estimated by several noninvasive methods including direct transcutaneous measurement, cutaneous photometric measurement, or sampling of expired gases. Of these, only the later method is in common use in the ED.

Expired gases can be directly sampled to determine their CO_2 content. The carbon dioxide content of expired gases at the end of the expiration phase of respiration ($Etco_2$) proportionally approximates the $Paco_2$ content in healthy individuals because CO_2 rapidly diffuses into the alveolar space along its pressure gradient, and arterial levels are typically only about 5 mm Hg higher than alveolar samples when pulmonary ventilation and perfusion are functioning normally. The CO_2 content of the entire volume of expired gas can be photometrically assessed by means of a **mainstream** detector, or a sample of the expired gases can be aspirated from airway via a **side stream** detector. Mainstream detectors are larger and must be inserted into the ventilator loop, either in a ventilator circuit or with the patient breathing through a mask or other tube. Side stream detectors are smaller and have the advantage of ease of use in nonintubated patients. Interpretation of the capnogram is not necessarily intuitive. A summary of typical capnogram waveforms is described in **Figure 16-2.**

End-tidal CO_2 measurements ($PEtco_2$) do not accurately represent $Paco_2$. Mainstream and side stream sampling may each include air that has not been involved in the gas exchange process, either from physiologic dead space or via environmental air that enters the sample. In either case the $PEtco_2$ value will be lower than the arterial value. End-tidal CO_2 measurement is not as useful in obstructive pulmonary disease due to incomplete expiration of gases secondary to air trapping. In a study of ED patients with chronic obstructive pulmonary disease, end-tidal measurements did not significantly vary from presentation to admission and were not clinically different for patients discharged home as compared to those requiring admission.[31] Studies assessing the accuracy of $Etco_2$ measurements compared to arterial sampling are mixed. In one study of patients presenting to the ED with undifferentiated dyspnea, mainstream $PEtco_2$ did correlate closely with $Paco_2$.[32] In a comparison of healthy individuals, neither mainstream nor side stream sampling accurately predicted the arterial Pco_2.[33] A convenience sample of ED patients with an indication for arterial blood gas did not have a close correlation of side stream $Etco_2$ with the $Paco_2$.[34] The precise role

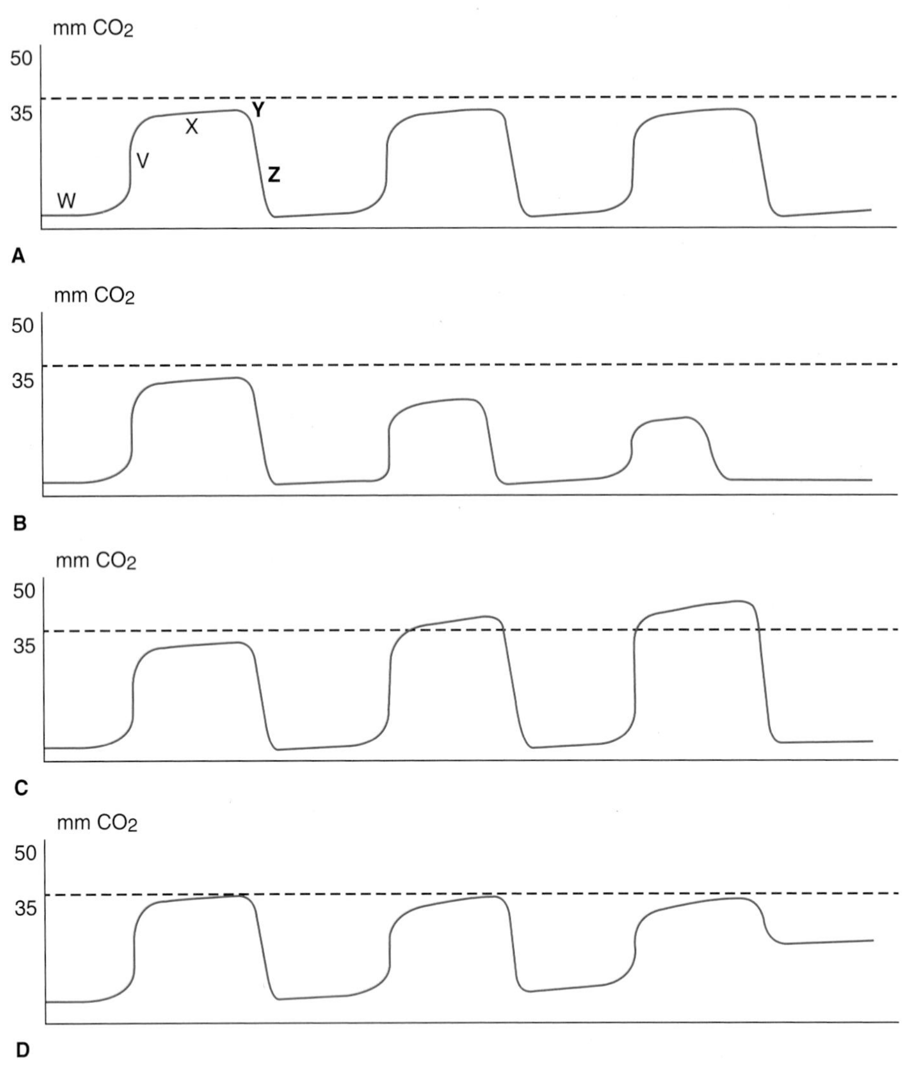

FIGURE 16-2. End-tidal capnogram. Capnogram A depicts a normal capnogram with inspiratory baseline (V), expiratory upstroke (W), expiratory plateau (X), end-tidal concentration (Y), and inspiratory downstroke (Z). Capnogram B represents apnea, which appears as serially decreasing end-tidal concentrations as little gas is expired. Capnogram C represents hypoventilation, which appears as an upward trend in the plateau and end-tidal concentration. Capnogram D represents rebreathing or air trapping, which appears as an increase in the baseline phase of the capnogram.

for $Etco_2$ measurements in the management of critically ill patients in the ED or intensive care unit is still to be determined.[35]

REFERENCES

The complete reference list is available online at www.TintinalliEM.com.

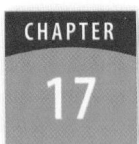

Fluids and Electrolytes

Roberta Petrino
Roberta Marino

FLUIDS AND SODIUM

PATHOPHYSIOLOGY

Total body water (TBW), which accounts for approximately 60% of total body weight, can be divided into intracellular fluid (ICF) and extracellular fluid (ECF) compartments. The ECF is comprised of intravascular fluid and extravascular, or interstitial, fluid. Body fluid compartment proportions for an adult are diagrammed in **Figure 17-1**. **Figure 17-2** presents the individual characteristics of each compartment. Three fundamental homeostatic equilibriums govern the behavior of fluids: the osmotic equilibrium, the electric equilibrium, and the acid-base equilibrium.

The key point is that sodium is much more concentrated in the ECF (~140 mEq/L) than in the ICF (~10 mEq/L) but is equal in both compartments of the ECF because the capillary membrane between intravascular fluid and interstitial fluid is permeable to water and electrolytes. In contrast, the cell membrane is permeable to water but not to electrolytes, which are moved through ionic pumps against gradient to keep the intracellular sodium concentration constant around 10 mEq/L and potassium at 150 mEq/L. **Table 17-1** lists the electrolyte concentration of body fluids and the most commonly used therapeutic solutions. **Table 17-2** defines commonly used terms that describe measures or characteristics of electrolytes and/or disorders.

When two solutions are separated by a membrane that is permeable only to water, water crosses into the compartment with the more concentrated solution to equalize the ion concentration in each. The force driving this movement is "osmotic pressure."[1] In human fluids, the substances that contribute the most to osmotic pressure in ECF are Na^+ and the anions HCO_3^- and Cl^-, plus glucose. In physiology, this force is called *effective osmolality* or *tonicity*. This force is not affected by molecules like urea that may enter freely into the cells. The formula to calculate **effective osmolality** or **tonicity** is

2 × [Na] + glucose/18 (normal range, 275–290 mOsm/L)

If values are in SI units, these are already molar (mmol/L, for example), so these do not need to be divided by their molecular weight.

As a function of	TBW	ICF	ECF	IF	IVF
Total weight	60%	40%	20%	15%	5%
TBW		67%	33%	25%	8%
ECF compartment				75%	25%

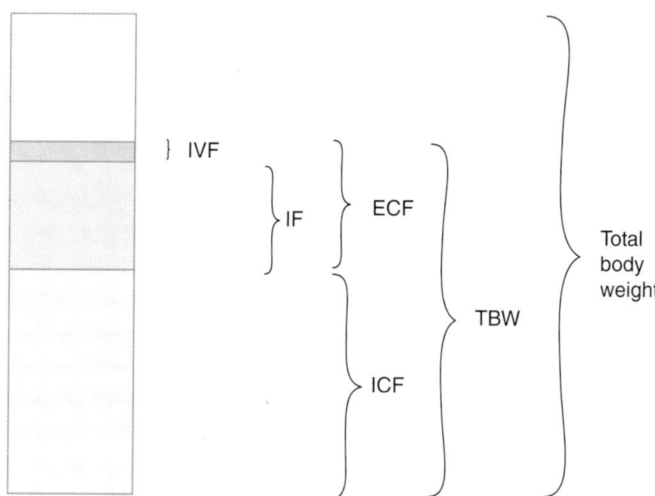

FIGURE 17-1. Relation of fluid compartments to body weight and each other. ECF = extracellular fluid; ICF = intracellular fluid; IF = interstitial (extravascular) fluid; IVF = intravascular fluid; TBW = total body water.

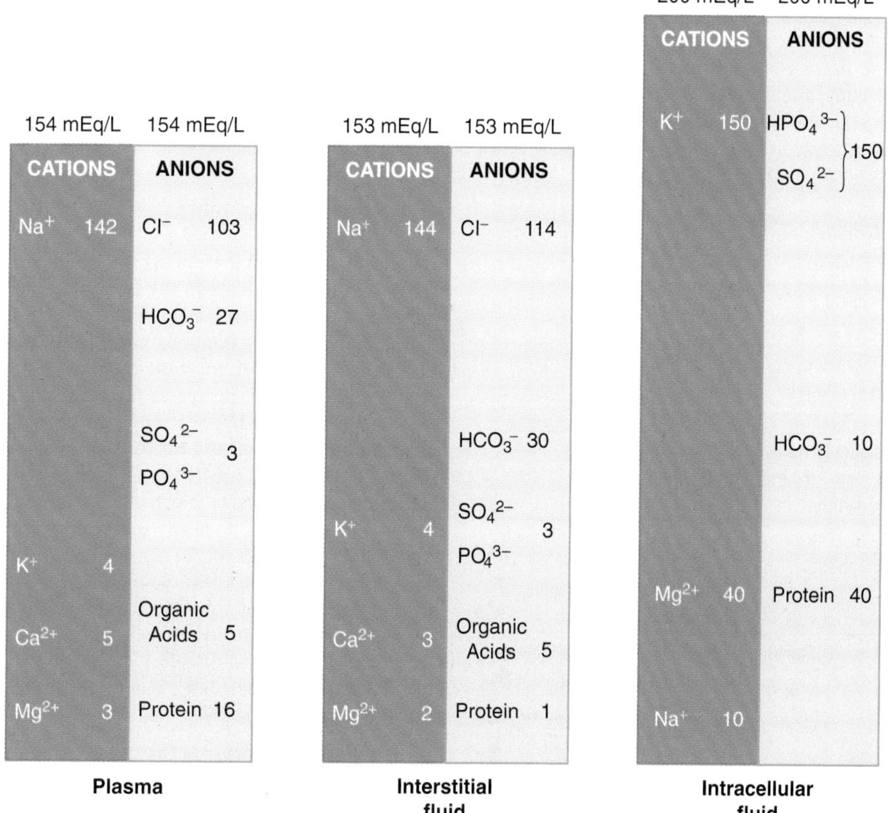

FIGURE 17-2. Chemical composition of body fluid compartments. [Reproduced with permission from Brunicardi FC, Andersen DK, Billiar TR, et al (eds): *Schwartz's Principles of Surgery*, 10th ed. McGraw-Hill, Inc., 2015. Fig 3-2, p. 67.]

TABLE 17-1 Electrolyte Concentrations of Fluids (mEq/L)

Solution	Plasma	Interstitial	Intracellular	Normal Saline	Lactated Ringer's Solution
Cations					
Sodium	142	144	10	154	130
Potassium	4	4.5	150	—	4
Magnesium*	2	1	40	—	—
Calcium†	5	2.5	—	—	3
Total cations	153	152	200	154	137
Anions					
Chloride	104	113	—	154	109
Lactate‡	—	—	—	—	28
Phosphates	2	2	120	—	—
Sulfates	1	1	30	—	—
Bicarbonate	27	30	10	—	—
Proteins	13	1	40	—	—
Organic acids	6	5	—	—	—
Total anions	153	152	200	154	137

*Multiply by 0.411 to convert to International System of Units (SI) units in mmol/L.
†Multiply by 0.25 to convert to SI units in mmol/L.
‡Multiply by 0.323 to convert to SI units in mmol/L.

When 1 L of free water is added to the ECF it crosses the cell membrane into the ICF to equalize ECF osmolality. The result is TBW expansion and slight reduction in osmolality (**Figure 17-3**). When 1 L of isotonic saline solution 0.9% is added to the ECF, there is no movement of water into the cells, and the final result is ECF expansion only[2] (Figure 17-3).

In contrast, when there is a fluid loss and a consequent increase in osmolality, the subject feels thirsty and the antidiuretic hormone (ADH) is secreted by the pituitary gland stimulated by baroreceptors and osmoreceptors, with a consequent urine water reabsorption and vasoconstriction.[1-3]

TABLE 17-2 Definition of Terms

Term	Definition	Comments
Mole	6.02×10^{23} molecules of a substance	Unit measure used in International System of Units format.
Equivalent	Mass (in grams) of a mole of a substance divided by charge of substance	Unit of measure used in conventional lab values.
Osmole	Amount of a substance (in moles) that dissociates to form 1 mole of osmotically active particles	
Osmolarity	Measure of solute concentration per unit *volume* of solvent	Osmolarity varies with changing temperature, because water changes its volume according to temperature.
Osmolality	Measure of solute concentration per unit *mass* of solvent	Osmolality is the preferred term because it remains constant with changes in temperature.
Tonicity or effective osmolality	Measure of the osmotic pressure gradient between two solutions, across a semipermeable membrane	Tonicity is affected only by solutes that cannot cross a semipermeable membrane. For example, tonicity is not affected by urea or glucose as they cross semipermeable membranes

A useful index to roughly evaluate Na^+ balance and the ability of the kidney to concentrate or dilute the urine is the **electrolyte free water clearance ($_CH_2Oe$)**.[2] It is expressed with the formula:

$$_CH_2Oe = V_{urine}(1 - U_{Na+} + U_{K+}/P_{Na+})$$

where V_{urine} is urine volume, U_{Na+} is the urine sodium level, U_{K+} is the urine potassium level, and P_{Na+} is the plasma sodium level. When more water is reabsorbed, $_CH_2Oe$ is negative and hyponatremia will develop. When more water is excreted, $_CH_2Oe$ is positive and hypernatremia will be present. The $_CH_2Oe$ is calculated using a 24-hour urine collection, which is not possible in the ED. The spot urine calculation of the ratio, $U_{Na+} + U_{K+}/P_{Na+}$, is a reliable compromise. In hyponatremia, the ratio is >1, and in hypernatremia it is ≤0.5. A ratio between 0.5 and 1 is considered normal.

HYPONATREMIA

The human body tightly maintains serum [Na^+] between 138 and 142 mEq/L despite what may be marked changes in daily intake depending on the person's diet. Hyponatremia is a condition of excess water relative to Na^+ and is defined as a serum [Na^+] <138 mEq/L. However, symptomatic hyponatremia rarely occurs until [Na^+] falls below 135 mEq/L or lower. In the setting of normal water intake, high circulating levels of ADH with subsequent water retention is a prerequisite for the development of hyponatremia.[3] Urine osmolality is always >100 mOsm/L H_2O with the exception of samples from patients with psychogenic polydipsia, which drives down urine osmolality below the typical minimum.

EPIDEMIOLOGY

Mild hyponatremia is common, with an incidence of 15% to 30% in hospitalized patients; only 1% to 4% of patients have sodium levels below 130 mEq/L.[4,5] Approximately 50% of cases are iatrogenic from administration of hypotonic fluids.[4,5]

CLASSIFICATION AND ETIOLOGY

The concentration of Na^+ does not give information regarding volume status. **Therefore, the first step in the evaluation should include a clinical evaluation of ECF volume status plus measured and calculated plasma osmolarities.** In *true* hyponatremia, plasma osmolality is reduced; in *factitious* hyponatremic states, it is normal or increased as shown in **Table 17-3**.[2]

HYPEROSMOLAR HYPONATREMIA (P_{osm} >295 mOsm/kg H_2O)

Hyperosmolar hyponatremia occurs when large quantities of osmotically active solutes accumulate in the ECF space. In this setting, there is a net movement of water from the ICF to the ECF, thereby effectively diluting the ECF [Na^+]. **This happens commonly with severe hyperglycemia.** Each 100 milligram/dL increase in plasma glucose above the normal level of 100 milligrams/dL decreases the serum [Na^+] by 1.6 mEq/L.[1-4] Other causes of hypertonic hyponatremia are administration of osmotic agents like mannitol, glycerol, and maltose, causing an osmolar gap and hyponatremia. The osmolar gap is the difference between measured osmolality and calculated osmolality. Normally the difference is around 10 mOsm/L; if it is >15 mOsm/L it means that a nondetectable agent with osmotic activity is present, causing an osmolar gap. A consequent osmotic diuresis will cause [Na^+] deficit with volume depletion that must be treated with saline solution. Other substances like methanol, alcohol, ethylene glycol, and urea, although causing an osmolar gap, do not cause water movement across membranes and therefore do not cause hyponatremia (see chapter 185, "Alcohols" in Toxicology section for more details).[2]

ISO-OSMOLAR HYPONATREMIA (P_{osm} 275 TO 295 mOsm/kg H_2O)

Pseudohyponatremia is a factitiously low value of [Na^+] that may occur in the setting of severe hyperproteinemia or hyperlipidemia. This phenomena is due to displacement of serum water by an elevated concentration of lipids or protein creating laboratory misinterpretation

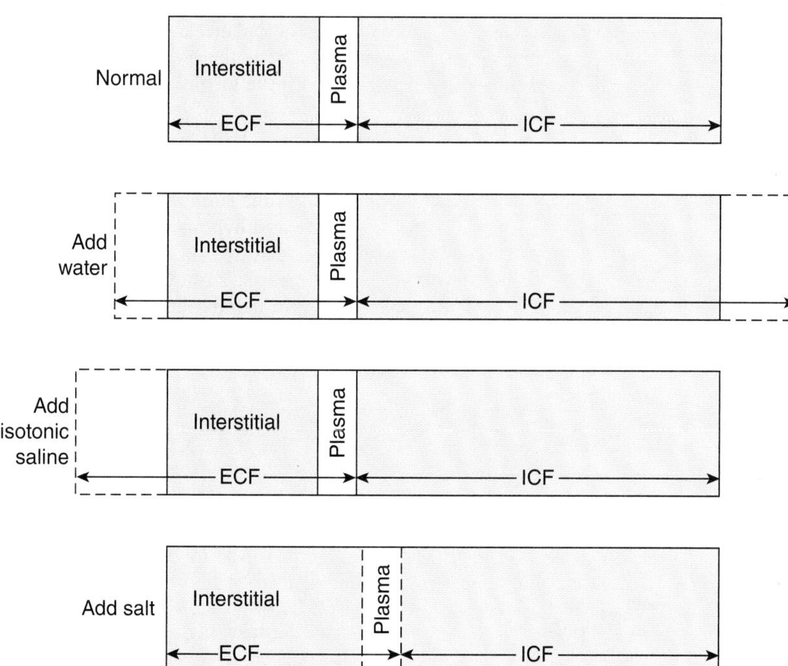

FIGURE 17-3. Distribution of total body water into the intracellular fluid (ICF) and extracellular fluid (ECF) compartments. Addition of water expands both compartments. Addition of isotonic saline expands only the ECF, whereas addition of salt without water expands the ECF at the expense of the ICF. [Reproduced with permission from Eaton DC, Poole JP (eds): *Vander's Renal Physiology*, 8th ed. McGraw-Hill, Inc., 2013. Fig 6-1.]

of normal [Na+]; some laboratories use instruments that avoid this laboratory error; check with your laboratory administrator. Patients are asymptomatic; treatment is not needed.

HYPO-OSMOLAR HYPONATREMIA (P_{osm} <275 mOsm/kg H_2O)

In **Table 17-4**,[6] the different causes of hypo-osmolar (hypotonic) hyponatremia according to volume status are listed.[2,3] Hyponatremia develops due to an increase in ADH secretion and activity, which causes impaired water excretion and increased water reabsorption. In situations like heart failure,[7,8] cirrhosis,[9] and nephrotic syndrome, the effective arterial blood volume is decreased because water is mainly distributed to the interstitial space. Thus Na^+ and water reabsorption are increased, and water excretion is reduced.

Two important hyponatremic disorders are the **syndrome of inappropriate ADH secretion** and the less common **cerebral salt-wasting syndrome.**[1,2] Both conditions are diagnoses of exclusion after dismissing other causes of hyponatremia. The onset of both syndromes is linked to chronic cerebral disease, but syndrome of inappropriate ADH secretion may also be caused by many other diseases and conditions as described in **Table 17-5**. In syndrome of inappropriate ADH secretion, volume status is normal, whereas in cerebral salt-wasting syndrome, there is hypovolemia; therefore, these two disorders are treated differently (see treatment section below).

Methylenedioxymethamphetamine (MDMA or Ecstasy) intoxication is an uncommon but important cause of hyponatremia that may be profound. This "club drug" induces inappropriate secretion of ADH and causes increased gut water absorption[10] (see also chapter 188, "Hallucinogens").

TABLE 17-3 Classification of Hyponatremia According to Serum Osmolality

Serum Osmolality	Clinical Conditions	Mechanisms
Hyperosmolality (Hypertonic hyponatremia)	Hyperglycemia Mannitol administration Glycerol administration Maltose administration	Hyponatremia due to osmotic diuresis
Iso-osmolality (Pseudohyponatremia)	Hyperproteinemia Hyperlipidemia	Displacement of serum water by elevated concentration of lipids or protein creating laboratory misinterpretation of normal [Na+]
Hypo-osmolality (Hypotonic hyponatremia)	See Table 17-4	Hypervolemic Normovolemic Hypovolemic

CLINICAL FEATURES

The most important symptoms of hyponatremia are due to its effects on the brain; symptoms can be divided into moderately severe and severe, according to a European clinical practice guideline.[3,4] Moderately severe symptoms often start when a plasma [Na] is <130 mEq/L and consist of headache, nausea, disorientation, confusion, agitation, ataxia, and areflexia. When [Na^+] reach levels <120 mEq/L, severe symptoms may develop including intractable vomiting, seizures, coma, and ultimately respiratory arrest due to brainstem herniation. Brain injury may become irreversible. The symptoms of hyponatremia can be due to many other conditions, and clinicians are cautioned to consider other etiologies before making treatment decisions.[4] The presence of hyponatremia-related symptoms is directly related to the rapidity of onset. After a certain period, brain cells begin to adapt to hyponatremia. Initially the hypo-osmolality drives water into the brain cells yielding swelling.[2,3] Due to the rigid skull, intracranial hypertension occurs and the described symptoms begin. After 48 hours, the brain cells start to adapt by extruding Na^+, K^+, Cl^-, and organic osmolytes like glycine and taurine from the cells, reducing cell osmolality and preventing further water uptake. In several clinical or physiologic conditions, this adaptation mechanism is impaired, as in the syndrome of inappropriate ADH secretion, in children, in menstruating women, and in hypoxia. In such cases, symptoms are more severe and persistent.

DIAGNOSIS

The diagnosis of hyponatremia and its subtypes is based on the clinical findings of volume status in association with specific laboratory values including serum [Na^+], serum osmolality, volume status, urinary sodium (U_{Na+}), and urine osmolality (U_{osm}). Acute and chronic hyponatremia are defined by an onset time of less than (acute) or greater than (chronic) 24 to 48 hours. Experts recommend that when duration is unknown, the hyponatremia should be assumed to be chronic and treated as chronic with a longer correction time. If urine osmolality is not readily available from the laboratory, it can be estimated using urinary specific gravity (π). Consider the numerals in the hundredths and thousandths decimal places of the π as whole numbers and multiply them by 35 to obtain U_{osm}. As an example, for a π of 1.0<u>05</u>, U_{osm} = 05 ×

TABLE 17-4 Classification, Differential Diagnosis, and Features of Hyponatremia According to Volume Status

	Clinical Conditions	Orthostatic Hypotension	Edema	$U_{[Na^+]}$, mEq/L*	U_{osm}, mOsm/L*
Hypervolemic hypernatremia	CHF Cirrhosis Nephrotic syndrome Acute and chronic kidney disease	Absent	Yes	Compensated: >20 Decompensated: <10	Compensated: <100 Decompensated: >100
Normovolemic hyponatremia	Psychogenic polydipsia Glucocorticoid deficit Hypokalemia Drugs SIADH	Absent	No	>20	>100
Renal hypovolemic hyponatremia	Diuretics Mineralocorticoid deficit Salt-losing nephropathy	Normally present	No	>20	>100
Extrarenal hypovolemic hyponatremia	Vomiting Diarrhea	Normally present	No	<10	>100

Abbreviations: CHF = congestive heart failure; SIADH = syndrome of inappropriate ADH excretion.

35 = 175 mOsm/L.[1] Table 17-4 lists the values of U_{Na+} and U_{osm} in different classifications of hyponatremia according to volume status and the differential diagnosis for each classification. As a rule, only in patients with edematous syndromes and in patients with vomiting and diarrhea will U_{Na+} be found to be <10 mEq/L.[6] The diagnostic criteria for syndrome of inappropriate ADH secretion are listed in **Table 17-6.**

Use care when assessing patients with potential exercise-associated hyponatremia. Since the worldwide effort to encourage consuming fluids during endurance exercise beginning in the early 1980s, overhydration with hypotonic fluids is now being seen. If a postexercise athlete presents with bloating, nausea, vomiting, and edema (check wrists and fingers), consider hyponatremia; dehydration presents with excessive thirst, sunken eyes, poor skin turgor, and postural hypotension.

TABLE 17-5 Causes of Syndrome of Inappropriate Antidiuretic Hormone Secretion

1. Neurologic and psychiatric disorders
   a. Infections: meningitis, encephalitis, brain abscess
   b. Vascular: thrombosis, subarachnoid or subdural hemorrhage, temporal arteritis, cavernous sinus thrombosis, stroke
   c. Malignancy: primary or metastatic
   d. Traumatic brain injury
   e. Psychosis, delirium tremens
   f. Other: Guillain-Barré syndrome, neurosurgery
2. Drugs
   a. Cyclophosphamide
   b. Carbamazepine
   c. Vinca alkaloids
   d. Thioridazine, other phenothiazines, haloperidol
   e. Selective serotonin reuptake inhibitors and selective serotonin and norepinephrine reuptake inhibitors
   f. Bromocriptine
   g. Narcotics, opiate derivatives
   h. Amiodarone
   i. Desmopressin overtreatment of DI or enuresis
3. Lung diseases
   a. Tuberculosis
   b. Lung abscess, empyema
   c. Acute respiratory failure
4. Non-CNS tumors with ectopic production of vasopressin
   a. Carcinoma of lung (small cell, bronchogenic), duodenum, pancreas, thymus, olfactory neuroblastoma, bladder, prostate, uterus
   b. Lymphoma, leukemia
   c. Sarcoma

Abbreviations: DI = diabetes insipidus.

TREATMENT

Treatment of hyponatremia is guided by four variables: severity of symptoms, rate of onset, volume status, and the current serum [Na⁺]. **When [Na⁺] is <120 mEg/L, the patient presents with severe neurologic symptoms, and hyponatremia is acute, the initial treatment includes infusion of 3% hypertonic saline** as recommended by European guidelines,[4] and U.S. experts[5,11] (**Table 17-7**).

Raising serum sodium by 4 to 6 mEq/L is typically all that is required to see an improvement in severe neurologic symptoms.[4,11,12] The volume of a saline solution required to raise the serum sodium the desired amount can be calculated. First calculate the expected change in serum sodium from the infusion of a liter of saline solution. Second, determine the portion of the liter required to raise the sodium the desired amount. To calculate the expected change in serum sodium after an infusion of 1 L IV saline, use the following formula:

$$\textbf{Expected change in serum Na}^+ \textbf{ (mEq/L)} =$$

$$\textbf{Infusate Na}^+ \textbf{ (mEq/L)} - \textbf{serum Na}^+ \textbf{ (mEq/L)/(TBW + 1)}$$

Estimate TBW based on age, sex, and weight of the patient. For children and adult males <65 years old, TBW is 60% of the weight; for adult females <65 years old and elderly males, TBW is 50% of the weight; for elderly females, TBW is 45% of weight. Three percent hypertonic saline contains 513 mEq/L of sodium. As an example, a clinician desires to

TABLE 17-6 Syndrome of Inappropriate Secretion of Antidiuretic Hormone Diagnostic Criteria

Diagnostic Criteria
Hypotonic hyponatremia with (P_{osm} <275 mOsm/kg H_2O)
Inappropriately elevated urinary osmolality (usually >200 mOsm/kg)
Elevated urinary [Na⁺] (typically >20 mEq/L)
Clinical euvolemia
Normal adrenal, renal, cardiac, hepatic, and thyroid functions

TABLE 17-7 Treatment for Hyponatremia Symptomatic with Seizures or Coma

Step 1	Assess for indication for 3% hypertonic saline: severe symptoms of hyponatremia such as seizures or coma with suspected impending brainstem herniation in setting of acute* or chronic† hyponatremia
Step 2	Infuse 100 mL of 3% hypertonic saline IV over 10–15 min‡
Step 3	Measure serum sodium level after each 3% hypertonic saline infusion
Step 4	Stop infusion when symptoms improve, or a target of 5 mEq/L (range 4–6 mEq/L) increase in serum sodium concentration is achieved.
Step 5	May repeat 100 mL of 3% hypertonic saline up to three total doses, or a total of 300 mL IV of 3% hypertonic saline.
Step 6	Keep the IV line open with minimal volume of 0.9% normal saline until cause-specific treatment is started. Limit increase in sodium level to no more than 8 mEq/L during the first 24 h.

*Both European guidelines and U.S. expert panel recommend 3% hypertonic saline infusion for acute life-threatening hyponatremia, which is most commonly due to self-induced water intoxication during endurance exercise, psychiatric illness, in association with methylenedioxymethamphetamine intoxication, or intracranial pathology or increased intracranial pressure.

†European guidelines state that regardless of onset of acute or chronic hyponatremia, presence of seizures or coma is an indication for brief infusion of hypertonic saline to improve symptoms.

‡European guidelines recommend a prompt 150-mL 3% hypertonic saline infusion over 20 minutes, then checking the serum sodium concentration after 20 minutes while repeating an infusion of 150 mL 3% hypertonic saline for the next 20 minutes, repeating this sequence up to twice more, and stopping with clinical improvement or when target sodium level is reached.

raise the sodium level of a 68-year-old male having seizures secondary to a [Na^+] of 108 mEq/L, using 3% hypertonic saline. The man weighs 70 kg; therefore, the calculated TBW would be [$0.5_{\text{correction factor}} \times 70$ kg] = 35 L. Change in [Na^+] expected = (513 – 108)/(35 + 1) = 11.25 mEq rise in serum sodium if the man was given 1000 mL of 3% hypertonic saline. The fraction of the liter of 3% hypertonic saline required to raise serum sodium 5 mEq/L would be 444 mL of 3% hypertonic saline.

After clinical improvement in severe symptoms, the 3% hypertonic saline must be stopped and either continued at a slower rate or with a different [Na^+] in the solution. For patients with acute hyponatremia with mild or moderate symptoms, 3% hypertonic saline infusion at 0.5 to 2 mL/kg/h can be given with frequent [Na^+] checks every 2 hours. Na^+ and K^+ lost in urine should be replaced with the appropriate solution.[1,2]

In chronic hyponatremia, the [Na^+] correction should be slower than for acute hyponatremia. Rapid correction increases risk for the most dangerous complication of treatment, the osmotic demyelination syndrome. For **chronic hyponatremia [Na^+], the correction rate should not exceed 6 mEq/24 h** in high-risk patients and 12 mEq/24 h in low-risk patients (see "Osmotic Demyelination Syndrome" section below for risks).[3,4] Hypertonic (3%) saline can be given at a low infusion rate, 0.5 to 1 mL/kg/h, with frequent [Na^+] checks. Isotonic (0.9%) saline is frequently used (sometimes before the [Na^+] is known), especially for the treatment of mild hyponatremia; however, the additional fluid load must be accounted for in treatment calculations. Loop diuretics (primarily furosemide, starting with a small dose of 20 milligrams IV) may be used in addition to treatment with saline infusions. Urine volume and [Na^+] should be strictly measured. Specific recommendations for hyponatremia treatment are summarized in **Table 17-8**.[2]

COMPLICATIONS OF TREATMENT

Osmotic Demyelination Syndrome Osmotic demyelination syndrome is caused by rapid correction of hyponatremia (>12 mEq/L/24 h) as water moves from cells to ECF yielding intracellular dehydration (**Figure 17-4**). Risk factors for osmotic demyelination syndrome include [Na^+] <120 mEq/L, chronic heart failure, alcoholism, cirrhosis, hypokalemia, malnutrition, and treatment with vasopressin antagonists such as tolvaptan. Main symptoms are dysarthria, dysphagia, lethargy, paraparesis or quadriparesis, seizures, coma, and death. The treatment of [Na^+] overcorrection is rarely done in the ED but consists of giving 5% dextrose in water at 3 mL/kg/h, loop diuretics, and desmopressin.[3,4]

HYPERNATREMIA

Hypernatremia is defined as serum or plasma **[Na^+] >145 mEq/L and hyperosmolality** (serum osmolality >295 mOsm/L).

TABLE 17-8 Cause-Specific Treatment for Hyponatremia

Clinical Condition	Therapy	Cautions/Comments
Chronic heart failure and cirrhosis	Loop diuretics, water restriction. Consider vasopressin antagonists* if the above therapies fail for patients with chronic heart failure.	When vasopressin antagonists* are used serum [Na^+] should be frequently measured to avoid hypernatremia. FDA recommends against vasopressin antagonists in patients with liver disease.
Nephrotic syndrome	Water restriction	
Acute or chronic kidney disease	Water restriction	Frequent assessment of creatinine
Psychogenic polydipsia	Water restriction	Treat the underlying psychiatric disease
Hypothyroidism	Levothyroxine	Several days of therapy are typically required to correct hyponatremia.
Glucocorticoid deficiency	Hydrocortisone. If neurologic symptoms, consider vasopressin antagonists* if resistant to hydrocortisone.	When vasopressin antagonists* are used, [Na^+] should be frequently measured.
SIADH	Water restriction. Enhanced Na^+ and protein intake + furosemide. Vasopressin antagonists* can be used for [Na^+] <125 mEq/L. Demeclocycline. Lithium.	Isotonic (0.9%) NaCl may worsen hyponatremia; when vasopressin antagonists* are used, [Na^+] should be frequently measured.
Diarrhea and vomiting	Isotonic (0.9%) NaCl. Add KCl if hypokalemia is present.	Treat the cause, monitor hemodynamic status
Diuretics (most commonly thiazides)	Stop diuretic. KCl may be sufficient in patients with coexistent potassium depletion and normal dietary sodium intake. NaCl can be given orally.	Slow correction is recommended. Do not overcorrect K^+ deficit.
Mineralocorticoid deficiency	Replace volume deficit. Fludrocortisone therapy is indicated once diagnosis is confirmed.	Mechanism: volume depletion → ↑ ADH → decreases water excretion, ↑ Na loss
Salt losing nephropathies	Isotonic (0.9%) NaCl.	
Cerebral salt wasting	Isotonic (0.9%) NaCl. Fludrocortisone may be considered after the diagnosis is confirmed.	NaCl orally at home

Abbreviations: ADH = antidiuretic hormone; FDA = Food and Drug Administration; SIADH = syndrome of inappropriate antidiuretic hormone secretion.

*Vasopressin antagonists or vaptans are rarely started in the ED; they are not indicated unless [Na^+] <125 mEq/L; starting doses are tolvaptan, 15 milligrams PO daily; and conivaptan, 20 milligrams loading dose IV over 30 minutes, then continuous infusion of 20 milligrams over 24 hours for 2 to 4 days.

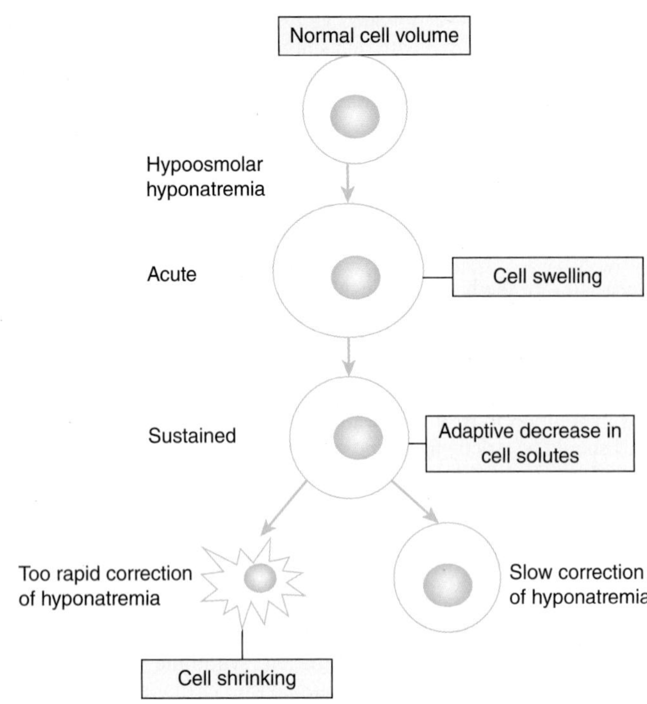

FIGURE 17-4. Adaptation of brain volume to hyponatremia and effect of correction.

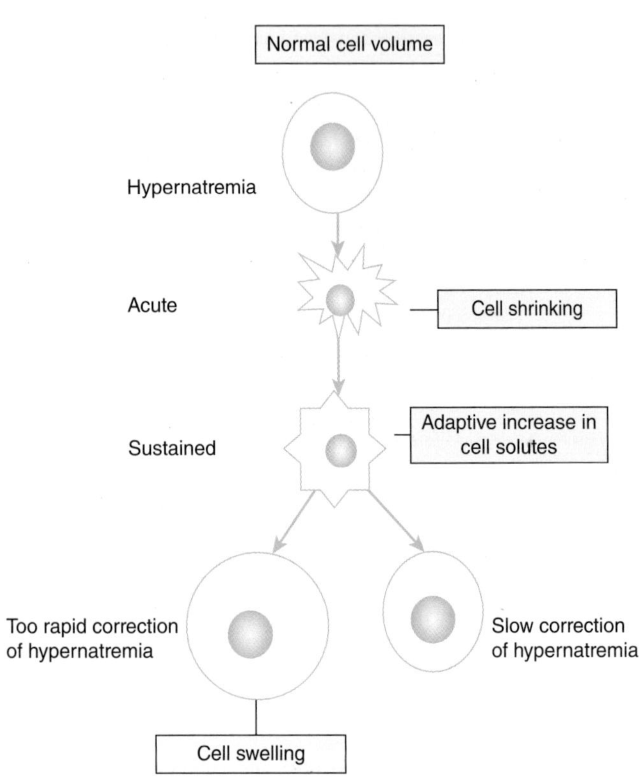

FIGURE 17-5. Adaptation of brain volume to hypernatremia and effect of correction.

PATHOPHYSIOLOGY

Hypernatremia results from a deficit in TBW and/or a net gain of Na^+ (less common). When $[Na^+]$ and osmolality increase, normal subjects become thirsty, drink free water, and the Na^+ level returns toward normal. Any clinical situation that impairs the patient's sense of thirst, limits the availability of water, limits the kidney's ability to concentrate urine, or results in increased salt intake predisposes the patient to hypernatremia. Elderly patients, decompensated diabetics, infants, and hospitalized patients are at particular risk of developing hypernatremia. In addition, hypernatremia may be the result of loss of free water in diarrheal stools or in the urine.[13]

As in hyponatremia, symptoms will be more severe and evident when the onset is rapid; after the first 48 hours, there is an adaptation of brain cells with an increase in electrolytes and organic osmolytes and thus increased intracellular water partly correcting the initial cell shrinking (**Figure 17-5**).

If severe hypernatremia develops in the course of minutes to hours, such as from a massive salt overdose in a suicide attempt, a suddenly shrinking brain may prompt intracranial hemorrhage. While the causes of hypernatremia are many, leading to varied signs and symptoms, the most serious manifestations are related to changes in the brain. If hypernatremia is corrected too rapidly, cerebral edema and potentially central herniation may occur.

CLASSIFICATION AND ETIOLOGY

Based on volume status, hypernatremia may be classified as hypovolemic hypernatremia (decreased TBW and total body Na^+ with a relatively greater decrease in TBW), hypervolemic hypernatremia (increased total body Na^+ with normal or increased TBW), or normovolemic hypernatremia (near normal total body sodium and decreased TBW)[1,2] (**Table 17-9**).

CLINICAL FEATURES

History depends on hypernatremia type and may reveal nausea and vomiting, lethargy, weakness, increased thirst, low water intake, salt intake, polyuria (>3000 mL of urine/24 h), diabetes, hypercalcemia, hypokalemia, medications such as lactulose, loop diuretics, lithium, demeclocycline (may cause nephrogenic diabetes insipidus), or nonsteroidal anti-inflammatory drugs (may cause interstitial nephritis). Physical exam may reveal hypotension, tachycardia, orthostatic blood pressures, sunken eyes, dry mucous membranes (symptoms of hypovolemia) altered mental status (may be present in any the hypernatremia classifications), poor skin turgor, or edema in hypervolemic hypernatremia (Table 17-9). Without intervention, coma, seizures, and shock may occur. Signs of Cushing's syndrome may be present, including moon facies, fatty deposits between the shoulders and upper back, and thinning of the skin.

DIAGNOSIS

The diagnosis of hypernatremia and its classification are based on the clinical evaluation including volume status and specific laboratory tests, including serum electrolytes and osmolality, urine osmolality, urea/creatinine ratio, and free water deficit. A BUN/creatinine ratio >40 is indicative of hyperosmolar dehydration. The free water deficit[1,2] may be calculated with the formula:

$$\textbf{Free water deficit} = \textbf{TBW} \times \textbf{P}_{\textbf{osm}} - \textbf{285/P}_{\textbf{osm}}$$

where TBW is calculated using age and sex (giving a correction factor for body water) times weight in kilograms (see hyponatremia treatment section for scale), $P_{osm} = 2 \times [Na^+] + \text{glucose}/18$, and 285 is used as normal plasma osmolality. As an example, a 60-kg woman with a $[Na^+]$ of 165 mEq/L and glucose of 130 milligrams/dL has a free water deficit calculated as follows: TBW = 0.5 × 60 = 30; P_{osm} = (2 × 165 = 330) + (130/18 = 7.2) = 337.2 mOsm/kg H_2O; free water deficit = 30 × (337.2 − 285)/337.2 = 4.64 L. Urine osmolality can be used to suggest the type of hypernatremia (**Table 17-10**). If urine osmolality is not readily available, it can be estimated using urine specific gravity (π). Consider the numerals in the hundredths and thousandths decimal places of the π as whole numbers and multiply them by 35 to estimate U_{osm}.

TREATMENT

First, shock, hypoperfusion, or volume deficits should be treated with isotonic (0.9%) saline. Second, treat any existing underlying cause,

TABLE 17-9 Hypernatremia Classification and Features According to Volume Status

	Clinical Conditions	Orthostatic Hypotension	Edema	$U_{[Na^+]}$, mEq/L	U_{osm}, mOsm/kg H_2O
Hypervolemic hypernatremia	Cushing's syndrome Primary hyperaldosteronism Salt water intake Iatrogenic	Absent unless treated with diuretics	Yes	Compensated >20	>100
Normovolemic hypernatremia	DI Central DI Partial DI Gestational DI Nephrogenic DI Hypodipsia	Absent	No	>20	Central DI <300 Partial DI >300 but <800
Renal hypovolemic hypernatremia	Osmotic diuretics Loop diuretics Postobstructive diuresis	Normally present	No	>20	>100
Extrarenal hypovolemic hypernatremia	Vomiting Diarrhea GI fistulas Sweating Burns	Normally present	No	<10	>800

Abbreviation: DI = diabetes insipidus.

such as diabetes insipidus (see "Diabetes Insipidus" section below) vomiting, diarrhea, or fever. Third, correct the patient's free water deficit at a rate reflecting the acuity or duration time of the hypernatremia onset (**Table 17-11**).[11,14,15] In cases of a lethal sodium chloride ingestion/load (0.75 to 3.0 grams/kg) less than 6 hours prior to presentation, FWD may be replaced rapidly with no reported adverse events.[11,14] Management requires evaluating volume status and the free water deficit (see formula above in diagnosis section). When the adaptation of brain cells is incomplete (onset over <48 hours), the correction rate of acute hypernatremia can be performed at a rate of 1 mEq/L/h. In an alert patient capable of safely drinking water, the route of administration should be two-thirds free water orally and one-third IV. If hypernatremia is chronic (onset over >48 hours), the rate of correction should be slower, to avoid the risk of cerebral edema, at no more than 0.5 mEq/L/h or 10 to 12 mEq/24 h.[11,16]

DIABETES INSIPIDUS

Diabetes insipidus is a disease where the ability of the kidney to reabsorb free water is compromised.[2,17] The disorder is characterized by polyuria, polydipsia, and an increased volume of hypo-osmolar urine. Hypernatremia is present only when the thirst center is impaired or water intake is reduced. Diabetes insipidus can be central (also called neurogenic), due to inadequate ADH secretion, or renal (also called nephrogenic), when ADH secretion is normal or increased but the v2R receptors of the kidney's collecting duct cells do not respond appropriately to ADH. Diabetes insipidus may be congenital or acquired. In **Table 17-12**, the main causes of diabetes insipidus are listed. Congenital forms of diabetes insipidus present during infancy. Eventually, recurrent cellular dehydration causes cerebral calcifications that manifest as delayed intellectual advancement.

TABLE 17-10 Urine Osmolality Findings in Selected Hypernatremic States

Urine Osmolality (U_{osm})	Potential Hypernatremic State
U_{osm} <300 mOsm/kg H_2O	Central or nephrogenic diabetes insipidus
U_{osm} >300, <800 mOsm/kg H_2O	Partial diabetes insipidus or osmotic diuresis
U_{osm} >800 mOsm/kg H_2O	Hypertonic dehydration

Central diabetes insipidus is acquired in most cases, associated with various disorders that cause destruction of ADH-secreting neurons. When a diagnosis is not possible, despite imaging and other diagnostic tests, diabetes insipidus will be defined as idiopathic diabetes insipidus.

The most common clinical symptoms and signs are excessive thirst, polydipsia, and polyuria plus several nonspecific symptoms including weakness, lethargy, myalgias, and irritability. In infancy, congenital forms of diabetes insipidus present with fatigue and weakness often manifested by less activity or tiring with feeding, vomiting, polyuria, and sometimes fever. Diagnosis can be suspected in the ED by clinical presentation, but the diagnosis requires a prolonged test, requiring 4 to 18 hours. Urine osmolality is assessed after water deprivation; many cases require another assessment after a dose of desmopressin, the "water deprivation test." A spot check in the ED without water deprivation will typically reveal a U_{osm} of <300 mOsm/L. In central diabetes insipidus, a

TABLE 17-11 Treatment of Hypernatremia

Treatment	Indication and Comments
Isotonic (0.9%) saline	Use for correction of volumn deficits.
Etiology-specific therapy	Treat fever with antipyretics, vomiting with antiemetics, and diabetes insipidus with desmopressin (see "Diabetes Insipidus" section below).
D_5W to replace free water deficit over 2-3 days	In cases of chronic hypernatremia, it is suggested that correcting (lowering) the sodium level should occur at a rate of no more than 0.5 mEq/L/h or 10 to 12 mEq/24 h.
0.45% normal saline at 100 mL/hour	Correct volume defects first. A commonly used infusion for mild to moderate hypernatremia, but this therapy adds to total body sodium.
D_5W to replace free water deficit over 1-2 hours	Reserved only for those cases where acuity is known to be <6 h and the salt load is known to be lethal (0.75–3.0 grams/kg of body weight).
Hemodialysis	An alternative or as a suppliment to D_5W to replace free water deficit in life-threatenting acute cases of salt ingestion.

Abbreviation: D_5W = 5% dextrose in water.

TABLE 17-12 Classification of Diabetes Insipidus

Class	Acquisition	Pathophysiology
Central or neurogenic diabetes insipidus	Congenital	Structural malformations affecting the hypothalamus or pituitary
		Autosomal dominant (or rarely recessive) mutations in the gene encoding AVP-NPII precursor protein
	Acquired	Primary tumors (craniopharyngioma) or metastases
		Infection (e.g., meningitis, encephalitis)
		Histiocytosis and granulomatous diseases
		Trauma
		Surgery
		Idiopathic
Nephrogenic diabetes insipidus	Congenital	X-linked: inactivating mutations in *AVPR2* gene
		Autosomal: recessive or dominant mutations in *AQP-2* gene
	Acquired	Primary renal disease
		Obstructive uropathy
		Metabolic causes (e.g., hypokalemia, hypercalcemia)
		Sickle cell disease
		Drugs (e.g., lithium, demeclocycline)
Primary polydipsia or dipsogenic diabetes insipidus	Acquired	Psychogenic illness characterized by excessive fluid intake. Treatment is aimed at the psychiatric disease.

cerebral MRI is indicated (on a nonurgent outpatient basis) to evaluate the hypothalamic–pituitary area (**Figure 17-6**).

Central diabetes insipidus is treated with the synthetic hormone desmopressin, as a nasal spray, 10 micrograms (0.1 mL) every 12 hours, or PO, 0.05 milligrams every 12 hours, as starting doses. Therapy of nephrogenic diabetes insipidus includes a low-salt, low-protein diet, adequate hydration, and the careful use of one to three agents that act together to concentrate urine in these patients: a thiazide diuretic, the potassium-sparing diuretic amiloride, and indomethacin. Exogenous ADH, 5 to 10 micrograms subcutaneously, two to four times daily, is also used in noncongenital nephrogenic diabetes insipidus, as these patients have a partial response to ADH. Patients with significant electrolyte abnormalities should be admitted to the hospital, whereas stable patients suspected of having diabetes insipidus should be referred for testing.

POTASSIUM

PATHOPHYSIOLOGY

Potassium (K^+) is the major intracellular cation of the body: 98% of total body potassium in healthy subjects is intracellular, and 70% to 75% of total K^+ is in muscle tissues. The normal intracellular concentration averages 150 mEq/L, and the normal extracellular concentration is 3.5 to 5.0 mEq/L. The total body K^+ store is approximately 55 mEq/kg or 3500 mEq in a healthy 70-kg adult. Daily intake of K^+ ranges from 50 to 150 mEq. Foods rich in potassium include vegetables, fruits, dry fruits, nuts, and meat. Potassium is excreted predominantly by the kidneys (80% to 90%). Potassium is filtered freely through the renal glomerulus and then reabsorbed in the proximal and ascending tubules. It is secreted in the distal tubule in exchange for Na^+. In healthy individuals, the kidneys are able to excrete up to 6 mEq/kg/d. The several mechanisms of potassium handling along the nephron are the targets of diuretic therapy.

Extracellular [K^+] represents about 2% of total body K^+ and is influenced by two important variables: total body K^+ stores and distribution between the ICF and ECF spaces. Being mostly intracellular, an accurate calculation of total body K^+ is difficult, but an estimation of the K^+ deficit can be determined with the following equation: **estimated K^+ deficit in mEq/L = (expected serum [K^+] in mEq/L − measured serum [K^+] in mEq/L) × ICF** (calculated as 40% of total body weight).[1]

However, this equation is only reliable for healthy subjects, because critical patients sustain significant and rapid intracellular to extracellular shifting in response to severe injury (i.e., surgical stress, trauma, or burns), acid-base imbalance, catabolic states, increased extracellular osmolality, or insulin deficiency. So it is possible to have hyperkalemia in patients with a total body K^+ deficit (e.g., diabetic ketoacidosis) and hypokalemia with total body K^+ surplus.[2] These shifts are crucial considering the role of potassium in maintaining the resting membrane potential, as the ratio of intracellular to extracellular K^+ is the most important determinate of neuromuscular and cardiovascular excitability.[18,19]

Acid-base imbalance plays an important role in critically ill patients: there is an inverse proportionality between serum pH and [K^+], with [K^+] rising about 0.6 mEq/L for every 0.1 decrease in pH and vice versa, through an exchange between H^+ and K^+.[1,20]

Also the duration of both hypo- and hyperkalemia influences the clinical response: chronic potassium depletion or surplus allows adaptation through shifts in intra-/extracellular K^+ concentration to maintain the resting membrane potential, thus mitigating neuromuscular and cardiac electrophysiologic effects.

HYPOKALEMIA

PATHOPHYSIOLOGY

Hypokalemia is defined as a serum [K^+] of <3.5 mEq/L. The most frequent causes of hypokalemia are insufficient dietary intake (e.g., fasting, eating disorders, alcoholism), intracellular shifts (e.g., alkalosis, insulin, β_2-agonists, hypokalemic periodic paralysis), and increased losses, mainly GI (vomiting, nasogastric suction, diarrhea) or renal (diuretics,[5] hyperaldosteronism, osmotic diuresis, toxins)[21] (**Table 17-13**).

The clinical manifestations result from abnormalities in membrane polarization and affect almost every body system, but are particularly dangerous in the excitable myocardium. Hypokalemia makes the resting potential more electronegative, thus enhancing depolarization; the reduction in [K^+] conduction delays repolarization, causing prolonged QT_c, flattened T waves, and the appearance of U waves in the ECG (**Figure 17-7**).

CLINICAL FEATURES

Symptoms of hypokalemia (**Table 17-14**) usually start when serum concentrations reach 2.5 mEq/L, although they may appear sooner with rapid decreases in concentration or appear later (i.e., at even lower [K^+]) for chronic depletion.

Particular attention must be paid to cardiac arrhythmias, usually tachyarrhythmias (atrial fibrillation,[22] torsade de pointes, ventricular tachycardia, and ventricular fibrillation), that can be life threatening.

DIAGNOSIS

Diagnosis of hypokalemia is made with serum chemistry measurement; the etiology is investigated with additional testing. An ECG should be obtained from hypokalemic patients in the ED (Figure 17-7). Obtain blood gas analysis when alkalosis is suspected. If the cause of hypokalemia is not apparent from history, spot urinary electrolytes can be obtained before starting K^+ replacement (see **Table 17-15** for interpretation of urine K^+ values[1]); also U_{Na+}, U_{osm}, and P_{osm} should be measured, because a U_{Na+} value <30 mEq/L and a U_{osm} value less than P_{osm} suggest polyuria. Polyuria can increase K^+ excretion even if total body K^+ is depleted; thus U_{K+} may be misleading for diagnosis in the setting of polyuria.[2]

Another useful tool for differential diagnosis is **transtubular K^+ gradient (TTKG) = $(U_{K+} \times P_{osm})/(U_{osm} \times P_{K+})$** with normal values of 8 to 9 mEq/L. Values lower than 5 mEq/L suggest hyperaldosteronism; if paralysis is present, values lower than 3 mEq/L suggest hypokalemic periodic paralysis. A calcium/phosphate ratio >1.7 on a spot urine is 100% sensitive and 96% specific for thyrotoxic hypokalemic periodic paralysis.[23,24]

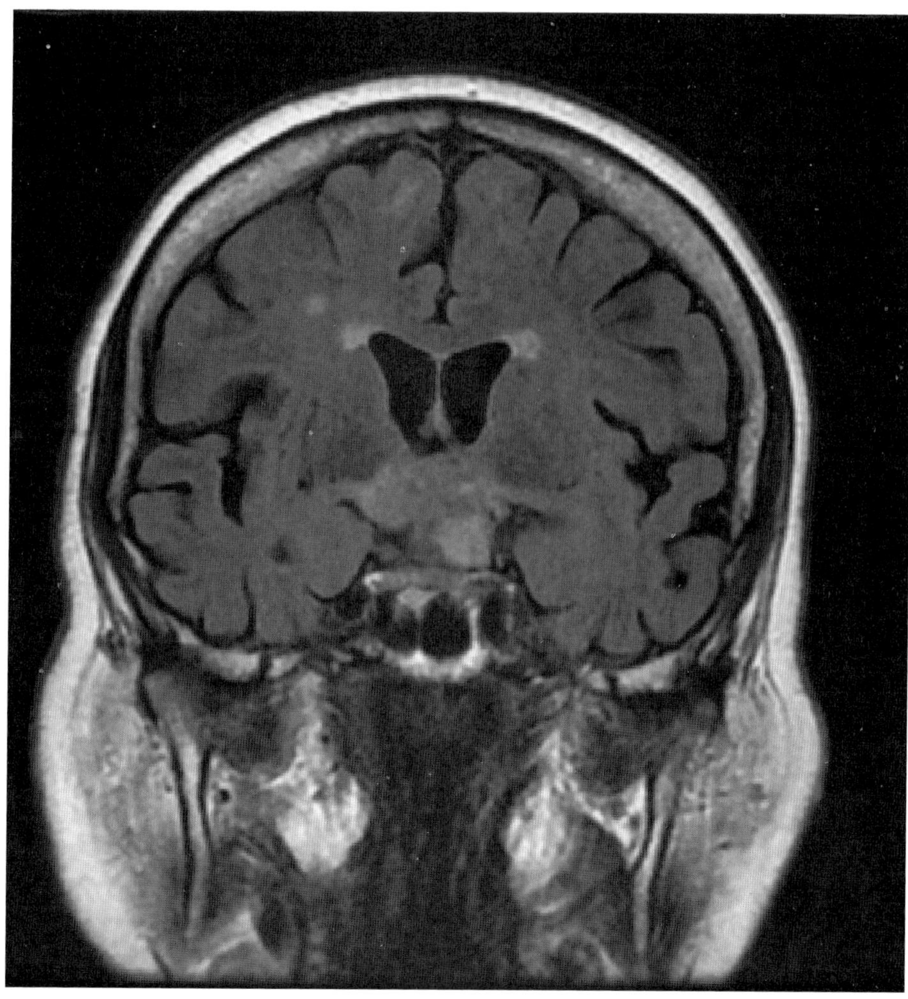

FIGURE 17-6. MRI image of a craniopharyngioma that caused diabetes insipidus in a 46-year-old patient.

TREATMENT

The treatment of hypokalemia is replacement of K^+. This should be done orally in stable patients with mild hypokalemia (>3.0 mEq/L) who are able to tolerate oral intake.[2] Foods rich in K^+ (fruits, dried fruits, vegetables) can be suggested at discharge from ED, as well as salt substitutes or K^+ supplements that should be prescribed with abundant fluids and/or food to prevent gastric irritation. Additional treatment targeted to the underlying cause should be considered. For example, it is possible to treat (and prevent) chronic hypokalemia induced by loop or thiazide diuretics by adding an adequate amount of spironolactone to the patient's chronic therapy[25]; however, the primary care physician should be aware of or guide such a change in medication. Whenever modifying diuretics or other drugs at ED discharge, recommend follow-up within 1 week for repeat assessment of renal function and [K^+]. In hypokalemia secondary to respiratory alkalosis (as caused by an acute anxiety disorder), the simple correction of the acid-base imbalance (through reassurance or anxiolytics) can correct [K^+] without administering exogenous potassium.

Intravenous replacement is indicated in patients with severe (<2.5 mEq/L) hypokalemia and in symptomatic patients with moderate (2.5 to 3 mEq/L) hypokalemia. Treat patients with cardiac arrhythmias, prolonged QT_c, or when oral replacement is not tolerated or not feasible (see **Table 17-16** for common medications known to prolong QT_c). Monitor the patient's rhythm when treating with intravenous K^+.

Monitor closely those patients who sustain rapid [K^+] changes due to their illness (e.g., postobstructive polyuria) or intravenous treatment. An example is diabetic ketoacidosis treatment, where rapid hypokalemia (including life-threatening arrhythmias) should be prevented by adequate IV K^+ administration prior to the detection of a rapid fall in serum potassium.

The following are **general principles in hypokalemia correction:**

1. Use KCl and avoid administering K^+ in glucose solutions, to reduce insulin-induced K^+ transfer into cells.
2. Potassium is irritating to the endothelium; adequate dilution is mandatory to prevent pain and phlebitis (maximum recommended [K^+] in 500 mL of a saline solution is 40 mEq, to be infused in 4 to 6 hours in a peripheral line. If a more aggressive correction is needed, an identical solution can be administered in a second peripheral line. Higher concentrations can be administered through a central line, but infusion rates should never exceed 20 mEq/h).
3. Reassessing serum [K^+] should be adjusted to infusion rate and coexisting factors (e.g., concomitant acid-base imbalance, volume depletion, cardiac arrhythmias).
4. ECG monitoring is recommended.
5. In most cases, hypokalemic patients are also hypomagnesemic. So Mg^{2+} (20 to 60 mEq/24 h) may be added to the infusion both to optimize tubular reuptake of potassium and to contrast proarrhythmic effect of hypokalemia.[1]

HYPERKALEMIA

PATHOPHYSIOLOGY

Hyperkalemia is defined as measured serum [K^+] of >5.5 mEq/L. The most common cause is factitious hyperkalemia due to release of intracellular potassium caused by hemolysis during phlebotomy. Other causes are listed in **Table 17-17**.

Clinical manifestations of hyperkalemia result from disordered membrane polarization (**Figure 17-8**). Cardiac manifestations are the most

TABLE 17-13 Causes of Hypokalemia

Transcellular shifts	Alkalosis*
	Increased plasma insulin (treatment of diabetic ketoacidosis)
	β-Adrenergic agonists
	Hypokalemic periodic paralysis (congenital)
	Thyrotoxic hypokalemic periodic paralysis
Decreased intake	Fasting
	Alcoholism (worsened by hypomagnesemia)
	Eating disorders
GI loss	Vomiting*, nasogastric suction
	Diarrhea* (including laxative, enema abuse)
	Malabsorption
	Ureterosigmoidostomy
	Enteric fistula
	Villous adenoma
Renal loss	Diuretics (carbonic anhydrase inhibitors, loop diuretics, and thiazide-like diuretics)*
	Primary hyperaldosteronism
	Secondary hyperaldosteronism
	Licorice ingestion
	Excessive use of chewing tobacco
	Renal tubular acidosis
	Postobstructive diuresis
	Osmotic diuresis
	Bartter's syndrome (mimics loop diuretic use)
	Gitelman's syndrome (mimics thiazide diuretic use)
	Apparent mineralocorticoid excess and related syndromes (Conn's, Liddle's)
	Drugs and toxins (aminoglycosides, echinocandins, carbenicillin, penicillins, amphotericin B, levodopa, lithium, thallium, cesium, barium, toluene, theophylline, chloroquine, steroids, etc.)
Sweat loss	Heavy exercise
	Heat stroke
	Fever
Other	Hypomagnesemia
	Acute leukemia and lymphomas
	IV hyperalimentation
	Recovery from megaloblastic anemia
	Hypothermia (accidental or induced)

*Frequently encountered etiologies in the ED.

serious. In hyperkalemia the resting potential of the excitable myocardium becomes less electronegative, with a consequent partial depolarization that reduces the activation of voltage-dependent sodium channels; this results in a slower and reduced amplitude of action potential. **Table 17-18** summarizes the ECG effects that may lead to arrhythmic complications, such as sinoatrial and atrioventricular blocks and atrial paralysis (Figure 17-8). Calcium administration does not affect potassium levels; rather, calcium antagonizes the effects of hyperkalemia at the level of the cell membrane, raising the threshold potential, thus restoring the membrane potential and myocyte excitability close to normal[1] (**Figure 17-9**).

CLINICAL FEATURES

Cardiac dysrhythmias, such as ventricular fibrillation, sinoatrial and atrioventricular blocks until complete heart block, and asystole, may occur. Death from hyperkalemia is usually the result of diastolic arrest or ventricular fibrillation. Other common symptoms include neuromuscular dysfunctional weakness, paresthesias, areflexia, ascending paralysis, and GI effects (nausea, vomiting, and diarrhea).[26,27]

TREATMENT

A stat ECG is essential in all hyperkalemic patients (Table 17-18); **if ECG changes are present, emergency treatment of hyperkalemia should start immediately.** In addition, if ECG changes are detected in a patient whose electrolyte levels are not yet known (e.g., a dialysis patient), hyperkalemia should be suspected and treated. A symptomatic patient with a relatively small elevation of [K^+] (5.0 to 6.0 mEq/L) requires identification and treatment of the underlying cause. A spot urine potassium may identify the diagnosis. An elevated spot urine potassium (>20 mEq/L) suggests an extrarenal cause (and will more likely be responsive to therapy). A low urine K^+ output (<10 mEq/L) suggests oliguric kidney failure or drug effect, such as angiotensin-converting enzyme inhibitors or angiotensin II receptor blockers.

Emergency treatment includes continuous ECG monitoring and immediate intervention with several therapeutic medications, which based on the action mechanism, can be divided into three modalities: membrane stabilization (crucial for cardiac tissue, must be done immediately), intracellular shift of K^+, and removal/excretion of K^+ from the body. All three modalities should be administered sequentially in rapid succession. Each mode has a different onset time and duration[28] (**Table 17-19**).

A blood gas is essential if acidosis is present; treatment should correct the underlying cause of the acid-base imbalance. If pH is normal or alkaline, the therapeutic measures that act to promote an intra- to extracellular shift of [K^+] will be less effective, and treatment should be aimed to improve renal excretion.

Until recently, sodium polystyrene sulfonate was the only oral agent that lowered potassium levels by enhancing excretion (rather than shifting potassium into cells). This agent has an unpleasant taste and may cause diarrhea. Two new oral agents currently in development, **patiromer** and **sodium zirconium cyclosilicate**, may prove useful to lower potassium levels for patients with mild hyperkalemia if confirmatory studies support the initial randomized controlled trials[29,30]; however, the onset of action for these new drugs is too slow to be of benefit in life-threatening hyperkalemia.

The following are **general principles in treatment of hyperkalemia:**

1. Immediate cessation of further K^+ administration, reduction of dietary intake, and suspension of drugs impairing K^+ renal excretion directly (angiotensin-converting enzyme inhibitors, angiotensin receptor blockers, K^+-sparing diuretics) or indirectly through worsening of renal function (e.g., nonsteroidal anti-inflammatory drugs, iodine contrast, antibiotics).
2. Fluid administration enhances K^+ renal excretion through increasing urine output.
3. If a patient is on digitalis,[31] hypercalcemia enhances the toxic cardiac effects of digitalis. However, in severe hyperkalemia secondary to digitalis intoxication with advanced intraventricular conduction impairment (wide, low-voltage QRS complexes), calcium administration must be considered, in association with antidigoxin antibodies.[1,32]
4. ECG continuous monitoring should be used to confirm the effects of therapy, thus reducing the frequency of rechecking [K^+].

MAGNESIUM

The total body content of magnesium (Mg^{2+}) is 24 grams, or 2000 mEq, 50% to 70% of which is fixed in bone and only slowly exchangeable. Most of the remaining Mg^{2+} is found in the ICF space, with a concentration of approximately 40 mEq/L. The distribution of Mg^{2+} is similar to that of K^+, with the major portion being intracellular. It is the second most abundant intracellular cation. Normal serum [Mg^{2+}] ranges between 1.5 and 2.5 mEq/L (0.7 to 1.1 mmol/L or 1.7 to 2.7 milligrams/dL). Circulating Mg^{2+} is 25% to 35% bound to proteins (mainly albumin), 10% to 15% complexed, and 50% to 60% ionized, which is the active portion. The normal dietary intake of Mg^{2+} is approximately 240 to 336 milligrams/d

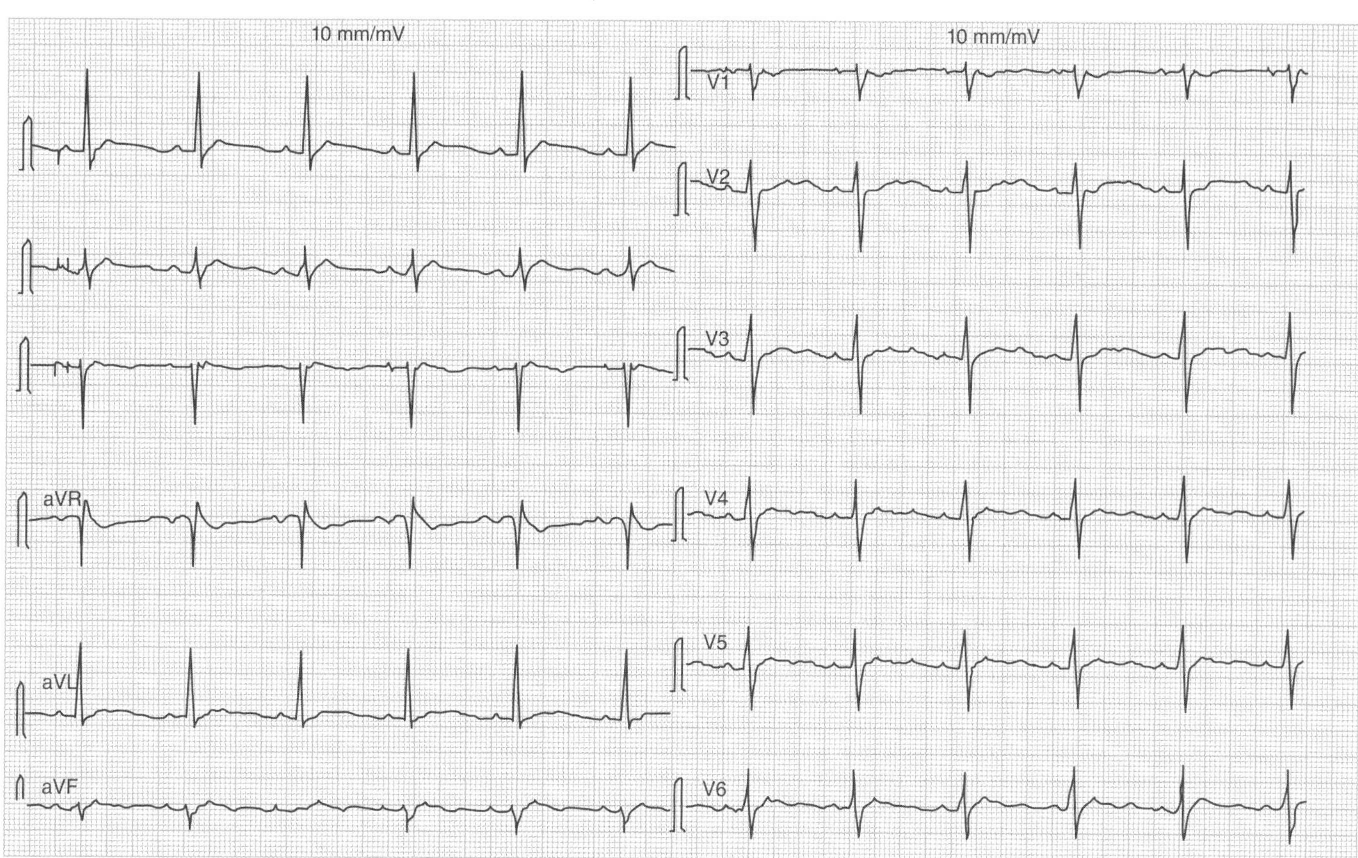

FIGURE 17-7. ECG of a patient with K^+ of 1.4 mEq/L, with leg paralysis and deep fatigue. The patient had been taking a thiazide-like diuretic for hypertension. Notice the prolonged QT_c and a flattened T wave with a U wave visible in V_2-V_5.

and is found in vegetables such as dry beans and leafy greens, meat, and cereals. Sixty percent of excreted Mg^{2+} is through stool, with the remainder via the urine. Renal reabsorption is carried out with sodium and water and is unidirectional; that means that it is impaired by volume overload, osmotic diuresis, and diuretics. About 300 enzymes have their activities regulated by Mg^{2+}; it assists the production of adenosine triphosphate, participates in nucleic acid and protein synthesis, and is involved in coagulation, platelet aggregation, and neuromuscular activity, as well as in cardiac action potential.[1,2,33]

Magnesium homeostasis is very complex and finely regulated by many factors, such as parathyroid hormone, calcitonin, ADH, glucose, insulin, glucagon, catecholamines, sodium, potassium, calcium, and phosphorus levels. Magnesium is effective therapy in severe asthma when added to standard therapy[34] (see chapter 69, "Acute Asthma").

TABLE 17-14 Symptoms and Signs of Hypokalemia

Cardiovascular	Hypertension
	Orthostatic hypotension
	Potentiation of digitalis toxicity
	Dysrhythmias (usually tachyarrhythmias)
	T-wave flattening, QT prolongation, U waves, ST depression
Neuromuscular	Malaise, weakness, fatigue
	Hyporeflexia
	Cramps
	Paresthesias
	Paralysis
	Rhabdomyolysis
GI	Nausea, vomiting
	Abdominal distension
	Ileus
Renal	Increased ammonia production
	Urinary concentrating defects
	Metabolic alkalemia, paradoxical aciduria
	Nephrogenic diabetes insipidus
Endocrine	Glucose intolerance

TABLE 17-15 Interpretation of Urinary Potassium

Spot Urinary Potassium	Mechanism
U_{K+} <10 mEq/L	*Decreased K^+ intake, nonrenal losses*
	GI losses
	Sweat losses
	Nasogastric suction ($\downarrow U_{Cl-}$)
	Transcellular shift
	Alkalosis ($\downarrow U_{Cl-}$)
	Hypomagnesemia ($\uparrow U_{Cl-}$)
	Hypokalemic periodic paralysis
	Thyrotoxic hypokalemic periodic paralysis (calculate TTKG)
U_{K+} >20 mEq/L	*Renal losses*
	If hypernatremia coexists consider:
	Hyperaldosteronism (calculate TTKG)
	Massive GI losses (secondary to metabolic alkalosis)

Abbreviation: TTKG = transtubular K^+ gradient.

TABLE 17-16 Common Medications Known to Prolong QTc

Antiarrhythmics	Amiodarone, sotalol, flecainide, quinidine, dronedarone, dofetilide
Vasopressors/inotropes	Epinephrine, norepinephrine, dopamine, dobutamine
Neuroleptics	Haloperidol, droperidol, chlorpromazine, olanzapine, quetiapine, risperidone, paliperidone, clozapine, aripiprazole
Antidepressants	Amitriptyline, nortriptyline citalopram, escitalopram, fluoxetine, paroxetine, sertraline, venlafaxine
Antibiotics	Macrolides, quinolones, metronidazole, cotrimoxazole
GI prokinetics	Domperidone, cisapride, metoclopramide
Antiemetics	Ondansetron, granisetron, dolasetron, promethazine
Antifungals	Fluconazole, itraconazole, voriconazole, ketoconazole, posaconazole
Antivirals	Foscarnet, amantadine, atazanavir, nelfinavir, rilpivirine, ritonavir, saquinavir, telaprevir
Antiparasitics	Chloroquine, mefloquine, quinine, hydroxychloroquine, pentamidine
Antihistaminics	Terfenadine, hydroxyzine, diphenhydramine
Others	Cocaine, lithium, methadone, tamoxifen, vardenafil, tacrolimus, pseudoephedrine

TABLE 17-17 Causes of Hyperkalemia

Pseudohyperkalemia	Tourniquet use
	Hemolysis (in vitro)*
	Leukocytosis
	Thrombocytosis
Intra- to extracellular potassium shift	Acidosis*
	Heavy exercise
	β-Blockade
	Insulin deficiency
	Digitalis intoxication
	Hyperkalemic periodic paralysis
Potassium load	Potassium supplements
	Potassium-rich foods
	IV potassium
	Potassium-containing drugs
	Transfusion of aged blood
	Hemolysis (in vivo)
	GI bleeding
	Cell destruction after chemotherapy
	Rhabdomyolysis/crush injury*
	Extensive tissue necrosis
Decreased potassium excretion	Renal failure*
	Drugs—potassium-sparing diuretics,* β-blockade, nonsteroidal anti-inflammatory drugs, angiotensin-converting enzyme inhibitors, angiotensin II receptor blockers, cyclosporine, tacrolimus
	Aldosterone deficiency*
	Selective defect in renal potassium excretion (pseudohypoaldosteronism, systemic lupus erythematosus, sickle cell disease, obstructive uropathy, renal transplantation, type IV renal tubular acidosis)

*Frequent or important ED diagnostic considerations.

HYPOMAGNESEMIA

PATHOPHYSIOLOGY

Table 17-20 lists the different causes of hypomagnesemia. The major causes are alcoholism, malnutrition, cirrhosis, pancreatitis, and excessive GI fluid losses.

IV hyperalimentation or treatment of diabetic ketoacidosis without adequate provision of Mg^{2+}, especially in a previously malnourished patient, can cause an abrupt fall in plasma magnesium levels. Acid-base imbalance affects the levels of ionized magnesium; a typical example is respiratory alkalosis that enhances neuromuscular activity (thus provoking tremors and cramps) by rapidly decreasing ionized [Mg^{2+}] and [Ca^{2+}] at the same time.

Among the iatrogenic causes, **proton pump inhibitors** may cause hypomagnesemia,[35,36] especially in association with **diuretic therapy**, probably through the inhibition of intestinal absorption. Concomitant hypomagnesemia and hypokalemia may coexist.

CLINICAL FEATURES

Magnesium is essential to a large number of enzymes, including membrane-bound adenosine triphosphatase. Consequently, hypomagnesemia may result in a wide variety of neuromuscular, GI, and cardiovascular effects (**Table 17-21**).

DIAGNOSIS

Hypomagnesemia is common in acute illness; it has been found in 12% of hospitalized patients and in up to 65% of medical intensive care patients.[37,38] It is likely underdiagnosed because few hospitalized patients have levels drawn.[39]

The diagnosis of hypomagnesemia in the presence of normal serum calcium levels is suggested by increased neuromuscular irritability, shown by hyperreflexia tremor, tetany, or even convulsions. Chvostek sign and Trousseau sign, findings traditionally associated with hypocalcemia, may be elicited in hypomagnesemic patients. Hypomagnesemia should be suspected in patients with alcoholism, cirrhosis, or those requiring IV fluids or hyperalimentation for prolonged periods.

The ECG changes may be similar to those caused by hypokalemia and/or hypocalcemia because they may be due to Mg^{2+} deficiency altering cardiac intracellular potassium content. As for hypokalemia, low [Mg^{2+}] levels enhance digitalis toxicity, so hypomagnesemia should be searched in ECG disturbances associated with digoxin intake, especially when both digoxin and potassium levels are normal.[40]

Low total [Mg^{2+}] can also be secondary to hypoalbuminemia; if it is not possible to measure ionized magnesium, which is unaffected by hypoalbuminemia, the following two formulas can be used to correct magnesemia for albumin level. If reference lab reports [Mg^{2+}] in mmol/L: corrected serum [Mg^{2+}] (mmol/L) = measured total [Mg^{2+}] + [0.005 × (40 − serum albumin in grams/L)]. If reference lab reports [Mg^{2+}] in milligrams/dL, use the following conversion: corrected serum [Mg^{2+}] (mEq/L) = measured total [Mg^{2+}] × 0.42 + 0.05 (4 − serum albumin in grams/dL).

TREATMENT

Hypokalemia, hypocalcemia, and hypophosphatemia are often present with severe hypomagnesemia and must be monitored carefully. Hypocalcemia does not develop until [Mg^{2+}] falls below 1.2 milligrams/dL.

The following are **general principles in treatment of hypomagnesemia:**

1. Treat or stop the cause of hypomagnesemia.
2. For asymptomatic patients (including ECG changes), magnesium supplements should be administered orally, in multiple low doses during the day, to avoid diarrhea. Magnesium lactate, chloride, gluconate, and proteinate are the formulations with minimum effect on intestinal motility.
3. For severe and symptomatic hypomagnesemia, urgent IV replacement is mandatory. The formulation most commonly used is

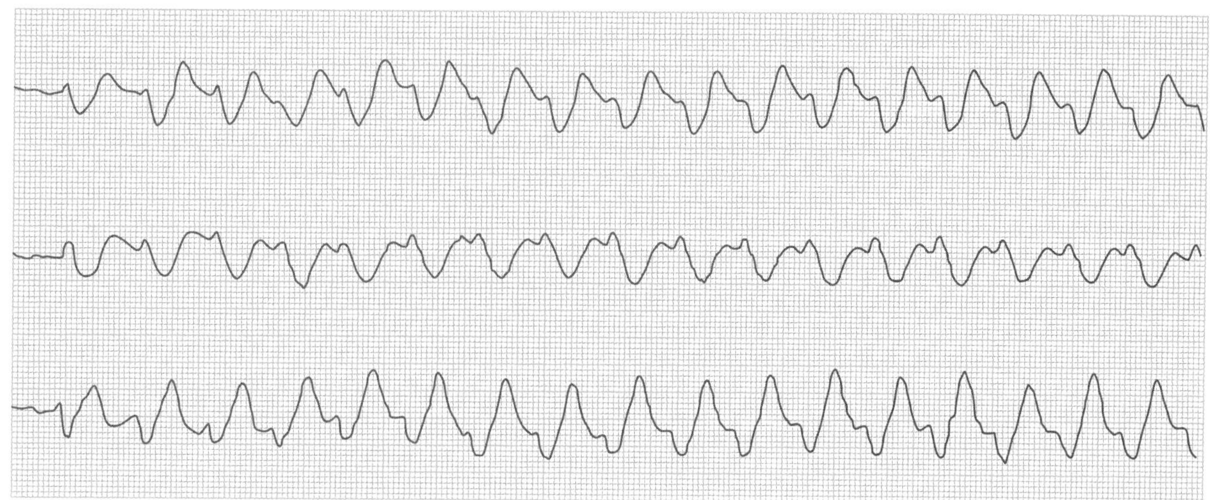

FIGURE 17-8. Monitor strip (V_1–V_3) of a 35-year-old patient in critical condition, who was hypotensive and fatigued and rapidly deteriorated into cardiac arrest. Potassium level was 9.1 mEq/L. She was on spironolactone and steroid therapy.

TABLE 17-18 ECG Changes Associated with Hyperkalemia

$[K^+]$ (mEq/L)	ECG Changes*
6.5–7.5	Prolonged PR interval, tall peaked T waves, short QT interval
7.5–8.0	Flattening of the P wave, QRS widening
10–12	QRS complex degradation into a sinusoidal pattern

*In chronic or slowly developing hyperkalemia, ECG changes may not occur until higher $[K^+]$ levels are reached.

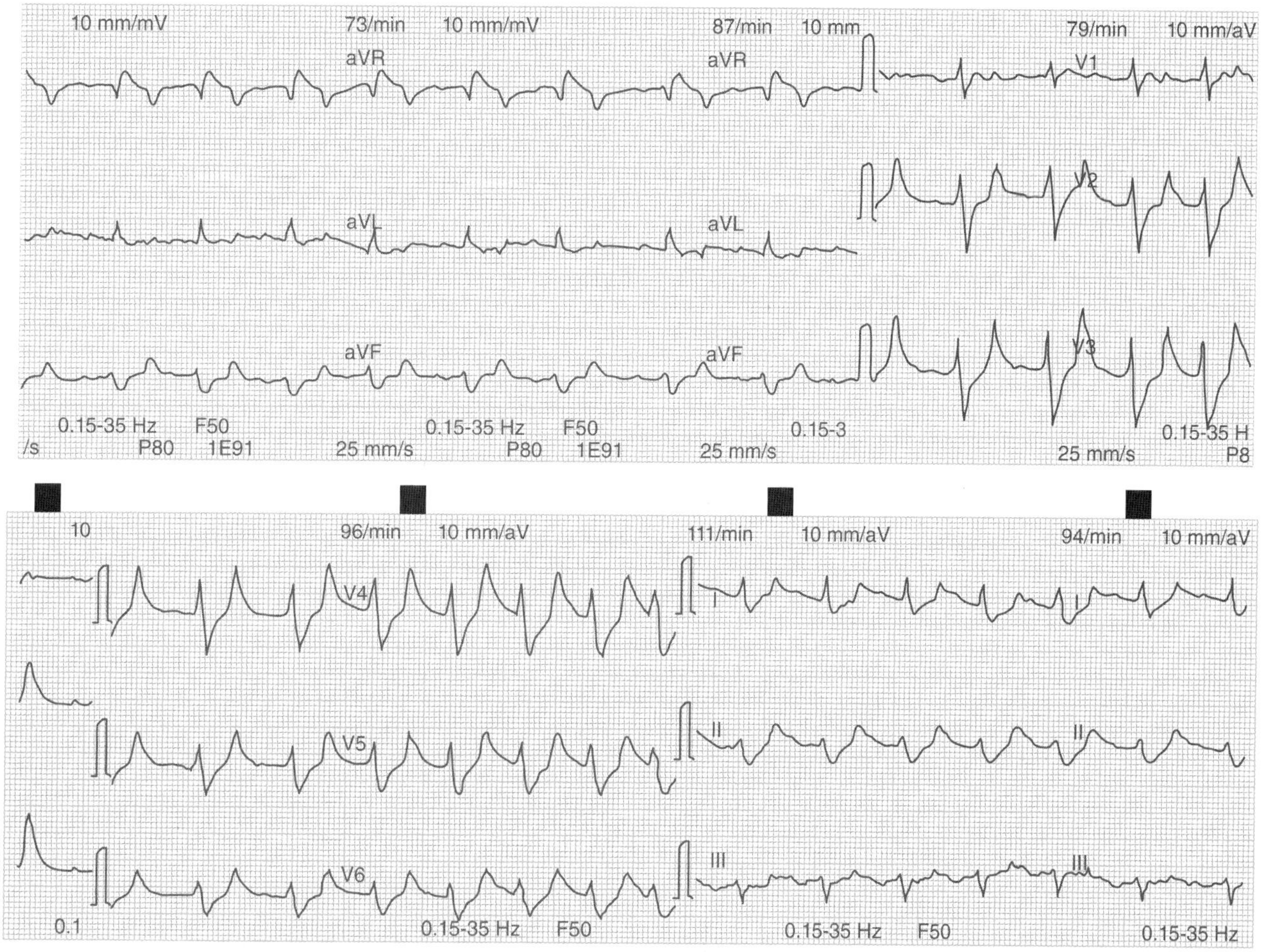

FIGURE 17-9. The same patient as in Figure 17-8 during calcium chloride infusion. She regained a pulse and became conscious. The QRS and T wave narrowed, as compared with Figure 17-8.

TABLE 17-19 Emergency Therapy of Hyperkalemia

Therapy	Dose and Route	Onset of Action	Duration of Effect	Mechanism
Calcium chloride (10%)*	5–10 mL IV	1–3 min	30–50 min	Membrane stabilization
Calcium gluconate (10%)*	10–20 mL IV	1–3 min	30–50 min	Membrane stabilization
$NaHCO_3$	50–150 mEq IV	5–10 min	1–2 h	Shifts $[K^+]$ into cell
Albuterol (nebulized)	10–20 milligrams in 4 mL of normal saline, nebulized over 10 min	15–30 min	2–4 h	Upregulates cyclic adenosine monophosphate, shifts $[K^+]$ into cell
Insulin† and glucose‡	5–10 units regular insulin IV Glucose 25 grams (50% solution) IV	30 min	4–6 h	Shifts $[K^+]$ into cell
Furosemide	40–80 milligrams IV	Varies	Varies	Renal $[K^+]$ excretion
Sodium polystyrene sulfonate	25–50 grams PO or PR	1–2 h	4–6 h	GI $[K^+]$ excretion
Hemodialysis	—	Minutes	Varies	Removes $[K^+]$

*Calcium chloride has three times the elemental calcium when compared to calcium gluconate. 10% calcium chloride = 27.2 milligrams $[Ca^{2+}]$/mL; 10% calcium gluconate = 9 milligrams $[Ca^{2+}]$/mL. Due to its short duration, calcium administration (both chloride and gluconate) can be repeated up to four times per hour.
†Reduce dose of insulin in patients with renal failure.
‡Glucose infusion should be administered after initial bolus to prevent hypoglycemia. Glucose should not be administered in hyperglycemic patients.

TABLE 17-20 Causes of Hypomagnesemia

Redistribution	IV glucose
	Correction of diabetic ketoacidosis
	IV hyperalimentation
	Refeeding after starvation
	Acute pancreatitis
	Postparathyroidectomy (hungry bone syndrome)
	Osteoblastic metastasis (hungry bone syndrome)
Extrarenal loss	Nasogastric suction (infrequent)
	Lactation
	Profuse sweating, burns, sepsis
	Intestinal or biliary fistula
	Diarrhea
Decreased intake	Alcoholism (cirrhosis)
	Malnutrition, poor intake
	Small bowel resection
	Malabsorption (steatorrhea)
Renal loss	Ketoacidosis
	Saline or osmotic diuresis
	Potassium depletion
	Phosphorus depletion
	Familial hypophosphatemia
	Tubulointerstitial renal disease
Drugs	Loop diuretics
	Aminoglycosides
	Amphotericin B
	Vitamin D intoxication
	Alcohol
	Cisplatin
	Theophylline
	Proton pump inhibitors
	Calcineurin inhibitors (cyclosporine, tacrolimus)
Endocrine disorders	Syndrome of inappropriate antidiuretic hormone secretion
	Hyperthyroidism
	Hyperparathyroidism
	Hypercalcemic states
	Primary or secondary aldosteronism

magnesium sulfate ($MgSO_4$). In life-threatening conditions (torsade de pointes, eclampsia), 1 to 4 grams or 8 to 32 mEq diluted in at least 100 mL of 5% dextrose or normal saline (0.9%) solution can be administered in 10 to 60 minutes under continuous monitoring: ECG (risk of hypokinetic arrhythmias), noninvasive blood pressure (risk of hypotension), and ventilatory pattern (risk of respiratory depression, usually preceded by areflexia, that can be monitored as an alarm sign). As a minor side effect, flushing due to vasodilatation is common.

4. Patients with chronic Mg^{2+} deficiency may require >50 mEq of oral Mg^{2+} (6 grams of $[MgSO_4]$ per day). In chronic alcoholics with delirium tremens and in patients with severe hypomagnesemia, up to 8 to 12 grams of $MgSO_4$ may be given IM (possible, but very painful) or IV the first day. The first 10 to 15 mEq (1.5 to 2.0 grams) of IV $MgSO_4$ can be given over 1 to 2 hours. This may be followed by up to 4 to 6 grams/d. Approximately half of the administered Mg^{2+} will be lost in the urine.
5. Spironolactone is effective in maintaining $[Mg^{2+}]$ homeostasis as well as in reducing the incidence of arrhythmias in congestive heart failure patients.[41]

TABLE 17-21 Symptoms and Signs of Hypomagnesemia

Neuromuscular	Tetany
	Muscle weakness
	Chvostek and Trousseau signs
	Cerebellar (ataxia, nystagmus, vertigo)
	Confusion, obtundation, coma
	Seizures
	Apathy, depression
	Irritability
	Paresthesias
GI	Dysphagia
	Anorexia, nausea
Cardiovascular	Heart failure
	Dysrhythmias
	Hypotension
Miscellaneous	Hypokalemia
	Hypocalcemia
	Anemia

TABLE 17-22 Causes of Hypermagnesemia

Renal Failure	Acute or Chronic
Increased magnesium load	Magnesium-containing laxatives, antacids, or enemas*
	Treatment of pre-eclampsia/eclampsia (mothers and neonates)
	Diabetic ketoacidosis (untreated)*
	Tumor lysis
	Rhabdomyolysis*
Increased renal magnesium absorption	Hyperparathyroidism
	Familial hypocalciuric hypercalcemia
	Hypothyroidism
	Mineralocorticoid deficiency, adrenal insufficiency (Addison's disease)

*Most likely presentation relevant to the ED.

HYPERMAGNESEMIA

PATHOPHYSIOLOGY

Hypermagnesemia is rarely encountered in emergency medicine practice, because the kidney can increase the fractional excretion of magnesium up to nearly 100%. A small elevation in serum concentration has little clinical significance. The most common cause for hypermagnesemia can be found in patients with renal insufficiency or renal failure who ingest Mg^{2+}-containing drugs.[42] Hypermagnesemia is more commonly seen in the perinatal setting secondary to the treatment of pre-eclampsia or eclampsia. It has been described as a serious, life-threatening consequence of magnesium-containing laxative abuse in patients with normal renal function.[43,44] Other causes of hypermagnesemia include lithium ingestion, volume depletion, or familial hypocalciuric hypercalcemia (**Table 17-22**).

CLINICAL FEATURES

Hypermagnesemia rarely produces symptoms. Magnesium decreases the transmission of neuromuscular messages and thus acts as a CNS depressant and decreases neuromuscular activity. Signs and symptoms related to [Mg^{2+}] can be found in **Table 17-23**.

DIAGNOSIS

Serum [Mg^{2+}] is usually diagnostic. **The possibility of hypermagnesemia should be considered in patients with hyperkalemia or hypercalcemia.** Hypermagnesemia also should be suspected in patients with renal failure, particularly in those who are taking magnesium-containing antacids or laxatives.

TREATMENT

Immediate cessation of Mg^{2+} administration is required. If renal failure is not evident, dilution by IV fluids followed by furosemide (40 to 80 milligrams IV) may be indicated. Calcium directly antagonizes the cardiac effects of magnesium because it reverts the calcium channel blockade provoked by elevated [Mg^{2+}]. Severe symptomatic hypermagnesemia can be treated with 10 mL of 10% $CaCl_2$ IV over 2 to 3 minutes. Further infusion of 40 to 60 mL during the next 24 hours can be administered. Patients with renal failure may benefit from dialysis using a decreased [Mg^{2+}] bath that lowers serum [Mg^{2+}].

TABLE 17-23 Symptoms and Signs of Hypermagnesemia

Level (mEq/L)	Clinical Manifestations
2.0–3.0	Nausea
3.0–4.0	Somnolence
4.0–8.0	Loss of deep tendon reflexes
8.0–12.0	Respiratory depression
12.0–15.0	Hypotension, heart block, cardiac arrest

CALCIUM

PATHOPHYSIOLOGY

Calcium is the most abundant mineral in the body. The total body [Ca^{2+}] is 15 grams/kg of body weight, or about 1 kg in an average-sized adult. Calcium is 99% bound in bone as phosphate and carbonate (mineral apatite), with the remainder in the teeth, soft tissues, plasma, and cells. The normal daily intake of Ca^{2+} is 800 to 3000 milligrams, one third of which is absorbed primarily in the small bowel by active (vitamin D–dependent) and passive (concentration-dependent) absorption. Excretion of Ca^{2+} is primarily via the stool.

The cell content of Ca^{2+} is 10,000 times lower than the plasma content, and this gradient is maintained by Ca-ATPase, Ca^{2+}-specific channels and by Na/Ca exchangers.

Plasma [Ca^{2+}] is between 8.5 and 10.5 milligrams/dL (4.3 to 5.3 mEq/L or 2.2 to 2.7 mmol/L) and is present in three different forms: ionized calcium, 50% of total (4.5 to 5.6 milligrams/dL; 1.1 to 1.4 mmol/L), which is the only active fraction; protein bound calcium, 40% of total, which is inactive and not filtered by glomerulus; and complexed calcium, 10% of total, which is bound to anions like phosphate, carbonate, and citrate.

It is necessary to be aware of **standard units** used by different laboratories to express calcium value: **1 mEq/L = 2 milligrams/dL = 0.5 mmol/L.** The ionized fraction is the only biologically active fraction; a decrease in albumin decreases the total [Ca^{2+}] but does not change the ionized fraction. On average, 0.8 milligram of Ca^{2+} binds to 1 gram of protein. Therefore, total serum [Ca^{2+}] is equal to ionized [Ca^{2+}] plus the product of 0.8 and total protein. Alkalosis produces a decrease in ionized fraction with no change in the total serum [Ca^{2+}]. Each 0.1 rise in pH lowers ionized [Ca^{2+}] by about 3% to 8%. The opposite effect is produced by acidosis.

The role of Ca^{2+} is crucial for muscle and cardiac contraction, nerve conduction, cell growth, enzyme activation, and coagulation, and consequently, any hypo- or hypercalcemia leads to severe dysfunctions.

HOMEOSTASIS OF CALCIUM

The organs involved in the homeostasis of calcium are bones, kidneys, and the intestines, whereas the major determinates are three hormones and one receptor.[1,2,44,45]

1. **1,25-Dihydroxycholecalciferol (active vitamin D_3)**[45] is formed in the distal tubule. It promotes Ca^{2+} absorption from intestine, but this activity is modulated by physiologic conditions that may enhance it (pregnancy and growth) or reduce it (oxalates and phytates in food and aging).
2. **Parathyroid hormone (PTH)** is secreted by parathyroid glands when [Ca^{2+}] is low and is regulated by Ca^{2+}-sensing receptor, vitamin D_3, and Mg^{2+} (hypomagnesemia inhibits PTH secretion). PTH stimulates bone demineralization by activating osteoclasts and by increasing the synthesis of vitamin D_3 and increasing Ca^{2+} reabsorption from kidney.
3. **Calcitonin** is a peptide secreted by C-cells of the thyroid gland when [Ca^{2+}] is high. It inhibits the activity of osteoclasts and thus bone resorption.
4. **Ca^{2+}-sensing receptor**[46,47] is mainly present on plasma membranes of parathyroids, kidney, bones, and thyroid. It becomes active in case of hypercalcemia and inhibits the production of PTH. In the kidney, activated Ca^{2+}-sensing receptor provokes hypercalciuria and polyuria preventing nephrocalcinosis. The activation of the receptor also stimulates the secretion of calcitonin and inhibits osteoclast formation.

Urinary secretion of calcium is variable and influenced by many different factors. Hypercalcemia, metabolic acidosis, hypervolemia, and loop diuretics increase urinary secretion of [Ca^{2+}]. PTH, vitamin D_3,

TABLE 17-24 Some Causes of Hypocalcemia

Cause	Mechanism
Decreased calcium absorption	
Vitamin D deficiency	
Decreased oral intake	Malnutrition
Decreased intestinal absorption	Intestinal bypass, gastrectomy
Decreased production of $25(OH)D_3$	Liver failure
Decreased synthesis of $1,25(OH2)D_3$	Renal failure, hyperphosphatemia
Malabsorption syndromes	
Increased calcium excretion/reduced bone resorption	
Alcoholism	Hypomagnesemia causing inhibition of PTH secretion, PTH resistance to bone resorption
Hypoparathyroidism	Genetic, autoimmune, surgical, tumoral
Pseudohypoparathyroidism	Resistance to PTH action
Hypomagnesemia	Inhibition of PTH secretion, PTH resistance to bone resorption
Drugs (Table 17-25)	
Miscellaneous	
Sepsis	
Acute pancreatitis	Fatty acids combine with [Ca^{2+}] to form insoluble Ca^{2+} soaps and lead to a reduction of serum [Ca^{2+}]
Massive transfusions	
Rhabdomyolysis	

Abbreviations: $25(OH)D_3$ = 25-hydroxyvitamin D_3; $1,25(OH2)D_3$ = 1,25-dihydroxyvitamin D3; PTH = parathyroid hormone.

TABLE 17-25 Drugs That Can Cause Hypocalcemia

Phosphates (e.g., enemas, laxatives)
Phenytoin, phenobarbital
Gentamicin, tobramycin, dactinomycin, foscarnet
Cisplatin
Citrate
Loop diuretics
Glucocorticoids
Magnesium sulfate
Bisphosphonates, calcitonin, denosumab
Cinacalcet

metabolic alkalosis, hypovolemia, and the chronic use of thiazides reduce secretion.

HYPOCALCEMIA

PATHOPHYSIOLOGY

Hypocalcemia is defined by an ionized [Ca^{2+}] level <2.0 mEq/L (<4 milligrams/dL; or <1.1 mmol/L). Homeostasis is regulated by the maintenance of the gradient between cells and ECF, is controlled by the above described mechanism, and is mediated intracellularly by phosphates, cyclic adenosine monophosphate, and ion pumps.[44] Any process that interferes with cell metabolism, such as shock or sepsis, will tend to reduce ionized [Ca^{2+}] by allowing increased net movement of Ca^{2+} across the cell membrane into the cytoplasm of the poorly functioning cells. As an example, serum [Ca^{2+}] may be low after trauma, especially with the fat embolism syndrome, not only due to cell dysfunction and binding of calcium to free fatty acids but also because of fatty inhibition of cell membrane calcium pumps.

ETIOLOGY

Table 17-24[1,2,47,48] lists the most common causes of hypocalcemia and the primary mechanism of each. **Table 17-25** lists the principal drugs that cause hypocalcemia.[2]

CLINICAL FEATURES

The severity of signs and symptoms depends greatly on the rapidity of the decrease in [Ca^{2+}]. **Table 17-26** lists the different signs and symptoms that can be seen in the course of hypocalcemia.[1,2]

Neuromuscular and cardiovascular signs and symptoms predominate. As serum [Ca^{2+}] falls, neuronal membranes become increasingly more permeable to sodium, thereby enhancing excitation, causing smooth and skeletal muscle contractions. Irritability, confusion, dementia, extrapyramidal symptoms, seizures, and hallucination may occur.

Decreased ionized [Ca^{2+}] reduces the strength of myocardial contraction primarily by inhibiting relaxation. The most characteristic ECG finding in hypocalcemia is a prolonged QT_c interval.[18,19] The T wave may be of normal width, and it is the ST segment that is actually prolonged. In very severe hypocalcemia, T waves may present abnormalities that may mimic ischemia (**Figure 17-10**). This finding is usually seen with total serum calcium levels <6.0 milligrams/dL.

A positive Chvostek sign (twitch at the corner of the mouth when the examiner taps over the facial nerve just in front of the ear) and Trousseau sign (carpal spasm produced when the examiner applies a blood pressure cuff to the upper arm and maintains a pressure above systolic for 2 to 3 minutes; the fingers are spastically extended at the interphalangeal joints and flexed at the metacarpophalangeal joints with wrist flexion and forearm pronation) are classically associated with hypocalcemia (but also may occur in respiratory alkalosis, which shifts ionized calcium to the protein-bound form). These diagnostic signs have not been subjected to rigorous assessment, and there is no agreement on sensitivity or specificity.[49,50]

DIAGNOSIS

In addition to total serum [Ca^{2+}], a full electrolyte panel, renal function tests, ionized [Ca^{2+}], and magnesium levels aid in the diagnosis. An albumin level should be obtained because hypoalbuminemia may falsify the diagnosis.

In cases where acid-base abnormalities are suspected, a blood gas analysis to evaluate pH should be obtained. Also consider a phosphate

TABLE 17-26 Symptoms and Signs of Hypocalcemia

Muscular	Weakness, fatigue Spasms, cramps
Neurologic	Tetany Chvostek sign, Trousseau sign Circumoral and digital paresthesias Impaired memory, confusion Hallucinations, dementia, seizures Extrapyramidal disorders
Dermatologic	Hyperpigmentation Coarse, brittle hair Dry, scaly skin
Cardiovascular	Heart failure Ventricular arrhythmias, torsade de pointes Vasoconstriction
Skeletal	Osteodystrophy Rickets Osteomalacia
Miscellaneous	Dental hypoplasia Cataracts Decreased insulin secretion

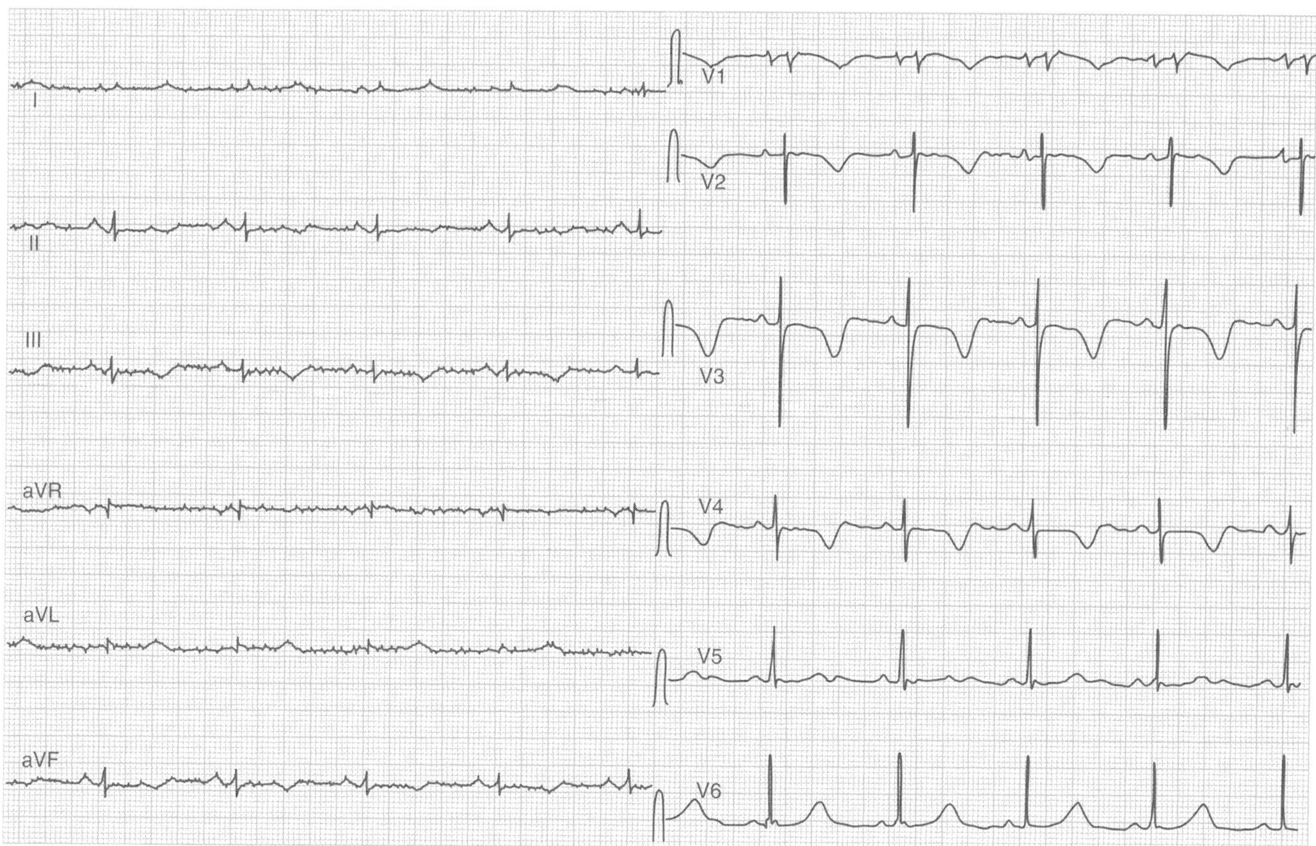

FIGURE 17-10. ECG of a patient with severe hypocalcemia (Ca^{2+} 4.5 milligrams/dL) who was complaining of chest and abdominal pain, pain in the legs, and Trousseau sign. A very long QT_c and T wave abnormalities mimicking ischemia are evident.

level. Blood samples for PTH and vitamin D_3 levels should be drawn (but results are not required) before starting therapy.

TREATMENT

Treatment of hypocalcemia is tailored to the individual patient and directed toward the underlying cause. If a patient is asymptomatic or if the hypocalcemia is not severe or prolonged for >10 to 14 days, oral Ca^{2+} therapy with or without vitamin D may be sufficient. Ca^{2+} lactate, ascorbate, carbonate, and gluconate are available in oral preparations and contain variable percentages of elemental calcium; 1 mEq of elemental calcium is equal to 20 milligrams of elemental calcium. **Regimens can be 500 to 3000 milligrams of elemental calcium by mouth daily, in one dose or up to three divided doses. The dose must be individualized for each patient, according to the cause and severity of hypocalcemia.**

IV calcium is recommended only in cases of symptomatic or severe hypocalcemia[2] (ionized [Ca^{2+}] <1.9 mEq/L or <0.95 mmol/L), because IV Ca^{2+} administration causes vasoconstriction and possible ischemia, especially in patients with low cardiac output who already have significant peripheral vasoconstriction. **IV calcium gluconate is preferred over IV calcium chloride** in nonemergency settings due to the dangers of extravasation with calcium chloride (calcinosis cutis). **With severe acute hypocalcemia, 10 mL of 10% $CaCl_2$ (or 10 to 30 mL of 10% Ca^{2+} gluconate) may be given IV over 10 to 20 minutes and repeated every 60 minutes until symptoms resolve or followed by a continuous IV infusion of 10% $CaCl_2$ at 0.02 to 0.08 mL/kg/h (1.4 to 5.6 mL/h in a 70-kg patient).**[51] The serum [Ca^{2+}] should then be rechecked before continuing parenteral Ca^{2+}. **IV Ca^{2+} should be used with caution in patients taking digitalis, because hypercalcemia can potentiate digitalis toxicity.**[52] Symptomatic patients after thyroid or parathyroid surgery are often treated with parenteral Ca^{2+}.

During massive transfusions, if the blood is being given faster than 1 unit every 5 minutes, 10 mL of 10% $CaCl_2$ can be given after every 4 to 6 units of blood if a patient is in shock or has heart failure despite adequate volume replacement therapy.

Hypocalcemia is difficult to correct if hypomagnesemia is also present because of reduction of PTH and Ca^{2+} releases from bone. Therefore, magnesium should be replaced before, or in conjunction with, Ca^{2+} replacement.[44,45]

HYPERCALCEMIA

Hypercalcemia is relatively common. It is defined as a total [Ca^{2+}] >10.5 milligrams/dL or an ionized [Ca^{2+}] level >2.7 mEq/L.

PATHOPHYSIOLOGY

Because calcium is necessary for cellular functions, every organ and system is affected by hypercalcemia, and clinical manifestations are dependent on the level of [Ca2+]: mild hypercalcemia, 10.5 to 11.9 milligrams/dL; moderate, 12 to 13.9 milligrams/dL; severe, >14 milligrams/dL.[2,4,53]

Neuromuscular changes include decreased sensitivity, responsiveness, and strength of muscular contraction and nerve conduction. The conduction of the heart is slowed and automaticity is decreased with a shortening of the refractory period. Increased sensitivity to cardiac glycosides may be seen.

Loss of concentrating ability is the most frequent renal effect of hypercalcemia. This is a reversible tubular defect, which results in polyuria and volume depletion even in the presence of thirst. Potassium wasting resulting in hypokalemia may occur in up to one third of patients. Nephrocalcinosis and nephrolithiasis may result from hypercalcemia and can be exacerbated by volume depletion. As the hypercalcemia persists, increasing microscopic Ca^{2+} deposits in the kidney can lead to progressive renal insufficiency.

TABLE 17-27 Causes of Hypercalcemia

Cause	Mechanism
Hypercalcemia due to increased bone Ca^{2+} resorption	
Primary hyperparathyroidism	↑ PTH
Malignancy	Osteolysis, PTH-related protein (PTHrP) production
Pseudohyperparathyroidism	PTH
Renal failure	Secondary and tertiary hyper-PTH due to chronic hypocalcemia
Addison's disease	↑ Albumin, bone reabsorption
Hyperthyroidism	Osteoclast activation
Immobilization	
Hypercalcemia due to decreased urinary Ca^{2+} excretion	
Familial hypercalcemic hypocalciuria	Mutation of CaSR
Thiazides	Increased kidney Ca^{2+} reabsorption in proximal tubule
Hypercalcemia due to increased GI Ca^{2+} absorption	
Granulomatous diseases (sarcoidosis, tuberculosis, coccidioidomycosis, histoplasmosis)	1α-Hydroxylase activity
Milk (calcium)-alkali syndrome	Vitamin D_3
Vitamin D intoxication	↑Ca^{2+} intake and absorption, ↑renal reabsorption due to nephrogenic diabetes insipidus

Abbreviations: CaSR = Ca^{2+}-sensing receptor; PTH = parathyroid hormone.

TABLE 17-28 Signs and Symptoms of Hypercalcemia

General	*Cardiovascular*
Malaise, weakness	Hypertension
Polydipsia, dehydration	Dysrhythmias
Neurologic	Vascular calcifications
Confusion	ECG abnormalities
Apathy, depression, stupor	QT shortening
Decreased memory	Coving of ST-T wave
Irritability	Widening of T wave
Hallucinations	Digitalis sensitivity
Headache	*Gastrointestinal*
Ataxia	Anorexia, weight loss
Hyporeflexia, hypotonia	Nausea, vomiting
Mental retardation (infants)	Constipation
Metastatic calcification	Abdominal pain
Band keratopathy	Peptic ulcer disease
Conjunctivitis	Pancreatitis
Pruritus	*Urologic*
Skeletal	Polyuria, nocturia
Fractures	Renal insufficiency
Bone pain	Nephrolithiasis
Deformities	

ETIOLOGY

More than 90% of occurrences are associated with hyperparathyroidism[2,54] or malignancy, the latter being the most likely presentation in the ED. A list of potential causes of hypercalcemia and the relative mechanism of onset is provided in **Table 17-27**.[2]

CLINICAL FEATURES

Hypercalcemic patients with plasma total [Ca^{2+}] below 12.0 milligrams/dL are usually asymptomatic, but higher levels can cause a wide variety of symptoms (**Table 17-28**).

Patients with total [Ca^{2+}] >14 to 16 milligrams/dL are usually very weak, lethargic, and confused. Polyuria and polydipsia are due to impaired renal tubular reabsorption of water and result in volume depletion. Total [Ca^{2+}] >15.0 milligrams/dL may cause somnolence, stupor, and even coma. A mnemonic sometimes used for the signs and symptoms of hypercalcemia is *stones* (renal calculi), *bones* (osteolysis), *moans* (psychiatric disorders), and *groans* (peptic ulcer disease, pancreatitis, and constipation).

Hypercalcemia should be investigated in patients with extensive metastatic bone disease, particularly if the primary site involves the breast, lungs, or kidneys, and in individuals with combinations of clinical problems, such as renal calculi, pancreatitis, or ulcer disease.

On ECG, hypercalcemia may be associated with depressed ST segments, widened T waves, and shortened ST segments and QT intervals. Bradyarrhythmias may occur, with bundle-branch patterns that may progress to second-degree block or complete heart block. Levels of [Ca^{2+}] above 20 milligrams/dL may cause cardiac arrest.

DIAGNOSIS

True hypercalcemia must be confirmed by measuring ionized [Ca^{2+}][55]; then electrolytes, CBC, phosphate, magnesium, BUN, creatinine, and alkaline phosphatase will help determine the cause. The acuity of hypercalcemia can be determined or suggested using the medical history together with an ECG, chest x-ray, and laboratory investigation. The need for other studies such as serum or urine protein electrophoresis, PTH and vitamin D levels, thyroid tests, or bone scans should be individualized and will not determine what is done in the ED. Normally, acute, severe hypercalcemia is not caused by hyperparathyroidism. Malignancies, in particular lymphoma, leukemia, and metastatic bone cancer, are common causes of severe, acute hypercalcemia. A corrected calcium level should be calculated if albumin is not in the normal range: Corrected Ca^{2+} (milligrams/dL) = measured total Ca^{2+} (milligrams/dL) + 0.8 (4.0 − serum albumin [grams/dL]), where 4.0 represents the average albumin level in grams/dL. If the reference lab reports values in mmol/L, use the following formula: Corrected Ca^{2+} (mmol/L) = measured total Ca^{2+} (mmol/L) + 0.02 (40 − serum albumin [grams/L]), where 40 represents the average albumin level in grams/L. If the values listed in the corrected calcium formulas for normal albumin do not match your institution's lab, adjust this value accordingly.

TREATMENT

Symptomatic patients or asymptomatic patients with [Ca^{2+}] levels above 14 milligrams/dL should receive treatment starting with volume repletion. Administer **0.9% normal saline at 500 to 1000 mL/h for 2 to 4 hours** as tolerated by the patient. In general, 3 to 4 L should be given over the first 24 hours, then 2 to 3 L per 24 hours until a urine output of 2 L/d is achieved.[56] Furosemide is recommended to promote a diuresis of 150 to 200 mL/h, which increases the calciuric effect,[1,56] with an initial dose of 20 to 40 milligrams. Larger doses may be required. Hypokalemia and/or hypomagnesemia should be assessed and treated, especially if furosemide is being used.

Decreased mobilization of [Ca^{2+}] from bone through reduction of osteoclastic activity can be obtained with **corticosteroids,** such as prednisone, 1 to 2 milligrams/kg PO, or hydrocortisone, 200 to 300 milligrams IV initial dose, in Addison's disease or in steroid-responsive malignancies.

In very severe cases, it will be necessary to receive **hemodialysis** to quickly remove calcium from blood.[53] In the ED, initiating bisphosphonates or calcitonin is not mandatory. However, for hypercalcemia associated with malignancy, intravenous bisphosphonates are now considered first-line therapy;[56] examples are pamidronate or zoledronate (zoledronic acid). Zoledronic acid is recommended;[56] for a corrected [Ca^{2+}] level of 12 milligrams/dL or higher, 4 milligrams as a single dose can be given IV over 15 minutes. Calcitonin works more rapidly than bisphosphonates and can be given at a dose of 4 units/kg SC or IM.

PHOSPHORUS

Phosphorus (PO_4^{3-}) is an essential mineral that exists mainly as hydroxyapatite (85%) or as an intracellular constituent (10% to 15%). Only about 1% is in the ECF, so serum measurements may not accurately reflect total body stores. It is involved in oxidative phosphorylation and mitochondrial respiration, and it is the essential component of adenosine triphosphate, a requirement for cellular energy metabolism.[2,57] Serum [PO_4^{3-}] decreases with age from a range of 4.0 to 7.0 milligrams/dL in newborns to 2.5 to 5.0 milligrams/dL in adults. The total body phosphorus store in a normal man is approximately 700 grams (10 to 15 grams/kg). Metabolism of phosphorus is strictly linked to that of calcium. The only active status of PO_4^{3-} is in biological fluids. Homeostasis of PO_4^{3-} is mainly regulated by gut absorption and urine excretion. Gut absorption is localized in two different sites. The first is the duodenum, which is inhibited by calcitonin and is stimulated by a vitamin D_3 and low phosphate intake. The second is the jejunum and ileum, where absorption is passive and dependent on PO_4^{3-} concentration in the gut.

Excretion is predominantly in the urine by the glomerulus, with the majority reabsorbed in the proximal tubules. Excretion is regulated by PTH, which lowers serum phosphate by increasing renal excretion, and by a hormone secreted by osteoclasts and osteoblasts, the fibroblast growth factor-23, that increases PO_4^{3-} excretion and inhibits intestinal absorption. Proximal tubule absorption increases when serum [PO_4^{3-}] levels drop and with hypoparathyroidism, volume depletion, hypocalcemia, or the presence of growth hormone. Excretion increases in the presence of volume expansion, hypercalcemia, acidosis, hypomagnesemia, hypokalemia, glucocorticoids, diuretics, calcitonin, or PTH.[57]

TABLE 17-29 Causes of Hypophosphatemia

Shift from ECF to ICF without depletion of PO_4^{3-}	Glucose Insulin Catecholamines Respiratory alkalosis
Shift from ECF to ICF with depletion of PO_4^{3-}	Hyperalimentation Refeeding syndrome
Decreased intestinal absorption	Low intake Malabsorption Chronic use of calcium acetate or bicarbonate, aluminum hydroxide Vitamin D deficiency
Increased renal loss	Hyperparathyroidism Increased fibroblast growth factor (FGF-23) Genetic hypophosphatemia mutations Tubular acidosis Fanconi's syndrome Hypokalemia Hypomagnesemia Polyuria Acidosis
Miscellaneous causes	Alcoholism (poor intake, vitamin D deficiency) Diabetic ketoacidosis (osmotic diuresis) Toxic shock syndrome
Drugs	See **Table 17-30**

HYPOPHOSPHATEMIA

PATHOPHYSIOLOGY

Hypophosphatemia is defined as serum [PO_4^{3-}] <2.5 milligrams/dL, but severe symptoms may not occur until the [PO_4^{3-}] level drops to <1 milligram/dL. Because phosphorus is abundant in many foods and readily absorbed, hypophosphatemia is relatively unusual. Mechanisms include a shift of phosphate into cells, increased renal excretion, and decreased GI absorption (**Table 17-29**). Only when depletion is present will clinical manifestations occur and require treatment. It is important to understand pseudohypophosphatemia, which occurs when a patient is treated with mannitol, which binds to molybdate in the serum, causing an artificially low value when [PO_4^{3-}] is measured by the laboratory.

Severe hypophosphatemia can occur in patients with prolonged use of antacids, such as aluminum hydroxide, magnesium hydroxide, or calcium carbonate. Several other drugs may cause hypophosphatemia with different mechanism (**Table 17-30**).

Critically ill patients are particularly at risk for hypophosphatemia, which occurs in up to 30% of those admitted to the intensive care unit with sepsis, trauma, and pulmonary diseases. The mechanism is glucose infusions, starvation, refeeding, shock, acidosis, alkalosis, diuretics, and catecholamine treatment.

TABLE 17-30 Drugs That Cause Hypophosphatemia and Underlying Mechanism

Osmotic diuretics, loop diuretics, carbonic anhydrase inhibitor	↓ Renal reabsorption and phosphaturia
Acyclovir	Inhibition of Na/Pi-IIa cotransporter
Acetaminophen	↓ Renal reabsorption and phosphaturia
Tyrosine kinase inhibitors	Ca^{2+} and phosphate reabsorption and secondary hyperparathyroidism
Bisphosphonates	Inhibits bone resorption
Aminoglycosides, tetracyclines ,valproic acid	Induction of Fanconi's syndrome
Cyclophosphamide, cisplatin	↑ Phosphaturia
Corticosteroids	↓ Intestinal phosphate absorption and phosphaturia

CLINICAL FEATURES

Symptoms are due to the depletion of adenosine triphosphate and the reduction of erythrocyte 2,3-diphosphoglycerate. The final outcome will be cellular dysfunction and hypoxia. The main symptoms of hypophosphatemia are listed in **Table 17-31**.[58]

TABLE 17-31 Symptoms and Signs of Hypophosphatemia

Hematologic

Reduced survival and function of platelets and red and white blood cells

Impaired macrophage function

Neuromuscular

Weakness, tremors, circumoral and fingertip paresthesias, decreased deep tendon reflexes, decreased mental status, anorexia

Cardiac

Impaired myocardial function

Metabolic

Insulin resistance

TREATMENT

When symptomatic, hypophosphatemia can be corrected both orally and IV. Possible adverse effects of IV therapy include hypocalcemia with consequent myocardial depression, arrhythmias, acute kidney injury, and calcifications. The suggested doses for PO_4^{3-} replacement are listed in **Table 17-32**, and the commonly used preparations are described in **Table 17-33**.[2,58]

TABLE 17-32 IV PO_4^{3-} Replacement Dose (6–72 h)

Serum $[PO_4^{3-}]$ (milligrams/dL)	Dose (mmol/kg)	Duration (h)
<1	0.6	6–72
1–1.7	0.3–0.4	6–72
1.8–2.2	0.15–0.2	6–72

TABLE 17-33 PO_4^{3-} Preparations

Preparation	PO_4^{3-} Content	Na^+ Content	K^+ Content
Neutral Na/K PO_4 (PO)	8 mmol	7.1 mEq	7.1 mEq
Sodium PO_4^{3-} (IV)	3 mmol/mL	4 mEq/mL	0
Potassium PO_4^{3-} (IV)	3 mmol/mL	0	4.4 mEq/mL

TABLE 17-34 Causes of Hyperphosphatemia

Decrease in renal excretion of PO_4^{3-}	Acute and chronic renal failure* Hypoparathyroidism, pseudohypoparathyroidism
Shift of PO_4^{3-} from ICF to ECF	Hemolysis* Rhabdomyolysis* Tumor lysis syndrome Respiratory acidosis Diabetic ketoacidosis
Addition of PO_4^{3-} exogenous to the ECF	Oral or IV treatment of hypophosphatemia Phosphate-containing laxatives, antacids*
Drugs	Excess of vitamin D Growth hormone Bisphosphonates

*Most likely presentation relevant to the ED.

In asymptomatic or mildly symptomatic patients, hypophosphatemia may be treated orally with skimmed milk ($[PO_4^{3-}]$ 1 gram/L) or oral preparations like Neutra-Phos®, one to two tabs PO four times daily, or K-Phos®, one tab PO four times daily, which contain 150 to 250 milligrams per tablet (PO_4^{3-}: 1 mmol/L = 3.1 milligrams/dL). A treatment regimen of 50 mmol/d for 7 to 10 days is sufficient to replace deficits, but in severe hypophosphatemia, higher doses may be necessary.

HYPERPHOSPHATEMIA

Hyperphosphatemia is defined as serum $[PO_4^{3-}]$ >4.5 milligrams/dL and is rarely encountered in emergency medicine practice. The causes can be divided in three groups according to mechanism: decrease in renal excretion of PO_4^{3-}, addition or movement of PO_4^{3-} from ICF to ECF, and drugs (**Table 17-34**).[57] In clinical practice, the most important cause of hyperphosphatemia is acute or chronic renal failure.

Hyperphosphatemia worsens renal tubulointerstitial disease, renal osteodystrophies, and cardiovascular disease. The acute symptoms are due to renal failure, hypocalcemia, and hypomagnesemia.

It is important to lower phosphorus intake with a careful protein-containing diet and to avoid excessive vitamin D intake to limit intestinal absorption.[59] In very high PO_4^{3-} levels, it is necessary to remove it with hemodialysis. Phosphate binders like calcium carbonate or calcium acetate bind intestinal phosphate, decreasing its absorption.[60]

REFERENCES

The complete reference list is available online at www.TintinalliEM.com.

CHAPTER 18

Cardiac Rhythm Disturbances

William J. Brady
Thomas S. Laughrey
Chris A. Ghaemmaghami

GENERAL CONSIDERATIONS

INITIAL APPROACH TO THE STABLE PATIENT

The focused evaluation of the patient includes determining the presenting complaint(s), obtaining the medical history, identifying medication use, performing a physical examination, initiating continuous cardiac rhythm monitoring, reviewing the 12-lead ECG, and analyzing the cardiac rhythm on the rhythm monitor, a printer strip, or the ECG.

Presenting symptoms may include palpitations, lightheadedness, fatigue, or weakness. Ischemic symptoms, such as chest pain, nausea, dyspnea, or lightheadedness, may be due to dysrhythmia-induced ischemia.

The medication history includes prescribed medications, herbals, recreational drugs, and caffeine-containing beverages. Especially note recently started new medications or increased medication doses. Symptoms of hyperthyroidism should be sought. Patients with a family history of sudden death, syncope, or dysrhythmias and those with organic heart disease have a higher risk of cardiac dysrhythmias and complications. Panic or anxiety is a diagnosis of exclusion in tachycardic ED patients.

INITIAL APPROACH TO THE UNSTABLE PATIENT

An unstable patient needs rapid assessment and treatment to prevent cardiovascular collapse. Instability means that the dysrhythmia is (1) impairing cardiac output and threatening vital organ function or (2) has the potential to suddenly deteriorate into cardiac arrest (**Table 18-1**).[1] Establish an IV line, initiate cardiac rhythm monitoring, obtain an ECG, and be prepared for drug or electrical therapy.

Dysrhythmia-induced chest pain results from coronary hypoperfusion, and dyspnea results from pulmonary edema, usually with objective evidence: ST segment abnormalities, rales on examination, or low oxygen saturation. As the ventricular rate exceeds 200 beats/min, severe systemic hypoperfusion often results and the RR interval narrows proportionally, increasing the opportunity for malignant ventricular dysrhythmias.

GENERAL APPROACH TO BRADYDYSRHYTHMIAS

Bradydysrhythmia describes rhythms with a ventricular rate slower than 60 beats/min in the adult. Age-appropriate heart rates define pediatric bradydysrhythmia. Bradydysrhythmias can be broadly categorized as bradycardias (atria and ventricles beat at the same slow rate) and atrioventricular (AV) blocks (ventricles beat slower than the atria).[1] The bradycardias include sinus bradycardia, junctional rhythm, idioventricular rhythm, and hyperkalemia-related sinoventricular rhythm. Bradydysrhythmias due to AV blocks include second-degree (usually type II) and third-degree AV block, as well as atrial fibrillation and atrial flutter with a slow ventricular response.

The most common bradycardia is sinus bradycardia, followed by junctional rhythm, and less commonly idioventricular rhythm. These

TABLE 18-1 Instability Indicators in the Patient with Cardiac Dysrhythmias

Hypotension: e.g., systolic blood pressure <90 mm Hg (<12 kPa)
Systemic hypoperfusion
Altered mentation
Ischemic chest pain
Respiratory distress
Extremely rapid ventricular rate: e.g., rate over 200 beats/min in adult

dysrhythmias are found in both stable and unstable patients. Atrial fibrillation and flutter with slow ventricular response are uncommon. If the patient is unstable, the vast majority of AV blocks are third-degree heart block followed much less frequently by second-degree AV block. If the patient is stable, second-degree type I AV block is most frequently seen, third-degree AV block is less common, whereas second-degree type II AV block is quite rare.[2-4]

Bradydysrhythmias result from conditions that affect the automaticity and refractoriness of cardiac cells as well as the conduction of impulses within the cardiac electrical system.[1,4] About 80% of bradydysrhythmias are caused by factors external to the cardiac electrical system including acute coronary syndrome, drug effects or overdose, and hypoxia with cardiac hypoperfusion.[2,3]

Emergent treatment of bradydysrhythmia is not required unless (1) the heart rate is slower than 50 beats/min accompanied by hypotension or hypoperfusion and/or (2) the bradydysrhythmia is due to structural disease of the infranodal conduction system. This first group requires resuscitative treatment while evaluating the cause. The second group of patients does not require immediate treatment but should be closely monitored, with pacing readily available while arranging definitive care.

Medications used to increase heart rate in symptomatic bradycardias include atropine, β-adrenergic agonists, and glucagon (**Table 18-2**; see

TABLE 18-2 Drug Treatment for Cardiac Dysrhythmias in Adults

Drug	Dose	Comments
Drugs for Bradydysrhythmias		
Atropine	0.5-milligram IV push, may repeat every 3–5 min until desired heart rate is achieved or to total dose of 3 milligrams (0.04 milligram/kg)	Most effective for bradydysrhythmias due to sinus and AV nodal disease
Dopamine	IV infusion at rate 2–20 micrograms/kg per min, titrate to desired heart rate	May precipitate myocardial ischemia and ectopy
Epinephrine	IV infusion at rate 2–10 micrograms/min, titrate to desired heart rate	May precipitate myocardial ischemia and ectopy
Glucagon	3–10 milligrams IV infused over 1–2 min, followed by an IV continuous infusion of 1–5 milligrams/h	Used for cardiotoxicity associated with β-blocker and calcium channel blocker overdose Nausea and vomiting are often limiting side effects Tachyphylaxis may develop during infusion
Drugs to Block AV Nodal Conduction		
Adenosine	6-milligram rapid IV push; if after 2 min the dysrhythmia persists, repeat rapid IV push with 12 milligrams; may repeat once more if dysrhythmia persists	Effective in terminating narrow QRS complex reentrant tachydysrhythmias involving the AV node
Verapamil	2.5–5 milligrams IV bolus over 2–3 min; if after 15 min the dysrhythmia persists, may repeat with dose of 5–10 milligrams	Effective in terminating narrow QRS complex reentrant tachydysrhythmias involving the AV node and reducing ventricular rate in atrial fibrillation or flutter
Diltiazem	15–20 milligrams IV bolus over 2 min, followed by IV infusion at 5–10 milligrams/h	
Esmolol	500 micrograms/kg IV bolus over 1 min, followed by IV infusion starting at 50 micrograms/kg per min; titrate infusion to desired heart rate	
Metoprolol	5-milligram IV bolus; may repeat 5 milligrams IV every 5 min up to total dose of 15 milligrams	
Propranolol	30 micrograms/kg IV over 1 min; may repeat same dose every 2 min, up to total dose of 100 micrograms/kg	
Drugs to Terminate Tachydysrhythmias		
Procainamide	15–17 milligrams/kg IV over 30 min, followed by IV infusion at 1–4 milligrams (20–80 micrograms/kg) per min; or 20-50 milligrams/min; or 100 milligrams IV q 5 min	Used in wide-complex tachydysrhythmias and new-onset atrial fibrillation Median time to conversion of new-onset atrial fibrillation about 1 h Caution in patients with AMI and LV dysfunction Infuse initial dose at rate of 20 milligrams/min to reduce adverse effects
Amiodarone	Stable patient: 150 milligrams IV over 10 min; may repeat same dose every 10 min up to total dose of 2 grams OR use IV infusion 0.5 milligram/min Ventricular fibrillation or pulseless ventricular tachycardia: 300 milligrams IV bolus; may repeat with additional dose of 150 milligrams IV bolus	Used in wide-complex tachydysrhythmias and new-onset atrial fibrillation Preferred in setting of AMI or LV dysfunction Contraindicated in pregnancy
Lidocaine	1 milligram/kg IV over 60 s; may repeat 0.5 milligram/kg IV every 5–10 min, up to 300 milligrams in a 1 h period; followed by infusion of 1–4 milligrams/min	Third-line agent for ventricular tachycardia and ventricular fibrillation
Magnesium sulfate	2 grams IV over 2 min, followed by infusion of 1–2 grams/h	Used in torsades de pointes with long QT interval
Ibutilide	Weight <60 kg: 10 micrograms/kg IV over 10 min Weight >60 kg: 1 milligram IV over 10 min	Used for conversion of new-onset atrial fibrillation or flutter Median time to conversion 20–30 min
Flecainide	200 milligrams PO < 70 kg 300 milligrams PO > 70 kg ; or 2 milligrams/kg IV over 10 min*	Used for conversion of new-onset atrial fibrillation or flutter Median time to conversion up to 4 h Avoid in patients with ACS or cardiomyopathy
Propafenone	450 milligrams PO < 70 kg 600 milligrams PO > 70 kg ; or 2 milligrams IV over 10 min*	Used for conversion of new-onset atrial fibrillation or flutter Median time to conversion 2 h Avoid in patients with ACS, cardiomyopathy, or severe COPD
Vernakalant*	3 milligrams/kg IV infusion over 10 min; if dysrhythmia persists after 15 min, a second infusion of 2 milligrams/kg IV over 10 min can be given	Used for conversion of new-onset atrial fibrillation or flutter Median time to conversion 8–11 min Avoid in patients with hypotension, ACS within 30 days, severe aortic stenosis, and prolonged QT interval

Abbreviations: ACS = acute coronary syndrome; AMI = acute myocardial infarction; AV = atrioventricular; COPD = chronic obstructive pulmonary disease; LV = left ventricle.

*Not available in the United States.

chapter 19, "Pharmacology of Antiarrhythmics and Antihypertensives").[1,4] Atropine enhances the automaticity of the sinoatrial (SA) node and potentiates conduction through the AV node by direct vagolytic activity. Atropine is usually effective for sinus bradycardia and junctional rhythms but is not useful (nor particularly harmful) in idioventricular rhythms and second-degree type II and third-degree AV block.[2,3] β-Adrenergic agents stimulate both chronotropic and inotropic cardiac activity, as well as enhancing electrical conduction within the AV node and infranodal system, thus their potential to produce ischemia and ectopy. Glucagon stimulates inotropic and chronotropic cardiac activity independent of the β-adrenergic receptors. Glucagon is primarily used for bradycardias due to cardiotoxicity from β-blocker or calcium channel blocker overdose. Effectiveness of drug treatment for bradycardia varies, and in general, these agents are best used as a temporary bridge to cardiac pacing.

Transcutaneous pacing can be applied quickly and is the most appropriate pacing method for the acutely symptomatic patient (see chapter 33, "Cardiac Pacing and Implanted Defibrillation"). Transvenous pacing requires considerable physician expertise and specialized equipment for insertion and proper placement. Disease-specific therapies can also be effective in reversing a toxin-induced bradycardia (e.g., treatment of hyperkalemia or toxicity from calcium channel blockers, β-blockers, or digitalis).

GENERAL APPROACH TO TACHYDYSRHYTHMIAS

Tachydysrhythmia describes rhythms with a ventricular rate greater than 100 beats/min in an adult, with age-appropriate limits in children. Tachycardias are categorized as supraventricular or ventricular (**Figure 18-1**). Supraventricular tachycardias originate from a focus within or above the AV node and most often present with a narrow QRS complex; thus, they are termed *narrow-complex tachycardias*. Ventricular tachycardias, resulting from a focus below the AV node in the ventricular myocardium, usually demonstrate a widened QRS complex and are referred to as *wide-complex tachycardias*. This classification scheme does have limitations; a supraventricular rhythm can present with a widened QRS complex due to aberrant ventricular conduction, the widened QRS complex resulting from a fixed (i.e., preexisting) bundle-branch block, rate-related conduction block, ventricular preexcitation syndrome (i.e., Wolff-Parkinson-White [WPW] syndrome), or toxic-metabolic condition.[5] The normal QRS complex duration is less than 120 milliseconds for older children and adults; therefore, a wide-complex tachycardia possesses a QRS complex width greater than 120 milliseconds.

Common narrow-complex tachycardias include sinus tachycardia, atrial fibrillation, atrial flutter, and paroxysmal supraventricular tachycardia; less common narrow-complex tachycardias include multifocal atrial tachycardia, atrial tachycardias, and preexcited tachycardias seen in accessory pathway syndromes including WPW syndrome.[6] Wide-complex tachycardias include ventricular tachycardia and supraventricular tachycardia with aberrant conduction.[5,7] Ventricular tachycardia further is subdivided into monomorphic and polymorphic forms; the polymorphic category includes the subtype called *torsade de pointes*.[8]

Treatment for symptomatic tachycardia is primarily intravenous medications for the stable patient and electrical therapy for the unstable patient (see chapter 23, "Defibrillation and Cardioversion"). The QRS width, often indicating the portion of the heart where the dysrhythmia originates, guides therapeutic choices.

Narrow-Complex Tachycardia Sinus tachycardia and multifocal atrial tachycardia are best managed by treating the underlying cause, rather than the dysrhythmia specifically. Other narrow-complex tachycardias require specific antidysrhythmic treatment by a combination of vagal maneuvers (**Table 18-3**), medications (Table 18-2), and electrical cardioversion (**Figure 18-2**).[9] Basic supportive therapy in most patients involves an IV fluid bolus to expand the circulating intravascular volume and supplemental oxygen.

Vagal maneuvers heighten parasympathetic tone and may slow electrical conduction in the heart to a degree that abolishes sustained reentry. If applied early, vagal maneuvers can convert about 20% of patients presenting with reentrant tachycardias, such as paroxysmal supraventricular tachycardia and narrow-complex tachycardia associated with WPW syndrome. Effective vagal maneuvers include carotid sinus massage, the release phase of the Valsalva maneuver, and the diving reflex; the response to these vagal maneuvers is enhanced by placing the patient supine.[10-12]

Adenosine is a very-short-acting agent that blocks conduction through the AV node and can interrupt sustained reentry when the AV node is part of the circuit (Table 18-2). The AV nodal blocking effect of adenosine is very transient, although quite profound, so a brief period of AV nodal blockade with near-immediate recurrence of the reentrant supraventricular tachycardia is not a treatment failure but a consequence of the medication's short duration of effect. In such situations, repeat adenosine with a higher dose (12 milligrams).[13]

β-Blockers and calcium channel blockers slow conduction through the AV node and can convert some supraventricular tachycardias, such as reentrant supraventricular tachycardias, and slow the ventricular response in others, such as atrial fibrillation or flutter. Esmolol, an intravenous β-blocker with a short duration of effect, can be used when temporary AV nodal blockade is desired and a longer period of action is not anticipated (as in conversion of paroxysmal supraventricular tachycardia) or

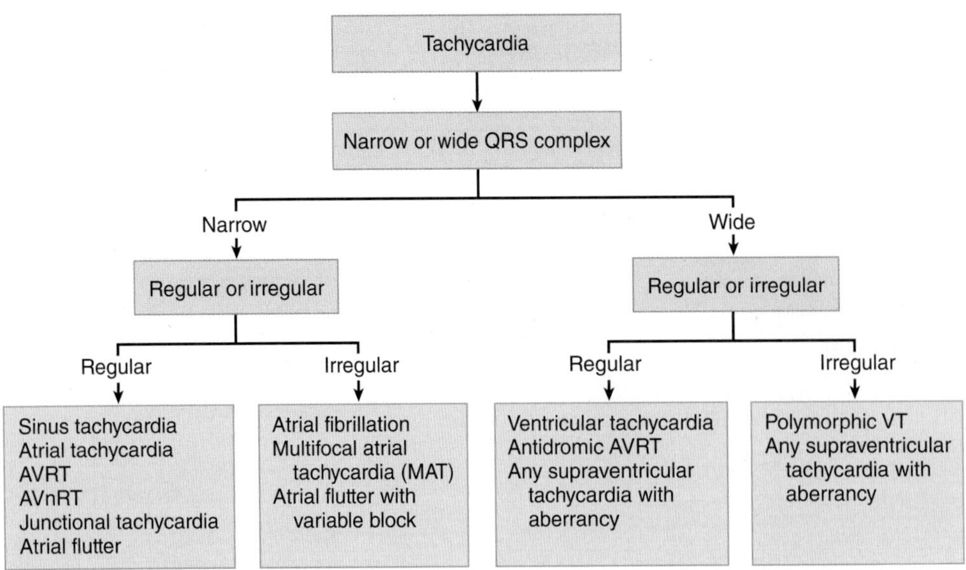

FIGURE 18-1. Tachycardia classification. AVnRT = atrioventricular nodal reentrant tachycardia; AVRT = atrioventricular reentrant tachycardia; VT = ventricular tachycardia.

TABLE 18-3 Vagal Maneuvers

Carotid sinus massage	Listen for bruit first; do not massage an artery with a bruit Massage only one side at a time Massage for 20 s or less
Valsalva maneuver	Have patient hold breath and strain against closed glottis while tightening abdominal wall muscles Hold for as long as practical, ideally >20 s Increased vagal tone seen during release phase after breath hold
Diving reflex	More effective in infants than adults Place bag of ice and water on face for 15–30 s

when the patient is unstable and the ability to titrate the degree of drug effect is important. Metoprolol is a longer acting β-blocker used in more stable patients, typically for ventricular rate control in patients with atrial fibrillation. Verapamil is a calcium channel blocker used for conversion of reentrant supraventricular tachycardias, and although it can be used for ventricular rate control, there is potential for hypotension, so diltiazem, which does not have as much potential to induce hypotension, is the calcium channel blocker recommended for ventricular rate control.

Synchronized electrical cardioversion can be used in narrow-complex tachycardias when patients are unstable or do not respond to pharmacologic measures (see chapter 23).

Wide-Complex Tachycardia In the stable patient, pharmacologic agents used to terminate a wide-complex tachycardia include procainamide, amiodarone, lidocaine, and magnesium (Table 18-2 and **Figure 18-3**). **For rapid treatment, amiodarone is the antiarrhythmic of choice, given as an IV bolus.** Procainamide is effective for stable ventricular tachycardia in patients with preserved left ventricular dysfunction, given as an IV infusion.[14] Lidocaine is a less effective alternative.[14] Magnesium is used for tachydysrhythmias associated with QT interval prolongation, such as torsade de pointes.

Electrical cardioversion is the preferred treatment for wide-complex tachycardia with hemodynamic instability, myocardial ischemia, or failure of pharmacologic treatment (see chapter 23).[7,8]

NON-TACHYCARDIC IRREGULAR DYSRHYTHMIAS

SINUS ARRHYTHMIA

Description While some variation in the rate of sinus (or SA) node electrical discharge is normal, sinus arrhythmia is present when the variation in the SA node discharge rate is greater than 120 milliseconds between the longest and shortest P to P wave intervals (**Figure 18-4**). There should be a consistent P-wave morphology indicating that the electrical impulses are all originating from the same atrial pacemaker, usually the SA node (**Table 18-4**). Two or more different P wave morphologies suggest atrial ectopy, wandering atrial pacemaker, or other nonsinus focus.

Clinical Significance Sinus arrhythmia is a normal finding in children and young adults but is less common in the middle-aged and elderly. Sinus arrhythmia is most commonly a respiro-phasic phenomenon; the sinus node rate accelerates during inspiration and decelerates during expiration. This variation is thought to be due to changes in vagal tone occurring with respiration, termed *the Bainbridge reflex*. Any condition or medication that alters vagal tone may exaggerate an underlying sinus arrhythmia. During long intervals of sinus arrhythmia, junctional escape beats may occur.

Treatment None is required.

SINOATRIAL BLOCK

Description The SA node electrical discharge must be conducted into the atria to pace the heart during sinus rhythm. If sinus node discharges are delayed or blocked in their outward propagation (exit block), then SA block is present. SA block is divided into first-, second-, and third-degree varieties, much like the classification system used for AV nodal blockade.

In **first-degree SA block,** the impulse is delayed in its conduction out of the sinus node into the atria, a condition that cannot be recognized on the clinical 12-lead ECG; this entity is diagnosed in the electrophysiology laboratory. In **second-degree SA block,** some impulses get through and some are blocked. **Second-degree SA block** can be suspected whenever an expected P wave and the corresponding QRS complex are absent. Usually, the interval between normal P waves encompassing the missing beat is a simple multiple of the existing P to P rate. **Third-degree SA block** occurs when the sinus node discharge is completely blocked and no P wave originating from the sinus is seen. In addition to

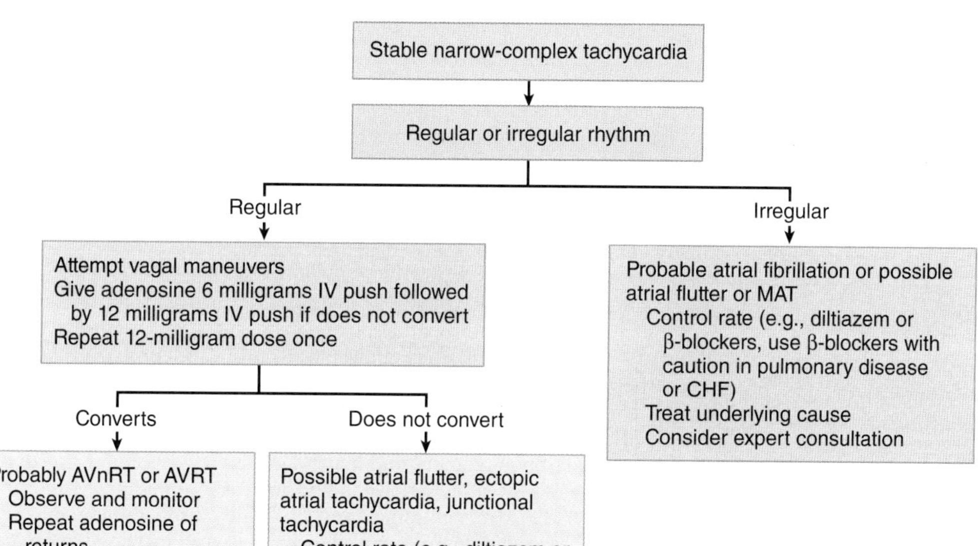

FIGURE 18-2. Treatment of narrow-complex tachycardia. AV = atrioventricular; AVnRT = atrioventricular nodal reentrant tachycardia; AVRT = atrioventricular reentrant tachycardia; CHF = congestive heart failure; MAT = multifocal atrial tachycardia; VT = ventricular tachycardia.

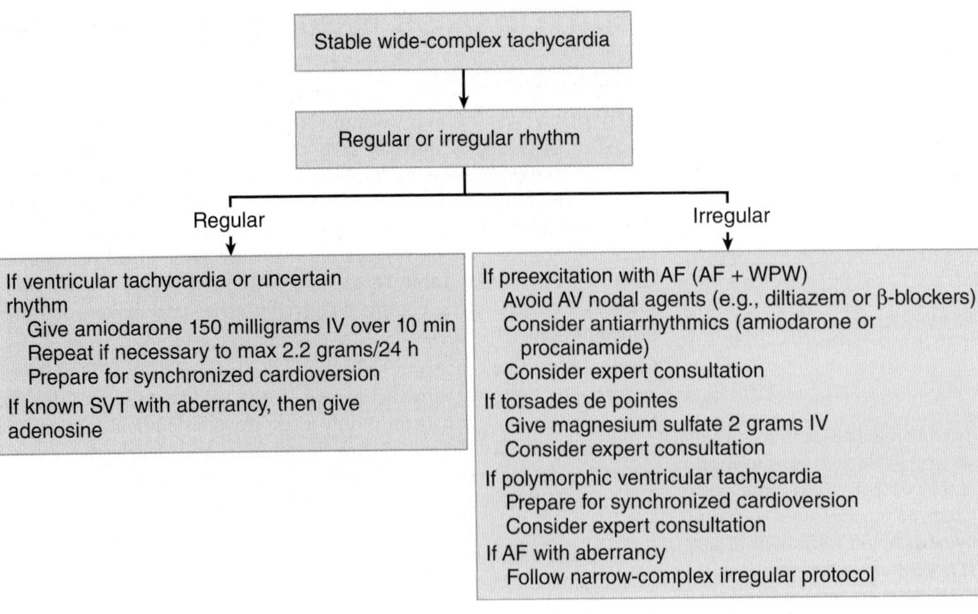

FIGURE 18-3. Treatment of wide-complex tachycardia. AF = atrial fibrillation; AV = atrioventricular; SVT = supraventricular tachycardia; WPW = Wolff-Parkinson-White syndrome.

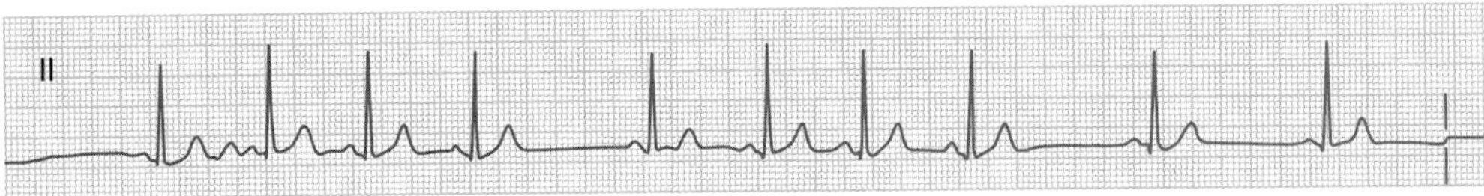

FIGURE 18-4. Sinus arrhythmia.

third-degree SA block, absence of a P wave may also be caused by (1) sinus node failure, (2) a sinus node stimulus inadequate to activate the atria, and (3) atrial unresponsiveness.

Clinical Significance SA block usually arises from myocardial disease (acute rheumatic fever, acute inferior MI, or other causes of myocarditis) or drug toxicity (digoxin, quinidine, salicylates, β-blockers, or calcium channel blockers). In rare individuals, vagal stimulation can produce SA block.

Treatment Treatment depends on the underlying cause, associated dysrhythmias, and whether symptoms of hypoperfusion are present. Sinus node discharge rate and SA conduction can be facilitated by atropine when clinically required; however, ischemia may result from a rhythm that is accelerated. Cardiac pacing is indicated for recurrent or persistent symptomatic bradycardia.

SINUS ARREST (PAUSE)

Description Sinus pause is a failure of impulse formation within the sinus node. In sinus arrest, the P to P wave interval encompassing the missing beat has no relation to the underlying SA node discharge rate (**Figure 18-5**).

Clinical Significance The same conditions that produce SA block produce sinus arrest, especially digoxin toxicity and aging disease of the SA node. Brief periods of sinus arrest may occur in healthy individuals due to increased vagal tone. If sinus arrest is prolonged, AV junctional escape beats often occur.

TABLE 18-4 ECG Features of Sinus Arrhythmia

Upright P waves in leads I, II, and III
Consistent P wave–QRS complex relationship
Consistent P-wave morphology from beat-to-beat
Variation in the sinus node discharge rate >120 ms between longest and shortest P to P wave intervals

Treatment Treatment is often unneeded and when considered depends on the underlying cause, associated dysrhythmias, and whether symptoms of hypoperfusion are present. If sinus arrest is symptomatic, atropine usually will increase the SA node discharge rate. Cardiac pacing is indicated for recurrent or persistent symptomatic bradycardia.

SICK SINUS SYNDROME

Description Sick sinus syndrome (sometimes referred to as the *tachycardia-bradycardia syndrome*) is a heterogeneous disorder consisting of abnormalities of supraventricular impulse generation and conduction that produce a wide variety of intermittent supraventricular tachy- and bradydysrhythmias (**Table 18-5**). The tachydysrhythmias are usually atrial fibrillation, junctional tachycardia, paroxysmal supraventricular tachycardia, and atrial flutter. The bradydysrhythmias are marked sinus bradycardia, prolonged sinus arrest, and SA block, usually associated with AV nodal conduction abnormalities and inadequate junctional escape rhythms.

Clinical Significance Sick sinus syndrome is most commonly seen in elderly patients and is associated with a variety of cardiac diseases that can affect the SA and AV nodes, including ischemic disorders, myocarditis and pericarditis, rheumatologic disease, metastatic tumors, surgical damage, or cardiomyopathies.

Symptoms of sick sinus syndrome are due to the effects of fast or slow heart rate. Common symptoms include syncope or near-syncope, palpitations, dyspnea, chest pain, and cerebrovascular ischemic events. Conditions that increase vagal tone (abdominal pain, increased intracranial pressure), thyrotoxicosis, and hyperkalemia may exacerbate the abnormalities of sick sinus syndrome and increase symptoms. Medications such as digoxin, quinidine, procainamide, disopyramide, nicotine, β-blockers, and calcium channel blockers also can increase symptoms.

Ambulatory ECG monitoring or electrophysiologic studies are usually necessary for diagnosis, because intermittent dysrhythmias may not be evident during the examination.

Treatment By definition, symptomatic patients will have both tachy- and bradydysrhythmias, and each of the elements may need to be

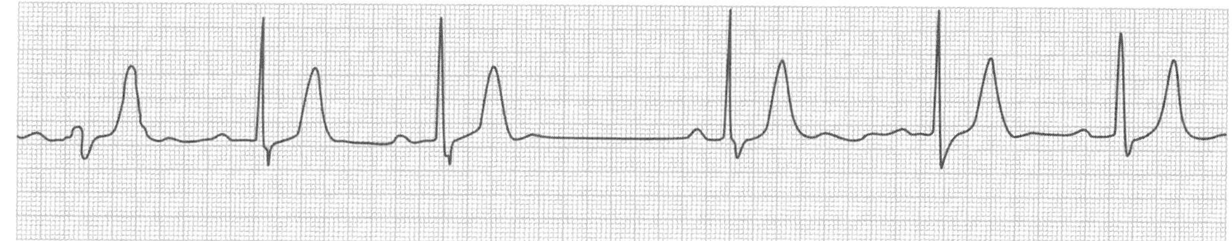

FIGURE 18-5. Sinus pause.

addressed. Aggressive pharmacologic treatments and ablation procedures to reduce tachycardia carry risks of worsening bradycardia, AV block, and pauses. Transcutaneous pacing may be required if the patient is being pharmacologically treated for atrial tachydysrhythmias in the setting of sick sinus syndrome. Permanent pacemaker implantation is frequently indicated.

PREMATURE ATRIAL CONTRACTIONS

Description Premature atrial contractions originate from ectopic pacemakers anywhere in the atrium other than the SA node (**Figure 18-6**) with characteristic ECG features (**Table 18-6**). The ectopic P wave may not be conducted through the AV node if the premature atrial contraction reaches the AV node during the absolute refractory period. When a premature atrial contraction reaches the AV node during the relative refractory period, it may be conducted with a delay, as demonstrated on the ECG by a longer PR interval than seen with a sinus beat. Nonconducted premature atrial contractions are the most common cause of pauses in cardiac rhythm. Premature atrial contractions may occur in a pattern, such as every other beat (atrial bigeminy), every third beat (atrial trigeminy), and so on.

Most premature atrial contractions are conducted with baseline QRS complexes, but some may be conducted aberrantly through the infranodal system, particularly if they reach a bundle branch during the refractory period. The premature atrial contraction will often depolarize the SA node ("reset"), so the interval between normal P waves encompassing the premature atrial contraction will not be twice the existing P to P interval, creating a shorter pause than the fully compensatory pauses seen after most premature ventricular contractions.

Clinical Significance Premature atrial contractions are common at all ages and usually do not indicate underlying heart disease. Increased rates of premature atrial contractions are seen in patients with chronic heart or lung disease. Chemical agents that enhance either sympathetic tone (e.g., cocaine, amphetamines, caffeine, nicotine) or parasympathetic tone (e.g., digoxin) may lead to a higher frequency of premature atrial contractions in an individual patient. Premature atrial contractions can precipitate sustained atrial tachycardia, flutter, or fibrillation under certain circumstances.

Treatment No specific treatment is necessary. If the premature atrial contractions are symptomatic, discontinue any precipitating toxins and treat any underlying disorder that is contributing to symptoms.

TABLE 18-5 ECG Features of Sick Sinus Syndrome

Intermittent combination of bradydysrhythmias and tachydysrhythmias
Bradydysrhythmias
Sinus bradycardia
Sinus arrest
SA block
Tachydysrhythymias
Atrial fibrillation
Atrial flutter
Paroxysmal supraventricular tachycardia

Abbreviation: SA = sinoatrial.

TABLE 18-6 ECG Features of Premature Atrial Contractions

P waves that appear sooner (prematurely) than expected sinus beat
Ectopic P waves
With different shape and axis than the SA node–initiated P wave
That may or may not be conducted through the AV node
Interval between normal P waves encompassing the premature atrial contraction is less than twice the existing P to P cycle length (a noncompensatory pause)

Abbreviations: AV = atrioventricular; SA = sinoatrial.

TABLE 18-7 ECG Features of Premature Junctional Contractions

Ectopic P wave
With different shape, axis, and amplitude from SA node–initiated P waves
That may occur before or after QRS complex
QRS complex with similar morphology to SA node–initiated QRS complex

Abbreviation: SA = sinoatrial.

PREMATURE JUNCTIONAL CONTRACTIONS

Description Premature junctional contractions are due to an ectopic pacemaker within the AV node or common AV bundle with characteristic ECG features (**Table 18-7**).

Because the premature junctional contraction is usually conducted back into the atria, the SA node is usually affected by the ectopic depolarization, and the postectopic pause is noncompensatory, but a compensatory pause is seen if the premature junctional contraction is not conducted in retrograde fashion. Premature junctional contraction may be isolated, multiple (as in bigeminy or trigeminy), or multifocal.

Clinical Significance Premature junctional contractions are uncommon in healthy hearts and are typically seen in patients with heart failure, digitalis toxicity, ischemic heart disease, and myocardial ischemia (especially of the inferior wall).

Treatment No specific treatment is usually required. Treatment of the underlying disorder is appropriate.

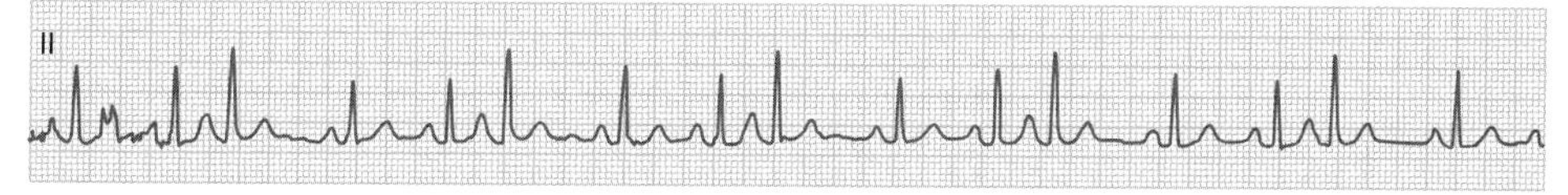

FIGURE 18-6. Premature atrial contractions in an atrial trigeminy pattern.

PREMATURE VENTRICULAR CONTRACTIONS

Description Premature ventricular contractions occur when electrical impulses originate from single or multiple areas in the ventricles. ECG characteristics (**Figure 18-7** and **Table 18-8**) are used to differentiate premature ventricular contractions from other premature beats.

Most premature ventricular contractions do not affect the spontaneous discharge of the SA node, so the interval between normal sinus P waves encompassing the premature ventricular contraction is twice the previous P to P interval, termed a fully compensatory postectopic pause. This fully compensatory pause occurs because the SA node discharges during the refractory period of either the AV node or His bundles induced by the premature ventricular contraction. Less commonly, a premature ventricular contraction may be interpolated between two sinus beats. Many premature ventricular contractions occurring in a bigeminal or trigeminal pattern have a fixed coupling interval (within 40 milliseconds) from the preceding sinus beat (**Figure 18-8**). Occasionally, a **ventricular fusion beat** occurs when both supraventricular and ventricular impulses depolarize the ventricular myocardium almost simultaneously. The QRS configuration of a fusion beat has characteristics of both the normally conducted beat and the ectopic one.

The degree (quantity and quality) of the premature ventricular contractions is categorized as follows: (1) an occasional premature ventricular contraction seen on the rhythm strip is called an isolated premature ventricular contraction (Figure 18-7A), (2) multiple premature ventricular contractions of similar morphology are called unifocal premature ventricular contractions (Figure 18-7B), and (3) multiple premature ventricular contractions with different morphology are called multifocal premature ventricular contractions (Figure 18-7C), implying more than one ventricular focus is producing ectopy. Periods of sustained unifocal premature ventricular contractions may occasionally be seen, often with a fixed ratio and coupling interval to sinus beats.

Clinical Significance Premature ventricular contractions are very common and related to factors that alter the electrophysiology of cardiac tissue or to pathologic conditions of the myocardium itself. Sometimes, infrequent or rare premature ventricular contractions may be observed in patients without any evidence of heart disease. Premature ventricular contractions may trigger sustained runs of ventricular tachycardia (**Figure 18-9**).[15]

There is a correlation between the severity of underlying coronary artery disease and the degree of ventricular ectopy, and in addition, ventricular ectopy is an independent risk factor for sudden cardiac death.[16,17] In acute coronary syndrome, premature ventricular contractions indicate the underlying electrical instability of the heart, but patterns of premature ventricular contractions ("warning dysrhythmias") are not reliable predictors of subsequent ventricular fibrillation.

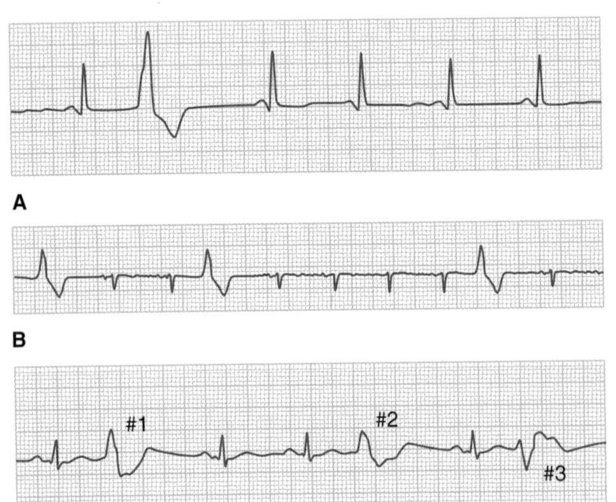

FIGURE 18-7. Sinus rhythm with premature ventricular contractions (PVCs). **A.** Sinus rhythm with a single PVC. **B.** Sinus rhythm with multiple unifocal PVCs. **C.** Sinus rhythm with multifocal PVCs (three different PVC morphologies in this single lead, indicated by #1, #2, and #3).

TABLE 18-8 ECG Features of Premature Ventricular Contractions

Absence of P wave prior to the QRS complex
Occasional retrograde P wave following QRS complex
Abnormally widened QRS complex with different morphology from SA node–initiated QRS complex
Commonly a compensatory postectopic pause following the premature ventricular contraction to next SA node–initiated beat
ST segments and T waves that are directed opposite the major QRS complex deflection

Abbreviation: SA = sinoatrial.

Treatment Review the ECG for evidence of ischemia or infarction, chamber enlargement, QT interval prolongation, or Brugada syndrome. Assess for potentially reversible conditions such as hypoxia, drug effect, or electrolyte abnormalities. In general, treat the underlying cause.[18,19] Typical recommendations for stress reduction and elimination of stimulants such as caffeine or nicotine are not consistently effective.[19] Patients with greater than three premature ventricular contractions in a row are considered to have nonsustained ventricular tachycardia, which can be a marker for sustained tachydysrhythmias and sudden cardiac death. If this is a new dysrhythmia, initiate emergency cardiac investigation.

Pharmacologic suppression of isolated premature ventricular contractions with antiarrhythmic medications in the acute setting does not confer improved survival for the acute condition. Attempts to suppress premature ventricular contractions with long-term oral antidysrhythmics increase mortality due to the dangerous prodysrhythmic properties of the medications themselves.[18,19] Implantable cardioverter defibrillators are used in patients with premature ventricular contractions that have potential to trigger malignant ventricular dysrhythmias or cardiac arrest.

BRADYDYSRHYTHMIAS

SINUS BRADYCARDIA

Description Sinus bradycardia is when the SA node discharge rate falls below 60 beats/min and AV conduction remains intact with a constant PR interval (**Figure 18-10**). The ECG characteristics are identical to sinus rhythm with the exception of a slow heart rate (**Table 18-9**).

Clinical Significance Sinus bradycardia represents a reduction of the SA node discharge rate. Sinus bradycardia can be (1) physiologic (in well-conditioned athletes, during sleep, or with vagal stimulation), (2) pharmacologic (β-blockers, digoxin, opioids, calcium channel blockers), or (3) pathologic (hypoxia, acute inferior wall myocardial ischemia or infarction, increased intracranial pressure, carotid sinus hypersensitivity, hypothyroidism).

Treatment Sinus bradycardia usually does not require specific treatment unless the heart rate is slower than 50 beats/min and there is evidence of hypoperfusion. Correct underlying causes. Use atropine in the unstable patient, followed by transcutaneous cardiac pacing and infusions of dopamine or epinephrine if there is no response to atropine.[1]

JUNCTIONAL RHYTHM

Description Under normal circumstances, the SA node discharges at a faster rate than the AV node, so the pacemaker function of the AV node and all other slower pacemakers are suppressed. If SA node discharges slow or fail to reach the AV node, junctional escape beats will produce a rhythm (**Figure 18-11**) usually at a rate between 40 and 60 beats/min. If the junctional beats continue in sequence, then a junctional rhythm is present. In most cases, junctional escape beats do not conduct retrograde into the atria, so a QRS complex without a P wave is usually seen (Figure 18-11A); rarely, the junctional escape beat does

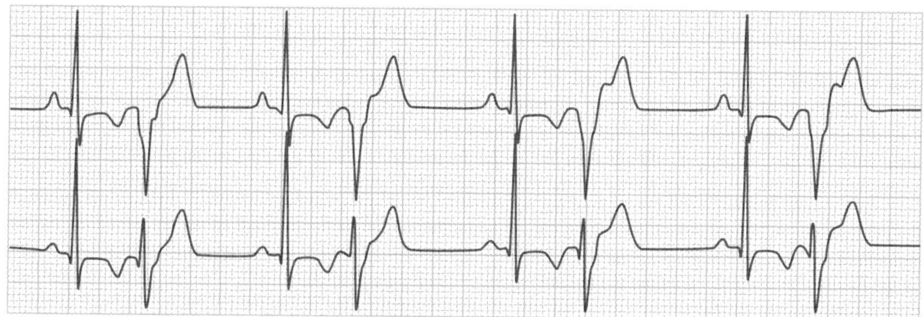

FIGURE 18-8. Premature ventricular contractions producing ventricular bigeminy.

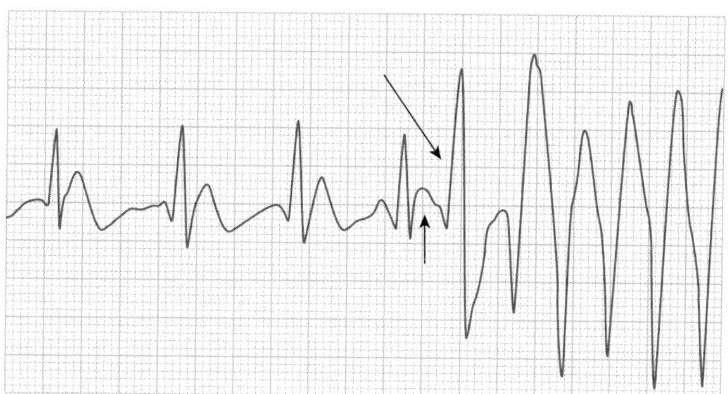

FIGURE 18-9. Sinus rhythm in an ST-segment elevation myocardial infarction patient with a premature ventricular contraction (PVC) initiating ventricular tachycardia. Note the R wave (*large arrow*) of a PVC falling on the T wave (*small arrow*) of the last sinus beat. This R-on-T event produces ventricular tachycardia.

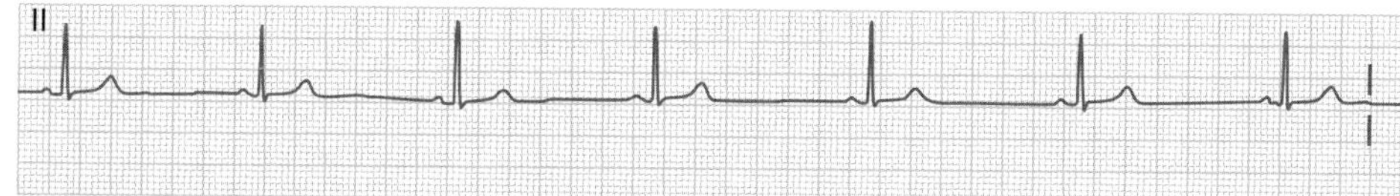

FIGURE 18-10. Sinus bradycardia.

TABLE 18-9 ECG Features of Sinus Bradycardia

ECG Features of Sinus Bradycardia
Normal SA node–initiated P waves: consistent morphology among all P waves with upright amplitude in leads I, II, and III
Normal PR interval: 120–200 milliseconds
1:1 atrioventricular conduction: a QRS complex for each P wave with consistent association
Rate <60 beats/min and regular

Abbreviation: SA = sinoatrial.

conduct retrograde into the atria, producing the retrograde P wave; a P wave usually inverted and found immediately prior to or following the QRS complex (Figure 18-11B).

At times, enhanced AV nodal automaticity overrides the sinus node and produces an accelerated junctional rhythm with a rate of 60 to 100 beats/min or junctional tachycardia with a rate greater than 100 beats/min. Usually, the enhanced junctional pacemaker captures both the atria and ventricles.

Clinical Significance Junctional escape beats may occur whenever there is a long enough pause in the impulses reaching the AV node, as with sinus bradycardia, slow phase of sinus arrhythmia, or during the

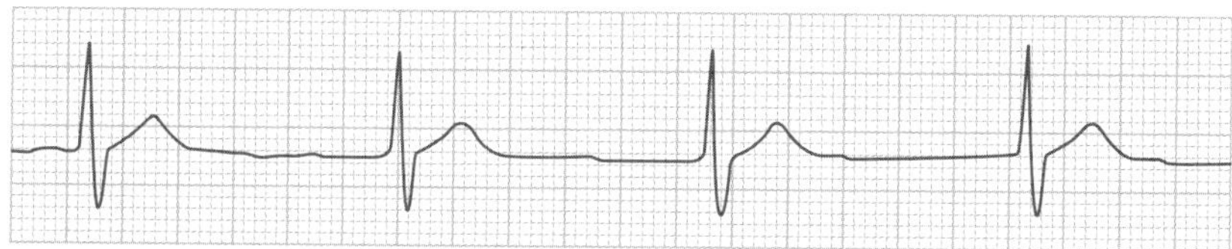

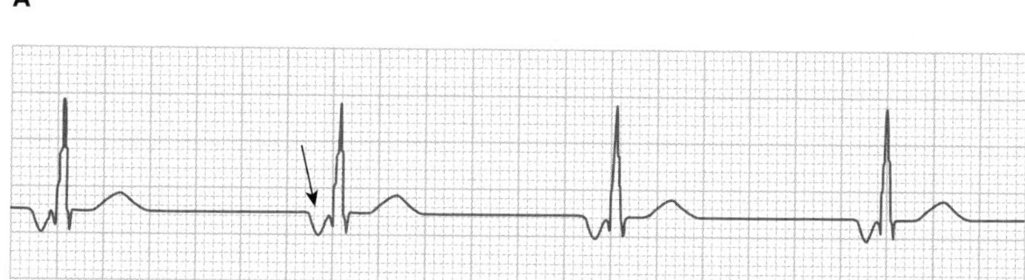

FIGURE 18-11. Junctional rhythm. **A.** Junctional rhythm. **B.** Junctional rhythm with retrograde P waves (*arrow*).

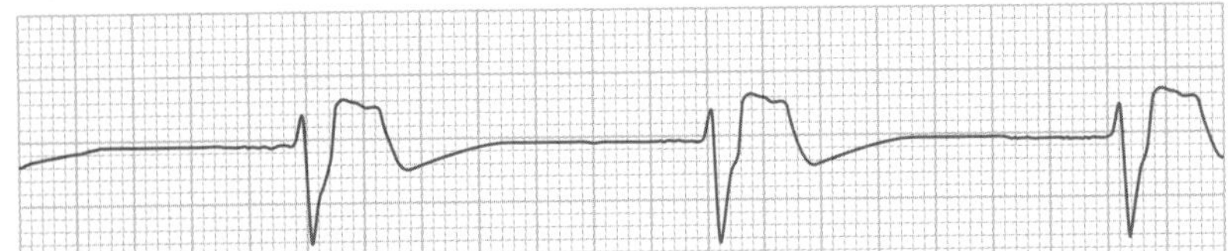

FIGURE 18-12. Idioventricular rhythm with a ventricular rate of approximately 30 beats/min.

pause after premature beats. Sustained junctional escape rhythms may be seen with heart failure, myocarditis, hypokalemia, or digitalis toxicity.

Accelerated junctional rhythm, including junctional tachycardia, may occur from medication toxicity, acute rheumatic fever, or inferior myocardial ischemia. With medication toxicity (particularly digitalis compounds) in a patient being treated for atrial fibrillation, the rate is usually between 70 and 130 beats/min and the ECG is characterized by regular QRS complexes superimposed on atrial fibrillatory waves.

Treatment Isolated, infrequent junctional escape beats usually do not require specific treatment. If sustained junctional escape rhythms are producing symptoms, the underlying cause should be treated. Atropine can be used to accelerate the SA node discharge rate and enhance AV nodal conduction. Accelerated junctional rhythm and junctional tachycardia usually do not produce significant symptoms.

IDIOVENTRICULAR RHYTHMS

Description Idioventricular rhythms are of ventricular origin (**Figure 18-12**), manifesting as regular widened QRS complexes without evidence of atrial activity (**Table 18-11**). An idioventricular rhythm has a ventricular rate of 30 to 50 beats/min, and the accelerated idioventricular rhythm has a ventricular rate of 50 to 75 beats/min. Idioventricular rhythm tends to appear in nonsustained fashion with runs of short duration, ranging from 3 to 30 consecutive beats, and will typically begin with a fusion beat.

Clinical Significance Idioventricular rhythm is seen most commonly in the setting of an ST-segment elevation myocardial infarction. An accelerated idioventricular rhythm that appears during successful fibrinolysis of an occluded coronary artery is termed a *reperfusion dysrhythmia*. Although there is some association with ventricular tachycardia, there is no apparent association with ventricular fibrillation. Idioventricular rhythms, particularly the slower versions, can produce dizziness, weakness, syncope, chest pain, and dyspnea; profound hypoperfusion may occur. Accelerated idioventricular rhythm itself usually produces no symptoms, but the loss of atrial contraction and subsequent fall in cardiac output can produce hemodynamic deterioration.

Treatment With idioventricular rhythm producing hypoperfuson, drugs to increase the heart rate are appropriate. Atropine is recommended, although the likelihood of successful treatment is low. Cardiac pacing is often needed, starting via the transcutaneous route. In most cases of accelerated idioventricular rhythm, treatment is not necessary. If accelerated idioventricular rhythm is the only functioning pacemaker, **suppression with antiarrhythmic agents may lead to asystole**. If sustained accelerated idioventricular rhythm produces symptoms secondary to a decrease in cardiac output, pacing is recommended.

TABLE 18-10 ECG Features of Junctional Rhythm
Absence of normal (sinus-mediated) P waves with normal PR interval
Rare retrograde P wave (usually an inverted P wave and immediately adjacent to QRS complex, pre or post)
Narrow QRS complex
Regular rate
Ventricular rate
Between 40 and 60 beats/min for junctional rhythm
Between 60 and 100 beats/min for accelerated junctional rhythm
>100 beats/min for junctional tachycardia

ATRIOVENTRICULAR BLOCKS

First-degree AV block is characterized by a delay in AV conduction manifested by a prolonged PR interval. Second-degree AV block is characterized by intermittent AV conduction: some atrial impulses reach the ventricles, and others are blocked. Third-degree AV block is characterized by the complete blockage of atrial impulses to the ventricles.

AV blocks are divided into nodal and infranodal blocks because of the clinical significance and prognostic differences.[1] Nodal AV block (block within the AV node) is usually due to reversible depression of conduction, is often self-limited, and generally has a stable infranodal escape pacemaker pacing the ventricles. Infranodal blocks (block below the AV node) usually are due to organic disease of the His bundle or bundle branches; often the damage is irreversible. They generally have a slow and unstable ventricular escape rhythm pacing the ventricles, and they frequently have a bad prognosis.

FIRST-DEGREE ATRIOVENTRICULAR BLOCK

Description In first-degree AV block, each atrial impulse is conducted to the ventricles but less rapidly than normal, as noted by a prolonged PR interval, greater than 200 milliseconds. There is a P wave for each QRS complex; this association is consistent from one beat to the next (**Figure 18-13** and **Table 18-12**). The AV node is usually the site of conduction delay, although this block may occur at an infranodal level.

Clinical Significance First-degree AV block occasionally is found in normal hearts. Other common causes include increased vagal tone of any cause, medication toxicity, inferior myocardial infarction, and myocarditis. Patients with first-degree AV block without evidence of organic heart disease appear to have no difference in mortality compared with matched controls. In the setting of an acute coronary syndrome event, its appearance can indicate an increased chance of progression to complete heart block.

Treatment Usually none is required. Close monitoring in the patient with acute myocardial ischemia is indicated due to the potential for progression to complete heart block.

SECOND-DEGREE MOBITZ TYPE I (WENCKEBACH) ATRIOVENTRICULAR BLOCK

Description In second-degree Mobitz type I (Wenckebach) block, there is progressive prolongation of AV conduction (and the PR interval) until an atrial impulse is completely blocked; when an atrial impulse is blocked, no accompanying QRS complex is seen (**Figure 18-14** and **Table 18-13**). Conduction ratios indicate the ratio of atrial to ventricular depolarizations; for instance, a 4:3 ratio indicates that three of four atrial impulses are conducted into the ventricles. Usually, only one atrial

TABLE 18-11 ECG Features of Idioventricular Rhythm
Widened QRS complex
QRS complexes occurring regularly
No evidence of atrial activity: no P waves
Ventricular rate
30–50 beats/min for idioventricular rhythm
50–75 beats/min for accelerated idioventricular rhythm
Often in nonsustained fashion with runs of short duration: 3–30 consecutive beats

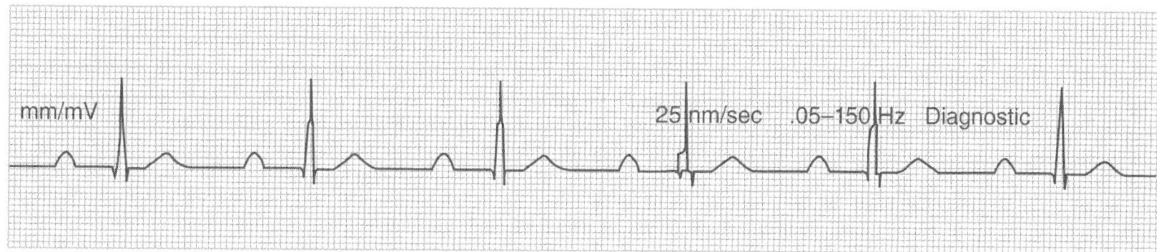

FIGURE 18-13. Sinus rhythm with first-degree atrioventricular block (PR interval, 300 milliseconds).

impulse is blocked. After the dropped beat, the AV conduction returns to normal, and the cycle usually repeats itself with the same conduction ratio (fixed ratio) or a different conduction ratio (variable ratio). This type of block almost always occurs at the level of the AV node and is often due to reversible depression of AV nodal conduction.

Second-degree type I, or Wenckebach, block occurs because each successive depolarization produces prolongation of the refractory period of the AV node. When the next atrial impulse comes upon the node, it is earlier in the relative refractory period, and conduction occurs more slowly relative to the previous stimulus. This process is progressive until an atrial impulse reaches the AV node during the absolute refractory period, and conduction is blocked altogether. The pause allows the AV node to recover, and the cycle repeats. This cyclic occurrence produces a pattern of "grouped beating" and is apparent over successive cycles (**Figure 18-15**).

Clinical Significance This block is often transient and usually associated with an inferior myocardial ischemia, medication toxicity, or myocarditis, or after cardiac surgery. It may occur when a normal AV node is exposed to very rapid atrial rates. This block can also be a normal variant, not indicative of acute or chronic heart disease.

Treatment Specific treatment is usually not necessary unless very slow ventricular rates produce signs of hypoperfusion, where most patients will respond to atropine. The need for an increased rate and increased perfusion must be balanced with the increased myocardial work in the acutely ischemic patient.

SECOND-DEGREE MOBITZ TYPE II ATRIOVENTRICULAR BLOCK

Description In second-degree Mobitz type II block, the PR interval remains constant across the rhythm strip, both before and after the nonconducted atrial beats (**Figure 18-16** and **Table 18-14**). Each P wave is associated with a QRS complex until a nonconducted atrial depolarization (i.e., P wave) is noted without accompanying QRS complex. Mobitz II blocks usually occur in the infranodal conducting system, often with coexistent fascicular or bundle-branch blocks, and the QRS complexes therefore are usually wide. Even if the QRS complexes are narrow, the block is generally in the infranodal system. High-grade AV block is noted when more than one consecutive P wave is not conducted (Figure 18-16C).

TABLE 18-12 ECG Features of First-Degree Atrioventricular Block

Consistent P wave to QRS complex relationship
Prolongation of PR interval >200 ms

When second-degree AV block occurs with a fixed conduction ratio of 2:1, it is not possible to differentiate between type I (Wenckebach) or type II block. If the QRS complex is wide, the block is more likely to be in the infranodal system. If the QRS complex is narrow, then the block is in the AV node or infranodal system with about equal incidence; it is recommended that the "worst case scenario" be assumed in such presentations and to consider the "untypable" second-degree AV block a type II blockage.

Clinical Significance Type II blocks imply structural damage to the infranodal conducting system, are usually permanent, and may progress suddenly to complete heart block, notably with concomitant acute myocardial ischemia.

Treatment Patients should have transcutaneous cardiac pacing pads applied in the ED in anticipation of possible need. Start emergent pacing when slow ventricular rates produce symptoms of hypoperfusion. Atropine can be tried but the effect is inconsistent.[2,3] Most patients, especially in the setting of acute myocardial ischemia, will require eventual transvenous cardiac pacing.

THIRD-DEGREE ATRIOVENTRICULAR BLOCK (COMPLETE HEART BLOCK)

Description In third-degree AV block, there is no AV conduction (**Figure 18-17** and **Table 18-15**). An escape pacemaker (manifested by the QRS complex) paces the ventricles at a rate slower than the atrial rate manifested by the P wave. When third-degree AV block occurs in the AV node, a junctional escape pacemaker takes over with a ventricular rate of 40 to 60 beats/min. The QRS complexes are narrow because the rhythm originates above the bifurcation of the bundle of His. When third-degree AV block occurs at the infranodal level, the ventricles are driven by a ventricular escape rhythm at a rate slower than 40 beats/min. Third-degree AV blocks at the His bundle level can have a narrow or wide QRS complex, whereas blocks in the bundle branches or elsewhere in the Purkinje system invariably have escape rhythms with wide QRS complexes.

TABLE 18-13 ECG Features of Second-Degree Mobitz Type I (Wenckebach's) Atrioventricular Block

Progressive prolongation of PR interval until an atrial impulse is completely blocked: a P wave without accompanying QRS complex
After the nonconducted beat, cycle repeats
Grouped beating

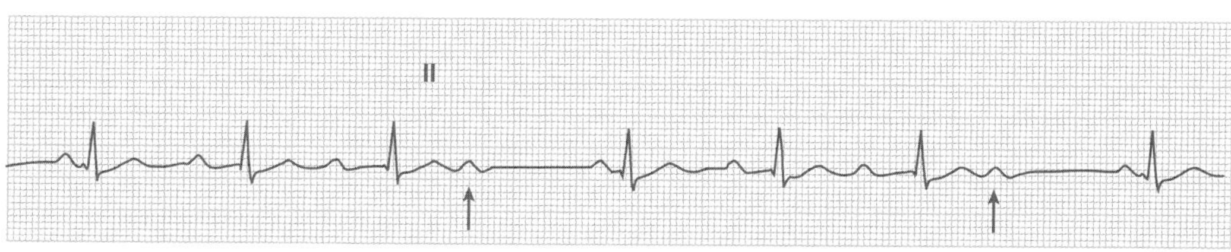

FIGURE 18-14. Second-degree, type I atrioventricular block. Note the nonconducted P waves (*arrows*).

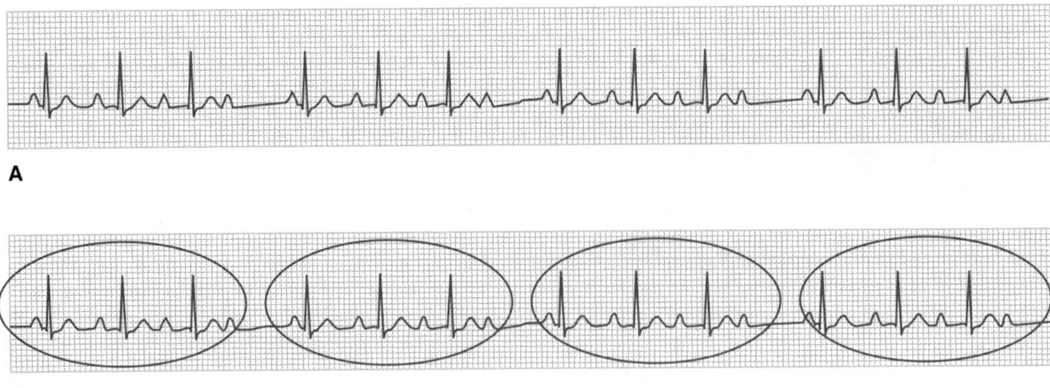

FIGURE 18-15. **A.** Second-degree, type I atrioventricular block. **B.** The cardiac rhythm strip illustrates the concept of grouped beating, or clustering of QRS complexes indicated by the ovals in the rhythm strip.

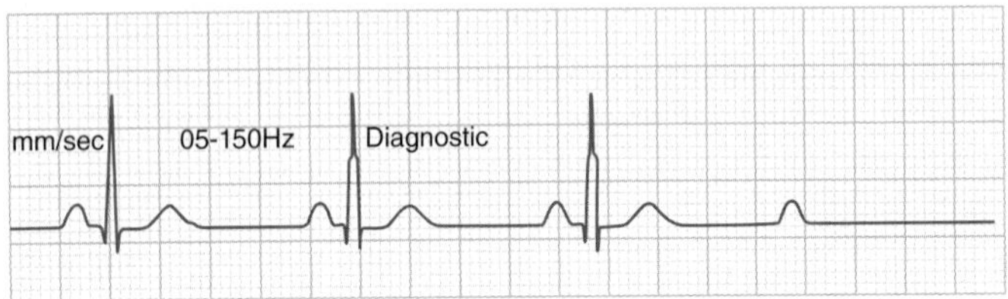

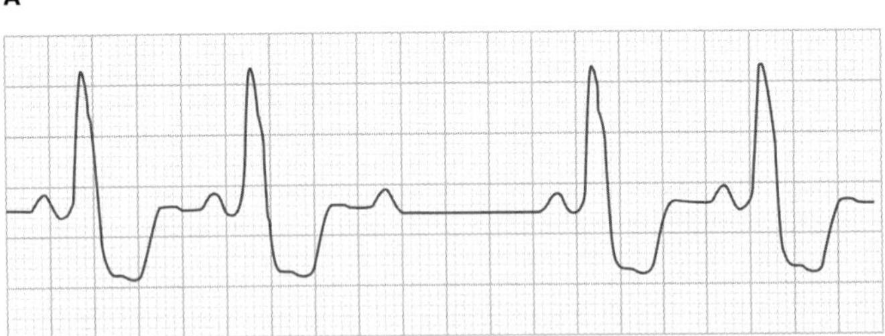

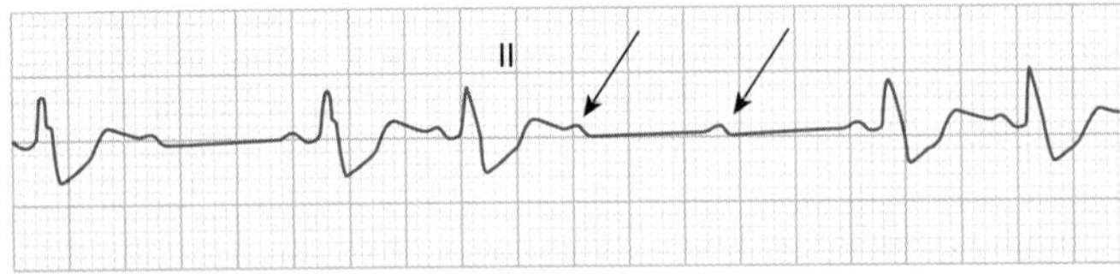

FIGURE 18-16. Three examples of second-degree, type II atrioventricular (AV) block: **(A)** with narrow QRS complex rhythm; **(B)** with wide QRS complex rhythm; and **(C)** with wide QRS complex rhythm and high-grade AV block indicated by two or more consecutive nonconducted P waves (*arrows*).

TABLE 18-14 ECG Features of Second-Degree Mobitz Type II Atrioventricular Block (AVB)

PR interval remains constant
Each P wave is associated with a QRS complex until a non-conducted atrial depolarization (i.e., P wave) is noted without accompanying QRS complex
QRS complexes are usually widened though a narrow complex is occasionally seen
High grade AVB is noted when more than one consecutive P wave is not conducted

TABLE 18-15 ECG Features of Third-Degree Atrioventricular Block (Complete Heart Block)

No association of P wave with QRS complexes
Atrial rate greater than ventricular rate
QRS complexes are usually widened; occasional narrow QRS complexes are seen
Ventricular rate is regular

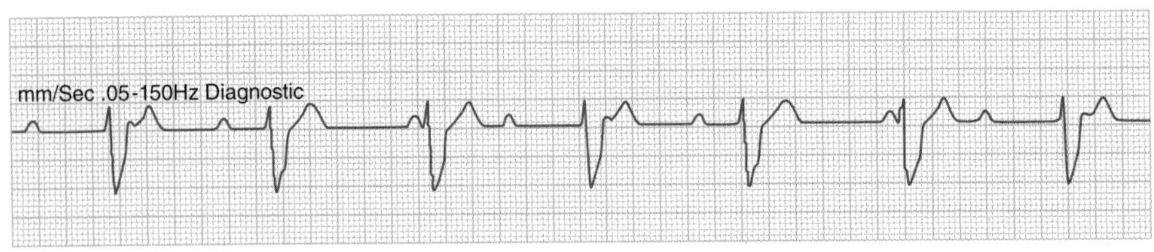

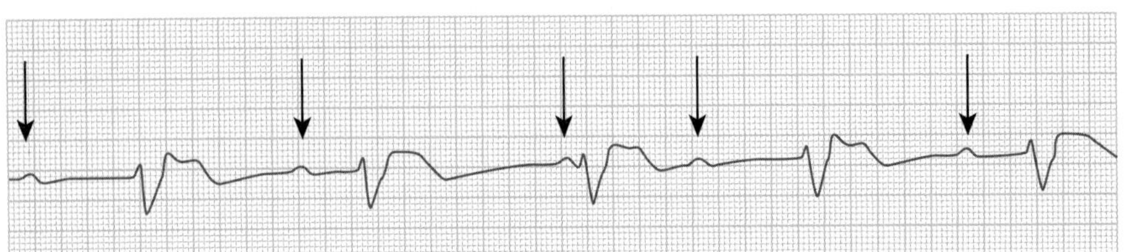

FIGURE 18-17. Two examples of third-degree atrioventricular block. Both have an atrial rate of 83 with ventricular escape rate of 50. Not all P waves are visible; some are hidden by the QRS complex or T wave.

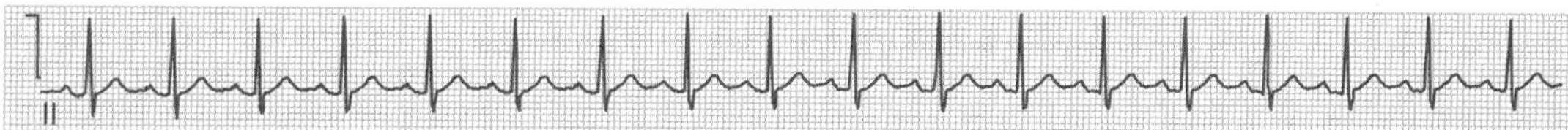

FIGURE 18-18. Sinus tachycardia at a rate of 110 beats/min.

Clinical Significance Nodal third-degree AV block (i.e., with a narrow QRS complex) develops in up to 8% of inferior acute myocardial infarction patients and may last for several days. Infranodal third-degree AV blocks (i.e., with a wide QRS complex) indicate structural damage to the infranodal conducting system, as seen with an extensive anterior acute myocardial infarction. The ventricular escape pacemaker is usually inadequate to maintain cardiac output and the patient is unstable, with periods of ventricular asystole. When third-degree block is seen in acute myocardial infarction, mortality is increased even with pacing.

Treatment Infrequently, patients with complete heart block will present with minimal to no symptomatology; these patients require monitoring and admission. Manage the symptomatic patient with either medication and/or pacing. Nodal blocks may respond to atropine; infranodal blocks are unlikely to respond to atropine or other medications that can enhance AV nodal conduction. Patients should have transcutaneous cardiac pacer pads applied in the ED. If there is no or incomplete response to atropine, use transcutaneous cardiac pacing, recognizing that transvenous pacing is eventually necessary in most patients.

NARROW-COMPLEX TACHYCARDIAS

SINUS TACHYCARDIA

Description Sinus tachycardia (**Figure 18-18** and **Table 18-16**), the most common narrow-complex tachycardia encountered in the ED, is defined as sinus rhythm with rates greater than 100 beats/min.

Clinical Significance Sinus tachycardia should be considered a reactive rhythm, occurring in response to a triggering condition. Generally, sinus tachycardia is a benign rhythm without any end-organ dysfunction.

Treatment Because sinus tachycardia is often a compensatory mechanism resulting from a physiologic stress, address the underlying cause, not the rhythm.

ATRIAL FIBRILLATION AND ATRIAL FLUTTER

Description After sinus tachycardia, atrial fibrillation is the next most frequent narrow-complex tachycardia encountered in the ED; atrial flutter is a less common dysrhythmia. Atrial fibrillation occurs when there are multiple, small areas of atrial myocardium continuously discharging and contracting.[20] There is no uniform atrial depolarization and contraction but, rather, only a quivering of the atrial chamber walls, resulting in less than effective ventricular filling and diminished cardiac output.

The ECG hallmarks of atrial fibrillation (**Figure 18-19** and **Table 18-17**) include the absence of discernible P waves and an irregularly irregular ventricular rhythm. With the chaotic atrial activity, distinct P waves are not noted; rather either a flat or chaotic baseline is seen, most prominent in lead V_1. The irregularly irregular ventricular rhythm results from the atrial chaos and the variable conduction of impulses through the AV node to the ventricle. The atrial rate in atrial fibrillation is often greater than 600 beats/min, whereas the ventricular rate is markedly lower due to the refractory period of the AV node; in atrial fibrillation where the AV node is unaffected by disease or medications,

TABLE 18-16 ECG Features of Sinus Tachycardia
Normal sinus P waves and PR interval
1:1 atrioventricular conduction
Atrial rate usually between 100 and 160 beats/min

TABLE 18-17 ECG Features of Atrial Fibrillation
Absence of discernible P waves with flat or chaotic isoelectric baseline
QRS complexes narrow unless preexisting bundle-branch block or preexcitation syndrome
Irregularly irregular ventricular rhythm

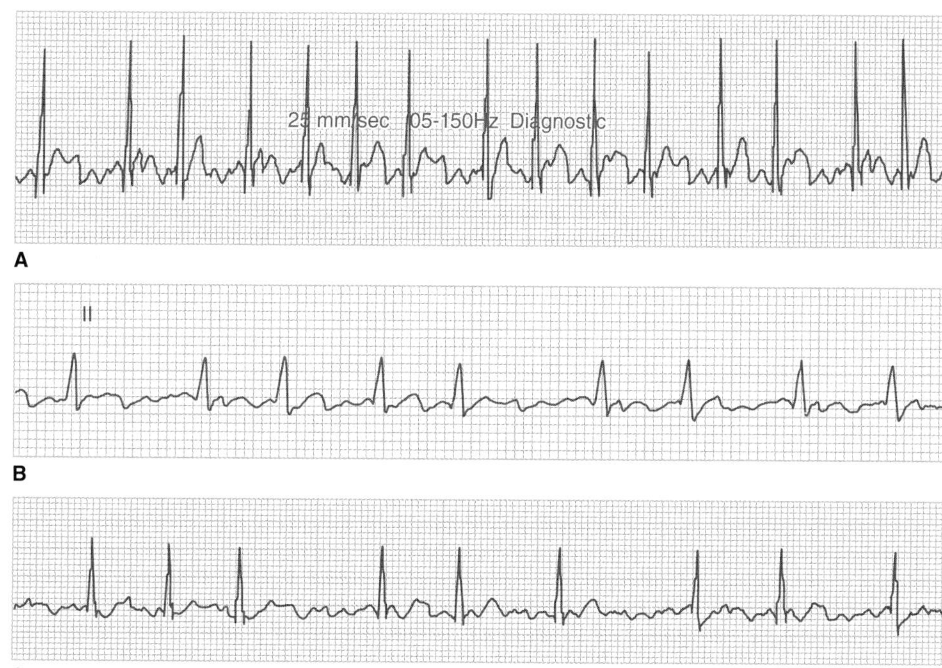

FIGURE 18-19. Three examples of atrial fibrillation with irregular ventricular response.

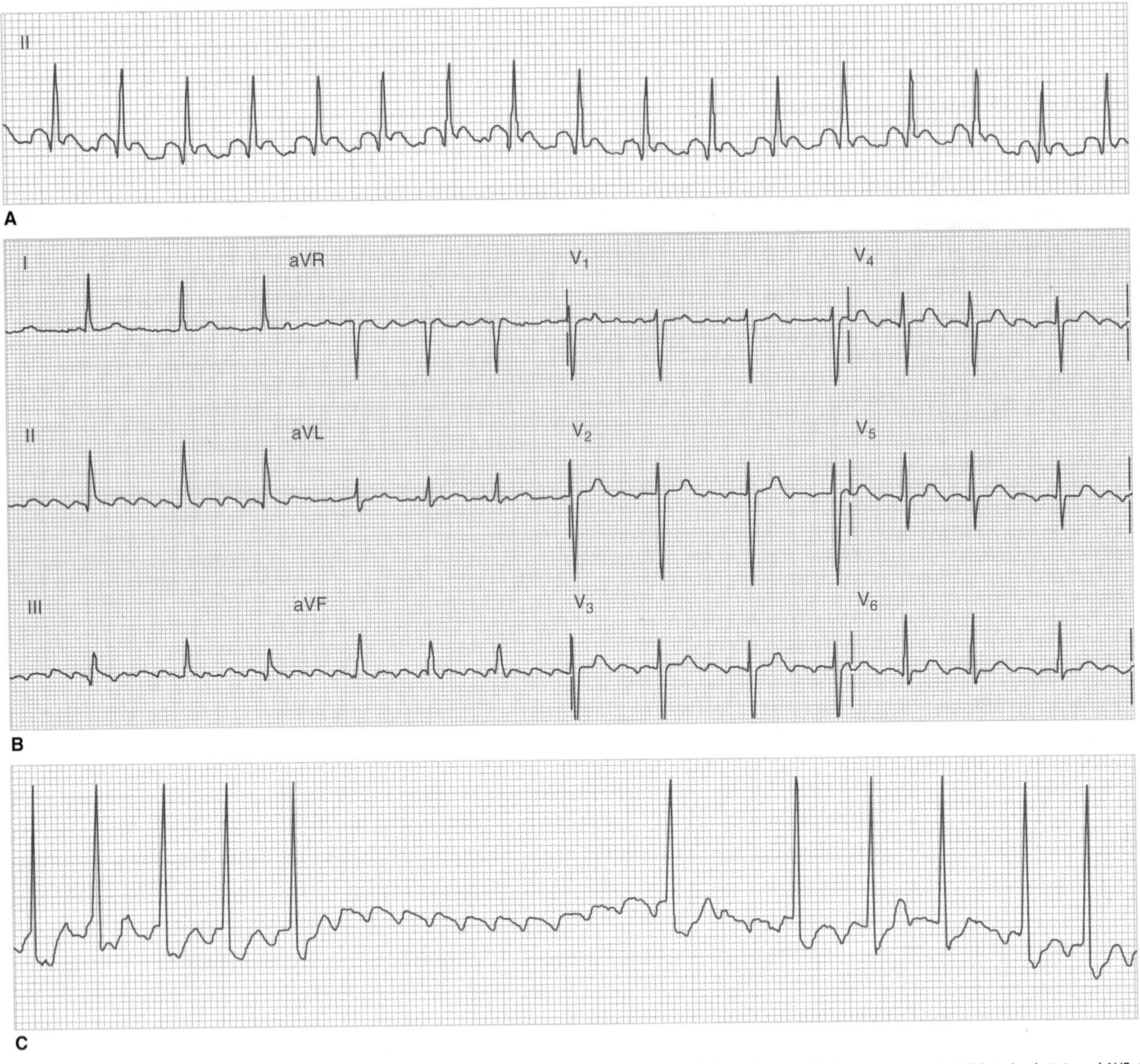

FIGURE 18-20. Atrial flutter. **A.** Regular, narrow-complex tachycardia at a ventricular rate of 155 beats/min. **B.** Atrial flutter with flutter waves most visible in leads 2, 3, and AVF. **C.** Atrial flutter response to carotid sinus massage inducing transient AV block and unmasking flutter waves.

the ventricular rate is typically 120 to 170 beats/min. Illnesses or medications may reduce AV node conduction and markedly slow ventricular response. A very rapid ventricular response (>200 beats/min) may be seen in patients with accessory or bypass tracts (discussed later in this chapter).

In contrast to atrial fibrillation, atrial flutter most often is a regular rhythm (**Figure 18-20** and **Table 18-18**); in rare cases, it can be irregular. P waves are present and of a single morphology, typically a downward deflection, called *flutter waves* resembling a saw blade with a "sawtooth" pattern, best seen in the inferior ECG leads and lead V_1. Most commonly, the atrial rate is regular, classically around 300 beats/min, varying between 250 and 350 beats/min. The ventricular rhythm is frequently regular and is a function of the AV block. AV ratios of 2:1 are common and produce a ventricular rate around 150 beats/min, whereas a 3:1 AV ratio will result in a ventricular rate of 100 beats/min. Although the degree of AV conduction is often fixed, it may also be variable and create an irregular ventricular response. **A regular narrow-complex tachycardia at an approximate rate of 150 beats/min strongly suggests atrial flutter with 2:1 conduction.**

TABLE 18-18 ECG Features of Atrial Flutter
Identifiable P waves
Single morphology
Negative amplitude ("flutter waves" in "sawtooth pattern") best seen in inferior ECG leads and V1
Atrial rate is regular, usually at 300 beats/min
QRS complexes narrow unless preexisting bundle-branch block
Ventricular rate regular although occasional irregularity can be seen
Ventricular rate often 150 beats/min

Clinical Significance Atrial fibrillation is usually associated with ischemic or valvular heart disease; less common causes include congestive cardiomyopathy, myocarditis, alcohol binge ("holiday heart"), thyrotoxicosis, and blunt chest trauma.[20,21] Left atrial enlargement is a common feature of patients with chronic atrial fibrillation. Atrial fibrillation can be paroxysmal (lasting less than 7 days, terminating either spontaneously or with treatment), persistent (sustained longer than 7 days or requiring treatment to terminate), long-standing persistent (lasting continuously longer than 1 year), or permanent (long-standing where a decision has been made not to try to restore normal sinus rhythm).[20]

New or recent onset is applied to symptomatic patients presenting to the ED without a prior history of atrial fibrillation.

The clinical consequences of atrial fibrillation include loss of atrial contraction, potential for rapid ventricular rates, and risk of arterial embolism. In patients with compromised cardiac function, left atrial contraction contributes significantly to left ventricular filling, so the loss of effective atrial contraction, as in atrial fibrillation, may produce heart failure in these patients. A rapid ventricular rate can impact ventricular filling as well as coronary and systemic perfusion. Atrial fibrillation increases the risk of venous and atrial thrombosis, with potential for pulmonary and systemic arterial embolism. If an atrial thrombus has formed, conversion from atrial fibrillation to sinus rhythm can propel a portion of the thrombosis out into the systemic circulation, and this risk increases with duration of the dysrhythmia. Observational studies note that conversion from new-onset atrial fibrillation that has been present for 12 hours or less carries a 0.3% risk of arterial embolism, whereas that risk is about 1% for durations of 12 to 48 hours before conversion.[22] For patients with heart failure and diabetes mellitus, conversion from new-onset (duration <48 hours) atrial fibrillation carries a risk of thromboembolic events as high as 9.8%.[23] Conversely, the incidence of thromboembolic events is 0.2% in patients age <60 years and no heart failure.[23] After a duration of >48 hours, the risk of conversion-induced thromboembolic events is increased across all patient groups and a period of anticoagulation is recommended prior to conversion.[20,24]

Treatment Treatment of atrial fibrillation in the ED involves three issues: ventricular rate control, rhythm conversion, and anticoagulation to prevent arterial embolism.[24-26] Treatment varies according to patient stability, duration of symptoms, and chronicity of atrial fibrillation (paroxysmal, persistent, or permanent). Review prior records to identify past episodes or treatment for atrial fibrillation. For new-onset atrial fibrillation, consider checking thyroid function.[27] For patients on warfarin, check the prothrombin time. Calculate either the $CHADS_2$ or CHA_2DS_2-VASc score to risk-stratify the potential for future arterial embolic complications; a $CHADS_2$ score of 0 or a CHA_2DS_2-VASc score of 0 or 1 identify low-risk patients (**Table 18-19**).[20,21]

For patients with paroxysmal atrial fibrillation or acute medical conditions producing atrial fibrillation, a period of observation and treatment in the ED is appropriate as the atrial fibrillation may spontaneously convert.[12,28] Up to 70% of otherwise healthy ED patients evaluated for acute-onset atrial fibrillation will spontaneously convert within 48 to 72 hours.[29] Ventricular rate control may help control symptoms until conversion. Also, it is more difficult to achieve rate or rhythm control of atrial fibrillation in patients with acute underlying medical illness, and such attempts are associated with an increased incidence of adverse events.[30]

For patients with recent-onset atrial fibrillation and a rapid ventricular response that is producing hypotension, myocardial ischemia, or pulmonary edema, treat with urgent electrical cardioversion.[20,24,25,31] When possible, first determine if the patient has long-standing atrial fibrillation because electrical cardioversion is not likely to succeed, and instead, initiate ventricular rate control treatment. If the patient is at increased risk for embolic complications ($CHADS_2$ or CHA_2DS_2-VASc scores ≥1, mechanical heart value, or rheumatic valvular disease), consider anticoagulation with heparin before or immediately after electrical cardioversion and continue that as a bridge to oral anticoagulants.[31]

TABLE 18-19 $CHADS_2$ and CHA_2DS_2-VASc scores

Criteria	$CHADS_2$	CHA_2DS_2-VASc
Congestive heart failure	1	1
Hypertension	1	1
Age ≥75 y	1	2
Diabetes mellitus	1	1
Stroke, TIA, or thromboembolism	2	2
Vascular disease (CAD, PAD)	–	1
Age 65–74 y	–	1
Sex (female)	–	1
Range	0–6	0–9

Abbreviations: CAD = coronary artery disease; PAD = peripheral artery disease; TIA = transient ischemic attack.

TABLE 18-20 ED Management of New-Onset Atrial Fibrillation in Stable Patients*

Clinical Circumstance	Treatment	Follow-Up Therapy
Duration <48 h Low-risk for embolism†	Chemical or electrical cardioversion to sinus rhythm	If successful conversion, no antithrombotic therapy
Duration <48 h Low-risk for embolism†	Ventricular rate control <100 beats/min	No antithrombotic therapy Close follow-up
Duration >48 h	Ventricular rate control <100 beats/min	Therapeutic anticoagulation for 3–4 wk
High-risk for embolic complications‡	Ventricular rate control <100 beats/min	Therapeutic anticoagulation for 3–4 wk

*See Table 18-2 for drug treatment.

†Low risk = $CHADS_2$ score of 0 or a CHA_2DS_2-VASc score of 0 or 1.

‡High risk = $CHADS_2$ score ≥1 or a CHA_2DS_2-VASc score ≥2.

For stable low-risk patients in the ED with new-onset atrial fibrillation, either rate-control or rhythm-conversion strategies are appropriate (**Table 18-20**).[20,24,25] The rate-control approach consists of initiating medications that block the AV node to control the ventricular response, initiating oral anticoagulants to prevent thromboembolism (if appropriate), and re-evaluation after 3 to 4 weeks for elective cardioversion. The rhythm-conversion approach uses electrical or pharmacologic methods to convert the patient back into sinus rhythm while in the ED.

Control of the ventricular response is done using a calcium channel blocker (diltiazem) or β-blockers (metoprolol and esmolol) with limited data favoring more effective acute rate control with diltiazem.[32] If β-blockers or calcium channel blockers are ineffective, intravenous procainamide or amiodarone is an option to slow the ventricular response. The goal for rate control is a ventricular rate of <100 beats/min at rest.[25]

Electrical cardioversion using 150 to 200 J can terminate atrial fibrillation allowing for sinus rhythm to resume.[24,31] Conversion to and retention of sinus rhythm is more likely when atrial fibrillation is of short duration (<48 hours) and the atria are not greatly dilated. Observational analysis also notes that administration of rate-control or rhythm-conversion medications prior to electrical cardioversion attempts is associated with a reduced rate of successful conversion to sinus rhythm.[33] Although ED electrical cardioversion is effective in many atrial fibrillation patients[34] and observational studies indicate shorter ED length of stay,[26] there has been mixed acceptance of this approach.[35-37] As noted above, a significant portion of patients with new-onset atrial fibrillation will spontaneously convert to sinus rhythm within 24 hours of onset and evaluation.[12,28,29,38,39] This rate of spontaneous conversion coupled with the results of atrial fibrillation trials demonstrating that rate-control is similar to rhythm-control in terms of several key endpoints indicates no proven benefit for conversion of all new atrial fibrillation patients to sinus rhythm while in the ED.[24,38,39] The patient with new-onset atrial fibrillation who is stable can certainly be managed with rate-control alone, either as an inpatient or outpatient depending overall clinical condition.

The antiarrhythmics procainamide, ibutilide, flecainide, propafenone, and vernakalant can chemically convert atrial fibrillation to sinus rhythm.[24,40,41] Of the five, ibutilide has the highest consistent success rate for conversion. Ibutilide should not be given in the presence of hypokalemia, prolonged QT interval, or history of heart failure, as torsade de pointes may be initiated. This risk of torsade de pointes persists for 4 to 6 hours after the ibutilide is given. Pharmacologic conversion therapy is best avoided if duration is unknown or greater than 48 hours, allowing for heart clot detection and anticoagulation prior to any attempt.

Patients with recurrent paroxysmal atrial fibrillation are sometimes given oral medications (usually flecainide or propafenone) to be taken at the onset of the dysrhythmia; this "pill in a pocket" approach is successful in selected outpatients.[24] This approach should only be used in patients with paroxysmal episodes after SA or AV node dysfunction,

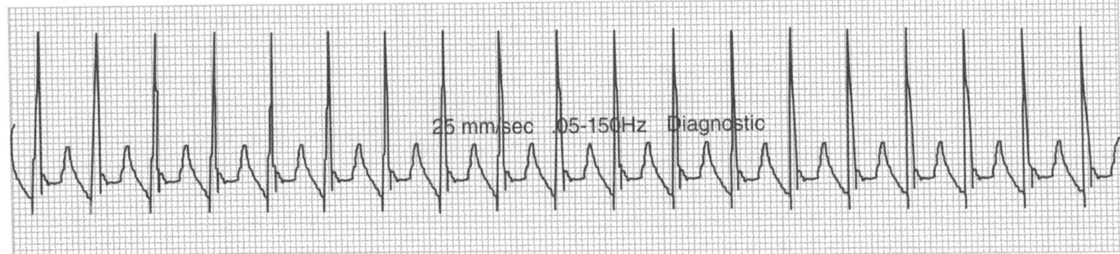

FIGURE 18-21. Paroxysmal supraventricular tachycardia.

conduction disturbance (bundle branch block, Brugada syndrome), and structural heart disease have been excluded.[2]

Atrial flutter is managed in the same fashion as atrial fibrillation: either rhythm conversion or ventricular rate-control with β-blockers or calcium channel blockers.[24] Atrial flutter is very responsive to electrical cardioversion; as little as 25 to 50 J is often effective. In general, patients in atrial flutter tend to better tolerate the dysrhythmia hemodynamically than patients with atrial fibrillation. This "hemodynamic toleration" results from the organized atrial contraction seen with atrial flutter, as opposed to the lack of organized atrial contraction with atrial fibrillation. Despite organized atrial activity, there is a risk of arterial embolism with atrial flutter,[42] and corresponding recommendations for anticoagulation are based on the same criteria used for atrial fibrillation.[25]

Patients with chronic atrial fibrillation and planned cardioversion should be anticoagulated for 3 to 4 weeks, assuming clinical stability allows such an approach.[20] Patients with permanent atrial fibrillation are at increased risk for embolic stroke, and oral anticoagulation can reduce that occurrence. The benefits of oral anticoagulation are counterbalanced by the potential adverse effects, usually hemorrhagic events. Clinical scoring tools, such as the CHA_2DS_2-VASc, can be used to guide the decision to initiate long-term oral anticoagulation therapy in atrial fibrillation patients.[20,21]

PAROXYSMAL SUPRAVENTRICULAR TACHYCARDIA

Description Paroxysmal supraventricular tachycardia most frequently results from sustained reentry occurring with the AV node, with an ectopic atrial focus accounting for the remaining 15% to 20%. In paroxysmal supraventricular tachycardia (**Figure 18-21** and **Table 18-21**), the QRS complex is of normal width, rapid, and regular. P waves are "buried" within the QRS complex in about 70% of cases. In the others, a P wave (so-called "retrograde" P wave) is found immediately adjacent before, during, or after the QRS complex without a measurable PR interval.

Clinical Significance Paroxysmal supraventricular tachycardia is seen more frequently in females, with a peak in the late teenage and young adult years. The majority of patients are without active cardiovascular disease.[43] Patients may be able to describe the abrupt onset of this reentrant dysrhythmia and also note when it self-terminates. Palpitations, lightheadedness, and dyspnea are common symptoms.

Treatment If applied early in the dysrhythmia course, vagal maneuvers are often effective (Table 18-3).[10,11] Attention to technique is important to maximize success rate. If there is no response to vagal maneuvers, adenosine IV is recommended to convert to sinus rhythm.[9] It is the rare patient who requires β-blocker or calcium channel blocker. In patients with recalcitrant paroxysmal supraventricular tachycardia or who are unstable, use electrical cardioversion to convert the dysrhythmia.

TABLE 18-21 ECG Features of Paroxysmal Supraventricular Tachycardia
Absence of normal (sinus-mediated) P waves with normal PR interval
Rare retrograde P wave (usually inverted P wave and immediately adjacent to QRS complex, pre or post)
Narrow QRS complex, usually <100 ms in duration
Ventricular rate usually 170–180 beats/min; the rate can range from as low as 130 beats/min to as high as 300 beats/min

MULTIFOCAL ATRIAL TACHYCARDIA

Description Multifocal atrial tachycardia is an irregular rhythm resulting from at least three different atrial ectopic foci competing to pace the heart. The electrocardiographic characteristics (**Figure 18-22** and **Table 18-22**) require at least three distinct P-wave morphologies. Due to irregularity and the chaotic appearance of atrial depolarization, multifocal atrial tachycardia is often confused with atrial fibrillation or atrial flutter.

Clinical Significance Multifocal atrial tachycardia is found most often in elderly patients with decompensated chronic lung disease, but may also complicate heart failure or sepsis.

Treatment Treatment is directed toward the underlying disorder. With decompensated lung disease, oxygen and bronchodilators improve pulmonary function and arterial oxygenation and decrease atrial ectopy. Antidysrhythmic treatment is not indicated, and cardioversion has no effect.

WIDE-COMPLEX TACHYDYSRHYTHMIAS

Wide-complex tachydysrhythmias are defined as a rhythm with a QRS complex duration greater than 120 milliseconds and a rate over 100 beats/min. Both ventricular tachycardia and supraventricular tachydysrhythmias with aberrant ventricular conduction present as wide-complex tachydysrhythmias (**Figure 18-23**).[5]

Traditional teaching, derived largely from coronary care units and electrophysiology laboratories, presents that 80% of wide-complex tachycardias are ventricular tachycardia.[44] However, in the ED, there is a range of pathophysiologic conditions that can produce delayed ventricular depolarization that when combined with a sinus tachycardia induced by acute illness result in a wide-complex tachycardia.[7] The conduction abnormality can be the result of a bundle-branch block (new-onset, preexisting, or rate-related), metabolic abnormality (e.g., hyperkalemia), adverse medication effect (e.g., sodium channel blockade), or ventricular preexcitation syndrome. All supraventricular tachycardias can present as a wide-complex tachycardia if intraventricular conduction is abnormal. In addition, two tachydysrhythmias seen in WPW syndrome will present with a widened QRS complex: the antidromic version of the AV nodal reentrant tachycardia and atrial fibrillation or flutter with ventricular depolarization predominantly or exclusively via the accessory tract.

VENTRICULAR TACHYCARDIA

Description Ventricular tachycardia is the occurrence of three or more consecutive depolarizations from a ventricular ectopic pacemaker at a rate faster than 100 beats/min.[8] Ventricular tachycardia can occur in a nonsustained manner,[45] with short episodes, lasting several beats, with spontaneous termination, or it can occur in a sustained fashion, with longer episodes that typically require treatment.[8] Ventricular tachycardia

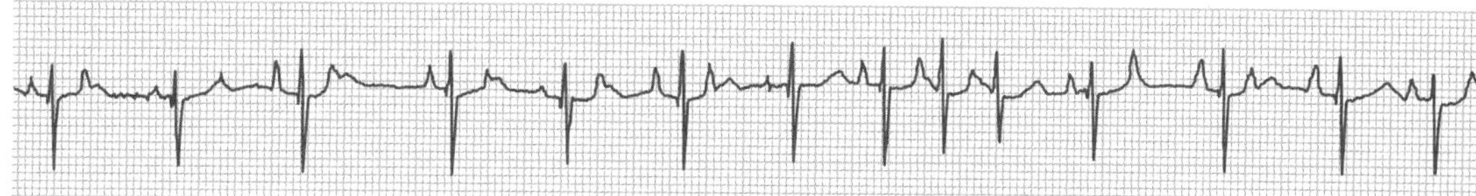

FIGURE 18-22. Multifocal atrial tachycardia. Note multiple P-wave morphologies with irregular tachycardia rhythm.

can be further characterized according to hemodynamic effect (stable vs unstable), morphology (monomorphic vs polymorphic), or clinical presentation (perfusing vs pulseless as during cardiac arrest).

The electrocardiographic features (**Figure 18-24** and **Table 18-23**) vary between the monomorphic and polymorphic varieties. Morphologic ventricular tachycardia is the most commonly encountered form of ventricular tachycardia, accounting for about 70% of cases, and is usually very regular with rates most often in the 140 to 180 beats/min range. Medications, such as amiodarone, may slow the rate of ventricular tachycardia; such patients may present with ventricular rates of 110 to 130 beats/min. On rare occasions, monomorphic ventricular tachycardia may present with an irregular rhythm, but only minimally irregular as compared to an aberrantly conducted atrial fibrillation, which ordinarily manifests marked irregularity.

TABLE 18-22 ECG Features of Multifocal Atrial Tachycardia

At least 3 distinct P-wave morphologies in a single ECG lead
No consistent P to P, PR, or R to R intervals
Irregularly irregular rhythm with rates usually 100–180 beats/min
Normal QRS complex unless preexisting bundle-branch blocks
Frequently confused with atrial fibrillation or flutter

Polymorphic ventricular tachycardia has varying QRS morphology in any single ECG lead (**Figure 18-25** and Table 18-23). Variations in both the RR interval and electrical axis are also features of this form of ventricular tachycardia. Torsade de pointes, a specific subtype of polymorphic ventricular tachycardia, occurs in the setting of delayed myocardial repolarization manifested on the sinus rhythm ECG by a prolongation of the QT interval.[46] The French term *torsade de pointes* means "twisting of the points" and describes the appearance of the QRS complex as it varies in appearance (Figure 18-25B).

Clinical Significance Ventricular tachycardia is rare in patients without underlying heart disease.[5] The most common causes of ventricular tachycardia are chronic ischemic heart disease and acute myocardial infarction, comprising about 50% of all cases of symptomatic ventricular tachycardia. Less common causes of ventricular tachycardia include dilated or hypertrophic cardiomyopathy, valvular heart disease (including mitral valve prolapse), inherited ion channel abnormalities, and drug toxicity. Hypoxia,

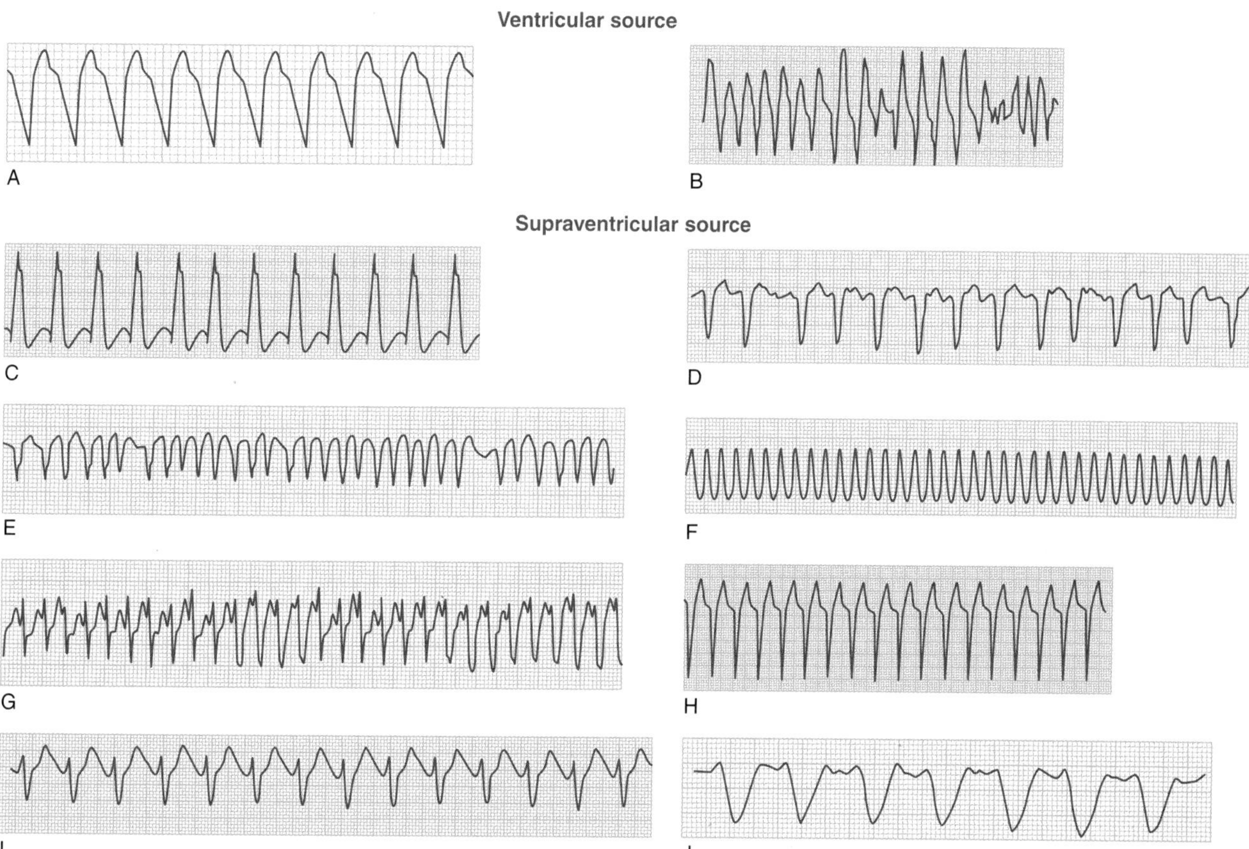

FIGURE 18-23. Wide complex tachydysrhythmias. **A.** Ventricular tachycardia (monomorphic). **B.** Ventricular tachycardia (polymorphic). **C.** Sinus tachycardia with bundle-branch block. **D.** Atrial fibrillation with preexisting bundle-branch block. **E.** Preexcited atrial fibrillation in the Wolff-Parkinson-White syndrome. **F.** Atrioventricular reentrant tachycardia in the Wolff-Parkinson-White syndrome. **G.** Paroxysmal supraventricular tachycardia with rate-related bundle-branch block in an infant. **H.** Paroxysmal supraventricular tachycardia with fixed (preexisting) bundle branch block. **I.** Sodium channel blocker toxicity with wide-complex tachycardia. **J.** Wide-complex tachycardia in patient with severe hyperkalemia.

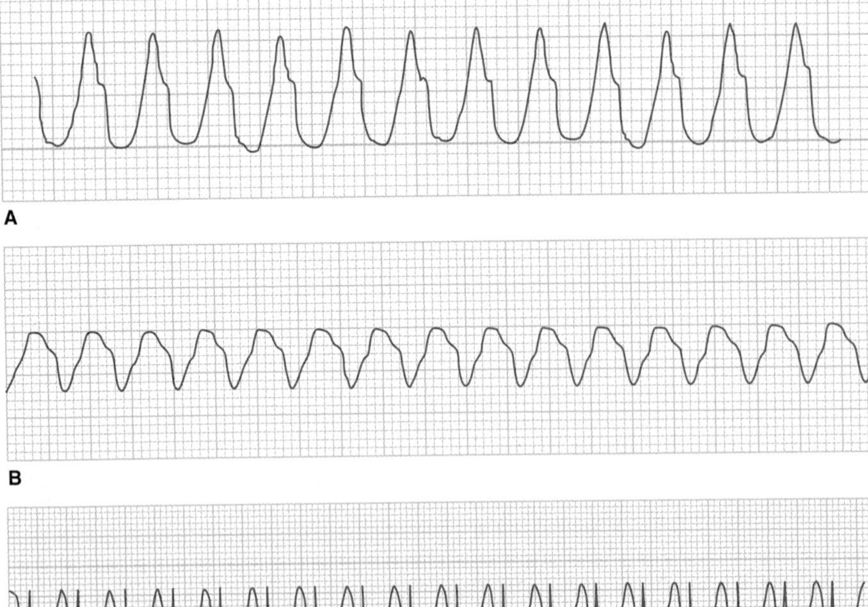

FIGURE 18-24. Three examples of monomorphic ventricular tachycardia. **A.** Ventricular tachycardia with a rate of 270 beats/min. **B.** Ventricular tachycardia with a rate of 220 beats/min. **C.** Ventricular tachycardia with a rate of 180 beats/min.

TABLE 18-23 ECG Features of Monomorphic and Polymorphic Ventricular Tachycardia

Monomorphic
No P waves associated with QRS complex, occasional dissociated P wave
Rapid and regular rhythm
Rate usually 140–180 beats/min (range, 120–300 beats/min)
Widened QRS complex >100–120 ms with consistent beat-to-beat morphology
Polymorphic
No P waves associated with QRS complex; may have occasional dissociated P wave
Rapid and irregular rhythm
Rate 140–180 bpm (range, 120–300 beats/min)
Widened QRS complex >100–120 ms with inconsistent beat-to-beat morphology

alkalosis, and electrolyte abnormalities, especially hyperkalemia, exacerbate the propensity for ventricular ectopy and tachycardia.

Torsade de pointes occurs when repolarization is delayed, and cardiac after-potentials can initiate this form of polymorphic ventricular tachycardia. Delayed repolarization is seen in inherited (congenital long QT syndrome) and acquired (primarily drug toxicity) circumstances.[46] Torsade de pointes often occurs in bursts of up to 30 cycles before spontaneously stopping. Sustained torsade de pointes is uncommon and can potentially degenerate into ventricular fibrillation.

It is a misconception that patients with ventricular tachycardia are clinically unstable. Ventricular tachycardia cannot be reliably differentiated from supraventricular tachycardia with aberrant

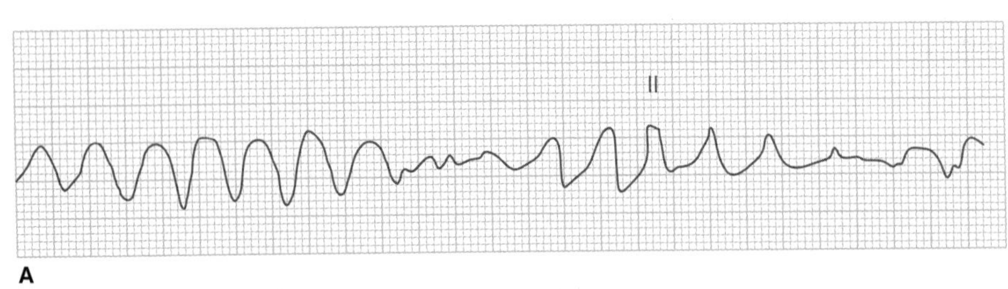

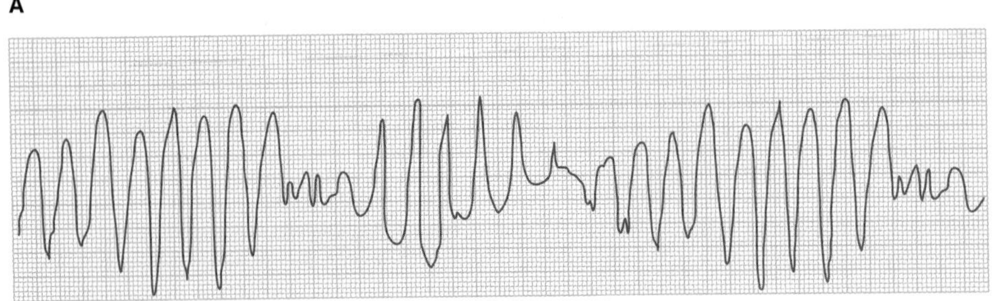

FIGURE 18-25. Two examples of polymorphic ventricular tachycardia. **A.** Polymorphic ventricular tachycardia. **B.** Polymorphic ventricular tachycardia of the torsade de pointes subtype, with the characteristic pattern of progressively changing QRS complex amplitude and direction.

conduction on the basis of clinical symptoms or vital signs. Differentiation using the 12-lead ECG can be challenging and, at times, impossible (see discussion in next section).

Treatment The management of ventricular tachycardia is based on the patient's clinical stability. The most extreme form of instability is cardiac arrest; these patients should receive prompt electrical defibrillation, chest compressions, and other advanced life support measures. Patients with a pulse but compromised by the ventricular tachycardia should undergo electrical cardioversion coupled with administration of a procedural analgesia and sedation if clinical status allows time to administer. In the stable patient, pharmacologic agents are first-line therapy.[47]

Drug therapy for ventricular tachycardia includes procainamide, amiodarone, lidocaine, and magnesium. Procainamide is an effective agent for stable ventricular tachycardia in patients with preserved left ventricular dysfunction.[14] Based on limited human comparative studies, procainamide is superior to lidocaine for converting patients with stable ventricular tachycardia.[14] The primary disadvantage of procainamide is the relatively slow dosing because rapid infusions can cause hypotension.

For patients with tenuous hemodynamic status, amiodarone is the antiarrhythmic of choice with lidocaine as the less effective alternative. If pharmacologic interventions are unsuccessful, then sedation-assisted electrical (synchronized) cardioversion is the next option.

Magnesium is primarily used as an antiarrhythmic agent in patients with known hypomagnesemia, QT interval prolongation, polymorphic ventricular tachycardia, or torsade de pointes.[48] Case reports describe the benefits of isoproterenol or phenytoin in torsade de pointes, but controlled studies are lacking.[49-51] Definitive treatment of torsade de pointes is ventricular pacing at a rate necessary to prevent the bursts of polymorphous ventricular tachycardia. Pacing is continued until the cause of QT prolongation (drug toxicity, electrolyte abnormality) is ameliorated.

UNDIFFERENTIATED WIDE-COMPLEX TACHYCARDIA

Description A regular, wide-complex tachycardia can be either of ventricular origin (ventricular tachycardia) or due to a supraventricular tachycardia with aberrant conduction of the electrical impulse through the ventricles. The differentiation between ectopic beats of ventricular origin and those of aberrantly conducted supraventricular origin can be difficult, more so in sustained tachycardias with widened QRS complexes.

Clinical Features Traditional teaching emphasizes five electrocardiographic features as helpful in differentiating ventricular tachycardia from supraventricular tachycardia with aberrant conduction: irregularity, AV dissociation, fusion and capture beats, QRS duration, and QRS complex concordance (**Figure 18-26**).[5,7] Ventricular tachycardia is usually very regular; if irregular, the degree of irregularity is minimal (Figures 18-23A and 18-26C). Marked irregularity is strongly suggestive of atrial fibrillation with bundle-branch block; of course, torsade de pointes is also irregular, but the changing polarity of the QRS complex is usually quite apparent.

AV dissociation, where the atria and ventricles have separate independent pacemakers (Figure 18-26C), if noted, is strongly suggestive of ventricular tachycardia. In cases of ventricular tachycardia without retrograde conduction to the atria, the SA node continues to initiate atrial depolarization. Because atrial depolarization is completely independent of ventricular activity, the resulting P waves will be dissociated from the QRS complexes. AV dissociation is not common; it is noted in only approximately 10% of ventricular tachycardia patients.

Capture and fusion beats (Figure 18-26D) are potentially useful and suggest ventricular tachycardia. In the patient with ventricular tachycardia, an independent atrial impulse may occasionally cause ventricular depolarization via the normal conducting system; such a supraventricular impulse, if conducted and able to trigger a depolarization within the ventricle, will result in a different QRS complex morphology—different than the other wide QRS complex beats. If the resulting QRS complex occurs earlier than expected and is narrow, the complex

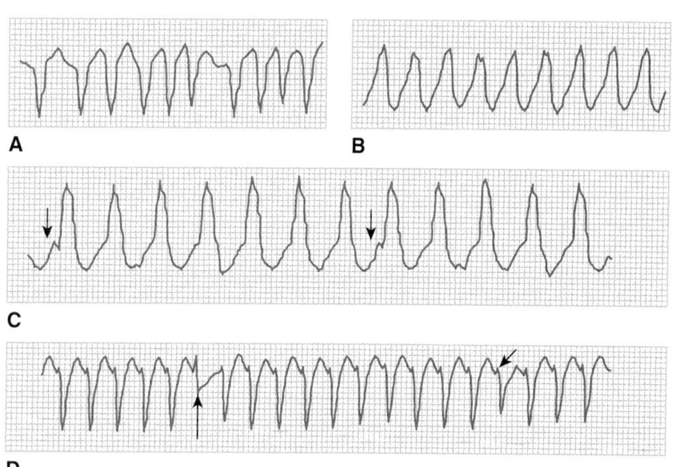

FIGURE 18-26. ECG considerations in the distinction of supraventricular tachycardia with aberrant ventricular conduction from ventricular tachycardia. **A.** Irregular rhythm in Wolff-Parkinson-White–related atrial fibrillation. **B.** Regular rhythm in ventricular tachycardia. **C.** Atrioventricular dissociation in ventricular tachycardia. The *arrows* indicate P waves, indicative of atrioventricular dissociation, which is strongly suggestive of ventricular tachycardia. **D.** Capture (*large arrow*) and fusion (*small arrow*) beats that are indicative of ventricular tachycardia.

is called a capture beat; the supraventricular impulse electrically captures the ventricle, producing a narrow complex. The presence of capture beats strongly supports a diagnosis of ventricular tachycardia. Fusion beats occur when a sinus beat conducts to the ventricles via the AV node and joins, or fuses, with a ventricular beat originating from the abnormal ectopic focus. These two electrical "beats" combine, resulting in a QRS complex of intermediate width and differing morphology when compared to the other beats of ventricular tachycardia. As with capture beats, the presence of fusion beats is strongly suggestive of ventricular tachycardia. Fusion and capture beats occur infrequently and are seen in fewer than 10% of patients with ventricular tachycardia.

Ventricular tachycardia usually has a wider QRS complex than does supraventricular tachycardia with aberrancy, so extreme QRS durations >160 milliseconds argue in favor of ventricular tachycardia. Concordance describes that the polarity of the QRS complexes is consistent across the precordium, either all negative or positive from leads V_1 to V_6. Negative concordance, with all the precordial QRS complexes having a negative or downward deflection, suggests ventricular tachycardia.

In addition to these traditional characteristic, features of the QRS complex on the 12-lead ECG have been analyzed as differentiators of ventricular tachycardia versus supraventricular tachycardia with aberrancy. Since 1991, five different algorithms have been created, studied, and compared (**Table 18-24**).[52-56] The approach varies: the Brugada, Griffith, and Lau approaches use multiple leads and criteria; the Vereckei algorithm uses only lead aVR, although with four criteria; and the Pava algorithm only uses lead II and only one criterion. The Griffith approach is reversed from the other four; it assumes that the wide-complex tachycardia is ventricular in origin and then looks for evidence that favors supraventricular with aberrancy. Published comparisons are mixed regarding the sensitivity and specificity of these different algorithms, and neither has proven consistently superior.[57-61] Simplicity favors the Vereckei or Pava approaches.

Treatment **When in doubt, it is safer to assume a new and symptomatic wide-complex tachycardia is ventricular in origin than the converse. Maintain a focus on treating the entire patient, not solely the ECG.** If rapid treatment is needed, use IV amiodarone. In stable patients, response to adenosine can be helpful in differentiating ventricular from supraventricular wide-complex tachycardias.[62] Not all wide-complex tachycardias require antiarrhythmic agents or urgent electrical therapy. Treatment of the causative syndrome is often the most appropriate action.

TABLE 18-24 Methods for Wide-Complex Tachycardia Differentiation

Author and Year	Favors Ventricular Tachycardia (VT)	Favors Supraventricular Tachycardia with Aberrant Conduction (SVTAC)
Brugada, 1991[52]	VT diagnosed if, analyzed in sequence, any one of these 4 criteria is present: Absence of RS complexes in all precordial leads R to S interval >100 ms in one or more precordial leads AV dissociation Morphologic criteria for VT in leads V_1 and V_6 (V_1: monophasic R, qR, QS, or RS; and V_6: rS, QS, qR, or S > R)	SVTAC diagnosed if no to all 4 criteria for VT
Griffith, 1994[53]	VT diagnosed if no to either criteria for SVTAC	SVTAC diagnosed if both criteria are present: QRS morphology classic for bundle-branch block: LBBB (rS or QS in leads V_1 and V_2; time to S wave nadir in lead V_1 or V_2 >70 ms; R wave and no Q wave in V_6) *or* RBBB (rSR′ in lead V_1; RS in lead V_6; R wave larger than S wave in V_6) No atrioventricular dissociation is seen
Lau, 2000[54]	Bayesian analysis starting with pretest odds for VT then multiply by likelihood ratio for VT associated with each of these factors: QRS duration QRS frontal plane axis V_1 morphology with a RBBB pattern V_1 and V_2 morphology with a LBBB pattern Interval of initial R-wave deflection in V_6 V_6 morphology VT diagnosed if posttest odds >3	SVTAC diagnosed if posttest odds <0.33
Vereckei, 2008[55]	VT diagnosed if, analyzed in sequence, any of these 4 criteria are present in lead aVR: Initial R wave Initial r or q wave >40 ms Notch present on the initial descending limb of a predominately negative QRS Slow conduction at beginning of QRS: ratio of vertical distance travelled in voltage during the initial 40 ms (v_i) and terminal 40 ms (v_t); ratio of v_i/v_t <1	SVTAC diagnosed if none of the 4 criteria for VT are present
Pava, 2010[56]	VT diagnosed if time from isoelectric to peak of R wave in lead II is >50 ms	SVTAC diagnosed if not

Abbreviations: LBBB = left bundle-branch block; RBBB = right bundle-branch block.

VENTRICULAR FIBRILLATION

Description Ventricular fibrillation is disorganized depolarization and chaotic contraction of small areas of ventricular myocardium absent any effective mechanical cardiac activity; there is no cardiac output. The ECG of ventricular fibrillation shows a fine, irregular pattern without discernible P waves or organized QRS complexes. The irregular pattern itself can be coarse, intermediate, or fine in amplitude (**Figure 18-27**).

Clinical Significance Ventricular fibrillation is seen most commonly in patients with severe ischemic heart disease, with or without an acute myocardial infarction. Primary ventricular fibrillation occurs suddenly and without preceding hemodynamic deterioration, whereas secondary ventricular fibrillation occurs after a prolonged period of left ventricular failure and/or circulatory shock. In addition, direct stimulation of the myocardium by catheters or other instruments, electrocution, and direct blunt chest trauma (also known as *comotio cordis*) can induce ventricular fibrillation.

Treatment Treatment of pulseless ventricular tachycardia or fibrillation is with electrical defibrillation along with chest compressions and other advanced life support measures. If resuscitation is successful at restoring spontaneous circulation, address any dysrhythmic triggers including acute ischemia, metabolic derangements, or toxicologic insult.

DYSRHYTHMIA ASSOCIATED CONDUCTION ABNORMALITIES

WOLFF-PARKINSON-WHITE SYNDROME

Description WPW syndrome is a form of ventricular preexcitation involving an accessory conduction pathway that bypasses the AV node

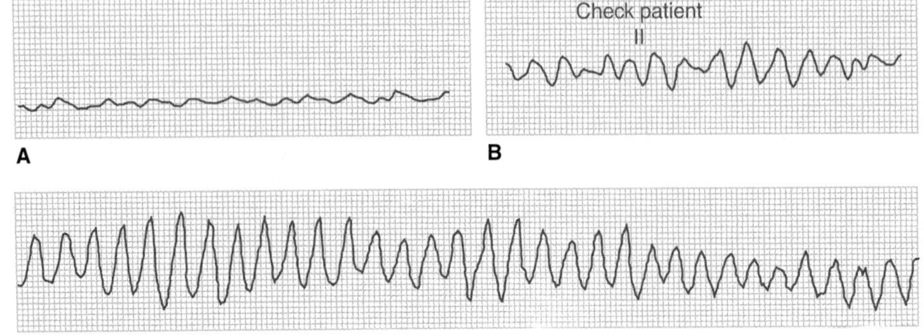

FIGURE 18-27. Three examples of ventricular fibrillation. **A.** Coarse amplitude. **B.** Fine amplitude. **C.** Coarse amplitude mimicking ventricular tachycardia.

TABLE 18-25 Dysrhythmias Seen in Symptomatic Wolff-Parkinson-White Syndrome

Atrioventricular reciprocating tachycardia (AVRT)
Narrow QRS complex tachycardia (orthodromic AVRT) – 65%
No P wave
Narrow QRS complexes
No delta wave
Rapid and regular
Ventricular rates ranging from 160–220 beats/min
Difficult to distinguish from paroxysmal supraventricular tachycardia
Wide QRS complex tachycardia (antidromic AVRT) – 10%
No P wave
Widened QRS complexes with consistent QRS complex morphology
Delta wave
Rapid and regular
Ventricular rates ranging from 160–220 beats/min
Difficult to distinguish from ventricular tachycardia
Atrial fibrillation – 25%
No P wave
Widened QRS complexes with varying, bizarre QRS complex morphologies
Delta wave
Rapid and irregular
Ventricular rates consistently >200 beats/min

and creates a direct electrical connection between the atria and ventricles.[63] WPW patients are prone to a variety of supraventricular tachydysrhythmias (**Table 18-25**). Ventricular fibrillation is very rare and usually only occurs in the setting of therapeutic misadventure.

Clinical Features The classic triad of ECG findings (**Figure 18-28** and **Table 18-26**) seen in WPW is visible during sinus rhythm and is usually not detectable during tachydysrhythmias. The PR interval is shortened in sinus rhythm because the impulse moving through the accessory pathway is not subject to the physiologic slowing within the AV node. The ventricle is activated by two separate pathways, resulting in a fused, or widened, QRS complex. The initial part of the complex, the delta wave, represents aberrant activation through the accessory pathway, while the terminal portion of the QRS complex represents normal activation through the His-Purkinje system from impulses traveling through the AV node. Due to altered ventricular depolarization, secondary repolarization changes reflected in altered ST segments and T waves that are generally directed opposite (discordant) to the major delta wave and QRS complex. The delta wave may create Q waves that can mimic ECG changes associated with ischemic heart disease.

An incidental ECG may identify WPW in an otherwise asymptomatic individual. While such asymptomatic individuals will never develop tachydysrhythmias, a portion of patients do, and some rare patients experience ventricular fibrillation and cardiac arrest.[64] Electrophysiologic studies can identify patients with multiple accessory tracts and short refractory periods in those tracts and, thus, who are at increased risk for ventricular fibrillation and cardiac arrest.[65]

The most frequent dysrhythmia seen in the WPW patient is a reentrant tachycardia termed AV reciprocating tachycardia. In AV reciprocating tachycardia, the reentry circuit involves the AV node and the accessory pathway. AV reciprocating tachycardia is either orthodromic (anterograde conduction through the AV node) or antidromic (retrograde conduction through the AV node). During orthodromic or anterograde AV reciprocating tachycardia (**Figure 18-29** and Table 18-26), the atrial stimulus is conducted to the ventricle through the AV node with a return of the impulse back to the atria through the accessory pathway. Since the ventricles are stimulated solely via the normal His-Purkinje system, the QRS complexes are narrow and there is no delta wave. Orthodromic AV reciprocating tachycardia accounts for approximately 65% of dysrhythmias seen in WPW patients and is difficult to distinguish from AV nodal reentrant tachycardia (i.e., typical paroxysmal supraventricular tachycardia).

In approximately 10% of symptomatic WPW patients, an antidromic (retrograde) AV reciprocating tachycardia occurs (**Figure 18-30** and Table 18-25). In antidromic AV reciprocating tachycardia, the reentrant

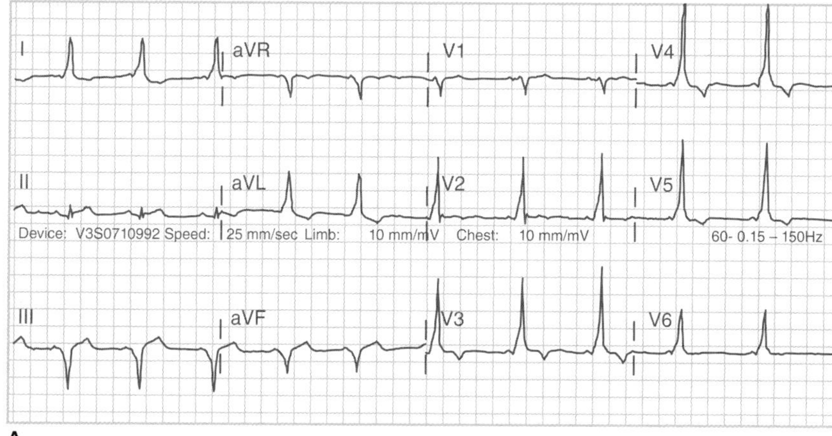

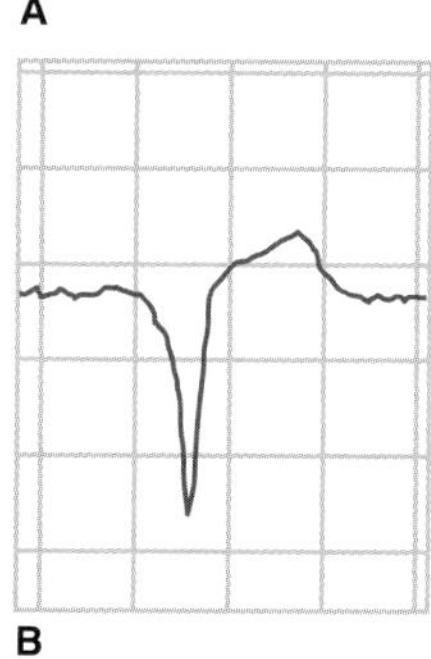

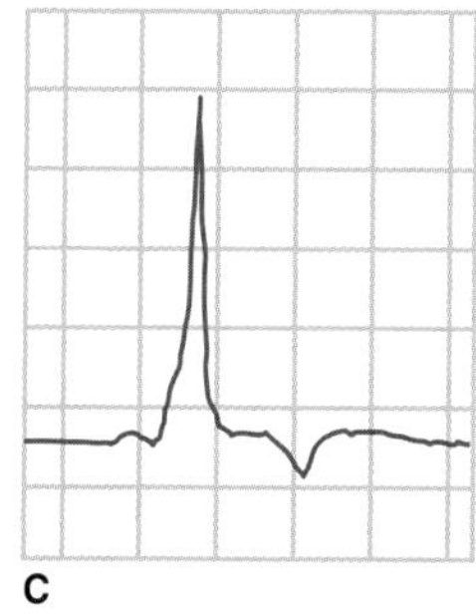

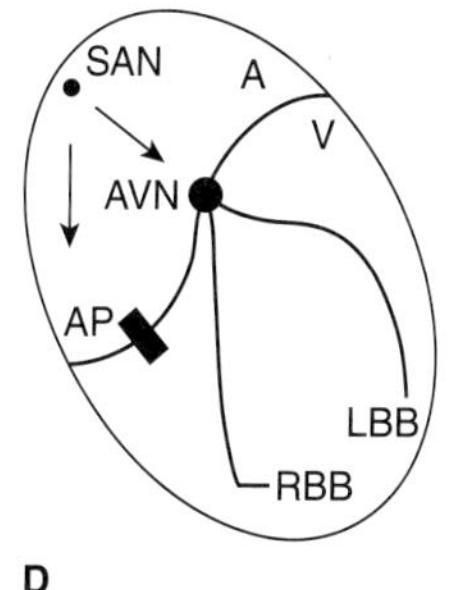

FIGURE 18-28. **A.** A 12-lead ECG of patient with the Wolff-Parkinson-White (WPW) syndrome in sinus rhythm. **B** and **C.** Single P-QRS-T complex; note the shortened PR interval, delta wave, and widened QRS complex. **D.** The direction of cardiac impulse conduction in the WPW syndrome patient in sinus rhythm. The *two arrows* indicate the direction of the impulse, moving from atrial (A) tissues to ventricular (V) tissues via the accessory pathway (AP) and atrioventricular node (AVN). The impulse arrives at the ventricular tissues via the AVN and moves through ventricular tissues via the right bundle branch (RBB) and left bundle branch (LBB); the impulse also arrives at ventricular tissues via the AP and moves through ventricular tissues using cell-to-cell conduction. SAN = sinoatrial node.

TABLE 18-26 The ECG Triad of Wolff-Parkinson-White Syndrome During Sinus Rhythm

PR interval <120 ms
Slurring of the initial QRS complex, known as a delta wave
Widened QRS complex

circuit conducts in the opposite direction, with anterograde conduction down the accessory pathway and return of the impulse retrograde to the atria via the AV node. With this pathway, the QRS complexes are wide; the ECG displays a very rapid, wide-complex tachycardia that looks like ventricular tachycardia.

Atrial fibrillation occurs in up to 25% of WPW patients with symptomatic dysrhythmias. The electrocardiographic features (**Figure 18-31** and Table 18-25) of atrial fibrillation with WPW syndrome are a very fast ventricular rate due to the ability of the accessory pathway to conduct impulses into the ventricle faster than through the AV node and significant beat-to-beat variation in the QRS complex morphology resulting from a combination of the two impulses arriving at the ventricle and fusing to form a composite depolarization. This wide-complex dysrhythmia may appear relatively regular and can be misdiagnosed as ventricular tachycardia.[66]

Treatment Treat all three tachydysrhythmias in the WPW patient according to the patient's clinical stability and the electrocardiographic features of the dysrhythmia. Use electrical cardioversion in patients with hemodynamic instability.

In the stable patient, therapy is guided by the QRS complex width and the regularity of the rhythm. In patients with a regular, narrow QRS complex tachycardia (i.e., orthodromic AV reciprocating tachycardia),

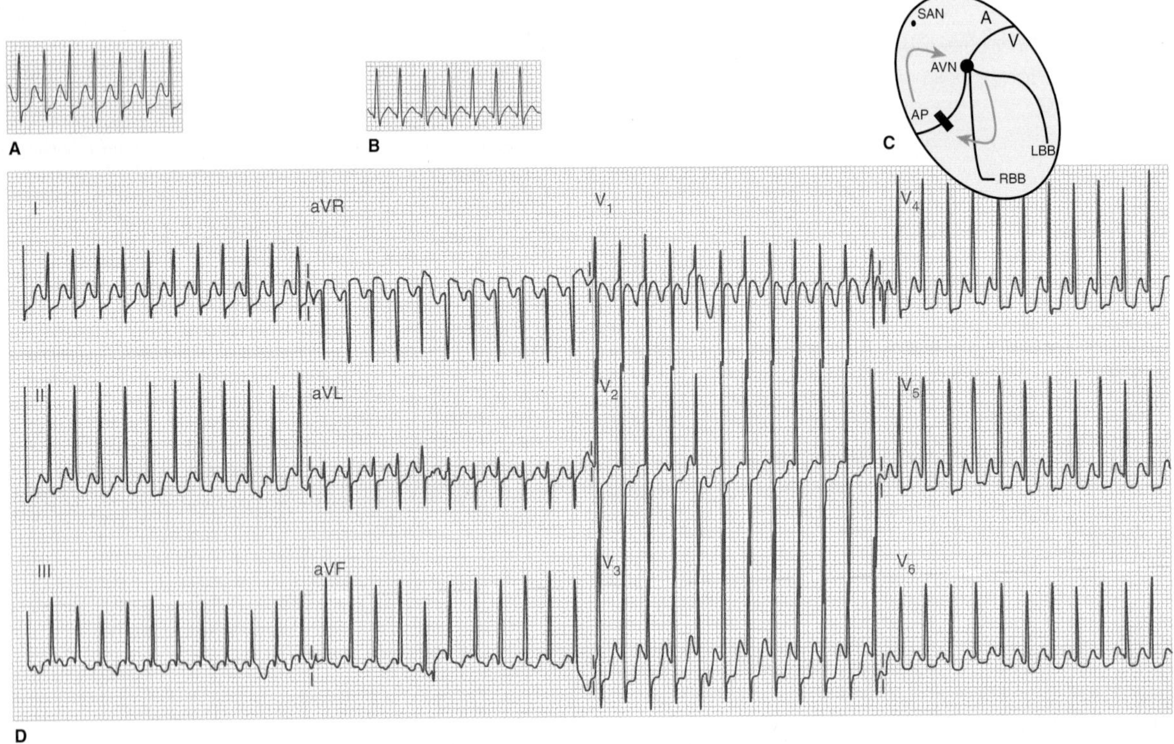

FIGURE 18-29. Narrow-complex tachycardia (orthodromic atrioventricular [AV] reciprocating tachycardia [AVRT]), the most common dysrhythmia of the Wolff-Parkinson-White syndrome. **A** and **B.** Rapid, regular, narrow QRS complexes without delta waves. **C.** The direction of cardiac impulse conduction in orthodromic AVRT; anterograde from atrial (A) tissues to ventricular (V) tissues through the AV node (AVN) and returning to the atrial tissues from ventricular tissues via the accessory pathway (AP). **D.** A 12-lead ECG demonstrating orthodromic AVRT. AP = accessory pathway; LBB = left bundle branch; RBB = right bundle branch; SAN = sinoatrial node.

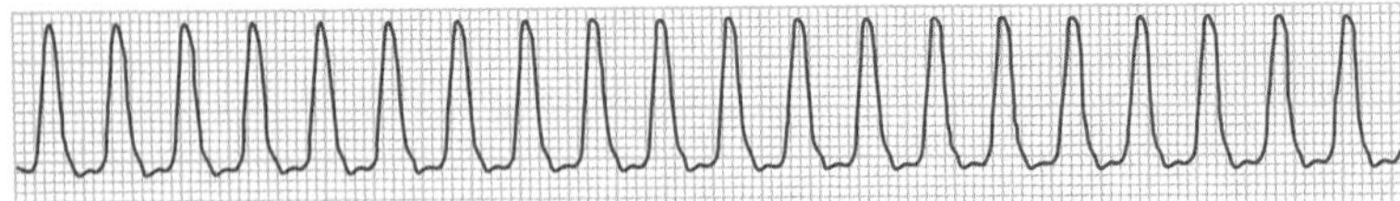

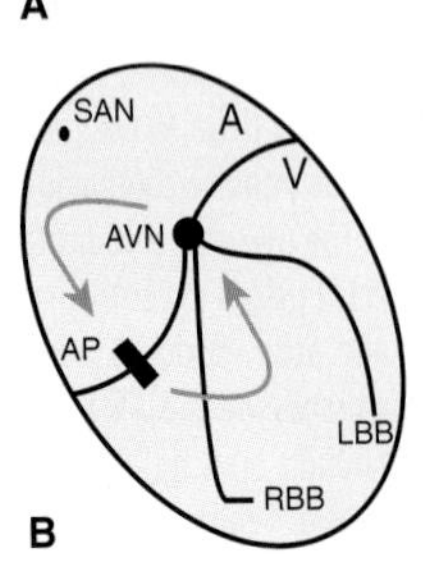

FIGURE 18-30. Antidromic atrioventricular (AV) reciprocating tachycardia (AVRT; wide-complex tachycardia). **A.** Wide-complex tachycardia that mimics ventricular tachycardia. **B.** The direction of cardiac impulse conduction in a Wolff-Parkinson-White syndrome patient during antidromic AVRT. The *two arrows* indicate the direction of the impulse movement, anterograde from atrial (A) tissues to ventricular (V) tissues through the accessory pathway (AP) and returning to the atrial tissues from ventricular tissues via the AV node (AVN). LBB = left bundle branch; RBB = right bundle branch; SAN = sinoatrial node.

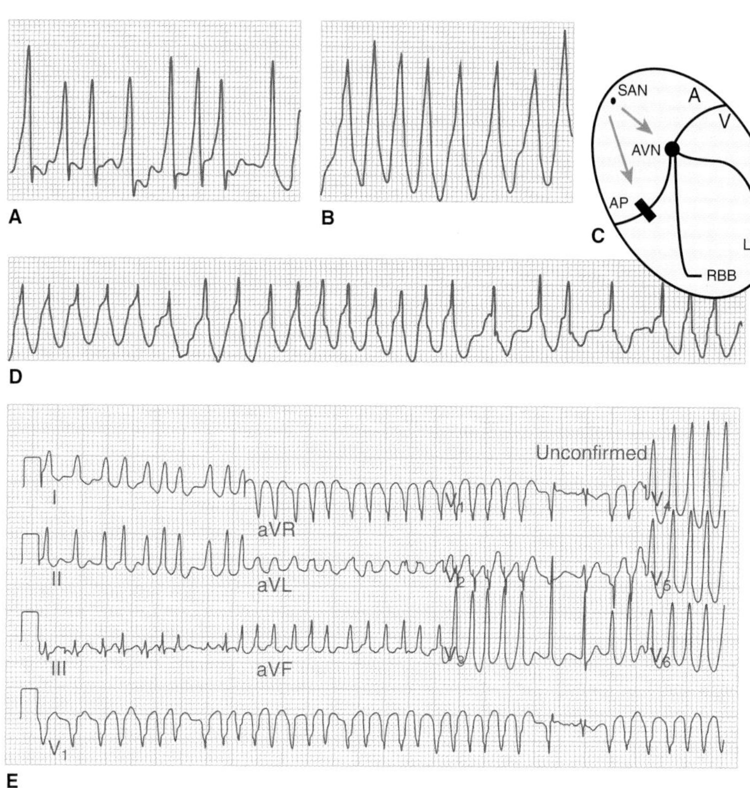

FIGURE 18-31. Atrial fibrillation in Wolff-Parkinson-White (WPW) syndrome. **A, B,** and **D.** Rapid, wide, irregular QRS complex tachycardia with varying QRS complex morphologies. **C.** The direction of cardiac impulse conduction in a WPW syndrome patient during atrial fibrillation. The *two arrows* indicate the direction of the impulse movement, both anterograde from atrial (A) tissues to ventricular (V) tissues through both the accessory pathway (AP) and the atrioventricular node (AVN). The larger of the two arrows indicates that the majority of impulses travel to the ventricular via the AP. **E.** A 12-lead ECG demonstrating a rapid, wide, irregular QRS complex tachycardia with varying QRS complex morphologies. LBB = left bundle branch; RBB = right bundle branch; SAN = sinoatrial node.

the first intervention is vagal maneuver (Table 18-3). If this intervention fails, the next step would be intravenous adenosine (Table 18-2). If adenosine fails, then longer acting AV nodal blocking agents, such as β-blockers and calcium channel blockers are indicated. In refractory cases, procainamide is an effective agent that blocks conduction in the accessory conduction pathway and can terminate this reentrant tachycardia. If all medications are unsuccessful, the patient can be electrically cardioverted with appropriate sedation.

In stable patients with a wide QRS complex tachycardia, either regular (i.e., orthodromic AV reciprocating tachycardia) or irregular (atrial fibrillation), procainamide should be administered.[67] If unsuccessful, electrical cardioversion with appropriate sedation should be considered. Some antiarrhythmic medications can paradoxically enhance condition via the accessory tract, potentially enabling excessively rapid atrial activity to trigger ventricular fibrillation. Also, by blocking conduction through the AV node in WPW patients with atrial fibrillation, more of the rapid atrial depolarizations are able to initiate ventricular depolarization because competition from the normal conducting pathway is impaired, although evidence of adverse clinical outcome by such action is weak.[68] **Agents that can enhance conduction in the accessory tract and/or block conduction in the AV node should be avoided in WPW patients with wide-complex irregular tachycardias; these include adenosine, amiodarone, β-blockers, and calcium channel blockers.**[20]

After conversion, observe the patient with continuous cardiac rhythm monitoring and a repeat ECG. In general, patients who have rare episodes of tachydysrhythmias and who are stable after conversion can be discharged home with routine follow-up. Patients with frequent tachydysrhythmia episodes or who have an episode of atrial fibrillation with a very rapid ventricular response should be promptly referred for ablation of the accessory pathway. Patients who experience loss of consciousness during a known or possible tachydysrhythmia should be kept for observation due to the potential for repeat episode or cardiac arrest. Asymptomatic patients in whom WPW appears as an incidental finding should be referred to a cardiologist for further evaluation.[69]

BRUGADA SYNDROME

Description Brugada syndrome is an inherited disorder of myocardial depolarization that predisposes young individuals to malignant ventricular dysrhythmias and sudden death.[70-72] Congenital Brugada syndrome is due to mutations in the genes responsible for transmembrane sodium, calcium, or potassium ion channels in the heart.[73] Eight genetic mutations have been identified as producing a *channelopathy* that results in the Brugada syndrome. The prevalence of Brugada syndrome varies dramatically among different ethnic groups; it is highest in East and Southeast Asian populations and relatively lower in groups originating from Western Europe.

Clinical Features The majority of patients with Brugada syndrome are asymptomatic and are only found via an incidental ECG. Symptomatic patients present with palpitations, near to complete syncope, or seizures due to ventricular tachydysrhythmias. Characteristic ECG changes are necessary for the diagnosis, but such changes are variable and not always evident (**Table 18-27** and **Figure 18-32**).[74] Fever and provocative testing with a sodium channel blocker (e.g., flecainide) may provoke surface ECG abnormalities associated with Brugada syndrome. The type 1 pattern is considered diagnostic when combined with appropriate clinical

TABLE 18-27	**ECG Patterns Associated with Brugada Syndrome in ECG Leads V_1 to V_3**
Type 1	Coved-shaped ST-segment elevation >2 mm Followed by an inverted T wave
Type 2	ST segment elevation >2 mm With a trough in the ST segment at least 1 mm deep Followed by a positive or biphasic T wave Producing a "saddleback" pattern
Type 3	Coved-shaped or saddleback pattern ST segment With 1- to 2-mm elevation

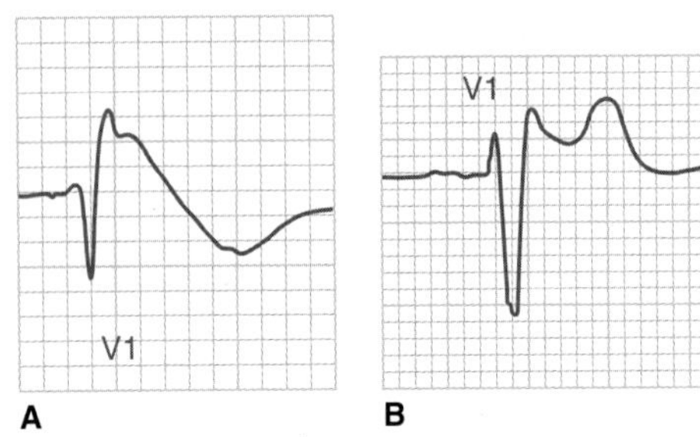

FIGURE 18-32. Brugada ECG pattern. **A.** Type 1. **B.** Type 2.

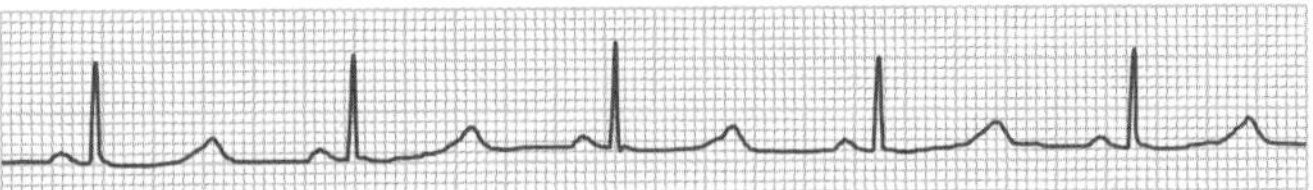

FIGURE 18-33. Long QT interval; QTc is 550 milliseconds.

TABLE 18-29 Diagnostic Score for Congenital Long QT Syndrome

Feature		Points
ECG*		
QTc	≥480 ms	3
	460–479 ms	2
	450–459 (male) ms	1
QTc ≥480 ms at 4th min of recovery from exercise stress test		1
T-wave alternans		1
Notched T waves in three ECG leads		1
Heart rate <2nd percentile for age (<50 in adult age 20–60)		0.5
Clinical history		
Syncope *or* episode of torsade de pointes (not both)	Torsade de pointes	2
	Syncope provoked by stress	2
	Syncope not provoked by stress	1
Congenital deafness		0.5
Family history		
Family members with definite long QT syndrome		1
Immediate family member <30 years old with unexplained sudden cardiac death		0.5
Scoring: Range, 0 to 10; 1.5 to 3 points = intermediate probability; ≥3.5 points = high probability		

*In absence of medications or conditions known to affect QT interval or T wave.

or family history (**Table 18-28**). Types 2 and 3 are considered suggestive but not diagnostic of Brugada syndrome. Because types 2 and 3 may convert to type 1, either spontaneously or with provocative testing, further evaluation is recommended if there is an appropriate history.

Risk stratification is done to identify patients with Brugada syndrome at significant risk for malignant ventricular tachydysrhythmias.[75] In patients with aborted sudden cardiac death, the risk of recurrence of ventricular fibrillation is over 50% within 5 years.

Treatment An important role for the emergency provider is to recognize this ECG pattern, especially in patients who present with symptoms, and to refer to for appropriate follow up.[76] Avoid exacerbating the underlying pathophysiology; do not use medications that possess sodium channel blockade effects (http://www.brugadadrugs.org). Educate the patient on the importance of treating fever, with even minor infections. The only proven therapy to terminate malignant ventricular arrhythmias and prevent sudden death is implantable cardioverter defibrillator placement. Quinidine, a class Ia antiarrhythmic, is sometimes used as an adjunct with implantable cardioverter defibrillator placement to reduce the incidence of dysrhythmias. Side effects (hepatitis, thrombocytopenia, and diarrhea) and the potential to induce torsade de pointes are cautions to quinidine's routine use.

LONG QT SYNDROME

Description The long QT syndromes are characterized by prolongation of the QT interval (**Figure 18-33**) and a predisposition to ventricular tachydysrhythmias, including torsade de pointes and sudden cardiac death.[77-79] Congenital long QT syndrome is an inherited disorder due to mutations in cation channel genes (*channelopathies*). Of the 13 described variants of congenital long QT syndrome, the three most common, accounting for about 90% of all cases, are mutations in a cardiac potassium channel for long QT syndrome types 1 and 2 and the sodium ion channel for long QT syndrome type 3.[79] With increased awareness and identification, the prevalence of congenital long QT syndrome is estimated to be 1 in 2000 live births. Acquired long QT syndrome can occur from electrolyte abnormalities (hypokalemia, hypomagnesemia), medication effects, and other disease states, such as acute coronary syndrome and severe left ventricular dysfunction.[80,81]

Clinical Features The normal QT interval corrected for heart rate (QTc) is up 440 milliseconds in adult males and 460 milliseconds in adult females. The risk of dysrhythmias associated with long QT syndrome increases as the QTc prolongs, with moderate risk when the QTc is between 480 and 499 milliseconds and significantly higher risk when the QTc is greater than 500 milliseconds.[27] Syncope is the most common symptom, and torsade de pointes is the most common dysrhythmia. A diagnostic scoring system has been created to assist in identifying patients with congenital long QT syndrome (**Table 18-29**).[82]

TABLE 18-28 Risk Stratification in Brugada Syndrome

Personal history	Near or complete syncope Seizure Nocturnal agonal respiration
Aborted sudden cardiac death	Polymorphous ventricular tachycardia Ventricular fibrillation
Family history	Family history of unexplained sudden cardiac death Family history of coved-shaped ST segment (type 1) ECG pattern
Electrophysiologic study	Inducibility of ventricular tachycardia or fibrillation with programmed stimulation

Treatment An important role for the emergency provider is to recognize this ECG pattern, especially in patients who present with syncope, and to refer for appropriate follow-up.[76] Avoid exacerbating the underlying pathophysiology; do not use medications that possess channel blockade effects, impair cardiac repolarization, prolong the QT interval, and provoke tachydysrhythmias (https://crediblemeds.org/healthcare-providers/).[83] Correct underlying electrolyte abnormalities, especially those of potassium and magnesium. β-Blockers are the initial treatment for symptomatic patients with congenital long QT syndrome.[84] Propranolol and nadolol are the most effective β-blockers, and patients with congenital long QT syndrome type 1 are the most responsive.

Lifestyle modifications are beneficial in congenital long QT syndrome.[85] Exercise is a trigger for lethal dysrhythmic events, especially in patients with congenital long QT syndrome type 1, where swimming is notably dangerous. Patients with congenital long QT syndrome type 2 are sensitive to decreased serum potassium and are at risk for lethal cardiac events triggered by emotions or being startled, as being roughly aroused from rest or sleep.

REFERENCES

The complete reference list is available online at www.TintinalliEM.com.

CHAPTER 19 Pharmacology of Antiarrhythmics and Antihypertensives

Sara H. Shields
Rachel M. Holland
R. Dustin Pippin
Benjamin Small

This chapter reviews the pharmacology of selected antiarrhythmics and antihypertensives (β-blockers and calcium channel blockers) used in the ED. Discussion of additional antihypertensives can be found in chapter 57, "Systemic Hypertension."

Antiarrhythmic medications treat cardiac rhythm abnormalities by modifying autonomic function or myocardial ion channels, leading to changes in conduction velocity or duration of the effective refractory period.[1] Failure to reduce mortality has been a criticism of many agents in this class of drugs.[2-5] In general, electrical cardioversion is preferable to pharmacologic conversion in patients who are hemodynamically unstable. The majority of antiarrhythmics are organized based on the Vaughan-Williams classification system (Classes I to IV) (**Table 19-1**). Other medications used to treat arrhythmias include digoxin, atropine, adenosine, magnesium, and isoproterenol.

CLASS I ANTIARRHYTHMICS: FAST SODIUM CHANNEL BLOCKERS

Class I agents block fast sodium channels (I_{Na}) and are further subcategorized based on their degree of blockade into Classes Ia (moderate blockade), Ib (weak blockage), and Ic (strong blockade). Sodium channel blockers increase the excitability threshold, requiring more sodium channels to open in order to overcome the potassium current and generate an action potential. This effect increases refractoriness and can be useful in terminating reentry currents. In addition, some Class I agents block potassium channels (I_K) and exhibit antimuscarinic effects.

CLASS Ia AGENTS

Class Ia antiarrhythmics block open sodium channels and have a slow dissociation from their target, causing an increase in the refractory period. The use of these agents is limited by their side effect profile and proarrhythmic nature. Quinidine and disopyramide are Class Ia agents but are not discussed here because they are infrequently used in the ED. Quinidine can cause **torsades de pointes**. Disopyramide is used orally in patients with hypertrophic cardiomyopathy due to its negative inotropic properties; however, its association with heart failure and hypotension and its anticholinergic effects, including urinary retention, limit its use.

TABLE 19-1 Vaughan-Williams Classification of Antiarrhythmic Medications

Action	Class	Example Medications
Sodium channel blockers	Class Ia	Disopyramide, quinidine, procainamide
	Class Ib	Lidocaine, mexiletine, phenytoin,
	Class Ic	Flecainide, propafenone
β-Blockers	Class II	Esmolol, labetalol, metoprolol, propranolol
Potassium channel blockers	Class III	Amiodarone, dronedarone, dofetilide*, ibutilide, sotalol†, vernakalant‡
Calcium channel blockers	Class IV	Diltiazem, verapamil
Unclassified agents#		Adenosine, atropine, digoxin, isoproterenol, magnesium

*Only available by prescription by specifically trained physicians.

†Also a β-blocker.

‡Not available in the United States.

#Not classified by Vaughan-Williams system.

TABLE 19-2 Procainamide Pharmacokinetics

Distribution	Metabolism	Excretion	Half-Life	Onset/Duration of Action
2 L/kg	Hepatic and renal	Urine, feces	Procainamide: 2.5–4.7 h	Onset: 5–10 min
	Active metabolite: NAPA (renally eliminated)		NAPA: 6–8 h	Duration: 1–2 h

PROCAINAMIDE

Actions Procainamide is a Class Ia agent that increases the refractory period, decreases automaticity and conduction, and prolongs cardiac action potentials through intermediate blockade of open sodium and potassium channels. NAPA, the active metabolite of procainamide, lacks sodium channel effects but does block potassium channels, which can lead to QT prolongation.

Pharmacokinetics See **Table 19-2**.[6]

Indications Procainamide is indicated for life-threatening ventricular arrhythmias and supraventricular arrhythmias. Although it can be used to treat supraventricular tachycardia, the proarrhythmic nature of this agent (including torsades de pointes) and the risk of toxicity make procainamide less desirable for this indication. For hemodynamically stable ventricular tachycardias, procainamide can be considered as a therapeutic option; however it should be avoided in patients with prolonged QT intervals or congestive heart failure.[7]

Dosing and Administration See **Table 19-3**.[6]

Adverse Effects The most common adverse effects associated with procainamide are hypotension, cardiac conduction abnormalities, and rash. Serious adverse effects include prolonged QT interval, torsades de pointes, ventricular fibrillation, paradoxical increase in ventricular rate in atrial fibrillation/flutter, hepatotoxicity, and congestive heart failure.

CLASS Ib AGENTS

Class Ib agents have weak sodium channel–blocking properties and a high affinity for both open and inactive sodium channels with very rapid dissociation. The cumulative effects of these agents result in decreased automaticity due to an increase in the threshold for excitability. Because of their quick dissociation, these drugs are less effective on myocardial tissues with rapid conduction, such as atrial tissue.

LIDOCAINE

Actions Lidocaine is a Class Ib agent with weak sodium channel blocker properties that preferentially acts on ischemic myocardial tissue to decrease conduction; in addition, it has local anesthetic properties. Effects exerted on the cardiac action potential are negligible, with very

TABLE 19-3 Procainamide Dosing and Administration

Advanced Cardiac Life Support (ACLS)–Ventricular Arrhythmia
Initial: 20–50* milligrams/min IV until the arrhythmia is suppressed, hypotension ensues, or the QRS complex is prolonged by 50% from its original duration (maximum dose: 17 milligrams/kg)
Maintenance infusion rate: 1–4 milligrams/min
OR
100 milligrams IV every 5 min until the arrhythmia is controlled or one of the above conditions is met

*Slower administration preferred if patient is stable.

TABLE 19-4 Lidocaine Pharmacokinetics

Distribution	Metabolism	Excretion	Half-Life	Onset/Duration of Action
1.1–2.1 L/kg	Hepatic Active metabolites	Urine	Initial: 7–30 min Terminal: 1.5–2 h	Onset: 45–90 s Duration: 10–20 min

minimal decrease to no effect on the QT interval and the refractory period.

Pharmacokinetics See **Table 19-4**.[6]

Indications Lidocaine is indicated in the acute management of ventricular arrhythmias. Per advanced cardiac life support guidelines, lidocaine is considered a second-line therapy, if amiodarone is unavailable, in patients with ventricular fibrillation or pulseless ventricular tachycardia due to the failure of clinical studies to show improved rates of return of spontaneous circulation when compared to amiodarone.[5]

Dosing and Administration See **Table 19-5**.[6]

Adverse Effects Adverse effects of lidocaine are typically dose dependent, with few hemodynamic effects at lower infusion rates. Patients should be monitored for CNS effects, including numbness, speech impairment, somnolence, dizziness, and seizures.

CLASS Ic AGENTS

Class Ic agents are most commonly used for the treatment of supraventricular tachycardia. They have the highest degree of fast sodium channel blockade, resulting in marked prolongation of the QRS interval without QT prolongation. These agents act only on open sodium channels and demonstrate slow dissociation from their targets, leading to increased refractoriness and decreased conduction. They have a high proarrhythmic potential that can be amplified in cases of diseased myocardial tissue, increased sympathetic tone, and higher heart rates. Large clinical studies have associated several Class Ic agents with increased mortality when used in patients with cardiovascular disease or after myocardial infarction.[8,9]

PROPAFENONE

Propafenone is a Class Ic agent with additional β-adrenergic–blocking properties; therefore, it can cause bradycardia and bronchospasm. It is more selective for cells with high rates of conduction. Propafenone is indicated for the conversion of recent-onset atrial fibrillation (<7 days) to sinus rhythm.[10] Under continuous cardiac monitoring, the patient can be given a one-time oral dose of 450 milligrams (weight <70 kg) or 600 milligrams (weight ≥70 kg). Adverse effects include hypotension, bradycardia, bronchospasm, atrial flutter with 1:1 atrioventricular conduction, and ventricular proarrhythmia. This drug should be avoided in patients with coronary artery disease or significant structural heart disease, and should be given with caution to patients with asthma, hepatic dysfunction, or congestive heart failure. Although propafenone carries an indication for paroxysmal supraventricular tachycardia and ventricular tachycardia, it is rarely used for these indications in the ED.

TABLE 19-5 Lidocaine Dosing and Administration

Ventricular Arrhythmia	Ventricular Fibrillation
Loading dose: 50–100 milligrams (0.7–1.4 milligrams/kg) IV over 2–3 min. May repeat in 5 min (up to 300 milligrams in any 1-h period) Maintenance: 1–4 milligrams/min IV (0.014–0.057 milligrams/kg/min)	Initial dose: 1–1.5 milligrams/kg IV If VF/pulseless VT persists, additional doses of 0.5–0.75 milligrams/kg IV every 5–10 min (maximum total dose: 3 milligrams/kg)

Abbreviations: VF = ventricular fibrillation; VT = ventricular tachycardia.

FLECAINIDE

Flecainide is a Class 1c agent that reduces excitability, primarily in the His-Purkinje system and ventricular myocardium. Flecainide is indicated for the conversion of recent-onset atrial fibrillation (<7 days) to sinus rhythm.[10] Under continuous cardiac monitoring, the patient can be given a one-time oral dose of 200 milligrams (weight <70 kg) or 300 milligrams (weight ≥70 kg). Adverse effects include hypotension, atrial flutter with 1:1 atrioventricular conduction, and ventricular proarrhythmia. This drug should be avoided in patients with coronary artery disease, significant structural heart disease, congestive heart failure, or hypokalemia. Although flecainide carries an indication for paroxysmal supraventricular tachycardia and ventricular tachycardia, it is rarely used for these indications in the ED.

CLASS II ANTIARRHYTHMICS: β-BLOCKERS

β-Blockers are used for the treatment of various indications including hypertension, supraventricular tachycardia and ventricular arrhythmias, recurrent atrial fibrillation (rate control), and thyrotoxicosis (symptom control). Although these medications share the principal characteristic of blocking catecholamine effects on β-receptors, individual agents differ with respect to their cardioselectivity, α-adrenergic blocking activity, intrinsic sympathomimetic activity, membrane-stabilizing effect, and pharmacokinetic properties (**Table 19-6**). β-Receptors are divided into two subtypes. β_1-Receptors are found in heart muscle, and β_2-receptors are found in bronchial and vascular smooth muscle. Nonselective β-blocking medications target all β-receptors, thereby affecting heart rate, conduction, and contractility, as well as smooth muscle contraction, thus increasing the risk of bronchospasm. In contrast, cardioselective agents have relative selectivity for β_1-receptors and decrease heart rate and blood pressure. These agents may be a better option for patients with a history of asthma, chronic obstructive pulmonary disease, or insulin-dependent diabetes because they are less likely to act on β_2-receptors. Because cardioselectivity is dose-dependent, it decreases or is lost at higher doses. This is variable between agents, and the dose at which this occurs has not been clearly established.

With the exception of sotalol, all listed β-blockers are indicated for the treatment of hypertension. These agents are also used for ventricular rate control in atrial fibrillation as they slow atrioventricular nodal conduction by decreasing sympathetic tone.

PROPRANOLOL

Actions Propranolol is a nonselective antagonist of β_1- and β_2-receptors.

Pharmacokinetics See Table 19-6.

Indications See Table 19-6.

Dosing and Administration See Table 19-6.

Adverse Effects Serious adverse effects associated with IV propranolol administration include bradycardia, heart block, hypotension, worsening heart failure, and bronchospasm.

ESMOLOL

Actions Esmolol is a short-acting, selective β_1-antagonist that exhibits negative inotropic and chronotropic effects. By blocking β_1-receptors, esmolol prevents excessive adrenergic stimulation of the myocardium, thus causing an increase in sinus cycle length, prolongation of sinoatrial nodal recovery time, and a decrease in conduction through the atrioventricular node.

Pharmacokinetics See Table 19-6.[6] Esmolol is available as a parenteral formulation only and has a rapid onset of action and short duration of action, with complete reversal of medication effects seen within 10 to 30 minutes after discontinuation.

Indications See Table 19-6.[4]

Dosing and Administration All listed doses are in micrograms. For the treatment of supraventricular tachycardia, the dose of esmolol is a 500 microgram/kg bolus (optional) over 1 minute, followed by an

TABLE 19-6 Class II Antiarrhythmics: β-Blockers

Generic Name	Onset of Action	Duration of Action	Metabolism	Half-Life	IV Dose (Adult)	Indications
Noncardioselective						
Propranolol	Oral: 1–2 h IV: ≤1 min	Oral: IR: 6–12 h ER: 24–27 h IV: 4–6 h	Hepatic, extensive first-pass elimination	3–6 h ER formulations: 8–10 h	Tachyarrhythmias: 1–3 milligrams/dose slow IVP; may repeat every 2–5 min up to a total of 5 milligrams *OR* 0.5–1 milligrams over 1 min; may repeat, if necessary, up to a total maximum dose of 0.1 milligram/kg	HTN, SVT arrhythmias, VT
Cardioselective						
Esmolol	IV: 2–10 min	IV: 10–30 min	In blood by RBC esterases	9 min	See text	HTN, SVT arrhythmias, AFib/AFlut (rate control)
Metoprolol	Oral: 1–2 h IV: 20 min	Oral: IR: variable ER: 24 h IV: 5–8 h	Hepatic, extensive first-pass elimination	3–4 h	Initial: 1.25–5 milligrams IV every 5 min up to 15 milligrams initial dose (titrate to response)	HTN, acute MI (oral), angina, rate control in AFib/AFlut
Vasodilatory, Nonselective						
Labetalol	Oral: 20 min–2 h IV: 2–5 min	Oral: 8–12 h IV: 2–18 h	Hepatic, extensive first-pass elimination	Oral: 6–8 h IV: 5.5 h	IV bolus (initial): 20 milligrams IVP over 2 min; may administer 40–80 milligrams at 10-min intervals (up to 300 milligrams total cumulative dose) IV infusion (acute loading): Initial: 2 milligrams/min, titrate to response (up to 300 milligrams total cumulative dose)	HTN

Abbreviations: AFib = atrial fibrillation; AFlut = atrial flutter; ER = extended release; HTN = hypertension; IR = immediate release; IVP = IV push; MI = myocardial infarction; RBC = red blood cell; SVT = supraventricular tachycardia; VT = ventricular tachycardia.

infusion starting at 50 micrograms/kg/min titrated to therapeutic effect in 50 microgram/kg/min increments every 4 minutes. To achieve a more rapid response, two additional 500 microgram/kg bolus doses may be given prior to increasing the infusion rate to 100 micrograms/kg/min (after second bolus) and 150 micrograms/kg/min (after third bolus), as required. After 4 minutes at the rate of 150 micrograms/kg/min, the infusion rate may be increased to a maximum rate of 200 micrograms/kg/min (without an additional bolus dose).

Adverse Effects Cardiovascular adverse effects of esmolol include hypotension (most common), bradycardia, and heart block. Abrupt discontinuation may cause rebound hypertension or angina. Other adverse effects may include injection site reaction, nausea, bronchospasm, and pulmonary edema.

METOPROLOL

Actions Metoprolol is a selective antagonist of β_1-receptors and exerts its antihypertensive effects by decreasing cardiac output, reducing sympathetic outflow, and suppressing renin activity.

Pharmacokinetics See Table 19-6.

Indications See Table 19-6.

Dosing and Administration See Table 19-6 and **Table 19-7**.

Adverse Effects Significant adverse effects associated with metoprolol include bradycardia, heart block, hypotension, and bronchospasm.

LABETALOL

Actions Labetalol is a combined selective α_1-blocking and nonselective β-blocking agent with direct vasodilatory action. The β-blocking effects of labetalol are greater than the α_1-blocking effects, with ratios of 3:1 in the oral and 7:1 in the parenteral formulation. Labetalol is useful as an antihypertensive agent because it decreases heart rate, contractility, cardiac output, and total peripheral resistance.

TABLE 19-7 IV to PO Conversion of Metoprolol

Medication	IV to PO Conversion
Metoprolol	5 milligrams IV = 12.5 milligrams PO

Pharmacokinetics See Table 19-6.

Indications Labetalol is used primarily for its antihypertensive effects. It is used in patients with acute hypertensive emergencies where rapid blood pressure reduction is indicated (see chapter 57, "Systemic Hypertension") and is considered safe for use in the treatment of hypertension in pregnancy (see chapters 99, "Comorbid Disorders in Pregnancy" and 100, "Maternal Emergencies after 20 Weeks of Pregnancy and in the Postpartum Period").

Dosing and Administration See Table 19-6 and **Table 19-8**. Labetalol can be administered IV by multiple boluses or as a continuous infusion. Once control of blood pressure has been established, patients may transition to oral labetalol (Table 19-8).[6]

Adverse Effects The most common adverse effect of labetalol is orthostatic hypotension, which occurs primarily with IV administration. Other common adverse effects include nausea, dizziness, and fatigue. Serious adverse effects include heart failure, hyperkalemia, hepatotoxicity, and bronchospasm.

CLASS III ANTIARRHYTHMICS

Class III antiarrhythmic medications inhibit inward potassium currents (**Table 19-9**),[6] which leads to a significantly longer refractory period. Myocardial tissue in a refractory state is resistant to reentrant conduction

TABLE 19-8 IV to PO Conversion of Labetalol

Medication	IV to PO Conversion
Labetalol	Upon discontinuation of IV infusion, initiate 200 milligrams orally, followed in 6–12 h with an additional dose of 200–400 milligrams. Thereafter, dose patients with 400–2400 milligrams/d in divided doses depending on blood pressure response.

TABLE 19-9 Pharmacology of Class III Antiarrhythmic Agents

	Ion Channels and Receptors Antagonized				
	K^+ Channels	Na^+ Channels	Ca^{2+} Channels	β-Adrenergic	α-Adrenergic
Amiodarone	+	+	+	+	+
Dronedarone	+	+	+	+	+
Sotalol	+			+	
Dofetilide	+				
Ibutilide	+ Lesser effect	Activates a slow inward Na^+ current			
Vernakalant	+*	+†			

*Ultrarapid and acetylcholine K^+ currents.

†Lesser effect.

circuits that may produce arrhythmia. These agents prolong the QT interval, which is associated with significant risk for torsades de pointes. Clinical indications for Class III antiarrhythmics are contrasted in **Table 19-10**.

AMIODARONE

Amiodarone is a highly effective "broad-spectrum" antiarrhythmic indicated in the acute management and chronic suppression of supraventricular tachycardia and ventricular arrhythmias. Potential benefits of amiodarone must be weighed against an array of potentially serious adverse effects, and clinical use is further complicated by distinctive pharmacokinetics and significant drug interactions.

Actions Amiodarone possesses properties of all four classes of antiarrhythmics (**Table 19-11**).[6,11]

Pharmacokinetics The pharmacokinetics of amiodarone are listed in **Table 19-12**.[6] Amiodarone is highly lipophilic and extensively distributed to bodily tissues.[12] Although IV amiodarone produces a rapid antiarrhythmic effect, it quickly redistributes from the serum into tissue, causing a precipitous drop in serum concentration.[13] Therefore, large oral or IV loading doses, generally given over a week or more, are needed to fill this large tissue reservoir and achieve sustained serum concentrations. As tissue stores become saturated after long-term oral therapy, terminal-phase elimination dominates and is characterized by a long half-life (≤55 days) and duration of action (≤50 days). Amiodarone is eliminated primarily by hepatic metabolism and biliary excretion.

Indications Specific indications for amiodarone are listed in **Table 19-13**.[7,10,14-16]

Dosing and Administration Amiodarone dosing is detailed in **Table 19-14**.[6] Intravenous amiodarone is associated with bradycardia, hypotension, and phlebitis. Hypotension may be dose and infusion rate dependent; therefore, infusion rates should not exceed 30 milligrams/min, and total daily doses should not exceed 2.2 grams. Preparations of IV amiodarone should be mixed in 5% dextrose in water, as amiodarone has precipitated in compatibility studies with normal saline.[17] Dose adjustments are not required for renal insufficiency but should be considered for severe hepatic dysfunction.

Adverse Effects Adverse effects of amiodarone are listed in **Table 19-15**.[6,18] Long-term amiodarone has many common, serious, and potentially fatal adverse effects that limit widespread clinical use and require regular monitoring of liver, pulmonary, thyroid, and ocular function. As a result, patients should be regularly monitored for these toxicities. Although amiodarone prolongs the QT interval, it has a relatively low incidence of torsades de pointes even in patients with structural heart disease.

Amiodarone is responsible for many clinically significant drug interactions. As a strong inhibitor of liver enzymes, amiodarone increases serum concentrations of many other medications. Amiodarone may also augment the effects of medications that concomitantly prolong the QT_c interval or cause bradycardia. Specific dose reductions are required for digoxin, warfarin, procainamide, quinidine, simvastatin, and lovastatin when used concomitantly with amiodarone. Given amiodarone's extremely long half-life, drug interactions may persist for months after discontinuation of therapy.

TABLE 19-10 Class III Antiarrhythmic Indications

	Clinical Indications	
	Supraventricular Arrhythmias	Ventricular Arrhythmias
Amiodarone	Acute rate control or cardioversion and maintenance of sinus rhythm*	Acute management of life-threatening arrhythmias; chronic suppression
Dronedarone	AFib (history of paroxysmal or persistent, but currently in sinus rhythm) to reduce risk of hospitalization	No
Sotalol	AFib or AFlut	Monomorphic VT†
Dofetilide	AFib or AFlut; conversion to and maintenance of sinus rhythm	No
Ibutilide	Acute cardioversion of AFib or AFlut	No
Vernakalant	Acute cardioversion of AFib‡	No

Abbreviations: AFib = atrial fibrillation; AFlut = atrial flutter; VT = ventricular tachycardia.

*Off label.

†Off label in United States, but guideline recommended with IV formulation if available.

‡Approved in Europe, not in United States.

DRONEDARONE

Actions Dronedarone is a noniodinated, less lipophilic derivative of amiodarone, designed to have a more favorable adverse effect profile than its predecessor. Dronedarone is categorized as a Class III antiarrhythmic

TABLE 19-11 Electrophysiologic and Electrocardiographic Effects of Amiodarone

Ion Channels and Receptors	Effects on Cardiac Electrophysiology	Effects on the ECG
Blocks inactivated Na^+ channels Noncompetitive blockade of α- and β-adrenergic receptors Blocks inward K^+ channel rectifier Blocks myocardial Ca^+ channels	Prolongs the refractory period Decreases sinoatrial node function Slows atrioventricular node conduction Modifies automaticity of Purkinje fibers	Decreases heart rate and may cause sinus bradycardia Prolongs: PR interval QRS interval* QT interval*

*More common with chronic oral administration than with acute IV use.

TABLE 19-12 Amiodarone Pharmacokinetics

Absorption	Distribution	Metabolism	Excretion	Half-Life	Onset/Peak/Duration of Action
Oral BA: 35%–65% Slow and variable GI absorption	Vd: 66 L/kg (range: 18-148 L/kg) Plasma protein binding: ~96%	Hepatic (CYP450 3A4 and 2C8) Active metabolite	Primarily biliary Urinary <1%, as unchanged drug	After IV administration: 25 d After chronic oral therapy: 40–55 d	Onset Oral: 2 d–3 wk IV: initial effects rapid Peak 1 wk–5 mo Duration 7- 50 days

Abbreviations: BA = bioavailability; Vd = volume of distribution.

TABLE 19-13 Acute Intravenous Amiodarone Clinical Indications

Indication	Comments and Cautions
Atrial fibrillation Ventricular rate control	Consider the potential risks of cardioversion (thromboembolic complications)* Consider when other measures are ineffective or contraindicated† Can be used in hemodynamically stable atrial fibrillation with conduction over an accessory pathway such as Wolff-Parkinson-White syndrome† Considered a first-line option in patients with HF†
Atrial fibrillation Cardioversion	Not first line, considered a reasonable option for pharmacologic cardioversion of atrial fibrillation† Slow onset, average time to cardioversion is 24 h Consider risk of thromboembolic complications
VT Monomorphic, sustained	A first-line agent for hemodynamically stable VT*
VT Polymorphic, not associated with long QT interval	If not associated with long QT interval (i.e., torsades)* Polymorphic VT with normal QT interval may be associated with myocardial ischemia, and amiodarone may be effective in arrhythmia suppression*
ACLS Pulseless VT or VF	Antiarrhythmic of choice in ACLS algorithm*

Abbreviations: ACLS = advanced cardiac life support; HF = heart failure; VF = ventricular fibrillation; VT = ventricular tachycardia.

*2010 ACLS guideline recommendation.

†2011 American College of Cardiology Foundation/American Heart Association/Heart Rhythm Society atrial fibrillation management guideline recommendation.

TABLE 19-14 Amiodarone Intravenous Dosing and Administration by Indication

Indications	Dosing and Administration
ACLS Pulseless VT VF (refractory to defibrillation)	300-milligram IV rapid bolus (may give undiluted) May give a single repeat 150-milligram bolus IV if needed
VT Stable monomorphic VT Polymorphic VT with normal QT interval **SVT** Conversion of atrial fibrillation to sinus rhythm To control rapid ventricular rate due to accessory pathway conduction in pre-excited atrial arrhythmias	150 milligrams IV in 100 mL of D5W over 10 min, followed by infusion at 1 mg/min for 6 h, then 0.5 mg/min for the next 18 h If breakthrough arrhythmia occurs, may give repeat 150-milligram IV boluses over 10 min Maximum total daily dose is 2.2 grams

Abbreviations: ACLS = advanced cardiac life support; D5W = dextrose in 5% water; SVT = supraventricular tachycardia; VF = ventricular fibrillation; VT = ventricular tachycardia.

but has all four antiarrhythmic class effects and blocks α-adrenergic receptors. Electrophysiologic action is primarily mediated through Class III antiarrhythmic effects by prolonging the refractory period.[6]

Pharmacokinetics Pharmacokinetics of dronedarone are listed in **Table 19-16**. Dronedarone is ≤94% absorbed, but significant first-pass metabolism decreases the overall bioavailability to ≤15%. With sustained oral dosing, the half-life increases to 27 to 32 hours, and steady-state concentrations are achieved in 4 to 8 days. Dronedarone displays

TABLE 19-15 Amiodarone Adverse Effects*

Cardiovascular	Sinus bradycardia (5% with oral) Ventricular arrhythmias Torsades de pointes (<1%) Increased risk with: Concomitant QT_c prolonging agent Hypokalemia, hypomagnesemia Female gender Thrombophlebitis Atrioventricular nodal block Hypotension (16% with IV); may be related to infusion rate with IV therapy or the IV solution emulsifier polysorbate 80
CNS	Disorders of gait and movement Paresthesias and peripheral neuropathy Dizziness
GI	Nausea/vomiting, anorexia, constipation (10%–33%) Usually responds to a dose reduction or divided doses
Hepatic	Increased liver enzymes (15%–50%) Hepatic injury is typically mild and reversible, but liver failure and death have been reported Monitor baseline LFTs and LFTs every 6 months thereafter
Pulmonary	Pulmonary toxicity (2%–7%, as high as 17%) May be most serious adverse effect other than cardiac. Often reversible, but fatalities have been reported after only 8–14 d of treatment Various manifestations Pulmonary fibrosis, eosinophilia, interstitial pneumonia, allergic alveolitis Monitor baseline PFTs and chest x-ray; repeat chest x-ray annually
Thyroid	Hypothyroidism, more common (4%–22% in some studies) Hyperthyroidism (3%–10%) Hyperthyroidism may diminish antiarrhythmic effect Monitor thyroid function at baseline and every 3–6 months thereafter

Abbreviations: LFTs = liver function tests; PFTs = pulmonary function tests.

*Incomplete listing; excludes nonacute/non–life-threatening dermatologic, ocular, and other effects.

TABLE 19-16 Dronedarone Pharmacokinetics

Absorption	Distribution	Metabolism	Excretion	Half-Life
Bioavailability Fasting: 4% High-fat meal: 15%	**Volume** 1400 L Plasma protein binding: >98%	Hepatic (cytochrome P450 3A) Active metabolite	**Primarily as metabolites** Feces: 84% Renal: 6%	**Single dose** 13–19 h **Sustained oral dosing** 27–32 h

nonlinear kinetics, so doubling a dose may increase plasma concentrations by 2.5- to 3-fold.

Indications Dronedarone is indicated to reduce the risk of hospitalization for atrial fibrillation in patients in sinus rhythm with a history of paroxysmal or persistent atrial fibrillation. It is less efficacious than amiodarone for maintenance of sinus rhythm.

Dosing and Administration The dose of dronedarone is 400 milligrams orally twice daily and should be given with the morning and evening meal to increase bioavailability. Coadministration with grapefruit or grapefruit juice is contraindicated, as this may increase serum concentrations.

Adverse Effects Contraindications and significant adverse effects of dronedarone are highlighted in **Table 19-17**. Compared to amiodarone, dronedarone has lower rates of pulmonary toxicity and has not demonstrated adverse effects on thyroid function. Two clinical trials with dronedarone were prematurely discontinued due to significantly higher rates of serious adverse events in the dronedarone treatment groups, prompting black box warnings that dronedarone is contraindicated in severe or decompensated heart failure and in patients with permanent atrial fibrillation.[5,19] ECGs should be monitored at least every 3 months while on dronedarone. If the patient is found to be in atrial fibrillation, he or she should be cardioverted (if clinically indicated) or dronedarone should be discontinued. Liver function should also be monitored periodically, especially during the first 6 months of therapy.

SOTALOL

Actions Sotalol is a unique, noncardioselective β-blocker that exhibits electrophysiologic characteristics of Class III antiarrhythmics, thus prolonging repolarization and refractoriness without affecting conduction.

TABLE 19-17 Contraindications and Significant Adverse Effects of Dronedarone

Contraindications	In patients with NYHA Class IV HF or NYHA Class II–III HF with recent decompensation requiring referral to a specialized HF clinic
	Permanent atrial fibrillation (in patients in whom sinus rhythm will not or cannot be restored)
	Severe hepatic impairment or previous liver or lung toxicity with amiodarone
	Bradycardia <50 beats/min, QT_c ≥500 ms or PR interval >280 ms, second-degree or third-degree AV block or sick sinus syndrome (except when used in conjunction with a pacemaker)
	Drug–drug interactions with strong cytochrome P450 inhibitors and QT_c prolonging medications
Significant adverse effects	Cardiovascular
	New-onset or worsening HF; QT_c prolongation
	Hepatic
	Severe liver injury, including acute liver failure
	Renal
	Upon initiation, serum creatinine may increase ~0.1 milligram/dL
	Respiratory
	Interstitial lung disease; pulmonary fibrosis and pneumonitis

Abbreviations: AV = atrioventricular; HF = heart failure, NYHA = New York Heart Association.

Pharmacokinetics The onset of action of sotalol is 1 to 2 hours for the oral formulation and 5 to 10 hours after IV administration, with a duration of action of 8 to 16 hours after one dose. The elimination half-life is 12 hours and increases with renal dysfunction. No metabolites are formed, and the drug is primarily eliminated unchanged in the urine.

Indications Sotalol is an effective agent for the suppression of life-threatening ventricular arrhythmias refractory to other antiarrhythmic drugs. It can suppress supraventricular tachycardia and atrial fibrillation but is not indicated for cardioversion of atrial fibrillation.[10]

Dosing and Administration The usual starting dose is 80 milligrams PO twice daily (which can be titrated), and the usual maintenance dose is 160 to 320 milligrams/d; the dose should be reduced by 50% or more in patients with renal insufficiency (creatinine clearance <60 mL/min), and sotalol should not be used (except in special cases) if creatinine clearance is <40 mL/min. IV sotalol is indicated in the current advanced cardiac life support guidelines for hemodynamically stable monomorphic ventricular tachycardia at 1.5 milligrams/kg infused over 5 min. Monitoring of cardiac and renal function is recommended when sotalol is started. During initiation of sotalol therapy (pretreatment QT_c should be <450 milliseconds), QT_c intervals are measured 2 to 4 hours after each oral dose or at the end of an infusion, and therapy is discontinued if QT_c measures ≥500 milliseconds.

Adverse Effects The most common adverse effects of sotalol are bradycardia and hypotension. Sotalol does possess a significant proarrhythmic effect with a 4.3% rate of new or worsened ventricular arrhythmias and a 2.4% rate of torsades de pointes.[20]

DOFETILIDE

Actions/Indications/Dosing Dofetilide is a pure Class III antiarrhythmic and is indicated for the conversion to, and maintenance of, normal sinus rhythm in patients with atrial fibrillation or flutter. Because dofetilide has a significant proarrhythmic effect, it is reserved for patients in whom atrial fibrillation or flutter is highly symptomatic. Dofetilide prescribing is restricted to physicians who have received specific education on dosing and administration and, therefore, is not covered here in detail.[21]

Adverse Effects Serious adverse effects of dofetilide are ventricular tachycardia and QT_c interval prolongation, which can result in torsades de pointes. The risk of developing torsades de pointes is associated with higher dofetilide doses, initiation of therapy, and electrolyte abnormalities.

IBUTILIDE

Actions/Pharmacokinetics Ibutilide prolongs the refractory period in atrial and ventricular cardiac tissues. This action is caused by activation of a slow inward sodium current, as opposed to inhibition of outward potassium currents. Blockade of the delayed rectifier potassium current, which slows repolarization, may also contribute to its clinical effects. The onset of action of ibutilide is ~90 minutes after starting the infusion. Ibutilide is metabolized in the liver, is excreted in the urine and feces, and has a half-life of 2 to 12 hours after IV administration.

Indications/Dosing and Administration/Adverse Effects Ibutilide is indicated for the rapid conversion of recent-onset atrial fibrillation or flutter (greater efficacy) to sinus rhythm.[10] If effective, cardioversion is expected to occur within 1 hour of administration. For patients with atrial fibrillation and an accessory pathway, ibutilide is considered a reasonable option for pharmacologic cardioversion.[16] Serum magnesium and potassium levels should be evaluated and resuscitation equipment made available before ibutilide administration. The loading dose is 1 milligram IV (weight ≥60 kg) or 0.01 milligram/kg IV (weight <60 kg) over 10 minutes and may be repeated once every 10 minutes after completion of the first dose. Electrocardiographic monitoring is continued for at least 4 hours or until the QT_c interval returns to baseline (longer if arrhythmias are observed). Cardiovascular adverse effects of ibutilide include hypotension, hypertension, bradycardia, sinus arrest, syncope, QT_c interval prolongation, congestive heart failure, and torsades de pointes.

TABLE 19-18 Diltiazem and Verapamil Pharmacokinetics

	Absorption	Distribution	Metabolism	Excretion	Half-Life	Onset/Peak/Duration of Action
Diltiazem	Oral BA: IR: 40% ER: 93%–95%	Volume: 5.3 L/kg Plasma protein binding: 70%–80%	Hepatic (cytochrome P450) Active metabolites	Fecal: 60%–65% Renal: 30%	IV/IR 3.4–4.9 h ER: 5–10 h	Onset: IV: 2–3 min PO: 15–60 min Peak: IV: 2–7 min IR: 2–4 h ER: 11–18 h Duration: IV: 1–3 h
Verapamil	Oral BA: 20%–35%	Vd: 3.89 L/kg Plasma protein binding: ~90%	Hepatic (cytochrome P450) Active metabolites	Renal: 70% (as metabolites) Fecal: 16%	3–7 h	Onset/Peak: IV: 1–5 min Duration: IV: 10–20 min

Abbreviations: BA = bioavailability; ER = extended release (controlled release); IR = immediate release; Vd = volume of distribution.

VERNAKALANT

Vernakalant is a Class III antiarrhythmic that inhibits sodium and potassium currents. The atria are more susceptible to vernakalant-induced refractory period prolongation. Vernakalant is not U.S. Food and Drug Administration approved for use in the United States. In Europe, vernakalant is indicated for rapid conversion of recent-onset atrial fibrillation in adults.[22]

CLASS IV ANTIARRHYTHMICS: CALCIUM CHANNEL BLOCKERS

Calcium channel blockers inhibit L-type calcium channels, resulting in slowing of atrioventricular nodal conduction and an increase in the refractory period of nodal tissue. In the myocardium, calcium channels primarily affect the action potential plateau and modulate the strength of muscle contraction. Calcium channel blockers are divided into two categories, dihydropyridine and nondihydropyridine. Nondihydropyridine calcium channel blockers have greater cardioselectivity and are generally used for paroxysmal supraventricular tachycardia and rate control in atrial fibrillation, whereas dihydropyridine calcium channel blockers are more selective for the vasculature and are used to treat hypertension.

DILTIAZEM/VERAPAMIL

Actions Diltiazem and verapamil are nondihydropyridine calcium channel blockers that slow atrioventricular nodal conduction, increase the atrioventricular node's refractory period, decrease automaticity, and prolong the PR interval. Verapamil is more potent than diltiazem resulting in greater atrioventricular nodal depression; therefore, verapamil is used more frequently to abort supraventricular tachycardia than diltiazem.

Pharmacokinetics See **Table 19-18**. Oral diltiazem has a relatively rapid onset of action (15 to 60 minutes); therefore, transitioning from an IV infusion to an oral preparation can be accomplished with relative ease. In addition, diltiazem has a short duration of action (1 to 3 hours), necessitating either a continuous infusion or repeat oral doses. Compared to diltiazem, verapamil has a longer half-life and duration of action. Verapamil also has active metabolites that can accumulate if renal or hepatic disease is present.

Indications Diltiazem and verapamil are indicated for paroxysmal supraventricular tachycardia as well as for rate control in atrial fibrillation[10]; however, verapamil is used more commonly to abort supraventricular tachycardia with a conversion rate to sinus similar to adenosine (90%),[23] whereas diltiazem is used more commonly to control rapid ventricular rate in atrial fibrillation.[10] Both agents are contraindicated for wide-complex tachyarrhythmias, which may be a result of Wolff-Parkinson-White syndrome, due to the high risk of life-threatening ventricular arrhythmia when given to these patients. Other contraindications include sick sinus syndrome, second- or third-degree atrioventricular block, severe hypotension, cardiogenic shock, administration concomitantly or within a few hours of IV β-blockers, and ventricular tachycardia.

Diltiazem Dosing and Administration When initiating diltiazem, an IV bolus of 0.25 milligram/kg over 2 minutes is given, and a continuous infusion is started at 5 to 10 milligrams/h (if bolus is effective). A repeat bolus of 0.35 milligram/kg over 2 minutes may be given if there is inadequate response to initial bolus. The continuous infusion may be increased in 5 milligram/h increments until rate control is achieved to a maximum rate of 15 milligrams/h. Once rate control is achieved, patients may be transitioned to oral diltiazem (**Table 19-19**).

Immediate-release formulations should be used when initially converting the patient to oral diltiazem. Once stable on immediate-release diltiazem, patients can be transitioned to an extended-release formulation by giving an equivalent daily dose.

Verapamil Dosing and Administration For treatment of supraventricular tachycardia, give 2.5 to 5 milligrams IV over 2 minutes. A second dose of 5 to 10 milligrams (~0.15 milligram/kg) may be given 15 to 30 minutes after the initial dose if the patient does not respond to the initial dose and can tolerate a second dose (maximum total dose: 20 to 30 milligrams).[6]

Adverse Effects Diltiazem is generally well tolerated by patients and has a favorable safety profile when compared to other antiarrhythmic agents. Adverse effects associated with diltiazem and verapamil administration are bradyarrhythmia, asystole, fatigue, headache, hypotension, atrioventricular block, peripheral edema, syncope, and dizziness.

NICARDIPINE

Actions Nicardipine is a dihydropyridine calcium channel antagonist that causes relaxation of smooth muscle, thereby lowering blood

TABLE 19-19 IV to PO Conversion of Diltiazem

Medication	IV to PO Conversion	
Diltiazem	After maintenance drip at typical rate of 5–15 milligrams/h has heart rate controlled, may convert to PO. Discontinue infusion 2–3 h after oral dose is given.	
	Diltiazem Drip Rate	**Equivalent PO Dose (Immediate Release)**
	5 milligrams/h	60 milligrams PO every 6 h
	10 milligrams/h	90 milligrams PO every 6 h
	15 milligrams/h	120 milligrams PO every 6 h

TABLE 19-20 Nicardipine Pharmacokinetics

Distribution	Metabolism	Excretion	Half-Life	Onset/Peak/ Duration of Action
Volume: 8.3 L/kg Plasma protein binding: 95%	Hepatic (cytochrome P450)	Fecal: 43% Renal: 49%	2–4 h	Onset: 1 min Peak: 10 min Duration: 3 h

pressure. It has no antiarrhythmic properties and little to no effect on the myocardium.

Pharmacokinetics See **Table 19-20**.

Indications Nicardipine is primarily used for the treatment of hypertension and is contraindicated in patients with aortic stenosis. It is especially useful in patients with acute neurologic emergencies where progressive rapid blood pressure reduction over 15 to 30 minutes is indicated.

Dosing and Administration Nicardipine is administered as an IV infusion with an initial rate of 5 milligrams/h. The infusion may be titrated in 2.5 milligram/h increments every 5 to 15 minutes based on blood pressure response with a maximum infusion rate of 15 milligrams/h.

Adverse Effect Profile Nicardipine is generally well tolerated by patients. Common side effects associated with nicardipine administration include hypotension/orthostatic hypotension, edema, flushing, tachycardia, palpitations, and nausea.

OTHER ANTIARRHYTHMIC MEDICATIONS

DIGOXIN

Actions Digoxin, a cardiac glycoside, has positive inotropic, negative chronotropic, and negative dromotropic effects on the myocardium due to inhibition of the sodium-potassium ATPase.

Pharmacokinetics See **Table 19-21**.[6] Many disease states such as congestive heart failure, hypokalemia, renal failure, and thyroid disease can have a substantial effect on the pharmacokinetics of digoxin. It has a narrow therapeutic index (therapeutic range, 0.5 to 2 nanograms/mL), and toxicity can develop at levels greater than 2 nanograms/mL. In addition, digoxin has numerous drug interactions that can be clinically significant.

Indications Digoxin is indicated for rate control in atrial fibrillation (not first line)[10] and for symptom reduction in congestive heart failure unrelieved by diuretics and angiotensin-converting enzyme inhibitors. Although digoxin is only contraindicated in patients with ventricular arrhythmias, its use should be avoided in patients with Wolff-Parkinson-White syndrome (potential for ventricular fibrillation), acute myocardial infarction, beri-beri heart disease, electrolyte imbalances, sinus node disease, atrioventricular block, and renal impairment. Studies on the mortality associated with digoxin use report conflicting results.[24-28]

Dosing and Administration There are many dosing strategies for digoxin initiation. For atrial fibrillation, current guidelines recommend 0.25 milligram IV every 2 hours up to 1.5 milligrams total. Repeat dosing is necessary when loading digoxin due to the prolonged distribution phase. Maintenance dosing is 0.125 to 0.375 milligram daily. Dose adjustments are often necessary based on age, comorbidities, concomitant medications, and renal dysfunction. Digoxin levels should be monitored for safety and efficacy.

TABLE 19-21 Digoxin IV Pharmacokinetics

Distribution	Metabolism	Excretion	Half-Life	Onset/Peak/ Duration of Action
Volume: 6–7 L/kg Plasma protein binding: ~25%	GI tract Hepatic	Urine: 50%–70% as unchanged drug	38 h	Onset: 5–60 min Peak: 1–6 h Duration: 3–4 d

Adverse Effects Adverse effects of digoxin are generally GI. Other more rare adverse effects may include gynecomastia, skin rash, eosinophilia, and thrombocytopenia. Digoxin can also cause cardiac arrhythmias, such as sinus bradycardia, atrioventricular or sinoatrial nodal block, and ventricular arrhythmias.

Symptoms of digoxin toxicity include mental status changes, visual disturbances, delirium, and seizures. Many types of arrhythmias can occur as a result of digoxin toxicity, and the clinician must be able to recognize the signs and symptoms associated with toxicity and treat accordingly.

ATROPINE

TABLE 19-22 Atropine Drug Information

Generic Name	Onset of Action	Metabolism	Half-Life	IV Dose (Adult)	Indications
Atropine	Rapid	Hepatic	2–3 h	0.5 milligram IV every 3–5 min (maximum total dose: 3 milligrams or 0.04 milligram/kg)	Sinus bradycardia (symptomatic)

Use is no longer recommended in the management of asystole or pulseless electrical activity.

Actions Atropine blocks the effects of acetylcholine at parasympathetic sites in smooth muscle thus increasing cardiac output.[6]

Pharmacokinetics See **Table 19-22**.

Indications Atropine is considered first-line therapy for the treatment of symptomatic bradycardia. Based on the current advanced cardiac life support treatment guidelines, it is no longer recommended for the treatment of asystole or pulseless electrical activity.[7] Atropine should be used with caution in patients with coronary heart disease, acute myocardial ischemia, congestive heart failure, tachycardia, and hypertension.[6]

Dosing and Administration See Table 19-22.[6,7] Doses <0.5 milligram and slow injection have been associated with paradoxical bradycardia.

Adverse Effects The most common adverse effects of atropine include tachyarrhythmia, constipation, xerostomia, blurred vision, and photophobia.

ADENOSINE

Actions Adenosine is an endogenous nucleoside that exerts multiple effects mediated by binding adenosine receptors and inhibiting adenylate cyclase, resulting in the decreased flow of calcium ions in the atrioventricular node. It also decreases sinoatrial nodal depolarization by activation of acetylcholine-sensitive potassium currents. These effects result in hyperpolarization and automaticity in cardiac nodal tissue. Adenosine is a first-line agent used in the treatment of narrow-complex supraventricular tachycardia in patients who have failed vagal maneuvers, and it may also be used in the setting of stable monomorphic, wide-complex tachycardias as a diagnostic tool.

Pharmacokinetics See **Table 19-23**.

Indications Adenosine is used for the treatment of supraventricular tachycardia with or without reentry pathways, after failure of vagal maneuvers. It is ineffective for the treatment of atrial fibrillation and flutter and ventricular tachycardias.

TABLE 19-23 Adenosine Pharmacokinetics

Metabolism	Half-Life	Onset/Duration of Action
Blood, tissue	<10 s	Onset: rapid Duration: very brief

TABLE 19-24 Adenosine Intravenous Dosing and Administration

Indication	Dosing and Administration
Paroxysmal supraventricular tachycardia	Initial dose: 6 milligrams IV If ineffective after 1–2 min, may give second dose of 12 milligrams IV May repeat 12 milligrams IV if needed

Rapid IV push over 1–2 seconds via peripheral line. Flush line after each dose with 20 mL of normal saline. Patients usually experience transient asystole (<5 seconds).

The initial adenosine dose should be reduced to 3 milligrams in patients on concomitant therapy with dipyridamole or carbamazepine, in heart transplant patients, or for central line administration.

Adenosine effects are antagonized by caffeine and theophylline, and patients may require higher doses.

Dosing and Administration See **Table 19-24.**[6]

Adverse Effects The most common adverse effects associated with adenosine administration include transient asystole (treatment goal), chest discomfort/pressure, headache, flushing, and nausea. The adverse effects are usually temporary due to the short half-life of the drug. Bronchospasm and atrial fibrillation can also occur, but the incidence is rare. Severe adverse effects, including cardiac conduction abnormalities and hypotension, are more common with continuous infusion adenosine used in stress testing.

MAGNESIUM SULFATE

Actions/Indications/Dosing and Administration Intravenous magnesium sulfate exerts antiarrhythmic effects in the treatment of torsades de pointes. Its antiarrhythmic activity is mediated by inhibiting calcium currents that cause pathologic early after-depolarizations and thereby cardiac dyssynchrony. Magnesium slows sinoatrial node activity, prolongs myocardial conduction time, stabilizes excitable membranes, and is a cofactor in ion movement.[29] IV magnesium sulfate has a rapid onset of action and is indicated in the treatment of torsades de pointes, polymorphic ventricular tachycardia associated with a prolonged QT interval, and cardiac arrest when ventricular fibrillation/pulseless ventricular tachycardia is associated with torsades de pointes. In patients with a pulse, 1 to 2 grams IV is diluted in normal saline or 5% dextrose in water and administered as a rapid bolus. Rapid IV administration of magnesium sulfate is associated with vasodilation, flushing, and hypotension.

ISOPROTERENOL

Actions/Pharmacokinetics/Indications Isoproterenol exerts antiarrhythmic effects by stimulating β_1- and β_2-receptors. The β_1-receptor interaction results in increased chronotropic and inotropic activities in the myocardium and vasodilation by β_2-receptor–mediated relaxation of smooth muscle. Isoproterenol has an immediate onset of action, a half-life of 2.5 to 5 minutes, and a duration of 10 to 15 minutes. It is indicated for refractory bradyarrhythmias, atrioventricular nodal block, and refractory torsades de pointes. Isoproterenol is contraindicated in patients with angina, preexisting ventricular arrhythmias, tachyarrhythmias, or digoxin toxicity.

Dosing and Administration Isoproterenol should be initiated at 2 micrograms/min (maximum rate, 10 micrograms/min) and titrated every 5 to 10 minutes based on patient response.

Adverse Effect Profile Serious adverse effects of isoproterenol include hypotension, premature ventricular beats, tachyarrhythmia, ventricular arrhythmia, dyspnea, and pulmonary edema.

REFERENCES

The complete reference list is available online at www.TintinalliEM.com.

CHAPTER 20 Pharmacology of Vasopressors and Inotropes

Sara H. Shields
Rachel M. Holland

INTRODUCTION

Vasopressors are potent pharmacologic agents that are used to increase blood pressure and mean arterial pressure by vasoconstriction, thus increasing systemic vascular resistance. As such, they should be reserved for cases of persistent hypotension and tissue hypoperfusion after volume resuscitation has failed. Most vasopressors have multiple actions on the heart and vasculature and have a propensity to cause arrhythmias. Some vasopressors are also inotropes and are used to improve cardiac output, particularly in patients with left ventricular pump failure or cardiogenic shock. **Table 20-1**[1-3] provides a summary of common vasopressor and inotropic agent doses, effects, and uses.

VASOPRESSORS

DOPAMINE

Actions Dopamine is an endogenous catecholamine and a metabolic precursor of norepinephrine and epinephrine that acts on dopaminergic, α_1, β_1, and β_2 receptors in a dose-dependent fashion. At intermediate doses (5 to 15 micrograms/kg/min), dopamine increases renal blood flow, heart rate, cardiac contractility, and cardiac output. At high doses (>15 micrograms/kg/min), the α-adrenergic effects of dopamine dominate, leading to vasoconstriction and increased blood pressure. Low-dose (renal dose) dopamine is no longer recommended for renal protection due to lack of data support.[4]

Pharmacokinetics See **Table 20-2.**[3]

Indications Dopamine increases cardiac output, blood pressure, and peripheral perfusion and is indicated for reversing hemodynamically significant hypotension caused by myocardial infarction, trauma, heart failure, and renal failure, when fluid resuscitation is unsuccessful or inappropriate. Based on the 2012 Surviving Sepsis Campaign guidelines, dopamine is no longer recommended as an initial vasopressor of choice for septic shock, based on data showing lower short-term mortality and arrhythmias in patients receiving norepinephrine versus dopamine.[5] Dopamine can be considered as an alternative vasopressor agent to norepinephrine only in highly selected patients (i.e., patients with low risk of tachyarrhythmias and absolute or relative bradycardia).[4] Although not considered a first-line agent, dopamine can also be used for the treatment of symptomatic bradycardia (particularly if associated with hypotension) that is unresponsive to atropine.[5]

Dosing and Administration See Table 20-1. Dopamine is administered as a continuous IV infusion (central line recommended) and should be titrated to desired response. When discontinuing the infusion, the dose should be gradually decreased to avoid hypotension.

Adverse Effects Adverse effects of dopamine include chest pain, hypotension (low doses), hypertension (higher doses), ectopic beats, palpitations, nausea, vomiting, headache, gangrene, and tachycardia. Extravasation of dopamine may cause tissue necrosis and sloughing and can be treated by local infiltration with phentolamine. Dopamine is contraindicated in patients with pheochromocytoma or tachyarrhythmias/ventricular fibrillation.

EPINEPHRINE

Actions Epinephrine, an endogenous catecholamine, is a nonselective α- and β-adrenergic agonist that causes increases in systemic vascular resistance, heart rate, cardiac output, and blood pressure. It is used as a

TABLE 20-1 Summary of Common Vasopressor Doses, Effects, and Uses

Drug	Dose Range	Receptor Activation	Cardiovascular Effects	Use
Dopamine	2–20 micrograms/kg/min	Dose dependent <5 micrograms/kg/min: DA_1, DA_2 5–10 micrograms/kg/min: β_1 >10 micrograms/kg/min: α_1	*↑HR, BP, CO, SVR	Cardiogenic shock, vasodilatory shock
Epinephrine	2–10 micrograms/min or 0.05–0.5 micrograms/kg/min	α_1, β_1, β_2	↑HR, BP, MAP, SV, SVR, CO	Cardiogenic shock, vasodilatory shock, ACLS
Norepinephrine	2–50 micrograms/min or 0.02–2 micrograms/kg/min	α_1, β_1	↑BP, MAP, SVR, CO	Cardiogenic shock, vasodilatory shock
Phenylephrine	50–300 micrograms/min or 0.02–2 micrograms/kg/min	α_1	↑BP, MAP, SVR	Vasodilatory shock, obstructive shock
Vasopressin	0.01–0.04 units/min	V_1	↑BP, SVR	Cardiogenic shock, vasodilatory shock, ACLS
Dobutamine	2–20 micrograms/kg/min	β_1, β_2	↑HR, BP, MAP, CO; ↓SVR	ADHF, cardiogenic shock, vasodilatory shock
Milrinone	50 micrograms/kg bolus (optional); 0.25–0.75 micrograms/kg/min†	N/A	↑HR, BP, MAP, CO; ↓SVR	ADHF

Abbreviations: ACLS = advanced cardiac life support; ADHF = acute decompensated heart failure; BP = blood pressure; CO = cardiac output; HR = heart rate; MAP = mean arterial pressure; SV = stroke volume; SVR = systemic vascular resistance; ↑ = increased; ↓ = decreased.

*Dose dependent.

†Renal adjustment required.

bronchodilator in acute asthma and for the treatment of anaphylactic reactions. Epinephrine also increases cerebral and coronary perfusion and cerebral perfusion pressure during resuscitation and is therefore used in various advanced cardiac life support algorithms including cardiac arrest.

Pharmacokinetics See **Table 20-3**.[3,6]

Indications Epinephrine is indicated for the treatment of anaphylaxis, hypersensitivity reactions, and acute asthma exacerbations. Based on current advanced cardiac life support guidelines, it is indicated in the treatment of cardiac arrest (i.e., pulseless ventricular tachycardia/ventricular fibrillation, pulseless electrical activity, and asystole) because it improves return of spontaneous circulation (but does not improve survival or function), and it can also be used for symptomatic bradycardia unresponsive to atropine or pacing.[5] In addition, the 2012 Surviving Sepsis Campaign guidelines recommend epinephrine (added to and potentially substituted for norepinephrine) when an additional agent is needed to maintain adequate blood pressure in patients with severe sepsis or septic shock.[4]

Dosing and Administration See **Table 20-4**.[3]

Adverse Effects Adverse effects of epinephrine include angina, palpitations, arrhythmias, hypertension, tachycardia, nausea, vomiting, headache, anxiety, and pulmonary edema. Extravasation of epinephrine may cause tissue necrosis and sloughing and can be treated by local infiltration with phentolamine.

NOREPINEPHRINE

Actions Norepinephrine is an endogenous catecholamine that stimulates α-adrenergic receptors, resulting in peripheral vasoconstriction and increased blood pressure, as well as β-adrenergic receptors ($\beta_1 > \beta_2$), leading to inotropic stimulation of the heart and coronary artery vasodilation. It is used for the treatment of sepsis and septic shock refractory to fluid resuscitation and in severe hypotension.

Pharmacokinetics See **Table 20-5**.[3,6]

Indications Norepinephrine is indicated for the treatment of acute hypotension and profound hypotension in post–cardiac arrest patients. Based on the 2012 Surviving Sepsis Campaign guidelines, it is also considered the initial vasopressor of choice for the treatment of severe sepsis and septic shock refractory to adequate fluid resuscitation.[4]

Dosing and Administration See **Table 20-6**.[3,6]

Adverse Effects Adverse effects of norepinephrine include bradycardia, arrhythmias, peripheral (digital) ischemia, hypertension, nausea, vomiting, headache, anxiety, and cardiac arrest. Extravasation of norepinephrine may cause tissue necrosis and sloughing and can be treated by local infiltration with phentolamine.

PHENYLEPHRINE

Actions Phenylephrine is a selective α_1-adrenergic agonist that essentially lacks β-adrenergic activity. The cumulative effect of phenylephrine results in systemic arterial vasoconstriction, leading to increased systemic vascular resistance and dose-dependent elevations in systolic and diastolic blood pressure. Phenylephrine has no direct effects on heart rate; however, reflex bradycardia and reduced cardiac output may occur, especially in patients with heart failure or cardiogenic shock.[6,7]

Pharmacokinetics See **Table 20-7**.[3]

Indications Phenylephrine is indicated for the treatment of hypotension and shock. Use of phenylephrine is not recommended for the treatment of cardiogenic or septic shock.

Dosing and Administration Phenylephrine is administered as a continuous IV infusion. The typical starting dose of phenylephrine is 50 to 150 micrograms/min or 0.02 to 2 micrograms/kg/min and should be titrated based on hemodynamic parameters and clinical effect. The com-

TABLE 20-2 Dopamine Pharmacokinetics (IV)

Metabolism	Excretion	Half-Life	Onset/Duration of Action
Renal, hepatic, plasma; 75% to inactive metabolites by monoamine oxidase and 25% to norepinephrine	Urine (as metabolites)	~2 min	Onset: ≤5 min Duration: <10 min

TABLE 20-3 Epinephrine Pharmacokinetics (IV)

Metabolism	Excretion	Half-Life	Onset/Duration of Action
Hepatic, other tissues: rapidly inactivated and degraded by enzymes Hepatic: metabolized by monoamine oxidase and catechol-o-methyltransferase	Urine (mostly as inactive metabolites)	2 min	Onset: 1–2 min Duration: 2–10 min

TABLE 20-4 Epinephrine Dosing and Administration

ACLS (asystole, pulseless arrest, pulseless VT/VF)†	Bradycardia	Hypotension/Shock	Anaphylaxis
1 milligram IV/IO every 3–5 min until ROSC (1:1000 solution) **2–2.5 milligrams ET every 3–5 min until IV/IO access established or ROSC (dilute in 5–10 mL NS or SW)**	IV infusion: 2–10 micrograms/min *or* 0.05–0.5 micrograms/kg/min (titrate to desired effect)	IV infusion: 0.05–0.5 micrograms/kg/min (titrate to desired response)	0.2–0.5 milligrams IM/SC every 5 min as needed (1:1000 solution) 0.1 milligram IV (1:10,000 solution) over 5 min; may infuse at 1–4 micrograms/min to prevent frequent repeat injections *or* may initiate with an infusion at 5–15 micrograms/min (with crystalloid administration)*

Abbreviations: ET = endotracheal; IO = intraosseous; NS = normal saline; ROSC = return of spontaneous circulation; SW = sterile water; **VT = ventricular tachycardia; VF = ventricular fibrillation.**

*In general, IV administration should be reserved for patients who are profoundly hypotensive or are in cardiopulmonary arrest refractory to volume resuscitation and several epinephrine injections. **When administering as a continuous IV infusion, central line administration is preferred.**

†Current at the time of publication, epinephrine is recommended in ACLS guidelines for pulseless rhythms, however, some studies have shown worse outcomes, while others have shown no improvement in long term survival or neurologic function.

mon maintenance infusion range is 40 to 60 micrograms/min to maintain blood pressure. Phenylephrine can also be given as an IV bolus for acute blood pressure management. The normal bolus dose range is 100 to 500 micrograms/dose IV every 10 to 15 minutes as needed.

Adverse Effects Adverse effects of phenylephrine include hypertension, decreased cardiac output, reflex bradycardia, and arrhythmias (rare). Phenylephrine use can also lead to renal, mesenteric, and myocardial ischemia, as well as ischemia and necrosis to the extremities. Because phenylephrine is a vesicant, IV extravasation can result in local necrosis and sloughing of affected tissue. If extravasation occurs, the infusion should be stopped immediately and phentolamine should be administered.

Phenylephrine should be used with caution in patients with bradycardia, hyperthyroidism, heart block, and coronary artery disease. The use of phenylephrine is not recommended for cardiogenic shock because it can further worsen cardiac output due to reflex bradycardia.[6] The 2012 Surviving Sepsis Campaign guidelines recommend against the use of phenylephrine for septic shock unless a trial of norepinephrine was associated with serious arrhythmias, cardiac output is known to be high, or it is used as add-on therapy when other first-line vasopressor agents fail to achieve goal mean arterial pressure.[4] Appropriate volume resuscitation should occur before phenylephrine is used in hypotensive patients.

TABLE 20-5 Norepinephrine Pharmacokinetics (IV)

Metabolism	Excretion	Half-Life	Onset/Duration of Action
Via monoamine oxidase and catechol-o-methyltransferase	Urine (84%–96% as inactive metabolites)	3 min	Onset: 1–2 min Duration: 5–10 min

TABLE 20-6 Norepinephrine Dosing and Administration

Hypotension	Post–Cardiac Arrest Care (Advanced Cardiac Life Support)	Sepsis/Septic Shock
Initial: 8–12 micrograms/min (titrate to desired response) Maintenance: 2–4 micrograms/min	Initial: 0.05–0.5 micrograms/kg/min (titrate to desired response)	0.02–2 micrograms/kg/min

Administer as a continuous IV infusion (central line recommended).

Do not discontinue infusion abruptly. Slowly taper the dose to avoid rebound hypertension.

TABLE 20-7 Phenylephrine Pharmacokinetics (IV)

Metabolism	Excretion	Half-Life	Onset/Duration of Action
Hepatic via oxidative deamination (50%); undergoes sulfation (8%) and some glucuronidation; forms inactive metabolites	Urine (mostly as inactive metabolites)	Alpha phase: ~5 min Terminal phase: 2–3 h	Onset: immediate Duration: ~15–20 min

VASOPRESSIN

Actions Vasopressin, an endogenous nonadrenergic vasopressor, stimulates V_1 receptors in vascular smooth muscle, causing direct peripheral vasoconstriction and subsequent increases in systemic vascular resistance and blood pressure, as well as improved cerebral and cardiac perfusion. It does not exhibit inotropic or chronotropic effects on the heart and can cause a decrease in heart rate and cardiac output. Vasopressin also acts on V_2 receptors in the kidneys causing an antidiuretic effect.

Pharmacokinetics See **Table 20-8**.[3,6]

Indications Vasopressin is indicated for the treatment of diabetes insipidus. Based on current advanced cardiac life support guidelines, a single dose of vasopressin can be used to replace the first or second dose of epinephrine in the treatment of cardiac arrest (i.e., pulseless ventricular tachycardia/ventricular fibrillation, asystole, and pulseless electrical activity) to improve return of spontaneous circulation.[5] According to the 2012 Surviving Sepsis Campaign guidelines, vasopressin (up to 0.03 unit/min) may be added to norepinephrine to either raise mean arterial pressure to target or to decrease norepinephrine dose but should not be used as the single initial vasopressor for treatment of sepsis-induced hypotension. Doses higher than 0.03 to 0.04 unit/min should be reserved for salvage therapy (failure to achieve adequate mean arterial pressure with other vasopressor agents).[6]

Dosing and Administration See **Table 20-9**.[3]

Adverse Effects Adverse effects of vasopressin include diaphoresis, nausea, vomiting, headache, urticaria, gangrenous disorder, arrhythmias, mesenteric ischemia, chest pain, myocardial infarction, bronchial

TABLE 20-8 Vasopressin Pharmacokinetics (IV)

Metabolism	Excretion	Half-Life	Onset/Duration of Action
Hepatic, renal	Renal (5%–15%)	10–20 min	Onset: immediate Duration: 10–0 min

TABLE 20-9 Vasopressin Dosing and Administration

Cardiac Arrest	Septic Shock
40 units IV/IO to replace first or second dose of epinephrine (single dose) May give endotracheally if no IV/IO access	IV infusion: 0.01–0.04 unit/min (in combination with 1–2 additional catecholamines)

constriction, venous thrombosis, and cardiac arrest. Extravasation of vasopressin may cause tissue necrosis and sloughing and can be treated by local infiltration with phentolamine.

INOTROPES

DOBUTAMINE

Actions Dobutamine is a synthetic dopamine analog with potent inotropic and mild vasodilatory and chronotropic effects. It competitively binds and stimulates α- and β-receptors ($\beta_1 > \beta_2 > \alpha$), resulting in the major effects of increased contractility and heart rate, with mostly neutral effects on blood pressure.

Pharmacokinetics See **Table 20-10**.[3]

Indications Dobutamine is indicated for the short-term management of patients with acute cardiac decompensation, particularly in patients presenting with cardiogenic shock. Dobutamine can also be used for septic shock as monotherapy or in addition to vasopressors in patients presenting with myocardial dysfunction, low cardiac output, or persistent signs of hypoperfusion.[4]

Dosing and Administration Dobutamine is administered as a continuous infusion with a normal starting dose of 2 micrograms/kg/min titrated up to a maximum dose of 40 micrograms/kg/min based on clinical effect. The maximum recommended dose for septic shock is 20 micrograms/kg/min.[4]

Adverse Effects Adverse effects associated with dobutamine include hypertension, hypotension, tachycardia, arrhythmias, myocardial ischemia, angina, and hypokalemia. Dobutamine IV extravasation can cause phlebitis, local inflammation, and rarely tissue necrosis.

The use of dobutamine in patients with atrial fibrillation is cautioned due to the potential to increase ventricular response. It should also be used with caution in post–myocardial infarction patients because of increased myocardial oxygen demand. Dobutamine is ineffective in the presence of aortic stenosis and should be avoided. Concomitant use of monoamine oxidase inhibitors may result in prolonged hypertension and should be avoided. Dobutamine should be limited to short-term use when possible. Prolonged inotrope therapy has been associated with increased mortality.[8]

MILRINONE

Actions Milrinone is an inotrope with vasodilator properties ("inodilator") that selectively inhibits the phosphodiesterase type III enzyme, resulting in the inhibition of the breakdown of cyclic adenosine monophosphate in myocardial and vascular smooth muscle cells. Increased cyclic adenosine monophosphate levels result in increased cardiac contractility as well as peripheral arterial and venous vasodilation. The cumulative effects of milrinone include increased cardiac output and reduced systemic vascular resistance .[9]

Pharmacokinetics See **Table 20-11**.

Indications Milrinone is indicated for the short-term treatment of acute decompensated heart failure.

Dosing and Administration Milrinone is administered as an optional IV loading dose and a continuous infusion. The typical loading dose of milrinone is 50 micrograms/kg IV over 10 minutes, while the maintenance infusion should be started at 0.25 to 0.75 micrograms/kg/min and titrated to effect. The loading dose is commonly omitted, particularly in patients who are hypotensive. Milrinone must be renally adjusted if the creatinine clearance is less than 50 mL/min.

TABLE 20-10 Dobutamine Pharmacokinetics (IV)

Metabolism	Excretion	Half-Life	Onset of Action/ Peak Effect
In tissues and hepatically to inactive metabolites	Urine (as metabolites)	2 min	Onset: 1–10 min Peak: 10–20 min

TABLE 20-11 Milrinone Pharmacokinetics (IV)

Metabolism	Excretion	Half-Life	Onset of Action
Hepatic (12%)	Urine (85% as unchanged drug)	~2.5 h, prolonged in renal dysfunction	Onset: 5–15 min

Adverse Effects Adverse effects associated with milrinone use include ventricular and supraventricular arrhythmias, hypotension, angina, and headache. Thrombocytopenia and abnormal liver function tests are rare but may also occur.

Unlike dobutamine, milrinone use is not recommended for use in septic shock. Milrinone can exacerbate hypotension and arrhythmias; consequently, extreme caution is warranted when used in these circumstances. Fluid resuscitation and electrolyte correction should occur before initiating milrinone. Long-term treatment of inotropic therapy has been associated with increased mortality and should be limited to short-term therapy in most cases.

REFERENCES

The complete reference list is available online at www.TintinalliEM.com.

CHAPTER 21 Hyperbaric Oxygen Therapy

David S. Lambert
Stephen R. Thom

INTRODUCTION

Hyperbaric oxygen (HBO) therapy involves breathing oxygen with the body exposed to an ambient pressure greater than that of sea level. HBO therapy results in the systemic delivery of oxygen that produces supraphysiologic oxygen tension in perfused tissues. The effects of HBO therapy are due to the combined effects of both increased ambient pressure and increased oxygen tension.[1]

HBO therapy is delivered in a hyperbaric chamber. Monoplace chambers accommodate a single occupant and are typically clear, acrylic, plastic, cylindrical units with a door at one end (**Figure 21-1**). An attendant monitors the patient from the outside and communicates via intercom. Specially designed cardiopulmonary monitoring devices, intravenous infusion pumps, and ventilators enable critically ill patients to be treated in most monoplace chambers. Multiplace chambers can simultaneously treat multiple patients and will accommodate medical personnel inside the chamber (chamber tender or assistant) to perform hands-on patient assessment and care (**Figure 21-2**). Monoplace chambers generally use 100% oxygen for pressurization, whereas multiplace units are pressurized with air and patients breathe oxygen using tight-fitting facemasks, a hood, or endotracheal tube while inside. Most HBO chamber facilities have equipment and treatment protocols analogous to an intensive care unit.

Ambient pressure is an important concept in HBO therapy. At sea level, the pressure exerted by the air column (the atmosphere) above is quantified as 1 atmospheres absolute of pressure (1 ATA), 14.7 lb per square inch, 760 mm Hg, or 760 torr. Once a patient is placed inside a chamber, the ambient pressure is increased by the gradual inflow of compressed gas, either oxygen or air. Most HBO therapy takes place with an ambient pressure between 2.0 and 3.0 ATA.

In hyperbaric and diving medicine, the increased ambient pressure was originally described as of feet of sea water (fsw) or meters of sea water (msw) for both HBO treatment and during scuba diving. One atmosphere is equal to the pressure exerted by 33 fsw (10 msw), so starting at sea level, the ambient pressure is 1 ATA, and at a depth of 33 fsw,

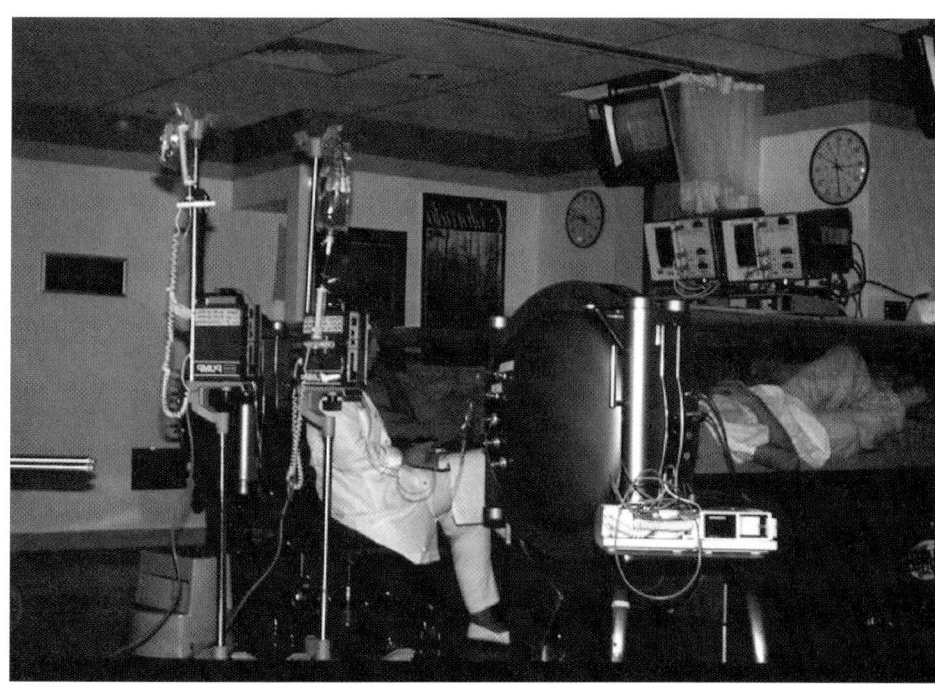

FIGURE 21-1. Monoplace hyperbaric chamber.

the ambient pressure would be 2 ATA. Describing an HBO treatment at either 2 ATA or 33 fsw communicates equivalent pressure.

A typical HBO treatment lasts 90 to 120 minutes. The initial pressurization phase is done over 10 to 15 minutes to allow for equalization of pressures within the sinuses and middle ear as ambient pressure increases. Pressure is then maintained at the desired levels for 40 to 90 minutes, followed by depressurization over 5 to 10 minutes. In a monoplace chamber, the patient is surrounded by and breathes 100% oxygen during the entire treatment. If desired, air breaks are done for 5 to 10 minutes with the patient breathing air from a mask while in the chamber. In a multiplace chamber, the patient is surrounded by air during the entire treatment and breathes 100% oxygen via a face mask or hood. Air breaks in a multiplace chamber are accomplished by removing the mask or hood and breathing the surrounding air. HBO treatments are done using preset protocols that define the level of pressurization, duration of each individual treatment, the use of air breaks, and the number of individual sessions in a course of therapy.

GAS LAWS

The physics of HBO therapy are governed by the ideal gas laws. Boyle's law states that for gases kept at a constant temperature, the volume of that gas is inversely proportional to the pressure exerted on it. If pressure doubles, then the volume is halved. Boyle's law is the principal behind HBO treatment of decompression sickness and air or gas embolism—

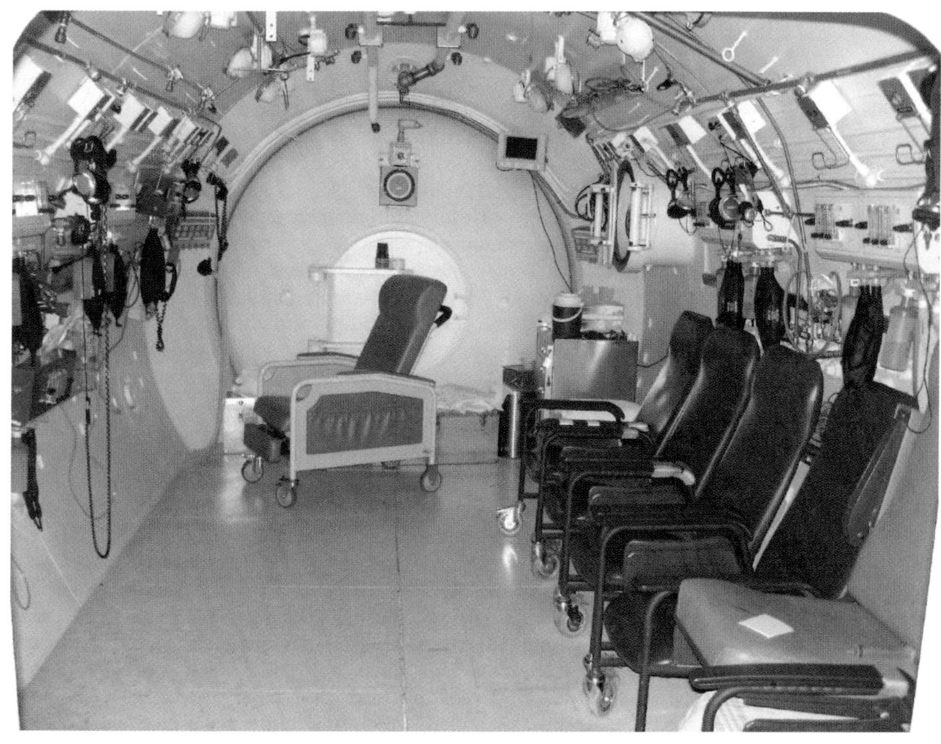

FIGURE 21-2. Multiplace hyperbaric chamber.

reducing the size of gas bubbles within tissues and circulation by increasing ambient pressure. Boyle's law also explains the occurrence of pain in the sinuses and ears during pressurization and decompression, as trapped pockets of gas contract or expand as ambient pressure changes.

Gay-Lussac's law states that at a constant volume (e.g., a hyperbaric chamber) the absolute pressure is directly proportional to the absolute temperature. This explains why the ambient temperature inside a chamber increases transiently as it is pressurized and cools with decompression.

Henry's law specifies that the partial pressure of a gas dissolved in a liquid is proportional to the pressure exerted on that gas. HBO therapy increases the ambient partial pressure of oxygen (Po_2), producing an increase in the amount of dissolved oxygen carried by the blood. A patient in a hyperbaric chamber compressed to 2 ATA (equivalent to a diver at 33 fsw) breathing 21% oxygen is exposed to a Po_2 of 320 mm Hg, twice the Po_2 at ambient pressure before starting the treatment. Although the percentage of oxygen at 2 ATA is still 21%, the patient is inhaling twice as many molecules of oxygen with each breath. This is functionally equivalent to breathing 42% oxygen at sea level or 1 ATA.

The oxygen content of the blood is the sum of the oxygen carried by hemoglobin and oxygen dissolved in the plasma. Hemoglobin becomes fully saturated around a Po_2 of 100 mm Hg; fully saturated hemoglobin carries approximately 20 mL of oxygen per 100 mL of blood, which is expressed as 20 vol%. At 1 ATA breathing room air, dissolved oxygen in the plasma is typically only 0.3 vol%. At a pressure of 3 ATA inside an HBO chamber pressurized with 100% oxygen, the arterial oxygen tension (Pao_2) will approach 2200 mm Hg, which will bring the dissolved oxygen content up to about 5.4 vol%.[2] This amount of dissolved oxygen can sustain basal metabolic functions in the complete absence of hemoglobin.

PHYSIOLOGIC EFFECTS

HBO therapy should be viewed as a drug and the hyperbaric chamber as a delivery device. HBO affects tissues in two ways: there are effects related to mechanical forces of increased pressure and effects due to hyperoxygenation. Of the two, elevating tissue oxygen tension is the primary effect.

Hyperoxygenation induces the formation of reactive oxygen species (superoxide, hydrogen peroxide, hypochlorous acid, and hydroxyl) and reactive nitrogen species (primarily nitric oxide). Levels generated during HBO therapy have beneficial effects seen after tissue oxygen levels return to normal (**Table 21-1**). Reactive oxygen species are natural byproducts of metabolism that can oxidize proteins and membrane lipids, damage DNA, and mediate tissue and organ damage seen in oxygen toxicity. The body has scavenger antioxidant systems to reverse the oxidative damage caused by reactive oxygen species generated during a typical HBO treatment of about 2 hours, so that oxygen toxicity is rare.

INDICATIONS

The Undersea and Hyperbaric Medical Society has defined clinical indications for HBO therapy, some of which are within the scope of emergency medicine practice (**Table 21-2**).[3]

TABLE 21-1 Beneficial Effects of Reactive Oxygen and Nitrogen Species
Inhibit microbial endotoxin and exotoxin production
Enhance oxygen-dependent transport of antibiotics across cell walls
Improve neutrophil oxygen-dependent peroxidase bactericidal activity
Induce vasoconstriction that reduces posttraumatic tissue edema
Stimulate angiogenesis by promoting the production of oxygen-dependent collagen matrix
Promote wound healing by amplifying oxygen gradients at the periphery of ischemic wounds
Blunt endothelial ischemia-reperfusion injury

TABLE 21-2 Indications for Hyperbaric Oxygen Therapy
Arterial gas embolism with neurologic symptoms*
Decompression sickness*
Carbon monoxide poisoning*
Crush injury, compartment syndrome, and other acute traumatic ischemias*
Exceptional blood loss anemia*
Delayed radiation injury (osteoradionecrosis and soft tissue)
Compromised skin grafts and flaps
Acute thermal burns*
Arterial insufficiencies (enhancement of healing in selected problem wounds, central retinal artery occlusion)
Necrotizing soft tissue infections*
Clostridial myonecrosis (gas gangrene)*
Osteomyelitis (refractory)
Intracranial abscesses

*Conditions that lend themselves to emergency medicine practice.

AIR OR GAS EMBOLISM

Air or gas embolism can occur as a consequence of a deep sea dive–related accident[4] or as the result of a medical procedure.[5] Iatrogenic air or gas embolism has been reported in association with cardiovascular, obstetric/gynecologic, neurosurgical, and orthopedic procedures, generally associated with disruption of a vascular wall.[6] Nonsurgical processes reported to cause air or gas embolism include overexpansion during mechanical ventilation, hemodialysis, and after accidental opening of central venous catheters. Air or gas embolism can occur either on the venous or arterial side of the circulatory system.

The consequences of an arterial gas embolism depend on location and magnitude of arterial occlusion. Often skeletal muscle, connective tissue, and skin can tolerate small emboli, but bubbles entering the coronary or cerebral arteries can precipitate acute coronary syndrome or stroke. Air entering the spinal cord circulation can produce weakness or paralysis. Any diver who surfaces with sudden onset of neurologic symptoms, such as confusion, speech difficulty, focal weakness, or paralysis, in less than 5 to 10 minutes should be assumed to have arterial gas embolism unless proven otherwise. Imaging with CT or MRI may help exclude an ischemic stroke or intracerebral hemorrhage. CT scan of the brain may show air in the cerebral vessels; however, this finding is variable and can be difficult to recognize (**Figure 21-3**).

Venous gas embolism is common after compressed-gas diving and surgical procedures.[6] The amount of gas is typically small, and the bubbles are trapped in the pulmonary capillaries and resorbed without symptoms. Large quantities of gas in the pulmonary vasculature can stimulate cough, dyspnea, and pulmonary edema. A paradoxical arterial gas embolism may develop when a venous gas embolism travels to the arterial system by way of an intrapulmonary shunt or through an atrial septal defect or patent foramen ovale.

Administer oxygen to support arterial oxygenation and hasten bubble resorption. Place the patient in the supine position; there is no proven benefit to a head-down position to lower the risk of additional cerebral air embolization or a left lateral decubitus position to trap gas within the apex of the right ventricle and minimize migration. Catheter aspiration of trapped air in the right ventricle may be attempted in those rare instances when it is visualized.

HBO is recommended for air or gas embolism with neurologic or cardiovascular impairment.[3] The faster the patient receives HBO, the greater is the chance for complete neurologic recovery. Various protocols are used for air or gas embolism. A standard one is Treatment Table 6 from the U.S. Navy Diving Manual, which uses compression to 2.8 ATA for 75 minutes (with three air breaks), following by decompression to 1.8 ATA for 150 minutes (with two air breaks) for a total treatment time of 285 minutes. For patients whose symptoms are not improved or worsen, a protocol using pressurization up to 6 ATA (Treatment Table 6A) is recommended. For patients with residual symptoms after the initial HBO treatment, additional treatments are recommended until there is no further neurologic improvement, typically one to two additional treatments.

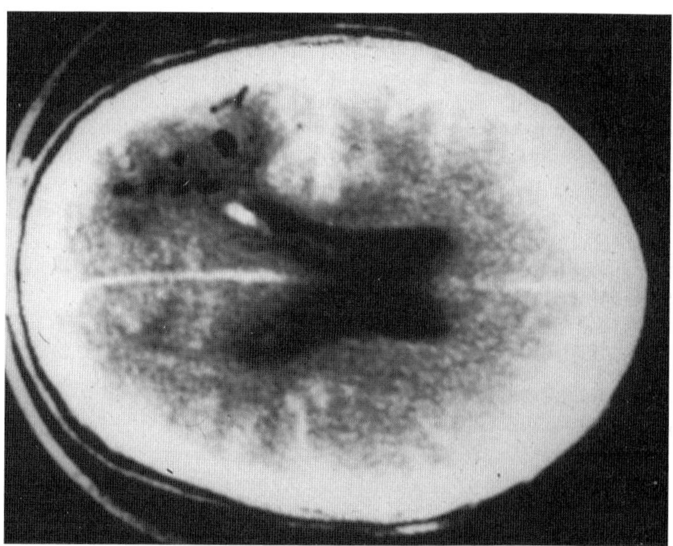

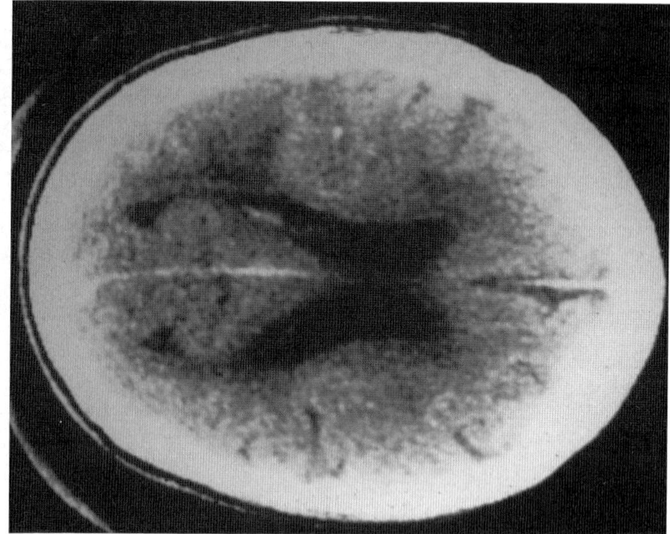

FIGURE 21-3. Head CT demonstrating air in cerebral vessels before hyperbaric oxygen treatment (*left*) and eradication after treatment (*right*).

DECOMPRESSION SICKNESS

Decompression sickness is due to the formation of nitrogen bubbles in body tissue and circulation during decompression (see chapter 214, "Diving Disorders").[7] During pressurization, inert gas (nitrogen if breathing air) is dissolved in body fluids. Upon reduction in ambient pressure, the dissolved gas comes out of solution and forms small bubbles in the tissue and circulation. HBO is an effective treatment because the increase in ambient pressure reduces gas bubble volume and the supplemental oxygen hastens inert gas diffusion out of the body.

Decompression sickness should be treated with HBO when such therapy is available and no contraindication exists. If HBO therapy is not available, patients with mild symptoms and neurologic stability for longer than 24 hours may be treated with supplemental oxygen therapy alone. If a patient must be transported by air to a hyperbaric facility, use pressurized aircraft to maintain sea-level pressure or transport at the lowest possible altitude in a nonpressurized craft, such a helicopter.

A variety of HBO regimens are used to treat decompression sickness,[8] but most have in common pressurization to 2.8 ATA for 60 to 90 minutes, followed by stepwise decompression, similar to U.S. Navy Diving Manual Treatment Table 6. Most patients respond to a single treatment. Gas bubbles can persist for several days, and HBO may be beneficial even when begun after long delays.[8]

CARBON MONOXIDE POISONING

Carbon monoxide (CO) toxicity develops from impairment of hemoglobin function and direct CO-mediated cellular damage (see chapter 222, "Carbon Monoxide"). The affinity of CO for hemoglobin, forming carboxyhemoglobin, is more than 200-fold greater than that of oxygen. Carboxyhemoglobin cannot carry oxygen, so as the level rises, the oxygen-carrying capacity of blood decreases, inducing hypoxic stress initially on organs most dependent on oxidative metabolism—the brain and heart. After removal from continued CO exposure, the CO slowly dissociates from the hemoglobin and is metabolized or exhaled, and the carboxyhemoglobin levels fall. Treatment with HBO enhances the decline of carboxyhemoglobin levels, more rapidly restoring oxygen-carrying capacity of the blood. In animal models of CO poisoning, HBO treatment ameliorates pathophysiologic events associated with CNS injuries mediated by CO, such as improvement in mitochondrial oxidative processes,[9] inhibition of lipid peroxidation,[10] and impairment of leukocyte adhesion to injured microvasculature.[11] Animals poisoned with CO and treated with HBO have more rapid improvement in cardiovascular status,[12] lower mortality,[13] and lower incidence of neurologic sequelae.[14]

Five prospective, randomized trials have assessed clinical efficacy of HBO for acute human CO poisoning.[15-19] Three did not find benefit,[15,17,18] but have been criticized for methodologic weaknesses that may have affected results.[20-23] The clinical trial from Salt Lake City found a significant reduction in neuropsychological sequelae at 6 weeks in HBO-treated patients.[19] This study has been analyzed and debated by advocates and critics of HBO treatment.[24] The results have been considered an outlier by meta-analysis that concluded there is no evidence that HBO reduces incidence of adverse CO-mediated neurologic outcomes.[25,26] Despite the uncertainties, HBO treatment should at least be considered in cases of serious acute CO poisoning because 1) the neurologic sequelae can be severe, 2) retrospective analysis found that HBO was associated with diminished acute mortality,[20] and the Salt Lake City trial found benefit.[27]

The Salt Lake City protocol for CO poisoning uses pressurization to 3 ATA for 60 minutes, with two air breaks, followed by a reduction in pressure to 2 ATA for 65 minutes with one air break.[19] Two additional treatments are given in 6- to 12-hour intervals. An alternative protocol uses 2.8 ATA for 30 minutes followed by 2.0 ATA for 90 minutes.

CYANIDE POISONING

Concomitant cyanide and CO poisoning may be seen in patients rescued from closed-space fires in which synthetic materials are burned. Experimental evidence suggests that cyanide and CO can produce synergistic toxicity.[28-30] HBO may directly reduce cyanide toxicity[31,32] or augment other antidote treatments.[33] However, clinical experience with HBO for cyanide toxicity is sparse.[34-38]

Cyanide is among the most lethal poisons, and toxicity is rapid, so standard antidotal therapy for isolated cyanide poisoning is of primary importance. HBO can be considered in case of dual CO and cyanide poisoning and in cyanide poisoning when vital signs and mental status do not improve with antidote treatment.

EXCEPTIONAL BLOOD LOSS ANEMIA

In cases of severe anemia where transfusion cannot effectively improve oxygen content to sustainable levels (e.g., Jehovah's Witness, Rh incompatibility/transfusion reactions, patient refusal), HBO aids in sustaining life.[39] Anecdotal reports describe using 100% oxygen at 2.5 to 3.0 ATA to raise Pao_2 in plasma to meet metabolic needs.[40-43] Treatments are administered for 3 to 4 hours, with air breaks, with sessions up to four times per day, and continued until red blood cell concentration improves.

ACUTE THERMAL BURN INJURY

Some burn centers use adjunctive HBO for severe burns. This is not a universal practice, and controversy persists.[44] Animal models have documented benefits with HBO in reducing partial- to full-thickness skin loss, hastening epithelialization, and lowering mortality.[2] Randomized clinical trials with small patient numbers have reported improved rates of healing with shorter hospitalization stays.[45-48] Uncontrolled series have reported mixed results.[49-51] A typical HBO protocol for thermal burns uses pressurization to 2.4 ATA for 100 minutes with two air breaks. Treatments are initiated at three sessions a day, then decreased to twice a day as healing occurs, and continued up to a total of 45 sessions.

NECROTIZING SOFT TISSUE INFECTIONS

Necrotizing soft tissue infections, such as necrotizing fasciitis and Fournier's gangrene, are typically mixed aerobic-anaerobic infections. HBO is potentially beneficial due to its ability to suppress growth of anaerobic microorganisms and improve bactericidal action of leukocytes that function poorly in hypoxic conditions.[52-55]

Variation in time of diagnosis and clinical status at time of admission make analysis of the six nonrandomized comparisons and four case series using HBO to treat necrotizing soft tissue infection too complex to yield a straightforward conclusion.[56-65] Most studies have reported that when HBO is added to surgery and antibiotic therapy, mortality is reduced. Typical HBO therapy for necrotizing soft tissue infection uses pressurization to 2.4 ATA for 100 minutes with two air breaks, with treatments started at two sessions per day and then decreased to once a day for up to a total of 30 sessions.

CLOSTRIDIAL MYONECROSIS (GAS GANGRENE)

Gas gangrene is a serious infection with high morbidity and mortality. When tissue Po_2 reaches about 250 mm Hg, α toxin production stops. Once production is halted, α toxin is rapidly cleared.[66] In addition, HBO suppresses the growth of clostridial organisms.[66] HBO therapy of gas gangrene has been the subject of five retrospective comparisons and 13 case series, along with separate analysis.[2,67-69] Assessment of HBO therapy efficacy based on mortality or "tissue salvage" rates is difficult due to variation in patients and clinical practice. Most authors report clinical benefit from treatment, especially the often dramatic temporal improvement of vital signs. A typical HBO therapy protocol for gas gangrene follows the U.S. Navy Diving Manual Treatment Table 21-5: pressurization to 2.8 ATA for 45 minutes with one air break, followed by a slow reduction in pressure over 30 minutes to 1.8 ATA, maintaining pressure there for 30 minutes with two air breaks, followed by decompression, for a total treatment time of 135 minutes. Three treatments are done the first day, and two treatments are done each day for 4 to 5 days more.

CRUSH INJURY, COMPARTMENT SYNDROME, AND OTHER ACUTE TRAUMATIC ISCHEMIAS

The rationale for considering HBO therapy in crushed and ischemic tissues is to temporarily improve oxygenation to hypoperfused tissues and promote arterial hyperoxia, which will cause vasoconstriction and diminish edema formation.[70] This latter mechanism has been convincingly demonstrated in experimental compartment syndrome.[71] A single randomized controlled trial (involving 36 patients) with crushed limbs found that HBO therapy improved healing and reduced infection and wound dehiscence.[72] In a case series of 23 patients, HBO resulted in limb preservation.[73] Comparative evaluation of HBO treatment for complex extremity wounds sustained from bullets or explosions also showed considerable benefit.[74] HBO therapy can be considered when complications or poor outcomes are thought to be likely despite appropriate surgical and medical care.

A typical HBO protocol for these injuries is pressurization to 2.4 ATA for 100 minutes, with two air breaks. Treatments are started at three sessions per day for 2 days, then decreased to twice a day for 2 days and then once a day for 2 days, for a total of 12 sessions.

CENTRAL RETINAL ARTERY OCCLUSION

Central retinal artery occlusion is rare yet devastating and can result in permanent vision loss. There is fair to good evidence based on retrospective case series that HBO therapy started with 24 hours after the onset of symptoms will improve outcome.[3,75] Standard therapies, such as supplemental oxygen and lowering intraocular pressure, are recommended until HBO can be initiated.[1,3]

A typical HBO therapy protocol would be pressurization to 2.0 ATA; if vision improves with this pressure, the patient is treated for 90 minutes with two air breaks. Treatments are done twice a day and continued until there is no improvement in vision after 3 consecutive days. If pressurization to 2.0 ATA does not produce improvement, pressurization to 2.8 ATA is used.

COMPLICATIONS

BAROTRAUMA

Middle ear barotrauma is the most common adverse effect of HBO treatment.[76] As the ambient pressure within the hyperbaric chamber increases, a patient must be able to equalize the pressure within the middle ear by auto-insufflation (pinching the nose while trying to blow through the nose) or else ear pain, tympanic hemorrhage, serous effusion, or rupture will develop. Standard protocols include instruction of patients on auto-insufflation techniques and adding oral or topical decongestants when needed. When these interventions fail, tympanostomy tubes must be placed in order for HBO therapy to continue. The reported overall incidence of aural barotrauma is between 1.2% and 7% of patients who undergo a course of treatment.[77,78] One series reported a 4% incidence of tympanostomy tube placement.[79]

Pulmonary barotrauma during HBO treatment is extremely rare but should be suspected when significant chest or hemodynamic symptoms occur during, or shortly after, decompression. If symptoms develop and the patient is in a multiplace chamber, stop decompression and evaluate for pneumothorax. If the patient is in a monoplace chamber, slowly decompress and provide supplemental oxygen upon returning to ambient pressure.

OXYGEN TOXICITY

Biochemical oxygen toxicity can injure the brain, lungs, and eyes. Acute oxygen toxicity manifests as a grand mal seizure, reported to occur approximately 1 to 4 times per 10,000 patient treatments.[77,80-82] The risk of seizure is higher in hypercapnic patients and possibly those who are acidotic or septic. One case series of HBO therapy for gas gangrene reported a seizure incidence of 7%.[67] Seizures are managed by reducing the inspired oxygen tension while leaving the patient at the same pressure (to avoid pulmonary overexpansion injury when a patient is in tonic convulsion phase).

Chronic oxygen toxicity can impair lung mechanics (elasticity), vital capacity, and gas exchange.[2] These changes are typically observed only when treatment duration and pressures exceed typical therapeutic protocols.[83-85]

Progressive myopia has been reported in patients who undergo prolonged daily therapy, but this typically reverses within 6 weeks after termination of treatments.[86] There is a risk for nuclear cataract development, most typically when treatments exceed a total of 150 to 200 hours, but they may arise with less provocative exposures.[87,88] Current experimental and clinical evidence does not indicate that typical HBO therapy protocols have detrimental effects on neonates or the unborn fetus.[89] This is likely due to the relatively short duration of hyperoxia.

MISCELLANEOUS COMPLICATIONS

Confinement anxiety may occur and is typically managed with sedating agents. Any environment with an elevated concentration of oxygen presents a risk for fire. Scrupulous avoidance of an ignition source is standard in HBO therapy programs.[90]

REFERENCES

The complete reference list is available online at www.TintinalliEM.com.

SECTION 4

Resuscitative Procedures

Basic Cardiopulmonary Resuscitation

Adam D. Friedlander
Jon Mark Hirshon

INTRODUCTION

The purpose of CPR is to temporarily provide effective oxygenation of vital organs, especially the brain and heart, through artificial circulation of oxygenated blood until the restoration of normal cardiac and respiratory activity occurs. The intended effect is to stop the degenerative processes of ischemia and anoxia caused by inadequate circulation and inadequate oxygenation.[1] A key component of the 2005 American Heart Association guidelines was the recognition that immediate high-quality CPR is crucial for optimal patient outcome after sudden cardiac arrest.[2] However, the **2010 American Heart Association guidelines** identify several barriers to providing immediate high-quality CPR and address them.[3] Furthermore, even after defibrillation, most victims demonstrate asystole or pulseless electrical activity for several minutes, and high-quality CPR immediately following defibrillation can convert nonperfusing rhythms to perfusing rhythms.[2,3] The time sensitivity of CPR in sudden cardiac death is emphasized in the American Heart Association **"Chain of Survival"** (**Table 22-1**).

This chapter reviews basic CPR for adults and children ≥8 years old, including the approach to an unresponsive patient; the physiology and mechanics of closed chest compression techniques; and basic airway opening procedures, including initial management of an obstructed airway. This chapter is specifically directed toward healthcare providers, although key updates for lay rescuers are noted, given the healthcare provider's role in layperson education.

SUMMARY OF KEY UPDATES TO PREVIOUS ALGORITHMS[3]

1. "Look, listen, and feel" has been removed from all algorithms. Simply put, subjectivity plays too large a role in this step and has been shown to lead to delays. ***Immediate* high-quality CPR is strongly emphasized**, and should begin in any person who is unresponsive without respirations or with abnormal breathing.
2. Lone rescuers no longer follow the "ABCs." **The sequence "CAB" has been adopted instead.** Two rescue breaths are no longer recommended prior to initiating chest compressions.
3. **Compression rate should be *at least* 100/minute**, not approximately 100/minute.
4. **Compression depth should be *at least* 2 inches**, not 1½ to 2 inches.
5. Untrained bystanders should begin **"compression only" CPR**, "hard and fast" in the center of the chest. They may be directed to do so by EMS or by a healthcare provider. This effectively removes the barrier of lack of training or fear of having to perform mouth-to-mouth resuscitation on a stranger.
6. **Pulse checks** are deemphasized for all rescuers, with a **maximum of 10 seconds allowable** for a pulse check. End-tidal carbon dioxide monitoring, when available, is superior to pulse checks, showing an abrupt rise in end-tidal carbon dioxide when spontaneous circulation has returned.
7. For trained rescuers delivering breaths, cricoid pressure is no longer recommended.
8. Postresuscitation care, including therapeutic hypothermia, consideration of cardiac catheterization, and hemodynamic optimization, is emphasized.

Table 22-2 outlines the sequence of steps to be taken when someone is found unresponsive.

STEP 1 AND STEP 2 IN BASIC CPR

Before approaching a collapsed individual, assess the scene for risks to healthcare providers. Potential risks include the presence of hazardous materials, an unstable physical environment, or personal violence. Once the patient is reached, determine the patient's level of responsiveness to noxious stimuli. If the patient is without normal breathing, get help first before starting chest compressions. In a hospital, this may mean calling for the arrest team and requesting the arrest cart. Outside the hospital, this is likely to mean asking a bystander to activate the local EMS system. Look around to see if an automatic external defibrillator is nearby. Rapid application of defibrillation for unstable ventricular tachycardia or ventricular fibrillation is critical for patient survival.

STEP 3 IN BASIC CPR (HEALTHCARE PROVIDER ONLY)

The carotid artery is generally the most reliable and accessible location to palpate a pulse. The artery is located by placing two fingers on the trachea and then sliding them down to the groove between the trachea and the sternocleidomastoid muscle. Simultaneous palpation of both carotid arteries should not be performed because, in low-pressure states, this could obstruct cerebral blood flow and may interfere with the ability to detect a pulse. The femoral artery may be used as an alternative site to palpate a pulse. This can be found just below the inguinal ligament approximately halfway between the anterior superior iliac spine and the pubic tubercle. If no definite pulse is felt within 10 seconds, chest compression should begin.

STEP 4 IN BASIC CPR

Physiology of Closed Chest Compressions There has been an active debate as to the exact mechanism that causes blood flow since the technique of closed chest compressions was put forth in the 1960s.[4,5] In a closed system, liquid flows when pressure gradients develop. There are three basic theories for how pressure gradients and flow are produced during **closed chest cardiac massage**.[6,7] The conventional theory of blood flow during compressions is called the **cardiac pump theory**. The pump theory postulates that direct compression of the heart between the spine and the sternum leads to increased pressure in the ventricles. This causes closure of the mitral and tricuspid valves, leading to blood flow into the aorta and the pulmonary arteries. The **thoracic pump theory** postulates that compressions lead to an increase in pressure throughout the thoracic cavity, leading to a pressure gradient from intrathoracic to extrathoracic arteries. The third mechanism described is the **abdominal pump theory**, which has both an arterial and a venous component. The arterial component postulates blood flow into the peripheral arterial system from increased arterial pressure caused by abdominal compressions that forces blood from the abdominal aorta against the closed aortic valve. The venous component leads to blood return via the inferior vena cava from abdominal pressure. However, regardless of the mechanism, conventional chest compressions generate one fourth to one third of physiologic cardiac output. Lower ratios can

TABLE 22-1 American Heart Association Chain of Survival

Links in Chain	Comment
Immediate recognition/ early access	Phone 911 (or local emergency medical telephone number).* Early recognition of the emergency and activation of the EMS or local emergency response system.
Early CPR	Immediate bystander CPR can double or triple the victim's chance of survival from ventricular fibrillation.
Early defibrillation	CPR plus defibrillation within 3 to 5 min of collapse can produce survival rates as high as 49%–75%.
Early advanced care	Postresuscitation care delivered by healthcare providers.
Postarrest care	High-quality, integrated post–cardiac arrest clinical care.

*For a global list of emergency numbers and mobile phone use, see http://en.wikipedia.org/wiki/Emergency_telephone_number.

TABLE 22-3 Techniques of Closed Chest Compression

Closed chest compressions	Depth: *At least* 5 cm (*at least* 2 in.). Rate: *At least* 100/min. Allow complete recoil of the chest between compressions, with approximately equal compression and relaxation times. Minimize interruptions.
Ventilations	Single rescuer or two rescuers, nonintubated patient: give two breaths after every 30 compressions. Two rescuers, intubated patient: give breaths at a rate of 8–10 breaths/min. Do not pause chest compressions during ventilations.

be expected with delays in initiating compressions. The techniques of closed chest compression are detailed in **Table 22-3**.

When the lack of a pulse is confirmed, begin serial rhythmic closed chest compressions. Place the victim supine on a firm surface, with the rescuer at the victim's side. Place the heel of one hand midline on the lower half of the sternum, 4 to 5 cm (~2 in.) cephalad of the xiphoid process (**Figure 22-1**). The heel of the hand should be parallel with the long axis of the patient's body. Then place the second hand on top of the first hand, so the hands are parallel with each other. The fingers of the two hands may be interlaced if desired, but they should not be touching the chest. Keep the arms straight and the elbows locked. The vector of the compression force should start from the rescuer's shoulders and be directed downward. Lateral compressive forces will decrease the efficiency of the compressions and increase the likelihood of complications. **Depress the sternum *at least* 5 cm (*at least* 2 in.) in an adult, at a rate of *at least* 100 compressions per minute.** Rates lower than this are inadequate. The compression-release phases should be roughly equal in length. **With a single rescuer or with two rescuers if the patient is not intubated, give two ventilations after every 30 compressions. With two rescuers assisting an intubated patient, ventilate at a rate of 8 to 10 per minute, without interrupting chest compressions.** Of note, although assisting ventilation is important, not everyone is willing to perform mouth-to-mouth breathing due to concerns over infectious disease transmission. **Chest compressions alone can be effective and should be provided even if rescue breathing is not being performed.**[8,9]

TABLE 22-2 Systematic Approach to CPR

CPR Steps	Comments
Step 1: Recognition	Assess for responsiveness, lack of breathing, or presence of abnormal breathing/gasping. Continue to step 2.
Step 2: Phone 911 and get an automatic external defibrillator	If possible, call for an assistant to do so. If no assistant is available and underlying etiology is asphyxia (e.g., drowning), call 911.* Automatic external defibrillator may be delayed to provide five cycles (or 2 min) of CPR.
Step 3: Assess circulation (*healthcare provider only*)	If no pulse after 10-second maximum check, go to step 4. (*Pulse checks are for healthcare providers only.*)
Step 4: Begin cycle of 30 closed chest compressions and two breaths	Compressions: "Push hard and fast." *At least* 100 compressions/min. Compress *at least* 5 cm (*at least* 2 in.). Allow for complete chest recoil, and minimize frequency and duration of interruptions. Ratio of 30 compressions to two breaths.
Step 5: Use the defibrillator when available and indicated	Healthcare provider to consider providing five cycles (or 2 min) of CPR before defibrillation for unwitnessed arrest. This recommendation is especially important when the interval from the call to scene response is >4 min. Provide five cycles (or 2 min) of CPR between rhythm checks during treatment of pulseless arrest.
Step 6: Rescue breathing	Rescue breaths can be initiated once chest compressions have been started. Deliver each breath over 1 second with sufficient tidal volume to see a visible chest rise. Continue 30 closed chest compressions and two breaths, minimizing interruptions.

*For a global list of emergency numbers and mobile phone use, see http://en.wikipedia.org/wiki/Emergency_telephone_number.

Open Chest Cardiac Compressions Open chest cardiac massage is an alternative to standard CPR and improves blood flow in animal models. Although there are no data showing improved clinical outcomes with the use of open chest cardiac massage versus closed chest cardiac massage, this technique may be considered in a number of situations, including (1) after penetrating chest trauma; (2) the perioperative period before or after cardiothoracic surgery; (3) cardiac arrest caused by hypothermia, pulmonary embolism, pericardial tamponade, or abdominal hemorrhage; (4) cases of chest deformity in which closed chest CPR is ineffective; (5) penetrating abdominal trauma with deterioration and cardiac arrest; and (6) blunt trauma with cardiac arrest.[10] However, the use of this technique requires a well-coordinated multidisciplinary team (see chapter 262, Cardiac Trauma).

STEP 5 IN BASIC CPR

Defibrillation is discussed in chapter 23, Defibrillation and Cardioversion.

COMPLICATIONS OF CPR

Ventilations can cause insufflation of the stomach, leading to regurgitation and aspiration and possibly to gastric rupture. Closed chest compressions can lead to fractures of the sternum or the ribs, separation of the ribs from the sternum, pulmonary contusion, pneumothorax, myocardial contusion, hemorrhagic pericardial effusions, splenic laceration, or liver laceration. Proper techniques can minimize these complications but cannot totally prevent them. Late complications include pulmonary edema, GI hemorrhage, pneumonia, and recurrent cardiopulmonary arrest. Anoxic brain injury can occur in a resuscitated individual subjected to prolonged hypoxia; it is the most common cause of death in resuscitated patients.

STEP 6 IN BASIC CPR

The sixth step is to **assess the upper airway of the victim**. This usually requires positioning the individual supine on a flat, firm surface with the arms along the sides of the body. Unless trauma can be definitely excluded, any movement of the victim should consider the possibility of a spine injury. As the patient is placed supine, stabilize the cervical spine by maintaining the head, neck, and trunk in a straight line. If the neck is not already straight, then it should be moved as little as possible

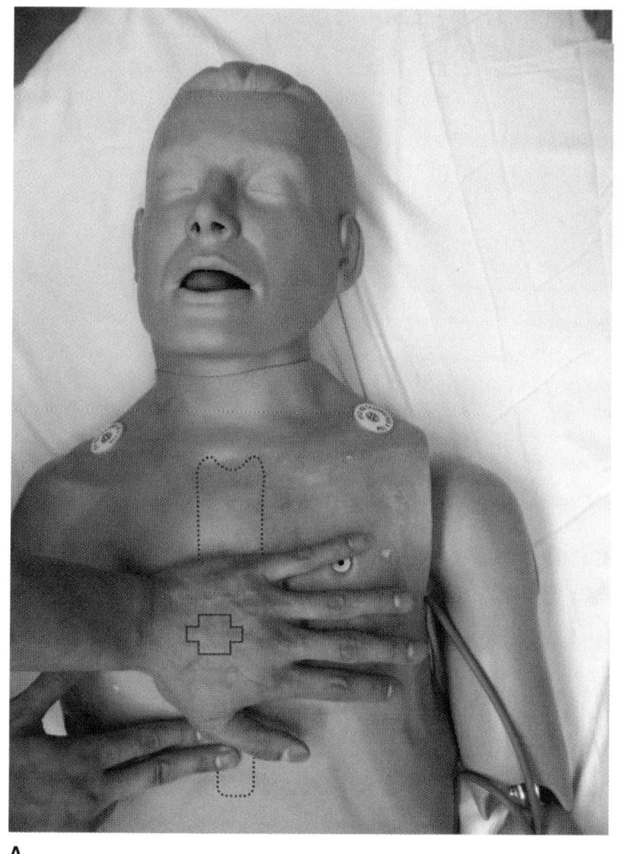
A

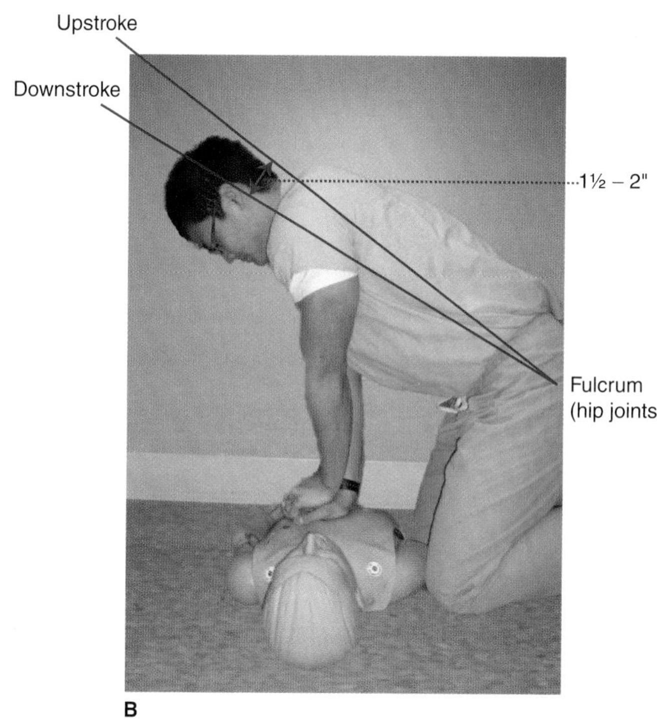

B

FIGURE 22-1. Proper hand (**A**) and rescuer (**B**) positioning for chest compression. [Image used with permission of Rita K. Cydulka, MD, MS, MetroHealth Medical Center.]

to establish the airway. If the patient cannot be placed supine, the jaw thrust maneuver (see "Jaw Thrust Maneuver" section) can be applied with the rescuer at the victim's side. **Common causes of airway obstruction in an unconscious patient are occlusion of the oropharynx by the tongue and laxity of the epiglottis.** With loss of muscle tone, the tongue or the epiglottis can be forced back into the oropharynx upon inspiration. This can create the effect of a one-way valve at the entrance to the trachea, leading to airway obstruction. After positioning the patient, inspect the mouth and oropharynx for secretions, foreign objects, loose (floppy) dentures, partial dentures, or broken teeth. If dentures fit properly, keep them in place if possible, as they will allow for a better seal. If secretions are present, they can be removed with the use of oropharyngeal suction if available; a visualized foreign body may be dislodged by use of a finger sweep and then manually removed. **In contrast to earlier recommendations, a blind finger sweep should never be performed as there is a risk of worsening airway obstruction** (see "Finger Sweep" section).

Once the oropharynx has been cleared, two basic maneuvers for opening the airway may be tried. These are the head tilt–chin lift and the jaw thrust. These maneuvers help to open the airway by mechanically displacing the mandible and the attached tongue out of the oropharynx.

Head Tilt–Chin Lift Maneuver To perform the **head tilt–chin lift maneuver**, gently extend the patient's neck by placing one hand under the patient's neck and the other on the forehead and extending the head in relation to the neck. This maneuver should place the patient's head in the sniffing position, with the nose pointing up. In conjunction with the head tilt, perform the chin lift. The chin lift is done by carefully placing the hand that had been supporting the neck for the head tilt under the symphysis of the mandible, taking care not to compress the soft tissues of the submental triangle and the base of the tongue. Then lift the mandible forward and up, until the teeth barely touch. This supports the jaw and helps tilt the head back.

Jaw Thrust Maneuver The **jaw thrust** is the safest method for opening the airway if there is the possibility of cervical spine injury. This maneuver helps to maintain the cervical spine in a neutral position. The rescuer, who is positioned at the head of the patient, places the hands at the sides of the victim's face, grasps the mandible at its angle, and lifts the mandible forward (**Figure 22-2**). This lifts the jaw and opens the airway with minimal head movement.

After opening the airway, assess respiratory effort and air movement. Look for chest expansion, and listen and feel for airflow. The simple act of opening the airway may be adequate for the return of spontaneous respirations. However, if the victim remains without adequate respiratory effort, then further intervention is required. **If rescuers are reluctant to**

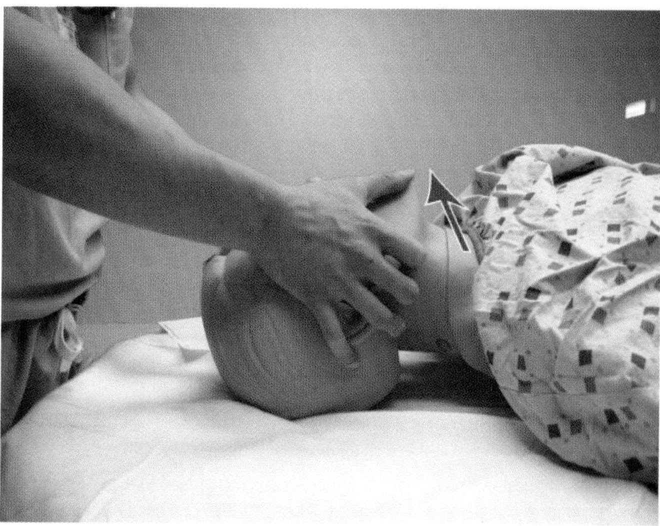

FIGURE 22-2. Jaw thrust maneuver. [Image used with permission of Rita K. Cydulka, MD, MS, MetroHealth Medical Center.]

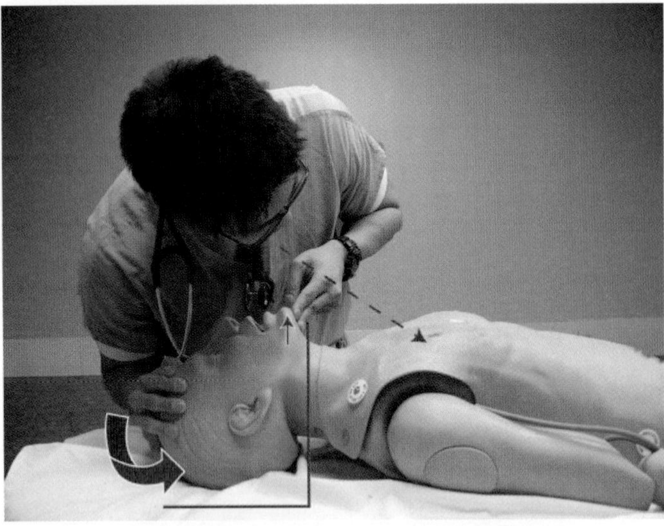

FIGURE 22-3. Determine breathlessness. [Image used with permission of Rita K. Cydulka, MD, MS, MetroHealth Medical Center.]

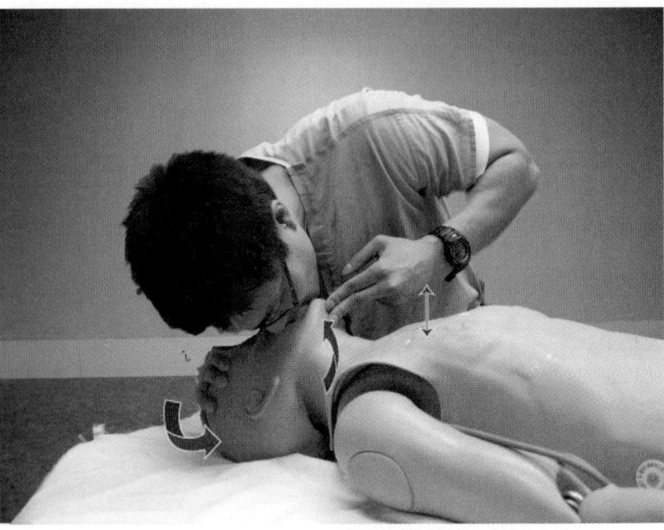

FIGURE 22-4. Mouth-to-mouth rescue breathing. [Image used with permission of Rita K. Cydulka, MD, MS, MetroHealth Medical Center.]

perform mouth-to-mouth ventilation and the patient is in cardiac arrest, chest compressions alone can be effective (Table 22-3).

Two breaths over 1 second each should be given with sufficient volume to cause visible chest rise. At this point, if a foreign body obstruction is noted, as indicated by a lack of chest rise or airflow on ventilation, the obstruction requires removal (**Figure 22-3**). Agonal respirations in an individual who has just suffered a cardiac arrest are not considered adequate for ventilation. Intermittent positive-pressure ventilation, with oxygen-enriched air if possible, should be initiated.

Ventilation Techniques Table 22-4 outlines the recommendations for delivery of rescue breaths during cardiac arrest.[3] When an advanced airway (e.g., endotracheal tube, Combitube, or laryngeal mask airway) is in place during two-person CPR, ventilate at a rate of 8 to 10 breaths per minute without attempting to synchronize breaths between compressions. There should be no pause in chest compressions for delivery of ventilations.[2]

In an adult with normal perfusion, 8 to 10 mL/kg tidal volume is required for adequate oxygenation and ventilation. However, in the setting of CPR, where cardiac output is only 25% to 33% of normal, a lower minute ventilation, and thus tidal volume, can be satisfactory. **Approximately 6 to 7 mL/kg will suffice.** Use an appropriately sized bag for bag-valve mask ventilation. A pediatric bag will provide inadequate tidal volumes for an adult.

There are a number of techniques for ventilating an individual, including mouth to mouth, mouth to nose, mouth to stoma, and mouth to mask. **Rescue breaths with an inspiratory time of 1 second each should be given at a rate of 8 to 10 per minute, with a volume adequate to make the chest rise visibly (approximately 6 to 7 mL/kg; 500 to 600 mL in adults). Supplemental oxygen should be delivered as soon as possible.** Expired air has a fraction of expired oxygen of 16% to 17%. Too large a volume or too rapid an inspiratory flow rate can cause gastric distention, which can lead to regurgitation and aspiration.

Mouth-to-Mouth Ventilation With the airway open, gently pinch the patient's nose shut with the thumb and index finger (**Figure 22-4**). This prevents air escape. After taking a deep breath, place the lips around the patient's mouth, forming an airtight seal. Slowly exhale. Release the seal and allow adequate time for passive exhalation by the victim, and then repeat the procedure. Protective devices such as face shields decrease the risks to the provider of contracting an infectious disease and can be purchased from most medical equipment stores.

Mouth-to-Nose Ventilation In some cases, as with severe maxillofacial trauma, mouth-to-nose ventilation may be effective. With the airway open, lift the patient's jaw, closing the patient's mouth. After a deep breath, place the lips around the patient's nose, forming an airtight seal. Slowly exhale.

Mouth-to-Stoma or Tracheostomy Ventilation After laryngectomy or tracheotomy, the stoma or tracheostomy becomes the patient's airway. As with the other techniques, a seal is made around the stoma or tracheostomy tube, and the rescuer slowly exhales.

Mouth-to-Mask Ventilation Proper and secure placement of the mask on a victim's face is important when using a mask for ventilation, either with a bag or via mouth to mask. Place the mask over the bridge of the patient's nose and around the mouth. Place the thumb on the part of the mask that is sitting on the patient's nose and place the index finger of the same hand on the part of the mask sitting on the patient's chin (**Figure 22-5**). The

TABLE 22-4 Delivery of Rescue Breaths During CPR

Deliver each rescue breath over 1 s (Class IIA recommendation).
Give a sufficient tidal volume (by mouth-to-mouth/mask or bag-mask with or without supplementary oxygen) to produce visible chest rise (Class IIA recommendation).
Avoid rapid or forceful breaths.
Avoid hyperventilation.

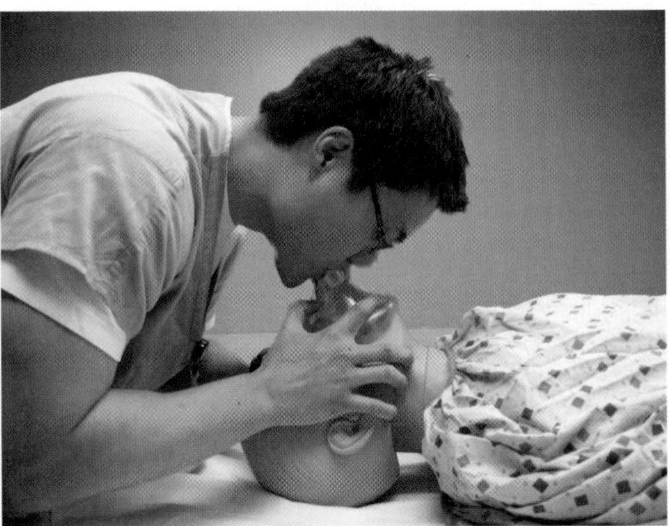

FIGURE 22-5. Mouth-to-mask rescue breathing with proper mask placement. [Image used with permission of Rita K. Cydulka, MD, MS, MetroHealth Medical Center.]

three other fingers of the same hand are then placed along the bony margin of the jaw. The mask can then be firmly sealed to the patient's face. Two hands may be used for this technique if a second rescuer is available. Ventilations are then performed through the mask. Some masks also allow for supplemental oxygenation.

Foreign Body Obstruction It is important to recognize and be able to assist someone with an airway obstruction due to a foreign body.[11] An individual in distress from a compromised airway is likely to use the **universal sign for an airway obstruction**, which is for the individual to grab his or her neck with both hands. Foreign bodies can cause partial or complete obstruction. With a partial airway obstruction, air exchange may be adequate or inadequate. If the victim is able to speak, cough, and exchange air, then he or she should be encouraged to continue spontaneous efforts. Obtain assistance, such as activation of the local EMS system. Do not interfere with the patient's attempts to cough or expel the foreign body **and do not perform a blind finger sweep**. If air exchange becomes inadequate, as indicated by an inability to speak, increased difficulty breathing, weak and ineffective cough, worsening stridor, or cyanosis, immediate medical intervention is needed (see next section, "Obstruction-Relieving Maneuvers"). Inadequate air exchange from a severe partial or a complete airway obstruction should be managed the same way. In an unconscious person, the presence of airway obstruction may be ascertained by noting inadequate airflow and poor chest rise with efforts to ventilate.

Obstruction-Relieving Maneuvers Maneuvers used to relieve foreign body obstructions include the **Heimlich maneuver** (subdiaphragmatic abdominal thrusts), **chest thrusts**, and the finger sweep. In a conscious individual, the obstructed airway (Heimlich) maneuver is the recommended maneuver in most adults for relieving airway obstruction due to a solid object. It is not useful for liquids. In an unconscious individual suspected of having an aspirated foreign body and in whom the foreign body is visualized, the recommended first step is the finger sweep. **A blind finger sweep is no longer recommended** as it may worsen airway obstruction by pushing an unseen object into an even less favorable position. Otherwise, in an unconscious patient, the recommended sequence is to perform the obstructed airway maneuver up to five times, open the mouth and perform a finger sweep if a foreign body has become visible, and then attempt to ventilate. This sequence may be repeated as often as needed until the patient recovers or additional assistance arrives.

Obstructed Airway (Heimlich) Maneuver The **Heimlich maneuver** creates an artificial cough by forcefully elevating the diaphragm and forcing air from the lungs.[12] It may be repeated multiple times. Each individual thrust should be performed aggressively, with the intention of removing the obstruction. The maneuver can be performed with the victim standing, sitting, or lying down, or it can be self-administered (**Figure 22-6**). To perform the maneuver with the patient standing or sitting, stand behind the patient and place the thumb side of a fist against the victim's abdomen midline just above the umbilicus and well below the xiphoid process (**Figure 22-6**). Grasp the fist with the other hand, and forcefully push the fist into the victim's abdomen with a quick upward thrust. Repeat until the item is dislodged or the patient becomes unconscious. For an unconscious patient, place the victim supine on a firm surface and sit astride the victim's thighs (**Figure 22-7**). Place the heel of the dominant hand midline just above the patient's umbilicus, and the other hand directly on top of the first. Then deliver quick upward thrusts. To self-administer thrusts, the individual can either use his or her own fist to deliver the thrusts or lean forcibly against a firm object, such as a porch rail or the back of a chair. Potential complications of the Heimlich maneuver include injury or rupture of abdominal or thoracic viscera and regurgitation of stomach contents.

Chest Thrusts The **chest thrust** maneuver is used primarily if someone is morbidly obese or in the late stages of pregnancy, and the rescuer cannot reach around the patient's abdomen to perform abdominal thrusts (**Figure 22-8**). To perform chest thrusts with the patient standing or sitting, stand behind the patient and place the thumb side of a fist against the victim's sternum, avoiding the costal margins and the xiphoid process. Grasp the fist with the other hand, and press the fist into the victim's chest with a quick backward thrust. Repeat until the item is dislodged or the patient becomes unconscious. For an unconscious patient, place the victim supine on a firm surface and kneel close to the victim's side. Place the hands in the same position as for chest compression (i.e., the lower sternum), and deliver quick thrusts.

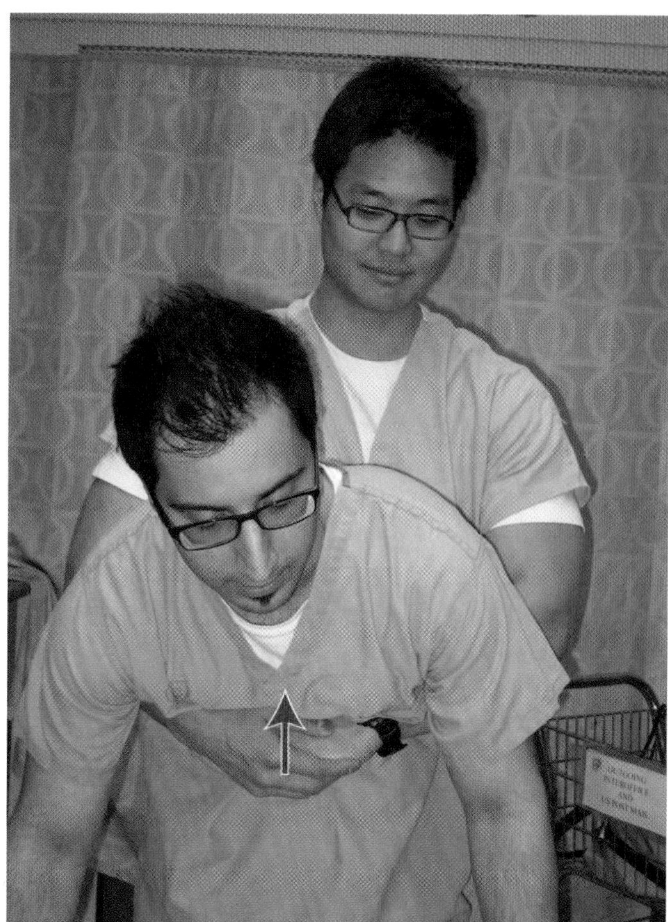

FIGURE 22-6. Standing Heimlich maneuver administered to conscious victim of foreign body airway obstruction. [Image used with permission of Rita K. Cydulka, MD, MS, MetroHealth Medical Center.]

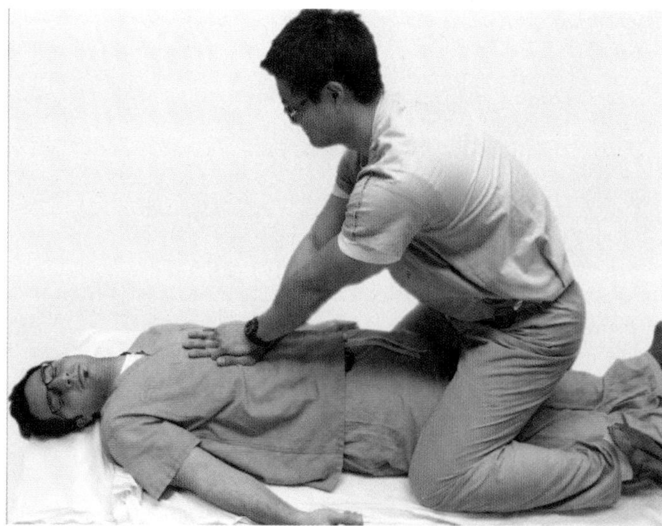

FIGURE 22-7. Prone Heimlich maneuver administered to unconscious victim of foreign body airway obstruction. [Image used with permission of Rita K. Cydulka, MD, MS, MetroHealth Medical Center.]

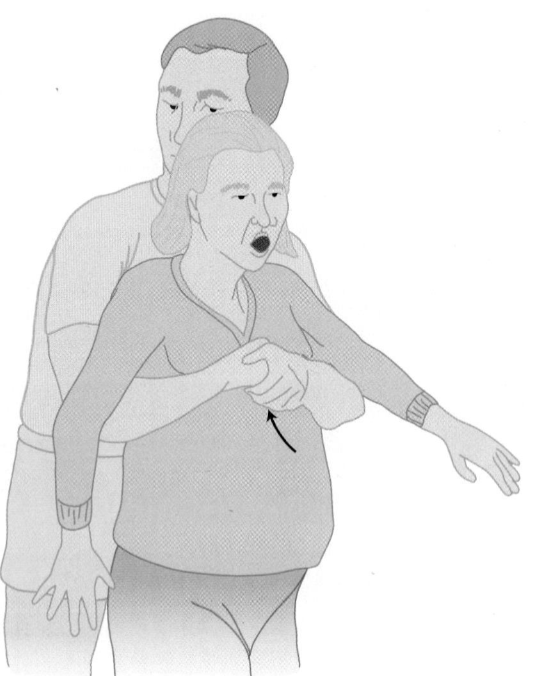

FIGURE 22-8. Standing chest thrust maneuver administered to conscious victim of foreign body airway obstruction.

Finger Sweep The **finger sweep** maneuver is used only in unconscious patients (**Figure 22-9**). Using the thumb and fingers of one hand, grasp both the tongue and the mandible and lift them. This may partially relieve the obstruction by lifting the tongue away from the back of the throat. With the other hand, insert the index finger into the back of the throat, and use a hooking action in an attempt to dislodge the foreign body to move it into the mouth for manual removal. Use care so the foreign object is not pushed deeper into the throat.

EXPERIMENTAL TECHNIQUES AND NEW DIRECTIONS

There are currently several experimental techniques and devices for improving the effectiveness of closed chest cardiac massage. To date, none have consistently proven to be superior to the use of manual CPR and a defibrillator.[2,3,13] Devices that deliver real-time audiovisual feedback to rescuers may improve CPR performance.[14] Studies evaluating adjuncts, such as hypothermia during resuscitation and extracorporeal circulation plus CPR, are also ongoing (see chapter 21, Hyperbaric Oxygen Therapy).[15-17]

One observational study reported that the addition of extracorporeal life support to CPR in patients requiring CPR for >10 minutes was associated with an increased short-term and 1-year survival in patients who experienced in-hospital cardiac arrest.[16] The success of this method is best explained by the presumption that coronary blood flow and thus myocardial viability are enhanced by extracorporeal circulation. Another advantage of this technique is that hypothermia can be easily induced in situations in which doing so may be beneficial, such as hypoxic brain injury[17] (see chapter 21, Hyperbaric Oxygen Therapy).

A final new direction is cardiocerebral resuscitation, which emphasizes current American Heart Association guidelines of high-quality chest compression, but further delays airway intervention. Data indicate that patients receiving hands-only CPR have similar 30-day and 1-year neurologic outcomes as those receiving conventional CPR. These outcomes, combined with the reluctance of bystanders to perform the mouth-to-mouth component of CPR at all, resulted in a 2008 "call to action" (distinct from a recommendation) by the American Heart Association calling for "hands-only" CPR in certain scenarios and is now a formal component of the 2010 guidelines.[3] Animal studies and extrapolation from clinical evidence suggest that rescue breathing during the first 5 minutes of CPR for ventricular fibrillation or sudden cardiac death may not be necessary. The suggestion is that occasional gasps and chest recoil between compressions likely provide sufficient ventilation in a setting where a normal ventilation–perfusion ratio requires a lower than normal minute ventilation.[2] Further studies suggest that withholding airway intervention for 5 to 10 minutes, in favor of continuous, high-quality check compressions, improves both resuscitation rates and neurologic survival.[18-20] Expert opinion has strongly suggested the incorporation of cardiocerebral resuscitation into current guidelines.[21]

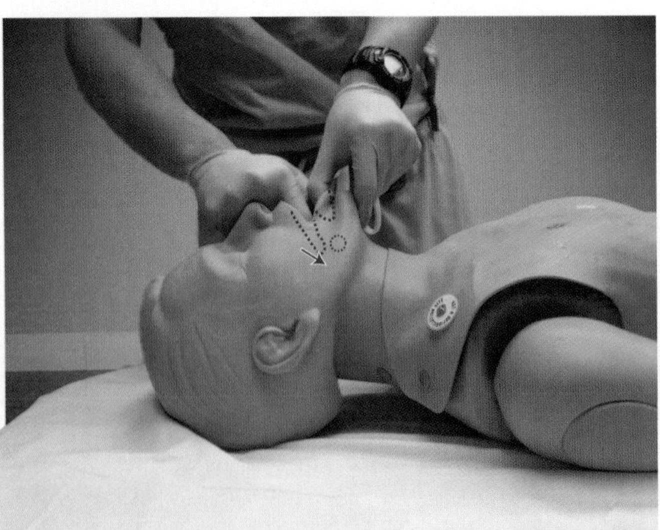

FIGURE 22-9. Finger sweep maneuver administered to unconscious victim of foreign body airway obstruction. [Image used with permission of Rita K. Cydulka, MD, MS, MetroHealth Medical Center.]

TERMINATING RESUSCITATION

Efforts at resuscitation should be continued until the patient recovers spontaneous respirations and cardiac output, the rescuer becomes exhausted, or the patient is pronounced dead. An atraumatic individual who recovers spontaneous respirations and circulation should be placed on his or her side—the ***recovery position***. Recovery from cardiac arrest depends on time to CPR and rhythm-specific intervention. Resuscitation and long-term outcome in normothermic patients with arrest times of 20 minutes or more are very poor.

ETHICAL CONSIDERATIONS IN RESUSCITATION

During the initiation of resuscitation attempts, try to discover whether or not the victim has advance directives that prohibit CPR.[22] Family members may wish to be present during resuscitation attempts,[22] and support from social services and clergy should be sought early (see chapter 27, Ethical Issues of Resuscitation).

REFERENCES

The complete reference list is available online at www.TintinalliEM.com.

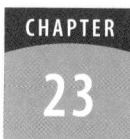

Defibrillation and Cardioversion

Marcus E. H. Ong
Swee Han Lim
Anantharaman Venkataraman

PURPOSE OF PROCEDURE

Defibrillation is the therapeutic use of electricity to depolarize the myocardium so coordinated contractions can occur. The term *defibrillation* is usually applied to an attempt to terminate a nonperfusing rhythm (e.g., ventricular fibrillation or pulseless ventricular tachycardia).

Cardioversion is the application of electricity to terminate a still perfusing rhythm (e.g., ventricular tachycardia with a pulse, supraventricular tachycardias including atrial arrhythmias) to allow a normal sinus rhythm to restart. By this definition, cardioversion is a less urgent procedure compared to defibrillation, although the patient requiring cardioversion may be hypotensive or hemodynamically unstable, rather than in cardiac arrest.

PATIENT SELECTION

Indications for defibrillation include ventricular fibrillation (VF) (**Figure 23-1**) and pulseless ventricular tachycardia (VT) (**Figure 23-2**). Defibrillation is not indicated for asystole and pulseless electrical activity and is contraindicated for sinus rhythm, a conscious patient with a pulse, or when there is danger to the operator or others (e.g., from a wet patient or wet surroundings).

Cardioversion is indicated for a hemodynamically unstable patient with VT, supraventricular tachycardia, atrial flutter, or atrial fibrillation. It is also possibly indicated after failed pharmacologic therapy for the previously mentioned arrhythmias, especially if the patient becomes hemodynamically unstable. **Cardioversion should be synchronized, which means the electric current will be timed with the patient's intrinsic QRS complexes**, to minimize the risk of inducing VF.

RISKS AND PRECAUTIONS

Electrical energy can terminate an abnormal rhythm, but if inappropriately delivered, it can also induce VF. This can happen if the electric shock is delivered during the relative refractory portion of the cardiac electrical activity.[1]

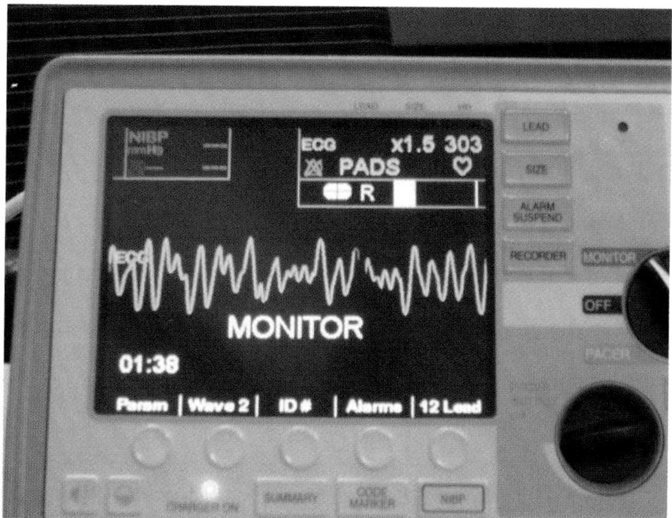

FIGURE 23-1. Ventricular fibrillation.

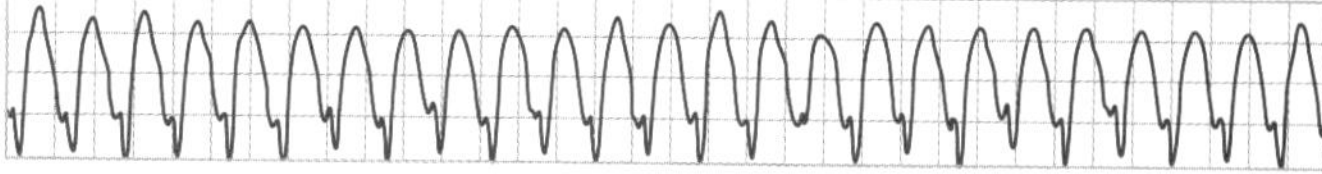

FIGURE 23-2. Ventricular tachycardia.

When preparing for defibrillation, check the patient and rhythm to ensure that a shock is truly indicated. Movement artifacts or loose leads may look like VF. New defibrillator technology is available that can filter compression or movement artifacts to "see through" the underlying rhythm. **However, when using automated external defibrillators (AEDs), all manufacturers currently still recommend stopping all compressions and patient movement (e.g., during transport) before initiating analysis mode.**

Make sure that no rescuer is inadvertently in contact with the patient when a shock is delivered. Neither single nor double gloves provide the rescuer with complete safety from current,[2] so we still recommend "stand clear" drills during defibrillator training, "stand clear" practice during actual defibrillation, and minimizing rather than eliminating the pause in compressions for defibrillation. **If the patient is on a wet or conducting surface, move the patient to a safe area and dry the body before delivering the shock.** When using manual defibrillation paddles, make sure that the paddles are either on the defibrillator cradle or on the patient's chest, with minimal time in transit from one position to the other. To prevent inadvertent discharges, always point the paddles downward and never wave the paddles around or face them toward each other, especially when charged. This is to prevent inadvertent discharges or "sparking."

To avoid skin burns, remove all metallic objects and nitroglycerin patches from the patient. Ensure correct placement of defibrillation paddles/pads and **remove all direct sources of oxygen to avoid fire.**[3,4] If paddles are used, do not allow the conducting gel to spread to within 5 cm of the other paddle. In patients with an internal pacemaker requiring defibrillation, ensure that the paddles/pads are placed well away (12.5 cm or 5 inches) from the pacemaker before discharging.

Avoid prolonged pauses (>10 seconds) to CPR when performing defibrillation.[5,6] Thus, the emphasis is on minimal interruptions to CPR for analysis, a single shock instead of three "stacked" shocks, and immediate resumption of CPR without a pulse or rhythm check immediately after defibrillation. In addition, if a mechanical CPR device is being used, defibrillation can be safely performed without stopping ongoing mechanical compressions to reduce unnecessary pauses.

EQUIPMENT

1. Defibrillator: This can be a manual, semi-automated, or fully automated external defibrillator.
2. Paddles or self-adhesive defibrillation pads.
3. Conductive gel or gel pads for defibrillation paddles.
4. Related resuscitation equipment (e.g., bag-valve mask device, airway devices, suction, IV cannulation, drugs).

Defibrillators should be properly maintained and in a constant state of readiness. We recommend the use of checklists[7] to identify defibrillator malfunction and ensure proper maintenance of batteries. Users should be trained in the proper use of checklists, and checks should be performed frequently (as often as every shift). Perform cardioversion in a resuscitation area with appropriate monitoring and standby resuscitation equipment, in case the patient deteriorates or develops cardiac arrest.

PATIENT POSITIONING

Place the patient in the supine position. Expose the chest, and remove jewelry and medication patches. If the chest is very hairy in the areas where electrodes are to be placed, quickly shave the hair to ensure the electrodes stick onto the chest. If the chest is wet (because of sweat or because the patient has been in water), wipe dry immediately. Sweat or moisture on the chest will reduce adhesion of the electrodes.

ANESTHESIA AND PROCEDURAL MONITORING

For a patient in cardiac arrest, defibrillation is part of the immediate resuscitation process. However, for an elective or semi-elective cardioversion, procedural sedation and monitoring—before, during, and after the procedure—are essential. Provide cardiac, blood pressure, and pulse oximetry monitoring; place an IV line; and make sure airway equipment, suction, and oxygen are immediately available. Obtain informed consent when possible. Sedation is typically provided with an IV agent such as etomidate, propofol, or midazolam.

STEP-BY-STEP TECHNIQUE

PLACEMENT OF PADDLES/PADS

Regarding placement of defibrillation paddles or pads, there are several alternative positions:

1. **Antero-apical position:** Place one paddle/pad to the right of the upper half of the sternum (breastbone), just below the patient's right clavicle (collarbone), and place the other pad just below and to the left of the left nipple (in the axilla). With a female patient, place the paddle/pad just below and to the left side of the breast. Do not place it over the breast (**Figure 23-3**).

   This is the preferred position for a supine patient and when using defibrillation paddles. The idea is to maximize current flow through the cardiac chambers rather than along the chest wall.

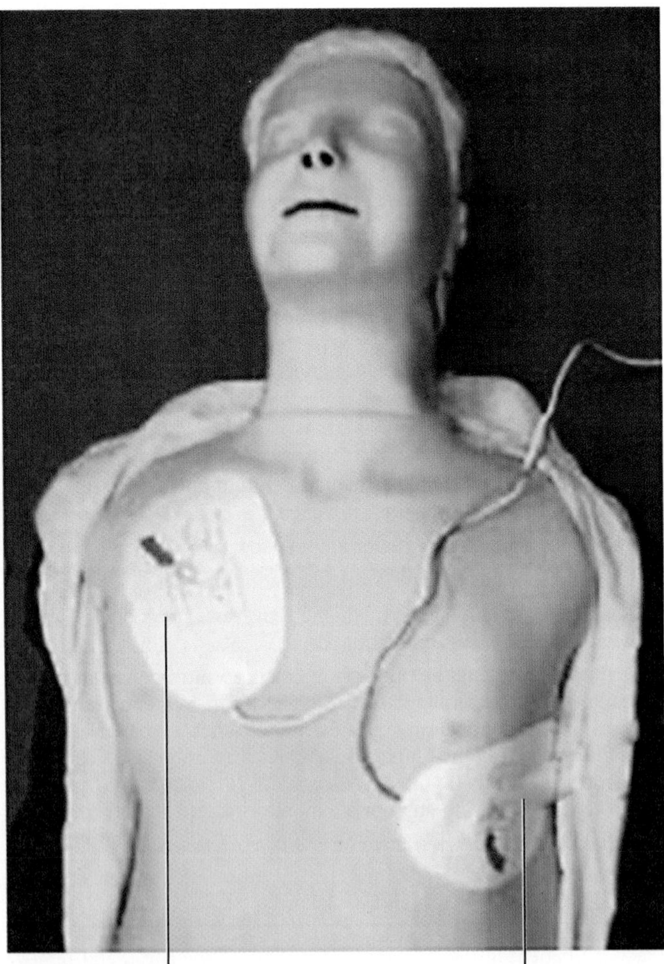

FIGURE 23-3. Antero-apical positioning of defibrillation pads. [Image used with permission of Institute for Medical Simulation & Education.]

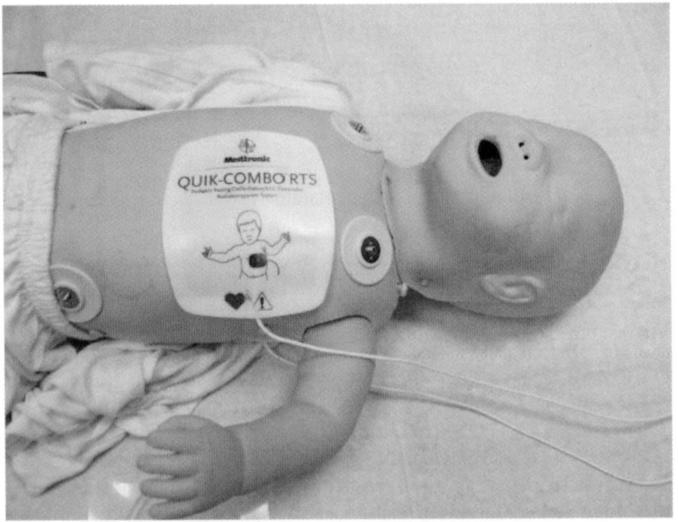

A

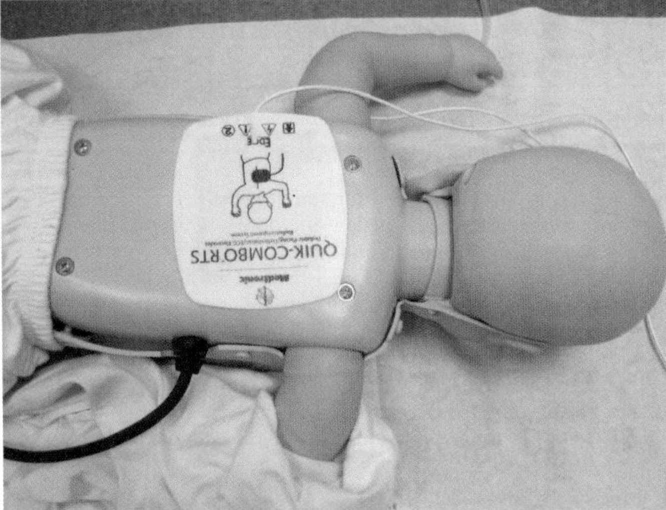

B

FIGURE 23-4. Anteroposterior positioning of defibrillation pads in an infant. [Reproduced, with permission, from Children's Emergency, KK Women's and Children's Hospital, Singapore.]

2. **Anteroposterior position:** Place one pad/paddle at the left lower sternal border and the posterior pad/paddle below the left scapula (**Figure 23-4, A and B**).
3. **Apex-posterior position:** Place one pad/paddle at the apex, just below and to the left of the left nipple, and the posterior pad/paddle below the left scapula.

When using paddles (**Figure 23-5**), apply conducting gel or a gel pad and firmly place the paddles onto the chest wall (25 lb/square inch or 2 cm^2 of pressure). When using defibrillation pads, ensure the electrodes are firmly attached and there is good contact by pressing gently with fingers over the center and around the edges to check for good adhesion. Good contact increases shock efficiency. In the AED mode, if contact is insufficient for the defibrillator to operate, the "Check Electrodes" message will also be heard. Outcomes are better with larger electrodes (12 cm) than with smaller electrodes (≤8 cm).

MANUAL DEFIBRILLATION

1. Prepare the patient and equipment as described earlier. CPR should be ongoing.
2. Check that the rhythm is VF or pulseless VT.
3. Check that the defibrillator is in *unsynchronized* mode.

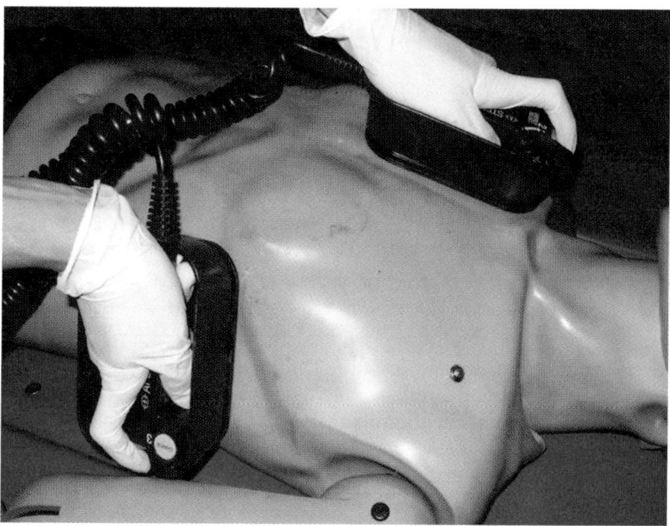

FIGURE 23-5. Antero-apical positioning of defibrillation paddles in an adult.

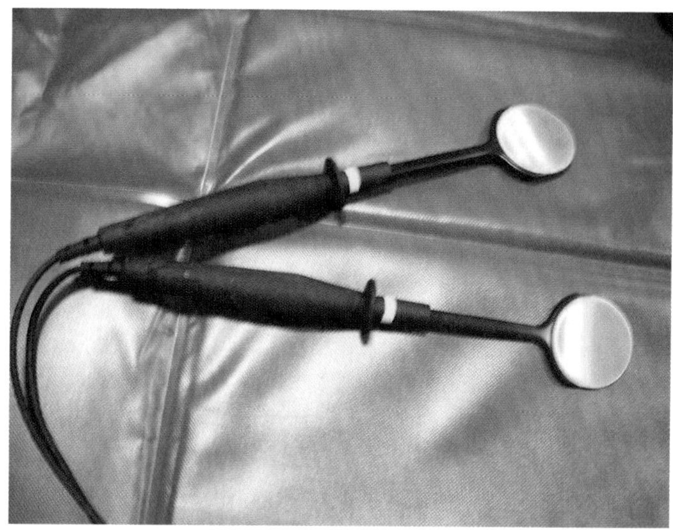

FIGURE 23-6. Internal defibrillation paddles.

4. Select the appropriate energy level. For biphasic machines, select according to the manufacturer's recommendation (150 to 200 J with biphasic truncated exponential waveforms and 120 J for rectilinear biphasic waveforms). For monophasic defibrillators, it is reasonable to begin with an initial 360-J shock.[6]
5. Apply the paddles or pads (may be applied beforehand) and charge.
6. Check that no one is in contact with the patient or trolley and call out, "Stand clear."
7. Discharge the shock.
8. Continue CPR and manage according to the local resuscitation protocol. The advanced cardiac life support universal cardiac arrest algorithm is shown in Figure 23-2.

AUTOMATED EXTERNAL DEFIBRILLATION

1. Prepare the patient and equipment as described earlier. **CPR should be ongoing.**
2. Open the package containing the defibrillation pads with attached cable and connector. With the chest prepared, carefully pull off the protective backing from the pads. Attach the pads.
3. Turn on the device (follow the voice prompts according to your device).
4. Initiate analysis of the rhythm, and ensure there is no movement during analysis. If a shock is indicated, the device will automatically charge up to a preset level.
5. Check that no one is in contact with the patient or trolley and call out, "Stand clear."
6. Discharge the shock (note that fully automated defibrillators do not require the operator's input to discharge a shock).
7. Continue CPR and manage according to the local resuscitation protocol. The advanced cardiac life support universal cardiac arrest algorithm is shown in Figure 23-2.

CARDIOVERSION

1. Prepare the patient and equipment as described earlier. Ensure the patient has adequate monitoring and that there is resuscitation equipment on standby.
2. Check the patient and the rhythm.
3. Check that the defibrillator is in *synchronized* mode.
4. Select the appropriate energy level. For monophasic defibrillators, start at 50 J for paroxysmal supraventricular tachycardia and atrial flutter and at 100 J for VT and atrial fibrillation. For biphasic defibrillators, follow the manufacturer's recommendations.
5. Provide sedation with an appropriate agent when ready.
6. Apply the paddles or pads (may be applied beforehand) and charge.
7. Check that no one is in contact with the patient or trolley and call out, "Stand clear."
8. Discharge the shock.
9. Continue to monitor and manage according to local protocols.

INTERNAL DEFIBRILLATION

Internal defibrillation is indicated in a patient with VF or pulseless VT with an open thoracotomy. This could be in a patient with traumatic cardiac arrest, for example, or during open heart surgery. The procedure requires a special set of internal defibrillator paddles (**Figure 23-6**), which should be connected to the defibrillator.

Moisten the internal defibrillator paddles with saline, and then place one paddle posteriorly over the left ventricle and the other anteriorly over the right ventricle. Hold the paddles firmly against the myocardium to ensure good contact. Begin with 10 J for defibrillation and increase as needed.

PEDIATRIC DEFIBRILLATION

VF in children is relatively uncommon, and the most frequent cause of cardiac arrest is usually respiratory. Thus, treatment should be directed toward preventing cardiac arrest by supporting ventilation and respiration. In the event of VF, use a weight-related dose of 4 J/kg body weight for the first and any subsequent shocks. For VT with a pulse, cardiovert with 1 J/kg synchronized. This can be increased to 4 J/kg subsequently if needed. Special pediatric paddles (**Figure 23-7, A and B**) or pads are available. Some AEDs also come with pediatric attenuator pads. In an infant, it is possible to defibrillate with the patient propped on the side using anteroposterior paddle placement.

OUTCOMES ASSESSMENT

The aim of defibrillation or cardioversion is termination of the abnormal rhythm and restoration of a normal perfusing rhythm.

COMPLICATIONS

Possible complications include skin burns, inadvertent electric shock to others, and defibrillation-induced myocardial damage. However, these complications are minimal compared to the ultimate complication of patient death if defibrillation is unsuccessful or not attempted.

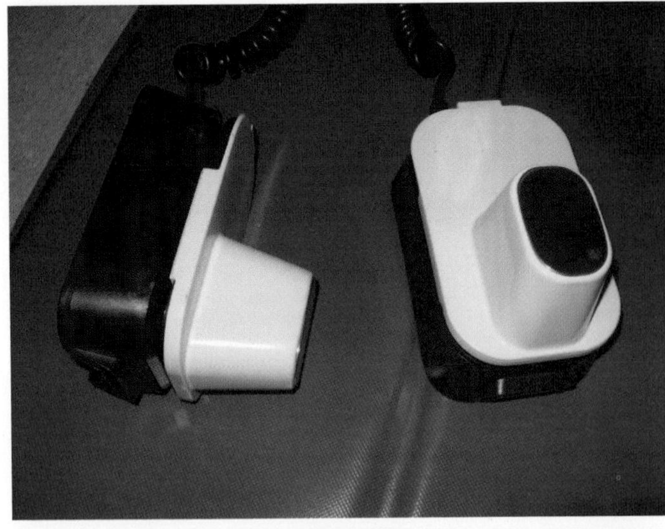

A

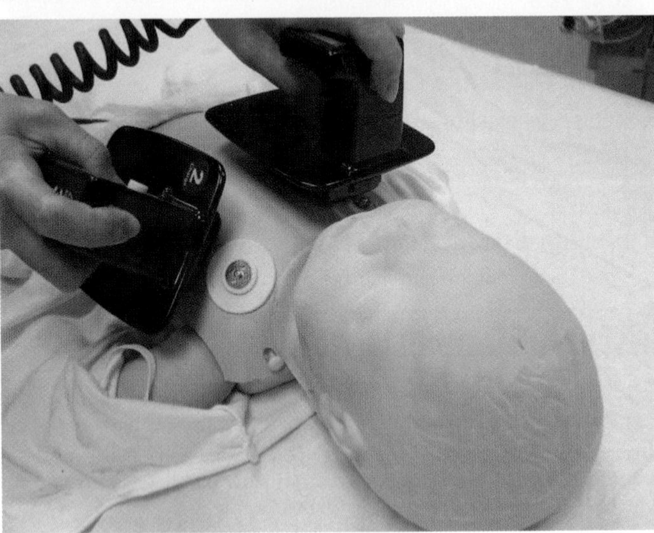

B

FIGURE 23-7. (**A**) Pediatric defibrillation paddles. (**B**) Antero-apical positioning of defibrillation paddles in an infant. [Reproduced, with permission, from Children's Emergency, KK Women's and Children's Hospital, Singapore.]

FOLLOW-UP

Patients requiring defibrillation or cardioversion will require intensive monitoring and close postresuscitation care.

Acknowledgments: Dr. Tham Lai Peng, Senior Consultant, Children's Emergency, KK Women's and Children's Hospital, Singapore; Madhavi Suppiah, Manager, Life Support Training Center, Singapore General Hospital, Singapore; Susan Yap, Research Nurse, Department of Emergency Medicine, Singapore General Hospital, Singapore; Garion Koh ZhiXiong, Research Associate, Department of Emergency Medicine, Singapore General Hospital, Singapore.

REFERENCES

The complete reference list is available online at www.TintinalliEM.com.

Advanced Cardiac Life Support

Anantharaman Venkataraman
Swee Han Lim
Marcus E. H. Ong
Kenneth B. K. Tan

INTRODUCTION AND EPIDEMIOLOGY

Every year, approximately 6.8 to 8.5 million persons throughout the world[1] sustain cardiac arrest. About 70% of cardiac arrests occur out of hospital. The proportion of cardiac arrest patients who are treated varies from about 54.6% (United States) to about 28.3% (Asia). The proportions with ventricular fibrillation (VF) and survival vary from 11% and 2%, respectively, in Asia, to 28% and 6% in North America, 35% and 9% in Europe, and 40% and 11% in Australia.[2] About half of cardiac arrest victims are <65 years old.

Ventricular tachyarrhythmias are the initiating event in about 80% of patients with out-of-hospital primary cardiac arrest. During ambulatory electrocardiogram (ECG) monitoring of 157 witnessed cardiac arrests, Bayés de Luna et al[3] documented 70% with ventricular tachycardia (VT) and VF, 13% with torsades de pointes, and 17% with bradyarrhythmias. Untreated VF deteriorates to asystole in about 15 minutes.[4] For patients with sudden cardiac arrest, the rate of survival declines rapidly by about 7% to 10% for each minute without defibrillation.[5] If delay to defibrillation exceeds 12 minutes,[6] survival is of the order of 0% to 5%.

THE CHAIN OF SURVIVAL

The structured emergency care system concept for treatment of cardiac arrest is called the **Chain of Survival and includes four components: Early Access, Early CPR, Early Defibrillation, and Early Advanced Care**. If a community's prehospital EMS can be activated promptly, reach the patient within 5 minutes of collapse, and deliver the first shock shortly thereafter, survival in excess of 15% to 20% can be expected, with recent reports of >30% survival.[7,8] With delayed initiation of CPR, defibrillation, and access to the patient by the emergency services, the impact of advanced life support measures is small (**Figure 24-1**). Improved survival can only occur if structured emergency care systems allow trained providers to access the patient rapidly and deliver the appropriate treatment in a timely fashion. Delays in initiating the various links weaken the chain and adversely affect the next link, resulting in a decreased chance of a good outcome for the patient.

ADVANCED CARDIAC LIFE SUPPORT (ACLS)

The basic life support assessments and interventions are often called the **Primary ABCD Survey**, and the advanced life support assessments and interventions are often called the **Secondary ABCD Survey**.

An organized approach to resuscitation begins with the Primary ABCD and blends smoothly with the Secondary ABCD. These are summarized in the **Universal ACLS Algorithm** (**Figure 24-2**). This method helps any ACLS provider remember the sequence of resuscitation actions and, therefore, be less likely to miss any of the vital steps in the care of the patient.

PRIMARY ABCD SURVEY

The **Primary ABCD Survey** addresses the identification of cardiac arrest and performance of good-quality CPR (including ventilation) and defibrillation. The procedures for the ABCs of the primary ABCD are described in chapters 22 and 23.

For ventilation, bag-valve masks deliver 21% oxygen if using room air, 60% oxygen when connected to an oxygen source with flow at 12 L/min,

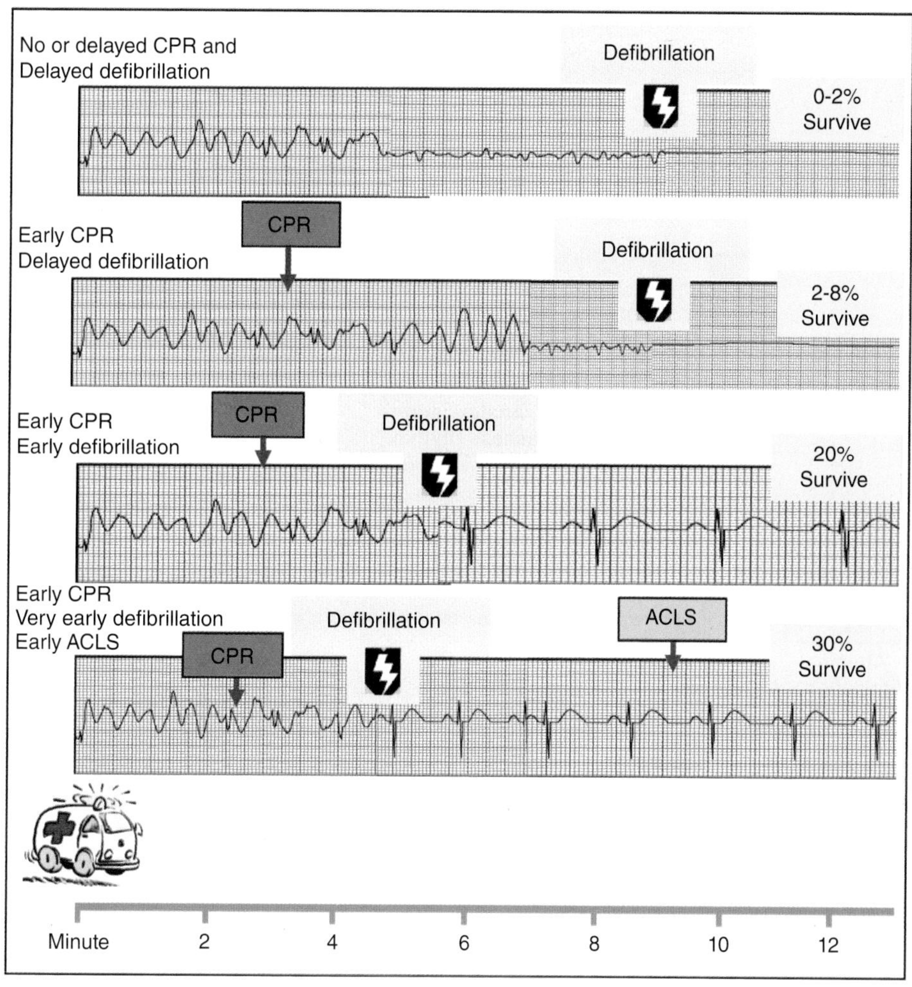

FIGURE 24-1. Incremental survival benefits by the links in the Chain of Survival. ACLS, advanced cardiac life support. [Reproduced, with permission, from the National Resuscitation Council, Singapore.]

and 90% to 95% with a reservoir bag. Chest compressions need not be stopped to initiate or continue ventilation.

The rescuer also needs to focus on providing good chest compressions (30 compressions for every 2 ventilations [30:2] with compression rate of ≥100/min, compression depth of at least 5 cm or 2 inches, and relaxation of pressure on the chest wall to allow unrestricted chest recoil). Feedback devices are available for the rescuer to provide improved standards of chest compressions.

Mechanical CPR devices may also be used. The two most common types of mechanical CPR devices employed in clinical practice are the LUCAS-2 with a piston attached to an active compression-decompression cup (**Figure 24-3**) and the load-distributing band Autopulse (**Figure 24-4**). Defibrillator pads must be applied to the bare chest before application of the mechanical CPR devices. These devices allow provision of either 30:2 CPR or continuous chest compressions with interposed manual ventilations.

The critical rhythms associated with cardiac arrest are **VF** (**Figure 24-5**), pulseless **VT** (**Figure 24-6**), asystole (**Figure 24-7**), and pulseless electrical activity (**PEA**) (**Figure 24-8**).

Defibrillation may be done with either an automated external defibrillator (**AED**) or a manual defibrillator (see chapter 23). **Deliver shocks for VF or pulseless VT with minimal interruption of chest compressions only during actual shock delivery.** Make sure that the position of the defibrillator pads (**Figure 24-9**) does not interfere with monitoring leads.

After delivery of the first shock, resume CPR (**Figure 24-10**) immediately for up to about 2 minutes before reviewing the ECG monitor for a rhythm diagnosis. If a viable rhythm has returned, check for pulse and breathing. If breathing and pulse have returned, begin care for post–return of spontaneous circulation (**ROSC**) management. If breathing is absent, continue rescue breathing with a bag-valve mask at the rate of about 6 to 10 breaths per minute; if pulse is not present, continue CPR and move to the **Secondary ABCD Survey**.

SECONDARY ABCD SURVEY

Components of the Secondary ABCD Survey are listed in **Table 24-1**.

The Secondary ABCD Survey includes endotracheal intubation or the placement of another airway adjunct, assessment of ventilatory status, gaining intravenous access, identifying ECG rhythms, delivering drugs to enhance circulation, and addressing the reasons for the occurrence or persistence of cardiac arrest. While the secondary ABCDs are in progress, continue the basic resuscitative actions of the primary ABCDs. Usually, defibrillation pads placed carefully left of the apex and to the right of the sternum just below the right clavicle (Figure 24-9) can also act as monitoring leads. Otherwise, true monitoring leads may be placed at the front of the right and left shoulders and over the left iliac crest. Such placement does not interfere with defibrillation or cardiac pacing procedures. Further management is based on the cardiac rhythm.

VASCULAR ACCESS

Vascular access techniques are discussed in Chapter 31, "Vascular Access." A large peripheral vein allows a rapid rate of fluid administration, if needed. If unable to cannulate a peripheral vein, establish intraosseous access. Central venous lines take time to establish and, because of the length of the cannula, cannot deliver fluids as rapidly as a

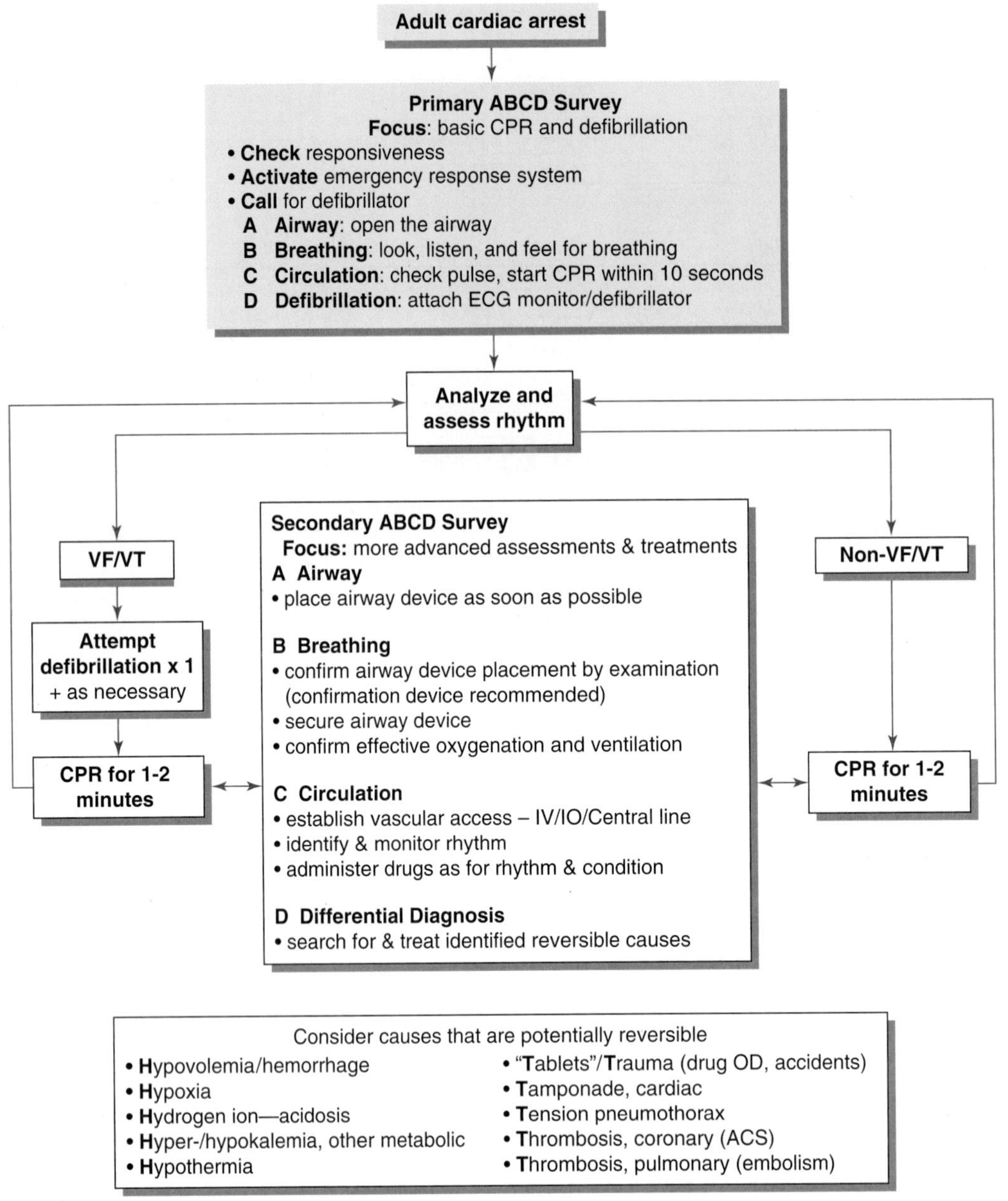

FIGURE 24-2. Universal ACLS Algorithm. ACS, acute coronary syndrome; OD, overdose. [Reproduced, with permission, from National Resuscitation Council, Singapore.]

peripheral line, and every bolus dose of drugs requires flushing with at least 20 mL of normal saline. Central lines are useful for central venous pressure monitoring to guide fluid resuscitation and circulatory management.

In cardiac arrest, circulation of blood grinds to a halt. With good-quality CPR, one can expect to generate up to about 30% of normal cardiac output, which is just about what is required to supply vital organs such as the heart, brain, and kidneys. The reduced circulation is associated with a slower circulation time. Therefore, drugs given during cardiac resuscitation are best administered via a proximal peripheral vein. Once drugs are given, flush the line with normal saline, and continue CPR for at least 30 to 60 seconds before repeat external defibrillation, so that the heart is optimally primed to respond.

The optimal infusion fluid is normal saline and not dextrose, Ringer's lactate, or sodium bicarbonate. However, unless hypovolemia is a contributing factor to cardiac arrest, fluid infusion should be slow, if at all necessary. Drug dosages are the same whether given by the intraosseous, IV, or central line routes. The endotracheal tube route is no longer recommended for drug administration because drug absorption is limited if the airway is filled with pulmonary edema fluid.

DRUGS USED IN RESUSCITATION TO ROSC FROM CARDIAC ARREST

Drugs available for cardiac resuscitation and cardiac dysrhythmia management are also described in chapters 19 and 20. This section will cover those drugs specifically used for resuscitation from cardiac arrest to ROSC. Drugs are an adjunct in the management of cardiac arrest patients. Good CPR, ventilation, and early defibrillation are the cornerstones of management of cardiac arrest. The effectiveness of standard resuscitative drugs on ROSC and survival to hospital discharge has not been well demonstrated.[9-11] However, consensus documents recommend the standard resuscitative drugs described below with the presumptive rationale that drugs help "restart" the heart and preserve coronary and cerebral circulation.

EPINEPHRINE

Epinephrine (adrenaline) is an endogenous catecholamine. It has an important role in cardiac arrest, although the evidence base for improved outcomes in humans is weak.[12] Epinephrine seems to improve short-term

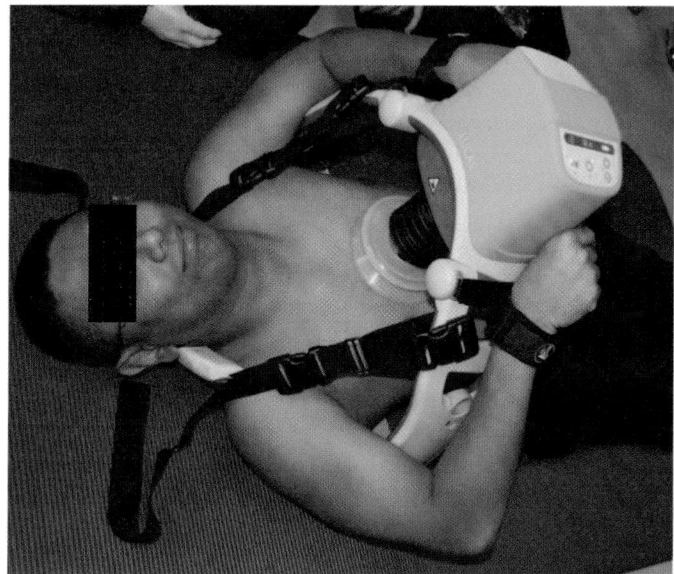

FIGURE 24-3. The LUCAS-2 chest compression gadget with its attached active compression-decompression device.

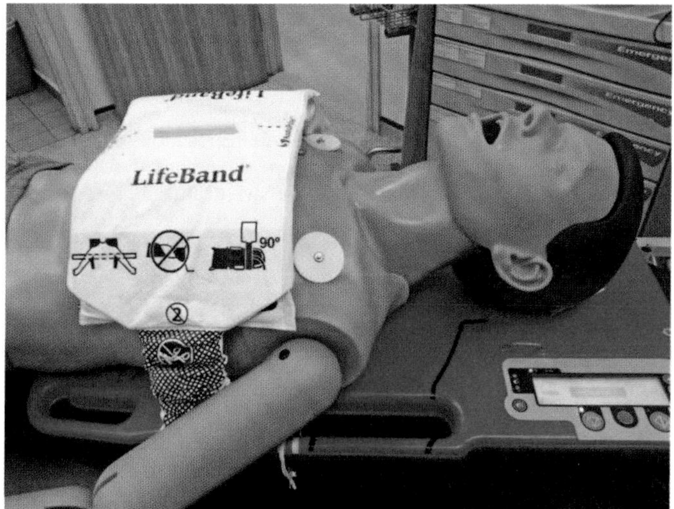

FIGURE 24-4. The Autopulse mechanical CPR device with its load-distributing band.

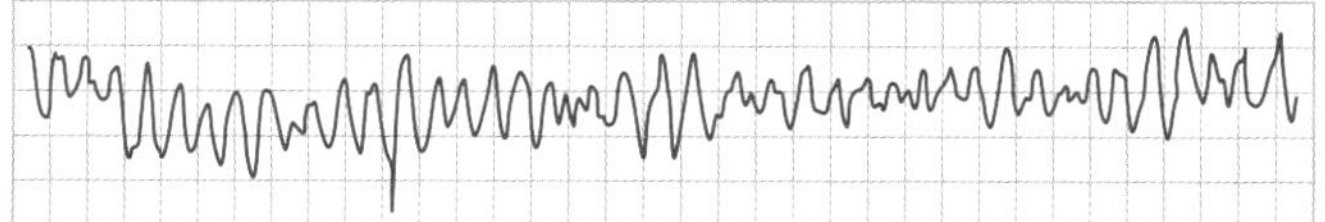

FIGURE 24-5. Ventricular fibrillation.

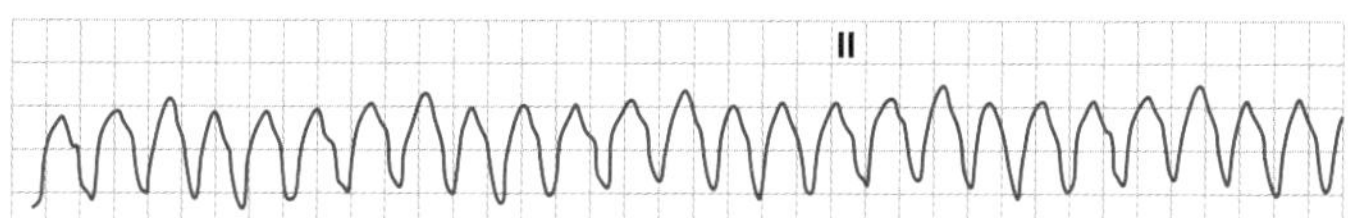

FIGURE 24-6. Pulseless ventricular tachycardia.

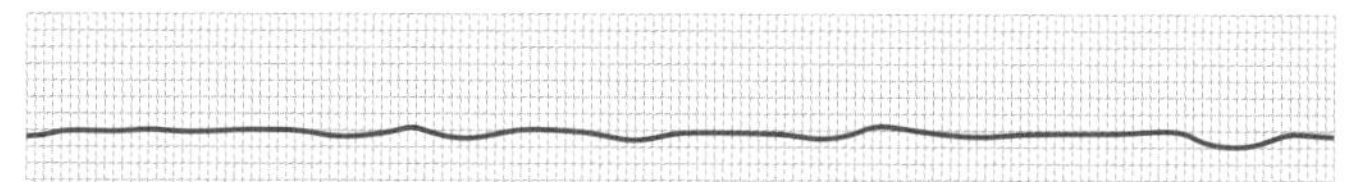

FIGURE 24-7. Asystole.

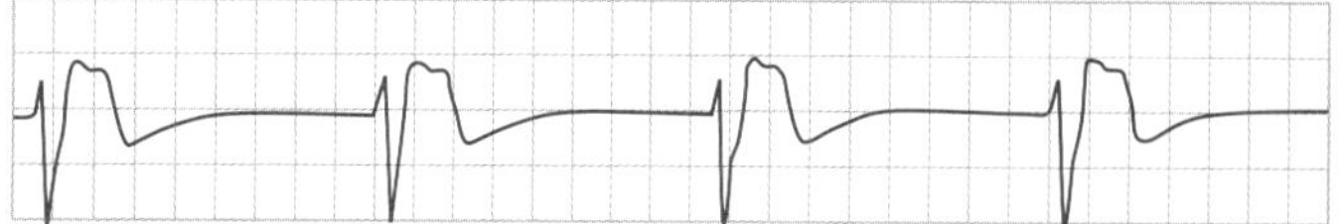

FIGURE 24-8. Pulseless electrical activity.

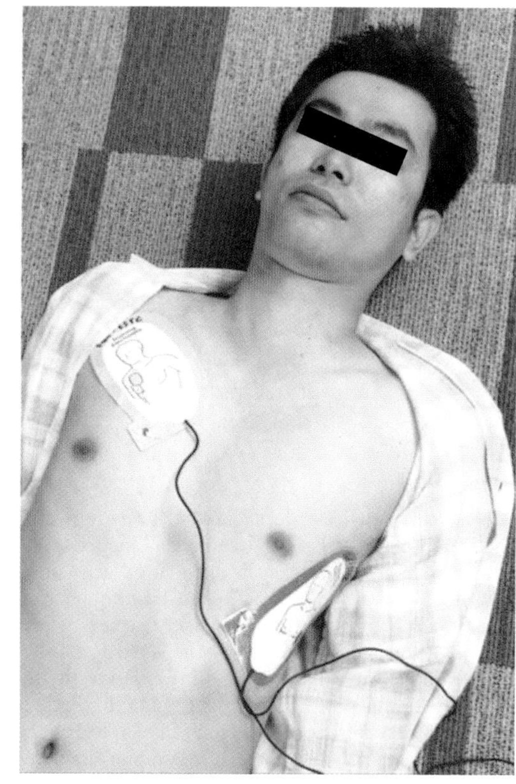

FIGURE 24-9. Placement of defibrillator pads.

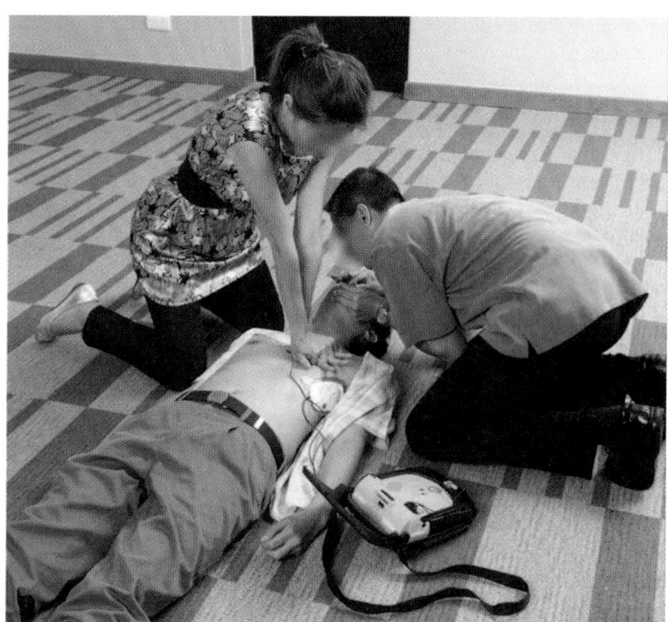

FIGURE 24-10. Continuing CPR after shock using an AED.

TABLE 24-1 Components of the Secondary ABCD Survey

Component and Function	Detailed Components
A: Securing the Airway	Endotracheal intubation or other supraglottic airway, eg, Laryngeal Mask Airway
B: Breathing (Ventilation)	1. Ventilation with Bag-Valve Mask 2. Oxygen 3. Mechanical ventilation
C: Maintaining the Circulation	1. Continue CPR 2. Provide defibrillation and cardioversion to correct life threatening 'shockable' rhythms 3. Continuous ECG monitoring to monitor the circulation's rhythm and identify arrhythmias that need to be corrected 4. Gain vascular access through IV/IO line 5. Provide drugs to help maintain circulation 6. Consider use of ECMO
D: Differential diagnosis	1. Determine why the patient is not responding to the resuscitative efforts 2. Look for correctible causes of collapse and provide necessary interventions
Specialized Care after ROSC*	Therapeutic hypothermia, glycemic control, early goal directed therapy, percutaneous coronary interventions

* ROSC, return of spontaneous circulation

survival.[13] The primary beneficial effect appears to be peripheral vasoconstriction, which improves cerebral and coronary blood flow. Potential adverse effects include an increase in myocardial oxygen consumption and an increase in pulmonary shunting. The most common adverse reaction is tachycardia. Epinephrine may worsen myocardial ischemia and induce ventricular ectopy and VT. **Epinephrine is used mainly to treat cardiac arrest from VF or pulseless VT unresponsive to the initial shock, asystole, PEA, and profoundly symptomatic bradycardia.** The standard dose in cardiac arrest is 1.0 milligram diluted to 10 mL (10 mL of 1:10,000) given IV. Repeat if needed at 3- to 5-minute intervals. There is no maximum dose. Escalating doses at 2 to 5 milligrams IV every 3 to 5 minutes (high-dose epinephrine) have not resulted in increased long-term survival.[12] For IV infusion in patients with cardiogenic shock or symptomatic bradycardia, the dose is 1 milligram in 500 mL normal saline beginning at 2 to 10 micrograms/min, escalating as needed at 3- to 5-minute intervals. Do not add epinephrine to infusions that contain alkaline solutions because epinephrine has ineffective clinical activity in alkaline solutions.

AMIODARONE

Amiodarone is generally considered a Class III antiarrhythmic drug, but it possesses electrophysiologic characteristics of all four Vaughn-Williams classes. It causes coronary and peripheral artery vasodilation. It is more effective than lidocaine for improving short-term survival.[14] **Its main use in cardiac arrest is for persistent VT or VF after defibrillation and epinephrine.** It can also be used for hemodynamically stable VT, hemodynamically stable polymorphic VT, and hemodynamically stable wide-complex tachycardia of uncertain origin. Amiodarone is also used for the pharmacologic conversion of atrial fibrillation, control of rapid ventricular rate in preexcitation supraventricular dysrhythmias, and as an adjunct to electrical cardioversion of refractory paroxysmal supraventricular tachycardia/atrial tachycardia. For pulseless VT or VF, the dose is a bolus of 300 milligrams IV followed by a 20-mL flush with 5% dextrose in water or saline. Give another 150-milligram bolus if there is no response to the first dose. For stable ventricular and supraventricular dysrhythmias, administer amiodarone IV 150 milligrams over 10 to 15 minutes (not to exceed 30 milligrams/min), followed by a maintenance infusion of 1 milligram/min for 6 hours and then 0.5 milligrams/min for the next 18 hours. Infusions exceeding 2 hours should be administered in glass or polyolefin bottles because the drug precipitates in plastic tubing. Hypotension and bradycardia are the most common unwanted effects. These may be addressed by slowing the infusion rate, giving an IV fluid challenge, or using pressors or positive chronotropic agents. Occasionally, temporary pacing for refractory bradycardia from amiodarone may be required, especially if other measures are ineffective.

LIDOCAINE (LIGNOCAINE)

Lidocaine (lignocaine) (see also chapter 12, Approach to Shock) is a Class I antiarrhythmic drug. It reduces automaticity, suppresses ventricular ectopy, and is used for hemodynamically stable VT and refractory VF/pulseless VT. **Lidocaine is a second-choice drug after amiodarone or is used if amiodarone is not available.** In cardiac arrest, the dose is an IV bolus of 1 to 1.5 milligrams/kg body weight. Give a second bolus of 0.5 to 0.75 milligrams/kg if the rhythm persists. Upon restoration of spontaneous circulation, give lidocaine as an infusion at a rate of 1 to 4 milligrams/min. If dysrhythmia reappears during the infusion of lidocaine, give a bolus of 0.5 milligrams/kg and increase the infusion rate to 4 milligrams/min. Toxicity may occur with doses exceeding 3 milligrams/kg body weight bolus or in patients with liver disease, since the drug is hepatically metabolized. Symptoms include neurologic changes such as drowsiness, disorientation, reduced hearing ability, perioral paresthesia, muscle tremors, and seizures. Myocardial depression and circulatory depression are also features of toxicity, and these may be illustrated by widening QRS complexes and falling blood pressures. In patients with known impaired liver function or patients >70 years old, give the same recommended bolus doses, but decrease the normal infusion rate by 50%.

MAGNESIUM

Magnesium is a cofactor in numerous enzymatic reactions. It is essential for the function of the Na-K-ATPase pump. Magnesium deficiency may be associated with cardiac arrhythmias, sudden death, and precipitation of VF. Magnesium is used to treat hypomagnesemia, with or without dysrhythmias.

Magnesium is initial treatment for torsades de pointes and dysrhythmias secondary to hypomagnesemia, cardiac arrest from QT_c prolongation, or cardiac glycoside toxicity.[9,15] For patients in VF or pulseless VT due to the above conditions, give 1 to 2 grams in 10mL 5% dextrose in water IV over 1 minute. Magnesium provides no benefit for routine use in cardiac arrest. For patients with a pulse, the dose is 1 to 4 grams in 50 mL 5% dextrose in water over 60 minutes. Adverse reactions include flushing, sweating, mild bradycardia, hypotension, asystole with circulatory collapse (with too rapid administration), and respiratory depression. Hypermagnesemia may produce depressed reflexes, flaccid paralysis, diarrhea, respiratory depression, and circulatory collapse.

OTHER DRUGS IN CARDIAC ARREST

Atropine **Atropine** is a parasympatholytic agent that enhances sinus node automaticity and atrioventricular conduction by direct vagolytic action. **It is not recommended for PEA or for treatment of cardiac arrest.** It is indicated for symptomatic bradycardia. The dose is 0.5 or 0.6 milligrams IV (dose depends on formulation in country of use) and may be repeated at 5- to 10-minute intervals up to a maximum of 0.04 milligrams/kg body weight. Atropine may induce tachycardia or premature ventricular contractions and cause worsening of myocardial ischemia. Symptoms of overdosage include tachycardia, delirium, coma, flushed and hot skin, ataxia, and blurred vision. Administration of low doses less than 0.5 milligrams IV may produce paradoxical bradycardia and precipitate VF.

Calcium **Calcium is given during resuscitation only for cardiac arrest from hyperkalemia, hypocalcemia, or calcium channel blocker overdose.** Calcium is not recommended for routine administration for VF/pulseless VT or PEA.[9,16] The dose of calcium chloride is 0.2 mL/kg of 10% calcium chloride, given as a slow IV bolus.

Sodium Bicarbonate The use of sodium bicarbonate during cardiac arrest was advocated in the past to treat presumptive acidosis, because severe acidosis decreases myocardial contractility.[17] However, **routine use during cardiac arrest is no longer recommended** due to a number of potential adverse effects. Sodium bicarbonate causes hypernatremia, hyperosmolality, and alkalosis (which in turn induces a left shift of the oxyhemoglobin dissociation curve), and IV sodium bicarbonate produces carbon dioxide, resulting in hypercarbia unless ventilation is increased. It does not appear to improve defibrillation success. **It may be given in cardiac arrest from hyperkalemia or cyclic antidepressant overdose.** It is also acceptable and possibly helpful for intubated patients with a long arrest interval until ROSC and with persistent severe metabolic acidosis. The dose is 1 to 1.5 mEq/kg IV bolus, followed by 0.75 mEq/kg every 10 to 15 minutes as needed. If continuous infusion of sodium bicarbonate is used, check pH to guide therapy.

VASOPRESSIN

Vasopressin, also called antidiuretic hormone, is a naturally occurring neurohypophysial peptide hormone synthesized in the hypothalamus and stored in the pituitary gland. It increases water absorption in the nephron and increases peripheral vascular resistance. Vasopressin levels elevate during cardiac arrest, and this observation led to investigation of its role in resuscitation. Vasopressin has a longer duration of action and, in laboratory studies, maintains coronary perfusion pressure, myocardial blood flow, and cerebral blood flow better than epinephrine. However, most studies do not show superiority of vasopressin over epinephrine.[12,16] Vasopressin as a first-line agent in cardiac arrest (40-milligram dose) does not improve long-term survival when compared to epinephrine,[18] although vasopressin might improve short-term survival in patients with prolonged cardiac arrest.[18] Combining vasopressin (40 milligrams) with epinephrine does not appear to improve outcomes.[12]

COMMON CARDIAC ARREST ALGORITHMS

The algorithmic approach to cardiac arrest management allows a structured decision-making process when managing cardiac arrest victims. The cardiac arrest rhythms discussed here are pulseless VT/VF, asystole, and PEA.

VENTRICULAR FIBRILLATION (VF)/PULSELESS VENTRICULAR TACHYCARDIA (VT)

Once VF or pulseless VT is diagnosed, prepare for electrical conversion while CPR is in progress. If ROSC does not occur after the first shock, move to the mega-VF approach (**Figure 24-11**). Continue CPR for 1 to 2 minutes followed by rhythm analysis, and if VF persists or recurs, deliver electrical shocks, usually biphasic, beginning usually at 150 J and escalating, if needed, to 360 J. For monophasic defibrillators, begin at 360 J. After delivery of shock, follow with CPR again for 1 to 2 minutes before rhythm analysis. Maintain good-quality CPR for optimal coronary and vital organ perfusion. Parallel to the CPR-analysis-shock-CPR-analysis-shock-CPR cycle, begin secondary ABCDs and give drugs that may help to lower defibrillation thresholds, such as epinephrine (adrenaline), amiodarone, and/or lidocaine (lignocaine). Any or all of these drugs may be administered in any combination and repeated at roughly 3- to 5-minute intervals. After administration of any of these drugs, provide at least 30 to 60 seconds of effective CPR to allow the injected drug to reach the central circulation before the next shock. Continue the resuscitation cycle for as long as the rhythm remains as VF or pulseless VT.

ASYSTOLE/PULSELESS ELECTRICAL ACTIVITY (PEA)

For asystole or PEA, (a condition in which cardiac contractions are absent in the presence of coordinated electrical activity), continue CPR and institute the secondary ABCDs. Give drugs to enhance the chances of ROSC (**Figure 24-12**). Epinephrine (adrenaline) 1.0 milligram as a bolus dose in 10 mL is the drug of choice. Vasopressin alone or in combination with epinephrine is no more effective than epinephrine alone. Repeat epinephrine as needed in 3- to 5-minute intervals. Consider other possible causes of asystole or PEA, and identify and correct them. It is currently assumed that narrow-complex PEA[19]

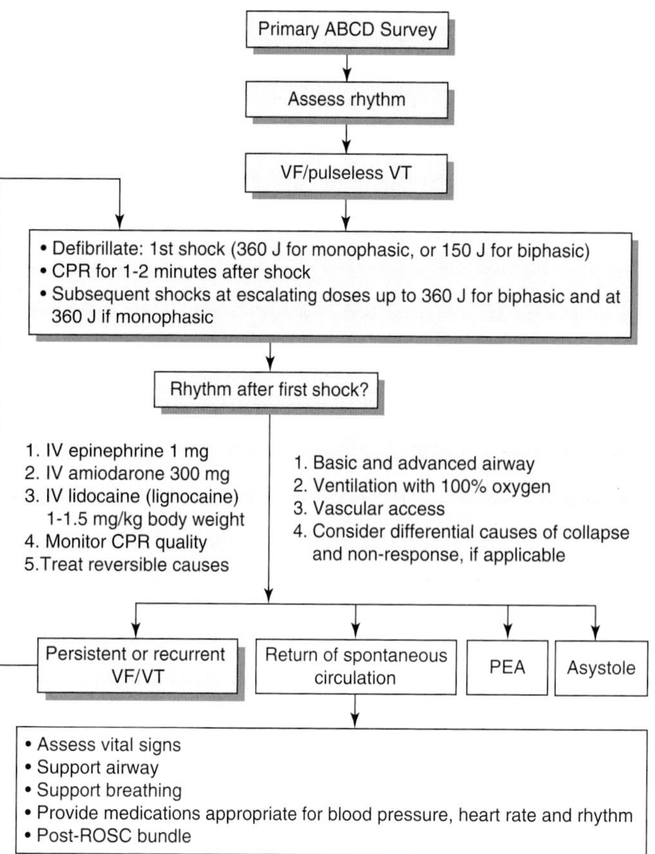

FIGURE 24-11. Management of VF/pulseless VT. [Reproduced, with permission, from National Resuscitation Council, Singapore.]

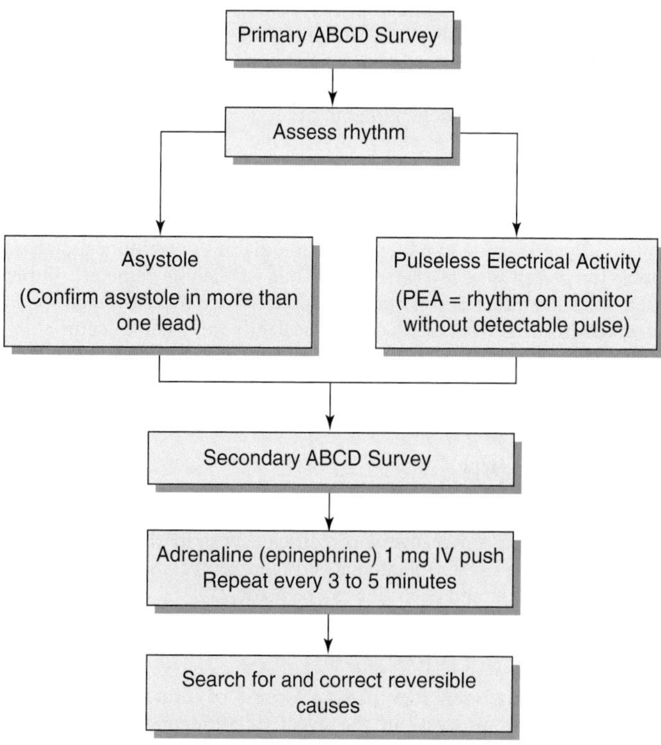

FIGURE 24-12. Asystole/PEA management algorithm. [Reproduced, with permission, from National Resuscitation Council, Singapore.]

could be the result of mechanical problems such as cardiac tamponade, pneumothorax, mechanical hyperinflation, pulmonary embolism, or myocardial rupture. Point-of-care US and assessment of the clinical scenario can direct specific treatment. Wide-complex PEA,[19] on the other hand, can result from a metabolic problem (ie, hyperkalemia), drug toxicity (ie, sodium channel blocker toxicity), or cardiac ischemia, and left ventricular failure and should be treated as appropriate. Survival is low if patients in asystole do not achieve ROSC in the field or convert to a shockable rhythm.[20-22]

DIFFERENTIAL DIAGNOSES OF CARDIAC ARREST

In every resuscitation, it is useful to identify important causes of cardiac arrest and reasons for lack of response to standard resuscitation algorithms. Causes can be grouped as the **5 H's—hypovolemia or hemorrhage, hypoxia, hydrogen ion (acidosis), hypo- or hyperkalemia, and hypothermia**—and the **5 T's—trauma + tablets (overdose), cardiac tamponade, coronary thrombosis, tension pneumothorax, and thrombosis (pulmonary embolism)**.

H: HYPOVOLEMIA OR HEMORRHAGE

History of fluid or blood loss may be available. Rectal examination can identify massive lower GI bleeding; nasogastric intubation can identify massive upper GI bleeding; and bedside FAST can diagnose massive intraperitoneal bleeding. Treat with fluids and blood products.

H: HYPOXIA

Hypoxia occurs with lack of oxygen and alveolar ventilation. Make sure that the airway adjunct is placed correctly. Check breath sounds at intervals to ensure that the endotracheal tube has not slipped out of the trachea or to identify pneumothorax. Verify the source of oxygen—an oxygen cylinder or the piped oxygen supply.

H: HYDROGEN ION (ACIDOSIS)

The acidosis of cardiac arrest is a combination of respiratory and metabolic acidosis. Respiratory acidosis is addressed by early endotracheal intubation and alveolar ventilation. Metabolic acidosis can be somewhat addressed by good-quality CPR. Sodium bicarbonate is administered for severe metabolic acidosis from prolonged or poor initial resuscitation, at a dose of 1 to 1.5 mEq/kg. Half the initial dose can be readministered after 10 to 15 minutes, depending on pH.

H: HYPER- OR HYPOKALEMIA, OTHER METABOLIC DISORDERS

Suspect hyperkalemia in patients on hemodialysis or peritoneal dialysis (look for presence of arteriovenous fistula or dialysis catheter). Other metabolic disorders are extremely difficult to confidently identify in cardiac arrest. If hyperkalemia is suspected, administer calcium chloride, sodium bicarbonate, insulin, and glucose. Treat hyperkalemia from suspected digitalis toxicity with IV magnesium sulfate or digoxin-specific Fab fragments (Digibind®).

H: HYPOTHERMIA

Treat hypothermia with gradual rewarming with blankets and warm IV fluids. If there is no recovery of consciousness in the hypothermic patient following ROSC, maintain a body core temperature of 33°C until further assessment and decisions can be made.

T: "TABLETS" (DRUG OVERDOSE)

Drug overdose is rarely identified as a cause of cardiac arrest during the resuscitation process. In the event of antidepressant overdose, administer IV sodium bicarbonate. Lipid emulsion infusion may be useful in cardiac arrest associated with cyclic antidepressants or local anesthetics.[24-28]

T: CARDIAC TAMPONADE

Cardiac tamponade is best identified during resuscitation by bedside transthoracic US. This requires brief interruption of chest compressions. Treatment of tamponade causing cardiac arrest is bedside pericardiocentesis.

T: TENSION PNEUMOTHORAX

Suspect tension pneumothorax during cardiac resuscitation if breath sounds are unequal on chest auscultation after verifying correct endotracheal tube placement. Treatment is immediate needle decompression.

T: CORONARY THROMBOSIS

Acute coronary thrombosis or acute myocardial infarction is one of the most common causes of cardiac arrest. Risk factors are a history of coronary artery disease and initial rhythm of VF/VT.[24-28] Cardiac catheterization after resuscitation is an underused procedure.[29] A 12-lead ECG in the immediate post–cardiac arrest state can identify an ST-elevation acute myocardial infarction and allow arrangements for immediate coronary angiography. Myocardial and neurologic function can improve after percutaneous coronary intervention following cardiac arrest.[30] Thus, after ROSC, especially in the face of post-ROSC ECG evidence of acute myocardial infarction, advocate for cardiac catheterization and percutaneous coronary revascularization if available and appropriate. A few case reports describe fibrinolysis during CPR with resultant ROSC and good neurologic outcome.[31] Reports are too few to determine whether thrombolysis together with CPR results in more severe bleeding than thrombolysis without CPR.[31]

T: THROMBOSIS (PULMONARY EMBOLISM)

Pulmonary embolism causing cardiac arrest requires fibrinolysis or embolectomy. However, the diagnosis is rarely made at time of collapse, and even then, most systems are not geared to make such prompt diagnosis and initiate the necessary procedures for embolectomy. Fibrinolytic agents could be considered during cardiac arrest from suspected pulmonary embolism on a case-by-case basis.[32] Factors suggestive of pulmonary embolism causing cardiac arrest include two of three signs/symptoms (prearrest respiratory distress, altered mental status, or shock); arrest witnessed by a physician or emergency medical technician; and PEA as the first or primary arrest rhythm.[33]

POST-ROSC COMPLICATIONS

After ROSC, many factors affect survival: anoxic brain injury, post–cardiac arrest myocardial dysfunction, the systemic reperfusion response, and the cause of cardiac arrest. Ischemic-reperfusion injury is discussed in chapter 26, Post-Cardiac Arrest Syndrome. Anoxic brain injury results in disturbance of cerebral microvascular hemostasis and manifests as coma, seizures, myoclonus, and varying degrees of neurocognitive dysfunction, including brain death. Post–cardiac arrest myocardial dysfunction results from myocardial stunning with cardiac hypokinesis and a low left ventricular ejection fraction. Clinical manifestations include tachycardia and elevated left ventricular end-diastolic pressures progressing to hypotension and reduced cardiac output. The systemic ischemia-reperfusion response consists of inflammation, endothelial activation, and disturbed vasoregulation with generalized activation of immunologic and coagulation pathways, causing increased risk of multiple organ failure and infection. Clinical manifestations of the systemic ischemia-reperfusion response include impaired oxygen delivery and utilization and increased susceptibility to infection.

OXYGENATION AND VENTILATION

Hyperoxia during the early phase of reperfusion after ROSC harms postischemic neurons and increases brain lipid peroxidation.[34,35] After ROSC, adjust the rate of ventilation and tidal volume to maintain arterial oxyhemoglobin saturation at 94% to 98%.[36] Hyperventilation is not recommended because it can increase intrathoracic pressures and decrease venous return and cardiac output. In addition, hypocarbia resulting from hyperventilation decreases cerebral blood flow and aggravates anoxic brain damage. The suggested ventilator parameters during the post-ROSC phase[34-36] are as follows: Pa_{CO_2} between 35 and 45 mm Hg (5 to 6 kPa); Sa_{O_2} between 94% and 98%; tidal volume between 6 and 8 mL/kg ideal body weight; P_{ETCO_2} between 35 and 40 mm Hg; and 10 to 12 ventilations per minute.

HEMODYNAMIC MANAGEMENT

Obtain 12-lead ECG after ROSC and repeat at 8 hours or as needed. Administer IV fluids and drugs to optimize blood pressure, cardiac output, and urine output. The target for blood pressure is a mean arterial pressure of 65 to 100 mm Hg, and the target for blood oxygenation is an S_{CVO_2} of ≥70%.[37,38] Pharmaceutical agents to support the circulation include epinephrine, norepinephrine, dopamine, dobutamine, nitroglycerine, and esmolol. Obtain an echocardiogram at 24 hours after ROSC to detect regional wall motion abnormalities and determine ejection fractions.

TARGETED TEMPERATURE MANAGEMENT (THERAPEUTIC HYPOTHERMIA)

Brain cooling decreases cerebral oxygen demand, reduces cellular effects of reperfusion, and decreases the production of reactive oxide radicals. Targeted temperature management (cooling to 32 to 36°C; temperature goal is controversial) during the first 24 hours after ROSC improves survival and neurologic recovery[39-42] in patients who remain comatose soon after ROSC. Hyperpyrexia during the first 48 hours is usually associated with a lowered chance of optimal neurologic recovery.[43] See chapter 26, Post-Cardiac Arrest Syndrome, for detailed discussion.

GLYCEMIC CONTROL

Post-ROSC hyperglycemia is associated with increased mortality and worse neurologic outcomes.[44] Hypoglycemia, similarly, is also associated with poor outcomes in critically ill patients.[45] Maintain blood sugar levels between 100 and 180 milligrams/dL (6 and 10 mmol/L).

NEUROLOGIC ASSESSMENT

Features of brain injury after ROSC include coma, seizures, myoclonus, and various degrees of neurocognitive dysfunction ranging from memory deficits to a persistent vegetative state and finally brain death. Treat seizures promptly. The neurologic prognosis in the majority of comatose cardiac arrest survivors undergoing therapeutic hypothermia cannot be reliably predicted in the ED.

REFERENCES

The complete reference list is available online at www.TintinalliEM.com.

ECPR (ECMO) in Cardiac Arrest

Extracorporeal Membrane Oxygenation (ECMO), also known as Extracorporeal Life Support (ECLS) is a recent introduction in the management of cardiac arrest. Its use is well-documented in the neonatal and paediatric population,[1] and in adults, for refractory respiratory failure, and cardiogenic shock. Use in refractory cardiac arrest is also known as ECPR. ECPR is a bridging therapy to definitive treatments, such as percutaneous coronary interventions, cardiac bypass surgery, or heart transplant.

The ECMO equipment consists of a blood pump, a venous reservoir, an oxygenator for exchanging both oxygen and carbon dioxide, and a heat exchanger to warm the blood used. The whole system is monitored through pressure, oxygen saturation, and temperature monitors. Three types of ECMO circuits are available:

1. A veno-arterial ECMO (VA-ECMO) pumps blood from the venous side to the arterial side to facilitate gas exchange and provide hemodynamic support. The blood is pumped from the venous circulation through a cannula inserted in either the inferior vena cava or right atrium, through the oxygenator where gas exchange occurs, then warmed and returned to the patient through a cannula placed in either the aortic arch or femoral artery into the arterial circulation. This is the modality that is used to support cardiac arrest patients.
2. A veno-venous (VV) ECMO removes blood from the right atrium, passes it through the gas exchanger, and returns it across the tricuspid valve into the right ventricle. It does not provide hemodynamic support. This modality is used mainly for refractory respiratory failure.
3. An arterio-venous ECMO (AV-ECMO) makes use of the patient's own arterial pressure to pump the blood from the arterial to the venous side and facilitates gas exchange in the process. This does not require the use of a separate blood pump.

The ECMO circuit is initially primed with fresh blood, which is then pumped through the circuit. During maintenance of ECMO, haemodynamic parameters, urinary output, hematological indices, fluids, and electrolytes are monitored.

ECPR complications can be mechanical or medical, or both. Mechanical complications consist of clots in the circuit, mediastinal bleeding from tears to the great vessels, oxygenator failure and malfunction of the blood pump, oxygenator, heat exchanger and sensors. Medical complications include intracranial and systemic hemorrhage, initial cardiac stunning that may occur soon after initiation of ECMO, pneumothorax, acute kidney injury, gastrointestinal bleeding, sepsis, and metabolic derangement.

ECPR must also be accompanied by good post-cardiac arrest management, to include targeted temperature and hemodynamic management, and early coronary angiography for definitive treatment.[3] At the present time, survival rates are low, but can be improved with EMS and ED training, appropriate patient selection, and more widespread application of the technique.[2,3]

TABLE 1 General Indications and Contraindications for ECPR (ECMO in Cardiac Arrest)

Indications	Contraindications
Good pre-morbid status before cardiac arrest	Advanced age; advanced malignancy; poor baseline neurologic function; baseline inability to perform activities of daily living; pre-exisitng 'do not resuscitate' order
Intervention to be curative, not palliative	Suspect aortic dissection or severe aortic regurgitation; traumatic cardiac arrest
Reversible trigger event for cardiac arrest (dysrhythmia, STEMI, etc.)	Unwitnessed cardiac arrest and no bystander CPR Long prehospital transport time Prolonged cardiac arrest unless good perfusion and metabolic support is documented[2]

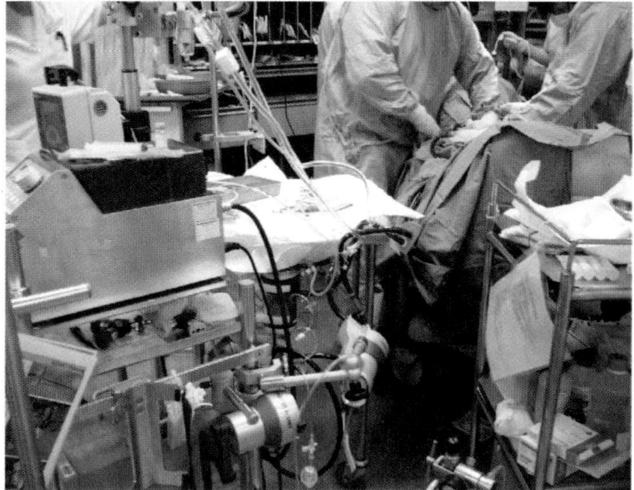

FIGURE 1. ECPR in the emergency department, Singapore General Hospital.

REFERENCES

The complete reference list is available online at www.TintinalliEM.com

CHAPTER 25

Resuscitation in Pregnancy

Boyd Burns

INTRODUCTION AND EPIDEMIOLOGY

Cardiac arrest in pregnancy is rare, and resuscitation of a pregnant woman is typically an unexpected and chaotic event, which ideally involves multiple consultants from different specialties with different levels and types of skills. Emergency care and lifesaving procedures for resuscitation and cardiac arrest should not be delayed if specialists are not available. Contact the closest center providing neonatal and maternal services as soon as possible to facilitate rapid transport and continued care of the newly delivered infant and the mother.

The World Health Organization defines maternal deaths as deaths while pregnant or within 42 days of the end of pregnancy, related to or aggravated by pregnancy or pregnancy management, regardless of the duration or site of the pregnancy and irrespective of the cause of death.[1] Factors associated with pregnancy-related deaths in the United States include advanced maternal age, African American race, increasing live birth order, and lack of prenatal care.[2]

Management of emergencies during labor and delivery and diagnosis and management of pulmonary embolism and eclampsia are discussed in the chapters 101, "Emergency Delivery" and 100, "Maternal Emergencies after 20 Weeks of Pregnancy and in the Postpartum Period."

PHYSIOLOGY OF PREGNANCY

Beginning early in pregnancy, virtually all major organ systems undergo changes (**Table 25-1**) that affect patient management.

CARDIOVASCULAR CHANGES

Uterine blood flow is not autoregulated but is directly proportional to the maternal mean arterial pressure and inversely proportional to the resistance of the uterine vasculature. Conditions that decrease uterine blood flow during pregnancy include maternal hypovolemia, hypotension, uterine vasoconstriction, tetanic uterine contractions and aortocaval compression.

As the uterus enlarges throughout pregnancy, compression of the pelvic and abdominal vasculature can occur, especially when the patient is supine. Compression of the inferior vena cava can decrease maternal venous return and reduce cardiac output from 10% to 30% (**Figure 25-1**).[4] This can contribute to supine hypotension syndrome, which is a constellation of findings including hypotension, tachycardia, dizziness, pallor, and nausea. It is reported to occur after 30 minutes in the supine position.[4] Therefore, place any patient in the third trimester of pregnancy in the full left lateral tilt position when in hemodynamic distress or exhibiting hypotension.[5] Left lateral tilt can be achieved by placing a roll under the patient's right hip, insertion of a Cardiff wedge, or full left lateral tilt of the patient while on a backboard (**Figure 25-2**).

TABLE 25-1 Physiologic Changes in Pregnancy Affecting Resuscitation

System	Parameters	Comment
Cardiovascular	Cardiac output	Increases 30%–50%
	Peripheral resistance	Decreases 20%
	Blood pressure	Decreases 10–15 mm Hg systolic in first half of pregnancy; then back to baseline
	Blood volume	100 cc/kg or 6–7 L
	Central venous pressure	May be increased up to 10 mm Hg
	Central venous oxygen saturation	Increases as high as 80%[3]
	Plasma volume	Increases 30%–50%
Hematologic	Fibrinogen, factors V, VII, VIII, X, von Willebrand factor	Increase, with heightened risk for venous thromboembolism in second half of pregnancy
Respiratory and pulmonary	Upper airway edema, hyperemia, and friability	Estrogen and volume effects; can result in difficult airway
	Diaphragm elevation	Higher thoracostomy tube insertion site during pregnancy
	Hemoglobin F has greater affinity for oxygen than maternal hemoglobin	Fetal oxygen maintained at expense of maternal oxygenation; maintain maternal oxygen saturation <95%
	Respiratory rate	No change
	Tidal volume, minute ventilation	Increase
Renal and urinary	Progesterone dilates renal collecting system; ureteral peristalsis decreases	Renal US may show mild hydronephrosis; increased risk for ascending infection
GI	Alkaline phosphatase rises from placental production; bile is more lithogenic	Increased risk of cholecystitis/cholelithiasis
	Decreased lower esophageal tone; decreased gastric emptying	Increased likelihood of aspiration of gastric contents
Uteroplacental unit	25% of blood flow directed to uteroplacental unit; no autoregulation of blood flow; enlarging uterus can compress vena cava and vessels below the diaphragm; supine hypotension syndrome can occur after 30 min of supine position	Place patient in left lateral tilt position during third trimester; replace volume adequately to account for increased blood and plasma volume in pregnancy; avoid femoral and lower extremity site for blood and volume delivery in second half of pregnancy

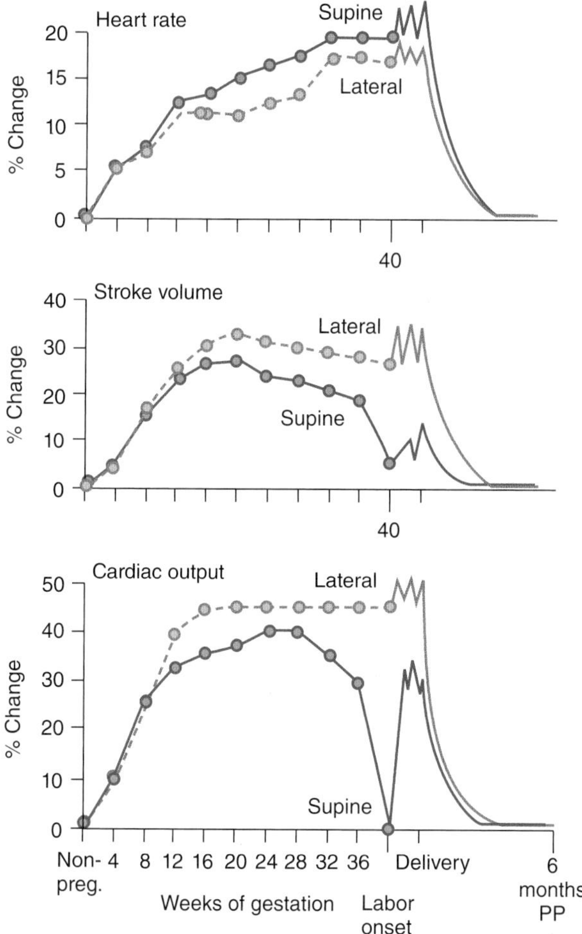

FIGURE 25-1. Changes in maternal heart rate, stroke volume, and cardiac output during pregnancy (preg.), with the gravida in the supine and lateral positions. PP = postpartum. [Reproduced with permission from Barclay ML: Critical physiologic alterations in pregnancy, in Pearlman MD, Tintinalli JE (eds): *Emergency Care of the Woman*. New York, The McGraw-Hill Companies, Inc., 1998, Chapter 2, Figure 2-3, p. 14. Copyright © 1998 by The McGraw-Hill Companies, Inc. All rights reserved.]

The Cardiff wedge provides a tilt of 27 degrees from the horizontal. Foam or hard wedges are better for maintaining the left lateral tilt position than are pillows or manual tilting.[6] Because compression of the abdominal vasculature can compromise intravascular delivery of medications through sites below the diaphragm, avoid femoral or saphenous venous sites for IV access during the resuscitation of a pregnant woman at >20 weeks of gestation. The negative effects of great vessel compression on uteroplacental blood flow increase in the presence of maternal hypotension and uterine contractions.

RESPIRATORY AND PULMONARY CHANGES

Respiratory changes occur early to help optimize fetal oxygenation. Progesterone drives an increase in resting minute ventilation and tidal volume. The respiratory rate, however, remains relatively unchanged, so **do not dismiss tachypnea as a normal part of pregnancy**. As pregnancy progresses, the diaphragm elevates approximately 4 cm with an increase of the transverse diameter of the thoracic cage by 2 cm.[7] Changes in pulmonary physiology and increased metabolic oxygen consumption can result in the rapid development of hypoxia during respiratory illnesses or as a result of respiratory arrest.

Because the fetal oxyhemoglobin dissociation curve is shifted to the left relative to the maternal oxyhemoglobin dissociation curve, the bond of fetal hemoglobin to oxygen is stronger than maternal hemoglobin, which results in preservation and optimization of fetal oxygen delivery at any given Po_2. Strive to maintain maternal pulse oximetry readings >95% to maintain a Pao_2 of >70 mm Hg to optimize maternal oxygenation and oxygen delivery to the placenta.[7]

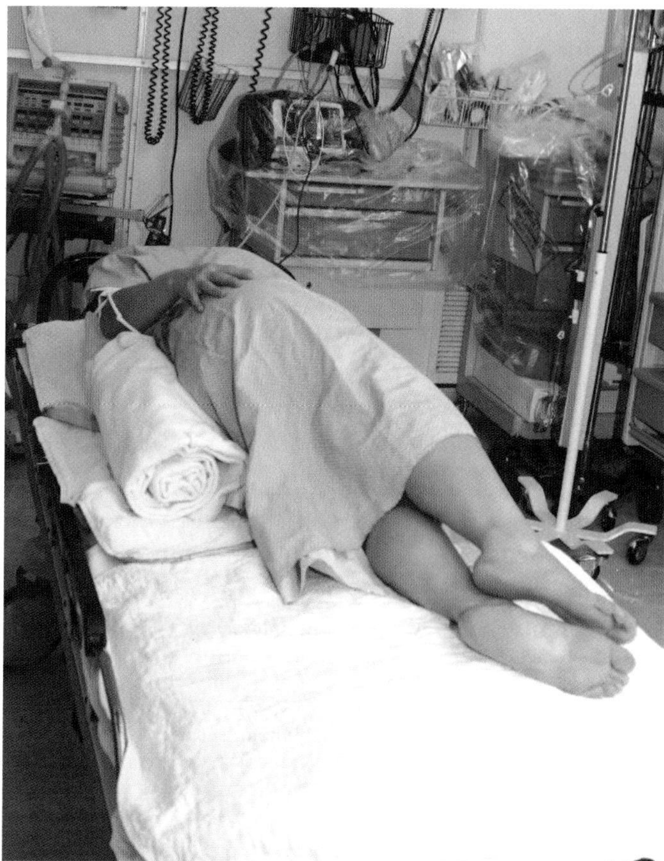

FIGURE 25-2. Left lateral tilt position.

The fetus exists in a physiologically acidemic state relative to the mother, which allows preferential oxygen transfer at the fetal tissue level.[8] Acidemia favors a rightward shift of the oxyhemoglobin dissociation curve, resulting in a greater amount of oxygen supplied to fetal tissues. Fetal cardiac output protects against brief periods of hypoxia, with increases in umbilical blood flow, placental gas exchange, and preferential redistribution to vital tissues.

RESUSCITATION IN PREGNANCY

The most common causes of pregnancy-related deaths in the United States are cardiovascular disease, cardiomyopathy, hemorrhage, infection/sepsis, hypertensive disorders of pregnancy, and thrombotic pulmonary embolism.[2,9,10] Major trauma is the greatest risk for nonobstetric cause of death. Motor vehicle collisions account for almost half of trauma, followed by falls and assaults.[11]

The best maternal care will provide the best fetal care, so follow general principles of resuscitation when treating pregnant women. **To accommodate the increase in blood and plasma volume that develops during pregnancy, make sure that the volume of resuscitative fluids increases by 50% above that required by the nonpregnant patient.** Place two large-bore IVs, and provide rapid infusions of isotonic saline. Volume must be adequately replaced before considering vasopressors, especially in pregnancy, because the uterine arteries are maximally dilated and blood flow is pressure dependent.

Select a vasopressor by the desired effects in the mother and the least harmful effects on the fetus (see Table 25-4). Because of variable effects of vasopressors on fetomaternal circulation, obtain critical care and obstetrical consultation if possible, before selecting vasopressors.

Studies of vasopressors in pregnancy focus on the treatment of hypotension with pseudoephedrine or ephedrine during spinal anesthesia for cesarean section or involve animal models, and data are difficult to extrapolate to other human hypotensive situations. **Phenylephrine** (pregnancy risk factor C) is an α_1 selective agent without any β activity, so it raises blood pressure but decreases heart rate. It crosses the placenta and is excreted in breast milk but has a favorable fetal acid-base profile. **Ephedrine** (pregnancy risk factor C) is a mixed α and β stimulator. It crosses the placenta and can induce fetal acidosis.[12,13] The vasopressors norepinephrine, dopamine, and vasopressin are all pregnancy risk factor C with limited data available on use in pregnancy.

SEPSIS

Sepsis is a systemic inflammatory response to infection, leading to acute organ dysfunction. Currently there are no sepsis guidelines specifically for pregnant women, because this population has been excluded from early landmark sepsis studies. Pregnant women, when compared with nongravid women, are more likely to develop complications from serious infections. Maintain a high index of suspicion for sepsis in pregnant women, because signs and symptoms of sepsis may not be as apparent when compared to the nonpregnant population.[14] The clinical features of sepsis in pregnancy include fever or rigors, diarrhea or vomiting, rash, abdominal or pelvic pain, vaginal discharge, productive cough, or urinary symptoms.[15]

Septic shock in pregnancy is rare, occurring in a small number (0.002% to 0.01%) of deliveries and in only 0.3% to 0.6% of pregnant women (**Table 25-2**). However, sepsis as a cause of mortality can vary between 2.7% in developed countries to 11.6% in developing countries.[16] Common causes of sepsis are pyelonephritis, pneumonia, chorioamnionitis, and septic abortion.[17] Malaria, human immunodeficiency virus, and community-acquired pneumonia are causes of sepsis in developing countries.[18]

Pyelonephritis is the most common cause of septic shock in pregnancy.[17] Progesterone produces dilatation of the ureters, and mechanical compression of the urinary system by the enlarging uterus results in relative obstruction of the urinary tract. The most common causative agent is *Escherichia coli*, with *Klebsiella*, *Proteus*, and *Enterobacter* responsible for most other cases. Consider renal US to assess for renal/ureteral stones and to assess for renal complications.[19] Hospitalize pregnant women with pyelonephritis, because bacteremia is likely and the physiologic changes of pregnancy can rapidly cause hypoxia.[20,21] Begin empiric antibiotics. Treatment needs to consider local resistance patterns. In general, for mild to moderate disease, standard regimens are amoxicillin/clavulanate, ampicillin plus gentamicin, ceftriaxone, or cefepime. For severe disease with immunocompromise, consider ticarcillin/clavulanate or piperacillin/tazobactam.

Pneumonia in pregnancy can be particularly severe because a rapid decline in oxygen saturation can complicate the course whether or not sepsis is present.[20,21] Follow standard community-acquired pneumonia protocols for pneumonia treatment[22] (see chapter 65, "Pneumonia and Pulmonary Infiltrates" for further discussion). All antibiotics cross the placenta. Select pregnancy risk category B agents for treatment.

TABLE 25-2 Some Causes of Maternal Sepsis
Pyelonephritis
Chorioamnionitis
Endometritis
Septic abortion
Pelvic abscess
Pneumonia
Influenza
Herpes
Varicella
Wound infection/abscess
Necrotizing cellulitis/fasciitis
Appendicitis
Cholecystitis
Pancreatitis
Malaria or HIV in developing countries

AIRWAY IN PREGNANCY

ANATOMIC CHANGES AFFECTING INTUBATION

Fluid retention causes edema within the structures of the upper airway,[23,24] and weight gain with adipose deposition can contribute to landmark distortion. Anticipate difficulty with mask ventilation, laryngoscopy, glottic visualization, and endotracheal intubation. Desaturation occurs quickly as a result of maternal increased oxygen consumption and decreased functional residual capacity.

During pregnancy, the incidence of **Mallampati Class III** airways increases (only the soft palate and base of the uvula are seen when the mouth is open and the tongue is protruding), making intubation more difficult (see Figure 29-8 in chapter titled "Intubation and Mechanical Ventilation"). Increased Mallampati scores correlate with gains in body weight,[25] and because obesity in pregnancy is more common than in the nonpregnant state, this contributes to the likelihood of a difficult airway.[26]

Mucosal engorgement and increased capillary friability make airway bleeding and swelling likely. Due to the engorgement and friability of the nasal mucosa, avoid blind nasotracheal intubation if possible. Pregnant women are likely to have full and intact dentition, and there may be little interdental distance in which to maneuver a laryngoscope. In addition, there are often redundant pharyngeal and palatal folds in the airways of obese gravid women. The rates of difficult intubation are reported to range from 1% to 6% and the incidence of failed intubation from 0.1% to 0.6%.[26,27] Decreased lower esophageal tone, increased intra-abdominal pressure, decreased gastric emptying, and a full stomach increase the likelihood of gastric aspiration.

INTUBATION

The most experienced physician should undertake the intubation with adjunctive airway equipment, smaller-sized endotracheal tubes, a gum elastic bougie, short laryngoscope handles, and stylets readily available. A video laryngoscope system facilitates first-pass success and direct visualization and decreases complications and prolonged hypoxia.[28-30]

Preoxygenate to 95% oxygen saturation to prevent hypoxia during intubation. Provide high-flow supplemental oxygenation by nasal cannula set to deliver 15 L/min during the procedure, even after paralysis, to continue oxygen delivery to the alveoli (passive apneic oxygenation).[31]

Place the patient in the supine position; manually displace the uterus to the left. Elevate the head and shoulders with a pillow or folded sheets to achieve the sniffing position. This maneuver is particularly important in obese patients.

For rapid-sequence induction, use standard doses of induction agents and paralytics (see chapter 29). The laryngeal mask airway was described as safe and effective in healthy selected patients undergoing elective cesarean section[32] and has been used as a rescue device after failed intubation.[33]

The determination of the initial ventilator settings should be the same as in the nonpregnant patient, with a P_{CO_2} goal of 28 to 35 mm Hg. Avoid respiratory alkalosis, as in animal models, this decreases uteroplacental flow.[34]

CARDIAC ARREST IN PREGNANCY

Pregnant women are typically younger than the traditional cardiac arrest patient but often have poor outcomes, with survival rates reported as low as 6.9%.[2,9,10] The causes of cardiac arrest in pregnancy are listed in **Table 25-3**.[35,36]

Cardiopulmonary arrest in pregnancy is broken down into two categories: before and after fetal viability. Typically, the onset of fetal viability varies between 22 and 26 weeks, with some institutional variation considering backup and available resources. By 20 weeks, the uterine fundus is palpable at the umbilicus; then from 20 to 32 weeks, the fundal height (in centimeters) approximates the gestational age (for singleton pregnancies). If the fundal height is at or below the umbilicus, resuscitative effort should focus on the mother with no modifications of CPR. If the uterus is palpable above the umbilicus, one person should provide

Perimortem Cesarean Section

Michael A. Bohrn
Jaylaine Ghoubrial

If maternal cardiac arrest occurs and the fetus is presumed to be of viable gestational age (**estimated beyond 24 weeks**), then perform a perimortem cesarean section. The prognosis of intact neonatal survival is best if delivery occurs <5 minutes after the maternal arrest.[1-3] If maternal arrest has exceeded5 minutes, still proceed with the perimortem cesarean section, because there is at least one case report of neonatal survival with good neurologic function after perimortem cesarean section at 30 minutes after maternal death.[4] Current Advanced Cardiovascular Life Support guidelines also recommend proceeding with cesarean delivery in this situation.[5]

Plan the procedure prior to the patient's arrival if advanced warning is available. Consider activation of a multidisciplinary code-type team, if this resource is available.[6] The chance of a neurologically intact neonate is increased with a more rapid delivery. Maternal pulses can return after delivery, once aortocaval compression is relieved.[7,8]

In an ideal setting, an emergency physician, nurses or technicians to assist with CPR, an obstetrician, a surgical assistant, and a neonatologist or pediatrician would be the team assembled to meet the patient immediately on arrival, but the reality is that the emergency physician and a nurse may be the only individuals present. **Shift focus from a typical cardiac arrest scenario to one that focuses both on maternal CPR and rapid delivery of the baby.** Once the baby is delivered, the resuscitation of the mother and baby can continue. The perimortem cesarean section should occur in the ED. Time to transport to the operating room only delays a potentially lifesaving procedure.

EQUIPMENT REQUIRED FOR EMERGENCY PERIMORTEM CESAREAN SECTION

- Scalpel
- Mayo scissors
- Bandage scissors (if available)
- Toothed forceps
- Needle holders
- 0 or 1 vicryl or chromic sutures
- 0 or 1 permanent suture
- Richardson retractors
- Bladder blade (may substitute another retractor if not available)
- IM oxytocin (Pitocin) administration: 10 units/mL oxytocin vials and a 10-mL syringe with IM needle
- *Or* IV oxytocin administration: 1 L of IV fluids with 20 units of oxytocin per liter
- Sponges and/or towel
- Wall or other suction (wall suction preferred as large amounts of amniotic fluid may need to be cleared)
- Clamps × 2
- Equipment for neonatal resuscitation

PROCEDURE FOR PERIMORTEM CESAREAN SECTION

MATERNAL CPR

Continue maternal CPR during the procedure. Remember personnel need to step away from the table if defibrillating the patient during the resuscitation. Keep the patient in left lateral tilt position if good compressions can be performed with the patient in that position; otherwise, keep the patient supine.

MATERNAL PREPARATION

Splash the abdomen with povidone-iodine or other antiseptic if it is readily available, but to avoid unnecessary delay, do not prep, drape, or give preoperative IV antibiotics. Place a Foley catheter only if it will not delay the delivery procedure. Draining the bladder will allow better visualization for the procedure and can decrease the risk of bladder injury.

STEPS FOR CESAREAN SECTION

1. Make a vertical incision with the scalpel from just below the umbilicus to the symphysis pubis (**Figure 25-1**). Some authors advocate a xiphoid to symphysis pubis incision (**Figure 25-2**), but umbilicus to symphysis pubis is typically adequate. The pigmented **linea nigra** is your guide for the midline. The incision should penetrate the skin, subcutaneous layer, and fascia (white layer).
2. Use your fingers to bluntly separate the rectus muscles laterally.
3. Sharply (using the scalpel) or bluntly (using your fingers) enter the peritoneum.
4. Once the uterus is exposed, have an assistant retract from above and place a bladder blade or other retractor inside the inferior aspect of the incision to aid with visualization.

   Make a vertical incision in the midline of the uterus (Figure 25-3). Continue incising with the scalpel to the level of the intrauterine cavity; the uterine muscle wall is thick. Enter the uterine cavity bluntly (using your fingers) or sharply and extend the incision with bandage scissors. **Keep the incision in the midline** of the uterus because the uterine vessels enter laterally. If an anterior placenta is encountered upon entry, go through the placenta and rapidly proceed with delivery of the baby. Expect some increased bleeding, but this is only temporary.
5. Rupture the amniotic sac with a sharp instrument if it has not occurred spontaneously. **Have wall suction ready to evacuate the fluid.**

FETAL DELIVERY

1. Place your hand into the uterine cavity between the symphysis pubis and the fetal vertex (or buttocks if breech) (**Figure 25-4**). Elevate the vertex (or buttocks) out of the pelvis, and then the physician or assistant should remove the bladder blade.

Once the head (or buttocks) is to the level of the uterine incision, have the assistant **apply steady pressure to the fundus** to assist in delivery of the baby's vertex (or buttocks) through the incision followed by shoulders and body.

In a **breech** presentation, deliver the buttocks first, followed by both legs, and then the body of the baby to the level of the shoulders. When one arm is delivered, rotate and deliver the contralateral arm, flex the head, and deliver the baby.

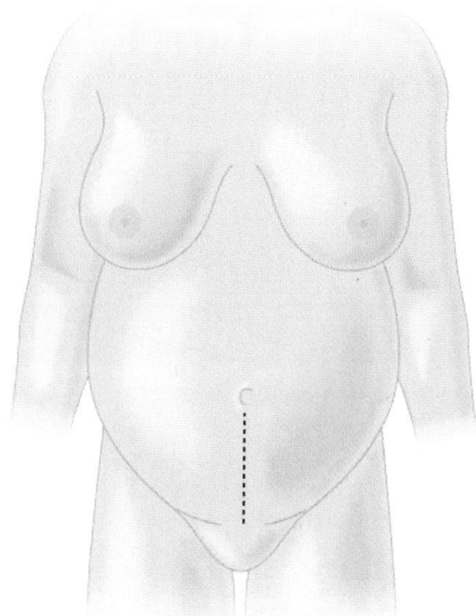

FIGURE 25-1. Midline vertical incision from umbilicus to symphysis pubis.

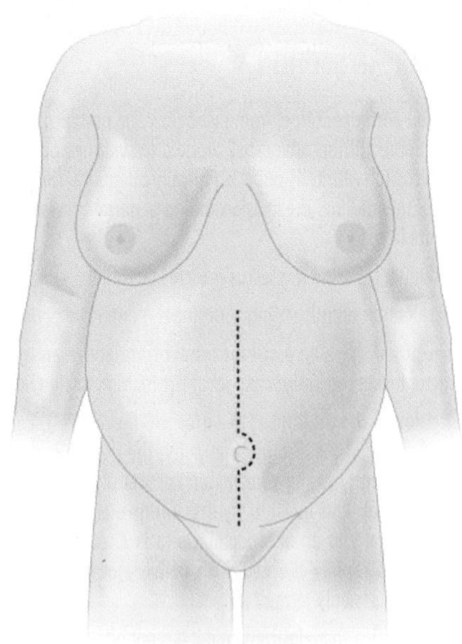

FIGURE 25-2. Midline vertical incision from xiphoid to symphysis pubis.

If a **footling breech** is encountered, gently grasp both feet and deliver to the level of the baby's shoulder and continue as a breech extraction as noted earlier.

2. Once the baby is delivered, **doubly clamp the cord, cut the cord between the clamps**, and take the baby to the providers who will be performing additional evaluation and resuscitation (if additional providers are available). There is some debate about delayed clamping of the umbilical cord. Delaying clamping for longer than 60 seconds (or beyond when cord pulsations cease) may provide the benefit of increased hemoglobin and iron stores in the newborn.[9] However, this is primarily based on studies of healthy babies, so **do not delay cord clamping if the baby requires immediate resuscitation.** If no additional providers are present, quickly determine the emergency physician's greatest benefit for resuscitation and proceed accordingly (i.e., lead/aid ongoing resuscitation of the mother or proceed to lead/aid resuscitation of the newborn baby).

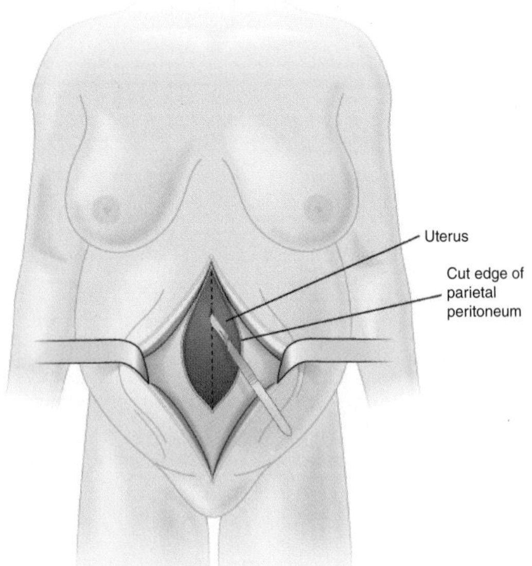

FIGURE 25-3. Uterine midline vertical incision.

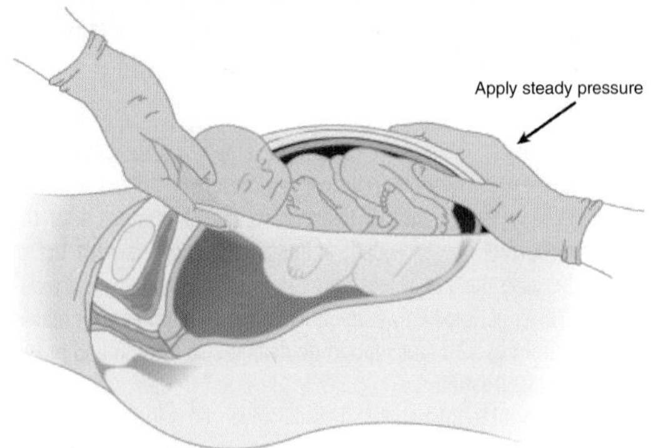

FIGURE 25-4. Delivering the fetus.

PLACENTAL DELIVERY AND UTERINE CARE

1. **Manually remove the placenta** and begin an infusion of 20 units of oxytocin (Pitocin) in 1 L NS wide open or 10 units of oxytocin (Pitocin) IM to help the uterus contract and decrease bleeding. **Uterine massage** will also aid in uterine contraction and decrease blood loss. The average estimated blood loss for a cesarean section is 1000 mL.

2A. **If an obstetrician or surgeon is available** to complete the closure, once the placenta is delivered, clean out the uterine cavity with sponges until it is completely cleared. Temporarily pack the uterus and abdomen with moistened laparotomy sponges until the obstetrician or surgeon arrives.

2B. **If a surgeon or obstetrician is not available,** then exteriorize the uterus and clean out the uterine cavity with sponges until it is completely cleared.

3. Close the uterus with one or two layers with a locked running stitch of number 0 or 1 vicryl or chromic suture on a large needle. Close the fascia with number 0 or 1 permanent suture in a running fashion.
4. Finally, close the skin with staples or suture.

Informed consent for perimortem cesarean section is not necessary because it is part of resuscitation. Perimortem cesarean section during cardiac arrest fulfills the criteria for absence of malfeasance and beneficence for the mother and the fetus, and as yet, there has not been a physician charged with criminal or civil malfeasance for the procedure.

REFERENCES

1. Katz VL, Dotters DJ, Droegemueller W: Perimortem cesarean delivery. *Obstet Gynecol* 68: 571, 1986. [PMID: 3528956]
2. Katz VL: Perimortem cesarean delivery: its role in maternal mortality. *Semin Perinatol* 36: 68, 2012. [PMID: 22280869]
3. Katz V, Balderston K, DeFreest M: Perimortem cesarean delivery: were our assumptions correct? *Am J Obstet Gynecol* 192: 1916, 2005. [PMID: 15970850]
4. Capobianco G, Balata A, Mannazzu MC, et al: Perimortem cesarean delivery 30 minutes after a laboring patient jumped from a fourth-floor window: baby survives and is normal at age 4 years. *Am J Obstet Gynecol* 198: e15, 2008. [PMID: 18166293]
5. Vanden Hoek TL, Morrison LJ, Shuster M, et al: Part 12: cardiac arrest in special situations: 2010 American Heart Association Guidelines for Cardiopulmonary Resuscitation and Emergency Cardiovascular Care. *Circulation* 122(18 Suppl 3): S829, 2010. [PMID: 20956228]
6. Mathur D, Leong SB: Perimortem caesarean section: rethinking the resuscitation codes? *J Obstet Anaesth Crit Care* 3: 35, 2013. [No PMID.]
7. Dijkman A, Huisman CM, Smit M, et al: Cardiac arrest in pregnancy: increasing use of perimortem caesarean section due to emergency skills training? *BJOG* 117: 282, 2010. [PMID: 20078586]
8. McDonnell NJ: Cardiopulmonary arrest in pregnancy: two case reports of successful outcomes in association with perimortem caesarean delivery. *Br J Anaesth* 103: 406, 2009. [PMID: 19561013]
9. McDonald SJ, Middleton P, Dowswell T, Morris PS: Effect of timing of umbilical cord clamping of term infants on maternal and neonatal outcomes. *Cochrane Database Syst Rev* 7: CD004074, 2013. [PMID: 23843134]

TABLE 25-3 Pregnancy-Related Causes of Maternal Cardiopulmonary Arrest

Obstetric complications
- Hemorrhage (17.2%)
  - Uterine atony
  - Placental abruption
  - Placenta previa, accreta, increta, or percreta
  - Disseminated intravascular coagulopathy
- Severe pregnancy-induced hypertension (15.7%)
- Amniotic fluid embolism
- Idiopathic peripartum cardiomyopathy (8.3%)
- Iatrogenic events
- Failed intubation
- Pulmonary aspiration
- Intravascular local anesthetic overdose (1.6%)
- Drug error, overdose, or allergy
- Hypermagnesemia

Pulmonary embolism (19.6%)
- Thrombus
- Air
- Fat

Stroke (5%)

Trauma
- Homicide
- Suicide
- Motor vehicle accident

Infection or sepsis (12.6%)

Other (19.2%) (cardiovascular, pulmonary, and neurologic comorbidities)

Reproduced with permission from Chang J, Elam-Evans LD, Berg CJ, et al: Pregnancy-related mortality surveillance—United States, 1991–1999. *MMWR Surveill Summ* 52: 1, 2003.

manual left lateral displacement of the uterus while another is performing CPR.[5,36]

Make preparations for completion of perimortem cesarean section if time from arrest is short and the fetus is of survivable gestational age. The following factors are associated with an increased chance of fetal survival after maternal cardiac arrest: gestational age >28 weeks or fetal weight >1 kg, short interval between maternal death and delivery, cause of maternal death not related to chronic hypoxia, healthy fetal status before maternal death, availability of neonatal intensive care facilities, and quality of maternal resuscitation.[37]

DEFIBRILLATION AND VASOACTIVE MEDICATIONS

Treat pregnant women in cardiac arrest according to current Advanced Cardiovascular Life Support guidelines (**Table 25-4**). Perform defibrillation at recommended adult doses. Despite an increase in plasma volume and glomerular filtration rate, there is no evidence that the standard doses of Advanced Cardiovascular Life Support medications should be altered. Place IV sites above the diaphragm secondary to aortocaval compression.

POST–CARDIAC ARREST HYPOTHERMIA

Case reports describe successful use of post–cardiac arrest hypothermia during pregnancy. The 2010 American Heart Association guidelines, Cardiac Arrest in Special Situations, recommend hypothermia in early pregnancy without emergency cesarean section (with fetal heart monitoring). Hypothermia can be used on a case-by-case basis based on the current recommendations for the nonpregnant patient.[38-40]

REFERENCES

The complete reference list is available online at www.TintinalliEM.com.

TABLE 25-4 Medications Used during Resuscitation—Considerations in Pregnancy

Drug	Indications	Pregnancy Risk Category
Epinephrine	Potentially beneficial in all forms of cardiac arrest	Category C. Teratogenic in animals in large doses; may induce uteroplacental vasoconstriction and fetal anoxia.
Lidocaine	Ventricular ectopy, tachycardia, and fibrillation	Category B. Use during pregnancy is not well studied; crosses the placenta, but in therapeutic doses has no teratogenic effect on the fetus; may cause fetal bradycardia.
Atropine	Symptomatic bradycardia	Category B. Crosses placenta but results in no fetal abnormalities; can cause fetal tachycardia.
Sodium bicarbonate	Cardiac arrest unresponsive to other measures; documented preexisting metabolic acidosis	Category C. No studies of risk. Use for hyperkalemia and selected toxic overdoses.
Dopamine	Hemodynamically significant hypotension in the absence of hypovolemia	Category C. No teratogenic effects in animals, but sufficient studies in humans are lacking; use only when clearly indicated.
Dobutamine	Short-term inotropic support of patients with depressed myocardial contractility	Category B. Not teratogenic in animal studies.
Norepinephrine	Vasopressor for septic shock after adequate volume replacement	Category C. No animal reproductive studies done. Crosses the placenta.
Amiodarone	Ventricular fibrillation, tachycardia, and supraventricular tachycardia	**Category D. Do not use in pregnancy;** serious fetal adverse effects of congenital goiter and hypothyroidism.
Adenosine	Supraventricular tachycardia	Class C. Multiple case reports of the safe use of adenosine to treat maternal and fetal supraventricular tachycardia.
Magnesium sulfate	Torsades de pointes	Class B. This drug is commonly used in pregnancy for toxemia and tocolysis with no reports of congenital defects; neonatal neurologic depression may occur with respiratory depression, muscle weakness, and loss of reflexes.
Ephedrine	Hypotension related to spinal anesthesia or unresponsive to fluids	Class C. Multiple reports of use during anesthesia-related hypotension in pregnancy. Maintains uterine blood flow. May cause dose-dependent increase in fetal acidosis, tachycardia, and abnormal variability in fetal heart rate (indicative of fetal stress), or an increase in metabolic activity.
Phenylephrine	Hypotension related to spinal anesthesia or unresponsive to fluids	Class C. Superior to ephedrine for management of hypotension after spinal anesthesia with a decrease in fetal acidosis.[12]
Vasopressin	Cardiac arrest	Class C. There are no controlled data in human pregnancy. Current data suggest no benefit over epinephrine in cardiac arrest.

Post-Cardiac Arrest Syndrome

Benjamin S. Abella
Bentley J. Bobrow

INTRODUCTION AND EPIDEMIOLOGY

Sudden cardiac arrest represents one of the most time-sensitive diseases in the practice of emergency medicine, requiring prompt recognition and rapid delivery of resuscitative care, including high-quality CPR, early defibrillation when appropriate, and appropriate airway management.[1] Even with these interventions, aggregate survival to hospital discharge is less than 20% in most communities and hospital systems.[2,3] Among survivors, neurologic injury is common (present in up to 50% of survivors) and widely varied, ranging from subtle memory deficits to persistent vegetative state.[4,5] This chapter focuses on the pathophysiology of ischemia-reperfusion injury and the provision of targeted temperature management, also called therapeutic hypothermia.[6]

PATHOPHYSIOLOGY OF ISCHEMIA-REPERFUSION INJURY

The brain is exquisitely sensitive to ischemia, such that disruption of blood flow for several minutes is sufficient to initiate a set of injury mechanisms that may lead to irreversible disabilities.[7,8] The complete loss of blood flow, followed by the abrupt return of spontaneous circulation (**ROSC**), rapidly leads to a complex pathophysiologic process known as ischemia-reperfusion injury, also known specifically in the sudden cardiac arrest setting as postresuscitation syndrome.[8,9]

When blood flow is abruptly stopped and then restored, a number of overlapping mechanisms lead to clinical injury (**Figure 26-1**).

CELLULAR RESPONSES TO ROSC

At the cellular level, mitochondrial integrity and function become damaged, with release of crucial enzymatic machinery such as cytochrome c and disruption of oxidative phosphorylation.[9,10] Mitochondrial injury is implicated in the increased concentration of oxygen free radicals and downstream activation of programmed cell death pathways.[10,11] At the humoral level, reperfusion triggers a broad array of immune activation, including increased blood levels of cytokines including interleukin-6 and tumor necrosis factor alpha.[12] In addition, aberrant neutrophil and platelet activation can occur. These immune phenomena have led Adrie et al[13] to describe the postresuscitation condition as a "sepsis-like syndrome," in which inflammation plays a crucial role in injury. Immune activation, in turn, can lead to additional production of oxygen free radicals such as superoxide and hydrogen peroxide. These molecules, produced in small quantities during normal cellular function, are usually converted to oxygen and water by the enzymes catalase and superoxide dismutase. However, enzyme systems become overwhelmed with the dramatic increase of free radical species generated during postresuscitation syndrome. Different tissues exhibit varying sensitivity to ischemia-reperfusion processes, with brain tissue and vascular endothelium appearing to be particularly vulnerable.[8,9]

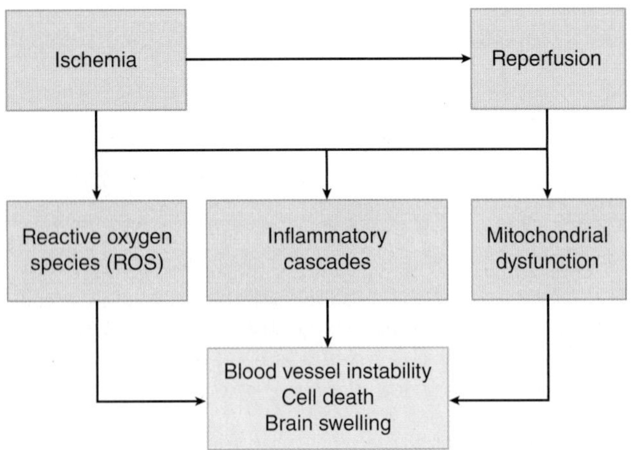

FIGURE 26-1. Schematic of postarrest pathophysiology, also called ischemia-reperfusion injury. The concepts shown here represent processes that occur at the subcellular, cellular, tissue, and organismal levels. The kinetics of these processes following cardiac arrest and the extent to which they affect clinical outcomes are still unclear.

ORGAN SYSTEM EFFECTS OF ROSC

The biochemical and cellular phenomena described earlier lead to diverse clinical manifestations of injury in the minutes to hours following resuscitation. Inflammatory changes and immune cellular activation can lead to vascular leak and a drop in peripheral vascular resistance, with concomitant loss of fluid from the intravascular compartment and hypotension.[14] Cellular injury in the brain, combined with endothelial damage, can trigger cerebral edema, a common and dangerous component of postresuscitation syndrome.[15] Cerebral edema and increased intracranial pressure can cause cerebral herniation and serve as the cause of death, often in the initial 72 hours following resuscitation. Myocardial stunning is clinically evident on echocardiography as global hypokinesis and markedly reduced ejection fraction.[16,17] Myocardial depression is usually transient and typically resolves over the first few days following resuscitation with appropriate hemodynamic support.[17,18] Postresuscitation infection may be related to bacterial translocation into the bloodstream from loss of intestinal tissue integrity.[19] Adrenal injury from ischemia may cause adrenal insufficiency as a further cause of clinical deterioration.[20]

CLINICAL FEATURES AFTER ROSC

Following initial resuscitation, the clinical condition of patients varies considerably. Some patients with prompt recovery after only brief periods of CPR can be awake and responsive; however, most patients are initially comatose or markedly obtunded following resuscitation. Neurologic assessment is highly limited in most cases, as in the course of clinical resuscitation care, patients are intubated and sedated and/or pharmacologically paralyzed. Patients may be hypotensive or hypertensive, depending on factors such as myocardial stunning, degree of vascular leak, and preexisting hypertensive disease. Patients are most frequently tachycardic following resuscitation; bradycardia may reflect underlying myocardial ischemia and damage to the conduction system.

Physical examination is limited in the immediate postresuscitation period as well. Most patients exhibit absent or abnormal papillary responses and absent gag reflex or doll's eyes responses. **Clinical neurologic reflexes are not predictive of cardiac arrest outcomes.**[21] **The bedside neurologic examination should not influence decisions for continued care in the hours following successful resuscitation.** Focus the physical examination after resuscitation on identifying clues to determine the possible cause of cardiac arrest, such as the presence or absence of asymmetric lower extremity edema that might suggest thromboembolic disease, absent or decreased lung sounds that might implicate pneumothorax, or jugular venous distension and muted heart sounds that might suggest cardiac tamponade. An ECG should be obtained and if ST segment elevation consistent with an acute myocardial infarction is present, coronary reperfusion with percutaneous coronary intervention is recommended.

DIAGNOSIS OF ANOXIC BRAIN INJURY AFTER ROSC

Neuroprognostication after sudden cardiac arrest is a crucial issue for healthcare providers in the critical care setting but persists as a challenging and inexact process. A variety of radiographic, biochemical, and neurophysiologic tools are available to assess brain injury following sudden cardiac arrest, but most are poorly validated and require additional research to determine clinical utility.

In the ED, perform head CT in survivors as soon as feasible. Head CT can identify subarachnoid hemorrhage[21,22] or epidural and subdural hematomas. The degree of cerebral edema can also be assessed by head CT.[22-24] Because cerebral edema often peaks several days after resuscitation, swelling that is radiographically apparent on initial CT is a worrisome sign. Brain MRI is generally neither practical nor useful during initial ED management.[25]

Marked elevations of nerve-specific enolase or S100 calcium-binding protein B are often associated with a poor neurologic prognosis,[26] and a nerve-specific enolase level >33 micrograms/L has been used as a cut-off with very high sensitivity for severe brain injury and poor prognosis. The biomarker glial fibrillary acidic protein is under current investigation.[27] At present, biomarker measurement is not part of standard emergency medicine practice.

Many protocols for postarrest care involve the early institution of continuous electroencephalogram monitoring to assess for electrical convulsive activity, which is present in up to 25% of patients after resuscitation.[28] The presence of seizures generally augurs a poor prognosis, but not all patients with electrical seizure activity sustain severe long-term injury. Bispectral index monitoring, a simple approach to electrical brain monitoring relative to electroencephalography, can be useful to predict neurologic outcome.[29,30] Measurement of somatosensory evoked potentials, a bedside test of neuronal connectivity and function, can be performed several days following cardiac arrest and may also be useful to predict outcome.[31]

TABLE 26-2 Suggested Inclusion and Exclusion Criteria for Postarrest Targeted Temperature Management[40A]

Inclusion criteria	Pulse ROSC and GCS motor score <6
	No other reason for coma
	No DNR or DNI status
	Adult (age >17 years)*
Exclusion criteria	Awake/alert after cardiac arrest
	Arrest of traumatic etiology
	Arrest associated with significant bleeding
	Cerebral Performance Score 4–5 before arrest†
	Pregnancy*
	DNR/DNI status
Not an exclusion criterion	Patient on warfarin or heparin
	Arrest rhythm was nonshockable
	Long QT syndrome

Note the inclusion of a category of clinical items that would NOT preclude the use of therapeutic hypothermia. These represent issues commonly asked about by practitioners but should not represent exclusion criteria.

*Criteria that are controversial and may vary from hospital to hospital.

†See Cerebral Performance Scores in **Table 26-1**.

Abbreviations: DNI = do not intubate; DNR = do not resuscitate; GCS = Glasgow Coma Scale; ROSC = return of spontaneous circulation.

TARGETED TEMPERATURE MANAGEMENT (OR THERAPEUTIC HYPOTHERMIA)

The key ED intervention for postresuscitation syndrome is the prompt delivery of systemic cooling therapy, also called therapeutic hypothermia or targeted temperature management. Cooling of resuscitated adult cardiac arrest patients to a core body temperature of 32 to 36°C (89.6 to 96.8°F) for 24 hours following arrest and ROSC can dramatically improve survival and neurologic outcomes.[32-34] The ideal temperature is not clear. Neurologic outcome after ROSC can be assessed by the Cerebral Performance Score (**Table 26-1**),[35] where a score of 4 or 5 predicts poor quality of life with a sensitivity of 55.6% (95% confidence interval 42-67%) and specificity of 96.8% (95% confidence interval 94-98%). A European study[33] demonstrated that therapeutic hypothermia instituted for 24 hours following cardiac arrest and ROSC resulted in a Cerebral Performance Score of 1 or 2 in 55% of hypothermia-treated patients, whereas only 39% of patients in the control group achieved a score of 1 or 2. Six-month mortality was 41% in the hypothermia group and 55% in controls. The trial only enrolled out-of-hospital cardiac arrest patients with ventricular fibrillation/ventricular tachycardia (VF/VT) as an initial rhythm; no definitive trial has been performed for patients with either pulseless electrical activity (PEA) or asystole as the initial arrest rhythm. However, a body of clinical evidence suggests that therapeutic hypothermia also improves outcomes for patients with PEA or asystole.[36-39]

INCLUSION AND EXCLUSION CRITERIA FOR THERAPEUTIC HYPOTHERMIA

Patients who are awake and appropriately alert following ROSC are excluded from consideration (**Table 26-2**). Patients with very poor neurologic status before arrest and resuscitation are often not considered for therapeutic hypothermia, as treatment can at best only restore patients to their prearrest clinical state. Other inclusion and exclusion criteria are less well defined. For example, many hospital protocols for postarrest care exclude pregnant patients; however, several case reports have demonstrated good outcomes for postarrest pregnant patients.[41,42] Because coagulopathy and bleeding can result from lowering of core body temperature, patients with clinically significant bleeding at the time of arrest or who have arrested from penetrating trauma are generally excluded from therapeutic hypothermia. Anticoagulation is not considered a contraindication. Therapeutic hypothermia may benefit patients resuscitated from hanging-related asphyxial arrest.[43]

TABLE 26-1 Cerebral Performance Score[40]

Score	Description
1	Awake and alert; can work
2	Awake and alert; cannot work but can perform independent daily activities
3	Conscious but dependent on others
4	Coma or vegetative state
5	Brain death

PRACTICAL CONSIDERATIONS

The technique requires the coordination of care between the ED, critical care units, and cardiology intensive care units. A standing hospital protocol is a crucial step for hospital systems. Sample protocols are available on the Internet.[44] Protocols should delineate processes for hypothermia induction, maintenance, and rewarming, as well as adjunctive pharmacologic interventions (sedation, paralysis) and monitoring. Incorporation of these protocols into electronic order sets for postarrest care encourages uniformity of treatment. An overview of the time course of treatment is shown in **Figure 26-2**.

Cooling and Supportive Care **Table 26-3** outlines elements of cooling and supportive care. To lower core body temperature to 32 to 36°C (89.6 to 96.8°F), apply commercially available clinical cooling systems (both surface-wrap or catheter-based cooling solutions exist), or apply chilled saline or ice packs to the axillae and groin. The aim is to reach goal temperature within several hours of resuscitation, so a combination of these approaches is often employed.

Maintain hypothermia for 12 to 24 hours following lowering of core temperature. It is difficult to maintain a steady temperature with chilled saline or ice packs alone.[45,52,53] Commercial cooling devices take input from temperature probes to modify cooling power and carefully hold core temperature steady. During hypothermia maintenance, check serum electrolytes frequently (every 4 h) as hypokalemia can result from

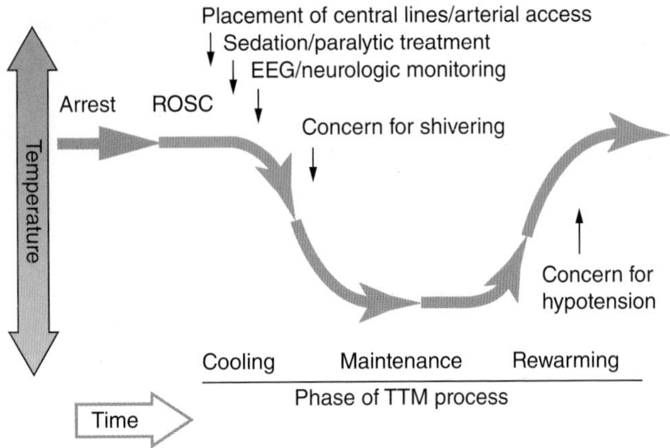

FIGURE 26-2. Timeline of postarrest therapeutic hypothermia induction, maintenance, and rewarming. Relevant clinical actions are shown in relation to these three phases of the treatment process. For further protocol details, consult the protocol repository at the University of Pennsylvania Internet resource site.[45] EEG = electroencephalographic; ROCS = return of spontaneous circulation; TTM = targeted temperature management.

cold-mediated diuresis.[53,54] Monitor hemodynamic parameters carefully to maintain a mean arterial pressure sufficient to enable cerebral perfusion (often a mean arterial pressure >60 mm Hg [>8kPa] is considered minimum).[55] After the maintenance phase, rewarm over 12 to 24 hours. More rapid rewarming can induce hypotension from vasodilation as well as electrolyte shifts.

Complications A number of possible adverse effects have been associated with temperature-targeted hypothermia (**Table 26-4**). Bradycardia is very common and often pronounced (heart rate <50 beats/min is common) with induction, but usually is of little clinical consequence and requires no treatment.[32] Tachydysrhythmias, atrial fibrillation, and nonsustained ventricular tachycardia are uncommon unless core body temperature is <32°C (89.6°F). QT_c prolongation has been observed, so continuous cardiac monitoring and interval electrocardiograms are necessary.[56]

Shivering can impede the lowering of body temperature. A variety of treatment approaches to shivering exist, the most definitive being neuromuscular blockade. Bleeding can be exacerbated by lowered core temperature but occurs in <5% of cases.[32,57] Hypokalemia and hypomagnesemia can result from intracellular shifts and diuresis mediated by lowered core temperature.

TABLE 26-3 Components of Cooling and Supportive Care

Lower core body temperature to 32–36°C (89.6–96.8°F) as soon as possible but within 4–6 h after ROSC[46]
Surface cooling:
Chilled saline or ice packs to the axillae, neck, and groin
Cooling blankets, vests, and leg wraps[47]
Cooling helmet[48,49]
Intravascular cooling[50]
IV 30 mL/kg normal saline at 4°C over 30 min[51]
Intubation and mechanical ventilation
Obtain electrocardiogram and provide continuous cardiac monitoring, pulse oximetry, and capnometry
Sedation and neuromuscular blockade
Central venous and arterial access
Continuous core temperature monitoring; use bladder catheter, central venous catheter, or esophageal probe
Maintain mean arterial pressure >60 mm Hg
Check electrolytes every 4 h
Maintain hypothermia for 12–24 h
Do not let core temperature drop to <32°C (89.6°F); avoid fever

TABLE 26-4 Potential Adverse Effects of Targeted Temperature Management (Therapeutic Hypothermia)

More Common	Less Common
Bradycardia	Nonsustained ventricular tachycardia
Prolongation of QT interval	Significant bleeding
Coagulopathy with PTT prolongation	Skin injury/ulceration from surface cooling
Hypokalemia during cooling	
Hyperkalemia during rewarming	
Shivering	

Abbreviation: PTT = partial thromboplastin time.

SPECIAL CONSIDERATIONS FOR TARGETED TEMPERATURE MANAGEMENT (THERAPEUTIC HYPOTHERMIA)

Children The indications for therapeutic hypothermia after cardiac arrest in children are not well established. Although hypothermia improves outcomes after neonatal hypoxic ischemic encephalopathy, no supporting randomized trial evidence exists for its use after pediatric sudden cardiac arrest.[58] Regardless, some hospitals use hypothermia protocols for resuscitated children.

Prehospital Application Therapeutic hypothermia could have maximal benefit when begun immediately after ROSC.[59,60] Although effective hospital-based interventions exist, they may be used infrequently due to multiple barriers such as lack of knowledge, experience, resources, and infrastructure.[61] These barriers and the safety and relative ease of inducing hypothermia in the prehospital setting have led some EMS systems to implement protocols directed at induction of cooling prior to hospital arrival.[62-64] Although this strategy has logical validity, the impact of prehospital hypothermia induction on outcomes is not well established.[65-67]

REFERENCES

The complete reference list is available online at www.TintinalliEM.com.

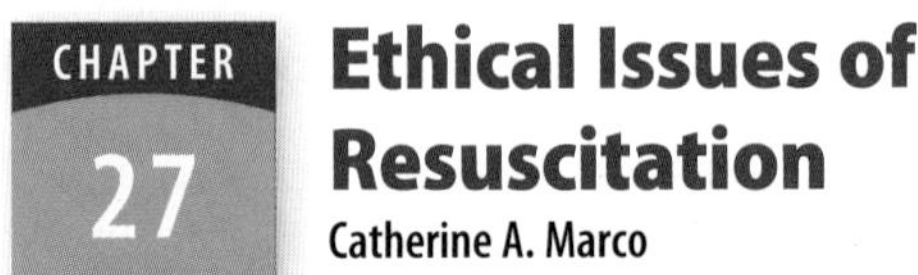

CHAPTER 27

Ethical Issues of Resuscitation

Catherine A. Marco

GENERAL PRINCIPLES OF MEDICAL ETHICS

The study of ethics is an effort to *understand and examine the moral life.*[1] The Hippocratic Oath is revered as one of the oldest codes of medical ethics. More recently, the American Medical Association Code of Ethics (earliest version in 1847)[2,3] and the American College of Emergency Physicians Code of Ethics (1997 and 2008)[4,5] have provided guidance to emergency physicians in the application of ethical principles to clinical practice. Most ethical codes share common tenets such as *beneficence* (doing good); *nonmaleficence* (*primum non nocere*, or "do no harm"); respect for patient *autonomy, confidentiality, and honesty; distributive justice*; and *respect for the law.* Ethical dilemmas arise when there is a potential conflict between two principles or values. Physicians resolve these dilemmas by gathering additional information; conducting meetings with other healthcare professionals, patients, and families; and applying an informed judgment in individual situations. In some circumstances, physicians may seek the involvement of the institutional ethics committee or the judicial system.

CARDIAC RESUSCITATION AND OUTCOMES

There are approximately 300,000 sudden deaths in the United States annually.[6] The outcome of resuscitative efforts for victims of cardiac arrest is uniformly poor but varies depending on a variety of factors, including

TABLE 27-1 Proposed Prehospital Termination of Resuscitation Criteria

Unwitnessed arrest
No shock delivered
No bystander CPR
No return of spontaneous circulation in response to advanced cardiac life support protocols
Initial rhythm of asystole or pulseless electrical activity

time elapsed since arrest (down time), presenting rhythm, bystander CPR, and response to prehospital advanced cardiac life support protocols.

Physicians should consider the patient's potential outcome including quality of life when initiating a resuscitation effort. Patients who receive early advanced cardiac life support have improved outcomes.[7,8] Patients presenting with ventricular fibrillation or ventricular tachycardia have higher survival rates than patients with asystole or pulseless electrical activity.[9,10] Many studies of cardiac arrest victims have estimated survival to hospital discharge to be between 0% and 13%.[6,8-19] Advanced resuscitative techniques, such as therapeutic hypothermia and advanced cardiac life support protocols, have improved the survival rate for patients with cardiac arrest.[9]

Based on such data, several authors have proposed criteria for withholding resuscitative efforts for patients with a low likelihood of successful resuscitation. Several validated decision rules incorporate related factors predictive of dismal outcome[20-29] (**Table 27-1**).

RISKS AND BENEFITS OF RESUSCITATIVE EFFORTS

When considering offering or withholding resuscitative efforts, the physician must take into account the risks and benefits of resuscitation. The primary goals of resuscitative efforts are to restore the patient's circulation and, ideally, normal function. Another less tangible benefit may be providing additional time for survivors to accept the distressing news of imminent death of their loved one.

Resuscitative measures are frequently undertaken in clinical situations where physiologic survival with meaningful neurologic function is very unlikely. Patients may be left with significant anoxic brain injury, persistent vegetative state, or dementia with poor quality of life.

Substantial resources are consumed in resuscitative efforts, and clinicians are taken away from other patients (a violation of distributive justice). Another benefit in limiting resuscitative efforts is the freeing of time and resources for family counseling and communication.

FUTILITY AND NONBENEFICIAL INTERVENTIONS

The term *futility* is subject to interpretation.[30] Healthcare professionals may determine futile interventions to be those that carry an absolute impossibility of successful outcome, a low likelihood of return to spontaneous circulation, a low likelihood of survival to discharge from the hospital, or a low likelihood of restoration of meaningful quality of life. *Futility* can be defined as "any effort to achieve a result that is possible, but that reasoning or experience suggests is highly improbable and that cannot be systematically produced."[31] There is no consensus among physicians about the meaning of the term. It is probably more accurate to use terminology such as *nonbeneficial, ineffectual*, or *low likelihood of success* when discussing resuscitation with patients or families.

Many ethicists agree that physicians are not required to provide treatments that they estimate will provide little or no benefit to the patient.[32,33] The American Medical Association Council on Ethical and Judicial Affairs stated that CPR may be withheld, even if requested by the patient, "when efforts to resuscitate a patient are judged by the treating physician to be futile."[34] Dilemmas regarding nonbeneficial interventions often arise due to inadequate or ineffective communication between the physician, patient, and family. This is of particular concern in emergency medicine, in which previous relationships with patients and family rarely exist and time is often inadequate to establish effective relationships. Thus, initial efforts should be directed to improve communication, education, and joint decision making.

TABLE 27-2 Ethical Issues at the End of Life: The American College of Emergency Physicians Policy

The American College of Emergency Physicians believes that:

- Emergency physicians play an important role in providing care at the end of life.
- Helping patients and their families achieve greater control over the dying process will improve end-of-life care.
- Advance care planning can help patients formulate and express individual wishes for end-of-life care and communicate those wishes to their healthcare providers by means of advance directives (including state-approved advance directives, do not attempt resuscitation [DNAR] orders, living wills, and durable powers of attorney for health care).

To enhance end-of-life care in the ED, the American College of Emergency Physicians believes that emergency physicians should:

- Respect the dying patient's needs for care, comfort, and compassion.
- Communicate promptly and appropriately with patients and their families about end-of-life care choices, avoiding medical jargon.
- Elicit the patient's goals for care before initiating treatment, recognizing that end-of-life care includes a broad range of therapeutic and palliative options.
- Respect the wishes of dying patients including those expressed in advance directives.
- Assist surrogates who make care choices for patients who lack decision-making capacity, based on the patient's own preferences, values, and goals.
- Encourage the presence of family and friends at the patient's bedside near the end of life, if desired by the patient.
- Protect the privacy of patients and families near the end of life.
- Promote liaisons with individuals and organizations in order to help patients and families honor end-of-life cultural and religious traditions.
- Develop skill at communicating sensitive information, including poor prognoses and the death of a loved one.
- Comply with institutional policies regarding recovery of organs for transplantation.
- Obtain informed consent from surrogates for postmortem procedures.

The American College of Emergency Physicians states that "physicians are under no ethical obligation to render treatments that they judge have no realistic likelihood of medical benefit to the patient" (**Table 27-2**). Emergency physicians' judgments should be unbiased, based on available scientific evidence, mindful of societal and professional standards, and sensitive to differences of opinion regarding the value of medical intervention in various situations.[35]

Ultimately, the decision regarding CPR and its likelihood of benefit to the patient and decisions to provide, limit, or withhold resuscitative efforts are to be made by the emergency physician in the context of well-accepted research results, patient and family wishes, and professional judgment. Individual bias regarding quality of life or other related issues should be avoided. There are many situations in which dying can be accepted as a natural process, even in an emergency setting.

ADVANCE DIRECTIVES

An **advance directive** is any proactive document stating the patient's wishes in various situations should the patient be unable to do so. The **living will** is a document suitable for terminally ill individuals, and the treating physician should accept the provisions. Many advance directives state that no life support should be applied in situations in which meaningful recovery is improbable. **Durable power of attorney** specifies a surrogate decision maker in the event that the patient no longer has the capacity to make medical decisions. The U.S. Federal Patient Self-Determination Act mandates that the opportunity to sign an advance directive is provided for all patients admitted to a hospital.

Despite widespread advocacy and legal mandates for the increased use of advance directives, only a minority of patients have completed an advance directive, and an even smaller minority arrive in the ED with the necessary documentation.[36] Advance directives and code status are especially important in emergency care medical decision making.[32,37,38]

FAMILY PRESENCE DURING RESUSCITATION

Family presence during resuscitation may serve to improve understanding and relieve family member guilt or disappointment and may be a helpful part of the grieving process.[39-45] Physicians should be sensitive to the possibility that this option may be difficult for certain family members or staff.[46] If family members are invited to be present, provide a liaison to assist with communication and education about procedures and other medical issues.[42]

PROCEDURES ON RECENTLY DECEASED PATIENTS

The practices of teaching and performing procedures on recently deceased patients are controversial. The most important benefit of these practices is the opportunity for hands-on practice for students, house staff, and even experienced physicians.[47] However, some consider performing procedures without informed consent to be disrespectful, deceptive, or unethical.[48] Obtaining consent from families or surrogates is recommended before such practice.[49,50]

RESUSCITATION RESEARCH

Research on resuscitation techniques and pharmaceuticals has been problematic due to the frequent inability to obtain informed consent and the constraints of the decision-making process. Ordinarily, the informed consent procedure for human subject research is designed to ensure protection and autonomy of the subject. However, this process is time-consuming and requires decisional capacity in the subject. Because of these difficulties, the U.S. Food and Drug Administration issued guidelines under which resuscitation research may be performed, with a **waiver of informed consent** under certain conditions.[51] When designing such research protocols, relevant factors include the patient's wishes (if known), expected safety of the study protocol, expected benefit of the therapeutic intervention, overall predicted benefit to society by improved knowledge regarding resuscitation, related animal data, feasibility of surrogate consent, local institutional review board opinion, and local general public opinion, if available. Waiver of consent is available through application with the Food and Drug Administration with local institutional review board approval.

COMMUNICATION AND COUNSELING FOR SURVIVORS

Counseling should be available for families and friends of those patients who have died in the ED. See chapter 300, "Death Notification and Advance Directives": Delivering Effective Death Notifications in the Emergency Department, for detailed discussion on communication strategies. **Table 27-3** provides a summary of practical advice for resuscitation scenarios.

TABLE 27-3 Practical Advice for Resuscitation Scenarios

Assess patient wishes (advance directive, prior communications).
Communicate with family and loved ones throughout resuscitative efforts.
Allow family to be present during resuscitative efforts, if appropriate.
Assess likely outcome, based on scientific evidence.
Weigh risks and benefits of resuscitation, in conjunction with family and primary care provider, if available.
Enroll in research trials, with surrogate consent, or using U.S. Food and Drug Administration waiver of consent rule, as appropriate.
Consider teaching procedures, with consent of patient or surrogate.
Use a multidisciplinary approach to family communications.
Provide spiritual, psychosocial, and educational support to family and loved ones throughout and after termination of resuscitative effort.

REFERENCES

The complete reference list is available online at www.TintinalliEM.com.

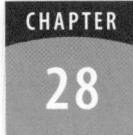

CHAPTER 28 Noninvasive Airway Management

Jestin N. Carlson
Henry E. Wang

INTRODUCTION

Airway management is a critical need in many acutely ill and injured patients. Optimal strategies seek to assist with airway patency, oxygen delivery, and carbon dioxide excretion. Commonly, many classify airway management techniques into two categories: noninvasive (passive oxygenation, bag-valve mask ventilation, supraglottic airways, and noninvasive positive-pressure ventilation) and invasive (endotracheal intubation, cricothyroidotomy, transcutaneous needle jet ventilation, and tracheostomy). This chapter discusses noninvasive airway management strategies. Detailed discussion of invasive airway management strategies is found in the chapters 29, Intubation and Mechanical Ventilation and chapter 111, Intubation and Ventilation in Infants and Children.

ASSESSMENT OF THE AIRWAY AND VENTILATORY EFFORT

The decision to initiate airway support must often be made rapidly based on the patient's clinical condition. Laboratory testing or other studies should not delay the decision to initiate airway management strategies.

First, assess every patient for airway obstruction, which can be functional (e.g., unconscious patient) or mechanical (e.g., foreign body). The ability to spontaneously swallow and speak provides a basic indication of airway patency, and the absence is a potential sign of obstruction. Other potential signs of airway obstruction include anxiety, wheezing or stridor, and coughing. Many conditions can cause airway obstruction (**Table 28-1**).

Some obstructions, such as foreign bodies or masses, are subglottic, or below the vocal cords.

Laryngospasm is obstructive closure of the glottis by constriction of laryngeal muscles. Laryngospasm may result from stimulation of the upper airway receptors on the tongue, palate, and oropharynx. Other causes include chemical irritation, secretions, blood, water, and vomitus in the upper airway and traction on the pelvic/abdominal viscera. Laryngospasm can persist after the causative stimulus has departed.

TABLE 28-1 Causes of Upper Airway Obstruction

Congenital/ Genetic	Infectious	Medical	Trauma/Tumor
Large tonsils	Tonsillitis	Cystic fibrosis	Laryngeal trauma
Macroglossia	Peritonsillar abscess	Angioedema	Hematoma/masses
Micrognathia	Pretracheal abscess	Laryngospasm	Smoke inhalation
Neck masses	Epiglottitis	Inflammatory	Thermal injuries
Large adenoids	Laryngitis/respiratory syncytial virus Ludwig angina Retropharyngeal abscess	Airway muscle relaxation	Foreign body/ hemorrhage

SIGNS AND SYMPTOMS OF RESPIRATORY FAILURE

Patients with hypoventilation (inadequate carbon dioxide excretion) and hypoxia (inadequate alveolar oxygen content) can present with a variety of symptoms including weakness, fatigue, chest pain, or shortness of breath. Inadequate oxygenation and ventilation can lead to altered mentation, including anxiety, confusion, obtundation, or coma. Patients with respiratory distress can present with audible wheezing, stridor, or a silent chest. A subjective gauge of respiratory distress is the patient's respiratory effort or "work of breathing."[1] Dyspnea, tachypnea, hyperpnea, or hypopnea, accessory muscle use, and cyanosis are signs of increased work of breathing.

TYPES OF RESPIRATORY FAILURE

There are two types of respiratory failure. **Type 1 respiratory failure** is characterized by hypoxia *without* hypercapnia. Type 1 respiratory failure may be the result of conditions that affect oxygenation but not necessarily ventilation (e.g., pneumonia, pulmonary embolism). Patients with type 1 respiratory failure require assistance with oxygenation. Treatment of type 1 failure focuses on optimizing oxygenation. **Type 2 respiratory failure** is characterized by hypoxia *with* hypercapnia. Type 2 respiratory failure is often the result of conditions that affect ventilation (e.g., chronic obstructive pulmonary disease). Treatment of type 2 failure requires not only optimizing oxygenation but also supporting ventilation.

PREPARATION FOR AIRWAY MANAGEMENT

AIRWAY EQUIPMENT

Having key equipment at the bedside is a fundamental requirement for optimal airway management. **Table 28-2** provides a model list of equipment.

PREDICTING THE DIFFICULT AIRWAY

Anticipating challenges with airway management is best done before any attempts to intervene. **Table 28-3** lists some factors that may complicate noninvasive airway management.

TABLE 28-2 Sample List of Equipment for Noninvasive Airway Management

Oxygen source and tubing
Tongue blade
Bag-valve mask device
Clear facemasks—various sizes and shapes
Oropharyngeal airways—small, medium, large
Nasopharyngeal airways—small, medium, large
Suction catheter
Suction source
Pulse oximetry
End tidal carbon dioxide detector
Laryngoscope blades and handles
Syringes
Magill forceps
Water-soluble lubricant or anesthetic jelly
CPAP/BiPAP mask and machine
Supraglottic airways: laryngeal mask airway, intubating laryngeal mask airway, Shiley™ esophageal tracheal airway (Covidien, Boulder, CO), King LT® (King Systems, Noblesville, IN)
Backup equipment in the case of unsuccessful NIPPV*†

*See chapter 29, "Intubation and Mechanical Ventilation."

†See chapter 30, "Surgical Airways."

Abbreviations: BiPAP = bilevel positive airway pressure; CPAP = continuous positive airway pressure; NIPPV = noninvasive positive-pressure ventilation.

TABLE 28-3 Predictors of Difficult Noninvasive Airway Management Techniques[2]

BVM ventilation			
	M	Mask seal	Beard, trauma, or other situations that may cause BVM to not seal
	O	Obesity or Obstruction	
	A	Age	Age >55 years
	N	No teeth	
	S	Stiff lungs or chest wall	
Supraglottic airway			
	R	Restricted mouth opening	
	O	Obesity or Obstruction	
	D	Disrupted or Distorted airway	
	S	Stiff lungs or cervical spine	

Abbreviation: BVM: bag-valve mask ventilation.

OXYGENATION

Provide supplemental oxygen to all critically ill patients requiring airway management. The method of oxygenation used depends on the patient's clinical condition and oxygen requirement (**Table 28-4**). Even if the patient is apneic, providing supplemental oxygenation with nasal cannulae can extend the time to hypoxia and hypoxemia, allowing providers additional time to prepare for or attempt airway maneuvers.[3]

PATIENT POSITIONING

The first step in airway management is to optimize patient positioning to facilitate airway patency and subsequent airway management efforts.

Upper airway obstruction occurs in the unconscious patient as the intrinsic muscles of the neck and upper airway relax, causing the epiglottis to obstruct the laryngeal inlet. Although the tongue displaces posteriorly during anesthesia in supine patients, it may not always occlude the pharynx.[4]

The first relief step in upper airway obstructions is extension of the neck with anterior displacement of the mandible. This maneuver moves the hyoid bone anteriorly and, in turn, lifts the epiglottis away from the laryngeal inlet. Forward flexion of the neck in addition to extension ("sniffing" position) may also help to relieve upper airway obstructions and requires less neck extension. This can be accomplished by placing a *folded* towel (not rolled) or foam rubber device underneath the patient's occiput. Neither maneuver should be attempted in patients when there is concern for cervical spine injury.

Oropharyngeal (Oral) Airway An oropharyngeal or oral airway (**Figure 28-1**) is a curved, rigid instrument used to prevent the base of the tongue from occluding the hypopharynx. Use only in a comatose or deeply obtunded patient without a gag reflex. Properly sized oral airways should reach from the corner of the mouth to the angle of the mandible. Place an oral airway with the concave portion of the airway cephalad and rotated 180 degrees after passing the tongue. Alternatively, the concaved portion can be oriented horizontally and rotated 90 degrees, following the curvature of the tongue, after insertion.

Nasopharyngeal (Nasal) Airway A nasopharyngeal or nasal airway (**Figure 28-2**) is made of pliable material and is placed into the nostril, displacing the soft palate and posterior tongue. Nasal airways are helpful

TABLE 28-4 Oxygen delivery methods

	O_2 Flow	FiO_2 Delivered
Nasal cannulae	2–5 L/min	20%–40%
Simple face mask	6–10 L/min	40%–60%
Non-rebreather mask	10–15 L/min	Near 100%

Abbreviation: FiO_2 = inhaled fraction of oxygen.

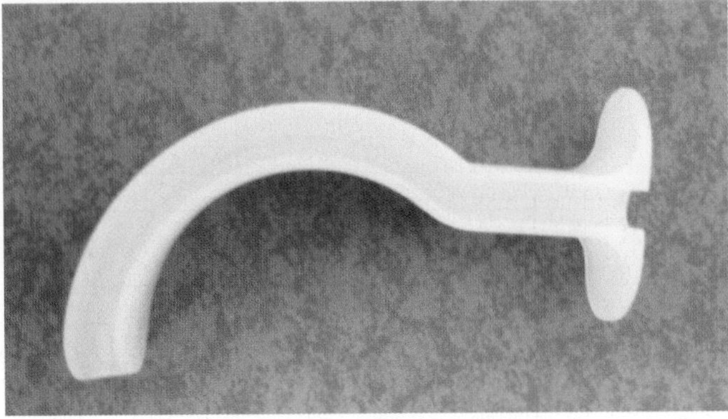

FIGURE 28-1. An oral airway.

in patients with an intact gag reflex absent any midface trauma. Properly sized nasal airways should reach from the corner of the mouth to the angle of the mandible. After lubrication, insert the nasopharyngeal airway in the most patent nostril and horizontal to the palate with the bevel oriented toward the nasal septum.

Bag-Valve Mask Bag-valve masks (BVMs) (**Figure 28-3**) contain a self-inflating insufflation bag coupled with a facemask and a valve to prevent re-inhalation of exhaled air. Effective BVM ventilation requires a good seal and a patent airway. Although typically used with supplemental oxygen, the BVM can aid even when used with room air. Most BVM systems deliver approximately 75% oxygen. A demand valve attached to the reservoir port of the ventilation bag may help to a deliver higher concentration of oxygen.[5] Adequate oxygenation and ventilation with a BVM require a good face–mask seal, which may be difficult in patients with facial trauma, facial hair, or anatomic anomalies or in those who are edentulous.

BVM ventilation is performed using one- or two-person techniques. Two-person techniques deliver greater tidal volumes than one-person techniques and are preferred if possible.[6]

With the one-person approach, the rescuer uses one hand to grasp and seal the mask and the other hand to squeeze the BVM reservoir bag. A common mask-sealing technique is to grasp the mask with the thumb and index finger in a "C" shape while placing the third, fourth and fifth digits in an "E" shape to lift the mandible. During mask ventilation, be careful to keep the fingers *on* the mandible, not compressing the soft tissue beneath (and hence compressing the airway) (**Figure 28-4A**).

In the two-operator approach, one rescuer seals the facemask using both hands, while the other squeezes the reservoir bag. The rescuer sealing the mask may use the same "E-C" approach but with both hands applied to the mask (**Figure 28-4B**). In an alternate modified two-handed technique, the practitioner places the thenar eminence and thumb of each hand on the mask while the remaining digits grasp the mandible (**Figure 28-4C**). Both two-handed techniques provide similar tidal volumes.[6]

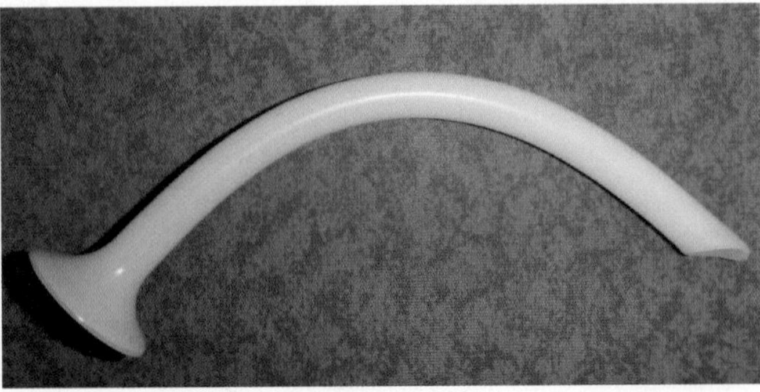

FIGURE 28-2. A nasal airway.

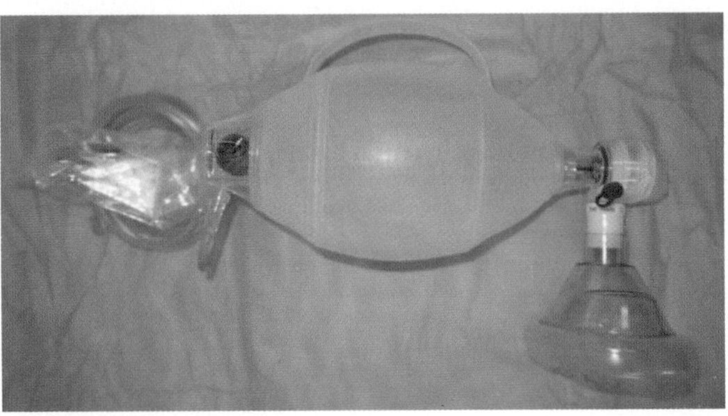

FIGURE 28-3. Bag-valve mask.

NONINVASIVE POSITIVE-PRESSURE VENTILATION

Noninvasive positive-pressure ventilation (NIPPV) provides positive-pressure airway support through a face or nasal mask without the use of an endotracheal tube or other airway device. NIPPV is an initial noninvasive airway management strategy. In adults, NIPPV includes continuous positive airway pressure (CPAP) and bilevel positive airway pressure (BiPAP).

NIPPV helps to augment spontaneous respirations. Ideal patients for NIPPV are cooperative, have protective airway reflexes, and have intact ventilatory efforts. NIPPV is not appropriate in patients who have absent or agonal respiratory effort, impaired or absent gag reflex, altered mental status, severe maxillofacial trauma, potential basilar skull fracture, life-threatening epistaxis, or bullous lung disease. Use NIPPV with caution in hypotensive patients because any volume depletion can be worsened from the positive pressure, triggering more hypotension (**Table 28-5**).

NIPPV reduces work of breathing through multiple mechanisms.[7,8] NIPPV improves pulmonary compliance and recruits and stabilizes collapsed alveoli, improving alveoli aeration and ventilation-perfusion mismatches.[1] NIPPV increases both intrathoracic and hydrostatic pressure, shifting pulmonary edema into the vasculature. Increased intrathoracic pressure can also decrease venous return, transmural pressure, and afterload, leading to improved cardiac function. NIPPV also increases tidal volume and minute ventilation, leading to increased $Pa{O_2}$ and reduction in $Pa{CO_2}$. NIPPV reduces work of breathing by 60% and dyspnea scores by 29% to 67%, while improving inspiratory muscle endurance by 14% to 95% over spontaneous respirations.[1] The ability of NIPPV to improve pulmonary function such as forced expiratory volume and forced vital capacity is unclear.[9-11]

CPAP delivers a constant positive pressure throughout the respiratory cycle. **BiPAP** provides different levels of positive airway pressure during inspiration (inspiratory positive airway pressure [IPAP]) and expiration (expiratory positive airway pressure [EPAP]). Although the terms EPAP and positive end-expiratory pressure are often used interchangeably, positive end-expiratory pressure is specific to the end of the respiratory cycle whereas EPAP refers to the pressure administered via the BiPAP machine during the entire expiratory phase. Both CPAP and BiPAP can be used in a variety of patient populations with limited data directly comparing the two methods.

Be aware that different NIPPV devices exist with differing operating mechanisms. Many standard ventilators can provide NIPPV, although in these devices, the inspiratory and expiratory pressures are additive. For example, if the IPAP is set at 5 cm H_2O and the IPAP is set at 15 cm H_2O, the total delivered IPAP may be 20 cm H_2O (5 + 15). There are standalone NIPPV units that can provide both CPAP and BiPAP, allowing for independent setting of inspiratory and expiratory pressures. For example, if the IPAP is set at 5 cm H_2O and the IPAP is set at 15 cm H_2O, the total delivered IPAP will be 15 cm H_2O. Specialized adapters that connect directly to oxygen tanks and wall-mounted oxygen units may provide CPAP for a brief period of time. These devices have a limited range of settings and should be used on a temporary basis.

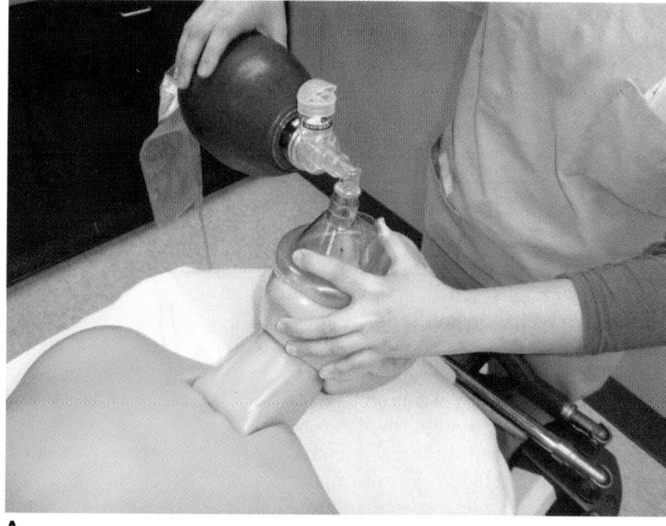

A

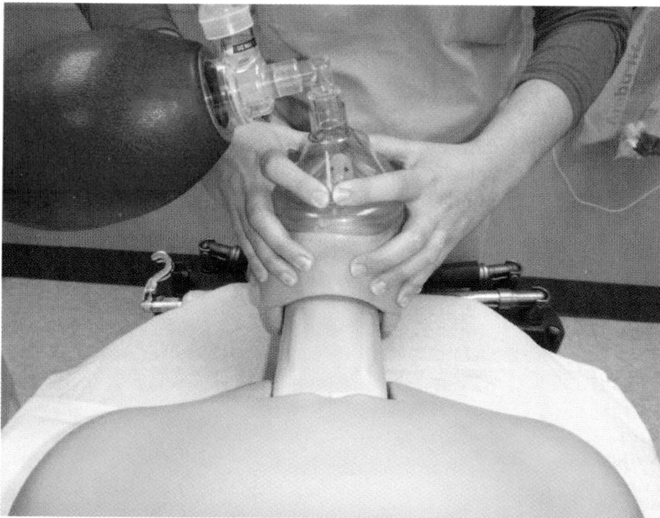

B

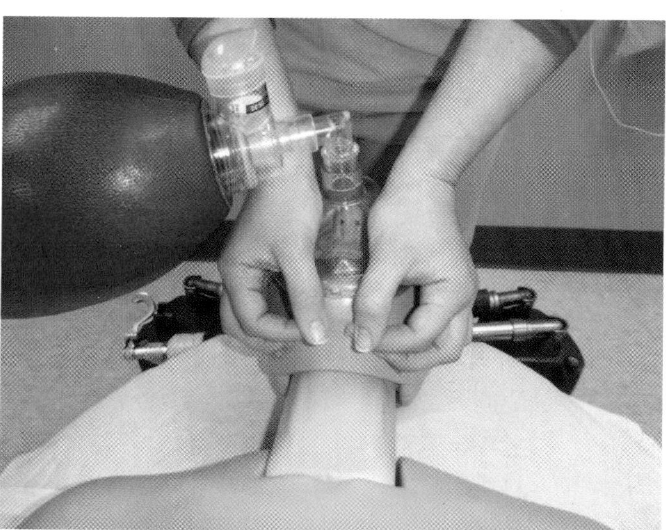

C

FIGURE 28-4. **A.** One-person bag-valve mask ventilation. **B.** Two-handed mask seal. **C.** Modified two-handed mask seal.

TABLE 28-5 Advantages and Adverse Effects of Noninvasive Positive Pressure Ventilation

Advantages	Disadvantages
Reduces work of breathing	Air trapping
Improves pulmonary compliance	Increased intrathoracic pressure leading to decreased venous return, afterload, and cardiac output, and hypotension
Recruits atelectatic alveoli	Pulmonary barotrauma leading to pneumothorax
Less sedation	Respiratory alkalosis
Shorter hospital stay	Abdominal compartment syndrome
Decreased rate of intubation without risks of endotracheal intubation	

INITIATING AND TITRATING NIPPV

Select the mask for NIPPV to create a tight seal while preserving patient comfort. Base the initial settings on the patient's condition and type of respiratory failure. Typical starting settings for CPAP are 5 to 15 cm H_2O. Typical starting setting for BiPAP include "spontaneous" mode with IPAP set to 8 to 10 cm H_2O and EPAP set to 3 to 5 cm H_2O. Be cautious when using NIPPV at pressures >15 cm H_2O because this may increase the intrathoracic pressure, leading to barotrauma along with decreased venous return, decreased preload and afterload, and eventually decreased cardiac output.

NIPPV requires frequent assessment for work of breathing, heart rate, respiratory rate, oxygen saturation, and blood pressure. Arterial blood gas analysis can aid in titrating NIPPV but is not mandatory. EPAP can help open and stabilize collapsed alveoli and reverse hypoxemia. In patients in whom ventilation is an issue, adjust the IPAP settings to help decrease the work of breathing and improve ventilation.

If the patient is not tolerating NIPPV, the first potential cause is an air leak. NIPPV is a flow-limited, pressure support system, and therefore, leaks prevent the machine from reaching the preprogrammed flow rate for a set pressure. As a result, the inspiratory time may be prolonged, making each breath cycle less comfortable for the patient. Potential solutions for air leaks include programming the machine to limit the inspiratory time or selecting alternative modes of ventilation including proportional assist ventilation.[1] Proportional assist ventilation is a form of synchronized ventilatory support where the NIPPV machine generates pressure in proportion to the patient's instantaneous effort such that as the patient generates a greater inspiratory effort, the machine generates greater IPAP. This allows the machine to adjust to air leaks that may impair ventilation and oxygenation with other modes (CPAP and BiPAP). Although proportional assist ventilation has not been shown to improve clinical outcomes, it is better tolerated by some patients.[12]

If the patient is not improving with NIPPV, consider endotracheal intubation and ventilation.

NIPPV Applications The most common use of NIPPV is for **cardiogenic pulmonary edema** where NIPPV may reduce rates of endotracheal intubation, hospital length of stay, and mortality.[13-20] In patients with **chronic obstructive pulmonary disease,** NIPPV is helpful in those with respiratory acidosis.[21] NIPPV may similarly benefit patients with moderate to severe **asthma** exacerbations, although data on effectiveness are limited.[22] Because of the bronchospastic nature of chronic obstructive pulmonary disease and asthma, be vigilant for air trapping and subsequent barotrauma when using NIPPV.

NIPPV may reduce the rate of intubation and in-hospital death in patients with **pneumonia.**[23-25] Exercise caution in this patient group because hypovolemia may coexist, with resultant NIPPV-induced hypotension.

There are reports of NIPPV use in **blunt chest wall trauma,** including **flail chest,** although it does not yet clearly decrease mortality or hospital length of stay.[26-28] NIPPV is also reported in burn patients. Do not use NIPPV in patients with suspected or confirmed high esophageal or tracheal injuries, maxillofacial or basilar skull fractures, or severe facial burns.[29,30]

Prehospital NIPPV Prehospital NIPPV in patients with cardiogenic pulmonary edema and chronic obstructive pulmonary disease decreases the rate of subsequent intubation and mortality.[31-34] When such patients arrive in the ED, assess the response to NIPPV and determine whether to discontinue NIPPV, adjust the NIPPV settings, or change to invasive airway strategies.

NIPPV Complications Complications of NIPPV include difficulty with mask seal, patient discomfort, aspiration (rare), air trapping, pulmonary barotrauma including pneumothorax, and increased intrathoracic pressure leading to decreased cardiac output and hypotension. Monitor patients carefully to determine NIPPV effectiveness and to identify the need to further secure the airway with intubation. Aspiration risk can be minimized by proper patient selection[35]; make sure patients have a gag reflex and do not have altered mental status. Gastric distension and increased intragastric pressure can lead to *abdominal compartment syndrome*, resulting in oliguria, hypoxia, hypercarbia, high peak inspiratory pressures, and even renal failure. A nasogastric tube can decompress the stomach and relieve this syndrome.[36] Although complications are uncommon, evaluate patients frequently to identify any of these complications early.

Occasionally, patients develop anxiety and agitation during NIPPV treatment due to the claustrophobic feeling of the mask or the discomfort of positive-pressure ventilation. Anxiety and agitation can increase the work of breathing and result in NIPPV asynchrony. Although often relieved with encouragement, verbal support, or hand restraints, anxiety and agitation may require the administration of sedatives or anxiolytics. There are no systematic studies of sedation during NIPPV, and sedation practices are typically based on physician preference.[35,37] Avoid agents or doses that cause excess sedation or respiratory depression. Dexmedetomidine, a centrally acting α_2 agent, can provide sedation without decreasing respiratory drive, but its expense and availability limit general use.[38] Benzodiazepines and opiates are commonly used but can be difficult to titrate and may cause respiratory depression.[35,37,38] Haloperidol in low doses may accomplish anxiolysis with less respiratory depression than opiates or benzodiazepines.[37]

SUPRAGLOTTIC AIRWAYS

Supraglottic airways (SGAs) are devices placed in the oropharynx, allowing for oxygenation and ventilation without the use of an endotracheal tube. SGAs are the initial bridge to endotracheal intubation or a rescue device after failed intubation efforts. Although SGAs provide adequate oxygenation and ventilation for short periods of time, they are not used for prolonged ventilation. SGA should not be the initial airway management strategy in any patient needing high inspiratory pressures (e.g., chronic obstructive pulmonary disease) given the seal issues and leak that occur.[39] Although these devices are often used during cardiac arrest care, an animal study suggests that the large cuffs of these devices can impair carotid blood flow during cardiac arrest.[40]

SGAs are most often placed in apneic, unconscious patients; their large cuffs can cause gagging and discomfort in awake patients. Another option is use after deploying a rapid sequence induction medication regimen.41 Providers must confirm proper position of any SGA with end-tidal carbon dioxide and then secure it with tape or commercial holders.[42,43] A number of SGAs are commercially available (**Figure 28-5A–C**).

SHILEY™ ESOPHAGEAL TRACHEAL AIRWAY

The Shiley™ esophageal tracheal airway (Covidien, Boulder, CO; Figure 28-5A) is a plastic double-lumen tube that is inserted blindly. It has a proximal low-pressure cuff that seals the pharyngeal area and a

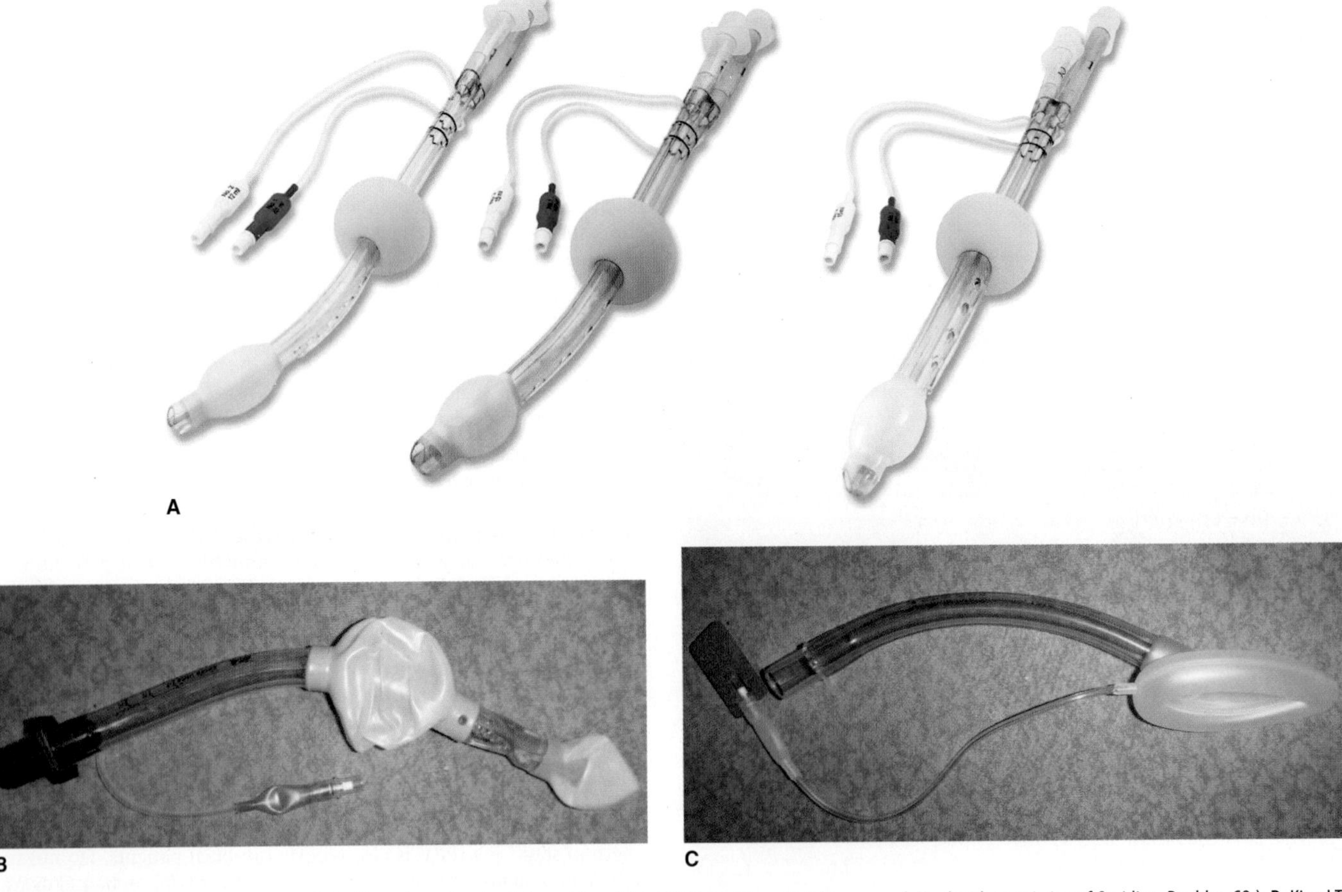

FIGURE 28-5. Esophageal airways. **A.** Shiley™ esophageal tracheal airway (Copyright ©2014 Covidien. All rights reserved. Used with permission of Covidien, Boulder, CO.). **B.** King LT. **C.** Laryngeal Mask Airway.

distal cuff that seals the esophagus. After placement, the proximal balloon is inflated with 80 cc of air while the distal balloon is inflated with 10 cc of air. During insertion, the device may rest in the esophagus or trachea. To determine the location of the device, first ventilate through the longer blue port; this allows oxygen to be delivered through fenestrations between the proximal and distal balloons. If chest rise is absent, the ETC is in the trachea; switch to ventilation to the shorter, clear/white port. The standard Shiley™ esophageal tracheal airway is sized for patients 5 feet, 6 inches or taller. The Shiley™ is used for patients 4 feet to 5 feet, 6 inches tall. Complication with the Shiley™ include hypoxia (from ventilating the incorrect port), esophageal perforation, and aspiration pneumonitis.[44]

KING LARYNGEAL TUBE (KING LT™)

The King LT™ (King Systems, Noblesville, IN) (Figure 28-5B) is similar to an ETC but has a *single* lumen. A proximal cuff seals the posterior oropharynx while a distal cuff occludes the esophagus. The King LT is placed blindly into the oropharynx until the lip aligns with the device lip line. The balloon is then inflated to a pressure of 60 cm H_2O. After placement, the provider may need to withdraw the King LT slightly to allow it to fully occlude the oropharynx. The King LT is placed in the esophagus >95% of the time, allowing ventilation of the trachea through the multiple fenestrations between the proximal pharyngeal and distal esophageal cuffs.[45] Complications with the King LT are similar to the Shiley™ but also include tongue engorgement whereby the proximal balloon can impair venous drainage of the tongue.[46] Removing the King LT will relieve this condition. The King LT is available in several sizes depending on the patient's height: 4 to 5 feet, size 3 (yellow); 5 to 6 feet, size 4 (red); and >6 feet, size 5 (purple).

LARYNGEAL MASK AIRWAY (LMA™)

The Laryngeal Mask Airway (LMA™; Teleflex, Research Triangle Park, NC; Figure 28-5C) is another SGA placed blindly through the mouth; it occludes the structures around the larynx. The LMA consists of a single cuff inflated with generally 20 to 30 mL of air. To insert the LMA, place a gloved index finger into the oropharynx to guide the device into the oropharynx and position the cuff around the larynx. The LMA is an alternative when the endotracheal tube fails, especially when the vocal cords cannot be visualized, and is successfully placed 88% to 100% of the time.[47,48] There are various models, including an intubating LMA, which allows an endotracheal tube to be passed through the lumen. This permits conversion from an SGA to an endotracheal tube without visualizing the glottis. Complications of the LMA include partial or complete airway obstruction and aspiration of gastric contents, although animal data suggest the LMA may prevent aspiration.[49] The LMA is available in several sizes based on the patient's estimated body weight: 50 to 70 kg, size 4; 70 to 100 kg, size 5; and >100 kg, size 6.

OTHER SUPRAGLOTTIC AIRWAYS

Other SGAs are available including the i-gel® (Intersurgical Inc., Liverpool, NY) and CobraPLA™ (Engineered Medical Systems, Indianapolis, IN). These have not been well studied for emergency care. The i-gel has a soft, gel-like cuff that seals the perilaryngeal structures without inflation. This limits tissue compression that may be caused by devices with large cuffs. Lubricate the gel-like cuff prior to insertion. The device is advanced into the poster pharynx until resistance is met and the lips align with the lip line on the i-gel. The i-gel is available in various sizes for patients from 2 to >90 kg.

The CobraPLA is a cuffed SGA that is inserted blindly similarly to the King LT. The potential advantage of the CobraPLA is that providers can pass an endotracheal tube through the lumen of the device, easing conversion to an endotracheal tube. Like all SGAs, neither of these is used for long-term ventilation or in conditions that may require elevated peak airway pressures, and neither has proven to prevent aspiration. The CobraPLA is available in various sizes for patients from 2.5 to >130 kg.

Converting a Supraglottic Airway to an Endotracheal Tube In general, SGAs may have a higher risk of aspiration than endotracheal tubes, and the large cuffs may cause hypopharyngeal mucosal damage. Thus, although SGAs may play an essential role during emergent airway management, endotracheal tubes are better suited for long-term ventilation. **SGAs do not need to be *immediately* changed to an endotracheal tube.** The urgency for conversion depends on the condition of the patient, the adequacy of oxygenation and ventilation through the SGA, and the reasons for SGA insertion. Strategies for converting an SGA to endotracheal tube include:

- **Remove the supraglottic device and perform direct laryngoscopy.** Determine why the SGA was initially inserted. If the SGA was placed because of intubation difficulty, removing the SGA and attempting direct laryngoscopy is risky, and alternative techniques should be strongly considered. When attempting direct visualization, use airway adjuncts (gum elastic bougie, video laryngoscopy, etc.) to help make laryngoscopy efforts successful.
- **Convert the SGA with a gum elastic bougie (King LT only).** To exchange the SGA over a gum elastic bougie, insert the gum elastic bougie blindly though the King LT into the trachea and then remove the King LT, leaving the gum elastic bougie in place. Then pass a standard endotracheal tube over the bougie. This is a "blind" exchange, meaning that the operator does not visualize the glottis during the conversion. This maneuver is not possible with the Shiley™ or standard LMA.
- **Convert the SGA with a fiberoptic bronchoscope (King LT or LMA).** To convert using a fiberoptic bronchoscope, one must use a special intubating catheter (Aintree; Cook Medical, Inc., Bloomington, IN), which is similar to a bougie but is hollow, allowing placement over a fiberoptic bronchoscope. First, place the catheter over the fiberoptic scope, and then direct the scope into the trachea. Next, remove the fiberoptic scope and SGA, leaving the catheter in the trachea. Finally, direct a standard endotracheal tube over the catheter into the trachea. This technique allows for visualization of the glottis but requires expertise in the use of a fiberoptic bronchoscope. This technique is not possible with the Shiley™.
- **Leave the SGA in place and perform a surgical airway (cricothyroidotomy or tracheostomy).** Providers may elect to convert directly to a surgical airway in cases where an SGA was placed due to difficulties with intubation and if the patient requires prolonged mechanical ventilation. This can be done either in the operating room or in the ED if needed depending on the patient's condition, available resources, and skills of the provider.

REFERENCES

The complete reference list is available online at www.TintinalliEM.com.

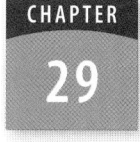

CHAPTER 29 Intubation and Mechanical Ventilation

Robert J. Vissers
Daniel F. Danzl

INTRODUCTION

The goals of emergency airway management are maintaining airway patency, assuring oxygenation and ventilation, and preventing aspiration. Tracheal intubation can achieve these goals. Sedation or paralysis after intubation can facilitate diagnostic testing. Extraglottic devices are discussed in detail in the chapter 28, "Noninvasive Airway Management."

Rapid-sequence intubation (RSI) is the sequential administration of an induction agent and neuromuscular blocking agent to facilitate endotracheal intubation. It is the method of choice for emergency airway management.[1] RSI allows the highest intubation success rate in properly selected emergency airway cases and is superior to sedation alone. Not all patients targeted for intubation are best managed with RSI; patients deeply comatose and those in cardiac or respiratory arrest will not likely have a response to laryngoscopy and may be intubated without pharmacologic assistance.

Whenever performing endotracheal intubation, anticipate airway difficulties and be facile with alternative airway techniques: bag-mask ventilation, rescue airway devices, and surgical access to the airway.[2] In addition, if bag-mask ventilation or rescue device deployment is not likely to succeed or if anatomic alterations exist that will not improve with RSI (edema, mass, bony disruption), do not extinguish intrinsic airway protection and respirations with paralysis.

Develop and discuss an intubation plan, and communicate responsibilities of the care team. Make sure medications are prepared. Have equipment for the difficult or failed airway available. Review proper patient positioning. Discuss the plan for postintubation hypoxia, hypotension, sedation, and ventilation. The use of a checklist may facilitate decision making and error prevention.[3]

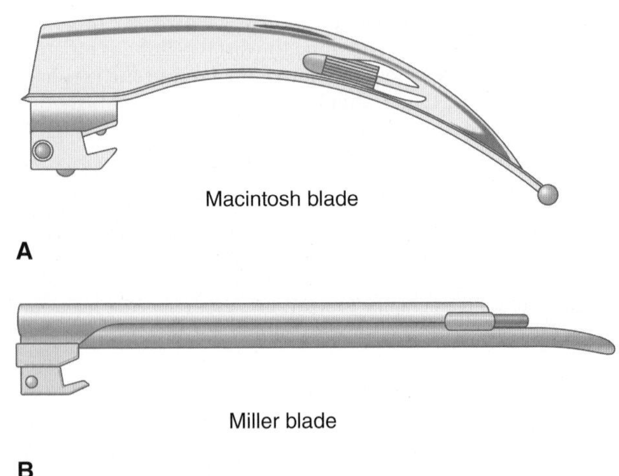

FIGURE 29-1. **A.** Curved or Macintosh blade. **B.** Straight or Miller blade.

OROTRACHEAL INTUBATION

PREPARATION

Clinical assessment, pulse oximetry, capnography, and the expected course of the patient all collectively guide decisions regarding the need for tracheal intubation. See the "Difficult Airway" section below for detailed discussion of airway assessment.

EQUIPMENT

Table 29-1 lists all equipment needed at the bedside before beginning intubation.

Rescue devices and a surgical airway option ideally are placed in a designated difficult airway cart in the ED and include pediatric sizes (see chapter 111, "Intubation and Ventilation in Infants and Children".)

When preparing for intubation, select the appropriate-size endotracheal tube (ETT) and an additional tube (0.5 to 1.0 mm smaller in diameter), and check the cuffs for air leaks with a 10-mL syringe. ETTs with high-volume, low-pressure cuffs are preferred. The approximate sizes for ETTs are 8.0- to 8.5-mm inner diameter for an average adult male and 7.5- to 8.0-mm inner diameter for an adult female. The second hole at the end of the tube above the bevel is called the **Murphy eye**. This hole permits some uninterrupted airflow if the tip is occluded. A stylet can aid emergent intubations, especially when using video laryngoscopy. Test the light on the laryngoscope after attaching the appropriate-size blade.

TABLE 29-1 Equipment Needed for Airway Management
Oxygen source and tubing
Ambu bag
Mask with valve, various sizes and shapes
Oropharyngeal airways—small, medium, large
Nasopharyngeal airways—small, medium, large
Suction catheter
Suction source
Pulse oximetry
Carbon dioxide detector
Endotracheal tubes—various sizes
Laryngoscope blades and handles
Syringes
Magill forceps
Stylets, assorted
Tongue blade
Intubating stylet (gum elastic bougie)
Water-soluble lubricant or anesthetic jelly
Alternative or rescue devices: video laryngoscopes, laryngeal mask airway, intubating laryngeal mask airway, Combitube® (Sheridan Catheter Corp., Argyle, NY), King LT® (King Systems, Noblesville, IN)
Surgical cricothyroidotomy kit
Medications for topical airway anesthesia, sedation, and rapid-sequence intubation

Laryngoscopes have straight or curved blades. The straight **Miller blade** physically lifts the epiglottis to visualize the larynx. The curved **Macintosh blade** tip is placed in the vallecula to indirectly lift the epiglottis off the larynx (**Figure 29-1**). The curved blade may cause less trauma and is less likely to stimulate an airway reflex when used properly, because it does not directly touch the larynx. It also allows more room for adequate visualization during tube placement and is helpful in the obese patient. The straight blade is mechanically easier to insert in many patients who do not have large central incisors. In adults, the curved Macintosh #3 is popular, and #4 is more useful in large patients. The straight Miller #2 and #3 are popular for the same purposes.

There are a variety of other straight and curved blades available; however, the Miller or Macintosh blades are most commonly used in direct laryngoscopy. Video laryngoscopes often use blades that have a much more acute angle to the blade because of the indirect visualization. **Video laryngoscopy** is an alternative to traditional direct laryngoscopy and preferred in some clinical scenarios including morbid obesity, difficult airway, or limited neck mobility.[4]

PROCEDURE

Preoxygenation Begin preoxygenation as soon as possible, even for patients with no apparent hypoxia/hypoxemia. Preoxygenation optimizes blood oxygen content and also displaces nitrogen in the alveoli, creating a potential reservoir of oxygen that may prevent hypoxia and hypoxemia during the first minutes of apnea. Even with adequate preoxygenation, hypoxia develops more quickly in children, pregnant women, and obese patients and in hyperdynamic states. **To preoxygenate, administer 100% oxygen for 3 minutes, using a non-rebreather mask supplied with 15 L/min of oxygen. Nasal cannulas alone do not provide optimal preoxygenation.** Non-rebreather masks typically deliver 60% to 70% oxygen. A bag-mask ventilator, appropriately applied, can deliver 90% to 97% oxygen. This requires a tight seal, with either active bagging or enough inspiratory pressure from the patient to open the one-way valve. There are a number of bag-mask devices that vary in their oxygen delivery; use a bag-valve mask device with one-way inspiratory and expiratory valves.

In patients who have arterial oxygen saturations that remain below 95% despite supplemental oxygen, a short period of noninvasive positive-pressure ventilation may improve the oxygen reservoir. This strategy is particularly effective in obese patients.[5] Elevating the head of the patient 20 to 30 degrees improves preoxygenation. Finally, providing high-flow nasal cannula oxygen (≥15 L/min) or the Optiflow™ oxygen delivery system (which allows even higher flow) throughout the apneic phase of RSI prolongs the period of safe apnea during paralysis and is wise in all patients undergoing emergent RSI.[5]

Patient Positioning Flex the lower neck and extend the atlanto-occipital joint (sniffing position) to align the oropharyngeal–laryngeal axis for a direct view of the larynx. Padding under the shoulders, not the neck, also improves visualization. For most airway maneuvers, the best position occurs when **the ear is horizontally aligned with the sternal notch**. Inadequate equipment preparation and poor patient positioning are common failure triggers; take the time to do these right before using the laryngoscope. Reposition the patient if initial attempts at viewing the larynx fail.

Sellick Maneuver The **Sellick or cricoid maneuver** (application of direct pressure on the cricoid ring in the unconscious or paralyzed patient) can impair bag-mask ventilation, worsen the laryngoscopic view, and hamper insertion of the tube.[6] Some practitioners still use it to prevent aspiration of gastric contents, although it may trigger vomiting. If the Sellick maneuver is used, apply *cricoid* (not thyroid) pressure and release if visualization does not improve. Aspiration occurs due to low esophageal sphincter tone, depressed protective laryngeal airway reflexes, or stimulation in the patient with upper airway fluids or stomach contents (**Table 29-2**).

Endotracheal Tube Insertion with Direct Laryngoscopy Instructions for ETT insertion are summarized in **Table 29-3**.

Suction at the bedside is critical. The Yankauer catheter is the most common device used, but any large-diameter suction system and tubing that allows for the removal of particulate matter or large clots is acceptable.

ETT insertion without clear cord visualization commonly leads to espohageal placement. Some techniques can help avoid esophageal placement: (1) retracting the right side of the mouth laterally by an assistant aids visualization; (2) using backward-upward-rightward pressure on the thyroid cartilage enhances visualization of the anterior glottis (**BURP maneuver**); and (3) bimanual laryngoscopy, where the intubator manipulates the larynx with the right hand until ideal visualization and then an assistant maintains this position, improves visualization of the vocal cords.[6] To avoid error, make sure you see the cuff of the ETT pass completely through the cords. Finally, abort the attempt if you cannot visualize the larynx.

The endotracheal introducer, also known as the "**gum elastic bougie**"[7] (**Figure 29-2**), may aid and is typically 70 cm in length and made of plastic. The angled tip facilitates insertion when the glottis cannot be fully visualized, although it is not helpful when no visualization exists. Once correctly inserted, you may feel the bougie tip moving over the tracheal rings. Thread the ETT over the introducer into the trachea and then remove the introducer. Never force the tube through the vocal cords, which can avulse the arytenoid cartilages or lacerate the vocal cords.

Most difficulties in passing the tube are a result of the failure to maintain the best possible laryngoscopic view, selecting too large a tube, applying cricoid pressure, or the formation of an undesirable curve on a semi-rigid stylet that is inserted into the ETT. A stylet angle of <35 degrees is more likely to pass through the glottis. Switching to a smaller tube, altering the curve of the stylet, or rotating the tube 90 degrees to align the bevel with the glottic opening are other techniques for eventual success. Do not apply cricoid pressure when inserting the ETT.

Advance the tube until the cuff disappears below the cords. Inflate the cuff with 5 to 7 cc of air. To avoid ischemia of the tracheal mucosa while limiting aspiration and maintaining a seal, target a cuff pressure of 25 to 40 cm H_2O. There is poor correlation between volume of air and tracheal cuff pressure, and if there is concern about cuff pressure, a manometer can be used to measure cuff pressure.

Tracheobronchial Suction After ETT insertion, use a well-lubricated, soft, curved-tip catheter to suction the tracheobronchial tree. Straight catheters usually will pass into the right mainstem bronchus. If a curved-tip

TABLE 29-3 Instructions for Endotracheal Tube Insertion

Step	Comments
1. Hold laryngoscope in left hand.	Holding the laryngoscope at the base, where the blade inserts to the handle, aids proper use and lift; do not hold further up the handle.
2. Use right hand to:	Remove dentures and any obscuring blood, secretions, or vomitus suctioned before insertion of the ETT.
Insert the ETT Operate suction catheter. Manipulate larynx externally to enhance the visualization.	Use a properly sized, semi-rigid, malleable, blunt-tipped, metal or plastic stylet to assist with tube placement. The tip of the stylet must not extend beyond the end of the ETT or exit the Murphy eye.
3. Insert blade into the right corner of the patient's mouth.	The flange of the curved Macintosh blade will push the tongue toward the left side of the oropharynx.
	If the blade is inserted directly down the middle, the tongue can force the line of sight posteriorly, impairing the view.
4. Visualize arytenoids.	—
5. Lift epiglottis.	Lift the epiglottis directly with the straight blade or indirectly with the curved blade.
6. Expose larynx.	Pull laryngoscope handle in the direction that it points (i.e., 90 degrees to the blade).
	Cocking the handle back, especially with the straight blade, risks fracturing central incisors and is ineffective at revealing the cords.
7. Advance blade incrementally.	Look for the arytenoid cartilages to avoid overly deep insertion of the blade, which is a common error. BURP maneuver may improve visualization.
8. Advance ETT.	Visualize tube *and* cuff passing through vocal cords.
	Correct tube placement is a minimum of 2 cm above the carina (approximately 23 cm in men and 21 cm in women).
	The base of the pilot tube (a tube with the adapter to inflate the cuff) is usually at the level of the teeth.
9. Check ETT placement.	Listen for bilateral breath sounds and the absence of epigastric sounds.
	Confirm placement with colorimetric carbon dioxide detector or capnography.
10. Inflate balloon.	Use 5–7 cc of air. Ask the technician to check cuff pressure to avoid tracheal injury from pressure (target 25–40 cm H_2O).
11. Secure ETT.	Do not impede cervical venous return with umbilical tape or a fixator; circumferential securing devices can cause skin breakdown if too tight or in place too long.
	Use a modified clove-hitch knot or a commercial fixator to avoid kinking the pilot tube.

Abbreviations: BURP = backward-upward-rightward pressure; ETT = endotracheal tube.

TABLE 29-2 Common Situations and Conditions Associated with Aspiration

Iatrogenic
Bag-valve mask ventilation
Nasogastric tube placement
Pharmacologic neuromuscular paralysis
Medical conditions
Trauma
Bowel obstruction
Obesity
Overdose
Pregnancy
Hiatus hernia
Seizures

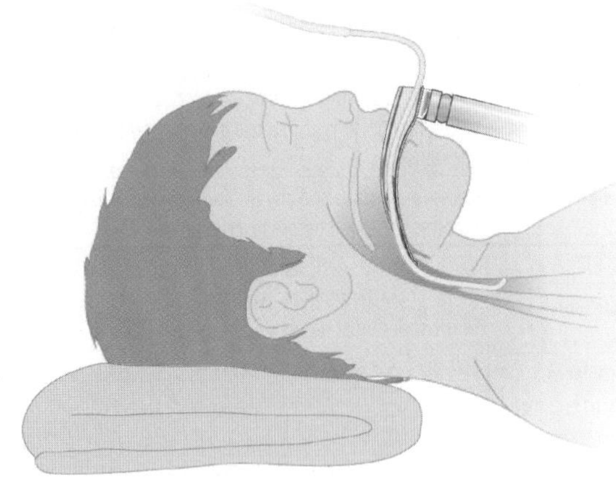

FIGURE 29-2. Depiction of a gum elastic bougie. Note the angled tip.

catheter is available, turn the head to the right and rotate the catheter to facilitate passage into the left bronchus. The suction catheter should be no larger than half the diameter of the ETT to prevent pulmonic collapse from insufficient ventilation during suctioning. Insert the catheter without suctioning and then slowly remove it while rotating and suctioning over 10 to 15 seconds.

Complications of suctioning include hypoxia/hypoxemia, cardiac dysrhythmias, hypotension, pulmonic collapse, and direct mucosal injury. Intracranial pressure may increase during suctioning due to coughing.

Confirm Endotracheal Tube Location **"When in doubt, take it out."** Mainstem bronchial or esophageal intubation results in hypoxia or hypoxemia and hypercarbia. There is no clinically reliable substitute for directly visualizing the tube passing through the vocal cords. Other clinical assessments, including chest and epigastric auscultation, tube condensation, or symmetric chest wall expansion, are not infallible. "Breath sounds" from the stomach can be transmitted through the chest after gastric insufflation. You should confirm intratracheal tube positioning with an objective measure.

The two basic categories of confirmatory adjuncts either assess expired (end-tidal) carbon dioxide ($ETco_2$) or assess misplacement by esophageal detection. Both have advantages provided that the operator knows the limits of each approach.

Capnometers and capnographs measure carbon dioxide in the expired air. The most commonly used capnometric devices in the ED are colorimetric, with a pH-sensitive purple filter paper. Hydrogen ions are formed by contact with carbon dioxide, resulting in color changes that vary with the concentration of carbon dioxide. For example, with the Nellcor Easy Cap II (Nellcor, Boulder, CO), the paper turns yellow after exposure to 2% to 5% $ETco_2$, which is equivalent to 15 to 38 mm Hg partial pressure of carbon dioxide (Pco_2). No color change occurs (the filter paper remains purple) if the $ETco_2$ is <0.5%, equivalent to <4 mm Hg Pco_2. Colorimetric capnometers are useful for assessing proper ETT placement but are not accurate enough for precise $ETco_2$ determinations and cannot exclude bronchial mainstem intubation.

Capnography displays real-time characteristic carbon dioxide waveforms. A persistent positive capnograph formation after clear and direct visualization of tube placement approaches certainty about tube placement. Rarely, a misplaced hypopharyngeal glottic tube tip may result in normal oximetry and capnography in a spontaneously breathing patient. This error is recognized by noting inadequate depth of tube insertion, inadequate ventilatory volumes, or incorrect tube placement on chest x-ray.

Table 29-4 notes conditions associated with false colorimetric or capnographic carbon dioxide readings.

Esophageal detection devices help determine initial tube location and do not depend on adequate cardiac output and pulmonary perfusion—an asset in the cardiac arrest patient. When the ETT is in the esophagus, the soft, noncartilaginous walls will collapse, and air cannot be easily aspirated with an esophageal detector. Esophageal detection devices use a syringe aspiration or a compressible bulb technique. The device is attached to the ETT adapter after intubation but before ventilation. The syringe is then rapidly retracted or the bulb is compressed. Taking advantage of the anatomic differences between the rigid cartilage of the trachea and the collapsible esophagus, syringe aspiration or bulb refilling is rapid when in the trachea. If the ETT tube is in the esophagus, the vacuum causes the esophagus to collapse around the tube, creating resistance to aspiration or preventing the bulb from refilling.

After intubation, obtain a chest x-ray to identify mainstem bronchus intubation and to locate the ETT tip. A chest x-ray does not reliably distinguish ETT placement in the trachea from the esophagus.

TABLE 29-4 Conditions Associated with False Colorimetric or False Capnographic Carbon Dioxide Readings

False-Negative Reading	Comments
Low pulmonary perfusion—cardiac arrest, inadequate chest compressions during CPR, massive pulmonary embolism	—
Massive obesity	—
Tube obstruction	Secretions, blood, foreign bodies
False-Positive Reading	**Comments**
Recent ingestion of carbonated beverage	Will not persist beyond 6 breaths
Heated humidifier, nebulizer, or endotracheal epinephrine	Transient

COMPLICATIONS OF ENDOTRACHEAL INTUBATION

Adverse events include unrecognized esophageal intubation, aspiration, oxygen desaturation, hypotension, dysrhythmia, and cardiac arrest. In the ED, first-attempt success is achieved 80% to 95% of the time.[1,8,9] Higher first-attempt success is associated with more experienced clinicians, trained emergency physicians, the use of RSI, the use of video laryngoscopy, and the absence of predictors of airway difficulty.[4,10] Multiple intubation attempts are associated with increased adverse events; this is why it is important to employ an intubation strategy most likely to lead to first-pass success.[9,11]

Immediate complications include unrecognized esophageal intubation or mainstem bronchus intubation. *Never assume correct positioning and patency after intubation if deterioration is seen.* **Tube displacement can occur during patient movement or if the tube is not properly secured.** Repeated suctioning helps prevent secretions from obstructing the tube or bronchus. Cuff displacement or overinflation obstructs or damages the airway. If tracheal ball-valve obstruction is suspected, deflate the cuff.

If the **ETT cuff leaks** after the intubation, check the inflation valve. A simple remedy for a leaking inflation valve is to attach a three-way stopcock to the valve, re-inflate the cuff, and turn off the stopcock. If the tube needs to be replaced, use a tube changer. Commercially available tube changers are semi-rigid catheters with 15-mm adaptors or connectors to permit ventilation during the tube exchange. Insert the changer into the ETT, withdraw the ETT, and then insert a new ETT over the catheter and reconfirm placement.

Although uncommon, soft tissue injury related to emergent endotracheal intubation does occur. Arytenoid cartilage avulsion or displacement, usually on the right, will prevent the patient from phonating properly after extubation. Other complications include intubation of the pyriform sinus, pharyngeal-esophageal perforation, and development of stenosis. Subglottic stenosis usually occurs in patients with poorly secured tubes who are combative or mechanically ventilated for extended intervals.

RAPID-SEQUENCE INTUBATION

RSI is the simultaneous administration of an induction and a neuromuscular blocking agent to facilitate tracheal intubation and is preferred for emergency intubation (**Table 29-5**).

TABLE 29-5 Rapid-Sequence Intubation Steps

1. Set up IV access, cardiac monitor, oximetry, and capnography/capnometry.
2. Plan procedure incorporating assessment of physiologic status and airway difficulty.
3. Prepare equipment, suction, and potential rescue devices.
4. Preoxygenate and denitrogenate.
5. Consider pretreatment agents based on underlying conditions.*
6. Induce with sedative agent.
7. Give neuromuscular blocking agent immediately after induction.
8. Bag-mask ventilate only if hypoxic; otherwise, provide high flow oxygen during apneic phase. Cricoid pressure during laryngoscopy only, if needed.
9. Intubate trachea after muscle relaxation has been achieved.
10. Confirm placement and secure tube.
11. Provide postintubation sedation and low tidal volume (6 cc/kg start) management.

*It is unclear if pretreatment improves outcome.[12]

Bag-mask ventilation may increase gastric distention and is best deferred in the well-oxygenated patient before laryngoscopy. Once the patient is adequately sedated and paralyzed, perform laryngoscopy and tracheal intubation. Contraindications to RSI are relative and primarily occur when the anticipated airway difficulties suggest that paralysis may lead to a "cannot intubate, cannot ventilate" predicament or when not needed or unlikely to aid (massive edema or fixed anatomic hindrances). Always be prepared for failure and have two alternatives ready, often including rescue airways.

PRETREATMENT AGENTS

Pretreatment agents attenuate adverse physiologic responses to laryngoscopy and intubation; however, data do not show a clear outcome benefit from pretreatment agents.[12,13] Adverse effects from laryngoscopy include a reflex sympathetic response that causes increases in heart rate and blood pressure; this may be harmful in patients with elevated intracranial pressure, myocardial ischemia, and aortic dissection. In children, the vagal response predominates and can result in bradycardia, even in the absence of succinylcholine. Patients without cerebral autoregulation can experience a centrally mediated increase in intracranial pressure. Laryngeal stimulation also can have respiratory effects, including laryngospasm, cough, and bronchospasm. Constraints on time, usually from worsening clinical status, often preclude pretreatment; if pretreatment agents are used, administer them 3 to 5 minutes before initiation of RSI (**Table 29-6**). Finally, the duration and nimbleness of laryngoscopy are the biggest factors in physiologic perturbations; quick and with minimal extraneous movement are best.

Fentanyl can attenuate the reflex sympathetic response to airway manipulation. It may aid in patients in whom a rise in blood pressure and heart rate could be detrimental, such as patients with elevated intracranial pressure and certain cardiovascular conditions (i.e., aortic dissection, ischemic heart disease, and aneurysms). Fentanyl is less likely to produce hypotension in the suggested dose (3 micrograms/kg IV) than other agents with similar effects and has a rapid onset of action. Adverse reactions, such as respiratory depression and chest rigidity, are rare when fentanyl is given in lower RSI doses (3 micrograms/kg IV) and over 30 to 60 seconds.

Pretreatment with atropine limits but does not universally prevent bradycardia in children. It is recommended for symptomatic bradycardia, and not as a routine agent.[13] **Pretreatment with a small dose of a nondepolarizing neuromuscular blocking agent, such as vecuronium or rocuronium in one tenth of full dose, is no longer recommended to alter side effects.**

TABLE 29-6 Pretreatment Agents Considered in Rapid-Sequence Intubation

Agent	Dose	Indications	Precautions
Lidocaine	1.5 milligrams/kg IV/topically	Elevated ICP	Lack of evidence-based studies on effectiveness in ICP[12]
		Bronchospasm	No evidence of improved outcome and may not be better than inhaled albuterol
		Asthma	
Fentanyl	3 micrograms/kg IV	Elevated ICP	Respiratory depression
		Cardiac ischemia	Hypotension
		Aortic dissection	Chest wall rigidity
Atropine	0.02 milligram/kg IV	Children <5 y with bradycardia	Minimal dose 0.10 milligram
		Children <10 y receiving succinylcholine and with bradycardia	Recommend giving in response to bradycardia, not as routine agent[13]
	0.01 milligram/kg IV	Bradycardia from repeat succinylcholine in adults	

Abbreviation: ICP = intracranial pressure.

INDUCTION AGENTS

There is no single agent of choice for achieving adequate sedation during RSI in the ED. All of the commonly used agents offer advantages and risks in specific clinical conditions (**Table 29-7**).

Etomidate Etomidate, a nonbarbiturate hypnotic, is a popular agent for ED RSI. It protects from myocardial and cerebral ischemia, causes minimal histamine release, has little hemodynamic depression in most patients, and has short duration of action. Myoclonus, nausea, and vomiting can occur in awake patients, but clinically important effects are rare. Etomidate is not an analgesic, and it does not blunt the sympathetic response to intubation. There is no evidence that a single dose of etomidate given in the ED for RSI worsens patient outcomes through cortisol inhibition, even in septic shock, although this can be measured and is key to recognize after use.[14]

Propofol Propofol is a highly lipophilic, rapid-acting sedative that is effective for emergent RSI. Propofol has a more rapid onset of action than etomidate and a shorter duration of action. It has anticonvulsant and antiemetic properties, and it may lower intracranial pressure without triggering histamine release. Propofol can cause hypotension through myocardial depression and vasodilation; for this reason, avoid it in trauma patients and any patient with hypovolemia or hypotension. Trismus and dystonic reactions are rare side effects of propofol.

Ketamine Ketamine, a phencyclidine derivative, is a dissociative induction agent that provides analgesia and amnesia. Ketamine preserves the respiratory drive, an ideal feature for sedation during awake intubation. It causes an increase in blood pressure and heart rate through catecholamine

TABLE 29-7 Preferred Rapid-Sequence Intubation Induction Agents

Agent	Dose	Onset	Duration	Benefits	Caveats
Etomidate	0.3–0.5 milligram/kg IV	<1 min	10–20 min	↓ ICP	Myoclonic jerking or seizures and vomiting in awake patients
				↓ Intraocular pressure	No analgesia
				Neutral BP	↓ Cortisol
Propofol	0.5–1.5 milligrams/kg IV	20–40 s	8–15 min	Antiemetic	Apnea
				Anticonvulsant	↓ BP
				↓ ICP	No analgesia
Ketamine	1–2 milligrams/kg IV	1 min	10–20 min	Bronchodilator	↑ Secretions
				"Dissociative" amnesia	↑ BP
				Analgesia	Emergence phenomenon

Abbreviations: BP = blood pressure; ICP = intracranial pressure.

release, which is useful in hypovolemic or hypotensive patients. Ketamine causes direct smooth muscle relaxation and bronchodilation and is often used in those with refractory status asthmaticus.

Ketamine does not cause consistent increased intracranial pressure in sedated and ventilated patients, and some studies suggest that the drug has possible cerebroprotective effects.[15] Despite previous theoretic concerns about γ-aminobutyric acid–altering effects that could worsen CNS function, ketamine is a good option in patients with head injury and hypotension. Ketamine is not a preferred agent for the elderly or for patients with a potential for cardiac ischemia, because of the potential for associated tachycardia and hypertension.

Other Agents **Barbiturates** commonly cause hypotension from myocardial depression and venous dilatation; they have been largely replaced with etomidate or propofol. Benzodiazepines may be used when other agents are contraindicated or unavailable, with **midazolam** being the common choice.

PARALYTIC AGENTS

Depolarizing and nondepolarizing neuromuscular blocking agents facilitate RSI (**Table 29-8**). Depolarizing neuromuscular blocking agents have high affinity for cholinergic receptors of the motor end plate and are resistant to acetylcholinesterase. Depolarizing blockade is not antagonized and may be enhanced by anticholinesterase agents. Succinylcholine is the common depolarizing agent.

Nondepolarizing neuromuscular blocking agents compete with acetylcholine for the cholinergic receptors and usually can be antagonized by anticholinesterase agents. **Rocuronium** and **vecuronium** are nondepolarizing agents used in the emergency setting; rocuronium is the most common alternative to succinylcholine in RSI due to its shorter duration of action and its ability to achieve intubating conditions closest to those of succinylcholine (**Table 29-9**).[16] Vecuronium has a longer time of onset, even with the high-dose approaches, making it a less favorable choice in RSI; it is primarily used for ongoing paralysis after intubation.

In the ED, neuromuscular blockade can facilitate tracheal intubation, improve mechanical ventilation, and help control intracranial hypertension. Paralysis improves oxygenation and decreases peak airway pressures in a variety of disorders, including refractory pulmonary edema and respiratory distress syndrome. Neuromuscular blockade limits assessments of neurologic status, and long-term use increases critical illness polyneuropathy and posttraumatic stress disorder. Neuromuscular blockers are neither anxiolytics nor analgesics, so agents targeting these are needed. **Maintain sedation during initial paralysis to avoid patient awareness;** later, some patients can be managed with less or little sedation, but this is not ideal in the emergent setting.

Depolarizing Agent: Succinylcholine Succinylcholine is the most commonly used agent for neuromuscular blockade in ED RSI. Succinylcholine is two joined acetylcholine molecules and is rapidly hydrolyzed by plasma cholinesterase. It has a rapid onset after IV dosing and a shorter duration of action than do the nondepolarizing agents. After brief fasciculation, complete relaxation occurs at 60 seconds, with maximal paralysis at 2 to 3 minutes.[17] Effective respirations resume in 8 to 12 minutes. IM succinylcholine (4 milligrams/kg) will act more slowly and last longer; however, this is best reserved for the rare setting where paralysis is required absent IV access.

TABLE 29-8 Succinylcholine Complications and Contraindications

Clinically important hyperkalemia in patients with:
Burns >5 d old
Denervation injury >5 d old
Significant crush injuries >5 d old
Severe infection >5 d old
Preexisting myopathies
Preexisting hyperkalemia
Fasciculations
Transient increased intragastric, intraocular, and intracranial pressure (? impact)
Masseter spasm alone or with malignant hyperthermia
Bradycardia
Prolonged apnea with pseudocholinesterase deficiency or myasthenia gravis

TABLE 29-9 Paralytic Agents in RSI

Agent	Adult Intubating IV Dose	Onset	Duration	Comments
Rocuronium (intermediate/long)	1 milligram/kg	1–3 min	30–45 min	Tachycardia. Longer duration of action and onset compared to succinylcholine. Most common alternative to succinylcholine in RSI.[15]
Vecuronium (intermediate/long)	0.08–0.15 milligram/kg	2–4 min	25–40 min	Prolonged recovery time in obese or elderly, or if there is hepatorenal dysfunction.
	0.15–0.28 milligram/kg (high-dose protocol)		60–120 min	
Succinylcholine	1.5 milligrams/kg	45–60 s	5–9 min	Provides optimal intubating conditions most quickly. There are several rare but important contraindications (see Table 29-8).

Succinylcholine provides excellent intubation conditions and is the preferred agent for RSI in the ED.[16] In the event of a failed airway, mask ventilation may be required for up to 12 minutes, until the return of spontaneous ventilation. Give the induction agent immediately before succinylcholine to avoid awareness and enhance intubating conditions.

Serum potassium will transiently rise an average of 0.5 mEq/L with succinylcholine, usually without any clinical impact (Table 29-9). A clinically significant or exaggerated hyperkalemic response can occur 5 or more days after a burn, denervation, or crush injury. The exaggerated hyperkalemic response is due to acetylcholine receptor upregulation at the neuromuscular junction, which requires time to occur and thus is not an immediate factor. Patients with preexisting myopathies are at particular risk for a life-threatening hyperkalemic response. **Do not use succinylcholine in patients with suspected preexisting significant hyperkalemia (especially renal failure), myopathies, or myasthenia gravis.**

Other succinylcholine complications are rare. Genetically susceptible individuals may develop malignant hyperthermia after succinylcholine (or after a volatile inhaled anesthetic). Suspect malignant hyperthermia if unexplained rapid fever with muscle rigidity, acidosis, or hyperkalemia occurs after succinylcholine, and treat with IV dantrolene sodium (2.5 milligrams/kg) and temperature control. Patients with acquired or genetic atypical or low plasma cholinesterase may have prolonged paralysis. Cocaine is metabolized by plasma cholinesterase, which reduces the amount of enzyme available for succinylcholine metabolism. **If known plasma cholinesterase deficiency is suspected, use a nondepolarizing agent (usually rocuronium) instead of succinylcholine.**

Nondepolarizing Agents: **Rocuronium** is an intermediate-duration nondepolarizing agent that is an excellent alternative to succinylcholine for RSI.[16] By increasing the dose of rocuronium to 0.9 to 1.2 milligrams/kg, the onset of action approximates that of succinylcholine, but the duration of action is prolonged. There are fewer side effects and contraindications with rocuronium than with vecuronium (Table 29-8).

Vecuronium bromide is an intermediate- to long-acting nondepolarizing agent (Table 29-8). Vecuronium has no cardiac effects. Hypersensitivity reactions are rare, doses are only minimally cumulative, and excretion is biliary. Despite the lack of histamine release, hypotension may occur through other mechanisms that include sympathetic ganglia block and less venous return from altered absent muscle tone and positive-pressure ventilation.

Sugammadex is a reversal agent that encapsulates the molecules of the nondepolarizing agent that are circulating in plasma. It reverses blockade from rocuronium or vecuronium within minutes. It is not yet approved by the Food and Drug Administration in the United States but is available in Europe. The dose is 2 to 4 milligrams/kg, depending on the intensity of neuromuscular paralysis.[18] Neostigmine, a cholinesterase inhibitor, has cardiac and cholinergic side effects that make its use undesirable, and reversal is not effective anyway until there is evidence of some spontaneous recovery.

VIDEO LARYNGOSCOPY

Video laryngoscopes use an integrated monitor, antifogging mechanisms, and a high-resolution camera to indirectly visualize the glottis. ETT advancement and position are viewed through the video screen. All of the other elements of preparation, preoxygenation, and confirmation of intubation are unchanged.

Video laryngoscopy is either a rescue technique for failed direct intubation or the primary technique for routine and difficult airways. Video laryngoscopy improves glottic visualization and first-pass and overall intubation success rates compared to direct laryngoscopy in the emergency setting.[4,19] It may require a longer first attempt to intubation interval. Success rates as a rescue device in patients who have failed direct laryngoscopy are reported as greater than 90%.[20] Video laryngoscopy is useful in those with potentially difficult airways, notably obese patients and those with limited neck mobility.[21] Avoid video approaches and use direct laryngoscopy if the camera could be obscured by blood or emesis.

Although the video laryngoscope handle has the familiarity of the traditional laryngoscope, the operator performs the intubation watching a video screen rather than looking into the oropharynx. The angle of the blade and transmission to the monitor creates a magnified view and provides views that cannot be obtained through direct laryngoscopy. The device can be used in patients with limited oral opening and with the neck in neutral position. These are advantages in patients with difficult airways or restricted cervical spine mobility. These devices also allow shared visualization and video recording useful for quality review, education, and training.

The two most studied video laryngoscopes are the **GlideScope Video Laryngoscope**® (Verathon, Bothell, WA) and the **C-MAC Video Laryngoscope**® (Karl Storz, Tuttlingen, Germany). Both devices offer a sharp-angled blade that is best used with malleable stylets or rigid stylets designed specifically for this purpose. Blades similar in shape to Macintosh and Miller blades, pediatric sizes, and disposable blades are available. Comparative studies between devices are limited, and no significant difference in success has been clearly demonstrated.

The technique for both blades differs from traditional laryngoscopy, in that a midline insertion is preferred and a tongue sweep is not needed. Once past the teeth, the operator identifies the midline by finding the uvula. The blade is then slowly advanced down the tongue until the epiglottis is seen. The ideal view is usually obtained by insertion into the vallecula, much like a Macintosh blade. The handle is then gently tilted forward until visualization of the glottis opening is obtained.

FIBEROPTIC LARYNGOSCOPY

The flexible fiberoptic laryngoscope is a valuable adjunct when anatomic limitations prevent visualization of the vocal cords.[21] Clinical examples include conditions that prevent opening or movement of the mandible, massive tongue swelling from angioedema, upper airway infections, congenital anatomic abnormalities, and cervical spine immobility. Flexible fiberoptic scopes allow visualization of the posterior pharynx, glottis, and laryngeal structures (**Figure 29-3**).

Use of a fiberoptic scope requires instruction, facility, and practice, often initially in the simulation lab. Fiberoptic scopes allow airway assessment in select patients before attempting intubation. If equipment or expertise is not available in the ED, consult an expert with fiberoptic skills and tools.

Contraindications to fiberoptic intubation are relative. The procedure requires time to set up and usually a compliant, spontaneously breathing patient. Patients needing an immediate airway, with near-complete obstruction, with large bleeding or vomitus, and who cannot be ventilated to maintain saturation, are poor candidates.

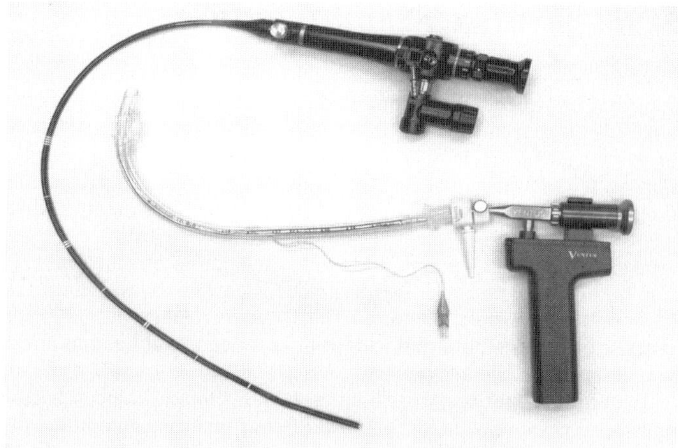

FIGURE 29-3. A fiberoptic laryngoscope and a Shikani endoscope [Clarus Medical LLC, Minneapolis, MN].

Topical anesthesia is essential to fiberoptic intubation success. Use atomized or nebulized topical anesthetics, such as lidocaine or tetracaine. An antisialagogue, such as glycopyrrolate, 0.01 milligram/kg, reduces secretions and enhances topical anesthesia but should be given 20 minutes prior for best effect. Sedation is often required because most patients are spontaneously breathing and aware. If using the nasal route, instill a topical vasoconstrictor such as phenylephrine or oxymetazoline. Nasal viscous lidocaine followed by a nasal airway allows topical anesthesia and enhanced passage of the scope through the airway, although remember to remove the nasal tube prior to the passage of an ETT.

The nasal route allows easier midline airway positioning, and the optic tip enters the glottis at a less acute angle. Oral obstruction, such as tongue or posterior pharyngeal swelling, is a common indication for nasal fiberoptic intubation. If using the oral route, tongue extrusion and anterior mandibular displacement help. Fiberoptic equipment is more frequently damaged transorally, so use a bite block. In the emergent setting, the nasal approach is preferred to the oral route in an upright, awake patient.

To begin the procedure, focus the eyepiece and lubricate the flexible shaft. Immerse the lens at the tip of the laryngoscope in warm water or apply antifogging solution. Newer flexible scopes use video technology, not fiberoptics, and interface directly with video laryngoscope monitors.

Continuously monitor pulse oximetry, and reduce the gag reflex with topical anesthetic. After attaching the oxygen tubing to the suction port, intermittent insufflation of oxygen at 10 to 15 L/min will keep the optic tip clear.

The adapter initially is removed from an ETT. If possible, use a tube that is at least 7.5 mm in inner diameter; slip the lubricated tube over the shaft up to the handle. The distal end of the fiberoptic laryngoscope must extend beyond the end of the ETT. Hold the laryngoscope in the left hand to control tip deflection while advancing it through the cords. The laryngoscope will function as a stylet for the tube. After the laryngoscope is in the trachea, the ETT is advanced, and the laryngoscope is removed.

Another option is to insert a warmed nasotracheal tube into the nasopharynx, stopping just proximal to the posterior pharynx. Dilating with lubricated nasopharyngeal airways before placement can be helpful. Then insert the scope through the ETT, and direct the fiberoptic tip into the glottis. This technique provides the assurance that the tube can be passed and allows the scope to bypass the secretion-laden anterior nares. Advancing the scope through the cords is the greatest technical challenge and requires good glottic anesthesia. Spraying 4% lidocaine through the working channel when the scope is over the glottic opening provides further suppression of the gag or cough reflex. Once the scope is through the cords, the tube is gently passed over the scope in a Seldinger technique. Resistance at the cords is best overcome with tube rotation rather than forceful insertion.

BLIND NASOTRACHEAL INTUBATION

Blind nasotracheal intubation is helpful in situations in which laryngoscopy may be difficult, RSI is contraindicated, and flexible fiberoptics are not available to facilitate nasal intubation. This technique is particularly useful in patients in whom oral intubation is impossible due to obstruction, such as severe angioedema, or with limited oral opening, such as fracture or recent surgery. Severely dyspneic patients with congestive heart failure, chronic obstructive pulmonary disease, or asthma who are awake often cannot remain supine but may tolerate nasotracheal intubation in the sitting position. This technique is now rarely used given the other options available; do not try this in an emergency without prior practice or unless a physician with prior experience is at hand to direct you in the procedure to avoid failure.

To minimize epistaxis, spray both nares with a topical vasoconstrictor anesthetic. Select a cuffed ETT 0.5 to 1.0 mm smaller than optimal for oral intubation. Verify the integrity of the cuff and the tube adapter to ensure a snug fit. Use universal precautions. Insert a nasal airway, first in one nare and then in the other, to determine which is more patent. Select the nare for intubation that is the largest and easiest to maneuver.

Have an assistant immobilize the patient's head and maintain it in a neutral or slightly extended position ("sniffing position"). The intubator stands at the side of the patient, with one hand on the tube and with the thumb and index finger of the other hand straddling the larynx. Advance the lubricated tube along the nasal floor on the more patent side. Facing the bevel against the septum helps minimize abrasions of the Kiesselbach plexus. Steady, gentle pressure or slow rotation of the tube usually bypasses small obstructions. Pass the tube *straight back toward the occiput* (not upward), and then advance it while rotating it medially 15 to 30 degrees until maximal airflow is heard through the tube. Then, gently, but swiftly, advance the tube at the *initiation (upswing) of inspiration*. Entrance into the larynx may initiate a cough, and most expired air should exit through the tube even though the cuff is uninflated. **If the patient can speak, the trachea was not intubated; remove the tube.**

You may palpate or externally see the tube enter the trachea toward the carina. The normal distance from the external nares to the carina is 32 cm in the adult male and 27 to 28 cm in the adult female. Therefore, **the optimal initial depth of tube placement for nasotracheal intubation in adults at the nares exit is 28 cm in men and 26 cm in women.** Confirm the tube placement as with oral intubation, and suction the tube before initiating positive-pressure ventilation.

If nasotracheal intubation is unsuccessful, carefully inspect the neck to identify tube malposition. Most commonly, the tube is in the pyriform fossa on the same side as the nostril used. A lateral neck bulge may be seen or palpated. Withdraw the tube into the retropharynx until breath sounds are heard. Then redirect the tube while manually displacing the larynx toward the side of the previous bulge. If there is no contraindication, flexing and rotating the neck to the ipsilateral side while the tube is rotated medially often is effective. If the tube hangs up on the vocal cords, shrill, turbulent air noises will be heard. The tube can be rotated slightly to realign the bevel with the cords.

The risk of inadvertent intracranial passage of a nasotracheal tube is extremely low. Severe traumatic nasal or pharyngeal hemorrhages are relative contraindications to nasotracheal intubation.

Serious complications of nasotracheal intubation are rare. The most common complication is epistaxis from inadequate topical vasoconstriction, excessive tube size, poor technique, or anatomic defects. Excessive force can damage the nasal septum or turbinates. Retropharyngeal lacerations, abscesses, and nasal necrosis are reported. Once the patient is stabilized, the nasotracheal tube can be electively replaced with an oral tube. If left in place for more than 48 hours, virtually all patients will have evidence of sinus blockage on imaging and many develop clinical infection.

DIFFICULT AIRWAY

The difficult airway is one in which mask ventilation or tracheal intubation fails or is likely to fail. Approximately 1% to 3% of attempts at tracheal intubation fail with standard techniques. *Difficult mask ventilation* is the inability to maintain oxygen saturation above 90% despite optimal positioning and airway adjuncts. *A failed airway* is defined as three unsuccessful attempts at intubation by an experienced operator or failure to maintain oxygenation.[22] The key to difficult airway management is expecting it to happen, preparing with a plan and expertise, and placing the appropriate airway equipment ready in one location at the bedside (**Table 29-10**).

TABLE 29-10 Suggested Difficult-Airway Cart Equipment

Endotracheal tubes: assorted sizes, designs, tip control, fiberoptic
Laryngoscope blades: alternate sizes and designs, fiberoptic (extra bulbs)
Laryngoscope handles: extra batteries
Stylets: Eschmann bougie, semi-rigid, hollow, light wand
Syringes, fixators, and Magill forceps
4% lidocaine, viscous lidocaine
1% phenylephrine (Neo-Synephrine), oxymetazoline
Suction catheters
Rescue devices:
Laryngeal mask airways
Combitube® (Sheridan Catheter Corp., Argyle, NY)
King LT® (King Systems, Noblesville, IN)
A surgical airway option:
Transtracheal jet ventilation equipment
Cricothyrotomy equipment
Tracheostomy tubes
Video laryngoscopy
Diagnostic flexible nasopharyngoscope
Intubating flexible scope

Before any attempt at intubation, assess potential difficulties for bag-valve mask ventilation and laryngoscopy. The presence of two of the following factors increases the likelihood of difficult bag-valve mask ventilation: facial hair, obesity, edentulous patient, advanced age, and snoring. An inability to adequately ventilate with a bag-valve mask is usually solved by better positioning, jaw thrust, a tighter seal with two-person bagging, and the use of oral and nasal airways.[23] A lubricant may improve the seal in a bearded patient; dentures left in place facilitate bag-valve mask ventilation, but remove dentures before any intubation attempt. External features associated with difficult intubation include obesity, a short neck, small or large chin, buckteeth, high arched palate, and any airway deformity due to trauma, tumor, or inflammation.

Most studies of airway difficulty use a grading system identified through laryngoscopic view. Such methods are not practical in the ED. A simple, systematic, and rapid evaluation of the airway is used to predict a potentially poor laryngoscopic view before RSI and neuromuscular blockade.[22,24] The mandibular opening in an adult should be at least 4 cm, or **two to three fingerbreadths**. The ability of the mandible to accommodate the tongue can be estimated by the distance between the mentum and the hyoid bone, which should be **three to four fingerbreadths**. A small mandible is more likely to have a tongue obstruction impairing visualization during laryngoscopy. An unusually large mandible also may impair visualization by elongating the oral axis. A high, anterior larynx is possible if the space between the mandible and top of the thyroid cartilage is narrower than two fingerbreadths. The degree to which the tongue obstructs the visualization of the posterior pharynx on mouth opening has some correlation with the visualization of the glottis. Assess this with the **Mallampati criteria**, with classes III and IV being associated with poor visualization and higher failure rates (up to 5% and 20%, respectively; **Figure 29-4**). The *Mallampati approach is limited in that it requires an upright patient who can open his/her mouth spontaneously*; attempting this in a supine patient or with a tongue depressor will not accurately predict laryngoscopic views.

Neck immobility interferes with the ability to align the visual axes by preventing the desired "sniffing position." Neck immobility can occur

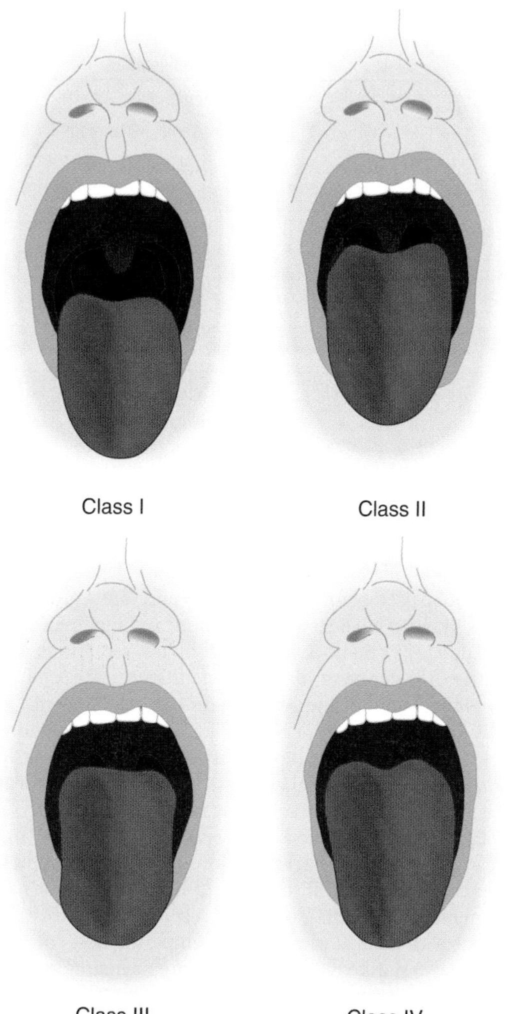

FIGURE 29-4. Classification of tongue size relative to the size of the oral cavity as described by Mallampati and colleagues. Class I: Faucial pillars, soft palate, and uvula can be visualized. Class II: Faucial pillars and soft palate can be visualized, but the uvula is masked by the base of the tongue. Class III: Only the base of the uvula can be visualized. Class IV: None of the three structures can be visualized.

from a cervical collar or structural changes that include fracture, dislocation, or arthritis. If there is no suspicion of cervical injury, assess atlanto-occipital extension; if unimpeded, laryngoscopy will likely be easier.

Airway obstruction presents another challenge to airway management. If evidence of obstruction is present, consider the location of the obstruction, whether it is fixed (e.g., tumor) or mobile (e.g., epiglottis), and how rapidly it is progressing. The location may determine which approach or rescue device can be used. Oral airway obstruction from angioedema of the tongue may limit the physician to nasal techniques or a surgical airway (see chapter 30, "Surgical Airways"). Bag-valve mask ventilation is more likely to be successful in mobile as opposed to fixed obstruction. The speed of progression determines whether the patient can await alternative management elsewhere.

MECHANICAL VENTILATORY SUPPORT

Ventilators are pressure or volume cycled. Volume-cycled ventilators are used routinely in EDs. Decisions with regard to mechanical ventilatory support in the ED include the rate, mode, fraction of inspired oxygen, minute ventilation, and use of positive end-expiratory pressure.

There are three common ventilator methods for providing the tidal volume: continuous mechanical ventilation, assist-control, and synchronized intermittent mandatory ventilation. Continuous mechanical

TABLE 29-11 Initial Ventilator Settings and Goals

Ventilator Parameters	Ventilator Settings
Mode	Assist-control
FIO_2	Begin with 100% oxygen
Tidal volume	6 mL/kg (ideal body weight) to start
Respiratory rate	12 breaths/min
Inspiratory flow rate	60 L/min
Inspiratory:expiratory ratio	1:2 or 1:3 ratio
Positive end-expiratory pressure	Begin with 5 cm H_2O, titrate to 10 cm H_2O
Ventilation goals	PaO_2: 60–90 mm Hg $PaCO_2$: 40 mm Hg pH: 7.35–7.45 FIO_2 of 40%–60% Inspiratory peak pressure <35 cm H_2O

Abbreviations: FIO_2 = fraction of inspired oxygen; $PaCO_2$ = partial pressure of arterial carbon dioxide; PaO_2 = partial pressure of arterial oxygen.

ventilation is most commonly used in the operating room for heavily sedated or paralyzed apneic patients. The **assist-control mode** is preferred initially for patients in respiratory distress, allowing inspiration triggered by either the intrinsic effort or an elapsed time interval. The ventilator provides a "controlled" breath at a predetermined tidal volume during the selected time cycle or sooner if triggered by the patient's effort. In the **synchronized intermittent mode**, a predetermined number of ventilator-generated tidal volumes exists, and ventilation is synchronized to patient effort. If the intrinsic respiratory rate is below the set rate, synchronized intermittent mode acts like the assist-control mode. However, if the patient is breathing above the set respiratory rate, the efforts are not assisted; this increases the work of breathing, making synchronized intermittent mode undesirable in the ED. Initial ventilator settings and goals can be found in **Table 29-11**. Obtain an arterial blood gas after initiation of mechanical ventilation to ensure proper ventilation.

Adjust initial mechanical ventilation based on responses to oximetry, capnography, and plateau pressures.[25] Minimize plateau pressures and tidal volumes to reduce the risk of lung injury. Tidal volumes of 6 cc/kg are best for lung protection. In some cases, such as obstructive airway disease, hypercapnia is tolerated to achieve lower plateau pressures. Positive end-expiratory pressure, starting at 5 cm H_2O and titrating to 10 cm H_2O if tolerated, can prevent alveolar collapse and improve oxygenation. Unless a contraindication exists, elevate the head of the bed 30 degrees to prevent aspiration and ventilator-associated pneumonia and improve lung recruitment. A prone position aids to improve lung segment recruitment, although this is not often started in the ED and is usually deployed after paralysis and the other measures fail. When possible, titrate oxygen to less than 60% to prevent oxygen toxicity.

Maintain patient sedation and analgesia initially during mechanical ventilation, particularly if the patient is paralyzed.[26] This is usually best achieved with an initial bolus followed by an IV infusion titrated to need. Intermittent boluses are reserved for anticipated short-term mechanical ventilation (**Table 29-12**). The goal is the optimal sedation (not deeper or longer than needed) for comfort and to allow recovery; targeting clinical assessments of sedation, blood pressure, and heart rate are common. The goals include amnesia, pain control, and the ability to ventilate without neuromuscular blockade if possible. Later, sedation withdrawal is an option based on response and can limit postextubation cognitive changes.

EXTUBATION

This maneuver is not common in the ED but may be required in settings of rapid recovery or after prolonged ED care. Before extubation, assess respiratory sufficiency by determining inspiratory capacity—it should be at least 15 mL/kg. Ideally, there should be no intercostal or suprasternal reactions, and the patient hand grip should be firm.

TABLE 29-12 Sedation During Mechanical Ventilation

Drug	Initial Bolus	Starting Infusion	Comments
Fentanyl	1-2 micrograms/kg IV	0.5–1 microgram/kg/h	Often combined with midazolam
Remifentanil	1.5 micrograms/kg IV	0.5–1 microgram/kg/h	Ultra-short-acting
Midazolam	0.05 milligram/kg IV	0.025 milligram/kg/h	Often combined with fentanyl
Propofol	0.5 milligram/kg IV	20-50 micrograms/kg/min	Can cause hypotension
Ketamine	0.5–1 milligram/kg IV	0.5 milligram/kg/h	May provide broncho-dilation; sympathetic stimulation

After suctioning secretions and ensuring ongoing adequate oxygenation, explain the procedure to the patient. Positive-pressure ventilation with a mask will help while the cuff is deflated. *Remove the tube at the end of a deep inspiration.* Continue giving oxygen by mask to prevent secretory reaccumulation.

Observe closely for stridor after extubation. Postextubation laryngospasm is treated initially with positive-pressure oxygen or using a high-flow oxygen (including an Optiflow™) delivery system. If necessary, nebulized racemic epinephrine (0.5 mL of 2.25% epinephrine in 4 mL of saline) helps when stridor suggests laryngospasm or upper airway edema secondary to tube placement and removal.

REFERENCES

The complete reference list is available online at www.TintinalliEM.com.

Surgical Airways

Michael D. Smith
Donald M. Yealy

INTRODUCTION

Establishing an airway by means of a surgical approach—incision or percutaneous insertion—is a challenging procedure deployed at high-risk and high-stress moments when basic airway maneuvers have failed. **The key is preparation and practice, which means having all equipment ready and available** (often in a common cart to ensure consistency) **and prior practice** in laboratory settings if not recently performed in clinical care. Knowing what options are available and then choosing one and implementing it before respiratory collapse will improve the outcome. The success rates depend largely on the preparedness of the ED and the training of the staff.[1,2]

Surgical cricothyrotomy refers to incision of the cricothyroid membrane under direct visualization and insertion of a tracheostomy tube either directly through the incision or by using the Seldinger technique. **Needle cricothyrotomy** is a dated term referring to insertion of a 12- to 16-gauge needle catheter into the trachea and connected to either a bag-valve device or wall oxygen. **We do not recommend needle cricothyrotomy. Percutaneous transtracheal jet ventilation** uses a 12- to 16-gauge catheter inserted into the cricothyroid membrane and connected to a high-pressure (35 to 50 psi) oxygen source for both oxygenation and ventilation.

PATIENT SELECTION

The primary indication for surgical airway placement is a "can't intubate, can't ventilate" scenario. Most emergency surgical airways follow a failed attempt to establish an oral endotracheal airway. Cricothyrotomy or jet ventilation can be used before laryngoscopy and direct glottic intubation if the latter is likely to fail because of anatomic impingement or any other cause that impedes visualization, notable blood, secretions, swelling, or foreign matter. *It is not necessary to try to intubate once before moving to cricothyrotomy*; this often simply enhances the risk of harm.

TABLE 30-1 Clinical Manifestations Associated with Acute Airway Obstruction

Etiology	Manifestation
Vascular	Hematoma External hemorrhage Hypotension Hemoptysis
Laryngotracheal	Stridor Subcutaneous air (massive) Hoarseness Dysphonia Hemoptysis
Pharyngeal and/or hypopharyngeal	Subcutaneous air Hematemesis Dysphagia Sucking wound

Difficulty in establishing an airway may be due to anatomy (short, obese neck), a disease state (epiglottitis, laryngeal edema, paralyzed vocal cords, or retropharyngeal abscess), trauma from distortion of the neck by hematoma (cervical fracture or major vessel injury), aspiration of blood (facial trauma), or loss of supporting structures (mandibular fractures). Assess for these factors before any laryngoscopic attempts, have a surgical airway plan in mind, and have equipment ready at the bedside to manage impending or actual respiratory failure.

In a patient with a failed intubation attempt, the best course of action is to use bag-valve mask ventilation to restore or maintain gas exchange while regrouping. If bag mask ventilation is successful, try another attempt at laryngoscopy with a different operator and approach, rather than performing immediate cricothyrotomy. Clinical signs and symptoms of airway obstruction—one common reason to choose a surgical airway—are listed in **Table 30-1**.

PATIENT AGE

Most children do not require advanced airway management, especially a surgical airway. In children under 12 years, the larynx is more easily damaged by cricothyrotomy, and placement is challenged by compressible structures and less distinction between cartilages. Late airway complications, especially stenosis, occur more often in children.[3] **For children under 12 years old, especially those under 8 years, tracheotomy is preferred**; the difficulty is that few emergency physicians have experience performing this successfully, making it an unavailable practical option. Alternatively, a 14- to 16-gauge catheter inserted percutaneously through the cricothyroid membrane to either oxygenate (temporizing for minutes, done by connecting the catheter to high-flow wall oxygen) or jet ventilate (connecting to 0.5 psi/kg compressed gas source, using a 1:3 second insufflation/expiration ratio) is an option while awaiting tracheotomy. Neither technique is well studied, although jet ventilation offers wider capabilities but requires specific equipment ready in advance. Again, the key to success is advance thought, planning, and equipment preparation coupled with training for this specific event. Needle/jet approaches are discussed in more detail later.

INJURIES REQUIRING OPEN OR PERCUTANEOUS CRICOTHYROTOMY

Penetrating trauma to the neck affecting a major artery (carotid, vertebral, or thyroid) may create an expanding hematoma and obstruct the

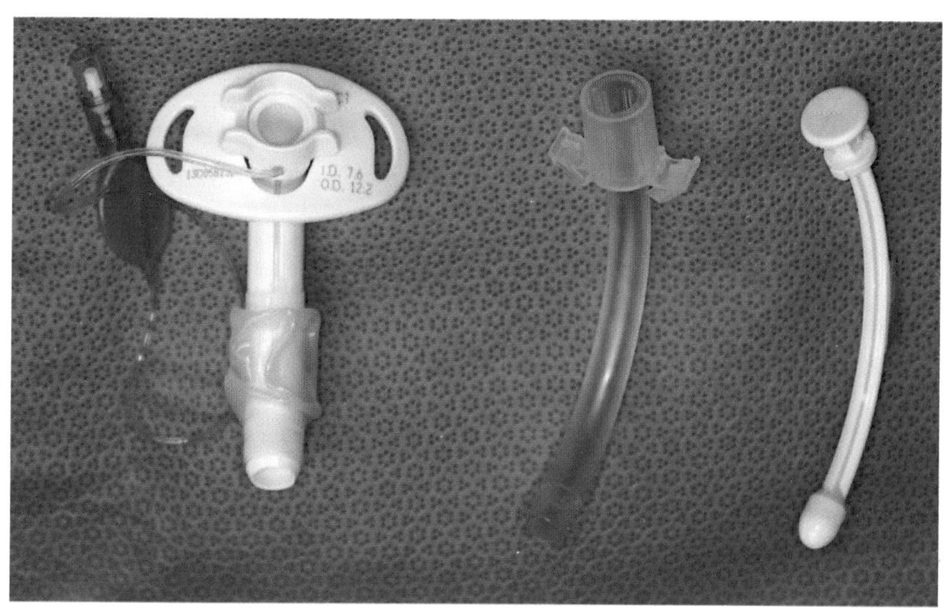

FIGURE 30-1. Tracheostomy tube with obturator. [Photo used with permission of David Effron, MD.]

airway. If free blood spills into the oro- or hypopharynx, direct visualization for intubation is often not possible. Placing a cuffed tracheostomy tube after cricothyrotomy is the best option to restore gas exchange and limit aspiration. Difficulty in establishing an airway occurs in approximately 10% of patients with penetrating cervical trauma.[4]

Blunt trauma to the neck or face may cause hemorrhage of the soft tissues or injury to the trachea/larynx, including rupture. **If the trachea or larynx is disrupted, *do not* attempt cricothyrotomy**; in this rare setting, an emergency tracheostomy is needed. In blunt facial trauma, the principal cause of death is airway obstruction from bleeding (often from fractures) or soft tissue swelling; a surgical airway can prevent death and harm if deployed quickly and with skill.

TYPE OF EMERGENCY AIRWAY AND TUBE SELECTION

Cricothyrotomy is preferred over percutaneous approaches (except for children <12 years old). The most skilled provider should perform this procedure to optimize success and limit harm.

Although any large-bore tube is adequate, we suggest using a **tracheostomy tube** because it has an obturator to ease insertion, is shorter and easier to suction, and secures well by using the flanges on each side and a cloth ribbon around the neck or suturing to nearby skin (**Figure 30-1**). When an endotracheal tube is placed during cricothyrotomy, the tube is difficult to secure and may be advanced too deeply; it also may be inadvertently directed cephalad (the wrong way) when placed through the cricothyrotomy incision. To avoid this, many use a gum elastic bougie to ensure tracheal placement and the correct tube direction.[5] If a standard endotracheal tube is used and then designated for change to a tracheostomy tube, use the Seldinger (change over a guide device) technique. Use a suction catheter with the suction vent cut off at one end as an obturator for endotracheal tube removal and tracheostomy tube insertion.

The diameter of the tube inserted is crucial. A common choice for an adult is a **6-mm tracheostomy or 6- to 7-mm endotracheal tube. Do not choose a larger (≥7 mm) tube or one smaller than 4 mm.** Larger tubes are difficult to insert in the narrow space between the cricoid and thyroid cartilages. If airway pressures are high with the small-diameter tube or ventilation is inadequate, consider changing to a larger diameter tube. Ventilation problems may occur when a smaller tube is used (3-mm internal diameter or less.) Any tube with a 4- or 5-mm internal diameter will allow adequate volume ventilation in most patients, although at 4 mm there is limited area for suctioning and aggressive minute ventilation; for that reason, select a 4- to 5-mm size only if a 6-mm tube is unavailable or cannot be placed.

SURGICAL CRICOTHYROTOMY

ANATOMY

The cricothyroid membrane is located between the thyroid and cricoid cartilages (**Figure 30-2A**). Both structures are easily palpated but are not directly seen because they are covered with the pretracheal fascia. In men, the thyroid cartilage is prominent and creates the "Adam's apple"; in women and children, the thyroid and cricoid cartilages can be hard to distinguish from each other.

The cricothyroid membrane is found approximately one-third the distance from the manubrium to the chin in the midline in patients with normal habitus (**Figure 30-2B**). In a patient with a short, obese neck, the membrane may be hidden at the level of the manubrium. In a patient with a thin, long neck, it may be midway between the chin and the manubrium. The thyroid gland overlies the trachea; both structures are difficult to palpate. One easy way to find the cricoid membrane is to slowly palpate the trachea as you move up toward the head from the sternal notch; when your fingers "fall off" after a firm structure, you have palpated the thyroid cartilage. Next, slowly palpate downward toward the feet, and the first "soft spot" after that thyroid cartilage is the cricoid membrane.

The vascular structure potentially injured during the course of a properly performed cricothyrotomy is a thyroid artery, a branch of the aorta running up to the thyroid gland in the midline. This vessel infrequently reaches the level of the cricothyroid membrane. A carotid injury is potential when landmarks are not seen or not adhered to or when technique is poor; this can be catastrophic and requires immediate direct pressure to avoid harm.

EQUIPMENT

The equipment needed to perform a surgical cricothyrotomy is listed in **Table 30-2**.

PATIENT PREPARATION AND POSITIONING

Place the patient supine, with the neck slightly hyperextended if no cervical trauma is present (neutral if there is suspected trauma) so neck structures can be palpated and identified. If time permits, apply antiseptic solution to the skin. Ventilate with a bag-valve mask connected to 100% oxygen while preparing.

PROCEDURE

The procedure for performing a surgical cricothyrotomy is summarized in **Table 30-3**.

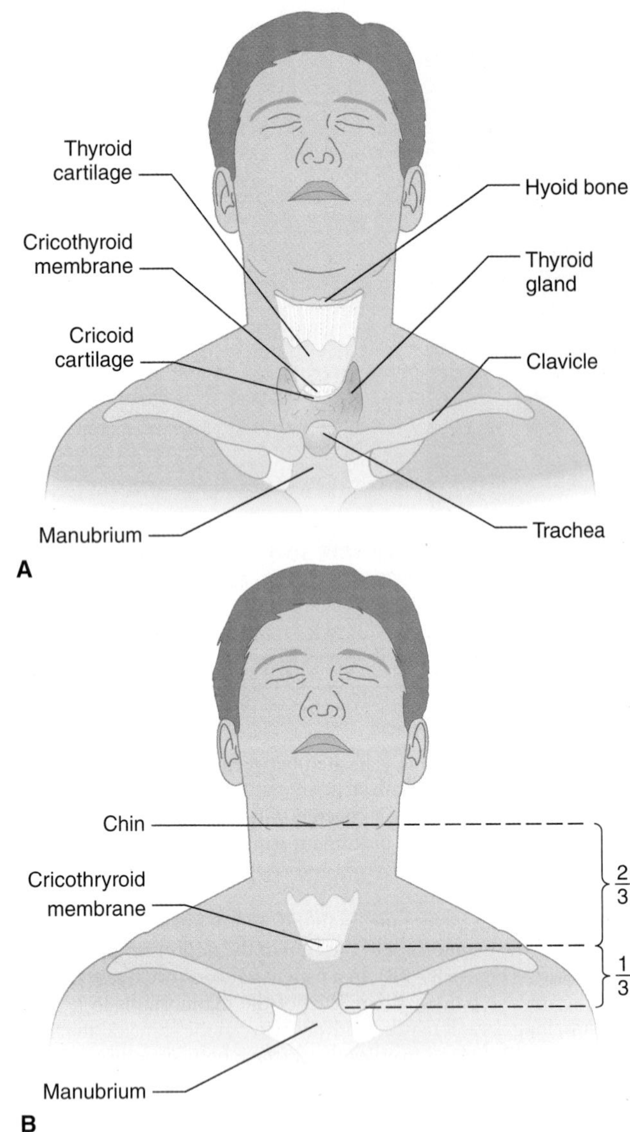

FIGURE 30-2. A. Neck anatomy. B. Location of the cricothyroid membrane.

SURGICAL CRICOTHYROTOMY USING SELDINGER TECHNIQUE

This method uses the Seldinger technique (**Figure 30-8**). Make a small vertical incision through the skin at the cricothyroid membrane. Insert the needle and aspirate air to make sure the needle is in the trachea. Next, pass the guide wire through the needle, directing the guide wire caudally. Place a tracheostomy tube over the dilator, and make a "nick"

TABLE 30-2 Equipment Needed to Perform a Surgical Cricothyrotomy

Personal protective equipment
Scalpel with a #10 (preferable because of its greater width) or #11 blade
A 6-mm endotracheal tube or tracheostomy tube (latter preferred), plus a smaller one available
Tape to secure the tube in place
Cloth ribbon and sutures to secure tracheostomy tube in place
Bag-valve mask device and oxygen source
Gum elastic bougie for guiding tube
Suction devices

TABLE 30-3 Performing a Surgical Cricothyrotomy

Step	Comment
1. Stand to one side of the patient at the level of the neck.	Right-handed practitioner—stand on the patient's right side. Left-handed practitioner—stand on the patient's left side.
2. Locate the cricothyroid membrane.	Locate the cricoid ring. Place the index finger at the sternal notch and palpate cephalad until the first rigid structure is felt (cricoid ring), or use "fall off and return" approach noted earlier. Roll the index finger one finger breadth above to locate the membrane between the cricoid and thyroid cartilages (**Figure 30-3**).
3. Using the thumb and middle finger of the nondominant hand, stabilize the two cartilages.	—
4. Use the scalpel to make a vertical incision in the midline between the two cartilages, extending if needed.	Incise through the skin and subcutaneous tissues. The structures are superficial, so do not incise deep to avoid damage to the cricoid or thyroid cartilage or vascular structures (**Figure 30-4**). The membrane is felt, not directly seen, after incision.
5. With the scalpel blade positioned horizontally, perforate the cricothyroid membrane so that the blade goes in approximately half its length.	The horizontal orientation is in anatomic alignment with the membranes to avoid vascular injury (**Figure 30-5**). **Once the membrane is perforated, do not leave it empty**; slide forceps or dilator around the blade or place a bougie before removing the scalpel.
6. Widen the incision opening.	A dilator or mosquito or Kelly clamp may be used (**Figure 30-6**).
7. Place the tube in the opening.	Although instinct may guide you to direct the tracheostomy tube posterior, remember that the trachea is superficial and the tube should follow the tracheal axis (**Figure 30-7**).
8. Connect to a bag-valve mask device for ventilation. Check for breath sounds with ventilation.	If no ventilation is heard bilaterally, pull the tube out and reinsert it. Recheck for breath sounds to ensure that the endotracheal tube is correctly positioned after any manipulation. When inserting a standard endotracheal tube, listen for asymmetry of breath sounds. If breath sounds are absent on the left side, then the tube has been inserted down the right mainstem bronchus and needs to be pulled back a few centimeters. If using an endotracheal tube, insert no more than 2–3 cm to avoid mainstem bronchus placement.
9. Secure the tube carefully with a ribbon and/or adhesive tape.	More challenging with a standard endotracheal tube.
10. Apply dressing and further secure the tube.	If a tracheostomy tube has been used, fashion a simple dressing by cutting a slit halfway down the middle of a 4×4 gauze dressing and placing it under the tracheostomy tube. Secure the tube with a ribbon placed through the flanges of the tracheostomy tube. For added security, use 2-0 nylon sutures to fix the tube to the skin. Consider changing endotracheal tubes to tracheostomy tubes whenever possible.

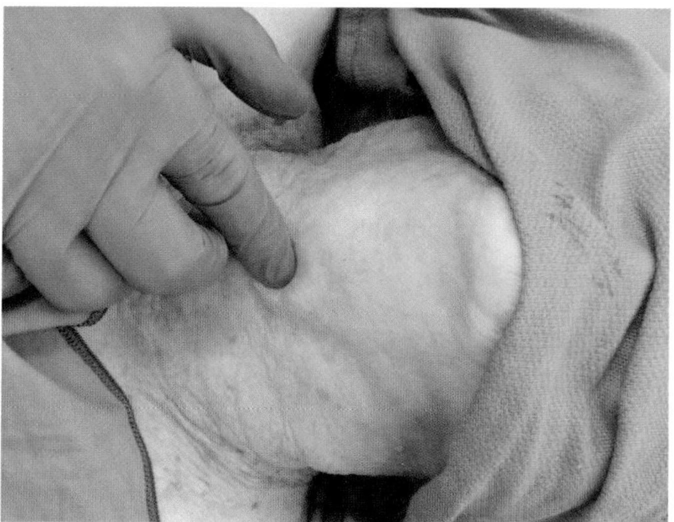

FIGURE 30-3. Locate the cricothyroid membrane. [Photo used with permission of Jennifer McBride, PhD, and Michael D. Smith, MD.]

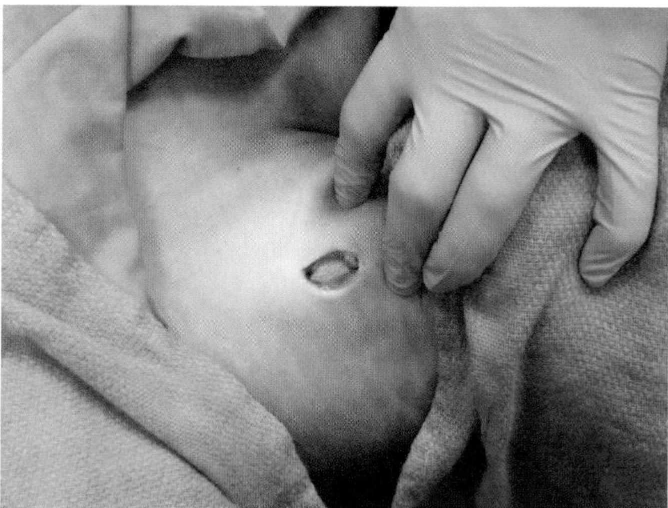

FIGURE 30-4. Make a midline vertical incision. The pretracheal fascia is seen through the incision. Bleeding is less likely with a vertical incision. [Photo used with permission of Jennifer McBride, PhD, and Michael Phelan, MD.]

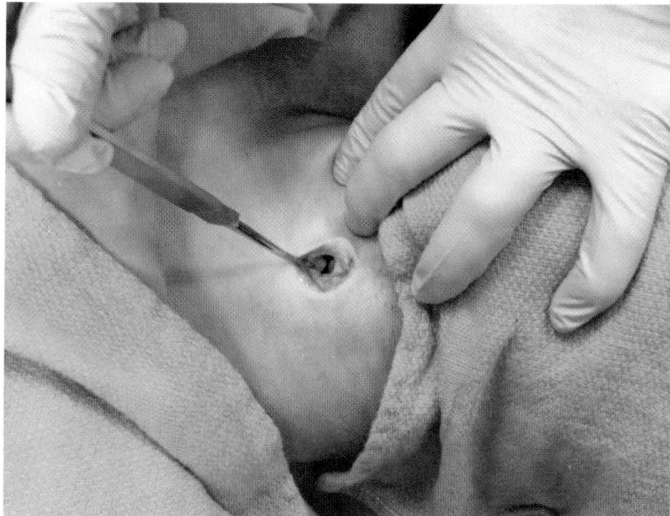

FIGURE 30-5. Perforate the cricoid membrane with a horizontal incision. [Photo used with permission of Jennifer McBride, PhD, and Michael Phelan, MD.]

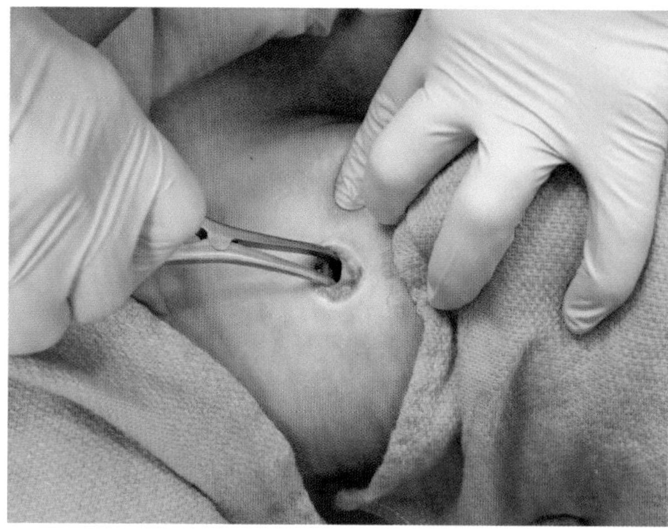

FIGURE 30-6. Widen the opening. [Photo used with permission of Jennifer McBride, PhD, and Michael Phelan, MD.]

in the skin to ease penetration. Then pass the dilator, with the tracheostomy tube, over the guide wire into the trachea. Once the dilator is in the trachea, remove the guide wire, direct the tracheostomy tube into the trachea, and verify correct placement. Indications and complications are similar to the open method, and direct comparisons in real use do not exist. Multiple commercial kits exist, but proper use requires deliberate, repetitive training.

COMPLICATIONS

Acute complications after emergency cricothyrotomy occur in up to 15% of cases.[6] Venous bleeding usually occurs from small veins and stops spontaneously. Using a vertical neck incision that is not too long decreases the chance of ongoing bleeding. Arterial bleeding can be from the thyroid artery or from a small artery at the base of the cricothyroid membrane. The first step in controlling ongoing bleeding is to apply gentle pressure. If bleeding persists, topical hemostatic agents or ligation may be necessary. A small amount of bleeding usually creates no hemodynamic concerns, but it can make the procedure more challenging.

In an obese patient, it is possible to place the tube anterior to the larynx and trachea into the mediastinum, making ventilation impossible.

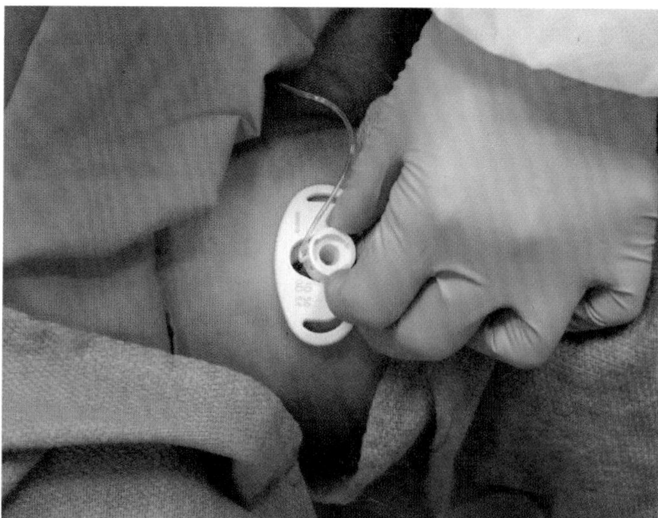

FIGURE 30-7. Insert a tracheostomy tube with obturator. [Photo used with permission of Jennifer McBride, PhD, and Michael Phelan, MD.]

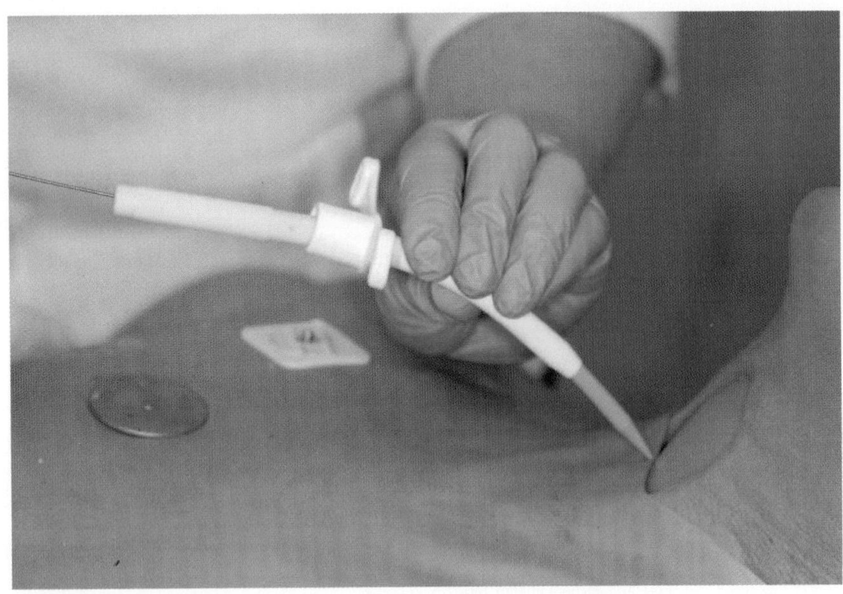

FIGURE 30-8. Placement of a percutaneous cricothyrotomy with a commercial kit and the Seldinger technique. [Photo used with permission of David Effron, MD.]

Signs of an incorrectly positioned tube are high airway pressures, absent breath sounds, and massive subcutaneous emphysema. If this complication is suspected, remove the tube and make a second attempt at insertion. Endotracheal tubes passed through the cricoid membrane may curl toward the mouth, making ventilation impossible. A gum elastic bougie can help direct the endotracheal tube.[5]

Laceration of the trachea, esophagus, or recurrent laryngeal nerves is rare and is more likely to occur if one is unfamiliar with the neck anatomy. Pneumothorax is usually secondary to barotrauma caused by ventilation initiated immediately after tube placement.

A tube left in the narrow space between the cricoid and thyroid cartilages can erode both cartilages, and bacterial chondritis may occur. The cartilages will be destroyed and eventually scar, leading to stenosis and loss of the function of the larynx. Because cricothyrotomy has a high incidence of airway stenosis,[6] a change to tracheostomy is common after 2 to 3 days.

PERCUTANEOUS CRICOTHYROTOMY AND TRANSTRACHEAL JET INSUFFLATION

We do not recommend "needle cricothyrotomy"—defined as a 12- to 16-gauge needle catheter inserted into the trachea and connected to either a bag-valve device or wall oxygen—as a rescue technique. Although many texts and general guidelines discuss this approach, it **will not** reverse ventilation gaps and will only modestly aid oxygen delivery.[7,8] In addition, the use of needle cricothyrotomy requires rapid reestablishment of a proper airway.

The only small catheter option is ***correctly performed jet ventilation***. The proper equipment must be procured and maintained and the procedure must be practiced, because many physicians lack the proper equipment and knowledge of the procedure.[9] **Do not perform jet ventilation without the correct high-pressure equipment ready in advance and without antecedent practice**; one cannot simply "put this together" at the time of critical need.

Jet ventilation uses a small catheter but also a pressured oxygen source—35 to 50 psi (much high than exiting standard bag-valve devices and oxygen wall outlets) to deliver 500 to 12,000 cc of gas. In jet ventilation, the catheter and high-pressure gas provide volume inhalation, and the native airway is the *passive* exhalation route. **With proper jet ventilation, adequate oxygenation and ventilation occur.**[10] Duration is limited only by airway desiccation from nonhumidified gas, an effect that takes hours to a day to occur. **Properly performed jet ventilation does not create hypercarbia** or the need for *rapid* reestablishment of another airway; only poorly performed or "needle cricothyrotomy" low-pressure techniques create that situation.

Jet ventilation does not harm the lower airways because the high pressure dissipates rapidly; it also allows some aspiration control as the expelled gas clears the upper airway. The only absolute contraindication is complete, including expiratory, airway obstruction; this is exceptionally rare because most upper airway obstruction is inspiratory, including obstruction from masses. Relative contraindications are unfamiliarity, not having the equipment ready, and local infection at puncture site.

ANATOMY, INDICATIONS, AND CONTRAINDICATIONS

The anatomy and general indications are listed in earlier in "Surgical Cricothyrotomy."

EQUIPMENT NEEDED

Equipment needed for transtracheal jet ventilation is listed in **Table 30-4**. The key is having this prepared in advance; **trying to use standard oxygen tubing, three-way stopcocks, or bag-valve devices or attaching to wall outlets turned to highest liter flow will not allow for proper jet ventilation**.

PROCEDURE

The steps of performing jet ventilation are summarized in **Table 30-5**. Optimize preprocedural oxygenation and ventilation if possible (although often failure is the reason for the procedure).

TABLE 30-4 Equipment Needed to Perform Jet Ventilation
Personal protective equipment
A 16 gauge or larger sheathed needle catheter or a commercial jet catheter
A 3-mL syringe
Connective tubing and connectors designed for high pressure (not standard oxygen tubing/securing attachments; these will not allow jet ventilation)
High-flow regulator with insufflation control
A high-pressure oxygen source; your respiratory technician can have the jet insufflator attached to an E cylinder or wall unit before downregulation to ensure high-pressure (35–50 psi) gas

TABLE 30-5 Performing Jet Ventilation

Step	Comment
1. Stand to one side of the patient at the level of the neck.	Right-handed practitioner—stand on the patient's right side. Left-handed practitioner—stand on the patient's left side.
2. Locate the cricothyroid membrane.	Locate the cricoid ring. Place the index finger at the sternal notch and palpate cephalad until the first rigid structure is felt (cricoid ring). Roll the index finger one finger breadth above to locate the "hollow" between the cricoid and thyroid cartilages, locating the cricothyroid membrane (Figure 30-3).
3. Attach a 3-mL syringe to the catheter.	Smaller catheters tend to kink easily, as noted in photos, and limit gas flow. Use of a 16-gauge or larger, commercial catheter is preferred (13 gauge).
4. Introduce the catheter into the subcutaneous tissue at a 45-degree angle to the skin, aiming toward the patient's feet.	**Figure 30-9.**
5. Aspirate gently while advancing the catheter over the needle.	
6. When air suddenly returns (indicating entry into the airway), advance the catheter over the needle into the larynx.	Free air aspiration = intratracheal placement; any resistance means not clearly in trachea.
7. Once fully inserted, remove the needle and reaspirate to ensure ongoing free air aspiration.	If resistance to air aspiration occurs after advancement, remove catheter and retry. **Once the catheter is fully inserted, a stabilizing hand *must* always be present**; do not ever let the proximal end be unsecured.
8. Attach the high-flow regulator via connective tubing to the catheter and start ventilation with a 100% oxygen source. If a child, use 0.5 psi/kg to start and a 16-gauge catheter (**Figure 30-10**).	Connect to a high-pressure source (35–50 psi); bag-valve devices and **standard wall oxygen valves opened to 15 L/min do *not* deliver 35–50 psi**. The jet device is attached directly to wall unit before standard regulators or directly to E cylinder (latter will allow >30 min of ventilation if full). Insufflate by holding valve down (open) for maximum of 1 s, and then release the occlusion for 4 s. Listen for symmetric breath sounds, watch the chest rise and fall, and measure exhaled CO_2 if desired.
9. Hold the catheter securely to avoid dislodgement. The catheter tends to kink easily, so maintain care with positioning.	The inspiration:expiration of 1:4 allows passive exhalation and avoids over ventilation. Monitor like any volume ventilation technique.
10. Stabilization is similar to cricothyrotomy, and plan for next airway; gas exchange will be adequate for a prolonged interval, allowing a careful and controlled approach.	Dressings are not necessary, and commercial kits have straps like tracheostomy tubes. The exhaled gas offers some aspiration protection.

COMPLICATIONS

Complications from the jet ventilation procedure are infrequent. Failure to properly secure the catheter can lead to displacement. Bleeding at the puncture site and infection may occur. Inadvertent perforation of the esophagus or back wall of the trachea or larynx is rare. Massive subcutaneous emphysema can develop during ventilation. The catheter also may be misplaced in the soft tissues of the neck. Even if the cricoid membrane is not used (from misidentification), jet punctures rarely cause long-term airway complications, an advantage over cricothyrotomy.

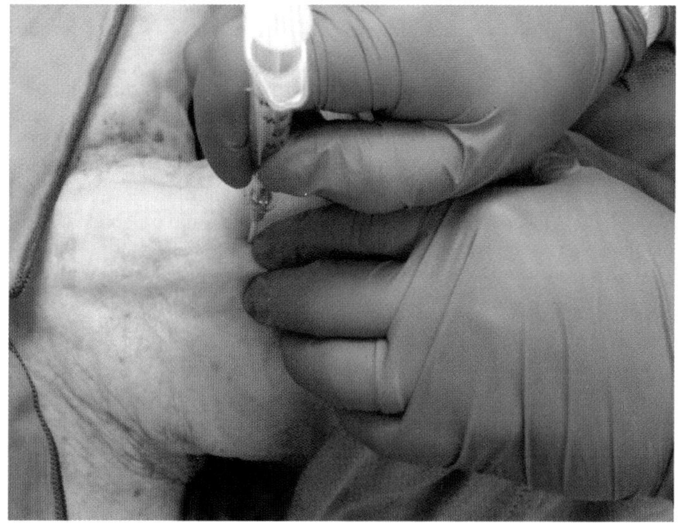

A

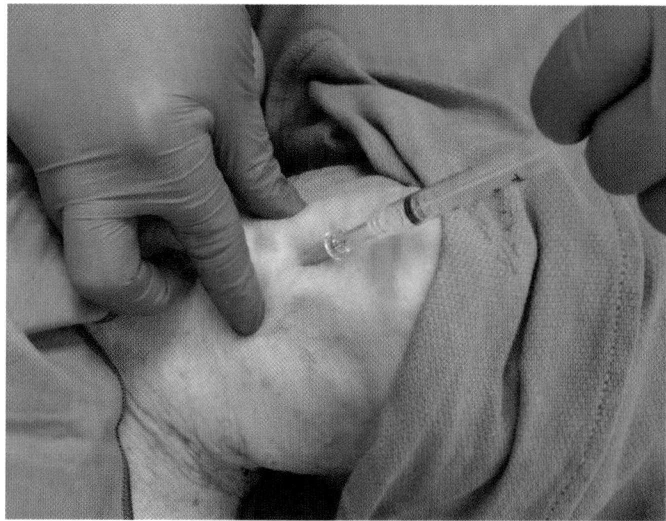

B

FIGURE 30-9. Introduce the catheter into the larynx. A. Introduce the catheter into the larynx skin at a 90-degree angle to the skin. B. When air returns, change the angle to 45 degrees. [Photo used with permission of Jennifer McBride, PhD, and Michael D. Smith, MD.]

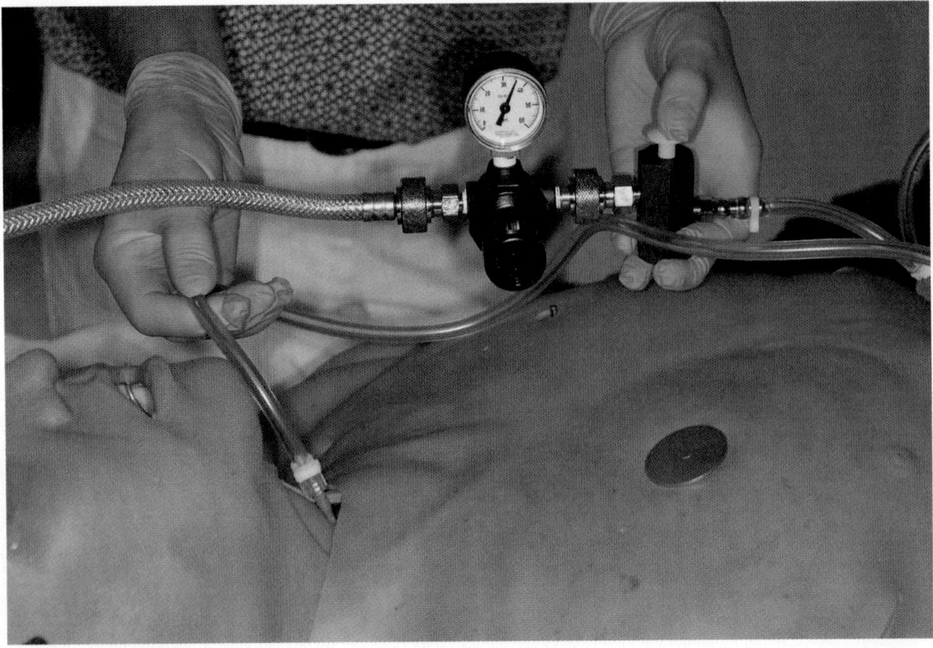

FIGURE 30-10. Attach the high-flow regulator via connective tubing to the catheter and start ventilation with high-pressure 100% oxygen source. Note: Stabilize catheter at the base to avoid dislodgement (not done in figure for display purposes). [Photo used with permission of David Effron, MD.]

DEVICE REMOVAL

Jet ventilation allows a more controlled approach to airway management; plan the next step(s) carefully and without fear of ventilation failure if done properly, avoiding any rush to another procedure. Often, a better laryngoscopic attempt or a formal tracheostomy can occur once time pressures are abated with jet ventilation.

REFERENCES

The complete reference list is available online at www.TintinalliEM.com.

CHAPTER 31

Vascular Access

Chris Wyatt

Multiple factors determine the route and site for vascular access, and knowing the basic anatomy, techniques, indications, and contraindications is essential to emergency care.

Infusion rate is key in the resuscitation of those with severe hypovolemia or hemorrhage.[1] Infusion rates through a medical catheter behave according to Poiseuille's law:

$$\text{Rate of flow} = \frac{\pi \times (\text{catheter radius}^4) \times \text{pressure gradient}}{8 \times \text{viscosity} \times \text{length of catheter}}$$

The rate of flow is directly proportional to the catheter radius and the pressure gradient, and inversely proportional to the dynamic fluid viscosity and catheter length. Flow rates increase with larger catheter radius, use of more pressure (gravity, manual push-pull devices, pressure bag application, or commercial rapid infusing devices), decreasing viscosity (co-administration of crystalloid with viscous blood products), or decreasing catheter length (peripheral angiocatheter vs triple-lumen catheter). **Flow rates are maximized by using the largest internal diameter catheter possible.**

PERIPHERAL VENOUS ACCESS SITES

PERIPHERAL VENOUS ANATOMY OF THE UPPER EXTREMITY

The most commonly accessed veins for peripheral catheterization of the upper extremity are the dorsal hand veins and the veins of the antecubital fossa (**Figure 31-1**).

Peripheral catheterization of the superficial veins of the lower extremity can require cutdown of the great and small saphenous veins. The femoral vein is the primary deep vein of the lower extremity. It is located medial to the femoral artery.

TECHNIQUE FOR PERIPHERAL VENOUS ACCESS

Gather all equipment before beginning the procedure (**Table 31-1**). Observe universal precautions. The procedure for peripheral IV line insertion is summarized in **Table 31-2**.

Avoid venous access through or distal to areas of infection, injury, or sites of potential vascular disruption (e.g., injury to the inferior vena cava from abdominal trauma). Also avoid using extremities with arteriovenous fistulas or grafts or those in which there have been previous lymph node dissections. If possible, avoid IV access of the lower extremity in diabetics due to an increased risk of infection and phlebitis. Do not use peripheral venous access to administer vasopressors for infusion, sclerosing solutions, concentrated electrolyte or glucose solutions, or cytotoxic chemotherapeutic agents.

POSTPROCEDURE CARE

Flush peripheral catheters with normal saline every 8 hours; change dressings that are damp or soiled, and change the catheter site every 72 to 96 hours.[2] Risk of infection and thrombophlebitis increases with time. Assess the skin for signs of infection (erythema) or infiltration (induration, edema). Reassess catheter function and neurovascular status of the distal extremity frequently.

Complications The complications of peripheral venous access are listed in **Table 31-3**. **The first step in treating all complications is catheter removal.**

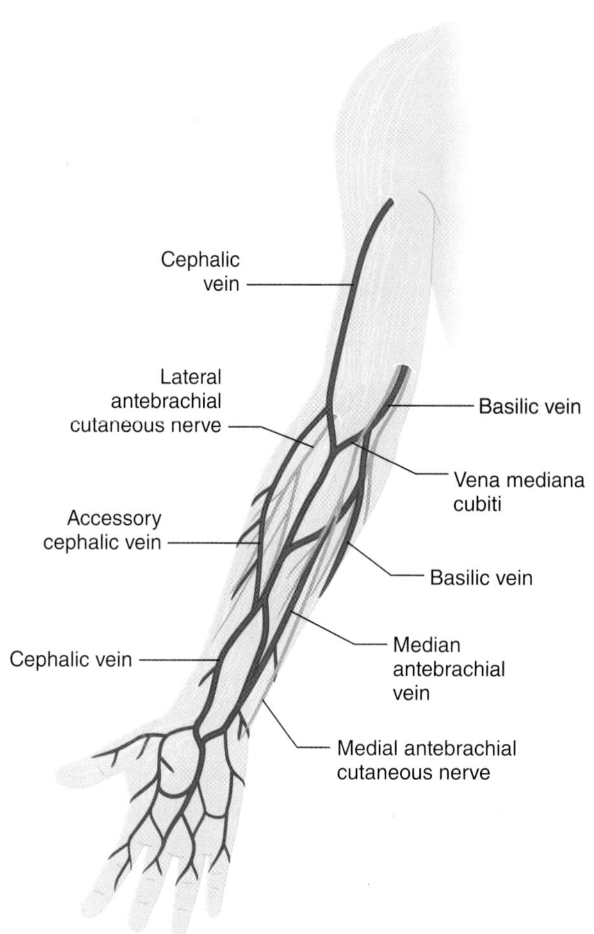

FIGURE 31-1. Venous anatomy of the upper extremity.

TABLE 31-2 Peripheral IV Line Insertion

Step	Comment
1. Apply tourniquet.	Apply tourniquet tightly enough to facilitate adequate venous filling and distention without causing patient discomfort or ischemia.
2. Locate vein.	Inspect and palpate the vein. Warm the skin, tap the vein, or apply topical nitroglycerin ointment to ease identification.
3. Clean area with either an alcohol swab or povidone iodine solution.	—
4. Apply gentle traction with the nondominant hand to anchor the vein.	—
5. Insert catheter needle into skin and vessel at a 15- to 30-degree angle with dominant hand.	Peripheral veins are easiest to access at the apex of the "Y" formed by merging veins or where veins are straight for several centimeters. Use a more obtuse (60-degree) angle for deeper veins.
6. Observe for blood flash in catheter hub.	This indicates successful vessel penetration.
7. Gently advance catheter into vessel lumen until the hub is flush against the skin.	See **Figure 31-2**. If you meet resistance, withdraw the catheter slightly, as it may have penetrated the posterior vessel wall.
8. Remove tourniquet.	—
9. Attach IV tubing and monitor for flow.	—
10. Secure catheter with tape and a sterile transparent dressing.	—

US-GUIDED PERIPHERAL ACCESS

US can localize veins with inconsistent anatomic relationships or those too deep to palpate. US-guided peripheral IV placement results in high success rates, few complications, and a decreased need for central vein cannulation.[5,6] The cephalic and brachial veins, which are not readily palpable, are easily located and cannulated using US guidance.

When inserting an IV using US guidance, use a high-frequency linear transducer. Vascular structures are anechoic (black) in US imaging. Key sonographic characteristics help distinguish veins from arteries. Veins are more easily compressed, have thinner walls, and have no arterial pulsation. Color flow may also help differentiate between the two structures. A centimeter scale on the US monitor indicates the depth of the vessel.

To locate a vessel, view it in short axis (transverse plane) and long axis (sagittal plane), then center the vessel on the screen. The midpoint of the screen correlates with the midpoint of the transducer. Introduce the catheter into the skin at the transducer's midpoint and direct it toward the vessel lumen. Use a longer catheter (2.5 in. or 6.4 cm) for deeper vessels. Watch the screen as the catheter enters the vessel lumen. Secure the catheter and apply a sterile dressing to the IV line.

TABLE 31-1 Materials for Peripheral IV Line Placement

Personal protective equipment (gloves, face shield)
Tourniquet
Alcohol swabs or povidone iodine
Appropriate-sized venous catheter
IV solution and tubing (if indicated)
2 × 2 gauze
Tape
Sterile transparent dressing

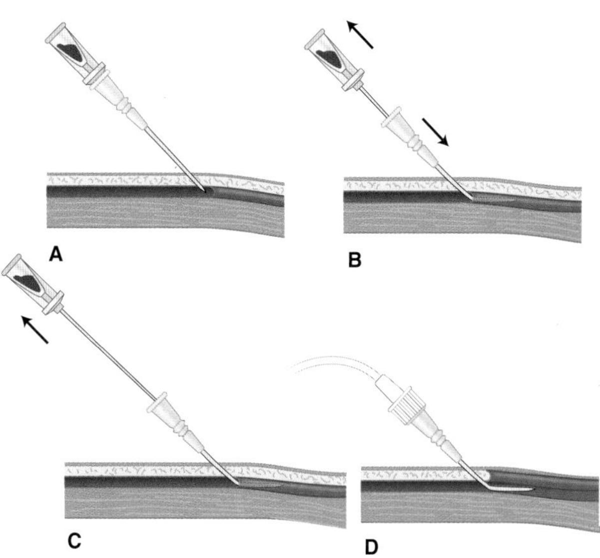

FIGURE 31-2. Catheter-over-needle technique for venous access. A. Catheter needle is inserted into skin and vessel until blood flash. B. Catheter is advanced. C. Needle is withdrawn. D. Catheter is attached to IV tubing and secured.

CENTRAL VENOUS ACCESS

The indications for central venous catheterization are listed in **Table 31-4**. The indication for direct central venous access in the setting of resuscitation of cardiac arrest is debated.

CENTRAL VENOUS ANATOMY

The most frequent sites used for central venous access are the internal jugular, subclavian, and femoral veins (**Figures 31-3 and 31-4**). The external jugular vein, a superficial structure, also provides a route to the central circulation but is technically a peripheral site.

The clavicles, first ribs, sternum, sternocleidomastoid, platysma, and other strap muscles of the neck overlie the internal jugular and subclavian veins (Figure 31-3). The internal jugular vein lies lateral to the internal carotid artery inside the carotid sheath. The internal jugular vein joins the subclavian vein to form the brachiocephalic vein.

The subclavian vein crosses under the clavicle at the medial to proximal third of the clavicle. The subclavian artery lies posterior and superior to the brachiocephalic vein. The thoracic duct joins the left subclavian vein at its junction with the left internal jugular vein. The domes of the pleura lie posterior and inferior to the subclavian veins and medial to the anterior scalene muscles.

The femoral vein is the most accessible central vein below the waist. It travels in the femoral sheath with the femoral artery, nerve, and lymphatics deep to the medial third of the inguinal ligament. A mnemonic for the anatomy of the femoral structures from lateral to medial is NAVEL: nerve, artery, vein, empty space, and lymphatics.

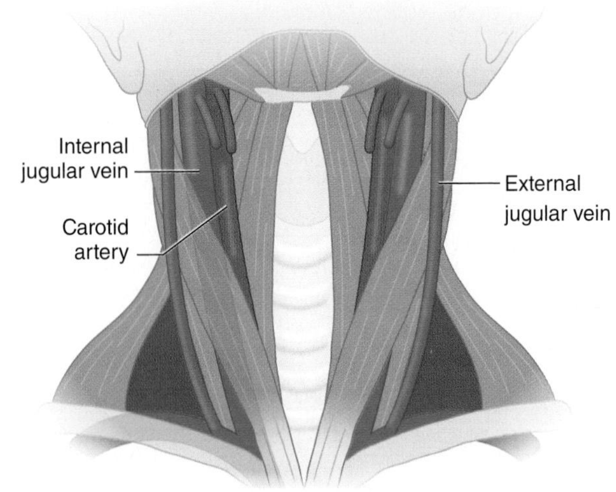

FIGURE 31-3. Vascular anatomy of the neck.

TABLE 31-3 Complications of Peripheral Venous Access

Complication	Comment
Hematoma formation and pain	Prevent hematomas by removing the tourniquet before needle removal and applying direct pressure to site after removal.
Extravasation of fluids	Apply cool or warm compresses and elevate extremity. Monitor site for tissue damage and necrosis.
Phlebitis (vein inflammation)	Occurs in 2%–13% of catheterized veins.[3,4] Presents as discomfort or pain at the catheter site with warmth, erythema, and tenderness along the vein. A palpable cord may also be present. Give anti-inflammatory medications. Apply warm compresses.
Cellulitis	Infection rates with peripheral IVs are relatively low. Typical organisms include *Staphylococcus epidermidis*, *S. aureus*, and *Candida*. Treat with antibiotics effective against suspected pathogens. Infection can be reduced by using sterile technique during IV placement and routine handling.
Neurovascular injury	—
Bacteremia/sepsis	—
Deep vein thrombosis	—
Tissue necrosis	—

TABLE 31-4 Indications for Central Venous Catheterization

Inability to obtain peripheral access
Access to central circulation needed for procedures (pulmonary artery catheter placement, transvenous pacemaker placement, or urgent hemodialysis)
Measurement of central venous pressure (sepsis, congestive heart failure, pericardial effusion)
Administration of sclerosing medications, continuous vasopressors, concentrated ionic solutions, or cytotoxic chemotherapeutic agents

TECHNIQUE FOR CENTRAL VENOUS ACCESS

After gaining consent if possible, identify the access site and approach and position the patient. Prepare all materials before the procedure (**Table 31-5**). Use a procedure checklist to optimize infection prevention practices.

The technique for all approaches is summarized in **Table 31-6** and depicted in **Figure 31-5**.

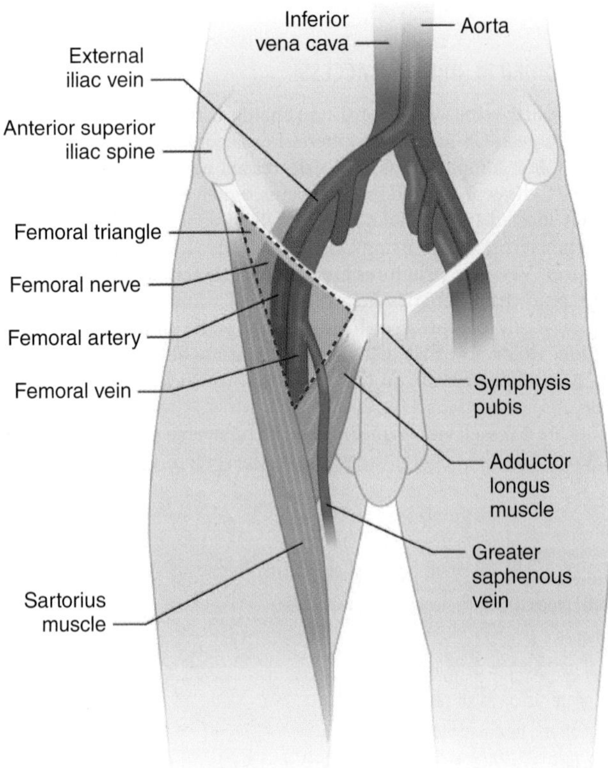

FIGURE 31-4. Vascular anatomy of the torso and lower extremities.

TABLE 31-5 Materials for Central Venous Catheterization

Sterile personal protective gear (gloves, gown, mask, hair cover)
Sterile drape and towels
Sterile prep solution (povidone-iodine or chlorhexidine)
3 × 10-mL syringes containing sterile normal saline flush
Central venous catheter set containing:
1% Lidocaine, small-gauge needle and syringe
18-Gauge introducer needle
Guidewire
#11 Blade scalpel
Venodilator
Single- or multilumen catheter
4 × 4 gauze pads
3-0 or 4-0 silk suture with straight needle or with needle driver
Sterile transparent dressing

COMPLICATIONS

Complications of central venous catheterization are listed in **Table 31-7**.

Complication rates increase with each additional attempt or percutaneous puncture. Accidental arterial puncture during internal jugular cannulation can lead to hematoma formation and airway compromise. Carotid arterial puncture may result in acute plaque rupture and stroke in patients with known carotid artery stenosis or atherosclerosis. Femoral lines often become infected and thrombose (nearly 20% each in some studies) and so are avoided for longer use. Do not use the subclavian approach in patients with coagulopathy because accidental subclavian arterial puncture or injury is not amenable to direct vascular compression.

US-GUIDED CENTRAL VENOUS ACCESS

US-guided central venous access increases first attempt success rates and decreases the number of attempts needed for success when compared to the unassisted standard method. Complication rates are similar in both techniques. The technique of US-guided central venous access is similar to peripheral venous access described previously.

TECHNIQUES OF COMMONLY USED APPROACHES

External Jugular Vein The external jugular vein is readily available due to its superficial location in the subcutaneous tissue overlying the sternocleidomastoid muscle. Place the patient in the head-down position or use Valsalva maneuvers to distend the vein and improve visualization. Entering a central vein via the external jugular vein is difficult and rarely successful without using a J wire; it is often not required because the site accommodates large-volume flow. Puncture the skin at a 10-degree angle. Placement is aided by tilting the head to the contralateral side, applying skin traction to "straighten" the course of the vein, and by rotating the guidewire 180 degrees before re-advancement if the first pass fails.

Internal Jugular Vein • *US-Guided Approach* The internal jugular vein is easily located with US guidance.

Place the probe on the sternocleidomastoid muscle (**Figure 31-6**). Identify the thyroid gland and carotid artery in addition to the internal jugular vein. Do not attempt needle insertion before visualizing all three structures.

Traditional Approaches The three traditional approaches to internal jugular vein catheterization are central, posterior, and anterior. The right internal jugular has a shorter, straighter course to the superior vena cava and avoids injury to the thoracic duct on the left; use this site unless contraindications exist.

Central Approach Place the patient in Trendelenburg position, head slightly tilted to the contralateral side. The landmark for the central approach is the triangle created by the clavicle and the sternal and clavicular heads of the sternocleidomastoid. The internal jugular vein lies just deep to this triangle. Insert the needle at a 30- to 45-degree angle to the skin, 1 cm below the apex of the triangle, parallel to the carotid artery located medially, and directed toward the ipsilateral nipple (**Figure 31-7**). Successful venous return typically occurs within 1 to 3 cm of needle advancement.

Posterior Approach The landmark for the posterior approach is the lateral aspect of the clavicular portion of the sternocleidomastoid, one third of the distance from the clavicle to the mastoid process. The needle is directed toward the sternal notch (**Figure 31-8**). Successful venous return typically occurs within 3 to 5 cm of needle advancement.

Anterior Approach Identify the pulse and course of the carotid artery, which lies just medial to the site of entry for the anterior approach. Hold the carotid artery with fingers of the nondominant hand. Hold the needle and syringe in the dominant hand at an angle of 30 to 45 degrees and enter at the midpoint of the medial aspect of the sternal portion of the sternocleidomastoid muscle. Aim the needle toward the ipsilateral nipple (**Figure 31-9**). Successful venous return typically occurs within 3 to 5 cm of needle advancement.

See **Table 31-8** for a summary of traditional approaches to internal jugular vein catheterization.

Subclavian Vein The location of the subclavian vein allows patient mobility and is an excellent choice for longer-term use.

US-Guided Approach The supraclavicular approach allows good sonographic visualization of the proximal subclavian vein anatomy. The infraclavicular approach to US-guided subclavian vein catheter placement is limited by the large acoustic shadow created by the clavicle (**Figure 31-10**).

Traditional Approaches The two traditional approaches to the catheterization of the subclavian vein are the infraclavicular and supraclavicular (**Figure 31-11**).

Infraclavicular Approach Place the patient head down and in a neutral position with a small towel under the thoracic spine to help identify the clavicle. The landmark for the site of entry is the junction of the middle and medial thirds of the clavicle. Orient the bevel of the needle inferomedially to direct the guidewire to the brachiocephalic trunk rather than the internal jugular vein. Align the numbered markings on the syringe with the bevel of the needle to guide the orientation of the bevel once the needle has breached the skin. Place the index finger of the nondominant hand at the suprasternal notch and the thumb at the midpoint of the clavicle. Direct the needle toward the suprasternal notch at a 10-degree angle parallel to the surface of the chest (**Figure 31-12**). If the clavicle is encountered, "walk" the needle down the clavicle until the needle is posterior to it. Successful venous return occurs typically at a depth of 3 to 5 cm.

Supraclavicular Approach The supraclavicular approach is often referred to as the "pocket-shot." The supraclavicular approach has fewer failures, fewer catheter malpositions, and less interference with CPR than the

Preprocedure Checklist for Central Line Access

Before the procedure, did the provider:

- Perform a time out to ensure right patient, right location/side?
- Cleanse hands immediately prior?
- Sterilize procedure site and allow site to dry?
  - 30 s for dry site
  - 2 min for moist site (femoral)
- Drape the patient from head to toe with a large sterile drape?

During the procedure:

- Did the provider wear sterile gloves, cap, mask, and gown?
- Did assisting physician(s) follow the above precautions?
- Did the provider maintain sterility of tray, site, field, and gloves at all times?
- Did ALL staff in room wear a mask?
- Was unnecessary traffic in and out of the room prevented during the procedure (did the door remain closed)?

After the procedure, did the provider:

- Apply a dated sterile dressing?

TABLE 31-6 Seldinger Technique* for Insertion of Central Venous Line

Step	Comments
1. Gown in sterile fashion.	Use sterile gloves and gown. Wear mask and hair covering.
2. Identify vessel—US guidance preferred over landmarks.	—
3. Prep and drape patient using standard sterile procedure.	Prep a wide area so an alternate site can be used if initial attempts fail. Prep the entire ipsilateral neck and upper chest when preparing to insert an internal jugular or subclavian catheter.
4. Open the central catheter kit. Inspect for content in a sterile fashion. Place kit close to bedside and operator. Maintain sterile conditions.	—
5. Anesthetize area in all conscious patients.	Inject area with 1%–2% lidocaine. Anesthetize the periosteum of the clavicle if using the subclavian approach. Reorient to landmarks after injection.
6. Hold the 18-gauge introducer needle on a 10-mL syringe in the dominant hand and align the needle to the target.	—
7. Advance the needle slowly though the skin and subcutaneous tissue until a flash of dark venous blood appears.	Maintain steady constant aspiration of syringe.
8. Stabilize the needle with the nondominant hand.	—
9. Check for continued free venous flow with aspiration.	If no flow is noted, withdraw the needle slightly, as the needle may have breached the posterior vessel wall.
10. Remove the syringe attached to the needle and immediately occlude the catheter with a finger.	This maneuver helps to prevent introducing air in the catheter and subsequent central system air embolism.
11. Insert the guidewire gently through the needle. Always maintain a firm grip on the wire—do not let go of the wire for any reason.	The wire should advance with minimal resistance. Do not force the wire for any reason. If the wire does not pass easily, reattach the syringe and aspirate to confirm continued venous flow. Reposition the needle as needed. Premature ventricular contractions or dysrhythmias during wire advancement may indicate that the wire is in the right atrium or beyond.
12. Remove the needle over the wire when the guidewire is inserted at least 10 cm into the vessel.	—
13. Incise the skin with a #11 blade scalpel at the entry site to accommodate the venodilator or catheter.	Do not cut the guidewire.
14. Advance the dilator or catheter over the guidewire into the vessel lumen with a gentle twisting motion.	—
15. Remove the dilator (if used), and advance the catheter over the wire until the wire is advanced through the distal port.	Maintain a grip on the guidewire during this procedure.
16. Grab the end of the guidewire.	—
17. Advance the catheter to the appropriate depth.	—
18. Remove the guidewire.	It is easy to "lose" the wire; if you cannot find it after a procedure, immediately obtain an x-ray to seek retention.
19. Aspirate and flush all ports to confirm catheter function.	—
20. Secure catheter with suture and apply a sterile transparent dressing.	—
21. Confirm catheter placement in the superior vena cava with chest x-ray.	A catheter tip in the right atrium can perforate the right atrium and cause hemothorax or hemomediastinum with pericardial tamponade. Examine the chest x-ray for signs of complications.

infraclavicular approach. It may also be performed in the upright position in patients unable to lay supine in the setting of severe orthopnea.

The landmark for entry is 1 cm lateral to the clavicular head of the sternocleidomastoid and 1 cm posterior to the clavicle. Enter at an angle of 10 degrees above horizontal. Orient the bevel of the needle medially, bisecting the angle formed by the clavicle and sternocleidomastoid toward the contralateral nipple. Successful venous return typically occurs at a depth of 2 to 3 cm (**Figure 31-13**).

COMPLICATIONS

The risk of pneumothorax is higher when cannulating the subclavian vein. If attempts at subclavian venous access fail on one side, assess for pneumothorax using chest x-ray or US before attempting cannulation on the contralateral side.

Femoral Vein The femoral vein is the most accessible central access site during critical illness, notably cardiac arrest.

US-Guided Approach Place the transducer in a transverse position just below the midportion of the inguinal ligament. Identify the femoral vein just below the inguinal ligament and medial to the femoral arterial pulsation. The vein is more easily compressed than the artery. The relationship among the vessels varies depending on limb position (**Figure 31-14**).

Traditional Approach Place the patient supine in reverse Trendelenburg position with the hip slightly abducted and leg slightly externally

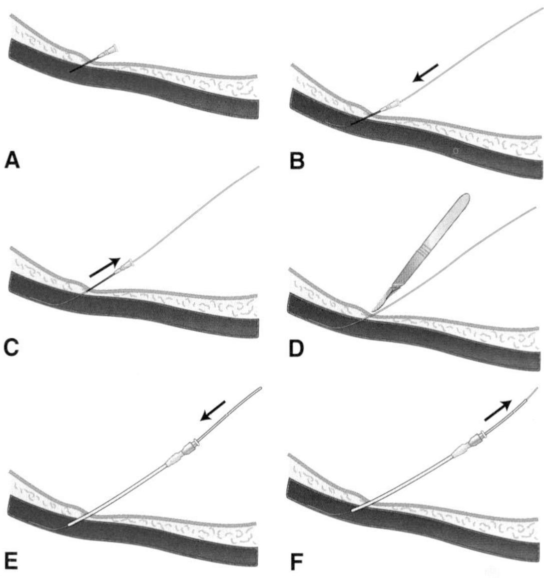

FIGURE 31-5. Seldinger technique. A. Needle is inserted through skin and vessel until venous blood is aspirated. B. Guidewire is inserted gently through the needle and advanced. C. Needle is removed over guidewire. D. The skin is incised. E. Dilator or catheter is inserted over the guidewire. F. The guidewire is removed.

TABLE 31-7 Complications of Central Venous Catheterization
Pneumothorax
Arterial puncture
Malpositioning
Catheter-associated infection
Thrombosis
Chylothorax (injury to the thoracic duct on left-sided attempts)
Hydrothorax/hydromediastinum (infusion into the pleural space)
Air emboli
Great vessel or right atrial perforation (hemothorax, tamponade)
Airway compromise (tracheal injury, hematoma with airway compression)

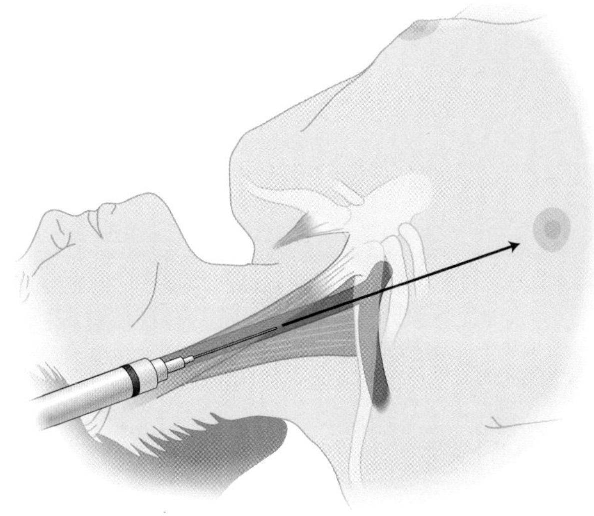

FIGURE 31-7. Central approach to the internal jugular vein.

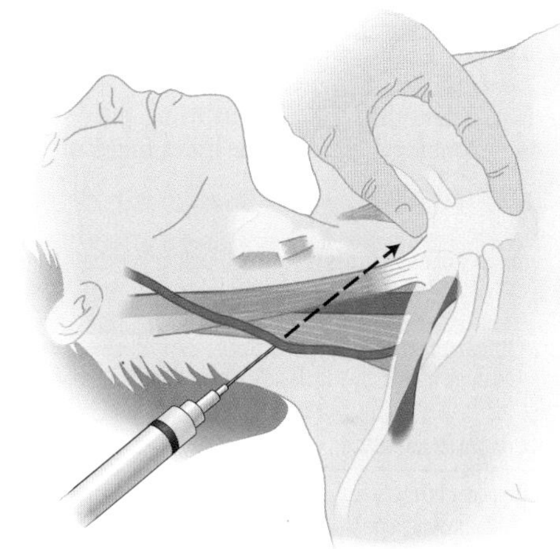

FIGURE 31-8. Posterior approach to the internal jugular vein.

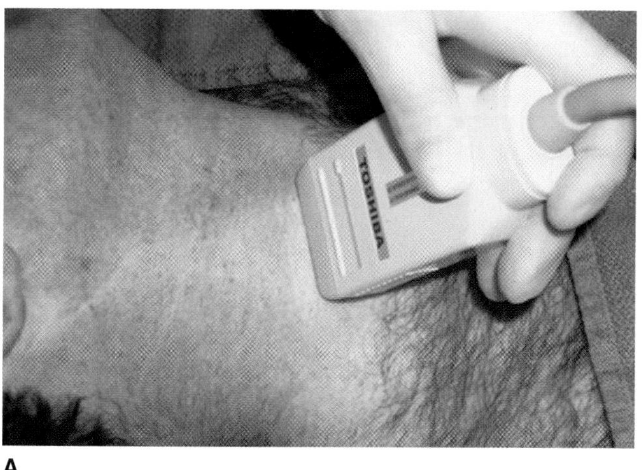

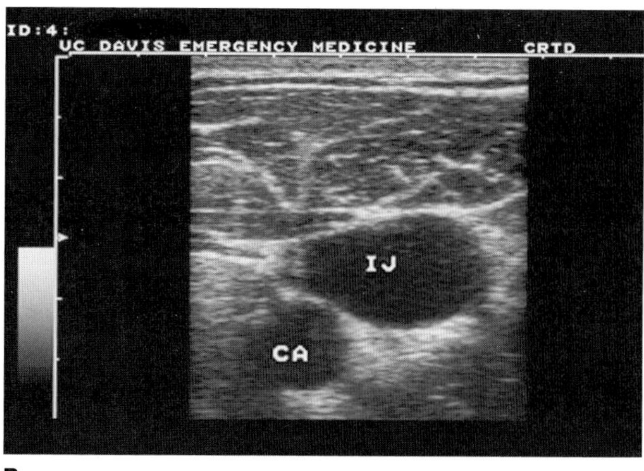

FIGURE 31-6. US-guided localization of the internal jugular vein. US image of the large internal jugular vein and deeper carotid artery. Probe position (A) and corresponding US image (B). CA = carotid artery; IJ = internal jugular vein.

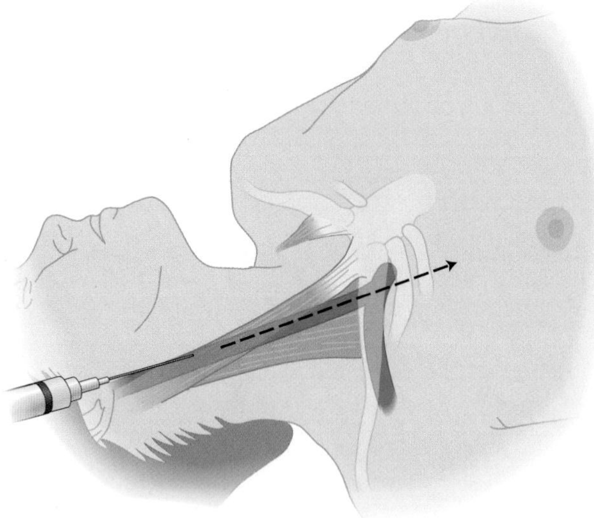

FIGURE 31-9. Anterior approach to the internal jugular vein.

rotated.[7,8] Palpate the femoral artery, if possible. Classically, the femoral vein is just medial to the femoral artery and 1 to 2 cm below the inguinal ligament, although US often demonstrates an anomalous position, which is one reason why landmark-based insertions are less successful (**Figure 31-15**). Use a 45-degree angle of approach.

In pulseless arrest, locate the femoral vein using the "V" technique. Place the thumb on the pubic tubercle and the index finger on the anterior superior iliac spine. The femoral vein is typically located at the interdigital space (the "V" of the finger and thumb) just inferior to the inguinal ligament.

Always insert the needle below the inguinal ligament, because vascular injury above the inguinal ligament may cause severe hidden hemorrhage into the retroperitoneal space.

Limit femoral vein cannulation because of the higher complication rates (notably infection and thrombosis) and the limits it places on patient mobility.

TABLE 31-8 Summary of Approaches to Internal Jugular Vein Catheterization

	Landmarks	Direction of Aim	Depth of Vein (cm)
Central	Apex of triangle formed by the clavicle and sternal and clavicular components of the sternocleidomastoid muscle	Ipsilateral nipple	1–3
Posterior	Lateral aspect of the clavicular portion of the sternocleidomastoid, one third of the distance from the clavicle to the mastoid process	Sternal notch	3–5
Anterior	Midpoint of the medial aspect of the sternal portion of the sternocleidomastoid, lateral to the carotid artery	Ipsilateral nipple	3–5

VENOUS CUTDOWN

Venous cutdown is typically performed on the saphenous vein, anterior and superior to the medial malleolus.

IO VASCULAR ACCESS

IO vascular access is used in patients of all ages when venous access cannot be quickly and reliably established during circulatory collapse.[8] The commercial EZ-IO® (Vidacare Corp., San Antonio, TX) eases procedure performance (**Figure 31-16**). Contraindications to IO access include proximal ipsilateral fracture, ipsilateral vascular injury, and severe osteoporosis or osteogenesis imperfecta.

TECHNIQUE FOR IO ACCESS

Use either a standard bone marrow aspiration needle or specialized IO infusion needle. In children, the site of entry is two finger-widths (2 cm) below the tibial tuberosity on the medial, flat surface of the proximal tibia (**Figure 31-17**). Use other sites, such as the medial malleolus, distal femur, sternum, humerus, and ileum, in adults, because the tibia is thick and difficult to penetrate.

The procedure for manual insertion of IO venous needles is summarized in **Table 31-9** and illustrated in **Figure 31-18**.

COMPLICATIONS

Complications of IO access include cellulitis, osteomyelitis, iatrogenic fracture or physeal plate injury, and fat embolism (rare).

ENDOTRACHEAL SUBSTITUTION FOR VASCULAR ACCESS

A number of medications can be administered via the endotracheal tube in the critical minutes of resuscitation before IV access is obtained. These medications include lidocaine, epinephrine, atropine,

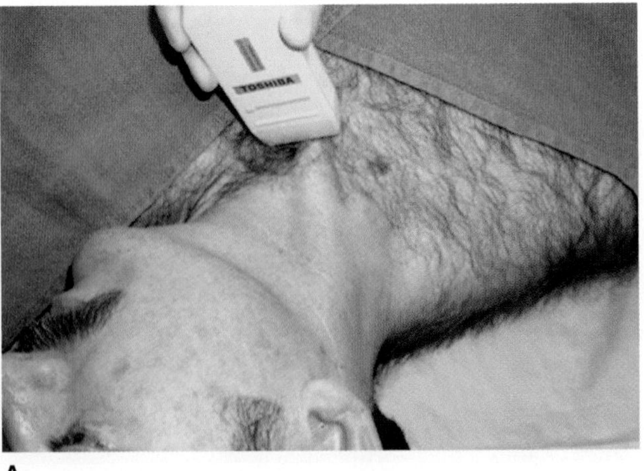

A

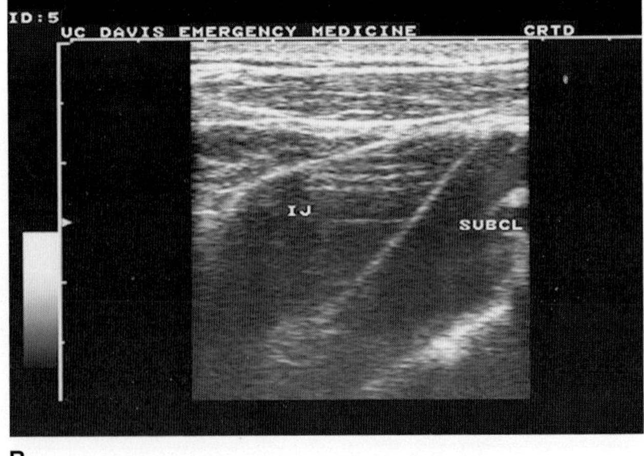

B

FIGURE 31-10. US-guided localization of the subclavian vein. A. Placement of the transducer to facilitate visualization of the internal jugular/subclavian vein junction using a supraclavicular approach. In some patients, a more lateral probe position is required. B. Transverse view of the "venous lake" created by the combined subclavian (SUBCL) vein and internal jugular (IJ) vein.

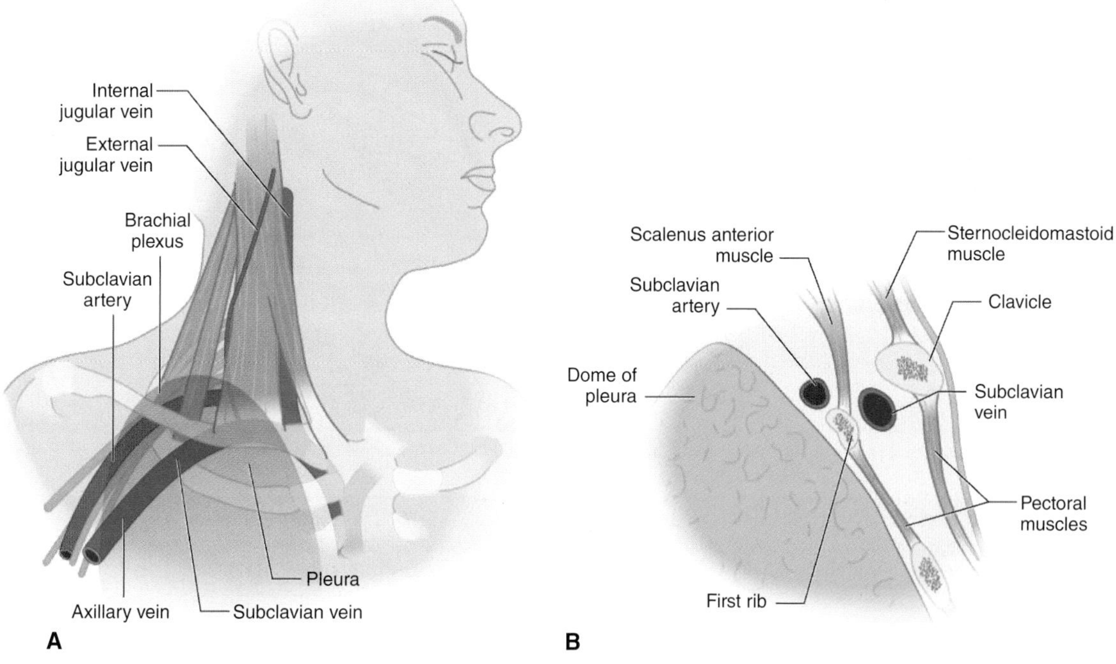

FIGURE 31-11. Anatomy of the subclavian vein. A. Anatomy of the subclavian vein. B. Cross-section of the subclavian vein with its relation to the clavicle.

and naloxone (mnemonic LEAN). The most commonly administered medication is epinephrine, given as a high-concentration preparation of 1 milligram/mL (1:1000) with a recommended dose of 2 to 2.5 milligrams in adults.[9]

Dosage recommendations are empirical and usually double or triple the standard IV dose[9] diluted in 3 to 5 mL of normal saline. After injecting the medication down the tube, administer several positive-pressure ventilations with a bag-to-tube device.

Outcomes after endotracheal drug administration during cardiac arrest are inferior to IV administration.[10] With other access techniques possible, notably IO, this route has little utility even in cardiac arrest.

ARTERIAL ACCESS

The indications for arterial line placement are listed in **Table 31-10**.

RADIAL ARTERY ANATOMY

The most common site for arterial line placement is the radial artery due to the ease of identifying its location and its accessibility at the wrist. The collateral artery blood supply provided by the arterial artery lowers the risk of complications (**Figure 31-19**). The anatomic landmarks for the radial artery are medial to the radial styloid process and lateral to the flexor carpi radialis tendon at the proximal flexor crease of the wrist. **A palpable radial pulse should be felt, and radial and ulnar artery compression tests (release of latter to assess collateral circulation, looking for hand to "pink up" rapidly—called the Allen test) are done prior to any puncture**, although the latter test has a limited ability to predict later ischemic complications.

FEMORAL ARTERY ANATOMY

As discussed in the section on femoral central venous access, the femoral artery lies in the femoral triangle inferior to the inguinal ligament, midway between the pubic symphysis and the anterior superior iliac spine (Figure 31-4). A longer catheter is typically needed to cannulate the deeper femoral artery compared to the radial artery.

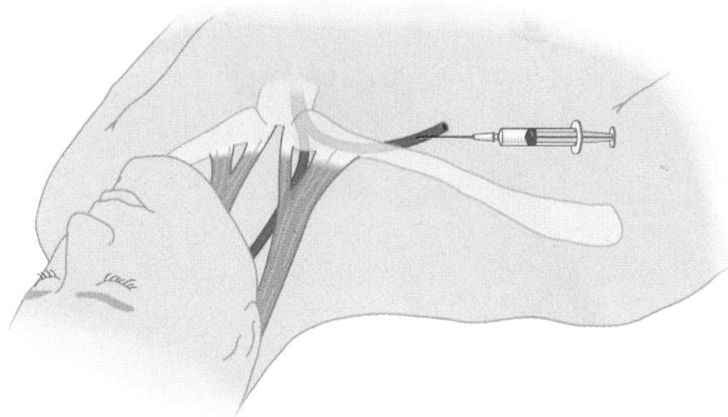

FIGURE 31-12. Infraclavicular approach to the subclavian vein.

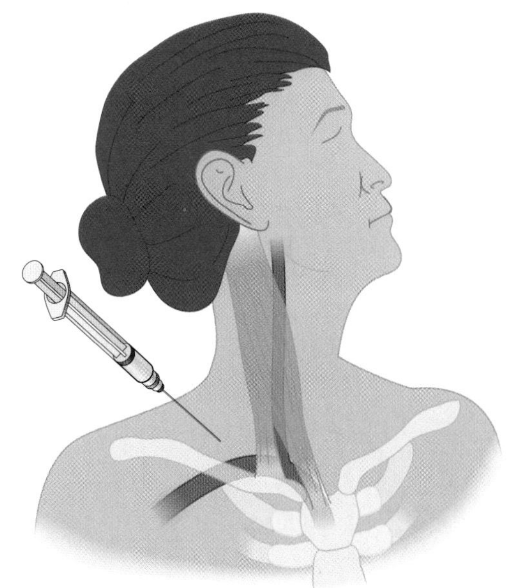

FIGURE 31-13. Supraclavicular approach to the subclavian vein.

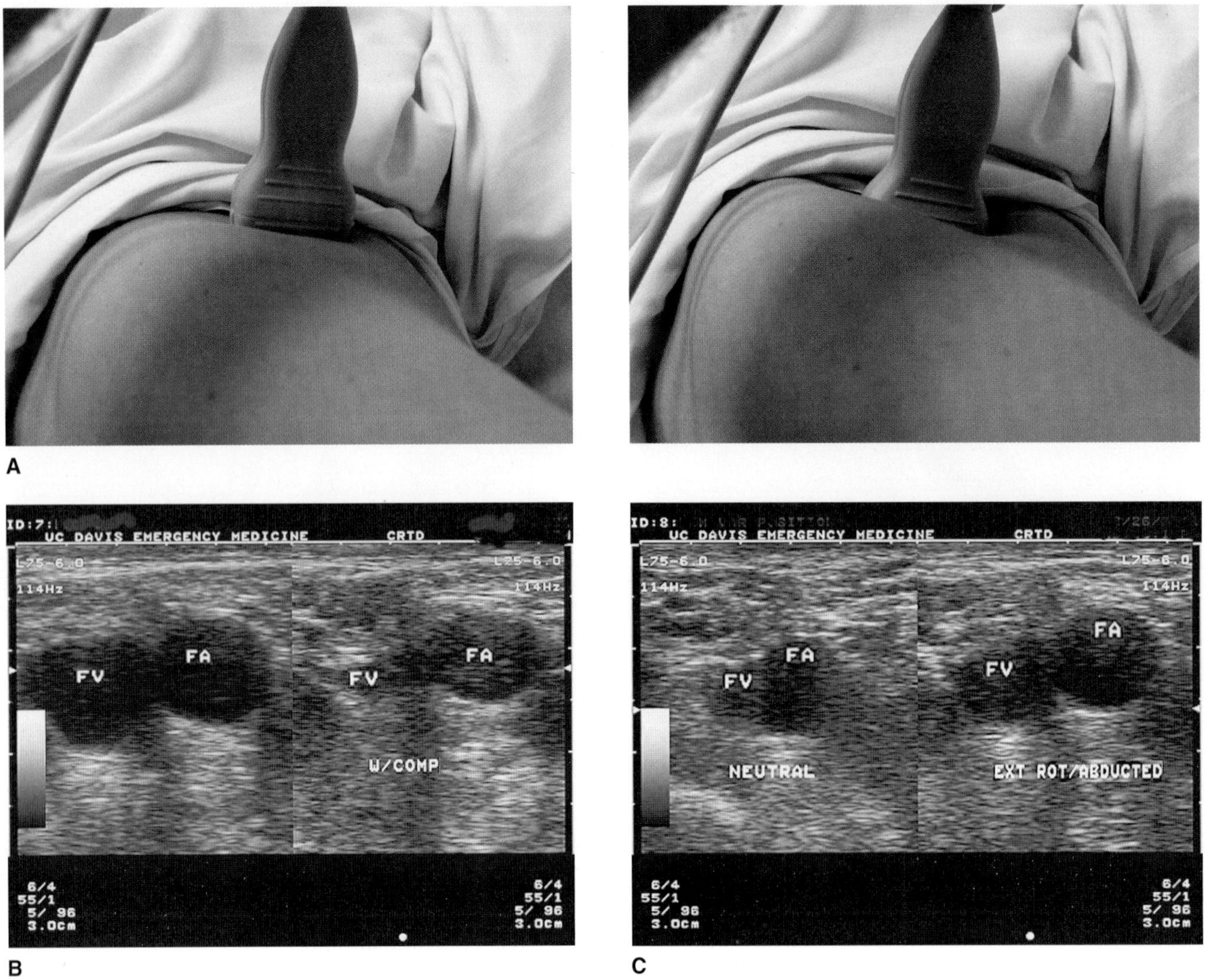

A

B

C

FIGURE 31-14. US-guided localization of the femoral vein. A. Gentle pressure is applied to the transducer to identify venous structures by their easy compressibility. B. Femoral vein (FV) collapses with compression, and the femoral artery (FA) retains its shape even with compression. C. FV position is seen to vary with hip abduction and external rotation. In neutral position (*left frame*), the vein is closely opposed to the FA; however, when the hip is abducted and rotated, the vein is displaced from the artery (*right frame*). [Part A used with permission of Michael Blaivas, MD.]

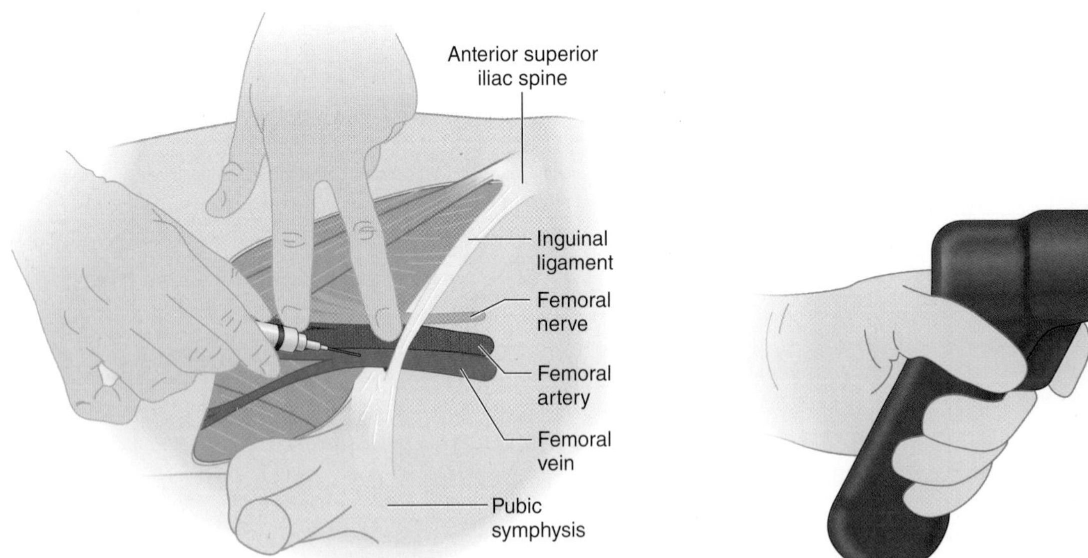

FIGURE 31-15. Technique for femoral vein access.

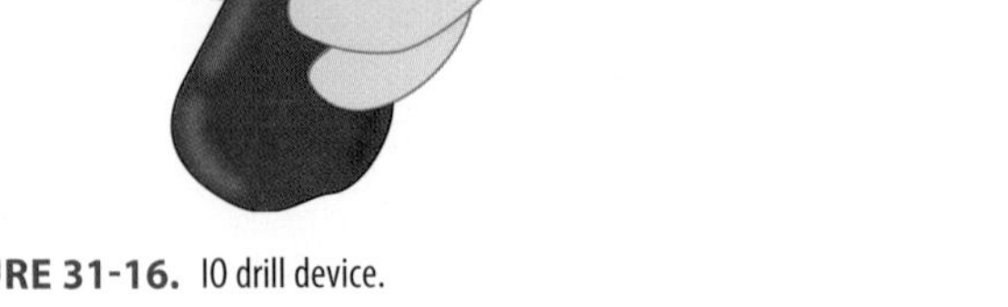

FIGURE 31-16. IO drill device.

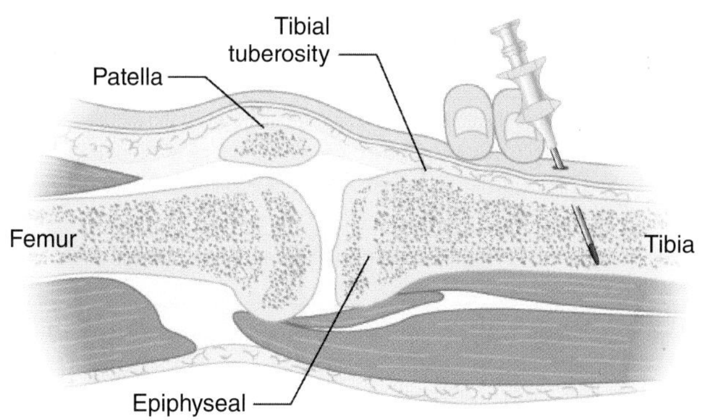

FIGURE 31-17. Location for IO placement in the proximal tibia.

TABLE 31-9 Procedure for Manual IO Venous Access

Prepare site using routine sterile fashion.
Infiltrate area with 1%–2% lidocaine to anesthetize the skin and periosteum if the patient is conscious.
Support and stabilize the leg with the nondominant hand.
Grasp the needle in the palm of the dominant hand.
Direct the needle perpendicular to the bone and away from the joint space (to avoid injury to the physeal plate in pediatric patients).
Twist and apply constant pressure until resistance is abruptly decreased and the marrow cavity is breached.
Remove the stylet.
Confirm placement by either aspiration or continuous infusion.
Observe for signs of extravasation (Figure 31-18).
Secure the IO needle with gauze and a bulky dressing.
Confirm placement and exclude iatrogenic fracture with x-ray after stabilizing the patient.

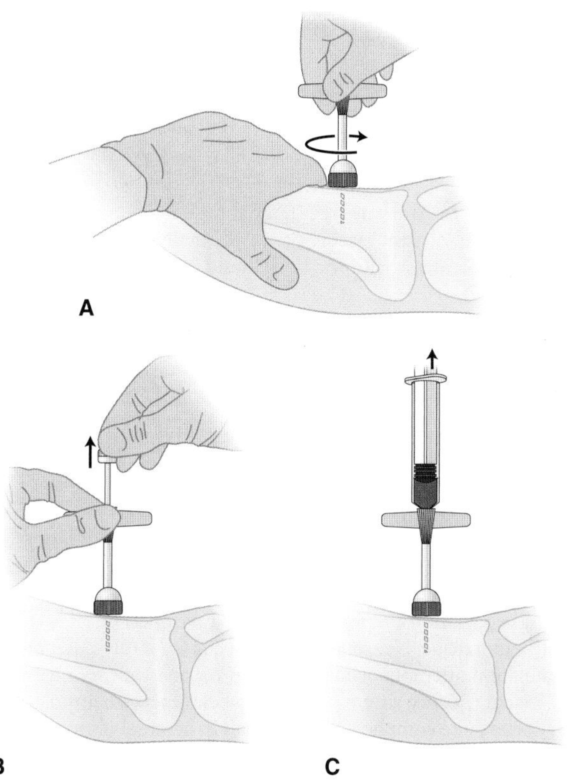

FIGURE 31-18. Technique for IO placement. A. Needle is directed perpendicular to the bone with constant pressure and a twisting motion. B. Stylet is removed. C. Placement is confirmed with successful aspiration.

TABLE 31-10 Indications for Arterial Catheter Placement

Frequent laboratory testing, including arterial blood gas sampling for acid-base status or monitoring of oxygen saturations and carbon dioxide levels in patients with respiratory failure
Need for accurate, moment-to-moment blood pressure monitoring in hypotensive patients, patients on vasopressors, or hypertensive patients with intracranial hemorrhages or vascular catastrophes (i.e., aortic dissections, abdominal aortic aneurysms)

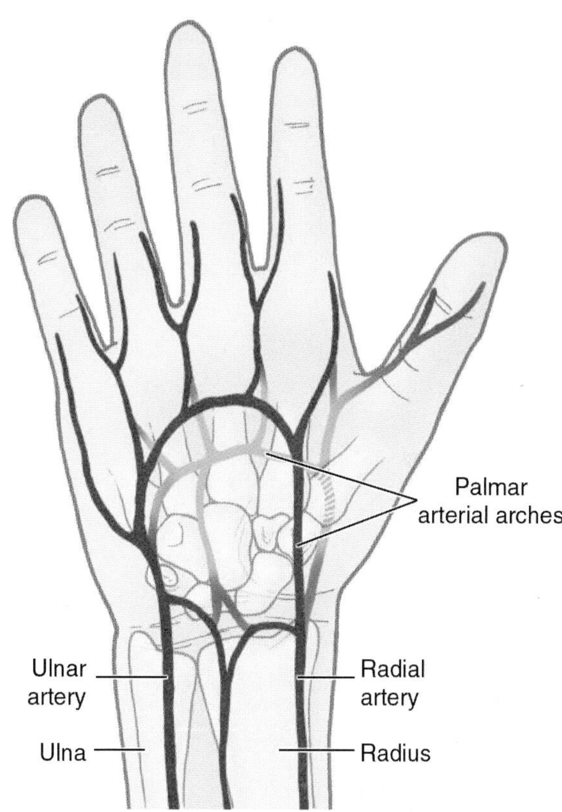

FIGURE 31-19. Arterial anatomy of the wrist and hand. [Reproduced with permission from Reichman EF: *Emergency Medicine Procedures*, 2nd ed. Chapter 57. Arterial Puncture and Cannulation. McGraw-Hill, Inc., 2013, Figure 57-1.]

ALTERNATIVE ARTERIAL SITES

Other sites for arterial catheter placement include the dorsalis pedis artery and the brachial artery. Similar to the radial artery, the dorsalis pedis artery is superficial and easy to identify, and the foot has collateral circulation similar to the hand. The brachial artery is located just medial to the biceps brachii muscle in the antecubital fossa adjacent to the medial nerve. The lack of collateral blood flow at the level of the brachial

TABLE 31-11 Materials for Arterial Access

Sterile personal protective gear (gloves, gown, mask, hair covering)
Sterile towels
Povidone-iodine or chlorhexidine cleaning solution
1% Lidocaine, small-gauge needle, and syringe (e.g., a 1-mL tuberculin syringe)
20-Gauge angiocatheter or integral-guidewire arterial catheter
4 × 4 gauze
3-0 or 4-0 nylon suture with straight needle or needle driver
Sterile transparent dressing
Arterial line setup (pressure bag, saline, tubing, transducer, and flushing system)

TABLE 31-12 Technique for Artery Cannulation

Step	Comments
1. Position the patient for the procedure.	For radial artery approach, the wrist is extended. A towel roll under the dorsal wrist can maintain this position. See Figure 31-20. For femoral artery approach, the hip is slightly abducted and leg slightly externally rotated. See Figure 31-4.
2. Gown in standard sterile fashion.	Use sterile gloves and gown. Wear mask and hair covering. **Do not stand in direct line of the catheter.**
3. Identify artery using either landmarks or US guidance.	A palpable pulse is a must for landmark approach. Palpate pulse with 2 fingers of nondominant hand.
4. Prep and drape patient using standard sterile procedure.	Improper sterile technique increases risk of infection.
5. Anesthetize area in all conscious patients.	Inject 1% lidocaine with 1-mL tuberculin syringe.
6. Hold the 20-gauge angiocatheter or integral-guidewire catheter in the dominant hand at a 30- to 45-degree angle to the skin surface.	For direct angiocatheter cannulation, see Figure 31-21. For use of an integral-guidewire catheter see Figure 31-22.
7. Advance the needle slowly through the skin and subcutaneous tissue until pulsatile red blood return is obtained.	—
8. Stabilize the needle with the nondominant hand.	—
9. If an integral-guidewire catheter is used, advance the wire with the dominant hand.	If resistance is encountered, STOP advancing the guidewire immediately, withdraw the entire unit, and apply pressure to the puncture site.
10. Advance the catheter over the needle (or needle and guidewire if used).	A gentle rotating motion of the catheter may be helpful.
11. Remove the needle or needle-guidewire unit and *immediately occlude the catheter with a finger.*	Occlusion prevents arterial blood loss and air embolism.
12. Attach arterial line setup/IV tubing to the catheter.	Be sure to have arterial line setup prepared prior to start of the procedure.
13. Secure catheter with suture and apply a sterile transparent dressing.	—
14. "Zero" the transducer.	Align the stopcock to the level of the heart. Turn the stopcock off to the patient and open to air. Adjust the monitor display to zero.
15. Monitor for signs of bleeding, hematoma, or infection.	Assess the continued need for the arterial line daily.

artery increases the risk of upper extremity ischemia and is avoided for this reason.

TECHNIQUE FOR ARTERIAL ACCESS

After explaining the procedure and gaining consent, identify the access site and approach and position the patient with all materials at the bedside (**Table 31-11**).

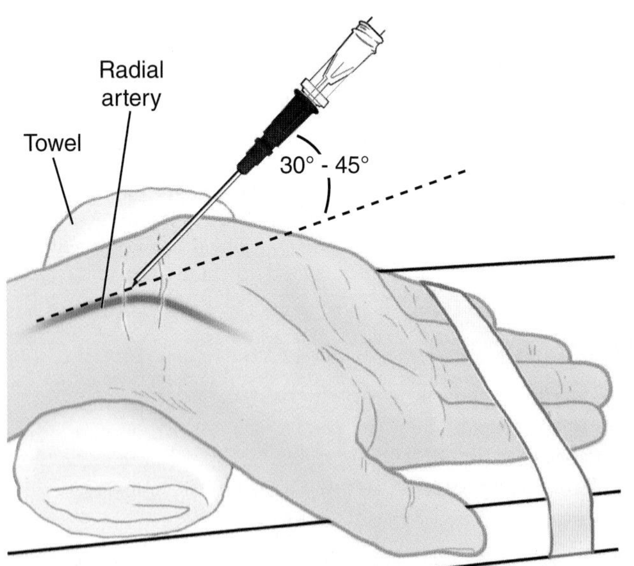

FIGURE 31-20. Correct positioning for radial artery cannulation. Flexion of the wrist is supported by a dorsal towel roll. [Reproduced with permission from Reichman EF: *Emergency Medicine Procedures*, 2nd ed. Chapter 57. Arterial Puncture and Cannulation. McGraw-Hill, Inc., 2013, Figure 57-5.]

The technique for all approaches is summarized in **Table 31-12** and **Figures 31-20, 31-21,** and **31-22**. The direct puncture approach is less likely successful, takes longer, and requires more puncture attempts than the integral wire approach.

POSTPROCEDURE CARE

Secure the arterial catheter to the skin either by suture or adhesive catheter locking device with a sterile transparent protective dressing placed over the site. An arm board or wrist splint may aid securing a radial artery line. Monitor the site regularly for dislodgment, hematoma, bleeding, infection, or distal ischemia. The dressing should be changed regularly, and the necessity for the line should be determined daily.

COMPLICATIONS

The complications of peripheral venous access are listed in **Table 31-13. The first step in treating all complications is catheter removal. Direct pressure should be applied a minimum of 3 to 5 minutes after removal at all peripheral sites and 10 minutes for a femoral site.**

Air embolization from an arterial catheter is more likely to have adverse sequelae than from venous catheterization because of no pulmonary filtration. Infection rates increase with poor aseptic technique and duration of catheter use. Thrombosis occurs in up to 25% of patients who have an arterial catheter, although clinical morbidity occurs in less than 1%. Femoral artery catheterization can lead to concealed retroperitoneal hematoma and major hemorrhage. Neuropathies can occur from direct nerve injury from cannulation attempts or hematoma formation causing nerve compression. Brachial artery sites can lead to median nerve neuropathy, and an axillary artery site complication can result in brachial plexopathy.

US-GUIDED ARTERIAL ACCESS

US-guided arterial puncture aids cannulation, especially when a palpable pulse is difficult to identify.[11] Key sonographic characteristics to

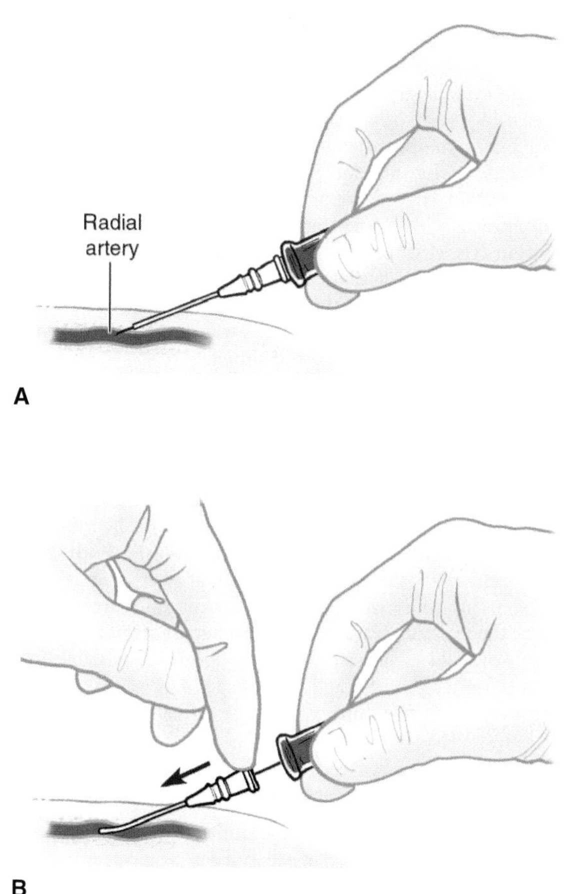

FIGURE 31-21. Direct angiocatheter technique for arterial cannulation. A. The angiocatheter and needle are held at a 30- to 45-degree angle to the skin with the dominant hand and advanced into the artery. B. The catheter is advanced over the needle and into the artery with the nondominant hand. [Reproduced with permission from Reichman EF: *Emergency Medicine Procedures*, 2nd ed. Chapter 57. Arterial Puncture and Cannulation. McGraw-Hill, Inc., 2013, Figure 57-7.]

TABLE 31-13 Complications of Arterial Access and Cannulation
Pain at site
Hematoma formation
Hemorrhage
Artery laceration/injury
Arterial vasospasm
Pseudoaneurysm formation
Arteriovenous fistula
Infection
Limb ischemia
Thrombosis/embolization
Nerve damage/neuropathy

identify arteries include round, pulsatile, thick-walled vessels that are difficult to compress.

REFERENCES

The complete reference list is available online at www.TintinalliEM.com.

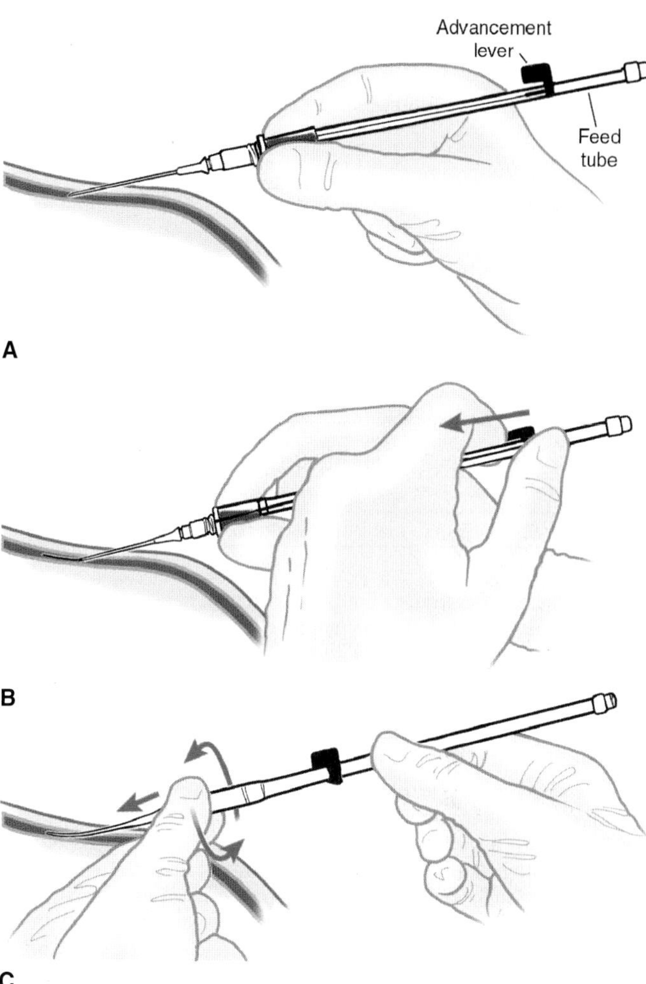

FIGURE 31-22. Integral-guidewire technique for arterial cannulation. A. The integral-catheter unit is held at a 30- to 45-degree angle to the skin and slowly advanced into the artery. B. The guidewire is advanced through the needle and into the artery with the nondominant hand. C. The catheter is advanced over the guidewire and into the artery with a gentle twisting motion. [Reproduced with permission from Reichman EF: *Emergency Medicine Procedures*, 2nd ed. Chapter 57. Arterial Puncture and Cannulation. McGraw-Hill, Inc., 2013, Figure 57-8.]

CHAPTER 32 Hemodynamic Monitoring

H. Bryant Nguyen
David T. Huang
Michael R. Pinsky

INTRODUCTION

Hemodynamic monitoring can identify cardiovascular insufficiency and ensure optimal treatment of the critically ill. Advanced techniques help identify and prioritize various causes of hemodynamic instability and can enable tailored interventions.

Hemodynamic monitoring changes therapeutic decisions in more than 50% of patients and can detect cryptic cardiovascular compromise. We will focus on techniques applicable to the ED: blood pressure monitoring, central venous pressure (CVP) monitoring, cardiac output (CO) monitoring, and blood oxygenation and organ perfusion monitoring (**Table 32-1**). Use of any technology must be associated with a therapy and a response to therapy—*functional hemodynamic monitoring*. Applying a technology

TABLE 32-1 Hemodynamic Variables Obtainable in the ED

Hemodynamic Variable	Method of Measurement
Hemoglobin oxygen saturation, %	Pulse oximetry, arterial blood gas analysis
Heart rate, beats/min	Physical examination, pulse oximetry, electrocardiography
Blood pressure, mm Hg	Sphygmomanometry, oscillometry, intra-arterial catheterization
Central venous pressure, mm Hg	Jugular venous pulsation, US, central venous catheterization
Cardiac output, L/min	Thoracic bioimpedance or bioreactance, esophageal Doppler US, transcutaneous Doppler US, pulse contour analysis, lithium dilution, transpulmonary (arterial) thermodilution, pulmonary artery thermodilution
Central venous oxygen saturation, %	Central venous catheterization for intermittent venous blood sampling or continuous measurement
Lactate, mmol/L	Arterial, venous, or capillary sampling
Tissue oxygen saturation, %	Near-infrared spectroscopy

without a therapeutic strategy limits any potential benefit. In practice, it is best to use more than one approach and monitor therapeutic responses (**Table 32-2**).[1]

ARTERIAL BLOOD PRESSURE

Blood pressure is the force exerted by the circulating blood through a blood vessel. Assessing arterial pressure is very important, as hypotension implies tissue hypoperfusion; shock is a state of organ hypoperfusion but is not always associated with hypotension. **Hypotension is always pathologic and reflects a failure of normal circulatory homeostatic mechanisms, whereas normotension does not necessarily indicate cardiovascular stability.** Normal blood pressure can occur in the setting of profound circulatory shock in the face of significant vasoconstriction or in a patient with antecedent high arterial pressure. For example, a patient in cardiogenic or hypovolemic shock may remain normotensive because of a marked increase in vascular resistance.

OPTIMAL BLOOD PRESSURE

Arterial pressure is the input pressure for organ perfusion and is a function of peripheral vascular resistance and blood flow. There is no absolute level of normal CO in the unstable, metabolically active patient because CO is proportional to metabolic demand. However, organ perfusion pressure becomes compromised as mean arterial pressure (MAP) decreases below 60 mm Hg and/or cardiac index (CO/body surface area) decreases below 2.0 L/min/m^2.

Optimal MAP varies depending on the underlying cause of hemodynamic instability. In distributive shock, such as refractory septic shock, increasing MAP >65 mm Hg with fluids and vasopressors increases oxygen delivery but does not improve outcome, indices of organ perfusion, or survival.[2]

TABLE 32-2 Hemodynamic Monitoring Principles[1]

No hemodynamic monitoring technique can improve outcome by itself.
Monitoring requirements may vary over time and can depend on local equipment availability and training.
There are no optimal hemodynamic values that are applicable to all patients.
We need to combine and integrate hemodynamic variables.
Measurements of Svo_2 can be helpful.
A high cardiac output and a high Svo_2 are not always best.
Cardiac output is estimated, not measured.
Monitoring hemodynamic changes over short periods of time is important.
Continuous measurement of all hemodynamic variables is preferable.
Noninvasiveness is not the only issue.

Abbreviation: Svo_2 = venous oxygen saturation.

The American College of Cardiology/American Heart Association guidelines in 2004 recommend targeting a systolic pressure of at least 80 mm Hg in patients with acute myocardial infarction. In traumatic brain injury, a systolic pressure <90 mm Hg is an independent predictor for increased morbidity and mortality. A higher blood pressure may be required to maintain optimal cerebral perfusion pressure of 50 to 70 mm Hg (cerebral perfusion pressure = MAP – intracranial pressure), such that MAP <80 mm Hg may be an independent predictor of worse outcome.[3] In patients with hemorrhagic shock, delayed fluid resuscitation and toleration of a MAP of 40 mm Hg until definitive surgical intervention may improve survival.[4] **The International Consensus Conference recommends a target MAP of 40 mm Hg in uncontrolled hemorrhage due to trauma, a MAP of 90 mm Hg for traumatic brain injury, and a MAP >65 mm Hg for other forms of shock.**[5]

NONINVASIVE BLOOD PRESSURE MEASUREMENT

Blood pressure varies with each heartbeat. The *systolic pressure* is the maximum pressure during ventricular ejection, and the *diastolic pressure* is the lowest pressure in the blood vessels between heartbeats during ventricular filling. Because the vascular circuit is elastic, both systolic and diastolic pressures vary throughout the vascular system. Systolic pressure can increase by up to 20 mm Hg, while the diastolic pressure similarly decreases as the pressure wave moves peripherally from the aorta. However, MAP (**Formula 1**) varies by only 1 to 2 mm Hg, whether measured centrally or peripherally; in practice, estimate MAP using the sum of the diastolic pressure and one third of the pulse pressure (Formula 1).[6]

Mean arterial blood pressure =
Diastolic blood pressure + [Pulse pressure/3]

FORMULA 1. Mean arterial pressure.

PALPATION

Ability to palpate the radial, femoral, or carotid pulse in an emergency situation is traditionally thought to represent a minimum systolic pressure of 80, 70, or 60 mm Hg, respectively. However, confirmatory data are lacking, and these estimates may overestimate systolic pressure when compared to invasive measurements in patients with hypovolemic shock.

SPHYGMOMANOMETRY

Auscultation for blood pressure began with the invention of the sphygmomanometer by Scipione Riva-Rocci in 1896 and was later refined by Nicolai Korotkoff in 1905. To auscultate for blood pressure, place a cuff around the upper arm. Hold the bell of the stethoscope over the brachial artery as the cuff is gradually inflated to at least 30 mm Hg above the point at which the radial pulse disappears. Next, deflate the cuff at a rate of 2 to 3 mm Hg per second. The appearance of tapping sounds (Korotkoff sounds) corresponds to the systolic pressure. The diastolic pressure corresponds to the disappearance of Korotkoff sounds. Appropriate cuff size, cuff placement, proper placement of the stethoscope bell, appropriate cuff deflation rate, auscultation of Korotkoff sounds, dysrhythmia, observer bias, and faulty equipment all contribute to variability in the auscultatory method. Ideal cuff sizes are noted in **Table 32-3**.

An inappropriately small cuff for the size of the arm results in falsely elevated blood pressure measurements. A cuff too large for the size of the arm results in falsely low measurements.

TABLE 32-3 Blood Pressure Cuff Sizes

Arm Circumference Measurement (cm)	Cuff Size: Cuff Measurement
22–26	Small adult: 12 × 22 cm
27–34	Adult: 16 × 30 cm
35–44	Large adult: 16 × 36 cm
45–52	Adult thigh: 16 × 42 cm

Sphygmomanometric measurements of blood pressure often report slightly higher systolic pressure and lower diastolic pressure than those reported from simultaneous direct measurement using an intra-arterial catheter. This is because the reflected pressure waves summate with cuff inflation and increase systolic pressure, whereas the ischemic vasodilation downstream from the occluded cuff decreases cuff opening diastolic pressure.

OSCILLOMETRY

Most clinical blood pressure monitors use oscillometry. The amplitude of the fluctuations (or oscillations) in blood pressure in a sphygmomanometer cuff is analyzed and converted to pressure measurements by a computer device without the need for auscultation with the stethoscope. With gradual deflation of the cuff, oscillations begin above systolic pressure. The point of maximum oscillation corresponds to MAP. The systolic and diastolic pressures are estimated by an empiric algorithm. Despite widespread use, controversy exists regarding the accuracy of oscillometric blood pressure monitors. **When in doubt, use manual sphygmomanometric measurement of blood pressure.**

PHOTOPLETHYSMOGRAPHY

To measure the beat-to-beat blood pressure and thus provide continuous blood pressure monitoring, Penaz developed a technique with a small finger cuff containing a photoplethysmograph.[7] This device estimates blood volume in the finger with a light source on one side of the cuff and an infrared detector on the opposite side. The pressure in the blood vessels is proportional to the pressure in the cuff required to keep the blood volume constant. Special proprietary algorithms adjust for potential measurement errors caused by cold temperature or vasoactive agents.

INVASIVE BLOOD PRESSURE MEASUREMENT

In the vasoconstricted patient, noninvasive blood pressure measurements can underestimate systolic pressure by more than 30 mm Hg. MAP, however, is generally similar, whether measured noninvasively or invasively.[8]

The arterial catheter can be used for measuring MAP and pulse pressure, for estimating CO, and for repeated blood sampling. The International Consensus Conference for Hemodynamic Monitoring in Shock recommends invasive blood pressure monitoring for patients with refractory shock receiving vasoactive agents.[5] Uses for arterial catheterization are described in **Table 32-4**.

The radial artery is used most frequently for arterial catheterization. The femoral artery is an alternative in emergent situations, and often easier to access than the radial artery, especially in hypotensive patients. Other potential sites include the axillary, brachial, dorsalis pedis, ulnar, tibialis posterior, and temporal arteries, although these sites are rarely used (see chapter 31, "Vascular Access.")

In the presence of vasoconstriction, femoral arterial blood pressure measurements are more accurate than radial artery measurements. The risk for infection and limb ischemia is similar between radial and femoral artery cannulation (**Table 32-5**).[9] The primary risk of emergent femoral arterial catheterization is trauma to the artery during catheter insertion, with potential development of a pseudoaneurysm or retroperitoneal hematoma.

Placement of an intra-arterial catheter requires knowledge of the anatomic landmarks of the selected site. US guidance may be used.

The catheter can be inserted directly over a needle or by using the Seldinger technique over a guidewire. The Allen test, used to confirm collateral blood flow before radial artery catheterization, is inaccurate in predicting postcatheterization hand ischemia. In patients with profound hypotension, a cutdown may be required to cannulate the artery. After successful arterial catheterization, connection of the catheter to the pressure transducer should reveal an arterial waveform. The square wave flush test is applied to determine if artifacts in the tubing and recording system are damping the pressure measurements. See **Figure 32-1** for the square wave flush test with intra-arterial blood pressure measurement.

TABLE 32-4 Uses for Arterial Catheterization in the ED

Uses for arterial catheterization in the ED
Guides management of vasodilator or vasopressor drug to maintain target mean arterial pressure and avoid hypotension
Provides access port for the repetitive sampling of arterial blood in patients
Allows monitoring of cardiovascular deterioration in patients at risk for cardiovascular instability
Allows calculation of pulse pressure variation and cardiac output via pulse contour analysis
Useful applications of arterial catheterization in the diagnosis of cardiovascular insufficiency
Differentiate cardiac tamponade (pulsus paradoxus) from respiration-induced swings in systolic pressure
Tamponade reduces the pulse pressure but keeps diastolic pressure constant.
Respiration reduces systolic and diastolic pressure equally, such that the pulse pressure is constant.
Differentiate hypovolemia from cardiac dysfunction as the cause of hemodynamic instability
Systolic pressure decreases after a positive-pressure breath as compared to an apneic baseline during hypovolemia.
Systolic pressure increases during positive-pressure inspiration when left ventricular contractility is reduced.

TABLE 32-5 Complications of Intra-Arterial Catheterization

	Radial Artery (%)	Femoral Artery (%)	Axillary Artery (%)
Permanent ischemia	0.1	0.2	0.2
Temporary occlusion	19.7	1.5	1.2
Sepsis	0.1	0.4	0.5
Local infection	0.7	0.8	2.2
Pseudoaneurysm	0.1	0.3	0.1
Hematoma	14.4	6.1	2.3
Bleeding	0.5	1.6	1.4

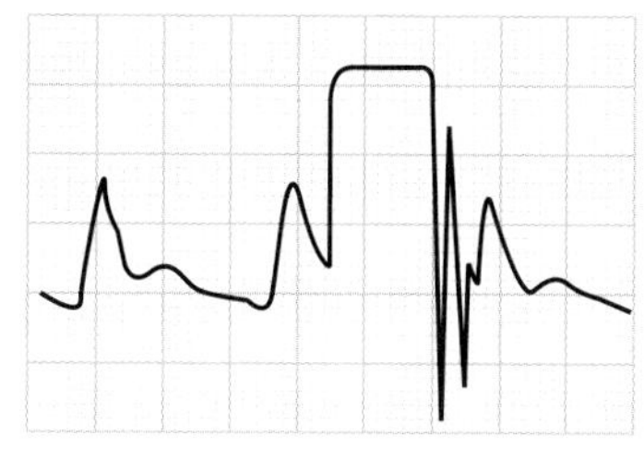

Optimally damped:
1.5–2 oscillations before returning to tracing. Values obtained are accurate.

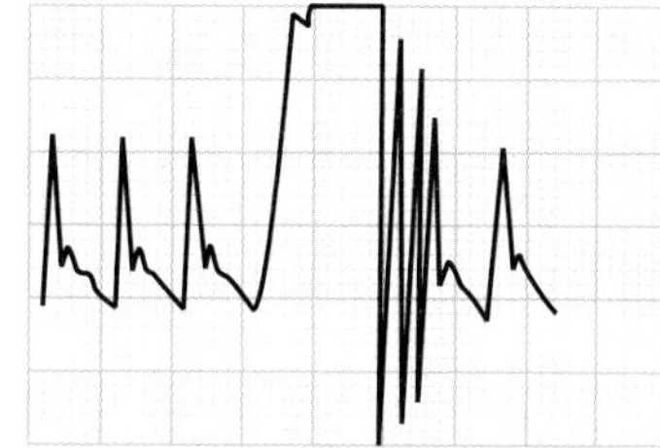

Underdamped:
>2 oscillations. Overestimated systolic pressure, diastolic pressure may be underestimated.

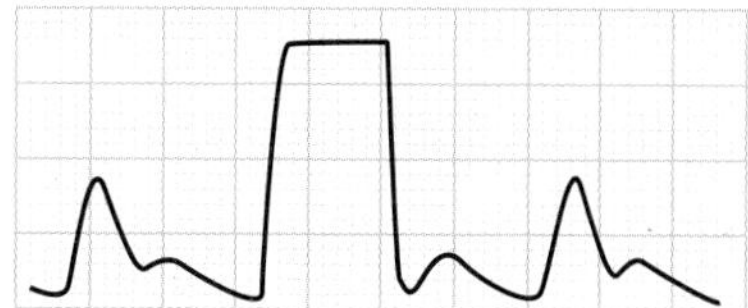

Overdamped:
<1.5 oscillations. Underestimation of systolic pressure, diastolic may not be affected.

FIGURE 32-1. Square wave flush test with intra-arterial blood pressure measurement. During a flush bolus of the catheter tubing, a square wave is observed. The number of oscillations after the square wave at the end of the bolus and prior to returning of the blood pressure tracing may result in an overestimated or underestimated blood pressure.

An overdamped system suggests that trapped air bubbles in the tubing are falsely lowering pressure measurements. An underdamped system will overestimate systolic pressure and underestimate diastolic pressure. Of note, in both situations, MAP is the most accurate measure. Flushing the system should remove the air bubbles. If this does not fix the problem, replace the tubing.

CENTRAL VENOUS PRESSURE MONITORING

By definition, CVP is the back pressure to systemic venous return, with high values indicating larger than normal volume returning to the heart from the systemic circulation. A number of factors contribute to the CVP value (**Table 32-6**). The use of CVP monitoring as a guide to resuscitation in critically ill patients is a subject of debate.

OPTIMAL CENTRAL VENOUS PRESSURE

CVP measurements range from 2 to 8 mm Hg in normal healthy individuals and are affected by multiple factors (Table 32-6).[10] A single absolute CVP value helps most when very low (such as to exclude right heart failure in a patient with a normal MAP) or very high (such as to suggest right heart failure and/or volume overload). **In general, a CVP <4 mm Hg in the critically ill patient should prompt fluid resuscitation with careful monitoring.**[5] However, CVP measures do not correlate with circulating blood volume or changes in blood volume.

Volume expansion in a healthy volunteer with normal diastolic compliance will immediately increase blood volume, whereas the CVP remains relatively normal. On the contrary, the same volume expansion in an elderly patient with cardiomyopathy, decreased diastolic compliance, and low circulating volume will elevate CVP (**Figure 32-2**).

Despite the limitations of CVP as a measure of blood volume, the classic "5-2 rule" can still provide a rapid estimation in the ED of volume status.[11] **After initial CVP measurement, infuse 250 mL normal saline IV over 15 minutes (10 to 20 mL/min bolus). An increase in CVP >5 mm Hg indicates volume overload and discontinuation of fluid. An increase in CVP of ≤2 mm Hg indicates hypovolemia and justifies additional fluid challenge.** "Volume responsiveness" is the best use of CVP in resuscitation. A target CVP of 8 to 12 mm Hg during resuscitation of the critically ill patient has been advocated, but the relative response will better guide therapy than any target alone.[12]

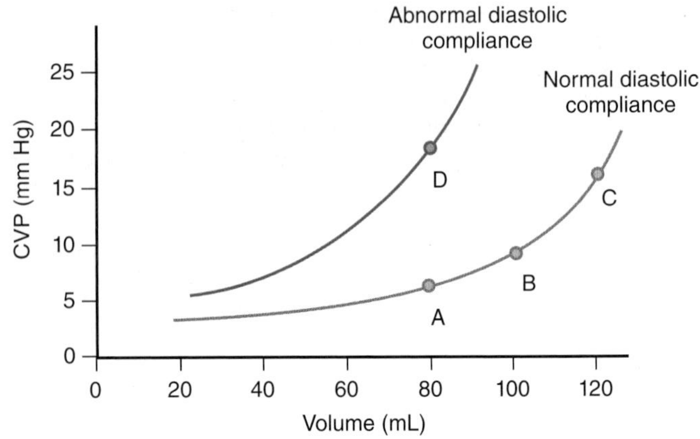

FIGURE 32-2. Right ventricular end-diastolic volume versus central venous pressure (CVP) varies with cardiac compliance. The same volume (80 mL) may result in different CVP measurements depending on diastolic compliance. The letters A-D designate response after small fluid bolus of same size in these groups.

Always measure CVP at end-expiration in both spontaneously breathing and mechanically ventilated patients. During spontaneous inspiration, the decreased intrathoracic pressure decreases transmural pressure in the heart, resulting in a decreased CVP. Conversely, intrathoracic pressure increases during an inspiratory breath of mechanical ventilation, resulting in an increase in CVP. Significant variation in inspiratory and expiratory CVP measurements suggests a compliant heart wall that will most likely respond to volume infusion. Conversely, the lack of respiratory variation in CVP may indicate that the heart is on the flat part of the cardiac function curve and will no longer respond to fluids.

TABLE 32-6 Contributors to Central Venous Pressure Values

Central venous blood volume
Venous return
Cardiac output
Total blood volume
Compliance of the central compartment
Vascular tone
Right ventricular compliance
Myocardial disease
Pericardial disease
Tamponade
Tricuspid valve disease
Stenosis
Regurgitation
Dysrhythmia
Junctional rhythm
Atrial fibrillation
Atrioventricular dissociation
Reference level of transducer
Positioning of patient
Intrathoracic pressure
Respiratory changes
Intermittent positive pressure ventilation
Positive end-expiratory pressure
Tension pneumothorax

NONINVASIVE CVP MEASUREMENT

JUGULAR VENOUS PULSATION

Observing internal jugular venous pulsation is a method to estimate right atrial pressure. The sternal angle is roughly 5 cm above the center of the right atrium regardless of the patient's position. With the patient sitting at a 45-degree angle, add 5 cm (distance from the sternal angle to the right atrium) to the vertical distance between the jugular pulsation and the sternal angle to estimate CVP in cm of water (cm H_2O). **A pulsation >4.5 cm vertically above the sternal angle when the patient is sitting at 45 degrees indicates a CVP of >9.5 cm H_2O (Figure 32-3).** In patients with heart failure, an elevated jugular venous pressure is independently associated with adverse outcomes, such as hospitalization and death.[13] Visualization of the internal jugular vein pulsation by physical examination is not always possible in the ED in obese or uncooperative patients.

ULTRASONOGRAPHY

US is a valuable tool to visualize the neck veins for central venous catheterization. It can also be used to determine elevated jugular venous pressure and provide a noninvasive method for measuring CVP. The right jugular vein is examined using a high-frequency linear transducer (7 to 9 MHz). The jugular venous pulse is the site where the vein tapers, resembling the neck of a wine bottle (**Figure 32-4**). Measure the vertical distance in centimeters between this point of vein collapse and the sternal angle and add 5 cm to obtain a CVP measurement in cm H_2O.

If the jugular vein is distended and larger than the adjacent common carotid artery when viewed in the transverse plane with the patient in a semi-upright position, then the CVP is >10 cm H_2O.

A nearly collapsed internal jugular vein on the transverse view in the supine position indicates a very low CVP. Correlation between US and echocardiogram is very good at high measurements.[14] Bedside US

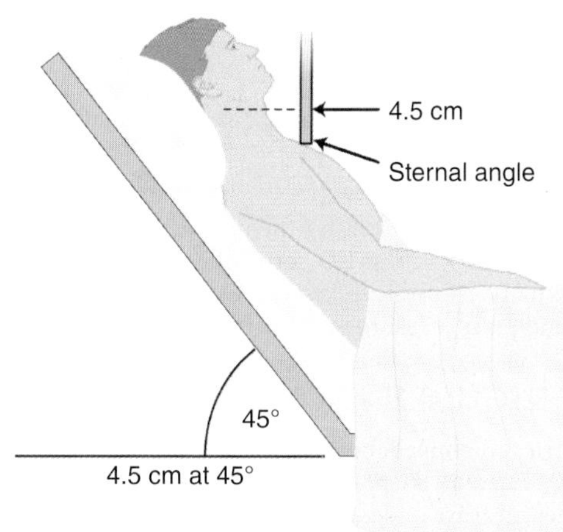

FIGURE 32-3. Internal jugular venous pulsation as an estimate of central venous pressure (CVP; or right atrial pressure). With the patient's head slightly turned to the left, shine a light tangentially in front of the neck to obtain a jugular shadow. The oscillations observed reflect the changing pressures within the right atrium and the various wave components of the CVP. The first elevation in the jugular pulse indicates the a-wave, or atrial contraction. The venous pressure is more accurately seen on the right side than the left because the right internal jugular vein has a more direct path to the right atrium. If the jugular pulse is higher than 4.5 cm at a 45-degree angle, it indicates an elevated CVP.

interpretations agree with formal echocardiographic estimates, with 83% for high, 67% for moderate, and 20% for low CVP measurements.

INVASIVE CVP MEASUREMENT

Traditionally, CVP is monitored with a fluid-filled catheter inserted in the internal jugular or subclavian vein proximal to the right atrium. The distal tip sits in the superior vena cava. Indications for central venous catheterization include fluid and vasopressor administration, unsuccessful or inadequate peripheral venous access, central venous oxygenation ($Scvo_2$) measurement, pulmonary artery catheterization, and transvenous pacemaker placement. Further details regarding central venous cannulation are provided in chapter 31.

After successful catheter insertion and radiographic verification, connect the catheter to a manometer or a pressure transducer of a monitor for continuous CVP waveform display. Place the transducer at the level of the right atrium, approximately 5 cm below the sternal angle. An acceptable

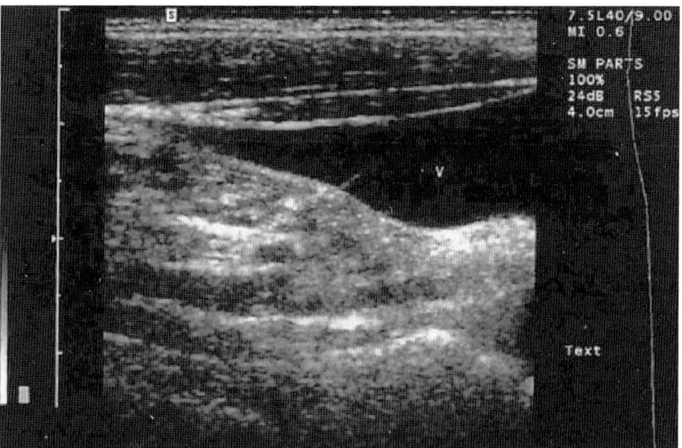

FIGURE 32-4. US longitudinal view of the neck showing the internal jugular vein tapering at the point of the jugular venous pulsation. v = vein. [Reproduced with permission from Lipton B: Estimation of central venous pressure by US of the internal jugular vein. *Am J Emerg Med* 18: 432, 2000. Copyright Elsevier.]

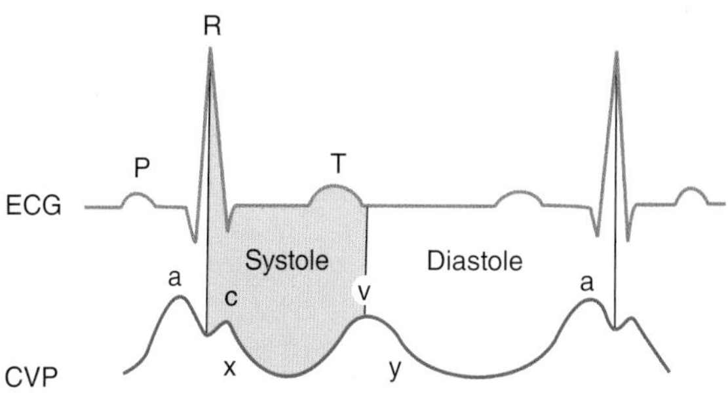

FIGURE 32-5. Central venous pressure (CVP) waveform and its relationship to the ECG. a = a-wave due to atrial contraction during diastole, which is absent in atrial fibrillation, but enlarged in tricuspid stenosis, pulmonary stenosis, and pulmonary hypertension; c = c-wave due to bulging of tricuspid valve back into the right atrium at the onset of systole; v = v-wave due to rise in atrial pressure from venous return through the vena cavae during systole and before the tricuspid valve opens at the onset of diastole, which is enlarged in tricuspid regurgitation; x = x-descent due to atrial relaxation; y = y-descent due to atrial emptying into the ventricle during diastole.

CVP waveform is needed to accurately interpret the measured values (**Figure 32-5**). The *c-wave* represents bulging of the tricuspid valve into the right atrium and occurs at the onset of systole. The base of the *c-wave* is used to determine a CVP value because it is the final pressure in the ventricle before the onset of contraction, reflecting *preload*.

Measurement of CVP from the internal jugular or subclavian vein is ideal. However, at times, measurement using femoral vein catheterization is required, such as in patients with coagulopathy, patients in whom subclavian and/or internal jugular vein catheterization is unsuccessful or has resulted in a complication, or when immediate central venous access is required. While not preferred, femoral CVP measurements are reliable.[15]

CARDIAC OUTPUT MONITORING

Oxygen delivery is a function of arterial oxygen content and CO. Perfusion pressure is the most important driving force determining regional blood flow, which in the aggregate defines CO. Because the primary goal of resuscitation from shock is to reverse tissue hypoperfusion, CO is often considered the ideal indicator of perfusion and oxygen delivery.

OPTIMAL CARDIAC OUTPUT AND DETERMINING FLUID RESPONSIVENESS

Traditionally, Starling's law (**Figure 32-6**) guided resuscitation care, with an increase in CO of greater than 15% after a fluid challenge considered the standard for assessing ideal fluid replacement. The most important contributor to increasing CO is increasing preload by successive fluid challenges.

VOLUME RESPONSIVENESS IN MECHANICALLY VENTILATED PATIENTS

Respiratory variations in blood pressure may aid in assessing volume status in the mechanically ventilated patient. Positive-pressure mechanical ventilation alters venous return and induces several predictable cyclic changes in vena caval diameters, pulmonary blood flow, and left ventricular output (**Figure 32-7**). In the volume-responsive patient, increasing intrathoracic pressure during positive-pressure inspiration will decrease venous return by decreasing the pressure gradient, which causes superior and inferior vena cava narrowing, decreased pulmonary blood flow, and a three- to four-beat phase lag decrease in left ventricular stroke volume and arterial pulse pressure.[16] A pulse pressure variation >13% predicts a >15% increase in CO in response to a 500-mL crystalloid bolus.[17]

Continuing fluid administration until the pulse pressure variation between inspiration and expiration decreases to <10% improves outcomes.[18] Because arterial pressure is directly proportional to stroke volume,

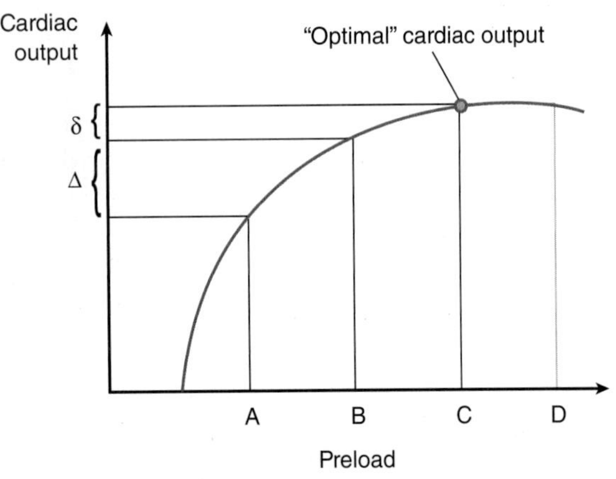

FIGURE 32-6. Starling cardiac function curve illustrating the effects of increased preload on cardiac output. As illustrated in the Starling cardiac function curve, the first increase in preload (from A to B) results in a large increase in cardiac output (Δ) as the cardiovascular system operates in the "preload-dependent" portion of the curve. The second increase in preload (from B to C) only results in a small increase in cardiac output (δ), and further increase in preload (from C to D) does not yield any increase in cardiac output as the cardiovascular system is now considered "volume resuscitated" or preload independent.

stroke volume variation strongly predicts fluid responsiveness, with a sensitivity of 81% and specificity of 80%.[19] A disadvantage of this technique is that the patient must be fully in synchrony with the positive-pressure mechanical breaths and without vigorous spontaneous breathing or dysrhythmia for stroke volume variation to be accurate. Nonetheless, this technique is useful to assess volume responsiveness in the sedated and ventilated patient.

VOLUME RESPONSIVENESS IN SPONTANEOUSLY BREATHING PATIENTS

Volume responsiveness in spontaneously breathing patients and those with dysrhythmias may be assessed by passive leg raising. Postural changes transiently increase venous return when the legs are raised to 30 degrees above the chest and held for 1 minute. This maneuver approximates giving a 300-mL blood bolus to a 70-kg patient. Changes in heart rate, blood pressure, CVP, or CO persist for approximately 2 to 3 minutes after passive leg raising. The dynamic increases in CO induced by passive leg raising are as sensitive and specific to predicting volume responsiveness as pulse pressure variation during positive-pressure mechanical ventilation.[20]

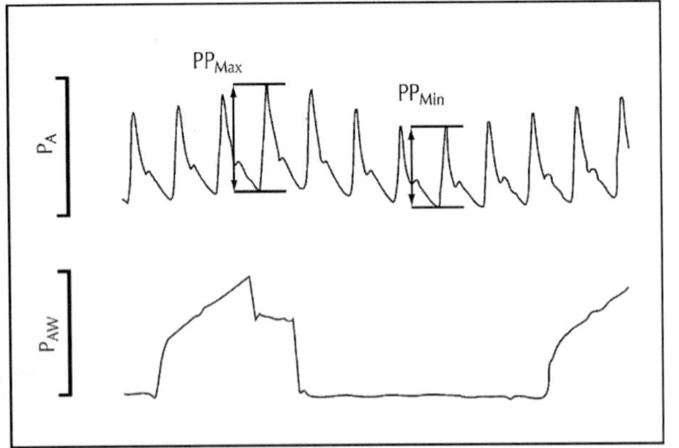

FIGURE 32-7. Pulse pressure variation (PPV) on positive-pressure mechanical ventilation. PPV is defined as the maximal pulse pressure (PP_{Max}) during inspiration minus the minimum pulse pressure (PP_{Min}) during expiration, divided by the average of these two pressures. P_A = arterial pressure; P_{AW} = airway pressure. [Reproduced with permission from Gunn SR, Pinsky MR: Implications of arterial pressure variation in patients in the intensive care unit. *Curr Opin Crit Care* 7: 212, 2001. Lippincott Williams & Wilkins, Inc. Copyright Wolters Kluwer Health.]

NONINVASIVE CARDIAC OUTPUT MEASUREMENT

Minimally invasive or noninvasive hemodynamic monitoring techniques to measure CO in the ED setting include thoracic electrical bioimpedance/bioreactance, esophageal Doppler US, transcutaneous Doppler US, and pulse pressure waveform analysis.

THORACIC ELECTRICAL BIOIMPEDANCE AND BIOREACTANCE

Thoracic electrical bioimpedance measures total blood flow within the aorta (or CO). Current is applied between the outer electrodes. The inner electrodes measure impedance to current flow through the thorax. Maximal current flow is along the path of least resistance (i.e., the great vessels). The change in impedance is proportional to change in volume and CO (**Figure 32-8**).[21]

Thoracic electrical bioimpedance was first used clinically to monitor CO in astronauts. CO measured with thoracic electrical bioimpedance correlates well with invasive measurements. It can also be used to differentiate cardiac from noncardiac causes of dyspnea and guide treatment in the ED.[22] A limit of this technique is that patient movement decreases signal reliability and accuracy.

Bioreactance is a modification of bioimpedance. Bioreactance applies a signal filter to analyze frequency shifts traversing the thoracic cavity creating a greater signal-to-noise ratio than bioimpedance. It is less sensitive to patient movement and external interference, although the accuracy in measuring CO is debated.[23]

ESOPHAGEAL DOPPLER US

Esophageal Doppler US measures instantaneous blood flow velocity in the descending aorta to determine stroke volume and CO (i.e., CO = stroke volume × heart rate). A Doppler transducer probe is inserted through the mouth or nose into the esophagus until its tip is at the midthoracic level. The probe is then rotated until the transducer faces the aorta to detect the characteristic aortic velocity signal profile (**Figure 32-9**).

Esophageal Doppler US CO readings correlate well with pulmonary artery catheter measurements.[24] However, this technique is operator dependent and often not well tolerated in awake patients, limiting ED use.

TRANSCUTANEOUS DOPPLER US

Transcutaneous Doppler US uses the same principles to measure CO as esophageal Doppler US. Measurements are obtained by applying the Doppler US probe at the sternal notch, with the US beam aimed at the ascending aorta. Significant operator training is required, again limiting the ED utility.[25]

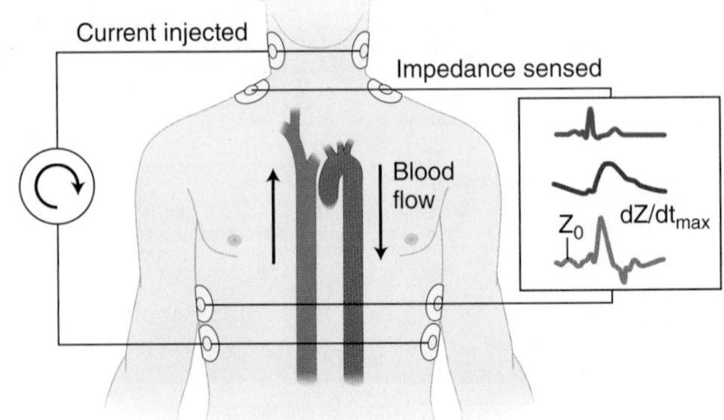

FIGURE 32-8. Thoracic bioimpedance cardiac output measurement. Z_0 = baseline impedance; dZ/dt_{max} = peak ejection velocity.

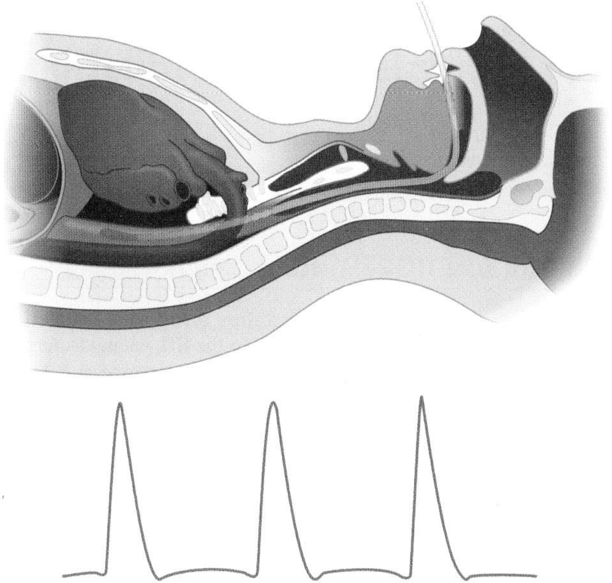

FIGURE 32-9. Esophageal Doppler cardiac output measurement. Cardiac output is proportional to the area under the curve of the aortic velocity and the aortic cross-sectional area. The tracing has been redrawn from the original.

PULSE PRESSURE WAVEFORM ANALYSIS

Pulse pressure waveform analysis uses an indwelling intra-arterial catheter to measure CO. Proprietary algorithms use arterial pressure waveform (or the pulse contour) and arterial vascular compliance to derive CO. Depending on the manufacturer, the measured CO may have to be regularly calibrated with another reference standard, such as lithium. Other systems may require the patient's specific physical characteristics for calibration. This technology has not yet been tested within a treatment protocol for the ED setting.

INVASIVE CO MEASUREMENT

CO is most commonly measured invasively with pulmonary artery catheterization using the thermodilution method. The benefit of using the pulmonary artery catheter for hemodynamic monitoring in the ED setting has not been investigated. Current expert consensus does not recommend the routine use of the pulmonary artery catheter in the management of the critically ill patient.[5,26] Given all this, pulmonary artery catheterization is usually avoided in the ED.

ORGAN OXYGENATION AND PERFUSION MONITORING

Blood pressure, CVP, and CO serve as macro-hemodynamic parameters. To assess tissue oxygenation or perfusion, venous oxygen saturation, serum lactate level, and tissue oxygenation provide further guidance during resuscitation.

CENTRAL VENOUS OXYGEN SATURATION

Venous oxygen saturation monitoring is a method to assess the relationship between tissue oxygen extraction, oxygen delivery, and oxygen consumption. A normal oxygen extraction ratio of 25% to 35% results in a *venous* oxygen delivery (reflected in venous oxygen saturation) of approximately 70% of arterial oxygen delivery. Venous oxygen saturation (SvO_2) is ideally measured in the pulmonary artery as a mixed venous sample ($Smvo_2$); this access point is generally not practical in the ED. Clinically, venous oxygen saturation reflects the balance between oxygen delivery and oxygen consumption, with low values reflecting inadequate delivery and/or excessive consumption.

Central venous oxygen saturation ($Scvo_2$) measurement only requires placement of a central venous catheter in the jugular or subclavian vein, making it an attractive alternative to $Smvo_2$. $Scvo_2$ can be easily measured by drawing a standard venous blood gas from the distal port of the central line and obtaining a *measured* oxygen saturation. Also, a special catheter allows continuous measurement if desired.

In healthy individuals, $Scvo_2$ is 2% to 3% less than $Smvo_2$; in shock states, $Scvo_2$ is typically 5% to 10% *higher* than $Smvo_2$ as blood flow is redistributed from the abdominal vascular beds to the cerebral and coronary circulation.[27] Although absolute values of $Scvo_2$ and $Smvo_2$ may be different, low values of either measurement reflect an imbalance in oxygen transport and portend worse outcomes. Most important, the two measures typically change in parallel and thus *trends* in $Scvo_2$ closely reflect trends in $Smvo_2$.[28]

Clinical Use of Central Venous Oxygen Saturation The principal value of $Scvo_2$ is its ability to detect occult inadequate oxygen delivery. During initial management, low $Scvo_2$ points to global tissue hypoxia despite normal vital signs and urine output. Left untreated, tissue hypoxia can lead to organ failure and death. Thus, regardless of the underlying pathophysiologic state (e.g., heart failure, septic shock, trauma), a low $Scvo_2$ value represents inadequate oxygen delivery relative to oxygen consumption. Troubleshooting a low $Scvo_2$ then focuses on the determinants of oxygen delivery (Is the patient hypoxic? Anemic? Is CO impaired, and if so, why? For example, low contractility, hypovolemia, or tamponade.). On the demand side, is oxygen consumption increased due to heightened metabolic demand such as from fever, pain, or seizure (**Table 32-7**)? Clinically, hypoxia and anemia are generally easily diagnosed and treated. A low $Scvo_2$ can detect occult low CO, prompting further investigation and therapy.

Normal (approximately 70%) or high $Scvo_2$ values do not necessarily mean that the patient is hemodynamically stable. $Scvo_2$ is a global measure of oxygen transport, and regional areas of tissue hypoperfusion can be present even with normal $Scvo_2$ values, particularly in the lower half of the body. In several disease states (e.g., hypothermia, terminal shock, cyanide poisoning), the ability of the tissues to extract oxygen from the blood is impaired, leading to "arterialization" of the venous blood with high $Scvo_2$.

Using $Scvo_2$ monitoring in a treatment protocol—targeting CVP 8 to 12 mm Hg, MAP >65 mm Hg, and $Scvo_2$ >70%—for septic shock patients early after arrival to the ED (or *early goal-directed therapy*) decreased mortality in single-center studies.[12,29-32] However, new data showed this invasive approach had no improved outcome compared to usual care in a multicenter study enrolling patients after early recognition, fluid boluses, and antibiotics have occured.[33] These results show

TABLE 32-7 Contributors to Abnormal Central Venous Oxygen Saturation ($Scvo_2$)

Low $Scvo_2$ (<70%)		High $Scvo_2$ (>70%)	
Low Do_2	High $\dot{V}o_2$	High Do_2	Low $\dot{V}o_2$
Hypoxia, suctioning (low Sao_2)	Exercise	Hyperoxia (high Fio_2)	Hypothermia
Anemia, hemorrhage (low Hgb)	Pain	Erythrocytosis (high Hgb)	Anesthesia, pharmacologic paralysis
Cardiac dysfunction, hypovolemia, shock, arrhythmia (low CO)	Hyperthermia, shivering, seizure	Hyperdynamic state (high CO)	Arteriovenous shunting, mitochondria defect, terminal shock

Note: Determining the causes of and treating a low or high $Scvo_2$ clinical state involves troubleshooting for conditions resulting in abnormal oxygen delivery (Do_2) and oxygen consumption ($\dot{V}o_2$).

Abbreviations: CO = cardiac output; Fio_2 = fraction of inspired oxygen; Hgb = hemoglobin; Sao_2 = arterial oxygen saturation.

that CVP and $Scvo_2$-guided care may be an appropriate option in patients where shock is failing to resolve despite efforts to identify.

LACTATE

In critical illness, an oxygen debt develops when oxygen delivery is inadequate to meet tissue oxygen demand and compensatory mechanisms are exhausted. This results in global tissue hypoxia, anaerobic metabolism, and lactate production. High lactate is a well-established prognostic marker in critically ill patients with various forms of shock, a fact identified in the 1800s.[34]

In addition to shock, causes of elevated lactate include seizure, diabetic ketoacidosis, malignancy, thiamine deficiency, malaria, human immunodeficiency virus infection, carbon monoxide or cyanide poisoning, and mitochondrial myopathies. Commonly used drugs, such as metformin, simvastatin, lactulose, antiretrovirals, niacin, isoniazid, and linezolid, can also cause a lactate elevation.[35]

Blood lactate concentrations also reflect the interaction between its production and elimination. During critical illness, a patient with hepatic dysfunction may have a higher lactate level compared with another patient without liver disease due to impaired hepatic clearance. However, lactate elevation in a patient with chronic liver disease still portends a poor prognosis, because patients with liver disease do not commonly have a high lactate level in the absence of shock.[36]

Clinical Use of Lactate Hyperlactatemia is not always accompanied by hypotension or a low bicarbonate level and/or elevated anion gap; thus, the lactate level must be separately measured. Venous lactate levels correlate well with arterial lactate levels.[37] However, repeat any elevated venous lactate level if inconsistent with the clinical condition, preferably with an arterial measurement.

A lactate level ≥4 mmol/L in normotensive patients requires further attention, because this cutoff is associated with increased intensive care unit admission rates and mortality. Furthermore, persistent elevation in lactate for >24 hours is associated with increased mortality as high as 90%.[38] Lactate clearance (or the ability to decrease serum lactate levels) as early as 6 hours in patients with septic shock improves 60-day survival.[39] When included in a treatment protocol, lactate clearance is noninferior to $Scvo_2$-guided care in the ED.[40] However, targeting both lactate clearance and optimal $Scvo_2$ may result in better outcomes than either alone.[41]

TISSUE OXYGEN SATURATION

Tissue oxygen saturation (Sto_2) can be measured by near-infrared spectroscopy, a noninvasive technique capable of continuous measurement using the varying light absorption properties of deoxygenated and oxygenated blood. Near-infrared light (680 to 800 nm) is largely transparent to biologic tissue, absorbed primarily by hemoglobin, and minimally affected by skin blood flow. Importantly, the near-infrared spectroscopy signal primarily reflects hemoglobin in the small end vessels and approximates the oxygen saturation of venous blood. Near-infrared spectroscopy Sto_2 measurements correlate and trend with $Smvo_2$ and $Scvo_2$ and can detect occult regional hypoxia even when $Smvo_2$ and vital signs have normalized.[42] However, darkly pigmented skin may impair measurement accuracy.

Clinical Use of Tissue Oxygen Saturation Sto_2 values reflect resuscitation adequacy and the magnitude of traumatic injury, as well as organ failure in critically ill patients.[43] An Sto_2 <75% measured at the thenar eminence distinguishes severe shock patients from healthy volunteers. Dynamic measurements using a brief vascular occlusion test to measure changes in Sto_2 may offer greater value than static Sto_2 measurements.[44]

Changes in Sto_2 during the vascular occlusion test are associated with the need for emergency operation or transfusion within the first 24 hours of hospitalization in trauma patients.[45] However, Sto_2 as a hemodynamic goal incorporated in an ED treatment protocol is still investigative.

REFERENCES

The complete reference list is available online at www.TintinalliEM.com.

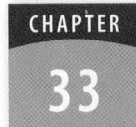

Cardiac Pacing and Implanted Defibrillation

Swee Han Lim
Wee Siong Teo
Anantharaman Venkataraman

PURPOSE OF PROCEDURE

Cardiac pacing serves to maintain or restore myocardial depolarization and thus ensure adequate cardiac output. In the ED, pacing is performed therapeutically to correct an ongoing rhythm disturbance or in anticipation of the onset of a conduction problem with hemodynamic impact.[1]

Indications for emergency pacing are listed in **Table 33-1**.

The indications for emergency cardiac pacing are found in chapter 18, "Cardiac Rhythm Disturbances."

GENERAL EQUIPMENT

All cardiac pacemakers deliver an electrical stimulus to the heart by electrodes that cause depolarization and subsequent cardiac contraction.[2] The modern pacemaker only stimulates the heart chamber if it does not recognize (sense) intrinsic electrical activity from that chamber after a selected time interval. Impulses are delivered to either the atria or ventricles, or to both.

Components of a cardiac pacemaker include:

- Pulse generator
- Electronic circuitry for sensing and pacing
- Lead system that connects the pulse generator to the electrode(s) and stimulates the myocardium

Relevant clinical details of these components are listed in **Table 33-2**.

TRANSCUTANEOUS PACING

Transcutaneous pacing is the emergency technique of choice because of its easy application. It uses externally applied electrodes to deliver an electric impulse directly across the intact chest wall to stimulate the

TABLE 33-1 Indications for Emergency Pacing

Indication	Comments
Symptomatic or hemodynamically unstable bradycardia/AV block	Symptoms include hypotension, change in mental status, angina, and pulmonary edema. Pharmacologic therapy may be used to temporize while preparing to pace.
Severe sick sinus syndrome with prolonged asystole (generally >3 s) and syncope	—
Ventricular standstill due to complete heart block or Mobitz type II AV block	—
Torsade de pointes	Overdrive pacing.
Recurrent monomorphic ventricular tachycardia	Overdrive pacing. The technique is limited by: Maximum pacing rate of the pacing device (usually 180 beats/min). Potential of accelerating the ventricular tachycardia and inducing ventricular fibrillation.
Unstable supraventricular tachycardia	Overdrive pacing should only be used after pharmacologic intervention and cardioversion have failed.

Abbreviation: AV = atrioventricular.

TABLE 33-2 Pacemaker Component Details

Pacemaker Type	Pulse Generator Location	Electrode Location
Transcutaneous	External	Skin of anterior chest wall and back or Anterior chest wall below right clavicle and apex
Transvenous	External	Venous catheter with tip in right ventricle and/or right atrium
Transesophageal	External	Esophagus
Epicardial	External or Internal	Epicardium Electrodes are usually placed on heart's surface during surgery
Permanent	Internal (subcutaneous in the prepectoral region)	Venous or epicardial

myocardium. Transcutaneous pacers differ from standard pulse generators in several important ways. The pulse duration of the stimulating impulse is longer and the current output higher than in internal pacing. Muscle contraction (usually the chest wall or diaphragm) is notable during pacing, especially at high outputs, and may be painful. Severe twitching makes palpation of the radial, carotid, or femoral pulse difficult. Cardiac monitoring with standard ECG monitors is difficult due to interference from the large current outputs that create large-amplitude pacing spikes. Most of the newer transcutaneous pacing units have a monitor that filters pacing spikes, allowing simultaneous monitoring.

RISKS AND PRECAUTIONS

There is little risk of electrical injury to healthcare providers during transcutaneous pacing. The electrodes are insulated, and closed chest compressions can be done over pads while pacing. Inadvertent contact with the active pacing surface results only in a mild shock.

EQUIPMENT

Table 33-3 lists the equipment needed to perform transcutaneous pacing.

TABLE 33-3 Transcutaneous Pacing Equipment

Pulse generator and monitor (usually a combination defibrillator/cardioversion/pacemaker unit)
Pacing cables
Pacemaker pads
ECG electrode pads
ECG monitor and cables
Medications for sedation and analgesia

TECHNIQUE

If time and conditions allow, explain the procedure to the patient and administer IV sedation and analgesia.

Apply the external pacing pads as shown in **Figure 33-1**. The same pads and electrodes are used for pacing, cardioversion, and defibrillation in most of the newer defibrillator units. If separate defibrillator pads or paddles are used, place them at least 2 to 3 cm from the pacing pads.

In bradyasystolic arrest, turn the stimulating current to maximum output and then decrease the output after capture is achieved; after restoring pulses, you may titrate energy to a level just above loss of capture. In a patient with a hemodynamically compromising bradycardia outside of cardiac arrest, slowly increase the output from the minimum setting until capture is achieved—usually between 50 and 100 mA. Continue pacing at about 1.25 times the threshold of initial electrical capture.

Transcutaneous pacing may be fixed rate (asynchronous) or demand (synchronous). **Asynchronous pacing** delivers an electrical impulse at a regular interval without regard to intrinsic cardiac pacemaker activity. This creates the potential risk of precipitating a dysrhythmia if the pacing stimulus occurs during the vulnerable period of ventricular repolarization. While many state a preference for synchronous pacing, there are little outcome or safety data to support that preference.

OUTCOMES ASSESSMENT

Assess capture using the ECG on the filtered monitor of the pacing unit. Look for the presence of a consistent ST segment and T wave after each pacer spike. Palpate for carotid and femoral pulses. Bedside US can be used to assess external pacer capture. If these appear favorable, assess blood pressure by cuff or arterial catheter.

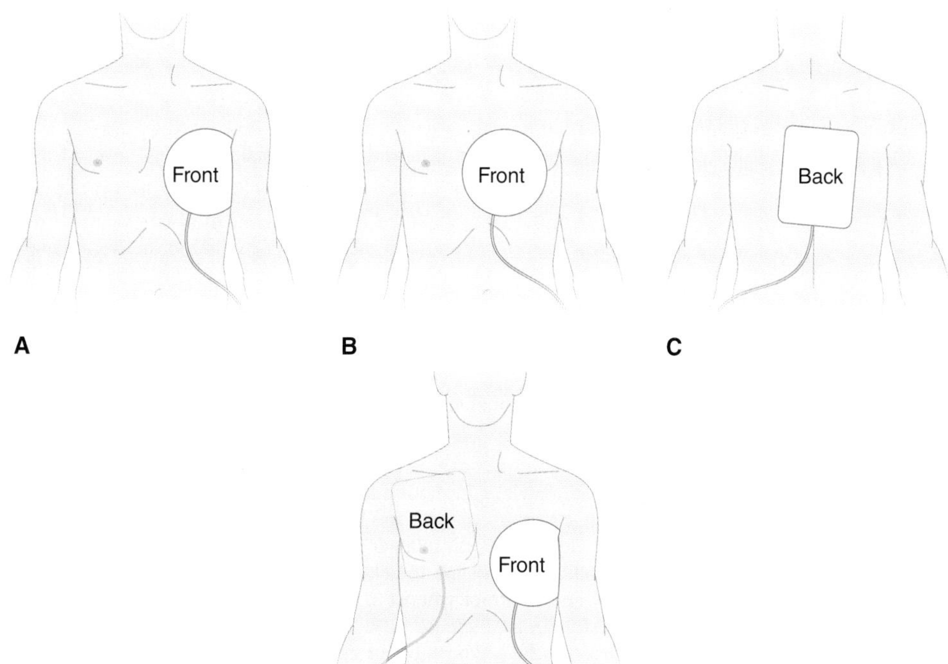

FIGURE 33-1. Placement of the transcutaneous pacing electrodes. **A.** Anterior (negative) electrode position centered over the cardiac apex. **B.** Anterior (negative) electrode position centered over the V_3 lead position. **C.** Posterior (positive) electrode position. [Reproduced with permission from Doukky R, Rajanahally RS: Transcutaneous cardiac pacing, in Reichman EF, Simon RR (eds): *Emergency Medicine Procedures*. Figures 20-2 and 20-3. Copyright © 2004. The McGraw-Hill Companies, Inc., all rights reserved.]

Failure to capture with transcutaneous pacing may be related to faulty electrical contact, electrode placement, patient size, or underlying pathology. Recheck the lead connections, skin–electrode contact, and electrode placement. On occasion, pneumothorax, pericardial effusion or tamponade, severe myocardial ischemia, and metabolic derangements limit capture. No clinical myocardial damage results from properly performed transcutaneous pacing. Unless an easily resolved trigger exists, arrange for temporary transvenous pacing as soon as possible since ongoing pacing is likely needed.

TRANSVENOUS PACING

The indications for transvenous pacing are the same as for other methods of cardiac pacing.

Gather all equipment needed, including that to insert a central venous catheter (see chapter 31, "Vascular Access.") Resuscitation equipment and drugs, and the pacing needs listed in **Table 33-4**.

TECHNIQUE

You should know the equipment and practiced or done the procedure before starting. If conditions permit, explain the procedure to the patient and obtain informed consent. Next, identify the access site and approach and position the patient. The primary **sites of catheter insertion in the ED are the right internal jugular vein (preferred)** and the left subclavian vein. The right internal jugular vein allows a relatively straight line of access through the superior vena cava and right atrium into the right ventricle.

The steps for transvenous pacemaker insertion are listed in **Table 33-5**.

The most commonly encountered difficulties with transvenous pacing are securing venous access and obtaining proper placement of the stimulating electrode in the right ventricle, both of which can be time-consuming. Placement of the catheter tip into the apex of the right ventricle is the key to successful transvenous pacing.

When patients have decreased or no forward blood flow, positioning of the pacer tip within the right ventricle is difficult. Balloon-tipped catheters do not aid during low- or no-flow states. In an emergency, connect the pacemaker electrodes to the power source and advance the catheter until the tip encounters the endocardium of the right ventricle and creates capture.

Set the initial rate between 80 to 100 beats/min, using the asynchronous mode (sensitivity off) initially in patients requiring emergency pacing for hemodynamically unstable bradycardias. Follow the ECG to determine the presence or absence of capture (**Figure 33-3**). Adjust subsequent rate and sensitivity settings as clinically indicated by the response and underlying rhythm disturbance.

Transvenous pacing is best used in urgent rather than emergent situations (with transcutaneous serving as the bridge), allowing fluoroscopy.

COMPLICATIONS

Complications include perforation of the myocardium, cardiac arrhythmias, air embolism, failure of the circuit, catheter dislodgement, and delayed infection, in addition to the complications possible with central venous access (see chapter 31).

TABLE 33-4 Equipment Needed for Transvenous Pacing

Central catheter kit—introducer sheath must be one size larger than the pacer catheter
Flexible transvenous cardiac pacing catheter
Pacemaker generator and battery (and spare battery)
Cardiac monitor
Insulated connecting wire with alligator clamps at both ends

PERMANENT PACING

Permanent pacing is not performed in the ED.[1] Permanent pacemaker pulse generators (battery) are placed subcutaneously on the side of the patient's nondominant hand (thus, usually in the left prepectoral region below the left clavicle). The endocardial transvenous leads are positioned in the right ventricle at the apex, septum, or right ventricular outflow tract, and in the case of a dual-chamber device, also in the right atrium. A subclavian or cephalic vein approach is common. An epicardial lead may be implanted during concomitant open heart surgery.

Pacemaker leads are either bipolar or unipolar in configuration; unipolar leads are prone to oversensing myopotential and electromagnetic interference. The disadvantage of the bipolar configuration is that it is larger and more prone to lead fractures.

PACEMAKER NOMENCLATURE

A five-letter code is used to describe the features of the pacemaker[3] (**Table 33-6**). The first three code letters are used most commonly. The first letter refers to the chamber or chambers in which the pacing occurs: **A = atrium, V = ventricle**, and **D = dual chamber** or both A and V. The second letter refers to the chamber or chambers in which sensing occurs. The letters are the same as those for the first letter code. "**I**" indicates that a sense event inhibits the output pulse and causes the pacemaker to recycle the timing cycles, "**T**" means that an output pulse is triggered in response to a sensed event. "**D**" means that both "**T**" and "**I**" response can occur. The most common pacemakers are **VVI** and **DDD**. The fourth letter is used to indicate the presence or absence of an adaptive-rate mechanism (rate modulation). Pacemakers are then indicated as VVIR or DDDR. The fifth letter is used to indicate whether multisite pacing is present and is rarely used. See **Figures 33-4 and 33-5** for examples of ECGs with pacemaker spikes.

RESUSCITATION IN PATIENTS WITH PERMANENT PACEMAKER

If a patient who has a permanent pacemaker requires countershock, place the pads or paddles at least 8 cm from the pulse generator. The current normal positioning of the paddles—below the right clavicle and apex of the heart—is safe because the majority of pulse generators are below the left clavicle. Alternatively, place adhesive electrodes in an anteroposterior configuration. After countershock, interrogate the pacemaker to ensure that it is still functioning normally.

Potential problems after defibrillation include:

- Pacemaker inhibition due to reversion to noise mode
- Deletion (reprogramming)
- Circuit damage
- Myocardial damage adjacent to the lead tip caused by current transmission via the electrode to the myocardial interface

Another reason that immediate return of pacing (capture) fails after defibrillation is that global myocardial ischemia increases pacing threshold. If this occurs, try transcutaneous pacing at higher delivered energy settings.

PACEMAKER COMPLICATIONS

Complications for which a patient may seek care in the ED in the early period after pacemaker insertion are listed in **Table 33-7**. Two are discussed in detail.

Pacemaker Syndrome Atrioventricular synchrony and the presence of ventriculoatrial conduction are most common in the setting of VVI pacing but may occur with the DDI mode. With VVI pacing, the ventricle is electrically stimulated, resulting in ventricular contraction. If sinus node functions are intact, the atria can be depolarized by a sinus impulse and contract when the tricuspid and mitral valves are closed. This results in an increase in jugular and pulmonary venous pressures and may produce symptoms of congestive heart failure. Atrial distention can result in reflex vasodepressor effects mediated by the central

TABLE 33-5 Transvenous Pacemaker Insertion

Step	Comments
1. Gown in standard sterile fashion.	Use sterile gloves and gown. Wear mask and hair covering.
2. Identify vessel using either US guidance or landmarks.	—
3. Prep and drape patient using standard sterile procedure.	Prep a wide area in case initial attempts fail and an alternate site is needed. Prep the entire ipsilateral neck and upper chest when preparing to insert an internal jugular or subclavian catheter.
4. Open a central catheter kit that contains an introducer catheter. Inspect for content in a sterile fashion. Place kit close to bedside and operator. Maintain sterile conditions.	The introducer catheter should be one size larger than the pacing catheter.
5. Open pacing catheter and pacing kit (if available).	Pulmonary artery catheters with dedicated atrial and ventricular ports may also be used. Assess integrity of the pacing catheter balloon by inflating it with 1.5 mL of air and immersing it in sterile saline. Air bubbles indicate a leaky balloon.
6. Attach the pacemaker to any of the V leads and ensure it is recording.	—
7. Anesthetize area in all conscious patients.	Inject area with 1%–2% lidocaine. Anesthetize the periosteum of the clavicle if using the subclavian approach. Reorient to landmarks after injection.
8. Hold the 18-gauge introducer needle on a 10-mL syringe in the dominant hand and align the needle to the target.	—
9. Advance the needle slowly though the skin and subcutaneous tissue until a flash of dark venous blood appears.	Maintain steady constant aspiration of syringe.
10. Stabilize the needle with the nondominant hand.	—
11. Check for continued free venous flow with aspiration.	If no flow is noted, withdraw the needle slightly, as the needle may have breached the posterior vessel wall.
12. Remove the syringe attached to the needle, and immediately occlude the catheter with a finger.	This maneuver helps to prevent introducing air in the catheter and subsequent central system air embolism.
13. Insert the guidewire gently through the needle. Always maintain a firm grip on the wire—do not let go of the wire for any reason.	The wire should advance with minimal resistance. Do not force the wire for any reason. If the wire does not pass easily, reattach the syringe and aspirate to confirm continued venous flow. Reposition the needle as needed. Premature ventricular contractions (PVCs) or dysrhythmias during wire advancement may indicate that the wire is in the right atrium or beyond.
14. Remove the needle over the wire when the guidewire is inserted at least 10 cm into the vessel.	—
15. Incise the skin with a #11 blade scalpel at the entry site to accommodate the introducer.	Do not cut the guidewire.
16. Advance the introducer over the guidewire into the vessel lumen with a gentle twisting motion.	Maintain a grip on the guidewire during this procedure.
17. Remove the guidewire.	—
18. Insert and advance the pacing catheter approximately 10 cm.	This ensures that the balloon is past the introducer catheter and within the vascular system. Inflate the balloon with 1.5 mL of sterile saline.
19. Slowly advance the catheter into the right ventricle.	Use fluoroscopy or bedside US to guide placement. The ECG tracing recorded from the electrode also helps localize the position of the catheter tip. Inflate the balloon after the catheter enters the superior vena cava. Stop advancing when the pacing catheter is in the apex of the right ventricle. See **Figure 33-2**.
20. Reassess balloon integrity.	—
21. Connect the pacemaker generator to the catheter.	—
22. Disconnect the negative terminal of the pacemaker catheter from the ECG lead.	—
23. Connect the proximal pacemaker catheter terminals to the terminals of the pacemaker generator.	—
24. Set the pacemaker generator on demand mode with a rate of 80–100 beats/min.	Start with 5 mA of energy on the output dial.
25. Turn on the pacemaker.	With optimal tip position, capture should occur at <2 mA. Pacing spikes and a wide QRS complex in lead V_1 reflect capture.
26. After capture, decrease the pacemaker generator output to just below where pacing stops.	Continue pacing at 1.5–2.0 times the threshold output required for capture
27. Examine the chest x-ray for catheter tip placement and signs of complications.	—
28. Secure catheter and apply a sterile transparent dressing.	—

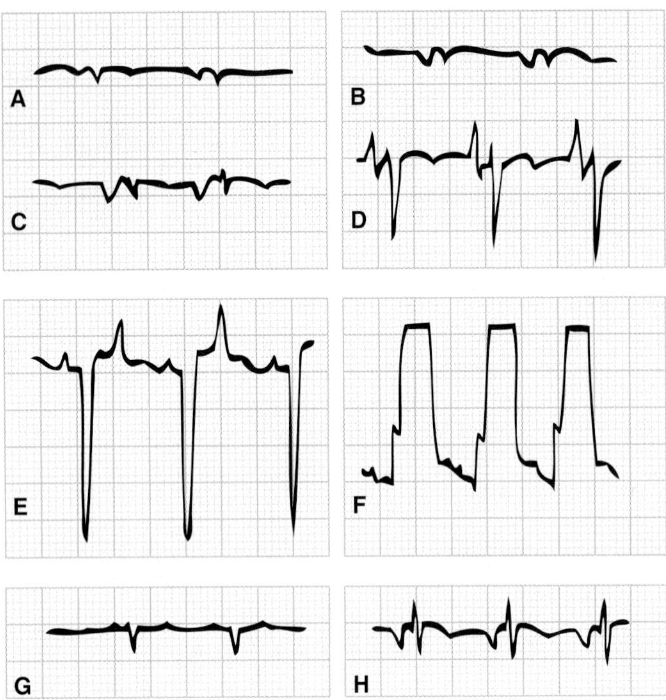

FIGURE 33-2. Typical ECG tracings seen with a transvenous pacing catheter within the different anatomic sites. **A.** The subclavian or internal jugular vein. **B.** The superior vena cava. **C.** The high right atrium. **D.** The low right atrium. **E.** Free-floating in the right ventricle. **F.** Abutting the right ventricular wall. **G.** The inferior vena cava. **H.** The pulmonary artery. [Reproduced with permission from Wilson DD, Reichman EF: Transvenous cardiac pacing, in Reichman EF, Simon RR (eds): *Emergency Medicine Procedures.* Figure 22-6. Copyright © 2004. The McGraw-Hill Companies, Inc., all rights reserved.]

nervous system. If the contribution of atrial contraction to late diastolic ventricular filling is important in maintaining an adequate cardiac output, orthostatic hypotension may occur. DDI pacing in a patient with atrioventricular block can result in pacemaker syndrome if the sinus node discharge rate exceeds the programmed rate of the pacemaker.

In most instances, symptoms are mild and patients adapt to them. In about one third of these patients, symptoms are severe. Treatment usually requires upgrading a VVI pacemaker to a dual-chamber pacemaker or lowering the pacing rate of the VVI unit, so that ventricular pacing does not occur but provided intrinsic conduction occurs. If symptoms occur in a patient paced in the DDI mode, optimizing the timing of atrial and ventricular pacing is usually required. Consult with a cardiologist.

PACEMAKER MALFUNCTION

Pacemaker malfunction is divided into four areas: failure to sense, failure to pace, failure to capture, or overpacing or pacemaker-associated tachycardia.[4]

Failure to Sense (Undersensing) Undersensing occurs when the pacemaker cannot adequately detect the intrinsic electrical cardiac activity. This results from lead placement in an area of the heart with poor or variable conductivity, or if a lead is loose, dislodged, or physically broken. Sensing failure can occur if the programmed sensing threshold is set too high. With undersensing, if the pacer is set in an inhibit mode, it will fire at a set rate that is not coordinated with the patients underlying cardiac cycle (**Figure 33-6A**).

Failure to Pace (Oversensing) Oversensing occurs when the pacemaker experiences interference from electrical signals within the body (i.e., skeletal or smooth muscle myopotentials) that are not related to the normal cardiac cycle. Sources of interference may include skeletal muscle, the diaphragm, nerve stimulators, broken pacer leads, and uncommonly, coarse atrial fibrillation. When electrical activity is oversensed, the pacemaker erroneously inhibits the pulse generator and the patient may develop bradycardic rhythms (**Figure 33-6B**).

Failure to Capture Failure to capture occurs when the pulse generator fires but the current delivered to the endocardium is too low to initiate depolarization and wavefront propagation. Dislodged leads, poor cardiac conductivity due to myocardial disease (e.g., ischemia, acidosis, fibrosis), and programming problems are the most common reasons for this malfunction. Failure to capture can be intermittent (**Figure 33-6C**).

PACEMAKER-ASSOCIATED TACHYCARDIA

Occasionally the patient with an implanted device may present with a rapid paced rhythm. This may be due to:

- Rapid atrial arrhythmia triggering an upper rate response in a patient with complete heart block
- Pacemaker-mediated tachycardia
- Runaway pacemaker

Unless preprogrammed to mode switch, pacemakers detect rapid atrial rhythms and track them, resulting in pacing at the upper rate limit. Pacemaker-mediated tachycardia can occur in a *dual-chamber pacemaker* when a premature ventricular ectopic beat triggers a retrogradely conducted atrial depolarization outside the atrial refractory period, which is then sensed by the pacemaker, initiating ventricular pacing. If this continues, it can cause an endless loop tachycardia. Rarely the pacemaker may malfunction with acceleration of pacing (runaway pacemaker). This occur when the pulse generator discharges at a rapid rate above its preset upper limit and is most commonly associated with a battery failure or damage from external interference. Placing a magnet over the pacemaker may help in the pacemaker-mediated tachycardia or runaway pacemaker. However, interrogation of the device is usually required, and the device must be replaced if programming is not successful.

PACEMAKER PROGRAMMING ERRORS

Pacemakers are computer-controlled devices with complex software that requires adjustment and maintenance. Reprogramming is accomplished

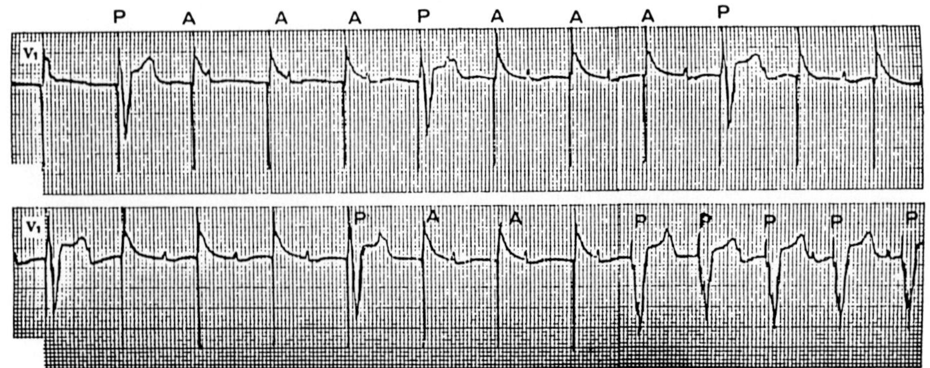

FIGURE 33-3. Pacing with intermittent capture. "P" indicates paced beats, and "A" indicates pacer artifact without capture.

TABLE 33-6 The Five-Letter Code System for Implanted Cardiac Pacemakers: The NASPE/BPEG Generic Pacemaker Code

Letter Position	1	II	III	IV	V
Category	Chamber(s) Paced	Chamber(s) Sensed	Response to Sensing	Programmability, Rate	Antitachyarrhythmic Function(s)
	0, none	0, none	0, none	0, none	0, none
	A, atrium	A, atrium	T, triggered	P, simple programmable	P, pacing
	V, ventricle	V, ventricle	1, inhibited	M, multiprogrammable	S, shock
	D, dual (A + V)*	D, dual (A + V)*	D, dual (D + I)†	C, Communicating (telemetry)	D, dual (P + S)‡
	S, single chamber	S, single chamber	—	R, rate modulation	—

Abbreviation: NASPE/BPEG = North American Society for Pacing and Electrophysiology/British Pacing and Electrophysiology Group.

*Atrial and ventricular.

†Dual (atrial and ventricular) and inhibited.

‡Pacing and shock.

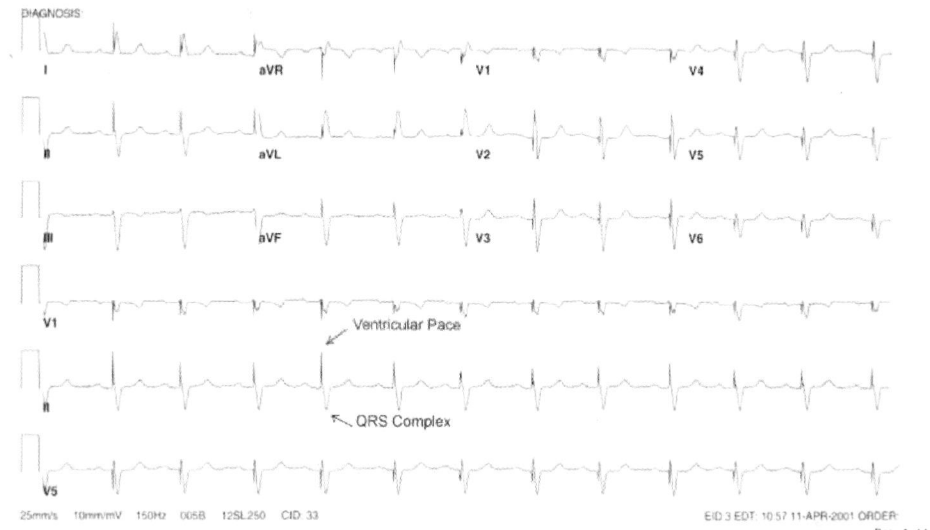

FIGURE 33-4. Single-lead pacemaker. Only the ventricle is paced.

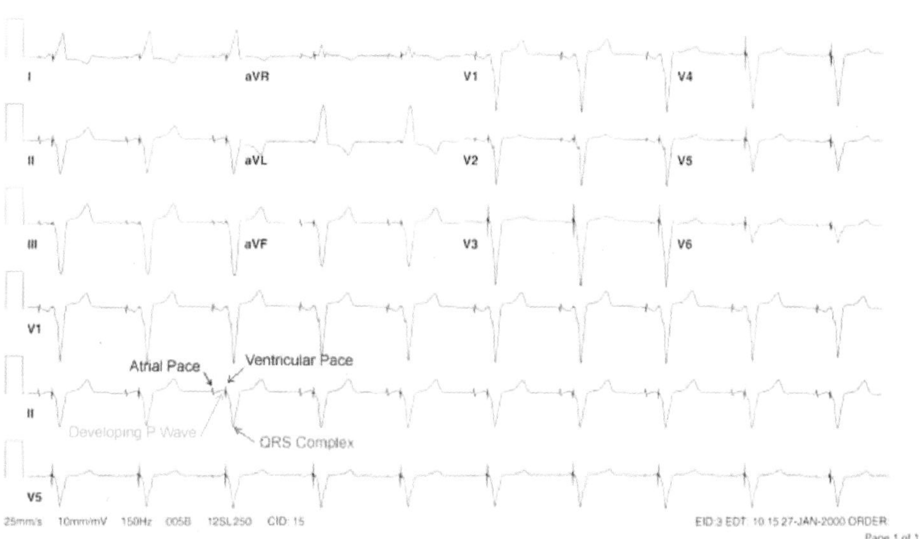

FIGURE 33-5. Atrioventricular pacer spikes seen best in leads II and aVF.

TABLE 33-7 Complications Seen after Pacemaker Insertion

Complication	Comment
Infection	Infection rate is <1%. Infections are more common in patients after pacemaker replacement or prolonged procedure. Early infections are most commonly caused by *Staphylococcus aureus or Staphylococcus epidermidis.* Pacemaker infection presents as: Local inflammation or abscess formation in the pacemaker pocket, as evidenced by pain, tenderness, or redness at the site. Skin adherence to the device, especially with discoloration of the skin over it, is highly indicative of localized infection. Do not aspirate the pocket because this can worsen the infection. If only a superficial infection is suspected, antibiotics and analgesics may be given with an early referral to the device implanter to review. Erosion of the device or lead through the skin resulting in the leads or pulse generator being exposed. Complete device and lead removal is almost always required. Cardiac device–related infective endocarditis involving the lead or valves. Patient may present with sepsis and positive blood culture without sign of local inflammation.
Thrombophlebitis and venous obstruction	Symptomatic thrombosis of the upper extremities and central veins is uncommon, possibly because of extensive venous collaterals (0.3%–3.0% of patients). Site of insertion does affect incidence. Symptoms include edema, pain, or venous engorgement of the arm ipsilateral to lead insertion. Treatment includes IV heparin therapy followed by long-term warfarin administration.
Pneumothorax	1% of patients. More common with subclavian introducer technique. Hemothorax and pneumomediastinum are rare.
Pacemaker syndrome	20% of patients. New or worsening of symptoms such as syncope or near-syncope, orthostatic dizziness, exercise intolerance, dizziness, uncomfortable pulsation over the neck and abdomen, right upper quadrant pain, etc.

noninvasively with devices that communicate to the pacemaker through radiofrequencies. Occasional settings can be inadvertently altered, and software, as with any computer, can fail. Software changes may occur in set rates, sensing thresholds, and current outputs.

IMPLANTABLE CARDIOVERTER-DEFIBRILLATORS

Implantable cardioverter-defibrillators are the treatment of choice for sudden cardiac death, reducing mortality from approximately 30% to 45% per year to <2% per year.[5] This remarkable efficacy, coupled with the failure (and potentially proarrhythmic effects) of pharmacologic therapy and the increasing sophistication and miniaturization of the devices, has led to an explosion in implantable cardioverter-defibrillator use. Expanding indications for implantable cardioverter-defibrillator implantation make it likely that emergency physicians will regularly see patients with these devices.

An implantable cardioverter-defibrillator consists of a pulse generator, a lead system with both sensing and shocking electrodes, circuitry to analyze the cardiac rhythm and trigger defibrillation, and a power supply.

In the past, these devices generally were placed by thoracotomy or sternotomy, and defibrillation occurred through electrodes positioned inside or outside the pericardium. Rate-sensing electrodes were placed epicardially or transvenously. Roughly one third of patients with second-generation implantable cardioverter-defibrillators received inappropriate shock(s) triggered by a supraventricular tachycardia during the working life of the device.

In newer implantable cardioverter-defibrillators, sensing-pacing-defibrillation electrodes are placed transvenously, and the device itself is generally implanted subcutaneously in the subpectoral region or in an abdominal pocket. Newer implantable cardioverter-defibrillators are better at discriminating supraventricular tachycardia and are capable of a variety of responses to ventricular tachycardia and fibrillation. Most are programmed to follow a tiered approach to ventricular dysrhythmias: antitachycardia pacing, low-energy cardioversion, and finally defibrillation. Depending on the frequency of discharge and whether the pacemaker function is used, the latest implantable cardioverter-defibrillators have a projected life span of approximately 6 to 9 years, depending on whether they are single- or dual-chamber devices.

Implantable cardioverter-defibrillators are remarkably effective in preventing sudden cardiac death. The most common cause of death in patients with implantable cardioverter-defibrillators is congestive heart failure, which should be managed in standard fashion in the ED.

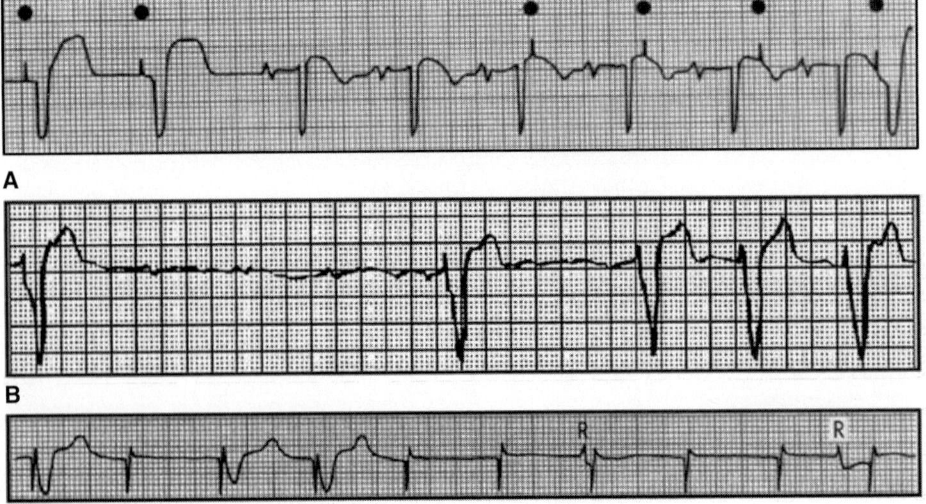

FIGURE 33-6. Various pacemaker malfunctions. **A.** Undersensing. **B.** Oversensing. **C.** Failure to capture.

TABLE 33-8 Potential Causes of Inappropriate Implantable Cardioverter-Defibrillator (ICD) Shock Delivery

False sensing
Supraventricular tachycardia with rapid ventricular response
Muscular activity (shivering, diaphragmatic contraction)
Extraneous source (tapping of chest wall, vibrations, pacer spikes)
Sensing T waves as QRS complex (double counting)
Sensing lead fracture or migration
Unsustained tachyarrhythmia
ICD–pacemaker interactions
Component failure

ED EVALUATION

The most common reason an patient with an implantable cardioverter-defibrillator comes to the ED is evaluation after a delivered shock. Causes of inappropriate shock delivery are summarized in **Table 33-8**. Determine the number of shocks delivered, the activity of the patient at the time of shock, and any prodromal symptoms or postshock trauma. Ask about any recent changes in rhythm-directed drug therapy. Focus the physical examination on the vital signs, the cardiovascular status, the generator pocket, and evidence of incidental trauma. Place each patient on a continuous ECG monitor, and **obtain a 12-lead ECG; any shock-related ST-segment elevations or depressions should resolve within 15 minutes; ongoing changes suggest new ischemia.** Examine a chest radiograph for electrode migration, displacement, or fracture. Obtain rhythm-related drug levels and serum electrolyte levels.[6,7]

If the patient is receiving repeated inappropriate shocks for a non-lethal rhythm, temporarily deactivate the implantable cardioverter-defibrillator by placing a magnet over the device. Defibrillation can be re-enabled by removing the magnet. All implantable cardioverter-defibrillators should be evaluated by a cardiologist after exposure to a magnet.

For a patient with an implantable cardioverter-defibrillator in cardiac arrest, follow all normal resuscitation measures. **If defibrillation is necessary, do not place either the paddle or pad directly over the implantable cardioverter-defibrillator pulse generator.** Perform CPR in the usual fashion. If the implantable cardioverter-defibrillator discharges during CPR, the CPR provider may perceive a small electrical shock, but the shock is neither uncomfortable nor dangerous.

DISPOSITION AND FOLLOW-UP

Admission criteria depend on the reason for shock delivery; consultation with the treating cardiologist is key. The ICD can be interrogated by external telemetry devices that are manufacturer and model specific. General admission recommendations include any sign of cardiovascular instability, a history of two or more shocks in a 1-week period, correctable causes of dysrhythmia, and any sign of infection or mechanical disruption of the implantable cardioverter-defibrillator or lead system.

Acknowledgment: The authors thank Edward S. Bessman, author of this chapter in the previous edition.

REFERENCES

The complete reference list is available online at www.TintinalliEM.com.

Pericardiocentesis

Carolyn K. Synovitz
Eric J. Brown

INTRODUCTION AND EPIDEMIOLOGY

Cardiac tamponade is a relatively rare condition. **If a pericardial effusion compromises hemodynamics, pericardiocentesis can be lifesaving.** The cause of cardiac tamponade may be determined by fluid analysis after pericardiocentesis (**Table 34-1**).[1-4]

In a small study of medical cardiac tamponade, the mean volume drained was 593 ± 313 mL. When the primary cause was malignancy, the 1-year mortality was almost 80%.[5] In Africa, up to 70% of pericardial effusions in patients with human immunodeficiency virus are caused by tuberculosis.[6]

Maintain a high degree of suspicion of cardiac tamponade for oncology patients who fit the clinical signs and symptoms of tamponade.

Blunt cardiac rupture is rare, occurring approximately in 1 in 2400 blunt trauma patients. Of this subgroup, 89% arrive alive to the ED.[7] Those who arrive alive may benefit from a bedside US examination to detect a traumatic effusion. **Tamponade, as a result of trauma, may require a temporizing pericardiocentesis while the patient is prepared for definitive surgical repair.**

In a South African study, the mortality rates from gunshot wounds and stab wounds were 81% and 15.6%, respectively.[8] This comparison underlines the probability that patients with stab wounds to the heart are more likely to survive to the ED and may benefit from pericardiocentesis.

PATHOPHYSIOLOGY

The pericardium is a fibrocollagenous sac covering the heart that contains a small amount of physiologic serous fluid. The fibrocollagenous pericardium has elastic properties and will stretch in response to increases in intrapericardial fluid. Accumulation of fluid that exceeds the stretch capacity of the pericardium precipitates hemodynamic compromise and results in pericardial tamponade.

The initial portion of the pericardial volume–pressure curve is flat, so early on, relatively large increases in volume result in comparatively small changes in intrapericardial pressure. The pericardium becomes less elastic as the slope of the curve marches upward. As fluid continues to accumulate, intrapericardial pressure rises to a level greater than that of the filling pressures of the right atrium and ventricle. When this occurs, ventricular filling is restricted and results in cardiac tamponade.[9]

Pulsus paradoxus is commonly seen with cardiac tamponade and is defined as an abnormal decrease in systolic blood pressure and pulse wave amplitude. During normal respirations, systolic blood pressure drops less than 10 mm Hg. In pulsus paradoxus, systolic blood pressure drops >10 mm Hg, resulting in a cardiac contraction that does not result in a normal radial pulse. This causes a paradoxical pulse.[10]

In blunt trauma, forces within the thorax can compress the right atrium, resulting in rupture of the atrium or the right atrial appendage. This occurs when blood continues to fill the relatively inelastic pericardial sac. Deceleration injuries can lead to a cardiac or pericardial rupture, herniation, or a myocardial contusion with intrapericardial hemorrhage. Blast injuries can cause acute cardiac tamponade.[11] **During an acute rapidly expanding pericardial effusion, stroke volume will increase with removal of even a small amount of fluid (as little as 50 mL) from the pericardial sac (Figure 34-1).**

CLINICAL FEATURES

HISTORY

Trauma as a cause of pericardial tamponade is generally evident from history and clinical presentation. Oncology patients comprise the largest

TABLE 34-1 Causes of Pericardial Effusions

Cause	Sagrista-Sauleda et al[1] (n = 322) (%)	Corey et al[2] (n = 75) (%)	Levy et al[3] (n = 204) (%)	Kil et al[4] (n = 116) (%)
Acute idiopathic	20	7	48	—
Idiopathic	16	7	—	4
Malignancy	13	23	15	52
Chronic	9	—	—	—
Post–myocardial infarction	8	—	—	—
Uremia	6	12	2	7
Autoimmune	5	12	10	5
Radiation	—	14	—	—
Infection	—	27	16	4
Hypothyroidism	—	—	10	3
Tuberculosis	—	—	—	14

group with pericardial effusions leading to hemodynamic compromise. Other conditions that may predispose a patient to pericardial effusion and tamponade include acute infection (viral, bacterial, mycoplasma, fungal, parasitic, or endocarditis) or radiation exposure. Other chronic conditions in which this diagnosis may be considered include tuberculosis, renal failure, autoimmune diseases, drugs that induce a lupus-like syndrome, hypothyroidism, or ovarian hyperstimulation syndrome.[12] Many cases are idiopathic.

The **key symptoms of tamponade** are dyspnea and chest pain. Trauma patients may or may not exhibit pleuritic pain, tachypnea, and dyspnea before becoming confused, losing consciousness, or developing shock.[13] Other symptoms include chest fullness, nausea, esophageal pain, or abdominal pain from hepatic and visceral congestion. Other nonspecific symptoms include lethargy, fever, weakness, fatigue, anorexia, palpitations, and shock. Be aware of these symptoms and accordingly focus the examination to exclude life-threatening conditions, such as cardiac tamponade.

PHYSICAL EXAMINATION

Common clinical signs of cardiac tamponade may resemble other severe cardiopulmonary disease processes, such as tension pneumothorax or decompensated congestive heart failure. The sensitivities of examination findings are pulsus paradoxus >10 mm Hg (82%), tachycardia (77%), jugular venous distention (76%), diminished heart sounds (28%), and hypotension (26%). These findings are not surprising because the **Beck triad** includes low blood pressure, elevated jugular venous distention, and decreased heart sounds.[10] Detection of jugular distention may be difficult to appreciate in patients with a short, thick neck or if working under levels of low lighting. **The combination of pulsus paradoxus and elements of the Beck triad should prompt imaging with bedside US to search for a pericardial effusion.** Any disorder that increases intrathoracic pressure may result in pulsus paradoxus, including chronic obstructive pulmonary disease, obesity, tense ascites, severe asthma, congestive heart failure, mitral stenosis, and massive pulmonary embolism.

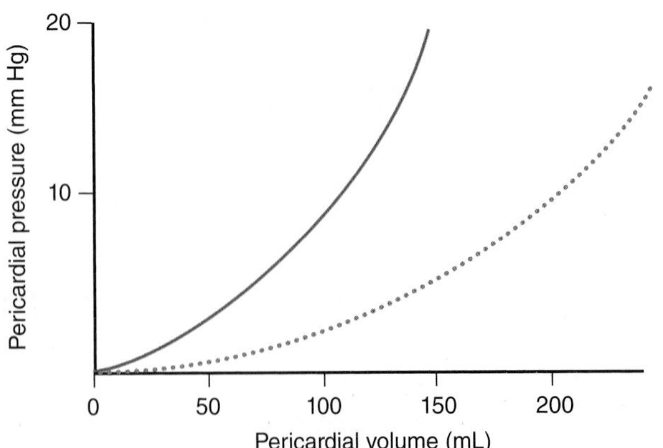

FIGURE 34-1. Acute versus chronic pericardial effusion. Pericardial volume–pressure curve with acute (*solid line*) versus chronic effusion (*dotted line*). [Reproduced with permission from Reardon RF, Joing SA: Cardiac, in Ma OJ, Mateer J, Blavais M (eds): *Emergency Ultrasound*, 2nd ed. New York: McGraw-Hill, 2004.]

DIAGNOSIS

The diagnosis in an undifferentiated patient relies on clinical suspicion using the signs and symptoms of cardiac tamponade, with confirmation by bedside US (see discussion in "Echocardiography" section, below).

The ECG can be normal. The classic ECG finding is electrical alternans. Electrical alternans is alternating high- and low-voltage QRS complexes as the heart swings toward and then away from the ECG leads on the chest wall with each contraction (**Figure 34-2**). Other findings can include nonspecific ST-T wave changes or bradycardia, which can be seen in the late stages of cardiac tamponade progressing to pulseless electrical activity (PEA). In the absence of hypotension and tension pneumothorax in a patient with PEA, consider the diagnosis of cardiac tamponade.

IMAGING

Chest radiographs may show a normal or enlarged cardiac silhouette with clear lungs, as demonstrated in **Figure 34-3**. On lateral chest radiographs, a double lucency sign demonstrates the epicardial fat pad.

Echocardiography Cardiac tamponade can be imaged at the bedside with two-dimensional echocardiography and Doppler echocardiography. This allows for visualization of a pericardial effusion and the compression of the ventricles. The most characteristic sign on echocardiogram is right-sided heart collapse. During diastole, the right ventricle presses inward (**Figure 34-4**), and during systole, the right atrium presses inward. Right-sided collapse portends rapid development of cardiac tamponade. Right atrial collapse during at least 30% of the cardiac cycle is more sensitive than the finding of right ventricular collapse for cardiac tamponade. In 25% of patients with tamponade, a late finding is left atrium collapse. Doppler US can be used to monitor the respiratory changes in flow between ventricle and atrium.[9]

PROCEDURE: EMERGENCY PERICARDIOCENTESIS

When hemodynamic compromise is present, infusion of a normal saline fluid bolus can be temporizing by improving right ventricular volume while preparations are made for emergency pericardiocentesis.[1]

PURPOSE AND INDICATIONS

The purpose of emergency pericardiocentesis is treatment of hemodynamic compromise from cardiac tamponade. Emergency pericardiocentesis is also indicated during resuscitation from PEA after other causes of PEA have been excluded.

Postoperative or penetrating trauma patients may develop tamponade 2 weeks or more after surgery.[7] In one study of traumatic tamponade, the most common indications for pericardiocentesis were clinical tamponade (83%), with echocardiographic findings of ventricular diastolic collapse (69%) and right atrial collapse (33%).[14] Pericardiocentesis for a traumatic effusion from penetrating cardiac trauma may be performed during resuscitation to stabilize a patient until surgery for definitive repair is available, but surgical drainage is preferred in traumatic effusions and purulent pericarditis.[15] **If the patient is hemodynamically compromised and on the verge of cardiac arrest, perform emergency pericardiocentesis in the ED, rather than delay treatment by transporting to the OR.**

BEDSIDE US

If bedside US is available, two-dimensional echocardiographic imaging is preferred to guide pericardiocentesis[16-19] and can also evaluate the size of the effusion and its effect on cardiac output. The 2010 Focused Cardiac Ultrasound in the Emergent Setting guidelines state: "When emergency pericardiocentesis is indicated ultrasound can provide guidance by first imaging the fluid collection from the subxiphoid/subcostal or other transthoracic windows to define the best trajectory for needle insertion."[20] The guidelines further emphasize that bedside US results in fewer complications and greater success in performance of pericardiocentesis.[20] The European Society of Cardiology's 2004 Guidelines on the Diagnosis and Management of Pericardial Disease has evidence-based guidelines on pericardiocentesis. Pericardiocentesis is lifesaving in cardiac tamponade (level of evidence B, Class I indication) and indicated in effusions >20 mm in echocardiography but also in smaller effusions for diagnostic purposes (pericardial fluid and tissue analyses, pericardioscopy, and epicardial/pericardial biopsy; level of evidence B, Class IIa indication). American College of Cardiology/American Heart Association 2005 guidelines for the use of echocardiography gives Class I recommendations to using this methodology for visualizing effusions and detecting hemodynamic compromise secondary to tamponade. The European Society of Cardiology 2004 guidelines recommend that practitioners use US guidance rather than blind approaches and the ECG-alone guided approach for pericardiocentesis.[21] Using echocardiographic-guided pericardiocentesis reduces radiation associated with fluoroscopy and allows the procedure to be performed safely at the bedside.[22]

CONTRAINDICATIONS TO PERICARDIOCENTESIS

Some authors list aortic dissection as an absolute contraindication. Relative contraindications include uncorrected coagulopathy, anticoagulant therapy, thrombocytopenia, and small posterior loculated effusions.

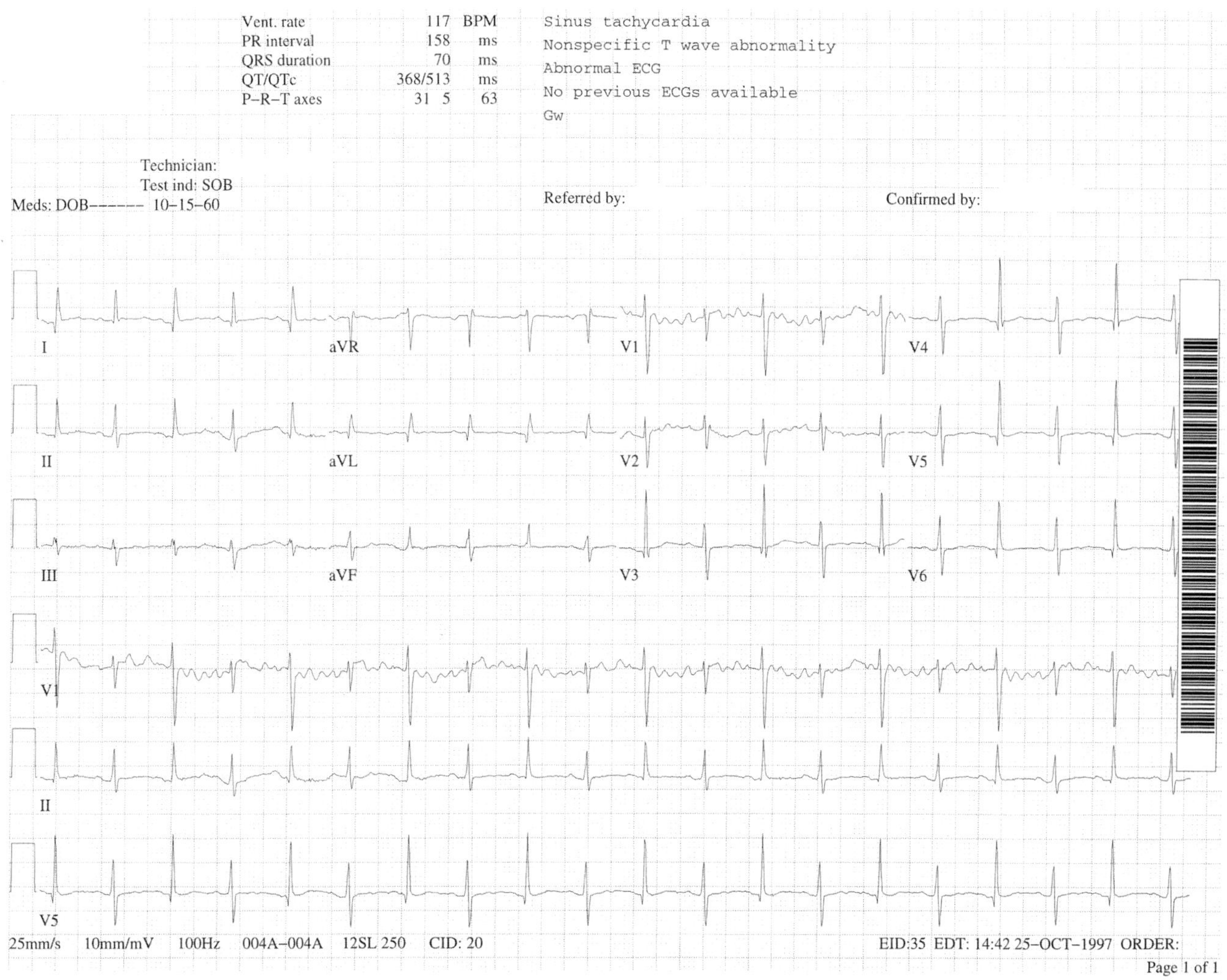

A

FIGURE 34-2. ECG of electrical alternans, with alternating higher and lower voltage QRS complexes. **A.** Initial ECG in the ED. Bedside echocardiography revealed a large pericardial effusion with right ventricular diastolic collapse. **B.** Resolution of electrical alternans after pericardiocentesis. [Reproduced with permission from Smith RF: Pericardiocentesis, in Reichman EF, Simon RR (eds): *Emergency Medicine Procedures.* New York: McGraw-Hill, 2004.]

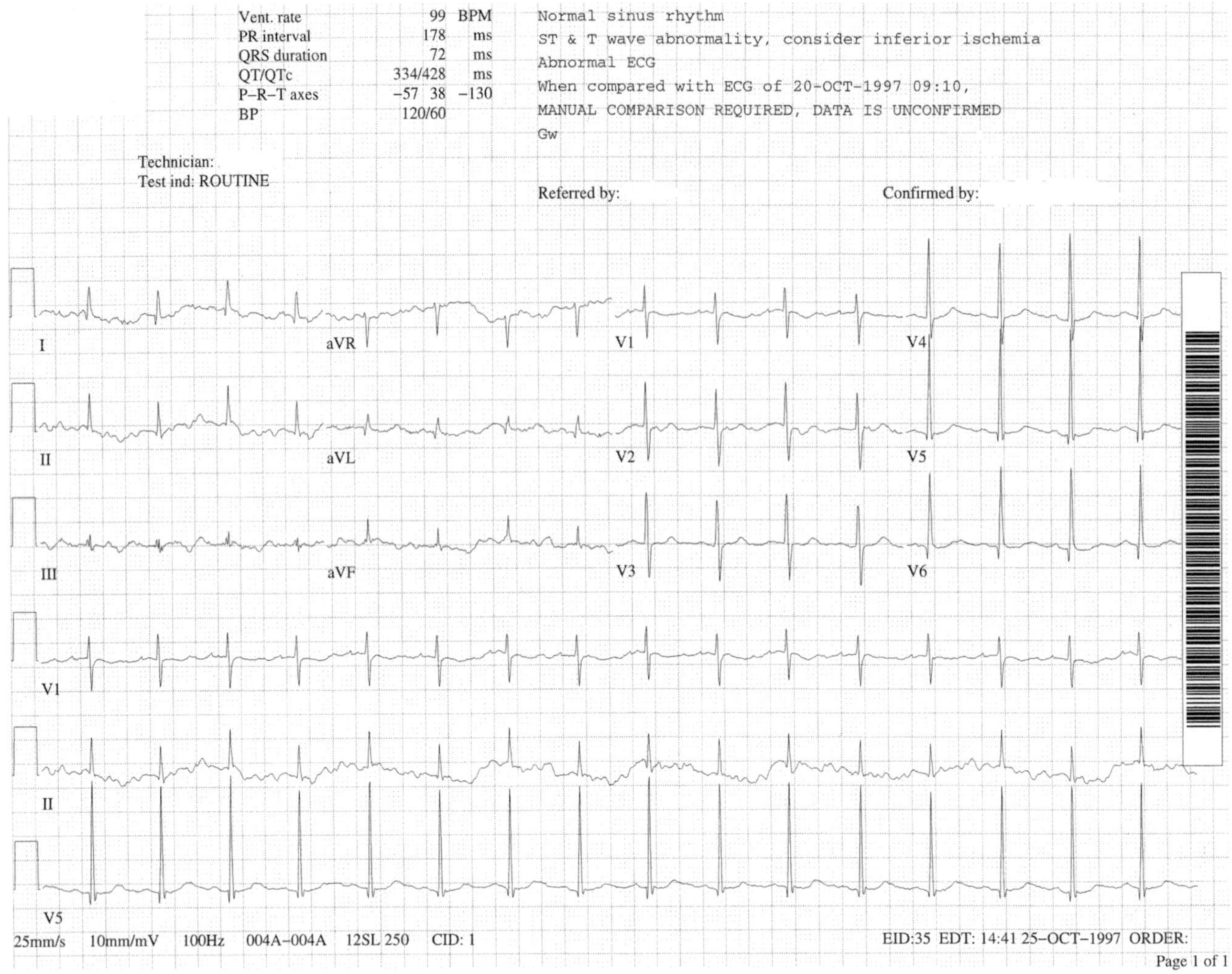

Vent. rate 99 BPM
PR interval 178 ms
QRS duration 72 ms
QT/QTc 334/428 ms
P–R–T axes –57 38 –130
BP 120/60

Normal sinus rhythm
ST & T wave abnormality, consider inferior ischemia
Abnormal ECG
When compared with ECG of 20-OCT-1997 09:10,
MANUAL COMPARISON REQUIRED, DATA IS UNCONFIRMED
Gw

Technician:
Test ind: ROUTINE

Referred by: Confirmed by:

I aVR V1 V4
II aVL V2 V5
III aVF V3 V6
V1
II
V5

25mm/s 10mm/mV 100Hz 004A–004A 12SL 250 CID: 1 EID:35 EDT: 14:41 25–OCT–1997 ORDER:
Page 1 of 1

B

FIGURE 34-2. (*Continued*) ECG of electrical alternans, with alternating higher and lower voltage QRS complexes. **A.** Initial ECG in the ED. Bedside echocardiography revealed a large pericardial effusion with right ventricular diastolic collapse. **B.** Resolution of electrical alternans after pericardiocentesis. [Reproduced with permission from Smith RF: Pericardiocentesis, in Reichman EF, Simon RR (eds): *Emergency Medicine Procedures*. New York: McGraw-Hill, 2004.]

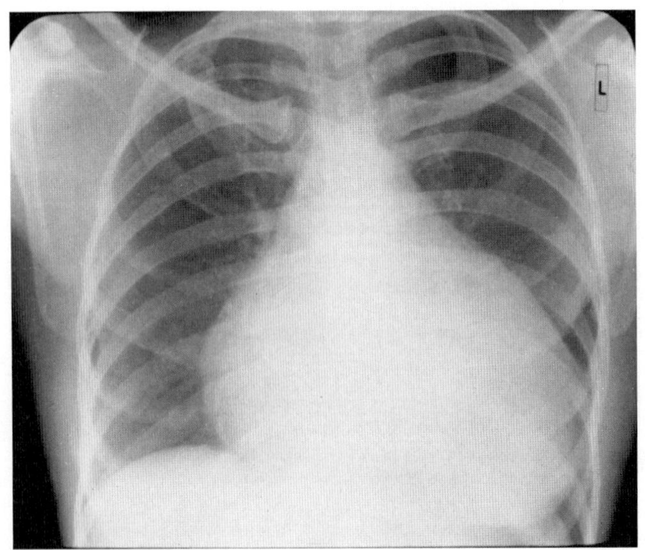

FIGURE 34-3. Pericardial effusion on posteroanterior chest film. Note how the cardiac silhouette is rounded in its lower portion and tapers at the base of the heart, resembling a plastic bag filled with water sitting on a table. [Reproduced with permission from Belenkie I: Pericardial disease, in Hall JB, Schmidt GA, Wood LDH (eds): *Principles of Critical Care*, 3rd ed. New York: McGraw-Hill, 2005.]

RISKS AND PRECAUTIONS

Traditional blind subxiphoid approaches increase risk of damage to adjacent structures, such as the liver, lung, diaphragm, and GI tract. The cardiovascular system may also sustain injuries during the procedure, including chamber puncture, myocardial damage, and laceration of coronary arteries/veins. Resultant arrhythmias may develop as well, secondary to myocardial damage. Although risks must be considered, use of specific techniques and imaging can significantly reduce injury from the procedure itself. If bedside US is not available and the patient has cardiac or hemodynamic compromise, the blind subxiphoid approach for cardiac tamponade for acute hemopericardium can be used.[23] See **Table 34-2** for a list of equipment needed.

PATIENT PREPARATION AND POSITIONING

If time and conditions permit, obtain and review a stat portable chest x-ray to identify mediastinal shift or pneumothorax. Traditional positioning for pericardiocentesis is with the head of the bed elevated to approximately 30 to 45 degrees, but in cardiac arrest or near-arrest, this position may not be feasible. Therefore, the procedure is often performed with the patient supine. Before choosing the needle insertion site, it must be noted if the patient has mediastinal shift, as this can displace structures and alter normal anatomic locations. In some instances, very small effusion volumes (50 to 100 mL) precipitate cardiac tamponade, and therefore, fluid may collect in dependent portions of the pericardial space. If the size of the effusion is small, rolling a patient to the

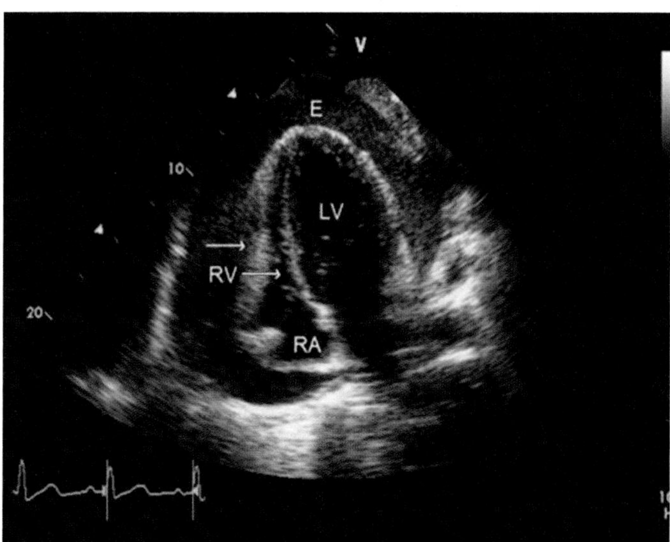

FIGURE 34-4. RV compression (*arrow*) in cardiac tamponade (apical four-chamber plane). E = effusion; LV = left ventricle; RA = right atrium; RV = right ventricle. [Reproduced with permission from Fuster V, O'Rourke RA, Walsh RA, Poole-Wilson P: *Hurst's the Heart*, 12th ed. New York: McGraw-Hill Inc.; 2008. Figure 16-135B.]

left lateral decubitus position allows fluid to collect around the apex and provides easier access. This positioning also allows the left lung to move laterally, thereby increasing cardiac exposure.

ANESTHESIA AND MONITORING

Patients undergoing emergency pericardiocentesis in the ED are often in significant distress and are being resuscitated. They may therefore already be sedated or paralyzed, or both. If local anesthesia is needed, immediately before the procedure, administer 1% to 2% lidocaine SC and along the plane of expected needle insertion. Aspirate during infiltration to avoid injection of lidocaine directly into vascular structures.

Institute cardiac monitoring and pulse oximetry, and provide supplemental oxygen. Assistants can monitor the pulse amplitude.

TABLE 34-2 Equipment for Emergency Pericardiocentesis

Antiseptic (e.g., povidone-iodine, ChloraPrep)
Local anesthetic (1%–2% lidocaine)
25-gauge needle, $^5/_8$ in. long
18-gauge catheter-type needle, $1^1/_2$ in. long (for parasternal or apical approaches)
Syringes (10, 20, and 60 mL)
4 × 4 gauze squares
Plastic tubing
Collection system or basin
US machine
Sterile US probe cover (can be sterile glove)
Sterile drapes
Yankauer suction catheter
Suction tubing
Cardiac monitoring
Optional
18-Gauge spinal needle $3^1/_2$ in. long (if needed for subxiphoid blind approach)
Alligator clips connected by wire (for ECG approach)
Bedside ECG
Nasogastric tube
Variable angle needle guide attachment for US
Towel clips
#11 scalpel blade
J-tipped guidewire 0.035 mm diameter
6F–8F pigtail catheter
Three-way stopcock

STEP-BY-STEP TECHNIQUE

1. Use universal precautions.
2. Organize needed materials.
3. Position patient as needed.
4. Identify point of maximal effusion with US (i.e., closest to transducer/skin and where accumulation is maximal). Pericardial effusions are dark, or anechoic, areas surrounding the heart. Usually the pericardium can be seen overlying the effusion. In addition, paradoxical motion of the right ventricular wall with collapse during diastole is noted in states of tamponade. Distance from the skin surface to the effusion border can be measured with most US models to better assess expected needle depth.
5. Choose needle trajectory. Trajectory should be chosen to coincide with the plane of the US beam. Identify any anatomic structure between the skin and pericardial space that lies within the expected needle path. Although many approaches can be used, the best approach should aim for the point of maximal effusion with the fewest intervening structures. For most patients, the optimal approach is the left chest wall. Most common is the left parasternal approach or the apical approach, both at the fifth intercostal space (**Figure 34-5**), or the subxiphoid approach. If using the left parasternal approach, select a site approximately 3 to 5 cm from the sternal edge to avoid the left internal mammary artery. Direct the needle over the superior margin of the rib to avoid injuring the neurovascular bundle on the inferior margin of each rib. The site may be marked with a surgical pen for easier location after sterile preparation.
6. Sterile preparation. Prepare area with povidone-iodine or equivalent antiseptic. Drape the surrounding area with sterile towels or a premade drape (clear drapes available commercially).
7. Inject local anesthetic. Inject 1% to 2% lidocaine with a 25-gauge, $^5/_8$ inch needle at the selected site before the procedure. Produce a subcutaneous wheal, and then inject into deeper tissues while avoiding entry into the chest cavity. Aspirate before injection to avoid injection of anesthetic into vascular structures.

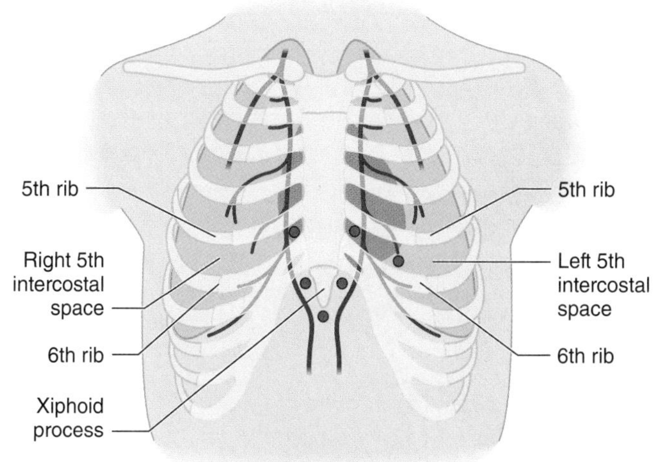

FIGURE 34-5. Potential sites to perform a pericardiocentesis. [Adapted with permission from Smith RF: Pericardiocentesis, in Reichman EF, Simon RR (eds): *Emergency Medicine Procedures*. New York: McGraw-Hill, 2004.]

8. Preparation of US. Using the cardiac probe, place a sterile cover over the probe (may use sterile glove) after placing US gel on the probe tip. Place sterile US gel over the planned site of entry. Using the nondominant hand, hold the US probe in the plane of planned needle insertion. A second operator technique may be used.
9. Pericardial needle insertion. Under direct US guidance, insert needle at the predetermined site at an approximately 45-degree angle to the skin at the transducer. Visualize the needle "tenting" the pericardium. Upon entry into the pericardial sac, a return of blood, serous fluid, pus, and so on, should be obtained. Clotted blood may prevent aspiration. Blood can clot within the needle or may have clotted within the pericardial space. Often, clotted blood within the pericardial space can be identified on US examination as echogenic material. If you suspect needle obstruction, attempt flushing the needle with 1 to 2 mL of normal saline to cleanse the needle. If aspiration is too easy, suspect ventricular puncture. To decrease complications of needle insertion, do not redirect the needle within the pericardium while aspirating. This may reduce the number of occurrences of inadvertent coronary artery lacerations or penetrating the pericardium.
10. Fluid collection. Fluid may be collected for diagnostic testing to assess for protein or albumin, cell counts, Gram stain, and cultures, among others.
11. Catheter removal. Once adequate fluid has been withdrawn from the pericardial space and hemodynamic equilibrium has returned, the catheter may be removed. The site should be dressed as with any needle insertion site. Alternatively, an optional indwelling flexible J-tip catheter may be placed as in step 2 under "Optional Steps." Although recurrence rates have been shown to decrease significantly with indwelling or extended catheter drainage, this is not routinely performed in the ED secondary to patient acuity and ongoing resuscitative measures. Once hemodynamics have been returned to normal and the patient stabilized, evaluation and possible indwelling catheter placement can be performed by the cardiologist.

OPTIONAL STEPS

1. Saline echo-contrast technique. When confirmation of the needle tip is necessary, agitated saline solution can be used. Using a three-way stopcock, attach one end to the catheter. Attach one syringe with 3 mL of normal saline and one syringe with an equivalent amount of air to the remaining two ports. Quickly mix the saline and air together and then inject into the pericardial sac under US visualization. Alternatively, the saline may be agitated by simply shaking a 10-mL syringe filled with 3 to 5 mL of normal saline and then injecting this into the pericardial space. An echo-contrasted medium should appear in the pericardial space. If the contrast disappears quickly after injection, suspect tip placement in ventricle. Rather than attempting to reinsert needle into the catheter, it is best to start again with a new needle should this complication arise.
2. Catheter placement. Using the standard Seldinger technique, a flexible J-tip guidewire is introduced through the catheter. The catheter is then removed. Next, a small "stab" incision is made at the needle entry site. A 6- to 8-French dilator is introduced over the guidewire and then removed. A 6- to 8-French pigtail catheter is then introduced over the guidewire. The guidewire is then removed. Confirmation of placement can be done by saline echo-contrast as in step 1 above. Catheter is then placed to suction.
3. Dressing. Secure catheter to chest wall with suture, dressing, or both.
4. Catheter drainage and maintenance. Pericardial fluid should be aspirated intermittently approximately every 4 to 6 hours. To prevent catheter blockage, continuous drainage is avoided. Flushing of the catheter with saline after drainage will ensure patency. Strict inputs and outputs should be measured by staff.
5. Catheter removal. Although not routinely done by ED staff, the catheter may be removed once drainage has decreased to <30 mL in 24 hours. In addition, follow-up two-dimensional echocardiography should confirm resolution of the effusion.

BLIND SUBXIPHOID APPROACH

The blind subxiphoid approach starts with similar preparation and anesthetic. The point of needle insertion starts either directly below or adjacent to the xiphoid process. An 18-gauge needle is inserted at a 45-degree angle to the patient's skin, and the needle tip is directed to *either* the left or right shoulder (**Figure 34-6**). Some authors advocate using the right shoulder as the direction of choice because this direction is parallel to the ventricular wall (in contrast to perpendicular for left shoulder direction), thereby theoretically reducing the chance of myocardial injury. In either approach, the needle is aimed toward the heart with continuous aspiration of the syringe until return of pericardial fluid.

ECG MONITORING TECHNIQUE

The ECG monitoring technique uses ECG monitoring to detect myocardial injury patterns and localize needle location. However, ECG injury monitoring alone is not an adequate safeguard.[17] The approach is similar to the blind approach in orientation. Attach the V_1 monitor lead to the needle. Watch the monitor while introducing the needle. ST elevation on

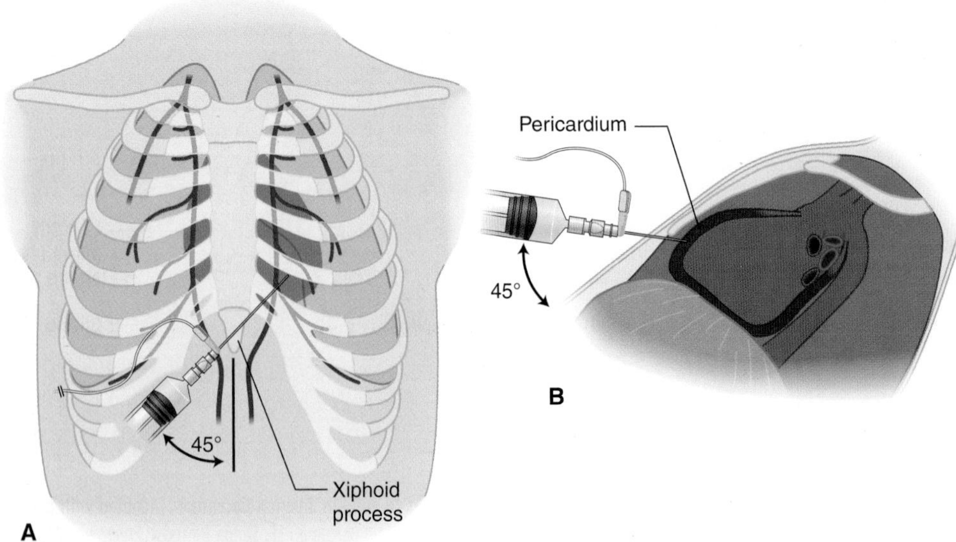

FIGURE 34-6. The subxiphoid approach. The needle is inserted at a 45-degree angle to the midsagittal plane **(A)** and at a 45-degree angle to the abdominal wall **(B)**. [Adapted with permission from Smith RF: Pericardiocentesis, in Reichman EF, Simon RR (eds): *Emergency Medicine Procedures*. New York: McGraw-Hill, 2004.]

the monitor indicates that the needle tip has contacted the myocardium. Withdraw the needle slightly and aspirate. This technique is rarely used currently due to complexity in the emergent setting and advances in US allowing for safer alternatives.

OUTCOME ASSESSMENT

A favorable outcome is the restoration of hemodynamic stability with return of normal blood pressure and heart rate. Two-dimensional echocardiography should also show decreased effusion, increased cardiac contractility, and increased cardiac output.

COMPLICATIONS

Complications may vary widely, dependent on approach and the underlying cause of tamponade. Traditional blind techniques have been associated with morbidity of 20%, with mortality as high as 6%. The overall complication rate of US-guided approaches is <5%.[16]

Major complications include chamber lacerations requiring surgery, intercostal vessel injury requiring surgery, pneumothorax requiring chest tube placement, ventricular tachycardia, and bacteremia. Minor complications include transient chamber entries, small pneumothorax not requiring intervention, hypotension secondary to vasovagal response, sinus tachycardia, pericardial catheter occlusion, and possible pleuropericardial fistulas.[16] Cardiac arrhythmias, such as atrial fibrillation, ventricular tachycardia, or asystole, may occur when the needle penetrates the pericardium. Monitor the patient closely for reaccumulation of pericardial fluid after pericardiocentesis.

DISPOSITION AND FOLLOW-UP

All patients undergoing pericardiocentesis in the ED require admission to the intensive care unit. Consult the trauma surgeon, cardiologist, or cardiothoracic surgeon, as appropriate, early in patient evaluation.

REFERENCES

The complete reference list is available online at www.TintinalliEM.com.

Analgesia, Anesthesia, and Procedural Sedation

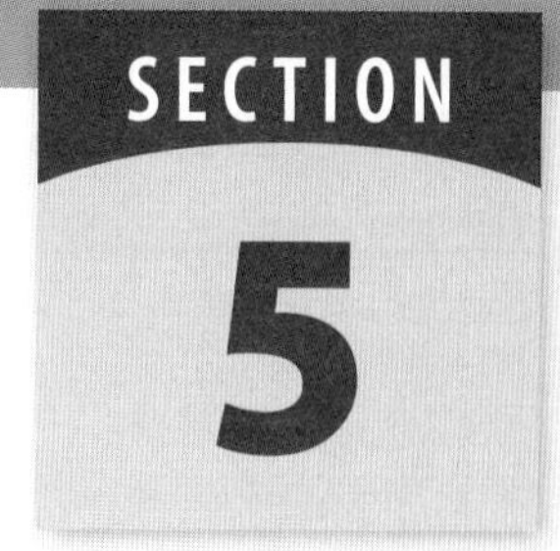

CHAPTER 35 Acute Pain Management

James Ducharme

INTRODUCTION

Pain is the most common presenting symptom for patients coming to the ED, with 75% to 80% of all patients having pain as their primary complaint.[1] Despite increasing research and information about pain management, oligoanalgesia, or the under treatment of pain, persists.[2-5] While all patients are susceptible to oligoanalgesia, certain subgroups, such as ethnic minorities, the aged, the very young, and those with diminished cognitive function, are more at risk (**Table 35-1**).[6-9] Pain management is further influenced by concerns of prescription opioid misuse, a rising concern in all age groups but most notably in adolescents and young adults. Pain and addiction are not mutually exclusive,[10] and appropriate treatment of acute pain should not be withheld for fear of facilitating drug misuse.

Specific measures to treat pain should occur *in addition* to, and at the same time as, treatment of the underlying illness or injury. **It is not possible to generalize the extent and quality of pain control needed for a specific patient.** For example, pain is an indicator of ongoing cardiac ischemia, and the goal should be to eliminate all pain. On the other hand, a patient with a traumatic injury may choose to endure more pain out of personal or cultural beliefs. Physicians may limit analgesics in those with head injuries to perform serial neurologic examinations. Whenever possible, medications that act on specific sites that initiate the pain signal—a mechanistic approach—are preferred to agents such as opioids that mask pain, which is a symptomatic approach. Current migraine treatment is an excellent example of the mechanistic approach; preferred treatment includes a serotonin agonist (triptan)[11] or a dopamine antagonist (phenothiazine),[12] rather than opiates.[13,14]

PATHOPHYSIOLOGY

Pain is the physiologic response to a noxious stimulus, whereas suffering—the expression of pain—is modified by the complex interaction of cognitive, behavioral, and sociocultural dimensions. Individual pain experience is therefore not static, but varies depending on current and past medical history, physical and emotional maturity, cognitive state, meaning of pain, family attitudes, culture, and environment. Emotions can modify pain either negatively or positively: fear and anxiety may accentuate pain, or pain can be suppressed completely if an essential task must be performed or if there is acute concern about a loved one.

The peripheral nervous system (e.g., nociceptors, C fibers, A-δ fibers, and free nerve endings) initiates the sensation of somatic pain by responding to a noxious stimulus and sending a neuronal discharge to the dorsal horn of the spinal cord.[15] Neurons in the dorsal horn of the spinal cord integrate and modulate input from multiple peripheral nerves and other sensory stimuli. Transmission then proceeds up the spinal cord to the CNS (e.g., hypothalamus, thalamic nuclei, limbic system, and reticular activating system) where further integration and processing generate the perception of pain. Identification and localization of pain, cognitive interpretation, and triggering of emotional and physiologic reactions also occur at these central sites. Unlike somatic pain, which is easily localized, visceral pain pathways are more complex and differ in structure from somatic pain pathways, which may explain the poor localization of visceral pain.

Opioid analgesics work by binding to receptors in the spinal cord and brain. There are four types of **opioid receptors**: three classic families (**delta, kappa, and mu**, each with identified subtypes) and nociceptin, a receptor with significant structural homology. These receptors are found in the brain, spinal cord, and GI tract where their physiologic function is to interact with endogenous dynorphins, enkephalins, endomorphins, endorphins, and nociceptin. Opioid analgesics interact with these receptors in varying degrees, accounting for the difference in desired and adverse effects among the drugs in this class. Stimulation of the mu-1 (μ_1) receptor produces supraspinal analgesia. Stimulation of the mu-2 (μ_2) receptor results in euphoria, miosis, respiratory depression, and depressed GI motility. Stimulation of the delta (δ) receptor produces analgesia, but less than the μ_1 receptor, and also exerts an antidepressant effect. Stimulation of the kappa (κ) receptor produces dysphoria, along with dissociation, delirium, and diuresis by inhibiting antidiuretic hormone release.

EVALUATION

Document the degree of pain on initial assessment. This process serves to identify patients with severe pain, facilitates treatment, and meets the mandates of regulatory agencies that promote assessing and treating pain. ED pain assessment should determine duration, location, quality, severity, and exacerbating and relieving factors. **The patient's subjective reporting of pain, not the physician's impression, is the basis for pain assessment and treatment.** There is at best a weak correlation between nonverbal signs, such as tachycardia, tachypnea, and changes in patient expression and movements, and the patient's report of pain, so do ***not*** rely on these to determine the severity of a patient's pain[16,17] or response to treatment.[18] Because pain is dynamic and changes with time, periodic pain reassessment is needed.

Although standardized scales for measuring reported pain are commonly used, their impact on effective pain control is uncertain.[19,20] The primary value of pain scales is their essential role in research enabling reproducible comparisons of interventions. Some studies have suggested that the use of pain scales may actually *decrease* the provision of analgesics. Given the subjectivity both of pain reporting and the provider's interpretation of such reporting, the use of simple descriptors such as "a little" or "an awful lot" is equally valid in the clinical setting. What *is* important is that the patient's subjective reporting should be the basis for assessment and management. For most, but not all, painful conditions, the goal is to control pain to the level the patient desires. **Asking if the patient requires more analgesic may even be simpler and accomplish more than using any standardized pain evaluation tool.**[21,22]

PAIN SCALES

The purpose of pain scales is to quantitate pain severity, guide the selection and administration of an analgesic agent, and reassess the pain response to determine the need for repeated doses or more effective analgesics. Several self-report instruments are valid in patients with acute pain, and some require only a verbal response (**Table 35-2**). Each tool has advantages and specific limitations. ED personnel in any one location should use the same tool so information collected is standardized. **A value assigned by a patient is not an absolute value but rather a reference point *based on past personal experience.***[23]

PAIN SCALE PERFORMANCE IN SPECIAL PATIENT POPULATIONS

The elderly often report pain differently from younger patients because of physiologic, psychological, and cultural changes associated with aging. Visual, hearing, motor, and cognitive impairments can be barriers to effective pain assessment. Using a numerical pain scale, the elderly may also experience a decrease in the minimum clinically significant

TABLE 35-1 Barriers to Adequate ED Pain Control

Patient Related	Provider Related	System Related
Ethnicity, gender, age (very young, very old) Diminished cognitive function Fear of medications: addiction, side effects Acceptance of pain as being inevitable Unwillingness to bother healthcare providers	Inadequate education No objective measuring tool for pain Accepting only pain reports that conform to our expectations Perception of addiction and drug-seeking behavior	Lack of clearly articulated standards Paucity of treatment guidelines Fear of regulatory sanctions Lack of healthcare provider accountability

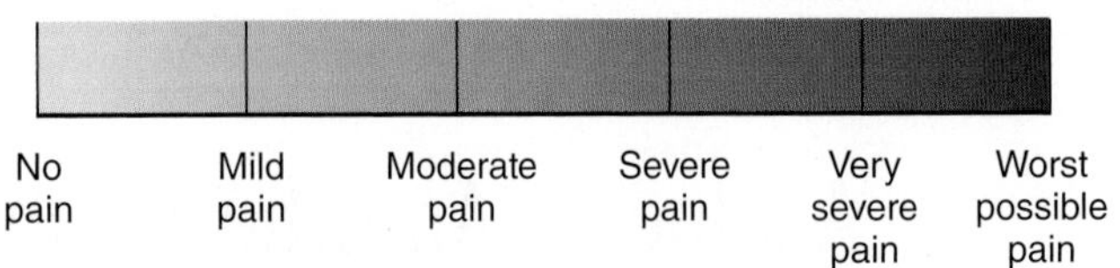

FIGURE 35-1. Pain scale: Adjective rating scale.

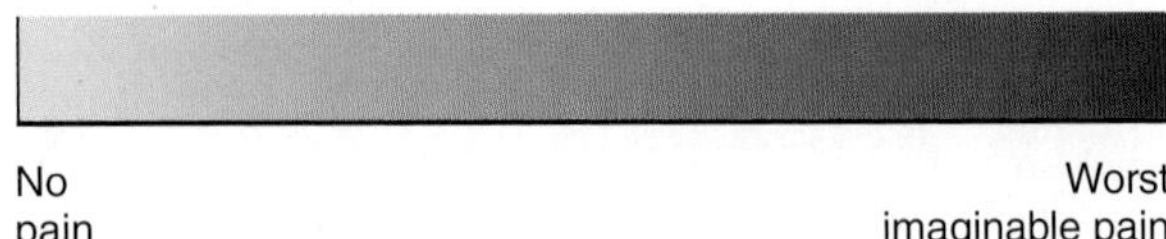

FIGURE 35-2. Pain scale: Visual analog scale (VAS).

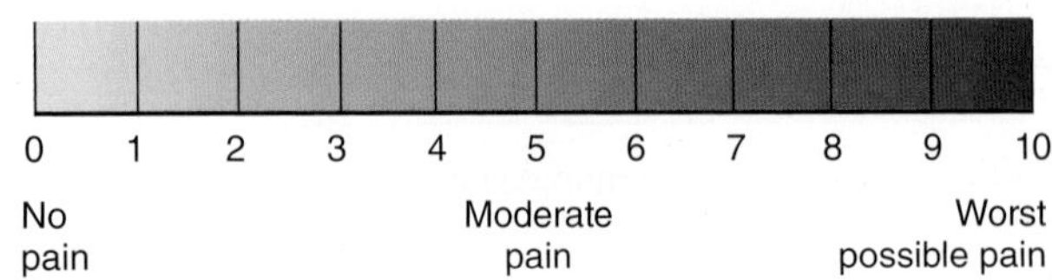

FIGURE 35-3. Pain scale: Numeric rating scale.

noticeable difference in acute pain over time.[24,25] Family members and caregivers are often able to judge nonverbal actions of the patient as representing pain or distress, so they should be used if available to help with pain assessment in the noncommunicating elderly patient.

Trauma patients and those with acute intoxication do not perform as well on pain scales.[26] Women are more likely to express pain and to actively seek treatment for pain,[27,28] yet there is a tendency to underestimate and undertreat pain in women. Ethnicity of both the patient and the physician has a bearing on different cultural concepts of pain and on the characteristics of culturally appropriate pain-related behaviors.[7] Translators and family members should be asked to provide assistance. There is also interplay between the ethnicity of the patient and that of the physician.[7] **When there are language difficulties or cross-cultural differences, the visual analog scale is the preferred pain assessment tool because it is the least affected by these factors.**

TABLE 35-3 Pain Severity with VAS or NRS

Pain Severity	VAS (0 to 100 mm) or NRS (0 to 10)
Mild	VAS: 0 to 30–40 mm or NRS: 0 to 3–4
Moderate	VAS: 40 to 60–70 mm or NRS: 4 to 6–7
Severe	VAS: >60–70 mm or NRS: >6–7

Abbreviations: NRS = numeric rating scale; VAS = visual analog scale.

PHARMACOLOGIC PAIN TREATMENT

The administration of pharmacologic agents is the mainstay of acute pain management. **The key to effective pharmacologic pain management in the ED is selection of an agent appropriate for the intensity of pain and it's time to onset of analgesic activity, ease of administration, safety, and efficacy.**[29] Acute pain is usually accompanied by anxiety and feelings of loss of control. If verbal reassurance combined with an analgesic does not suffice, an anxiolytic may be useful.

The "tiered approach" to pain management starts with an agent of low potency regardless of pain intensity, assesses the response after a clinically relevant period, and sequentially changes to agents of higher potency if pain persists. **The tiered approach for acute pain management unnecessarily subjects the patient to more prolonged suffering. It is preferable to select initial analgesics that are appropriate to treat the intensity (mild, moderate, or severe) of the patient's pain.** Agents such as nonsteroidal anti-inflammatory drugs should be considered for mild to moderate pain, and systemic opioids for moderate to severe pain (**Table 35-3**). In specific instances such as renal and

TABLE 35-2 Pain Scales[29A]

Scale	Method	Comments
Adjective rating scale (**Figure 35-1**)	Patient rates pain by choosing from an ordered list of pain descriptors, ranging from *no pain* to *worst possible pain*, with allowance for marks between discrete labels.	Easy to administer.
Visual analog scale (VAS) (**Figure 35-2**)	Patient places a mark that best describes pain intensity along a 10-cm linear scale marked at one end with a term such as *no pain* and at the other end with *worst imaginable pain*.	Pain intensity measured in millimeters from the no-pain end. A difference of 13 mm is the minimum clinically significant change *noticeable* by patients, whereas an average decrease of 30 mm appears to be the minimum *acceptable* change for pain control.*
Numeric rating scale (**Figure 35-3**)	The patient is asked to self-report pain on a scale of 0 to 10 with descriptors.	Can be used in patients with visual, speech, or manual dexterity difficulties by using upheld fingers. Not as discriminating as the VAS.
5-Point global scale	Patient rates pain as: 0 = none 1 = a little 2 = some 3 = a lot 4 = worst possible	A decrease of 1 point is a large change; scales with more choices allow monitoring of small changes in pain and may be more sensitive to changes.
Verbal quantitative scale	The patient is asked to self-report pain on a scale of 0 to 10 without descriptors.	Most commonly used scale; easy to administer.

TABLE 35-4 Pain Treatment: Comparison of Pharmacologic Classes

Class	Route	Advantages	Disadvantages
Nonsteroidal anti-inflammatory drugs	PO	Mild/moderate somatic pain plus severe colicky pain	Use caution in the elderly and in those with renal, GI, and hematologic disorders
	Parenteral	Does not require GI absorption	No more effective than PO More costly
Opioids	PO	Can be effective if adequately dosed	Variable absorption, somewhat slower onset
	IM	No IV access required	Painful injections Unreliable absorption
	IV	Ideal for titrated dosing	Need for IV access
Local anesthetics	Infiltration	Technical ease	Limited duration of action
	Peripheral nerve block	Opioid sparing	Technically difficult at some sites Facilitated with use of US guidance

biliary colic, a parenteral nonsteroidal anti-inflammatory drug may control severe pain, although combination therapy with an opioid is usually superior.

When possible, local anesthesia is a useful adjunct (**Table 35-4**). Peripheral nerve blockade for pain control and for procedures is a useful option, especially if guided by US (see chapter 36, Local and Regional Anesthesia).[30,31]

OPIOID ANALGESICS

Opioid analgesics are the cornerstone of pharmacologic management of moderate to severe acute pain (**Table 35-5**). The term *opiate* refers to agents that are structurally related to natural alkaloids found in opium, the dried resin of the opium poppy. The term *opioid* describes any compound with pharmacologic activity similar to an opiate, regardless of

TABLE 35-5 Pain Treatment: Initial Opioid Dosing

Drug [Class]	Typical Initial Adult Dose	Pharmacokinetics	Comments
Morphine [natural alkaloid]	0.1 milligram/kg IV 10 milligrams IM/SC 0.3 milligram/kg PO	Onset: 1–2 min (IV) and 10–15 min (IM/SC) Peak effect: 3–5 min (IV) and 15–30 min (IM) Duration: 1–2 h (IV) and 3–4 h (IM/SC)	Histamine release may produce transient hypotension or nausea and emesis; neither require routine adjunctive treatment.
Hydromorphone [semi-synthetic alkaloid]	0.015 milligram/kg IV 1–2 milligrams IM	Onset: 3–5 min (IV) Peak effect: 7–10 min (IV) Duration: 2–4 h (IV)	More euphoria inducing than morphine.
Fentanyl [synthetic piperidine]	1.0 microgram/kg IV	Onset: <1 min (IV) Peak effect: 2–5 min (IV) Duration: 30–60 min (IV)	Less cardiovascular depression than morphine. High doses can cause chest wall rigidity (>5 micrograms/kg IV).
	100-microgram nasal spray in 1 nostril		Used for breakthrough pain in opioid-tolerant cancer patients. Wait >2 h before treating another episode. May increase dose by 100 micrograms per episode.
	100-microgram buccal mucosa tablet		Used for breakthrough pain in opioid-tolerant cancer patients. May repeat after 30 min. Wait >4 h before treating another episode. May increase dose by 100 micrograms per episode. Available transmucosal forms not bioequivalent.
Meperidine (pethidine) [synthetic piperidine]	1.0–1.5 milligrams/kg IV/IM	Onset: 5 min (IV) Peak effect: 5–10 min (IV) Duration: 2–3 h (IV)	Contraindicated when patient is taking a monoamine oxidase inhibitor. Neurotoxicity may occur when multiple doses are given in the presence of renal failure.
Oxycodone [semi-synthetic alkaloid]	5–10 milligrams PO OR 0.125 milligram/kg PO 30 milligrams PR	Onset: 10–15 min (PO) Duration: 3–6 h (PO)	Lower incidence of nausea. Possible inadvertent acetaminophen overdose with combination agents.
Hydrocodone [semi-synthetic alkaloid]	5–10 milligrams PO	Onset: 30–60 min (PO) Duration: 4–6 h (PO)	Lower incidence of nausea. Possible inadvertent acetaminophen overdose with combination agents.
Codeine [natural alkaloid]	30–60 milligrams PO 30–100 milligrams IM	Onset: 30–60 min (PO) Duration: 4–6 h (PO)	High incidence of GI side effects. Some patients cannot convert to codeine-6-glucuronide and morphine. Possible inadvertent acetaminophen overdose with combination agents.
Tramadol [other]	50–100 milligrams PO	Onset: 10–15 min (PO) Duration: 4–6 h (PO)	CNS side effects common.

TABLE 35-6 Equipotent Opioid Doses

Drug	Equipotent IV Dose (milligrams)	Equipotent PO Dose (milligrams)	Equipotent IM Dose (milligrams)
Morphine	10	60 (acute) and 30 (chronic)	10
Hydromorphone	1.5	7.5	1.5
Fentanyl	0.1	0.2 (transmucosal)	0.1
Meperidine (pethidine)	75	300	75
Oxycodone	15	30	15
Hydrocodone	—	30	—
Codeine	130	200	130
Tramadol	—	350	—

chemical structure. Opioid use in the ED is often affected by concern for the precipitation of adverse events, such as respiratory depression or hypotension, or for facilitating drug-seeking behavior. As noted, a greater concern is oligoanalgesia and inadequate dosing of opioids when used. Considerations for use of opioids include (1) desired onset of action, (2) available routes of administration, (3) achievable frequency of administration, (4) concurrent use of nonopioid analgesics and adjunctive agents, (5) possible incidence and severity of side effects, and (6) continuation of the agent in an inpatient or ambulatory setting

Opioids need to be titrated to effect; patients differ greatly in their response to opioid analgesics.[32-34] Variation in pain reduction is related to age, initial pain severity, and previous or chronic exposure to opioids, but not body mass[35,36] or gender.[37] Relative potency estimates provide a rational basis for selecting the appropriate starting dose to initiate analgesic therapy,[38] changing the route of administration (e.g., from parenteral to PO), or switching to another opioid (**Table 35-6**), but undue reliance on these ratios is an oversimplification with potential for over- or underdosing.[39]

Opioid hypersensitivity is uncommon, and true allergic reactions are extremely rare. There is minimal evidence of clinical cross-sensitivity within opioid classes, with the possible exception that cross-sensitivity has been suggested among the piperidines (fentanyl, alfentanil, sufentanil, and meperidine). **Until more is known, it would be prudent to switch to a drug from a different opioid class if a patient develops a hypersensitivity reaction.** When used in equianalgesic doses, there is no compelling evidence to recommend one opioid over another. As much as possible, avoid using multiple agents, and titrate a single drug to the desired effect.

The use of **meperidine** is discouraged for several reasons: it is often underdosed; meperidine can interact with many drugs to precipitate a serotonin syndrome; and the parent drug is metabolized to normeperidine, which has neuroexcitatory properties and a long elimination half-life (24 to 48 hours).[40] Normeperidine can accumulate and produce toxicity in the elderly and those with renal failure, although this is a rare event.

Codeine is not a reliable analgesic, and it produces more nausea, vomiting, and dysphoria than other opioids. The analgesic effect of codeine is highly dependent on the metabolic conversion to the active metabolites codeine-6-glucuronide and morphine. Up to 10% of the U.S. population is deficient in the relevant enzymes for this conversion and, therefore, has an inadequate analgesic response to codeine. Conversely, there are case reports of neonatal deaths as a result of breastfeeding from mothers who were hypermetabolizers of codeine. In addition, the standard PO dose of 30 to 60 milligrams produces little analgesic effect above that of acetaminophen or nonsteroidal anti-inflammatory drugs.[41]

Tramadol binds to mu-receptors and weakly inhibits the reuptake of norepinephrine and serotonin producing a central opioid analgesic effect. Common side effects include dizziness, nausea, constipation and headache. Tramadol can induce the serotonin syndrome. Severe toxicity can include agitation and seizures. It is one of the many substances that can produce a false-positive result on the urine phencyclidine screen.[42]

Adverse effects of opioids include nausea, vomiting, constipation, pruritus, urinary retention, confusion, and respiratory depression. Pruritus, urinary retention, confusion, and respiratory depression are more common with IV, transmucosal, and epidural administrations as opposed to PO administration.

Adjuncts are sometimes used to enhance the analgesic effect, reduce the amount of opioid required, and prevent side effects (**Table 35-7**). Depending on the agent, amount, route, and setting, a beneficial effect can be seen. However, appropriate titration with opioids in the ED is highly effective, and there are few data to support the routine use of adjuncts with opioids in the ED.[43] Pretreatment with antiemetics is not necessary given the low risk of emesis,[44] but symptom-targeted therapy is sometimes necessary.

Transdermal formulations are not useful for acute pain treatment because of delayed onset and prolonged duration of action. **Transdermal fentanyl** and **transdermal buprenorphine** preparations are used for chronic pain, particularly in cancer patients. When such patients are treated for acute pain in the ED, it is best to remove the delayed-release transdermal opioid patches to better titrate the acute opioid dose and to minimize adverse reactions from the combination of agents.

OPIOID AGONISTS-ANTAGONISTS

Opioid agonists-antagonists are used to minimize some of the adverse effects of pure opioid agonists (**Table 35-8**). The major benefit claimed is a ceiling on respiratory depression (no further reduction in respiration with increasing doses past a set amount). It is not clear if there is a ceiling effect for analgesia. The variability in efficacy relates to each particular agent's affinity for the various central opioid receptors. **Because of the antagonistic effects, these agents should be used with extreme caution in patients with opioid addiction as they may precipitate withdrawal symptoms.**

NONOPIOID AGENTS

Acetaminophen (paracetamol) is an effective analgesic for mild to moderate pain (**Table 35-9**).[45] Acetaminophen does not affect platelet aggregation and does not have anti-inflammatory properties. No change is required for renal or mild hepatic impairment (see chapter 190, Acetaminophen).

Aspirin and the *nonsteroidal anti-inflammatory drugs* are both anti-inflammatory agents and analgesics. As anti-inflammatory agents, aspirin and nonsteroidal anti-inflammatory drugs decrease the production of prostanoids and arachidonic acid–mediated inflammatory peptides generated at the site of tissue injury, diminishing the inflammatory

TABLE 35-7 Pain Management: Adjunctive Medications

Drug	Initial Dosing	Pharmacokinetics	Comments
Prochlorperazine	5–10 milligrams IV/IM	Duration: 4–6 h	Can cause extrapyramidal reactions
Promethazine	25–50 milligrams IV/IM	Duration: 4–6 h	Can cause extrapyramidal reactions
Metoclopramide	5–10 milligrams IV/IM	Duration: 4–6 h	Can cause extrapyramidal reactions

TABLE 35-8 Pain Management: Initial Opioid Agonist-Antagonist Dosing

Drug [Class]	Initial Dosing	Pharmacokinetics	Comments
Buprenorphine [synthetic oripavine]	0.3 milligram IV/IM every 6 h 0.4 milligram sublingually every 6-8 h	Onset: rapid Duration: 4–10 h	Sedation, dizziness, nausea
Butorphanol [synthetic morphinan]	0.5–2.0 milligrams IV every 3–4 h 1–4 milligrams IM every 3–4 h	Onset: <1 min Duration: 2–4 h	Sedation, dizziness, nausea
Dezocine [synthetic benzomorphan]	2.5–10.0 milligrams IV every 4 h 5–20 milligrams IM every 6 h	Onset: 15 min (IV) and 30 min (IM) Duration: 4–6 h	Dizziness, respiratory depression
Nalbuphine [synthetic morphinan]	10–20 milligrams IV/IM/SC every 3–6 h	Onset: 2–3 min (IV) and 30 min (IM) Duration: 3–6 h	Sedation, headache, dizziness
Pentazocine [synthetic benzomorphan]	30 milligrams IV/IM/SC every 3–6 h	Onset: 2–3 min (IV) and 15–20 min (IM) Duration: 2–3 h	CNS side effects

response seen with some noxious stimuli. As analgesics, inhibition of the cyclooxygenase-2 enzyme in the spinal cord decreases the excitability of dorsal horn neurons that produce hyperalgesia and allodynia. These agents do not cause sedation or respiratory depression or interfere with bowel or bladder function. Nonsteroidal anti-inflammatory drugs have significant opioid dose-sparing effects.

Adverse effects of nonsteroidal anti-inflammatory drugs include platelet dysfunction, GI irritation and mucosal bleeding, nephropathy, headaches, and dizziness. All nonsteroidal anti-inflammatory drugs increase the risk of cardiac death in patients with ischemic heart disease,[46,47] although the cyclooxygenase-2-specific agents appear to carry higher risk than the nonselective agents.[48,49] Nonsteroidal anti-inflammatory drug–induced acute renal failure is more common in elderly patients and in those who are volume depleted, have preexisting renal or cardiac disease, or are taking loop diuretics.

OTHER PHARMACOLOGIC AGENTS

Ketamine A phencyclidine derivative, ketamine produces analgesia and/or dissociative anesthesia with the advantage of causing minimal respiratory depression with usual doses (see chapter 37, Procedural Sedation). Low-dose (subdissociative) infusions of ketamine are effective in combination with opioids for patients in severe pain.[50-52] Ketamine dosing for analgesia is typically a loading dose of 0.15 to 0.4 milligrams/kg IV over 10 minutes followed by an infusion if desired. Ketamine can be used in trauma patients, resulting in a lower opioid requirement for pain control, and is also effective in controlling acute flare-ups of neuropathic pain. Ketamine is also useful as an SC infusion in palliative care patients. Adverse effects include hypersalivation and reemergence phenomena (disagreeable dreams or hallucinations upon awakening), especially when larger induction doses are used (1.5 milligrams/kg IV).

TABLE 35-9 Pain Management: Nonopioid Analgesics

Drug	Adult Dosage	Comments
Acetaminophen (paracetamol)	325–1000 milligrams PO every 4–6 h 325–650 milligrams PR every 4–6 h If >50 kg: 1 gram IV every 6 h If <50 kg: 15 milligrams/kg IV every 6 h	Liver dysfunction and necrosis. Maximum oral dose is 3.9 grams per day when using the 325-milligram oral preparation and 3 grams per day when using the 500-milligram oral preparation. Maximum IV dose is 4 g per day.
Aspirin	325–650 milligrams PO every 4 h 300–600 milligrams PR every 4–6 h	GI irritation and mucosal bleeding. Platelet dysfunction. Tinnitus, CNS toxicity, metabolic acidosis. Maximum dose is 4 g per day.
Ibuprofen	400–800 milligrams PO every 4–6 h 400–800 milligrams IV every 6 h	GI upset, platelet dysfunction, renal dysfunction, bronchospasm. Maximum dose is 2400 milligrams per day.
Naproxen	250–500 milligrams PO every 8–12 h	GI upset, platelet dysfunction, renal dysfunction, bronchospasm. Maximum dose is 1250 milligrams per day for acute therapy.
Indomethacin	25–50 milligrams PO every 8 h 50 milligrams PR every 6 h	GI upset, platelet dysfunction, renal dysfunction, bronchospasm. Maximum dose is 200 milligrams per day.
Ketorolac	Multiple dose therapy: 30 milligrams IV/IM every 6 h, 15 milligrams IV/IM every 6 h if age >65 y or weight <50 kg Single dose therapy: 60 milligrams IM or 30 milligrams IV, 30 milligrams IM or 15 milligrams IV if age >65 y or weight <50 kg 10 milligrams PO every 4-6 h	GI upset, platelet dysfunction, renal dysfunction, bronchospasm. Greater risk of GI bleeding than ibuprofen. Use limited to 3 d IV and 5 d PO. Maximum IV/IM dose is 120 milligrams per day, but if age >65 y or weight <50 kg, then maximum dose is 60 milligrams per day. Maximum PO dose is 40 milligrams per day.
Ketamine	0.15–0.4 milligrams/kg IV over 10 min; can follow by IV infusion 0.1–0.2 milligrams/kg/h	No renal or hepatic adjustment; adverse effects uncommon with single doses; dizziness, agitation, hallucinations possible with higher doses.

TABLE 35-10 Pain Management: Neuropathic Pain Syndromes

Drug	Use	Initial Dosage	Titrate	Typical Effective Dosage (Maximum Daily Dose)
Amitriptyline or nortriptyline	Chronic pain	0.1 milligram/kg PO once in the evening	Increase over 2–3 wk	0.5–2.0 milligrams/kg per day PO (maximum 150 milligrams per day)
Carbamazepine	Trigeminal neuralgia	100 milligrams PO twice per day	Increase 100–200 milligrams per day	200–400 milligrams PO twice per day (1200 milligrams per day)
Oxcarbazepine	Trigeminal neuralgia	300 milligrams PO twice per day	Increase 300–600 milligrams per day every week	450–1200 milligrams PO twice per day
Duloxetine	Diabetic neuropathic pain	30 milligrams PO once per day	Increase after 1 wk on initial dose	60 milligrams PO once per day (maximum 120 milligrams per day)
Gabapentin	Neuropathic pain, postherpetic neuralgia	300 milligrams PO per day	Increase up to 300 milligrams per day	300–1200 milligrams PO three times per day (maximum 3600 milligrams per day)
Pregabalin	Neuropathic pain, postherpetic neuralgia	50 milligrams PO three times per day	Increase over 1 wk	150 milligrams PO twice per day to 100 milligrams PO three times per day (maximum 600 milligrams per day)

Nitrous Oxide Nitrous oxide is a fast-onset, short-acting analgesic and sedative inhalational agent useful for brief, minor procedures (see chapter 37) and for prehospital analgesia.[53] The primary adverse effects are nausea and vomiting. Nitrous oxide is usually supplied as a preblended 50% mixture with oxygen and administered to the patient by face mask, but if available, the 70/30 nitrous oxide/oxygen mixture is more effective. Barriers to ED use of nitrous oxide include the need for patient cooperation and an effective scavenging system. In addition, nitrous oxide is contraindicated in patients with altered mental status, head injury, suspected pneumothorax, or perforated abdominal viscus. Severe pulmonary disease also may alter the respiratory elimination of nitrous oxide.

Cyclic Antidepressants and Anticonvulsants Patients with acute-onset neuropathic pain, such as postherpetic or trigeminal neuralgia, are difficult to treat with short-acting opioid analgesics. It may be difficult to identify neuropathic causes of pain in ED patients, but if suspected, more specific therapy and follow-up instructions are needed. ***Long-acting* opioids, cyclic antidepressants, serotonin-norepinephrine reuptake inhibitors, and anticonvulsants are effective for neuropathic pain (Table 35-10).** When initiating an agent for patients with new-onset neuropathic pain, close follow-up with the primary care physician is important so that titration to effect may continue.[54,55] Patients already taking one of these agents for chronic neuropathic pain may require either titration upward of their medication or addition of a second agent; this should be discussed with the patient's regular physician.

Topical Medications Topical administration of medications at the site of injury or inflammation can provide pain relief with reduced systemic drug absorption and a lower risk of adverse drug reactions (**Table 35-11**).[56] This approach differs from the transdermal drug administration to achieve systemic effects, typically with opioids (see Route of Administration). Topical nonsteroidal anti-inflammatory drugs are effective for treating acute soft tissue injuries such as sprains and strains and also for chronic joint pain from osteoarthritis. Topical lidocaine therapy is effective for patients with postherpetic neuralgia and diabetic neuropathy. Topical capsaicin has produced variable results depending on the treatment population and dose applied; regular use appears necessary for prolonged pain relief. A single 60-minute application of a high-dose preparation (8% capsaicin topical patch) is effective for postherpetic neuralgia but requires professional application and removal to minimize side effects.

The primary adverse reaction of topical medications is local burning, particularly seen with capsaicin, which is derived from chili peppers. Rare cases of localized burns have been reported with topical muscle and joint pain relievers.[57] Most of the serious burns were associated with agents containing menthol (>3% concentration) and/or methyl salicylate (>10% concentration).

ROUTE OF ADMINISTRATION

Systemic pain medications can be given by multiple routes (**Table 35-12**). Oral administration is convenient, inexpensive, and appropriate once the patient can tolerate oral intake; it is a mainstay of pain management in the ambulatory ED population.

IV opioids are suitable for bolus administration or continuous infusion and are preferred to intermittent IM injections. IM injections are painful, do not allow for easy titration, and have no clinically relevant advantage over PO medications. Absorption can be variable, especially in sickle cell patients (due to scarring) and hypotensive or volume-depleted patients. Patient-controlled IV analgesic systems are particularly effective for ED patients with acute abdominal pain and in addicts

TABLE 35-11 Pain Management: Topical Analgesic Agents

Agent	Preparation	Comments
Diclofenac	1% gel 1.3% topical patch	Gel: apply using dosing card—4 grams for knees, ankles, and feet, and 2 grams for elbows, wrists, and hands. Lightly rub until absorbed. Use up to 4 times a day. Maximum total daily dose 32 grams. Patch: apply to intact skin at most painful site twice a day.
Ibuprofen*	5% gel	Squeeze 50–125 milligrams (4–10 cm) of the gel from the tube and lightly rub into the affected area until absorbed. Apply up to 4 times per day.
Ketoprofen*	2.5% gel	Squeeze 2–4 grams (5–10 cm) of the gel from the tube and lightly rub into the affected area until absorbed. Apply 2–4 times per day.
Lidocaine	5% gel 5% topical patch	Gel: apply a moderately thick layer to the affected area (approximately 1/8 inch thick). Allow time for numbness to develop. Best results obtained 20 min to 1 hour after application. Patch: apply to intact skin to cover the most painful area. Use only once for up to 12 h within a 24-h period.
Capsaicin	0.025% cream 0.075% cream 0.1% gel 8% patch	Cream and gel: apply to affected area not more than 3–4 times daily. Massage into area until thoroughly absorbed. Patch: only for postherpetic neuralgia. Requires physician or healthcare professional application. Applied for 60 min. Treatment may be repeated every 3 months.

*Not available in the United States.

TABLE 35-12 Delivery Routes of Systemic Analgesia

Method	Advantages	Disadvantages
PO	Ease Painless Minimal cost No technical skill required Patient acceptability	Unreliable GI absorption Requires gastric motility Slow onset Titration less reliable
IV	Rapid onset Titratable Usually easier to reverse	Venous access required Potential for overdose
IM or SC	Convenient	Painful Titration difficult and requires repeated injections Absorption variable More expensive than PO route
PR (transmucosal)	No first-pass hepatic metabolism No reliance on gastric motility	Requires patient acceptance and cooperation Variable absorption
Buccal/nasal (transmucosal)	Ease Painless	Difficult to control dose Can irritate nasal mucosa Available buccal mucosal fentanyl preparations are no bioequivalent
Transdermal	Ease Painless	Variable dose and duration Difficult to titrate Slow onset Prolonged duration after removal
Inhalational	Rapid onset and offset	Requires patient cooperation Scavenger equipment required
Intra-articular	Direct action No systemic side effects Can last up to 48 h	Only in major joints Risk of joint infection

with pain when compared with the usual approach of intermittent nurse-administered parenteral medications.[58-60] Intra-articular analgesia using opioids or bupivacaine can provide sustained relief during the immediate postoperative period following hip and knee surgery.[61-63] Nasal and buccal preparations of fentanyl are available primarily for breakthrough pain in opioid-tolerant cancer patients, and these routes may have a role in prehospital and ED acute pain management.[64] Sublingual buprenorphine is described as effective for ED management of acute pain from fractures.[65]

DOSAGE AND PRECAUTIONS

Safe and effective use of opioids is facilitated by choosing an appropriate initial dose[66] and subsequently titrating additional doses toward the desired effect, thus avoiding overmedication and minimizing unwanted effects. In unmonitored opioid-naïve patients, excessive doses of opioids can result in respiratory depression and decreased levels of consciousness. Hypotension is infrequent, is almost always due to histamine release with the first dose of medication, and is usually of short duration. With comorbidities, such as altered mental status, hemodynamic instability, respiratory dysfunction, or multisystem trauma, initial dosing should be decreased, and dose titration is important for achieving satisfactory pain relief.

The Elderly Acute pain management for the elderly can be a challenge; these patients may have more than one source of pain and/or multiple comorbidities and are at increased risk for drug–drug and drug–disease interactions.[67] Opioid-naïve elderly patients are more sensitive to the analgesic effects of opioid drugs, because they experience a higher peak and longer duration of pain relief. Moreover, they are more sensitive to sedation, respiratory depression, and cognitive and neuropsychiatric dysfunction. Initial IV opioid doses in the elderly are typically half those used in younger adults (e.g., morphine 0.05 milligram/kg and hydromorphone 0.0075 milligram/kg), although single doses may not achieve adequate pain control for elderly patients with acute severe pain.[68]

Addiction and Dependence Addiction is the misuse of a medication or drug to the detriment of the patient's well-being. Dependence infers that abrupt cessation of a medication will result in acute withdrawal symptoms. Dependence on opioids requires regular daily usage for 4 to 6 weeks in most patients, whereas addiction may occur after one use of heroin. Care should be taken to assess a patient's risk for addiction or diversion of prescription medications, but when uncertainty exists, the general approach is to err on the side of acute pain control, although management in opioid-tolerant patients can be a challenge.[69] Contemporary and rigorous evidence is that dependence and addiction occur in up to one-third of patients on chronic opioid therapy,[70] but there is little knowledge regarding the risk of short-term (<2 weeks) opioid therapy following an ED visit for an acute injury or temporary illness. Although EDs are not where most cases of opioid abuse originate, they are perceived as a potential perpetuator of misuse.[71] Distinguishing patient requests for medications because of oligoanalgesia from addiction often requires multiple patient assessments over time; subjective assessment in the ED during a single visit is usually inaccurate for identifying addiction versus aberrant behavior due to oligoanalgesia.[72] Use of an assessment tool such as the Drug Abuse Screening Test may provide a more objective means of screening for addiction.[73]

Renal and Hepatic Dysfunction Because most analgesics are metabolized by the liver or kidney, take care when using opioids in patients with impaired hepatic or renal function. Renal excretion is a major route of elimination for such pharmacologically active opioid metabolites such as norpropoxyphene, normeperidine, morphine-6-glucuronide, and dihydrocodeine. Mild renal failure can impede excretion of the metabolites of many opioids, resulting in clinically significant narcosis and respiratory depression. **In patients with renal failure, hydromorphone and fentanyl are the preferred opioids.** Mild hepatic dysfunction has little effect on opioid metabolism. In patients with severe hepatic dysfunction, titration with low doses of analgesics will minimize the risk of overdose.

Respiratory Insufficiency Patients with respiratory insufficiency and those with chronic obstructive pulmonary disease, cystic fibrosis, and neuromuscular disorders affecting respiratory effort (e.g., muscular dystrophy and myasthenia gravis) are particularly vulnerable to the respiratory depressant effects of opioids and nitrous oxide. Careful dose titration and monitoring of oxygenation and ventilation are necessary. Ketamine may be a useful alternative agent in such cases.

Drug Interactions Opioids may have adverse synergistic sedative effects in patients with psychiatric illnesses taking anxiolytics or other psychoactive drugs. **The use of monoamine oxidase inhibitors with meperidine is associated with severe adverse reactions, including death as the result of precipitating a serotonin syndrome (see chapter 178, Atypical and Serotonergic Antidepressants).** The cyclic antidepressants clomipramine and amitriptyline may increase morphine levels and potentiate the opioid effects.

NONPHARMACOLOGIC MODALITIES

Traditionally, nonpharmacologic techniques of pain management in the ED have been limited to application of heat or cold and immobilization and elevation of injured extremities. Other techniques may be useful in the ED and after discharge. Cognitive-behavioral techniques can be effective in reducing pain and anxiety, may control mild pain when used alone, and can enhance patient satisfaction. Such techniques include reassurance, explanation, relaxation, music, psychoprophylaxis, biofeedback, guided imagery, hypnosis, and distraction. They are a useful adjunct to pharmacologic management of moderate to severe pain. Successful application of these therapies requires a cognitively intact patient and skilled personnel, but many of the techniques require only a few minutes to teach the patient.

Physical nonpharmacologic agents are becoming increasingly relevant to acute pain management. In addition to the traditional techniques noted above, less commonly used physical modalities, such as transcutaneous electrical nerve stimulation and acupuncture, may have some potential role in the ED. Although specific technical skills and equipment are required, there is no need for IV access, and there is no systemic effect such as respiratory depression or altered mental status.

SPECIFIC SITUATIONS

ABDOMINAL PAIN

Early administration of IV opioids is safe for the treatment of acute abdominal pain in the ED and does not affect the accuracy of the evaluation, diagnosis, or management.[74-77] The dogma against the use of opioids for patients with acute abdominal pain stated in previous editions of *Cope's Early Diagnosis of the Acute Abdomen* was revised in 2000.[78] The one valid concern regarding analgesia and abdominal pain is that reduction in pain does not indicate improvement in pathophysiology. Analgesia without proper evaluation is as inappropriate as proper evaluation without analgesia.

MIGRAINE

There is no one, consistent, best analgesic agent for the management of a patient with migraine headache in the ED.[11,12,14] Opioid use for acute migraine treatment has lost favor due to poor performance in clinical trials, but can be considered if other agents have been ineffective.[14] The high success rates with promethazine, chlorpromazine, and prochlorperazine are tempered by the extrapyramidal side effects, seen in as many as 45% of patients, and occasional intense dysphoria (see chapter 165, Headache).[13]

TRAUMA

Patients in shock and those with trauma, burns, and hemodynamic or respiratory instability need judicious use of opioids.[2] Fentanyl, first as a bolus and then as an infusion, may be the opioid of choice due to its lesser impact on hemodynamic function. Use of regional analgesia is encouraged.[29] Nonsteroidal anti-inflammatory drugs should not be given to patients with major trauma due to the risks of excessive bleeding from platelet dysfunction and gastric stress ulcers and the potential for acute renal failure in a volume-depleted patient.

DISPOSITION

Although rare, intractable acute pain can be a primary reason for hospital admission. Otherwise, most patients may be safely discharged with a plan for pain management that includes instructions for use of short-acting analgesics (i.e., those with a duration of action of up to 6 hours). Persistent pain after ED discharge is common.[79-81] Prescriptions for long-acting agents (e.g., methadone, controlled-release preparations of morphine or oxycodone) are generally avoided upon ED discharge but are sometimes used for special patients, such as those with cancer in whom short-acting agents are no longer effective (see chapter 38, Chronic Pain).

Patients should be counseled to take subsequent doses on a regular basis or when their pain begins to return, rather than when it approaches its peak. Patients with recurrence of severe pain or changes in the quality of pain should be told to return to the ED for reassessment. It is best to prescribe only a few days' worth of analgesics, because conditions with a longer duration of pain require follow-up with the primary care physician. If opioids are prescribed to the elderly or those naïve to narcotics, home observation by a responsible adult is recommended so that adverse effects can be quickly recognized. **Discharge instructions for those given opioids should include instructions to avoid making important decisions while medicated and to avoid driving, operating machinery, climbing or working from heights, and so on, and should also include instructions for treatment of constipation.** Education about securing opioid prescriptions is important because up to 85% of prescription opioids misused by adolescents come from their parents' medication cabinet.

REFERENCES

The complete reference list is available online at www.TintinalliEM.com.

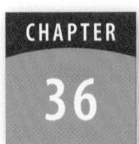

Local and Regional Anesthesia

Douglas C. Dillon
Michael A. Gibbs

INTRODUCTION

Before the availability of local anesthetics, local pain control for lacerations, fractures, and minor surgery was achieved by minimizing the pain response centrally, typically with opiates or alcohol. Procaine, which entered clinical use in 1904, was the only local anesthetic available for almost 40 years, but the short duration of action and high rate of allergic reactions limited its effectiveness. Lidocaine was introduced in 1943 and continues to be the local anesthetic most commonly used in the ED.[1,2] Additional local anesthetics are available for both topical and injectable use (**Tables 36-1** and **36-2**). Emergency physicians commonly use local and regional anesthetic techniques for potentially painful procedures performed in the ED.[3] Regional anesthesia can also be used to control the pain of acute injuries and reduce the utilization of systemic analgesics.[4,5]

LOCAL ANESTHESIA

PHARMACOLOGY

Local anesthetics are divided into two classes: **esters** and **amides**.[1,2] Both classes work by reversibly blocking sodium channels and inhibiting the propagation of nerve impulses.[1,2] Sodium channel blockade first affects the smaller nerve fibers, causing a reduction in pain and temperature sensation, followed by loss of touch, deep pressure sensation, and, finally, motor function. Esters are hydrolyzed by cholinesterase enzymes in plasma, whereas amides are metabolized by hepatic microsomal enzymes. Onset of action, duration of anesthesia, and potential for systemic toxicity are the three primary factors in selecting a local anesthetic.

The onset of action of a local anesthetic is dependent on the pK_a (the pH at which 50% of the drug is ionized and 50% of the drug is nonionized). If the ambient pH is higher than the pK_a of the agent, a greater percentage of the drug will be in the nonionized form, which diffuses more rapidly across lipid membranes, and the onset of action is shorter. Thus, drugs with a lower pK_a have a more rapid onset of action. The pH of available local anesthetic solutions is acidic, varying from 3.3 to 6.8, depending on the agent, additives, and buffers. The duration of action of the local anesthetics is a function of receptor affinity. Agents with a higher receptor affinity (e.g., bupivacaine, ropivacaine, levobupivacaine) have a longer duration of action than those with lower receptor affinity (e.g., lidocaine, prilocaine).[6] Selecting agents with a longer duration of action provides superior results for long procedures or for those in which postprocedure analgesia is desired. Longer-acting agents also offer continued analgesia when providers are pulled away from the procedure. The downside of long-acting agents is the greater risk of systemic toxicity.[7] Levobupivacaine[8] and ropivacaine[9] appear to have a lower risk of systemic toxicity than bupivacaine.

Systemic Toxicity of Local Anesthetics The systemic toxicity of local anesthetics occurs with dose-related clinical progression of sodium

TABLE 36-1 Topical Anesthetic Agents

Agent	Active Ingredients	Application	Time to Effectiveness
Intact Dermis			
Eutectic mixture of local anesthetic agents (EMLA®)	Lidocaine 2.5% Prilocaine 2.5%	Apply thick layer, 5–10 grams (maximum 20 grams), to area to be anesthetized; cover with semiocclusive dressing.	60 min
Tetracaine (amethocaine) gel (Ametop®)	Tetracaine 4%	Apply 1 gram (one tube) to area to be anesthetized; cover with occlusive dressing.	30 min
Liposome encapsulated tetracaine	Tetracaine 5%	Apply 0.5 gram to area to be anesthetized.	60 min
Liposome encapsulated lidocaine (LMX4® and LMX5®)	Lidocaine 4% or 5%	Apply 2.5 grams to area to be anesthetized.	30–60 min
Open Dermis			
Lidocaine, epinephrine, tetracaine (LET)	Lidocaine 4% Epinephrine 0.1% Tetracaine 0.5%	Apply 5 mL to gauze pad placed into wound; cover with semiocclusive dressing.	20–30 min
Mucosa			
Topical anesthetic gel (ZAP®)	Benzocaine 18% Tetracaine 2%	Apply 0.2 mL (one dispenser application) with cotton swab to area to be anesthetized.	5 min
Benzocaine spray (Hurricaine®)	Benzocaine 20%	Apply 1-s spray to area to be anesthetized; volume delivered is highly dependent on canister orientation and residual volume.	15–30 s
Viscous lidocaine	Lidocaine 2%	Apply 10–15 mL to area (e.g., topical anesthesia before upper airway procedures).	2–5 min

channel blockade in nontarget tissues, primarily the brain and heart.[10,11] Toxicity can range from subtle neurologic symptoms to refractory seizures and, ultimately, cardiovascular collapse (**Figure 36-1**).[12-14] The risk of systemic toxicity can be reduced by adherence to dose limitation and techniques to minimize systemic absorption.[15-18] Seizures due to neurologic toxicity should be treated with benzodiazepines.[19] Typical agents used to treat cardiac arrest (e.g., vasopressin) and tachyarrhythmias (e.g., β-blockers and calcium channel antagonists) should be avoided in the setting of local anesthetic systemic toxicity.[19] **IV 20% lipid emulsion** is an effective treatment for systemic toxicity from local anesthetics, especially if due to bupivacaine with its high lipid solubility.[19-27] Published reports have utilized different dosing protocols, but one consensus guideline recommends an initial dose of 20% lipid emulsion, 1.5 mL/kg infused over 1 minute with continuous infusion or repeat

TABLE 36-2 Local Anesthetic Agents

Agent	Lipid Solubility*	Protein Binding	Duration† (min)	Onset‡ (min)	Maximum Dose (milligrams/kg, with epinephrine)	Concentration (subdermal use)	Concentration (regional anesthesia use)
Amides							
Bupivacaine	High	High	200+	10–15	3 (5)	0.50%–0.75%	0.25%–0.50%
Lidocaine	Medium	Medium	30–60	5	4 (7)	0.5%–1.0%	1%–2%
Levobupivacaine	High	High	200+	10–15	2	0.25%	0.50%
Mepivacaine	Low	Low	45–90	3	4	0.5%–1.0%	1%–2%
Prilocaine	Medium	Medium	30–90	5	5	4%	NA
Ropivacaine	Medium	Medium	200+	5–15	3	0.5%	0.5%
Esters							
Procaine	Low	Low	40	15–20	7	0.25%–0.5%	0.5%–2.0%
Chloroprocaine	Low	Low	45	5	8	1%–2%	1%–2%
Tetracaine (amethocaine)	High	High	200	15	1.5	NA	0.2%–0.3%
Alternatives for patients with reactions to amides and esters							
Diphenhydramine#			25			1%	NA
Benzyl alcohol with epinephrine*ƒ*			15–25			0.9%	NA

Abbreviation: NA = not applicable.

*Lipid solubility determines the potency of the anesthetic, with the more lipophilic anesthetics having enhanced potency compared with less lipophilic agents.

†The more an anesthetic is bound to proteins, generally, the longer the duration of action.

‡The onset of action of an anesthetic is determined by the total dose of anesthetic given and the pH at which 50% of the drug is ionized and 50% of the drug is nonionized.

#Diphenhydramine 1% or 10 milligrams/mL (created by mixing 4 parts normal saline and 1 part 5% diphenhydramine).

*ƒ*Benzyl alcohol 0.9% solution (created by mixing 0.2 mL of epinephrine 1:1000 with a 20-mL vial of normal saline containing benzyl alcohol 0.9%).

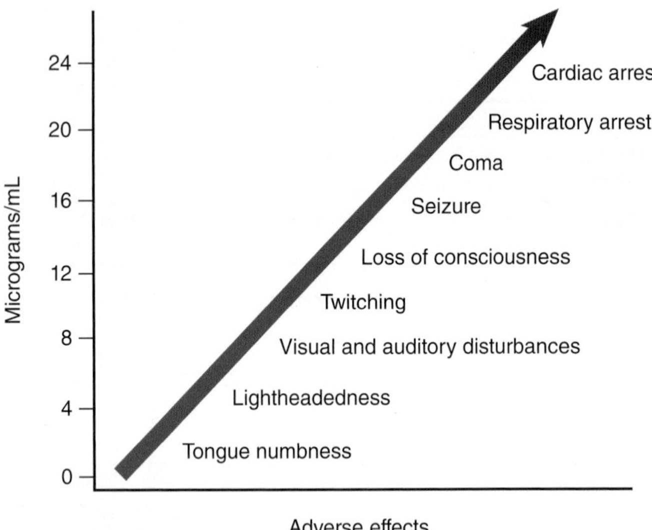

FIGURE 36-1. Adverse effects of local anesthetics. Plasma concentration of local anesthetics versus toxic effects.

doses according to the clinical condition.[19] The recommended maximum dose is about 10 mL/kg over the initial 30 minutes.[19]

Prilocaine and benzocaine can cause the oxidation of the ferric form of hemoglobin to the ferrous form, creating methemoglobin that becomes visible as cyanosis when methemoglobin concentration exceeds 1.5 grams/dL.

GENERAL PRINCIPLES OF LOCAL ANESTHETIC USE

When using any local anesthetic, calculate the volume and concentration of drug used, especially when treating smaller patients or tending to large wounds (**Table 36-2**). Aspiration before injection helps to avoid inadvertent deposit of local anesthetic in a vein or artery. When the use of a large quantity of local anesthetic seems unavoidable, procedural sedation or alternative regional blocking techniques and supplementation with systemic analgesics or anxiolytics should be considered (see chapter 37, Procedural Sedation).

The addition of **epinephrine** to the injected local anesthetic solution increases the duration of anesthesia, helps to control wound bleeding, and slows the systemic absorption.[28] The use of local anesthetic with epinephrine is safe for use in end-arterial fields (fingers, toes, etc.) in selected healthy patients,[29-34] but probably should be avoided in suspected digital vascular injury; patients with vascular disease, such as Raynaud's or Berger's disease; or other conditions in which end-arterial vascular supply is problematic. An alternative to epinephrine is clonidine (U.S. Food and Drug Administration unlabeled use), an α-adrenergic agonist, which can also be used in combination with a local anesthetic to prolong the duration of anesthesia.[35-37] A dose of 0.5 micrograms/kg of clonidine (maximal dose 150 micrograms) can be mixed with the anesthetic to prolong the duration of anesthesia by >50%. Do not exceed a maximal dose of 150 micrograms because sedation, hypotension, and bradycardia can result.[36,37]

Adverse reactions to local anesthetics are most often local reactions to preservatives or the epinephrine in the solution, and true allergic reactions are extremely rare.[38,39] In patients with true allergies to local anesthetics, two nontraditional agents can be used for wound repair via local injection—**diphenhydramine** and **benzyl alcohol** (**Table 36-2**).[40-42]

The addition of **sodium bicarbonate** to local anesthetics shortens the onset of action by raising tissue pH and reduces the pain of injection.[3,43-45] Lidocaine can be buffered by adding 1 mL of sodium bicarbonate 8.4% (1 mEq/mL) to 9 mL of 1% lidocaine. Bupivacaine can be buffered by adding 1 mL of sodium bicarbonate 8.4% (1 mEq/mL) to 29 mL of bupivacaine 0.25%. However, the addition of bicarbonate can cause precipitation of the anesthetic agent (most prominently bupivacaine) and accelerate the degradation of epinephrine in the solution, so **bicarbonate should not be added to the anesthetic unless it can be used immediately**. Additional means of reducing the pain of infiltration include the use of a 27- to 30-gauge needle, slow injection, warming the solution to body temperature, and injecting through the margins of a wound rather than through intact skin surrounding the wound.[3,43-48]

Local anesthetics can be administered topically, intradermally, subdermally, or infiltrated near peripheral nerves. When considering which approach best meets the patient's needs, many factors should be considered. In the setting of wound management, these include patient factors (age, anticipated pain tolerance, comorbidities), wound factors (location, depth, presence or absence of contamination, and/or neurovascular injury), and technical factors (time required, clinician experience). Clinical judgment combined with individual patient needs should dictate the best approach.

TOPICAL ANESTHESIA

Topical anesthetics are used in three major situations: on *intact skin* before dermal instrumentation, applied to *intact mucosa*, and placed on *open skin* for pain control or before wound repair.[49-51] Topical anesthetics are probably as effective as local anesthetic infiltration for suturing of many dermal lacerations, although the comparison studies are of modest quality.[52]

An alkaline (pH approximately 9) cream mixture of lidocaine and prilocaine [eutectic mixture of local anesthetics (**EMLA®**)] was the first topical anesthetic formulated to penetrate intact skin. When applied for at least 60 minutes under a semiocclusive dressing before dermal instrumentation, this lidocaine/prilocaine mixture is as efficacious as the infiltration of local anesthetic and is ideal for venous catheter insertion and lumbar puncture. Liposome-encapsulated tetracaine, liposome-encapsulated lidocaine, and tetracaine gel have all been compared to the lidocaine/prilocaine mixture and found to be equally efficacious (**Table 36-1**).[53-57]

The tetracaine, epinephrine, and cocaine mixture is a topical anesthetic used on open dermis. Due to the potential for CNS and cardiovascular toxicity, the cocaine component of this combination has been replaced with lidocaine. This mixture—**lidocaine, epinephrine, and tetracaine**—has a variety of formulations and is usually compounded by the hospital pharmacy in accordance with the concentration preferences of local clinicians. A common version is 4% lidocaine, 0.1% epinephrine, and 0.5% tetracaine prepared in 5-mL vials.

INTRADERMAL AND SUBDERMAL ANESTHESIA

Intradermal injection produces a visible wheal, whereas subdermal injection does not. Intradermal injection produces more immediate pain upon injection due to stretching of the compact dermal structure, but can enhance the anesthetic effect by applying pressure to and numbing the cutaneous pain sensors. Intradermal injection raises the skin surface and is useful when shaving off a cutaneous lesion. Subdermal injections have a slower onset of action, are less painful, and are the most commonly used method of achieving local anesthesia in the ED and for office-based surgery.[3,58] Local anesthetics may be delivered directly into the subdermal space in most clean lacerations or as a field block for contaminated wounds.

In addition to modifying the injected solution, a variety of techniques are used to reduce the pain of needle puncture and local anesthetic injection[43-45,59]: application of a topical anesthetic prior to injection,[60,61] warming the local anesthetic agent,[46-48] stretching the skin at the puncture site, vibrating the skin adjacent to the area,[62,63] talking during the process to distract the patient, inserting the needle through enlarged pores or hair follicles, inserting the needle with bevel up position,[64] or numbing the skin with an aerosol refrigerant.[65-69]

REGIONAL ANESTHESIA

Regional anesthesia is a technique that infiltrates local anesthetic agents adjacent to peripheral nerves ("nerve blocks") and is typically used for complicated lacerations, abscesses, fractures, and dislocations.[70-72]

Providing adequate anesthesia quells patient anxiety, provides greater patient satisfaction, and increases the likelihood of an optimal result when treating complex injuries. With careful technique, serious complications from peripheral nerve blocks are uncommon.[73-75] Assess and document distal neurovascular status before application of a regional nerve block to prevent masking a primary traumatic neurovascular injury. Distal vascular function is assessed by noting skin color and temperature, measuring capillary refill time, and palpating pulses. Distal neurologic function is assessed by noting cutaneous sensation (pain, touch) and motor function (active movement, strength). For digital injuries, assess digital nerves by determining two-point discrimination on the volar pad before anesthetic injection. **Normal two-point discrimination is <6 mm at the fingertips and is often <2 mm. Compare the injured digit with the contralateral normal digit.**

Regional anesthesia for laceration repair eliminates wound distortion caused by large-volume subdermal injection. Regional anesthesia on the extremities provides superior pain control when compared with subdermal infiltration of anesthetic.[70] Topical anesthetic before peripheral nerve blocks can minimize the pain associated with the block.[53-57,60,61]

When selecting a local anesthetic for regional anesthesia, consider the onset of clinical effects, duration of analgesia, and risk of toxicity.[70] Although lidocaine continues to be the most popular agent, bupivacaine, levobupivacaine, and ropivacaine offer a longer duration of action, with levobupivacaine and ropivacaine being significantly less cardiotoxic.[6,8,9] Peripheral nerve blocks require time to achieve optimal analgesia, approximately 10 to 20 minutes for lidocaine and 15 to 30 minutes for bupivacaine. Pain and temperature sensation are affected first, followed by loss of touch, deep pressure, and then motor function. Intraneural injection of anesthetic causes significant pain.[76] Thus, if excessive pain upon injection is noted, withdraw the needle a few millimeters, and after pain abates, resume the injection.

The regional nerve blocks commonly performed by emergency physicians are often done using the "landmark" technique to identify the site of local anesthetic injection.[70] The major disadvantage of the landmark approach is anatomic variation. Large volumes of anesthetic are typically administered, in case the needle tip is not close to the desired nerve. Two devices in common use help localize and direct the needle to maximize the rate of successful anesthesia: a peripheral nerve stimulator using electrically insulated needles and US guidance to localize the nerve.[77-81] US guidance shortens the block performance time, reduces the number of needle passes, and enables blocks to be performed using lower anesthetic doses.[82-84] Training to use US-guided regional anesthesia in the ED typically involves a didactic session, supervised practice in ultrasonographic identification of the relevant structures, and procedural practice on simulation mannequin.[85,86] The use of US is recommended when performing more complex nerve blocks.

The performance of peripheral nerve blocks requires an element of hand–eye coordination that is difficult to display in words and photographs.

DIGITAL BLOCKS

Digital Nerve Block • *Purpose* A digital nerve block provides anesthesia to the entire digit and is an excellent block when tending to lacerations of the fingers or toes, drainage of paronychia, finger or toenail removal or repair, and reduction of fractured or dislocated fingers or toes.[87] Use of topical anesthesia before instrumentation can quell anxiety about the procedure and minimize pain. Assess distal capillary refill and two-point discrimination (normal <6 mm) on the volar pad before application of the block. For digital blocks, there is less pain with injection using lidocaine 1% with epinephrine compared to bupivacaine 0.5%, but the duration of anesthesia is only about half as long.[88]

Patient Positioning and Anatomy The hand and wrist are placed in a prone (palm down) position. The common digital nerves are derived from the median and ulnar nerves. In the distal palm, the common digital nerve divides into paired palmar branches that travel on both sides of the flexor tendon sheath and innervate the lateral and palmar aspect of each digit. The dorsal digital nerves are smaller, derived from the radial and ulnar nerves, and travel on the dorsal lateral aspect of each finger to provide sensation to the back of the finger.

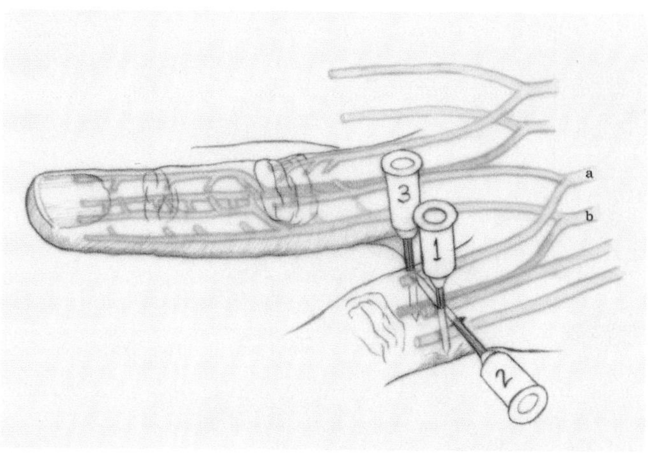

FIGURE 36-2. Digital nerve block. Anesthetic placed as shown blocks both the dorsal (a) and palmar (b) digital nerves, ensuring circumferential anesthesia of the finger. By using the sequence shown, the prior injection provides relief from the injection to follow. See Digital Nerve Block section for further details. [Illustration used with permission of Timothy Sweeney, MD.]

Technique Insert the needle on the dorsal surface of the proximal phalanx, advance toward the volar surface staying tangential to the phalanx, aspirate to ensure no inadvertent vascular puncture has occurred, deposit 1 mL of anesthetic solution, and inject an additional 1 mL while withdrawing the needle back to the skin surface (**Figure 36-2**). Reinsert the needle in the same location, but direct it across the dorsum of the digit to the other side, and inject a 1-mL band of anesthetic solution into the subcutaneous space across the dorsum of the digit. Repeat the initial injection process on the other side of the digit.

Transthecal or Flexor Tendon Sheath Digital Nerve Block • *Purpose* A transthecal or flexor tendon sheath digital nerve block provides anesthesia to the entire digit by utilizing the flexor tendon sheath to apply anesthetic to the digital nerves.[89] This procedure can be performed in addition or as an alternative to a digital nerve block. However, **flexor tendon sheath block may not fully anesthetize the distal fingertip**.

Patient Positioning and Anatomy The hand and wrist are placed in a supine (palm up) position. The flexor tendon sheath surrounds the flexor tendon on the palmar side of the digit.

Technique Identify the distal palmar crease on the palmar aspect of the hand. Have the patient flex the finger against resistance to improve visualization of the flexor tendon. Identify the distal palmar crease of the digit to be blocked, and insert the needle at a 45-degree angle to the palmar plane with the tip pointed distally (**Figure 36-3**). Advance the needle until a "pop" is felt, indicating penetration of the flexor tendon sheath. Inject 2 to 3 mL of anesthetic solution. If bone is struck before the "pop" is felt, withdraw the needle 2 to 3 mm and inject the solution.

A modification of the transthecal approach is to inject into the flexor tendon sheath at the base of the digit in the metacarpal crease[90,91] or into the midportion of the proximal phalanx.[92]

HAND AND WRIST BLOCKS

The median, radial, and ulnar nerves supply the sensory innervation to the hand and can be used in part or in combination to provide anesthesia for lacerations, puncture wounds, or fracture/dislocation reductions (**Figures 36-4** and **36-5**).

Median Nerve Block • *Purpose* A median nerve block provides anesthesia to the thumb, index, long, and half of the ring finger distal to the proximal interphalangeal joint, but not the dorsum of the thumb (**Figures 36-4** and **36-5**).

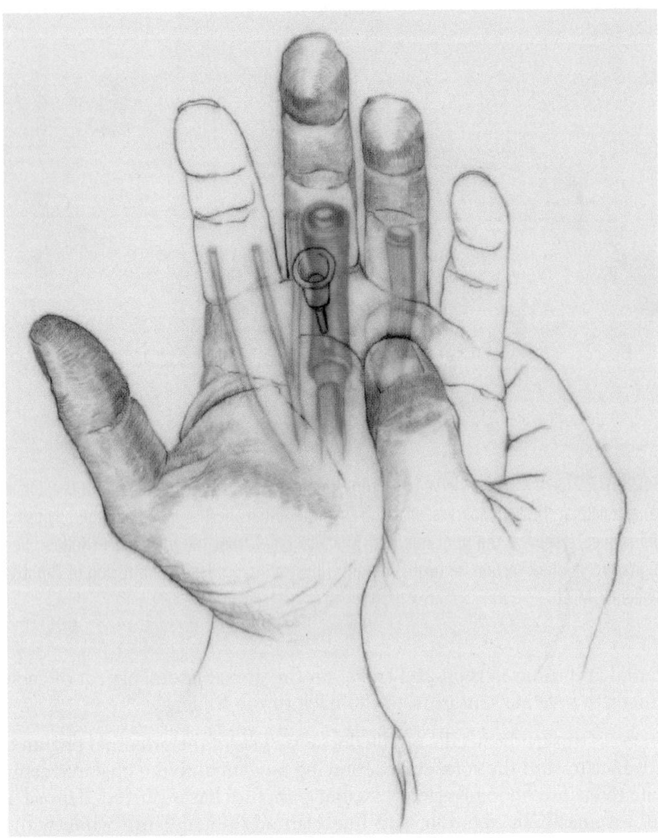

FIGURE 36-3. Transthecal (flexor tendon sheath) digital nerve block. The point of injection is in the middle of the flexor tendon sheath at the level of the distal palmar crease. A 25-gauge needle is advanced at 45 degrees, with tip directed distally until it enters the flexor tendon sheath (shown in blue) or until bone is encountered. When the needle is properly placed within the flexor tendon sheath, the anesthetic solution is injected. Diffusion out of the tendon sheath blocks adjacent palmar digital nerves. See Transthecal or Flexor Tendon Sheath Digital Nerve Block section for further details. [Illustration used with permission of Timothy Sweeney, MD.]

Patient Positioning and Anatomy The hand and wrist are placed in a supine (palm up) position. The median nerve traverses between the flexor carpi radialis and the palmaris longus tendon at the proximal wrist crease. With the hand and wrist in a supine position, the flexor carpi radialis is lateral (radial direction) and the palmaris longus is medial (ulnar direction) to the nerve. When the patient makes a fist and flexes the wrist, the

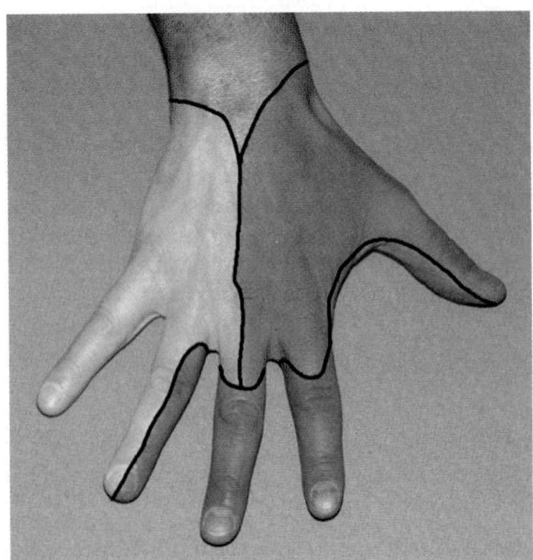

FIGURE 36-4. Hand innervation, dorsal view. Dorsal hand distribution of ulnar nerve (yellow), radial nerve (red), and median nerve (blue).

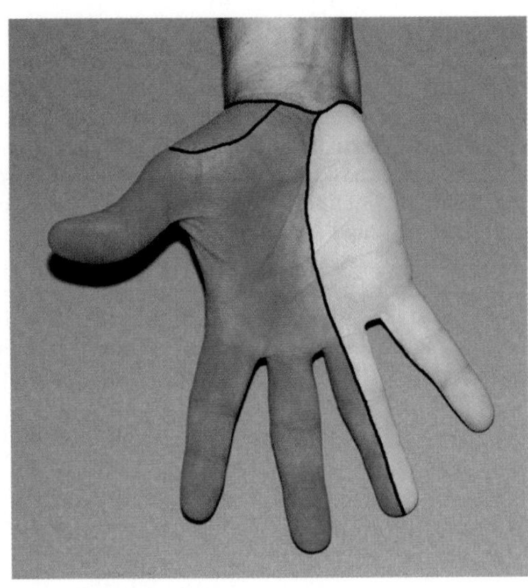

FIGURE 36-5. Hand innervation, palmar view. Palmar hand distribution of ulnar nerve (yellow), radial nerve (red), and median nerve (blue).

palmaris longus tendon is usually the more prominent of the two tendons (**Figure 36-6**, top left).

Technique Raise a wheal of anesthetic in the subcutaneous space between the palmaris longus and flexor carpi radialis at the level of the proximal palmar crease (**Figure 36-6**, right). Insert the needle until the "pop" of

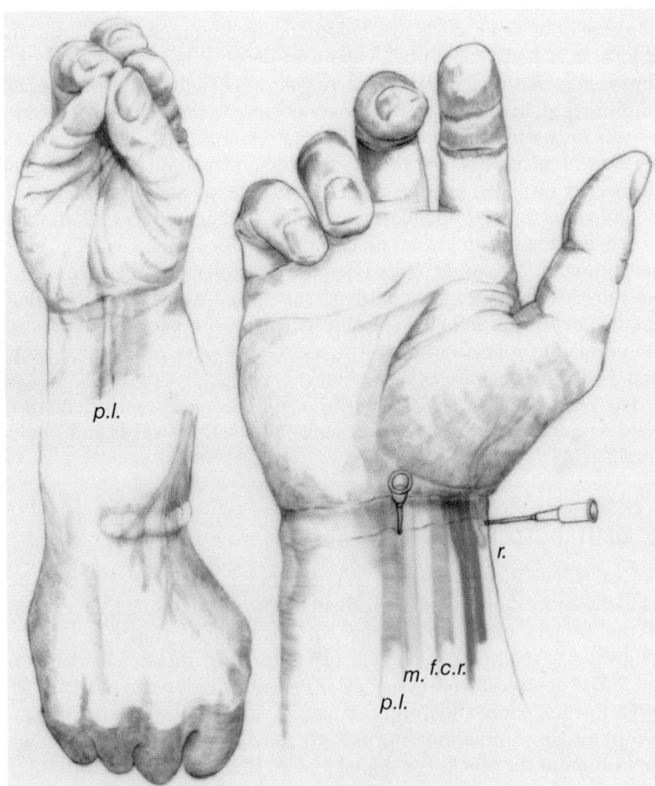

FIGURE 36-6. Median and radial nerve block. *Top left:* Technique for identification of the palmaris longus tendon (p.l.) through wrist flexion using finger and thumb opposition. *Right:* The median nerve (m.) is blocked by inserting the needle between the palmaris longus and flexor carpi radialis (f.c.r.) tendons. The radial nerve (r.) block begins with an injection over the lateral aspect of the radial styloid. *Lower left:* The radial nerve block continues dorsally as a subcutaneous field block extending to the dorsal mid wrist. See Median Nerve Block section for further details. [Illustration used with permission of Timothy Sweeney, MD.]

the deep fascia can be felt, and inject 3 to 5 mL of anesthetic. If bone is contacted before the "pop" is felt, withdraw the needle 2 to 3 mm and inject the solution. To increase the probability of a successful block, withdraw the needle back to the skin and reinsert, directing the needle 30 degrees medially and laterally, and inject an additional 1 to 2 mL of anesthetic solution. The palmar branch of the medial nerve is superficial and can be blocked by withdrawing the needle to the subcutaneous space and injecting 2 to 3 mL of anesthetic solution.

Radial Nerve Block • *Purpose* A radial nerve block provides anesthesia to the dorsal lateral half of the hand and dorsal aspect of the thumb.

Patient Positioning and Anatomy The hand and wrist start in a neutral position (thumb side up) and then rotate into a prone (palm down) position. The superficial branch of the radial nerve traverses above the styloid process of the radius and provides sensation to the dorsum of the thumb, index finger, and lateral half of the middle finger (**Figures 36-4** and **36-5**). Other branches of the radial nerve traverse over the anatomic snuff box. The anatomic snuff box is formed by the extensor tendons of the pollicis brevis and longus and the radial styloid.

Technique Raise a wheal of anesthetic in the subcutaneous space just proximal to the anatomic snuffbox. Inject 5 mL of anesthetic solution into the subcutaneous tissue overlying the radial styloid (**Figure 36-6**, right). Then, reinsert the needle and direct it through the subcutaneous space in a lateral (ulnar) direction, injecting a band of an additional 5 mL of anesthetic solution to ensure blockage of the smaller branches of the radial nerve (**Figure 36-6**, lower left). The distribution of the radial nerve is less predictable; therefore, a generous amount of anesthesia should be injected.

Ulnar Nerve Block • *Purpose* An ulnar nerve block provides anesthesia to the entire fifth digit, half of the fourth digit, and the medial aspect of the hand and wrist.

Patient Positioning and Anatomy The hand and wrist are placed in a supine (palm up) position. The ulnar nerve travels with the corresponding vein and nerve and can be located underneath (deep) to the flexor carpi ulnaris. To identify the flexor carpi ulnaris, have the patient make a fist and tense the wrist. The flexor carpi ulnaris is the most prominent tendon on the ulnar side at the wrist (**Figure 36-7A**).

Technique Raise a wheal of anesthetic in the subcutaneous space just proximal (1 to 2 cm) to the most distal wrist crease. Insert the needle under the flexor carpi ulnaris tendon to an additional 5 to 10 mm past the edge of the tendon (**Figure 36-7C**). Aspirate before injection to ensure that inadvertent arterial/venous puncture has not occurred, and inject 3 to 5 mL of anesthetic solution. To block the dorsal branches of the ulnar nerve, inject 2 to 3 mL of anesthetic solution in the subcutaneous space just above the tendon of the extensor carpi ulnaris (**Figure 36-7B**). US guidance can be useful when anatomic landmarks are not easy to discern.[93]

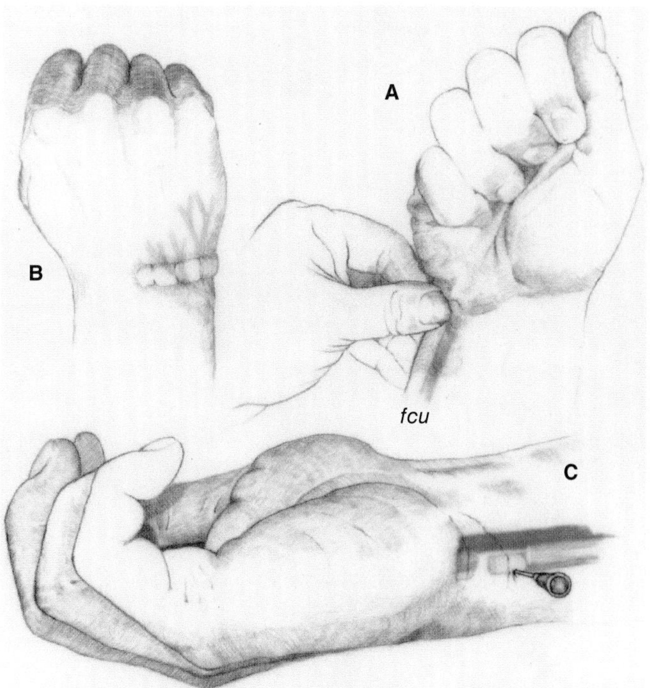

FIGURE 36-7. Ulnar nerve block. **A.** Technique for identifying the flexor carpi ulnaris tendon (fcu) by making a fist and tensing the wrist. **B.** The subcutaneous field block of the dorsal ulnar nerve branches, extending from the site of insertion of the ulnar block to the midline dorsal wrist. **C.** The needle is oriented horizontally beneath the flexor carpi ulnaris tendon and inserted to a depth of 5 to 10 mm past the tendon edge where the anesthetic solution is injected after a negative aspiration. See Ulnar Nerve Block section for further details. [Illustration used with permission of Timothy Sweeney, MD.]

FOOT AND ANKLE BLOCKS

The five nerves that provide sensation to the foot are four branches of the sciatic nerve (deep and superficial peroneal, tibial, and sural nerves) and one cutaneous branch of the femoral nerve (saphenous nerve; **Figures 36-8** through **36-11**). These are excellent blocks to use alone or in combination for lacerations, fracture reductions, and exploring wounds. The deep peroneal nerve and the posterior tibial nerves are deep nerves and can be more consistently found by anatomic landmarks. The superficial peroneal, sural, and saphenous nerves are superficial and located in the subcutaneous tissue encircling the ankle. Due to the anatomic variability of these three nerves, no single injection point can reliably provide adequate anesthesia, so these nerves are blocked by depositing the local anesthetic agent as a field block in the subcutaneous space in the area through which the nerve travels. The pertinent landmarks for performing all of the ankle blocks are the extensor hallucis longus, tibialis anterior tendon, Achilles tendon, and the medial and lateral malleolus (**Figure 36-12**).

When all five blocks are used for complete foot anesthesia, the deep nerves (deep peroneal and posterior tibial) should be anesthetized before the surface anatomy is distorted by the superficial field blocks of

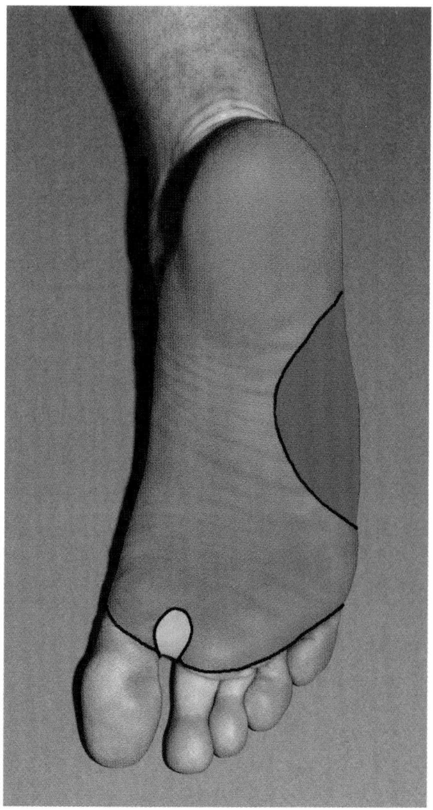

FIGURE 36-8. Foot innervation plantar view. Plantar foot distribution of deep peroneal nerve (green), posterior tibial nerve (red), and sural nerve (blue).

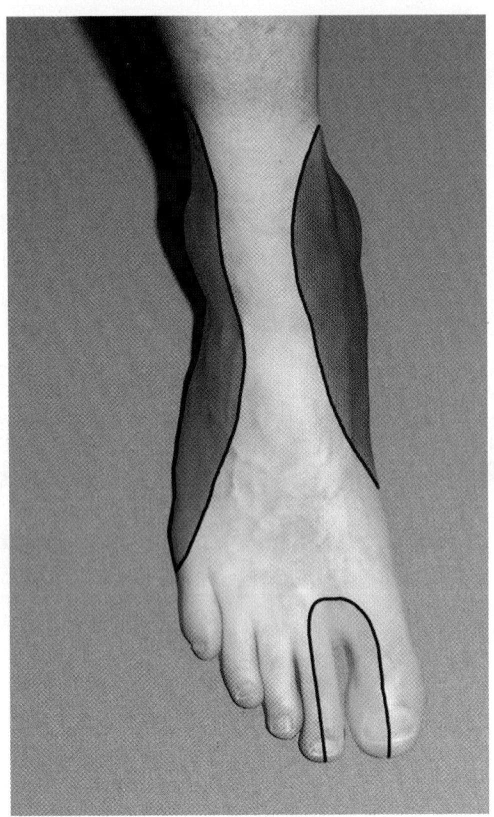

FIGURE 36-9. Foot innervation dorsal view. Dorsal foot distribution of deep peroneal nerve (green), superficial peroneal nerve (yellow), saphenous nerve (brown), and sural nerve (blue).

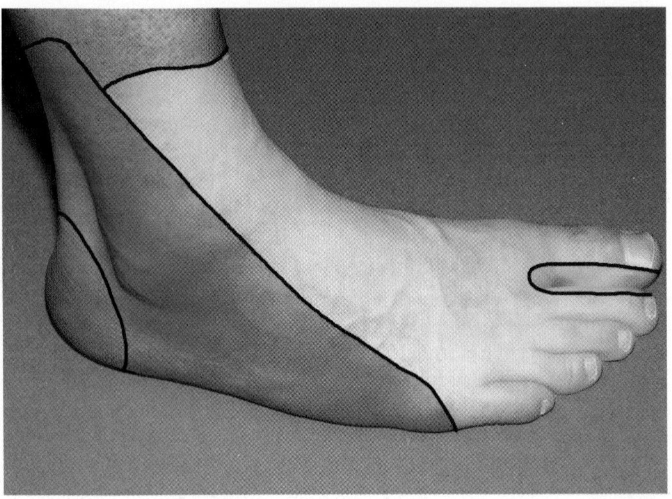

FIGURE 36-11. Foot innervation lateral view. Lateral foot distribution of deep peroneal nerve (green), superficial peroneal nerve (yellow), posterior tibial nerve (red), and sural nerve (blue).

the other three. An additional tip is to prepare and clean the entire foot before starting so that the physician can change his or her body position and reposition the patient's foot as needed to avoid awkward reaches when accessing all five sites.

Deep Peroneal Nerve Block • *Purpose* A deep peroneal nerve block provides anesthesia to the web space between the first and second toe and a small area just proximal to the first and second toe on the plantar aspect of the foot.

Patient Positioning and Anatomy The foot is placed in a neutral position. At the level of the medial malleolus, the deep peroneal nerve can be found

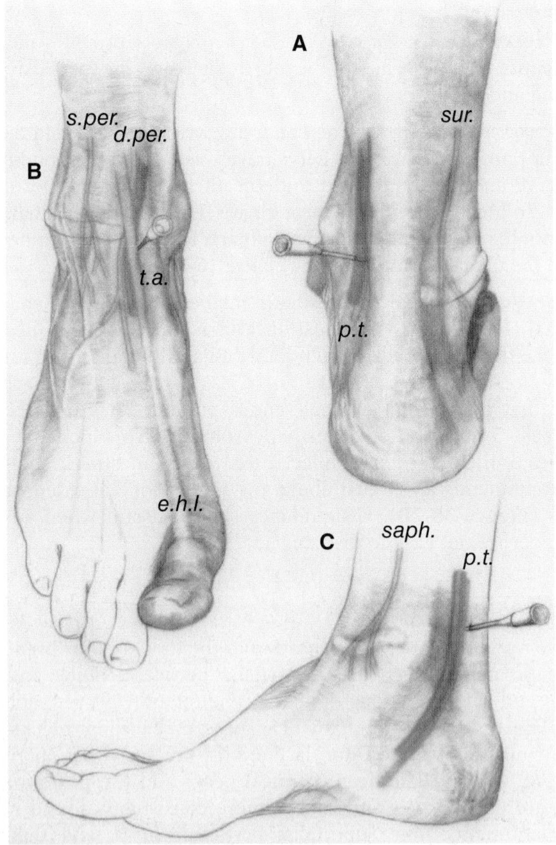

FIGURE 36-12. Ankle nerve blocks. **A.** The subcutaneous field block of the sural nerve (sur.) extends from the Achilles tendon to the lateral malleolus. The posterior tibial nerve (p.t.) is blocked just behind the posterior tibial artery. **B.** The deep peroneal nerve (d.per.) block is blocked at the level of the medial malleolus between the anterior tibial tendon (t.a.) and extensor hallucis longus tendon (e.h.l.). The subcutaneous field block of the superficial peroneal nerve (s.per.) extends from the lateral malleolus to the anterior tibial tendon. **C.** The posterior tibial nerve is blocked posteriorly to the posterior tibial artery. The subcutaneous field block of the saphenous nerve (saph.) extends from the medial malleolus to the anterior tibial tendon. See Foot and Ankle Blocks section for further details. [Illustration used with permission of Timothy Sweeney, MD.]

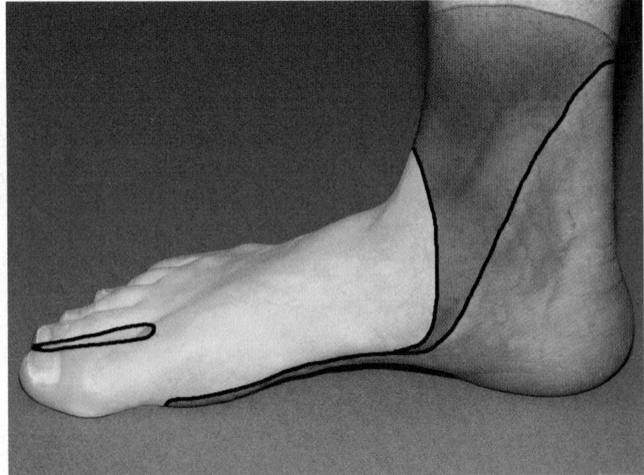

FIGURE 36-10. Foot innervation medial view. Medial foot distribution of superficial peroneal nerve (yellow), saphenous nerve (brown), and posterior tibial nerve (red).

between the extensor hallucis longus and the tibialis anterior tendon. Extension of the big toe against resistance will help to identify the extensor hallucis longus. Dorsiflexion and inversion of the ankle will help to identify the tibialis anterior tendon.

Technique Raise a wheal of anesthesia in the subcutaneous space between the extensor hallucis longus and the tibialis anterior tendon at the level of the medial malleolus (**Figure 36-12B**). With the syringe perpendicular to the skin, insert the needle until the extensor retinaculum is penetrated or bone is struck. If bone is struck, withdraw the needle 2 mm. After aspirating to verify that no vascular structure has been entered, inject approximately 2 to 3 mL of anesthetic solution. To increase the chance of a successful block, withdraw the needle back to the skin and reinsert, direct the needle 30 degrees medially and laterally, and deposit an additional 2 mL of anesthetic solution on each side.

Posterior Tibial Nerve Block • *Purpose* A posterior tibial nerve block provides anesthesia to the plantar aspect of the foot. This is an excellent block when repairing a laceration on the bottom of the foot.

Patient Positioning and Anatomy The patient can be either supine with the foot rotated outward or prone with the foot rotated inward. The posterior tibial nerve, artery, and vein can be found just posterior to the medial malleolus. The nerve is deep to the fascia and superficial/posterior to the artery.

Technique Raise a wheal of anesthesia posterior to the medial malleolus. Palpate the posterior tibial artery and insert the needle just posterior to the artery until it is deep to the fascia or bone is struck (**Figure 36-12A** and **C**). If bone is struck, withdraw the needle 2 mm. Inject 2 to 3 mL of local anesthetic solution after aspirating to ensure that inadvertent arterial/venous puncture has not occurred. To increase the chance of a successful block, withdraw the needle back to the skin and reinsert, directing the needle 30 degrees medially and laterally, and deposit an additional 2 mL of anesthetic solution on each side. US guidance can be used to guide the needle and increase the completeness of a posterior tibial nerve block.[94]

Superficial Peroneal Nerve Block • *Purpose* A superficial peroneal nerve block provides anesthesia to the dorsal lateral aspect of the foot.

Patient Positioning and Anatomy The patient is supine, and the foot is rotated inward. The superficial peroneal nerve traverses the lateral portion of the ankle in the subcutaneous space between the lateral malleolus and the tibialis anterior tendon.

Technique Prepare a sterile site between the superior border of the lateral malleolus and the tibialis anterior tendon. Dorsiflexion and inversion of the ankle will help to identify the tibialis anterior tendon. In the subcutaneous space, inject 5 mL of anesthetic, tracking from the tibialis anterior tendon to the superior portion of the lateral malleolus (**Figure 36-12B**). Creation of a subcutaneous wheal indicates proper anesthetic placement.

Sural Nerve Block • *Purpose* A sural nerve block provides anesthesia to the lateral aspect of the ankle with some extension of anesthesia to the plantar aspect of the foot.

Patient Positioning and Anatomy The patient can be either supine with the foot rotated inward or prone with the foot rotated outward. The sural nerve traverses the posterior lateral portion of the ankle in the subcutaneous space between the Achilles tendon and the lateral malleolus.

Technique Identify the space between the Achilles tendon and the superior border of the lateral malleolus. In the subcutaneous space, inject 5 to 6 mL of anesthetic solution in a band running from the superior portion of the lateral malleolus to the Achilles tendon (**Figure 36-12A**). Creation of a subcutaneous wheal indicates proper anesthetic placement. US guidance by injecting the local anesthetic around the lesser saphenous vein may facilitate a more complete and longer duration block.[95]

Saphenous Nerve Block • *Purpose* A saphenous nerve block provides anesthesia to the medial aspect of the ankle.

Patient Positioning and Anatomy The foot is in a neutral position. The saphenous nerve traverses the anterior medial portion of the ankle in the subcutaneous space between the tibialis anterior tendon and the medial malleolus.

Technique Identify the space between the tibialis anterior tendon and the superior border of the medial malleolus. In the subcutaneous space, inject 5 to 6 mL of anesthetic solution from the tibialis anterior tendon to the superior portion of the medial malleolus (**Figure 36-12C**). Creation of a subcutaneous wheal indicates proper anesthetic placement.

FACIAL NERVE BLOCKS

Facial nerve blocks provide excellent analgesia and little to no distortion of the forehead, cheek, and chin (**Figure 36-13**).[70,96] **Topical anesthetic applied to the mucosa should be used before the intraoral approach for infraorbital and mental nerve blocks.** It is important to assess neurovascular status before application of the block to prevent masking a primary traumatic neurovascular injury.

Supraorbital and Supratrochlear Nerve Blocks • *Purpose* Supraorbital and supratrochlear nerve blocks provide anesthesia to the entire forehead up to the vertex of the scalp and down the bridge of the nose.

Patient Positioning and Anatomy The patient is either supine or sitting. The supraorbital nerve exits the supraorbital foramen, which is in line with the pupil and above the superior orbital rim. The supratrochlear nerve exits from under the superior orbital rim 5 to 10 mm medial to the supraorbital foramen. The supraorbital nerve supplies most of the forehead, whereas the supratrochlear nerve supplies the area along the bridge of the nose (**Figure 36-13**).

Technique Raise a wheal of anesthesia in the subcutaneous space just superior to the eyebrow and in line with the pupil. Deposit 2 to 3 mL of anesthetic solution in the subcutaneous space, and then direct the needle medially to raise a horizontal wheal reaching to the medial border of the eyebrow using an additional 5 mL of anesthetic solution (**Figure 36-14**).

Infraorbital Nerve Block • *Purpose* An infraorbital nerve block provides anesthesia to the lower lid, medial cheek, ipsilateral side of the nose, and the ipsilateral upper lip (**Figure 36-13**).

Patient Positioning and Anatomy The patient is either supine or sitting. The infraorbital nerve exits the infraorbital foramen 5 to 10 mm inferior to the midportion of the orbital rim and just cranial (superior) to the

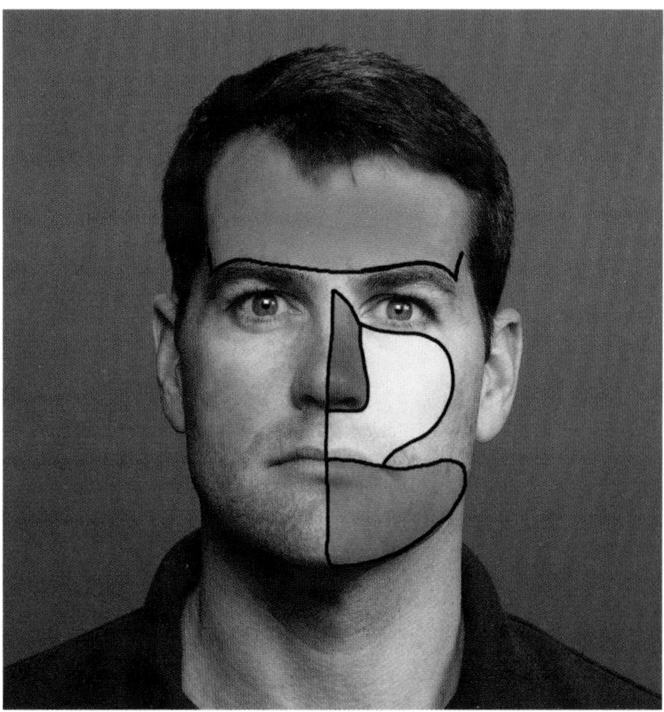

FIGURE 36-13. Face innervation frontal view. Nerve distribution to the face with supraorbital nerve (red), supratrochlear nerve (brown), infraorbital nerve (yellow), and mental nerve (blue).

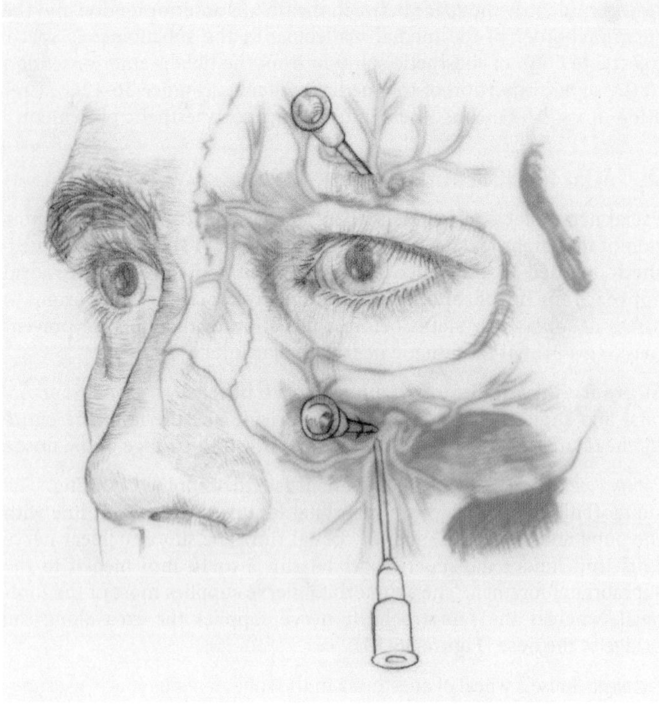

FIGURE 36-14. Supraorbital and infraorbital nerve blocks. Palpation of the subtle supraorbital foramen may be difficult, although identification is achieved when forehead paresthesias are elicited. A subcutaneous field block extending horizontally above the eyebrow is a useful addition. Palpation of the infraorbital foramen, especially via the intraoral approach, is typically easier. See Supraorbital and Infraorbital Nerve Blocks section for further details. [Illustration used with permission of Timothy Sweeney, MD.]

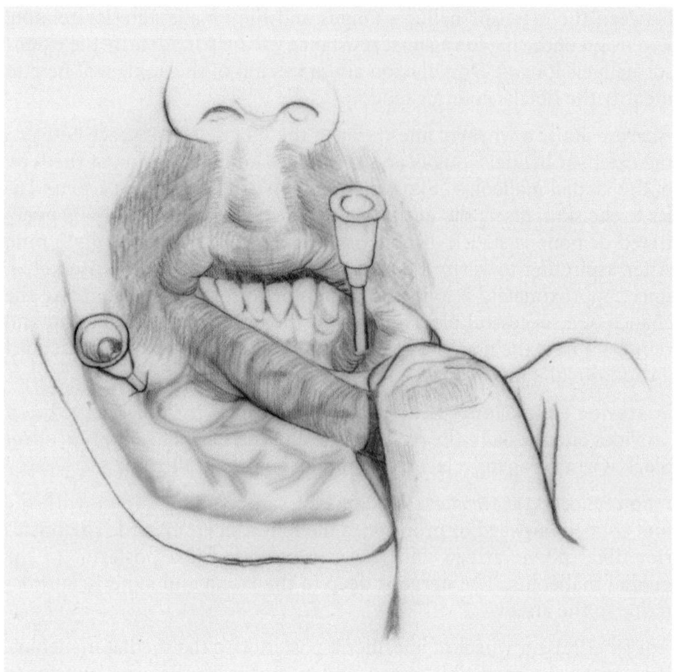

FIGURE 36-15. Mental nerve block. Infiltration of anesthetic around the mental foramen from an intraoral (*right needle*) or transcutaneous (*left needle*) approach. See Mental Nerve Block section for further details. [Illustration used with permission of Timothy Sweeney, MD.]

maxillary canine teeth (tooth #6 on the patient's right and #11 on the patient's left).

Technique After adequately providing topical anesthetic to the mucosa superior to the maxillary canine, dry the mucosa and retract the upper lip. The recommended technique involves placing the index finger and middle finger of the noninjecting hand on the inferior optic rim and everting the upper lip with the thumb. Insert the needle at the gingival reflection above the maxillary canine, direct the needle superiorly, advance approximately half the distance from the entry site to the orbital rim, and inject 3 to 5 mL of anesthetic solution (**Figure 36-14**). Depending on the patient's anatomy, it may be possible for the physician's index or middle finger to palpate the infraorbital foramen through the skin and direct the needle to this site.

Mental Nerve Block • *Purpose* A mental nerve block provides anesthesia to the labial mucosa, gingiva, and lower lip adjacent to the incisors and canines.

Patient Positioning and Anatomy The patient can be either supine or sitting. The inferior alveolar nerve gives rise to the mental nerve, which exits the mental foramen, located inferior to the mandibular canines and first premolars (teeth #21 and #22 on the patient's left, and #27 and #28 on the patient's right).

Technique After adequately providing topical anesthetic to the mucosa inferior to the canine and first premolars, dry the mucosa and evert the lower lip. Insert the needle at the gingival reflection at this site, direct the needle inferiorly, advance approximately 1 cm, and inject 3 to 5 mL of anesthetic solution (**Figure 36-15**). Depending on the patient's anatomy, it may be possible for the physician's finger to palpate the mental foramen through the skin and direct the needle to this site.

Auricular Block • *Purpose* An auricular block provides anesthesia to the entire ear.

Patient Positioning and Anatomy Patient can either be supine or sitting. The sensation to the ear is provided anteriorly by the auriculotemporal nerve and posteriorly by the greater auricular nerve and the mastoid branch of the lesser occipital nerve.

Technique Raise a wheal in the subcutaneous space inferior to the auricle. From this site, direct the needle in the subcutaneous space anterior and superior, and inject 2 to 3 mL of anesthetic while withdrawing the needle (**Figure 36-16**). From the original injection point, redirect the needle posteriorly and superiorly and deposit 2 to 3 mL in the subcutaneous space while withdrawing the needle. Repeat this process from the superior aspect of the ear, injecting 2 to 3 mL of local anesthetic in the subcutaneous space both anterior and posterior to the ear to complete the field block around the ear.

INTERCOSTAL NERVE BLOCK

Purpose An intercostal nerve block provides analgesia to the intercostal nerve above and below the affected rib in a band-like fashion around the chest wall. These blocks provide an alternative to parenteral analgesia for controlling pain from rib fractures that make movement and normal respiration quite painful[97,98] and for placement of tube thoracostomy.[99] Although controlled trials comparing parenteral analgesia with intercostal nerve blocks are lacking, clinical observations suggest better pain control and increased lung function associated with intercostal blocks.[100] A good intercostal block will provide anesthesia duration between 8 and 18 hours.

Patient Positioning and Anatomy Patient is sitting upright, with the ipsilateral arm raised at the shoulder and the wrist rested on top of the head. Within the subcostal groove of the rib, the intercostal nerve originates from the thoracic nerve and runs inferior to the artery and vein ("vein, artery, nerve"). Ribs 1 through 6 are difficult to block due to the position of the scapula and rhomboid muscles. With both anterior and posterior rib fractures, the optimal block site is at the "rib angle," approximately 6 cm lateral to the midline, or just lateral to the paraspinous muscles. **Blocking posterior to the midaxillary line ensures analgesia to the lateral cutaneous and anterior branch of the intercostal nerve (Figure 36-17, right).**

Technique Palpate the inferior border of the rib to be blocked with the noninjecting hand, and retract the skin cephalad at a location about

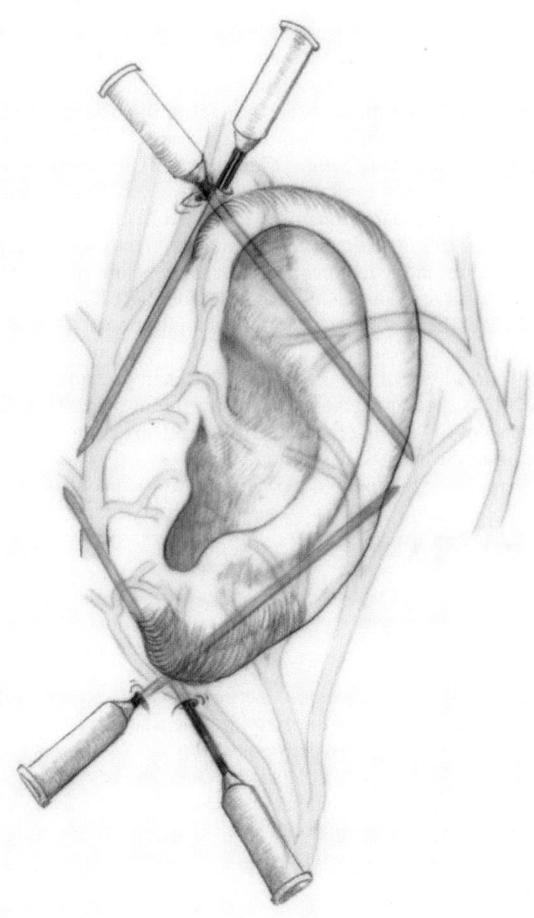

FIGURE 36-16. Auricular field block. The auricular block is a simple field block around the base of the external ear. [Illustration used with permission of Timothy Sweeney, MD.]

6 cm from the midline. Raise a wheal in the subcutaneous space, and insert the needle bevel up with the syringe lower than the entry site. The optimal angle is approximately 10 to 15 degrees off the perpendicular with the needle tip angled cephalad (**Figure 36-17**, top). Continue inserting the needle until it contacts bone. The needle should be resting at the inferior border of the rib to be blocked. Release the skin being retracted with the noninjecting hand, walk the needle caudally until it drops off the inferior edge of the rib, and advance the needle approximately 3 mm. This is the subcostal groove. Aspirate before injection, and deposit 2 to 5 mL of anesthetic.

The patient should be monitored for 30 minutes after the procedure to watch for clinical signs of pneumothorax. A postprocedure chest x-ray is not routinely indicated unless clinical signs of pneumothorax, including coughing, shortness of breath, or hypoxia, occur. Pneumothorax occurs in 8% to 9% of patients, or at a rate of about 1.4% for each individual intercostal block.[101]

FEMORAL NERVE BLOCK

Purpose Regional anesthesia in the femoral region can result in an isolated femoral nerve block or a larger block involving the femoral, obturator, and lateral femoral cutaneous nerves. These blocks provide good to excellent pain control for patients with proximal femur and hip fractures and are especially useful in the elderly.[102-105] The "three-in-one" block uses the same injection location as a femoral nerve block but applies distal pressure to promote cephalad distribution of the anesthetic agent to block the obturator and lateral femoral cutaneous nerves.[106] It is important to assess distal neurovascular status before application of the block to prevent masking a primary traumatic neurovascular injury.

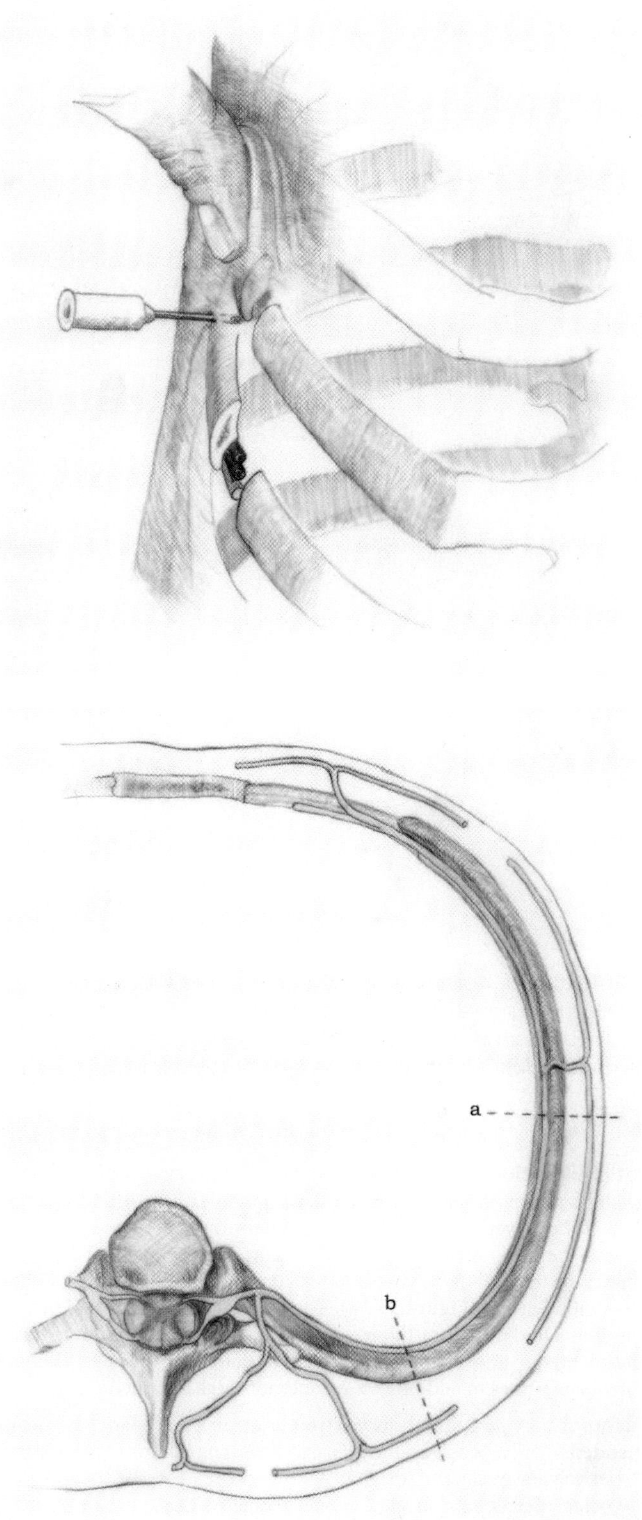

FIGURE 36-17. Intercostal block. *Top:* Cross-section of the chest shows the relevant branching of a typical intercostal nerve. Intercostal nerve blocks are commonly performed at the midaxillary line (a) or the posterior axillary "rib angle" line (b). *Bottom:* Retraction of the skin cephalad from the lower edge of the rib exposes the site of entry. The needle is inserted at a 10-degree angle off perpendicular, tip cephalad until contact is made with the lower rib edge. When the skin is released, the needle is allowed to slide caudad to the lowermost rib border. There, the needle is advanced 3 mm, aspiration is attempted, and the anesthetic solution is injected. See Intercostal Nerve Block section for further details. [Illustration used with permission of Timothy Sweeney, MD.]

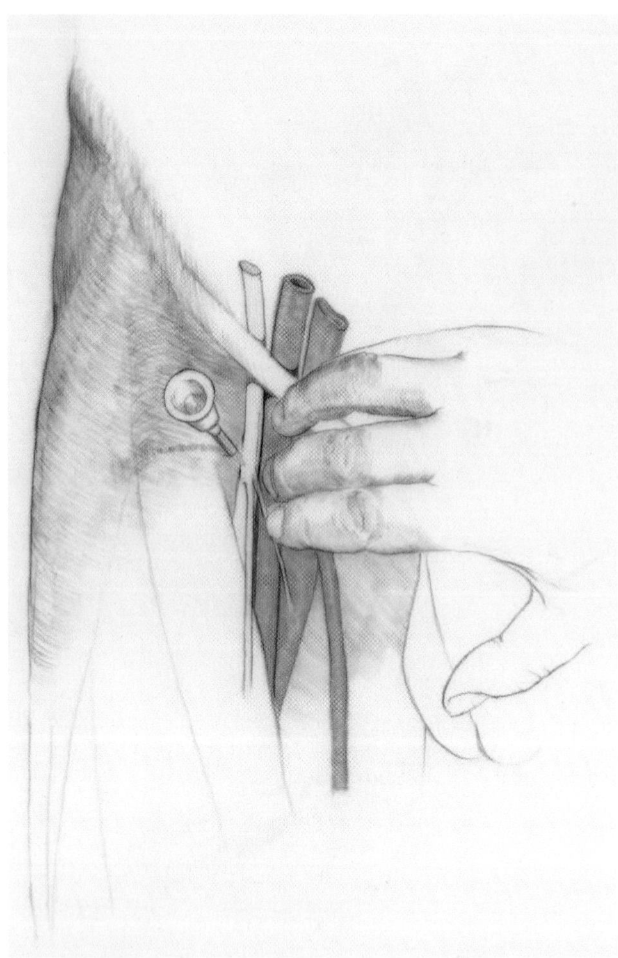

FIGURE 36-18. Femoral nerve block. The area 1 cm lateral to the femoral artery and at the level of the inguinal crease provides the point of insertion. The needle enters directly slightly cephalad and advances until paresthesia is felt. See Femoral Nerve Block section for further details. [Illustration used with permission of Timothy Sweeney, MD.]

Patient Positioning and Anatomy The patient is in a supine position. In obese patients, placement of a pillow underneath the hip and retraction of the lower abdominal pannus superiorly and laterally will help expose the area. At the inguinal ligament and the inguinal (femoral) crease, the femoral nerve is positioned lateral to and slightly deeper than the femoral artery (**Figure 36-18**). The femoral nerve block will provide anesthesia to the anterior thigh and medial leg. The "three-in-one" block anesthetizes regions innervated by the obturator and the lateral femoral cutaneous nerves in addition to the anterior thigh and medial leg.

Technique A peripheral nerve stimulator or US guidance is recommended.[77-84,107,108] Ropivacaine is an excellent long-acting anesthetic with a relatively lower cardiac toxicity.[6,8,9]

Locate the femoral artery on the affected side at the level of the inguinal crease. Palpate the femoral artery with the noninjecting hand, and raise a wheal of anesthetic in the subcutaneous space at the level of the inguinal crease and 1 cm lateral to the femoral artery. Insert the needle at this site and directed slightly cephalad (**Figure 36-18**). The femoral nerve is a relatively superficial nerve, typically 2 to 3 cm below the skin.

If a peripheral nerve stimulator is being used, needle position is confirmed by contraction of the quadriceps muscle and subsequent patellar movement. If the sartorius muscle contracts, the needle should be repositioned slightly lateral and deeper. The sartorius muscle may mimic the quadriceps contractions, but the patella will only move with quadriceps contractions. US guidance can also be used to accurately place the anesthetic agent for a femoral nerve block.[108]

If a peripheral nerve stimulator is not being used, correct positioning of the needle is confirmed by the patient reporting paresthesia over the anterior thigh as the needle impacts the femoral nerve. Back the needle off slightly and inject approximately 20 mL of the anesthetic solution into the perineural space. If paresthesia over the anterior thigh cannot be elicited, the needle should be withdrawn to the skin, redirected 10 to 15 degrees laterally, and advanced as before. More lateral skin insertions may be required to locate the femoral nerve. Alternatively, a "blind" attempt can be made by injecting a larger quantity (30 to 40 mL) of anesthetic solution in and around the original site in an effort to spread the anesthetic through the region and reach the femoral nerve. Aspirate before each injection to avoid inadvertent arterial puncture, and do not inject if resistance is felt, as this indicates the possibility for intraneural injection.

To perform a "three-in-one" block, needle position should be confirmed by paresthesia or preferably by US.[107] Firm pressure distal to the injection site is then applied and held for 5 minutes as 20 to 30 mL of anesthetic solution is delivered. This distal pressure promotes cephalad distribution of the anesthetic solution.

An alternative to the femoral nerve block for pain control in patients with hip and femoral neck fractures is the fascia iliaca compartment block that has been recently studied in ED patients.[109,110]

HEMATOMA BLOCK

PURPOSE

Hematoma blocks are commonly performed for fracture reduction, utilizing the hematoma formation around the fracture to deliver anesthetic to the fracture site, most commonly for Colles' fractures.[111-113] This block has waned in use due to the rising popularity of procedural sedation and the misconception that hematoma blocks dramatically increase the risk of infection. The hematoma block remains a staple in the armamentarium of fracture analgesia, because it is simple, fast, and requires no special tools or personnel.

PATIENT POSITIONING

The patient is usually supine with the limb placed to access the fracture hematoma.

TECHNIQUE

Prepare a sterile block site over the bony fracture site and insert the needle directly into the hematoma (**Figure 36-19**). Positioning the needle in the hematoma can be difficult at times. Aspiration of blood aids in confirmation of needle position. Inject 5 to 15 mL of local anesthetic solution into the fracture site. **When performing this block, ensure that the maximum dose of local anesthetic is not exceeded. This procedure should not be performed through a contaminated wound or an open fracture.**

INTRAVENOUS REGIONAL ANESTHESIA (BIER BLOCK)

PURPOSE

The Bier block provides dense anesthesia in a limb for up to 60 minutes without the risks of general anesthesia. It is an excellent block for large complex lacerations, fracture reductions, and surgical procedures of <1 hour duration on the extremities[114] and does not require fasting for safe performance.[115] **Although this block is relatively easy to perform, it does require a specialized pneumatic tourniquet and provides no postprocedure pain control.** Because the local anesthetic solution is directly infused into the venous system, careful attention to technique is important to prevent systemic toxicity.[116] It is important to assess neurovascular status in the involved limb before application of the block to prevent masking a primary traumatic neurovascular injury.

TECHNIQUE

Place two IV catheters, one small gauge in the affected extremity and the other in the unaffected extremity for fluid administration and sedation,

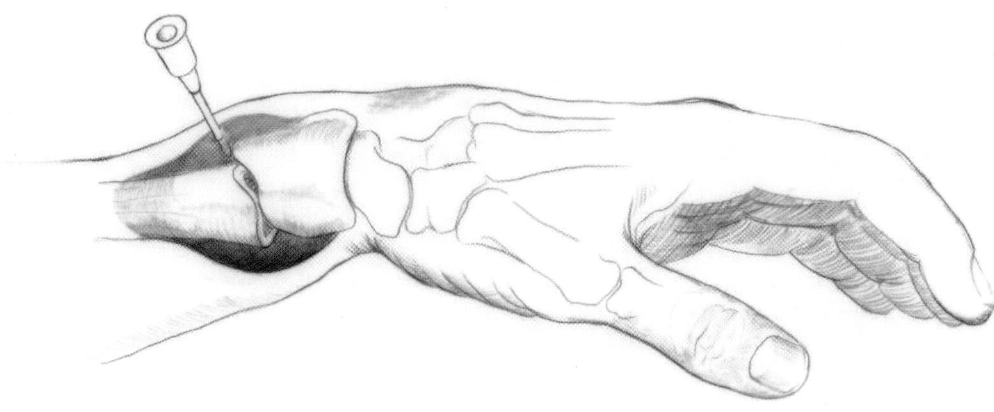

FIGURE 36-19. Hematoma block. After careful palpation for the fracture edge, the needle is inserted directly into the hematoma, with care taken to avoid regional vessels. See Hematoma Block section for further details. [Illustration used with permission of Timothy Sweeney, MD.]

if needed. Apply the specialized double-cuff pneumatic tourniquet to the affected upper arm or thigh. **The standard blood pressure cuff is not an acceptable alternative.** Provide adequate padding beneath the cuff, as this is often the site of maximal discomfort during the procedure.

Exsanguinate the affected extremity by either elevating it for 3 to 4 minutes or wrapping the extremity with a compression bandage from distal to proximal. The cuffs are then inflated in the following sequence: Inflate the distal cuff first, followed by inflating the proximal cuff and, finally, deflating the distal cuff. In the upper extremity, inflate the pneumatic tourniquet to 250 to 300 mm Hg (30 to 45 kPa) or 100 mm Hg (15 kPa) above the patient's systolic blood pressure. In the leg, cuff inflation pressures are 350 to 400 mm Hg (45 to 55 kPa). The compression bandage should be removed if used. The limb should be pale, and pulses should not be palpable.

Infuse the anesthetic via the small catheter of the affected limb. Most authors recommend diluting standard 1% lidocaine with equal parts normal saline to create a 0.5% (5 milligrams/mL) solution. The amount infused varies according to physician preference in the range of 1.5 to 3.0 milligrams/kg (3 to 6 mL of the 0.5% lidocaine solution for every 10 kg of body weight).[114] Onset of anesthesia is usually within 5 minutes. If inadequate anesthesia occurs when using a minidose (1.5 milligrams/kg), infuse additional lidocaine up to 3 milligrams/kg. If adequate anesthesia is not obtained with the maximum dose of lidocaine, infuse additional normal saline to help circulate the anesthetic.

The patient may report a sensation of warmth or cold, and the skin will become mottled. The smaller nerve fibers are affected first, causing a reduction in pain and temperature sensation followed by loss of touch, deep pressure, and, finally, motor function. An ideal Bier block will provide complete anesthesia and muscle relaxation, but patients may retain varying degrees of intact touch, deep pressure sensation, and motor function. Remove the IV in the affected extremity once adequate analgesia is obtained. Many patients will describe pain or pressure at the tourniquet site, usually within 30 minutes or so. This is handled by reinflating the previously deflated distal cuff. After ensuring that the distal cuff is inflated to the proper level and will hold pressure, the proximal cuff is slowly deflated. Dexmedetomidine mixed with the local anesthetic can also be used to control the pain of tourniquet inflation and provide postprocedure analgesia.[117]

The cuff should not be released until a minimum of 30 minutes after the initial lidocaine infusion; premature release of the cuff increases the chance of systemic toxicity from the anesthetic. Upon completion of the procedure, the pneumatic tourniquet should be cycled by lowering the cuff pressure for 5 to 10 seconds and then reinflating it for 1 to 2 minutes. This cycling should be repeated three to five times to prevent any possible bolus of anesthetic into the central circulation. Additional analgesia is usually required after completion of the procedure because anesthesia rapidly dissipates after release of the tourniquet. The patient should be monitored for approximately 30 minutes to ensure that no adverse reaction to the anesthetic has occurred.[114]

REFERENCES

The complete reference list is available online at www.TintinalliEM.com.

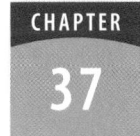

Procedural Sedation

Chris Weaver

INTRODUCTION

Procedural sedation is the administration of sedatives or dissociative anesthetics to induce a depressed level of consciousness while maintaining cardiorespiratory function so that a medical procedure can be performed with little or no patient reaction or memory.[1] Procedural sedation and analgesia is the addition of agents to reduce or eliminate pain.[1] Levels of sedation are defined by the patient's level of responsiveness and cardiopulmonary function, not by the agents used (**Table 37-1**).[2] By definition, patients receiving procedural sedation do not require routine airway protection with endotracheal intubation or other airway adjuncts, as opposed to general anesthesia, which typically requires airway protection. Procedural sedation is commonly done for scheduled outpatient medical procedures by nonanesthesiologists[3,4] and is an accepted technique in emergency medicine.[5-8] Procedural sedation performed in the ED presents different issues to the practitioner than scheduled outpatient sedation (**Table 37-2**).[1,7,8]

SEDATION LEVEL

There are several key principles that must be followed to safely perform procedural sedation and analgesia (**Table 37-3**).[1,2,7,8] Despite careful planning and performance, the depth of sedation needed or achieved cannot always be predicted. It is therefore important to prepare for managing deeper levels of sedation than anticipated. Most of the agents used can produce variable levels of sedation, so pay particular attention to dosing and to the patient's responses to the medications.

TABLE 37-1 Levels of Sedation and Analgesia

	Responsiveness	Airway	Breathing	Circulation
Minimal sedation (aka "anxiolysis")	Normal but slowed response to verbal stimulation	Unaffected	Unaffected	Unaffected
Moderate sedation (aka "conscious sedation")	Purposeful response to verbal or physical stimulation	Usually maintained	Usually adequate	Usually maintained
Deep sedation	Purposeful response after repeated or painful physical stimulation	May be impaired	May be suppressed	Usually maintained

Minimal sedation is characterized by anxiolysis but with normal, although sometimes slowed, response to verbal stimuli. Minimal sedation is typically used for procedures that require patient cooperation and those in which pain is controlled by local or regional anesthesia. Minimal sedation procedures might include abscess incision and drainage, lumbar puncture, simple fracture reductions, and laceration repair. During minimal sedation, ventilatory function is usually maintained with a low risk of hypoxia or hypoventilation. Agents typically used for minimal sedation in adults include nitrous oxide, midazolam, fentanyl, pentobarbital, and low-dose ketamine.

Moderate sedation is characterized by a depressed level of consciousness and a slower but purposeful motor response to simple verbal or tactile stimuli. Moderate sedation most closely matches the formerly used term "conscious sedation." Patients at this level generally have their eyes closed and respond slowly to verbal commands. Moderate sedation can be used for procedures in which detailed patient cooperation is not necessary, and muscular relaxation with diminished pain reaction is desired. During moderate sedation, the patient is usually able to maintain a patent airway with adequate respirations.[9] Depending on the agent, the incidence of hypoxia and/or hypoventilation during moderate sedation is 10% to 30%.[10-12] Procedures performed using moderate sedation include reduction of dislocated joints, thoracostomy tube insertion, and synchronized cardioversion. Agents used for moderate sedation in adults include propofol, etomidate, ketamine, methohexital, and the combination of fentanyl and midazolam.

Dissociative sedation is a type of moderate sedation. Dissociation is a state in which the cortical centers are prevented from receiving sensory stimuli, but cardiopulmonary activity and responses are preserved. Ketamine is the agent most commonly used for dissociative sedation.[13]

Deep sedation is characterized by a profoundly depressed level of consciousness, with a purposeful motor response elicited only after repeated or painful stimuli. Deep sedation may be required with procedures that are painful and require muscular relaxation with minimal patient reaction. The risk of losing airway patency or developing hypoxia or hypoventilation is greater with deep sedation than with moderate or minimal sedation.[10,14,15] Examples of ED procedures sometimes requiring deep sedation are reducing fracture dislocations, open fracture reductions, and burn wound care. Deep sedation generally is achieved in the ED with the same agents as moderate sedation, but with larger or more frequent doses.

RISK ASSESSMENT AND PATIENT SAFETY

Complications are primarily determined by the interaction of the depth of sedation and the patient's current medical condition. A common tool for assessing the patient's underlying medical condition is the American Society of Anesthesiologists' physical status classification system.[16] The risk of a significant complication from ED procedural sedation and analgesia in American Society of Anesthesiologists class I (healthy normal patient) and II (patient with mild systemic disease) is low, usually less than 5%.[1,5-8] The risk of an adverse procedural sedation and analgesia event is correspondingly higher in patients with an American Society of Anesthesiologists class of III (patient with severe systemic disease) or IV (severe systemic disease that is a constant threat to life).[17,18]

PATIENT EVALUATION

To prepare for procedural sedation, perform a focused history and physical examination.[1,3,4,8] The focused history should determine the fasting state, prior experiences with sedation or anesthesia, current medications, and allergies. The focused physical examination identifies a potentially difficult airway or cardiorespiratory problems. A potentially difficult airway should be anticipated when the following findings or conditions are present: short neck, micrognathia, large tongue, trismus, morbid obesity, a history of difficult intubation, or anatomic anomalies of the airway and neck. The implications of these individual factors vary,[19-21] partially due to the weak interobserver reproducibility.[22] Additionally, studies on the association between these findings and difficult intubation are usually done on patients going to the operating room for general anesthesia, and these findings may not be entirely relevant to the ED patient.[23] If time allows and an anesthesiologist is available, consultation may be advisable before undertaking procedural sedation in a patient with a potentially difficult airway. At a minimum, difficult airway equipment should be present and available.

Cardiorespiratory conditions increase the complication rate. Most agents can cause vasodilatation and hypotension, particularly in patients with preexisting hypovolemia. Clinically active obstructive pulmonary disease and active upper respiratory infections may predispose the patient to heightened airway reactivity during the procedure and promote hypoventilation. Drug or alcohol intoxication or reduced level of consciousness increases the risk of hypoxemia and hypoventilation. If possible, delay procedural sedation in intoxicated patients until mental status improves.

Routine laboratory studies are not necessary in otherwise healthy patients. Directed ancillary testing may be useful in patients with conditions such as airway abnormalities, infections, advanced age, hepatic or renal disease, dehydration, fever, or hypovolemia. Such conditions may increase the risk of hypotension, prolonged sedation, or hypoxemia. These should be corrected if possible. If correction before procedural sedation is not possible, either delay the procedure or use the lowest possible level of sedation.

The need for sedation is sometimes more urgent than a full preprocedure evaluation. Emergent indications include cardioversion for life-threatening arrhythmias, neuroimaging for head trauma, reduction of

TABLE 37-2 Comparison of Outpatient and ED Procedural Sedation

	Outpatient	ED
Occurrence	Scheduled	Unpredictable
Timing	Not time dependent, can be rescheduled	More time dependent, sometimes emergent
Gastric state	Fasting	Variable
Preprocedure pain	Minimal to none	Often moderate to severe
Patient selection	Preselected for little to no systemic disease to reduce sedation risk	Unselected, may have moderate systemic disease

TABLE 37-3 Key Principles of Procedural Sedation and Analgesia

Determine appropriate level of sedation desired
Have appropriate monitoring and rescue equipment
Administer analgesic before sedative
Titrate agents to desired level of sedation
Observe and monitor until recovery to baseline mental status

fractures or dislocations with soft tissue or vascular compromise, care of contaminated wounds, or intractable pain. Stable fractures, abscess incision and drainage, care of clean wounds, foreign body removal, and laceration repair require less urgent procedural sedation. Nonurgent indications for sedation include the removal of a soft tissue foreign body, placing splints on fractures that require minimal manipulation, or changing splints on fractures that have already been reduced.

RISKS AND PRECAUTIONS

FASTING STATE

There is no primary evidence that the risk of aspiration during procedural sedation is increased with recent oral intake.[24-26] Current guidelines regarding the safe fasting period prior to procedural sedation were developed by expert consensus,[27] and the American Society of Anesthesiologists guidelines for fasting prior to general anesthesia are of limited relevance to the risk of aspiration with ED procedural sedation.[25] Thus recent food intake is not a contraindication.[27] If the risk of aspiration is concerning, waiting 3 hours after the last oral intake before performing procedural sedation is associated with a low risk of aspiration, regardless of the level of sedation.[27]

NUMBER OF PHYSICIANS NEEDED

The anesthesia model for procedural sedation consists of two physicians, one to perform sedation and monitor the patient and the other to perform the procedure. In theory, if one physician is dedicated to administering procedural sedation, it should be possible to monitor the level of sedation, titrate the medication carefully, and identify adverse events earlier. Despite such potential benefits, clinical experience indicates that one emergency physician—providing sedation and performing the procedure—may achieve the same low risk of adverse events as having two physicians.[1,28] Thus, for minimal and moderate levels of sedation, one emergency physician simultaneously administering sedation and performing the procedure with a nurse monitoring the patient appears to be an appropriate practice. If available, a clinical pharmacist can provide useful information and assist during procedural sedation, with the potential to reduce the likelihood for medication errors.[29]

EQUIPMENT

The sedation area should include all necessary size-appropriate equipment for airway management and resuscitation, including oxygen, a bag-mask ventilation device, suction, oral/nasal airway(s), and intubation equipment.[1,3,4,8] A defibrillator should be available. Reversal agents, such as opioid receptor and benzodiazepine receptor antagonists, should also be readily available.

PROCEDURAL SEDATION MONITORING

Two types of monitoring are used for ED procedural sedation: interactive monitoring by dedicated observers and electronic monitoring with equipment connected to the patient. The recommended extent of monitoring is determined by the level of sedation (**Table 37-4**). **No matter which method is used, patients must be checked after each dose of medication to assess the response, determine the need for further doses, and make appropriate interventions if adverse events arise.**

INTERACTIVE MONITORING

Interactive monitoring is the direct observation of the patient to assess the depth of sedation and observe for hypoventilation or apnea, upper airway obstruction, laryngospasm, vomiting, or aspiration. Thus interactive monitoring requires an unobstructed view of the patient's face, mouth, and chest wall.

For minimal sedation, the risk of adverse events is so low that observation by the physician performing the procedure is usually adequate. For moderate and deep sedation, a dedicated observer—typically a nurse in the one-physician model—should continuously monitor the patient while the physician oversees drug administration and performs theprocedure.

ELECTRONIC MONITORING

Electronic monitoring uses equipment to assess arterial oxygenation, ventilation, blood pressure, and cardiac rate and rhythm. Moderate and deep sedation require constant observation and continuous monitoring. Cardiac monitoring is particularly recommended for patients with preexisting cardiac disease or dysrhythmias or during procedures in which the cardiac rhythm is of interest, such as during cardioversion. Arterial oxygen saturation is monitored with pulse oximetry. For almost all patients undergoing minimal sedation and many undergoing moderate sedation, pulse oximetry is adequate as the sole mechanical monitoring modality. However, pulse oximetry is not a substitute for monitoring ventilation, as hypoventilation or apnea develop before oxygen saturation decreases, especially in patients who receive supplemental oxygen.[30-33]

Ventilation can be electronically monitored using capnography, the measurement of the partial pressure of carbon dioxide in exhaled breath.[32,33] Many experts suggest that capnography should be used to monitor procedural sedation.[34-36] The capnography device uses an infrared carbon dioxide detector placed at the nares to sample inhaled and exhaled gases. The partial pressure of carbon dioxide detected at the nares during the respiratory cycle is represented by the carbon dioxide waveform (capnogram) that can be displayed on the monitor (**Figure 37-1**). A value commonly reported on the capnography device is the end-tidal carbon dioxide: the maximum carbon dioxide concentration at the end of each tidal breath. The end-tidal carbon dioxide correlates with arterial partial pressure of carbon dioxide so that an end-tidal car-

TABLE 37-4 Recommendations for Procedural Sedation and Analgesia Monitoring by Target Sedation Level

Target Level of Sedation	Level of Consciousness	Heart Rate	Respiratory Rate	Blood Pressure	Oxygen Saturation	Capnography End-Tidal CO_2
Minimal	Observe frequently	Measure every 15 min	Measure every 15 min	Measure every 15 min and after sedative boluses	Monitor continuously	No recommendation
Moderate or dissociative	Observe constantly	Monitor continuously	Continuous direct observation	Record every 5 min and after sedative boluses	Monitor continuously	Consider continuous monitoring
Deep	Observe constantly	Monitor continuously	Continuous direct observation	Record every 5 min and after sedative boluses	Monitor continuously	Recommend continuous monitoring for prolonged procedures

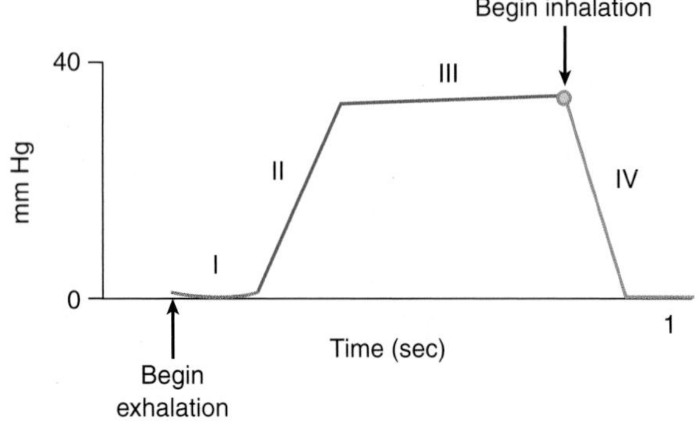

FIGURE 37-1. Normal capnogram. Phase I: At the start of exhalation, carbon dioxide concentration in the exhaled gas is essentially zero, representing gas from the anatomic dead space that does not participate in gas exchange. Phase II: As the anatomic dead space is exhaled, carbon dioxide concentration rises as alveolar gas exits the airway. Phase III: For most of exhalation, carbon dioxide concentration is constant and reflects the concentration of carbon dioxide in alveolar gas. Phase IV: During inhalation, carbon dioxide concentration decreases to zero as atmospheric air enters the airway. [Reproduced with permission from Krauss B, Hess DR: Capnography for procedural sedation and analgesia in the emergency department. *Ann Emerg Med* 50: 172, 2007 (Table 1, p. 176). Copyright Elsevier.]

bon dioxide above 50 mm Hg or an increase in end-tidal carbon dioxide >10 mm Hg indicates hypoventilation. Capnography can assess the severity of ventilatory abnormalities and the response to interventions. Most importantly, capnography can detect changes in ventilation before clinical observation.[32,33]

Variations in the capnogram can identify specific conditions, such as apnea, upper airway obstruction, laryngospasm, bronchospasm, and respiratory failure.[32] A flat-line capnogram can be due to apnea, upper airway obstruction, or complete laryngospasm. Normalization of the waveform after airway alignment maneuvers (chin lift, jaw thrust, or oral airway placement) confirms that apnea was due to upper airway obstruction.

Capnography during procedural sedation allows the early recognition of adverse events.[1,32,33] Because the risk of respiratory depression increases with the depth of sedation, capnography should be considered for moderate sedation and is recommended for prolonged deep sedation.

FREQUENCY OF MONITORING

Vital signs (pulse, blood pressure, and respiratory rate) and oxygen saturation should be obtained and recorded before the procedure, after each dose of medication, upon completion of the procedure, at the beginning of the recovery period, and before discharge.[1,3,4,8] For mild sedation, intermittent measurements are sufficient. For moderate and deep sedation, it is recommended that blood pressure be assessed every 5 minutes and heart rate and pulse oximetry be continuously monitored. Patients are at the highest risk of hypoxia and hypoventilation during the period immediately after IV medication administration (until the peak effect of the medication has been reached) and during the immediate postprocedure period (when external stimuli are discontinued and the stimulating pain of the procedure has subsided).

DOCUMENTATION

Predesigned documentation forms are a good practice because such forms can guide the providers through the procedure, improve the quality of the documentation of the procedure,[37] and better tabulate sedation-related events for quality-auditing purposes.[38]

SCALES FOR MONITORING DEPTH OF SEDATION

The level of sedation can be assessed using structured scoring techniques, such as the Ramsay Sedation Scale© and the Observer's Assessment of Alertness/Sedation Scale©. However, regular patient monitoring is more important than the application of scales. Specific central nervous system monitoring, such as the bispectral index scale that uses processed electroencephalogram signals to measure the depth of sedation, is primarily a research tool for procedural sedation.[11,15,39,40]

STEP-BY-STEP TECHNIQUE

PREPROCEDURE PAIN MANAGEMENT

The administration of morphine or fentanyl for pain control before the start of procedural sedation will provide the patient with analgesia during the procedure. Pain should be controlled so the patient is comfortable, but if preprocedure pain is intractable and if the procedure itself will result in pain relief, do not wait for complete pain control to begin.

Begin procedural sedation after the last dose of analgesic has reached its peak effect (3 to 5 minutes for IV morphine and 2 to 3 minutes for IV fentanyl). The administration of propofol or etomidate concurrently with analgesics may increase the likelihood of adverse events, so these medications should be titrated separately.[18,41]

The opioid dose needed before a procedure is typically more than the amount required after the procedure. Shorter-acting agents are preferred to drugs with a longer duration of action to minimize postprocedure respiratory depression. (See chapter 35, Acute Pain Management, for further discussion).

SUPPLEMENTAL OXYGEN

The incidence of oxygen desaturation during ED procedural sedation ranges from 6% to 40% without supplemental oxygen.[10-12,30,42,43] Supplemental oxygen reduces the incidence of hypoxemia[30,31,42,43] and has no adverse clinical effects. However, the administration of supplemental oxygen can delay the recognition of respiratory suppression, because oxygen saturation is maintained despite rising carbon dioxide noted by capnography.[32,33,42] In morbidly obese patients, bilevel positive airway pressure may be useful to facilitate adequate sedation while averting hypoventilation.[44]

SEDATION MANAGEMENT

After the patient has been evaluated, the appropriate sedation target level is selected, the monitoring modalities are applied, and preparations are made for possible adverse events, then procedural sedation can begin (**Table 37-5**). Observe and monitor the patient until the peak effect of the initial sedative dose has been reached. If necessary, titrate with additional medications to the desired sedation level. Once the patient has achieved the target sedation level, the actual procedure may begin. If the

TABLE 37-5 Procedural Sedation and Analgesia Workflow by Procedural Urgency

Emergent procedure
Sedate with single-bolus agent, moderate sedation, if possible.
Perform procedure.
Begin analgesia therapy after sedation recovery.
Repeat sedation for further procedures, if necessary, with single-bolus agent after complete recovery from first procedure.
Urgent and semi-urgent procedure
Analgesia.
Single-bolus or titrated agent based on estimated complexity of the procedure.
Choose level based on need for relaxation; moderate and deep sedation are the same to the patient.
Analgesia, as needed.
Non-urgent procedure
Analgesia.
Minimal sedation.
Repeat analgesia, as needed.

patient begins to regain alertness before completion of the procedure, additional sedative doses may be required. However, additional sedative doses given to extend procedural sedation are associated with an increased risk of respiratory depression. As larger cumulative doses of the drug are given, the half-life of each bolus will increase. After the patient recovers from sedation, analgesics are administered as needed, for patient comfort.

SEDATION AGENTS

NITROUS OXIDE

Nitrous oxide is typically supplied in a 50:50 mixture with oxygen (**Table 37-6**). Nitrous oxide can be used alone for minimal sedation or as an adjunct with IV medications for moderate sedation (**Table 37-6**).[45,46] Technical aspects of nitrous oxide administration include the use of a demand delivery system triggered by the patient's inspiratory force and a disposal or scavenger system to prevent accumulation of nitrous oxide in the room. Nitrous oxide has a rapid onset (1 to 2 minutes) and a rapid recovery (3 to 5 minutes) when inhalation of the gas is discontinued.

Nitrous oxide has few adverse side effects.[47] Nitrous oxide is a mild cardiac depressant and pulmonary vasoconstrictor so it is relatively contraindicated in patients with pulmonary hypertension. Nitrous oxide is an inhibitor of folate metabolism and is therefore contraindicated in pregnant women. Nitrous oxide may promote expansion of internal gas-filled structures and should be avoided in patients with pneumothorax, pneumocephalus, and vascular air embolism.

MIDAZOLAM

Midazolam is a short-acting benzodiazepine commonly used as a sole agent for minimal sedation.[48] After IV administration, peak effect is seen within 2 to 3 minutes, and duration of retrograde amnesia is 20 to 30 minutes (**Table 37-6**). Midazolam can be combined with an opioid for moderate or deep procedural sedation, but when given with an opioid, there is an increased risk of respiratory depression.

Midazolam causes mild cardiovascular depression, and hypotension can result when this agent is given to hypovolemic patients. Paradoxical agitation has been reported with the use of midazolam in 1% to 15% of patients, and flumazenil can be given for reversal.[48]

Midazolam can be administered IV, PO, IM, PR, or intranasally. The IV route has the most predictable onset and duration of action. The PO route can result in unreliable levels of sedation as a result of first-pass hepatic metabolism. Because the agent has a low pH and benzyl alcohol is added as a preservative, intranasal midazolam irritates the nasal mucosa, which can be painful and provoke anxiety. Buffering the solution does not decrease the irritation. Both the PR and IM routes have unreliable onset and depth of sedation, but can be easier to administer in some patients.

FENTANYL AND ALFENTANIL

Fentanyl is a potent, relatively short-acting opioid. A single IV dose has rapid onset of <1 minute, peak effect in 2 to 3 minutes, and duration of 30 to 60 minutes. It is easily titratable when used alone for minimal sedation and can be used in combination with midazolam for moderate and deep procedural sedation and analgesia.

Rigid chest syndrome, a rare complication characterized by spasm of the respiratory muscles leading to respiratory depression or apnea, is seen when high doses (>5 micrograms/kg) of fentanyl are given by rapid IV bolus. In small children, this syndrome may be precipitated by rapidly flushing the IV line. Rigid chest syndrome is not reversible with opioid receptor antagonists. Intubation with rapid-sequence induction and pharmacologic paralysis is usually required to ventilate the patient in this situation. **Slow administration of fentanyl (1 to 3 micrograms/kg over 5 minutes) followed by slow and careful flushing of the IV line can prevent rigid chest syndrome.**

Alfentanil is an effective agent but is associated with a 30% to 40% rate of airway and respiratory adverse effects,[49,50] a rate typically higher than that seen with fentanyl or propofol alone.

METHOHEXITAL

Methohexital is an ultra-short-acting barbiturate that produces sedation within 1 minute of IV administration and has an effective duration of

TABLE 37-6 Sedation Agents for Adult Procedural Sedation and Analgesia

Medication	Recommended Dosage	Route of Administration	Peak Effect	Approximate Duration	Use
Nitrous oxide	50:50 mixture with oxygen	Inhalational	1–2 min	3–5 min	Minimal sedation
Midazolam	0.05–0.1 milligram/kg. May repeat 0.05 milligram/kg every 2 min until adequately sedated	IV	2–3 min	20–30 min	Minimal or moderate sedation
	0.1 milligram/kg	IM	15–30 min	1–2 h	Minimal sedation
Fentanyl	1–3 micrograms/kg, can be titrated up to 5 micrograms/kg	IV	2–3 min	30–60 min	Minimal sedation
Fentanyl and midazolam	1–2 micrograms/kg fentanyl plus 0.1 milligram/kg midazolam	IV	2–3 min	1 h	Moderate and deep sedation
Methohexital	1 milligram/kg	IV	1 min	3–5 min	Moderate or deep sedation
Pentobarbital	2.5 milligrams/kg followed by 1.25 milligram/kg, as needed, up to two times	IV rate should be <50 milligrams/min	3–5 min	15 min	Minimal and moderate sedation. Frequently used for radiologic procedures.
Ketamine	1 milligram/kg	IV	1–3 min	15–30 min	Dissociative sedation
	2–5 milligrams/kg	IM	5–20 min	30–60 min	Dissociative sedation
Ketamine and midazolam	Ketamine as above plus midazolam, 0.03 to 0.05 milligram/kg	IV	1–3 min	30–60 min	Dissociative sedation
Etomidate	0.15 milligram/kg, followed by 0.1 milligram/kg every 2 min, if needed	IV	15–30 s	3–8 min	Moderate and deep sedation
Propofol	0.5–1.0 milligram/kg, followed by 0.5 milligram/kg every 3 min, if needed	IV	30–60 s	5–6 min	Moderate and deep sedation
Ketamine and propofol "ketofol"	Ketamine 0.125–0.5 milligram/kg and Propofol 0.5 milligram/kg	IV	30–60 s	15 min	Moderate and deep sedation

3 to 5 minutes. Methohexital is best used for brief moderate and deep sedation, such as that needed for joint dislocation reduction. The major adverse effect of methohexital is respiratory depression; the risk increases if additional boluses are given after the initial dose.[12]

PENTOBARBITAL

Pentobarbital is a short-acting barbiturate that is useful when the procedure itself is painless, but the associated circumstances may cause anxiety (e.g., radiologic procedures). Pentobarbital produces sedation within 3 to 5 minutes of IV administration and lasts approximately 15 minutes, and complete recovery occurs in 30 to 40 minutes.

KETAMINE

Ketamine produces a state of dissociation characterized by profound analgesia, sedation, and amnesia. Unlike other agents used for procedural sedation, ketamine possesses both analgesic and anxiolytic properties.[13] Ketamine is an effective agent for ED procedural sedation[13,51-55] and for prehospital analgesia and sedation when used by physicians.[55]

Ketamine does not have a typical dose-response continuum with progressive titration. At doses lower than a threshold, analgesia and sedation occur. Once a critical dosing threshold is exceeded (about 1.0 to 1.5 milligrams/kg IV or 3 to 4 milligrams/kg IM), the characteristic dissociative state abruptly appears. This dissociation has no observable levels of depth. The only value of additional ketamine is to prolong the dissociative state for extended procedures.

Ketamine can be given either IV or IM. The IM route allows for approximately 40 minutes of sedation, compared with 10 minutes by the IV route. **Ketamine is the only sedative agent that typically preserves a patient's ventilatory effort and has minimal effect on blood pressure.** Ketamine can induce hypersalivation. Anticholinergics, such as atropine 10 micrograms/kg IV or glycopyrrolate 4 micrograms/kg IV, are often administered to counter this effect. However, studies evaluating this practice of coadministering anticholinergics fail to demonstrate tangible benefit or harm. Thus anticholinergics can be reserved for the treatment of clinically significant hypersalivation or for patients with an impaired ability to mobilize secretions.[13] Other adverse effects also include laryngospasm, vomiting (most often in the late recovery phase), and emergence reactions. Laryngospasm has been reported primarily in children, with reported rates of occurrence of <1.0% to 2.5%. It is typically transient and responds to positive pressure ventilation with a bag-valve mask. Children with significant upper respiratory tract infectious symptoms and patients who will undergo major stimulation of the oropharynx (e.g., endoscopy) should not receive ketamine due to a possible increased risk of laryngospasm.[13]

Emergence reactions are common with ketamine and range from mild agitation to recurrent nightmares and hallucinations.[53,54] Midazolam can be given along with ketamine to blunt the occurrence of emergence reactions.[56,57] However, the overall clinical benefit of such prophylaxis has not been demonstrated.[13] It is sufficient to give ketamine without midazolam and then treat patients who develop emergence reactions with midazolam as they occur. Because of these emergence reactions, ketamine should not be used in patients with schizophrenia and psychosis.[13]

It is commonly stated that ketamine increases intracranial pressure, which potentially limits its use in many emergent situations.[58] The experimental data from animal studies and human observations are conflicting, depending on the specific circumstances.[58,59] Thus there is no clear evidence that ketamine is harmful as an induction or sedation agent in patients with potential head injury. Ketamine does increase intraocular pressure and should be avoided in patients with eye injuries or glaucoma.[60]

ETOMIDATE

Etomidate is a nonbarbiturate sedative-hypnotic with a rapid onset (15 to 30 seconds) and a short duration of effect (3 to 8 minutes). Compared with the other sedative agents, etomidate causes less cardiovascular depression but a similar degree of respiratory depression. Etomidate is an effective agent for ED procedural sedation, with a reported complication rate of 10% to 15%, most complications being minor.[61-64]

Myoclonic jerking occurs in up to 20% of patients and can interfere with the procedure for which the patient was sedated.[64] Etomidate causes suppression of the adrenal-cortical axis, and when used for rapid sequence induction in critically ill patients, it is associated with adrenal insufficiency and increased mortality.[65-68] However, no clinically significant adverse event related to adrenal suppression has been detected from etomidate used during ED procedural sedation in stable patients.

PROPOFOL

Propofol is frequently used for moderate and deep procedural sedation in the ED.[18,69-77] Propofol is associated with fewer complications than etomidate or methohexital in patients who received multiple doses and is much easier to titrate.[12,64] Because of the short duration of action, propofol results in a shorter recovery time and ED length of stay.[76-79]

The most serious adverse effect of propofol is sudden respiratory depression and apnea,[24,41] so ventilatory support equipment should be at the bedside when using propofol. Propofol can produce hypotension as a result of both negative inotropy and vasodilatation. Hypotension is more common in hypovolemic patients and those with American Society of Anesthesiologists physical status scores of III or IV.[70] **Hypovolemia should be corrected before propofol administration.**

Sedation from propofol occurs within 30 to 60 seconds after injection and lasts for about 5 to 6 minutes. Propofol is rapidly distributed into tissues, and once tissues are saturated, subsequent doses will have a greater effect than the initial bolus. The recommended dose for ED procedural sedation in healthy nonelderly adults is 0.5 to 1.0 milligram/kg IV, followed by 0.5 milligram/kg IV every 3 minutes if needed. Higher doses are associated with more respiratory depression.

Propofol is formulated in a soybean oil, glycerol, and egg lecithin emulsion and is contraindicated in patients who are allergic to eggs or soy protein. Propofol causes local pain at the IV site during administration. Methods to reduce the pain of propofol administration include placing a tourniquet proximal to the IV and injecting 0.05 milligram/kg of lidocaine through the IV approximately 60 seconds before injecting the propofol, mixing the propofol with lidocaine, or coadministering the short-acting opioid alfentanil at 10 micrograms/kg.[80,81]

KETAMINE AND PROPOFOL

The combination of ketamine and propofol for ED procedural sedation has a well-documented safety and efficacy profile.[82,83-92] Propofol is an excellent sedative, but respiratory depression and hypotension are its principal adverse events. The sympathomimetic properties of ketamine may mitigate these, in addition to adding analgesia. Ketamine causes emergence reactions and vomiting as adverse events, whereas propofol has antiemetic and hypnotic properties. This combination is safe and effective for ED procedural sedation and analgesia.[83-92] Published "ketofol" ED procedural sedation studies have used a variety of combinations, from equal mixtures of propofol and ketamine to normal doses of propofol with sub-dissociative doses of ketamine for its analgesic properties. Adding ketamine to propofol promotes hemodynamic stability, which is reassuring in patients with known or potentially reduced cardiac function.[88] There is also evidence of synergism between the two drugs, and data indicate that ketofol provides less erratic sedation depth than propofol alone.[87] The analgesic properties of ketamine preclude the need for and risks of opioids administered with propofol.[84,88] When the total dose of ketamine administered during ketofol use is less than the reliable dissociative dose (<1.5 milligram/kg), clinical observation suggests that recovery time is longer than that for full doses of propofol (1.6 to 1.8 milligrams/kg) alone[82,86] but shorter than that of full dissociative doses of ketamine (1.0 to 1.5 milligrams/kg) alone.[82] However, despite the theoretical benefit for decreasing complications, studies to date have failed to demonstrate a consistent difference in complications between ketofol (mixtures of ketamine and propofol from 1:1 to 1:4) compared with propofol alone.[89,90] The advantage of ketofol is that it may be able to achieve adequate sedation with lower total doses compared with when either drug alone is used, and ketofol prolongs the duration of sedation more than propofol alone, which is useful for procedures anticipated to take more time, and without the need for additional doses of propofol.

OUTCOME ASSESSMENT/COMPLICATIONS

Reported complication rates for ED procedural sedation range from 2.3% to 11%.[28,69,93-95] Most of these are minor. Factors associated with an increased rate of complications include age >65 years,[93,94] level of sedation,[94,95] premedication with fentanyl,[94] use of short-acting agents,[94] and procedural sedation and analgesia performed at night, when procedural sedation and analgesia could be administered by physicians with varying levels of training and experience and when consultant-level supervision is not always physically present.[95] Serious adverse events include the need for assisted ventilation, endotracheal intubation, or treatment of hypotension or cardiac dysrhythmias. Minor adverse events resolve spontaneously and include sedation to a deeper level than intended, transient hypoxia, or emesis. Complications can occur unexpectedly, so careful preparation, appropriate procedural monitoring, and careful selection of the target sedation level will minimize the rate of occurrence and severity of adverse events.

Failure to successfully complete a procedure during ED procedural sedation occurs in about 5% and is more common with some joint reductions (hips, mandibles) and with patient body weight >100 kg.[96]

FOLLOW-UP AND PATIENT INSTRUCTIONS

At the completion of sedation and the procedure, patients should be monitored until they return to baseline mental status and cardiopulmonary function. A structured assessment, such as the Aldrete Score©,[97] can be used to assess the patient's recovery and safety for discharge. Such assessment tools are typically part of procedural sedation documentation forms.

The duration of observation before discharge is variable. It depends on the quantity of sedatives given, the patient's response, the duration of the procedure, and the occurrence of any adverse events. Generally, patients who have returned to a baseline level of consciousness are unlikely to have further negative changes in level of consciousness. Most adverse events occur during procedural sedation itself, typically within a few minutes of sedative administration. The occurrence of adverse events >5 minutes after completion of the procedure is rare (<1%).[98] The occurrence of adverse events after discharge of an ED patient who has undergone procedural sedation has not been reported. Patients should be instructed to return if they develop respiratory complaints or nausea or vomiting. The follow-up interval required for patients who undergo ED procedural sedation is usually related to the procedure rather than the sedation itself.

SPECIAL CIRCUMSTANCES

PROCEDURAL SEDATION AND ANALGESIA IN CRITICALLY ILL PATIENTS

Etomidate might arguably be the drug of choice for hypotensive patients who require sedation for an emergency procedure because it produces less cardiovascular suppression than other agents.[17] However, etomidate suppresses the adrenal-cortical axis, and when used for rapid-sequence induction in critically ill patients, it is associated with adrenal insufficiency and increased mortality.[65-68] Thus other sedation agents should be used in critically ill patients. Patients undergoing extended complex procedures are likely to require sedation longer than can be achieved with a single bolus of methohexital or propofol, or etomidate, and are at a higher risk of complications.[12,17,64] Critically ill patients who require prolonged sedation should be referred for general anesthesia in the operating room.

PROCEDURAL SEDATION AND ANALGESIA IN THE ELDERLY

Procedural sedation in the elderly is associated with increased technical and pharmacologic adverse events.[93,94] Ventilatory drive and the ability to maintain a patent airway are reduced. Remove false teeth or partial dentures before sedation to prevent aspiration of the devices. Risk of pulmonary aspiration increases as a result of reduced gag reflex and gastroesophageal sphincter incompetence. Underlying comorbidities or hepatic or renal insufficiency affect the response to sedatives. The risk of respiratory depression from all agents is increased. All these factors indicate a need for more planning, monitoring, and slow titration of sedative agents in the elderly. With such preparation, procedural sedation of the elderly is safe.[93]

Etomidate is a good sedative agent in the elderly because of its minimal cardiovascular effects.[63] For painful procedures, opioids may be necessary, as etomidate has no analgesic effect. In elderly patients with underlying clonus, etomidate should be avoided, as it can exacerbate that symptom.

Propofol produces greater peak plasma concentrations after a specific IV bolus dose in the elderly, therefore producing a greater risk of respiratory depression and apnea. **To counteract this, the initial and subsequent doses should be 50% (0.25 to 0.5 milligrams/kg) of those recommended for younger adults, and more cautious titration is needed.** Lower dosing of the sedative with increased age and American Society of Anesthesiologists score may lead to similar complication rates as those for younger patients.[93]

The elderly, especially those with underlying cerebral disease or dementia, are more sensitive to the neurologic side effects of benzodiazepines and barbiturates. These agents should be used with caution, particularly if opioid analgesics are also given.

PROCEDURAL SEDATION AND ANALGESIA FOR EMERGENCY ENDOSCOPY

Procedural sedation is a standard part of outpatient endoscopy. If an ED patient requires emergency endoscopy, the emergency physician may be asked to perform procedural sedation. Ideally, a protocol during emergency endoscopy should be jointly developed by emergency medicine and gastroenterology. Sedation during endoscopy presents some unique challenges related to the medications used and the performance of the procedure itself.[99-101]

Endoscopy increases the risk for vasovagal reactions, with bradycardia and hypotension. These reactions can occur with upper gastrointestinal endoscopy during passage of the endoscope through the pharynx or gaseous distention of the small bowel, or with colonoscopy during gaseous distention of the colon. Most reactions are transient, and treatment with atropine should be reserved for rare cases of persistent bradycardia.

Passage of the endoscope through the pharynx into the stomach can exacerbate the risks for hypoxia, apnea, and aspiration. The endoscope can interfere with ventilation and can induce vomiting. Topical agents (benzocaine, lidocaine) are used for pharyngeal anesthesia. The occurrence of methemoglobinemia after benzocaine topical spray can interfere with pulse oximetry monitoring.

Antiemetic agents used during the procedure, such as promethazine or droperidol, can cause complications during the performance of procedural sedation. Promethazine exerts an α-adrenergic blocking effect and may produce hypotension. In addition, the sedative effect of promethazine may last >2 hours, so a prolonged recovery should be anticipated. Droperidol, which is occasionally used, increases the risk of transient hypotension and may also prolong the recovery phase (up to 3 to 6 hours). Ondansetron is an antiemetic without these potential effects and is a reasonable alternative.

REFERENCES

The complete reference list is available online at www.TintinalliEM.com.

CHAPTER 38

Chronic Pain

David M. Cline

CHRONIC PAIN

INTRODUCTION

Chronic pain is a painful condition that lasts >3 months, pain that persists beyond the reasonable time for an injury to heal, or pain that persists 1 month beyond the usual course of an acute disease. Chronic pain lacks the essential function of acute pain. Whereas acute pain is a vital biologic signal to stop the individual from a potentially injurious activity or to pursue medical care, chronic pain serves no obvious biologic function. Complete pain relief is unrealistic in cases of chronic pain. Rather, the goal of therapy is pain reduction and return to functional status. Chronic pain syndromes discussed in this chapter are divided into neuropathic and nonneuropathic conditions. Aberrant drug-related behavior, also called drug-seeking behavior, is discussed.

Chronic pain is a common problem affecting 30.7% of the U.S. population and is more prevalent in women (34.3%) than in men (26.7%).[1] Back pain is the most common site for chronic pain, followed by the knee and neck.[1] The prevalence of neuropathic pain is 6.9% to 10% of the population.[2] Risk factors for chronic pain include increasing age, female gender, higher body mass, and chronic illness.[3] An exacerbation of chronic pain is part of the presentation of 11% to 15% of ED visits.[4] Compared to patients with acute pain, chronic pain patients are more likely to report their pain as severe and more likely to be frequent visitors to the ED.[5]

PATHOPHYSIOLOGY

The pathophysiology of chronic pain is incompletely understood. Many chronic pain syndromes follow nerve or tissue injury, producing nerve dysfunction secondary to the mechanical injury or in response to chemical mediators released from adjacent cell injury. Peripheral nerves, the CNS, or both become abnormally sensitive and develop pathologic spontaneous activity through upregulation of sodium channels and receptors.[6] Neuroplastic changes in the central descending pain modulatory systems, inhibitory or facilitatory, may lead to further hyperexcitability. These changes lead to **hyperalgesia** (exaggerated response to a normally painful stimulus) and **allodynia** (pain from a normally nonpainful stimulus). In several disorders, a history of injury may be lacking, such as for fibromyalgia, where central sensitization is thought to play a key role.[7] Psychological factors frequently precede or follow the onset of chronic pain and frequently predispose individuals to physiologic changes, through the fear-avoidance model. The fear of pain may lead to disuse disability, which leads to nerve hyperexcitability and dysfunction, and ultimately, may result in a chronic pain syndrome.[8]

CLINICAL FEATURES

The nonneuropathic syndromes share certain characteristics, the most common feature being muscle-related pain (**Table 38-1**). A feature common to most neuropathic syndromes is allodynia (**Table 38-2**).

Clinical assessment should be appropriate to the circumstances, and can be focused or comprehensive. A comprehensive evaluation starts with assessing the quality and character of the patient's current pain, including initiating, exacerbating, or relieving factors. Compare and quantify prior episodes to the current episode. Determine sources, modes, and success or failure of prior treatment, including medications and dosages for physician-prescribed, over-the-counter, or alternative medications. Determine the patient's functional status across the course of the illness and treatment. Treatments that have provided pain relief yet have led to disability cannot be considered a success. Assess any history of alcohol or drug addiction, need for prior detoxification, or psychiatric illness that may impact decisions about choice of medication. A review of systems should assess for potential life- or limb-threatening conditions.

Objective findings of acute pain include tachycardia, hypertension, diaphoresis, and muscle spasms on stimulation. Objective evidence of chronic pain includes muscle atrophy in the distribution of pain due to disuse and skin temperature changes due to the effects of the sympathetic nervous system after disuse or secondary to nerve injury. Trigger points, another objective sign, are focal points of muscle tenderness and tension that, when stimulated with pressure, provoke referred pain, typically in the distribution of the involved muscle. Trigger points are differentiated from simple focal tender portions of the muscle, as trigger points provoke referred pain throughout the affected muscle. Trigger points lack a biologic basis and interexaminer agreement, yet they remain an essential feature of the diagnosis of myofascial pain syndromes.[9] Objective evidence of pain is not observed for the pain to be factual. For ED patients, there is no observed correlation between numeric pain scores and vital signs.[10]

CLINICAL FEATURES OF SELECTED CHRONIC PAIN SYNDROMES

Further discussion including treatment of chronic back pain, neck pain, and sciatica is found in chapter 279, Neck and Back Pain. Migraine headaches and tension headaches are discussed in chapter 165, Headache.

Transformed migraine is a syndrome in which classic or common migraine headaches change over time and develop into a chronic pain syndrome, most commonly from medication overuse.[11] Chronic migraine (15 or more migraine days a month) is a precursor to transformed migraine. Medications implicated in this transition are barbiturates taken 5 or more days per month, opioids taken 8 or more days per

TABLE 38-1 Symptoms and Signs of Nonneuropathic Pain Syndromes

Disorder	Pain Symptoms	Signs
Myofascial headache	Constant dull pain, occasionally shooting pain	Trigger points on scalp, muscle tenderness and tension
Chronic tension headache	Constant dull pain	Diffuse tenderness of the scalp and associated tension
Transformed migraine	Initially migraine-like, becomes constant, dull; nausea, vomiting	Muscle tenderness and tension, normal neurologic exam
Myofascial neck pain	Constant dull pain, occasionally shooting pain; pain does not typically follow nerve distribution	Trigger points in area of pain, usually no muscle atrophy, poor ROM in involved muscle
Chronic neck pain	Constant dull pain, occasionally shooting pain; pain does not follow nerve distribution	No trigger points, poor ROM in involved muscle due to pain
Chronic back pain	Constant dull pain, occasionally shooting pain; pain does not follow nerve distribution	No trigger points, poor ROM in involved muscle due to pain
Myofascial back pain syndrome	Constant dull pain, occasionally shooting pain; pain does not typically follow nerve distribution	Trigger points in area of pain, usually no muscle atrophy, poor ROM in involved muscle

Abbreviation: ROM = range of motion.

TABLE 38-2 Symptoms and Signs of Neuropathic Pain Syndromes

Disorder	Pain Symptoms	Signs
Painful diabetic neuropathy	Symmetric numbness and burning or stabbing pain in lower extremities; allodynia may occur	Sensory loss in lower extremities
Phantom limb pain	Variable: aching, cramping, burning, squeezing, or tearing sensation	May have peri-incisional sensory loss
Trigeminal neuralgia	Paroxysmal, short bursts of sharp, electric-like pain in nerve distribution	Tearing or red eye may be present
HIV-associated sensory neuropathy	Symmetric pain and paresthesias, most prominent in toes and feet	Sensory loss in areas of greatest pain symptoms
Postherpetic neuralgia	Allodynia; shooting, lancinating pain	Sensory changes in the involved dermatome
Fibromyalgia	Widespread muscular pain and stiffness, fatigue, sleep disturbance, and cognitive dysfunction (forgetfulness, inability to concentrate or recall simple words or numbers, confusion)	Muscle tenderness in >6 body areas out of 19 total regions
Poststroke pain	Same side as weakness; throbbing, shooting pain; allodynia	Loss of hot and cold differentiation
Sciatica (neurogenic back pain)	Constant or intermittent, burning or aching, shooting or electric shock–like pain; may follow dermatome; leg pain > back pain	Possible muscle atrophy in area of pain, possible reflex changes
Complex regional pain type I	Burning persistent pain, allodynia, associated with immobilization or disuse, not associated with nerve injury	Early: edema, warmth, local sweating Late: above alternates with cold, pale, cyanosis, eventually atrophic changes
Complex regional pain type II	Burning persistent pain, allodynia, associated with peripheral nerve injury, associated with nerve injury, usually more painful and difficult to control than Type I	Early: edema, warmth, local sweating Late: above alternates with cold, pale, cyanosis, eventually atrophic changes

Abbreviation: HIV = human immunodeficiency syndrome.

month, and triptans or nonsteroidal anti-inflammatory drugs (NSAIDs) taken 10 or more days per month.[11] Patients with chronic migraine may have more symptoms similar to tension headache with tenderness and tension of scalp musculature. Nausea and vomiting or failure of an oral antimigraine medication often prompts an ED visit. In addition to increased headache frequency, headache duration is longer in chronic migraine.

Fibromyalgia is widespread muscular pain involving greater than six body areas out of 19 total regions and a symptom severity score of 5 or more, rating four areas: fatigue, sleep disturbance, and cognitive dysfunction (e.g., forgetfulness, inability to concentrate or recall simple words or numbers, confusion and associated non-muscle pain symptoms).[12,13] Prevalence is thought to be 5.4% of the population.[14]

The symptoms of **painful diabetic neuropathy** are symmetric numbness associated with burning, electrical, or stabbing pain in lower extremities. Patients may have hyperesthesia, dysesthesias, and/or deep aching pain. Pain may be provoked with a gentle touch to the skin in the areas of abnormal sensation.

Postherpetic neuralgia may follow the course of an acute episode of herpes zoster in 5% to 30% of cases; pain lasts more than 1 year for 30% of patients.[15] Pain is characterized by allodynia and shooting, lancinating (tearing or sharply cutting) pain. Often, patients have hyperesthesia in the involved dermatome. Occasionally there are pigmentation changes in the distribution of the involved dermatome, but this is not unique to postherpetic neuralgia.

Typical symptoms of **trigeminal neuralgia** include paroxysmal, short bursts of sharp, electric shock–like pain in the nerve distribution of the trigeminal nerve. Pain is often triggered by chewing, speaking, washing, brushing teeth, or something touching the face. Tearing of the eyes or red eye may be present.

Phantom limb pain is quite variable in presentation but is more frequent in patients who had pain in the extremity before amputation. Pain may be aching, cramping, burning, tearing, or squeezing. Phantom limb pain occurs in 30% to 81% of amputations and changes over years, becoming less "knife-like" and more "burning" in character.[16]

There are two types of **complex regional pain syndrome**: type I, from prolonged immobilization or disuse, as after stroke; and type II, from a peripheral nerve injury (e.g., due to fracture or gunshot). Symptoms include allodynia and a persistent burning or shooting pain on the affected side or limb. Associated signs early in the course of the disease include edema, warmth, and localized abnormal sweating. It may be difficult to distinguish this stage from an underlying wound infection or osteomyelitis. Later signs include periods of edema and warmth that alternate with cold, pale, cyanotic skin, and, eventually, atrophic changes.

Patients with **acquired immunodeficiency syndrome** can develop distal sensory polyneuropathy characterized by shooting pain, numbness, and burning sensations primarily on the soles, dorsum of the feet, and toes. This human immunodeficiency virus–associated sensory neuropathy is associated with antiretroviral therapy, but not with low CD4 counts.[17] Sensory loss is common in the areas of greatest pain symptoms. As the neuropathy progresses, walking becomes difficult, and quality of life is diminished.

DIAGNOSIS

The most important task is to distinguish an exacerbation of chronic pain from a life- or limb-threatening condition. The history and physical examination should either confirm the chronic condition or point to the need for further evaluation when unexpected signs or symptoms are elicited. Because patients with chronic pain may be frequent visitors to the ED, the entire staff may prejudge complaints as simply chronic or even factitious. Follow routine procedures, including a standard triage assessment and a complete set of vital signs.

After eliminating potential conditions that require emergent treatment, clinical judgment determines if focused management of pain is an appropriate course of action in the ED. The principles of focused management are to identify that symptoms are an exacerbation or continuation of a chronic pain pattern, provide appropriate rescue therapy for pain relief, and reinforce the need for a single provider (physician or clinic) for ongoing pain management.

Rarely is a provisional diagnosis of a chronic pain condition made for the first time in the ED. Definitive assessment for chronic pain conditions is difficult and requires expert opinion and often advanced procedures such as MRI, CT, and thermography. Furthermore, abnormal results do not confirm with certainty the cause of pain. For example, abnormalities on MRI of the spine and extremities are common in both asymptomatic and symptomatic patients. Therefore, referral back to the primary source of care is warranted to confirm the diagnosis.

TREATMENT

OPIOIDS FOR CHRONIC PAIN

In 1986, Portenoy and Foley[18] reported a case series of 38 patients treated with long-acting opioids for chronic, noncancer pain claiming that this therapy was safe and effective and that the risk of addiction was less than 1%, citing unrelated data. Without randomized controlled trials to support their assertions, the use of opioids to treat chronic, noncancer pain rapidly gained popularity with physicians who were twice as likely to prescribe an opioid for chronic pain in 2000, compared to 1980, and with prescriptions for strong opioids (oxycodone compared to codeine) quadrupled.[19] From 2001 to 2010, the percentage of patients receiving an opioid prescription at ED discharge increased from 20.8% to 31.0%, while the percentage of visits for painful conditions increased only 4.0%.[20] ED visits for nonmedical use of opioids (adverse events including nonfatal overdose) increased 111% from 2004 to 2008.[21] The age-adjusted rate for opioid-analgesic poisoning deaths nearly quadrupled from 1.4 per 100,000 in 1999 to 5.4 per 100,000 in 2011;[22] poisoning is now the most common cause of injury-related death in the United States, surpassing motor vehicle–related death.

In response to the dramatic increase in opioid-analgesic poisoning, state agencies created statewide prescription drug monitoring programs accessible by the Internet for registered medical providers to view controlled substance prescriptions that a patient has received.[23] As of June 2014, 48 states had operational prescription drug monitoring programs.[24] Many state medical boards have issued guidelines for the prescription of controlled substances by physicians licensed in that state with specific recommendations for emergency care providers, including Arizona, Arkansas, California, New York, North Carolina, Ohio, Oklahoma, and Washington State;[25] additional state guidelines are pending. The American College of Emergency Physicians issued a policy on the prescription of opioids for patients discharged from the ED.[26] **Table 38-3** summarizes key guideline statements from the American College of Emergency Physicians policy[26] and Washington State guidelines.[25]

TABLE 38-3 Guidelines for Prescribing Opioids for Adults in the ED

*For the treatment of back pain, given a lack of demonstrated evidence of superior efficacy of either opioid or nonopioid analgesics, and the individual and community risks associated with opioid use, misuse, and abuse, opioids should be reserved for more severe pain or pain refractory to other analgesics rather than routinely prescribed.

*If opioids are indicated, the prescription should be for the lowest practical dose for a limited duration (e.g., <1 week), and the prescriber should consider the patient's risk for opioid misuse, abuse, or diversion.

*Avoid the routine prescribing of outpatient opioids for a patient with an acute exacerbation of chronic noncancer pain seen in the ED.

*Honor existing patient-physician pain contracts/treatment agreements.

*Consider past prescription patterns from information sources such as prescription drug monitoring programs.

†The administration of intravenous and intramuscular opioids in the ED for the relief of acute exacerbations of chronic pain is discouraged.

†Do not provide replacement prescriptions for controlled substances that were lost, destroyed, or stolen.

†Long-acting or controlled-release opioids (such as OxyContin®, fentanyl patches, and methadone) should not be prescribed from the ED.

†Prescriptions for controlled substances from the ED should state that the patient is required to provide a government-issued picture identification (ID) to the pharmacy filling the prescription.

†Do not provide replacement doses of methadone for patients in a methadone treatment program.

†If opioids are prescribed to a patient with chronic pain, prescribe only enough pills to last until the office of the patient's primary opioid prescriber opens.

*2012 American College of Emergency Physicians policy

†Washington State Opioid Prescribing Guidelines

TREATMENT OF CHRONIC NONNEUROPATHIC PAIN SYNDROMES

Evidence-based treatment for chronic nonneuropathic pain syndromes is divided into primary and secondary treatment modalities (**Table 38-4**).[27-33] For management in the ED, an acute exacerbation of a chronic migraine can be treated like an exacerbation of episodic migraine.[27] When selecting a standard NSAID, adding a proton pump inhibitor reduces GI complications, and the combination is less expensive than daily use of the cyclooxygenase-2 inhibitors.[34]

Treatment in the ED should never be regarded as definitive, and follow-up care is essential. Many emergency providers will elect to prescribe short-acting nonspecific pain medications (**Table 38-3**) for patients with chronic pain, deferring initiating of more specific therapy for the primary care physician or pain specialist. Specialty referral may provide optimization of therapy, trigger point injections, and novel treatments, such as onabotulinumtoxinA injections.

TREATMENT OF CHRONIC NEUROPATHIC PAIN SYNDROMES

Evidence-based treatment for chronic neuropathic pain syndromes is divided into primary and secondary treatment modalities (**Table 38-5**).[35-44]

There is no convincing unbiased evidence to support the use of opioids (specifically oxycodone) in the treatment of neuropathic pain including fibromyalgia.[45] Duloxetine is favored over pregabalin and gabapentin in the treatment of painful diabetic neuropathy.[40] Human immunodeficiency syndrome–related neuropathy is resistant to many therapies commonly used for neuropathic pain; although topical capsaicin is effective,[38] it is best directed by a specialist because pain increases at first application and pretreatment with topical lidocaine may be required.

Tramadol reduces pain in most neuropathic pain syndromes but is considered secondary treatment because it is less effective than the primary treatments (**Table 38-5**).[40,46] Complex regional pain syndrome is the most resistant to pharmacotherapy of all neuropathic pain conditions.[44] An IV infusion of ketamine may reduce pain for up to 12 weeks,[44] but does not improve function. Corticosteroids (prednisone, 60 milligrams PO once a day) have been recommended at the time of first diagnosis when signs of inflammation are present,[44] but steroids do not affect the course of illness. Patients should be informed that NSAIDs and strong opioids are generally ineffective in neuropathic pain. Although considered second line, cyclic antidepressants are effective therapy for most patients with neuropathic pain, except spinal cord injury pain, phantom limb pain, human immunodeficiency syndrome–related neuropathy, and chronic regional pain syndrome. Amitriptyline can be started at 25 milligrams PO nightly, and escalated by the follow-up clinician. Complete relief of pain is an unrealistic goal for patients with chronic pain, both for the ED visit and for follow-up care; patients should be informed of this limitation early in their ED course.

DISPOSITION AND FOLLOW-UP

Referral to an appropriate specialist is one of the most productive means of aiding in the care of chronic pain patients who present to the ED. Chronic pain clinics have been successful in changing the lives of patients by eliminating opioid use, decreasing medication use, reducing pain levels, and increasing work hours. Patients' compliance with pain clinics may improve if these benefits are explained. Admission to the hospital is rarely indicated. However, occasionally patients may be admitted for pain control, possibly using self-controlled analgesic administration.

SPECIAL POPULATIONS

ELDERLY PATIENTS

The prevalence of chronic pain increases with age.[1] Opioid analgesic alternatives, such as NSAIDs, have side effects that may limit their use in the elderly who are prone to GI and renal complications; however, when compared to opioids, NSAIDs have fewer side effects overall and are less likely to lead to premature death in the elderly.[47] GI bleeding rates are similar for patients treated with opiates or nonselective NSAIDs and lower

TABLE 38-4 Management of Nonneuropathic Chronic Pain Syndromes

Disorder	Primary Treatment	Secondary Treatment	Possible Referral Outcome
Myofascial pain syndromes	Nonsteroidal anti-inflammatory drugs orally, topical diclofenac patch for single site of pain	Amitriptyline	Trigger point injections or dry needling, US treatments, optimization of medical therapy, recommendations for exercise
Chronic migraine headache	See chapter 165 for treatment of acute exacerbations	Prophylaxis with sodium valproate or topiramate	Optimization of medical therapy, evaluation for use of prophylactic onabotulinumtoxinA
Transformed migraine/medication overuse headache	Stop prior medications	Celecoxib or prednisone taper during withdrawal period	Optimization of medical therapy, withdrawal of prior medications, evaluation for use of prophylactic onabotulinumtoxinA

Note: Medication dosing for above indications: **amitriptyline**, 25 milligrams at bedtime; **celecoxib**, 400 milligrams/d for the first 5 days, then decreased at a rate of 100 mg every 5 days; **diclofenac**, 1.3% patch every 12 hours over single site of focal pain; **prednisone**, 60 milligrams/d orally for the first 5 days, then taper down dose by 20 milligrams every 5 days; **sodium valproate**, 250 milligrams two times daily; **topiramate**, 25 milligrams at bedtime in first week, 25 milligrams two times daily in second week, and further dose adjustments at follow-up.

for those treated with cyclooxygenase-2 inhibitors.[47] NSAIDs should not be given to patients with renal dysfunction. Topical analgesics (lidocaine 5%, capsaicin 8%) are effective[48] and can be given alone or as adjuncts. Topical NSAIDs provide excellent joint and tissue levels with low plasma levels and are available as diclofenac gel, patch, or topical solution.[48]

Cognitively and mentally impaired adults with chronic pain are at risk for inadequate pain control due to barriers in communicating the nature and intensity of their pain. Be alert to these potential barriers and look for nonverbal signs of pain: agitation, irregular breathing, facial expressions of pain, stiffened body positioning, and reports of irregular sleep patterns. The ability to monitor undesired side effects, such as sedation, may limit the use of certain pain medications in this population.

ABERRANT DRUG-RELATED BEHAVIOR

INTRODUCTION AND EPIDEMIOLOGY

The term *drug-seeking behavior* is imperfect, and its definition varies among clinicians. A more accurate term is *aberrant drug-related behavior*, which raises concern for addiction and opioid misuse (**Table 38-6**). The spectrum of people seeking controlled drugs includes those who have chronic pain and have been prescribed limited opioids, the drug addict who is trying to supplement a habit, and the "hustler" who is obtaining prescription drugs to sell on the street. However, the ability of the physician to correctly identify individuals in any of these three categories is difficult and imperfect.

The prevalence of aberrant drug-related behaviors is not known; however, there is considerable indirect evidence of the problem. A systematic review of the literature found that the only consistent predictor of aberrant drug-related behaviors in chronic pain patients is a personal history of illicit drug and alcohol abuse.[49] A separate systematic review of chronic nonmalignant pain patients exposed to chronic opioid analgesic therapy found that 20.4% of patients had negative urine tests for prescribed opioids despite filling regular prescriptions, and 14.5% tested positive for illicit drugs.[50] In 2012, 17% of the teens trying illicit drugs for the first time used prescription opioids, second only to marijuana.[51]

Individuals attempting to secure opioids from emergency providers are successful through persistence. A 1996 study found that the average aberrant drug-related behavior patient presented to an ED 12.6 times per year, visited 4.1 different hospitals, and used 2.2 different aliases.[52] Patients who were refused opioids at one facility were successful in obtaining opioids at another facility 93% of the time and were later successful at obtaining opioids from the original facility 71% of the time.[52]

CLINICAL FEATURES

Because of the spectrum of aberrant drug-related behaviors, the history given may be factual or fraudulent. Patients may be demanding, intimidating, or flattering. The most common complaints of patients who attempt to obtain opioids from the ED are (in decreasing order): back pain, headache, extremity pain, and dental pain.[52] Patients may complain of panic disorder or drug withdrawal symptoms and request benzodiazepines. In some cases, observation of vital signs and physical examination findings will help the physician identify factitious illness, but even experienced clinicians are frequently misled.

TABLE 38-5 Management of Neuropathic Chronic Pain

Disorder	Primary Treatment	Secondary Treatment	Possible Referral Outcome
Fibromyalgia	Pregabalin	Duloxetine	Exercise program, optimization of medical therapy
Trigeminal neuralgia	Carbamazepine	Oxcarbazepine	Optimization of medical therapy, consideration for surgery or radiation
Human immunodeficiency virus neuropathy pain	Topical capsaicin	Gabapentin	Optimization of medical therapy
Spinal cord pain	Pregabalin	Tramadol	Optimization of medical therapy
Painful diabetic neuropathy	Duloxetine	Gabapentin or Pregabalin	Optimization of medical therapy
Postherpetic neuralgia	Pregabalin or gabapentin	Tramadol	Optimization of medical therapy, regional nerve blockade
Phantom limb pain	Gabapentin	Tramadol	Optimization of medical therapy, ketamine infusion
Poststroke pain	Pregabalin	Gabapentin	Optimization of medical therapy
Complex regional pain syndrome types I and II (reflex sympathetic dystrophy and causalgia)	Acute phase: prednisone	Chronic: intermittent infusions of low-dose ketamine by specialist	Physical therapy, individualized therapy based on neurologic testing

Note: Dosing for above indications can be started as follow: **capsaicin** is best started at follow-up because pain increases before it decreases; **carbamazepine**, 100 milligrams PO two times daily; **duloxetine**, 30 to 60 milligrams daily; **gabapentin**, 300 milligrams PO, once on day 1, two times on day 2, then three times daily, eventually increasing to 1200 milligrams/d guided by follow-up clinician; **oxcarbazepine**, 300 milligrams PO two times daily for 3 days, 300 milligrams in morning and 600 milligrams in evening for 3 days, then 600 milligrams two times daily; **prednisone**, 60 milligrams daily for 7 days to be adjusted by follow-up physician; **pregabalin**, 50 milligrams three time per day; **tramadol**, 50 milligrams every 6 hours as needed.

TABLE 38-6 Aberrant Drug-Related Behaviors
Forges/alters prescriptions*
Sells controlled drugs*
Uses aliases to receive opioids*
Current illicit drug use*
Factitious illness, requests opioids
Conceals multiple physicians prescribing opioids
Abusive when refused
Conceals multiple ED visits for opioids

*Unlawful behaviors in many states.

Patients should be examined for signs of injection drug use, including needle marks, and the heart should be examined for evidence of a regurgitant murmur indicative of valve damage from prior endocarditis. Look for key characteristics of patients attempting to falsify illness (**Table 38-7**). Patients most commonly have completely normal physical examination findings. Widespread anecdotal experience of ED personnel has indicated that such patients will relate an allergy to alternative pharmacotherapy and insist that only one or two specific opioids are effective.

DIAGNOSIS

The diagnosis of drug-seeking behavior may not be possible in the ED. The medical record can provide a wealth of information about the patient, including documentation proving that the patient is supplying false information. Often the diagnosis is suspected in the ED but cannot be confirmed. In such cases, the clinical impression should be documented in the chart listing the provider's concerns, but physicians should be careful when using terms such as *drug-seeking behavior* without solid evidence. A listing or card file at the nurses' desk of "drug-seekers" violates confidentiality between patient and physician unless it is part of the patient's permanent medical record and subject to the same controls restricting access. However, electronic medical records can be programmed to flag charts with alerts for patient safety; accidental overdose is always a concern in such patients.

Do not miss a true emergency in patients suspected of aberrant drug-related behaviors because the negotiation over pain medicine can distract the entire team from a subtle yet life-threatening medical or surgical illness.

Prescription drug monitoring programs and other computerized tracking systems may help identify patients who are abusing or overusing prescription drugs. Practitioners are encouraged to review the prescription drug monitoring program database before prescribing a discharge medication, because that information is likely to change the intended discharge plan.[53]

TREATMENT, DISPOSITION, AND FOLLOW-UP

The treatment of definite aberrant drug-related behavior is to refuse the controlled substance, consider the need for alternative medication or treatment, and refer for drug counseling (**Table 38-7**). The patient who complains of multiple drug allergies can be difficult. Occasionally the medical record will show previous administration of the drug in question (usually an opioid substitute) with no adverse reaction. When confronted, patients hoping to acquire opioids may become verbally abusive, and hospital security may be required to control the situation and, if necessary, escort the patient out of the ED. A nonjudgmental attitude facilitates communication; avoid using labels such as "narcotics addict" or "drug-seeker." Stick to the facts, inform the patient that you are not able to prescribe or administrate the medication they seek, and offer a substitute.

When aberrant drug-related behavior is confirmed or suspected in the ED, it should be documented in the chart, stating only the facts. Concerns about opioid overuse can be documented without diagnosing the patient with "drug-seeking behavior," which may not be appropriate without evidence of illegal behavior. When physicians are notified by a pharmacist of forged or altered prescriptions, law enforcement authorities should be called, and physicians should cooperate with the legal investigation. The prosecution of fraudulent behaviors, such as using

TABLE 38-7 Recommendations to Manage Fraudulent Techniques Used by Patients Attempting to Obtain Narcotics for Illicit Use

Technique	Characteristics	Management
Lost prescription	Calls or returns stating that opioid prescription was lost before being filled.	Establish a policy: no lost opioid prescriptions refilled. Notify patients of policy at discharge as they receive prescriptions.
"Stolen" prescription or pill bottle	Police have not been called.	Inform patient this is a police issue and recommend calling police to rectify matter. Establish a policy: no stolen opioid prescriptions refilled.
Impending surgery	Wants temporizing opioids, doctor "unavailable," previous surgery, patient from out of town.	Use Internet and phone calls to check validity of information. Check medical records. Offer substitute for opioid.
Carries own records and x-rays	Suspicious or forged records, doctor's written permission to receive opioids, patient from out of town.	Use Internet and phone calls to check validity of information. Check records. Offer substitute for opioid.
Factitious hematuria with complaint of kidney stones	Appears comfortable or overacting, pricked finger dipped in urine, lip/cheek bitten and blood spitted into the urine.	Examine fingers and mouth. Obtain witnessed urinalysis. Offer nonopioid pain medicine. Obtain confirmatory test before giving opioid.
Self-mutilation	Done with dominant hand, requests opioids for pain.	Use bupivacaine for local block. Do not prescribe opioids without indications. Offer substitute for opioids.
Dental pain	Dental caries only.	Give local nerve block with bupivacaine. Refer to dentist.
Factitious injury	Old injury, old deformity, self-massaged to produce erythema, patient from out of town.	X-ray before treatment. Check records. Check for erythema that dissipates over time.

aliases to obtain opioids, requires the involvement of the state bureau of investigation or a similar state agency.

SPECIAL CONSIDERATIONS: LEGAL ISSUES

The U.S. Drug Enforcement Agency (in addition to state agencies) licenses physicians to administer or dispense controlled substances. However, state law determines most prescribing regulations. Physicians should be aware of state laws regulating controlled substances prescribed in their practice setting. The prescribing of opioids to a known drug addict could result in restriction of the physician's medical license in some states, although this is rarely prosecuted for isolated incidents. If a patient refuses to acknowledge an addiction, the physician cannot be held accountable unless medical records at the facility where the patient presents document the addiction. In all states, it is illegal for patients to forge or alter prescriptions. In some states, it is illegal for patients to use aliases or factitious illness to obtain opioids. Furthermore, in some states, concealing previous or recent prescriptions for opioids when requesting opioids from a new practitioner is illegal.

REFERENCES

The complete reference list is available online at www.TintinalliEM.com.

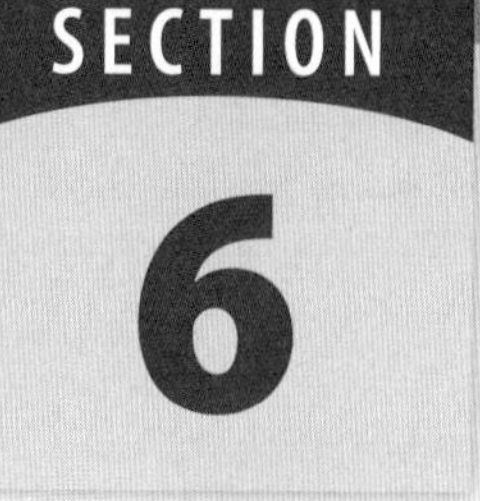

Wound Management

CHAPTER 39 Wound Evaluation

Adam J. Singer
Judd E. Hollander

PRINCIPLES OF INITIAL EVALUATION

Evaluation of the patient with a traumatic wound begins with overall patient assessment.[1,2] Less obvious but more serious life-threatening injuries need care before directing attention to wound management. Determine the patient's past medical history and circumstances surrounding the injury.[1,2] Remove rings or other circumferential jewelry as soon as possible so they do not act as constricting bands when swelling progresses. Remove clothing over the injured area to reduce the potential for contamination.

External bleeding can usually be controlled by direct pressure over the bleeding site. When possible, replace skin flaps to their original position before applying pressure in order to avoid exacerbating vascular compromise. Tourniquet application may be necessary to stop life-threatening exsanguination or when needed for a short period to create a "bloodless" field for wound inspection.[3-5] Amputated fingers or extremities should be wrapped with a moist, sterile, protective dressing, placed in a waterproof bag, and then placed in a container of ice water for preservation and consideration for future reattachment. Before wound exploration, cleansing, and repair, most patients will need some form of anesthesia.[6] Systemic analgesia or procedural sedation may be required (see chapter 35, Acute Pain Management, and chapter 37, Procedural Sedation).

RISK ASSESSMENT

Proper wound management begins with a pertinent patient history (**Table 39-1**).[1,2] A variety of patient factors have adverse effects on wound healing and increase the rate of wound infection—extremes of age, diabetes mellitus, chronic renal failure, obesity, malnutrition, the use of immunosuppressive medications, the presence of connective tissue disorders, and protein and vitamin C deficiencies.[1] Predictive factors for infection are the wound characteristics of location, age, depth, configuration, and contamination.[7,8]

Ascertain the tendency of patients to form hypertrophic scars or keloids by both history and examination, as past experience may predict poor scar formation. Black and Asian patients are more prone to keloid formation than whites. Hypertrophic scars are due to tissue tension during wound healing, and these scars stay within the original wound boundaries and tend to undergo partial spontaneous regression within 1 to 2 years. Keloids are genetically linked variations in wound healing, resulting in the production of excess collagen beyond the original wound boundaries (**Figure 39-1**). Once they form, keloids rarely decrease in size.

Obtain a detailed history of allergies or prior adverse reactions to anesthetic agents or antibiotics. **Review any prior allergies to latex.**[9] **Determine the status of prior tetanus immunization and the need for further tetanus vaccination** (see chapter 156, Tetanus).

Review the mechanism of injury to identify the presence of potential wound contaminants and foreign bodies. Bite wounds are at high risk for infection and are generally managed differently than other lacerations (see chapter 46, Puncture Wounds and Bites). Foreign bodies are common in puncture wounds, wounds associated with broken glass, and motor vehicle collisions.[10-13] Ask about the presence of a foreign body sensation. In adults, those reporting a foreign body sensation are more likely to have a retained foreign body than those who do not (positive likelihood ratio = 2.49 and negative likelihood ratio = 0.69).[14] This question has little utility in children.[15]

Both foreign body retention and visible contamination increase the risk of infection.[7,8] Organic and inorganic components of soil can cause infection even from very small doses of bacterial inoculum. Clay is the major inorganic soil component responsible for infection. Conversely, sand grains and black dirt from roadways are relatively inert.

The likelihood of wound infection varies according to the forces applied at the time of injury.[7,8] The most common mechanism for traumatic wounds is blunt force. The skin is crushed against underlying bone and tears or splits from the subsequent tension. Sharp objects produce shear forces that cut skin cleanly. Crush injuries produce more tissue devitalization and are more susceptible to infection than wounds from shear forces.

Low-energy impact injuries may not result in lacerations, but instead may disrupt vessels, leading to ecchymosis or hematoma formation. Some hematomas spontaneously resorb. Those that become encapsulated may eventually require aspiration or incision and drainage.

Determine the time that the injury occurred. Although the growth of the bacterial inoculum is directly related to the time interval from injury to laceration repair,[1,7] **there is no clearly defined relationship of time to closure to clinical infection**[16-18] **(Table 39-2). Therefore, time from injury until presentation is only one element to be considered, in addition to the wound etiology, location, degree of contamination, host risk factors, and the importance of cosmetic appearance, before determining whether or not to perform primary wound closure.** Wounds that are not closed primarily because of a high risk of infection should be considered for delayed primary closure after 4 days. The clinical consensus of wound care experts is that after 4 days of open wound management, the risk of infection after closure substantially decreases, although this approach has not been subjected to randomized controlled trials.[19]

Determine whether the wound was the result of an intentional, unintentional, or workplace event. Most states have regulations that require the reporting of intentional injuries, and patients with self-inflicted injuries may need psychiatric evaluation. Occupational injuries may require alternative follow-up arrangements.

The anatomic location of the injury helps predict the clinical outcome, both in terms of infection risk and cosmetic result[7,8,15,20] (**Table 39-3**). The risk of infection is determined largely by the interplay between baseline bacterial colonization and vascular blood supply. With respect to bacterial colonization, the density of the bacterial population is low on the upper arms, legs, and torso. Conversely, moist areas of the body, such as the axilla, perineum, toe webs, and intertriginous areas, harbor millions of bacteria per square centimeter, including anaerobes. Obviously, any wounds with human or animal fecal contaminants run a high risk of infection, even with therapeutic intervention.

Wounds located on highly vascular areas, such as the face or scalp, are less likely to be infected than wounds located in less vascular areas.[7,8,15,17,20] The increased vascularity of the area more than offsets the high bacterial inoculum found in the scalp, and lacerations of the scalp and face have a very low infection rate regardless of the intensity of cleansing.[21] While prophylactic oral antibiotics have traditionally been considered as warranted for intra-oral lacerations, there is inconclusive evidence to support their use.[22]

TABLE 39-1 Pertinent Medical History

Symptoms
- Pain, swelling, paresthesias, muscle weakness

Type of force causing injury
- Crush (blunt) or shear (sharp)
- Bite or puncture

Elements of contamination
- Time elapsed from injury until initial cleansing
- Time elapsed from injury until presentation
- Wound care performed prior to ED arrival
- Object that caused injury (glass, wood, etc.)
- Cleanliness of body and environment at time of injury and afterward

Factors resulting in injury
- Intentional or unintentional
- Occupation or nonoccupation related
- Assault or self-inflicted

Foreign body potential
- Did the object break or shatter?
- Foreign body sensation
- Removal of portion of object

Function
- Occupation and handedness

Allergies
- Anesthetics, analgesics, antibiotics, and latex

Medications

Chronic medical conditions that increase risk of infection

Chronic medical conditions that increase likelihood of poor wound healing

Previous scar formation (hypertrophic scars or keloids)

WOUND EXAMINATION

Thorough wound examination should be conducted when the patient is calm and cooperative and positioned appropriately, with optimal lighting conditions, and with little or no residual bleeding (**Figure 39-2**).

Cursory examination under poor lighting or when the depths of the wound are obscured by blood will occasionally result in poor detection of foreign bodies and tendon, nerve, and vascular injuries. If bleeding is a problem, epinephrine-containing anesthetic solutions may be helpful, when not contraindicated. **Tourniquets may be used to obtain a bloodless field, but they should not be used for more than 30 minutes.**[3-5] Lacerations over joints may have penetrated the joint capsule, and sometimes it is necessary to inject the joint to ensure that there is no communication between the joint space and the laceration. Evaluate the wound in neutral position and also in the position present during injury. Chain-saw knee wounds, for example, are often sustained with the knee in flexed position. **Repositioning the joint or extremity in the position assumed during injury can better reconstruct the mechanism of injury and identify injured structures.** Lacerations over the metacarpophalangeal joints are suspicious for having occurred during a fight (clenched fist injury) and should be treated as though they are human bites.

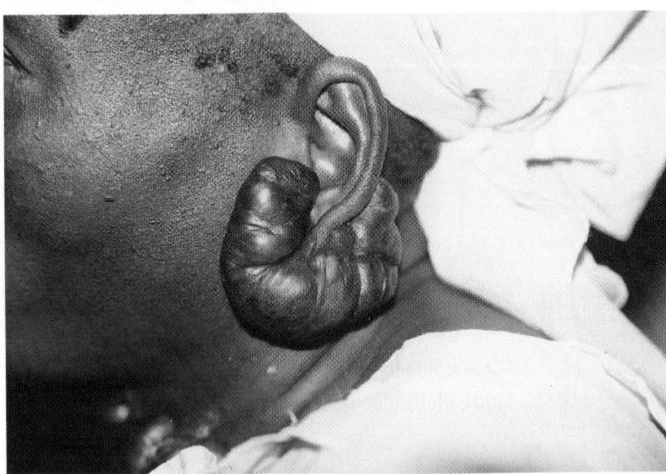

FIGURE 39-1. A large keloid extending beyond the original wound margins. [Reproduced with permission from Sztajnkrycer MD, Trott AD: Wounds and soft tissue injuries, in Knoop KJ, Stack LB, Storrow AB (eds): *Atlas of Emergency Medicine, 2nd ed*. Figure 18-37. Copyright © 2002, 1997, by The McGraw-Hill Companies, Inc. All rights reserved.]

IMAGING

Although most lacerations will not require any diagnostic testing, on occasion, wound imaging for detection of foreign bodies may be necessary (see chapter 45, Soft Tissue Foreign Bodies). Most foreign bodies commonly found in wounds are much denser than the surrounding tissue and are readily apparent on plain radiographs. Metal, bone, teeth, pencil graphite, certain plastics, glass, gravel, sand, some fish bones, some painted wood, and most aluminum are visible on plain radiographs.

CT and MRI are useful for identifying and locating objects that have densities similar to soft tissue. US may also be useful, particularly for wooden foreign bodies, although the sensitivity of US is inadequate to reliably exclude small (<2.5 mm) wood fragments.

PATIENT EDUCATION

Patients should be carefully educated regarding the expected cosmetic outcome. They should be informed that there will be some scarring and, if predisposed, possible keloid formation.[1] Some indication of the maximal width of the scar can be predicted based on wound location,

TABLE 39-2 Risk of Wound Infection as Function of Time From Injury to Closure

Reference	Comments	Distinction Between Early and Late Closure (h)	Infection Rate/Inadequate Healing With Early Closure	Infection Rate/Inadequate Healing With Late Closure	Percent age Difference (95% CI)
Morgan et al., 1980[16]	Hand and forearm; all patients received IM penicillin and half received PO clindamycin	4	10/148 (7%)	14/69 (21%)	13.5% (3.2% to 23.9%)
Baker and Lanuti, 1990[18]	Children, 59% head and neck location	6	32/2665 (1.2%)	2/147 (1.3%)	0.16% (−1.76% to 2.08%)
Berk et al., 1988[17]	All locations	19	8/97 (8.2%)	25/107 (23.4%)	15.1% (5.4% to 24.8%)
	Head	19	2/44 (5%)	1/36 (3%)	−1.8% (−9.9% to 6.4%)
	Trunk and extremities	19	6/53 (11.3%)	24/71 (33.8%)	22.5% (8.6% to 36.4%)

TABLE 39-3 Risk of Wound Infection After ED Closure

Location	Risk of Infection (%)
Head and neck	1–2
Upper extremity	4
Lower extremity	7

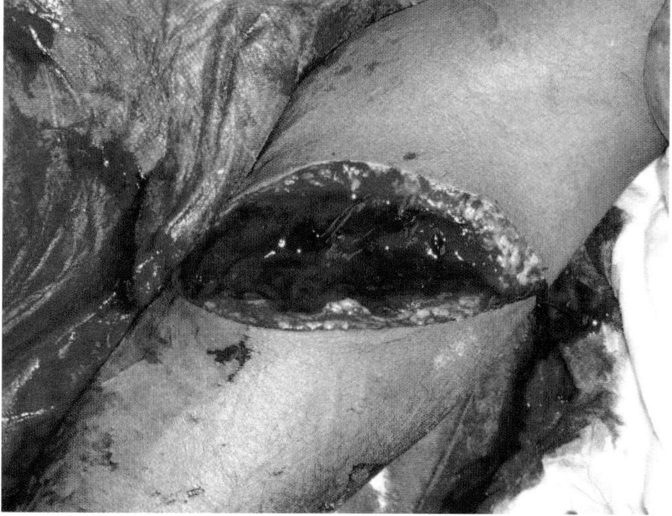

FIGURE 39-2. This deep antecubital laceration could involve arterial, venous, nerve, and tendon injury. Such wounds require careful and complete exploration. Proximal arterial control is important for visual inspection in a "bloodless" field. [Image used with permission of J. Stephan Stapczynski, MD.]

whether the laceration is aligned parallel or perpendicular with lines of minimal tension, and how gaping the wound is while at rest (static tension) or when put through a range of motion (dynamic tension).[20,23] Lacerations over joints (which have more dynamic tension) will have wider scars than similar lacerations subject to less tension. Wounds that deviate from the lines of skin tension will also be prone to greater scar formation after suturing than wounds that are more closely aligned with skin tension.[23] The most important determinant of cosmetic outcome under control of the treating physician is meticulous wound repair with approximation of viable wound edges under little tension. Patients should be clearly educated that all lacerations result in some scarring.

REFERENCES

The complete reference list is available online at www.TintinalliEM.com.

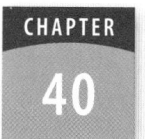

Wound Preparation

Aleksandr M. Tichter
Wallace A. Carter
Susan C. Stone

INTRODUCTION

The common methods of wound care are reasonably effective, resulting in a good outcome for the vast majority of cutaneous wounds treated in the ED.[1-3] Wound preparation is the most important step in restoring tissue integrity and function, minimizing infection risk, and achieving the best possible cosmetic result. However, there is surprisingly little scientific validation for most of these methods.[4-7] With some patient and wound characteristics (**Table 40-1**), the risk of improper healing increases, and the importance of careful wound preparation becomes more important.[4,5,8-10]

TABLE 40-1 Risk Factors for Poor Wound Repair Outcome

Patient Factors	Wound Factors
Immunosuppression: diabetes, chemotherapeutic agents, chronic steroid therapy, chronic renal failure, hematologic malignancies, congenital immunodeficiencies	Crush injuries
Tissue ischemia: peripheral vascular disease, anemia, vasculitis	Tissue loss
Poor wound healing: elderly, cigarette smoking, malnourished, connective tissue disorders	Contamination
	Foreign bodies
	Peripheral location

ANESTHESIA

Thorough cleansing and meticulous wound evaluation and repair can be painful procedures, so adequate anesthesia is important for patient comfort and cooperation. Choice of anesthetic agent and route varies according to wound location and size (see chapter 36, Local and Regional Anesthesia). The sensory, motor, and vascular examination should be performed at and distal to the wound site prior to the administration of local or regional anesthetic.

Sensory examination should include evaluation of pain or touch. If a wound involves the hand or fingers, additional assessment for digital nerve injury using **two-point discrimination (normal <6 mm)** on the volar pads should be performed prior to local or regional anesthesia administration. Motor examination should assess movement and strength of tendons and muscles around the wound site as well as muscles that are innervated by nerves traversing the site. Vascular examination should assess distal perfusion by noting skin color, temperature, capillary refill time, and quality of pulses. Comparison of the systolic blood pressure in the injured extremity with the noninjured one (using a Doppler stethoscope and pneumatic cuff) assesses for hemodynamically significant arterial compromise. While performing the sensory examination prior to the administration of an anesthetic is important, adequate motor examination can be occasionally limited by pain, with improved strength testing following achievement of pain control.

IRRIGATION

Wound irrigation is widely considered to be the most important step in the management of acute wounds; it decreases bacterial count and helps to remove debris and foreign bodies, thereby reducing the risk of wound infection.[1,3,11] Choices in the performance of wound irrigation include solution composition, temperature of the irrigant, pressure with which it is applied, and the total volume used.

In most medical settings, wound irrigation is performed with sterile normal saline, but potable tap water is as effective and may be superior when taking into account time, resources, cost, and the potential for occupational exposures during clinician-performed irrigation techniques.[12-17] Limited studies indicate that dilute solutions containing povidone-iodine or hydrogen peroxide do not appear to confer greater benefit than water alone.[18-20] **Polyhexanide** (a chlorhexidine polymer) is an antiseptic that, when used for wound irrigation of dirty and contaminated soft tissue wounds, reduced the rate of postrepair wound infections compared to Ringer's lactate, povidone-iodine, or hydrogen peroxide irrigation.[21-23] One small clinical trial suggests that warmed solution may be more comfortable than room temperature irrigant.[24]

High-pressure irrigation is defined as approximately 7 psi (50 kPa) or greater, and is achieved using any combination of a 30- to 65-mL syringe and a 19-gauge catheter or needle hub, or commercially available splashguard, with forceful depression of the syringe piston.[3,25-28] **Low-pressure irrigation** is defined as approximately 0.5 psi (3.5 kPa) or lower, and is achieved with a slow, gentle wash.[29] Low-pressure irrigation may be sufficient for cleansing simple, nonbite, uncontaminated wounds in highly vascular areas such as the scalp and face.[30]

However, high-pressure irrigation is generally regarded as more effective for clearance of debris and reduction of infection.[11,16,31]

Wound soaking is not effective in cleansing contaminated wounds and may actually increase wound bacterial counts.[32] Routine scrubbing of traumatic wounds with a sponge is also ineffective, inflicting trauma and impairing resistance to infection.

Many wounds and lacerations seen in the ED have little visible contamination, and there is no strong evidence regarding the amount of irrigation effective to minimize postrepair infection. Common sense dictates that the higher the volume of irrigation, the more thoroughly cleansed the wound and the less likely infection will ensue. Typical recommendations by wound care experts range from 25 to 100 mL/cm of wound length for "clean"-appearing wounds.[11] Additional volumes should be based on anatomic location, mechanism of injury, degree of contamination, and patient factors that lower resistance to infection.

High-pressure wound irrigation risks mucous membrane exposure of the healthcare worker to contaminated body fluids. Irrigation shields provide some measure of safety,[28] but universal precautions, including barrier protection with face mask/shield, should be employed as a matter of routine.

SKIN DISINFECTION

A common practice is to disinfect intact skin around the wound with either a povidone-iodine–based or chlorhexidine-containing agent. These agents suppress bacterial growth on intact skin and are thus favorable antiseptics prior to surgical incision,[33-35] but within the environment of an already open wound, they can impair host defenses and promote bacterial growth. Both povidone-iodine[36,37] and chlorhexidine[38] can produce chemical burns on intact skin and in the eyes. Apply disinfectants from the wound edges outward in order to avoid cytotoxic exposure of nonintact skin.[10,11,20]

STERILE TECHNIQUE

Although observing sterile technique has been well demonstrated to have a beneficial effect on patient outcomes in several settings, the extent to which its routine employment in the ED treatment of traumatically contaminated wounds reduces infection rates is unclear. Adherence to full aseptic methods (cap, gown, mask, and gloves) does not appear to be of substantial benefit,[39] nor does hand antisepsis prior to initiation of wound repair.[40] Although recommendations exist for the use of sterile gloves in the repair of uncomplicated lacerations, supportive evidence is lacking, if not refutative.[41] These findings suggest that aspects of the sterile technique may be curbed, leading to time and cost savings per laceration by using common-sense cleanliness.

HEMOSTASIS

To adequately evaluate a wound, hemostasis is needed to prepare a clear visual field. The most common sources of wound-related bleeding are the subdermal plexus and superficial veins. Oozing from these sources can usually be controlled with the application of direct pressure using saline-soaked sponges or gauze.

In the event of continual bleeding, the next step is typically an attempt at chemical hemostasis using **epinephrine mixed with local anesthetics** in concentrations of 1:100,000 or 1:200,000 and injected into the wound area. Local epinephrine induces vasoconstriction that will additionally allow a longer duration of anesthesia and a larger total local anesthetic dose due to the depot effect of the vasoconstriction.[42-45] Despite the theoretical risk of end-organ ischemia (i.e., fingers, nose, ears, toes), when mixed with local anesthetics, the safety of epinephrine use in these regions has been well documented.[46-52] Use caution in patients with small vessel disease, where end-organ epinephrine injection remains ill advised. Although epinephrine interferes with wound healing in experimental animal models,[4,5] no increase in wound infection has been observed with the addition of epinephrine to local anesthetics used in the ED.

Physical means of applying pressure to bleeding include the use of **gelatin**, **cellulose**, or **collagen** sponges placed directly into the wound.

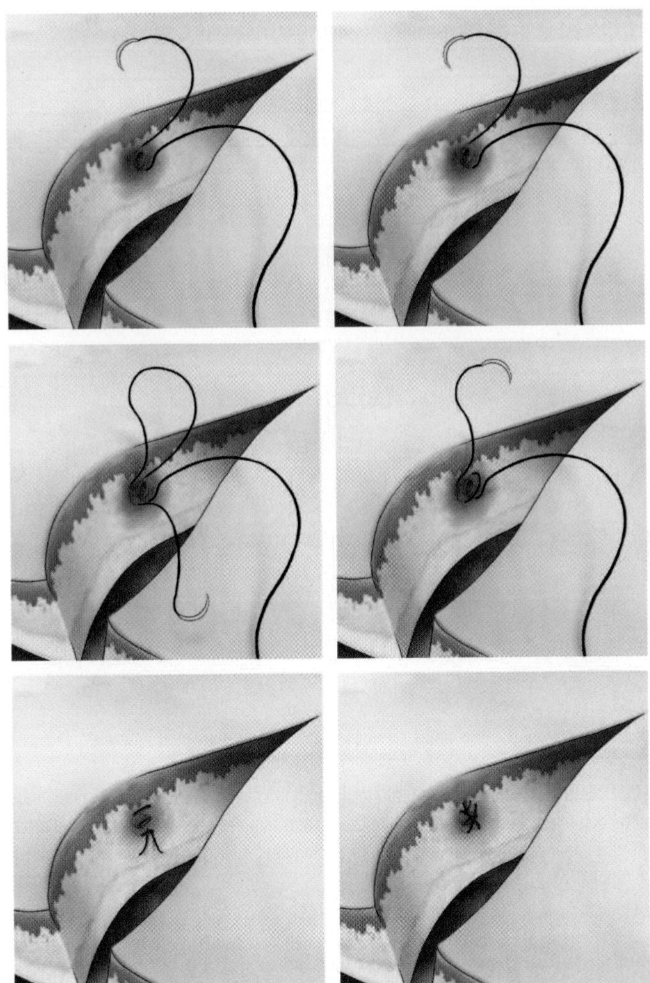

FIGURE 40-1. Suture to control bleeding wound edges where the involved vessel is not visible. **Left column:** Standard horizontal mattress suture. **Right column:** Figure-of-eight suture. [Image used with permission of Nicholas Hatch, MD.]

Denatured gelatin (Gelfoam®; Pfizer, Inc., New York, NY) has no intrinsic hemostatic properties and works by the pressure it exerts as it expands. A cellulose derivative (Oxycel®; Becton Dickinson Infusion Therapy Systems, Inc., Sandy, UT) or a collagen (Actifoam®; Med-Chem Products, Inc., Woburn, MA) sponge reacts with blood, forming an artificial clot. These products are not particularly effective for actively bleeding wounds, as the blood flowing into the wound can wash them out.

If the source of bleeding is a small vessel that has been lacerated but can be easily visualized, control may be achieved through direct pressure applied with a gloved fingertip directly on the vessel. Once bleeding has ceased, more permanent control can be obtained by clamping the vessel, isolating a short length, and ligating it with absorbable synthetic suture (typically 5-0). Take care to avoid clamping or ensnaring adjacent structures (i.e., nerves and tendons), particularly when working with wounds of the face.

For bleeding wound edges where the involved vessel is not visible, a figure-of-eight or horizontal mattress suture (**Figure 40-1**) applied adjacent to the site of bleeding will sometimes achieve control. However, this technique may impair blood flow and leave nonviable tissue in the wound.

Bipolar **electrocautery** can achieve hemostasis in blood vessels <2 mm in diameter, but if improperly or too extensively applied, it can result in tissue necrosis. Electrocautery units are not routinely available in many EDs. Battery-powered, hand-held cautery devices (**Figure 40-2**), although more accessible, do not generate sufficient heat to produce coagulation in vessels larger than capillaries. Low-temperature units, identified where the wire loop does not glow when heated, are recommended for ED use.

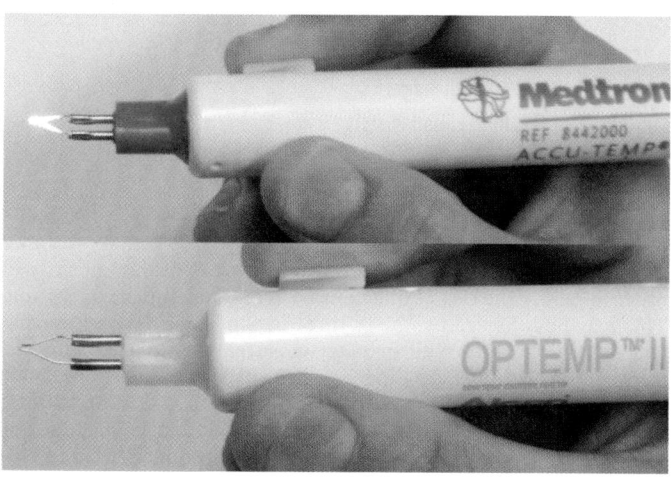

FIGURE 40-2. Battery-powered, hand-held thermal cautery units commonly used in the ED. **Top:** High-temperature unit (1200°C); wire loop glows when heated. **Bottom:** Low-temperature unit (690°C); wire loop does not glow when heated. [Image used with permission of J. Stephan Stapczynski, MD.]

Scalp lacerations can bleed extensively from the wound edges due to the highly vascular subcutaneous layer. If traditional methods of hemostasis fail, scalp bleeding can be controlled by the use of specially designed clips applied along the wound edges (**Figure 40-3**). If the source of bleeding is determined to be a major artery, do not ligate the vessel. Maintain direct pressure on the vessel and obtain surgical consultation.

Extremity wounds that are refractory to direct pressure, ligation, or cautery may require an arterial tourniquet.[53] **Tourniquets** may compress and damage underlying blood vessels and nerves, reducing tissue viability, and therefore should not be left in place for greater than 20 to 30 minutes at a time. The simplest tourniquet to use in an ED is a blood pressure cuff placed proximal to the wound and inflated to 20 to 30 mm Hg (2.7 to 3 kPa) above the patient's systolic pressure. Elevating the extremity to reduce venous blood volume prior to cuff inflation may be useful. If an extremity tourniquet is needed to control bleeding, the best course of action is exploration and repair in the operating room.

FOREIGN BODY REMOVAL

Retained foreign bodies are a frequent concern in the management of traumatic wounds. The risk for retained foreign bodies is increased in patients with head or foot wounds, wounds sustained in motor vehicle collisions, and puncture wounds. Clinical clues to their presence include foreign body sensation, point tenderness, or increased pain on range of motion.

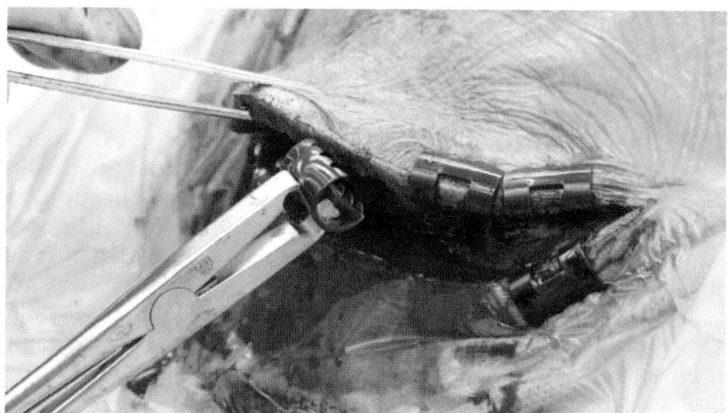

FIGURE 40-3. Raney clips are used to control bleeding from the wound edges of scalp lacerations. An applicator is used to apply the open clip. When the applicator is released, the clip closes and pinches onto the wound edges. [Image used with permission of J. Stephan Stapczynski, MD.]

Visual wound inspection, down to the full depth and along the full course of the wound, is the most important method of detection. Carefully remove obvious foreign debris, using forceps to avoid injury to the physician from sharp edges or points. Probing wounds with a gloved fingertip to detect foreign bodies by palpation is discouraged. Despite thorough exploration, some reports suggest that up to 4% of superficial wounds have retained foreign bodies missed on exam.[54]

Imaging modalities may be used as a diagnostic adjunct. These include plain radiographs, which are most sensitive for radiopaque foreign bodies (e.g., metal, gravel), and high-frequency US, which is most sensitive for radiolucent foreign bodies (e.g., rubber, wood), as well as CT and MRI (see chapter 45, Soft Tissue Foreign Bodies).[55]

HAIR REMOVAL

Although the presence of hair around a wound can interfere with wound closure, obstruct field of view, become entangled in sutures or staples, and complicate the application of adhesive dressings following repair, routine hair removal does not appear to have an effect on the rate of skin and soft tissue infections following neurosurgery[56-63] or scalp laceration repair.[64] Rather, shaving may increase the rate of postoperative skin and soft tissue infection.[65,66] Hair removal prior to wound repair may also result in irregular and cosmetically undesirable regrowth in certain anatomic locations (e.g., eyebrows and hairline). In the event that hair is interfering with wound care, it is best removed by clipping it 1 to 2 mm above the skin with scissors.[1,3,11] An alternative method to clipping is to use ointment or saline to allow the hair to be parted away from the wound edges.

DEBRIDEMENT

Nonviable tissue in the wound increases the risk of infection and delays healing by simultaneously acting as a culture medium and inhibiting host defenses.[1,3,8] Debridement serves the dual purposes of removing foreign matter, bacteria, and devitalized tissue, and creating a clean wound edge that is easier to repair.[67]

Excisional debridement targets tissue that has a narrow base, has irregular devitalized edges, or lacks capillary refill, and is performed using a standard surgical blade or scissors (**Figure 40-4**), with the goal of converting a contaminated wound into a clean surgical edge and

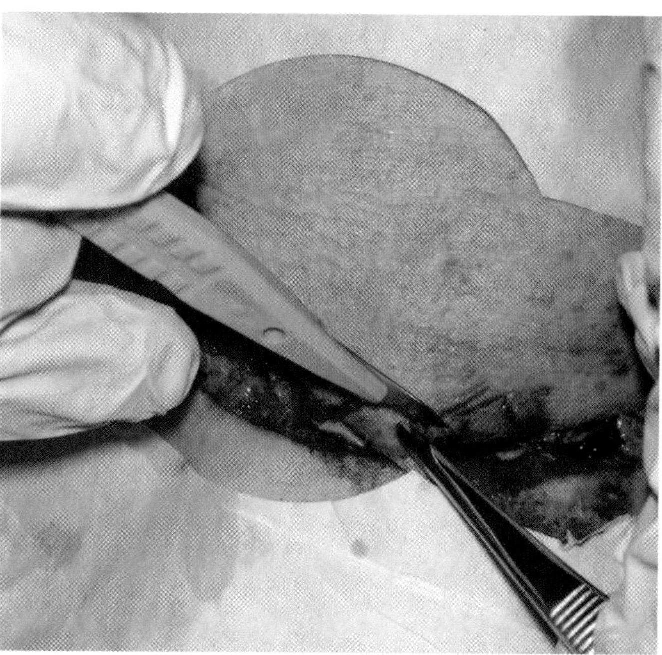

FIGURE 40-4. Sharp debridement of the contused and jagged edge of a 10-cm infrapatellar knee laceration sustained from a fall onto gravel. [Image used with permission of J. Stephan Stapczynski, MD.]

re-establishing a margin of normal healthy tissue.[67] The easiest technique for excisional debridement is to mark an elliptical area around the sides of the wound and then use a scalpel to cut only through the epidermis. Relaxed skin tension lines should be respected, and extensive excision should be avoided. Certain types of wounds with devitalized tissue (e.g., low-velocity civilian gunshot wounds to the extremities) can be successfully managed without debridement, using conservative wound care techniques (irrigation and cleaning) alone.[68,69]

Wounds with an extensive amount of nonviable tissue or heavy contamination are more problematic. They may require operative debridement and need more delayed wound closure or grafting. In general, a surgeon should be consulted to assist in their management.[11]

PROPHYLACTIC ANTIBIOTICS

Infections occur in approximately 2% to 5% of traumatic wounds repaired in EDs, although this rate varies widely according to mechanism, location, and patient factors (**Table 40-1**).[2,9] Less vascular, moist (axilla and perineum), and exposed areas (feet and hands) tend to be at higher risk for infection. Crush or puncture wounds are more prone to infection due to the tensile and compressive forces generated that increase the potential for devitalized tissue. With current methods for ED wound care, **the time from injury until wound closure for simple lacerations does not have much influence on the occurrence of postrepair infection.**[70-72] The most important step in the prevention of a wound infection is adequate irrigation and debridement.

There is no clear evidence that routine antibiotic prophylaxis prevents infections in most patients whose wounds are closed in the ED (see chapter 47, Postrepair Wound Care).[9,73-76] Certain types of injuries that have historically been considered high risk, specifically, uncomplicated hand lacerations[77] and mammalian bites,[78-82] appear to have no clear benefit from routine prophylaxis either.

If antibiotic prophylaxis is chosen, the principles learned from the surgical literature suggest that effectiveness requires the achievement of antimicrobial blood levels prior to, or rapidly after, wound contamination.[82-85] Antibiotic prophylaxis for traumatic wounds in an ED should be (1) initiated before significant tissue manipulation is done, (2) performed with agents that are effective against predicted pathogens, and (3) administered by routes that rapidly achieve desired blood levels. There are no studies that compare the common practice of IV administration of the initial dose of prophylactic antibiotics with PO administration. Based on the above principles, the PO route may be as effective if administered before manipulation using an agent with an appropriate spectrum and rapid PO absorption.

Most nonbite wound infections are due to staphylococci or streptococci, and despite the increase in methicillin-resistant *Staphylococcus aureus* skin infections, prophylactic coverage with a β-lactam remains adequate (see chapter 47).[86] The duration for adequate antibiotic prophylaxis is unknown; most experts recommend only 3 to 5 days.[87] Patients with established wound infections require longer treatment.

Prophylactic antibiotics are recommended for all human bites to the hands and feet, as well as to those overlying joints or cartilage.[80] *Eikenella* is the target organism, and adequate prophylaxis can be attained with amoxicillin-clavulanate.

Prophylactic antibiotics are recommended for all mammalian bites to the hand.[78,79,81] The studies of mammalian bites have not been of adequate size to draw conclusions regarding the benefit of antibiotic prophylaxis in locations other than the hand. *Pasteurella* is the target organism, and adequate prophylaxis can be attained with amoxicillin-clavulanate.

Wounds contaminated by fresh water or plantar puncture wounds through athletic shoes carry the theoretical risk of *Pseudomonas* infection, and although there is little evidence for prophylactic antibiotics, agents should be chosen whose spectrum includes this pathogen (see chapter 46, Puncture Wounds and Bites).

REFERENCES

The complete reference list is available online at www.TintinalliEM.com.

CHAPTER 41

Wound Closure

Adam J. Singer
Judd E. Hollander

INTRODUCTION

The major goal of wound closure is to restore the skin's integrity in order to reduce the risk of infection, scarring, and impaired function. This may be achieved by one of three methods: primary, secondary, and delayed closure. With **primary closure**, the wound is immediately closed by approximating its edges, with the main advantage being a reduction in healing time in comparison with other closure methods. Primary wound closure also may reduce bleeding and discomfort often associated with open wounds. **Secondary wound closure**, in which the wound is left open and allowed to close on its own, is particularly well suited for highly contaminated or infected wounds as well as in patients at high risk of infection. Although this method may reduce the risk of infection, it is relatively slow and uncomfortable and leaves a larger scar than primary closure. With **delayed (or tertiary) closure**, the wound is initially cleansed and then packed with dry sterile gauze covered by a sterile covering. The dressing is left undisturbed unless signs of infection—fever, purulent exudate, or spreading cellulitis—develop. After 4 to 5 days, the dressing is removed, and the wound edges can be closed if no infection has supervened. This approach may be useful for highly contaminated wounds and animal bites, and while commonly described and recommended, there is little evidence documenting the effectiveness for traumatic wounds seen in the ED.[1]

OVERVIEW OF WOUND CLOSURE METHODS

Lacerations may be closed by one of five commonly available methods or devices: sutures, staples, adhesive tapes, tissue adhesives, and hair apposition. Each method has advantages and disadvantages (**Table 41-1**). Choice of the wound closure method and timing should take into account both patient and wound characteristics.[2] Cosmetic outcome is more closely related to practitioner technique and the patient's own healing characteristics than to any specific closure method or device. Many of the principles discussed in this chapter are based on experience and observation rather than on controlled trials.

One of the most important considerations when choosing a wound closure method is the amount of tension on the wound, both *static* (at rest) and *dynamic* (with motion). *Linear lacerations subject to little tension* can usually be closed by any one of the five closure methods. For low-tension lacerations, consider patient characteristics and preferences such as compliance, the availability to return for follow-up and device removal, and overall level of patient anxiety. *With low-tension irregular lacerations,* sutures may be the best alternative, allowing the greatest degree of precision for accurate wound edge approximation. Conversely, some small lacerations that would typically be closed may not actually benefit from primary closure. For example, simple (**<2 cm**) uncomplicated hand and finger lacerations, when treated with antibiotic ointment and gauze dressing, heal as fast and with no notable differences in appearance or function as those closed primarily with sutures.[3] But note that this technique is limited to small, superficial hand lacerations; it cannot be recommended for larger lacerations and in other sites.

With *lacerations subject to high tension* (static and/or dynamic) one can relieve the amount of tension on the wound in order to avoid early dehiscence or gradual widening of the scar. Relief of tension is best achieved by careful undermining, placement of deep dermal sutures, and wound immobilization (when appropriate). After placement of deep, tension-relieving sutures, the superficial epidermal layer may be closed by any of the aforementioned closure methods. Reinforcement with adhesive skin tape is useful when the skin is thin, as in pretibial lacerations.[4-6]

TABLE 41-1 Advantages and Disadvantages of Wound Closure Techniques

Technique	Advantages	Disadvantages
Sutures	Time honored Meticulous closure Greatest tensile strength Lowest dehiscence rate	Requires removal (if using nonabsorbable material) Requires anesthesia Risk of needle stick to physician Greatest tissue reactivity Highest cost Slowest application
Staples	Rapid application Low tissue reactivity Low cost Low risk of needle stick	Less meticulous closure May interfere with some imaging techniques (CT, MRI) Requires removal
Tissue adhesives	Rapid application Patient comfort Resistant to bacterial growth No need for removal Low cost No risk of needle stick Microbial barrier Occlusive dressing	Lower tensile strength than 5-0 or larger sutures Dehiscence over high-tension areas (joints) Not useful on hands Cannot bathe or swim (can shower)
Adhesive tapes	Least reactive Lowest infection rates Rapid application Patient comfort Low cost No risk of needle stick	Frequently fall off Lower tensile strength than sutures or tissue adhesives Highest rate of dehiscence Often requires use of toxic adjuncts Cannot be used in areas with hair Cannot get wet
Hair apposition	Simple Low cost No foreign body placed in wound No risk of needle stick	Can only be used on the scalp Can only approximate simple nongaping lacerations

With patients at risk of **keloid** formation, it makes logical sense to relieve tension and minimize the amount of foreign material introduced into the wound. Skin tapes or tissue adhesives, instead of sutures, can minimize the amount of foreign material and inflammation that may increase the likelihood of excessive scar formation.

SUTURES

Sutures are the strongest of all the closure devices and allow the most accurate approximation of the wound edges, regardless of their shape or configuration. However, sutures are the most time-consuming and operator dependent of all wound closure methods and have the risk of inadvertent needle-stick injury. Using forceps to handle the needle during suturing can reduce this risk. A needle-catcher device is reported to be useful in reducing needle-stick injury during skin suturing.[7-9]

Sutures may be classified as absorbable and nonabsorbable. ***Nonabsorbable sutures*** **retain their tensile strength for at least 60 days.** They are most often used to close the outermost layer of the skin (where they can be removed) or for repair of tendons (where prolonged strength is necessary due to very high tension). In general, nonabsorbable sutures are avoided in deep vascularized tissues where their presence stimulates a foreign body response with fibroblastic proliferation. Nonabsorbable sutures are differentiated by their origin and structure (**Table 41-2**). Due to their strength, handling, and relatively low tissue reactivity, synthetic monofilament sutures (such as nylon or polypropylene) are preferred. Polybutester sutures have the ability to elongate in response to external forces and possess elasticity to return to the original size once the load is removed. This property may be useful in wounds where swelling is anticipated. Less distensible sutures, such as nylon or polypropylene, cannot expand, and instead may lacerate the wound edges as the tissue swells.

Absorbable sutures **lose most of their tensile strength in less than 60 days.** As a result, they are well suited for closure of deep structures such as the dermis and fascia (**Table 41-3**). Poliglecaprone 25 has handling characteristics that are similar to nonabsorbable sutures (such as nylon) and is particularly useful for intracuticular or subcuticular closure. Due to its rapid absorption, poliglecaprone 25 should probably be limited to relatively low-tension wounds. With high-tension wounds, a suture with more sustained tensile strength is preferred. Absorbable sutures that incorporate the antibacterial agent triclosan are also available and may be especially indicated in contaminated wounds.[10,11] Rapidly absorbing sutures can also be used to close the superficial skin layers, especially when avoidance of suture removal is desirable.[12-15]

For most ED use, the choice between absorbable and nonabsorbable material for percutaneous sutures is clinically irrelevant.[12-15] The cosmetic outcomes and complications of traumatic lacerations and surgical incisions closed with absorbable or nonabsorbable sutures have similar short- (infection, dehiscence) and long-term (cosmesis) outcomes.[16] Absorbable sutures, like rapidly absorbing gut, are especially useful for skin closure in children who are not candidates for wound repair with skin tapes or tissue adhesives.

Suture material is categorized by the U.S. Pharmacopeia gauge size. The larger the suture size number, the thinner the suture, so that, for example, a 6-0 suture is thinner than a 5-0 suture. **A general principle is that larger-diameter material produces more damage to the tissues and leaves larger holes in the skin, so generally thinner suture material is used**

TABLE 41-2 Nonabsorbable Suture Characteristics

Suture	Structure	Raw Material	Tensile Strength Retention Profile	Tissue Reactivity	Common ED Uses
Silk	Braided	Organic protein fibroin	Degradation of fiber results in loss of strength over many months	Significant inflammatory reaction	Intraoral mucosal surfaces for comfort
Nylon (Ethilon®, Dermalon®)	Braided and monofilament	Polyamide polymer	Hydrolysis results in 20% loss in strength per year	Minimal	Soft tissue and skin reapproximation
Polypropylene (Prolene®, Surgipro®)	Monofilament	Polypropylene polymer	Indefinite	Least	Soft tissue and skin reapproximation
Polyester (Mersilene®, Ti-Cron®)	Braided and monofilament	Polyethylene terephthalate polymer	Indefinite	Minimal	Tendon repair using undyed (white) color
Polybutester (Novafil®)	Monofilament	Copolymer of butylene terephthalate and polytetramethylene ether glycol	Indefinite	Minimal	Soft tissue approximation

TABLE 41-3 Absorbable Sutures

Suture	Structure	Raw Material	Tensile Strength Retention Profile	Absorption Rate	Tissue Reactivity	Common ED Uses
Surgical gut	Monofilament	Collagen derived from beef serosa or sheep submucosa	7–10 d	Absorbed by proteolytic processes in 70 d	Moderate reactivity	Intraoral wounds
Chromic gut	Monofilament with chromic salt coating	Collagen derived from beef serosa or sheep submucosa	21–28 d	Absorbed by proteolytic processes in 90 d	Moderate reactivity	Subcutaneous approximation and intraoral wounds
Fast-absorbing gut	Monofilament heat treated to facilitate absorption	Collagen derived from beef serosa or sheep submucosa	5–7 d	Absorbed by proteolytic processes in 21–42 d	Moderate reactivity	Facial wounds and skin grafts
Polyglycolic acid (Dexon®)	Braided	Glycolic acid polymer	65% at 14 d and 35% at 21 d	Absorbed by hydrolysis, complete by 60–90 d	Minimal	Subcutaneous approximation and ligation of vessels
Coated polyglactin 910 (Vicryl®)	Braided	Copolymer of lactide and glycolide, coated with polyglactin 370 and calcium stearate	75% at 14 d and 40% at 21 d	Absorbed by hydrolysis, complete by 56–70 d	Minimal	Subcutaneous approximation and ligation of vessels
Coated polyglactin 910 with triclosan (Vicryl PLUS®)	Braided	Copolymer of lactide and glycolide, coated with polyglactin 370 and calcium stearate; incorporates antibacterial agent triclosan	75% at 14 d, 50% at 21 d, and 25% at 28 d	Absorbed by hydrolysis, complete by 56–70 d	Minimal	Subcutaneous approximation and ligation of vessels, especially useful in contaminated wounds
Coated polyglactin 910 rapid absorption (Vicryl Rapide®)	Braided	Copolymer of glycolide and lactide, coated with polyglactin 370 and calcium stearate	50% by 5 d and 0% at 14 d	Absorbed by hydrolysis, complete by 42 d	Minimal to moderate	Skin approximation when absorbable sutures are used
Coated glycolide and lactide (Polysorb®)	Braided	Copolymer of glycolide and lactide, coated with mixture of caprolactone, glycolide copolymer, and calcium stearoyl lactylate	80% at 14 d and 30% at 21 d	Absorbed by hydrolysis, complete by 56–70 d	Minimal	Subcutaneous soft tissue approximation
Polydioxanone (PDS II®)	Monofilament	Polyester polymer	70% at 14 d, 50% at 28 d, and 25% at 42 d	Absorbed by hydrolysis, complete at 180–210 d	Slight	Subcutaneous soft tissue approximation where more prolonged strength is needed
Poliglecaprone 25 (Monocryl®)	Monofilament	Copolymer of glycolide and epsilon-caprolactone	50–70% at 7 d and 20–40% at 14 d	Absorbed by hydrolysis, complete by 91–119 d	Minimal	Subcutaneous soft tissue approximation
Poliglecaprone 25 with triclosan (Monocryl PLUS®)	Monofilament	Copolymer of glycolide and epsilon-caprolactone; incorporates antibacterial agent triclosan	50–70% at 7 d and 20–40% at 14 d	Absorbed by hydrolysis, complete by 91–119 d	Minimal	Subcutaneous soft tissue approximation; especially in contaminated wounds
Glycomer 631 (Biosyn®)	Monofilament	Polyester composed of glycolide, dioxanone, and trimethylene carbonate	75% at 14 d and 40% at 21 d	Absorbed by hydrolysis, complete by 90–110 d	Slight	Subcutaneous soft tissue approximation where extended strength is not needed
Polyglyconate (Maxon®)	Monofilament	Copolymer of glycolic acid and trimethylene carbonate	80% at 7 d, 75% at 14 d, 65% at 21 d, 50% at 28 d, and 25% at 42 d	Absorbed by hydrolysis, complete by 180 d	Slight	Subcutaneous soft tissue approximation where more prolonged strength is needed

whenever possible. Because smaller-diameter material has less strength, the trade-off is that more individual sutures closer together are sometimes needed to close a wound. Where cosmetic appearance is important, as on the face, smaller-diameter material is preferred (**Table 41-4**).

Improper tissue handling further traumatizes the tissues and results in an increased risk of infection and poor scarring.[17] Gentle tissue handling using either skin hooks or the open limb of fine forceps is encouraged (**Figure 41-1**). Magnifying lenses such as surgical loupes can assist in accurate placement of sutures. While there are many types of **surgical loupes** available, a version useful in the ED is a magnifying power of 2.5× with the Keplerian lens system, which will provide a bright, clear image out to a field of view of 10 cm. Hemostasis is best achieved by direct pressure. Topical vasoconstrictors (such as epinephrine) applied to the wound edges and bed or mixed with the local anesthetic injected into the wound may help control bleeding in traumatic lacerations treated in the ED. With bleeding from vessels >2 mm in diameter, careful and selective placement of a ligature tie is often necessary. Electrocautery increases the risk of wound infection and scarring.[17] The technique requires training and policies for its use, to ensure patient and healthcare professional safety.

The best cosmetic outcome is achieved by carefully matching each layer of the wound with its corresponding counterpart on the opposite side, ensuring eversion of the wound edges and minimizing the amount of tension on the wound. As the wound heals and the swelling subsides, the wound will eventually flatten, becoming flush with the surrounding skin surface. Inadvertent inversion of the wound edges may result in an

TABLE 41-4 Recommended Suture Size Based on Laceration Location

Location	Suture Size
Scalp	3-0 or 4-0
Face	6-0
Trunk	4-0
Extremities	4-0
Digits	5-0

unsightly depressed scar. A variety of suture techniques can be used to handle wounds of nearly all shapes, irregularities, and depths (**Table 41-5**).

SIMPLE INTERRUPTED PERCUTANEOUS SUTURES

Individual simple interrupted percutaneous sutures are the most basic and most commonly used approach to close lacerations. Introduce the needle through the outer layer of the skin, and exit at the level of the dermis on one side of the wound. Then, reinsert the needle through the opposite wound edge starting at the level of the dermis and exit superficially (**Figure 41-2**). In order to ensure proper wound edge eversion, the needle should enter and exit the skin at equal distances from the wound and at an angle of 90 degrees. Wound edge eversion is achieved by taking a larger bite through the depth of the wound than through the more superficial layers (**Figure 41-3**).

The entrance and exit of the suture should be close enough to the wound edges that they are not puckered when the knot is tied but far enough away to allow the suture material a firm hold on the tissue. **Sutures are tied using square knots, and, generally, the number of knot ties should correspond to the suture size** (i.e., four ties for a 4-0 suture, five ties for a 5-0 suture, etc.). Additional ties do not increase the strength of a properly tied square knot; they only add to its bulk. The extra ties are to increase knot security and prevent unraveling. Once the knot is completed, it should be moved to one side of the wound so as to not rest directly over the edges. For simple linear lacerations, a useful approach is to place the first suture in the middle of the wound, creating

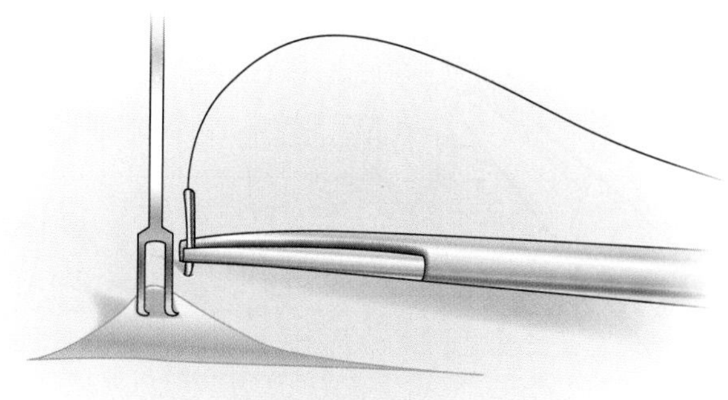

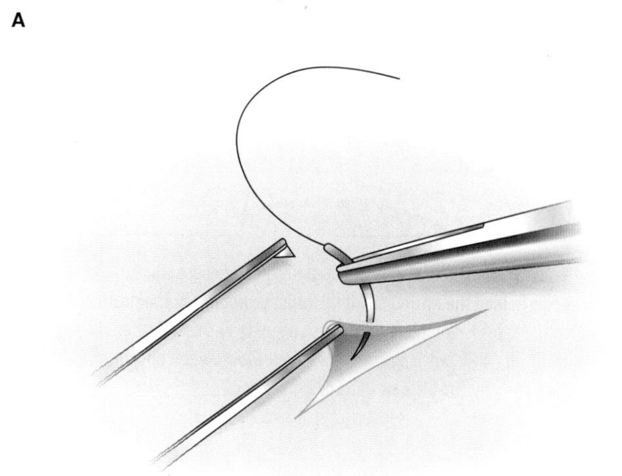

FIGURE 41-1. The skin hook (A) or one limb of a tissue forceps with teeth (B) is used to elevate the wound edge to facilitate placement of the percutaneous suture.

TABLE 41-5 Suture Techniques Based on Wound Type

Suture Type	Advantages	Disadvantages	Frequent Uses
Interrupted percutaneous	Excellent approximation for irregular and complex lacerations	Time-consuming May strangulate tissues	Low-tension wounds May be used with deep sutures for high-tension wounds
Continuous percutaneous	Rapid closure Accommodates edema	Less meticulous closure than interrupted sutures Wound may dehisce if a single knot unravels and no deep sutures were placed	Percutaneous closure in conjunction with deep sutures
Deep dermal	Reduces tension on wound surface Allows early removal of percutaneous sutures, avoiding hatch marking May reduce scar width	May increase infection in contaminated wounds	High-tension wounds Closure of dead space
Continuous subcuticular	Rapid Reduces tension on wound surface Reduces or eliminates need for percutaneous sutures May reduce scar width	Technically difficult Less accurate approximation than interrupted sutures Wound may dehisce if a single knot unravels	Cosmetically visible areas to reduce scarring
Vertical mattress	Excellent wound edge eversion Combines advantages of deep and superficial sutures	May cause tissue strangulation	Thin or lax skin with little dermal or fascial tissue High-tension areas (e.g., extremities)
Horizontal mattress	More rapid than simple interrupted sutures Avoids punctures close to wound edges that may impair perfusion Accommodates wound swelling	Requires skill to achieve wound edge eversion	Volar wounds of the hands Initial approximation of high-tension wounds
Half-buried horizontal mattress	Less compromising to flap tip perfusion and stellate lacerations	Technically difficult	Corner stitches and flaps Stellate lacerations

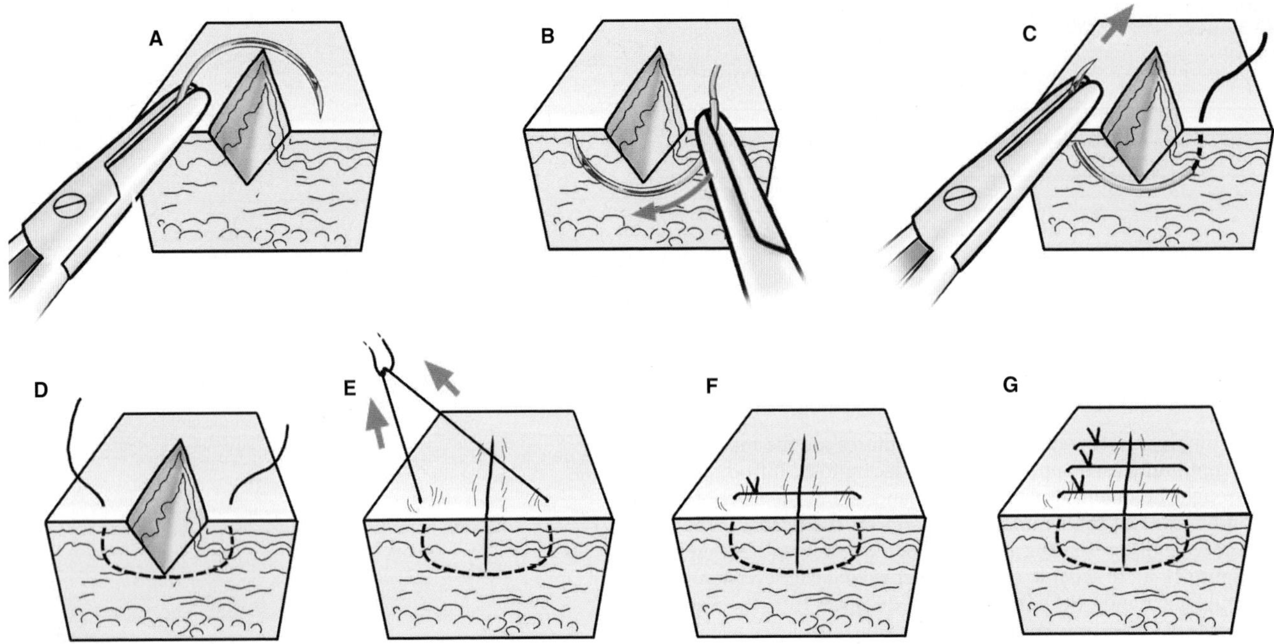

FIGURE 41-2. Placement of simple interrupted percutaneous sutures. **A.** Insert the needle at a 90-degree angle to the skin. **B.** Drive the needle through the tissue until the tip exits the skin. **C.** Grasp the needle behind the tip and pull it through the wound. **D.** The suture should enter and exit the skin equidistant from the wound edges. **E.** Pull the suture to oppose the wound edges and cinch down the knot. **F.** Complete the knot to one side of the laceration. **G.** Apply additional sutures equidistant from each other until the wound is closed. [Reproduced with permission from Reichman EF, Simon RR (eds): *Emergency Medicine Procedures*. Copyright © 2004 by Eric F. Reichman, PhD, MD, and Robert R. Simon, MD. All rights reserved. Printed in the United States of America, Figure 78-6. By The McGraw-Hill Companies, Inc.]

two smaller segments that are sequentially bisected into smaller segments until adequate coaptation of the edges is achieved.

CONTINUOUS (RUNNING) PERCUTANEOUS SUTURES

The major advantage of this method is its rapidity, as the entire wound is closed before any of the suture material is cut. This technique is most appropriate for long linear lacerations. Because it does not allow for precise wound edge apposition, it should be avoided in irregularly shaped lacerations. With this method, the first suture is placed at one end of the laceration similarly to an interrupted percutaneous suture. After the knot is tied, the suture material is not cut, and the needle is reintroduced into the skin on the opposite side, pulling the suture across the wound at a 65-degree angle (**Figure 41-4**). The needle then crosses the depth of the wound in a circular motion perpendicular to the wound, exiting on the opposite side approximately 3 to 5 mm from the wound edge. This process is repeated as needed until the entire wound is approximated and a second knot is tied.

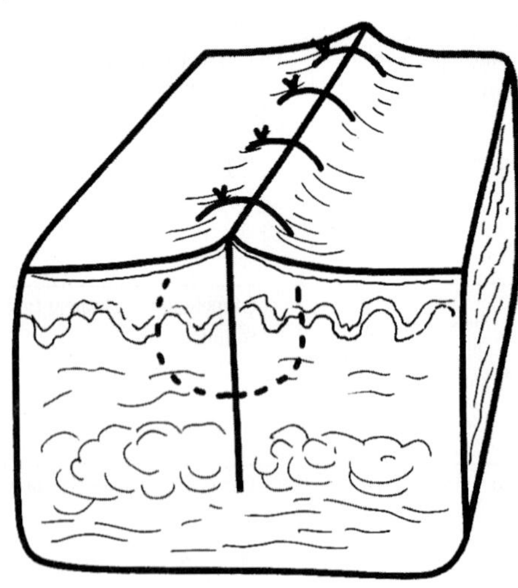

FIGURE 41-3. Wound edge eversion. The distance of the suture from the wound edge is greater at the depth of the wound than at the surface, promoting wound edge eversion when tightened. [Reproduced with permission from Reichman EF, Simon RR (eds): *Emergency Medicine Procedures*. Copyright © 2004 by Eric F. Reichman, PhD, MD, and Robert R. Simon, MD. All rights reserved. Printed in the United States of America, Figure 41-77-8. By The McGraw-Hill Companies, Inc.]

BURIED DERMAL SUTURES

Deep dermal sutures are used to reduce tension on the wound and to close dead spaces. Placement of buried dermal sutures requires judgment because the benefits for nongaping small wounds are unproven and their presence may increase the risk of infection in contaminated wounds.[18,19] Sutures through adipose tissue do not hold tension, are unnecessary in clean surgical cases, and only promote infection in contaminated wounds.[19,20]

With buried dermal sutures, the needle is first inserted at the level of the mid dermis on one side of the wound and then exits more superficially below the dermal–epidermal junction (**Figure 41-5**). The needle is then introduced below the dermal–epidermal junction on the opposite wound side and exits at the level of the mid dermis. Thus the knot becomes buried in the depth of the tissue when tying of the suture is completed. The first suture is placed at the center of the laceration, followed by additional sutures that sequentially bisect the wound. The number of buried sutures should be minimized.

CONTINUOUS SUBCUTICULAR SUTURES

The continuous subcuticular suture is one of the more complex methods of wound closure. The major advantage of this method is that it results in fairly good wound approximation, often without requiring any percutaneous sutures. For this technique, after anchoring the absorbable suture at one end of the wound, sequential, horizontally oriented "bites" are taken immediately below the dermal–epidermal junction, working toward the other end until the wound is adequately

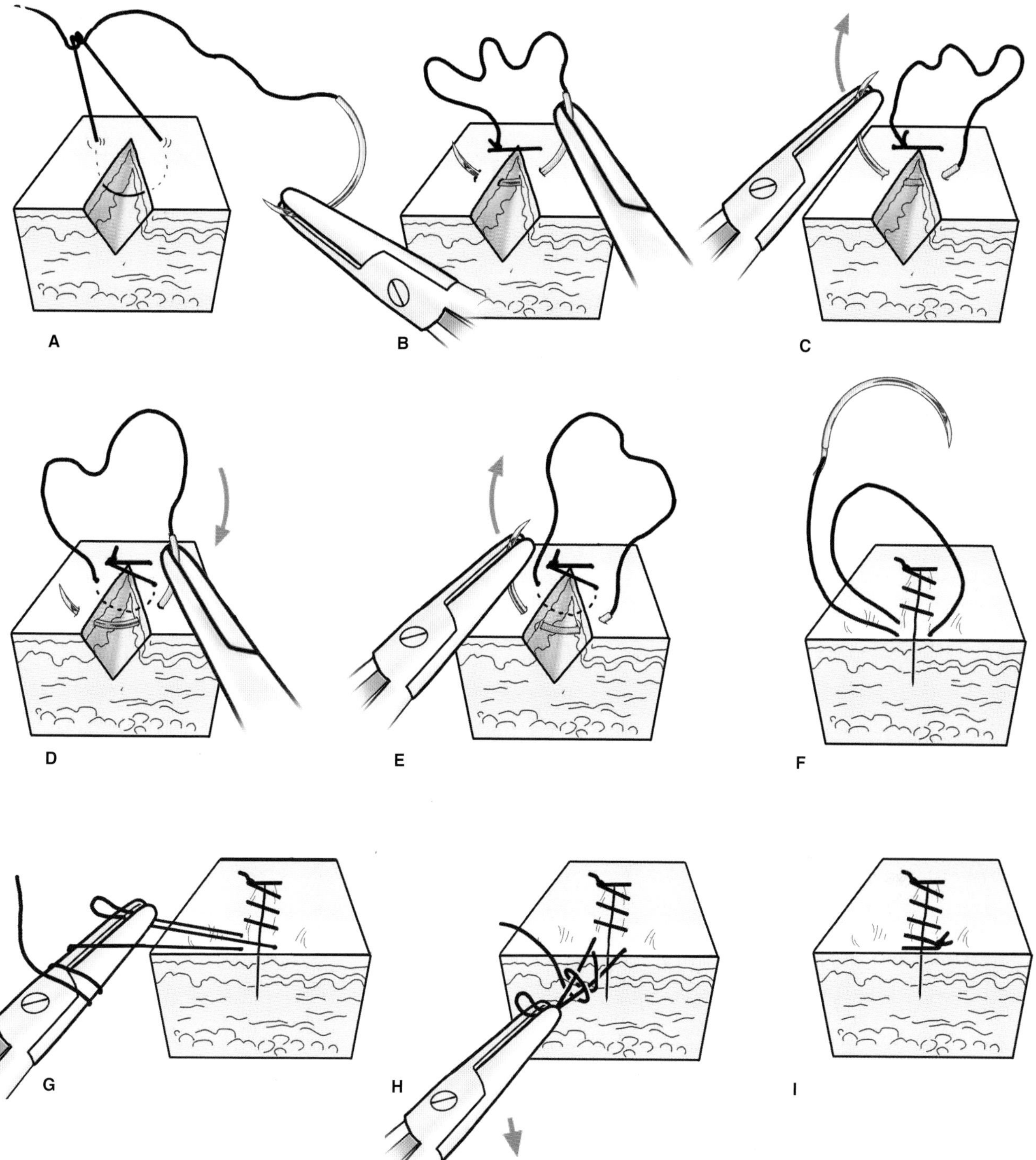

FIGURE 41-4. Continuous or running percutaneous suture. **A.** Place the initial stitch as a simple interrupted stitch, but do not cut the suture after the knot is securely tied. **B** and **C.** Place a second stitch 3 to 5 mm from the first stitch as if placing another simple interrupted stitch. **D** and **E.** Place a third stitch 3 to 5 mm from the second stitch and continue to place additional stitches until the end of the laceration is reached. **F.** Do not pull the last throw taut against the skin; the loop will act as the tail end of the suture for knot tying. **G.** Loop the needle end of the suture twice around the tip of the needle driver and grasp the last throw with the tips of the needle driver. **H.** Pull the last throw through the loops until the knot is against the skin. **I.** Perform three to five more instrument ties to secure the knot, and then cut off the excess suture. [Reproduced with permission from Reichman EF, Simon RR (eds): *Emergency Medicine Procedures*. Copyright © 2004 by Eric F. Reichman, PhD, MD, and Robert R. Simon, MD. All rights reserved. Printed in the United States of America, Figure 78-9. By The McGraw-Hill Companies, Inc.]

approximated (**Figure 41-6**). The second knot is tied with the tails cut short so as to remain buried.

VERTICAL MATTRESS SUTURES

Vertical mattress sutures combine some of the advantages of deep and percutaneous sutures. They also result in excellent wound edge eversion. Vertical mattress sutures are particularly useful in very thin or lax skin and in areas where the deep subcutaneous tissues are too fragile to be used for anchoring tension-reducing sutures (e.g., over the shin). After taking a large, deep bite from both sides of the wound ("far to far"), the direction of the needle is reversed, and a smaller superficial bite is taken from both sides ("near to near") of the laceration (**Figure 41-7**). Vertical mattress sutures may result in excessive tension on the more superficial

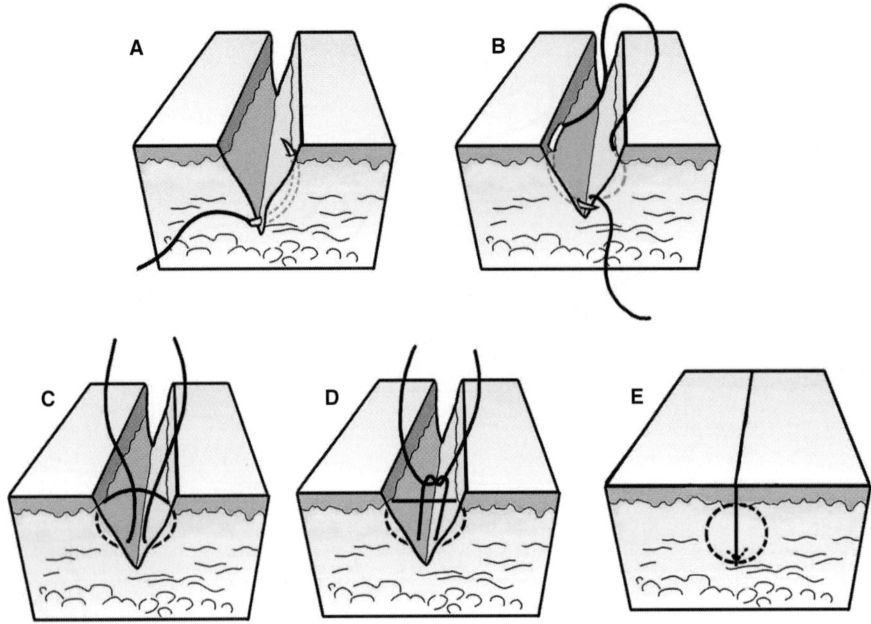

FIGURE 41-5. Buried dermal suture. **A.** Insert the needle into one side of the base of the wound, and drive the needle from deep to superficial and exiting at the dermal–epidermal junction. **B.** Insert the needle through the dermal–epidermal junction on the opposite side of the wound and drive it through the base of the wound. The suture should exit the base of the wound across from and level with the entrance site of the first throw. **C.** Pull both free ends of the suture up and out through the laceration. **D.** Tie a knot in the suture. **E.** Pull both free ends of the suture to lower the knot to the base of the wound and oppose the tissue. Tie two additional knots to secure the suture. Cut off any excess suture. [Reproduced with permission from Reichman EF, Simon RR (eds): *Emergency Medicine Procedures*. Copyright © 2004 by Eric F. Reichman, PhD, MD, and Robert R. Simon, MD. All rights reserved. Printed in the United States of America, Figure 78-19. By The McGraw-Hill Companies, Inc.]

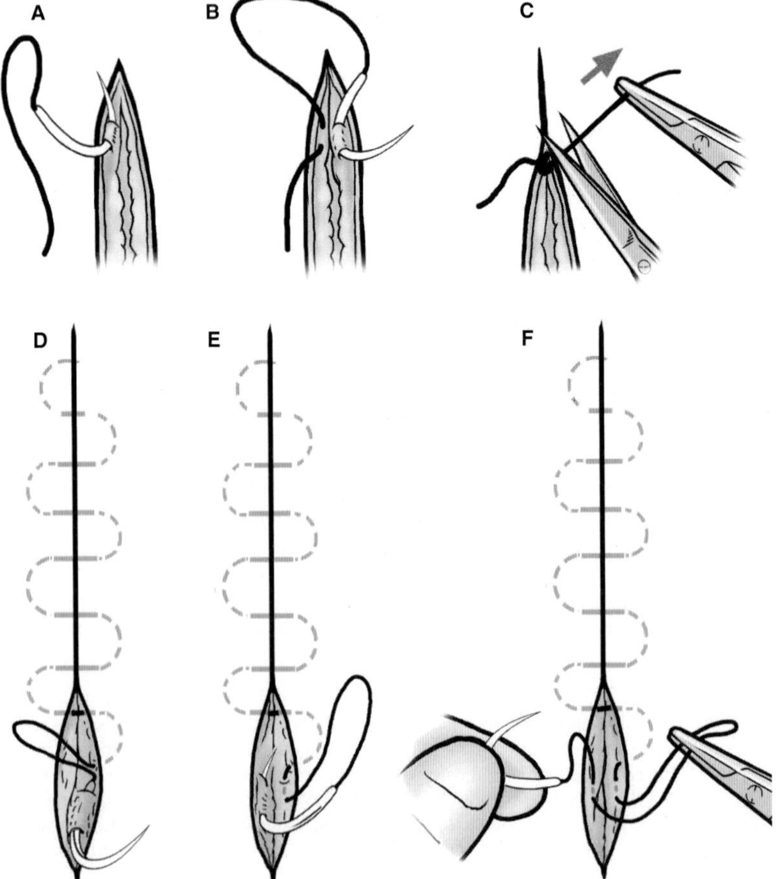

FIGURE 41-6. Continuous subcuticular sutures. **A, B,** and **C.** Place the first stitch into the dermis, just inside the laceration edge, as a buried knot. **D.** Place the continuous suture until the opposite end of the laceration is reached. **E.** The final throw should be left lax with a trailing loop of suture. **F.** The loop should be used as the "tail end" to perform an instrument tie. Tie three or four knots in the suture. Lift the free ends of the suture and cut them just above the knot. Apply adhesive tape across the laceration to help maintain the apposition of the wound. [Reproduced with permission from Reichman EF, Simon RR (eds): *Emergency Medicine Procedures*. Copyright © 2004 by Eric F. Reichman, PhD, MD, and Robert R. Simon, MD. All rights reserved. Printed in the United States of America, Figure 78-18. By The McGraw-Hill Companies, Inc.]

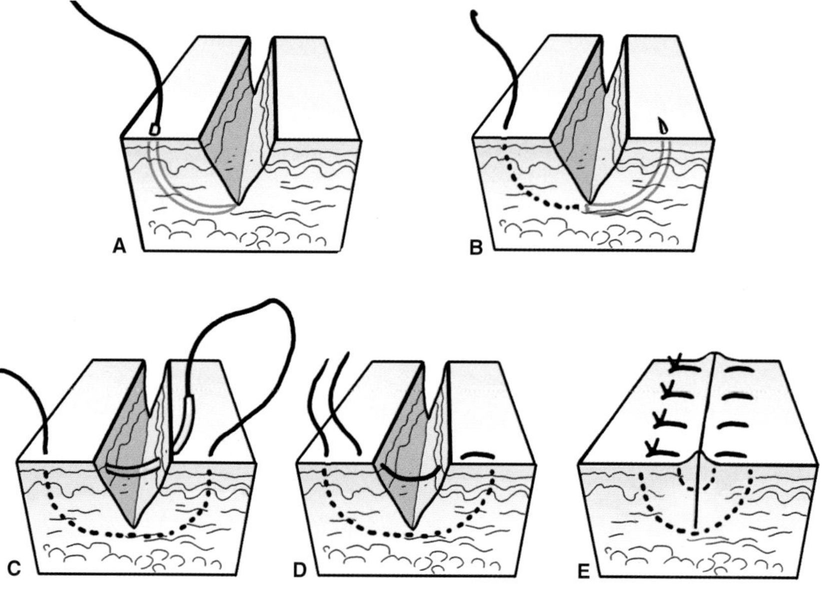

FIGURE 41-7. Vertical mattress suture. **A.** The needle should enter and exit the skin 1.0 to 1.5 cm from the wound edge. **B.** The needle should traverse the base of the wound and grasp a large amount of tissue. **C** and **D.** Reverse the needle. The second throw should enter and exit the skin approximately 2 to 3 mm from the wound edge. The first and second throws must be directly over each other and parallel. **E.** Tie the suture to approximate the wound edges. The first throw will close the wound base and relieve the tension at the skin surface. The second throw approximates and everts the skin edges. [Reproduced with permission from Reichman EF, Simon RR (eds): *Emergency Medicine Procedures*. Copyright © 2004 by Eric F. Reichman, PhD, MD, and Robert R. Simon, MD. All rights reserved. Printed in the United States of America, Figure 78-11. By The McGraw-Hill Companies, Inc.]

skin edges, which reduces blood supply to the skin and may result in necrosis of the wound margins.

A modification of the standard vertical mattress suture is the shorthand version. In this approach, the first throw is close to the wound edges ("near to near"); the suture is then grasped and pulled away from the wound, elevating the wound edges while a second throw is performed farther away from the wound ("far to far") (**Figure 41-8**).[21] This shorthand version can be performed in less time with the same outcome; however, blind placement of the larger bite may injure underlying structures.

HORIZONTAL MATTRESS SUTURES

The horizontal mattress is a good suture technique to close wounds with poor circulation to the wound edges because no percutaneous punctures

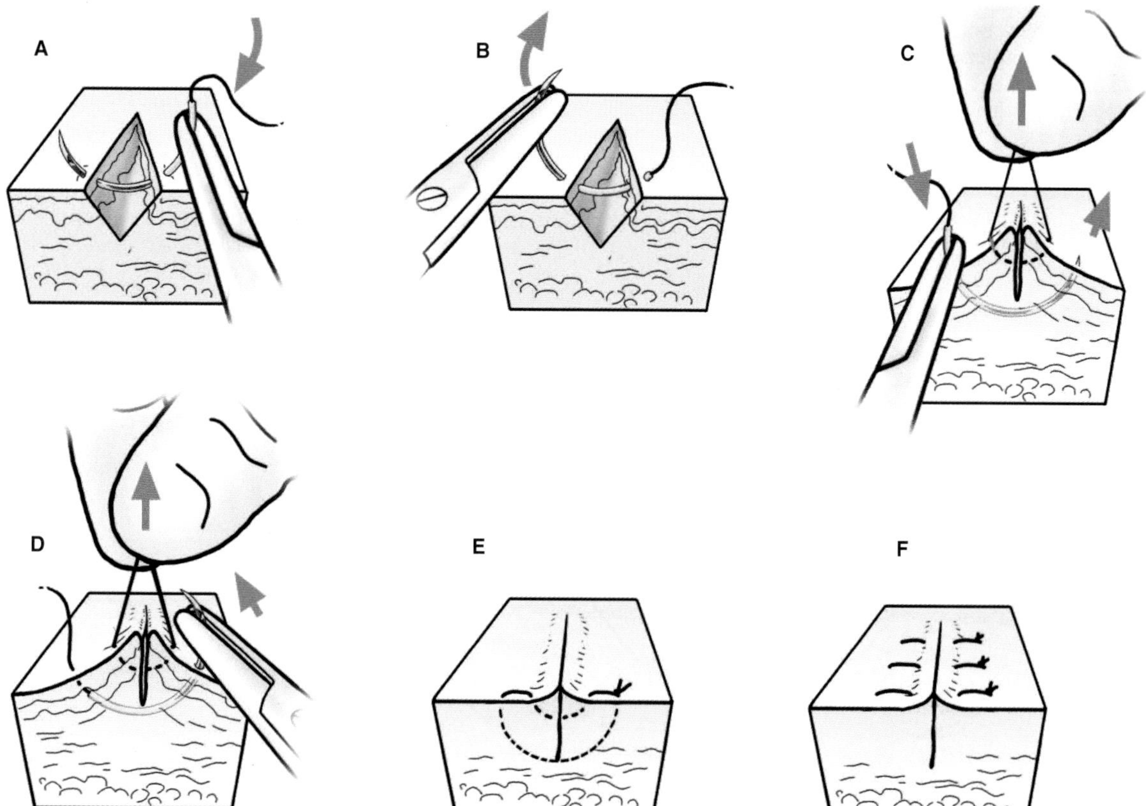

FIGURE 41-8. The "shorthand" vertical mattress suture. **A** and **B.** Place the first throw close to the lacerated wound edge to approximate the skin edges. **C.** Grasp and pull the suture to elevate the wound edges. This allows the needle to more easily take a large bite of tissue on the second throw. **D.** Place the second throw 1.0 to 1.5 cm from the wound edge. Release the suture. **E.** Tie the suture to approximate the wound edges and evert the skin surface. **F.** The final product looks exactly the same as the traditional vertical mattress suture. [Reproduced with permission from Reichman EF, Simon RR (eds): *Emergency Medicine Procedures*. Copyright © 2004 by Eric F. Reichman, PhD, MD, and Robert R. Simon, MD. All rights reserved. Printed in the United States of America, Figure 78-12. By The McGraw-Hill Companies, Inc.]

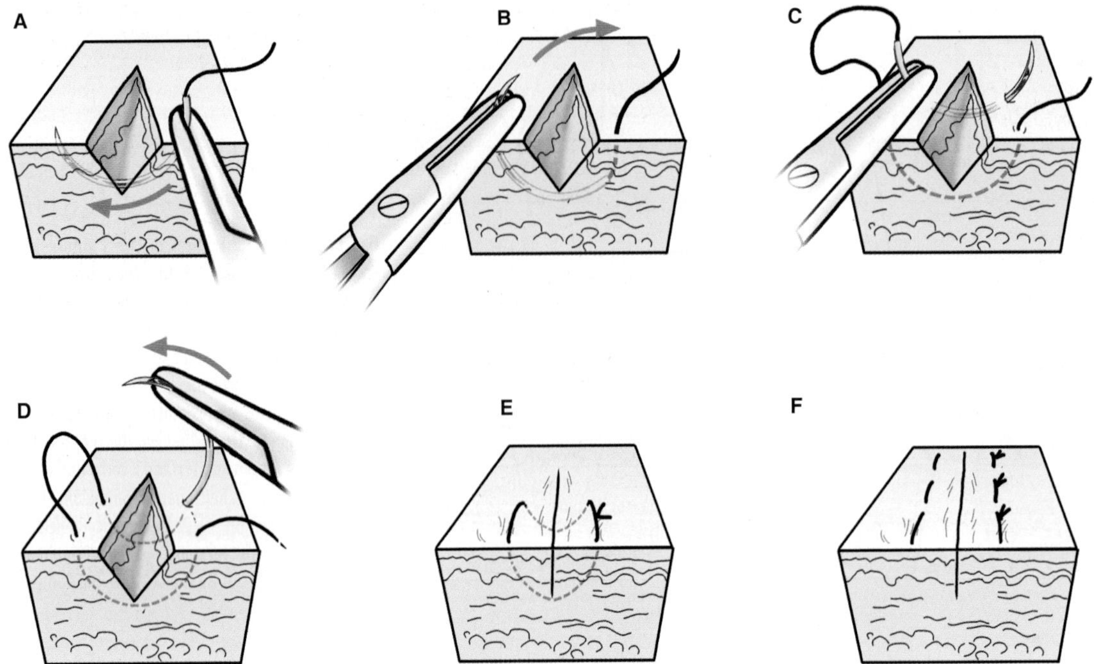

FIGURE 41-9. Horizontal mattress suture. **A.** The needle should enter and exit the skin 0.5 to 1.0 cm from the wound edge. **B.** The needle should traverse the base of the wound. **C.** Reverse the needle and make a second throw 0.5 cm from the first. **D.** The needle must enter and exit the skin and the wound edges so that the first and second throws are parallel to each other. **E.** Pull the free ends of the suture taut to oppose and evert the wound edges. **F.** The final result. [Reproduced with permission from Reichman EF, Simon RR (eds): *Emergency Medicine Procedures*. Copyright © 2004 by Eric F. Reichman, PhD, MD, and Robert R. Simon, MD. All rights reserved. Printed in the United States of America, Figure 78-14. By The McGraw-Hill Companies, Inc.]

that could further disrupt skin perfusion are placed close to the wound edges. This suture also reduces tension at the wound edges and reduces the potential for subsequent local necrosis. Horizontal mattress sutures can close a wound with fewer individual stitches because each stitch encases more tissue than other techniques (**Figure 41-9**). This suture is useful on the volar surfaces of the hands and fingers, because these delicate skin areas may swell but the skin edges are not easily cut due to the placement of the skin punctures far from the wound. The main disadvantage of the horizontal mattress stitch is the skill required to place the suture to achieve wound eversion.

HORIZONTAL HALF-BURIED MATTRESS SUTURES

Horizontal half-buried mattress sutures are particularly well suited for closing the tip of skin flaps and stellate lacerations because they minimize strangulation of the blood supply to the tip. **The key to this stitch is that the needle and suture pass through the dermis of the tip and not the epidermis.** The needle is introduced percutaneously through one side of the wound, then horizontally through the tip at the level of the dermis. The suture is completed by exiting the skin through the other side and tying the knot (**Figure 41-10**).

STAPLES

The major advantages of staples are their speed and relative ease of use.[22-26] They are also cost-effective, especially when devices containing fewer staples are used in the ED, where most lacerations are relatively short. However, of all closure techniques, staples allow the least precision in wound approximation. As a result, **their use should be limited to linear, nonfacial lacerations**. Staples are particularly useful for scalp lacerations because the hair does not require clipping and staples are easier to locate than sutures for removal.[22-25] However, deep sutures may be required to

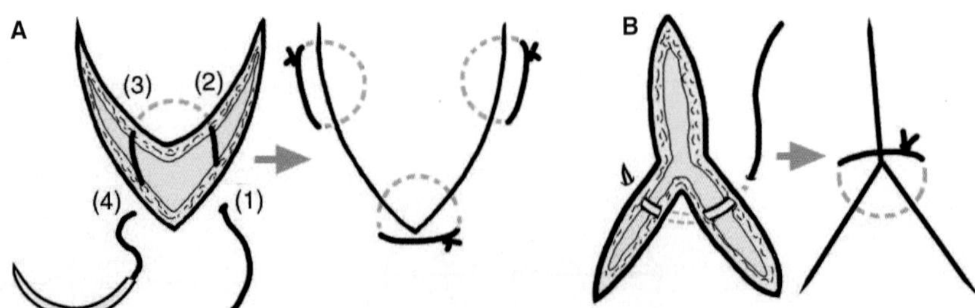

FIGURE 41-10. Half-buried horizontal mattress suture. **A.** To close a flap tip, place the first stitch percutaneously through the skin adjacent to the tip of the flap. Advance the needle through the dermal layer of the flap, the dermal layer of the skin adjacent to the tip of the flap, and out the skin adjacent to the tip of the flap opposite to where the stitch began. The needle must traverse the dermis of the flap and adjacent tissue at the same level of the dermis to properly approximate the wound edges. Gently pull on the free ends of the suture to approximate the flap against the adjacent skin edges. Tie and secure the suture in the usual manner. **B.** To close a stellate laceration, insert the needle through the skin of the largest flap. Advance the needle so that its tip exits the dermis. Continue to advance the needle through the dermis of each flap. The half-buried horizontal mattress stitch should encompass the tips of all the flaps. [Reproduced with permission from Reichman EF, Simon RR (eds): *Emergency Medicine Procedures*. Copyright © 2004 by Eric F. Reichman, PhD, MD, and Robert R. Simon, MD. All rights reserved. Printed in the United States of America, Figure 78-15. By The McGraw-Hill Companies, Inc.]

close lacerations of the galea aponeurotica, whereas percutaneous sutures are always desirable when hemostasis is difficult. In appropriate patients, staples have infection rates and cosmetic outcomes similar to sutures. Staple removal is more painful than removal of sutures.[27]

Although a variety of stapling devices are commercially available, there are few practical differences between them from the standpoint of the emergency practitioner. The key principle is to approximate the wound edges and align the centerline indicator of the head of the stapler so that the legs of the staple will straddle the wound an equal distance on each side (**Figure 41-11**). Touch the stapler lightly to the skin so that the staple comes out and pinches the wound edges together with eversion. **Pressing firmly downward can cause depression of the wound edges.** After the staple is set, pull the stapler slightly backward to disengage. New stapling devices that allow placement of deep staples are available, but they have not been studied in the ED.

ADHESIVE TAPES

Adhesive tapes are the least reactive and most cost-effective of all wound closure devices.[28] Their application is simple, painless, and rapid, and they also do not require formal removal. However, adhesive tapes tend to slough off when exposed to any tension or moisture. As a result, their use is limited to very low-tension simple wounds or for closure of fragile skin subject to low tension, like superficial skin tears. They are also of little use in noncompliant patients because they are so easy to remove.

In order to increase their adhesiveness, skin tapes should be used in conjunction with an adhesive adjunct, such as tincture of benzoin or Mastisol®, that is gently painted on either side of the wound edges and allowed to dry until tacky. Because these adhesive adjuncts are toxic to wounds, avoid their introduction into the wound itself.

The tapes should be placed perpendicular to the wound edges approximately 2 to 3 mm apart. With long lacerations, the first strip of tape should be placed across the center of the wound followed by additional strips on either side of the wound center (**Figure 41-12**). To reduce the possibility of skin blistering or premature dislodgement, additional strips should be placed over the ends of the other strips, parallel to the laceration.

Simple skin tapes may also be used to reinforce lacerations after suture or staple removal. The cosmetic results and dehiscence rates after closure of small (<4 cm) and superficial facial lacerations with tapes are similar to those with cyanoacrylate tissue adhesives.[29] A version of skin tape comprised of two independent parts, each with an adhesive underside and multiple interlocking filaments attached to pulling ends, is useful for simple wound closure (Steri-Strip™ S Surgical Skin Closure; 3M, St. Paul, MN; **Figure 41-13**).[30,31]

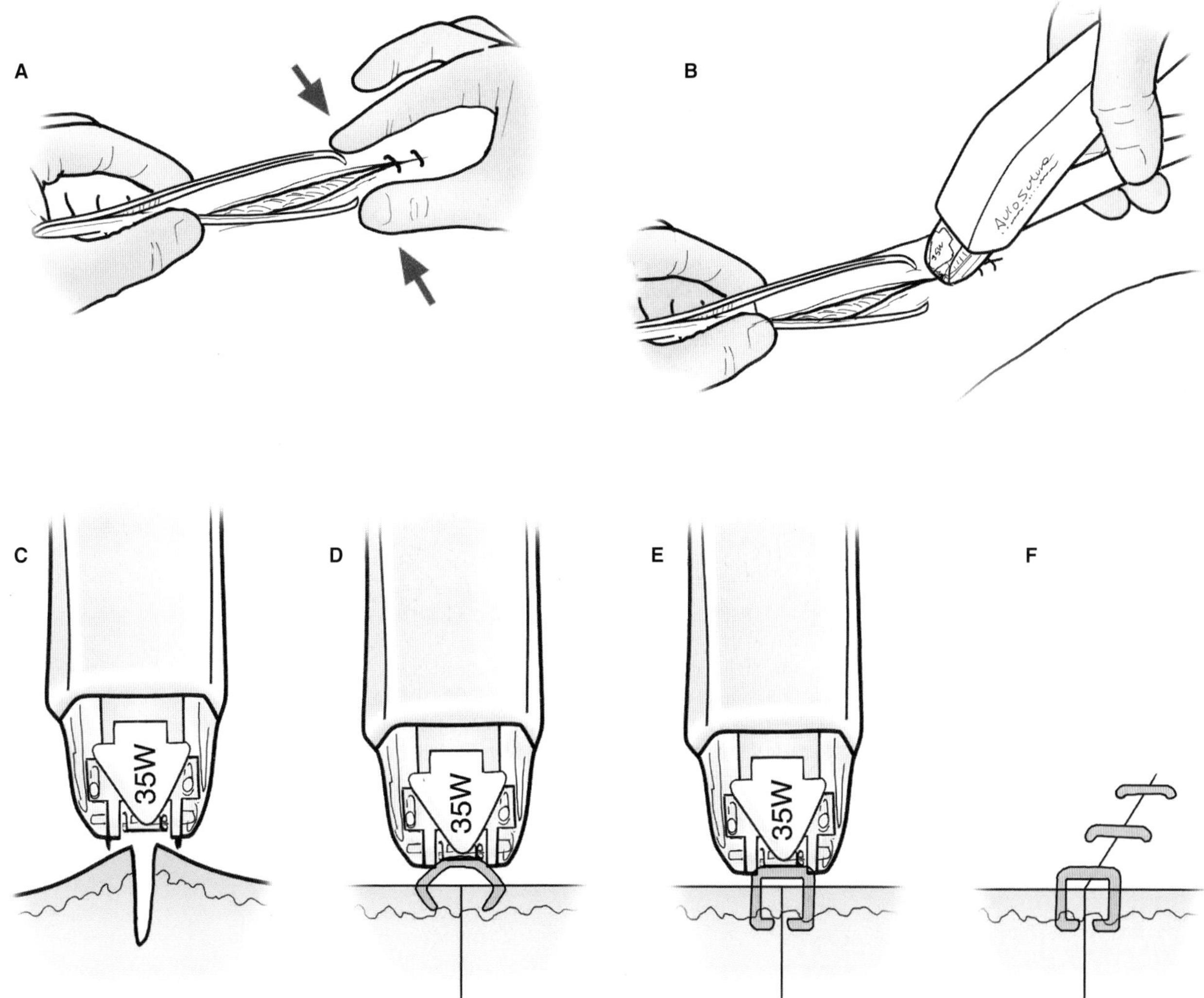

FIGURE 41-11. Laceration repair with staple closure. **A.** The wound edges are opposed and everted. **B.** The stapler is applied over the laceration. **C.** The stapler is applied over the everted wound edges. **D.** The plunger advances the staple into the wound margins. **E.** The anvil bends the staple into shape. **F.** The final result. [Reproduced with permission from Reichman EF, Simon RR (eds): *Emergency Medicine Procedures*. Copyright © 2004 by Eric F. Reichman, PhD, MD, and Robert R. Simon, MD. All rights reserved. Printed in the United States of America, Figure 78-26. By The McGraw-Hill Companies, Inc.]

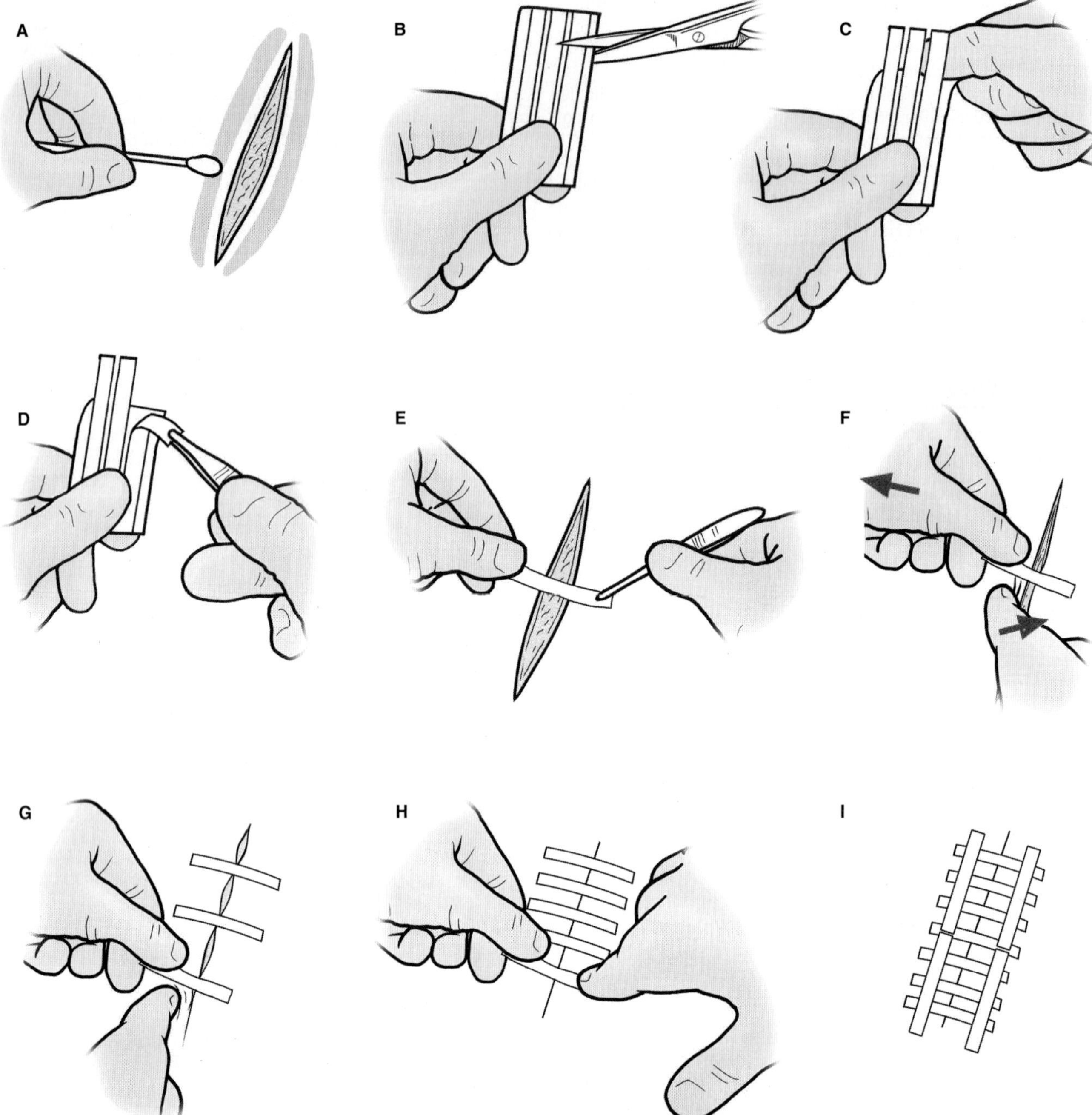

FIGURE 41-12. Laceration repair with adhesive tapes. **A.** After the initial cleansing of the skin, clean the skin surface with acetone or alcohol to remove any surface oils. Allow the skin to dry. Apply benzoin solution to the skin on both sides of the wound with a cotton applicator. **B.** Cut the skin closure tapes to the proper length. **C.** Gently tear the end-tab off the back of the card to prevent the strips from deforming. **D.** Remove a strip from the card. **E.** Firmly secure the tape to one side of the wound. **F.** Use the nondominant hand to oppose the wound edges as the tape is brought over and secured to the skin on the opposite wound edge. **G** and **H.** Place additional tapes at 2- to 3-mm intervals until the wound edges are opposed. **I.** Place pieces of tape across the tape edges to prevent premature removal and skin blistering from the tape ends. [Reproduced with permission from Reichman EF, Simon RR (eds): *Emergency Medicine Procedures*. Copyright © 2004 by Eric F. Reichman, PhD, MD, and Robert R. Simon, MD. All rights reserved. Printed in the United States of America, Figure 78-23. By The McGraw-Hill Companies, Inc.]

CYANOACRYLATE TISSUE ADHESIVES

The cyanoacrylate tissue adhesives are liquid monomers that polymerize into a stable bond when they come into contact with moisture.[32] The adhesive is applied topically to the epidermis across the apposed wound edges, forming a strong bridge that holds the wound closed. The adhesive is sloughed off in 5 to 10 days as the skin renews itself. The tissue adhesives offer many advantages over other wound closure methods. They may be applied rapidly and painlessly to any easily approximated laceration. Because they slough off spontaneously, they do not require removal. The cyanoacrylates form an occlusive dressing that serves as a barrier to microbial penetration. They have antibacterial effects in vitro and reduce infection rates in experimental contaminated wound models in animals.[33]

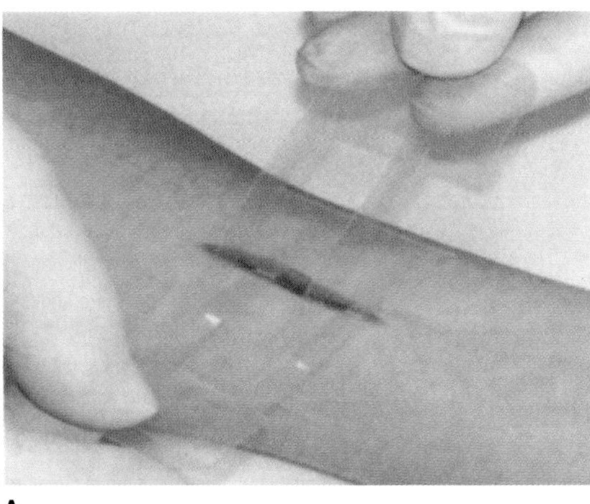

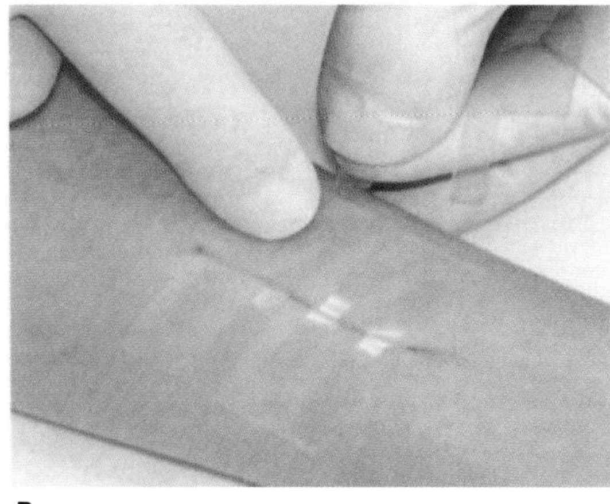

FIGURE 41-13. Application of Steri-Strip™ S Surgical Skin Closure (3M, St. Paul, MN). **A.** The two adhesive pads are applied to the two sides of the wound approximately 1 to 2 mm from the wound edges. **B.** The skin edges are drawn together by pulling on the clear pulling tabs across the wound at a 45-degree angle in opposite directions approximating and aligning the wound edges.

The cyanoacrylate tissue adhesives are similar in strength to 4-0 poliglecaprone subcuticular sutures, but weaker than staples.[34] Tissue adhesives should not be used alone for high-tension wounds nor should they be used for wounds subjected to varying dynamic tension, like over a moving joint. However, they can be used in conjunction with deep dermal sutures and/or immobilization aimed at reducing wound tension. A variety of octyl- and butyl-based cyanoacrylate adhesives are now commercially available. The tensile strength and surface characteristics of octyl- and butyl-cyanoacrylate differ (**Table 41-6**).[35] Octyl-cyanoacrylate is generally stronger and more flexible than butyl-cyanoacrylate, allowing its use on irregular surfaces and long lacerations. The mechanical characteristics of the adhesive are also determined by a number of additives such as chemical initiators and plasticizers.

Wound closure with the tissue adhesives is faster than with other wound closure methods, is cost-effective compared with sutures, and has comparable rates of infection and ultimate cosmetic appearance.[36-41] Patient-reported pain scores and physician-reported procedure time are lower with tissue adhesives.[42,43] However, there is a small increase, about 4%, in wound dehiscence using tissue adhesives, emphasizing the need to limit the use of adhesives to low-tension wounds.

TABLE 41-6 Comparison of Butyl- and Octyl-Cyanoacrylate

	Octyl-Cyanoacrylate	Butyl-Cyanoacrylate
Number of carbons in side chain	8	4
Bursting strength	High	Moderate
Plasticizers that enhance flexibility	Present	Absent
Water resistance	Moderate	Minimal
Need for refrigeration	No	Yes
Clinical experience	Short and long incisions and lacerations	Limited to incisions and lacerations up to 8 cm
Viscosity	High	Low
Cost	Moderate	Slightly less than octyl-cyanoacrylate
Polymerization time	30–45 s	5–10 s
Working time once applicator opened	2–3 min	Unlimited

Few studies have directly compared the various cyanoacrylate tissue adhesives against each other. For closure of short, simple facial lacerations in children, comparable results are seen with either type of cyanoacrylate.[44] For closure of pediatric operative wounds, octyl-cyanoacrylate had a lower wound dehiscence rate.[45]

To ensure optimal results, tissue adhesives should only be used when laceration edges are easily approximated with the practitioner's hands, forceps, or tape. An assistant can maintain constant and meticulous wound edge apposition while the adhesive is applied. With octyl-cyanoacrylate, the adhesive is carefully expressed through the tip of the applicator and gently brushed over the wound surface parallel to the wound edges in a continuous, steady motion (**Figure 41-14A**). **The adhesive should cover the entire wound and extend 5 to 10 mm on either side of the wound edges.** After allowing the first layer of the adhesive to polymerize for 30 to 45 seconds, apply a second layer of adhesive. With butyl-cyanoacrylate, the adhesive is applied from the tip of the applicator in discrete drops along the wound edges, similar to "spot welds" (**Figure 41-14B**), or as a thin single layer.

With long or complex lacerations, adhesive tape can be used to approximate the wound edges, making closure with an adhesive easier (**Figure 41-15**). Application of a tissue adhesive *on top of adhesive tape* also results in greater wound-bursting strength than either device alone.[46] A combination of a mesh tape and tissue adhesive has recently become available and may be especially useful on very long lacerations.[47] Care in application will reduce some of the common problems associated with tissue adhesives (**Table 41-7**).

HAIR APPOSITION

Simple scalp wounds, without contamination or active bleeding, may be closed via the hair apposition technique.[48,49] This technique is an efficient alternative to more traditional methods of closure, with potentially fewer complications, less pain to the patient, and less overall cost.[50-52] Contraindications to hair apposition closure include large lacerations (e.g., >10 cm), grossly contaminated wounds, uncontrolled bleeding, wounds that gape open and cannot be closed without significant tension, and hair strands adjacent to the wound that are less than 3 cm in length.

After wound irrigation and control of bleeding, select and twist together three to seven stands of hair at least 3 cm in length that lie close to the edge on one side of the wound. Repeat this process directly opposite on the other side of the wound. Then twist these two hair bundles in a full 360-degree revolution and secure the intertwined hair bundles by applying a few drops of tissue adhesive. Repeat this process

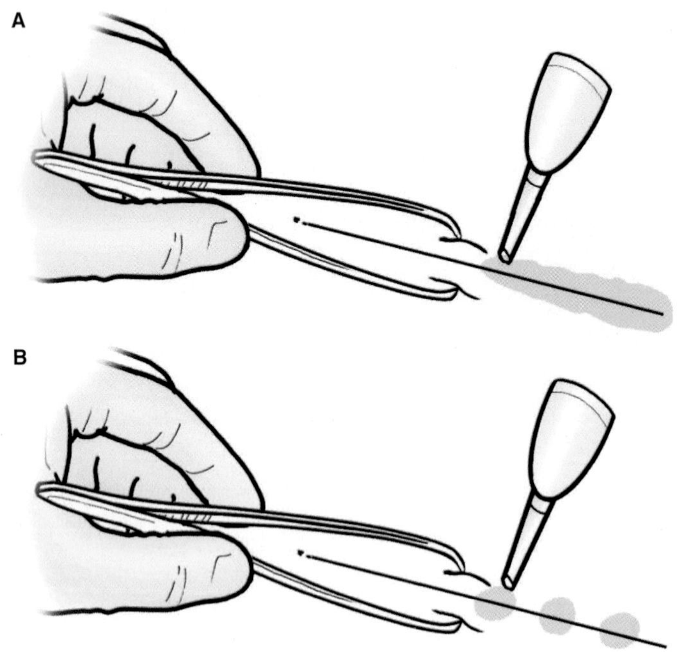

FIGURE 41-14. Laceration repair with tissue adhesives. **A.** Apply the adhesive in two or three layers along the wound edge. **B.** The adhesive may also be applied in spots over the laceration. [Reproduced with modification and permission from Reichman EF, Simon RR (eds): *Emergency Medicine Procedures*. Copyright © 2004 by Eric F. Reichman, PhD, MD, and Robert R. Simon, MD. All rights reserved. Printed in the United States of America, Figure 78-22 Parts C & D. By The McGraw-Hill Companies, Inc.]

TABLE 41-7 Avoiding Potential Pitfalls of Tissue Adhesives

Problem	Ways to Avoid the Problem
Runoff	Position patient with wound parallel to floor. Use high-viscosity adhesive. Apply small, controlled amount of adhesive.
Spillage into eyes	Cover eyes with moist gauze barrier. Position patient so adhesive will not run into the eye. For eyebrow and forehead lacerations, place the patient in the Trendelenburg position. For lacerations on the cheek and lower face, place the patient in the reverse Trendelenburg position. Apply petrolatum-based ointment on the eyelashes before applying adhesive.
Wound dehiscence	Avoid adhesive use for high-tension wounds. Reduce exposure to friction or moisture. Use deep sutures or immobilization for high-tension wounds. Do not introduce adhesive into wound.
Wound infection	Use adhesives only for properly selected wounds. Use proper wound preparation, including irrigation, exploration, and, when necessary, debridement. Use proper application technique.
Getting stuck to the wound	Practice expressing small amounts of adhesive and controlling runoff. Alternate the hand used to oppose wound edges prior to complete polymerization of the adhesive.

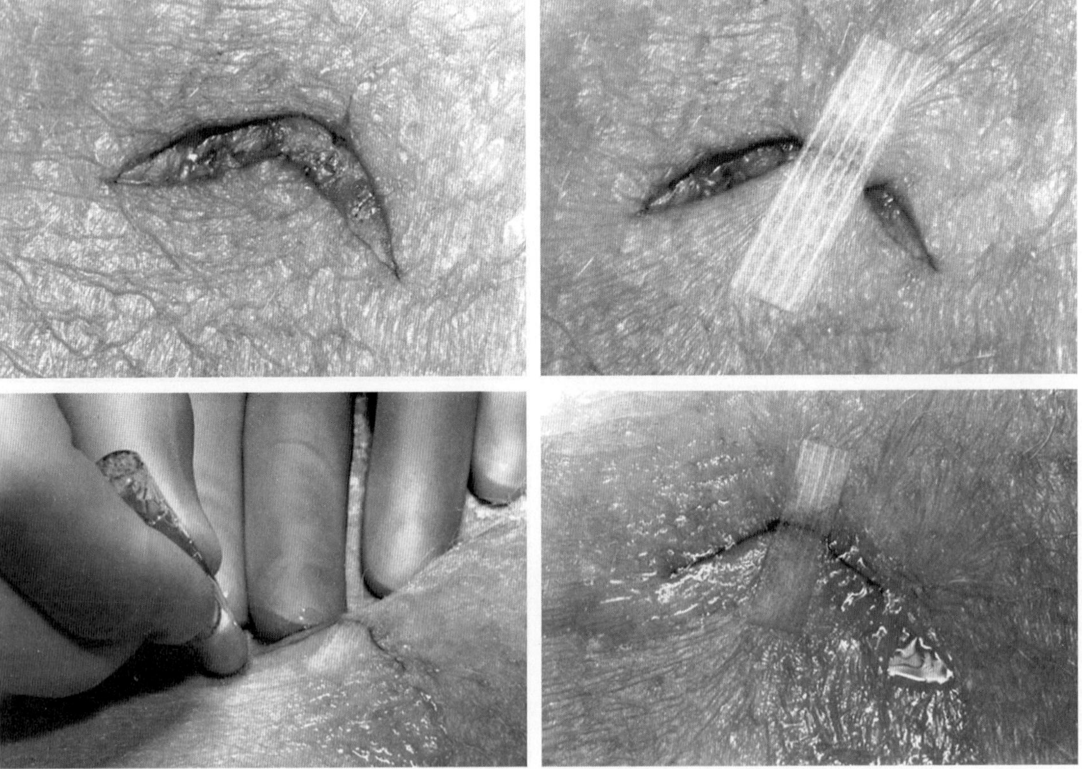

FIGURE 41-15. Closure of a long or complex laceration is achieved by applying adhesive tape to approximate the wound edges followed by application of the tissue adhesive over the approximated wound and tape.

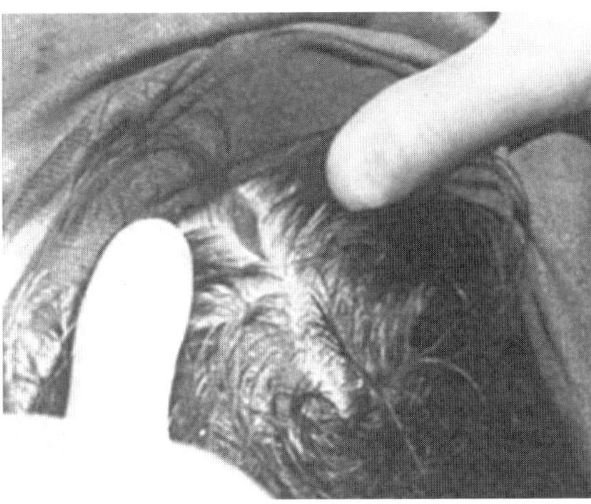

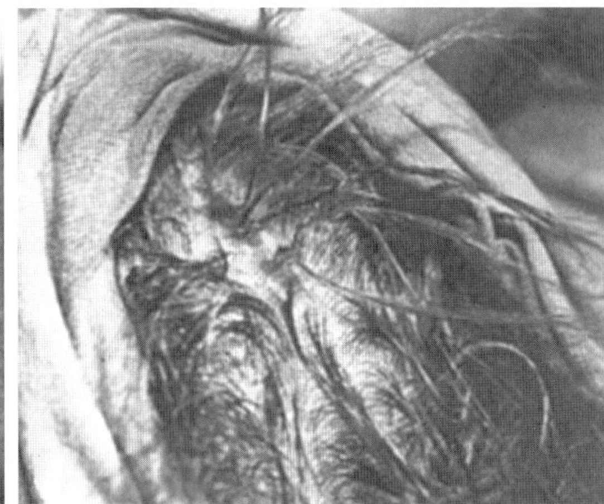

FIGURE 41-16. Hair apposition technique. **A.** Simple linear scalp wound. **B.** Three to seven hair strands on each side of the laceration are separately twisted into bundles. The two bundles on the opposite side of the wound are then twisted in a full 360-degree revolution and secured by applying a few drops of tissue adhesive. The process is repeated as needed to close the full length of the laceration. [Reproduced with permission from Roberts JR, Hedges JR: *Clinical Procedures in Emergency Medicine*, 4th ed. Copyright © 2004. Saunders, An Imprint of Elsevier.]

as needed to close the full length of the laceration (**Figure 41-16**). The patient will not need routine return because the tissue adhesive will flake off and the hair will unravel in about a week.

REFERENCES

The complete reference list is available online at www.TintinalliEM.com.

CHAPTER 42 Face and Scalp Lacerations

Wendy C. Coates

INTRODUCTION AND EPIDEMIOLOGY

Lacerations of the face and scalp are proximate in location but have important differences regarding repair. Facial wounds are the most cosmetically apparent of all wounds and therefore warrant careful evaluation and meticulous repair technique for the best possible outcome. Scalp wounds are less visible and are typically closed with less attention to detail. Most facial and scalp lacerations can be closed by the emergency physician, but consult with specialists if the technical aspects of closure are complex.

Three common principles guide repair of facial and scalp lacerations.[1] First, cleanse, irrigate, and remove foreign material to minimize infection. Second, limit debridement of skin edges because the excellent blood supply enables tissues to recover that initially appear nonviable. And third, if local anesthetic infiltration distorts anatomy and hinders wound edge alignment, use regional nerve blocks (see chapter 36, "Local and Regional Anesthesia").[2]

Use nonabsorbable monofilament suture for facial skin. Rapidly absorbable suture and tissue adhesives are alternatives in selected locations and for children.[3,4] Use absorbable suture for mucosa and facial layers. To minimize scarring, place percutaneous sutures on the face 1 to 2 mm from the wound edges, 3 to 4 mm apart, with everted edges. Place mucosal sutures 2 to 3 mm from the wound edges, 5 to 7 mm apart, and superficial so as to only include the mucosa and not the underlying muscle or fascia. Use of magnification with surgical loupes may facilitate more accurate suture placement in facial wounds.

Ask about the possibility of domestic violence in patients with facial injuries, and notify appropriate authorities if violence is suspected (**Table 42-1**).[5-7]

PATHOPHYSIOLOGY

Facial and scalp wounds are most often caused by a combination of sharp and blunt mechanisms. Lacerations caused by sharp objects likely have discrete edges but may extend deeply and involve underlying structures, such as the muscles of facial expression, nerves, and arteries. Wounds caused by blunt forces burst the skin open, damage cells, and produce tissue edema, all of which slow the wound-healing process. As a result, it takes an average of 10 times fewer bacteria to cause an infection in a blunt wound compared with a sharp wound. Blunt forces are also more likely to cause diffuse underlying damage, such as fractures of the facial bones or skull.

In most patients with isolated facial trauma resulting in lacerations, the incidence of facial fractures is low, especially in children.[8] However, in multiply injured patients, suspect underlying fracture in facial lacerations involving the infraorbital area, zygoma, nose, lips, and intraoral mucosa, so perform careful physical examination and obtain facial CT scans.[9,10]

Facial and scalp lacerations have a low incidence of postrepair infection, so **primary closure can usually be done in wounds that are not obviously infected, regardless of the duration of time since the injury[11-13] or even if injury was from a bite.**[14,15] The presence of foreign bodies, such as soil, glass, or wood fragments, complicates wound healing.[13]

SCALP AND FOREHEAD

ANATOMY

Both the scalp and forehead overlie bone with little cushioning fat and have thick skin (**Figure 42-1**). The one difference is that the scalp has

TABLE 42-1 Maxillofacial Injuries and Domestic Violence in the ED
Most victims of domestic violence have maxillofacial injuries.
Women are more commonly affected than men.
Fist is most common weapon.
Left side of face is most common site of injury (from right-hand-dominant assailants).
Nasal bone is commonly fractured.

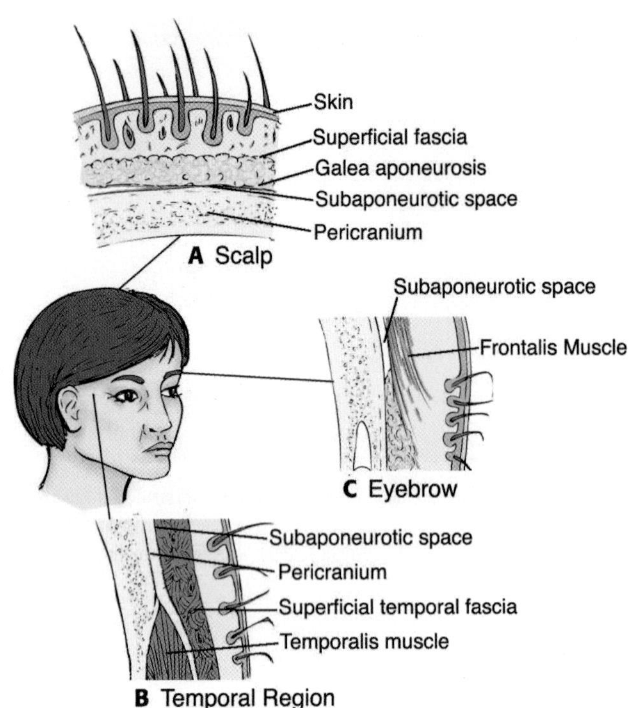

FIGURE 42-1. Layers of the scalp.

abundant hair follicles and sebaceous glands. Three branches of the external carotid artery (occipital, superficial temporal, and posterior auricular arteries) and two branches from the internal carotid artery (supraorbital and supratrochlear arteries) provide a rich blood supply to the scalp and forehead. The fibrous dermal tissue limits vessel retraction after injury, so significant hemorrhage can result from an arterial laceration. The potential space between the pericranium (periosteum covering the external surface of the skull bones) and the galea aponeurosis that allows for easy movement of the scalp over the cranium also enables hematoma and infection to collect in this subaponeurotic space and spread to involve the entire forehead and scalp. This high degree of mobility sometimes leads to a scalping injury, in which a large segment of the scalp is torn off in one piece.

CLINICAL FEATURES

For some patients with scalp and forehead lacerations, the wound may be only a minor part of the overall injury. Perform a focused assessment looking for intracranial injury before definitive wound care. Control scalp hemorrhage by applying direct pressure or clamping the involved vessel(s) at the wound edges (e.g., using Raney clips; see chapter 40) until the assessment is completed.[16]

Inspect scalp lacerations, and gently palpate with a gloved finger to determine depth and to identify galeal laceration or depressed skull fracture. Evaluate palpable depressions with a CT scan. Orientation of forehead lacerations has important cosmetic implications. In general, forehead wounds that fall parallel to the lines of skin tension have better cosmetic results than wounds that are perpendicular. The horizontal lines seen on the forehead when the brow is raised are perpendicular to the frontalis muscle underneath (**Figure 42-2**).

TREATMENT

Children may need sedation for wound repair (see chapter 113, "Pain Management and Procedural Sedation in Infants and Children"). Anesthesia can be provided by topical, local, or regional infiltration. Topical agents alone, such as lidocaine-epinephrine-tetracaine, provide adequate anesthesia in about half of patients and reduce the pain of local anesthetic injection.[17-20] Local anesthetics containing epinephrine are often used in highly vascular wounds to help control hemorrhage from small vessels.

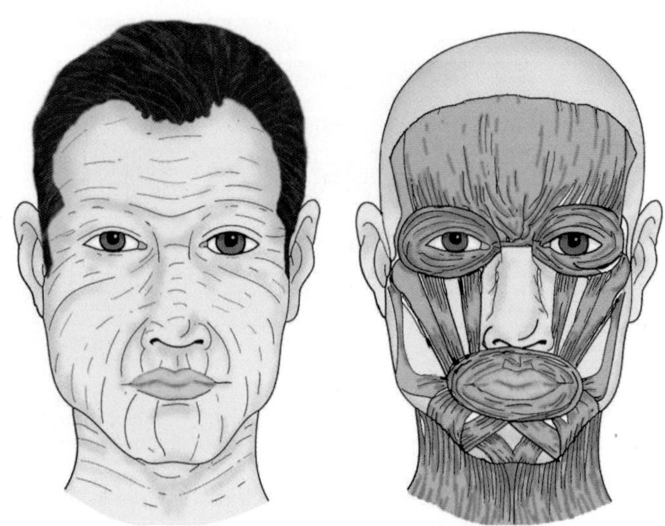

FIGURE 42-2. Skin tension lines. Skin tension lines are perpendicular to underlying muscles.

Irrigate (see chapter 40, "Wound Preparation") to reduce contamination and lessen the risk of wound infection. Appropriate pressure for irrigation can be accomplished with a 30-mL syringe and 18-gauge IV catheter or commercially available irrigation device. However, in resource-poor situations, because the face and scalp are highly vascular, clean-appearing wounds have been repaired using adhesive strips, without prior cleansing and irrigation.[21]

Repair of Scalp Lacerations Do not shave hair before wound closure, because shaving increases the risk of infection.[22] To visualize the injured area, brush the hair aside or matt it down with an ointment, such as bacitracin zinc or petrolatum.[23] If visualization is still difficult, trim the adjacent scalp hair with scissors.

Suture accessible lacerations of the galea[24] to prevent formation of a subgaleal hematoma (**Table 42-2**).[25]

Close scalp skin with surgical staples or simple interrupted percutaneous sutures using nonabsorbable monofilament or rapidly absorbable material.[26-29] Leave suture tails long, and use sutures of a color different than the hair for easy suture removal.

Hair braiding is a technique combining hair apposition and tissue adhesive.[30-32] In this technique, bring together four to five strands of hair from opposite sides of the wound, twist the strands once, and secure them with a drop of tissue adhesive. This technique requires the wound edges to approximate with little tension, so subcutaneous sutures are sometimes necessary before hair apposition is used to close the skin.

Consider a pressure dressing over a deep scalp laceration for the first 24 hours after repair, to prevent wound hematoma formation.

Repair of Forehead Lacerations Forehead lacerations are categorized as either superficial, meaning the **frontalis muscle** is not injured, or deep, meaning the frontalis muscle is involved. For superficial lacerations, close the skin with 6-0 nonabsorbable interrupted suture, rapidly absorbable suture, or tissue adhesive.[24,33,34] For deep lacerations, close the muscle layer to avoid noticeable defects, especially when the facial muscles of expression are involved. Close the muscle layer with buried 5-0 absorbable suture. Close the epidermal layer with 6-0 nonabsorbable sutures in a simple, interrupted fashion; with skin closure strips; or with tissue adhesive (**Table 42-3**).[35] Strips or adhesives are especially attractive if the patient is at risk for keloids or hypertrophic scars. Use key stitches to align skin tension lines and the hairline (**Figure 42-3**).

Repair of Eyebrow Lacerations Do not clip or shave eyebrows because their delicate contour and form are valuable landmarks for wound edge reapproximation. Debridement of loose or nonviable skin in the eyebrow region should be minimal and, if necessary, done so that the remaining hairs preserve as much as possible of the original length, width, and curve of the eyebrow. Use care to align the hair margins. Use sutures that are a different color from the hair and leave long tails to facilitate removal.

TABLE 42-2 Suturing Guidelines for the Face and Scalp

Area	Suture	Size	Anesthetic	Removal
Scalp				
Galea	Absorbable	4-0	Local	Not removed
Skin	Staples	Standard	Local	14 d
	Nonabsorbable monofilament	4-0	Local	14 d
	Rapidly absorbing	4-0	Local	Not removed
Forehead				
Frontalis muscle	Absorbable	4-0	Local or supraorbital nerve block	Not removed
Skin	Nonabsorbable monofilament	5-0 or 6-0	Local or supraorbital nerve block	5 d
	Tissue adhesive	May need deep layer	—	Not removed
Cheek and face				
Muscle fascia	Absorbable	4-0	Local or infraorbital nerve block	Not removed
Skin	Nonabsorbable monofilament	6-0	Local or infraorbital nerve block	5 d
	Rapidly absorbing	6-0	Local or infraorbital nerve block	Not removed
	Tissue adhesive	May need facial layer closure	—	Not removed
Eyelids				
Skin	Nonabsorbable monofilament	6-0 or 7-0	Supra- or infraorbital nerve block	3 d
Nose				
Mucosa	Rapidly absorbing	4-0	Intranasal	Not removed
Cartilage	Nonabsorbable (if necessary)	5-0	Intranasal	Not removed
Skin	Nonabsorbable monofilament	6-0	Local or intranasal	3–5 d
Ears				
Skin	Nonabsorbable monofilament	6-0	Auricular block	5 d
Cartilage	Nonabsorbable monofilament	5-0	Auricular block	Not removed
Lips				
Mucosa	Rapidly absorbing	5-0	Local, infraorbital, mandibular, or mental nerve block	Not removed
Muscle fascia	Absorbable	4-0 or 5-0	Local, infraorbital, submandibular, or mental nerve block	Not removed
Skin	Nonabsorbable monofilament	6-0	Local, infraorbital, or mental nerve block	3–5 d

EYELIDS

ANATOMY

The eyelid is composed of five layers: skin, subcutaneous tissue, orbicularis oculi muscle, tarsal plate, and conjunctiva. The muscular layer controls lid closure and forms both the medial and lateral canthus. Fibers of the orbicularis oculi wrap around the lacrimal system. Nerve supply to the eyelid arises from the temporal and zygomatic branches of the facial nerve. The tarsal plate forms the main body of the lower half of the lid and consists of elastic tissue in a dense matrix of connective tissue. Embedded in the tarsal plate are the meibomian glands, which open onto the white line just in front of the conjunctival edge of the lid margin. In the lid margin, the eyelashes are arranged in three irregular rows with their follicles extending obliquely into the tarsal plate.

The lacrimal system begins at the upper and lower puncta that transition into the canaliculi. The canaliculi travel medially into the lacrimal sac that extends inferiorly to the nasolacrimal duct responsible for tear drainage into the nose (**Figure 42-4**).

TABLE 42-3 Indications for Tissue Adhesives on the Face

Minimal tension
Not a hair-covered area
Epidermal closure only (no mucosa)

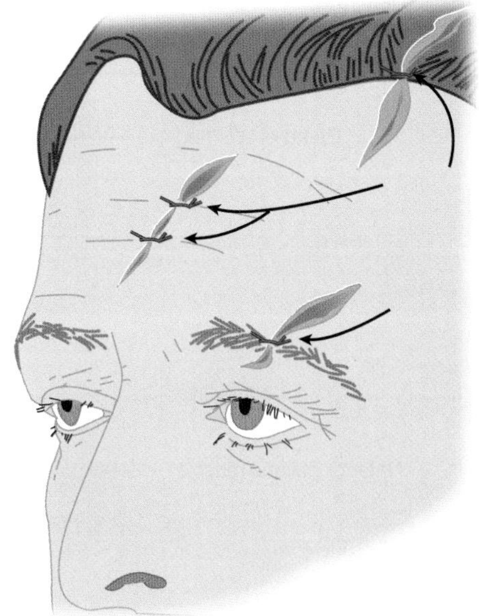

FIGURE 42-3. Key stitches in the forehead to align natural skin tension lines and cosmetically important landmarks.

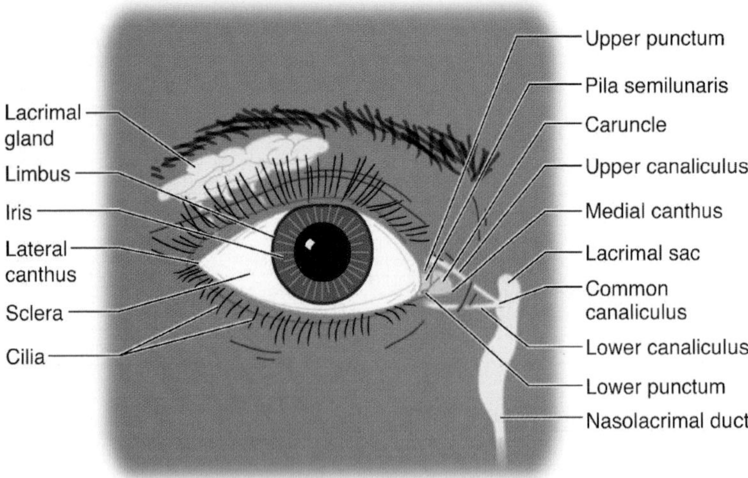

FIGURE 42-4. Periorbital anatomy.

CLINICAL FEATURES

The structures surrounding the eye and eyelids are delicate as well as cosmetically and functionally important. The eyelids are thin and offer limited protection from injuries to the globe, so **examine the eye's structure and function before laceration repair**. Once the integrity and function of the globe and orbital structures are verified, examine the lid for involvement of the canthi, the lacrimal system, or penetration through the tarsal plate or lid margin. **Eyelid injuries within 6 to 8 mm of the medial canthus are at risk for canalicular laceration, especially if associated with medal wall blow-out fractures.**[36] Refer the following injuries to an ophthalmologist or oculoplastic specialist: (1) injuries involving the inner surface of the lid, (2) wounds across lid margins, (3) injuries to the lacrimal duct, (4) wounds associated with ptosis, or (5) injuries extending into the tarsal plate (**Figure 42-5**).

Poor repair of the inside surface of the eyelid can lead to scar formation and persistent corneal irritation. Imprecise approximation of the lid margins leads to notching. Failure to recognize and properly repair the lacrimal system can result in chronic tearing (epiphora). Wounds through the tarsal plate or with ptosis require careful closure of the orbicularis oculi to preserve normal eyelid appearance. In general, wounds that are superficial, and especially those parallel to the lid margins, may be carefully repaired by the emergency physician.

TREATMENT

After topical anesthesia, gently irrigate the wound with normal saline. For closure, use 6-0 or 7-0 nonabsorbable monofilament for simple interrupted percutaneous sutures. Avoid deep penetration of the needle through the lid and into the underlying globe. **Do not use tissue**

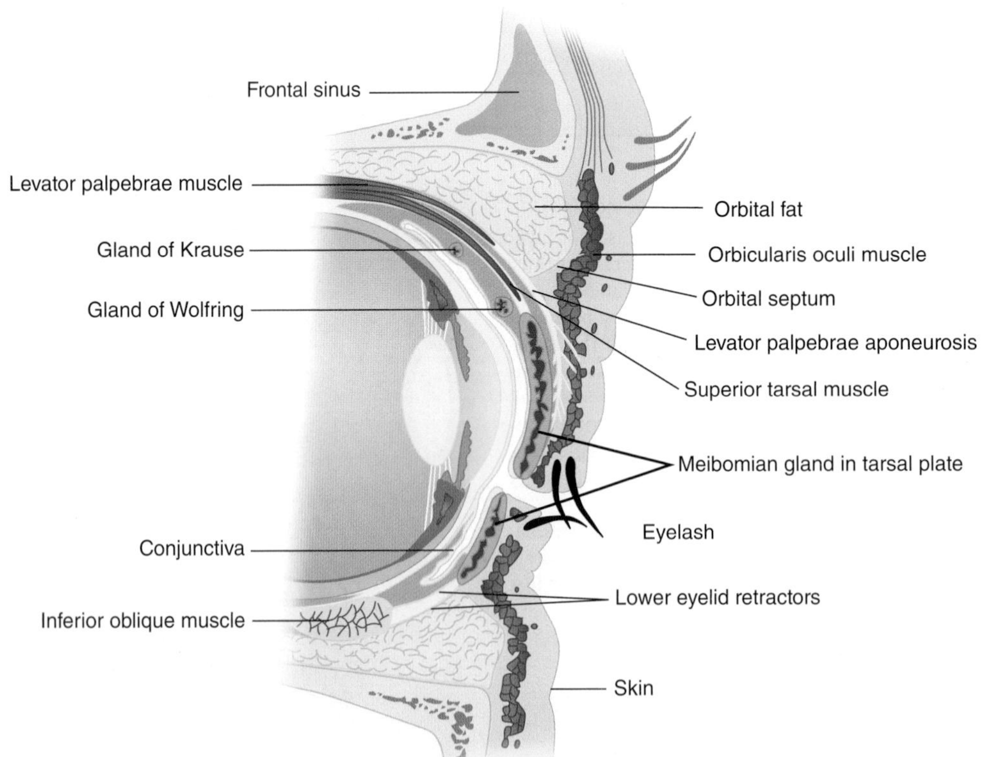

FIGURE 42-5. Cross-section of the eyelid. [Reproduced with permission from Riordan-Eva P, Whitcher J: *Vaughn & Asbury's General Ophthalmology*, 17th ed. New York: Lange Medical Books/Mcgraw-Hill, 2008.]

adhesive near the eye, as adhesives may abrade the cornea or bond the lids together.[37] If tissue adhesive inadvertently finds its way onto the cornea, apply ophthalmic ointment to dissolve the adhesive. If the eyelids are unintentionally bonded, petroleum jelly can dissolve the bond.

Lacerations <1 mm at the lid edge do not need suturing and heal spontaneously. See the chapter 241, "Eye Emergencies" for additional discussion.

NOSE

ANATOMY

The nose is especially vulnerable to blunt trauma, and nasal fracture is the most common fracture in victims of domestic violence and assault.[7] The nose is composed of cartilaginous and osseous structures that support the overlying skin and musculature and the underlying mucosa. It is separated into halves by the septum. Two C-shaped alar cartilages that are covered directly by skin form the tip of the nose. The interior of the nose is covered by specialized skin with mucus-producing cells and thick, long hairs near the end, whereas the proximal portion of the nasal lining is made up of ciliated pseudostratified columnar epithelial cells.

CLINICAL FEATURES

The most important assessment of nasal lacerations is to determine their depth and the involvement of the deeper tissue layers.[38] Exposed cartilage or penetration through all tissue layers increases the risk of infection. Inspect the nasal septum and look for discolored lateral budging indicating a septal hematoma. This hematoma develops between the cartilage and its protective mucoperichondrial layer and may produce complications such as (1) permanent thickening of the septum, causing partial airway obstruction of the nasal passage; (2) necrosis and subsequent erosion of the septum, resulting in communication between the nasal passageways; or (3) septal erosion leading to a saddle-nose deformity. With direct blunt trauma to the nose, assess for a cribriform plate fracture with cerebrospinal fluid rhinorrhea.

TREATMENT

Epinephrine-containing local anesthetics are acceptable for infiltrative anesthesia on the nose.[39] Topical application of lidocaine into the nasal cavity may provide sufficient anesthesia for local wound repair. Insertion of multiple cotton-tipped swabs or plain nasal packing gauze soaked in 4% lidocaine solution is usually sufficient (**Figure 42-6A**). After several minutes in place and before repair, remove the swabs or gauze.

Close superficial lacerations to the skin layer with 6-0 nonabsorbable monofilament simple interrupted sutures. Close lacerations over exposed cartilage promptly. Preserve any small pieces of loose cartilage under the skin for use in future revision by a plastic surgeon.

If the laceration extends through all tissue layers and involves the nostril, begin closure with a 5-0 nonabsorbable monofilament suture that aligns the skin surrounding the entrance to the nasal canals at the alar margin (**Figure 42-6B**). Initially, leave the ends untied and long to facilitate the closure of the deeper structures. *Gentle* traction on this suture facilitates alignment of the mucosa and cartilage layers during placement of subsequent sutures. Close the mucosal layer with 5-0 rapidly absorbable interrupted sutures, and reirrigate the area gently from the outside. Placement of sutures directly into the cartilage is not recommended; in most cases, closure of the overlying skin is usually sufficient to align the cartilage. If necessary to align cartilage pieces, place a minimal number of 5-0 nonabsorbable sutures through the cartilage. Reevaluate the initial stitch at the alar margin, and then tie it. Finally, suture the remainder of the skin with 6-0 nonabsorbable monofilament material close to the wound edges. With extensive wounds, consider a loose anterior nasal pack with antibiotic-impregnated gauze to prevent scar contracture.

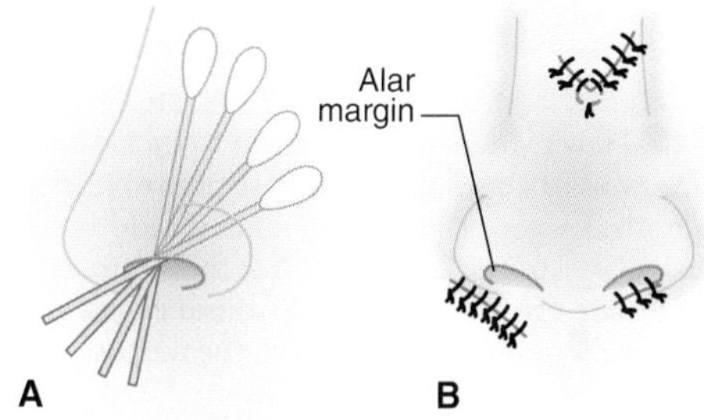

FIGURE 42-6. The nose. A. Nasal anesthetic technique using cotton-tipped applicators. B. Frontal view showing closure of skin edges.

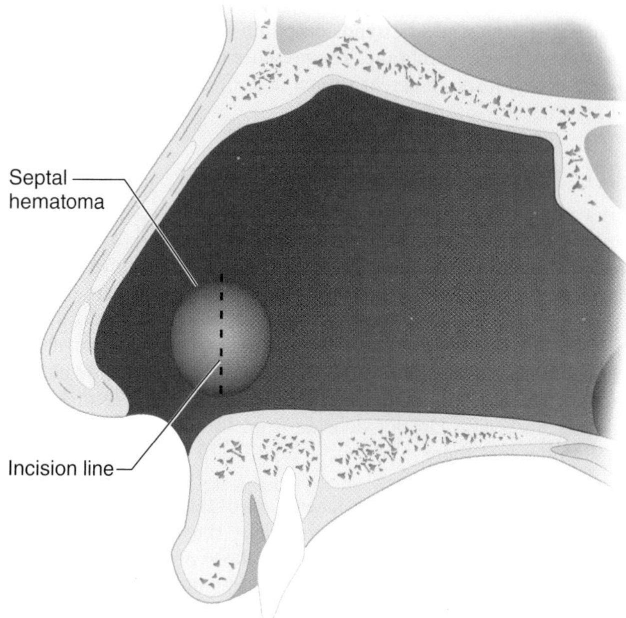

FIGURE 42-7. Incision for drainage of septal hematoma. Septal hematoma with markings for a vertical incision through the mucoperichondrium. [Reproduced with permission from Reichman EF, (ed): Emergency Medicine Procedures, 2ed. Figure 171-5. Copyright © 2013 The McGraw-Hill Companies, Inc. All rights reserved.]

Drain septal hematomas. For a small, unilateral hematoma, the clot can often be aspirated through an 18-gauge needle. Larger hematomas require an incision in the septal mucoperichondrium overlying the hematoma (**Figure 42-7**).[40] After hematoma evacuation, place an anterior nasal pack to discourage reaccumulation of the hematoma. After trauma, it is common practice to prescribe antibiotics to prevent infection of the cartilage and infection after nasal packing.[41] Bilateral hematomas are often drained in the operating room.

EARS

ANATOMY

The external ear begins with the external auditory canal and extends to the fibrocartilaginous framework of the auricle and the soft fatty tissue of the earlobe. The blood supply to the ear arises from the superficial temporal and posterior auricular arteries. The majority of the sensory innervation is from the anterior and posterior branches of the greater auricular nerve. **The auricular branches of the vagus nerve supply the posterior wall of the external auditory canal, so lacerations that involve this area cannot be anesthetized with auricular nerve blocks.**

CLINICAL FEATURES

Lacerations caused by blunt forces to the ear can rupture the tympanic membrane or produce a subchondral hematoma even in the absence of a laceration. Lacerations caused by blunt or shear forces may also involve the cartilage.[1,42] If a wound extends deep into the canal, verify the integrity of the tympanic membrane. The presence of hemotympanum, mastoid area ecchymoses, or cerebrospinal fluid otorrhea suggests a basilar skull fracture.

TREATMENT

Insert a cotton plug into the ear canal during wound preparation and irrigation. Regional anesthesia by auricular field block is ideal (see chapter 36, "Local and Regional Anesthesia"). Hemostasis before repair of an auricular laceration is important to prevent the formation of a hematoma.

Close superficial lacerations to the skin with 6-0 nonabsorbable monofilament interrupted sutures.[43] Cover any exposed cartilage to prevent subsequent infection. Do not remove crushed or loose pieces of cartilage under the skin, as the pieces may be beneficial if reconstructive surgery is necessary. Do not debride from the edges of an auricular laceration because there is very little excess skin available to cover the existing cartilage.

In most through-and-through lacerations of the auricle, skin approximation will adequately support and align the underlying cartilage (**Figure 42-8A**). Include the thin layer of loose material overlying the cartilage (perichondrium) when placing percutaneous sutures to assist in bringing the cartilage together (**Figure 42-8B**). If the overlying skin is avulsed, refer to a plastic surgeon for repair.[1,42] Complete avulsion of the ear requires immediate plastic surgery consultation.

A perichondral hematoma is a potentially damaging complication after repair of auricular lacerations. The collection of blood and build up of pressure may damage the cartilage and create a deformed external ear. A postrepair **auricular pressure dressing** can prevent hematoma formation. Pressure dressing placement involves several steps (**Figure 42-9**). Start by applying a nonadherent dressing over the repair site—either a piece of gauze with antibiotic ointment or other nonadherent wound dressing. Conform this dressing to the shape of the ear using gentle pressure. Then open and fluff up gauze pads, placing them behind the ear to fill the space between the skull and pinna and in front of the ear to fill the interior contours. Wrap the head and ear with gauze wrap covered with a light (not tight) elastic bandage wrap. **Reevaluate the dressing and the ear in 24 hours. If there is no hematoma, there is no need to reapply the pressure dressing.**

An **auricular hematoma** may develop within the first few days after injury. The patient typically presents with pain and swelling; the ear may look purplish; and the repair site is swollen, warm, and mushy to touch, and blood often oozes when the area is squeezed. Consult with a plastic surgeon or otolaryngologist. Proper treatment requires evacuation of the hematoma and bleeding control. If a specialist is not available, the emergency physician may choose to drain the hematoma. The initial step is to remove all the sutures, drain the blood, and thoroughly irrigate the wound.[40] Then resuture the wound and apply a pressure dressing.

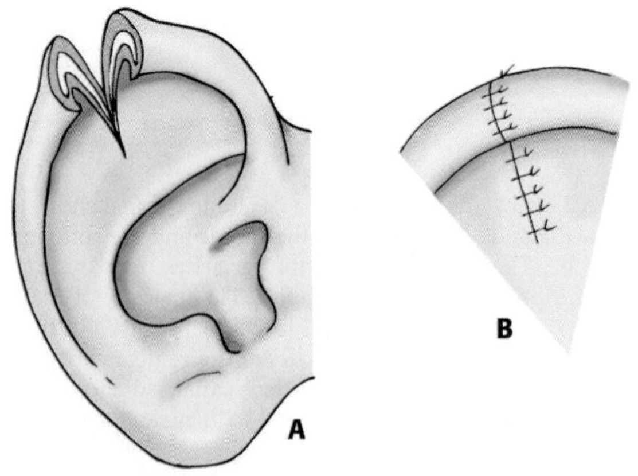

FIGURE 42-8. Repair of auricular laceration. A. Laceration through auricle. B. Interrupted 6-0 nonabsorbable sutures approximate the skin edges.

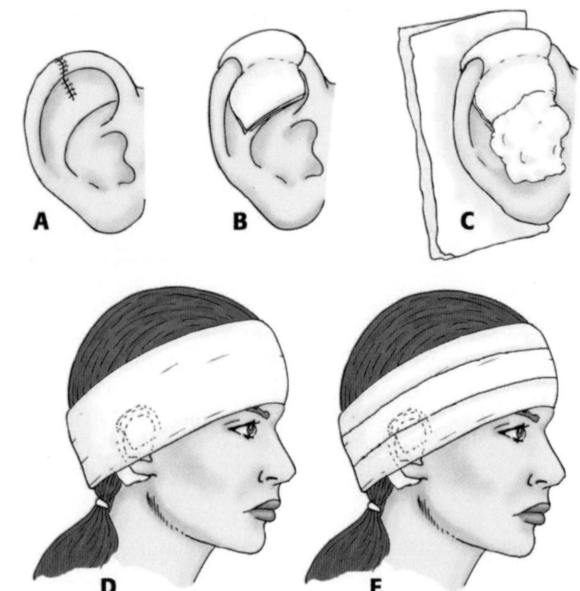

FIGURE 42-9. Auricular pressure dressing. **A.** Apply a nonadherent dressing over the repair site. **B.** Conform this dressing to the shape of the ear using gentle pressure. **C.** Place opened and fluffed gauze pads behind the ear to fill the space between the skull and pinna and in front of the ear to fill the interior contours. **D.** Wrap the head and ear with gauze wrap. **E.** Cover with a light (not tight) elastic bandage wrap. Do not enclose opposite external ear.

LIPS

ANATOMY

The external surfaces of the lips have three distinct regions: the skin, the vermilion, and the oral mucosa. The cosmetically important junction of the skin and the red portion of the lip is the **vermilion border**. The orbicularis oris muscle surrounds the mouth. Its integrity is responsible for retaining the saliva inside the mouth, producing the bilabial sounds of speech, and providing important facial expressions. The infraorbital nerve supplies the upper lip, and the submandibular nerve supplies the lower lip. Both are branches of the trigeminal nerve and can easily be blocked by regional anesthetic techniques. The lips are richly supplied by the labial arteries.

CLINICAL FEATURES

External and intraoral examination is required to appreciate the complete injury. Fully explore lacerations, teeth, and mucosa. Identify missing, impacted, or fractured teeth (see Figure 245-2 in the chapter titled "Oral and Dental Emergencies") or exposed bone of the maxilla or mandible. If portions of the teeth are missing, after adequate anesthesia, explore the wound fully because broken off pieces may become imbedded in the laceration.[44-46] Note if lacerations cross the vermilion-skin and/or the vermilion-mucosal borders.

TREATMENT

Intraoral mucosal lacerations may not need to be sutured if they are isolated and the wound edges spontaneously approximate, especially if <1 cm in length. Larger or gaping wounds should be closed with a rapidly absorbable 5-0 suture. Carefully place the suture to include only mucosa with entrance 2 to 3 mm from the wound edges, and use care to evert the edges. Larger tissue bites can bunch the mucosa and pucker the outside skin.

Through-and-through lacerations that do not include the vermilion border should be closed in layers. Close the mucosal layer with a 5-0 rapidly absorbable suture as described in the previous paragraph, followed by gentle reirrigation from the outside. Next, approximate the

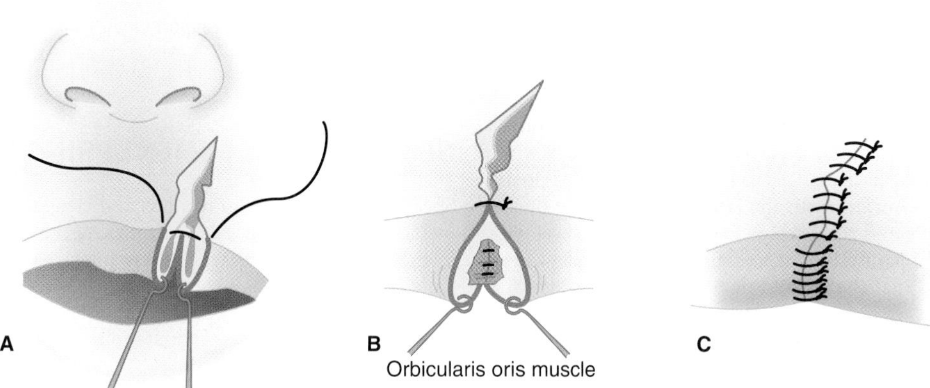

FIGURE 42-10. Lip laceration repair. **A.** The first suture is placed to align the vermilion skin junction. **B.** The orbicularis oris muscle is then repaired with 5-0 absorbable sutures. **C.** The irregular edges of the skin are then approximated with 6-0 nonabsorbable sutures.

orbicularis oris muscle with 4-0 or 5-0 absorbable suture material with a simple interrupted or horizontal mattress technique. Finally, after repeat irrigation, suture the skin with 6-0 nonabsorbable monofilament sutures in a simple interrupted fashion. Alternatively, the skin can be approximated with tissue adhesive.

Wounds that cross the vermilion border should be repaired by placing the first stitch with 6-0 nonabsorbable monofilament suture to precisely align the edges of the vermilion border (**Figure 42-10**). Even 1 mm of step-off will be cosmetically unappealing.[47] After this first stitch, repair the vermilion and skin with the same 6-0 material, and repair the mucosa with 5-0 rapidly absorbable suture. A useful technique in some cases is to leave the initial alignment suture untied and apply gentle traction on the ends to help approximate and align the underlying tissue as the skin and vermilion are closed. Use gentle traction to avoid pulling the suture through the skin in this delicate area. Use clinical judgment for the prescription of antibiotics. Contaminated wounds and through-and-through lacerations likely benefit from antibiotics.

INTRAORAL MUCOSAL LACERATIONS

ANATOMY

Two types of intraoral mucosal lacerations are common: those involving the buccal mucosa and those at the mucosal reflections. Buccal mucosal lacerations near the parotid duct opening, identified as a small papilla adjacent to the upper second molar, may injure that structure. Intraoral mucosal reflections are located at the transition from the cheek to the outside surface of the maxilla or mandible. Because of the loose attachment of the mucosa in this area, lacerations may have great depth and extend deeper than initially suspected.

CLINICAL FEATURES

Visualize and explore intraoral lacerations to determine their depth and extent. **Lacerations of the mucosal reflections are easily missed unless the lips are manipulated to see into all the recesses.** Evaluate the adjacent teeth for fracture or avulsion, because missing tooth fragments may be embedded in the wound, swallowed, or aspirated into the airway.

TREATMENT

Small intraoral lacerations (<1 cm) do not need routine repair and can be allowed to heal naturally. **Suture closure of intraoral lacerations is usually indicated when wounds are large enough to trap food particles or have a tissue flap that interferes with chewing.** Use 4-0 absorbable suture to close the mucosa. To avoid bunching of the mucosa as the suture knot is tied, insert the needle about 2 to 3 mm from the edge of the wound. Include only the mucosa in the suture because an external pucker may be created if the underlying muscle is ensnared in the suture loop. Be sure to evert the edges. Close suture placement is not necessary; typically, sutures placed 5 to 7 mm apart are adequate.

CHEEKS AND FACE

ANATOMY

The cheek area has two structures that influence wound repair: the parotid duct and branches of the facial nerve (**Figure 42-11**).[1] The opening of the parotid duct is adjacent to the upper second molar; wounds in this region can lacerate the parotid duct. As the facial nerve traverses the parotid gland, it divides into five major segments, the precise courses of

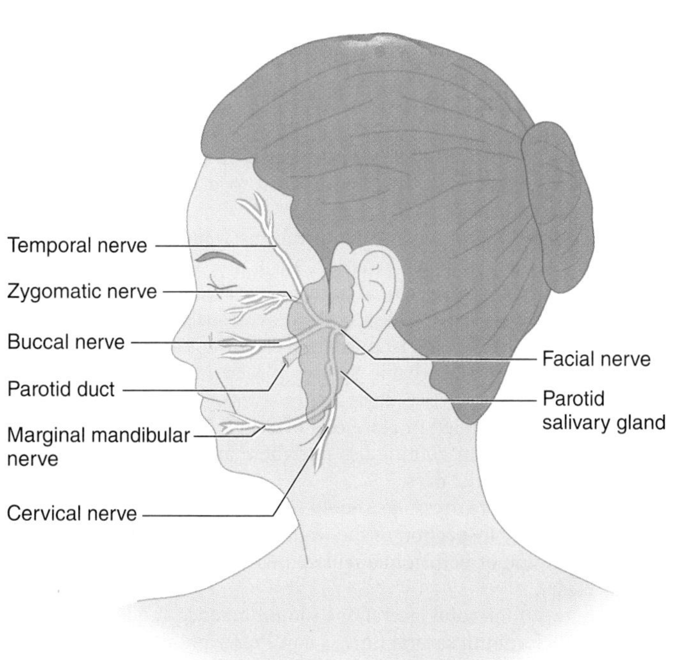

FIGURE 42-11. Cheek anatomy. The course of the parotid duct is within 1.5 cm of the midportion of a line drawn from the lower border of the tragus to the cheilion.[48] The five branches of the facial nerve are the temporal, zygomatic, buccal, marginal mandibular, and cervical.

which are difficult to predict. Therefore, lacerations or deeply placed sutures may ensnare one of these branches.

CLINICAL FEATURES

Evaluate wound depth and assess for damage to the parotid gland, parotid duct, and facial nerve. Assess the teeth for fracture, avulsion, or fragments embedded in the wound. Suspect parotid duct injury when the wound crosses a line from the tragus to the frenulum and is posterior to a vertical line downward from the lateral canthus. The buccal branch of the facial nerve and a branch of the facial artery travel with the parotid duct, so facial paralysis or arterial bleeding from the wound should arouse suspicion that the parotid duct is also injured. Parotid duct laceration can be confirmed by inserting a 19-gauge silastic tube into the intraoral parotid duct papilla and seeing if the catheter is visible in the wound. Alternatively, a small amount of saline can be injected into the tube while observing for flow in the wound. These procedures require patient cooperation and are usually performed by the consulting specialist.

TREATMENT

Repair superficial lacerations that involve the cheek and surface of the face with 6-0 nonabsorbable monofilament, simple, interrupted, percutaneous sutures. Alternatives include rapidly absorbable sutures or tissue adhesives. If there is significant skin tension, place intradermal 4-0 absorbable sutures, and make sure the parotid duct is not caught in the suture (Figure 42-11). If the parotid duct is injured, operative repair is indicated.

A full-thickness cheek laceration traverses the skin and the underlying subcutaneous tissue/muscle and penetrates through the intraoral mucosa. Such wounds are repaired in layers, starting with the intraoral mucosa. Once the mucosa is closed, reirrigate the wound before closure of the skin and subcutaneous layers. The skin and subcutaneous layers can often be brought together with percutaneous sutures using 5-0 or 6-0 material. If this does not allow the subcutaneous tissue to fill in the wound, use a small number of 4-0 absorbable simple sutures to approximate the muscle or subcutaneous tissue.

DISPOSITION AND FOLLOW-UP

Where possible, the wound should be dressed with either an antibiotic ointment or nonadherent dressing material to maintain moisture and encourage wound healing.[49-51]

Patients should be discharged with routine wound-care instructions (see chapter 47, "Postrepair Wound Care") and, if the injury resulted from a major blunt impact, closed head injury precautions. Remove scalp sutures or staples in 10 to 14 days, and remove nonabsorbable percutaneous sutures in the forehead, face, external ear, or lips in 5 to 7 days.

Percutaneous nonabsorbable sutures placed in the eyelid or nose should be removed in 3 to 5 days. A thin layer of ophthalmic antibiotic ointment may be applied in place of a dressing; do not apply antibiotic ointment intended for routine use elsewhere around the eye. Remove intranasal packing in 2 days.

Auricular pressure dressings should be left on for 24 to 48 hours and then removed for inspection of the wound site. If the wound is healing without infection or hematoma, replacement of the pressure dressing is not necessary.

Patients with intraoral lacerations should practice good oral hygiene and rinse their mouth several times a day. Prescription of antibiotics for intraoral lacerations and through-and-through facial wounds is a matter of physician preference.[52]

REFERENCES

The complete reference list is available online at www.TintinalliEM.com.

CHAPTER 43

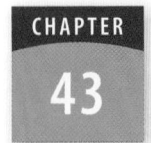

Arm and Hand Lacerations

Moira Davenport

GENERAL MANAGEMENT PRINCIPLES

Specific issues relative to wounds and lacerations of the arm and hand include potential injury to the arteries, nerves, and tendons that lie close to the skin and the impact of these injuries on the use of the hands in daily and occupational life. Injuries may be classified as either isolated or combinations of closed crush, simple lacerations, open crush, partial amputation, and complete amputation.

HISTORY AND EXAMINATION

Specific considerations in the history include patient age, occupation, mechanism of injury, and hand dominance. Age is important because the potential for bony injury increases with decreasing bone density, and the likelihood for healing and functional recovery decrease because of loss of elasticity. Mechanism of injury identifies wounds that are more prone to infections. Note the time from injury to repair. There is no distinct threshold for infection from time from injury to closure, but wounds sutured >12 hours after injury could be more prone to infection.[1,2]

Examination of arm and hand injuries begins with inspection and continues with evaluation of motor and sensory nerve function, tendon/ligament integrity, and assessment of perfusion. During inspection, observe the position and stance of the arm, hand, and digits. Identify exposed tendon or bone, and note the location of the wound relative to major arteries, nerves, and tendons. Explore the wound carefully for possible foreign body, debris, or other visible contaminants. Note significant soft tissue avulsion or loss of length of the injured part, as these findings may be indications for operative repair.

Active and Passive Movement Examine active motion and resistance to passive movement. Patients with a painful injury may be unwilling to move the affected extremity. After checking sensory function, local anesthesia may be required to obtain an adequate motor exam. The long-held belief that a local anesthetic with epinephrine should not be used for digital nerve blocks has been disproven, and agents containing epinephrine are acceptable for digital nerve blocks.[3-5]

Because there are several muscles with cross innervations, the most distal pure motor function of each major nerve should be tested against resistance (**Table 43-1**).

Individually assess each tendon in, and adjacent to, the injured area. For injuries to the hand and fingers individually examine the extensor digitorum, flexor digitorum profundus, and the flexor digitorum superficialis of each digit. The flexor digitorum superficialis, which splits and inserts at the proximal interphalangeal joint, can be examined by holding all other digits in extension and flexing the proximal interphalangeal joint against resistance. The flexor digitorum profundus, which runs below the flexor digitorum superficialis past the split to attach at the distal interphalangeal joint, can be examined by holding the proximal interphalangeal joint in extension and flexing the distal interphalangeal joint against resistance. The extensor digitorum can be assessed by sequentially flexing the digit at the metacarpophalangeal, proximal interphalangeal, and distal interphalangeal joints and having the patient

TABLE 43-1 Motor Testing of the Peripheral Nerves of the Upper Extremity

Nerve	Motor Exam
Radial	Dorsiflexion of wrist
Median	Thumb abduction away from the palm
	Thumb interphalangeal joint flexion
Ulnar	Adduction/abduction of digits

TABLE 43-2 Sensory Testing of Peripheral Nerves in the Upper Extremity

Sensory Nerve	Area of Test
Radial	First dorsal web space
Median	Volar tip of index finger
Ulnar	Volar tip of little finger

extend the digit. Extension should be performed first against gravity and then against resistance applied by the examiner. **Weak, limited, or painful movement suggests partial involvement of a tendon.** Abnormality in motor nerve or tendon function testing warrants a more in-depth examination, including visual inspection and appropriate consultation.

Sensation and Two-Point Discrimination Assess pain and touch in the median, ulnar, and radial nerve distributions (**Table 43-2** and **Figure 43-1**). For injuries distal to the midpalm, assess the digital nerves by static two-point discrimination, testing longitudinally along the ulnar and radial aspect of the volar pad of the potentially involved digits. Static two-point discrimination is evaluated by using electrocardiogram calipers or a paper clip bent into a "V" shape with the two ends separated by approximately 5 to 6 mm. During testing, the two points should not cross the midline, and each stimulus should be timed 3 to 4 seconds apart. **Normal two-point discrimination is defined as <6 mm**; good is 6 to 10 mm, fair is 11 to 15 mm, and poor is >15 mm. Two-point spatial acuity of touch diminishes with age. Young (18 to 33 years) patients have a mean two-point acuity of 2 mm, whereas elderly (>66 years old) patients have a mean acuity of 5 mm.[6] The two most important areas to maintain sensation are the ulnar side of the distal thumb and the radial side of the index volar pad to preserve pinch sensation.

Vascular Assessment Intact radial and ulnar pulses and capillary refill are usually adequate to exclude significant vascular injury. However, an arterial injury proximal to the wrist may not be obvious as a result of collateral circulation. To better assess the integrity of the radial and ulnar arteries, perform **Allen's test**. The test is performed by first instructing the patient to make a fist as tight as possible. Then, apply digital pressure to both the radial and ulnar artery at the volar aspect of the wrist. Next, while maintaining compression of the radial and ulnar artery, have the patient open the hand—a blanched palm indicates that arterial inflow is occluded. Now release the radial artery, and note the time for the hand to return to normal color. Repeat the entire process, this time releasing and assessing flow from the ulnar artery. If the patient cannot make a fist, occlusion of both arteries will still blanch the hand, but the color change will not be as evident or pronounced. **Refill times >3 seconds raise suspicion for a significant vascular injury.**

A Doppler probe is useful to detect a diminished pulse, detect flow in digital arteries, and to calculate an arterial pressure index. The **arterial pressure index** is the ratio of the systolic blood pressure between the injured and the uninjured side. It is useful to assess the vascular integrity of an injured arm or leg. To obtain the index, place a blood pressure cuff proximal to the ankle or wrist of the injured limb and distal to the wound. Then use a Doppler probe to determine the systolic pressure at the dorsalis pedis or posterior tibial artery, or the radial or ulnar artery. In the absence of a diminished pulse or an arterial pressure index ratio <1.0, the likelihood of a clinically significant occult arterial injury is exceedingly small (sensitivity 95%, specificity 97%).[7,8] Lack of obvious arterial bleeding does not rule out arterial injury because cleanly transected arteries may contract and prevent obvious bleeding. Any abnormal findings warrant consultation with a vascular surgeon as well as with a hand surgeon.

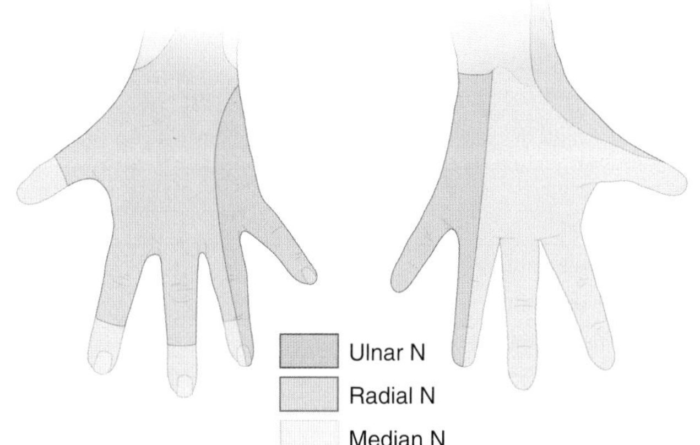

FIGURE 43-1. Sensory innervation to the hand.

IMAGING

Obtain radiographs with anteroposterior, oblique, and lateral views if bony injuries, foreign bodies, or joint penetration are suspected. Additional oblique views of the hand and digits are useful to visualize small areas with overlapping bones. For isolated finger injuries, dedicated anteroposterior and lateral radiographs of the involved digit(s) are preferred, as the detail on hand films alone is often not adequate for complete visualization of small, subtle fractures. **Plain radiography visualizes radiopaque objects as small as 1 mm.** When there is suspicion for a radiolucent-retained foreign body, especially wood, other imaging modalities (US, CT, or MRI) may be necessary (see chapter 45, Soft Tissue Foreign Bodies).

WOUND VISUALIZATION AND TOURNIQUET APPLICATION

Because wounds and the affected structures are often small, patient positioning, bright lighting, and a bloodless field are necessary for wound evaluation. For some injuries, a bloodless field may require a proximal tourniquet to temporarily halt arterial inflow and allow adequate visualization of the injury. Penrose (rubber) drains are typically used to tourniquet an injured finger, and pneumatic tourniquets placed around the arm are used with forearm and wrist injuries. To tourniquet a digital injury, place a 1-in. Penrose drain around the base of the finger, stretch the drain away from the hand, and secure the drain with a clamp or hemostat. If time allows, the digit can be exsanguinated before tourniquet placement by wrapping the digit with the Penrose drain from distal to proximal, then carefully removing the drain from distal to proximal before securing it around the base of the digit. **Excessively high pressures and tourniquet times >15 to 20 minutes can cause neurovascular damage and may be avoided by limiting the stretch of the drain to no more than 50% of the original length.**[9]

For more proximal injuries, especially those with brisk arterial bleeding, an inflated manual blood pressure cuff is used. **Esmarch's technique** is as follows: Elevate the injured extremity and apply an elastic bandage starting distally and proceeding proximally to the area where the cuff will be applied. This will help to exsanguinate the limb and prevent backflow bleeding. The cuff is applied around the upper arm and inflated to pressures above the systolic blood pressure of the patient, but not to exceed 250 mm Hg. The cuff tubing is clamped with a hemostat instead of closing the air release valve to prevent slow air leakage. The maximum cuff inflation time is limited to 30 minutes to limit ischemic damage to the distal muscles and nerves.

Once adequate visualization is obtained, examine the area for foreign bodies and tendon and joint capsule injuries. **Examine the arm and hand in a variety of positions, including the position of injury and a full, passive range of motion, to avoid missing injuries that may move out of the field of view when the extremity is examined in a neutral position.** Examine lacerations near a joint carefully to identify violation of the joint capsule. If the location and depth of the injury raise the question of extension into the joint capsule, joint injection for a **saline load test** should be done. After standard sterile preparation of the area, inject the joint with normal saline at an area away from the laceration. Inject 5 mL in the wrist and 1 to 2 mL in finger joints.[10] Inject sufficient amounts of saline to adequately stress the capsule. False-negative results may be obtained if too little fluid is injected.[11,12] Fluid dripping from the joint indicates an open joint capsule and requires specialty consultation. For small joints or questionable exams, a few drops of sterile fluorescein for

IV use (Ak-Flor®) may be added to the injected saline and the joint examined with a Wood's lamp for evidence of fluorescent effluent. **Do not use methylene blue because it stains the intra-articular surfaces** and may affect operative management of intra-articular injuries.

WOUND DRESSING AND POSTREPAIR CARE

After the injury is repaired, apply antibiotic ointment to the repaired incision/sutures and cover the wound with a nonadherent dressing. Wrap the area loosely with a soft dressing to allow for adequate circulation. A small portion of the fingernail or volar pad should remain visible to allow serial assessment of capillary refill in patients with digital injuries. Certain injuries, especially large lacerations in close proximity to a joint and those with tendon involvement, may be splinted for protection and limitation of pain. A padded aluminum splint is satisfactory for isolated digital lacerations. Provide adequate analgesia and remind the patient to keep the injured extremity elevated above the level of the heart to reduce edema. A follow-up wound check is recommended within 48 to 72 hours. Sutures are usually removed 8 to 10 days after the injury.

Prophylactic antibiotics are not needed for uncomplicated hand lacerations.[2] The definition of an uncomplicated hand laceration is as follows: (1) not caused by a human or animal bite; (2) not associated with a burn; (3) not complicated by a fracture through bone or a joint; (4) not involving tendons, bones, large vessels or nerves; (5) no severe soft tissue damage or maceration.[2] Antibiotics are generally given for complicated hand lacerations, mammalian bite wounds, injuries >12 hours old, contaminated wounds, injuries with exposed bone, or injuries occurring in patients with concurrent medical problems that may affect wound healing (i.e., diabetes, renal or peripheral vascular disease, immunocompromise).[13-15] Antibiotics should be chosen to cover suspected contaminants and pathogens and should be given early in the ED by a route that quickly achieves high blood and tissue concentrations.

Provide tetanus immunization or booster as needed.

Indications for admission to the hospital include injuries that require repair in the operating room, those that require a course of IV antibiotics, or the presence of social issues such as abuse cases, homelessness, or other factors affecting the patient's ability to follow basic aftercare instructions.

INJURIES IN CHILDREN

Because of the presence of an open epiphysis in children, a fracture can be difficult to identify using plain radiographs. It is often necessary to obtain radiographs of the unaffected side for comparison. If a complicated repair is indicated and the child is unable to tolerate the procedure after local anesthesia alone, procedural sedation may be required. The continuous high activity level of children makes keeping dressings intact a problem, rendering routine hand dressings and protective finger splints ineffective. If the dressing and immobilization is essential to wound healing, the child should be placed in a bi-valved long arm cast.

DORSAL FOREARM, WRIST, AND HAND LACERATIONS

The forearm has six extensor compartments located dorsally, all of which are innervated by the radial nerve (**Table 43-3**). Tendons and nerves distal to the wound should be individually examined.

The skin on the dorsum of the forearm and hand is thin and lacks underlying tissue, which allows skin avulsion to occur easily and makes wound edge approximation sometimes difficult.[16] For most lacerations, simple 5-0 nonabsorbable percutaneous sutures should be adequate for closure. To provide better cosmesis for injuries to the dorsum of the hand, we recommend subcuticular stitches with 5-0 absorbable material. A pull-through subcuticular closure with nonabsorbable suture is preferred for linear lacerations (**Figure 43-2**).[16] For deep wounds that penetrate through the muscle fascia and lacerate the muscle belly, closure of the fascial defect with 4-0 absorbable suture is generally recommended. However, deep sutures increase the potential for infection in a contaminated wound.

CLENCHED FIST INJURIES

Patients with lacerations to the dorsum of the hand should be questioned about the possibility of a **clenched fist injury or "fight bite,"** wounds created by the patient throwing a punch and impacting the front teeth of the intended target and producing a small laceration (3 to 5 mm) over the dorsal metacarpophalangeal joint.[17] Extension of the hand after the fight deeply inoculates oral bacteria into the wound. *Staphylococcus aureus* is the most common bacterial species isolated from human bite wounds, followed by *Streptococcus* spp., *Corynebacterium* spp., and *Eikenella corrodens*. In clenched fist injury infections, polymicrobial involvement is the rule. Human bites can also transmit herpes, actinomycosis, syphilis, tetanus, and hepatitis B and C.[17] Bites are not the only way to inoculate the hand with human oral flora; significant hand and finger infections have been reported after toothpick injuries. Patients sustaining such puncture wounds should receive antibiotics to protect against the above-mentioned bacteria.[18]

Obtain radiographs on clenched fist injuries to evaluate for embedded teeth, air in the joint/soft tissues, and fractures. Patients who delay evaluation and develop obvious infection require exploration, open irrigation, and debridement in the operating room followed by admission for IV antibiotics and elevation. If the patient presents soon after the injury and without evident infection, then evaluation, exploration, irrigation, and debridement can be done in the ED with appropriate equipment and physician expertise. It is important to visualize the full extent of the wound, evaluate the hand through full range of motion, and exclude injury to the extensor tendon and joint capsule. If no injury to these structures is seen, the wound should be copiously irrigated and covered with a nonadherent dressing. **Lacerations resulting from clenched fist injuries should not be sutured, but rather allowed to heal by secondary intention.**

Splint the hand in a position of function (**Figure 43-3**). A 3- to 5-day course of prophylactic antibiotics should be prescribed, usually amoxicillin-clavulanic acid. Give the first antibiotic dose in the ED. Instruct the

TABLE 43-3 Extensor Compartments in the Forearm

Compartment	Muscle	Function
First compartment	Abductor pollicis longus	Abducts and extends thumb
	Extensor pollicis brevis	Extends thumb at MCP joint
Second compartment	Extensor carpi radialis longus	Extends and radially deviates wrist
	Extensor carpi radialis brevis	Extends and radially deviates wrist
Third compartment	Extensor pollicis longus	Extends thumb at interphalangeal joint
Fourth compartment	Extensor digitorum communis	Splits into four tendons at level of the wrist; extends index, long, ring, and little digits
	Extensor indicis proprius	Extends index finger
Fifth compartment	Extensor digiti minimi	Extends little finger at MCP joint
Sixth compartment	Extensor carpi ulnaris	Extends and radially deviates wrist

Abbreviation: MCP = metacarpophalangeal.

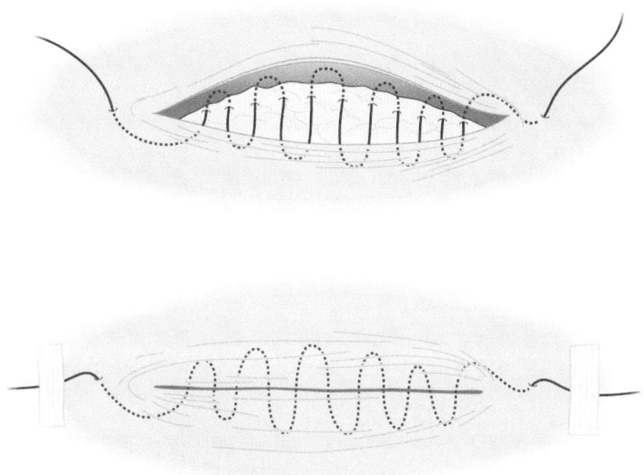

FIGURE 43-2. Pull-through subcuticular suture.

patient to elevate the extremity and return for reevaluation in 24 to 48 hours. If there is already evidence of infection or joint/tendon involvement, consult a hand surgeon and consider admission for observation and IV antibiotics, typically ampicillin-sulbactam or cefoxitin.

EXTENSOR TENDON LACERATIONS

The dorsal skin of the hand is thin and freely mobile, allowing for extensive range of motion for all joints. Because of this mobility and the superficial nature of the extensor tendons, a careful examination through a full range of motion at the site of injury in a neutral position and in the position of injury is necessary to avoid missing a tendon injury. Refer extensor tendon injuries of the thumb or those with severe contamination to a hand surgeon. An experienced emergency physician can repair extensor tendon injuries between the distal wrist and metacarpophalangeal joints. In this case, it is recommended to consult the hand surgeon for treatment preferences and ensure continuity of care. Small partial extensor tendon injuries (<50% transected) should be repaired with absorbable synthetic material.[19] Larger partial tendon injuries (>50% transected) and complete extensor tendon lacerations should be sutured with 4-0 (5-0 for smaller tendons) colorless nonabsorbable material, such as polypropylene or nylon, and the skin closed with 5-0 nonabsorbable suture material.[19] A figure-of-eight stitch with the knot placed at the edge of the tendon is recommended to repair lacerated extensors (**Figure 43-4**).

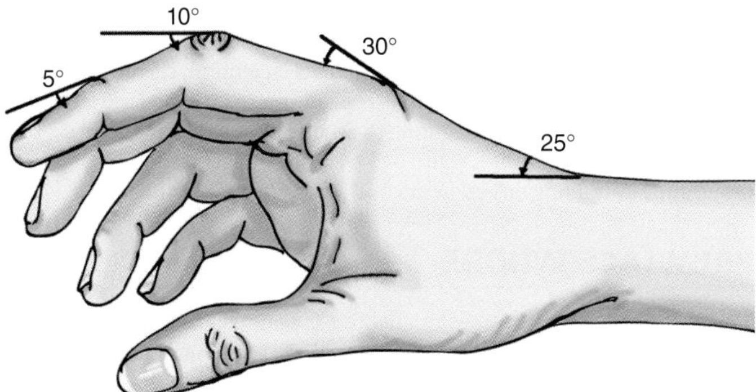

FIGURE 43-3. Wrist and hand position when splinted in "position of function." The wrist is extended 25 degrees so that the thumb metacarpal is in alignment with the forearm. The thumb is abducted away from the palm. Metacarpophalangeal joints are flexed to 30 degrees. Proximal interphalangeal joints are flexed to 10 degrees. Distal interphalangeal joints are flexed to 5 degrees.

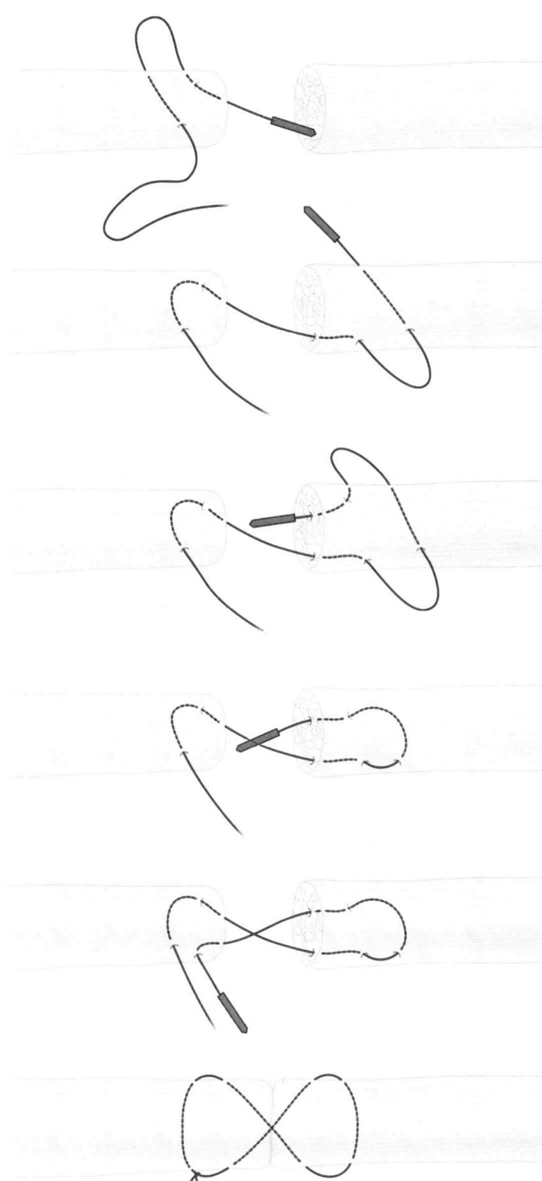

FIGURE 43-4. Extensor tendon laceration repair with a figure-of-eight stitch.

After repair of the tendon and overlying skin, **splint the hand or digit in a position of function** with instructions to maintain elevation of the extremity (**Figure 43-3**). Follow-up with a hand surgeon is recommended within 7 days.

Complications can be seen with disrupted extensor mechanisms. The **mallet finger deformity** (inability to extend the distal interphalangeal joint, resulting in the joint being held in flexion) and **swan neck deformity** (hyperextension of the proximal interphalangeal joint resulting from unrepaired mallet finger deformity) are caused by the complete disruption of the terminal extensor mechanism and subsequent proximal and dorsal displacement of the lateral bands (**Figures 5A** and **5B**). A **boutonniere deformity** (hyperflexion of the proximal interphalangeal joint with hyperextension of the distal interphalangeal joint) is usually a delayed complication after injury to the proximal interphalangeal joint. The central slip of the extensor tendon is disrupted, allowing the lateral bands to move volarly and operate as flexors at the proximal interphalangeal joint while still producing extension at the distal interphalangeal joint (**Figure 43-5C**). If these injuries are open, operative repair is required. Closed injuries may be treated by splinting the digit in extension (distal interphalangeal joint for mallet finger and both proximal interphalangeal and distal interphalangeal joints for Boutonniere's deformity)

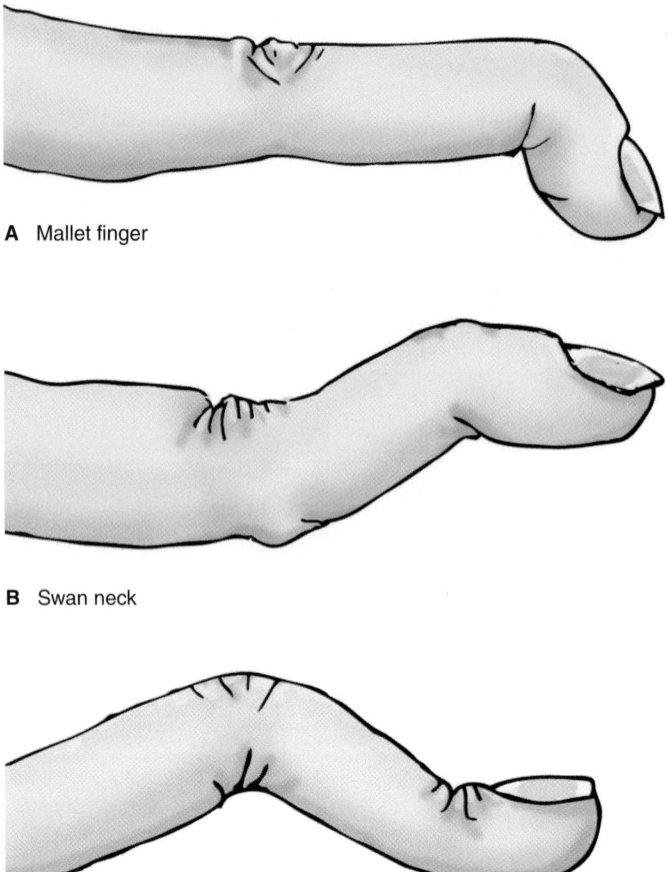

A Mallet finger

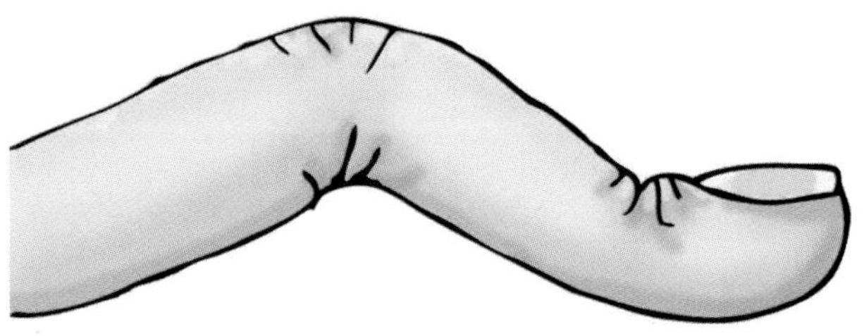

B Swan neck

C Boutonniere

FIGURE 43-5. **A.** Mallet finger. **B.** Swan neck finger. **C.** Boutonniere's deformity.

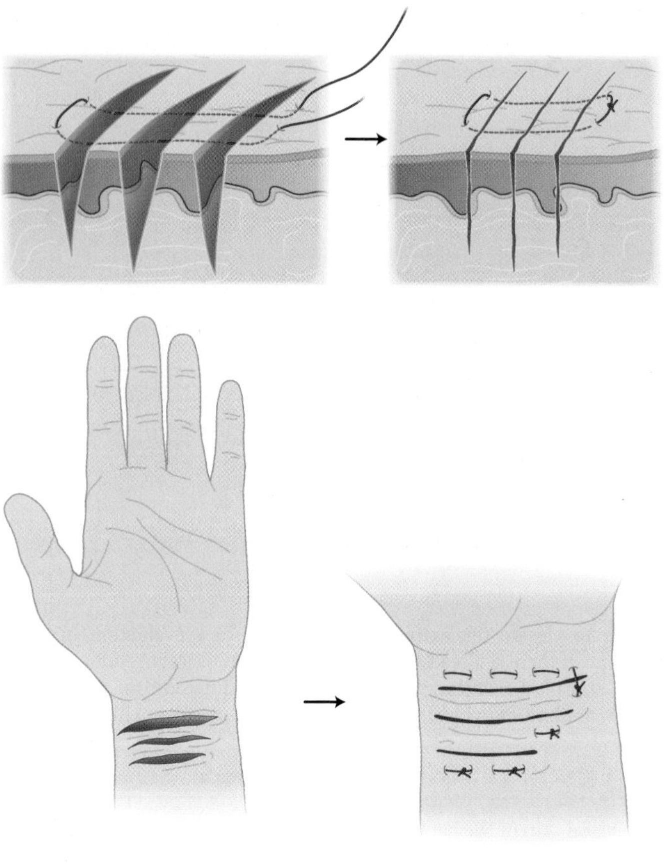

for up to 6 weeks or until operative repair. All cases should be referred to a hand surgeon for follow-up.[20,21]

VOLAR FOREARM, WRIST, AND HAND LACERATIONS

Patients with volar wrist lacerations should be questioned about suicidal attempts, and potentially suicidal patients require psychiatric evaluation after wound repair.[22] There are 12 flexor tendons innervated by the median and ulnar nerves located on the volar surface of the forearm that cross the wrist (**Table 43-4**). Tendons and nerves distal to the wound should be individually examined.

Injuries in the elbow region may affect the radial and ulnar nerves, which run in close proximity to the lateral and medial epicondyles, respectively. The radial nerve emanates from the spiral groove in the humerus approximately 10 cm proximal to the lateral epicondyle. The ulnar nerve travels behind the medial epicondyle as it runs between the two heads of the flexor carpi ulnaris into the forearm. The median nerve in the elbow region is more protected, as it runs in close proximity to the brachial artery and crosses anteriorly to the ulnar artery at the origin of the anterior interosseous nerve in the forearm. Although injuries to these nerves are more common with fractures and dislocations, simple soft tissue injuries at the elbow may result in nerve damage due to the superficial location and lack of overlying protective soft tissue in this area.

For most simple lacerations to the volar surface of the forearm and wrist, 4-0 or 5-0 nonabsorbable monofilament percutaneous sutures, such as nylon or polypropylene, should be used. For gaping injuries or injuries under high stress, a layer of deep sutures using 4-0 absorbable material may be required. Alternatively, mattress sutures can be used as well. For deep wounds that penetrate through the muscle fascia and lacerate the muscle belly, closure of the fascial defect with 4-0 absorbable suture is generally recommended.

Injuries that involve more than one parallel laceration, classic for suicide attempts, may require horizontal mattress sutures to cross all lacerations for closure to prevent compromising the vascular supply of the island of skin located between incisions (**Figure 43-6**). Alternatively, adhesive tapes or tissue adhesives alone or in conjunction with sutures may be used.[16]

TABLE 43-4 Flexor Tendons in the Forearm

Flexor Tendon	Function
Flexor carpi radialis	Flexes and radially deviates wrist
Flexor carpi ulnaris	Flexes and ulnarly deviates wrist
Palmaris longus	Flexes wrist
Flexor pollicis longus	Flexes thumb at MCP and interphalangeal joints
Flexor digitorum superficialis	Flexes index, long, ring, and little digits at MCP and PIP joints
Flexor digitorum profundus	Flexes index, long, ring, and little digits at MCP, PIP, and DIP joints

Abbreviations: DIP = distal interphalangeal; MCP = metacarpophalangeal; PIP = proximal interphalangeal.

FIGURE 43-6. Horizontal mattress sutures for multiple parallel lacerations.

PALM LACERATIONS

The palmar skin surface is well adapted for contact with objects in the environment. Palmar skin is thicker than dorsal skin and has an underlying connective tissue fascial layer, making it much more adherent to bone. The thenar, palmar, and digital creases are connections between the skin and underlying fascia, and these areas have no intervening adipose tissue. Because tendons, nerves, and arteries course through this area, palm lacerations have great potential to damage these deep structures through small and innocuous-appearing lacerations.[23,24] **Carefully assess digital flexor tendon function and two-point discrimination.**

Carefully approximate creases during skin closure. The thickness of palmar skin makes eversion of the edges especially difficult. For this reason, interrupted horizontal mattress sutures with 5-0 nonabsorbable monofilament are recommended to ensure that sutures do not pull through the skin.[16]

FLEXOR TENDON LACERATIONS

Flexor tendon injuries are usually repaired in the operating room by a hand surgeon because of the complexity of the anatomy and the reparative procedures required. Early consultation is important, as many surgeons prefer to repair complete flexor tendon lacerations within 24 hours after injury. If operative repair of the flexor tendon is going to be delayed, the wound should be appropriately cleaned, the skin closed, and the affected extremity splinted. **Splint with the wrist and metacarpophalangeal joint flexed and the proximal interphalangeal and distal interphalangeal joints in extension to prevent contraction of the surrounding muscles.**[25] The hand surgeon can follow up the patient in 2 to 3 days to schedule the flexor tendon repair within 7 days of the injury. **Timely repair is important, as postinjury scarring and tendon retraction make flexor tendon repairs more difficult after 10 to 14 days.** Rapid repair is also recommended to restore vascular and synovial flow to the area and maximize biologic properties of healing.[25] Patients with suspected partial flexor tendon lacerations should also have follow-up with a hand surgeon because unrepaired partial flexor digitorum superficialis disruption can produce a trigger finger.[26]

FINGER LACERATIONS

In general, isolated finger lacerations are straightforward injuries to examine and repair. Vascular status is checked by capillary refill, and sensory nerve status is checked by static two-point discrimination. Assess motor function of the extensor and flexor mechanisms. Careful examination and wound exploration of hand and digit lacerations is important, regardless of size. A prospective study of patients with metacarpal or digit lacerations <2 cm in size found that more than half had an associated deep structure injury, most commonly a tendon, with extensor tendon defects more common than flexor tendon injuries.[24]

Simple interrupted sutures with 5-0 nonabsorbable suture provide adequate closure for most digital lacerations.[16] Alternatively, small, <2 cm, clean, and uncomplicated hand and digit lacerations can be treated conservatively without wound closure.[27] Although there appears to be no difference in cosmetic appearance or time to return to normal function without wound closure compared with wound closure, this practice has not been widely adopted.

DIGIT AMPUTATIONS

Deep finger lacerations may include partial or complete amputations of the digit. Amputations should involve the consultation of a hand surgeon to discuss the possibility of replantation. Relative indications for replantation are injuries in children, injuries to the thumb, multiple digit amputation, and single digit amputation proximal to the insertion of the flexor digitorum superficialis.[28,29] Goals of replantation are to "preserve 2 sensate digits able to oppose each other"[30] with "motion preferred over strength."[31]

The strongest contraindications to replantation are crush and avulsion injuries because neurovascular damage to the amputated digit is significant and functional outcome is poor. Other relative contraindications include multiple levels of injury to the amputated part, prolonged ischemia time (>24 hours) of the amputated part, patients in poor health, or significant comorbid factors, such as diabetes or severe pulmonary or cardiac disease that may lead to significant perioperative mortality.[28] Another relative contraindication is a smoking history, as replants in smokers are prone to profound vasospasm, leading to loss of the replanted digit. The final relative contraindication for replantation is injuries between the metacarpophalangeal joint and the midlevel of the middle phalanx. Fingers replanted at this level are often stiff due to recurrent tendon adhesions between the flexor digitorum superficialis and flexor digitorum profundus tendons, limiting the function of the adjacent uninjured fingers as well as the reattached finger.

DIGITAL NERVE INJURIES

Suspect digital nerve injuries when static two-point discrimination is distinctly greater on one side of the volar pad than the other, or when it is >10 mm. Digital nerve injuries can be repaired using microsurgical techniques either acutely or days to weeks after the injury. Concomitant injuries and wound contamination are the most common indications for delayed repair. Prognosis depends on the specific injury and the age of the patient. Nerve contusions have variable healing, with a range of 12 days to 6 months. Nerve transection injuries do slightly better than crush injuries, but even with microsurgical repair, recovery is often incomplete.

FINGERTIP INJURIES

Fingertip injuries occur distal to the insertion of the deep flexor and extensor tendons at about the level of the lunula. This location is among the most frequently injured parts of the hand. Such injuries may involve the skin, pulp tissue, distal phalanx, and the perionychium (the nail, nail bed, and surrounding structures) (**Figure 43-7**).[32] The goals of healing are to maintain length and cosmetic appearance and have the fingertip approach normal sensation and function.

DIGITAL TIP INJURIES WITH SKIN AND PULP TISSUE LOSS ONLY

Distal fingertip amputations that are 1 cm^2 or less in size without exposed bone or nail bed involvement can usually be treated conservatively with serial dressing changes alone (Figure 43-8, line A).[32] The key to this technique is the use of nonadherent dressing on the wound itself; this initial dressing is then covered with standard gauze for additional wound protection. Ideally, apply the nonadherent dressing only to the wound itself so that the surrounding intact skin does not become macerated. Provide a follow-up wound check in 2 days. Wound care is vital for proper healing. Instruct the patient to soak the injured fingertip for 10 minutes a day in warm water to which an antibacterial soap has been added, followed by tap-water irrigation and application of a new sterile nonadherent dressing. Change dressings daily for the first 10 to15 days and every other day thereafter. Complete healing may take 4 to 8 weeks. Conservative management of fingertip injuries without bone exposure appears to be superior in terms of cosmetic appearance, improved function, and sensibility of the involved digit.[32] Conservative management is advocated in children <12 years of age, as there is greater regenerative potential in this age group than in adults.

An alternative, but less favored technique, is to use a viable amputated portion as a full-thickness skin graft. The amputated tissue is cleaned and debrided of nonviable tissue, the undersurface of the skin is then defatted with sharp scissors, and the graft is sutured to the defect using

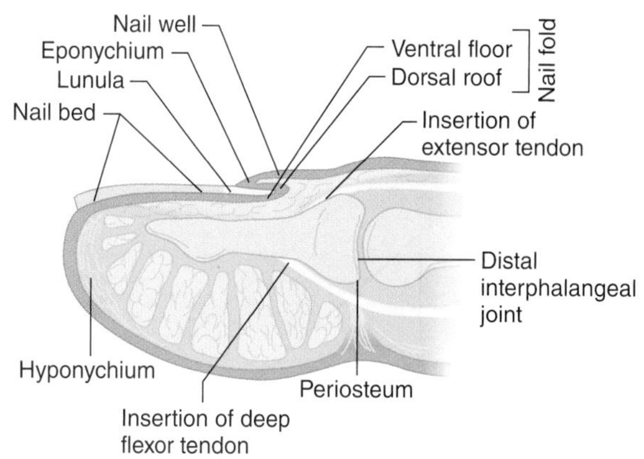

FIGURE 43-7. Anatomy of the perionychium.

percutaneous nylon sutures. Suture ends are left long and tied over a 2×2-cm gauze stent dressing to compress the graft firmly against the fingertip. Unless obvious infection develops, the stented dressing is left undisturbed for 7 to 12 days until follow-up with a hand surgeon. A split- or full-thickness skin graft harvested from a distant site is another means of wound closure in situations in which the severed skin tip is either not available or nonviable, significant pulp tissue loss is >1 cm^2, or the patient's desire to have full use of the hand precludes waiting the 4 to 8 weeks necessary for healing by secondary intention. In these cases, consultation with a hand specialist is appropriate.

DIGITAL TIP INJURIES WITH EXPOSED BONE

Skin grafting will be unsuccessful if a significant loss of tissue at the fingertip exposes the distal phalanx tuft, as bone does not provide adequate vascularity to support donor tissue.[29] Several treatment options exist, and the method used should be based on the best way to preserve the digit length and maintain the sensitivity and functionality of the fingertip. The size and geometry of the injury, the angle of the amputation, and the availability of the amputated tip will determine the options available for repair.[33]

If the bony protuberance is <0.5 cm in length and the soft tissue defect is <1 cm^2, the bone may be trimmed back using a rongeur and the wound left to heal by secondary intention with wound care, as described in Digital Tip Injuries With Skin and Pulp Tissue Loss Only. A dorsal, obliquely angulated wound may be treated in the ED with bone shortening followed by primary closure of the wound using the adjacent volar tissue (**Figure 43-8**, line D). Fat from the local tissue may need to be trimmed to allow wound closure without tension. The nail should be removed, and the nail bed and surrounding structures should be repaired. Although results are comparable to those following conservative management, shortcomings include loss of length as well as tenderness of the fingertip and some degree of functional disability.

Amputations that are angled either in a transverse or volar direction have less favorable outcomes, as there is not always adequate soft tissue and skin coverage to allow for primary closure and preservation of length (**Figure 43-8**, lines B, C, and D). Consultation with a hand surgeon is necessary, as these injuries often require techniques beyond the scope of practice of most emergency physicians.

Incomplete digital tip amputations, defined by the retention of the neurovascular bundle as well as portions of the underlying bone, are among the most difficult injuries to reconstruct and require consultation with a specialist. If adequate circulation is retained in the tip, the injury is treated with fracture reduction, internal pin fixation, and repair of the soft tissue injury. This procedure is optimally performed in the operating room.

Consult a hand surgeon for a complete digital tip amputation occurring proximal to the lunula, to evaluate the potential for replantation in the operating room.[28] Replantation of a complete amputation distal to the lunula is not usually advocated for adults because the procedure is technically demanding and has a generally poor prognosis.

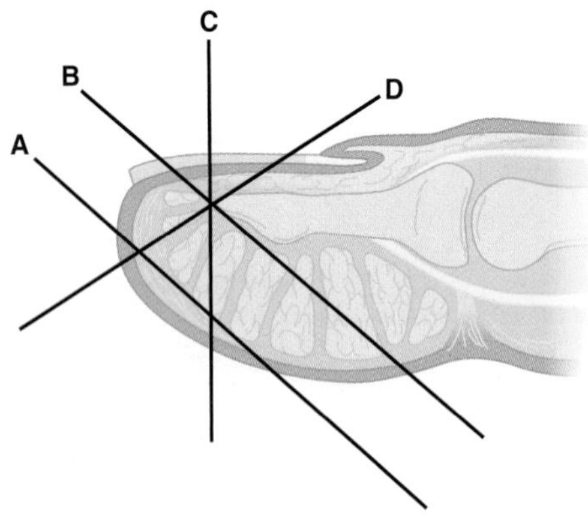

FIGURE 43-8. Fingertip amputations. (**A**) Volar angulation without bone exposure. (**B**) Volar angulation with bone exposure. (**C**) Transverse or perpendicular angulation with bone exposure. (**D**) Dorsal angulation with bone exposure.

However, specialist consultation is indicated in patients with specific occupational concerns and when the affected digit is the thumb or index finger.

Although fingertip injuries are quite common in children, most require only conservative management owing to the rapid healing ability of the young. Repairs in young children should be done using absorbable sutures to eliminate the need for suture removal, as suture removal often requires repeat procedural sedation. Surgical procedures such as grafts and advancement flaps should be avoided. A completely amputated composite tip may be reattached to serve solely as a biologic dressing, and parents should be informed that the tip might necrose, dry up, and turn black as the underlying wound continues to heal. In children <6 years of age, the hand specialist may opt for replantation and revascularization of the composite tip.

INJURIES INVOLVING THE NAIL AND NAIL BED

The nail, nail bed, and surrounding soft tissue make up the perionychium (**Figure 43-7**). The nail bed is made up of the germinal and sterile matrices. The germinal matrix begins at the proximal base of the nail (typically 3 to 5 mm proximal to the eponychium) and extends to the lunula. From there, the sterile matrix extends distally to the hyponychium. Nail injuries can be described as simple nail bed laceration, stellate laceration, severe crush, and complete avulsion. Injury to the perionychium is most commonly due to closure of the fingertip in a door and is usually located at the distal portion of the nail bed. The mechanism of injury is a force directed to the dorsum of the nail, causing it to bend or break, and crushing the nail bed against the unyielding distal phalanx. Distal tuft or phalanx fractures are associated with approximately 50% of nail bed injuries, so imaging of the involved digit(s) is needed, as discussed in the Imaging Studies section. Nail plate deformity permanently affecting nail growth is the most common complication resulting from inadequate treatment.

SUBUNGUAL HEMATOMA

Disruption of the blood vessels of the nail bed without fracture of the nail results in accumulation of blood under the nail. A subungual hematoma that covers >50% is treated with trephination of the nail plate to allow decompression and drainage of the hematoma. Various tools for this purpose include a heated paper clip, electric nail drill, electrocautery, 18-gauge needle, or scalpel. The disadvantages of the heated paper clip include coagulation of the hematoma and introduction of carbon particles into the nail bed, which may delay healing and cause tattooing. Use of a needle, scalpel, or nail drill can be painful and may necessitate a digital nerve block. A hand-held electrocautery device provides rapid and painless trephination. Do not apply alcohol or other flammables to the fingertip before electrocautery, because flames result when electrocautery is then applied. **Simple trephination produces a good to excellent outcome in most patients regardless of subungual hematoma size, injury mechanism, or the presence of fracture.**[34,35] After drainage, instruct patients to soak the affected finger in warm water containing antibacterial soap two to three times a day for 7 days and to follow basic wound-care principles.

NAIL BED INJURIES

Nail removal is recommended only if there is associated partial nail avulsion or surrounding nail fold disruption. Nail removal can be accomplished with adequate anesthesia, elevation of the nail off the nail bed using iris scissors, elevation of the eponychium off the nail, and then removal by gentle longitudinal traction with a hemostat. Tourniquet application to the digit with or without exsanguination may be required to adequately visualize the extent of nail bed laceration. Lacerations of the nail bed should be carefully repaired using 6-0 absorbable sutures to provide a smooth surface so the nail can grow without cosmetic deformity. Tissue adhesives can also be used to repair small nail bed lacerations. The use of tissue adhesives facilitates nail replacement by providing an additional structural anchor and minimizes venous bleeding associated with suturing the delicate nail bed tissue. Crush injuries often result in stellate lacerations, which may require extensive, meticulous repair using magnifying loupes for visualization. Nail bed injuries in children can also be repaired with a good outcome.[36]

Gently cleanse the removed nail with saline, taking care to avoid damage to the germinal matrix. Once the nail is clean, trephinate the nail to prevent the development of a postrepair subungual hematoma, and secure the nail in its anatomic position. To secure the nail, place a 5-0 nonabsorbable suture through the proximal end of the nail plate, and then pass the suture underneath and through the center of the eponychial fold. Once the nail plate is secured in its anatomic position, tie the suture down over the nail. The replaced nail acts as a natural splint to the terminal phalanx, prevents formation of synechiae, and protects the sensitive nail bed. If the nail is not available, nonbiologic stents or a sterile piece of aluminum foil (such as that used to wrap suture materials) may be fashioned to resemble the avulsed nail, inserted under the eponychium, and sutured in place similar to a replaced nail.

Then dress the fingertip with nonadherent gauze, and apply a volar splint to limit distal interphalangeal joint movement. Provide postoperative wound-care instructions (e.g., regarding hand elevation as well as neurovascular checks) and adequate pain relief. Unless obvious purulence is noted, leave the dressing undisturbed for 5 to 7 days. At that time, examine the site for new hematoma formation. The suture attached to the nail can be removed after 3 weeks. The existing nail will be dislodged by the new (growing) nail after an additional 1 to 3 months of growth.

If an associated distal phalanx or tuft fracture coexists with a nail bed laceration, it usually manifests as an avulsion of the nail out of the proximal eponychial fold. In this case, remove the nail, stabilize the fracture by manual reduction, and repair the nail bed as described previously. Once replaced in its anatomic position, the nail serves as a biologic splint to maintain fracture reduction owing to its proximity to the underlying bone. Unstable reductions require consultation with a hand surgeon for internal fixation using Kirschner wires to prevent deformity of the nail bed.

NAIL BED AVULSION INJURIES

Avulsion injuries to the nail bed have the poorest prognosis of any fingertip injury. An avulsion or crush injury may tear the nail completely away from the digit, with fragments of germinal matrix tissue left on the underside of the avulsed nail. These matrix fragments should be preserved for use as free grafts and, when possible, reattached to the nail bed using 6-0 or 7-0 absorbable sutures. When the nail or avulsed nail bed fragments are not available, or if the nail bed defect is large, a full-thickness nail bed graft can be harvested from the patient's toe and sutured into the nail bed of the affected finger. Consultation with a hand surgeon is needed, as these injuries are complex, and repair is technically challenging.

Avulsion injuries may also incompletely tear the proximal portion of the nail out from under the eponychium. Management entails replacement of the nail root into its anatomic position using a series of three horizontal mattress sutures (**Figure 43-9**). One suture is placed through the center and one in each corner of the eponychial fold. The sutures are then passed through the proximal portion of the corresponding segment of avulsed germinal matrix and then back out through the nail fold, pulling the matrix back to its anatomic position.

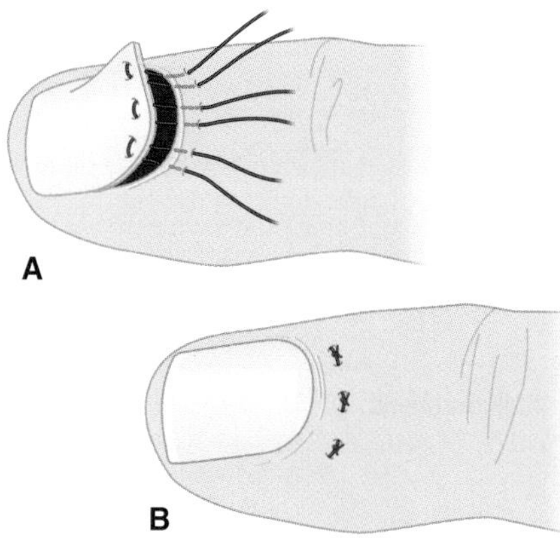

FIGURE 43-9. A and B. Technique for repair of an avulsion of the germinal matrix using three horizontal mattress sutures.

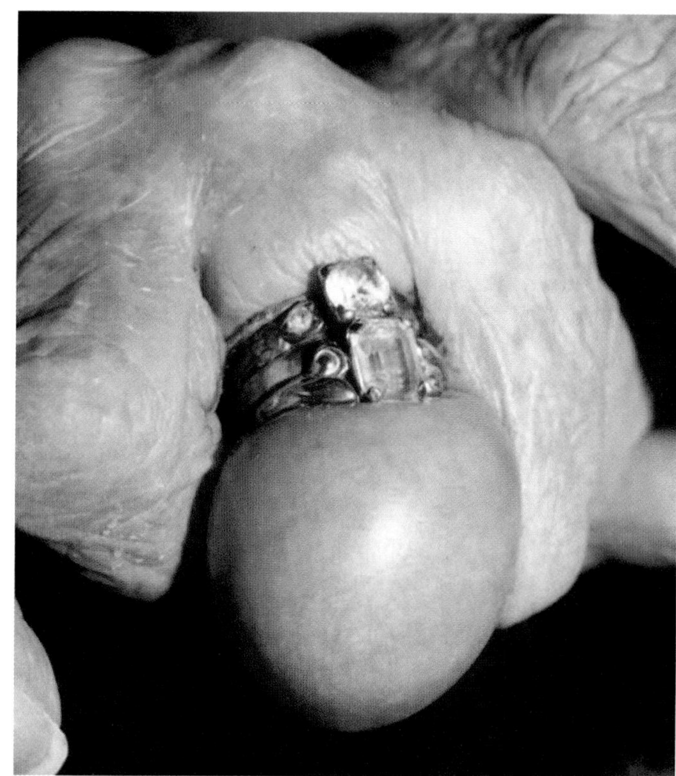

FIGURE 43-10. Tight ring with swollen finger tightly flexed at proximal interphalangeal joint. (Image used with permission of J. Stephan Stapczynski, MD.)

RING TOURNIQUET SYNDROME

A tight ring encircling the proximal phalanx may become entrapped as a result of distal swelling (**Figure 43-10**). As the digit expands, venous outflow is restricted by the tight ring, producing more swelling. This vicious cycle may lead to nerve damage, ischemia, and digital gangrene. The presence of impaired sensation (diminished static two-point discrimination) or diminished perfusion (delayed capillary refill) indicates significant constriction. Rapid ring removal is then warranted, typically cutting the ring. If sensation and perfusion are intact, removal can be attempted with slower techniques that preserve the ring. However, if there is an underlying phalangeal fracture, it is prudent to cut the ring.

In all ring-preservation methods (string technique, rubber band technique), the hand should be elevated to encourage venous and lymphatic drainage and thus reduce swelling. Additionally, the finger can be circumferentially wrapped with a $^1/_2$- to 1-in. elastic band (e.g., Penrose drain), starting from the distal tip and winding the band tightly around the finger, progressing toward the proximal phalanx to reduce swelling. Leave the wrap in place for several minutes before it is unwrapped and the ring is removed. A digital nerve block or other method of regional anesthesia is often required prior to ring removal. A metacarpal or tendon sheath block produces less swelling of the finger but may not provide as much anesthesia as a digital block.[37] After ring removal, reassess sensation and perfusion.

REFERENCES

The complete reference list is available online at www.TintinalliEM.com.

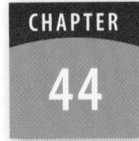

Leg and Foot Lacerations

Annabella Salvador-Kelly
Nancy Kwon

INTRODUCTION

Lower extremity injuries most frequently involve the lower leg and ankle, followed by the foot and toes, hip, and then knee.[1] Lacerations and wounds occur from sports and recreational activity,[2-8] tools and equipment,[9-11] occupational activity,[12] and explosions.[13]

ANATOMY

In the foot, the plantar epidermis and dermis are thick, except in the arch area. This thick skin is able to withstand the force produced by a moving body but is also quite sensitive to two-point discrimination and pressure. The heel has an 18-mm-thick modified pad of fat separated into chambers by fibrous septae. There is an additional broad internal fibrous arch, called the *inner cup ligament*, which helps maintain the shape of the heel. The skin of the sole readily hypertrophies and can become quite thickened, especially in people who walk barefoot. The dense fibrous fatty tissue of the ball of the foot and heel makes wound exploration and visualization difficult in the ED.

In contrast to the protective plantar surface, skin on the dorsal aspect of the foot and the entire ankle provides little protection for underlying tendons, nerves, and blood vessels. The dorsum of the foot, the ankle, and the pretibial surface are particularly vulnerable to blunt-force injuries. Most lacerations on the dorsal foot and in the ankle area are easily explored, except for posterior ankle lacerations, a limitation when partial laceration of the Achilles tendon is considered. Lacerations involving the shin, calf, and thigh usually present few problems regarding wound exploration and visualization.

Several important tendons in the leg are at risk for injury. The fibularis longus and fibularis brevis (also known as the peroneus longus and peroneus brevis) tendons, which contribute to foot plantar flexion and eversion, run behind the lateral malleolus and can be lacerated at this location (**Figure 44-1**). The extensor hallucis longus tendon, which extends the first toe, runs along the top of the first metatarsal and may be injured when heavy objects are dropped on the foot. The Achilles tendon, the primary contributor to foot plantar flexion, may be severed by penetrating injuries to the posterior ankle. Lacerations of the shin rarely involve vital nerves or tendons. Infrapatellar lacerations can transect the patellar tendon, resulting in inability to extend the leg. Suprapatellar lacerations may involve the quadriceps tendon, also resulting in impaired knee extension.

Sensory nerves predominate in the foot, with most motor control of the foot being performed by nerves and muscles in the lower leg (**Figures 44-2 and 44-3**). **The exceptions to this generalization are that the posterior tibial nerve innervates the intrinsic foot musculature, and the deep peroneal nerve innervates the extensor digitorum brevis and extensor hallucis brevis muscles; injuries to these nerves may result in toe clawing.**[14] The common peroneal nerve can be injured in complex fractures, sharp injuries, or lacerations of the lower extremity resulting in foot drop (**Figure 44-4**).[15]

Arterial injury resulting from penetrating and blast wounds most commonly affects the superficial femoral, popliteal, crural, common femoral, and deep femoral arteries (**Figure 44-5**).[16] Arterial injuries are at high risk for limb loss.[17]

ASSESSMENT

HISTORY

Obtain a description of the mechanism of injury, assessing the potential for damage to underlying tissue, the risk of a retained foreign body, and degree of potential contamination. Determine the time interval from injury to evaluation, because delayed presentations can increase the incidence of infection. Inquire about foreign body sensation, paresthesias, anesthesia, weakness, or loss of function suggesting a nerve, vascular, or tendon injury.

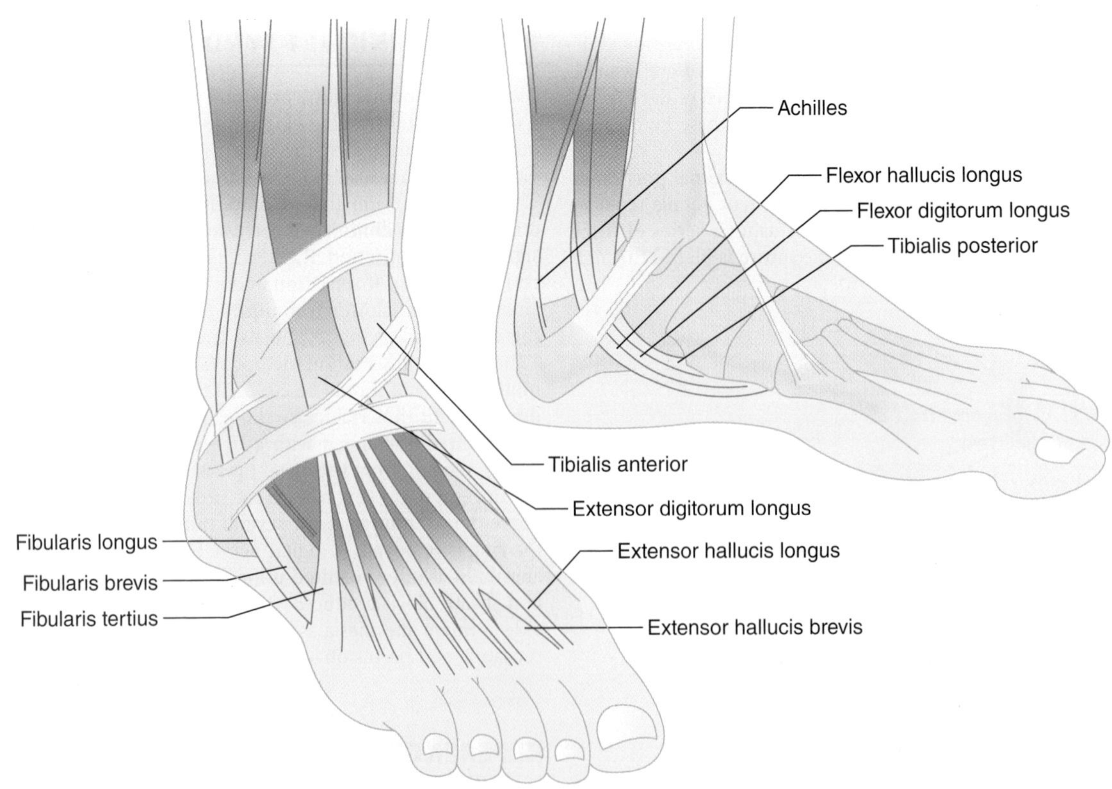

FIGURE 44-1. Tendons of the foot.

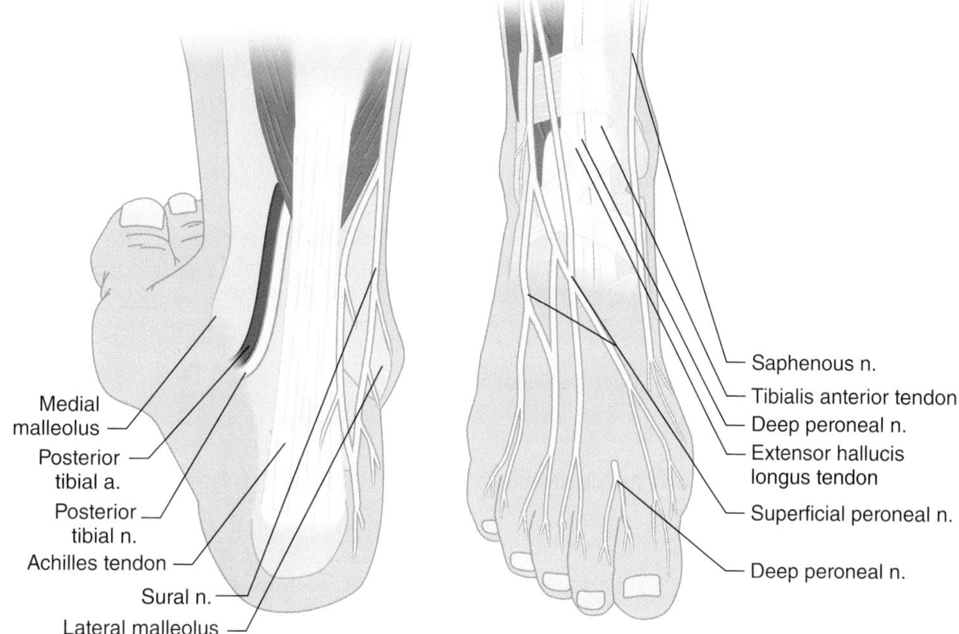

FIGURE 44-2. Nerves of the foot. a. = artery; n. = nerve.

The patient's age influences wound healing and functional status following the injury. Ask about tetanus immunization status and conditions that increase the risk for infection or delayed wound healing such as diabetes, immunosuppression, or vascular disease. Note the social history, because patients who smoke, consume alcohol, or use illicit substances may be at additional risk of poor healing secondary to vascular disease.

PHYSICAL EXAMINATION

Inspect the wound, noting its location and proximity to underlying nerves or arteries. General appearance, obvious injuries, or visible foreign bodies should be noted; more detailed wound exploration typically waits until after anesthesia and radiographs, if needed. If a nerve laceration is suspected, light touch and/or static two-point

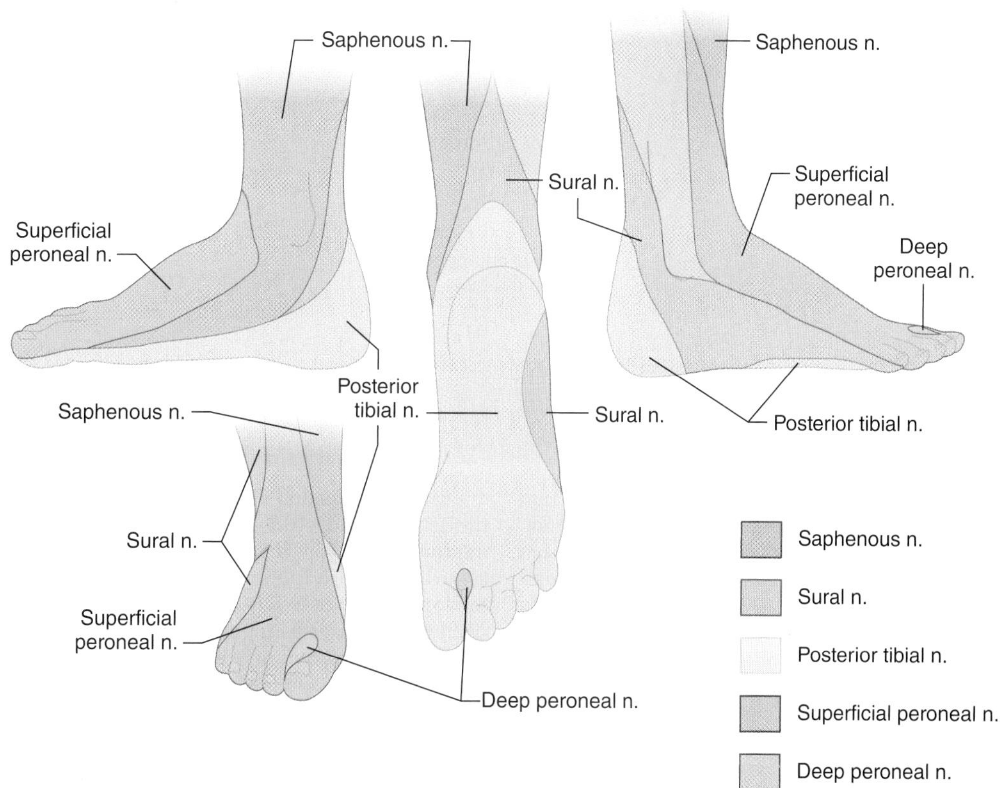

FIGURE 44-3. Sensory innervation of the foot. n. = nerve.

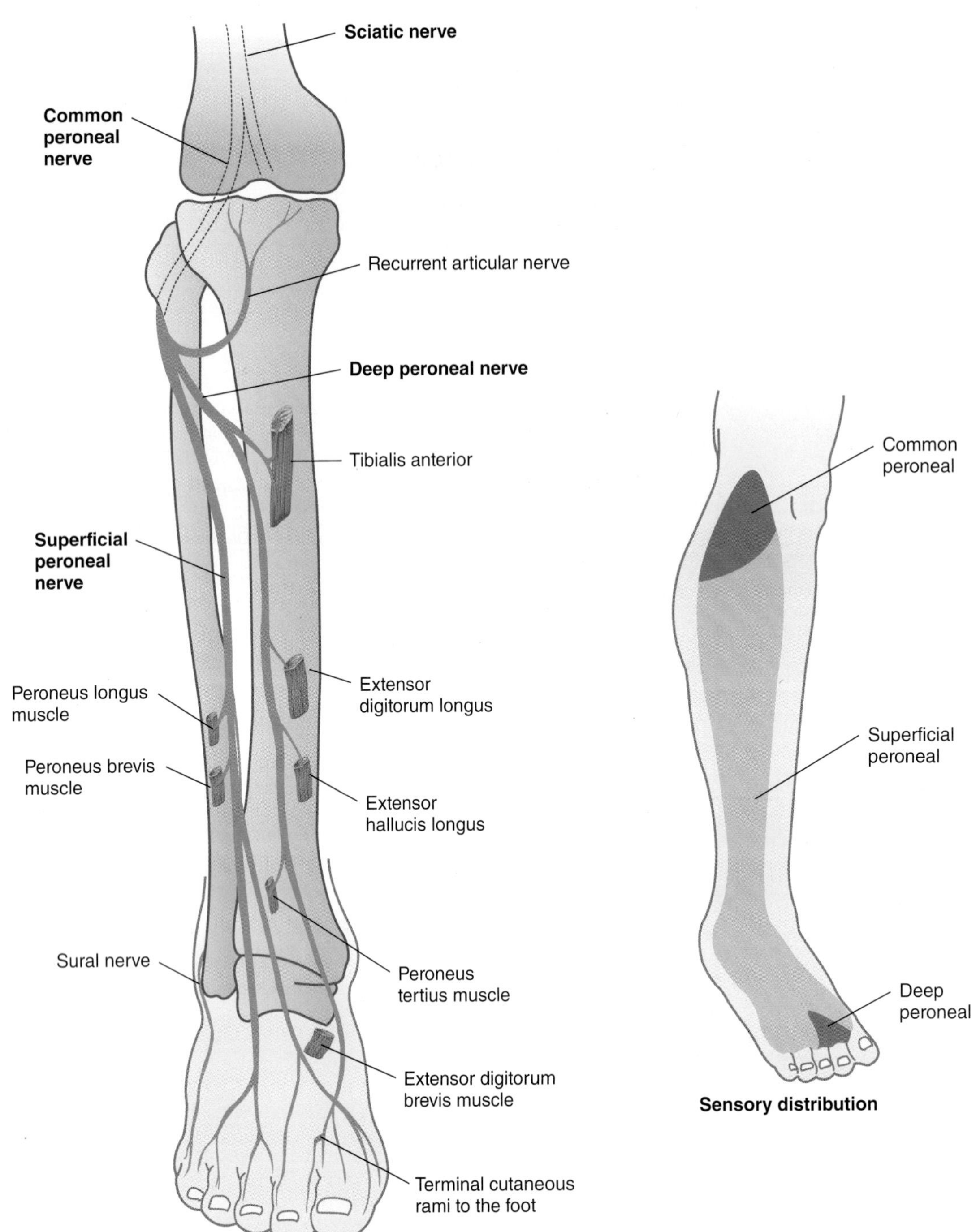

FIGURE 44-4. Common peroneal nerve. [Reproduced with permission from: Waxman SG: Appendix C. Spinal nerves and plexuses. In: Waxman SG (ed): *Clinical Neuroanatomy,* 27th ed. New York, NY: McGraw-Hill; 2013. Figure C-16.]

discrimination should be tested in the foot and toes and compared with the uninjured side. Two-point discrimination varies in the foot, with normal values of 1.5 cm in the hind, mid, and forefoot, and <1 cm in the big toe, but these measures are not reliable in patients with diabetes or peripheral vascular disease.[18] Sensory deficits to the foot can result in significant long-term morbidity. Motor function may be easier to assess after anesthesia or reduction of an associated fracture or dislocation. Obtain prompt surgical consultation if motor nerve or major sensory nerve injury is identified because primary repair may be indicated.[14] Nerve injuries caused by open blunt injuries are not typically repaired at the time of injury, in part because of the risk of infection and in part because of the possibility that a contused nerve will regain function without surgical intervention.

Evaluate for tendon injuries by assessing motor function, palpating the tendon, and observing the tendon through its entire range of motion. A partially injured tendon may be noted to "catch" on the synovial sheath during range of motion. Lacerations of the Achilles tendon may be easily visualized with simple exploration through the open wound, by palpating a defect in the tendon, or by US. Sometimes, the tendon laceration may not be visible or palpable, and presence of active plantar flexion of the foot cannot be used to exclude the injury. The Achilles tendon is not the only structure responsible for plantar flexion of the foot—the tibialis posterior muscle flexes the foot at the ankle. The Thompson test can assist in detecting an Achilles tendon rupture. The patient lies prone on the examination cart with the feet hanging over the edge of the bed, and the examiner places one hand on

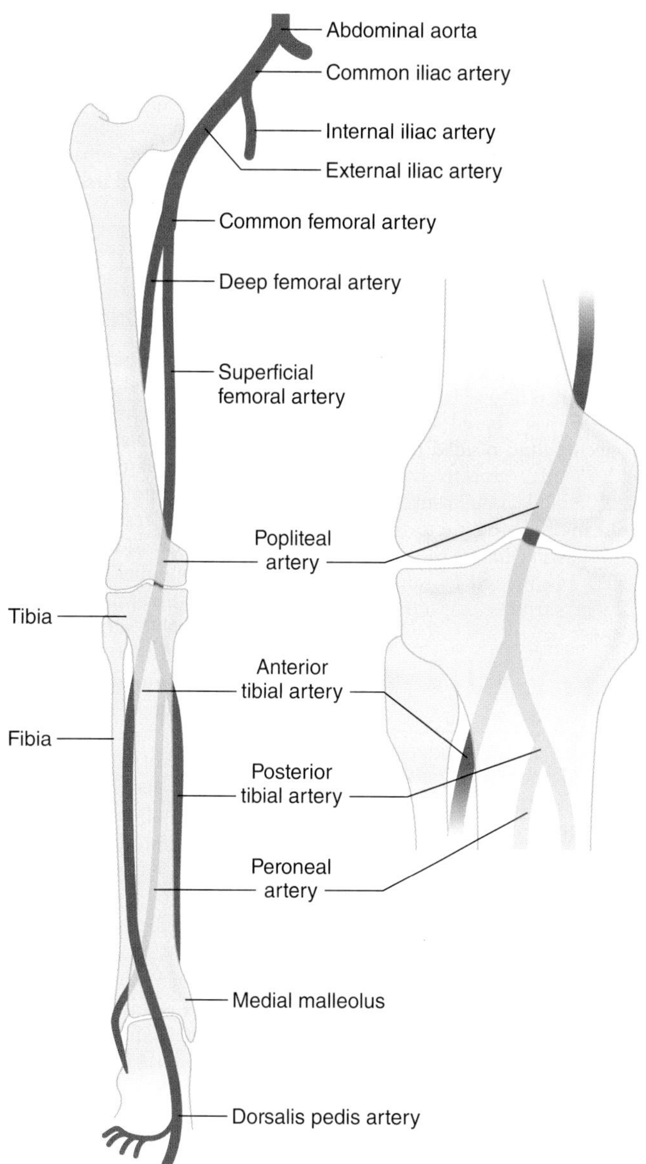

FIGURE 44-5. Major arteries of the leg.

each mid-calf (**Figure 44-6**). If the Achilles tendon is intact, the foot plantar flexes when the calf is squeezed, and comparison with the unaffected side is helpful to detect subtle movement. A positive Thompson test is when the affected foot does not flex, indicative of an Achilles tendon rupture.[19]

Document the location, length, estimated depth, and general shape of the wound. Provide anesthesia, cleanse the wound, and carefully inspect the full extent of the wound for foreign bodies. The loose, thin skin over the dorsum of the foot allows for adequate visual, digital, and instrument exploration for tendon lacerations, as well as for foreign body discovery. The dense tissue of the plantar surface of the foot limits wound visualization, and the risk of creating further injury limits exploration. An exception to this general rule of limited exploration on the weight-bearing plantar surface is in an infected wound with suspected foreign body. With significant injury to the leg, like a crush injury, consider compartment syndrome and evaluate accordingly.

ANCILLARY STUDIES

Obtain radiographs when a fracture, radiopaque foreign body, or joint penetration is suspected.[20,21] Foregoing radiographs and using wound exploration alone to exclude a foreign body is a reasonable approach, but carries a

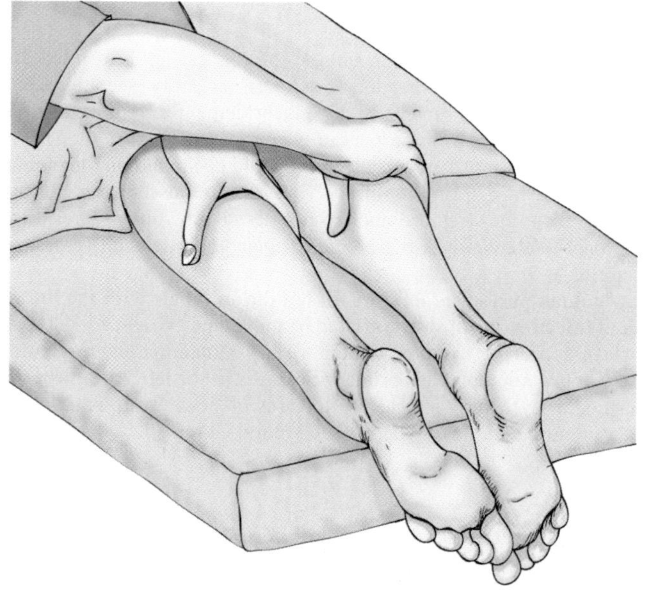

FIGURE 44-6. Thompson test.

small risk of missing a retained object.[22-24] CT or MRI can detect retained organic material. Bedside US may identify retained foreign bodies and detect tendon lacerations and fractures (see chapter 45, "Soft Tissue Foreign Bodies"). Fluoroscopy is a useful dynamic imaging modality that may assist in identifying and removing foreign bodies. No single imaging modality or wound exploration will identify every foreign body; emphasize close follow-up if the mechanism of injury suggests a potential for a foreign body but none was identified on imaging or wound exploration.

Lacerations in proximity to joint spaces may penetrate the articular space. Detecting joint penetration by physical examination alone is often difficult. Intra-articular gas on plain radiograph is a sign of joint penetration. **If the radiograph does not display intra-articular gas, use the saline load test to determine joint integrity, especially in the knee and ankle.**[25,26] Inject sufficient amounts of saline to adequately stress the capsule, because false-negative results may be obtained if too little fluid is injected.[27,28] Volumes injected into the knee may vary based on the location of the approach; mean volumes of injected fluid needed for a positive result are approximately 65 mL and 95 mL, respectively, at the inferomedial and superomedial locations.[26-28] Fluid leaking from the wound indicates joint penetration. **Do not add methylene blue** to the injected saline to aid in visualization of fluid existing in the wound because it does not increase diagnostic accuracy compared to saline alone and the resultant staining of the articular surfaces may affect operative management of intra-articular injuries.[29]

TREATMENT

ANESTHESIA

Anesthesia can be administered by topical, local, or regional routes. The toes can be anesthetized using standard digital blocks. Epinephrine-containing local anesthetics can be safely used for digital blocks in toes (see chapter 36, "Local and Regional Anesthesia").

Lacerations to the dorsum of the foot can be sufficiently anesthetized by infiltration of local anesthetic. The plantar surface of the foot is sensitive to the infiltration of a local anesthetic, so regional nerve blocks may be helpful. The sural nerve block and the posterior tibial nerve block (see chapter 36) are the two most commonly used nerve blocks for the foot. Topical local anesthetic preparations can achieve adequate anesthesia on the dorsum of the foot and leg, but may be ineffective on the dense epidermis of the plantar surface of the foot. In children, distraction techniques, use of child-life specialists, anxiolytics, and conscious sedation may help alleviate anxiety and pain response (see chapter 113, "Pain Management and Procedural Sedation in Infants and Children").

WOUND PREPARATION

Wound irrigation with copious amounts of saline is recommended due to the increased risk of infection with lower extremity lacerations (see chapter 40, "Wound Preparation").[30-32] Debridement to remove devitalized tissue is an important aspect of wound care to reduce the risk of wound complications, but debridement should be limited on the plantar surface of the foot or on the shin because skin in those areas is not pliable enough to be stretched and cover a defect. Any opening resulting from debridement would then require repair under tension across the laceration.

A "golden period" of 6 hours for laceration repair with the lowest risk of infection is not substantiated by published evidence.[32-34] Repair of clean-appearing wounds without visible contamination presenting after 6 hours is acceptable if primary closure is felt beneficial. Otherwise, consider delayed primary closure in cases of delayed presentation or heavy contamination (see chapter 41 "Wound Closure").

WOUND CLOSURE

Wound location, size, and shape guide the decision to close with adhesive strips, sutures, or staples. Staples are acceptable for linear lacerations through the dermis as long as the wound is sharp with straight and accurately aligned wound edges, minimizing the potential for scar formation. Most foot and leg lacerations do not have these characteristics, so using staples will often result in less aesthetic wound healing.[31] Staples should not be used on the foot because they are uncomfortable when attempting to walk during recovery. Lacerations of the lower extremity can be under increased wound tension compared with other anatomic sites, so these lacerations are frequently repaired using techniques such as multiple-layered closure or horizontal mattress closure.

FOOT AND ANKLE LACERATIONS

DIGITAL LACERATIONS

Digital lacerations frequently require special attention. Nail bed injuries often accompany digital fractures. Clinical signs such as bleeding from the eponychium and a laceration proximal to the nail bed suggest a possible open fracture.[35] Nail bed lacerations place the underlying bone at risk for bacterial contamination because the skin is directly attached to the periosteum with no intervening layer of subcutaneous tissue. Missed open fractures have resulted in osteomyelitis and growth delay of the digit in children. Consider removal of the nail to evaluate for nail bed laceration if a subungual hematoma occupies a large portion of the nail plate or if there is disruption of the nail or nail folds.[36] Repair the nail bed with either absorbable sutures or tissue adhesives.[37] Nail bed lacerations are considered to be open fractures of the distal phalanx, so prophylactic antibiotics are recommended.[35] Conversely, simple nail trephination is adequate for drainage of subungual hematomas without nail or nail fold deformities.

Tendon injuries of the digits may require consultation, especially when the extensor hallucis longus is involved, because injury to this tendon impairs functionality during the swing phase of the gait cycle. Surgery is often recommended for patients with extensor hallucis longus tendon lacerations, and grafting may be needed.[38,39]

INTERDIGITAL LACERATIONS

Lacerations between the toes are difficult to repair because the confined interdigital space is difficult to access for suturing. An assistant gently separating the toes enhances the exploration and repair of interdigital lacerations. Simple interrupted sutures often lead to skin inversion and risk of failure of the initial wound repair with interdigital lacerations. The more effective closure technique, albeit somewhat more difficult to perform, is to place horizontal or vertical mattress sutures. Use 5-0 monofilament nonabsorbable sutures on a small cutting needle. Use monofilament absorbable sutures in young children, thus avoiding suture removal. When a web space laceration involves the neurovascular bundle, the skin is usually closed without attempting to repair the neurovascular injury, followed by subsequent referral to a specialist.

HAIR-THREAD TOURNIQUET SYNDROME

Hair-thread tourniquet syndrome, also referred to as *acquired constriction ring syndrome*, is an unusual type of toe injury usually seen during infancy[40] and rarely seen in older children.[41] A long strand of hair or thread becomes wrapped around a toe, often producing strangulation and digital ischemia. This can be an occult source of irritability for infants.[40] Complete removal is required to restore perfusion and allow skin healing. Two standard approaches to salvage the compromised digit are to either unwind the hair or thread if possible or, otherwise, make a midline longitudinal incision along the extensor surface of the toe to cut the hair or thread.[42] To cut the hair, it will often be necessary to split the fibers of the extensor ligament, but avoid transecting the fibers. The multiple strands of hair or thread are then removed using fine forceps without teeth. The toe often retains the initial appearance, making the physician uncertain whether all of the strands have been removed or cut. A novel but unvalidated method is to apply hair-dissolving compounds.[43] Hair-thread tourniquet syndrome can cause deep cutaneous lacerations that result in tendon lacerations requiring operative repair.[44] Hair-thread tourniquet syndrome is not the result of intentional injury and does not warrant reporting as suspected child abuse.[45]

PLANTAR FOOT LACERATIONS

Repairing a laceration on the plantar surface is best done with the patient placed in a prone position, with the foot overhanging the cart or elevated by placing a pillow beneath the ankle. A large suture needle with thick thread is required to penetrate the hypertrophied epidermis and dermis of the sole of the foot. If there is tissue loss or the site is under tension, vertical mattress sutures may be required. In the arch area, achieving tissue eversion can be difficult. Do not use adhesive tapes, tissue adhesives, and staples on the plantar surface. Small or superficial wounds to the plantar surface typically heal rapidly without sutures. Repair small plantar lacerations if the wound gapes open or there is a risk for infection.

DORSAL FOOT AND ANKLE LACERATIONS

Dorsal surface lacerations are repaired almost exclusively with nonabsorbable, monofilament suture material, most commonly 4-0 or 5-0 for small lacerations. Use careful technique suturing the skin to avoid vessels, nerves, and tendons that lie just under the surface. Deep sutures are not recommended for the same reason. Running sutures are acceptable on the dorsal surface, and smaller lacerations may be closed with adhesive tapes or tissue adhesives. For lacerations under tension, consider applying a splint to restrict movement, allowing for healing during the first 5 to 7 days.

The decision to repair tendon lacerations in the foot depends on the functional impairment caused by the injury compared with the benefits of repair. Many extensor tendon lacerations involving the mid-foot and forefoot can go unrepaired without compromising foot function. The skin is closed and the foot splinted, leaving the injured tendon alone. Lacerations of the extensor hallucis longus or tibialis anterior require consultation with an orthopedist or podiatrist because dorsiflexion of the great toe and foot are important in walking and running.[39,46] Closure without tendon suturing and with immediate mobilization is acceptable in patients with partial lacerations of the extensor hallucis longus tendon.[39]

Flexor tendon lacerations across the toes (excluding the great toe) can usually be left unrepaired without significant functional sequelae, but occasionally a hammer toe or claw toe deformity develops. Lacerations of the flexor hallucis longus are frequently repaired, although long-term benefit is unproven, even in athletes.[46]

LEG LACERATIONS

PRETIBIAL LACERATIONS

Managing pretibial skin lacerations, especially in the elderly patient with comorbidities, is challenging. These wounds often occur on the distal third of the pretibial region, which is poorly vascularized and slow to heal. Pretibial wounds are approached according to the type and severity (**Table 44-1**).[47,48]

Wounds where the edges can be approximated without tension can be closed with adhesive tapes or simple sutures. Wounds with tension can be closed using horizontal mattress sutures with 4-0 nonabsorbable sutures. Occasionally, the 4-0 suture is too fine and cuts through the skin, so use 3-0 sutures. The natural contraction of the thin skin makes closure more difficult because sutures often cut through the fragile skin when attempting to approximate the wound edges. A technique to overcome this problem is to re-enforce the wound edges with adhesive tape applied along the edges before closure with placement of percutaneous sutures penetrating through the adhesive tape.[49-51] Additionally, to minimize tension across the wound, tincture of benzoin can be applied over the sutures, and then broad adhesive tape strips (1/2 in.) can be placed over the sutures to minimize tension across the wound. Alternatively, the wound edges can be held in place by adhesive strips perpendicular to the wound, with sutures placed through the strips, thereby removing the shear force of the strip on the skin.

Flap lacerations with significant skin loss are best repaired with primary excision and skin grafting.[48,52] Apply a foam adhesive dressing (such as 3M™ Tegaderm™; 3M, St. Paul, MN) to absorb exudate and reduce healing time.[53] Patients should remain ambulatory during the healing of pretibial injuries, even after skin grafting.[54] Protecting the repair from the tension created by foot plantarflexion is useful; consider using a lightweight plastic ankle-foot orthosis.[55]

TABLE 44-1 Pretibial Lacerations

Classification	Description	Management
Ia	Simple linear laceration not under tension	Primary closure with adhesive strips or sutures
Ib	Simple linear laceration under tension	Primary closure using methods to reduce skin tension
IIa	Flap laceration with no skin loss and/or wound hematoma	Close with adhesive strips
IIb	Flap laceration with some necrosis and/or hematoma	Excise small nonviable areas; close with adhesive strips
III	Flap laceration with significant skin loss or necrosis	Primary excision and skin grafting under local anesthesia
IV	Degloving injury	Plastic surgery consult

KNEE LACERATIONS

Close simple lacerations in the knee area with 4-0 nonabsorbable sutures, using interrupted or horizontal mattress sutures because of the marked active skin tension in this area. **As already noted, assess for joint capsule penetration and laceration of the patellar and quadriceps tendons.** The common peroneal nerve is prone to injury as it runs over the head of the fibula laterally, so distal limb motor function should be assessed (foot eversion and dorsiflexion). Deep popliteal wounds can injure the popliteal artery and tibial nerve. Popliteal artery injuries typically require emergent repair because, in most individuals, there is minimal collateral circulation at the level of the knee (Figure 44-5).

The knee should be splinted or placed in a knee immobilizer to decrease active tension and promote better wound healing. Knee area lacerations in children can be closed with tissue adhesives and splints to restrict movement.

PROXIMAL LOWER EXTREMITY LACERATIONS

Proximal lower extremity lacerations are usually straightforward, and thickness of the soft tissue layers helps to prevent injury to vital structures. Lacerations to the proximal lower extremity also have less tension on them, allowing for easier exploration, debridement, and repair. Assess lacerations to the proximal femoral area for injuries to the femoral artery, vein, and nerve. Although acute traumatic femoral artery injuries are uncommon, they are associated with a high incidence of limb loss and morbidity.[17]

DISPOSITION AND FOLLOW-UP

Most patients with lower extremity lacerations will be able to go home after ED evaluation and treatment. Patients at high risk for compartment syndrome, those with limited mobility and inadequate home assistance, and patients requiring operative repair should be admitted. Patients may require ancillary devices such as crutches, walkers, and wheelchairs. Elevation of the extremity decreases swelling and infection risk. Sutures are typically removed in 10 to 14 days.

Significant tendon lacerations of the lower extremity are usually repaired a few days to weeks after the initial injury. Treatment in the ED consists of skin closure; splinting of the foot, ankle, and leg; initiation of prophylactic antibiotics; instruction for non–weight-bearing crutch use; and arrangement for the patient to follow up with an orthopedist or podiatrist.

SPECIAL CONSIDERATIONS

AGE CONSIDERATIONS

The preverbal child may have particular difficulty limiting movement of the injured extremity and is more likely to contaminate the wound.

Generous dressings aid in protecting any lower extremity laceration; the general rule is **"the smaller the child, the larger the dressing."**

Elderly patients tend to have thin skin and decreased subcutaneous fat, especially over the pretibial surface, making wound edges more difficult to appose, resulting in closure under tension. Additionally, fragile skin in elderly patients predisposes sutures to tear through the skin. Adhesive tapes may be needed to reinforce the closure. Elderly patients are more likely to have medical conditions that can delay wound healing and are less likely to be adequately immunized against tetanus. Assess for fall risk and the ability to perform daily tasks after repair and immobilization of the injured leg.

AMPUTATION

Reimplantation of a severed toe is not typically performed. Reattachment of an amputated great toe, forefoot, or entire foot is occasionally done, although it is extremely complex. Immediate consultation with a reimplantation surgeon is essential in such circumstances. Any severed part should be gently washed (not scrubbed) with sterile saline to remove gross debris, wrapped in saline-soaked gauze, and placed in a plastic bag that is then closed and placed in an ice water bath.

RETAINED FOREIGN BODIES

Retained (nonreactive) foreign bodies, such as glass, can pose a problem. Chronic pain, especially during walking, can occur if the material is not removed. In the absence of chronic discomfort, inert foreign bodies can remain in the foot, where they typically become encapsulated without causing injury or infection. Conversely, reactive organic material does not become encapsulated and does promote infection. Therefore, reactive organic material should be aggressively identified and removed. Fluoroscopy may be useful to help locate and remove radiopaque foreign bodies. Deep foreign bodies in the foot can be extremely difficult to remove in the ED, and such cases are best referred to the surgeon for location and removal in the operating room.

PROPHYLACTIC ANTIBIOTICS

Although infection occurs in 3% to 8% of lower extremity lacerations, and up to 34% of plantar lacerations, there is no evidence to support routine antibiotic prophylaxis in uncomplicated lacerations (see chapter 47, "Postrepair Wound Care"). However, use prophylactic antibiotics for complicated lacerations in the setting of bites, open fractures, tendon or joint involvement, presence of foreign debris, and obvious infections.[56] Diabetes and other predisposing medical conditions, wound contamination, and laceration length greater than 5 cm are factors that predispose to wound infection.[32]

Similar to wound infections in other parts of the body, most lower extremity wound infections are due to either *Staphylococcus* and/or *Streptococcus* species. Animal bites to the leg and foot require coverage against *Staphylococcus, Streptococcus,* and *Pasteurella.* Asplenic or immunocompromised patients who sustain a dog bite should receive coverage against *Capnocytophaga canimorsus.* Amoxicillin-clavulanate will cover all four organisms

The most common organisms causing soft tissue infections in plantar puncture wounds are *Staphylococcus* and *Streptococcus. Pseudomonas aeruginosa* is a frequent cause of osteomyelitis and osteochondritis when the puncture occurs through the sole of a shoe.[57] **Open fractures should receive antibiotic prophylaxis. Consensus practice guidelines typically recommend coverage for gram-positive organisms for grade I and II open fractures, with added coverage for grade III injuries.**[58]

Acknowledgment: The authors gratefully acknowledge the contributions of Timothy F. Platts-Mills and the authors of this chapter in the previous editions.

REFERENCES

The complete reference list is available online at www.TintinalliEM.com.

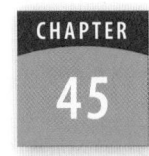

Soft Tissue Foreign Bodies

Richard L. Lammers

INTRODUCTION

Soft tissue foreign bodies may be encountered when managing new wounds or evaluating complications of old wounds. This chapter discusses methods of detecting and removing them.

Methodically search fresh wounds for contamination by foreign material. If a foreign body is discovered within a wound cavity or deeply embedded in tissue, decide if removal of the material is urgent, can be delayed, or is even necessary. The decision to remove foreign bodies located below the dermal layer of skin depends on the size, location, composition, accessibility, and anticipated mechanical and inflammatory effects of the object. Many foreign bodies should be removed in the ED. For example, all foreign material within the cavities of fresh lacerations should be irrigated away, debrided, or extracted with instruments. Occasionally, patients with subcutaneous foreign bodies should be referred to appropriate specialists for delayed removal.

Most foreign bodies are detectable during clinical examination.[1,2] Imaging studies are used to evaluate wounds when a concealed object is possibly present.[3]

PATHOPHYSIOLOGY

Transient inflammation is an integral part of normal wound healing. A small amount of foreign debris in a wound provokes an inflammatory response in an effort to eliminate or contain the invader. Large quantities of devitalized tissue, foreign debris, bacteria, or other irritants present within a wound intensify this protective response. Excessive or prolonged inflammation delays wound healing and destroys surrounding soft tissue and bone, producing periosteal reactions, osteolytic lesions, synovitis, and arthritis. If the body fails to dissolve or extrude foreign material, it may become encapsulated within a fibrous capsule. Once a retained foreign body is encapsulated, inflammation subsides.

The type, timing, and intensity of an inflammatory reaction are determined primarily by the chemical composition and physical form of the foreign object. Material that is inert—such as glass, metal, or plastic—may not elicit any abnormal tissue response. Objects with smooth, nonporous surfaces produce less inflammation and fibrosis than those with rough surfaces. Most metals are inert, but those that oxidize will cause mild to moderate inflammation. Earrings with studs dipped in gold paint cause earlobe swelling and inflammation when the paint flakes off. Vegetative foreign bodies, such as wood, thorns, and spines, trigger the most severe inflammatory reactions. Sea urchin spines, other marine foreign bodies, and hair may cause chronic inflammation with granuloma formation.

In some cases, inflammation is caused by a local toxic reaction. For example, blackthorns contain an alkaloid that produces intense inflammation. The oils and resins in redwood and cedar splinters also cause considerable inflammation. Sea urchin spines and catfish spines contain venom that causes severe burning pain at the puncture site and a variety of systemic symptoms (see chapter 213, "Marine Trauma and Envenomation"). A sudden, local inflammatory reaction from a rose thorn or cactus spine may be an allergic response to fungi on the plant. Some cacti cause a delayed hypersensitivity reaction. Systemic toxic and allergic reactions are unusual but serious complications of foreign bodies. Although toxicity is unlikely, foreign bodies containing lead, such as bullets, have the potential to produce systemic lead poisoning, particularly if they are in contact with pleural, peritoneal, cerebrospinal, or joint fluid.[4,5]

Infections are the most common complication of retained foreign bodies, producing local wound infection, cellulitis, abscess formation, lymphangitis, tenosynovitis, bursitis, septic arthritis, and osteomyelitis.[6,7] Infections associated with retained soft tissue foreign bodies are characteristically resistant to therapy; antibiotics, anti-inflammatory drugs, and steroids may produce a partial regression but seldom eradicate the infection.[8]

Some infections will resolve spontaneously once the foreign bodies are removed. Bacteria are infrequently detected after plant thorn injuries, possibly due to the empiric use of antibiotics, but when bacteria are found, *Pantoea agglomerans* is the most commonly reported isolate.[9,10] Vegetative foreign bodies may also cause fungal infections, particularly in immunosuppressed patients.

Foreign objects can also cause mechanical damage by compressing or lacerating anatomic structures or occluding vessels. Repeated movement of tissue containing a foreign object increases the fibrous reaction.

CLINICAL FEATURES

HISTORY

Every wound has the potential for concealing a foreign body, but only a small percentage of lacerations and puncture wounds actually contain them.[1,2,11] Historical factors associated with a higher risk for a retained foreign body include the mechanism of injury, composition and shape of the wounding object, and the shape and location of the resulting wound. Blows to the mouth may fracture teeth, embedding fragments in the lip, tongue, or buccal mucosa of the patient or in the hand of the assailant.[12-14] Objects that shatter, splinter, or break in the process of causing a wound often leave remnants behind. Thorns, spines, and sharp wooden branches are usually brittle and tend to penetrate deeply into puncture wounds before breaking. Wood splinters are notorious for fragmenting, especially when they are pulled out of a puncture wound.

Patients impaled by long, thin metallic objects, such as hypodermic or sewing needles, may remove them without realizing that a portion of the object broke off beneath the skin surface. Both remnants of a needle and impurities in street drugs can cause persistent pain or abscess formation at the site of IV drug use. Nails that penetrate socks and shoes may drive leather, rubber, or cloth into the plantar surface of a patient's foot. Blunt objects with a diameter >4.5 mm may push a plug of skin deep into a wound, resulting in an epidermal inclusion cyst. If any object pulled from a wound does not appear intact, the wound should be explored for further contaminants.

The patient's description of a foreign body sensation in a fresh wound is a useful sign in adults—the perception of a foreign body more than doubles the likelihood of one being present.[11] However, foreign body sensation is less useful in verbal-age children.[15] If a patient reports a sudden, sharp pain on the bottom of the foot while walking barefoot, consider the possibility of impalement with a needle, toothpick, splinter, or shard of glass.

Patients with retained foreign bodies may present to the ED after a wound heals complaining of sharp pain with movement or with pressure over the site. Failure of a wound to heal also may be evidence of a retained irritant. Chronic, delayed, and recurrent infections are associated with retained foreign bodies (**Figure 45-1**). New puncture wounds that become infected and infections that are resistant to antibiotic therapy suggest a retained foreign body. Arthritis in a joint near an old puncture wound may be plant thorn–induced synovitis.[7,8] Unsuspected foreign bodies may present as soft tissue masses.[16]

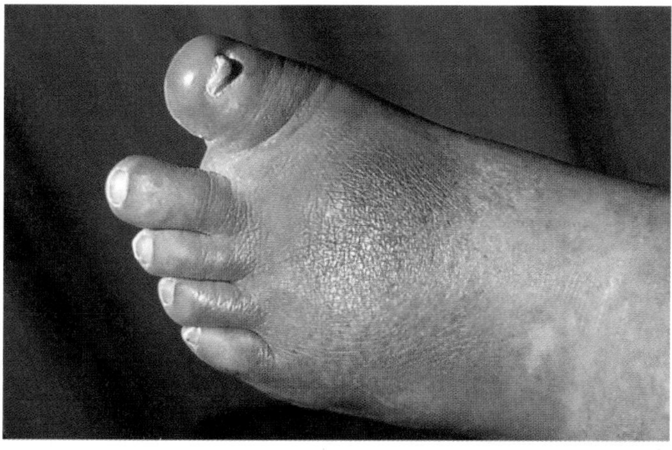

A

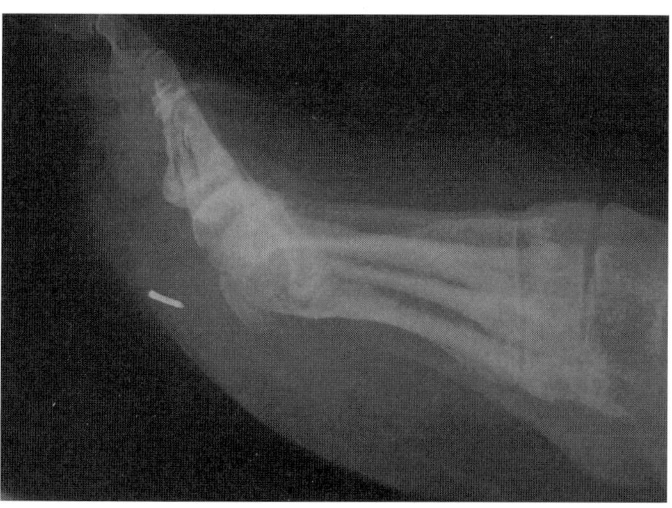
C

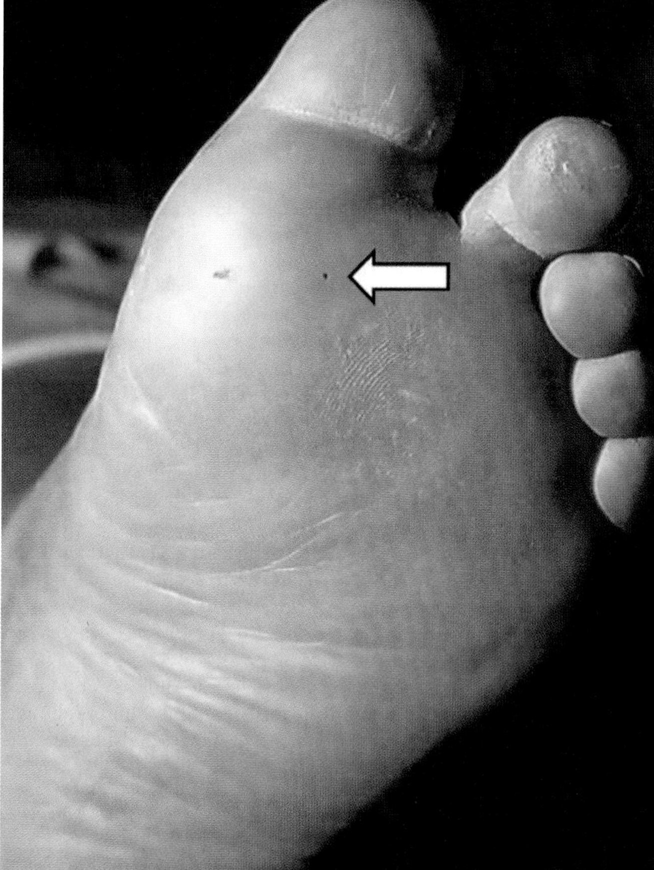
B

FIGURE 45-1. **A.** A diabetic patient presented with redness, swelling, and mild pain of her left foot. Although she admitted to walking barefoot on occasion, she had no recollection of stepping on a sharp object. **B.** A small, healing puncture wound was visible on the plantar surface of her foot. **C.** Lateral radiographic view.

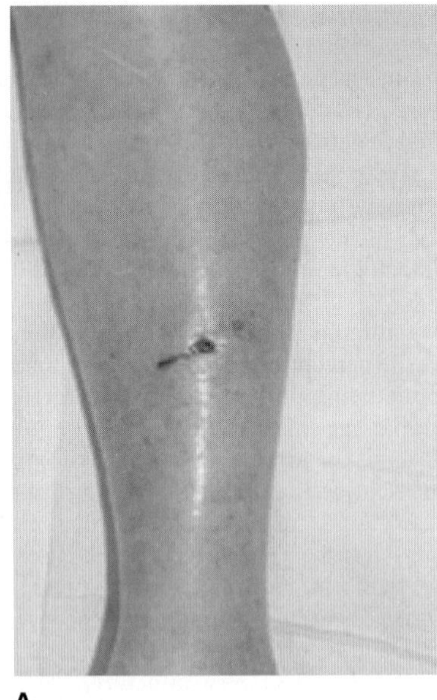
A

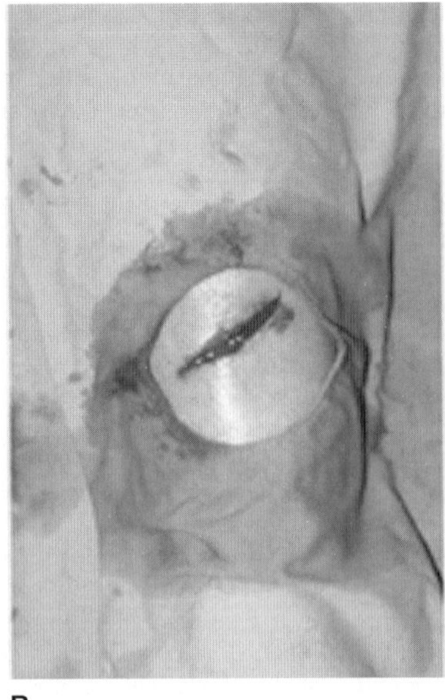
B

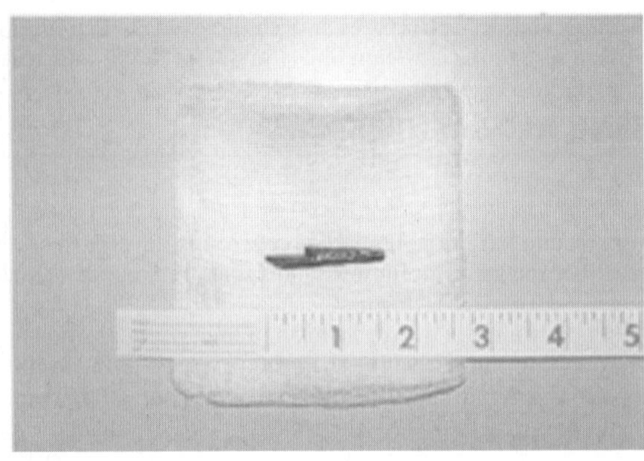

C

FIGURE 45-2. This patient's leg was punctured by a wooden stake 2 days before presentation. **A.** Surrounding cellulitis and point tenderness lateral to the wound indicated the probability of a retained foreign body. **B.** The entrance to the wound was extended. **C.** A 3.7-cm piece of wood was removed.

PHYSICAL EXAMINATION

Physicians are occasionally surprised by foreign bodies that are embedded in small or seemingly superficial wounds. Physical findings that are associated with the presence of a foreign body include a discoloration or visible mass under the epidermis, palpation of a mass, sharp well-localized pain with palpation over or adjacent to a wound, and limitation of passive range of movement of a joint near a wound.

Old wounds with retained foreign bodies may have a persistent purulent drainage, a chronic draining sinus, or a chronic granulomatous reaction. A sterile abscess that complicates wound healing may be the result of a foreign body.

Some foreign bodies are discovered in wounds unexpectedly, but most are found during a deliberate and careful exploration of wounds considered to be at risk.[1,2,11] Adequate lighting, good hemostasis, appropriate anesthesia, and patient cooperation are essential. Magnifying loupes can enhance visualization of small debris fragments or foreign bodies. Make effort to visually inspect all recesses of a wound. **Wounds deeper than 5 mm and wounds whose depth cannot be visualized have a higher association with foreign bodies.** If punctures and other narrow wounds make direct visualization difficult and there is concern about a foreign body below the surface, the wound margins should be extended with a scalpel (**Figure 45-2**).

Wounds that penetrate deeply into adipose tissue are difficult to explore and easily hide foreign material. Blind and gentle probing with a hemostat is a less effective but sometimes acceptable alternative to wound exploration when the wound is narrow and deep and extending the wound is not desirable. This method is used frequently to evaluate plantar puncture wounds caused by nails and to search for clear glass, which is difficult to see in a wound. A closed hemostat should be introduced into the wound and either used as a probe or spread open and then withdrawn. If an instrument strikes a metallic or glass foreign body, it will produce a grating sensation. The instrument should not be used to grasp blindly in hopes of clamping an unseen object. Blind probing is especially dangerous in hands, feet, or face, where direct visualization is the preferred method of exploration.

DIAGNOSIS

Imaging studies should be ordered in most cases in which a retained foreign body is suspected but not found during wound exploration or when exploration of the entire wound is technically impossible.[3,17] Imaging is also useful after initial removal of multiple foreign bodies to determine if all the pieces were found.

Four imaging modalities are available: plain radiography, US, CT, and MRI.[18] The sensitivity and specificity of each imaging modality depend on the object's size, shape, density, and orientation relative to the imaging beam (**Table 45-1**).[3,18] Materials that are the same density as surrounding soft tissue are difficult to see with any type of radiographic or sonographic technique.

LOCALIZATION METHODS

Accurate localization of a foreign body before removal is important because blind searching is time consuming and can cause further injury. However, it is usually easier to detect the presence of a foreign body than to locate its exact position. If a foreign body is radiopaque, one can estimate its location and depth by taping radiopaque skin markers, such as lead circles, paper clips, or a grid, on the skin at the wound entrance or directly over the object.[19] With multiple projections, the object can be seen in relation to the markers. Hypodermic needles can be used as skin markers. Two or three needles are inserted into the skin near the object at approximately 90 degrees to each other to provide a frame of reference around the object. Plain films taken in multiple projections allow the physician to gauge the distance of the object from the closest needle or its distance between two needles (**Figures 45-3** and **45-4**).

The limitations of this technique are that it does not provide a true three-dimensional view and that images on radiographs are distorted by divergence and parallax. Tendons and other structures may block the most direct path to the foreign body.

TABLE 45-1 Imaging Modalities for Detection of Soft Tissue Foreign Bodies[20–23]

Material	Plain Radiographs	High-Resolution US	CT	MRI
Wood	Poor	Good	Moderate to good	Moderate
Metal	Excellent	Good	Excellent	Poor
Glass	Excellent	Good	Excellent	Good
Organic (most plant thorns and cactus spines)	Poor	Good	Good	Good
Plastic	Moderate	Moderate to good	Good	Good
Palm thorn	Poor	Moderate	Good	Good

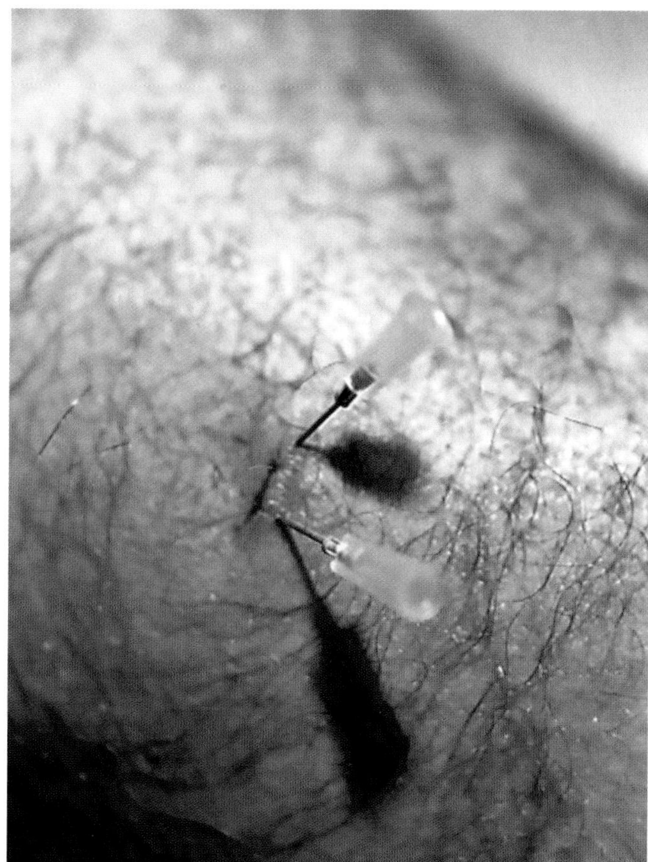

FIGURE 45-3. Hypodermic needles used as skin markers.

IMAGE STUDY SELECTION

Unless a foreign body is embedded at a relatively superficial level or lies within the cavity of a fresh wound, it will not be easily detected or located by physical examination. If a foreign body is suspected based on the mechanism of injury but not found during exploration of a wound, a radiograph should be ordered first, because plain radiography will detect as many as 80% to 90% of all foreign bodies. It is also prudent to order films if a patient believes there is a retained object.[11,15,17] If the wound was caused by metal, glass, or gravel and no foreign body was found on plain films or wound exploration, the physician can end the search. For objects not routinely visible (or not found) on plain radiography, like wood, sonography is the modality of choice, with CT or MRI as alternatives.[18] **The bottom line is that no single imaging modality is ideal for all types of foreign bodies.**

PLAIN RADIOGRAPHY

Most foreign bodies that can be missed during the initial clinical evaluation can be seen on plain radiographs, but the images must be inspected carefully to detect small and faint objects.[3] **Metal, mammalian bone, some types of fish bones (cod, haddock, grey mullet, red snapper, and sole), teeth, pencil graphite, certain plastics, glass, gravel, sand, and aluminum are visible on plain radiographs.** Almost all glass is visible on radiographs if it is 2 mm or larger, and glass does not have to contain lead to be visible on plain films (**Figure 45-5**).[24] A radiopaque fragment is more easily seen if its long axis is positioned parallel to the central ray of the x-ray beam, increasing its apparent density; thus a foreign body may be evident on one radiographic view but not another.

Obtain plain film radiographs using an underpenetrated soft tissue technique, producing a lighter image that increases the contrast between the foreign body and surrounding tissue. **If the radiograph is displayed on a digital imaging system, the contrast and brightness of the image can be adjusted to achieve the same effect as an underpenetrated film.** Digital edge enhancement adjustments may make the foreign object stand out from the background. Radiographs should be taken in multiple projections to separate the shadow of the foreign body from underlying bone and to help gauge the depth of the object in the tissue (**Figure 45-6**). Chronic inflammatory changes may create secondary bony changes, such as osteolytic and osteoblastic lesions, pseudotumor formation, and periosteal reaction, revealing the object's location.

Many common or highly reactive materials, such as wood, thorns, cactus spines, some fish bones, other organic matter, and most plastics, are not visible on plain radiographs.[3,18,25] Sometimes, there is indirect evidence of their presence. A radiolucent filling defect may occur when the object is less dense than surrounding tissue. However, even

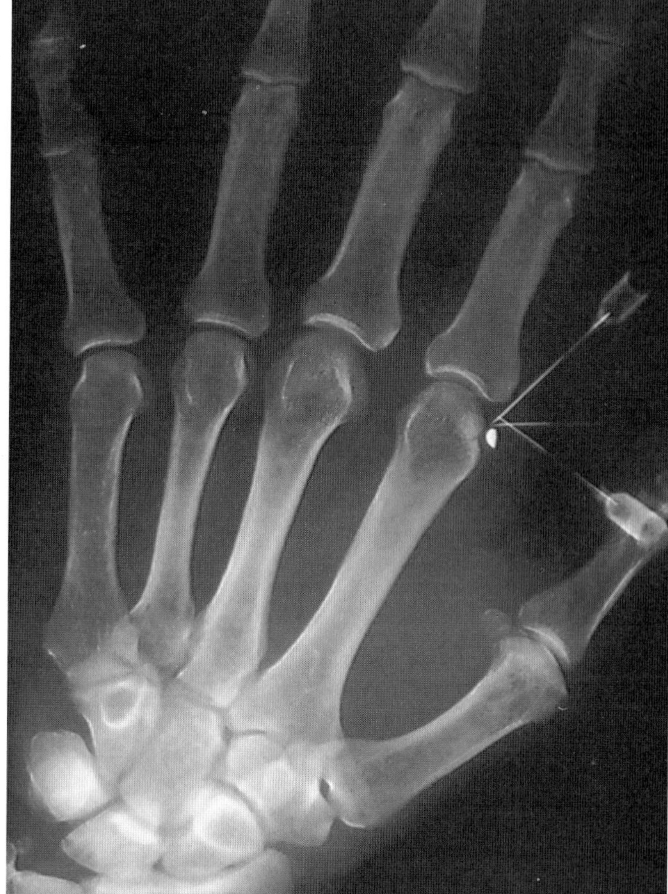

A

B

FIGURE 45-4. Needle markers are used to triangulate the location of a radiopaque foreign body. **A.** Plain radiograph, anteroposterior view. **B.** Oblique view.

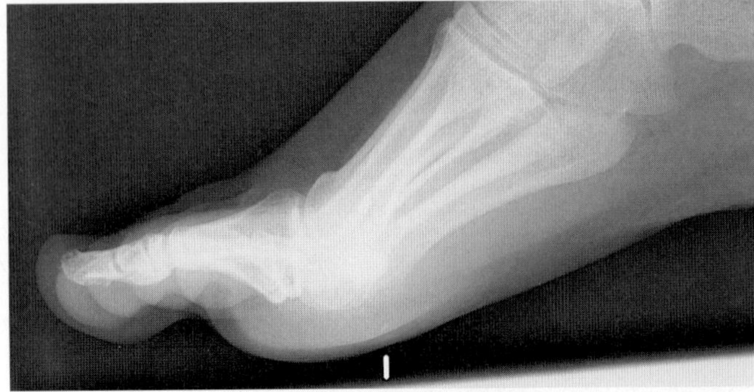

A

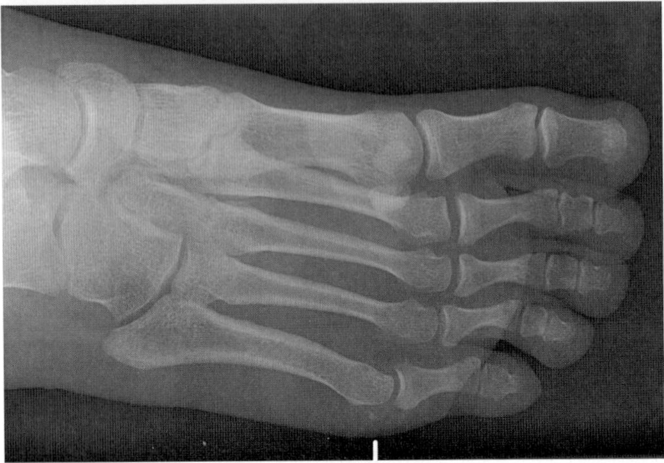

B

FIGURE 45-5. **A.** The marker points to a glass fragment in the plantar surface of this patient's foot on the lateral view of this radiograph. **B.** Oblique view.

radiopaque foreign bodies may be invisible on plain films if they are obscured by, or impacted in, bone.

CT

CT is capable of detecting more types of foreign materials than plain film radiography because it is 100 times more sensitive in differentiating densities (**Figure 45-7**).[18] Subtle density differences can be distinguished with a narrow radiographic density window adjustment, particularly if a computer workstation is used to vary the gain and contrast settings. **Thorns, spines, wood splinters and toothpicks, fish bones, and plastic foreign bodies can be identified with CT.**[3] In dry wood, the interstices between the fibers are filled with air, imparting reduced radiodensity and making dry wood less visible on CT.[18] Water-rich wood, either fresh from a tree or as occurs when dry wood has been imbedded in tissue long enough to absorb serohematic fluid, is more visible as a slightly hyperdense object on CT.[26]

CT will often detect the inflammatory response to an object that has been in place long enough to elicit the reaction. CT may detect objects embedded in bone, and isodense objects may be outlined by surrounding air within the wound. Digital edge enhancement can further improve the visibility of these objects. CT images can be created in multiple planes and can demonstrate the relationship of a foreign object to important anatomic structures. The principal disadvantages of CT are its cost, higher radiation dose, and the fact that wood and other organic material have radiographic density close to water, making them difficult to distinguish from surrounding tissue. **Another pitfall of CT is that wood foreign bodies may initially mimic air bubbles on CT images.**[27]

US

US is useful for directing exploration and foreign body removal.[28-30] **US can identify a wide variety of soft tissue foreign bodies such as wood,**

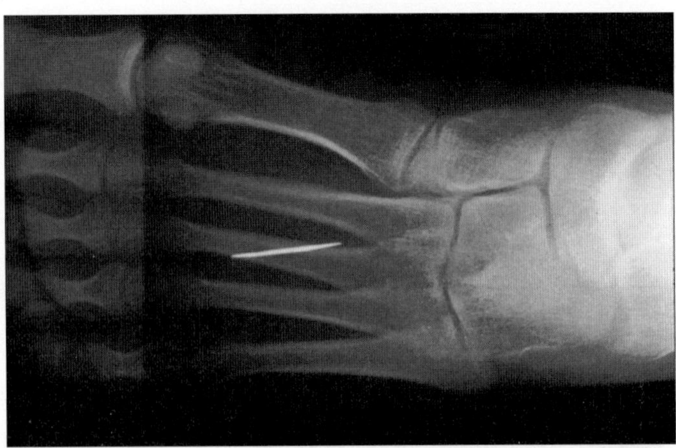

A

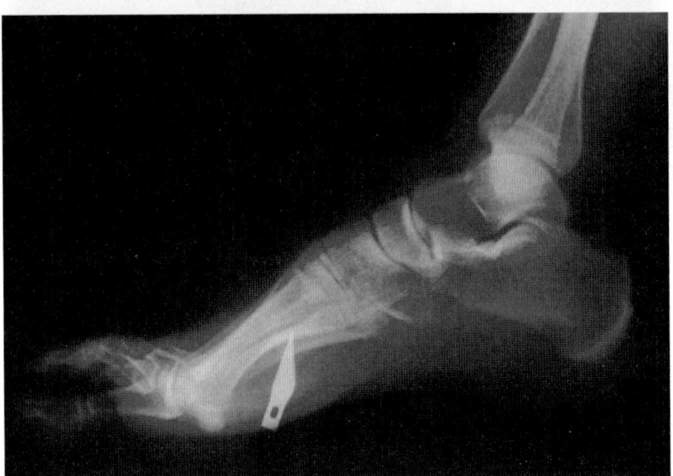

B

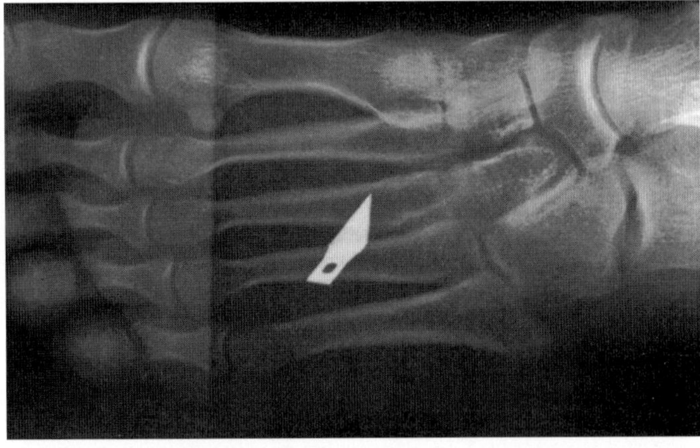

C

FIGURE 45-6. **A.** The identity of this metallic foreign body is not apparent on the anteroposterior view of this radiograph. **B.** The shape and depth of the blade are best seen on the lateral view. **C.** Oblique view.

fish bones, sea urchin spines, other organic material, fiber, and plastic, with >90% sensitivity for foreign bodies >4 to 5 mm (Figure 45-8).[31-36] Detection rates may be less due to the size and sonographic nature of the foreign body, the number of foreign bodies, the presence of confounding factors (e.g., bone, blood, purulence, scars, old sutures) associated with the foreign body, and operator skill and experience. Foreign bodies appear as hyperechoic foci, usually with acoustic shadowing extending distally.[37] A hyperechoic rim, or **halo sign**, indicates an abscess or granuloma around the object. Sonography can estimate the depth of a foreign body below the skin surface.[34]

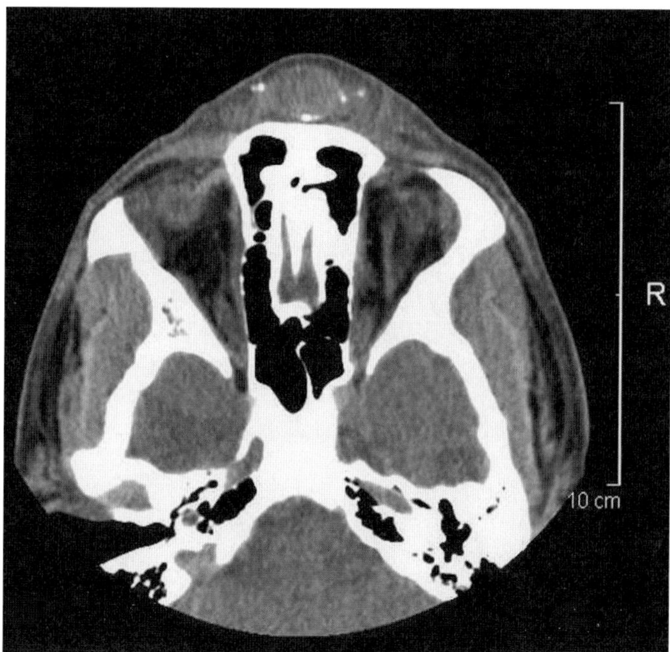

FIGURE 45-7. This patient sustained forehead lacerations when he struck his head on a car windshield. Glass foreign bodies were not identified before wound closure and were not visible on plain films, but were evident on CT.

With experience, sonography can be applied to body areas previously difficult to image for soft tissue foreign bodies, such as the hands and feet.[38-41] Soft tissue gas does not appear to reduce the ability to detect a foreign body but does decrease the ability to discriminate between metal and wood.[42]

An important technical aspect of US for soft tissue foreign body detection is the transducer frequency.[43] **Higher frequencies have a reduced effective depth of penetration for the US wave. A 3.5-MHz transducer will locate foreign bodies that are as deep as 10 cm, a 5-MHz transducer at depths of approximately 7 cm, a 7.5-MHz transducer at depths of 5 cm, and a 12.5-MHz transducer at depths of 2.0 to 0.2 cm.** Conversely, the resolution of the image—ability to distinguish two adjacent objects and detect small objects—is greatest with higher frequencies. Thus, low frequencies can detect larger objects at greater depth but may miss smaller objects and may not be able to discriminate multiple objects. Higher frequencies will detect smaller and multiple objects, but only at shallower depths, and may miss deeper objects. **Use both low and high transducer frequencies for best advantage.**

US has a unique set of limitations. Areas with many echogenic structures, such as calcifications, sesamoid bones, and tendons, may hide foreign bodies within their acoustic shadows, so these areas must be scanned slowly to detect foreign bodies that are small or oriented perpendicular to the skin surface. Some areas of the body that are prone to foreign body penetration, such as the web spaces of the hands or toes, may not accommodate a US probe using standard gel. In this circumstance, a water-bath interface between the probe and body part is useful.[38-40,43,44] False-positive findings result in an unnecessary surgical dissection. False-positive rates for sonography vary from 3% to 15% in clinical case series, depending on the material being studied.[34,36,45,46]

Once a foreign body is confirmed by plain films or CT studies, US can be used in place of fluoroscopy to guide an instrument to the object during retrieval.[28-30,38,39] The scanning beam should be oriented parallel to the long axis of a hemostat, which can be directed toward the long axis of the foreign body (**Figure 45-9**). Transverse and longitudinal scans provide views in multiple planes. A 7.5-MHz linear-array transducer can be used to find objects that are small and superficial (up to 5 cm deep), and a 5.0-MHz transducer can be used for larger and deeper objects. The linear scan is preferred for localization, and the sector scan for retrieval.[28] The primary advantage of sonography is the avoidance of radiation exposure.

MRI

MRI can detect nonmetallic radiolucent foreign bodies and, in comparison studies, is more accurate (less sensitive than US but fewer false-positive interpretations) than any other modality in identifying wood, plastic, spines, and thorns.[3,18,47] **MRI should not be used with gravel or metal-containing foreign bodies because ferromagnetic streaks obscure visualization.** MRI may provide more information than CT about the position of a foreign body relative to (and its effects on) nearby structures, such as tendons, neurovascular bundles, joints, and muscles.

FLUOROSCOPY

Bedside fluoroscopy accurately detects radiopaque (metal, gravel, glass, and pencil graphite) foreign bodies as small as 3 mm.[48,49] Using fluoroscopy to accurately detect glass foreign bodies can be accomplished in a brief training session.[50,51] Advantages are convenience, reduced cost, shortened ED time, and, if done with brief intermittent imaging and appropriate shielding, less radiation exposure than CT. An important limitation is that the body part must be able to fit within the fluoroscopic beam path and be thin enough that a viewable image can be obtained. For most adult patients, this limits fluoroscopy to the limbs. Fluoroscopy can be used to assist foreign body removal by helping guide the instrument, as the body part (usually extremity) can be rotated during fluoroscopic imaging to provide a real-time, three-dimensional view of the object relative to the physician's instruments, skin surface, or skin markers.[48,49] An incision is made between needles or markers, or dissection is carried along the path of the closest needle.

GENERAL TREATMENT PRINCIPLES

Once a soft tissue foreign body is discovered, weigh the risk of leaving the foreign body in place against the potential harm of attempting to remove it. Not all foreign bodies must be removed, and not all that require removal must be extracted in the ED. General indications for foreign body removal include potential for later infection, toxicity, injury, and functional problems (**Table 45-2**). Usually, objects that are small, inert, deeply embedded, and causing no symptoms can be left in place. Bullets that come to rest deep within a muscle belly are usually not removed because the procedure can cause more damage than leaving the foreign object in place. However, projectiles may drag bits of clothing or skin into the wound, so the entrance wound deserves cleaning and debridement. Bullet migration and embolization are rare but possible complications. Bullets near vessels can enter the systemic circulation. Bullets that cause distal ischemia, thrombus formation, or wall erosion or that lie within the lumen of a blood vessel require immediate removal in the operating room.

Thorns, spines, wood splinters, and other vegetative materials should be promptly removed because they cause intense and excessive inflammation. Foreign objects that are heavily contaminated, such as fractured teeth and soil-covered objects, should be removed as soon as possible. Antibiotic treatment cannot replace foreign body removal. Glass, metal, and plastic are relatively inert, and removal can be postponed, if necessary. Glass foreign bodies in hands or feet can cause persistent pain with gripping or walking, and they can sever nerves or tendons years after the initial injury. Patients with deep, sharp foreign bodies in these locations should be referred to appropriate specialists for eventual removal.

Sometimes, harmless foreign bodies are psychologically distressing to patients, particularly when they are visible under the skin surface or produce a lump. Patient concern may be a justification for elective removal.[52]

The techniques for soft tissue foreign body removal are based on clinical experience; there are no controlled or randomized studies comparing different approaches or techniques.[53,54] Successful removal of foreign bodies requires adequate local or regional anesthesia and good lighting. Depending on location and depth, tourniquet control of bleeding and assistance may be needed. Depth and accessibility of the object and physician time are the limiting factors for removal of foreign bodies by the emergency physician. Foreign bodies buried deeply in adipose tissue or muscles are difficult to locate. Although most foreign bodies in hands should be removed because the hand is mobile and sensitive, deep exploration of the hand by the emergency physician is not recommended because knowledge and experience are needed to avoid injury

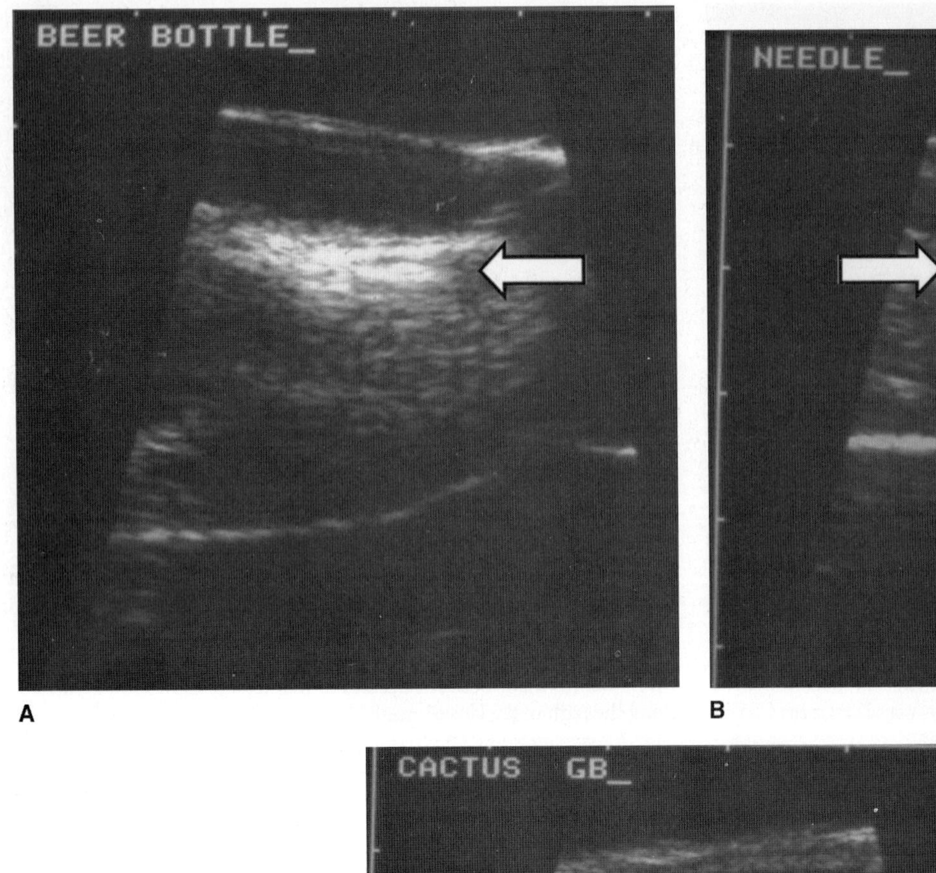

A

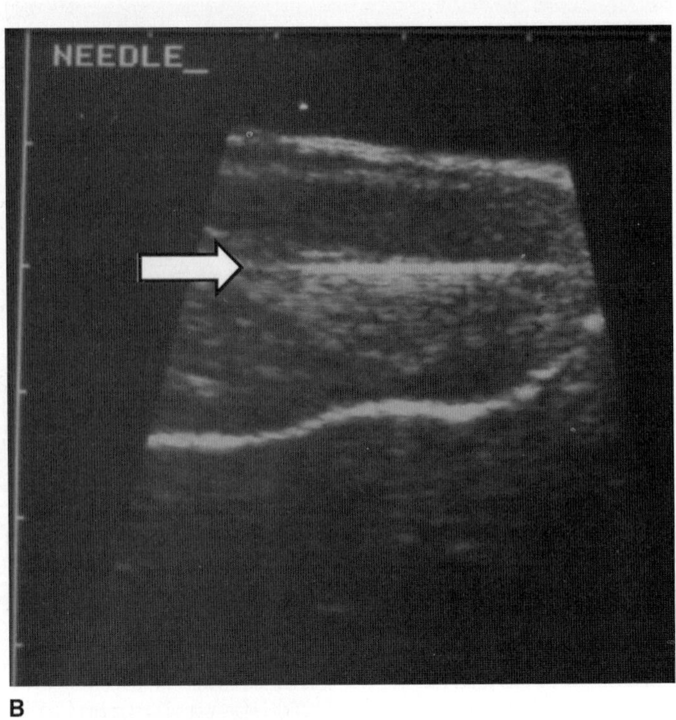

B

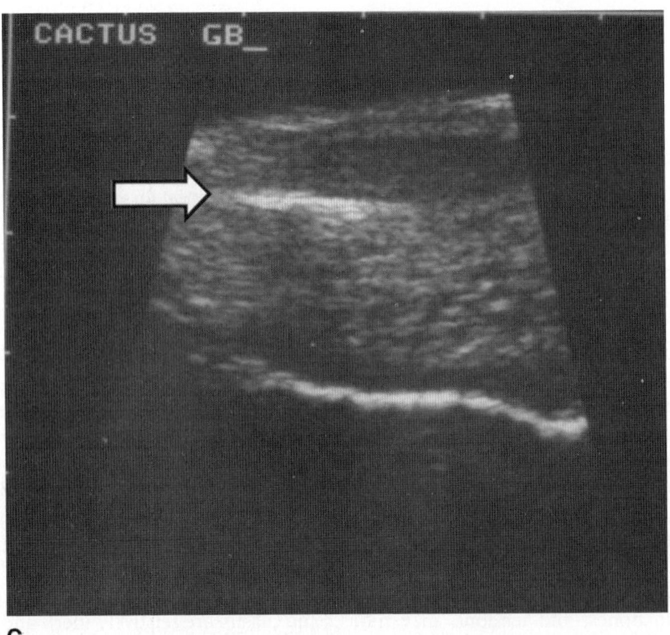

C

FIGURE 45-8. Sonographic images of (**A**) beer bottle glass (*arrow*), (**B**) sewing needle with long axis parallel to the scan plane (*arrow*), and (**C**) cactus spine (*arrow*), in a tissue model. All objects appear as bright, hyperechoic foci.

to numerous closely spaced vital structures. The "No Man's Land" of the hand (see Figure 268-10 in chapter titled "Injuries to the Hand and Digits") should not be explored either.

In a busy ED, it may only be possible to devote 15 to 30 minutes to a removal procedure, particularly when other patients demand attention. This amount of time is sufficient for locating most foreign bodies. Inform the patient before the procedure that the duration of the exploration will be limited and a best effort will be made to locate and remove the foreign body. If unsuccessful, referral to an appropriate specialist will be made.

POSTREMOVAL TREATMENT

After removal of a foreign body, irrigate the wound thoroughly with standard wound irrigation techniques (see chapter 40, "Wound Preparation"). A puncture wound is difficult to clean adequately because either the small wound diameter prevents the irrigation fluid from reaching the wounded tissue or the fluid enters the wound but does not completely drain (see chapter 46, "Puncture Wounds and Bites"). In general, if the puncture site is contaminated, the entrance wound can be enlarged to allow more effective cleaning, and if foreign debris is impregnated in tissue, the contaminated area can be debrided or excised. **If multiple radiopaque objects were removed, obtain a postprocedure plain radiograph.**

The decision to close lacerations, incisions, and block excisions depends on the potential for infection. **Wounds in which all foreign contaminants can be removed and those in locations with good blood supply can be closed primarily. Otherwise, delayed primary closure is preferred.** Provide necessary tetanus immunization. There is no proven

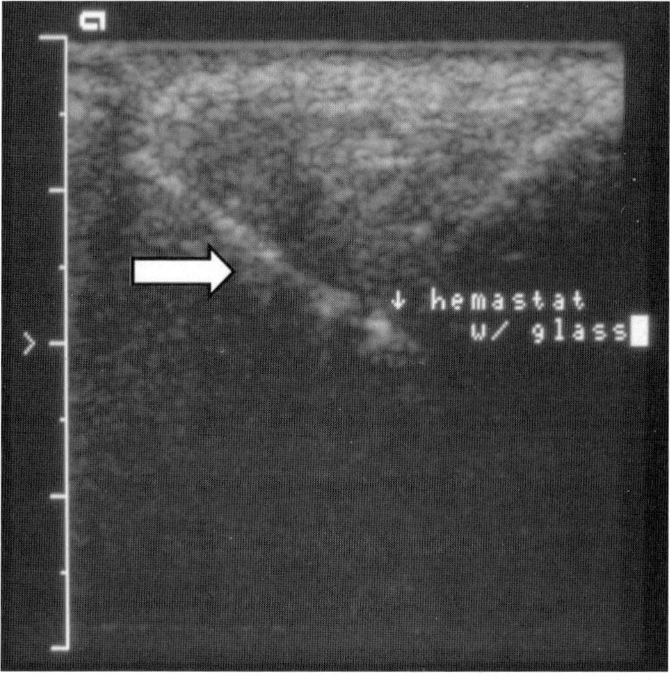

A

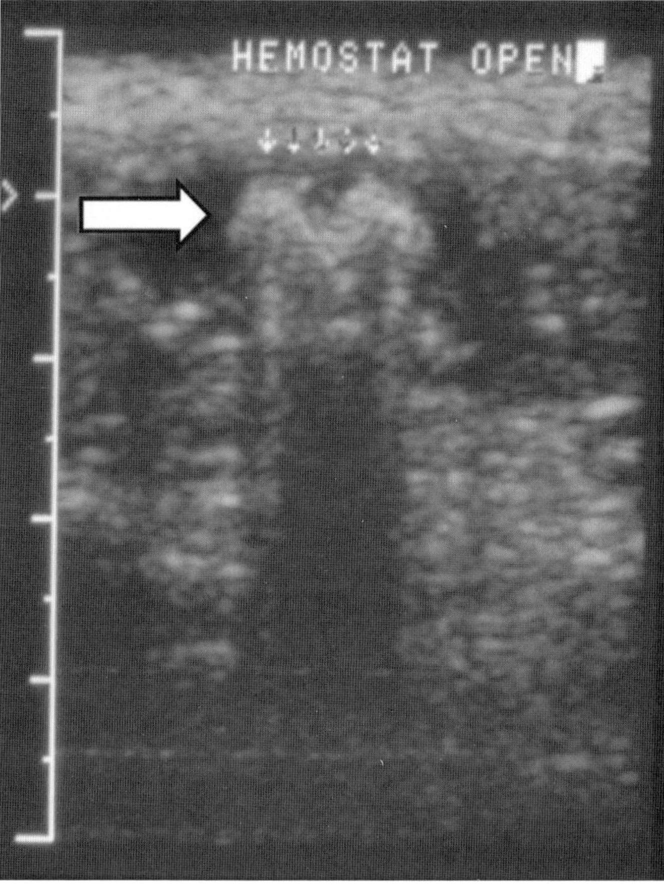

B

FIGURE 45-9. **A.** Sonographic image of the long axis of a hemostat grasping a piece of glass (*arrow*). **B.** Sonographic image of the tips of a hemostat surrounding a piece of glass (*arrow*).

TABLE 45-2 Indications for Foreign Body Removal
Potential for inflammation or infection
Vegetative or chemically reactive material
Heavy bacterial contamination (e.g., teeth, soil)
Proximity to fractured bone
Established infection
Allergic reaction
Potential for toxicity, as with heavy metals
Spines with venom
Impingement on nerves, vessels, or tendons
Intra-articular or intravascular location

benefit for prophylactic antibiotics for uninfected wounds containing foreign bodies.[55] Antibiotics are justified for infected wounds, particularly when removal must be postponed.

If a foreign body is deliberately left in place, inform the patient of the proposed plan and necessary follow-up. If foreign material was removed, warn the patient that there is always a possibility that not all pieces were found despite careful exploration and imaging studies.

DELAYED REMOVAL

Refer patients to surgeons or interventional radiologists for delayed removal of foreign bodies.[56-58] Inform the patient that the object is present but unlikely to cause harm before it is removed. **If a foreign body is near a joint or highly mobile region, the affected area should be splinted before removal to prevent further injury or migration of the object.**

SPECIFIC FOREIGN BODIES AND REMOVAL PROCEDURES

METALLIC NEEDLES

Long, thin foreign bodies, such as sewing and hypodermic needles, may be difficult to locate in soft tissue. Two techniques are available for removing needles that are parallel to the surface of the skin. If the needle is superficial enough to be palpable, make an incision at one end to expose and grasp it with a hemostat. If the needle is deep, make an incision perpendicular to the needle at its midpoint, where it can be clamped with a hemostat and pushed out of the entrance of the original wound (**Figure 45-10**). Sometimes application of a magnet may attract the foreign body to the magnet for removal. Do not apply magnets in patients with pacemakers or implanted defibrillators.

Long, thin foreign bodies that are oriented perpendicular to the skin surface can be elusive. If a needle or nail can be reached with an alligator

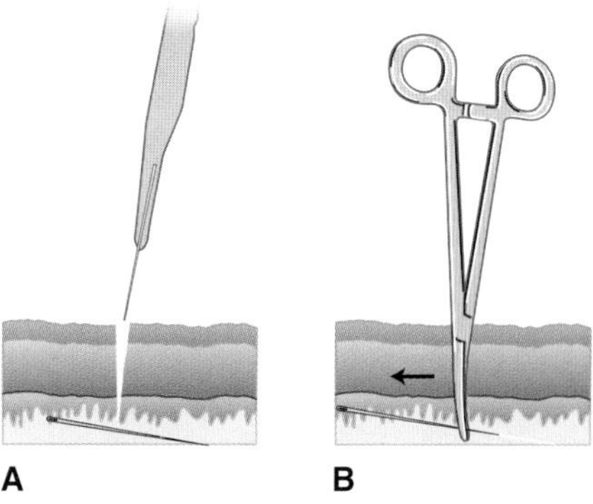

FIGURE 45-10. **A.** An incision is made perpendicular to the needle at its midpoint. **B.** The needle is grasped through the incision with a hemostat and backed out of the puncture wound.

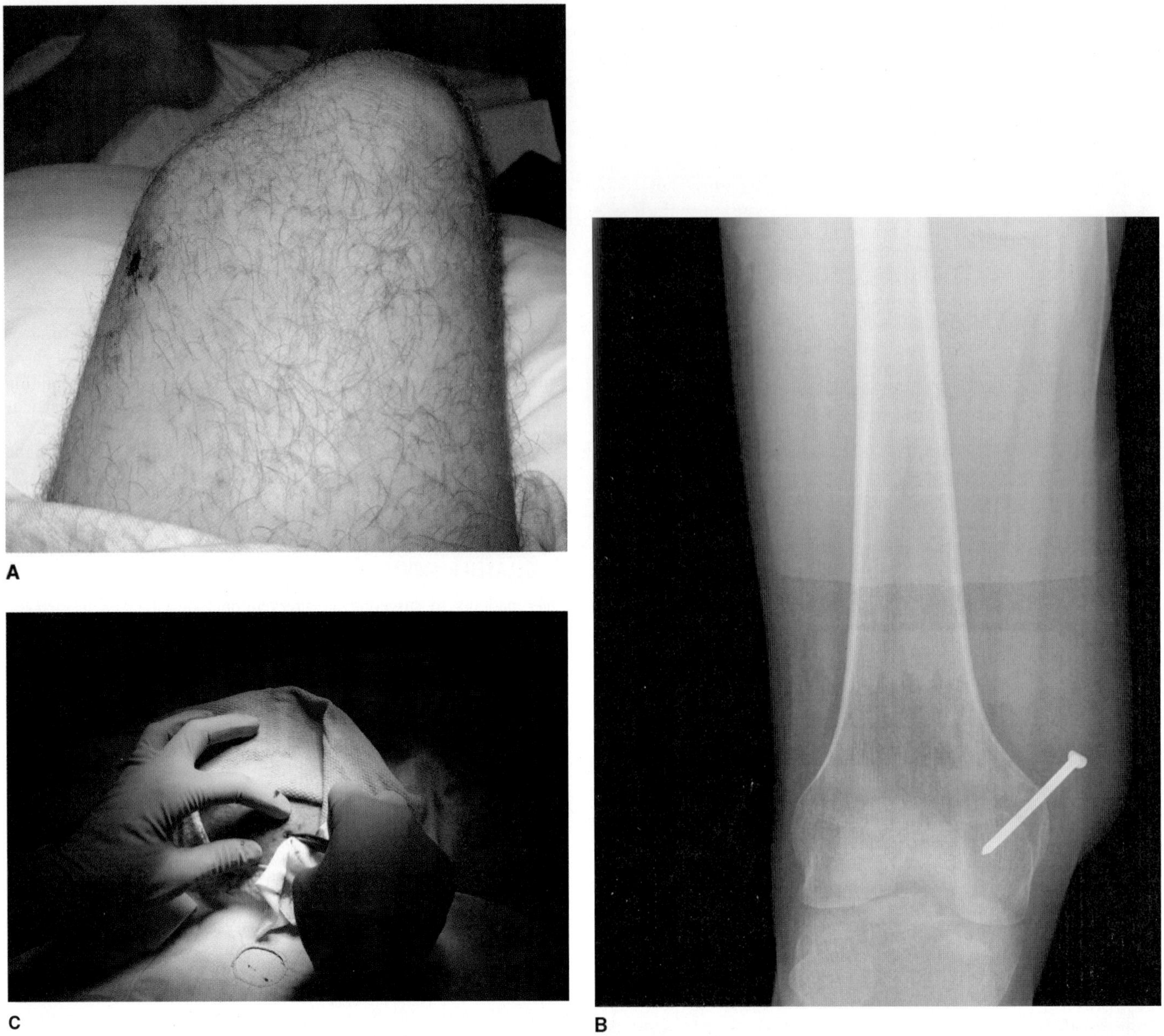

A

C

B

FIGURE 45-11. **A.** Nail gun injury to the medial aspect of the distal right thigh. **B.** Anteroposterior radiographic view. **C.** Extraction of nail through the entrance wound.

forceps or hemostat, it can be pulled straight out (**Figure 45-11**). If a needle lies beyond the reach of an instrument, the entrance wound can be enlarged with a skin incision (**Figure 45-12**). However, the incision may easily pass to the side of the object, so undermine the skin edges and apply pressure on the skin edges that will displace the foreign body into the center of the wound, where it can be seen and grasped. Once removed, the needle and the wound should be inspected to ensure that the object was removed in its entirety.

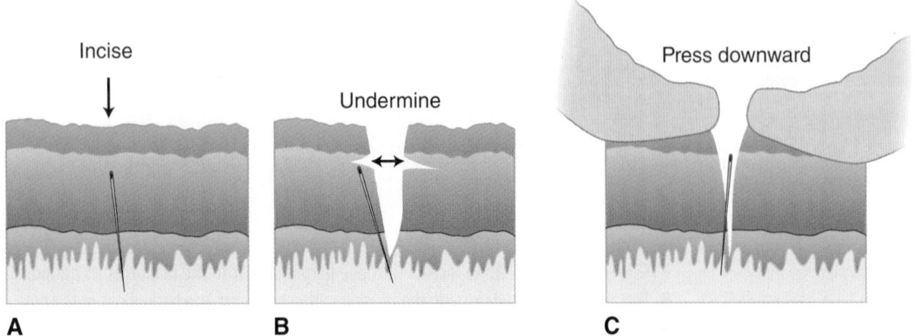

FIGURE 45-12. **A.** The entrance site is enlarged with a skin incision. **B.** If the incision passes to the side of the object, the skin is undermined. **C.** Pressure on the skin edges displaces the foreign body into the center of the wound.

WOOD SPLINTERS AND ORGANIC SPINES

Solid foreign bodies can be pulled out of puncture wounds with forceps, but wood splinters and organic spines (e.g., cactus, sea urchin, and fish) may disintegrate with this technique. Only superficial splinters that are a few millimeters long can be grasped and removed with a fine-point splinter forceps. A splinter parallel to the skin surface should be lifted out of the wound after incising the skin along the long axis of the object (**Figure 45-13**). If the splinter is lodged in the subcutaneous tissue, the entrance wound should be enlarged with a skin incision so the foreign body can be grasped under direct visualization. Wood fragments may be impossible to locate precisely. One solution is to create an elliptical incision around the puncture wound and extract the fragment in a block of tissue (**Figure 45-14**). Avoid incorporating nerves, vessels, or tendons within the excised block. Either technique creates a larger wound but allows a better inspection and more thorough cleaning after removal.

Subungual splinters should be removed because of the risk of subsequent infection with the possibility for distal phalanx osteomyelitis. If the splinter is underneath the distal end of the nail, it can be grasped by a splinter forceps or hooked by a hypodermic needle bent at its tip. More proximal splinters can be reached by anesthetizing the finger and removing a wedge of the nail overlying part of the foreign body (**Figure 45-15**). If there are multiple splinters, the entire nail can be removed in one piece, the foreign bodies extracted, and the nail placed back under the cuticle and tacked down on to the nail bed (see chapter 43, "Arm and Hand Lacerations").

Numerous, tiny cactus spines in the dermis can be plucked out individually with forceps or extracted together with depilatory wax, professional-quality facial gel, rubber cement, or household glue. Larger spines and thorns should be removed with incision or excision techniques.

FISHHOOKS

Fishhooks have a variety of sizes and shapes based on a common pattern (**Figure 45-16**). The barb, which is a projection extending backward from the point of the hook, keeps the point embedded in the fish's mouth and makes removal from skin a challenging task. Most fishhook injuries involve the hands, head, or face (**Figure 45-17**).

There are several methods for removing fishhooks imbedded in skin. The best strategy depends primarily on the depth of the hook. If the hook has multiple barbs, take precautions to avoid impaling the treating physician, bystanders, or the patient (a second time) during removal by taping or cutting off the exposed barbs. With any technique, the skin should be cleaned and anesthetized at the entry site. If the hook is superficial, use the **retrograde technique** by applying gentle downward pressure on the shank while the hook is simply pulled back out along the path of entry (**Figure 45-18**).

The **string-pull method** is a variation on the retrograde technique. Wrap string around the bend of the hook where it enters the skin. Depress the end of the shank with one hand to disengage the barb from deeper tissue. With the other hand, give a quick pull on the string, extracting the hook (**Figure 45-19**). The disadvantages of this technique

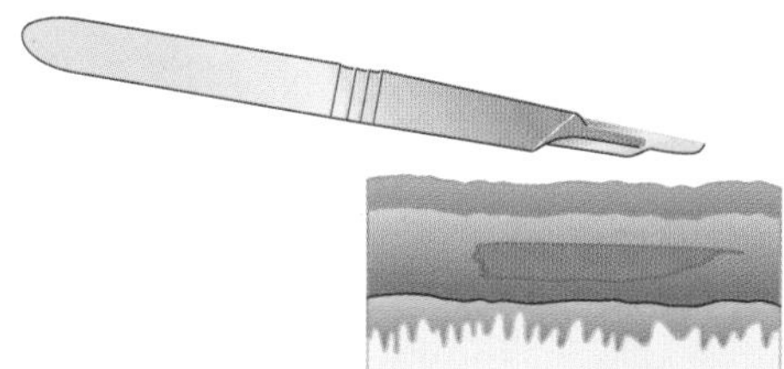

FIGURE 45-13. To remove a friable foreign body such as a wood splinter that is parallel to the skin surface, an incision is made along its long axis. The object can be lifted out and the entire length of the wound inspected for remnants.

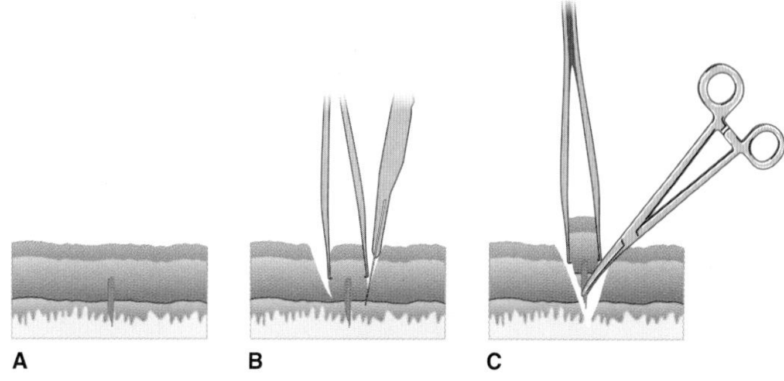

FIGURE 45-14. Block excision is effective for foreign bodies that are friable, difficult to find, buried in fatty tissue, or stain surrounding tissue. **A.** A small, elliptical incision is made around the original wound. **B.** The incision is undercut until contact is made with the foreign body. **C.** The block of tissue is grasped with a forceps, the foreign body is clamped with a hemostat, and both are removed.

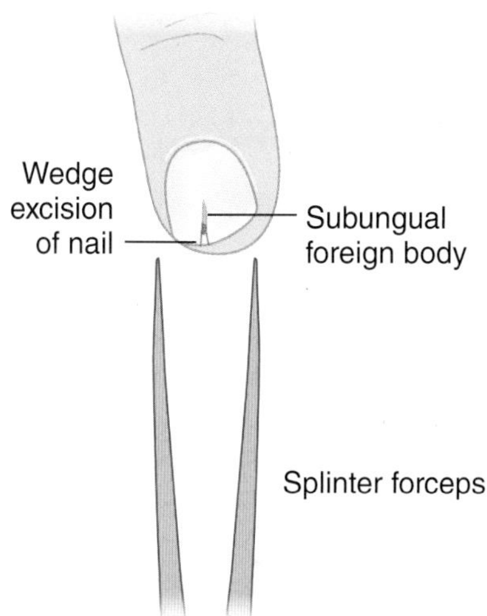

FIGURE 45-15. Subungual foreign bodies that are beyond the reach of a splinter forceps can be exposed by excising a wedge of the overlying nail.

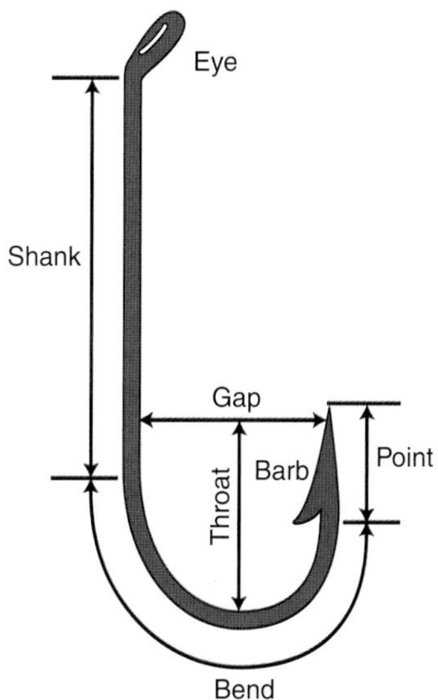

FIGURE 45-16. Anatomy of a fishhook.

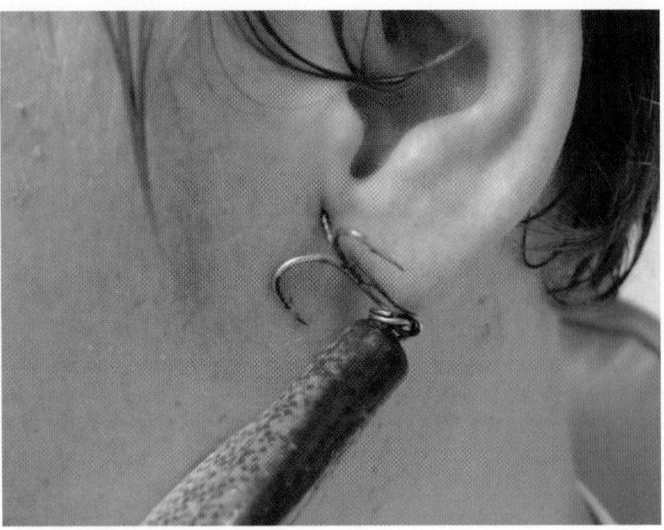

FIGURE 45-17. Fishhook in ear.

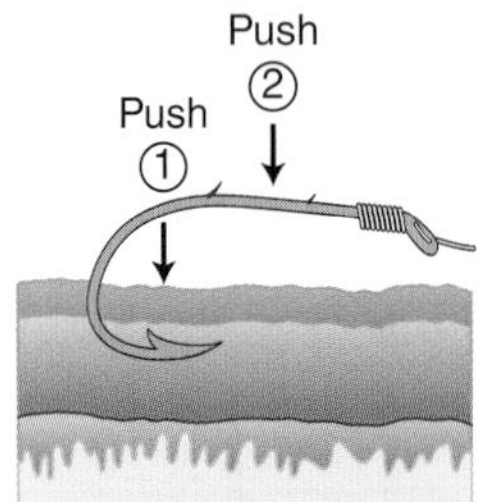

FIGURE 45-18. Simple retrograde technique for fishhook removal. While pressing the skin over the tip of the hook to disengage the barb and applying gentle downward pressure on the shank, back the hook out of the skin. If the barb catches on skin fibers, other techniques must be used.

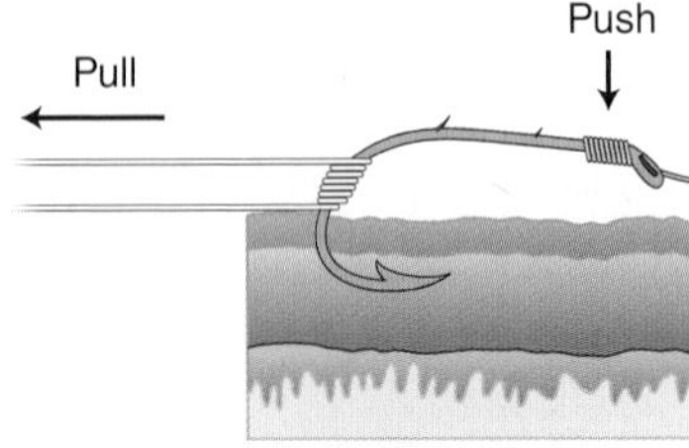

FIGURE 45-19. String-pull technique for fishhook removal. String or suture material is tied to the curve of the hook. The hook is positioned as described in the simple retrograde technique (Figure 45-18), and a quick pull on the string will dislodge the hook.

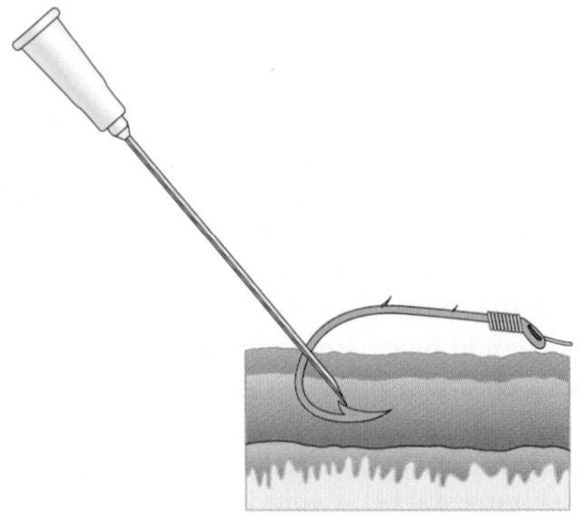

FIGURE 45-20. Needle-cover technique for fishhook removal. The area is anesthetized, and an 18-gauge needle is inserted into the entrance wound along the hook. The lumen of the needle is placed over the barb to cover it, and both the hook and needle are backed out of the wound.

are that failure can cause further pain to the patient and success can result in ripped tissue or a sharp, blood-contaminated object flying uncontrollably across the room.

The **needle-cover technique** is commonly described but rarely successful. The technique requires physician dexterity and is only useful if the hook is superficial. Insert an 18-gauge needle into the entrance wound alongside the shank of the hook. Have the needle follow the bend of the hook until the lumen of the needle can be placed over the barb to sheathe it. The hook and needle are then withdrawn from the wound as a unit (**Figure 45-20**).

The **advance-and-cut technique** is useful for deeply penetrated and larger fishhooks (**Figure 45-21**). Advance the tip of the hook through the skin surface. Once exposed, the point and barb are cut with wire cutters, and the remaining part of the hook is rotated back out of the original wound. If barbs along the shank are embedded beneath the dermis, the shank can be clipped near the hook's eye. The remaining part of the hook is then passed antegrade through the skin. The advance-and-cut method traumatizes and contaminates tissue but is an effective method in the ED if the barb has nearly or already penetrated the surface of the skin.

The **incision technique** is nearly always successful in removing fishhooks. Enlarge the entrance wound 2 to 3 mm with a #11 scalpel blade. Continue the incision along the bend of the hook to the barb until the barb is disengaged from the soft tissue. The hook can then be withdrawn easily through the larger entrance (**Figure 45-22**). If necessary, the barb can be grasped with a hemostat to prevent it from snagging tissue on the way out. There are two major benefits to enlarging puncture wounds containing foreign bodies. First, the wound is more easily inspected for additional foreign bodies. In the case of fishhook impalement, the wound may be harboring the bait that was on the hook. Second, the

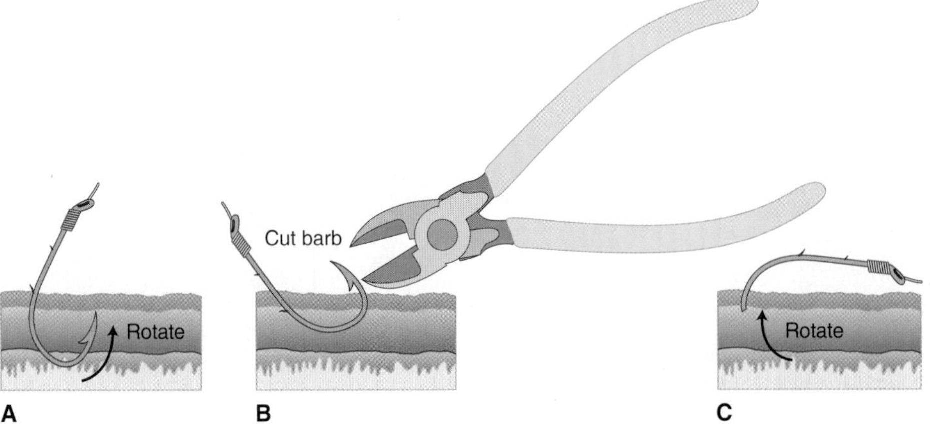

FIGURE 45-21. Advance-and-cut technique for fishhook removal. The area is anesthetized, and the tip of the hook is advanced through the skin surface (**A**), the barb is cut (**B**), and the hook is rotated back out of the original wound (**C**).

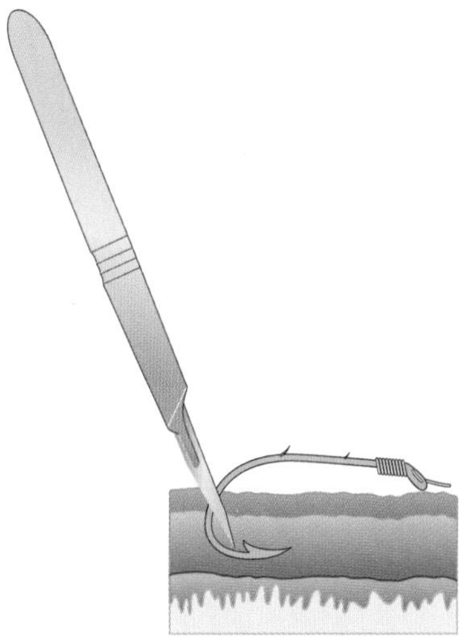

FIGURE 45-22. Incision technique for fishhook removal. The area is anesthetized, and a small incision is made along the shaft of the hook to the barb. The hook is withdrawn through the incision.

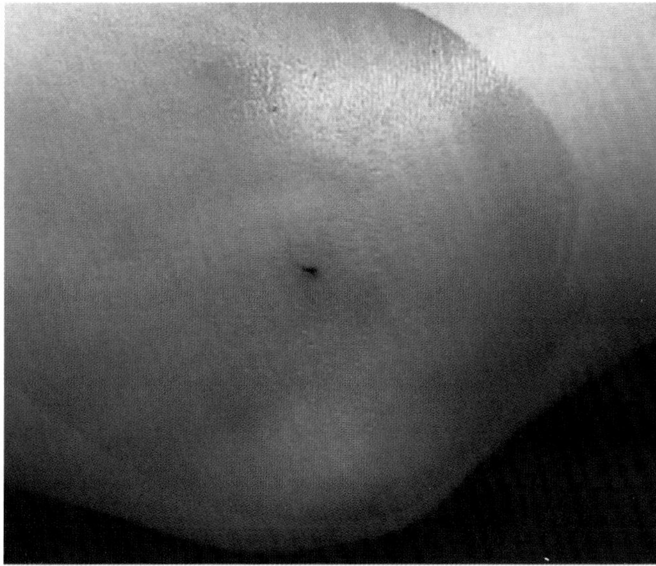

A

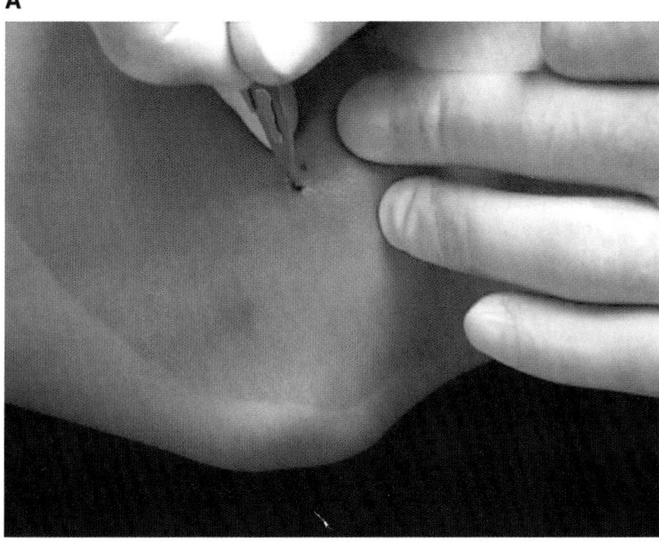

B

FIGURE 45-23. A. Graphite foreign body (pencil lead) embedded near knee. B. Excision of foreign body.

wound tract is more easily irrigated through a larger opening. However, the incising scalpel can easily injure tendons, nerves, and vessels.

TRAUMATIC DERMAL TATTOOING

Foreign particulates may be embedded in the epidermal and dermal layers of skin by an abrasion, which permanently stains or "tattoos" the surrounding tissue. If vigorous scrubbing does not remove the particulates, refer the patient to specialists for dermabrasion or block excision. The graphite from pencil lead can produce a pigmentation that may never dissolve; therefore, graphite should be excised in cosmetic areas (**Figure 45-23**).

REFERENCES

The complete reference list is available online at www.TintinalliEM.com.

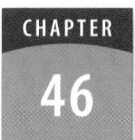

CHAPTER 46 Puncture Wounds and Bites

James Quinn

PUNCTURE WOUNDS

A puncture wound is defined as a wound whose depth is greater than its width. These injuries most commonly occur on the plantar surface of the foot after stepping on a sharp object.[1,2] Despite the relatively innocuous-appearing skin wound, there is significant risk of infection and injury to underlying structures. Puncture wounds caused by high-pressure injection equipment and animal bites, and those involving exposure to body fluids have the potential for unique complications.

PATHOPHYSIOLOGY

With puncture wounds, shear forces between the penetrating object and tissue result in tissue disruption, producing hemorrhage and devitalization of skin and underlying tissues. Inoculation of infectious organisms into the deeper tissues can occur from the penetrating object (with or without leaving behind a foreign body from the object or material that has been pierced)[3] or from the skin surface. When the penetrating object is removed, closure of the small skin wound creates a favorable environment for the development of infection. The reported infection rate from plantar puncture wounds is approximately 6% to 11%.[4,5] Furthermore, exploration of infected plantar puncture wounds finds foreign material in about 25% of patients.[6]

Most soft tissue infections from puncture wounds are caused by gram-positive organisms. *Staphylococcus aureus* predominates, followed by other staphylococcal and streptococcal species.[4,7-10] Puncture wounds over joints can penetrate the joint capsule and produce septic arthritis. Those that penetrate cartilage, periosteum, and bone can lead to osteomyelitis. *Pseudomonas aeruginosa* is the most frequent pathogen isolated from plantar puncture wound–related osteomyelitis, particularly when the injury occurs through the rubber sole of an athletic shoe.[6,9-11] The source appears to be *Pseudomonas* that colonizes the foam lining of athletic shoes.

Difficulty in visualizing and cleaning to the full depth of the injury contributes to the higher risk for infection for puncture wounds compared with other traumatic lacerations. Other host and wound factors are associated with delayed healing and/or infection (**Table 46-1**).[12,13]

Plantar puncture wounds of the forefoot are at risk for foreign body deposition and infection,[6] and because most of the body weight is transmitted to the metatarsal heads during walking, a puncture in this area might penetrate more deeply than elsewhere on the sole and produce a higher rate of infection. However, case series of patients hospitalized with infected plantar puncture wounds both support[9,14] and refute[10] this theory.

TABLE 46-1 Risk Factors for Puncture Wound Complications

Patient characteristics
Elderly
Diabetes with or without microvascular complications
Immunocompromised (acquired immune deficiency syndrome, steroids, chemotherapy)
Peripheral vascular disease
Wound characteristics
Contaminated with soil or debris
Containing foreign body
Occurring outdoors
Occurring through a shoe and/or sock
Deeper penetration (jumping, falling, running)

RISK ASSESSMENT

The patient should be asked about the time of injury and circumstances involved. Wounds greater than 6 hours old with increasing pain and redness are likely infected. Falling or jumping onto an object suggests deeper penetration with potential for greater injury. Footwear (for plantar injuries) or clothing through which the object passed increases the potential for foreign body retention and infection. The patient should be asked to estimate the depth of penetration and about a foreign body sensation in the wound. Ask about postinjury care rendered before presentation and about host factors predisposing to infection.

Ask about the penetrating object. Materials such as wood, glass, or plastic are prone to break or splinter, leaving retained fragments in the wound and increasing the risk for infection. Thin objects, such as needles or pins, can break off cleanly beneath the skin surface, leaving a fragment behind.

Examine the puncture wound site and the function of underlying structures. Note the size and location of the wound, condition of surrounding skin, and presence of foreign matter or devitalized tissue. Assess the puncture wound for proximity to underlying structures. Assess distal function of tendons and nerves and the integrity of distal perfusion, especially with puncture wounds of the hand and wrist.[15]

Because the entire depth of a puncture wound cannot be reliably explored, assessment for a possible foreign body is complicated. Patient perception of a foreign body is modestly useful in predicting the presence of one.[16,17] The practice of probing the wound with a blunt instrument to assess depth and the presence of a foreign body is of unproven utility.

DIAGNOSIS

Plain-film radiographs using soft tissue visualization techniques are indicated in all infected puncture wounds, in wounds caused by materials prone to fragment, and whenever the patient reports a foreign body sensation (**Table 46-2**) (see chapter 45, Soft Tissue Foreign Bodies).[18]

TABLE 46-2 Indications for Imaging in Puncture Wounds

Plain radiographs
Suspicion of fracture
Infected wound
Wound caused by materials prone to fragment (wood, glass, etc.)
Foreign body sensation reported by patient
CT or MRI
Suspected deep-space infection
Persistent pain after injury
Failure to respond to treatment

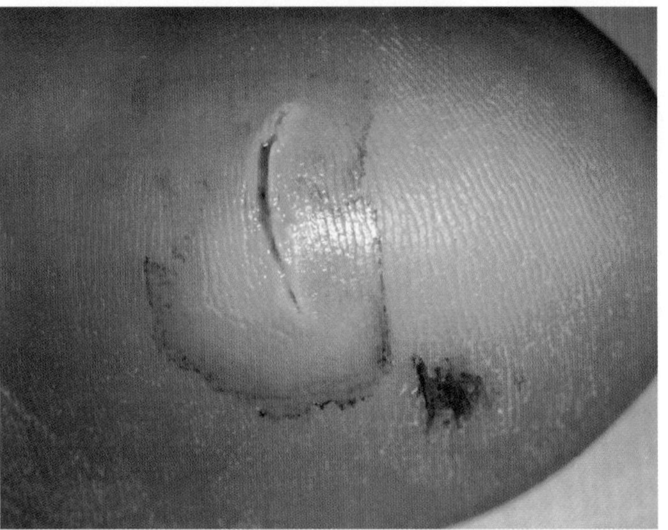

A

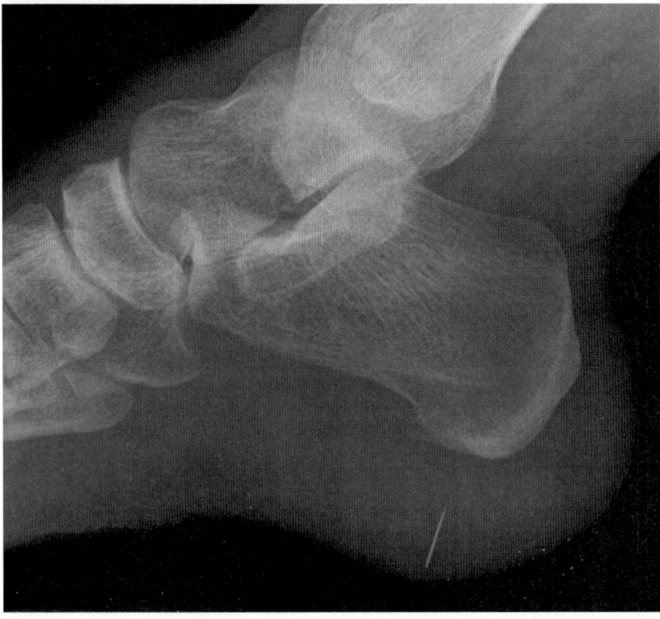

B

FIGURE 46-1. Puncture wound to heel. **A.** Physician enlarged the wound in an unsuccessful attempt to locate and remove foreign body. **B.** Radiograph showing retained foreign body.

Plain radiographs will detect >90% of radiopaque foreign bodies >1 mm in diameter (**Figure 46-1**). Most organic substances, such as wood, thorns, and other plant matter, have radiodensities close to that of soft tissue and cannot reliably be detected in puncture wounds with plain radiographs.

US can identify soft tissue foreign bodies, but the ability to detect small objects that might have been introduced through a puncture wound is limited. US can be helpful in imaging puncture wounds with increasing pain when an abscess is suspected. CT can accurately detect most radiolucent foreign bodies and is the imaging modality to use when a retained foreign body is suspected but the plain radiograph does not show one. MRI provides excellent visualization of foreign bodies but cannot be used to image metallic objects or objects containing certain minerals due to the production of ferromagnetic artifacts. CT or MRI is indicated in patients with deep-space infection, persistent pain after a puncture wound, or when superficial infections fail to respond to therapy (**Table 46-2**). Rubber from athletic shoes is difficult to visualize with any imaging modality.[3]

TREATMENT

Treatment recommendations for puncture wounds are largely based on anecdotal evidence and reviews of uncontrolled case series.[4,7-12] Traditional wound cleaning techniques are largely ineffective as a result of the small entrance wound that has often spontaneously sealed by the time of presentation. The occurrence of serious infections after puncture wounds leads some clinicians to recommend more aggressive wound debridement and irrigation, although there is no evidence that this treatment reduces the rate or severity of post–puncture wound infections. The majority of puncture wounds have a benign course, and potentially catastrophic complications are uncommon.[1,4,5]

Wound Cleansing, Irrigation, and Debridement Uncomplicated clean punctures presenting <6 hours after injury require superficial wound cleansing and tetanus prophylaxis as indicated.[10] Soaking of the wound in an antiseptic solution has no proven benefit. Low-pressure (e.g., approximately 0.5 psi) irrigation of wounds will assist in surface cleansing and allow visualization of the entrance site, but will not penetrate the puncture tract. High-pressure (e.g., approximately 7 psi) injection of irrigation fluid into the wound might penetrate the tract, but has no proven benefit and theoretically could force foreign matter and bacteria deeper into the surrounding tissue.[19]

Debridement or coring of the wound tract in clean wounds does not reduce infection or facilitate accurate diagnosis of deeper structural injury. Adverse effects from debridement or coring include increased pain and a wound that is larger than the initial injury.

Antibiotics The role for prophylactic antibiotics in the management of puncture wounds is controversial, especially for plantar puncture wounds.[7-9] **There is no proven benefit of prophylactic antibiotics in any type of puncture, although antibiotic prophylaxis is recommended for use in high-risk patients with plantar puncture wounds.**[20] "High-risk" includes patients with diabetes[13] and impaired host defenses and may also include forefoot injuries and patients sustaining punctures through athletic shoes.[6] There is only one published study comparing patients receiving prophylactic antibiotics for plantar puncture wounds with untreated patients, and a variety of oral antibiotics were used.[21] There were many confounders with this observational study, and a subsequent review concluded that no evidence-based recommendations can be made regarding the use of prophylactic antibiotics for plantar puncture wounds.[22]

If prophylactic antibiotics are used, agents typically used for established wound infection are recommended—such as a first-generation oral cephalosporin, antistaphylococcal penicillin, or macrolide.[20] Although methicillin-resistant *S. aureus* has become a common cause of skin and soft tissue infections, postinjury antibiotic prophylaxis to cover this pathogen is not necessary.[20] **For plantar puncture wounds through athletic shoes, an oral fluoroquinolone with antipseudomonal activity, such as ciprofloxacin, seems sensible.** Agents such as trimethoprim-sulfamethoxazole and tetracycline can provide antistaphylococcal coverage but lack antipseudomonal activity. If antipseudomonal coverage is desired and oral fluoroquinolones are contraindicated, a combination of oral antistaphylococcal and parenteral antipseudomonal antibiotics (e.g., ticarcillin, ceftazidime, or cefepime) would be an acceptable albeit inconvenient choice.

COMPLICATIONS

Infectious complications of puncture wounds include cellulitis, localized abscess, deep soft tissue infection, and osteomyelitis. The hallmark of all complications is persistent pain. Patients with continued or increasing pain >48 hours postinjury should undergo an evaluation for retained foreign body or abscess.

Cellulitis Cellulitis usually presents within 4 days after injury. The patient typically notes pain with or without swelling and redness. Physical examination may demonstrate tenderness, erythema at the site of injury, warmth, and swelling. Postinjury cellulitis is an indication for imaging to evaluate for a retained foreign body. Cellulitis is generally caused by streptococcal and staphylococcal skin flora and usually responds to a 7- to 10-day course of a first-generation cephalosporin, antistaphylococcal penicillin, trimethoprim-sulfamethoxazole, or clindamycin.

Abscess Localized abscess is usually associated with a retained foreign body. Patients may note swelling and possibly drainage. A tender, warm, fluctuant mass can be palpated and further defined with US. Standard incision and drainage is generally curative. Where possible, the incision should be longitudinal or parallel to underlying tendons, vessels, or nerves. A short course of antibiotics is indicated if there is surrounding cellulitis.

Deep soft tissue infection is generally more painful than that of cellulitis or localized abscess. The key physical examination finding is tenderness, redness, or swelling remote from the puncture site. With plantar or palmar injuries, redness on the dorsum of the foot or hand, respectively, suggests a deep space infection. CT or MRI studies are indicated. Treatment requires parenteral antibiotics and surgical exploration with drainage, excision of necrotic tissue, and irrigation of infected areas.

Osteomyelitis Osteomyelitis is the most disastrous consequence of puncture wounds, occurring in 0.1% to 2.0% of all plantar puncture wounds and perhaps with a greater prevalence in forefoot punctures occurring through athletic shoes.[7-11] Patients with osteomyelitis present later than patients with other infections, often >7 days after injury and sometimes after a period of symptomatic improvement.[10] Pain is present in nearly every case, but the examination may be deceptively normal. Radiographs are normal in the early stages of osteomyelitis. Elevated erythrocyte sedimentation rate or C-reactive protein supports the diagnosis, but a normal value does not exclude osteomyelitis.[10,23,24] Imaging modalities most helpful in the diagnosis of osteomyelitis are nuclear medicine (either a triple-phase radionuclide bone scan with planar scintigraphy or with single-photon emission CT) or MRI.[25-27] Once the diagnosis is made, immediate surgical referral should be made. Antibiotic administration should be withheld pending discussion with the consultant, as pathogen identification is best done from cultures obtained during operative debridement. If antibiotics are administered before surgery, staphylococcal and pseudomonal coverage is recommended.

Disposition and Follow-Up of Complications Cellulitis and localized abscesses are almost always treated on an outpatient basis with incision and drainage, with oral antibiotics added in the case of surrounding cellulitis or fever. Follow-up is recommended in 48 hours to assess response.[10] Inpatient therapy is indicated when the patient has a significant systemic response to this localized infection, the infection is extensive, comorbidities or drug allergies preclude safe oral therapy, patients cannot tolerate oral medications, or patients cannot reliably care for the infection outside of the hospital setting. Deep soft tissue infection and osteomyelitis require admission, surgical intervention, and IV antibiotics.

SPECIAL CONSIDERATIONS FOR PUNCTURE WOUNDS

Needle-Stick Injuries **Needle-stick injuries** are common among healthcare professionals, especially in nurses and physicians who perform invasive procedures.[28,29] Mechanical damage from needle-stick injuries is essentially negligible. The major concerns are the risk of infection with hepatitis viruses and human immunodeficiency virus. **The risk of infection in a nonimmune recipient after an inadvertent needle stick contaminated from an infectious source has been estimated to be negligible for hepatitis A, 6% for hepatitis B, 2% for hepatitis C, and 0.3% for HIV.**[30]

Postexposure prophylaxis is available for hepatitis B and HIV, but is not for hepatitis C.[30] Recommendations for the assessment and management of occupational exposures to blood and body fluids (such as needle sticks) are complex and change frequently. Hospitals should have predetermined protocols endorsed by local infectious diseases specialists that are readily available and periodically reviewed. Consensus recommendations for postexposure prophylaxis of human immunodeficiency virus are updated regularly by the Centers for Disease Control and Prevention and are available from the National HIV/AIDS Clinicians' Consultation Center, accessible via the Internet at http://www.nccc.ucsf.edu/home/ or by phone at the National Clinicians' Post-Exposure Prophylaxis Hotline (PEPline) at

1-888-448-4911. When available, the use of rapid human immunodeficiency virus testing on the source (patient, blood, or fluid) can reduce the need for unnecessary prophylaxis on the exposed individual.

High-Pressure Injection Injuries **High-pressure injection injuries** are caused by industrial equipment designed to force grease, paint, or other liquids through a small-diameter nozzle at high pressures.[31-35] When the nozzle is applied close to or directly on the skin surface, the high pressure results in penetration of intact skin, forcing the material deep into the underlying structures and along fascial planes. The nozzle pressures for these devices are typically 5000 to 10,000 psi for grease guns, 2000 to 6000 psi for diesel fuel injectors, and up to 5000 psi for paint and water sprayers. Such extreme pressure can lacerate skin and fracture bones (**Figure 46-2**). The type, amount, and viscosity of material injected will determine the degree of tissue inflammatory response, and in less distensible tissue compartments, sudden pressure elevations can produce vascular injuries, ischemic necrosis, and gangrene.[32,35]

Most high-pressure injection injuries occur in the nondominant hand of an operator using a trigger-activated gun. The initial injury may cause little pain and appear relatively innocuous, leading to delays in presentation and under-appreciation of the extent of injury. Within hours, pain typically becomes severe, with evidence of ischemia or spreading inflammation. Delays in initial management increase the risk of amputation or disability.[32-35]

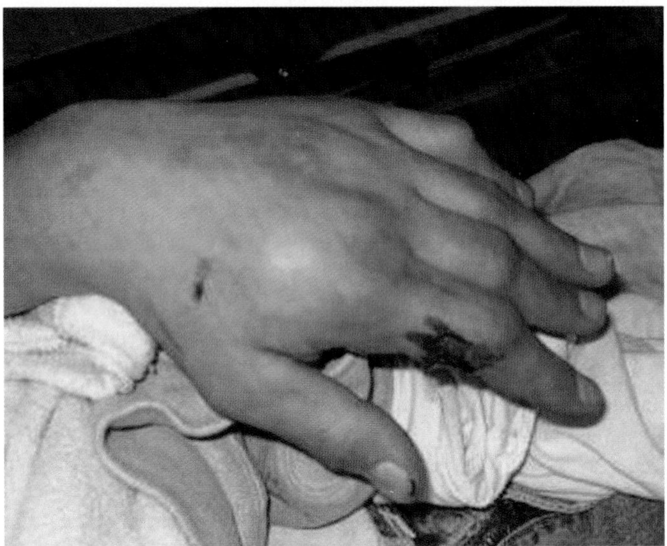

A

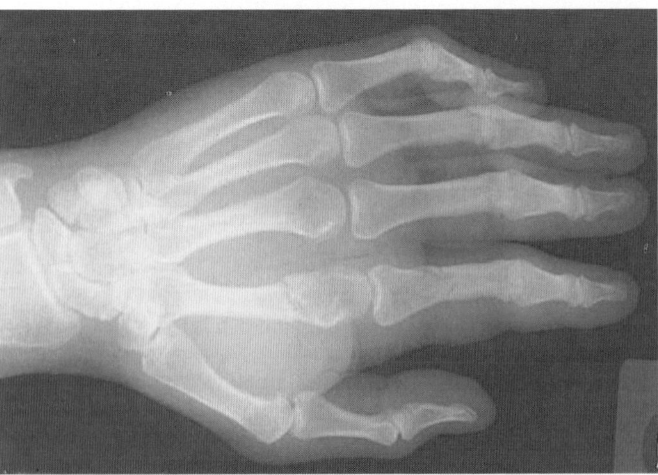

B

FIGURE 46-2. **A.** Skin and soft tissue injury of left index finger due to high-pressure water device. **B.** Radiograph showing fractures of metacarpal and proximal phalanx as well as subcutaneous air. [Photo contributed by J. S. Stapczynski, MD.]

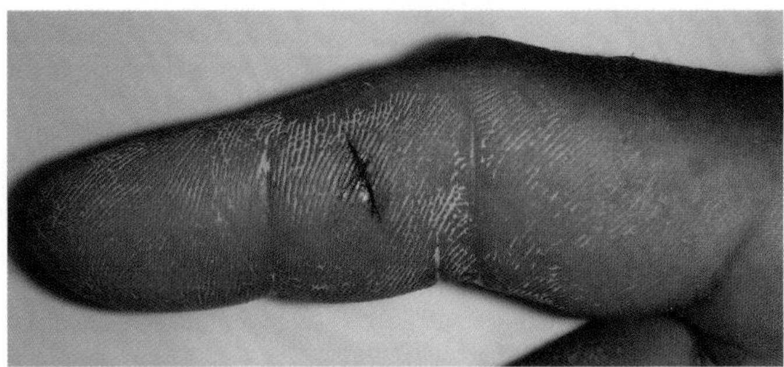

A

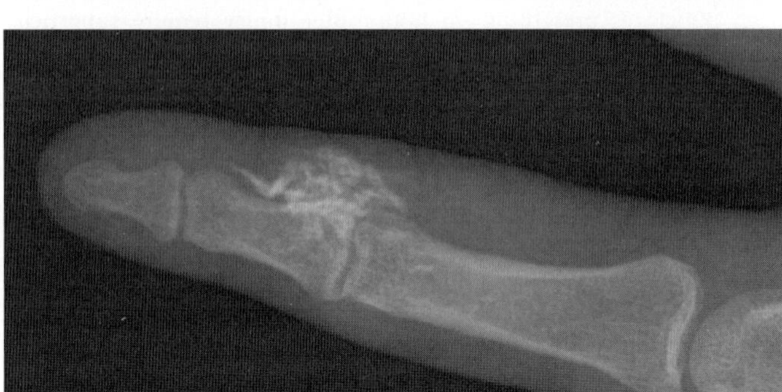

B

FIGURE 46-3. **A.** High-pressure injection paint injury to index finger. **B.** Radiograph showing radiopaque material. [Photo contributed by J. S. Stapczynski, MD.]

Despite an initial appearance that suggests only a minor injury (**Figure 46-3**), the history of high-pressure injection device use alone should prompt immediate consultation with a hand surgeon.[32-35]

ED evaluation includes assessment of neurovascular integrity and tendon function, pain management using IV opioids, prophylactic antibiotic coverage against skin flora, and tetanus prophylaxis as indicated. Radiographs will often demonstrate wide dissemination of radiopaque material as well as injected air along fascial planes (**Figures 46-2** and **44-3**). **Digital nerve blocks should be avoided, as they may further increase pressure in finger compartments. The risk of subsequent amputation is reduced if surgical debridement is performed within 6 hours of the injury, especially in cases of organic solvents.**[32,33,35] For patients with high-pressure injection of water only into the hand, it may be possible to forego exploration and manage with antibiotics, analgesics, and elevation, but that decision should be made in consultation with a hand specialist.[35,36]

Epinephrine Autoinjector Injuries **Epinephrine autoinjector injuries** occur most often to the finger (**Figure 46-4**). The typical scenario involves a patient who is unfamiliar with the proper use of the autoinjector or who errs as a result of the stress of the situation.[37,38] Patients present with pain due to the needle stick, paresthesias, and epinephrine-induced vasospasm to the injected area. In the extreme, the entire digit can be blanched and cold.[39,40] The intensity of digital ischemia and response to treatment can be assessed with digital pulse oximetry of the involved finger. The natural history of this injury is spontaneous resolution over several hours, with a reported range of resolution from 6 to 13 hours.[37-41] The published case reports sometimes express concern that the intense vasospasm can lead to tissue loss or gangrene, although the chance of this occurring appears rare.[42,43] Additionally, patients sustaining accidental injection without acute symptoms or signs of ischemia do well.[41,43] **There is no clear evidence that active treatment is better than observation alone,**[43] although patients and physicians may be uncomfortable with a prolonged ischemic and painful finger.

Attempts to increase blood flow to the ischemic digit with massage, warm water immersion, amyl nitrite inhalations, metacarpal nerve

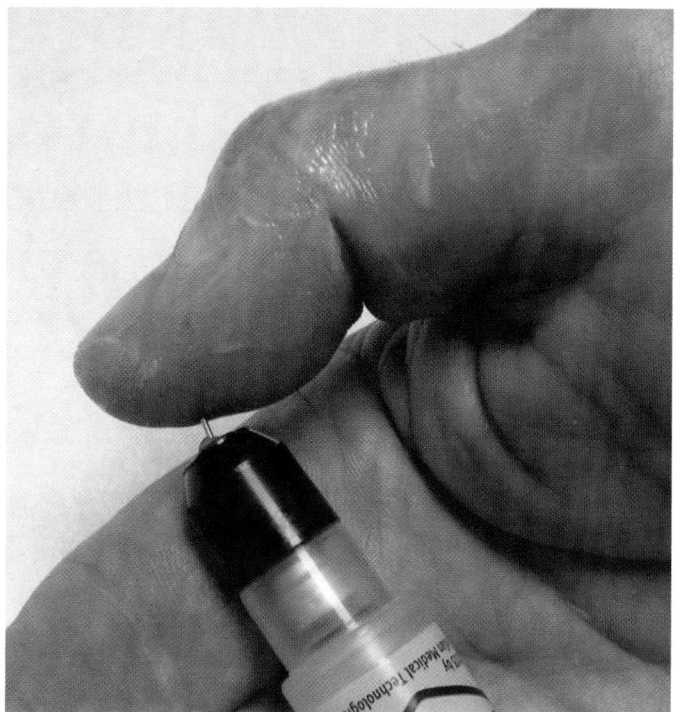

FIGURE 46-4. Accidental epinephrine autoinjector injury to thumb. [Photo contributed by Sean Donahue, DO.]

block, or topical nitroglycerin paste application have no proven value.[37,42] Subcutaneous phentolamine injection into the affected area is the one treatment consistently described that rapidly reverses digital ischemia from accidental epinephrine injection.[37,39-42] Phentolamine doses described range from 1.5 to 3.0 milligrams, and response is usually seen within minutes. A mixture of 0.5 mL of standard phentolamine solution (5 milligrams/mL concentration) and 0.5 mL of 1% lidocaine solution will produce a 1 mL total volume containing 2.5 milligrams of phentolamine that can be subcutaneously injected directly through the site of autoinjector puncture. Once the ischemia is resolved, the patient can be discharged, as relapse appears very unlikely.

MAMMALIAN BITES

Most patients presenting for ED care of bite injuries have been bitten by domestic dogs or cats. In the United States, an estimated nearly 4 million people are bitten each year, approximately 800,000 seek medical attention, and 10 to 20 will die of their injuries.[44] Because of their size, children have greater potential for serious injuries and seek care for bites more often than adults.[45-47] Dogs that are specifically bred or trained for guard duty cause a disproportionate number of serious injuries and deaths.[45,47]

GENERAL PRINCIPLES OF BITE WOUND MANAGEMENT

Complications from bite wounds include the mechanical injury inflicted by the bite itself, local bacterial infection, and systemic infection or illness.[48] A large animal or multiple animals attacking a child or small adult can inflict severe injuries, including vascular damage and blunt or penetrating trauma. Standard assessment and resuscitation protocols for trauma victims should be employed if the patient is seriously injured. Take particular care when assessing children with facial and scalp bites from large dogs, as there are numerous case reports of innocuous-looking wounds associated with skull penetration resulting in brain abscess.[49,50] In most animal bite wounds, there is an isolated soft tissue injury and wound management and prevention of infection are the key issues.[48]

Meticulous examination and cleansing measures, including aggressive irrigation and debridement of devitalized tissue, are important.

TABLE 46-3 Indications for Primary Closure of Mammalian Bite Wounds
Location: face or scalp
Wound characteristics: simple and appropriate for single-layer closure, no devitalized tissue
Lack of underlying injury: no underlying fracture
Host: no systemic immunocompromising conditions

Determine the extent of underlying tissue damage, with special attention to the potential for penetration into joint spaces and tendon sheaths. Management of wounds involving the face, hands, or perineum can be challenging due to the close proximity of delicate structures. If there is suspicion of retained foreign material in the wound, such as animal teeth, imaging is needed.[51]

Some bite lacerations can safely undergo primary repair (**Table 46-3**). If desired for cosmetic or functional reasons, a skilled practitioner can primarily close the wound with percutaneous sutures with a risk of postrepair wound infection of less than 5%.[52-58] Delayed primary closure is applicable for the management of contaminated bite injuries, especially in areas other than the face (see chapter 41, Wound Closure).

Case reports have described the occurrence of bacteremia, sepsis, and death after dog bites in immunocompromised individuals, most often due to *Capnocytophaga canimorsus*.[59,60] **Wound closure is associated with a small increased risk of local wound infection but is unlikely to enhance the risk of serious systemic infection from *Capnocytophaga*, unless the patient is immunodeficient or the wound is at high risk of infection. The current practice is to avoid primary wound closure in patients with systemic immunodeficiencies and higher risk wounds (Table 46-4).**[61] High-risk wounds should be cleaned and debrided of devitalized tissue, closure avoided, and dressed with a nonadherent wound dressing to maintain a moist environment for epithelial regeneration, with re-evaluation in 24 to 48 hours. Prophylactic antibiotics are recommended for higher risk wounds, especially if primarily closed (**Table 46-5**).[61]

MICROBIOLOGY AND THERAPY OF INFECTIONS FROM CAT AND DOG BITES

Mammalian saliva contains large concentrations of microorganisms, and bite wounds should be considered to be contaminated with pathogenic bacteria.[62] The force of a bite, especially a clenching bite, can inoculate bacteria deep into the underlying tissue, leading to cellulitis, tenosynovitis, and septic arthritis. **Most dog bite wounds are relatively superficial, and despite the inoculation of bacteria, only approximately 5% of untreated dog bites will become infected.** Cats have narrower, sharper teeth than dogs, giving them the ability to deliver infectious agents deeper into a small-bore puncture wound. Thus **up to 80% of cat bites that present for care will become infected,** although the true rate of infection is unknown since most patients with cat bites do not present for care unless the bite appears infected (**Figure 46-5**).[62,63]

TABLE 46-4 Bite Wounds at Higher Risk of Infection
Cat or human bites
Livestock bites
Monkey bites
Puncture wounds
Hand or foot wounds
Bites in immunosuppressed patients
Signs of local infection when first evaluated
Heavily contaminated wounds that are older with devitalized tissue
Diabetes

TABLE 46-5 Common Bites and First-Line Treatment

Animal	Organism	First-Line Antibiotic
Cat	*Pasteurella multocida*	Amoxicillin-clavulanate
	Bartonella henselae (cat-scratch fever)	Azithromycin
Dog	*Pasteurella*, streptococci, staphylococci, *Capnocytophaga canimorsus*	Amoxicillin-clavulanate
Human	*Eikenella*, staphylococci, streptococci	Amoxicillin-clavulanate
	Herpes simplex (herpetic whitlow)	Acyclovir or valacyclovir
Rats, mice, squirrels, gerbils	*Streptobacillus moniliformis* (North America) or *Spirillum minus/minor* (Asia)	Amoxicillin-clavulanate
Livestock, large game animals	Multiple organisms	Amoxicillin-clavulanate or specific agent for disease
	Brucella, Leptospira, Francisella tularensis	
Bats, monkeys, dogs, skunks, raccoons, foxes (all carnivores and omnivores)	Rabies	Rabies immune globulin, rabies vaccine
Monkeys	Herpes B virus (*Cercopithecine herpesvirus*)	Acyclovir or valacyclovir
Freshwater fish	*Aeromonas*, staphylococci, streptococci	Fluoroquinolone or trimethoprim-sulfamethoxazole
Saltwater fish	*Vibrio*, staphylococci, streptococci	Fluoroquinolone

Infection after a cat bite is often due to *Pasteurella multocida*, particularly if the infection develops with 24 hours.[64-66] Infected dog bites are just as likely to contain *Pasteurella*, as well as anaerobes, streptococcal, and staphylococcal species.[64,66] Postexposure antibiotic prophylaxis of most bite wounds to prevent infection is controversial.[20,67] The only evidence-based benefit for prophylactic antibiotics is with dog or cat bites of the hands.[67,68]

A prudent approach is to use prophylactic antibiotics for higher-risk uninfected wounds. These include all cat bites, all bites in immunocompromised hosts, deep dog bite puncture wounds, hand wounds, and any injury undergoing surgical repair.[20] A 3- to 5-day course of an appropriate antimicrobial (**Table 46-5**) should be sufficient. Routine follow-up wound check is recommended in all but the most trivial cases. In lower-risk situations, counseling and advice regarding the lack of benefit from prophylactic antibiotics in addition to wound-care precautions are warranted.

Amoxicillin-clavulanate is the antibiotic most commonly recommended for prophylaxis of uninfected wounds and for treatment of local infections following dog, cat, or human bites.[20,48,54,63,67,68] However, penicillin V or ampicillin should be adequate for *Pasteurella multocida* infections and represent logical lower-cost alternatives for prophylaxis of cat bites.[68] Penicillin-allergic patients should receive doxycycline or cefuroxime for cat bites and clindamycin plus a fluoroquinolone for dog bites. **Cephalexin, dicloxacillin, erythromycin, or clindamycin should not be used alone for dog or cat bites, as they do not reliably cover *Pasteurella* species.**

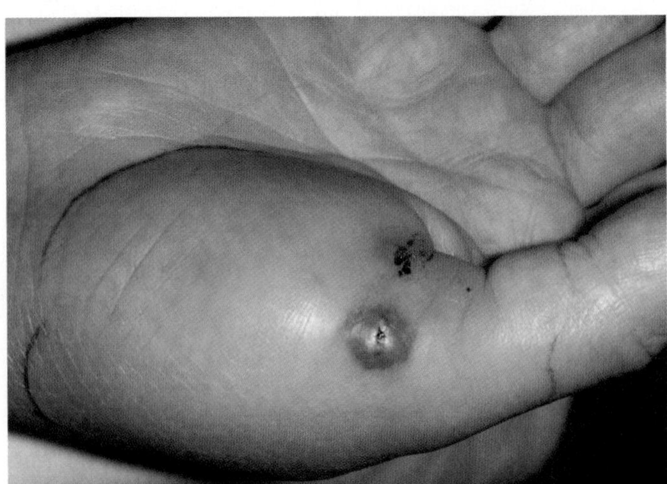

FIGURE 46-5. Hand infection after a cat bite. Wound fluid culture grew *Pasteurella multocida*. [Photo contributed by J. S. Stapczynski, MD.]

SYSTEMIC BACTERIAL INFECTIONS AFTER DOG AND CAT BITES

Capnocytophaga Serious systemic infection after dog or cat bites is rare, but can develop days after the bite and is not necessarily accompanied by local bite wound infection.[60,69] *Capnocytophaga canimorsus* produces a rare but fulminant bacteremic illness after a dog bite, with fatal multiorgan failure, particularly in splenectomized patients and those with alcoholism or other immunosuppressive disorders.[59] Broad-spectrum therapy with penicillin and other agents is indicated in concert with aggressive resuscitation.[59] The virulence of this rare infection provides some justification for the prophylactic use of a penicillin-class agent in all immunocompromised patients bitten by dogs.

Cat-Scratch Disease Cat-scratch disease is a clinical syndrome of regional lymphadenopathy developing 7 to 12 days after a cat bite or scratch.[70-72] This chronic indolent infection caused by *Bartonella henselae* can result in painful, matted masses of lymph nodes.[71] Mild constitutional symptoms are common, and nonlymphoid organs may be affected in approximately 10% of cases (**Table 46-6**). The causative bacteria cannot be easily cultured from human lymph node tissue, so the diagnosis is usually made using a combination of epidemiologic, clinical, histologic, and/or serologic criteria.[70-72]

Most cases with only lymph node involvement resolve in 2 to 5 months, and therapy consists primarily of pain relief and reassurance. Large, painful, fluctuant nodes can be aspirated for symptomatic relief. Incision and drainage is to be avoided, as persistent fistula and scarring

TABLE 46-6 Organ Involvement in Cat Scratch Disease

Constitutional symptoms
Low-grade fever
Malaise and fatigue
Headache
Nausea and anorexia
Nonlymphoid organ involvement—often with prolonged fever
CNS: encephalopathy with headache, seizures, confusion, or altered mental status
Musculoskeletal: synovitis with joint pain and swelling
Lungs: pneumonitis with dyspnea and cough
Abdomen: granulomatous hepatitis or splenitis producing abdominal pain
Eyes: retinitis with vision loss

have been reported. Antibiotics are not indicated in most cases, but in patients with severe painful lymphadenopathy, a 5-day course of azithromycin may speed resolution of adenopathy.[73] Patients with systemic immunodeficiencies are susceptible to severe infection and bacteremia from *B. henselae*, so it is reasonable to treat immunodeficient patients with a 7- to 10-day course of trimethoprim-sulfamethoxazole, ciprofloxacin, or rifampin. Patients with nonlymphoid organ involvement usually require admission for definitive evaluation and parenteral antibiotic treatment. The vast majority of patients, even those with multiorgan involvement, recover without sequelae.

HUMAN BITES

Human bites tend to be more serious than bites from domestic animals.[74-76] The reasons are likely due to the nature of the event, location of the bite, and potential bacteria inoculated into the wound. Treatment recommendations are based on experience. All human bites should be treated as contaminated wounds. Patients with human bites often present for care late after injury.[75] The **closed-fist injury**, incurred when a flexed knuckle strikes a human tooth in the course of an altercation, is a common human bite injury (see chapter 43, Arm and Hand Lacerations). Most human bite wounds should not undergo primary closure, with the possible exception of wounds to the face, where primary closure is associated with a postrepair wound infection rate of approximately 10%.[56,76]

Human bite wound infections are usually polymicrobial, and the most common organisms isolated are staphylococcal and streptococcal species. Other pathogens include the species-specific gram-negative rod *Eikenella corrodens*. **Amoxicillin-clavulanate is recommended for prophylaxis after all but the most trivial human bites.**[20,63] For established infections, parenteral agents of choice include ampicillin-sulbactam, cefoxitin, or piperacillin-tazobactam.

Herpes simplex virus can cause local infection, termed **herpetic whitlow**, after a human bite or contact with infected saliva.[77] The appearance is usually a painful coalescence of vesicles, typically on the distal phalanx (**Figure 46-6**). Vesicles usually resolve in 3 to 4 weeks. Treatment with oral acyclovir for 7 to 10 days or topical acyclovir ointment for 7 to 14 days may shorten the duration of the symptoms.

RODENTS, LIVESTOCK, EXOTIC AND WILD ANIMALS

Rodents Patients often seek care or consultation after being bitten by a rodent. The injury is usually trivial, the risk of local wound infection is low, and rodents are not known to carry or transmit rabies, so standard wound care and reassurance should suffice. Of more concern is the potential zoonotic systemic infections carried by mice and rats.[78] **Rat-bite fever** consists of two similar febrile illnesses occurring after a small percentage of bites from rats, mice, squirrels, or gerbils due to either *Streptobacillus moniliformis* (more common in North America) or *Spirillum minus/minor* (more common in Asia).[79] Infection can also result from exposure to rat feces or urine. The incubation period for the streptobacillary form is typically 3 to 7 days, whereas it is usually longer than 10 days for the spirillary variety. Onset is typically with rigors and fevers and progresses to migratory polyarthralgia and a maculopapular petechial or purpuric rash. Infection can spread to the heart, brain, arteries, liver, kidneys, and lungs. The mortality rate for untreated infection is 10% to 15%. Treatment is with IV penicillin for 5 to 7 days followed by oral penicillin for an additional 7 days. Doxycycline or tetracycline is used for penicillin-allergic patients.

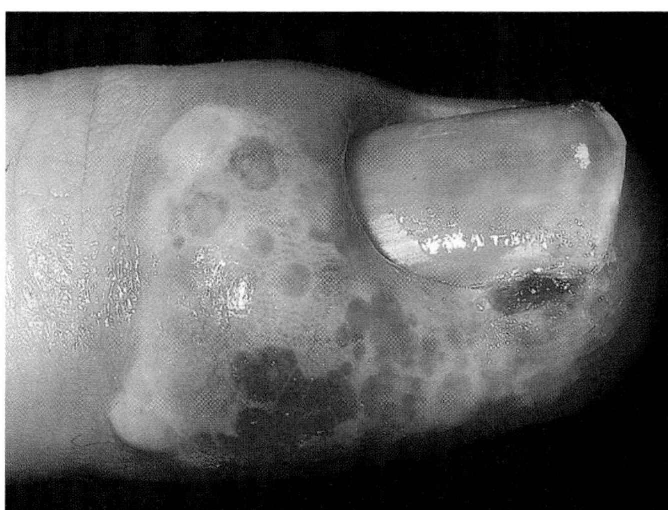

FIGURE 46-6. Herpes simplex virus infection: herpetic whitlow. Painful, grouped, confluent vesicles on an erythematous edematous base on the distal finger were the first (and presumed primary) symptomatic infection. [Reproduced with permission from Wolff K, Johnson RA: *Fitzpatrick's Color Atlas and Synopsis of Clinical Dermatology, 6th ed.* New York. McGraw-Hill; 2009, p. 821.]

Livestock and Large Game Animals Livestock and large game animals can inflict serious tissue injury with their powerful jaws and grinding teeth.[80] The risk of wound infection is significant, and systemic illnesses, such as brucellosis, leptospirosis, or tularemia, can follow the injury. Aggressive wound care, imaging to detect fractures, and prophylactic broad-spectrum antibiotics are recommended. A febrile illness after such a bite usually requires inpatient antibiotic therapy guided by blood culture results.[60]

Fish Bites Freshwater fish bite infections can be due to *Aeromonas*, streptococci, and staphylococci, and treatment is with a fluoroquinolone or trimethoprim-sulfamethoxazole. Saltwater fish bite infections require coverage for *Vibrio*, usually with a fluoroquinolone.

SYSTEMIC INFECTIONS: SPIROCHETES, RABIES, AND OTHER VIRUSES

Disseminated spirochetal and viral illnesses resulting from mammalian bites include syphilis, rabies, hepatitis, herpes B virus, or human immunodeficiency virus. The risk of infection is variable depending on the amount of infectious organisms in the saliva of the biting animal.

Most human rabies cases identified in the United States were acquired from contact with domestic bats or from dog bites sustained while traveling abroad (see chapter 157, Rabies). In South Asia, monkeys are presumed to be at high risk for carriage and transmission of rabies. North American reservoirs of animal rabies exist in bats, skunks, raccoons, and foxes. **All carnivores and omnivores can transmit rabies, whereas rodents, hares, and rabbits are extremely unlikely to harbor the disease.** Local public health agencies or the state veterinarian are a good source of information regarding the rabies risk from contact with specific indigenous animals and recommended postexposure prophylaxis with immunoglobulin and vaccine.

B virus, also called herpes B, is caused by *Macacine herpesvirus* 1 and can be transmitted by bites from monkeys and other nonhuman primates.[81,82] Human infection with B virus causes myelitis and hemorrhagic encephalitis, with a case fatality rate of 70%. Immediate and thorough wound cleaning after a bite reduces the chance of infection, and acyclovir or valacyclovir given immediately after injury can prevent or ameliorate this illness.[83] Consultation with an infectious disease expert is strongly advised. The Centers for Disease Control and Prevention maintains a Web site with current B virus information at http://www.cdc.gov/herpesbvirus/index.html.

Viral hepatitis and human immunodeficiency virus can both be transmitted by a human bite, although human immunodeficiency virus concentration in nonbloody saliva is thought to be relatively low. **A protocol similar to that for an occupational needle-stick injury should be used when a patient sustains a bite from a high-risk source** (see chapter 154, Human Immunodeficiency Virus Infection).

REFERENCES

The complete reference list is available online at www.TintinalliEM.com.

CHAPTER 47

Postrepair Wound Care

Adam J. Singer
Judd E. Hollander

INTRODUCTION

Postoperative care begins immediately after laceration repair in the ED with gentle cleansing using normal saline or clean (tap) water to remove any residual blood products or contamination. Additional considerations include dressings, topical antibiotics, edema reduction techniques, prophylactic antibiotics, tetanus prophylaxis, and wound drains. Before ED release, give the patient instructions regarding wound care and cleansing, pain control, signs of infection, follow-up dates, and short-term and long-term cosmetic expectations.

WOUND DRESSINGS

Postoperative wound dressing should be tailored to both the type of wound and method of wound closure. Most sutured or stapled lacerations should be covered with a protective, nonadherent dressing for 24 to 48 hours. Maintaining a moist environment increases the rate of re-epithelialization, and occluded wounds heal faster than those exposed to air.[1-3] Conversely, leaving lacerations exposed to air may result in a slightly lower healing rate but does not result in an increased rate of infection.[4]

Useful dressings are semipermeable films manufactured from transparent polyurethane or similar synthetic films coated on one surface with a water-resistant hypoallergenic adhesive. They are highly elastic, conform easily to body parts, and are generally resistant to shear and tear. They are permeable to moisture vapor and oxygen but impermeable to water and bacteria. Common brands of semipermeable wound dressings are OpSite Post-Op® (Smith & Nephew PLC, London, UK), Bioclusive® (Johnson & Johnson, New Brunswick, NJ), and Tegaderm® (3M, St. Paul, MN). The disadvantages of these products are that they cannot absorb large amounts of fluid and exudate, and they do not adhere well to very moist wounds.

Topical antibiotic creams and ointments are an alternative to the use of commercial dressings to maintain a moist environment. As an added benefit, topical antibiotics may help reduce infection rates and may also prevent scab formation.[5-7] **However, patients whose lacerations are closed with tissue adhesives should not use topical ointments or creams because they will loosen the adhesive and may result in dehiscence.** Tissue adhesives serve as their own antimicrobial barrier and occlusive dressing; wounds closed with tissue adhesives do not require supplementary dressings.

EDEMA REDUCTION AFTER WOUND REPAIR

Wounds with associated soft tissue contusion should have the injury site elevated above the patient's heart for 24 to 48 hours to limit accumulation of fluid in the wound interstitial spaces. Wounds with little edema heal more rapidly than those with marked edema. Pressure dressings can be used to minimize the accumulation of intercellular fluid in the subcutaneous space. Pressure dressings are useful for ear and scalp lacerations (see chapter 42, "Face and Scalp Lacerations"). Pressure dressing applied to the ear can prevent auricular hematoma formation and reduce the subsequent likelihood of a cauliflower deformity. Vaseline gauze or Xeroform® (Kendall Healthcare, Mansfield, MA) dressings are easy to mold around the ear. For large scalp lacerations that have a tendency to bleed, short-term use of a pressure dressing will limit subcutaneous hematoma formation. However, excessive pressure should be avoided in all pressure dressings, especially in the extremities where they may compromise circulation. Consider a short period of splinting with large lacerations over joints to reduce pain, limit tension on the wound, minimize swelling, and promote healing.

PROPHYLACTIC ANTIBIOTICS

Prophylactic oral antibiotics are not recommended except for select circumstances[8-11] based on guiding principles: the degree of bacterial contamination, the presence of infection-potentiating factors (e.g., soil), the mechanism of injury, and the presence or absence of host predisposition to infection.[12-14] **Compulsive wound cleansing is far more important than antibiotics to reduce postrepair wound infection.**[15,16]

Prophylactic antibiotics are recommended for human bites, cat bites, deep dog bite puncture wounds, bite wounds to the hand, open fractures, and wounds with exposed joints or tendon.[12-17] Also, consider prophylactic antibiotics after wound closure in a lymphedematous area.[18,19]

The risk of bacteremia during care of grossly contaminated lacerations in the ED is unknown, but is likely to be small.[20] However, some patients who have structural heart disease, arteriovenous hemodialysis fistulas, prosthetic joints, cerebrospinal fluid shunts, vascular grafts, or other permanent indwelling "hardware" may trap bacteria from the blood stream and develop infections in the above-mentioned organs or devices. There is no evidence for preprocedure antibiotic prophylaxis to prevent bacteremic spread of infection from manipulation of a contaminated site. If the physician chooses to use antibiotic prophylaxis for the management of a heavily contaminated wound in a patient with these conditions or devices, give a single dose of an IV antibiotic before the wound is manipulated.

Antibiotics used for postrepair prophylaxis are similar to those used for treatment of established infections (**Table 47-1**).[8] For most patients, a first-generation cephalosporin or antistaphylococcal penicillin (e.g., dicloxacillin) is reasonable. Although methicillin-resistant *Staphylococcus aureus* has become a common cause of skin and soft tissue infections, postinjury antibiotic prophylaxis to cover this pathogen does not appear necessary.[8] Amoxicillin-clavulanate is the preferred prophylactic treatment for high-risk mammalian bite wounds.[12,13] For open fractures or joints, a parenteral antistaphylococcal agent and an aminoglycoside should be used.[17] There is no evidence that patients who receive antibiotic prophylaxis benefit from an initial IV dose. Antibiotic prophylaxis

TABLE 47-1 Postrepair Oral Antibiotic Prophylaxis

Situation	Primary Recommendation	Alternative Recommendation
Uncomplicated patient	First-generation cephalosporin or antistaphylococcal penicillin	Macrolide Clindamycin
Grossly contaminated wounds and/or retained foreign body	Amoxicillin/clavulanate or second-generation cephalosporin	Clindamycin plus a fluoroquinolone
Bite wounds	Amoxicillin/clavulanate	Clindamycin plus either a fluoroquinolone or trimethoprim-sulfamethoxazole
Plantar puncture wounds	Ciprofloxacin	First-generation cephalosporin or antistaphylococcal penicillin
Underlying systemic immunodeficiency (AIDS, chronic steroid use, poorly controlled diabetes mellitus)	Amoxicillin/clavulanate or second-generation cephalosporin	Clindamycin plus a fluoroquinolone
Impaired local defenses (peripheral arterial disease, lymphedema)	Amoxicillin/clavulanate	Clindamycin or erythromycin

TABLE 47-2 Recommendations for Tetanus Prophylaxis

	Clean Minor Wounds		All Other Wounds*	
History of Tetanus Immunization	Administer Tetanus Toxoid†	Administer TIG‡	Administer Tetanus Toxoid	Administer TIG
<3 or uncertain doses	Yes	No	Yes	Yes
≥3 doses				
Last dose within 5 y	No	No	No	No
Last dose within 5–10 y	No	No	Yes	No
Last dose >10 y	Yes	No	Yes	No

*Especially if wound care delayed (>6 h), deep (>1 cm), grossly contaminated, exposed to saliva or feces, stellate, ischemic or infected, avulsions, punctures, or crush injuries.

†Tetanus toxoid: Tdap if adult and no prior record of administration; otherwise, tetanus-diphtheria toxoid if >7 years and diphtheria-tetanus toxoid if <7 years, preferably administered into the deltoid.

‡Tetanus immune globulin: adult dose, 250–500 IU administered into deltoid opposite the tetanus-diphtheria toxoid immunization site.

continues for 3 to 5 days for nonbite injuries and 5 to 7 days for bite wounds. Patients at high risk for infection should be told to return for a wound check in 24 to 48 hours.

TETANUS PROPHYLAXIS

Two thirds of the recent tetanus cases in the United States follow lacerations, puncture wounds, and crush injuries (see chapter 156, "Tetanus"),[21] so, as part of wound care, ask about previous tetanus immunizations. Recommendations for tetanus prophylaxis are based on the condition of the wound and the patient's immunization history (**Table 47-2**). Consider passive immunization with tetanus immune globulin for those without a history of a primary series of three tetanus immunizations. Because of the emergence of pertussis infections, Tdap (containing the acellular pertussis vaccine) should replace a single dose of tetanus and diphtheria toxoids for adults who have not previously received a dose of Tdap (either in the primary series, as a booster, or for wound management).[22] The 2013 Advisory Committee on Immunization practices recommend either Tdap or Boostrix® for those >65 years old.

The only contraindication to tetanus toxoid is a history of neurologic or severe systemic reaction after a previous dose. Local self-limited reactions, such as erythema, induration, and pain at the injection site, are common after tetanus vaccination. These local side effects do not preclude future tetanus immunization. Exaggerated local reactions occur occasionally after tetanus toxoid and involve extensive pain and swelling of the entire extremity. Exaggerated local reactions occur most often in adults with high serum tetanus antitoxin levels who have received frequent doses of tetanus toxoid. Such patients should not receive tetanus toxoid more frequently than every 10 years. Severe systemic reactions to tetanus immunization include generalized urticaria, anaphylaxis, or neurologic complications, including peripheral neuropathy and Guillain-Barré syndrome. A severe allergic reaction, including acute respiratory distress or cardiovascular collapse after a dose of tetanus toxoid, is a contraindication to further immunization. A moderate or severe acute illness is also a reason to defer routine immunization, although a minor illness is not. If the use of a tetanus toxoid is contraindicated, consider passive immunization with tetanus immune globulin in a tetanus-prone wound.

WOUND CLEANSING

Sutured or stapled wounds can be gently washed and cleansed with tap water as early as 8 hours after closure without an increase in infection rate.[23,24] Using soap and tap water to cleanse lacerations will not increase the infection rate.[25] Use gentle blotting to dry the area; aggressive wiping could cause wound dehiscence. For routine wounds, tell patients to remove dressings after 24 hours, cleanse the wound, and examine it for signs of infections. In certain special situations, the dressing should remain undisturbed for 4 to 5 days until the patient is reevaluated by the physician.

Thereafter, daily cleansing ensures that the patient examines the laceration for early signs of infection. Patients should observe the wound for redness, warmth, swelling, and drainage, and contact a physician if such signs develop. Standardized wound-care instructions improve patient compliance and understanding.[26]

Reapplication of topical antibiotics for 3 to 5 days will decrease scab formation, thereby preventing wound edge separation. Patients with tissue adhesives may shower but should avoid bathing and swimming because prolonged moisture will loosen the adhesive bond and result in slightly earlier sloughing of the adhesive.[27]

WOUND DRAINS

Drains are placed in wounds and surgical incisions under three circumstances: (1) to drain interstitial fluid or blood and prevent accumulation into a seroma or hematoma, respectively; (2) to maintain a tract so pus can drain from an infected area; or (3) to allow for drainage from a contaminated location and prevent an abscess from forming.[28] Drains allow for near-complete wound closure in circumstances where closure would otherwise be impeded by fluid, pus, or blood accumulation. Drains can be categorized as (1) gauze packing to maintain open drainage and collect the exudate, (2) open systems using soft rubber (e.g., Penrose drain) or silicone tubing to direct drainage onto external gauze dressings, or (3) closed systems using silicone tubing and attached fluid collection reservoirs. Drains can be placed either through the suture line of the initial wound or incision or through an adjacent incision made specifically for drain access.

The most common type of wound drain placed in the ED is $^1/_4$- to 1-in. (0.6- to 2.5-cm) ribbon gauze used to pack an abscess cavity after incision and drainage. Dressings over draining abscesses may initially require frequent changes. **The internal packing should be replaced daily as long as the wound continues to produce exudate. Once the purulence stops, internal packing is no longer required, and daily cleaning with external dressing changes should continue until enough granulation tissue forms and the wound stops draining.** Maintaining a moist, clean environment promotes wound healing. Equivalent outcomes in otherwise healthy patients with subcutaneous abscesses can be obtained with alternatives to traditional packing: no packing,[29-31] incision and loop drainage,[32-35] modified Pezzar catheter,[36] and silver-containing hydrofiber dressing.[37]

Open drainage using soft rubber tubing (e.g., Penrose drains) has been used for years to drain infected or contaminated wounds that have been partially or completely closed. A safety pin placed through the tubing can prevent the drain from inappropriately advancing into the wound. As the exudate diminishes and the wound heals, the Penrose drain can be pulled out a portion each day to allow the wound to heal from the "bottom up." The disadvantage of open drains, such as the Penrose, is the access they provide for bacteria into the wound.

For many wounds, especially postsurgical wounds, closed drainage systems have replaced open wound drains. The collection reservoir for closed drainage systems often has a self-inflating ability so it can be squeezed before attachment to the tubing in order to place vacuum suction in the wound to enhance drainage (e.g., Jackson-Pratt®, Cardinal Health, Dublin, OH; Hemovac®, Zimmer, Inc., Warsaw, IN; ConstaVac®, Stryker Corp., Kalamazoo, MI). Assessment of the tubing and emptying of the reservoir should be done with sterile technique (similar to dressing changes for indwelling lines). The reservoir may require emptying several times per day, depending on the drainage volume. It is common practice to remove closed drains when the amount of fluid drained each day reaches low levels (typically 30 to 40 mL per day). If a drainage tube is accidentally pulled out, it should not be reinserted. In many surgical settings, the benefit of closed drainage systems is unproven.[38-47]

Vacuum-assisted closure or negative-pressure wound therapy is a method used to close difficult wounds.[48-51] The vacuum-assisted closure technique consists of insertion of an open-cell foam sponge into the wound, sealing with an adhesive drape, and subsequent application of negative, subatmospheric pressure, usually at 125 mm Hg.[50] Vacuum-assisted closure promotes wound healing by removing localized edema, which improves vascular and lymphatic flow by reducing bacteria density, by promoting angiogenesis, and by increasing granulation tissue formation.[48-50] There is no proven role for vacuum-assisted closure in the management of lacerations closed in the ED.

PAIN CONTROL

Abrasions and some lacerations can be quite painful. Patients should be educated regarding the expected degree of pain and measures that may help reduce pain. Splints can be used to reduce swelling and pain for extremity lacerations. Appropriate analgesic medications and anti-inflammatory agents will help control pain. The pain from lacerations generally decreases after the initial 48 hours, and opioid analgesics are rarely necessary after that time. Patients with concurrent contusions (such as victims of motor vehicle crashes) will often report worsening pain 24 to 48 hours after the initial injury.

FOLLOW-UP

Tell patients when and with whom to follow up for suture removal or wound examination.[26] Sutures or staples in most locations should be removed after approximately 7 to 10 days (**Table 47-3**). Remove facial sutures in 3 to 5 days to avoid formation of unsightly sinus tracts and hatch marks.[52] Sutures over the joints or in the hands should be left in place for 10 to 14 days, as they may be subject to increased tension during movement. When removing sutures, avoid applying tension in a direction that would tend to cause dehiscence. Debride any scab or crusting over the sutures before suture removal by gently applying gauze soaked with hydrogen peroxide. Then, grasp the suture at the knot with the forceps for removal (**Figure 47-1**). Use scissors or a #12 blade to cut the sutures. Skin staples are removed with a specific device that deforms the center and extracts the legs from the skin (**Figure 47-2**).

Tissue adhesives will slough off, typically within 5 to 10 days of application, and do not usually require removal. Tell the patient to avoid picking at the tissue adhesive or scrubbing the area or exposing it to water for more than brief periods. If tissue adhesives remain on the skin for prolonged periods, antibiotic ointment, petroleum jelly, or bathing can accelerate removal. When adhesive tapes are used, they can be removed by gentle peeling away from the skin, starting at one end of the laceration and proceeding along and parallel to the wound, avoiding pulling across or perpendicular to the wound.

Scheduled "wound checks" might be useful in high-risk patients, high-risk wounds, or patients unable to identify signs of infection. Because many healing wounds may develop erythema and patients are not able to correctly identify wound infections, do not prescribe antibiotics

TABLE 47-3 Suture and Staple Removal Recommendations

Location	Days
Face	3–4 (child), 3–5 (adult)
Neck	2–3 (child), 3–4 (adult)
Upper extremity	7–10
Hand	10–14
Chest	7–10
Back	10–14
Buttocks	10–14
Legs	8–10
Foot	10–14
Delayed closure	8–12
Retention sutures	14–30
Overlying joints	10–14

Source: Reproduced with permission from Reichman EF: *Emergency Medicine Procedures*, 2nd ed. McGraw-Hill, Inc., 2013, Chapter 92. General Principles of Wound Management, Table 92-4.

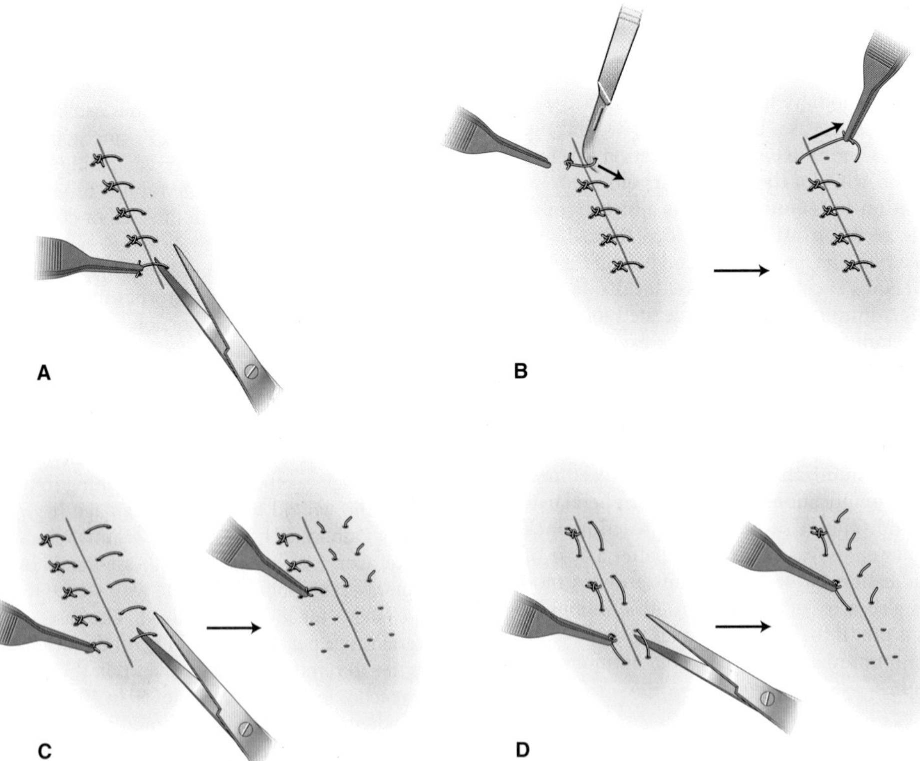

FIGURE 47-1. Suture removal. A. For simple interrupted percutaneous sutures, grasp the suture with the forceps at the knot, cut the suture with scissors on the side of the wound opposite the knot, and pull the knot across the wound. B. Alternatively, cut the suture with a curved #12 blade on the side of the wound opposite the knot (*left*) and pull the knot across the wound (*right*). C. For vertical mattress sutures, cut the suture on the side opposite the knot and pull the knot with forceps. D. For horizontal mattress sutures, cut the suture on the side opposite the knot and pull the knot with forceps. [A, C, and D reproduced with permission from Flippin AL, Cebrun H, Reichman ER: Basic wound closure techniques, in Reichman ER, Simon RR (eds): *Emergency Medical Procedures*. New York, McGraw-Hill, 2004, p. 730.]

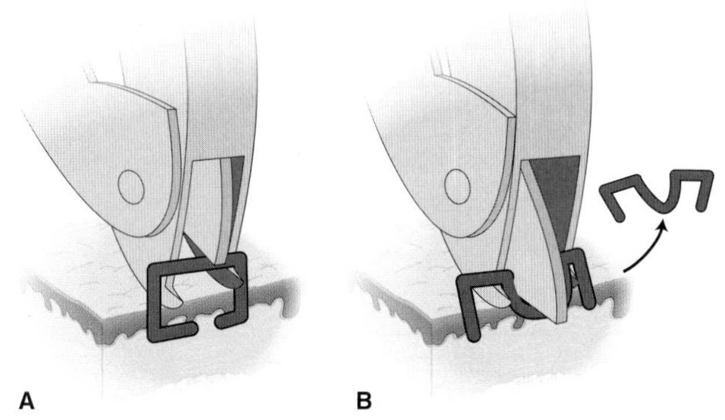

FIGURE 47-2. Skin staple removal. A. Place the lower jaw of the staple remover under the horizontal portion of the staple. B. The upper jaw deforms the center of the staple and extracts the vertical legs from the skin. [Reproduced with permission from Flippin AL, Cebrun H, Reichman ER: Basic wound closure techniques, in Reichman ER, Simon RR (eds): *Emergency Medical Procedures*. New York, McGraw-Hill, 2004, p. 735.]

without a reevaluation.[53] Patients who require further tetanus immunization to complete their primary series should have the second dose 1 to 2 months after the first dose, and the third dose 6 to 12 months after the second dose.

LONG-TERM COSMETIC OUTCOME

Educate patients about the expected outcome before wound closure. Re-enforce the message at the time of suture or staple removal or wound follow-up. Tell patients that all traumatic lacerations result in some scarring and that short-term cosmetic appearance is not highly predictive of the ultimate cosmetic outcome.[54] Healing lacerations and abrasions should not be exposed to direct sunlight, because sun exposure can result in permanent hyperpigmentation.[55] Protect injured skin with a sun-blocking agent for 6 to 12 months after injury.

REFERENCES

The complete reference list is available online at www.TintinalliEM.com.

SECTION 7

Cardiovascular Disease

CHAPTER 48

Chest Pain

Simon A. Mahler

INTRODUCTION AND EPIDEMIOLOGY

About 8 million patients with chest pain present to a U.S. ED each year.[1] Of these, 50% to 70% are placed into an observation unit or admitted to the hospital, yet only about 10% are eventually diagnosed with an acute coronary syndrome.[2-5] Still, 2% to 5% of patients with acute myocardial infarctions are missed on initial presentation and discharged from the ED.[2] We discuss the features and approach that help differentiate acute coronary syndrome from other causes of chest pain. The chapters titled "Acute Coronary Syndromes" and "Low Probability Acute Coronary Syndromes" discuss management of these specific syndromes.

Acute chest pain is the recent onset of pain, pressure, or tightness in the anterior thorax between the xiphoid, suprasternal notch, and both midaxillary lines. **Acute coronary syndrome** includes **acute myocardial infarction** and acute ischemia (unstable angina). Acute myocardial infarction is defined by myocardial necrosis with elevation of cardiac biomarkers and is classified by ECG findings as **ST-segment elevation myocardial infarction** or **non-ST-segment elevation myocardial infarction**. Unstable angina is a clinical diagnosis defined by chest pain or an equivalent (neck or upper extremity pain) from inadequate myocardial perfusion that is new, occurring with greater frequency, less activity, or at rest. Patients with unstable angina do not have pathologic ST-segment elevation on ECG or cardiac biomarker elevation, but they are at risk of eventual myocardial damage absent recognition and treatment.

PATHOPHYSIOLOGY

The chest wall, from the dermis to the parietal pleura, is innervated by somatic pain fibers. Neurons enter the spinal cord at specific levels corresponding to the skin dermatomes. Visceral pain fibers are found in internal organs, such as the heart, blood vessels, esophagus, and visceral pleura. Visceral pain fibers enter the spinal cord and map to areas on the parietal cortex corresponding to cord levels shared with somatic fibers. Stimulation of visceral or somatic afferent pain fibers results in two distinct pain syndromes. Pain from somatic fibers is usually easily described, precisely located, and often experienced as a sharp sensation. Pain from visceral fibers is generally more difficult to describe and imprecisely localized. Patients with visceral pain are more likely to use terms such as *discomfort, heaviness, pressure, tightness*, or *aching*. Visceral pain is often referred to an area of the body corresponding to adjacent somatic nerves, which explains why pain from an acute myocardial infarction may radiate to the neck, jaw, or arms. Factors such as age, sex, comorbid illnesses, medications, drugs, and alcohol may interact with psychological and cultural factors to alter pain perception and communication.

CLINICAL FEATURES

RISK ASSESSMENT

Patients with abnormal vital signs, concerning ECG findings (if available initially), a history of prior coronary artery disease, multiple atherosclerotic risk factors, or any abrupt, new, or severe chest pain or dyspnea should be quickly placed into a treatment bed. Initiate cardiac monitoring and IV access, and obtain an ECG, ideally within 10 minutes of arrival. Identify and treat immediate life needs like supporting the airway, breathing, and circulation. Measure vital signs promptly and at regular intervals. Administer oxygen if ambient saturation is <95%.

Once the patient is stable, focus on history, physical exam, and laboratory findings associated with cardiac (acute coronary syndrome) versus noncardiac chest pain causes. Obtain a focused history that includes symptoms, abridged past medical history, and review of systems, seeking features of life-threatening causes of chest pain, such as acute coronary syndrome, aortic dissection, pulmonary embolism, severe pneumonia, and esophageal rupture. Ask about the onset, timing, severity, radiation, and character of the chest pain; alleviating and exacerbating factors; and presence of associated symptoms, such as diaphoresis, dyspnea, nausea, vomiting, palpitations, and dizziness.

Focus the physical examination on findings pertinent to life-threatening causes of chest pain. Inspect the thorax for prior surgical incisions, chest wall deformities, and symmetric rise and fall with respiration. Palpate the chest wall for tenderness, masses, or crepitus. Auscultate to identify chest consolidation or pneumothorax, murmurs, gallops, or friction rubs, and obtain a chest x-ray immediately to identify immediate life-threatening processes.

HISTORY

Patients with serious and life-threatening intrathoracic disorders, including acute coronary syndrome, may report pain outside the chest, such as in the epigastrium, neck, jaw, shoulders, or arms. Some patients never experience chest pain or have migratory pain that is no longer in the chest at the time of medical evaluation. Patients with acute myocardial infarction who present without chest pain have diagnostic and treatment delays and have an in-hospital mortality rate more than twice that of acute myocardial infarction patients with chest pain.[6]

Classic Chest Pain Terms such as "typical" and "atypical" symptoms are misleading because symptoms among patients with acute coronary syndrome vary and may not include classic findings. **Classic cardiac chest pain** is retrosternal left anterior chest crushing, squeezing, tightness, or pressure. Cardiac chest pain is often brought on or exacerbated by exertion and relieved by rest. Traditional teaching is that anginal pain lasts 2 to 10 minutes, unstable angina pain lasts 10 to 30 minutes, and pain from acute myocardial infarction often lasts longer than 30 minutes, but great overlap exists. Other classic features of acute coronary syndrome presentation include radiation of the pain to the arms, neck, or jaw; diaphoresis; dyspnea; and nausea or vomiting.[7]

Nonclassic Chest Pain Patients with acute coronary syndrome frequently present without a "classic" chest pain story. The absence of classic symptoms contributes to delays in seeking care and in evaluation once they reach the ED.

Nonclassic presentations include chest pain lasting for seconds, constant pains lasting for 12 to 24 hours or more without waxing and waning intensity, or pain worsened by specific body movements or positions, such as twisting and turning of the thorax. Reports of stabbing, well-localized, positional, or pleuritic chest pain are uncommon with acute coronary syndrome but do not exclude it with certainty. The Multicenter Chest Pain Study reported that 22% of patients with acute myocardial infarction described their chest pain as sharp or stabbing.[8] **Nonclassic presentations of acute coronary syndrome occur more frequently in women, racial minorities, diabetics, the elderly, and patients with**

TABLE 48-1 Acute Myocardial Infarction Symptoms: Positive Likelihood Ratios[22,24,25]

Pain Descriptor	Study	No. of Patients Studied	Positive Likelihood Ratio (95% Confidence Interval)
Radiation to right arm or shoulder	Chun et al.	770	4.7 (1.9–12.0)
Radiation to both arms or shoulders	Goodacre et al.	893	4.1 (2.5–6.5)
Associated with exertion	Goodacre et al.	893	2.4 (1.5–3.8)
Radiation to left arm	Panju et al.	278	2.3 (1.7–3.1)
Associated with diaphoresis	Panju et al.	8426	2.0 (1.9–2.2)
Associated with nausea or vomiting	Panju et al.	970	1.9 (1.7–2.3)
Worse than previous angina or similar to previous myocardial infarction	Chun et al.	7734	1.8 (1.6–2.0)
Described as pressure	Chun et al.	11,504	1.3 (1.2–1.5)

psychiatric disease or altered mental status than in other patient groups.[6,9,10] Multiple prescription medications, drugs, alcohol, patient or provider sex, and cultural differences can impact the pain perception or reporting of symptoms.[11-13] For example, the term "sharp" in some cultures is interpreted to mean "severe," rather than knife-like.[14]

Premenopausal and early menopausal women with acute coronary syndrome are more likely to present with pain unrelated to exercise, pain not relieved by rest or nitroglycerin, pain relieved by antacids, palpitations without chest pain, or a chief complaint of fatigue.[15] Associated symptoms of nausea, emesis, jaw pain, neck pain, and back pain are more common in women with acute coronary syndrome, while diaphoresis is more common among men.[15]

Anginal Equivalents One large public hospital reported that 47% of 721 consecutive patients with myocardial infarction presented complaining of symptoms other than chest pain.[10] This means ED physicians must consider potential **anginal-equivalent symptoms** like dyspnea at rest or with exertion, nausea, light-headedness, generalized weakness, acute changes in mental status, diaphoresis, or shoulder, arm, or jaw discomfort. Patients with dyspnea alone have a fourfold increased risk of sudden death from cardiac causes compared with asymptomatic patients, and a twofold increased risk compared with patients with classic angina.[16]

Epigastric or upper abdominal discomfort, even when relieved with antacids, should raise suspicion for acute coronary syndrome, especially for patients >50 years old and those with known coronary artery disease. In these two high-risk groups, include an ECG in routine evaluation of abdominal pain. Consider acute coronary syndrome in patients presenting with palpitations, because myocardial ischemia may increase automaticity and irritability, leading to dysrhythmias. Furthermore, tachycardia can cause an increase in myocardial oxygen demand, triggering myocardial ischemia.

Risk Factors Major risk factors for coronary artery disease include age >40 years old, male or postmenopausal female, hypertension, tobacco use, hypercholesterolemia, diabetes, truncal obesity, family history, and a sedentary lifestyle.[17,18] **Cocaine** use is associated with acute myocardial infarction even in young people with minimal or no coronary artery disease. Chronic cocaine use may accelerate atherosclerosis and severe coronary artery disease,[19] although some suggest no relationship once controlling for other cardiovascular risk factors.[20] **Human immunodeficiency virus** infection and treatment with highly active antiretroviral therapy can accelerate atherosclerosis.[21]

Although cardiac risk factors are useful in predicting coronary artery disease risk within a given population, they are less useful for diagnosing the presence or absence of acute coronary syndrome in an individual patient.[7,22,23] Patients with known coronary artery disease and prior acute coronary syndrome are at risk for another acute coronary syndrome event. So, identify previous episodes of chest pain, prior echocardiography, stress testing or coronary angiography, or prior revascularization (stent placement or coronary artery bypass graft surgery).

ACUTE MYOCARDIAL INFARCTION SIGNS AND SYMPTOMS: LIKELIHOOD RATIOS

There are no historical features with sufficient sensitivity and specificity to either diagnose or exclude acute coronary syndrome. Radiation to the arms and shoulders, particularly to the right arm or both arms, is the historical feature most strongly associated with acute coronary syndrome (likelihood ratio range of 2.3–4.7).[22,24,25] Chest pain with exertion or associated symptoms of dyspnea, diaphoresis, nausea, or vomiting are associated with twofold likelihood of acute coronary syndrome.[24,25] Pressure-like chest sensation has limited value in the prediction of acute coronary syndrome.[22] Sharp, pleuritic, positional chest pain is associated with a decreased likelihood of acute coronary syndrome but cannot eliminate the diagnosis.[22] Lack of exertional pain or pain radiation has no diagnostic value for exclusion of acute coronary syndrome.[22,25] Since classic cardiac ischemic pain is not universal and men and women both present with nonclassic symptoms, the diagnostic utility of specific chest pain descriptions does not differ significantly between men and women.[26] **Tables 48-1** and **48-2** summarize the chest pain characteristics associated with increased or decreased likelihood ratios of acute myocardial infarction.

TABLE 48-2 AMI Symptoms: Negative Likelihood Ratios[22,25,27]

Pain Descriptor	Study	No. of Patients Studied	Positive Likelihood Ratio (95% Confidence Interval)
Described as pleuritic	Chun et al.	8822	0.2 (0.1–0.3)
Described as positional	Chun et al.	8330	0.3 (0.2–0.5)
Described as sharp	Chun et al.	1088	0.3 (0.2–0.5)
Reproducible with palpation	Chun et al.	8822	0.3 (0.2–0.4)
Reproducible with positioning	Chun et al.	8330	0.3 (0.2–0.5)
Inframammary location	Everts et al.	903	0.8 (0.7–0.9)
Not associated with exertion	Goodacre et al.	893	0.8 (0.6–0.9)

PHYSICAL EXAMINATION

The examination of patients with acute coronary syndrome is often normal, and there are no exam findings that are sensitive or specific enough to exclude or diagnose acute coronary syndrome. Use the exam in conjunction with history to identify or exclude other causes of chest pain and to guide therapy.

Vital sign abnormalities from acute coronary syndrome may include hyper- or hypotension, tachycardia, or bradycardia. Tachycardia may result from increased sympathetic tone and decreased left ventricular stroke volume. Bradycardia may occur due to ischemia or infarction involving the conduction system or alterations in sympathetic and parasympathetic activation of the sinoatrial or atrioventricular nodes. Patients with acute myocardial ischemia or infarction may have abnormal heart sounds due to changes in ventricular function or compliance, such as an S_3 or S_4 gallop, diminished S_1, or a paradoxically split S_2. New murmurs in patients with chest pain may be associated with acute myocardial infarction with chordae tendineae rupture or aortic root dissection. Ischemia-induced congestive heart failure may produce crackles on auscultation of the lungs.

Physical examination findings most strongly associated with acute myocardial infarction in patients presenting with acute chest pain are hypotension, S_3 gallop, and diaphoresis, although the frequency, interrater reliability, and added diagnostic value are limited.[22] Reproducible chest wall tenderness is suggestive of a musculoskeletal etiology but is reported in up to 15% of patients with confirmed acute myocardial infarction and cannot alone exclude the diagnosis of acute coronary syndrome.[28]

RESPONSE TO THERAPY

Response to medications poorly discriminates between cardiac and noncardiac chest pain. While nitroglycerin reduces anginal pain, it may also relieve the pain from noncardiac conditions such as esophageal spasm.[22,29-31] Similarly, relief from antacid or combination "GI cocktail" therapy does not represent a noncardiac cause of chest pain.[32,33] Combine the above responses with other features to best assess the likely presence or absence of acute coronary syndrome.

DIAGNOSIS

Life-threatening concerns in acute chest pain are acute coronary syndrome, aortic dissection, pulmonary embolism, pneumonia, tension pneumothorax, and esophageal rupture. Other diagnoses with the potential for morbidity and mortality include simple pneumothorax, myocarditis, pericarditis, aortic stenosis, perforated ulcer, and cholecystitis. Benign causes of chest pain include anxiety, musculoskeletal pain, esophagitis, and gastritis. Common causes of chest pain are listed in **Table 48-3**. **Table 48-4** summarizes the classic symptoms of the life-threatening causes of acute chest pain.

TABLE 48-3 Common Causes of Acute Chest Pain

Visceral Pain	Pleuritic Pain	Chest Wall Pain
Typical angina	**Pulmonary embolism**	Costosternal syndrome
Unstable angina	**Pneumonia**	Costochondritis (Tietze's syndrome)
Acute myocardial infarction	Spontaneous pneumothorax	Precordial catch syndrome
Aortic dissection	Pericarditis	Xiphodynia
Esophageal rupture	Pleurisy	Radicular syndromes
Esophageal reflux or spasm		Intercostal nerve syndromes
Mitral valve prolapse		Fibromyalgia

PULMONARY EMBOLISM

Symptoms of pulmonary embolism include sharp chest pain (may worsen with inspiration, called "pleuritic"), dyspnea, hypoxemia, syncope, or shock. There may be associated cough or hemoptysis. Patients with pulmonary embolism may be febrile and have leg swelling or pain, and some patients will report chest wall tenderness. Common physical examination findings include tachypnea, tachycardia, and hypoxemia. Pulmonary embolism risk factors include recent surgery, trauma, prolonged immobility, active cancer, estrogens from birth control pills or hormone replacement therapy (particularly when combined with smoking), procoagulant syndromes, or a history of prior pulmonary embolism or deep venous thrombosis.[34,35]

Clinical decision aids, such as the **Wells and Revised Geneva Scores,** can risk stratify patients with possible pulmonary embolism.[36,37] The **Pulmonary Embolism Rule-Out Criteria** exclude pulmonary embolism in patients with a low pretest probability without further diagnostic testing.[38] Normal **D-dimer** testing, measured by a sensitive enzyme-linked immunosorbent assay, in a hemodynamically stable low- to intermediate-risk patient (with a Revised Geneva Criteria Score of 0 to 10) makes pulmonary embolism exceptionally unlikely; in those with higher risk assessment, a negative D-dimer has limited value.[39,40] In patients with pulmonary embolism, elevated cardiac troponin (cTn) indicates ventricular dysfunction and identifies patients with an elevated risk of death and complications.[41]

In pulmonary embolism, ECG findings are nonspecific, with the most common finding being sinus tachycardia. Chest radiographs are usually normal, but in rare cases may show signs of pulmonary infarction. CT pulmonary angiography is the test of choice and is highly sensitive for the detection of large to medium-sized pulmonary emboli. See more details on pulmonary embolism in the chapter 46, "Venous Thromboembolism."

AORTIC DISSECTION

Pain from aortic dissection is classically described as a ripping or tearing sensation radiating to the interscapular area of the back. The pain is often sudden in onset, maximal at the time of symptom onset, and may migrate or be noted above and below the diaphragm. Lack of sudden-onset pain decreases the probability of aortic dissection but cannot exclude it.[42] Secondary symptoms of aortic dissection result from arterial branch occlusions and include stroke, acute myocardial infarction, or limb ischemia. Risk factors include male sex, age over 50 years, poorly controlled hypertension, cocaine or amphetamine use, a bicuspid aortic valve or prior aortic valve replacement, connective tissue disorders (Marfan's syndrome and Ehlers-Danlos syndrome), and pregnancy.[43]

Physical exam findings for aortic dissection lack sensitivity and specificity. A unilateral pulse deficit of the carotid, radial, or femoral arteries is suggestive of aortic dissection (likelihood ratio 5.7; 95% confidence interval, 1.4–23).[42] Focal neurologic deficits are rare, occurring in only 17% of patients with aortic dissection, but the combination of chest pain and a focal neurologic deficit greatly increase the likelihood of aortic dissection.[42] While a completely normal chest radiograph lowers the likelihood of aortic dissection being present, it does not exclude dissection. A negative **D-dimer** lowers the probability of aortic dissection (detecting the clotting/declotting expected), but it also cannot exclude the disease.[44] ECG changes are common among patients with aortic dissection, with up to 40% to 50% presenting with ST-segment or T-wave changes.[45,46] Elevated cTn among patients with aortic dissection is associated with increased mortality.[47] If aortic dissection is suspected, obtain a CT aortogram or transesophageal echocardiogram. See chapter 59, "Aortic Dissection and Related Aortic Syndromes."

PNEUMONIA

Pneumonia is potentially life threatening in the elderly, immunocompromised, or patients with multiple comorbid conditions. Chest pain from pneumonia is usually described as sharp, pleuritic, and associated

TABLE 48-4 Classic Symptoms of Potentially Life-Threatening Causes of Chest Pain*

Disorder	Pain Location	Pain Character	Radiation	Associated Signs and Symptoms
Acute coronary syndrome	Retrosternal, L chest, or epigastric	Crushing, tightness, squeezing, pressure	R or L shoulder, R or L arm/hand, jaw	Dyspnea, diaphoresis, nausea
Pulmonary embolism	Focal chest	Pleuritic	None	Tachycardia, tachypnea, hypoxia, may have hemoptysis
Aortic dissection	Midline, substernal	Ripping, tearing	Intrascapular area of back	Secondary arterial branch occlusion
Pneumonia	Focal chest	Sharp, pleuritic	None	Fever, hypoxia, may see signs of sepsis
Esophageal rupture	Substernal	Sudden, sharp, after forceful vomiting	Back	Dyspnea, diaphoresis, may see signs of sepsis
Pneumothorax	One side of chest	Sudden, sharp, lancinating, pleuritic	Shoulder, back	Dyspnea
Pericarditis	Substernal	Sharp, constant or pleuritic	Back, neck, shoulder	Fever, pericardial friction rub
Perforated peptic ulcer	Epigastric	Severe, sharp	Back, up into chest	Acute distress, diaphoresis

Abbreviations: L = left; R = right.

*Atypical presentations are common.

with fever, cough, sputum production, and possibly hypoxemia.[48] Auscultation may reveal decreased breath sounds, rales, or bronchial breath sounds over the affected areas of consolidation. A chest radiograph usually confirms the diagnosis. See chapter 65, "Pneumonia and Pulmonary Infiltrates."

ESOPHAGEAL RUPTURE (BOERHAAVE'S SYNDROME)

Patients classically present with a history of sudden-onset, sharp, substernal chest pain following forceful vomiting. Patients with esophageal rupture are usually ill-appearing and may be tachycardic, febrile, dyspneic, or diaphoretic. Physical examination may reveal crepitus in the neck or chest from subcutaneous emphysema. **Hamman's crunch**, audible crepitus that varies with the heartbeat on auscultation of the precordium, is a rare finding associated with pneumomediastinum. Chest radiography may demonstrate a pleural effusion (left more common than right), pneumothorax, pneumomediastinum, pneumoperitoneum, or subcutaneous air, although a normal x-ray cannot exclude esophageal rupture. If esophageal rupture is suspected, obtain a CT with oral water-soluble contrast. See chapter 77, "Esophageal Emergencies."

SPONTANEOUS PNEUMOTHORAX

The symptoms of spontaneous pneumothorax are sudden-onset, sharp, pleuritic chest pain with dyspnea. Classically, spontaneous pneumothorax occurs in tall, slender males. Risk factors for spontaneous pneumothorax include smoking and chronic lung diseases such as asthma and chronic obstructive pulmonary disease. Approximately 1% to 3% of patients with a spontaneous pneumothorax progress to develop a tension pneumothorax.[49] Auscultation may reveal decreased breath sounds and hyperresonance to percussion on the ipsilateral side. However, the physical exam findings of a simple pneumothorax are inconstant and cannot be used to exclude presence, with the diagnosis made by chest radiography. See chapter 68, "Pneumothorax."

ACUTE PERICARDITIS

Pain from acute pericarditis is classically described as a sharp, severe, constant pain with a substernal location. The pain may radiate to the back, neck, or shoulders; worsens by lying flat and by inspiration; and is relieved by sitting up and leaning forward. A pericardial friction rub is the most specific physical exam finding but is not always evident. The classic ECG findings are diffuse ST-segment elevation with PR depression.[50] See chapter 55, "Cardiomyopathies and Pericardial Disease."

MITRAL VALVE PROLAPSE

Symptoms attributed to mitral valve prolapse include sharp chest pain, palpitations, fatigue, anxiety, and dyspnea unrelated to exertion. A midsystolic click may be heard on auscultation. However, most patients are asymptomatic and have no consistent association of chest pain, dyspnea, or anxiety with the disorder.[51,52] See chapter 54, "Valvular Emergencies."

CHEST WALL PAIN

Musculoskeletal or chest wall pain is characterized by sharp, highly localized, and positional pain. The pain should be completely reproducible by light to moderate palpation or by specific movements and may be increased by inspiration or coughing. However, chest wall tenderness is also reported by some patients with acute coronary syndrome and pulmonary embolism. **Costochondritis (Tietze's syndrome)** is an inflammation of the costal cartilages or their sternal articulations and causes chest pain that is variably sharp, dull, and often increased with respirations. **Xiphodynia** is inflammation of the xiphoid process that causes sharp, pleuritic chest pain reproduced by light palpation. **Precordial catch syndrome** is a short, lancinating chest pain occurring in bunches lasting 1 to 2 minutes near the cardiac apex and is associated with inspiration, poor posture, and inactivity. *Pleurisy* is inflammation of the parietal pleura resulting in sharp pleuritic chest pain.

GI PAIN

GI disorders often cannot be reliably differentiated from acute coronary syndrome by history and physical examination alone.[25,53] **Gastritis** and **esophageal reflux** typically produce burning or gnawing pain in the lower half of the chest, with a brackish or acidic taste in the back of the mouth. The pain may be lessened with antacids and exacerbated by recumbency. **Peptic ulcer disease** is classically described as a postprandial, dull, boring pain in the epigastric region. Patients often describe being awakened from sleep by discomfort. Duodenal ulcer pain may be relieved after eating food, whereas gastric ulcer pain is often exacerbated by eating. Antacid medications usually provide symptomatic relief. **Acute pancreatitis** and **biliary disease** typically present with right upper quadrant or epigastric pain and tenderness but can also cause chest pain. *Esophageal spasm* is often associated with reflux disease and is characterized by a sudden onset of dull or tight substernal chest pain. The pain is frequently precipitated by consumption of hot or cold liquids or a large food bolus and may be relieved by nitroglycerin. See chapter 77, "Esophageal Emergencies" and 78, "Peptic Ulcer Disease and Gastritis."

PANIC DISORDER

Panic disorder is characterized by recurrent, unexpected, and discrete periods of intense fear or discomfort (panic attacks) with at least four of the following symptoms: chest pain, dyspnea, palpitations, diaphoresis, nausea, tremor, choking, dizziness, fear of losing control or dying, paresthesias, chills, or hot flashes. In one study, 25% of ED patients with chest pain met diagnostic criteria for panic disorder. Conversely, 9% of the patients identified as having panic disorder were ultimately diagnosed with acute coronary syndrome on hospital discharge.[54] This means panic disorder is at best a diagnosis of exclusion or a co-diagnosis with acute coronary syndrome (or another cause). Do not assume panic disorder in a patient with chest pain in the ED until further testing allows better risk stratification. See chapter 289, "Mood and Anxiety Disorders."

DIAGNOSTIC TESTING

Focus initial diagnostic testing for patients with chest pain on the exclusion or confirmation of serious pathology based on the differential diagnosis drawn from the history and physical examination. When history and exam make acute coronary syndrome a potential cause, testing commonly includes an ECG, chest x-ray, and cardiac biomarkers. Stress testing, advanced cardiac imaging, serial or continuous ECG monitoring, and serial cardiac biomarker measurements are discussed in chapter 49, "Acute Coronary Syndromes."

IMAGING

Chest radiography is commonly performed in the evaluation of ED patients with chest pain. Most patients with acute coronary syndrome have a normal chest x-ray, but the images are useful to diagnose or exclude other conditions such as pneumonia and pneumothorax.[55] Other imaging modalities such as CT help evaluate conditions such as aortic dissection or pulmonary embolism.

ECG

Guidelines recommend a screening ECG within 10 minutes of ED arrival on patients with chest pain or other symptoms concerning for acute coronary syndrome.[56] Rapid ECG screening is essential because delay in identification of an ST-segment elevation myocardial infarction is associated with increased mortality.[57] Routine triage ECG testing and prehospital ECG transmission reduce delays to ST-segment elevation myocardial infarction identification, decrease door-to-balloon or door-to-needle time, and improve patient outcomes.[58-61]

Less than 5% of patients presenting to the ED with chest pain have evidence of an ST-segment elevation myocardial infarction on ECG.[62,63] However, new ST-segment elevation of ≥1 mm in at least two contiguous leads represents an acute myocardial infarction that will benefit from rapid reperfusion interventions.[22,64] ST-segment elevation also occurs in patients with pericarditis, myocarditis, early repolarization, left ventricular hypertrophy, and ventricular aneurysms. ST-segment depression and T-wave inversions are also associated with an increase in risk of acute myocardial infarction.[22,65]

A normal ECG lacks the sensitivity to exclude acute coronary syndrome, notably unstable angina, or non-ST-segment elevation myocardial infarction. In a large multicenter observational study of 391,208 patients with an evaluable ECG and diagnosis of acute myocardial infarction, 57% had "diagnostic" ECG changes, 35% had nonspecific changes, and 8% had normal ECGs. Diagnostic changes were defined as ST-segment elevation, ST-segment depression, or left bundle-branch block.[66] Other studies document normal or near normal ECGs in 5% to 10% of patients with acute myocardial infarction.[67-70] A normal ECG is also an independent risk factor for missed acute myocardial infarction and inappropriate ED discharge (odds ratio 7.7; 95% confidence interval, 2.9–20.2).[2] However, among young patients (<40 years old) without known coronary artery disease, a normal ECG is associated with a cardiovascular event rate of less than 1% at 30 days.[71]

Misinterpretation of ECGs (i.e., failure to detect ischemic changes that are present) occurs in up to 40% of missed acute myocardial infarction cases.[70] In addition, the initial ECG represents only a single time point in a dynamic pathophysiologic process; the diagnostic value of an ECG is improved by comparing it to a prior ECG or repeating it.[72]

CARDIAC BIOMARKERS

Cardiac Troponins Cardiac cTns are proteins essential to cardiac muscle contraction, which are complexed with actin and myosin filaments within cardiac myofibrils and are present within cardiac myocyte cytoplasm.[73] Myocardial injury resulting in the disruption of myocyte cell membrane integrity or myofibril destruction results in extracellular cTn leak, which can be detected in the patient's peripheral blood and used to identify and quantify myocardial damage.[74] Due to its high sensitivity and nearly complete cardiac specificity, cTn is the biomarker of choice for the detection of myocardial injury.[75]

Although cTn elevation is specific for myocardial necrosis, elevation does not indicate the mechanism of injury, nor does it necessarily indicate acute myocardial infarction. There are numerous nonischemic causes of cTn elevations, which are summarized in **Table 48-5**. Acute myocardial infarction can be differentiated from nonischemic cTn elevations based on the pattern of cTn elevation and the clinical context. The diagnostic criteria for acute myocardial infarction include a gradual rise and fall of cTn with a maximum value above the 99th percentile of a reference population (the upper reference limit), combined with any of the following: symptoms consistent with ischemia, characteristic acute ECG changes (ST- and T-wave changes, new left bundle-branch block, or new Q waves), or imaging evidence of a new regional wall motion abnormality or new loss of viable myocardium.[76]

Immunoassays have been developed for the isoforms of cTnI and cTnT. Isoforms I and T provide nearly identical information, and selection between them is driven mainly by central laboratory vendor and equipment preference.[77] A single manufacturer produces the cTnT assay;

TABLE 48-5 Conditions Associated with Elevated Cardiac Troponin Levels in the Absence of Ischemic Heart Disease
Cardiac contusion
Cardiac procedures (surgery, ablation, pacing, stenting)
Acute or chronic congestive heart failure
Aortic dissection
Aortic valve disease
Hypertrophic cardiomyopathy
Arrhythmias (tachyarrhythmia or bradyarrhythmia)
Apical ballooning syndrome
Rhabdomyolysis with cardiac injury
Pulmonary hypertension
Pulmonary embolism
Acute neurologic disease (e.g., stroke, subarachnoid hemorrhage)
Myocardial infiltrative diseases (amyloid, sarcoid, hemochromatosis, scleroderma)
Inflammatory cardiac diseases (myocarditis, endocarditis, pericarditis)
Drug toxicity
Respiratory failure
Sepsis
Burns
Extreme exertion (e.g., endurance athletes)

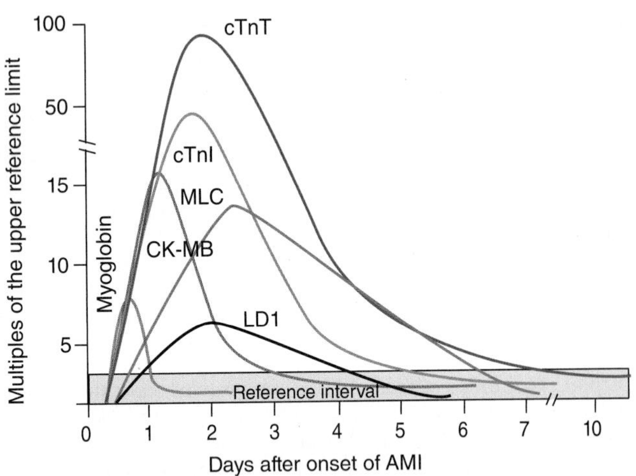

FIGURE 48-1. Typical pattern of contemporary serum marker elevation after acute myocardial infarction (AMI). CK-MB = MB fraction of creatine kinase; cTnI = cardiac troponin I; cTnT = cardiac troponin T; LD1 = lactate dehydrogenase isoenzyme 1; MLC = myosin light chain.

however, multiple manufacturers produce cTnI assays, which differ in their upper reference limits (the cTn value above the 99th percentile of a reference population), coefficients of variability, and lower limits of detection.

Over the past 25 years, cTn assays have become more analytically sensitive, pushing down the upper reference limits (URLs) and limits of detection. For example, a "first-generation" assay, available in 1995, had a URL of 0.4 nanograms/mL, whereas a commonly used contemporary (current-generation) assay has a 10-fold lower URL (0.04 nanograms/mL).[78,79] Current commercially available contemporary cTn assays have URLs ranging from 0.023 to 0.20 nanograms/mL and lower limits of detection ranging from 0.006 to 0.15 nanograms/mL.[80] Point-of-care assays offer a shorter turnaround time but with slightly lower analytic sensitivities than conventional assays.[76,81]

With contemporary assays, cTn is detected in serum as early as 2 hours after symptom onset of an acute myocardial infarction, but elevations are not reliably present until 6 hours or more.[82] Elevations peak at approximately 48 hours from symptom onset unless repeat injury occurs, and cTns remain elevated for up to 10 days (**Figure 48-1**). This persistence makes cTn a good tool in diagnosing acute myocardial infarction in patients with delayed presentations. However, in patients with intermittent symptoms over a period of days, an elevated cTn could represent a remote or new infarct. In this rare setting, the concomitant use of creatine kinase-MB fraction, which returns to normal sooner, can help differentiate acute from remote infarction.

Obtain cardiac cTn levels in all patients with suspected acute coronary syndrome.[55] Contemporary cTn assays will identify most patients (approximately 80%) with acute myocardial infarction within 2 to 3 hours of ED arrival.[82-84] Patients with early presentations (within 6 hours of symptom onset) or those with intermittent symptoms should have serial measurements of cTn over time. In patients with constant symptoms for >8 to 12 hours, a single cTn may be sufficient to exclude acute myocardial infarction.[56,85] Measurement of cTn at short time intervals, such as 2 to 4 hours, to evaluate for serial change (delta cTn) is more sensitive for acute myocardial infarction than a single cTn approach.[55]

Newer high-sensitivity cTn assays have a 10-fold higher analytical sensitivity compared to contemporary assays; these are currently pending U.S. Food and Drug Administration approval.[80,87,88] Compared with contemporary assays, high-sensitivity cTn assays are more sensitive for the detection of acute myocardial infarction in all patients (94% to 96% vs. 85% to 90%) and increase the early detection of myocardial injury.[83,84] Among patients presenting within 3 hours of chest pain onset, high-sensitivity cTn assays are 92% to 94% sensitive for acute myocardial infarction compared to 76% for a contemporary assay.[83] However, the increased sensitivity of high-sensitivity cTn assays for acute myocardial infarction is balanced by the detection of more patients with non–acute myocardial infarction cTn elevations.[83,88] The overall impact on ED decision making and ultimate outcome is not yet defined or shown to be clearly superior to previous assay use.

An elevated cTn is associated with an increased risk of cardiac death or acute myocardial infarction at 30 days (odds ratio 3.4; 95% confidence interval, 2.9–4.0).[89] This elevated risk of death or cardiovascular complications is independent of ECG findings or creatine kinase-MB levels.[90] Higher cTn elevations also are associated with more adverse events, even with minimal elevations.[91]

Patients with **renal disease** often have an elevated cTnT (15% to 50%), whereas cTnI elevations are less common (<10%). After dialysis, serum levels of cTnT generally increase while cTnI levels decrease.[92] Despite these features, cTnT and cTnI assays remain highly sensitive for acute myocardial infarction in patients with renal failure, particularly when new measures can be compared with baseline measures. Furthermore, renal failure patients with elevated cTn levels are at higher risk for death and adverse events than patients with normal cTn levels.[93]

Creatine Kinase-MB and Myoglobin Troponin testing has made these markers almost obsolete in acute coronary syndrome care. **Creatine kinase-MB** fraction levels elevate within 4 to 8 hours after acute myocardial infarction, peak between 12 and 24 hours, and return to normal between 36 and 72 hours (Figure 48-1). When used with cTn, creatine kinase-MB provides little additional information.[94] Creatine kinase-MB testing may be useful in a small subset of patients in whom the timing of infarction is unclear. Elevated creatine kinase-MB and cTn indicate an acute infarct, whereas a negative creatine kinase-MB with an elevated cTn suggests a remote or subacute infarction.

Myoglobin is a small heme-containing protein found in skeletal and cardiac muscle. After acute myocardial infarction, serum myoglobin levels rise within 3 hours of symptoms, peak at 4 to 9 hours, and return to baseline within 24 hours (Figure 48-1). False-positive results are common, and false-negative results may occur in patients with delayed presentations. Due to the improved sensitivity of contemporary cTn assays, myoglobin does not appear to have added value in the early detection of acute myocardial infarction.[95]

B-Type Natriuretic Peptide Natriuretic peptide elevations are not specific to myocardial ischemia or infarction and will rise with any ventricular dysfunction. Patients with acute coronary syndrome and an elevated natriuretic peptide level have higher short-term mortality, although the lab test does not aid in specific patient management actions.

Other Biomarkers High-sensitivity C-reactive protein aids long-term cardiac event prediction, but this test is not recommended for ED care.[54] A variety of other assays have been studied as cardiac biomarkers, such as ischemia-modified albumin, interleukin-6, vascular cell adhesion molecule, intercellular adhesion molecule, E-selectin, P-selectin, pregnancy-associated plasma protein A, and myeloperoxidase. Current evidence does not support the use of these novel biomarkers for ED chest pain evaluations.

CLINICAL RISK SCORES AND DECISION AIDS

The **Thrombosis in Myocardial Infarction** risk score or **Global Registry of Acute Coronary Events** score can aid acute coronary syndrome risk stratification (**Figure 48-2**).[56] The Thrombosis in Myocardial Infarction and Global Registry of Acute Coronary Events scores were drawn from groups with acute coronary syndrome present or strongly suspected, and then were applied to a wider population. Each stratifies patients into low-, intermediate-, or high-risk groups for acute coronary syndrome. However, a low-risk score is not sensitive enough to exclude acute coronary syndrome or identify patients for early discharge without further evaluation.[96,97]

The **HEART** score, **ADAPT**, and the **North American Chest Pain Rule** (**Figure 48-3**) combine clinical information to risk stratify patients and guide key decisions, notably discharge with follow-up for the lowest

TIMI Score	Yes 1 point	No 0 points
Age ≥65		
≥3 Risk factors for ACS; hypertension, hyperlipidemia, smoking, diabetes, family history		
Use of aspirin in last 7 days		
Prior coronary stenosis >50%		
≥2 angina events in 24 hours or persisting discomfort		
ST-segment deviation of ≥0.05 mV on initial ECG		
Elevated cardiac biomarkers		
Total Score		

Low Risk	0-2
Intermediate Risk	3-4
High Risk	5-7

GRACE Score									
Age	Points	**HR**	Points	**SBP**	Points	**Cr**	Points	**Killip Class**	Points
<39	0	<70	0	<80	40	0.0-0.39	1	I	0
40-49	18	70-89	5	80-99	37	0.4-0.79	4	II	15
50-59	36	90-109	10	100-119	30	0.8-1.19	7	III	29
60-69	55	110-149	17	120-139	23	1.2-159	10	IV	44
70-79	73	150-199	26	140-159	17	1.6-1.99	13	**Cardiac arrest**	30
80-89	91	≥200	34	160-199	7	2.0-3.99	21	**Elevated cardiac markers**	13
>90	100	-	-	≥200	0	≥4	28	**St-segment deviation**	17

Low Risk	1-88
Intermediate Risk	89-118
High Risk	≥119

FIGURE 48-2. Thrombosis in Myocardial Infarction (TIMI) score and the Global Registry of Acute Coronary Events (GRACE) score. ACS = acute coronary syndrome; Cr = creatinine; HR = heart rate; SBP = systolic blood pressure.

ADAPT		
High risk criteria	**Yes**	**No**
1. TIMI Score >0		
a. Age ≥65		
b. ≥3 Risk factors		
c. Use of aspirin in last 7 days		
d. Significant coronary stenosis (prior stenosis ≥50%)		
e. ≥2 angina events in 24 hours or persisting discomfort		
f. ST-segment deviation of ≥0.05 mV on initial ECG		
g. Increased initial troponin		
2. Positive troponin test at 0 or 2 hours		
3. New ischemic ECG changes		

HEART Score		**Points**
History	Highly Suspicious	2
	Moderately Suspicious	1
	Slightly Suspicious	0
ECG	Significant ST-depression	2
	Non-specific repolarization abnormality	1
	Normal	0
Age	≥65	2
	45-65	1
	≤45	0
Risk factors	3 or more risk factors	2
	1-2 risk factors	1
	No risk factors	0
Troponin	≥3× normal limit	2
	1-3× normal limit	1
	≤ normal limit	0
Total		

North American Chest Pain Rule		
High risk criteria	**Yes**	**No**
Age ≥50		
Acute ischemic ECG changes		
Known coronary artery disease		
Pain typical for ACS		
Any troponin >99th percentile		

FIGURE 48-3. ADAPT, the North American Chest Pain Rule (NACPR), and the HEART score. With ADAPT and NACPR, a patient is considered low risk if the patient has none of the high-risk criteria. For ADAPT, risk factors include family history of coronary disease, hypertension, hypercholesterolemia, diabetes mellitus, and current smoker. With the HEART score, low risk is a score of 0 to 3, and high risk is a score of 4 or greater. Risk factors include currently treated diabetes mellitus, current or recent (<90 days) smoker, diagnosed and/or treated hypertension, diagnosed hypercholesterolemia, family history of coronary artery disease, obesity (body mass index >30), or a history of significant atherosclerosis (coronary revascularization, myocardial infarction, stroke, or peripheral arterial disease). ACS = acute coronary syndrome; TIMI = Thrombosis in Myocardial Infarction score.

risk patients or observation/admission for the remaining patients. Although these decision support tools may improve the quality and efficiency of chest pain care in the ED, they require further impact assessment before routine use.[98-100]

REFERENCES

The complete reference list is available online at www.TintinalliEM.com.

CHAPTER 49 Acute Coronary Syndromes

Judd E. Hollander
Deborah B. Diercks

EPIDEMIOLOGY

Ischemic heart disease is the leading cause of death among adults in the United States, with more than 405,000 people dying annually. Atherosclerotic disease of the epicardial coronary arteries—termed *coronary artery disease* (CAD)—accounts for the vast majority of patients with ischemic heart disease. The predominant symptom of CAD is chest pain, and patient concern over potential acute heart disease contributes to the >8 million visits each year to U.S. EDs. In a typical adult ED population with acute chest pain, about 15% of patients will have an acute coronary syndrome (ACS). ACS encompasses unstable angina through acute myocardial infarction (AMI). Of patients with an ACS, approximately one third have an AMI, and the remainder have unstable angina.

TABLE 49-1 Three Principal Presentations of Unstable Angina

Class	Presentation
Rest angina*	Angina occurring at rest and that is prolonged, usually >20 min
New-onset angina	New-onset angina that markedly limits ordinary physical activity, such as walking 1–2 blocks or climbing 1 flight of stairs or performing lighter activity
Increasing angina	Previously diagnosed angina that has become distinctly more frequent, has a longer duration, or is lower in threshold, limiting ability to walk 1–2 blocks or climb 1 flight of stairs or perform lighter activity

*Patients with non-ST-elevated myocardial infarction usually present with angina at rest.

The three principal presentations of unstable angina are listed in **Table 49-1**.[1] These definitions assume that the anginal chest pain is due to ischemia, and this categorization does not apply to patients presenting to the ED with chest pain from other causes. During the initial ED assessment, it may not be possible to determine whether the patient has or will sustain permanent damage to the myocardium, has reversible ischemia (injury or unstable angina), or has a noncardiac cause of symptoms.

The American College of Cardiology and American Heart Association have a tool for estimating the short-term risk for death or AMI in patients with unstable angina (**Table 49-2**).[1]

ANATOMY

The left coronary artery divides into the left circumflex and the left anterior descending branches (**Figure 49-1**). The left anterior descending branch courses down the anterior aspect of the heart providing the

TABLE 49-2 Short-Term Risk of Death or Nonfatal Myocardial Infarction by Risk Stratification in Patients with Unstable Angina

Feature	High Likelihood (at least one of the following features must be present)	Intermediate Likelihood (no high-risk feature, but must have one of the following)	Low Likelihood (no high- or intermediate-risk feature, but may have any of the following)
History	Accelerating tempo of ischemic symptoms in preceding 48 h	Prior myocardial infarction, peripheral or cerebrovascular disease, or coronary artery bypass grafting; prior aspirin use	
Character of the pain	Prolonged, ongoing (>20 min) rest pain	Prolonged (>20 min) rest angina, now resolved, with moderate or high likelihood of CAD Rest angina (>20 min) or relieved with rest or sublingual nitroglycerin Nocturnal angina New-onset or progressive angina in the past 2 wk without prolonged (>20 min) rest pain but with intermediate or high likelihood of CAD (see Table 49-3)	Increased angina frequency, severity, or duration Angina provoked at a lower threshold New-onset angina with onset 2 wk to 2 mo before presentation
Clinical findings	Pulmonary edema, most likely due to ischemia New or worsening mitral regurgitation murmur S_3 or new/worsening rales Hypotension, bradycardia, tachycardia Age >75 y old	Age >70 y old	Chest discomfort reproduced by palpation
ECG	Angina at rest with transient ST-segment changes >0.5 mm Bundle-branch block, new or presumed new Sustained ventricular tachycardia	T-wave changes, pathologic Q waves, or resting ST depression <1 mm in multiple lead groups (anterior, inferior, lateral)	Normal or unchanged ECG
Cardiac markers	Elevated cardiac TnT, TnI (e.g., TnT or TnI >0.1 nanogram/mL)	Slightly elevated cardiac TnT, TnI (e.g., TnT >0.01 but <0.1 nanogram/mL)	Normal

Abbreviations: CAD = coronary artery disease; TnI = troponin I; TnT = troponin T.

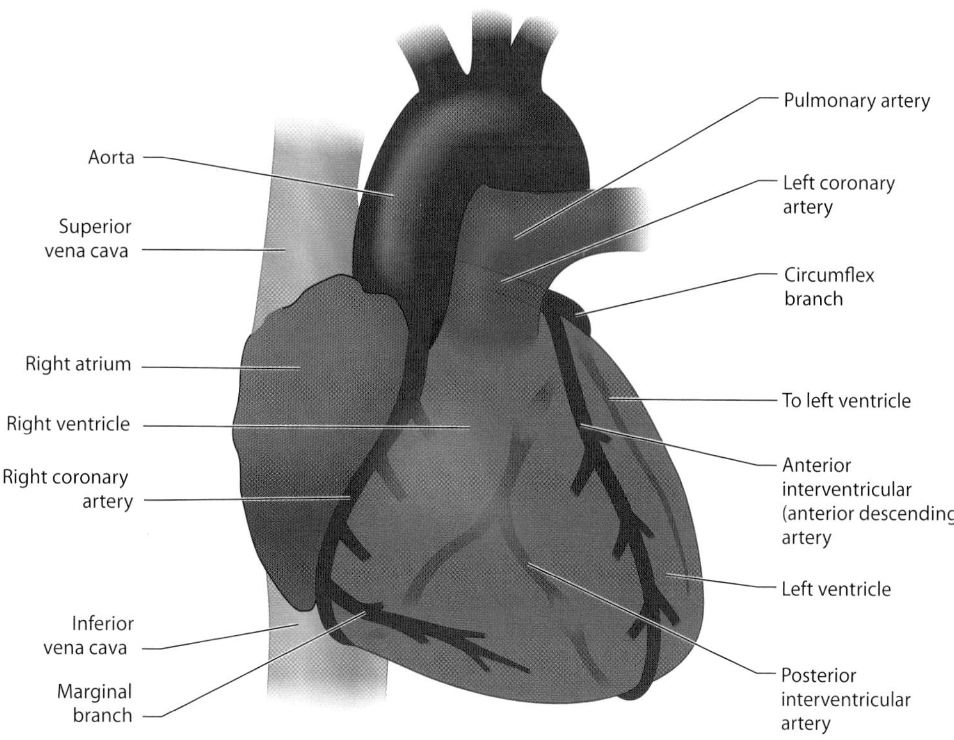

FIGURE 49-1. Schematic diagram of the coronary arteries.

main blood supply to the anterior and septal regions of the heart. The circumflex branch supplies blood to some of the anterior wall and a large portion of the lateral wall of the heart. The right coronary artery supplies the right side of the heart and provides some perfusion to the inferior aspect of the left ventricle through its continuation as the right posterior descending artery.

The atrioventricular conduction system receives blood supply from the atrioventricular branch of the right coronary artery and the septal perforating branch of the left anterior descending coronary artery. Similarly, the right bundle branch and the posterior division of the left bundle branch each obtain blood flow from both the left anterior descending and right coronary arteries. The posteromedial papillary muscle receives blood supply from one coronary artery, usually the right coronary artery.

PATHOPHYSIOLOGY

Ischemia occurs when there is an imbalance between oxygen (O_2) demand and O_2 supply. O_2 supply is influenced by the O_2-carrying capacity of the blood and the coronary artery blood flow. The O_2-carrying capacity of the blood is determined by the amount of hemoglobin present and O_2 saturation. Coronary artery blood flow is determined by the duration of diastolic relaxation of the heart and peripheral vascular resistance. Humoral, neural, metabolic, and extravascular compressive forces and local autoregulation mechanisms determine the coronary vascular resistance.

Exercise-induced myocardial ischemia and its sequelae usually occur as a result of fixed atherosclerotic lesions. ACS may be caused by secondary reduction in myocardial blood flow due to coronary arterial spasm, disruption or erosion of atherosclerotic plaques, and platelet aggregation or thrombus formation at the site of an atherosclerotic lesion. Secondary causes of myocardial ischemia are less common and prompted by factors extrinsic to the coronary arteries such as increased myocardial O_2 demand (i.e., fever, tachycardia, thyrotoxicosis), reduced blood flow (i.e., hypotension), or reduced O_2 delivery (i.e., anemia, hypoxemia). In the event of a secondary cause, global ischemia may occur widely or focally.

Atherosclerotic plaque forms through repetitive injury to the vessel wall. Macrophages and smooth muscle cells are the main cellular elements in plaque development, whereas lipids are predominant in the extracellular milieu. Plaque fissuring and rupture are affected by features inherent to the plaque, such as its composition and shape; local factors, such as shear forces, coronary arterial tone, and coronary arterial perfusion pressure; and movements of the artery in response to myocardial contractions. When plaque rupture occurs, potent thrombogenic substances activate circulating platelets.

The platelet response involves adhesion, activation, and aggregation. Platelet adhesion occurs through the weak platelet interactions with subendothelial adhesion molecules, such as collagen, fibronectin, and laminin, and the binding of the glycoprotein IIb receptor to the subendothelial form of von Willebrand factor. Adherent platelets are strongly thrombogenic. Lipid-laden macrophages in the plaque core and adventitia of the vessel wall release tissue factor, which stimulates the conversion of prothrombin to thrombin. Thrombin and the local shear forces are also potent platelet activators. Platelet secretion of adenosine diphosphate, thromboxane A_2, and serotonin are autostimulatory agonists of platelet activation. Activated platelet glycoprotein IIb/IIIa receptors become cross-linked by fibrinogen or von Willebrand factor in the final common pathway of platelet aggregation.

The extent of O_2 deprivation and the clinical presentation of ACS depend on the limitation of O_2 delivery imposed by thrombus adhering to a plaque. In stable angina, ischemia occurs only when activity induces O_2 demands beyond the supply restrictions imposed by a partially occluded coronary vessel. Ischemia occurs at a relatively fixed point and changes slowly over time. In this scenario, the atherosclerotic plaque has not ruptured, and there is little or no superimposed thrombus. In ACS, atherosclerotic plaque rupture and platelet-rich thrombus develop. Coronary blood flow is reduced suddenly, and myocardial ischemia occurs. The degree and duration of the O_2 supply–demand mismatch determines whether the patient develops reversible myocardial ischemia without necrosis (unstable angina) or myocardial ischemia with necrosis (AMI). More severe and prolonged obstruction increases the likelihood of infarction.

AMI may inhibit myocardial contractility and impair both central and peripheral perfusion. When an area of the myocardium does not receive adequate O_2, the functional deterioration progresses; as the size of the infarcted myocardium increases, left ventricular pump function decreases. This creates increased left ventricular end-diastolic pressure and end-systolic volume. Cardiac output, stroke volume, and blood pressure may decrease. When left atrial and pulmonary capillary pressures increase, heart failure or pulmonary edema may develop.

Poor perfusion to the brain and kidneys can result in altered mental status and impaired renal function, respectively.

CLINICAL FEATURES

HISTORY AND ASSOCIATED SYMPTOMS

The main symptom of ischemic heart disease is chest discomfort or pain, and the history should characterize its severity, location, radiation, duration, and quality. In addition, the presence of associated symptoms such as nausea, vomiting, diaphoresis, dyspnea, light-headedness, syncope, and palpitations may help detect myocardial ischemia (see Tables 48-1 and 48-2 in chapter 48 “Chest Pain”). Obtain information regarding the onset and duration of symptoms, activities that precipitate symptoms, and prior evaluations for similar symptoms to assess the possibility of acute myocardial ischemia.

Symptoms of acute myocardial ischemia often will be described as *discomfort* rather than pain; look for descriptions of chest pressure, heaviness, tightness, fullness, or squeezing. Less commonly, patients will describe their symptoms as knife-like, sharp, or stabbing. The classic pain or discomfort location is substernal or in the left chest, with radiation to the arm (either), neck, or jaw. Reproducible chest wall tenderness is noted in some.

Exercise, stress, and a cold environment classically precipitate angina. Angina typically has a duration of symptoms of <10 minutes, occasionally lasting up to 10 to 20 minutes, and usually improves within 2 to 5 minutes after rest or nitroglycerin. In contrast, acute myocardial ischemia is usually accompanied by more prolonged and severe chest discomfort, more prominent associated symptoms (e.g., nausea, diaphoresis, shortness of breath), and little response to initial sublingual nitroglycerin. Easy fatigability may be a prominent symptom of ACS, especially in women.[2]

Ask about the frequency of anginal episodes and any change in frequency of episodes over the past months. Determine if there is any increase in severity or duration of symptoms, or whether less effort is required to precipitate symptoms.

Advanced age, female gender, and a history of diabetes mellitus are associated with more nonclassic ACS presentations. Presentations with nonclassic features or silent myocardial ischemia are common; for example, as many as 37.5% of women and 27.4% of men present without chest pain.[3] Up to 30% of patients with acute myocardial ischemia identified in large longitudinal studies are clinically unrecognized, often not seeking medical care or not recalling any symptoms. The prognosis for patients with nonclassic symptoms (e.g., fatigue, weakness, not feeling well, vague discomfort) at the time of infarction is worse than that of patients with more classic symptoms. Women and the elderly are more likely to have presentations that differ from classic ones in the younger patients; across all age groups, those with unstable angina have nonclassic features nearly half the time. This is why the term *atypical chest pain* is misleading, because nonclassic presentations are common despite being often called atypical.

Cardiac risk factors are poor predictors of risk for AMI or other ACSs.[4] Traditional cardiac risk factors for CAD, such as hypertension, diabetes mellitus, tobacco use, family history at an early age, and hypercholesterolemia, are not helpful to predict ACS in ED patients >40 years old.[4] The cardiac risk factors predict risk of CAD over time, not likelihood of presence at one moment.

PHYSICAL EXAMINATION

Patients with ACS may appear well, without any clinical signs of distress, or may be uncomfortable, pale, cyanotic, or in respiratory distress. The pulse rate may be normal or display bradycardia, tachycardia, or irregular pulses. Bradycardic rhythms are more common with inferior wall myocardial ischemia; in the setting of an acute anterior wall infarction, bradycardia or new heart block is a poor prognostic sign. Blood pressure can be normal, elevated (due to baseline hypertension, sympathetic stimulation, and anxiety), or decreased (due to pump failure or inadequate preload), although extremes of blood pressure are associated with a worse prognosis.

An S_3 is present in 15% to 20% of patients with AMI; if detected, an S_3 may indicate a failing myocardium. **The presence of a new systolic murmur is an ominous sign, because it may signify papillary muscle dysfunction, a flail leaflet of the mitral valve with resultant mitral regurgitation, or a ventricular septal defect.**

The presence of rales, with or without an S_3 gallop, indicates left ventricular dysfunction and left-sided heart failure. Jugular venous distention, hepatojugular reflex, and peripheral edema suggest right-sided heart failure.

DIAGNOSIS

The diagnosis of ST-segment elevation myocardial infarction (**STEMI**) depends on the ECG in the setting of symptoms suggestive of myocardial infarction. The diagnosis of non-ST-segment elevation myocardial infarction (**NSTEMI**) depends on abnormal elevation of cardiac biomarkers but may include ECG changes not meeting criteria for STEMI. The diagnosis of **unstable angina** is based on history (Table 49-1) because the ECG and cardiac injury biomarkers are nondiagnostic. Early risk assessment for the likelihood of myocardial infarction uses all of these data to aid decision making (**Tables 49-3** and **49-4**).

TABLE 49-3 Likelihood That Signs and Symptoms Represent Acute Coronary Syndrome Secondary to Coronary Artery Disease

Feature	High Likelihood (any of the following)	Intermediate Likelihood (absence of high-likelihood features and presence of any of the following)	Low Likelihood (absence of high- or intermediate-likelihood features but may have the following)
History	Chest or left arm pain or discomfort as chief symptom reproducing prior documented angina Known history of coronary artery disease, including myocardial infarction	Chest or left arm pain or discomfort as chief symptom Age >70 y old Male sex Diabetes mellitus	Probable ischemic symptoms in absence of any of the intermediate-likelihood characteristics Recent cocaine use
Examination	Transient mitral regurgitation murmur, hypotension, diaphoresis, pulmonary edema, or rales	Extracardiac vascular disease	Chest discomfort reproduced by palpation
ECG	New, or presumably new, transient ST-segment deviation (≥1 mm) or T-wave inversion in multiple precordial leads	Fixed Q waves ST depression 0.5–1.0 mm or T-wave inversion >1 mm	T-wave flattening or inversion <1 mm in leads with dominant R waves Normal ECG
Cardiac markers	Elevated cardiac troponin I, troponin T, or MB fraction of creatine kinase	Normal	Normal

Note: Estimation of the likelihood of significant coronary artery disease is a complex, multivariable problem that cannot be fully specified in a table such as this. Therefore, the table is meant to illustrate major relationships rather than offer rigid algorithms.

TABLE 49-4 Thrombosis in Myocardial Infarction (TIMI) Score for Unstable Angina

Age 65 y or older
3 or more traditional risk factors for coronary artery disease
Prior coronary stenosis of 50% or more
ST-segment deviation on presenting electrocardiogram
2 or more anginal events in prior 24 h
Aspirin use within the 7 d prior to presentation
Elevated cardiac markers
The presence of each of the above is assigned 1 point. The maximum possible score is 7.

TABLE 49-5 Electrocardiographic ST-Segment–Based Criteria for Acute Myocardial Infarction

Location	Electrocardiographic Findings
Anteroseptal	ST-segment elevations in V_1, V_2, and possibly, V_3
Anterior	ST-segment elevations in V_1, V_2, V_3, and V_4
Anterolateral	ST-segment elevations in V_1–V_6, I, and aVL
Lateral	ST-segment elevations in I and aVL
Inferior	ST-segment elevations in II, III, and aVF
Inferolateral	ST-segment elevations in II, III, aVF, and V_5 and V_6
True posterior*	Initial R waves in V_1 and V_2 >0.04 s and R/S ratio ≥1
Right ventricular	ST-segment elevations in II, III, and aVF and ST elevation in right-side V_4

*Posterior wall infarction does not produce Q-wave abnormalities in conventional leads and is diagnosed in the presence of tall R waves in V_1 and V_2.

The **Thrombosis in Myocardial Infarction (TIMI) score** is a seven-item tool that helps stratify patients with potential ACSs in the ED. Patients with a score of 0 to 2 have a 2% to 9% 30-day risk of death, myocardial infarction, or revascularization. Patients with higher scores have higher risks.

ELECTROCARDIOGRAPHY

The standard 12-lead ECG is the single best test—although it can be fallible—to identify patients with AMI upon ED presentation.[1] **Obtain the initial 12-lead ECG and interpret the tracing quickly, ideally within 10 minutes of presentation in those patients with symptoms suggestive of myocardial ischemia.** Prehospital ECGs reduce the time from symptom onset to reperfusion therapy in STEMI patients and are an optimal tool when possible.[5,6]

ST-segment–based diagnostic ECG criteria for AMI are shown in **Table 49-5**. STEMI in the listed distributions suggests acute transmural injury. ST-segment depressions in these distributions suggest ischemia. **Inferior wall AMIs should have a right-sided lead V_4 (V_4R) obtained,** because ST-segment elevation in V_4R is highly suggestive of right ventricular infarction. For patients with a nondiagnostic tracing and persistent symptoms who have a high risk of ACS, repeat the ECG to detect developing changes.[1,5,7] Early studies of fibrinolytic therapy identified an increased risk of mortality in patients with new bundle-branch block; this led to interpreting a new left bundle-branch block as being a "STEMI equivalent." However, <10% of patients with new or possibly new left bundle-branch block have AMI.[8]

Reciprocal ST-segment changes—those in leads away from or opposite the elevation area—are from subendocardial ischemia and denote a larger area of injury risk, an increased severity of underlying CAD, more severe pump failure, a higher likelihood of cardiovascular complications, and increased mortality. In general, **the more elevated the ST segments and the more ST segments that are elevated, the more extensive is the injury.**

The ECG changes correlate often with the infarct-related vessel (**Table 49-6**). Inferior wall AMIs can result from occlusion of the left circumflex artery or the right coronary artery. In the setting of an inferior wall AMI, ST-segment elevation in at least one lateral lead (V_5, V_6, or aVL) with an isoelectric or elevated ST segment in lead I is strongly suggestive of a left circumflex lesion (**Figure 49-2**). The presence of ST-segment elevation in lead III greater than that in lead II predicts a right coronary artery occlusion (**Figure 49-3**). When accompanied by ST-segment elevation in V_1 or a V_4R, it predicts a proximal right coronary artery lesion with accompanying right ventricular infarction (**Figure 49-4**). Reciprocal anterior ST-segment depressions in V_1 through V_4 are equally prevalent in right coronary and left circumflex inferior wall AMIs. **Figure 49-5** shows anterior myocardial infarction from distal left anterior descending artery

TABLE 49-6 ECG Findings and Culprit Coronary Artery[9–13]

ECG Findings	Culprit Artery	Sensitivity (%)	Specificity (%)	Positive Predictive Value (%)	Negative Predictive Value (%)
ECG findings for inferior ST-segment elevation myocardial infarction					
ST-segment elevation in lead III greater than in lead II plus ST-segment depression of >1 mm in lead I, lead aVL, or both	Right coronary artery	90	71	94	70
In addition to the findings immediately above, ST-segment elevation on V_1, V_4R, or both	Proximal right coronary artery	79	100	100	88
Absence of the above findings plus ST-segment elevation in leads I, aVL, V_5, and V_6 and ST-segment depression in leads V_1, V_2, and V_3	Left circumflex coronary artery	83	96	91	93
ECG findings for anterior ST-segment elevation myocardial infarction					
ST-segment elevation in leads V_1, V_2, and V_3 plus any of the features below:					
ST-segment elevation of >2.5 mm in lead V_1, or right bundle-branch block with Q wave, or both	Proximal left anterior descending coronary artery	12	100	100	61
ST-segment depression of >1 mm in leads II, III, and aVF	Proximal left anterior descending coronary artery	34	98	93	68
ST-segment depression of ≤1 mm, or ST-segment elevation in leads II, III, and aVF	Distal left anterior descending coronary artery	66	73	78	62

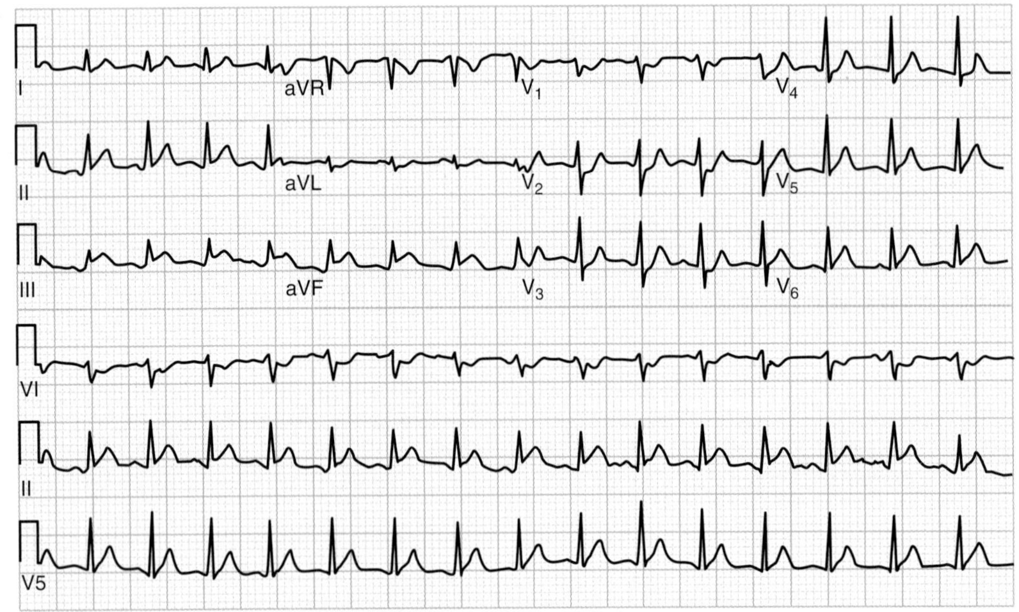

FIGURE 49-2. ECG showing inferior-lateral myocardial infarction from left circumflex coronary artery occlusion. ECG from a 42-year-old man presenting with chest pain. ECG shows ST-segment elevation in limb leads II, III (inferior), and aVF, as well as lead V_6 (lateral). ST-segment depression is evident in leads V_1, V_2, and V_3, reflecting reciprocal changes in the anterior leads. The patient was found to have 100% occlusion of the left circumflex coronary artery at cardiac catheterization. [Used with permission of David M. Cline, MD, Wake Forest University.]

occlusion, whereas **Figure 49-6** shows anterior myocardial infarction from proximal left anterior descending artery occlusion.

ECGs are frequently misinterpreted, with a low of 5.9% to as many as 29% being misinterpreted.[14] False-positive interpretations of the ECG, indicating STEMI when no injury exists, occur between 11% and 14% of the time.[13] Balancing this is the observation that **even patients with normal or nonspecific ECGs have a 1% to 5% incidence of AMI and a 4% to 23% incidence of unstable angina**. Patients with nondiagnostic ECGs or evidence of ischemia that is age-indeterminate have a 4% to 7% incidence of AMI and a 21% to 48% incidence of unstable angina. Demonstration of new ischemia in ECG increases the risk of AMI from 25% to 73% and the unstable angina risk from 14% to 43%. Thus, the standard 12-lead ECG is useful for cardiovascular risk stratification of patients with ACSs. The only guideline-recommended addition to the standard 12-lead ECG is the use of right-sided precordial lead, V_4R, in the setting of acute inferior myocardial infarction to detect right ventricular involvement.[1,5,6]

There are several clinical conditions in which ECG interpretation is difficult (**Table 49-7**). In the setting of paced rhythms or left bundle-branch block, acute myocardial ischemia can be identified (**Figure 49-7**) with select findings. **In those with a preexisting left bundle-branch block, the following patterns are indicative of AMI:** (1) ST-segment elevation of 1 mm or greater and concordant (in the same direction as the main deflection) with the QRS complex (odds ratio, 25.2; 95% confidence interval [CI], 11.6% to 54.7%) seen in Figure 49-7C; (2) ST-segment depression of 1 mm or more in leads V_1, V_2, or V_3 (odds ratio, 6.0; 95% CI, 1.9% to 19.3%) seen in Figure 49-7D; and (3) ST-segment elevation of 5 mm or greater and discordant (in the opposite direction) with the QRS complex (odds ratio, 4.3; 95% CI, 1.8% to 10.6%) seen in Figure 49-7E.[14]

Right ventricular pacing, the common pacemaker lead location, causes secondary repolarization changes of opposing polarity to that of the predominant QRS complex. Most leads have predominant negative QRS complexes followed by ST-segment elevation and positive T waves. ST-segment elevation of at least 5 mm is most indicative of AMI in leads with predominantly negative QRS complexes.[15] Any ST-segment elevation concordant to the QRS complex in a predominantly positive QRS complex is highly specific for AMI. The QRS complex is predominantly

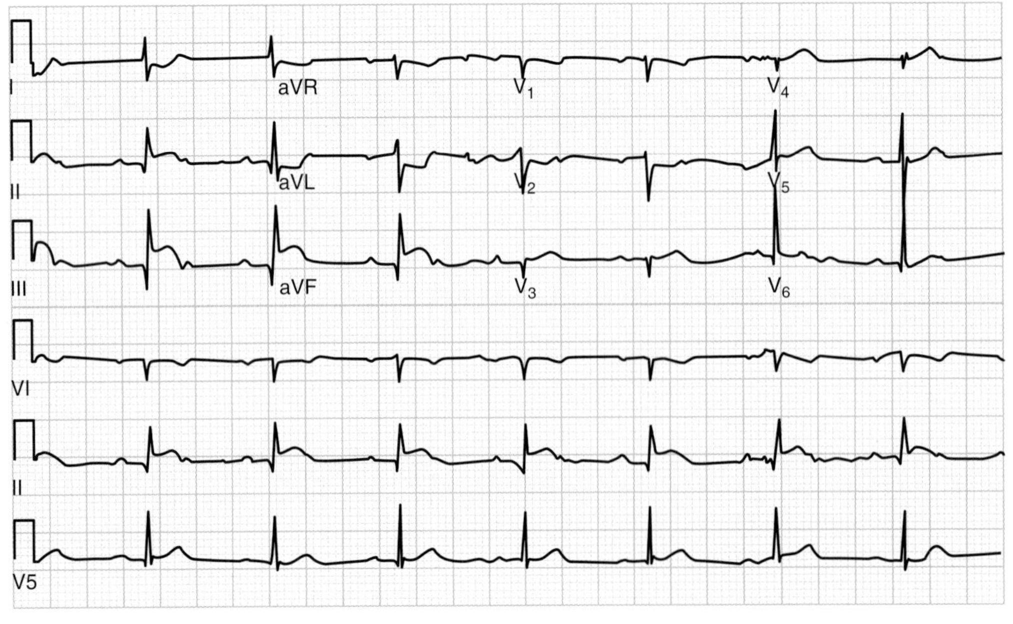

FIGURE 49-3. ECG showing inferior myocardial infarction from right coronary artery occlusion. ECG from an 80-year-old man presenting with acute chest pain. The ECG shows ST-segment elevation in lead III greater than in lead II plus ST-segment depression of >1 mm in lead I and lead aVL. The patient was found to have 100% occlusion of the right coronary artery at cardiac catheterization. [Used with permission of David M. Cline, MD, Wake Forest University.]

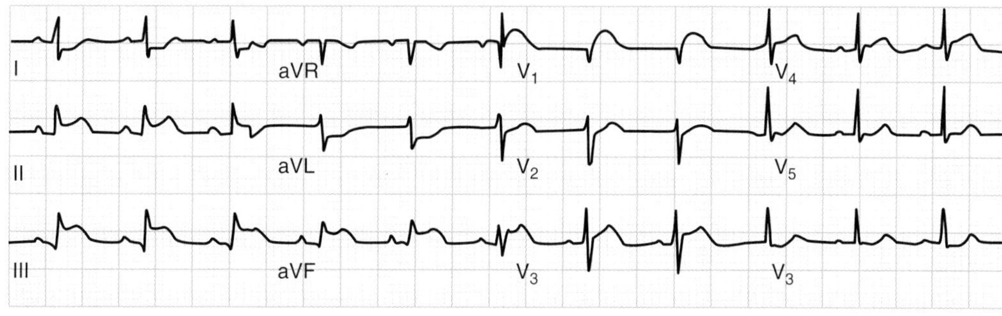

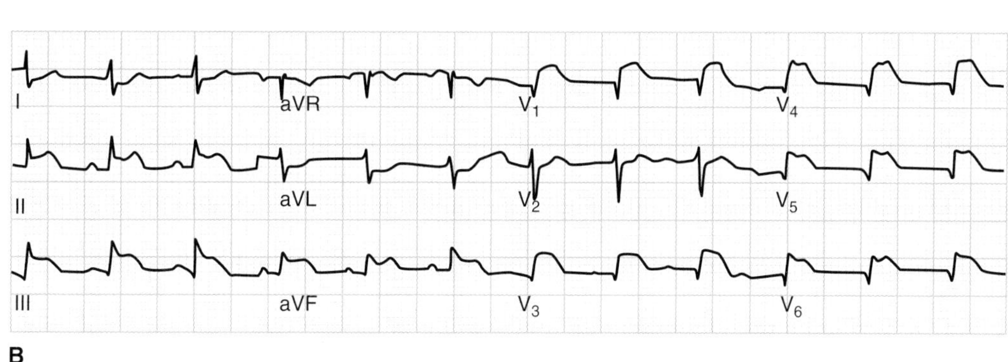

FIGURE 49-4. A. Inferior wall myocardial infarction with ST elevation in lead V_1. ECG showing inferior ST-segment elevation myocardial infarction and ST-segment elevation in lead V_1 suggestive of right ventricular infarction. **B.** Inferior wall myocardial infarction with right ventricular leads. Same patient with placement of right ventricular leads, showing ST-segment elevation in V_3R, V_4R, V_5R, and V_6R compatible with right ventricular infarction. [Used with permission of J. Stephan Stapczynski, Maricopa Medical Center.]

negative in leads V_1 to V_3 with right ventricular pacing. ST-segment depression in these leads has 80% specificity for AMI.[15]

SERUM MARKERS OF MYOCARDIAL INJURY

Patients with diagnostic ST-segment elevation on their initial ECG do not require serum marker measurement to make treatment and disposition decisions. Conversely, serum markers are useful in patients with nondiagnostic ECGs for diagnosis of NSTEMI and risk stratification of patients with STEMI, NSTEMI, and unstable angina. Even low-level cardiac marker elevations are independent risk factors for acute (<30 days) cardiac complications and short-term (<1 year) prognosis in unstable angina.[16] A rise in serum troponin I or T, with at least one value above the 99th percentile, is diagnostic for AMI in patients with symptoms consistent with ACS.[17] Low-level elevations in either troponin correlate with risk for cardiovascular complications in unstable angina, CAD, and renal failure.[16] Troponin is sensitive and specific for cardiac myocardial necrosis, but there are many causes of myocardial necrosis unrelated to ACS (see Table 48-5). Minor elevations in cardiac troponin I and cardiac troponin T identify patients more likely to benefit from treatment with glycoprotein IIb/IIIa inhibitors, enoxaparin, and early invasive treatment strategy (catheterization within 24 to 48 hours).[18]

New high-sensitivity cardiac troponins have improved ability to detect ischemia. First-generation single assays of cardiac troponin I at the time of presentation had an AMI sensitivity of 39%. Serial sampling increased sensitivity to 90% to 100%, with specificity of 83% to 96% for cardiac troponin I and 76% to 91% for cardiac troponin T. The high-sensitivity troponins, initially used in Europe, identify 90% to 100% of patients with AMI at the time of arrival using the lowest cut point, albeit with limited specificity (between 34% and 80% depending on the cut-off used).[19-21] The concern regarding use of high-sensitivity assays focuses on the frequency of false-positive results that lead to unnecessary procedures

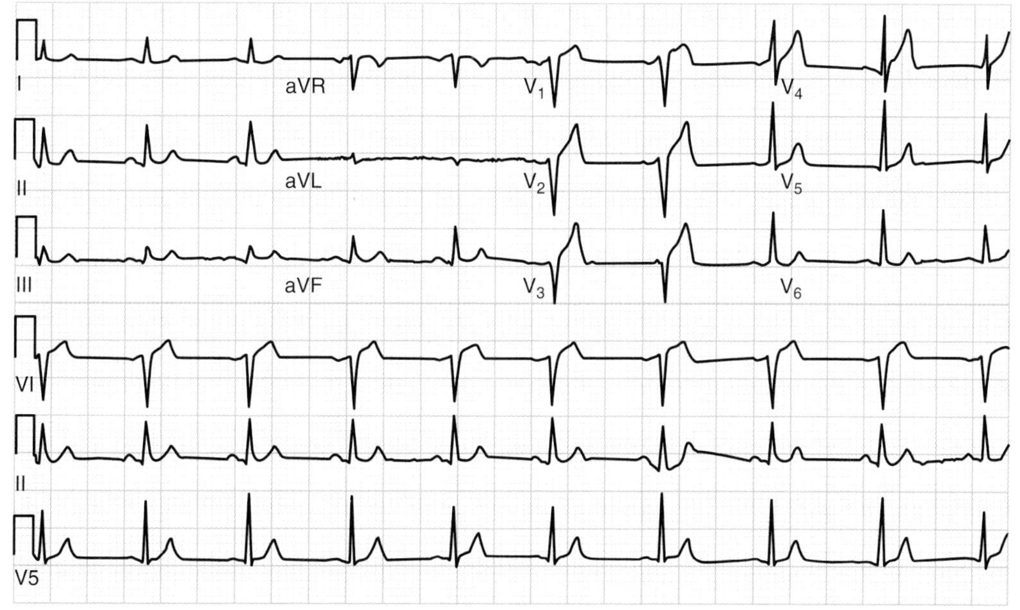

FIGURE 49-5. ECG showing anterior myocardial infarction from distal left anterior descending coronary artery occlusion. ECG from a 52-year-old man presenting with chest pain. ECG shows ST-segment elevation in V_1, V_2, and V_3, with the absence of ST-segment depression in leads II, III, and aVF. The patient was found to have 100% occlusion of the distal left anterior descending coronary artery at cardiac catheterization. [Used with permission of David M. Cline, MD, Wake Forest University.]

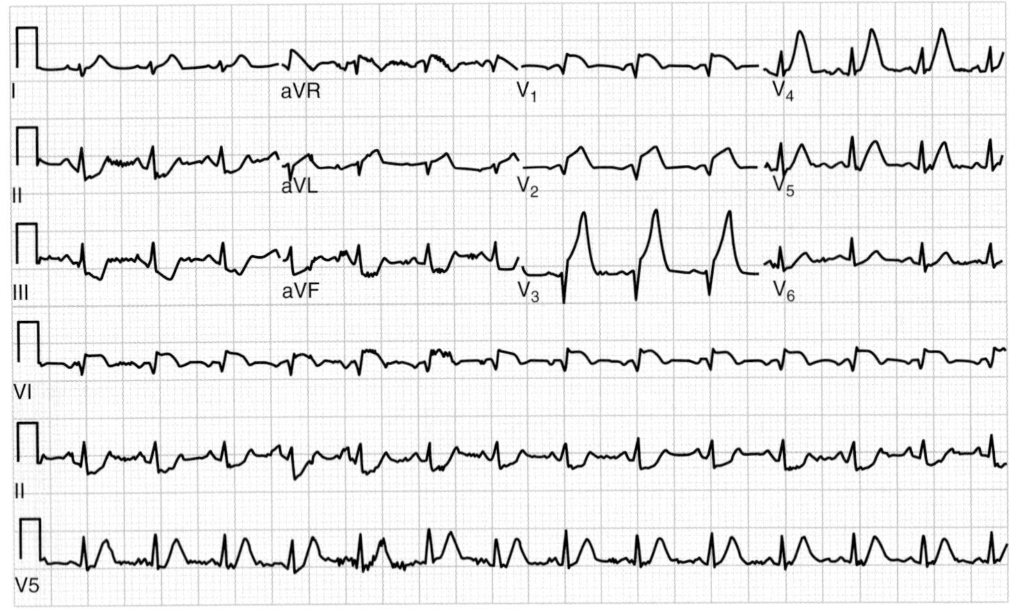

FIGURE 49-6. ECG showing anterior myocardial infarction from proximal left anterior descending coronary artery occlusion. ECG from a 65-year-old man presenting with chest pain. ECG shows ST-segment elevation in V_1, V_2, and V_3, and >1 mm of ST-segment depression in leads II, III, and aVF. The patient was found to have 100% occlusion of the proximal left anterior descending coronary artery at cardiac catheterization. [Used with permission of David M. Cline, MD, Wake Forest University.]

TABLE 49-7 Conditions in Which ECG Interpretation Can Be Difficult

May have ST-segment elevation in the absence of acute myocardial infarction
Early repolarization
Left ventricular hypertrophy
Pericarditis
Myocarditis
Left ventricular aneurysm
Hypertrophic cardiomyopathy
Hypothermia
Ventricular paced rhythms
Left bundle-branch block
May have ST-segment depressions in the absence of ischemia
Hypokalemia
Digoxin effect
Cor pulmonale and right heart strain
Early repolarization
Left ventricular hypertrophy
Ventricular-paced rhythms
Left bundle-branch block
May have T-wave inversions in the absence of ischemia
Persistent juvenile pattern
Stokes-Adams syncope or seizures
Posttachycardia T-wave inversion
Postpacemaker T-wave inversion
Intracranial pathology (CNS hemorrhage)
Mitral valve prolapse
Pericarditis
Primary or secondary myocardial diseases
Pulmonary embolism or cor pulmonale from other causes
Spontaneous pneumothorax
Myocardial contusion
Left ventricular hypertrophy
Ventricular-paced rhythms
Left bundle-branch block
Right bundle-branch block

and hospital admissions or no benefit. Authors of a large observational study advocated using a single undetectable high-sensitivity troponin plus no ECG evidence of ischemia as a decision point to discharge chest pain patients from the ED.

Despite the new sensitive assays, guidelines[1,5,6] and experts[22] recommend serial troponin testing to identify acute disease. A serial high-sensitivity troponin interval as short as 2 hours coupled with a low TIMI risk score (<2) virtually excludes AMI.[23] The European Society of Cardiology recommends a 3-hour serial interval when high-sensitivity troponins are used.[24]

Elevated levels of the cardiac troponins in patients with NSTEMI increase the short-term risk of death 3.1-fold (1.6% vs 5.2%).[19] Although patients with elevated troponins in the absence of ACS may be "false positive" for AMI, elevated troponin of any amount is associated with a high frequency of worse outcomes. Taken together, the data strongly support the claim that **any measurable elevated troponin is always worse than no elevated troponin and that more troponin elevation is always worse than less troponin elevation with respect to prognosis.**

B-type natriuretic peptide, an established marker for patients with heart failure, is also elevated in patients with ACS and can identify ACS patients who are at higher risk for adverse cardiovascular events, heart failure, or death.[5] When used in conjunction with other markers, the addition of B-type natriuretic peptide increases sensitivity at the cost of decreased specificity, with only a slightly increase in overall diagnostic accuracy.

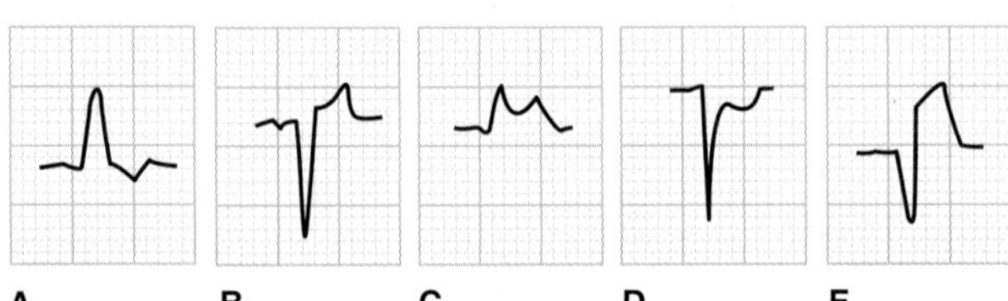

FIGURE 49-7. Discordant and concordant ST elevation and depression in the setting of left bundle-branch block. ST-segment abnormalities in left bundle-branch block. **A.** Discordant ST-segment depression ("normal"). **B.** Discordant ST-segment elevation ("normal"). **C.** Concordant ST-segment elevation (strongly suggestive of acute myocardial infarction [AMI]). **D.** Concordant ST-segment depression (suggestive of AMI). **E.** Excessive (>5 mm) discordant ST-segment elevation (weakly suggestive of AMI). [Used with permission of William Brady, MD, University of Virginia.]

For this reason, B-type natriuretic peptide is not routinely needed in those with suspected ACS.

GENERAL TREATMENT

The treatment of ACSs is based on duration and persistence of symptoms, cardiac history, and findings on physical examination and the initial ECG (see **Figure 49-8**). Establish IV access, give aspirin if not already given by EMS, and, as long as there are no contraindications, provide ECG monitoring. Many recommend supplemental O_2[6]; however, there is little evidence for benefit in patients without hypoxemia, and small studies have shown a negative effect with high-flow O_2.[25] The key treatment strategies aim to achieve immediate reperfusion and limit infarct size (**Tables 49-8** and **49-9**).

Patients with persistent symptoms and STEMI should receive reperfusion attempts. Reperfusion therapies can be mechanical or pharmacologic. **Percutaneous coronary intervention (PCI)** with or without stent placement is the dominant current approach to mechanical reperfusion.[5] Pharmacologic reperfusion is accomplished with fibrinolytic therapy, which is improved with adjuvant antiplatelet and antithrombin therapy.

American Heart Association/American College of Cardiology guidelines target a treatment goal of ≤90 minutes for a patient who arrives at a hospital with PCI capability or of ≤120 minutes for patients arriving at a hospital without PCI capability to account for transfer time.[5,6] Fibrinolysis should be given within 30 minutes of ED arrival if PCI cannot be accomplished within these time frames.[6] The concept of "first medical contact to device/balloon time" replaces the "door to needle" or "door to balloon" time.[6] Each health system and institution treating ACS patients should develop protocols to drive optimal methods of

TABLE 49-8 Drugs Used in the Emergency Treatment of STEMI

Antiplatelet Agents		
Aspirin	162–325 milligrams.	
Clopidogrel	Loading dose of 600 milligrams PO followed by 75 milligrams/d. No loading dose is administered in patients >75 y old receiving fibrinolytics.	
Prasugrel	Loading dose of 60 milligrams promptly and no more than 1 h after PCI once coronary anatomy is defined and a decision is made to proceed with PCI.	
Ticagrelor	Loading dose is 180 milligrams PO followed by 90 milligrams twice a day.	
Antithrombins		
Unfractionated heparin	Bolus of 60 units/kg (maximum, 4000 units) followed by infusion of 12 units/kg/h (maximum, 1000 units/h) titrated to a partial thromboplastin time 1.5–2.5 × control.	
Enoxaparin	30 milligrams IV bolus followed by 1 milligram/kg SC every 12 h.	
Fondaparinux	2.5 milligrams SC.*	
Fibrinolytic Agents		
Streptokinase	1.5 million units over 60 min.	
Anistreplase	30 units IV over 2–5 min.	
Alteplase	Body weight >67 kg: 15 milligrams initial IV bolus; 50 milligrams infused over next 30 min; 35 milligrams infused over next 60 min.	
	Body weight <67 kg: 15 milligrams initial IV bolus; 0.75 milligrams/kg infused over next 30 min; 0.5 milligram/kg infused over next 60 min.	
Reteplase	10 units IV over 2 min followed by 10 units IV bolus 30 min later.	
Tenecteplase	Weight	Dose (total dose not to exceed 50 milligrams)
	<60 kg	30 milligrams
	≥60 but <70 kg	35 milligrams
	≥70 but <80 kg	40 milligrams
	≥80 but <90	45 milligrams
	≥90	50 milligrams
Glycoprotein IIb/IIIa Inhibitors†		
Abciximab	0.25 milligram/kg bolus followed by infusion of 0.125 microgram/kg/min (maximum, 10 micrograms/min) for 12–24 h.	
Eptifibatide	180 micrograms/kg bolus followed by infusion of 2.0 micrograms/kg/min for 72–96 h.	
Tirofiban	0.4 micrograms/kg/min for 30 min followed by infusion of 0.1 microgram/kg/min for 48–96 h.	
Other Anti-Ischemic Therapies		
Nitroglycerin	Sublingual: 0.4 milligram every 5 min × 3 PRN pain.	
	IV: Start at 10 micrograms/min, titrate to 10% reduction in MAP if normotensive, 30% reduction in MAP if hypertensive.	
Morphine	2–5 milligrams IV every 5–15 min PRN pain.	
Metoprolol	50 milligrams PO every 12 h on first day, unless significant hypertension, may consider 5 milligrams IV over 2 min every 5 min up to 15 milligrams; withhold β-blockers initially if the patient is at risk for cardiogenic shock/adverse effects.‡	
Atenolol	25–50 milligrams PO, unless significant hypertension, may consider 5 milligrams IV over 5 min, repeat once 10 min later; withhold β-blockers initially if the patient is at risk for cardiogenic shock/adverse effects.‡	

Abbreviations: MAP = mean arterial pressure; PCI = percutaneous coronary intervention; PRN = as needed; STEMI= ST-segment elevation myocardial infarction.

*Fondaparinux should not be used as monotherapy for PCI; if used, addition of unfractionated heparin or bivalirudin is recommended before PCI.

†American College of Cardiology/American Heart Association 2009 focused update for STEMI patients recommended glycoprotein IIB/IIa inhibitors be given at the time of PCI; benefit prior to arrival in the cardiac catheterization laboratory is uncertain.

‡Risk factors for cardiogenic shock/adverse effects: 1. Signs of heart failure; 2. evidence of a low cardiac output state; 3. increased risk for cardiogenic shock (cumulatively: age >70 y old, systolic blood pressure <120 mm Hg, sinus tachycardia >110 beats/min or bradycardia <60 beats/min, and longer duration of STEMI symptoms before diagnosis and treatment); or 4. standard relative contraindications to β-blockade (PR interval >0.24 s, second- or third-degree heart block, active asthma, or reactive airway disease).

TABLE 49-9 Drugs Used in the Emergency Treatment of Unstable Angina or NSTEMI

Drug	Dosage
Antiplatelet Agents	
Aspirin	162–325 milligrams
Clopidogrel	Loading dose of 300–600 milligrams PO followed by 75 milligrams/d
Prasugrel	Loading dose of 60 milligrams promptly and no more than 1 h after PCI once coronary anatomy is defined and a decision is made to proceed with PCI
Ticagrelor	Loading dose of 180 milligrams PO followed by 90 milligrams twice a day
Antithrombins	
Heparin	Bolus of 60 units/kg (maximum, 4000 units) followed by infusion of 12 units/kg/h (maximum, 1000 units/h) titrated to a partial thromboplastin time 1.5–2.5 × control
Enoxaparin	1 milligram/kg SC every 12 h
Fondaparinux	2.5 milligrams SC
Direct Thrombin Inhibitor	
Bivalirudin	0.75 milligram/kg IV bolus followed by 1.75 milligrams/kg/h infusion for duration of procedure
Glycoprotein IIb/IIIa Inhibitors	
Abciximab	0.25 milligram/kg bolus followed by infusion of 0.125 microgram/kg/min (maximum, 10 micrograms/min) for 12–24 h
Eptifibatide	180 micrograms/kg bolus followed by infusion of 2.0 micrograms/kg/min for 72–96 h
Tirofiban	0.4 microgram/kg/min for 30 min followed by infusion of 0.1 microgram/kg/min for 48–96 h
Other Anti-Ischemic Therapies	
Nitroglycerin	Sublingual: 0.4 milligram every 5 min × 3 PRN pain IV: Start at 10 micrograms/min, titrate to 10% reduction in MAP if normotensive, 30% reduction in MAP if hypertensive
Metoprolol	50 milligrams PO every 12 h first day, unless significant hypertension, may consider 5 milligrams IV over 2 min every 5 min up to 15 milligrams; withhold β-blockers initially if the patient is at risk for cardiogenic shock/adverse effects*
Atenolol	25–50 milligrams PO, unless significant hypertension, may consider 5 milligrams IV over 5 min, repeat once 10 min later; withhold β-blockers initially if the patient is at risk for cardiogenic shock/adverse effects*

Abbreviations: MAP = mean arterial pressure; NSTEMI = non-ST-segment elevation myocardial infarction; PRN = as needed.

*Risk factors for cardiogenic shock/adverse effects: 1. Signs of heart failure; 2. evidence of a low cardiac output state; 3. increased risk for cardiogenic shock (cumulatively: age >70 years old, systolic blood pressure <120 mm Hg, sinus tachycardia >110 beats/min or bradycardia <60 beats/min, and longer duration of ST-segment elevation myocardial infarction symptoms before diagnosis and treatment); or 4. standard relative contraindications to β-blockade (PR interval >0.24 s, second- or third-degree heart block, active asthma, or reactive airway disease).

reperfusion, determining which strategy it will use depending on its capabilities.

Most STEMI patients receive antiplatelet agents, antithrombins, and nitrates in the ED. Treat patients with unstable angina or NSTEMI with antiplatelet agents, antithrombins, and nitrates.[1] Those with unstable angina or NSTEMI refractory to these therapies or those scheduled to undergo PCI also may benefit from the use of glycoprotein IIb/IIIa antagonists (Tables 49-8 and 49-9).[1]

NSTEMI TREATMENT

For patients with NSTEMI (which by definition requires the time for biomarkers to become elevated and the clinical laboratory to perform the measurement), an invasive approach within 24 to 48 hours using PCI reduces the composite of death, MI, or recurrent ACS by 19% in women and 27% in men.[26] Therefore, the **very early** invasive approach deployed in STEMI is recommended in NSTEMI patients only with refractory angina or hemodynamic or electrical instability, or in patients at increased risk for clinical events.[1] Although the proportion of myocardial infarction patients with NSTEMI has increased from 52.8% in 2002 to 68.6% in 2011, utilization of the early invasive approach increased from 27.8% to 41.4% while in-hospital mortality dropped.[27]

Based on the results of these trials and a meta-analysis,[28] the American Heart Association/American College of Cardiology guidelines for the management of unstable angina/NSTEMI patients recommend early (within 48 hours) invasive therapy in patients with recurrent angina/ischemia with or without symptoms of congestive heart failure, elevated cardiac troponins, new or presumably new ST-segment depression, high-risk findings on noninvasive stress testing, depressed left ventricular function, hemodynamic instability, sustained ventricular tachycardia, PCIs within the previous 6 months, or prior coronary artery bypass grafting.[1] More aggressive and earlier PCI in these patients has not proven beneficial compared to the within 48 hours approach.[29,30]

PERCUTANEOUS CORONARY INTERVENTION

The American College of Cardiology, the American Heart Association, and the European Society of Cardiology recommend PCI as the preferred method of reperfusion therapy if the first medical contact to first balloon inflation time is less than 90 to 120 minutes.[5,6,31] In the early presenting cohort (within 3 hours of symptom onset), the decision to use primary PCI rather than fibrinolysis is based on institutional expertise, availability of the cardiac catheterization team, and the individual patient risk of complications from fibrinolysis.

Coronary angioplasty with or without stent placement is the most common PCI; alternatives include atherectomy and laser angioplasty. Balloon angioplasty increases the size of the arterial lumen through endothelial denudation; cracking, splitting, and disruption of atherosclerotic plaque; dehiscence of intima and plaque from underlying media; and stretching or tearing of underlying media and adventitia. With successful dilatation, small amounts of arterial wall dissection and aneurysmal expansion may be seen. The greater the increase in luminal size, the lower is the risk of restenosis. However, more aggressive balloon inflation can augment dissection, platelet deposition, thrombus formation, and plaque hemorrhage.

Alternative PCI procedures attempt to limit complications. Directional and rotational coronary atherectomy extract atherosclerotic tissue from the coronary artery. Excimer laser atherectomy vaporizes atheromatous tissue. It results in larger luminal diameters but has not reduced rates of restenosis or other complications associated with percutaneous angioplasty procedures.

Coronary stents are fenestrated stainless steel tubes that are expanded by a balloon to provide scaffolding within the coronary arteries.

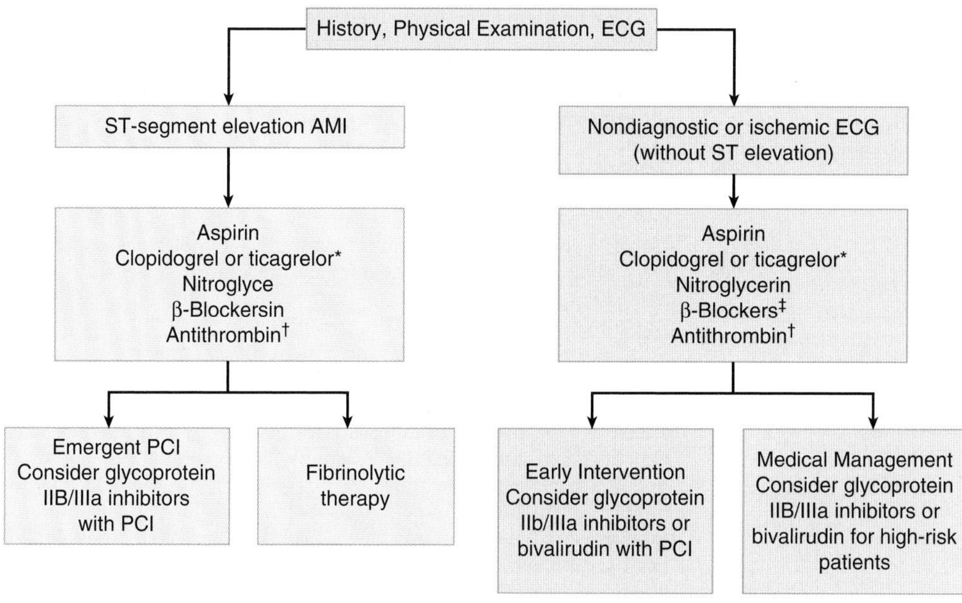

*Prasugrel should be considered at the time of PCI in patients who have not yet received either clopidogrel or ticagrelor.

†Enoxaparin, unfractionated heparin, or fondaparinux. Note:See text for discussion of individual treatment options, indications, and contraindications.

‡Risk factors for cardiogenic shock/adverse effects: 1. Signs of heart failure; 2. evidence of a low cardiac output state; 3. increased risk for cardiogenic shock (cumulatively: age >70 y old, systolic blood pressure <120 mm Hg, sinus tachycardia >110 beats/min or bradycardia <60 beats/min, and longer duration of ST-segment elevation myocardial infarction symptoms before diagnosis and treatment); or 4. standard relative contraindications to β-blockade (PR interval >0.24 s, second- or third-degree heart block, active asthma, or reactive airway disease).

AMI = acute myocardial infarction; PCI = percutaneous coronary intervention.

FIGURE 49-8. Treatment considerations for acute coronary syndrome patients. *Prasugrel should be considered at the time of PCI in patients who have not yet received either clopidogrel or ticagrelor. †Enoxaparin, unfractionated heparin, or fondaparinux. Note: See text for discussion of individual treatment options, indications, and contraindications. ‡Risk factors for cardiogenic shock/adverse effects: 1. Signs of heart failure; 2. evidence of a low cardiac output state; 3. increased risk for cardiogenic shock (cumulatively: age >70 y old, systolic blood pressure <120 mm Hg, sinus tachycardia >110 beats/min or bradycardia <60 beats/min, and longer duration of ST-segment elevation myocardial infarction symptoms before diagnosis and treatment); or 4. standard relative contraindications to β-blockade (PR interval >0.24 s, second- or third-degree heart block, active asthma, or reactive airway disease). AMI = acute myocardial infarction; PCI = percutaneous coronary intervention.

Adding antiplatelet therapy (in particular, thienopyridines and glycoprotein IIb/IIIa inhibitors) results in lower adverse events at 6 months. Drug-eluting stents are associated with **decreased early** (within months) vessel closure but a **higher delayed** closure, particularly once antiplatelet agents (clopidogrel) are stopped.

In centers with expertise in direct angioplasty, primary PCI reduces the cardiovascular complication rate in patients with AMI compared to fibrinolysis.[5,32,33] The longer the duration of symptoms, the greater is the benefit to primary PCI over fibrinolysis. PCI is more effective in establishing flow and reducing reocclusion in the infarct-related artery than fibrinolytic therapy and is associated with a decreased incidence of short- and long-term death, nonfatal reinfarction, and intracranial hemorrhage compared with fibrinolytic therapy.[6]

Registry data show that the targeted reperfusion time goal is met less than half the time.[31,34] Strategies[35] to optimize door to balloon time include: EMS direct or emergency physician activation of the catheterization laboratory without cardiologist consultation by a one call system (similar to trauma activations); having a trained catheterization team ready in 20 minutes; a feedback loop providing the EMS provider and emergency physician with data on the individual case; quality assurance processes in place to measure and report back times; and continually enhancing the team-based approach.

FIBRINOLYTICS

Fibrinolytic agents (tissue plasminogen activator, recombinant tissue plasminogen activator, tenecteplase, streptokinase, and anistreplase) act on the acute thrombosis directly or indirectly as plasminogen activators. Plasminogen, an inactive proteolytic enzyme, binds directly to fibrin during thrombus formation to form a plasminogen–fibrin complex. This plasminogen–fibrin complex incorporated into the clot is more susceptible than circulating plasma plasminogen to activation—thus, the concept that fibrinolytic agents are to a varying degree "clot specific," promoting fibrin proteolysis.

Fibrinolytic therapy improves left ventricular function and short-term and long-term mortality. A meta-analysis found that the net benefit of fibrinolytic treatment in the first 3 hours was >30 lives saved per 1000 patients.[36] The loss of benefit per hour delay in fibrinolytic administration was 1.6 lives per 1000 patients per hour.

Fibrinolytic therapy is indicated for patients with STEMI (as a reperfusion option) if time to treatment is <6 to 12 hours from symptom onset and the ECG has at least 1 mm of ST-segment elevation in two or more contiguous leads.[5,6] Therapy is more beneficial if given early and for larger infarctions and anterior infarctions than for smaller or inferior infarctions. In the elderly, the overall risk of mortality from AMI is high. The proportionate reduction in mortality rate appears to be less in patients >75 years old, but the absolute number of patients who may be saved is still considerable.

After failed fibrinolytic administration, rescue PCI is recommended for patients in cardiogenic shock who are <75 years old, patients with severe heart failure or pulmonary edema, patients with hemodynamically compromising ventricular arrhythmias, and patients in whom fibrinolytic therapy has failed and a moderate or large area of myocardium is at risk.[5]

Because tissue plasminogen activator, recombinant tissue plasminogen activator, and tenecteplase have similar efficacy and safety profiles, the choice of which to use is usually based on ease of administration, cost, and the local preferences.

TABLE 49-10 Contraindications to Fibrinolytic Therapy in ST-Segment Elevation Myocardial Infarction

Absolute contraindications
Any prior intracranial hemorrhage
Known structural cerebral vascular lesion (e.g., arteriovenous malformation)
Known intracranial neoplasm
Ischemic stroke within 3 mo
Active internal bleeding (excluding menses)
Suspected aortic dissection or pericarditis
Relative contraindications
Severe uncontrolled blood pressure (>180/100 mm Hg)
History of chronic, severe, poorly controlled hypertension
History of prior ischemic stroke >3 mo or known intracranial pathology not covered in contraindications
Current use of anticoagulants with known INR >2–3
Known bleeding diathesis
Recent trauma (past 2 wk)
Prolonged CPR (>10 min)
Major surgery (<3 wk)
Noncompressible vascular punctures (including subclavian and internal jugular central lines)
Recent internal bleeding (within 2–4 wk)
Patients treated previously with streptokinase should not receive streptokinase a second time
Pregnancy
Active peptic ulcer disease
Other medical conditions likely to increase risk of bleeding (e.g., diabetic retinopathy)

Contraindications to fibrinolytic therapy are those that increase the risk of hemorrhage (**Table 49-10**). The most catastrophic complication is intracranial bleeding. Clinical variables that can be assessed in the ED and predict an increased risk of intracranial hemorrhage are age (>65 years old), low body mass (<70 kg), and hypertension on presentation.[5] Intracranial hemorrhage is more common with tissue plasminogen activator than with streptokinase (odds ratio of 1.6). Patients with relative contraindications may still receive fibrinolytic therapy when the benefits of therapy outweigh the risks of the complications.

Patients treated with fibrinolytics benefit from early follow-up invasive intervention, called *pharmacoinvasive therapy*. In the TRANSFER-AMI study, high-risk patients treated with fibrinolytics for STEMI at non–PCI-capable centers were randomized to standard care or immediate transfer for PCI within 6 hours after fibrinolysis.[37] The patients who underwent the pharmacoinvasive strategy had a 6.2% absolute reduction in the composite endpoint of death, reinfarction, recurrent ischemia, new or worsening heart failure, or cardiogenic shock at 30 days.

Facilitated PCI refers to a planned initial pharmacologic treatment followed by PCI for treatment of STEMI. The ASSENT-4 PCI trial found no benefit and a higher incidence of death, congestive heart failure, or shock at 90 days in the group receiving fibrinolytics compared with the PCI-only group. Current guidelines state that a facilitated approach might be considered in high-risk patients with low bleeding risk with long duration to PCI.[5] However, no clear benefits are apparent for this method.

Fibrinolytic therapy in STEMI is limited in several ways. First, even the most potent fibrinolytic agents do not achieve early and complete restoration of coronary blood flow in 40% to 50% of patients. Fibrinolytics are plasminogen activators. When fibrin is lysed, thrombin is exposed. The exposed thrombin is a potent biologic platelet activator. As a result, the more fibrin that is lysed, the more thrombin is exposed, and the more prothrombotic substrate is engendered. This may be one reason why optimal antithrombin therapy (enoxaparin rather than unfractionated heparin) and dual antiplatelet therapy (both aspirin and clopidogrel) lead to improved outcomes. The second limitation of fibrinolytic therapy is that approximately 0.5% to 1.0% of patients have intracranial hemorrhage, which usually results in death or disabling stroke.

STEMI patients who have received fibrinolytics should receive full-dose anticoagulants for a minimum of 48 hours.[5] Recommended therapies include unfractionated heparin, enoxaparin, or fondaparinux.[5,6]

STREPTOKINASE AND ANISTREPLASE

Streptokinase is a polypeptide derived from β-hemolytic *Streptococcus* cultures. It binds 1:1 to plasminogen, causing a conformational change that activates the plasminogen–streptokinase complex. This complex cleaves peptide bonds on other plasminogen molecules to activate them. This activated complex does not have fibrin specificity with a corresponding potential for marked systemic fibrinogen depletion. Anistreplase is a modified active plasminogen–streptokinase complex. Streptokinase compared with placebo reduces mortality rate and improves left ventricular function in patients with STEMI.

Allergic reactions occur in about 5% of patients treated with streptokinase for the first time, especially those with a recent *Streptococcus* infection. Self-limited allergic reactions usually respond to antihistamines. Anaphylactic reactions are rare. During IV administration, a minority of patients will experience hypotension, which usually responds to decreasing the rate of infusion and volume expansion. Streptokinase has a serum half-life of approximately 23 minutes but produces a fibrinolytic state for up to 24 hours. Antibodies may develop after streptokinase use, so retreatment is generally avoided. Streptokinase is less costly than other fibrinolytic agents. As a result, it is the most widely used fibrinolytic in some countries.[38,39]

ALTEPLASE/TISSUE PLASMINOGEN ACTIVATOR

Alteplase (also called *tissue plasminogen activator*) is a naturally occurring enzyme produced by the vascular endothelium and other tissues. It has a binding site for fibrin that allows it to attach to a formed thrombus and trigger fibrinolysis (fibrin specificity) with only mild systemic fibrinogen depletion. Tissue plasminogen activator achieves higher infarct-related artery patency rates than streptokinase (about 75% vs 50%, respectively). However, the choice of which fibrinolytic agent to use is probably less relevant than quick door-to-needle time (which saves an additional 1.6 per 1000 lives per hour earlier when treatment is provided). The mechanism of improved benefit of tissue plasminogen activator is early patency of the infarct-related vessel, which predicts short- and long-term survival.

RETEPLASE

Reteplase (recombinant tissue plasminogen activator) is a genetically engineered modification of tissue plasminogen activator that has a longer half-life (18 minutes vs 3 minutes) but reduced fibrin binding with potential for moderate systemic fibrinogen depletion. The third Global Use of Strategies to Open Occluded Coronary Arteries III trial showed no clinical difference in outcomes (mortality and stroke) between tissue plasminogen activator and reteplase. Reteplase can be given as a double slow-IV bolus, 10 milligrams each, 30 minutes apart. The easy double-bolus administration is an advantage in the ED.

TENECTEPLASE

Tenecteplase is another tissue plasminogen activator variant with a prolonged half-life (about 20 minutes), is resistant to endogenous plasminogen activator inhibitor 1 inactivation, and has high fibrin specificity and binding with minimal systemic fibrinogen depletion. There is no difference in 30-day mortality or intracranial hemorrhage rates between tenecteplase and tissue plasminogen activator. Single-bolus administration makes this an easy fibrinolytic agent to administer, but tenecteplase requires weight-based dosing, which may not always be practical.

ANTIPLATELET AGENTS

The glycoprotein IIb/IIIa antagonists are stronger antiplatelet agents than aspirin, interrupting platelet activation regardless of the agonist. In contrast, aspirin only inhibits platelet aggregation stimulated through thromboxane A_2 and mediated through the arachidonic acid pathway.

ASPIRIN

Give aspirin, ≥162 milligrams and preferably 325 milligrams if naïve of aspirin, as soon as possible to all patients with STEMI, NSTEMI, and unstable angina. Aspirin prevents formation of thromboxane A_2, an agonist of platelet aggregation. This inhibition persists for the 8- to 12-day life of the platelet, because platelets are unable to generate new cyclooxygenase. In patients with STEMI, aspirin alone reduces relative mortality rate by 23%.[5] The estimated number needed to treat to aid is 41 patients, with the number needed to harm (nondangerous bleeding) being 167 patients.[40] Aspirin used in conjunction with fibrinolytic therapy further reduces ischemic events and coronary artery reocclusion. Aspirin doses >162 milligrams cause immediate, near-complete inhibition of thromboxane A_2. Smaller doses may not be effective for acute use. Aspirin reduces vascular events in patients with AMI and patients with unstable angina, especially in those with prior myocardial infarction or stroke (decrease by about 4%).

The side effects of aspirin are mainly GI, accumulative, and dose related. They can be reduced by using diluted or buffered aspirin solutions, lowest possible doses, or concurrent antacid or H_2 antagonist administration. Due to the substantial benefits of aspirin therapy during ACS, do not withhold this agent from patients with minor contraindications (vague allergy, history of remote peptic ulcer, or GI bleeding).[5] Other antiplatelet agents such as clopidogrel are alternatives if true aspirin allergy or active peptic ulcer disease exists.

ADENOSINE DIPHOSPHATE RECEPTOR ANTAGONISTS

Prasugrel Prasugrel is an irreversible, potent platelet receptor antagonist in this class. In the TRITON-TIMI 38 trial, prasugrel compared favorably with clopidogrel,[41] reducing the primary composite outcome by an absolute 2.2%, although with an increased frequency of bleeding. In post hoc analysis, this increased bleeding risk was greatest in patients with a history of stroke and patients age ≥75 years. The **U.S. Food and Drug Administration issued a boxed warning for prasugrel, indicating use is contraindicated in patients with a prior cerebrovascular accident or transient ischemic attack or with pathologic bleeding. Additional risk factors for bleeding are age ≥75 years, propensity for bleeding, and concomitant use of medications that increase the risk of bleeding.** Prasugrel has only been studied in patients with known coronary anatomy, so it has limited generalizability to ED patients.[42]

Ticagrelor Ticagrelor is a reversible nonthienopyridine P2Y12 receptor antagonist, with the effect gone within 3 days of stopping the agent. The PLATO study compared ticagrelor to clopidogrel[43] in patients with ACS (with or without ST elevation). The composite primary outcome in those treated with ticagrelor was 1.9% absolute frequency lower without any difference in major bleeding. In the patients with STEMI undergoing PCI, there was an increase in stroke in patients receiving ticagrelor (1.7% vs 1.0%, $P = 0.02$)

Clopidogrel The addition of clopidogrel to aspirin and antithrombin therapy improves cardiovascular outcomes in patients receiving fibrinolysis for STEMI. The CLARITY-TIMI 28 trial[44] and the COMMIT Trial[45] both demonstrated improvements in hospital and 30-day outcomes with the addition of clopidogrel to standard therapy. The American College of Cardiology/American Heart Association STEMI guidelines consider this dual therapy a Class I, level of evidence A recommendation.[5]

Clopidogrel reduces a composite outcome of death, AMI, and stroke in patients with unstable angina/NSTEMI. The CURE trial randomized patients with unstable angina/NSTEMI to clopidogrel (300-milligram loading dose and 75-milligram daily dose) or placebo,[46] with all patients receiving aspirin. The clopidogrel group had a 20% reduction in death, AMI, or stroke between 3 and 12 months. There was an excess of bleeding in the clopidogrel group compared with controls; however, this was reduced in patients who received lower doses of aspirin.

Give clopidogrel to patients with true aspirin allergy. Early administration is recommended in patients with ACS regardless of whether noninvasive management or PCI is planned.[47] For patients undergoing urgent PCI, 600 milligrams is superior to 300 milligrams in preventing postprocedure MI.[48,49] However, the results of the CURRENT-OASIS-7 trial reported that although increasing the clopidogrel dose to 600 milligrams caused a decrease in ischemic events, there was also an increased rate of bleeding.[50] Therefore, the current guidelines still provide a clopidogrel dose range of 300 to 600 milligrams in patients with unstable angina/NSTEMI.[1]

In late 2009 and early 2010, the U.S. Food and Drug Administration issued warnings on the efficacy of clopidogrel in two selected patient groups. First, patients taking omeprazole experience an approximately 50% reduction in the antiplatelet aggregation effects of clopidogrel. Second, patients with the variant *CYP2C19* gene have impaired metabolism of clopidogrel and hence a reduced ability to convert the drug to its active form, leading to an increase in stent thromboses and recurrent ischemic events. Consider alternative antiplatelet agents in this group of patients.

Because of an increased bleeding risk, withhold clopidogrel for 5 days before coronary artery bypass grafting when possible. About 5% to 20% of patients with unstable angina/NSTEMI eventually have near-term coronary artery bypass grafting; do not withhold clopidogrel unless coronary artery bypass grafting is imminent.

GLYCOPROTEIN IIB/IIIA INHIBITORS

Abciximab is a chimeric antibody that binds irreversibly to the glycoprotein IIb/IIIa antagonists. The duration of action is longer than that of the smaller peptide molecules. **Eptifibatide** is a synthetic heptapeptide that binds reversibly to the glycoprotein IIb/IIIa receptor. **Tirofiban** is a synthetic small molecule with reversible binding to the glycoprotein IIb/IIIa receptor. All require an IV infusion to demonstrate sustained benefits. Reversal of platelet inhibition after cessation of infusion is more rapid with the polypeptide or small-molecule agents eptifibatide or tirofiban, an advantage when bleeding complications occur.

Despite potential benefits, routine initiation of a glycoprotein IIb/IIIa inhibitor in the ED is not recommended due to conflicting information about the timing of PCI after administration and potential for bleeding.[51]

The glycoprotein IIb/IIIa inhibitor recommendations include patients with high-risk features, such as positive troponins, or patients who are likely to receive PCI, but initiation prior to catheterization does not have proven benefit over initiation in the catheterization laboratory. Six large trials together enrolled more than 10,000 PCI patients and found that patients treated with glycoprotein IIb/IIIa inhibitors (in addition to aspirin and an antithrombin) have an approximately 40% reduced risk of death or AMI in 30 days.[51] Some of this benefit was sustained for up to 3 years (13% reduction).

Four large trials evaluated glycoprotein IIb/IIIa antagonists for the medical stabilization of patients with unstable angina/NSTEMI. Tirofiban and eptifibatide reduced the rates of the triple composite endpoint of death, AMI, and recurrent ischemia. However, abciximab was not a benefit in patients who did not undergo coronary angiography within 48 hours. In a meta-analysis of six randomized placebo-controlled trials, a small reduction in the composite (but not individual) endpoint of death or AMI occurred in patients receiving glycoprotein IIb/IIIa inhibitors (11.8% vs 10.8%), with the most benefit and bleeding in patients undergoing PCI.[51] Thus, **the American Heart Association/American College of Cardiology guidelines for the management of unstable angina/NSTEMI patients make administration of glycoprotein IIb/IIIa inhibitors to patients in whom a PCI is planned a Class IIb recommendation.**[1] Abciximab is not recommended for patients who will be receiving medical management without PCI. A trial by Giugliano et al[52] published in 2009 found that for NSTEMI patients taken to PCI (invasive strategy), eptifibatide delayed to the time of PCI resulted in less bleeding with otherwise similar outcomes, suggesting that the preferred time for administration of glycoprotein IIb/IIa inhibitors to this group of patients is at the time of PCI.[53]

ANTITHROMBINS

UNFRACTIONATED HEPARIN

Unfractionated heparin reduces the risk of AMI and death during the acute phase of unstable angina. The combination therapy of aspirin and heparin reduces the short-term risk of death or AMI by 56% compared with aspirin alone. When unfractionated heparin is used in combination with aspirin, recurrence of ischemia is diminished after cessation of the infusion. **Thus, combination therapy with aspirin and heparin is indicated for patients with ACS.**

Unfractionated heparin has an unpredictable anticoagulant response because the bioavailability of heparin is variable. Even in clinical trials, less than half of patients are appropriately anticoagulated within 24 hours. Unfractionated heparin requires careful laboratory monitoring and dose adjustment. The weight-adjusted regimen is recommended, with an initial bolus of 60 units/kg (maximum of 4000 units per American Heart Association/American College of Cardiology guidelines[1,5]) and an infusion of 12 units/kg/h (maximum, 1000 units/h[1,5]). Unfractionated heparin dosing according to the European Society of Cardiology is 70 to 100 units/kg IV bolus when no glycoprotein IIb/IIIa inhibitor is planned and 50 to 60 units/kg IV bolus when given with glycoprotein IIb/IIIa inhibitors.[6] Optimally, cease unfractionated heparin after 48 hours of therapy to reduce the risk of developing heparin-induced thrombocytopenia.[5] Use other agents if ongoing anticoagulation is needed.

LOW-MOLECULAR-WEIGHT HEPARINS

The low-molecular-weight heparins have greater bioavailability, lower protein binding, and a longer half-life, and achieve a more reliable anticoagulant effect. As a result, they are given in a fixed dose subcutaneously once or twice a day and achieve a stable therapeutic response without the need for monitoring anticoagulation.

Large clinical trials show that enoxaparin, rather than unfractionated heparin, improved outcome in STEMI patients treated with aspirin and fibrinolysis.[54] **Enoxaparin is not considered a first-line antithrombin for patients receiving primary PCI for treatment of STEMI**[5]; however, in the event that a patient previously started on enoxaparin goes for PCI, enoxaparin should be continued.

A meta-analysis of six trials comparing enoxaparin with unfractionated heparin demonstrates a 0.9% reduction in death or recurrent AMI in patients receiving enoxaparin rather than unfractionated heparin, in addition to other standard therapies.[55] The benefit of enoxaparin is greater in patients with higher risk, with a significant decrease in the composite endpoint of death, AMI, and recurrent ischemia requiring PCI at 14 days in patients with a TIMI risk score >3. Trials with high rates of PCI have demonstrated the safety and efficacy of low-molecular-weight heparins in patients receiving PCI. The SYNERGY trial demonstrated improved outcomes in patients with consistent therapy (use of a single antithrombin from the ED through the catheterization laboratory) and increased bleeding when the patient was changed from one antithrombin to another. **The best approach is for the emergency physician and cardiologist to work in collaboration** to choose the antithrombin agent used from ED through PCI and aftercare. If coronary artery bypass grafting is planned, hold low-molecular-weight heparin for 12 to 24 hours, bridging with unfractionated heparin.

FONDAPARINUX

Fondaparinux is a synthetic pentasaccharide that binds to antithrombin-III to form an antithrombic complex, but unlike heparin, this complex is very specific for factor Xa inhibition. Fondaparinux has been evaluated in two large clinical trials. In STEMI patients, it has similar efficacy to unfractionated heparin in patients receiving fibrinolytics or primary PCI. However, the European Society of Cardiology does not recommend fondaparinux in patients going for PCI.[6] American College of Cardiology/American Heart Association guidelines make the following caution: **fondaparinux is not a monotherapy for PCI; if used, add unfractionated heparin or bivalirudin before PCI.**[5]

In unstable angina/NSTEMI patients, bleeding was lower in fondaparinux- versus enoxaparin-treated patients. For NSTEMI patients in whom a conservative management is to be used, the American College of Chest Physicians Evidence-Based Clinical Practice Guidelines recommended fondaparinux over enoxaparin,[56] as did the European Society of Cardiology,[24] but it is not yet U.S. Food and Drug Administration approved for this indication.

DIRECT THROMBIN INHIBITOR: BIVALIRUDIN

Direct thrombin inhibitors bind to the catalytic site of thrombin, bind to thrombin in clot, and are resistant to agents that degrade heparin. Bivalirudin reduces the short-term risk of postischemic complications relative to high-dose unfractionated heparin in patients undergoing PCI for unstable or postinfarction angina. The ACUITY trial demonstrated that bivalirudin is safe and effective for intermediate- to high-risk unstable angina/NSTEMI patients receiving PCI.[57] The HORIZONS-AMI trial showed that, in patients with STEMI who are undergoing PCI, anticoagulation with bivalirudin alone, as compared with unfractionated heparin plus glycoprotein IIb/IIIa inhibitors, resulted in significantly reduced 30-day rates of major bleeding.[58]

LIMITING INFARCT SIZE

NITRATES

Nitrates relax vascular smooth muscle in arteries, arterioles, and veins through the metabolic conversion of organic nitrates to nitric oxide. The pulmonary capillary wedge pressure, systemic arterial pressure, and left ventricular end-systolic and end-diastolic volumes decrease. Reduction in right and left ventricular filling pressures that result from peripheral dilatation combined with afterload reduction that results from arterial dilatation decrease cardiac work and myocardial O_2 requirements. Nitroglycerin has direct vasodilator effects on the coronary vascular bed and increases global and regional myocardial blood flows. When obstructing atherosclerotic lesions contain intact vascular smooth muscle, nitrates may dilate these vessels, thereby improving blood flow. Platelet aggregation is also inhibited by nitroglycerin.

When nitroglycerin is used in AMI patients not treated with thrombolytics, it reduces infarct size, improves regional function, and decreases the rate of cardiovascular complications. The mortality rate is lowered by 35% with the use of nitrates. It is important to note that in most studies, IV nitroglycerin titration to 10% reduction in mean arterial pressure for normotensive patients and to 30% reduction in mean arterial pressure for hypertensive patients occurred, not for symptom resolution. **In AMI, titrate IV nitroglycerin to blood pressure reduction rather than to symptom (chest pain) resolution.** Data are confounded regarding a benefit of nitroglycerin in those receiving fibrinolytic therapy.

The American College of Cardiology/American Heart Association recommends the use of IV nitroglycerin for the first 24 to 48 hours for patients with STEMI and recurrent ischemia, congestive heart failure, or hypertension.[5] Benefits are likely to be greatest in patients not receiving concurrent fibrinolytic therapy. For unstable angina/NSTEMI, IV nitroglycerin is used in patients who are not responsive to sublingual nitroglycerin tablets.[1]

The most serious side effect of nitroglycerin is hypotension, which may result in reflex tachycardia and worsening ischemia; paradoxical bradycardia can also follow nitrate use. **Use nitroglycerin cautiously for patients with inferior wall ischemia**, because one third of such patients might have right ventricular involvement and hence are volume dependent; nitrates reduce preload and commonly trigger hypotension in this setting, worsening infarct. If nitroglycerin results in hypotension, stop the drug and administer fluid for blood pressure. Avoid nitrates in patients with ACS who recently received a phosphodiesterase inhibitor for erectile dysfunction (within 24 hours of sildenafil use or within 48 hours of tadalafil use).

BLOCKERS

β-Adrenergic antagonists have antidysrhythmic, anti-ischemic, and antihypertensive properties. During AMI, they diminish myocardial O_2 demand by decreasing heart rate, systemic arterial pressure, and myocardial contractility. Prolongation of diastole may augment perfusion to ischemic myocardium.

Contemporary trials show no benefit from early β-blocker therapy, and data from one large trial have changed the guideline recommendations for β-antagonists.[59] The COMMIT/CCS-2 trial randomized 45,852 patients within 24 hours of myocardial infarction symptom onset to receive either IV metoprolol followed by oral metoprolol or placebo. **Metoprolol reduced the absolute risks of reinfarction by 5 per 1000 and of ventricular fibrillation by 5 per 1000, but importantly, it increased the risk of cardiogenic shock by 11 per 1000.** Overall, metoprolol did not significantly reduce mortality in the hospital.[59] **American College of Cardiology/American Heart Association recommendations are to start PO (not IV) β-antagonists in patients with STEMI or NSTEMI within 24 hours provided the patient has none of the following**: (1) signs of heart failure, (2) evidence of a low cardiac output state, (3) increased risk for cardiogenic shock (cumulatively: age >70 years old, systolic blood pressure <120 mm Hg, sinus tachycardia >110 beats/min or bradycardia <60 beats/min, and longer duration of STEMI symptoms before diagnosis and treatment), or (4) standard relative contraindications to β-blockade (PR interval >0.24 seconds, second- or third-degree heart block, active asthma, or reactive airway disease).[1,5] IV therapy is reserved for patients with significant hypertension.

ANGIOTENSIN-CONVERTING ENZYME INHIBITORS

Angiotensin-converting enzyme inhibitors reduce left ventricular dysfunction and left ventricular dilatation and slow the development of congestive heart failure during AMI. Oral angiotensin-converting enzyme therapy lowers mortality after AMI.[60]

The American College of Cardiology/American Heart Association recommends that patients with STEMI or heart failure receive treatment with oral angiotensin-converting enzyme inhibitors within the first 24 hours (**not necessarily in the ED**).[5] For unstable angina/NSTEMI, angiotensin-converting enzyme inhibitors should be administered within the first 24 hours in patients with pulmonary congestion or a left ventricular ejection fraction <40%, in the absence of hypotension or contraindications.[1]

Contraindications to angiotensin-converting enzyme inhibitors include hypotension, bilateral renal artery stenosis, renal failure, or history of cough or angioedema due to prior angiotensin-converting enzyme inhibitor use. The efficacy of angiotensin-converting enzyme inhibitors in unstable angina has not been well evaluated.

MAGNESIUM

Magnesium produces systemic and coronary vasodilatation, possesses antiplatelet activity, suppresses automaticity, and protects myocytes from calcium influx during reperfusion. However, studies are conflicting: some have found that the mortality rate is reduced, whereas others have shown no benefit at all. In light of these conflicting data, correct documented hypomagnesemia during AMI and give magnesium for torsades-type ventricular tachycardia with a prolonged QT interval.[5] Magnesium bolus and infusion in high-risk patients, such as the elderly and those in whom reperfusion therapy is not suitable, are considered possibly beneficial.[5]

CALCIUM CHANNEL ANTAGONISTS

Calcium channel blockers have antianginal, vasodilatory, and antihypertensive properties. **Calcium antagonists do *not* reduce mortality rate after AMI, and they may be harmful to some patients with cardiovascular disease.**[5]

Verapamil and diltiazem are potentially beneficial in patients with ongoing ischemia or atrial fibrillation with rapid ventricular response who do not have congestive heart failure, left ventricular dysfunction, or atrioventricular block, and when β-adrenergic antagonists are contraindicated.

COMPLICATIONS OF ACUTE CORONARY SYNDROME

Myocardial perfusion and cardiac function affect blood flow to the entire body. As a result, any end organ can be damaged when cardiac pump function is decreased. In this section, discussion of the complications of ACS is limited to the direct effects on the heart. The systemic effects of cardiac function are discussed in organ-appropriate chapters of this book.

DYSRHYTHMIAS AND CONDUCTION DISTURBANCES

The genesis, diagnosis, and treatment of dysrhythmias are presented in chapter 18, "Cardiac Rhythm Disturbances." The effect dysrhythmias have in complicating the course of patients with ACS is the subject of this section.

Dysrhythmias occur in 72% to 100% of AMI patients treated in the coronary care unit. **Table 49-11** shows the approximate frequency of the various dysrhythmias observed in patients with AMI. Many dysrhythmias occur in the prehospital and ED settings. The main consequences of dysrhythmias are impaired hemodynamic performance, compromised myocardial viability due to increased myocardial O_2 requirements, and predisposition to even more serious rhythm disturbances due to diminished ventricular fibrillation threshold.

The hemodynamic consequences of dysrhythmias are dependent on ventricular function. Patients with left ventricular dysfunction have a relatively fixed stroke volume. They depend on changes in heart rate to alter cardiac output. The range of heart rate that is optimal becomes narrowed with increasing dysfunction. Slower or faster heart rates may further depress cardiac output.

In addition, maintenance of the atrial filling of the ventricle (or "the atrial kick") is important for patients with AMI. Patients with normal hearts have a loss of 10% to 20% of left ventricular output when the atrial kick is eliminated. Patients with reduced left ventricular compliance, common in AMI, have up to 35% reduction in stroke volume when the atrial systole is eliminated. "Pump" failure with resultant increased sympathetic stimulation can also result in sinus tachycardia, atrial fibrillation or flutter, and supraventricular tachycardias.

TABLE 49-11 Early Dysrhythmias after Acute Myocardial Infarction

Dysrhythmia	Frequency of Occurrence (%)
Bradydysrhythmias	
Sinus bradycardia	35–40
First-degree AV block	4–15
Second-degree AV block, type I	4–10
Second-degree AV block, type II	0.5–1.0
Third-degree AV block	5–8
Asystole	1–5
Tachydysrhythmias	
Sinus tachycardia	30–35
Atrial premature contractions	50
Supraventricular tachycardia	2–9
Atrial fibrillation	4–10
Atrial flutter	1–2
Ventricular premature beats	99
Accelerated idioventricular rhythm	50–70
Ventricular tachycardia, nonsustained	60–69
Ventricular tachycardia, sustained	2–6
Ventricular fibrillation	4–7

Abbreviation: AV = atrioventricular.

Sinus tachycardia is quite prominent in patients with anterior wall AMI. Because of increased myocardial O_2 use, **persistent sinus tachycardia is associated with a poor prognosis in AMI; seek the cause and resolve it**. Causes may include anxiety, pain, left ventricular failure, fever, pericarditis, hypovolemia, atrial infarction, pulmonary emboli, or use of medications that accelerate heart rate. Similarly, paroxysmal supraventricular tachycardia, atrial fibrillation, and atrial flutter are associated with an increased mortality.

Atrial fibrillation associated with AMI most typically occurs in the first 24 hours and is usually transient. It more often occurs in patients with excess catecholamine release, hypokalemia, hypomagnesemia, hypoxia, chronic lung disease, and sinus node or left circumflex ischemia. Patients with supraventricular tachycardia, atrial fibrillation, or atrial flutter who have hemodynamic compromise are best treated with direct current cardioversion (see chapter 18). Patients who are partially/fully compensated or who do not respond to cardioversion can receive amiodarone or-β-adrenergic antagonists to slow the ventricular rate[61] absent any contraindications. Patients with ongoing ischemia but without hemodynamic compromise, clinical left ventricular dysfunction, reactive airway disease, or heart block should have rate control with β-adrenergic antagonists, such as atenolol (2.5 to 5.0 milligrams over 2 minutes to a total of 10 milligrams) or metoprolol (2.5 to 5.0 milligrams every 2 to 5 minutes to a total of 15 milligrams). Patients with contraindications to β-adrenergic antagonists can be treated with digoxin (0.3- to 0.5-milligram initial bolus with a repeat dose in 4 hours) or a calcium channel antagonist.[5] Anticoagulate patients with atrial fibrillation and AMI to limit systemic embolization.

Sinus bradycardia without hypotension does not appear to increase mortality during AMI. Prognosis is related to the site of infarction, the site of the block (intranodal vs infranodal), the type of escape rhythm, and the hemodynamic response to the rhythm. Atropine is used for sinus bradycardia when it results in hypotension, ischemia, or ventricular escape rhythms and for treatment of symptomatic atrioventricular block occurring at the atrioventricular nodal level (such as second-degree type I). Atropine can improve heart rate, systemic vascular resistance, and blood pressure; use it with caution in the setting of AMI since the parasympathetic tone is protective against infarct extension, ventricular fibrillation, and excessive myocardial O_2 demand.

Complete heart block can occur in patients with anterior and inferior AMI, because the AV conduction system receives blood supply from the atrioventricular branch of the right coronary artery and the septal perforating branch of the left anterior descending coronary artery. In the absence of right ventricular involvement, the mortality is approximately 15%. It rises to >30% when right ventricular involvement is present. Complete heart block in the setting of an anterior myocardial infarction portends a grave prognosis. Junctional rhythms are usually transient and occur within 48 hours of infarction.

The increased mortality in patients with heart block during AMI is related to more extensive myocardial damage and not to the heart block itself. As a result, pacing does not reduce mortality in patients with atrioventricular block or intraventricular conduction delay. Nonetheless, pacing is recommended to protect against sudden hypotension, acute ischemia, and precipitation of ventricular dysrhythmias in certain patients.

Use temporary **transcutaneous** pacers in patients at moderate to high risk of progression to atrioventricular block (see Table 49-12). **Transvenous** pacing follows for patients with a high likelihood (>30%) of requiring permanent pacing (**Table 49-12**). Patients with right ventricular infarction who are very dependent on atrial systole may require atrioventricular sequential pacing to maintain cardiac output.

Ventricular premature contractions are common in patients with AMI and are benign. **Accelerated idioventricular rhythms** in patients with AMI do not affect prognosis or require treatment. **Ventricular tachycardia** shortly after AMI is often transient and does not confer a poor prognosis. When ventricular tachycardia occurs late in the course of AMI, it is usually associated with transmural infarction and left ventricular dysfunction, induces hemodynamic deterioration, and is associated with a mortality rate approaching 50%. Primary **ventricular fibrillation** occurring shortly after symptom onset does not appear to have a large effect on mortality and prognosis, as long as it is quickly and effectively treated. Delayed or secondary ventricular fibrillation during hospitalization is associated with severe ventricular dysfunction and 75% in-hospital mortality.

TABLE 49-12 Indications for Temporary Pacemaker Placement

Temporary transcutaneous pacemaker indications
Unresponsive symptomatic bradycardia
Mobitz II or higher AV blocks
New LBBB and bifascicular blocks
RBBB or LBBB with first-degree block
Some cases with stable bradycardia and new or indeterminate-age RBBB
Temporary transvenous pacemaker indications
Asystole
Unresponsive symptomatic bradycardia
Mobitz II or higher AV blocks
New or indeterminate-age LBBB
Alternating bundle-branch block
RBBB or LBBB with first-degree block
Consider in RBBB with left anterior or posterior hemiblocks
Overdrive pacing in unresponsive ventricular tachycardia
Unresponsive recurrent sinus pauses (>3 s)

Abbreviations: AV = atrioventricular; LBBB = left bundle-branch block; RBBB = right bundle-branch block.

New right bundle-branch block occurs in approximately 2% of AMI patients, most commonly with anteroseptal AMI; it is associated with an increased mortality and complete atrioventricular block. **New left bundle-branch block** occurs in <10% of patients with AMI and is also associated with a higher mortality than in patients without left bundle-branch block. Recognizing STEMI in the presence of left bundle-branch block is difficult,[8] and due to this uncertainty and false catheterization lab activation, new or suspected new left bundle-branch block alone has been removed from the most recent recommendations for emergency perfusion.[5] The left posterior fascicle is larger than the left anterior fascicle. Thus, left posterior hemiblock is associated with a higher mortality than is isolated left anterior hemiblock, because it represents a larger area of infarction. Bifascicular block (right bundle-branch block and a left hemiblock) has an increased likelihood of progression to complete heart block; it represents a large infarction and has more frequent pump failure and greater mortality.[20] See chapter 18, "Cardiac Rhythm Disturbances" for more detail.

HEART FAILURE

Some 15% to 20% of patients with AMI present with some degree of heart failure. One third of these patients have circulatory shock. In AMI, heart failure occurs from diastolic dysfunction alone or a combination of systolic and diastolic dysfunction. Left ventricular diastolic dysfunction leads to pulmonary congestion. Systolic dysfunction is responsible for decreased forward flow, reduced cardiac output, and reduced ejection fraction. In general, the more severe the degree of left ventricular dysfunction, the higher is the mortality. The degree of left ventricular dysfunction in any single patient depends on the net effect of prior myocardial dysfunction (prior myocardial infarction or cardiomyopathy), baseline myocardial hypertrophy, acute myocardial necrosis, and acute reversible myocardial dysfunction ("stunned myocardium"). For further discussion, see chapters 53, "Acute Heart Failure" and 50, "Cardiogenic Shock."

Mortality for patients with AMI increases as cardiac output decreases or pulmonary congestion increases, with mortality rates as follows: no heart failure, 10%; mild heart failure, 15% to 20%; frank pulmonary edema, 40%; and cardiogenic shock, 50% to 80%. Elevated levels of B-type natriuretic peptide or pro-B-type natriuretic peptide early in the hospital course portend a worse 30-day outcome.

The presence of shock in AMI results in a complex spiral relationship. Coronary obstruction leads to myocardial ischemia, which impairs myocardial contractility and ventricular outflow. The resulting reduction in arterial blood pressure leads to further decreases in coronary arterial perfusion, resulting in worsening myocardial ischemia and more severe myocardial necrosis. Interruption of this downward spiral requires careful attention to fluid management and the use of inotropic agents. Resolution of ischemia and preventing or minimizing the area of stunned myocardium that progresses to infarction are imperative; guidelines recommend that patients with STEMI and cardiogenic shock who are <75 years of age should be considered for PCI.[5] For further discussion, see chapters 50 and 53.

MECHANICAL COMPLICATIONS

Sudden decompensation of previously stable patients should raise concern for the mechanical complications of AMI. These complications usually involve the tearing or rupture of **infarcted** tissue, not seen in unstable angina. The clinical presentation of these entities depends on the site of rupture (papillary muscles, interventricular septum, or ventricular free wall).

Ventricular free wall rupture occurs in 10% of AMI fatalities, usually 1 to 5 days after infarction. Rupture of the left ventricular free wall usually leads to pericardial tamponade and death (in >90% of cases). Patients may complain of tearing pain or sudden onset of severe pain. They will be hypotensive and tachycardic and may have onset of confusion and agitation. Increased neck veins, decreased heart sounds, and pulsus paradoxus may be present. In the ED, echocardiography is the diagnostic test of choice. Near equalization of right atrial, right ventricular mid-diastolic, and right ventricular systolic pressures on pulmonary artery catheterization is also useful but seldom available in the ED. Treatment is surgical.

Rupture of the interventricular septum is more often detected clinically than rupture of the ventricular free wall. The size of the defect determines the degree of left-to-right shunt and the ultimate prognosis. Clinically, interventricular septal rupture presents with chest pain, dyspnea, and sudden appearance of a new holosystolic murmur. The murmur is usually accompanied by a palpable thrill and is heard best at the lower left sternal border. Doppler echocardiography is the diagnostic procedure of choice. Demonstration of left-to-right shunt by pulmonary catheter blood sampling may be useful. An O_2 step-up of >10% from right atrial to right ventricular samples is diagnostic. Rupture of the interventricular septum is more common in patients with anterior wall myocardial infarction and patients with extensive (three-vessel) coronary artery disease. Treatment is surgical.

Papillary muscle rupture occurs in approximately 1% of patients with AMI, is more common with inferior myocardial infarction, and usually occurs 3 to 5 days after AMI. In contrast to rupture of the interventricular septum, papillary muscle rupture often occurs with a small- to modest-sized AMI. Patients present with acute onset of dyspnea, increasing heart failure and pulmonary edema, and a new holosystolic murmur consistent with mitral regurgitation. The posteromedial papillary muscle is most commonly ruptured, because it receives blood supply from one coronary artery, usually the right coronary artery. Echocardiography often can distinguish rupture of a portion of the papillary muscle from other etiologies of mitral regurgitation. Treatment is surgical.[5,6]

PERICARDITIS

In the era of PCI intervention, early post-AMI pericarditis occurs in less than 5% of patients,[62] a drop from 20% since the 1980s. It is more common in patients with transmural AMI and delayed initial presentations. Pericarditis results from inflammation adjacent on the epicardial surface of a transmural infarction, often 2 to 4 days after AMI. Pericardial friction rubs are detected more often with inferior wall and right ventricular infarction, because the right ventricle lies immediately beneath the chest wall. The pain of pericarditis can be confused with that of infarct extension or post-AMI angina. Classically, the discomfort of pericarditis becomes worse with a deep inspiration and may be relieved by sitting forward.

Echocardiography may demonstrate a pericardial effusion, but pericardial effusions are much more common than pericarditis and often are present in the absence of pericarditis. Similarly, pericarditis can be present in the absence of a pericardial effusion. The resorption rate of post-AMI pericardial effusions is slow, often taking several months. Treatment is symptomatic with aspirin, 650 milligrams PO every 4 to 6 hours, or colchicine, 0.6 mg twice daily. Ibuprofen is not recommended because it interferes with the antiplatelet effect of aspirin and can cause myocardial scar thinning and infarct expansion. **Dressler's syndrome** (late post-AMI syndrome) occurs 2 to 10 weeks after AMI and presents with chest pain, fever, and pleuropericarditis. Dressler's syndrome is treated with aspirin and colchicine.[63]

RIGHT VENTRICULAR INFARCTION

Isolated right ventricular infarction is extremely rare and is usually seen as a complication of an inferior infarction. The right ventricle most commonly receives its blood supply from the right coronary artery. In patients with left dominant systems, the blood supply may come from the left circumflex. The anterior portion of the right ventricle is supplied by branches of the left anterior diagonal artery. Approximately 30% of inferior wall myocardial infarction involves the right ventricle. The presence of right ventricular infarction is associated with a significant increase in mortality and cardiovascular complications. Right ventricular infarction can be diagnosed by the presence of ST-segment elevation in the precordial V_4R lead in the setting of an inferior wall myocardial infarction (Figure 49-4). The presence of elevated neck veins or hypotension in response to nitroglycerin is also suggestive. Echocardiography or nuclear imaging can be diagnostic, but they are less readily available in the ED.

The most serious complication of right ventricular infarction is shock. The severity of the hemodynamic derangement in the setting of right ventricular infarction is related to the extent of right ventricular dysfunction, the interaction between the ventricles (the right and left ventricles share the interventricular septum), and the interaction between the pericardium and the right ventricle. Right ventricular infarction results in a reduction in right ventricular end-systolic pressure, left ventricular end-diastolic size, cardiac output, and aortic pressure as the right ventricle becomes more of a passive conduit to blood flow. Left ventricular contraction causes bulging of the interventricular septum into the right ventricle, with resultant ejection of blood into the pulmonary circulation. As a result, right ventricular infarction with concurrent left ventricular infarction has a particularly devastating effect on hemodynamic function. Fluid balance and maintenance of adequate preload are critical in the treatment of right ventricular infarction. Factors that reduce preload (volume depletion, diuretics, and nitrates) or decrease right atrial contraction (atrial infarction and loss of atrioventricular synchrony) and factors that increase right ventricular afterload (left ventricular failure) can lead to significant hemodynamic derangements.

Treatment of right ventricular infarction includes maintenance of preload, reduction of right ventricular afterload, and inotropic support of the ischemic right ventricle, in addition to early reperfusion. Patients with right ventricular infarction should not be treated with drugs, such as nitrates, that reduce preload. **In the setting of right ventricular infarction, nitrates often will reduce cardiac output and produce hypotension.** Instead, patients with marginal preload or hypotension should be treated with volume loading (normal saline). The increased preload will improve right ventricular cardiac output. **If cardiac output is not improved after 1 to 2 L of normal saline, begin inotropic support with dobutamine.**

High-degree heart block is very common in patients with right ventricular infarction. The loss of right atrial contraction can greatly compromise right ventricular cardiac output. Restitution of atrioventricular synchrony is important. Patients who do not attain hemodynamic improvement after placement of a ventricular pacer may still improve with atrioventricular sequential pacing.

When right ventricular infarction is accompanied by left ventricular dysfunction, the use of nitroprusside to reduce afterload or intra-aortic balloon counterpulsation may be of benefit. Reduction in left ventricular afterload may help passive movement of blood through the right ventricle.

OTHER COMPLICATIONS

Other complications of AMI that occur but are not usually seen in the ED include left ventricular thrombus formation, arterial embolization, venous thrombosis, pulmonary embolism, postinfarction angina, and infarct extension. With the more rapid discharge of uncomplicated AMI patients, keep these possibilities in mind for patients who return to the ED shortly after hospital discharge.

RECURRENT OR REFRACTORY ISCHEMIA

Patients unresponsive to medical management with continued ischemia require an individualized approach to treatment. Depending on the infarct distribution and coronary anatomy, decisions could be made regarding continued medical management, rescue angioplasty, or coronary artery bypass grafting. Refractory ischemia is investigated with coronary catheterization. Treat patients with ACS after stent placement with antithrombin and antiplatelet therapy, and these patients may require urgent coronary catheterization.

In situations where emergent catheterization is not available or the patient is hemodynamically unstable, an **intra-aortic balloon pump** may be used. Intra-aortic balloon counterpulsation delivers phased pulsations synchronized to the electrocardiograph, so that balloon inflation will occur at the time of aortic valve closure and deflation occurs just before onset of systole. The augmented coronary perfusion pressure during diastole enhances coronary blood flow. Balloon deflation during systole allows the left ventricle to eject blood against a lower resistance. The net effect of intra-aortic balloon counterpulsation is an increase in cardiac output, reduction in systolic arterial pressure, increase in diastolic arterial pressure, little change in mean arterial pressure, and reduction in heart rate. The reduction in left ventricular afterload leads to reduced myocardial O_2 consumption, thereby decreasing the amount of myocardial ischemia. Intra-aortic balloon counterpulsation is recommended for patients with ACS who are refractory to aggressive medical management or are hemodynamically unstable as a means to bridge a patient's stability en route to definitive treatment.

SPECIAL POPULATIONS

POSTPROCEDURE CHEST PAIN

Patients who present with symptoms of an ACS shortly after PCIs, such as angioplasty or stent placement, should be assumed to have had abrupt vessel closure, until proven otherwise. Subacute thrombotic occlusion after stent placement occurs in approximately 4% of patients 2 to 14 days postprocedure. **Bare metal stents are more likely to restenose in the short term. Drug-eluting stents are more likely to present with late stent thrombosis after cessation of daily clopidogrel, 9 to 12 months later.** Treat patients aggressively for an ACS, and obtain emergent cardiology consultation. Patients with chest pain syndromes after coronary artery bypass grafting also may have abrupt vessel closure. However, symptoms of recurrent ischemia can be confused with post-AMI pericarditis, as discussed above.

COCAINE- AND AMPHETAMINE-INDUCED ACUTE CORONARY SYNDROME

AMI occurs in approximately 6% of patients who present to the ED with chest pain after cocaine use. Cocaine-associated myocardial infarction occurs in younger patients, but over the past two decades, the average age has increased from 38 years[64] to 50 years,[65] highlighting the increased use of cocaine in middle-age patients. The initial evaluation of the patient with suspected cocaine-associated myocardial infarction should begin as recommended in the "History and Associated Symptoms" and "Physical Examination" sections of this chapter. The sensitivity, specificity, positive predictive value, and negative predictive value of the ECG to identify cocaine-associated MI are 36%, 89.9%, 17.9%, and 95.8%, respectively.[66] Cardiac troponin is the most sensitive biomarker for cocaine-associated myocardial infarction. Aspirin, nitrates, and benzodiazepines are the mainstays of therapy for initial stabilization; β-blockers are contraindicated in the first 24 hours.[66] Patients with cocaine-associated STEMI are best managed with PCI.[66] Antithrombotic and antiplatelet therapy may be given according to current guidelines for non–cocaine-related ACS.

There are fewer cases of amphetamine-induced MI to guide therapy and no care guidelines. The initial ECG may be unreliable in the setting of methamphetamine-related ACS, with false-positive ST-segment elevation prompting unneeded thrombolytic therapy. In one case series of 33 patients admitted for chest pain who were methamphetamine positive, nine (25%) were diagnosed with ACS (positive markers or required revascularization). Three patients (8%) (two ACS and one non-ACS) suffered cardiac complications (ventricular fibrillation, ventricular tachycardia, and supraventricular tachycardia, respectively). Only one patient had Q-wave myocardial infarction treated with PCI. Medical management was the mainstay of therapy.

ACUTE MEDICAL DISORDERS ASSOCIATED WITH ACUTE CORONARY SYNDROME

Those with GI bleeding,[67] stroke,[68,69] and severe infection have a higher frequency of ACS[70]; even those with disorders considered otherwise benign, such as acute anxiety or emotional upset, have a higher frequency of MI.[71] In the case of stroke and GI bleeding, the primary disease process (which came first) is sometimes unclear or underdiagnosed until late in the patient's course. In a group of patients admitted to the intensive care unit for GI bleeding, approximately 13% sustained MI; however, this did not affect mortality in this intensive care unit population. A case-control study found increased risk of death in patients with GI bleeding meeting criteria for myocardial infarction when compared with those with negative markers (33% vs 8%).[67] In general, treatment of the GI bleed takes priority, which precludes the major treatments for AMI. **For patients with acute ischemic stroke, 17% have positive troponin assessment, which is associated with 3.2 relative risk of death compared with patients with normal troponin.** The risk of stroke complicating the course of AMI has been formerly reported as 2.4% to 3.5%,[72] but with improved treatments for AMI, the risk has dropped to 0.6% to 1.8%. Hospital mortality in patients with stroke after AMI is high (17% to 27%). ECG abnormalities are common in patients with subarachnoid hemorrhage, and elevated troponin levels occur in 28%, with over half of these demonstrating transient left ventricular dysfunction. However, simultaneous STEMI is not common with a subarachnoid hemorrhage. Approximately 50% of patients with severe sepsis and septic shock have impairment of left ventricular systolic function, frequently with an elevated troponin level.[71] AMI occurs in 5.3% of patients hospitalized with community-acquired pneumonia, with the risk increasing to 15% in those with severe pneumonia.[73]

For all patients with dual or multiple acute medical issues, individualize management and weigh the risks of AMI guideline therapies. When indicated, use PCI over thrombolysis to identify the lesion and need for additional therapy.

AFTER HOURS AND WEEKEND PRESENTATIONS

The management of patients with ACS is time sensitive and intensive. Patients who present "after hours" and on weekends wait longer for interventions, and this has an adverse impact on outcome. Patients who present when the ED is busy with other ill patients (e.g., trauma patients) or in settings with increased health system dysfunction and high levels of ED boarding, as well as patients who are not expeditiously transferred to an inpatient bed, have worse outcomes.[74-76] Systems solutions to improve hospital flow for patients with ACS will help optimize the care of patients with ACSs.

REFERENCES

The complete reference list is available online at www.TintinalliEM.com.

CHAPTER 50

Cardiogenic Shock

Casey Glass
David Manthey

INTRODUCTION AND EPIDEMIOLOGY

Cardiogenic shock is an acute state of decreased cardiac output resulting in inadequate tissue perfusion despite adequate circulating volume. Cardiogenic shock is the leading cause of in-hospital death in patients with acute myocardial infarction (AMI).[1] The true incidence of cardiogenic shock is unknown because many patients die before arrival and escape estimates. Cardiogenic shock is seen in 4% to 8% of patients with ST-segment elevation myocardial infarction (STEMI).[2,3] The incidence is declining in part as a result of the increased use of percutaneous intervention for AMI.[3-6] Cardiogenic shock occurs less frequently (2.5%) in those with non–ST-segment elevation myocardial infarction (NSTEMI) compared with those with STEMI.[7,8] Only ~10% of AMI patients who will develop cardiogenic shock have it at ED presentation, with the median time of onset after arrival being approximately 6 hours.[2,9] This underscores the therapeutic opportunity that exists by thwarting ongoing myocardial ischemia.

During the past decade, a strategy of early revascularization by percutaneous coronary intervention or coronary artery bypass surgery improved survival of cardiogenic shock patients with acute ischemia compared to medical therapy alone.[3,10-12] Despite these advances, the mortality remains high (~50%), with half of the deaths occurring within the first 48 hours after presentation.[3,13-15] **Early recognition of cardiogenic shock or ongoing myocardial ischemia is the key for emergency physicians. Prompt and successful efforts to restore perfusion optimize patient outcomes.**

The more risk factors that are present (**Table 50-1**), the greater is the amount of vulnerable myocardium and the greater is the likelihood of cardiogenic shock.

PATHOPHYSIOLOGY

The most common cause of cardiogenic shock is extensive myocardial infarction that depresses myocardial contractility. Additional causes are listed in **Table 50-2**. Regardless of the precipitating cause, cardiogenic shock is primarily "pump failure," which results in reduced cardiac output. The systolic blood pressure drops due to poor cardiac output, and vital organ perfusion is limited. Absent a rise in systemic vascular resistance, the diastolic blood pressure also drops, resulting in coronary artery hypoperfusion. This creates a cycle of worsening myocardial ischemia and pump dysfunction, and eventual decompensation.

Historically, many believed cardiogenic shock was associated with a reflex compensatory vasoconstriction that would increase systemic vascular resistance. Contemporary data refute this belief, showing the average systemic vascular resistance was not elevated in cardiogenic shock patients, even with vasopressor use.[16] Furthermore, the average left ventricular ejection fraction (EF) was only moderately depressed (~30%),[17] and diastolic dysfunction was seen early and frequently, and was associated with greater depression of EF and an increased need for mechanical support.[18,19]

A systemic inflammatory response syndrome occurs after AMI and in cardiogenic shock, due to complement system activation and release of systemic inflammatory mediators, including cytokines and inducible nitric oxide synthase.[20,21] The inflammatory response also depresses pump function, dilates the peripheral vasculature, and increases the risk of death.[22] However, targeting nitric oxide with tilarginine does not alter mortality, although it improves blood pressure.[23] The monoclonal c5 antibody pexelizumab has been studied as an adjunct to percutaneous intervention in an effort to blunt the activation of the complement cascade associated with infarction. The largest trial of pexelizumab failed to show a mortality benefit compared to placebo.[24]

Resolution of severe ischemia, neurohormonal, and inflammatory abnormalities may explain the reversible nature of cardiogenic shock in some patients. The wide variations in EF, ventricular size, and vascular resistance suggest that the pathophysiology of cardiogenic shock is diverse and poorly understood.

TABLE 50-1 Risk Factors for Cardiogenic Shock

Elderly
Female
Acute or prior ischemic event associated with the following:
Impaired ejection fraction
Extensive infarct (evidence of large myocellular leak)
Proximal left anterior descending coronary artery occlusion
Anterior myocardial infarction
Multivessel coronary artery disease
Prior medical history:
Previous myocardial infarction
Congestive heart failure
Diabetes

TABLE 50-2 Causes of Cardiogenic Shock

Mechanical complications:
Acute mitral regurgitation secondary to papillary muscle dysfunction or chordal rupture
Ventricular septal defect
Free wall rupture
Right ventricular infarction
Acute aortic insufficiency (aortic dissection)
Severe depression of cardiac contractility:
Acute myocardial infarction
Sepsis
Myocarditis
Myocardial contusion
Cardiomyopathy
Medication toxicity (e.g., β-blocker overdose, calcium channel blocker overdose)
Unstable dysrhythmia
Mechanical obstruction to forward blood flow:
Aortic stenosis
Hypertrophic cardiomyopathy
Mitral stenosis
Left atrial myxoma
Pericardial tamponade

CLINICAL FEATURES

HISTORY

History can be difficult to obtain if the patient is severely ill. EMS personnel, family, or the medical record may offer additional historical information, notably of existing ischemic heart disease. Patients commonly complain of shortness of breath, chest pain, or weakness. Through history, try to exclude other causes of shock, such as sepsis, massive pulmonary embolism, hemorrhage, or a viral prodrome suggesting myocarditis. Ask about a history of preexisting valvular disease, recent illnesses, hypercoagulable states, substance abuse, or other risk factors for cardiogenic shock as outlined in Table 50-1. Assess for other causes of shock because treatment differs depending on the cause of cardiovascular system failure (**Table 50-3**).

TABLE 50-3 Cardiogenic Shock: A Limited Differential Diagnosis

Acute pulmonary decompensation:
Chronic obstructive pulmonary disease exacerbation
Cor pulmonale
Massive pulmonary embolism
Distributive shock:
Sepsis
Anaphylaxis
Neurogenic shock (spinal cord injury)
Hypovolemic shock:
Hemorrhage
Severe dehydration
Dissociative shock:
Toxins/drugs of abuse (cyanide)

PHYSICAL EXAMINATION

Cardiogenic shock is characterized by hypoperfusion; this is not always accompanied by hypotension.[9] Systolic blood pressure is usually <90 mm Hg, although it can be higher with preexisting hypertension. A pulse pressure <20 mm Hg is another finding if systemic resistance has not plummeted, and sinus tachycardia is common unless the patient is on medications that block a tachycardic response. Unless the patient has advanced to the stage of respiratory fatigue or agonal respirations, tachypnea is common. The lung examination demonstrates rales due to the presence of pulmonary edema, except in cases of isolated right-sided failure. Jugular venous distention and a positive hepatojugular reflex are usually present. Patients are usually pale or cyanotic and may have cool skin and mottled extremities or other signs of hypoperfusion. Peripheral edema suggests preexisting heart failure. Diaphoresis indicates activation of the sympathetic nervous system. Cerebral hypoperfusion may result in altered mental status, and renal hypoperfusion may decrease urine output.

If the cardiac point of maximal impulse is normally located, shock is likely due to an acute event. If the point of maximal impulse is laterally shifted and diffuse from cardiac remodeling and enlargement, long-standing cardiac disease with acute decompensation can be presumed. **About 10% of cardiogenic shock after AMI is caused by mechanical complications.**[14] A new murmur may be the only physical exam finding of mechanical catastrophe; carefully seek any loud or new systolic murmurs. **Acute mitral regurgitation** can occur from chordae tendineae rupture or papillary muscle dysfunction, accompanied by a soft holosystolic murmur at the apex radiating to the axilla with rales. With papillary muscle dysfunction, the murmur starts with the first heart sound but terminates before the second. An **acute ventral septal defect** is associated with a new loud holosystolic left parasternal murmur, often with a palpable thrill, that decreases in intensity as the intraventricular pressures equalize. **Acute aortic insufficiency** is characterized by a soft diastolic murmur and a softer S_1 sound.

DIAGNOSIS

Clinical signs of cardiogenic shock include evidence of poor cardiac output with tissue hypoperfusion (hypotension, mental status changes, cool mottled skin) and evidence of volume overload (dyspnea, rales, jugular venous distention). Hemodynamic criteria for cardiogenic shock include (1) sustained hypotension (systolic blood pressure <90 mm Hg), (2) reduced cardiac index (<2.2 L/min/m^2), and (3) an elevated (>18 mm Hg) pulmonary artery occlusion pressure. The causes and differential diagnosis of cardiogenic shock are listed in Tables 50-2 and 50-3.

LABORATORY TESTING

There are no laboratory markers specific for the diagnosis of cardiogenic shock. Cardiac biomarkers (primarily troponin) may not be elevated upon initial presentation from an acute myocardial ischemic triggering event, but will eventually elevate. A CBC excludes anemia, which can contribute to cardiac ischemia. The clinical presentation guides the need for specific drug levels (e.g., digoxin, ethanol, or illicit drugs). Hypoperfusion commonly results in an elevated serum lactate, so checking serum lactate may aid diagnosis when overt hypotension is absent. Serum electrolytes and renal and hepatic studies can identify end-organ dysfunction.

The level of **serum B-type natriuretic peptide (BNP)** is an indicator of left ventricular dysfunction. Because of its high negative predictive value, a normal BNP level (<100 picograms/mL) eliminates cardiogenic shock as the cause of hypoperfusion unless very early after onset or with isolated right heart failure. Conversely, an elevated BNP does not diagnose cardiogenic shock.[25,26]

Although elevated inflammatory markers such as C-reactive protein have some prognostic value, these are rarely needed in the acute phase of care.[27] Arterial blood gas measurements help identify those at risk of carbon dioxide retention, quantify the presence and severity of acidosis, and determine the contribution of metabolic or respiratory components to acidosis.

IMAGING AND ANCILLARY STUDIES

Electrocardiogram The ECG helps detect ischemia or STEMI, evaluates for rhythm abnormalities, and provides evidence of electrolytic abnormalities (e.g., hypokalemia) or drug toxicity (e.g., digoxin).

It is important to assess for right ventricle (RV) involvement whenever ischemia is considered because RV infarction is associated with an increased risk for cardiogenic shock and death.[28] **RV infarction is best evaluated by obtaining right-sided ECG leads (usually V_4R and V_5R) (Figure 50-1).** RV infarction complicating inferior myocardial infarction is detected by ST elevation in lead V_1 with depression in V_2.

Chest Radiography Obtain a portable chest radiograph in all patients. Chest x-ray typically shows pulmonary congestion or edema, alveolar infiltrates, and pleural effusion. These findings may lag by hours, so their absence does not exclude cardiogenic shock. Another confounder to interpreting the chest radiograph is underlying preexisting cardiopulmonary disease; pulmonary edema is difficult to detect on chest radiography in patients with severe chronic obstructive lung disease or interstitial lung disease. Cardiomegaly is the end result of long-standing myocardial remodeling, and its presence may not explain the acute symptoms. The chest radiograph can suggest alternative or confounding diagnoses, such as pneumonia, pneumothorax, aortic dissection, or progressive pericardial effusion (globular cardiac shape).

Bedside Echocardiography In the setting of cardiogenic shock, emergency bedside echocardiography can help exclude alternative etiologies of shock, identify some mechanical complications, and guide therapy. Assessment should include evaluation of the inferior vena cava (IVC) to determine volume status and estimate right atrial pressure. A subcostal four-chamber view is helpful to visualize pericardial effusion and identify cardiac tamponade. When tamponade is present, there is a pericardial effusion with associated dilation of the IVC and diastolic collapse of the RV with systolic collapse of the right atrium. When cardiac rupture has occurred, there may be a visible clot in the pericardial space. Subcostal, parasternal, and apical views together can help estimate EF and cardiac contractility. An aortic root measurement greater than 3 cm is concerning for ascending aortic dissection, especially when associated with a pericardial effusion. Also assess mitral valve morphology and motion. Apical four-chamber views are helpful for evaluating chamber size. In cases of acute right heart failure due to ischemia, the RV will be dilated and the left ventricle (LV) will appear to be smaller than expected due to low filling pressures. In left heart failure there will be dilation of the LV secondary to decreased cardiac output and increased filling pressure.

Bedside echocardiography is not a substitute for emergent formal transthoracic echocardiography. Formal echocardiography is better able to use color and spectral Doppler to identify mechanical complications and to characterize the nature of cardiac impairment. Echocardiography can detect regional wall motion abnormalities and identify a lack of compensatory hyperkinesis in uninvolved cardiac segments. Loss of RV contractility, RV dilatation, and normal estimated pulmonary pressures occur more commonly with RV infarction.

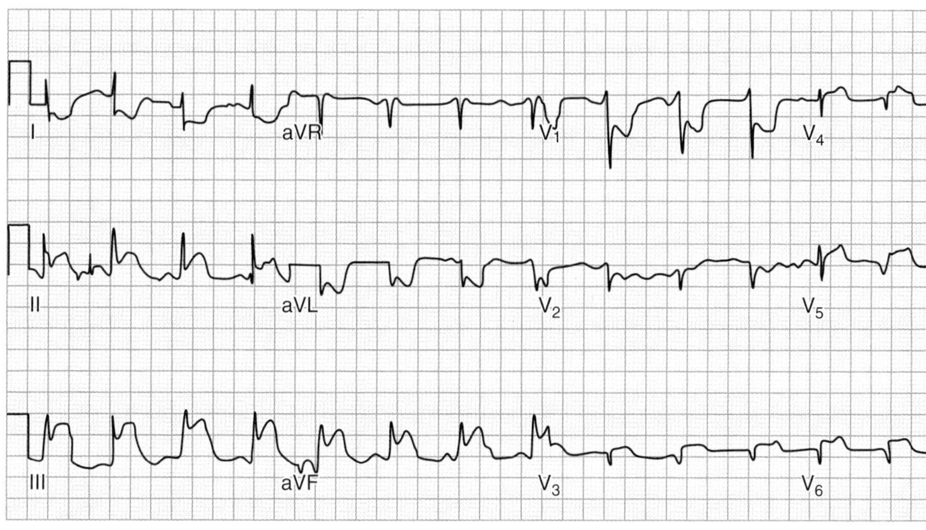

FIGURE 50-1. Right-sided leads demonstrating right ventricular infarction associated with inferior wall myocardial infarction. Right sided leads have replaced the normal left-sided V leads. In this example, the ST-segment elevation is prominent in leads VR_{3-6}.

Color flow Doppler transthoracic echocardiography can identify mechanical causes of cardiogenic shock, such as acute mitral regurgitation or ventricular septal defect. Echocardiography can detect other causes of decreased cardiac output, notably pulmonary embolism. Acute RV dilatation, tricuspid insufficiency, paradoxical systolic septal motion, and high estimated pulmonary artery and RV pressures suggest pulmonary hypertension from an acute pulmonary embolus.

Mechanical Catastrophe Diagnosis If mechanical catastrophe is suspected, consult cardiothoracic surgery immediately while obtaining a bedside echocardiogram. In the case of **myocardial free wall rupture**, death is probable unless a pseudoaneurysm forms. Pseudoaneurysm is detected as an acute pericardial effusion on echocardiography. An acute **ventricular septal defect** is confirmed by color Doppler echocardiography or right heart catheterization demonstrating oxygen saturation step-up from the right atrium to the RV. **Acute mitral regurgitation**, from papillary muscle rupture or dysfunction, can complicate AMI.

Hemodynamic Monitoring Patients in cardiogenic shock typically have low cardiac index (<2.2 L/min/m^2) and elevated LV end-diastolic pressure (pulmonary artery occlusion pressure >18 mm Hg).[29] Invasive hemodynamic monitoring with a pulmonary artery catheter can provide data and guide treatment but is unavailable in most EDs.[29] Central venous pressure measurements can help guide fluid resuscitation, with the trend in venous pressures being more important than absolute values. Most patients will require continuous blood pressure monitoring, often with an indwelling catheter.

TREATMENT

The most important intervention for ischemic-related cardiogenic shock is emergent revascularization.[10,11,14,30] **ED stabilization is a temporizing measure while arranging for definitive therapy such as revascularization in the cardiac catheterization laboratory or surgical intervention for mechanical catastrophe.** In the prehospital setting, EMS should direct any suspected cardiogenic shock patient to a facility that has 24-hour emergency cardiac revascularization capability (i.e., cardiac bypass team).[31]

Initial management focuses on airway stability and improving myocardial pump function to maintain end-organ perfusion. Diagnosis, therapy, and arrangements for definitive cardiac care must proceed simultaneously.

AIRWAY

Give supplemental oxygen, and monitor closely for impending or acute respiratory failure that will require immediate mechanical ventilation. Continuous positive airway pressure or bilevel positive airway pressure can provide temporary airway support, but these methods require a hemodynamically stable, cooperative patient—a set of conditions rare in those with cardiogenic shock.

Endotracheal intubation is often necessary to maintain oxygenation and ventilation. However, **the change to positive pressure ventilation may further decrease preload and cardiac output and worsen hypotension.** Be prepared to administer a fluid bolus in the absence of pulmonary congestion, initiate an appropriate inotrope if congested with a compensated blood pressure, or start a vasopressor if hypotension exists.

STABILIZATION

Cardiac monitoring and IV access are necessary. Correct any hypoxemia, hypovolemia, rhythm disturbances, electrolyte abnormalities, and acid-base alterations rapidly. Place a urinary drainage catheter to monitor urine output in response to therapy.

In AMI, give aspirin early (if not already taking long term) unless there is an absolute contraindication.[32] If blood pressure is >90 mm Hg systolic, chest pain may be relieved by careful use of IV nitroglycerin or morphine. **Do not use β-blockers in patients with myocardial infarction in cardiogenic shock or who are at risk for cardiogenic shock** (Table 50-1).[32] Withhold angiotensin-converting enzyme inhibitors or other vasodilators.

HYPOTENSION

Initial therapy is guided by clinical findings. Give crystalloid fluid boluses (250 to 500 cc) for an RV infarct with hypotension, if pulmonary congestion is absent. If there is no improvement with the fluid bolus or if pulmonary congestion develops, vasopressors or inotropes are indicated (**Table 50-4**).

TABLE 50-4 Inotropic Medications Used in Cardiogenic Shock

Drug	Dose	Comments
Dobutamine	2–5 micrograms/kg/min, titrated up to 20 micrograms/kg/min	Inotrope and potential vasodilator; lowers blood pressure; give as individual agent as long as systolic blood pressure (SBP) ≥90. Can use with dopamine.
Dopamine	3–5 micrograms/kg/min, titrated up to 20–50 micrograms/kg/min as needed	Inotrope and vasoconstrictor; increases left ventricular end-diastolic pressure and causes tachycardia. Can use with dobutamine.
Norepinephrine	2 micrograms/min, titrate to response	Vasoconstrictor and inotrope; preferred as a single agent over dobutamine if SBP <70. Can use combined with dobutamine.
Epinephrine	0.1–0.5 micrograms/kg/min	Inotrope and vasoconstrictor; second-tier choice because it causes acidosis and dysrhythmias.
Milrinone	0.5 micrograms/kg/min	Inotrope and vasodilator; lowers blood pressure. Second tier to dobutamine.

Inotropes do not change outcome alone but can temporize while ED personnel arrange interventions to restore coronary artery perfusion and LV function.[33] In the absence of profound hypotension, **dobutamine** is a mainstay of initial pharmacologic treatment. Dobutamine may increase cardiac contractility and should be considered as an individual agent if systolic blood pressure is ≥90 mm Hg without signs of overt shock or organ dysfunction. Avoid the use of dobutamine alone when the systolic blood pressure is <90 mm Hg because of its vasodilatory potential. Often, a vasoconstrictor is needed in addition to dobutamine. **Dopamine** may increase cardiac work by increasing heart rate and may also increase LV end-diastolic pressure by its β-agonist effect. Combination therapy with a vasopressor (dopamine) and an inotrope (dobutamine) may be more effective than either agent alone. **Norepinephrine** when combined with dobutamine may have more of an effect on peripheral vasoconstriction than dopamine when combined with dobutamine. If the systolic blood pressure is <70 mm Hg, norepinephrine is preferred over dobutamine due to its antithrombotic effect.[34] If shock persists despite use of these agents, an intra-aortic balloon pump is typically placed, although long-term evidence of benefit is lacking.[25,35-39]

Epinephrine is an alternative to norepinephrine/dobutamine when dobutamine is not available; however, it is associated with increased systemic acidosis, tachycardia, and dysrhythmias compared to the combination of norepinephrine and dobutamine.[40]

Patients on β-blocker therapy may have an attenuated response to dobutamine, making norepinephrine a better choice. **Milrinone** (a selective phosphodiesterase inhibitor) **can be substituted for the catecholamine if dobutamine is ineffective.**

Pure vasoconstrictors and α_1-adrenergic receptor agonists, such as phenylephrine, are contraindicated because they increase cardiac afterload without augmenting cardiac contractility.

EARLY REVASCULARIZATION

In ischemic cardiogenic shock, early revascularization by percutaneous coronary intervention or coronary artery bypass grafting is the treatment of choice. The greatest short-term benefit is reported in patients <75 years old, those without previous myocardial infarction, and those treated within 6 hours of symptom onset. However, patients >75 years old who receive revascularization have improved survival over those >75 years old who have delayed or no revascularization, even though those >75 years old are less likely to receive revascularization.[41] Coronary artery bypass grafting requires extensive surgical and medical resources and poses operative risk for seriously ill patients. The cardiac surgeon will make an overall judgment, with operative intervention chosen often for those with good prior functional status and less severe, early presentation of shock. Survival is higher in those receiving early revascularization compared with medical stabilization, even when elderly.[41] Current guidelines do not have an age cutoff for percutaneous coronary intervention.[27,38,39,42]

THROMBOLYTIC THERAPY

Emergency coronary intervention in the catheterization laboratory or operating suite is the preferred definitive treatment for cardiogenic shock.[43,44] Thrombolytic therapy is not as effective in establishing reperfusion in AMI with cardiogenic shock as it is in uncomplicated AMI. Survival from cardiogenic shock is highest with emergency coronary intervention, followed by intra-aortic balloon pump combined with thrombolytic therapy; thrombolytic therapy alone is least effective in reducing mortality. Rescue percutaneous coronary intervention does not convey the same mortality benefit as primary percutaneous coronary intervention for these patients.[45] If no other definitive treatment modalities for cardiogenic shock are available, if the hospital does not have a catheterization laboratory, or if there is prolonged transport time for coronary intervention, thrombolytic therapy should be given to reduce mortality compared to supportive treatment alone.

INTRA-AORTIC BALLOON PUMP COUNTERPULSATION

Intra-aortic balloon pump counterpulsation provides hemodynamic support by decreasing afterload (which lowers myocardial oxygen consumption) and increasing diastolic blood pressure (which augments coronary perfusion).[38,42] Intra-aortic balloon pump improves survival after thrombolytic therapy by augmenting diastolic perfusion pressure and unloading the LV.[11,46,47] Outside of those receiving reperfusion, the long-term benefits of intra-aortic balloon pump use are not clear.[36,37]

Resolution of hemodynamic instability with intra-aortic balloon pump support has positive prognostic value.[48] In hospitals without direct angioplasty capability, stabilization with intra-aortic balloon pump and thrombolysis followed by transfer to a tertiary care facility may be the best management option.[38,42]

PERCUTANEOUS LEFT VENTRICULAR ASSIST DEVICES

If cardiogenic shock persists despite revascularization and maximal medical therapy, a left ventricular assist device may augment cardiac output. This device is currently approved by the U.S. Food and Drug Administration only as a bridge to transplantation, and most cardiogenic shock patients are not such candidates. Case studies have described successful support and weaning of patients suffering from cardiogenic shock in the setting of acute infarction.[49-53] A recent meta-analysis failed to demonstrate a mortality benefit for left ventricular assist devices compared with intra-aortic balloon pumps in patients with cardiogenic shock refractory to inotropic and vasopressor support.[54]

EXTRACORPOREAL MEMBRANE OXYGENATION

Extracorporeal membrane oxygenation can provide almost total circulatory support for a failing heart. Extracorporeal membrane oxygenation is typically instituted in emergency situations when maximum medical therapy has failed. The treating physician must consider the likelihood of recovery before instituting extracorporeal membrane oxygenation; patients with a very poor prognosis are not appropriate for extracorporeal membrane oxygenation. In the best cases, extracorporeal membrane oxygenation can provide support until percutaneous coronary intervention can be performed or until the heart begins to recover after intervention. In other cases, it can provide a "bridge to decision" for transplant or permanent left ventricular assist device placement.

DISPOSITION AND FOLLOW-UP

All patients with cardiogenic shock require admission to the intensive care unit at an institution with invasive revascularization capability.[10,30] In noncapable institutions, transfer should be accomplished as quickly as possible.[55,56] If no other definitive treatment modalities for cardiogenic shock are available, if the hospital does not have a catheterization laboratory, or if there is prolonged transport time for coronary intervention, thrombolytic therapy should be given.

SPECIAL CONSIDERATIONS

Compliance with guidelines for AMI has improved over the last two decades, although compliance in patients with cardiogenic shock may be less.[3,57,58] Some populations continue to face barriers to effective care, especially the elderly and minorities.[58,59] Compliance with recommended guidelines is needed in order to improve outcomes. The most recent American College of Cardiology/American Heart Association guidelines from 2011 recommend aggressive management of patients in cardiogenic shock. Class 1 recommendations include percutaneous coronary intervention or coronary artery bypass graft for STEMI patients in shock (level of evidence B), percutaneous coronary intervention or coronary artery bypass graft for NSTEMI patients in shock (level of evidence B), and transfer for rescue or facilitated percutaneous coronary intervention in patients with persistent ischemia or shock despite lytic therapy (level of evidence B). European guidelines reflect the same treatment priorities.[60]

Acknowledgment: We thank Jim Edward Weber and W. Frank Peacock for their contributions to the prior edition of this chapter.

REFERENCES

The complete reference list is available online at www.TintinalliEM.com.

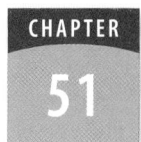

Low-Probability Acute Coronary Syndrome

Kathleen A. Hosmer
Chadwick D. Miller

INTRODUCTION AND EPIDEMIOLOGY

This chapter discusses the features of *low-probability or possible acute coronary syndrome (ACS)*, which includes patients who have chest pain or another equivalent ischemic symptom but no objective evidence of acute coronary ischemia or infarction—that is, no characteristic ECG ST-segment elevation or depression and normal levels of cardiac markers. Patients with diagnostic ECG or cardiac marker levels or with other high-risk features are discussed in chapter 49, "Acute Coronary Syndromes."

Of ED patients with undifferentiated chest pain, 7% will have ECG findings consistent with acute ischemia or infarction, and 6% to 10% of those in whom cardiac markers are ordered will have initially positive results.[1] The remaining patients who do not have diagnostic ECG changes or initially positive cardiac marker results have *low-probability* or *possible ACS*. The evaluation of those with possible or actual ACS costs approximately $10 billion to $12 billion each year in the United States.[2]

Of all patients with *possible ACS*, 5% to 15% ultimately prove to have ACS.[3] The rate of discharge from the ED for patients with ACS remains approximately 4%. Patients with ACS who are discharged home from the ED have worse clinical outcomes and higher mortality compared with patients who are initially hospitalized. The clinical data readily available to the emergency physician, such as historical features, examination findings, and ECG results, cannot exclude ACS among most patients, because 3% to 6% of patients thought to have noncardiac chest pain or a clear-cut alternative diagnosis will have a short-term adverse cardiac event.[4,5] Therefore, most patients with *possible ACS* undergo further observation and testing.

PATHOPHYSIOLOGY

ACS is a constellation of signs and symptoms resulting from an imbalance of myocardial oxygen supply and demand. There are three general ACS classifications: unstable angina, non–ST-segment elevation myocardial infarction (NSTEMI), and ST-segment elevation myocardial infarction (STEMI). Unstable angina is a type of ACS with no elevation of biomarkers and no pathologic ST-segment elevation, resulting in ischemia but not infarction. Acute myocardial infarction (AMI) occurs when myocardial tissue is devoid of oxygen and substrate for a sufficient period of time to cause myocyte death. NSTEMI is characterized by biomarker elevation and no pathologic ST-segment elevation. STEMI is characterized by ST-segment elevation and biomarker elevation (STEMI), although biomarker elevation is not required at onset to make this diagnosis. Detailed discussion is in chapter 49.

The distinction between NSTEMI and unstable angina is based on elevated cardiac markers of necrosis in the case of NSTEMI. Troponin I and troponin T are the most specific cardiac markers of cell injury or death available. These biomarkers may not reach detectable thresholds for up to 6 hours after infarction. Patients presenting soon after infarction may have normal biomarker results and initially be categorized as having *possible ACS*. Patients with evolving myocardial infarctions represent approximately 4% of patients undergoing serial cardiac markers and generally have other high-risk features of ACS such as ST-segment depression.[6,7]

CLINICAL FEATURES

HISTORY AND COMORBIDITIES

The history is one tool to help assess patients with suspected or possible ACS but cannot be used to exclude ACS. Obtain detailed information, including symptom quality, location, duration, severity, associated symptoms, precipitating and relieving factors, and similarity to prior episodes. Consider other noncardiac but life-threatening causes of chest pain (see Tables 48-3 and 48-4 in chapter "Chest Pain").

Among patients with possible ACS, historical features can be categorized as low risk, probable low risk, probable high risk, and high risk. **However, even patients with low-risk features or in a low-risk category have a residual risk of ACS.**[8] Lowest risk features include pleuritic, positional, reproducible, or sharp/stabbing pain. Another low-risk feature is pain that is not exertional or located in a small inframammary area. Higher risk features include chest pressure (positive likelihood ratio [LR+] 1.3), pain similar to or worse than prior cardiac pain (LR+ 1.8), and associated nausea/vomiting or diaphoresis (LR+ 1.9 and 2.0, respectively). The highest risk features include radiation to the right arm or shoulder (LR+ 4.7), left arm (LR+ 2.3), or both arms or shoulders (LR+ 4.1), and exertional chest pain (LR+ 2.4).

Traditional cardiac risk factors, such as hypertension, diabetes mellitus, tobacco use, family history of coronary artery disease (CAD) at an early age, and hypercholesterolemia, are modestly predictive of the presence of CAD in asymptomatic patients. In acute decision making, **cardiac risk factors are poor predictors of cardiac risk for myocardial infarction or other ACS.**[9] CAD is rare in patients <30 years old, but possible and usually accompanied by other risk(s).

Although a true alternative diagnosis decreases the likelihood of ACS, many patients with ACS are mistakenly diagnosed with gastric reflux or musculoskeletal pain.[5] Clinical response to treatment with antacids (18% to 45% of ACS patients have relief of pain with antacids), viscous lidocaine, or nonsteroidal anti-inflammatory medications cannot exclude ACS. Lack of pain relief with nitroglycerin is similarly unreliable, because 65% of patients with an ACS in one study failed to have relief of pain.

Prior cardiac testing (previous ECG tracings, echocardiograms, cardiac catheterization reports, and stress testing reports) aids the ED evaluation. ECG changes offer strong bedside evidence of new disease. Recent cardiac catheterization reports are especially useful, because a truly negative (defined as no luminal irregularities) result is associated with a very low incidence of subsequent infarction or ACS in the next 2 years. Although a prior positive stress test increases the likelihood of a subsequent acute cardiac event,[10] a prior negative stress test provides little reassurance that a current chest pain event is benign. Patients with a recent negative evaluation for ACS that included objective cardiac testing (mostly stress testing) have a 6-month incidence of ACS as high as 14%. Furthermore, patients with a prior negative stress test have a similar incidence of ACS compared with those with no prior stress testing when presenting with chest pain to the ED.[11] Overall, previous stress test results add evidence but cannot confirm disease presence or absence.

PHYSICAL EXAMINATION

Usually, the exam in the low-risk or possible ACS patient seeks complications or alternative causes of the symptoms. When an alternate diagnosis is not clear, the physical examination alone cannot distinguish between those with and without ACS. However, pay special attention to examination findings that make ACS more or less likely. High-risk features on physical examination are uncommon and include signs of cardiac failure such as hypotension, diaphoresis, pulmonary rales, jugular venous distention, new mitral regurgitation, bradycardia, tachycardia, and an S_3 cardiac gallop.[12] Cardiac rate abnormalities are also a high-risk feature, including either bradycardia (seen with ischemia, especially in the inferior myocardium, or infarction that has led to disturbance of the conduction system) or tachycardia (may signify pump failure, pain, or stress, or could be a clue to an alternative diagnosis such as pulmonary embolism). Positional changes in the pain severity can be easily assessed at the bedside and may suggest pericarditis or another pleural-based syndrome as a cause of pain.

CARDINAL FEATURES

The classic patient with possible ACS has chest pain or another symptom (weakness, dyspnea, other upper body pain), no clear alternative

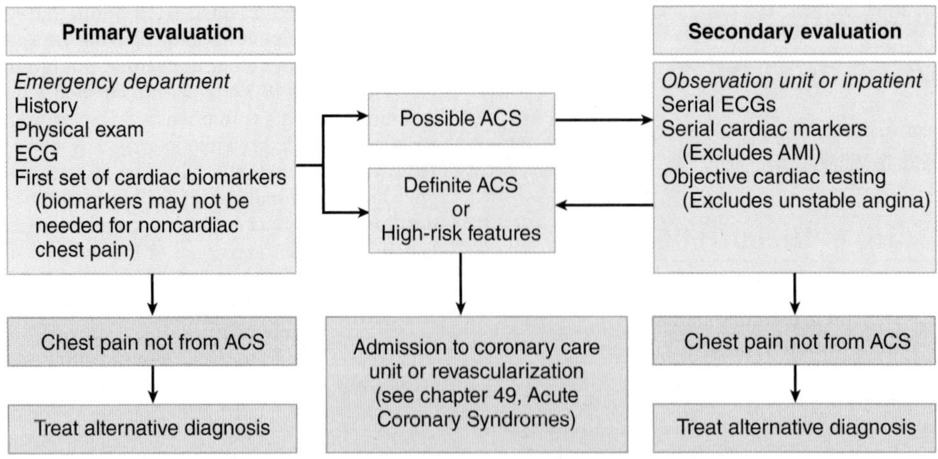

FIGURE 51-1. Evaluation process for patients with possible acute coronary syndrome (ACS). AMI = acute myocardial infarction

cause, and no clear evidence of cardiac injury or stress on ECG and biomarker tests. **In this group, the likelihood of ACS is >2% but still low, making the diagnosis of *possible ACS*.**

DIAGNOSIS

The diagnostic process is conceptually split into a primary and secondary evaluation (**Figure 51-1**).

PRIMARY EVALUATION

The goal during the primary evaluation is to distinguish patients with definite ACS from those with possible ACS and those with symptoms that are definitely not from ACS. This process involves gathering information from the history, physical examination, ECG, chest radiography, and medical record. This information is used to produce an initial risk assessment that guides the subsequent laboratory testing and initial treatment.

ECG

For adult patients with chest pain in whom cardiac causes are possible, obtain a 12-lead ECG rapidly[12,13] and compare to any previous tracings. Patients with ST-segment elevation, a new left bundle-branch block, or ST-segment depression have an ACS and are treated as outlined in chapter 49. Between 1% and 6% of patients with a normal ECG will ultimately prove to have NSTEMI, and at least another 4% will prove to have unstable angina.[12] Obtaining follow-up ECG(s) in patients with ongoing or worsening symptoms helps detect changes diagnostic of ACS, or it can show reversal of previous ST-segment or T-wave changes thought to be old—both define *dynamic changes* and the high likelihood of ACS. In the setting of dynamic ECG changes, incidence of CAD is 84% with classic anginal symptoms and 8% with nonclassic anginal symptoms as assessed by coronary angiography.[14]

CHEST RADIOGRAPH

Chest radiography provides additional cardiovascular information, including cardiac silhouette size, pulmonary edema, and aortic contour. Additional causes of chest pain, such as pneumothorax, bony metastasis, rib fracture, and pneumonia, may also be detected on chest radiography. Patients presenting with anterior chest pain have findings on chest radiography that influence management 14% of the time.

RISK ASSESSMENT

The goal of early decision making is to determine if the patient actually belongs in the *possible ACS* cohort and is at high enough risk to warrant cardiac testing. All available data are used to create a composite picture for decision making. **Some posit that when the pretest probability of ACS is ≤2%, further testing is not indicated[15]; others have suggested a threshold of <1% to stop testing.[16] Detecting patients with a zero chance of any ACS in the presence of ACS-like symptoms is virtually impossible.**

Most computer algorithms, risk scores, and clinical decision rules have been unsuccessful at identifying a very-low-risk (<2%) cohort that does not require further testing. The HEART score is one tool that identifies low-risk patients who are eligible for evaluation and possible early discharge home from the ED (**Table 51-1**). Large-scale validation data are lacking, although current evidence suggests that patients with a

TABLE 51-1 The HEART Score

	Points
History	
Highly suspicious	2
Moderately suspicious	1
Slightly suspicious	0
ECG	
Significant ST-segment depression	2
Nonspecific repolarization abnormality	1
Normal	0
Age	
≥65	2
45–65	1
≤45	0
Risk factors[a]	
3 or more risk factors	2
1–2 risk factors	1
No risk factors	0
Troponin	
≥3 × normal limit	2
1–3 × normal limit	1
≤ normal limit	0
Total	

Low risk = 0–3, high risk ≥4.

[a]Risk factors include currently treated diabetes mellitus, current or recent (<90 days) smoker, diagnosed and/or treated hypertension, diagnosed hypercholesterolemia, family history of coronary artery disease, obesity (body mass index >30), or a history of significant atherosclerosis (coronary revascularization, myocardial infarction, stroke, or peripheral arterial disease).

TABLE 51-2 Thrombolysis in Acute Myocardial Infarction Score

Age ≥65 years?
≥3 Risk factors for coronary artery disease (CAD)?*
Known CAD (stenosis ≥50%)?
Aspirin use in last 7 d?
Severe angina (≥2 episodes in last 24 h)?
ST changes ≥0.5 mm?
Positive cardiac marker?

Calculate total score giving 1 point for each positive answer.

*Risk factors for CAD include diabetes, cigarette smoking, hypertension (≥140/90 mm Hg or on antihypertensive medication), low high-density lipoprotein cholesterol (<40 mg/dL), family history of premature CAD (CAD in male first-degree relative age <55, or female first-degree relative <65).

HEART score of 0 to 3 have a 1% to 2% risk for major adverse cardiac events within 6 weeks of presentation.[17,18]

The Heart Pathway involves using the HEART score with the addition of a 4- to 6-hour repeat troponin to increase the sensitivity for major adverse cardiac events.[19] Preliminary data note 100% sensitivity for major adverse cardiac events while decreasing the amount of index visit cardiac testing (CT or stress imaging).

The Accelerated Diagnostic Protocol uses Thrombolysis in Acute Myocardial Infarction (TIMI) study[20] risk scores and ED testing to stratify risk (**Table 51-2**). Patients with ACS-consistent pain, a Thrombolysis in Acute Myocardial Infarction score of 0, no new ischemic changes on ECG, and negative troponins at 0 and 2 hours have a very low risk of subsequent cardiac events and may be discharged. In a prospective observational study, the Accelerated Diagnostic Protocol was 99.7% sensitive (95% confidence interval [CI] 98.1% to 99.9%) for major adverse cardiac events at 30 days.[21] A subsequent randomized trial demonstrated that 19.3% of patients were discharged within 6 hours using the Accelerated Diagnostic Protocol compared to 11.0% of control group patients (P = 0.008), and 1.9% (95% CI 0% to 10%) of patients had a major adverse cardiac event in 30 days.[22] This method also needs wider impact testing to determine safety and utility before mainstream implementation.

When risk-stratifying patients with possible ACS, be wary of overconfidence in an alternative diagnosis, because the rate of ACS is as high as 4% among patients with chest pain and a "clear-cut" noncardiac alternative diagnosis.[5] Reserve determinations of noncardiac chest pain to patients with a very low likelihood of coronary disease (<1%) and clear evidence of an alternative diagnosis or with atypical historical features. The rest of patients with ACS-consistent symptoms should have further testing.

After determination that the patient is appropriately categorized as possible ACS, further stratification occurs (**Table 51-3**).[12,13,23] Patients in category I (AMI) and category II (probable acute ischemia) are discussed in chapter 49. Patients in category III (possible ischemia) and IV (probably not ischemia or stable angina pectoris) undergo primary and secondary assessments as detailed below.

CARDIAC MARKERS

Laboratory testing during the primary evaluation focuses on two goals: detecting myocardial cellular necrosis and excluding alternative causes of chest pain. Usual testing includes a CBC, serum electrolytes with renal function, and serum cardiac markers. Other testing is guided by the history and physical examination.

Serum markers of necrosis are used to diagnose AMI. AMI is one component of ACS, which also includes unstable angina. The difference between these two clinical syndromes is the presence of myocardial necrosis. **Thus, although serum markers performed over a period of time can exclude AMI, they cannot exclude unstable angina.**

See chapter 48, "Chest Pain" for an introduction to the use of cardiac markers for the diagnosis of myocardial infarction. In that chapter, Figure 48-1 shows the typical pattern of serum marker elevation after AMI; Table 51-5 lists conditions associated with elevation of troponin; and Table 51-6 lists conditions that elevate CK-MB, the isoform of the MB fraction of creatine kinase. The unique release kinetics of each marker should be evaluated in the context of the patient's time of symptom onset, compared with the time of presentation. **Patients with positive troponin results *have* ACS.**

Other markers such as C-reactive protein, ischemia-modified albumin, myeloperoxidase, and B-type natriuretic peptide are not robust enough for incorporation into standard ED decision making.

Single-Marker Measurement Although single-sample normal myocardial marker measurements cannot exclude the diagnosis of AMI in the ED, very-low-risk (Table 51-3) patients may benefit from at least one myocardial marker measurement before discharge, especially if pain is present and unremitting for >6 hours. This area is evolving with the introduction of higher sensitivity troponin assays.

Change in Marker Measurements In AMI, the initial CK-MB measurement obtained is elevated in about 30% to 50% of patients. Seeking a change in values, referred to as the *delta CK-MB* (ΔCK-MB), helps detect ACS even if threshold positive values are not reached.[24] ΔCK-MB

TABLE 51-3 Prognosis-Based Classification System for ED Chest Pain Patients*

I.	**Acute myocardial infarction: immediate revascularization candidate**
II.	**Probable acute ischemia: high risk for adverse events (any of the following):**
	Evidence of clinical instability (i.e., pulmonary edema, hypotension, arrhythmia, transient mitral regurgitation murmur, diaphoresis)
	Ongoing pain thought to be ischemic (consider chest pain or discomfort as chief symptom, reproducing documented angina, or pain in setting of known coronary artery disease, including myocardial infarction)
	Pain at rest associated with ischemic ECG changes (consider new, or presumably new, transient, ST-segment deviation, 1 mm or greater, or T-wave inversion in multiple precordial leads)
	One or more positive myocardial marker measurements
	Positive perfusion imaging study
III.	**Possible acute ischemia: intermediate risk for adverse events. History suggestive of ischemia with absence of high-risk features, and any of the following:**
	Rest pain, now resolved
	New onset of pain
	Crescendo pattern of pain
	Ischemic pattern on ECG not associated with pain (may include ST-segment depression <1 mm or T-wave inversion >1 mm)
IV.	**Possible acute ischemia: low risk for adverse events. Requires all of the following:**
	History not strongly suggestive of ischemia
	ECG normal, unchanged from previous, or nonspecific changes
	Negative myocardial marker measurement
	or (requires all of the following)
	>2 wk of unchanged symptom pattern or long-standing symptoms with only mild change in exertional pain threshold
	ECG normal, unchanged from previous, or nonspecific changes
	Negative initial myocardial marker measurement
V.	**Definitely not ischemia: very low risk for adverse events. Requires all of the following:**
	Clear objective evidence of nonischemic symptom etiology
	ECG normal, unchanged from previous, or nonspecific changes
	Negative initial myocardial marker measurement†
	or
	Unstructured clinician estimate of acute coronary syndrome ≤2%

*Authors' analyses from multiple sources.[12,13,23]

†Literature not conclusive.

also outperforms Δ myoglobin for early AMI diagnosis. The same principle can be applied with serial measurements of troponin.

SECONDARY EVALUATION

RISK REASSESSMENT

Patient risk is reevaluated as results from diagnostic tests become available. At the beginning of the secondary evaluation, review the results of the initial and any subsequent ECGs and cardiac markers, chest radiography, and previous cardiac evaluations. After data collection, stratify patients into one of five classifications (Table 51-3).

THE DIAGNOSTIC PLAN

Base the diagnostic plan for patients with possible ACS after the primary evaluation on the clinical data and the available resources at each facility. This may include inpatient secondary testing, hospital-based observation testing, or ED-based observation testing. Once ACS is determined to be present or likely, admission and care by an internist or cardiologist are started.

Serial Marker Approach Patients with possible ACS require serial serum markers to detect necrosis. The purpose of serial markers is twofold. First, evidence of myocardial necrosis confirms the diagnosis of ACS and should change treatment. Second, the presence of necrosis places the patient at higher risk for an adverse event during provocative cardiac testing. Most facilities use a traditional protocol for serial marker timing, whereas some use an accelerated testing protocol in concert with early myocardial imaging. Traditional testing protocols for patients with possible ACS involve obtaining serial troponin and/or serial creatine kinase and CK-MB at presentation and after 6 hours of observation. Accelerated protocols may have similar efficacy. ΔCK-MB measurements over a 2-hour period have 93% sensitivity for AMI.[24] Similarly, changes in myoglobin over 90 minutes when used with troponin results may also have high sensitivity.[25] However, given the imperfect sensitivity and inability to exclude unstable angina, accelerated cardiac marker protocols are not the sole determination to exclude ACS but are used in combination with cardiac imaging.

INDICATIONS FOR ADVANCED CARDIAC TESTING

Normal serial ECGs and myocardial marker measurements reduce the likelihood of AMI but do not exclude unstable angina, which still puts the patient at high risk for a subsequent adverse cardiac event. Therefore, patients with possible ACS should undergo some form of direct cardiac testing to evaluate coronary anatomy, cardiac function, or both. Common modalities used include stress electrocardiography, stress echocardiography, resting and/or stress nuclear medicine testing, stress cardiac MRI, and CT coronary angiography (CTCA).

Advanced cardiac testing is performed after normal biomarkers are present and no clear ischemic ECG changes exist; this happens either as an inpatient or during an observation unit stay, with the latter being less expensive. Another option proffered by the American College of Cardiology/American Heart Association guidelines is to do the advanced testing as an outpatient and within 72 hours of ED discharge if patients are at low risk for ACS, are pain free without recurrent symptoms, have no evidence of ischemia on their ECG, and have normal serial cardiac markers over 6 to 8 hours.[12] This latter approach simply uses the ED stay as the observational interval.

Available data suggest that low-risk patients may safely undergo immediate stress testing. One center performed over 3000 immediate exercise stress tests in low-risk patients who had at least one negative serum cardiac marker, noting no adverse events.[26]

CARDIAC TESTING MODALITIES

ECG-Based Exercise Treadmill Testing The accuracy of ED stress testing is particularly difficult to quantify, because test sensitivity and specificity are greatly influenced by characteristics of the population

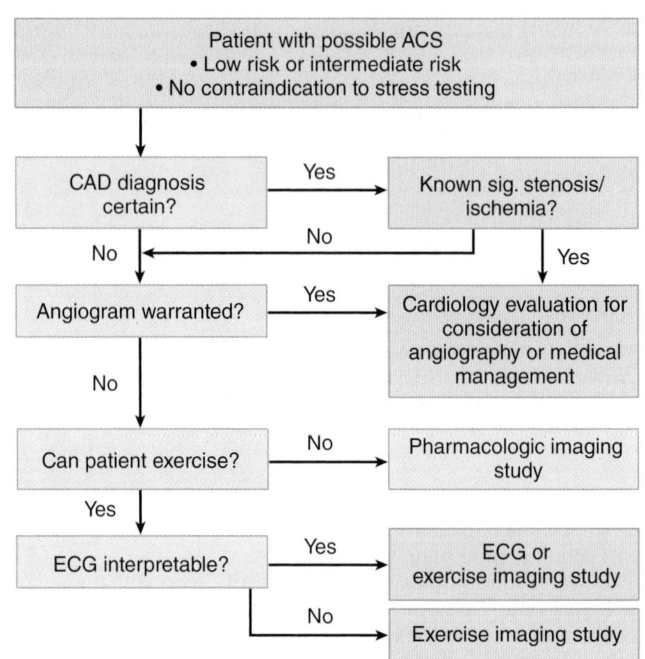

FIGURE 51-2. Stress testing decision making for patients with possible acute coronary syndrome (ACS). CAD = coronary artery disease; sig = significant.

being tested. As the pretest probability of CAD increases, the likelihood of a false-negative test also increases. Conversely, when a population with a very low pretest probability of disease is tested, the likelihood of a false-positive result increases. **Based on current data, diagnostic stress testing is recommended for patients with a low to moderate pretest probability of CAD but is unlikely to be helpful in those at very low risk or at high risk.** Guidelines to assist with stress test selection are summarized in **Figure 51-2.**[27]

ECG-based exercise treadmill testing is commonly used for patients without known coronary disease who are placed in an observation unit. Subjects exercise, most commonly on a treadmill, until a predetermined percentage of predicted maximum heart rate or other end points are reached. The most commonly used definition of a positive exercise test result from an ECG standpoint is ≥1 mm of horizontal or downsloping ST-segment depression or elevation for at least 60 to 80 milliseconds after the end of the QRS complex; ST-segment elevation is not sought because it defines acute ischemia.

Sensitivity of exercise treadmill testing depends on the risk and severity of disease of the patient population to which it is applied. Meta-analysis of 24,000 patient encounters notes that the sensitivity and specificity for significant coronary disease are 68% and 77%, respectively.[27] Advantages of exercise treadmill testing are low cost, wide availability, and short test performance time. Exercise stress testing is contraindicated for various reasons (**Table 51-4**).[27] Exercise testing may not be safe for patients at high risk for acute ischemia or those with other uncontrolled cardiovascular or pulmonary pathologies. Furthermore, patients with an abnormal baseline ECG, such as those with left ventricular hypertrophy, bundle-branch block, or digoxin effect, are less likely to benefit from standard exercise testing due to difficulties in interpretation of exercise-induced ECG changes.

Echocardiography Echocardiography to evaluate wall motion at rest and while under stress (either exercise or pharmacologically induced) is widely used in patients with possible ACS. Advantages of stress echocardiography over exercise treadmill testing are improved accuracy for coronary disease and nondependence on the ECG. Compared with other cardiac imaging techniques, echocardiography is noninvasive, delivers no ionizing radiation, and provides information on myocardial function.

Detection of wall-thickening abnormalities defines acute ischemia; this is dependent on imaging technique and interpretative skills, with

TABLE 51-4 Contraindications to Exercise Testing

Absolute
Acute myocardial infarction (within 2 d)
High-risk unstable angina
Uncontrolled cardiac dysrhythmias causing symptoms or hemodynamic compromise
Symptomatic severe aortic stenosis
Uncontrolled symptomatic heart failure
Acute pulmonary embolus or pulmonary infarction
Acute myocarditis or pericarditis
Acute aortic dissection
Relative*
Left main coronary stenosis
Moderate stenotic valvular heart disease
Electrolyte abnormalities
Severe arterial hypertension (>200 mm Hg systolic, >110 mm Hg diastolic)
Tachydysrhythmias or bradydysrhythmias
Hypertrophic cardiomyopathy and other forms of outflow tract obstruction
Mental or physical impairment leading to inability to exercise adequately
High-degree atrioventricular block

*Relative contraindications can be superseded if the benefits of exercise outweigh the risks.

up to 10% of tests being technically inadequate. The echocardiogram cannot distinguish between myocardial ischemia and acute infarction, cannot reliably detect subendocardial ischemia, and may be falsely interpreted as positive in the presence of several conditions (notably conduction disturbances, volume overload, heart surgery, or trauma). Timing of the test relative to the onset of symptoms is critical, because transient wall motion abnormalities may resolve within minutes of an ischemic episode. Resting echocardiography within 12 hours of ED arrival does not provide additional predictive value for myocardial infarction over myocardial markers alone. **Thus, a normal resting echocardiogram in the ED cannot exclude ACS, although it lowers the likelihood.**

Stress echocardiography combines a standard ECG stress test with cardiac imaging at rest and after exercise or pharmacologically induced tachycardia. Overall, stress echocardiography is 80% sensitive and 84% specific for significant coronary disease, superior to ECG-based stress testing. In low-risk ED patients, three studies have reported negative predictive values for subsequent cardiac events to be 97% to 100%, comparable to that of stress testing using nuclear imaging techniques.

Nuclear Medicine Nuclear medicine techniques use an IV-injected radioactive tracer. Local myocardial uptake and images depend on regional coronary flow and myocardial cell integrity. Tracer uptake occurs in direct proportion to regional myocardial blood flow.

Thallium-201 has been in use longest and is rapidly redistributed after initial uptake. The image generated after thallium injection represents blood flow at the moment of imaging. Areas of positive uptake reflect adequate coronary flow and viable myocardium, whereas areas without uptake represent infarcted or ischemic myocardium. On repeat imaging several hours later, continued lack of perfusion ("irreversible defect") indicates an area of infarction, and tracer uptake only on delayed images ("reversible defect") represents ischemic but not infarcted myocardium. Combined with conventional ECG-based stress testing, thallium imaging offers improved sensitivity and specificity for detection of significant CAD over ECG-based testing alone, and it is not hampered by baseline ECG abnormalities. Thallium-based imaging must be performed soon after injection, making it impractical for use in patients with ongoing chest pain. Also, the long half-life requires a lower injected dose to avoid excessive radiation exposure. This may impair imaging and create false-negative and false-positive results, especially in women and obese patients. Due to these limitations and the lack of ED-based outcome studies, thallium-201 imaging alone is not an ideal agent for use in the ED.

Myocardial perfusion imaging using technetium-99m (^{99m}Tc)-labeled agents such as **sestamibi** offers advantages over thallium for ED use. Because the half-life of ^{99m}Tc is much shorter than that of thallium (6 vs 73 hours), a larger dose is possible without harm to the patient. This produces superior image quality, decreased tissue attenuation–related artifacts, and higher ACS detection specificity for sestamibi imaging. In contrast to thallium, ^{99m}Tc is stable for several hours, allowing accurate imaging up to 3 hours after injection; the image represents the blood flow at the moment of injection. By using "gated" image acquisition technology, sestamibi scanning also estimates ejection fraction. As with thallium, resting and stress (exercise or pharmacologic) images can be compared to yield additional data.

Perfusion sestamibi imaging of patients *with current or recent* (within 30 minutes of injection) *pain* and no cardiac ischemia on ECG and biomarker analysis is very sensitive in detecting physiologic ischemia; a negative test would allow discharge to home. This latter approach requires broader study but is promising in select patients.

Dual-isotope stress testing using thallium and sestamibi is an increasingly common component of ED ACS evaluation protocols. In this technique, a resting thallium scan is first performed. Patients without resting defects can then immediately undergo stress testing with sestamibi imaging, thereby avoiding the delay usually required for isotope "washout" in single-isotope techniques. Dual-isotope stress testing in one trial reliably identified or excluded ACS.

Cardiac MRI Cardiac MRI assesses wall motion, perfusion, and coronary anatomy, either at rest or after pharmacologic stress. It is noninvasive and does not expose the patients to radiation. However, cardiac MRI cannot be performed on approximately 11% of ED patients with chest pain due to contraindications such as claustrophobia and implanted metallic objects. Another limit is the longer test performance time, although this is improving with newer scanners and software. Cardiac magnetic resonance stress imaging has excellent test performance but currently is not a common tool for early ACS evaluation.

CT Coronary Angiography CTCA allows gated images of the coronary arteries after rapid, peripheral (not central) IV contrast. Images are improved when the heart rate is <65 beats/min in 16-slice CT scanners, sometimes necessitating β-blocking medications; dual-source scanners (128-slice) can image adequately at higher heart rates but are less available. The advantages of CTCA are ready access to necessary equipment, rapid image acquisition, and the ability to image coronary structure. Notable disadvantages include ionizing radiation exposure, IV contrast exposure (and risk of allergy or kidney injury), need for specially trained technicians, and nondiagnostic scans due to nonvisualization of coronary segments. Additionally, CTCA provides a limited assessment of cardiac function. CTCA-detected lesions of >50% stenosis correlate with lesions on standard left-heart angiography; this means the test offers limited information in those with known coronary disease. Patients with positive scans require confirmation either with a cardiac catheterization or a functional advanced cardiac test.

Two recent clinical trials evaluated the usefulness of CTCA in decreasing ED length of stay and assessing for serious cardiac events within 30 days of discharge.[28,29] Both studies included patients with low to intermediate risk for ACS and considered CTCA results of <50% stenosis as negative. These trials found that patients randomized to CTCA versus traditional care had a higher rate of discharge from the ED and a decreased overall length of stay. No significant coronary disease was missed on CTCA evaluation versus traditional stress testing, although one study found that patients with positive CTCA findings had more overall testing and increased radiation exposure. The cost of care was similar for both groups of patients. Overall, these studies provide evidence that CTCA allows for faster and safe discharge of patients from the ED.[28,29]

CTCA findings also have a strong correlation with 1-year prognosis as demonstrated in a meta-analysis that included 18 studies with 9592 patients. Researchers evaluated for major adverse cardiac events, including death, myocardial infarction, and need for revascularization. The overall event rate for patients with positive CTCA (>50% stenosis of any vessel) versus normal CTCA was 8.8% versus 0.17% per year, thus demonstrating that major adverse events in patients with negative CTCA imaging are rare.[30]

While ED CTCA helps deliver a prompt, safe disposition of patients in the ED, up to 24% of patients will have nondiagnostic CTCA imaging.[2] The ideal approach to these patients is undefined and usually reverts to the previous strategies for evaluating low-risk ACS patients.

DIAGNOSTIC PATHWAYS FOR PATIENTS WITH POSSIBLE ACUTE CORONARY SYNDROME

INPATIENT ADMISSION

In settings without an observation unit, all patients with low or higher risk of ACS are admitted to an inpatient bed. Specific destinations and care level are driven by stratification; those with a prior history of CAD, evidence of congestive heart failure on physical examination, recurrent chest pain, or new or presumed new ischemic ECG changes are at higher short-term risk and may be more appropriately managed in an intermediate-care (step-down) unit.

ED OBSERVATION AND TESTING

ED observation unit management decreases hospital admissions, length of stay, and hospital cost while providing a high level of care. The traditional observation unit chest pain protocol was refined by Lateef and colleagues,[32] with patients observed for 9 hours with continuous 12-lead ST-segment ECG monitoring and serial CK-MB testing at 0, 3, 6, and 9 hours after presentation. Those who completed a negative 9-hour evaluation subsequently underwent echocardiography followed by graded exercise stress testing in the ED before discharge. With this approach, 82.1% of patients were released home from the cardiac evaluation unit. The approach of **serial cardiac markers followed by objective cardiac testing remains the foundation of ED and other observation unit protocols**. Although early observation unit protocols focused on low-risk patients, more recent investigations successfully studied patients with intermediate-risk chest pain.

Figure 51-3 describes alternative approaches to the observation unit management of patients with possible ACS. For approach 3,[33] patients with intermediate- and low-risk chest pain underwent immediate resting myocardial perfusion imaging and serial cardiac markers. Patients with negative results were discharged for outpatient evaluation and stress testing. At 30 days, no patients with normal perfusion imaging experienced AMI, and 2% required revascularization. Based on this work, immediate perfusion imaging, serial cardiac markers, and outpatient stress testing are diagnostic options for patients with possible ACS.

After identification of patients as having possible ACS, immediate exercise stress testing is a safe option (Approach 4, Figure 51-3).[26] This approach had no stress testing–related adverse outcomes and allowed discharge of approximately two thirds of evaluated patients.[26] Immediate exercise stress testing has also been successfully extended to patients with known coronary disease.

The Erlanger chest pain evaluation protocol[34] (Approach 5, Figure 51-3) incorporates baseline and 2-hour marker determinations along with continuous ST-segment monitoring and serial ECGs. Those with positive results or any increase in markers are admitted for further evaluation.

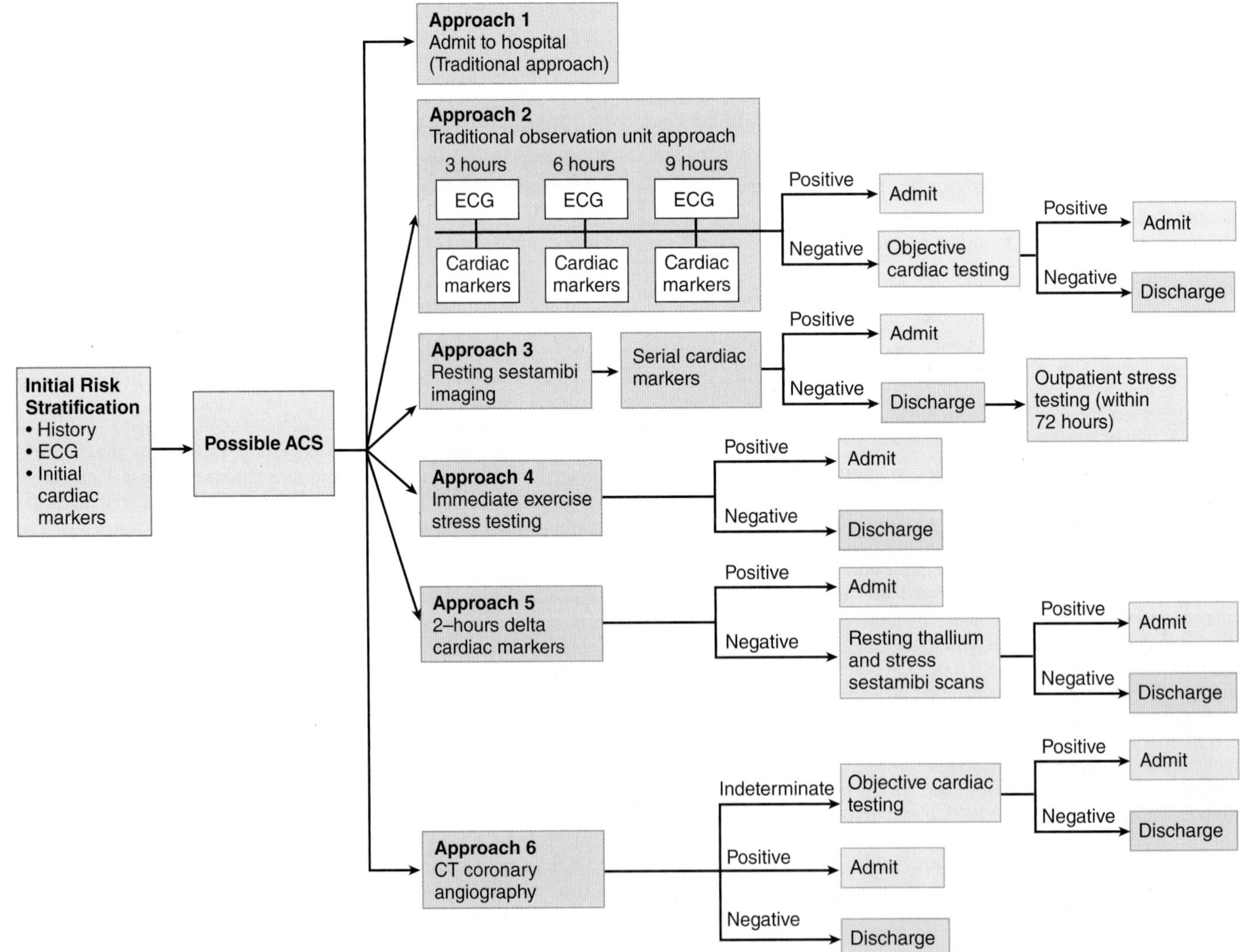

FIGURE 51-3. Pathways for secondary assessment of patients with possible acute coronary syndrome (ACS).

Patients thought to be at very low risk for ACS do not undergo stress testing and are discharged home, whereas those with low-risk chest pain undergo cardiac imaging with resting thallium and stress sestamibi scans. This protocol demonstrated a sensitivity of 99% and specificity of 87% for ACS at 30 days.

Some observation units adequately manage patients at intermediate risk for ACS, whereas some facilities manage these patients in the hospital. Any protocol that treats all patients with possible ACS equally should incorporate serial cardiac markers and stress testing. Second, no data exist to support exclusion of ACS based on cardiac markers without cardiac imaging except possibly in very-low-risk patients. Third, early stress testing after a negative ultra-short cardiac marker testing strategy, or exercise stress testing after one negative cardiac marker in patients with possible ACS, appears safe in low- and intermediate-risk patients. Fourth, outpatient stress testing is an option for low-risk patients in whom AMI has been excluded in reliable patients presenting to a facility where a mechanism exists to arrange this testing. Compliance with follow-up testing is better when scheduled before discharge.[35]

TREATMENT

STANDARD TREATMENT

Clinical trials often do not include patients with possible ACS and instead focus on the higher risk patients with positive cardiac markers or ST-segment changes on their ECG. Therefore, treatment recommendations for patients with possible ACS are derived from reviewing the risk-to-benefit profile suggested from clinical trial results in the higher risk patient populations. Additional information on the mechanisms of action and data from clinical trials are discussed in chapter 49.

Therapy for patients with possible ACS is linked to the patient's stratification level (Table 51-3). In general, patients at low risk of adverse events (Level IV) receive aspirin, anti-ischemic therapy with nitroglycerin, and β-blockers. Patients at intermediate risk (Level III) additionally receive antithrombin therapy and dual antiplatelet therapy (**Table 51-5**).[12]

Contraindications to aspirin include allergy, active bleeding, hemophilia, active retinal bleeding, severe untreated hypertension, an active peptic ulcer, or other serious causes of GI or GU bleeding.[12] Use clopidogrel in patients who are unable to tolerate aspirin due to allergy or GI intolerance.[12]

Very little data are available to support or refute β-blocker use in patients with possible ACS. No evidence suggests superiority of one β-blocker medication over another; however, cardioselective β_1 antagonism is often preferred over the nonselective effects of other agents, making metoprolol, esmolol, and atenolol common choices. β-Blocker medications also offset reflex tachycardia that can be seen with nitrates, and thus, these medications should be administered simultaneously.[12] The first dose of β-blockers can be administered PO or IV, with oral administration preferred and IV administration reserved for patients with hypertension at the time of treatment.[12] Do not use β-blockers with in those with signs of acute heart failure, low cardiac output, heart blocks, active asthma, or reactive airway disease, or in those at risk for cardiogenic shock (age >70 years old, systolic blood pressure <120 mm Hg systolic, sinus tachycardia >110 beats/min).[12]

DISPOSITION AND FOLLOW-UP

ADMISSION AND DISCHARGE CRITERIA

Disposition after the Primary Evaluation After the primary evaluation, if the treating physician estimates that the probability of ACS is <2%, further testing for ACS is not warranted. After exclusion of other life-threatening causes of chest pain, these patients may be discharged home. These patients may benefit from primary care follow-up or care from

TABLE 51-5 Recommended Treatment for Patients with Possible Acute Coronary Syndrome (ACS)

Class	Common Dosing	Common Contraindications (all include known hypersensitivity)
Core Therapy for Patients with Possible ACS		
Oxygen	As needed to keep O_2 saturation >95%	Not applicable
Aspirin	160–325 milligrams PO	Active bleeding; see text for further details
Nitroglycerin	0.4 milligram sublingual or spray	Right ventricular infarction, phosphodiesterase use, hypotension
Morphine sulfate	1–5 milligrams IV	—
β-Blockers (metoprolol, esmolol)	Metoprolol: 25–50 milligrams PO in the first 24 h	Bradycardia, heart block, hypotension, chronic obstructive pulmonary disease, severe left ventricular dysfunction, active reactive airway disease, PR interval >0.24 s, at risk for cardiogenic shock (age >70 y old, systolic blood pressure <120 mm Hg systolic, sinus tachycardia >110 beats/min)
Adjunctive Therapy for Patients at Intermediate Risk for Adverse Events*		
Dual antiplatelet therapy		
Clopidogrel (in addition to aspirin)	300–600 milligrams PO (loading dose)	Active bleeding
Antithrombin therapy		
Unfractionated heparin	60 units/kg IV bolus (maximum bolus 4000 units) 12 units/kg/h IV infusion (maximum infusion 1000 units/h)	Active bleeding, history of heparin-induced thrombocytopenia
Low-molecular-weight heparin	Enoxaparin, 1 milligram/kg SC every 12 h	
Direct thrombin inhibitors	Bivalirudin (only for patients undergoing an initial invasive approach), 0.1 milligram/kg IV bolus, 0.25 milligram/kg/h IV infusion	Active bleeding
Factor Xa inhibitor	Fondaparinux, 2.5 milligrams SC once daily	Active bleeding, creatine clearance <30 mL/min, body weight <50 kg

*See text for discussion; information is the author's interpretation of clinical trial data and guidelines from Anderson JL, Adams CD, Antman EM, et al: ACC/AHA 2007 Guidelines for the Management of Patients with Unstable Angina/Non ST-Elevation Myocardial Infarction. A report of the American College of Cardiology/American Heart Association Task Force on Practice Guidelines (Writing Committee to Revise the 2002 Guidelines for the Management of Patients with Unstable Angina/Non ST-Elevation Myocardial Infarction). *J Am Coll Cardiol* 50: e1, 2007.

another specialty physician depending on the suspected cause (e.g., GI, pulmonary).

Disposition after the Secondary Evaluation Most patients with possible ACS undergo further evaluation to diagnose or exclude ACS. Upon completion of these protocols, those with negative cardiac markers, no dynamic ECG changes, and negative objective cardiac testing can be safely discharged home. Patients with positive cardiac markers, diagnostic ECG changes, or diagnostic testing supporting ACS are admitted to the hospital for cardiac care. Those with nondiagnostic cardiac testing are handled on a case-by-case basis after discussion with a cardiologist.

SUGGESTED FOLLOW-UP INTERVAL

Despite advanced testing, a negative evaluation does not entirely exclude ACS. Patients discharged after exclusion of ACS should be given detailed precautions describing reasons to return to the ED. Ideally, patients should follow up with their primary care physician within the next 2 to 3 days.

SPECIAL POPULATIONS

Age, ethnic, racial, and gender differences are well described in patients presenting with ACSs. Most current knowledge of ACS-related symptoms and risk factors comes from population-based studies. Studies have suggested that women are more likely to present without chest pain and often have a prodrome of fatigue. Similarly, the elderly less often present with a chief complaint of chest pain and, less frequently, have typical chest pain. Other studies have noted delayed presentation for ACS in black women[36] and less frequent chest pain with ACS in those of Asian descent.[37] The Framingham criteria overestimate the risk of coronary disease when applied to Chinese patients,[38] and these patients are less likely to experience classic symptoms of ACS. Be aware of all these confounders as you assess the clinical likelihood of ACS.

COCAINE-ASSOCIATED CHEST PAIN

In a study of 130 patients with cocaine-associated myocardial infarction, the mean age was 38 years. AMI occurs in approximately 6% of patients who present to the ED with chest pain after cocaine use. The initial evaluation of the patient with cocaine-associated chest pain is the same as outlined earlier, using the history, exam, ECG, and cardiac biomarkers as the foundation. The sensitivity, specificity, positive predictive value, and negative predictive value of the ECG to identify cocaine-associated myocardial infarction are 36%, 89.9%, 17.9%, and 95.8%, respectively. Cardiac troponin is the most sensitive biomarker for cocaine-associated myocardial infarction. Aspirin, nitrates, and benzodiazepines are the mainstays of therapy for chest pain; β-blockers are contraindicated. Thrombolysis in Acute Myocardial Infarction scoring has little predictive value in patients with cocaine-associated chest pain,[39] but patients with nondiagnostic initial ECGs can be managed in an observation unit using serial ECGs and biomarkers over 6 to 12 hours. There is no difference in the outcomes of patients managed with or without stress testing. The American Heart Association guideline recommends stress testing as an option for patients with cocaine-associated chest pain absent other higher risk factors or features.[40] In one study, the 1-year rate of myocardial infarction after a negative chest pain observation evaluation for patients with cocaine-associated chest pain was <1%, despite a 66% rate of ongoing cocaine use.[41]

PRACTICE GUIDELINES

The American College of Cardiology and American Heart Association offer guidance for the management of patients with unstable angina and NSTEMI.[12]

REFERENCES

The complete reference list is available online at www.TintinalliEM.com.

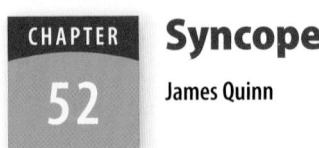

CHAPTER 52 Syncope

James Quinn

INTRODUCTION AND EPIDEMIOLOGY

Syncope or fainting is a symptom complex consisting of a brief loss of consciousness associated with an inability to maintain postural tone that spontaneously resolves without medical intervention. Syncope accounts for approximately 1% to 2% of ED visits each year and up to 6% of hospital admissions.[1-3] In the **Framingham Heart Study**, 7814 patients were followed for 17 years, and 10.5% reported syncope.[4] Syncope in the preceding year is the best predictor of recurrence.[5] It can affect the young and the old, with the elderly having the greatest morbidity.[6] **Near-syncope**, a premonition of fainting without loss of consciousness, shares the same basic pathophysiologic process as syncope and may carry the same risks.[7,8]

PATHOPHYSIOLOGY

The final common pathway of syncope is the same regardless of the underlying cause: about 10 seconds of complete disruption of blood flow or nutrient delivery to both cerebral cortices or to the brainstem reticular activating system, or reduction of cerebral perfusion by 35% to 50%. Most commonly, an inciting event causes a drop in cardiac output, which decreases oxygen and substrate delivery to the brain. Less commonly, vasospasm reduces CNS blood flow. Cerebral perfusion and consciousness are restored by the supine position, the response of autonomic autoregulatory centers, or restoration of a perfusing cardiac rhythm.

The causes of syncope are numerous (**Table 52-1**). The major causes of syncope identified in the Framingham Heart Study were vasovagal (reflex mediated, 21%), cardiac (10%), orthostatic (9%), medication related (7%), neurologic (4%), and unknown (37%).[4] In most studies, even with exhaustive patient evaluation, the cause remains unknown in about 40% of individuals.[9,10] After ED investigation, the unknown proportion may be 50% to 60%. Diagnosis is important, because each diagnostic classification carries with it prognostic risk. In the Framingham study, cardiac syncope doubled the risk of death, neurologic syncope increased the risk of death by 50%, and syncope of unknown cause increased the risk of death by 30%, compared to the general population cohort of the study. Individuals with neurally/reflex-mediated or vasovagal syncope had no increased risk of death compared with the general population cohort.[4]

CLINICAL FEATURES

CARDIAC-RELATED SYNCOPE

Cardiac-related syncope is the most dangerous type and is a risk for sudden death. Because patients with documented cardiac syncope have a 6-month mortality rate that exceeds 10%, timely and thorough evaluation is warranted.[4,10] Well-appearing patients with undiagnosed cardiac disease are the most challenging group. The causes of cardiac syncope are divided into two categories: structural disease and dysrhythmias (**Table 52-1**). In both settings, the heart is unable to provide adequate cardiac output to maintain cerebral perfusion.

Syncope can occur if **structural disease** limits the heart's ability to increase cardiac output to meet demand. Examples of structural cardiac disease associated with syncope include aortic stenosis, hypertrophic cardiomyopathy, pulmonary embolism, and myocardial infarction. **Consider aortic stenosis as a structural cardiac cause of syncope in the elderly.** The classic symptom constellation of aortic stenosis is chest pain, dyspnea on exertion, and syncope. **Hypertrophic cardiomyopathy** is characterized by a stiff noncompliant left ventricle, diastolic dysfunction, and outflow tract obstruction. It is the most common cause

TABLE 52-1 Causes of Syncope

Cardiac*	Neural/Reflex Mediated
Structural cardiopulmonary disease	*Vasovagal*
Valvular heart disease	*Situational*
Aortic stenosis	Cough
Tricuspid stenosis	Micturition
Mitral stenosis	Defecation
Cardiomyopathy	Swallow
Pulmonary hypertension	Neuralgia
Congenital heart disease	*Carotid sinus syndrome*
Myxoma	Other
Pericardial disease	**Orthostatic hypotension** (see text)
Aortic dissection	**Psychiatric**
Pulmonary embolism	**Neurologic**
Myocardial ischemia	Transient ischemic attacks
Myocardial infarction	Subclavian steal
Dysrhythmias	Migraine
Bradydysrhythmias	**Medications (Table 52-2)**
Short or long QT syndromes	**Breath holding** (pediatric)*
Stokes-Adams attack	
Sinus node disease	
Second- or third-degree heart block	
Pacemaker malfunction	
Tachydysrhythmias	
Ventricular tachycardia	
Torsade de pointes	
Supraventricular tachycardia	
Atrial fibrillation or flutter	

*See chapter 131, Seizures and Status Epilepticus in Children, and chapter 165, Seizures and Status Epilepticus in Adults.

of sudden cardiac death in young adults, but the disorder may be first recognized in those >60 years old.[11] Massive acute **pulmonary embolism** may cause syncope due to obstruction of the pulmonary vascular bed and reduction in cardiac output.[12] **Acute myocardial infarction** may cause syncope if myocardial dyskinesia reduces cardiac output. Individual chapters in the Cardiovascular Disease section of this text provide more discussion on structural cardiopulmonary disorders that may cause syncope.

Although both **brady- and tachydysrhythmias** may lead to transient cerebral hypoperfusion (**Table 52-1**), there is no absolute high or low heart rate that will predictably produce syncope. Symptoms depend on both the autonomic nervous system's ability to compensate for a decrease in cardiac output and the degree of underlying cerebrovascular disease. Dysrhythmias may also result from of a primary electrolyte imbalance, as in hypomagnesemia (e.g., torsade de pointes). Dysrhythmias can occasionally occur in structurally normal hearts, such as in the familial disorders of **Brugada syndrome**, long or short **QT syndromes**, and catecholamine-associated polymorphic ventricular tachycardia. **Syncope from dysrhythmias is typically sudden and usually without prodromal symptoms.**

TABLE 52-2 Drugs Commonly Implicated in Syncope

Erectile dysfunction drugs
Antihypertensives
β-Blockers
Cardiac glycosides
Diuretics
Antidysrhythmics
Antipsychotics
Antiparkinsonism drugs
Antidepressants
Phenothiazines
Nitrates
Alcohol
Cocaine

VASOVAGAL AND NEURALLY/REFLEX-MEDIATED SYNCOPE

Vasovagal syncope, a form of reflex-mediated or neurally mediated syncope, is associated with inappropriate vasodilatation, bradycardia, or both, as a result of inappropriate vagal or sympathetic tone.[13,14] A prodrome of lightheadedness, with or without nausea, pallor, and/or sweating, and an associated feeling of warmth may accompany vasovagal syncope. **A slow, progressive onset with associated prodrome suggests vasovagal syncope**. Vasovagal syncope may occur after exposure to an unexpected or unpleasant sight, sound, or smell; fear; severe pain; emotional distress; or instrumentation. It may also occur in association with prolonged standing or kneeling in a crowded or warm place. **Situational syncope** occurs during or immediately after coughing, micturition, defecation, or swallowing.

Carotid sinus hypersensitivity, characterized by bradycardia or hypotension, is another type of reflex-mediated syncope. The carotid body, located at the carotid bifurcation, contains pressure-sensitive receptors. The stimulation of an abnormally sensitive carotid body by external pressure may lead to two autonomic responses. Most commonly, there is an abnormal vagal response, leading to bradycardia and asystole of >3 seconds. Less commonly, there is a vasodepressor response, leading to a decrease in blood pressure of >50 mm Hg without a significant change in heart rate. Both responses may occur simultaneously. Carotid sinus hypersensitivity is more common in men, the elderly, and among those with ischemic heart disease, hypertension, and certain head and neck malignancies. Although some patients may demonstrate a hypersensitive carotid sinus response on provocative testing, unless this response culminates in syncope or recurrence of prodromal symptoms, and unless it is associated with an inciting event, such as shaving or turning of the head, it cannot be definitely diagnosed as the cause of syncope. About 25% of patients with carotid sinus hypersensitivity have true carotid sinus syndrome with spontaneous symptoms.[5] **Consider carotid sinus hypersensitivity in older patients with recurrent syncope and negative cardiac evaluations.**

ORTHOSTATIC SYNCOPE

Orthostatic syncope is suggested when postural hypotension is associated with syncope or presyncope.[15] When a person assumes an upright posture, gravity shifts blood to the lower part of the body, and cardiac output drops. This change triggers the healthy autonomic nervous system to increase sympathetic output and decrease parasympathetic output, increasing heart rate and peripheral vascular resistance, and thus increasing cardiac output and blood pressure.[16,17] If the autonomic response is insufficient to counter the drop in cardiac output upon standing, decreased cerebral perfusion and syncope may follow. Symptom onset is usually within the first 3 minutes after assuming the upright posture, but may be more delayed in some patients. However, positive orthostatic changes have been documented in up to 40% of asymptomatic patients >70 years old and in about a quarter of those <60 years old, so orthostasis does not always result in syncope.[14,18] Causes of orthostatic syncope include intravascular volume loss and poor vascular tone caused by α-receptor disorders or medications. **Many serious causes of syncope may be associated with orthostatic changes, so consider other life-threatening causes before attributing syncope to orthostasis, especially in the elderly.**

PSYCHIATRIC DISORDERS

Psychiatric disorders are found in a modest percentage of patients with syncope[19]—up to 40% of those with vasovagal syncope and up to 62% of those with unexplained syncope.[20] In one study, the most frequent psychiatric diagnoses associated with syncope were generalized anxiety disorder and major depressive disorder.[21] Hyperventilation has been used as a provocative maneuver in diagnosing panic disorder and generalized anxiety disorders and can lead to hypocarbia, cerebral vasoconstriction, and syncope.[22] Hyperventilation may not be obvious to the observer but can be documented by end-tidal carbon dioxide monitoring. In general, a patient with syncope and a psychiatric disorder is likely to be young, with repeated episodes of syncope and multiple prodromal symptoms.[21] A psychiatric cause for syncope should be one of exclusion, assigned only after organic causes have been excluded.

NEUROLOGIC SYNCOPE

Neurologic causes of syncope are rare. To meet the definition of syncope, symptoms must be transient and with no persistent neurologic deficits. **Thus, patients with loss of consciousness with persistent neurologic deficits or altered mental status do not have true syncope.** Brainstem ischemia, vertebrobasilar atherosclerotic disease, or basilar artery migraine may result in a decrease in blood flow to the reticular activating system, leading to sudden, brief episodes of loss of consciousness. Loss of consciousness is typically preceded by other signs or symptoms, such as diplopia, vertigo, focal neurologic deficits, or nausea. **Subclavian steal syndrome** is a rare cause of brainstem ischemia. It is characterized by an abnormal narrowing of the subclavian artery proximal to the origin of the vertebral artery, so that with exercise of the ipsilateral arm, blood is shunted, or "stolen," from the vertebrobasilar system to the subclavian artery supplying the arm muscles. Anatomically, narrowing is more common on the left. Physical examination may identify decreased pulse volume and diminished blood pressure in the affected arm.

Subarachnoid hemorrhage may present with syncope but is usually accompanied by other symptoms such as focal neurologic deficits, headache, or persistent altered mental status. The mechanism for syncope is thought to be an increase in intracranial pressure with a decrease in cerebral perfusion pressure. **Subarachnoid hemorrhage can also follow a fall and head injury from syncope secondary to another cause.** See chapter 166, Spontaneous Subarachnoid and Intracerebral Hemorrhage, for further discussion.

Seizure may be confused with syncope, because brief tonic-clonic movements are often associated with syncope. However, confusion (postictal state) lasting several minutes, tongue biting, incontinence, or an epileptic aura suggests a seizure.

MEDICATION-INDUCED SYNCOPE

Medications may contribute to syncope by a variety of means (**Table 52-2**), but the most common is orthostasis.[23] β-Blockers or calcium channel blockers may lead to a blunted heart rate response after orthostatic stress. Diuretics may produce volume depletion, and some medications have proarrhythmic properties, increasing the concern for dysrhythmia as the cause of syncope.

PRINCIPLES OF EVALUATION

The goal of ED evaluation is to identify those at risk for immediate and future morbidity or sudden death. For patients with a specific diagnosis, the diagnosis directs the disposition plan. For patients without a specific diagnosis, risk stratification is based on a careful history, thorough physical examination, and electrocardiogram interpretation, with additional testing as needed.

HISTORY

Obtain clinical history from the patient and any witnesses of the event. Begin with a detailed description of the events preceding the loss of consciousness, including patient position, environmental stimuli, strenuous activity, or arm exercise. Record premonitory symptoms such as headache, diplopia, vertigo, or focal weakness. Ask about chest pain and palpitations. Clarify the duration of loss of consciousness and symptoms occurring after regaining consciousness. Symptoms associated with syncope that should raise concern of an immediately life-threatening diagnosis include **chest pain** (acute myocardial infarction, aortic dissection, pulmonary embolism, aortic stenosis), **palpitations** (dysrhythmia), shortness of breath (pulmonary embolism, congestive heart failure), **headache** (subarachnoid hemorrhage), and **abdominal or back pain** (leaking abdominal aortic aneurysm, ruptured ectopic pregnancy). A sudden event without warning and events associated with exertion raise suspicion for a cardiac dysrhythmia or structural cardiopulmonary lesion.[24] Ask about antecedent illness and alcohol ingestion or substance abuse. The past medical history should include questions regarding underlying structural heart disease, including congenital heart disease, valvular heart disease, coronary artery disease, congestive heart failure, pulmonary embolism, and ventricular dysrhythmias. Document any prior history of syncope, as patients with more than five syncopal episodes in 1 year are more likely to have vasovagal syncope or a psychiatric diagnosis than dysrhythmia as the cause.[5] All medications should be recorded, including over-the-counter medications such as laxatives. Patients aggressively dieting to lose weight may have electrolyte disturbances or may be taking amphetamine-like medications. The family history is important in regard to history of prolonged QT syndrome, dysrhythmias, sudden cardiac death, or other cardiac risks.

Special attention should be paid to patients presenting after single-car motor vehicle crashes (frequently with a history of driving off the road), particularly if the patients are elderly. Clinicians may become preoccupied by the trauma evaluation and miss the possibility of a syncopal event.

Seizure is the most common event mistaken as syncope. Mild, brief, tonic-clonic activity ("convulsive syncope") may accompany syncope of any etiology. The two conditions do not share the same pathophysiologic mechanisms. History is very important in differentiating syncope from seizure.[25] Premonitory and postevent symptoms may assist in differentiation. A classic aura or postictal confusion and muscle pain indicate seizure, whereas characteristic prodromal symptoms of nausea and diaphoresis suggest reflex-mediated (vasovagal) syncope. Witness information of the event may also be useful. Witnessed head turning or unusual posture during the event is consistent with seizure. A prolonged postictal phase is more common with seizure. Urinary incontinence is not useful in the distinction.

PHYSICAL EXAMINATION

Evidence of trauma without defensive injuries to the hands or knees should raise suspicion of a sudden event without warning, such as a dysrhythmia, but patients with noncardiac syncope are also just as likely to suffer significant facial and head trauma. The physical examination should focus on both the cardiovascular and neurologic systems. Obtain blood pressure measurements in both arms. Unequal blood pressures should increase suspicion of aortic dissection or subclavian steal. Take orthostatic blood pressures after 5 minutes in the supine position. Repeat measurements after 1 and 3 minutes of standing. A symptomatic decrease of >20 mm Hg in the systolic pressure is considered abnormal, as is a drop in pressure below 90 mm Hg independent of the development of symptoms. Cardiac examination may reveal the murmur of hypertrophic cardiomyopathy or aortic stenosis. The neurologic examination may uncover findings of focal neurologic disease or evidence of autonomic instability such as peripheral neuropathy. Perform rectal examination to check stool guaiac to evaluate for GI bleeding.

DIAGNOSIS

The diagnosis of syncope is clinical, with careful evaluation of the presentation and selected use of diagnostic tests. History is most important, and most diagnostic tests have low diagnostic yield.[26] The differential diagnosis is presented in **Tables 52-1** and **52-2**.

ELECTROCARDIOGRAM

Obtain a 12-lead electrocardiogram. Even though the electrocardiogram leads to a diagnosis in only a few patients, it is a simple, noninvasive test and is important for risk stratification.[27] Assess the electrocardiogram for evidence of prior cardiopulmonary disease, acute ischemia or new electrocardiogram changes, dysrhythmia, heart block, and prolonged or short QTc interval. A prolonged QTc interval has a variable definition, but the literature suggests it is defined as >470 milliseconds, with >500 milliseconds associated with significant outcomes,[28-30] whereas a short QTc interval <350 milliseconds is concerning as well.[31] New or old left bundle conduction abnormalities (left bundle-branch block, posterior or anterior fascicular block, QRS widening) are 3.5 times more likely to be associated with morbidity than electrocardiograms lacking these findings. Non-sinus rhythms are 2.5 times more likely to be associated with morbidity than sinus rhythms.[32] For further discussion, see chapter 18, Cardiac Rhythm Disturbances.

LABORATORY TESTING

Laboratory testing is directed by results of the history and physical examination. For example, a patient with orthostatic symptoms and a heme-positive stool test warrants at least a CBC. A reproductive-age female should have a urine pregnancy test. A transitory, wide anion gap acidosis follows a generalized seizure but is not present in simple syncope. Serum electrolytes rarely determine the cause of syncope. B-type natriuretic peptide or pro–B-type natriuretic peptide levels appear to be predictive of those at risk for morbidity. One study suggests that a level >300 pg/mL in the setting of syncope indicates risk,[33] but whether this adds any value over a history of congestive heart failure or structural disease is unclear.[34,35] See chapter 53, Acute Heart Failure, for a discussion of the diagnostic use of B-type natriuretic peptide.

ANCILLARY TESTING

Carotid Massage Carotid massage is used to diagnose carotid sinus hypersensitivity in the patient with a history suggestive of carotid sinus syndrome. Although not generally used in emergency medicine at this time, carotid massage can be done at the bedside in the ED with continuous electrocardiographic and blood pressure monitoring, after obtaining informed consent. Each carotid body is separately massaged for 5 to 10 seconds. The test is considered positive if symptoms are reproduced in the presence of asystole >3 seconds or a decrease in systolic blood pressure of >50 mm Hg. **Do not perform carotid massage if the patient has known carotid stenosis, if bruits are present, if there is history of recent (<3 months) stroke or myocardial infarction, or if there is a history of ventricular tachycardia or fibrillation.** Neurologic deficits resulting from cardiac massage are rare, with deficits lasting more than 24 hours in approximately 0.1% of patients.[36] Only a small number of patients with carotid hypersensitivity will have the true carotid sinus syndrome. Given the small benefit of the maneuver and that the rare potential adverse events are catastrophic, most physicians do not routinely perform carotid massage.

Hyperventilation Maneuver A hyperventilation maneuver (open-mouthed, slow, deep breaths at a rate of 20 to 30 breaths per minute for 2 to 3 minutes) can be very useful in the young patient with undiagnosed syncope and suspected psychiatric illness. This test can easily be performed in the ED. A recurrence of prodromal symptoms or syncope significantly correlates with psychiatric (anxiety-provoking) causes of syncope.[21]

Neurologic Testing When the history or physical examination does not suggest trauma or a neurologic cause for syncope, the clinical yield of routine CT scanning, electroencephalogram, or lumbar puncture is very low. Consequently, in asymptomatic patients who have experienced an isolated syncopal event, and in those without head trauma from the event, a head CT scan or MRI scan is not warranted.

DECISION MAKING AND RISK ASSESSMENT

DIAGNOSIS ESTABLISHED

If a cause of syncope can be determined by the initial history, physical examination, and ECG, the disposition is simple. Patients with cardiac or neurologic syncope should be admitted. Patients with vasovagal, orthostatic, and medication-related syncope have no increased risk of cardiovascular morbidity or mortality[6] and do not need admission as long as deficits are corrected.

UNEXPLAINED SYNCOPE

Despite best efforts, a diagnosis will not be established in about 40% of the patients with syncope. Several studies have assessed risk stratification variables to identify patients at risk of both short-term and 1-year morbidity and mortality. Martin et al[37] performed derivation and validation studies on cohorts of consecutive ED patients with syncope to identify predictors of arrhythmia and death at 1 year. Important risk factors were a history of arrhythmia, an abnormal electrocardiogram, a history of congestive heart failure, and age >45 years. Quinn et al[2,38] assessed adverse outcomes at 7 and 30 days in their derivation and validation of the **San Francisco Syncope Rule**. Significant predictors of adverse events (primarily arrhythmia) included (1) a history of congestive heart failure, (2) an abnormal electrocardiogram (a rhythm other than sinus, including those on rhythm strips or monitoring, conduction delays or new changes as minimal as first-degree atrioventricular block, or any morphologic changes to the QRS complex or ST segment that could not be proven to be old by prior tracings), (3) a hematocrit of <30, (4) a complaint of shortness of breath, and (5) a systolic blood pressure of <90 mm Hg in the ED. There have been inconsistent findings when validating the San Francisco Syncope Rule, which have been primarily related to definitions of syncope and when applying variables.[39] The Osservatorio Epidemiologico sulla Sincope nel Lazio study group developed a risk score based on predictors of death at 1 year, which they found to be an abnormal electrocardiogram, a history of cardiovascular disease (including congestive heart failure), age >65 years, and syncope without prodrome.[40] Sarasin et al[41] developed a prediction score for subsequent arrhythmia in patients with unexplained syncope after a standard ED evaluation; they found the significant variables to be an abnormal electrocardiogram, a history of congestive heart failure, and age >65 years. Continued analysis of the San Francisco syncope cohort, assessing 1418 consecutive patients with syncope, found the death rate to be 1.4% at 30 days, 4.3% at 6 months, and 7.6% at 1 year. The five high-risk criteria listed earlier had an 89% sensitivity and 52% specificity for death at 1 year.[42]

Using the risk factors identified in these studies can help clinicians determine patient risk and appropriate disposition. Although each study may be limited by the size of the cohort, the number of adverse events, and the definition of these events, there is a consistent theme that patients with an abnormal electrocardiogram on presentation and/or a history of heart disease, particularly structural heart disease especially characterized by a history of congestive heart failure, are clearly at increased risk.

GENERAL MANAGEMENT ALGORITHM

A general management algorithm is shown in **Figure 52-1**, which follows the recommendations of the American College of Emergency Medicine guidelines for the disposition of patients with syncope presenting to the ED and lists essential risk factors.[43]

Risk factors not included in Figure 52-1, but suggested by guidelines[44,45] as factors that could be used for admission or expedited follow-up decision making, include **syncope while supine, syncope during exercise, syncope without prodromal symptoms, palpations preceding syncope, and the specific age cut points of >60 or >65 years.**

TREATMENT

Treatment should be guided by the diagnosis. Patients with or at risk for life-threatening dysrhythmias can be treated with pacemakers or automatic implantable defibrillators as indicated. For patients with suspected medication causes, remove the offending agent. Rehydrate those with orthostasis and dehydration. Educate patients with vasovagal syncope; episodes are likely to recur, and patients should lie or sit down when they sense a prodrome. β-Blockers do not decrease episodes of vasovagal syncope.[46]

DISPOSITION AND FOLLOW-UP

INPATIENT EVALUATION

With the exception of patients with acute life-threatening diagnoses (e.g., stroke, aortic dissection), the core of the inpatient evaluation is focused on identification of underlying heart disease and detection of

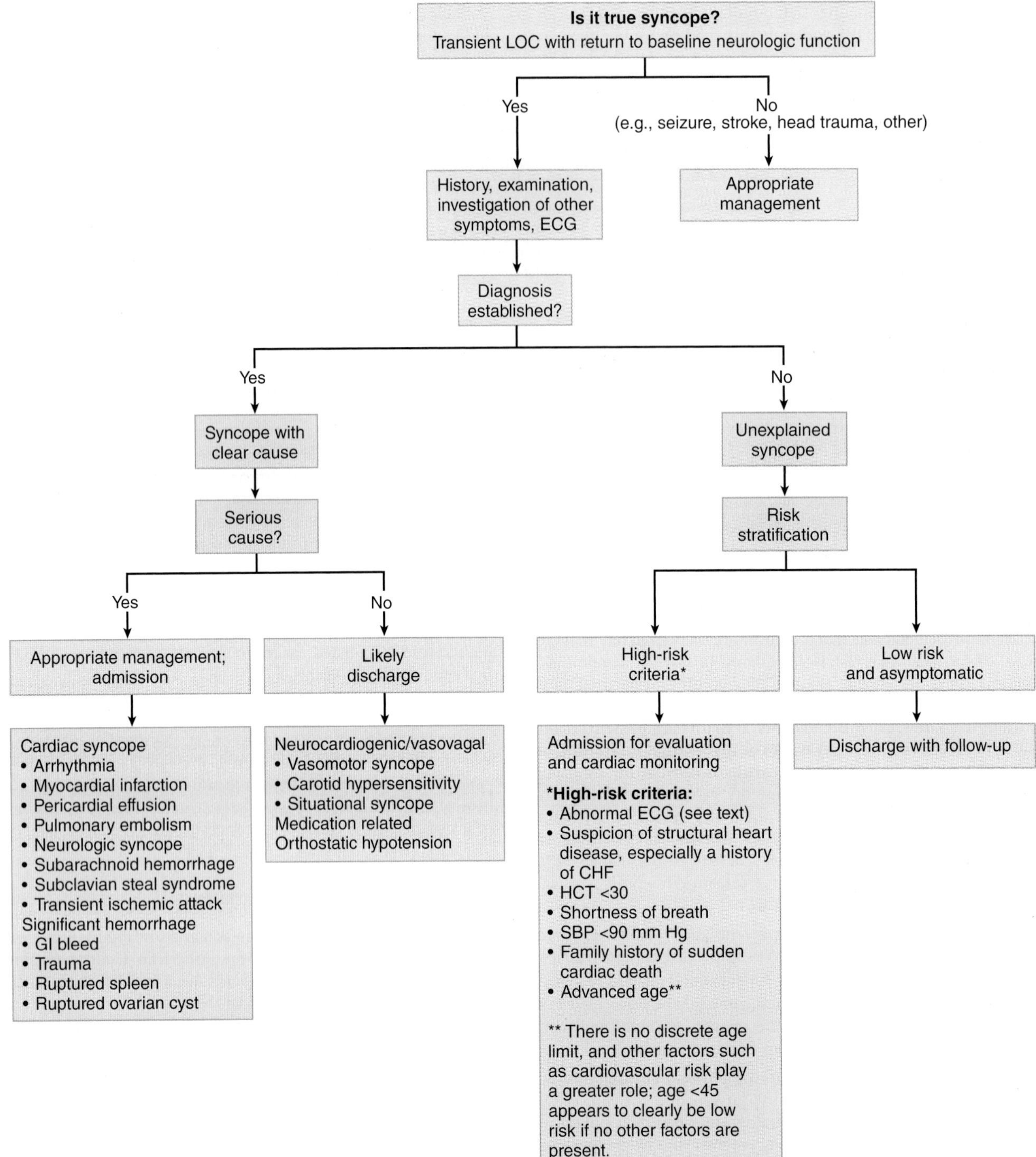

FIGURE 52-1. ED evaluation of syncope provides a general management strategy. CHF = congestive heart failure; ECG = electrocardiogram; HCT = hematocrit; LOC = loss of consciousness; SBP = systolic blood pressure.

dysrhythmias (**Table 52-3**). Although admitted patients undergo continuous electrocardiographic monitoring, the utility of admission and monitoring is questioned.[26,47] Dysrhythmia as the cause of syncope is confirmed in the patient with recurrent symptoms during a monitored dysrhythmia and excluded in the patient with recurrent symptoms and sinus rhythm. An echocardiogram should be performed on patients with known or suspected heart disease to evaluate for valvular disorders, congenital anomalies, and cardiomyopathies and to determine overall cardiac function. Echocardiogram abnormalities are usually clinically apparent and will seldom be found in patients with a normal cardiac examination and electrocardiogram. Stress testing is used to identify exercise-induced dysrhythmias or ischemia or to reproduce exertional syncope once hypertrophic cardiomyopathy has been excluded by echocardiography. Electrophysiology testing is typically reserved for patients with documented dysrhythmia, preexcitation, or underlying heart disease. Electrophysiology testing involves invasive electrical stimulation and cardiac monitoring to uncover possible conduction abnormalities that predispose to tachydysrhythmias (both ventricular and supraventricular) or bradydysrhythmias.

OUTPATIENT EVALUATION

Patients directed to outpatient syncope evaluation should be at low risk for serious cardiac dysrhythmias. Long-term cardiac monitoring, which

TABLE 52-3 Post-ED Testing for Syncope/Syncope Mimics

Test	Indication	Utility
Cardiac syncope		
Electrocardiographic monitoring	Admission Outpatient ambulatory monitoring if no significant cardiac disease suspected	Cardiac syncope confirmed if recurrent symptoms occur during monitored dysrhythmia; excluded if recurrent symptoms reported during sinus rhythm
Implantable loop recorder	Recurrent syncope after admission evaluation	Long-term use with diagnostic yield of >50% in patients with recurrent syncope
Echocardiography	History, examination, or electrocardiogram suggestive of structural heart disease	Confirms and quantifies suspected structural heart disease
Electrophysiology testing	Documented dysrhythmia or serious underlying heart disease	Identifies inducible tachydysrhythmias and some bradydysrhythmias
Stress testing	Exercise-related syncope	Identifies exercise-induced dysrhythmias and postexercise syncope
Neurologic syncope		
CT/magnetic resonance angiography/ carotid Doppler	Neurologic signs or symptoms	Identifies cerebrovascular abnormality or subclavian stenosis
Electroencephalography	Suspected seizure	Documents underlying seizure disorder
Reflex-mediated syncope		
Tilt-table testing	Recurrent syncope, cardiac etiology excluded	Positive test establishes diagnosis of neurocardiogenic syncope
Psychogenic		
Psychiatric testing	Young patient, no underlying heart disease	Identifies underlying psychiatric disorder predisposing to syncope

includes ambulatory or event monitors, is useful to identify dysrhythmias (**Table 52-3**). The duration one should wear an ambulatory monitor is debatable, but monitors are now more portable and can be worn for long periods.[48] Long-term use of implantable loop recorders have a diagnostic yield of >50% in patients with recurrent syncope.[49-51] Tilt-table testing is also suggested for patients with recurrent, unexplained syncope. This test is designed to identify reflex-mediated syncope by rapidly moving the patient from a supine position on the tilt table to an upright position of 60 degrees for 45 minutes. A positive end-point is reached if syncope, hypotension, or the patient's typical symptoms are reproduced. Repeat testing with isoproterenol or sublingual nitroglycerin is performed if the initial evaluation is negative. Recurrent reflex-mediated syncope resistant to conservative therapies can be treated with a cardiac pacemaker. Psychiatric referral is recommended for young patients without underlying heart disease who have frequent syncopal events. Generalized anxiety and depressive disorders are the most commonly assigned diagnoses. Patients with a prolonged QT segment should be referred for genetic testing for the *LQTS* gene. Those who are gene negative have very little risk for fatal syncope.[52]

SPECIAL POPULATIONS

THE ELDERLY

Because of both normal physiologic changes with aging and age-related disease processes, the elderly are at increased risk for syncope and adverse outcomes.[8] Syncope in the elderly is often multifactorial, and the cause is often difficult to establish, particularly in the ED.

Various specified ages have been studied as risk factors for fatal or serious outcomes after syncope; however, there is a gradual continuum of increasing risk with increasing age. Cardiovascular risk factors appear to be better predictors than age itself. As a person ages, the blood vessels become calcified and less compliant, leading to diminished flow rates. The left ventricle also becomes less compliant, resulting in increased diastolic filling pressures and an increased dependence on the "atrial kick." There is a general decrease in adrenergic receptor responsiveness of both the heart and the peripheral blood vessels. Decreased adrenergic responsiveness contributes to the diminished chronotropic response seen after orthostatic stresses in the elderly. The incidence of vasovagal syncope actually decreases with age, in part as a consequence of the decreased responsiveness of the autonomic nervous systems. The elderly also have a less sensitive thirst mechanism and a decreased endocrine response to volume depletion, exacerbating orthostatic hypotension. Postprandial hypotension is more common in the elderly, especially in nursing home patients, and is thought to be due to a rapid rate of nutrient delivery from the stomach into the small intestine. Pathophysiologic processes that may contribute to diminished cerebral perfusion include disorders such as hypertension, atherosclerosis, and valvular disease. Atherosclerotic disease leads to ischemia, myocardial infarction, congestive heart failure, and dysrhythmias. Aortic stenosis is the most common obstructive cardiac lesion in the elderly, producing a fixed cardiac output. Diabetes may lead to autonomic dysfunction and peripheral neuropathy. Finally, medication usage is much more common in the elderly population, increasing the risk of orthostasis and decreasing autonomic responsiveness to orthostatic stress.[18]

PREGNANT WOMEN

Pregnancy is associated with numerous physiologic changes, including increased heart rate, decreased peripheral resistance, and increased stroke volume. In late pregnancy, the enlarged uterus may compress the inferior vena cava, decreasing venous return. The incidence of cardiac dysrhythmias, especially premature ventricular contractions, increases during normal pregnancy in young healthy women. However, there is no positive correlation between symptoms of presyncope or syncope and cardiac dysrhythmia in pregnant women. Important considerations for syncope in pregnancy include ruptured ectopic pregnancy and pulmonary embolism, although these disorders typically have other associated symptoms such as abdominal or dyspnea.

CHILDREN

Syncope in children is discussed in chapter 127, "Syncope, Dysrhythmias, and ECG Interpretation in Children."

PRACTICE GUIDELINES

Guidelines for the management of patients sustaining syncope have been published by the American College of Emergency Physicians,[43] the European Society of Cardiology,[44] the Canadian Cardiovascular Society,[45] and the American Heart Association/American College of Cardiology Foundation.[53]

REFERENCES

The complete reference list is available online at www.TintinalliEM.com.

Acute Heart Failure

Sean P. Collins
Alan B. Storrow

INTRODUCTION AND EPIDEMIOLOGY

Acute heart failure covers a wide spectrum of illness, ranging from a gradual increase in leg swelling, shortness of breath, or decreased exercise tolerance to the abrupt onset of pulmonary edema. While alternative terms such as *decompensated heart failure, acute heart failure syndrome,* or *hospitalized with heart failure* have been used nearly interchangeably over the last decade, we refer to patients with either an acute exacerbation of chronic heart failure or a new-onset heart failure as having *acute heart failure.* The term *congestive heart failure* is outdated and describes patients with signs and symptoms of fluid accumulation.

Most ED visits for acute heart failure result in hospital admission.[1] With the aging population, increased survival from acute myocardial infarction, and evidence-based outpatient treatment options, the prevalence of heart failure is expected to increase over the next decade.[2-4] ED physicians drive most disposition decisions.[5,6] There have been tremendous advances in outpatient management of heart failure patients. While long-term heart failure management has improved through the use of β-blockers, angiotensin-converting enzyme inhibitors, spironolactone, and cardiac resynchronization therapy,[2,3] acute therapy is largely unchanged. Acute therapies include nitrates, diuretics, and positive-pressure ventilation, the same as in 1974.[7] Only one therapy, nesiritide, has been approved for heart failure treatment in the last three decades, but it is not significantly better than standard treatment.[8]

Heart failure has a poor prognosis, with approximately 50% of patients diagnosed dying within 5 years.[9] Hospitalization also marks an inflection point in a patient's HF trajectory, with those hospitalized having higher mortality than a matched nonhospitalized cohort.[10]

PATHOPHYSIOLOGY

Heart failure is a complicated syndrome manifested by cardinal symptoms (shortness of breath, edema, and fatigue) occurring from functional or structural cardiac damage, impairing the ability of the heart to act as an efficient pump. A clinically useful definition of heart failure is as follows: a complex clinical syndrome that results from any structural or functional impairment of ventricular filling or ejection of blood. The cardinal manifestations of heart failure are dyspnea and fatigue, which may limit exercise tolerance, and fluid retention, which may lead to pulmonary and/or splanchnic congestion and/or peripheral edema.[2] There are numerous responsive adaptations in the kidney, peripheral circulation, skeletal muscle, and other organs to maintain short-term circulatory function. Eventually, these responses may become maladaptive, contribute to long-term disease progression, and contribute to acute exacerbations.

Threats to cardiac output from myocardial injury or stress trigger a neurohormonally mediated cascade that includes activation of the renin-angiotensin-aldosterone system and the sympathetic nervous systems. Levels of norepinephrine, vasopressin, endothelin (a potent vasoconstrictor), and tumor necrosis factor-α are increased. Although not measured in routine care, elevated levels of these hormones correlate with higher mortality.

The combined clinical effects of neurohormonal activation are sodium and water retention coupled with increased systemic vascular resistance. These maintain blood pressure and perfusion, but at the cost of increasing myocardial workload, wall tension, and myocardial oxygen demand. Although some patients are initially asymptomatic, a secondary pathologic process called cardiac remodeling begins to occur, eventually triggering more dysfunction.

Natriuretic peptides are the endogenous counterregulatory response to neurohormonal activation in heart failure. Three types are recognized: atrial natriuretic peptide, primarily secreted from the atria; B-type natriuretic peptide, secreted mainly from the cardiac ventricle; and C-type natriuretic peptide, localized in the endothelium. Natriuretic peptides produce vasodilation, natriuresis, decreased levels of endothelin, and inhibition of the renin-angiotensin-aldosterone system and the sympathetic nervous systems. B-type natriuretic peptide is synthesized as N-terminal pre–pro-B-type natriuretic peptide, which is cleaved into two substances, inactive N-terminal pro-B-type natriuretic peptide, with a half-life of approximately 2 hours, and physiologically active B-type natriuretic peptide, with a half-life of about 20 minutes. Assays for both B-type natriuretic peptide and N-terminal pro-B-type natriuretic peptide are available for ED use. Because elevated levels of neurohormones portend a worse prognosis in heart failure, their attenuation provides the basis for most chronic therapies proven to delay heart failure morbidity and mortality. These include treatment with angiotensin-converting enzyme inhibitors, angiotensin receptor blockers, aldosterone antagonists, and β-blockers.

Heart failure may also result from pump dysfunction from acute myocardial infarction. Mechanistically, loss of a critical mass of myocardium results in immediate symptoms. If there is symptomatic hypotension with inadequate perfusion, cardiogenic shock is present (see chapter 50 "Cardiogenic Shock"). Acute pulmonary edema may be precipitous and is the clinical manifestation of a downward spiral of rapidly decreasing cardiac output and rising systemic vascular resistance on top of underlying cardiac dysfunction. Even relatively small elevations of blood pressure can result in decreased cardiac output. Decreasing cardiac output triggers increasing systemic vascular resistance, which further decreases cardiac output. Acute pulmonary edema can present acutely with severe symptoms, and if not promptly reversed, it may be a terminal event.

ACUTE HEART FAILURE CLASSIFICATION

There are many causes for heart failure (**Table 53-1**).

Patients can be categorized into six phenotypes to assist with investigating the causes and precipitants for the acute presentation, as well as directing initial therapy (**Table 53-2**).[11] Those with acute heart failure and hypertension often have a precipitous presentation and may have significant pulmonary edema and hypoxia. Symptoms may be due to fluid redistribution more than fluid overload, and treatment initially focuses on antihypertensive therapy.[12,13] Pulmonary edema may benefit from noninvasive ventilation to decrease the work of breathing and avoid intubation.[14,15] For heart failure accompanied by hypotension or poor perfusion without another cause, think of an ischemic or structural heart trigger creating cardiogenic shock; patients often benefit from inotropic agents and invasive hemodynamic monitoring to guide other therapies.

Patients with acute-on-chronic heart failure tend to present with gradual symptoms and weight gain over days to weeks. High-output heart failure is distinguished by a relatively normal ejection fraction and is often caused by anemia or thyrotoxicosis. Isolated right heart failure is characterized by lower extremity edema and jugular venous distension but little or no pulmonary congestion, and the cause is usually from pulmonary disease, valvular disease such as tricuspid regurgitation, or obstructive sleep apnea. Treatment approaches center on identifying and treating the underlying cause, often without volume removal because low-output states may coexist.

SYSTOLIC AND DIASTOLIC HEART FAILURE

Heart failure is classified as systolic or diastolic by ejection fraction, which is normally 60%. **Systolic dysfunction**, or heart failure with reduced ejection fraction, is defined as an ejection fraction <50%. Mechanistically, the ventricle has difficulty ejecting blood, leading to increased intracardiac volume and *afterload sensitivity.* With circulatory stress (e.g., walking), failure to improve contractility despite increasing venous return results in increased cardiac pressures, pulmonary congestion, and edema.

Diastolic dysfunction, or heart failure with is preserved ejection fraction, is characterized by impaired ventricular relaxation, causing an abnormal relation between diastolic pressure and volume. This results in a

TABLE 53-1 Common Causes of Heart Failure and Pulmonary Edema

Myocardial ischemia: acute and chronic*
Systemic hypertension*
Cardiac dysrhythmias (especially atrial fibrillation with rapid ventricular response)*
Valvular dysfunction
  Aortic valve disease
    Aortic stenosis
    Aortic insufficiency
      Aortic dissection
      Infectious endocarditis
  Mitral valve disease
    Mitral stenosis
    Mitral regurgitation
      Papillary muscle dysfunction or rupture
      Ruptured chordae tendineae
      Infectious endocarditis
  Prosthetic valve malfunction
Other causes of left ventricular outflow obstruction
  Supravalvular aortic stenosis
  Membranous subvalvular aortic stenosis
Cardiomyopathy*
  Hypertrophic cardiomyopathy
  Dilated†
  Restrictive
Acquired cardiomyopathy
  Toxic: alcohol, cocaine, doxorubicin
  Metabolic: thyrotoxicosis, myxedema
Myocarditis: radiation, infection
Constrictive pericarditis
Cardiac tamponade
Anemia

*Seen in the ED with higher frequency.

†Includes idiopathic (see chapter 55, "Cardiomyopathies and Pericardial Disease").

TABLE 53-2 Classification of Acute Heart Failure

Classification	Characteristics
Hypertensive AHF	Signs and symptoms of AHF with relatively preserved left ventricular function, systolic blood pressure >140 mm Hg, typically with a chest radiograph compatible with pulmonary edema and symptom onset less than 48 h
Pulmonary edema	Respiratory distress, rales on chest auscultation, reduced oxygen saturation from baseline, verified by chest radiograph findings
Cardiogenic shock (see chapter 50)	Evidence of tissue hypoperfusion (systolic blood pressure typically <90 mm Hg)
Acute-on-chronic HF	Signs and symptoms of AHF that are mild to moderate and do not meet criteria for hypertensive HF, pulmonary edema, or cardiogenic shock, systolic blood pressure <140 mm Hg and >90 mm Hg, typically associated with increased peripheral edema and symptom onset over several days
High-output failure	High cardiac output, typically with tachycardia, warm extremities, and pulmonary congestion
Right heart failure	Low-output syndrome with jugular venous distention, hepatomegaly, and may have hypotension

Abbreviations: AHF = acute heart failure; HF = heart failure.

left ventricle that has difficulty receiving blood. Decreased left ventricular compliance necessitates higher atrial pressures to ensure adequate left ventricular diastolic filling, creating a *preload sensitivity*. The frequency of diastolic dysfunction increases with age and is more common in chronic hypertension, which leads to left ventricular hypertrophy. Coronary artery disease also contributes, as diastolic dysfunction is an early event in the ischemic cascade.

DIAGNOSIS

Most hospitalized patients with heart failure are admitted through the ED. Commonly, patients will present with dyspnea, which has a large differential diagnosis including heart failure, chronic obstructive pulmonary disease, asthma, pneumonia, and acute coronary syndrome. Misdiagnosis increases mortality, prolongs hospital stay, and increases treatment costs.[16-20] **Table 53-3** lists common causes of dyspnea in ED patients. ***There is no single diagnostic test*** for heart failure; it is a clinical diagnosis based on the history and physical examination. Having an understanding of the diagnostic certainty regarding the history, physical examination, and laboratory and radiographic testing is extremely important when caring for ED patients with undifferentiated dyspnea.

HISTORY AND PHYSICAL EXAMINATION

There is ***no singular historical or physical* examination finding** that achieves both 70% sensitivity and 70% specificity for the diagnosis of acute heart failure.[19] The initial global clinical judgment has a sensitivity of 61% and specificity of 86%. A history of heart failure is the most useful historical parameter, but only has a sensitivity of 60% and specificity of 90% (positive likelihood ratio [LR+] = 5.8; negative likelihood ratio [LR–] = 0.45). Risk factors for acute heart failure sometimes may be helpful, including hypertension, diabetes, valvular heart disease, old age, male sex, and obesity. The symptom with the highest sensitivity for diag-

TABLE 53-3 Common Causes of Dyspnea

Dyspneic states
  Heart failure
  Asthma exacerbation
  Chronic obstructive pulmonary disease exacerbation
  Pleural effusion
  Pneumonia or other pulmonary infection
  Pneumothorax
  Pulmonary embolus
  Physical deconditioning or obesity
Fluid retentive states
  Dependent edema or deep vein thrombosis
  Hypoproteinemia
  Liver failure or cirrhosis
  Portal vein thrombosis
  Renal failure or nephrotic syndrome
Impaired cardiac output states
  Acute myocardial infarction
  Acute valvular insufficiency
  Drug overdose/effect
  Dysrhythmias
  Pericardial tamponade
  Tension pneumothorax
  High-output states
  Sepsis
  Anemia
  Thyroid dysfunction

TABLE 53-4 Precipitants of AHF

Nonadherence
Excess salt or fluid intake*
Medication nonadherence*
Renal failure (especially missed dialysis)*
Substance abuse—cocaine, methamphetamines, ethanol
Poorly controlled hypertension
Iatrogenic
Recent addition of negative inotropic drugs (e.g., calcium channel blocker, β-blocker)
Initiation of salt-retaining drugs (e.g., NSAID, steroids, thiazolidinediones)
Inappropriate therapy reduction
New antiarrhythmic agents

*Common in ED patients

Abbreviations: AHF = acute heart failure; NSAID = nonsteroidal anti-inflammatory drug.

TABLE 53-5 Natriuretic Peptide Cut Points for Clinical Decision Making

	Low Cut Point (rule out HF)	High Cut Point (HF likely)		
BNP	100 pg/mL	500 pg/mL		
	Sensitivity 90%	Sensitivity 75%		
	Specificity 73%	Specificity 90%		
N-terminal pro-BNP[29]	300 pg/mL	450 pg/mL if <50 years old	900 pg/mL if 50–75 years old	1800 pg/mL
	Sensitivity 99%	Sensitivity 97%	Sensitivity 90%	Sensitivity 85%
	Specificity 60%	Specificity 93%	Specificity 82%	Specificity 73%

Abbreviations: BNP = B-type natriuretic peptide; HF = heart failure.

nosis is dyspnea on exertion (84%).[19,20] The most specific symptoms are paroxysmal nocturnal dyspnea, orthopnea, and edema (76% to 84%).[19,20] Evaluation for historical precipitating factors (**Table 53-4**) is also useful.

On exam, an S_3 has the highest LR+ for acute heart failure (11), but its absence is not useful as a negative predictor (0.88).[19] However, the interrater reliability of an S_3 is not good,[21-23] and the ambient noise in a busy ED may interfere with S_3 detection. Abdominojugular reflux (LR+ = 6.4) and jugular venous distension (LR+ = 5.1) are the only other two physical examination findings that have an LR+ greater than 5. Increased neck size, obesity, and rapid breathing may diminish the ability to accurately measure jugular venous distension at the bedside in the ED.

When clinicians are 80% confident of the diagnosis of acute heart failure, the "clinical gestalt" outperforms diagnostic tests available in the ED for the diagnosis[19]; however, clinical gestalt may be about 50% accurate in an outpatient setting.[24] Data from the Breathing Not Proper Trial found that clinical judgment and a single B-type natriuretic peptide value had a similar accuracy performance.[25]

CHEST RADIOGRAPHY

Chest radiographs showing pulmonary venous congestion, cardiomegaly, and interstitial edema are most specific for a final diagnosis of acute heart failure,[18,19] but the absence of these does not rule it out, because up to 20% of patients subsequently diagnosed with heart failure have chest radiographs without signs of congestion at the time of prior ED evaluation.[26] Particularly in late-stage heart failure, patients may have few radiographic signs, despite symptoms and elevated pulmonary capillary wedge pressure.[18]

ECG

The ECG is not useful for diagnosis, but it may reveal an underlying cause or precipitant. ECG signs of ischemia, acute myocardial infarction, or dysrhythmias may point to the precipitating cause. The presence of atrial fibrillation has the highest LR+ for a diagnosis of heart failure; however, new T-wave changes were also associated with the diagnosis.[19]

BIOMARKERS

The most widely investigated markers have been the natriuretic peptides, B-type natriuretic peptide, and N-terminal pro-B-type natriuretic peptide. Other novel biomarkers have been explored for both diagnosis and prognosis, such as ST2, galectin 3, and neutrophil gelatinase-associated lipocalin. Their role in the ED is not established; B-type natriuretic peptide and N-terminal pro-B-type natriuretic peptide remain the most important biomarkers in clinical use. Natriuretic peptide tests may add value in the setting of undifferentiated dyspnea in the ED, improving diagnostic discrimination in a variety of settings[25,27] and correlating with cardiac filling pressures and ventricular stretch.[28] As a result, B-type natriuretic peptide or N-terminal pro-B-type natriuretic peptide testing is recommended and helpful when the cause of dyspnea is unclear after standard evaluation (**Table 53-5**).

Despite the established value of natriuretic peptide testing, there are many situations where interpretation of results is unclear. Levels can be affected by age, gender, and body mass, and may elevate later in patients who present with flash pulmonary edema.[30] Dyspnea and modest B-type natriuretic peptide elevation are evident in conditions such as pulmonary hypertension, pulmonary embolism, pneumonia, sepsis, and renal failure. As many as 25% of patients will fall into the diagnostic "grey zone" (100 to 500 pg/mL for B-type natriuretic peptide), complicating test interpretation. **B-type natriuretic peptide/N-terminal B-type natriuretic peptide testing is best used when diagnostic uncertainty exists and as an addition to the physician assessment, rather than as a routine measurement.**[27] Similarly, while marked natriuretic peptide elevations are associated with worse short-term outcomes, even low elevations have increased mortality risk, limiting usefulness in bedside prognostication in the ED.[31,32]

POINT-OF-CARE ULTRASOUND (US)

Point-of-care cardiopulmonary US can help to determine the cause of dyspnea, including cardiac tamponade, and can determine left ventricular function and volume status, but is not a substitute for comprehensive echocardiography.[31,32] Bedside cardiopulmonary US can also address three questions (**Figure 53-1**): (1) Are there signs of pulmonary congestion? (2) Are there signs of volume overload by measuring the size of the inferior vena cava and its collapsibility? (3) Is the left ventricular ejection fraction low or normal?

Pulmonary US is used first to determine if pulmonary congestion is present by looking for B lines. **Sonographic B lines** (**Figure 53-2**) are ring-down artifacts that arise from the interface of the visceral and parietal pleura when there is swelling of the lung's interlobular septa due to lymphatic congestion as is seen in pulmonary edema.[33] They are the sonographic equivalent of Kerley B lines seen on chest radiography.[34] More than two B lines in any one sonographic window along the anterior and anterolateral chest are pathologic and highly specific for alveolar and interstitial edema.[35]

Because bilateral B lines can be present in other conditions not caused by pulmonary edema (e.g., pulmonary fibrosis, pulmonary contusion, bilateral pneumonia), rapid assessment for elevated central venous pressure as a marker of right heart congestion is needed.[36] An inferior vena cava size greater than 2 cm or collapsibility index of <50% is indicative of elevated central venous pressure. In the absence of significant pulmonary disease, these measures are highly correlated with pulmonary capillary wedge pressure and are specific for acute heart failure. One should also use US to look for other clinical conditions that cause an elevation in right heart pressure, including pulmonary embolism or clinically significant tricuspid regurgitation, because both conditions could cause inferior vena cava changes consistent with heart failure.

Determination of left ventricular ejection fraction is the final piece of ED-based bedside ultrasonography. Many of the methods for measuring left ventricular ejection fraction are highly technical and are not

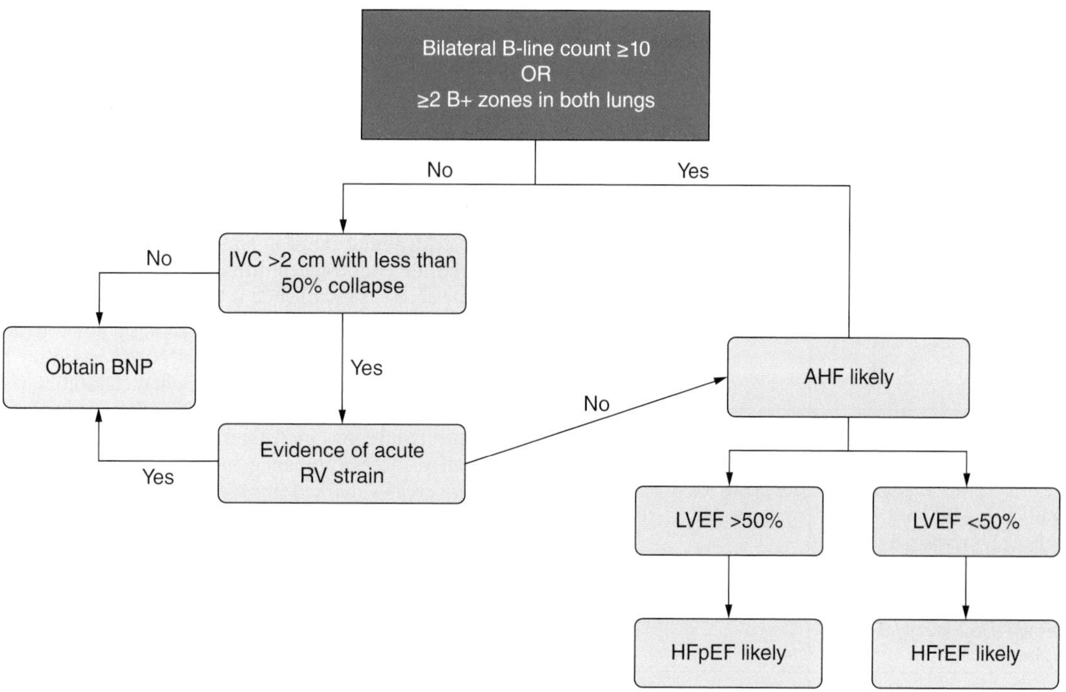

FIGURE 53-1. Bedside US use to identify acute heart failure (AHF) in dyspneic ED patients. BNP = B-type natriuretic peptide; IVC = inferior vena cava; HFpEF = heart failure with preserved ejection fraction; HFrEF = heart failure with reduced ejection fraction; LVEF = left ventricular ejection fraction; RV = right ventricle.

compatible with the need for rapid left ventricular ejection fraction determination during the initial ED evaluation of the dyspneic patient. However, with limited training, emergency physicians trained in focused cardiac US have reasonable agreement with expert cardiology interpretations by using a visual estimation of left ventricular ejection fraction into broad categories of normal, moderately reduced, and severely reduced.[37,38] Other markers that have been suggested, such as E-point septal separation and fractional shortening, are less reliable markers and may be more time-consuming.[39]

TREATMENT

The initial approach is driven by the acuity at presentation, hemodynamics, and volume status. In critically ill patients, airway management is the first priority to ensure adequate oxygenation and ventilation. In those less acutely ill, a focused evaluation ensues next, followed by treatment.

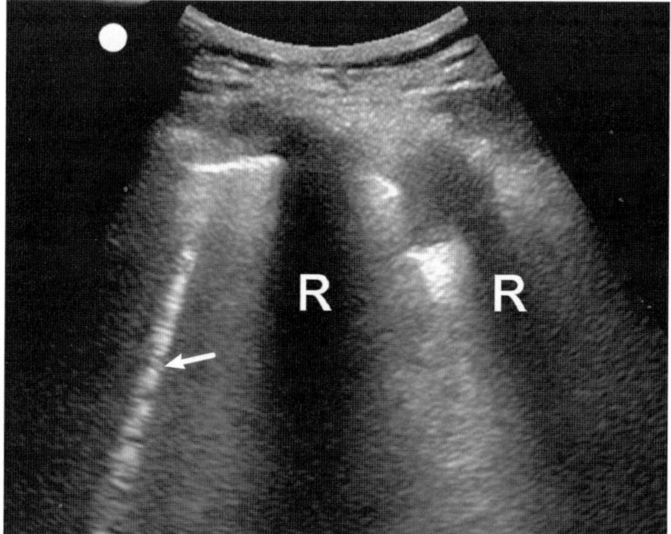

FIGURE 53-2. B lines representing thickened inter-alveolar/interlobular septa. R = rib; arrow = B line. [Reproduced with permission from Ma, Mateer, Reardon, and Joing (eds): *Emergency Ultrasound*, 3rd ed. McGraw-Hill, Inc., 2014. Fig. 7-5, Part C only.]

Supplemental oxygen use is guided by pulse oximetry, seeking saturations above 95%. Because hypoxemia is a greater risk than hypercarbia, do not withhold oxygen even when there is concern about carbon dioxide retention. Capnometry and arterial blood gas measurements can later help titrate therapy in the critically ill or if carbon dioxide retention is likely. In those with extreme findings, endotracheal intubation with mechanical ventilation is indicated.

Noninvasive ventilation may improve the symptoms in patients presenting with heart failure or pulmonary edema.[14,40] Successful noninvasive ventilation requires close monitoring, hemodynamic stability, facial anatomy that allows an adequate facemask seal, and patient cooperation. Using either a facemask or a nasal device, noninvasive ventilation can be delivered with continuous positive airway pressure throughout the respiratory cycle or with bilevel positive airway pressure (see chapter 28, "Noninvasive Airway Management"). Noninvasive ventilation plus standard medical therapy appears to reduce the need for intubation and improves respiratory distress and metabolic disturbance versus standard therapy alone.[14,15] Whether it decreases hospital mortality is unclear.[14]

Acute heart failure with hypotension occurs in approximately 3% of patients.[41] Consider acute coronary syndrome, and management may require reperfusion therapy (see chapters 49, "Acute Coronary Syndromes and 50, "Cardiogenic Shock"). Treatment includes the initiation of inotropic therapy (commonly norepinephrine, dopamine, or dobutamine) and admission to an intensive care unit.

Other standard initial measures include cardiac monitoring, pulse oximetry, IV access, and frequent vital sign assessments. A urinary drainage catheter may aid in monitoring fluid status in the severely ill or incontinent, but this is best reserved for those with extreme illness or an inability to void (to avoid catheter-related complications later.).

HYPERTENSIVE ACUTE HEART FAILURE

The failing heart is sensitive to increases in afterload, with some patients developing pulmonary edema with a systolic blood pressure as low as 150 mm Hg. Prompt recognition and afterload reduction with vasodilators can avoid the need for intubation.[42]

TABLE 53-6 Management of Hypertensive Acute Heart Failure*

Stepwise Approach	Comments
Administer oxygen as needed for saturation ≥95%; give sublingual nitroglycerin.	Sublingual nitroglycerin may be repeated up to one per minute.
If severe dyspnea, consider NIV or intubation.	
If BP >150/100 mm Hg, add IV nitroglycerin or nitroprusside; if BP falls below 100 mm Hg, stop nitrates, and monitor for persistent hypotension or symptoms (see chapter 50, "Cardiogenic Shock"). If BP <150/100 mm Hg after sublingual administration and if improved, consider transdermal nitroglycerin.	See chapter 58, "Pulmonary Hypertension"; see text for discussion of these agents.
Start IV loop diuretic (furosemide or bumetanide) in the setting of volume overload.	Initiate nitrates before diuretics.
Assess for severity of illness/high risk: altered mental status persistent, hypoxia despite NIV, hypotension, troponin elevation, ischemic ECG changes, blood urea nitrogen >43, creatinine >2.75, tachycardia, tachypnea, or inadequate urine output.	See chapter 49, "Acute Coronary Syndromes" for ECG criteria.
Admit to intensive care unit if high severity of illness or risk of decompensation.	
Choose discharge or ED observation unit admission if good response to therapy, no high-risk features, and good social support. Admit the rest. Admit to ICU if any ongoing cardiorespiratory compromise or acute ischemia.	Scoring systems may not reliably identify all patients at risk.

*Inclusion: SBP >140 mm Hg.

Abbreviations: BP = blood pressure; ICU = intensive care unit; NIV = noninvasive ventilation; SBP = systolic blood pressure.

Nitroglycerin A short-acting, rapid-onset, systemic venous and arterial dilator, **nitroglycerin** decreases mean arterial pressure by reducing preload and, at high doses initially, afterload. Nitroglycerin may have coronary vasodilatory effects, decreasing myocardial ischemia and improving cardiac function. The routes chosen—IV, sublingual, or transdermal—are often based on severity of symptoms. Sublingual nitroglycerin is easily administered, rapidly bioavailable, and can be given as often as needed to reach a desired clinical end point provided there is adequate blood pressure. An initial approach is repeated sublingual administration of nitroglycerin, 0.4 milligrams, at a rate of up to one per minute, until relief or replacement with IV nitroglycerin. When using the latter (often for those most symptomatic), a starting dose of 0.5 to 0.7 micrograms/kg/min is common and titrated every few minutes up to 200 micrograms/min based on the blood pressure (avoiding large drops) and symptoms (**Table 53-6**; see also Table 53-8). High doses may be beneficial in the acute setting, and adverse events are uncommon.[43] Apply transdermal nitroglycerine (0.5–2 inches to the chest wall based on blood pressure) **only** after initial therapy has improved conditions, or if symptoms are minor, because of the slow onset of action by this route.

The most important nitroglycerin complication is hypotension, often only lasting transiently and at times even seen with overall clinical improvement. Hypotension usually resolves after cessation of nitroglycerin. If persistent, think of concomitant volume depletion or right ventricular infarct, and deliver a normal saline fluid bolus (250 to 1000 mL). Headache is frequent, but acetaminophen usually is adequate therapy. Methemoglobinemia is a theoretic possibility but not a concern unless high doses are used for extended intervals. Despite broad uptake into regular clinical practice, nitroglycerin has been subject to surprisingly little prospective study.

Nitroprusside If further afterload reduction is required (i.e., continued high systemic vascular resistance usually manifested by persistent elevated blood pressure and continued symptoms despite nitroglycerin doses >200 micrograms/min), use IV **nitroprusside**. This drug is a more potent arterial vasodilator than nitroglycerin; its hemodynamic effects include decreased blood pressure, left ventricular filling pressure reduction, and increased cardiac output. The initial dose of nitroprusside is 0.3 micrograms/kg/min, titrated upward every 5 to 10 minutes based on blood pressure and clinical response (maximum 10 micrograms/kg/min). The major complication is hypotension. It is also associated with thiocyanate toxicity, especially with high doses, prolonged (longer than 3 days) use, and hepatic or renal impairment.

The critical end point is rapidly lowering filling pressure to prevent the need for endotracheal intubation. Give IV vasodilators as soon as vascular access is established if the blood pressure remains elevated.

Loop Diuretics After vasodilator therapy, some patients may require diuretics (see Table 53-8 and next section) based on continued symptoms after blood pressure is controlled. Diuretics (**furosemide** most commonly used) administered alone without vasodilators for hypertensive heart failure may increase mortality[44] and worsen renal dysfunction. Ultimately, successful management of blood pressure and cardiac filling pressure creates marked improvement in respiratory status long before any diuresis.

Contraindications and Alternatives to Vasodilation in Select Settings Because all vasodilators exert hypotensive effects, do not use if there are signs of hypoperfusion or existing hypotension. **Flow-limiting, preload-dependent states such as right ventricular infarction, aortic stenosis, hypertrophic obstructive cardiomyopathy, or volume depletion increase the risk of vasodilator-associated hypotension (Table 53-7).** Combined with acute pulmonary edema, the latter preload-dependent states are very difficult to manage. Therapy is aimed at decreasing the outflow gradient by slowing heart rate and cardiac contractility. Although this can be accomplished with IV β-blockers, treatment is best done in the intensive care unit with invasive hemodynamic guidance. If there is coexistent shock in the setting of hypertrophic obstructive cardiomyopathy, phenylephrine (40 to 100 micrograms/min IV) is a good choice because it creates peripheral vasoconstriction without increasing cardiac contractility.

NORMOTENSIVE HEART FAILURE

Shortness of breath, orthopnea, jugular venous distension, rales, and possibly an S_3 may still be evident even in the presence of normal vital signs, oxygenation, and ventilation. In this situation, treat with diuresis first, with further treatment based on response to therapy (**Table 53-8**).

Diuretics Loop diuretics provide rapid symptomatic relief of congestive symptoms and improve the effects of angiotensin-converting enzyme inhibitors by decreasing intravascular volume. Most ED patients require IV dosing, because bowel wall edema may prevent proper GI absorption. Dosing is guided by symptoms and prior usage (Table 53-8). In general, dose loop diuretics at the lowest possible dose that relieves congestion. Once congestion is resolved, a fixed maintenance dose is continued to prevent recurrence.

Loop diuretics promote water and sodium excretion and are effective except in severe renal dysfunction. Furosemide is inexpensive and effective. Alternatives are bumetanide (1 milligram equivalent to 40 milligrams of furosemide) or torsemide (20 milligrams equivalent to 40 milligrams of furosemide). All trigger rapid diuresis after an IV dose, often within 10 to 15 minutes.

TABLE 53-7 Causes of Hypotension after Vasodilator Use

Excessive vasodilation
Hypertrophic obstructive cardiomyopathy
Intravascular volume depletion
Right ventricular infarction
Cardiogenic shock/myocardial infarction
Aortic stenosis
Anaphylaxis
Unsuspected sepsis

TABLE 53-8 Medications for Acute Heart Failure

Vasodilators for Acute Heart Failure

Vasodilator	Dose	Titration End Point	Complications
Sublingual NTG	0.4 milligram every 1–5 min	Blood pressure	Hypotension
IV NTG	0.2–0.4 microgram/kg/min (starting dose)	Symptoms	Headache, hypotension
Nitroprusside	0.3 microgram/kg/min (starting dose), 10 micrograms/kg/min (maximum)	Blood pressure	Hypotension, cyanide/thiocyanate toxicity, coronary steal
		Symptoms	

Diuretics for Heart Failure

Diuretic	Dose (IV)	Effect	Complications
Furosemide	No prior use: 20–40 milligrams IVP	Diuresis starts within 15–20 min	↓K+, ↓Mg^{2+}, hyperuricemia, hypovolemia
	If prior use: total daily IV dose 1 to 2.5 times the patient's previous total daily oral dose, divided in half and given IV bolus every 12 h	Duration of action is 4–6 h	Ototoxicity, prerenal azotemia
	If no effect by 20–30 min, increase subsequent dose		
Bumetanide	1–3 milligrams IV	Diuresis starts within 10 min	Same as above
		Peak action at 60 min	
Torsemide	10–20 milligrams IV	Diuresis starts within 10 min	Same as above
		Peak action in 1–2 h	

Abbreviations: IVP = IV push; NTG = nitroglycerin; ↓ = decreased.

The DOSE trial suggests a total daily IV dose 1 to 2.5 times the patient's previous total daily oral dose, divided in half and administered by IV bolus every 12 hours.[45] For example, if the patient is on furosemide 80 milligrams PO twice a day, then an initial ED dose is 80 to 200 milligrams IV bolus. Higher doses are associated with more rapid symptom improvement but a slight decrease in renal function. For patients who are loop diuretic naïve, a reasonable starting dose is furosemide 40 milligrams IV. Bolus and continuous infusion therapy are equivalent, but the latter is more challenging in the ED and hence often eschewed. Ethacrynic acid (0.5 to 1 milligram/kg; maximum 100 milligrams) is another option. Sulfa allergy is generally not a concern with nonantibiotic drugs such as diuretics that contain a sulfa moiety (see chapter 206 "Antimicrobials" for more discussion).

Diuretics may worsen renal function and create hypokalemia. An increasing QT interval should trigger a search for hypocalcemia, hypokalemia, or hypomagnesemia. Ototoxicity is rare but may occur if diuretics are used in conjunction with aminoglycoside antibiotics. Potassium-sparing diuretics, such as spironolactone (25 to 50 milligrams PO), are generally reserved for advanced chronic heart failure; these are used more for their mortality benefit than diuretic effect.

Urinary diuretic response requires monitoring. With greater symptoms or less response to initial IV diuretics, double the dose and repeat in 30 to 60 minutes or as needed based on urine output. Ongoing congestion or dyspnea after a loop diuretic may signal the need for another therapy, such as a vasodilator.

Other Treatments **Ultrafiltration** allows the extracorporeal removal of plasma water from whole blood across a semipermeable membrane with a transmembrane pressure gradient.[46] Ultrafiltration has advantages over diuresis including more precise regulation of fluid removal, avoidance of diuretic-associated electrolyte abnormalities, a higher level of sodium removal for a given amount of volume, and attenuation of significant fluctuations in intravascular volume.[47] While initial studies provided promising safety and efficacy data,[48,49] subsequent study in patients with cardiorenal syndrome and persistent congestion did not demonstrate an advantage of ultrafiltration over bolus diuretic therapy.[50] If all diuretic and medical strategies are unsuccessful, consider ultrafiltration for patients with obvious volume overload to alleviate congestive symptoms and excess weight.[2] Ultrafiltration is unlikely to be deployed in the ED given the need to optimize other approaches first.

Morphine (2 to 5 milligrams IV) relieves congestion and anxiety, but it is associated with adverse events, including the need for mechanical ventilation, prolonged hospitalization, ICU admission, and mortality.[51] If desired for its venodilation properties or pain control, use morphine in small, titrated doses (2 to 4 milligrams IV) and with close monitoring. The trial noting harm did not set out to study morphine use, so selection bias may explain some or much of the findings. Only those failing standard therapy or with severe symptoms received the drug, multiplying the negative outcomes. Nonetheless, morphine has a role secondary to nitrates and loop diuretics and is not needed routinely.

Nesiritide is a vasodilator whose formulation uses recombinant human B-type natriuretic peptide. Several small studies suggested a benefit of adding nesiritide to standard therapy on patient-reported relief of dyspnea, but additional studies, including the pivotal mortality trial ASCEND-HF,[8] found no significant difference in the frequency of rehospitalization or mortality. ASCEND-HF reported an increased risk of both symptomatic and asymptomatic hypotension among patients randomized to nesiritide.[8] Nesiritide does not result in substantial clinical improvement when added to standard care and is a second-line agent when nitroglycerin is ineffective or contraindicated.

Angiotensin-converting enzyme inhibitors and angiotensin receptor blockers are given for hypertension and chronic heart failure, but there is little data to recommend use in the ED for acute heart failure.

Oral angiotensin-converting enzyme inhibitors decrease mortality and hospitalizations in patients with reduced ejection fraction[2]; these are often used after observation care if no contraindications exist after contact with a primary care physician or cardiologist. Oral angiotensin receptor blockers are alternatives to or can be added to angiotensin-converting enzyme inhibitors in select heart failure patients with reduced ejection fraction.[2] Their use may also be considered after consultation and the conclusion of treatment. Treatment of angiotensin-converting enzyme inhibitor–induced angioedema is outlined in the chapter 14, "Anaphylaxis, Allergies, and Angioedema."

β-Blockers are not usually initiated in the acute setting, except perhaps to control rate-related heart failure. They are generally reserved for stable patients. The rationale for β-blockers rests on the fact that norepinephrine levels are elevated in heart failure, contribute to myocardial hypertrophy, increase afterload and coronary vasoconstriction, and are associated with mortality. β-Blockers reduce sympathetic nervous system activity and are used for mortality reduction and symptom relief.

Drugs to Avoid in Acute Heart Failure Oral **calcium channel blockers** have myocardial depressant activity and are not routine treatment for acute heart failure, with trials demonstrating either no benefit or worse outcomes. If necessary, amlodipine may be used for compelling clinical reasons (e.g., as an antianginal agent despite maximal therapy with nitrates and β-blockers).

Avoid selective or nonselective **nonsteroidal anti-inflammatory drugs** in patients with acute heart failure. They can cause sodium and water retention and blunt the effects of diuretics,[2] and may increase morbidity and mortality.

DISPOSITION DECISIONS

While risk-stratification tools are commonplace in other ED disease processes such as chest pain and pneumonia, we lack a readily available and validated ED-based risk-stratification tool that has been compared to physician judgment.

Thus, disposition decisions in ED patients with acute heart failure are often based on physician judgment, a physiologic risk assessment, and an assessment of barriers to successful outpatient care such as caregiver support, access to medications, and timely follow-up (**Figure 53-3**). High-risk physiologic markers in ED patients with acute heart failure associated with morbidity and mortality (**Table 53-9**)[52] include renal dysfunction, low blood pressure, low serum sodium, and elevated natriuretic peptides or cardiac troponin. Unfortunately, high-risk markers are not present in up to 50% of ED patients, limiting the impact in disposition decisions.[53] Prospective testing of four acute heart failure prediction rules suggests they would not be useful in the ED.[54]

The unpredictability of postdischarge behavior and care limits, coupled with the elevated overall risk of harm or repeated care events, limits the ability to discharge patients directly from the ED. Admit patients with high-risk features to the hospital (**Table 53-10**).[55] Those who require invasive monitoring or procedures require intensive care unit admission. Others may be appropriate for non–intensive care unit level care. Observation unit management is an option in others with lower risk features. Many patients do not have high-risk features at initial ED evaluation and experience improvement in dyspnea during their ED stay as a result of standard therapy.[56] Many have complete symptom resolution within 12 to 24 hours of initial therapy, a typical time period of observation. The monitoring of blood pressure, heart rate, urine output, and body weight is easily accomplished in the observation setting, and any diagnostic testing (labs, echocardiography) needed can occur. Finally, an extended observation interval allows patients to receive heart failure education, confirm outpatient medications, and arrange follow-up prior to discharge. Ideally, outpatient follow-up within 5 days can decrease readmissions.[57] Prior studies suggest 75% of patients will respond to therapy, will have no identifiable high-risk features, and will be discharged home. Their rates of readmission

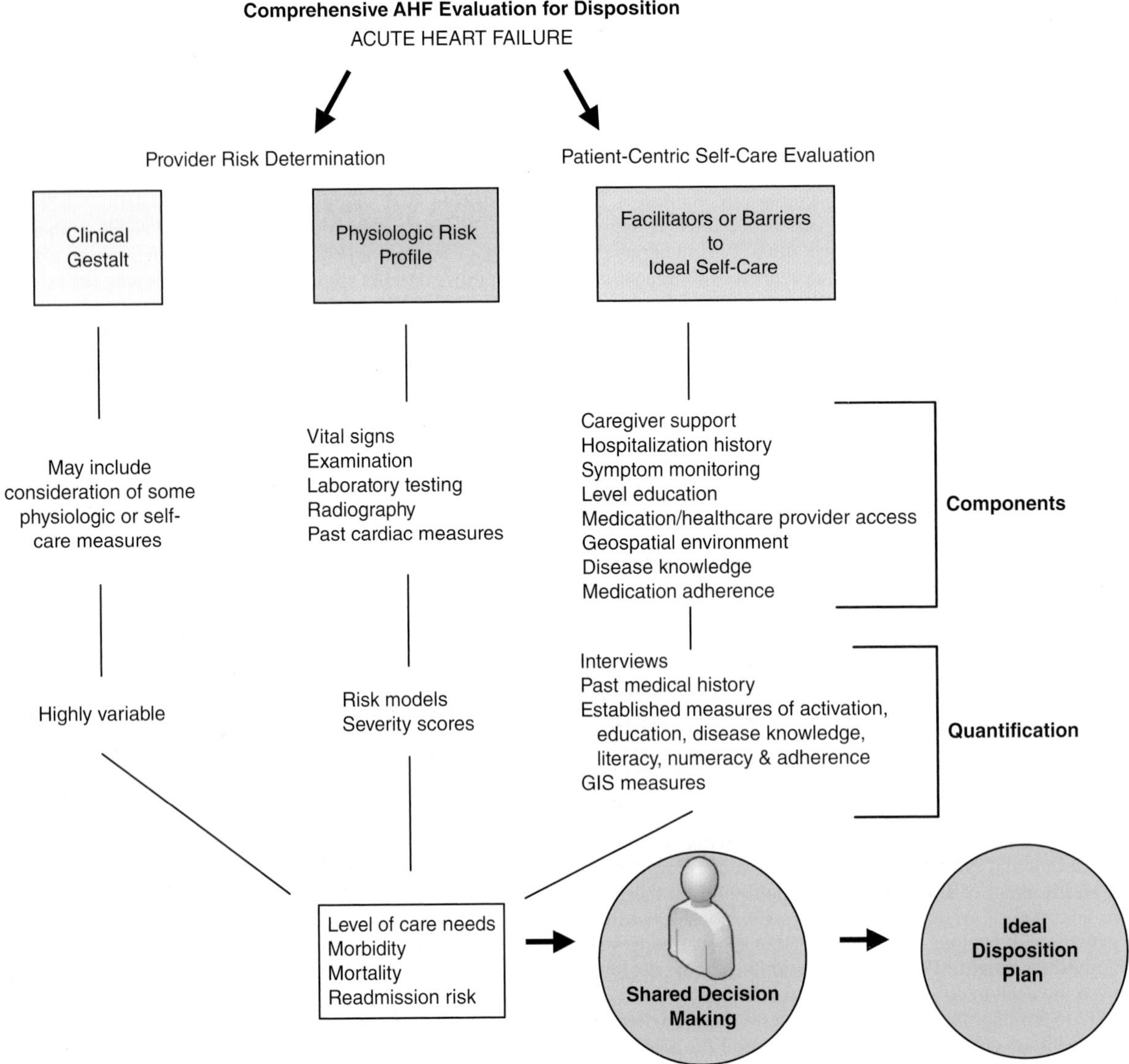

FIGURE 53-3. Factors impacting disposition decisions in ED patients with acute heart failure (AHF).

TABLE 53-9 Selected ED-Based Risk-Stratification Studies from the Last 8 Years that Examine Events within 30 Days or Less of Index ED Presentation

Author/Year	N	Predicted Outcome	Variables in Final Model	Low-Risk Markers
Lassus/2013	441–4450 (pooled analysis, total n varied by biomarker evaluated)	30-d and 1-y mortality	ST2, MR-proADM, CRP, NT-proBNP, BNP, MR-proANP in addition to clinical model (age, gender, blood pressure on admission, estimated glomerular filtration rate <60 mL/min/1.73 m^2, sodium and hemoglobin levels, and heart rate)	No
Stiell/2013	559	30-d death and 14-d serious nonfatal events	History of TIA/CVA, vital signs, ECG and lab findings	No
Lee/2012	15,164	7-d mortality	Creatinine, BP, O_2 saturation, Tn, history of cancer, home metolazone, EMS transport	Yes
Hsieh/2008	8384	Inpatient mortality or serious medical complications, 30-d mortality	pH, pulse, renal function, WBC, glucose, sodium	Yes
Lee/2003	2624/1407	30-d mortality	Age, RR, BP, BUN, sodium, cerebrovascular disease, dementia, COPD, cirrhosis, cancer, hemoglobin	Yes
Auble/2005	33,533	Inpatient mortality or serious medical complications, 30-d mortality and AHF readmission	pH, pulse, renal function, WBC, glucose, sodium	Yes
Fonarow/2005	65,275	In-hospital mortality	BUN, systolic BP, creatinine	No

Abbreviations: AHF = acute heart failure; ANP = atrial natriuretic peptide; BNP = B-type natriuretic peptide; BP = blood pressure; COPD = chronic obstructive pulmonary disease; CRP = C-reactive protein; CVA = cerebrovascular accident; RR = respiratory rate; TIA = transient ischemic attack; Tn = troponin.

TABLE 53-10 Heart Failure Observation Unit/Short Stay Exclusion Criteria

Recommended Exclusions
- Positive troponin
- Blood urea nitrogen >40 milligrams/dL
- Creatinine >3.0 milligrams/dL
- Sodium <135 mEq/L
- New ischemic changes on ECG
- New onset of acute heart failure*
- IV vasoactive infusions being actively titrated
- Significant comorbidities requiring acute interventions
- Respiratory rate ≥32 breaths/min and/or requiring noninvasive ventilation at the time of OU consideration
- Signs of poor perfusion at the time of OU consideration

Suggested Exclusions
- Poor social support
- Poor follow-up

*Although part of the published guidelines, many institutions admit patients to OUs with new-onset heart failure.

Abbreviation: OU = observation unit.

are similar to or better than those who are managed in an inpatient setting.[58,59] Patients with an inadequate response to initial therapy or with high-risk features identified during their observation stay are admitted to the hospital for further management. An observation unit strategy can help reduce costs while delivering quality care for select lower risk ED patients with acute heart failure.[58]

Acknowledgments: The authors wish to acknowledge Dr. W. Franklin Peacock, IV, for his contributions to the previous edition and to thank Amy Diatikar for her assistance with chapter preparation.

REFERENCES

The complete reference list is available online at www.TintinalliEM.com.

Valvular Emergencies

William D. Alley
Simon A. Mahler

INTRODUCTION

In contrast to the dramatic symptoms associated with acute valvular dysfunction, most valvular heart disease encountered in the ED is chronic and incidentally noted on exam. Adaptive responses preserve cardiac function and can delay the diagnosis of chronic valvular disease for decades but contribute to eventual cardiac dysfunction. Compared with the general population, patients with clinically evident valvular heart disease have a 2.5-fold higher death rate and a 3-fold increased rate of stroke.[1]

THE NEWLY DISCOVERED MURMUR

After discovering a new murmur, the first step in the ED is to determine the clinical significance. Benign or physiologic murmurs do not cause symptoms or findings compatible with cardiovascular disease; they are generally soft systolic ejection murmurs that begin after S_1, end before S_2, and are not associated with abnormal heart sounds. Systolic murmurs may be associated with anemia, sepsis, volume overload, or other conditions causing an increased cardiac output. Evaluation and treatment are focused on the underlying trigger rather than the murmur itself. Patients without chest pain, dyspnea, fever, or other signs attributable to valvular disease do not need emergent echocardiography but should be referred for eventual imaging.

Any diastolic murmur or new systolic murmur with symptoms at rest is pathologic and warrants emergent echocardiographic imaging. Patients with syncope from suspected aortic stenosis require admission for monitoring and echocardiography (**Figure 54-1**). **Table 54-1** presents a grading system for murmurs. Another consideration in the newly diagnosed murmur is the possibility of endocarditis, especially in suspected valvular insufficiency (see chapter 155, "Endocarditis").

MITRAL STENOSIS

EPIDEMIOLOGY AND PATHOPHYSIOLOGY

Mitral stenosis prevents normal diastolic filling of the left ventricle. Despite declining frequency, rheumatic heart disease remains the most

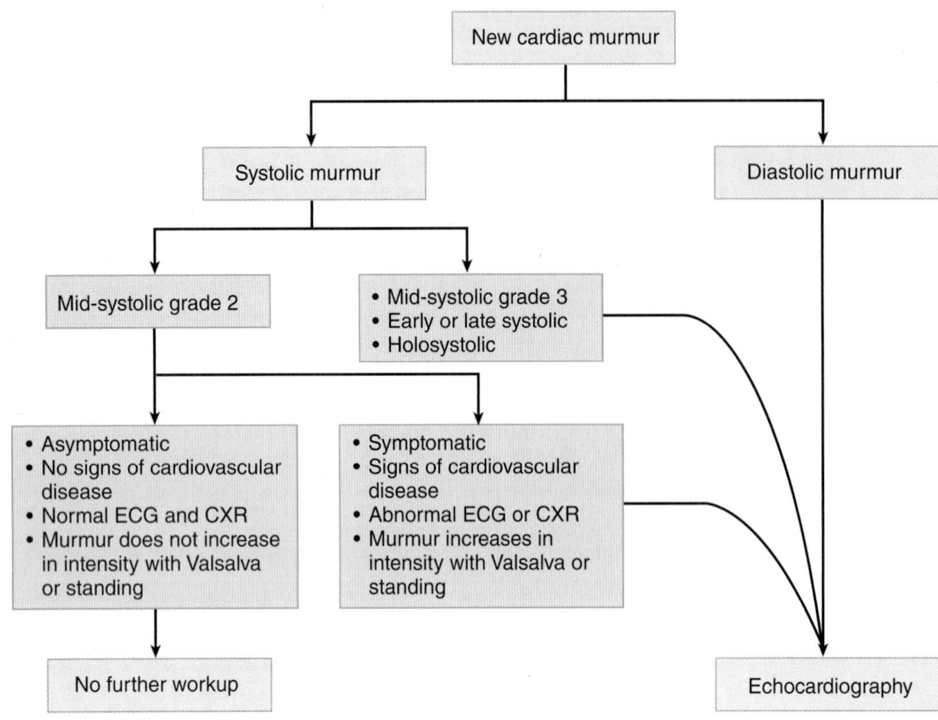

FIGURE 54-1. Algorithm for evaluation of newly discovered systolic murmur. CXR = chest x-ray.

common cause worldwide. Rheumatic carditis causes fusion of valvular commissures, matting of chordae tendineae, and eventual calcification and limited mobility of the valve. Valvular obstruction is slowly progressive, often with 20 to 40 years before onset of symptoms. Mitral valve obstruction causes left atrial pressure to rise, resulting in left atrial enlargement, pulmonary congestion, pulmonary hypertension, and frequently atrial fibrillation. In severe disease, pulmonary hypertension may lead to pulmonic and tricuspid valve incompetence, pulmonary edema, right-sided heart failure, and bronchial vein rupture.

Mitral annular calcification is a slowly progressive nonrheumatic cause of mitral stenosis. It is more common among women, elderly, and those with hypertension or with chronic renal failure.[2] Due to its slow progression, mitral annular calcification rarely causes severe symptoms.

CLINICAL FEATURES

Exertional dyspnea is the most frequent presenting complaint in patients with mitral stenosis. It is often precipitated by anemia or infection, which increases cardiac demand. Orthopnea and premature atrial contractions are also common. Symptoms associated with left- or right-sided heart failure may occur with more severe obstruction. Systemic emboli are a risk, especially when accompanied by atrial fibrillation. Due to earlier recognition and treatment, hemoptysis is a rare presenting symptom, although it can be massive.

Signs of mitral stenosis include a mid-diastolic rumbling murmur with crescendo toward S_2. With the onset of atrial fibrillation, the presystolic accentuation of the murmur disappears. Typically, the S_1 is loud and is followed by a loud opening snap that is high-pitched and best heard to the right of the apex (**Table 54-2**). The apical impulse is small and tapping due to an underfilled left ventricle. Systemic blood pressure is typically normal or low. If pulmonary hypertension is present, signs may include a thin body habitus, peripheral cyanosis, and cool extremities due to compromised cardiac output. Auscultatory findings are less obvious.

TABLE 54-1 A Grading System for Murmurs

Grade	Description
1	Faint, may not be heard in all positions
2	Quiet, but heard immediately with stethoscope placement onto the chest wall
3	Moderately loud
4	Loud
5	Heard with stethoscope partly off the chest wall
6	Heard when stethoscope is entirely off the chest wall

DIAGNOSIS AND TREATMENT

The ECG may demonstrate notched or biphasic P waves and right axis deviation in patients with mitral stenosis (**Figure 54-2**). On chest radiograph, straightening of the left heart border, indicating left atrial enlargement, is a typical and early radiographic finding. Eventually, findings of pulmonary congestion are noted.

The diagnosis is confirmed with echocardiography (**Figure 54-3**). In candidates for surgical repair, transesophageal echocardiography best

TABLE 54-2 Comparison of Heart Murmurs, Sounds, and Signs

Valve Disorder	Murmur	Heart Sounds and Signs
Mitral stenosis	Mid-diastolic rumble, crescendos into S_2	Loud snapping S_1, small apical impulse, tapping due to underfilled ventricle
Mitral regurgitation	Acute: harsh apical systolic murmur starts with S_1 and may end before S_2 Chronic: high-pitched apical holosystolic murmur radiating into S_2	S_3 and S_4 may be heard
Mitral valve prolapse	Click may be followed by a late systolic murmur that crescendos into S_2	Mid-systolic click; S_2 may be diminished by the late systolic murmur
Aortic stenosis	Harsh systolic ejection murmur	Paradoxical splitting of S_2, S_3, and S_4 may be present; pulse of small amplitude with a slow rise and sustained peak
Aortic regurgitation	High-pitched blowing diastolic murmur immediately after S_2	S_3 may be present; wide pulse pressure

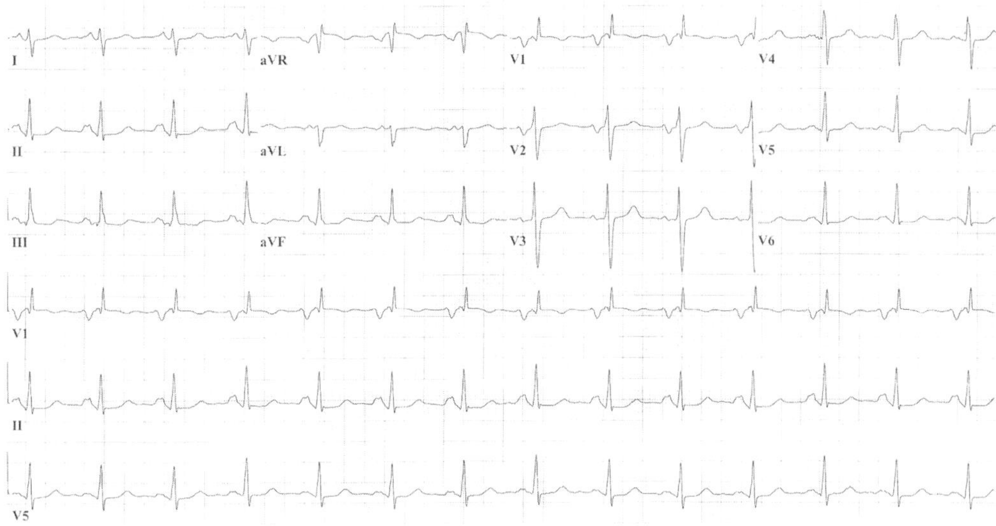

FIGURE 54-2. The ECG in mitral stenosis, demonstrating left atrial enlargement and right axis deviation. Note abnormal P waves in lead V_2.

assesses the degree of mitral regurgitation and the presence of a left atrial thrombus.[3]

Medical management focuses primarily on symptom control and anticoagulation. Patients in atrial fibrillation with rapid ventricular response or with dyspnea on exertion may benefit from heart rate control (see chapter 18, "Cardiac Rhythm Disturbances"). Experts recommend anticoagulation if the left atrial diameter is greater than 55 mm or the patient has atrial fibrillation, a left atrial thrombus, or history of systemic emboli. In patients who present with hemoptysis from mitral stenosis–induced pulmonary hypertension, bleeding may be severe enough to require blood transfusion, emergent bronchoscopy, and consultation with a thoracic surgeon.

The most important ED action for patients with suspected but asymptomatic mitral stenosis is recognition and referral. The primary treatment for symptomatic disease is mechanical intervention, by balloon valvotomy, valve repair, or valve replacement, all optimally performed before the onset of severe pulmonary hypertension.

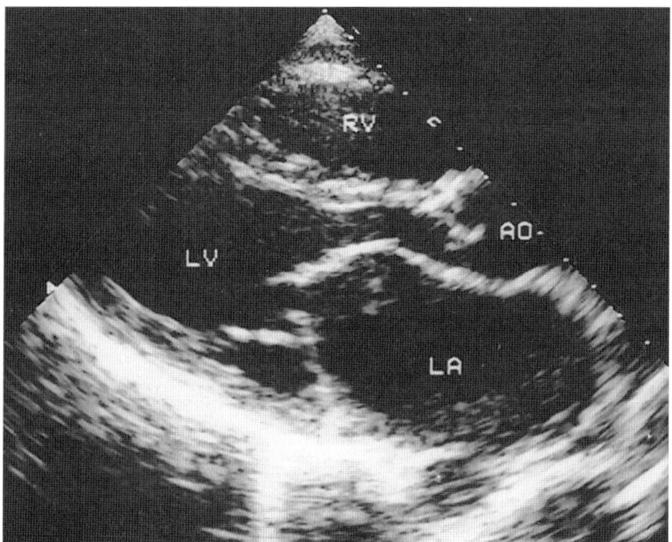

FIGURE 54-3. Parasternal long-axis view of mitral stenosis. The left atrium is enlarged, mitral opening is limited, and doming of the anterior mitral leaflet is present. AO = aorta; LA = left atrium; LV = left ventricle; RV = right ventricle. [Reproduced with permission from Fuster V, O'Rourke RA, Walsh RA, Poole-Wilson P (eds): *Hurst's the Heart*, 12th ed. © 2008, McGraw-Hill, New York.]

MITRAL REGURGITATION

EPIDEMIOLOGY AND PATHOPHYSIOLOGY

Mitral regurgitation occurs when a dysfunctional valve allows retrograde blood flow from the left ventricle into the left atrium during systole. Most patients with mitral regurgitation follow a chronic and slowly progressive course. The most common cause is fibroelastic deficiency syndrome, seen primarily in the elderly.[4] **Mitral valve prolapse** is another cause of mitral regurgitation and is typically found in younger patients. Secondary mitral regurgitation occurs when a dilated left ventricle causes papillary muscle displacement and valve dysfunction.

In chronic mitral regurgitation, the left atrium dilates to accommodate increasing regurgitant flow to keep left atrial pressure near normal. Stroke volume is augmented, maintaining effective forward flow despite a large regurgitant volume. In contrast, acute mitral regurgitation results in new-onset pulmonary vascular congestion and peripheral edema. Cardiogenic shock may also exist from impaired forward blood flow. **Acute mitral regurgitation** is typically caused by papillary muscle or chordae tendineae rupture from myocardial infarction or valve leaflet perforation from infective endocarditis. Blunt thoracic trauma and spontaneous chordae tendineae rupture are other rare causes.

CLINICAL FEATURES

Symptoms of acute mitral regurgitation are severe dyspnea, tachycardia, and pulmonary edema. Cardiogenic shock or cardiac arrest can develop rapidly. Typical signs include an S_4 gallop and a harsh apical systolic murmur loudest in early or mid-systole, diminishing before S_2 (Table 54-2). Even with severe symptoms, the murmur may not be audible over breath sounds in the noisy ED environment. A hyperactive apical impulse may be apparent. In the setting of ischemia, chest pain may be masked by overwhelming dyspnea.

Chronic mitral regurgitation can be tolerated for years without symptoms. Eventually exertional dyspnea develops, sometimes associated with palpitations or atrial fibrillation. Signs include a late systolic left parasternal lift and lateral displacement of the apical impulse. A high-pitched holosystolic murmur is best heard in the fifth intercostal space and mid-left thorax and radiates to the axilla. The first heart sound is soft and often obscured by the murmur. An S_3 is usually heard and is followed by a short diastolic rumble, indicating increased flow into the left ventricle. Given its slowly progressive course, signs of systemic thromboembolism may be the first suggestion of mitral regurgitation associated with atrial fibrillation.

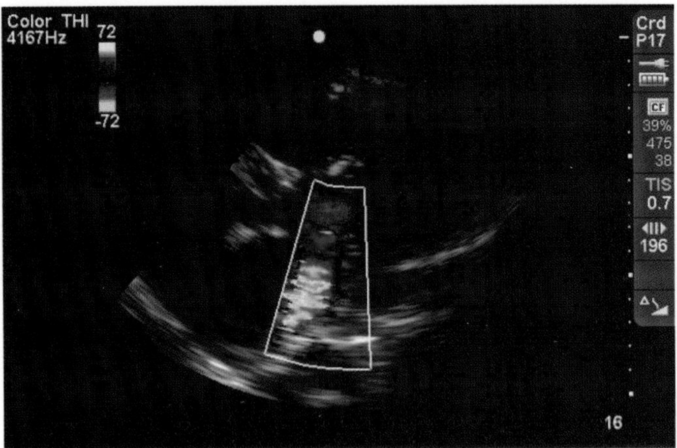

FIGURE 54-4. An echocardiogram demonstrating severe mitral regurgitation. Color flow Doppler shows regurgitant flow back into the left atrium.

DIAGNOSIS AND TREATMENT

Think of acute mitral regurgitation in any patient with new-onset and marked pulmonary edema, especially in patients with near-normal heart size on chest radiograph or in those who do not respond to conventional therapy. Obtain an ECG to look for signs of ischemia, frequently in the inferior or anterior walls. In chronic mitral regurgitation, the ECG may demonstrate left atrial enlargement and left ventricular hypertrophy, and the chest x-ray shows left atrial and ventricular enlargement that is proportional to the severity of the regurgitant volume. Transthoracic echocardiography (**Figure 54-4**) diagnoses mitral regurgitation, but may underestimate the severity of regurgitation. If transthoracic echocardiography is nondiagnostic, cardiac MRI or transesophageal echocardiography may be undertaken.[3] Exercise stress echocardiography may also be useful.

For acute mitral regurgitation due to papillary muscle rupture, emergency surgery is the treatment of choice. In the ED, start therapy with oxygen and positive-pressure ventilation for respiratory failure (see chapter 53, "Acute Heart Failure"). Nitrates provide afterload reduction, which results in increased forward flow into the aorta and partially restores mitral valve competence as left ventricular size diminishes. Inotropic therapy with dobutamine may be necessary. Aortic balloon counterpulsation increases forward flow and mean arterial pressure while diminishing regurgitant volume and left ventricular filling pressure.

Treatment of severe mitral regurgitation from acute myocardial infarction includes emergent revascularization.[5] Endocarditis as a cause of acute mitral valve insufficiency requires specific evaluation and treatment (see chapter 155, "Endocarditis").

Medical therapy may improve regurgitant flow and allow a delay to surgery. The key is emergency cardiology and surgical consultation while medically optimizing care.

In patients with chronic mitral regurgitation, treat acute symptoms. Control atrial fibrillation with rapid ventricular response with β-blockers or calcium channel blockers, and start anticoagulation to avoid embolization. Long-term management is best decided by the primary care provider or a cardiologist.

MITRAL VALVE PROLAPSE

EPIDEMIOLOGY AND PATHOPHYSIOLOGY

Mitral valve prolapse is a systolic billowing of one or both leaflets into the left atrium occurring with or without mitral regurgitation. It is characterized by myxomatous degeneration of the valve caused by heritable defects in connective tissue proteins. It is the most common valvular heart disease in industrialized countries, affecting approximately 2.4% of the population.[6] Morbidity and mortality are greatly influenced by the presence of concomitant mitral regurgitation.[7]

CLINICAL FEATURES

Most patients with mitral valve prolapse are asymptomatic. Associated symptoms can include nonclassic chest pain, palpitations, fatigue, anxiety, and dyspnea unrelated to exertion. Signs such as scoliosis, pectus excavatum, and low body weight can also be associated. If exercise induces symptoms, morbidity increases.[8]

The classic auscultatory finding is a mid-systolic click (Table 54-2). Maneuvers that decrease preload, such as Valsalva or standing, will cause the click to occur earlier in diastole. Increasing preload by squatting or afterload by hand grips causes the systolic click to move later in systole. A late systolic murmur that crescendos into S_2 is present in some patients.

DIAGNOSIS AND TREATMENT

The diagnosis is unlikely to be made in the ED. The emergency evaluation focuses on late complications such as atrial fibrillation or heart failure. The ECG is usually normal, as is the chest radiograph unless scoliosis or pectus excavatum is seen. If mitral valve prolapse is suspected, refer the patient to a cardiologist for outpatient echocardiography to confirm the diagnosis and to identify any associated mitral regurgitation.[9]

ED treatment is rarely required. Patients with palpitations attributed to mitral valve prolapse may respond to oral β-blockers, but that treatment is typically left to the cardiologist or primary care physician. Antithrombotic therapy is not routinely recommended unless complicated by transient ischemic attacks, stroke, or atrial fibrillation.[10,11] Patients with mitral valve prolapse *and* concomitant mitral regurgitation require endocarditis prophylaxis (see chapter 155, "Endocarditis").[9]

AORTIC STENOSIS

EPIDEMIOLOGY AND PATHOPHYSIOLOGY

Aortic stenosis is a structural abnormality of the aortic valve that prevents left ventricular outflow. In the United States, the most common cause of adult aortic stenosis is degenerative calcification (calcific aortic stenosis), associated with increasing age, hypertension, smoking, elevated cholesterol, and diabetes.[12] Rheumatic heart disease is a major cause of aortic valve disease worldwide. Bicuspid aortic valves and congenital heart disease are causes as well, especially in younger patients. The prevalence of aortic stenosis is about 3% of patients >74 years old.[13]

The typical course involves a long asymptomatic period, during which the left ventricle hypertrophies to preserve ejection fraction. Ventricular hypertrophy eventually impairs diastolic filling and increases myocardial oxygen demand. Slowly, aortic valve obstruction worsens, cardiac output diminishes, and systemic blood flow and coronary blood flow are impaired.

CLINICAL FEATURES

The classic triad of aortic stenosis is dyspnea, chest pain, and syncope. However, many patients with severe stenosis (aortic valve area <1.0 cm^2) are asymptomatic. Often, a long asymptomatic period is followed by stepwise onset of symptoms starting with dyspnea followed by chest pain, then syncope, and finally signs of heart failure. Once symptoms start, mortality increases.[14] Decreased exercise tolerance and exertional dyspnea or dizziness may be unnoticed or unreported prior to more ominous symptoms.

Classic physical examination findings are a late peaking systolic murmur at the right second intercostal space, radiating to the carotids, a single or paradoxically split S_2, an S_4 gallop, and a diminished carotid pulse with a delayed upstroke (pulsus parvus et tardus; Table 54-2). Brachioradial delay may also be a useful early finding. Simultaneously palpate the patient's right brachial artery and right radial artery. Any palpable delay between the brachial and radial pulses is abnormal. A narrowed pulse pressure, with or without hypotension, is another important clinical finding.

Aortic stenosis with atrial fibrillation can have dire consequences. Patients with AS typically have diastolic dysfunction and are dependent on preload from atrial contraction to maintain cardiac output. Without effective atrial contraction, cardiac output drops dramatically, especially if the patient is given nitroglycerin to treat chest pain or dyspnea.

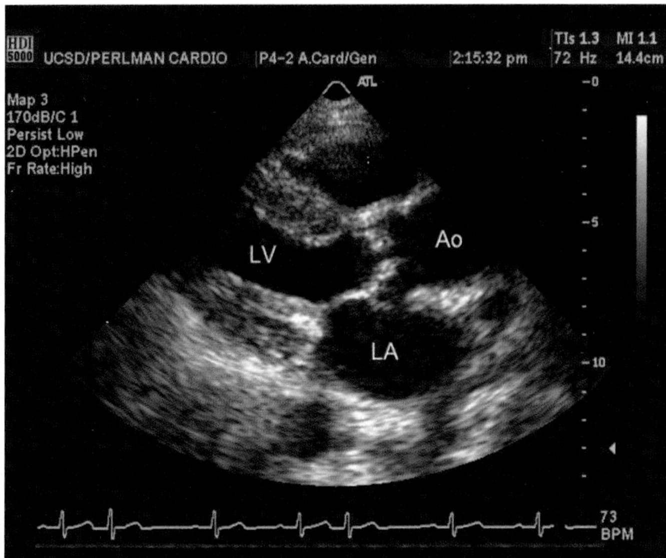

FIGURE 54-5. Parasternal long-axis plane demonstrating a thickened, stenotic aortic valve. Ao = aorta; LA = left atrium; LV = left ventricle. [Reproduced with permission from Fuster V, O'Rourke RA, Walsh RA, Poole-Wilson P (eds): *Hurst's the Heart*, 12th ed. © 2008, McGraw-Hill, New York.]

DIAGNOSIS AND TREATMENT

ECG and chest radiograph findings lack sensitivity and specificity. The ECG usually demonstrates left ventricular hypertrophy, and a left or right bundle-branch block may be present in up to 10% of patients. The chest radiograph is normal early in the disease, but eventually signs of left ventricular hypertrophy and congestive heart failure develop. Transthoracic echocardiography confirms the diagnosis and determines severity (**Figure 54-5**). Low-dose dobutamine stress echocardiography may be useful to identify patients with severe aortic stenosis prior to the development of classic symptoms.[3]

Treat pulmonary edema with oxygen and positive-pressure ventilation as necessary. Negative inotropic drugs, such as β-blockers or calcium channel blockers, are often poorly tolerated. **Use nitrates, vasodilators, and diuretics with caution** because reducing preload or afterload may cause significant hypotension. New-onset atrial fibrillation may require cardioversion to maintain cardiac output.

Most patients with newly symptomatic aortic stenosis are admitted. Without surgery, 40% to 50% of patients with classic symptoms die within 1 year.[15,16] Patients discharged from the ED should avoid vigorous physical activity and be seen promptly by a cardiologist. Endocarditis in isolated aortic stenosis is uncommon, and antibiotic prophylaxis is not recommended routinely (see chapter 155, "Endocarditis").[9]

AORTIC REGURGITATION

EPIDEMIOLOGY AND PATHOPHYSIOLOGY

Aortic regurgitation occurs when valve leaflets fail to close fully, causing blood to flow from the aorta into the left ventricle during diastole. The course is usually slowly progressive, with many patients remaining asymptomatic for decades. Over time, aortic regurgitation increases left ventricular wall stress, leading to hypertrophy. Increased stroke volume followed by a rapid pressure drop during diastole causes wide pulse pressures. Tachycardia shortens diastole, which decreases regurgitant volume and mutes symptoms early in the disease. In contrast, increased afterload during stress or isometric exercise exacerbates regurgitant flow and may precipitate symptoms. Over time, the combination of increasing left ventricular dilatation and hypertrophy compromises systolic function, and reduced cardiac output results in symptoms of heart failure.

Among patients in the Framingham Heart Study receiving echocardiography, aortic insufficiency was documented in 13% of men and 8.5% of women, mostly of trace or minor severity.[17] Approximately half of cases are due to valvular leaflet problems from bicuspid aortic valves, infective endocarditis, or rheumatic disease. Nonvalvular causes include aortic dissection, Marfan's syndrome, or aortitis.[18] Aortic regurgitation is also frequently associated with aortic stenosis, and at times, associated regurgitation may be severe.

CLINICAL FEATURES

Acute aortic regurgitation generally presents rapidly, with dyspnea and pulmonary edema being the most common presenting symptoms. To maintain cardiac output, tachycardia develops, but is often inadequate, resulting in cardiogenic shock or cardiac arrest. Sudden-onset ripping or tearing interscapular pain suggests **aortic dissection**. Fever or a history of IV drug abuse suggests endocarditis.

On physical exam, aortic regurgitation is associated with a high-pitched blowing diastolic murmur heard immediately after S_2, in the second or third intercostal space at the left sternal border (Table 54-2). In acute disease, the murmur may be inaudible due to tachycardia, tachypnea, and rales. A systolic ejection murmur due to increased stroke volume and an S_3 due to ventricular dilatation may also be heard. In the left lateral decubitus position, a mid-diastolic rumble (Austin Flint murmur) may be appreciated using the bell of the stethoscope at the cardiac apex. Patients often have a widened pulse pressure. The classic "water hammer pulse" (Corrigan pulse) is a peripheral pulse with a quick rise in upstroke due to increased stroke volume followed by collapse from a rapid fall in diastolic pressure. Other classic findings include accentuated precordial apical thrust, pulsus bisferiens, Duroziez sign (a "to-and-fro" femoral murmur), de Musset sign (pulsatile head bobbing), and Quincke sign (capillary pulsations visible at the proximal nail bed while pressure is applied at the tip).

Patients with chronic aortic regurgitation typically present with exertional dyspnea or fatigue. Chest pain may occur from myocardial ischemia due to low diastolic pressures that decrease coronary blood flow. Palpitations may be caused by large stroke volume or premature ventricular contractions. Symptoms of left ventricular failure may occur late in the course of the disease, but greater than one quarter of patients with chronic aortic regurgitation who die or develop left heart dysfunction do so before symptoms occur.[9]

DIAGNOSIS AND TREATMENT

Echocardiography confirms the diagnosis and determines the cause and severity of regurgitation.[3] Unstable patients require bedside transthoracic echocardiography (**Figure 54-6**). Chest x-ray may show acute

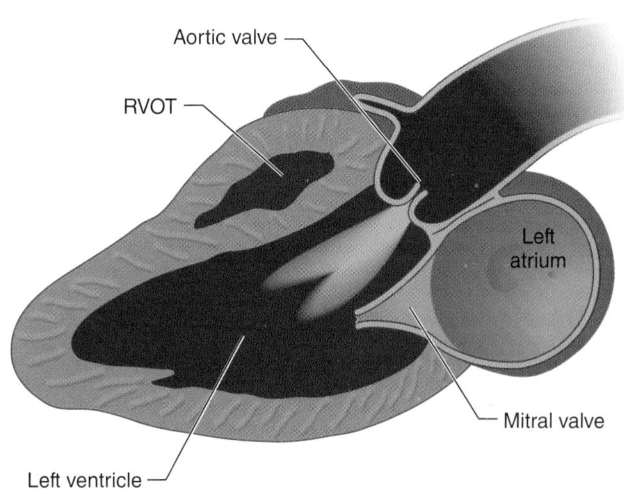

FIGURE 54-6. An illustration of an echocardiogram demonstrating aortic regurgitation. Note regurgitant flow back into the left ventricle. RVOT = right ventricular outflow tract. [Courtesy of P. Lynch, MD, Yale Cardiology Department and Cancer Imaging Program, with permission.]

pulmonary edema without cardiac enlargement. In aortic regurgitation due to aortic dissection, the chest x-ray may have additional findings associated with dissection such as a widened mediastinum (see chapter 59, "Aortic Dissection and Related Aortic Syndromes"). If aortic dissection is suspected, CT with contrast is needed to assess the aorta, and transesophageal echocardiography is needed to assess valvular function. ECG findings in patients include sinus tachycardia and are generally nonspecific. Ischemic changes or ST elevation may be seen from aortic dissection involving the coronary arteries. In chronic aortic regurgitation, the chest x-ray reveals cardiomegaly, aortic dilatation, and, possibly, evidence of congestive heart failure. The most common ECG abnormality is left ventricular hypertrophy.

Acute aortic regurgitation requires immediate surgical intervention. Treat pulmonary edema with oxygen and intubation for respiratory failure. Nitroprusside, combined with inotropic agents such as dobutamine or dopamine, can augment forward flow and reduce left ventricular end-diastolic pressure. Diuretics and nitrates are usually ineffective. **Although β-blockers are commonly used in aortic dissection, avoid these in acute aortic regurgitation** because they block the compensatory tachycardia that is critical in maintaining cardiac output. Intra-aortic balloon counterpulsation is also contraindicated because it worsens regurgitant flow. Despite intensive medical management, death from ventricular dysrhythmias, pulmonary edema, or cardiogenic shock is common. In patients with only mild acute aortic regurgitation due to endocarditis, antibiotics may be adequate treatment without acute surgical intervention (see chapter 155).

Chronic aortic regurgitation is usually treated with vasodilators such as angiotensin-converting enzyme inhibitors or dihydropyridine calcium channel blockers.[3] If acute symptoms such as pulmonary edema or chest pain occur, admit the patient for stabilization and further management. Patients who become symptomatic, have a low ejection fraction, or have significant left ventricular dilatation are candidates for aortic valve replacement.

RIGHT-SIDED VALVULAR HEART DISEASE

EPIDEMIOLOGY AND PATHOPHYSIOLOGY

The incidence of true right-sided valvular heart disease is not known because normal subjects frequently have a small amount of tricuspid and pulmonary valve regurgitation at baseline. Pathologic **tricuspid regurgitation** is usually due to elevated right heart pressure or volume overload, such as from pulmonary hypertension, chronic lung disease, pulmonary embolism, or atrial septal defects. **Tricuspid stenosis** is rare and is generally accompanied by regurgitation. The **pulmonic valve** is the least likely valve to be affected by acquired disease. Most pulmonic valvular disease is congenital (see chapter 126, "Congenital and Acquired Pediatric Heart Disease"), although pulmonary hypertension, rheumatic heart disease, and carcinoid syndrome can rarely cause some degree of pulmonic valve disease. Acute onset of symptomatic tricuspid disease is most often due to endocarditis. Tricuspid valve endocarditis typically involves aggressive organisms, such as *Staphylococcus aureus,* which can cause rapid valve destruction.

CLINICAL FEATURES

Clinically significant right-sided valvular disease causes signs and symptoms of right heart failure such as jugular venous distention, peripheral edema, hepatomegaly, splenomegaly, and ascites. Exertional dyspnea is often the first symptom in patients with right-sided valvular disease associated with pulmonary hypertension. Patients with tricuspid valve regurgitation from endocarditis are often acutely ill with signs of sepsis. The murmur of tricuspid valve regurgitation is soft, blowing, and holosystolic. It is best heard along the lower left sternal border and increases with inspiration. A systolic waveform in the jugular vein, hepatic pulsations, and systolic eyeball propulsion may be seen in severe tricuspid incompetence. Tricuspid valve stenosis is associated with a rumbling crescendo-decrescendo diastolic murmur occurring just before S_1. This murmur is best heard along the lower left sternal border, increases with inspiration, and is often preceded by an opening snap.

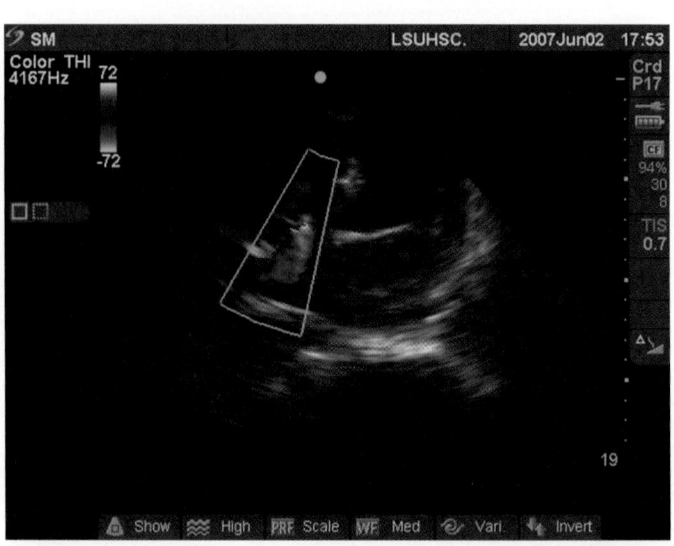

FIGURE 54-7. An echocardiogram demonstrating tricuspid regurgitation. Note regurgitant flow into the right atrium.

Pulmonic stenosis often presents with exertional dyspnea, syncope, chest pain, and the signs and symptoms of right heart failure. There is a harsh systolic murmur, best heard in the left second intercostal space, which increases with inspiration. A loud ejection click may precede the murmur, and an S_4 is often heard. Pulmonic regurgitation is associated with a high-pitched and blowing diastolic murmur (Graham Steell murmur), which increases in intensity during inspiration and is best heard over the left second and third intercostal spaces. An S_3 gallop is often present. Patients with severe right-sided valvular disease typically have a palpable right ventricle thrill or heave.

DIAGNOSIS AND TREATMENT

The diagnosis of right-sided valvular heart disease requires echocardiography (**Figure 54-7**), with transesophageal echocardiography being more sensitive than transthoracic studies. Chest radiography and ECG findings lack sensitivity or specificity. Chest radiography may show signs of right atrial and ventricular enlargement. In pulmonic stenosis, there may be dilatation of the left pulmonary artery. ECG may demonstrate right atrial enlargement and signs of right ventricular hypertrophy.

Treatment of right-sided valvular heart disease is aimed at the underlying cause. Treat those with endocarditis with antibiotics. Patients with functional tricuspid or pulmonic regurgitation should receive treatment aimed at the underlying cause of the pulmonary hypertension or right-sided failure. Diuretics treat the effects of elevated venous pressure, such as lower extremity edema, ascites, and hepatic congestion, but use with caution to avoid volume depletion or electrolyte abnormalities.[19] Patients with symptomatic pulmonic or tricuspid stenosis may be candidates for balloon valvotomy, and those with severe tricuspid regurgitation due to a structural valve abnormality may require valve replacement.

PROSTHETIC VALVE DISEASE

PATHOPHYSIOLOGY

Prosthetic valves are divided into two basic groups: mechanical and bioprosthetic. Mechanical valves are more durable with lower failure rates but have a higher risk for thromboembolic complications. Life-long anticoagulation is necessary to reduce the thrombotic risk. Bioprosthetic valves, from porcine, bovine, or human sources, are less thrombogenic but are more likely to fail and require repeat surgery.

Systemic thromboembolism is a common complication of mechanical heart valves. Without anticoagulation, the risk of valve thrombosis or thromboembolism is about 8%, and falls to 1% to 2% per year with anticoagulation.[20,21] Embolic risk is highest during the first 3 postoperative months, and emboli are more common from mitral rather than from aortic valves. Antiplatelet therapy is recommended for all patients with prosthetic valves. In all patients with mechanical valves, lifelong anticoagulation is recommended.[10] The rate of bleeding complications is dependent on the type and intensity of anticoagulation. Major bleeding complications from warfarin occur in approximately 1.4% of prosthetic valve patients per year.[22]

Prosthetic valves may malfunction in a number of ways, including thrombosis, dehiscence of sutures, gradual degeneration, or even sudden fracture. Symptoms are often slowly progressive, but in acute failures, severe symptoms and death may occur before corrective surgery can be accomplished.

Prosthetic valve endocarditis occurs in up to 6% of patients within 5 years of surgery.[23] Early cases (within the first year) are more commonly caused by *Staphylococcus epidermidis* and *S. aureus*.[24] Late cases of endocarditis are caused by similar organisms as those affecting native valves.[24] The most frequent organism is *Streptococcus viridans,* but *Serratia* and *Pseudomonas* are also implicated. Regardless of source, prosthetic valve endocarditis carries a high mortality rate.[25]

CLINICAL FEATURES

Although valve replacement relieves valvular obstruction and regurgitation, cardiac remodeling persists, and many patients have persistent cardiac symptoms after valve replacement. Long-standing volume or pressure overload leads to ventricular dysfunction, and many patients continue to have dyspnea and symptoms of heart failure. Patients are also likely to have concomitant coronary artery disease, systemic hypertension, or atrial fibrillation.

Symptoms of prosthetic valve dysfunction depend on the type and location of the valve. Patients with prosthetic valves experience some symptoms specific to the presence of the artificial valve. Thromboembolism may cause systemic symptoms such as transient neurologic symptoms, amaurosis fugax, or self-limited ischemic episodes in the extremities or organs. Major embolic events include stroke, mesenteric infarction, or sudden death. Prophylaxis against thrombotic complications of prosthetic valves with systemic anticoagulation may cause major bleeding, with hemorrhagic stroke being the most common lethal bleeding complication.

Acute onset of respiratory distress, pulmonary edema, and cardiogenic shock may be associated with mechanical valve failure, tearing of a bioprosthesis, or a large clot obstructing the valve or preventing closure. Failures often result in sudden death before corrective surgery can be done. A paravalvular leak also presents with congestive heart failure. The severity of symptoms is dependent on leak size and how rapidly the leak develops. Slowly progressive development of heart failure may occur with gradual accumulation of a prosthetic valve thrombus.

Patients with bioprostheses usually have a normal S_1 and S_2, with no abnormal opening sounds. Mechanical valves normally have a loud, clicking, metallic sound associated with valve closure. Systolic murmurs of prosthetic aortic valves are common, but loud diastolic murmurs should be considered pathologic. A "quiet" mechanical valve is concerning. A loud holosystolic murmur indicates prosthetic mitral valve dysfunction. Aortic bioprostheses usually cause a short mid-systolic murmur, and mitral bioprostheses may cause a short diastolic rumble.

DIAGNOSIS OF PROSTHETIC VALVE DYSFUNCTION OR COMPLICATIONS

Think of potential prosthetic valve dysfunction in any patient with a valve replacement and new or progressive dyspnea, congestive heart failure, decreased exercise tolerance, or chest pain. Suspect thromboembolism, septic embolism, or intracranial hemorrhage in any patient with a prosthetic valve and new focal neurologic deficit. Finally, consider endocarditis in prosthetic valve patients with persistent fever or fever without a clear source.

Echocardiography is the diagnostic test of choice. Chest radiography lacks sensitivity and specificity but may show a change in valve position or signs of heart failure. Obtain a head CT in patients with focal neurologic deficits to evaluate for hemorrhage or embolic stroke. Patients on warfarin may require a complete blood count and coagulation studies. Obtain blood cultures for suspected endocarditis.

TREATMENT AND DISPOSITION

Emergency treatment for acute prosthetic valve dysfunction requires cardiology and cardiothoracic surgery consultation. Emergent surgery and thrombolytic therapy are potential therapies for acute valve thrombosis. Lesser degrees of obstruction should be treated by optimizing anticoagulation. Obtain consultation before discharging a patient with suspected prosthetic valve dysfunction.

REVERSAL OF ANTICOAGULATION WITH PROSTHETIC VALVES

Management of patients with prosthetic valves in the ED requires knowledge of the recommendations on anticoagulation and reversal of excessive anticoagulation. Mechanical mitral valves require an INR of 2.5 to 3.5, whereas bileaflet mechanical valves in the aortic position require an INR of 2.0 to 3.0.[3,10] Aspirin is recommended for all patients with prosthetic valves—mechanical or bioprosthetic.[10]

For the emergency physician, the greatest dilemma regarding anticoagulation is not who should be on anticoagulation, but how to treat supratherapeutic anticoagulation with or without bleeding. An INR >5 poses a significant risk of excess bleeding, but rapid changes in anticoagulation pose an equally ominous risk of valve thrombosis and thromboembolism. Patients with an INR of 5 to 10 without bleeding may be treated by withholding warfarin or administering 1.0 to 2.5 milligrams of oral vitamin K. **Patients with severe bleeding complications are best treated with fresh frozen plasma or prothrombin complex concentrate.[3] Avoid parenteral, high-dose vitamin K due to risk of overcorrection.**[9]

PREGNANT WOMEN WITH VALVULAR DISEASE

The changes in cardiovascular physiology during pregnancy may be poorly tolerated by patients with underlying valvular disease. Increases in cardiac output and blood volume accentuate the murmurs associated with mitral or aortic stenosis. Regurgitant aortic or mitral murmurs may be attenuated due to pregnancy-associated decreases in systemic vascular resistance. In general, asymptomatic mild lesions are well tolerated and pose low maternal and fetal risks. However, more pronounced disease that produces symptoms or is associated with pulmonary hypertension or left ventricular dysfunction is risky and requires high-risk obstetric follow-up. Neonatal complications associated with symptomatic maternal valvular lesions include prematurity, intrauterine growth retardation, respiratory distress syndrome, intraventricular hemorrhage, and death.[26]

Patients with mild valvular heart disease can often be managed medically during pregnancy. Those with moderate or severe stenotic valvular heart disease may require balloon valvotomy or surgery. Patients with aortic or mitral regurgitation who have severe symptoms refractory to medical management may also require surgery. Endocarditis prophylaxis is unnecessary in patients with valvular heart disease when undergoing vaginal or cesarean delivery.[9]

Pregnant women with valvular heart disease may present in extremis, with dyspnea, pulmonary edema, angina, or syncope. These are generally treated in a similar fashion as discussed above. Pregnancy is associated with a hypercoagulable state due to changes in circulating hormone levels as well as venous stasis. Pregnant patients with valvular heart disease or prosthetic valves are at increased risk for thromboembolic events, and anticoagulation is recommended.[3] Warfarin in pregnancy is associated with teratogenic effects, spontaneous abortion, prematurity, and stillbirth. Unfractionated and low-molecular-weight heparins are safe in pregnancy, but require close monitoring. Heparin therapy should be targeted to a partial thromboplastin time ratio of at least twice the control. However, the effectiveness of heparin thromboembolic prophylaxis is not well established in pregnant women despite being a common path.[9,26] Low-dose aspirin (81 to 162 milligrams) once daily is recommended during the second and third trimesters for pregnant patients with mechanical or bioprosthetic valves.

PRACTICE GUIDELINES

Practice guidelines include the 2014 American College of Cardiology/American Heart Association Guidelines for the Management of Patients with Valvular Heart Disease[3] and the Joint Task Force on the Management of Valvular Heart Disease of the European Society of Cardiology and the European Association for Cardio-Thoracic Surgery Guidelines on the Management of Valvular Heart Disease.[19]

REFERENCES

The complete reference list is available online at www.TintinalliEM.com.

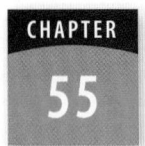

Cardiomyopathies and Pericardial Disease

James T. Niemann

INTRODUCTION

The term cardiomyopathy describes a heterogeneous group of diseases that directly alter cardiac structure, impair myocardial function, or alter myocardial electrical properties. Discoveries in molecular genetics and the description of (ion) channelopathies as diseases have prompted new definitions and classification of cardiomyopathies.[1] Primary cardiomyopathies are diseases that solely or predominantly involve the myocardium[1]; the most common disorders are listed in **Table 55-1**. Secondary cardiomyopathies include heart muscle diseases associated with specific systemic disorders. At present, no classification method perfectly distinguishes all forms of cardiomyopathy, and overlap exists between categories.[2,3] Secondary cardiomyopathies often present with hemodynamic findings similar to those of the idiopathic dilated or restrictive forms of cardiomyopathy. The most common causes of secondary cardiomyopathies are listed in **Table 55-2**. As a group, the cardiomyopathies are the third most common form of cardiac disease encountered in the United States, following coronary (ischemic) heart disease and hypertensive heart disease. **Hypertrophic cardiomyopathy** is the second most common cause of sudden cardiac death in the adolescent population and the leading cause of sudden death in competitive athletes.[4]

An in-depth discussion of each of the primary and secondary cardiomyopathies is beyond the scope of this chapter, and one is unlikely to make a specific diagnosis in the ED. This chapter discusses selected cardiomyopathies (**Table 55-3**). The cardiomyopathies usually present with signs of systolic and diastolic ventricular dysfunction. The ED evaluation will generally guide the need for urgent treatment, admission, or referral for further diagnostic evaluation, based on the severity of symptoms.

CARDIOMYOPATHIES WITH SYSTOLIC AND DIASTOLIC DYSFUNCTION

DILATED CARDIOMYOPATHY

Epidemiology and Pathophysiology Dilated cardiomyopathy is the most common cardiomyopathy and is usually idiopathic but may be familial or occur with specific cardiac or systemic disorders (**Tables 55-1** and **53-2**). **Peripartum cardiomyopathy** most commonly manifests as dilated cardiomyopathy and is discussed in chapter 100, "Maternal Emergencies after 20 Weeks of Pregnancy and in the Postpartum Period." The idiopathic form of dilated cardiomyopathy causes approximately 25% of all cases of congestive heart failure (CHF) and is the primary indication for cardiac transplantation in the United States. The prevalence of **idiopathic dilated cardiomyopathy** is about 36 cases per 100,000 population. Blacks and males have a 2.5-fold increase in risk compared with whites and females. Most patients are diagnosed between the ages of 20 and 50 years, and the majority have advanced symptoms of CHF at the time of initial presentation.[5]

TABLE 55-1 The Primary Cardiomyopathies

Genetic
Hypertrophic cardiomyopathy
Arrhythmogenic right ventricular cardiomyopathy/dysplasia
Left ventricular noncompaction
Conduction system disease
Long QT syndrome
Brugada syndrome
Catecholaminergic polymorphic ventricular tachycardia
Short QT syndrome
Idiopathic ventricular fibrillation
Mixed (genetic and nongenetic)
Dilated cardiomyopathy
Primary restrictive nonhypertrophied cardiomyopathy
Acquired
Myocarditis (inflammatory cardiomyopathy)
Stress (Takotsubo) cardiomyopathy
Peripartum cardiomyopathy

Dilated cardiomyopathy is characterized by systolic and diastolic dysfunction and diminished left ventricular (LV) and, often, right ventricular (RV) contractile force, resulting in a low cardiac output and increased end-systolic and end-diastolic ventricular volumes. A decrease in ventricular compliance leads to an increase in intracavitary pressures. LV and, often, RV dilatation accompanied by normal LV wall thickness are the hallmarks of dilated cardiomyopathy.

Clinical Features As a result of systolic pump failure, the patient presents with signs and symptoms of CHF: dyspnea on exertion, orthopnea, paroxysmal nocturnal dyspnea, bibasilar rales, and dependent edema. Depressed ventricular contractile function and dilatation may result in the formation of mural thrombi, and the patient may develop signs of peripheral embolization (e.g., an acute neurologic deficit, flank pain, and hematuria or a pulseless, cyanotic extremity). Chest pain is felt to be

TABLE 55-2 Common Causes of Secondary Cardiomyopathies

Toxins
Ethanol
Chemotherapeutic agents (doxorubicin)
Antiretroviral agents (zidovudine, didanosine)
Phenothiazines
Cocaine
Methamphetamine
Infiltrative diseases
Amyloidosis
Storage diseases
Hemochromatosis
Autoimmune disorders
Scleroderma
Systemic lupus erythematosus
Rheumatoid arthritis
Dermatomyositis
Metabolic
Nutritional deficiency (thiamine, selenium)
Endocrine (diabetes mellitus, hypothyroidism, hyperthyroidism)
Electrolytic disturbance (hypophosphatemia, hypocalcemia)
Neuromuscular disorders
Muscular dystrophy
Friedreich's ataxia

TABLE 55-3 Features of Selected Cardiomyopathies

Type	Name	Clinical Features	ECG
Systolic and diastolic dysfunction	Dilated cardiomyopathy	Congestive heart failure Chest pain Regurgitant murmurs	LVH Poor R-wave progression
	Myocarditis	Fever Tachycardia Myalgias Chest pain	Nonspecific ST-T wave changes, often with pericarditis
Diastolic dysfunction	Hypertrophic cardiomyopathy	Dyspnea on exertion Chest pain Palpitations Syncope Prominent J wave Pulsus bisferiens Systolic ejection murmur, increases with Valsalva and decreases with squatting	LVH Large septal Q waves
	Restrictive cardiomyopathies	"Square root sign" of left ventricular filling pressures; easily confused with constrictive pericarditis	In some, low voltage of QRS; conduction disturbances; atrial fibrillation

Abbreviations: ECG = electrocardiogram; LVH = left ventricular hypertrophy.

due to limited coronary vascular reserve rather than atherosclerotic coronary artery disease, but the cause cannot be distinguished clinically.

Murmurs do not necessarily indicate primary valvular disease. Annular dilatation and displacement of the papillary muscles of the atrioventricular valves inhibit complete valve closure. Holosystolic mitral or tricuspid regurgitant murmurs are frequently heard at the apex or lower left sternal border. An apical diastolic rumble may be heard and is due either to accentuated, early diastolic atrial-to-ventricular flow (the result of mitral regurgitation and left atrial overload) or to a loud summation gallop. The liver will be enlarged and pulsatile if tricuspid insufficiency is significant.

Diagnosis The diagnosis may be suspected in patients with typical radiographic and electrocardiographic findings, but the diagnosis is typically made at follow-up with echocardiography and additional testing as indicated by individual characteristics. The chest radiograph invariably shows an enlarged cardiac silhouette and increased cardiothoracic ratio. Biventricular enlargement is common. Evidence of pulmonary venous hypertension ("cephalization" of flow and enlarged hila) is also frequent and may serve to differentiate cardiac enlargement due to myocardial failure from that due to a large pericardial effusion.

The electrocardiogram is almost always abnormal. LV hypertrophy and left atrial enlargement are the most common findings. Q or QS waves and poor R-wave progression across the anterior precordium may produce a pseudoinfarction pattern. Atrial fibrillation and ventricular ectopy are common rhythm disturbances.

Echocardiographic studies in a symptomatic patient demonstrate a decreased ejection fraction, increased systolic and diastolic volumes, and ventricular and atrial enlargement.[6] Echocardiography is indicated when the cause of heart failure is uncertain to exclude known causes of heart failure that may be correctable (e.g., pericardial effusion or valvular disease), to estimate ejection fraction, and to rule out other potential complications (e.g., mural thrombi) that may be amenable to therapy. The acuity of the patient's presentation determines the urgency of echocardiography.

Treatment and Disposition For the treatment of acute decompensated heart failure, see chapter 53, "Acute Heart Failure." Chronic therapy may include diuretics and digoxin, but these drugs do not appear to improve survival rates.[7] Guidelines from the American College of Cardiology for the management of heart failure (and other cardiovascular disorders) are available online at http://www.cardiosource.org/Science-And-Quality/Practice-Guidelines-and-Quality-Standards.aspx. The use of angiotensin-converting enzyme inhibitors and blockers, specifically carvedilol, improves survival in patients with dilated cardiomyopathy and CHF.[8] Selected patients benefit from cardiac resynchronization therapy.[9-11] Patients with complex ventricular ectopy who are found to be at risk for sudden cardiac death may benefit from amiodarone therapy or an implanted cardioverter-defibrillator.[12]

Patients with a known dilated cardiomyopathy and chronic CHF may present to the ED with a mild to moderate worsening of symptoms.[13] If the cause is noncompliance with medical therapy or diet, ED treatment with nitrates, IV diuretics, reinstitution of prescribed medications, patient counseling, and timely referral to the primary care physician are appropriate. However, life-threatening causes of acute exacerbations, such as cardiac ischemia, should be considered before assuming benign causes. Acutely symptomatic patients require hospitalization for definitive diagnosis and management. Important subsets of patients with dilated cardiomyopathy are treated with left ventricular assist devices while awaiting heart transplantation or as destination therapy.[14,15] Principles of patient assessment and management and device complications are described in **Left Ventricular Assist Devices** (see next page).

MYOCARDITIS (INFLAMMATORY CARDIOMYOPATHY)

Pathophysiology Myocarditis is a common cause of dilated cardiomyopathy but is discussed separately to highlight its acute presentation and individual therapy. Myocarditis is inflammation of the heart muscle and is most frequently characterized pathologically by focal infiltration of the myocardium by lymphocytes, plasma cells, and histiocytes. Varying amounts of myocytolysis and destruction of the interstitial reticulin network are also seen.[16] Because many episodes are mild, they do not always come to medical attention. **Table 55-4** lists some common infectious causes of myocarditis. Myocarditis is frequently accompanied by pericarditis.

TABLE 55-4 Common Infectious Causes of Myocarditis

Viral Agents	Bacteria
Coxsackie B virus	*Corynebacterium diphtheriae*
Echovirus	*Neisseria meningitidis*
Influenza virus	*Mycoplasma pneumoniae*
Parainfluenza virus	β-Hemolytic streptococci (rheumatic fever)
Epstein-Barr virus	Lyme disease
Hepatitis B virus	
Human immunodeficiency virus	

LEFT VENTRICULAR ASSIST DEVICES (LVADs)

Daniel Renner, Heather Heaton, and Jason N. Katz

Left ventricular assist devices (LVADs) augment left ventricular output in patients with severe cardiomyopathy. Right ventricular assist devices and biventricular assist devices also exist, though these are much less common and are used only for temporary circulatory support. There are several models of LVADs in current use which share many similar features.

In all LVADs, the implanted pump transfers blood from the apex of the left ventricle to the proximal aorta (Figure 1). The pump is powered by an external power source (battery or bedside unit), which is connected to a controller. Both the battery and controller reside outside of the body and can be carried or worn by the patient. The controller drives the pump through a driveline, which connects the implanted pump to the external controller through a surgical incision in the abdominal wall.

Most contemporary LVADs use pumps that drive blood through a continuous-flow mechanism (e.g. axial or centrifugal flow), maintaining a normal mean arterial blood pressure in the absence of a palpable pulse. However, many patients may still retain some cardiac contractility; in these individuals the LVAD serves to assist (and not replace) normal physiologic cardiac output, and a pulse may be present. Because the LVAD can (in some patients) maintain systemic perfusion even with minimal cardiac function, an LVAD patient can sometimes be clinically stable even in the setting of ventricular fibrillation. LVAD patients still rely upon reasonable right ventricular function to pump blood to the lungs.

Patients and families are thoroughly trained on the management of the LVAD and its complications, and they should be involved during patient assessment and management. It is important to call the patient's LVAD coordinator as soon as possible to assist with management decisions--this information should be present in the patient's travel bag, along with a spare controller and batteries.

CLINICAL FEATURES

LVAD patients should have a normal mean arterial pressure. Blood pressure can be assessed by a mechanical cuff or by doppler ultrasound. If using a doppler, remember that blood flow can be continuous and not pulsatile. When auscultating the heart, the continuous whirr of the pump is heard.

The ECG should have discernible QRS complexes (Figure 2).

The LVAD is visible on a chest radiograph (Figure 3). Bedside US can be used to assess RV function and to evaluate for pericardial effusion/tamponade. Plain imaging and CT scans are safe, but MRIs are contraindicated.

THE HEMODYNAMICALLY UNSTABLE LVAD PATIENT

NEVER PERFORM CHEST COMPRESSIONS ON AN LVAD PATIENT. Chest compressions can dislodge the LVAD from the heart and aorta, causing LV rupture and intractable hemorrhage.

Immediately auscultate the precordium -- an audible "whirr" indicates that the pump is functioning. If nothing is heard, search for a cause of mechanical LVAD failure. With the help of family or the patient, check and/or change the batteries and/or controller. **Do not disconnect anything.**

If the pump is audible and functioning, obtain a blood pressure (by automatic cuff or manual doppler) and place the patient on a cardiac monitor and continuous pulse oximetry. If the LVAD model does not provide pulsatile flow, it is difficult to obtain a reading by pulse oximetry.

For **hypotension**, give a bolus of normal saline. Assess for bleeding, especially from GI hemorrhage. **If hypotension persists despite adequate fluid resuscitation, or in the presence of right ventricular failure or LVAD malfunction, initiate IV pressors.** Dopamine is a reasonable first line therapy. **Obtain an ECG** to rule out right ventricular myocardial infarction or strain. Obtain standard laboratory studies as clinically indicated. **Bedside US** can assess for right ventricular dilatation or failure. If there is right ventricular strain, consider pulmonary hypertension or pulmonary embolism. Give heparin if **pulmonary embolism or device thrombosis** is suspected and bleeding is excluded.

VF or VT in an unstable patient requires defibrillation/cardioversion, using standard ACLS energy recommendations. Do not place defibrillator pads over the driveline. If the patient is clinically stable, give amiodarone according to ACLS protocols.

MEDICAL COMPLICATIONS

Medical complications include anemia, bleeding, thromboembolism, or infection. **Anemia** can be caused by hemolysis (erythrocyte destruction from the pump) or bleeding. LVAD patients are typically anticoagulated with warfarin to an INR target of 2-3. **Bleeding and coagulopathy** are investigated and treated with standard measures. LVAD patients are also at risk for **thromboembolism**, such as pulmonary embolism, stroke and mesenteric ischemia, especially in the setting of suboptimal anticoagulation. Heparin is safe and indicated for such events once bleeding has been ruled out. **Infection** is a common complication, especially at the driveline exit site. Treat sepsis with volume resuscitation, blood cultures, and antibiotics.

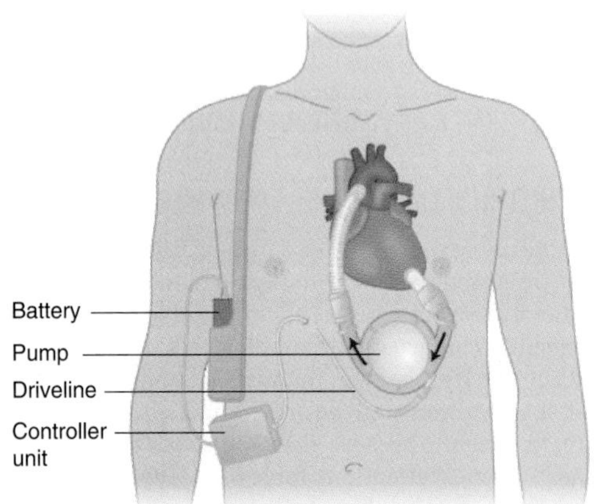

FIGURE 1. LVAD carries blood from the left ventricle to the aorta.

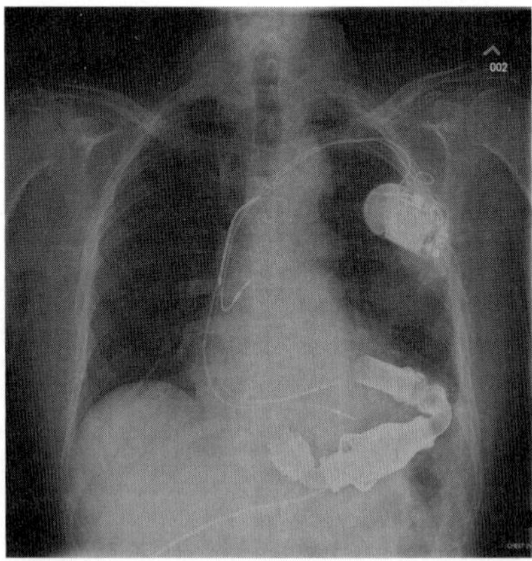

FIGURE 3. Posteroanterior chest radiograph of a patient with an LVAD and an implantable defibrillator. The outflow conduit to the proximal aorta is not radiographically visible. [ECG used with permission of Daniel Renner, MD.]

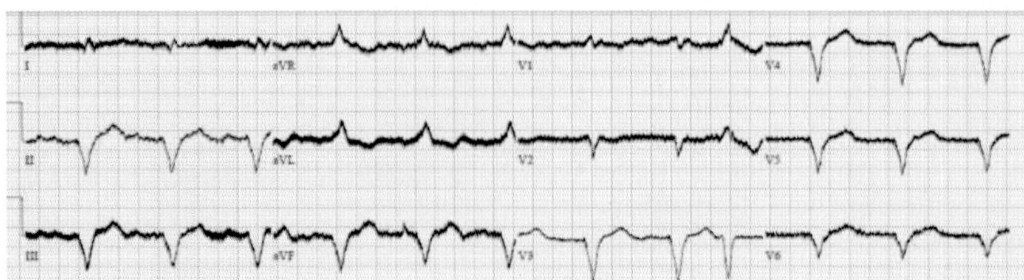

FIGURE 2. ECG of a patient with an LVAD. QRS is evident and baseline shows some electrical interference from the pump. [ECG used with permission of Daniel Renner, MD.]

Clinical Features Fever, myalgias, headache, and sinus tachycardia usually out of proportion with fever are common signs and symptoms. Other signs and symptoms depend on the extent of myocardial involvement and myocardial depression. In severe cases, heart failure can develop. With less extensive myocardial involvement, pericarditis and the clinical manifestations of systemic illness (fever, myalgias, headache, and rigors) may overshadow clinical signs of myocardial dysfunction, and myocarditis may not be suspected. Retrosternal or precordial angina-type chest pain is frequent and is usually due to pericardial inflammation **(myopericarditis)**. A pericardial friction rub is commonly heard.

Diagnosis The gold standard for diagnosis of myocarditis is endocardial biopsy, but this invasive modality is uncommonly used.[17] The diagnosis is more commonly made clinically based on symptoms with supportive testing. The chest radiograph is usually normal or nondiagnostic. Cardiomegaly and pulmonary venous hypertension or pulmonary edema are present with severe disease. Electrocardiogram changes include nonspecific ST-T–wave changes, ST-segment elevation or PR depression from associated pericarditis, atrioventricular block, and QRS interval prolongation. Cardiac enzymes may be elevated.[18] Echocardiographic studies are also nonspecific, with myocardial depression and wall motion abnormalities in severe cases. Newer imaging modalities include nuclear imaging with gallium-67– or indium-111–labeled antimyosin antibodies and cardiac MRI.[19-21]

Treatment and Disposition Treatment for idiopathic or viral myocarditis is supportive. Antibiotics are needed for myocarditis complicating rheumatic fever, diphtheria, or meningococcemia. Immunosuppressive therapy (e.g., prednisone, azathioprine, and others) may be of value in selected patients, but large trials have not consistently demonstrated benefit.[19] Immunosuppressive therapy is usually reserved for more severe cases and is rarely begun in the ED. Admission is usually indicated if the patient presents with CHF.

CARDIOMYOPATHIES WITH DIASTOLIC DYSFUNCTION

HYPERTROPHIC CARDIOMYOPATHY

Epidemiology and Pathophysiology **Hypertrophic cardiomyopathy** is characterized by LV and/or RV hypertrophy that is usually asymmetric and involves primarily the interventricular septum. The diagnostic hallmarks of the disease remain echocardiographic asymmetric septal hypertrophy and histologic hypertrophy associated with myocardial fiber disarray surrounding areas of increased loose connective tissue.[22] The underlying pathophysiology appears to be microvascular dysfunction with mechanico-energetic uncoupling. The disorder can be familial, with autosomal dominant inheritance, or it can occur sporadically. There is no apparent sex or ethnic predilection. Hypertrophic cardiomyopathy is a heterogeneous disease of the sarcomere with many mutations. The most common mutation involves the beta-myosin heavy chain. Particular genotypes have more rapidly progressive courses. The prevalence in the general population is approximately 1 in 500. The annual mortality rate in the overall hypertrophic cardiomyopathy population is about 1% per annum, but is up to 4% to 6% in childhood and adolescence.

Hemodynamically, hypertrophic cardiomyopathy is characterized by abnormal LV diastolic function due to reduced compliance of the hypertrophied left ventricle. Decreased compliance is reflected by an increase in LV filling pressure. Cardiac output, ejection fraction, and end-systolic and end-diastolic volumes are usually normal. During cardiac catheterization and hemodynamic monitoring, a systolic pressure gradient between the body of the left ventricle and the subvalvular outflow tract can be recorded in some patients at rest or after provocation (e.g., exercise or isoproterenol infusion). Most clinical symptoms are the result of impaired diastolic relaxation and restricted LV filling.

Clinical Features Severity of symptoms in most instances is related to the patient's age; the older the patient, the more severe are the symptoms. Dyspnea on exertion is the most frequent initial complaint and is due to exercise-induced sinus tachycardia, which results in an abrupt elevated LV diastolic pressure and pulmonary venous hypertension. Additional symptoms include chest pain, palpitations, and syncope. A family history of death due to cardiac disease, frequently described as "massive heart attack" or "heart failure," is not uncommon.

Chest pain in hypertrophic cardiomyopathy patients is due to an imbalance between the oxygen demand of the hypertrophied left ventricle and the available myocardial blood flow.[15] In older patients, associated atherosclerotic coronary artery disease may further limit myocardial perfusion. Precordial or retrosternal chest discomfort in hypertrophic cardiomyopathy may mimic angina pectoris or may be "atypical." Response to nitroglycerin administration is poor and highly variable.

The hypertrophic cardiomyopathy patient may be aware of forceful ventricular contraction and complain of an abnormal heartbeat or "palpitations." Atrial fibrillation is poorly tolerated because of the increased importance of the atrial contribution to LV filling.

Jugular venous pressure is usually not elevated. However, a prominent a (atrial) wave may be noted on close inspection of the neck veins. The upstroke of the carotid arterial pulse is rapid and frequently biphasic or bifid (pulsus bisferiens). The apical impulse is sustained and hyperdynamic, and a presystolic lift is common.

The first and second heart sounds are usually normal, with an S_4 heard in most patients. The systolic ejection murmur of hypertrophic cardiomyopathy is heard best at the lower left sternal border or at the apex and rarely radiates to the carotid arteries. Easily performed bedside maneuvers can be used to increase the intensity and duration of the murmur (**Table 55-5**). **Interventions that decrease LV filling and the distending pressure in the LV outflow tract or that increase the force of myocardial contraction accentuate the murmur of hypertrophic cardiomyopathy.** Such interventions include standing and the strain phase of the Valsalva maneuver. The murmur is also louder with the first sinus beat after a premature ventricular contraction. **Maneuvers that increase LV filling (squatting, passive leg elevation, and hand grip) decrease the murmur.** The murmurs of hypertrophic cardiomyopathy and mitral valve prolapse, when associated with murmur, are similar and are compared in **Table 55-5**.

Diagnosis The diagnosis may be suspected in the ED based on symptoms and supportive testing, but typically is confirmed at follow-up with echocardiography or cardiac MRI, frequently followed by genetic testing. The resting ECG is nonspecific in most patients with hypertrophic cardiomyopathy, often demonstrating LV hypertrophy and left atrial enlargement. Evidence of chamber enlargement is most common in patients with large gradients across the LV outflow tract. Q waves >0.3 mV, termed septal Q waves, may be seen in anterior, lateral, or inferior leads. Q waves may mimic those seen after myocardial infarction (pseudoinfarction pattern). The polarity of the T wave can differentiate between hypertrophic cardiomyopathy septal Q waves from Q waves due to myocardial infarction. Upright T waves in those leads with QS or QR complexes are usually found in hypertrophic cardiomyopathy, whereas

TABLE 55-5 Effect of Bedside Interventions on the Murmur of Hypertrophic Cardiomyopathy Compared to Mitral Valve Prolapse

Intervention	Hypertrophic Cardiomyopathy	Mitral Valve Prolapse
Valsalva maneuver (strain phase)	Murmur increased	Click closer to S_1, murmur increased
Standing after squatting	Murmur increased	Click closer to S_1, murmur increased
Passive leg elevation in supine patient	Murmur decreased	Click closer to S_2, murmur decreased
Hand grip	Murmur decreased	Click closer to S_1, murmur increased
Squatting	Murmur decreased	Click closer to S_2, murmur decreased

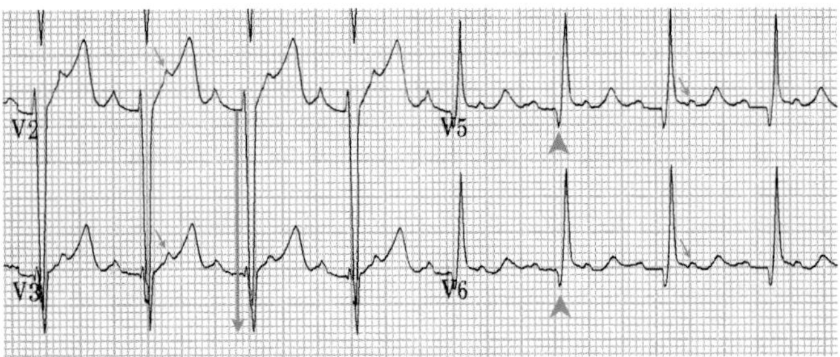

FIGURE 55-1. Deep S-wave voltage (28 mm S in V_2, *large arrow*) signifies LV hypertrophy, and narrow septal Q waves in V_5 and V_6 (*arrowheads*) are noted. T waves are upright in the leads with the septal Q waves, typical of hypertrophic cardiomyopathy. This patient also has atrial flutter with 2:1 block. The additional P waves appear in the ST segments (*small arrows*). [Reproduced with permission from Knoop KJ, Stack LB, Storrow AB, Thurman RJ (eds): *The Atlas of Emergency Medicine,* 3rd ed. New York: McGraw-Hill, 2010; Fig 23.40B.]

T-wave inversion in such leads is highly suggestive of ischemic heart disease. From a patient with hypertrophic cardiomyopathy, **Figure 55-1** demonstrates evidence of LV hypertrophy as shown by deep S waves in V_2 and septal Q waves with upright T waves in leads V_5 and V_6. The chest radiograph is usually normal or nonspecific.

Echocardiography plays a substantial role in the diagnosis of hypertrophic cardiomyopathy, in the correlation of the auscultatory and hemodynamic events with LV anatomic changes, and in defining inheritance patterns. The characteristic echocardiographic finding is disproportionate septal hypertrophy. Other echocardiographic abnormalities include reduced LV end-diastolic dimensions, systolic anterior motion of the mitral valve, and mid-systolic closure of the aortic valve. Cardiac MRI is recommended when echocardiography is inconclusive in patients clinically suspected of having the disease.[22]

Treatment and Disposition The majority of patients with hypertrophic cardiomyopathy who seek medical care typically do so because of declining exercise tolerance, chest pain, or syncope.[22] The patient who presents complaining of exercise intolerance or chest pain in whom the typical murmur of hypertrophic cardiomyopathy is heard should be referred for echocardiographic evaluation. Syncope in patients with hypertrophic cardiomyopathy typically occurs during or immediately after exercise. **If hypertrophic cardiomyopathy is suspected in a patient with syncope, hospitalization is indicated.** The diagnostic evaluation in such cases is extensive and includes echocardiographic studies as well as extended ambulatory (Holter) monitoring, exercise stress testing to assess blood pressure response, and tilt testing. **Syncope in patients with hypertrophic cardiomyopathy may presage sudden cardiac death.** β-Blockers are the mainstay of therapy for patients with chest pain.[22] Preparticipation screening guidelines for athletes advocated in the United States include personal and family medical history, and careful physical examination.[23] At this time, routine electrocardiography or echocardiography is not recommended in the United States[24,25] because evidence does not yet support universal testing.[25,26]

RESTRICTIVE CARDIOMYOPATHY

Epidemiology and Pathophysiology Restrictive cardiomyopathy may result from systemic disorders (amyloidosis, sarcoidosis, hemochromatosis, progressive systemic sclerosis [scleroderma], carcinoid heart disease, endomyocardial fibrosis, or hypereosinophilic syndrome), but in most cases, it is idiopathic. The idiopathic form is sometimes familial, with autosomal dominant transmission. There has been no clearly demonstrated predilection for gender or ethnicity.

Restrictive cardiomyopathy is heart muscle disease that results in "restricted" ventricular filling, with normal or decreased diastolic volume of one or both ventricles. Systolic function is usually normal, and ventricular wall thickness may be normal or increased, depending on the underlying cause. The hemodynamic hallmarks include (1) elevated LV and RV end-diastolic pressure, (2) normal LV systolic function (ejection fraction >50%), and (3) a marked decrease followed by a rapid rise and plateau in early diastolic ventricular pressure. The rapid rise and abrupt plateau in the early diastolic ventricular pressure trace produce a characteristic "square root sign" or "dip-and-plateau" filling pattern due to increased myocardial stiffness. This pattern is not diagnostic, however, and may be seen in constrictive pericarditis, with which restrictive cardiomyopathy is commonly confused. Differentiation between the two is critical because constrictive pericarditis can be cured surgically. The diagnosis of restrictive cardiomyopathy should be considered in a patient presenting with CHF but no evidence of cardiomegaly or systolic dysfunction.[27]

Clinical Features and Diagnosis Symptoms are typical of CHF and include dyspnea, orthopnea, and pedal edema. Right-sided heart failure may predominate and results in hepatomegaly, right upper quadrant pain, and ascites. Chest pain is uncommon, except in amyloidosis.

Findings on physical examination depend on the stage or severity of myocardial involvement. An S_3 and an S_4 are often heard. Pulmonary rales, jugular venous distention, Kussmaul sign (jugular venous pulse rises during inspiration rather than falling), hepatomegaly, pedal edema, and ascites are also typical findings. On chest x-ray, there may be signs of CHF but a normal heart size. Chamber enlargement due to wall thickening, but not dilatation, and nonspecific ST-T–wave changes are usually noted on the electrocardiogram. Cardiac conduction disturbances are common in amyloidosis and sarcoidosis. Atrial fibrillation may occur in the setting of atrial enlargement. Low-voltage QRS complexes (QRS amplitude <0.7 mV) are frequently described in patients with restrictive cardiomyopathy secondary to amyloidosis and hemochromatosis. The differential diagnosis includes constrictive pericarditis or diastolic LV dysfunction (most commonly due to ischemic heart disease, hypertension, or age-related changes in ventricular diastolic compliance). Doppler echocardiographic studies and cardiac catheterization with hemodynamic assessment are often required for specific diagnosis.

Treatment and Disposition CT and MRI of the heart can differentiate constrictive pericarditis from restrictive cardiomyopathy.[28] Correct diagnosis is important because constrictive pericarditis can be surgically corrected, and diastolic LV dysfunction usually responds well to β-blockers or calcium channel blockers. The medical management of restrictive cardiomyopathy is less effective and symptom directed (diuretics and angiotensin-converting enzyme inhibitors) unless due to sarcoidosis (corticosteroid therapy) or hemochromatosis (chelation therapy). The need for admission is usually determined by the severity of symptoms and the availability of diagnostics.

PERICARDIAL DISEASE

The pericardium consists of a serous or loose fibrous membrane (visceral pericardium) overlying the epicardium and a dense collagenous sac (parietal pericardium) surrounding the heart. The space between the visceral and parietal pericardium may normally contain up to 50 mL of fluid.[28] Because its layers are serosal surfaces and because of its proximity and attachments to other structures, the pericardium may be involved in a number of disease processes (**Table 55-6**). In this section, the clinical manifestations and evaluation of acute and constrictive pericarditis and nontraumatic cardiac tamponade are discussed.

ACUTE PERICARDITIS

Clinical Features The most common symptom of acute pericarditis is sharp or stabbing precordial or retrosternal chest pain. Pain may be of sudden or gradual onset and radiates to the back, neck, left shoulder, or arm, and may be aggravated by inspiration or movement. Referral of pain to the left trapezial ridge (due to inflammation of the joining diaphragmatic pleura) is a particular distinguishing feature. Chest pain due

TABLE 55-6 Common Causes of Acute Pericarditis

Idiopathic

Infectious

- Viral (coxsackie virus, echovirus, human immunodeficiency virus)
- Bacterial (especially *Staphylococcus, Streptococcus pneumoniae*, β-hemolytic streptococci [acute rheumatic fever], *Mycobacterium tuberculosis*)
- Fungal (especially *Histoplasma capsulatum*)

Malignancy (leukemia, lymphoma, metastatic breast and lung carcinoma, melanoma)

Drug induced (procainamide, hydralazine)

Systemic rheumatic diseases (systemic lupus erythematosus, rheumatoid arthritis, scleroderma, polyarteritis nodosa, dermatomyositis)

Radiation induced

Postmyocardial infarction (Dressler's syndrome)

Uremia

Myxedema

to acute pericarditis may be aggravated by inspiration or movement. Typically, chest pain is most severe when the patient is supine and is relieved when the patient sits up and leans forward.[29,30] Associated symptoms include fever, dyspnea due to accentuated pain with inspiration, and dysphagia from irritation of the esophagus by the posterior pericardium.

A pericardial friction rub is the most common and important physical finding in pericarditis but may be difficult to appreciate in a noisy ED. It is best heard with the diaphragm of the stethoscope at the lower left sternal border or apex when the patient is sitting and leaning forward. It may be audible only during a certain phase of respiration and characteristically is intermittent. A pericardial friction rub is most often triphasic, with a systolic component due to ventricular contraction, an early diastolic component during the early phase of ventricular filling, and a presystolic component synchronous with atrial systole. It is less commonly biphasic, with a systolic component with either an early diastolic or presystolic component. A monophasic rub is less common but is most often systolic.

Diagnosis • *Electrocardiogram* Serial electrocardiogram changes during acute pericarditis and its convalescence are characterized by four stages (**Table 55-7** and **Figure 55-2**).

If a large pericardial effusion develops during the course of acute pericarditis, low-voltage QRS complexes and electrical alternans may be evident. Pericardial fluid attenuates myocardial electrical signals, and the pendular motion of the heart within the fluid-filled pericardial space results in electrical alternans (see **Figure 55-5** in the Nontraumatic Cardiac Tamponade section of this chapter).

Although serial ECG tracings are of diagnostic value in acute pericarditis, sequential ECG assessment is not a diagnostic luxury afforded the emergency physician. Differentiating pericarditis from the normal variant with "early repolarization" is a common problem and can be difficult when only a single 12-lead electrocardiogram is available. The ST-T-wave changes present in the early repolarization or normal variant electrocardiogram mimic those of pericarditis and have been reported in 2% of healthy young adults. However, the ST-segment/T-wave amplitude ratio in leads V_5, V_6, or I can differentiate pericarditis from early repolarization.[31,32] Using the end of the PR segment as a baseline, or 0 mV, the amplitude or height of the ST segment at its onset is measured in V_5, V_6, or lead I and recorded in millivolts. The height of the T wave in the same lead is measured from the baseline to the T-wave peak. If the ratio of ST amplitude (in millivolts) to T-wave amplitude (in millivolts) is >0.25, acute pericarditis is likely, and if the ratio is <0.25, acute pericarditis is unlikely (**Figure 55-2**). Sensitivity at an ST/T ratio >0.25 for acute pericarditis is >0.85, and the specificity is >0.8 (positive likelihood ratio of about 4 and negative likelihood ratio of about 0.2). Pericarditis alone does not cause significant cardiac rhythm disturbances.

TABLE 55-7 Serial Electrocardiogram Changes of Acute Pericarditis

Stage	PR Segment	ST Segment	T Wave
1 (acute)	Depression, especially in II, aVF, and V_4–V_6	Elevation, especially in I, V_5, and V_6; ST amplitude: T-wave amplitude >0.25	—
2	Isoelectric or depressed	Returns to isoelectric line	Amplitude decreases, inversion rare
3	Isoelectric or depressed	Isoelectric	T-wave inversion, especially in I, V_5, and V_6
4	Isoelectric	Isoelectric	Normal

Radiographic Assessment Chest radiographs are of limited value. The cardiac silhouette may be of normal size and contour in acute pericarditis and, in some instances, the setting of cardiac tamponade. If previous chest radiographs are available for comparison, a recent increase in the size of the cardiac silhouette or an increase in the cardiothoracic ratio without radiographic evidence of pulmonary venous hypertension can distinguish an expanding pericardial effusion from left heart failure. The "epicardial fat-pad sign" is rarely seen on the lateral chest radiograph and has been reported in only 15% of cases of acute pericarditis during fluoroscopy with image intensification. If acute pericarditis is suspected on the basis of history, physical examination, or ECG, a chest radiograph may help establish an underlying cause, such as neoplasm or infection.

Echocardiographic Studies Echocardiography is the procedure of choice for the detection, confirmation, and serial follow-up of patients with acute pericarditis and a pericardial effusion.[33] (See http://www.cardiosource.org/Science-And-Quality/Practice-Guidelines-and-Quality-Standards.aspx for more information.)

Normally, the pericardial sac is only a "potential" space, and the myocardium is echocardiographically in direct contact with surrounding thoracic structures. The anterior RV wall is in contact with the chest wall, and the posterior LV wall is in contact with the posterior pericardium and adjacent pleura. When a pericardial effusion is present, the pericardial space fills with echo-free fluid (**Figure 55-3**).

Echocardiographically, a separation is seen between the right ventricle and the chest wall and between the left ventricle and the posterior pericardium. Quantitation of the size of the effusion is arbitrary and is determined by where the echo-free space is seen (anterior or posterior) and when in the cardiac cycle it occurs. For example, when an echo-free space is seen only posteriorly and only during systole, a small effusion is said to be present. The sensitivity of CT for detecting pericardial effusion is similar to that of echocardiography (**Figure 55-4**).

Ancillary Laboratory Evaluation Suggested laboratory studies are listed in **Table 55-8**. **Serum creatine kinase–MB fraction and troponins may be elevated in acute pericarditis due to associated myocarditis.**[11]

Treatment and Disposition Treatment of pericarditis depends on the cause.[34] Most patients with idiopathic or presumed viral pericarditis have a benign course lasting 1 to 2 weeks. Symptoms respond well to nonsteroidal anti-inflammatory agents administered for 7 days to 3 weeks. Ibuprofen, 300 to 800 milligrams orally every 6 to 8 hours, may be preferred because of fewer side effects, limited impact on coronary artery blood flow, and large dose range. Colchicine, 0.5 milligram orally twice a day, may be a beneficial adjuvant and may prevent recurrent episodes.[35,36] Hospitalization is not necessary in most cases, unless there is associated myocarditis, and follow-up or repeat echocardiography is not needed unless symptoms fail to resolve or reappear or new symptoms are noted.[37] Indicators of a poor prognosis include temperature >38°C (100.4°F), subacute onset over weeks, immunosuppression, history of oral anticoagulant use, associated myocarditis (elevated cardiac biomarkers, symptoms of CHF), and a large pericardial effusion (an echo-free space >20 mm).[38] In general, patients with these risk factors or with an enlarged cardiac silhouette on chest radiograph should be admitted for echocardiography to assess the extent of the effusion and degree of hemodynamic compromise and cardiac dysfunction.

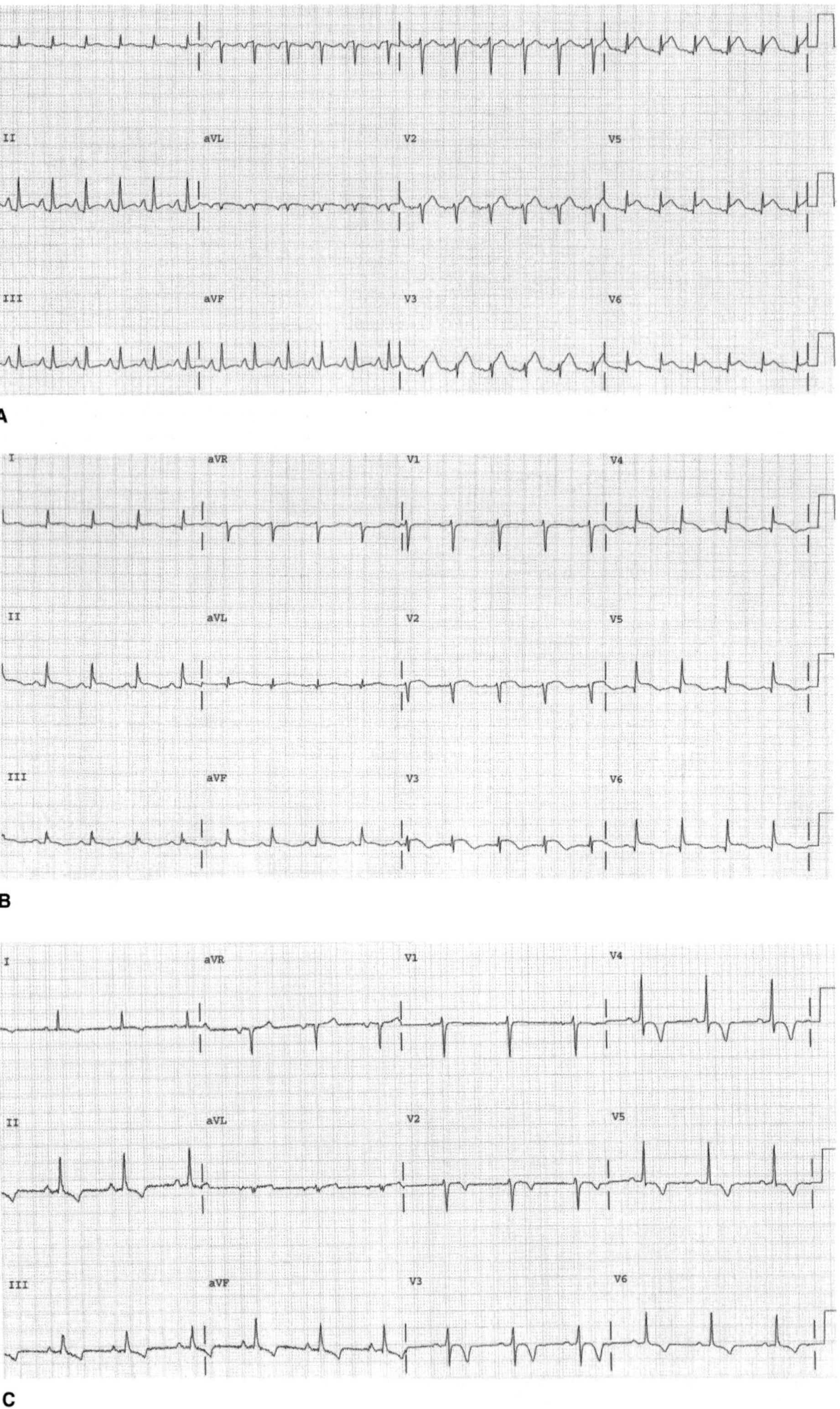

FIGURE 55-2. This series of three electrocardiograms (ECGs) shows the typical progression of changes associated with acute pericarditis. **A.** In stage I pericarditis, the ECG shows diffuse ST-segment elevation and PR depression in leads I, II, III, and avF. The ST-segment to T-wave amplitude ratio measured in V_6 is 2 mm/4 mm, or 0.50, thus meeting criteria for pericarditis rather than early repolarization (see the text under Diagnosis, Electrocardiogram). **B.** In stage II pericarditis, ST segments are returning toward the isoelectric point in most leads in which they had been elevated. **C.** In stage III pericarditis, we see resolution of ST changes and the appearance of diffuse T-wave inversion. These evolutionary changes are typical of and diagnostic for pericarditis and usually occur over several weeks.

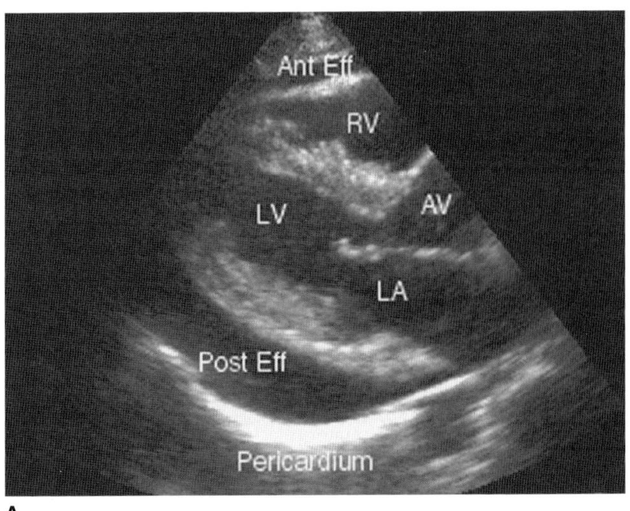

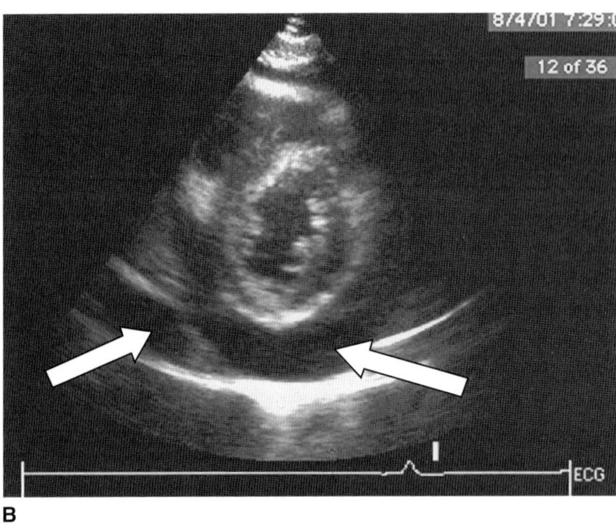

FIGURE 55-3. **A.** Pericardial effusion on parasternal long-axis view. Ant Eff = anterior effusion; AV = aortic valve; LA = left atrium; LV = left ventricle; Post Eff = posterior effusion; RV = right ventricle. **B.** Pericardial effusion on (*arrows*) parasternal short-axis view. [Reprinted with permission from Reardon RF, Joing SA: Cardiac, in Ma OJ, Mateer JR, Blaivas M (eds): *Emergency Ultrasound*, 2nd ed. Copyright © 2008, The McGraw-Hill Companies, Inc., all rights reserved, Figure 6-24.]

NONTRAUMATIC CARDIAC TAMPONADE

Pathophysiology An increase in the amount of fluid within the pericardial sac results in an increase in intrapericardial pressure. The normal fibrocollagenous parietal pericardium has elastic properties and stretches to accommodate increases in intrapericardial fluid. The initial portion of the pericardial volume-pressure curve is flat: Relatively large increases in volume result in comparatively small changes in intrapericardial pressure. The curve becomes steeper as the parietal pericardium reaches the limits of its distensibility.[39] If fluid continues to accumulate, intrapericardial pressure rises to a level greater than that of the normal filling pressures of the right heart chambers. When this occurs, ventricular filling is restricted and results in cardiac tamponade. The point at which this occurs is determined by the rate of fluid accumulation, pericardial compliance (a thickened parietal pericardium is less distensible), and intravascular volume (hypovolemia lowers ventricular filling pressure). Common causes of cardiac tamponade in nontrauma patients are listed in **Table 55-9**.

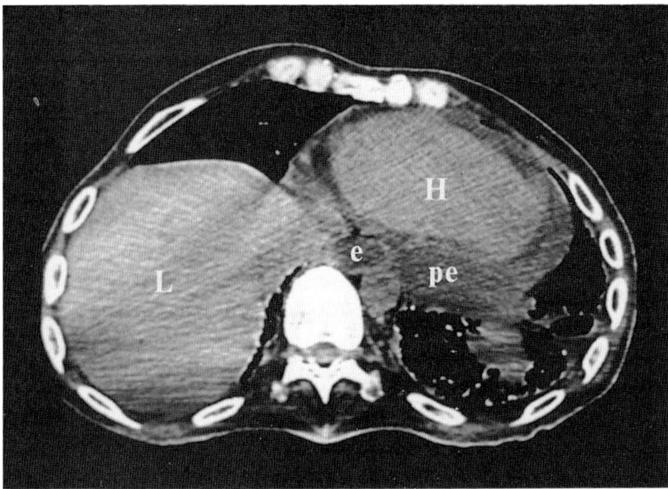

FIGURE 55-4. This CT scan of the chest shows a large pericardial effusion (pe) predominantly posteriorly located in a patient with scleroderma and pericarditis. No pericardial thickening or calcification was detected. Esophageal (e) dilatation is noted. Cardiac function cannot be evaluated. H = heart; L = liver. [Reprinted with permission from Roldan CA: Connective tissue diseases & the heart, in Crawford MH (ed): *Current Diagnosis & Treatment in Cardiology*, 3rd ed. Copyright © 2009, The McGraw-Hill Companies, Inc., all rights reserved, Figure 33-5.]

TABLE 55-8 Ancillary Diagnostic Studies in Acute Pericarditis

Diagnostic Study	Considerations
Cardiac markers	Indicate myocardial involvement
CBC and differential WBC count	May suggest infection or leukemia
BUN/creatinine	May suggest a diagnosis of uremic pericarditis
Streptococcal serologic testing (antistreptolysin O, anti-DNAse, antihyaluronidase)	Particularly in patients with a history of rheumatic heart disease or pharyngitis
Blood cultures	If bacterial infection suspected
Serologic studies	Antinuclear antibodies, anti-DNA titers, or rheumatoid factor in patients with systemic symptoms
Erythrocyte sedimentation rate	Will not determine specific diagnosis, but can confirm clinical suspicion of pericarditis and can be followed serially to assess response to therapy
Acute and convalescent viral antibody titers	Measuring viral titers would not be expected to change the course of treatment
Thyroid function studies	Thyrotoxicosis is a rare cause of pericarditis; thyrotoxicosis can cause pericardial effusion without the typical electrocardiogram changes and symptoms of pericarditis

TABLE 55-9 Common Causes of Cardiac Tamponade in Medical (Nontrauma) Patients

Cause	Approximate Frequency (%)
Metastatic malignancy	40
Acute idiopathic pericarditis	15
Uremia	10
Bacterial or tubercular pericarditis	10
Chronic idiopathic pericarditis	10
Hemorrhage (anticoagulant)	5
Other (systemic lupus erythematosus, postradiation, myxedema, etc.)	10

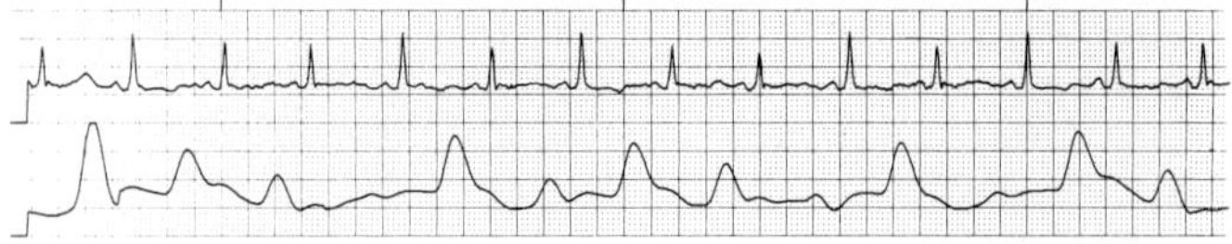

FIGURE 55-5. This rhythm strip (lead II, top tracing) and plethysmograph (bottom tracing) were recorded in a patient who presented with dyspnea, hypotension, and clinical and echocardiographic evidence of cardiac tamponade. A paradoxical pulse was noted on palpation of the radial artery. The amplitude of the R waves varies from beat to beat (electrical alternans).

Clinical Features Symptoms are nonspecific, and patients most commonly complain of dyspnea at rest and with exertion. Additional symptoms may be due to the underlying disease (e.g., uremia or tuberculous pericarditis).

Physical examination may reveal tachycardia and low systolic arterial blood pressure with a narrow pulse pressure. **Pulsus paradoxus** may also be present. A paradoxical arterial pulse is said to be present when the cardiac rhythm is regular and there are apparent dropped beats in the peripheral pulse during inspiration. There is usually a <10 mm Hg decrease in systolic blood pressure during inspiration in the supine position. A value >10 mm Hg usually separates true tamponade from lesser degrees of restricted cardiac filling.[28,40] Pulsus paradoxus is not diagnostic of cardiac tamponade and may be noted in other cardiopulmonary processes. In cardiac tamponade, the neck veins may be distended with an absent "y" descent. The apical impulse is indistinct or tapping in quality. Cardiac auscultation may reveal "distant" or soft heart sounds. Pulmonary rales are usually absent, and there may be right upper quadrant tenderness from hepatic venous congestion.

Diagnosis The chest radiograph may or may not reveal an enlarged cardiac silhouette because this finding depends on the amount of intrapericardial fluid accumulation. The pulmonary vasculature typically appears normal. An epicardial fat-pad sign may occasionally be seen within the cardiac silhouette.

The ECG usually shows low-voltage QRS complexes (<0.7 mV) and ST-segment elevation (due to the inflammation of the epicardium) with PR-segment depression, as in pericarditis. Electrical alternans (beat-to-beat variation in the amplitude of the P and R waves unrelated to the respiratory cycles; **Figure 55-5**) is a classic but uncommon finding.

The diagnosis should be suspected based on the clinical examination and chest radiograph findings. Echocardiography is the diagnostic test of choice. In addition to a large pericardial fluid volume, typical echocardiographic findings described in cardiac tamponade are right atrial compression, RV diastolic collapse, abnormal respiratory variation in tricuspid and mitral flow velocities, and dilated inferior vena cava with lack of inspiratory collapse.

Treatment and Disposition Volume expansion with a bolus of normal saline solution (500 to 1000 mL) will increase intravascular volume, facilitate right heart filling, and increase cardiac output and arterial pressure. However, it is a temporary measure. Pericardiocentesis is necessary for definitive therapy and for specific diagnosis.

If there is hemodynamic instability, emergency pericardiocentesis is indicated in the ED. The technique is described in Section 4, Resuscitative Procedures, chapter 34, Pericardiocentesis. However, pericardiocentesis is optimally performed in the cardiac catheterization laboratory using echocardiographic guidance to avoid cardiac perforation and coronary artery laceration. In addition, a pigtail catheter can be inserted to allow continuous fluid drainage and prevention of reaccumulation.

CONSTRICTIVE PERICARDITIS

Pathophysiology Constrictive pericarditis results from pericardial injury and inflammation, resulting in fibrous thickening of the layers of the pericardium, which prevents passive diastolic filling of the cardiac chambers.[16] Some causes include postcardiac trauma with intrapericardial hemorrhage, after pericardiotomy (open-heart surgery, including coronary revascularization), in fungal or tuberculous pericarditis, and in chronic renal failure (uremic pericarditis), but in most cases, a specific cause is not determined.

Clinical Features The symptoms of constrictive pericarditis usually develop gradually and may mimic those of CHF and restrictive cardiomyopathy. However, clinical signs may occur early if fluid also accumulates within the thickened, noncompliant pericardial sac (effusive constrictive pericarditis).

Common signs and symptoms include exertional dyspnea, pedal edema, hepatomegaly, and ascites. Examination of the neck veins with the patient at a 45-degree angle from horizontal will reveal jugular venous distention and a rapid "y" descent of the cervical venous pulse. Elevated venous pressure is also seen in CHF, but a rapid "y" descent is infrequently encountered. The Kussmaul sign (inspiratory neck vein distention) is frequent in constrictive pericarditis but rare in CHF. A paradoxical pulse is uncommon, and its absence does not exclude constrictive pericarditis. On cardiac auscultation, an early diastolic sound, a pericardial "knock," may be heard at the apex 60 to 120 milliseconds after the second heart sound. The pericardial knock sounds like a ventricular gallop but occurs earlier than the S_3 of CHF, which it may mimic. The knock is due to accelerated RV inflow in early diastole and early myocardial distention, followed by an abrupt slowing of further ventricular expansion.

Diagnosis • *Electrocardiogram* Low-voltage QRS complexes and inverted T waves are common, but there are no specific diagnostic electrocardiogram signs.

Radiographic Assessment Chest radiographs most commonly demonstrate a normal or slightly enlarged cardiac silhouette, clear lung fields, and little or no evidence of pulmonary venous congestion. Pericardial calcification may be seen. Thoracic CT and MRI may also demonstrate a thickened pericardium.

Echocardiographic Studies On occasion, two-dimensional echocardiography may demonstrate pericardial thickening and abnormal ventricular septal motion in a patient with suspected constrictive pericarditis. However, its diagnostic utility is much less than that in a patient with acute pericarditis. Doppler echocardiography, cardiac CT, and MRI are preferred.

Cardiac Catheterization In many instances cardiac catheterization with measurement of intraventricular pressures will be required to confirm the diagnosis. A characteristic dip and plateau (the "square root sign") of the right ventricular pressure trace is characteristic of the disease.[41]

Treatment and Disposition In cases of significant constriction and impaired ventricular filling, admission for pericardiectomy is the treatment of choice.

REFERENCES

The complete reference list is available online at www.TintinalliEM.com.

Venous Thromboembolism

Jeffrey A. Kline

INTRODUCTION AND EPIDEMIOLOGY

Pulmonary embolism (PE) occurs when clotted blood enters the pulmonary arterial circulation. Most PEs result from deep vein thrombosis (DVT) in the legs, arms, or pelvis and occasionally from the jugular vein or inferior vena cava. The term *venous thromboembolism* (VTE) includes PE and DVT.

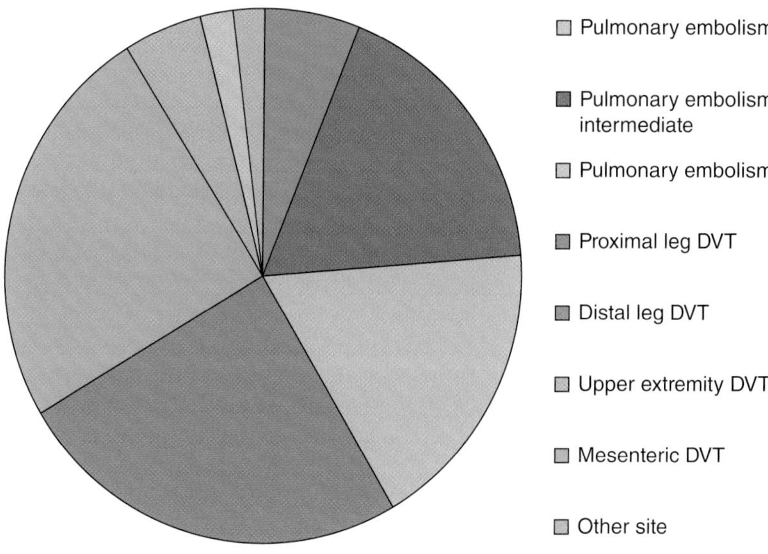

FIGURE 56-1. Distribution of the frequency of clots diagnosed by emergency physicians by severity and location. Major refers to pulmonary embolism (PE) with hypotension, intermediate is PE with right ventricular dysfunction, and minor is small PE without hemodynamic effect. Distal deep vein thrombosis (DVT) refers to calf vein and saphenous vein thrombosis, and other sites include inferior vena cava, pelvic, jugular, ovarian, cerebral, and retinal veins.

In the United States, approximately 200,000 people will have new or recurrent PE diagnosed each year, and twice that many will have DVT without confirmed PE.[1] VTE collectively affects about 1 in 500 persons per year in North America, and about 1 in every 300 adult ED patients receive the diagnosis (**Figure 56-1**). The incidence of VTE increases with age, peaking at 1 in 100 per year at age 80. Based on autopsy data, PE is the second leading cause of sudden, unexpected, nontraumatic death in outpatients.[2] The case fatality rate from PE depends on the hemodynamic severity of the PE, age, and comorbid conditions; the case fatality rate is 45% for PE with circulatory shock, but only about 4% to 5% of patients with PE have shock. In patients with hemodynamically stable PE who are less than 50 years old and without other comorbidities, the case fatality rate is 1%.[3]

Morbidity from DVT includes PE and the postthrombotic syndrome. The latter is manifested as chronic leg swelling and pain and occurs in about 20% of all ED patients with proximal DVT.[4] Both DVT and PE present across a spectrum of severity, with recognition of minor forms of the disease, including distal PE (called subsegmental) and distal DVT, usually in the calf or saphenous veins.[5]

PATHOPHYSIOLOGY

Blood clots occur when coagulation exceeds the removal by fibrinolysis. *Thrombophilias* are conditions that tip the balance of coagulation-fibrinolysis toward excessive clotting. Most guidelines categorize VTE as provoked (or secondary) or unprovoked (idiopathic).[6] Provoked VTEs are *acquired* and often time-limited conditions, generally often following recent surgery, trauma, or any condition associated with limb or body immobility; active cancer is a VTE provoker that often persists. Other provoking factors generally include diseases or conditions that impede venous blood flow, infection, chronic disease, estrogen use, pregnancy or initial postpartum interval, and age >50 years (each year after 50 increases the risk). Unprovoked VTE patients have no known risk factors, suggesting an increased tendency to clot.

Most VTEs diagnosed in the ED are unprovoked.[3,7] Patients with unprovoked VTE have a 15% chance of recurrence in the next year compared with 5% for those with a provoked episode. For this reason, those with unprovoked VTE usually receive longer treatment than patients with provoked VTE.[8] Those with provoked VTE have a higher 1-year death rate, likely from the comorbid conditions (notably cancer).[9]

Venous thrombi that are large enough to cause clinically important PE can form in the popliteal, common femoral, superficial femoral, pelvic, axillary, jugular, and great veins. At least one third of patients with DVT have concomitant PE, even when the patient lacks symptoms of PE.[10] Although 75% to 80% of hospitalized patients with PE have image-demonstrated DVT, only 40% of ambulatory ED patients with PE have concomitant DVT.[11]

Blood clots that form in the large veins of the legs, especially the femoral and iliofemoral veins, usually begin on the valves, leading to scarring and poor function of the venous valves. This causes pooling of venous blood in the legs, leading to varicose veins, pain, swelling, skin hyperpigmentation, and ulcers, known as the postthrombotic syndrome.[4] With PE, the correlation between the degree of initial pulmonary vascular obstruction and clinical severity is weak, but patients without prior heart or lung disease generally begin to experience symptoms from PE when approximately 20% of lung vasculature becomes occluded.[12] With larger clot burden, the pulmonary arterial pressure increases, leading to right ventricular dilation and myocardial damage, causing the release of troponin and B-type natriuretic peptide. Right ventricular dilation or injury, as evidenced on CT or echocardiography or suggested by elevated troponin or B-type natriuretic peptide, indicates right heart failure and increased risk of circulatory shock and death.[13] The two principle mechanisms of death from PE appear to be abrupt near-total pulmonary artery occlusion that leads to pulseless electrical activity and asystole from ischemic effect on the His-Purkinje conduction system. Approximately one third of survivors of large PEs go on to have persistent right heart dysfunction and severe symptoms.[14] Approximately 5% of patients with PE go on to experience chronic pulmonary vascular obstruction, leading to progressive damage to the lung vessels and right heart with disabling dyspnea and pulmonary hypertension, called *chronic thromboembolic pulmonary hypertension.*

Inherited thrombophilias increase risk of first-time VTE, although most of these patients are unaware of this condition until a clot occurs. The risk of recurrent VTE in those with a known thrombophilia is the same as in those who have had a prior unprovoked VTE absent that condition.[15]

With limb immobility, the risk *increases* depending on joint, as follows: elbow (least), shoulder, ankle, knee, and hip (most). Acute immobilization of the hip and knee in one leg with non–weight bearing causes the greatest risk for VTE, whereas immobilization of the wrist alone probably causes no risk. In addition to the presence of limb immobility, risk of VTE increases with whole-body immobility or neurologic immobility, but not by travel, even if >8 hours.[16]

Over half of patients with postoperative PE receive the diagnosis after hospital discharge, and the average time from surgery to PE diagnosis is >10 days. Risk increases with patient age, longer surgery, open surgery, and surgery in which thromboprophylaxis is not used. The highest-risk surgeries include abdominal surgery to remove cancer, joint replacement surgery, and surgery on the brain or spinal cord in the setting of neurologic deficits. However, the risk of recurrence after surgery-provoked VTE is generally lower than for unprovoked VTE, although the 4-year risk of recurrence ranges from 5% to 11% per year depending on the surgical procedure.[17]

Thrombogenic potential of cancer varies with host factors, tumor stage, and tumor type. In general, the more undifferentiated the cell type and the larger the tumor burden (especially distant metastasis), the higher is the risk. Cancers that are particularly thrombogenic include adenocarcinoma, glioblastoma, metastatic melanoma, lymphoma, and multiple myeloma.[18] Pancreatic, stomach, ovarian, and renal cell cancers carry notoriously high risk.

Cancers with minimal risk of VTE include localized breast, cervical, prostate, and nonmelanomatous localized skin cancers such as squamous cell carcinoma and basal cell carcinoma not treated with chemotherapy. However, about 10% of patients with advanced-stage breast cancer or with breast cancer undergoing chemotherapy develop symptomatic VTE. VTE risk is high during the induction phase of chemotherapy, especially if treated with L-asparaginase and bolus fluorouracil or tamoxifen. Concomitant treatment with red blood cell growth factors such as erythropoietin increases risk of thrombosis, regardless of tumor type or stage.[18] Similarly, multiple myeloma patients treated with lenalidomide or thalidomide are at high risk of VTE.[19]

A family history of VTE increases longitudinal risk of VTE,[20] although this has no impact on outcomes.[7] Although sex does not play a role in first-time VTE, men have more recurrent VTE.[8]

Table 56-1 presents a list of risk factors for VTE relevant to ED practice.

Although smoking causes conditions that increase risk (e.g., cancer) and acts synergistically with obesity and possibly oral contraceptive use, smoking is not an independent risk factor for VTE.[7]

TABLE 56-1 Risk Factors for Venous Thromboembolism (VTE) That are Generally Relevant to Emergency Medicine

Factor	Comment
Age	Risk becomes significant at 50 y and increases with each year of life until age 80 y.
Obesity	In the general population, VTE risk starts at BMI >35 kg/m^2 and increases with increasing BMI.
Pregnancy and postpartum state	70% of all peripartum PEs occur postpartum. Risk increases with trimester (but overall risk remains low throughout pregnancy).
Prior VTE	Highest risk of recurrence is for unprovoked VTE in men, particularly if D-dimer remains elevated
Solid cancers	Risk greatest with adenocarcinomas and metastatic disease. A history of remote, inactive cancer probably does not increase risk.
Hematologic cancers	Acute leukemias and myeloma confer the greatest risk, particularly when treated with L-asparaginase and the thalidomide derivatives.
Thrombophilias	Non-O blood type, lupus anticoagulant, shortened aPTT, factor V Leiden, and familial protein C and S and antithrombin deficiency have the strongest risk.
Recent surgery or major trauma	Risk increased with endotracheal intubation or epidural anesthesia and continues at least 4 weeks after exposure. Risk varies with type of surgery.
Immobility	Acute limb immobility of two contiguous joints confers the highest risk.
Bed rest	Becomes a risk factor at approximately 72 h.
Indwelling catheters	Cause approximately one half of arm deep venous thromboses.
Long-distance travel	Published data are controversial. In general, risk becomes significant after 6 h of continuous travel.
Smoking	A population risk factor, but not a factor that increases probability of VTE in the ED setting. May increase risk of other factors such as obesity.
Congestive heart failure	Related primarily to severity of systolic dysfunction.
Stroke	Risk greatest in first month after deficit.
Estrogen	Highest-risk period is in the first few months. All contraceptives containing estrogen increase risk of VTE including transdermal and transvaginal preparations.
Noninfectious inflammatory conditions	Examples are inflammatory bowel disease, lupus, and nephrotic syndrome. Risk of VTE increases roughly in proportion to severity of underlying disease.

Abbreviations: aPTT = activated partial thromboplastin time; BMI = body mass index; PE = pulmonary embolism.

CLINICAL FEATURES OF PULMONARY EMBOLISM

PE symptoms range from none to sudden death. Patients with similar comorbidities and clot burden may have drastically different clinical presentations. **Table 56-2** lists factors that affect symptoms.

The hallmark of PE is dyspnea unexplained by auscultatory findings, ECG changes, or clear alternative diagnosis on chest radiograph. Chest pain with pleuritic features is the second most common symptom of PE, although about one half of all patients diagnosed with PE in the ED have no complaint of chest pain.[7] The classic PE pain is in the thorax between the clavicles and the costal margin that increases with cough or breathing; it is not purely substernal and not manifested from the skin or muscle. Pulmonary infarction can inflict severe focal pain, although most patients with PE and pleuritic chest pain have no radiographic evidence of pulmonary infarction. Pulmonary infarction in basilar lung segments can manifest as referred pain to either shoulder or mimic biliary or ureteral colic. Proximal PE without infarction can also cause pleuritic chest pain without focal pain.

HISTORY

In addition to the common symptoms of chest pain and dyspnea, approximately 3% to 4% of ED patients with PE have syncope, and another 1% to 2% present with new-onset seizure (or convulsion-like activity) or confusion.[3] Because about 20% of people have a patent foramen ovale, PE that increases right-sided pressures can lead to right-to-left transit of thrombotic material in the atria and showers into the brain circulation, producing stroke-like symptoms called the **paradoxical embolism syndrome**. Neurologic symptoms can vary widely, from classic localized findings to staring spells, transient altered mental status, and atypical myelopathy symptoms (e.g., numbness below the waist), all of which can fluctuate.[21] Presence of a patent foramen ovale worsens the prognosis in PE.

PHYSICAL EXAMINATION

On physical examination, abnormal vital signs suggest acute cardiopulmonary stress in a patient with PE: tachycardia, tachypnea, a low pulse oximetry reading, and sometimes mild fever. Unfortunately, PE does not predictably alter any vital sign; approximately one half of patients with proven PE have a heart rate of <100 beats/min at diagnosis, and approximately one third have abnormal early vital signs that normalize in the ED.[22] The mechanism of altered vital signs results in obstruction to blood flow and clot-derived autacoids, which together stimulate adrenergic efferent fibers to the heart and cause ventilation–perfusion mismatch on the lungs. The amount of clot burden does not predict vital sign changes reliably, with no clear correlation between measured clot and initial heart rate or oximetry. Although approximately 10% of patients with PE have an oral temperature of >38°C (100.4°F), <2% of patients with PE have a temperature of >39.2°C (102.5°F).

Most patients with PE have clear lungs on auscultation. Wheezes or bilateral rales make an alternative diagnosis of bronchospasm or pneumonia possible but do not exclude PE. For example, pulmonary infarction may produce rales over the affected lung segment. On heart

TABLE 56-2 Factors That Can Affect the Clinical Presentation of Patients with Pulmonary Embolism (PE)

Cofactor	Clinical Impact	Comment
Previously healthy and young age	Less severe signs and symptoms	One half of previously healthy patients with first-time PE have normal vital sign values at diagnosis.
Prior cardiopulmonary disease	Can either amplify or obscure history and findings	Most patients with PE complicating baseline cardiopulmonary disease describe dyspnea with PE as "worse than usual."
Patient cognitive dysfunction	Causes the history to be less reliable	Approximately 20% of patients with PE missed by ED clinicians had baseline dementia.
Clot size and location	Affects severity of dyspnea, pain, and signs	Proximal clots cause ventilation–perfusion mismatch and dyspnea; distal clots cause infarction with pain.
Gradual loading of PE over time	Gradual onset of dyspnea on exertion and fatigue	Has symptom overlap with left ventricular dysfunction. Fewer than one half of patients with PE describe symptom onset as sudden.

examination, one may hear a right ventricular S_3 or a split S_2 with a loud second sound. The presence of a percutaneous indwelling catheters in the arm increases the probability of axillary vein thrombosis, although it is less clear whether these lines, dialysis catheters, or pacemaker wires also increase the risk of symptomatic PE.

CLINICAL FEATURES OF DEEP VEIN THROMBOSIS

Patients with DVT complain of extremity pain, swelling, or cramping. A difference of ≥2 cm between right and left leg diameter at 10 cm below the tibial tubercle doubles the likelihood of DVT. Patients presenting with upper extremity catheter-related DVT often complain of hand swelling or tightness around finger rings. About one quarter of patients with DVT have tenderness and redness in the swollen extremity, findings that are similar to those of cellulitis. Calf or saphenous vein clots are more likely to cause thrombophlebitis, defined formally as inflammation (pain, tenderness, redness, and swelling) over a vein secondary to the presence of thrombotic material in the vein. Signs and symptoms of thrombophlebitis can persist after the vein has recannulated and the clot has dissolved entirely. Calf vein thrombosis may cause **Homan's sign**, which is calf pain elicited by passive foot dorsiflexion; this test has such low sensitivity and specificity that it has no predictive value.

Proximal DVT that causes complete venous obstruction leads to increased compartmental pressures, manifested as an extremely painful, swollen extremity. A swollen, painful, and pale or white limb with a proximal venous thrombosis is termed **phlegmasia alba dolens**, whereas a limb with a dusky or blue color is called **phlegmasia cerulea dolens**. Either condition poses the threat of limb loss, demanding aggressive treatment that can include thrombolysis or catheter-directed thrombectomy.

DIAGNOSIS

Routine cardiopulmonary testing in the ED generally demonstrates nonspecific findings in patients with PE. The mean pulse oximetry reading is lower in patients with proven PE than in those without PE (93 ± 2% vs 95 ± 3%), although this one signal may be absent in those with PE. Similarly, the mean partial pressure of oxygen in arterial blood (Pao_2) is lower (73 ± 19 mm Hg vs 80 ± 21 mm Hg), and the difference between the estimated partial pressure of oxygen in the alveoli (PAO_2) and the measured Pao_2, the alveolar-arterial gradient [$P(A\text{-}a)O_2$], is increased. The arterial partial pressure of carbon dioxide ($Paco_2$) is usually low, reflecting a 20% to 50% increase in minute ventilation to compensate for loss of lung efficiency secondary to the increased dead space. Spontaneously breathing patients with PE also demonstrate a lower end-tidal carbon dioxide compared with healthy individuals.[23]

Most patients with PE have a chest radiograph with one or more abnormalities, including cardiomegaly, basilar atelectasis, infiltrate, or pleural effusion; all are nonspecific for PE. In <5% of patients, a wedge-shaped area of lung oligemia (Westermark sign—usually from complete lobar artery obstruction) or peripheral dome-shaped dense opacification (Hampton hump—always indicative of pulmonary infarction) exists. **The presence of hypoxemia or dyspnea with clear lungs on physical exam and imaging suggests PE.**

The 12-lead ECG is usually nonspecific, with sinus tachycardia or nonspecific ST- and T-wave changes. When PE causes the right ventricular systolic pressure to exceed 40 mm Hg, the ECG can be more specific, including T-wave inversion in leads V_1 to V_4, incomplete or complete right bundle-branch block, and the classic but uncommon S_1-Q_3-T_3 pattern (**Figure 56-2**).[24] A clinical ECG score allows severity assessment in those with diagnosed PE (higher score equates to higher mortality, **Table 56-3**).[25]

DIAGNOSTIC TESTING FOR VENOUS THROMBOEMBOLISM

DECISION RULES AND CLINICAL ASSESSMENT

Estimating the pretest probability for VTE in a patient is the first step in selecting a diagnostic pathway. Figure 56-3 shows one diagnostic algorithm; **no singular diagnostic test or algorithm perfectly excludes or diagnoses VTE.** Aggressive diagnostic searches can cause harm disproportionate to benefit from hemorrhage associated with anticoagulation for a false-positive result or self-limited small clot diagnosis or from contrast nephropathy. One approach is to test further only in those with pretest probabilities of >2.5%[26]; those with a pretest probability of PE <2.5% are more likely to be harmed than helped by a diagnostic test, even a D-dimer assay.

The PE rule-out criteria (**Table 56-4**) reliably forecast a probability of PE that is below the 2.0% test threshold in patients *with a gestalt low clinical suspicion*.[27,28] The American College of Emergency Physicians' Clinical Guidelines committee provided a 2b recommendation for the PE rule-out criteria rule.[29] The PE rule-out criteria rule had an apparently high failure rate in one secondary analysis done in a European population with a prevalence of disease of 27% in conjunction with a low-risk Geneva score.[30] However, the subsequent published erratum to the work showed that the PE rule-out criteria rule had 100% sensitivity in the same population *when combined with low gestalt pretest probability* as designed, which was also the case in other studies.[28,31] Thus, taken together, the weight of the available information indicates that PE can be reliably excluded by the combination of a low gestalt pretest probability plus a negative PE rule-out criteria rule. However, not all patients who have any positive PE rule-out criteria must undergo an objective test for PE, since anyone over 50 years old would be tested with any finding even if suspicion was low. The key is generating a clinical gestalt first and, if low, using the PE rule-out criteria to guide further testing.

Most validated PE prediction systems categorize the patient into one of two (low or above low probability) or three (low, moderate, or higher probability) categories.[33] One method uses a computerized database-derived method based on the method of attribute matching to estimate a discrete numerical percentage probability of PE.[26] The **Wells' score** is the most robust scoring system for categorizing the pretest probability for both PE (**Table 56-5**) and DVT (**Table 56-6**).

The Wells' original rules separate patients into low-, moderate-, and high-probability groups. The Wells' DVT and PE scoring systems both reliably produce a stepwise increase in probability of clot presence with higher scores. The Wells' scoring system has been modified to classify patients being evaluated for possible PE into a low-risk (score ≤4) or a non–low-risk group (score >4), which has become a mainstream method of use.[34] The **Charlotte rule** is designed to categorize patients into either a low-risk or non–low-risk group (designated "safe" or "unsafe" in **Figure 56-4**).

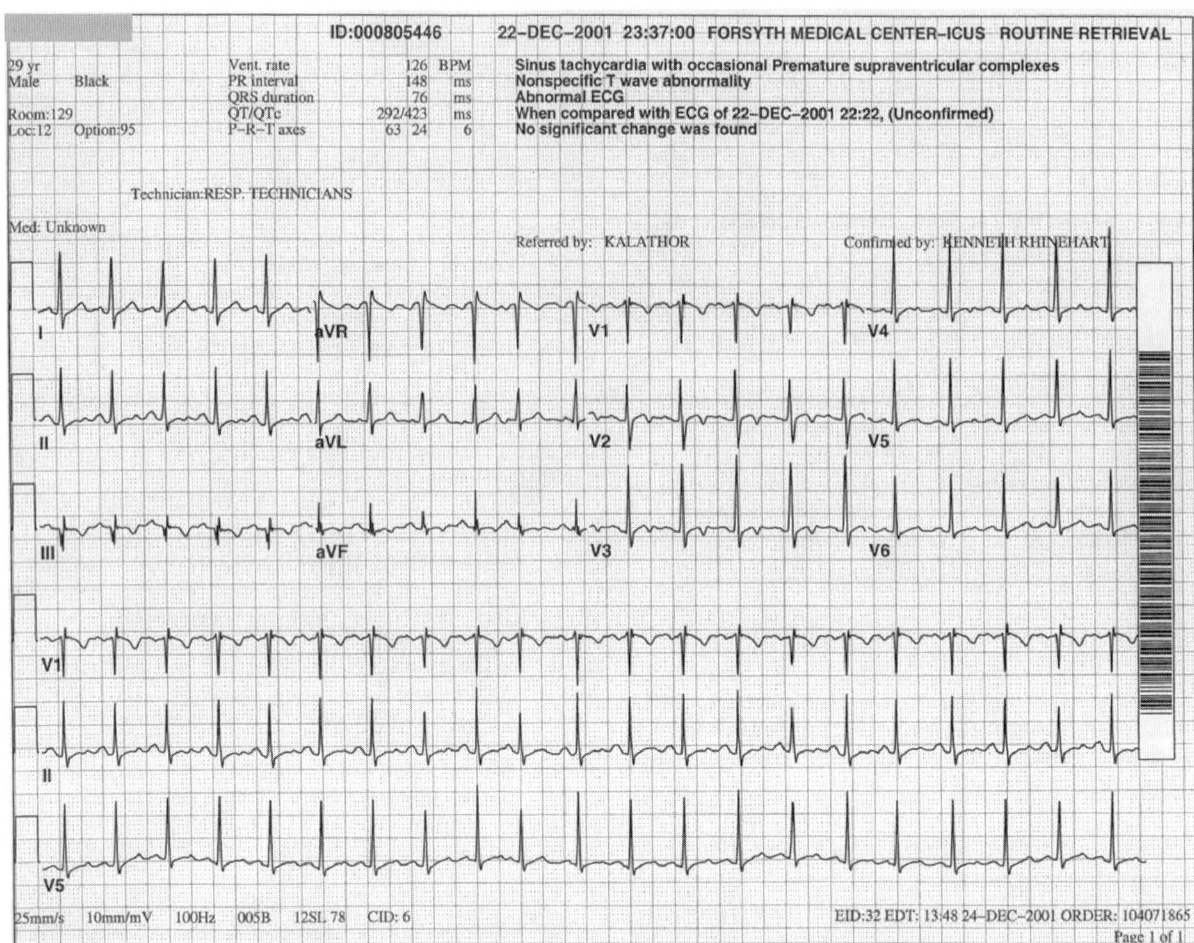

FIGURE 56-2. This 12-lead ECG shows many features of a severe PE: tachycardia, an incomplete right bundle-branch block, an S_1-Q_3-T_3 pattern, and T-wave inversion in the anterior leads.

TABLE 56-3 ECG Scoring Method to Assess Severity of Pulmonary Embolism

Characteristics	Score
Tachycardia (>100 beats/min)	2
Incomplete right bundle-branch block	2
Complete right bundle-branch block	3
T-wave inversion in leads V_1 through V_4	4
T-wave inversion in lead V_1*	
<1 mm	0
1–2 mm	1
>2 mm	2
T-wave inversion in lead V_2*	
<1 mm	1
1–2 mm	2
>2 mm	3
T-wave inversion in lead V_3*	
<1 mm	1
1–2 mm	2
>2 mm	3
S wave in lead 1	0
Q wave in lead 3	1
Inverted T wave in lead 3	1
If all S_1-Q_3-T_3 pattern, add	2
Total score (maximum: 21)	

*If present, check maximum only.

The Wells' rule has a subjective component—clinical judgment of the likelihood of an alternative diagnosis. Both the Charlotte rule and the revised **Geneva score** (**Table 56-7**) exclude subjective assessments.

Runyon et al[35] studied the accuracy of unstructured, gestalt estimation of pretest probability for PE, grouping patients into low-, moderate-, and high-risk categories (where the cutoffs suggested to the clinicians were <15%, 15% to 40%, and >40%); the measured frequencies of PE were similar when stratified by Wells' or Geneva scores.[33] Moreover, the interobserver agreement for gestalt classification was good (κ = 0.60), and gestalt estimation did not show a decrease in sensitivity based on training level.[35] Gestalt estimation is a viable method to estimate pretest probability and is preferred over no estimation.

D-DIMER TESTING

The D-dimer assay is the best blood test to exclude VTE, working on the principle that clots contain fibrin that is degraded naturally through the action of plasmin. Fibrin breakdown liberates the D-dimer protein into the blood. Multiple manufacturers each produce a slightly different assay, but the D-dimer test can be broadly classified as either qualitative or quantitative. Qualitative tests generally have lower diagnostic sensitivity but higher specificity compared with quantitative tests. Quantitative tests are usually done in the central hospital laboratory and require a turnaround time of at least 1 hour. Different D-dimer assays have different thresholds for normal because of different capture antibodies and optical methods of detection. Some laboratories report results in D-dimer mass concentration (e.g., nanograms per milliliter or micrograms per milliliter), and others report fibrinogen equivalent units. Two fibrinogen molecules produce one D-dimer unit, so that the fibrinogen equivalent unit number is twice the D-dimer number for the same measurement. For PE and DVT, the diagnostic sensitivity of automated

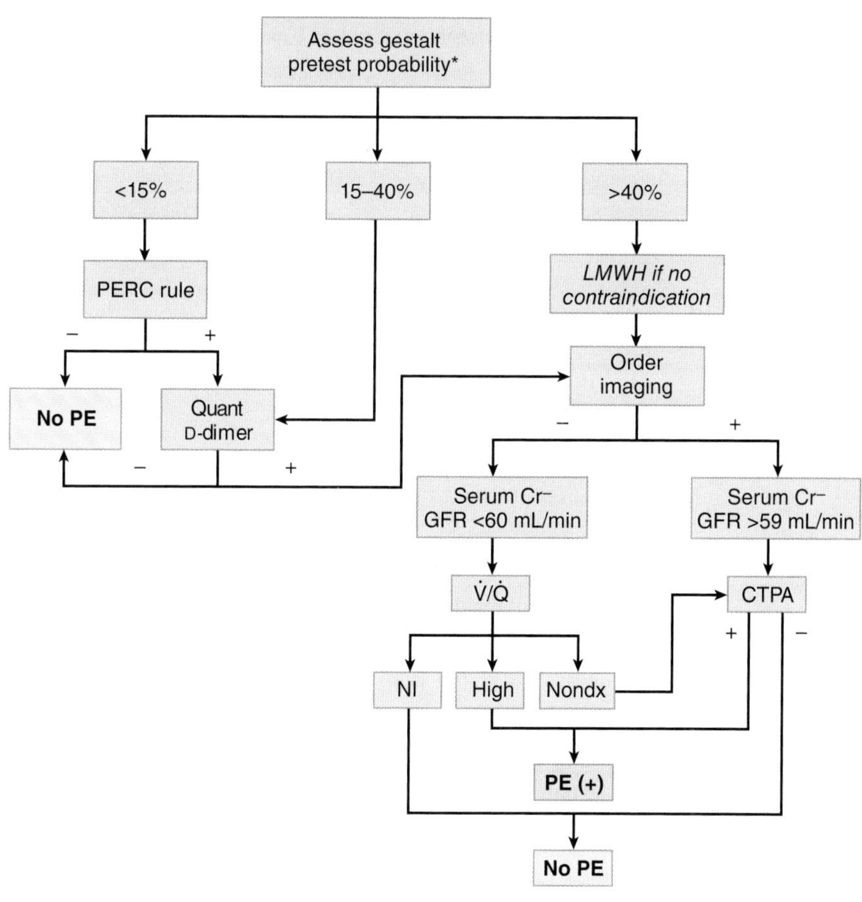

FIGURE 56-3. Pulmonary embolism rule-out criteria (PERC) rule—diagnostic algorithm for pulmonary embolism (PE). *Some physicians prefer to start with a clinical decision rule such as the Wells' score (where <2, 2–6, and >6 are used instead of <15%, 15%–40%, and >40%, respectively). Note: Determine renal function by clinical picture (healthy, no risk factors for reduced glomerular filtration rate [GFR]) or calculated GFR. Nondiagnostic ventilation–perfusion (V̇/Q̇) scan findings require confirmation from results of another test, such as CT pulmonary angiography (CTPA), if benefits outweigh risks. + = positive for PE; – = negative for PE; Cr = creatinine; High = high probability scan findings; LMWH = low-molecular-weight heparin; Nl = normal; Nondx = nondiagnostic (any reading other than normal or high probability); quant = quantitative.

TABLE 56-4 Pulmonary Embolism Rule-Out Criteria Rule (all nine factors must be present to exclude pulmonary embolism)[32]

Clinical low probability (<15% probability of pulmonary embolism based on gestalt assessment)
Age <50 years
Pulse <100 beats/min during entire stay in ED
Pulse oximetry >94% at near sea level (>92% at altitudes near 5000 feet above sea level)
No hemoptysis
No prior venous thromboembolism history
No surgery or trauma requiring endotracheal or epidural anesthesia within the last 4 weeks
No estrogen use
No unilateral leg swelling, defined as asymmetrical calves on visual inspection with patient's heels raised off the bed

TABLE 56-5 Wells' Score for Pulmonary Embolism

Factor	Points*
Suspected deep venous thrombosis	3
Alternative diagnosis less likely than PE	3
Heart rate >100 beats/min	1.5
Prior venous thromboembolism	1.5
Immobilization within prior 4 wk	1.5
Active malignancy	1
Hemoptysis	1

*Risk score interpretation (probability of PE): >6 points = high risk (78.4%); 2–6 points = moderate risk (27.8%); and <2 points = low risk (3.4%).

Source: Adapted with permission from Wells PS, Anderson DR, Rodger M, et al: Derivation of a simple clinical model to categorize patients' probability of pulmonary embolism: increasing the model utility with the SimpliRED D-dimer. *Thromb Haemost* 83: 418, 2000.

TABLE 56-6 Wells' Score for Deep Vein Thrombosis

Clinical Feature	Points*
Active cancer (treatment within 6 mo, or palliation)	1
Paralysis, paresis, or immobilization of lower extremity	1
Bedridden for >3 d because of surgery (within 12 wk)	1
Localized tenderness along distribution of deep veins	1
Entire leg swollen	1
Unilateral calf swelling of >3 cm (below tibial tuberosity)	1
Unilateral pitting edema	1
Collateral superficial veins	1
Alternative diagnosis as likely as or more likely than deep venous thrombosis	–2
Prior history of DVT or PE†	1

*Risk score interpretation (probability of deep venous thrombosis) in original Wells DVT model: ≥3 points: high risk (75%); 1 or 2 points: moderate risk (17%); <1 point: low risk (3%).

†Only awarded in the modified (dichotomized) Wells DVT model: ≤1 point DVT unlikely >1 point DVT likely.

Source: Adapted from Geersing GJ, Zuithoff NP, Kearon C, et al. Exclusion of deep vein thrombosis using the Wells rule in clinically important subgroups: individual patient data meta-analysis. BMJ. 2014 348:g1340 (1-13).

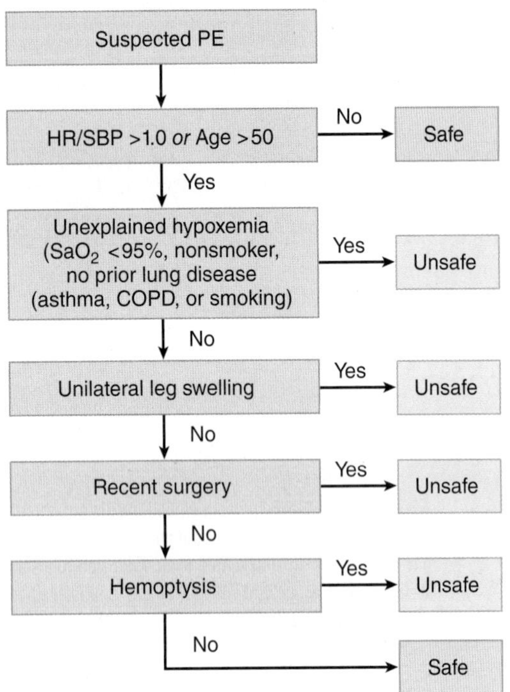

FIGURE 56-4. Charlotte rule for patients with suspected pulmonary embolism (PE). Patients for whom the decision tree leads to the "safe" boxes have a sufficiently low pretest probability to permit PE to be ruled out solely on the basis of a normal quantitative D-Dimer test result. COPD = chronic obstructive pulmonary disease; HR = heart rate; Sa_{O_2} = arterial oxygen saturation; SBP = systolic blood pressure.

quantitative D-dimer assays ranges from 94% to 98% and the specificity ranges from 50% to 60%. **The D-dimer has a half-life of approximately 8 hours and can be elevated for at least 3 days after symptomatic VTE.**

The most common causes of a false-negative or positive D-dimer result are listed in **Table 56-8**; notably, all risk factors for VTE may elevate the D-dimer level. D-Dimer increases with age and should be adjusted upward for age to maintain adequate exclusionary ability. The most common formula studied is age × 10 nanograms/mL (e.g., an 80-year-old patient would have an adjusted threshold for abnormal at 800 nanograms/mL).[34] This assumes the conventional D-dimer cutoff of 500 nanograms/mL; in a large multicenter study, this adjusted approach resulted in a very low false-negative rate (0.3%) when used in conjunction with a Wells' score ≤4 or a simplified revised Geneva score <5.[34]

TABLE 56-7 Revised Geneva Score for Pulmonary Embolism

Clinical Variable	Points*
Age >65 y	1
Previous venous thromboembolism	3
Surgery requiring anesthesia or fracture of lower limb in past month	2
Active malignancy	2
Unilateral leg pain	3
Hemoptysis	2
Unilateral leg edema	4
Heart rate	
75–94 beats/min	3
>95 beats/min	5

*Total score of 0–3 indicates low probability, score of 4–10 indicates moderate probability, and score of >10 indicates high probability of pulmonary embolism.

TABLE 56-8 Factors Known to Alter the D-Dimer Level from Expected Values

Potential False-Positive Levels	Potential False-Negative Levels
Age >70 y	Warfarin treatment
Pregnancy	Symptoms lasting over 5 d
Active malignancy or metastasis	Presence of small clots
Surgical procedure in previous week	Isolated small pulmonary infarction
Liver disease	Isolated calf vein thrombosis
Rheumatoid arthritis	Lipemia
Infections	
Trauma	

IMAGING

Chest CT Angiography **Chest CT angiography** is the most common imaging modality for PE, identifying a clot as a filling defect in contrast-enhanced pulmonary arteries (**Figure 56-5**). Equipment with more detector heads (e.g., 64- or 128-head scanners) allows better resolution and observation of filling defects in subsegmental pulmonary arteries. The diagnostic sensitivity and specificity of a technically adequate mutidetector CT scan are about 90%.[36] Most CT pulmonary angiography protocols require the patient to lie supine and hold their breath for a few seconds, and the scan requires injection of approximately 120 mL of contrast by a computer-controlled injection device. In most centers, the patient must have a peripheral IV catheter (20 gauge or larger) or an approved indwelling line to allow injection of the contrast, and a central catheter cannot be used for injection.

In addition to clot recognition, a CT scan can detect alternative diagnoses, often pneumonia (8% to 22% of cases).[37] Interobserver agreement in identifying segmental or larger filling defects is very good, but interobserver agreement for subsegmental clots is poor. In practice, approximately 10% of CT scans are inadequate from secondary motion artifact or poor pulmonary artery opacification, commonly in obese or

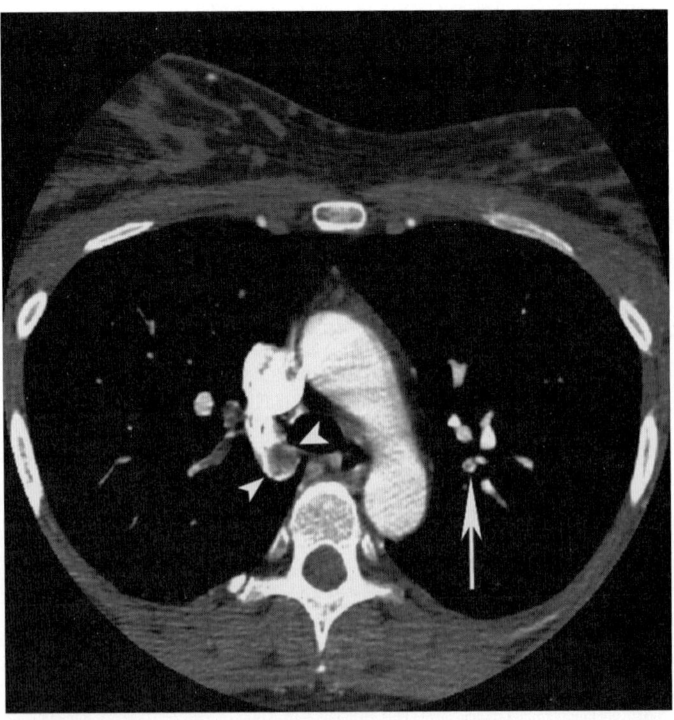

FIGURE 56-5. Axial image from a chest CT angiogram demonstrating a filling defect consistent with acute pulmonary embolism. Two *white arrowheads* outline a circular filling defect in the right middle lobar pulmonary artery. The *long white arrow* projecting in the left lung points to a filling defect in a segmental artery in the posterior medial segmental artery.

very tachypneic patients. Acute life-threatening contrast-triggered anaphylaxis or pulmonary edema is very rare, occurring in about 1 in 1000 patients.[38] About 15% of patients undergoing contrast-enhanced chest CT scan develop contrast nephropathy, defined as a 25% or greater increase in the serum creatinine concentration within 2 to 7 days of the examination.[39,40] **At present, the only clearly helpful prophylactic measure to reduce contrast nephropathy is hydration with intravenous balanced crystalloid solutions.**[41] Other complications from CT scanning include contrast extravasation into a limb that can cause pain or compartment syndrome, and creation of a secondary thrombophlebitis.

Ventilation-Perfusion Lung Scanning **Ventilation–perfusion ($\dot{V}/\dot{Q}$) lung scanning** can identify a perfusion defect when ventilation is normal. $\dot{V}/\dot{Q}$ scanning measures scintillation produced from a gamma ray–emitting atom and yields an image that plots the density of scintillations emitted from the chest using two phases. The perfusion images are usually obtained first and require a peripheral IV catheter for injection and the ability of the patient to sit up and lie down during the procedure. The ventilation component requires the patient to breathe into a nebulizer to inhale an aerosol that contains the isotope. A $\dot{V}/\dot{Q}$ scan with homogeneous scintillation throughout the lung in the perfusion portion has nearly 100% sensitivity in excluding PE, regardless of the appearance of the ventilation portion. A $\dot{V}/\dot{Q}$ scan with two or more apex central wedge-shaped defects in the perfusion phase (**Figure 56-6**) with normal ventilation in these regions indicates >80% probability of PE. All other $\dot{V}/\dot{Q}$ scan findings are nondiagnostic; taken alone, these cannot exclude or diagnose PE.

PULMONARY ANGIOGRAPHY Direct **pulmonary angiography** identifies a clot as a filling defect within the pulmonary artery. This test requires placement of a catheter into the pulmonary artery, usually through the femoral vein, followed by injection of 150 to 300 mL of contrast material. Advantages of direct pulmonary angiography include the ability to demonstrate filling defects in 3-mm or smaller vessels; the ability to measure pulmonary artery pressures; and the potential to treat PE with intrapulmonary catheter–directed modalities or to deploy a vena caval filter. Disadvantages of pulmonary angiography include lack of availability, radiation exposure, and the possibility of contrast-related complications, cardiac dysrhythmias, and rare cardiac or pulmonary arterial perforation.

Venous US **Venous US** is the imaging test of choice in DVT; it can be done quickly and does not use ionizing radiation. When performed by experienced ultrasonographers, it has a diagnostic sensitivity of 90% to 95% and a specificity of 95% for DVT, and venous US has a sensitivity of about 40% as a surrogate method to diagnose PE. The mean sensitivity for DVT of US performed by a trained emergency physician compared with the reference imaging test is 96.1% (95% CI, 90.6% to 98.5%), with a weighted mean specificity of 96.8% (95% CI. 94.6% to 98.1%).[42] However, the details of test performance and training remain important, as two-point compression US may miss some clots and new users require experience with at least 10 examinations before gaining adequate skill.

Compression ultrasonography operates on the principle that normal veins compress but thrombosed veins do not. A 7.5-MHz probe is used to visualize the common femoral, superficial femoral, and popliteal veins for comparison with the adjacent femoral and popliteal arteries. The sonographer manually compresses the probe and compares the flattening of the vein with that of the artery. If the vein compresses completely whereas the artery remains patent, this finding indicates "normal compressibility," and the absence of a thrombus is inferred (**Figure 56-7**). Conversely, if the vein does not compress, the examination is considered positive for a thrombus. The practice of examining the saphenous, tibial, and peroneal veins varies among centers.

The disadvantages of formal US include the need for specialized equipment and a qualified sonographer and radiologist. The examination can be difficult to perform in obese patients, and the probability of an indeterminate result increases with higher patient body mass index. The compression component of the examination causes pain in some patients and could promote clot embolization. Prior history of DVT can make it difficult to determine if venous noncompressibility represents an old or new clot. Color flow Doppler US can help identify recannulization, suggesting a chronic clot, which may not need anticoagulation.

Venography Indirect **CT venography** acquires axial images of the leg veins during the venous return phase minutes after the contrast is injected for chest CT angiography. At present, the low rate of clinical utility, increased gonadal radiation, poor technical resolution, and low interobserver reliability for distal DVT all point away from the value of routine CT venography in the workup of an ED patient with suspected PE.[43]

Planar venography requires injection of contrast material into a small vein in the foot with a proximal venous tourniquet. Subsequent images detail the entire leg venous system, identifying filling defects

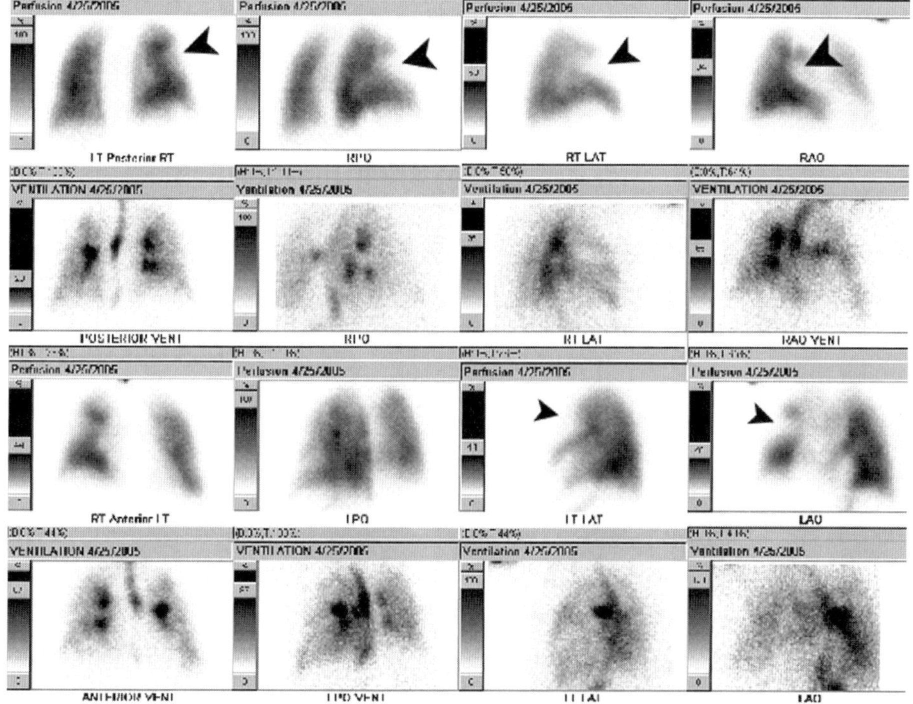

FIGURE 56-6. Ventilation–perfusion lung scan series consistent with a high probability of acute pulmonary embolism (PE) using standard criteria. The first and third rows project the perfusion phases of the examination, and the second and fourth rows show the ventilation phases. The *black arrowheads* point to wedge-shaped defects in the perfusion images. Comparison with the corresponding ventilation view immediately below shows relatively homogeneous scintillation activity in the anatomic segments that lack perfusion. These defects are consistent with an acute PE.

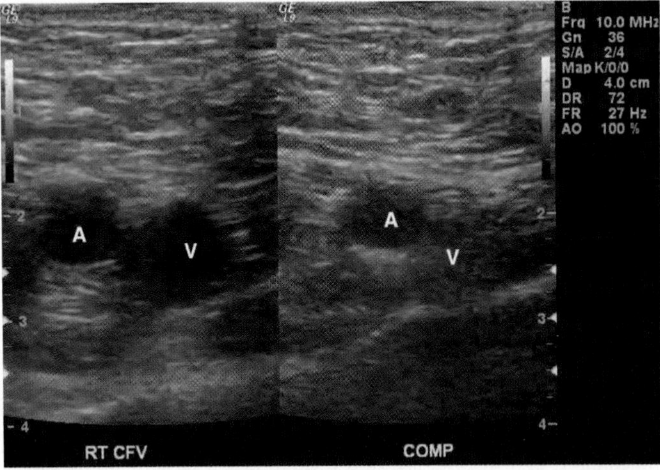

A

B

FIGURE 56-7. Compression venous US images showing normal findings and findings indicating deep venous thrombosis. **A.** Compression venous US of the common femoral vein and femoral artery. The left view shows a sonographic image of the right femoral artery (A) and common femoral vein (V) obtained immediately inferior to the inguinal ligament. The image on the right shows the same view after manual compression by the operator. The image demonstrates obliteration of the vein while the artery remains open. This is a normal US finding for the vein. **B.** Venous US image showing evidence of common left femoral vein thrombosis after compression (right panel). The common femoral vein (V) does not compress. Echogenic thrombolytic material can be observed within the vein.

anywhere from the distal calf up to the iliac vein. Because alternative diagnostic imaging is readily available and a contrast-induced leg clot can result from the test in 10% to 15% of uses, venography is now rarely performed.

INTEGRATED APPROACH TO DIAGNOSIS AND TREATMENT

STEP ONE

For a patient to enter a PE testing regimen, he or she should have at least one physiologic manifestation of PE. This may be a symptom (e.g., pain in the chest or torso, a breathing problem, or altered mental status) or a finding (e.g., an abnormal vital sign) that could be produced by a clot in the lung. The physiologic manifestation must be placed in the context of the given patient—an untreated asthmatic patient with shortness of breath and wheezing should be treated first for bronchospasm and reevaluated and not immediately tested for PE. A risk factor for PE in the absence of a known sign or symptom ***does not*** mandate testing for PE or DVT.

STEP TWO

After finding a physiologic manifestation of PE, the next step is to ask, "Do I have more than a low initial suspicion for PE?" Low suspicion means that the physician's gestalt interpretation of the overall clinical picture is PE presence of <15%. If the answer to this question is yes, then a diagnostic test is needed. If the answer is no, then it remains possible that PE can be excluded using the PE rule-out criteria rule. If all eight criteria of the PE rule-out criteria rule are met in the setting of a gestalt-based low suspicion, then no further testing is necessary.[27] In general, if any one of the eight criteria is not met or a prominent finding exists, order a diagnostic test for PE.

STEP THREE

If PE cannot be excluded with the PE rule-out criteria rule, choose a diagnostic test result that can produce a posttest probability of <2.0%. An age-adjusted quantitative D-dimer assay is the best diagnostic test in patients for whom clinical suspicion is low or moderate based on either gestalt estimation, a Wells' score of ≤4, or a "safe" designation according to the Charlotte rule. Before ordering a D-dimer assay, consider factors could separately elevate the D-dimer concentration and impair the utility (**Table 56-9**).

STEP FOUR

Test further only those with a positive D-dimer result; base the choice of the next test on patient and facility factors. The algorithm presented in Figure 56-2 is one path. In general, the next best step for a patient with suspected PE and a positive D-dimer result is chest CT angiography. $\dot{V}/\dot{Q}$ scan is an option in a pregnant patient or a patients with renal insufficiency or prior adverse reaction to contrast material. Performing lower extremity venous US is another option; it lacks ionizing radiation and its ability to diagnose DVT in a patient with PE symptoms is tantamount to diagnosing PE directly. However, **the diagnostic sensitivity of lower extremity US for PE is <40%,** so all patients suspected of having PE for whom US findings are negative require pulmonary vascular imaging.

To diagnose VTE, the clinical assessment and diagnostic tests usually must have a probability of 80% or greater, which is achievable with

TABLE 56-9 Likelihood Ratios (LRs) of Diagnostic Tests and Pretest Probabilities Required to Diagnose or Exclude Pulmonary Embolism (PE)

Test	LR for PE if Test Result Is Negative	LR for PE if Test Result Is Positive*	Examples of Scores on Published Methods That Would Allow Pretest Probability to Rule Out VTE if Test Result Is Negative
Qualitative D-dimer	0.25	2	Wells' score <2, all pulmonary embolism rule-out criteria negative
Quantitative D-dimer†	0.1	2	Gestalt estimate low, Wells' score ≤4, or Charlotte rule negative ("safe") Age-adjustment of the D-dimer cutoff using the formula age × 10 nanograms/mL
CT angiography	0.12	12	Gestalt estimate low, Wells' score ≤4, or Charlotte rule negative ("safe")
$\dot{V}/\dot{Q}$ scan: normal	0.05	NA	Any
$\dot{V}/\dot{Q}$ scan: high probability	NA	12	NA

Abbreviations: NA = not applicable; $\dot{V}/\dot{Q}$ = ventilation–perfusion; VTE = venous thromboembolism.

*A positive D-dimer result should not be used to rule in VTE.

†Assumes a US Food and Drug Administration–cleared assay with cutoff of 500 nanograms/mL as threshold.

positive CT findings or high-probability $\dot{V}/\dot{Q}$ scan results or venous US with findings indicative of DVT. Lesser probability means VTE may be present but is still clinically uncertain.

A low-risk patient with a CT scan demonstrating a large filling defect in the main pulmonary artery surely has a PE. In contrast, a low-risk patient with a CT image that is partially obscured by motion artifact and an eccentric filling defect in a segmental artery with lung consolidation needs more testing. With an indeterminate CT scan, options are venous US and a quantitative D-dimer assay. If the venous US results are positive, assume and treat for PE. If the US results are negative but the D-dimer concentration is eightfold higher than the upper limit of normal, the likelihood of acute VTE is high and supports therapy.

If the patient has no image-detected DVT or PE and has a normal or marginally elevated D-dimer concentration, then further imaging before anticoagulation is started is an option, especially if the patient has any increased risk of bleeding complications. The combination of a small, irregular filling defect on a suboptimal-quality CT angiogram, together with evidence of no DVT, a normal or even marginally elevated D-dimer concentration (<150% of the threshold), and a low-probability $\dot{V}/\dot{Q}$ scan result, supports a decision not to initiate anticoagulation in a patient with normal or near-normal vital signs and oxygenation. Commonly, a repeat venous US within 2 to 7 days can help exclude VTE.

Patients with PE detected until after admission from the ED have a higher frequency of altered mental status and preexisting heart or lung diseases.[44-47] Of those discharged home with PE detected later, the clinical features often are a lack of dyspnea, sharp chest pain or hemoptysis with a pulmonary infiltrate on imaging (an infarct masquerading as infection), or a lower D-dimer concentration and a small distal clot seen on pulmonary vascular imaging.[46] More evidence is needed to determine if these patients actually benefit from systemic anticoagulation absent concomitant DVT.

Figure 56-8 is one algorithm describing the diagnostic decision making for DVT. Evaluate first using the Wells' criteria for pretest probability of DVT (Table 56-6). Patients with a low pretest probability (score <1) or patients without cancer, a modified Wells DVT score ≤1, and a normal D-dimer result are safely considered negative for DVT; any positive result requires US in this group. Patients with moderate to high Wells' scores or DVT likely (modified Wells DVT score) should undergo US testing, assessing D-dimer only if the US result is negative. In these subjects, assume no clot exists if both US and D-dimer tests are negative; if they have negative US findings and positive D-dimer results, repeat the US 2 to 7 days later.

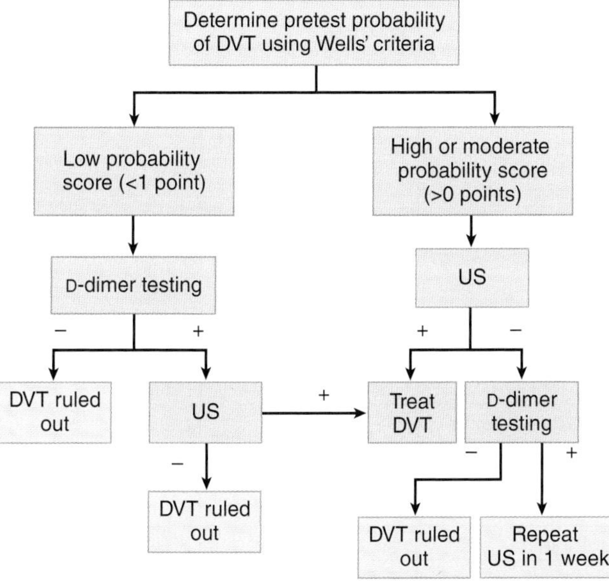

FIGURE 56-8. Diagnostic algorithm for deep vein thrombosis (DVT), applied in patients with leg symptoms compatible with DVT. + = positive test result; – = negative test result.

VENOUS THROMBOEMBOLISM TREATMENT

TREATMENT OF PULMONARY EMBOLISM AND DEEP AND SUPERFICIAL EXTREMITY THROMBOSES

Treatment of VTE requires systemic anticoagulation to prevent further clot formation and allow endogenous fibrinolysis to proceed. In many cases, the initial treatment for VTE is heparin or heparin-like drug. The two most common options are unfractionated heparin or a low-molecular-weight heparin (**Table 56-10**).[6] Initial anticoagulation treatment for VTE can also include oral rivaroxaban.[6] It is anticipated that apixaban will soon have US Food and Drug Administration approval for VTE. Dabigatran can also be used but requires anticoagulation with heparin for several days.

Current data favor the use of low-molecular-weight heparins over unfractionated heparin for treatment of both PE and DVT in terms of composite outcomes (bleeding and death) and cost, although the magnitude of benefit is not large.[6] If uncertain about PE presence, the likelihood can guide anticoagulation therapy; the benefit of empiric anticoagulation for 24 hours exceeds the risks (bleeding and heparin-induced thrombocytopenia) for any patient with a pretest probability of PE of >20%.[48] Delay in administration of heparin to patients with PE is associated with increased mortality, but no study has found that heparin, administered early and prior to imaging, improves morbidity or mortality.

In patients with severe renal insufficiency and acute DVT or PE, most experts recommend unfractionated heparin over low-molecular-weight heparin.[6] **Treat upper extremity DVT the same as lower extremity DVT**, and remove any indwelling catheters associated with clot. Heparin interferes with a few of the assays of enzymatic activity (lupus anticoagulant and endogenous proteases) used to diagnose thrombophilia; however, **do not delay unfractionated heparin for any added**

TABLE 56-10 Antithrombotic Therapy for Deep Venous Thrombosis (DVT) and Pulmonary Embolism (PE)

	Dosage	Comments
Unfractionated heparin	80 units/kg bolus, then 18 units/kg/h infusion	Recommended if outpatient therapy not appropriate or in cases of severe renal failure
LMWHs		Outpatient treatment with LMWH preferred
Dalteparin	100 IU/kg SC every 12 h or 200 IU/kg SC every day	
Enoxaparin	1 milligram/kg SC every 12 h or 1.5 milligrams/kg SC every day	
Tinzaparin	175 IU/kg SC every day	
Factor Xa inhibitors		
Fondaparinux	<50 kg, 5 milligrams SC every day; 50–100 kg, 7.5 milligrams SC every day; >100 kg, 10 milligrams SC every day	Do not use in renal failure
Target-specific anticoagulants		
Rivaroxaban (Xarelto®)	15 milligrams BID for 21 d, then 20 milligrams every day with food	No heparin requirement; good choice for outpatient treatment
Apixaban (Eliquis®)	10 milligrams BID for 7 days then 5 mg BID	No heparin requirement; good choice for outpatient treatment
Dabigatran (Pradaxa®)	150 milligrams BID	Requires run in of heparin for 5–10 d; renal excretion
Thrombolytic therapy	Tissue plasminogen activator or alteplase (Activase®), 10-milligram IV bolus followed by 90 milligrams infused over 2 h	For PE with hemodynamic compromise; after infusion, begin unfractionated heparin or LMWH

Abbreviations: BID = twice a day; FDA = Food and Drug Administration; LMWH = low-molecular-weight heparin; VTE = venous thromboembolism.

thrombophilia testing when VTE is clearly present, because the evaluation can be postponed to the future. No evidence demonstrates any clinical benefit to a thrombophilia evaluation in guiding the intensity or duration of anticoagulation.[49]

DVT that causes **phlegmasia cerulea dolens** requires rapid action to reduce the venous pressure. In addition to initiating anticoagulation, place the affected limb at a neutral level; remove constrictive clothing, cast, or dressing; and arrange for consultant-delivered catheter-directed thrombolysis. If no such service is available and emergency transfer cannot be arranged within 6 hours, consider systemic fibrinolytics if there are no absolute contraindications. One regimen is 50 to 100 milligrams of alteplase infused IV over 4 hours.

TREATMENT FOR SUPERFICIAL THROMBOPHLEBITIS

Treatment for localized superficial thrombophlebitis is an oral nonsteroidal anti-inflammatory drug or topical diclofenac gel until symptoms resolve; there is no need for systemic anticoagulation. For extensive superficial vein involvement, full-dose anticoagulation is recommended.[6] Compression stockings do not aid this condition.[50]

TREATMENT FOR ISOLATED CALF VEIN THROMBOSIS

There are no universally accepted treatment guidelines for thromboses isolated to the calf veins (soleal or gastrocnemius) or the saphenous vein, although many use 3 months of oral anticoagulation. Alternatives include no acute treatment with repeat US in 1 week to identify progression of clot, or outpatient treatment with low-molecular-weight heparin (Table 56-10). Patients with a history of VTE or risk factors for VTE (Table 56-1) should receive 3 months of full-dose anticoagulation when calf thrombosis exists unless contraindications are present.[6]

OUTPATIENT TREATMENT OF PULMONARY EMBOLISM

Patients with DVT diagnosed in the ED are typically discharged after receiving the first dose of low-molecular-weight heparin (Table 56-10) and with anticoagulation continued as an outpatient. More recently, many centers have begun the same practice for carefully selected low-risk patients with PE. Patients with PE and a low risk of death plus adequate home support can qualify for outpatient anticoagulation. The incidence of short-term mortality and the bleeding risk are very low with outpatient treatment, the overall cost of care is less, and the experience is preferred by patients.[51,52] Select low-risk patients using either the Hestia criteria or the Simplified PE Severity Index criteria (**Table 56-11**).[13,53] If low risk, assess the patient's wishes and ability to comply; if no high-risk features exist (elevated troponin, a B-type natriuretic peptide >100 picograms/mL, pulmonary arterial hypertension on ECG, or bleeding risks), outpatient care after an ED stay (up to 23 hours) is an option; otherwise, short-term hospitalization is a good choice.

In practice, the biggest barrier to ED discharge of any VTE patient is ensuring access to anticoagulation. If warfarin is the long-term anticoagulant, the patient must receive low-molecular-weight heparin until the prothrombin time is adequately prolonged *and* for at least 5 days.[6] For low-molecular-weight heparin, patients or their families must learn how to administer subcutaneous injections, have access to drug, have a follow-up appointment where the prothrombin time can be monitored, and have dosing advice given, which are all challenges in some EDs. At this time, only one newer oral anticoagulant, rivaroxaban (Xarelto®), is approved for both DVT and PE. This drug does not require blood monitoring or dosing adjustment for body size. The primary limitation to rivaroxaban is cost, although the manufacturer offers a patient assistance program, and it is on Medicaid and Medicare formularies.

FIBRINOLYSIS FOR PULMONARY EMBOLISM

PE is classified into three categories based on severity: massive, submassive, and less severe PE. **Massive PE** patients have a systolic blood pressure of <90 mm Hg for >15 minutes, a systolic blood pressure of <100 mm Hg with a history of hypertension, or a >40% reduction in baseline systolic blood pressure. **Submassive PE** patients have normal or near-normal blood pressure, but with other evidence of cardiopulmonary stress (**Table 56-12**).

All other PE cases are classified as "less severe." Patients with low-risk PE should not receive fibrinolysis; those with massive PE (defined as a systolic blood pressure <90 mm Hg or an observed decrease of 40 mm Hg) benefit from fibrinolysis. Patients with more severe submassive PE (i.e., causing right ventricular dilation or hypokinesis, elevated troponin or B-type natriuretic peptide, or persistent hypoxemia with distress) may also benefit from fibrinolysis, including higher survival and better quality of life although at a higher bleeding risk.[54-55]

Systemic Fibrinolysis The best evidence suggests **considering systemic fibrinolysis in patients with no contraindications to fibrinolysis**

TABLE 56-11 Two Prognostic Systems That Can Select Low-Risk Patients for Outpatient Treatment

Simplified PE Severity Index Score

0 = low risk; ^{3}1 = high risk

- Age >80
- History of cancer
- History of heart failure or chronic lung disease
- Pulse >110 beats/min
- SBP <100 mm Hg
- O_2 saturation <90%

Hestia Criteria

Identifies low-risk PE if:

- SBP >100 mm Hg
- No thrombolysis needed
- No active bleeding
- No O_2 required >24 h to maintain saturation >90%
- Not already anticoagulated
- Absence of severe pain requiring IV narcotics for >24 h
- Absence of other medical or social reasons to admit
- Creatinine clearance >30 mL/min
- Not pregnant, no severe liver disease or HIT

Abbreviations: HIT = heparin-induced thrombocytopenia; PE = pulmonary embolism; SBP = systolic blood pressure.

TABLE 56-12 Modalities to Risk-Stratify Pulmonary Embolism (PE)

Test	Less Severe PE	More Severe PE (massive and some submassive PE)
Hestia criteria	All negative	Any positive
PE Severity Index score	<80	>120
Simplified PE Severity Index criteria	All negative	Any positive
Shock index (heart rate/systolic blood pressure)	<1.0	≥1.0
Pulse oximetry reading	>94%	<95%
Echocardiography	Normal RV systolic function Normal RV size No tricuspid regurgitation	RV hypokinesis RV dilation RVSP >40 mm Hg
Troponin I or T level	Normal	Elevated
B-type natriuretic peptide level	<90 picograms/mL	≥90 picograms/mL
N-terminal pro-B-type natriuretic peptide	<900 picograms/mL	≥900 picograms/mL
D-Dimer level	<4000 nanograms/mL	>8000 nanograms/mL
Serum sodium concentration	<125 mEq/L	≥125 mEq/L

Abbreviations: RV = right ventricular; RVSP = right ventricular systolic pressure.

and any of the following: cardiac arrest; hypotension; respiratory failure, evidenced by severe hypoxemia (pulse oximetry reading <90%) despite oxygen administration, together with evidence of increased work of breathing; or evidence of right-sided heart strain on echocardiography or elevated levels of troponin T or I, or both (**Table 56-12**). **Major contraindications to thrombolytic therapy** include intracranial disease, uncontrolled hypertension at presentation, recent major surgery or trauma (past 3 weeks), and metastatic cancer. Any patient with head trauma from syncope should have a CT scan prior to therapy to detect hemorrhage. **Alteplase** (tissue plasminogen activator) is the only currently approved agent for PE, dosed 100 milligrams IV over 2 hours. Either enoxaparin (1 milligram/kg SC) or unfractionated heparin (80 units/kg IV bolus followed by 18 units/kg/h) is the anticoagulant, with the activated partial thromboplastin time kept at <120 seconds for unfractionated heparin. Heparin or low-molecular-weight heparin is typically started after the thrombolytic infusion. For further discussion of fibrinolytic agents, see the chapter 239, "Thrombotics and Antithrombotics."

Catheter-Directed Thrombolysis Two randomized trials have tested the utility of catheter-directed, intrapulmonary delivery of tissue plasminogen activator and found better outcomes than heparin alone, but not better than systemic tissue plasminogen activator.[56] In view of these study results, as well as the risks of pulmonary arterial catheterization and associated drug delivery delay due to the need to activate the vascular intervention suite, intrapulmonary fibrinolytic delivery is not used in most patients with massive PE.[57] However, catheter-directed thrombolysis for PE requires a far lower dose of alteplase (approximately 10 milligrams total), which may confer a lower bleeding risk. Thus, catheter-directed thrombolysis is an option for patients over 65 years old, where intracranial bleeding risk is highest.[54] Alternatively, 50 milligrams of systemic IV alteplase—half of the Food and Drug Administration–approved dose—is an option with safety advantages.[58] Tiered-dose tenecteplase (TNKase®: <60 kg: 30-milligram dose; ≥60 to <70 kg: 35-milligram dose; ≥70 to <80 kg: 40-milligram dose; ≥80 to <90 kg: 45-milligram dose; ≥90 kg: 50-milligram dose) appears to offer similar effectiveness as alteplase, although it is not yet approved by the Food and Drug Administration for PE.

Surgical Embolectomy If available, surgical embolectomy is an option in young patients with large, proximal PE accompanied by hypotension. Because surgical embolectomy is often delayed, the reported mortality rate is approximately 30%. The amount of clot that can be extracted is often extensive, and removal may help limit later cardiopulmonary complications.

DISPOSITION AND FOLLOW-UP

Patients with severe PE or receiving any thrombolysis/extraction generally are placed in an intensive care unit (**Table 56-13**). Outpatient treatment of DVT and PE is favored in low-risk patients who can adhere to therapy. Indications for admission in patients with DVT are listed in Table 56-13.

SPECIAL POPULATIONS

PREGNANCY

If the general patient has a high pretest probability by Wells' or the revised Geneva score, then proceed to pulmonary vascular imaging.[60] However, in pregnant women, limiting fetal exposure to radiation and iodinated contrast is preferred.[61] One study measured D-dimer levels in 228 pregnant women with suspected DVT and found a prevalence of DVT in the study population of 6.6%.[62] See chapter 100, "Maternal Emergencies after 20 Weeks of Pregnancy and in the Postpartum Period" especially the section on thromboembolic disease of pregnancy.

ISOLATED SUBSEGMENTAL PULMONARY EMBOLISM

Isolated subsegmental PE refers to a filling defect seen in one small pulmonary artery, usually <3 mm in diameter and in the absence of DVT; radiologists often do not agree when viewing these images separately.

TABLE 56-13 Indications for Hospital Admission in Patients with Deep Venous Thrombosis[59]
An extensive iliofemoral deep venous thrombosis with circulatory compromise
An increased risk of bleeding (coagulopathy, active peptic ulcer disease, liver disease) that requires close monitoring of therapy
A limited cardiorespiratory reserve that suggests need for additional care such as monitoring for hypoxemia
A risk of poor compliance with home therapy regimen or inadequate support (i.e., community, social, or medical), or concern with ability to arrange follow-up
A contraindication to use of low-molecular-weight heparin, and inability to use an oral target-specific anticoagulant, which would necessitate IV heparin therapy
Known or suspected coexistent pulmonary embolism with a Simplified Pulmonary Embolism Severity Index score >0 or Hestia criteria positive
A high suspicion of heparin-induced thrombocytopenia without or with thrombosis
Renal insufficiency requiring monitoring of anti–factor Xa level, or use of unfractionated heparin

The incidence of subsegmental PE identification has increased sharply with increased resolution of multidetector-row CT scanning, but the clinical significance is unclear.[63] This raises concern that subsegmental PE may be a radiographic artifact rather than a true disease. Most experts agree that treatment is best in those with subsegmental PE and active cancer; no strong data support the safety of withholding anticoagulation in others with this finding; most still receive standard anticoagulation for 3 to 6 months.[6] It is best to discuss the risks and benefits of treatment of subsegmental PE with patients and their physicians to help make the best decision about anticoagulation.

CANCER PATIENTS WITH VENOUS THROMBOEMBOLISM

Current data and guidelines recommend treatment of patients with active cancer with low-molecular-weight heparin for at least 6 months.[64] Some patients cannot give themselves injections for prolonged periods of time, forcing the choice between oral warfarin versus an oral newer anticoagulant. Pooled data from four newer agent trials in cancer-related VTE (dabigatran, rivaroxaban, and edoxaban) show better outcomes with thrombin or factor Xa inhibitors compared with warfarin.[65] About 2% of cancer patients undergoing staging and surveillance CT scanning have incidental PE detected. These patients are treated with anticoagulation, often at home if low risk.[66,67]

REFERENCES

The complete reference list is available online at www.TintinalliEM.com.

CHAPTER 57 Systemic Hypertension

Brigitte M. Baumann

INTRODUCTION AND EPIDEMIOLOGY

Hypertension affects approximately 30% of the U.S. population, and 1% to 6% of all ED patients will present with severe hypertension.[1-5] Of the latter, between a third and one half will have end-organ damage.[2-5] Risk factors for the development of hypertensive crisis include obesity, cigarette smoking, and older age.[6]

Chronic hypertension is categorized into three classifications: prehypertension, stage 1 hypertension, and stage 2 hypertension[7] (**Table 57-1**).

Hypertensive emergency is an acute elevation of blood pressure (≥180/120 mm Hg) associated with end-organ damage; the targeted end organs include the brain, heart, aorta, kidneys, or eyes[7] (**Table 57-2**). Acute hypertensive emergencies are more common in

TABLE 57-1 JNC7 Classification of Hypertension

Class	Systolic BP (mm Hg)		Diastolic BP (mm Hg)
Normal	<120	and	<80
Prehypertension	120–139	or	80–89
Stage 1	140–159	or	90–99
Stage 2	≥160	or	≥100

Abbreviations: BP = blood pressure; JNC7 = Seventh Report of the Joint National Committee on Prevention, Detection, Evaluation, and Treatment of High Blood Pressure.

TABLE 57-2 Hypertensive Emergencies

Diagnostic Category	Signs and Symptoms	Evidence of Acute End-Organ Damage
Acute aortic dissection	Chest pain, back pain Unequal blood pressures (>20 mm Hg difference) in upper extremities	Abnormal CT angiogram of chest and abdomen/pelvis or transesophageal echocardiogram of the aorta
Acute pulmonary edema	Shortness of breath	Interstitial edema on chest radiograph
Acute myocardial infarction	Chest pain, nausea, vomiting, diaphoresis	Changes on ECG or elevated levels of cardiac biomarkers
Acute coronary syndrome	Chest pain, nausea, vomiting, diaphoresis	Clinical diagnosis, changes on ECG, or elevated levels of cardiac biomarkers
Acute renal failure	May have systolic or diastolic abdominal bruit	Elevated serum creatinine level, proteinuria
Severe pre-eclampsia, HELLP syndrome, eclampsia	Seizures	Proteinuria, hemolysis, elevated liver enzyme levels, low platelet counts
Hypertensive retinopathy	Blurred vision	Retinal hemorrhages and cotton-wool spots (**Figure 57-1**), hard exudates, and sausage-shaped veins
Hypertensive encephalopathy	Altered mental status, nausea, vomiting, headache	May see papilledema or arteriolar hemorrhage or exudates on funduscopic examination, may note cerebral edema with a predilection for the posterior white matter of the brain on MRI
Subarachnoid hemorrhage	Headache, focal neurologic deficits	Abnormal CT of the brain; red blood cells on lumbar puncture
Intracranial hemorrhage	Headache, new neurologic deficits	Abnormal CT of the brain
Acute ischemic stroke	New neurologic deficits	Abnormal MRI or CT of the brain
Acute perioperative hypertension	Bleeding unresponsive to direct pressure	Clinical diagnosis; manifestations of other hypertensive emergencies
Sympathetic crisis*	Anxiety, palpitations, tachycardia, diaphoresis	Clinical diagnosis in the setting of sympathomimetic drug use (i.e., cocaine or amphetamines) or pheochromocytoma (24-h urine assay for catecholamines and metanephrine or plasma fractionated metanephrines)

Abbreviation: HELLP = hemolysis, elevated liver enzymes, low platelets.

*In this syndrome, acute end-organ dysfunction may not be measurable, but complications affecting the brain, heart, or kidneys may occur in the absence of acute treatment.

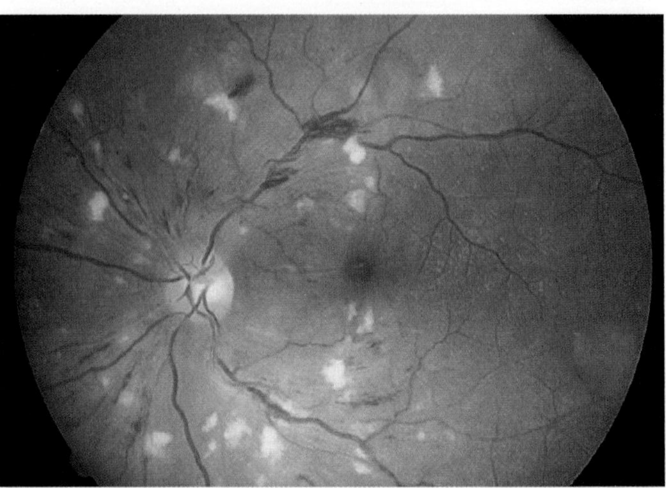

FIGURE 57-1. Hypertensive retinopathy. Scattered flame (splinter) hemorrhages and cotton-wool spots (nerve fiber layer infarcts) in a patient with headache and a blood pressure of 234/120 mm Hg.

chronic hypertensive patients who fail to adhere to their antihypertensive therapy regimens and those who are unable to access outpatient health care.[6]

Hypertensive urgency is a term for profound elevations in blood pressure without acute target organ dysfunction.[7] An arbitrary blood pressure of ≥180/120 mm Hg is often cited as an urgency and an indication for rapid pharmacologic intervention (often parenteral) to reduce blood pressure within hours; however, no clear clinical benefit of such treatment exists, and risk can occur from precipitous drops in blood pressure.[8,9] Hypertensive urgency is better seen as another form of severe hypertension where prompt therapy with oral agent(s) is the best path, seeking reduction in blood pressure over days to weeks.

PATHOPHYSIOLOGY

At baseline, chronic hypertensive patients have biochemical and structural changes in the arterial walls that shift the vascular autoregulatory curve, requiring higher arterial pressures to maintain end-organ blood flow, notably in the brain.[10-12] Eventually, the ability to adapt is passed. The resultant mechanical wall stress and endothelial injury lead to increased permeability, and excessive perfusion of the cerebral, cardiac, and renal vascular beds results. This can be followed by activation of the coagulation cascade and platelets, and deposition of fibrin results in fibrinoid necrosis of the arterioles. Clinically, this is manifested by hematuria (involvement of the renal vasculature) or arterial hemorrhages or exudates on funduscopic examination. Further contributing to the damage are prostaglandins, free radicals, cytokines, and mitogenic, chemoattractant, and proliferation factors, which result in endothelial damage, smooth muscle proliferation, and thrombosis.[10,12] The renin-angiotensin system may also be activated, which leads to vasoconstriction. Pressure natriuresis occurs, leading to volume depletion, prompting additional release of vasoconstrictors from the kidney. These combined effects produce hypoperfusion, ischemia, and dysfunction of end organs. Endothelial dysfunction from such crises can persist for years after the acute event.[13]

CLINICAL FEATURES

Measure blood pressure in both arms quickly and consecutively, while the patient is quietly resting. Check blood pressure several times before starting antihypertensive therapy. Blood pressure differences can result from aortic dissection, coarctation, peripheral vascular disease, and some unilateral neurologic and musculoskeletal abnormalities.

TABLE 57-3 Specific Diseases Associated with Elevated Blood Pressures

Disease	Threshold Value Raising Risk	% of Patients with Elevated Pressures
Subarachnoid hemorrhage[20]	≥140 mm Hg SBP	100%
Ischemic stroke[20,21]	≥140 mm Hg SBP ≥160 mm Hg SBP	77%–82% 47%–54%
Intracerebral hemorrhage[20]	≥140 mm Hg SBP ≥160 mm Hg SBP	75% 27%
Type B aortic dissection[22,23]	≥140 mm Hg SBP or ≥90 mm Hg DBP	67%–77%
Type A aortic dissection[24]	>150 mm Hg SBP	36%–74%
Acute heart failure[25]	>140 mm Hg SBP	54%
NSTEMI-ACS[25,26]	≥140 mm Hg SBP ≥160 mm Hg SBP	57%–59% 31%

Abbreviations: BP = diastolic blood pressure; NSTEMI-ACS = non-ST-segment elevation myocardial infarction acute coronary syndrome; SBP = systolic blood pressure.

However, interarm blood pressure differences are also reported in "normal" individuals. The most important factor in blood pressure difference is increasing age, with the thought that loss of vascular elasticity or asymmetrical atheromatous narrowing of subclavian or brachial arteries might be causative. Although there are no guidelines or standards for determining the significance of blood pressure measurement disparities, a between-arm difference >10 to 20 mm Hg is suggested as meaningful,[14,15] and each 10-mm Hg difference carries an increasing mortality hazard. **When a blood pressure difference is detected, treat the higher blood pressure and make sure that subsequent measurements are made on the same arm.**[15] Blood pressure measurements with wrist oscillometric devices give lower readings than arm measurements, so arm measurements are preferred.[16] Use the same device for repeat blood pressure measurements.

After careful blood pressure measurement, the next question in a patient with severely elevated blood pressure is whether this constitutes a hypertensive crisis. Although a modest drop (4 to 12 mm Hg) in systolic and diastolic blood pressures can be expected in patients presenting with elevated blood pressures,[17-19] do not discount a diagnosis of hypertensive emergency simply because the patient has no prior history of hypertension. Up to 16% of patients presenting with hypertensive emergency have no known history of hypertension.[4] The key is to seek acute end-organ involvement.

Table 57-3 lists the proportion of patients who present with elevated blood pressure by stroke subtypes, aortic dissection subtypes, heart failure, and acute coronary syndrome. Although elevations in blood pressure accompany the majority of these presentations, note that **severe** elevations of blood pressure are far less common in presentations typically labeled as hypertensive emergencies (Table 57-2).

CHEST PAIN AND SEVERE HYPERTENSION

Rapid diagnosis and treatment of acute aortic dissection are critical because delays increase mortality. Differentiating the relatively uncommon aortic dissection from the more common acute coronary syndromes is important because blood pressure management is different in these two disorders, and anticoagulation can prove catastrophic in a patient with acute aortic dissection.[27]

Acute aortic dissection presents with abrupt, sudden onset of pain, usually in the chest, often described as tearing or ripping, and radiating to the interscapular region[23,28] (see chapter 59, "Aortic Dissection and Related Aortic Syndromes"). Less than a quarter of patients with acute aortic dissection have a neurologic deficit or pulse deficits based on blood pressure differentials ≥20 mm Hg, and only about a third have a diastolic murmur. Chest radiograph is abnormal in most but usually nonspecific, and only 25% of radiographs demonstrate the classic widened mediastinum,[24] so CT of the chest is needed for the diagnosis. ECG changes are nonspecific, but <10% demonstrate findings consistent with a myocardial infarction.[24] D-Dimer testing cannot be used in isolation to exclude the diagnosis, but elevated D-dimer and C-reactive protein levels are associated with higher in-hospital mortality.[29,30]

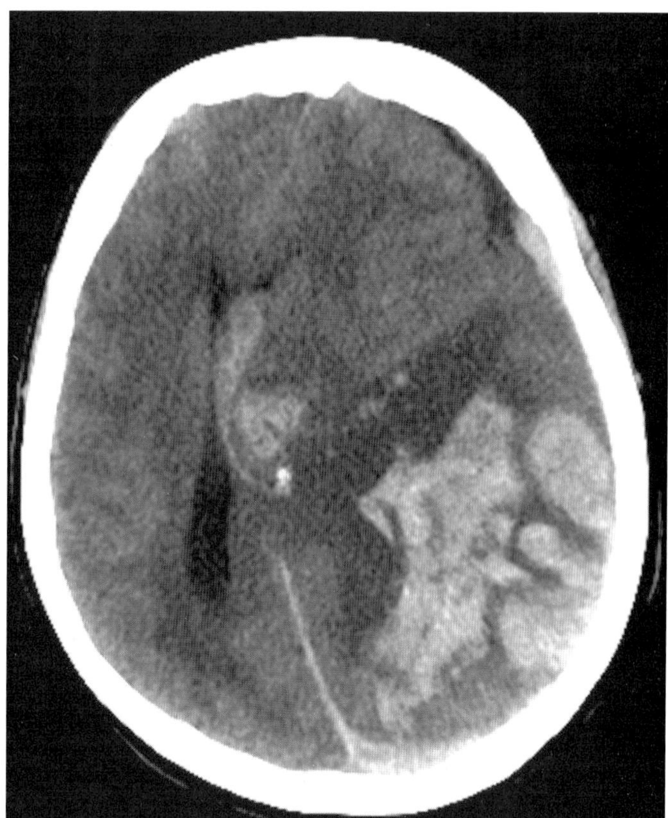

FIGURE 57-2. Intracerebral hypertensive hemorrhage. Noncontrast head CT scan with acute intraparenchymal hemorrhage, mass effect, midline shift, and intraventricular extension. [Image used with permission of Todd Siegal, MD.]

ACUTE NEUROLOGIC SYMPTOMS AND SEVERE HYPERTENSION

Elevated blood pressure, headache, and focal neurologic deficits are associated with either ischemic or hemorrhagic strokes. Acute ischemic strokes may be diagnosed with MRI, and cerebral hemorrhage is identified on head CT (see chapter 167, "Stroke Syndromes") (**Figure 57-2**).

Hypertensive encephalopathy is a clinical diagnosis after excluding focal ischemia or bleeding. It is characterized by altered mental status, headache, vomiting, seizures, or visual disturbances, and most patients will have papilledema. When MRI findings demonstrate reversible edema that is primarily focused posteriorly (occipital vs frontal regions), this is referred to as **posterior reversible encephalopathy syndrome** (**Figure 57-3**).

ACUTE RENAL FAILURE, PERIPHERAL EDEMA, AND SEVERE HYPERTENSION

Patients with new-onset renal failure may have peripheral edema, oliguria, loss of appetite, nausea and vomiting, orthostatic changes, or confusion. However, some patients have few or no specific symptoms (see chapter 88, "Acute Kidney Injury"). Elevated serum creatinine confirms the diagnosis, and urinary sediment is also abnormal.

Pre-eclampsia is associated with hypertension, peripheral edema, and proteinuria. These patients may also develop hemolysis, elevated liver enzyme levels, and low platelet counts (HELLP syndrome) (see chapter 100, "Maternal Emergencies after 20 Weeks of Pregnancy and in the Postpartum Period").

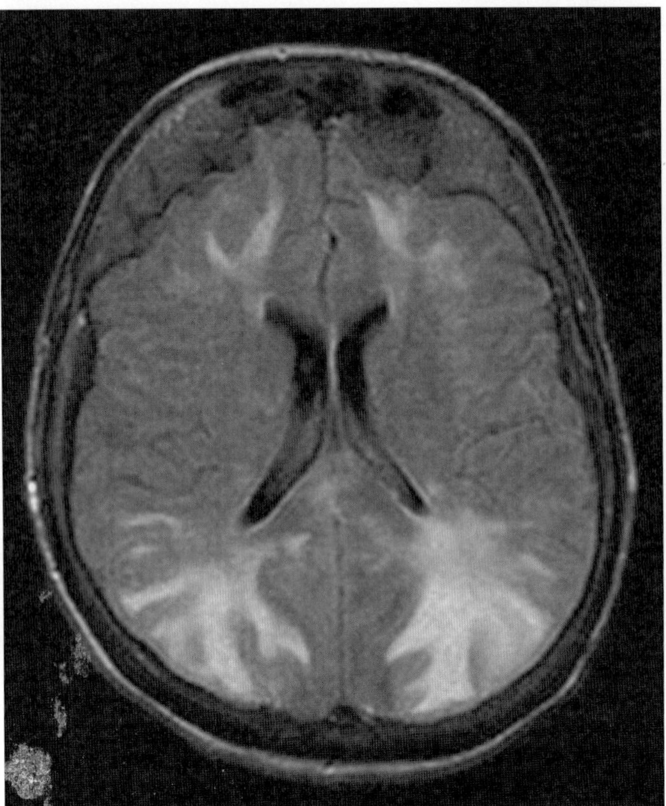

FIGURE 57-3. Axial fluid-attenuated inversion recovery MRI showing white matter hyperintensity in the occipital lobes bilaterally consistent with posterior reversible encephalopathy syndrome. The patient's confusion improved with blood pressure control. Repeat MRI after several days of therapy demonstrated remarkable improvement. [Image used with permission of Michael Farner, MD.]

SYMPATHETIC CRISIS AND SEVERE HYPERTENSION

There are four settings in which an excess of catecholamines can result in a hypertensive emergency. An acute catecholaminergic syndrome may occur with abrupt discontinuation of oral or transdermal **clonidine**. The withdrawal syndrome is potentiated by concomitant β-blocker therapy due to unopposed α-mediated vasoconstriction.

Pheochromocytoma is rare, and between 5% and 20% of tumors are malignant. Patients may experience life-threatening hypertension.[31] Signs of pheochromocytoma include headache, alternating periods of normal and elevated blood pressure, tachycardia, and flushed skin, punctuated by asymptomatic periods.

Sympathomimetic drugs such as cocaine, amphetamines, phencyclidine hydrochloride (PCP), and lysergic acid diethylamide (LSD), can precipitate a hypertensive emergency, with tachycardia, diaphoresis, chest pain, and, depending on the agent, mental status changes.[32] Patients receiving **monoamine oxidase inhibitor** therapy who consume tyramine-containing foods may develop a hyperadrenergic state.[33] **Autonomic dysfunction** due to spinal cord or severe head injury or abnormalities such as spina bifida may also present as a hypertensive emergency, with the diagnosis made clinically based on the existing injury.

ASYMPTOMATIC PATIENTS WITH SEVERE HYPERTENSION

Formal recommendations for the evaluation of an ED patient presenting with asymptomatic but severe hypertension do not exist.[9] Commonly ordered tests include basic metabolic panel (73%), ECG (53%), chest radiograph (46%), and urinalysis (43%).[3] In a prospective study of over 100 ED patients with asymptomatic severe hypertension, clinically meaningful results existed in only 6% of patients, with only 5% of patients thought to have abnormal results attributable to acute hypertensive target organ injury.[34] Until more data are available, base ED evaluation on the patient complaint, history, and review of systems, and perform selected testing.

TREATMENT

Table 57-4 lists agents for the management of hypertensive emergencies categorized by diagnosis. Hypertensive emergencies in pregnancy are discussed in chapter 100. In selecting therapy, be familiar with the use of the selected agent, and establish a target range for blood pressure reduction. The goal is to minimize end-organ damage by initial blood pressure reduction while avoiding hypoperfusion of cerebral, coronary, and renovascular beds. **Acute aortic dissection is the exception, because the risk of morbidity and mortality due to inadequate blood pressure and heart rate control outweighs the risk of hypoperfusion syndromes.**

AORTIC DISSECTION

The therapeutic goal in acute aortic dissection is a systolic blood pressure between 100 and 140 mm Hg and a heart rate ≤60 beats/min.[23,35-37] The resultant reduction in tachycardia decreases the shearing forces and aortic wall stress, limiting the progression of the dissection.[37] Pain control with opioids helps to decrease sympathetic tone.

ACUTE HYPERTENSIVE PULMONARY EDEMA

The treatment of hypertensive pulmonary edema is tailored to the underlying pathophysiology, which could be due to transient left ventricular systolic or diastolic dysfunction, acute dyssynchrony, or ischemic mitral regurgitation. Occasionally, the left ventricular ejection fraction may be normal during the acute episode with only a decrease in systolic function and increased diastolic stiffness and filling pressures, suggesting decreased myocardial capacity to adapt to changes in loading.[39,67] For these reasons, there are no clear evidence-based guidelines for the single best treatment of hypertensive pulmonary edema.

The mainstay of therapy is vasodilators and intravenous diuretics.[39] Intravenous, sublingual, and topical nitrates reduce blood pressure, decrease myocardial oxygen consumption, and improve coronary blood flow.[39,40,68] Diuretics improve symptoms within 6 hours of administration but may not ultimately affect mortality. Be careful using loop diuretics in combination with **nesiritide**, or to a lesser degree **nitroglycerin**, because together these might worsen renal function.[40,69] In patients with systolic dysfunction, intravenous **nicardipine** is an option that increases both stroke volume and coronary blood flow, a potential benefit.[70] When hypertensive pulmonary edema is a result of acute coronary syndrome or atrial fibrillation with rapid ventricular response, **β-blockers** are an appropriate choice.[71]

ACUTE MYOCARDIAL INFARCTION

Patients presenting with severely elevated blood pressure and ischemic changes on ECG should be treated with sublingual or intravenous **nitrates.**[42-44] Routine intravenous β-blockade has fallen out of favor due to conflicting reports of mortality benefits. Currently, intravenous β-blockade is only recommended for patients presenting with severe hypertension. Oral β-blockade in patients presenting with ST-segment elevation myocardial infarctions and non–ST-segment elevation myocardial infarctions remains part of early care, but this route may not provide sufficient or rapid enough blood pressure control in a hypertensive emergency.[42,44]

ACUTE SYMPATHETIC CRISIS

Patients in acute sympathetic crisis due to either cocaine or amphetamines should initially be managed with an IV benzodiazepine, such as lorazepam or diazepam, to decrease adrenergic stimulation.[32,45]

TABLE 57-4 Treatment of Hypertensive Emergencies by Diagnosis

Diagnosis	Therapy Goals	Agents	Risks	Comments
Aortic dissection	Reduce shear forces by ↓ BP and PR; lower SBP to 100–120 mm Hg[35-37]; or lower SBP to <140 mm Hg[23]; ↓ PR <60 beats/min			Measure BP in both arms and treat higher BP
		Labetalol[35-37] IV continuous infusion or **esmolol**[35-37] IV bolus, then continuous infusion	Respiratory distress in COPD, asthma patients; test dose of esmolol recommended, switch to diltiazem if esmolol intolerant[36]	
		Nicardipine[38] IV continuous infusion (after β-blocker)		Always use β-blocker prior to vasodilators
		Nitroprusside[36,37] continuous infusion (after β-blocker)		Always use β-blocker prior to vasodilators; nitroprusside alone increases wall stress from reflex tachycardia; cyanide and thiocyanate toxicity in patients with reduced renal function or therapy >24–48 h
Acute hypertensive pulmonary edema	Reduce BP by 20%–30%; diuresis through vasodilation; symptomatic relief			
		Nitroglycerin SL, topical, or IV continuous infusion[39,40]		IV nitrates dilate capacitance vessels at low doses; higher doses dilate arterioles and lower BP
		Enalaprilat IV[40]	ACE inhibitor, can worsen renal function	Avoid hypotension
		Nicardipine IV continuous infusion		Use with caution; some patients experience a negative inotropic effect
		Nitroprusside IV continuous infusion[39,40]		Cyanide and thiocyanate toxicity in patients with reduced renal function or therapy >24–48 h
		Nesiritide IV[39,40]	Mixed outcomes (favorable and unfavorable) with nesiritide, with most recent ASCEND-HF trial showing no difference in dyspnea and mortality when compared to placebo[41]	Nesiritide lowers PCWP more than nitroglycerin[39]
Acute myocardial infarction	Reduce ischemia; avoid ≤25% reduction of MAP[42]		BP >180/110 mm Hg is a relative contraindication for thrombolytics[43,44]	
		Nitroglycerin SL, topical, or IV continuous infusion[42-44]	Do not give nitrates in patients who have taken phosphodiesterase inhibitors for erectile dysfunction ≤24 h (48 h for tadalafil)[43]	
		Metoprolol or **labetalol** IV bolus[42-44]	Do not give β-blockers in CHF, low-output states, or other contraindications to β-blockers	Monitor for hypotension; consider RV infarct and volume depletion
Acute sympathetic crisis (cocaine, amphetamines, MAOI toxicity)	Reduce excessive sympathetic drive and symptomatic relief			Labetalol is controversial; if given, administer along with a nitrate[42]
		Benzodiazepine[32,45] IV bolus		Benzodiazepines are first-line agents; observe for respiratory depression
		Nitroglycerin SL, topical, or IV continuous infusion[42,45]		
		Phentolamine[45] IV or IM		
		Nicardipine IV continuous infusion[42,45]		
Acute renal failure	Reduce BP by no more than 20% acutely[11]			Do not give nitroprusside, as it results in cyanide and thiocyanate toxicity; avoid ACE inhibitor acutely (some authors contradict this caution)[11]
		Nicardipine[46] IV continuous infusion		

(Continued)

TABLE 57-4 Treatment of Hypertensive Emergencies by Diagnosis (*Continued*)

Diagnosis	Therapy Goals	Agents	Risks	Comments
		Clevidipine IV continuous infusion		
		Fenoldopam[46] IV continuous infusion		
Hypertensive encephalopathy	Decrease MAP 20%–25% in the first hour of presentation[47]; more aggressive lowering may lead to ischemic infarction			Autoregulation of cerebral perfusion may be significantly impaired, so avoid rapid BP lowering; do not give nitroglycerin[48] as it may worsen cerebral autoregulation
		Nicardipine[49] IV continuous infusion		
		Labetalol[50] IV continuous infusion		Avoid in sympathetic crisis from drugs
		Fenoldopam[50] IV continuous infusion		
		Clevidipine IV continuous infusion[51]		
Subarachnoid hemorrhage	SBP <160 mm Hg to prevent rebleeding[52]; avoid hypotension to preserve cerebral perfusion; BP parameters have not yet been defined[52]			Nimodipine is used to decrease mortality. BP control is not its primary goal, but some decrease in BP may be seen.[52] Clazosentan is used with success in lieu of nimodipine and has similar hypotensive effects.[53]
		Nicardipine[54-56] IV continuous infusion		
		Labetalol[52,56] IV bolus, 10–20 milligrams IV, or continuous infusion		
		Esmolol IV bolus, then continuous infusion		
		Clevidipine[52] IV continuous infusion		
Intracerebral hemorrhage	If SBP >200 or MAP >150 mm Hg, consider aggressive management, IV infusion.[57] If SBP >180 or MAP >130 mm Hg and possibly elevated ICP*, use infusions or IV boluses while maintaining CPP ≥60 mm Hg.[57] If SBP >180 or MAP >130 mm Hg and no elevated ICP, goal MAP is 110 mm Hg (160/90 mm Hg).[57]			Drops in SBP <150 mm Hg are not associated with increased morbidity.[58] Early hemorrhage growth often occurs in first 6 h. Recent data suggest that during this time, aggressive BP control (SBP 120–160 mm Hg) diminishes hematoma growth, morbidity, and mortality.[58-60]
		Labetalol[56,61] IV bolus or continuous infusion		
		Nicardipine[56,61-63] IV continuous infusion		
		Esmolol[64] IV bolus, then continuous infusion		
Acute ischemic stroke, rtPA candidate (BP ≤185/110 mm Hg)	If fibrinolytic therapy planned, treat if BP remains >185/110 mm Hg after 3 measurements[65]; SBP goal is between 141 and 150 mm Hg[66]		Excess BP Lowering may worsen ischemia	Elevated BP spontaneously decreases within 90 min after onset of acute stroke symptoms
		Labetalol[65] 10–20 milligrams IV bolus; may repeat one time		
		Nicardipine[65] IV continuous infusion 5 milligrams/h, titrate up by 2.5 milligrams/h every 5–15 min; maximum 15 milligrams/h; adjust when desired BP is reached		
		Nitroprusside[65] may be used if BP is not controlled with above agents or DBP >140 mm Hg		

(*Continued*)

TABLE 57-4 Treatment of Hypertensive Emergencies by Diagnosis (*Continued*)

Diagnosis	Therapy Goals	Agents	Risks	Comments
Acute ischemic stroke, hypertension excludes rtPA (BP >185/110 mm Hg)	Treat if >220/120 mm Hg on third of 3 measurements, spaced 15 min apart[65]			Do not lower SBP by >10%–15% in first 24 h.[65] BP that is lower during the acute ischemic stroke than the premorbid pressure could be considered hypotension. Be careful with BP control efforts in patients taking oral β-blockers or clonidine; antihypertensive withdrawal syndrome may occur.
		Labetalol[65] 10 milligrams IV bolus, followed by IV continuous infusion 2–8 milligrams/min		
		Nicardipine[65] 5 milligrams/h IV continuous infusion, titrate up to desired effect by 2.5 milligrams/h every 5–15 min; maximum 15 milligrams/h		

Abbreviations: ACE = angiotensin-converting enzyme; BP = blood pressure; CCP = cerebral perfusion pressure; CHF = congestive heart failure; COPD = chronic obstructive pulmonary disease; DBP = diastolic blood pressure; ICP = intracranial pressure; MAP = mean arterial pressure; MAOI = monoamine oxidase inhibitor; PCWP = pulmonary capillary wedge pressure; PR = pulse rate; rtPA= recombinant tissue-type plasminogen activator; RV = right ventricular; SBP = systolic blood pressure; SL = sublingual.

*Clinical and CT predictors of elevated ICP include decreased level of consciousness, evidence of midline shift, and hematoma volume >30 mL.

Monitor for respiratory depression and sedation. If benzodiazepines are not effective, nitroglycerin or phentolamine may be used next. A calcium channel blocker can serve as a third-line agent.[42,45,72] β-Blockers can result in unopposed α-blockade, which then can worsen coronary vasoconstriction and increase blood pressure.[45] If a β-blocker is used, labetalol is the adrenergic blocking agent in conjunction with a vasodilator.[42]

In patients with pheochromocytoma and a hypertensive emergency, intravenous phentolamine is recommended (intramuscular if venous access is impaired).[73,74] In the preoperative setting, patients who are hypertensive but not in crisis may be managed and prepared for resection with oral phenoxybenzamine, a long-acting adrenergic α-receptor blocker. Another option before resection is urapidil, a selective α_1-receptor antagonist and 5-HT_{1a} receptor agonist that is available in Europe but is not yet approved by the U.S. Food and Drug Administration.[75]

Patients with monoamine oxidase inhibitor toxicity often respond to an intravenous benzodiazepine; if more therapy is needed, use phentolamine, nitroglycerin, or nitroprusside. Nitroglycerin is indicated for associated chest pain or cardiac ischemia. Monitor closely after reaching a targeted blood pressure, because the hypertensive phase is often followed by a hypotensive phase.

ACUTE RENAL FAILURE

Fenoldopam, nicardipine, and clevidipine are all suitable for acute hypertension-induced renal failure, because they reduce systemic vascular resistance while preserving renal blood flow.[46] Nitroprusside is an alternative, although cyanide toxicity with high or prolonged use dampens enthusiasm in practice. Fenoldopam is considered by some to be a first-line agent because it improves natriuresis and creatinine clearance in patients with elevated blood pressure and impaired renal function.[46]

ECLAMPSIA AND PRE-ECLAMPSIA

Obstetrical hypertensive emergencies can occur well below the blood pressure threshold for other hypertensive emergencies. Treatment is discussed in detail in Section 11, "Obstetrics and Gynecology," in chapter 100, "Maternal Emergencies after 20 Weeks of Pregnancy and in the Postpartum Period."

NEUROLOGIC EMERGENCIES

Hypertensive encephalopathy (defined as a change in sensorium or seizure from the blood pressure elevation) is a clear indication for rapid blood pressure reduction, once other neurologic emergencies, notably ischemic or hemorrhagic stroke, are excluded.[47,76]

Appropriate agents for the management of hypertensive encephalopathy include intravenous nicardipine, labetalol, fenoldopam, and clevidipine.[49-51,77] Do not use nitroglycerin because it dilates cerebral arteries and alters both global and regional blood flow, which may worsen the autoregulation failure.[48]

The ideal targets for blood pressure control in subarachnoid hemorrhage and ischemic stroke are not clear and should be balanced to avoid worsening ischemia or rebleeding. For **subarachnoid hemorrhage,**[78] recommended agents include intravenous nicardipine, labetalol, and clevidipine[54-56] without one superior agent to date.[52] Oral nimodipine is a good choice for those with modest blood pressure elevations because it lowers blood pressure and reduces vasospasm and subsequent cerebral infarction rates, improving neurologic outcomes.[52,79,80] Clazosentan can also decrease the incidence of vasospasm-related delayed ischemic neurologic deficits and has similar blood pressure–lowering effects as nimodipine.[53] If an anticonvulsant is used and an agent that may further reduce blood pressure is selected, such as intravenous phenytoin (rate dependent) or a benzodiazepine, caution must be exercised with additional blood pressure reduction attempts.

The treatment of hypertension in patients with **intracerebral hemorrhage** includes labetalol, nicardipine, and esmolol.[56,57,61-64] Enalaprilat may also be used, but due to concerns of precipitous blood pressure drop, start with a smaller test dose (0.625 mg).[64] Lowering systolic blood pressures from >180 mm Hg to 120 to 160 mm Hg may improve clinical outcomes.[58-60]

In **ischemic stroke**, moderately elevated blood pressure may be beneficial in preserving cerebral perfusion of ischemic areas. Conversely, it may also worsen edema and contribute to hemorrhagic transformation. It is likely that ideal blood pressure ranges exist for ischemic stroke subtypes, but at this time, such ranges have not yet been determined. For the treatment of ischemic stroke, labetalol and nicardipine are the recommended agents; however, the route and degree of blood pressure reduction depend on whether the patient is a candidate for reperfusion therapy (Table 57-4).[65] **Fibrinolytic therapy is contraindicated in patients who maintain a blood pressure >185/110 mm Hg *after* antihypertensive therapy**. In patients who maintain blood pressures ≤185/110 mm Hg (with or without antihypertensive therapy) and undergo fibrinolytic therapy, blood pressure goal is at or below 180/105 mm Hg. Blood pressure should be monitored every 15 minutes for 2 hours from the start of recombinant tissue plasminogen activator therapy, then every 30 minutes for 6 hours, and then every hour for 16 hours. Specific antihypertensive agents and blood pressure recommendations for severely hypertensive patients presenting with ischemic stroke are presented in Table 57-4.

PHARMACOLOGIC AGENTS

Parenteral agents used for hypertensive emergencies, including dosage, mechanisms, and warnings, are listed in **Table 57-5**. Refer to Table 57-4 for indications. Other considerations for drug choice include ability to monitor the patient and comorbidities, including respiratory and vascular disease.

β-BLOCKERS

Labetalol is unique among commonly used β-blockers because it also has modest selective α_1-inhibitory effects, with an α- to β-blocking ratio of 1:7.[82] It recommended for nearly all hypertensive emergencies with the exception of cocaine intoxication and systolic dysfunction in association with decompensated heart failure. In the latter, nicardipine is preferred when nitroglycerin fails. Oral **metoprolol** is indicated in the majority of patients presenting with acute coronary syndromes: Oral β-blockers have a clear benefit in terms of survival, whereas mortality data are conflicting with intravenous formulations.[42,44] However, if blood pressure control is needed in a patient with acute coronary syndrome, the intravenous formulation should be used. Esmolol has a short duration of action and is titrable, an advantage in patients at risk for the adverse effects of β-blockers, such as those with severe asthma and chronic obstructive pulmonary disease.

CALCIUM CHANNEL BLOCKERS

Clevidipine is a third-generation dihydropyridine calcium channel blocker with ultra-short-acting selective arteriolar vasodilator properties.[82] It has been studied in the perioperative setting and in patients with renal dysfunction.[83-85] Its advantage is its ability to be titrated with a half-life less than a minute. **Nicardipine** has an onset of action of 5 to 15 minutes and can be titrated at 15-minute intervals. It has been found to be safe and effective in neurologic hypertensive emergencies and has a favorable effect on myocardial oxygen balance increasing both stroke index and coronary blood flow. When compared to labetalol, patients were more likely to reach physician-specified target blood pressure goal in the initial 30 minutes of therapy.[81] **Nifedipine** use (10 milligrams PO) is discouraged in hypertensive emergencies except in peripartum patients.[86,87]

VASODILATORS

Nitroglycerin is a potent venodilator, showing arterial dilatation only at very high doses. Use may cause hypotension and reflex tachycardia, both worsened by the volume depletion characteristic of hypertensive emergencies. **Nitroglycerin is recommended as a first-line agent only in the treatment of heart failure and acute coronary syndromes** due to its favorable effects on coronary blood flow and cardiac workload. Its hypotensive effects are due to its reduction of preload and cardiac output, which makes it a poor choice in other hypertensive emergencies.

Sodium nitroprusside is best used when other agents fail. It requires more titration than nicardipine in hypertensive neurosurgical patients[88] and has higher mortality rates in cardiac surgery patients when compared to clevidipine.[89] Concerns about cyanide toxicity, heightened in patients with renal or hepatic insufficiency, and the need for invasive monitoring further curtail its use.[90] Combination therapy is the most common current use, as in aortic dissection patients who also receive esmolol to achieve blood pressure targets at lower doses.

OTHER AGENTS

Fenoldopam is a unique peripheral dopaminergic-1 receptor agonist, and due to its ability to promote diuresis, natriuresis, and creatinine clearance, its primary application is in renal hypertensive emergencies.[82] **Phentolamine** is used successfully in cocaine-, amphetamine-, and pheochromocytoma-related hypertensive emergencies.[73,74,82] **Enalaprilat**, the only available IV angiotensin-converting enzyme inhibitor, has special application in patients with heart failure or acute coronary syndrome, but caution should be exercised because of common first-dose hypotension.[64]

Clonidine, a central α_2-agonist, generally does not have a role in the treatment of patients with hypertensive emergencies with the exception of those who have recently stopped taking the drug. An abrupt cessation of clonidine can induce a rebound hypertension, which may be difficult to control with other agents. It can be given orally, at 0.2 to 0.3 milligram initially, with blood pressure reduction starting within 30 to 60 minutes and peaking at 2 to 4 hours.[82] In patients who are unable to take oral medications, a clonidine patch for dermal delivery may be used. However, the onset action may be delayed by 2 to 3 days, and titration is challenging. For maximum absorption, apply the patch to the chest or upper arm.[82,91] Although abrupt cessation of either clonidine or a β-blocker may result in rebound hypertension, clonidine withdrawal tends to be more severe and often will not respond to therapy without reinstitution.

TREATMENT OF ASYMPTOMATIC SEVERE HYPERTENSION

Acute treatment of asymptomatic severe hypertension does not prevent or reduce short-term patient morbidity or mortality.[8] Nevertheless, a small study demonstrated increased risk of cardiovascular events within 4 years of ED presentation in hypertensive urgency patients (systolic blood pressure >220 mm Hg and/or diastolic blood pressure >120 mm Hg) compared to control patients with systolic blood pressures between 135 and 180 mm Hg and diastolic blood pressures between 85 and 110 mm Hg.[92] These data, combined with the evidence that uncontrolled blood pressure is a major risk factor for cardiovascular disease, renal failure, and cerebrovascular accidents, are reasons to initiate outpatient blood pressure reduction regimens prior to discharge. **Table 57-6** lists oral agents commonly used for hypertension. The drugs listed are chosen for their relatively rapid onset of action and their potential use for ongoing control of chronic hypertension. Choosing an agent that can be used once daily and is inexpensive is often an ideal plan (e.g., generic lisinopril, started at 10 milligrams daily). If choosing an angiotensin-converting enzyme inhibitor or angiotensin II receptor antagonist, check the creatinine and potassium first.

DISPOSITION AND FOLLOW-UP OF ASYMPTOMATIC HYPERTENSION

Table 57-7 provides consensus-based and the newer, focused Eighth Report of the Joint National Committee recommendations.[9,93-95] Many ED patients who present with elevated blood pressure have a reduction after approximately 90 minutes; however, patients whose blood pressures remain persistently elevated (systolic blood pressure >140 mm Hg or diastolic blood pressure >90 mm Hg, age <60 years, no medical problems **or** systolic blood pressure >150 mm Hg or diastolic blood pressure >90 mm Hg, age ≥60 years or a history of diabetes or chronic kidney disease) should have clear follow-up and can benefit from starting oral therapy, because only 6% have normal blood pressure values later.[93] Reinforce the need for outpatient follow-up, with or without ED-initiated oral therapy, even if elevated blood pressure was not part of the chief complaint.[95]

Initial therapy recommendations for nonblack individuals are a thiazide diuretic (e.g., hydrochlorothiazide, 25 milligrams daily), an angiotensin-converting enzyme inhibitor (e.g., lisinopril, 10 milligrams daily), or

TABLE 57-5 Intravenous Agents Used for Hypertensive Emergencies

Drug	Dosage	Mechanism/Comments	Warnings
β-Blockers			
Labetalol	Bolus: 10–20 milligrams (0.25 milligram/kg for an 80-kg patient) IV over 2 min; may administer 40–80 milligrams at 10-min intervals, up to 300 milligrams total dose. Continuous infusion: initially, 2 milligrams/min; titrate to response up to 300 milligrams total dose, if needed.	Combined selective α_1-adrenergic and nonselective β-adrenergic receptor blocker with an α- to β-blocking ratio of 1:7.[81] Effect in 2–5 min, peaking by 15 min, duration 2–4 h. Renal, cerebral, and coronary blood flow maintained; minimal placental transfer. **Pregnancy category C**	Avoid use in patients with bradycardia, >first-degree heart block, uncompensated cardiac failure, or active bronchospasm, and in patients receiving IV verapamil or diltiazem. Caution in patients with liver impairment (effects may be prolonged); the elderly have a less predictable response and more toxicity.
Esmolol	Loading dose: 250–500 micrograms/kg infused over 1–3 min IV, follow with: Maintenance infusion: 50 micrograms/kg/min IV over 4 min; if adequate effect not observed, repeat loading dose and increase infusion rate using increments of 50 micrograms/kg/min IV (for 4 min). This regimen can be repeated ×4 bolus doses and to an infusion rate of 300 micrograms/kg/min.	Ultra-short-acting, cardioselective, β-adrenergic receptor blocker. Onset within 60 s, duration 10–20 min. Ideal for use in patients at risk for complications from β-blockers, especially patients with mild to moderately severe left ventricular dysfunction or peripheral vascular disease. Duration 10–20 min; easily stopped. **Pregnancy category C**	Avoid use in patients with bradycardia, heart block, cardiogenic shock, decompensated cardiac failure, or active bronchospasm, and in patients receiving IV verapamil or diltiazem. Caution in patients with asthma, COPD, uncompensated cardiac failure; extravasation can lead to skin necrosis and sloughing; anemic patients will have a prolonged half-life, because drug is metabolized by red blood cell esterases.
Calcium Channel Blockers			
Nicardipine	Continuous infusion: start at rate of 5 milligrams/h. If target BP not achieved in 15 min, increase dose by 2.5 milligrams/h every 15 min until target pressure or the maximum dose of 15 milligrams/h is reached.	Second-generation dihydropyridine calcium channel blocker with vascular selectivity for the cerebral and coronary arteries. Onset of action is 5–10 min, duration is 1-4 h. **Pregnancy category C**	Avoid in patients with advanced aortic stenosis. Caution in decompensated heart failure. Avoid in patients receiving IV β-blockers. Common side effects are headache, hypotension, vomiting, and tachycardia.
Clevidipine	Continuous infusion: initiate IV infusion at 1–2 milligrams/h. Dose titration: double dose at short (90-s) intervals initially. As BP approaches goal, increase dose by less than doubling and lengthen time between dose adjustments to every 5–10 min.	Very rapid onset and offset of effect due to its ultra-short half-life, approximately 2–4 min. Clevidipine is rapidly hydrolyzed to its inactive metabolite in blood and extravascular tissues. It exerts a selective vasodilating action on arteriolar resistance vessels, but has no effect on venous capacitance vessels. Its metabolism is independent of the kidney or liver. **Pregnancy category C**	Cautions: Clevidipine contains approximately 0.2 gram of lipid per mL (2.0 kcal). Lipid intake restrictions may be necessary for patients with significant disorders of lipid metabolism. Clevidipine may produce systemic hypotension and reflex tachycardia. Contraindicated in patients with severe aortic stenosis and egg or soy hypersensitivity
Vasodilators			
Nitroglycerin	Sublingual: 0.4 milligrams. Paste: 1–2 inches. Continuous infusion: start 5 micrograms/min, increase by 5 micrograms/min every 3–5 min to 20 micrograms/min; if no response at 20 micrograms/min, increase by 10 micrograms/min every 3–5 min, up to 200 micrograms/min (note: many clinicians initiate with a higher infusion rate).	Potent venodilator and only at high doses affects arterial tone. Onset begins at 2 min, duration is 10–20 min (paste duration 3–4 h, unless removed). Reduces BP by reducing preload and cardiac output. Decreases coronary vasospasm and cardiac workload. **Pregnancy category C**	Avoid in cases of compromised cerebral and renal perfusion; avoid concurrent use (within past 24–48 h) with phosphodiesterase 5 inhibitors (sildenafil, tadalafil, or vardenafil). Caution: may cause hypotension with reflex tachycardia, which is exacerbated by volume depletion.
Nitroprusside	Continuous infusion: 0.5 microgram/kg/min IV initial infusion, increase in increments of 0.5 microgram/kg/min; titrate to desired effect. Rates >2 micrograms/kg/min may lead to cyanide toxicity. Use lowest possible dose. For infusions of 4–10 micrograms/kg/min, institute a thiosulfate infusion.	Arterial and venous vasodilator due to its interaction with oxyhemoglobin to produce nitric oxide. It decreases preload and afterload. Onset of action is in seconds, duration is 1–2 min. Cerebral blood flow is decreased, whereas intracranial pressure is increased. **Pregnancy category C**	Avoid in patients with kidney or hepatic failure, arteriovenous shunts, hereditary optic nerve atrophy (increases nerve ischemia), or elevated ICP. Caution: intra-arterial monitoring is recommended; must be protected from light. Nitroprusside is recommended only when other agents fail. Coronary steal syndrome may occur.
Other Agents			
Phentolamine	Bolus load: 1–5 milligrams IV. Continuous infusion: 0.2–0.5 milligram/min.	α_1- and α_2-adrenergic blocking agent, effective for pheochromocytoma and hypercatecholaminergic-induced hypertension. **Pregnancy category C**	Myocardial infarction, cerebrovascular spasm, and cerebrovascular occlusion have occurred after administration.
Fenoldopam	Continuous infusion: start 0.1 microgram/kg/min, titrate to desired effect every 15 min, range 0.1–1.6 micrograms/kg/min.	Dopamine 1 receptor agonist. Onset of action in 5 min, peak effect at 15 min, duration 30–60 min. Metabolized by liver, without P-450 system. Improves creatinine clearance, urine flow, and sodium excretion. **Pregnancy category B**	Caution: causes reflex tachycardia at higher dosages. Concurrent use of acetaminophen may increase fenoldopam levels. May cause flushing, dizziness, vomiting. Caution in patients with increased ocular pressures and ICP; caution in patients who have sulfite sensitivity (it is contained in a solution of sodium metabisulfite).
Enalaprilat	Bolus: 1.25 milligrams IV over 5 min every 4–6 h, titrate at increments of 1.25 milligrams every 12–24 h, with a maximum of 5 milligrams every 6 h.	Angiotensin-converting enzyme inhibitor. Test dose of 0.625 milligrams recommended when concern for first-dose hypotension exists.[64] **Pregnancy category D**	Avoid in pregnancy. Caution: first-dose hypotension is common, especially in high renin states; may cause dizziness and headache.

Abbreviations: BP = blood pressure; COPD = chronic obstructive pulmonary disease; ICP = intracranial pressure.

TABLE 57-6 Oral Agents for Hypertensive Urgencies

Agent	Mechanism of Action	Dosage	Onset of Action	Duration	Contraindications	Adverse Effects
Labetalol	α_1-, β-Adrenergic blocker	200–400 milligrams PO, repeat every 2–3 h	30–120 min	6–12 h	Asthma, chronic obstructive pulmonary disease, bradycardia, heart block, heart failure	Bronchoconstriction, bradycardia Pregnancy category C
Captopril	Angiotensin-converting enzyme inhibitor	12.5–25 milligrams PO	15–30 min	4–6 h	Renal artery stenosis, pregnancy	Acute renal failure, angioedema, side effect of chronic cough Pregnancy category D
Losartan	Angiotensin II antagonist	50 milligrams PO	60 min	12–24 h	Second and third trimesters of pregnancy	Allergic reaction (rare) Pregnancy category C in first trimester Category D in second and third trimesters
Nifedipine (extended release) **Indicated for pre-eclampsia only**	Calcium channel blocker	10 milligrams PO, may repeat every 30–60 min	5–15 min	3–6 h	Angina, acute hypertension	Myocardial infarction, cerebrovascular accident, syncope, heart block, CHF Pregnancy category C
Clonidine **Primary indication for rebound hypertension**	Central α_2-agonist	0.1–0.2 milligram PO	30–60 min	6–8 h	CHF, second- or third-degree heart block Would not recommend as a new or singular antihypertensive agent	Drowsiness, sedation, tachycardia, dry mouth Pregnancy category C

Abbreviation: CHF = congestive heart failure.

a calcium channel blocker. In blacks, initiate a thiazide diuretic or a calcium channel blocker, alone or in combination.[95] In patients with chronic kidney disease, with or without diabetes, initiate an angiotensin-converting enzyme inhibitor or an angiotensin receptor blocker.[7,93,95] **Table 57-8** lists indications for recommended oral antihypertensive classes based on trial data, as put forward in the Seventh and Eighth Reports of Joint National Committee.[7,95]

Consider and teach patients about potential adverse effects when prescribing an antihypertensive medication to a patient at discharge. A list of the most common side effects stratified by drug class appears in **Table 57-9**.

HYPERTENSIVE EMERGENCIES IN CHILDREN

The epidemiology, presentation, and management of hypertensive emergencies in children is less well documented than in adults. A formal definition of hypertension crisis does not exist for children.[96] Hypertension in children is defined as systolic and/or diastolic blood pressure measurement that exceeds the 95th percentile for that child's age, sex, and weight on three or more occasions, and this determination can be made using the pediatric nomograms found at http://www.nhlbi.nih.gov/health-pro/guidelines/current/hypertension-pediatric-jnc-4/blood-pressure-tables; a single elevated blood pressure in the ED is insufficient to diagnose hypertension. Severe blood pressure elevation can be considered any blood pressure that exceeds the 95th to 99th percentile for that child's age, sex, and weight by an additional 20 mm Hg or more.[97] As in adults, hypertensive emergencies in children refer to severely elevated blood pressures accompanied by target organ damage. Neonates may present with apnea, cyanosis, irritability, and poor feeding, whereas older children may have symptoms that more closely approximate adult presentations, such as headache, confusion or encephalopathy, focal neurologic deficits, vision changes, shortness of breath, peripheral edema, and decreased renal output.[96]

TABLE 57-7 Recommended Treatment Protocol for ED Patients with Increased Blood Pressure (BP)

Systolic BP (mm Hg)		Diastolic BP (mm Hg)	Follow-Up/Treatment
120–160	*or*	80–100	Advise follow-up within 2 months
>160	*or*	>100	Advise follow-up within 1 month
>180	*or*	>110	Consider initiating therapy at discharge; follow up within 1 week
>200	*or*	>120	Begin antihypertensive therapy at discharge; follow up within 1 week

In children who are noted to have severely elevated blood pressures but no evidence of target organ damage, consult the child's pediatrician for outpatient follow-up or initiation of an antihypertensive agent prior to discharge. In children who present with a hypertensive emergency, immediate blood pressure control is needed, along with consultation with the pediatric intensivist or nephrologist, with admission to the pediatric intensive care unit. Blood pressure control should be initiated in the ED, with the primary aim of therapy to reduce the blood pressure to <95th percentile and to <90th percentile in the presence of comorbid conditions like diabetes or cardiac or renal disease. The mean arterial blood pressure should be lowered no more than ≤25% of the initial value in the first hour, with normalization of blood pressure gradually over the next 24 to 48 hours. Preferred first-line medications for hypertensive emergencies in children include labetalol, 0.2 to 1.0 milligram/kg per dose up to 40 milligrams/dose, or an infusion of 0.25 to 3.0 mg/kg/h; or nicardipine, 0.5 to 3 microgram/kg/min infusion. Second-line agents include hydralazine, 0.2 to 0.6 milligram/kg administered as a bolus to a maximum of 20 milligrams; esmolol administered as a 100 to 500 microgram/kg loading dose followed by an infusion of 50 to 150 micrograms/kg/min to a maximum of 1000 micrograms/kg/min; and clevidipine 0.5 to 3.5 micrograms/kg/min infusion; if prior drugs fail, use IV nitroprusside, 0.5 to 10.0 microgram/kg/min.[96,98,99] Phentolamine, 0.1 milligram/kg to a maximum of 5 milligrams, is the drug of choice for conditions associated with high circulating catecholamines, such as cocaine or pseudoephedrine overdose.

PRACTICE GUIDELINES

The American College of Emergency Physicians policy document titled "Clinical Policy: Critical Issues in the Evaluation and Management of Adult Patients in the Emergency Department with Asymptomatic Elevated Blood Pressure" can be found at http://www.acep.org/Content.aspx?id=30060.

TABLE 57-8 Indications for Specific Antihypertensive Therapy

	Heart Failure	Post–Myocardial Infarction	High Coronary Artery Disease Risk	Recurrent Stroke Prevention	Diabetes	Chronic Kidney Disease
Blood pressure goal	<140/90 mm Hg	<140/90 mm Hg	<140/90 mm Hg	<140/90 mm Hg	<140/90 mm Hg	<140/90 mm Hg
First-line therapy	Diuretic with ACE inhibitor	β-Blocker or ACE inhibitor	β-Blocker	Diuretic with ACE inhibitor or ARB	Nonblack: Thiazide diuretic, ACE inhibitor, ARB or CCB Black: Thiazide diuretic or CCB	ACE inhibitor or ARB
Second-line therapy	β-Blocker	Aldosterone antagonist	ACE inhibitor, calcium channel blocker, or diuretic	—	Above alone or in combination	Above alone or in combination with other drug class

Abbreviations: ACE = angiotensin-converting enzyme; ARB = angiotensin receptor blocker; CCB = calcium channel blocker.

TABLE 57-9 Common Adverse Effects of Antihypertensive Drugs

Antihypertensive Class	Recommended Ancillary Testing prior to Therapy	Most Common Adverse Effects
Diuretic	Chemistry panel: renal function and electrolytes	Hypokalemia, hypomagnesemia, hyperglycemia, hypercalcemia, hyperuremia, hyponatremia
Angiotensin-converting enzyme inhibitor	Chemistry panel: renal function and electrolytes Pregnancy test	Cough, hyperkalemia, acute renal failure, angioedema, myopathy, fetal abnormalities
Angiotensin receptor blocker	Chemistry panel: renal function and electrolytes Pregnancy test	Hyperkalemia, acute renal failure, angioedema, myopathy, fetal abnormalities
β-Blocker	ECG	Bronchospasm, bradycardia, depression, erectile dysfunction
Calcium channel blocker	ECG	Bradycardia, constipation, lower extremity edema
Aldosterone antagonist	Chemistry panel: renal function and electrolytes Pregnancy test	Hyperkalemia, gynecomastia, feminization of male fetuses

The full 2003 Seventh Report of the Joint National Committee can be found at http://www.nhlbi.nih.gov/guidelines/hypertension/jnc7full.htm. The 2013 update, the Eighth Report of the Joint National Committee, focuses primarily on blood pressure goals and initial therapies.[95]

Acknowledgments: The author gratefully acknowledges the contributions of David M. Cline, the author of this chapter in the previous edition.

REFERENCES

The complete reference list is available online at www.TintinalliEM.com.

Pulmonary Hypertension

Michael E. Winters

INTRODUCTION AND EPIDEMIOLOGY

Normally, the pulmonary vascular system is a high-flow, low-resistance circuit, with a mean pulmonary arterial pressure that constitutes approximately 15% to 20% of the systemic circulation.[1] Normal pulmonary arterial systolic pressures range from 15 to 30 mm Hg, whereas diastolic pulmonary arterial pressures range from 4 to 12 mm Hg.[1] Pulmonary hypertension is defined as a mean pulmonary arterial pressure >25 mm Hg at rest or >30 mm Hg during exertion.[1,2]

Pulmonary hypertension is classified based on measurements of pulmonary capillary wedge pressure (PCWP) and pulmonary vascular resistance. Patients with pulmonary arterial hypertension have a mean pulmonary arterial pressure >25 mm Hg, a pulmonary vascular resistance >240 dynes/s/cm^5, and a PCWP <15 mm Hg.[2] In contrast, patients with pulmonary hypertension caused by left heart disease, the most common cause of pulmonary hypertension, have a PCWP >15 mm Hg.[2] Although echocardiography can estimate pulmonary arterial pressure in a patient with suspected pulmonary hypertension, definitive diagnosis requires right heart catheterization.

The World Health Organization classifies pulmonary hypertension into five categories based on cause and response to treatment (**Table 58-1**).[1,3] Some patients have features of multiple categories, but the majority have one predominant type of pulmonary hypertension.[4] Accurate classification of pulmonary hypertension is key to directing treatments, which vary among the categories. Pulmonary venous hypertension is the most common cause of pulmonary hypertension, affecting almost 4 million patients in the United States.[4] In contrast, pulmonary arterial hypertension is the least common cause of pulmonary hypertension, with an estimated prevalence of 15 patients per million.[4,5] Pulmonary hypertension develops in up to 4% of patients with chronic thromboembolic disease.[4,6,7] Regardless of

TABLE 58-1 World Health Organization Classification of Pulmonary Hypertension

Group 1: Pulmonary Arterial Hypertension
- Idiopathic
- Genetic/heritable abnormalities
- Drug or toxin induced
- Associated with known risk factors for pulmonary arterial hypertension (human immunodeficiency virus, liver disease, collagen vascular disorders)

Group 2: Pulmonary Venous Hypertension (left heart disease)
- Systolic or diastolic dysfunction
- Mitral or aortic valve disease

Group 3: Chronic Hypoxemic Lung Disease
- Obstructive lung disorders (chronic obstructive pulmonary disease)
- Interstitial lung disease
  - Idiopathic pulmonary fibrosis
  - Collagen vascular disorders
- Sleep-disordered breathing (obstructive sleep apnea)
- Chronic exposure to high altitude

Group 4: Embolic Disease

Group 5: Miscellaneous
- Lymphatic obstruction
- Hematologic disorders: myeloproliferative disorders
- Systemic disorders: sarcoidosis, neurofibromatosis
- Metabolic disorders: glycogen storage disease, thyroid disorders

the cause, patients with pulmonary hypertension have high morbidity and mortality rates,[4,8] with a 5-year mortality rate for patients with idiopathic pulmonary arterial hypertension exceeding 30%.[5]

PATHOPHYSIOLOGY

The exact pathophysiology of all forms of pulmonary hypertension remains unknown. In **pulmonary arterial hypertension**, the initial abnormality is endothelial dysfunction, which results in an imbalance between endogenous vasodilators (e.g., prostacyclin) and vasoconstrictors (e.g., endothelin-1). The net effect is vasoconstriction and the formation of in situ thrombi. Additional pathologic processes include alterations in microvascular permeability, abnormal hypoxic vasoconstriction, microvascular thrombosis, and the formation of plexiform lesions, leading to vascular remodeling. Ultimately, these abnormalities result in sustained elevations of pulmonary vascular resistance and impairment of pulmonary blood flow.

With persistent elevations in pulmonary vascular resistance, the right ventricle (RV) dilates to maintain an adequate stroke volume. RV dilation increases the ventricular wall tension, increases oxygen consumption, and eventually decreases contractility. With progressive RV dilation, the intraventricular septum is displaced toward the left ventricle. This displacement inhibits left ventricular filling and ultimately impairs cardiac output and systemic perfusion.

Perfusion of the **right coronary artery (RCA)** depends on the gradient between the aorta and RV. Normally, the RCA is perfused during both systole and diastole. In patients with advanced pulmonary hypertension, RCA perfusion occurs almost exclusively during diastole.[9,10] Decreased perfusion results in right ventricular ischemia and further impairment of left ventricular output. Eventually, this cycle results in right ventricular failure and cardiovascular collapse.

CLINICAL FEATURES

The most common symptom of pulmonary hypertension is dyspnea, either at rest or with exertion, which is present in over 50% of patients.[1,11] Other symptoms include fatigue, chest pain, near syncope, syncope, and exertional lightheadedness.[3,11,12] Since these initial symptoms are nonspecific, it is not surprising that delays in diagnosis are common, with an average interval between symptom onset and diagnosis of pulmonary hypertension of 2 years.[13] As pulmonary arterial pressure increases, patients can develop early satiety, anorexia, orthopnea, paroxysmal nocturnal dyspnea, and peripheral edema.

The physical examination is often normal in the early stages of pulmonary hypertension.[1] As pulmonary hypertension worsens, findings of right ventricular failure emerge (e.g., a holosystolic tricuspid regurgitation murmur, jugular venous distention, hepatomegaly, ascites, and lower extremity edema).[1,4] Additional findings include an increased intensity of the pulmonary component of the second heart sound (P_2), a parasternal heave, and a subxiphoid thrust in patients with right ventricular hypertrophy.[1,4]

DIAGNOSTIC TESTING

ELECTROCARDIOGRAM

The most common ECG abnormality seen in pulmonary hypertension patients is right axis deviation.[12] Additional findings associated with pulmonary hypertension include an R/S ratio >1 in lead V_1, an R/S ratio <1 in leads V_5 and V_6, a qR complex in lead V_1, an $S_1Q_3T_3$, right atrial enlargement in the inferior leads, and an incomplete or complete right bundle branch block[14] (**Figure 58-1**). These findings are neither sensitive nor specific for the identification of pulmonary hypertension.

The ECG may show signs of right ventricular ischemia or dysrhythmia. The most common dysrhythmias in patients with pulmonary hypertension are atrial fibrillation, atrial flutter, and atrioventricular nodal reentrant tachycardia.[15,16] Of these, atrial fibrillation is associated with the highest mortality rate.[15]

LABORATORY TESTING

Routine laboratory testing (e.g., CBC, comprehensive metabolic panel) is often nonspecific in the initial evaluation of the pulmonary hypertension patient with dyspnea. **B-type natriuretic peptide** and **N-terminal B-type natriuretic peptide** are often elevated and correlate with outcomes in patients with pulmonary hypertension but have limited impact in ED care.[17-19] Elevations in troponin from myocardial ischemia or a strain-induced leak can be seen and are associated with higher morbidity and mortality.[20,21]

IMAGING

Common chest radiographic abnormalities associated with pulmonary hypertension include enlargement of the right atrium, RV, and hilar pulmonary arteries.[12,22] Depending on the cause of the pulmonary hypertension, additional radiographic findings might include pulmonary edema, hyperinflation, or interstitial lung disease. In most patients presenting with dyspnea, a chest radiograph is obtained to identify other causes of dyspnea, such as pneumonia or pneumothorax.

Transthoracic echocardiography is the best initial diagnostic test to assess pulmonary hypertension in the ED. It allows estimation of the

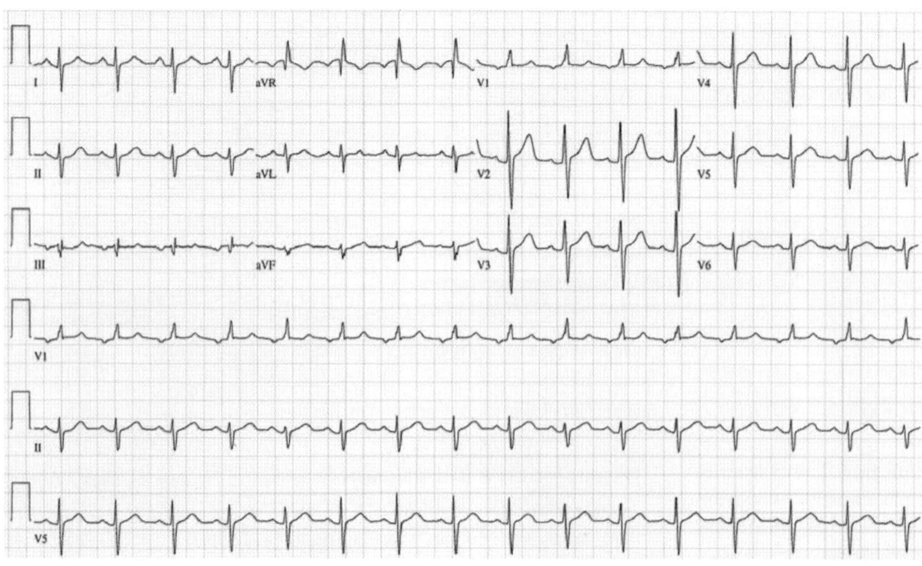

FIGURE 58-1. ECG with findings predictive of pulmonary hypertension: S wave in V_1 <2 mm, R/S ratio in V_1 >1, R/S ratio in V_6 <1, and QRS axis >110 degrees.

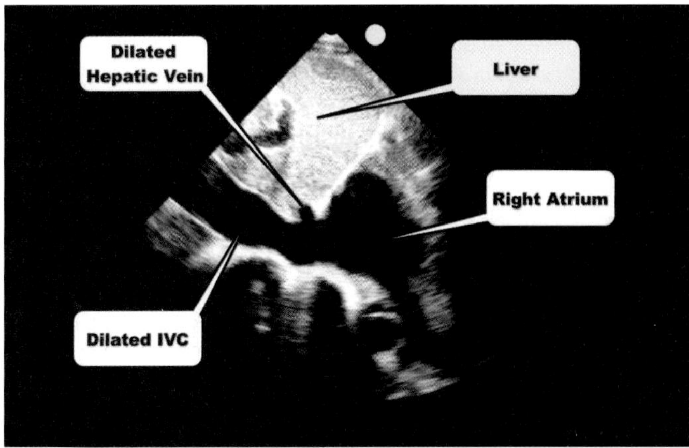

FIGURE 58-2. US of elevated right atrial pressures. Inferior vena cava (IVC) and hepatic vein dilation. [Image used with permission of Haney Mallemat, MD, in the Department of Emergency Medicine at the University of Maryland School of Medicine.]

pulmonary artery systolic pressure[4] and detection of decreased RV function, right atrial hypertrophy, and right ventricular hypertrophy, each of which is indicative of more severe disease.[1] Additional echocardiographic findings in patients with severe pulmonary hypertension include leftward deviation of the intraventricular septum and a right ventricle-to-left ventricle end-diastolic diameter >1 in the four-chamber view.[1,23] **Figures 58-2, 58-3, and 58-4** demonstrate typical echocardiographic findings in patients with pulmonary hypertension.

Echocardiography can also detect precipitating factors for right ventricular failure, including pericardial effusion, regional wall motion abnormalities of the RV or left ventricle, and acute valvular abnormalities.[24]

TREATMENT

No consensus guidelines exist for the management of critically ill patients with pulmonary hypertension in the ED. The mainstays of ED therapy include supplemental oxygen, optimizing intravascular volume, augmenting right ventricular function, maintaining coronary artery perfusion, and decreasing right ventricular afterload (**Table 58-2**).[25]

OXYGEN AND MECHANICAL VENTILATION

While the optimal oxygen saturation is unknown, consensus opinion is to titrate supplemental oxygen to maintain a level >90%.[25] Although intubation and mechanical ventilation are common ED therapies for the

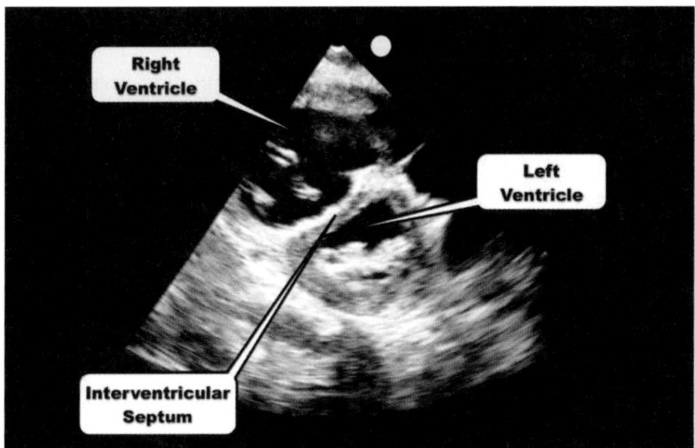

FIGURE 58-3. Cardiac US, parasternal short-axis view of right and left ventricles. Notice the flattening of the interventricular septum occurring in systole, suggesting elevated right ventricular systolic pressures. This is also known as a D-shaped septum. IVC = inferior vena cava. [Image used with permission of Haney Mallemat, MD, in the Department of Emergency Medicine at the University of Maryland School of Medicine.]

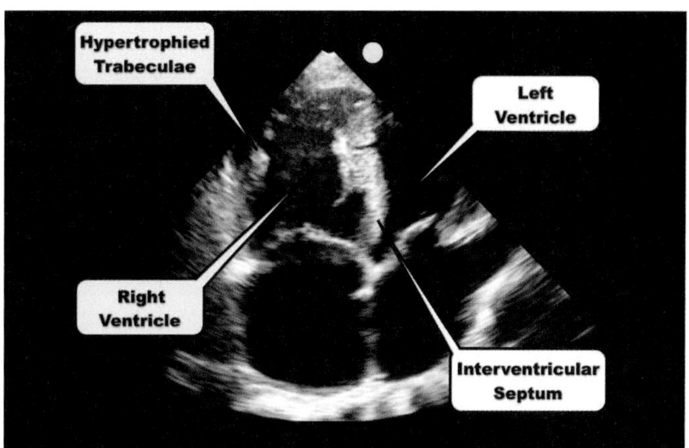

FIGURE 58-4. Apical four-chamber view of right and left ventricles. The right ventricle is dilated with hypertrophy of the right ventricular trabeculae, indicating chronic right ventricular overload. The interventricular septum is also shifted toward the left ventricle in systole, suggesting right ventricular pressure overload. IVC = inferior vena cava. [Image used with permission of Haney Mallemat, MD, in the Department of Emergency Medicine at the University of Maryland School of Medicine.]

patient with acute respiratory failure, be wary of the complications. **In patients with severe pulmonary hypertension, intubation and ventilation can cause rapid cardiovascular collapse due to increased intrathoracic pressure from positive-pressure ventilation and effects of sedative medications on right ventricular function and systemic vascular resistance.**

When mechanical ventilation is needed, set the ventilator to maintain low airway pressure,[25] using lung-protective settings (i.e., a tidal volume of 6 mL/kg of ideal body weight and the lowest positive end-expiratory pressure to maintain the oxygen saturation above 90%). Monitor serial plateau pressure measurements and target pressures to <30 cm H_2O. Adjust the respiratory rate to avoid hypercapnia, which can increase pulmonary vascular resistance, pulmonary artery pressure, and RV strain.[26]

INTRAVASCULAR VOLUME

Volume overload can cause RV dilation, displacing the intraventricular septum, impairing left ventricular output, and ultimately compromising tissue perfusion.[3] For patients who are hypovolemic, give serial boluses of an isotonic crystalloid solution in 250- to 500-mL aliquots with close monitoring. As a result of baseline elevations in right-sided pressures, common methods used to monitor volume responsiveness, such as absolute values of central venous pressure and respiratory variation of the inferior vena cava with US, are less reliable in the patient with pulmonary hypertension.

RIGHT VENTRICULAR FUNCTION

For RV failure, start an inotropic medication to augment function and improve cardiac output. **Dobutamine is preferred**,[25,27,28] starting at

TABLE 58-2 Drugs for Pulmonary Hypertension

Condition	Drug	Comments
RV failure	Dobutamine 2–10 micrograms/kg/min *OR*	Avoid >10 micrograms/kg/min
	Milrinone 0.375 micrograms/kg/min	Higher doses can cause hypotension
RCA perfusion	Norepinephrine 0.05–0.75 micrograms/kg/min	Avoid high doses of norepinephrine; avoid dopamine and phenylephrine
RV afterload	Prostanoids	Rarely initiated in ED

Abbreviations: RCA = right coronary artery; RV = right ventricle.

2 micrograms/kg/min and titrated to 10 micrograms/kg/min. Avoid doses >10 micrograms/kg/min, because large doses can increase pulmonary vascular resistance and cause tachydysrhythmias and hypotension.[29,30] For patients unable to tolerate dobutamine, **milrinone** is an alternative. Milrinone is a phosphodiesterase-3 inhibitor and can indirectly augment right ventricular function through a reduction in pulmonary vascular resistance.[25] Start milrinone at 0.375 micrograms/kg/min and titrate to a maximum of 0.75 micrograms/kg/min. Higher doses of milrinone can cause hypotension.

RIGHT CORONARY ARTERY PERFUSION

Adequate perfusion of the RCA is necessary to maintain right ventricular function and cardiac output. To maintain RCA blood flow, arterial pressure at the aortic root must be higher than the pulmonary artery pressure. For the hypotensive pulmonary hypertension patient, use a vasopressor to increase aortic root pressure and maintain RCA perfusion. Although there are limited data regarding a singular superior agent, norepinephrine is recommended.[25] **Norepinephrine** improves cardiac output and is initiated at a dose of 0.05 micrograms/kg/min. Avoid high doses of norepinephrine because it can increase pulmonary vascular resistance and impair right ventricular output. Avoid dopamine and phenylephrine because these drugs can cause tachydysrhythmias and can elevate pulmonary artery pressure and pulmonary vascular resistance.

RIGHT VENTRICULAR AFTERLOAD

Reducing right ventricular afterload with pulmonary vasodilators is a critical component in the management of stable patients with pulmonary hypertension. The most commonly used pulmonary vasodilators are prostanoids, endothelin receptor antagonists, and phosphodiesterase-5 (PDE-5) inhibitors. These medications are used primarily in the treatment of patients with pulmonary arterial hypertension; they are rarely, if ever, administered in the ED, but understanding the therapeutic agents is important. **Prostanoids** (epoprostenol, treprostinil, and iloprost) are potent vasodilators and are the initial treatment of choice in patients with pulmonary arterial hypertension and right ventricular failure. These medications have antiplatelet and antiproliferative properties.[1] Epoprostenol is the only therapy proven to improve survival.[25] It has a half-life of just 2 to 5 minutes and must be given by continuous IV infusion.[31,32] In contrast, treprostinil has a half-life of 4 to 5 hours and is approved for both IV and SC administration.

For the acutely ill pulmonary hypertension patient receiving ongoing IV prostanoid, the first step is to confirm catheter and pump function. If occlusion or malfunction is detected, consult with the primary provider. Both epoprostenol and treprostinil can be administered by peripheral IV. Iloprost is given as an aerosol and is usually reserved for patients unable to tolerate a parenteral prostanoid.[25] Side effects of prostanoids include headache, nausea, vomiting, flushing, diarrhea, and jaw pain.[1]

Endothelin receptor antagonists are administered orally and increase exercise capacity, improve hemodynamics, and can delay the time to clinical worsening in pulmonary hypertension patients.[1,33-37] Currently, bosentan and ambrisentan are the only available endothelin receptor antagonists, but neither drug has been evaluated in the acutely decompensating pulmonary hypertension patient with right ventricular failure.[25] Side effects of these medications include an elevation in liver transaminase levels and a decrease in hemoglobin concentration.[1]

The **PDE-5 inhibitors** sildenafil and tadalafil are approved for use in patients with pulmonary hypertension. They are administered orally, seeking to improve hemodynamics and exercise capacity in patients with pulmonary arterial hypertension.[1,38-43] Like the endothelin receptor antagonists, they are not currently used in acutely ill pulmonary hypertension patients. Side effects of the PDE-5 inhibitors include headache, flushing, dyspepsia, and hypotension when used concomitantly with nitrates.[1]

DISPOSITION AND FOLLOW-UP

When patients with pulmonary hypertension present to an ED, they are often critically ill, with signs and symptoms of acute right heart failure. As a result, nearly all require admission, often to an intensive care or coronary care unit with expertise in pulmonary hypertension. On rare occasions, a mildly symptomatic patient may be discharged home after consultation, care plan development, and close follow-up with the primary provider.

PRACTICE GUIDELINES

No consensus guidelines exist for the evaluation and management of critically ill ED patients with pulmonary hypertension. Current recommendations are based on expert opinion.

Acknowledgment: The author gratefully acknowledges the contributions of David M. Cline and Alberto J. Machado to this chapter in the previous edition.

REFERENCES

The complete reference list is available online at www.TintinalliEM.com.

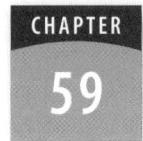

Aortic Dissection and Related Aortic Syndromes

Gary A. Johnson
Louise A. Prince

INTRODUCTION AND EPIDEMIOLOGY

Acute aortic syndromes encompass a number of life-threatening aortic emergencies. These include aortic dissection, penetrating atherosclerotic ulcer, intramural hematoma, and aortic aneurysmal leakage or ruptured abdominal aortic aneurysm (see chapter 60, Aneurysmal Disease).

Acute aortic syndromes are uncommon but frequently fatal. The incidence ranges from 2.9 to 4.7 cases per 100,000 people per year.[1-4] The 1-year, 5-year, and 10-year actuarial survival rates are 92%, 77%, and 57%, respectively, for operative patients.[4] Twenty-two percent of cases are undiagnosed prior to death.[5] The most common cardiovascular complication of Marfan's syndrome is aortic root disease and type A dissection (ascending aorta). The identification of gene mutations associated with Marfan's syndrome, such as *TGFBR2* and *FBN1*, combined with regular follow-up can reduce fatal outcomes.[6]

PATHOPHYSIOLOGY

Acute aortic syndromes occur in the setting of chronic hypertension and other factors that lead to degeneration of the media of the aortic wall. Bicuspid aortic valve, Marfan's syndrome, Ehlers-Danlos syndrome, and familial history of aortic dissection all predispose to aortic syndromes. Chronic cocaine or amphetamine use accelerates atherosclerosis, increasing the risk for dissection.[7] Prior cardiac surgery is another risk factor for aortic dissection. All mechanisms involve weakening of the medial layer and intimal wall stress. Response to stress may include aortic dilation, aneurysm formation, development of a penetrating ulcer, intramural hemorrhage, aortic dissection, and aortic rupture.

Aortic dissection occurs after a violation of the intima allows blood to enter the media and dissect between the intimal and adventitial layers. The dissecting column of blood forms a false lumen and may extend proximally, distally, or in both directions. Blood may dissect and reenter the intima, and this may clinically suggest a spontaneous cure. Alternatively, the blood may dissect through the adventitia, which nearly always proves rapidly fatal.

Aortic dissection has a bimodal age distribution.[4] The first peak involves younger patients with specific predisposing conditions such as connective tissue disorders. The second peak includes those aged >50 years with chronic hypertension. Other atherosclerotic risk factors appear to be only minor contributors to pathogenesis of acute aortic syndromes.

Aortic dissections are classified using two separate systems, the Stanford and DeBakey systems. The **Stanford classification** considers any involvement of the ascending aorta a type A dissection. Stanford type B dissections are restricted to only the descending aorta. **DeBakey** type 1 dissections simultaneously involve the ascending aorta, the arch, and the descending aorta. DeBakey type 2 dissections involve only the ascending aorta, and type 3 involve only the descending aorta.

An **aortic intramural hematoma** results from infarction of the aortic media, usually from injury to the vasa vasorum.[8] An intramural hematoma may resolve spontaneously or may lead to dissection.[9] **Penetrating atherosclerotic ulcer** can lead to intramural hematoma, aortic dissection, or perforation of the aorta.[8,10]

CLINICAL FEATURES

HISTORY

The site of initial intimal disruption predicts the initial symptoms.[11] Symptoms may change as the dissection extends along the aorta or involves other arteries or organs. Classically, dissection presents with abrupt and severe pain in the chest that radiates to an area between the scapulae and may be accompanied by a feeling of impending doom. In a case series of 464 dissections,[5] 60% of patients had anterior chest pain (more common in Stanford type A); abdominal pain is more common in Stanford type B. Most patients describe the pain as severe or the worst they have ever experienced. Sixty-four percent describe it as sharp pain and 50% as tearing or ripping pain. Syncope occurs almost 10% of the time (more common in Stanford type A). Twenty-two percent of dissections occur in patients with prior cardiac surgery.[5]

Dissection in or near a carotid artery may present as a classic **stroke**, and 20% of patients with type A dissection display neurologic findings, which predicts a poorer prognosis.[12,13] Interruption of blood supply to the spinal cord may lead to paraplegia. Further distal dissection may present as back, flank, or abdominal pain. A proximal dissection to the aortic root may lead to **cardiac tamponade** and is generally fatal.

PHYSICAL EXAMINATION

For most patients with aortic dissection, examination findings are relatively normal. An aortic insufficiency murmur may occur (32%), and a pulse deficit in radial arteries or femoral arteries can be found (15%).[9] Hypertension is common (49%), but hypotension occurs in 18% to 25% and worsens prognosis.[5,9,14] Aneurysmal dilation of the aorta may compress regional structures such as the esophagus, the recurrent laryngeal nerve, or the superior cervical sympathetic ganglion, causing dysphagia, hoarseness, or Horner syndrome.

Using retrospective data from the International Registry of Acute Aortic Dissection,[15,16] three clinical categories (underlying condition; pain quality and location; examination findings) were parsed into 12 features[15,16] associated with acute aortic dissection (**Table 59-1**).

TABLE 59-1 Acute Aortic Dissection: Features From the International Registry of Acute Aortic Dissection

Category 1: Underlying Condition	Category 2: Pain in Chest, Back, or Abdomen	Category 3: Abnormal Examination
Marfan's syndrome	Abrupt onset	Systolic blood pressure differential in extremities or pulse amplitude difference
Family history of aortic disease	Severe in intensity	Focal neurologic deficit and chest, back, or abdominal pain
Aortic valvular disease	Ripping or tearing	New murmur of aortic insufficiency and chest, back, or abdominal pain
Recent aortic manipulation		Shock or hypotension
Thoracic aortic aneurysm		

TABLE 59-2 Differential Diagnosis of Aortic Dissection

Myocardial infarction or acute coronary syndromes
Pericardial disease
Stroke
Musculoskeletal disease of the extremity
Spinal cord injuries and disorders
Intra-abdominal disorders
Pulmonary disorders, including pulmonary embolus, pneumonia, pleurisy, pneumothorax

DIAGNOSIS

The large differential diagnosis for chest pain plus the many end-organ ischemic manifestations associated with aortic dissections make the diagnosis challenging. The most important differential diagnoses are listed in **Table 59-2**.

Ischemic manifestations may change with time (as the dissection progresses), and this may distract the physician from making the correct diagnosis. Rupture of the dissection into the true aortic lumen may cause a cessation of symptoms, and the correct diagnosis may then be inappropriately dismissed. History, physical examination, and chest radiography can suggest the diagnosis, but only if one is alert to aortic dissection as one of the diagnostic possibilities in a patient with acute chest pain, syncope, or acute focal neurologic signs. Factors associated with misdiagnosis include walk-in mode of admission, normal mediastinal width/aortic contour on chest radiograph, absent extremity pulse amplitude differences, and nonspecific symptoms.[17-19]

ECG

It may be difficult to differentiate aortic dissection from acute coronary syndromes on ECG, because both conditions are associated with ECG changes; dissection may limit or obstruct coronary artery blood flow. Abnormal ECG findings include new Q waves or ST-segment elevation in 3% to 4%, ST depression in 15% to 22%, and nonspecific ST and T-wave changes in 41% to 62%.[5,9,20] The ECG is normal in only 19% to 31% of patients.[5,20]

BIOMARKERS

Several potential biomarkers have been investigated for their utility to identify or exclude aortic dissection.[21] **D-Dimer** is the marker most thoroughly investigated. A meta-analysis of seven studies involving 298 subjects with acute aortic dissection and 436 without found a sensitivity of 97% (95% confidence interval, 94% to 99%) and negative predictive value of 96% (95% confidence interval, 93% to 98%) using a D-dimer cut point of 500 ng/mL (1620 nmol/L).[22] The specificity was low at 56% (95% confidence interval, 51% to 60%). Guidelines do not endorse the use of D-dimer as the sole means of excluding aortic dissection,[15] and several authors have cautioned against this practice.[23-26] One report found that young adult patients with short dissection length and thrombosed false lumen were likely to have a false-negative D-dimer.[24] The false-negative rate using D-dimer is as high at 18%.[25]

IMAGING

A plain chest radiograph may provide important clues for the diagnosis. However, from 12% to 37% of patients have no abnormality, and this study should not be used to exclude dissection.[5,27] The most common radiographic abnormality is a widened mediastinum or abnormal aortic contour. Other possible findings include pleural effusion, displacement of aortic intimal calcification, and deviation of the trachea, mainstream bronchi, or esophagus (**Figure 59-1**).

CT (especially multidetector-row CT) is the imaging modality of choice for diagnosis of dissection.[11,15,28] CT can reliably identify a false lumen (**Figure 59-2**) and can provide additional details such as the anatomy of the dissection, the location of the dissection flap, extension of the flap into great vessels (**Figure 59-3**), signs of aortic rupture, and

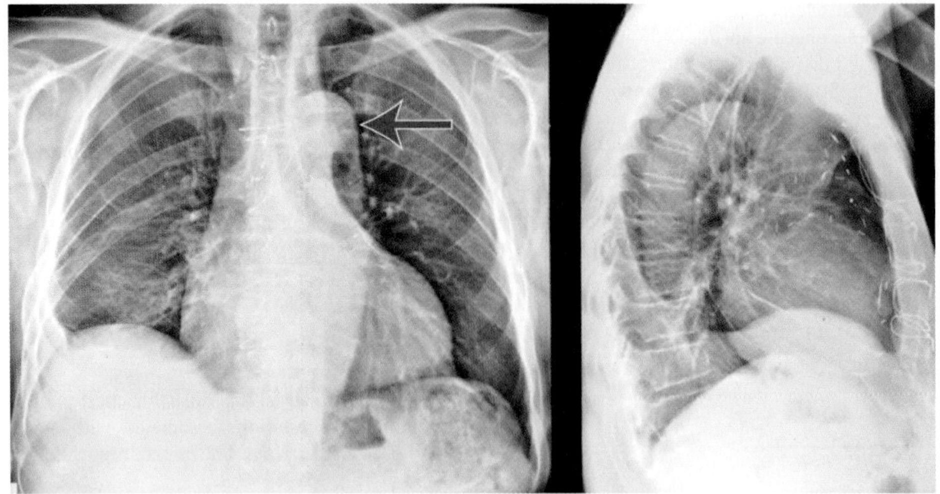

FIGURE 59-1. Abnormal aortic contour on chest radiography. Frontal and lateral radiographs of the chest in a patient with type B aortic dissection reveal an abnormal aortic contour (*arrow*). A right pleural effusion is present, and multiple postoperative clips and wires are also seen.

signs of end-organ damage. CT protocols should be both with and without IV contrast. Invasive catheter angiography is rarely necessary.

CT may also diagnose intramural hematoma and penetrating atherosclerotic ulcer.[28] Penetrating atherosclerotic ulcer can be difficult to distinguish from large atheromatous plaques (**Figure 59-4**). CT diagnosis of penetrating atherosclerotic ulcer depends on extension of the ulcer past the intima. Ulcers often have overhanging edges and focal outpouchings of the aorta itself. Intramural hematoma is often identified by a high-signal mass in the aorta on CT (**Figure 59-5**). This often appears as a crescent and is best seen on noncontrasted images.

In experienced hands, **transesophageal echocardiography** may be as sensitive and specific as CT. The procedure generally has to be performed under moderate sedation or even general anesthesia. Known esophageal disease is a relative contraindication. Sound transmission is disrupted by air in the trachea or left bronchia, which may make evaluation of the ascending aorta difficult. The accuracy and precision of transesophageal echocardiography are highly operator dependent. **MRI** has been used to evaluate stable patients with suspected aortic disease.[28]

Coronary CT angiography, or the "**triple rule-out**," can diagnose and differentiate coronary artery disease, pulmonary embolism, and acute aortic dissection.[29,30] However, it requires a specialized contrast infusion protocol to image the three vascular beds of interest and an increased radiation dosage.[31] Furthermore, the "triple rule-out" study has not been shown to improve diagnostic yield, reduce clinical events, or diminish downstream resource use.[32]

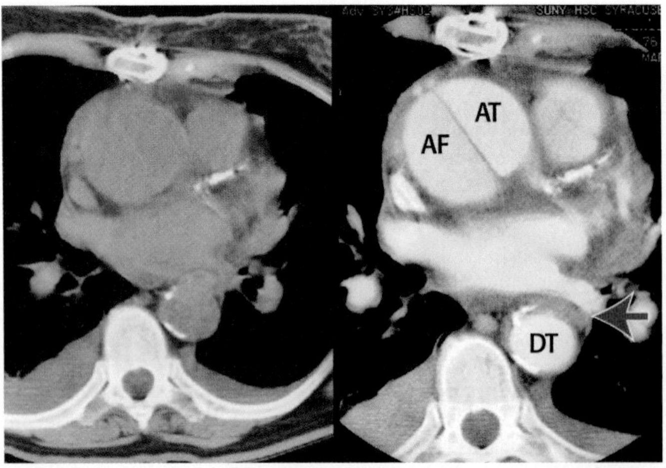

FIGURE 59-2. CT image of a type A aortic dissection. True and false lumens are present in the ascending aorta and descending aorta (descending false lumen at arrow) on noncontrast (*left*) and contrast (*right*) images. AF = ascending false lumen; AT = ascending true lumen; DT = descending true lumen.

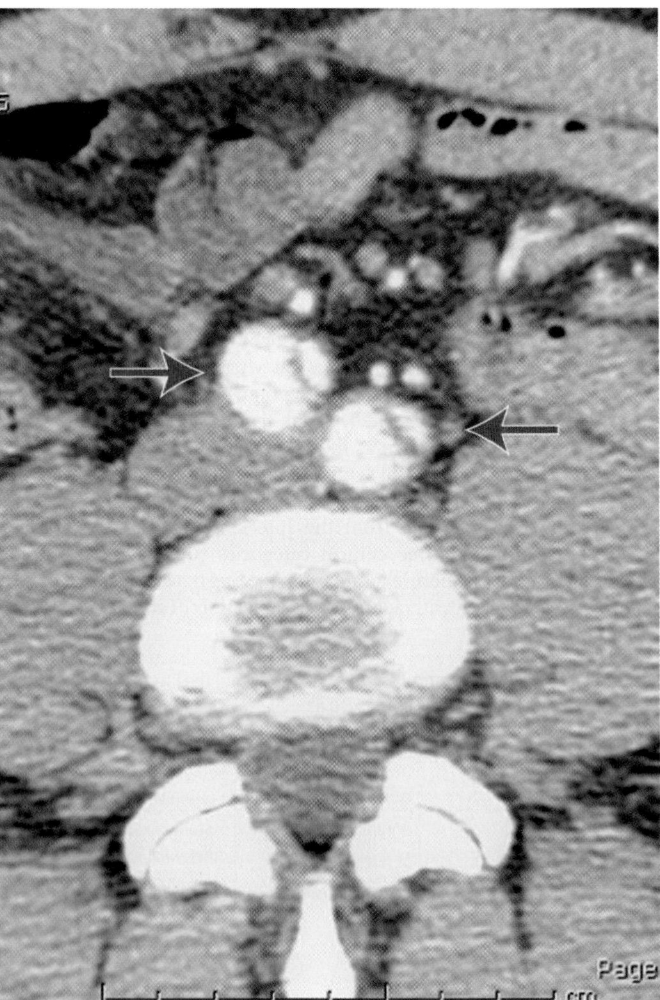

FIGURE 59-3. Type B dissection into the iliac arteries. Contrast CT image of dissection extending into the iliac arteries (anterior to vertebral body). True and false lumens are visible in both arteries (*arrows*).

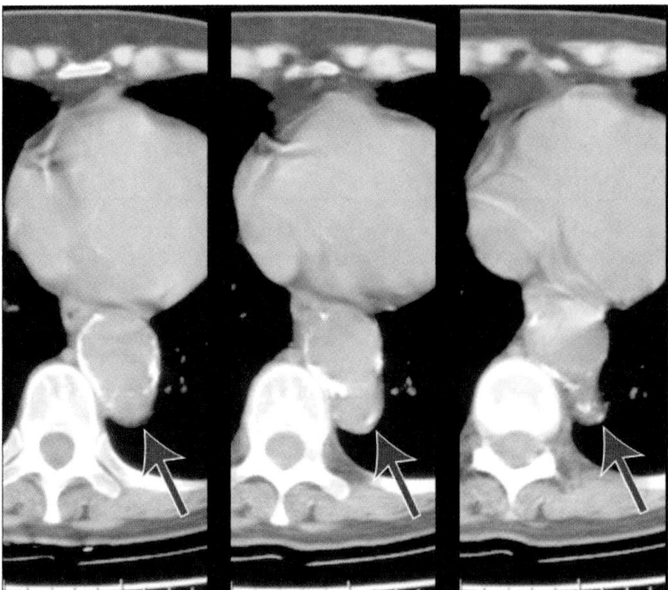

FIGURE 59-4. Noncontrast CT image of a penetrating aortic ulcer in the descending aorta (*arrows*), demonstrating an outpouched, abnormal contour of the aorta in three sections. [Image used with permission of Dr. Ernest Scalzetti, MD.]

TREATMENT

ANTIHYPERTENSIVES: NEGATIVE INOTROPIC AGENTS

While aortic dissections may cause hypotension that requires fluid or blood product resuscitation, suspected aortic dissection commonly requires antihypertensive treatment. Initial treatment is with a negative inotropic agent in order to lower blood pressure without increasing the shear force on the intimal flap of the aorta. β-Blockade is ideal, and short-acting β-blockers such as propranolol, labetalol, or esmolol are preferred over long-acting β-blockers. The ideal target blood pressure is undefined by controlled trials and must be tailored to each patient (see chapters 57, "Systemic Hypertension" and 58, "Pulmonary Hypertension"). However, **a systolic pressure of 120 to 130 mm Hg is a reasonable starting point; guidelines suggest a goal of 100 to 120 mm Hg.**[15]

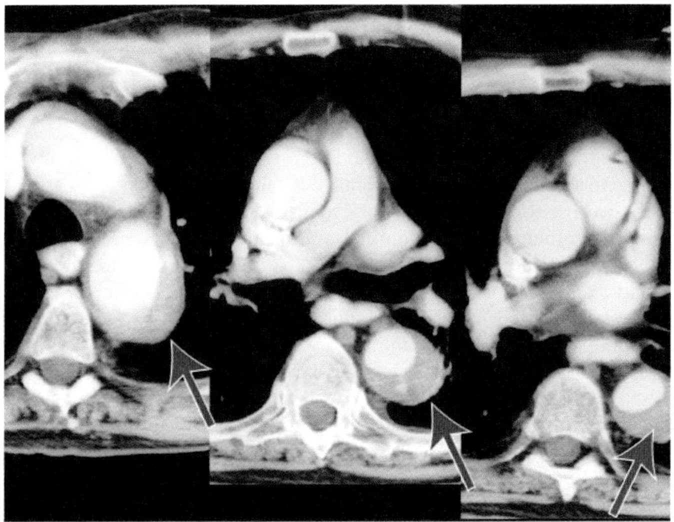

FIGURE 59-5. Contrast CT image of an intramural hematoma (*arrows* point to the crescent-shaped lesion along the posterior lateral aortic wall) in the descending aorta. [Image used with permission of Dr. Ernest Scalzetti, MD.]

Esmolol may be given as an initial bolus of 0.1 to 0.5 milligram/kg IV over 1 minute followed by an infusion of 0.025 to 0.2 milligram/kg/min. **Labetalol** (a β-blocker with limited α-blocking characteristics in a 7:1 ratio) also may be used at an initial dose of 10 to 20 milligrams IV with repeat doses of 20 to 40 milligrams every 10 minutes to desired effect or a maximum dose of 300 milligrams. Calcium channel blockers may be used in the event of a contraindication to β-blockade, but experience with their use in the setting of aortic dissection is limited. β-Blocker use has been associated with improved survival in the International Registry of Acute Aortic Dissection (IRAD) database.[33,34]

VASODILATORS

Vasodilators such as **nitroprusside** may be added for further antihypertensive treatment after successful administration of a negative inotrope. Adequate β-receptor or calcium channel blockade should be achieved prior to starting a vasodilator (see chapters 57 and 58). **Nicardipine,** a parenteral dihydropyridine calcium channel blocker, has been used with success as a replacement for nitroprusside.[35]

DEFINITIVE REPAIR

Rapid referral to a surgeon is mandatory. Dissection with involvement of the ascending aorta requires prompt surgical repair.

Endovascular repair treats some aortic type A and complicated type B[36] dissections (patients with malperfusion, persistent severe pain, persistent false lumen, resistant hypertension, or expanding aortic diameter), penetrating ulcers,[37] and intramural hematomas.[38] Stenting has been combined with fenestration for patients with malperfusion.[39] Endovascular therapy has uncertain long-term effects but has shown short-term benefit.[36] Endovascular treatment is minimally invasive and avoids sternotomy and circulatory arrest. In treating dissection, goals of therapy include expansion and stabilization of the true lumen and passive resorption of thrombosis of the false lumen. In addition, visceral artery blood flow can be restored passively or by fenestration of the initial flap. Refractory pain in patients treated medically with type B dissection may be an indication for invasive intervention.[40]

DISPOSITION AND FOLLOW-UP

Patients with acute aortic syndromes are likely to require admission to an intensive care unit for hemodynamic therapy and careful monitoring. Acute intermural hematomas and penetrating ulcers have an unclear clinical course and natural history. Therefore, the management of patients with these disorders remains controversial.[41] Clearly no patient with an acute aortic syndrome should be discharged without consultation with a cardiovascular or vascular surgeon.

SPECIAL CONSIDERATIONS

AORTIC DISSECTION COMPLICATING PREGNANCY

Aortic dissection in pregnancy is rare and usually occurs in the third trimester and postpartum period.[41] Risk factors are bicuspid aortic valve, connective tissue disorders, hypertension, and a family history. Pregnancy increases the risk of dissection in patients with Marfan's syndrome, complicating 4.4% of pregnancies in women with the syndrome.[42] Depending on the gestational age[43] of the fetus, cesarean section with concomitant aortic repair is recommended for type A dissection. Simultaneous consultation with obstetrics and cardiovascular surgery is needed if the diagnosis is considered.

PRACTICE GUIDELINES

Guidelines have been published on the management of thoracic aortic disease, including type A dissection, by the American College of Cardiology/American Heart Association Task Force on Practice Guidelines, American Association for Thoracic Surgery, American College of Radiology, American Stroke Association, Society of Cardiovascular Anesthesiologists, Society for Cardiovascular Angiography and Interventions, Society of Interventional Radiology, Society of Thoracic Surgeons, and Society for Vascular Medicine.[15] Because of the relative infrequency of this condition, most of the recommendations are consensus based.

REFERENCES

The complete reference list is available online at www.TintinalliEM.com.

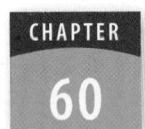

Aneurysmal Disease

Louise A. Prince
Gary A. Johnson

INTRODUCTION

An aneurysm is dilation of the arterial wall to >1.5 times its normal diameter. Aneurysms have been classically distinguished as true aneurysms, pseudoaneurysms, and mycotic aneurysms. The wall of a **true aneurysm** involves of all layers of the vessel. Risk factors for these include connective tissue disorders, familial history of aneurysm, and atherosclerotic risk factors (i.e., age, smoking, hypertension, and hyperlipidemia). A progressive decrease in elastin, collagen, and fibrolamellar units results in thinning of the media of the vascular wall and a decrease in its tensile strength. In aortic true aneurysm, the dilatation and increased wall force are intertwined, creating more dilatation (Laplace law: wall tension = pressure × radius). The rate of aneurysmal dilatation is variable and predictable, with larger aneurysms expanding more quickly and changing a mean 0.25 to 0.5 cm per year. However, abrupt expansion occurs and is not predictable, with larger aneurysm more likely to rupture. Rupture is catastrophic, occurring once the stress on the vessel wall exceeds its tensile strength.

The wall of a **pseudoaneurysm** consists partly of the vessel wall and partly of fibrous or other surrounding tissue. A pseudoaneurysm can develop at the site of previous vessel catheterization and at anastomoses from prior vascular reconstruction, trauma, or infection.[1] Small pseudoaneurysms may eventually spontaneously thrombose.

A **mycotic aneurysm** develops as a result of infection in the vessel wall, often in an immunocompromised patient. The source can be direct extension from a neighboring infection or embolization from valvular endocarditis.

Peripheral and visceral aneurysms are less frequent but an important subset of arterial aneurysmal disease. Popliteal artery aneurysms are the most common peripheral aneurysm; they often co-exist with contralateral popliteal aneurysms or abdominal aortic aneurysms.[2] Aneurysms of the femoral artery are uncommon and often accompany aneurysmal disease at other sites. Visceral artery aneurysms may occur anywhere but are most common in the renal, splenic, and hepatic arteries. Most visceral aneurysms remain silent and undetected until a complication such as rupture occurs. All but splenic artery aneurysms are more common in elderly men. Complications of aneurysms include rupture, which has an 80% mortality rate,[3] and thrombosis, creating ischemia in the perfused organ.[4,5]

GENERAL CLINICAL FEATURES OF ANEURYSMS

Clinical signs and symptoms can be nonspecific; often, the symptoms are driven by location, the pressure exerted upon neighboring structures, or the signs of peripheral embolization from an intramural thrombus. Visceral aneurysms are often detected after an abdominal CT scan for abdominal or flank complaints; similarly, lower extremity aneurysms are often detected during an extremity Doppler US examination in a search for deep venous thrombosis. Once rupture occurs in any truncal aneurysm, hemorrhagic shock develops and mortality is high without prompt surgical intervention.

SYMPTOMATIC ABDOMINAL AORTIC ANEURYSMS

An abdominal aortic aneurysm is defined as an aorta ≥3.0 cm in diameter; repair is considered for an aneurysm ≥5.0 cm in diameter. Patients with an abdominal aortic aneurysm often (18%) have a first-degree relative with an aortic aneurysm, compared with <3% of those without aneurysm. Most patients are >60 years old, and males have an increased risk of the disease. Patients with aneurysms involving other major arteries and those with peripheral arterial disease are also at increased risk for aortic aneurysmal disease. The risk increases with the number of years of smoking and decreases with the number of years since quitting smoking.[6] As smoking becomes less prevalent in the United States, abdominal aortic aneurysm deaths have decreased.[7]

CLINICAL FEATURES

Symptomatic abdominal aortic aneurysms may present with a variety of signs or symptoms that can mimic other primary diagnoses: syncope; flank, back, or abdominal pain; GI bleeding from an aortoduodenal fistula; extremity ischemia from embolization of a thrombus in the aneurysm; shock; or sudden death. Sudden death most commonly occurs from intraperitoneal rupture of the aneurysm, which leads to massive, rapid blood loss. Syncope without warning symptoms followed by severe abdominal or back pain suggests rupture of an abdominal aortic or visceral aneurysm with some temporary containment. Syncope is caused by rapid blood loss and a lack of cerebral perfusion. Patients may regain consciousness, but irreversible hemorrhagic shock follows without prompt diagnosis and intervention.

Back or abdominal pain is the most common presenting symptom with aortic aneurysm or rupture. The pain is classically severe and abrupt in onset, with about half of patients describing a ripping or tearing pain. Syncope occurs in about 10%. Many patients present with nonclassic sites of pain: flank, groin, isolated quadrants of the abdomen, and hip. Other common symptoms exist, such as nausea, vomiting, bladder pain, hip pain, or tenesmus.

DIAGNOSIS

Physical examination has only a moderate ability to detect a large abdominal aortic aneurysm. The sensitivity of abdominal palpation increases with aortic aneurysm diameter, ranging from 29% for a diameter of 3.0 to 3.9 cm to 50% for a diameter of 4.0 to 4.9 cm and 76% for a diameter of ≥5.0 cm.[8] Tenderness to palpation of an aneurysm is commonly interpreted as a sign of aneurysmal expansion or rupture. However, a lack of tenderness does not indicate an intact aorta. Examination is difficult in the obese and the very thin.

The differential diagnoses include the causes of syncope, abdominal pain, chest pain, back pain, and shock. When seeing patient with abrupt back pain with syncope or shock, consider aortic aneurysm rupture. However, other cardiac, abdominal, and retroperitoneal diseases may be the cause, including renal disorders, hepatobiliary disorders, and pancreatic disease. If symptoms are insidious, it is possible that some patients may appear well enough and receive benign diagnoses, such as musculoskeletal back pain, and are discharged from the ED.

Diagnosis is confounded by coexisting pathology. Coronary artery disease and chronic lung disease are often present, and signs and symptoms of these disorders may distract the physician from the diagnosis of aneurysmal disease. This is especially true in patients without severe pain or with findings that seem congruent with another cause (e.g., ECG changes or dyspnea).

External signs of acute rupture are rare and include periumbilical ecchymosis (**Cullen sign**) or flank ecchymosis (**Grey Turner sign**). Retroperitoneal blood may dissect into the perineum or groin, causing scrotal or vulvar hematomas, or inguinal masses. Retroperitoneal blood may irritate the psoas muscle, triggering an "iliopsoas sign" (pain upon extension of the hip, typically with the patient lying on the opposite side). Blood may compress the femoral nerve and present as a neuropathy. The presence or rupture of an abdominal aortic aneurysm typically does not alter femoral arterial pulsations.[9]

Think of **aortoenteric fistulas** in patients with unexplained or high-volume upper or lower GI bleeding, especially in patients without liver disease. A history of aortic graft placement increases the risk of fistula. Fistulas most frequently involve the duodenum, with hematemesis, melenemesis, melena, or hematochezia. While massive, life-threatening bleeding is common, mild sentinel bleeding may be the first sign. Aortic aneurysms also may erode into the venous vasculature and form **aortovenous fistulas**, which cause high-output cardiac failure, decreased arterial blood flow distal to the fistula, and increased central venous volume.

Contained chronic abdominal aortic aneurysmal ruptures are not common. A retroperitoneal rupture may cause enough fibrosis to limit blood loss, and the patient may look well. The inflammatory response commonly causes pain, with pain continuing for an extended interval, clouding the diagnosis.

Imaging Imaging performed away from the bedside can delay emergency consultation and operative repair, so consult a surgeon early and before any transport for imaging when a symptomatic aneurysm is suspected.

Radiologic evaluation may include plain radiography (**Figure 60-1**), US (**Figure 60-2**), CT scanning (**Figure 60-3**), or MRI. Plain abdominal films may show a calcified and bulging aortic contour, implying the presence of an aneurysm (Figure 60-1). Approximately 65% of patients with symptomatic aortic aneurysmal disease have a calcified aorta, often better seen on a lateral view. An anteroposterior projection may show an arch of calcification, most commonly on the patient's left. Rarely, a chronic aneurysm may erode into a vertebral body and be seen on plain film. Plain film radiographs do not exclude the presence of

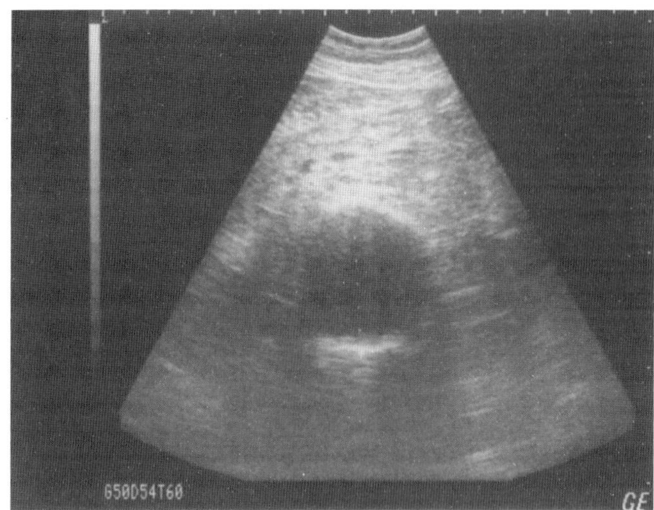

FIGURE 60-2. Bedside US image of an abdominal aortic aneurysm. This aneurysm measures 6.5 cm.

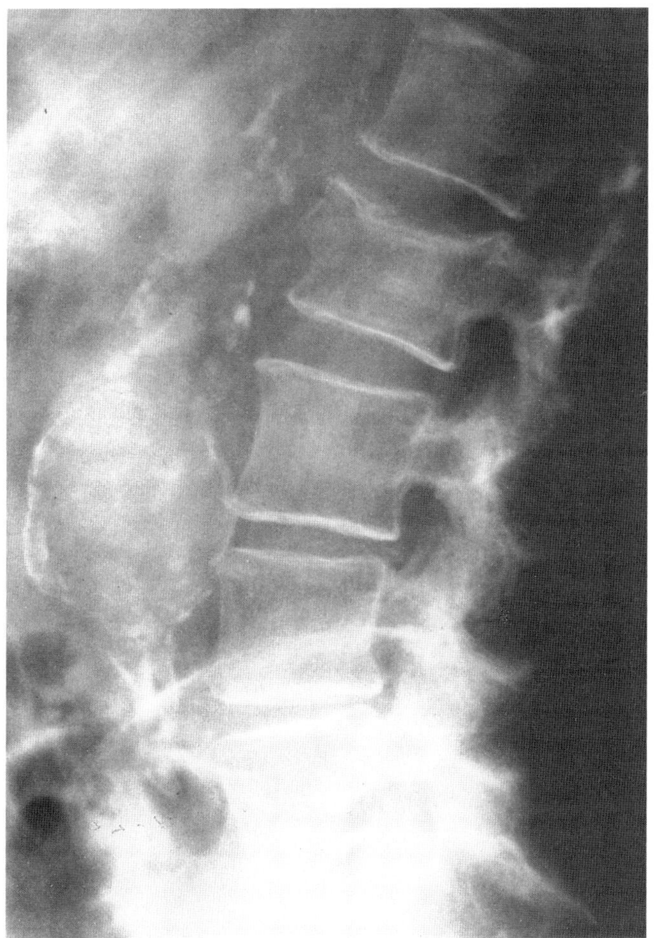

A

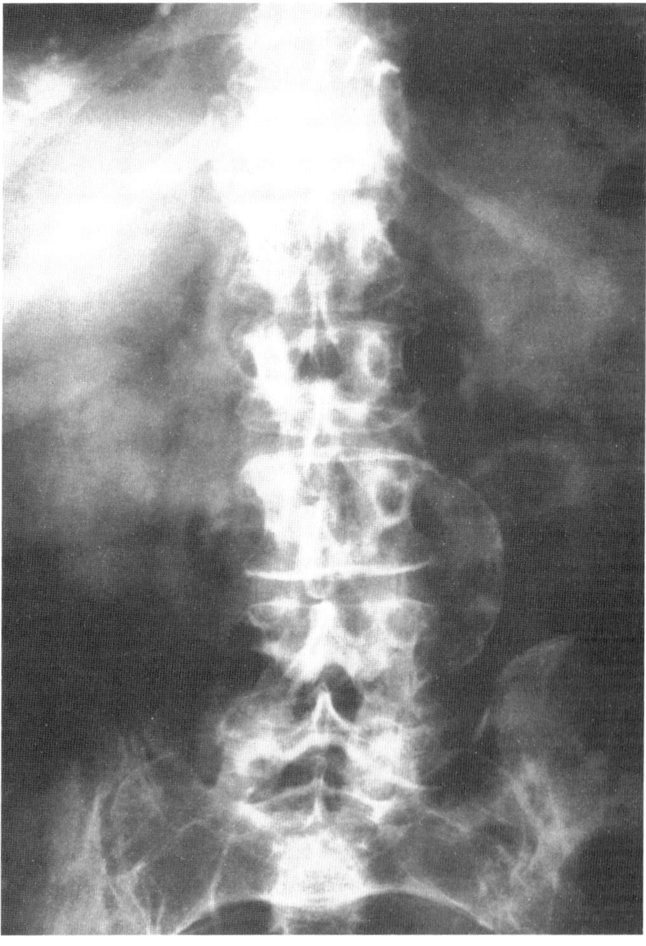

B

FIGURE 60-1. Plain radiographic images of an abdominal aortic aneurysm. **A.** Lateral view of a calcified infrarenal aortic aneurysm. **B.** Posteroanterior view of a calcified infrarenal aortic aneurysm.

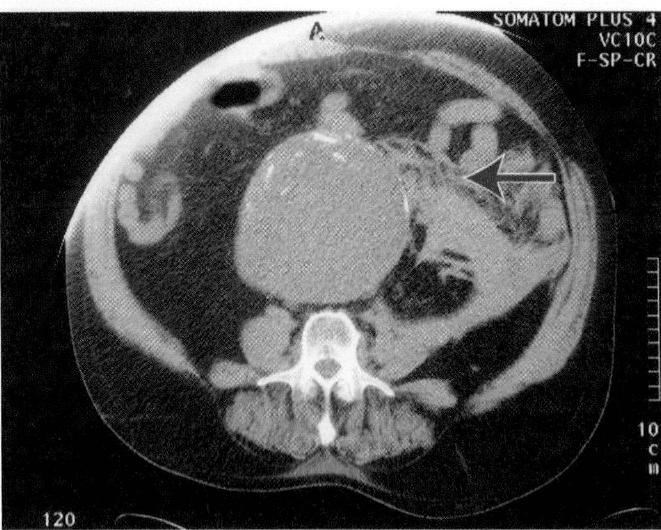

FIGURE 60-3. CT scan of a patient with a 12-cm abdominal aortic aneurysm. Calcification of the aortic wall is seen in the anterior aspect of the aneurysm. Evidence of hemorrhage and surrounding inflammation (*arrow*) is seen in the left side of the abdomen.

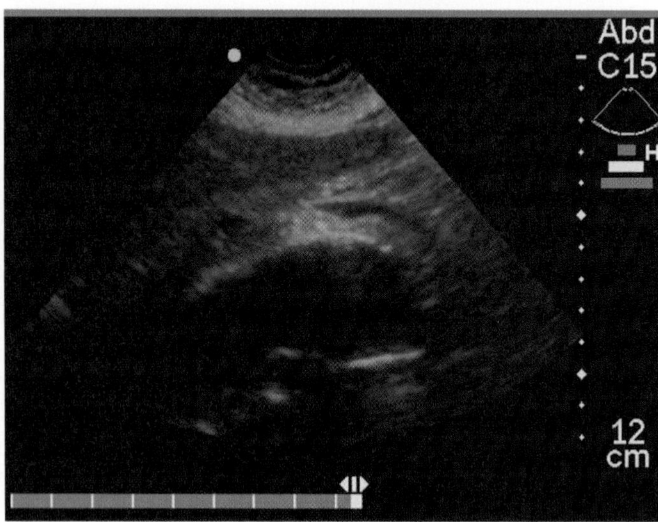

FIGURE 60-5. US image of an abdominal aortic aneurysm in the longitudinal plane.

abdominal aortic aneurysm or detect rupture and can be omitted in most patients.

Bedside US (Figure 60-2) is ideal for initial screening and for patients with any hemodynamic compromise. Emergency US is noninvasive, easily deployed, and does not entail removal of the patient from the resuscitation area.[10] **A technically adequate US study has >90% sensitivity for demonstrating the presence of an aneurysm and measuring its diameter.**[10] Obesity, bowel gas, and abdominal tenderness may make the study difficult to perform. Measure aneurysms from the outside margin of one wall to the outside margin of the opposite wall in both the transverse (**Figure 60-4**) and longitudinal (**Figure 60-5**) planes. Identifying the superior mesenteric artery (**Figure 60-6**) allows distinguishing the aorta from the vena cava. **An aortic diameter <3.0 cm excludes acute aneurysmal disease.**

CT scanning with IV contrast (Figure 60-3) best detects the anatomic details of the aneurysm and associated hemorrhage. Scan all stable patients with suspected abdominal aneurysmal disease or rupture. For those who cannot have IV contrast, unenhanced CT can reveal aneurysm size and retroperitoneal hemorrhage.

TREATMENT

ED interventions are listed in **Table 60-1**.

All asymptomatic aortic aneurysms should be referred for follow-up. **Abdominal aortic aneurysms ≥5 cm in diameter are at an increased risk of rupture (size is measured from outer wall to outer wall) and require prompt (days) follow-up.** Aneurysms of 3 to 5 cm are less likely to rupture and can be followed by their primary care physicians or surgeons. The management of patients with small, asymptomatic aneurysms (including the timing of surgery) varies. **Symptomatic aneurysms of any size are considered emergent.**

All symptomatic aortic aneurysms require emergency surgical consultation or transfer to an institution capable of performing emergency repair. If at a site without appropriate surgical ability, initiate patient resuscitation and arrange for immediate transfer to a medical center that can provide emergency repair. Outcomes are better if prompt transfer occurs rather than local diagnostics (aside from bedside US).[11,12] Immediate transfer with providers able to recognize and treat shock (having fluid, blood, and blood products available) is the best option for patients in unstable condition.

In the ED, detection and arranging rapid care for hemorrhage control are key. Consult a surgeon early while evaluating any patient with the triad of abdominal and/or back pain, a pulsatile abdominal mass, and

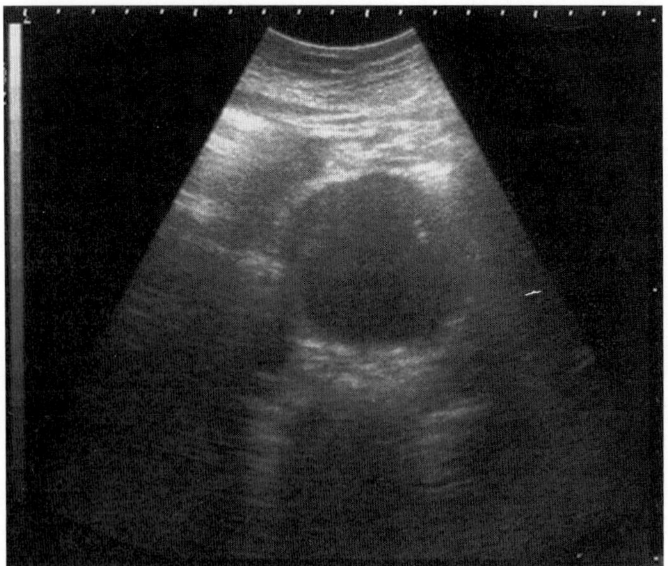

FIGURE 60-4. US image of an abdominal aortic aneurysm in the transverse plane.

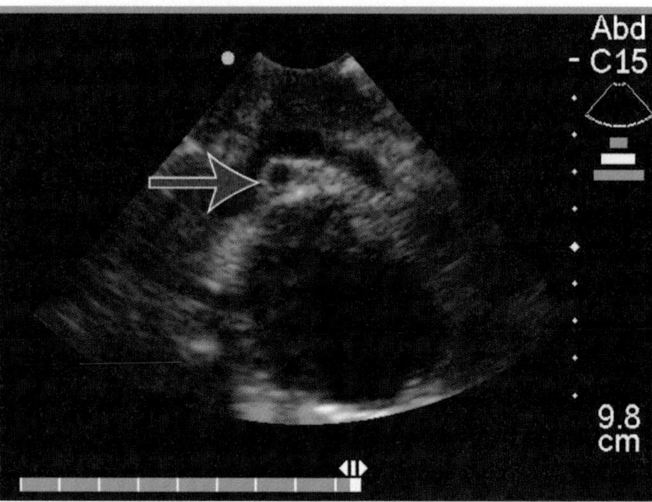

FIGURE 60-6. US image of an abdominal aortic aneurysm in the transverse plane showing the superior mesenteric artery (*arrow*) coursing parallel to the aorta.

TABLE 60-1 ED Interventions for Symptomatic Abdominal Aortic Aneurysms

Intervention	Comments
Consultation	As soon as diagnosis is suspected, consult with vascular or general surgeon or transfer to an institution capable of emergency repair.
Blood and fluids	Targets unclear; restoring normal blood pressure may worsen outcomes; often, permissive hypotension seeking a blood pressure of 90 mm Hg is best. Level of consciousness is another target for volume replacement.[14]
Pain control	Be careful to avoid hypotension or depressed respiratory drive.

hypotension[13]; however, this triad occurs in only one third of patients with ruptured abdominal aortic aneurysm.[8] Never delay consultation for imaging if hypotension or acute end-organ perfusion deficit is evident; often, bedside US can aid in quick tentative diagnosis.[13]

Any ruptured aortic aneurysm requires prompt operative repair. Use imaging only in those **fully** compensated or unlikely to have a ruptured abdominal aortic aneurysm. Standard resuscitative actions include insertion of two large-bore IV catheters, initiation of cardiac monitoring, and supplemental oxygen. Vigorous fluid resuscitation may be harmful; there are limited data, but animal research and anecdote support limiting resuscitation to a target of 90 mm Hg blood pressure and intact mentation until surgical control occurs.[15] Perioperative administration of β-blockers in nonruptured aneurysms reduces dysrhythmias and myocardial ischemia but does not appear to affect the rate of myocardial infarction, mortality, or length of hospitalization.[13] When used, esmolol (a short-acting β-blocker) is a common choice.

Endovascular techniques for the repair of ruptured abdominal aortic aneurysm are a feasible alternative to an open repair.[16] This intervention requires a skilled provider and appropriate facilities and team members.

Refer any patient with asymptomatic aortic abdominal aneurysms to a vascular surgeon and a primary care provider, the latter for blood pressure control.[17] Repairing aortic abdominal aneurysms smaller than 5.5 cm does not improve survival in men,[17] but may be indicated in women.[14]

THORACIC AORTIC ANEURYSMS

Thoracic aortic aneurysms may compress or erode into adjacent structures. Presenting symptoms include esophageal, tracheal, bronchial, or even neurologic complaints. A thoracic aneurysm that erodes into an adjacent structure is generally immediately fatal unless in the presence of rapid hemodynamic resuscitation. Refer any asymptomatic thoracic aortic aneurysm patient to a surgeon and primary care provider for management, including blood pressure control. Repair may involve open or endovascular methods, with controversy over the best long-term outcomes between these approaches.[18]

EXTREMITY AND VISCERAL ANEURYSMS

Aneurysms of arteries other than the aorta cause symptoms by expansion or rupture. **Table 60-2** lists the risk factors, clinical presentation, and management of nonaortic large-artery aneurysms. Aneurysms of peripheral arteries, such as the popliteal, subclavian, or femoral, may present with limb-threatening complications, including rupture, thrombosis, and peripheral embolization. Visceral artery aneurysms remain silent until a complication occurs. Complications include renovascular hypertension, renal artery thrombosis, organ infarction from distal embolization, arteriovenous fistula formation, and rupture.[19,20] Consider visceral artery aneurysms in the differential diagnosis of a patient with sudden acute abdominal pain and evidence for intraperitoneal hemorrhage.[4,5,13,21]

A **popliteal aneurysm** is a localized dilation of the popliteal artery of >2 cm or >150% of the normal arterial caliber. Symptoms include discomfort behind the knee, leg swelling with or without deep venous thrombosis, or claudication. Rupture is rare. Sudden acute limb ischemia caused by thrombosis or embolization from the aneurysm is the most serious common complication.[2] On physical examination, a firm mass or a palpable pulsatile mass is evident in the popliteal fossa. Confirm the diagnosis with arterial US, and assess both extremities since popliteal aneurysms can be bilateral.

Femoral or iliac artery aneurysms present as a pulsatile mass in the groin or upper thigh, scrotal hematoma, or acute limb ischemia. Iliac artery aneurysms are notoriously difficult to suspect clinically because the iliac artery cannot be examined directly, and symptoms suggest urologic, bowel, or groin disorders.

Hepatic artery aneurysms result from atherosclerosis or trauma and present as acute hemorrhagic shock with intraperitoneal or retroperitoneal rupture. **Quincke's triad** (jaundice, biliary colic, and upper GI bleeding) is seen when hemobilia from a leaking hepatic artery aneurysm occurs.

Splenic artery aneurysms present with left upper quadrant pain, undifferentiated shock, or intra-abdominal hemorrhage. A rupture of

TABLE 60-2 Nonaortic Large-Artery Aneurysms

Artery	Risk Factors	Clinical Presentation	Management
Popliteal (>2 cm or >150% of normal caliber)	Advanced age, male gender, trauma, congenital disorders	Most common peripheral aneurysm; discomfort behind knee with swelling with or without deep venous thrombosis	Thrombolysis, ligation, arterial bypass, endovascular repair
Subclavian	Arteriosclerosis, thoracic outlet obstruction	Pulsatile mass above or below clavicle, dysphagia, stridor, chest pain, hoarseness, upper extremity fatigue or numbness and tingling, limb ischemic symptoms	Surgical repair
Femoral	Advanced age, male gender, trauma, congenital disorders	Pulsatile mass with or without pain, limb ischemic symptoms, peripheral embolic symptoms	Thrombolysis, ligation, arterial bypass, endovascular repair
Femoral pseudoaneurysm	Prior femoral artery catheterization, trauma, infection	Pulsatile mass with or without pain	Surgical repair
Iliac		Pain in groin, scrotum, or lower abdomen; sciatica; vulvar or groin hematoma with rupture	Surgical repair
Renal	Age 40–60 y, no gender preference, HTN, fibrodysplasia, arteriosclerosis	Flank pain, hematuria, collecting system obstruction, shock if ruptured	Surgical repair, nephrectomy
Splenic	Advanced age, female gender, HTN, congenital, arteriosclerosis, liver disease, multiparous, rupture increased in pregnancy	Rapid symptom onset; epigastric or left upper quadrant pain first, then diffuse abdominal pain with rupture, shock	Surgical repair, splenectomy, embolization if unruptured
Hepatic	Infection, arteriosclerosis, trauma, vasculitis	Obstructive jaundice, hemobilia from rupture into common bile duct, right upper quadrant pain, peritonitis, upper GI bleed	Surgical ligation, embolization

Abbreviation: HTN = hypertension.

the splenic artery has a poor prognosis because of its intraperitoneal location and nondescript presentation; be wary of these in the third trimester of pregnancy.[21]

Symptomatic **subclavian and innominate artery aneurysms** can lead to limb ischemia. When evaluating a patient with upper extremity pain, weakness, pallor, or nondermatome sensory changes, think of this as a possible cause.

Anastomotic aneurysms may occur in the aortic, iliac, or femoral arteries. These aneurysms cause catastrophic bleeding if they rupture; however, they may present with smaller sentinel hemorrhages noted as pain or transient hypotension. Anastomotic aneurysms may erode into the adjacent intestine and form an aortoenteric fistula. Severe lower GI bleeding in a patient with a history of abdominal aortic aneurysm repair is a classic presentation of this event.

Doppler US is the initial noninvasive diagnostic study for peripheral aneurysmal disease of the femoral, popliteal, and subclavian artery. If ischemia and thrombosis exist, emergent arteriography is usually performed for both diagnosis and potential treatment.

Symptomatic peripheral artery aneurysms require rapid diagnosis and consultation, especially in light of the potential for rupture, thrombosis, and limb ischemia (Table 60-2). For patients with clinical extremity ischemia, consult immediately with a vascular surgeon to expedite repair and limb salvage. Asymptomatic peripheral aneurysms are managed by a vascular consultant as an outpatient.

PRACTICE GUIDELINES

The 2011 American Heart Association guidelines are available at http://circ.ahajournals.org/content/124/18/2020.

REFERENCES

The complete reference list is available online at www.TintinalliEM.com.

Arterial Occlusion

Anil Chopra
David Carr

INTRODUCTION AND EPIDEMIOLOGY

Acute limb ischemia requires rapid recognition and therapy for limb salvage. *Critical limb ischemia* occurs in chronic progressive peripheral arterial disease when pain at rest, ulceration, or gangrene exists. Despite improvements in the management of peripheral arterial disease, current 1-year mortality after the onset of critical limb ischemia is 25%, and 25% of survivors require amputation.[1,2]

The prevalence of peripheral arterial disease (defined as an ankle-brachial index of <0.9) in the United States is 4.3% for those >40 years old and 15.5% for those >70 years old.[3] This prevalence increases to 29% in high-risk populations in those >70 years old and those >50 years old with diabetes or a smoking history.[4] In the elderly, both sexes are affected equally, although symptoms are present two to four times more commonly in men. Smoking and diabetes are the most important risk factors for arterial insufficiency.[5] Additional risk factors include hyperlipidemia, hypertension, hyperhomocysteinemia, and an elevated C-reactive protein level.

Between 40% and 60% of patients with occlusive arterial disease have either coronary or cerebrovascular disease.[6] The severity of peripheral vascular disease is closely linked to the risk of myocardial infarction, ischemic stroke, and death from vascular disease.[7] The most frequently diseased arteries leading to limb ischemia are, in order of occurrence, the femoropopliteal, tibial, aortoiliac, and brachiocephalic vessels.

PATHOPHYSIOLOGY

Acute limb ischemia results from a lack of blood supply to meet tissue oxygen and nutrient requirements. As time proceeds, cell death or irreversible tissue damage occurs. Peripheral nerves and skeletal muscle are more sensitive to ischemia, and irreversible changes occur in these tissues within 6 hours.

After restoration of the blood flow, **reperfusion injury** can occur, noted by the presence of muscle pain and swelling, renal failure, and peripheral muscle infarction. Often, hyperkalemia, myoglobinemia, metabolic acidosis, and an elevation in creatine kinase level exist. The extent of reperfusion injury depends on the duration and location of the arterial blockage, the amount of collateral flow, and the previous health of the involved limb. Approximately one third of all deaths from occlusive arterial disease are secondary to metabolic complications after revascularization.[8]

Disorders that can lead to arterial occlusion are compared in **Table 61-1**.

THROMBOSIS

Thrombotic occlusion is the most common cause of *acute* limb ischemia. Both native vessels and bypass grafts can thrombose. In the lower limbs, thrombotic occlusion accounts for >80% of cases.[14] In the upper limbs, about half of all cases of acute limb ischemia are due to thrombosis, one third are due to embolism, and one fourth are secondary to arteritis.[15] The distinction between a thrombosis and an embolism in any given patient is not always clear.

Nonembolic limb ischemia is secondary to atherosclerosis in most patients. Complete or high-grade obstruction occurs from plaque rupture or endothelial erosion followed by thrombus formation. Acute limb ischemia from plaque rupture obstructs flow completely, triggering symptoms. However, most nonembolic ischemia is characterized by chronic occlusion that may be clinically silent or muted depending on the collateral network.

Other than plaque rupture, progression of ischemic injury occurs through several mechanisms: (1) propagation of clot to occlude collateral vessels, (2) ischemia-related distal edema leading to high compartment pressures (compartment syndrome), (3) fragmentation of clot into the microcirculation, and (4) edema of the microvasculature cells. Large-vessel reperfusion may not resolve obstruction of the microvasculature.

Uncommonly, arterial thrombosis can develop in an apparently normal vessel without an atherosclerotic plaque; if seen, seek an underlying hypercoagulable condition. Subclinical vessel injury (from injections, catheters, or other mechanical events) or early atherosclerosis may still underlie these events.

EMBOLISM

Occlusion from embolism is less common than occlusion from thrombosis, in part due to the decline in the incidence of rheumatic heart disease and the treatment of **atrial fibrillation** with anticoagulants. Emboli originate from the heart in most cases. Atrial fibrillation is associated with at least two thirds of all peripheral emboli, and the clot most commonly originates in the left atrial appendage. The second most frequent source is a **mural thrombus** in the ventricle after recent myocardial infarction, accounting for about 20% of all limb emboli. Both atrial fibrillation and acute myocardial infarction predispose to poor cardiac wall motion and stagnant blood flow that promote clot formation. The mean time to development of a clot after myocardial infarction is 14 days (range, 3 to 28 days).[16] The incidence of emboli originating from a mechanical valve has been lowered by advances in anticoagulation. Rare cardiac sources of emboli include tumor emboli from atrial myxomas, vegetations from valve leaflets, and parts of prosthetic cardiac devices.

Noncardiac sources of arterial emboli include thrombi from aneurysms and atheromatous plaques. Mural thrombi in aneurysms of aortoiliac, femoral, popliteal, and subclavian arteries are the most notable sources. Atheroemboli result from plaque fragmentation and cause obstruction of the microcirculation, producing symptoms in the hands, feet (blue toe syndrome), or cerebral circulation (transient ischemic attack). Atheroemboli consist of cholesterol-laden debris and

TABLE 61-1 Disorders Associated with Acute Arterial Occlusion

Disorder	Cause	Symptoms/Signs	Management
Thrombus	Atherosclerosis or thrombosis of bypass grafts	Intermittent claudication	Medical first, then consider interventional
Embolism	Cardiac source: atrial fibrillation, rheumatic heart disease, mechanical valves, post–myocardial infarction thrombus, atrial myxomas and leaflet vegetations	Sudden onset of territorial arterial symptoms	Preventative anticoagulation, embolectomy
Catheterization complication (brachial or femoral)	Can occur during standard angioplasty, angiography, or arterial blood gas	Expanding hematoma, pain, temperature and pulse changes	Conservative vs. operative repair
Trash foot or blue toe syndrome	Cholesterol/platelet aggregate emboli	Painful cyanotic discoloration of isolated portion of foot; remainder of the foot is warm	Conservative therapy
Vasculitis: rheumatoid arthritis, lupus, polyarteritis nodosa	Autoimmune inflammation of small arteries	Systemic symptoms and multiorgan ischemia	Steroids, immunosuppressive agents
Raynaud's disease	Vasospasm in small arteries or arterioles provoked by cold or stressors	Local pain, pallor, cyanosis, numbness, paresthesias in hands usually resolving in 30–60 min	Rewarming, medications: calcium channel blockers, α-blockers, vasodilators
Takayasu's arteritis	Autoimmune vasculitis of aortic arch and branches	Young Asian women: peripheral ischemia and necrosis leading to pulseless phase; may have fever, rash, muscle aches, arthritis	Steroids, immunosuppressive agents
Thromboangiitis obliterans (Buerger's disease)	Nonatherosclerotic segmental inflammation of small/medium vessels; typically, only seen in smokers	Painful nodules, ulceration, and gangrenous digits in young adults (age 20–40 y)	Smoking cessation
HIV arteritis[9]	Chronic inflammation of arteries associated with low CD4 counts	Intermittent claudication	Optimization of HIV management, angioplasty, or vein graft
Hypothenar hammer syndrome	Repeated trauma to the hypothenar area with hammering in laborers, as well as those using vibrational tools, causing narrowing of ulnar artery or aneurysmal degeneration	Painful discoloration of one or more ulnar fingers with sparing of thumb	Aspirin, nifedipine, intra-arterial fibrinolysis, interposition vein graft
Popliteal artery entrapment (young males) and popliteal aneurysms (older males)[10]	Anatomic crowding of popliteal fossa with anomalous relationships between popliteal artery and surrounding muscle and fascia or luminal narrowing and thrombosis of aneurysm	Pain in anterior aspect of lower one third of leg with exercise, reproducible with active ankle plantar flexion or passive dorsiflexion	Surgical repair of popliteal fossa or aneurysm and grafting
External iliac artery endofibrosis[11]	External iliac artery fibrosis secondary to prolonged hip flexion	Thigh pain and numbness in cyclists and triathletes: measure pre- and postcycling ankle-brachial indexes	Surgical management or catheter dilatation
Local arterial trauma[12,13]	Penetrating or blunt damage to vessel	Suspect in patients with knee dislocation or penetrating extremity trauma	Surgical repair
Shock-related arterial ischemia	Low cardiac output states: congestive heart failure, sepsis, cardiogenic or hypovolemic shock	Generalized hypoperfusion	Resuscitation with fluids, blood products, vasopressors, inotropes; treat infection
Thoracic aortic dissection	False lumen of dissection occludes arteries	Chest or back pain	Surgical repair

Abbreviation: HIV = human immunodeficiency virus (infection).

platelet aggregates that can disseminate to multiple sites in the body. Paradoxical embolization can occur when a venous clot passes from the right to the left side of the heart through an intracardiac shunt, most commonly a patent foramen ovale.

The natural history of an embolus is either to fragment and embolize distally or to propagate locally into a larger clot. Two thirds of all noncerebral emboli enter vessels of the lower limbs and lodge where vessels branch or taper. The most common location for an embolus in the leg is the bifurcation of the common femoral artery, followed by the popliteal artery. In the upper limb, the brachial artery is the vessel most commonly affected by an embolism.

OTHER CAUSES

Intentional or accidental **intra-arterial drug injections** by medical personnel or those taking illicit drugs can result in local vasospasm, infectious arteritis, thrombosis, pseudoaneurysm, and mycotic aneurysm. Inert particles or drug crystals can embolize to obstruct end arteries, which can lead to gangrene of the digits. The prolonged use of vasopressor medications may result in arterial ischemia and occlusion, and their use requires close observation of extremity perfusion, particularly in patients with known pre-existing vascular disease.

Limb ischemia may also occur with nonembolic central causes. A **thoracic aortic dissection** can propagate into the subclavian and iliofemoral systems and present with neurologic and/or extremity findings. The false lumen created by the dissection occludes flow in the involved artery.

CLINICAL FEATURES

Patients with acute limb ischemia exhibit one or more of the **"six Ps": pain, pallor, paralysis, pulselessness, paresthesias, and polar**

TABLE 61-2 Rutherford Criteria for Acute Limb Ischemia

		Findings		Doppler Signals	
Category	Description/Prognosis	Sensory Loss	Muscle Weakness	Arterial	Venous
I. Viable	Not immediately threatened	None	None	Audible	Audible
II. Threatened					
a. Marginally	Salvageable if promptly treated	Minimal (toes) or none	None	Inaudible	Audible
b. Immediately	Salvageable with immediate revascularization	More than toes, associated with rest pain	Mild, moderate	Inaudible	Audible
III. Irreversible	Major tissue loss or permanent nerve damage inevitable	Profound, anesthetic	Profound, paralysis (rigor)	Inaudible	Inaudible

Source: Reproduced with permission from Rutherford RB, Baker JD, Ernst C, et al: Recommended standards for reports dealing with lower extremity ischemia: revised edition. *J Vasc Surg* 26: 517, 1997. Copyright Elsevier.

(for cold). A lack of one or more of these findings does not exclude ischemia. Furthermore, total occlusion of a severely diseased artery in patients with peripheral vascular disease with well-developed collateral blood supply may not be a dramatic event and can be silent. Pain alone may be the earliest symptom of ischemia, localized in the limb distal to the site of obstruction.

Skin changes include pallor first, followed by blotchy and mottled areas of cyanosis, and then associated petechiae and blisters. Late findings consist of skin and fat necrosis.

With vessel occlusion, severe and steady pain in the involved extremity associated with decreased skin temperature is common. Hypoesthesia or hyperesthesia due to ischemic neuropathy is typically an early finding, as is muscle weakness. Two-point discrimination, vibratory sensation, and proprioception are often diminished prior to the loss of deep sensation. Absence of a palpable distal pulse is not a particularly helpful sign in a patient with long-standing vascular disease unless accompanied by skin changes compatible with acute arterial obstruction. An abrupt loss of a previously strong pulse is suggestive of acute embolization.

As ischemic injury progresses, anesthesia and paralysis become evident and foreshadow impending gangrene and the loss of limb viability. Preservation of light touch on skin testing is a good guide to tissue viability. A patient with an acute ischemic limb with signs of muscle paralysis, sensory loss, and prolonged ischemia has a limb that is likely nonviable. The **Rutherford criteria** (**Table 61-2**) provide a more formal prognostic stratification of the clinical stages of acute limb ischemia.

The time limit for limb viability is dependent on the effectiveness of collateral circulation. Therefore, no arbitrary time period should be used to rule out treatment options despite the common belief that "treatment must occur in 4 to 6 hours."

Microemboli present clinically with pain and cyanosis in the involved digit, petechiae, and local muscle pain and tenderness at the site of infarction. Showering of these emboli creates several different small areas of involvement. Although mottling and decreased function may occur, pulses are preserved, assuming they were present to start, which is unusual in this population. Table 61-1 notes symptoms of related disorders.

ACUTE VERSUS CHRONIC ARTERIAL DISEASE

Acute limb ischemia is defined as symptoms starting within a 2-week period. Pain over the distal forefoot waking the patient at night or requiring the patient to hang his or her feet over the bed is suggestive of severe arterial occlusion and requires prompt consultation and treatment.

Claudication is a cramp-like pain, ache, or tiredness that is brought on by exercise and relieved by rest. It is reproducible, resolves within 2 to 5 minutes of rest, and recurs at consistent walking distances. The pain of acute limb ischemia is not well localized, is not relieved by rest or gravity, and can be a worsening of chronic pain (if it is caused by a thrombotic event).

Chronic obstructive arterial disease is characterized by intermittent claudication, which may progress to intermittent ischemic pain at rest. Femoropopliteal disease and aortoiliac disease often cause reproducible calf pain with activity that is relieved with rest. Pain at rest typically localizes to the foot and is aggravated by leg elevation, improves with standing, and is poorly controlled with analgesics. Classical teaching suggests that single-level disease in one of the segments noted in **Table 61-3** may result in claudication, whereas multilevel disease results in rest pain or tissue loss. Table 61-3 lists symptom sites of commonly compromised arteries.

The pain associated with intermittent vascular claudication can be confused with leg pain from many causes (**Table 61-4**) including spinal stenosis or lumbosacral radiculopathy.

Uncommon presentations of deep venous thrombosis—**phlegmasia cerulea dolens** (painful blue inflammation) and **phlegmasia alba dolens**, or "milk leg"—can be confused with obstructive arterial disease. In phlegmasia cerulea dolens, the leg is markedly swollen and cyanotic from venous engorgement due to massive iliofemoral thrombosis. This high-grade obstruction can compromise perfusion to the foot from high compartment pressures and lead to venous gangrene.[17] Phlegmasia alba dolens is usually seen during pregnancy and is a result of iliofemoral thrombosis with concomitant leg pallor from arterial spasm. Dorsalis pedis and posterior tibial pulses may be diminished or absent, which can lead to a false diagnosis of arterial occlusion. The arterial spasm with milk leg is transient and often followed by venous engorgement, which aids diagnosis. For a more complete list of the differential diagnoses for intermittent claudication, see Table 61-4.

On physical examination, examine the skin and all peripheral pulses of both extremities. Compare the unaffected to the affected limb. Shiny, hyperpigmented skin with hair loss and ulceration, thickened nails, muscle atrophy, vascular bruits, and poor pulses are the hallmark of chronic obstructive arterial disease. In contrast to the common medial malleolar location of venous insufficiency ulcers, arterial ulcers tend to occur on the foot and toes and are typically more painful. When evaluating someone with a chronic, nonhealing ulcer, consider the possibility of both venous and arterial insufficiency. Perform a cardiovascular and abdominal examination, including auscultation for bruits, search for murmurs, and palpation of the abdominal aorta.

DIAGNOSIS

The clinical exam guides initial decisions and causes (**Table 61-5**); if severe or limb-threating new ischemia of any cause is suspected, promptly consult

TABLE 61-3 Artery-Specific Claudication Sites

Artery Involved	Claudication Site
Iliac artery	Buttocks, thigh, and sometimes calf (if bilateral, may cause impotence in men)
Common femoral artery	Thigh
Superficial femoral artery	Upper two thirds of calf
Popliteal artery	Lower one third of calf
Infrapopliteal (tibial and peroneal) artery	Foot

TABLE 61-4 Differential Diagnoses of Intermittent Claudication (IC)

Condition	Location	Prevalence	Characteristic	Effect of Exercise	Effect of Rest	Effect of Position	Other Characteristics
Calf IC	Calf muscles	3%–5% of adult population	Cramping, aching discomfort	Reproducible onset	Quickly relieved	None	May have atypical limb symptoms on exercise
Thigh and buttock IC	Buttocks, hip, thigh	Rare	Cramping, aching discomfort	Reproducible onset	Quickly relieved	None	Impotence May have normal pedal pulses with isolated iliac artery disease
Foot IC	Foot arch	Rare	Severe pain on exercise	Reproducible onset	Quickly relieved	None	Also may present as numbness
Chronic compartment syndrome	Calf muscles	Rare	Tight, bursting pain	After much exercise (jogging)	Subsides very slowly	Relief with elevation	Typically heavily muscled athletes
Venous claudication	Entire leg, worse in calf	Rare	Tight, bursting pain	After walking	Subsides slowly	Relief speeded by elevation	History of iliofemoral deep venous thrombosis, signs of venous congestion, edema
Nerve root compression	Radiates down leg	Common	Sharp lancinating pain	Induced by sitting, standing, or walking	Often present at rest	Improved by change in position	History of back problems Worse with sitting Relief when supine
Symptomatic Baker's cyst	Behind knee, down calf	Rare	Swelling, tenderness	With exercise	Present at rest	None	Not intermittent
Hip arthritis	Lateral hip, thigh	Common	Aching discomfort	After variable degree of exercise	Not quickly relieved	Improved when not weight bearing	Symptoms variable History of degenerative arthritis
Spinal stenosis	Often bilateral buttocks, posterior leg	Common	Pain and weakness	May mimic IC	Variable relief but can take a long time to recover	Relief by lumbar spine flexion	Worse with standing and extending spine
Foot/ankle arthritis	Ankle, foot, arch	Common	Aching pain	After variable degree of exercise	Not quickly relieved	May be relieved by not bearing weight	Variable, may relate to activity level and be present at rest

Source: Reproduced with permission from Norgren L, Hiatt WR, Dormandy JA, et al: Inter-society consensus for the management of peripheral arterial disease (TASC II). *J Vasc Surg* 45: S5A, 2007. Copyright Elsevier.

a vascular surgeon prior to performing confirmatory imaging. Other features guide care; a history of an abruptly ischemic limb in a patient with atrial fibrillation or recent myocardial infarction strongly suggests an embolus. Acute ischemia in the limb of a patient known to have advanced obstructive arterial disease is more likely due to thrombosis or a low cardiac output state. In patients without antecedent claudication and a normal uninvolved limb, embolic occlusion is likely present. If there are ischemic changes, an arterial thrombotic cause is more likely than an embolism.

For a more detailed comparison of acute embolism and thrombosis, see Table 61-5.

Decreased perfusion is detected by blanching the involved extremity with finger pressure and noting a delay in the return of blood compared with the uninvolved extremity; 2 to 3 seconds is considered normal. The test is influenced by many other factors, so it alone cannot determine perfusion status.

TABLE 61-5 Embolic versus Thrombotic Occlusion

Factor	Embolism	Thrombosis
History of claudication	No	Yes
Physical examination	Normal contralateral limb	Marked signs of occlusive arterial disease bilaterally
Source identified	Often	None
Timing	Sudden, exact time known	More gradual
Radiologic features	Sudden abrupt cutoff in blood flow with no collateral circulation and minimal diseased vessel	Widespread disease with collaterals present and gradual narrowing of blood flow seen

Use a hand-held Doppler ultrasound device over pulse areas to detect presence or absence of blood flow and the amplitude. Approximately 10% of patients have only one pedal or ankle pulse present secondary to an anatomic variation. If Doppler flow is detected in the affected limb, check the **ankle-brachial index** and segmental leg pressures. The ankle-brachial index is the ratio of the systolic blood pressure with the cuff just above the malleolus (with the Doppler probe over the posterior tibial or dorsalis pedis artery) to the highest brachial pressure in either arm (**Figure 61-1**). Patients with chronic obstructive arterial disease have an ankle-brachial index of <0.9. Values of <0.25 suggest potentially limb-threatening vascular disease. An ankle-brachial index of >1.3 is likely secondary to a noncompressible vessel; it may be seen in patients with severe vascular calcification, especially diabetics, and is notoriously unreliable in this patient population. In such cases, toe-brachial pressures can be measured, but the technique requires specialized equipment. Segmental blood pressures measured with the Doppler device on the posterior tibial or dorsalis pedis artery and the cuff placed below the knee, above the knee, and on the high thigh can aid assessment. **A difference of 30 mm Hg or more between any two adjacent levels localizes the site of obstruction.** With successful reperfusion, the ankle-brachial index and segmental pressures begin to return to baseline or normalize if no residual obstruction remains after clot dissolution.

LABORATORY EVALUATION

Aside from seeking markers of cellular death (e.g., creatine kinase or myoglobin and serum lactate), obtain other tests to assess metabolic

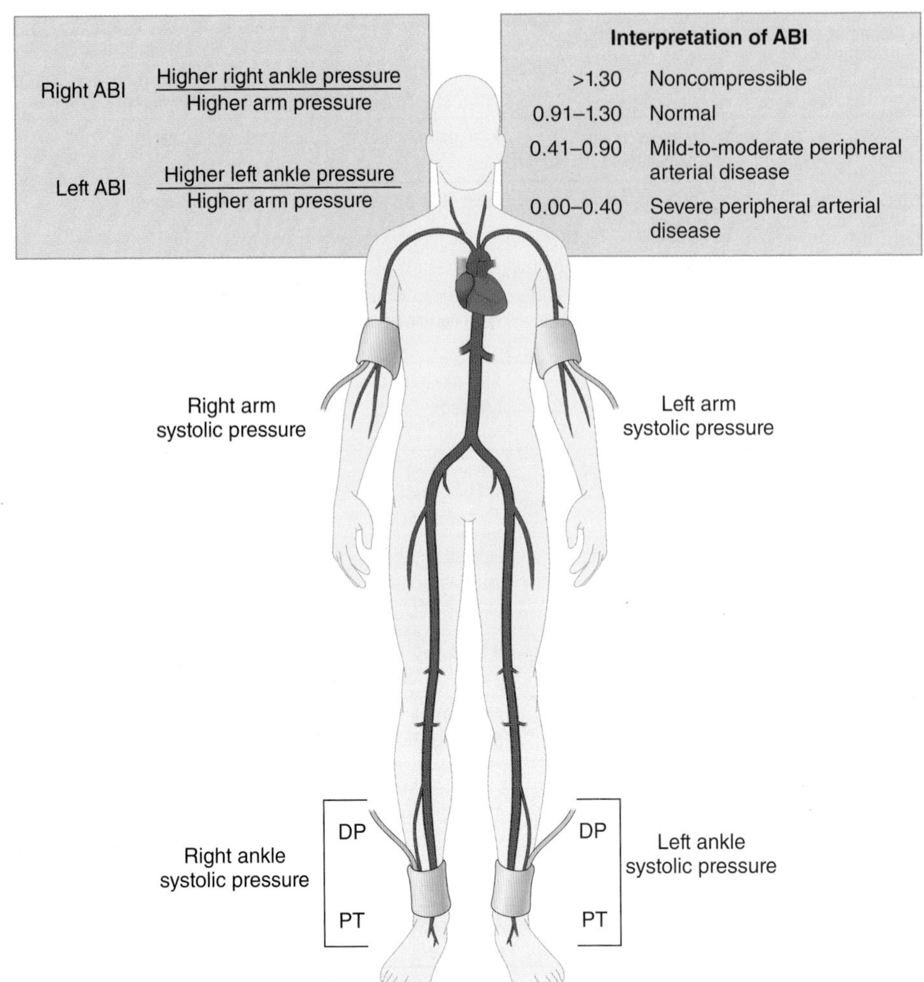

FIGURE 61-1. Measurement of the ankle-brachial index (ABI). Measure the systolic blood pressure using Doppler US in each arm and in the dorsalis pedis (DP) and posterior tibial (PT) arteries in each ankle. Select the higher of the two arm pressures (right vs. left) and the higher of the two pressures in the ankle (DP vs. PT). Determine the right and left ABI values by dividing the higher ankle pressure in each leg by the higher arm pressure. The ranges of the ABI and the interpretation are shown in the figure. In the case of a noncompressible calcified vessel, the true pressure at that location cannot be obtained, and alternative tests are required to diagnose peripheral arterial disease. Patients with claudication typically have ABI values ranging from 0.41 to 0.90, and those with critical leg ischemia have values <0.41.

status (electrolytes and glucose), renal function (BUN and creatinine plus urinalysis), anemia and infection (CBC), and bleeding tendency (prothrombin and partial thromboplastin times). Levels of cardiac markers and ECG may identify associated cardiac triggers (including infarction or rhythm change).

IMAGING

If the diagnosis of arterial occlusion is in question, duplex US is very accurate for detecting complete or incomplete obstruction. Sensitivity declines for localization of thromboembolic occlusion at or below the calf level. Transthoracic cardiac echocardiography can help detect embolic sources, and transesophageal approaches add the ability to detect aortic root pathology.

Arteriography is often obtained prior to surgical intervention[1] or to direct therapy. Embolic occlusion displays an abrupt cutoff of blood flow in a disease-free or minimally diseased vessel. Arteriography requires the administration of contrast material, so assess renal function and hydrate before the study.

CT with contrast is the most readily available added study in the ED and has a sensitivity similar to that of conventional contrast studies in large vessels. MRI has higher sensitivity and specificity but is less readily available.

TREATMENT

The objectives of therapy for acute arterial obstruction are restoration of blood flow to preserve limb and life, and prevention of recurrent thrombosis or embolism (**Table 61-6**).

IV unfractionated heparin (weight-based 80 units/kg bolus followed by an infusion of 18 units/kg/h) is common initial therapy. Anticoagulation may prevent clot extension, recurrent embolization, venous thrombosis, microthrombi distal to the obstruction, and reocclusion after reperfusion.[19] It is still unclear whether heparin administration improves outcome in the clinical circumstance of thrombosis in a plaque-laden artery.

TABLE 61-6 ED Medical Therapy for Acute Limb Ischemia

Intervention	Comments
Unfractionated heparin[18]	80 units/kg bolus followed by infusion of 18 units/kg/h
Aspirin[18]	325 milligrams PO first dose (82 milligrams daily thereafter)
Pain control	As needed for patient comfort and cooperation
Environment protection	Protect ischemic limb from temperature extremes

Enoxaparin (1 milligram/kg SC) is an alternative, although heparin remains the common choice. Aspirin (325 milligrams in naïve patients) may enhance clot reduction through antiplatelet actions.

Even before starting anticoagulation, start seeking vascular consultation, transferring if needed. Stratifying patients with acute limb ischemia by Rutherford criteria (Table 61-1) can guide initial care. Patients with stage I and stage IIa limb ischemia may undergo diagnostic imaging workup prior to more definitive treatments. Patients with stage IIb ischemia often require immediate revascularization without additional diagnostic imaging modalities prior to operative or interventional treatment. Patients with stage III ischemia have suffered irreversible damage and likely require amputation. Provide adequate analgesia and fluid resuscitation and treat heart failure (if existing) to help improve limb perfusion.

The vascular surgeon determines definitive treatment, which can include catheter-directed thrombolysis, percutaneous mechanical thrombectomy, revision of an occluded bypass graft, and revascularization with either percutaneous transluminal angioplasty or standard surgery.[2,18] Catheter-directed intra-arterial thrombolysis is now often chosen over systemic thrombolysis for peripheral artery embolic or thrombotic disease.[18,19] In a subacute thrombotic occlusion with a well-developed collateral blood supply, medical management is common.

The longer-term nonsurgical management of chronic obstructive arterial disease focuses on the combination of smoking cessation, exercise, and pharmacotherapy. Daily aspirin (81 to 162 milligrams) reduces mortality by 25%.[4,20-23] Anticoagulants, such as warfarin, factor Xa, or thrombin inhibitors, are used when clot formation is severe or recurrent.[20] Lowering cholesterol and blood pressure and improving glycemic control also are key secondary modifiers.[4]

The American College of Cardiology/American Heart Association 2005 guidelines include cilostazol, a phosphodiesterase inhibitor, as a Class I recommendation for the treatment of claudication in patients with obstructive arterial disease[2] (avoid in patients with heart failure). Pentoxifylline is a second-line therapy for the treatment of claudication (Class IIb).[2,24]

DISPOSITION AND FOLLOW-UP

Patients with acute or worsening chronic ischemia require further assessment and hospital admission or transfer to a center with vascular surgery capability. Patients with chronic peripheral arterial disease without an immediate threat to limb viability absent other acute illness can be discharged home to follow up with a vascular surgeon or primary care physician. Instruct patients to return immediately for worsening of symptoms. Prescribe aspirin (81 milligrams daily after first dose of 325 milligrams) if there are no contraindications.

PRACTICE GUIDELINES

Guidelines for the management of patients with peripheral arterial disease (lower extremity, renal, mesenteric, and abdominal aortic)[2] are available at http://circ.ahajournals.org/cgi/reprint/113/11/e463.

SPECIAL CONSIDERATIONS

UPPER EXTREMITY ISCHEMIA

Acute arterial occlusion in the upper extremities is much less common than in the lower limbs, and due to well-developed collateral circulation around the shoulder and elbow, is better tolerated. Ischemic pain at rest and gangrene, in the absence of distal embolization, are rare in the upper limb. Causes of upper limb ischemia include vasospasm, arteritis, trauma, atherosclerotic plaque rupture, embolism, iatrogenic injury (e.g., during brachial artery access for cardiac catheterization), thoracic outlet syndromes, aneurysms, and hypercoagulable states. After clinical examination, further investigation of suspected ischemia is done with segmental blood pressure measurements above and below the elbow, Doppler evaluation, duplex US, and arteriography. Treatment of acute limb-threatening ischemia of the hand and forearm includes heparin (Table 61-6) and emergent surgical thromboembolectomy.

REFERENCES

The complete reference list is available online at www.TintinalliEM.com.

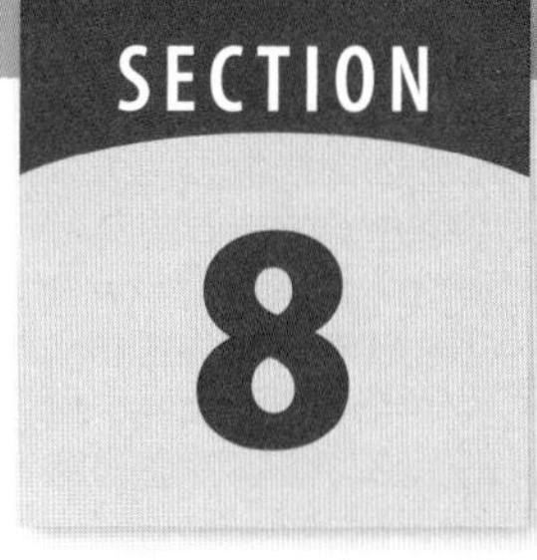

Pulmonary Disorders

SECTION 8

CHAPTER 62 Respiratory Distress

John Sarko
J. Stephan Stapczynski

GENERAL APPROACH TO RESPIRATORY DISTRESS

INTRODUCTION

Dyspnea is a subjective feeling of difficult, labored, or uncomfortable breathing, which patients often describe as "shortness of breath," "breathlessness," or "not getting enough air."[1] Dyspnea is frequently associated with other respiratory symptoms or signs. **Tachypnea** is rapid breathing. **Orthopnea** is dyspnea in the recumbent position. It is most often the result of left ventricular failure, but can also be seen with diaphragmatic paralysis or chronic obstructive pulmonary disease. **Paroxysmal nocturnal dyspnea** is orthopnea that awakens the patient from sleep, prompting an upright posture in order to resolve breathlessness. **Trepopnea** is dyspnea associated with only one of several recumbent positions. Trepopnea can occur with unilateral diaphragmatic paralysis, with ball-valve airway obstruction, or after surgical pneumonectomy. **Platypnea** is the opposite of orthopnea: dyspnea in the upright position. Platypnea results from the loss of abdominal wall muscular tone and, in rare cases, from right-to-left intracardiac shunting, as occurs from a patent foramen ovale. **Hyperpnea** is essentially hyperventilation and is defined as minute ventilation in excess of metabolic demand. **Respiratory distress** is a term used by the physician, combining the patient's subjective sensation of dyspnea with signs indicating difficulty breathing. **Ventilatory or respiratory failure** occurs when the lungs and ventilatory muscles cannot move enough air in and out of the alveoli to adequately oxygenate arterial blood and eliminate carbon dioxide.

PATHOPHYSIOLOGY

Dyspnea is a complex sensation that arises from the interaction of multiple pathophysiologic mechanisms.[1,2] Sensory information about respiratory activity generated by multiple afferent receptors is integrated within the CNS at both the subcortical and cortical levels. The current explanation for the sensation of dyspnea is when imbalance exists among the inspiratory drive, efferent activity to the respiratory muscles, and feedback from these afferent receptors.

CLINICAL FEATURES

Dyspnea is a feature of several disorders seen in the ED (**Table 62-1**). The presence or degree of dyspnea is difficult to measure, although categorical scales (e.g., the Borg or Fletcher scales) and visual analog scales can be used to gauge response to therapy.[1,3] Assess for evidence of impending respiratory failure: marked tachypnea and tachycardia; stridor; use of the accessory respiratory muscles, including the sternocleidomastoid, sternoclavicular, and intercostals; inability to speak normally as a consequence of breathlessness; agitation or lethargy as a consequence of hypoxemia; depressed consciousness due to hypercapnia; and paradoxical abdominal wall movement when the abdominal wall retracts inward with inspiration, indicating diaphragmatic fatigue. In patients with these signs, give oxygen and be prepared for more advanced measures (discussed elsewhere). Lesser degrees of dyspnea allow for a more detailed medical history, physical examination, and indicated ancillary tests.

DIAGNOSIS

Ask about recent infectious and environmental exposures that may impair respiratory function. Carefully question patients who require daily medications for symptom control about compliance and possible drug interactions.

Dyspnea is a prominent symptom of heart failure,[4] and differentiating heart failure from pulmonary causes of dyspnea is an important and frequently difficult task. Treatment and prognosis differ, and embarking down the wrong pathway of treatment can have adverse consequences.[5] Several findings can assist in this differentiation, although few of them are definitive by themselves (**Table 62-2**).[6-8]

An S_3 gallop on physical examination or pulmonary venous congestion/interstitial edema (especially with concomitant cardiomegaly) on chest x-ray strongly suggest heart failure as the cause of the dyspnea (**Figure 62-1**).[6] The physician's overall gestalt of the diagnosis, the presence of jugular venous distention on examination, and alveolar edema on chest x-ray suggest heart failure. Wheezing, dyspnea on exertion, orthopnea, paroxysmal nocturnal dyspnea, and leg edema are not useful in discriminating between cardiac and pulmonary causes. Conversely, the absence of these findings does not exclude heart failure.

LABORATORY TESTING AND IMAGING

Pulse oximetry provides a rapid assessment of arterial oxygen saturation but is an insensitive screening test for disorders of gas exchange. Arterial blood gas analysis is more sensitive for detecting impaired gas exchange but cannot evaluate the work of breathing. Arterial blood gas testing can find the rare patient with dyspnea or tachypnea who exhibits no evidence of hypoxemia or pulmonary disease, suggesting hyperventilating from metabolic acidosis.

Bedside spirometric analysis (e.g., peak expiratory flow), especially if performed before and after bronchodilator therapy, can be used to diagnose dyspnea resulting from asthma or chronic obstructive pulmonary disease, but spirometry requires voluntary effort that might be difficult for dyspneic patients.

Negative inspiratory force can assess strength of the diaphragm and inspiratory muscles. Other potentially useful tests include an ECG and measuring the hemoglobin level. In most ED patients, the cause of dyspnea can be identified by the history, the physical examination, and these ancillary tests.

B-type natriuretic peptide (BNP) is a polypeptide secreted by ventricular myocytes in response to volume expansion and pressure overload; BNP elevates with any cause of overload, including heart failure, myocardial ischemia, pulmonary embolism, sepsis, chronic obstructive pulmonary disease, or any right heart strain. Serum levels of BNP or its precursor, N-terminal pro-BNP, are measured using two methods: an enzyme-linked immunosorbent assay and a radioimmunoassay; the enzyme-linked immunosorbent assay is more accurate than the radioimmunoassay.[9]

A normal BNP (<100 picograms/mL) or N-terminal pro-BNP (<500 picograms/mL) excludes heart failure in low and moderate pretest probability patients outside of "flash" settings.[6,9,10] A high level (BNP >500 picograms/mL or N-terminal pro-BNP >2000 picograms/mL)

TABLE 62-1 Common Causes of Dyspnea in the ED

Most Common Causes	Most Immediately Life-Threatening Causes
Obstructive airway disease: asthma, chronic obstructive pulmonary disease	Upper airway obstruction: foreign body, angioedema, hemorrhage
Decompensated heart failure/ cardiogenic pulmonary edema	Tension pneumothorax
Ischemic heart disease: unstable angina and myocardial infarction	Pulmonary embolism
Pneumonia	Neuromuscular weakness: myasthenia gravis, Guillain-Barré syndrome, botulism
Psychogenic	Fat embolism

is moderately useful for establishing the diagnosis of heart failure, although these elevations are rarely unsuspected after a careful history, exam, and chest radiograph.[10,11] Overall, BNP measurement offers limited real help in assessing dyspneic patients,[12] especially when values between 100 and 500 picograms/mL occur, which is common in the patient without a clear clinical syndrome.[11,13,14]

A chest radiograph may find a pulmonary abnormality, infiltrate, effusion, and pneumothorax.

Bedside lung US is an important tool in the assessment of acute dyspnea. It can differentiate acute decompensated heart failure from noncardiac causes of acute dyspnea with a sensitivity and specificity of about 97% and is superior to chest x-ray and natriuretic peptide determination.[15,16] Bedside US can identify pleural effusion, pneumothorax, cardiac tamponade, cardiac functional abnormalities, pulmonary consolidation, and intravascular volume status (**Figures 62-2 to 62-4**).[17,18]

TREATMENT

In severe dyspnea, the initial treatment goal is maintenance of the airway and oxygenation, seeking a partial pressure of alveolar oxygen (Pao_2) > 60 mm Hg and/or arterial oxygen saturation (Sao_2) ≥90%. Next, or in those with lesser dyspnea, treat the underlying disorder. Rarely are opioids or benzodiazepines used as dyspnea therapy, except in near terminal states for patient comfort.[1,19]

TABLE 62-2 Factors Supporting Heart Failure as the Cause of Dyspnea[6]

Finding	LR+ (95% CI)	LR– (95% CI)
Clinical gestalt	4.4 (1.8–10.0)	0.45 (0.28–0.73)
History		
Heart failure	5.8 (4.1–8.0)	0.45 (0.38–0.53)
Myocardial infarction	3.1 (2.0–4.9)	0.69 (0.58–0.82)
Coronary artery disease	1.8 (1.1–2.8)	0.68 (0.48–0.96)
Symptoms		
Paroxysmal nocturnal dyspnea	2.6 (1.5–4.5)	0.70 (0.54–0.91)
Orthopnea	2.2 (1.2–3.9)	0.65 (0.45–0.92)
Edema	2.1 (0.92–5.00)	0.64 (0.39–1.10)
Dyspnea on exertion	1.3 (1.2–1.4)	0.48 (0.35–0.67)
Physical examination		
S_3 gallop	11.0 (4.9–25.0)	0.88 (0.83–0.94)
Jugular venous distention	5.1 (3.2–7.9)	0.66 (0.57–0.77)
Hepatojugular reflex	6.4 (0.81–51.00)	0.79 (0.62–1.00)
S4	1.6 (0.47–5.50)	0.98 (0.93–1.00)
Wheezing	0.52 (0.38–0.71)	1.3 (1.1–1.7)
Chest x-ray		
Pulmonary venous congestion	12.0 (6.8–21.0)	0.48 (0.28–0.83)
Interstitial edema	12.0 (5.2–27.0)	0.68 (0.54–0.85)
Alveolar edema	6.0 (2.2–16.0)	0.95 (0.93–0.94)
Cardiomegaly	3.3 (2.4–4.7)	0.33 (0.23–0.48)
ECG		
Atrial fibrillation	3.8 (1.7–8.8)	0.79 (0.65–0.96)
Any abnormal finding	2.2 (1.6–3.1)	0.64 (0.47–0.88)

Abbreviations: CI = confidence interval; LR = likelihood ratio.

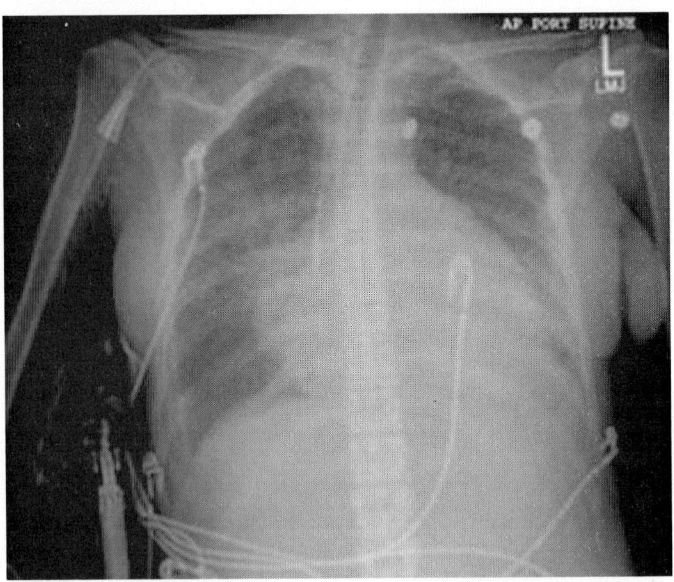

FIGURE 62-1. Pulmonary edema. Cardiomegaly is present, the pulmonary vasculature is engorged, and cephalization of flow is present.

HYPOXIA AND HYPOXEMIA

Hypoxia is insufficient delivery of oxygen to the tissues. The amount of oxygen available to the tissues is a function of the arterial oxygen content (Cao_2) comprising a small portion dissolved in plasma and a larger portion bound to Hb:

$$Cao_2 = 0.0031 \times Pao_2 + 1.38 \times Hb \times Sao_2 \quad \text{[Formula 1]}$$

Oxygen delivery (Do_2) is a product of arterial oxygen content and cardiac output (CO):

$$Do_2 = Cao_2 \times CO \quad \text{[Formula 2]}$$

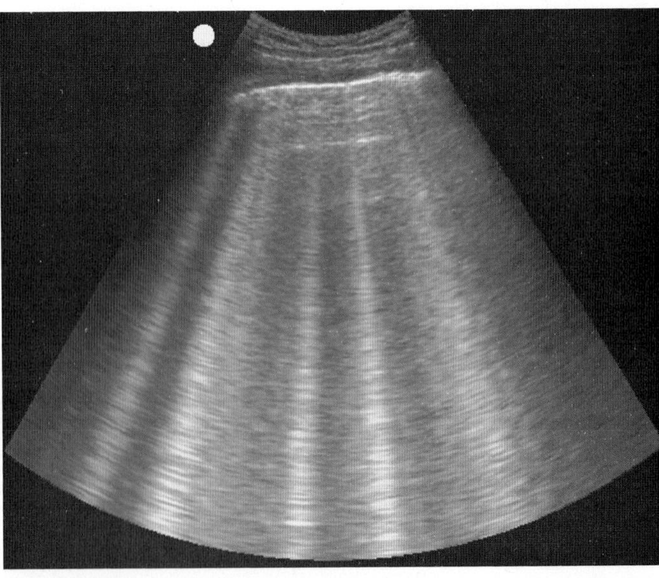

FIGURE 62-2. B lines of pulmonary edema. [Reproduced with permission from Silva FR, Mills L: Chapter 7. Pulmonary, in Ma OJ, Mateer JR, Reardon RF, et al (eds): *Ma and Mateer's Emergency Ultrasound*, 3rd ed. New York: McGraw-Hill Education; 2014. Fig. 7-4, Part B, p. 176.]

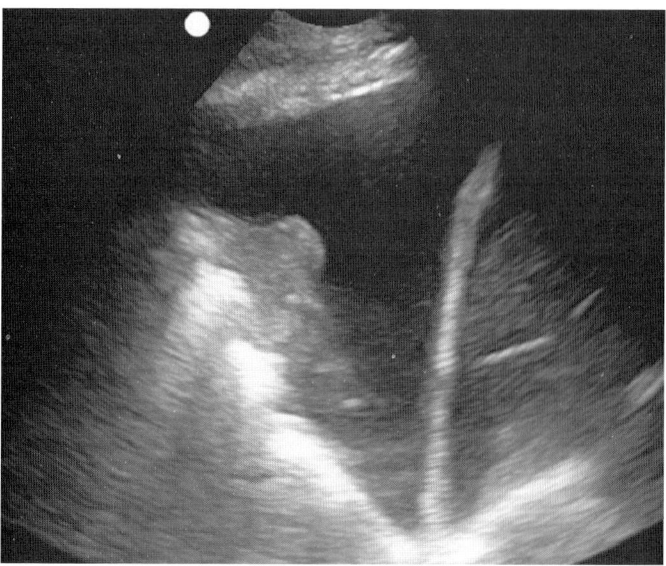

FIGURE 62-3. Pleural effusion. [Reproduced with permission from Silva FR, Mills L: Chapter 7. Pulmonary, in Ma OJ, Mateer JR, Reardon RF, et al (eds): *Ma and Mateer's Emergency Ultrasound*, 3rd ed. New York: McGraw-Hill Education; 2014. Fig. 7-4, Part D, p. 177.]

Tissue hypoxia occurs in states of low cardiac output, low Hb concentration, or low Sa_{O_2}. The level of oxygen saturation in arterial Hb is, in turn, dependent on the Pa_{O_2}, as determined by the oxygen-Hb dissociation curve. **Hypoxemia** is an abnormally low arterial oxygen tension (defined as a Pa_{O_2} <60 mm Hg). While hypoxemia is the most common cause of hypoxia, *hypoxia* and *hypoxemia* are not interchangeable; one can occur without the other. For example, in states of low Pa_{O_2} (hypoxemia) with concomitant polycythemia, the patient may have no tissue hypoxia. Alternatively, severely anemic patients may suffer tissue hypoxia despite a normal Pa_{O_2}.

Relative hypoxemia is the term used when the arterial oxygen tension is lower than expected for a given level of inhaled oxygen. The degree of relative hypoxemia can be assessed by calculating the alveolar arterial (A-a) oxygen partial pressure gradient, [$P(A\text{-}a)_{O_2}$], which measures efficiency of oxygen transfer from the lungs to the circulation. Alveolar oxygen partial pressure is determined by the inhaled oxygen concentration (21% for room air), atmospheric pressure (760 mm Hg at sea level), and displacement by water vapor (47 mm Hg for full saturation) and carbon dioxide (CO_2). Gas in the alveolus is fully saturated with water vapor, and the amount of alveolar oxygen is further reduced by CO_2 that freely diffuses from the pulmonary capillaries in an amount determined by the ratio between oxygen consumption and CO_2 production, termed the *respiratory quotient* (R), which is affected by diet. On a typical mixed diet, the R is 0.8. Alveolar oxygen breathing room air at sea level has a:

$$P_{A_{O_2}} = 0.21 \times (760 - 47) - Pa_{CO_2}/0.8 \qquad \textbf{[Formula 3]}$$

The A-a gradient at sea level for room air is a:

$$P(A\text{-}a)_{O_2} = 149 - Pa_{CO_2}/0.8 - Pa_{O_2} \qquad \textbf{[Formula 4]}$$

A simplified formula often used is:

$$P(A\text{-}a)_{O_2} = 145 - Pa_{CO_2} - Pa_{O_2} \qquad \textbf{[Formula 5]}$$

A normal $P(A\text{-}a)_{O_2}$ is <10 mm Hg in young, healthy patients and increases with age, predicted by the formula:

$$P(A\text{-}a)_{O_2} = 2.5 + 0.21 \text{ (age in years) } (\pm 11) \qquad \textbf{[Formula 6]}$$

This normal A-a gradient is for healthy, asymptomatic individuals measured in an upright or sitting position. The supine position alone, as well as many chronic cardiac or pulmonary diseases, may raise the A-a gradient. The supine position is a common ED patient position, impairing the assessment.

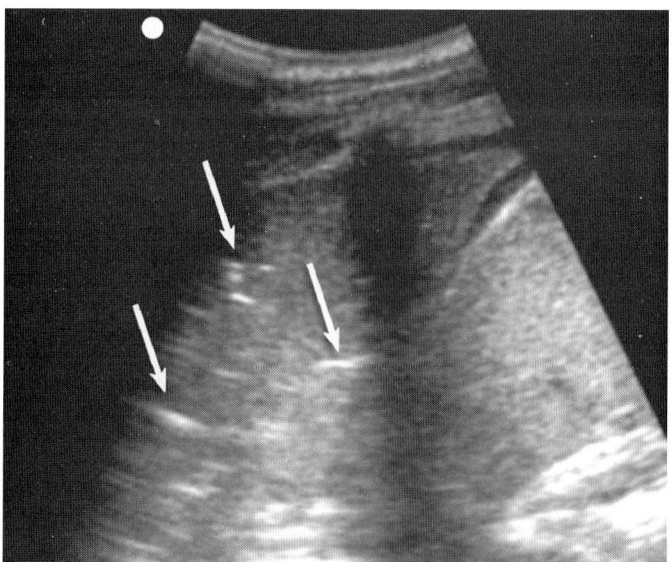

FIGURE 62-4. *Arrows* point to areas of pulmonary consolidation. [Reproduced with permission from Silva FR, Mills L: Chapter 7. Pulmonary, in Ma OJ, Mateer JR, Reardon RF, et al (eds): *Ma and Mateer's Emergency Ultrasound*, 3rd ed. New York: McGraw-Hill Education; 2014. Fig. 7-4, Part C, p. 177.]

PATHOPHYSIOLOGY

Hypoxemia results from any combination of five mechanisms.

1. *Hypoventilation.* Hypoxemia from hypoventilation alone has an increased Pa_{CO_2} and a normal A-a O_2 gradient. The additional CO_2 displaces inhaled oxygen in the alveolus. However, the remaining alveolar oxygen diffuses and mixes normally into the arterial blood, displaying a normal A-a O_2 gradient as long as there is no alveolar or interstitial disease.
2. *Right-to-left shunt.* Right-to-left shunting occurs when blood enters the systemic circulation without traversing ventilated lung. There is always a small degree of right-to-left shunting because of the direct left atrial return of deoxygenated blood from both the coronary veins and the bronchial arteries. Increased right-to-left shunting occurs in a variety of conditions, including congenital cardiac malformation and acquired pulmonary disorders (pulmonary consolidation, pulmonary atelectasis). Regardless of the specific cause of the right-to-left shunt, it is always associated with an increase in the A-a O_2 gradient. **A hallmark of significant right-to-left shunting is the failure of arterial oxygen levels to increase in response to supplemental oxygen.** Although a small improvement may be observed with supplemental oxygen, hypoxemia is never fully eliminated because of the mixing of deoxygenated blood in the systemic circulation.
3. *Ventilation-perfusion ($\dot{V}/\dot{Q}$) mismatch.* Ideal pulmonary gas exchange depends on a balance of ventilation and perfusion. Any abnormality resulting in a regional alteration of either ventilation or perfusion can adversely affect pulmonary gas exchange, resulting in hypoxemia. There are many causes of $\dot{V}/\dot{Q}$ mismatch, including pulmonary emboli, pneumonia, asthma, chronic obstructive pulmonary disease, and even extrinsic vascular compression. Regardless of cause, hypoxemia from ventilation-perfusion mismatch is associated with an increased A-a O_2 gradient, and hypoxemia improves with supplemental oxygen.

4. *Diffusion impairment.* Pulmonary gas exchange requires diffusion across the alveolar–blood barrier. Regardless of the specific cause of the diffusion impairment, the A-a O_2 gradient is increased, and hypoxemia improves with supplemental oxygen.
5. *Low inspired oxygen.* Decreased ambient oxygen pressure results in hypoxemia. This is commonly seen at high altitude (including commercial air travel) or in nonobstructive asphyxia. The A-a O_2 gradient is normal, and hypoxemia improves with supplemental oxygen. For example, Denver, at 5400 ft (1646 m) above sea level, has an atmospheric pressure of 620 mm Hg and an inhaled Po_2 of only $0.21 \times 620 = 130$ mm Hg, as opposed to 160 mm Hg at sea level.

There are three distinct acute compensatory mechanisms for hypoxemia. Initially, minute ventilation increases. Next, pulmonary arterial vasoconstriction decreases perfusion to hypoxic alveoli. Although vasoconstriction balances ventilation and perfusion to restore arterial oxygenation, it may also cause acute right heart failure and is ineffective with diffuse lung disease. Finally, sympathetic tone increases and improves oxygen delivery by increasing cardiac output, usually with an increased heart rate. Chronic compensatory mechanisms include an increased red blood cell mass and decreased tissue oxygen demands. These compensatory mechanisms appear to be activated at different levels of hypoxemia among different individuals. However, the acute compensatory mechanisms are always activated when Pao_2 reaches 60 mm Hg, and compensatory mechanisms fail when Pao_2 falls below 20 mm Hg.

CLINICAL FEATURES

The signs and symptoms of hypoxemia are nonspecific. CNS manifestations include agitation, headache, somnolence, coma, and seizures. Although tachypnea and hyperventilation are often present, by the time Pao_2 is <20 mm Hg, there is a central depression of respiration. **Cyanosis, the blood or tissue discoloration associated with a lowered arterial oxygenation saturation, is not a sensitive or specific indicator of hypoxemia.** Patients with chronic compensatory mechanisms may display polycythemia or alterations in body habitus (e.g., pulmonary cachexia).

DIAGNOSIS AND TREATMENT

Hypoxemia is defined as a Pao_2 <60 mm Hg, so formal diagnosis requires arterial blood gas analysis. Although pulse oximetry is useful for screening purposes and decreased Sao_2 readings accurately predict significant hypoxemia, clinically acceptable pulse oximetry saturation readings (>90%) do not exclude hypoxemia. If certain hemoglobin abnormalities exist (e.g., methemoglobin or carboxyhemoglobin), pulse oximetry analysis may overestimate oxygen saturation and under measure the response to supplemental oxygen (see the section "Cyanosis," below). Regardless of the specific cause of hypoxemia, the initial approach remains the same: ensuring a patent airway and providing supplemental oxygenation with a goal of maintaining a Pao_2 >60 mm Hg. **Except in patients with right-to-left shunts, arterial oxygenation responds to supplemental oxygen.**

HYPERCAPNIA

Hypercapnia is exclusively caused by alveolar hypoventilation and is defined as a $Paco_2$ >45 mm Hg. Alveolar hypoventilation has many causes, including rapid shallow breathing, small tidal volumes, underventilation of the lung, or reduced respiratory drive. **Hypercapnia never results from increased CO_2 production alone (Table 62-3).**

TABLE 62-3 Causes of Hypercapnia

Causes of Hypercapnia
Depressed central respiratory drive
Structural CNS disease: brainstem lesions
Drug depression of respiratory center: opioids, sedatives, anesthetics
Endogenous toxins: tetanus
Thoracic cage disorders
Kyphoscoliosis
Morbid obesity
Neuromuscular impairment
Neuromuscular disease: myasthenia gravis, Guillain-Barré syndrome
Neuromuscular toxin: organophosphate poisoning, botulism
Intrinsic lung disease associated with increased dead space
Chronic obstructive pulmonary disease
Upper airway obstruction

PATHOPHYSIOLOGY

A portion of each tidal volume remains in the non–gas-exchange portion of the respiratory system—termed the *dead space*—that is determined by the anatomic size of the conducting airways (trachea and bronchi). The portion of the tidal volume that reaches the alveoli is that which remains after the dead space volume is subtracted:

$$\text{Ta (alveolar volume)} = \text{V}_\text{T} \text{ (tidal volume)} - \text{Td (dead space)} \quad \textbf{[Formula 7]}$$

Alveolar ventilation (VA) per minute is the alveolar volume multiplied by the respiratory rate:

$$\text{V}_\text{A} = \text{Ta} \times \text{R} = (\text{V}_\text{T} - \text{Td}) \times \text{R} \quad \textbf{[Formula 8]}$$

Alveolar hypoventilation can result from a decrease in respiratory rate, a decrease in VT, or an increase in dead space. Dead space volume can increase above that due to the anatomic size of the conducting airways, such as seen as a result of ventilation of lung portions with deficient or absent perfusion; these ventilated portions do not participate fully in gas exchange because of inadequate blood flow.

Medullary chemoreceptors stimulate both respiratory rate and VT in response to increased CO_2, so that alveolar ventilation is finely controlled relative to CO_2 production and $Paco_2$ is maintained within a narrow range. Decreased respiratory drive is associated with CNS lesions and toxic depression (Table 62-3). Thoracic cage and neuromuscular disorders produce hypoventilation by slowing respiratory rate and/or decreasing VT relative to the production of CO_2. Intrinsic lung diseases, such as chronic obstructive pulmonary disease, produce alveolar hypoventilation because of an increase in dead space.

CLINICAL FEATURES

The signs and symptoms of hypercapnia depend on the absolute value of $Paco_2$ and its rate of change. Acute elevations result in increased intracranial pressure, and patients may complain of headache, confusion, or lethargy. Severe hypercapnia can produce seizures and coma. Extreme hypercapnia can result in cardiovascular collapse, but this is usually seen only with acute elevations of $Paco_2$ >100 mm Hg. As opposed to acute hypercapnia, chronic hypercapnia, even >80 mm Hg, may be well tolerated.

DIAGNOSIS

Diagnosis of hypercapnia requires arterial blood gas analysis, and pulse oximetry assessment can be normal. With acute hypercapnia, the serum bicarbonate level increases slightly as a result of mass action through the CO_2–bicarbonate (HCO_3^-) equilibrium: HCO_3^- increases about 1 mEq/L for each increase of 10 mm Hg in the $Paco_2$. Patients with chronic hypercapnia have an elevated serum HCO_3^- concentration and normal pH due to the renal retention of bicarbonate in response to increased $Paco_2$: the serum HCO_3^- concentration increases about 3.5 mEq/L for each increase of 10 mm Hg in the $Paco_2$.

TREATMENT

Hypercapnia is treated by increasing minute ventilation, both the respiratory rate and the VT, as appropriate. This involves ensuring a patent airway and may require noninvasive ventilation, mechanical ventilation, the use of an antidote to reverse drug toxicity, or, rarely, the use of a respiratory stimulant such as doxapram.[20] **Do not withhold oxygen required to maintain minimum saturation levels in any chronic lung disease patient in an effort to stimulate ventilation and reduce hypercapnia.**

The disposition of hypercapnic patients depends primarily on the underlying cause and severity. In general, patients with hypercapnia with new acidosis or that causes CNS symptoms should be hospitalized. Also, patients with neuromuscular disease—either congenital or acquired—who present with acute hypercapnia should be hospitalized. Some chronic obstructive pulmonary disease patients have chronic hypercapnia and do not require admission provided they are stable. Conversely, patients with chronic obstructive pulmonary disease who display worsening hypercapnia despite maximal outpatient therapy require hospital admission.

WHEEZING

Wheezes are "musical" adventitious lung sounds produced by airflow through the central and distal airways.[21] The duration is prolonged, typically >80 milliseconds. Wheezes differ from the other two main adventitial lung sounds: rhonchi and crackles (rales). Rhonchi are a series of damped sinusoidal sounds of lower frequency (<300 Hz) and prolonged duration (>100 milliseconds). Crackles or rales are a series of intermittent individual sounds, typically <20 milliseconds in duration. Wheezing is usually more prominent on exhalation, in contrast to upper airway stridor, which is more prominent during inspiration.

The current theory is that wheezes are produced by airway flutter and vortex shedding from the central and distal airways, although movement of airway secretions may play a small role. Airway obstruction comes from bronchial smooth muscle contraction (bronchospasm), smooth muscle hypertrophy, increased mucus secretion, and peribronchial inflammation.

Wheezing is usually associated lower airway disease such as with asthma or other obstructive pulmonary diseases with muscular spasm and inflammation (**Table 62-4**). Upper airway obstruction causes stridor, which is loudest during inspiration. An occasional wheeze is normal during forced expiration in some normal children and adults, and conversely, patients with severe airflow obstruction may not have audible wheezes.

Diagnosis and treatment of the different causes of wheezing are discussed in specific chapters in the Adult and Pediatric sections of this book. Treatment of wheezing is directed to the underlying disorder.

TABLE 62-4 Differential Diagnosis of Wheezing

Upper airway (more likely to be stridor, may be hard to separate from wheezing)
Angioedema: allergic, angiotensin-converting enzyme inhibitor, idiopathic
Foreign body
Infection: croup, epiglottis, tracheitis
Lower airway
Asthma
Transient airway hyperreactivity (usually caused by infection or irritation)
Bronchiolitis
Chronic obstructive pulmonary disease
Foreign body
Cardiovascular
Cardiogenic pulmonary edema ("cardiac asthma")
Noncardiogenic pulmonary edema (acute respiratory distress syndrome)
Pulmonary embolus (rare)
Psychogenic

COUGH

Cough is a protective reflex for clearing secretions and foreign debris from the tracheobronchial tree.[22] Coughing is initiated by stimulation of irritant receptors located largely in the larynx, trachea, and major bronchi. These receptors are stimulated by inhaled irritants (e.g., dust), allergens (e.g., ragweed pollen), toxic substances (e.g., gastric acid), hypo- or hyperosmotic liquids, inflammation (e.g., asthma), cold air, instrumentation, and excess pulmonary secretions. Minor cough receptors located in the upper respiratory tract (sinuses and pharynx) and chest (pleura, pericardium, and diaphragm) may stimulate coughing. Signals from these receptors travel by means of the vagus, phrenic, and other nerves to the cough center in the medulla.

Once stimulated, the cough center initiates the stereotypical cough pattern: a deep inspiration followed by attempted expiration against a closed glottis that suddenly opens, providing for a forceful exhalation of gas, secretions, and foreign debris from the tracheobronchial tree. The coughing sound is generated at the larynx and resonates in the nasal cavity and the lungs.

CLINICAL FEATURES

Acute cough is cough lasting <3 weeks and is usually associated with self-limited infectious upper respiratory or bronchial infections (Table 62-5).[23] Subacute cough lasts 3 to 8 weeks and is most commonly postinfectious, but causes of subacute cough overlap with causes of acute and chronic cough. **Chronic cough is cough present for >8 weeks.**[23]

ACUTE COUGH

Acute cough is most often caused by upper respiratory tract infection, lower respiratory tract infection, and allergic reactions.[23] Common upper respiratory infections are associated with a combination of rhinorrhea, sinusitis, pharyngitis, and laryngitis, with the cough a result of drainage from the nasopharynx onto cough receptors in the pharynx and larynx. A productive cough is the hallmark of acute bronchitis. Although pneumonia generally produces a cough, pulmonary secretions may be scant and the cough nonproductive. Pertussis in adults has been associated with acute cough lasting 1 to 6 weeks.[24] The observed increased incidence of pertussis in adolescents and young adults is thought to be due to waning vaccine immunity with increasing age.

SUBACUTE COUGH

Postinfectious cough is the most likely cause of subacute cough. The mechanisms include postviral airway inflammation with bronchial hyperresponsiveness, mucus hypersecretion, upper airway cough syndrome (postnasal discharge), or asthma.

TABLE 62-5 Differential Diagnosis of Cough

Acute	Chronic	Chronic: Less Common
Upper respiratory infection: rhinitis, sinusitis, pertussis	Smoking and/or chronic bronchitis	Heart failure
Lower respiratory tract infection: bronchitis, pneumonia	Upper airway cough syndrome (postnasal discharge syndrome)	Bronchiectasis
Allergic reaction	Asthma: reactive airways disease	Lung cancer or other intrathoracic mass
Asthma	Gastroesophageal reflux	Emphysema
Environmental irritants	Angiotensin-converting enzyme inhibitor	Occupational and environmental irritants
Transient airway hyperresponsiveness	Angiotensin II receptor blocker	Recurrent aspiration or chronic foreign body
Foreign body	Postinfectious; pertussis	Psychiatric
		Miscellaneous: cystic fibrosis, interstitial lung disease

CHRONIC COUGH

The most common causes of chronic cough are (1) smoking, often with chronic bronchitis; (2) upper airway cough syndrome (formerly postnasal discharge); (3) asthma; (4) gastroesophageal reflux; and (5) angiotensin-converting enzyme (ACE) inhibitor or angiotensin II receptor blocker (ARB) therapy (Table 62-5).[25,26] Smoking-induced coughing is usually worse in the morning and, with chronic bronchitis, usually productive. Upper airway cough syndrome, formerly called *postnasal discharge syndrome*, is associated with mucus drainage from the nose, a history of "allergies or sinus problems," and frequent clearing of the throat or swallowing of mucus.[27] The postnasal drainage itself may not only directly stimulate a cough, but the conditions producing postnasal drainage (e.g., allergic rhinitis) may also cause irritation or inflammation of upper airway structures that directly stimulates cough receptors independently of the drainage. Chronic cough associated with asthma is usually worse at night, exacerbated by irritants, and associated with episodic wheezing and dyspnea.[28] Asthma can be exacerbated by β-blocker therapy and also presents with nocturnal coughing. Cough associated with gastroesophageal reflux often has a history of heartburn, is worse when lying down, and improves with anti-acid therapy (antacids, H_2 blockers, or proton pump blockers).[29]

The incidence of ACE inhibitor cough is approximately 10% to 12%, although higher values have been reported.[30] All ACE inhibitors and ARBs can induce cough, although ARBs appear to have a lower reported incidence.[31] ACE inhibitor cough is thought to result when the blockade of ACE leads to accumulation of bradykinin and substance P, which stimulate the pulmonary cough receptors and enhance the formation of irritating prostaglandin metabolites. ACE inhibitor cough is highly variable in (1) onset (as early as 1 week to as late as 1 year after starting treatment), (2) severity (only slightly bothersome to debilitating symptoms), and (3) variation during the day. Cough typically resolves in 1 to 4 weeks after ACE or ARB therapy is stopped but may linger up to 3 months.[30] See chapter 14, "Anaphylaxis, Allergies, and Angioedema," for further discussion.

DIAGNOSIS AND TREATMENT

Most causes of acute cough do not warrant ancillary tests. A chest radiograph is wise for patients with purulent sputum and/or fever, and spirometry can document the presence of airflow obstruction in patients with asthma. Pertussis is a clinical diagnosis in patients with subacute cough as the commonly available culture, and polymerase chain reaction tests have decreasing sensitivity after the third week of coughing.[14]

ACUTE COUGH

In addition to disease-specific therapy,[32] patients with acute cough may benefit from antitussives, which block the cough reflex at various locations.[33,34] Demulcents, part of most proprietary cough preparations, soothe the pharynx and somewhat suppress the cough reflex. Of the herbal agents, menthol and the pungent spices (e.g., pepper, mustard, garlic, radish, and onions) have an antitussive effect.[35] Naproxen reduces coughing in patients with acute bronchitis.[36,37] In both children and adults, acute coughing illnesses can last up to 3 weeks.[38,39] For intractable coughing paroxysms in the ED, some patients respond to 4 mL of 1% or 2% preservative-free lidocaine (40 or 80 milligrams) by nebulization. This will cause transient suppression of the gag reflex due to posterior pharyngeal anesthesia.

SUBACUTE AND CHRONIC COUGH

Determine if the subacute cough is postinfectious—one following a recent respiratory infection. If postinfectious, then assess for transient bronchial hyperresponsiveness, asthma, pertussis, upper airway cough syndrome, pneumonia, or an acute exacerbation of chronic bronchitis. Treatment is then directed at the presumed cause. If subacute cough is not postinfectious, it is evaluated and treated in the same manner as a chronic cough.

Chronic cough is most often the result of a few common disorders, so an algorithmic approach to treatment using sequential steps is effective[25,26,40] (**Figure 62-5**):

- Reduce exposure to lung irritants (e.g., smoking) and discontinue ACE inhibitors, ARBs, and β-blockers.

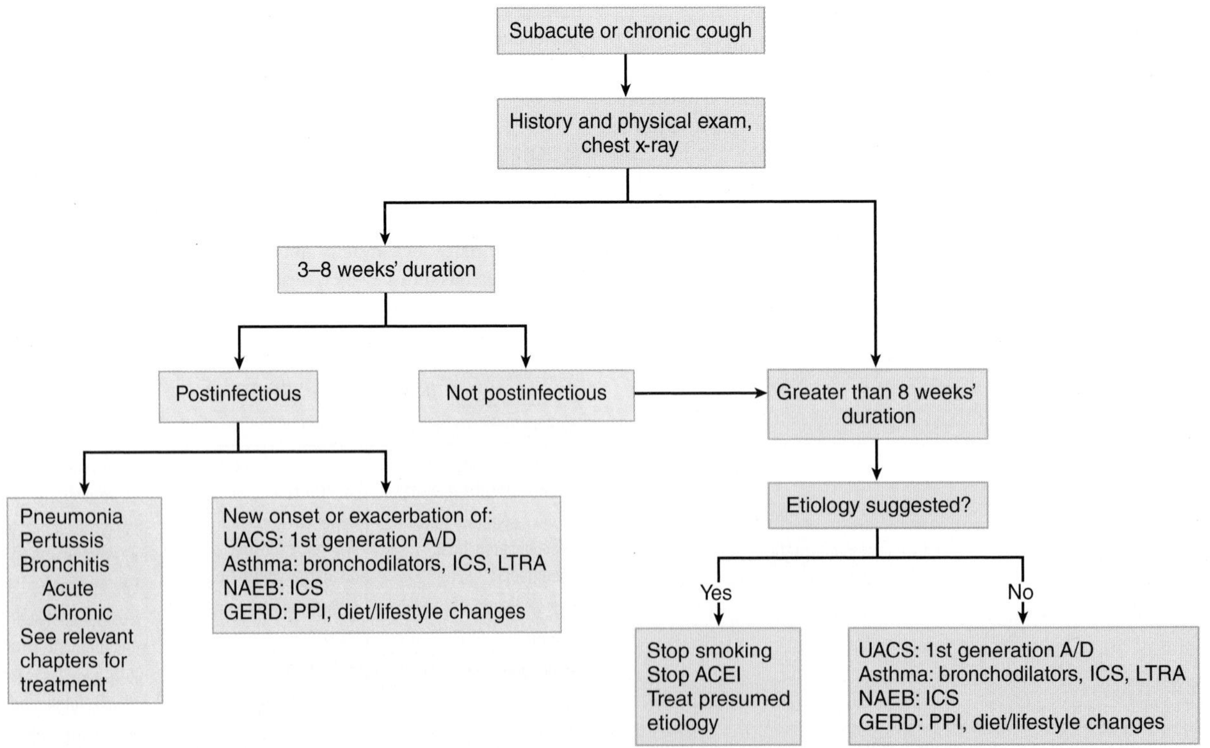

FIGURE 62-5. Evaluation of subacute and chronic cough for patients 15 years of age and older.[23] ACEI = angiotensin-converting enzyme inhibitor; A/D = antihistamine/decongestant; GERD = gastroesophageal reflux disease; ICS = inhaled corticosteroids; LTRA = leukotriene receptor antagonist; NAEB = nonasthmatic eosinophilic bronchitis; PPI = proton pump inhibitor; UACS = upper airway cough syndrome.

- Treat for postnasal discharge with an oral first-generation antihistamine/decongestant with or without an inhaled nasal steroid. If the cough improves, continue treatment and evaluate for sinus disease with imaging studies.
- Evaluate and treat for asthma.
- Obtain chest and sinus imaging if not already done.
- Evaluate and treat for gastroesophageal reflux.
- Refer the patient for specialist evaluation, for CT of the chest and evaluation for pulmonary and nonpulmonary causes of cough, or bronchoscopy.

By using a sequential approach, >95% of patients achieve resolution of their cough.[40] Opioid and nonopioid antitussives may help some patients who remain symptomatic.[41]

HICCUPS

Hiccup, or singultus, is involuntary spastic contraction of the inspiratory muscles. Hiccups have no specific protective purpose.[42]

PATHOPHYSIOLOGY

The afferent arm of the hiccup reflex consists of the phrenic and vagus nerves as well as the thoracic sympathetic chain. Normally, glottis closure inhibits inspiration and prevents aspiration during swallowing. Conversely, inspiration normally inhibits glottic closure and maintains an open airway. The hiccup reflex disrupts the connection between these two processes so that 30 to 40 milliseconds after the onset of inspiration, glottic closure is stimulated. In most cases in which a specific cause can be assigned, hiccups appear to result from stimulation, inflammation, or injury to one of the nerves of the reflex arc.

CLINICAL FEATURES

Hiccups are classified as benign and self-limited or persistent and intractable (**Table 62-6**).[42]

Benign hiccups are generally initiated by gastric distention from food, drinking (especially carbonated beverages), or air. Alcohol ingestion appears to precipitate hiccups by relaxing the relationship between inspiration and glottic closure, making it easier for other stimuli to trigger the reflex.

Persistent hiccups are usually a result of injury or irritation to a branch of the vagus or phrenic nerves. One rare but readily treatable stimulus is a foreign body (often a hair) in the external auditory canal that is pressing against the tympanic membrane and stimulating the auricular branch of the vagus nerve. Several drugs—usually steroids and benzodiazepines—are implicated in inducing hiccups, but the evidence is weak.[43]

DIAGNOSIS AND TREATMENT

Determine whether a specific triggering event exists (Table 62-6). Ask if the hiccups persist during sleep; resolution during sleep suggests a psychogenic cause, although this distinction is not absolute. Look in the external auditory canal for a foreign body. A chest radiograph should be done to evaluate for intrathoracic pathology. Fluoroscopy can evaluate for unilateral versus bilateral diaphragmatic movement during hiccups but is not part of the ED evaluation. Unilateral movement suggests focal injury to the phrenic nerve on the affected side.

A variety of physical maneuvers and medications have been used to terminate an acute episode of hiccups (**Tables 62-7 and 62-8**).[44,45]

Many of these physical maneuvers are based on the concept that stimulating the pharynx will block the vagal portion of the reflex arc and abolish the hiccups.[44] No one method appears to be more effective than another. Swallowing a teaspoon of dry granulated sugar is about as effective as others and does not involve the infliction of noxious or painful stimulation.

Drug treatment (Table 62-8) also works by inhibiting the reflex arc.[44] Several agents are described as effective, but mostly only through case reports.[45] Of the recommended drugs, only chlorpromazine has U.S. Food and Drug Administration approval for treatment of intractable hiccups. Chlorpromazine and metoclopramide take effect within 30 minutes. Adverse effects include extrapyramidal symptoms with both agents and hypotension with chlorpromazine. Nifedipine, valproate, baclofen, and gabapentin[46] are second-line outpatient options usually started by the primary care physician.

TABLE 62-6 Differential Diagnosis of Consequence: Hiccups

Acute: Benign, Self-Limited	Chronic: Persistent, Intractable
Gastric distention	CNS structural lesions
Alcohol intoxication	Vagal or phrenic nerve irritation
Excessive smoking	Metabolic: uremia, hyperglycemia
Abrupt change in environmental temperature	General anesthesia
Psychogenic	Surgical procedures: thoracic, abdominal, prostate and urinary tract, craniotomy
	Foreign body in ear touching tympanic membrane (especially hair)

TABLE 62-7 Treatment of Hiccups: Physical Maneuvers

Remove foreign body from ear
Swallow a teaspoon of sugar
Sip ice water
Drink water quickly

CYANOSIS

Cyanosis is a bluish color of the skin and mucous membranes resulting from an increased amount of reduced Hb (deoxyhemoglobin) or Hb derivatives. The detection of cyanosis is subjective and is not a sensitive indicator of the state of arterial oxygenation; cyanosis is determined by the absolute amount of deoxygenated Hb in the blood, not the amount of oxygenated Hb. Cyanosis is divided into central or peripheral categories (**Table 62-9**). **Central cyanosis is cyanosis of mucous membranes and tongue due to inadequate pulmonary oxygenation or an abnormal Hb. Peripheral cyanosis is cyanosis of the fingers or extremities from vasoconstriction and diminished peripheral blood flow.** All conditions that cause central cyanosis also result in peripheral cyanosis.

TABLE 62-8 Treatment of Hiccups: Drug Treatment

Drug	Initial Dose	Maintenance Dose
Chlorpromazine	25–50 milligrams IV, repeat in 2–4 h if needed	25–50 milligrams PO three to four times a day
Metoclopramide	10 milligrams IV or IM	10–20 milligrams PO three times a day for 10 d
Haloperidol	2–5 milligrams IM	1–4 milligrams PO three times a day
Nifedipine	10–20 milligrams PO	10–20 milligrams PO three to four times a day
Valproate	15 milligrams/kg PO	15 milligrams/kg PO three times a day
Baclofen	10 milligrams PO	10 milligrams PO three times a day
Gabapentin	100 milligrams	100 milligrams PO three times a day

TABLE 62-9 Differential Diagnosis of Cyanosis

Central Cyanosis	Peripheral Cyanosis
Hypoxemia Decreased fraction of inspired oxygen: high altitude Hypoventilation Ventilation–perfusion mismatch Right-to-left shunt: congenital heart disease, pulmonary arteriovenous fistulas, multiple intrapulmonary shunts	Reduced cardiac output Cold extremities Maldistribution of blood flow: distributive forms of shock Arterial or venous obstruction
Abnormal hemoglobin Methemoglobinemia: hereditary, acquired Sulfhemoglobinemia: acquired Carboxyhemoglobinemia	

CLINICAL FEATURES

Cyanosis is usually visible when deoxygenated Hb exceeds 5 grams/dL, but individuals with sensitive vision in ideal circumstances may detect central cyanosis with deoxyhemoglobin concentration as low as 1.5 grams/dL. Various physiologic, anatomic, and physical factors other than the amount of reduced Hb may influence the appearance of cyanosis, making an accurate clinical detection of the degree or even the presence of cyanosis difficult (**Table 62-10**).

The tongue and buccal mucosa are thought to be sensitive sites for observing central cyanosis. Peripheral cyanosis is caused by the slowing of blood flow to an area and an abnormally large extraction of oxygen from normally saturated arterial blood. Peripheral vascular disease, shock states, heart failure, and cold exposure all create states of vasoconstriction and decreased peripheral blood flow, with cyanosis of the nail beds. Massage or gentle warming of a cyanotic extremity will increase peripheral blood flow and abolish peripheral, but not central, cyanosis.

Pseudocyanosis is a bluish or slate-gray skin discoloration due to drugs (chlorpromazine, minocycline, amiodarone, nicorandil) or heavy metals (gold, silver).[47,48] In pseudocyanosis, the lips and mucous membranes are of normal color, the abnormal skin discoloration does not blanch with pressure, and the discoloration tends to be more intense in sun-exposed areas. Focal areas of pseudocyanosis may be due to local contact with color dyes, gold, or silver.

DIAGNOSIS AND TREATMENT

Pulse oximetry can detect hypoxemia and provide an accurate oxygen saturation measurement. However, with hemoglobinopathy, standard pulse oximetry is often inaccurate. In methemoglobinemia, pulse oximetry will read 80% to 85% regardless of the oxygen level, thereby often overestimating the true oxygen saturation (it may be lower, but pulse oximetry will not read lower). **With carboxyhemoglobinemia, the pulse oximetry reads carboxyhemoglobin as oxyhemoglobin** reporting a higher percentage for oxygen saturation (see chapters 207, "Dyshemoglobinemias," and 222, "Carbon Monoxide"). **Arterial blood gas analysis using co-oximetry (a specific multi-wavelength measurement of oxygen saturation) is needed in the assessment of any patient with suspected cyanosis.** In central cyanosis, the oxygen saturation measured from the arterial blood gas is decreased because of the underlying hypoxemia. In peripheral cyanosis, the oxygen saturation should be normal. With methemoglobinemia or carboxyhemoglobinemia, arterial blood gas co-oximetry will show a normal Pao_2 (reflecting a normal amount of dissolved oxygen in the plasma), a normal calculated oxygen saturation (from the normal Pao_2), and a decreased measured oxygen saturation (because of a decreased number of oxygen-binding sites).

Give oxygen to all patients with central cyanosis; failure to improve suggests impaired circulation (shock), abnormal Hb, or pseudocyanosis.

TABLE 62-10 Factors Influencing the Physical Appearance of Cyanosis

Physiologic factors
Oxygen content of blood
Degree of oxygen extraction
Oxyhemoglobin dissociation curve
Anatomic factors
Status of microcirculation
Skin pigmentation
Skin thickness
Physical factors
Quality/intensity of light in examination area
Skill of examining physician

PLEURAL EFFUSION

Pleural effusions result from fluid accumulating in the potential space between the visceral and parietal pleurae. Although pleural effusions can result from many causes, in developed countries, the most common causes are heart failure, pneumonia, and cancer (**Table 62-11**).[49-51]

PATHOPHYSIOLOGY

A continuous amount of fluid is secreted from the parietal pleura into the pleural space where it is absorbed by the visceral pleural microcirculation, averaging about 8 L/d in an adult. This fluid reduces friction between the pleural layers and allows for smooth lung expansion and contraction with respiration. Any process that increases fluid production or interferes with fluid absorption will result in accumulation in the pleural space. Pleural effusions are traditionally divided into exudates or transudates.[49-51] Exudative effusions result from pleural disease, usually inflammation or neoplasia that produces active fluid secretion or leakage with high protein content. Transudative effusions result from an imbalance between hydrostatic and oncotic pressures. This imbalance results in the production of an ultrafiltrate with low protein content into the pleural space.

CLINICAL FEATURES

A pleural effusion may be clinically silent or come to detection from either symptoms of an underlying disease, an increase in volume of the effusion with the production of dyspnea, or the development of inflammation and associated pain with respiration. Physical findings of a pleural effusion include percussion dullness and decreased breath sounds. Because pleural fluid typically pools in the dependent portions of the hemithorax, small or

TABLE 62-11 Differential Diagnosis of Pleural Effusion

Common	Less Common
Transudates	
Heart failure	Cirrhosis with ascites Peritoneal dialysis Nephrotic syndrome
Exudates	
Cancer: primary or metastatic	Viral, fungal, mycobacterial, or parasitic infection
Bacterial pneumonia with parapneumonic effusion	Systemic rheumatologic disorders: systemic lupus erythematosus, rheumatoid arthritis
Pulmonary embolism	Uremia, pancreatitis Postcardiac surgery or radiotherapy Drug-related: amiodarone
Either transudates or exudates	
Transudates after diuretic therapy	Pulmonary embolism

moderate-size effusions have percussion dullness and decreased breath sounds at the lung base with relatively normal lung findings above the level of fluid. With large or massive effusions, it may be impossible to distinguish a fluid level on clinical examination.

DIAGNOSIS

In an adult, 150 to 200 mL of pleural fluid in the hemithorax is required to be detectable on upright chest radiography. Supine chest radiographs may demonstrate only a hazy appearance of pleural fluid in the posterior pleural space (**Figure 62-6A**). CT scanning of the chest may clarify uncertain findings on chest radiograph (**Figure 62-6B**). Small free-flowing pleural effusions are better visualized on decubitus radiographic views (**Figure 62-7**). US can also identify a pleural effusion (Figure 62-3). **A significant pleural effusion is large enough to produce a pleural fluid strip >10 mm wide on lateral decubitus radiographic views or by ultrasonography.**[49]

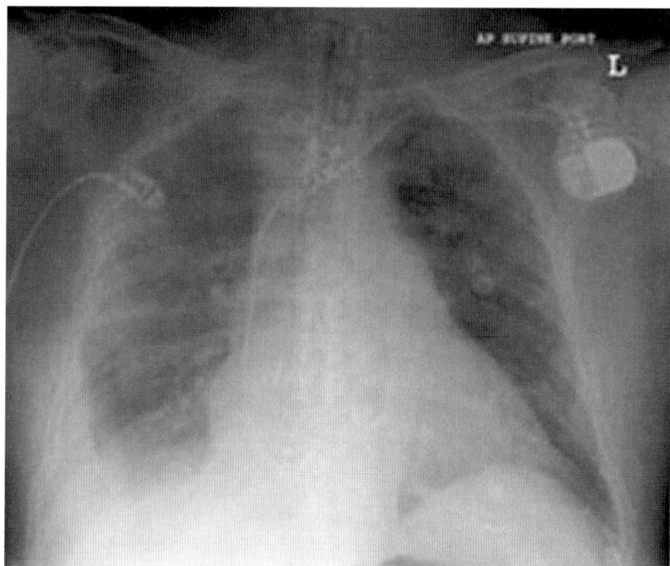

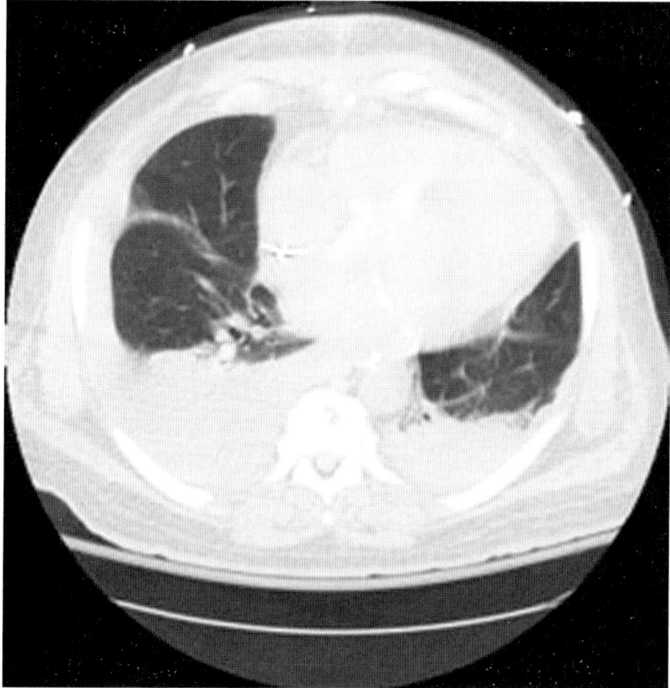

B

FIGURE 62-6. **A.** Supine radiograph showing a right-sided pleural effusion. The right lung field is hazy compared to the left, and a small layer of fluid is noted inferiorly. **B.** CT scan of the same patient. A moderate pleural effusion is seen in the right lung field, and a small effusion not seen in the left lung field of the plain radiograph is present on the CT scan.

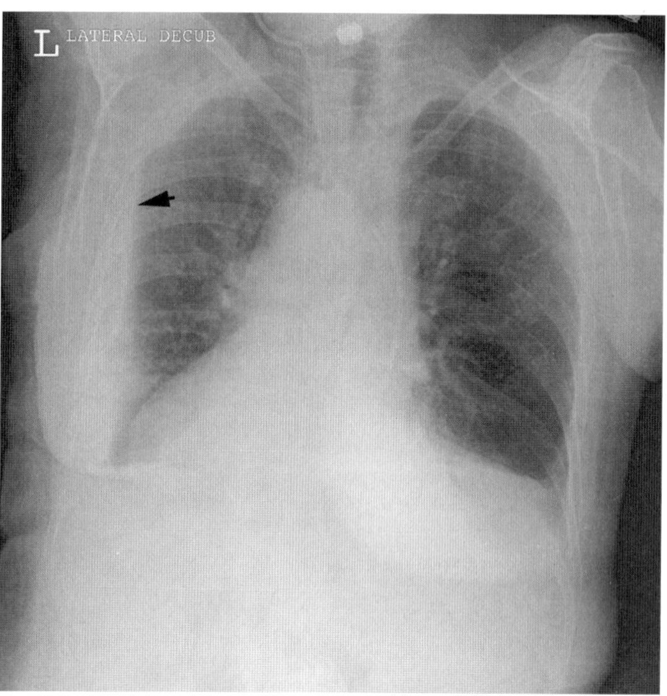

FIGURE 62-7. Left lateral decubitus radiograph showing a layering of a small pleural effusion. *Arrowhead* points to the layer of fluid.

Diagnostic thoracentesis is done to obtain pleural fluid for analysis in cases without a clearly evident cause, to confirm a suspected diagnosis, or to detect pleural space infection. For example, because the largest single cause of pleural effusion is heart failure, if a patient presents with a typical appearance (cardiomegaly, roughly equal in size bilateral effusions), then a period of treatment with monitoring for pleural fluid resolution is indicated, and routine thoracentesis is reserved for patients who do not experience resolution in 3 to 4 days. Otherwise, diagnostic thoracentesis and pleural fluid analysis are indicated.

Light developed the most widely used criteria to differentiate transudates from exudates using serum and pleural fluid protein and lactate dehydrogenase levels (**Table 62-12**).[52] Modifications to the original criteria have been proposed,[51,53] but the overall sensitivity for the detection of an exudative pleural effusion remains 98% to 99% with specificity from 65% to 86%. If the clinical circumstances suggest that the effusion is likely to be transudative, the only tests indicated are pleural fluid and serum protein content and lactate dehydrogenase levels. If the pleural effusion is exudative, additional tests are indicated (Table 62-12).[49-51]

The distinction between exudates and transudates may be obscured by the effect of diuretic therapy in patients with transudative pleural effusions.[49,50] During diuresis, the resorption of water is faster than that of protein, so the protein concentration rises into the range consistent with an exudative etiology. A serum to pleural albumin difference of >1.2 grams/dL has been proposed to help in this scenario, but this approach will reduce the sensitivity of exudative pleural effusion detection by >10%.[49,50,52]

TREATMENT

Therapeutic thoracentesis with drainage of 1.0 to 1.5 L of fluid is indicated if the patient has dyspnea at rest. Acute drainage of larger volumes is associated with reexpansion pulmonary edema, so large-volume

TABLE 62-12 Pleural Fluid Diagnostic Tests

Detection of exudative pleural effusion
Light criteria for pleural exudate: one or more of the following present:[49]
Pleural fluid/serum protein ratio >0.5
or
Pleural fluid/serum LDH ratio >0.6
or
Pleural fluid LDH greater than two thirds of the upper limit for serum LDH
Additional tests on exudative effusions
Gram stain and culture to detect bacterial infection
Cell count
Neutrophil predominance: parapneumonic, pulmonary embolism, pancreatitis
Lymphocytic predominance: cancer, tuberculosis, postcardiac surgery
Glucose: low glucose seen in parapneumonic, malignant, tuberculosis, and rheumatoid arthritis causes of pleural effusions
Cytology for malignancy: highest yield is with adenocarcinoma, much lower with squamous cell, lymphoma, or mesothelioma
Pleural fluid pH: normal pleural fluid pH around 7.64. In parapneumonic effusions, a pleural fluid pH <7.10 predicts development of empyema or persistence and indicates need for thoracostomy tube drainage.
Pleural fluid amylase: elevated in pleural effusions due to pancreatitis or esophageal rupture
Mycobacterial and fungal stains and cultures: as suggested clinically
Tuberculosis pleural fluid markers: polymerase chain reaction for mycobacterial DNA, pleural fluid adenosine deaminase, or pleural fluid interferon-γ

Abbreviation: LDH = lactate dehydrogenase.

drainage is to be avoided. Diuretic therapy typically resolves >75% of effusions due to heart failure within 2 to 3 days.

Patients with pleural empyema (gross pus or organisms on Gram stain) require drainage with large-bore thoracostomy tubes. Treatment of parapneumonic effusions is controversial (see chapter 66, "Lung Empyema and Abscess").[54-56] Clinical findings that suggest the need for thoracostomy tube drainage for parapneumonic effusion include comorbid disease, failure to respond to antibiotic therapy, anaerobic organisms, pleural fluid pH <7.10, and effusion involving >50% of the thorax or air-fluid level on the chest radiograph.[54]

REFERENCES

The complete reference list is available online at www.TintinalliEM.com.

CHAPTER 63 Hemoptysis

Troy Sims

INTRODUCTION AND EPIDEMIOLOGY

Hemoptysis is the expectoration of blood from the lungs or tracheobronchial tree. Severity ranges from mild to severe, and it can be difficult to stop. The challenge is to stabilize the patient while simultaneously determining the source and providing treatment. Most cases of hemoptysis are mild and resolve spontaneously; predicting which individual will develop large-volume bleeding is difficult. Determining the cause, location, and extent of hemoptysis requires a multidisciplinary approach.[1]

Assessing the amount of expectorated blood is difficult, because patients may either exaggerate or be unable to quantify the amount. The definition of **"massive" or "severe" hemoptysis** varies, with reported ranges from 100 mL per 24 hours to >1000 mL per 24 hours,[2,3] with a midpoint value of 600 mL per 24 hours accepted by many.[4] However, because even small volumes of blood can cause asphyxiation, any hemoptysis requires prompt attention.[5] Morbidity and mortality depend on the rate of bleeding, the ability of the patient to clear the blood, and the presence of underlying lung disease, which potentiates the effects of blood in the airways. We define **"minor" hemoptysis** as small-volume expectoration of blood in a patient with no comorbid lung disease, normal/stable oxygenation and ventilation, normal vital signs, and no risk factors for continued bleeding.

PATHOPHYSIOLOGY

Hemoptysis results from disruption of blood vessels within the walls of the airways, from trachea to bronchi, bronchioles, and the lung parenchyma (**Table 63-1**). The pulmonary arteries account for 99% of the

TABLE 63-1 Causes of Hemoptysis

Infectious
Acute bronchitis
Tuberculosis
Lung parasites (paragonimiasis, echinococcus, schistosomiasis)
Mycetoma (aspergilloma)
Structural
Bronchiectasis (cystic fibrosis, organizing pneumonia, chronic bronchitis)
Tracheoarterial fistula (tracheostomy)
Aortobronchial fistula (aortic aneurysm erosion)
Hypersensitivity pneumonitis (occupational exposure)
Vasculitides
Goodpasture's syndrome (also known as antiglomerular basement membrane disease)
Granulomatosis with polyangiitis (formerly Wegener's granulomatosis)
Systemic lupus erythematosus
Behçet's syndrome
Cardiovascular
Pulmonary embolism with infarction
Pulmonary hypertension (mitral stenosis, congestive heart failure, left-sided endocarditis)
Neoplastic
Bronchogenic carcinoma
Bronchial adenoma
Iatrogenic
Bronchoscopy
Lung biopsy
Pulmonary artery catheter injury
Traumatic
Ruptured bronchus from deceleration injury
Lung contusion from blunt injury
Penetrating trauma
Miscellaneous
Nitrogen dioxide inhalation (ice arenas)
Cocaine inhalation
Catamenial (pulmonary endometriosis)

arterial blood flow to the lungs but are a low-pressure system and rarely the source of hemoptysis. The bronchial circulation accounts for only about 1% of the arterial blood flow to the lungs but 90% of the cases of hemoptysis because it is a high-pressure system.[6] The bronchial arteries typically branch off the thoracic aorta and are responsible for supplying oxygenated blood to the bronchi, pulmonary arteries and veins, and lung parenchyma. They follow the course of bronchi along their tortuous paths. Once the bronchial arteries reach the level of capillaries, three anastomoses occur: the larger bronchial arteries can merge directly with the alveolar microvasculature; the smaller bronchial arteries can merge with the veins of the pleural and pulmonary drainage system; and bronchial capillaries can merge directly with pulmonary capillaries.[7] These connections produce a physiological right-to-left shunt comprising 5% of the total cardiac output.

Many inflammatory and infectious processes can lead to hemoptysis. Coughing in the setting of transient airway inflammation (e.g., acute bronchitis) can lead to minor bleeding even in otherwise healthy lungs. In chronic inflammatory states like tuberculosis, cystic fibrosis, or chronic obstructive pulmonary disease (COPD), the bronchial arteries can proliferate and enlarge to enhance the delivery of blood to the alveoli. Such neoangiogenesis creates thin-walled, fragile vessels prone to rupture. Chronic disease states can lead to bronchiectasis (chronic bronchial wall inflammation), resulting in dilatation and destruction of the cartilaginous support, predisposing blood vessels to rupture. In the case of *Aspergillus* infection, there can be necrotic destruction of tissue, but more often there is a colonization of a previous area of pulmonary decay, resulting in cavitary **fungal balls**. Neoangiogenesis from bronchial artery branches occurs in the cavity walls.[5] A **Rasmussen's aneurysm** is a false aneurysm of dilated, tortuous branches of pulmonary arteries crossing the wall of a tuberculosis cavity. Although tumors can directly invade the bronchial and pulmonary arteries, they also promote neoangiogenesis. In particular, squamous cell carcinoma accounts for a large number of cases of massive hemoptysis.[5]

Traumatic causes of hemoptysis include deceleration injuries and penetrating trauma to the chest. Iatrogenic causes include direct arterial injury by pulmonary artery catheterization or biopsy of lung tissue during bronchoscopy. Biopsy of a carcinoid tumor can be associated with impressive hemoptysis.[5]

Hemoptysis secondary to fistulae between an aortic aneurysm or aortic inflammation and its primary branches can precipitate catastrophic hemoptysis. Tracheo-innominate fistulae result from erosion of a tracheostomy into the innominate artery that courses posterior to the upper sternum.

Arteriovenous fistulas forming between the low-pressure pulmonary arteries and pulmonary veins have thin walls that are easily ruptured. Osler-Weber-Rendu disease is associated with hemorrhagic telangiectasias of pulmonary arteriovenous fistulas as well as telangiectasias of the skin or mucous membranes.

Cardiac disease processes that elevate pulmonary pressure, such as mitral stenosis and congenital heart disease, can trigger hemoptysis. Distal pulmonary embolism can lead to infarction of lung tissue that results in edema and hemorrhage, which can be exacerbated by the use of anticoagulants.

Vasculitis and collagen vascular diseases such as Goodpasture's syndrome, systemic lupus erythematosus, and granulomatosis with polyangiitis (formerly Wegener's granulomatosis) damage the lung parenchyma predisposing to alveolar hemorrhage. Anemia can result from chronic diffuse alveolar hemorrhage.[9]

The cause of hemoptysis in up to 30% of the cases is undetermined.[1]

CLINICAL FEATURES

First, identify if the condition is truly hemoptysis, and exclude hematemesis and epistaxis. Upper GI (UGI) bleeding is identified by a history of dark stools, nausea or abdominal pain, and positive stool guaiac test. Epistaxis can be identified on examination. Expectorated blood is bright colored if the source is the upper airway or lungs.

HISTORY

If hemoptysis resolves prior to ED evaluation, history is then paramount for evaluation.

Patients give an accurate history regarding the source of bleeding about half the time. Ask about risk factors for hemoptysis; for example, smoking predisposes to chronic lung inflammation and vascular disruption and increases the risk of bronchogenic carcinoma. Tuberculosis is a leading cause of hemoptysis worldwide, so ask about a history of tuberculosis or emigration/travel from an endemic area. High-prevalence tuberculosis areas are Africa, inner-city New York, the Middle East, and Southeast Asia. Patients with previous venous thrombotic disease may have a pulmonary embolism as a cause. Ask about hematuria or known renal insufficiency given the link to Goodpasture's syndrome. Individuals with a connective tissue disease or suggestive symptoms such as arthralgias, myalgias, recurrent fevers, or rash may develop vasculitis and hemoptysis. Granulomatosis with polyangiitis is a more insidious vasculitis; look for saddle nose deformity from septal perforation. The lung fluke, *Paragonimus* spp., infects humans after eating infected crab and crayfish and can cause hemoptysis in chronic infection. The tapeworm, *Echinococcosis* spp., can lead to hydatid cysts within the lungs. Cyclical hemoptysis coordinating with a woman's menstrual cycle could indicate a catamenial source from pulmonary endometriosis.

Cocaine and heroin inhalation can trigger diffuse alveolar hemorrhage. Nitrogen dioxide exposure in indoor ice arenas may cause hemoptysis in hockey players. Finally, ask about use of anticoagulants and recent procedures such as Swan-Ganz catheter insertion and bronchoscopy.

PHYSICAL EXAMINATION

Examine the sputum to see if it is just blood-streaked or contains clots of blood. Patients often bring a sample of expectorated sputum to the ED, which helps assessment. Look for signs suggestive of major hemoptysis or underlying lung disease, such as tachypnea, tachycardia, hypotension, labored respirations, and hypoxemia.

If airway, breathing, and circulation are maintained, then focus on the physical exam. Evaluate the nares and posterior pharynx for evidence of epistaxis. Next, assess airway patency and potential difficulty of intubation. Auscultate the lungs for any wheezing suggesting airway inflammation or focally reduced breath sounds indicating a location of bleeding. Occasionally, crackles may be present, suggesting diffuse alveolar hemorrhage or heart failure. On the cardiac exam, auscultate for murmurs of valvular disease. Check for telangiectasia and petechiae on the skin exam.

DIAGNOSIS

Most patients with minor hemoptysis need no specific tests unless on anticoagulation medication. For patients with massive hemoptysis or recurring hemoptysis, obtain a metabolic assessment including electrolytes and renal function studies, CBC, coagulation studies, and urinalysis. Baseline hemoglobin concentration is often falsely elevated in acute, rapid bleeding, as equilibration may not occur for 6 hours. Thrombocytopenia and coagulopathy increase recurrence risk and morbidity from hemoptysis. Urinalysis and renal function tests help narrow the differential diagnosis that includes Goodpasture's syndrome and granulomatosis with polyangiitis, and can also identify those at risk for contrast nephropathy if imaging is contemplated.

IMAGING

Chest x-ray is the initial imaging modality and yields a diagnosis up to 50% of the time[1]; in massive hemoptysis, x-ray is rarely normal.

Diffuse alveolar hemorrhage manifests as scattered alveolar infiltrates on chest x-ray, whereas infiltrates, atelectasis, masses, and cavitation are localized as potential sources of hemoptysis.

Multidetector row CT delineates abnormal bronchial and nonbronchial arteries using reformatted images while limiting scan time and respiratory motion artifact. It can also identify bleeding from a pulmonary artery as in Rasmussen's aneurysm or from an anomalous vessel as in Dieulafoy's disease, a tortuous dysplastic artery within the submucosa. Bronchial arterial bleeding is almost always detected on multidetector row CT, whereas nonbronchial arterial sources can be identified more than half of the time.[10] Multidetector row CT is preferred over CT angiography. The limitation of CT evaluation for hemoptysis is that areas of bleeding can appear similar to infiltrate and tumor, and active bleeding can obscure a mass within the parenchyma.

TREATMENT: MILD HEMOPTYSIS

Hemoptysis promotes anxiety in the patient and their family members, so the goal is to identify the cause, reassure those with minor features and no threat of imminent harm, and provide an appropriate ED disposition. The amount of blood expectorated, respiratory status, and risk factors for continued bleeding dictate the disposition. Patients with mild hemoptysis can be assessed as described in **Figure 63-1**.

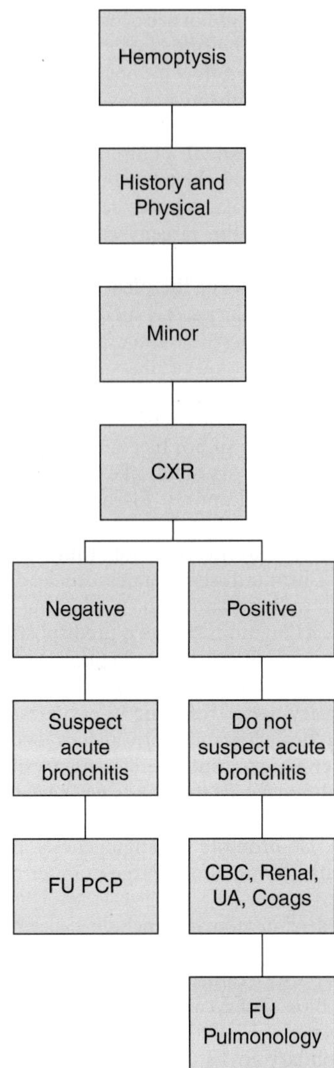

FIGURE 63-1. Diagnosis and management of minor hemoptysis. CXR = chest x-ray; FU = follow-up; PCP = primary care physician; UA = urinalysis.

DISPOSITION AND FOLLOW-UP

Most cases of hemoptysis are mild and self-limited. For mild hemoptysis, arrange follow-up with a primary care physician, otolaryngologist, or pulmonologist. Choose a pulmonologist if lung cancer or structural disease is suspected. Treat acute bronchitis with appropriate antibiotics.

TREATMENT: SEVERE HEMOPTYSIS

Massive hemoptysis requires airway control and emergency bronchoscopy and often requires consultation with cardiothoracic surgery and interventional radiology (**Figure 63-2**) for definitive control of bleeding.

AIRWAY CONTROL

In patients with more severe bleeding, assessing and ensuring the airway patency and ongoing oxygenation are key. If the patient has a tracheostomy, look for a trachea-innominate fistula; this can be controlled with direct digital pressure on the anterior portion of the trachea against the posterior aspect of the sternum using the tracheostomy as the point of access. If the patient does not have a tracheostomy and requires airway control, proceed immediately with rapid sequence intubation,[10] using a larger-diameter endotracheal tube to allow for bronchoscopy. Once intubation is successful, place the patient so the affected lung is in a dependent position to prevent spilling of blood into the unaffected side. If bleeding is uncontrollable, you may preferentially intubate the main bronchus of the unaffected lung; and alternatively, to stop bleeding, some use a Fogarty catheter (14 French/100 cm) to tamponade the bronchus of the affected lung.[5] The latter can be accomplished by passing the Fogarty catheter adjacent to the endotracheal tube once the patient is intubated (**Figure 63-3**). If attempts at intubation fail, cricothyrotomy is an option.

Once the airway is stabilized, restore volume with crystalloid and transfusion of blood products to correct for anemia and coagulopathy as indicated.

BRONCHOSCOPY

Urgent bronchoscopy is needed in massive hemoptysis to identify the origin of bleeding and provide stabilizing treatment. Bronchoscopy may be performed in the ED by a consultant if the patient is unstable. Awake flexible, fiberoptic bronchoscopy provides visualization of the more peripheral and upper lobes but does not provide optimal suctioning and does not allow for local treatment. Rigid bronchoscopy usually requires general anesthesia but can be performed with deep sedation in skilled hands. Rigid bronchoscopy cannot fully view the upper lobes and peripheral lesions, but it offers greater suctioning ability than fiberoptic bronchoscopy and can provide treatment, such as the passage of Fogarty balloon catheters for tamponade of bleeding, epinephrine instillation, and ice water lavage. After rigid bronchoscopy, a flexible bronchoscope can be passed down the lumen of a rigid bronchoscope for more detailed inspection.

DEFINITIVE BLEEDING CONTROL

Definitive bleeding control may involve consultation with a cardiothoracic surgeon or an interventional radiologist.[9,11,12] Emergency surgery is often reserved for massive hemoptysis resulting from leaking aortic aneurysm, iatrogenic pulmonary artery injury, thoracic trauma, or

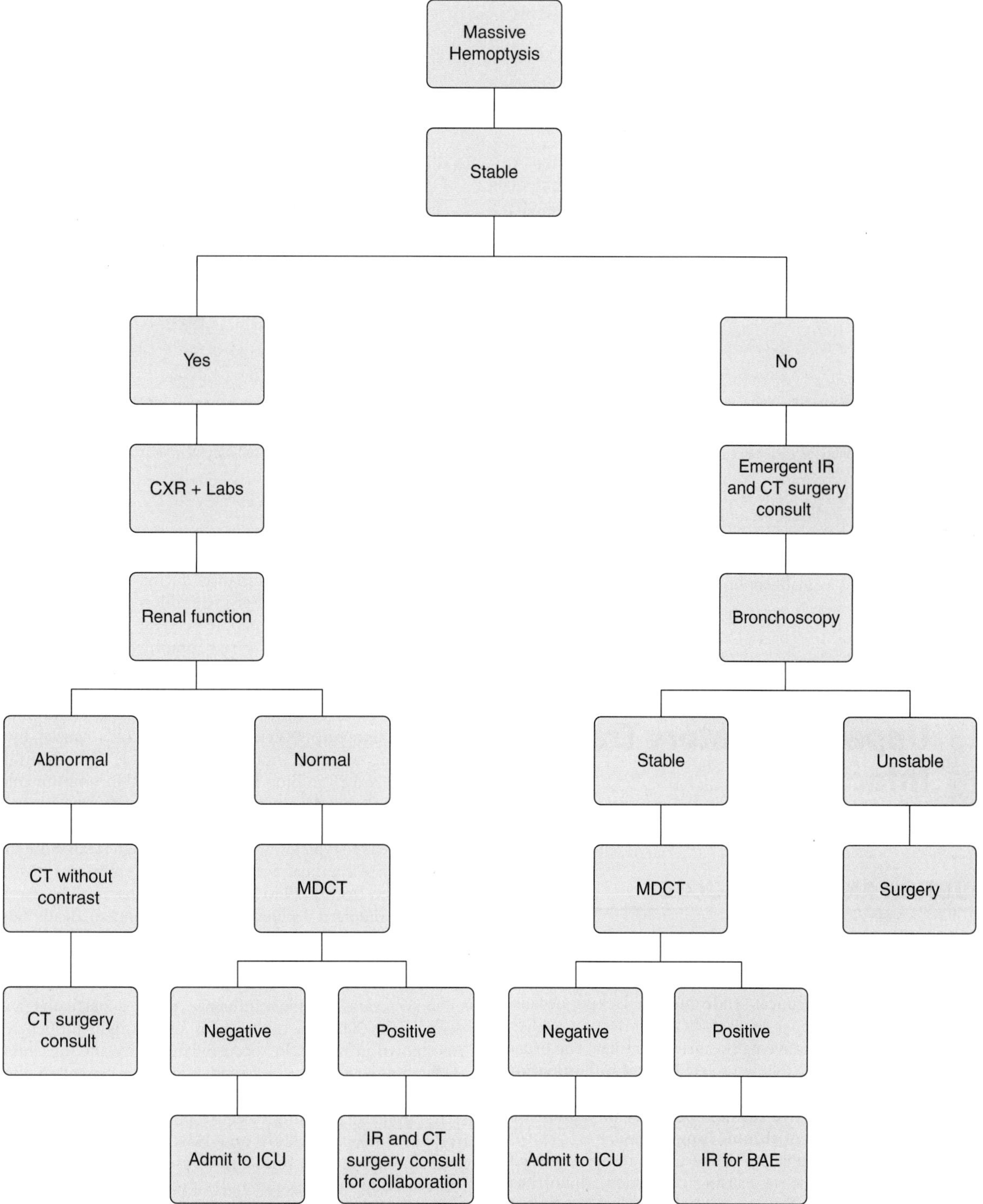

FIGURE 63-2. Algorithm for massive hemoptysis. Determine whether patient is stable based on history provided by patient, rate of ongoing bleeding, ability of patient to clear the blood, and comorbidities. BAE = bronchial artery embolization; CT surgery = cardiothoracic surgery; CXR = chest x-ray; ICU = intensive care unit; IR = interventional radiology; MDCT = multidetector computed tomography.

bleeding from a tracheo-innominate artery fistula at a tracheostomy site.[9,12] In other causes of hemoptysis or if cause is uncertain, bronchial artery embolization is a common treatment of massive and recurrent hemoptysis.[9] Even in cases of mycetoma from aspergillosis, adenoma, hydatid cyst, and active tuberculosis, where surgery is still indicated as the ultimate treatment, embolization can temporize bleeding and stabilize patients for elective surgery.[12] Risks of bronchial artery embolization include transverse myelitis due to spinal cord ischemia and pulmonary artery infarction from spread of embolic material beyond its intended site.[10]

DISPOSITION

Admission to an intensive care setting or transfer to a tertiary care center is necessary for management of severe hemoptysis.

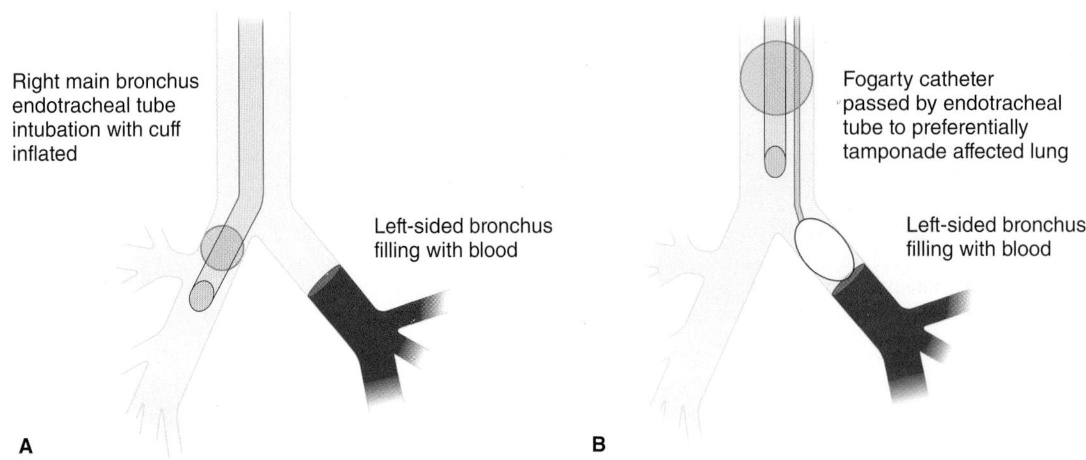

FIGURE 63-3. These are examples of techniques to control bleeding from the left lung. A. Selective right main bronchus intubation for left-sided massive hemoptysis. B. Using Fogarty catheter to direct control of hemoptysis coming from affected lung. The same techniques are used to control bleeding from the right lung. [Adapted with permission from Lordan JL, Gascoigne A, Corris PA. The pulmonary physician in critical care. Illustrative case 7: Assessment and management of massive haemoptysis. *Thorax* 2003; 58: 814-819. Copyright BMJ Publishing Group.]

REFERENCES

The complete reference list is available online at www.TintinalliEM.com.

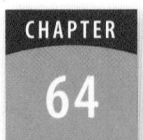

Acute Bronchitis and Upper Respiratory Tract Infections

Cedric W. Lefebvre

INTRODUCTION AND EPIDEMIOLOGY

Bacterial and viral infections of the respiratory tract can result in a wide range of clinical syndromes including acute bronchitis, the common cold, influenza, and respiratory distress syndromes. Uniform definitions for the most common of these clinical syndromes are lacking because the symptoms associated with upper respiratory tract infections (URIs) frequently overlap and their causative pathogens are similar. The broad definition of acute bronchitis is as follows: **a self-limited inflammation of the large airways characterized by cough without evidence of pneumonia, without an alternative medical disorder to explain the symptoms, or without a history of chronic lung disease.**[1]

The **common cold** is a viral infection of the upper respiratory tract, primarily affecting the nasal mucosa, causing congestion, rhinorrhea, and sneezing. **Influenza**, or the "flu," is a respiratory illness caused by influenza viruses. Symptoms of influenza infection range from mild to severe and include fever, chills, myalgias, headache, malaise, cough, and fatigue. **Severe acute respiratory syndrome** is a unique respiratory illness that has clinical characteristics similar to other URIs but confers a high rate of mortality. Reported in 2012, **Middle East respiratory syndrome coronavirus** is novel viral respiratory infection that became a concern to the World Health Organization due to its fatality rate. Infections of the upper respiratory tract also cause specific clinical conditions like otitis media, pharyngitis, epiglottitis, bronchiolitis, laryngitis, tracheitis, and sinusitis (see corresponding chapters that discuss these diseases).

EPIDEMIOLOGY

In ambulatory care settings nationwide, URIs are the third most common diagnosis.[2] Annually, the estimated direct costs of noninfluenza viral URI in the United States is $17 billion, with indirect costs exceeding $22 billion.[3] Acute bronchitis is among the most commonly diagnosed outpatient illnesses in the United States every year, with an annual incidence of about 5%,[4] predominantly during fall and winter.[1] The disorder accounts for approximately 10 million office visits per year, or 10 ambulatory visits per 1000 people per year. Symptom relief is the primary reason for office visits among adults within the first 2 weeks of illness, and many of these visits result in the unnecessary prescription of antibiotics by clinicians.[5] The common cold afflicts adults three or three times every year, whereas children suffer up to eight colds annually.[6-8] The incidence of colds caused by rhinovirus peaks during autumn months.[9] Responsible for 22 million missed school days and 23 million lost work days, the common cold generates an enormous economic burden.[4]

Influenza affects millions of people worldwide every year during seasonal outbreaks (typically November through March in the northern hemisphere). An annual average of 41,000 Americans died from influenza infection from 1979 to 2001.[10] The Centers for Disease Control and Prevention reported influenza-associated annual death rates between 1976 and 2007 that ranged from 1.4 to 16.7 deaths per 100,000 persons. Deaths associated with influenza have increased in recent decades in the United States. With 90% of influenza-associated deaths occurring among people 65 years or older, influenza poses a particular threat to the elderly.[11,12] In 2009, an outbreak of swine-origin influenza A (H1N1) virus, known as "**swine flu**," occurred in Mexico and the United States.[13,14]

Influenza viruses are classified into three genera: A, B, and C. Of these, influenza A has the greatest impact on human populations and has the greatest potential to cause pandemics. Influenza A has many serotypes, including H1N1 and H3N2, both of which are currently active among humans. Influenza viruses are unique pathogens because their evolution involves a complex process of antigenic shifts and sporadic cross-species transmissions between humans, swine, and birds. The intensity of seasonal influenza varies from one year to the next, and localized influenza outbreaks can occur during interpandemic years.[15] Furthermore, seasonal influenza outbreaks tend to occur simultaneously in countries on similar latitudes. Population immunity against influenza can be achieved by natural infection or vaccination; however, antigenic shifts allow influenza viruses to survive from year to year and preserve their capacity to cause global pandemics.

ACUTE BRONCHITIS

PATHOPHYSIOLOGY

Etiologic studies of acute bronchitis are difficult to interpret because the disease lacks a precise definition and the cause is undetermined in 31% to 84% of cases vigorously tested.[16-23] Respiratory viruses are the most common causative agents, with confirmed cases in 9% to 63% of patients studied, depending on the criteria used to make the diagnosis and the population.[16-23] Influenza A and B viruses are the most common cause, accounting for 6% to 35% of cases.[16-23] Parainfluenza virus, respiratory syncytial virus, coronavirus, adenovirus, rhinovirus, and human metapneumovirus combined account for another third of cases.[16-23] Bacterial causes of acute bronchitis range from less than 10%[16] to as much as 44% of cases in studies of older populations with comorbidities and severe symptoms.[21] *Streptococcus pneumoniae* (0% to 30% of cases), *Haemophilus influenzae* (0% to 9% of cases), and *Moraxella catarrhalis* (0% to 2% of cases) have been isolated in patients with acute bronchitis.[16-23] Atypical bacterial species such as *Bordetella pertussis* (0% to 1%),[24] *Chlamydia pneumoniae* (0% to 17%), and *Mycoplasma pneumoniae* (1% to 10%) also cause acute bronchitis.[16-23]

There are two overlapping sequential phases in the pathophysiology of acute bronchitis.[25] The first phase results from the direct inoculation of the tracheobronchial epithelium, yielding variable constitutional symptoms of fever, myalgias, malaise, and organism-specific upper respiratory symptoms, lasting 1 to 5 days, the severity of which depends on the infectious agent. The second phase is characterized by hypersensitivity of the tracheobronchial epithelium and airway receptors resulting in persistent, productive cough and lasting 1 to 3 weeks, peaking at 7 to 14 days. It is this second phase that best characterizes the illness. Sloughed epithelial cells and increased mucus produce sputum in most patients; sputum is not an indication of ongoing bacterial infection as frequently suspected by clinicians.[25] Inflammation and thickening of the bronchial and tracheal mucosa (**Figure 64-1**) result in airflow obstruction and decreased forced expiratory volume in 1 second, manifesting as wheezing and dyspnea in many patients.

CLINICAL FEATURES

The clinical manifestations of acute bronchitis depend on the infectious agent, especially in the first phase of the illness. Therefore, the initial symptoms are variable and may include fever, dyspnea, myalgias, malaise, sore throat, nasal congestion, and cough. The hallmark of acute bronchitis is cough (with or without phlegm production) persisting into the second phase of the illness lasing more than 5 days and up to 3 or 4 weeks.[1,25] The mean duration of cough is 18 days.[26] During this phase, the patient may or may not have dyspnea and/or chest discomfort. Physical exam may be completely normal, or the patient may have tachypnea, tachycardia, fever, wheezing, rhonchi, or rales. One important etiology of acute bronchitis to identify is *Bordetella pertussis,* because antibiotic treatment is recommended (see later discussion).[25,27] Suspect pertussis in patients with posttussive emesis or inspiratory whoop[27]; consider pertussis in any patient with cough lasting greater than 2 weeks if exposed to a known case or presenting during an epidemic.[1,25]

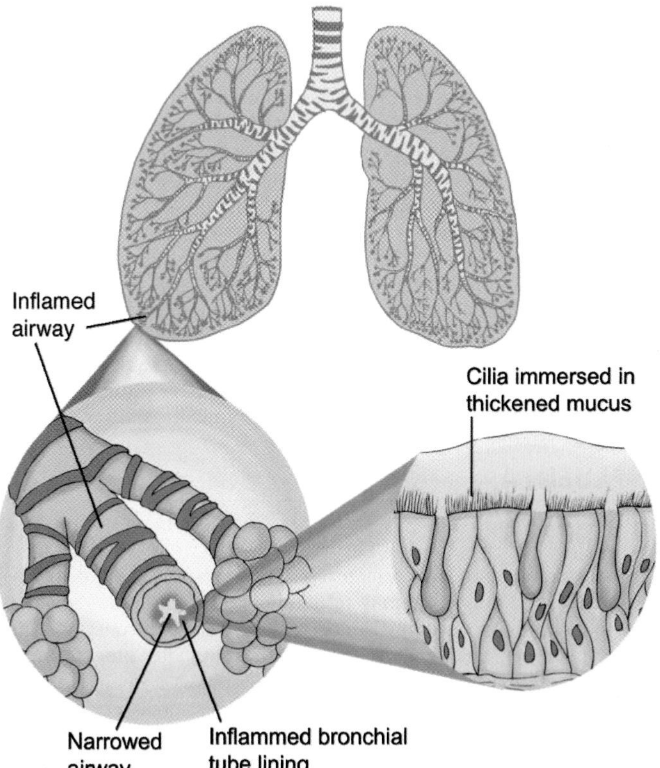

FIGURE 64-1. The respiratory epithelial infection of acute bronchitis leads to inflammation, thickening, and increased mucus production in the airways.

DIAGNOSIS

The diagnosis of acute bronchitis is made using clinical findings and historical information: when acute cough (dry or productive) is present for more than 5 days and when evidence of pneumonia, acute asthma, or an alternative explanation for the symptoms is are absent. Patients with chronic obstructive pulmonary disease are excluded from the diagnosis (see chapter 70, Chronic Obstructive Pulmonary Disease).

The primary objective in patient evaluation is carefully excluding pneumonia, either clinically or radiographically. Physicians are poor at differentiating patients with pneumonia from patients with bronchitis based on history and physical exam.[28-31] The addition of C-reactive protein testing does not improve diagnostic accuracy.[29,32] Identification of patients at low risk for pneumonia may be accomplished based on the absence of vital sign abnormalities and physical exam findings.[30,31,33] See **Table 64-1** for criteria suggesting pneumonia; patients meeting none of these criteria have a probability of pneumonia of 5% or less, and further testing is not required provided the patient has follow-up in the next 3 days and is able to return to the ED if symptoms worsen.[30,31,33] Patients with hypoxia or unstable vital signs (in the setting of respiratory symptoms) are at high risk for pneumonia and require further testing and treatment (see chapter 65, Pneumonia and Pulmonary Infiltrates). Obtain a chest radiograph in patients at intermediate risk for pneumonia. Although chest radiography remains the most common confirmatory test for pneumonia,[34,35] the sensitivity of a standard two-view chest film ranges from 69% in symptomatic patients suspected of pneumonia in the community,[36] to as low as 43.5% in patients being evaluated for pulmonary embolism in the ED[37] (both studies using high-resolution CT scan as the criterion reference). Therefore, if pneumonia is suspected on clinical grounds, treat accordingly regardless of a negative chest radiograph (see chapter 65) especially in the elderly, among whom distinctive signs and symptoms of pneumonia may be lacking.[1] Laboratory tests should be obtained if treatment for *B. pertussis* is being planned; tests include a culture, using a Dacron swab specimen, collected from the posterior nasopharynx; performing direct fluorescent antibody staining; collecting a polymerase chain reaction test; or testing for serum antibodies by enzyme-linked immunosorbent assays or Western blot.[27] Otherwise, further testing for acute bronchitis is not necessary unless alternative diagnoses require investigation. The differential diagnosis of cough is broad; see Table 64-5, Differential of Consequence: Cough, in chapter 62, Respiratory Distress.

TABLE 64-1 Clinical Criteria Suggesting Possible Pneumonia

Criteria	Clinical Finding
1	Heart rate >100 beats/min
2	Respiratory rate >24 breaths/min
3	Temperature of >38°C (100.4°F)
4	Chest examination findings of focal consolidation, egophony (increased resonance of voice sounds heard when auscultating the lungs), or fremitus (tactile vibrations felt over the chest when the patient repeats "boy oh boy")
5	Age > 64 y old

All five criteria must be absent in an individual patient to lower the probability of pneumonia to 5% or less.

TREATMENT

Case definitions of acute bronchitis that specify constitutional or respiratory symptoms including characteristics of sputum are used by research investigators and can define the spectrum of microbiologic causes but have not identified a patient subset that clearly benefits from antibiotics (see Acute Bronchitis, Treatment, later in this chapter).

Despite the fact that some patients with acute bronchitis have evidence of a bacterial infection in epidemiologic studies, antibiotics are not beneficial and are not indicated except in isolated cases.[1,5,38,39] A Cochrane analysis reviewed 15 randomized controlled trials, involving 2618 patients, including smokers and nonsmokers, comparing any antibiotic versus placebo or no treatment for acute bronchitis. At follow-up, patients receiving antibiotics were less likely to have cough (relative risk 0.64; 95% confidence interval 0.49 to 0.85), were less likely to have abnormal lung exam findings (relative risk 0.54; 95% confidence interval 0.41 to 0.70), experienced fewer days of feeling ill (mean difference −0.64; 95% confidence interval −1.16 to −0.13), and had fewer days with limited activity (mean difference −0.49; 95% CI −0.94 to −0.04).[39] Although the differences between these outcome measures reached statistical significance, the benefits demonstrated were modest (less than 1-day benefit in an illness lasting 10 to 21 days). Consider potential medication side effects, cost, and the potential for microbial resistance when using antibiotics to achieve these modest benefits for an otherwise self-limiting illness. Despite the lack of evidence supporting their use, the majority of acute bronchitis patients receive antibiotics, especially elderly patients and smokers.[1,5,38,40-42]

To counter public perception and patients' prior experiences with antibiotics, offer patient education.[43] Both printed and computer-assisted patient educational intervention reduce antibiotic prescriptions in the primary care setting.[44] Give azithromycin (500 milligrams on day 1, 250 milligrams on days 2 to 5) or similar macrolide for patients with presumed or confirmed *B. pertussis* infection to prevent transmission to contacts.[1,5,27] For influenza, if the patient presents very early in the course and influenza is suspected as the cause, consider influenza-specific antiviral therapy (see later section, Influenza).

There is little evidence to support the routine use of β_2-agonists for acute bronchitis in the absence of wheezing on physical exam.[1,5,39] A Cochrane Review reported no significant differences in daily cough scores or in duration of cough among adults with acute bronchitis who received β_2-agonists versus placebo or no treatment. Adults treated with β_2-agonists were more likely to report adverse effects such as tremor, shakiness, and nervousness (relative risk 7.94; 95% confidence interval 1.17 to 53.94).[45] However, among patients with evidence of airflow obstruction, β_2-agonists result in lower symptom scores and faster cough resolution.[45] Therefore, consider bronchodilators in acute bronchitis patients with wheezing.[46] Antihistamines do not reduce mean cough scores in acute bronchitis. Limited data are available on the efficacy of antitussives for acute bronchitis, and no data exist on the value of oral corticosteroids in nonasthmatics with acute bronchitis.[47] Dextromethorphan and codeine preparations may be no more effective than placebo in improving symptoms or reducing cough severity in acute bronchitis.[38] If used, limit antitussive therapy to those patients with a cough causing discomfort where inhibition of airway secretion clearance will not compromise breathing.[46]

COMMON COLD

PATHOPHYSIOLOGY

The pathogens responsible for causing the common cold include rhinovirus, adenovirus, parainfluenza virus, respiratory syncytial virus, enterovirus, and coronavirus. The rhinovirus, a species of the *Enterovirus* genus of the *Picornaviridae* family, is the most common cause of the common cold and causes up to 80% of all respiratory infections during peak seasons.[8,9,48] Dozens of rhinovirus serotypes and frequent antigenic changes among them make identification, characterization, and eradication exceedingly complex. After deposition in the anterior nasal mucosa, rhinovirus replication and infection are thought to begin upon mucociliary transport to the posterior nasopharynx and adenoids. As soon as 10 to 12 hours after inoculation, symptoms may begin. The mean duration of symptoms is 7 to 10 days, but symptoms can persist for as long as 3 weeks.[9] Nasal mucosal infection and the host's subsequent inflammatory response cause vasodilation and increased vascular permeability. These events result in nasal obstruction and rhinorrhea, whereas cholinergic stimulation prompts mucus production and sneezing.

CLINICAL FEATURES

Patients afflicted with the common cold can experience nasal congestion, rhinorrhea, sneezing, sore throat, cough, and malaise.[6] Clinical signs of rhinovirus infection include nasal discharge and hoarse voice. The consistency and purulence of nasal discharge in patients with the common cold do not necessarily indicate a bacterial infection. The high incidence of sinus abnormalities in patients with uncomplicated colds makes the identification of true bacterial sinusitis challenging. Sinusitis is estimated to complicate rhinovirus illness in 0.5% to 2% of cases (see chapter 244, Nose and Sinuses). Although fever is a common finding in children with rhinovirus infection, fever is uncommon in adults. Middle ear effusions may be noted, particularly among children, in whom acute otitis media occurs in up to 20% of viral URIs.[9]

DIAGNOSIS

The presence of classical features for rhinovirus infection, coupled with the absence of signs of bacterial infection or serious respiratory illness, is sufficient to make the diagnosis of the common cold. The common cold is a clinical diagnosis, and diagnostic testing is not necessary.

TREATMENT

The goal of treatment for the common cold is symptom relief. Decongestants and combination antihistamine/decongestant preparations can decrease cough, congestion, and other symptoms in adults.[43,49] Avoid cough preparations in children.[50,51] H_1-receptor antagonists may offer a modest reduction of rhinorrhea and sneezing during the first 2 days of a cold in adults.[6] First-generation antihistamines are sedating, so advise the patient about caution during their use. Topical and oral nasal decongestants (i.e., topical oxymetazoline, oral pseudoephedrine) have moderate benefit in adults and adolescents in reducing nasal airway resistance.[6,51] Evidence-based data do not support the use of antibiotics in the treatment of the common cold because they do not improve symptoms or shorten the course of illness.[6,51,52] There is also a lack of compelling evidence supporting the use of dextromethorphan for acute cough.

According to a Cochrane Review,[53] **vitamin C** used as daily prophylaxis at doses of ≥0.2 grams or more had a "modest but consistent effect" on the duration and severity of common cold symptoms (8% and 13% decreases in duration for adults and children, respectively). When taken therapeutically after the onset of symptoms, however, high-dose vitamin C has not shown clear benefit in trials.[53] *Echinacea* is an herbal remedy commonly used for treating the common cold; at this time, there is no clear evidence that echinacea is effective. Zinc has also been proposed for the treatment of common cold symptoms, and a meta-analysis found that oral zinc lozenges may shorten the course of symptoms in adults (no benefit in children), but nausea and altered taste were common, and the authors cautioned against a generalized recommendation.[54]

INFLUENZA

PATHOPHYSIOLOGY

The incubation period for influenza is 1 to 4 days, and the time interval between symptom onset among related household cases is estimated to be 3 to 4 days. Viral shedding can occur 1 day before the onset of symptoms. Shedding generally decreases by 3 to 5 days after illness in adults but can continue for more than 10 days after illness onset in children.[55] Understanding the routes of influenza transmission is critical to the development of effective infection control guidelines and for the planning of global, regional, and local pandemic responses. A debate exists over the route(s) of influenza virus transmission in mammals. It is believed that influenza can be transferred among humans by direct contact, indirect contact, droplets, or aerosolization. Short distances (<1 m) are generally required for contact and droplet transmission to occur between the source person and the susceptible individual. Airborne transmission may occur over longer distances (>1 m). Experimental and observational studies support the possibility of influenza transmission by all of these routes. However, most evidence-based data suggest that direct contact and droplet transfer are the predominant modes of transmission for influenza.[56]

CLINICAL FEATURES

Influenza infection is characterized by abrupt onset of fever, headache, dry cough, sore throat, myalgias, and rhinitis. Oropharyngeal irritation and mild cervical lymphadenopathy may be present. Although the presence of fever can help distinguish influenza from the common cold, up to one third of H1N1 influenza cases in 2009 demonstrated flu symptoms without fever.[55] Hence, influenza can be difficult to distinguish from other viral URIs. Fever and intense myalgias are generally more prevalent in influenza infection than other viral URIs. Healthy individuals with uncomplicated influenza illness will generally experience resolution of symptoms in 3 to 7 days, although cough and malaise may persist beyond 2 weeks (see earlier section, Acute Bronchitis).

DIAGNOSIS

During seasonal influenza outbreaks, most cases of influenza can be diagnosed on clinical grounds alone. A retrospective analysis of 3744 subjects showed that the development of cough and fever are the best multivariate predictors of influenza infection with a positive predictive value of 79% (P <0.001).[57] During interpandemic periods, clinical signs and symptoms may be less predictive of sporadic influenza infection, and management decisions may be aided by diagnostic testing.

If the diagnostic test result for influenza will influence management decisions, certain patients should undergo testing. When signs of influenza infection are present *during an influenza outbreak*, perform testing on hospitalized patients, patients with high-risk conditions, and patients for whom a positive result would impact clinical care decisions. When a patient presents with signs of influenza infection at *any time of year*, consider testing for (1) healthcare personnel or visitors linked to an influenza outbreak presenting within 5 days of illness and (2) patients who are epidemiologically linked to an influenza outbreak presenting within 5 days of symptom onset.[58]

When testing for influenza, obtain specimens as close to symptom onset as possible. Nasal aspirates and swabs are the best specimens to obtain when testing infants and young children. For older children and adults, swabs and aspirates from the nasopharynx are preferred. Additional specimens from endotracheal aspirates and/or bronchoalveolar lavage fluid should be obtained from ventilated patients to allow testing of the lower respiratory tract.[58] Several influenza tests are available for clinical use (**Table 64-2**). Given their ability to provide results rapidly (<30 minutes), commercially available rapid influenza diagnostic tests are most practical in the ED. However, with reported sensitivities of these kits ranging from 10% to 80% (specificity 85% to 100%), negative rapid influenza tests do not completely exclude infection.[58,59]

TABLE 64-2 Influenza Testing Modalities

Test	Time to Results	Comments
Rapid influenza test–antigen detection (EIA)	10–20 min	70%–90% sensitivity in children, <40%–60% sensitivity in adults, follow-up testing with RT-PCR should be considered to confirm negative result
Rapid influenza test–neuraminidase detection assay	20–30 min	Detects but does not distinguish between influenza A and B
RT-PCR	2 h	High sensitivity and specificity, highly recommended test for influenza
Immunofluorescence	2–4 h	Direct and indirect immunofluorescent antibody staining detects and distinguishes between influenza A/B and other viruses
Viral culture–shell vial Viral culture–cell culture isolation	48–72 h 3–10 d	Viral isolation/cultures are not screening tests; highest specificity, moderately high sensitivity; useful for confirming screening tests and surveillance purposes

Abbreviations: EIA, enzyme immunoassay, RT-PCR, reverse transcription polymerase chain reaction.

Adapted with permission from Harper S, Bradley J, Englund J, et al: Seasonal influenza in adults and children—diagnosis, treatment, chemoprophylaxis, and institutional outbreak management: clinical practice guidelines of the Infectious Diseases Society of America. *Clin Infect Dis* 48: 1003, 2009. Copyright Oxford University Press.

TREATMENT

Early antiviral treatment for influenza infection shortens the duration of influenza symptoms, decreases the length of hospital stays, and reduces the risk of complications.[60] Recommendations for the treatment of influenza are updated frequently by the Centers for Disease Control and Prevention based on epidemiologic data and antiviral resistance patterns. The treatment of influenza infection is recommended as early as possible for any patient with confirmed or suspected influenza who (1) is at high risk for influenza complications (**Table 64-3**), (2) has severe, complicated or progressive illness, or (3) is hospitalized.[55,60]

A patient who does not meet the above criteria may still require treatment depending on clinical circumstances and clinician concern. Give antiviral therapy for influenza within 48 hours of symptom onset (or earlier), and do not delay treatment for laboratory confirmation if a rapid test is not available. Antiviral treatment can provide benefit even after 48 hours in pregnant and other high-risk patients.[61,62] Therefore, consider antiviral treatment even 3 or 4 days after onset of illness in certain high-risk populations.[60]

For the 2012 to 2013 influenza season, the neuraminidase inhibitors zanamivir and oseltamivir were recommended by the Centers for Disease Control and Prevention for the prevention and treatment of influenza infection[55,60] (see **Table 64-4** for dosing recommendations). The recent development of resistance among several influenza strains to the neuraminidase inhibitors emphasizes the importance of following updated epidemiologic reports and recommendations by the Centers for Disease Control and Prevention and other health agencies.

Vaccination is the most effective method of preventing influenza illness. Antiviral chemoprophylaxis is also helpful in preventing influenza (70% to 90% effective) and should be considered as an adjunct to vaccination in certain scenarios or when vaccination is unavailable or not possible. Generally, antiviral chemoprophylaxis is used during periods of influenza activity for (1) high-risk persons who cannot receive vaccination (due to contraindications) or in whom recent vaccination does not, or is not expected to, afford a sufficient immune response; (2) controlling outbreaks among high-risk persons in institutional settings; and (3) high-risk persons with influenza exposures.[58,60] For more information about the indications for antiviral chemoprophylaxis, consult the Centers for Disease Control and Prevention website

TABLE 64-3 Persons at Higher Risk for Complications of Influenza Infection[34]

Children <5 y (especially <2 y)
Adults ≥65 y
Persons with chronic illnesses and/or conditions*
Persons with immunosuppression, including secondary to human immunodeficiency virus infection or medications
Women who are pregnant or postpartum (within 2 weeks of delivery)
Persons <18 y receiving long-term aspirin therapy
Residents of nursing homes and other chronic care facilities
Persons who are morbidly obese (body mass index ≥40)
American Indians/Alaska Natives

*Includes persons with chronic pulmonary (including asthma, cystic fibrosis), cardiovascular (except hypertension alone), renal, hematologic (including sickle cell disease), and hepatic diseases; metabolic disorders (including diabetes mellitus); cancers; or neurologic and neurodevelopment conditions including disorders of the brain, spinal cord, peripheral nerve, and muscle such as cerebral palsy, epilepsy (seizure disorders), stroke, intellectual disability (mental retardation), moderate to severe developmental delay, muscular dystrophy, or spinal cord injury.

TABLE 64-4 Neuraminidase Inhibitor Dosing Recommendations[60]

Oseltamivir (Tamiflu®)		
	Treatment	Chemoprophylaxis
Adults	75 milligrams twice daily × 5 d*	75 milligrams once daily × 7 d†
Children‡		
<15 kg	30 milligrams twice daily × 5 d*	30 milligrams once daily × 7 d
15–23 kg	45 milligrams twice daily × 5 d*	45 milligrams once daily × 7 d
24–40 kg	60 milligrams twice daily × 5 d*	60 milligrams once daily × 7 d
>40 kg	75 milligrams twice daily × 5 d*	75 milligrams once daily × 7 d
Zanamivir (Relenza®)		
	Treatment	Chemoprophylaxis
Adults	10 milligrams (2 inhalations) twice daily × 5 d*	10 milligrams (2 inhalations) once daily × 7 d†
Children‡		
≥5 y old#	N/A	10 milligrams (2 inhalations) once daily
≥7 y old	10 milligrams (2 inhalations) twice daily × 5 d*	10 milligrams (2 inhalations) once daily × 7 d†

*Longer courses can be considered for patients who remain severely ill after 5 days of treatment.

†For controlling outbreaks in long-term care facilities, the Centers for Disease Control and Prevention recommend a minimum of 2 weeks of chemoprophylaxis and up to 1 week after the last identified case, and 7 days after most recent known exposure in other cases.

‡Antiviral medications are not Food and Drug Administration approved for treatment or prophylaxis of influenza in children age <12 months. Limited data are available in this age group. Oseltamivir was used in infants during the 2009 influenza A (H1N1) pandemic under Emergency Use Authorization (expired June 2010).

#Zanamivir is approved for treatment of influenza in children age ≥7 years and for influenza chemoprophylaxis in children age ≥5 years.

(http://www.cdc.gov/flu). Widespread and routine use of chemoprophylaxis is discouraged due to the possibility of promoting resistance and depleting supplies for high-risk or critically ill patients during influenza outbreaks.

DISEASE COMPLICATIONS

Complications of influenza infection include primary influenza viral pneumonia; secondary bacterial pneumonia; sinusitis; otitis media; coinfection with bacterial agents; and exacerbation of preexisting medical conditions, particularly asthma and chronic obstructive pulmonary disease. Pneumonia is one of the most common complications of influenza illness in children and contributes significantly to morbidity and mortality. Children with influenza-associated pneumonia are more likely than children admitted for influenza illness to develop respiratory failure (11% vs. 3%), require intensive care unit admission (21% vs. 11%), and die (0.9% vs. 0.3%).[63]

SEVERE ACUTE RESPIRATORY SYNDROME (SARS)

Severe acute respiratory syndrome is a rapidly progressive illness caused by a coronavirus, the severe acute respiratory syndrome coronavirus. Emerging in China in November 2002, severe acute respiratory syndrome quickly became a global health concern by early 2003. The World Health Organization reported 8096 probable severe acute respiratory syndrome cases worldwide through April 21, 2004. Deaths attributed to severe acute respiratory syndrome totaled 774 during that time period (9.6% case fatality rate).[64] Isolation procedures for suspected severe acute respiratory syndrome patients include airborne, droplet, and contact isolation. Healthcare providers should wear an N95 or higher respiratory facemask when caring for patients with severe acute respiratory syndrome, in addition to glove, gown, and eye protection.

Although severe acute respiratory syndrome shares many clinical features with viral URIs, its clinical characteristics are ill-defined, and case definitions were updated frequently during its emergence. The clinical features of coronavirus infection include fever (99% frequency), nonproductive cough, dyspnea, myalgias, headache, and diarrhea. Many cases progress to a moderate-severe condition characterized by hypoxia and dyspnea at rest. Respiratory failure requiring mechanical ventilation occurs in 10% to 20% of hospitalized patients with severe acute respiratory syndrome. Risk factors for death in coronavirus infection include age >60 years, diabetes mellitus, and hepatitis B infection.[65]

Consider the diagnosis of severe acute respiratory syndrome on clinical grounds when the patient has been exposed to known cases or has traveled to regions with severe acute respiratory syndrome activity. Chest radiographs may show subtle peripheral pulmonary infiltrates. Chest CT demonstrates ground-glass consolidation during early phases of illness. Lymphopenia, thrombocytopenia, elevated lactic dehydrogenase, liver enzymes, and creatine phosphokinase levels have been reported but are not pathognomonic for severe acute respiratory syndrome.[66] When severe acute respiratory syndrome is suspected, collect two specimens (from different locations) for polymerase chain reaction testing and obtain serum for serologic testing. To date, several diagnostic tests are available to detect coronavirus, but each has substantial limitations in sensitivity, specificity, or clinical practicality. Treatment for severe acute respiratory syndrome is largely supportive. When lopinavir-ritonavir was added to standard therapy (ribavirin and corticosteroids) for severe acute respiratory syndrome during a nonrandomized, open-label study in Hong Kong, a significant reduction in death rate was noted. Limitations in this study, however, make it difficult to derive definitive conclusions about its efficacy.[65]

MIDDLE EAST RESPIRATORY SYNDROME CORONAVIRUS (MERS)

In the summer of 2012, in Jeddah, Saudi Arabia, a novel coronavirus was isolated from the sputum of a patient with pneumonia and renal failure.[67] Since that time, the virus has been named the Middle East respiratory syndrome coronavirus. As of August 30, 2013, there have been 108 reported cases (several still hospitalized at that time) and 50 deaths.[68] All cases have been directly or indirectly linked to one of four countries: Saudi Arabia, Qatar, Jordan, and the United Arab Emirates, with the largest number from Saudi Arabia.[69] The original source is suspected to have come from bats.[70] Median age of patients is 56 years (range 2 to 94 years). All patients had respiratory symptoms, and some had GI symptoms including abdominal pain and diarrhea. The majority of patients experience severe acute respiratory disease requiring hospitalization; the case fatality rate has been reported as 56%. In addition to respiratory failure, renal failure and septic shock are common causes of death. Several patients had significant preexisting comorbidities, including immunosuppression. Cases have included healthcare workers and family contacts. A documented patient-to-patient nosocomial transmission has been reported in France.[71] Treatment is supportive and frequently requires mechanical ventilation, dialysis, and extracorporeal membrane oxygenation. Nonspecific antiviral drugs have been used, such as ribavirin, lopinavir, and type I interferon, but their efficiency is still unclear.[72] Patients should be isolated in an airborne infection isolation room.[73] Healthcare workers should wear personal protective equipment including gloves, gown, eye protection, and a fit-tested N95 respirator facemask.[73]

PERTUSSIS

Pertussis, or "whooping cough," is an acute respiratory infection in humans caused by the aerobic gram-negative rod, *B. pertussis*. Pertussis toxins cause respiratory epithelial and mucosal injury and interfere with immune cell function. Pertussis pneumonia can occur in children, but in school-age children, adolescents, and adults, URIs are the rule.

IMMUNIZATION

Although pertussis is often considered a disease of infants (primarily in those <1 year old who have not completed three doses of vaccination) and a disease in developing countries where immunization is not universal, in North America, the disease is now more common in school-age children and adults. School-age children are the usual sources of infection, and adults may serve as carriers of disease. Cyclical outbreaks occur every 3 to 5 years despite widespread immunization practices.

There are two types of vaccines, whole-cell and acellular. Whole-cell pertussis vaccination is effective for about 10 years and is used in developing nations. The acellular diphtheria, tetanus, and pertussis vaccine (DTaP), developed to remove toxins from the cell membrane, does not protect as long as the whole-cell vaccine and is typically used in the developed world.[74] The typical immunization schedule is at 2, 4, 6, and 18 months of age and a booster at age 5. Adolescents should receive a DTaP booster. **Pregnant women** should receive a booster of DTaP to protect neonates and infants and to prevent infection in the mother. For the unimmunized elderly (>65 years old), one dose of DTaP is recommended.[75] Although the vaccine is specifically not registered for the elderly,[76] a study of nearly 120,000 individuals ≥65 years old did not demonstrate any increase in inflammatory or allergic events in those receiving DTaP compared with those receiving only the tetanus and diphtheria vaccine.[77] There is no lifelong immunity after a clinical episode of pertussis.

CLINICAL FEATURES

Clinical features in adults are those of the common cold, but after 1 week, prolonged, paroxysmal, and sleep-disturbing cough develops. Whooping is uncommon in adults. Consider pertussis in situations of chronic cough >2 weeks in duration. Cough may last for several months. Since pertussis is highly communicable, with an attack rate of about 20% even in the immunized, suspect pertussis if there is contact with other individuals with prolonged cough. Except in the elderly, pertussis in adults is not associated with pneumonia. Clinical or radiologic evidence of pneumonia in adults or the elderly suggests secondary bacterial infection.

DIAGNOSIS

Diagnosis is often clinical, especially during epidemics. Definitive diagnosis is usually by polymerase chain reaction of nasopharyngeal secretions or serologic detection of antibodies. Other causes of respiratory illnesses with prolonged cough include *Mycoplasma*, *Chlamydophila*, influenza virus, and other respiratory viruses. In adults, chronic cough can be associated with angiotensin-converting enzyme inhibitors, gastroesophageal reflux, or asthma.

TREATMENT

Treatment of pertussis is azithromycin, 500 milligrams PO on day 1 and 250 milligrams PO on days 2 to 5. Trimethoprim-sulfamethoxazole, 160 milligrams/800 milligrams twice a day for 14 days (check renal dosing), is an alternative to those allergic to, or unable to tolerate, macrolides. Treatment is best if started early, in the first week. After that, antibiotic treatment does not alter the duration of cough. Chemoprophylaxis is typically given for household contacts, although the evidence base for such treatment is weak.

REFERENCES

The complete reference list is available online at www.TintinalliEM.com.

CHAPTER 65 Pneumonia and Pulmonary Infiltrates

Gerald Maloney
Eric Anderson
Donald M. Yealy

PNEUMONIA

EPIDEMIOLOGY

Pneumonia is an infection of the alveoli (the gas-exchanging portion of the lung) emanating from different pathogens, notably bacteria and viruses, but also fungi. Community-acquired pneumonia occurs in 4 million people and results in 1 million hospitalizations per year in the United States.[1,2] Pneumonia is the eighth leading cause of death, particularly among older adults,[3] and is the most common trigger for sepsis. Those who develop hospital- or other healthcare-associated pneumonia (acquired after placement in a care facility) often have infection from resistant organisms (**Table 65-1**).[4,5]

TABLE 65-1 Acquisition Environment Classification for Pneumonia

Classification	Criteria
Community-acquired pneumonia	Acute pulmonary infection in a patient who is not hospitalized or residing in a long-term care facility 14 or more days before presentation
Hospital-acquired pneumonia	New infection occurring 48 or more hours after hospital admission
Ventilator-acquired pneumonia	New infection occurring 48 or more hours after starting mechanical ventilation
Healthcare-associated pneumonia	Patients hospitalized for 2 or more days within the past 90 days
	Nursing home/long-term care residents
	Patients receiving home IV antibiotic therapy
	Dialysis patients
	Patients receiving chronic wound care
	Patients receiving chemotherapy
	Immunocompromised patients

PATHOPHYSIOLOGY

Pathogenic lung organisms are usually aspirated, especially in the hospital or healthcare setting (where eating is often not done sitting upright for dubious reasons), although inhalation is another potential route. *Staphylococcus aureus* and *Streptococcus pneumoniae* can produce pneumonia from hematogenous seeding. Patients most at risk for pneumonia are those with a predisposition to aspiration, impaired mucociliary clearance, or risk of bacteremia (**Table 65-2**).

Some forms of pneumonia produce an intense inflammatory response within the alveoli that leads to filling of the air space with exudate and white blood cells. Bacterial pneumonia results in an intense inflammatory response and tends to cause a productive cough. Atypical organisms often trigger a less intense inflammatory response and create a milder or nonproductive cough.

In about half of patients with community-acquired pneumonia, no specific pathogen is identified. When an organism is identified, the pneumococcus is still the most common, followed by viruses and the atypical agents *Mycoplasma*, *Chlamydia*, and *Legionella*. Most patients with severe community-acquired pneumonia who were otherwise healthy have *S. pneumoniae* and *Legionella* as pathogens.

In up to 5% of cases, more than one pathogen exists. In nursing home residents, alcoholics, and those with human immunodeficiency virus (HIV) infection and depressed CD4 counts, all the common pathogens exist along with others rarely seen in other patients.

CLINICAL FEATURES

Patients with pneumonia frequently will present with cough (79% to 91%), fatigue (90%), fever (71% to 75%), dyspnea (67% to 75%), sputum production (60% to 65%), and pleuritic chest pain (39% to 49%).[6] Despite described patterns of presentation, the variability in the individual symptoms and physical findings can make clinical diagnosis and differentiation from bronchitis and other upper respiratory tract disease difficult.[7,8] Many types of pneumonia do not have a sudden and characteristic presentation, and many patients with pneumonia have an antecedent viral upper respiratory infection with coryza, low-grade fever, rhinorrhea, or nonproductive cough. Weight loss, malaise, dizziness, and weakness may be associated with pneumonia. Some of the atypical agents are associated with headache or GI illness. Occasionally, pneumonia is associated with

TABLE 65-2 Risk Factors for Pneumonia

Risk Factors for Pneumonia
Aspiration risk
Swallowing and esophageal motility disorders
Stroke
Nasogastric tube
Intubation
Seizure and syncope
Bacteremia risk
Indwelling vascular devices
Intrathoracic devices (e.g., chest tube)
Debilitation
Alcoholism
Extremes of age
Neoplasia
Immunosuppression
Chronic diseases
Diabetes
Renal failure
Liver failure
Valvular heart disease
Congestive heart failure
Pulmonary disorders
Chronic obstructive pulmonary disease
Chest wall disorders
Skeletal muscle disorders
Bronchial obstruction
Bronchoscopy
Viral lung infections

extrapulmonary symptoms, including joint pain, hematuria, or skin rashes. **Table 65-3** lists common pathogen and clinical feature correlations, all of which can vary or be absent in an individual patient.

The physical examination in a patient with acute pneumonia may show evidence of alveolar fluid (rales), consolidation (bronchial breath sounds), pleural effusion (dullness and decreased breath sounds), or bronchial congestion (rhonchi and wheezing).[7,8] Radiologic findings in pneumonia sometimes provide a specific pathogenic diagnosis (Table 65-3).

Pneumococcal Pneumonia The elderly, children <2 years old, minorities, children who attend group day care centers, and those with immune-depressing comorbid conditions (e.g., previous splenectomy, transplantation, HIV infection, sickle cell disease) are at highest risk for pneumococcal pneumonia. Classically, patients with pneumococcal pneumonia present with sudden onset of disease with rigors, bloody sputum, high fever, and chest pain with lobar infiltrates (**Figure 65-1**); 25% will have parapneumonic pleural effusions. Patients with chronic lung disease, nursing home patients, or otherwise healthy elderly patients tend to have a slower progression of pneumonia, with symptoms of malaise with minimal cough or sputum production.

Laboratory findings in pneumonia include leukocytosis, elevation of the serum bilirubin or hepatic enzymes, and hyponatremia; none is diagnostic of the infection, but all detail the other organ involvement that can occur.

Pneumococcal pneumonia responds to a variety of antibiotics, although there is an increased incidence of penicillin-, macrolide-, and fluoroquinolone-resistant pneumococci.[9] Penicillin resistance ranges from 5% to 80%, depending on location, with increasing resistance reported in Spain, Italy, and Eastern Europe. Resistance is also increasing to tetracycline and trimethoprim-sulfamethoxazole. Patients with intermediate penicillin-resistant pneumococci may still be effectively treated with routine antibiotics so long as an adequate dose is administered.[10] However, the bacteriologic agent is rarely known to clinicians at the start of therapy. Patients with highly penicillin-resistant pneumococci require treatment with vancomycin, imipenem, a newer respiratory fluoroquinolone, or ketolide.

TABLE 65-3 Clinical Characteristics of Common Bacterial Pneumonias

Organism	Symptoms	Sputum	Chest X-Ray
Streptococcus pneumoniae	Sudden onset, fever, rigors, pleuritic chest pain, productive cough, dyspnea	Rust-colored; gram-positive encapsulated diplococci	Lobar infiltrate, occasionally patchy, occasional pleural effusion
Staphylococcus aureus	Gradual onset of productive cough, fever, dyspnea, especially just after viral illness	Purulent; gram-positive cocci in clusters	Patchy, multilobar infiltrate; empyema, lung abscess
Klebsiella pneumoniae	Sudden onset, rigors, dyspnea, chest pain, bloody sputum; especially in alcoholics or nursing home patients	Brown "currant jelly"; thick, short, plump, gram-negative, encapsulated, paired coccobacilli	Upper lobe infiltrate, bulging fissure sign, abscess formation
Pseudomonas aeruginosa	Recently hospitalized, debilitated, or immunocompromised patient with fever, dyspnea, cough	Gram-negative coccobacilli	Patchy infiltrate with frequent abscess formation
Haemophilus influenzae	Gradual onset, fever, dyspnea, pleuritic chest pain; especially in elderly and COPD patients	Short, tiny, gram-negative encapsulated coccobacilli	Patchy, frequently basilar infiltrate, occasional pleural effusion
Legionella pneumophila	Fever, chills, headache, malaise, dry cough, dyspnea, anorexia, diarrhea, nausea, vomiting	Few neutrophils and no predominant bacterial species	Multiple patchy nonsegmented infiltrates, progresses to consolidation, occasional cavitation and pleural effusion
Moraxella catarrhalis	Indolent course of cough, fever, sputum, and chest pain; more common in COPD patients	Gram-negative diplococci found in sputum	Diffuse infiltrates
Chlamydophila pneumoniae	Gradual onset, fever, dry cough, wheezing, occasionally sinus symptoms	Few neutrophils, organisms not visible	Patchy subsegmental infiltrates
Mycoplasma pneumoniae	Upper and lower respiratory tract symptoms, nonproductive cough, headache, malaise, fever	Few neutrophils, organisms not visible	Interstitial infiltrates, (reticulonodular pattern), patchy densities, occasional consolidation
Anaerobic organisms	Gradual onset, putrid sputum, especially in alcoholics	Purulent; multiple neutrophils and mixed organisms	Consolidation of dependent portion of lung; abscess formation

Abbreviation: COPD = chronic obstructive pulmonary disease.

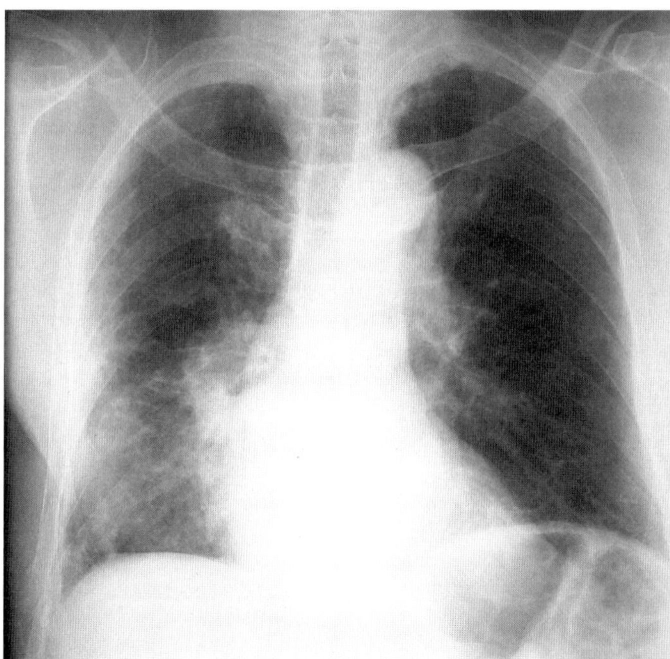

FIGURE 65-1. Lobar pneumonia.

Other Bacterial Pneumonias ***S. aureus*** pneumonia is a consideration in patients with chronic lung disease, patients with laryngeal cancer, immunosuppressed patients, nursing home patients, or others at risk for aspiration pneumonia. *S. aureus* pneumonia may occur in otherwise healthy patients after viral illness, such as during an influenza epidemic, although pneumococcal pneumonia is still more common. Patients with staphylococcal pneumonia typically have an insidious onset of disease with low-grade fever, sputum production, and dyspnea. The chest radiograph usually demonstrates extensive disease with empyema, pleural effusions, and multiple areas of infiltrate (**Figure 65-2**). If leucocidin excretion by the organism accompanies this infection (rare and not predictable), rapid progression and death are common even with adequate therapy. Patients with healthcare-acquired pneumonia are at risk for infection with methicillin-resistant *S. aureus*.[5,11]

Klebsiella pneumonia often occurs in compromised patients: those at risk of aspiration, alcoholics, the elderly, and those with chronic lung disease. In contrast to *S. aureus*, patients with *Klebsiella* have acute onset of severe disease with fever, rigors, and chest pain. Patients with *Klebsiella* may develop pulmonary abscesses, although more commonly radiographs show a lobar infiltrate.

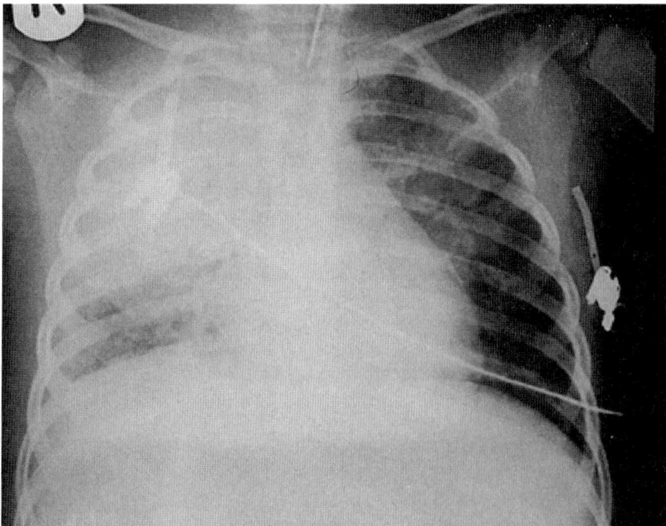

FIGURE 65-2. Staphylococcal pneumonia with extensive infiltration and effusion or empyema.

Pseudomonas causes a severe pneumonia with cyanosis, confusion, and other signs of systemic illness. The chest radiograph may show bilateral lower lobe infiltrates, occasionally associated with empyema. *Pseudomonas* is not a typical cause of community-acquired pneumonia, more often seen in patients with a prolonged hospitalization, who have received broad-spectrum antibiotics or high-dose steroid therapy, who have structural lung disease (including cystic fibrosis), or who are nursing home residents.

Haemophilus influenzae pneumonia occurs in any age, although it most commonly occurs in the elderly, or in those with chronic lung disease, sickle cell disease, or immunocompromised disorders and in alcoholics and diabetics. Since the onset of routine vaccination of children, the incidence of *H. influenzae* pneumonia in children has markedly dropped. Patients with this type of community-acquired pneumonia may either have a gradual progression of disease with low-grade fever and sputum production or occasionally the sudden onset of chest pain, dyspnea, and sputum production. Bacteremia may be seen in older adults. Pleural effusions and multilobar infiltrates are common findings in *H. influenzae* pneumonia.

Moraxella catarrhalis pneumonia has clinical features similar in spectrum to those of *H. influenzae*. Typically, patients with *M. catarrhalis* present with an indolent course of cough and sputum production, with fever and pleuritic chest pain are common. The chest radiograph usually shows diffuse infiltrates.

Pneumonia from Atypical Bacteria and Viruses The atypical bacteria are *Legionella*, *Chlamydophila*, and *Mycoplasma*. Because these agents lack a cell wall, they do not respond to β-lactam antibiotics but respond to macrolides or a respiratory fluoroquinolone.

Legionella can cause a range of illness from benign self-limited disease to multisystem organ failure with acute respiratory distress syndrome. Patients at particular risk include cigarette smokers, patients with chronic lung disease, transplant patients, and the immunosuppressed. **There is no seasonality to *Legionella* pneumonia, making it a more prominent cause of pneumonia in the summer when other pathogens decline in frequency.** *Legionella* pneumonia is commonly complicated by GI symptoms, including abdominal pain, vomiting, and diarrhea. In addition, *Legionella* can affect other organ systems, causing sinusitis, pancreatitis, myocarditis, and pyelonephritis. The chest radiograph frequently shows a patchy infiltrate, with the occasional appearance of hilar adenopathy and pleural effusions (**Figure 65-3**).

Infection with *Chlamydophila* usually causes a mild illness with sore throat, low-grade fever, and nonproductive cough, although occasionally patients have a more severe course. Patients with *Chlamydophila* pneumonia frequently have rales or rhonchi. The chest radiograph usually shows a patchy subsegmental infiltrate, overlapping with the appearance of *Legionella* pneumonia. Chlamydial infection is linked to adult-onset asthma.

Mycoplasma pneumonia also occurs year-round, although it tends to cluster in epidemics every 4 to 8 years. *Mycoplasma* may cause a subacute respiratory illness with cough, sore throat, and headache. *Mycoplasma* pneumonia is also frequently associated with retrosternal chest pain. Unlike *Legionella*, *Mycoplasma* usually is not associated with GI symptoms. Like the other atypical pathogens, chest radiograph often shows patchy infiltrates, commonly with hilar adenopathy or pleural effusions. *Mycoplasma* occasionally causes extrapulmonary symptoms, including rash, neurologic symptoms, arthralgia, hematologic abnormalities, or rarely acute kidney injury. Bullous myringitis is not at all specific for *Mycoplasma* infection but is associated with many other causes of otitis media.

Viruses cause pneumonia, often severe; influenza is the most common viral pneumonia and is seasonal. The outbreak of severe acute respiratory syndrome and the Middle East respiratory syndrome, both from coronaviruses, demonstrates how a local infection can be rapidly transmitted worldwide.[12] The most recent pandemic viral infection has been H1N1 in 2009. Varicella, typically benign in most childhood infections, can lead to a virulent pneumonia in pregnant patients.

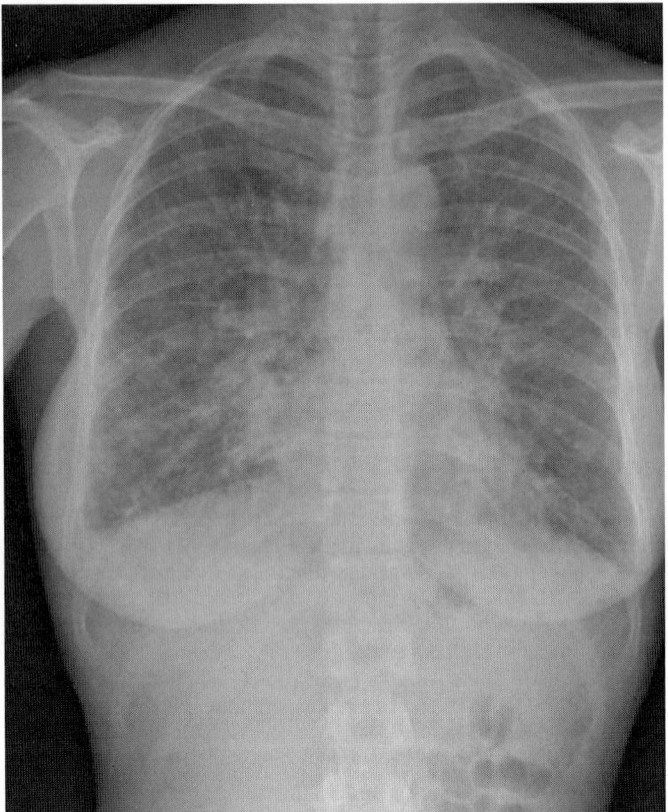

FIGURE 65-3. Classic diffuse, patchy infiltrates seen with *Legionella pneumonia*.

Further discussion of life-threatening viral infections is covered elsewhere (see chapter 153, "Serious Viral Infections").

DIAGNOSIS

Suspect pneumonia from symptoms and signs (often fever, cough, dyspnea, or weakness with rales or rhonchi), while recognizing that each individual symptom or finding lacks high accuracy. When symptoms suggest a possibility, order a chest radiograph; if clinical findings suggest pneumonia (with or without an infiltrate on chest x-ray), treat emprically.[13] No single set of recommendations for diagnostic testing applies to all patients, requiring clinical judgment. In otherwise healthy, mildly ill, ambulatory patients, no further ancillary testing may be necessary. To optimally risk-stratify anyone over 50 years old or more than mildly ill, seek evidence of other organ affliction; this is done by including CBC, serum electrolytes, BUN, creatinine, and glucose levels. Pulse oximetry is needed in all cases because a saturation on room air of <91% is associated with more complications. An arterial blood gas analysis is reserved for those appearing ill, with underlying lung disease, with oxygen desaturation, or in respiratory distress.

Most patients do not require identification of a specific organism through blood or sputum analysis to direct antibiotic treatment. The incidence of positive blood cultures in nonhospitalized patients with community-acquired pneumonia is low, pathogen identification usually does not alter treatment, and the majority of patients respond to empiric antibiotic treatment. The value of sputum culture is similar to the value of blood cultures and often limited by poor sampling, with less than 15% being adequate and helpful.[14] Atypical agents may be detected by evaluation of titers from acute and convalescence sera or by direct fluorescent antibody testing.

In hospitalized community-acquired pneumonia patients, the incidence of positive blood cultures increases along with increasing disease severity.[15] For this reason, **obtain blood cultures in those admitted to the intensive care unit and in those with leukopenia, cavitary lesions, severe liver disease, alcohol abuse, asplenia, or pleural effusions.**[16] In any admitted patient, a **sputum culture and Gram stain are options if an adequate sample can be obtained.** *Legionella* urine antigen tests are useful in intensive care unit patients, alcoholics, those with classic findings, and those with a recent (within the past 2 weeks) travel history.

The differential diagnosis of patients with cough and radiographic abnormality includes lung cancer, tuberculosis, pulmonary embolism, chemical or hypersensitivity pneumonitis, connective tissue disorders, granulomatous disease, and fungal infections. Because radiographic signs of pneumonia vary, it is difficult to predict the causative microorganism by its radiographic appearance. In general, patients with bacterial pneumonia are more likely to have unilobar or focal infiltrates than patients with viral or atypical pneumonia. Hilar adenopathy is more common in patients with atypical pneumonia. Pleural effusions can accompany bacterial, viral, or atypical pneumonia. Cavitary lesions occur in patients with bacterial pneumonia or tuberculosis. Lung abscesses are rare complications of pneumonia in the antibiotic era, usually due to *S. aureus* or *Klebsiella*. Pneumococcal and staphylococcal pneumonia may mimic a lung mass, along with other atypical pneumonias, such as Q fever and tularemia.

PNEUMONIA IN SPECIAL POPULATIONS

Pneumonia in Alcoholics Alcoholics have a higher risk than the normal population for many lung diseases, including pneumonia, tuberculosis, pleurisy, bronchitis, empyema, and chronic obstructive pulmonary disease. Alcoholics are more likely than the general population to be undernourished, to develop aspiration pneumonitis, to be heavy smokers, and to have sequelae of alcoholic cirrhosis and portal hypertension. Compared with the nonalcoholic, the alcoholic has greater oropharyngeal colonization with gram-negative bacteria, and also has depressed granulocyte and lymphocyte counts with impaired neutrophil delivery.

***S. pneumoniae* is the most common pathogen causing pneumonia in alcoholics, but *Klebsiella* species and *Haemophilus* species are also important agents of infection.** In general, rates of pneumonia and subsequent mortality are higher in alcoholics compared with nonalcoholic patients.

Pneumonia in Diabetics Diabetic patients between the ages of 25 and 64 years old are four times more likely to have pneumonia and influenza, and diabetics are two to three times more likely than nondiabetics to die with pneumonia and influenza as an underlying cause of death. **Pathogens that occur with increased frequency in diabetic patients include *S. aureus*, gram-negative bacteria, mucormycosis, and *Mycobacterium tuberculosis*.** Infections due to *S. pneumoniae*, *Legionella pneumophila*, and influenza are associated with increased morbidity and mortality in diabetic patients.

Pneumonia in Pregnant Women Community-acquired pneumonia in pregnancy is one of the most serious nonobstetric infections, with maternal mortality of approximately 3%. Pregnancy does not alter the course of bacterial pneumonia, but the prognosis of viral pneumonia during pregnancy is more serious than in the nonpregnant patient. Pregnant woman are at risk for developing severe influenza-associated pneumonia, and antivirals are often used in this patient group (see chapter 153, "Serious Viral Infections").

Pregnant women who develop varicella pneumonia are more often smokers and have skin lesions suggestive of the disease on exam. **Obtain a chest radiograph and pulse oximetry measure in any pregnant woman with symptoms of respiratory tract infection and varicella exposure.** Empiric IV acyclovir is often used, although there is little evidence that the timing of administration affects outcome.

Pneumocystis jiroveci pneumonia is the most common cause of acquired immunodeficiency syndrome–related death in pregnant women in the United States, with a mortality of approximately 50%; over half receive mechanical ventilation during hospitalization. Combination treatment with pentamidine, steroids, and eflornithine improves survival compared with patients treated with trimethoprim-sulfamethoxazole alone.

Pneumonia in the Elderly Pneumonia is the most common serious elderly infection, representing the fifth leading cause of death.[17] The incidence of lower respiratory tract infection in the elderly ranges from 25 to 44 cases per 1000 in the general population, with a mortality rate approaching 40%. Chronic obstructive pulmonary disease, congestive heart failure, cardiovascular and cerebrovascular disease, lung cancer, dementia, diminished gag reflex, and other aspiration risks make the elderly susceptible to infection.

Those over age 65 years are three times more likely to have pneumococcal bacteremia than younger patients. Atypical pathogens are still more common in younger populations but occur in the elderly. *Legionella* is the most common atypical agent in the elderly and is responsible for up to 10% of cases of community-acquired pneumonia. **Influenza is the most common serious viral infection in the elderly. Postinfluenza bacterial pneumonia, whether following H1N1 or other seasonal influenza, is most commonly caused by *S. pneumoniae*, *S. aureus*, or *H. influenzae*.** This usually presents as a worsening of respiratory symptoms after days of improvement.

Elderly patients with pneumonia may present with nonpulmonary symptoms like falls, weakness, tremulousness, functional decline, abdominal complaints, delirium, or confusion. Elderly patients are more likely to be afebrile on presentation but are more likely than younger adults to have a serious bacterial infection when the temperature is higher than 38.3°C (100.9°F).

Age alone does not confer a poor prognosis until extremes (over 85 years), but age does interact with other organ dysfunction to increase mortality and morbidity. Up to one third of elderly patients with community-acquired pneumonia will not manifest leukocytosis. Poor prognostic indicators for pneumonia in the elderly include hypothermia or a temperature >38.3°C (100.9°F), leukopenia, immunosuppression, gram-negative or staphylococcal infection, cardiac disease, bilateral infiltrates, and extrapulmonary disease. Elderly pneumonia patients frequently require hospitalization, and 10% receive intensive care.

Pneumonia in Nursing Home Patients Pneumonia is a major cause of morbidity, mortality, and hospitalization among nursing home residents.[17,18] Nursing home patients are less likely than those living independently to have a productive cough or pleuritic chest pain, but more likely to be confused and have poorer functional status and more severe disease.[18] Eight findings are independent predictors of pneumonia in nursing home patients: increased pulse rate, respiratory rate ≥30 breaths/min, temperature ≥38°C (100.4°F), somnolence or decreased alertness, presence of acute confusion, lung crackles on auscultation, the absence of wheezes, and an increased leukocyte count.[19] A patient with one of these features has a 33% chance of having pneumonia, whereas three or more features suggest a 50% likelihood of pneumonia.[19] Fewer than 10% of nursing home patients with pneumonia will have no respiratory symptoms. Fever, although nonspecific, is present in approximately 40% of cases of nursing home–acquired pneumonia.

The most frequently reported pathogens among patients with nursing home–acquired pneumonia are *S. pneumoniae*, gram-negative bacilli, and *H. influenzae*. Because nursing home patients live in close proximity to each other, residents are subject to outbreaks of influenza. Vaccination against influenza is 33% to 55% effective in preventing postinfluenzal pneumonia in nursing home patients. *M. pneumoniae* and *Legionella* are uncommon causes of pneumonia in nursing home patients.

Nursing home–acquired pneumonia is often treated in the hospital, but some patients can be treated in nursing homes with either intramuscular or oral antibiotics.[20] **Nursing home patients are at risk for the organisms linked to health care–associated pneumonia, so therapy should include coverage for gram-negative bacteria and methicillin-resistant *S. aureus*.**[4]

Pneumonia in Human Immunodeficiency Virus Patients Community-acquired pneumonia accounts for roughly three fourths of bacterial pneumonia diagnosed in patients hospitalized with HIV infection. Compared with HIV-seropositive patients hospitalized *without* pneumonia, those admitted *with* pneumonia generally have a lower CD4+ T-cell count, a higher Acute Physiology and Chronic Health Evaluation II score, a longer length of hospital stay, a greater chance of intensive care unit admission, and a higher case fatality rate.

***S. pneumoniae* is the most common cause of bacterial pneumonia in patients with HIV. *Pseudomonas aeruginosa* is also a common cause of bacterial pneumonia in HIV-positive patients.** HIV-positive patients with *P. aeruginosa* pneumonia, compared with HIV-negative patients, are more likely to have a lower leukocyte and CD4+ T-cell count and a longer hospital stay but a similar case fatality rate. (See chapter 154, "Human Immunodeficiency Virus Infection.")

Pneumonia in Transplant Patients Bacterial pneumonia is more common in patients receiving liver, heart, or lung transplants during the first 3 months after surgery, compared with other transplant and surgical patients. Gram-negative bacilli (especially *P. aeruginosa* associated with mechanical ventilation), *S. aureus*, and *Legionella* predominate in the first 3 months posttransplantation. *K. pneumoniae*, *Escherichia coli*, and fungi may also cause pneumonia in this time period. These early-onset nosocomial bacterial pneumonias carry a substantial mortality rate, approximately 33%. Cytomegalovirus, *P. jiroveci*, and fungal infections, especially *Aspergillus* species, are opportunistic infections, which may be seen in the first 6 months after surgery. **After 6 months posttransplantation, typical community-acquired pneumonia bacteria (*S. pneumoniae*, *H. influenzae*) are common and less often fatal than earlier infections** (see chapter 297, "The Transplant Patient").

TREATMENT

Emergency physicians start community-acquired pneumonia therapy usually based on bedside features rather than culture data; the Infectious Diseases Society of America and the American Thoracic Society guidelines, along with the American College of Emergency Physicians (ACEP) Clinical Policy, help care decisions.[21] Pediatric recommendations are provided in the chapter 125, "Pneumonia in Infants and Children."

The drugs listed in Tables 65-4 through 65-9[4,16,22] are based on site acquisition and comorbidities but do not represent a comprehensive list. Other antibiotic regimens are effective and guided by local resistance patterns and availbility.[16] Outpatient treatments are listed in **Tables 65-4** and **65-5**. Inpatient treatments are listed in **Tables 65-6** through **65-9**.

TABLE 65-4 Therapy for Outpatient Treatment of Uncomplicated Patients*

Class	Examples	Comments
Macrolide	Azithromycin, 500 milligrams PO on day 1 and 250 milligrams on days 2–5	Respiratory fluoroquinolones reserved for those who cannot tolerate or have failed other therapy
	or	
	Clarithromycin XL, 1000 milligrams PO each day for 7 d	
Tetracycline-like macrolide	Doxycycline, 100 milligrams twice a day for 10–14 d	Second-line choice

*Other drugs may also be effective.

TABLE 65-5 Therapy for Outpatient Management of Patients with Significant Comorbidities* without Criteria for Healthcare-Associated Pneumonia

Class	Examples	Comments
Fluoroquinolone	Levofloxacin, 750 milligrams daily for 5 d	Other respiratory fluoroquinolones may also be used.
	or	
	Moxifloxacin, 400 milligrams daily for 7–14 d	
β-Lactamase inhibitor penicillin derivative	Amoxicillin-clavulanate, 2 grams twice daily	A third-generation cephalosporin may be used instead of the aminopenicillin.
plus	*plus*	
Macrolide	Azithromycin, 500 milligrams PO on day 1 and 250 milligrams on days 2–5	

*Significant comorbidities include chronic heart, lung, liver, or renal disease; diabetes mellitus; alcoholism; malignancies; and asplenia. See text. Dosing may need adjustment for patients with renal insufficiency. Other therapies may also be effective.

TABLE 65-6 Inpatient Therapy for Non–Intensive Care Unit Patients* with Community-Acquired Pneumonia

Class	Examples	Comments
Fluoroquinolone	Levofloxacin, 750 milligrams IV	Other respiratory fluoroquinolones may also be used.
	or	
	Moxifloxacin, 400 milligrams IV	
Cephalosporin or penicillin class with β-lactamase inhibitor	Ceftriaxone, 1 gram IV or ampicillin/sulbactam 1.5 gram IV	Other third-generation cephalosporins may also be used in combination with other macrolides or doxycycline.
plus	*plus*	
Macrolide	Azithromycin, 500 milligrams IV	

*Other drugs may also be effective; dosing may need adjustment for patients with renal insufficiency. Oral therapy with selected drugs may be acceptable for non–intensive care unit patients.

TABLE 65-7 Empiric Therapy for Patients with Suspected Healthcare-Associated Pneumonia

Three-Drug Regimen Recommended

Class	Examples	Comments
Antipseudomonal cephalosporin	Cefepime, 1–2 grams every 8–12 h	An aminoglycoside may be substituted in place of the fluoroquinolone. Levofloxacin, 750 milligrams every 8 h, may be substituted for ciprofloxacin. Linezolid, 600 milligrams every 12 h, may be substituted for vancomycin.
	or	
	Ceftazidime, 2 grams every 8 h	
plus	*plus*	
Fluoroquinolone	Ciprofloxacin, 400 milligrams every 8 h*	
plus	*plus*	
Anti-MRSA drug	Vancomycin, 15 milligrams/kg every 12 h	
Antipseudomonal carbapenem	Imipenem, 500 milligrams every 6 h	An aminoglycoside may be substituted in place of the fluoroquinolone. Levofloxacin, 750 milligrams every 8 h, may be substituted for ciprofloxacin. Linezolid, 600 milligrams every 12 h, may be substituted for vancomycin.
	or	
	Meropenem, 1 gram every 8 h	
plus	*plus*	
Fluoroquinolone	Ciprofloxacin, 400 milligrams every 8 h*	
plus	*plus*	
Anti-MRSA drug	Vancomycin, 15 milligrams/kg every12 h	
β-Lactam/β-lactamase inhibitor	Piperacillin-tazobactam, 4.5 grams every 6 h	An aminoglycoside may be substituted in place of the fluoroquinolone. Levofloxacin, 750 milligrams every 8 h, may be substituted for ciprofloxacin. Linezolid, 600 milligrams every 12 h, may be substituted for vancomycin.
plus	*plus*	
Antipseudomonal fluoroquinolone	Ciprofloxacin, 400 milligrams every 8 h*	
plus	*plus*	
Anti-MRSA drug	Vancomycin, 15 milligrams/kg every 12 h	

Note: Healthcare-associated pneumonia risks include (1) patients hospitalized for 2 or more days within the past 90 days, (2) nursing home/long-term care residents, (3) patients receiving home IV antibiotic therapy, (4) dialysis patients, (5) patients receiving chronic wound care, (6) patients receiving chemotherapy, and (7) immunocompromised patients.

Abbreviation: MRSA = methicillin-resistant *Staphylococcus aureus*.

*See text. Dosing may need adjustment for patients with renal insufficiency.

TABLE 65-8 Inpatient Therapy for Intensive Care Unit Patients*

Class	Example	Comments
Cephalosporin	Ceftriaxone, 1 gram IV	Other β-lactams may also be used in place of ceftriaxone. See Table 65-9 for additional recommendations.
plus	*plus*	
Macrolide	Azithromycin, 500 milligrams IV	
Cephalosporin	Ceftriaxone, 1 gram	Other β-lactams may also be used in place of ceftriaxone. See Table 65-9 for additional recommendations.
plus	*plus*	
Fluoroquinolone	Either moxifloxacin, 400 milligrams IV	
	or	
	Levofloxacin, 750 milligrams IV	
Fluoroquinolone	Moxifloxacin, 400 milligrams IV	Aztreonam is generally well tolerated in penicillin-allergic patients.
plus	*or*	
Either a monobactam	Levofloxacin, 750 milligrams IV	
or	*plus*	
Lincosamide	Either aztreonam, 1–2 grams IV	
	or	
	Clindamycin, 600 milligrams IV	
Anti-MRSA drug (add if HCAP or MRSA risk)	Vancomycin, 10–15 milligrams/kg IV	To be added to one of the above regimens for patients with MRSA or HCAP risk.
	or	
	Linezolid, 600 milligrams IV	

Abbreviations: HCAP = healthcare-associated pneumonia; MRSA = methicillin-resistant *Staphylococcus aureus*.

*Other combinations may also be used. Dosing may need adjustment for patients with renal insufficiency.

TABLE 65-9 Inpatient Therapy for Patients with Higher *Pseudomonas* Risk*

Class	Example	Comments
β-Lactam/β-lactamase inhibitor	Piperacillin-tazobactam, 3.375 milligrams IV	Other antipseudomonal cephalosporins or quinolones may be used. Carbapenems are also appropriate. Consider adding an aminoglycoside if substituting a macrolide.
plus	*plus*	
Fluoroquinolone	Ciprofloxacin, 400 milligrams IV	
Monobactam	Aztreonam, 1 gram IV	May be used for patients with penicillin allergy. Carbapenems and aminoglycosides may also be appropriate.
plus	*plus*	
Fluoroquinolone	*either* Moxifloxacin, 400 milligrams IV	
	or	
	Levofloxacin, 750 milligrams IV	
Anti-MRSA drug (add if HCAP or MRSA risk)	Vancomycin, 10–15 milligrams/kg IV	To be added to one of the above regimens for patients with MRSA or HCAP risk.
	or	
	Linezolid, 600 milligrams IV	

Abbreviations: HCAP = healthcare-associated pneumonia; MRSA = methicillin-resistant *Staphylococcus aureus*.

*Other combinations may also be used. Dosing may need adjustment for patients with renal insufficiency.

In **outpatients,** single-drug therapy is the common first choice, using a macrolide or a respiratory fluoroquinolone, with doxycycline as an alternative. Erythromycin is a cost-effective agent for community-acquired pneumonia but is associated with GI side effects in about 25% of adult patients and also causes photosensitivity. Clarithromycin has fewer GI side effects, although some patients may complain about a metallic taste. Azithromycin has the advantage of once-a-day dosing or single-dose therapy with the newer formulations. The newer fluoroquinolone agents, including moxifloxacin, levofloxacin, and gemifloxacin, extend coverage to both common bacterial agents and atypical agents, along with the advantage of once-a-day dosing. However, given concerns about resistance developing, **the Centers for Disease Control and Prevention recommends that fluoroquinolones be reserved for patients who cannot tolerate other agents, have documented pneumococcal resistance, or have failed other therapies. Fluoroquinolones should not be used in patients with myasthenia gravis.**

Patients who received broad-spectrum antibiotics within the previous 3 months are at risk for drug-resistant infection. In these patients, consider a respiratory fluoroquinolone or combination therapy using an aminopenicillin or a third-generation cephalosporin with a macrolide (including doxycycline). Patients with chronic cardiac, pulmonary, renal, or hepatic disease, severe diabetics, chronic alcoholics, patients on immunosuppressive therapy, or patients with asplenia may require therapy with more than one agent.

Inpatients not admitted to the intensive care unit benefit from coverage for both atypical and common organisms. Often, monotherapy using a respiratory fluoroquinolone is an option, although single-agent therapy with a macrolide or doxycycline is avoided. An aminopenicillin/β-lactamase or cephalosporin in combination with a macrolide or with a respiratory fluoroquinolone is common.

Treat patients admitted to the intensive care unit with a combination of agents, including an aminopenicillin or cephalosporin with either a respiratory fluoroquinolone or a macrolide. Penicillin-allergic patients could be treated with a respiratory fluoroquinolone with either aztreonam or clindamycin. For patients at risk for *Pseudomonas* infection, add at least two agents active against the organism. This may include an antipseudomonal β-lactam such as piperacillin-tazobactam or cefepime with a respiratory fluoroquinolone. Alternatively, a carbapenem, such as imipenem, along with either a fluoroquinolone or aminoglycoside is appropriate. In penicillin-allergic patients, use a monobactam along with a fluoroquinolone. If the combination does not include two drugs with antipseudomonal activity, consider adding an aminoglycoside. Patients admitted to the intensive care unit with healthcare-associated pneumonia should have coverage for methicillin-resistant *S. aureus* with drugs such as vancomycin or linezolid.[22]

Emergency physicians play a prominent role in the initiation of treatment for patients being hospitalized with community-acquired pneumonia, although the effect of delays in care are debated.[16,23,24] The Joint Commission currently recommends starting antibiotics within 6 hours of diagnosis. Although it is reasonable to not delay therapy, there is no single best time frame to optimize outcomes without overuse.

DISPOSITION AND FOLLOW-UP

Most patients with community-acquired pneumonia do not require hospitalization.[25] In general, physicians tend to overestimate the risk of pneumonia mortality. **It is best to use an illness severity or prognostic tool to better aid care site decisions.**

The best-tested tool is the **Pneumonia Severity Index (PSI),** which estimates the risk of short-term death and intensive care unit need in those with community-acquired pneumonia.[25-27] With the Pneumonia Severity Index, patients are assigned to one of five risk categories (class I to V) based on points (starting with age, adjusted for sex) and bedside features; **the lowest risk patients (<50 years old with minimal x-ray and vital sign/concomitant condition threats) need no further testing;** all others have labs tested to better assess prognosis and organ function. Nonhypoxemic (room air saturation of 91% or higher) Pneumonia Severity Index class I to III patients have <4% mortality and are candidates for outpatient therapy. The Pneumonia Severity Index was not designed to determine prognosis in patients with severe HIV, patients with other forms of pneumonia (ventilator or hospital-acquired), or pregnant patients. Other factors, such as social situation or unusual medical conditions, play a role in the admission decision. Also, one profound derangement should drive care (e.g., blood pressure <60 mm Hg systolic or presence of coma), irrespective of the class assigned. A brief hospitalization or observation is an alternative for class III patients with mild hypoxemia, and class IV and V patients are usually treated as inpatients. A free online Pneumonia Severity Index calculator is available at http://pda.ahrq.gov/clinic/psi/psicalc.asp, and a version that can be downloaded to a hand-held computer is obtainable from http://pda.ahrq.gov/clinic/psi/psi.htm.

The **CURB-65 rule** looks at the presence of *c*onfusion, *u*remia >7 mmol/L, *r*espiratory rate ≥30 breaths/min, age ≥65 years old, or abnormal *b*lood pressure (systolic <90 mm Hg or diastolic <60 mm Hg), with 1 point assigned for each factor.[20] The CRB-65 uses the same variables but eliminates the uremia measurement. Patients with a CURB-65 or CRB-65 score of <2 have a low mortality rate and are candidates for outpatient therapy.

The Pneumonia Severity Index and CURB scoring systems *inform* but do not *determine* care location. Some patients are better served based on social or medical factors not assessed by these scores. Nonetheless, the validated scoring tools help safely increase the number of appropriate patients treated on an outpatient basis and to limit unnecessary admissions.[26] Absent a structured approach, admission decision patterns for patients with community-acquired pneumonia among emergency physicians can vary widely, often unrelated to disease severity and socioeconomic states.

Once the decision to admit the patient is made, the next decision is to determine which patients require admission to the intensive care unit. Patients in septic shock or those requiring mechanical ventilation will be placed in an intensive care unit setting. Other criteria for intensive care unit admission include a markedly elevated respiratory rate, a partial pressure of arterial oxygen/fraction of inspired oxygen ratio ≤250, multilobar infiltrates, confusion, uremia with a BUN >20 milligrams/dL, leukopenia, thrombocytopenia, hypothermia, hyponatremia, lactic acidosis, and asplenia. No single criterion will mandate intensive care unit admission; consider intensive care unit or intermediate-care admission for patients with three or more of the criteria in **Tables 65-10** through **65-12.** Those with a PSI class of V or a CURB-65 of ≥3 often require intensive care.[20,25]

Most patients will achieve some resolution within 3 to 5 days after the initiation of antibiotics. Many hospitalized patients can be switched to oral antibiotics at approximately 3 days and then subsequently discharged to complete a course of therapy. After ED or hospital discharge, contact within 3 to 5 days may help avoid a need for repeat care. However, up to half of patients are still symptomatic at 30 days,

TABLE 65-10 Step 1 of Pneumonia Severity Index (PSI)

Step 1: Assess initial factors
Age (if <50 y old, move on to next features; if ≥50 y, go to Step 2)
Comorbid conditions—ask about:
Neoplastic disease
Cerebrovascular disease
Congestive heart failure
Renal disease
Liver disease
Physical examination
No altered mental status
Pulse <125 beats/min
Respiratory rate <30 breaths/min
Systolic blood pressure >90 mm Hg
Temperature >35°C (95°F) or <40°C (104°F)

If all negative, then assign to risk class I (lowest risk); if over 50 y or *any* abnormality present, go on to Step 2 testing and classification in Table 65-11.

TABLE 65-11 Step 2 of Pneumonia Severity Index: Assignment to Risk Classes II to V

Criteria	Points Given
Demographics	
Age	Men: Age (in years)
	Women: Age (in years) − 10
Nursing home resident	10
Coexistent illness (same as Step 1)	
Neoplastic disease	30
Congestive heart failure	10
Cerebrovascular accident	10
Renal disease	10
Liver disease	20
Physical examination (same as Step 1)	
Abnormal mental status	20
Pulse ≥125 beats/min	10
Respiratory rate >30 breaths/min	20
Systolic blood pressure (<90 mm Hg)	20
Temperature <35°C (95°F) or >40°C (104°F)	15
Ancillary studies	
Arterial pH <7.35 (may assume normal if clinical condition suggests)	30
BUN ≥30 milligrams/dL (11 mmol/liter)	20
Na <130 mEq/L	20
Glucose >250 milligrams/dL (14 mmol/liter)	10
Hematocrit <30%	10
Pa_{O_2} <60 mm Hg or O_2 saturation on room air <91%	10
Pleural effusion	10
Summary points risk assignment	
Sum of points <70 = risk class II	
Sum of points 71–90 = risk class III	
Sum of points 91–130 = risk class IV	
Sum of points >130 = risk class V	

with a significant minority of patients experiencing chest pain, malaise, or mild dyspnea even 2 to 3 months after treatment. Educate patients about smoking cessation and moderation of alcohol use, and provide information about rest, nutrition, hydration, follow-up, and the importance of pneumococcal and influenza vaccination.

Finally, not all radiographic infiltrates result from an infection. Congestive heart failure may present a radiographic picture that overlaps with pneumonia, and pulmonary embolism can be associated with segmental or lobar densities. A variety of cancers may mimic pneumonia, best detected by CT scan or repeat radiographs after therapy. Eosinophilic or fungal diseases often have transient or recurring infiltrates. Finally, obtain an occupational history to identify patients with hypersensitivity disorders or chemical pneumonitis.

TABLE 65-12 Prediction of Mortality from Pneumonia

Class	Points	Mortality (%)	Treatment Recommendation
I	No predictors	0.1	Outpatient
II	<70	0.6	Outpatient
III	71–90	2.8	Individualized; nonhypoxemic may be candidate for home therapy
IV	91–130	8.2	Inpatient
V	>130	29.2	Inpatient (often intensive care unit)

ASPIRATION PNEUMONIA

DEFINITIONS AND EPIDEMIOLOGY

Aspiration pneumonia results from the swallowing of colonized oropharyngeal contents into the lower respiratory tract with subsequent inflammation and infection. Aspiration pneumonitis is from exposure of sterile gastric contents into the lower respiratory tract. This results in a rapid chemical pneumonitis due to irritation of the pulmonary tissues from the acidic material. Aspiration pneumonia—infection occurring from the exposure—is often unwitnessed, especially in the elderly. Other aspiration syndromes include drowning, solid foreign body aspiration with or without asphyxia, and lipoid pneumonia. Sterile pneumonitis and aspiration pneumonia are difficult to distinguish from one another, even with bronchial lavage. When certain, the treatment of aspiration pneumonitis is largely supportive.[28]

Aspiration of small amounts of oropharyngeal content is common. Approximately half of healthy adults aspirate small amounts oropharyngeal secretions during sleep.[28] Silent aspiration is more common in patients with community-acquired pneumonia. Aspiration occurred in 71% of patients with pneumonia compared to 10% of control subjects.[29] Approximately 5% to 15% of community-acquired pneumonia cases result from aspiration,[30-32] and 30% of those in continuing care facilities with pneumonia have aspiration pneumonia.[30,33] Mortality rates differ for aspiration based on location, with mortality higher in nursing home patients with aspiration pneumonia (28.2%) compared with those with community-acquired aspiration pneumonia (19.4%).[30,33] The incidence of aspiration pneumonia in those who aspirate with acute stroke or chronic degenerative neurologic conditions is higher than in patients without those conditions.[30]

Risks for aspiration pneumonia include conditions that promote oropharyngeal colonization with pathogenic bacteria or conditions that impair the swallowing or gag mechanism (**Table 65-13**). The incidence of aspiration is highest in patients with dementia or stroke. The risk of

TABLE 65-13 Risk Factors for Aspiration Pneumonia

Intoxicants
Alcohol and illicit drugs
Therapeutic drug overdose
Sedative drug use
Procedural sedation
General anesthesia
Neurologic
Stroke, especially brainstem involvement with dysphagia
Seizure
Head trauma
Chronic debilitating neurologic condition, especially dementia
Oropharyngeal
Impaired glottic functions
Emergent intubation
Periodontal disease and poor oral hygiene
GI
High gastric pressures: prior meal, bag-mask ventilation
Gastroesophageal reflux
Esophageal dysmotility or obstruction
Nasogastric, orogastric, percutaneous gastric tube
Tracheobronchial fistula
Other
Chronic supine position
Rapid sequence intubation
Advanced age
Chronic debility
Extension neck contractures

infection is compounded by poor oral care, which leads to oropharyngeal colonization of the oral cavity. Placement of nasogastric or gastric feeding tubes and the use of sedative and neuroleptic drugs also increase the risk of aspiration.[34-38] Aspiration pneumonia is the most common cause of death in gastric tube–fed patients.[39]

Although many patients have clinical evidence of aspiration, along with dysphagia, emesis, or coughing while eating, up to one third of those who aspirate have "silent aspiration" without evidence of cough or gagging. Small bowel obstruction, gastroesophageal reflux, esophageal dysmotility, esophageal obstruction, and tracheoesophageal fistula are GI risk factors for aspiration. Chronic degenerative neurologic conditions such as Parkinson's disease, myasthenia gravis, amyotrophic lateral sclerosis, acute stroke, encephalopathy, seizures, and alteration of consciousness increase the risk of aspiration.

PATHOPHYSIOLOGY

The development of pneumonitis depends on the volume and pH of the aspirate, with consensus that gastric contents with pH <2.5 and an aspirated volume of 0.3 to 0.4 mL/kg (20 to 30 mL in adults) are required to develop aspiration pneumonitis.[32] The injury produced by acid aspiration is initially a direct caustic effect followed by an inflammatory response that peaks in 4 to 6 hours. Proinflammatory cytokines increase capillary permeability and cause fluid and inflammatory cells to enter the area of irritation. These reactions may manifest clinically as cough, pleuritic chest pain, fever, and radiographic findings. Aspiration of solid or viscous material blocking the airway may result in precipitous asphyxiation.

Typical bacterial species involved in aspiration pneumonia include *S. pneumoniae, S. aureus, H. influenzae*, and Enterobacteriaceae in community-acquired aspiration pneumonia.[32] Common bacterial species in hospital-acquired aspiration pneumonia include *P. aeruginosa* and gram-negative organisms.[32] Antibiotic therapy for typical aspiration syndromes should include coverage for anaerobic organisms.[40,41]

The posterior portions of the upper lobes and the upper portions of the lower lobes are most commonly involved in recumbent aspiration. In upright patients, the most dependent portions of the lungs are the basal segments of the lower lobes. The inflammatory injury may include bilateral patchy, interstitial or alveolar infiltrates, particularly in aspiration of large volumes seen with near drowning.[42]

CLINICAL FEATURES

Witnessed aspiration is a key feature in the diagnosis of aspiration pneumonitis or pneumonia. Typically those with noninfectious aspiration are younger, and the aspiration is witnessed. These patients will present giving a history of aspiration and coughing immediately afterward. "Silent aspirators" are typically older and have a chronic neurologic disorder and will present with a cough or fever or general malaise. Silent aspirators are more likely to be from a chronic care facility and have a history of prior pneumonia episodes. Historical features that suggest silent aspiration include general debility, recurrent cough, hoarseness, or dysphagia. History may be difficult to obtain in chronically debilitated or otherwise noncommunicative patients.

The clinical symptoms of aspiration pneumonia include fever, dyspnea, and productive cough. Other symptoms of systemic infection in the elderly and debilitated may be present, including a change in mental status, lethargy, and nausea or vomiting.[43] The physical examination may reveal signs classic for pneumonia, including tachycardia, tachypnea, fever, rales, or decreased breath sounds in an ill-appearing patient. Patients with underlying pulmonary disease may decompensate rapidly and have more symptoms and signs of respiratory distress.

DIAGNOSIS

Chest radiographs in aspiration pneumonia usually show unilateral focal or patchy consolidations in the dependent lung segments (**Figure 65-4**). Occasionally, a bilateral or interstitial pattern can be seen. The right lower lobe is the most common area of consolidation if the aspiration occurs when the patient is upright.

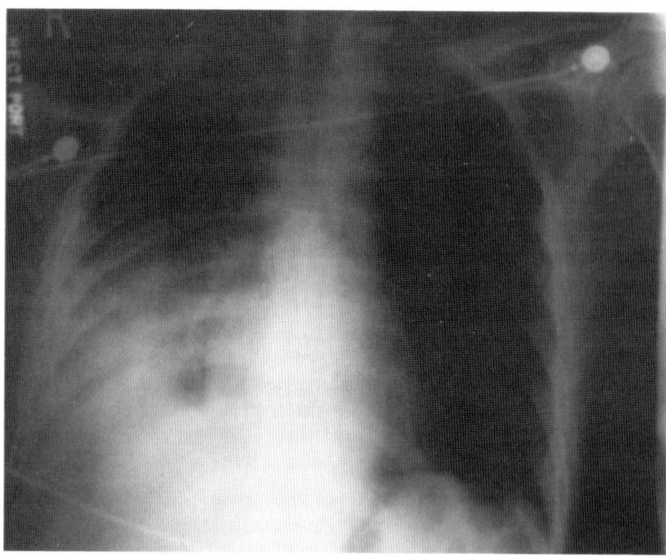

FIGURE 65-4. Aspiration pneumonia of the right lower lobe.

Early in the course, the white blood cell count may not be elevated. Arterial blood gases to identify hypoxemia or hypoventilation aid care and are best compared to previous values if chronic lung disease exists.

TREATMENT

Aspiration of large volumes of solid material, foods, nonfood objects, or very tenacious liquids may require suctioning of the tracheobronchial tree or bronchoalveolar lavage to clear the airway. Bronchodilators aid aspiration-induced bronchospasm.

Choice of antibiotics depends on the circumstances of the aspiration and the suspected bacterial etiology of the infection (**Table 65-14**).[32,44,45] Most patients with aspiration pneumonia are infected by gram-negative organisms and require broad-spectrum antibiotics, such as third-generation cephalosporins, fluoroquinolones, piperacillin-tazobactam, or carbapenems.[28] When methicillin-resistant *S. aureus* is suspected, consider the addition of vancomycin or linezolid.[28] In community-acquired aspiration pneumonia where the usual organisms are *S. aureus, S. pneumoniae*, and *H. influenzae*, levofloxacin and ceftriaxone are recommended.[46] Patients with severe periodontal disease, putrid sputum, or lung abscess require anaerobic coverage, such as piperacillin-tazobactam or imipenem or a combination of two drugs (levofloxacin, ciprofloxacin, or ceftriaxone plus clindamycin or metronidazole).[46]

TABLE 65-14 Initial Treatment for Presumed Aspiration Pneumonia

Acquisition Site	Empiric Therapy	Empiric Therapy for Penicillin Allergy
Community acquired	Ampicillin/sublactam *or* Amoxicillin/clavulanate *or* Levofloxacin *or* Moxifloxacin	Clindamycin
Hospital acquired or Severe periodontal disease, putrid sputum or alcoholism	Pipracillin-tazobactam +/– Vancomycin +/– gentamicin *or* Cefepime or ceftazidime *plus* Clindamycin or metronidazole *or* Levofloxacin + clindamycin	Ciprofloxacin + vancomycin

TABLE 65-15 Noninfectious Causes of Pulmonary Infiltrates

Disease	Pathophysiology	Chest Radiography Findings	Symptoms
Congestive heart failure	As pulmonary capillary hydrostatic pressure rises, fluid crosses into the interstitium. When the capacity of lymphatic drainage is exceeded, fluid accumulates in the interstitium and eventually collects in the alveoli.	With increasing atrial pressures, chest x-ray reveals cephalization, Kerley B lines (thickening of the interlobular septa), interstitial edema, thickening of fissures, and, ultimately, alveolar edema and pleural effusions.	See chapter 53, Acute Heart Failure.
Pulmonary embolism	Pulmonary artery occlusion, typically at multiple sites, with its secondary effects, including infarction.	Chest x-ray nonspecific or normal: cardiac enlargement (27%), normal (24%), pleural effusion (23%), elevated hemidiaphragm (20%).	See chapter 56, "Venous Thromboembolism."
Aspiration pneumonitis	After aspiration of gastric contents, an intense inflammatory reaction occurs; biphasic pattern, at 1–2 h, caustic effect of low pH of the aspirate on alveolar cells; at 4–6 h, infiltration of neutrophils into the alveoli and lung interstitium.	Alveolar infiltrates in the posterior segments of the upper lobes if aspiration occurs while the patient is in the supine position; infiltrates in the basal segments of the lower lobes if aspiration occurs while the patient is upright.	See "Aspiration Pneumonia" section earlier in this chapter.
Allergic bronchopulmonary aspergillosis	Allergic lung reaction to *Aspergillus fumigatus* that occurs most commonly in patients with asthma or cystic fibrosis. Eosinophils fill small airways and alveolar spaces due to inflammation. Bronchiectasis.	Branching band-like opacities may be seen, or may see alveolar infiltrates, peripheral and migratory.	Dyspnea, wheezing, productive cough; may have hemoptysis and occasionally fever.
Eosinophilic lung disease; chronic (Löffler's syndrome) and acute forms exist	The acute form leads to rapidly progressive respiratory failure. This is a reaction to the presence of infection, such as ascariasis, or in association with chronic conditions, such as asthma or atopic disease. Eosinophils accumulate in distal airways and alveolar and interstitial spaces.	Alveolar and interstitial infiltrates; classically, these are peripheral, but findings are proximal in equal numbers.	Mild or severe symptoms; dyspnea, fever, cough, and wheezing. In acute forms, hypoxia and potential for progression to respiratory failure.
Hypersensitivity pneumonitis (also called extrinsic allergic alveolitis)	Inflammation of the alveoli secondary to hypersensitivity in response to inhaled organic dust.	Diffuse micronodular interstitial infiltrates, may see ground-glass densities in the lower or mid-lung fields.	Fever, chills, malaise, cough, chest tightness, dyspnea, and headache.
Acute interstitial pneumonitis	Idiopathic.	Bilateral interstitial infiltrates, sometimes patchy alveolar densities and ground-glass appearance.	Progressive dyspnea over days to weeks.
Acute respiratory distress syndrome	Reaction of the lung to a number of precipitating causes, including sepsis, trauma, surgeries, transfusions, and therapeutically induced immunosuppression.	Classically, patchy peripheral infiltrates that extend to the lateral lung margins suggest the diagnosis.	Hypoxia, tachypnea, rales.
Drug-induced pneumonitis	Causes include chemotherapeutic, immunosuppressive, antimicrobial, and herbal agents.	Typically, bilateral interstitial infiltrates.	Cough, mild fever, dyspnea, and, potentially, hypoxia.
Sarcoidosis	Systemic granulomatous disease of unknown etiology.	Hilar lymph node enlargement and/or diffuse parenchymal interstitial pulmonary infiltrates. Occasionally may be peripheral.	Dyspnea, cough, weight loss; skin lesions may also be found. May be asymptomatic.
Bronchiolitis obliterans with organizing pneumonia	Inflammation of the bronchioles and surrounding tissues, leading to loss of the integrity of the bronchioles and organizing pneumonia without infection. Occurs in association with immunocompromise and connective tissue diseases, such as SLE.	Patchy alveolar infiltrates and, occasionally, cavitation.	Cough, dyspnea, fever.
Wegener's granulomatosis (granulomatosis with polyangiitis)	Inflammatory and granulomatosis disease involving the blood vessels of unknown etiology. The upper respiratory tract, lung parenchyma, and kidneys are typically affected.	Alveolar infiltrates, nodules, or cavities.	Cough and dyspnea; may see epistaxis and sinusitis.
Goodpasture's syndrome (antiglomerular basement antibody disease)	Autoimmune disease affecting the lungs and kidney.	Diffuse, bilateral, predominately alveolar densities.	Fatigue, dyspnea, cough with hemoptysis; may have simultaneous hematuria.
Churg-Strauss vasculitis (eosinophilic granulomatosis with polyangiitis)	Systemic vasculitis of unknown cause primarily affecting the lung and may eventually involve the skin, nervous system, kidney, GI tract, and heart.	Bilateral peripheral, patchy, alveolar infiltrates. May see nodules.	Cough, dyspnea, allergic rhinitis, may see symptoms related to skin, coronary, or intestinal involvement.
Radiation pneumonitis	Interstitial pulmonary inflammation seen in 5%–15% of patients with thoracic radiation treatment.	Subtle hazy ground-glass densities to marked patchy infiltrates or homogenous consolidation. Air bronchograms are commonly present.	Symptoms occur 1–6 mo after treatment: low-grade fever, cough, fullness in the chest.

(*Continued*)

TABLE 65-15 Noninfectious Causes of Pulmonary Infiltrates (*Continued*)

Disease	Pathophysiology	Chest Radiography Findings	Symptoms
Chemical pneumonitis	Inflammatory reaction to the presence of foreign substance, such as barium, petroleum distillates, pesticide, or irritating gases.	Diffuse, alveolar, and interstitial infiltrates.	History of exposure or aspiration of substance; acute dyspnea, cough, and, possibly, wheezing.
Alveolar cell carcinoma, often called bronchiolar carcinoma	Malignant pulmonary cancer originating in a bronchiole and spreading across the alveolar walls.	Classically, a butterfly distribution of alveolar infiltrates, but may be unilateral.	Often severe coughing, dyspnea, and copious sputum production.
Bronchoalveolar cell carcinoma	Adenocarcinoma that typically originates in the lung periphery and grows along alveolar walls.	Peripheral alveolar infiltrates that do not respond to antibiotics; may see a peripheral nodule or mass.	Symptoms like pneumonia but fails to respond to antibiotics. May lack fever or leukocytosis.
Fat emboli	ED presentations are typically after trauma, associated with long-bone fracture.	Interstitial prominence, suggesting interstitial edema. Radiographic findings may be delayed 1–2 d after trauma.	Dyspnea, cough, hemoptysis, and pleural pain. May be associated with confusion, stupor, delirium, and a petechial skin rash, most commonly on the chest.
Alveolar hemorrhage	In the setting of chemotherapy induction for leukemia and thrombocytopenia (<20,000/mL), hemorrhage filling alveoli is common from endobrachial and interstitial sources. Also seen with SLE.	Focal or diffuse alveolar infiltrates.	Dyspnea, hemoptysis; symptoms are frequently less severe than radiographic appearance would predict.
Leukemic infiltrates	Most common in myeloid leukemia when peripheral blast cell counts exceed 100,000/mL. Primitive myeloid leukemic cells invade through the endothelium of the lung capillary beds, yielding hemorrhage.	Interstitial or alveolar infiltrates. Diffuse infiltrates associated with hypoxia and need for intubation; focal infiltrates associated with coexistent pneumonia.	Respiratory distress, hypoxemia, and may progress to respiratory failure.

Abbreviation: SLE = systemic lupus erythematosus.

DISPOSITION

Healthy persons who aspirate small volumes of nontoxic material may be observed and, if stable and reliable, discharged to return for worsening symptoms. Antibiotic treatment is generally not needed for witnessed aspiration of a small amount of nontoxic liquid provided the patient's symptoms (cough, low-grade fever) resolve within 24 to 48 hours.[28] Patients should be able to identify worsening symptoms and have the ability to follow up if symptoms worsen.

Stable patients at risk for worsening (e.g., diabetes, advanced age, renal dialysis, recent stroke, chronic pulmonary disease, active cancer and HIV) are usually admitted to the hospital or an observation unit. Start antibiotics in the ED in those who have definite evidence of infection. Deliver supplemental oxygen as needed, and treat cardiopulmonary compromise. Noninvasive positive-pressure ventilation and endotracheal intubation are options if gas exchange is impaired (see chapters 28 "Noninvasive Airway Management" and 29 "Intubation and Mechanical Ventilation"). Admit all unstable patients to an intensive care unit.

NONINFECTIOUS PULMONARY INFILTRATES

Commonly, a noninfectious cause is suspected by the appearance of the chest radiograph or after antibiotics fail to improve the patient's symptoms. Noninfectious infiltrates occur in response to a wide variety of pathophysiologic processes involving the respiratory, cardiovascular, and immune systems or may be due to the infiltration of malignant cells.

CLINICAL FEATURES

The most important symptom of noninfectious pulmonary infiltrates is dyspnea, but some disorders present with hemoptysis, cough, chest pain, or fatigue. Fever can also be a symptom of autoimmune disease exacerbation; however, it may be impossible to clinically differentiate a noninfectious source from an infectious source of fever in the ED.

Table 65-15 lists the most common causes of noninfectious pulmonary infiltrates, their pathophysiology, chest radiograph findings, and symptoms.[45,47-52] Typical radiographic appearances help to prioritize the differential diagnosis. An interstitial infiltrate is classically described as fine, diffuse, linear density representing fluid or the accumulation of cells in the interstitial spaces. An alveolar infiltrate is a small ill-defined or reticular density representing fluid or abnormal cells in the alveoli. A ground-glass appearance is defined as multiple finely granular densities. Table 65-15 lists diseases that produce acute radiographic change, not diseases that produce chronic densities, such as fibrosis or scarring.

Patients with connective tissue diseases or on immunosuppression are at risk for bronchiolitis obliterans, organizing pneumonia, pneumonitis, and alveolar hemorrhage, often from therapy. Patients with atopic disease or asthma are at risk for eosinophilic lung disease.

DIAGNOSIS

Assess critically ill patients with CBC, renal function assessment, electrolytes, chest radiograph, and liver function tests, and add specimen cultures to look for complications of the acute disease process rather than establishing a new disease diagnosis. Newer high-sensitivity procalcitonin assays help differentiate infection from an exacerbation of a systemic inflammatory condition (very low values suggest a nonbacterial cause).[53] In many patients, an infectious cause of pulmonary infiltration cannot be excluded until bronchoscopy or lung biopsy. Therefore, the diagnostic plan can rarely be completed in the ED.

TREATMENT

Assess gas exchange with pulse oximetry in all, and use selective arterial blood gas analysis in those ill, hypoxemic, or with underlying chronic lung disease; use noninvasive or mechanical ventilation as needed. Prepare for possible subglottic stenosis with difficult airway equipment in patients with systemic inflammatory disease.[52] Broad-spectrum antibiotics, such as piperacillin-tazobactam (3.375 to 4.5 grams IV) and vancomycin (1 gram IV), or similar coverage, are recommended for critically ill patients with pneumonia and systemic inflammatory disease or immunocompromise.[48] Definitive treatment for noninfectious pulmonary diseases will occur after ED stabilization. Many of the disorders listed in Table 65-15 are treated acutely with corticosteroids such as methylprednisolone (0.5 to 1 gram IV).[52] Additional immunosuppressive drugs may be initiated by the admitting physician.

DISPOSITION AND FOLLOW-UP

Patients suspected of having a noninfectious cause of pulmonary infiltrate require testing beyond the capabilities of the ED. Hospitalization should be based on the severity of the medical illness, with attention to hypoxemia, hypercapnia, and work of breathing. In stable patients with mild symptoms, outpatient referral to a pulmonologist or another specialist is best.

PRACTICE GUIDELINES

Guidelines concerning the management of community-acquired pneumonia[16] and healthcare-associated pneumonia[4] are undergoing revision, but will be available online at the following address: http://www.thoracic.org/professionals/clinical-resources/disease-related-resources/pneumonia.php.

REFERENCES

The complete reference list is available online at www.TintinalliEM.com.

Lung Empyema and Abscess

Eric Anderson
Sharon E. Mace

EMPYEMA

INTRODUCTION AND EPIDEMIOLOGY

Empyema is a pleural space infection with pus, a positive Gram stain or culture, or parapneumonic effusions without pleural fluid sampling. Causes of empyema include pulmonary infections, most commonly bacterial pneumonia (56%), complications of chest surgery (22%), trauma (4%), esophageal perforation (4%), complications of chest tube/thoracentesis (4%), an extension from a subdiaphramatic infection (3%), and other causes (7%), such as osteomyelitis or other near pleural infections or a hemothorax, chylothorax, or hydrothorax that becomes infected.[1]

Predisposing factors for empyema include aspiration pneumonia (and the conditions causing this event, notably neurologic disease altering swallowing), respiratory disease impairing ciliary function, immunocompromise, malignancy, and alcoholism. The common organisms in empyema stratified by associated pathology are listed in **Table 66-1**.[1]

CLINICAL FEATURES

Suspect empyema if symptoms of pneumonia (fever, cough, dyspnea, pleuritic chest pain, and malaise) do not resolve. The onset of empyema may be insidious, with patients appearing chronically ill with weight loss, anemia, and night sweats.

Physical examination findings include decreased breath sounds, dullness to percussion, decreased tactile fremitus, and on occasion a friction rub. Pain from an underlying effusion or empyema may cause splinting with respiration. If there is an underlying pulmonary infection, rales or rhonchi may be heard.

TABLE 66-1 Common Organisms in Empyema and Associated Pathology

Pathology	Organisms
Pneumonia	*Streptococcus pneumonia* *Staphylococcus aureus*
Pneumonia (unimmunized with *Haemophilus influenza* type B vaccine)	*Haemophilus influenza*
Lung abscess	Mixed oropharyngeal anaerobes
Aspiration pneumonia	*S. aureus*
Recent thoracotomy	Gram-negative bacilli
Pneumonia in the setting of human immunodeficiency virus	Tuberculosis Fungal infections
Chest trauma	*S. aureus* Gram-negative bacilli
Contiguous abdominal infection	Gram-negative bacilli Anaerobes
Esophageal rupture	Mixed oropharyngeal organisms

DIAGNOSIS

Diagnostic criteria for empyema are aspiration of grossly purulent material on thoracentesis and at least one of the following: thoracentesis fluid with a positive Gram stain or culture, pleural fluid glucose <40 milligrams/dL, pH <7.1, or lactate dehydrogenase >1000 IU/L. In countries where tuberculosis is a common cause of exudative effusions, the negative predictive value of adenosine deaminase is 99.9% and can exclude the disease.[2-4]

Empyema has three stages that impact treatment:

1. Exudative (may be very short, <48 hours; the free-flowing pleural effusion that is present is amenable to chest tube drainage)
2. Fibrinopurulent (fibrin strands form in the pleural fluid causing loculations; resolution of the empyema with single chest tube drainage is unlikely)
3. Organizational (takes several weeks; more extensive fibrosis; "pleural peel" restricts lung expansion)

TREATMENT

Treat any trigger, especially pneumonia or heart failure. Nonsteroidal anti-inflammatory drugs or opioids can aid the pleuritic pain. Thoracentesis can aid in therapy in a patient with respiratory or cardiac distress and can be used as symptomatic treatment in patients with dyspnea. The definitive treatment of an empyema is drainage and antibiotics.[1]

Initial antibiotic therapy for empyema targets the presumptive underlying pneumonia, lung abscess, or bronchiectasis. Recommended therapy includes piperacillin-tazobactam 3.375 to 4.5 grams every 6 hours IV or imipenem 0.5 to 1.0 gram IV every 6 hours. Add vancomycin for methicillin-resistant *Staphylococcus aureus* in those at risk. Those at risk for methicillin-resistant *S. aureus* include patients recently hospitalized, patients who have an invasive medical device, and patients residing in a long-term care facility. Those at risk of community-acquired methicillin-resistant *S. aureus* include participants in contact sports, those who live in crowded or unsanitary conditions, and men who have sex with men. Tailor antibiotics once culture results are available and the clinical course is apparent.[1]

Treat exudative empyema with chest tube thoracostomy in addition to antibiotics.[5] Consider intrapleural fibrinolytic agents for empyema in the fibropurulent stage in consultation with a thoracic surgeon or pulmonologist. Streptokinase, urokinase, and more recently, deoxyribonuclease (either streptococcal deoxyribonuclease or human recombinant deoxyribonuclease) and alteplase all have some reported success.[5,6] The decrease in the percentage of hemothorax occupied by pleural fluid is significantly greater for tissue plasminogen activator plus deoxyribonuclease (29.7%) versus tissue plasminogen activator alone (15.1%), saline (17%), or deoxyribonuclease alone (17.1%).[7] Video-assisted thoracoscopic surgery is useful in the treatment of loculated empyemas.[5] Surgical removal of the fibrous peel is required to treat empyema in the organizational stage.

LUNG ABSCESS

INTRODUCTION AND EPIDEMIOLOGY

Lung abscess is defined as a localized necrosis of the lung parenchyma, typically caused by suppurative microbial infection. This initial infection is usually caused by aspiration of oral contents. Lung abscess may also develop as a result of hematogenous spread of infectious material to the lung parenchyma or lung infarct. Other less common causes of pulmonary abscess include infection as a result of penetrating chest trauma, fungal and parasitic infections, primary and metastatic neoplasms, and inflammatory conditions such as Wegener's granulomatosis and sarcoidosis.

Primary lung abscess occurs in individuals in good health or in those prone to aspiration. Approximately 80% of lung abscesses are primary.[1] The in-hospital mortality rate is 10% to 15%. Secondary lung abscess is associated with malignancy, immunosuppression, extrapulmonary infection or sepsis, or complication of surgery; the mortality is higher than seen in primary lung abscess, often over 50%. Lung abscesses present for less than 1 month are acute, with the rest being considered chronic.[1]

The incidence of lung abscess and short-term mortality have both declined over the last four decades, presumably secondary to improved treatment regimens for pneumonia. The mortality rate for community-acquired (anaerobic) lung abscess is considerably lower than that of hospital-acquired (aerobic) lung abscess.

PATHOPHYSIOLOGY

Lung abscess typically is caused by a breakdown or overwhelming of the usual pulmonary defense mechanisms. This allows a parenchymal infection to evolve into an abscess. It takes approximately 7 to 14 days for aspiration pneumonia to develop into an abscess. Anaerobic bacteria are the most common isolates from lung abscess in immunocompetent patients.[8] Generally, both aerobic and anaerobic bacteria cause lung abscess, but anaerobes are more common.[1,9] Aerobic bacteria are found more commonly in lung abscesses in immunocompromised patients and include *S. aureus, Escherichia coli, Klebsiella pneumoniae, Pseudomonas aeruginosa, Streptococcus pyogenes, Burkholderia pseudomallei, Haemophilus influenzae, Legionella pneumophila, Nocardia asteroides, Actinomyces* species, and rarely pneumococci. Aerobic infections are often hospital-acquired and have a higher mortality rate; anaerobic infections usually are community-acquired and associated with aspiration. Typical anaerobic lung abscess pathogens are pigmented *Prevotella, Porphyromonas, Bacteroides, Fusobacterium*, and *Peptostreptococcus* species.

Aspiration predisposes patients to developing pneumonia and lung abscesses. Conditions increasing the frequency of aspiration are chronic alcoholism, chronic debility with extension neck contractures, chronically depressed mental status, poor dentition and gingival disease, therapeutic or recreational drug overdose, and gastric and jejunostomy tubes. These risk factors are covered in more detail in the chapter on aspiration pneumonia.

Lung abscesses caused by hematogenous spread tend to be multilobar; risk factors include IV drug use, endocarditis, and tricuspid valve endocarditis. Jugular vein suppurative thrombophlebitis (Lemierre's syndrome) is a complication of tonsillitis that can spread to the lungs with *Fusobacterium necrophorum* bacterial seeding.[10,11]

Lung abscesses typically occur in the basal segments of the lower lobes or the posterior segment of the upper lobes. When abscesses occur in the anterior lung, a neoplasm often underpins the infection. Cancer is associated with 8% to 18% of all lung abscesses; this rate increases to 30% in those older than 45 years.

CLINICAL FEATURES

Patients with lung abscess classically present with an indolent course of cough, fever, pleuritic chest pain, weight loss, and night sweats, often for 2 or more weeks. There may be cough productive of putrid sputum that layers out when allowed to stand. Hemoptysis occurs in up to 25% of cases. Because the infection is more indolent, tachycardia, tachypnea, and fever are often absent. Laboratory findings usually are nonspecific but commonly include an elevated WBC count and erythrocyte sedimentation rate.

DIAGNOSIS

The diagnosis is usually made by a chest radiograph showing an area of dense consolidation with an air-fluid level inside of a cavitary lesion, indicating that the abscess cavity communicated with a bronchiole. Bronchiole communication occurs in about three fourths of patients with lung abscesses (**Figure 66-1**). In the remaining quarter of patients, chest CT detects the cavitary lesion (**Figure 66-2**). Multiple abscesses are unusual but can be seen in septic emboli or Lemierre's syndrome (streptococcal sepsis from peritonsillar abscess).[10]

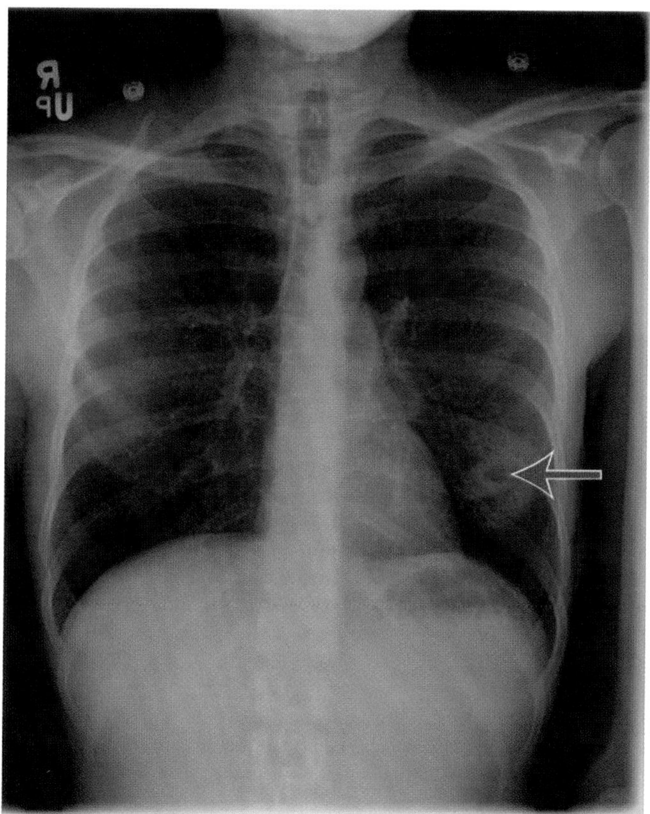

A

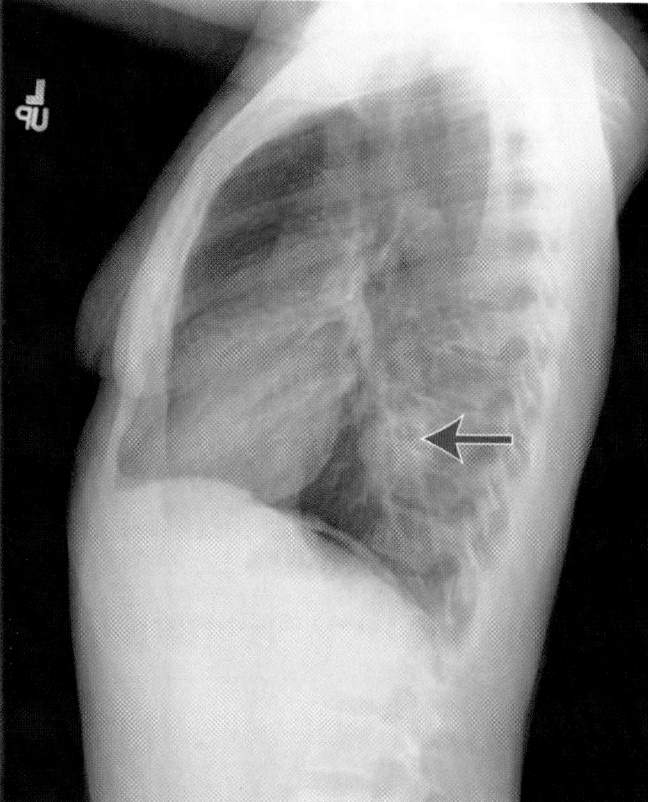

B

FIGURE 66-1. Posteroanterior and lateral chest x-ray. **A.** Chest radiograph demonstrating air-fluid level of abscess cavity at arrow. **B.** Lateral chest radiograph showing air-fluid level of abscess cavity at *arrow*.

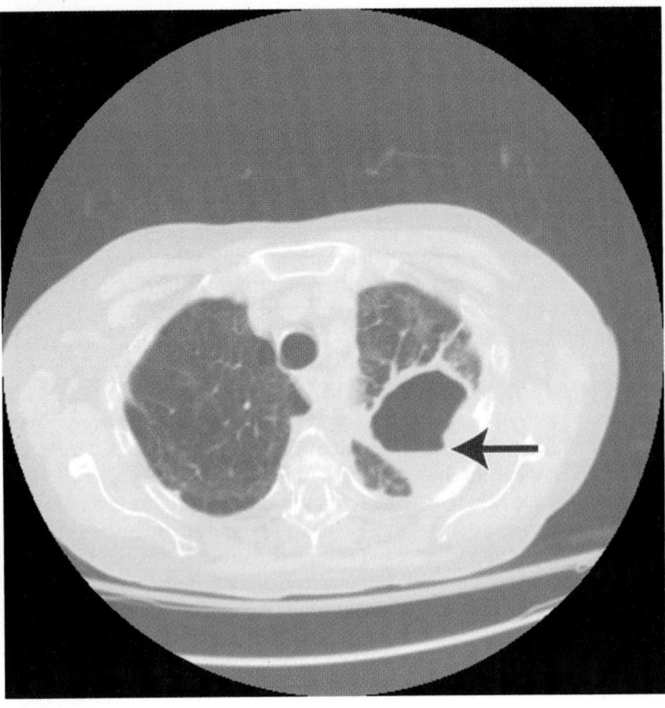

FIGURE 66-2. CT of the chest, demonstrating air-fluid level of abscess cavity at *arrow*.

TABLE 66-2 Cavitary Lung Lesions	
Infectious	
Bacterial	Anaerobic abscess (immunocompetent)
	Aerobic abscess (immunocompromised)
	Infected bullae
	Tuberculosis
	Actinomycosis
	Pleural empyema
Fungal	Coccidioidomycosis
	Histoplasmosis
	Blastomycosis
	Aspergillosis
	Cryptococcus
Parasitic	Echinococcosis
	Amebiasis
Neoplastic	Bronchogenic carcinoma (squamous cell or adenocarcinoma)
	Metastatic cancer (colorectal or renal)
	Lymphoma or Hodgkin's disease
Inflammatory	Wegener's granulomatosis
	Sarcoidosis

The differential diagnosis of cavitary lesions includes infected bullae, pleural fluid collection with bronchopleural fistula, and loop of bowel extending through a diaphragmatic hernia. Infected bullae have thin walls. Pleural fluid collection with bronchopleural fistula will demonstrate an air-fluid level that extends to the chest wall and tapers at the apex. A loop of bowel extending through a diaphragmatic hernia may result in nausea, vomiting, and abdominal pain due to incarceration or audible bowel sounds in the chest on the side on the hernia (**Figure 66-3**). **Table 66-2** lists different causes of cavitary lung lesions.

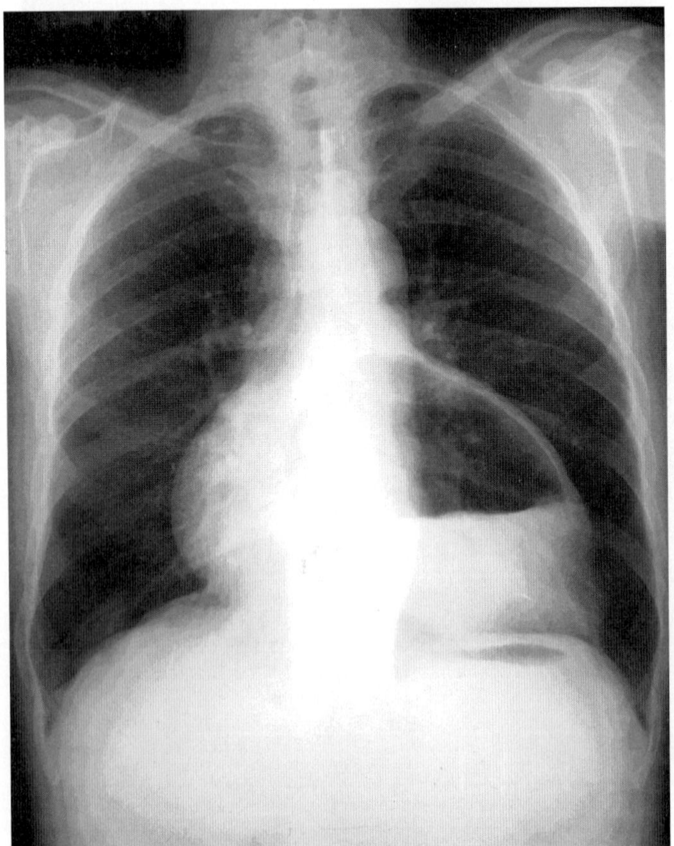

FIGURE 66-3. Hiatal hernia mimicking the appearance of cavity lesion.

TREATMENT

Medical management will resolve most lung abscesses. Initial treatment consists of clindamycin, 600 milligrams IV every 8 hours, or ampicillin-sulbactam, 1.5 to 3.0 grams IV every 6 hours, for those who cannot take clindamycin.[1,11] Alternative treatments include piperacillin-tazobactam, 3.375 grams IV every 6 hours, or meropenem or doripenem. Methicillin-resistant *S. aureus* infections are treated with linezolid, 600 milligrams IV every 12 hours, or vancomycin, 15 milligrams/kg IV every 12 hours (target trough level 15 to 20 μg/mL).[12]

Drainage usually occurs spontaneously from communication of the abscess cavity with the tracheobronchial tree. This is signaled by the development of an air-fluid level on the chest radiograph. Reasons for poor outcomes include aerobic infection, large abscess cavity, advanced age, debilitation, immunosuppression, malignancy, malnutrition, and sepsis. Reasons for failure of medical treatment include bronchial obstruction, nonbacterial cause of abscess, large cavity size, and concomitant empyema.

Surgical treatments for a nondraining lung abscess include image-guided percutaneous drainage or thoracotomy with pulmonary resection.

DISPOSITION

Admit patients with new lung abscess; hospitalization usually lasts several weeks. After resolution of symptoms, patients can be discharged on oral antibiotics for 4 to 8 weeks. Chest radiographic findings will lag behind clinical progress and will take more than 2 months to resolve.

COMPLICATIONS

Complications of lung abscess include empyema, massive hemoptysis, contamination of the uninvolved lung, and failure of the abscess cavity to resolve. Approximately 10% of bacterial lung abscesses require surgical intervention.[13]

REFERENCES

The complete reference list is available online at www.TintinalliEM.com.

CHAPTER 67 Tuberculosis

Vu D. Phan
Janet M. Poponick

INTRODUCTION AND EPIDEMIOLOGY

Tuberculosis remains an important worldwide infection, with more than one third of the overall population harboring the bacterium. It is the second leading cause of death among infectious diseases and a major cause of death among those with human immunodeficiency disease (HIV), especially in countries with limited resources.[1,2] Despite therapeutic progress over the past 20 years, drug resistance and HIV coinfection continue to challenge the global control of tuberculosis.[2]

Tuberculosis has been on the decline in the United States, with an average 3.8% decrease each year from 2000 to 2010.[3] This reduction is primarily due to tuberculosis control programs targeting high-risk individuals. In addition, improved infection control policies, increased vigilance among physicians, implementation of directly observed therapy, and standardized drug regimens all contributed to the decline of tuberculosis rates. Although overall national cases have decreased, the incidence in foreign-born patients remains 12 times that of U.S.-born persons.[3] In foreign-born patients, clinical tuberculosis is usually from reactivation of latent disease. Overall, reactivation of latent tuberculosis is responsible for 70% of active tuberculosis cases.[4]

Continued improvement in tuberculosis control and prevention requires recognition and treatment of high-risk populations (**Table 67-1**). Screening and treatment of latent infection in high-risk individuals are key to reducing tuberculosis in the United States.[4]

PATHOPHYSIOLOGY

Mycobacterium tuberculosis is a slow-growing aerobic rod that has a multilayered cell wall containing lipids that account for its acid-fast staining property. Because the organism is an obligate aerobe, it settles in areas of high oxygen content and blood flow. Transmission from person to person occurs through inhalation of droplet nuclei into the lungs. Persons with active tuberculosis who excrete mycobacteria in saliva or sputum are the most infectious.[5] Only 30% of patients actually become infected after a droplet exposure.[6]

PRIMARY AND LATENT INFECTION

Once the organisms reach the lungs, host defenses are activated. Some organisms survive and are transported to the regional lymph nodes, where the host cell-mediated immunity is activated to contain the infection. Granulomas, known as *tubercles*, form as a result of this process, which involves activated macrophages and T lymphocytes in addition to active bacteria in most cases. Tubercles are a sign of primary infection and may progress to caseation necrosis and calcification. In the lung, the **Ghon complex** (**Figure 67-1**) is a manifestation, appearing as calcified hilar lymph nodes.

If the tubercle fails to contain the infection, the mycobacteria may spread by hematogenous, lymphatic, or direct mechanical routes. The tendency is for survival in areas of high oxygen content or blood flow, such as the apical and posterior segments of the upper lobe and the superior segment of the lower lobe of the lung, the renal cortex, the meninges, the epiphyses of long bones, and the vertebrae. In these areas, the mycobacteria can remain dormant for years. During dormancy (or latent infection), the disease is detected by a positive tuberculin skin test. **The skin test generally becomes positive 1 to 2 months after initial exposure.** Only 1% to 13% of otherwise healthy patients will go on to develop active postprimary disease. However, children and HIV patients have a higher risk, approaching a 20% frequency of postprimary infection.[5,7]

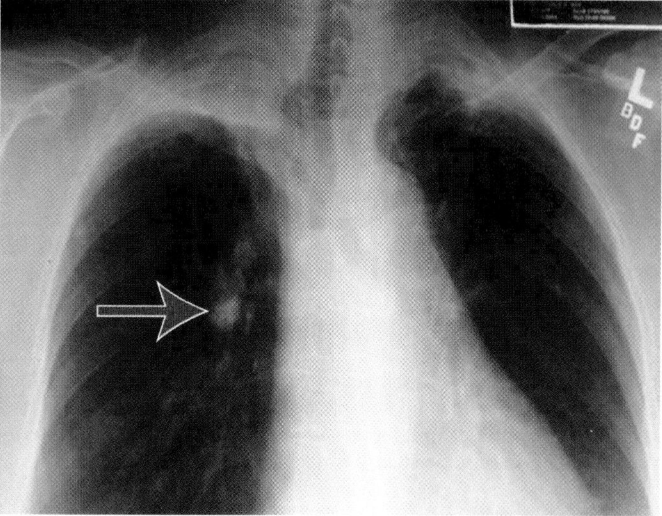

FIGURE 67-1. Primary Ghon complex (*arrow*).

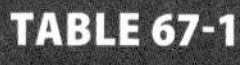

TABLE 67-1 Patients with a High Prevalence of Tuberculosis (Highest to Lowest Risk)

Immigrants from high-prevalence countries
Patients with the human immunodeficiency virus
Residents and staff of prisons or shelters for the homeless
Alcoholics and illicit drug users
Elderly and nursing home patients

REACTIVATION TUBERCULOSIS

Whether latent infection progresses to recurrently active (or "reactivation") tuberculosis is dependent on the immune status of the host.[5,6] As the host defense system weakens, it is no longer capable of containing the foci of previous hematogenous spread, and active tuberculosis may develop. The risk for reactivation is higher among HIV-infected persons and those more than 50 years old.[6] In 5% of persons, latent infection may progress to active disease within 2 years after initial exposure, with another 5% developing disease later in life.[5,7] In immunocompromised hosts, spread often occurs rapidly, and progression of early active disease is more frequent. HIV-infected patients are at particularly high risk, with progression reported at 7% to 10% per year.[5] Other groups at risk for developing tuberculosis activation include those immunocompromised from carcinoma of solid organs, leukemia, transplantation, or medications such as antagonists of tumor necrosis factor-α (etanercept or infliximab) or corticosteroids. Those with select chronic diseases such as diabetes, chronic renal failure requiring hemodialysis, psoriasis, and silicosis are also at increased risk for tuberculosis activation.[5,8]

CLINICAL FEATURES

PRIMARY TUBERCULOSIS

The initial infection is usually asymptomatic, often detected only by a positive screening tuberculin skin test or by abnormalities on chest radiograph. When the infection is primary and active, common symptoms include fever, malaise, weight loss, and chest pain.[5] Infrequently, a pneumonitis that is similar to a viral or bacterial infection appears. Hilar adenopathy is present but rarely massive. In some cases, especially in immunocompromised patients, the primary infection may be rapidly progressive and fatal.

REACTIVATION TUBERCULOSIS

When latent infection progresses to tuberculosis reactivation, symptoms may be systemic or pulmonary. The most common reactivation symptoms are similar to those of primary tuberculosis and include fever, night sweats, malaise, fatigue, and weight loss. Productive cough, hemoptysis, dyspnea, and pleuritic chest pain develop as the infection spreads within the lungs. Physical examination is generally unremarkable, although rales may be noted in areas of pulmonary infection.

Although most cases of active tuberculosis involve the lungs, up to 20% of cases will have extrapulmonary manifestations.[5] The most common extrapulmonary site of tuberculosis is the lymphatic system—painless lymphadenopathy (i.e., scrofula, cervical lymphadenitis). Other extrapulmonary manifestations include abdominal pain due to hepatosplenomegaly, peritoneal tubercles, prostatitis, epididymitis, or orchitis; adrenal insufficiency; bone pain with arthritis, osteomyelitis, or Pott's disease (bony destruction, often in the spine); hematuria and sterile puree; and meningitis. Tuberculosis can also cause pericarditis, which can lead to tamponade and constrictive symptoms. One key extrapulmonary tuberculosis axiom is that it can mimic many other common diseases, especially in the elderly and HIV patients.

DIAGNOSIS AND DIFFERENTIAL DIAGNOSIS

With the aging population, consider tuberculosis in all patients over 50 years old with a pneumonia-like presentation or prominent respiratory complaint.[5,6] Similarly, consider the disease in those with HIV or on immunosuppressive medications (notably after transplantation or with a connective tissue disease). The variable clinical presentation and the time required to culture the organism make diagnosis in the ED challenging. The goal is to have considered and begun testing for tuberculosis and to start respiratory precautions while awaiting results.

The ED is the point of entry into the healthcare system for many patients.[9] Prehospital and ED personnel should think of potential tuberculosis in higher-risk patients with lung symptoms, institute appropriate respiratory precautions, and notify healthcare providers about the possibility of tuberculosis. Place patients with suspected tuberculosis in separate waiting areas, provide them with surgical masks, and instruct them to cover the mouth and nose when coughing. Immunocompromised patients with respiratory symptoms should be evaluated promptly and isolated until tuberculosis can be excluded based on a chest radiograph.[10] A negative-pressure room is ideal for isolation when available.

During triage or initial assessment, consider the diagnosis of tuberculosis in any patient with a persistent cough (weeks or months) that has not improved despite appropriate treatment. Tuberculosis can mimic community-acquired pneumonia; clues that suggest tuberculosis include hemoptysis, night sweats, and weight loss. On chest radiograph, look carefully for upper lung field involvement, fibrocalcific changes, pleural capping, or a calcified Ghon complex.[5]

Once tuberculosis is suspected, give empiric antibiotics for pneumonia, admit the patient to an isolation bed, and institute airborne precautions. The evaluation should include sputum culture and tuberculosis skin testing and should also include HIV testing if the patient's HIV status is unknown.

MANTOUX OR TUBERCULIN SKIN TEST

The most common method for screening for exposure to *M. tuberculosis* is a skin test. The Mantoux test uses intracutaneous injection of 0.1 mL of **purified protein derivative** into the forearm. The test relies on a delayed-type hypersensitivity reaction that is triggered in those with past infection or those with a significant recent exposure to tuberculosis. The test is read between 48 and 72 hours after administration by measuring the extent of skin induration at the test site; erythema or other skin changes are not assessed (**Table 67-2**).[10] All persons with a new positive skin test or recent conversion should be referred for treatment of latent tuberculosis.

In a few situations, a positive skin test is not diagnostic of tuberculosis. Those who received **Bacillus Calmette-Guérin (BCG)** immunization for tuberculosis prevention will often have a positive skin test response in absence of infection. Exposure to nontuberculosis mycobacteria also can result in a false-positive test. False-negative skin test

TABLE 67-2 Interpretation of a Purified Protein Derivative Skin Test*

≥5-mm induration is positive in:
Patients with the human immunodeficiency virus
Patients with close contact with a tuberculosis-infected individual
Patients with abnormal chest radiograph suggestive of healed tuberculosis
Patients with organ transplants and other immunosuppressed patients receiving the equivalent of prednisone >15 milligrams per day for >1 month
≥10-mm induration is positive in patients not meeting the above criteria but who have other risks:
Injection drug users
High-prevalence groups (immigrants, long-term care facility residents, persons in local high-risk areas)
Patients with conditions that increase the risk of progression to active disease (silicosis, diabetes, carcinoma of the head, neck, or lung)
Children <4 y of age
≥15-mm induration is positive in all others
Detection of newly infected persons in a screening program:
≥10-mm induration increase within any 2-y period is positive if <35 y
≥15-mm induration increase within any 2-y period is positive if >35 y
If the patient is anergic, other epidemiologic factors must be considered

*A positive reaction does not necessarily indicate disease.

results occur with improper administration or reading, very early in the disease, or with profound underlying immunosuppression (notably in HIV).[7,8,11]

BLOOD TESTS

Interferon-gamma release assays (IGRA) are blood tests that indirectly assess for tuberculosis. The test seeks the response to peptides present in all *M. tuberculosis* proteins, which trigger the release of interferon-gamma by the infected host.[11] These proteins are absent in the BCG vaccine and in most nontuberculous mycobacteria, making IGRA more specific than skin testing.[8,11] IGRA is used in conjunction with a history, chest radiograph, and culture in those with suspected active tuberculosis.[11,12] Currently used IGRA tests give results in 16 to 24 hours. These tests are especially helpful when follow-up care compliance is a concern, notably in the homeless or drug-abusing patient, and can aid in those patients in whom skin testing is not helpful for the previously mentioned reasons or with known previous exposure (e.g., a healthcare worker).[8,11]

CHEST RADIOGRAPH

The chest radiograph is used to identify disease in those with pulmonary symptoms or after a positive skin test. No singular findings are pathognomonic for primary tuberculosis,[13] and the most common finding is a normal chest radiograph.[5] In primary infection, parenchymal infiltrates in any area of the lung may be found (**Figure 67-2**). Isolated ipsilateral hilar or mediastinal adenopathy is sometimes the only finding. Pleural effusions are usually unilateral and occur alone or in association with parenchymal disease. During primary infection, younger patients are more likely to have enlarged hilar lymph nodes, whereas adults more frequently have parenchymal abnormalities and effusions. The enlarged lymph nodes commonly encountered in children may cause external compression, leading to bronchial obstruction, atelectasis, and postobstructive hyperinflation. Because tuberculosis has a wide variety of appearances on chest radiographs, comparison with previous films is extremely helpful in determining the significance of an abnormal or unusual finding.[5,13]

In **latent tuberculosis**, nonspecific findings include upper lobe or hilar nodules and fibrotic lesions, which may be calcified. Other findings are bronchiectasis, volume loss, and pleural scarring. Healed primary areas of infection appear as Ghon foci, areas of scarring, and calcification (see Figure 67-1).

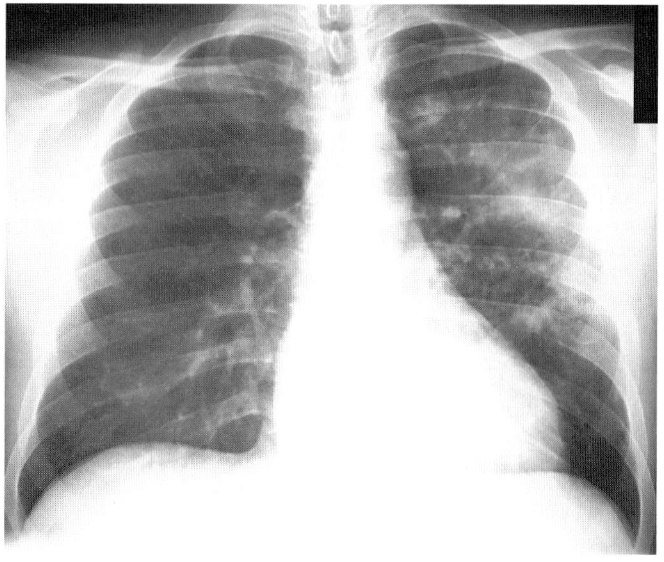

A

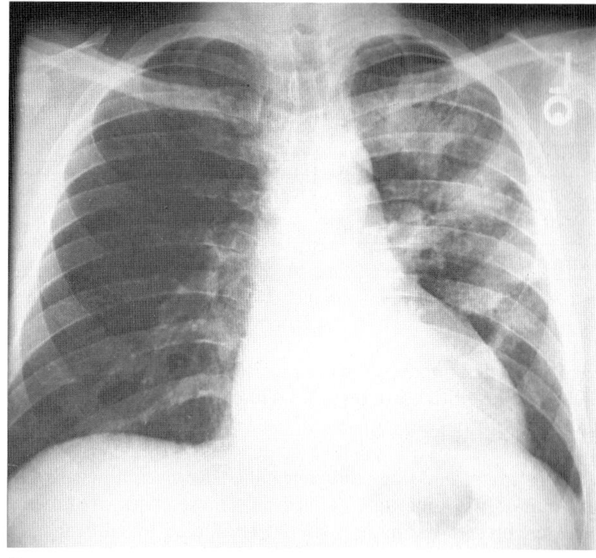

B

FIGURE 67-2. Reactivation tuberculosis. **A.** This elderly patient was treated with antibiotics for community-acquired pneumonia. **B.** When the patient did not respond, a past history of asymptomatic exposure to tuberculosis was elicited. Infiltrates were noted to be worse on hospital day 5 when tuberculosis skin test turned positive, diagnosing reactivation pulmonary tuberculosis.

Reactivation infections often have the classic findings of tuberculosis: cavitary or noncavitary lesions in the upper lobe or superior segment of the lower lobe of the lungs (**Figures 67-3 and 67-4**).

The radiographic appearance of tuberculosis is often dependent on the integrity of the immune system rather than the stage of tuberculous disease, with classic findings seen in the immunocompetent patient. Thus, immunocompromised patients are more likely to have radiographic findings traditionally considered findings of primary disease.[13,14] The frequency of classic findings on chest radiographs is directly related to the degree of immunosuppression; those HIV patients with low CD4 counts have more atypical findings on radiographs. Normal radiographs occur in up to 22% of tuberculosis patients with advanced HIV.[14,15]

FIGURE 67-3. Cavitary tuberculosis of the right upper lobe.

MICROSCOPY/CULTURES

Sputum is normally collected to detect the presence of *M. tuberculosis*. In the absence of a satisfactory sputum sample, gastric aspirates, pleural and other body fluids, or tissue samples may be used for culture and other diagnostic tests. The samples are typically stained with either a Ziehl-Neelsen stain or a fluorochrome procedure followed by exposure to an acidic agent. Mycobacteria will not lose the stain despite being rinsed with an acidic chemical. Hence, the term "**acid-fast bacilli**" is used to describe the appearance on microscopic smears. Unfortunately, the staining procedure is not sufficiently sensitive or specific to confirm or exclude the diagnosis of tuberculosis.[2] Negative smears are found in approximately 60% of culture-positive cases of tuberculosis. This number may be even higher in children and HIV patients.[13,15]

Cultures for *M. tuberculosis* are the best method of confirming diagnosis. Cultures also can aid detecting resistance to treatment regimens.

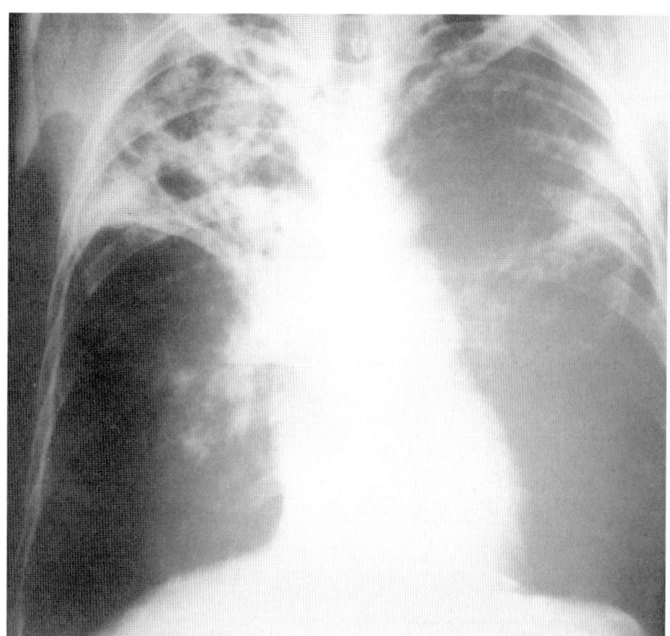

FIGURE 67-4. Advanced pulmonary tuberculosis involving apex and upper lobe.

TABLE 67-3 Antituberculous Medications

First-Line	Second-Line
Isoniazid	Cycloserine
Rifampin	Ethionamide
Rifapentine	Fluoroquinolones
Ethambutol	Streptomycin
Pyrazinamide	Amikacin
Rifabutin	Capreomycin

However, culture results are not available for weeks, thus creating the need for newer adjunctive tests to expedite diagnosis and treatment. The **nucleic acid amplification test (NAAT)** can yield results within 1 day. In patients with positive smears, it has a reported sensitivity of greater than 95%. Patients with positive smears and positive NAAT should receive treatment pending culture results.[2] However, a negative NAAT result cannot rule out tuberculosis. For these cases, treatment may depend on further testing and should be guided by clinical suspicion and culture results.[13]

TREATMENT

TREATMENT OF ACTIVE TUBERCULOSIS

Active tuberculosis treatment requires the use of a combination of antituberculous medications to overcome resistance (**Table 67-3**).[12] Initial therapy includes first-line medications (isoniazid [INH], rifampin [RIF], pyrazinamide [PZA], ethambutol) for 8 weeks, followed by two-drug continuation treatment for 18 to 31 weeks based on culture results. Second-line medications are used for drug-resistant cases or when side effects from initial therapy are not tolerable. In the ED, patients are either admitted to the hospital to determine the need for antituberculous medications or referred to specialists in the community for follow-up if compliance is likely. In most cases, antituberculous medications will not be started in the ED unless done in consultation and for classic cases. The recommended Centers for Disease Control and Prevention regimens are as follows[12]:

- Daily four-drug (INH, RIF, PZA, ethambutol) therapy for 8 weeks, followed by either INH/RIF or INH/rifapentine for 18 weeks *OR*
- Daily four-drug therapy for 2 weeks, followed by two times per week for 6 weeks, with subsequent INH/RIF or INH/rifapentine for 18 weeks *OR*
- Three times weekly four-drug therapy for 8 weeks, followed by INH/RIF three times weekly for 18 weeks *OR*
- Daily three-drug therapy (INH, RIF, ethambutol) for 8 weeks followed by INH/RIF for 31 weeks

More prolonged therapy is recommended for immunocompromised patients or for those with extrapulmonary disease. Initial therapy may be modified once drug susceptibilities are available. The importance of directly observed therapy is paramount in select patients where compliance is a concern; the Centers for Disease Control and Prevention recommends that all regimens of two or three times per week be given by directly observed therapy.[2,12]

Although the standard medications used to treat tuberculosis are generally effective and safe, side effects or drug interactions may occur (**Table 67-4**). Hepatotoxicity, or hepatitis, is the major adverse effect of INH. Preexisting liver disease, pregnancy, ethanol use, HIV, and hepatitis C infection have been associated with an increased risk for hepatotoxicity from INH. Those with preexisting medical conditions requiring multiple medications may be at higher risk for drug interactions with antituberculous agents.[2,12,15]

A portion of patients being treated for tuberculosis will clinically worsen after the initiation of antituberculous medications.[10,15,16] This effect is called a ***paradoxical reaction*** or ***immune reconstitution syndrome*** and can be seen in any patient receiving treatment for tuberculosis, although it is more commonly seen in those with HIV infection. Signs and symptoms include fever, worsening respiratory status, lymphadenopathy, hepatosplenomegaly, ascites, meningitis, and new or worsening CNS lesions. **Hypercalcemia** is a unique finding in paradoxical reactions. Because treatment of tuberculosis and HIV both improve immune function, the paradoxical reaction is thought to be a result of improvement in the body's ability to mount an inflammatory response as mycobacteria are cleared. The dilemma is differentiating this from treatment failures, drug resistance, and medication noncompliance. (See the Special Populations section.)

TREATMENT OF LATENT TUBERCULOSIS

Treatment of latent infection with INH alone is started in those with recent asymptomatic skin test conversion (see Table 67-2), any person in close contact with an actively infected patient, and anergic patients with known tuberculosis contact.[11,12] Unless contraindicated, therapy is for a minimum of 9 months for adults, children, and HIV-infected persons. Monitor those at risk for INH hepatotoxicity by serial laboratory assessment. For those exposed to INH-resistant strains or those who are intolerant, use RIF and PZA for 2 months with hepatotoxicity monitoring.[12]

TABLE 67-4 Treatment of Tuberculosis (Adults)*

Drug	Daily (maximum)	Three Times Weekly DOT (maximum)	Two Times Weekly DOT (maximum)	Potential Side Effects and Comments
Isoniazid	5 milligrams/kg PO* (300 milligrams)	15 milligrams/kg PO (900 milligrams)	15 milligrams/kg PO (900 milligrams)	Hepatitis, peripheral neuropathy, drug interactions.
Rifampin (RIF)	10 milligrams/kg PO* (600 milligrams)	10 milligrams/kg PO (600 milligrams)	10 milligrams/kg PO (600 milligrams)	Hepatitis, thrombocytopenia, GI disturbances, drug interactions.
Rifapentine	Not given daily	Not given 3 times weekly	600 milligrams PO twice weekly in adults; not approved in children <12 y old	Hepatitis, thrombocytopenia, exacerbation of porphyria. Recommended by Centers for Disease Control and Prevention for continuation therapy only for human immunodeficiency virus–negative patients.
Rifabutin	5 milligrams/kg PO (300 milligrams)	5 milligrams/kg PO (300 milligrams)	5 milligrams/kg PO (300 milligrams)	Similar to RIF; used for patients who cannot tolerate RIF.
Ethambutol	15–20 milligrams/kg PO (1.6 grams)	25–30 milligrams/kg PO (2.5 grams)	50 milligrams/kg PO (2.5 grams)	Retrobulbar neuritis, peripheral neuropathy.
Pyrazinamide	15–30 milligrams/kg PO (2 grams)	50 milligrams/kg PO (3 grams)	50 milligrams/kg PO (2 grams)	Hepatitis, arthralgia, hyperuricemia.

Abbreviation: DOT = directly observed therapy.

*See http://www.cdc.gov/tb for more accurate weight-based protocols and dosages for children.

TABLE 67-5 Engineering Controls to Reduce the Transmission of Tuberculosis

High airflow (at least 6 room air changes per hour) with external exhaust
High-efficiency particulate filters on ventilation system
Ultraviolet germicidal irradiation
Negative-pressure isolation rooms
Personal respiratory protection: high-efficiency particulate filter masks or respirators

DISPOSITION AND FOLLOW-UP

OUTPATIENT CARE

Most patients with tuberculosis can be treated initially as outpatients. If planning discharge or transfer for other nonmedical care, start or maintain therapy while awaiting smear and culture results on all with suspicious findings of active tuberculosis, notably cavitary lesions or known previous infection with new weakness or fevers.

Contact primary care physicians or public health services and arrange for long-term care before patient discharge. Discharge instructions include home isolation procedures and follow-up at the appropriate clinic to receive medication and ongoing care. **Antituberculosis medications should not be instituted in the ED unless there is joint agreement with the consultant and follow-up providers.**

HOSPITAL ADMISSION

Hospital admission should be done for the following cases: ill-appearing, hypoxemic, or dyspneic patients; if the diagnosis is uncertain; if noncompliance is likely or if the social situation makes it difficult to complete evaluation and start care; or patients with active drug-resistant tuberculosis. Hospitalized patients with suspected tuberculosis require respiratory isolation in a negative-pressure room (**Table 67-5**). An alternative to admission for therapy compliance alone is a court-ordered drug observation program (if available), where scheduled outpatient contacts to ensure medication use occur for the course of therapy.[2]

SPECIAL POPULATIONS

PATIENTS WITH TUBERCULOSIS AND HUMAN IMMUNODEFICIENCY VIRUS

HIV infection is the strongest known risk factor for tuberculosis, and the incidence of tuberculosis in HIV-positive patients is much higher than in the general population. Patients with a new diagnosis of tuberculosis are almost 20 times more likely to have HIV, and HIV patients are 20 to 30 times more likely to develop tuberculosis. Tuberculosis (pulmonary and extrapulmonary) often can be the initial clinical manifestation of immunodeficiency and is a defining event in the acquired immunodeficiency syndrome. Once active tuberculosis has developed, the risk of rapid progression and drug resistance is much higher in the HIV patient. Successful treatment with antiretroviral therapy lowers the rate of tuberculosis and reduces the incidence of extrapulmonary involvement.[17] **For these reasons, physicians considering a diagnosis of tuberculosis should obtain HIV testing to provide early diagnosis and therapy.**

Treatment of tuberculosis in HIV-positive patients is generally effective and not markedly different from others with the infection. However, due to the number of medications taken by patients with HIV, potential drug interactions are common, and compliance may become an issue. There is no consensus statement on the timing of antiretroviral therapy when treating both diseases. Recent studies support early antiretroviral therapy in combination with antituberculous medications, especially in those who are severely immunocompromised.[1,18]

Immune reconstitution inflammatory syndrome or paradoxical reaction (see Treatment of Active Tuberculosis) is a condition in which HIV patients clinically worsen as the immune system recovers after the initiation of antiretroviral therapy or antituberculous medications. The ideal timing of antiretroviral therapy in those with active tuberculosis is uncertain.[1,18] See chapter 154, Human Immunodeficiency Virus Infection.

MULTIDRUG-RESISTANT TUBERCULOSIS

Multidrug-resistant tuberculosis is defined as tuberculosis with isolates that demonstrate resistance to at least INH and RIF. *M. tuberculosis* becomes resistant by spontaneous genetic mutation, often as a result of inadequate drug therapy or noncompliance with initial treatment. While resistance is usually not confirmed until culture and sensitivity data are available, certain historical and clinical features raise the level of suspicion for multidrug-resistant tuberculosis. These include a history of tuberculosis treatment in the past, exposure to multidrug-resistant tuberculosis, known INH resistance in the community above 4%, and persistent symptoms or persistently positive sputum cultures despite 4 months of standard treatment.[19]

Extensive drug-resistant tuberculosis is a more intense worldwide threat to public health and tuberculosis control. Extensive drug-resistant tuberculosis is defined as disease resistant to INH and RIF, plus resistance to any fluoroquinolone, and resistance to at least one injectable second-line medication. It is associated with poor outcomes and higher mortality.

Treatment of multidrug-resistant tuberculosis depends on sensitivity patterns from culture. Some countries may use standardized regimens based on known local resistance patterns. Usually a combination therapy with four to six medications, including the more toxic and less potent second-line medications, is administered for up to 2 years. Success rates rarely exceed 75%.[20] In refractory cases, resectional surgery may be necessary in addition to ongoing medical therapy.[19]

The "Global Plan to Stop Tuberculosis" calls for new medications to fight against the problem of multidrug-resistant tuberculosis. In addition to testing and better current therapy compliance, new medications show promise, especially **delamanid**.[20]

CHILDREN

Tuberculosis in children occurs in the same risk groups as in the adult population (see Table 67-1). The clinical course and disease manifestations in children have several unique aspects. Although children are at greater risk for developing rapidly progressive and disseminated disease, their presenting signs and symptoms can be subtle. Primary tuberculosis in children is often asymptomatic and only identified through screening programs or contact tracing.[21] Children may be asymptomatic even with abnormal radiographs. Or, children may present with fever, cough, wheezing, poor feeding, and fatigue. The classic symptoms of fever, night sweats, and weight loss may be seen in older children; however, in those younger than 5 years, presentation may be that of miliary tuberculosis (see below), meningitis, or a pneumonia that does not respond to therapy. The most common extrapulmonary presentation is **cervical lymphadenitis,** but other regions may be involved including the meninges, pericardium, abdomen, bone, joints, kidneys, skin, and eyes.

The yield of sputum smears and cultures is lower in children because of difficulty in obtaining adequate samples in addition to the lower incidence of cavitary disease.[22,23] Traditionally, obtaining three early morning consecutive gastric lavage or gastric aspirate samples has been standard procedure. However, this is invasive, unpleasant, and often requires an overnight admission and trained staff. Sputum induction using bronchodilators, followed by nebulized saline and expectoration of mucus, can improve sampling.[23]

The diagnosis of tuberculosis in children is confirmed by culture in only 30% to 40% of cases.[13] The newer tests, IGRA and NAAT, are not recommended for children less than 5 years old. The immune response differs in this age group, making the tests less reliable.[11] Often, treatment is initiated based on a skin test or on clinical grounds (symptoms, a history of exposure, or abnormal radiographs), and the diagnosis is presumed based on response to treatment.[22] Multidrug therapy is currently recommended for all children considered to have active disease, whereas monotherapy is used for latent infections.

MILIARY TUBERCULOSIS

Miliary tuberculosis is a historic term used in reference to the gross appearance of the lung during disseminated tuberculosis. In such cases, the lung is often covered with multiple small lesions resembling millet seeds. Classic miliary tuberculosis shows diffuse nodules on radiographs (1 to 3 mm) in a patient with positive laboratory testing or by demonstration of mycobacteria in multiple organs. The classic radiographic findings may not appear on films until the disease has progressed over time. A miliary pattern on radiographs can be found in conditions other than tuberculosis including histoplasmosis, malignancy, siderosis, and sarcoidosis.[24]

Today, miliary tuberculosis refers to wide hematogenous spread during the primary or reactivation disease, and it is associated with higher mortality. Children, the elderly, and immunocompromised patients are all at increased risk of developing miliary disease.

Miliary disease during primary tuberculosis is generally more rapid and severe, often presenting with multiorgan failure, shock, and acute respiratory distress syndrome. Conversely, miliary reactivation often manifests with a chronic, nonspecific clinical course affecting any number of organ systems. Fever, anorexia, night sweats, cough, weight loss, splenomegaly, lymphadenopathy, and signs of multisystem illness should cause one to suspect miliary disease. Cutaneous involvement, seen more often in HIV patients, manifests as papules or vesiculopapules (*tuberculosis cutis miliaris disseminata* or *tuberculosis cutis acuta generalisata*). Choroidal tubercles found on ocular exam are pathognomonic for miliary tuberculosis.

TUBERCULOUS MENINGITIS

Tuberculous meningitis is often seen in children, although those with HIV or others who are immunocompromised may also be afflicted. The challenge is the subtle and subacute presentation over days to weeks, with gradual fever, headache, and cognition or sensorium changes that often are not accompanied by neck stiffness or irritation, in contrast with those seen in other forms of bacterial meningitis. Focal neurologic deficits or cranial nerve palsies may also be evident. Suspecting the infection and requesting tuberculosis cultures and smear are key to making a diagnosis, because other diagnostics are not helpful.[25] Long-term neurologic dysfunction is common, with ventriculoperitoneal shunting needed in 25% of patients for hydrocephalus. Tuberculous meningitis often seeds after a miliary infection. Treatment parallels other forms of tuberculosis.

PRACTICE GUIDELINES

The American Thoracic Society, Infectious Disease Society (http://www.idsociety.org), and Centers for Disease Control and Prevention (http://www.cdc.gov) have issued recent joint guidelines for the management of tuberculosis.

REFERENCES

The complete reference list is available online at www.TintinalliEM.com.

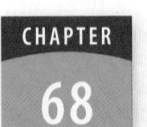

CHAPTER 68 Pneumothorax

Bret A. Nicks
David Manthey

INTRODUCTION AND EPIDEMIOLOGY

Pneumothorax occurs when free air enters the potential space between the visceral and parietal pleura. **Primary pneumothoraces** occur without clinically apparent lung disease, either spontaneously or from penetration of the intrapleural space by trauma. **Secondary pneumothoraces** occur in patients with underlying lung disease.

TABLE 68-1 Causes of Secondary Pneumothorax

Airway disease
Chronic obstructive pulmonary disease
Asthma
Cystic fibrosis (8%–20% will develop one in lifetime)
Interstitial lung disease
Sarcoidosis
Pulmonary fibrosis
Tuberous sclerosis
Infection
Human immunodeficiency virus infection, *Pneumocystis* pneumonia
Tuberculosis
Bacterial pneumonia, necrotizing
Lung abscess
Connective tissue disease
Marfan's syndrome
Ehlers-Danlos syndrome
Scleroderma
Rheumatoid arthritis
Cancer
Primary lung or metastatic disease
Catamenial pneumothorax

The incidence of **primary spontaneous pneumothorax** is 10 to 18 cases for men and 2 to 5 cases for women per 100,000 population.[1] Associated factors include cigarette smoking, male gender, mitral valve prolapse, Marfan's syndrome, and changes in ambient pressure. Familial patterns also suggest an inherited association.[2] Physical activity or exertion can precipitate but is not a common pneumothorax-triggering factor. **Traumatic pneumothoraces** are subdivided into iatrogenic and noniatrogenic. Noniatrogenic pneumothoraces will be further discussed in the chapter 261, "Pulmonary Trauma."

Causes of **secondary spontaneous pneumothorax** are listed in **Table 68-1**. Chronic obstructive pulmonary disease remains the most common cause.[3] Pneumothorax occurs in 5% of patients with acquired immunodeficiency syndrome, is associated with subpleural necrosis by *Pneumocystis* infection, and carries a high mortality. Because of necrosis of lung tissue and continued air leak, simple aspiration fails in this group of patients. Hemopneumothorax occurs in 2% to 7% of patients with secondary pneumothorax and, if associated with a large amount of blood in the pleural cavity, can be life threatening.[4-7] Treating the underlying disease may help decrease the risk of future pneumothorax.

PATHOPHYSIOLOGY

Under normal conditions, the parietal and visceral pleura are in close apposition. The pleural space is negatively pressured at −5 mm Hg with fluctuations of 6 to 8 mm Hg between inspiration and expiration. The inherent tendency of the chest wall is to expand and for the lungs to collapse from elastic recoil. With the loss of the normal negative pressure in the pleural space that "adheres" the visceral pleura (lungs) to the parietal pleura (ribs), the affected lung collapses. A primary spontaneous pneumothorax occurs when a subpleural bleb ruptures, disrupting pleural integrity. Rupture in primary spontaneous pneumothoraces usually involves the lung apex.[6-8] In secondary spontaneous pneumothoraces, disruption of the visceral pleura occurs secondary to underlying pulmonary disease processes.

Once there is a break in the visceral pleura, air travels down a pressure gradient into the intrapleural space, until pressure equilibrium occurs with partial or total lung collapse. Altered ventilation–perfusion relationships and decreased vital capacity contribute to dyspnea and hypoxemia. If air continues to enter the pleural space, intrapleural pressure becomes positive. **Tension pneumothorax** develops as inhaled air accumulates in the pleural space but cannot exit due to a check-valve system.

As intrathoracic pressure (>15 to 20 mm Hg) increases, the great vessels and heart are compressed and shifted contralaterally, severely restricting venous return, diastolic filling, and cardiac output causing ventilation-perfusion mismatch, and resulting in hypoxia and shock.[8] Tension pneumothorax can develop in the presence of a chest tube if gas egress is obstructed, including from the adjacent lung.

CLINICAL FEATURES

Classic symptoms of primary spontaneous pneumothorax are sudden onset of dyspnea and ipsilateral, pleuritic chest pain. The pleuritic component of the pneumothorax may resolve within the first 24 hours. Profound dyspnea is rare, unless the patient has poor reserve due to underlying parenchymal disease or develops a tension pneumothorax. Sinus tachycardia is the most common physical finding. Because many pneumothoraces are small, other classic findings like ipsilateral decreased breath sounds, hyperresonance to percussion, and decreased or absent tactile fremitus are absent. In *traumatic pneumothorax*, the positive predictive value of ipsilateral decreased breath sounds is 86% to 97% for the diagnosis.[9] Cough and exertional complaints are not common signs or symptoms.[2] Except for trauma, physical exam alone is not sensitive enough to exclude the diagnosis.

The clinical hallmarks of **tension pneumothorax** are tracheal deviation away from the involved side, hyperresonance of the affected side, hypotension, and significant dyspnea.[8]

DIAGNOSIS

Pneumothorax is an important differential consideration in patients with chest pain, especially in those with underlying lung disease. Patients with pleurisy, pleural effusions, infiltrates, or shingles can present with pain similar to those with pneumothorax.

IMAGING

Chest X-Ray A standard erect posteroanterior chest radiograph is the usual initial test and demonstrates loss of lung markings in the periphery and a pleural line that runs parallel to the chest wall (**Figure 68-1**).

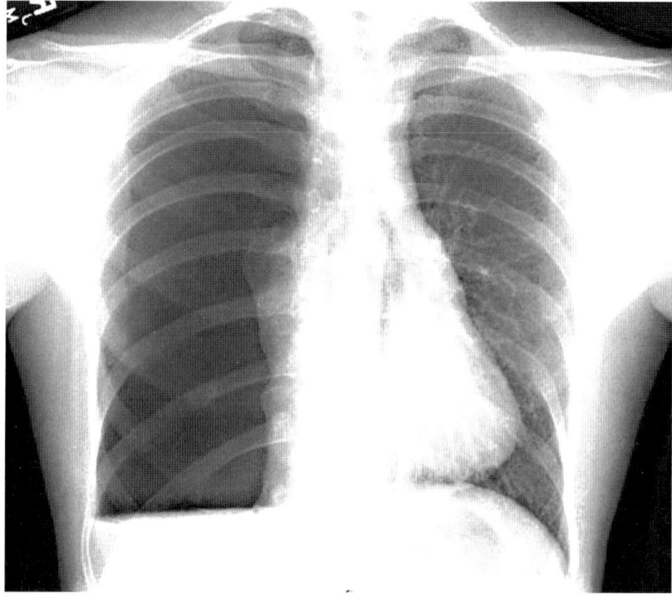

FIGURE 68-1. Spontaneous hemopneumothorax. Upright chest radiograph of a 19-year-old male college student with spontaneous hemopneumothorax. Note the large air-fluid level in the inferior portion of the right hemithorax in addition to the complete collapse of the entire right lung.

Ensure that the line does not extend outside of the chest cavity, suggesting a confluence of shadows or skin line. A lateral radiograph will identify a pneumothorax in an additional 14% of cases.[10] An expiratory radiograph does not identify many additional pneumothoraces. The sensitivity of anteroposterior chest radiography, when compared with CT, was 75.5% (95% confidence interval, 61.7% to 86.2%), with a specificity of 100% (95% confidence interval, 97.1% to 100%).[10-12] In critically ill patients, when they cannot be moved to an erect position, look for the **deep sulcus sign**, a deep lateral costophrenic angle, on the affected side.

Large bullae in patients with chronic obstructive pulmonary disease may look like a pneumothorax, although a pneumothorax pleural line will run parallel with the chest wall, whereas bullae will have a medially concave appearance. Pneumothoraces usually cross more than one lung segment, whereas bullae are limited to a single lobe. A chest CT can differentiate the two. A thoracostomy with the chest tube inserted into a bulla mistaken for a pneumothorax results in a large pneumothorax, associated bronchopulmonary fistula, and its complications.[12] Pleural adhesions cement the visceral and parietal pleura together, changing the appearance of the pneumothorax.

Pneumothorax size may be calculated by the Light index or Collins or Rhea methods, but most published formulae show only a modest correlation to actual pneumothorax size.[13-16] The American College of Chest Physicians supports a method of measurement from the apex of the lung to the cupula of the thoracic cavity on an upright posteroanterior film.[17] A measurement of less than 3 cm in this cephalad area is considered a small pneumothorax. Another method is to measure the interpleural distance at the level of the hilum; in this area, a distance of 2 cm correlates with a pneumothorax of approximately 50% by volume.[18] The British Thoracic Society defines a small pneumothorax as one with a <2-cm rim between the lung edge and chest wall and a large pneumothorax as one with a ≥2-cm rim.[18]

US US detects traumatic pneumothorax, with a reported sensitivity of 98.1% (95% confidence interval, 89.9% to 99.9%) and specificity of 99.2% (95% confidence interval, 95.6% to 99.9%).[13] The movement of the lung (ocean) against the stationary chest wall (shore) is often referred to as the "seashore." In a normal lung, there is commonly a sonographic reverberation distal to the pleura that looks like a **comet tail** and a **sliding sign** of the movement of the visceral pleura along the parietal pleura (**Figure 68-2**). In the presence of intrapleural air, pleural adhesions, effusions, and parenchymal disease, small pneumothoraces may be loculated, and therefore, the sliding sign and the comet tail reverberation are lost, limiting the specificity for pneumothorax.[14,15]

Chest CT Chest CT detects between 25% and 40% of pneumothoraces not visualized on a postprocedure chest radiograph.[12] CT can detect other pathology such as pulmonary blebs. If a chest radiograph does not demonstrate pneumothorax but there is clinical suspicion for the condition (e.g., in symptomatic high-risk patients, those with underlying lung disease or positive-pressure ventilation, or after lung biopsy), obtain a chest CT (**Figure 68-3**).

TREATMENT

The ED treatment goal is the elimination of intrapleural air. **Tension pneumothorax should be diagnosed clinically—before a radiograph—and *immediately* treated by needle decompression followed by tube thoracostomy.**

Treatment options are oxygen, observation, needle or catheter aspiration (either single or sequential aspirations), and tube thoracostomy (either small-size or standard chest tube) (see Tables 68-2 and 68-3). **Oxygen** administration (>28%) increases pleural air resorption three- to fourfold over the base 1.25% reabsorbed per day, by creating a nitrogen gas pressure gradient between the alveolus and trapped air.[19-21] Without supplemental oxygen, a 25% pneumothorax would take approximately 20 days to resolve. Recommended dosing ranges from 3 L/min nasal cannula to 10 L/min by mask and should be guided by the patient's status. Monitor for hypercapnia in patients with chronic obstructive pulmonary disease.

Observation is appropriate for small, stable pneumothoraces only. If this option is selected, observe the patient for at least 4 hours on

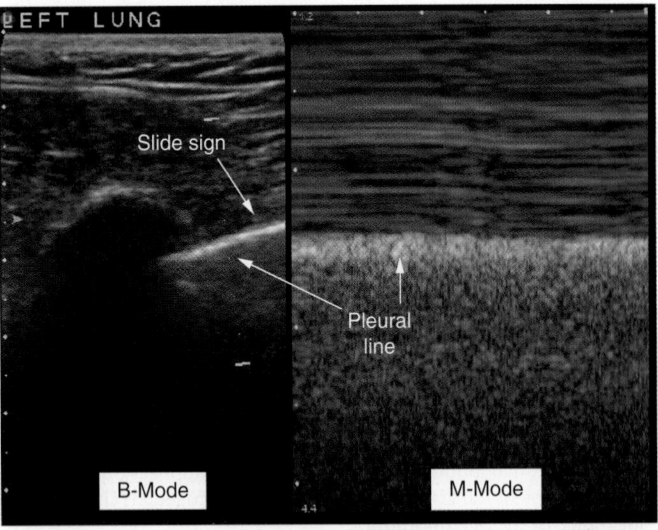

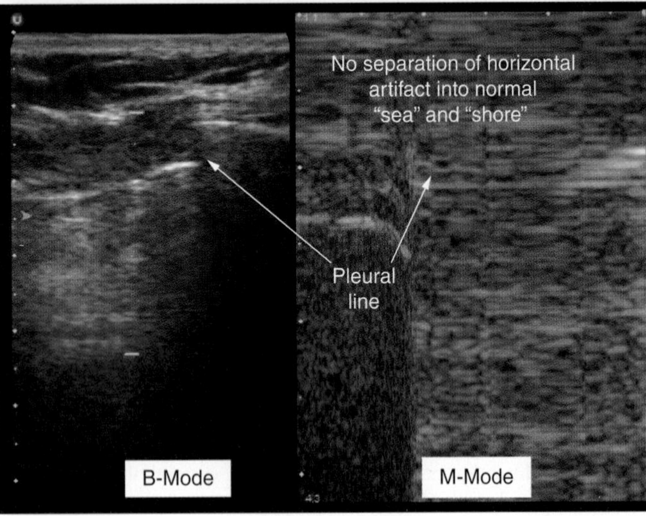

FIGURE 68-2. US with M-mode and B-mode imaging of normal (**A**) and abnormal (**B**) pleura. [Image used with permission of Casey Glass, MD, Wake Forest School of Medicine.]

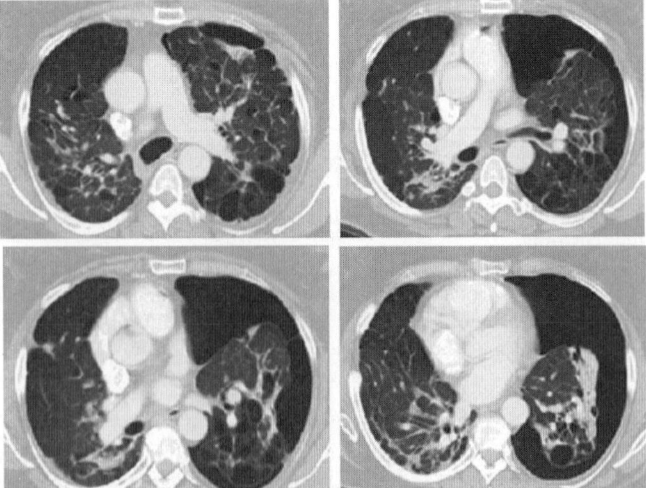

FIGURE 68-3. Secondary spontaneous pneumothorax. CT of a large, left-sided secondary spontaneous pneumothorax. Note diffuse bullous emphysema.

TABLE 68-2 Criteria for Stable Patient with Pneumothorax
Respiratory rate <24 breaths/min
No dyspnea at rest, speaks in full sentences
Pulse >60 and <120 beats/min
Normal blood pressure for patient
Room air oxygen saturation >90%
Absence of hemothorax

supplemental oxygen, and then repeat the chest radiograph. If symptoms and chest radiograph improve, the patient should return in 24 hours for repeat examination. First-time spontaneous pneumothorax of <20% lung volume in a stable, healthy adult may be treated initially with oxygen therapy and observation.[19-24]

Aspiration or tube thoracostomy is selected based on likelihood of recurrence and likelihood of spontaneous resolution. Pneumothoraces in patients with underlying pulmonary disease are likely to recur. Large pneumothoraces and those with an air leak are unlikely to resolve without drainage. Inability to return for care or to tolerate any pneumothorax increase (i.e., those with poor cardiopulmonary reserve) should prompt drainage.

When deciding to intervene procedurally on a pneumothorax, the stability of the patient, the degree of symptoms, the size and relative change in size over time, the cause of the pneumothorax, the degree of underlying lung disease, the likelihood of recurrence and resolution, and the need for positive-pressure ventilation are factors to consider. In situations when the patient is clinically stable (**Table 68-2**), various treatment approaches can be considered (**Tables 68-3 and 68-4**).[18-27]

The selection of catheter or chest tube size is based on the flow rate of air that the device can accommodate. Select large-bore tubes for anticipated big leaks, as from mechanical ventilation. Tension pneumothorax can develop if a large air leak develops, and small-bore tubes or catheters cannot handle the air flow. Every chest tube has a proximal hole, called the sentinel eye, which is visible radiographically and helps ensure that all drainage holes are inside the pleural cavity. Table 68-3 provides definitions for terms and various devices used to treat pneumothorax.[26-30]

NEEDLE DECOMPRESSION

To decompress, wear protective clothing or at least a mask to prevent material from squirting onto the operator. Use a 14-gauge needle for adults and an 18-gauge needle for children. Select a needle at least 2 inches (5 cm) long to penetrate the pleural cavity. Two locations are recommended: into the second or third intercostal space just above the rib (to avoid the intercostal artery) at the midclavicular line, or in the fourth or fifth intercostal space just above the rib and at the anterior axillary line (**Figure 68-4**). One small postmortem study analyzing both approaches reported only a 59% success rate in entering the pleural cavity.[31] If the needle is inserted medial to the midclavicular line, mediastinal vessels can

TABLE 68-3 Aspiration and Thoracostomy Devices*	
Single aspiration	Insertion of a needle or catheter, aspiration of air using an attached syringe, and immediate removal of the device
Needle aspiration	18-gauge needle (provided in kits as an 8-French catheter over an 18-gauge needle)
Small-size catheter	≤14 French
Small-size chest tube	10–14 French
Pigtail catheter	14 French, placement using Seldinger technique
Moderate-size chest tube	16–22 French
Large-size chest tube	24–36 French

*The term "catheter" is used for a thin flexible tube; the term "chest tube" is used for a more rigid, larger tube. French sizes represent tube or catheter diameter (1 French = $^1/_3$-mm diameter), and the larger the French number, the larger the device.

TABLE 68-4 Treatment of Pneumothorax

Condition	Treatment Options
Small primary pneumothorax (<20% or 3 cm apex-cupula and asymptomatic)	Observation for >3 h on oxygen, repeat chest x-ray, discharge if no symptoms, and return for check if symptoms recur or in 24 h Or Small-size catheter aspiration with immediate catheter removal, then observe for >3 h, discharge if no symptoms, and return for check if symptoms recur or in 24 h Or Small-size catheter aspiration or small-size chest tube insertion, Heimlich valve, or water seal and admission
Small secondary pneumothorax	Small-size catheter or small-size chest tube insertion, Heimlich valve, or water seal and admission
Large pneumothorax, either primary or secondary, or bilateral pneumothoraces	Moderate-size chest tube and admission; large-size chest tube if fluid or hemothorax present; water seal and admission
Tension pneumothorax	Immediate needle decompression followed by moderate or large-size chest tube insertion, water seal drainage, and admission; immediate chest tube placement ideal

be injured. A finger cot cut at its distal end can then be placed over the needle to fabricate a one-way valve. The Heimlich valve is still occasionally used for ambulatory treatment of pneumothorax, and serious complications with its use are rare.[32]

NEEDLE OR CATHETER ASPIRATION

Needle or catheter aspiration is as effective as thoracostomy for treating the first episode of small primary or secondary spontaneous pneumothorax,[25] with success ranging from 37% to 75%, or higher in those with primary spontaneous pneumothorax.[26] Techniques include simple one-time aspiration with a large-gauge needle or a small-bore catheter, repeated aspirations through a small-size catheter, or chest tube attached to a one-way valve or water seal drainage. The catheter technique has the advantages of both aspiration and chest tube placement.[27]

Small-Size Catheters The catheter technique involves placing a small catheter either into the second anterior intercostal space in the midclavicular line or laterally at the fourth or fifth intercostal space in the anterior axillary line after local anesthesia and sterile preparation. Attach a three-way stopcock, and use a 60-mL syringe to aspirate the pleural space until resistance is met, often triggering a cough. Close the stopcock, secure the tube, and obtain a follow-up chest radiograph to ensure lung reexpansion. Aspiration of more than 4 L suggests continued air leak and failure of simple aspiration. Failure of the lung to fully expand warrants another aspiration attempt or formal tube thoracostomy and admission.

Pigtail Catheters Using Seldinger Technique Advantages of this technique are a smaller incision, less tissue dissection, and smaller scar.

Insert the needle into the pleural space, making sure placement is in the "triangle of safety" (**Figure 68-5**).[29,32] Aspirate fluid or air to verify location in the pleural space, and advance a guidewire through the needle. Place a dilator over the guidewire until the pleural space is entered. Remove the dilator and place the chest tube over the wire into the pleural space. Remove the stylet, secure the tube, and attach to suction.

Tube Thoracostomy Chest tube thoracostomy is used to treat a large pneumothorax, recurrent or bilateral pneumothorax, or coexistent hemothorax, or if there are abnormal vital signs or dyspnea. A chest tube is used in small spontaneous secondary pneumothoraces where large air leak is anticipated or noted. Standard chest tube thoracostomy with underwater seal drainage is the most commonly used approach, with a low complication rate and a success rate of 95%.[24,25] Most guidelines suggest a small 10- to 14-French chest tube for nontrauma, reserving larger 14- to 22-French chest tubes if a large air leak is probable, such as from mechanical ventilation or with underlying pulmonary disease.

The technique of tube thoracostomy is described in the chapter 261, "Pulmonary Trauma."

There is no clear difference between simple aspiration and intercostal tube drainage in overall short- and long-term outcomes,[24] and simple aspiration is as safe and effective as tube thoracostomy for small-volume air leak primary spontaneous pneumothorax.[25]

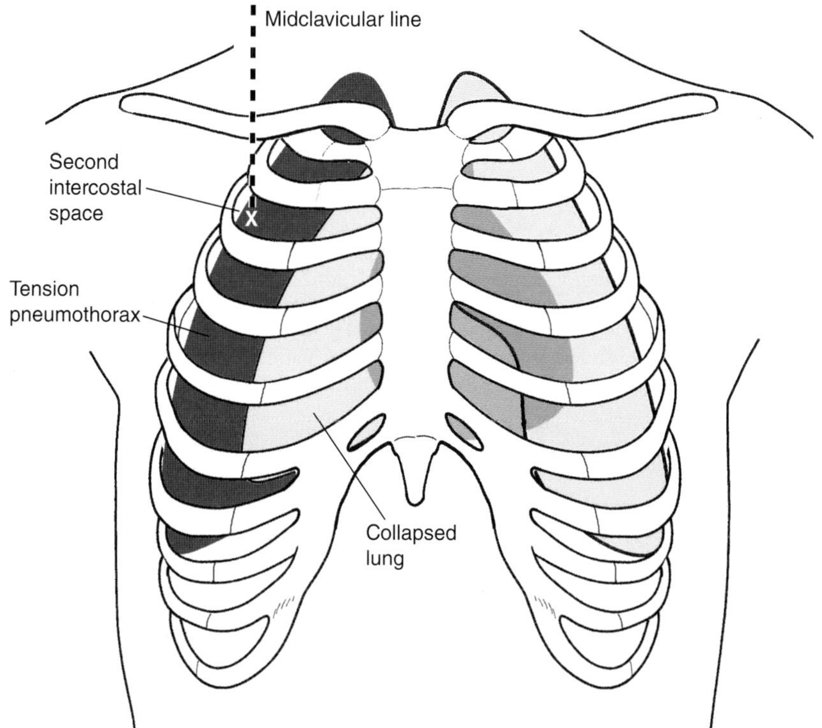

FIGURE 68-4. Needle placement for decompression of a right-sided tension pneumothorax. A site for a needle thoracostomy is the second intercostal space in the midclavicular line. [Reproduced with permission from Reichman EF, Simon RR: *Emergency Medicine Procedures*. © 2004, McGraw-Hill, New York.]

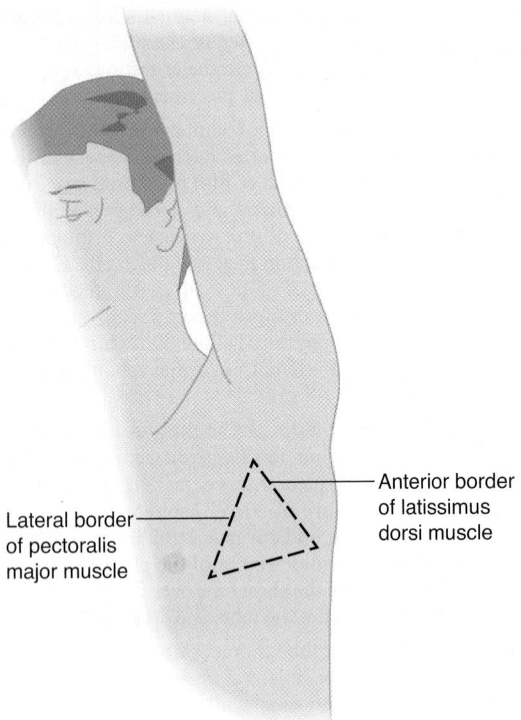

FIGURE 68-5. Safe location of chest tube, within a triangle bordered by the fifth intercostal space, pectoralis major, and latissimus dorsi.

TREATMENT COMPLICATIONS

Complications of the pneumothorax itself can include those due to hypoxia, hypercapnia, and hypotension. Reexpansion lung injury is uncommon and seen more often when there is collapse of the lung for greater than 72 hours, a large pneumothorax, rapid reexpansion, or negative pleural pressure suction of greater than 20 cm.[3,8] Most patients need no treatment for re-expansion injury aside from observation or oxygen, with virtually no adverse outcomes.[30]

Intervention complications include intercostal vessel hemorrhage, lung parenchymal injury, empyema, and tube malfunction (development of an air leak or tension pneumothorax). Pleurodesis for recurrence prevention is used in those with first spontaneous pneumothorax with a persistent air leak, second ipsilateral spontaneous pneumothorax, first contralateral pneumothorax, bilateral spontaneous pneumothoraces, first episode of a secondary pneumothorax, or recurrent high-risk activities (flying or diving).[3,8]

SPECIAL CONSIDERATIONS

IATROGENIC PNEUMOTHORAX

Iatrogenic pneumothorax is a subset of traumatic pneumothorax and occurs more often than spontaneous pneumothorax. Transthoracic needle procedures (needle biopsy and thoracentesis) account for approximately half of iatrogenic pneumothoraces, and subclavian vein catheterization accounts for one fourth. Given that one central venous line is placed every minute in the United States and that pneumothorax occurs after 0.5% to 3.0% of subclavian line attempts, iatrogenic pneumothorax is common, underdetected, and underreported.[28] Factors associated with the increasing frequency of iatrogenic pneumothorax include the patient population, underlying disease, body habitus, and experience of the operator. US guidance for central venous catheter insertion for thoracentesis reduces the pneumothorax complication rate.

Although it is routine to obtain a chest radiograph after central line placement or transthoracic needle procedures, chest radiograph may not identify a pneumothorax if supine or if there is inadequate time for the pneumothorax to develop, with up to one third detected later.[28]

Treatment for iatrogenic pneumothorax is generally the same as that for spontaneous pneumothorax. Patients with a small pneumothorax after a needle puncture and those not requiring positive-pressure ventilation can be observed or initially treated with simple catheter aspiration (with or without a Heimlich valve), which is adequate for 60% to 80% of patients.[28] Long-term recurrence is not a concern with iatrogenic pneumothorax.

AIR TRANSPORT WITH PNEUMOTHORAX

Increased elevation causes an increase in gas volume (Boyle's law), increasing the risk for tension pneumothorax in air transport patients with pneumothorax, particularly when transported in fixed-wing vehicles (airplane) given the altitudes reached.[21] High-altitude flying is not recommended for at least 7 to 14 days after pneumothorax resolution.

DIVING

Similarly, due to Boyle's law, development of a pneumothorax at depth may lead to a tension pneumothorax with ascent. Current guidelines suggest that a history of spontaneous pneumothorax is a contraindication to underwater diving unless treated by surgical pleurectomy and normal lung function exists.[21]

DISPOSITION

Patients with a primary spontaneous pneumothorax who have been treated with observation or with catheter aspiration can be discharged if the pneumothorax does not increase in size over 3 to 6 hours and symptoms resolve or do not worsen. The remaining patients are observed longer or admitted, with that decision based on the size, therapy, and clinical condition.

REFERENCES

The complete reference list is available online at www.TintinalliEM.com.

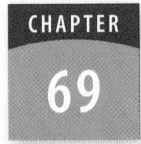

Acute Asthma

Rita K. Cydulka

INTRODUCTION AND EPIDEMIOLOGY

Asthma is a chronic inflammatory disorder characterized by increased responsiveness of the airways to multiple stimuli. In susceptible individuals, the inflammation causes recurrent episodes of wheezing, breathlessness, chest tightness, and coughing, particularly at night or in the early morning. These episodes usually are associated with widespread and varying airflow obstruction.

Although most acute attacks are reversible and improve spontaneously or within minutes to hours with treatment with symptom-free intervals in between, many asthmatic patients develop chronic airflow limitation. This impacts the diagnosis of, management of, and attempts to prevent acute exacerbations.

Asthma affects approximately 8% of the U.S. population, is the most common chronic disease of childhood (9% prevalence), affects 7% of the elderly, and has a similar prevalence in developed nations around the world.[1-3] Approximately one half of cases of asthma develop before the age of 10 years old, and another one third develop before the age of 40 years old.

PATHOPHYSIOLOGY

Asthma is characterized by an abnormal accumulation of eosinophils, lymphocytes, mast cells, macrophages, dendritic cells, and myofibroblasts in airways. The pathophysiologic hallmark of asthma is a reduction in

TABLE 69-1 Physiologic Consequences of Airflow Obstruction

Increased airway resistance
Decreased maximum expiratory flow rates
Air trapping
Increased airway pressure
Barotrauma
Adverse hemodynamic effects
Ventilation–perfusion imbalance
Hypoxemia
Hypercarbia
Increased work of breathing
Pulsus paradoxus
Respiratory muscle fatigue with ventilatory failure

airway diameter caused by smooth muscle contraction, vascular congestion, bronchial wall edema, and thick secretions. These changes are reflected in pulmonary function changes, increased work of breathing, and abnormal distribution of pulmonary blood flow (**Table 69-1**). Large and small airways contain plugs composed of mucus, serum proteins, inflammatory cells, and cellular debris. On a microscopic level, airways are infiltrated with eosinophils and mononuclear cells. Evidence of microvascular leakage, epithelial disruption, and vasodilation is frequently noted. The airway smooth muscle is hypertrophied and characterized by new vessel formation, an increased number of epithelial goblet cells, and deposition of interstitial collagen beneath the epithelium. Inflammation affects all bronchial pulmonary structures.

Asthma is a continuum from acute bronchospasm to airway inflammation to permanent airway remodeling. The structural changes associated with airway remodeling, such as sub-basement membrane thickening, subepithelial fibrosis, airway smooth muscle hypertrophy and hyperplasia, angiogenesis, and mucous gland hyperplasia and hypersecretion are associated with nonreversible loss of lung function.[4] Acute allergic bronchoconstriction results from immunoglobulin E–dependent release of mediators from mast cells. These mediators include histamine, leukotrienes, tryptase, and prostaglandins that directly contract airway smooth muscle.[4] Bronchospasm induced by aspirin and other nonsteroidal anti-inflammatory drugs also involves mediator release from airway cells.[4]

Inflammation plays a key role in the pathophysiology of asthma regardless of disease severity. Inhaled antigens activate immunoglobulin E, mast cells, and T helper cells in the airway and induce the production of inflammatory mediators and cytokines. In turn, this initiates a cascade of reactions involving lymphocytes, mast cells, eosinophils, dendritic cells, macrophages, resident airway cells, and epithelial cells that perpetuate the inflammatory response, with further release of chemokines, cytokines, cysteinyl leukotrienes, and nitric oxide. The inflammatory process is multicellular, redundant, and self-amplifying.

Numerous host and environmental factors, such as number and type of infections in childhood, frequent antibiotic use, Western lifestyle, and repeated exposures to allergens, may contribute to the development of allergic asthma. Viral respiratory infections are among the most common of the stimuli that invoke acute asthma exacerbation.[5] Increased airway responsiveness secondary to infection may last anywhere from 2 to 8 weeks.[5] Exercise is another common precipitant of acute asthma. Environmental conditions, such as atmospheric pollutants and antigens noted in heavy industrial or densely populated urban areas, or increased indoor antigens, such as mold, house dust mites, cockroaches, and animal dander, are associated with higher incidence and severity of asthma. Occupational exposures, such as metal salt, wood and vegetable dust, pharmaceuticals, industrial chemicals, plastics, biological enzymes, vapors, gases, and aerosols, also may stimulate an asthma attack. Agents such as aspirin, β-blockers (including topical β-blockers), nonsteroidal anti-inflammatory drugs, sulfating agents, tartrazine dyes, and food additives and preservatives may trigger acute asthma. Exposure to cold air alone can induce acute bronchospasm. Endocrine factors, such as changing levels of estradiol and progesterone during the normal menstrual cycle and pregnancy, contribute to the level of airway reactivity.[6] Emotional stress also can produce an asthma attack.

CLINICAL FEATURES

The symptoms of asthma include dyspnea, wheezing, and cough. Many, but not all, patients will relay the history of asthma upon presentation. Early in the attack, patients will complain of a sensation of chest constriction and cough. As the exacerbation progresses, wheezing becomes apparent, expiration becomes prolonged, and accessory muscle use may ensue. A thorough history can be helpful in guiding care for asthma exacerbations[7-10] (**Table 69-2**). Acute asthma exacerbations are categorized based on clinical features[7-10] (**Table 69-3**).

Physical examination findings are variable. Patients presenting with a severe asthma attack may be in respiratory distress, with rapid breathing and loud wheezing, whereas patients with mild exacerbation may present with only cough and end-expiratory wheezing. At times, wheezing may be audible without a stethoscope. Other conditions may present with wheezing and mimic asthma (**Table 69-4**). The use of accessory muscles of inspiration indicates diaphragmatic fatigue. The appearance of paradoxical respiration, which is chest deflation and abdominal protrusion during inspiration followed by chest expansion and abdominal deflation during expiration, is a sign of impending ventilatory failure. Alteration in the mental status (e.g., lethargy, exhaustion, agitation, or confusion) also heralds respiratory arrest.

Directed physical examination reveals hyperresonance to percussion, decreased intensity of breath sounds, and prolongation of the expiratory phase, usually with wheezing. Although wheezing results from the movement of air through narrowed airways, the intensity of the wheeze may not correlate with the severity of airflow obstruction. The "silent chest" reflects very severe airflow obstruction, with air movement insufficient to promote an audible wheeze. A **pulsus paradoxus** (change in blood pressure during inspiration) >20 mm Hg is also indicative of severe asthma, although it is not specific for asthma. Although tachycardia and tachypnea are usually seen with acute asthma, a normal heart rate, a normal respiratory rate, and the absence of a pulsus paradoxus do not indicate complete relief of airway obstruction.

TABLE 69-2 Key History Points for Acute Asthma Exacerbation[7-10]

Symptoms	Pattern	Disease History	Risk Factors for Death from Asthma
Cough	Perennial and/or seasonal	Age at onset	Past history of severe exacerbation
Wheezing	Continual or episodic	Present management and medications	≥2 hospitalizations for asthma in the past year
Shortness of breath	Onset	Medication regimen adherence	>3 ED visits for asthma in the past year
Chest tightness	Duration	History of corticosteroid use (chronic and/or intermittent)	>2 canisters per month of inhaled short-acting β_2-agonist
Sputum production	Frequency	Intensive care admissions	Difficulty perceiving airflow obstruction or its severity
Fever	Aggravating factors	History of intubation	Low socioeconomic status or inner-city resident
	Usual pattern of exacerbation and outcome	Best spirometry measures	Illicit drug use
			Psychiatric disease or medical comorbidities

TABLE 69-3 Classifying Severity of Asthma Exacerbations in Patients >12 Years Old and Adults*

	Symptoms and Signs	Initial PEF (or FEV_1)	Clinical Course
Mild	Dyspnea only with activity	PEF ≥70% predicted or personal best	Prompt relief with inhaled SABA.
Moderate	Dyspnea interferes with or limits usual activity	PEF 40%–69% predicted or personal best	Relief from frequent inhaled SABA. Symptoms for 1–2 d after oral corticosteroids begun.
Severe	Dyspnea at rest; interferes with conversation	PEF <40% predicted or personal best	Partial relief from frequent inhaled SABA. Symptoms for ≥3 d after oral corticosteroids begun.
Subset: life-threatening	Too dyspneic to speak; perspiring	PEF <25% predicted or personal best	Minimal or no relief from frequent inhaled SABA; IV steroids; adjunctive therapy; needs ED or intensive care unit.

*The presence of several parameters, but not necessarily all, indicates the general classification of the exacerbation. Many of these parameters have not been systemically studied, so they serve only as general guides.

Abbreviations: FEV_1 = forced expiratory volume in 1 second; PEF = peak expiratory flow; SABA = short-acting β_2 agonist.

Source: www.nhlbi.nih.gov/files/docs/guidelines/asthsumm.pdf (National Heart, Lung, and Blood Institute; National Institutes of Health; U.S. Department of Health and Human Services: NIH Publication Number 08-5846, October 2007, Fig. 20). Accessed November 18, 2014.

DIAGNOSIS AND PATIENT MONITORING

Bedside spirometry provides a rapid, objective assessment of patients and guides therapy. The forced expiratory volume in 1 second (FEV_1) and the peak expiratory flow rate (PEFR) rate directly measure the degree of large airway obstruction. Sequential measurements help assess severity and determine response to therapy. A flow-volume loop can help distinguish asthma from vocal cord dysfunction; the latter is often treated as asthma, sometimes with repeated visits. Vocal cord dysfunction responds to the moisture, *not* the drug, in a nebulized treatment, and "fails" metered-dose inhaler outpatient therapy because moisture is not a part of that delivery system. If not documented, obtain a full spirometry assessment only in patients with frequent outpatient failures.

Signs on physical examination and the subjective symptoms do not necessarily correlate well with the severity of airflow obstruction, making objective measures valuable. Patient cooperation is essential for these tests to be reliable, limiting the value of spirometry in severe exacerbations or in noncooperative patients.[7-10]

Pulse oximetry assesses oxygen saturation during treatment. Arterial blood gas measurement is not needed in most patients with mild to moderate asthma exacerbation, and it should be reserved for suspected hypoventilation with carbon dioxide retention and respiratory acidosis. With acute attacks, ventilation is stimulated, resulting in a decrease in partial pressure of arterial carbon dioxide ($Paco_2$). Therefore, a normal or slightly elevated $Paco_2$ (e.g., >42 mm Hg) indicates extreme airway obstruction and fatigue and may herald the onset of acute ventilatory failure. Patients with impending respiratory failure almost always have clinical evidence of severe attacks or spirometry demonstrating a PEFR or FEV_1 <25% predicted.[11] The use of capnography in acute asthma management is unclear. One small study reported good concordance between expired carbon dioxide levels measured by capnography and arterial carbon dioxide concentration,[12] but another reported differences of up to 10 mm Hg or more between the two measurements.[13]

TABLE 69-4 Important Asthma Mimickers

Acute heart failure ("cardiac asthma")
Upper airway obstruction
Multiple pulmonary emboli
Aspiration of foreign body or gastric acid
Tumors/disorders causing endobronchial obstruction
Interstitial lung disease
Vocal cord dysfunction

Radiography is indicated only if there is clinical suspicion of pneumothorax, pneumomediastinum, pneumonia, or other cause for symptoms (e.g., acute heart failure) or complication of asthma. For admitted asthma patients, less than one third of patients have an abnormal chest radiograph.[14]

A CBC is not routinely needed and likely will show modest leukocytosis secondary to administration of β-agonist therapy or corticosteroids. For those few patients taking theophylline, measure the serum level. Routine ECG is also unnecessary but may reveal right ventricular strain, abnormal P waves, or nonspecific ST- and T-wave abnormalities, which resolve with treatment. Older patients, especially those with coexisting heart disease, should have cardiac monitoring during treatment.

STANDARD TREATMENT

The goal is rapid reversal of airflow obstruction by repetitive or continuous administration of inhaled β_2-agonists, ensuring adequate oxygenation, and relieving inflammation.[7-10] **Figure 69-1** shows the National Asthma Education and Prevention Program Expert Panel ED treatment algorithm.[10] The following categories of medications are used in the treatment of acute asthma: β-adrenergic agonists, anticholinergics, and glucocorticoids. Treatments for impending or actual respiratory arrest are discussed below in "Status Asthmaticus."

ADRENERGIC AGENTS

β-Adrenergic agonists with rapid onset are the preferred initial rescue medication for acute bronchospasm (**Table 69-5**). Stimulation of β_1-receptors increases rate and force of cardiac contraction and decreases small intestine motility and tone, whereas β_2-adrenergic stimulation promotes bronchodilation, vasodilation, uterine relaxation, and skeletal muscle tremor.

β-Adrenergic drugs cause bronchodilation by stimulation of the enzyme adenyl cyclase, which converts intracellular adenosine triphosphate into cyclic adenosine monophosphate. This action enhances the binding of intracellular calcium to cell membranes, reducing the myoplasmic calcium concentration, and results in relaxation of bronchial smooth muscle. β-Adrenergic drugs also inhibit mediator release and promote mucociliary clearance.

The most common side effect of β-adrenergic drugs is skeletal muscle tremor. Patients also may experience nervousness, anxiety, insomnia, headache, hyperglycemia, palpitations, tachycardia, and hypertension. Clinical toxicity is rare and less common than undertreatment complications. Provoking dysrhythmias or myocardial ischemia is rare, especially in those without a prior history of coronary artery disease. The older catecholamine bronchodilators, such as epinephrine, are not β_2 specific and have a short duration of action.

Albuterol is a 50:50 racemic mixture (equal amounts of left and right isomers); it is now available in the hydrofluoroalkane formulation, which has increased the cost and the effectiveness. The *R* isomer has great binding affinity for the β_2-receptor and is responsible for bronchodilation. The *S* isomer has no bronchodilatory effect but has a long half-life (12 hours); this isomer may be responsible for late paradoxical bronchospasm in some patients. Levalbuterol (Xopenex®) is the pure *R* isomer form of the drug, intended to improve effectiveness and limit side effects such as tachycardia and rhythm change. Both racemic albuterol and levalbuterol can be given as intermittent or continuous nebulizations. Levalbuterol costs 5 to 25 times more than albuterol, and it has no clear advantage over albuterol regarding symptom change, admission, or tachycardia.[15-17]

Nonprescription racemic epinephrine (Asthmanefrin®) replaced Primatene® as an over-the-counter medication, and the cost is less than for prescription β_2-adrenergics. Asthmanefrin® contains 11.25 milligrams of racemic epinephrine/0.5 mL. In one study, subjects recruited through

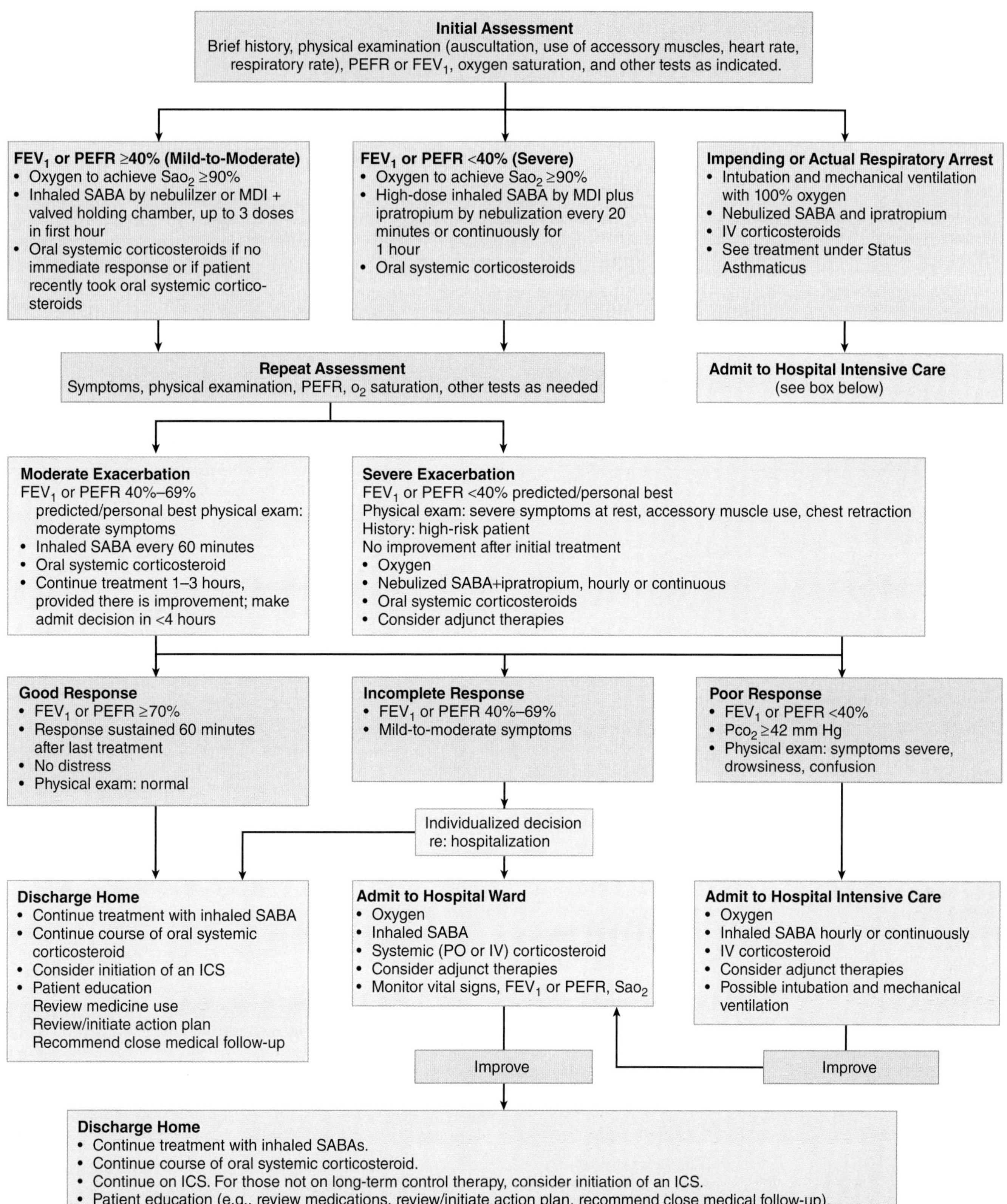

FIGURE 69-1. Management of asthma exacerbations: ED and hospital-based care. FEV_1 = forced expiratory volume in 1 second; ICS = inhaled corticosteroid; MDI = metered-dose inhaler; PEFR = peak expiratory flow rate; SABA = short-acting β_2-agonist; Sao_2 = oxygen saturation by pulse oximetry. [Source: http://www.nhlbi.nih.gov/guidelines/asthma/asthgdln.pdf (National Heart, Lung, and Blood Institute; National Institutes of Health; U.S. Department of Health and Human Services: National Asthma Education and Prevention Program, Expert Panel Report 3: Guidelines for the Diagnosis and Management of Asthma. Publication No. 08-4051. Bethesda, MD, National Institutes of Health, 2007.) Accessed November 18, 2014.]

TABLE 69-5 β-Adrenergic, Anticholinergic, and Steroid Dosages of Drugs for Asthma

Medication	Dose	Comments
Inhaled β_2-Agonists		
Albuterol		
Nebulizer solution (0.63 milligram/3 mL, 1.25 milligrams/3 mL, 2.5 milligrams/3 mL, 5.0 milligrams/mL)	2.5–5 milligrams every 20 min for three doses, then 2.5–10 milligrams every 1–4 h, as needed, or 10–15 milligrams/h as continuous nebulization.	Only selective β_2-agonists are recommended. For optimal delivery, dilute aerosols to minimum of 3 mL at gas flow of 6–8 L/min. Use large-volume nebulizers for continuous administration. May mix with ipratropium nebulizer solution.
MDI (90 micrograms/puff)	4–8 puffs every 20 min up to 4 h, then every 1–4 h as needed.	In mild-to-moderate exacerbations, MDI plus valved holding chamber is as effective as nebulized therapy with appropriate administration technique and coaching by trained personnel.
Bitolterol		
Nebulizer solution (2 milligrams/mL)	See albuterol dose.	Has not been studied in severe asthma exacerbations. Do not mix with other drugs.
MDI (370 micrograms/puff)	See albuterol MDI dose.	Has not been studied in severe asthma exacerbations.
Levalbuterol (R-albuterol)		
Nebulizer solution (0.63 milligram/3 mL, 1.25 milligrams/3 mL)	1.25–2.5 milligrams every 20 min for three doses, then 1.25–5 milligrams every 1–4 h, as needed.	Levalbuterol administered in one half the milligram dose of albuterol provides comparable efficacy and safety. Has not been evaluated by continuous nebulization.
MDI (45 micrograms/puff)	See albuterol MDI dose.	
Pirbuterol		
MDI (200 micrograms/puff)	See albuterol MDI dose.	Has not been studied in severe asthma exacerbations.
Systemic (Injected) β_2-Agonists		
Epinephrine		
1:1000 (1 milligram/mL)	0.3–0.5 milligram every 20 min for three doses SC.	No proven advantage of systemic therapy over aerosol.
Terbutaline		
(1 milligram/mL)	0.25 milligram every 20 min for three doses SC.	No proven advantage of systemic therapy over aerosol.
Anticholinergics/Combinations		
Ipratropium bromide		
Nebulizer solution (0.25 milligram/mL)	0.5 milligram every 20 min for three doses, then as needed.	May mix in same nebulizer with albuterol. Should not be used as first-line therapy; should be added to SABA therapy for severe exacerbations. The addition of ipratropium has not been shown to provide further benefit once the patient is hospitalized.
MDI (18 micrograms/puff)	Eight puffs every 20 min, as needed, up to 3 h.	Should use with valved holding chamber and face mask for children <4 y. Studies have examined ipratropium bromide MDI for up to 3 h.
Ipratropium with albuterol		
Nebulizer solution (each 3-mL vial contains 0.5 milligram of ipratropium bromide and 2.5 milligrams of albuterol.)	3 mL every 20 min for three doses, then as needed.	May be used for up to 3 h in the initial management of severe exacerbations. The addition of ipratropium has not been shown to provide further benefit once the patient is hospitalized.
MDI (each puff contains 18 micrograms of ipratropium bromide and 90 micrograms of albuterol.)	Eight puffs every 20 min as needed up to 3 h.	Should use with valved holding chamber and face mask for children <4 y.
Systemic Corticosteroids		Applies to all three corticosteroids for oral medications.
Prednisone	For inpatients: oral "burst," use 40–80 milligrams/d in one or two divided doses until PEFR reaches 70% of predicted or personal best.	For outpatients: oral "burst," use 40–60 milligrams in single or two divided doses for 5–10 d.
Methylprednisolone	IV: 1 milligram/kg every 4–6 h.	For outpatients: a single IM dose of 150 milligrams depot methylprednisolone may be used.[19]
Prednisolone	1–2 milligrams/kg/d for 5–10 d; may be divided twice daily.	More frequently used over prednisone in children due to increased palatably of available liquid formulations.

Notes: There is no known advantage for higher doses of corticosteroids in severe asthma exacerbations, nor is there any advantage for IV administration over oral therapy provided GI transit time or absorption is not impaired.

The course of systemic corticosteroids for an asthma exacerbation requiring an ED visit or hospitalization may last from 3 to 10 days. For corticosteroid courses of <1 week, there is no need to taper the dose. For slightly longer courses (e.g., up to 10 days), there probably is no need to taper, especially if patients are concurrently taking inhaled corticosteroids.

Inhaled corticosteroids can be started at any point in the treatment of an asthma exacerbation.

Abbreviations: MDI = metered-dose inhaler; PEFR = peak expiratory flow rate.

Source: http://www.nhlbi.nih.gov/guidelines/asthma/asthgdln.pdf (National Heart, Lung, and Blood Institute; National Institutes of Health; U.S. Department of Health and Human Services: National Asthma Education and Prevention Program, Expert Panel Report 3: Guidelines for the Diagnosis and Management of Asthma. Publication No. 08-4051. Bethesda, MD, National Institutes of Health, 2007.) Accessed November 18, 2014.

local pharmacies reported no worse asthma outcomes than individuals treated with prescription β-agonists.[18] No other data exist to guide use of Asthmanefrin® versus prescribed agents.

Aerosol therapy with β_2-adrenergic drugs produces excellent bronchodilation and is favored over oral or parenteral routes. The aerosol route achieves topical administration of a relatively small dose of drug, thereby producing local effects with minimum systemic absorption and fewer side effects. Aerosol delivery occurs with a metered-dose inhaler coupled to a spacing device or with a compressor-driven nebulizer.[20] A spacing device attached to the inhaler improves drug deposition; when optimally used, *metered-dose inhaler therapy delivers the most drug to target airways,* better than nebulized therapy. Even with optimum technique, a maximum of 15% of the drug dose is retained in the lungs, regardless of the aerosol method used.

Aerosol treatments may be administered every 15 to 20 minutes or on a continuous basis.[21] Subcutaneous epinephrine and terbutaline are options for patients unable to coordinate aerosolized or metered-dose inhaler treatments, seen often in severe airflow-limited states. IV β-agonist infusions offer no advantage over aerosolized or metered-dose inhaler–delivered agents and carry increased risk.[22]

Salmeterol xinafoate and formoterol are β_2-adrenoreceptor agonists that bind with greater affinity to the β_2-receptor site than albuterol. **They are indicated for twice-daily maintenance therapy. Neither drug should be used for acute asthma exacerbations.** Bronchodilator effects last at least 12 hours, and tachyphylaxis has not been reported with long-term use. The number of asthma-related deaths among patients receiving salmeterol, especially in African Americans, has increased for unknown reasons, although this may be due to failure to recognize the need for or use rescue short-acting agents and to seek care appropriately. Long-acting β_2-adrenoreceptor agonists are an effective treatment for long-term control of asthma, especially in conjunction with inhaled corticosteroids. Short-acting β_2-adrenoreceptor agonists are used for infrequent or breakthrough symptoms that occur despite the use of long-acting β_2-adrenoreceptor agonists.[7-10,21]

CORTICOSTEROIDS

Corticosteroids are a cornerstone of asthma treatment. Steroids produce beneficial effects by restoring β-adrenergic responsiveness and reducing inflammation. The peak anti-inflammatory effect occurs at least 4 to 8 hours after IV or PO administration, but early use is wise to enhance care quickly; corticosteroids given within 1 hour of arrival in the ED reduce the need for hospitalization.[23] Although there is disagreement over the optimal dose in acute asthma, an initial dose of **PO prednisone** of 40 to 60 milligrams or **IV methylprednisolone** of 1 milligram/kg is sufficient, and higher-dose corticosteroid therapy offers no advantage.[24] Admitted patients should receive additional daily corticosteroids until subjective and objective improvements are achieved. Patients who are being discharged home with an FEV_1 or PEF of <70% predicted after aggressive ED treatment should be prescribed a 5- to 10-day nontapering course of prednisone (40 to 60 milligrams/d in a single daily dose or its equivalent) or a 2-day course of oral dexamethasone (16 milligrams/d in a single daily dose).[7-10,19,25,26] A single dose of **depot methylprednisolone**, 150 milligrams IM, is another option if compliance is a concern.[27]

Current recommendations favor inhaled corticosteroids for all patients with mild persistent asthma or more severe asthma.[7-10] This means discharging patients with mild persistent or more severe asthma on maintenance inhaled corticosteroids in addition to any systemic bursts.[28-31] Inhaled corticosteroid options are beclomethasone, 80 to 240 micrograms/d; budesonide, 180 to 600 micrograms/d; flunisolide, 500 to 1000 micrograms/d; fluticasone, 88 to 264 micrograms/d; mometasone, 200 micrograms/d; and triamcinolone acetonide, 300 to 750 micrograms/d.

ANTICHOLINERGICS

The effects of anticholinergics used in combination with β-adrenergic agents are additive. Anticholinergics affect large, central airways, whereas β-adrenergic drugs dilate smaller airways. Anticholinergic drugs competitively antagonize acetylcholine at the postganglionic junction between the parasympathetic nerve terminal and effector cell. This process blocks the bronchoconstriction induced by vagal cholinergic-mediated innervation to the larger central airways. In addition, anticholinergics reduce concentrations of cyclic guanosine monophosphate in airway smooth muscle, further promoting bronchodilation.

The anticholinergic commonly used is inhaled ipratropium bromide. Ipratropium is available as a nebulized solution and a metered-dose inhaler or in combination with albuterol[7-10] (Table 69-5). Use an aerosolized ipratropium bromide solution, 0.5 milligrams, in patients with moderate to severe exacerbation.[7-10] **Adding multiple doses of ipratropium bromide to a short-acting selective β-agonist may improve bronchodilation and decrease the need for hospitalization among severely obstructed asthmatics,**[32] **although this benefit is not universal.**[33] Potential side effects with anticholinergics include dry mouth, thirst, and difficulty swallowing. Less commonly, tachycardia, restlessness, irritability, confusion, difficulty in micturition, ileus, blurring of vision, or an increase in intraocular pressure can occur. Long-acting anticholinergic agents have no role in acute care.

STATUS ASTHMATICUS (ACUTE SEVERE ASTHMA)

Status asthmaticus is an acute severe asthma attack that does not improve with usual doses of inhaled bronchodilators and steroids. Signs and symptoms include hypoxemia, tachypnea, tachycardia, accessory muscle use, and wheezing. Wheezing may be absent when airflow is severely reduced. Rapid treatment is the key to preventing cardiopulmonary arrest. In addition to usual and ongoing bronchodilators coupled with early steroids, other treatment adjuncts exist.

MAGNESIUM

IV magnesium sulfate is indicated in the management of acute, very severe asthma (FEV_1 <25% predicted).[34] The magnesium dose is 1 to 2 grams IV over 30 minutes. Nebulized magnesium is effective and may also improve pulmonary function in severe asthma when it follows aggressive β-agonist and steroid therapy.[34-36] Dosing regimens vary; one regimen is 95 milligrams of nebulized magnesium sulfate in four divided doses 20 minutes apart, and another is 384 milligrams of nebulized magnesium sulfate in sterile water.[37] When using magnesium in any form, monitor blood pressure and deep tendon reflexes during administration[37] because hypotension or neuromuscular blockade may occur, although this is exceptionally rare in the doses recommended.

NONINVASIVE POSITIVE-PRESSURE VENTILATION

Noninvasive positive-pressure ventilation (see chapter 28, "Noninvasive Airway Management") improves airflow and respirations compared with usual care, and despite little research, it is commonly used in clinical practice for acute life-threatening asthma.[38,39] Noninvasive positive-pressure ventilation decreases the need for intubation, results in clinical improvement, and decreases the need for hospitalization.[39] Do not institute noninvasive positive-pressure ventilation if intubation is indicated or in patients with suspected pneumothorax.

KETAMINE

Ketamine inhibits reuptake of noradrenaline and thus increases circulating catecholamines, aiding some with severe asthma. An IV bolus dose of 0.2 milligram/kg followed by an infusion of 0.5 milligram/kg/h is sometimes used;[40] higher doses are validated.[41] If intubation is needed, ketamine is a good agent to aid during the procedure and after mechanical ventilation starts. Controlled trials substantiating ketamine's efficacy in treating severe acute asthma are lacking.

EPINEPHRINE

Although epinephrine is standard treatment for anaphylactic asthma, it is overlooked as an adjunct to treat status asthmaticus. Epinephrine can be given SC or IM, 0.5 milligram in adults (standard adult EpiPen® dose), in refractory situations.[41]

MECHANICAL VENTILATION

If the patient manifests progressive hypercarbia or acidosis or becomes exhausted or confused, intubation and mechanical ventilation (see chapter 29, "Intubation and Mechanical Ventilation") are necessary to prevent respiratory arrest. **Mechanical ventilation does not relieve the airflow obstruction—it merely eliminates the work of breathing and enables the patient to rest while the airflow obstruction is resolved.**

The potential complications of mechanical ventilation in asthmatic patients include extremely high peak airway pressures with subsequent barotrauma and hemodynamic impairment. Mucous plugging is frequent, leading to increased airway resistance, atelectasis, and pulmonary infection. Due to the severity of airflow obstruction during the early phases of treatment, the tidal volume may be larger than the returned volume, leading to air trapping and increased residual volume (intrinsic positive end-expiratory pressure). Using rapid inspiratory flow rates at a reduced respiratory frequency (12 to 14 breaths/min) and allowing adequate time for the expiratory phase can mitigate these effects. Also, it is reasonable to target adequate arterial oxygen saturation (≥90%) without concern for "normalizing" the hypercarbic acidosis. This approach is called *controlled mechanical hypoventilation* or *permissive hypoventilation.*

Ventilation of asthmatic patients requires sedation. Neuromuscular blocking agents may be required, but extended use may cause postextubation muscle weakness.[42] See chapter 111, Intubation and Ventilation in Infants and Children for further discussion.

AGENTS OF UNCERTAIN OR NO BENEFIT IN STATUS ASTHMATICUS

Heliox A mixture of 80% helium and 20% oxygen (heliox) can lower airway resistance and act as an adjunct in the treatment of severe asthma exacerbations.[43] Heliox does not reliably avert tracheal intubation, change intensive care and hospital admission rates and duration, or decrease mortality in severe asthma.[43]

Methylxanthines Aminophylline is no longer a first- or second-line treatment for acute asthma.[44] The most common side effects of methylxanthines are nervousness, nausea, vomiting, anorexia, and headache. At plasma levels >30 milligrams/mL, there is a risk of seizures and cardiac arrhythmias.

Other Agents Mast cell modifiers, such as cromolyn and nedocromil, exert their anti-inflammatory action by blockage of chlorine channels, modulating mast cell mediator release and eosinophil recruitment. These agents also inhibit early and late responses to allergen challenge and exercise. Neither is indicated for treatment of acute bronchospasm.

Leukotrienes are potent proinflammatory mediators that contract airway smooth muscle, increase microvascular permeability, stimulate mucus secretion, decrease mucociliary clearance, and recruit eosinophils into the airway. Several leukotriene modifiers, namely montelukast, zafirlukast, and zileuton, are available as oral tablets for the treatment of asthma. Leukotriene modifiers improve lung function, diminish symptoms, and diminish the need for short-acting β_2-agonists. They may be used as an alternative to low-dose inhaled corticosteroid therapy in mild persistent asthmatics and as steroid-sparing agents with inhaled corticosteroids in moderate persistent asthmatics.[7-10] Despite one trial with adjuvant IV montelukast for acute asthma,[45] **there is no indication for the use of any of the leukotriene modifiers in the ED.**

DISPOSITION AND FOLLOW-UP

Disposition decisions should take into account a combination of subjective parameters, such as resolution of wheezing and improvement in air exchange, as assessed by auscultation and patient opinion; objective measures, such as normalization of FEV_1 or PEFR; and historical factors, such as compliance, history of ED use, and hospitalization. Some degree of residual airflow obstruction, airway lability, and inflammation persists after treatment and discharge from the ED.

Advise discharged patients to use a short-acting β-agonist on a scheduled basis for several days and to complete any oral corticosteroids regimens. Add inhaled corticosteroids in patients with a history of persistent asthma who are not already using this regimen.[28-30]

A good response to treatment resolves symptoms and results in a PEFR or FEV_1 of >70% predicted; these patients can be safely discharged home. **Patients with a poor response to treatment have persistent symptoms and FEV_1 or PEFR of <40% predicted; these patients are usually best observed or admitted.** An incomplete response to treatment, the middle ground, is defined as some persistence of symptoms and a PEF or FEV_1 between 40% and 69% predicted. Most asthmatics treated in the ED fall into this category and may be discharged home safely, although some benefit from prolonged observation or admission[7-10] (Table 69-2).

Patients who fail to improve adequately over a period of several hours because they are in the late phase of their exacerbation and those with significant risk factors for death from asthma are best placed in an observation unit or hospital bed. Many patients can be successfully treated in an ED observation unit with evidence-based care protocols.[46] Intubated patients require intensive care unit admission.

Arrange follow-up care to ensure resolution and to review the long-term medication plan for the chronic management of asthma. High previous relapse rates suggest the need for follow-up within 1 to 4 weeks of the ED visit.[7-10] Deliver an appropriate written discharge plan of action that addresses routine care and care of worsening symptoms (**Table 69-6**).

TABLE 69-6 Checklist for ED Discharge

Intervention	Dose/Timing	Education/Advice	MD/RN Initials
Inhaled medications (e.g., MDI with valved holding chamber; nebulizer)	Select agent, dose, and frequency (e.g., albuterol).	Teach purpose.	
Short-acting β_2-agonist	2–6 puffs every 4 h for __ days.	Teach and check technique.	
Corticosteroids	Low to medium dose for patients with chronic persistent asthma.	For MDIs, emphasize the importance of using a spacing device or holding chamber.	
Oral medications	Select agent, dose, and frequency (e.g., prednisone 40 milligrams once a day for 10 d).	Teach purpose. Teach side effects.	
Peak flow meter	For selected patients: measure a.m. and p.m. peak expiratory flow, and record best of three tries each time.	Teach purpose. Teach technique. Distribute peak flow diary.	
Follow-up visit	If possible, make appointment for follow-up care with primary clinician or asthma specialist or advise patient to make appointment.	Advise patient (or caregiver) of date, time, and location of appointment, ideally within 7 d of hospital discharge.	
Action plan	Before or at discharge.	Instruct patient (or caregiver) on simple plan for actions to be taken when symptoms, signs, and peak expiratory flow values suggest recurrent airflow obstruction.	

Abbreviation: MDI = metered dose inhaler.

Source: National Heart, Lung, and Blood Institute; National Institutes of Health; U.S. Department of Health and Human Services.

Educate patients on asthma triggers, and review all discharge medications and the correct use of the inhaler and a peak flow meter (for daily tracking).

REFERENCES

The complete reference list is available online at www.TintinalliEM.com.

Chronic Obstructive Pulmonary Disease

Rita K. Cydulka
Craig G. Bates

INTRODUCTION AND EPIDEMIOLOGY

Chronic obstructive pulmonary disease (COPD) is characterized by persistent airflow limitation that is generally progressive and associated with an abnormal inflammatory response to noxious particles or gases.[1-6] COPD has two main forms: *chronic bronchitis*, defined in clinical terms, and *emphysema*, defined in terms of anatomic pathology. This traditional categorization is often indistinct, limiting the clinical utility of the definitions.[2-6] **Chronic bronchitis** is the presence of chronic productive cough for 3 months in each of 2 successive years, where other causes of chronic cough have been excluded.[2-6] **Emphysema** results from destruction of bronchioles and alveoli. The World Health Organization's **Global Initiative for Chronic Obstructive Lung Disease** definition of COPD encompasses chronic bronchitis, emphysema, bronchiectasis, and asthma, and acknowledges that most patients have a combination of the different diseases.

COPD accounted for 715,000 U.S. hospitalizations in 2010,[7] with $49.9 billion estimated as the cost for care.[7] The prevalence of COPD in women has doubled in the past few decades, and women now account for >50% of COPD-related deaths; the prevalence has remained stable in men.[8] The prevalence of COPD is highest in those countries that have the greatest cigarette use.

CHRONICALLY COMPENSATED CHRONIC OBSTRUCTIVE PULMONARY DISEASE

PATHOPHYSIOLOGY

Although tobacco smoke is the major risk factor for developing COPD, only 15% of smokers will develop COPD. Occupational dust, chemical exposure, and air pollution are other risk factors for COPD. α_1-Antitrypsin deficiency accounts for <1% of COPD patients.

Irritants, notably tobacco smoke and air pollutants, trigger an increase in inflammatory cells in the airways, lung interstitium, and alveoli. Proteases eventually break down lung parenchyma and stimulate mucus secretion. Mucus-secreting cells replace cells that normally secrete surfactant and protease inhibitors. These changes result in a loss of elastic recoil, narrowing, and collapse of the smaller airways. Mucous stasis and bacterial colonization develop in the bronchi. The earliest objective changes in the evolution of COPD are clinically imperceptible; these early changes are small increases in peripheral airway resistance or lung compliance. Because dyspnea and hypersecretion often progress insidiously, it may take decades before COPD becomes clinically evident. The Global Initiative for Chronic Obstructive Lung Disease guidelines are helpful for the early diagnosis and treatment of COPD (**Table 70-1**),[6] although there is only a weak correlation between forced expiratory volume in 1 second (FEV_1), symptoms, and health-related quality of life.[6]

The central element of chronic lower airway obstruction is impedance to expiratory airflow due to increased resistance or decreased caliber of the small bronchi and bronchioles. Airflow obstruction results from a combination of airway secretions, mucosal edema, bronchospasm, and bronchoconstriction. Exaggerated airway resistance reduces total minute ventilation and increases respiratory work.

TABLE 70-1 Classification of COPD Severity[2-6]

Stage	In Patients with FEV_1/FVC <0.7:
Mild COPD	FEV_1 ≥80% predicted
Moderate COPD	FEV_1 between 50% and 79% predicted
Severe COPD	FEV_1 between 30% and 49% predicted
Very severe COPD	FEV_1 <30% predicted

Abbreviations: COPD = chronic obstructive pulmonary disease; FEV_1 = forced expiratory volume in 1 second; FVC = forced vital capacity.

In emphysema, alveolar and capillary surfaces are distorted or destroyed, resulting in alveolar hypoventilation and ventilation–perfusion mismatch. The result is hypoxemia and hypercarbia. Sleep may blunt the ventilatory response to hypercarbia. The right ventricle hypertrophies and dilates, resulting in pulmonary hypertension and right ventricular failure. Right ventricular pressure overload is associated with atrial and ventricular arrhythmias. (See chapters 57, "Systemic Hypertension and chapter 58, "Pulmonary Hypertension.")

CLINICAL FEATURES

The hallmark symptoms are chronic and progressive dyspnea, cough, and sputum production; these may vary from day to day.[2-6] Minor hemoptysis is frequent, especially in chronic bronchitis and bronchiectasis, although it may herald lung carcinoma. Physical findings may include tachypnea, accessory respiratory muscle use, or pursed-lip exhalation. Lower airway obstruction causes expiratory wheezing, especially during maximum forced exhalation, and prolongation of the expiratory time. Patients with chronic bronchitis exhibit coarse crackles as uncleared secretions move about the central airways. In patients with emphysematous disease, there is expansion of the thorax, impeded diaphragmatic motion, and global diminution of breath sounds. Poor dietary intake and excessive caloric expenditure for the work of breathing cause weight loss, notably in emphysema. In the early stages, arterial blood gas measurements reveal mild to moderate hypoxemia without hypercapnia.

As COPD advances, especially when the FEV_1 falls below 1 L, hypoxemia becomes more severe and hypercapnia develops. Arterial oxygenation worsens during acute exacerbations, exercise, and sleep. Clinical signs of severe COPD include facial vascular engorgement from secondary polycythemia, and tremor, somnolence, and confusion from hypercarbia. Right heart failure may occur and be seen as edema or ascites, and the signs are often disguised or underestimated by the seemingly more overwhelming signs of respiratory disease. If concomitant left heart failure exists, the cardiac auscultatory findings may be overshadowed by the pulmonary inflation abnormalities of COPD.

DIAGNOSIS

The diagnosis of chronic, compensated COPD is confirmed by spirometry: a postbronchodilator FEV_1 of <80% predicted, and a ratio of FEV_1 to forced vital capacity of <0.7.[6] Once the disease progresses, the percentage of predicted FEV_1 is a better measure of disease severity.[2-6]

Chronic bronchitis is not radiographically apparent unless bronchiectasis is present. In emphysema, radiographs show hyperaeration, seen as increased anteroposterior chest diameter, flattened diaphragms, increased parenchymal lucency, and attenuation of pulmonary arterial vascular shadows (**Figure 70-1**).

Distinguishing acute heart failure from COPD is difficult. A B-type natriuretic peptide level <100 picograms/mL supports a diagnosis of COPD; levels >500 picograms/mL have a sensitivity of 80% and positive predictive value of 47% for acute heart failure (see chapter 62, "Respiratory Distress").[9] The ECG detects dysrhythmias or ischemia but does not accurately assess the severity of pulmonary hypertension or right ventricular dysfunction.

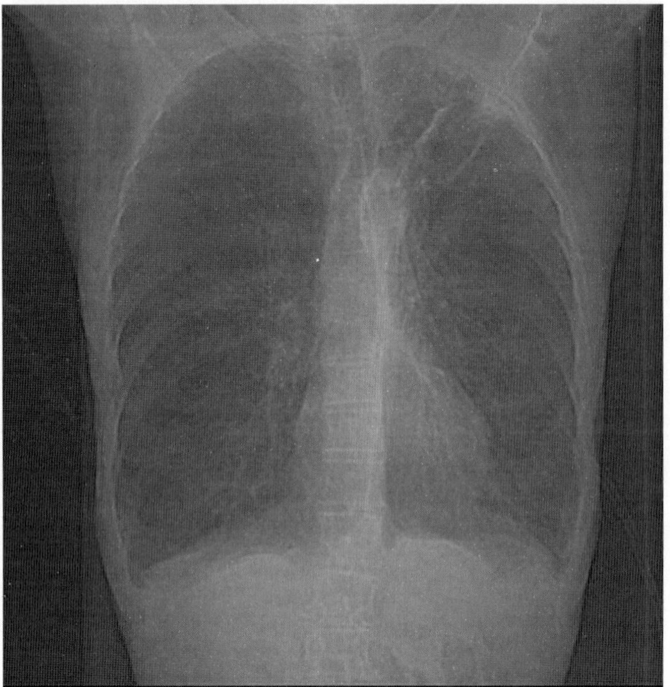

FIGURE 70-1. Posteroanterior chest radiograph in a patient with chronic obstructive pulmonary disease.

TREATMENT

Treatment for chronic compensated COPD includes oxygen, pharmacotherapy, measures to decrease mucus secretion, smoking cessation, and pulmonary rehabilitation.

Oxygen Long-term oxygen therapy reduces COPD mortality. The goal of long-term oxygen therapy is to increase the baseline partial pressure of arterial oxygen (Pao_2) to ≥60 mm Hg or the arterial oxygen saturation (Sao_2) to ≥90% at rest. Criteria for long-term oxygen therapy are a Pao_2 ≤55 mm Hg, a Sao_2 ≤88%, or a Pao_2 between 56 and 59 mm Hg when pulmonary hypertension, cor pulmonale (sustained right ventricular failure), or polycythemia is present.[6]

Pharmacotherapy Pharmacotherapy does not alter disease progression but provides symptomatic relief, controls exacerbations, improves quality of life, and improves exercise performance.[10] Inhaled long-acting β_2-agonists are preferred over short-acting formulations, coupled with anticholinergics. Combining bronchodilators with different mechanisms and duration of action may increase bronchodilation without increasing side effects.[11] Combination inhalers of short-acting β_2-agonists with anticholinergic agents include fenoterol/ipratropium and salbutamol/ipratropium. Long-acting inhaled β_2-agonists, such as salmeterol, formoterol, olodaterol, and indacaterol, are used on a regular basis, adding short-acting inhaled β_2-agonists, usually albuterol, as needed. Anticholinergic agents cause bronchodilation by blocking the effect of acetylcholine on muscarinic-3 receptors. Long-acting anticholinergic agents, such as tiotropium, aclidinium, and glycopyrronium, are preferred over short-acting agents, such as ipratropium bromide or oxitropium bromide.[12,13] Bronchodilators often only chronically improve FEV_1 by 10% .

Experts do not recommend long-term systemic corticosteroid therapy for all COPD patients,[14] because only about 20% to 30% improve. Short-term steroid use (days) aids in treating exacerbations. Regular treatment with inhaled corticosteroids is indicated for patients with a documented spirometric response to inhaled corticosteroids, those with an FEV_1 of <50%, or those with predicted and recurrent exacerbations requiring antibiotic treatment or systemic corticosteroids.[6] Long-term treatment with inhaled corticosteroids added to long-acting bronchodilators is recommended for patients at high risk of exacerbation. Combination inhalers with long-acting β_2-agonists plus corticosteroids include formoterol/budesonide, formoterol/mometasone, salmeterol/fluticasone, and vilanterol/fluticasone.[6]

Theophylline is relegated to an adjunct COPD therapy.[15] Theophylline inhibits phosphodiesterase and has an anti-inflammatory effect. It is not commonly used, but can be used in some patients not well controlled with inhaled corticosteroids or long-acting β_2-agonists. Although retrospective studies suggest that statins decrease the rate and severity of exacerbations, rate of hospitalization, and mortality, a large prospective trial failed to demonstrate benefit of daily simvastatin over placebo.[16] Daily azithromycin may decrease acute exacerbations in older patients and those with milder Global Initiative for Chronic Obstructive Lung Disease staging.[17]

Secretion Mobilization Respiratory secretions are kept mobilized by generous oral fluid intake and room humidification. Limit the use of antihistamines, antitussives, mucolytics, and decongestants. Expectorants are not of clear benefit.

Smoking Cessation and Pulmonary Rehabilitation Smoking cessation is the only intervention that can reduce both the rate of decline in lung function[6] and mortality from respiratory causes.[2-6] The ED is a site to attempt smoking cessation interventions.[18] A combination of nicotine replacement therapy or medications and behavioral interventions can assist patients with smoking cessation, especially with referral to a program.[19]

Pulmonary rehabilitation can improve exercise capacity and quality of life and is recommended in patients with moderate to severe COPD. Pneumococcal vaccination and influenza vaccination are key to dampen acute infections.[6]

ACUTE EXACERBATIONS OF CHRONIC OBSTRUCTIVE PULMONARY DISEASE

Acute exacerbations of COPD are characterized by worsening of respiratory symptoms beyond normal day-to-day variations[20] and are usually triggered by an infection or respiratory irritant. More than 75% of patients with acute exacerbations have evidence of viral or bacterial infection, with up to half specifically due to bacteria.[21,22] Other important triggers for exacerbations are hypoxia, cold weather,[23] β-blockers, narcotics, or sedative-hypnotic agents. The final common pathway for an exacerbation is the release of inflammatory mediators that result in bronchoconstriction, pulmonary vasoconstriction, and mucus hypersecretion. The work of breathing increases due to higher airway resistance and lung hyperinflation. The oxygen demand of respiratory muscles increases, generating additional carbon dioxide and causing hypercapnia, resulting in further physiologic stress.[23] Acute exacerbations of COPD are primarily due to ventilation–perfusion mismatch rather than the expiratory airflow limitation seen with asthma exacerbations.[24] Supplemental oxygen increases blood oxygen concentrations and can help reverse pulmonary vasoconstriction.

CLINICAL FEATURES

The most life-threatening feature of an acute exacerbation is hypoxemia (arterial saturation <90%). Signs of hypoxemia include tachypnea, tachycardia, systemic hypertension, cyanosis, and a change in mental status. With increased work of breathing, carbon dioxide production increases; alveolar hypoventilation creates arterial carbon dioxide retention and respiratory acidosis.

The patient tries to overcome severe dyspnea and orthopnea by sitting in an up-and-forward position, using pursed-lip exhalation, and engaging accessory muscles to breathe. Pulsus paradoxus (a drop of >10 mm Hg in systolic blood pressure during respiratory cycles) may be noted during palpation of the pulse or during blood pressure recording. **Complications, such as pneumonia, pneumothorax, pulmonary embolism, or an acute abdomen, may exacerbate COPD. Other acute triggers include asthma, congestive heart failure, pneumonia, pulmonary embolism, tuberculosis, and metabolic disturbances.**

DIAGNOSIS

With the history, seek causes for exacerbation and triggers plus sputum changes; then assess oxygenation and acid-base status, and perform a physical examination.

Pulse oximetry may identify hypoxemia, and capnography may identify hypercarbia. Arterial blood gas analysis is the best tool in acute evaluation for assessing oxygenation, ventilation, and acid-base disturbances. Arterial blood gases clarify the severity of exacerbation and the probable clinical course. Respiratory failure is characterized by an arterial Pa_{O_2} of <60 mm Hg or an arterial Sa_{O_2} <90% in room air. Respiratory acidosis is present if the partial pressure of carbon dioxide (P_{CO_2}) is >44 mm Hg. If the pH is <7.35, there is an acute and uncompensated component of respiratory or metabolic acidosis present.

In acute respiratory acidosis, the serum bicarbonate rises by 1 mEq/L for each 10-mm Hg increase in P_{CO_2}, and the pH will change by 0.008 × (40 − P_{CO_2}). In chronic respiratory acidosis, the bicarbonate rises by 3.5 mEq/L for each 10-mm Hg increase in P_{CO_2}, and the pH will change by 0.03 × (40 − P_{CO_2}) (Formulas 1 and 2). Changes outside of these ranges suggest an accompanying metabolic disorder (see chapters 15, "Acid-Base Disorders" and 62, "Respiratory Distress").

Frequently, patients with an acute COPD exacerbation are too dyspneic to perform bedside pulmonary function tests, and measurements are often inaccurate.[2-6] Similarly, physical examination and physician estimates of pulmonary function are inaccurate.[25]

Assessment of sputum includes questions about changes in volume and color, especially an increase in purulence. An increase in sputum volume and change in sputum color suggest a bacterial infection and the need for antibiotic therapy.[24,26] Sputum cultures usually contain mixed flora and do not help guide ED antibiotic selection.[2-6]

Ancillary Studies Radiographic abnormalities are common in COPD exacerbation and may identify the underlying cause of the exacerbation, such as pneumonia, or may identify an alternative diagnosis such as acute heart failure.[27]

The ECG can identify ischemia, acute myocardial infarction, cor pulmonale, and dysrhythmias. Measure levels in patients who take theophylline. Other tests, such as CBC, electrolytes, B-type natriuretic peptide, D-dimers, and CT angiography of the chest, are chosen based on clinical findings.

TREATMENT

The goals of treatment are to correct tissue oxygenation, alleviate reversible bronchospasm, and treat the underlying cause (**Table 70-2**). Factors that influence therapy in the ED include a patient's mental status changes; the degree of reversible bronchospasm; recent medication usage and assessment for drug toxicity; prior history of exacerbation courses, hospitalization, and intubation; presence of contraindications to any drug or drug class; and specific causes or complications from the exacerbation. Patients who do not respond as expected to standard therapy should prompt a reevaluation for other potentially life-threatening issues. See **Table 70-3** for an overview of the differential diagnosis of COPD exacerbations.

TABLE 70-2 ED Management of COPD Exacerbations[2-6]

Assess severity of symptoms
Administer controlled oxygen
Continuous cardiovascular status monitoring
Perform arterial blood gas measurement after 20–30 min if arterial oxygen saturation remains <90% or if concerned about symptomatic hypercapnia
Administer bronchodilators
β_2-Agonists and/or anticholinergic agents by nebulization or metered-dose inhaler with spacer
Add oral or IV corticosteroids
Consider antibiotics if increased sputum volume, change in sputum color, fever, or suspicion of infectious etiology of exacerbation
Consider adding IV methylxanthine if above treatments do not improve symptoms
Consider noninvasive mechanical ventilation
Evaluation may include chest radiograph, CBC with differential, basic metabolic panel, ECG
Address associated comorbidities

TABLE 70-3 Critical Differential Diagnosis of Chronic Obstructive Pulmonary Disease (COPD) Exacerbations[2-6]

Diagnosis	Clinical Features	Caveats
Asthma	Earlier onset Varying symptoms Family history Reversible airflow	Can coexist with COPD. Many patients diagnosed with asthma actually have COPD or mixed asthma-COPD
CHF	Presence of orthopnea (LR, 2.0) and dyspnea with exertion (LR, 1.3) slightly favors CHF Jugular venous distention, hepatojugular reflux, bibasilar rales Chest x-ray may show cardiomegaly or interstitial edema BNP <100 picograms/mL not likely to be CHF; BNP >500 picograms/mL more likely to be CHF	Can coexist with COPD. Shares some historical elements also found in COPD. Multiple conditions can falsely elevate or decrease the BNP level.
PE	Risk factors include older age, recent surgery or trauma, prior venous thromboembolic disease, hereditary thrombophilia, malignancy, smoking, and use of medications containing estrogen	20%–25% of patients with a severe COPD exacerbation with an unclear trigger have a PE.
	Patients with intermediate to high pretest probability may require further testing, such as CT angiography; D-dimer may be useful in ruling out PE in low-risk patients	Triad of PE (pleuritic chest pain, dyspnea, tachycardia, and hypoxemia) unusual.
ACS	Obtain ECG or troponin in those with chest pain or dyspnea and risk factors for ACS	Dyspnea may be the primary complaint in patients with ACS.
Pneumothorax	Obtain chest x-ray, US, or CT	COPD is a risk factor for spontaneous pneumothorax.
Pneumonia	Obtain chest x-ray	Frequently coexists with a COPD exacerbation.

Abbreviations: ACS = acute coronary syndrome; BNP = B-type natriuretic peptide; CHF = congestive heart failure; LR, likelihood ratio; PE = pulmonary embolism.

Oxygen **Administer oxygen to raise the Pa_{O_2} above 60 mm Hg or the Sa_{O_2} above 90%.** Use any of the following devices: standard dual-prong nasal cannula, simple facemask, Venturi mask, or nonrebreathing mask with reservoir and one-way valve. Because oxygen administration may produce hypercapnia, arterial blood gases and/or continuous end-tidal carbon dioxide and oxygen saturation monitoring with venous blood gases will allow optimal assessment of the P_{CO_2} and acid-base status. It may take 20 to 30 minutes from administration of supplemental oxygen for improvement to occur. If adequate oxygenation is not achieved or respiratory acidosis develops, assisted ventilation may be required.

β_2-Adrenergic Agonists Short-acting β_2-agonists and anticholinergic agents are first-line therapies in the management of acute, severe COPD.[2-6] Both lead to improved clinical outcomes and shorter ED lengths of stay, especially when used together.[2-6] Aerosolized forms, using nebulizer or metered-dose inhalers, deliver drug to the target area optimally and minimize systemic toxicity. β_2-Agonists are best given every 30 to 60 minutes if tolerated.[2-6] Nebulized aerosols every 20 minutes may result in more rapid improvement of FEV_1, but more frequent side effects,[28] including tremor, anxiety, and palpitations. Continuous cardiac monitoring is helpful, especially for patients with heart disease.

Anticholinergics Some guidelines favor β_2-agonists as a first-line therapy, whereas others favor anticholinergic agents. Ipratropium bromide given as a single dose by metered-dose inhaler with a spacer or as an inhalant solution by nebulization (0.5 milligram or 2.5 mL of the 0.02% inhalant solution) is the usual agent of choice, although aerosolized glycopyrrolate (2 milligrams in 10 mL of saline) is also effective. Side effects are minimal and appear to be limited to dry mouth and an occasional metallic taste.

Evidence regarding the efficacy of the combination of a β_2-adrenergic agent and an anticholinergic agent compared with a single agent alone is conflicting, although many physicians favor using this combination initially and some favor using it if the response to maximal doses of a single bronchodilator is poor. Long-acting inhaled anticholinergics, such as tiotropium, aclidinium, and glycopyrronium, are not used for the acute management of COPD.[2-6]

Corticosteroids The use of a short course (5 to 7 days) of systemic steroids improves lung function and hypoxemia and shortens recovery time in acute COPD exacerbations.[29] Use of corticosteroids in the ED does not affect the rate of hospitalization but does decrease the rate of return visits. The lack of effect on hospitalization rates is likely due to the approximately 6-hour delay before onset of action. There appears to be no clear benefit from a dose >40 to 60 milligrams of oral prednisone daily.[29] Hyperglycemia is the most common adverse effect.

Antibiotics Prescribe antibiotics if there is evidence of infection, such as change in volume of sputum and increased purulence of sputum.[26] **Choose agents directed at the most common pathogens associated with COPD exacerbation: *Streptococcus pneumoniae*, *Haemophilus influenzae*, and *Moraxella catarrhalis*.** There is no specific agent shown to be superior.[24,26] Initial antibiotics include macrolides (azithromycin), tetracyclines (doxycycline), or amoxicillin with or without clavulanic acid. There is little evidence regarding the duration of treatment, which ranges from 3 to 14 days.

Methylxanthines Methylxanthines, such as theophylline (oral) and aminophylline (parenteral), inhibit phosphodiesterases and may enhance respiration in two ways: by improving the mechanics of breathing (at the smooth muscle and diaphragm) and through an anti-inflammatory effect that happens at lower doses than used previously for bronchodilation and potentiating exogenous steroid effects. Data are conflicting on the value in acute COPD care, and these agents may induce nausea and vomiting.[30,31] The therapeutic index is narrow, so drug levels must be monitored. Methylxanthines (aminophylline 3 to 5 milligrams/kg IV over 20 minutes) are third-line options after inhaled therapies and steroids and when first-line therapies fail.

Noninvasive Ventilation Indications and relative contraindications of noninvasive ventilation are listed in **Table 70-4** Noninvasive ventilation can be delivered by nasal mask, full facemask, or mouthpiece. Patients with respiratory failure who receive noninvasive ventilation have better outcomes in terms of intubation rates, short-term mortality rates, symptomatic improvement, and length of hospitalization.[32] Disadvantages of noninvasive positive-pressure ventilation include slower correction of gas exchange abnormalities, risk of aspiration, inability to control airway secretions directly, and possible complications of gastric distention and skin necrosis. **Contraindications to noninvasive ventilation include an uncooperative or obtunded patient, inability of the patient to clear airway secretions, hemodynamic instability, respiratory arrest, recent facial or gastroesophageal surgery, burns, poor mask fit, or extreme obesity**. Noninvasive ventilation methods are discussed in detail elsewhere (see chapter 28, Noninvasive Airway Management).

All patients receiving noninvasive positive-pressure ventilation require continuous cardiorespiratory monitoring and frequent reassessment for setting changes and for tolerance of therapy.

Assisted Ventilation **Mechanical ventilation is indicated if there is evidence of respiratory muscle fatigue, worsening respiratory acidosis, deteriorating mental status, or refractory hypoxemia (Table 70-5).** The goals of assisted ventilation are to rest ventilatory muscles and to restore adequate gas exchange. After endotracheal intubation, the methods most commonly used are assist control ventilation, pressure support ventilation, or pressure support ventilation in combination with intermittent mandatory ventilation. Adverse events associated with invasive ventilation include pneumonia, barotrauma, and inability to wean the COPD patient from the ventilator.

Current evidence does not support the use of a mixture of helium and oxygen or magnesium in the treatment of an acute COPD exacerbation.

TABLE 70-4 Indications and Relative Contraindications for Noninvasive Ventilation[2-6]

Selection criteria	Acidosis (pH <7.36)/hypercapnia ($Paco_2$ >50 mm Hg)/ oxygenation deficit (Pao_2 <60 mm Hg or Sao_2 <90%)
	Severe dyspnea with clinical signs like respiratory muscle fatigue or increased work of breathing
Exclusion criteria (any)	Respiratory arrest
	Cardiovascular instability (hypotension, arrhythmias, myocardial infarction)
	Change in mental status; uncooperative patient
	High aspiration risk
	Viscous or copious secretions
	Recent facial or gastroesophageal surgery
	Craniofacial trauma
	Fixed nasopharyngeal abnormalities
	Burns
	Extreme obesity

Abbreviations: $Paco_2$ = partial pressure of arterial carbon dioxide; Pao_2 = partial pressure of arterial oxygen; Sao_2 = arterial oxygen saturation.

TABLE 70-5 Indications for Intubation with Mechanical Ventilation[2-6]

Unable to tolerate noninvasive ventilation (NIV) or NIV failure
Respiratory or cardiac arrest
Respiratory failure
Decreased consciousness or increased agitation
Massive aspiration
Persistent inability to remove respiratory secretions
Hypotension
Persistent hypoxemia despite optimal respiratory treatment
Hemodynamic instability

DISPOSITION AND FOLLOW-UP

Patients who fail to improve, those who deteriorate despite medical therapy, those with significant comorbidity, or those without an intact social support system are admitted. Objective criteria regarding hospital admission, observation unit stay, and ED discharge are lacking. The Global Initiative for Chronic Obstructive Lung Disease guidelines help guide the ED disposition decision-making process (**Tables 70-6** and **70-7**). Select patients without respiratory failure may avoid hospitalization with nurse-administered home care ("hospital at home care").[33] After ED discharge, 25% to 43% of patients with COPD exacerbation show ongoing or relapse of symptoms.[34-36]

The following are associated with a higher risk for relapse within 2 weeks after an ED visit: five or more ED or clinic visits in the past year,

TABLE 70-6 Indications for Hospital Admission[2-6]

Marked increase in intensity of symptoms, such as sudden development of resting dyspnea or inability to walk from room to room
Failure of exacerbation to respond to initial medical management
Significant comorbidities
Newly occurring dysrhythmias, heart failure
Frequent exacerbations and/or frequent relapse after ED treatment
Older age
Insufficient home support

TABLE 70-7 Indications for Intensive Care Admission[2-6]
Severe dyspnea that responds inadequately to initial emergency therapy
Respiratory or ventilatory failure (current or impending) despite supplemental oxygen and noninvasive positive-pressure ventilation
Decreasing level of consciousness or increasing confusion or agitation
Hemodynamic instability
Presence of comorbidities leading to end-organ failure

the amount of activity limitation (based on a 4-point scale), the initial respiratory rate (for each 5 breaths/min over 16 breaths/min), and use of oral corticosteroids before arrival in the ED.[34-36]

If discharging from the ED or observation unit, arrange the following: (1) a supply of home oxygen, if needed; (2) adequate and appropriate bronchodilator treatment (usually a metered-dose inhaler with a spacer *and* teaching; nebulized therapies are reserved for those who cannot use the metered-dose inhaler); (3) short course of oral corticosteroids[2-6]; and (4) a follow-up appointment with the primary care physician or pulmonologist, preferably within a week. Reassess inhaler technique, reinforce importance of completion of steroid therapy and antibiotics, if prescribed, and review management plan.

PRACTICE GUIDELINES

American Thoracic Society/European Respiratory Society guidelines—http://www.thoracic.org/clinical/copd-guidelines/resources/copddoc.pdf

Australian Lung Association Chronic Obstructive Pulmonary Disease checklist—http://www.copdx.org.au

Canadian Thoracic Society guidelines—http://www.respiratoryguidelines.ca/guideline/chronic-obstructive-pulmonary-disease#guidelines-and-standards

Global Initiative for Chronic Obstructive Lung Disease guidelines—http://www.goldcopd.org/guidelines-global-strategy-for-diagnosis-management.html

National Institute for Health and Care guidelines—http://www.nice.org.uk/guidance/CG101

REFERENCES

The complete reference list is available online at www.TintinalliEM.com.

SECTION 9

Gastrointestinal Disorders

Acute Abdominal Pain

Mary Claire O'Brien

INTRODUCTION AND EPIDEMIOLOGY

More adult patients visit the ED for "stomach and abdominal pain, cramps, or spasms" than for any other chief complaint. Demographics (age, gender, ethnicity, family history, sexual orientation, cultural practices, geography) influence both the incidence and the clinical expression of abdominal disease. History, physical examination, and laboratory studies can be helpful, but imaging is often required to make a specific diagnosis. Clinical suspicion for serious disease is especially important for patients in high-risk groups.

PATHOPHYSIOLOGY

Abdominal pain is divided into three neuroanatomic categories: visceral, parietal, and referred.

VISCERAL PAIN

Obstruction, ischemia, or inflammation can cause stretching of unmyelinated fibers that innervate the walls or capsules of organs, resulting in visceral pain. Visceral pain is often described as "crampy, dull, or achy," and it can be either steady or intermittent (colicky). Because the visceral afferent nerves follow a segmental distribution, visceral pain is localized by the sensory cortex to an approximate spinal cord level determined by the embryologic origin of the organ involved (**Table 71-1**).

Because intraperitoneal organs are bilaterally innervated, stimuli are sent to both sides of the spinal cord, causing intraperitoneal visceral pain to be felt in the midline, independent of its right- or left-sided anatomic origin. For example, stimuli from visceral fibers in the wall of the appendix enter the spinal cord at about T10. When obstruction causes appendiceal distention in early appendicitis, pain is initially perceived in the midline periumbilical area, corresponding roughly to the location of the T10 cutaneous dermatome.

PARIETAL PAIN

Parietal (somatic) abdominal pain is caused by irritation of myelinated fibers that innervate the parietal peritoneum, usually the portion covering the anterior abdominal wall. Because parietal afferent signals are sent from a specific area of peritoneum, parietal pain—in contrast to visceral pain—can be localized to the dermatome superficial to the site of the painful stimulus. As the underlying disease process evolves, the symptoms of visceral pain give way to the signs of parietal pain, causing tenderness and guarding. As localized peritonitis develops further, rigidity and rebound appear. Patients with peritonitis generally prefer to remain immobile.

REFERRED PAIN

Referred pain is felt at a location distant from the diseased organ. Referred pain patterns are also based on developmental embryology. For example, the ureter and the testes were once anatomically contiguous and therefore share the same segmental innervations. Thus acute ureteral obstruction is often associated with ipsilateral testicular pain. Referred pain is usually perceived on the same side as the involved organ, because it is not mediated by fibers that provide bilateral innervation to the cord. Referred pain is felt in the midline only if the pathologic process is also located in the midline.

CLINICAL FEATURES

CLINICAL RISK

To determine the urgency and method of the diagnostic approach, we recommend the use of a pragmatic scheme based on patient acuity and the identification of risk factors.

- Patient Acuity: Is this patient critically ill? If so, simultaneously resuscitate and evaluate.
- Risk Factors: Are there special conditions or risk factors that affect clinical risk or mask the disease process?

Patient Acuity: Is This Patient Critically Ill? Critically ill patients need immediate stabilization. Markers of high acuity include extremes of age, severe pain of rapid onset, abnormal vital signs, dehydration, and evidence of visceral involvement (e.g., pallor, diaphoresis, vomiting). The intensity of abdominal pain may bear no relationship to the severity of illness. Serious illness may be present even if vital signs are normal, particularly in high-risk groups such as the elderly and the immunocompromised. Shock that develops rapidly after the onset of acute abdominal pain is usually the consequence of intra-abdominal hemorrhage. Systolic pressure does not drop until blood loss reaches 30% to 40% of normal blood volume. Tachycardia is a useful parameter for the assessment of volume depletion, but its absence does not exclude blood/fluid loss. If pulse and blood pressure are in the normal range but there is reason to suspect intravascular volume depletion, obtain orthostatic vital signs. An increase in pulse rate of 30 beats/min after standing for 1 minute (or near-syncope that develops with a lesser increase) represents the loss of a liter of blood or its equivalent (a 20% blood loss for an average adult; roughly 3 L of normal saline).[1] The presence of orthostatic tachycardia is useful, but its absence does not exclude severe bleeding. Orthostatic hypotension is a later finding, representing the failure of sympathetic reflex tachycardia to maintain cardiac output. The threshold of 20 points of pulse change may not be applicable to patients on medications such as β-blockers, diabetic patients (who may have autonomic neuropathy), and the elderly (due to the effects of aging on the cardiac conduction system). "Orthostatics" should not be performed in patients who are already hypotensive. Tachypnea may indicate a cardiopulmonary process, metabolic acidosis, anxiety, or pain. Temperature is neither sensitive nor specific for disease process or patient condition. The presence or absence of fever cannot be used to distinguish surgical from medical disease.

Resuscitation of the critically ill patient with abdominal pain includes a cardiac monitor, oxygen (2 to 4 L/min via nasal cannula or mask), large-bore IV access, and an isotonic fluid bolus adjusted for age, weight, and cardiovascular status. For critically ill patients, blood samples should be drawn at the time of IV insertion, including, at a minimum, electrolytes, BUN and creatinine, CBC with platelets, clotting studies, and a type and antigen screen of blood. Order cross-matched blood if hemorrhage is suspected or if urgent transfusion is anticipated. In the presence of circulatory collapse, visualization of an enlarged aorta is

TABLE 71-1 Visceral Pain Features

Embryologic Origin	Involved Organs	Location of Visceral Pain
Foregut	Stomach, first/second parts of duodenum, liver, gallbladder, pancreas	Epigastric area
Midgut	Third/fourth parts of duodenum, jejunum, ileum, cecum, appendix, ascending colon, first two thirds of transverse colon	Periumbilical area
Hindgut	Last one third of transverse colon, descending colon, sigmoid, rectum, intraperitoneal GU organs	Suprapubic area

taken as de facto evidence of leakage or rupture, requiring immediate surgery. Bedside ED US can visualize and measure the abdominal aorta.[2,3] **Perform bedside US to identify abdominal aortic aneurysm and perform FAST if intra-abdominal hemorrhage is suspected.**[2,3]

Risk Factors: Are There Special Conditions or Risk Factors That Affect Clinical Risk or Mask the Disease Process? Identify pertinent past medical illness (diabetes, heart disease, hypertension, liver disease, renal disease, human immunodeficiency virus status, sexually transmitted diseases), previous abdominal surgeries, pregnancies and menstrual history (deliveries, abortions, ectopics), medications (steroids, immune suppressants, acetylsalicylic acid/nonsteroidal anti-inflammatory drugs, antibiotics, laxatives, narcotics, fertility agents, intrauterine devices, chemotherapeutic agents), allergies, and any recent trauma. Ask about previous episodes of similar abdominal pain, diagnostics, and treatments. Review previous medical records. Obtain a social history that includes habits (tobacco, alcohol, other drug use), occupation, possible toxic exposures, and living circumstances (homeless, dwelling heated, running water, living alone, other family members ill with similar symptoms).

A number of conditions camouflage critical illness in patients with acute abdominal pain. High-risk groups include patients with cognitive impairment secondary to dementia, intoxication, psychosis, mental retardation, or autism; patients who cannot communicate effectively because of aphasia or language barriers; patients in whom physical or laboratory findings may be minimal (the elderly) or obscured (patients with spinal cord injury); asplenic patients; neutropenic patients; transplant patients; patients whose immune systems are impaired by illness (human immunodeficiency virus; chronic renal disease; diabetes, cirrhosis, hemoglobinopathy; malnutrition, chronic malignancy, autoimmune disease, mycobacterial infection); and patients taking immune-suppressive or immune-modulating medications, such as steroids, calcineurin inhibitors, tumor necrosis factor inhibitors, antimetabolic agents, monoclonal and polyclonal antibodies, and chemotherapeutic agents.

In general, patients with mild to moderate immune dysfunction have delayed or atypical presentations of common diseases. Patients with severe immune dysfunction are more likely to present with opportunistic infections. The CD4 count is the most important measure of immune competency in patients with acquired immunodeficiency syndrome. **Patients with CD4 counts over 200/mm^3 are much less likely to have opportunistic infections.**

PHYSICAL EXAMINATION

Obtain a clear description of the pain itself **(PPQRSTT: provocative/palliative factors, quality, radiation, associated symptoms, timing, and what the patient has taken for the pain).**

Before the complete physical examination, take a few moments to gain the patient's trust by explaining what needs to be done, exposing only what needs to be seen, and re-covering exposed parts of the body sequentially. Provide patient privacy. Note the patient's skin (color, temperature, turgor, perfusion status), and perform a targeted heart and lung examination.

Inspection Inspect the abdomen for signs of distention (ascites, ileus, obstruction, volvulus), obvious masses (hernia, tumor, aneurysm, distended bladder), surgical scars (adhesions), ecchymoses (trauma, bleeding diathesis), and stigmata of liver disease (spider angiomata, caput medusa).

Auscultation of Bowel Sounds Bowel sounds are nonspecific diagnostic signs. Decreased bowel sounds suggest ileus, mesenteric infarction, narcotic use, or peritonitis. Hyperactive bowel sounds may be noted in small bowel obstruction.

Percussion Liver size can be estimated by the presence of percussion dullness in the midclavicular line, except in cases of severe bowel distention. A fluid wave may suggest ascites, and tympany may suggest dilated loops of bowel.

Palpation The vast majority of clinical information is acquired through gentle palpation, using the middle three fingers, and saving the painful area for last. Voluntary guarding (contraction of the abdominal musculature in anticipation of or in response to palpation) can be diminished by asking patients to flex the knees. Those who remain guarded after this maneuver will often relax if the clinician's hand is placed over the patient's, and the patient is then asked to use his or her own hand to palpate the abdomen. Distracting the patient with conversation may divert attention from the examination. Optimally, the patient's tenderness will be confined to one of the four traditional abdominal quadrants (right upper, right lower, left upper, left lower), and pain location can be used to generate a differential diagnosis. Often, this is not the case, and one finds more diffuse tenderness involving one or more of the four abdominal quadrants. Peritoneal irritation is suggested by rigidity (involuntary guarding or reflex spasm of abdominal muscles), as is pain referred to the point of maximum tenderness when palpating an adjacent quadrant. Rebound tenderness, often regarded as the *sine qua non* for peritonitis, has several important limitations. In patients with peritonitis, the combination of rigidity, referred tenderness, and pain with coughing usually provides sufficient diagnostic confirmation that little additional information is gained by eliciting the unnecessary pain of rebound. More than one third of patients with surgically proven appendicitis do not have rebound tenderness.[4] False positives occur without peritonitis, perhaps due to a nonspecific startle response. One might reasonably question whether rebound has sufficient predictive value to justify the discomfort it causes patients.

Evaluate the abdominal aorta, particularly in patients >50 years of age with acute abdominal, flank, or low back pain. Palpation cannot reliably exclude abdominal aortic aneurysm, and the presence or absence of femoral pulses is generally not helpful in the clinical diagnosis of abdominal aortic aneurysm.

It is wise to perform a pelvic examination in the evaluation of lower abdominal pain in women of reproductive age who have not had a complete hysterectomy. The presence of peritoneal signs, cervical motion tenderness, and unilateral or bilateral abdominal and/or pelvic tenderness suggests pelvic infection, or ectopic gestation in pregnant women. In males, hernia, testicular, and prostate examinations are indicated because disorders of these structures can cause lower abdominal pain.

The rectal examination does not increase diagnostic accuracy beyond what has already been obtained by other components of the physical examination. The main value of the rectal examination is the detection of grossly bloody, maroon, or melanotic stool.

One common approach to the evaluation of acute abdominal pain is to use the location of the pain (diffuse, right upper quadrant, right lower quadrant, left upper quadrant, left lower quadrant) to guide the generation of a differential diagnosis (**Figure 71-1**).[5]

Alternatively, abdominal crises may be grouped according to presenting symptomatology: pain, vomiting, abdominal distention, muscular rigidity, and/or shock (**Table 71-2**).

Although the location of the patient's pain and the grouping of symptoms can both help to differentiate among known diseases, clinical suspicion and an understanding of the individual is paramount, because the causes of acute abdominal pain vary considerably with patient demographics. For example, older adults are more likely than younger adults to have biliary disease, diverticulitis, and bowel obstruction. Appendicitis occurs more commonly in younger adults. In the words of Sir William Osler, it is important to know "what sort of patient has the disease."

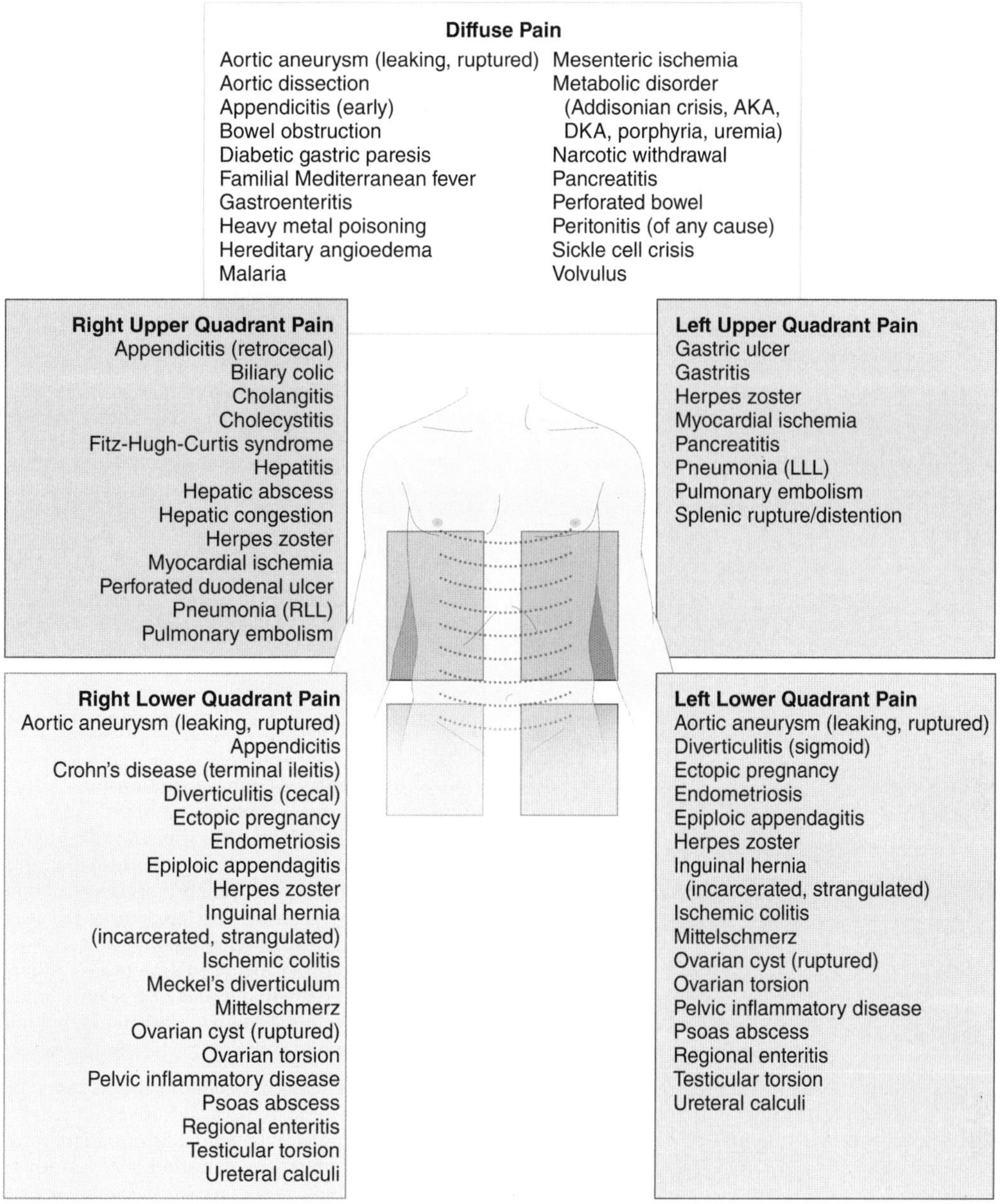

Diffuse Pain

Aortic aneurysm (leaking, ruptured)
Aortic dissection
Appendicitis (early)
Bowel obstruction
Diabetic gastric paresis
Familial Mediterranean fever
Gastroenteritis
Heavy metal poisoning
Hereditary angioedema
Malaria
Mesenteric ischemia
Metabolic disorder (Addisonian crisis, AKA, DKA, porphyria, uremia)
Narcotic withdrawal
Pancreatitis
Perforated bowel
Peritonitis (of any cause)
Sickle cell crisis
Volvulus

Right Upper Quadrant Pain

Appendicitis (retrocecal)
Biliary colic
Cholangitis
Cholecystitis
Fitz-Hugh-Curtis syndrome
Hepatitis
Hepatic abscess
Hepatic congestion
Herpes zoster
Myocardial ischemia
Perforated duodenal ulcer
Pneumonia (RLL)
Pulmonary embolism

Left Upper Quadrant Pain

Gastric ulcer
Gastritis
Herpes zoster
Myocardial ischemia
Pancreatitis
Pneumonia (LLL)
Pulmonary embolism
Splenic rupture/distention

Right Lower Quadrant Pain

Aortic aneurysm (leaking, ruptured)
Appendicitis
Crohn's disease (terminal ileitis)
Diverticulitis (cecal)
Ectopic pregnancy
Endometriosis
Epiploic appendagitis
Herpes zoster
Inguinal hernia (incarcerated, strangulated)
Ischemic colitis
Meckel's diverticulum
Mittelschmerz
Ovarian cyst (ruptured)
Ovarian torsion
Pelvic inflammatory disease
Psoas abscess
Regional enteritis
Testicular torsion
Ureteral calculi

Left Lower Quadrant Pain

Aortic aneurysm (leaking, ruptured)
Diverticulitis (sigmoid)
Ectopic pregnancy
Endometriosis
Epiploic appendagitis
Herpes zoster
Inguinal hernia (incarcerated, strangulated)
Ischemic colitis
Mittelschmerz
Ovarian cyst (ruptured)
Ovarian torsion
Pelvic inflammatory disease
Psoas abscess
Regional enteritis
Testicular torsion
Ureteral calculi

FIGURE 71-1. Differential diagnosis of acute abdominal pain by location. AKA = alcoholic ketoacidosis; DKA = diabetic ketoacidosis; LLL = left lower lobe; RLL = right lower lobe.

SYMPTOM TREATMENT AND FURTHER CLINICAL DIAGNOSIS

At this point, provide symptomatic relief. **Opioid analgesia relieves pain and will not obscure abdominal findings, delay diagnosis, or lead to increased morbidity/mortality.**[6,7] Do not withhold analgesia from patients with acute undifferentiated abdominal pain. The information on the safety of opioids cannot be extrapolated to nonsteroidal anti-inflammatory drugs such as parenteral ketorolac because nonsteroidal anti-inflammatory drugs are not pure analgesics and can mask early peritoneal inflammation.

Administer antiemetics as needed. A Cochrane review[8] reported that ondansetron and metoclopramide reduced postoperative nausea and vomiting.[8] Both drugs had equivalent effects. The dosage of IV ondansetron is 4 milligrams or 8 milligrams (0.45 milligram/kg total daily) to a maximum of 32 milligrams daily. Headache is a reported side effect. The dosage of IV metoclopramide is 10 milligrams, given slowly to minimize extrapyramidal side effects. Sometimes, 25 to 50 milligrams of IV diphenhydramine is administered as prophylaxis against dystonia. Patients with akathisia or dystonic reactions from metoclopramide cannot tolerate any other agents of the same class and should be given ondansetron. Such reactions are extremely rare from ondansetron. (See chapter 72, Nausea and Vomiting, for further discussion of antiemetics.)

Consider placement of nasogastric and urinary catheters. Nasogastric aspirate may confirm upper GI bleeding, and nasogastric suction may be used to decompress a bowel obstruction. A urinary catheter will relieve bladder obstruction, and hourly urine output helps to gauge renal perfusion.

LABORATORY TESTING

Laboratory testing does not take the place of a conscientious history and physical examination, and there is no evidence to support the usefulness of "routine abdominal labs." Information obtained by laboratory testing should help refine the differential diagnosis or alter the plan of treatment. **Table 71-3** lists laboratory studies that may be appropriate in

TABLE 71-2 Groupings of Known Abdominal Diseases by Symptoms

Pain/vomiting/± rigidity	Pain/vomiting/distention	Pain (± vomiting)
Acute pancreatitis	Bowel obstruction	Acute diverticulitis
Diabetic gastric paresis	Cecal volvulus	Adnexal torsion
Diabetic ketoacidosis		Mesenteric ischemia
Incarcerated hernia		Myocardial ischemia*
		Testicular torsion
Pain/shock	**Pain/shock/rigidity**	**Distention (± pain)**
Abdominal sepsis	Perforated appendix	Elderly with bowel obstruction/volvulus
Aortic dissection	Perforated diverticulum	
Hemorrhagic pancreatitis	Perforated ulcer	
Leaking/ruptured abdominal aortic aneurysm	Ruptured esophagus Splenic rupture	
Mesenteric ischemia (late)		
Myocardial ischemia*		
Ruptured ectopic pregnancy		

Note: These symptoms and etiologic groupings are a guideline and are not intended to be a rule.

*The symptoms of myocardial ischemia are variable.

TABLE 71-3 Suggested Laboratory Studies for Goal-Directed Clinical Testing in Acute Abdominal Pain

Laboratory Test	Clinical Suspicion
Amylase	Pancreatitis (if lipase is not available)
Lipase	Pancreatitis
β-Human chorionic gonadotrophin	Pregnancy Ectopic or molar pregnancy
Coagulation studies (prothrombin time/partial thromboplastin time)	GI bleeding End-stage liver disease Coagulopathy
Electrolytes	Dehydration Endocrine or metabolic disorder
Glucose	Diabetic ketoacidosis Pancreatitis
Gonococcal/chlamydia testing	Cervicitis/urethritis Pelvic inflammatory disease
Hemoglobin	GI bleeding
Lactate	Mesenteric ischemia
Liver function tests	Cholecystitis Cholelithiasis Hepatitis
Platelets	GI bleeding
Renal function tests	Dehydration Renal insufficiency Acute renal failure
Urinalysis	Urinary tract infection Pyelonephritis Nephrolithiasis
ECG	Myocardial ischemia or infarction

(Reproduced with permission from Fitch M: Utility and limitations of laboratory studies, in Cline DM, Stead LG (eds): *Abdominal Emergencies*. New York. McGraw-Hill Medical; 2008, p. 19.)

the evaluation of acute abdominal pain based on the clinical suspicions. Obtain an electrocardiogram for patients with upper abdominal pain, especially in elderly patients.

Be aware of the limitations of laboratory studies. The CBC does not offer sufficiently powerful likelihood ratios to revise disease probability. In a review of adult patients with appendicitis, only 65% had a serum WBC ≥12,000 mm^3.[9] A higher degree of leukocytosis was not associated with perforation. One approach to the use of the WBC is to take note only of high threshold abnormalities (e.g., a very elevated WBC [>20,000/mm^3]) and to resist the temptation to draw any reassurance from a "normal" WBC. **A single WBC cannot exclude serious or surgical disease.** Among patients with acute mesenteric ischemia, up to 25% have a normal serum lactate on initial presentation,[10] and studies on the utility of serum lactate values are limited by (among other things) varying intervals from the onset of symptoms to ED presentation. In a large study of patients with acute pancreatitis, serum lipase was 90% sensitive and 93% specific when drawn at the time of ED presentation.[11] Nineteen patients had pancreatitis with normal initial lipase levels; 14 of these had elevated lipase levels when the test was repeated later on the day of admission.[11]

DIAGNOSTIC IMAGING

Diagnostic imaging does not take the place of a conscientious history and physical examination. Not all patients with abdominal pain require imaging. Moreover, if the clinical impression suggests that the need for surgery is obvious, it is not necessary to wait for diagnostic imaging before surgical consultation.

Plain Radiographs In some institutions, an "abdominal series" includes an upright abdomen; in others, an upright chest; in still others, only a single supine film is obtained. If plain radiographs are obtained, make sure the inguinal region is included to help identify incarcerated hernia. Radiographic evidence of small bowel obstruction may be seen 6 to 12 hours before symptoms develop. However, signs may be absent in up to half of patients with developing small bowel obstruction.[12,13] Although an upright chest film is better to detect free air than an abdominal film, the sensitivity for small amounts of free air is only about 30%.[12,13] The use of plain abdominal radiographs should be limited to screening for obstruction, sigmoid volvulus, perforation, or severe constipation.

Ultrasound In adults, an abdominal US examination can visualize the gallbladder, pancreas, kidneys and ureters, urinary bladder volume, and aortic dimensions. Abdominal US is not useful for diagnosis of small or large bowel disorders. The detection of free air or appendicitis by US is operator dependent and limited by patient obesity and bowel gas.[14]

US is the preferred modality for the evaluation of biliary tract disease. When acute cholecystitis or biliary dyskinesia is strongly suspected but the US is normal, cholescintigraphy is recommended. Use bedside US to identify the urinary bladder and to determine whether acute urinary retention is the cause of acute lower abdominal pain and distention.

Abdominal-Pelvic CT Scanning CT scanning is a sensitive and specific diagnostic tool for many causes of abdominal pain. Its clinical usefulness is balanced by delays in surgical management and increase in ED throughput if oral contrast is used, and by radiation dose.[15] The radiation dose of abdominal CT is about 10 mSv, about 10 times that of plain abdominal radiographs.[12]

Options for CT scanning include noncontrast studies, or PO, PR, and/or IV contrast. Protocols vary depending on institutional, surgical, and radiology protocols; the prior probability of specific GI disorders in the patient population served; and individual radiologist preference. There are many contradictory studies on the best approach, especially for undifferentiated abdominal pain, for which the differential diagnosis is broad. Most studies have focused on the CT diagnosis of appendicitis.[16]

Noncontrast abdominopelvic CT has about 97% specificity for the diagnosis of acute appendicitis, with the possible exception of patients with a low BMI (<25). Noncontrast CT is the preferred imaging modality for the diagnosis of kidney and ureteral stones.

The use of oral contrast for the ED diagnosis of acute abdominal pain as a general protocol has been called into question.[16,17] Factors that affect the usefulness of oral contrast include patient vomiting, type and volume of oral contrast administered, transit time to the distal colon (variable, may be several hours), gastric emptying time (delayed induction of anesthesia, several hours), inadequate bowel opacification, and prolonged ED throughput time.[16] However, PO contrast CT is the imaging modality of choice in many institutions for suspected GI abscess, perforation, or fistula.

Rectal contrast CT can identify distal large bowel obstruction if that is the focused question.

IV contrast CT provides superior visualization of bowel mucosa, visceral organs, and vascular structures. It can identify small and large bowel obstruction and the transition point. It is the initial test of choice for suspected abdominal aortic aneurysm rupture or mesenteric ischemia. The risks of IV contrast are nephrotoxicity and allergic reactions. **If the serum creatinine is >1.5 or the glomerular filtration rate is <60, the use of IV contrast is generally not recommended except in life-threatening situations.** Patients receiving IV contrast should be hydrated with 1 to 2 L of normal saline as long as there are no contraindications to vigorous hydration. IV contrast is contraindicated in patients with a history of allergy to IV contrast or to iodine. There is no literature to support an allergy to shellfish as a contraindication to the use of IV contrast.

Common diagnoses for acute abdominal pain are listed in **Table 71-4**.

TREATMENT

ANTIBIOTICS

Antibiotics are indicated for suspected abdominal sepsis and peritonitis. Endogenous gut flora cause abdominal infections in the GI or GU tract. In all intra-abdominal nongynecologic infections, coverage should minimally be targeted at anaerobes and facultative aerobic gram negatives. An exception to this generalization is the need to provide additional coverage for gram-positive aerobes (e.g., *Pneumococcus*) in spontaneous (primary) bacterial peritonitis. Antibiotic treatment is summarized in **Table 71-5**.

The treatment of pelvic inflammatory disease (PID) requires different antibiotic combinations than do GI and GU infections. (For a detailed discussion, see chapter 103, Pelvic Inflammatory Disease.)

DISPOSITION AND FOLLOW-UP

Surgical consultation is required once a surgical diagnosis is made. Otherwise, consider hospital admission or observation for high-risk patients with acute abdominal pain. Patients who are elderly, immunocompromised, unable to communicate, or cognitively impaired are at especially high risk. Patients who appear ill, have intractable pain or vomiting, are unable to comply with discharge or follow-up instructions, or who lack appropriate social support should also be considered for admission. **Patients with an unclear diagnosis at discharge, even if the CT scan is "negative" (or for whom response to treatment is a concern) should be asked to return to the ED or their primary care physician for re-evaluation within 12 hours.** Discharge instructions should address diet (e.g., clear liquids only, push fluids, no fatty foods, no acidic foods) and medications (e.g., antacids, analgesics, avoid narcotics). The patient and the patient's family should understand that the diagnosis is uncertain, and they should know which symptoms warrant a return to the ED (e.g., increased/different pain, fever, vomiting, syncope, bleeding).

SPECIAL POPULATIONS

WOMEN

Gynecologic and nongynecologic disease can cause acute lower abdominal or pelvic pain in women (**Table 71-6**).

Hemorrhage from an ectopic gestation is the leading cause of pregnancy-related maternal death in the first trimester, despite improved diagnostic and treatment modalities. **Obtain a qualitative or quantitative urine or serum pregnancy test in women of childbearing age with acute abdominal pain who have not had a hysterectomy.** If the qualitative human chorionic gonadotropin is positive, transvaginal sonography should be the next diagnostic test to answer the question: Is this pregnancy in the uterus? Either inside or outside the uterus, a gestational sac is typically visible if the patient's serum β human chorionic gonadotropin is >1500 mIU/mL (the operator-dependent "discriminatory zone"). Detailed discussion of ectopic pregnancy is provided in chapter 98, Ectopic Pregnancy and Emergencies in the First 20 Weeks of Pregnancy. **Suspect ectopic pregnancy in a woman of reproductive age with hemodynamic collapse.** The presence of right lower quadrant pain in a woman who has an appendix is a common diagnostic dilemma. In general, the results of pelvic examination, consideration of patient risk factors for gynecologic versus gastrointestinal disease, and the clinician's best estimate of pretest probability for gynecologic versus gastrointestinal disease are the best guides for further imaging. If pretest probability favors gynecologic disease, a transvaginal ultrasound would be the next step. If pretest probability favors gastrointestinal disease or appendicitis, abdominopelvic CT scanning would be the next step.

ELDERLY PATIENTS

Symptoms in the elderly may be mild, vague, or underreported, and presentations may be late and atypical. Among those >80 years old, mortality almost doubles if the diagnosis is incorrect at the time of admission.[18] Poor hearing, decreased vision, and impaired cognition may affect the ability to give an adequate history. Surgical complications are more common: perforated viscus, gangrenous gallbladder, necrotizing pancreatitis, strangulated hernia, and infarcted bowel. Fever is not a reliable marker for serious disease, and the elderly may be hypothermic in the presence of serious abdominal infection. Fewer than 20% of elderly patients with perforated appendicitis have a "classic" presentation.[19] A WBC has a low predictive value for surgical disease in the elderly. **Although certain variables have been associated with poor outcome (age >84 years old, bandemia, free air) and others with the need for surgery (hypotension, abnormal bowel sounds, massively dilated loops of bowel, extreme leukocytosis), the absence of these variables does not preclude significant disease.**

Cholecystitis is the most common surgical entity in elderly patients with abdominal pain, followed by small bowel obstruction, perforated viscus, appendicitis, and large bowel obstruction. Viral gastroenteritis is uncommon among the elderly, but diarrhea occurs in 31% to 40% of patients with mesenteric ischemia.[10,20]

Any acute abdominal pain is important in an elderly patient. No single test can distinguish among patients who should be admitted and patients who can be safely discharged. **A liberal imaging/admission/observation policy is strongly advocated when the diagnosis is in doubt or follow-up is uncertain.**

BARIATRIC SURGERY PATIENTS

The purpose of bariatric surgery is to limit the absorption of nutrients from ingested food by reducing the size of the stomach, with or without a degree of associated malabsorption (**Table 71-7**). Detailed discussion of bariatric surgery complications is provided in chapter 298, The Patient With Morbid Obesity.

Staple breakdown after gastroplasty and band slippage after laparoscopic adjustable gastric banding may present as sudden intolerance to food or gastroesophageal reflux. Obstruction and erosion may also occur at the site of a gastric band. Diarrhea is a frequent complaint with predominantly malabsorptive procedures, and long-term malabsorption may result in protein depletion and vitamin deficiencies (particularly fat-soluble vitamins: A, D, and K).

Several specific problems can occur after successful Roux-en-Y gastric bypass (**Table 71-8**).

Bowel obstruction may be caused by internal hernia, anastomotic stenosis, or adhesions. Symptoms may be nonspecific (nausea, bloating, abdominal pain). Bowel obstruction in the immediate postoperative period after Roux-en-Y gastric bypass is a surgical emergency, as distention of biliopancreatic limb and distal stomach can result in gastric rupture and peritonitis. Bilious emesis after Roux-en-Y gastric bypass is pathognomonic for common channel obstruction, which requires immediate surgical intervention.[21] Gallstone formation is increased during the

TABLE 71-4 Common Diagnoses for Acute Abdominal Pain in Adults

Diagnosis	Epidemiology	Typical Location	Typical Radiation	Typical Quality	Helpful	Cautions	Laboratory	Imaging	Complications
Appendicitis	Peak age: adolescence and young adulthood	Early: periumbilical; late: RLQ. If retrocecal or third trimester pregnancy may be RUQ	—	Initially dull, becomes severe	RLQ pain; pain migrated from periumbilical area; pain before vomiting 100% sens, 66% spec; rigidity	Anorexia: 84% sens; vomiting 50% sens; fever: 67% sens; elevated WBC: 70%–90% sens	No single test is highly sensitive or specific; C-reactive protein may be helpful	CT preferred in adults and nonpregnant women	Perforation, abscess
Biliary colic	F >> M before age 60 y old, Hispanic > white > black	RUQ > epigastric	Right subscapular area	Initially colicky, becomes continuous; colic typically resolves <6 h	Bloating and dyspepsia are not related to gallstones	—	Suspect common bile duct stone if elevated bilirubin	US: 86%–96% sens, 78%–98% spec	Cholecystitis
Bladder outlet obstruction	Benign prostatic hypertrophy	Suprapubic	—	—	—	—	—	Bedside US	—
Bowel obstruction	History previous abdominal surgery	Diffuse	—	Colicky	Vomiting, distention	—	—	Plain films: 77% sens; 93% CT sens	Incarceration, strangulation
Cholecystitis	Most common surgical cause of abdominal pain in elderly	RUQ > epigastric	Right subscapular area	Continuous	(+) Murphy sign increases likelihood of cholecystitis (odds ratio 2.3–2.8); jaundice suggests obstruction	Up to 90% afebrile; elevated WBC only 63% sens and 57% spec. Cholangitis: elevated WBC only 80% sens	No single test can exclude diagnosis; elevated bilirubin/aspartate aminotransferase/alkaline phosphatase each only 70% sens and 42% spec	US: 91% sens; hepatobiliary iminodiacetic acid scan: 97% sens, 90% spec	Common bile duct obstruction; ascending cholangitis; gangrene
Diverticulitis	M > F before age 40 y old; incidence increases with age	Sigmoid (85%): LLQ; cecal/Meckel: RLQ	—	—	50% report previous episode of similar pain	Temperature may be normal; 25% (+) fecal occult blood	WBC may be normal	CT: sens 93%–100%; spec 100%	Perforation; abscess; fistula; obstruction
Epiploic appendagitis	Middle age; M > F	LLQ	—	—	Fever unusual; n/v infrequent; diarrhea 25%	In general, pts are not systemically ill	—	CT	—
Mesenteric arterial occlusion	Atrial fibrillation	Any	—	Severe	Pain out of proportion to physical findings; nausea: 56%–93%; vomiting: 38%–80%; diarrhea: 31%–48%	Atrial fibrillation	Lactate: 75%–90% sens; not specific; elevated WBC: 90%	Selective CT angiography: 96% sens	Metabolic acidosis
Mesenteric venous thrombosis	Hypercoagulable states, liver disease	Most commonly: generalized or epigastric	—	—	—	—	—	Contrast-enhanced CT	—
Mesenteric ischemia (nonocclusive)	Critically ill pts; vasoactive drugs	—	—	—	—	—	—	Angiography	—
Myocardial ischemia	—	Upper midline	—	Steady, dull	Abnormal ECG	ECG may be normal	Troponin: 80% sens at 4 h from symptom onset	—	—
Pancreatitis	M > F. Risks: alcohol; biliary disease; drugs; endoscopic retrograde cholangiopancreatography	Epigastric	Back	Severe, constant	Nausea and vomiting common	May have low-grade fever	Lipase: 90% sens first 24 h	US may show edema; CT: 78% sens, 86% spec	Hemorrhage; pseudocyst; adult respiratory distress syndrome; sepsis

PID	Sexually transmitted diseases; prior PID; multiple partners	RLQ and/or LLQ	—	—	Vaginal discharge; dyspareunia; cervical motion tenderness	Fever not necessary for diagnosis	Elevated WBC not necessary for diagnosis	—	Tubo-ovarian abscess; perihepatitis; infertility; ectopic pregnancy; chronic pain
Peptic ulcer disease	Peak age: 50s; M > F; chronic aspirin or NSAIDs; smoking; alcohol; *Helicobacter pylori*	Epigastric	—	Severe, persistent	Vomiting, tachycardia	Nonulcer dyspepsia more likely if: age <40 y old, no weight loss, no night pain, no vomiting	—	—	Perforation; bleeding
Perforated viscus	—	Any	—	Severe	—	—	—	Upright chest x-ray: 80% sens for free air	—
Ovarian torsion	—	RLQ or LLQ	Back, flank, or groin	Sudden onset, severe, sharp; may have nausea/vomiting	Adnexal mass	—	—	Pelvic US with Doppler flow	Ovarian salvage decreases with delay in diagnosis
Renal/ureteral colic	Average age: 30–40 y old; white > black; family history of stones	Right or left flank	Ipsilateral groin/ scrotum	Severe; colicky; nausea and vomiting common	85%–90% have hematuria; only 30% have gross hematuria	—	Urinalysis	CT	Obstruction; infection
Ruptured ectopic pregnancy	Previous ectopic; PID; infertility treatment; intrauterine device <1 y; tubal surgery	RUQ or LLQ	—	Sudden onset; severe pain	Pelvic mass	Pelvic exam may be normal	Pregnancy test	Transvaginal US	Shock
Ruptured/leaking abdominal aortic aneurysm	Older; male; atherosclerotic cardiovascular disease; smoker; (+) family history	Mid-abdomen or flank	Back, groin, or thigh	Severe; sudden onset; constant	Pulsatile mass detected: 22%–96% sens	Only 50% are hypotensive at presentation. Normal pulses do not exclude diagnosis	—	Bedside US 100% sens	Shock
Tubo-ovarian abscess	PID	Unilateral or bilateral pain	—	—	—	Fever may be absent	Leukocytosis may be absent	—	Rupture, peritonitis, shock

Abbreviations: > = more than; >> = much more than; < = less than; + = positive; F = female; LLQ = left lower quadrant; M = male; NSAIDs = nonsteroidal anti-inflammatory drugs; n/v = nausea and vomiting; PID = pelvic inflammatory disease; pts = patients; RLQ = right lower quadrant; RUQ = right upper quadrant; sens = sensitivity; spec = specificity.

TABLE 71-5 Antibiotic Regimens for Intra-abdominal Infections

Antibiotic	Comments
Aminoglycosides Gentamicin or tobramycin, 1.5 milligrams/kg IV every 8 h *or* Amikacin, 5 milligrams/kg IV every 8 h *and* Metronidazole, 1 gram IV followed by 500 milligrams IV every 6 h *or* Clindamycin, 900 milligrams IV every 8 h	Traditional therapy, if no reluctance for use of aminoglycoside; often selected for sicker, older, immunocompromised, or hypotensive patients; use ideal body weight for determining milligrams/kg/dose; adjust dosage for decreased glomerular filtration rate
Second-generation cephalosporins Cefoxitin, 2 grams IV every 6 h *or* Cefotetan, 2 grams IV every 12 h	Often selected for those less ill
Ampicillin-sulbactam, 3 grams IV every 6 h *or* Ticarcillin-clavulanate, 3.1 grams IV every 6 h	—
Piperacillin-tazobactam, 3.375 grams IV every 6 h *or* Imipenem-cilastatin, 1 gram IV every 8 h	Piperacillin-tazobactam often selected for suspected biliary sepsis
Aztreonam, 2 grams IV every 8 h maximum dose *and* Clindamycin or metronidazole (see above for dosages)	For patients with allergy to penicillins or cephalosporins
Ceftriaxone, 2 grams IV every 12 h maximum dose *or* Cefotaxime, 2 grams IV every 6 h	For spontaneous bacterial peritonitis, coverage for *Pneumococcus* as well as *Escherichia coli*

period of rapid weight loss after bariatric surgery. "Dumping syndrome" is caused by rapid postprandial gastric emptying, the release of gastric hormones, and splanchnic vasodilation. Patients with early dumping complain of nausea, vomiting, bloating, abdominal cramps, diarrhea, and sweating 30 to 60 minutes after a meal. Late dumping occurs 1 to 3 hours postprandially. It is a hyperinsulinemic and hypoglycemic state.

TABLE 71-6 Common Gynecologic Causes of Lower Abdominal/Pelvic Pain

Adnexal torsion*
Endometriosis
Endometritis/salpingitis (pelvic inflammatory disease)*
Myoma (degenerating)
Ruptured ectopic pregnancy*
Ruptured ovarian cyst*
Tubo-ovarian abscess*
Adnexal/uterine masses

*Potential threat to life.

TABLE 71-7 Types of Bariatric Surgical Procedures

Restrictive	Primarily Malabsorptive; Mildly Restrictive	Primarily Restrictive; Mildly Malabsorptive
Vertical banded gastroplasty ("stomach stapling")	Biliopancreatic diversion	Roux-en-Y gastric bypass
Laparoscopic adjustable gastric banding	Duodenal switch	

TABLE 71-8 Complications after Roux-en-Y Gastric Bypass

Anastomotic leak
Bowel obstruction (includes internal hernia and volvulus of Roux limb)
Cholelithiasis
Dumping syndrome
Enteric leak
Marginal ulcer
Metabolic complications (B_{12}, iron, thiamine, vitamin and mineral deficiencies; hyperoxaluria)
Stenosis of gastrojejunostomy site

Dietary modification is the initial treatment for dumping syndrome; patients should be advised to avoid highly concentrated foods and to separate eating and drinking. Severe cases of dumping syndrome have been successfully treated with subcutaneous octreotide.[22] The diagnosis of enteric leak requires a high index of suspicion, because the clinical presentation varies widely.[23] With Roux-en-Y gastric bypass, leaks occur most commonly at the gastrojejunostomy anastomosis. Patients with enteric leak typically present with features suggestive of sepsis (tachycardia, fever, abdominal pain). CT may show extravasation of oral contrast material, a finding highly suggestive of leak in the early postoperative period. Primary repair is the treatment of choice. The mortality for undiagnosed enteric leak is extremely high.

EPIPLOIC APPENDAGITIS

Epiploic (omental) appendages are fatty pedicular structures, typically 3 cm in length, that are found on the serosal surface of the normal colon. Their function is not known. It is estimated that each person has 50 to 100 epiploic appendages, most commonly on the sigmoid colon and cecum.[24] Acute epiploic appendagitis is a self-limited inflammatory condition usually caused by the torsion of an epiploic appendage. Spontaneous venous thrombosis and hernia incarceration of epiploic appendages have been more rarely reported. The cardinal sign is pain, which can mimic acute diverticulitis or acute appendicitis. In general, patients do not appear systemically ill, and fever is unusual. Nausea and vomiting are infrequent, but diarrhea has been reported in up to 25% of cases.[24] On US, epiploic appendagitis appears as an oval noncompressible hyperechoic mass at the site of maximal abdominal tenderness, with no color Doppler blood flow.[25] Normal epiploic appendages are not visualized on abdominal CT images in the absence of significant intraperitoneal fluid (e.g., hemoperitoneum, ascites).[25] Epiploic appendagitis appears on CT as an oval fatty mass with a slightly hyperdense rim and surrounding mesenteric stranding suggestive of inflammation.[25] Central calcification may occur from fatty necrosis. On occasion, the pedicle stalk of an epiploic appendage may break off, forming a free intraperitoneal body. The treatment is supportive and nonoperative. Pain control should be provided. Antibiotics are not indicated. Most cases resolve spontaneously within 1 to 2 weeks.

THE POSTOPERATIVE PATIENT WITH ACUTE ABDOMINAL PAIN

ILEUS AND EARLY POSTOPERATIVE BOWEL OBSTRUCTION

Anesthesia and surgical manipulation of the bowel decrease the normal propulsive activity of the gut. In the absence of precipitating factors, no specific treatment is necessary, and normal bowel function returns 2 to 3 days postoperatively. Mild cramps and flatus signal the return of peristalsis. A delay in the return of normal GI function may be caused by electrolyte abnormalities, intra-abdominal inflammation or infection, pancreatitis, or medications (particularly opioids, anticholinergics, phenothiazines, and psychotropics). The clinical findings of adynamic postoperative ileus are nausea, vomiting, abdominal distention, cramps, and obstipation. Plain radiographs of the abdomen demonstrate diffusely dilated loops of bowel, with air present in the distal colon and rectum. Adynamic ileus is treated supportively and by correction of precipitating factors.

The clinical differentiation of adynamic ileus and mechanical small bowel obstruction can be difficult. Patients with obstruction may report a temporary return of GI function postoperatively. The symptoms of obstruction are similar to those of adynamic ileus, but vary depending on the location and extent of the obstruction. Proximal obstruction is usually associated with early emesis and less abdominal distention, distal obstruction with later (sometimes bilious or feculent) emesis, and significant abdominal distention. High-pitched bowel sounds suggest mechanical obstruction. Plain abdominal radiographs show air-fluid levels (which suggest but are not pathognomonic for obstruction), thickened valvulae conniventes proximal to the obstruction, and little air in the bowel distal to the obstruction. The amount of dilated bowel is variable. Abdominal CT can reliably identify the transition point of normal to abnormal bowel, the degree of mechanical obstruction, and the presence of complications (perforation, abscess). In the absence of complications, partial small bowel obstruction is managed with observation. Surgery is generally required for high-grade obstruction or peritonitis. Mechanical small bowel obstruction is most often caused by adhesions.

ACUTE URINARY RETENTION

Acute urinary retention after ambulatory surgery should be an obvious diagnosis based on the patient's report of inability to urinate. Bedside bladder US confirms the diagnosis. Treatment is urinary bladder drainage.

REFERENCES

The complete reference list is available online at www.TintinalliEM.com.

CHAPTER 72 Nausea and Vomiting

Bophal Sarha Hang
Susan Bork
Jeff Ditkoff

INTRODUCTION AND EPIDEMIOLOGY

Nausea and vomiting accompany a variety of illnesses. Symptoms may be due to primary GI disorders such as bowel obstruction or gastroenteritis. However, symptoms may also represent pathology of the central nervous system (increased intracranial pressure, tumor), psychiatric conditions (bulimia nervosa, anxiety), endocrine or metabolic abnormalities (diabetic ketoacidosis, hyponatremia), or iatrogenic causes (medications, toxins). Also, nausea and vomiting may be the result of severe pain, myocardial infarction, sepsis, or other systemic illnesses. A comprehensive history and physical examination, as well as the use of various diagnostic modalities, are needed to determine the cause and its complications.

In the United States, the most common cause of acute nausea and vomiting is viral gastroenteritis. Other important considerations are side effects from medication and, in young women, pregnancy.[1]

PATHOPHYSIOLOGY

Multiple neurons in the medulla oblongata are activated in a sequential fashion to induce vomiting. The vomiting center is the chemoreceptor trigger zone, located in the area postrema of the fourth ventricle. Chemoreceptors in this area are outside the blood–brain barrier and are stimulated by circulating medications and toxins, including dopaminergic antagonists (levodopa, bromocriptine), nicotine, digoxin, and opiate analgesics. Another important peripheral pathway for emesis is mediated through vagal afferents. Vagal activation is triggered by direct gastric mucosal irritants (such as nonsteroidal inflammatory agents) or increased luminal distention (gastric outlet obstruction, gastroparesis). Vagus activation stimulates neurons in the area postrema and nucleus tractus solitarius. These areas are rich in serotonin receptors and are a major site of action of antiemetic drugs, such as granisetron and odansetron.[2] Similar receptors are found throughout the gastrointestinal tract, as well as the cortex and limbic system, vestibular system, heart, and genitalia. The anatomic locations and receptor-mediated triggering factors in emesis are shown in **Table 72-1**.

TABLE 72-1 Anatomic Locations of Receptor-Mediated Triggering Factors in Emesis

Anatomic Site	Chemoreceptors	Triggering Factor
Chemoreceptor trigger (area postrema)	Dopamine 5-HT_3 H_1 M_1 Vasopressin	Medications (dopamine agonists, digoxin, opiates, nicotine, chemotherapeutic drugs) Metabolic (uremia, diabetic ketoacidosis, hypercalcemia) Neuroendocrine (hyperemesis gravidum) Toxins
Peripheral vagal afferents	5-HT_3	Gastric irritants (salicylate, erythromycin, copper, ipecac) Bacterial toxins (*Staphylococcus* enterotoxin) Gastrointestinal distention (biliary colic, small bowel obstruction) Inflammation (peritonitis, cholecystitis) Chemotherapy Radiation
Vestibular system	H_1 M_1	Motion Labyrinth tumors or infections Benign position vertigo or Ménière's disease
Cerebral cortex and limbic system	Poorly characterized	Psychogenic (fear, anxiety) Noxious odors Visual stimuli

Abbreviations: 5-HT_3 = serotonin; H_1 = histamine; M_1 = muscarine.

Efferent pathways in the vagal, phrenic, and spinal nerves control the physiologic event of vomiting through coordinated muscle activity. Three stages of vomiting have been described: nausea, retching, and actual vomiting. Nausea is the unpleasant feeling that precedes vomiting. During nausea, there may be autonomic symptoms of hypersalivation, repetitive swallowing, and tachycardia. The exact physiologic pathway is not well understood but may be related to afferent abdominal vagal stimulation. During retching, there is gastric relaxation and repetitive simultaneous contraction of the diaphragm and abdominal muscles that allow for the development of a pressure gradient. Vomiting is the retrograde expulsion of gastric contents, and it is a response to changes in intra-abdominal and intrathoracic pressure generated by the contraction of the abdominal and respiratory muscles.[3]

CLINICAL FEATURES

The differential diagnosis of nausea and vomiting is exhaustive, as pathology of almost every organ system may lead to nausea and vomiting (**Table 72-2**). A thorough history and physical examination will help guide the diagnostic approach to the patient presenting with nausea and vomiting.

HISTORY

Identify the onset and duration of the symptoms. The evaluation for acute symptoms is quite different from the evaluation of a chronic problem.

TABLE 72-2 Differential Diagnosis of Nausea and Vomiting

Gastrointestinal	Neurologic	Infectious	Drugs/Toxins	Endocrine	Miscellaneous
Functional disorders	Head injury	Bacterial toxins	Digoxin	Pregnancy	Myocardial infarction
Psychogenic	Stroke	Pneumonia	Aspirin	Adrenal insufficiency	Acute glaucoma
Irritable bowel syndrome	Pseudotumor	Spontaneous bacterial peritonitis	NSAIDs	Diabetic ketoacidosis	Nephrolithiasis
Obstruction	Hydrocephalus	Urinary tract infection	Acetaminophen	Parathyroid disorders	Pain
Adhesions	Mass lesion	Viruses	Opiates	Thyroid disorders	Psychiatric disorders
Esophageal disorders	Meningitis	Adenovirus	Alcohol	Uremia	Anorexia nervosa
Achalasia	Migraines	Norwalk virus	Theophylline	Electrolyte disorders, especially hyponatremia	Bulimia
Intussusception	Labyrinthitis	Rotavirus	Chemotherapeutics		Conversion disorder
Tumor	Ménière's disease		Anticonvulsants		Depression
Pyloric stenosis	Motion sickness		Antibiotics		
Strangulated hernia			Antiarrhythmics		
Volvulus			Hormones		
Organic disorders			Illicit drugs		
Appendicitis			Radiation therapy		
Cholecystitis			Toxins		
Cholangitis			Arsenic		
Hepatitis			Organophosphates		
Irritable bowel disease			Carbon monoxide		
Mesenteric ischemia			Ricin		
Pancreatitis					
Peptic ulcer disease					
Peritonitis					

Abbreviation: NSAIDs = nonsteroidal anti-inflammatory drugs.

If the problem is chronic, asking the patient the results of any tests that have already been performed will help narrow the diagnostic possibilities. Chronic symptoms are defined as those symptoms present for >1 month.

Frequency of the episodes is helpful to gauge the severity of illness. Ask how many times vomiting occurred and the interval between episodes. Timing of the episodes, such as increased number of episodes in the morning, may suggest pregnancy or a central nervous system cause, whereas postprandial vomiting suggests gastroparesis or gastric outlet obstruction.

The content of the vomitus may be helpful to determine whether an obstruction is present and its location. Esophageal disorders produce vomitus with undigested food particles. Bile is often associated with a small bowel obstruction, whereas vomitus composed of food particles and devoid of bile often represents a gastric outlet obstruction. Large bowel obstruction often is composed of feculent material and has a foul odor.

Because of the number of organ systems that are the potential cause of pathology, it is important to ask the patient about associated symptoms. The presence or absence of abdominal pain is a focal starting point. If pain is present, elicit its location and quality. Pain preceding the nausea and vomiting is most particularly associated with an obstructive process.[2] Fever or, possibly, diarrhea suggests gastroenteritis. Ask about sick contacts or ingestion of food suspicious for a foodborne illness. A history of recent weight loss is associated with a malignancy or psychiatric component. Any central nervous system sign, such as headache, visual changes, vertigo, or neurologic deficits, may suggest a central cause for the nausea and vomiting. Obtain a thorough past medical history. Always ask about prior abdominal surgeries because the patient is at risk for bowel obstruction from adhesions. Review the patient's medication list to identify a medication with a common side effect of nausea and vomiting, such as nonsteroidal anti-inflammatory agents, cancer chemotherapeutic agents, various antibiotics, various antihypertensives and antiarrhythmics, and oral contraceptives. Other medications at toxic levels are known to cause nausea and vomiting. Examples include acetaminophen, salicylates, and digoxin.

PHYSICAL EXAMINATION

Assess vital signs for hypotension and tachycardia. Observe skin turgor, mucous membrane hydration, and capillary refill to assess for dehydration. In children, the most useful predictors of significant dehydration (>5% loss of body weight) are abnormal capillary refill, abnormal skin turgor, absent tears, and abnormal respiratory pattern.[4] The abdominal examination is particularly important to assess for an emergent problem, as well as to help narrow the differential diagnosis to a possible gastrointestinal cause.[5] Inspect, auscultate, and palpate the abdomen. (For further discussion of abdominal evaluation, see chapter 71, Acute Abdominal Pain.)

Investigate any other important examination findings particular to various organ systems, as findings may provide valuable information regarding the cause of the nausea and vomiting (**Table 72-3**).

DIAGNOSTIC TESTING

LABORATORY

After completing a proper history and physical examination, obtain serum and urine studies to help determine the cause of the symptoms and to evaluate for complications. Most often, a CBC as well as electrolyte testing is part of the basic evaluation. Obtain a pregnancy test in a woman in childbearing years who has not had a hysterectomy. Obtain liver function tests and a serum lipase in patients with upper abdominal pain or jaundice. Check thyroid function tests if thyrotoxicosis is suspected. Obtain specific drug levels for possible ingestions or suspected toxicity in patients taking acetaminophen, salicylates, digoxin, or theophylline. Also, obtain ethanol levels and narcotic drug screening tests in patients with suspected intoxication or withdrawal states.

TABLE 72-3 Differential Diagnosis Based on Physical Examination Findings

Physical Examination	Abnormal Signs or Symptoms	Some Diagnostic Considerations
General	Toxic appearing	Dehydration
	Generalized weakness	Chronic malnutrition
	Weight loss	Malignancy
Vital signs	Fever	Infection (gastroenteritis, appendicitis, cholecystitis)
	Tachycardia	Bowel perforation secondary peritonitis
	Hypotension	Severe volume depletion
	Hypertension	Intracranial hemorrhage or stroke
Head, eyes, ears, nose, throat	Nystagmus	Peripheral vs. central causes (benign positional vertigo, cerebellar infarct)
	Exophthalmos	Graves' disease
	Pin-point pupils	opiate abuse
	Fixed-dilated pupil, eye pain	Acute glaucoma
	Dry mucous membranes	Dehydration
		Bulimia
	Poor dental enamel, parotid gland enlargement	Bulimia
Abdomen	Distention, decreased bowel sounds, surgical scars	Small bowel obstruction, gastroparesis, gastric outlet obstruction, ileus
	Hernias or palpable masses	Incarcerated hernia, tumors
	Abdominal rigidity	Peritonitis
Neurologic	Mental status	Dehydration, intracranial lesion or pathology, brainstem tumor, elevated intracranial pressure
	Cranial nerve findings or neurologic deficits	
	Papilledema	
Extremities	Scarring on dorsal surface of the hands	Bulimia
Skin	Jaundice	Hepatobiliary disease (hepatitis, choledocholithiasis)
	Poor skin turgor	Dehydration
	Hyperpigmentation	Addison's disease
	Decreased elasticity	Scleroderma
	Skin track marks	Drug abuse/withdrawal

A urinalysis may be beneficial in several ways. The specific gravity may be used to help determine the degree of dehydration. The presence of ketones may suggest not only dehydration, but also diabetic ketoacidosis or hyperemesis gravidarum in a pregnant patient. The presence of bilirubinuria may suggest a biliary tract obstruction. Nitrites, leukocyte-esterase, bacteria, and white blood cells may indicate an upper or lower urinary tract infection. Also, red blood cells, in the proper clinical picture, may support a diagnosis of kidney stones. Lastly, an erythrocyte sedimentation rate may be evaluated to search for an inflammatory cause.

IMAGING

Flat and upright abdominal films are useful screening tests for bowel obstruction. Plain radiography is less sensitive than CT scanning, but the radiation dose is <1 mSv, about one tenth the radiation dose of an abdominal CT scan.[6,7] Abdominal CT with PO and IV contrast can diagnose a mechanical obstruction, identify the cause, and visualize visceral and vascular pathology. A noncontrast abdominopelvic CT or renal US are tests of choice if kidney stones are suspected. If the history or physical examination suggest a CNS cause, a CT of the head or MRI of the brain is ordered to evaluate for an intracranial mass or lesion. Other radiographic tests are available but are often ordered for a patient who requires admission to the hospital, or upon consultation with a gastroenterologist. These tests include esophagogastroduodenoscopy, upper GI radiography with barium contrast, small bowel follow-through, enteroclysis, gastric emptying scintigraphy, antroduodenal manometry, and cutaneous electrogastrography.

ANCILLARY TESTING

An abdominal US is helpful to evaluate a patient with associated right upper quadrant or epigastric pain to diagnose possible gallbladder, hepatic, or pancreatic pathology. Hepatobiliary iminodiacetic acid scans are sometimes performed in suspected cases of biliary dysfunction and/or cholecystitis. Suspected testicular torsion would also be diagnosed by US. Obtain an electrocardiogram for suspected myocardial infarction. Measure intraocular eye pressures if glaucoma is a part of the differential diagnosis.

TREATMENT

Stabilize the patient, paying attention to the ABCs: airway, breathing, and circulation. After stabilization, provide symptomatic relief (**Table 72-4**). Definitive management will often require disease-specific treatment. If no clear cause is noted at the outset, an H_1 histaminergic such as promethazine or a serotonin receptor antagonist such as ondansetron may be helpful for initial treatment, pending further workup.[8] However, promethazine is more sedating, with the potential side effect of vascular damage during IV administration. Recent studies have also compared the efficacy of selective serotonin receptor antagonist (tropisetron, ondansetron) versus other agents in treating nausea and vomiting for undifferentiated ED patients. Serotonin receptor blockers significantly lower the rates of vomiting when compared with metoclopramide.[9] Both ondansetron and prochlorperazine are equally effective.[10] Patients given either drug must be monitored for akathisia that may develop up to 48 hours after administration. Based on overall safety and efficacy, serotonin receptor antagonists such as ondansetron should be used as first-line therapy for undifferentiated nausea and vomiting in all age groups. For patients in the ED who have no response to ondansetron in 30 minutes, administration of another drug with activity at a different receptor site is more likely to be successful than repeat dosing of ondansetron.[11]

Acknowledgments: The authors gratefully acknowledge the contributions of Annie T. Sadosty and Jennifer J. Hess, the authors of this subject in the previous edition.

TABLE 72-4 Antiemetic Agents for the Treatment of Nausea and Vomiting

Medication Class	Route	Common Side Effects	Comments
Antihistamines		Drowsiness	Also show efficacy in prevention of motion sickness. Useful for migraines and vertigo.
Dimenhydrinate (Dramamine®)	PO		
Diphenhydramine (Benadryl®)*	IV, IM, PO		Used in migraines and vertigo, which are vestibular in origin.
Meclizine (Antivert®)	PO		
Benzodiazepines		Sedation	Adjunct for chemotherapy-induced nausea and vomiting.
Alprazolam (Xanax®)	PO		
Diazepam (Valium®)	PO, IV, PR		
Lorazepam (Ativan®)	PO, IV, IM		
Butyrophenones		Agitation, restlessness, sedation	Treatment of acute chemotherapy-induced symptoms.
Haloperidol (Haldol®)*	PO, IM		
Corticosteroids		Insomnia	Used as an adjunct in severe cases of chemotherapy-induced nausea and vomiting; reduces prostaglandin formation.
Dexamethasone	PO, IV, IM		
Serotonin antagonists		Constipation, dizziness	Well tolerated; uncommon side effects include headache, rare case report of anaphylaxis.
Ondansetron (Zofran®)*	PO, IV, SL		
Granisetron (Kytril®)*	PO, IV		
Dolasetron (Anzemet®)*	PO, IV		
Phenothiazines		Extrapyramidal symptoms,‡ sedation, orthostatic hypotension	Treatment in migraines, vertigo, and motion sickness; rare side effects include neuroleptic malignant syndrome, blood dyscrasias, and cholestatic jaundice.
Prochlorperazine (Compazine®)†	PO, IV, IM		
Promethazine (Phenergan®)†	PO, IV, IM, PR		
Benzamides		Extrapyramidal symptoms,‡ hyperprolactinemia	Used in treatment of gastroparesis and children with reflux.
Metoclopramide (Reglan®)	PO, IV, IM		
Trimethobenzamide (Tigan®)	PO		

*QT-interval prolongation reported.

†Nonspecific Q or T distortions reported.

‡Extrapyramidal symptoms: dystonia, tardive dyskinesia, oculogyric crisis, parkinsonism.

REFERENCES

The complete reference list is available online at www.TintinalliEM.com.

CHAPTER 73 Disorders Presenting Primarily With Diarrhea

Nicholas E. Kman
Howard A. Werman

GENERAL ASSESSMENT OF PATIENTS WITH DIARRHEA

INTRODUCTION AND EPIDEMIOLOGY

This chapter discusses the general assessment of patients with diarrhea and the special considerations of acute infectious and traveler's diarrhea, *Clostridium difficile* diarrhea and colitis, inflammatory bowel disease, ileitis and colitis, and ulcerative colitis.

Acute diarrhea is the sudden onset of an increase in the normal water content of stool. In general, humans lose approximately 10 mL/kg/day of fluids in stool. The increased water content of diarrhea results in an increased frequency of stools from 3 or more times daily to more than 20 bowel movements in a 24-hour period. Diarrhea is an increased frequency of defecation, usually greater than 3 bowel movements per day for a daily stool weight exceeding 200 grams.[1,2] Practically speaking, however, diarrhea is present when the patient is making more stools of lesser consistency more frequently.

PATHOPHYSIOLOGY

There are four basic mechanisms of diarrhea: increased intestinal secretion, decreased intestinal absorption, increased osmotic load, and abnormal intestinal motility. Normally, the jejunum receives between 6 and 8 L per day of fluid in the form of oral intake and gastric, pancreatic, and biliary secretions. Dietary intake actually constitutes a small portion of the jejunal load (1.5 L). A healthy small intestine absorbs nearly 75% of the fluid to which it is exposed. The 2 L of fluid not absorbed by the small intestine then enters the colon, where fluid is absorbed at an even higher rate. The absorptive power of the colon approaches 90% efficiency and far exceeds that of the small intestine. In fact, the colon can make up for a decrease in small intestinal absorption. Under normal conditions, very little fluid (<100 mL) is lost in the stool each day.[3]

In diarrheal states, normal intestinal physiology is disrupted. At a cellular level, intestinal absorption occurs through the villi, and secretion occurs through the crypts. Fluids are absorbed by two mechanisms: passively with the transport of sodium and actively with the absorption of glucose. Selected enterotoxins block the passive sodium resorption and specifically stimulate sodium excretion, resulting in a net loss of fluid. The glucose-dependent mechanism of water absorption, however, is unaffected by these toxins and can be exploited by including glucose in the rehydration treatments. The composition of oral rehydration therapies recommended by the World Health Organization is based largely on this physiology. In addition, diarrheal states, enterotoxins, inflammation, or ischemia disrupt the structure of the intestinal villi preferentially with less involvement in the crypts. As a result, diarrhea occurs because of diminished intestinal villi absorption *and* unopposed crypt secretion (the crypts are more resilient after injury).[4]

Another mechanism by which disease processes cause diarrhea is by the delivery of an osmotic load to the intestine. For example, administration of a laxative results in the collection of an osmotically active, nondigestible agent within the intestinal lumen. Other substances such as diet products and medications (e.g., colchicine) have similar effects.

Osmosis occurs, drawing fluid into the intestinal lumen, and results in diarrhea. Increased intestinal motility also causes diarrhea. This mechanism is responsible for diarrhea in patients with irritable bowel syndrome, neuropathies, or a shortened intestine secondary to surgery.

Diarrheal illness is primarily a viral infection (norovirus), but can also be caused by bacteria and parasites. Antibiotic and nosocomial diarrhea is most often caused by *C. difficile*. Many drugs affect gastrointestinal function. Erythromycin accelerates gastric emptying. Clavulanate stimulates small bowel motility. Other drugs that cause diarrhea are laxatives, sorbitol, lactose, nonsteroidal anti-inflammatory drugs, and cholinergics. Inflammatory bowel disease, ulcerative colitis, and Crohn's disease are characterized by diarrhea. **If patients have fecal evidence of inflammation and *Shigella*, *Salmonella*, *Campylobacter*, *C. difficile*, or *Entamoeba histolytica* have been excluded, suspect inflammatory bowel disease.** Less common causes of severe diarrhea include gastrointestinal bleeding, thyrotoxicosis, toxin exposure, and mesenteric ischemia, which are addressed elsewhere in the text.

CLINICAL FEATURES

History After confirming a diarrheal illness, focus on identifying the cause. Determine whether the diarrhea is acute (<3 weeks) or chronic (>3 weeks). The acute diarrheas are of greatest concern to the emergency physician as they are more apt to be a manifestation of an immediately life-threatening illness (infection, ischemia, intoxication, or inflammation).[2] In the United States, most infectious diarrheal illnesses are caused by noroviruses or rotaviruses and occur in the winter.[5]

Ask directed questions to characterize the diarrhea: Is the diarrhea bloody or melenic? Is it associated with possible food poisoning or the ingestion of certain foods, such as milk or sorbitol? Does it resolve or persist with fasting? If so, this can indicate an osmotic or secretory diarrhea, respectively. Are the stools of smaller volume, localizing to the large intestine, or of larger volume, indicating small intestine pathology? What symptoms accompany the diarrhea? Is there fever or abdominal pain, which may suggest diverticulitis, infectious gastroenteritis, or inflammatory bowel disease? Seizures accompanying diarrhea often point toward shigellosis but could also indicate theophylline toxicity or hyponatremia. Does the patient have heat intolerance and anxiety, suggesting thyrotoxicosis, or paresthesias and reverse temperature sensation, suggesting ciguatera poisoning?

Next, define the host by obtaining the medical and surgical history. The differential diagnosis for diarrhea is broadened if the patient is immunocompromised. Is the patient taking medication that may cause diarrhea? Has the patient recently traveled outside the United States or to a rural area? Rural hiking places the patient at risk for *Giardia,* particularly if water-purification procedures were not strictly followed, and travel to third-world countries increases the chances of parasitic infection and traveler's diarrhea. A patient's occupation may be a clue to a diagnosis of organophosphate poisoning.

Physical Examination Some examination findings helpful for diagnosis include thyroid enlargement, masses, oral ulcers, erythema nodosum, episcleritis, or an anal fissure, which would point toward inflammatory bowel disease. Reiter's syndrome, the triad of arthritis, conjunctivitis, and urethritis or cervicitis, should cause concern for *Salmonella, Shigella, Campylobacter,* or *Yersinia* infection.

Abdominal and rectal examinations are critical. Especially in the elderly, fecal impaction may result in diarrhea as liquid stool passes around the impaction. Pay attention to the presence or absence of surgical scars, tenderness, masses, or peritoneal signs. Check the stool for blood, because bloody diarrhea can be caused by inflammation, infection, or ischemia. An elderly patient with bloody diarrhea and abdominal pain out of proportion to the physical examination may have mesenteric ischemia—a true emergency.

DIAGNOSTIC STOOL EVALUATION

Diagnostic testing is rarely immediately helpful in the ED, but it can be helpful at patient follow-up. Since most diarrheal illnesses are self-limited, viral, or last less than 24 hours, most patients who present within 24 hours of onset need no microbiologic examination. **Patients who have severe abdominal pain, fever, and diarrhea that is voluminous, purulent, or bloody may have acute infectious diarrhea associated with the following pathogens: *Salmonella*, *Campylobacter*, *Shigella*, shiga toxin-producing *Escherichia coli*, *Yersinia*, *Vibrios*, or *C. difficile*.**[5] Patients fitting this subset will require microbiologic evaluation, as described next.

Wright's Stain When applied to a stool sample, Wright's stain allows detection of fecal leukocytes. A positive Wright's stain has a sensitivity of 52% to 82% and a specificity of 83% for the presence of bacterial pathogens by stool culture.[6] Historically, Wright's stain for fecal leukocytes has been used to differentiate invasive from noninvasive infectious diarrheas. In the past, this was an important distinction: physicians were reluctant to prescribe antibiotics for patients with infectious diarrhea because of the fear of prolonging the *Salmonella* carrier state. They therefore reserved antimicrobial treatment for the toxic patients who they felt *truly* had invasive diarrhea. Many physicians now treat patients with diarrheal illness with antibiotics regardless of whether or not the diarrhea is invasive or bacterial in origin.[7]

Bacterial Stool Culture Bacterial stool culture is expensive and labor intensive and plays a minor role in the ED evaluation of diarrhea. The diagnostic yield of stool cultures is probably <5%, unless there is careful patient selection.[1] Obtain stool cultures for bacteria in ill children; toxic, dehydrated, or febrile patients; patients with a diarrheal illness >3 days; patients with blood or pus in the stool; and the immunocompromised. For systemic illness, fever, or bloody stools, test for *Salmonella, Shigella, Campylobacter*, Shiga toxin-producing *E. coli*, or amoebic infection.[1,4,5] Many laboratories culture for only three common bacterial pathogens: *Salmonella, Shigella,* and *Campylobacter.* If other enteric pathogens are suspected, notify the laboratory so that appropriate testing may be performed.

Ova and Parasite Evaluation Suspect parasitic infection and evaluate stool for ova and parasites in travelers exposed to untreated water and those presenting with diarrhea for more than 7 days. Stool tests for ova and parasites lack sensitivity, because many parasites are fastidious, and shedding of the organisms is intermittent. Multiple samples may need to be collected for a positive result. Direct immunofluorescence staining improves the sensitivity for detecting *Giardia* and *Cryptosporidium.*[8]

***Clostridium difficile* Toxin Assay** *C. difficile* infection is the commonest cause of antibiotic-associated or nosocomial diarrhea. Diagnosis is by the *C. difficile* toxin assay. Unfortunately, this assay has a 10% false-negative rate, and the turnaround time on the test approaches 24 hours.[9]

Other Diagnostic Tests If diarrhea is not infectious in origin, data acquisition should be dictated by the differential diagnosis. Severely dehydrated patients need serum electrolyte and renal function measurements. Serum drug levels can assist the physician in making the diagnosis of theophylline, lithium, or heavy metal intoxication. In patients with a history of abdominal surgery, abdominal films may help rule out partial obstruction as a cause of diarrhea. A chest radiograph may help diagnose *Legionella* pneumonia in a patient with diarrhea and a cough. For patients in whom mesenteric ischemia is suspected, obtain a serum lactate, IV contrast CT scan, or mesenteric angiography.

Treatment Severely dehydrated patients need IV hydration. Oral rehydration with a glucose-based electrolyte solution can be initiated in patients without associated nausea or vomiting and without severe dehydration. Glucose-containing, caffeine-free beverages are the fluids of choice. The glucose transport mechanism is unaffected by enterotoxins, allowing for water absorption in the small intestine. For patients who can afford to buy it, Gatorade® is a good rehydration choice for patients with mild dehydration. The World Health Organization recommends a solution with a higher sodium concentration for more extensive dehydration. Mildly dehydrated patients should aim to drink 30 to 50 mL/kg over the first 4 hours. For moderate dehydration, patients should drink 100 mL/kg over the next 4 hours.[2]

Counsel patients to avoid caffeine, which stimulates gastric motility, and sorbitol-containing chewing gum or raw fruits, which can worsen osmotic diarrhea. Initially, avoid lactose until the colonic villi are able to recover and produce the necessary digestive enzymes. Encourage patients to attempt early solid food intake, but with the previously mentioned restrictions, because eating expedites the recovery from diarrheal illnesses.[10]

ACUTE INFECTIOUS AND TRAVELER'S DIARRHEA

INTRODUCTION AND EPIDEMIOLOGY

Viruses cause the vast majority of infectious diarrheas, followed by bacterial and parasitic organisms. **Norovirus causes 50% to 80% of all** infectious diarrhea in the United States, followed with much less frequency by non–Shiga toxin producing *E. coli*, *C. difficile*, invasive bacteria, Shiga toxin-producing *E. coli*, and protozoa.[1,5]

Approximately 40% of the 50 million Americans who travel annually to developing countries develop diarrhea in the first 2 weeks of travel.[11] **A history of foreign travel is associated with an 80% probability of bacterial diarrhea.**[5] The most important risk factor for traveler's diarrhea is the destination of travel, with the risk increasing with travel to areas of lower socioeconomic status. Countries in Asia, Africa, Latin America, and parts of the Middle East are considered high-risk destinations for traveler's diarrhea, with incidence rates ranging between 20% and 75%.[12] Other risk factors include the level of food contamination, the season of travel (rainy seasons are associated with a higher risk of traveler's diarrhea), use of a proton pump inhibitor, previous contraction of traveler's diarrhea (suggests genetic susceptibility), and the type of travel (adventure travel, camping, backpacking, and living with native inhabitants are associated with higher risk).[13] The major bacteria responsible are the toxin and non–toxin-producing strains of *E. coli*. These strains of *E. coli* make up most identifiable cases in Mexico and South America. The invasive bacteria, such as *Campylobacter jejuni*, *Shigella*, and *Salmonella*, are more commonly seen in travelers to southern Asia.[5,12]

CLINICAL FEATURES

The presence of severe abdominal pain, fever, or bloody stool requires microbiologic studies to rule out bacterial or amoebic infection.[11] Assess stool for polymorphonuclear white blood cells or fecal leukocytes by microscopy or by immunoassay for the neutrophil protein lactoferrin.[5] The presence of fecal leukocytes increases the likelihood of a bacterial pathogen. However, bloody stool without white blood cells is a common feature of Shiga toxin–producing *E. coli* or *E. coli* O157:H7 and colitis that is due to *E. histolytica*.[1,5]

Laboratory Testing Obtain stool culture for *Salmonella*, *Shigella*, *Campylobacter*, and *E. coli* O157:H7; assay for Shiga toxin; and obtain microscopy or antigen assay for *E. histolytica*.[5]

Exposure of a traveler or hiker to untreated water and illness that persists for more than 7 days should prompt evaluations for protozoal pathogens. Test stool for *E. histolytica* antigen, *Giardia intestinalis* antigen, and *Cryptosporidium parvum* antigen by enzyme immunoassay.[1,5] Rarely, helminthes such as *Ascaris*, *Enterobius*, and *Strongyloides* have been implicated.[14]

TREATMENT

Treatment of infectious diarrhea includes antibiotics, antimotility agents, restoration of fluid balance, and avoidance of agents that worsen diarrhea (**Table 73-1**). **Loperamide and antibiotics improve outcome.**[15,16]

For years, physicians avoided antibiotic use in the treatment of infectious diarrhea because of a fear of prolonging the *Salmonella* carrier state. This fear arose from an article published in 1969 in which the duration of *Salmonella* excretion was felt to be prolonged after antibiotic treatment.[17] Contemporary literature has put this to rest. Antibiotics shorten the duration of illness by about 24 hours.[7,17] Regardless of the causative agent, all patients—even those who had a negative Wright's stain, negative stool culture, and a low diarrheal illness score, suggesting less clinically significant disease and/or a viral cause—improve on ciprofloxacin.[18] Even though most cases of infectious diarrhea are self-limited, because of the inconveniencing and debilitating nature of the disease, **we recommend ciprofloxacin treatment for all patients believed to have an infectious diarrhea who do not have a contraindication to the drug** (e.g., children, allergy, pregnancy, or drug interaction). There are reports of growing fluoroquinolone resistance in bacterial pathogens.[19] Trimethoprim/sulfamethoxazole also shortens the duration of infectious diarrhea in adults but may be inferior to a course of ciprofloxacin because of resistant organisms.[18] Concerns remain about the impact of ciprofloxacin on the intestinal flora[20] and its side effect profile, and other non–gastrointestinal-absorbed agents such as rifaximin are an option.[21] (See **Table 73-2** for specific treatments.)

Loperamide shortens the duration of symptoms when combined with an antibiotic regimen. Loperamide, bismuth subsalicylate, and kaolin are the only agents that are labeled as antidiarrheals. **Do not use antimotility** agents in the subset of patients with bloody diarrhea or suspected inflammatory diarrhea because of the possibility of prolonged fever, toxic megacolon in *C. difficile* patients, and hemolytic uremic syndrome in children infected with Shiga-toxin producing *E. coli*.[1]

TABLE 73-1 Empiric Treatment of Traveler's Diarrhea in the Adult

	Trade Name	Dosage	Comments
Rehydration			
Fluids: chicken broth with fruit juices, Gatorade®, noncaffeinated sodas, packages of salts and glucose to be reconstituted with boiled or treated water, CeraLyte 90®, Pedialyte®			
Foods: complex carbohydrates (bananas, bread, rice, apple juice, and tortillas), potatoes, crackers, *Lactobacillus*-containing yogurt			
Antimotility Agents			
Bismuth subsalicylate	Pepto-Bismol®	30 mL or 2 tablets every 30 min for 8 doses; repeat on day 2	Salicylate toxicity may occur with excessive dosing; may cause bismuth encephalopathy in HIV-positive patients.
Loperamide	Imodium®	4 milligrams initially, then 2 milligrams after each unformed stool for no more than 2 days; maximum, 16 milligrams per day	Preferred first-line agent for antimotility, with minimal central opiate effects. Can be used with antibiotics.
Diphenoxylate and atropine	Lomotil®	4 milligrams four times a day for 2 days	Second-line agent with more central opiate effects (narcotic related to meperidine); may potentiate the action of barbiturates, tranquilizers, and alcohol.
Antibiotics			
Ciprofloxacin	Cipro®	500 milligrams single dose or 500 milligrams twice a day for 3 days	For moderately severe illness in adults; complete 3-day course if single dose fails; significant drug–drug interactions may occur.
Azithromycin	Zithromax®	1000 milligrams in a single dose	Safe for children and pregnant women
Trimethoprim/sulfamethoxazole (see sulfamethoxazole-trimethoprim)	Bactrim®	160 milligrams/800 milligrams for single dose, 160 milligrams/800 milligrams twice a day for 3 days	For moderately severe illness; resistance limits reliable effectiveness.
Rifaximin[13,22]	Xifaxan®, Salix®	200 milligrams PO three times daily for 3 days	For moderately severe illness; do not use for fever or bloody stools; class C in pregnancy.

Abbreviation: HIV = human immunodeficiency virus.

TABLE 73-2 Antimicrobial Recommendations for Infectious Pathogens in Adults

Organism	Primary Treatment	Alternative Treatment
Empiric treatment—but not for bloody diarrhea; not for Shiga toxin *E. coli* 0157:H7	Ciprofloxacin 500 milligrams PO twice a day for 5 days	Trimethoprim-sulfamethoxazole DS, 1 tab PO twice a day for 5 days
C. difficile	Metronidazole 500 milligrams PO 3 times a day for 14 days	Vancomycin, 125 milligrams PO four times a day for 14 days
E. coli 0157:H7	No antibiotics	No antibiotics
Listeria monocytogenes	No antibiotics	No antibiotics
Yersinia	No antibiotics; usually self-limited	Ciprofloxacin 500 milligrams PO twice a day for 3 days; or trimethoprim-sulfamethoxazole DS,1 tab PO twice a day for 3 days
Salmonella non-typhi	Ciprofloxacin 750 milligrams PO twice a day for 5 days	Azithromycin 500 milligrams PO once a day for 7 days
Shigella	Ciprofloxacin 750 milligrams PO twice a day for 3 days	Azithromycin 500 milligrams PO once a day for 3 days
V. cholerae	Doxycycline 500 milligrams PO for one dose *OR* Azithromycin 1 gram PO for one dose	Trimethoprim-sulfamethoxazole DS,1 tab PO twice a day for 3 days
E. histolytica	Metronidazole 750 milligrams PO three times a day for 10 days *AND* Paromomycin 10 milligrams/kg three times a day PO for 7 days	Metronidazole *AND* iodoquinol 650 milligrams PO three times a day for 20 days *OR* Tinidazole 2 grams PO once a day for three days *AND* paromomycin or iodoquinol
Cyclospora	Trimethoprim-sulfamethoxazole DS, 1 tab PO twice a day for 10 days	
Giardia	Tinidazole 2 grams PO for one dose	Nitazoxanide 500 milligrams PO twice a day for 3 days *OR* Metronidazole 750 milligrams PO three times a day for 10 days *OR* Paromomycin 10 milligrams/kg/day PO three times a day for 10 days

Note: Length of treatment often varies with different sources.

Probiotics are safe and beneficial when used alongside rehydration therapy.[23] Proton pump inhibitors are not effective.[15]

DISPOSITION

Admit the toxic patient and any patient who cannot comply with oral rehydration. Be conservative in admitting those at extremes of age. Most patients with diarrhea can be discharged home.

The best way to combat many infectious diarrheas is with prevention. Counsel families about frequent hand washing to minimize spread of disease. Counseling families about the proper selection and preparation of food and beverages consumed while traveling is a cornerstone of prevention.[12] Encourage the use of boiled, bottled, and carbonated water for drinking, brushing teeth, and preparing food and infant formula. Water can be made safe by boiling, treating it chemically, or filtering.[12] A quick phrase for prevention is, "Peel it, boil it, cook it, or forget it!"

In addition, vaccines against the most common etiologic agent, rotavirus, are now available.[24]

Provide work excuses for patients employed in the food, day-care, and healthcare industries.

CLOSTRIDIUM DIFFICILE-ASSOCIATED DIARRHEA AND COLITIS

INTRODUCTION AND EPIDEMIOLOGY

C. difficile is a spore-forming obligate anaerobic bacillus that causes infection ranging from mild diarrhea to severe pseudomembranous colitis. ***C. difficile* infection is the most common cause of bacterial diarrhea in hospitalized patients in Europe and North America.** The incidence and severity of disease has increased at an alarming rate of 25% per year since 2000.[25] A more virulent strain of *C. difficile* called North American pulsed-field type 1 or B1/NAP1/027 affects hospitalized patients, but can also occur in community-dwelling healthy adults.[26] This strain causes more severe disease that more often progresses to toxic megacolon.

The organism secretes two toxins, A and B, that cause a secretory diarrhea. At the most severe end of the spectrum, three different syndromes have been described: neonatal pseudomembranous enterocolitis, postoperative pseudomembranous enterocolitis, and antibiotic-associated pseudomembranous colitis. In pseudomembranous colitis, membrane-like yellowish exudative plaques overlie and replace necrotic intestinal mucosa. Recent antibiotic use, gastrointestinal surgery or manipulation, severe underlying medical illness, chemotherapy, and advancing age are risk factors for pseudomembranous colitis. Transmission of the organism is by direct human contact as well as contact with inanimate objects (commodes, telephones, rectal thermometers).

PATHOPHYSIOLOGY

Hospitalized patients are colonized with *C. difficile* in 10% to 25% of cases, so the development of diarrhea in recently discharged patients is suggestive of *C. difficile* infection. There is a linear relationship between the length of hospital stay, colonization with *C. difficile,* and the development of *C. difficile* diarrhea. Broad-spectrum antibiotics—most notably clindamycin, second- and third-generation cephalosporins, ampicillin/amoxicillin, and fluoroquinolones—reduce fecal anaerobes, which are needed for carbohydrate metabolism and bile acid breakdown. Accumulation of gut carbohydrates can cause osmotic diarrhea, and the accumulation of bile acids, which are colonic secretory agents, also results in diarrhea. Toxin-producing *C. difficile* then flourishes within the colon. Almost any antibiotic (including metronidazole and vancomycin) can lead to pseudomembranous colitis, and chemotherapeutic agents, proton pump inhibitors, and antiviral agents have also been implicated. Bowel ischemia, inflammatory bowel disease, recent bowel surgery, uremia, malnutrition, shock, advanced age, peripartum status, and Hirschsprung's disease also contribute to the development of *C. difficile* infection and pseudomembranous colitis.[26]

Most disease-producing strains of *C. difficile* produce two toxins: toxin A, an enterotoxin, and toxin B, a cytotoxin, that interact in a complex way to produce pseudomembranous colitis and its associated symptoms.

CLINICAL FEATURES

The disease typically begins 7 to 10 days after the institution of antibiotic therapy, although symptoms may occur up to 60 days after the antibiotic is discontinued. Pseudomembranous colitis results in a spectrum of clinical manifestations that vary from frequent, mucoid, watery stools to a toxic picture that includes profuse diarrhea (20 to 30 stools per day), crampy abdominal pain, fever, leukocytosis, and dehydration. Stool examination may demonstrate fecal leukocytes, which are not generally found in more benign forms of antibiotic-induced diarrhea.[27] In 1% to 3% of patients, toxic megacolon or colonic perforation may occur in patients with pseudomembranous colitis.[28]

DIAGNOSIS

The diagnosis is suggested by a history of diarrhea that develops during administration of antibiotics or within 2 weeks of their discontinuation.

Stool Assays The diagnosis is confirmed by the demonstration of *C. difficile* in the stool and by the detection of the toxin in stool filtrates. The organism is best identified by stool culture using a selective growth medium. This technique has a sensitivity approaching 100%, but lacks specificity because the presence of *C. difficile* does not necessarily implicate it in the cause of the disease.

Instead, *C. difficile* toxins are detected directly using a number of techniques including tissue-culture assay, enzyme-linked immunosorbent assays, latex agglutination, dot-immunobinding assays, and polymerase chain reaction. Tests vary in their sensitivity, specificity, and time to completion. Although tissue-culture assays are considered the gold standard, most laboratories use the enzyme-linked immunosorbent assay technique to detect the clostridial toxins; it has a sensitivity of 63% to 94% and a specificity of 75% to 100%.[28] Five to 20% of patients require more than one stool specimen to detect toxin.

Colonoscopy Colonoscopy reveals characteristic yellowish plaques within the intestinal lumen. Lesions may be seen throughout the entire alimentary tract, although they are typically limited to the right colon. Colonoscopy is not routinely needed to establish a diagnosis , but may be used in patients who require a rapid diagnosis and those who cannot produce a stool specimen due to ileus.

TREATMENT

Mild *C. difficile* infection in an otherwise healthy patient is treated by discontinuing the offending antibiotic.[25] This is effective in only about 20% of cases, however. Severely ill persons must be hospitalized. For specific antibiotic regimens, see **Table 73-3.**[29,30] Fidaxomicin (macrolide antibiotic) 200 milligrams PO twice a day for 10 days is also available for treatment.[31]

Rarely, emergency colectomy may be required for patients with severe *C. difficile* infection. Indications for emergency colectomy based on 30-day mortality include leukocytosis greater than 20,000 mm^3, lactate >5 mmoL/L, age >75 years, immunosuppression, shock, toxic megacolon, colonic perforation, or multiorgan system failure.

Relapses occur in 20% to 30% of patients.[29] Patients with prolonged antibiotic use, prolonged hospitalization, advanced age, diverticulosis, or multiple comorbidities are at increased risk for relapse.[26] The addition of monoclonal antibodies against the toxin to antibiotics reduces infection recurrence.[32] Probiotic treatment is not a useful adjunct for *C. difficile* infection.[33] The use of antidiarrheal agents is controversial.[34] Steroids are rarely needed.

Ensure contact isolation, use of personal protective equipment, and good hand washing with soap and water when caring for patients with suspected *C. difficile*–associated disease. Alcohol-based rubs are not effective in eliminating the spores of *C. difficile.*

TABLE 73-3 Treatment of *Clostridium difficile* Infection Based on Severity of Illness

Disease Severity	Treatment
Mild: WBC <15,000 mm^3	Metronidazole 500 milligrams PO three times a day for 14 days
Moderate: WBC >15,000 mm^3, patient able to tolerate PO	Vancomycin 125 milligrams PO four times a day for 14 days
First relapse	Metronidazole 500 milligrams PO three times a day for 14 days
Second relapse	Vancomycin 125 milligrams PO four times a day for 14 days; then taper dose over 4 weeks
Severe disease with toxic megacolon	Metronidazole 500 milligrams IV every 6 hours *and* vancomycin 500 milligrams PO every 6 hours (PO preferred to IV)

Note: Assume the offending antibiotic is discontinued.

DISPOSITION

Hospitalize patients with severe diarrhea, clinical toxicity, or symptoms that persist despite appropriate outpatient management. Consult the surgeon for suspected toxic megacolon or intestinal perforation for consideration of colectomy. For those patients who are discharged, discontinue antibiotics and encourage good oral hydration. Follow the antibiotic recommendations in **Table 73-3.**

INFLAMMATORY BOWEL DISEASE/ILEITIS/ COLITIS CROHN'S DISEASE

INTRODUCTION AND EPIDEMIOLOGY

Crohn's disease is a chronic granulomatous inflammatory disease of the gastrointestinal tract of unknown origin. **Crohn's disease can involve any part of the gastrointestinal tract from the mouth to the anus.** The ileum is involved in the majority of cases. In 20%, the disease is confined to the colon, making differentiation from ulcerative colitis difficult. The terms *regional enteritis, terminal ileitis, granulomatous ileocolitis,* and *Crohn's disease* are all used to describe the same disease process.

The peak incidence of Crohn's disease occurs between 15 and 22 years of age, with a secondary peak from 55 to 60 years. It is more common in women. The incidence is increasing, especially in children.[35] The disease is four times more common among Jews than non-Jews and is more common in whites than blacks, Asians, or Native Americans. A family history of inflammatory bowel disease is present in 10% to 15% of patients, particularly with early onset of disease. Ulcerative colitis as well as Crohn's disease may be present in other family members, and siblings of patients with Crohn's disease have a higher incidence of the disease. Smoking, oral contraceptive use, and the use of nonsteroidal anti-inflammatory agents worsen the course of the disease.

PATHOPHYSIOLOGY

The most important pathologic feature of Crohn's disease is the involvement of all the layers of the bowel and extension into mesenteric lymph nodes. The disease is discontinuous, with normal areas of bowel ("skip areas") located between one or more involved areas. Longitudinal, deep mucosal ulcerations are characteristic. If ulcerations penetrate the bowel wall, fissures, fistulas, and abscesses result. Late in the disease, a cobblestone appearance of the mucosa results from the criss-crossing of ulcers with intervening normal mucosa.

CLINICAL FEATURES

The clinical course of Crohn's disease varies and in the individual patient is unpredictable. Abdominal pain, anorexia, diarrhea, and weight loss are present in most cases. Chronic abdominal pain, fever, and diarrhea may be present for several years before definitive diagnosis is established. Perianal fissures or fistulas, hematochezia, abscesses, or rectal prolapse can develop, particularly with colonic involvement.[36,37] Patients may also present with complications of the disease, such as obstruction with vomiting, crampy abdominal pain, and obstipation, or an intra-abdominal abscess with fever, abdominal pain, and a palpable mass.

In 10% to 20% of patients, the extraintestinal manifestations of arthritis, uveitis, or liver disease may be presenting symptoms. Crohn's disease should also be considered in the differential diagnosis of patients with fever of unknown etiology.

The clinical course and manifestations of the disease appear to be related to its anatomic distribution: in 30% the disease involves only the small bowel, in 20% only the colon is involved, and in 50% both the small bowel and colon are involved. A small percentage of patients present with disease involving the mouth, esophagus, and stomach. Crohn's disease of the stomach may demonstrate symptoms of peptic ulcer disease.

Extraintestinal manifestations are seen in up to 40% of patients with Crohn's disease (**Table 73-4**),[38] and the incidence and types of extraintestinal complications are similar in patients with Crohn's disease and ulcerative colitis.

DIAGNOSIS

In most patients, the definitive diagnosis of Crohn's disease is established months or years after symptom onset. A provisional diagnosis of appendicitis or pelvic inflammatory disease may change to Crohn's disease after imaging or at the time of surgery. A detailed history asking about previous bowel symptoms that preceded the onset of acute right lower quadrant pain provides clues to the correct diagnosis.

ED evaluation focuses on determining the severity of the attack; identifying significant complications such as obstruction, intra-abdominal abscess, life-threatening hemorrhage, or toxic megacolon; and eliminating other possible causes of the patient's complaints.

Laboratory Testing Laboratory evaluation should include a CBC, serum electrolytes, BUN, creatinine, and a type and cross-match where appropriate. C-reactive protein levels can monitor disease activity.[39] Fecal markers of inflammation (calprotectin and lactoferrin) are other markers of disease activity.[40]

Imaging Plain radiographs of the abdomen may demonstrate obstruction, perforation, or toxic megacolon. Abdominal CT scanning with PO and IV contrast identifies bowel wall thickening, segmental narrowing, destruction of the normal mucosal pattern, mesenteric edema, fistulas, and abscesses, which suggest the diagnosis of Crohn's disease. Extraintestinal complications such as gallstones, renal calculi, sacroiliitis, and osteomyelitis can also be seen on CT scan. Diagnosis is confirmed by colonoscopy.

Differential Diagnosis The differential diagnosis of Crohn's disease includes lymphoma, ileocecal amebiasis, sarcoidosis, deep chronic mycotic infections involving the gastrointestinal tract, gastrointestinal tuberculosis, Kaposi's sarcoma, *Campylobacter* enteritis, and *Yersinia* ileocolitis. Fortunately, most of these are uncommon conditions and can be differentiated by appropriate laboratory tests. *Yersinia* ileocolitis and *Campylobacter* enteritis may cause chronic abdominal pain and diarrhea similar to Crohn's disease, but can be diagnosed by appropriate stool cultures. It is not uncommon that a bout of acute bacterial diarrhea may uncover a diagnosis of inflammatory bowel disease.[41] Acute ileitis should not be confused with Crohn's disease. Young patients with acute ileitis usually recover without sequelae and should not undergo surgery. When Crohn's disease is confined to the colon, ischemic bowel disease (particularly in the elderly) and pseudomembranous colitis as well as ulcerative colitis must be included in the differential diagnosis.

TREATMENT

The aim of therapy for this incurable disease includes relief of symptoms, induction of remission, maintenance of remission, prevention of complications, optimizing timing of surgery, and maintenance of nutrition.[42,43]

TABLE 73-4 Common Extraintestinal Manifestations of Inflammatory Bowel Disease

Manifestation	Description
Arthritic	
Peripheral arthritis	Migratory monoarticular or polyarticular pain in peripheral joints (hip, knee, ankle, wrist) with effusion
Ankylosing spondylitis	Pain and stiffness of spine, hips, neck, and rib cage with limitation in truncal motion, loss of lumbar lordosis; decreased chest expansion and forward cervical flexion in advanced disease
Sacroiliitis	Low back pain with morning stiffness, relieved by exercise; progressive joint sclerosis
Ocular	
Episcleritis	Eye burning or itching without visual changes or pain; scleral and conjunctival hyperemia
Uveitis	Acute blurring of vision, photophobia and pain; perilimbic scleral injection
Dermatologic	
Erythema nodosum	Painful, red, raised nodules on extensor surfaces of arms or legs
Pyoderma gangrenosum	Ulcerative lesions with a necrotic center and violaceous skin typically found in pretibial region or trunk
Hepatobiliary	
Cholelithiasis	Varies from asymptomatic stones to right upper quadrant pain, fever, vomiting
Fatty liver	Mild right upper quadrant pain; hepatomegaly
Pericholangitis	Mild elevation in serum alkaline phosphatase, asymptomatic
Chronic active hepatitis	Autoimmune elevation of liver aminotransferase enzymes, may progress to cirrhosis
Primary sclerosing cholangitis	Pruritus progressing to jaundice, fatigue, and lethargy; laboratory findings vary from mild elevations of alkaline phosphatase to cirrhosis, portal hypertension, and liver failure; male predominance
Cholangiocarcinoma	Extrahepatic biliary mass, evidence of biliary obstruction, jaundice, right upper quadrant pain, fever, malaise
Pancreatitis	Varies from painless elevation of serum amylase to clinically apparent central abdominal pain radiating to back; may be associated with drugs such as azathioprine, 6-mercaptopurine, sulfasalazine, mesalamine, olsalazine, metronidazole
Vascular	
Thromboembolic disease	Symptoms of deep venous thrombosis and pulmonary emboli; portal vein, mesenteric vein, and hepatic venous thrombosis reported
Other	
Malnutrition	Fatigue, malaise, muscular wasting, cachexia
Chronic anemia	Fatigue, malaise, pallor, dyspnea; may be microcytic (blood loss), macrocytic (B_{12} deficiency), or autoimmune hemolytic
Nephrolithiasis	Flank pain, nausea, vomiting, hematuria; stones result from increased dietary oxalate absorption (calcium oxalate stones) and dehydration (urate stones)

Initial treatment (**Table 73-5**) consists of adequate fluid resuscitation and restoration of electrolyte balance. Place a nasogastric tube for obstruction, peritonitis, or toxic megacolon. Administer broad-spectrum antibiotics for fulminant colitis or peritonitis. Patients with severe disease should receive IV steroids such as hydrocortisone 300 milligrams per day or an equivalent dose of methylprednisolone (48 milligrams per day) or prednisolone (60 milligrams per day).

Salicylates Sulfasalazine 3 to 5 grams per day is for mild to moderate Crohn's disease. Sulfapyridine is a byproduct of the colonic breakdown of sulfasalazine. Many of the toxic side effects of sulfasalazine (vomiting,

TABLE 73-5 Treatment of Fulminant Colitis

Restore fluid and electrolyte balance
Nothing by mouth
Nasogastric suction for
Obstruction
Adynamic ileus
Suspected toxic megacolon
Parenteral corticosteroids
Hydrocortisone 300 milligrams per day or methylprednisolone 48 milligrams per day or prednisolone 60 milligrams per day
Broad-spectrum antibiotics
Piperacillin-tazobactam 4.5 grams IV four times a day *OR*
Ampicillin 2 grams IV four times a day + metronidazole 500 milligrams IV three times a day + levofloxacin (Levaquin®) 750 milligrams IV once a day
Observe for complications
Obstruction
Perforation
Toxic megacolon
Life-threatening hemorrhage
Intra-abdominal abscess
Outpatient management (nontoxic patients)
Liquids only for first 48 h
Oral antibiotics
Ampicillin, trimethoprim-sulfamethoxazole, ciprofloxacin, cephalexin, or rifaximin
and
Metronidazole or clindamycin

anorexia, nausea, headache, diarrhea, epigastric distress, etc.) are attributable to sulfapyridine.

The active moiety in sulfasalazine is mesalamine. Many of the newer 5′-acetyl salicylic acid drugs feature a derivative of mesalamine without the sulfapyridine component. Pentasa®, Asacol®, Claversal®, Salofalk®, and Lialda® are mesalamine derivatives. Olsalazine (Dipentum®) and balsalazide (Colazide®) are 5-aminosalicylic molecules. The mesalamine formulations are most effective in patients with colonic disease and particularly in those with mild disease.

Corticosteroids Oral glucocorticoids such as prednisone (40 to 60 milligrams per day) have traditionally been reserved for more severely affected patients but are now used as induction therapy. An ileal-released form of budesonide (9 milligrams per day) may be beneficial in patients with ileal and right colon disease. Glucocorticoids are not preferred for maintaining remission because of their complications and concerns about effectiveness.

Immunosuppressives Immunosuppressive drugs such as 6-mercaptopurine, azathioprine, and thioguanine are useful in maintenance, as steroid-sparing agents, in healing fistulas, and in patients in whom there are serious contraindications to surgery.[44] Both agents have been associated with leukopenia, fever, hepatitis, and pancreatitis, necessitating the need for close follow-up, particularly during the initial phase of therapy. The response to immunosuppressives should not be expected before 3 to 6 months following the initiation of therapy. Parenteral methotrexate (15 to 25 milligrams per week) is considered third line and has been used following steroid and thiopurine metabolite failure.

Antibiotics Antibiotics are first-line agents for perianal disease and help induce remission. Ciprofloxacin (1.0 to 1.5 milligrams/kg per day) induces remission with rates (55%) similar to those in patients treated with mesalamine (4 grams per day).[45] Metronidazole (10 to 20 milligrams/kg per day) is also effective for perianal complications and fistulous disease. Combination therapies with antibiotics and biologic agents (see next section) have produced dramatic improvements in response.[46] Rifaximin is a broad-spectrum antibiotic that is not absorbed from the gastrointestinal tract. Rifaximin 800 milligrams twice daily for 12 weeks is effective for mild to moderate disease.[45] However, antibiotics raise concerns about precipitating *C. difficile* colitis infection.

Biologics Patients with medically resistant moderate to severe Crohn's disease may benefit from the antitumor necrosis factor antibody, infliximab (Remicade®) or adalimumab (Humira®).[45,47,48] All biologics increase the risk of infections, especially those caused by intracellular pathogens such as tuberculosis. Concern about the emergence of lymphomas and progressive multifocal leukoencephalopathy has limited the long-term use of these agents.

Maintenance therapy and the effectiveness of various therapeutic agents in Crohn's disease are variable. Glucocorticoids are not used for maintaining a remission because of the lack of sufficient evidence of their efficacy and the potential for long-term complications. A reduced dose of 5-aminosalicyclic acid derivatives is used for the maintenance of remission of colonic disease. The addition of sulfasalazine, azathioprine, and 6-mercaptopurine to prednisone does not improve the response rate and increases side effects. Infliximab or adalimumab and an immunosuppressive (azathioprine, 6-mercaptopurine, and methotrexate) can maintain remission.[45]

Antidiarrheal Agents Diarrhea can be controlled by loperamide (Imodium®) 4 to 16 milligrams per day, diphenoxylate (Lomotil®) 5 to 20 milligrams per day, and in some cases, cholestyramine (Questran®) 4 grams one to six times a day. The mechanism of action of cholestyramine is binding bile acids and eliminating their known cathartic action.

DISEASE COMPLICATIONS

More than three out of four patients with Crohn's disease will require surgery within the first 20 years of the onset of initial symptoms. **Abscess and fissure formation** is common. Abscesses can be characterized as intraperitoneal, visceral, retroperitoneal, interloop, or intramesenteric. Signs and symptoms are worsening abdominal pain and tenderness, fever, and possibly a palpable mass. Retroperitoneal abscesses may cause hip or back pain and difficulty ambulating.

Fistulas are the result of extension of the intestinal fissures seen in Crohn's disease into adjacent structures. The most common sites are between the ileum and the sigmoid colon, the cecum, another ileal segment, urinary bladder, vagina, or the skin. Suspect an internal fistula when there are changes in the patient's symptom complex, such as bowel movement frequency, amount of pain, or weight loss.

Obstruction is the result of both stricture formation due to the inflammatory process and of edema of the bowel wall. The distal small bowel is the most common site of obstruction. Symptoms include crampy abdominal pain, distention, nausea, and bloating.

Perianal complications include perianal or ischiorectal abscesses, fissures, fistulas, rectovaginal fistulas, and rectal prolapse. These are more commonly seen in patients with colonic involvement.

Major gastrointestinal bleeding is rare. Bleeding results from erosion into a vessel in the bowel wall. Toxic megacolon is also uncommon, but is associated with massive gastrointestinal bleeding in over half the cases.

When bowel symptoms are present, malnutrition, malabsorption, hypocalcemia, and vitamin deficiency can be severe. In addition to the complications of the disease itself are complications associated with the treatment of the disease with mesalamine, steroids, immunosuppressive agents, and antibiotics. These include leukopenia, thrombocytopenia, fever, infection, profuse diarrhea, pancreatitis, renal insufficiency, and liver failure.

The incidence of malignant neoplasm of the gastrointestinal tract is three times higher in patients with Crohn's disease than for the general population.

DISPOSITION

Patients with colitis, peritonitis, or complications such as obstruction, significant gastrointestinal hemorrhage, severe dehydration, or fluid/electrolyte imbalance should be hospitalized. Hospital admission should be considered in less severe cases that cannot be managed successfully with outpatient management. Surgical intervention is indicated in those patients with complications of the disease, including intestinal obstruction or hemorrhage, perforation, abscess or fistula formation, toxic megacolon, and perianal disease.

Before discharging patients with Crohn's disease, discuss alterations in the therapeutic regimen with the gastroenterologist. Assure close follow-up after discharge.

ULCERATIVE COLITIS

INTRODUCTION AND EPIDEMIOLOGY

Ulcerative colitis is a chronic inflammatory disease of the colon. The inflammation tends to be progressively more severe from the proximal to the distal colon. The rectum is involved nearly 100% of the time. The characteristic symptom is bloody diarrhea. The cause is unknown.

The disease is more prevalent in the United States and northern Europe than in other parts of the world, and peak incidence occurs in the second and third decades of life. It is more common in men. First-degree relatives of patients with ulcerative colitis have a 15-fold risk of developing ulcerative colitis and a 3.5-fold risk of developing Crohn's disease.

PATHOPHYSIOLOGY

Ulcerative colitis involves primarily the mucosa and submucosa. Microscopically, the disease is characterized by mucosal inflammation with the formation of crypt abscesses, epithelial necrosis, and mucosal ulceration. The submucosa, muscular layer, and serosa are usually spared. In the usual case, the disease increases in severity more distally, the rectosigmoid being involved in the vast majority of cases. In the early stages of the disease, the mucous membranes appear finely granular and friable. In more severe cases, the mucosa appears as a red, spongy surface dotted with small ulcerations oozing blood and purulent exudate. In very advanced disease, one sees large, oozing ulcerations, and pseudopolyps (areas of hyperplastic overgrowth surrounded by inflamed mucosa).

CLINICAL FEATURES

The clinical features and course of ulcerative colitis vary and depend on the anatomical distribution of the disease in the colon. Crampy abdominal pain, bloody diarrhea, and tenesmus are typical symptoms. The disease is classified as mild, moderate, or severe depending on the clinical manifestations. Patients with mild disease have fewer than four bowel movements per day, no systemic symptoms, and few extraintestinal manifestations. Of all patients with ulcerative colitis, 60% have mild disease; in 80% of cases, the disease is limited to the rectum. Occasionally, constipation and rectal bleeding are the presenting complaints. Progression to pancolitis occurs in 10% to 15% of patients with mild disease.

Moderate disease is seen in 25% of patients. Patients demonstrate a good response to therapy. These patients usually have colitis extending to the splenic flexure (left-sided colitis), but may develop pancolitis.

Patients with severe disease constitute 15% of those with ulcerative colitis. Severe disease is associated with frequent bowel movements, anemia, fever, weight loss, tachycardia, low serum albumin, and more frequent extraintestinal manifestations. Patients with severe disease account for 90% of the mortality from ulcerative colitis. Virtually all severely affected patients have pancolitis.

Ulcerative colitis is usually characterized by intermittent attacks of acute disease with complete remission between attacks. Sometimes, the first attack is followed by a prolonged period of inactivity, or the disease is chronically active. The factors associated with an unfavorable prognosis and increased mortality include higher severity and extent of disease, a short interval between attacks, systemic symptoms, and onset of the disease after 60 years of age.

Extraintestinal complications are listed in **Table 73-4**.

DIAGNOSIS

Laboratory findings in patients with ulcerative colitis are nonspecific and may include leukocytosis, anemia, thrombocytosis, decreased serum albumin, and abnormal liver function studies. There are many biomarkers for diagnosis and prognosis,[40] but none are available in the ED. Therefore, the diagnosis of ulcerative colitis rests on the following: a history of abdominal cramps and diarrhea, mucoid stools, stool examination negative for ova and parasites, stool cultures negative for enteric pathogens, and confirmation of diagnosis by colonoscopy.

Differential Diagnosis The major diseases that should be considered in the differential diagnosis of ulcerative colitis include infectious colitis, Crohn's colitis, ischemic colitis, radiation colitis, toxic colitis from antineoplastic agents, and pseudomembranous colitis. When the disease is limited to the rectum, consider rectal syphilis, gonococcal proctitis, lymphogranuloma venereum, and inflammations caused by herpes simplex virus, *Entamoeba histolytica, Shigella,* and *Campylobacter.*

TREATMENT

Patients with severe ulcerative colitis should be treated with IV steroids, replacement of fluids, correction of electrolyte abnormalities, broad-spectrum antibiotics, mesalamine, and steroids (**Table 73-5**). IV cyclosporine (4 milligrams/kg per day) or infliximab can be effective in fulminant colitis nonresponsive to IV corticosteroids.[45]

When toxic megacolon is suspected, place a nasogastric tube and obtain imaging and surgical consultation.

The majority of those with mild and moderate disease can be treated as outpatients. In the treatment of patients with mild active proctitis, proctosigmoiditis, and left-sided colitis (<60 cm of active disease), topical treatment with mesalamine suppositories or enemas is effective. Although not as effective for inducing remission as mesalamine, topical steroid preparations (beclomethasone, hydrocortisone, tixocortol, and budesonide) are successful and better tolerated.[45] If topical therapy is unsuccessful, glucocorticoids are effective in inducing a remission in the majority of cases. Daily doses of 40 to 60 milligrams of prednisone are usually sufficient and can be adjusted depending on the severity of the disease.

A combination of oral (2.4 grams/day) and topical mesalamine is used in the treatment of acute mild to moderate attacks but is inferior to steroids in the more severe cases. In addition to sulfasalazine, the newer 5-aminosalicylic derivatives are quite effective in inducing remission of ulcerative colitis as well as maintaining it. The choice of agents available for the treatment of ulcerative colitis is very similar to that in Crohn's disease (mesalamine [Pentasa®, Asacol®, Lialda®], olsalazine [Dipentum®], and balsalazide). Topical glucocorticoid enemas or 5-aminosalicylic enemas (Rowasa®, 2 to 4 grams/60 mL per day for 3 weeks) or suppositories (500 milligrams twice a day) are quite effective in distal proctosigmoiditis and have lower systemic side-effect profiles.

Infliximab (5 milligrams/kg) is the only biologic indicated for ulcerative colitis. It should be considered for use in patients with mild to moderate disease who are corticosteroid dependent or refractory and in patients who have immunomodulator refractory disease.[47]

Hydrophilic bulk agents such as psyllium (Metamucil®) can be used in some patients to improve stool consistency. Antidiarrheal agents are generally ineffective and may precipitate toxic megacolon.

DISEASE COMPLICATIONS

Blood loss from sustained hemorrhage is the most common complication, but toxic megacolon must not be missed.

Toxic megacolon develops in advanced cases of colitis when the disease process extends through all layers of the colon (**Figure 73-1**).The result is a loss of muscular tone within the colon, with dilatation and localized peritonitis. If the colon continues to dilate without treatment, signs of toxicity will develop. Plain radiography of the abdomen demonstrates a long, continuous segment of air-filled colon greater than 6 cm in diameter. Loss of colonic haustra and "thumb printing," representing bowel wall edema, may also be seen. The distended portion of the atonic colon can perforate, causing peritonitis and septicemia. Mortality is high.

A patient with toxic megacolon appears severely ill; the abdomen is distended, tender, and tympanic. Severe diarrhea (>10 bowel movements per day) is often seen but may have ceased. Fever, tachycardia, and hypotension are typically part of the clinical picture. Leukocytosis, anemia, electrolyte disturbances, and hypoalbuminemia are the supporting laboratory results.

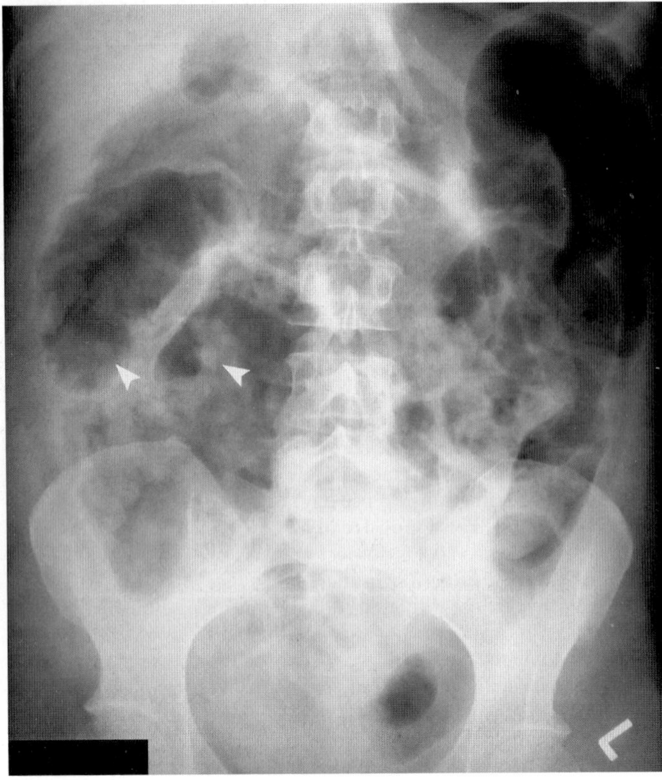

FIGURE 73-1. Abdominal distention due to toxic megacolon. Arrows point to mucosal nodules. [Reproduced with permission from Schwartz DT (Ed): *Emergency Radiology: Case Studies*. © McGraw-Hill, Inc., 2008. Chapter II-2, Fig. 23.]

Some of the more prominent features of toxic megacolon, such as leukocytosis and peritonitis, can be masked in the patient taking corticosteroids. Antidiarrheal agents, hypokalemia, narcotics, cathartics, pregnancy, enemas, and recent colonoscopy have been implicated as precipitating factors in toxic megacolon. Medical therapy with nasogastric suction, IV prednisolone 60 milligrams per day, or hydrocortisone 300 milligrams per day, parenteral broad-spectrum antibiotics active against coliforms and anaerobes, and IV fluids should be attempted as initial therapy, along with early surgical consultation.

Perirectal fistulas and abscesses may occur in up to 20% of patients with ulcerative colitis. Massive gastrointestinal hemorrhage, obstruction secondary to stricture formation, and acute perforation are other complications of the disease.

There is a 10- to 30-fold increase in the development of carcinoma of the colon in patients with ulcerative colitis. The major risk factors for the development of carcinoma of the colon are extensive involvement and prolonged duration of the disease. The cumulative risk of cancer after 20 and 30 years is 5% to 10% and 12% to 20%, respectively. Additional factors that constitute increased risk of cancer in patients with ulcerative colitis include early onset of the disease and a family history of colon cancer.

DISPOSITION

Patients with fulminant attacks of ulcerative colitis need hospitalization for aggressive fluid and electrolyte resuscitation and careful observation for the development of complications. Patients with complications such as gastrointestinal hemorrhage, toxic megacolon, and bowel perforation should also be admitted with consultation to both a gastroenterologist and a surgeon. In addition to toxic megacolon, the indications for surgery include colonic perforation, massive lower gastrointestinal bleeding, suspicion of colon cancer, and disease that is refractory to medical therapy (large doses of steroids required to control the disease).

Patients with mild to moderate disease can be discharged from the ED. Close follow-up should be arranged with the patient's physician or gastroenterologist, and any adjustment in medical therapy should be discussed prior to discharge.

Acknowledgments: The authors gratefully acknowledge the contributions of Hagop S. Mekhjian, Douglas A. Rund, Annie T. Sadosty, and Jennifer J. Hess, the authors of this topic in the prior edition.

REFERENCES

The complete reference list is available online at www.TintinalliEM.com.

CHAPTER 74 Constipation

Vito Rocco
Arash Armin

INTRODUCTION AND EPIDEMIOLOGY

Constipation is an extraordinarily common cause of patient morbidity in the United States.[1-4] The incidence of constipation increases with age, with 30% to 40% of persons >65 years old citing constipation as a problem.[4,5] Constipation affects as many as 80% of critically ill patients and is directly associated with patient mortality in this population.[6]

Physicians and patients define constipation differently. Physicians have traditionally defined constipation as fewer than three bowel movements per week. In contrast, patients commonly define constipation in terms such as abdominal discomfort, bloating, straining during bowel movements, or the sensation of incomplete evacuation. Consequently, constipation should not be defined simply by stool frequency alone, because doing so maximizes the potential to underdiagnose a significant number of patients who suffer from the condition.[7] The Rome criteria for the definition of constipation consist of two or more of the following signs or symptoms: (1) straining at defecation at least 25% of the time, (2) hard stools at least 25% of the time, (3) incomplete evacuation at least 25% of the time, (4) fewer than three bowel movements per week, (5) symptoms for at least 12 weeks (consecutive or nonconsecutive) in the preceding 12 months for chronic constipation.[8]

PATHOPHYSIOLOGY

Constipation is a complicated condition with multiple, often overlapping causes (**Table 74-1**). Gut motility is affected by diet, activity level, anatomic lesions, neurologic conditions, medications, toxins, hormone levels, rheumatologic conditions, microorganisms, and psychiatric conditions. Constipation is best thought of as either acute or chronic, as doing so helps formulate a differential diagnosis. Due to the rapidity of symptom onset, acute constipation is intestinal obstruction until proven otherwise. Common causes of intestinal obstruction include quickly growing tumors, strictures, hernias, adhesions, inflammatory conditions, and volvulus. Other causes of acute constipation include the addition of a new medicine (e.g., narcotic analgesic, antipsychotic, anticholinergic, antacid, antihistamine), change in exercise or diet (e.g., decreased level of exercise, fiber intake, or fluid intake), and painful rectal conditions (e.g., anal fissure, hemorrhoids, anorectal abscesses, proctitis). Chronic constipation can be caused by many of the same conditions that cause acute constipation. However, some specific causes of chronic constipation include neurologic conditions (e.g., neuropathies, Parkinson's disease, cerebral palsy, paraplegia), endocrine abnormalities (e.g., hypothyroidism, hyperparathyroidism, diabetes), electrolyte abnormalities (e.g., hypomagnesia, hypercalcemia, hypokalemia), rheumatologic conditions (e.g., amyloidosis, scleroderma), and toxicologic causes (e.g., iron, lead).

TABLE 74-1 Differential Diagnosis of Constipation
Acute causes
Gastrointestinal: quickly growing tumors, strictures, hernias, adhesions, inflammatory conditions, and volvulus
Medicinal: narcotic analgesic, antipsychotic, anticholinergic, antacid, antihistamine
Exercise and nutrition: decrease in level of exercise, fiber intake, fluid intake
Painful anal pathology: anal fissure, hemorrhoids, anorectal abscesses, proctitis
Chronic causes
Gastrointestinal: slowly growing tumor, colonic dysmotility, chronic anal pathology
Medicinal: chronic laxative abuse, narcotic analgesic, antipsychotic, anticholinergic, antacid, antihistamine
Neurologic: neuropathies, Parkinson's disease, cerebral palsy, paraplegia
Endocrine: hypothyroidism, hyperparathyroidism, diabetes
Electrolyte abnormalities: hypomagnesia, hypercalcemia, hypokalemia
Rheumatologic: amyloidosis, scleroderma
Toxicologic: lead, iron

CLINICAL FEATURES

HISTORY

The differential diagnosis of constipation is broad, so obtain a thorough history. Determine when the symptoms started and then determine whether there are any temporally related clues that can help narrow the differential diagnosis. Was a new medication or dietary supplement added at that time? Was there a decrease in fiber or fluid intake? Was there a change in activity level? Past medical and family history can help shed light on the cause of the constipation. Is there a history of hypothyroidism or diabetes? Does the patient have frequent kidney stones, which would point toward hyperparathyroidism? Although most patients who present with constipation do not have emergent conditions and may be treated symptomatically as outpatients, there are several historical elements that hint to a more ominous cause of symptoms, such as intestinal obstruction. Worrisome findings in addition to constipation include rapid onset, nausea or vomiting, inability to pass flatus, severe abdominal pain and distention, unexplained weight loss, rectal bleeding, unexplained iron-deficiency anemia, or a family history of colon cancer.[2] Any of these findings should prompt a more rigorous evaluation. Diarrhea alone does not rule out constipation/obstruction, as liquid stool can be passing past an obstructive source.

PHYSICAL EXAMINATION

In addition to a focused abdominal and pelvic examination, a rectal examination is essential. Examine the patient thoroughly for the presence of hernias and abdominal or pelvic masses. Bowel sounds will be decreased in cases of slow gut transit and increased in cases of obstruction. Ascites in the presence of constipation can be a sign of ovarian or uterine neoplasm in postmenopausal women. External rectal examination may demonstrate anal fissures, hemorrhoids, abscesses, or protruding masses. Digital rectal examination is useful in that it may demonstrate fecal impaction or an obstructing rectal mass. Especially common in the elderly is watery stool making its way around an overt impaction. Normal rectal tone is useful in ruling out neurologic causes of obstruction. Any stool retrieved from the rectal vault should be visually inspected and tested for occult blood. The finding of grossly bloody or guaiac-positive stool in the setting of constipation suggests concern for cancer, bowel ischemia, stercoral ulcer, or inflammatory bowel disease.

LABORATORY EVALUATION AND IMAGING

The evaluation of a constipated patient depends on the level of concern for an organic cause of constipation. If the patient is chronically

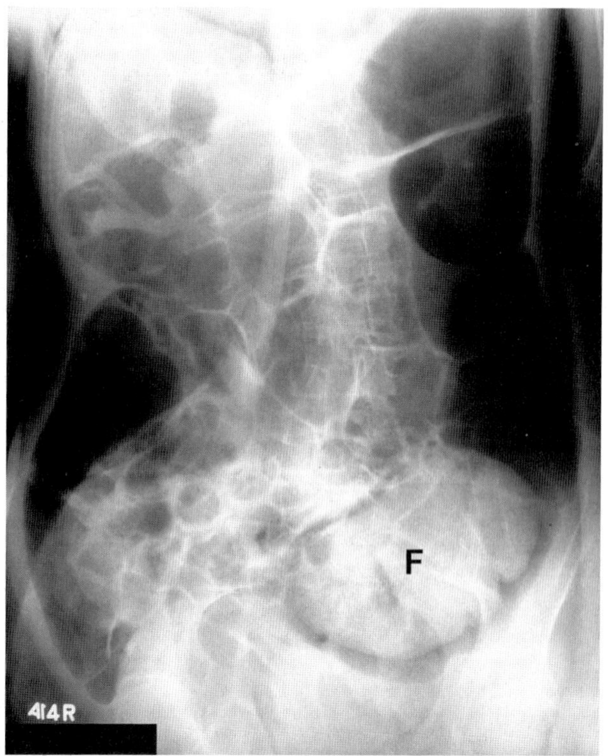

FIGURE 74-1. Large bowel obstruction due to fecal impaction (F). [Reused with permission from Schwartz DT (Ed): *Emergency Radiology: Case Studies*. © McGraw-Hill, Inc., 2008. Chapter II-2, Fig. 19.]

constipated, little is usually gained from any testing so long as the history and physical examination do not point toward an organic cause. If the patient has a history concerning for intestinal obstruction (e.g., acute onset of symptoms, vomiting, significant abdominal distention or pain), an upright chest film and abdominal flat and erect films are useful. In cases of complete or partial intestinal obstruction, these films may demonstrate air-fluid levels or dilated bowel. If there continues to be high clinical suspicion for intestinal obstruction despite a normal chest and abdominal series of radiographs, then abdominal CT with PO and IV contrast may be necessary to make the diagnosis. In cases of suspected fecal impaction, an abdominal film should be obtained (**Figure 74-1**). In a constipated patient, such a film will demonstrate colonic or rectal dilation with or without air-fluid levels. Normal maximum diameter of the colon is 6 cm, whereas normal maximum diameter of the rectum is 4 cm.[2] In all patients in whom an organic cause of constipation is suspected, laboratory evaluation should include a CBC and electrolytes. CBC is useful to screen for anemia, and electrolytes are useful to identify hypomagnesia, hypercalcemia, and hypokalemia. Obtain thyroid function tests for suspected hypothyroidism. Obtain serum lead and iron levels for suspected heavy metal toxicity.

SPECIAL CONSIDERATIONS

FUNCTIONAL CONSTIPATION

The treatment of chronic (functional) constipation requires a multidisciplinary approach. There is no quick medication fix to alleviate the problem. The most important thing a physician can do for the ED patient is to stress lifestyle and diet modification. A strict dietary and exercise regimen is important, because without adequate fluid (1.5 L per day), fiber (10 grams per day), and exercise, medicinal methods usually fail.[4] Both fiber and laxatives modestly improve bowel movement frequency in adults with chronic constipation. There is inadequate evidence to determine whether fiber is superior to laxatives or one laxative class is superior to another.[9]

TABLE 74-2 Medical Adjuncts for the Treatment of Constipation

Type	Generic Name	Trade Name	PRN Doses	Side Effects	Mechanism
Fiber	Bran	NA	1 cup daily	Bloating, flatulence	Increases stool bulk or transit time; increases gut motility
	Psyllium	Metamucil®	1 teaspoon three times a day	Bloating, flatulence	
Emollient	Docusate sodium	Colace®	100 milligrams daily/twice a day	Cramping	Facilitates mixture of stool fat and water
Stimulants	Bisacodyl	Dulcolax®	10 milligrams PR three times a day	Incontinence, rectal burning	Stimulates the myenteric plexus, thereby increasing intestinal motility
	Anthraquinones	Peri-Colace®	One to two tablets PO daily/twice a day	Melanosis coli, degeneration of myenteric plexus	
	Senna	Senokot®, Ex-lax®	Two tablets PO daily/twice a day or 15–30 mL daily/twice a day	Laxative abuse, nausea, melanosis coli, cramping	
Saline laxative	Magnesium	Milk of magnesia	15–30 mL daily/twice a day	Magnesium toxicity, especially in renal insufficiency	Decreased colonic transit time
		Magnesium citrate	100–240 mL daily/twice a day	Cramping, flatulence, hypermagnesemia	
Suppository	Glycerin suppository	NA	1 PR daily	Rectal irritation	Local rectal stimulation
Hyperosmolar agents	Lactulose	NA	15–30 mL daily/twice a day	Cramps, flatulence, belching, nausea	Osmotically active nonabsorbable sugars pull fluid into the gut
	Sorbitol	NA	15–30 mL daily/twice a day	Cramps, flatulence	
	Polyethylene glycol	GoLYTELY®	1 gallon/4 h	Nausea, cramping, anal irritation	
		MiraLAX®	17 grams daily, onset of effect 1-3 days		
Enemas	Mineral oil	NA	100–250 mL PR	Local trauma	Colonic distention encourages evacuation
	Tap water	NA	500 mL PR	Local trauma	
	Soap suds	NA	1500 mL PR	Local trauma	
	Monophosphate	Fleets®	1 unit PR	Local trauma, hyperphosphatemia (especially in patients with renal failure)	

Abbreviations: NA = not applicable; PRN = as needed.

Medications often employed in the treatment of constipation are listed in **Table 74-2**. Of note, insufficient evidence exists supporting that laxative treatment is better than placebo in children with constipation or probiotics as a natural alternative. No current recommendations support one laxative over another for childhood constipation.[10] Also, there is no "best" management of constipation in palliative care and no evidence to support the use of one laxative, or combinations of laxatives, over another.[11] There has been some promise recently with the subcutaneous use of methylnaltrexone in multiple studies.[12-14] The effectiveness of rectal irrigation for functional bowel disorders is not clear.[15] In its extreme form, functional constipation can result in a variety of potentially life-threatening complications, especially fecal impaction and intestinal pseudo-obstruction (Ogilvie's syndrome[13]).

OPIOID-INDUCED BOWEL DYSFUNCTION

Opioid-induced bowel dysfunction is a frequent condition in patients receiving opioids for chronic pain or even acute postoperative pain.[16] Nearly half of patients taking opioid therapy for pain of noncancerous origin report constipation related to opioid therapy (<3 complete bowel movements per week), compared with 7.6% in a control group.[17]

FECAL IMPACTION

Physician resistance to manual disimpaction does the patient a disservice, as enemas provide little or no relief. Diarrhea does not rule out fecal impaction, especially in the elderly, debilitated patient, and failure to perform a rectal examination will result in misdiagnosis. Manual disimpaction is a painful procedure for which patients may require sedation. After disimpaction, prescribe a regimen of medications and medical adjuncts to properly reestablish fecal flow.

INTESTINAL PSEUDO-OBSTRUCTION (OGILVIE'S SYNDROME)

Ogilvie's syndrome, or acute colonic pseudo-obstruction, is a clinical disorder with the signs, symptoms, and radiographic appearance of an acute large bowel obstruction with no evidence of distal colonic obstruction. The colon may become massively dilated >10 cm. If the bowel is not decompressed, the patient risks perforation, peritonitis, and death.[18,19] The exact mechanism is not known but is thought to be secondary to a dysregulation of colonic motor activity by the autonomic nervous system. Predisposing factors include recent surgery, underlying neurologic disorders, and critical illness.[20] Treatment is varied and determined with surgical consultation. The symptoms may resolve with conservative management but may require operative or colonoscopic decompression of the dilated intestine.

ORGANIC CONSTIPATION

Symptoms suggestive of organic constipation are acute onset, weight loss, rectal bleeding/melena, nausea/vomiting, fever, rectal pain, and change in stool caliber.[21] Intestinal obstruction or carcinoma is the primary consideration. If fecal impaction is the cause, manual disimpaction is the treatment.

DISPOSITION AND FOLLOW-UP

Many constipated patients can be safely discharged from the ED with the caveat that certain key aspects have been adequately addressed[22] (**Table 74-3**). Fecal impaction requires disimpaction before discharge. Patients with organic constipation of a nonobstructive cause also can be managed safely as outpatients. The primary care provider should be

TABLE 74-3 Key Aspects to Address Before Discharging a Constipated Patient
Possible obstructing lesion
Systemic illness
Medication interaction/effect
Electrolyte imbalance
Potential for intestinal perforation with self-administered enemas

contacted to ensure follow-up and to communicate concern for an organic process.

Referral to a gastroenterologist is warranted for patients with nonorganic constipation of recent onset; chronic constipation associated with weight loss, anemia, or change in stool caliber; refractory constipation; and constipation requiring chronic laxative use.[23] Patients with organic constipation of obstructive origin require hospitalization and surgical evaluation.

Acknowledgments: The authors would like to thank Annie T. Sadosty and Jennifer J. Hess, who were coauthors of the chapter in the previous edition.

REFERENCES

The complete reference list is available online at www.TintinalliEM.com.

Upper Gastrointestinal Bleeding

Christopher M. Ziebell
Andy Kitlowski
Janna M. Welch
Phillip A. Friesen

INTRODUCTION AND EPIDEMIOLOGY

Upper GI (UGI) bleeding is any GI bleeding originating proximal to the ligament of Treitz. The overall annual incidence of UGI bleeding ranges from 39 to 172 per 100,000 in Western countries.[1-3] Difference in prevalence between countries is attributed to variations in *Helicobacter pylori* rates, socioeconomic conditions, and prescription patterns of ulcer-healing and ulcer-promoting medications.[2] Increasing age, coexistent organ system disease, and recurrent hemorrhage are factors associated with increased morbidity and mortality.[3]

PATHOPHYSIOLOGY

PEPTIC ULCER DISEASE

Despite a downward trend in prevalence over the past 20 years, peptic ulcer disease, which includes gastric, duodenal, esophageal, and stomal ulcers, is still considered the most common cause of UGI bleeding.[2,4] However, the Analysis of Clinical Outcomes Research Initiative found gastric and duodenal ulcers in only 20.6% of 7822 endoscopies performed for suspected UGI bleeding.[4] This number is much lower than previous estimates of up to 50%.[5,6] Awareness that aspirin, nonsteroidal anti-inflammatory drugs (NSAIDs), and smoking cause bleeding and increased recognition and treatment of *H. pylori* infection may be responsible for decreased incidence.[7-10]

EROSIVE GASTRITIS AND ESOPHAGITIS

Erosive gastritis, esophagitis, and duodenitis are also common causes of GI hemorrhage.[11] Common predisposing factors include alcohol, salicylates, and NSAIDs. Infection, toxic ingestion, radiation, and stress from severe illness may also cause erosive gastritis. Stress-related mucosal disease occurs in patients with overwhelming sepsis, trauma, or respiratory failure requiring mechanical ventilation. *Candida*, herpes simplex virus, cytomegalovirus, and human immunodeficiency virus are potential sources of esophageal bleeding from infection.

ESOPHAGEAL AND GASTRIC VARICES

Esophageal and gastric varices result from portal hypertension and, in the United States, are most often a result of alcoholic liver disease.[12] Although varices account for a small percentage of all cases of UGI hemorrhage, they can rebleed and carry a high mortality rate. However, many patients with end-stage cirrhosis never develop varices; many patients with documented varices never bleed; and many patients with a documented history of varices presenting with UGI bleeding will actually bleed from nonvariceal sites. Variceal bleeding is the cause of UGI bleeding in cirrhotics 59% of the time, followed by peptic ulcer disease in 16% of cases.[13] In-hospital mortality rates for any type of GI bleed in cirrhotics are essentially double those of noncirrhotic patients.[14]

MALLORY-WEISS SYNDROME

Mallory-Weiss syndrome is bleeding secondary to a longitudinal mucosal tear at the gastroesophageal junction. The classic history is repeated vomiting followed by bright red hematemesis. The syndrome can be associated with alcoholic binge drinking, diabetic ketoacidosis, or chemotherapy administration. The Valsalva maneuver, such as from coughing or seizures, is also a reported cause.

DIEULAFOY LESIONS

Dieulafoy lesions are arteries of the GI tract that protrude through the submucosa. They are most commonly found in the lesser curvature of the stomach but may be found anywhere in the GI tract; 80% to 95% are found within 6 cm of the gastroesophageal junction.[15] These lesions are characterized by intermittent massive GI bleeding, without the standard predisposing factors of liver disease or NSAID use. Dieulafoy lesions are difficult to diagnose endoscopically, and sometimes patients report multiple previous diagnostic maneuvers with negative results.

OTHER CAUSES

Arteriovenous malformation and malignancy are other causes of UGI hemorrhage. Significant bleeding from ear, nose, and throat sources can also masquerade as GI hemorrhage. An aortoenteric fistula secondary to a preexisting aortic graft is an unusual but important cause of bleeding to keep in mind. Classically, this presents as a self-limited "herald" bleed with hematemesis or hematochezia, which precedes massive hemorrhage and exsanguination.

DIAGNOSIS

HISTORY

Ask about hematemesis, coffee-ground emesis, or melena. Classically, hematemesis and coffee-ground emesis suggest a UGI source. The presence of melena and age <50 years old more likely indicate an upper GI bleed versus a lower GI bleed, even in patients without hematemesis.[16] Vomiting and retching, followed by hematemesis, suggest a Mallory-Weiss tear. Be sure to ask about prior episodes of GI bleeding and any interventions performed. A history of an aortic graft should suggest bleeding from an aortoenteric fistula. Review the patient's medication list carefully. Salicylates, glucocorticoids, NSAIDs, and anticoagulants all place the patient at high risk for GI bleed. Alcohol abuse is strongly associated with a number of causes of bleeding, including peptic ulcer disease, erosive gastritis, and esophageal varices. Ingestion of iron or bismuth can simulate melena. Liquid medications with red dye, as well as certain foods, such as beets, can simulate hematochezia. In such cases, stool guaiac testing will be negative. Inquire about past history of GI bleeding, even though recurrent bleeding episodes may originate from different sources.

Although the medical history may suggest the source of bleeding, history can also be misleading. For instance, what initially appears to be lower GI bleeding may actually be a UGI bleed in disguise. **Bright red or maroon rectal bleeding unexpectedly originates from UGI sources about 14% of the time.**[16] Although patients volunteer complaints of hematemesis or melena, if there is no vomiting or the patient has not noted tarry stools, signs may be subtle. Patients with hypotension, tachycardia, angina, syncope, weakness, confusion, or cardiac arrest may have underlying GI hemorrhage.

PHYSICAL EXAMINATION

Visual inspection of the vomitus for a bloody, maroon, or coffee-ground appearance is the most reliable way to diagnose UGI bleeding in the ED. Consider keeping a sample of the vomitus or nasogastric (NG) aspirate at bedside for the gastroenterologist to view.

Vital signs may reveal obvious hypotension and tachycardia or more subtle findings such as decreased pulse pressure or tachypnea. Younger patients and those without comorbidities can tolerate substantial volume loss with minimal or no changes in vital signs. Paradoxical bradycardia may occur even in the face of profound hypovolemia. Remember that comorbid conditions and medications may mask the body's physiologic response to volume loss. β-Blockers, for example, will prevent tachycardia. Patients with baseline hypertension may have relatively normal blood pressure in the setting of hypovolemia.

Cool, clammy skin is an obvious sign of shock. Spider angiomas, palmar erythema, jaundice, and gynecomastia suggest liver disease. Petechiae and purpura suggest an underlying coagulopathy. Facial lesions, cutaneous macules, or telangiectasias may be suggestive of the Peutz-Jeghers, Rendu-Osler-Weber, or Gardner's syndromes. A careful ear, nose, and throat examination can reveal an occult bleeding source that has resulted in swallowed blood and subsequent coffee-ground emesis. Abdominal examination may disclose tenderness, masses, ascites, or organomegaly.

Perform rectal examination to detect the presence of blood and its appearance, whether bright red, maroon, or melanotic.

LABORATORY TESTING

In patients with significant bleeding, the single most important laboratory test is to obtain blood for type and cross-match in case transfusion is needed. A CBC is also important, although the initial hematocrit level may not reflect the actual amount of acute blood loss. In addition, consider BUN, creatinine, electrolyte, glucose, coagulation, and liver function studies. UGI hemorrhage will elevate BUN levels through digestion and absorption of hemoglobin. A BUN:creatinine ratio ≥30 suggests a UGI source of bleeding.[17] Coagulation studies, including INR, partial thromboplastin time, and platelet count, are useful in patients taking anticoagulants and those with underlying hepatic disease. Obtain an ECG in patients with underlying coronary artery disease. Silent cardiac or mesenteric ischemia can develop if bleeding decreases cardiac or mesenteric perfusion. A single elevated lactate level is a sentinel sign of severe illness. The success or failure of resuscitation efforts can be assessed by following dynamic lactate levels, because a rising lactate level in the hospital setting is a clear predictor of in-hospital mortality.[18]

Routine abdominal and chest radiographs are of limited value and are not needed in the absence of specific clinical indications. Barium contrast studies are contraindicated because barium may hinder subsequent endoscopy or angiography.

In cases where traditional endoscopy is unavailable or endoscopic visualization is unable to find the source, consider tagged red-cell scintigraphy or visceral angiography. Both of these tests will demonstrate the source only in cases of active bleeding. Scintigraphy and angiography help localize the source of bleeding to determine whether medical or surgical management is optimal.

NASOGASTRIC LAVAGE

NG intubation and aspiration are diagnostic and therapeutic.[19] In patients without a history of hematemesis, a positive aspirate provides strong evidence for a UGI source of bleeding. High-risk lesions are more likely in patients with bloody aspirates. Visual inspection of the aspirate to identify bloody, maroon, or coffee-ground material verifies UGI bleeding. Early NG lavage is associated with decreased time to endoscopy.[20] NG tube placement and lavage can confirm the diagnosis of UGI bleeding and stratify risk.

TABLE 75-1 Upper GI Bleeding Risk

Very Low Risk	High Risk
<60 y old	Advanced age
No major comorbidities	Comorbidities and prior endoscopic or transjugular intrahepatic portosystemic shunt procedures
No history of red hematemesis	Red hematemesis
No hematochezia	Hematochezia or melena
Negative nasogastric (NG) aspirate	Positive NG aspirate
Hemodynamically stable at ED presentation	Hemodynamically unstable
Normal laboratory studies	Abnormal laboratory studies

A negative NG aspirate does not conclusively exclude a UGI source. Intermittent bleeding, pyloric spasm, or edema preventing reflux of duodenal blood can cause false-negative results. Ultimately, NG aspiration yields a positive result in only 23% of patients without hematemesis who have occult UGI bleeding.[21]

Guaiac testing of NG aspirate can yield both false-negative and false-positive results. Conventional stool guaiac cards may be falsely negative. However, guaiac cards specifically designed for UGI sources are available. Conversely, even minimally traumatic NG intubation can result in positive guaiac testing even in the face of a clear aspirate. **Visual inspection of the aspirate for a bloody, maroon, or coffee-ground appearance is the most reliable way to diagnose UGI bleeding in the ED.**

If bright red blood or clots are found in the NG aspirate, perform gentle gastric lavage. Room temperature water is the preferred irrigant. Maintain the NG tube on mild, intermittent suction. Suction that is too vigorous may produce gastric erosions that can confuse findings on subsequent endoscopy.

As of this writing, there is no evidence to support concerns that NG tube passage may provoke bleeding in patients with varices.

RISK STRATIFICATION

Risk stratification depends on clinical judgment. There are no universally accepted pre-endoscopy risk stratification practice guidelines. However, the literature does seem to agree on those individuals that qualify as very low risk (**Table 75-1**). Pre-endoscopic predictors of higher risk include advanced age, comorbidities, red hematemesis, hematochezia, red blood on NG aspirate, hemodynamic instability, and abnormal laboratory studies.[22-26] Other high-risk factors include prior variceal banding, clamping or cauterization of an ulcer bed, or the transjugular intrahepatic portosystemic shunt procedure.

TREATMENT

Initial management is stabilization. Patients in hemorrhagic shock require emergent resuscitation, including two large-bore IVs, typed and cross-matched blood with the consideration of massive transfusion protocols, and in selected cases, early airway management. Intubating a patient with a UGI bleed who is hemodynamically unstable can be a perilous procedure. Aggressively resuscitate prior to intubation, and consider using smaller doses of the induction agent to minimize peri-intubation hypotension or arrest.[27] ED treatment is summarized in **Table 75-2.**

BLOOD TRANSFUSIONS

When UGI bleeding is severe, blood transfusions can be lifesaving. If a large amount of blood product is anticipated, use massive transfusion protocols.[28] See chapter 13, "Fluid and Blood Resuscitation in Traumatic Shock" for discussion of massive transfusion. In less severe

TABLE 75-2 Treatment of Upper GI Bleed

Treatment	Dose	Comments
Blood transfusion		Transfuse if ≤7 grams/dL in most; ≤9 grams/dL in older patients or patients with comorbidities
Correct coagulopathy		Correct if INR is elevated or platelets <50,000; or if bleeding severe, correct coagulopathy unless contraindications to correction (e.g., stents)
Omeprazole	80-milligram IV bolus then infusion of 8 milligrams/h	Labeled use for ulcer bleeding
Octreotide	50-microgram bolus then infusion of 25–50 micrograms/h	Unlabeled use for varices; for elderly, begin at lower dose range of 25-microgram bolus and infusion of 25 micrograms/h
Antibiotics	Ciprofloxacin 400 milligrams IV or ceftriaxone 1 gram IV	Antibiotics for cirrhotics with UGI bleeding

cases, the decision to transfuse can be difficult because hemoglobin concentrations do not fall until after hemodilution has occurred. Individualize thresholds for transfusion based on underlying comorbidities and hemodynamic status.[29] Liberally transfusing all bleeding patients using a high threshold (hemoglobin <9 grams/dL) can cause harm.[5] A restrictive transfusion threshold using hemoglobin concentrations of <7 grams/dL in most patients and <9 grams/dL in older patients with comorbidities who are not tolerating the acute anemia is recommended.[5,29]

COAGULOPATHY

In patients with life-threatening bleeding receiving anticoagulants, reverse the coagulopathy without concern for the INR unless there are contraindications to reversal, such as cardiac or vascular stents. In less severe bleeding, carefully consider the risks of reversal therapy. An INR ≥1.5 is a significant predictor of mortality in patients with a UGI bleed who are receiving anticoagulants.[30] International consensus guidelines recommend reversal of coagulopathy for UGI bleed patients who have an elevated INR or platelet counts <50,000/μL.[29,31] Coagulopathies from other causes such as the newer oral antithrombin and Xa inhibitors should be managed according to institutional protocols. See Figure 239-1 and Table 239-4 in chapter titled "Thrombotics and Antithrombotics" for recommendations for anticoagulant reversal. Reversal should not delay time to endoscopy. Tranexamic acid, an antifibrinolytic agent, has shown no benefit in the management UGI bleeding.[32]

PROTON PUMP INHIBITORS

Consensus guidelines continue to recommend proton pump inhibitors for patients with nonvariceal bleeding from peptic ulcer disease.[23] When proton pump inhibitors are given at high dose, the gastric pH remains neutral. Clot formation from platelet aggregation is dependent on a pH >6.0.[33] Administer a high-dose proton pump inhibitor such as omeprazole 80 milligrams IV bolus followed by infusion of 8 milligrams/h[34] because the cause of bleeding cannot be determined without endoscopy. In patients with peptic ulcer bleeding, proton pump inhibitors reduce the need for surgery, the length of stay in the hospital, and signs of bleeding.[35]

SOMATOSTATIN ANALOGS/OCTREOTIDE

Octreotide is a long-acting analog of somatostatin that elicits several actions in patients with UGI bleeding. It inhibits the secretion of gastric acid, reduces blood flow to the gastroduodenal mucosa, and causes splanchnic vasoconstriction.[36] The dose is a 50-microgram bolus followed by a continuous infusion of 25 to 50 micrograms/h. Despite its widespread use in the United States, octreotide does not appear to provide a clear benefit on mortality.[37] In contrast, terlipressin is preferred in countries where it is available because it is the only drug treatment associated with a reduction in mortality.[38]

ANTIBIOTICS

Patients with cirrhosis have an impaired immune system and have an increased risk of gut bacterial translocation during an acute bleeding episode. Prophylactic antibiotics (e.g., ciprofloxacin 400 milligrams IV or ceftriaxone 1 gram IV) reduce infectious complications, may decrease mortality,[39] and should be started as soon as possible.

PROMOTILITY AGENTS

Erythromycin and metoclopramide are examples of promotility agents used to enhance endoscopic visualization.[40] However, they are not recommended for routine use, but may be considered if the patient is undergoing endoscopy in the ED and the patient is suspected to have large amounts of blood in the UGI tract.[29]

ENDOSCOPY

UGI endoscopy is the diagnostic study of choice. Endoscopy allows visualization of the source of bleeding (in most cases) and administration of hemostatic therapy.[41] The optimal timing relates to the severity of the bleeding. Early endoscopy (within 24 hours of presentation) is recommended for most patients because it is associated with a significant cost reduction and decreased length of stay.[19,20,41-43] An unstable patient may benefit from emergent endoscopy immediately following resuscitation.

Endoscopic treatment options commonly used for variceal bleeding include variceal ligation and sclerotherapy. Clips, thermocoagulation, and sclerosant injections alone or in combination with epinephrine injections are commonly used in ulcerative lesions.

In some practices, the ED physician is asked to provide sedation for the endoscopist. Pretreat with an antiemetic such as ondansetron. Use short-acting titratable drugs with both analgesic properties (fentanyl) and sedative properties (versed or propofol). Ideal agents can be reversed if the patient's condition changes.[44-46] In unstable patients, one must consider using cardiovascular stable agents such as etomidate or ketamine. While providing sedation, consider that the most noxious part of the procedure is when the scope is passed around the tongue.

BALLOON TAMPONADE

Balloon tamponade is an effective short-term solution for life-threatening variceal bleeding. Because of the high rate of complications, it should be reserved for temporary stabilization of patients for transfer to an appropriate institution or until endoscopy can be done. The **Sengstaken-Blakemore tube** (which has a 250-cc gastric balloon, an esophageal balloon, and a single gastric suction port) (**Figure 75-1**) and the **Minnesota tube** (with an added esophageal suction port above the esophageal balloon) are examples of balloons that have been used. Adverse reactions include mucosal ulceration, esophageal or gastric rupture, asphyxiation from tracheal compression, and aspiration. Strongly consider intubation prior to balloon tamponade.

The device can be inserted either nasally or orally. The gastric balloon is inflated first. It is critical to know that one is in the stomach before fully inflating the gastric balloon. If bleeding does not stop, inflate the esophageal balloon while using a manometer to ensure the pressure does not exceed 50 mm Hg. Confirm tube placement by x-ray. To secure the tube, apply 1 kg of traction by attaching the distal end of the tube to a 1-L bag of saline hung from an IV pole. Alternatively, the tube can be secured directly to a football helmet.

SURGERY

Patients who do not respond to both pharmacologic and endoscopic treatments may require emergent surgery. In patients with variceal bleeding, there are two basic types of operations: shunt operations (transjugular intrahepatic portosystemic shunt procedure) and nonshunt operations (esophageal transection or gastroesophageal junction devascularization). In nonvariceal bleeding, percutaneous embolization or subtotal or total gastrectomy can be performed. Emergent surgical consultation is considered prudent in case of uncontrolled bleeding.

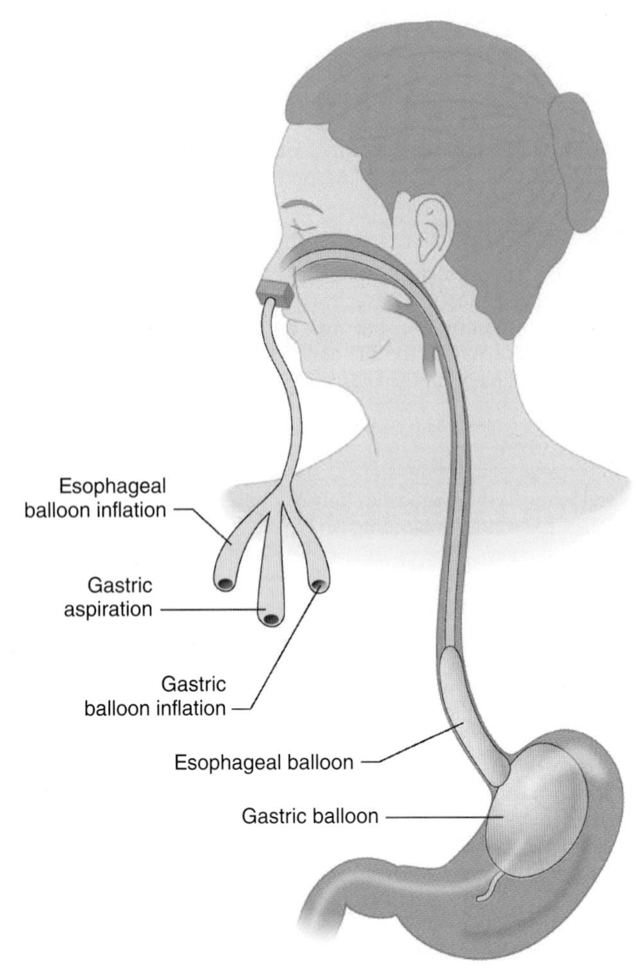

FIGURE 75-1. Sengstaken-Blakemore tube.

DISPOSITION AND FOLLOW-UP

Patients with significant UGI bleeding require intensive care unit admission and early endoscopy. Very-low-risk patients (Table 75-1) may be eligible for ED observation or be discharged home with adequate outpatient follow-up.

REFERENCES

The complete reference list is available online at www.TintinalliEM.com.

Lower Gastrointestinal Bleeding

Bruce M. Lo

INTRODUCTION AND EPIDEMIOLOGY

Lower GI (LGI) bleeding is the loss of blood from the GI tract distal to the ligament of Treitz. LGI bleeding is a common problem in emergency medicine and should be considered potentially life threatening until proven otherwise.

LGI bleeding occurs less often than upper GI (UGI) bleeding, with an annual incidence of approximately 36 per 100,000.[1] Because blood must travel through the UGI tract down to the LGI system, UGI bleeds are the most common source for all causes of blood detected in the LGI system. **Among patients with an established LGI source of bleeding (i.e., bleeding past the ligament of Treitz), the most common cause is diverticular disease, followed by colitis, adenomatous polyps, and malignancies.**[2,3] LGI bleeding is more common among females and increases significantly in the elderly.[1]

About 80% of episodes of LGI bleeding resolve spontaneously.[4] However, one cannot predict which episodes will spontaneously resolve or which episodes will result in complications. This is partly due to the difficulty in establishing a pathophysiologic diagnosis. In one study, a cause for bleeding was found in <50% of the cases.[5]

PATHOPHYSIOLOGY

Hematochezia is either bright red or maroon-colored rectal bleeding. If hematochezia originates from a UGI source, it indicates brisk UGI bleeding, which may be accompanied by hematemesis and hemodynamic instability. Approximately 10% of hematochezia episodes may be associated with UGI bleeding.[6] **Melena** is dark or black-colored stools and usually represents bleeding from a UGI source (proximal to the ligament of Treitz) but may also represent slow bleeding from an LGI source.

DIVERTICULOSIS

Diverticular bleeding is usually painless and results from erosion into the penetrating artery of the diverticulum. Diverticular bleeding may be massive, but up to 90% of episodes will resolve spontaneously. Bleeding can recur in up to half.[7,8] Although most diverticula are located on the left colon, right-sided diverticula are thought to be more likely to bleed.[9] Elderly patients with underlying medical illnesses, those with increased needs for transfusion, and those taking anticoagulants or nonsteroidal anti-inflammatory drugs have increased morbidity and mortality.[7]

VASCULAR ECTASIA

Vascular ectasia, which includes arteriovenous malformations and angiodysplasias of the colon, is a common cause of LGI bleeding. Vascular ectasia can also be present in the small bowel and is difficult to diagnose. The development of vascular ectasia in the large bowel seems to be due to a chronic process and increases with aging. Inherited conditions can also give rise to arteriovenous malformations. There is also a suggestion that valvular heart disease is a risk factor for developing bleeding vascular ectasias, although this is an area of debate.[4]

ISCHEMIC COLITIS AND MESENTERIC ISCHEMIA

Ischemic colitis is the most common cause of intestinal ischemia and is usually transient. The colon is predisposed to ischemia because of its poor vascular circulation and high bacterial content. Aneurysmal rupture, vasculitis, hypercoagulable states, prolonged strenuous exercise, cardiovascular insult, irritable bowel syndrome, and certain medications that cause vasoconstriction or slow bowel motility are known risk factors. Diagnosis is usually made by endoscopy. Although most cases will resolve on their own, up to 20% will require surgical intervention.[10]

Mesenteric ischemia can lead to bowel necrosis. Causes include thrombosis or embolism of the superior mesenteric artery, mesenteric venous thrombosis, and nonocclusive mesenteric ischemia associated with low arterial flow with vasoconstriction. Diagnosis is difficult, and the presentation can mimic other intra-abdominal pathologies. Diagnosis requires a high index of suspicion, especially in patients >60 years old and in those with atrial fibrillation, congestive heart failure, recent myocardial infarction, postprandial abdominal pain, or unexplained weight loss. CT has a specificity of 92% but only a sensitivity of 64%. Angiography remains the diagnostic study of choice. Despite aggressive treatment, prognosis is poor, with a survival of 50% if diagnosed within 24 hours.[11]

MECKEL'S DIVERTICULUM

Meckel's diverticulum consists of embryonic tissue, most commonly found in the terminal ileum. More than half of lesions contain ectopic

TABLE 76-1 Causes of Lower GI Bleeding

Upper GI bleed
Diverticulosis
GI carcinoma
Angiodysplasia
Arteriovenous malformations
Mesenteric ischemia
Ischemic colitis
Meckel's diverticulum
Hemorrhoids
Infectious colitis
Inflammatory bowel disease
Polyps
Radiation colitis
Rectal ulcers
Trauma
Foreign bodies
Carcinoma
Prostate biopsy sites
Endometriosis
Dieulafoy lesions
Colonic varices
Portal hypertensive enteropathy

gastric tissue, which can secrete gastric enzymes, eroding the mucosal wall and causing bleeding. It is a rare but important condition, especially in the younger population.

OTHER CAUSES OF LOWER GI BLEEDING

Numerous other lesions may result in LGI hemorrhage (**Table 76-1**), including infectious colitis, radiation colitis, rectal ulcers, trauma, and inflammatory bowel disease. Polyps and carcinomas can cause LGI bleeding and are usually a source of chronic anemia. Delayed hemorrhage can occur up to 3 weeks after polypectomy. Patients with left ventricular assist devices are prone to GI bleeding especially due to anticoagulation, risk of arteriovenous malformations, and acquired von Willebrand's disease.[12] Although hemorrhoids are the most common source of anorectal bleeding, massive hemorrhage is unusual.[10] For further discussion of hemorrhoids, see chapter 85, "Anorectal Disorders."

DIAGNOSIS

As with any emergency, the medical history, physical examination, and diagnostics often must be accomplished simultaneously with resuscitation and stabilization. **Factors associated with a high morbidity rate are hemodynamic instability, repeated hematochezia, gross blood on initial rectal examination, initial hematocrit <35%, syncope, nontender abdomen (predictive of severe bleeding), aspirin or nonsteroidal anti-inflammatory drug use (predictive of diverticular hemorrhage), and more than two comorbid conditions.**[2,3,13]

HISTORY

Although most patients will volunteer complaints of hematochezia or melena, signs and symptoms of hypotension, tachycardia, angina, syncope, weakness, or altered mental status can all occur as a result of LGI bleeding.

Ask about previous GI bleeding as well as a history of pain, trauma, ingestion or insertion of foreign bodies, and recent colonoscopies. Weight loss and changes in bowel habits may suggest malignancy. A history of an aortic graft may suggest the possibility of an aortoenteric fistula. Medications, such as salicylates, nonsteroidal anti-inflammatory drugs, and warfarin, increase the risk of LGI bleeding.[14-16] Ingestion of iron or bismuth can simulate melena, and certain foods, such as beets, can simulate hematochezia. However, stool guaiac testing in those cases will be negative.

PHYSICAL EXAMINATION

Hypotension and tachycardia, or decreased pulse pressure or tachypnea, develop with significant bleeding. However, changes in vital signs may be masked by concurrent medications, such as β-blockers, or medical conditions such as poorly controlled hypertension. Thus, relative tachycardia and hypotension may represent subtle clues to ongoing bleeding. Some patients can tolerate substantial volume losses with minimal or no changes in vital signs.

Cool, pale skin and an increase in capillary refill can be signs of shock. Physical findings of liver disease, as well as petechiae and purpura, suggest an underlying coagulopathy. The abdominal examination may disclose tenderness, masses, ascites, or organomegaly. In patients with LGI bleeding, a lack of abdominal tenderness suggests bleeding from disorders involving the vasculature, such as diverticulosis or angiodysplasia. Inflammatory bowel disorders with LGI bleeding are associated with abdominal tenderness on examination.

Thorough examination of the rectal area may reveal an obvious source of bleeding, such as a laceration, masses, trauma, anal fissures, or external hemorrhoids. A vaginal or urinary source of bleeding mistaken for a GI source will be identified by examination and testing. Perform a digital rectal examination to detect gross blood (either bright red or maroon) and for guaiac testing. Rectal examination can also detect the presence of masses.

Anoscopy can also be performed at the bedside. A source of bleeding such as hemorrhoids can sometimes be elucidated by anoscopy. However, blood originating beyond the level of visualization should raise the suspicion for other causes.[10]

LABORATORY TESTING

The most important laboratory tests are the CBC, coagulation studies, and typed and cross-matched blood. Coagulation studies, including prothrombin time, partial thromboplastin time, and platelet count, are of obvious benefit in patients taking anticoagulants or those with underlying hepatic disease. In addition, obtain blood urea nitrogen, creatinine, electrolytes, glucose, and liver function studies. In acute, brisk bleeding, the initial hematocrit level may not reflect the actual amount of blood loss. **Bleeding from a source higher in the GI tract may elevate blood urea nitrogen levels through digestion and absorption of hemoglobin.**

Obtain an ECG in patients with coronary artery disease. **Silent ischemia can occur secondary to the decreased oxygen delivery accompanying significant GI bleeding.**

IMAGING

Routine abdominal radiographs are of limited value without specific indications such as perforation, obstruction, or foreign bodies. Similarly, routine admission chest x-rays for patients with acute GI hemorrhage, even those admitted to the intensive care unit, are of limited utility in the absence of known pulmonary disease or abnormal findings on lung examination.[17] Barium contrast studies are not helpful and can interfere with subsequent emergent endoscopy or angiography.

The initial diagnostic procedure of choice—angiography, scintigraphy, or endoscopy—depends upon resource ability and consultant preference.[18-21] Angiography can sometimes detect the site of bleeding and help guide surgical management. Moreover, angiography permits therapeutic options such as transcatheter arterial embolization or the infusion of vasoconstrictive agents. However, **angiographic diagnosis and therapy require a relatively brisk bleeding rate (at least 0.5 mL/min). Serious complications can also occur with angiography in up to 10% of cases.**[10]

Technetium-labeled red cell scans can also localize the site of bleeding in obscure hemorrhage. Such localization can be used to help determine if angiography or surgery is the optimal approach. **Scintigraphy appears more sensitive than angiography and can localize the site of bleeding at as low a rate as 0.1 mL/min. It also has potential value over angiography if bleeding occurs intermittently but requires a minimum of 3 mL of blood to pool.**[22]

Multidetector CT angiography has a sensitivity and specificity of up to 100% and 99%, respectively, for detecting active or recent GI bleeding and is about 93% accurate in determining the site of bleeding.[23,24] It can be a useful tool prior to treatment with conventional angiography.

TREATMENT

Resuscitate unstable or actively bleeding patients. Administer oxygen and institute cardiac monitoring. Place two large-bore IV lines and replace volume with crystalloids. Correct coagulopathy. Blood transfusion should be based on the clinical findings of volume depletion or continued bleeding rather than on initial hematocrit values. In acute bleeding, hematocrit values may not represent true blood volume status, because it takes several hours for the hematocrit to decrease. **General guidelines for initiation of blood transfusion are continued active bleeding and failure to improve perfusion and vital signs after the infusion of 2 L of crystalloid.** The threshold for blood transfusion should be lower in the elderly.

Consider the placement of a nasogastric tube if LGI bleeding is significant. **Hematochezia unexpectedly originates from UGI sources approximately 10% to 14% of the time.**[6,25] Factors that suggest a UGI source for hematochezia include anemia and previous history of UGI bleeding.[6] Nasogastric aspiration has low sensitivity and negative predictive value for UGI bleeding.[26] In one study, 15% of patients with hematochezia had a negative nasogastric aspirate but had a UGI source of bleeding.[26] A nasogastric tube is likely beneficial only for those with significant ongoing UGI bleeding in whom immediate intervention will occur.[10,26]

Obtain early consultation for severe LGI bleeding to expedite the next steps of care. Surgical consultation along with consultation from the gastroenterologist is prudent for uncontrollable bleeding.

ENDOSCOPY AND SURGERY

Flexible sigmoidoscopy can evaluate possible distal colonic and rectal sources of bleeding but cannot identify more proximal sources of bleeding. Colonoscopy can diagnose various sources of LGI bleeding, such as diverticulosis or angiodysplasia, and may allow ablation of bleeding sites with various endoscopic hemostasis methods (injection sclerotherapy, electrocoagulation, heater probe therapy, banding, and clipping). If colonoscopy fails to determine the source of bleeding, the specialists may consider upper endoscopy to evaluate for a UGI source of bleeding, although upper endoscopy may be indicated first in certain situations.[27] Timing of endoscopy can vary. Some studies suggest that urgent colonoscopy is both safe and accurate within 12 to 24 hours of admission, but others report that delayed colonoscopy is appropriate in stable patients.[8-10,27]

Patients with continued bleeding and failure of endoscopic hemostasis may need emergency surgery. The reported proportion of patients requiring surgery varies from 5% to 25%.[10,18]

DISPOSITION AND FOLLOW-UP

Patients with LGI hemorrhage will often require hospital admission and early referral to an endoscopist. Those who are unstable or with active bleeding may require admission to the intensive care unit. Variables associated with morbidity include **hemodynamic instability, repeated hematochezia within 4 hours of evaluation, nontender abdomen, aspirin use, and more than two comorbid conditions.**[2,3] Although risk stratification scores have been developed for UGI bleeding for possible outpatient management, **no reliable scoring system exists to risk stratify which patients with LGI bleeding may be discharged home safely**. However, those with an obvious cause of mild bleeding (such as mild bleeding from hemorrhoids or anal fissures), or who have no bright red blood or maroon or melanotic stool on rectal examination and are hemodynamically stable and without major comorbidities, may be candidates for outpatient treatment.

REFERENCES

The complete reference list is available online at www.TintinalliEM.com.

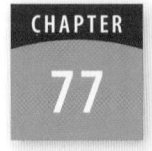

Esophageal Emergencies

Moss Mendelson

ESOPHAGEAL EMERGENCIES

The complaints of dysphagia, odynophagia, and ingested foreign body immediately implicate the esophagus. The esophagus also is often the site of pathology in patients who present with chest pain, upper GI bleeding (see chapter 75, "Upper Gastrointestinal Bleeding"), malignancy, and mediastinitis. Many diseases of the esophagus can be evaluated over time in an outpatient setting, but several, such as esophageal foreign body and esophageal perforation, require emergent intervention.

ANATOMY AND PATHOPHYSIOLOGY

The esophagus is a muscular tube approximately 20 to 25 cm long, primarily located in the mediastinum, posterior and slightly lateral to the trachea, with smaller cervical and abdominal components, as shown in **Figure 77-1**. There is an outer longitudinal muscle layer and an inner

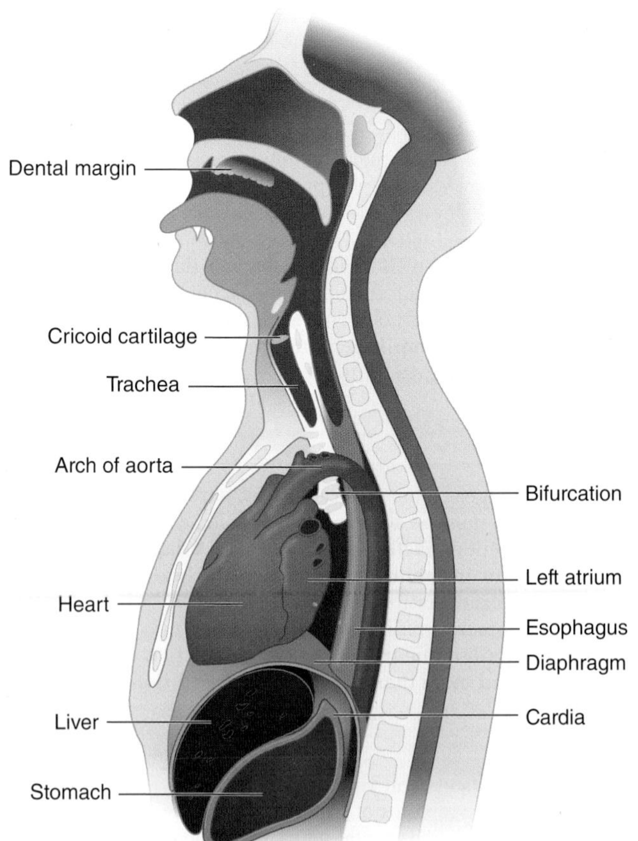

FIGURE 77-1. Anatomic relations of the esophagus (seen from the left side). The distance from the upper incisor teeth to the beginning of the esophagus (cricoid cartilage) is about 15 cm (6 in); from the upper incisors to the level of the bronchi, 22 to 23 cm (9 in); and to the cardia, 40 cm (16 in). Structures contiguous to the esophagus that affect esophageal function are shown.

circular muscle layer. The upper third of the esophagus is striated muscle, while the lower half is all smooth muscle (including the lower esophageal sphincter). The esophagus is lined with stratified squamous epithelial cells that have no secretory function.

Two sphincters regulate the passage of material into and out of the esophagus. The upper esophageal sphincter prevents air from entering the esophagus and food from refluxing into the pharynx. The lower esophageal sphincter regulates the passage of food into the stomach and prevents stomach contents from refluxing into the esophagus. The upper sphincter is composed primarily of the cricopharyngeus muscle, with a resting pressure of around 100 mm Hg. The lower sphincter is not anatomically discrete. The smooth muscle of the lower 1 to 2 cm of the esophagus, in combination with the skeletal muscle of the diaphragmatic hiatus, functions as the sphincter, with a lower resting pressure around 25 mm Hg. An empty esophagus collapses, but three anatomic constrictions affect the adult esophagus:

1. At the cricopharyngeus muscle (C6)
2. At the level of the aortic arch (T4)
3. At the gastroesophageal junction (T10 to T11)

The pediatric esophagus gets two additional areas of constriction:

1. At the thoracic inlet (T1)
2. At the tracheal bifurcation (T6)

The innervation of the heart mirrors that of the esophagus, with visceral and somatic stimuli converging within the sympathetic system. This anatomy makes pain of esophageal and cardiac origin similar. The esophageal venous circulation includes a submucosal plexus of veins that drains into a separate plexus of veins surrounding the esophagus. Blood flows from this outer plexus in part to the gastric venous system, an important link between portal and systemic circulation. Variceal dilatation of the submucosal system can lead to massive upper GI bleeding.

DYSPHAGIA

Dysphagia is difficulty with swallowing. Most patients with dysphagia have an identifiable, organic cause.

Oropharyngeal (transfer) and esophageal (transport) dysphagia describe two broad pathophysiologic types. **Transfer dysphagia** occurs very early in swallowing (as the food bolus moves from the oropharynx through the upper sphincter) and is often reported as difficulty in initiating a swallow. **Transport dysphagia** is impaired movement of the bolus down the esophagus and through the lower sphincter. Transport dysphagia is perceived later in the swallowing process, usually 2 to 4 seconds or longer after swallowing is initiated, and most commonly results in the feeling of the food "getting stuck." A history geared toward discerning transfer from transport dysphagia provides a differential of the likely underlying pathology (**Table 77-1**). Another useful classification scheme divides dysphagia into that due to obstructive disease and that due to motor dysfunction. Functional or motility disorders usually cause dysphagia that is intermittent and variable. Mechanical or obstructive disease is usually progressive (difficulty swallowing solids, then liquids).[1]

CLINICAL FEATURES

Although often an independent symptom, dysphagia can be associated with odynophagia, which is painful swallowing (suggesting an inflammatory process), or with chest pain that is esophageal in nature, suggesting gastroesophageal reflux disease (GERD) or a motility disorder. Question the patient regarding the course of symptoms (acute, subacute, or chronic, intermittent, progressive); food patterns (solids, liquids); location; and previous disease. Transport dysphagia that is present for solids only generally suggests a mechanical or obstructive process. Motility disorders typically cause transport dysphagia for solids and liquids.

Impaction of a poorly chewed meat bolus in the esophagus is a well-recognized complication of esophageal disease. A history of dysphagia may or may not be present. An impacted food bolus can be the presenting complaint for a variety of underlying esophageal pathologies. Patients are generally accurate in identifying location if the bolus is in

TABLE 77-1 Dysphagia

Transfer Dysphagia (Oropharyngeal)	Transport Dysphagia (Esophageal)
Discoordination in transferring bolus from pharynx to esophagus	Improper transfer of the bolus from the upper esophagus into the stomach
Swallowing symptoms—gagging, coughing, nasal regurgitation, inability to initiate swallow, need for repeated swallows	Swallowing symptoms—food "sticking," retrosternal fullness with solids (and eventually liquids), possibly odynophagia
Risk of aspiration present	Risk of aspiration present, generally less pronounced than in transfer dysphagia
Long term—weight loss, malnutrition, chronic bronchitis, asthma, multiple episodes of pneumonia	Long term—malnutrition, dehydration, weight loss, systemic effects of cancer
Neuromuscular disease (80%)—cerebrovascular accident, polymyositis and dermatomyositis, scleroderma, myasthenia gravis, tetanus, Parkinson's disease, botulism, lead poisoning, thyroid disease	Obstructive disease (85%)—foreign body, carcinoma, webs, strictures, thyroid enlargement, diverticulum, congenital or acquired large-vessel abnormalities
Localized disease—pharyngitis; aphthous ulcers; candidal infection; peritonsillar and retropharyngeal abscesses; carcinoma of tongue, pharynx, larynx; Zenker's diverticulum; cricopharyngeal bar; cervical osteophytes	Motor disorder—achalasia, peristaltic dysfunction (nutcracker esophagus), diffuse esophageal spasm, scleroderma
Inadequate lubrication—scleroderma	Inflammatory disease

the upper third of the esophagus. Esophageal filling proximal to the impacted bolus can cause inability to swallow secretions and can present an airway/aspiration risk.

Focus the physical examination on the head and neck and perform the neurologic examination. Assess for signs of previous stroke, muscle disease, or Parkinson's disease. Cachexia and cervical or supraclavicular nodes can be observed in patients with cancer of the esophagus. The physical findings are often normal in patients with dysphagia.[2] Watch the patient take a small sip of water. Inability to swallow water generally confirms at least a partial obstruction.

DIAGNOSIS

The diagnosis of the underlying pathology is most often made outside of the ED. Initial evaluation of dysphagia in the ED can include anteroposterior and lateral neck radiographs, which can be helpful in transfer dysphagia and cases in which the transport dysfunction seems proximal. Obtain a chest x-ray if considering transport dysphagia. Direct laryngoscopy can be used to identify proximal lesions.

Diagnosis of oropharyngeal dysphagia uses a variety of tools. Traditional barium swallow is often recommended as a first test. Video esophagography is a specialized form of barium swallow study in which videotaped images are played at low speed to allow detailed analysis. Manometry and esophagoscopy are also used, depending on the clinical picture.[2] If a foreign body is suspected, the diagnostic evaluation takes yet another path (see later section, "Swallowed Foreign Bodies and Food Impaction").

Neoplasm **Neoplasms** are a common cause of both transfer and transport dysphagia. The esophagus or surrounding structures can be the primary site. A large majority of esophageal neoplasms are squamous cell; the remaining are adenocarcinomas. Risk factors for squamous cell disease include alcohol, smoking, achalasia, and previous ingestion of caustic material with lye. Barrett's esophagus predisposes to adenocarcinoma. Surgery and radiation therapy for head and neck cancer are also important associations.[3]

There is usually a fairly rapid progression of dysphagia from solids to liquids (6 months). Bleeding is another sign suggesting neoplasm. Assume neoplasia in patients >40 years old with new-onset dysphagia. Definitive diagnosis is made by endoscopy with biopsy.

Anatomic Causes **Esophageal stricture** develops as a result of scarring from GERD or other chronic inflammation. Generally strictures occur in the distal esophagus proximal to the gastroesophageal junction and may interfere with lower sphincter function. Symptoms may build over years and are often noted solely with solids. Stricture can serve as a barrier to reflux, so heartburn may decrease as dysphagia increases. Evaluation involves ruling out malignancy, and treatment is dilatation.[4]

Schatzki ring is the most common cause of intermittent dysphagia with solids. This stricture near the gastroesophageal junction is present in up to 15% of the population, and most are asymptomatic. A ring may form over time in response to GERD. Food impaction in the esophagus is a frequent presenting event with a Schatzki ring. The treatment is dilatation.[4]

Esophageal webs are thin structures of mucosa and submucosa found most often in the middle or proximal esophagus. They can be congenital or acquired. Esophageal webs also occur as a component of Plummer-Vinson syndrome (along with iron deficiency anemia) and can be seen in patients with pemphigoid and epidermolysis bullosa. Treatment is dilatation.

Diverticula can be found throughout the esophagus. Pharyngoesophageal or Zenker's diverticulum is a progressive out-pouching of pharyngeal mucosa, just above the upper sphincter, caused by increased pressures during the hypopharyngeal phase of swallowing. Symptom onset is often after age 50, as most diverticula are acquired rather than congenital. Patients complain of typical transfer dysfunction or halitosis and the feeling of a neck mass. Diverticula can also be seen in the mid or distal esophagus, the latter usually in association with a motility disorder.[5]

Neuromuscular and Motility Disorders **Neuromuscular disorders** typically result in misdirection of food boluses with repeated swallowing attempts. Liquids, especially at the extremes of temperature, are generally more difficult to handle than solids, and symptoms are often intermittent. Stroke is the most common cause of this type of dysphagia. Oropharyngeal muscle weakness is often the mechanism, although upper sphincter dysfunction can also contribute. Polymyositis and dermatomyositis are also common causes of transfer dysphagia.

Achalasia is a dysmotility disorder of unknown cause and the most common motility disorder producing dysphagia. Impaired swallowing-induced relaxation of the lower sphincter is noted, along with the absence of esophageal peristalsis. Symptom onset is usually between 20 and 40 years of age. Achalasia may be associated with esophageal spasm and chest pain and with odynophagia. Associated symptoms can include regurgitation and weight loss. Dilation of the esophagus can be massive enough to impinge on the trachea and cause airway symptoms.[6] Therapy includes reduction of lower sphincter pressure by oral medications, endoscopic injection of botulinum toxin into the muscle of the sphincter, dilatations, or surgical myotomy.

Diffuse esophageal spasm is the intermittent interruption of normal peristalsis by nonperistaltic contraction. Dysphagia is intermittent and does not progress over time. Chest pain is a common symptom. Therapy involves control of acid reflux and consideration of smooth muscle relaxants and/or antidepressants, although effectiveness is unclear.[6]

Esophageal dysmotility is the excessive, uncoordinated contraction of esophageal smooth muscle. Clinically, chest pain is the usual presenting symptom of esophageal dysmotility. The onset is usually in the fifth decade. Pain often occurs at rest and is dull or colicky, and stress or ingestion of very hot or very cold liquids may serve as triggers. Acute pain may be followed by hours of dull, residual discomfort. Many patients also have dysphagia, usually intermittent. Pain from spasm may respond to nitroglycerin. Calcium channel blockers and anticholinergic agents can also be used. The other motility disorders commonly recognized include ineffective esophageal motility, hypertensive lower esophageal sphincter, and nutcracker esophagus. Nutcracker esophagus is a motility disorder in which there are high-amplitude, long-duration peristaltic contractions in the distal body of the esophagus or the lower sphincter. The cause is unknown.[6]

CHEST PAIN OF ESOPHAGEAL ORIGIN

Differentiating esophageal pain from ischemic chest pain is difficult at best and may be impossible in the ED. Patients with esophageal disease often report spontaneous onset of pain or pain at night, regurgitation, odynophagia, dysphagia, or meal-induced heartburn, but these symptoms are also found in patients with coronary artery disease, and there are no historical features with enough predictive value to allow accurate differentiation.

The ED working assumption is often that the pain is cardiac in nature. However, the incidence of esophageal disease in patients with chest pain and normal coronary arteries has been reported as up to 80%.[7] The use of ED observation units can help sort patients out with protocol-driven, rapid rule-out of infarction, followed by risk stratification for underlying acute coronary syndrome via a variety of modalities (see chapters 48, "Chest Pain" and 49, "Acute Coronary Syndrome" for further discussion). If a patient's presentation can be determined to be noncardiac in nature, treatment for reflux is often initiated empirically.[7]

GASTROESOPHAGEAL REFLUX DISEASE

Reflux of gastric contents into the esophagus causes a wide array of symptoms and long-term effects. Classically, a weak lower esophageal sphincter has been the mechanism held responsible for reflux, and this is seen in some patients. However, transient relaxation of the lower esophageal sphincter complex (with normal tone in between periods of relaxation) is the primary mechanism causing reflux. Hiatal hernia, prolonged gastric emptying, agents that decrease lower sphincter pressure, and impaired esophageal motility predispose to reflux.[8] **Table 77-2** highlights some common contributors.

Heartburn is the classic symptom of GERD, and chest discomfort may be the only symptom of the disease. The burning nature of the discomfort is probably due to localized lower esophageal mucosal inflammation. Many GERD patients report other associated GI symptoms, such as odynophagia, dysphagia, acid regurgitation, and hypersalivation. Pain and discomfort with meals point to GERD. Reflux symptoms can sometimes be dramatically exacerbated with a head-down position or an increase in intra-abdominal pressure. Symptoms are often relieved by antacids, but pain can return after the transient antacid effect wears off. Some patients with symptoms due to ischemic disease also report improvement with the same therapy. Unfortunately, like cardiac pain, GERD pain may be squeezing and pressure-like, and the history may include pain onset with exertion and offset with rest. Both types of pain may be accompanied by diaphoresis, pallor, and nausea and vomiting. Radiation of esophageal pain can occur to one or both arms, the neck, the shoulders, or the back. Given the serious outcome of unrecognized ischemic disease, a cautious approach is warranted.

Over time, GERD can cause complications including strictures, dysphagia, and inflammatory esophagitis. A severe consequence of GERD, Barrett's esophagus, is present in up to 10% of patients with GERD.[9,10] Less obvious presentations of GERD also occur such as asthma exacerbations, sore throat, and other ear, nose, and throat symptoms. GERD has also been implicated in dental erosion, vocal cord ulcers and granulomas, laryngitis with hoarseness, chronic sinusitis, and chronic cough.

Treatment of reflux disease involves decreasing acid production in the stomach, enhancing upper tract motility, and eliminating risk factors. Mild disease is often treated empirically. Histamine-2 blockers (histamine-2 antagonists) or proton pump inhibitors are mainstays of therapy. A prokinetic drug may help. ED discharge instructions given to patients thought to be experiencing reflux-related symptoms should include: avoid agents that exacerbate GERD (ethanol, caffeine,

TABLE 77-2 Causes of Gastroesophageal Reflux Disease

Decreased Pressure of Lower Esophageal Sphincter	Decreased Esophageal Motility	Prolonged Gastric Emptying
High-fat food	Achalasia	Medicines (anticholinergics)
Nicotine	Scleroderma	Outlet obstruction
Ethanol	Presbyesophagus	Diabetic gastroparesis
Caffeine	Diabetes mellitus	High-fat food
Medicines (nitrates, calcium channel blockers, anticholinergics, progesterone, estrogen)		
Pregnancy		

nicotine, chocolate, fatty foods), sleep with the head of the bed elevated (30 degrees), and avoid eating within 3 hours of going to bed at night. The need for additional testing can be determined at outpatient follow-up care.

ESOPHAGITIS

Esophagitis can cause prolonged periods of chest pain and almost always causes odynophagia as well. Diagnosis of more established esophagitis is by endoscopy. Low-grade disease can be seen by histopathologic examination.

INFLAMMATORY ESOPHAGITIS

GERD may induce an inflammatory response in the lower esophageal mucosa. Over time, esophageal ulcerations, scarring, and stricture formation can develop. The presence of reflux-induced esophagitis warrants aggressive pharmacologic therapy with acid-suppressive medications. If this treatment regimen is not sufficient, surgical options are considered.[8] Ingested medications can also be a source of inflammatory esophagitis, usually from prolonged contact of the medication with the esophageal mucosa. Ulcerations can form. Multiple medications have been implicated. Common offenders include nonsteroidal anti-inflammatory drugs and other anti-inflammatory drugs, potassium chloride, and some antibiotics (e.g., doxycycline, tetracycline, and clindamycin). Risk factors for pill-induced esophageal injury include swallowing position, fluid intake, capsule size, and age. Withdrawal of the offending agent is generally curative. Eosinophilic esophagitis is a chronic allergic-inflammatory condition in which eosinophils and other immune system cells infiltrate the esophagus and induce an inflammatory response.[10] Diagnosis is by endoscopy. Treatment is avoidance of allergens and swallowed liquid corticosteroids. Dilatation is necessary if strictures form.

INFECTIOUS ESOPHAGITIS

Patients with immunosuppression can develop infectious esophagitis. The diagnosis of infectious esophagitis in an otherwise seemingly healthy host should prompt an evaluation of immune status. Candidal species are the most common pathogens, often associated with dysphagia as a primary symptom. Herpes simplex or cytomegalovirus infection and aphthous ulceration are also seen and may be more frequently associated with odynophagia. Other causative agents are rare and include fungi, mycobacteria, and other viral pathogens such as varicella-zoster virus and Epstein-Barr virus. Endoscopy with biopsy and specimen culture is used to establish this diagnosis.[11]

ESOPHAGEAL PERFORATION

Perforation of the esophagus can occur secondary to a number of disparate processes (**Table 77-3**). Iatrogenic perforation is the most frequent.[12]

Boerhaave's syndrome is full-thickness perforation of the esophagus after a sudden rise in intraesophageal pressure. The mechanism is sudden, forceful emesis in about three fourths of the cases; coughing, straining, seizures, and childbirth have been reported as causing perforations as well. Alcohol consumption is frequently an antecedent to this syndrome. The perforation is usually in the distal esophagus on the left side.

Blunt or penetrating **neck trauma** can cause esophageal perforation. Rupture from blunt injury is rare. Penetrating esophageal wounds are often masked by injury to the airway and major vessels. A combination of esophagography and esophagoscopy is used to assess patients for potential esophageal injury.

Foreign-body ingestion or food impaction may result in perforation of the esophagus as well (see below).

The perforation rate from endoscopy is lower in an esophagus free of disease than in a diseased esophagus. Dilation of strictures increases the risk of perforation greatly. Other intraluminal procedures, such as variceal therapy and palliative laser treatment for cancer, are also associated with perforation. **Boerhaave's syndrome** is responsible for roughly 10% to 15% of esophageal perforations and is discussed above.

TABLE 77-3 Causes of Esophageal Perforation

Cause of Perforation	Description
Iatrogenic	Intraluminal procedures
	Endoscopy
	Dilatation
	Variceal therapy
	Gastric intubation
	Intraoperative injury
Boerhaave's syndrome	"Spontaneous," usually associated with transient increase in intraesophageal pressure
Trauma	Penetrating
	Blunt (rare)
	Caustic ingestion
Foreign body	Includes pill-related injury
Infection	Rare
Tumor	May be intrinsic or extrinsic cancer
Aortic pathology	Aneurysm
	Aberrant right subclavian artery
Miscellaneous	Barrett's esophagus
	Zollinger-Ellison syndrome

PATHOPHYSIOLOGY

Perforation causes a dramatic presentation if esophageal contents leak into the mediastinal, pleural, or peritoneal space. Fulminant, necrotizing mediastinitis, pneumonitis, or peritonitis can rapidly lead to shock. If the perforation is small and leakage is contained by contiguous structures, the course may be significantly more indolent. Most spontaneous perforations occur through the left posterolateral wall of the distal esophagus.[12] Proximal perforation, seen mostly with instrumentation, tends to be less severe than distal perforation and can form a periesophageal abscess with minimal systemic toxicity.

CLINICAL FEATURES

The pain of rupture is classically described as acute, severe, unrelenting, and diffuse, and is reported in the chest, neck, and abdomen. Pain can radiate to the back and shoulders. Back pain may be a very predominant symptom. The pain is often exacerbated by swallowing. Dysphagia, dyspnea, hematemesis, and cyanosis can be present as well.

Physical examination varies with the severity of the rupture and the elapsed time to presentation. Abdominal rigidity with hypotension and fever often occur early. Tachycardia and tachypnea are common. Cervical subcutaneous emphysema is common in cervical esophageal perforations. **Mediastinal emphysema takes time to develop. It is less commonly detected by examination or radiography in lower esophageal perforation, and its absence does not rule out perforation.** Hamman's crunch, caused by air in the mediastinum that is being moved by the beating heart, can sometimes be auscultated. Pleural effusion develops in half of patients with intrathoracic perforations but is uncommon in those with cervical perforations. Pleural fluid can be due to either direct contamination of the pleural space or a sympathetic serous effusion from mediastinitis.

DIAGNOSIS

Timely diagnosis in an ill patient with esophageal perforation requires suspicion on the clinician's part. Mistaking perforation for acute myocardial infarction, pulmonary embolism, or an acute abdomen can lead to delays in therapy. Chest radiographs can suggest the diagnosis. CT of the chest or emergency endoscopy is most often used to confirm the diagnosis. Perforation of the esophagus is associated with a high mortality rate regardless of the underlying cause. The pace of care and the location and etiology of the perforation all affect outcome. In the ED, resuscitate

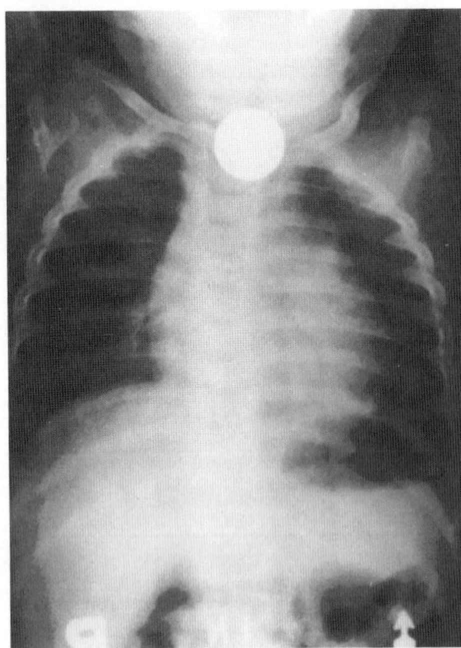

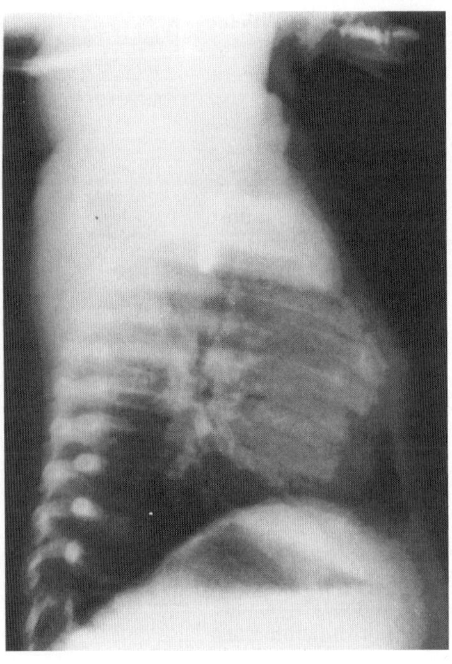

FIGURE 77-2. A coin lodged in a child's esophagus is visible on an anteroposterior radiograph. [Reproduced with permission from Effron D (ed): *Pediatric Photo and X-Ray Stimuli for Emergency Medicine*, vol II. Columbus, OH, Ohio Chapter of the American College of Emergency Physicians, 1997, case 27.]

the patient from shock, administer broad-spectrum parenteral antibiotics, and obtain emergency surgical consultation as soon as the diagnosis is seriously entertained. Patients with systemic symptoms and signs after perforation need operative management.[12]

SWALLOWED FOREIGN BODIES AND FOOD IMPACTION

PATHOPHYSIOLOGY

Children 18 to 48 months of age and those with mental illness account for most cases of ingested foreign bodies. Small objects, such as coins, toys, and crayons, typically lodge in the anatomically narrow proximal esophagus. In adults, dentures are sometimes swallowed, because diminished palatal sensitivity leads to unintentional ingestion. Adult candidates for swallowed foreign bodies are those with esophageal disease, prisoners, and psychiatric patients. In adults, most impactions are distal. In children and adults, once an object has traversed the pylorus, it usually continues through the GI tract and is passed without issue. If, however, the object has irregular or sharp edges or is particularly wide (>2.5 cm) or long (>6 cm), it may become lodged distal to the pylorous.[13] Esophageal impaction can result in airway obstruction, stricture, or perforation, the latter being the result of direct mechanical erosion (e.g., ingested bones) or chemical corrosion (e.g., ingested button batteries). Esophageal mucosal irritation (often mechanical from a swallowed bone, for example) can be perceived as a foreign body by the patient as well.

CLINICAL FEATURES

Adults with an esophageal foreign body generally provide unequivocal history. Patients often complain of retrosternal pain and may localize the object (often accurately in the upper third of the esophagus). Patients may have dysphagia, vomiting, and choking. If the patient attempts to wash down the object with liquid or if swallowed secretions pool proximal to the obstruction, coughing or aspiration can occur. **In children, the history can be unclear. Signs and symptoms can include refusal or inability to eat, vomiting, gagging and choking, stridor, neck or throat pain, and drooling. A high degree of suspicion is necessary for unwitnessed ingestions in children, especially in those <2 years of age.** Physical examination starts with an assessment of the airway. The nasopharynx, oropharynx, neck, and chest should also be examined but are often unremarkable. Occasionally, a foreign body can be directly visualized in the oropharynx.

DIAGNOSIS

Plain films are used to screen for radiopaque objects. Coins in the esophagus generally present their circular face on anteroposterior films (coronal alignment), as opposed to coins in the trachea, which show that face on lateral films (**Figure** 77-2). Obtaining plain films in patients with food impaction is rarely helpful and can generally be omitted. CT scanning is a very high-yield test for esophageal foreign body and has generally replaced the barium swallow test to evaluate ingestion of nonradiopaque objects. CT also delivers excellent information regarding perforation and subsequent infection.

TREATMENT

Endoscopy Patients in extremis or with pending airway compromise are resuscitated and often require active airway management. Complete obstruction of the esophagus (often distal esophageal food impactions) can lead to proximal pooling of secretions and aspiration. Emergent endoscopy is needed. **Table 77-4** lists other situations that require urgent endoscopy, even if patients are clinically stable. Some of these ingestions are discussed in more detail in the sections "Food Impaction," "Coin Ingestion," "Button Battery Ingestion," "Ingestion of Sharp Objects," and "Narcotics Ingestion" later in the chapter. In general, if endoscopy is clearly indicated, performing advanced imaging studies delays definitive intervention while adding little value to the care of the patient. In the vast majority of cases, the foreign body can be removed relatively easily with endoscopy without complication. Hospital admission is generally not needed.

Laryngoscopy In stable patients, indirect laryngoscopy or visualization of the oropharynx using a fiberoptic scope may allow removal of very proximal objects. For more distal objects, imaging studies are used

TABLE 77-4 Circumstances Warranting Urgent Endoscopy for Esophageal Foreign Bodies
Ingestion of sharp or elongated objects (including toothpicks, aluminum soda can tabs)
Ingestion of multiple foreign bodies
Ingestion of button batteries
Evidence of perforation
Coin at the level of the cricopharyngeus muscle in a child
Airway compromise
Presence of a foreign body for >24 h

to define the location and nature of the ingestion. Objects that persist over time or are in the upper half of the esophagus are less likely to pass, and consultation for endoscopy is prudent.

Expectant Treatment If the object is distal to the pylorus, has a benign shape and nature, and the patient is comfortable and tolerating intake by mouth, treatment is expectant. For worrisome foreign bodies that are in the more distal GI tract, surgery consultation may be necessary.

Foley Catheter Removal Alternatives to endoscopy have been advocated by some authors. These include use of a Foley catheter to remove coins (see section "Coin Ingestion" later in the chapter) and bougienage to advance the object from the esophagus into the stomach. Generally, the Foley catheter technique and bougienage should only be attempted in patients with blunt foreign bodies present for <24 hours and in patients without underlying esophageal disease. Provider comfort with the procedure likely influences the generally low complication rates in published series.[14]

Glucagon For distal esophageal objects, **glucagon, 1 to 2 mg IV in adults,** has been used to relax the lower sphincter and allow passage of the object. **Success rates of glucagon therapy are generally reported as poor, however, and it may be no better than watchful waiting without other intervention.**[15]

SPECIAL CONSIDERATIONS

FOOD IMPACTION

Meat is the food most commonly identified in food impaction. Food impaction with complete esophageal obstruction or impaction of food containing bony fragments requires emergency endoscopy. Uncomplicated food impaction may be treated expectantly. Time and sedation often allow the bolus to pass into the stomach, but the bolus should not be allowed to remain impacted for >12 to 24 hours. **The use of proteolytic enzymes (e.g., Adolph's Meat Tenderizer®, which contains papain) to dissolve a meat bolus is *contraindicated*, because of the potential for severe mucosal damage and esophageal perforation, and the availability of superior alternatives.** If **glucagon** therapy is attempted, an initial dose of 1 to 2 milligrams IV is given (for adults). If the food bolus is not passed in 20 minutes, an additional dose can given.[15]

COIN INGESTION

Many centers use endoscopy to remove esophageal coins in children. Removal with a Foley catheter is done under fluoroscopy, and advanced airway management should be immediately available. The patient is placed in the Trendelenburg position to prevent aspiration of the object. The catheter is passed down the esophagus beyond the object, the balloon inflated, and the catheter slowly withdrawn, bringing the object with it. Complications can include airway compromise and mucosal injury, although in experienced hands, the rate of these events is low.[14]

BUTTON BATTERY INGESTION

A button battery lodged in the esophagus is a true emergency requiring prompt removal, because the battery may quickly induce mucosal injury and necrosis. Perforation can occur within 6 hours of ingestion. Morbidity caused by the battery is likely related to the flow of electricity through a locally formed external circuit. Lithium cells are associated disproportionately with adverse outcome, probably due to higher voltage.[14]

Figure 77-3 outlines a management algorithm for button battery ingestion. Button batteries that have passed the esophagus can be managed expectantly, as long as follow-up in 24 hours can be assured. Repeat films should be obtained at 48 hours to ensure that the cell has passed through the pylorus (which may not occur if the battery is of large diameter and/or the patient is <6 years old). Most batteries pass completely through the body within 48 to 72 hours, although passage can take longer. Any patient with symptoms or signs of GI tract injury requires immediate surgical consultation. The National Button Battery Ingestion Hotline (National Capital Poison Center, Washington, DC) at 202-625-3333 is a 24-hour/7-day-a-week resource for help in management decisions.

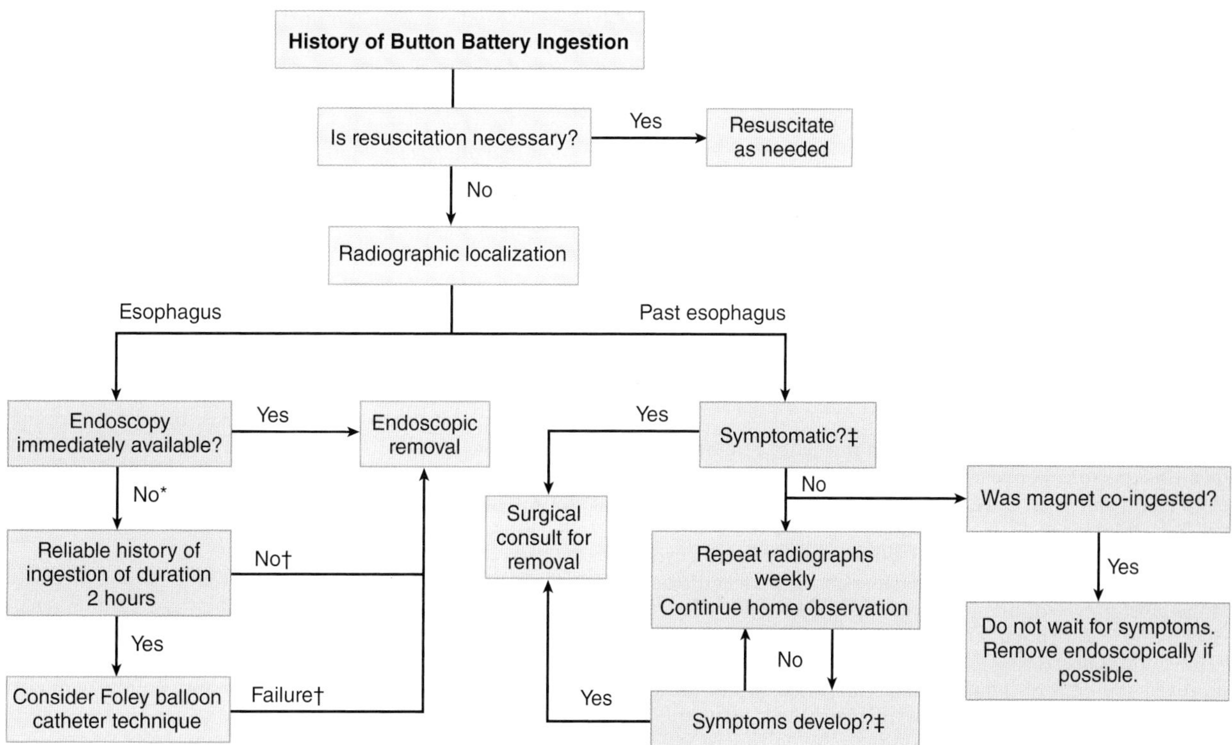

FIGURE 77-3. Algorithm for management of button battery ingestion. *Button batteries in the esophagus must be removed. Endoscopy should be used, if available. The balloon catheter technique can be used if the ingestion occurred ≤2 hours previously, but it should not be used after this period, because it may increase the amount of damage to the weakened esophagus. †When the Foley technique fails or is contraindicated because >2 hours have elapsed, the button battery should be removed endoscopically. This may require transfer of the patient. ‡Acute abdomen, tarry or bloody stools, fever,

INGESTION OF SHARP OBJECTS

Sharp objects in the esophagus need immediate removal. Sharp objects may pass into the stomach spontaneously. **Because intestinal perforation from ingested sharp objects that pass distal to the stomach is common, the American Society for Gastrointestinal Endoscopy guidelines recommend removal of sharp objects by endoscopy while they are in the stomach or duodenum.** If intestinal perforation occurs, it is usually at the ileocecal valve.

If the object is distal to the duodenum at presentation and the patient is asymptomatic, the object's passage should be documented with daily plain films. Surgical removal should be considered if 3 days elapse without passage. The development of symptoms or signs of intestinal injury (e.g., pain, emesis, fever, GI bleeding) requires immediate surgical consultation.[13]

NARCOTICS INGESTION

Narcotic couriers (body packers) ingest multiple small packets of a drug in order to conceal transport. A favored packet is the condom, which may hold up to 5 grams of narcotic. These packets are often visible on plain films. Rupture of even one such packet may be fatal, and endoscopy is contraindicated because of the risk of iatrogenic packet rupture. If the packet(s) appears to be passing intact through the intestinal tract, observation until the packet reaches the rectum is the favored treatment. Some authors advocate the use of whole-bowel irrigation to aid the process.

REFERENCES

The complete reference list is available online at www.TintinalliEM.com.

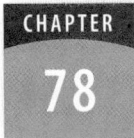

CHAPTER 78 Peptic Ulcer Disease and Gastritis

Matthew C. Gratton
Angela Bogle

INTRODUCTION AND EPIDEMIOLOGY

Peptic ulcer disease is a chronic illness manifested by recurrent ulcerations in the stomach and proximal duodenum. Acid and pepsin are thought to be crucial to ulcer development, but the great majority of peptic ulcers are directly related to infection with *Helicobacter pylori* or nonsteroidal anti-inflammatory drug (NSAID) use.[1,2] **Gastritis** is acute or chronic inflammation of the gastric mucosa and has various etiologies. **Dyspepsia** is continuous or recurrent upper abdominal pain or discomfort with or without associated symptoms (e.g., nausea, bloating).[3] Dyspepsia may be caused by a number of diseases or may be functional.

Uncomplicated peptic ulcer disease has an incidence of more than 5 cases per 1000 persons per year, and about 10% of people living in the Western world will experience a peptic ulcer at some point during their lives.[4,5] In the United States, peptic ulcer disease costs an estimated $5.65 billion per year in total direct and indirect costs.[6] *H. pylori* infection, one of the main risk factors of peptic ulcer disease, is one of the most prevalent human infections in the world, affecting at least 50% of the world's population.[7] The age-adjusted prevalence of *H. pylori* infection is decreasing in industrialized countries, likely due to an improved standard of living[7] and the increased use of proton pump inhibitors (PPIs) and antimicrobial therapy.[2,8] This may explain the decreasing incidence of peptic ulcer disease in the United States, but this may be partially offset by the widespread use of low-dose aspirin and NSAIDs.[2,9] Over 70 million prescriptions for NSAIDs are written, and over 30 billion tablets are sold over the counter annually in the United States.[10] Risk factors for ulcers not due to *H. pylori* or NSAIDs include antiplatelet agents, stress, *Helicobacter heilmannii*, cytomegalovirus infections, Behçet's disease, Zollinger-Ellison syndrome, Crohn's disease, cirrhosis with portal hypertension, older age, and African American ethnicity.[2]

Dyspepsia affects 20% to 40% of the world's population.[3] There is no consistent association with sex, age, socioeconomic status, smoking, or alcohol use; however, it is more common in people infected with *H. pylori* and who take NSAIDs, as well as some other medications.[3]

PATHOPHYSIOLOGY

Hydrochloric acid and pepsin destroy gastric and duodenal mucosa. Mucus and bicarbonate ion secretions protect mucosa. Prostaglandins protect mucosa by enhancing mucus and bicarbonate production and by enhancing mucosal blood flow, thereby supporting metabolism. The balance between these protective and destructive forces determines whether peptic ulcer disease occurs. *H. pylori* bacteria or NSAIDs are thought to be the causal agents of peptic ulcer disease in most cases.[1,2] Although traditional treatment of peptic ulcers by various modalities heals most ulcers, eradication of *H. pylori* cures peptic ulcers in over 80% of patients whose ulcers are not associated with the use of NSAIDs.[7,11]

H. pylori is a spiral, gram-negative, urease-producing, flagellated bacterium that is found living between the mucous gel and the mucosa. The bacterium's production of urease, cytotoxins, proteases, and other compounds is thought to disturb the mucous gel and cause tissue injury. In addition, increased gastrin levels and decreased mucus and bicarbonate production are associated with *H. pylori* infection. Chronic active (usually asymptomatic) gastritis is an almost universal finding with *H. pylori* infection, but only 1% to 10% of infected people develop peptic ulcer disease.[7] It is unclear why most infected persons do not develop symptomatic peptic ulcer disease, but it most likely reflects an interaction of factors, including characteristics of host and pathogen (different virulence of strains of bacteria). In 2005, Marshal and Warren were awarded the Nobel Prize in Physiology or Medicine for their discovery of *H. pylori* and its role in gastritis and peptic ulcer disease.

H. pylori is a causative agent of mucosa-associated lymphoid tissue lymphoma, and eradication of infection causes a remission in a sizable percentage of patients with low-grade tumors.[7] In addition, *H. pylori* infection is a risk factor for adenocarcinoma of the stomach, and as such, the World Health Organization has classified it as a human carcinogen.[7] However, because the prevalence of gastric cancer in the United States is very low and the *H. pylori* infection rate is high, other factors undoubtedly are involved. It is not clear whether eradication of the infection reduces the risk of gastric cancer.[7] *H. pylori* infection has been associated with the development of iron deficiency anemia, with possible mechanisms including decreased iron absorption and/or occult blood loss from chronic gastritis. A direct cause-and-effect relationship is yet to be determined.[12,13] Improvement in the platelet count in some patients with idiopathic thrombocytopenic purpura has been demonstrated with *H. pylori* eradication, but much more work remains to be done in this regard.[12,14]

NSAIDs inhibit prostaglandin synthesis, thereby decreasing mucus and bicarbonate production and mucosal blood flow, which allows ulcer formation. Gastrin-secreting tumors produce ulceration due to high levels of acid and pepsin production, but acid alone rarely causes ulceration. However, inhibition of acid secretion may allow ulcers to heal and is the basis for traditional ulcer treatments.

Hereditary factors cause a predisposition to peptic ulcer disease, as does smoking. There is an association between chronic renal failure, renal transplantation, cirrhosis, chronic obstructive pulmonary disease, and peptic ulceration, but the precise mechanism is unclear. Emotional stress may predispose to peptic ulcer disease, but diet and alcohol use do not.

Acute gastritis may be related to ischemia from severe illness (e.g., shock, trauma, severe burns, organ failure) or to the direct toxic effects of agents (e.g., NSAIDs, steroids, bile acids). *H. pylori* infection causes acute and chronic gastritis (both usually asymptomatic). Chronic gastritis may also be caused by autoimmune factors that destroy gastric parietal cells; this results in the loss of acid production and the loss of intrinsic factor production, which in turn cause malabsorption of vitamin B_{12} and, hence, pernicious anemia.

Dyspepsia has multiple causes. Endoscopy of patients with dyspepsia demonstrates that about 13% have erosive esophagitis, 8% have peptic ulcer disease, and less than 0.3% have gastric or esophageal cancer.[3] Other abnormalities such as gastritis, duodenitis, and gastric erosions may be present, but these may or may not be related to symptoms. About 70% to 80% of patients have no definite abnormal findings on endoscopy and are said to have "functional dyspepsia."[3] Patients with functional dyspepsia have evidence of abnormal gastric emptying, abnormal sensitivity to distention, abnormal ability of the stomach to distend with a meal, abnormalities in acid clearance, and abnormal duodenal sensitivity to acid. In addition, there appears to be an as yet poorly characterized interaction between the stomach and intestine and the central nervous system, which may contribute to symptoms.[3]

CLINICAL FEATURES

Burning epigastric pain is the most classic symptom of peptic ulcer disease. The pain also may be described as sharp, dull, an ache, or an "empty" or "hungry" feeling. Pain may be relieved by ingestion of milk, food, or antacids, presumably due to buffering and/or dilution of acid. **Pain recurs as the gastric contents empty, and the recurrent pain may classically awaken the patient at night.** Pain tends to occur daily for weeks, resolve, and then recur in weeks to months. Postprandial pain, food intolerance, nausea, retrosternal pain, and belching are not related to peptic ulcer disease. Atypical presentations are common in those >65 years old, including no pain, epigastric pain not relieved by eating, nausea, vomiting, anorexia, weight loss, and bleeding.

A change in the character of typical pain may herald a complication. Abrupt onset of severe or generalized pain may indicate perforation with peritoneal spillage of gastric or duodenal contents. Rapid onset of mid-back pain may be due to posterior penetration into the pancreas, resulting in pancreatitis. Nausea and vomiting may indicate gastric outlet obstruction from scarring or edema. Vomiting of bright red blood or coffee-ground emesis or passage of tarry or melanotic stool or hematochezia may indicate ulcer bleeding.

On physical examination, the only positive finding in patients with uncomplicated peptic ulcer disease may be epigastric tenderness. This finding is neither sensitive nor specific for the diagnosis. Other physical findings may be indicative of complications: a rigid abdomen consistent with peritonitis in perforation; abdominal distention or a succussion splash due to obstruction; or occult or gross rectal blood or blood in the nasogastric aspirate signaling ulcer bleeding.

Epigastric pain, nausea, and vomiting may be present with acute gastritis, but the most common presentation of gastritis is GI bleeding, ranging from occult blood loss in the stool to massive upper GI hemorrhage. Physical findings may be normal, may reflect only the GI bleeding, or may reflect a severe underlying associated illness (as listed earlier).

DIAGNOSIS

A definitive diagnosis of peptic ulcer disease cannot be made on clinical grounds alone. Uncomplicated peptic ulcer disease can be strongly suspected in the presence of a "classic" history, including epigastric burning pain; relief of pain with ingestion of milk, food, or antacids; and night pain accompanied by "benign" physical examination findings, including normal vital signs with or without mild epigastric tenderness. The differential diagnosis of epigastric pain is extensive and, in addition to peptic ulcer disease, includes gastritis, gastroesophageal reflux disease, cholelithiasis, pancreatitis, hepatitis, abdominal aortic aneurysm, gastroparesis, and functional dyspepsia. Careful history taking may elicit features that point away from peptic ulcer disease: burning pain radiating into the chest, water brash, and belching may suggest gastroesophageal reflux disease; more severe pain radiating to the right upper quadrant and around the right or left side suggests cholelithiasis; radiation through to the back indicates pancreatitis or abdominal aortic aneurysm; chronic pain, anorexia, or weight loss may indicate gastric cancer. Myocardial ischemic pain may also present as epigastric pain and should be strongly considered in the appropriate clinical setting.

Physical examination findings may suggest other diagnoses: right upper quadrant tenderness points to cholelithiasis or hepatitis, an epigastric mass to pancreatitis (pseudocyst) or pancreatic or gastric neoplasm, a pulsatile mass to abdominal aortic aneurysm, jaundice to hepatitis, and peritoneal findings to an acute abdomen.

ANCILLARY TESTING

Ancillary tests may help exclude peptic ulcer disease complications and narrow the differential diagnosis. Normal results for CBC rule out anemia from chronic GI bleeding due to peptic ulcer disease, gastritis, or cancer (but do not rule out acute blood loss). Elevated liver function test results may indicate hepatitis, and an elevated lipase level may indicate pancreatitis. An acute abdominal series may show free air associated with perforation. A limited ED US examination may show gallstones or an abdominal aortic aneurysm. An ECG and cardiac enzyme determination are indicated if there is a suspicion of myocardial ischemic pain.

The gold standard for diagnosis of peptic ulcer disease is visualization of an ulcer by **upper GI endoscopy**.[2,4] Although not all patients with undiagnosed dyspepsia require endoscopy, those with "alarm features" do[3,4] (**Table 78-1**). Alarm features raise the index of suspicion for gastric or esophageal cancer, as well as other potentially serious conditions, but the features are not specific.[3]

***H. pylori* Tests** Because most peptic ulcers are caused by *H. pylori* infection and eradication of *H. pylori* dramatically decreases the ulcer recurrence rate, it is important to know how to diagnose infection. *H. pylori* infection can be diagnosed by endoscopic tests, including the rapid urease test, histologic study, and culture, all of which rely on a biopsy of the gastric mucosa.[1,7,11] Noninvasive tests include serologic tests, urea breath tests, and stool antigen tests.[1,7,11]

The **rapid urease test** detects the presence of urease in a biopsy specimen (presumptive evidence of *H. pylori* infection) with >90% sensitivity and >95% specificity.[7] Histologic studies allow direct assessment of *H. pylori* infection and culture of the organism, but these tests require highly trained technicians and appropriate facilities and are not widely available.[7,11] The major disadvantage of all the aforementioned tests is the cost in time, dollars, and potential complications of endoscopy.

Serologic studies detect **immunoglobulin G antibodies to *H. pylori*** and are readily available, but the sensitivity and specificity are not very good (85% and 79%, respectively).[7,11] Serologic studies are not useful as a test of cure, because antibodies remain for several months to years after eradication of infection.

The **urea breath test** relies on the presence of urease produced by *H. pylori*. Urea labeled with carbon-13 or carbon-14 instead of carbon-12 is ingested and, in the presence of bacterial urease, is broken down into labeled carbon dioxide and ammonia. The labeled carbon dioxide is detected in the breath later. Sensitivity and specificity are >95%.[7,11] The urea breath test can be used to determine the presence of infection after eradication therapy.[11]

H. pylori antigens can be detected in the stool with >90% sensitivity and specificity.[1,7] Testing performed ≥4 weeks after completion of *H. pylori* eradication therapy is useful as a test of cure. The sensitivity of all tests that rely on active infection with *H. pylori* is decreased significantly by recent treatment with PPIs, histamine-2 (H_2) antagonists, antibiotics, and bismuth compounds.[7,11]

TABLE 78-1 "Alarm Features" for Endoscopy
Age >50 y, with new-onset symptoms
Unexplained weight loss
Persistent vomiting
Dysphagia or odynophagia
Iron deficiency anemia or GI bleeding
Abdominal mass or lymphadenopathy
Family history of upper GI malignancy

TREATMENT

After peptic ulcer disease is diagnosed, the goal of treatment is to heal the ulcer while relieving pain and preventing complications and recurrence. Traditional ulcer therapy heals the ulcer, relieves pain, and prevents complications, but does not prevent recurrence. Treatment of *H. pylori* infection, when present, dramatically decreases the recurrence rate.[7,11] If NSAID-associated ulcers are present, the offending agent should be stopped whenever possible. Traditional therapy includes PPIs, H_2 receptor antagonists (H_2RAs), sucralfate, and antacids.

Traditional ED treatment would entail initiating a trial of a PPI or an H_2RA, with antacids for breakthrough pain, and referring to a primary care provider to direct evaluation and subsequent treatment. This usually remains the best option. There is some evidence that a short course of a PPI provides better symptomatic relief than an H_2RA for undiagnosed dyspepsia, although the evidence is not from an ED setting.[3] Immediate referral for definite diagnosis is mandated if alarm features are present[3,4] (Table 78-1). Practice guidelines and reviews support treatment of *H. pylori*–positive dyspeptic patients with antimicrobial and antisecretory therapy followed by endoscopic study only in those with persistent symptoms.[3] It might be reasonable for the ED physician to begin symptomatic therapy, order a test for *H. pylori*, and refer the patient for early follow-up with a primary care provider for initiation of antibacterial therapy if the test results are positive. However, this strategy has not been tested.

PPIs

PPIs decrease acid production by irreversibly binding with an H^+K^+ ATPase molecule (proton pump) located on the gastric parietal cell, thus blocking hydrogen ion secretion.[1] PPIs are most effective if taken 30 to 60 minutes prior to a meal. **PPIs generally heal ulcers faster than do H_2RAs and also have some in vitro inhibitory effect against *H. pylori*.**[1] PPIs are metabolized in the liver by the cytochrome P-450 system and therefore may decrease the metabolism of many other drugs. In addition, PPIs may inhibit the absorption of drugs that rely on gastric acidity. PPIs are well tolerated by most patients.[1] There are six U.S. Food and Drug Administration–approved PPIs, and two (omeprazole and lansoprazole) have "over-the-counter" formulations.[1] If a patient develops an ulcer while taking NSAIDs and must continue therapy, PPIs heal ulcers faster than any other potential treatment.[1]

H_2RAs

H_2RAs competitively inhibit the actions of histamine on the H_2 receptors of the gastric parietal cells. All four H_2RAs (cimetidine, famotidine, nizatidine, and ranitidine) heal ulcers approximately equally and are available in over-the-counter preparations.[1] **Because of renal excretion, make dosage adjustments in patients with renal failure.** Side effects are uncommon but can include headache, confusion, lethargy, depression, and hallucinations.[1] Cimetidine has more significant drug interactions than do the other H_2RAs due to inhibition of cytochrome P-450 activity.[1]

OTHER AGENTS

Sucralfate, an aluminum hydroxide complex of sucrose, appears to protect the ulcer from acid exposure by forming a sticky gel that adheres to the ulcer crater and allows healing to occur but does not relieve pain as well as PPIs and H_2RAs.[1] Sucralfate has few side effects but can cause constipation and aluminum toxicity, as well as inhibit absorption of a number of medications.[1] **Antacids** heal ulcers by buffering gastric acid. Magnesium- and aluminum-containing antacids can inhibit absorption of drugs and should be avoided in patients with renal insufficiency or renal failure. In renal failure, aluminum can accumulate and cause osteoporosis and encephalopathy, and hypermagnesemia can also result. Due to the simplicity of PPI and H_2RA dosing requirements, antacids currently are used mainly on an as-needed basis for ulcer pain until healing occurs.

Although NSAIDs should be stopped in patients with peptic ulcer disease whenever possible, **misoprostol** may prevent ulcer formation in those concurrently receiving NSAID therapy. Misoprostol is a prostaglandin analog that may act by increasing mucus and bicarbonate production and by increasing mucosal blood flow. Because it is an abortifacient, do not use misoprostol in women who could become pregnant.[1]

H. PYLORI ERADICATION

If *H. pylori* infection is diagnosed in the presence of peptic ulcer disease, eradication is clearly indicated.[1,7,11] Multiple regimens have been proposed and studied, most commonly "triple therapy" with a PPI, clarithromycin, and either amoxicillin or metronidazole.[1,7,11] Authorities in the United States recommend 10- to 14-day regimens for the best cure rates.[1,7,11] In areas where clarithromycin resistance is high, quadruple therapy or sequential therapy may be the preferred option.[1,7,12]

Patients generally do not present to the ED with a definitive diagnosis of peptic ulcer disease but rather with a symptom, such as epigastric pain. If appropriate history, physical examination, and laboratory evaluation result in a physician's impression of "possible peptic ulcer disease" or "dyspepsia," the physician is left with three main options: empiric treatment with conventional antiulcer medication, immediate referral for definite diagnosis (endoscopic study), or noninvasive testing for *H. pylori* followed by antibiotic therapy for patients with positive test results.

COMPLICATIONS

HEMORRHAGE

About 400,000 patients per year are admitted to the hospital in the United States due to nonvariceal upper GI bleeding, and peptic ulcer disease is the most common cause.[15,16] As many as 15% of peptic ulcers bleed, resulting in an overall mortality rate of 10%.[2] Bleeding from peptic ulcers is most common in the elderly.

ED treatment for ulcer bleeding focuses on restoring hemodynamic stability by IV administration of isotonic saline solution and packed red blood cells (see chapter 75, "Upper Gastrointestinal Bleeding" for details of treatment). Early upper endoscopy is recommended in most patients to confirm the diagnosis and target endoscopic treatment.[8,15,16] Before endoscopy, a bolus dose of a PPI followed by a continuous infusion can be considered, as can use of a prokinetic agent, such as erythromycin, given IV. Neither has been consistently shown to improve clinical outcomes.[8,16] Nasogastric or orogastric lavage is not required for diagnosis. Up to 18% of upper GI bleeds may have clear or bile-stained aspirate.[16] Likewise neither is required for prognostic purposes, to improve visualization, or for specific therapy.[16]

Most patients should undergo upper GI endoscopy within 24 hours for diagnostic, prognostic, and treatment purposes.[8,15,16] Lesions can be described using the Forrest classification or descriptive terms.[16] Ranging from highest to lowest risk of rebleeding, these classifications include an ulcer with active spurting of blood; active oozing; nonbleeding visible vessel; adherent clot; flat pigmented spot; and an ulcer with a clean base.[16] Actively bleeding ulcers (including both active spurting and oozing ulcers) have a 55% risk of rebleeding and an 11% mortality rate, whereas those with a clean base have rates of 5% and 2%, respectively.[16] Treatment through endoscopy includes injection therapy (epinephrine, sclerosing agents), thermal therapy (electrocoagulation, heater probe), and mechanical clipping.[16] All of these treatments stop bleeding, prevent recurrences, and decrease transfusion rates and length of hospital stay. The technique chosen depends on the equipment available and the experience of the endoscopist.

Rebleeding after endoscopic therapy can be treated by repeat endoscopy.[16] If further bleeding occurs, then surgery or transcatheter arterial embolization should be considered.[16]

Hospitalization in an intensive care setting is indicated for patients with significant upper GI bleeding due to peptic ulcers. If clinical and endoscopic features suggest a low risk of rebleeding, a ward bed may be acceptable.

PERFORATION

Perforation is heralded by the abrupt onset of severe epigastric pain as gastric or duodenal contents spill into the peritoneal cavity, followed by the development of chemical and then bacterial peritonitis. Patients may not have a history of peptic ulcer disease and may in fact have no history of ulcer-like symptoms. Elderly patients may not have dramatic pain or impressive peritoneal findings.

When the diagnosis is suspected, obtain appropriate laboratory tests, including a CBC, type, and cross-match, and a lipase level determination; place two large-bore IV lines; provide oxygen for hypoxemia, and place a cardiac monitor; insert a nasogastric tube with suction; and obtain an acute abdominal series. Free air is not always evident. Give broad-spectrum antibiotics and obtain a surgical consult promptly. In some cases, nonsurgical therapy has been successful, but operative intervention is the standard in the United States.

OBSTRUCTION

Obstruction occurs because of scarring of the gastric outlet due to chronic peptic ulcer disease, edema due to an active ulcer, or some combination of both. Resulting symptoms include abdominal fullness, nausea, and vomiting, and signs may include abdominal distention and a succussion splash. Dehydration and electrolyte imbalances may occur. Treatment includes rehydration with IV fluids, correction of electrolyte abnormalities, and relief of distention with nasogastric suction. Hospitalization is almost always indicated. The outlet may open as edema subsides, but surgical correction is often necessary.

DISPOSITION AND FOLLOW-UP

Patients with complications always require consultation, and most require admission to an appropriate inpatient unit based on the diagnosis and hemodynamic stability. Most patients with epigastric pain or dyspepsia do not leave the ED with a definitive diagnosis, but, if critical diagnoses (e.g., abdominal aortic aneurysm or myocardial ischemia) are still in the differential, obtain consultation for admission, and further evaluation is indicated. When uncomplicated peptic ulcer disease, gastritis, or dyspepsia is strongly suspected, the great majority of patients can be discharged with acid-suppressive therapy with a PPI or an H_2RA and instructions to follow up with their primary care providers. If alarm features (indicating possible cancer or bleeding) are present, obtain consultation for early endoscopy.

Discharge instructions should include an explanation of the diagnosis and home treatment, specific follow-up instructions, and warning symptoms that should prompt immediate reevaluation. The explanation of the diagnosis should specify that peptic ulcer disease is a presumptive diagnosis and that more definitive diagnostic testing may be necessary. Instructions for home treatment should include a reminder to take medications as directed; a warning against use of alcohol, tobacco products, and aspirin or other NSAIDs; and a recommendation to avoid foods that appear to upset the individual's "stomach." Specific follow-up instructions should include the name and phone number of the appropriate provider whenever possible and a time frame for reevaluation, generally 24 to 48 hours if not improving or 1 to 2 weeks if improving. Warning symptoms that merit immediate reevaluation include those that may be attributed to ulcer complications or confounding illness: worsening pain, increased vomiting, hematemesis or melena, weakness or syncope, fever, chest pain, radiation of pain to the neck or back, and shortness of breath.

REFERENCES

The complete reference list is available online at www.TintinalliEM.com.

Pancreatitis and Cholecystitis

Bart Besinger
Christine R. Stehman

PANCREATITIS

INTRODUCTION/EPIDEMIOLOGY

Pancreatitis is an inflammatory process of the pancreas that may be limited to just the pancreas, may affect surrounding tissues, or may cause remote organ system dysfunction. Most patients will only have one episode of acute pancreatitis, whereas 15% to 30% will have at least one recurrence.[1-3] Between 5% and 25% of patients will ultimately develop chronic pancreatitis.[2,3]

Most cases (~80%) involve only mild inflammation of the pancreas, a disease state with a mortality rate of <1%, which generally resolves with only supportive care.[1,4] A small proportion of patients suffer from more severe disease that may involve pancreatic necrosis, inflammation of surrounding tissues, and organ failure, leading to a 30% mortality rate.[5,6]

The annual incidence of pancreatitis varies among nations and regions. Developed countries have a higher incidence of pancreatitis than developing countries. In general, men and women suffer from acute pancreatitis with equal frequency, although alcohol-associated acute pancreatitis is more common in men, while gallstone-induced pancreatitis is more common in women.[7] Blacks are affected two- to threefold more often than whites but have a mortality rate equal to the general population.[3,8] The incidence of acute pancreatitis varies with age, with a peak in middle age.[9] Other risk factors include smoking, obesity, and diabetes mellitus.[9,10]

Factors associated with acute pancreatitis are listed in **Table 79-1**. Most cases are related to either gallstones or alcohol consumption. About 5% of all patients who undergo endoscopic retrograde cholangiopancreatography for treatment of gallstones develop pancreatitis within 30 days.[11]

The nature of the association between alcohol use and acute pancreatitis is unclear. Some studies suggest that consumption of a large amount of alcohol over a short period of time is a more important factor than chronic alcohol use.[16] However, others suggest that at least 5 years of heavy alcohol use are required before alcohol can reliably be considered the cause.[17]

TABLE 79-1 Causes of Acute Pancreatitis

Common	Gallstones (35%–75%)[9,12]
	Alcohol (25%–35%)[9,12]
	Idiopathic (10%–20%)[13]
Uncommon	Hypertriglyceridemia (triglycerides >1000 milligrams/dL) (1%–4%)[14]
	Endoscopic retrograde cholangiopancreatography[11]
	Drugs (1.4%–2%)
More uncommon (total <8% of cases)	Abdominal trauma
	Postoperative complications
	Hyperparathyroidism
	Infection (bacterial, viral, or parasitic)
	Autoimmune disease
	Tumor (pancreatic, ampullary)
	Hypercalcemia
	Cystic fibrosis
Rare	Ischemia
	Posterior penetrating ulcer
	Toxin exposure
Unknown	Congenital abnormalities[15]

TABLE 79-2 Commonly Used Drugs Associated with Acute Pancreatitis[18,19]
Acetaminophen
Amiodarone
Cannabis
Carbamazepine
Chlorothiazide/hydrochlorothiazide
Codeine (and other opiates)
Dexamethasone (and other steroids)
Enalapril
Estrogens
Erythromycin
Furosemide
Losartan
Methimazole
Metronidazole
Pravastatin/simvastatin
Procainamide
Tetracycline
Trimethoprim-sulfamethoxazole
Tuberculosis antibiotics (dapsone, isoniazid, rifampin)

More than 120 drugs have been linked to acute pancreatitis but together account for fewer than 2% of cases. **Table 79-2** lists the commonly used drugs found by two sets of authors to be most well linked to acute pancreatitis based on number of case reports and recurrence after drug reexposure.[18,19]

PATHOPHYSIOLOGY

The pathophysiology of pancreatitis is not completely understood. Under normal circumstances, trypsinogen is produced in the pancreas and secreted into the duodenum where it is converted into the protease trypsin. In acute pancreatitis, for unclear reasons, trypsin is activated within the pancreatic acinar cells. Activation continues in an unregulated fashion and elimination of activated trypsin is inhibited, resulting in high pancreatic levels of activated trypsin. Activated trypsin in turn activates other digestive enzymes, complements, and kinins, leading to pancreatic autodigestion, injury, and inflammation. Pancreatic injury activates local production of inflammatory mediators, which cause further inflammation.[20,21] Fortunately, most cases never progress beyond local inflammation. However, in a minority of cases, termed necrotizing pancreatitis, pancreatic injury progresses to involve surrounding tissue or possibly remote organ systems.[22] The release of inflammatory mediators from the pancreas, in particular from the acinar cells, and extrapancreatic organs such as the liver leads to remote organ injury and failure, the systemic inflammatory response syndrome, multiorgan failure, and even death.[20-22]

CLINICAL FEATURES

HISTORY AND PHYSICAL EXAMINATION

Acute pancreatitis causes acute, severe, and persistent abdominal pain, usually associated with nausea, vomiting, anorexia, and decreased oral intake.[23] The pain is located in the epigastrium or occasionally in the left or right upper quadrants. Pain may radiate to the back, chest, or flanks. Pain may worsen with oral intake or laying supine and may improve with sitting up with the knees flexed.[24-26] Other symptoms include abdominal swelling, diaphoresis, hematemesis, and shortness of breath. **Pain described as lower abdominal pain or dull or colicky pain is highly unlikely to be pancreatitis.**[25]

The vital signs may be abnormal, with tachycardia, tachypnea, fever, or hypotension. Pain is confined to the epigastrium or upper abdomen, often with guarding and decreased bowel sounds.[23] Occasionally patients will be jaundiced, pale, or diaphoretic.

Rare physical findings associated with late, severe necrotizing pancreatitis include Cullen's sign (bluish discoloration around the umbilicus signifying hemoperitoneum), Grey-Turner sign (reddish-brown discoloration along the flanks signifying retroperitoneal blood or extravasation of pancreatic exudate), and erythematous skin nodules from focal subcutaneous fat necrosis.[26,27]

DIAGNOSIS

Formal diagnosis is based on at least two of three criteria: (1) clinical presentation consistent with acute pancreatitis, (2) a serum lipase or amylase value elevated above the upper limit of normal, or (3) imaging findings characteristic of acute pancreatitis (IV contrast-enhanced CT, MRI, or transabdominal US).[25,28] The differential diagnosis is wide and consists of all causes of upper abdominal pain, as detailed in chapter 71, "Acute Abdominal Pain."

LABORATORY STUDIES

There is no gold standard laboratory diagnosis for acute pancreatitis. Two current guidelines recommend that the amylase or lipase value be at least three times the upper limit of normal;[25,28] some recommend a lipase of two times normal or an amylase of three times normal in a patient with the appropriate clinical presentation;[29] and some recommend that any elevation above normal is consistent with the diagnosis.[23] Normal levels for amylase and lipase are based on values in young, healthy patients, making it difficult to determine applicable levels for older patients or those with multiple comorbidities.[29] Consequently, the combination of an elevated laboratory value with a clinical presentation consistent with pancreatitis is key for diagnosis.[25]

Amylase is not a good choice for diagnosis.[25] Amylase rises within a few hours after the onset of symptoms, peaks within 48 hours, and normalizes in 3 to 5 days.[29] About 20% of patients with pancreatitis, most of whom have alcohol- and hypertriglyceridemia-related disease, will have a normal amylase.[30] This fact, along with the rapid decrease in amylase after symptom onset, gives amylase a sensitivity of about 70%, with a positive predictive value ranging from 15% to 72%. [23] Amylase can be elevated in multiple non–pancreas-related diseases, such as renal insufficiency, salivary gland diseases, acute appendicitis, cholecystitis, intestinal obstruction or ischemia, and gynecologic diseases, lowering specificity for pancreatitis.[23,30]

Lipase is more specific to pancreatic injury and remains elevated for longer after onset of symptoms than amylase. Lipase may be elevated in diabetics at baseline and in other nonpancreatic diseases such as renal disease, appendicitis, and cholecystitis, but it is less associated with nonpancreatic diseases than amylase.[25,31] Lipase is more sensitive in patients with a delayed presentation and in cases of alcoholic or hypertriglyceridemic pancreatitis.[29]

When an elevation of both **lipase and amylase** is required to diagnose pancreatitis, specificity is increased and sensitivity is decreased compared to using either test alone, but there is no evidence that adding amylase to a nondiagnostic lipase improves diagnostic accuracy over lipase alone.[29]

The urine trypsinogen-2 dipstick test is a rapid, noninvasive test with high sensitivity (82%) and specificity (94%).[32] However, given its current limited availability, it is not included as part of the diagnostic criteria for pancreatitis.[28]

In addition to serum lipase and amylase, obtain blood studies to evaluate renal and liver function, electrolyte status, glucose level, WBC count, and hemoglobin/hematocrit. These lab results help the clinician predict disease severity and outcome (detailed below), optimize the clinical status of the patient, identify complications that need immediate treatment (cholangitis, organ failure), and assess effectiveness of treatment.

An **alanine aminotransferase** of >150 U/L within the first 48 hours of symptoms predicts gallstone pancreatitis with a greater than 85% positive predictive value.[33]

IMAGING

Imaging can identify the cause of pancreatitis and can identify complications and severity. For patients with acute pancreatitis where gallstones have not been excluded, obtain a transabdominal US in the ED to detect gallstone pancreatitis.[3,28,34] For any patient with respiratory complaints, obtain a chest radiograph to evaluate for pleural effusions and pulmonary infiltrates, both associated with more severe pancreatitis.

In patients who meet the clinical presentation and laboratory criteria, routine early CT, with or without IV or PO contrast, is not recommended for multiple reasons. Most patients have uncomplicated disease and are readily diagnosed by clinical and laboratory criteria. There is no evidence that early CT, with or without contrast, improves clinical outcomes.[28,35,36] Peripancreatic fluid collections or pancreatic necrosis detected by CT of any kind within the first few days of symptoms generally require no treatment, and the complete extent of these local complications is usually not appreciated until at least 3 days after onset of symptoms. The magnitude of morphologic change on imaging studies does not necessarily correlate with disease severity.[37] Finally, IV contrast infusion can cause allergic reactions, nephrotoxicity, and worsening of pancreatitis.[38]

If the clinical diagnosis of acute pancreatitis is in doubt, consider further evaluation with IV contrast **abdominal CT**. Characteristic findings include: (1) pancreatic parenchymal inflammation with or without peripancreatic fat inflammation; (2) pancreatic parenchymal necrosis or peripancreatic necrosis; (3) peripancreatic fluid collection; or (4) pancreatic pseudocyst.[25,39] **Figure 79-1A–D** compares CT image of a normal pancreas to images in various complications. Although noncontrast MRI is not readily available to the ED, this imaging modality can identify the complications of pancreatitis and choledocholithiasis. It can be an alternative for patients with renal failure, patients who are allergic to IV contrast, or pregnant patients.[40]

TREATMENT

Treatment is supportive and symptomatic therapy (Table 79-3). No specific medication effectively treats acute pancreatitis; however, early aggressive hydration decreases morbidity and mortality.[41-43] The benefit of fluid resuscitation may result from increased micro- and macrocirculatory support of the pancreas, which prevents complications such as pancreatic necrosis.[44]

Provide fluid resuscitation. Fluid loss results from vomiting, third spacing, increased insensible losses, and decreased oral intake. Patients generally need 2.5 to 4 L of fluid with at least one third delivered in the first 12 to 24 hours.[25,28] The specific rate of fluid delivery depends on the patient's clinical status. In the situation of renal or heart failure, deliver fluid more slowly to prevent complications such as volume overload, pulmonary edema, and abdominal compartment syndrome. Crystalloids are the resuscitation fluids of choice. Normal saline in large volumes may cause a nongap hyperchloremic acidosis and can worsen pancreatitis, possibly by activating trypsinogen and making acinar cells more susceptible to injury.[25,45] A single randomized study showed a decreased incidence of systemic inflammatory response syndrome in patients who received lactated Ringer's instead of 0.9% normal saline.[45] Regardless of which fluid is selected, monitor vital signs and urine output as responses to hydration.

Control pain and nausea. Pain control is best achieved with IV opioid analgesics. Initially, place patients on NPO (nothing by mouth) status and administer antiemetics. There is no benefit to nasogastric intubation.

Prolonged bowel and pancreas rest increases gut atrophy and bacterial translocation, leading to infection and increasing morbidity and mortality.[46] In the ED, if nausea and vomiting have resolved and pain has decreased, transition the patient to oral pain medications and small amounts of food.[47] A low-fat solid foods diet provides more calories than a clear liquid diet and is safe.[48]

Acute pancreatitis by itself is not a source of infection, and prophylactic use of antibiotics and antifungals is not recommended.[49] Administer antibiotics if a source of infection is demonstrated, such as cholangitis, urinary tract infection, pneumonia, or infected pancreatic necrosis.[49]

SEVERITY CLASSIFICATIONS OF ACUTE PANCREATITIS

Although most patients with acute pancreatitis have mild uncomplicated disease, a small percentage of patients have more severe disease. In the ED, it is difficult to distinguish disease severity, because most patients present so early in the disease course that complications that define moderately severe or severe disease are not evident. Moderately severe acute pancreatitis is characterized by transient organ failure (<48 hours), local complications, or systemic complications. Severe disease includes one or more local or systemic complications and persistent organ failure (>48 hours). Critical acute pancreatitis is persistent organ failure and infected pancreatic necrosis.[50]

Local complications involve the pancreas and surrounding tissues and include acute peripancreatic fluid collections, pancreatic pseudocyst, acute pancreatic or peripancreatic necrosis, walled off necrosis, gastric outlet dysfunction, splenic and portal vein thrombosis, and colonic inflammation/necrosis.[22] These are not usually well demonstrated on CT scan until at least 72 hours after the onset of symptoms. Suspect local complications in patients who have persistent or recurrent abdominal pain, an increase in pancreatic enzyme levels after an initial decrease, new or worsening organ dysfunction, or sepsis (fever, increased WBC count).

Organ failure can be seen in any system, but three organ systems are particularly susceptible: cardiovascular, respiratory, and renal. Because of the susceptibility of these three organ systems, pay special attention during the patient's initial evaluation.

Other possible complications of acute pancreatitis are listed in **Table 79-4.**

PREDICTION OF DISEASE SEVERITY

A number of different scoring systems exist, including the Ranson criteria, Acute Physiology and Chronic Health Examination-II, modified Glasgow score, Bedside Index for Severity in Acute Pancreatitis, and Balthazar CT Severity Index. These scoring systems include many data points, some of which are not collected until at least 48 hours after presentation, limiting their utility in the ED.[51] None of these scoring systems is superior to another.[52] **Systemic inflammatory response syndrome at admission and persistent at 48 hours predicts severe acute pancreatitis more simply and as accurately as the various scoring systems.[6,52,53] Besides systemic inflammatory response syndrome, a number of other clinical findings at initial assessment are associated with severe disease. These findings include patient characteristics (age >55 years, obesity, altered mental status, comorbidities), laboratory findings (BUN >20 milligrams/dL or rising; hematocrit >44% or rising; increased creatinine), and radiologic findings (many or large extrapancreatic fluid collections, pleural effusions, pulmonary infiltrates).[22,41,54]**

Overall, acute pancreatitis has a mortality rate of approximately 1%.[4] Moderately severe and severe disease mortality rates are 5% and 30%, respectively.[6,55] Most patients who die do so from multiorgan failure. The sensitivity of systemic inflammatory response syndrome on admission for mortality is 100% with a specificity of 31%, whereas the sensitivity and specificity of systemic inflammatory response syndrome at 48 hours (persistent systemic inflammatory response syndrome) are 77% to 89% and 79% to 86%, respectively.[6,53] Systemic inflammatory response syndrome at admission and 48 hours, combined with patient characteristics (age, comorbidities, and obesity) and response to treatment, helps predict outcome.

DISPOSITION AND FOLLOW-UP

Patients with nonbiliary pancreatitis whose pain can be controlled in the ED and who can tolerate oral feeding can be discharged. Patients who are discharged from the ED should be referred for appropriate follow-up to help prevent recurrence.

Consider **admission for a first bout of acute pancreatitis, for any case of biliary pancreatitis, and for patients needing frequent IV pain medication, not tolerating oral intake because of vomiting or increasing pain, with persistent abnormal vital signs, or with any signs of organ insufficiency (e.g., increased creatinine).**

Admit to the intensive care unit a patient with severe pancreatitis or anyone who meets local criteria for an intensive care unit admission. Any patient who has any signs, symptoms, laboratory values, or imaging results suggesting the need for intensive care should also receive consideration for intensive care unit admission or at least an intermediate care unit admission.

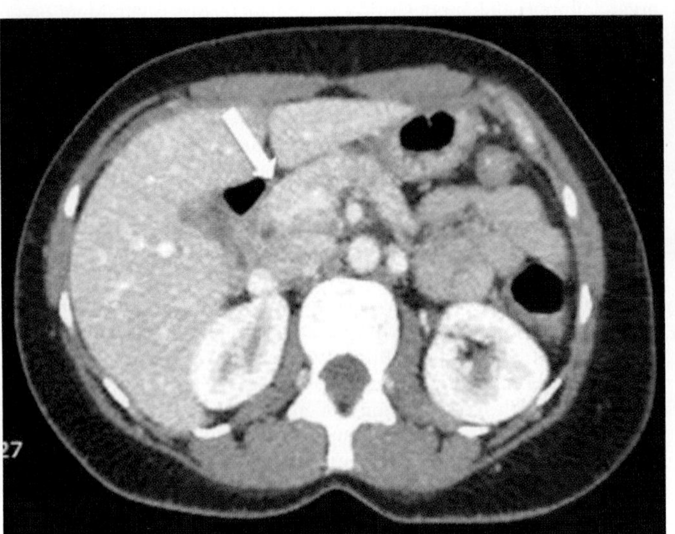

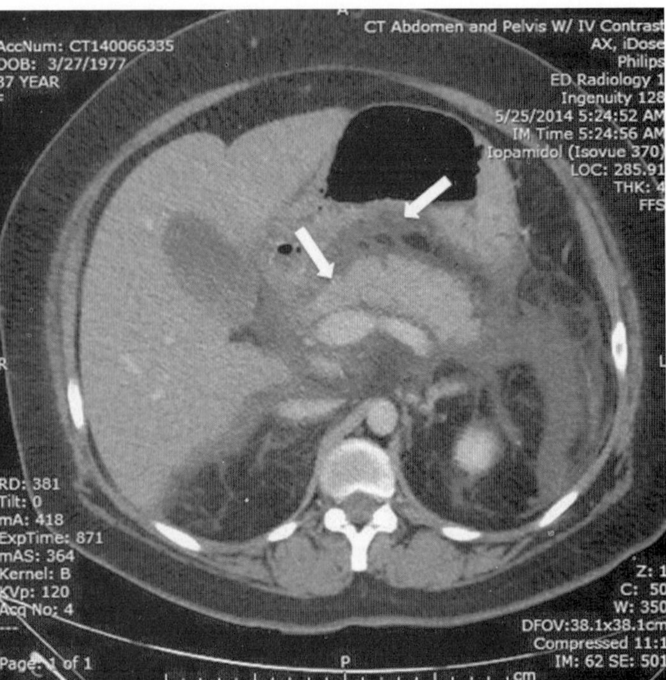

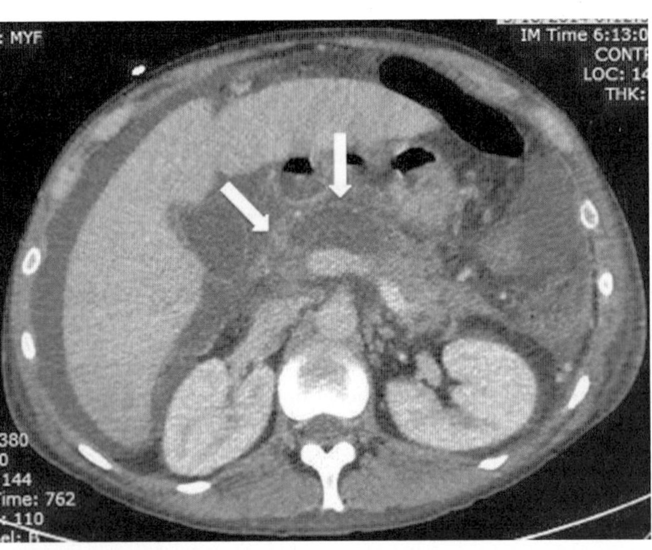

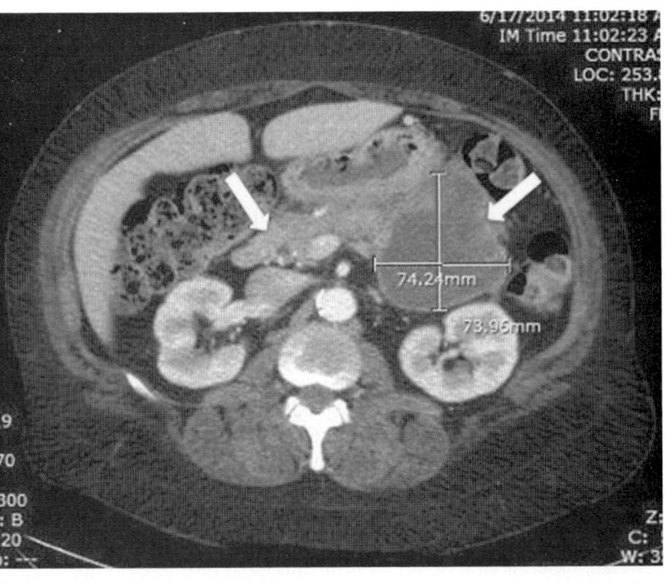

FIGURE 79-1. Abdominal IV contrast-enhanced CT scans showing: **A.** normal pancreas (*arrow*) with smooth outer contours, clear demarcation between pancreas and surrounding tissues, and without peripancreatic fluid; **B.** mild pancreatitis with indistinct pancreatic borders (*left arrow*), pancreatic edema, and peripancreatic fluid (*right arrow*); **C.** edematous pancreas with indistinct borders (*left arrow*) and area of nonenhancing parenchyma pancreatic necrosis with area of acute pancreatic necrosis (low attenuation representing nonenhancing parenchyma; *right arrow*); and **D.** edematous pancreas with indistinct pancreatic borders (*left arrow*) and a pseudocyst in the pancreatic tail (*right arrow*). [Images contributed by Bart Besinger, MD, FAAEM.]

Biliary pancreatitis requires either admission by surgeon or early surgical consultation for consideration of early cholecystectomy.[56] Cholecystectomies in patients not suffering from documented gallstone pancreatitis are associated with increased recurrence of acute pancreatitis.[57]

Patients with cholangitis or known biliary obstruction on admission may benefit from early endoscopic retrograde cholangiopancreatography.[58] Early routine endoscopic retrograde cholangiopancreatography in patients without one of these two complications does not improve mortality or modify or prevent local complications.[58]

SPECIAL CONSIDERATIONS

MEDICATIONS

Medications associated with acute pancreatitis can be categorized into three groups: antiretrovirals, chemotherapy, and immunosuppressants. Patients taking these medications are at particular risk of severe disease because of the underlying disease combined with the medication side effects. 2′,3′-Dideoxyinosine can cause potentially fatal pancreatitis, whereas patients receiving the antiretrovirals lamivudine and nelfinavir are at lower risk.[18,19]

TABLE 79-3 Treatment of Acute Pancreatitis

Treatment	Comments
Aggressive crystalloid therapy	Lactated Ringer's preferably 2.5–4 L, at least 250–500 mL/h or 5–10 mL/kg/h Use caution in congestive heart failure, renal insufficiency Monitor response: – Hematocrit 35%–44% – Maintain normal creatinine – Heart rate <120 beats/min – Mean arterial pressure 65–85 mm Hg – Urine output 0.5–1 mL/kg/h (if no renal failure)
Vital signs/pulse oximetry	Monitor closely/frequently; initially at least every 2 h, but patients may require more frequent monitoring
Electrolyte repletion	Correct low ionized calcium, hypomagnesemia Control hyperglycemia
Pain control	Parenteral narcotics
Supplemental oxygen	As needed for respiratory insufficiency
Antiemetics	Control nausea/vomiting NPO status Nasogastric tube/suction typically not indicated
Antibiotics	If known or strongly suspected infection, give appropriate antibiotics based on cause Prophylactic antibiotics and antibiotics for mild pancreatitis not indicated
Consultation for endoscopic retrograde cholangiopancreatography	In first 24 h for those with documented biliary obstruction or cholangitis

Abbreviation: NPO = nothing by mouth.

Cancer patients undergoing chemotherapy with one or more of seven medications have a risk of pancreatitis complicating the disease course. These medications are L-asparaginase, cisplatin, cytarabine, ifosfamide, mercaptopurine, pegaspargase, and tamoxifen.[18,19] These agents are used to treat leukemias, lymphomas, sarcomas, and breast, cervical, lung, ovarian, and testicular cancers.

Patients receiving azathioprine for posttransplantation immunosuppression or treatment of inflammatory diseases such as rheumatoid arthritis and inflammatory bowel disease are also at risk of developing pancreatitis.[18,19]

CHRONIC PANCREATITIS

Chronic pancreatitis is a continuum of acute pancreatitis. From 5% to 25% of patients can progress to chronic pancreatitis.[2,3] Progression is most common in alcohol-induced disease, but may happen in any situation.[2,3]

Attacks are similar to acute pancreatitis. The goal of treatment is hydration and pain and nausea control. The mortality risk of chronic pancreatitis recurrences is generally lower than that of acute pancreatitis.[2,3]

CHOLECYSTITIS

INTRODUCTION AND EPIDEMIOLOGY

Cholecystitis is inflammation of the gallbladder that is usually caused by an obstructing gallstone.

Gallstones produce disease states, including acute calculous cholecystitis, that vary considerably in their severity, clinical presentation, and management strategies. In the United States, the prevalence of gallstones is 8% among men and 17% among women.[59] Prevalence increases with age and with increasing body mass index. Bariatric surgery is also a risk factor for the development of gallstones.[60] The vast majority of gallstones are asymptomatic. *Asymptomatic gallstones* may be discovered incidentally on diagnostic imaging performed for another purpose. The risk of developing symptoms or complications is 1% to 4% per year.[61]

Biliary colic is the most common complication of gallstone disease. Patients experience recurrent attacks of steady upper abdominal pain that typically last no more than a few hours and resolve spontaneously when the gallstone moves from its obstructing position. If the obstructing stone remains in place, acute cholecystitis may develop over time as the gallbladder becomes distended, inflamed, and in some cases infected. As acute cholecystitis evolves, it may result in necrosis and gangrene of the gallbladder wall (**gangrenous cholecystitis**). **Emphysematous cholecystitis** occurs when the inflamed gallbladder becomes infected with gas-producing organisms. **Gallbladder perforation** is an uncommon but life-threatening complication of cholecystitis. Gangrenous cholecystitis, emphysematous cholecystitis, and gallbladder perforation may occur with or without the presence of gallstones.

Choledocholithiasis, gallstones within the common bile duct, may be either primary (arising from within the bile ducts) or, more commonly, secondary (forming in the gallbladder and then migrating to the common bile duct). Choledocholithiasis or other causes of common bile duct obstruction, such as stricture or tumor, may be complicated by *cholangitis*, an infection of the biliary tree. **Chronic cholecystitis** is a state of prolonged gallbladder inflammation typically caused by recurrent episodes of cystic duct obstruction by gallstones. Fibrotic thickening of the gallbladder wall develops. **Biliary sludge** is

TABLE 79-4 Complications of Acute Pancreatitis

Pancreatic	Peripancreatic	Extrapancreatic	
Fluid collection Necrosis Sterile or infected Acute or walled off Abscess Ascites	Fluid collection Necrosis Intra-abdominal or retroperitoneal hemorrhage Pseudoaneurysm (of contiguous visceral arteries, e.g., the splenic) Bowel inflammation, infarction, or necrosis Biliary obstruction with jaundice Splenic or portal vein thrombosis	*Cardiovascular* Hypotension Hypovolemia Myocardial depression Myocardial infarction Pericardial effusion *Pulmonary* Hypoxemia Atelectasis Pleural effusion (with or without fistula) Pulmonary infiltrates Acute respiratory distress syndrome Respiratory failure *Hematologic* Disseminated intravascular coagulation	*GI* Peptic ulcer disease/erosive gastritis GI perforation GI bleeding Duodenal or stomach obstruction Splenic infarction *Renal* Oliguria Azotemia Acute renal failure Thrombosis of renal artery or vein *Metabolic* Hyperglycemia Hypocalcemia Hypertriglyceridemia

TABLE 79-5 Gallstone Types

	Cholesterol Stones	Pigment Stones
Composition	Cholesterol monohydrate crystals	Black: Calcium bilirubinate Brown: Mixed composition; usually occur in setting of bacterial or helminthic infection of bile
Relative frequency	80%	20%
Radiographic appearance	Radiolucent	Radiopaque
Typical patients	Obese, female, elderly, rapid weight loss	Black: Chronic liver disease or hemolytic disease Brown: Bile duct stasis (sclerosing cholangitis, strictures); more common in Asia

microlithiasis composed of cholesterol crystals, calcium bilirubinate pigment, and other calcium salts. It may be seen on CT or US. The clinical course of biliary sludge is variable. It may resolve spontaneously or progress to cause complications including biliary colic, cholecystitis, cholangitis, or pancreatitis. **Acute acalculous cholecystitis** occurs in the absence of gallstones. It occurs much less commonly than calculous cholecystitis but is more likely to result in complications. It tends to occur in the setting of critical illness such as septic shock, burns, and major trauma or surgery. Old age, diabetes, and immunosuppression are also risk factors.

PATHOPHYSIOLOGY

Bile is produced by hepatocytes and transported via the biliary system to the small intestine where bile acids are necessary for the digestion and absorption of lipids. Bile is also the vehicle for eliminating a number of substances from the body including bile pigments (e.g., bilirubin), cholesterol, and some drugs. Bile is stored and concentrated in the gallbladder. When a meal is eaten, the gallbladder is provoked to contract by cholecystokinin and neural stimulation, resulting in the expulsion of bile into the cystic duct and then to the common bile duct, where it reaches the duodenum at the sphincter of Oddi.

Gallstone formation is a multifactorial process that involves supersaturation of bile components, crystal nucleation, and gallbladder dysmotility.[62] Gallstones are classified based on their composition into two categories: pigment stones and cholesterol stones. Pigment stones may be further divided into brown and black stones (**Table 79-5**).

Nonobstructing gallstones typically do not cause symptoms. As gallstones migrate through the biliary tree, they can obstruct the gallbladder neck, cystic duct, or common bile duct. The resultant distention and increased intraluminal pressure cause pain, nausea, and vomiting. Symptoms are relieved if the gallstone returns to a nonobstructing position within the gallbladder lumen or if it passes through the biliary tree into the duodenum. If the obstruction does not resolve, inflammation results from a complex process that involves mechanical distention, ischemia, and inflammatory mediators including prostaglandins. Interestingly, this long-held notion that gallbladder outlet obstruction is the inciting event in acute cholecystitis has been recently challenged.[63]

Bile cultures are positive in about half of patients with acute cholecystitis.[64-66] Gram-negative organisms predominate (*Escherichia coli*, 39%; *Klebsiella*, 35%), although gram-positive (*Streptococcus*, 18%; *Enterococcus*, 17%) and anaerobic (*Clostridia*, 14%; *Bacteroides*. 3%) infections occur as well.[65] Polymicrobial infections are common.

CLINICAL FEATURES

HISTORY

Biliary colic presents with pain in the epigastrium or right upper quadrant of the abdomen that occasionally radiates to the back. Despite its name, the pain of biliary colic is more often described as steady than colicky. The pain is often accompanied by nausea and vomiting. Its association with food intake is variable. Fatty food intolerance is not a reliable predictor of gallstone presence.[67,68] Biliary colic demonstrates significant circadian periodicity, with a peak in symptom occurrence around midnight.[69]

Symptoms of biliary colic typically last a few hours or less. If pain persists longer, gallstone complications of greater severity, such as acute cholecystitis or cholangitis, must be considered. In acute cholecystitis, pain becomes more localized to the right upper quadrant and increases in severity as peritoneal irritation occurs.[70]

PHYSICAL EXAMINATION

Patients with biliary colic typically have mild right upper quadrant tenderness without peritoneal signs. In acute cholecystitis, tenderness is more severe and may occasionally be accompanied by rigidity or rebound tenderness. Murphy's sign (the sudden cessation of deep inspiration due to pain when examining fingers reach the inflamed gallbladder upon palpation of the right subcostal region) is 65% sensitive and 87% specific for acute cholecystitis.[71] Patients with biliary colic are afebrile. Fever is classically described in acute cholecystitis but is in fact present in only about one third of cases.[71] Jaundice is rarely seen in acute cholecystitis. Jaundice in the setting of biliary tract stone disease implies an obstruction of the common bile duct from choledocholithiasis or extrinsic compression of the bile duct by an impacted cystic duct or gallbladder stone or adjacent inflammation (Mirizzi's syndrome).

DIAGNOSIS

The diagnosis of gallstones can be readily established with radiographic studies. However, it is incumbent upon the emergency physician to distinguish the patient with simple biliary colic from the patient with a more serious gallstone complication such as acute cholecystitis, choledocholithiasis, cholangitis, or gallstone pancreatitis.

Establishing the diagnosis of acute cholecystitis requires the integration of data from the history and physical examination with the results of laboratory and radiographic studies. There is no single clinical or laboratory finding that can be relied upon to rule in or rule out the diagnosis.[71] Diagnostic criteria for acute cholecystitis have been proposed (**Table 79-6**).[72]

The classic presentation of cholangitis is *Charcot's triad*: fever, right upper quadrant abdominal pain, and jaundice. It is present in slightly more than half of the cases.[73] Most patients will have a fever and right upper quadrant pain; the presence of jaundice is less common, occurring in about two thirds of patients. *Reynolds' pentad* adds altered mental status and shock to Charcot's triad.[74] It is seen in less than 10% of patients with cholangitis.[73]

The differential diagnosis of acute cholecystitis includes other diseases of the biliary tract such as biliary colic, choledocholithiasis, and

TABLE 79-6 Diagnostic Criteria for Acute Cholecystitis*

Local signs	Murphy's sign
	Right upper quadrant mass, pain, or tenderness
Systemic signs	Fever
	Elevated C-reactive protein
	Elevated WBC count
Imaging	Imaging findings characteristic of acute cholecystitis (see Table 79-7)
Diagnosis	Suspected: One local sign and one systemic sign Definite: One local sign, one systemic sign, and imaging findings of acute cholecystitis
Accuracy	Sensitivity 91.2%, specificity 96.9% for definite diagnosis criteria compared with surgical pathology gold standard

*Acute hepatitis, chronic cholecystitis, and other acute abdominal disorders should be excluded.

cholangitis and other conditions of the GI tract such as pancreatitis, hepatitis, peptic ulcer disease, gastritis, and functional dyspepsia. Appendicitis may occasionally present with right upper quadrant pain. Chest disease such as pneumonia, pleurisy, or pulmonary embolism may present with pain of the upper abdomen.

LABORATORY TESTING

Laboratory tests are typically normal in biliary colic. A leukocytosis may be seen in acute cholecystitis, but its absence does not exclude the diagnosis. A leukocyte count of >10,000/mm^3 has a 63% sensitivity, 57% specificity, positive likelihood ratio of 1.5, and negative likelihood ratio of 0.6.[71] The mean leukocyte count in cholecystitis is 12,600/mm^3.[75] Elevation of C-reactive protein is associated with acute cholecystitis but is nonspecific.[76]

Liver function tests, including bilirubin, alanine aminotransferase, aspartate aminotransferase, alkaline phosphatase, and γ-glutamyl transpeptidase, are often normal in acute cholecystitis. They are more likely to be elevated in the setting of choledocholithiasis or other cause of bile duct obstruction.[77,78] Abnormal γ-glutamyl transpeptidase is the most sensitive and specific serum marker of choledocholithiasis.[79] Marked elevations (>1000 IU/L) of alanine aminotransferase or aspartate aminotransferase can occur in the setting of choledocholithiasis but are more suggestive of a hepatocellular necrotic process.[80]

IMAGING

Plain radiography of the abdomen is of minimal value in assessing for biliary tract stone disease. Most gallstones do not contain sufficient amounts of calcium to be visible on plain x-rays. Plain radiography may demonstrate biliary tree air reflective of emphysematous cholecystitis or biliary-enteric fistula, but these are better and more reliably demonstrated with other imaging modalities.

Ultrasound **Abdominal US (Figure 79-2) is the imaging modality of choice for acute cholecystitis.**[81] Its sensitivity and specificity for acute cholecystitis are 81% and 83%, respectively.[82] Advantages of US include its availability, lack of ionizing radiation, short study time, excellent sensitivity for gallstones, and ability to elicit tenderness with placement of the US probe. Sonographic Murphy's sign, maximal tenderness over a sonographically identified gallbladder, is particularly important in the US diagnosis of cholecystitis. The presence of gallstones and a sonographic Murphy's sign has a positive predictive value of 92% for acute cholecystitis. The absence of both gallstones and the sonographic Murphy's sign has a negative predictive value of 95%.[83] Gallbladder wall thickening and pericholecystic fluid are relatively nonspecific for cholecystitis and may result instead from conditions such as ascites, heart failure, liver disease, or pancreatitis.

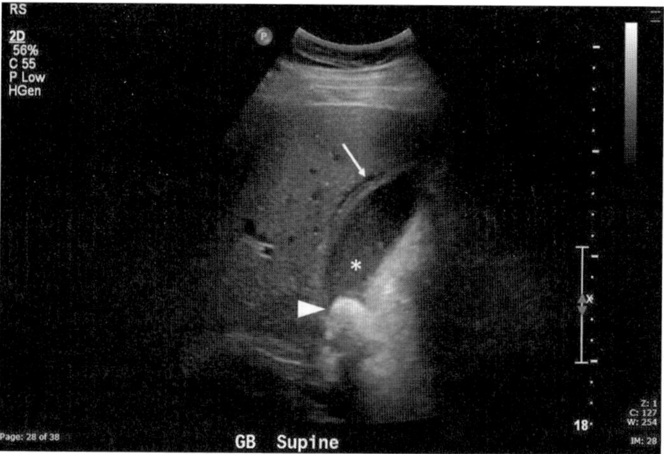

FIGURE 79-2. Abdominal US demonstrating acute cholecystitis with a gallstone (*arrowhead*), gallbladder sludge (*asterisk*), and pericholecystic fluid (*arrow*). [Image contributed by Bart Besinger, MD, FAAEM.]

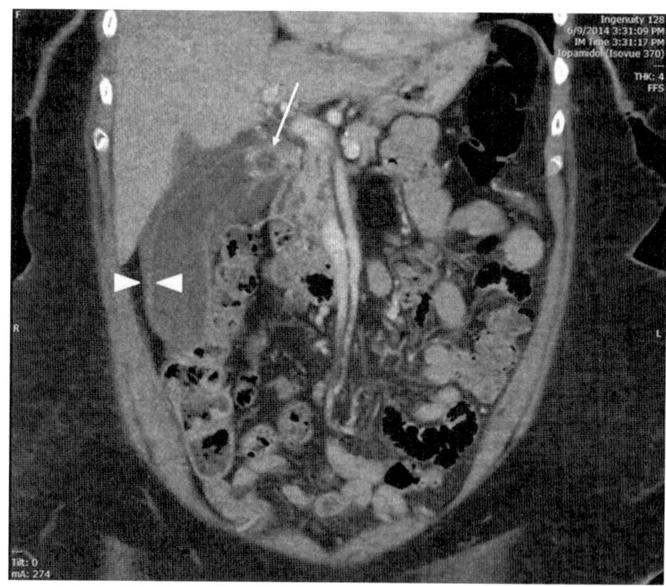

FIGURE 79-3. Enhanced abdominal CT showing acute cholecystitis with a radiodense gallstone at the gallbladder neck (*arrow*) and a thickened gallbladder wall (*arrowheads*). [Image contributed by Bart Besinger, MD, FAAEM.]

Bedside US of the right upper quadrant performed by emergency physicians is a useful modality for the diagnosis of cholelithiasis.[84] Its accuracy for diagnosing acute cholecystitis has been questioned.[85,86] However, in the hands of emergency physicians who are highly trained in its use, point-of-care US for cholecystitis is comparable to that performed by US technicians and interpreted by radiologists.[87]

CT, MRI, and Hepatobiliary Iminodiacetic Acid Scanning Acute cholecystitis may be demonstrated on IV contrast-enhanced **abdominal CT**, although the sensitivity and specificity of CT for cholecystitis are ill-defined (**Figure 79-3**). Limitations of CT include its relative insensitivity (~75%) for gallstones and its inability to detect a Murphy's sign.[88] IV contrast-enhanced CT may reveal complications of cholecystitis, such as gangrenous cholecystitis, emphysematous cholecystitis, gallstone ileus, and gallbladder perforation, that are not as reliably demonstrated on US.[89]

Technetium-99m hepatobiliary iminodiacetic acid cholescintigraphy is 96% sensitive and 90% specific for acute cholecystitis.[82] An injected radiotracer is excreted by the liver into bile, allowing visualization of the bile ducts and gallbladder. In acute cholecystitis, the obstructed cystic duct results in nonvisualization of the gallbladder. Cholescintigraphy may also reveal delayed gallbladder emptying (*biliary dyskinesia*). Cholescintigraphy requires hours to perform, limiting its use in the ED.

MRI, including magnetic resonance cholangiopancreatography, may be used to evaluate the gallbladder and biliary tree. The sensitivity and specificity of IV gadolinium-enhanced MRI for cholecystitis are similar to those of US.[82] MRI, however, demonstrates more consistent visualization of the biliary tree, has less interpreter variability, and is a useful alternative to those patients who are difficult to examine with US.[81]

Imaging for Choledocholithiasis Choledocholithiasis is difficult to exclude with US or CT. US fails to visualize the entire extrahepatic biliary tree in many patients and has a sensitivity for choledocholithiasis of about 60%.[90] CT, although limited by its inability to detect poorly calcified stones, performs somewhat better than US.[91,92] On either US or CT, the combined findings of gallbladder stones and common bile duct dilation provide indirect evidence of choledocholithiasis. Normal common bile duct diameter is <5 mm, although diameter is increased in patients with prior cholecystectomy and in the elderly. More definitive evaluation for choledocholithiasis can be accomplished by magnetic resonance cholangiopancreatography, endoscopic US, or endoscopic retrograde cholangiopancreatography.

Imaging findings in acute cholecystitis are summarized in **Table 79-7**.

TABLE 79-7 Imaging for Acute Cholecystitis

Modality	Findings	Comment
US	Sonographic Murphy's sign Gallbladder wall thickening >3 mm Pericholecystic fluid Gallbladder distention: short axis >40 mm	Preferred initial imaging test.
CT	Gallbladder wall thickening >3 mm Pericholecystic fluid Pericholecystic fat stranding Hyperdense gallbladder wall Gallbladder distention	Demonstrates complications such as gangrene, gas formation, and perforation. Insensitive for gallstones. Useful in evaluating alternative diagnoses.
HIDA	Nonvisualization of gallbladder	Excellent sensitivity and specificity. Time consuming, limited availability, ionizing radiation.
MRI/MRCP	Gallbladder wall thickening >3 mm Pericholecystic fluid Pericholecystic fat signal changes Gallbladder distention: short axis >40 mm	Specificity and sensitivity similar to US. Excellent visualization of biliary tree. Time consuming, limited availability.

Abbreviations: HIDA = hepatobiliary iminodiacetic acid cholescintigraphy; MRCP = magnetic resonance cholangiopancreatography.

TREATMENT

Asymptomatic gallstones generally require no treatment. Elective cholecystectomy is occasionally recommended for those at high risk for gallstone complications such as patients with sickle cell disease, patients with planned organ transplantation, or those belonging to ethnic groups at high risk for gallbladder cancer.

ED management of **biliary colic** includes symptom control and referral to a general surgeon for outpatient laparoscopic cholecystectomy. Symptom management in the ED includes antiemetics and analgesics. Nonsteroidal anti-inflammatory drugs are first-line therapy. The analgesic efficacy of parenteral nonsteroidal anti-inflammatory drugs is comparable to that of opioids in biliary colic. Additionally, nonsteroidal anti-inflammatory drugs decrease the frequency of short-term gallstone complications such as cholecystitis.[93] Opioid analgesics are often required for pain control. All opioids cause some degree of sphincter of Oddi spasm and increase in biliary pressure.[94] The clinical significance of this is unclear, and there is no evidence that any particular opioid drug is superior in treating the pain of biliary colic. Anticholinergic agents such as atropine and glycopyrrolate do not improve biliary colic pain.[95,96]

Acute cholecystitis and its complications are managed in the hospital with surgical consultation. Early laparoscopic cholecystectomy is often the treatment of choice. ED treatment includes the provision of analgesia, administration of antiemetics for nausea and vomiting, cessation of oral intake, volume and electrolyte replacement, and administration of antibiotics. Appropriate antibiotic regimens include second- and third-generation cephalosporins, carbapenems, β-lactam/β-lactamase inhibitor combinations, or the combination of metronidazole and a fluoroquinolone.[97-99] The value of antibiotics in mild acute cholecystitis has recently been questioned.[100]

Cholangitis can be a life-threatening disease that demands aggressive care including generous fluid resuscitation, the timely administration of antibiotics, and early biliary decompression. Endoscopic retrograde cholangiopancreatography is the decompression procedure of choice in most instances, and when cholangitis is suspected, emergency consultation with a GI surgeon or gastroenterologist is needed. Percutaneous or surgical drainage is an alternative when endoscopic retrograde cholangiopancreatography is not feasible or is unsuccessful.

DISPOSITION AND FOLLOW-UP

Once symptoms are adequately controlled, patients with biliary colic are typically discharged from the ED to follow up with a general surgeon. They should be instructed to return to the ED if symptoms of gallstone complications (e.g., prolonged pain, fever, jaundice) arise. Patients who present to the ED with acute cholecystitis or cholangitis require hospital admission. For suspected cholangitis, emergency consultation or transfer to an institution with treatment capabilities for endoscopic retrograde cholangiopancreatography is necessary. Patients with severe illness, including many with cholangitis, should be admitted to a critical care unit.

SPECIAL CONSIDERATIONS

Emphysematous cholecystitis is characterized by gas in the gallbladder wall or lumen resulting from infection with gas-producing organisms such as *Clostridium* species, *E. coli*, and *Klebsiella* species (**Figure 79-4**). It is associated with underlying diabetes and is more common in older patients. Its association with gallstones is variable. Gas occupying the gallbladder may be seen on plain x-rays, US, or, more reliably, IV contrast-enhanced CT. Emphysematous cholecystitis is notable for a 15% mortality, which is much higher than the mortality rate in uncomplicated cholecystitis.[101] In addition to broad-spectrum antibiotics, patients with emphysematous cholecystitis require prompt surgical consultation and consideration for urgent cholecystectomy. Percutaneous cholecystostomy is an alternative therapy for severely ill patients.

Gallstone ileus is a mechanical small bowel obstruction caused by an ectopic gallstone that has reached the intestinal lumen via a biliary-enteric fistula. Such a fistula may occur in the setting of inflammation secondary to cholecystitis. Gallstone ileus may be diagnosed on plain films of the abdomen or, more dependably, with CT. The classic radiographic appearance is Rigler's triad: a small bowel obstruction, pneumobilia, and an ectopic gallstone.[102] Operative therapy is typically indicated.

Acalculous cholecystitis represents a small minority of cholecystitis cases and most often occurs in the inpatient setting among patients with critical illness. Nevertheless, it may be occasionally encountered in the ED, particularly in immunocompromised patients. Diagnosis is challenging because the clinical presentation is variable and no test result is pathognomonic. US, IV contrast-enhanced CT, and cholescintigraphy are helpful in establishing the diagnosis, but sensitivity and specificity are less than for calculous cholecystitis. Acalculous cholecystitis runs a more fulminant course than cholecystitis associated with gallstones.

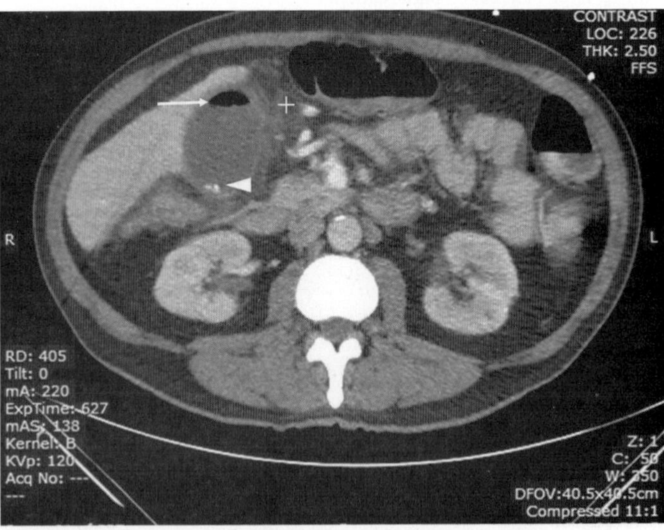

FIGURE 79-4. Contrast-enhanced abdominal CT showing emphysematous cholecystitis with gallstones (*arrowhead*), intraluminal gallbladder gas (*arrow*), and pericholecystic inflammatory changes (*plus sign*). [Images contributed by Bart Besinger, MD, FAAEM.]

Complications such as gangrene and perforation are common, and mortality is high.[103]

Chronic cholecystitis is gallbladder inflammation and scarring that occurs over time, usually secondary to intermittent cystic duct obstruction. It presents in a manner similar to biliary colic or acute cholecystitis, although symptoms and examination findings may be more subtle. Patients may report recurrent episodes of pain.

Postcholecystectomy syndrome refers to a heterogeneous group of disorders that present with persistent abdominal symptoms after removal of the gallbladder. In the early postcholecystectomy period, bile leak is the principal concern. Choledocholithiasis is a common cause of postcholecystectomy pain. Symptom-producing common bile duct stones may be "retained" (present at the time of surgery) or may develop postoperatively, formed primarily in the bile ducts often in the setting of bile stasis.[104] Postcholecystectomy syndrome may result from nonbiliary pain that was erroneously attributed to a biliary cause and therefore not remedied by cholecystectomy.

PRACTICE GUIDELINES

- Tenner S, Baillie J, DeWitt J, et al: American College of Gastroenterology guideline: management of acute pancreatitis. *Am J Gastroenterol* 108: 1400, 2013.
- Working Group IAP/APA Acute Pancreatitis Guidelines: IAP/APA evidence-based guidelines for the management of acute pancreatitis. *Pancreatology* 13: e1, 2013.
- Yarmish GM, Smith MP, Rosen MP, et al: ACR appropriateness criteria right upper quadrant pain. *J Am Coll Radiol* 11: 316, 2014.
- Yokoe M, Takada T, Strasberg S, et al: New diagnostic criteria and severity assessment of acute cholecystitis in revised Tokyo guidelines. *J Hepatobiliary Pancreat Sci* 19: 578, 2012.

REFERENCES

The complete reference list is available online at www.TintinalliEM.com.

Hepatic Disorders

Susan R. O'Mara
Kulleni Gebreyes

INTRODUCTION AND EPIDEMIOLOGY

This chapter discusses the ED presentation, evaluation, and treatment of acute and chronic liver disease as well as fulminant liver failure. Specific entities addressed in this chapter include viral and toxic hepatitis, nonalcoholic fatty liver disease (NAFLD), nonalcoholic steatohepatitis (NASH), and complications of cirrhosis including coagulopathy, ascites, spontaneous bacterial peritonitis, hepatorenal syndrome, and hepatic encephalopathy. Cholecystitis and biliary colic are addressed in chapter 79, "Pancreatitis and Cholecystitis." Variceal bleeding is addressed in chapter 75, "Upper Gastrointestinal Bleeding."

Liver disease is associated with many ED complaints: abdominal pain, vomiting, shortness of breath, altered mental status, GI bleeding, and even nonspecific malaise can all be attributed to malfunction of the liver. Globally, hepatitis A, B, C, D, and E are major public health problems. About two billion people are infected with hepatitis B and 150 million with hepatitis C, and cancer and cirrhosis resulting from these infections account for about 3% of deaths worldwide.[1] Cirrhosis is the 12th leading cause of death in the United States, and hepatitis C is the leading cause of cirrhosis in the United States, followed by alcoholic liver disease.[2] Acute, or fulminant, liver failure is uncommon and is caused primarily by acetaminophen poisoning (46%), with hepatitis B being the most common infectious cause.[3]

PATHOPHYSIOLOGY

Acute hepatitis is caused by an infectious, toxic, or metabolic injury to hepatocytes. The initial injury leads to inflammation, cellular death, and eventual scarring in the liver. In chronic disease, liver parenchyma is replaced by fibrous tissue, which separates the functioning hepatocytes into isolated nodules. This disruption of the normal tissue structure can become severe and lead to the central characteristics of liver failure: loss of metabolic and synthetic function at the cellular level, progressive development of portal hypertension, ascites formation, and portal-systemic shunting at the gross level.

The liver's synthetic functions include the production of **coagulation and anticoagulation factors.** The liver is responsible for production of the vitamin K–dependent clotting factors II, VII, IX, and X; proteins C and S; and other elements of the clotting and thrombolytic processes.[4] Inadequate production of these clotting factors makes uncontrolled bleeding one of the life-threatening features of liver disease and a potentially dramatic complication of hepatic failure.

Portal hypertension is increased hydrostatic pressure in the portal vein and its feeder vessels, caused by resistance to blood flow through the cirrhotic liver. It eventually causes esophageal and gastric varices and portal-systemic shunting. The increased hydrostatic pressure in the intraperitoneal veins, hypoalbuminemia, and poor renal management of sodium and water lead to ascites in the cirrhotic patient. Ascites can cause respiratory compromise and lead to spontaneous bacterial peritonitis (SBP), which occurs when normal flora translocate across an edematous bowel wall into the peritoneum. Bacteremia and infection of preexisting ascitic fluid ensue.[5]

Encephalopathy is a pivotal characteristic of chronic liver disease and is a hallmark of liver failure. Ammonia is often presumed to be the cause of confusion and lethargy in encephalopathic patients, but in fact, the pathophysiology is not completely understood. In cirrhosis, portal hypertension allows ammonia formed by colonic bacteria to enter the general circulation through portal-systemic shunting. Large intestinal protein loads, such as a high protein meal or GI bleeding, fuel this process. Although levels of ammonia do not reliably correlate with mental status, it is reasonable to think of ammonia as a contributing factor to alterations in mental status. In fulminant liver failure, cerebral edema and increased intracranial pressure can develop. In this end-stage state, loss of autoregulation of cerebral blood flow, ammonia-related edema, and a systemic inflammatory response are all thought to contribute to this deadly complication.[6]

Jaundice can be present in any stage of liver disease. Jaundice is caused by elevated levels of bilirubin in the circulation, leading to bile pigment deposits in the skin, sclerae, and mucous membranes. Hyperbilirubinemia can occur for one of three reasons: overproduction, inadequate cellular processing, or decreased excretion of bilirubin. Another way to think about this is prehepatic, hepatic, and posthepatic jaundice. Prehepatic jaundice is caused by any form of hemolysis, including inborn errors of bilirubin metabolism, which overwhelm the liver's ability to conjugate bilirubin. Viral infection and ingested toxins are typical causes of hepatic jaundice. When hepatocytes necrose, the liver's ability to conjugate bilirubin is impaired, and the level of unconjugated bilirubin rises in the blood. Unlike prehepatic and hepatic jaundice, which present with elevated unconjugated or indirect bilirubin, posthepatic jaundice produces a rise in conjugated bilirubin. Typical causes of posthepatic jaundice are a pancreatic tumor or a gallstone in the common bile duct. Parasitic infestation and biliary atresia are rare causes in the United States but are more common in other parts of the world.

CLINICAL FEATURES

Clinical features of hepatitis are listed in **Table 80-1**.

At ED presentation, a **chief complaint** of jaundice, nausea, vomiting, diarrhea, right upper quadrant or epigastric pain, pruritus, inappropriate bruising or bleeding, or altered mental status should raise the question of liver disease. In the **history of present illness**, pay attention to onset of symptoms after eating out or after ingestion of acetaminophen (in one-time overdose or chronically high doses), mushrooms,

TABLE 80-1 Clinical Features of Hepatitis

	Acute Hepatitis	Chronic Disease/ Cirrhosis	Acute Liver Failure
Symptoms			
Nausea/vomiting/diarrhea	+	±	+
Fever	+	–	–
Pain	+	±	±
Altered mental status	–	±	+
Bruising/bleeding	–	±	+
Physical examination			
Jaundice	+	+	+
Hepatomegaly	+	–	±
Ascites	–	+	+
Edema	–	+	–
Skin findings (bruising, vascular malformations)	–	+	+
Lab abnormalities			
Elevated ALT/AST	+	+	±
AST/ALT >2	+	±	±
Elevated PT/INR	–	±	+
Elevated ammonia	–	±	+
Low albumin	–	+	+
Direct bilirubinemia	–	+	±
Indirect bilirubinemia	+	+	±
Urobilinogen	+	+	+
Elevated blood urea nitrogen/ creatinine	–	–	±
Radiologic findings			
Ascites	–	+	+
Fatty liver	+	–	–
Cirrhosis	–	+	+

Abbreviations: ALT = alanine aminotransferase; AST = aspartate aminotransferase; PT = prothrombin time; + = typically present; – = typically absent; ± = variable.

or raw oysters. Note the duration of symptoms to characterize acuity. **Past medical history** can identify comorbidities or risk factors for liver disease. Risk factors include chronic hepatitis, transfusion of blood products, positive human immunodeficiency virus status, frequent use of pain medications, or depression. Obesity, type 2 diabetes, and hyperlipidemia are risk factors specific to NASH. High-risk medications include acetaminophen and acetaminophen-containing pain medications, vitamin A, isoniazid, propylthiouracil, phenytoin, and valproate, as well as a variety of herbal remedies.[7] Statins raise concern for hepatic toxicity but are rarely implicated in significant liver injury. Three percent of patients taking statins have mild transaminase elevations; clinically significant hepatotoxicity is rare.[8] A **social history** positive for injection drug use, chronic alcohol abuse, sexual promiscuity, or travel to countries with endemic parasitic liver diseases represents increased risk for liver disease.

The **review of systems** in the patient with suspected liver disease can identify important signs and symptoms. Cholestasis causes white (acholic) stools and brown or tea-colored urine. Stools can be black or bloody from variceal or other GI bleeding. Patients may notice yellow skin or sclerae, indicating elevated bilirubin. Ascites can increase abdominal girth or cause shortness of breath, and portal hypertension leads to generalized weakness, encephalopathic changes in mental status, and lower extremity edema. Lightheadedness or near-syncope can result from intravascular depletion and abnormalities in renal sodium and water excretion.

A number of findings on **physical examination** are hallmarks of liver disease. Liver enlargement and tenderness with or without jaundice are characteristic of acute hepatitis. Chronic liver disease is accompanied by a number of physical findings, including sallow or jaundiced complexion, extremity muscle atrophy, Dupuytren's contracture, palmar erythema, cutaneous spider nevi, distended abdomen with a fluid wave, enlarged veins on the surface of the abdomen (caput medusae), and asterixis. Extraordinary bruising or other signs of bleeding diathesis can be seen in liver failure.

ACUTE, CHRONIC, OR FULMINANT HEPATIC DISEASE

Liver disease can be categorized as acute, chronic, or fulminant. Accurately differentiating the acuity and severity of the disease process guides appropriate evaluation, treatment, and disposition.

Acute hepatitis typically presents with nausea, vomiting, and right upper quadrant abdominal pain. The patient with acute hepatitis can also have fever, jaundice, bilirubinuria, and an enlarged, tender liver. The most common causes are viral infection and toxic ingestion. Alcohol and acetaminophen are the most common toxic causes.

Patients with **chronic hepatitis** display evidence of long-standing hepatocellular damage. Cirrhotic patients with portal hypertension complain of abdominal pain and/or distention, abnormal bleeding (bruising, bleeding gums, epistaxis, blood in the stool), and lower body edema. They may also exhibit signs of infection, encephalopathy, ascites, and electrolyte derangement. Skin examination may reveal spider nevi, caput medusae, and other manifestations of abnormal shunting of blood to surface vessels.

Liver failure is the potential final common pathway for both acute and chronic liver disease. If there is a delay in seeking medical attention or a rapid acute course, **fulminant liver failure** can be the presenting disorder. For cirrhotic patients, the transition to liver failure is marked by the advent of coagulopathy, encephalopathy, abnormal fluid shifts, and hepatorenal syndrome.

ACUTE HEPATITIS—VIRAL

Hepatitis A virus, hepatitis B virus, and hepatitis C virus are the most prevalent forms of viral hepatitis encountered in the ED. **Hepatitis A virus** is transmitted by fecal-oral contamination. Although it is popularly associated with improper food handling or oyster consumption, the most common transmission occurs from asymptomatic children to adults. Implementation of the hepatitis A vaccine in children has dramatically decreased overall rates of infection. Hepatitis A virus infection has an incubation period of 15 to 50 days, followed by a prodrome of nausea, vomiting, and malaise. About a week into the illness, patients may note dark urine (bilirubinuria). A few days later, they develop clay-colored stools and jaundice. Hepatitis A virus does not have a chronic component, and death from hepatic failure is rare.[9]

Hepatitis B virus is transmitted sexually, by blood transfusion, by contaminated needles, and by perinatal transmission. Incubation period is 1 to 3 months, and patients can be infectious for 5 to 15 weeks after onset of symptoms if they clear the infection. Individuals who develop chronic disease will remain infectious indefinitely. Chronic infection occurs in only 6% to 10% of patients who contract hepatitis B virus as adults, whereas 90% of infants and 30% of children under the age of 5 progress to chronic status, which underlines the importance of vaccination of infants and women of childbearing age.[10] In the acute phase of hepatitis B virus, presentation to the ED is similar to that for hepatitis A virus, including complaints of malaise, nausea, vomiting, fever, abdominal pain, and jaundice.

Hepatitis C virus transmission occurs primarily through exposure to contaminated blood or blood products. In contrast to hepatitis A virus and hepatitis B virus, hepatitis C virus is most often asymptomatic in the acute phase of infection, and >75% of patients advance to the chronic stage. The rate of progression to liver failure varies and depends on the natural course of the virus and cofactors such as alcoholism and human immunodeficiency virus. Along with hepatitis B virus, hepatitis C virus is one of the most common causes of hepatocellular carcinoma. Of the patients who develop chronic hepatitis C virus, 1% to 5% will die of either cirrhosis or liver cancer.[11]

Hepatitis D virus is uncommon and is typically seen in people with preexisting chronic hepatitis B virus infection. Hepatitis D superinfection can result in a rapidly progressive or fulminant form of liver disease that carries a high short-term mortality rate. This variety of infection is most commonly associated with injection drug use.[11]

Acute illness with liver function test abnormalities also occurs with infection by other hepatotropic viruses such as cytomegalovirus, herpes simplex virus, Coxsackie virus, and Epstein-Barr virus. These agents are unlikely to cause clinically significant hepatitis in an otherwise healthy host.

ACUTE HEPATITIS—TOXIC

A toxic insult to the liver can cause acute hepatitis and/or fulminant liver failure. The most common of these is acetaminophen overdose. **Acetaminophen** accounts for >40% of liver failure cases in the United States and one third of deaths secondary to toxic ingestion. Patients develop nausea, vomiting, and abdominal pain. They may also give a history of an acute overdose of acetaminophen or chronic use of one or more acetaminophen-containing pain medicines. Up to 28% of patients with acetaminophen overdose will develop liver failure. The likelihood of liver failure depends on time from ingestion to presentation, the dose ingested, and the baseline health status of the patient.[12] Tylenol overdose is reviewed more completely in chapter 190, "Acetaminophen."

In addition to acetaminophen, there are a variety of **prescription medications** (antibiotics and statins prominent among them), **herbal remedies**, and **dietary supplements** that have been associated with acute hepatitis and liver failure. The list of prescription medications that have been implicated in liver disease is so long that it is prudent to refer to a pharmaceutical database to identify a potential culprit when toxic insult is suspected. Some of the most common herbal remedies that have been implicated in hepatic injury are listed in **Table 80-2**.

Alcoholic liver disease can range from asymptomatic, reversible fatty liver to acute alcoholic hepatitis, cirrhosis, or a combination of acute and cirrhotic features. The diagnosis of alcoholic liver disease carries a 35% 5-year survival rate. If a patient has asymptomatic liver disease (i.e., fatty liver seen on imaging), but the patient's drinking continues and acute alcoholic hepatitis develops, the mortality can be much higher.[13] A history of consistent heavy alcohol use (mean intake at presentation of 100 grams or more) is thought to be required for development of significant alcoholic liver disease.[14] However, information is often difficult to elicit from the patient or family, and the patient may have stopped drinking before ED presentation. Other nonhepatic features of alcohol abuse, such as malnutrition, stocking-glove neuropathy, pityriasis rosea, and cardiomyopathy, can be clues to alcohol-induced liver disease.

Mushroom poisoning is an uncommon but important cause of acute hepatitis with a high risk of liver failure. *Amanita phalloides* ("death cap") is the most lethal of the more than 50 types of mushrooms that are toxic to humans. For detailed discussion, see chapter 219, "Mushroom Poisoning."

CHRONIC HEPATITIS AND CIRRHOSIS

Most patients live for years with hepatitis B virus, hepatitis C virus, NASH, or alcoholic hepatitis without symptoms. During the asymptomatic period, normal liver parenchyma is being gradually replaced by scar tissue, and hepatic disease can manifest as mild transaminase elevation or, in cases of NASH and alcoholic hepatitis, as an incidental finding of fatty liver on abdominal imaging studies. When a critical amount of liver parenchyma is replaced by fibrotic tissue, symptoms of cirrhosis develop, such as abdominal pain, ascites, SBP, general weakness resulting from electrolyte derangement, or altered mental status due to hepatic encephalopathy.

Ascites One of the hallmarks of cirrhosis, ascites causes a protuberant abdomen, and a fluid wave is produced on physical exam. Intra-abdominal fluid can displace the diaphragm upward and produce sympathetic pleural effusion with the possibility of respiratory compromise. Smaller amounts of ascites can be difficult to identify on examination; bedside ultrasound can be particularly helpful in patients in whom the presence of ascites is uncertain (**Figure 80-1**).

Spontaneous Bacterial Peritonitis SBP is a subtle yet crucial complication of ascites. The survival rate for patients with a first episode of SBP is 68.1% at 1 month and 30.8% at 6 months. This is probably a result of acute infection occurring in the fragile setting of advanced liver disease.[15] Although common in cirrhotic patients—roughly 30% of ascitic patients will develop SBP in a given year—SBP is difficult to diagnose because signs of abdominal pain and fever are not always present, and physical examination does not always demonstrate abdominal tenderness. Consequently, patients who are diagnosed with ascites for

TABLE 80-2 Common Herbal Remedies Known to Cause Hepatic Toxicity

Herbal Remedy	Application	Nature of Injury
Black cohosh (*Actea racemosa/cimiifuga racemosa*)	Menopausal symptoms	Hepatic necrosis and bridging fibrosis
Chaparral (*Larrea ridentate*)	Antioxidant, health tonic	Cholestasis, chronic hepatitis, cholangitis, cirrhosis
Comfrey (*Symphytum*)	Broken bones, wound healing, reduce joint inflammation	Hepatic veno-occlusive disease
Echinacea (*E. angustifolia, E. pallida, E. purpurea*)	Respiratory infections, fever, immune booster	Acute cholestatic autoimmune hepatitis
Kava (*Piper methysticum*)	Anxiolytic, sleeping aid	Acute and chronic hepatitis, cholestasis, fulminant hepatic failure
Kombucha "mushroom" tea	Weight loss, increasing T-cell count, well-being, antiaging	Acute liver failure, hepatitis, acute renal failure with hyperthermia and lactic acidosis
Ma huang (*Ephedra sinica*)	Weight loss	Acute hepatitis
Mistletoe (*Viscum album*)	Hypertension, insomnia, epilepsy, asthma, infertility, urinary disorders	Acute hepatitis
Noni juice (*Morinda citrifolia*)	Health tonic	Subacute hepatic failure, acute hepatitis
Prostata (*Serenoa repens*); saw palmetto	Benign prostatic hyperplasia	Cholestatic hepatitis
Senna (*Cassia angustifolia*)	Laxative	Acute hepatitis, acute cholestatic hepatitis, acute liver failure
Skullcap (*Scutellaria baicalensis*)	Sedative, anti-inflammatory	Hepatic veno-occlusive disease, cholestasis, hepatitis
St John's wort (*Hypericum perforatum*)	Anti-depressant	Cytochrome P-450 induction, serotonin syndrome
Valerian (*Valeriana officinalis*)	Sedative, anxiolytic	Hepatitis

Source: Adapted with permission from Abdualmjid RJ, Sergi C: Hepatotoxic botanicals: an evidence-based systematic review. *J Pharm Pharm Sci* 16: 376, 2013.

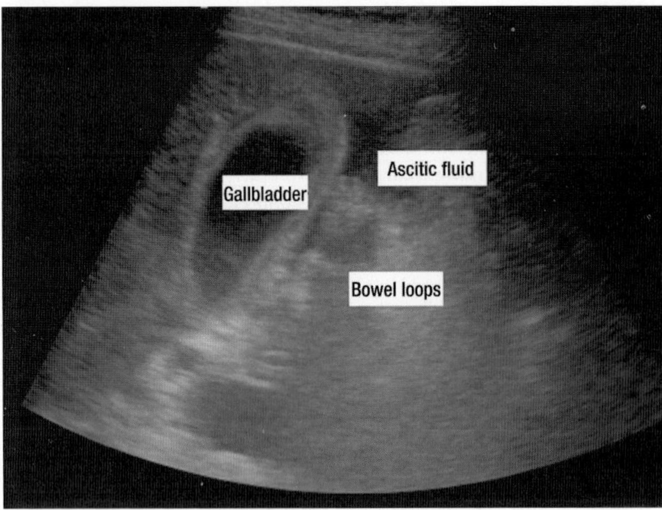

FIGURE 80-1. Sonographic image of ascitic fluid showing bowel loops and an edematous gallbladder wall, a common finding in patients with ascites. [Courtesy of and used with permission of Michael S. Antonis, DO, sonographer.]

the first time, or who have ascites and develop fever, abdominal pain, GI bleeding, or encephalopathy, should undergo paracentesis to check for SBP.

Hepatorenal Syndrome Hepatorenal syndrome is a complication of cirrhosis that often accompanies SBP. It is defined as acute renal failure in a patient with histologically normal kidneys in the presence of preexisting chronic or acute hepatic failure. The cause is not well understood. There are two types of hepatorenal syndrome. Type 1 is more serious and is identified by progressive oliguria and doubling of serum creatinine over a 2-week period. Type 2 is represented by a gradual impairment in renal function that may or may not advance beyond moderate dysfunction. The discovery of abrupt renal failure in a cirrhotic patient that cannot be attributed to any other cause should be viewed as a marker of extreme morbidity. Median survival for type 1 hepatorenal syndrome without medical treatment is 2 weeks.[16]

Hepatic Encephalopathy Hepatic encephalopathy is a poorly understood phenomenon attributed to the accumulation of nitrogenous waste products normally metabolized by the liver. Hepatic encephalopathy causes a spectrum of illness ranging from chronic fatigue or mild confusion to acute lethargy.

The development of hepatic encephalopathy suggests either that the liver is no longer able to metabolize the usual supply of nitrogenous waste or that the supply of such waste has increased. Sources of increased supply include protein loads from a large meal or from occult GI bleeding. In addition to progressive liver disease, constipation, hypo- or hyperglycemia, alcohol withdrawal, hypoperfusion states such as sepsis, and iatrogenic interventions can also compromise the liver's metabolic capacity. Hepatic encephalopathy is a common complication after **transjugular intrahepatic portosystemic shunt**, a procedure in which portal blood is shunted to the inferior vena cava, bypassing the liver. Although this procedure may succeed in reducing portal hypertension and variceal bleeding, it also slows metabolism of nitrogenous wastes by reducing hepatic blood flow. Adding or removing antibiotics from a patient's medicine regimen can also precipitate encephalopathy by changing the intestinal flora and altering the gut's ability to metabolize proteins.[17]

To appreciate the presence or worsening of encephalopathy, determine if there are changes in personality, worsening dementia, a decrease in levels of consciousness, or declining neuromuscular function. **Table 80-3** lists clinical stages of encephalopathy. Asterixis, which characterizes stage II, is elicited by having the patient hold the arms straight up and extending the wrists. The hands begin to flap repetitively. Another manifestation of asterixis is back-and-forth tongue movement when the tongue is extended. A patient with known encephalopathy in stage I or II who is otherwise well and has no other acute comorbidities may be managed as an outpatient after consultation with the primary care physician or gastroenterologist.

TABLE 80-3 Stages of Clinical Hepatic Encephalopathy

Stage	Features
I	General apathy
II	Lethargy, drowsiness, variable orientation, asterixis
III	Stupor with hyperreflexia, extensor plantar reflexes
IV	Coma

Hepatic encephalopathy is a diagnosis of exclusion. In the cirrhotic patient with altered mental status or lethargy, first exclude multiple other causes. This holds true even in the presence of an elevated serum ammonia level. Patients with end-stage liver disease are typically coagulopathic and may develop a spontaneous or traumatic subdural hematoma. Decreased hepatic gluconeogenesis and glycogen stores and poor nutritional status increase the risk of hypoglycemia and nutritional encephalopathies such as Wernicke-Korsakoff syndrome. Cirrhotic patients often are treated with diuretics and can develop hyper- or hyponatremia. Altered mental status can result form decreased hepatic clearance of drugs such as benzodiazepines and opiates, prolonging the effect and resulting in accidental overdose. Renal failure and sepsis are other considerations. Always exclude upper GI bleeding as a precipitant of hepatic encephalopathy, because the protein in the blood can translocate across the bowel of the cirrhotic patient.

Gastroesophageal varices and hemorrhage are complications of cirrhosis that are covered in chapter 75, "Upper Gastrointestinal Bleeding."

HEPATIC FAILURE

Liver failure is the final common pathway for several types of liver disease. Progression to liver failure is varied and depends largely on comorbid entities, such as human immunodeficiency virus/acquired immunodeficiency syndrome, diabetes, obesity, continued injection drug use, and alcohol intake. There are roughly 2000 cases per year in the United States. Patients who develop acute liver failure have an extremely poor prognosis, with survival rates of <30%.[18] Among the most common of the entities that present as acute liver failure in the United States are acetaminophen overdose (46%), indeterminate causes (14%), other drugs (11%), hepatitis B virus (7%), and autoimmune hepatitis.[3]

The clinical hallmarks of acute liver failure are hepatic encephalopathy, hepatorenal syndrome, and coagulopathy. The electrolyte imbalances seen in chronic liver disease can become extreme. Cerebral edema and intracranial hypertension are the most ominous complications. The catabolic nature of liver failure leads to negative nitrogen balance and immunodeficiency. Other clinical findings in acute liver failure include hypotension, hypoglycemia, and relative adrenal insufficiency. ED evaluation should include assessment for sepsis. Recognize when a patient has progressed from cirrhosis to failure or presents with acute hepatic failure, because transfer to a transplant center may be the most appropriate disposition.

GILBERT'S SYNDROME

Gilbert's syndrome is a familial liver disorder that produces occasional elevations in liver function tests and bilirubin. This syndrome does not cause cirrhosis or affect the synthetic or metabolic functions of the liver. Wilson's disease, hemochromatosis, and α_1-antitrypsin deficiency are familial disorders that can lead to severe chronic disease and liver failure. Autoimmune hepatitis is a progressive, chronic disease that is presumably triggered by viral hepatitis or by medications. Primary biliary cirrhosis is a presumably autoimmune disorder with a chronic or chronic-degenerative course.

PRE- AND POSTHEPATIC VENOUS THROMBOSIS

Vascular diseases of the liver are rare but important, because timely diagnosis and treatment can improve outcome. **Portal vein thrombosis** affects the prehepatic portal venous system and is associated with hypercoagulable states such as polycythemia vera; with deficiencies in proteins C and S, antithrombin 3, and factor V Leiden; and with abdominal trauma, sepsis, pancreatitis, cirrhosis, or hepatocellular carcinoma. The major symptom is abdominal pain; occasionally ascites can occur. Splenomegaly can occur without hepatomegaly on physical examination.[19] **Hepatic vein thrombosis (posthepatic), or Budd-Chiari syndrome**, has both acute and chronic presentations, including abdominal pain, hepatomegaly, and ascites. Associated conditions include coagulopathies, polycythemia vera, paroxysmal nocturnal hemoglobinuria, and congenital webs of the vena cava.[20]

LABORATORY EVALUATION AND IMAGING

Laboratory tests for hepatobiliary disease can be divided into four categories: (1) markers of acute hepatocyte injury or death, (2) measurements of hepatocyte synthetic function, (3) indicators of hepatocyte catabolic activity, and (4) tests to diagnose specific disease entities. Traditional liver function panels include a mix of markers of hepatocyte injury, usually including aspartate aminotransferase, alanine aminotransferase, and alkaline phosphatase, as well as indicators of hepatocyte catabolic activity (direct and indirect bilirubin). Tests that reflect hepatocyte synthetic function include prothrombin time and albumin. Ammonia reflects catabolic function of the liver. Viral hepatitis serologies are used to differentiate various types of hepatitis; acetaminophen levels can determine whether treatment for poisoning is appropriate; and various tests of ascitic fluid are used to diagnose SBP.

Bilirubin is a metabolite of heme proteins. The total level is usually reported along with the levels of conjugated (direct) and unconjugated (indirect) portions. In a functioning liver, unconjugated bilirubin is taken up by hepatocytes, conjugated, and then secreted into bile. Bilirubin is then excreted in the stool, with a small percentage being recirculated through the liver. An increased total and *indirect* bilirubin signifies either an overwhelming supply of unconjugated bilirubin to the hepatocytes (e.g., hemolytic anemia) or an injury to the hepatocytes themselves that damages their capacity to conjugate a normal supply of bilirubin (e.g., acute or chronic viral hepatitis). Total and *direct* bilirubin is increased when there is some obstruction preventing the secretion of the conjugated bilirubin that is produced by normally functioning hepatocytes (e.g., obstructing gallstone, pancreatic mass, or biliary atresia).

Transaminases (aspartate aminotransferase and alanine aminotransferase) are intracellular enzymes found in hepatocytes and some other cell types. Hepatocyte injury or necrosis releases these enzymes into the circulation. Elevations in the hundreds of units per liter suggest mild injury, or smoldering inflammation. Levels in the thousands suggest extensive acute hepatic necrosis. Less significant elevations, less than five times normal, are typical of alcoholic liver disease and NASH. Marked elevations are commonly seen with acute viral hepatitis. These enzyme levels may be near normal in end-stage liver failure, when the hepatocytes are beyond the stage of acute injury. An aspartate aminotransferase–to–alanine aminotransferase ratio of greater than 2 is common in alcoholic hepatitis because alcohol stimulates aspartate aminotransferase production.[1] Incidental findings of transaminase elevations of three to five times normal and alkaline phosphatase of up to twice normal in diabetic or obese patients suggest the presence of NASH in diabetic or obese patients.[21] Alanine aminotransferase is a more specific marker of hepatocyte injury than aspartate aminotransferase. Aspartate aminotransferase is found not only in liver but also in heart, smooth muscle, kidney, and brain. Elevated aspartate aminotransferase can be due to medications, including acetaminophen, nonsteroidal anti-inflammatory drugs (NSAIDs), angiotensin-converting enzyme inhibitors, nicotinic acid, isoniazid, sulfonamides, erythromycin, griseofulvin, and fluconazole.

γ-Glutamyl transpeptidase production is stimulated by alcohol consumption. It is also elevated by drugs inducing hepatic microsomal enzyme activity, such as phenobarbital and warfarin, and may rise in acute and chronic pancreatitis, acute myocardial infarction, uremia, chronic obstructive pulmonary disease, rheumatoid arthritis, and diabetes mellitus. An elevated γ-glutamyl transpeptidase in the setting of hepatitis suggests an alcoholic cause.

Alkaline phosphatase elevation is associated with biliary obstruction and cholestasis. Mild to moderate elevations accompany virtually all hepatobiliary disease, whereas elevations greater than four times normal strongly suggest cholestasis. Alkaline phosphatase is a nonspecific marker also derived from bone, placenta, intestine, kidneys, and leukocytes. A level of up to double the expected value is normal in pregnancy.

Lactate dehydrogenase is included in most liver test panels, but it is a nonspecific marker, which limits its utility. Moderate elevations are seen in all hepatocellular disorders and cirrhosis, whereas purely cholestatic conditions cause minimal elevations. Hemolysis can produce elevation of lactate dehydrogenase and unconjugated bilirubin. The isoenzyme lactate dehydrogenase-5 is specific to the liver. Tests for lactate dehydrogenase-5 are sometimes useful although not widely available.

Ammonia is generated by hepatic metabolism of nitrogen-containing compounds. The hepatic metabolic failure seen in acute and chronic liver disease can, therefore, cause an elevated serum ammonia level. Very high ammonia levels, seen in fulminant liver failure, contribute to overall toxicity and signify poor prognosis.

Prothrombin time prolongation in liver disease reflects the decreased synthesis of the vitamin K–dependent coagulation factors II, VII, IX, and X and, as such, serves as a true measure of liver function. Prolonged prothrombin time is a common complication of advancing cirrhosis, although it also occurs in acute hepatitis and exacerbations of chronic compensated liver disease. When present in acute viral hepatitis, prolonged prothrombin time often indicates severe disease with widespread hepatocellular necrosis. There is some correlation between the extent of prothrombin time prolongation and clinical outcome in fulminant liver disease. Although prothrombin time is useful as a marker of hepatic function, abnormal values may occur in the presence of a normal liver. Vitamin K deficiency from another entity (i.e., malabsorption of fat and, therefore, of fat-soluble vitamins) can be distinguished from liver synthetic dysfunction by administration of parenteral vitamin K (phytonadione, 10 milligrams IM). A 30% reduction in prothrombin time should occur within 24 hours in vitamin deficiency states.

Albumin also reflects the liver's synthetic function. It may decrease in advancing cirrhosis or severe acute hepatitis and suggests a poor short-term prognosis. Because its half-life is approximately 3 weeks, albumin is less useful than prothrombin time in evaluating fulminant liver disease. Prothrombin time becomes prolonged in a matter of days. Serum albumin levels are also low in malnutrition, so low albumin levels do not necessarily correlate with the degree of hepatic disease in a chronically ill patient.

Viral hepatitis serologies are often grouped into screening panels by hospital laboratories. The diagnosis of specific viral hepatitis entities is complicated by phase of illness, preexisting infections, and likelihood of a given type of infection. The patient who is acutely ill with hepatitis A virus will have positive immunoglobulin M anti–hepatitis A virus antibodies. Acute clinical illness in hepatitis B virus correlates with positive hepatitis B virus surface antigen. Positive immunoglobulin M antibodies correlate to the hepatitis B virus core antigen. Diagnosis of hepatitis C virus is initiated by ordering anti–hepatitis C virus antibodies. This diagnosis is sometimes masked by the 6- to 8-week delay between infection and antibody detection as well as by the acute asymptomatic phase of the hepatitis C virus infection.[22]

Ascitic fluid aspirate is tested for cell count, glucose and protein, Gram stain, and culture to identify bacterial peritonitis. The procedure for obtaining ascitic fluid, paracentesis, is explained in chapter 86, "Gastrointestinal Procedures and Devices." **A total WBC count >1000/mm^3 or a neutrophil count >250/mm^3 diagnoses SBP.** Low glucose or high protein values suggest infection. Gram stains and culture results can be falsely negative 30% to 40% of the time, so empiric antibiotics should be started in the ED based on clinical suspicion. Culture sensitivity increases by using 10 mL of ascitic fluid per blood culture bottle and by transferring the fluid to culture bottles at the patient's bedside. Additional studies of ascites that can help with inpatient evaluation are cytology, albumin, lactate dehydrogenase, and tumor markers.

NONHEPATIC CAUSES OF ABNORMAL LIVER TESTS

Multiple nonhepatic causes may lead to abnormal liver function tests. Abnormal liver test results occur in up to one third of those screened, and only 1% of these indicate clinically significant liver disease. Hypoalbuminemia accompanies protein-wasting enteropathies, malnutrition, and nephrotic syndrome. Alkaline phosphatase elevations occur with a variety of bone diseases, pregnancy, and malignancies. Aspartate aminotransferase elevations accompany acute myocardial infarction and rhabdomyolysis. Bilirubin elevations occur in severe hemolysis, sepsis, and syndromes involving abnormal erythropoiesis. Prothrombin time elevations occur in vitamin K deficiency, chronic antibiotic use, and warfarin therapy.[23,24]

Urine bilirubin and urobilinogen are sometimes used as screening tests for liver disease in the ED. The sensitivity of these urine assays is 70% to 74% for identifying elevated serum bilirubin. For correlation with other liver function tests, their sensitivity is in the 43% to 53% range. Specificity for showing either bilirubin or transaminase abnormality is 77% to 87%. Blood-tinged urine will give a false-positive urobilinogen on a urine dipstick test. Taken together, these statistics do not support screening for liver disease with urine dipstick testing.[25]

IMAGING

US and CT scanning are both useful for initial evaluation of liver disease. Bedside US can identify ascites and guide paracentesis, whereas formal US with duplex Doppler is the test of choice for identifying portal vein and hepatic vein thrombosis. Both sonogram and CT scan of the abdomen can be used to identify cancerous, vascular, or infectious lesions of the liver. CT scanning of the brain is used to identify intracranial hemorrhage in patients with liver disease and altered mental status.

TREATMENT

With the exception of acetaminophen poisoning (see chapter 190), treatment for acute hepatitis is supportive. Pay careful attention to associated conditions such as hyponatremia, alcohol or narcotic withdrawal, alcoholic ketoacidosis, and hypoglycemia. Treating chronic hepatitis in the ED means taking care of its many sequelae such as ascites, encephalopathy, coagulopathy, and variceal bleeding. Chronic hepatitis infection is typically treated by gastroenterologists in an outpatient setting. Liver failure requires critical care in the ED and consultation with a liver transplant center for disposition, including transfer if needed.

ASCITES

Mild- to moderate-volume ascites can be managed with a salt-restricted diet and diuretics, both of which create a negative sodium balance and encourage loss of ascitic fluid. Recommended diuretics include spironolactone, 50 to 200 milligrams per day, and amiloride, 5 to 10 milligrams per day. Furosemide can be problematic because it can lead to overdiuresis.[5] To facilitate monitoring for adverse side effects, diuretics for the cirrhotic patient should be prescribed in collaboration with his or her outpatient physician.

Paracentesis is recommended therapy for large-volume ascites. There are several important considerations when performing paracentesis on a cirrhotic patient. First, the patient's prothrombin time/INR is likely to be elevated. Second, the amount of fluid that can be removed without infusion of albumin to prevent intravascular collapse is controversial. For any tap, guidelines from the American Association for the Study of Liver Diseases state that paracentesis should be considered safe from a bleeding perspective unless there is evidence of fibrinolysis (i.e., three-dimensional bruising, oozing from IV start sites) or overt disseminated intravascular coagulation. For therapeutic paracentesis, American Association for the Study of Liver Diseases guidelines recommend the use of albumin, 6 to 8 milligrams/L of fluid removed, for amounts greater than 4 L.[5] One safe approach is to perform diagnostic paracentesis in the ED and defer large-volume therapeutic taps to the inpatient setting or the ED observation unit.

TABLE 80-4 Diagnosis and Treatment of Spontaneous Bacterial Peritonitis

Diagnosis	Ascitic fluid, obtain 50 cc for cell count, Gram stain, and culture (transfer blood to culture bottles at the bedside for best results)
	WBC count >1000/mm^3
	or
	Polymorphonuclear leukocytes >250/mL
	or
	Bacteria on Gram stain
Empiric treatment	Cefotaxime or other third-generation cephalosporin
	or
	IV fluoroquinolone (ineffective in patients who have received prophylactic quinolone treatment)
	or
	Oral fluoroquinolone in a very mild case with close follow-up

SPONTANEOUS BACTERIAL PERITONITIS

SBP is the most common life-threatening complication of ascites, classically presenting with fever and diffuse abdominal pain and tenderness. However, any or all of these features may be absent. In patients with known ascites, the 1-year incidence of SBP is 29%. Recurrence of SBP is as high as 44%, and survival in patients with a first episode of SBP is low (68.1% at 1 month and 30.8% at 6 months), probably a result of acute infection in the setting of advanced liver disease.[15]

Initial treatment is empiric antibiotic therapy to cover typical enteric flora. The most common isolates in SBP are *Escherichia coli, Klebsiella pneumoniae,* and *Streptococcal pneumoniae*. Empiric antibiotic treatment recommendations from the most recent (2012) guideline from the American Association for the Study of Liver Diseases are shown in **Table 80-4**.[5] Although there is no conclusive evidence proving that cefotaxime is superior to other choices, it is a widely accepted first-line parenteral treatment for SBP. Oral therapy with broad-spectrum quinolones is an option in patients with mild, uncomplicated disease and close follow-up.[26] Patients may have had prior infections with resistant organisms, so review microbiologic sensitivities from prior admissions, if available. The addition of IV albumin (1.5 grams/kg at diagnosis, 1 gram/kg on day 3) to antibiotic therapy may reduce renal failure and hospital mortality in patients with SBP.[27]

HEPATIC ENCEPHALOPATHY

To address hepatic encephalopathy, first consider other entities that could cause altered mental status, such as infection, intracranial hemorrhage, or hyponatremia. Once hepatic encephalopathy is diagnosed, treatment is aimed at reducing the production of nitrogenous wastes by reducing protein intake and suppressing the metabolic activity of intestinal bacteria.

Lactulose is the current mainstay of therapy for hepatic encephalopathy. Lactulose is a synthetic disaccharide containing one molecule of galactose and one of fructose. It is minimally absorbed into the bloodstream. In the colon, it degrades primarily into lactic acid. In the acidified environment, ammonia is trapped and excreted in the stool. Blood ammonia levels can decrease up to 50% using lactulose therapy. Lactulose also inhibits glutamine-dependent ammonia production in the gut wall. Lactulose is given PO or PR. The oral dose is 20 grams diluted in a glass of water, fruit juice, or carbonated drink. For rectal administration, dilute 300 mL of syrup with 700 mL of water or normal saline. The enema should be retained for 30 minutes.

Coagulopathy needs to be treated if the patient has uncontrolled bleeding or is scheduled to undergo a procedure with potential bleeding complications. Vitamin K deficiency can be treated with vitamin K, 10 milligrams IV or PO. Fresh frozen plasma can be given in doses appropriate for the patient's prothrombin level. Finally, decreased or malfunctioning platelets should be replaced with pooled donor platelets. Specific treatments for variceal bleeding are addressed in chapter 75.

METABOLIC AND RESPIRATORY FAILURE

Treatment of fulminant liver failure in the ED involves care of the patient's respiratory status, blood pressure, and encephalopathy; correction of electrolyte derangements; identification of cerebral edema or intracranial hemorrhage; attention to active bleeding; and careful disposition, ensuring that the patient will be assessed for liver transplant in a timely fashion.

Patients with respiratory failure due to ascites, effusions, or decreased alertness require intubation. Bilevel positive airway pressure is not typically an option in these cases because patients are too somnolent and at risk for aspiration. Blood pressure at this stage of liver disease is typically low due to malnutrition, bleeding, vomiting, diarrhea, and third spacing of fluid. Treat with judicious fluids, blood products, and vasopressors, as needed. Altered mental status at this stage can be from encephalopathy, metabolic abnormalities, intracranial bleeding, or brain edema with increased intracranial pressure. In the case of intracranial hemorrhage, treat coagulopathy. Consult neurosurgery or refer to a facility with neurosurgical services if the patient could benefit from hematoma evacuation or intracranial pressure monitoring. Mannitol is appropriate as a temporizing measure in cases of increased intracranial pressure caused by cerebral edema.[6]

DISPOSITION AND FOLLOW-UP

The disposition of a patient with acute or chronic hepatitis is complex and requires careful planning with the patient and caretakers. Discussion with the primary care physician and gastroenterologist can clarify a vague clinical picture. Patients with acute hepatitis require supportive treatment with pain management, antiemetic medication, and fluid resuscitation. Consider admission for high-risk patients, including the elderly and pregnant women, and patients who do not respond adequately to supportive care. Admit those who have a bilirubin ≥20 milligrams/dL, prothrombin time 50% above normal, hypoglycemia, low albumin, or GI bleeding, which requires further evaluation to determine the presence of varices.[28]

In patients with chronic hepatitis, admission may be indicated for patients with ascites if they have significant respiratory compromise or abdominal pain. In addition, admit the patient with fever, acidosis, or leukocytosis and for evaluation and treatment of SBP.[29] New-onset or worsening hepatic encephalopathy, hepatorenal syndrome, and coagulopathy with bleeding are also strong indications for admission.[30] Patients with severe hyponatremia and severe hyper- or hypovolemia should also be managed in the hospital.[31]

Consider patient safety in the disposition of patients with advanced cirrhosis. Weakness, muscle wasting, and mild encephalopathy are serious risks for falls, and coagulopathy is a risk for cerebral bleed. Patients must be stable on their feet or have supervised assistance for discharge to home.

Discharge planning should include follow-up care by a gastroenterologist or transplant specialist. Patients and family members can be referred to Alcoholics Anonymous, Al-Anon, or support groups for transplant or other special needs. Discharge medications may include antibiotics, diuretics, lactulose, antiemetics, and pain medications.

SPECIAL CONSIDERATIONS

PAIN CONTROL IN PATIENTS WITH HEPATIC DISEASE

It can be difficult to decide on appropriate pain medications and sedatives for patients with compromised liver function. Avoid NSAIDs in patients with chronic hepatitis and cirrhosis due to GI toxicity and possible potentiation of renal dysfunction. Acetaminophen has traditionally been avoided in patients with any type of liver disease, but there are several trials indicating it to be safe for short-term use, at a reduced dose of 2 grams total per day. Gabapentin and pregabalin are safe options for neuropathic pain. Avoid opioids whenever possible, because opioids are metabolized by the liver and their sedative effects can be unpredictable in patients with compromised liver function. Opioids are contraindicated in patients with a history of encephalopathy or substance use. If absolutely necessary, fentanyl and tramadol at reduced doses and increased dosing intervals are possible choices in select patients because they lack the toxic metabolites of traditional opioids.[32] When sedation or pain control is required for the critically ill patient with liver failure, a titratable infusion of a nonbenzodiazepine medication with a short half-life and no toxic metabolites is useful. Propofol has been well studied in the setting of endoscopy and is safe at least in the short term for patients with cirrhosis.[33] Fentanyl provides pain relief and some degree of sedation.

PREGNANCY

Pregnant women can present with various hepatic or cholestatic disorders not specific to pregnancy. HELLP syndrome (hemolysis, elevated liver enzymes, low platelets), however, stands apart as a life-threatening process that must not be missed in the ED. HELLP occurs as part of the pre-eclampsia–eclampsia spectrum in the late third trimester or in the postpartum period. It can present with symptoms resembling viral illness—headache, malaise, nausea, and vomiting. Hypertension, headache, and proteinuria are other associated findings. Eighty percent to 90% of patients present with relative hypertension, and proteinuria is present 85% to 100% of the time. Headache, usually considered a mainstay of the pre-eclampsia diagnosis, is not a sensitive or specific finding.[34]

Perinatal mortality in cases where HELLP complicates a pregnancy before 29 weeks can be as high as 20%. Check liver function studies, CBC, and lactate dehydrogenase in those who present with even vague symptoms of illness in their third trimester and in any third-trimester patient with relative hypertension. Definitive treatment in pregnancies later than 34 weeks is immediate delivery, whereas patients who are mildly ill with HELLP at <34 weeks of gestation may sometimes be managed expectantly. ED disposition of patients with elements of HELLP syndrome is admission to the obstetrics inpatient service.[34] Further discussion of HELLP is provided in chapter 100, "Maternal Emergencies after 20 Weeks of Pregnancy and in the Postpartum Period."

LIVER TRANSPLANT PATIENT

Liver transplant patients can develop a variety of illnesses, most commonly abdominal, infectious, and metabolic in nature. Febrile patients should be pan cultured, and broad-spectrum antibiotics should be initiated pending further inpatient evaluation. Metabolic derangements can include hyper- or hypoglycemia, sodium imbalance, and hypo- or hyperkalemia. Rejection of the transplant should be a concern even in the absence of abdominal pain and tenderness. Symptoms of rejection can be vague and can include nausea, vomiting, malaise, anorexia, abdominal pain, vomiting, and jaundice. In one series of 290 liver transplant patient visits to the ED, 69% resulted in hospitalization.[35] Further discussion is provided in the section on Special Situations in chapter 297, "The Transplant Patient."

NONALCOHOLIC FATTY LIVER DISEASE

NAFLD deserves particular mention in the discussion of chronic liver disease. It affects up to 30% of the U.S. population by some estimates and is now thought to be the third most common reason for transplantation after hepatitis C virus infection and alcoholic liver disease. Exact figures are unclear because NAFLD often goes undiagnosed through the phases of steatosis (fatty deposits in the liver) and steatohepatitis (fatty deposits with inflammation, also identified by the acronym NASH), and is often categorized as idiopathic cirrhosis by the time of diagnosis and consideration for transplantation. NAFLD is associated with obesity, type 2 diabetes, and hyperlipidemia. Many patients will have fatty liver seen incidentally on abdominal imaging, and few of these patients will go on to develop cirrhosis.[21] There is no specific treatment for NAFLD. The mainstays of treatment are weight loss and exercise, which have been shown to reduce fat deposition and inflammation of the liver parenchyma, but not fibrosis. The efficacy of diabetic medications and statins has not been well studied, but these are also used in the treatment of NAFLD. Patients with NAFLD found even incidentally during ED evaluation should be advised to avoid further injury by abstaining from alcohol.[21]

TRAVELERS AND GLOBAL CITIZENS

Travelers who have been outside the United States who present with abdominal pain, vomiting, diarrhea, or fever are at risk for having liver disease caused by parasitic infection. **Schistosomiasis** is a waterborne parasite that infects >200 million people worldwide and can cause portal hypertension by invading the portal venules. *Echinococcus* species cause multiple liver cysts. Ascariasis causes hepatobiliary obstruction. *Entamoeba histolytica* infects roughly 10% of the world's population and causes parasitic liver abscesses.[36] For further discussion, see chapter 161, "Global Travelers."

VENO-OCCLUSIVE DISEASE

Veno-occlusive disease of the liver is a potentially fatal adverse effect of herbal remedies, chemotherapy, or bone marrow transplant. It is associated with abdominal pain, the presence of hepatomegaly, ascites, weight gain, and jaundice in a patient with concerning history.[37]

PRACTICE GUIDELINES AND SOCIETY POSITION STATEMENTS

- Chalasani N, Younossi Z, Lavine JE, et al: The diagnosis and management of non-alcoholic fatty liver disease: practice guideline by the American Association for the Study of Liver Diseases (AASLD), American College of Gastroenterology, and the American Gastroenterological Association. *Hepatology* 55: 2005, 2012.
- Runyon BA: AASLD practice guideline: management of adult patients with ascites due to cirrhosis: update 2012. *Hepatology* 57: 1651, 2013.
- Lee WM, Larson AM, Stravitz RT; American Association for the Study of Liver Diseases: Position paper: the management of acute liver failure: update (2011). *Hepatology* 55: 965, 2012.
- American College of Obstetricians and Gynecologists (ACOG): Viral hepatitis in pregnancy. Washington, DC: American College of Obstetricians and Gynecologists, October 15, 2007, (ACOG Practice Bulletin, No. 86). *Reaffirmed 2012.*
- Wolf SJ, Heard K, Sloan EP, Jagoda AS: American College of Emergency Physicians (ACEP) clinical policy: critical issues in the management of patients presenting to the emergency department with acetaminophen overdose. *Ann Emerg Med* 50: 292, 2007.

Acknowledgments: The authors gratefully acknowledge the contributions of Richard O. Shields Jr., Joshua S. Broder, and Rawden Evans, the authors of the related chapter in the previous edition.

REFERENCES

The complete reference list is available online at www.TintinalliEM.com.

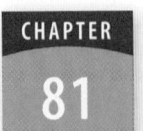

CHAPTER 81

Acute Appendicitis

E. Paul DeKoning

INTRODUCTION AND EPIDEMIOLOGY

Between 250,000 and 300,000 appendectomies for acute appendicitis are performed each year in the United States,[1] with an additional 700,000 patients affected in the European community.[2] The lifetime risk of acute appendicitis in the United States is an estimated 12% for males and 25% for females.[3] Yet, the epidemiology of this common ED diagnosis continues to change. Data suggest a reversal of a previous decline in incidence, with the annual rate increasing from 7.62 to 9.38 per 10,000 between 1993 and 2008,[4] whereas the rate of negative appendectomy has declined.[5] Similarly, between 2001 and 2008 the rate of perforation decreased, but this declining trend has not been consistent.[4,6] Acute appendicitis is most common in patients aged 10 to 19 years,[4] remains the most frequent cause of atraumatic abdominal pain in children >1 year old,[7] and is the most common nonobstetric surgical emergency in pregnancy, complicating up to 1 in 1500 pregnancies.[8,9] Despite advances in lab testing and imaging, accurate diagnosis is a challenge. Both "missed appendicitis" and unnecessary surgery for a false diagnosis are not without consequence. **Thus, consider appendicitis in any patient with acute atraumatic abdominal pain without prior appendectomy.**

PATHOPHYSIOLOGY

Appendicitis is caused by luminal obstruction of the vermiform appendix, typically by a fecalith. Other less frequent causes include obstruction by lymphatic tissue, gallstone, tumor, or parasites. Continued secretion from the luminal mucosa results in increased intraluminal pressure and appendiceal vascular insufficiency, leading ultimately to bacterial proliferation and inflammation. Left unchecked, perforation may occur.

Visceral innervation produces the vague, hard to localize periumbilical or central abdominal discomfort frequently observed early in the clinical course. Progressive inflammation and subsequent irritation of the somatically innervated parietal peritoneum produces the classic migration of pain to the right lower quadrant, to **McBurney's point**, located one third of the distance from the anterior superior iliac spine to the umbilicus. Up to 50% of patients may have an atypical presentation[10] due in part to anatomic variation. For example, a retrocecal appendix produces right flank or pelvic pain, whereas malrotation of the colon results in transposition of the appendix and, subsequently, pain to the left upper quadrant. Abdominal organ displacement from a gravid uterus may lead to right upper quadrant tenderness in pregnancy. Even so, a right lower quadrant location of pain remains the most common location of pain in pregnant women with appendicitis.[9]

CLINICAL FEATURES

The signs and symptoms of acute appendicitis lie along a spectrum that correlates with pathophysiology. Early on, patients classically complain of nonspecific symptoms of general malaise, indigestion, or bowel irregularity. Anorexia is common but not universally present. Alterations in bowel function are highly variable and can include constipation, diarrhea, and even obstruction as a late complication.[11] Periumbilical or central abdominal pain generally develop after nonspecific symptoms. If nausea develops, it typically follows the onset of pain.[12] Vomiting may or may not be present. Subjective or objective fever is frequent.

As the clinical course progresses, discomfort migrates to the right lower quadrant. Flank pain, dysuria, or hematuria can occur, given the typical proximity of the appendix to the urinary tract.[11]

Aggravating and alleviating features can help establish the diagnosis: worsening pain with deep inspiration may be present if there is peritoneal irritation, and individuals may state that the trip to the hospital was painful, particularly when encountering bumps in the road. Such features suggest a peritoneal process is under way. The release of intraluminal obstruction with perforation often results in sudden remittance of pain; consider appendiceal perforation if the patient's pain has suddenly improved.[11]

As the natural course progresses, examination findings likewise evolve. Progressive inflammation and peritoneal irritation yield reproducible tenderness to palpation in the right lower quadrant. The exception to right lower quadrant pain is a retrocecal appendix, which does not contact the anterior parietal peritoneum.[13] Rebound tenderness and involuntary guarding suggest peritonitis. Patients may have costovertebral tenderness, and percussion of the right heel or shaking of the hospital stretcher may elicit abdominal pain. There is no evidence that the digital rectal exam aids significantly in the diagnosis of acute appendicitis.[10] **Rovsing's sign** reproduces pain over McBurney's point as the clinician palpates the descending colon in the left lower quadrant. A positive psoas sign or obturator test suggests an inflammatory peritoneal process. The **psoas sign** is elicited if abdominal pain is produced with extension of the right leg at the hip while the patient lies on the left side. The **obturator test** elicits pain with internal and external rotation of the flexed right thigh at the hip. The presence of abdominal rigidity, a positive psoas sign, fever, or rebound tenderness increases the likelihood of acute appendicitis. Prior episodes of similar pain, the absence of right lower quadrant pain, and the absence of classic pain migration make appendicitis less likely. The presence or absence of any exam finding in isolation is neither sufficiently sensitive nor specific to rule out or rule in the diagnosis.

In a systematic review of 42 studies investigating appendicitis in patients aged 18 years or younger, fever was the single most useful sign with an LR(+) of 3.4 (95% confidence interval, 2.4 to 4.8), whereas its absence decreased the likelihood of appendicitis (LR(-), 0.32; 95% CI, 0.16 to 0.64). Rebound tenderness and pain migration to the right lower quadrant were also strong predictors.[14] In comparison, a classic study of exam findings in adult patients showed right lower quadrant pain as the single most useful sign (sensitivity, 0.81; specificity, 0.53; LR(+) 7.31-8.46; LR (-) 0-.28) followed by rigidity and migration of pain. Fever in adults had an LR(+) of 1.94 (95% CI, 0=0.28) of 1.94 (95% CI, 1.63 to 2.32) and a LR(-) of 0.58 (95% CI, 0.51 to 0.67).[15] **In both children and adults, however, no historical or physical examination finding is sufficient to rule in or rule out appendicitis.**[14,15]

DIAGNOSIS

Despite the advent of cross-sectional radiographic imaging and high-definition ultrasonography and a more than doubling of their use in recent years, detection rates for appendicitis have essentially remained the same.[16] There are numerous appendicitis mimics, and the differential diagnosis is broad (**Table 81-1**). Perform a complete physical examination, including a pelvic examination in women of childbearing age. Acute appendicitis is largely a clinical diagnosis, and no one adjunctive test is universally indicated.

Consider appendicitis in any patient with atraumatic right-sided abdominal, periumbilical, or flank pain who has not previously undergone appendectomy. Available diagnostic adjuncts include peripheral WBC and other acute inflammatory markers (e.g., C-reactive protein or erythrocyte sedimentation rate), urinalysis, and a pregnancy test. Diagnostic imaging should be considered in atypical presentations or if significant diagnostic uncertainty exists after thorough history and examination.

TABLE 81-1 Differential Diagnosis of Right Lower Quadrant Pain
GI
Cecal/Meckel's diverticulitis
Cecal volvulus
Colitis/terminal ileitis
Constipation/ileus/bowel obstruction
Crohn's/ulcerative colitis flair
Epiploic appendagitis
Functional abdominal pain
Incarcerated inguinal hernia
Intra-abdominal abscess
Intussusception
Malrotation
Mesenteric lymphadenitis
GU
Ectopic/heterotopic pregnancy
Ovarian torsion
Ovarian vein thrombosis
Pyelonephritis
Referred testicular pain
Renal colic
Tubo-ovarian abscess/salpingitis
MUSCULOSKELETAL
Abdominal wall/rectus sheath hematoma
Psoas abscess

SCORING SYSTEMS

Scoring systems, such as the Alvarado and Samuel scores, have been developed to aid in diagnosis. The modified **Alvarado score** for acute appendicitis ranks symptoms (migration, 1 point; anorexia or urinary acetone, 1 point; nausea or vomiting, 1 point), signs (right lower quadrant tenderness, 2 points; rebound, 1 point; fever, 1 point), and WBC count (>10,000/mm^3, 2 points) into low-risk appendicitis (score, 1 to 4) and possible or probable appendicitis (score, 5 to 9). However, the low-risk score (score, 1 to 4) was demonstrated as only 72% sensitive compared to 93% for clinical judgment when appendicitis was either the most likely or second most likely diagnosis.[17] Despite continued technologic advances and development of decision rules, different scoring systems often yield conflicting results and should not replace clinical judgment; the clinical impression of the experienced physician has the highest impact on patient outcome.[18-21]

LABORATORY TESTING

An increase in peripheral WBC may be the earliest marker of inflammation.[22] A study of 722 children identified both prospectively and retrospectively found acute appendicitis to be the most common diagnosis in children >4 years old with nontraumatic abdominal pain and leukocytosis.[23] However, a normal WBC is not uncommon, and leukopenic presentations have been documented.[24] **While numerous studies have evaluated the use of the WBC, there is no clear consensus on its utility.**[22,23,25-27] The WBC does not distinguish between simple and perforated appendicitis.[25] C-reactive protein and the erythrocyte sedimentation rate used alone lack the sensitivity and specificity to rule in or rule out the diagnosis. If the only diagnostic consideration is acute appendicitis (yes or no), the greatest utility of laboratory tests may be in combination: an elevated WBC and/or C-reactive protein may have a combined sensitivity as high as 98%. Normal values of both in patients with a low pretest probability of acute appendicitis make pathologically confirmed appendicitis very unlikely.[27-31] However, WBC and C-reactive protein levels are elevated in a number of other appendicitis mimics, so these markers are not useful if the differential diagnosis of pain is broad.[32,33]

Obtain a urinalysis because isolated microscopic hematuria may support a diagnosis of renal colic, and pyuria may suggest pyelonephritis. However, hematuria or sterile pyuria can be present in acute appendicitis.[11] Document a negative pregnancy test in females of reproductive age to rule out ectopic or heterotopic pregnancy. Other laboratory tests are not routinely indicated but may be beneficial when considering other diagnoses.

IMAGING

Obtain early surgical consultation before imaging in straightforward cases of suspected appendicitis in adults. Imaging is not universally necessary but may be of benefit in certain populations.[34-36] In children, some centers prefer pediatric surgery consultation prior to imaging with ionizing radiation.

When adjunctive imaging is indicated, early surgical consultation may aid guidance in imaging selection. The goal of imaging is to establish the diagnosis of appendicitis, avoid a negative appendectomy, identify perforation, and exclude other causes of abdominal pain with minimal radiation, cost, and time.

Plain radiography is not helpful. Findings are typically nonspecific but may demonstrate a nonspecific bowel gas pattern or adynamic ileus. An appendicolith may be visualized in up to 50% of children with appendicitis.[35]

US **Graded compression US should be the initial imaging modality of choice in both pregnant females[37] and children. It can likewise be considered in young, nonobese adults.** Reports of the effectiveness of US diagnosis of appendicitis in pregnancy are conflicting, with some reporting US as useful[38] and others reporting it as ineffective for diagnosis.[39] Regardless, US is safe, fast, well tolerated, and cost-effective.

The appendix is oval in the axial plane, ends blindly in the longitudinal plane, and should be compressible with a maximal diameter not exceeding 6 mm.[40] The normal appendix is typically differentiated from small bowel on US by the absence of peristalsis and the lack of change in configuration over time; its small size distinguishes it from large bowel. **Typical findings in appendicitis are a thickened, noncompressible appendix >6 mm in diameter (Figure 81-1).** Doppler US may illustrate hyperemia.[35] It is important to image the entire length of the appendix, because inflammation may be more pronounced at or localized to the distal end.[40] Given the highly operator-dependent nature of US, centers treating larger volumes of children may have greater reproducibility of high-quality studies. The diagnostic accuracy of abdominal US in children is better at ruling in acute appendicitis than excluding it.[41] Besides operator skill, other limitations to accuracy include cases of retrocecal appendicitis or perforation, excessive abdominal guarding or bowel gas, a gravid uterus or obese habitus, a decompressed bladder, and lack of patient cooperation. Perforation may lead to disappearance of specific imaging hallmarks and difficult visualization of the appendix on US. Pelvic US may be useful in cases of suspected appendicitis and a nondiagnostic abdominal US or CT,[42] or in the differentiation of appendicitis from pelvic inflammatory disease[43] (see chapter 97, "Abdominal and Pelvic Pain in the Nonpregnant Female").

Abdominopelvic CT In most adult males and nonpregnant females for whom the diagnosis of appendicitis is not sufficiently clear, consider abdominal CT that includes the abdomen and pelvis. Typical CT findings include a dilated appendix >6 mm with a thickened wall, periappendiceal inflammation, and potential visualization of an appendicolith or abscess.[44] Luminal obstruction and dilation may be relieved in cases of perforation, leading to disappearance of specific imaging hallmarks and difficult visualization of the appendix on CT.[11]

The accepted sensitivity of CT (composite studies using oral or IV contrast or no contrast) for the diagnosis of acute appendicitis is typically >94%, with a positive predictive value >95% (**Figure 81-2**).[34,36] In a comparison of CT versus US, the overall sensitivity of CT in patients >2 years old was 96%, with a 96% positive predictive value; graded compression US had an overall sensitivity of 86%, with a 95% positive predictive value.[36] In this same study,[36] women who had preoperative imaging had a statistically significant lower negative appendectomy rate than women who had no imaging, suggesting that women with suspected acute appendicitis derive the greatest benefit from preoperative imaging. **Appendiceal CT**, a less frequently used protocol, uses rectally administered contrast only with acquisition of thin cuts through the right iliac fossa. This avoids the difficulties of oral contrast administration in patients with active emesis and prevents potential adverse reactions of IV contrast. Time to acquisition of images is much shorter, typically around 15 minutes after administration of rectal contrast, but may produce significant patient discomfort.[45,46]

Oral and IV Contrast versus Nonenhanced CT Oral contrast medium has historically been recommended for CT of the abdomen and pelvis when investigating a broad differential of GI or pelvic diagnoses, and many centers continue to recommend CT imaging with both IV and oral contrast. Yet, a growing body of literature calls this practice into question. Multiple studies indicate that nonenhanced CT has excellent performance in the diagnosis of acute appendicitis.[47-53] The imaging evaluation of abdominal pain is time intensive and impacts ED overcrowding. Unenhanced studies can significantly decrease the time to diagnosis and eliminate patient discomfort from oral (especially in vomiting patients) or rectal contrast, and avoids altogether the risk of

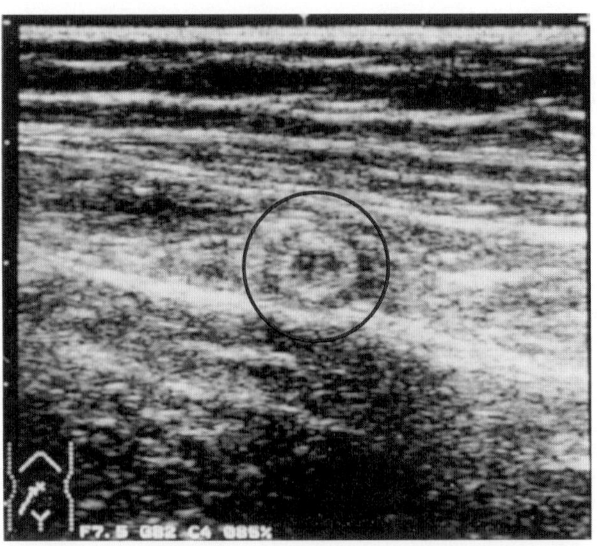

A

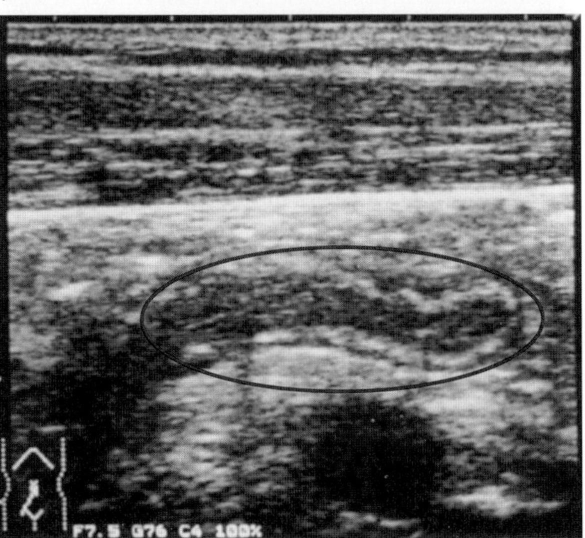

B

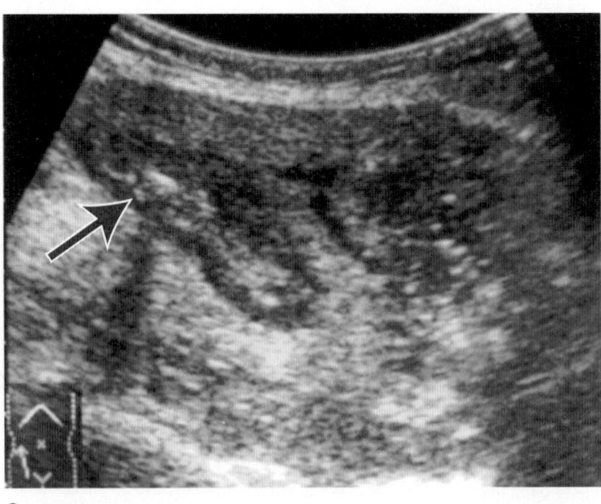

C

FIGURE 81-1. Ultrasonographic demonstration of acute appendicitis. A noncompressible, inflamed appendix (*red circles*) is shown in a cross-sectional view (A; 7.5 MHz) and a longitudinal section (B; 7.5 MHz). Mural lamination of the swollen appendix is maintained in the early stages of acute appendicitis. C. An appendicolith (*arrow*) with acoustic shadowing is demonstrated (5 MHz). [Reprinted with permission from Ma OJ, Mateer JR, Reardon RF, Blaivas M. *Emergency Ultrasound*. 3rd ed. Copyright © The McGraw-Hill Companies, 2014, All rights reserved. Chapter 11, General Surgery Applications, Figures 11-31A&B & 11-33.]

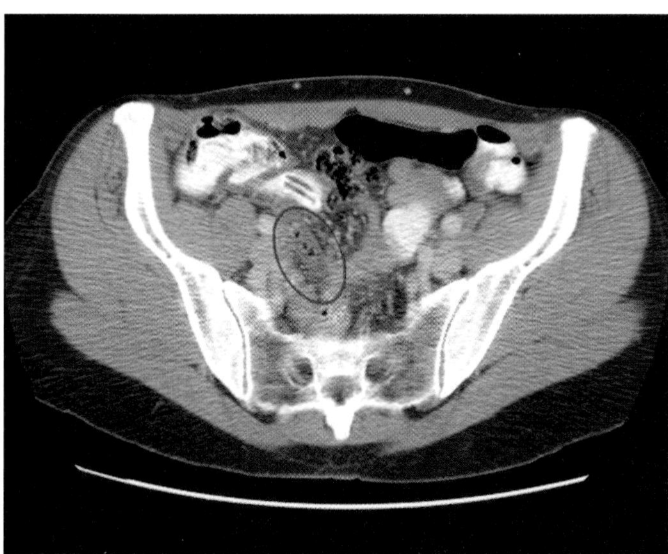

FIGURE 81-2. Acute appendicitis on contrast CT scan as evidenced by dilated and inflamed appendix (*red circle*).

renal injury from IV contrast. More than 52% of 462 patients who underwent CT imaging in at least one study had no oral, IV, or rectal contrast administered, with a combined sensitivity of 93% and a positive predictive value greater than 92%, supporting the suitability of nonenhanced CT imaging for making the diagnosis.[36] A comparison of nonenhanced CT with findings on laparoscopy reported 95% sensitivity with 100% specificity of nonenhanced CT in suspected appendicitis,[2] whereas another systematic review reported a pooled sensitivity of 92.7% (95% CI, 89.5% to 95.0%) and specificity of 96.1% (95% CI, 94.2% to 97.5%).[47] Another systematic review of 23 studies showed equivalent or improved diagnostic performance of nonenhanced CT when compared to oral contrast.[36] Oral contrast frequently does not reach the terminal ileum at the time of imaging, yet in this group of patients, at least one author has shown no diagnostic compromise in the performance of imaging.[52] Several studies attribute disagreement between nonenhanced CT and contrasted studies more to interobserver variability than contrast medium.[51,53] **Noncontrast CT should be considered an acceptable imaging modality in the workup of acute appendicitis.** In patients with renal insufficiency or dye allergy, administration of IV contrast is contraindicated. Body habitus may limit reproduction of noncontrast CT test characteristics; intraperitoneal fat serves as an intrinsic contrast medium in unenhanced CT, and its paucity in very thin patients can affect imaging interpretation.[44,45,54]

MRI Consider MRI as another reliable imaging technology in the evaluation of acute appendicitis, particularly in pregnant women. MRI avoids ionizing radiation and visualizes the entire abdomen in multiple planes. In a survey of U.S. academic medical centers with radiology residency programs, MRI was preferred over CT (39% vs. 32%) for evaluation of appendicitis in the first trimester of pregnancy. This preference reversed in the second and third trimesters.[37] **IV gadolinium crosses the placenta and is not used in pregnancy** given the teratogenic effects seen in animal studies.[55] **Gadolinium is not given to patients with renal insufficiency because it may cause nephrogenic fibrosing dermopathy.** Avoid MRI in the evaluation of the unstable patient given the time necessary for study acquisition. Sedation may be required for small children, rendering it impractical in many pediatric cases.

TREATMENT

Patients with acute appendicitis typically require appendectomy, so immediate surgical consultation is needed. Patients should be maintained as "nothing by mouth" to avoid operative delay. Provide resuscitation and maintenance IV fluids with appropriate antiemetics and analgesia. Initiate perioperative antibiotics upon diagnosis or if the patient exhibits signs of peritonitis. Appropriate choices should broadly cover aerobic and anaerobic gram-negative organisms. Acceptable regimens include ampicillin/sulbactam 3 grams IV (pediatric dose, 75 milligrams/kg IV); piperacillin/tazobactam 4.5 grams IV (100 milligrams/kg IV); cefoxitin 2 grams IV (40 milligrams/kg); or metronidazole 500 milligrams IV plus ciprofloxacin 400 milligrams IV.[56] Given the nonoperative management of uncomplicated diverticulitis, salpingitis, and neonatal enterocolitis with antibiotics, some suggest a similar nonoperative approach to uncomplicated acute appendicitis.[1] However, this is not yet considered the accepted standard of care.

DISPOSITION AND FOLLOW-UP

Surgery is the accepted standard of care for acute appendicitis. If the local surgical services are inadequate or unavailable, transfer the patient to an appropriate institution. For the patient in whom the diagnosis remains elusive despite a rigorous diagnostic evaluation, consider extended observation in the ED or hospital with serial examinations, allowing for evolution of the patient's condition. Alternatively, the stable, reliable patient without significant comorbidities may be a candidate for discharge provided they have a scheduled return visit to the ED or their primary physician (typically within 12 hours) for repeat examination. Patients must have adequate pain control and be able to tolerate oral hydration. Provide clear abdominal pain discharge instructions, including a list of concerning signs or symptoms that should prompt earlier return to the ED.

SPECIAL POPULATIONS

Uninsured/underinsured patients, individuals from low-income communities, and some ethnic minorities may be more likely to develop appendiceal perforation, but previously observed trends have been inconsistent in recent years.[6,57] The elderly are likely to have preexisting comorbidities that alter presentation, management, and outcomes. Institutionalized patients, those with communication difficulties, those with poor access to medical care, and the elderly may have more vague complaints, including diffuse pain, fever, or alteration in mental status. Such individuals commonly present later in the course of the disease and are more likely to have worse outcomes.[58] In such patients, an "atypical" presentation should be considered the norm. A low threshold for prolonged observation or admission can avoid unnecessary morbidity and mortality.

Pregnant women warrant special attention. Acute appendicitis is the most common surgical emergency in pregnancy, and delay in diagnosis is the greatest cause of increased morbidity in the pregnant woman with an acute abdomen.[8,9,59] Ovarian torsion and ectopic or heterotopic pregnancy are additional considerations. If abdominal US is nondiagnostic, consider pelvic US, CT, or MRI. Consult with the radiologist to select the most appropriate imaging study. Many radiologists avoid CT in the first trimester given teratogenic concerns of ionizing radiation.[37] In addition, although iodinated contrast material is safe in pregnancy, avoid IV gadolinium.[55]

Children are a diagnostic challenge, particularly if they cannot adequately verbalize their complaints. In such cases, physical examination, parallel history from the parent or guardian, and a high index of suspicion are the keys to accurate diagnosis. Pediatric imaging should begin with US, but many centers advise early surgical consultation before any imaging if appendicitis is a consideration.

REFERENCES

The complete reference list is available online at www.TintinalliEM.com.

Diverticulitis

Autumn Graham

INTRODUCTION AND EPIDEMIOLOGY

Although uncommon in developing countries, diverticular disease is increasingly prevalent in industrialized nations. Radiographic and autopsy data indicate that the prevalence of diverticulosis increases with age: 5% in patients age <40 years, 30% by age 60, and >70% by age 85.[1,2] One study noted a 26% jump in hospital admissions between 1998 and 2005, particularly in patients less than 45 years of age.[3]

In most patients, diverticular disease is an incidental finding. The natural history of the disease appears to be quite benign. One study followed 2366 Kaiser Permanente patients hospitalized with acute diverticulitis and treated nonoperatively. Of those, 86% required no further inpatient care for diverticulitis during a 9-year follow-up period. Only 4% had a second recurrence. No patient with a second recurrence required an operation.[4]

PATHOPHYSIOLOGY

Diverticula are small herniations at sites where the vasculature, called *vasa recta*, penetrates the circular muscle layer of the colon. Although *true diverticula* involve all layers of the colon wall, most acquired diverticula are considered *false diverticula*, involving only the mucosal and submucosal layers. Diverticula usually range from 5 to 10 mm, but can extend up to 20 mm in length. Diverticulitis occurs when inflammation develops and in complicated diverticulitis, leading to translocation of bacteria, microperforation, and abscess or phlegmon formation.[5]

There are similar chemical and histologic changes seen in inflammatory bowel disease and irritable bowel syndrome, but no unifying mechanism has been demonstrated.[5,6] The most common bacterial pathogens isolated are anaerobes, including *Bacteroides*, *Peptostreptococcus*, *Clostridium*, and *Fusobacterium* as well as gram-negative rods, such as *Escherichia coli*.

Altered bowel motility leads to high intraluminal colonic pressures and diverticula formation. The role of diet remains unclear. Smoking and obesity increase risk for diverticulitis, and an active lifestyle is said to decrease the risk. Nonsteroidal anti-inflammatory drugs, opioids, and steroids increase the risk of perforation.[5]

In the United States, diverticular disease is almost exclusively a left-sided colon disease, specifically the descending and sigmoid colon. Right-sided disease accounts for only 2% to 5% of cases and is found predominantly in Asian populations.[7]

CLINICAL FEATURES

Classically, diverticulitis presents with left lower quadrant abdominal pain, fever, and leukocytosis. Patients with a redundant sigmoid colon, of Asian descent, or with right-sided disease may complain of right lower quadrant or suprapubic pain. The pain may be intermittent or constant and often associated with a change of bowel habits, either diarrhea or constipation. Other associated symptoms include nausea/vomiting, anorexia, and urinary symptoms. On physical examination, patients may exhibit findings ranging from mild abdominal tenderness to moderate tenderness with a tender palpable mass to peritonitis with rebound and guarding.

DIAGNOSIS

In stable patients with a history of confirmed diverticulitis and a similar acute presentation, no further diagnostic evaluation is necessary unless the patient fails to improve with conservative medical treatment. If a prior diagnosis has not been confirmed or the current episode differs from the past episode, diagnostic imaging is required to exclude other intra-abdominal pathology and to evaluate for complications. The differential diagnosis of diverticulitis is extensive, including gynecologic emergencies, cancer, and inflammatory or infectious colitis (**Table 82-1**). Laboratory data are rarely diagnostic for diverticulitis, but liver function panels, CBC, renal panel, lipase, and urinalysis may aid in the exclusion of other disorders.

TABLE 82-1 Differential Diagnosis of Diverticulitis
Acute appendicitis
Colitis—ischemic or infectious
Inflammatory bowel disease (Crohn's disease, ulcerative colitis)
Colon cancer
Irritable bowel syndrome
Pseudomembranous colitis
Epiploic appendagitis
Gallbladder disease
Incarcerated hernia
Mesenteric infarction
Complicated ulcer disease
Peritonitis
Obstruction
Ovarian torsion
Ectopic pregnancy
Ovarian cyst or mass
Pelvic inflammatory disease
Cystitis
Kidney stone
Renal pathology
Pancreatic disease

IMAGING

CT is the preferred imaging modality because of its ability to evaluate the severity of disease and the presence of complications. CT with IV and oral contrast has documented sensitivities of 97% and specificities approaching 100%.[8] CT findings include increased soft tissue density within the pericolic fat, indicating inflammation; presence of diverticula; bowel wall thickening >4 mm; soft tissue masses, representing phlegmon; or pericolic fluid collections, representing abscesses.[8]

Compression US is operator dependent and limited based on the patient's body habitus. Sensitivity and specificity of US for diverticulitis vary but are >80% in experienced hands. CT is preferred to detect complications.[9]

TREATMENT

Treatment varies with disease severity (**Figure 82-1**). Uncomplicated diverticulitis is isolated to inflammation of the diverticula with or without phlegmon or small abscess confined to the bowel wall. Complicated diverticulitis includes diverticular inflammation associated with abscess, stricture, obstruction, fistula, or perforation.

Current treatment recommendations are provided in **Table 82-2**.

Uncomplicated diverticulitis is treated with bowel rest (liquid diet) and oral antibiotics (Table 82-2). Dietary restriction or modification is commonly recommended, but efficacy is not clear.[5] There is no advantage of IV antibiotics over oral antibiotics.[5] Admission is not necessary unless there are serious comorbidities or obstacles to outpatient care. If uncomplicated diverticulitis is confirmed with CT, the success rate of ambulatory treatment is about 98%.[10]

There is growing interest in the treatment of uncomplicated diverticulitis without antibiotics at all, due to questions about antibiotic efficacy and antibiotic adverse effects such as allergy, nausea and vomiting, and *Clostridium difficile* infection.[5,10-12]

One recent randomized controlled study in Sweden evaluated the need for antibiotics in uncomplicated diverticulitis confirmed by CT.

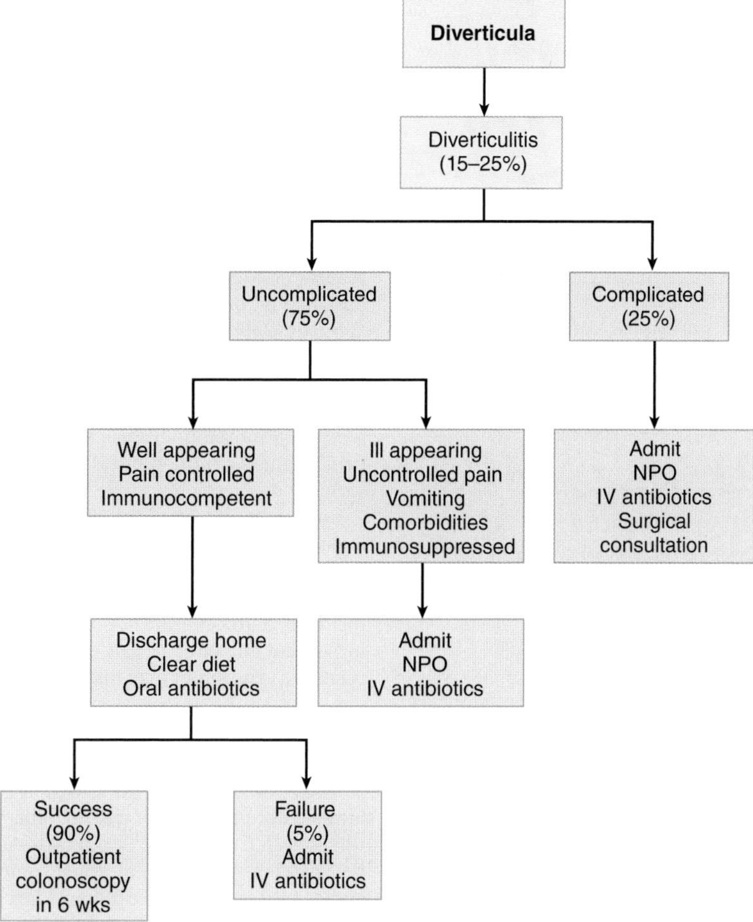

FIGURE 82-1. Algorithm for treatment of diverticulitis. NPO = nothing by mouth.

Of the 669 patients studied, 9 patients experienced complications: three abscesses and three perforations in the nonantibiotic group and three perforations in the antibiotic group. There were no differences in outcomes between the two groups, including symptoms at 30-day follow-up, need for emergency surgery, or median hospital stay.[10] The Infectious Diseases Society of America recommends a 4-day course of treatment.[13] As of this writing, there is no consensus on the omission of antibiotics.

Complicated diverticulitis generally requires admission. In addition to bowel rest and IV antibiotics, specific treatments are directed to complications. Complicated diverticulitis is often referred to by the Hinchey classification scheme[8]: Stage 1 is small, confined pericolic or mesenteric abscesses; stage 2 is larger abscesses, extending to the pelvis; stage 3 is perforated diverticulitis and purulent peritonitis; and stage 4 refers to free perforation with fecal contamination of the peritoneal cavity.

Abscesses and phlegmon are among the most common complications. Phlegmon is inflammation and infection of tissue without abscess. Advances in percutaneous drainage of abscesses have allowed many patients to undergo less invasive treatment. Abscesses that measure <4 cm and phlegmon (Hinchey stage 1) are often admitted for IV antibiotics and do not require percutaneous drainage. Perforation has a high mortality rate, and patients need volume resuscitation, IV antibiotics, and emergent exploratory surgery. For Hinchey stage 3, the mortality rate approaches 13% and increases to 43% for Hinchey stage 4.[8,14]

DISPOSITION AND FOLLOW-UP

ED discharge is appropriate for uncomplicated diverticulitis—that is, for a patient with stable vital signs, who is nontoxic appearing, in whom adequate analgesia can be maintained at home with oral narcotics, and with mild physical examination findings. Advise a clear diet to be advanced as tolerated, oral antibiotics, and instructions to follow up in 2 to 3 days with a primary care provider or return to the ED for recurring pain, high fevers, nausea/vomiting, or abdominal tenderness.

Patients with intractable nausea or vomiting, significant comorbid diseases,[15] poor support at home, high leukocytosis, or high fevers, as well as the elderly, the immunocompromised, and those with persistent pain should be admitted. The immunocompromised and those taking chronic steroids often present atypically and are at risk for morbidity and mortality. Patients with complicated diverticulitis or failed outpatient management should also be admitted. A failure of outpatient therapy is defined as symptoms or worsening radiographic imaging within 6 weeks of the initial episode.

SPECIAL CONSIDERATIONS

YOUNG PATIENTS

Patients <40 years old comprise a small proportion of patients with diverticulitis, but their numbers are growing. This trend may correlate with the growing obesity epidemic in the United States, because young diverticulitis patients tend to be overweight. Their disease is also thought to be more virulent than that of their older counterparts, with higher rates of recurrence, complicated presentation, and surgical intervention compared to patients >50 years old. Younger patients also seem to have higher rates of readmission.[16,17]

MECKEL'S DIVERTICULITIS

Meckel's diverticulum is a true congenital diverticulum that follows "the rule of 2's." It is present in approximately 2% of the population, 2 ft from the ileocecal valve, and symptomatic in 2% of patients. It generally presents with crampy abdominal pain, nausea/vomiting, and bleeding.

TABLE 82-2 Antibiotics for Diverticulitis		
Outpatient 4–7 days	First line	Metronidazole 500 milligrams PO q6h PLUS Ciprofloxacin 750 milligrams PO BID OR Levofloxacin 750 milligrams PO q24h OR Trimethoprim–sulfamethoxazole (Bactrim) 1 tab PO BID
	Alternate	Amoxicillin-clavulanate extended release 1000/62.5 milligrams 2 tabs PO BID
		Moxifloxacin 400 mg PO q24h
Inpatient		
Moderate disease	First line	Metronidazole 500 milligrams IV TID PLUS Ciprofloxacin 400 milligrams IV BID OR Levofloxacin 750 milligrams IV q24h OR Aztreonam 2 grams IV TID OR Ceftriaxone 1 gram IV q24h
	Alternative	Ertapenem 1 gram IV q24h
		Piperacillin-tazobactam 4.5 grams IV q8h
		Moxifloxacin 400 milligrams IV q24h
Severe, life-threatening	First line	Imipenem 500 milligrams IV q6h
		Meropenem 1 gram IV q8h
		Piperacillin-tazobactam 4.5 milligrams IV q8h
	Alternative	Ampicillin 2 grams IV q6h PLUS Metronidazole 500 milligrams IV q6h PLUS Ciprofloxacin 400 milligrams IV q12h OR Amikacin, gentamicin, or tobramycin (Penicillin allergy: Aztreonam 2 grams IV q6h PLUS metronidazole 500 milligrams IV q6h)

Definitive diagnosis is often difficult, but radionucleotide imaging or CT may be helpful. Due to overlapping signs and symptoms, Meckel's diverticulitis is often confused with acute appendicitis. Treatment is surgical.

EPIPLOIC APPENDAGITIS

Epiploic appendages are small fat-filled sacs situated near the lining of the colon that can become inflamed as a result of torsion or venous thrombosis. The typical presentation is sharp abdominal pain, nausea, and vomiting. The symptoms can be confused with acute appendicitis, diverticulitis, or cholecystitis. Epiploic appendagitis is usually an incidental finding on CT and follows a benign, self-limiting course. The treatment consists of pain management and follow-up in 1 week.

REFERENCES

The complete reference list is available online at www.TintinalliEM.com.

Bowel Obstruction

Timothy G. Price
Raymond J. Orthober

INTRODUCTION AND EPIDEMIOLOGY

Intestinal obstruction is the inability of the intestinal tract to allow for regular passage of food and bowel contents secondary to mechanical obstruction or adynamic ileus. Intestinal obstruction accounts for approximately 15% of all ED visits for acute abdominal pain.[1]

Mechanical obstruction can be caused by either intrinsic or extrinsic factors and generally requires definitive intervention in a relatively short period of time to determine the cause and minimize subsequent morbidity and mortality (**Tables 83-1 and 83-2**). Adynamic ileus (paralytic ileus) is more common but is usually self-limiting and does not require surgical intervention.

Both large and small intestines may be obstructed by various pathologic processes (Table 83-1). Extrinsic, intrinsic, or intraluminal processes precipitate mechanical obstruction. Differentiating small bowel obstruction from large bowel obstruction is important, because the incidence, clinical presentation, evaluation, and treatment vary depending on the anatomic site of obstruction. Intestinal pseudo-obstruction (Ogilvie's syndrome) may mimic bowel obstruction.

PATHOPHYSIOLOGY

Normal bowel contains gas as well as gastric secretions and food. Intraluminal accumulation of gastric, biliary, and pancreatic secretions continues even if there is no oral intake. As obstruction develops, the bowel becomes congested and intestinal contents fail to be absorbed. Vomiting and decreased oral intake follow. The combination of decreased absorption, vomiting, and reduced intake leads to volume depletion with hemoconcentration and electrolyte imbalance, and may lead to renal failure or shock.

Bowel distention often accompanies mechanical obstruction. Distention is due to the accumulation of fluids in the bowel lumen, an increase in intraluminal pressure with enhanced peristaltic contractions, and air swallowing. When intraluminal pressure exceeds capillary and venous pressure in the bowel wall, absorption and lymphatic drainage decrease, the bowel becomes ischemic, and septicemia and bowel necrosis can develop. Shock ensues rapidly. Mortality approaches 70% if bowel obstruction has progressed to this degree. This sequence of events may occur more rapidly in a closed-loop obstruction with no proximal escape for bowel contents. Examples of closed-loop obstruction include an incarcerated hernia and complete colon obstruction in the presence of a closed ileocecal valve.

SMALL BOWEL OBSTRUCTION

Small bowel obstruction is approximately four times more common than large bowel obstruction. The most common cause of small bowel obstruction is adhesions after abdominal surgery. Although in most

TABLE 83-1 Common Causes of Intestinal Obstruction

Duodenum	Small Bowel	Colon
Stenosis	Adhesions	Carcinoma
Foreign body (bezoars)	Hernia	Fecal impaction
Stricture	Intussusception	Ulcerative colitis
Superior mesenteric artery syndrome	Lymphoma	Volvulus
	Stricture	Diverticulitis (stricture, abscess)
		Intussusception
		Pseudo-obstruction

TABLE 83-2 Key Features of Ileus and Mechanical Bowel Obstruction

	Ileus	Bowel Obstruction
Pain	Mild to moderate	Moderate to severe
Location	Diffuse	May localize
Physical examination	Mild distention, ± tenderness, decreased bowel sounds	Mild distention, tenderness, high-pitched bowel sounds
Laboratory	Possible dehydration	Leukocytosis
Imaging	May be normal	Abnormal
Treatment	Observation, hydration	Nasogastric tube, surgery

cases several months to years have passed from the time of the previous surgery, small bowel obstruction may occur within the first few weeks after surgery. The second most common cause of small bowel obstruction is incarceration of a groin hernia (see chapter 84, "Hernias"). Other sites that occasionally are responsible for small bowel obstruction secondary to hernia include the umbilicus, femoral canal, and, rarely, the obturator foramen. Umbilical hernias are more readily apparent and occur in any age group. Obturator or femoral hernias are much less common. Elderly females are particularly susceptible to these hernias, which may present with femoral or medial thigh pain. Finally, a defect in the mesentery itself may cause intestinal obstruction. In the elderly population, adhesions and hernias are still common causes of small bowel obstruction, whereas carcinoma is the most likely cause of large bowel obstruction because of the increased likelihood of cancer as people age. Patients >60 years old are more likely to succumb secondary to complications of bowel obstruction.

Bariatric surgery may be complicated by internal hernias after Roux-en-Y gastric bypass.[2,3] Other causes of small bowel obstruction are much less common and generally are the result of intraluminal or intramural processes. Primary small bowel lesions include polyps, lymphoma, or adenocarcinoma. Hamartomatous polyps are common in Peutz-Jeghers syndrome; polyps occur in patients between the ages of 10 and 30 years and cause obstruction in about 40% of patients.[4] An unusual cause of intraluminal obstruction is gallstone ileus. In this situation, a gallstone has eroded from the gallbladder through the bowel wall and can cause obstruction at the ileocecal valve. Signs of gallstone ileus include bowel obstruction and air in the biliary tree. Lymphomas may be the leading point of intussusception and present as small bowel obstruction. Bezoars are most commonly composed of vegetable matter or pulp from persimmons. Patients who have undergone GI pyloroplasty or pyloric resection are most susceptible to intraluminal obstruction by bezoars.

Inflammatory bowel disease and infectious processes, including abscesses, may obstruct the small bowel at various sites. Radiation enteritis should be considered as a possible cause of small bowel obstruction in patients who have undergone radiation therapy. Blunt abdominal trauma may cause a duodenal hematoma. This condition is seen in children as a result of lap belt use and may present as intra-abdominal pain and vomiting similar to other causes of small bowel obstruction.

Visualization of the entire small bowel can be accomplished by capsule endoscopy. An important complication is capsule retention, with literature-reported frequencies of 1% to 20%.[5] Capsule retention can lead to obstruction and perforation, so patients with abdominal pain after capsule introduction should be carefully evaluated for these complications.[5]

LARGE BOWEL OBSTRUCTION

Neoplasms are by far the most common cause of large bowel obstruction. Colonic obstruction is almost never caused by hernia or surgical adhesions and should prompt an evaluation for a neoplasm. Diverticulitis may create significant mesenteric edema and secondary obstruction. Stricture formation may occur with chronic inflammation and scarring. Fecal impaction is a common problem in the elderly or debilitated and may present with symptoms of colonic obstruction.

The next most frequent cause of large bowel obstruction after cancer and diverticulitis is sigmoid volvulus. Elderly, bedridden, or psychiatric patients who are taking anticholinergic medication are most at risk for volvulus. A history of constipation may precede the development of volvulus. Radiographic appearance is usually classic (**Figure 83-1**). Cecal volvulus may cause large bowel obstruction. There is a higher incidence of cecal volvulus in gravid patients.[6]

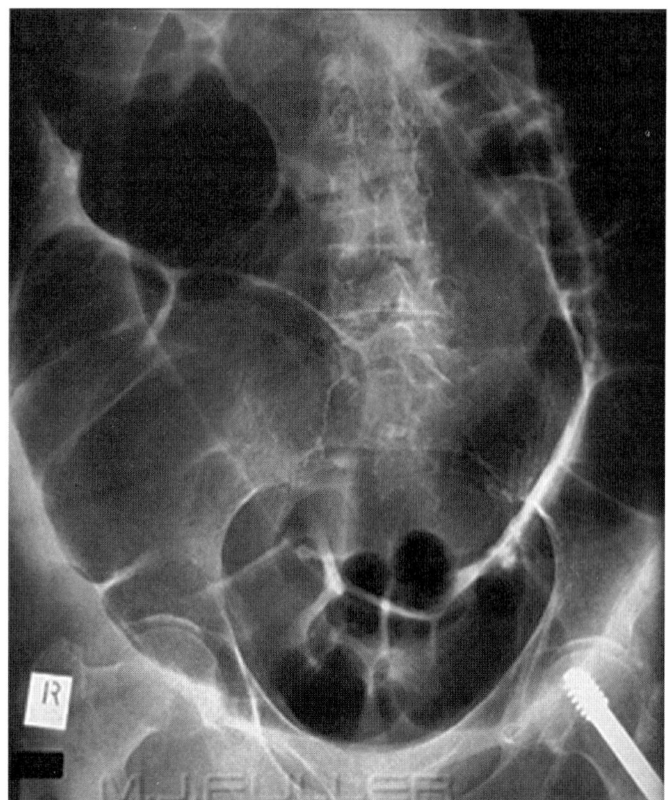

FIGURE 83-1. Sigmoid volvulus. Extends into the T10 area or higher. [Reproduced with permission from Wikiradiography.com.]

CLINICAL FEATURES

HISTORY

The site and nature of the obstruction and the preexisting condition of the patient will determine the clinical presentation. Although some generalizations are possible, there are no components of the history able to reliably predict small bowel obstruction.[7] Almost all patients will have abdominal pain. Pain generally is crampy and intermittent. Pain of mechanical small bowel obstruction is often episodic, lasting for a few minutes at a time, and may be periumbilical or diffuse. Pain tends to be less intense and more constant in adynamic ileus. Proximal obstruction usually causes vomiting. Vomitus is usually bilious in proximal obstruction but is feculent in distal ileal or large bowel obstruction. The pain of large bowel obstruction is usually hypogastric.

Other features that are consistently present with obstruction of small bowel or colon include the inability to have a bowel movement or pass flatus. "Constipation" is a common symptom of bowel obstruction. Partial bowel obstruction, however, is often associated with regular passage of stool and flatus. Additional risk factors are advanced age and anticholinergic or tricyclic antidepressants, which depress bowel motility.

PHYSICAL EXAMINATION

Physical findings vary depending on the site, duration, and etiology of the pathologic process. In small bowel obstruction, distention is the most reliable sign, and some distention is usually present early in the disease process.[7] Abdominal tenderness may be minimal to severe and localized or diffused. Peritonitis causes severe pain. The abdomen may be tympanitic to percussion. Mechanical obstruction produces active, high-pitched bowel sounds with occasional "rushes." If obstruction has been present for several hours, peristaltic waves and bowel sounds may be diminished. Patients with an adynamic ileus may have some abdominal distention associated with diminished or absent bowel sounds. Localized or rebound tenderness may be a sign of gangrenous or perforated bowel, which requires immediate surgical intervention.

Careful examination coupled with radiographic investigation will often distinguish bowel obstruction from ileus. Emptiness of the left iliac fossa has been reported to be a reliable sign of sigmoid volvulus. Organomegaly or masses may suggest a cause of the obstruction. The *absence* of stool or air in the rectal vault supports a diagnosis of obstruction and may aid in the diagnosis of bowel obstruction, but its *presence* does not eliminate a more proximal obstruction. A rectal examination may identify fecal impaction, rectal carcinoma, occult blood, or stricture. Consider a pelvic examination in women to identify gynecologic pathology causing obstruction (see chapter 97, "Abdominal and Pelvic Pain in the Nonpregnant Female"). A vaginal pessary can cause colonic obstruction due to extrinsic compression of the colon.[8] See Table 83-2 for the key causes of ileus and mechanical bowel obstruction.

DIAGNOSIS

Consider bowel obstruction or ileus in any patient with abdominal pain and distention. Numerous other pathologic processes may also cause these symptoms, but additional evaluation guided by the history and physical examination may be necessary to confirm or rule out obstruction or ileus. Although any segment of bowel may be affected, low colonic obstruction is the most common clinical presentation. Radiographs may demonstrate a massively dilated colon with well-defined septa and haustral markings and very little fluid, without air-fluid levels. A CT scan is the most reliable diagnostic modality and offers the advantage of detecting mucosal inflammation and evaluating mucosal viability.[9] Avoid barium studies because the patient may be unable to evacuate the barium.

LABORATORY TESTING

Laboratory studies usually include a CBC and electrolyte levels, the results of which may vary widely depending on the duration and site of obstruction and the presence of bowel necrosis. A leukocytosis of $>20,000/mm^3$ or left shift should make one suspect bowel gangrene, intra-abdominal abscess, or peritonitis. Extreme leukocytosis ($>40,000/mm^3$) suggests mesenteric vascular occlusion. The serum amylase and lipase levels may be mildly elevated. Increases in hematocrit, BUN, and creatinine are consistent with volume depletion and dehydration. Other indications of the severity of obstruction or secondary complications include increased urine specific gravity, ketonuria, elevated lactate levels, and metabolic acidosis. Small studies suggest that procalcitonin may predict bowel ischemia or failure of conservative management.[10]

IMAGING

In the ED, flat and upright abdominal radiographs with an upright chest x-ray or a lateral decubitus view can be used to confirm diagnostic suspicion for bowel obstruction, severe constipation, or free air. Plain x-rays can also localize the site of obstruction to large or small bowel (**Figure 83-2**). However, if clinical suspicion for obstruction is strong, CT scan with oral and IV contrast is the imaging method of choice in the ED. The CT scan is extremely sensitive in high-grade obstruction, providing information not only about the presence or absence of an obstruction but often its location, severity, and cause.[1] In the presence of renal insufficiency or contrast allergy, oral contrast alone may provide sufficient diagnostic information.

TREATMENT

Most patients with small bowel obstruction may be successfully managed nonoperatively, whereas most patients with large bowel obstruction will require surgery.[1] For colonic obstruction due to malignancy, resection of

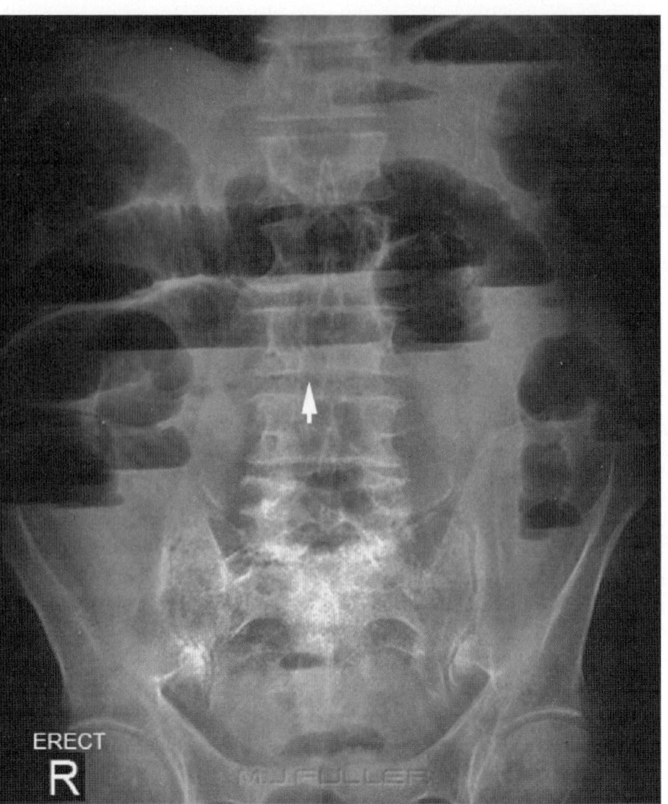

FIGURE 83-2. Small bowel obstruction. A. Multiple air-fluid levels. B. Coiled spring sign. [Reproduced with permission from Wikiradiography.com.]

the tumor has been the gold standard treatment. Self-expanding endoluminal stents can be used to relieve the obstruction and avoid emergent operation.[11] Use of a nasogastric tube is often unnecessary and is associated with potential benefit and potential risks. It should be considered in the presence of severe distention and vomiting. Local surgeon preference continues to dictate local practice with regard to nasogastric tube use. Vigorous IV fluid replacement is needed because of loss of absorptive capacity, decreased oral intake, and vomiting. Monitor adequacy of fluid resuscitation by the response of blood pressure, heart rate, and urine output. **Closed-loop obstruction, bowel necrosis, and cecal volvulus are surgical emergencies.** Administer preoperative broad-spectrum antibiotics in the ED. There are many possible regimens. Monotherapy could be tazobactam-piperacillin, 3.375 grams IV every 6 hours, ticarcillin-clavulanate, 3.1 grams IV every 6 hours, or a carbapenem.

If adynamic ileus is suspected or the diagnosis is uncertain, conservative inpatient management, including IV fluids and observation, generally is effective in allowing the bowel to resume normal activity and function. Any medication that inhibits bowel mobility should be discontinued.

DISPOSITION AND FOLLOW-UP

Admit patients with bowel obstruction to the hospital. Surgical consultation should generally be obtained in the ED or at the time of admission. Adynamic ileus should also be admitted for the treatment of the underlying cause and until resolution of the ileus.

REFERENCES

The complete reference list is available online at www.TintinalliEM.com.

Hernias

Donald Byars
Turan Kayagil

INTRODUCTION

With nearly 10% of the population developing some sort of hernia during their lifetime, this is among the most common of surgical problems.[1] Hernias are classified by anatomic location, hernia contents, and the status of those contents (e.g., reducible, strangulated, or incarcerated).[2]

A hernia is called **reducible** when the hernia sac itself is soft and easy to replace back through the hernia neck defect. A hernia is **incarcerated** when it is firm, often painful, and nonreducible by direct manual pressure. **Strangulation** develops as a consequence of incarceration and implies impairment of blood flow (arterial, venous, or both). A strangulated hernia presents as severe, exquisite pain at the hernia site, often with signs and symptoms of intestinal obstruction, toxic appearance, and, possibly, skin changes overlying the hernia sac. A strangulated hernia is an acute surgical emergency. This chapter discusses hernias in adults. Hernias in children are discussed in chapter 130, "Acute Abdominal Pain in Infants and Children."

ANATOMY OF COMMON HERNIAS

INGUINAL HERNIA

Seventy-five percent of all hernias occur in the inguinal region, making it the most common form of hernia, with two thirds of these being of the indirect type (**Figure 84-1**). Although there is a clear male predilection, inguinal hernias are also the most common hernias in women. Inguinal hernias present as a groin mass. Typically the mass has been present for some time, but may have recently become larger or the patient may have begun to develop symptoms of incarceration or strangulation. The differential diagnosis for a groin mass is somewhat broad and includes, in addition to hernia, hidradenitis, other abscess, sebaceous cyst, lymphoma, hydrocele, varicocele, femoral hernia, and femoral aneurysm. Thankfully, the physical examination for most hernias is fairly straightforward. Bedside US can be very helpful in the identification of an inguinal hernia if the diagnosis remains in question (**Figure 84-2**). One study reported 100% sensitivity and 100% specificity of bedside emergency US for the diagnosis of groin hernia.[3]

A **direct inguinal hernia** passes directly through a weakness in the transversalis fascia in the Hesselbach triangle. Hesselbach triangle is constructed with the lateral border of the inferior epigastric arteries, a medial border with the rectus sheath, and an inferior border of the inguinal ligament (**Figure 84-3**).[4]

The hernia sac from an **indirect inguinal hernia** passes from the internal to the external inguinal ring through the patent process vaginalis, and then to the scrotum (**Figure 84-4**).

VENTRAL AND INCISIONAL HERNIAS

Ventral hernias develop as a result of a defect in the anterior abdominal wall and can be either spontaneous or acquired. They are typically characterized by their anatomic location as epigastric, umbilical, incisional, or hypogastric (rare; **Figure 84-5**).[5]

Incisional hernias account for up to 20% of all abdominal wall hernias. They are often the result of excess wall tension or inadequate wound

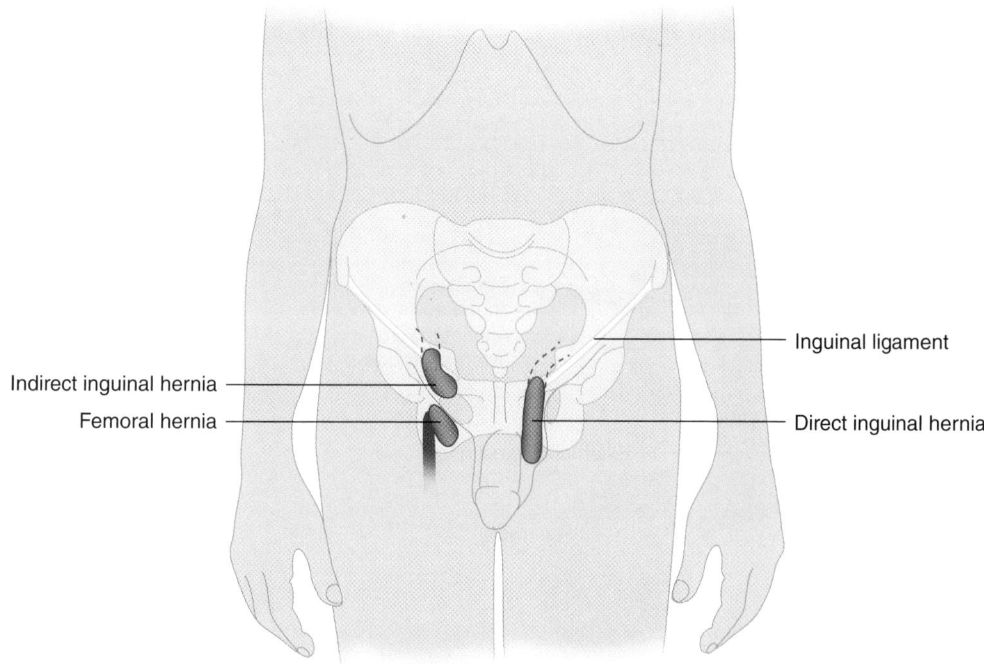

FIGURE 84-1. Groin hernia.

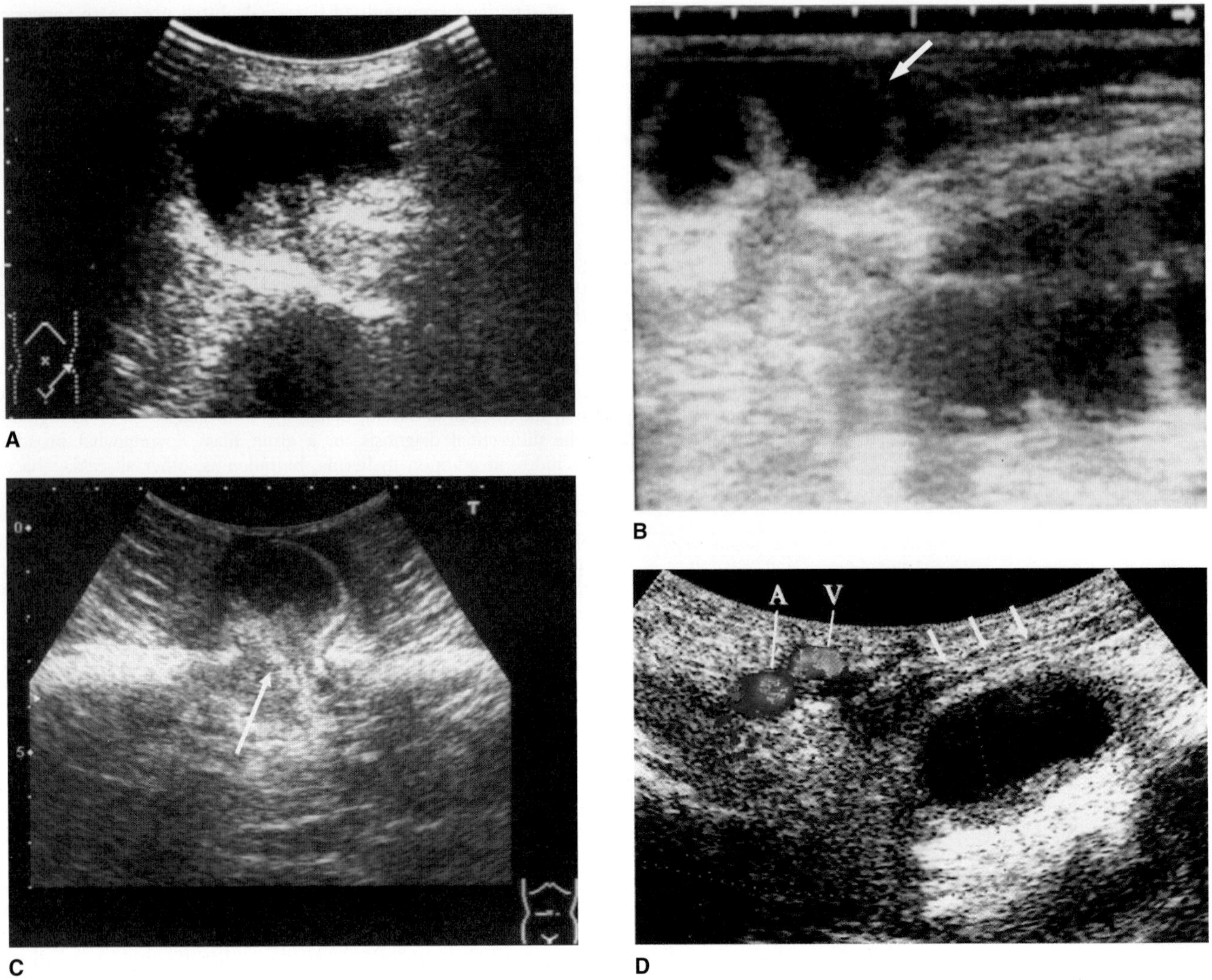

A

B

C

D

FIGURE 84-2. Incarcerated hernia. **A.** An incarcerated femoral hernia is demonstrated as a small-bowel segment herniated through the femoral canal. **B.** In an incarcerated incisional hernia, a small-bowel segment (*arrow*) is demonstrated as herniated through a small orifice in the abdominal wall. Dilated small-bowel loops are evident proximal to the incarceration. **C.** In an umbilical hernia, a herniated small-bowel segment is demonstrated within the fluid space in the hernia sac. The segment was softly strangulated at the hernia orifice (*arrow*) formed by a defect of the fascia and was easily reduced by manipulation in this case. **D.** An incarcerated obturator hernia is demonstrated deep in the femoral region. It locates posterior to the pectineus muscle (*arrows*) and medial to the femoral artery (A) and vein (V). [Reproduced with permission from Ma OJ, Mateer JR, Blaivas M (eds): *Emergency Ultrasound*, 2nd ed. Copyright © 2008 The McGraw-Hill Companies, All rights reserved. Chapter 9, General Surgery Applications, Common Abnormalities, Incarcerated Hernia. Figure 9-16.]

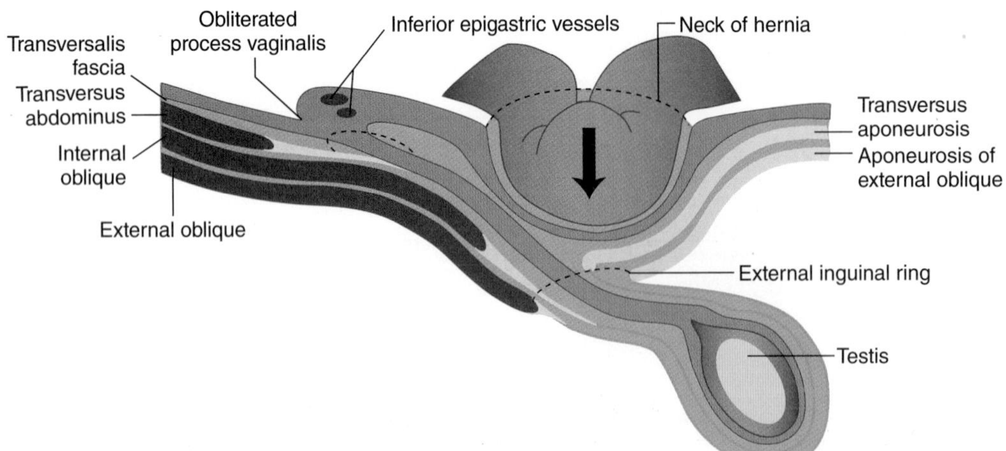

FIGURE 84-3. Direct inguinal hernia.

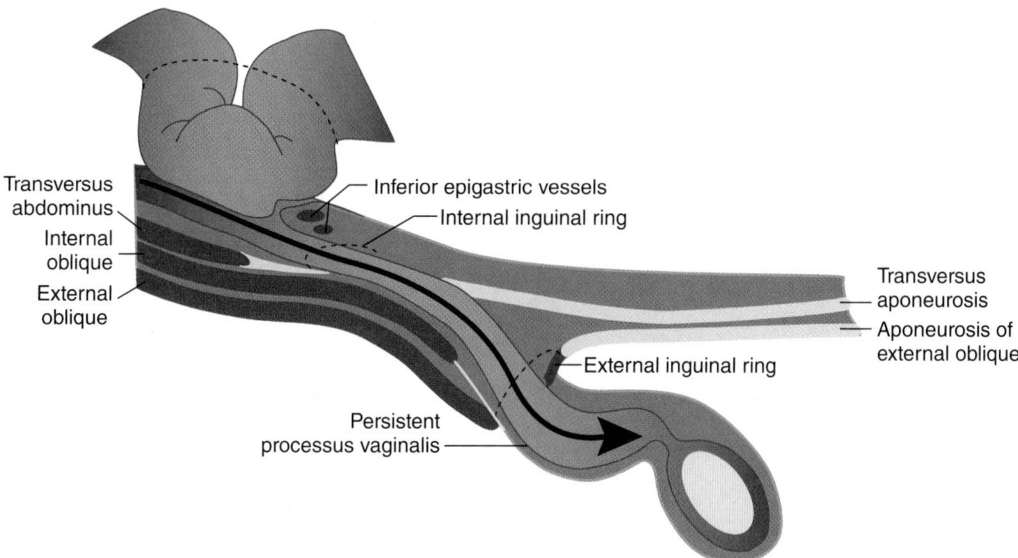

FIGURE 84-4. Indirect inguinal hernia.

healing. They are also associated with surgical wound infections. Risk factors for the development of incisional hernias include obesity, age, wound infection, and medical conditions (i.e., chronic obstructive pulmonary disease) that increase intra-abdominal pressure.[6] Incisional hernias can become quite large and produce symptoms varying from discomfort to extrusion of abdominal contents to incarceration and strangulation. Despite primary repair, the recurrence rate can be as high as 50%.

UMBILICAL HERNIA

The adult form of umbilical hernia is largely acquired and due to medical conditions that increase intra-abdominal pressure, including ascites, pregnancy, and obesity. Although strangulation is unusual in most patients, those with chronic ascites (i.e., cirrhotics) are at risk for umbilical hernia strangulation, rupture, and death from peritonitis.[7]

ANATOMY OF UNCOMMON HERNIAS

FEMORAL HERNIA

Femoral hernia (Figure 84-1) is so named because the hernia sac protrudes through the femoral canal and produces a mass that is typically below the inguinal ring. Femoral hernias are more common in women, with a 10 to 1 female predilection. The femoral hernia is particularly prone to complications, such as incarceration and strangulation. One study reported a 40% emergency surgery rate due to such complications in patients with a known femoral hernia.[8] All femoral hernias should be urgently referred for elective repair. Delays in femoral hernia repair lead to increasing rates of strangulation, reaching 45% at 21 months.[9] A small study by Malek et al[10] reported worrisome complication rates (31%) and surprising high mortality (13%) from delayed repair of femoral hernias.

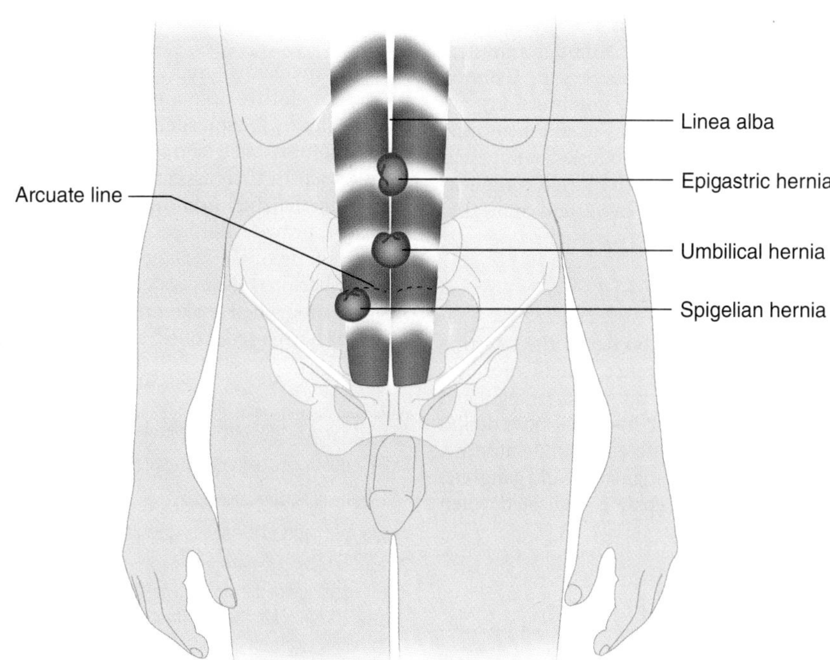

FIGURE 84-5. Anterior abdominal wall hernia.

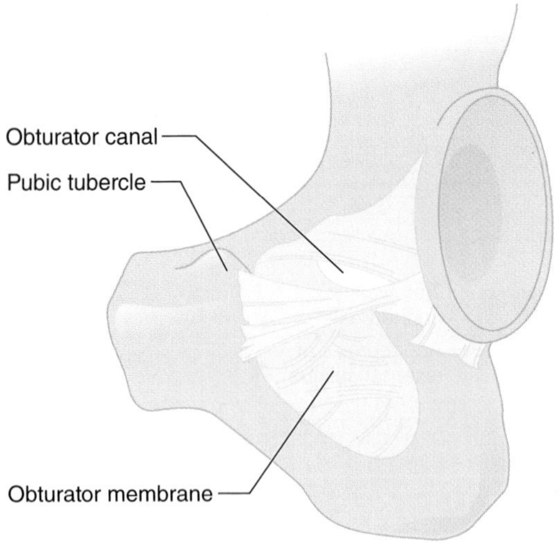

FIGURE 84-6. Obturator foramen. [Reproduced with permission from Pansky B: *Review of Gross Anatomy*, 6th ed, © 1995, The McGraw-Hill Companies, 1995, p. 511.]

SPIGELIAN HERNIA

Spigelian hernia (Figure 84-5), also known as a *lateral ventral hernia*, arises at the lateral edge of the rectus muscle and the arcuate (semilunar) line. Spigelian hernias are nearly always acquired conditions due to comorbidities that increase intra-abdominal pressure. These hernias are very difficult to diagnose, especially given the variability in presentation. The classic presentation is abdominal pain associated with an anterior lateral abdominal wall mass or bulge. Physical examination is unreliable,[11] and accurate diagnosis often requires diagnostic imaging. Bedside emergency US can accurately and quickly make the diagnosis.[12] CT scan remains the best radiologic test available but has the limitations of time, cost, and radiation exposure. Spigelian hernias should be surgically corrected given their high rates of incarceration.

OBTURATOR HERNIA

Obturator hernia is bowel herniation through the obturator canal (**Figure 84-6**) and nearly always presents as either a partial or complete bowel obstruction. The typical patient is an elderly frail female with signs and symptoms of intestinal obstruction. Although physical examination findings, such as the Howship-Romberg sign (pain in medial portion of the thigh due to obturator nerve compression), are well documented in the literature, the sign is not as useful in routine practice. Diagnosis is made by CT scanning of the abdomen and pelvis. It is important to properly diagnose this hernia given its high complication rate reported as perforation in >50% of cases and mortality approaching 20%.[13]

RICHTER HERNIA

Richter hernia involves only the antimesenteric border of the intestine and only involves a portion of the wall circumference. The Richter hernia presents differentially from a traditional incarcerated/strangulated hernia, as it often presents without vomiting or intestinal obstruction due to the incomplete involvement of the circumference of the intestine. Thus, the Richter hernia more often leads to strangulation and gangrene than other more standard hernias. Surgical repair is indicated when diagnosed.[14]

DIAGNOSIS

Traditional laboratory studies, such as a CBC, serum chemistries, and urinalysis, are routinely ordered but are of minimal value in the evaluation unless seeking an alternative diagnosis or for preoperative clearance.

IMAGING

Plain films are not required in hernia patients without significant symptoms. The acute abdominal series can reveal the presence of free air and signs of intestinal obstruction, but otherwise, plain films are usually indeterminate or nondiagnostic.

US has many advantages including low cost, no ionizing radiation, ready availability, no contrast agents used, and ability to be performed at the bedside. However, US is both operator and body habitus dependent. The primary role of US is the identification of the hernia itself. The **dynamic abdominal sonography for hernia** examination has good results in the hands of surgeons as compared to CT for the diagnosis of hernia.[15] When a hernia is identified by US, note hernia size, contents, reducibility, location of the facial defect, and tenderness.[16] In addition to determining whether bowel is present in a hernia sac, US can sometimes identify signs of incarceration and strangulation.[16-18] Strangulated bowel, by definition, has vascular compromise. In the natural history of an incarcerated hernia, the thin-walled veins and lymphatics become compressed and compromised before the thick-walled arterial supply. Doppler US can detect the arterial flow to the loop of bowel but is usually not sensitive enough to detect venous flow and cannot detect lymphatic flow. Thus, Doppler US can be insensitive for strangulation.[16-18] However, preservation of arterial inflow with obstruction of venous outflow causes increased intravascular pressure and extravasation of fluid into the extracellular space. This manifests itself as free fluid in the hernia sac on B-mode US, which is a sensitive finding for incarceration and strangulation. The specificity of free fluid in the hernia sac is good per se, but may be confounded by patients with ascites. Other US findings associated with incarceration and strangulation include hyperechoic fat, isoechoic thickening of the hernia sac, thickening of the wall of the herniated bowel, and free fluid within the herniated bowel loop.[16,18] Absence of peristalsis in a herniated bowel loop is suggestive of incarceration, and the presence of peristalsis implies that bowel resection is less likely to be necessary when the patient undergoes operative intervention.[18] US is most useful for diagnosis in children and pregnant women given its lack of ionizing radiation.[12]

It can be clinically difficult to differentiate hernia from hydrocele when assessing a scrotal mass. Obtaining a scrotal US in the standing position, with and without Valsalva maneuver, is a good way to demonstrate hernia.

CT is the best-performing radiographic test for hernia diagnosis and can identify uncommon hernia types (e.g., Spigelian or obturator) as well as demonstrate incarceration and strangulation.[19]

TREATMENT

If the hernia is easily reducible on physical examination, then refer the patient for elective outpatient surgical repair.

If the hernia is exquisitely tender and is associated with systemic signs and symptoms, such as intestinal obstruction, toxic appearance, peritonitis, or sepsis, then assume hernia strangulation. Consult general surgery immediately.[20] Administer broad-spectrum IV antibiotics, such as cefoxitin, provide fluid resuscitation and adequate narcotic analgesia, and obtain preoperative laboratory studies.

If the hernia is incarcerated but the patient does not yet show signs of strangulation, then make one or two attempts at reduction in the ED. Steps for hernia reduction[21] are listed in **Table 84-1**.

TABLE 84-1 Steps for Hernia Reduction
NPO status in case reduction attempts are unsuccessful.
Adequate IV narcotic analgesia.
Apply cold packs to the hernia site to reduce swelling and make reduction attempts easier.
Grasp and elongate the hernia neck with one hand, and with the other hand, apply firm, steady pressure to the proximal part of the hernia at the neck at the site of the fascial defect. US can aid in the identification of the fascial defect if it is not clinically obvious.
Applying pressure on the most distal part of the hernia can cause bulging (or ballooning) at the hernia neck and prevent reduction.
Consult surgery if the reduction is unsuccessful after one or two attempts.

After ED reduction of an incarcerated hernia, it is reasonable to observe the patient in the ED for a period of time for serial abdominal examinations. Persistent significant abdominal pain must raise clinical concern for "**reduction en mass**."[22] Although a rare complication of reduction attempts, it has been reported in the literature from the early 1900s to the present day.[23,24] A reduction en mass occurs when an incarcerated hernia is reduced back into the peritoneal cavity but a loop of bowel remains inside the hernia sac even after reduction, so that the retained bowel remains incarcerated.[22,24] In cases of reduction en masse, the patient will continue to exhibit signs and symptoms of incarceration despite apparent clinical reduction. Imaging can assist in the detection of this distinctly uncommon but serious diagnosis.

If there is any concern for strangulation, do not attempt hernia reduction. The reintroduction of ischemic, necrotic bowel back into the peritoneal cavity can result in subsequent perforation and sepsis.[25] Bedside US using a linear high-frequency probe with color or power Doppler of the hernia sac can be useful in borderline cases to establish the presence or absence of arterial blood flow.[12]

Acknowledgments: The author gratefully acknowledges the contributions of Frank W. Lavoie and Mary Harkins Becker, the coauthors of the chapter on hernias in adults and children in the previous edition. (Hernia in children is now discussed in chapter 130.)

REFERENCES

The complete reference list is available online at www.TintinalliEM.com.

Anorectal Disorders

Brian E. Burgess

INTRODUCTION

Anorectal disorders range from simple to complex and can manifest signs and symptoms of underlying serious local or systemic disorders that may be life threatening. Precise causes may be difficult to determine; thus a focused history and careful examination can narrow the differential diagnosis and aid timely and appropriate management.

ANATOMY

The rectum begins at the S3 vertebral body and descends for about 13 to 15 cm becoming the anus, comprised of the anal canal, anal verge, and anal margin. The rectum narrows and traverses through the muscular pelvic floor, at the level of the levator ani and coccygeal muscles, and becomes the anal canal, 4 cm in length, surrounded by the anal sphincter muscle (**Figure 85-1**).

The dentate line marks the junction of these two structures as the anal canal continues more distally joining the perianal skin at the anal verge (**Figure 85-2**). The anal canal mucosa consists of stratified squamous epithelium and contains no hair follicles or sweat glands. At the anal verge, the anoderm thickens and includes hair follicles and other cutaneous appendages. Proximal to the dentate line, the rectal ampulla narrows to conform to the opening of the anal canal. In doing so, its mucosa takes on a pleated appearance, forming 8 to 14 convoluted longitudinal folds: the columns of Morgagni. Each adjacent column is connected at the dentate line by a flap of mucosa that forms a small anal crypt, normally 1 to 3 mm deep. Anal sepsis, cryptitis, perianal abscesses, and fistulas result from inflammation, obstruction, and infection of the crypts and glands. The anal wall is a continuation of the usual layers of the wall of the colon and rectum, and the innermost mucosal lining continues to the anal verge. Just proximal to the dentate line, the mucosa transitions

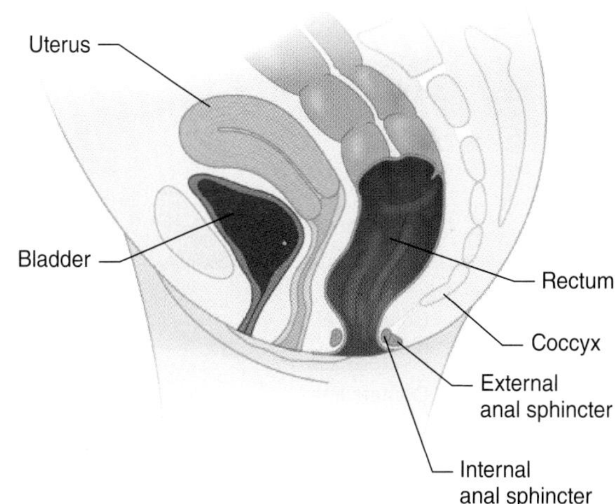

FIGURE 85-1. Midsagittal section, anorectum.

from rectal columnar to cuboidal to squamous epithelium. The submucosa, which normally contains the bulk of the bowel's blood vessels and autonomic nerves, thickens considerably proximal to the dentate line. The superior hemorrhoidal artery, from the internal mesenteric artery, supplies the proximal two thirds of the rectum, whereas the middle hemorrhoidal artery, from the internal iliac artery, supplies the distal one third of the rectum. The inferior hemorrhoidal artery supplies the anus but also supplies the rectum by a submucosal network. The venous and lymphatic system mirrors the arterial supply. The superior rectal vein drains into the portal system, whereas the middle rectal vein drains into the inferior vena cava. The inner circular muscle layer of the rectum thickens considerably as it terminates distally in the anorectum to form the involuntary internal sphincter muscles. The more attenuated longitudinal muscles of the rectum extend caudally, blending with fibers of voluntary skeletal muscles from the levator ani and external sphincter groups, to form the intersphincteric space (Figure 85-2).

The external sphincters are voluntary skeletal muscles and are actually a caudal extension of the puborectalis muscle, which interacts with the levator ani muscle, forming the pelvic floor. The puborectalis, the proximal external sphincters, and the internal sphincters form the ring of muscles that one palpates when performing a digital examination of the anorectum.

Lateral to the external sphincters is the ischiorectal space, and superior to the levator ani is the supralevator (pelvirectal) space, where deep, life-threatening infections can occur. Inferior mesenteric and para-aortic nodes drain the proximal two thirds of the rectum, whereas the lower one third of the rectum and proximal anal canal are drained by both the inferior mesenteric nodes and the internal iliac nodes. The inguinal nodes usually drain lymphatics distal to the dentate line. Proximal to the dentate line, the anus is supplied by the sympathetic and parasympathetic nerves, yet is devoid of somatic pain fibers, unlike distal to the dentate line, where somatic fibers are present. Parasympathetic nervous stimulation (S2 to S4) contracts the rectal wall and relaxes the internal anal sphincter, whereas sympathetic stimulation (L1 to L3) maintains continence through rectal wall inhibition and contraction of the internal anal sphincter.

PHYSICAL EXAMINATION

No matter how much historical information is obtained, no definitive diagnosis can be made without a careful examination of the anus and rectum. Patient education before and during the examination will be helpful in obtaining maximal cooperation. The lateral or Sims position is the most common position for routine digital rectal examination and anoscopy. This position is preferred for the elderly or pregnant women. Elevating the upper buttock provides better exposure of the perianal area. In debilitated patients, one may have to perform the examination

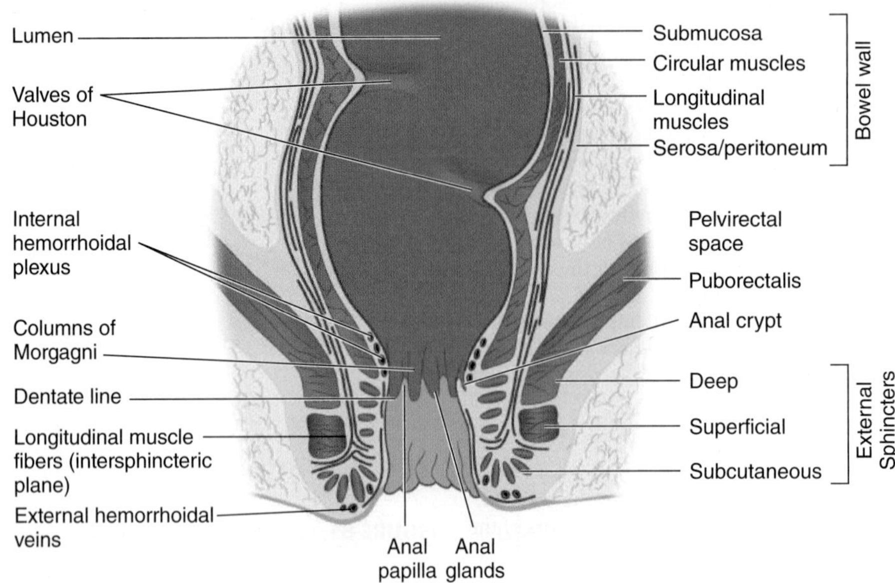

FIGURE 85-2. Coronal section, anorectum.

with the patient in a supine, lithotomy position. Examining a patient placed in the knee-chest position requires a cooperative patient who is not too ill or in too much distress.

A digital examination of the entire inner wall with a lubricated index finger should always be performed before doing any endoscopic procedure. In men, palpate the prostate to determine its size, texture, and tenderness or if masses are present. In women, palpate the posterior vaginal wall for a mass, rectocele, or rectovaginal fistula. Note anal tone and sensation. The anal mucosa, dentate line, both external and internal hemorrhoids, fistulas and fissures, condyloma, and distal rectal mucosa can be evaluated with the use of an anoscope (**Figure 85-3A**). No bowel preparation is needed for anoscopy, and cultures can be obtained. Suction and a good light source should be available. After performing a digital examination and determining that the patient will tolerate passage of an anoscope, introduce a well-lubricated, lighted anoscope with the obturator in place. Next, remove the obturator, and gently rotate as needed to view the anorectum circumferentially while withdrawing the anoscope (**Figure 85-3B**). After visual inspection, ask the patient to bear down to detect any rectal mucosal prolapse.

ANAL TAGS

Skin tags are minor projections of skin at the anal verge and are sometimes residuals of prior hemorrhoids (**Figure 85-4**).

CLINICAL FEATURES

Skin tags are usually asymptomatic, but inflammation may cause itching and pain. Skin tags covering anal crypts, fistulas, and fissures are called "sentinel tags." **Surgical referral for excision and/or biopsy is warranted because inflammatory bowel disease may be associated with sentinel tags.**

HEMORRHOIDS

ANATOMY

Hemorrhoids are vascular cushions that become enlarged and distally displaced within the anal canal. Current theory suggests that there is anal canal sliding and that hemorrhoidal formation occurs when the supporting tissues of these cushions deteriorate.[1] Consequently, the downward displacement of these cushions causes the internal and external hemorrhoidal plexuses to become excessively engorged, referred to as *hemorrhoids*—one of the most common problems afflicting human beings (**Figure 85-5**).

Hemorrhoids may become inflamed, thrombosed, prolapsed, ulcerated, or ischemic. Internal hemorrhoids originate proximal to the dentate line, from terminal branches of the superior rectal artery. They are constant in their location, coursing longitudinally at the right posterolateral, right anterolateral, and left lateral positions; 2-, 5-, and 9-o'clock positions, when the patient is viewed prone (**Figure 85-6A**). Commonly, they are single and are located at the 5-o'clock position. Internal hemorrhoids are not readily palpable and can best be visualized through an anoscope. Their appearance is consistent with the columnar epithelial surface of the surrounding anal canal (**Figure 85-6B**). **External hemorrhoids**, distal to the dentate line, are located anywhere along the anoderm, form as a result of dilatation of veins at the anal verge, and can be seen at external inspection. Their appearance is consistent with the stratified squamous epithelium of the surrounding anoderm, which has exquisite sensory innervation.

CLINICAL FEATURES

Enlarged hemorrhoids are associated with constipation and prolonged straining at stool, frequent diarrhea, and older age. Increased abdominal pressure may cause obstruction of venous return and engorgement of the hemorrhoidal plexus. Consider inflammatory bowel disease in patients with frequent diarrhea and hemorrhoids. Hemorrhoidal veins can have high resting pressures and are devoid of valves, and as patients age, the supportive connective tissue surrounding the vasculature diminishes. Hemorrhoids can develop during pregnancy and may be the result of sustained increased pressure on the venous drainage of the rectum. Increased portal pressure, from chronic liver disease, may produce marked dilatation and varix formation, distinct from true hemorrhoids, resulting in bleeding that can be extremely difficult to control. Tumors of the rectum and sigmoid colon, often associated with constipation, tenesmus, and incomplete evacuation, may cause hemorrhoids. **Although the most common cause of bright red rectal bleeding is hemorrhoids, tumors must be ruled out as a cause of rectal bleeding in patients >40 years of age.** Ascites, ovarian tumors, distended bladders, and excessive fibrosis from radiation therapy may contribute to the formation of external hemorrhoids. **Hemorrhoidal bleeding is usually limited, with the bright red blood on the surface of the stool, on the toilet tissue, or noted at the end of defecation, dripping into the toilet bowl. When patients describe the passage of blood clots, one should suspect colonic lesions. Chronic slow blood loss detected on fecal occult blood testing resulting in anemia requires further investigation.** Hemorrhoids themselves generally do not cause pain unless they are

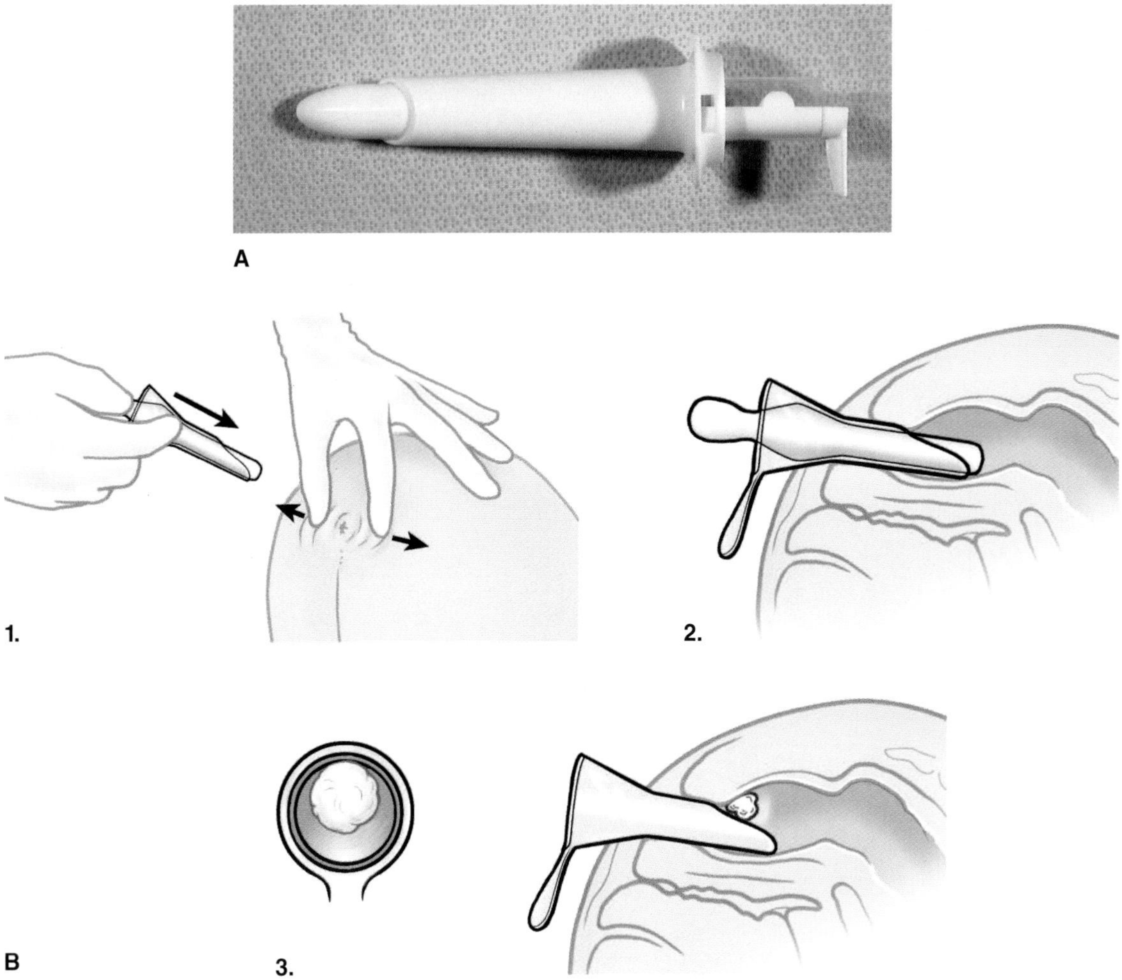

FIGURE 85-3. A. Anoscope. B. Anoscope insertion technique (1, 2, and 3). [Reproduced with permission from Reichman EF: *Emergency Medicine Procedures,* 2nd ed. McGraw-Hill, Inc., 2013. Figure 70-5A-C.]

thrombosed or are strangulated fourth-degree internal hemorrhoids. If the patient complains of pain, but on examination the hemorrhoids are not thrombosed, suspect perianal or intersphincteric abscesses or anal fissures. Thrombosed external hemorrhoids are painful and are often described as a burning perianal lump, and they usually exhibit a bluish-purple discoloration (**Figure 85-7**). Hemorrhoids may become more prominent with a Valsalva maneuver. As hemorrhoids increase in size, they may prolapse, requiring periodic reduction by the patient. Pain can be quite severe at the time of defecation and usually subsides with time.

Uncomplicated internal hemorrhoids are painless due to visceral innervation and lack of sensory innervation. Anoscopy reveals bulging, purple-colored veins at the distal rectum or anal canal (**Figure 85-8**). Often a chief complaint is painless, bright red rectal bleeding with defecation. Internal hemorrhoids may be palpable on digital examination

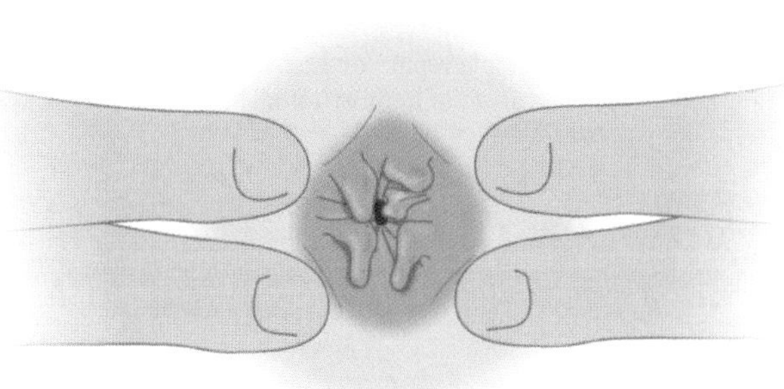

FIGURE 85-4. Anal skin tag.

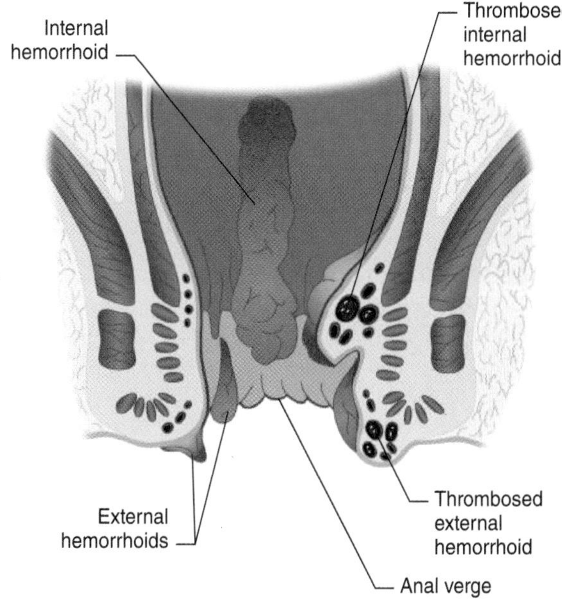

FIGURE 85-5. Coronal section of anorectum.

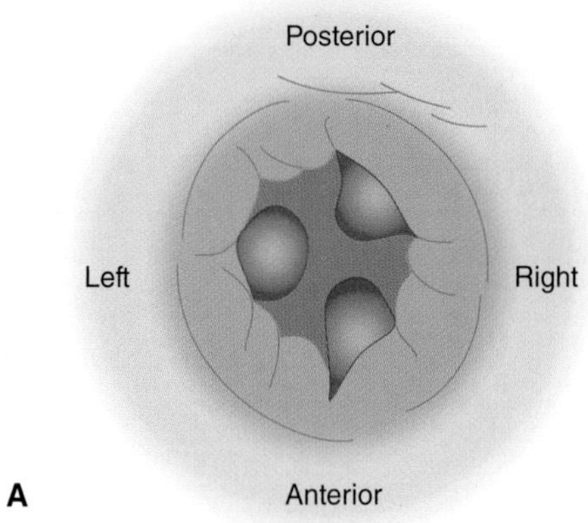

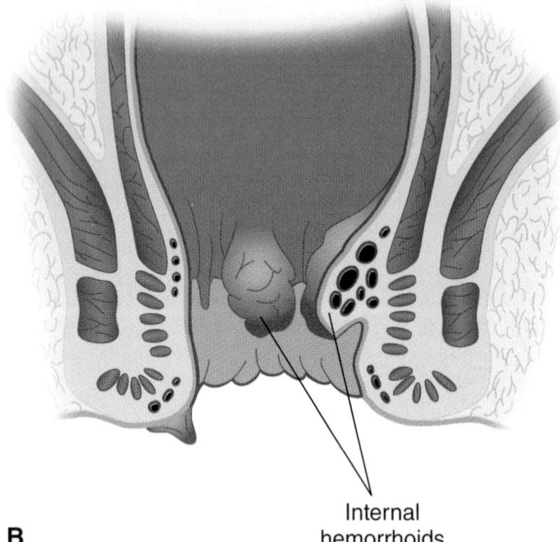

FIGURE 85-6. A. Internal hemorrhoids at 2, 5, and 9 o'clock. B. Protrusion of internal hemorrhoids.

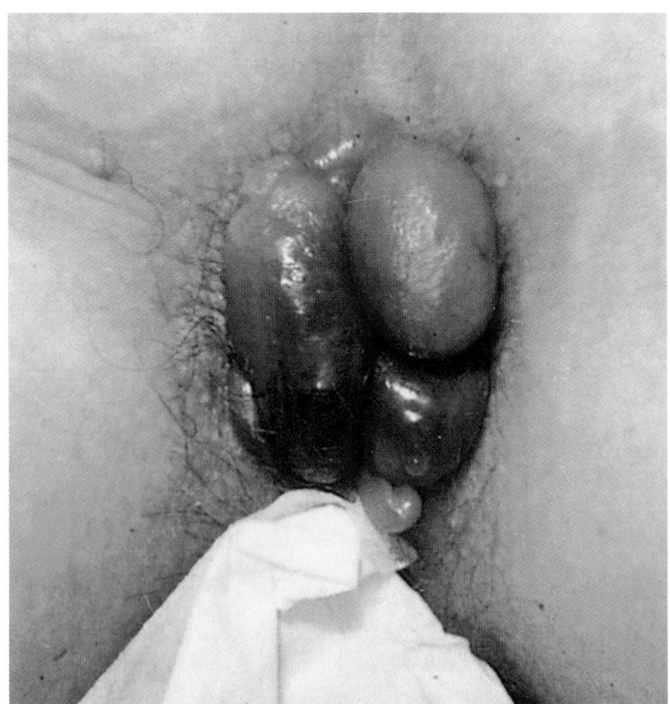

FIGURE 85-7. Nonthrombosed and thrombosed external hemorrhoids. [Reproduced with permission from Knoop K, Stack L, Storrow A, Thurman RJ: *Atlas of Emergency Medicine*, 2nd ed. © 2002, McGraw-Hill, New York.]

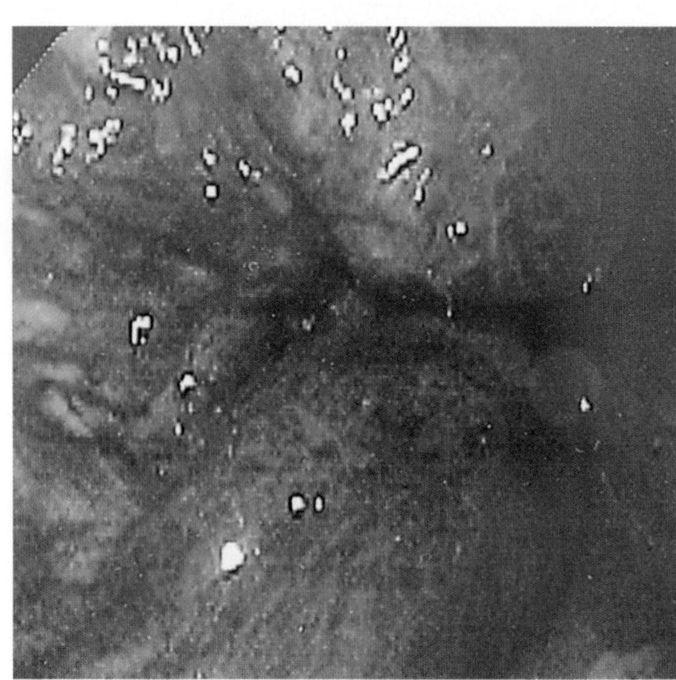

FIGURE 85-8. Grade I internal hemorrhoids. [Photo contributor: Virender K. Sharman, MD; reproduced with permission from Knoop K, Stack L, Storrow A, Thurman RJ: *Atlas of Emergency Medicine*, 3rd ed. © 2010, McGraw-Hill, New York.]

when thrombosed or prolapsed.[2] Nonreducible, prolapsed, internal hemorrhoids may become thrombosed and strangulated. They appear dark red, exhibit rectal bleeding, and cause exquisite pain and possibly urine retention. Ulceration, necrosis, gangrene, sepsis, and hepatic abscess formation may ensue. Internal hemorrhoids are classified by the amount of prolapse into the anal canal (**Table 85-1**).

Mucous discharge and pruritus ani may be seen with luminal prolapse[2] (Figure 85-8).

TREATMENT

Conservative therapy with warm baths is often successful for mild to moderate symptomatic grade I and II internal hemorrhoids. Manual reduction of grade III internal hemorrhoids and warm baths (which decrease sphincter pressures) for at least 15 minutes three times a day and after each bowel movement are the most effective ways to relieve symptoms. After the bath, the anus must be dried gently but thoroughly to avoid maceration of the perianal skin. Topical analgesics and steroid-containing ointments may provide relief. The patient should not sit on the commode for a prolonged period. Bulk laxatives and stool softeners should be used after the acute phase is treated. Avoid the use of laxatives causing liquid stool, because cryptitis and anal sepsis can result. A high-fiber, low-fat diet, with increased water consumption, regular exercise, and avoidance of constipating medications, should help prevent future problems. Recommend surgical referral for symptomatic hemorrhoids, because a variety of procedures (sclerosing injections, rubberband ligation, photocoagulation, cryotherapy, electrocautery, laser treatments, radiofrequency ablation, staple repair, or excision) can provide definitive treatment. A rare complication of hemorrhoidal banding is pelvic sepsis.[2]

TABLE 85-1 Grades of Internal Hemorrhoids

Grade I: Luminal protrusion above dentate line	Do not extend below dentate line and do not prolapse, cause painless bleeding
Grade II: Prolapse with spontaneous reduction	Prolapse during straining
Grade III: Prolapse requires manual reduction	Prolapse during straining
Grade IV: Prolapse-nonreducible	Can result in edema and strangulation

Obtain surgical evaluation in the ED for continued and severe bleeding, pain, incarceration, and/or strangulation (grade IV internal hemorrhoids). External hemorrhoidal thrombosis is usually self-limiting, with resolution in 1 week. Therapy for thrombosed external hemorrhoids depends on the severity of symptoms. If the thrombosis has been present for more than 48 hours, the swelling has started to shrink, the hemorrhoid is not tense, and the pain is tolerable, the patient may be treated with warm baths and bulk laxatives. Suppositories, which are placed proximal to the anorectal ring, are of no help. If, on the other hand, the thrombosis is acute, has lasted less than 48 hours, and is extremely painful, significant relief can be provided by clot excision.

Excision of Thrombosed External Hemorrhoid **Excision of thrombosed external hemorrhoids should not be performed in the ED on immunocompromised patients, children, pregnant women, patients with portal hypertension, and those who are anticoagulated or have a coagulopathy.** Obtain optimal exposure by placing the patient in the side-lying or prone position. The area of the overlying skin to be incised is infiltrated using a 30-gauge needle with a local anesthetic such as bupivacaine 0.5%, with epinephrine (1:200,000), and bicarbonate buffering. An elliptical incision distal to the anal verge in the overlying skin will expose the thrombosis. Remove the clot through the incision site. Because multiloculated clots can be present, the technique of unroofing a thrombosed hemorrhoid with an elliptical incision and removing the overlying skin gives far better results than the simple incision and evacuation of a clot (**Figure 85-9, A–C**).

Control the bleeding by tucking the corner of a small piece of gauze into the wound and leaving it in place for a few hours. A small pressure dressing may be applied external to the gauze and removed when the patient takes the first warm bath in 6 to 12 hours. Narcotics may be prescribed, but they cause constipation and may produce more problems. Complications, such as continued bleeding, recurrence, infection, fistula, and abscess formation, may occur; thus follow-up in 24 to 48 hours is recommended. Referral for definitive hemorrhoidectomy is prudent. Recently, small studies suggest that patients with acutely thrombosed internal or external hemorrhoids can be treated with topical nifedipine and 1.5% lidocaine ointment or isosorbide dinitrate ointment with surgical follow-up.[2,3]

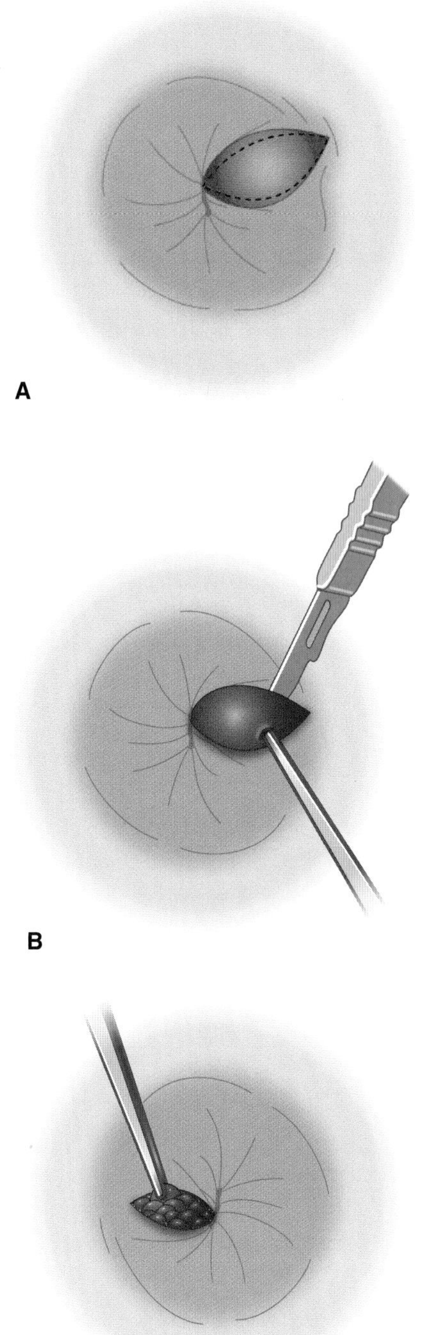

FIGURE 85-9. Excision of a thrombosed external hemorrhoid. **A.** Elliptical incision. **B.** Unroofing of thrombosed external hemorrhoid. **C.** Evacuation of clot.

ANAL FISSURES

ANATOMY

An anal fissure is the result of a superficial linear tear of the anal canal below the dentate line and extending distally to the anal verge (**Figure 85-10**). Acute fissures are present for less than 6 weeks; fissures are chronic if they persist longer. The mucosa of the anal canal has a rich supply of somatic sensory nerve fibers. Chronic anal fissures are pale in color with edema of the surrounding tissues. Fissures persist because of the severe, chronic, internal sphincter spasm that may occur along with development of a secondary infection at its base. The fissure edges become fibrotic and raised, possibly exposing sphincter fibers, hypertrophic papillae proximally, and the characteristic sentinel tag distally. The latter is frequently misdiagnosed as an external hemorrhoid when, in actuality, it is the result of edema and fibrosis secondary to the ulcerating fissure. The fissure may become inflamed and form a perianal or intersphincteric abscess that may drain into the anal canal or in the posterior midline externally.

CLINICAL FEATURES

Anal fissures are usually single and occur in the midline posteriorly in 80% to 90% of cases.[4] The posterior location of anal fissures may be because of the posterior angulation of the rectum on the anus where the posterior midline of the anorectal canal becomes the "lesser curvature" for the passage of stool. Anterior anal fissures are associated with younger age (33 years versus 41 years for posterior fissures), female sex, obstetric trauma, and occult external anal sphincter injury.[5] A chronic nonhealing fissure, lasting more than 6 weeks, or one not located in the midline should arouse suspicion that another, potentially serious cause may be involved. Such diagnostic possibilities include Crohn's disease, chronic ulcerative colitis, squamous cell carcinoma of the anus, adenocarcinoma of the rectum invading the anal canal, localized anal cancers such as Bowen's disease and extramammary Paget's disease, leukemia, lymphoma, syphilitic fissures, chlamydia, gonorrhea, human immunodeficiency virus, and a tuberculous ulcer. Consideration of these diagnoses requires referral for diagnostic biopsy of the ulcer edge, culture of the anal canal, and a systemic evaluation. Fissures due to Crohn's disease are multiple, off midline, and asymptomatic more commonly than the general population.[6] Most often, the traditional midline anal fissure is caused by the trauma produced by the passage of a particularly hard and large fecal mass, but it also may be seen after frequent acute episodes of diarrhea. Children with constipation will commonly complain of painful defecation only to find an anal fissure upon closer inspection (Figure 85-10A). Child abuse should be considered as a possible cause (Figure 85-10B).

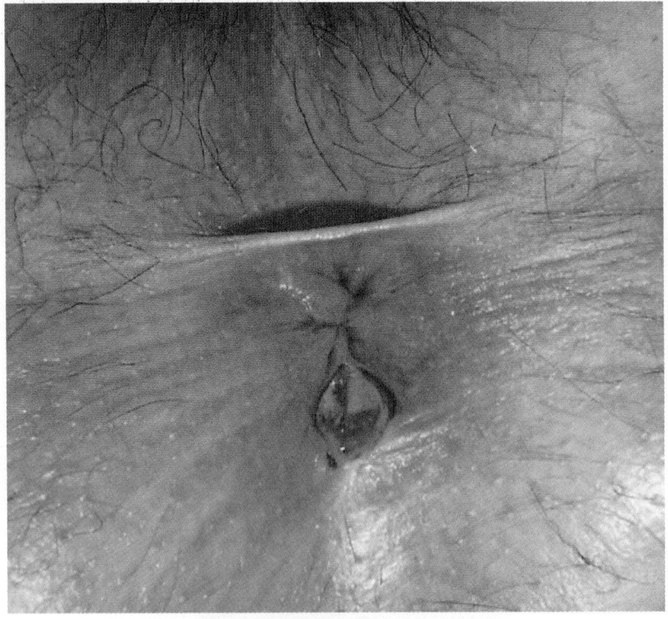

A

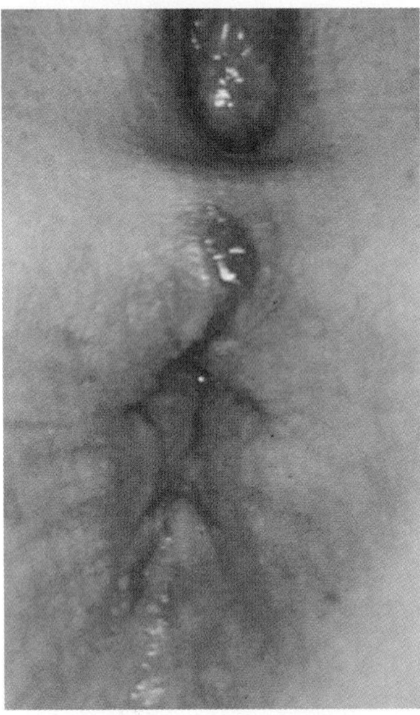

B

FIGURE 85-10. Anal mucosal fissures. A. Constipation. B. Sexual assault. [A: Photo contributor: Paul J. Kovalcik, MD. Reproduced with permission from Knoop K, Stack L, Storrow A, Thurman RJ: *Atlas of Emergency Medicine,* 3rd ed. © 2010, McGraw-Hill, New York. Figure 9-32; B: Reproduced with permission from Knoop K, Stack L, Storrow A, Thurman RJ: *Atlas of Emergency Medicine,* 3rd ed. © 2010, McGraw-Hill, New York.]

Anal fissures are characterized by tearing pain with defecation and rectal bleeding. The pain may persist as a dull ache and burning sensation for a few hours after each bowel movement. Invariably it subsides between movements, which is a feature that distinguishes fissures from other forms of painful anorectal disease. The bleeding is bright red and small in quantity, usually being noticed only on the toilet paper. In infants, the presence of small amounts of bright red blood on the stool or toilet paper is usually the presenting complaint from an anal fissure. Sphincter spasm and pain may be severe enough to make the patient retain stool and avoid defecation. The diagnosis of an anal fissure is usually suggested by the history, but the anal area must be examined in all cases. Fissures may often become more noticeable if the patient bears down as if having a bowel movement. With the patient relaxed, gentle separation of the buttocks will often expose the fissure. The mere retraction of the buttocks and the anal skin may cause considerable spasm and discomfort and may not permit digital examination. Topical 2% lidocaine jelly may provide some relief for examination, but severe pain may require sedation. If the fissure can be visualized and is present in the posterior midline, rectal examination can be deferred until the patient is having less spasm and pain.

TREATMENT

Healing is by the development of granulation tissue and the re-epithelialization of the ulcerated area. Most uncomplicated acute fissures will heal in a few weeks, but relapse can be as high as 50%. If healing does not occur within 6 weeks or relapses are frequent, surgical referral is recommended. Treatment is aimed at providing symptomatic relief, extinguishing the anal sphincter spasm, and preventing stricture formation. Warm baths for at least 15 minutes three to four times a day and after each bowel movement along with stool softeners may suffice. The addition of fiber to the diet will serve to prevent stricture formation by providing a bulky stool. Warm baths and increased fiber will result in healing in about half of all anal fissures.[6] Topical lidocaine ointments and 1% hydrocortisone creams may provide symptomatic relief. Medical therapies for anal fissure are generally no more effective than placebo, and for chronic fissures, all medical therapies are less effective than surgery.[7,8]

ANAL STENOSIS

Anal stenosis occurs when the pliable tissue is replaced by scarred fibrotic tissue. Congenital and primary causes may occur, yet secondary causes are more common. Stenosis most commonly occurs after surgical hemorrhoidectomy.[4] Other causes include radiation, fistulectomy, trauma, inflammatory bowel disease, chronic laxative use, sexually transmitted diseases, and chronic diarrhea.

CLINICAL FEATURES

Typical complaints include constipation, bleeding, pain with stool evacuation, and narrow-caliber stools. As stenosis progresses, performing a digital exam with the little finger is met with severe resistance. Incontinence secondary to overflow constipation may occur. Careful specialist examination, often with sedation, may be necessary.

TREATMENT

Treatment involves stool softeners, fiber supplementation, and daily gradual anal dilatation after initial dilatation in the operating room. Stricturotomy and stricturoplasty are used when conservative management has failed.

CRYPTITIS

Anal crypts are superficial mucosal pockets that lie between the columns of Morgagni. Formed by the puckering action of the sphincter muscles, crypts normally flatten out during the passage of a stool. Sphincter spasm and superficial trauma caused by repeated bouts of diarrhea or chronic constipation may cause breakdown in the mucosal lining of the crypts, leading to cryptitis. Infecting organisms enter crypt pockets, and inflammation extends into the lymphoid tissue of both the crypts and anal glands. Cryptitis could well be the common denominator for the development of fissure-in-ano, fistula-in-ano, and perirectal abscesses (**Figure 85-11, A and B**).

Visualized by anoscopy, the anal papillae appear as slight projections of pink epithelium that produce the serrated appearance of the dentate line. Initially, the locally inflamed crypts are asymptomatic, producing a bead-like spot of pus. Inflammation of the crypts extends to the adjacent papillae. Hypertrophied anal papillae may be palpated as small, hard nodules and are associated with cryptitis.

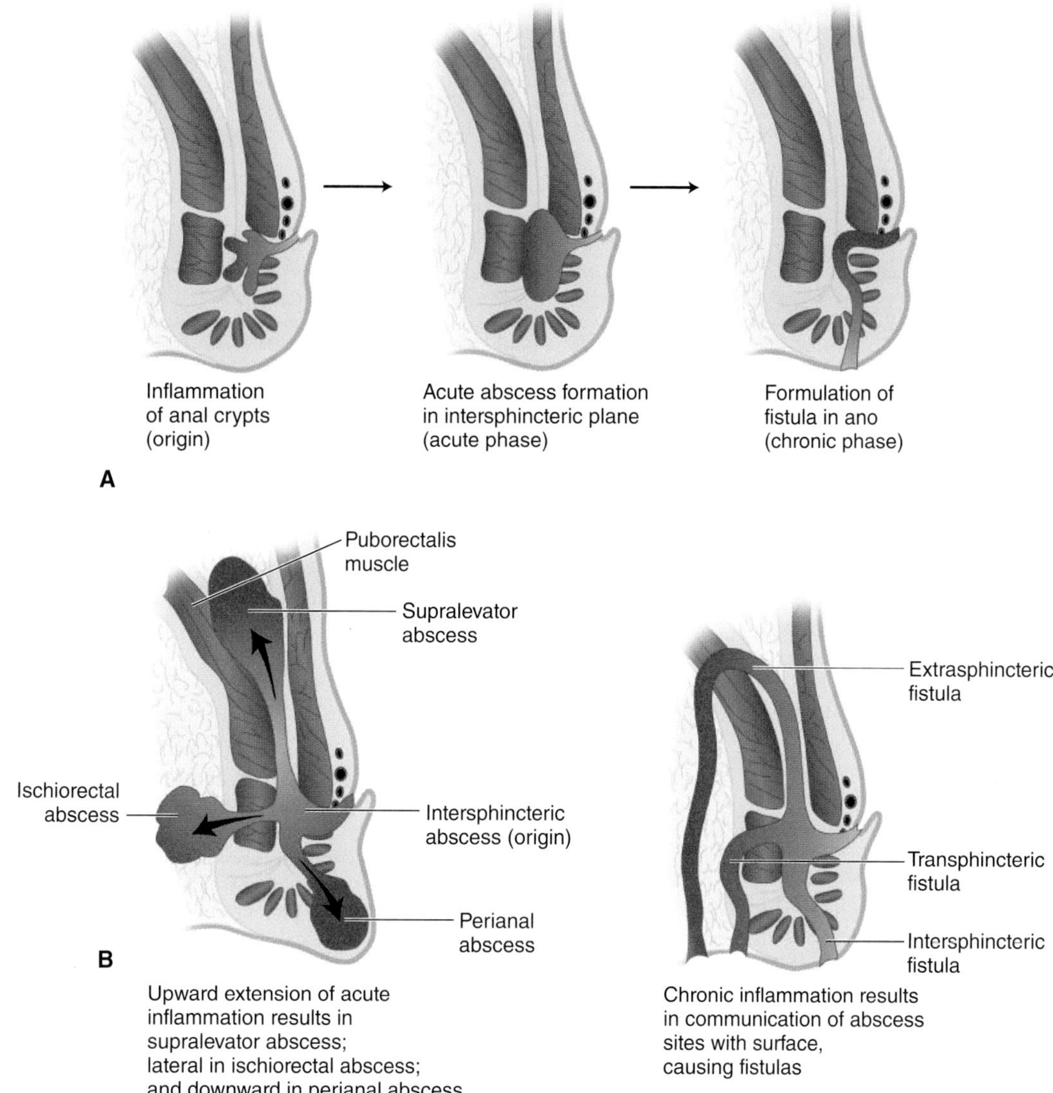

FIGURE 85-11. A, B. Illustration of the mechanism for anorectal abscess and fistula formation.

CLINICAL FEATURES

Anal pain, spasm, and itching with or without bleeding are the cardinal signs and symptoms of cryptitis. Rarely, papillae may hypertrophy and present as a prolapsing polypoid tumor. **The crypts most commonly involved are in the posterior half of the anal ring and, in most cases, in the posterior midline, the same location where anal fissures occur.** The definitive diagnosis of cryptitis is made by visualization of the erythema, inflammation, and pus during anoscopic examination.

TREATMENT

Treatment when the patient is symptomatic includes bulk laxatives and additional roughage added to the diet to produce formed, soft stools. Warm baths enhance healing by keeping the anus clean and the crypts empty. Refer to a surgeon for drainage when the infection has progressed and there is a deep, redundant crypt that will not drain adequately on its own. Cryptitis may be associated with underlying infections from parasites, inflammatory disorders, and localized trauma.

FISTULA-IN-ANO

Fistula-in-ano may result after drainage of an anorectal abscess. Fistulas may also be associated with ulcerative colitis, Crohn's disease, colonic malignancies, radiation, leukemia, sexually transmitted disease, actinomycosis, anal fissures, foreign bodies, or tuberculosis. Fistula-in-ano originates from an infected crypt and tracks to the skin. Fistulas are characterized according to the relationship to the anal sphincter: submucosal, intersphincteric, suprasphincteric, transsphincteric, or extrasphincteric (Figure 85-11). Goodsall's rule is used to help determine the location of the internal opening. Although anterior-opening fistulas tend to follow a simple, direct course to the anal canal, posterior-opening fistulas may follow a devious, curving path, including some that are horseshoe-shaped, opening in the posterior midline.

CLINICAL FEATURES

Open fistulous tracts may produce painless, blood-stained mucus, perianal itching, and malodorous discharge. If the tract becomes blocked, inflammation may be followed by spontaneous rupture or abscess formation. Abscess formation is associated with throbbing pain that is constant and worsened by sitting, moving, and defecation. Induration or a fibrous cord (more chronic fistula) may be palpated. A fistulous opening adjacent to the anal margin suggests a more superficial connection from the intersphincteric region. An opening more proximal to the anal margin suggests a deeper, more superior abscess. US using a 7.0-MHz endoprobe and enhanced with a hydrogen peroxide solution has been used to identify fistulas more easily.[9] In one study, endoscopic US was more accurate than CT scan (82% vs 24%) in the evaluation of perirectal fistulas, although it was comparable to MRI (91% vs 87%)[9] (**Figure 85-12, A and B**).

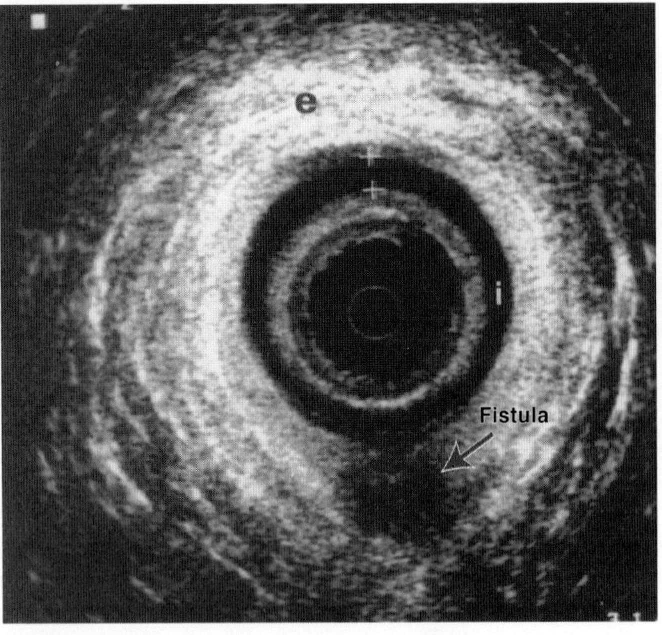

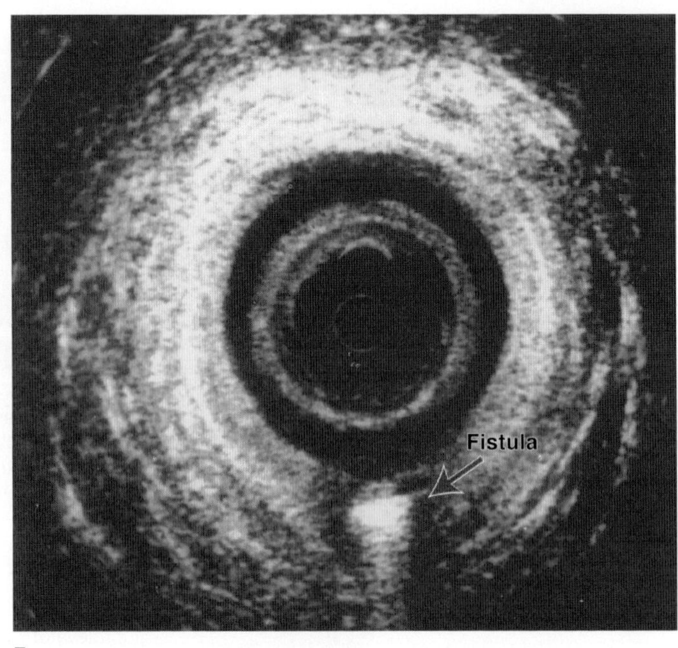

FIGURE 85-12. A. Transanal US, simple transsphincteric fistula. The dark hypoechoic area (*arrow*) is visible dorsally in the external anal sphincter. B. Transanal US after infusion of hydrogen peroxide revealing a hyperechoic fistula (*arrow*). e = external sphincter; i = internal sphincter.

TREATMENT

Give analgesics, IV fluids, antibiotics (ciprofloxacin and metronidazole), and antipyretics, and obtain surgical consultation to determine need for admission or to arrange surgical follow-up. Definitive treatment may involve placement of a drain through the fistula, fibrin glue (fibrinogen, thrombin, and calcium), fistulotomy, fistulectomy, or more complex procedures. Improperly excised fistulas may result in permanent fecal incontinence. Monoclonal antibody use may be considered in patients with Crohn's disease.

ANORECTAL ABSCESSES

Almost all abscesses begin with involvement of an anal crypt and its gland. Abscesses are typically polymicrobial with both aerobic and anaerobic bacteria. Infection with *Staphylococcus aureus, Streptococcus* and *Enterococcus* species, *Escherichia coli, Proteus,* and *Bacteroides* can progress to involve any of the potential spaces that are normally filled with fatty areolar tissue with little inherent resistance to the progression of infection. These spaces include the perianal, submucosal, intersphincteric, ischiorectal, and postanal (connecting the ischiorectal space on each side posteriorly), and the supralevator (pelvirectal) (**Figure 85-13, A and B**).

A variety of diseases and other conditions are less commonly associated with the development of abscesses, including Crohn's disease, carcinoma of the anorectum and adjacent organs, trauma, ulcerative colitis, radiation fibrosis, Hodgkin's disease, tuberculosis, gonococcal proctitis, *Chlamydia*, *Actinomyces*, herpes, lymphogranuloma venereum, and immunocompromised states. The perianal abscess occurs most commonly, and the supralevator abscess is the least common (**Figure 85-13, C and D**).

CLINICAL FEATURES

Located close to the anal verge, often posterior midline, the perianal abscess is a superficial tender mass, which may or may not be fluctuant (Figure 85-13, C and D). Ischiorectal abscesses, which are the second most common, traverse the external anal sphincter; tend to be larger, indurated, and well circumscribed; and are located more laterally on the medial aspect of the buttocks (Figure 85-13C). The patient may exhibit edema, fever, and anorexia. The deeper postanal abscess may not manifest cutaneous signs, but rectal pain and tenderness are invariably present (**Figure 85-14**). Anorectal abscesses are more common in early middle-aged males.

Isolated perianal abscesses are generally the only type of anorectal abscess that can be adequately treated in the ED (Figure 85-13, C and D). Surgical referral after drainage is suggested because fistula formation is not uncommon. Clinical evaluation of a perianal abscess is usually sufficient, but US localization may be helpful. If pain is out of proportion to physical findings or if the extent of the abscess is uncertain, CT or MRI is recommended. Ischiorectal abscesses can be problematic and complicated as the ischiorectal fossa forms a large potential space on either side of the rectum, communicating behind it through the deep postanal space. These abscesses may be palpable through the rectal wall or on the overlying skin. Intersphincteric, submucosal, postanal, and supralevator abscesses may not demonstrate edema but are often associated with constitutional symptoms. Infections in this area are insidious and extensive and can spread to an area some distance from the anal verge. If a complicated abscess is suspected, obtain CT or MRI (**Figure 85-15, A–D**). US may be useful to diagnose intersphincteric and submucosal abscesses, whereas CT and/or MRI are capable of detecting those as well as deeper abscess formations such as supralevator and ischiorectal rectal abscesses.

Perianal abscesses are easily palpable at the anal verge, whereas deeper perirectal abscesses may be palpated through the rectal wall or more lateral to the anal verge, on the buttocks. Initially, the patient notices a dull, aching, throbbing pain that becomes worse immediately before defecation, is lessened after defecation, but persists between bowel movements. Pain is exacerbated by movement and sitting. Perianal abscesses, unlike more complicated perirectal abscesses, are usually not accompanied by fever, leukocytosis, and sepsis in the immunocompetent patient. Pain is aggravated by straining or coughing, particularly when due to intersphincteric abscesses. **Ischiorectal abscesses** are often painful on rectal examination and are lateral to the anal verge. **Intersphincteric abscesses**, painful with defecation, may be associated with rectal discharge and fever, and a tender mass may be palpable on digital examination of the rectal canal, often in the posterior midline. **Supralevator abscesses**, often an extension of an intersphincteric abscess, frequently present with few outward signs. Generalized, nondistinct perirectal pain with fever, malaise, leukocytosis, and urinary retention may occur. Tender inguinal adenopathy is often a clue to these deeper abscesses. Supralevator abscesses may be palpable on vaginal examination.

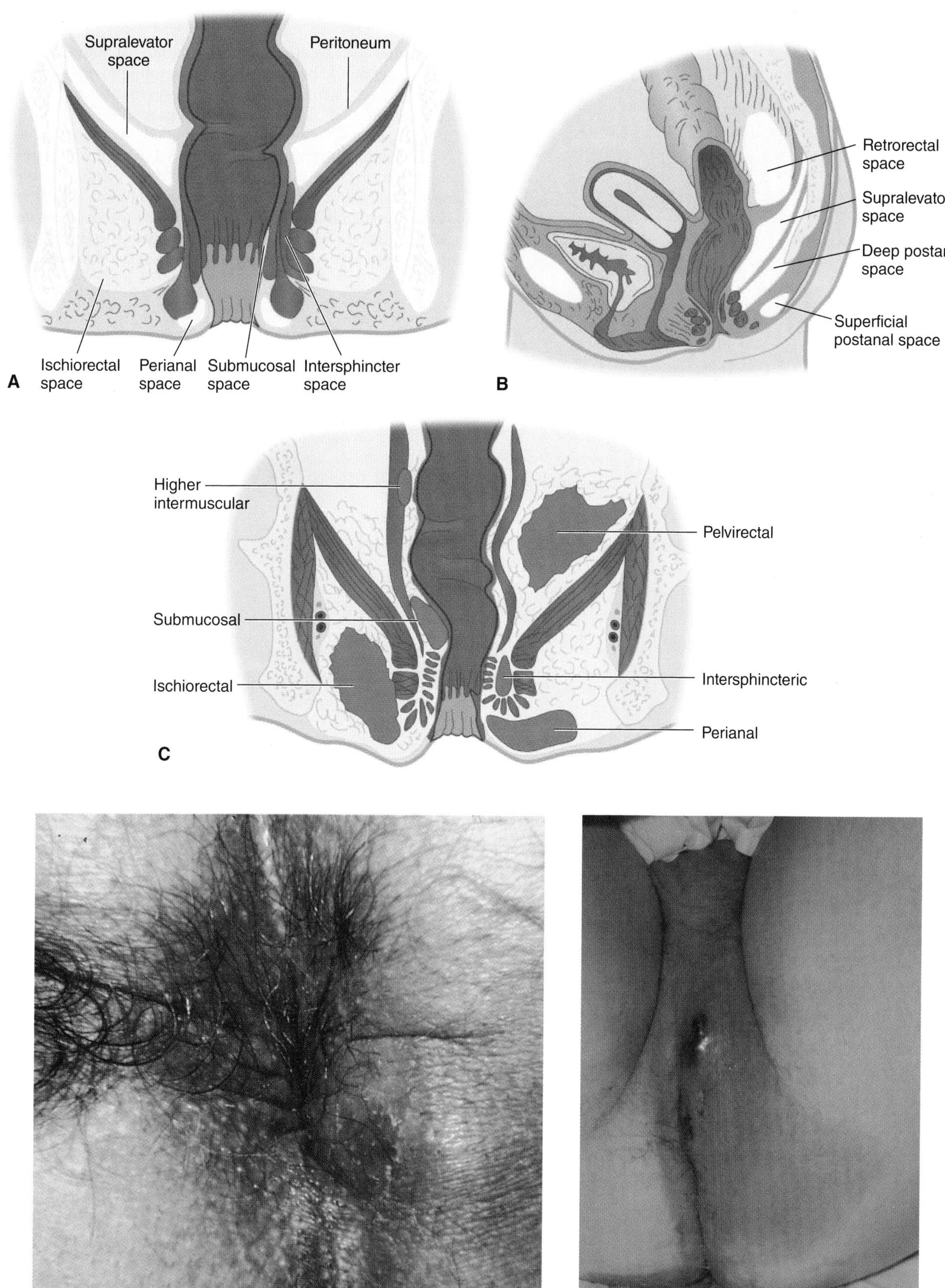

FIGURE 85-13. **A, B.** Anatomic classification of anorectal spaces. **C.** Anorectal abscesses. **D.** Perianal abscess. **E.** Complicated perirectal abscess. [A and B: Reproduced with permission from Reichman EF, Simon RR: *Emergency Medicine Procedures,* © 2010, McGraw-Hill, New York. D: Reproduced with permission from Knoop K, Stack L, Storrow A, Thurman RJ: *Atlas of Emergency Medicine,* 3rd ed. © 2010, McGraw-Hill, New York. E: Photo contributor: Lawrence B. Stack, MD. Reproduced with permission from Knoop K, Stack L, Storrow A, Thurman RJ: *Atlas of Emergency Medicine,* 3rd ed. © 2010, McGraw-Hill, New York. Figure 9-35.]

FIGURE 85-14. CT scan, postanal abscess (*arrow*).

TREATMENT

All perirectal abscesses (ischiorectal, submucosal, intersphincteric, and supralevator) should be drained in the operating room (Figure 85-13E). Simple, isolated, fluctuant perianal abscesses may be drained in the ED using local anesthetics and, occasionally, procedural sedation. Adequate patient positioning, preparation, and good exposure are necessary. Lidocaine with epinephrine should be administered with a small-gauge needle. Needle aspiration (18-gauge) over the painful region may be done to localize the purulent pocket. US can delineate the size and depth of the abscess. Drainage can be accomplished with a linear or cruciate incision. If using a linear incision, loosely pack the abscess cavity with strips of gauze to prevent premature closure of the skin edges. To ensure adequate drainage, a cruciate incision can be made over the fluctuant

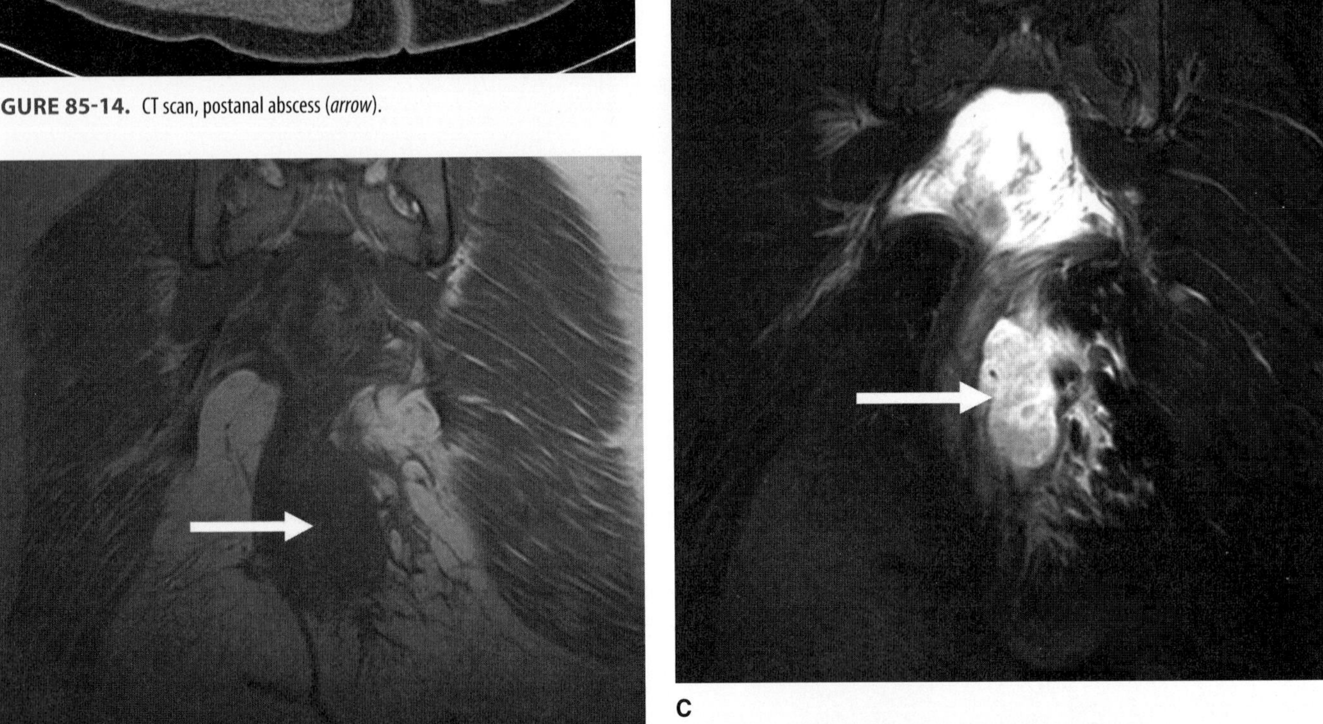

A

C

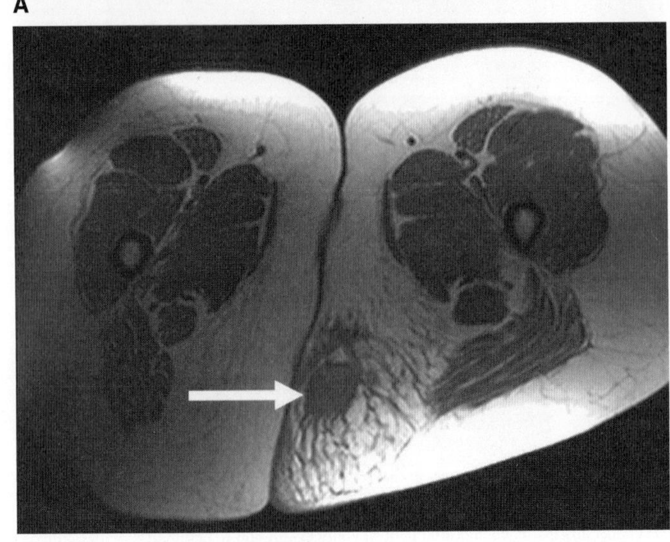

B

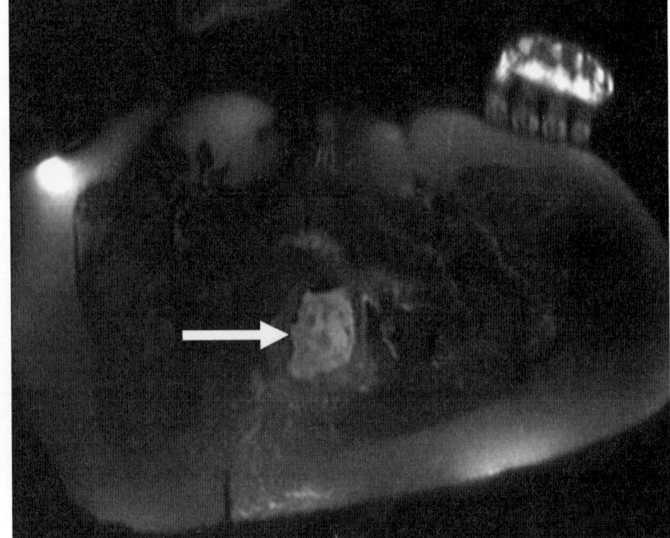

D

FIGURE 85-15. MRI of left ischiorectal abscess (*arrows*) in a pregnant woman, early second trimester. A. MRI of left ischiorectal abscess, T1 coronal view. B. MRI of left ischiorectal abscess, T1 axial view. C. MRI of left ischiorectal abscess, T2 coronal view. D. MRI of left ischiorectal abscess, T2 axial view.

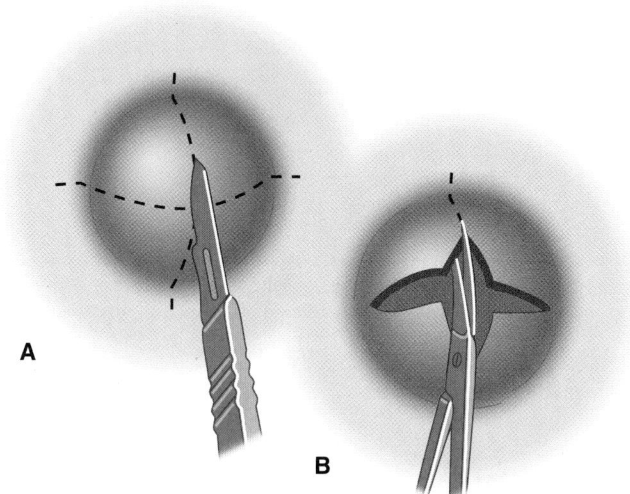

FIGURE 85-16. A and B. Technique to drain a perianal abscess.

part of the abscess. Trimming the flaps is suggested to prevent closure, and packing is not required (**Figure 85-16, A and B**).

Cover the wound with a bulky dressing, and have the patient take frequent warm baths starting the next day. Antibiotics are not necessary after adequate drainage in healthy patients. Provide ED follow-up in 24 hours, regardless of which type of incision is made, and consider surgical referral for definitive care. For the elderly or those with fever or leukocytosis, diabetes, valvular heart disease, cellulitis, or immunosuppression, give broad-spectrum antibiotics (piperacillin-tazobactam, 3.37 grams IV every 6 hours; or ampicillin-sulbactam, 3 grams IV every 6 hours), obtain surgical consultation, provide tetanus prophylaxis as needed, and admit to the hospital.

PROCTITIS

Proctitis is inflammation of the rectal mucosa. Clinical manifestations often include anorectal pain, itching, discharge, ulcers, diarrhea, bleeding, or lower abdominal cramping. Anoscopic examination may reveal mucosal inflammation, erythema, bleeding, ulcerations, and/or discharge. Proctitis may develop from prior radiation treatments, autoimmune disorders, vasculitis, ischemia, and infectious diseases (enteric pathogens and sexually transmitted infections (**Table 85-2**).

If the patient has an anorectal infection caused by one of the sexually transmitted infection organisms, assume that another may be present. Screen for other sexually transmitted infections; obtain appropriate blood tests, specimens from anoscopy for Gram stain, and viral and bacterial cultures; and start empiric therapy. For detailed discussion of sexually transmitted infections, see chapters 149, "Sexually Transmitted Infections" and 252, "Skin Disorders: Groin and Skinfolds."

CONDYLOMATA ACUMINATA

Condylomata acuminata, commonly known as *anal warts*, are often caused by human papillomavirus types 6 and 11.[10] Lesions begin as discrete, soft, fleshy growths on the perianal skin and the squamous epithelium of the anal canal. They may vary from dot-like to larger papilliform, cauliflower-like lesions. With time, pain, itching, bleeding, and anal discharge become part of the symptom complex. Perianal involvement is often associated with vulvovaginal and penile lesions. Optimal treatment is referral to an appropriate specialist for laser ablation, cryotherapy, electrocautery, immunotherapy, or surgical excision. **Anorectal carcinoma and cervical and orogenital cancer are associated with human papillomavirus types 16 and 18.**

TABLE 85-2 Anorectal Sexually Transmitted Infections

Bacteria	Viruses
*Neisseria gonorrhoeae**	Herpes simplex type 2*
*Chlamydia trachomatis**	Human immunodeficiency virus
*Treponema pallidum**	Human papillomavirus

**Most common sexually transmitted pathogens*

GONORRHEA

Surprisingly most women and about 50% of men with anorectal gonorrhea are asymptomatic.[10] Classically, patients experience tenesmus with profuse yellow, bloody discharge, which usually begins about 1 week after exposure. Patients in the acute phase generally have mild burning and/or pruritus with some purulent seepage. Anoscopic examination during this phase of the disease reveals marked hyperemia and edema of the rectal mucosa and diffuse inflammation with purulent discharge from the anal crypts. Unlike nonvenereal cryptitis, infection is not confined to the posterior crypt. Diagnosis is made by Gram stain, cultures, and nucleic acid amplification tests. Dissemination involving the heart, liver, CNS, and joints should be considered. Treatment is with ceftriaxone, 250 mg IM, and azithromycin, 1 gram PO once, or doxycycline, 100 milligrams PO twice a day for 7 days.

CHLAMYDIA

Chlamydia trachomatis causes both urogenital and anorectal infections. The lymphogranulomatous variety, serovars L1, L2, and L3, occurs mainly in the tropics. Infection can involve the rectum by perirectal lymphatic invasion from vaginal seeding or from direct anorectal mucosal infections. The nonlymphogranulomatous variety, serovars D to K, may infect the rectal mucosa, although it does not cause the extensive rectal scarring and stricturing that its lymph gland–invading cousin from the tropics does. A patient with chlamydial proctitis may be asymptomatic or may present with anal pruritus, pain, bleeding, tenesmus, and purulent discharge. The more severe form of proctitis occurring with this infection is usually due to the lymphogranulomatous type of chlamydia. Signs include fever, flulike symptoms, and prominent unilateral lymph node enlargement. Perirectal abscesses and chronic fistulas may develop. Red, friable mucosa and acutely painful anal ulcerations may be seen on anoscopy. Testing is not commonly available, and treatment is based on clinical findings. Treatment for nonlymphogranulomatous chlamydial proctitis includes azithromycin, 1 gram PO once, or doxycycline, 100 milligrams PO twice a day for 7 days. Treatment for lymphogranulomatous chlamydial infections includes doxycycline, 100 milligrams PO twice a day for 21 days, or erythromycin, 500 milligrams PO four times a day for 21 days.

SYPHILIS

The causative agent of syphilis is the spirochete *Treponema pallidum*. Chancres that form a few weeks after infection are the characteristic lesion of primary syphilis and usually manifest themselves at the anal verge or in the anal canal. Rectal mucosal involvement is uncommon, and at times, the chancre may be absent. **Syphilitic chancres may be misdiagnosed as a simple fissure because anal chancres are often very painful.** A symmetric lesion on the opposite side of the anal margin and inguinal adenopathy may be present. Condyloma lata are large, raised, flat, grey or white lesions. They appear in the perianal region as a manifestation of the secondary stage of syphilis. The rapid plasma reagin and the Venereal Disease Research Laboratory tests are commonly used for screening, with confirmation with a *T. pallidum*–specific immunoassay. Current treatments include benzathine penicillin G (Bicillin L-A), 2.4 million units IM for one dose, or doxycycline, 100 milligrams PO twice a day, or tetracycline, 500 milligrams PO four times a day for 14 days.

HERPES SIMPLEX VIRUS

Anorectal herpes is more commonly caused by the type 2 herpes simplex virus. Symptoms occur within a few weeks after exposure and consist of itching and soreness in the perianal area, progressing to severe anorectal

TABLE 85-3 Anorectal Acquired Immunodeficiency Syndrome–Related Infections

Herpes simplex virus types 1 and 2	*Campylobacter*
Mycobacterium avium-intracellulare	*Entamoeba*
Cytomegalovirus	*Cryptosporidium*
Salmonella enterocolitis	*Isospora*
Shigella	*Giardia*

pain. Early lesions are small, discrete vesicles on an erythematous base. Vesicles then enlarge, coalesce, and rupture, forming exquisitely tender ulcers on the perianal skin, the anoderm, and rectal mucosa. The pain and tenesmus from these lesions may be so intense that the patient develops severe constipation and difficulty urinating. The patient may develop a flulike illness with inguinal adenopathy noted on examination during the initial course of the illness. Symptoms persist for 1 to 2 weeks and are frequently recurrent, although less pronounced, during the ensuing year. Topical analgesia may be needed for adequate examination. Viral cultures, polymerase chain reaction, and immunofluorescent testing are helpful for diagnosis. Treatment consists of adequate pain medication, stool softeners, and acyclovir, 400 milligrams PO five times a day for 10 days for the initial episode, and 400 milligrams PO three times a day for 5 days for recurrent episodes. Suppression consists of acyclovir 400 milligrams PO twice a day. **Consider herpes simplex virus, syphilis, human immunodeficiency virus, chancroid, and donovanosis when anal ulcers are present.**

ANORECTAL ACQUIRED IMMUNODEFICIENCY SYNDROME–RELATED INFECTIONS

Patients rendered immunodeficient by human immunodeficiency virus are subject to a variety of opportunistic infections that affect the intestinal, anorectal, and other body systems (**Table 85-3**). Severe rectal pain, diarrhea, and hematochezia are common presenting symptoms. Anoscopy confirms anal canal ulcers and acute proctitis. Obtain serology for syphilis, and start antibiotic therapy.

Stool softeners, sitz baths, careful anal hygiene, and pain medications will provide some relief. Enteric pathogens may require antibiotics such as trimethoprim and sulfamethoxazole (*Isospora*), metronidazole (*Entamoeba, Giardia*), azithromycin (*Campylobacter*), acyclovir (herpes), or fluoroquinolones (*Salmonella, Shigella*). Provide empiric therapy against gonorrhea, nonlymphogranulomatous chlamydia, and incubating syphilis for human immunodeficiency virus–associated acute proctitis. Refer for appropriate follow-up, further evaluation, and definitive treatment.

RECTAL PROLAPSE

Rectal prolapse is the circumferential protrusion of part or all layers of the rectum through the anal canal. Basically, there are three types of rectal prolapse: (1) prolapse involving the rectal mucosa only, (2) prolapse involving all layers of the rectum (complete), and (3) intussusception of the upper rectum into and through the lower rectum so that the mucosal apex of the intussusception nearly extends to the anus (incomplete) (**Figure 85-17**).

Rectal prolapse in children is generally mucosal and occurs more commonly in males less than 3 years old. The prolapse may appear as a painless, maroon-colored, protruding mass with possible mucus and blood. The mucosal prolapse rarely protrudes more than 5 cm beyond the anal verge.[11] With children, parents often mistakenly believe that the prolapsed mucosa is a hemorrhoid. Mucosal prolapse is believed to occur due to a lack of the natural sacral curve reducing the anorectal angulation. With increased intra-abdominal pressure from coughing, diarrhea, vomiting, and straining, mucosal prolapse can develop. Incomplete and full-thickness prolapses occur because of the laxity of the pelvic fascia and muscles in addition to a generalized weakening of the anal sphincters.

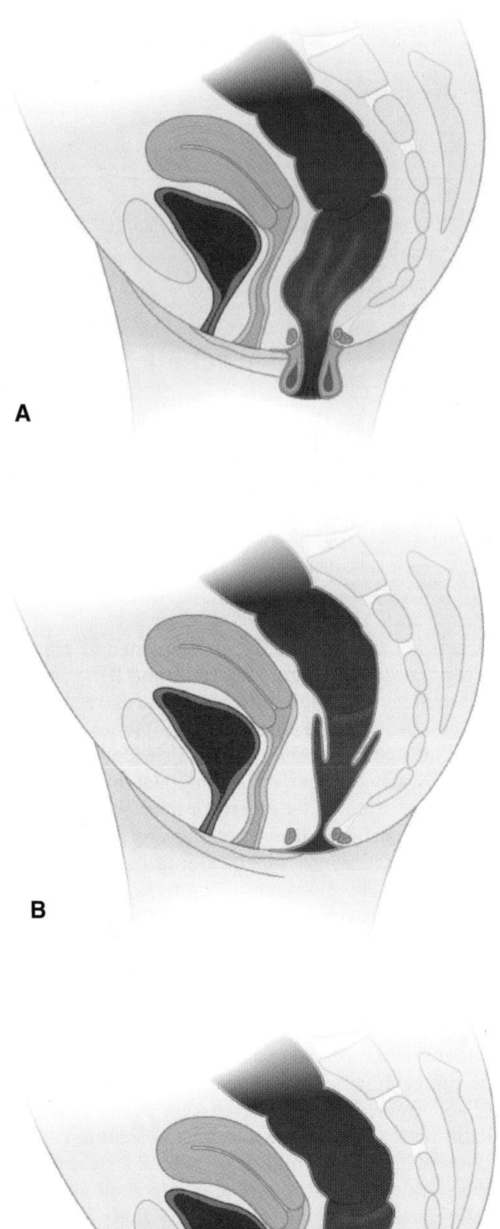

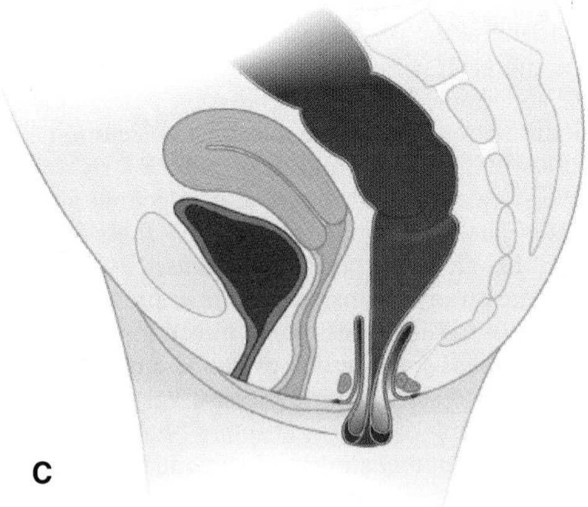

FIGURE 85-17. Rectal prolapse. A. Mucosal prolapse. B. Partial (incomplete) prolapse. C. Full-thickness prolapse.

CLINICAL FEATURES

Patients with partial prolapse may experience stool seepage or constipation. With more advanced cases, patients are able to detect the presence of a mass, especially after defecation or strenuous activity, or even with standing or walking. Irritation to the rectal mucosa caused by recurrent prolapse results in a mucous discharge along with bleeding. Associated anal sphincter weakness may result in fecal incontinence. With complete prolapse, the anus appears normal in contrast to a mucosal prolapse in which the anal edges appear everted. **Pain is not a significant feature with complete prolapse, but abdominal or pelvic discomfort may**

be present.[11] Digital rectal examination reveals a thick muscular wall with decreased tone, in contrast to a much thinner wall from a mucosal prolapse. Complete prolapse appears as a red, ball-like mass, with concentric folds in the protruding mucosa (**Figure 85-18, B and C**). Prolapsing internal hemorrhoids may be confused with mucosal or rectal prolapse. A distinguishing feature of prolapsed hemorrhoids are the radially directed folds (**Figure 85-18A**). With complete prolapse, a sulcus may be palpated between the extruded bowel and anus, compared to no sulcus with a mucosal prolapse.

TREATMENT

In young children, after appropriate analgesia and sedation, the prolapse can be reduced manually by first gently spreading the buttocks and then replacing the protruding mucosa, proximal to the anorectal ring of sphincter muscles, with a slow, steady pressure applied to the prolapsed segment. Digital rectal examination should then be performed. Every effort should be made to prevent constipation. **Refer the child for further evaluation due to a possible underlying condition such as cystic fibrosis, polyps, pelvic floor weakness, diarrhea, and malnutrition.**

In adults, a complete prolapsed rectum can sometimes be reduced with gentle continuous pressure, which may take several minutes. The buttocks may be taped apart while the prolapsed segment is grasped in such a way that the thumbs are placed over the luminal surfaces medially while the fingers grasp the outer walls laterally. Continuous pressure, starting with the thumbs followed by an internal rolling force of the fingers, will aid in reduction (**Figure 85-19**).

After reduction, perform a digital rectal examination to ensure that reduction is complete and to evaluate for a rectal mass or polyp. Obtain surgical consultation for repair, or refer for colonoscopy and dietary changes depending on the clinical circumstances.

Once the rectal walls become edematous, reduction is difficult. Prolonged prolapse may lead to venous engorgement, thrombosis, superficial ulcerations, rectal incarceration, strangulation, and ischemia. **An effective technique is the early application of generous amounts of granulated sugar over the entire prolapsed segment. Synthetic sweeteners are not effective. After 15 minutes or so of sugar application, the edema reduces, allowing for easier prolapse reduction.**[12] Gauze with lubricant can be placed over the anal verge after reduction and taped in place for a few hours. If the prolapse cannot be reduced, is severe, or recurs after reduction, or if ischemia or gangrene of the prolapsed segment is suspected, emergency surgical consultation and hospitalization are needed for reduction or surgical treatment (rectopexy).

ANORECTAL TUMORS

Carcinoma of the anal area is uncommon. Factors such as smoking, anal intercourse, human immunodeficiency virus, and human papillomavirus, particularly types 16 and 18, resulting in genital warts, have been associated with the development of anorectal cancer (**Figure 85-20**).

At the level of the dentate line and extending approximately 1 cm proximal is a transitional zone of epithelium connecting the squamous cell epithelium of the anoderm with the columnar epithelium of the rectum. This transition zone includes columnar, cuboidal, transitional, and squamous epithelial cells that represent the source for a variety of malignancies that arise in the anal canal. Anorectal malignancies can generally be divided into two regions: (1) malignancies of the portion proximal to the dentate line and including the transitional zone, which are referred to as *anal canal neoplasms*, and (2) tumors arising in the anoderm distal to the dentate line, which are referred to as *anal margin neoplasms* (**Table 85-4**).

Anal margin neoplasms have a low-grade malignant potential and are slow to metastasize, with the exception of melanoma. Anal canal neoplasms are far more virulent, metastasize early, and have a poor prognosis. Squamous cell carcinoma of the anal canal has a much poorer prognosis than its anal margin counterpart. Anal margin neoplasms generally metastasize to femoral and inguinal lymph nodes, whereas anal canal malignancies metastasize to the perirectal, mesenteric, and paravertebral lymph nodes via the portal circulation. **The anal canal is the third**

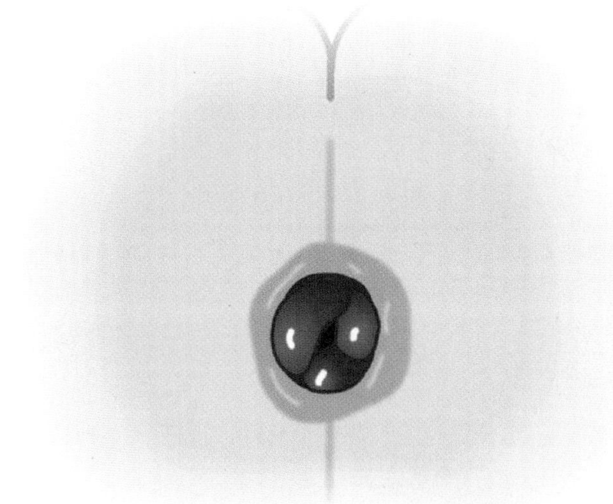

A

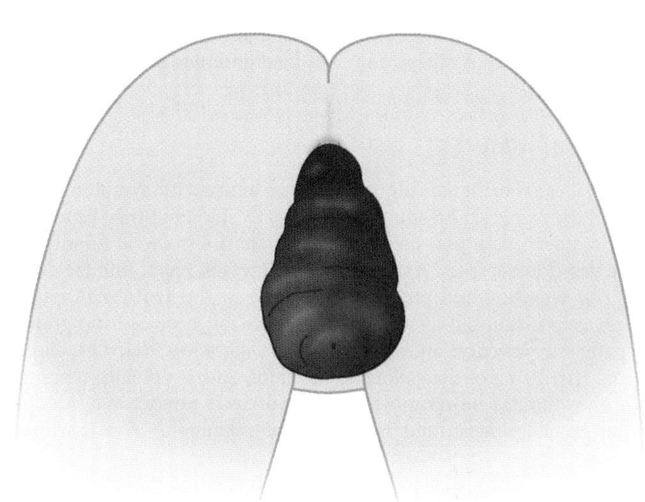

B

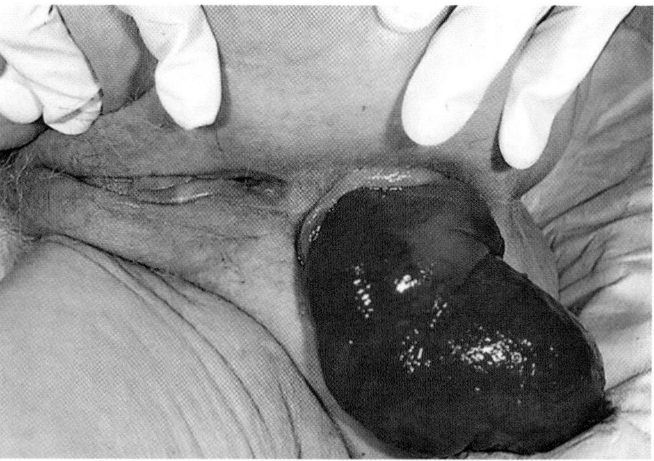

C

FIGURE 85-18. Differentiation: Prolapsed internal hemorrhoids from rectal prolapse. A. Prolapsing internal hemorrhoids with radial folds. B. Complete rectal prolapse with concentric folds. C. Complete rectal prolapse with a sulcus. [C: Photo contributor Alan B. Storrow, MD. Reproduced with permission from Knoop K, Stack L, Storrow A, Thurman RJ: *Atlas of Emergency Medicine*, 3rd ed. © 2010, McGraw-Hill, New York.]

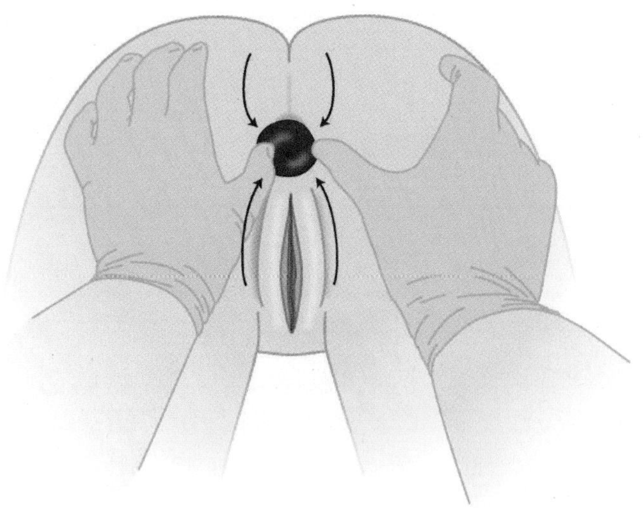

FIGURE 85-19. Reduction of complete rectal prolapse.

most common site of malignant melanoma (after the skin and the eye), which, when it occurs there, may not be pigmented and is frequently missed.

CLINICAL FEATURES

Early anal canal malignancies usually cause nonspecific symptoms, such as pruritus, pain, and bleeding admixed with stool, but may be asymptomatic. Rectal pain may also be referred from retrorectal tumors and pelvic vessel aneurysms. As the tumor progresses, rectal fullness develops. The sensation and presence of a lump in the anal canal may be erroneously diagnosed as a hemorrhoid. As the neoplasm progresses, the patient experiences anorexia, bloating, weight loss, diarrhea, constipation, narrowing of the caliber of the stool, and, eventually, tenesmus with or without a bowel movement. Anal canal tumors may produce partial rectal prolapse and hemorrhoidal dilatation. More advanced

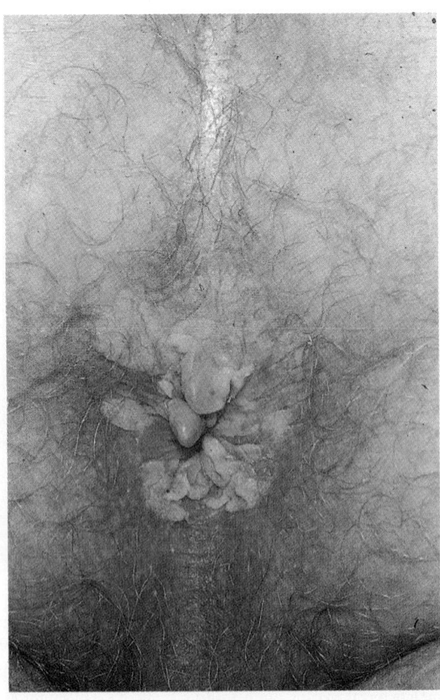

FIGURE 85-20. Perianal human papilloma virus–induced squamous cell carcinoma in situ. [Reproduced with permission from Wolff K, Johnson RA: *Color Atlas and Synopsis of Clinical Dermatology*, © 2009, McGraw-Hill, New York.]

TABLE 85-4 Anorectal Tumors

Anal Canal Neoplasms	Anal Margin Neoplasms
Adenocarcinoma of glands and ducts	Bowen's disease
Transitional cell carcinoma	Squamous cell carcinoma (SCC)
Melanoma, SCC	Basal cell carcinoma
Kaposi's sarcoma	Melanoma
Villous adenoma	Paget's disease

malignancies may present as perirectal abscesses, fistulas, and bloody mucous discharge. Villous adenomas, which arise from the rectal columnar epithelium, frequently produce clear, watery diarrhea and a profuse rectal discharge, with secondary excoriation of skin and pruritus. Watery diarrhea may cause hypokalemia or hyponatremia. Anal margin neoplasms tend to be circumferential and may present with bleeding, persistent ulcers, or chronic dermatologic conditions such as eczema or mycotic infections. Any ulcer that fails to heal within 30 days or any discrete skin lesion that fails to improve with appropriate therapy must be biopsied to rule out the presence of malignancy. **Virtually all anorectal tumors can be detected by careful visual examination of the perianal area, digital palpation of the distal rectum and anal canal, and proctoscopic or sigmoidoscopic examination.**

Specific diagnosis and treatment require surgical consultation and referral.

RECTAL FOREIGN BODIES

The medical literature is replete with the variety of foreign bodies that have been reported to have been inserted into the rectum (**Figure 85-21, A–D**).

CLINICAL FEATURES

Patients may complain of abdominal pain and cramping, anorectal bleeding, discharge, and discomfort and may not initially be forthcoming with an accurate history. Most foreign bodies are in the rectal ampulla and are therefore palpable through careful digital examination. Anoscopy may detect signs of trauma and should replace the digital exam when sharp objects are suspected. Foreign bodies lodged above the rectosigmoid junction are usually not palpable. Injuries may consist of hematoma formation, various lacerations with potential perforation, and ischemic segments (particularly a delayed presentation). X-rays of the abdomen may demonstrate not only the position, shapes, and number of foreign bodies, but also the possible presence of free air. Perforation of the rectum or colon, although uncommon, is a serious complication. Perforation of the rectum below the peritoneal reflection often causes retroperitoneal injuries, and plain radiographs may demonstrate extraperitoneal air along the psoas muscles. Perforation above the peritoneal reflection usually reveals intraperitoneal free air under the diaphragm noted on an upright chest x-ray. **CT scan is useful when the foreign body is radiolucent and for the detection of free air. Fever, leukocytosis, abdominal pain, rectal bleeding, and peritoneal signs are clinical manifestations suggestive of perforation.** Both can result in life-threatening sepsis, although perforation below the peritoneal reflection may be managed with more conservative therapy.

TREATMENT

Although some distal rectal foreign bodies can be removed by the emergency physician, many objects require surgical intervention, particularly if they are made of glass, have sharp edges, or show signs of perforation. Foreign bodies with greater success of being removed in the ED are those that are located in the mid to lower rectum. When assessing the likelihood of removal in the ED, determine the type of object inserted and likelihood of injury to the GI tract or sphincter from removal. Sims, lithotomy, or knee-chest position with application of suprapubic pressure while the examiner digitally grasps the foreign body may help expulse the foreign body. After anal lubrication and with the aid of obstetric forceps, ask the patient to assist extraction by bearing down

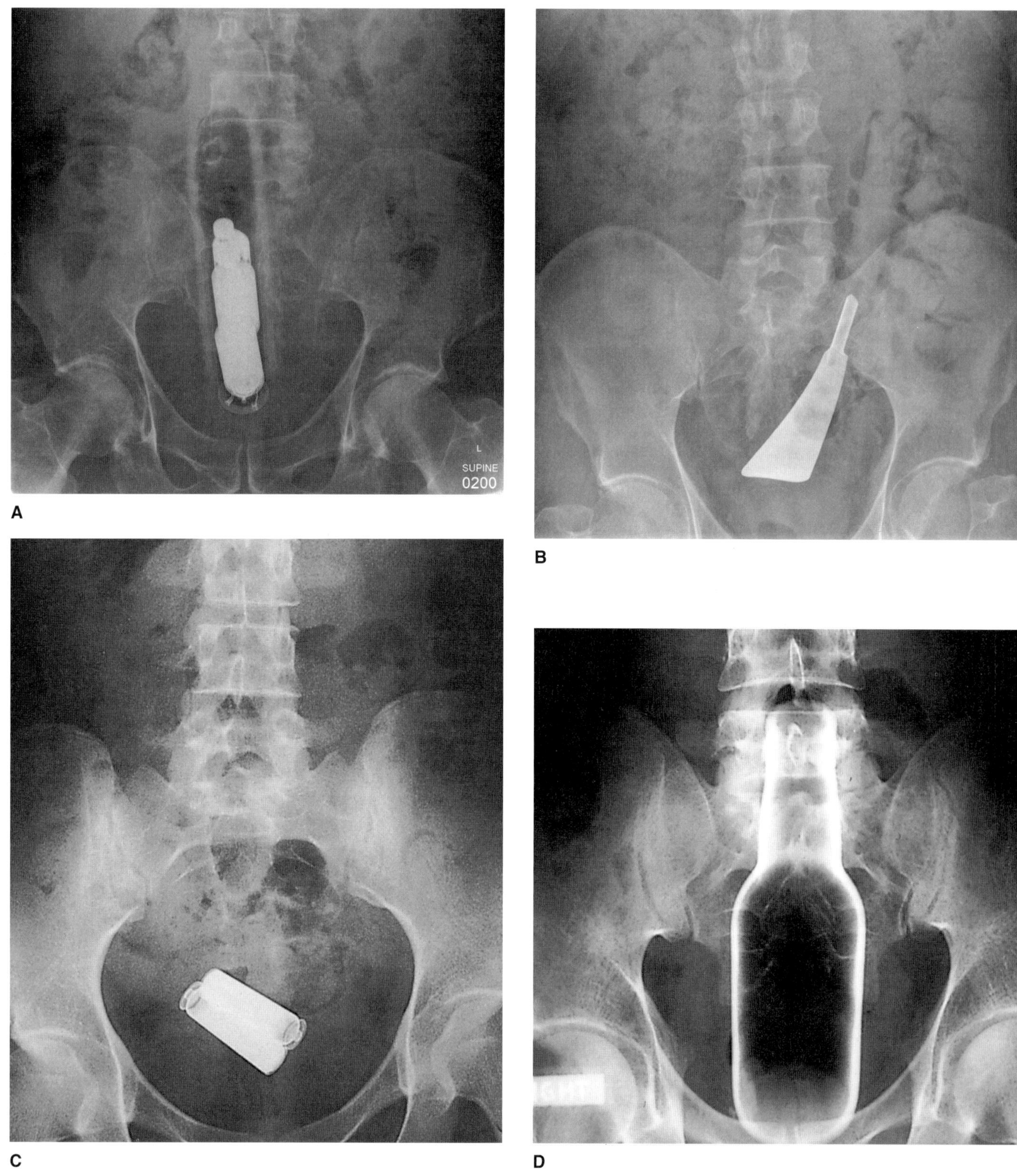

FIGURE 85-21. A–D. Rectal foreign bodies. [C and D: Photo contributor: Kevin J. Knoop, MD. Reproduced with permission from Knoop K, Stack L, Storrow A, Thurman RJ: *Atlas of Emergency Medicine,* 3rd ed. © 2010, McGraw-Hill, New York.]

(**Figure 85-22A**). If the foreign body is removed in the ED and is of a size or shape that could cause perforation or laceration, proctoscopic examination and x-ray studies must be performed. In questionable cases, observation for at least 12 hours should be done to ensure that perforation has not occurred. Rectal and anal lacerations may be present and require repair. For removal of large foreign bodies, surgical consultation or emergency colonoscopy by a gastroenterologist is usually required. Large bulbar objects create a vacuum-like effect in the rectal ampulla, making it difficult to retrieve the object by simple traction. The vacuum can be overcome by passing a 20- to 26-French, three-way catheter beyond the object and injecting up to 30 mL of air. Inserting Foley catheters around the foreign body may then be used as traction devices to deliver the foreign body or manipulate it into a more accessible position (**Figure 85-22B**). If there is a risk of sphincter injury, ischemia, or perforation, or if excess manipulation will be needed to remove the foreign body (potential for bacteremia), obtain emergent surgical evaluation and appropriate laboratory studies, initiate IV therapy with crystalloid solution, and administer a broad-spectrum antibiotic (i.e., piperacillin-tazobactam, 3.37 grams IV every 6 hours).

PRURITUS ANI

Pruritus ani is a symptom complex that occurs secondary to a variety of anal and systemic problems (**Table 85-5**). Primary or idiopathic disease occurs when no cause is identified. **Pruritus ani is the second most common anorectal condition after hemorrhoids.**[13] It affects 1% to 5% of the population; men are affected four times more often than women; and it most commonly occurs in the fourth to sixth decades of life.[14]

CLINICAL FEATURES

Symptoms are often worse at night. The skin becomes macerated by constant mucous and purulent discharge. Bacterial infections, such as staphylococci and streptococci, in addition to all sexually transmitted organisms, can cause pruritus.

Pinworms (*Enterobius vermicularis*) are a common cause of anal pruritus in children. Institutionalized adults may also develop pinworms.[13] *Candida albicans*, particularly in diabetic patients, is commonly found on the perianal skin but is not usually associated with pruritus; the *Trichophyton* species, on the other hand, are associated with pruritus. **Fecal contamination resulting from loose bowel movements, diarrhea, and poor anal hygiene is a frequent irritant to the perianal skin.** Excessive anal cleansing and wearing of synthetic, tight-fitting underwear that retains moisture can cause pruritus. Any of the anal margin neoplasms may initially cause pruritus. Systemic conditions, such as diabetes mellitus, psoriasis, pemphigus, leukemia, lymphoma, thyroid disorders, hepatic diseases, renal failure, iron deficiency anemia, and certain vitamin deficiencies (vitamins A and D and niacin), because of their secondary effect on the perianal skin, can cause pruritus. Lumbosacral radiculopathy has been associated with idiopathic pruritus ani.[13] The skin appears normal with early, mild cases. Superficial cracks seen on examination do not extend to the dentate line, as do fissures. With acute, more severe exacerbations, the perianal skin will appear reddened, edematous, excoriated, and moist. In chronic cases, the perianal skin takes on a thickened, almost leathery, depigmented appearance. The normal radiating folds of skin thicken into rugae and may produce factitiously induced superficial fissures.

TREATMENT

Diagnose and treat the underlying cause. Perianal streptococcal dermatitis (**Figure 85-23**) is well known in children, where it can cause

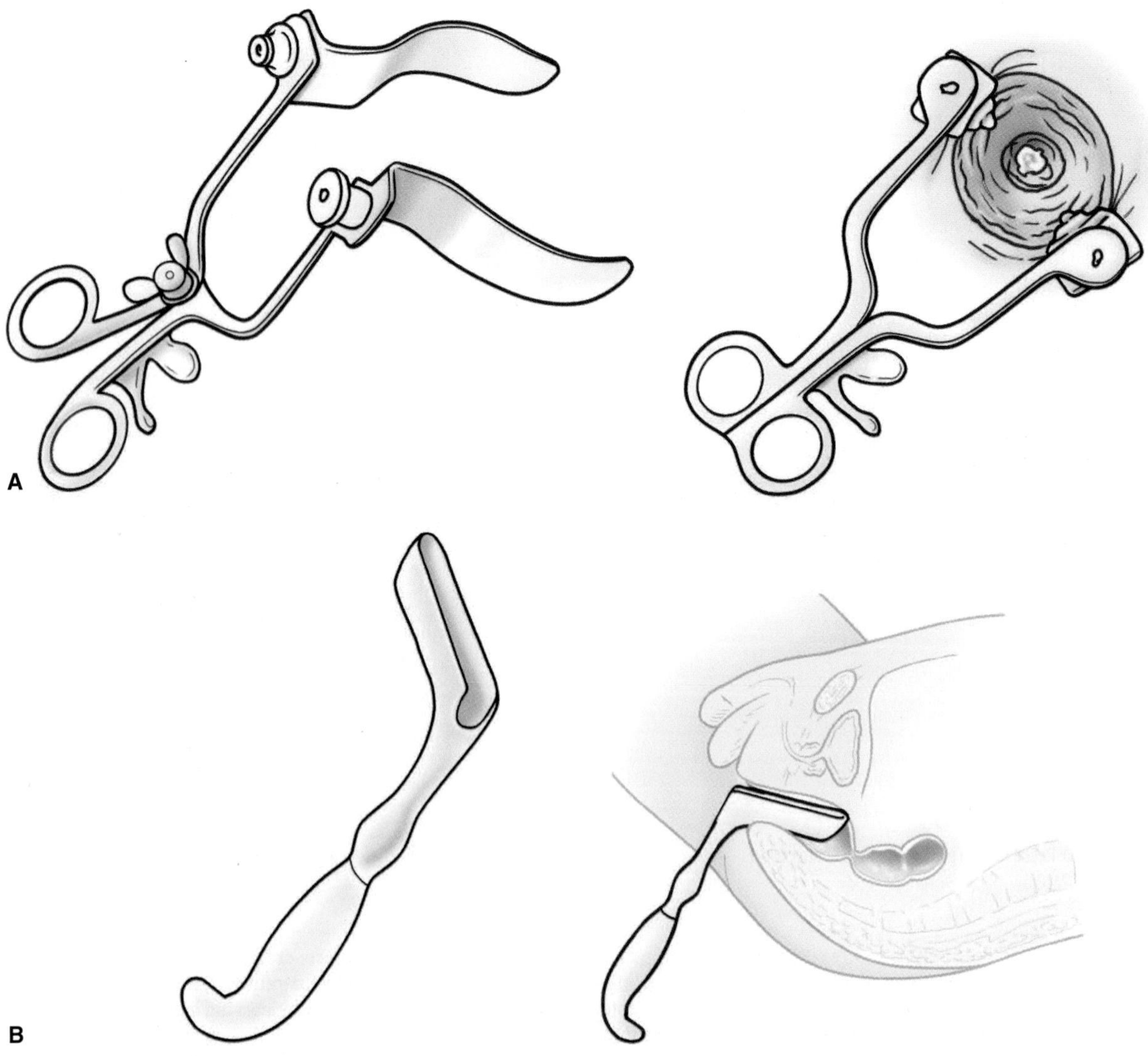

FIGURE 85-22. A. Foreign body exposure. B. Removal techniques. [Reproduced with permission from Reichman EF: *Emergency Medicine Procedures*, 2nd ed. McGraw-Hill, Inc., 2013. Figures 72-3, 72-4.]

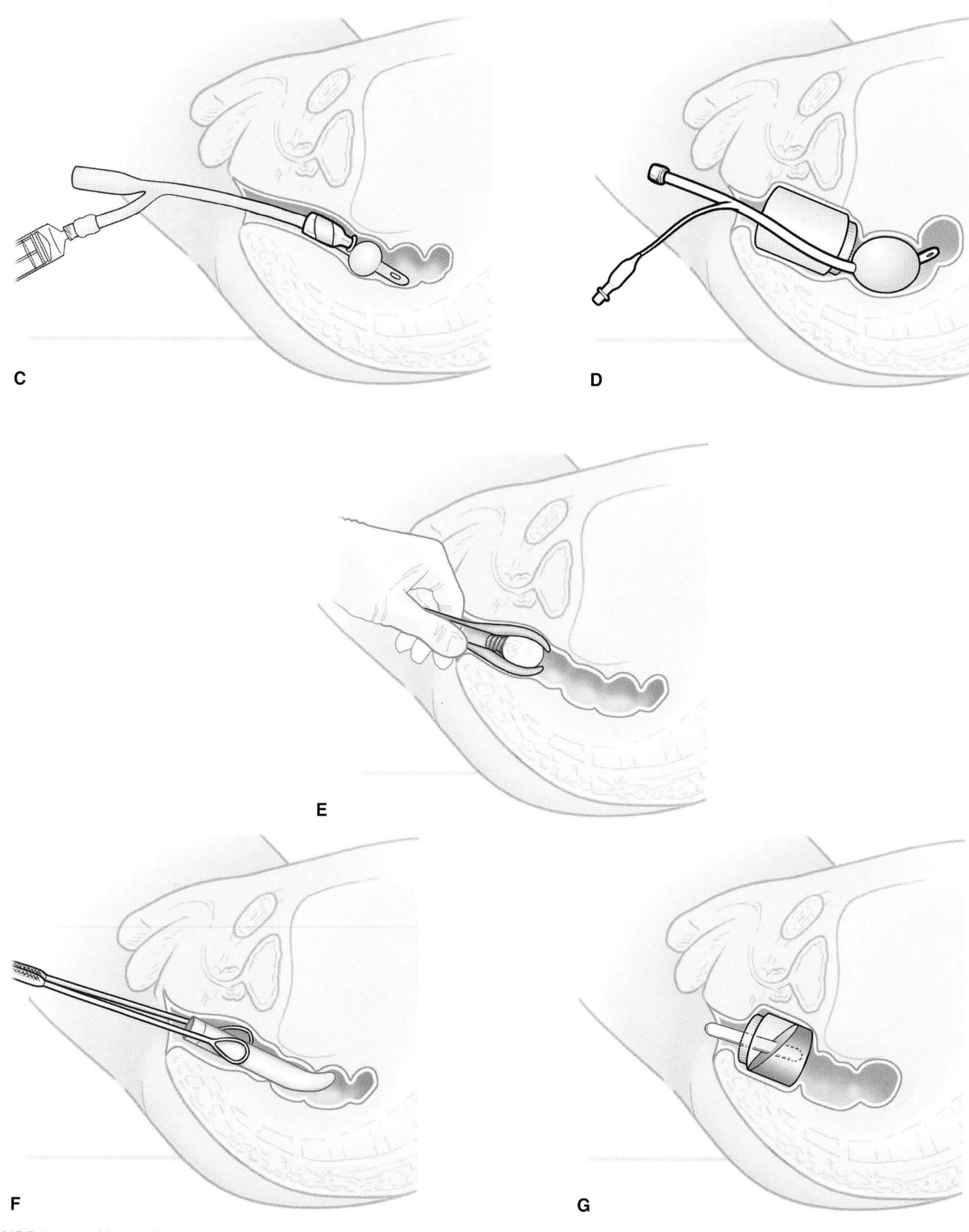

FIGURE 85-22. *(Continued)*

systemic infection, but is also recognized and can cause serious infection in adults. Obtain cultures and treat empirically with penicillin or erythromycin.[15] Pinworms can be identified by touching the perianal skin with transparent tape to collect the worm and then viewing under a microscope. Idiopathic causes may be treated by adding fiber to the diet, which can bulk the stools and help prevent persistent soiling and irritation when the patient is plagued by frequent loose stools. To avoid scratching at night, the patient can wear gloves at bedtime. Warm baths are recommended for at least 15 minutes two to three times a day for hygiene, instead of soap, followed by thorough drying. Zinc oxide ointment can provide a protective covering for the perianal skin and may promote healing, while athlete's foot powder may enhance drying.

TABLE 85-5 Some Secondary Causes of Pruritus Ani

Anorectal disease: Draining perirectal abscess, fissures, hemorrhoids, rectal prolapse, fistulas
Dietary factors: Caffeine, cola, calcium, chocolate, citrus, alcohol, tomatoes, spices, peanuts
Local infection: Bacteria, viruses, fungi, worms, lice, scabies, bed bugs, hidradenitis
Local irritants: Perfumed toilet tissue, soaps, detergents, hygiene sprays
Dermatologic: Atopic dermatitis, lichen planus, psoriasis, seborrheic dermatitis
Systemic illness: Diabetes, various malignancies, Crohn's disease, acanthosis
Psychogenic: Stress, obsessive compulsive disorder

One percent hydrocortisone cream is effective for the allergic component of the inflammation. Fungicidal creams, antibiotics, and antiviral and antiparasitic medications should be prescribed for patients with infectious causes. Hydroxyzine hydrochloride may be used as an effective bedtime sedative. Refer to a proctologist or dermatologist for resistant symptoms.

PILONIDAL SINUS

Pilonidal sinus is an acquired problem formed by the penetration of the skin by an ingrown hair, which causes a foreign body granuloma reaction. The sinus is perpetuated by the presence of the hair and repeated bouts of infection.

CLINICAL FEATURES

Pilonidal sinuses or cysts occur in the midline in the upper part of the natal cleft, which overlies the lower sacrum and coccyx. Because of their proximity to the anus, infected pilonidal cysts (abscesses) are sometimes mistakenly diagnosed as perirectal abscesses (**Figure 85-24, A–C**).

Occasionally, an inflamed cyst may refer pain to the coccygeal region. **An abscessed pilonidal sinus is almost always located in the posterior midline over the sacrum and coccyx.** Although there may be secondary fistulous openings on either side of the midline, they do not communicate with the anorectum. On the other hand, long, horseshoe-type fistulas emanating from a perirectal abscess may drain close to the location of a pilonidal sinus but not in the midline. Fistulous tracts most commonly ascend superiorly. Pilonidal disease may present as a painless cyst, an acute abscess, or chronic recurring cysts with draining sinuses. Alternate causes for draining fistulas should be considered, such as anal fistulas, syphilitic and tuberculous granulomas, simple furuncles, fungal infections, and sacral osteomyelitis. Carcinoma is a rare complication of

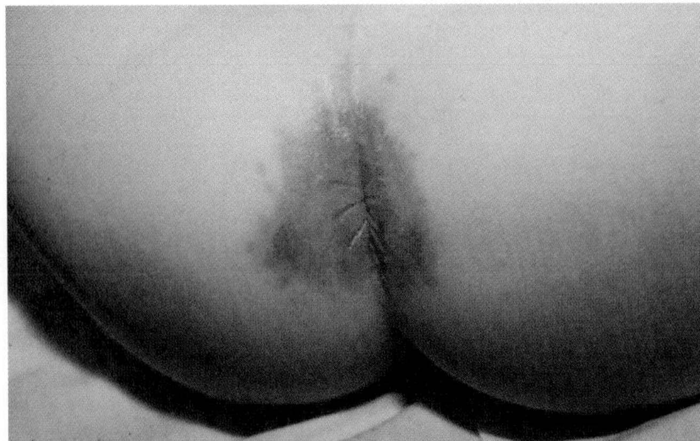

FIGURE 85-23. Example of pruritus ani. Pruritus ani from perianal strep infection. [Reproduced with permission from Knoop K, Stack L, Storrow A, Thurman RJ: *Atlas of Emergency Medicine,* 2nd ed. © 2002, McGraw-Hill, New York.]

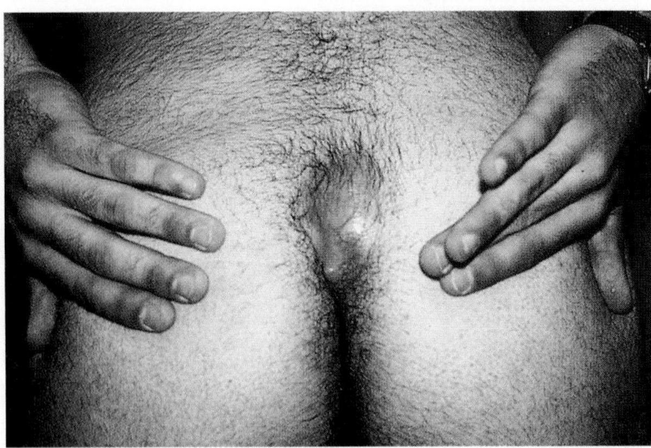

A

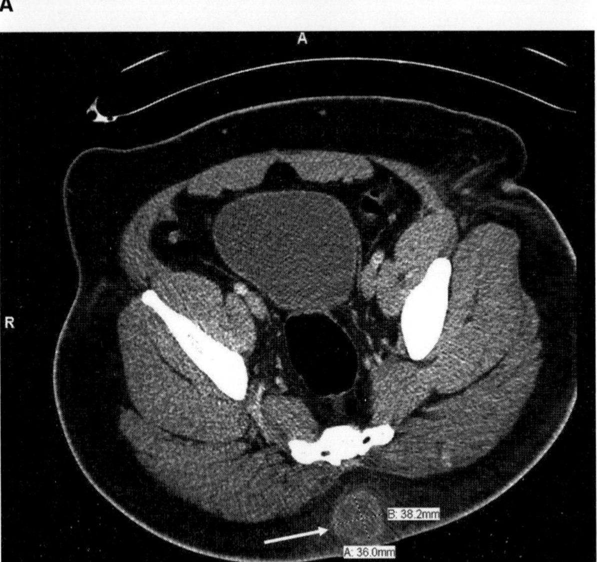

B

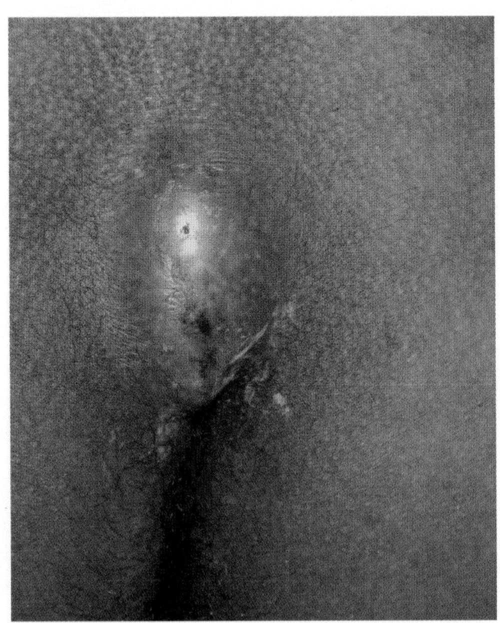

C

FIGURE 85-24. A. Pilonidal sinus. B. CT scan of a pilonidal sinus with abscess (*arrow*). C. Pilonidal sinus. [A: Reproduced with permission from Knoop K, Stack L, Storrow A, Thurman RJ: *Atlas of Emergency Medicine,* 3rd ed. © 2010, McGraw-Hill, New York. C: Photo contributor: Lawrence B. Stack, MD. Reproduced with permission from Knoop K, Stack L, Storrow A, Thurman RJ: *Atlas of Emergency Medicine,* 3rd ed. © 2010, McGraw-Hill, New York. Figure 9.43.]

chronic, recurring pilonidal sinus disease. It is more frequent in men and is usually a well-differentiated, dermal-type squamous cell carcinoma.

TREATMENT

Treatment is incision and drainage, and antibiotics are needed only if cellulitis is present. Ultrasonography can delineate the extent of the abscess. Following incision and drainage in the ED, refer to a surgeon for definitive care.

HIDRADENITIS SUPPURATIVA

In postpubertal males and females (the second to fourth decades of life), the perianal surface containing hair follicles and apocrine sweat glands may become blocked, which generally occurs in the perineal, groin, axillary, or inframammary regions. Perineal disease is more common in males, whereas axillary disease is more common in females.[16]

CLINICAL FEATURES

Fistulas with a malodorous discharge may develop but do not extend to the intersphincteric plane, and the abscesses are quite superficial and do not originate at the dentate line. Fistulas that extend above the dentate line may suggest coexisting cryptoglandular or Crohn's disease.[16] Chronic inflammation, edema, tissue induration, fibrosis, and significant pitted scarring may occur (**Figure 85-25**).

TREATMENT

Recurrence is common, particularly in the perineal region, resulting in scarring, edema, painful nodules, induration, and draining sinus tracts, all of which are difficult to treat. Small abscesses can be drained in the ED, but extensive lesions require surgical or dermatologic referral. Topical clindamycin or oral clindamycin with rifampin can be helpful.[16] Other treatments include erythromycin, tetracycline, and doxycycline as well as retinoids, hormones, and immunosuppressive and anti-inflammatory agents. Some success is seen with radiation, cryosurgery, and laser treatments. With advanced disease characterized by recurrent abscesses, multiple interconnecting fistulas, and scarring, resection of the skin and subcutaneous fat down to the fascia yields the lowest recurrence rate.[16]

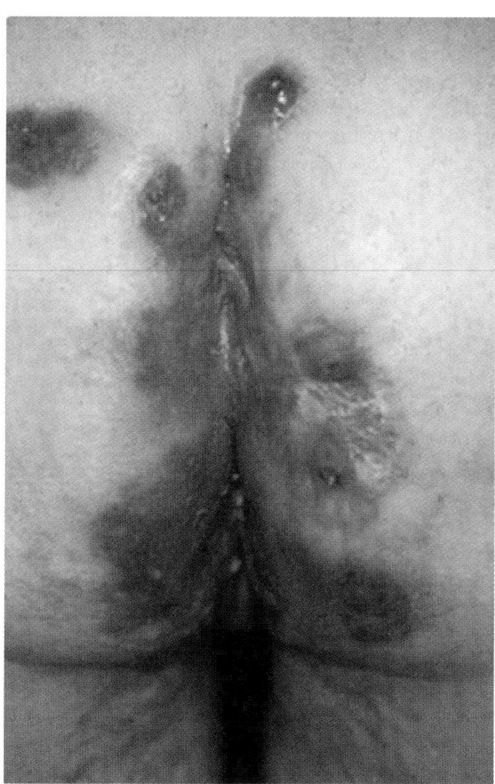

FIGURE 85-25. Perianal hidradenitis suppurativa in a 27-year-old man. Abscesses, draining sinuses, and scars are seen in the sacral region. [Reproduced with permission from Wolff K, Johnson RA: *Fitzpatrick's Color Atlas and Synopsis of Clinical Dermatology*, 6th ed. McGraw-Hill, New York, 2009.]

TABLE 85-6 Causes of Rectovaginal Fistulas

Gynecologic or surgical trauma or foreign body	Gynecologic malignancies
Pelvic irradiation	Leukemia
Local infection	Inflammatory bowel disease
Congenital	

RECTOVAGINAL FISTULA

The lower rectum and anal canal abut the posterior wall of the vagina, so the fistula may be located anywhere along this region.

CLINICAL FEATURES

The presenting complaint of patients with a rectovaginal fistula is usually flatulence and/or malodorous vaginal discharge or gross stool emanating from the vagina. They may note air or stool in the urine, or rectal urine. **Table 85-6** lists various causes. A rectovaginal fistula can arise from the rectum or small or large bowel. Usually, stool is seen during the pelvic examination. CT scan or MRI confirms the diagnosis. Surgical consultation is required.

REFERENCES

The complete reference list is available online at www.TintinalliEM.com.

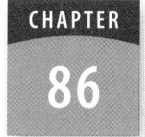

Gastrointestinal Procedures and Devices

Michael D. Witting

NASOGASTRIC ASPIRATION

Nasogastric (NG) aspiration is used to remove liquid contents from the stomach and decompress the stomach and small bowel. The need for NG aspiration often varies with the clinical presentation (**Table 86-1**). Gastric decompression is useful in small bowel obstruction, although some studies have shown that medical therapy with octreotide or somatostatin has allowed safe treatment of bowel obstruction associated with malignancy.[1,2] NG aspiration and decompression are no longer considered routine for the treatment of adynamic ileus.[3,4] **Removal of liquid contents is useful**

TABLE 86-1 Selection of Patients for Nasogastric Aspiration

Clinical Situation	Best Uses	Consider Withholding
GI bleeding with hematemesis	Rapid bleeding (large hematemesis, refractory hemodynamic instability)	Slow or mild bleeding (coffee grounds, blood-streaked emesis)
GI bleeding without hematemesis	Massive rectal bleeding with hemodynamic instability	Clinical picture suggests lower GI source (bright red blood per rectum, age >50 y, blood urea nitrogen/creatinine <30)[5]
Small bowel dilation	Small bowel obstruction	Ileus

TABLE 86-2 Complications of Placement of Nasogastric and Nasoenteric Tubes

Complications
Epistaxis
Intracranial placement
Bronchial placement
Pharyngeal placement
Esophageal obstruction or rupture
Bronchial or alveolar perforation
Pneumothorax
Charcoal instillation into the lungs and pleural cavity
Gastric or duodenal rupture
Vocal cord paralysis
Pneumomediastinum
Laryngeal injuries
Knotting (preventing removal)

in cases of GI bleeding, but not all patients with GI bleeding require NG aspiration.

In GI bleeding, a common and controversial situation for NG aspiration,[6] aspiration of stomach contents can localize the source of bleeding, indicate the rate of bleeding, and clear the stomach for endoscopy. Patients with hematemesis virtually always have an upper GI source, and NG aspiration is helpful to assess the rate of hemorrhage rather than identify the source. In significant upper GI bleeding, such as suggested by refractory hemodynamic instability or large quantities of bright red bloody emesis, the rate of bleeding can determine the success of medical interventions and the need for emergent endoscopy. When the clinical picture suggests a slower rate of bleeding, such as with coffee-ground emesis or blood-streaked emesis, the need for NG aspiration is less clear because less sensitive methods of assessing the rate of hemorrhage, such as observation of spontaneous bleeding, hemodynamic assessment, and serial hematocrit measurement, are often adequate.

In patients without hematemesis, NG aspiration lacks sensitivity to detect an upper GI source.[7,8] Although it has been reported that 10% of patients with hematochezia have an upper GI source, many of these are from a duodenal source and are beyond the reach of the NG tube.[9] Most patients with melena have an upper GI source and require upper endoscopy regardless of the results of NG aspiration. In severe, ongoing rectal bleeding with hemodynamic instability, NG aspiration is relatively useful because severe upper GI bleeding is generally easier to stop than severe lower GI bleeding.

The literature is riddled with case reports of bizarre mishaps resulting from the use of NG tubes, some of which are listed in **Table 86-2**. However, the rate of adverse effects has not been systematically addressed. The main morbidity from the procedure is probably related to pain, followed by epistaxis, both of which can be minimized by good technique.

The equipment required for NG tube insertion is listed in **Table 86-3**. The optimal positioning is with the patient seated upright with the neck slightly flexed. Topical application of anesthetic can reduce the pain of the procedure, and a vasoconstrictor can shrink the turbinates, creating a larger nasal opening, but use a vasoconstrictor with caution in hypertensive patients. One option is to mix 4% lidocaine with oxymetazoline and instill this solution using a nasal atomizer.[10] Nebulized lidocaine also provides effective analgesia.[11] Although it is tempting to use viscous lidocaine on the tip of the tube instead of premedication, this maneuver does not allow time for the lidocaine to be effective. A right-handed operator may choose the right side or the side of patient preference. Premedication with IV metoclopramide, in adults, or lingual 24% sucrose, in infants, may also decrease pain.[12,13]

TABLE 86-3 Equipment for Nasogastric Tube Insertion

Equipment
Absorbent pad (blue Chux®)
Kidney basin
Equipment for anesthesia and vasoconstriction
Nebulizer or nasal atomizer
Local anesthetic (4% lidocaine)
Vasoconstrictor (oxymetazoline, phenylephrine)
Water-soluble lubricant
Cup of water with straw
Nasogastric Salem sump tube—16 F
Catheter-tip syringe
Tubing connected to suction device, such as wall suction

TABLE 86-4 Techniques for Identifying Nasogastric and Nasointestinal Feeding Tube Placement

Technique
Indicates gastric placement
Epigastric auscultation of air insufflated through the tube
Aspiration of visually recognizable GI secretions
pH testing of aspirates (pH <6 indicates gastric placement)
Indicates tracheobronchial placement
Coughing or choking
Inability to speak
Air bubbles when proximal end of tube is placed in water

Describing the procedure to the patient in advance and talking to the patient during the procedure minimize anxiety. Insert the lubricated tube into the selected nostril. Direct the tube posteriorly, not superiorly, and it should naturally bend inferiorly toward the glottis. Resistance is expected at the level of the glottis. At this point, have the patient take a drink of water, and advance the tube at the time of swallowing. This step minimizes the potential for false passage at the level of the glottis. Warming the distal tip of the tube will make it more pliable and may further decrease the pain of the procedure. Once the tube is past the glottis, quickly advance the tube and aspirate stomach contents. If the patient coughs during the procedure, stop and make sure that the patient can speak clearly. Failure to aspirate stomach contents should prompt visualization of the pharynx to ensure the tube is not coiled in the posterior pharynx. If the appearance of the gastric aspirate is inconclusive, its pH can be tested, or air can be insufflated during auscultation over the stomach (**Table 86-4**). A chest x-ray can also be obtained to confirm tube placement. If the NG tube is to remain in place, it can be taped to the patient's nose and connected to low-intermittent suction.

Some situations make NG tube insertion more difficult, such as obstructed nares, lack of patient cooperation, or endotracheal intubation. In patients with obstructed nares, the orogastric route may be used, although this is often less comfortable than the NG route. In obtunded patients with a poor gag reflex, endotracheal intubation may prevent aspiration. In patients with endotracheal intubation, flexing the neck or cooling the tube in ice water to stiffen it may facilitate passage.

ANOSCOPY

Anoscopy can identify an anorectal cause of bleeding in patients with hematochezia. Although an uncomfortable test, it is safe if performed properly. Contraindications include rectal foreign bodies and suspected rectal perforation. Anoscopy requires only an anoscope (a hollow plastic tube with a blunt obturator), lubricant, 4 × 4 gauze pads, blue absorbent pads (Chux®), and a light source. Because both hands contact contaminated areas during anoscopy, an assistant can hold a hand-held light source, or the operator can use a forehead-mounted light.

Usually, the lateral decubitus position is least uncomfortable, although the knee-chest position is an alternative. The equipment can be assembled onto the blue absorbent pad on the bed. After a careful external visual inspection of the anus with retraction of the buttocks, the generously lubricated anoscope is gently inserted into the anus. Step-by-step verbal communication is essential. If resistance or pain is encountered, slowing the rate of insertion or redirecting can allow more comfortable passage. After insertion is completed, remove the obturator, obtain stool from the tip, and perform guaiac testing. Then peer through the anoscope as it is withdrawn, looking for potential sources of bleeding. Internal hemorrhoids are common sources of anorectal bleeding that are visible through the anoscope. After the procedure, the patient or operator may wipe off the lubricant with gauze and dispose of it in the blue absorbent pad.

OROGASTRIC LAVAGE

Orogastric lavage is used to remove pills and fragments from the stomach. It is only appropriate for patients presenting well within 1 hour after a potentially lethal ingestion.[14] Because an NG tube is too small to retrieve pill fragments, gastric lavage for solids is done orally with a large-bore tube. Gagging and vomiting during the procedure are common, and aspiration is a significant risk, particularly when airway protection is in doubt. Many other complications are possible, including tube misplacement into the bronchi, pharyngeal injury, and viscus perforation. Endotracheal intubation before this procedure can minimize these risks when a patient is or may become obtunded.

Equipment for the procedure includes a large-bore tube, such as the Ewald tube® or the Tum-E-Vac® (Ethox Corp, Buffalo, NY); lubricant; suction; emesis basin; blue absorbent pad; a catheter-tip syringe; irrigation fluid; and a bite block or oral airway to prevent patients from biting down on the tube. Patient positioning, tube advancement, and confirmation of placement are similar to NG tube insertion, but be especially sure to aim the proximal end away from others. After inserting a bite block in uncooperative patients, insert the gastric tube to the level of the glottis, and encourage the patient to swallow. Then pass the tube quickly into the stomach. Coughing or airflow from the tube raises concern for tracheal malpositioning. Have the patient vocalize to exclude tracheal placement. After suction and irrigation of gastric contents, charcoal and sorbitol can be instilled before withdrawal of the tube.

ESOPHAGEAL BALLOON (SENGSTAKEN-BLAKEMORE) TAMPONADE

The Sengstaken-Blakemore tube is designed to tamponade bleeding from esophageal varices (**Figure 86-1**). With the increasing availability of endoscopy and success of medical therapy with octreotide, somatostatin, and vasopressin, its use has declined. Nevertheless, it still has a role in cases in which endoscopy is unavailable or hemorrhage is refractory to endoscopic techniques. It is only useful in patients with esophageal varices that are known or suspected from the clinical picture, such as in patients with severe hematemesis and signs of cirrhosis. The procedure frequently provokes emesis, and aspiration can be minimized by endotracheal intubation. Other risks include gastric or esophageal rupture. Insert the tube orally after the same procedure described in the section "Orogastric Lavage." After confirming tube placement as described earlier, expand the distal balloon with water or normal saline and apply gentle traction to the tube. Because varices are often at the gastroesophageal junction, this often stops the bleeding. If not, expand the proximal balloon. To maintain traction, tape the proximal end of the tube to the face guard of a football or lacrosse helmet that the patient wears. The patient will not be able to swallow secretions with this in place, so proximal suction, whether from a proximal port in the device or an NG tube inserted proximally, will further minimize the risk of aspiration.

Once the tube is in place, maintain traction to the minimum amount necessary to stop the bleeding to minimize the risk of tissue ischemia. Maintain balloon tamponade until more definitive measures can be taken.

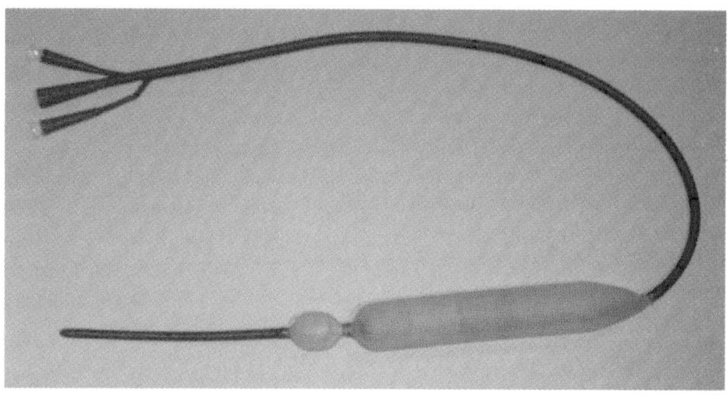

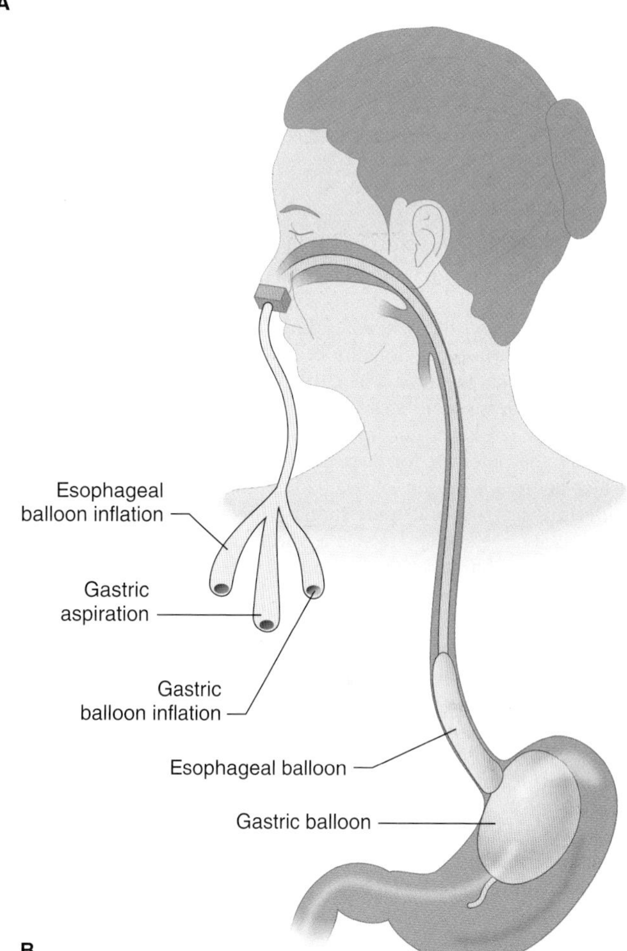

FIGURE 86-1. **A.** Sengstaken-Blakemore tube. **B.** Insertion of Sengstaken-Blakemore tube.

PARACENTESIS

In paracentesis, ascitic fluid is removed for diagnostic or therapeutic purposes. Patients with ascites and abdominal pain or other GI symptoms may have peritonitis, requiring diagnostic paracentesis. This may be true even if the abdominal pain is mild and unaccompanied by signs of systemic infection.[15] Patients with respiratory compromise or severe pain due to tense ascites require therapeutic paracentesis, in which a large quantity of fluid is removed. Large-volume therapeutic paracentesis is a lengthy procedure associated with complications such as hyponatremia, renal impairment, and encephalopathy, and many of these patients require other treatment.[16] Therefore, it is generally best reserved for the admitting team or ED observation unit, except in rare cases in which pain or respiratory compromise cannot be controlled in the ED with medications or supplemental oxygen. Other risks of paracentesis in general, whether diagnostic or therapeutic, include bowel perforation, ascitic fluid leak, hemorrhage, and introduction of infection.

Equipment for diagnostic paracentesis includes sterile drapes (both fenestrated and nonfenestrated), sterilizing solution (povidone-iodine or chlorhexidine), gauze, assorted syringes (3, 10, or 30 mL), a small-bore (27-gauge or smaller) needle, three medium-bore (21-gauge) needles, local anesthetic (lidocaine), and containers for cell count and culture for the laboratory. If paracentesis is also to be therapeutic, a three-way stopcock, sterile tubing, and a source of suction—either vacuum bottles or a setup for wall suction—are necessary, and a large-bore needle or plastic catheter (18- or 16-gauge) will speed the procedure. Ultrasonography can

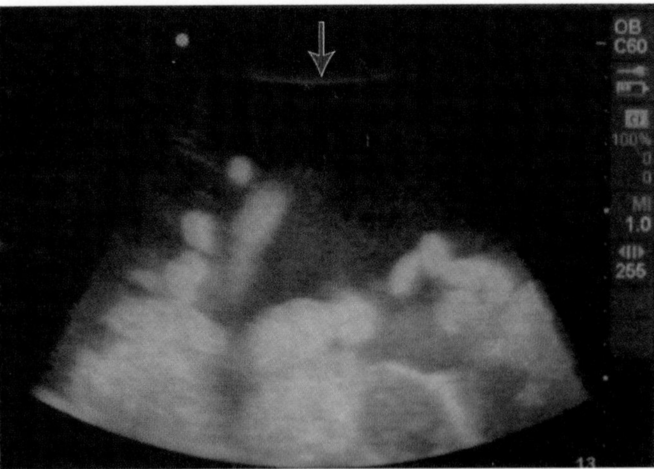

FIGURE 86-2. US view of a desirable puncture site for paracentesis (*arrow*).

confirm ascites and identify a target fluid collection to minimize the potential for bowel perforation (**Figure 86-2**). US guidance can also assist the operator in avoiding subcutaneous vessels dilated by portal hypertension, and it decreases the risk of bleeding.[17]

If the patient has coagulopathy or thrombocytopenia, correct deficiencies before paracentesis. Place the patient in a comfortable supine position, and cleanse and sterilely prepare the site of expected needle insertion. The left lower quadrant is generally a good area because this minimizes the potential for liver injury, but the right lower quadrant may also be used if the left lower quadrant has distorted anatomy, such as with prior scarring or ostomy surgery (**Figure 86-3**). Anesthetize the skin over the target area by raising a wheal, and then switch to a larger-bore needle to infiltrate to the level of the peritoneum. A Z-track technique, in which traction on the skin is used to create a displaced track to the peritoneum, can minimize the potential for infection and persistent leakage.[16] At a depth expected to be near the peritoneum, apply suction to the syringe and infiltrate lidocaine while advancing until peritoneal fluid is aspirated. Once the fluid is aspirated, change the syringe with the needle still in place, and then aspirate at least 50 cc of fluid into the fresh syringe for laboratory analysis. In therapeutic paracentesis, attach tubing to the needle, catheter, or stopcock, and connect to suction. Even if the goal is diagnosis, up to 1 L is unlikely to cause complications and may provide significant symptomatic relief. Then withdraw the needle or catheter and cover the insertion site with a dressing. A purse-string suture can be placed to minimize leakage. Recheck the patient in 30 minutes to identify persistent leakage or an increase in symptoms to suggest a complication. Patients with large-volume paracentesis should be monitored for hypotension for several hours after the procedure. Cover the puncture site with a dry dressing for 48 hours.

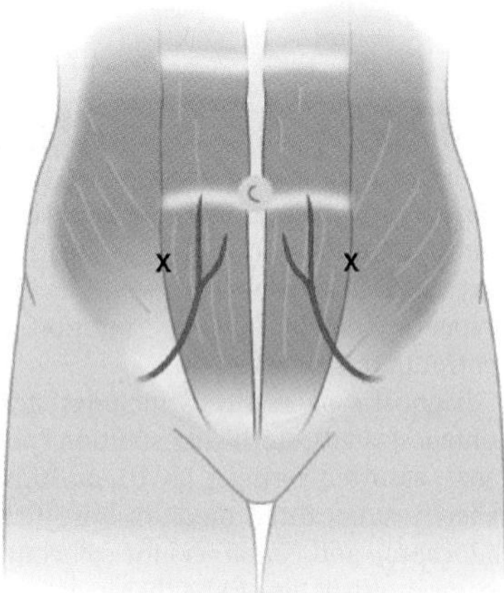

FIGURE 86-3. Sites for needle introduction in the left or right lower quadrant (x) for abdominal paracentesis.

TRANSABDOMINAL FEEDING TUBES

Although the techniques for the initial placement of transabdominal feeding tubes (gastrostomy [G-tube], jejunostomy [J-tube], and gastrojejunostomy) are beyond the scope of emergency physicians, complications related to these tubes need to be recognized (**Table 86-5**). These tubes can be placed by a surgeon using open technique, by a gastroenterologist using endoscopic technique (percutaneous endoscopic gastrostomy), or by a radiologist with percutaneous techniques. The radiographic technique has been associated with fewer complications than has open or endoscopically assisted placement.[18]

Frequent minor complications are associated with the use of these tubes, including purulent drainage and leakage around the stomal site, clogging, dislodgement, and vomiting and diarrhea.

Drainage from the stomal site is a common finding and represents a foreign-body reaction due to the catheter. As long as there is no evidence of cellulitis or necrotizing fasciitis, local skin care with hydrogen peroxide and warm water usually will clear up the problem. If there is granuloma

TABLE 86-5 Complications Seen with Transabdominal Feeding Tubes

Complication	Initial Considerations
Purulent drainage from stoma	Local care with hydrogen peroxide unless cellulitis is present.
Leakage from stoma	Carefully replace with larger tube.
Tube occlusion	Attempt irrigation; most often, just replace.
Dislodged tubes	Gently replace; confirm placement with x-rays.
Pneumothorax	High index of suspicion; consider needle aspiration.
Bacteremia	Consider as potential source in septic patient.
Bleeding from tract	If recently inserted, consider local injection, consult.
Bleeding from granuloma buildup	Local therapy with silver nitrate.
Infection of surrounding skin	Consultation, pull tube, IV antibiotics.
Necrotizing fasciitis	Consider MRI to help confirm; surgical debridement.
Peritonitis	Determine if fistula exists; consultation, IV antibiotics.
Pulmonary aspiration of feedings	Reduce flow rate, half-strength feeds, consider J-tube.
Vomiting or diarrhea	Reduce flow rate, half-strength feeds, stop feeds.
Gastroesophageal reflux	Reduce flow rate, half-strength feeds, consider J-tube.
Intestinal obstruction	Step feedings, NPO, admit, and observe.
Gastric outlet obstruction	Reposition tube.
Gastric volvulus	Surgical consult.
Gastric perforation	Surgical consult.
Esophageal perforation	Surgical consult.
Colonic perforation	Surgical consult.
Colocutaneous fistula	Surgical consult.
Electrolyte abnormalities	Change feedings or increase free water.
GI bleeding	Endoscopy and therapy directed at cause.
Bolster buried in abdominal wall	Surgical consult.

Abbreviations: J-tube = jejunostomy tube; NPO = nothing by mouth.

formation with localized bleeding from friable skin, local treatment with silver nitrate usually will help.

Leakage of gastric contents can become a problem. This is managed by careful insertion of a larger tube. Care should be used not to force too large a tube into the stoma, because this can cause separation of the stomach wall from the abdominal wall.

Prevention is the best treatment for clogging of gastrostomy and jejunostomy tubes. Frequent flushing with water and careful crushing of pills usually can prevent this problem. Vomiting and diarrhea can be relieved by decreasing the amount of the feedings and/or diluting the feedings. To unclog the tube, instill warm water or carbonated beverage (cola is most often used) and let it remain for 20 minutes. Then attempt flushing.[19] Alkalinized pancreatic enzymes (12,000 lipase units dissolved in 650 mL bicarbonate) have also proven effective in about 50% of cases.[20]

TUBE REPLACEMENT

If the tube cannot be unclogged or if it has fallen out, replacement will be necessary. If the tube was placed by a surgeon or gastroenterologist and has not been replaced, it probably will have a bolster (also called a *mushroom* or *bumper*) holding the tube in place (**Figure 86-4**). This will prevent the tube from being removed. The bolster must be removed endoscopically, or the tube may be cut off and the bolster allowed to pass through the GI tract.[21] The latter technique is generally safe in adults, but passage in children has complications,[22] and tube removal should be done by the endoscopist or surgeon. Tube removal should be done by the endoscopist or surgeon. Endoscopic removal in adults is advisable when there is suspected or potential obstructive disease of the GI tract, such as pyloric stenosis, intestinal pseudo-obstruction, and intestinal stricture (e.g., due to radiation, ischemia, or inflammatory bowel disease). If the tube is cut, an abdominal radiograph should be obtained 1 week later to confirm passage of the internal component. Most reported complications from a retained internal bolster have occurred when the bolster did not pass within 1 to 2 weeks.[23] If the bolster or bumper becomes buried in the abdominal wall, consult with the endoscopist or surgeon who placed the device. Do not attempt removal by traction. Some specially designed tubes have internal bumpers that can be removed by external traction, but consultation with the endoscopist or surgeon who placed the device is necessary before any traction is applied to verify the type of tube and the appropriate method of removal[24] (Figure 86-4).

If the tube has become dislodged or has fallen out, **replace it as quickly as possible (within a few hours) to prevent closure of the tract. Most tracts mature after 2 to 3 weeks. Do not attempt to replace a tube with an immature tract.**[19] First determine, if possible, which type of tube is being used. If the tube is available, replacement with the same size is usually possible. If the tube is not available, it can be difficult to determine whether the tract is for a jejunostomy or gastrostomy tube. Location site on the abdominal wall is not helpful to differentiate the two. A tract for a gastrostomy tube is usually larger. Old records may be useful and should be obtained, if possible. After determining the type of

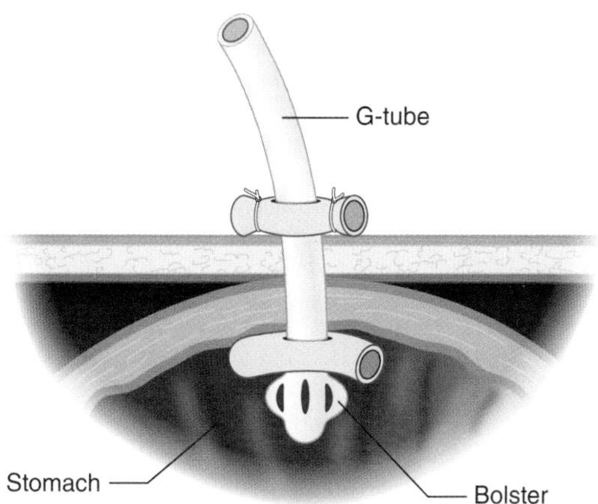

FIGURE 86-4. Percutaneous endoscopic gastrostomy tube (G-tube) with a mushroom bolster in place.

tract and size of tube used previously, insert the tube using a water-soluble lubricant. If the size of the tube being replaced is not known, it is reasonable to start with a 16- or 18-F replacement gastrostomy tube or Foley catheter. The lubricated tube should pass easily into the stoma without additional equipment. If resistance is met, abandon the attempt. A smaller tube can be tried to keep the tract open. After replacing the tube, instill a 20- to 30-mL bolus of a water-soluble contrast material (e.g., diatrizoate meglumine and diatrizoate sodium solution [Gastrografin]) through the tube, and obtain a supine abdominal x-ray within 1 to 2 minutes. The x-ray should demonstrate rugae of the stomach for a gastrostomy tube and flow into the small bowel for a jejunostomy tube. US can also be used to verify gastric placement. The tip of the tube can be visualized within the stomach, and confirmation of placement can be done by injecting 10 cc of normal saline into the tube and observing the fluid entering the stomach, using real-time US. Another way of determining placement is to withdraw gastric fluid and check pH to make sure it is acidic. If there is any question of improper placement, obtain immediate consultation.

A special caution regarding jejunostomy tubes should be noted. Jejunostomy tracts are smaller, and smaller tubes are used (8- to 14-F). These tubes usually are not sutured in place and frequently become dislodged. They can be replaced with catheters made specifically for jejunostomies or with Foley catheters. **If a Foley catheter is used to replace a lost jejunostomy catheter, the balloon should never be inflated** because it can cause a bowel obstruction or damage the jejunum. The tube is lubricated, inserted into the stoma, and advanced 20 cm. These tubes are easily replaced if the tract is mature; however, if resistance is met, referral to a radiologist for fluoroscopic placement using guidewires is recommended.

REFERENCES

The complete reference list is available online at www.TintinalliEM.com.

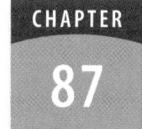

Complications of General Surgical Procedures

Edmond A. Hooker

INTRODUCTION

Outpatient surgical procedures are common, and with increasing pressure for cost containment, admitted patients are being discharged earlier in their postoperative course. As a result, more patients are coming to the ED with postoperative fever, respiratory complications, GU complaints, wound infections, vascular problems, and complications of drug therapy (**Table 87-1**). This chapter reviews the complications common to all surgical procedures and those specific to a single procedure.

The operating surgeon should be called when one of his or her patients appears in the ED with a surgical complication. This is not just a courtesy, but provides continuity of care important for the patient's well-being.

FEVER

Fever is a common presenting complaint (**Table 87-2**). A mnemonic for the common causes of postoperative fever is the "five Ws": *wind* (atelectasis or pneumonia), *water* (urinary tract infection), *wound*, *walking* (deep vein thrombosis), and *wonder drugs* (drug fever or pseudomembranous colitis).[1] Respiratory complications, such as atelectasis, and IV catheter–related problems, such as thrombophlebitis, are the predominant causes of fever in the first 72 hours. Necrotizing streptococcal and clostridial infections also occur in surgical wounds early in the postoperative course.

Urinary tract infections become evident 1 to 5 days postoperatively. Seven to 10 days postoperatively, clinical manifestations of wound

TABLE 87-1 Complications of General Surgical Procedures

Complication	Important Points
Fever	"Five Ws" (wind, water, wound, walking, wonder drugs) are common causes
Pulmonary complications	
Atelectasis	<24 h, treat with pulmonary toilet, discharge unless ill or hypoxemic
Pneumonia	2–7 d, polymicrobial, most require admission
Pneumothorax	Multiple causes, consider expiratory views, consider needle aspiration
Pulmonary embolism	Dyspnea is main symptom, high index of suspicion
GI complications	
Intestinal obstruction	Obtain radiographs, search for causes
Intra-abdominal abscess	CT diagnosis, early administration of broad-spectrum antibiotics
Pancreatitis	Always consider in postoperative patients with abdominal pain
Cholecystitis	Usually in older patients, can be acalculous
Fistulas	Can be high output, admit if concerns over output
GU complications	
Urinary tract infection	2–5 d, oral antibiotics, most discharged
Urinary retention	Rapid catheter drainage, most discharged
Acute renal failure	Prerenal, renal, and postrenal causes, most admitted
Wound complications	
Hematoma	Caused by poor hemostasis, can drain most, but be careful with neck hematomas and hematomas after vascular surgery
Seroma	Painless swelling, clear fluid, drain and discharge
Infection	Open, drain, and culture specimens; be careful with wounds associated with respiratory tract, GI tract, or GU tract, or secondary to trauma
Necrotizing fasciitis	Pain out of proportion to physical findings
Dehiscence	Be careful with abdominal incisions (potential for evisceration)
Vascular complications	
Superficial thrombophlebitis	Usually aseptic, provide local therapy and discharge
Deep venous thrombosis	Upper and lower extremity, perform Doppler studies
Complications of drug therapy	
Diarrhea	Consider pseudomembranous colitis
Drug fever	Many drugs implicated, requires admission
Tetanus	Can occur after GI surgery
Procedure-specific complications	See text

infections develop. Deep venous thrombosis can result in fever any time but usually not until the fifth postoperative day. Antibiotic-induced pseudomembranous colitis occurs up to 6 weeks postoperatively. An approach for evaluating and managing fever in postoperative patients is presented in **Table 87-3**.

RESPIRATORY COMPLICATIONS

ATELECTASIS

Atelectasis, the collapse of pulmonary alveoli, is very common. Contributing factors include inadequate clearance of secretions after general anesthesia, decreased intra-alveolar pressure, and postoperative pain, which results in hypoventilation. Although atelectasis can occur after any procedure, it frequently occurs after upper abdominal and thoracic surgery. The presentation varies from an isolated fever to tachypnea, dyspnea, and tachycardia.

Evaluation includes chest radiography, pulse oximetry, and a CBC. Chest radiographs may show normal findings or exhibit platelike linear densities, triangular densities, or lobar consolidation. Mild hypoxemia from ventilation and perfusion mismatch is common, but hypercarbia is uncommon. Patients with mild atelectasis and no evidence of hypoxemia may be managed as outpatients with pain control and increased deep breathing. Admission is indicated for aggressive pulmonary toilet and supplemental oxygenation in debilitated patients, patients with underlying lung disease, patients with hypoxemia, or those in whom the diagnosis is in question.

PNEUMONIA

Pneumonia usually becomes evident between 24 and 96 hours postoperatively. Predisposing factors include prolonged ventilatory support and atelectasis. Presenting symptoms can include dyspnea, chest pain, productive cough, fever, and tachypnea. Postoperative pneumonia is likely to be polymicrobial. After specimens of sputum and blood are obtained for culture, parenteral antimicrobial therapy is given. There are many options for polymicrobial coverage. One option is levofloxacin, 750 milligrams IV once daily, *and* vancomycin, 1 gram IV twice daily. Admission to the hospital is generally indicated.

PNEUMOTHORAX

Pneumothorax can occur as a complication of thoracic wall surgery, breast biopsy, laparoscopic abdominal surgery, abdominal paracentesis, nasogastric and feeding tube insertion, thoracic surgery, central venous catheter insertion, endoscopic procedures, shoulder arthroscopy, and tracheostomy. For further discussion, see chapter 68, "Pneumothorax."

TABLE 87-2 Common Causes of Postoperative Fevers in General Surgical Patients

Cause of Fever	Presentation	Signs and Symptoms	Diagnostic Test	Treatment
Atelectasis	First 24 h	Isolated fever; may have tachypnea, dyspnea, and/or tachycardia	Chest radiography	Pulmonary toilet; admission if unsure or patient is ill appearing
Pneumonia	3–7 d	Dyspnea, chest pain, productive cough, fever, and/or tachypnea	Chest radiography	Admission and coverage with broad-spectrum antibiotics
Urinary tract infections	2–5 d	Often none; possibly dysuria	Urinalysis	Admission if patient is elderly or toxic
Skin and soft tissue infection	5–10 d	Increasing pain, erythema, swelling, drainage, and tenderness at incision site	Examination, aspiration and/or opening of wound	Drainage, packing, and outpatient antibiotic therapy
Thrombophlebitis (septic and sterile)	<3 d	Warm, tender, and swollen vein	None	If not septic, warm soaks If septic, surgical removal
Deep vein thrombosis	4–6 d	Extremity swelling and pain	US	Admission and anticoagulation
Intra-abdominal abscesses	4–21 d	Fever and elevated WBC count without specific focal abdominal findings	CT	Admission and antibiotic administration
Pseudomembranous colitis	Anytime	Diarrhea	Stool testing using immunoassay	Vancomycin administration
Peritonitis	4–21 d	Tachycardia and abdominal pain, peritoneal irritation	CT	Admission and antibiotic administration
Pulmonary embolism	Anytime	Shortness of breath, tachypnea, and/or hemodynamic instability	CT or ventilation–perfusion scanning	Admission and anticoagulation
Transfusion reaction	First 24 h	Fever, chills	Transfusion check for incompatibility	Admission depending on condition of patient

PULMONARY EMBOLUS

Pulmonary embolism may present any time during the postoperative period. For further discussion of signs, symptoms, and treatment, see chapter 56, "Venous Thromboembolism."

TABLE 87-3 Evaluation and Management of Postoperative Fever

History
- Presenting signs and symptoms
- Onset of symptoms, time since procedure
- Procedures performed and complications
- Medications
- History of blood transfusion

Physical examination
- Particular attention to
  - Operative sites and contiguous areas
  - Sites of catheters and invasive monitors
  - Signs of deep venous thrombosis and pulmonary embolism
  - Decubitus ulcers
  - Lungs

Ancillary studies
- CBC with differential
- Chest radiograph
- Gram stain and culture of wound exudate
- Urinalysis (urine culture if infected)
- Sputum Gram stain and culture
- Blood cultures
- CT to exclude intra-abdominal pathology
- If diarrhea present, consider immunoassay of specimen for *Clostridium difficile* toxin
- Further tests as indicated (e.g., CT, radionuclide studies, venography, arteriography)

Treatment
- If source identified, start antibiotics; admission based on condition of patient
- If no source identified, consider admission, change all catheters and culture catheter specimens, stop all medication that might cause fever

GU COMPLICATIONS

URINARY TRACT INFECTION

Urinary tract infections can occur after any surgical procedure, but the incidence increases in patients who have undergone instrumentation of the GU tract or bladder catheterization. The cause is direct contamination of the urinary bladder, most commonly with *Escherichia coli*. Other organisms isolated include *Staphylococcus aureus*, *Staphylococcus epidermidis*, *Proteus mirabilis*, *Klebsiella*, *Pseudomonas*, and enterococci. Oral antibiotics (ciprofloxacin, 500 milligrams PO twice daily, or levofloxacin, 750 milligrams PO once daily) are appropriate for most infections, and choice of antibiotic should be based on local susceptibility patterns. Elderly or debilitated patients and those with sepsis require admission for parenteral administration of antibiotics (usually levofloxacin, 750 milligrams IV once daily).

URINARY RETENTION

Postoperative acute urinary retention is a common problem for surgical patients.[2] Urinary retention occurs as the result of catecholamine stimulation of α-adrenergic receptors in the bladder neck and urethral smooth muscle. Increased incidence of urinary retention is likely to occur in elderly men, patients receiving excessive fluid administration during surgery, those undergoing anorectal surgery, patients undergoing longer procedures (>2 hours), and those for whom spinal or epidural anesthesia was used.[3,4]

Patients with urinary retention present with lower abdominal discomfort, urinary urgency, and inability to void. The diagnosis is confirmed by use of a bladder scanner or placement of a Foley catheter. The bladder can be safely drained quickly, and there appears to be no foundation for the fears of hematuria, postobstructive diuresis, and hypotension. For patients with normal renal function and no anatomic obstruction, continued catheter drainage is not necessary. For patients with retention after GU procedures, a urologist should be consulted. Antibiotics can be given if the GU tract has been instrumented, if retention is prolonged, or if the patient is at risk for infection (see "Urinary Tract Infection" section above).

ACUTE RENAL FAILURE

Acute renal failure is classified according to the primary cause: prerenal, intrinsic, or postrenal. Volume depletion is the most common prerenal cause. The patient should be examined for signs of hypovolemia and a urinary catheter placed. Indwelling urinary catheters should be irrigated or replaced. A fluid bolus should be given. Intrinsic causes include acute tubular necrosis and drug nephrotoxicity. Obstructive uropathy is a common cause of postrenal failure. In patients with urinary outlet obstruction, placement of a urinary catheter is diagnostic and therapeutic. Renal US is needed to identify hydronephrosis or hydroureter.

WOUND COMPLICATIONS

Inform the operative surgeon about all postoperative wound complications.

HEMATOMAS

Wound hematomas result from unrecognized inadequate hemostasis. Patients have pain, pressure, and swelling within the wound. Patients with wound hematomas may be febrile and have sanguineous or serous wound drainage. Differentiating between hematoma and wound infection can be difficult. A few sutures should be removed to allow the hematoma to drain, and culture of wound specimens should be performed. If there is no evidence of infection and hemostasis can be maintained, the patient can be discharged. In patients who have a hematoma of the neck or who have undergone vascular surgery, extreme caution and consultation are appropriate.

SEROMAS

A seroma, a collection of serous fluid, is usually the result of inadequate control of lymphatics during dissection but can occur under split-thickness skin grafts and in areas with large dead spaces (e.g., axilla, groin, neck, or pelvis). Patients have painless swelling below the wound or graft, and needle aspiration yields a serous fluid. Aspiration confirms the diagnosis and alleviates the problem, although aspiration may have to be repeated later.

INFECTION

Systemic factors (e.g., extremes of age, poor nutrition, or diabetes) contribute to wound infections. However, local factors (e.g., necrotic tissue, poor perfusion, foreign bodies, and hematomas) are of greatest significance. In nontraumatic, uninfected operative wounds in which the respiratory, alimentary, and GU tracts were not entered, infection rates are low. In such cases, the infecting organism is usually from the skin but can originate from remote infected sources (e.g., urinary tract infection). If there is a remote infected source, the organism is probably the same in both infections. Wounds associated with entering the respiratory, alimentary, or GU tract or wounds secondary to trauma have a higher risk of infection.

Presenting signs and symptoms of wound infections include increasing pain, erythema, swelling, drainage, and tenderness at the incision site. Wounds not involving the perineum and not associated with entry into the GI or biliary tract are most often infected with *S. aureus* or streptococci. Such wounds can be safely managed with drainage, culture of a wound sample, irrigation, loose packing with gauze, and outpatient administration of antibiotics. Wounds involving the perineum or associated with the GI or biliary tract are often infected with multiple organisms, including gram-negative bacteria and anaerobes. Parenteral broad-spectrum antibiotics are administered, and hospital admission is necessary.

NECROTIZING FASCIITIS

Necrotizing fasciitis is a feared complication. The usual cause is direct contamination of the wound with group A streptococci or *S. aureus*. However, mixed aerobic and anaerobic infections have been reported. Risk factors include diabetes mellitus, alcoholism, immunosuppression, and peripheral vascular disease, but necrotizing fasciitis also occurs in young, otherwise healthy individuals. Early clinical differentiation from cellulitis can be difficult. CT may show asymmetric fascial thickening, gas tracking along fascial planes, or focal fluid collections. MRI is sensitive but not totally specific for necrotizing fasciitis and can be a useful adjunct.[5,6] Hallmarks of fasciitis are the presence of marked systemic toxicity and pain out of proportion to local findings. In more advanced cases, there may be deep pain with patchy areas of surface hypesthesia, crepitation, or bullae. Treatment should include antibiotics and immediate surgical debridement. Antibiotic choice is controversial, but triple antibiotic therapy with penicillin or a cephalosporin, an aminoglycoside, and clindamycin probably should be used.[7] For further discussion, see chapter 152, "Soft Tissue Infections."

WOUND DEHISCENCE

Wound dehiscence can be superficial or can extend into the deeper fascial planes. Dehiscence is caused by inadequate closure or intrinsic host factors, such as malnutrition, glucocorticoid use, or diabetes. Serosanguineous fluid may leak from the wound. Dehiscence of abdominal incisions has the potential for evisceration. If evisceration is not present, conservative management using abdominal binders is appropriate. However, if there is any uncertainty about the extent of dehiscence, operative exploration is indicated.

VASCULAR COMPLICATIONS

SUPERFICIAL THROMBOPHLEBITIS

Superficial thrombophlebitis of the lower extremities is most frequently secondary to stasis in varicose veins. It is usually aseptic. There is redness and warmth of the affected vein. If there is no evidence of surrounding cellulitis or lymphangitis and no evidence of deep vein involvement on US, treatment is local heat, elevation, and nonsteroidal anti-inflammatory drugs. Suppurative superficial thrombophlebitis is characterized by erythema, palpable tender cord, lymphangitis, and pain. Suppurative thrombophlebitis requires excision of the affected vein.

DEEP VENOUS THROMBOSIS

When lower extremity superficial thrombophlebitis is seen in a postoperative patient, the possibility of concurrent deep venous thrombosis should be considered. Deep venous thrombosis is typically characterized by leg pain or swelling, or both. For suspected deep venous thrombosis, Doppler US is the preferred diagnostic test. Patients with normal color flow Doppler study results should be treated with elevation and bed rest. Repeat color flow Doppler US studies should be performed in 3 days if symptoms persist, but sooner if symptoms worsen. For further discussion, see chapter 56, "Venous Thromboembolism."

COMPLICATIONS OF DRUG THERAPY

Complications of drug therapy are numerous, but the most commonly encountered problem in the ED is an allergic reaction.[8] Another common problem is antibiotic-associated diarrhea. Many antibiotics can cause diarrhea, but the greatest concern in postoperative patients is pseudomembranous colitis. Pseudomembranous colitis is due to the toxin produced by the bacterium *Clostridium difficile*. Pseudomembranous colitis is related to antibiotic use, which destroys the normal enteric bacterial flora, allowing an overgrowth of *C. difficile*. Even short courses of antibiotics have been associated with pseudomembranous colitis. Patients have watery and sometimes bloody diarrhea, fever, and crampy abdominal pain. There are three common ways to diagnose *C. difficile*: nucleic acid amplification tests, glutamate dehydrogenase, and enzyme immunoassay. The current recommendation for symptomatic patients is to use a nucleic acid amplification test technology like polymerase chain reaction.[9] For patients with moderate disease, discontinue the offending antibiotic and prescribe metronidazole. For severe disease, discontinue the offending antibiotic and give vancomycin.[9] For further discussion, see chapters 71, "Acute Abdominal Pain" and 73, "Disorders Presenting Primarily with Diarrhea."

Many medicines can cause drug fever, but antibiotics are the drug class most commonly implicated. The mechanisms proposed are hypersensitivity reactions, pyogenic effect, and disturbed thermoregulation. In patients in whom no source for fever can be found, it is appropriate to consider stopping medications known to cause drug fever. Most often, the patient will require admission to rule out this diagnosis.

COMPLICATIONS OF BREAST SURGERY

Complications of breast surgery are infrequent, but patients can develop minor wound infections and hematomas. Rarely, pneumothorax has been reported. Wound hematomas frequently require operative control for proper evacuation and hemostasis.

Early complications seen with mastectomies include wound infection, necrosis of skin flaps, and the accumulation of seromas. The incidence of postmastectomy lymphedema ranges from a low of 5.5% to a high of 80%.

COMPLICATIONS OF GI SURGERY

In addition to the complications already reviewed, patients who have undergone any GI surgery may have intestinal obstruction, intra-abdominal abscess, pancreatitis, cholecystitis, fistulas, and tetanus. Certain procedures, such as anastomoses, bariatric surgery, placement of gastrostomy tubes, biliary tract surgery, other laparoscopic surgery, stoma creation, colonoscopy, and rectal surgery, are associated with specific complications.

INTESTINAL OBSTRUCTION

Ileus, a functional obstruction of the bowel, is postulated to be the result of stimulation of the splanchnic nerves, leading to neuronal inhibition of coordinated intrinsic bowel wall motor activity. It is expected after any operation in which the peritoneal cavity is violated. After GI surgery, small bowel tone usually returns to normal within 24 hours, and colonic function returns within 3 to 5 days. Ileus can also occur after non-GI procedures and is usually secondary to anesthetic agents; function returns to normal after 24 hours. Prolonged ileus can be caused by peritonitis, intra-abdominal abscess, hemoperitoneum, pneumonia, electrolyte imbalance, sepsis, and medications.

Presenting symptoms of ileus include nausea, vomiting, obstipation, constipation, abdominal distention, and abdominal pain. When these symptoms are present in the first few days after surgery, they are most often due to adynamic ileus. The symptoms of adynamic ileus are most often mild and respond to nasogastric suction, bowel rest, and IV hydration. However, in cases of prolonged ileus, look for an underlying cause. Evaluation includes abdominal radiography to identify air-fluid levels, chest radiography, CBC, measurement of electrolyte levels, and urinalysis to search for secondary causes of ileus.

Mechanical ileus of the bowel is most often secondary to adhesions. Symptoms are abdominal distention and pain. Abdominal radiographs demonstrate multiple air-fluid levels and a paucity of gas in the colon; however, with high obstruction, above the ligament of Treitz, there may be no air-fluid levels. In the ED, differentiating between functional ileus and mechanical bowel obstruction can be difficult. Both disorders result in different degrees of abdominal pain, distention, nausea, vomiting, and failure to pass flatus and/or feces. Abdominal CT scanning is helpful to exclude obstruction due to bowel strangulation.[10] Results may have an impact on the decision to manage the obstruction expectantly or not. Once the diagnosis of mechanical obstruction is suspected or confirmed, surgical consultation is indicated.

INTRA-ABDOMINAL ABSCESS

Intra-abdominal abscess is caused most frequently by preoperative contamination, spillage of bowel contents during surgery, contamination of a hematoma, or postoperative anastomotic leaks. Patients may have abdominal pain, nausea, vomiting, ileus, abdominal distention, fever, chills, anorexia, and abdominal tenderness. If the diagnosis is suspected, obtain CT or US of the abdomen. The patient should receive broad-spectrum antibiotics (see chapter 71, "Acute Abdominal Pain"). Treatment is percutaneous drainage or surgical exploration.

PANCREATITIS

Pancreatitis after abdominal surgery is secondary to direct manipulation or retraction of the pancreatic duct. Pancreatitis most commonly occurs after gastric resection, biliary tract surgery, and endoscopic retrograde cholangiopancreatography. Clinical presentation varies from mild nausea, vomiting, and abdominal discomfort to intractable vomiting, leukocytosis, and left-sided pleural effusion. Severe hemorrhage can cause lumbar pain accompanied by blue-gray discoloration of the skin in the flank area (Turner sign) or similar changes around the umbilicus (Cullen sign). Although the serum amylase level rises in acute pancreatitis, it is also elevated in patients with severe cholecystitis, renal insufficiency, intestinal obstruction, perforated ulcer, or ischemic bowel. A serum lipase measurement may help to identify those with true pancreatitis, although it may be elevated in a patient with a perforated viscus and other conditions. Abdominal radiographs may show localized ileus in the region of the pancreas (sentinel loop). US and CT are useful in defining pancreatic fluid collections or abscesses. In general, the treatment of postoperative pancreatitis is similar to the treatment of nonoperative pancreatitis (see chapter 79, "Pancreatitis and Cholecystitis").

CHOLECYSTITIS

Postoperative complications related to the gallbladder include biliary colic, acute calculous cholecystitis, or acute acalculous cholecystitis. The cause of these disorders in the postoperative period is not clear. US studies of the gallbladder and pancreas should be performed to aid in the diagnosis.

Acalculous cholecystitis is of particular concern in the postoperative period. The disorder seems to be more common in elderly men, but can occur in any sex and age group. Signs and symptoms are similar to those for calculous cholecystitis. Results of liver function studies and the neutrophil count may be normal. Important findings on US include gallbladder enlargement, wall thickening, and pericholecystic fluid collection, but no gallstones. Hepatobiliary scintigraphy may be helpful. Early diagnosis is critical, because early operative intervention can reduce morbidity and mortality.

FISTULAS

Enterocutaneous fistulas can occur almost anywhere in the GI tract and are usually the result of technical complications or direct bowel injury. High-output fistulas can result in electrolyte abnormalities and volume depletion. Fistulas involving the proximal GI tract are frequently high output and are of the greatest concern. Sepsis is the other major complication. Most patients require admission, although many fistulas ultimately close spontaneously.

TETANUS

Although most cases of tetanus in the United States occur after minor trauma, there have been numerous reports of tetanus after general surgical procedures.[11] *Clostridium tetani* is found in the GI tract of 1% of the population. During GI surgery, there is spillage of *C. tetani*. Proliferation of the organism is facilitated by the presence of devitalized tissue, blood clots, and surgical suture. Incubation can take from 0 to 73 days, at which time the toxin leads to clinical tetanus. The classic symptoms of tetanus, trismus, and opisthotonos may not be evident initially. Patients may present with nonspecific symptoms of abdominal discomfort, fever, and abdominal wall rigidity. Diagnosis is based on physical examination and a history of inadequate immunization.

ANASTOMOTIC LEAKS

Anastomotic leaks occur most frequently after esophageal and colonic surgeries and least frequently after gastric and small-intestinal anastomoses. The cause of anastomotic leakage is related mainly to surgical technique.

Intrathoracic esophageal anastomotic leaks usually manifest within 10 days of surgery. The presentation is dramatic, with fever, chest pain, tachypnea, tachycardia, and possibly shock. Chest radiograph may reveal a pneumothorax with pleural effusion. Disruption can be confirmed by contrast esophagography using a water-soluble contrast agent. Even with immediate reoperation, morbidity and mortality rates are high.

The signs and symptoms of gastric anastomotic leaks include abdominal pain, fever, leukocytosis, gastric outlet obstruction, hyperamylasemia, hyperbilirubinemia, peritonitis, and shock. Plain radiographs may reveal pneumoperitoneum or air-fluid levels. Provide volume resuscitation, parenteral broad-spectrum antibiotics, and nasogastric tube drainage. Immediate surgery is required.

Small-intestinal anastomoses infrequently leak because of the excellent blood supply and rapid healing of the area. However, if a leak occurs, the patient usually presents with local abscess formation or peritonitis. Treatment is immediate reoperation.

Colorectal anastomoses are prone to disruption because of the large number of pathogenic bacteria found, the propensity for colonic distention, and the presence of only a single thin layer of circular muscle to support sutures. The patients usually present 7 to 14 days postoperatively with fever and abdominal pain. CT confirms the diagnosis. Patients should receive broad-spectrum parenteral antibiotics, nasogastric tube drainage, and adequate fluid resuscitation in preparation for surgery.

BARIATRIC SURGERY COMPLICATIONS

Four main bariatric procedures are currently being performed for morbid obesity: laparoscopic adjustable gastric banding using the LAP-BAND® device (Allergan, Inc., Irvine, CA), sleeve gastrectomy, Roux-en-Y gastric bypass, and biliopancreatic diversion with duodenal switch (see Figure 298-1 in chapter "The Patient With Morbid Obesity"). Overall operative mortality is <2%, but postoperative complications are common and are likely related to the technical skill of the surgeon.[12] Common complications are listed in **Table 87-4**.[13,14]

Nausea, vomiting, and abdominal pain are common symptoms in ED patients with a history of bariatric surgery. In the first few postoperative weeks, consider life-threatening problems like anastomotic leak and intra-abdominal bleeding. In patients with abdominal pain, tachycardia, or abdominal tenderness in the early postoperative period, a CT scan is often required to rule out these diagnoses.

A common complication of the Roux-en-Y gastric bypass is dumping syndrome, which can occur either right after the meal (early) or 2 to 4 hours later (late). Dumping symptoms occur when the pylorus is bypassed or removed. The hyperosmolar chyme contents of the stomach are dumped into the jejunum, causing rapid influx of extracellular fluid and an autonomic response. Patients experience nausea, epigastric discomfort, palpitations, colicky abdominal pain, diaphoresis, and, in some cases, dizziness and syncope. Patients with early dumping symptoms experience diarrhea, whereas those with late dumping symptoms, 2 to 4 hours postprandially, usually do not. The late dumping syndrome is believed to be due to a reactive hypoglycemia. The mainstay of treatment is dietary modification; consumption of small, dry meals; and separation of solids from liquids. In refractory cases, pyloroplasty can be tried. Most patients with dumping syndrome do not require hospital admission.

Patients with gastroesophageal reflux disease present with burning epigastric pain that is aggravated by meals and unrelieved by vomiting. The syndrome is caused by reflux of bile into the stomach. Diagnosis is made clinically, but other potential diagnoses are often ruled out with endoscopic examination.

Wernicke's encephalopathy is a rare, but serious, complication that must be considered in a patient with a history of bariatric surgery who presents with any cerebellar signs, ophthalmoplegia, weakness, and/or memory disturbances. Although vitamin deficiencies are common with both Roux-en-Y gastric bypass and biliopancreatic diversion, vitamin B_{12} deficiency is the only one that requires emergent intervention.

NONBARIATRIC GASTRIC SURGERY

Patients who have undergone partial or complete gastrectomy for nonbariatric reasons can present with a few distinct syndromes: dumping syndrome, alkaline reflux gastritis, afferent loop syndrome, and postvagotomy diarrhea. Although these complications are rare, the symptoms can be disabling. Dumping syndrome as a result of nonbariatric gastric surgery is treated in the same way as dumping syndrome after bariatric procedures.

Patients with afferent loop syndrome also develop severe epigastric pain 1 to 2 hours after eating, which is relieved by vomiting. The vomitus is bilious, without food. The syndrome occurs in patients who have undergone gastroenterostomy (Billroth II) reconstruction after partial gastrectomy. Diagnosis is made by contrast radiography or endoscopy. Operative reconstruction is required.

Truncal vagotomy usually results in increased bowel movements, but occasionally results in diarrhea. Diarrhea is variable in occurrence and not associated with food intake. It is often unpredictable and explosive, which can lead to weight loss, malnutrition, and severe social complications. The incidence of the diarrhea decreases with time, and treatment is mostly symptomatic.

Gastrostomy Tubes Most gastrostomy tubes are now placed by an endoscopist by percutaneous endoscopy or by a radiologist by percutaneous fluoroscopy. If the patient has undergone a laparotomy, the general surgeon may place a gastrostomy tube at the time of surgery.

TABLE 87-4 Complications of Gastric Bypass Procedures

Complication	Presentation	Signs and Symptoms	Diagnostic Test
Anastomotic leak	0–28 d	Tachycardia, fever, abdominal pain, nausea, vomiting, hypotension	Clinical suspicion. CT scan or upper GI study are useful, but may be negative
Intra-abdominal bleeding	0–28 d	Tachycardia, abdominal pain, hypotension	CT scan or upper GI study
Intraluminal GI bleeding	Hours to months	Melena, hematemesis, hypotension, altered mental status	Emergent endoscopy
Ventral hernia	Anytime	Pain at incision site or palpable hernia	Clinical diagnosis
Bowel obstruction	1 week to 8 months	Nausea, vomiting, abdominal pain	Plain radiography or CT looking for air-fluid levels
Stomal stenosis	2 months to 1 year	Postprandial abdominal pain, nausea, vomiting	Endoscopy or upper GI study
Stomal ulcer	Months to years	Abdominal pain, upper GI bleed	Endoscopy
Stomal obstruction	Months to years	Nausea and vomiting with solids and liquids	Endoscopy
Cholelithiasis/cholecystitis	Months to years	Abdominal pain with fatty foods, fever, tachycardia	US
Dumping syndrome	Anytime	Diarrhea, abdominal cramps, nausea, vomiting, tachycardia, palpitations, flushing, dizziness, syncope	Clinical diagnosis or endoscopy
Vitamin deficiencies	Months to years	Weakness, bone loss, anemia, fractures, neuropathy, hypercalcemia	CBC, iron studies, parathyroid hormone studies, vitamin levels
Gastric slippage	Days to years	Abdominal pain, dysphagia, food intolerance, reflux	Upper GI study
Esophageal, gastric pouch dilation	After band adjustment	Epigastric abdominal pain, dysphagia, reflux	Upper GI study
Gastric necrosis	Anytime	Abdominal pain	Upper GI study

TABLE 87-5 Complications of Cholecystectomy
Bile leak
Bile duct stricture
Bleeding
Bowel injury
Intra-abdominal abscess
Acute myocardial infarction
Pancreatitis
Peritonitis
Pulmonary complications
Retained common duct stones or stones spilled into peritoneum
Splenic injury
Umbilical hernia
Wound infection

If the tube was placed by the surgeon and has not been replaced, it will have a bumper holding the tube in place. The tube has to be cut and the bumper allowed to pass, or the bumper has to be removed by endoscopic technique. For further discussion, see chapter 86, "Gastrointestinal Procedures and Devices."

LAPAROSCOPIC SURGERY

BILIARY TRACT SURGERY

More than 90% of all cholecystectomies are now performed laparoscopically. Complications can occur after open and laparoscopic cholecystectomies (**Table 87-5**); complications can also be related to the laparoscopic technique (**Table 87-6**).[15]

The evaluation of abdominal pain after cholecystectomy depends on the clinical condition of the patient. If there are signs of peritoneal irritation or fever, an injury to the biliary system is likely. Obtain an abdominal CT in addition to a CBC, electrolyte measurements, liver function tests, and serum lipase level. A collection of bile can be seen on CT, but endoscopic retrograde cholangiopancreatography is required to identify the specific site of the injury. Depending on the endoscopic retrograde cholangiopancreatography results, reoperation may be necessary. Small collections of bile may require only observation or percutaneous drainage.

Patients presenting soon after cholecystectomy with pain, pancreatitis, and/or jaundice may have retained common duct stones. If US does not demonstrate a dilated common bile duct, or if CT does not reveal an intra-abdominal collection of fluid, an endoscopic retrograde cholangiopancreatography should be performed. Endoscopic sphincterotomy is usually an effective means of dealing with retained stones. Patients presenting late after cholecystectomy with fever, pain, and jaundice may have bile duct stricture. Diagnosis requires endoscopic retrograde cholangiopancreatography. Insertion of stents is usually tried first, but surgical repair may be necessary. A more recent concern has been the spillage of gallstones into the peritoneal cavity at the time of surgery. Initially, such stones were thought to be innocuous. However, they have been linked to abdominal pain, pelvic pain, dysmenorrhea, intra-abdominal abscess, colocutaneous fistula, and implantation into the ovary with subsequent infertility.

TABLE 87-6 Complications of Laparoscopy
Related to pneumoperitoneum
Cardiac arrhythmias during the procedure
Subcutaneous emphysema
Pneumothorax
Pneumomediastinum
Carbon dioxide embolization
Related to insertion of needle and trocar
Bleeding from trocar site
GI tract injuries
Laceration
Intestinal burns
GU tract injuries
Major vessel injuries
Hernia from trocar site
Wound infection
Miscellaneous
Retained intra-abdominal gallstones
Biliary cutaneous fistula
Chronic pain
Infertility
Cholelithiasis
Metastases to the trocar site

OTHER LAPAROSCOPIC SURGERIES

Laparoscopic techniques are used for cholecystectomy, appendectomy, colon resection, antireflux surgery, herniorrhaphy, fundoplication, and most gynecologic and urologic surgical procedures. As with any laparoscopic procedure, there are risks related to the pneumoperitoneum and insertion of the trocar (Table 87-6). In addition to the potential for bowel injury, major vessel injury, and splenic injury, gynecologic and urologic procedures carry a risk of injury to the urinary bladder and ureters.

STOMAS

The two most commonly placed stomas are the ileostomy and the colostomy. Problems with stomas can be quite debilitating. Most acute complications are related to technical errors of stoma placement. Other complications include the development of Crohn's disease or carcinoma at the stomal site, stomal ischemia and necrosis, peristomal skin irritation, peristomal hernia, and stomal prolapse.

Ischemia and stomal necrosis are manifested very early in the postoperative course. The cause is inadequate blood supply to the stoma. Normally, the stoma is pink, without evidence of cyanosis. Any evidence of compromised blood flow requires surgical evaluation.

Peristomal maceration and skin destruction are most likely secondary to a poor seal of the stomal appliance. Consult an enterostomal therapist for a properly fitting appliance.

Stomal prolapse can occur with ileostomies and colostomies. The cause is usually inadequate fixation of the intra-abdominal portion or too large an abdominal wall opening. Patients present with stoma protrusion, with or without pain. Examine the stoma for viability. It should be pink and painless. If the tissue is viable, attempt reduction and follow with surgical consultation. Definitive therapy requires surgical revision.

Parastomal hernias can develop if the abdominal wall opening is too large. Determine if the hernia is incarcerated, attempt reduction, and consult a surgeon. Definitive therapy requires local reconstruction of the orifice.

COLONOSCOPY

Potential complications of colonoscopy include hemorrhage, perforation, retroperitoneal abscess, pneumoscrotum, pneumothorax, volvulus, postcolonoscopy distention, splenic rupture, appendicitis, bacteremia, and infection.[16] Hemorrhage is the most common complication and can be secondary to polypectomy procedures, biopsies, laceration of the mucosa by the instrument, or tearing of the mesentery or spleen. If the bleeding is intraluminal, the patient will develop rectal bleeding. Patients with mesenteric or splenic injury have signs of intra-abdominal bleeding. Treatment of intraluminal bleeding depends on the magnitude of hemorrhage. Intra-abdominal bleeding requires emergency laparotomy. Colon perforation with pneumoperitoneum usually is evident immediately but can take several hours to manifest.[17] Perforation is usually secondary to intrinsic disease of the colon (e.g., diverticulitis) or to vigorous manipulation during the procedure. Most patients require immediate laparotomy, but in some patients presenting late (1 to 2 days later) without signs of peritonitis, hospital observation may be appropriate.

RECTAL SURGERY

Patients who have undergone hemorrhoidectomy frequently have problems with postoperative urinary retention, the management of which has been discussed previously in the section "Urinary Retention." Three other problems that can occur are constipation, rectal hemorrhage, and rectal prolapse.

The management of constipation in a patient who has undergone rectal surgery is no different from management in any other patient. Perform gentle rectal examination to identify fecal impaction, and if present, remove the impaction. Otherwise, enemas can be used. Posthemorrhoidectomy rectal hemorrhage can occur immediately postoperatively but may be delayed up to weeks after the surgery. Causes of delayed bleeding include sepsis of the pedicle, disruption of a clot, and sloughing of tissue. Bleeding can be scant or massive. Temporary balloon tamponade using a Foley catheter may temporize until surgical ligation of the involved vessel is performed.

Mucosal prolapse occurs when the surgeon has not removed all redundant mucosa during hemorrhoidectomy and is much more common than rectal prolapse. Local treatment by a surgeon is usually corrective. *Rectal prolapse* can occur after any anorectal surgical procedure and likely is related to injury of the puborectalis muscle. The diagnosis is obvious on examination. The treatment is reduction (see chapter 85, "Anorectal Disorders") and surgical consultation.

Infection after anorectal surgery is surprisingly uncommon. The patient usually complains of increasing pain and fever. Examination of the area is necessary to detect an abscess or cellulitis. Fournier's gangrene may follow anorectal surgery. If this is suspected, give broad-spectrum parenteral antibiotics immediately. The patient must undergo immediate surgical debridement.

REFERENCES

The complete reference list is available online at www.TintinalliEM.com.

SECTION 10

Renal and Genitourinary Disorders

CHAPTER 88

Acute Kidney Injury

Richard Sinert
Peter R. Peacock, Jr.

INTRODUCTION AND EPIDEMIOLOGY

Acute kidney injury is the deterioration of renal function over hours or days resulting in the accumulation of toxic wastes and the loss of internal homeostasis. Definitions based on renal function are listed in **Table 88-1**.[1]

Community- and hospital-acquired kidney injuries differ by cause, treatment, and outcome (**Table 88-2**). **Community-acquired renal failure** is diagnosed in only 1% of hospital admissions at the time of presentation[2,3] and is usually secondary to volume depletion; thus, the vast majority of cases presenting to the ED have a reversible cause.[3] Mortality among patients presenting to the ED with prerenal acute renal failure may be as low as 7%.[4]

Hospital-acquired renal failure is only apparent after admission.[5] Hospital factors include advanced patient age, potential nephrotoxic exposures in a hospital setting, sepsis,[6] and multiorgan system illness in hospitalized patients. There is an almost linear relationship between increasing severity of renal injury and mortality rate: no renal injury, 4.4%; *risk* category/stage 1, 15.1%; *injury* category/stage 2, 29.2%; and *failure* category/stage 3, 41.1%.[6]

TABLE 88-1 AKIN and RIFLE Criteria for Acute Kidney Injury

AKIN Stage	RIFLE Category	GFR Criteria	Urine Output Criteria
Stage 1	Risk	Serum Cr increased 1.5 times* *or* (AKIN only) Cr increase >0.3 milligrams/dL over <48 h* *or* GFR decrease 25%–50%*	0.5 mL/kg/h for 6 h
Stage 2	Injury	Serum Cr increased 2.0–3.0 times* *or* GFR decrease 50%–75%*	0.5 mL/kg/h for 12 h
Stage 3	Failure	Serum Cr increased >3.0 times* *or* Cr >4 milligrams/dL and acute increase >0.5 milligrams/dL* *or* GFR decrease >75%*	0.3 mL/kg/h for 24 h *or* Anuria for 12 h
N/A	Loss	Complete loss of kidney function for >4 wk	
	End-stage renal disease	Need for renal replacement therapy for >3 months	

Abbreviations: AKIN = Acute Kidney Injury Network; Cr = creatinine; GFR = glomerular filtration rate; N/A = not applicable; RIFLE = Risk, Injury, Failure, Loss, End Stage.
*All changes are relative to the patient's premorbid baseline.

PATHOPHYSIOLOGY

Renal insult is classified as **prerenal** (decreased perfusion of a normal kidney), **intrinsic** (pathologic change within the kidney itself), or **postobstructive** (obstruction to urine outflow).

The functions of the kidneys are glomerular filtration, tubular reabsorption, and secretion. Normal glomerular filtration rate (GFR) in early adulthood is approximately 120 mL/min/1.73 m^2 and typically decreases by 8 mL/min/1.73 m^2 every decade thereafter. The driving force for glomerular filtration is glomerular capillary pressure, which depends on renal blood flow and autoregulation. For most causes of acute renal failure, global or regional decrease in renal blood flow is the final common pathway. Recovery from acute renal failure first depends on restoration of renal blood flow.

In **prerenal failure**, tubular and glomerular functions are still maintained. Restoration of circulating blood volume is usually sufficient to restore function. **Postobstructive renal failure** initially results in an increase in tubular pressure, which decreases the driving force for filtration. This pressure gradient soon equalizes, and the maintenance of depressed GFR depends on vasoconstrictors. Rapid relief of urinary obstruction in **postrenal failure** results in a prompt decrease of vasoconstriction.

Intrinsic renal failure occurs with diseases of the glomerulus, small vessels, interstitium, or tubule and is associated with the release of renal vasoconstrictors. The most common cause of intrinsic renal failure is **ischemic injury or ischemic tubular necrosis** (also historically called **acute tubular necrosis**), when renal perfusion is decreased so much that the kidney parenchyma is affected.

During the period of depressed renal blood flow, the kidneys are especially vulnerable to further insults. Exposure at this time to known nephrotoxins such as radiocontrast agents and aminoglycosides causes iatrogenic acute renal failure. **Figure 88-1** illustrates the cellular and subcellular events leading to ischemic tubular necrosis.

In **intrinsic renal failure,** clearance of tubular toxins and initiation of therapy for glomerular diseases decrease vasoconstriction and help restore renal blood flow. Once the cause of injury is resolved, the remaining functional nephrons increase filtration and eventually hypertrophy. Depending on the size of the remnant nephron pool, GFR will proportionately recover. If the number of remaining nephrons is below some critical number, continued hyperfiltration results in progressive glomerular sclerosis, eventually leading to nephron loss. A vicious cycle then ensues until complete renal failure occurs. This sequence explains the commonly observed scenario in which progressive renal failure occurs after initial recovery from acute renal failure.

CLINICAL FEATURES

HISTORY AND COMORBIDITIES

Renal failure itself has few symptoms until severe uremia develops. Nausea, vomiting, drowsiness, fatigue, confusion, and coma are findings in uremia. Patients are more likely to present with symptoms related to the

TABLE 88-2 Causes of Community-Acquired and Hospital-Acquired Acute Renal Failure

Community Acquired		Hospital Acquired	
Prerenal	70%	Prerenal	20%
Intrinsic	20%	Acute tubular necrosis	70%
Postrenal	10%	Postrenal	10%

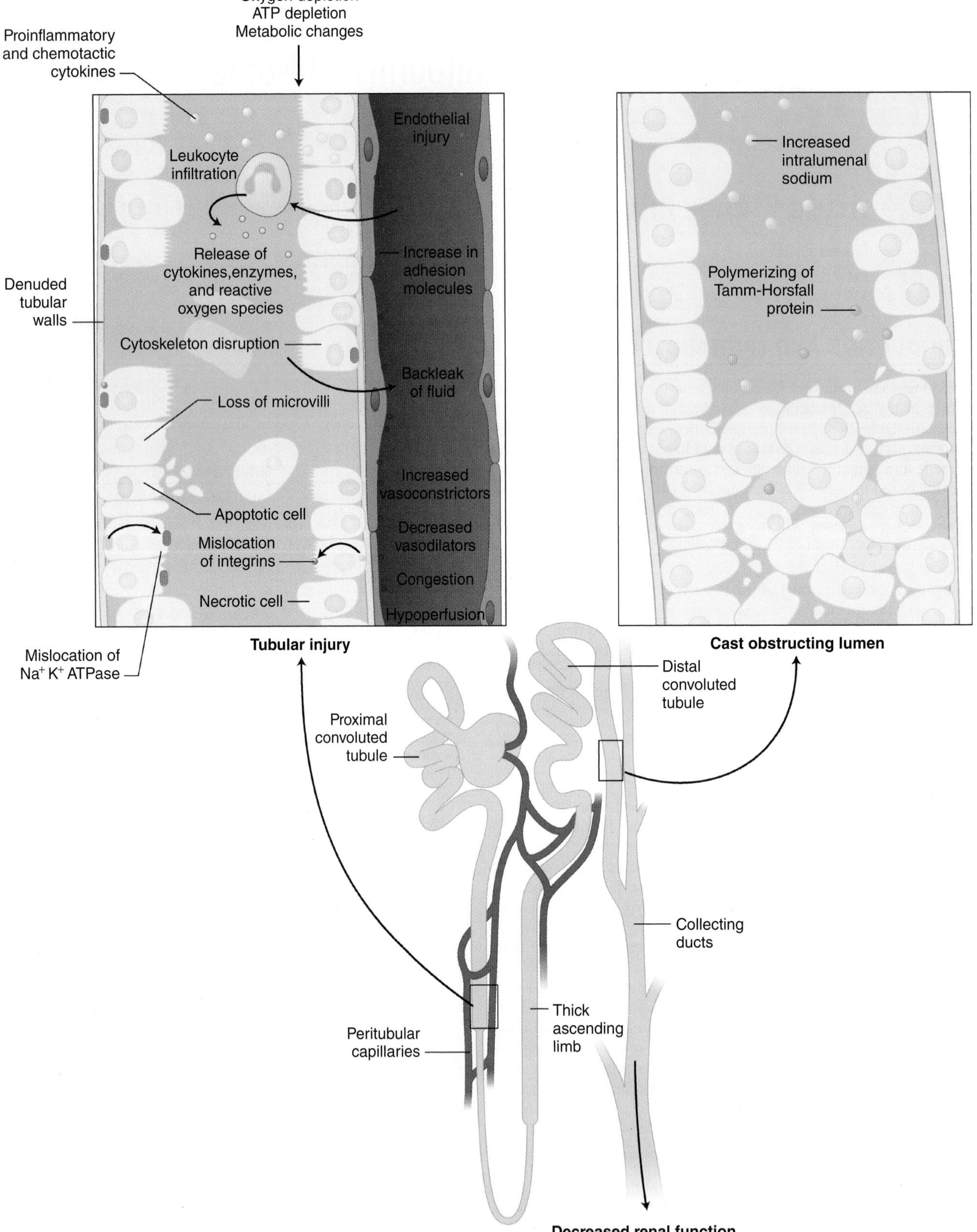

FIGURE 88-1. Ischemic tubular necrosis. Tubular injury is a direct consequence of vasoconstriction, inflammation, endothelial changes, disruption of cell-cell andcell-matrix connections, and apoptotic changes.

TABLE 88-3 Risk Factors for Renal Disease

Risk Factor	Comments
Medications	
COX-1 and COX-2 inhibitors	
ACE inhibitors	
Failure to dose medications for renal insufficiency	Antibiotics, metformin, proton pump inhibitors
Statins	Myopathy, rhabdomyolysis
Antiretroviral therapy	
Angiotensin receptor blockers	
Gabapentin, pregabalin, vigabatrin	>90% renal excretion
Levetiracetam	66% renal excretion
Topiramate	Low risk of renal tubular acidosis and nephrolithiasis
Eslicarbazepine	
Immunosuppressives	Tacrolimus, cyclosporine
Drugs of abuse	
Cocaine, ethanol, ethylene glycol	
Contrast agents	
Iodinated contrast media	
Gadolinium	Nephrogenic systemic fibrosis
Systemic disease	
Gout	
Coronary artery disease	
Hypertension	
Sepsis	
Hepatic disease	
Vascular disease	
Diabetes	
Outflow obstruction: prostatic/urethral disease	
Advanced age	
Heart failure	
Dehydration	
Multiple myeloma/hypercalcemia	
Vasculitis/autoimmune disease	
Systemic embolism: atrial fibrillation, endocarditis	
Malignancy	Drug effects; renal parenchymal invasion; bladder obstruction; light-chain proteins
Eclampsia and pre-eclampsia	
Kidney transplantation	Rejection, infection

Abbreviations: ACE = angiotensin-converting enzyme; COX = cyclooxygenase.

underlying cause of renal failure (**Table 88-3**), which should prompt assessment of renal function.[7]

Patients with **prerenal acute renal failure** commonly develop thirst, orthostatic light-headedness, and decreased urine output. Excessive vomiting, diarrhea, urination, hemorrhage, fever, or sweating can reduce circulating volume enough to precipitate acute renal failure. Causes of endothelial leak and third spacing, such as sepsis, pancreatitis, burns, and hepatic failure, can also result in prerenal failure, although these settings may also be associated with renal parenchymal injury. Progression of heart failure from any cause or overdiuresis of the patient with compensated congestive heart failure can result in renal failure. Decreased fluid intake from physical or cognitive disability can result in hypovolemia.

Intrinsic renal diseases can often be anticipated because of symptoms of the precipitating cause. Anticipate **ischemic acute kidney injury** after cardiac arrest, in severe sepsis, or with other causes of systemic hypotension. Renal failure from **crystal-induced nephropathy, nephrolithiasis, and papillary necrosis** can present as flank pain and hematuria. Suspect pigment-induced renal failure in **rhabdomyolysis**[8] (see chapter 89, "Rhabdomyolysis") or with hemolysis after recent blood transfusion. Darkening urine and edema with or without constitutional symptoms such as fever, malaise, and rash suggest **acute glomerulonephritis**, which may have been preceded by pharyngitis or cutaneous infection. Fever, arthralgia, and rash are common with **acute interstitial nephritis**. **Acute renal arterial occlusion** is usually marked by severe flank pain. Cough, dyspnea, and hemoptysis raise the possibility of **Goodpasture's syndrome** or **Wegener's granulomatosis**.

Suspect **postrenal failure** in men with prostatic disease or advanced age and patients with indwelling bladder catheters. Anuria strongly suggests obstruction, although vascular obstruction and fulminant renal disease are also possible. Alternating oliguria and polyuria is virtually pathognomonic of obstruction.

PHYSICAL EXAMINATION

Assess and correct volume status. Evaluate mucous membranes, jugular vein distention, lung auscultation, peripheral edema, and tissue turgor to identify dehydration. Base deficit, lactate level, central venous pressure and oxygen saturation, and US (see Imaging) can be reliable indicators of hypovolemia. Carefully assess for rashes, evidence of vasculitis, jaundice, abdominal or pelvic masses, or a distended palpable urinary bladder. On cardiac exam, check for atrial fibrillation, abdominal aortic aneurysm, and signs of heart failure, and assess extremity pulses.

DIAGNOSIS

In the ED, the goals are to identify patients at risk for acute kidney injury who aren't obviously ill and for those with diagnosed kidney injury to correct metabolic effects, decrease ongoing renal injury, and prevent iatrogenic injury. **Determine if kidney injury is prerenal, postrenal, or intrinsic.**

Obtain CBC, electrolyte levels including magnesium and phosphorus, and hepatic function tests and blood cultures if clinically appropriate. Obtain urinalysis, urine osmolality, and urine culture.

ECG is often the fastest screening test for **hyperkalemia**, but sensitivity for a level over 6.5 mmol/L ranges from 14% to 60%.[9,10] Although ECGs were read as "abnormal" in 83% of patients in one study, peaked T waves were only seen in 34%, which led to delayed therapy for most patients for whom peaked T waves were not evident[11] (see chapter 17, "Fluids and Electrolytes"). Chest radiography helps evaluate for increased volume, effusions, and pneumonia, all of which can result from or precipitate renal failure.

Obtain bedside US to assess urinary bladder volume. A large postvoid bladder residual volume (>125 mL) suggests bladder outlet obstruction for which you would place a urethral catheter. See chapter 92, "Acute Urinary Retention" for further discussion. Anuria is 100 mL urine per day and can be present with prerenal, postrenal, or intrinsic kidney disease. Alternating oliguria and polyuria is virtually pathognomonic of obstruction.

LABORATORY EVALUATION

Creatinine and Glomerular Filtration Rate Creatinine (Cr) is the mainstay for measuring renal function; it is a breakdown product of the skeletal muscle protein creatine, and its level is thus linked to muscle mass. **In patients with no renal function (GFR = 0), serum Cr level increases 1 to 3 milligrams/dL a day.** Lesser increases in Cr indicate residual renal function, whereas faster increases suggest rhabdomyolysis. Elevation of serum Cr may take 48 hours to accumulate after onset of decreased function, and a patient with a very low baseline Cr level can lose more than half of the functioning nephrons before serum Cr elevates to an abnormal level.

Cr clearance is used to estimate GFR, and although it is not perfect, it is a useful measure in the ED. Patients with lower muscle mass (e.g., older patients and women) have lower actual GFRs for any given Cr level. Glomerulonephritis increases tubular secretion of Cr, but trimethoprim, cimetidine, and salicylates decrease tubular secretion of Cr, thus altering the Cr level independently of the GFR.

GFR calculations are provided online, for hand-held devices, and in electronic medical record systems, and there are several formulas for GFR calculation. **Normal kidney function is a GFR >90 mL/min/1.73 m^2**, where 1.73 m^2 is used as the average body surface area. Stages of kidney disease are characterized by GFR: stage 1, GFR 90 mL/min/1.73 m^2; stage 2, GFR 60 to 89 mL/min/1.73 m^2; stage 3, GFR 30 to 59 mL/min/1.73 m^2; stage 4, GFR 15 to 29 mL/min/1.73 m^2; and stage 5, GFR <15 mL/min/1.73 m^2 (dialysis or transplant needed).

BUN:Cr Ratio The ratio of BUN to Cr can suggest hypovolemia because of differences in the way each is handled in the nephron. Both substances are passively filtered at the glomerulus, but whereas Cr remains within the tubule, the renal tubule is highly permeable to urea, which is passively reabsorbed with sodium. Therefore, in the setting of avid sodium retention, urea clearance is as low as 30% of GFR, whereas in the setting of adequate volume and sodium, urea clearance can increase to 70% to 100% of GFR. **Thus, if the patient has normal concentrating ability, in the setting of prerenal failure, the serum ratio of BUN to Cr is typically >10.** BUN level is depressed in patients with malnutrition and hepatic synthetic dysfunction and **can be increased in the setting of protein loading, GI hemorrhage, or trauma**. Although an elevated ratio of BUN to Cr had been assumed to suggest more reversible prerenal physiology, recent evidence has called that into question.[12]

Fractional Excretion of Sodium The fractional excretion of sodium ($Fe_{Na} = U_{Na}/P_{Na} \div U_{Cr}/P_{Cr}$, where U = urine and P = plasma) is another indicator that is commonly used to identify hypovolemia, but it has important limitations. For example, in the setting of intrinsic renal failure in which tubular concentrating capacity is retained, as in the case of glomerulonephritis, the fractional excretion of sodium may be depressed if there is concomitant volume depletion. With tubular injury such as ischemic acute tubular necrosis, the loss of concentrating ability results in a dilute urine, with a fractional excretion of sodium >1%, even if the patient is volume depleted (**Table 88-4**).

TABLE 88-4 Laboratory Findings in Conditions That Cause Acute Renal Failure

Category	Dipstick Test	Sediment Analysis	Urine Osmolality (mOsm/kg)	Fractional Excretion of Sodium (%)
Prerenal	Trace to no proteinuria, SG >1.015	A few hyaline casts possible	>500	<1
Renal				
Ischemia	Mild to moderate proteinuria	Pigmented granular casts, renal tubular epithelial cells	<350	>1
Nephrotoxins	Mild to moderate proteinuria	Pigmented granular casts	<350	>1
Acute interstitial nephritis	Mild to moderate proteinuria; hemoglobin, leukocytes	White cells, eosinophils, casts, red cells	<350	>1
Acute glomerulonephritis	Moderate to severe proteinuria; hemoglobin	Red cells and red cell casts; red cells can be dysmorphic	>500	Depends on volume status
Postrenal	Trace to no proteinuria; hemoglobin and leukocytes possible	Crystals, red cells, and white cells possible	<350	>1

Abbreviation: SG = specific gravity.

Urinalysis Microscopic examination of urine is useful in establishing the differential diagnosis. In acute glomerulonephritis, red blood cells enter the filtrate at the glomerulus and, on microscopic urinalysis, appear as casts and dysmorphic cells due to the increased tonicity of the renal medulla. In acute tubular necrosis, the tubular epithelium breaks down and allows protein to leak into the filtrate, and tubular epithelial cells may be seen in the sediment.

Hyaline casts are common in prerenal failure and can be a normal finding, but pigmented granular casts are common with ischemic or toxic tubular injury. Brown granular casts are common in hemoglobinuria or myoglobinuria. **The finding of hemoglobin on urine dipstick analysis with no red cells on microscopy suggests myoglobinuria.** Some crystals may be present in a normal urinalysis. Crystals are best seen with polarized light microscopy. Red cell casts and proteinuria suggest glomerulonephritis or an underlying autoimmune disease.

Imaging Renal US is the test of choice for urologic imaging in the setting of acute kidney injury. It has approximately 90% sensitivity and specificity for detecting hydronephrosis due to mechanical obstruction. **Figure 88-2** contrasts normal kidney US findings with US findings indicating hydronephrosis. If renal US detects hydronephrosis, a secondary imaging study to define the location of obstruction may be required.

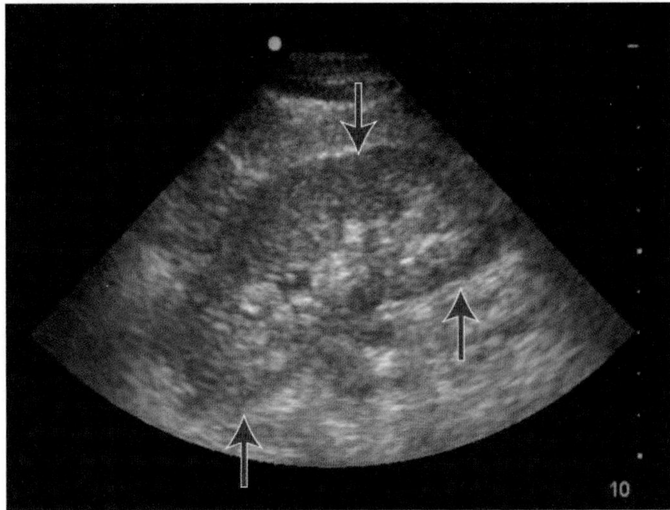

A

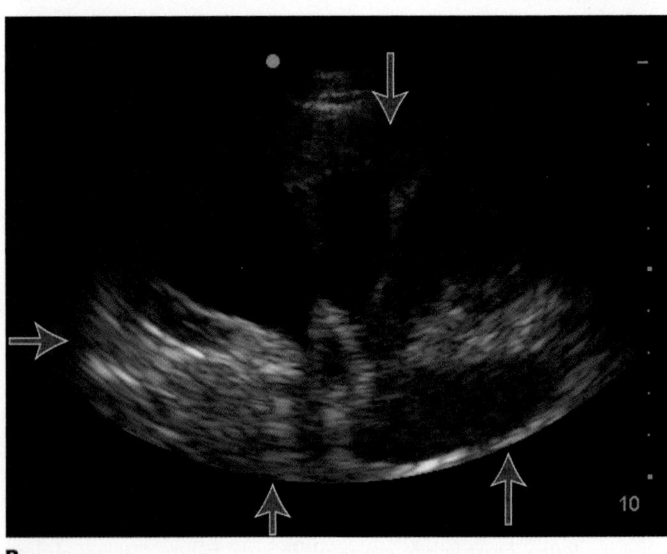

B

FIGURE 88-2. US of normal kidney and kidney showing hydronephrosis. A. Normal kidney, capsule margin at *arrows*. B. Hydronephrosis as would be expected in obstructive uropathy; the dilated kidney fills the majority of the screen, capsule at *arrows*. [Image used with permission of Michael B. Stone, MD, RDMS.]

Bipolar renal length is easy to assess by US, and **kidney dimension of <9 cm suggests chronic renal failure**. Renal parenchyma should be isoechoic or hypoechoic compared with that of the liver and spleen. Hyperechogenicity indicates diffuse parenchymal disease. Color flow Doppler US allows assessment of renal perfusion and can allow diagnosis of large-vessel causes of renal failure. Resistive index is the ratio of the difference between systolic and diastolic flow to systolic flow $[(V_{max} - V_{min})/V_{max}]$ as measured by color flow Doppler. In the vasoconstrictive phase of ischemic renal failure, in which there may be no diastolic flow, the ratio may be as high as 1.0. The normal ratio is <0.7.

In *intermittent or partial obstruction*, hydronephrosis may *not* be present, and it may even be *absent* in *complete obstruction* in the setting of retroperitoneal fibrosis. Furthermore, functional dilatation can occur in the setting of chronic reflux.

Noncontrast CT has sensitivity for hydronephrosis that is equivalent to that of US and has the added advantage of demonstrating the site and often the cause of obstruction. If functional obstruction is a consideration in the presence of a dilated GU tract, radionuclide scans and magnetic resonance urographs before and after administration of diuretics can be obtained.

TREATMENT

In the critically ill patient, resuscitation is the first priority, and multiple diagnostic and therapeutic processes advance simultaneously. Treat hypovolemia, and identify and treat sepsis, myocardial ischemia, and occult GI or retroperitoneal hemorrhage. Correct intravascular volume deficits with crystalloid. Crystalloid infusion is often sufficient to treat or improve many forms of acute renal failure, but accurate determination of volume status is essential to prevent volume overload, and often requires invasive hemodynamic monitoring, particularly in the setting of cardiac dysfunction. Bedside US can give some guidance for fluid resuscitation.[13] Inspiratory collapsibility of the intrahepatic segment of the inferior vena cava is one noninvasive measure of volume status and fluid responsiveness[14] (**Figure 88-3**).

Remember that most community-acquired acute kidney injury encountered in the ED is prerenal (see Table 88-2).

Make sure that renal dose adjustments are made for medication orders and prescriptions and that renal function is assessed before ordering radiographic contrast studies. In general, for IV contrast studies in patients with GFR of 30 to 59 mL/min/1.73 m², weigh benefits of the study against the risk of renal function decline. For patients with GFR <30 mL/min/1.73 m², avoid IV contrast studies if possible. Emergency contrast studies for major trauma, aortic dissection, or ST-segment elevation myocardial infarction are examples in which benefits typically outweigh risk. Make sure to avoid gadolinium for GFR <30 mL/min/1.73 m².

PRERENAL FAILURE

The causes of prerenal azotemia can be broken down into volume loss, hypotension, and diseases of the large and small renal arteries (**Table 88-5**). Prerenal failure is also a common precursor to ischemic and nephrotoxic conditions, leading to intrinsic renal failure.

POSTOBSTRUCTIVE RENAL FAILURE

Postrenal or postobstructive kidney injury accounts for 5% to 17% of all community-acquired disease, and in the elderly population, the rate is as high as 22% (**Table 88-6**). Risk factors include both extremes of age, male sex, malignancy, nephrolithiasis, retroperitoneal disease, GU surgery, and indwelling urinary catheters. Timely relief of obstruction is essential for the return of normal renal function. **Permanent loss of renal function develops over the course of 10 to 14 days in the setting of complete obstruction. The risk of permanent renal failure increases significantly if obstruction is complicated by urinary tract infection.** For more discussion of postobstructive renal failure, see chapter 92.

INTRINSIC RENAL FAILURE

Intrinsic kidney injury is not common in patients with community-acquired disease, but it is the most common cause in hospitalized patients. Intrinsic renal failure can result from injury to the glomerulus, tubule, interstitium, and vasculature. In community-acquired intrinsic renal failure, drugs (**Table 88-7**) and infection are common precipitants, whereas in the hospital, toxic and ischemic insults cause most cases.[2-4]

Radiocontrast-induced nephropathy can be provoked by imaging with an IV contrast agent in the ED (see discussion below). Incidence ranges from 2% to 12%, with some reporting an even higher incidence. The typical course is an increasing Cr level, 25% above baseline, over 3 to 5 days, followed by complete resolution. Risk factors include chronic renal insufficiency, diabetes, heart failure, liver disease, and hypertension.[15,16]

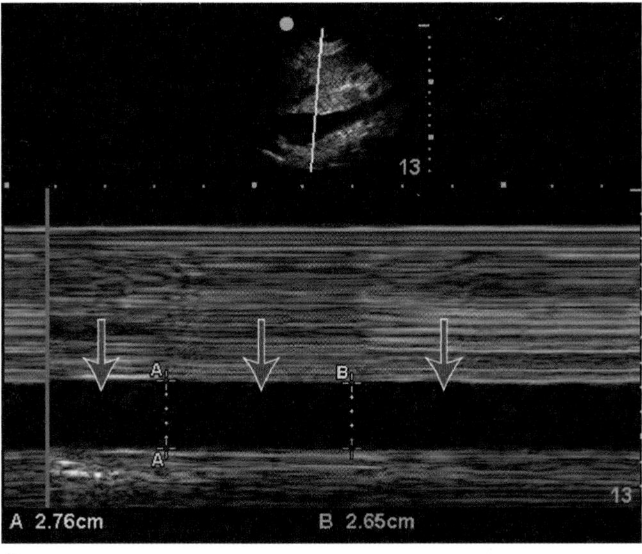

A

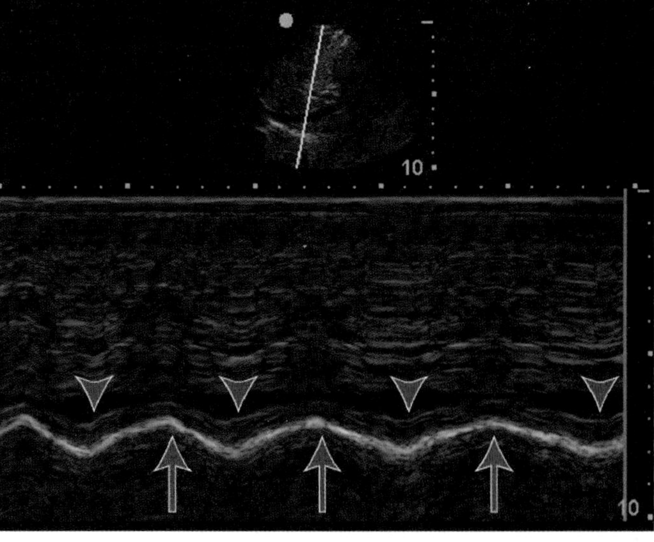

B

FIGURE 88-3. US of the inferior vena cava. A. Dilated inferior vena cava (*arrows*) with little respiratory variation as might be expected in volume overload. B. An almost fully collapsed inferior vena cava at inspiration (*arrows*) and expiration (*arrowheads*) as might be expected in prerenal acute kidney injury. [Image used with permission of Michael B. Stone, MD, RDMS.]

TABLE 88-5 Causes of Prerenal Failure

Hypovolemia
GI: decreased intake, vomiting and diarrhea
Pharmacologic: diuretics
Third spacing
Skin losses: fever, burns
Miscellaneous: hypoaldosteronism, salt-losing nephropathy, postobstructive diuresis
Hypotension (overt and relative)
Septic vasodilation
Hemorrhage
Decreased cardiac output: ischemia/infarction, valvulopathy, cardiomyopathy, tamponade
Pharmacologic: β-blockers, calcium channel blockers, other antihypertensive medications
High-output failure: thyrotoxicosis, thiamine deficiency, Paget's disease, arteriovenous fistula
Renal artery and small-vessel disease
Embolism: thrombotic, septic, cholesterol*
Thrombosis: atherosclerosis, vasculitis, sickle cell disease*
Dissection*
Pharmacologic: NSAIDs, angiotensin-converting enzyme inhibitors, angiotensin receptor blockers (these act on the microvasculature but have prerenal physiology)
Cyclosporine and tacrolimus
Microvascular thrombosis: pre-eclampsia, hemolytic-uremic syndrome, disseminated intravascular coagulation, vasculitis, sickle cell disease*
Hypercalcemia

Abbreviation: NSAIDs = nonsteroidal anti-inflammatory drugs.
*These causes include a component of ischemic acute kidney injury.

CRYSTAL-INDUCED NEPHROPATHY

Crystal-induced nephropathy is precipitation of crystals within the renal tubules, resulting in mechanical and inflammatory injuries of the tubular epithelium. Chronic renal insufficiency and hypovolemia predispose patients to this form of renal injury, and urinary pH affects the formation of many of these crystals. Elevated uric acid levels in the setting of **tumor lysis syndrome** and some medications—in particular, acyclovir, sulfonamides, indinavir, and triamterene—are the most common causes of crystal-induced acute kidney injury.

ANGIOTENSIN-CONVERTING ENZYME INHIBITORS

Angiotensin-converting enzyme (ACE) inhibitors can simultaneously decrease the GFR and increase renal blood flow. These changes naturally result in a modest (10% to 20%) increase in serum Cr, but in rare cases, the increase can be more dramatic. The increases in Cr are typically observed shortly after initiation of ACE inhibitor therapy.[17] Overt acute kidney injury in the setting of ACE inhibitor initiation should prompt consideration of **bilateral renal artery stenosis**. Volume depletion and concomitant use of vasoconstricting medications are other common precipitators of ACE inhibitor–induced renal failure. Angiotensin receptor blockers (ARBs) have similar effects. Hyperkalemia, usually mild, is a relatively common complication of ACE inhibitor administration. Because ACE inhibitors actually improve renal blood flow while decreasing GFR, renal insufficiency and renal failure are not contraindications to the use of ACE inhibitors in appropriate patients (e.g., those with acute congestive heart failure exacerbation).

NONSTEROIDAL ANTI-INFLAMMATORY DRUGS

Cyclooxygenase inhibitors (most nonsteroidal anti-inflammatory drugs [NSAIDs]) can also cause renal failure. This family of medications decreases synthesis of vasodilatory prostaglandins, which results in decreases of both GFR and renal blood flow. Renal effects of selective

TABLE 88-6 Causes of Postobstructive Renal Failure

Infants and children
Urethra and bladder outlet
Anatomic malformations: urethral atresia, meatal stenosis, anterior and posterior urethral valves (males)
Ureter
Anatomic malformations: vesicoureteral reflux (female preponderance), ureterovesical junction obstruction, ureterocele, megaureter (prune belly) syndrome, retrocaval ureter
Retroperitoneal tumor
All ages (various locations in the GU tract)
Trauma
Blood clot in bladder or urethra
Urethra and bladder outlet obstruction
Phimosis or urethral stricture (male preponderance)
Neurogenic bladder: diabetes mellitus, spinal cord disease, multiple sclerosis, Parkinson's disease; pharmacologic: anticholinergics, α-adrenergic antagonists, opiates
Calculus: in children in Southeast Asia, in adults typically a complication of mechanical intervention; in melamine-contaminated milk in China
Adults
Urethra and bladder outlet
Benign prostatic hypertrophy
Cancer of prostate, bladder, cervix, or colon
Obstructed catheters
Ureter obstruction
Calculi, uric acid crystals
Papillary necrosis: sickle cell disease, diabetes mellitus, pyelonephritis
Tumor: carcinoma of ureter, uterus, prostate, bladder, colon, rectum; retroperitoneal lymphoma; uterine leiomyomata
Retroperitoneal fibrosis: idiopathic, tuberculosis, sarcoidosis, methysergide, propranolol
Stricture: tuberculosis, radiation, schistosomiasis, nonsteroidal anti-inflammatory drugs
Miscellaneous: aortic aneurysm, pregnant uterus, inflammatory bowel disease, blood clot, trauma, accidental surgical ligation

cyclooxygenase-2 inhibitors seem to be very similar to those of nonselective inhibitors.[18] Risk factors for adverse reactions to these medications are older age, chronic renal insufficiency, congestive heart failure, diabetes, volume depletion, and use of diuretics or ACE inhibitors. Edema and renal insufficiency are typically observed early in the course

TABLE 88-7 Intrinsic Renal Failure Due to Drugs

Reduced renal perfusion by altered intrarenal hemodynamics	Amphotericin B, ACE inhibitors, cyclosporine, interleukin-2, NSAIDs, radiocontrast agents, tacrolimus
Direct tubular toxicity	Aminoglycoside antibiotics, amphotericin B, cisplatin, cyclosporine, foscarnet, heavy metals, IV immunoglobulin methotrexate, organic solvents, pentamidine, radiocontrast agents, tacrolimus
Rhabdomyolysis	Cocaine, ethanol, lovastatin
Intratubular obstruction	Acyclovir, chemotherapeutic agents, ethylene glycol, methotrexate, sulfonamides
Allergic interstitial nephritis	Allopurinol, cephalosporins, cimetidine, ciprofloxacin, furosemide, NSAIDs, phenytoin, penicillins, sulfonamides, rifampin, thiazide diuretics
Hemolytic-uremic syndrome	Cocaine, cyclosporine, conjugated estrogens, mitomycin, quinine, tacrolimus

Abbreviations: ACE = angiotensin-converting enzyme; NSAIDs = nonsteroidal anti-inflammatory drugs.

of treatment and are dose dependent. In reported cases, renal failure has resolved with discontinuation of the medication.

ANTIBIOTICS

Antibiotics and particularly **aminoglycosides** are another important cause of iatrogenic renal injury. Although peak concentration is typically most important for bactericidal activity, trough concentration appears to be more relevant in predicting renal injury, and once-daily dosing can reduce the incidence of nephrotoxicity.[19-22] Increased trough levels used with current **vancomycin** dosing for severe sepsis and septic shock are associated with increased rates of acute kidney injury. There is also evidence that **fluoroquinolones** may predispose to the condition.[23,24]

PIGMENTS

Hemoglobin and myoglobin from hemolysis or rhabdomyolysis are deposited and concentrated in the renal tubules. Renal injury occurs through tubular obstruction and direct toxicity. Large-volume crystalloid infusion is the cornerstone of treatment for rhabdomyolysis and hemoglobinuria (see chapter 89, "Rhabdomyolysis"). **Myeloma light-chain nephropathy** may also cause tubular obstruction.

TREATMENT OF INTRINSIC RENAL FAILURE

Low ("renal")-dose dopamine does not improve renal recovery or decrease mortality.[25] Fenoldopam is a potent dopamine D_1-selective receptor agonist that increases blood flow to the renal cortex and outer medulla while lowering systemic blood pressure. It reduces mortality and provides renal protection in critically ill patients with or at risk for renal failure.[26] Because it is titratable and reliably controls severe hypertension, **fenoldopam is considered by some to be the agent of choice for hypertensive emergencies with renal dysfunction** (see chapter 57, "Systemic Hypertension").

Venodilators (nitrates) and dialysis are the best treatment for volume overload. Diuretics may be helpful for volume overload, but high-dose **furosemide** can cause ototoxicity and otherwise provides no benefit to patients with acute kidney injury.[27,28] **Calcium channel blockers and mannitol have no role in the treatment of acute kidney injury.** Indications for emergency dialysis are listed in **Table 88-8**.

SPECIAL CONSIDERATIONS

RADIOCONTRAST-INDUCED NEPHROPATHY

Radiocontrast-induced nephropathy is an important consideration in the ED because of the high rate of use of radiocontrast-enhanced imaging (see **Table 88-9**). Risk for this condition is very closely related to existing renal insufficiency and the presence of concomitant renal insults, including diabetes, hypovolemia, sepsis, and use of nephrotoxic medications. Risk-scoring tools[29] have focused on coronary angiography. **Radiocontrast-induced nephropathy begins as a significant concern when GFR is <60 mL/min/1.73 m².[30] Do not give gadolinium-based contrast for MRI if the GFR is ≤30 mL/min/1.73 m² due to the risk of nephrogenic systemic fibrosis.**

The use of sodium bicarbonate appears promising and is translatable to the ED. A recent large meta-analysis reported that sodium bicarbonate–based hydration is superior to normal saline hydration with an odds ratio of 0.56 (confidence interval, 0.36 to 0.86) with a number needed to treat of 26.[31] However, the dosage, alkaline end points (blood versus urine pH), and mode of administration (single IV bolus versus continuous infusion) have not been defined.

TABLE 88-8 Indications for Emergent Dialysis

Indications for Emergent Dialysis
Uncontrolled hyperkalemia (K^+ >6.5 mmol/L or rising)
Intractable fluid overload in association with persistent hypoxia, or lack of response to conservative measures
Uremic pericarditis
Progressive uremic/metabolic encephalopathy; asterixis, seizures
Serum sodium level <115 or >165 mEq/L
Severe metabolic acidosis with concomitant acute kidney injury; treat underlying source of lactic acidosis and tolerate pH >7.2 in setting of permissive hypercapnia
Life-threatening poisoning with a dialyzable drug, such as lithium, aspirin, methanol, ethylene glycol, or theophylline
Bleeding dyscrasia secondary to uremia
Excessive BUN and Cr levels: trigger levels are arbitrary; it is generally advisable to keep BUN level <100 milligrams/dL, but each patient should be evaluated individually

TABLE 88-9 Minimizing Risk of Contrast-Induced Nephropathy

Identify patients at risk	Determine serum Cr and GFR before ordering contrast studies	Seriously consider risk of contrast if serum Cr >1.5 or GFR <60
Do not coadminister potentially nephrotoxic medications		Avoid parenteral NSAIDs
Provide hydration before and after test for at-risk patients	Before and after test as long as no congestive heart failure	Volume expansion improves renal blood flow, causes diuresis and dilutes contrast material within the tubules, and reduces activation of the renin-angiotensin system
Sodium bicarbonate	Seems to offer increased protection over normal saline[31]	Most commonly described dosing is 3 mL/kg bolus of a solution of 154 mmol/L $NaHCO_3$ in 5% dextrose in water, followed by 1 mL/kg/h (Merten Protocol)[32]
Use low- or iso-osmolar contrast agents		
Withhold metformin in diabetics	No metformin on day of test and for 48 h afterward	Risk of contrast nephropathy very low in diabetics with normal renal function; in patients with reduced renal function, clearance of metformin is decreased and lactic acidosis can result
N-Acetylcysteine	Value unproven; not recommended	

REFERENCES

The complete reference list is available online at www.TintinalliEM.com.

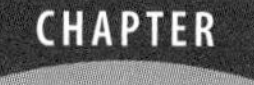

CHAPTER 89

Rhabdomyolysis

Francis L. Counselman
Bruce M. Lo

INTRODUCTION AND EPIDEMIOLOGY

Rhabdomyolysis is the destruction of skeletal muscle, caused by any mechanism that results in injury to myocytes and their membranes. Direct muscle injury and genetic and biochemical factors can predispose to rhabdomyolysis. Acute necrosis of skeletal muscle fibers and the leakage of cellular contents into the circulation result in myoglobinuria.

Several classification systems have been developed to characterize the numerous causes of rhabdomyolysis. None of these systems is universally recognized, and each has its limitations.

TABLE 89-1 Common Conditions Associated with Rhabdomyolysis in Adults

Trauma	Immunologic diseases involving muscle	Ischemic injury
Crush injury	Dermatomyositis	Compartment syndrome
Electrical or lightning injury	Polymyositis	Compression
Drugs of abuse	**Bacterial infection**	**Medications**
Amphetamines [including ecstasy (3,4-methylenedioxymethamphetamine)]	*Clostridium*	Antipsychotics
	Group A β-hemolytic streptococci	Barbiturates
Caffeine	*Legionella*	Benzodiazepines
Cocaine	*Salmonella*	Clofibrate
Ethanol	*Shigella*	Colchicine
Heroin	*Staphylococcus aureus*	Corticosteroids
Lysergic acid diethylamide	*Streptococcus pneumoniae*	Diphenhydramine
Methamphetamines	**Viral infection**	Isoniazid
Opiates	Coxsackievirus	Lithium
Phencyclidine	Cytomegalovirus	Monoamine oxidase inhibitors
Environment and excessive muscular activity	Epstein-Barr virus	Narcotics
Contact sports	Enterovirus	Neuroleptic agents
Delirium tremens	Hepatitis virus	Phenothiazines
Dystonia	Herpes simplex virus	Propofol
Psychosis	Human immunodeficiency virus	Salicylates
Seizures	Influenza virus (A and B)	Selective serotonin reuptake inhibitors
Marathons, military basic training	Rotavirus	Statins
Heat stroke	*Mycoplasma*	Theophylline
Genetic disorders		Tricyclic antidepressants
Glycolysis and glycogenolysis disorders		Zidovudine
Fatty acid oxidation disorders		Some novel cancer chemotherapeutic agents
Mitochondrial and respiratory chain metabolism disorders		

Table 89-1 lists commonly recognized conditions associated with rhabdomyolysis. **In general, the most common causes of rhabdomyolysis in adults appear to be alcohol and drugs of abuse, followed by medications, muscle diseases, trauma, neuroleptic malignant syndrome, seizures, immobility, infection, strenuous physical activity, and heat-related illness.**[1,2] A host of drugs and toxins have been identified that are associated with or causative of rhabdomyolysis.[3] Multiple causes are present in more than half of patients.[1] In children, rhabdomyolysis is less common and is thought to be more benign.[3] In one study of children, the most common causes of nonrecurrent rhabdomyolysis were trauma, viral myositis, and connective tissue disease.[4] For adults and children, inherited metabolic disorders should be suspected with recurrent episodes of rhabdomyolysis, especially if associated with exercise intolerance.

Patients in coma are at risk for rhabdomyolysis from unrelieved pressure on gravity-dependent body parts. Alcohol consumption can result in rhabdomyolysis secondary to coma-induced muscle compression and a direct toxic effect. Nutritional compromise, hypokalemia, hypomagnesemia, and hypophosphatemia, all common in alcoholics, increase the risk of rhabdomyolysis. Alcohol and drugs are thought to play a role in most cases of rhabdomyolysis in adults.[1] Drugs of abuse are commonly implicated in acute rhabdomyolysis, and many commonly prescribed medications have been associated as well.[2] **Statin-related myopathies** include myalgias with or without elevation of creatine kinase level, muscle weakness, and rhabdomyolysis. Statin-related rhabdomyolysis is rare, varies with the particular statin, and is also dose related. Drug combinations, including combinations with cyclosporine, macrolide antibiotics, warfarin, digoxin, and dual statin therapy, carry an increased risk for rhabdomyolysis.[3,5]

A number of bacterial and viral infections have been associated with rhabdomyolysis.[3] Strenuous physical activity, as seen in athletes, marathon runners, military recruits, and outdoor laborers, is a common cause. Physical activity that produces high-force eccentric contractions, such as strength training or heavy lifting, leads to greater breakdown in muscle and higher levels of creatine kinase than concentric contractions, such as endurance-based exercises.[6] Factors that increase the risk in this group of patients include poor physical conditioning, inadequate fluid intake, wearing of restrictive clothing, high ambient temperatures, and high humidity levels.[6]

PATHOPHYSIOLOGY

Rhabdomyolysis is a syndrome characterized by injury to skeletal muscle with subsequent effects from the release of intracellular contents. These contents include myoglobin, creatine kinase, aldolase, lactate dehydrogenase, aspartate aminotransferase, and potassium. Although numerous causes of rhabdomyolysis have been described, the common terminal event appears to involve the disruption of the $Na^{+}K^{+}ATPase$ pump and calcium transport, which results in increased intracellular calcium and subsequent muscle cell necrosis. In addition, calcium activates phospholipase A_2 and various vasoactive molecules and proteases and induces the production of free oxygen radicals.[3,7]

CLINICAL FEATURES

The presenting symptoms of rhabdomyolysis are usually acute in onset and include myalgias, stiffness, weakness, malaise, low-grade fever, and dark (usually brown) urine. Muscle symptoms, however, may be present in only half of cases.[4] Nausea, vomiting, abdominal pain, and tachycardia can occur in severe rhabdomyolysis. Mental status changes may develop from urea-induced encephalopathy. Swelling and tenderness of the involved muscle groups and hemorrhagic discoloration of overlying skin may be observed but are not common. Muscle involvement may be localized or diffuse, depending on the cause. Commonly, the postural muscles of the thighs, calves, and lower back are involved. Muscle swelling may not become apparent until after rehydration with IV fluids. An important point to remember is that acute rhabdomyolysis may be present without any of these signs or symptoms, and the patient may have normal findings on physical examination. For this reason, the diagnosis often is made only after soliciting a historical clue (e.g., recent cocaine use) or finding an elevated serum creatine kinase level or the presence of dark urine on routine laboratory testing.

DIAGNOSIS

An elevated **serum creatine kinase** is the most sensitive and reliable indicator of muscle injury. The degree of elevation correlates with the amount of muscle injury and the severity of illness, but not the development of renal failure or other morbidity. **Most investigators consider a fivefold or greater increase above the upper threshold of normal in serum creatine kinase level, in the absence of cardiac or brain injury, as the requirement for the diagnosis of rhabdomyolysis.** In general, the level begins to rise approximately 2 to 12 hours after the onset of muscle injury, peaks within 24 to 72 hours, and then declines at the relatively constant rate of 39% of the previous day's value. Ongoing muscle necrosis should be suspected in patients with elevated values that fail to decrease in this manner. The isoenzyme CK-MM (found in skeletal and cardiac muscle) is responsible in large part for the elevation in serum creatine kinase. The MB fraction of creatine kinase (found primarily in cardiac but also in skeletal muscle) also may be elevated but should not exceed 5% of the total creatine kinase.

Myoglobin is an oxygen-binding protein found in skeletal and cardiac muscle and is involved in oxidative metabolism. Myoglobinuria develops once skeletal muscle injury is >100 grams.[2] Myoglobin elevation occurs before creatine kinase elevation, and then is rapidly cleared from the plasma through renal excretion and metabolism to bilirubin. Myoglobin enters the urine when the plasma concentration is >1.5 milligrams/dL and causes the typical reddish brown discoloration when the urine myoglobin level is >100 milligrams/dL.[3,8] **Because myoglobin contains heme, qualitative tests such as the dipstick test (which uses the orthotoluidine reaction) do not differentiate among hemoglobin, myoglobin, and red blood cells.** Therefore, suspect myoglobinuria when the urine dipstick test is positive for blood but no red blood cells are present on microscopic examination. Radioimmunoassay is slightly more sensitive than the dipstick technique in identifying myoglobinuria, but usually is not necessary. Because myoglobin levels may return to normal within 1 to 6 hours after the onset of muscle necrosis, the absence of an elevated serum myoglobin level or of myoglobinuria does not exclude the diagnosis. In one study, only 19% of patients with rhabdomyolysis demonstrated myoglobinuria.[1]

Other laboratory studies may be useful to identify the common complications of rhabdomyolysis and the underlying cause. Serum electrolyte, calcium, phosphorus, and uric acid levels should be determined to identify hyperkalemia, abnormal calcium and phosphorus levels, and hyperuricemia. Urinalysis should be obtained for all patients. Serum creatinine and BUN levels are needed to identify acute renal failure. Because disseminated intravascular coagulation is a potential complication, a baseline CBC should be obtained and a coagulopathic screen considered [e.g., prothrombin time, partial thromboplastin time, fibrin split products, and fibrinogen level (see chapter 233, Acquired Bleeding Disorders)]. Other common laboratory findings in rhabdomyolysis include elevated levels of aldolase, lactate dehydrogenase, urea, creatine, and aminotransferases. Further laboratory testing to identify the underlying cause(s) of rhabdomyolysis should be based on the medical history and clinical presentation.

DIFFERENTIAL DIAGNOSIS

Other causes of muscle pain and weakness besides rhabdomyolysis should be considered in the appropriate clinical setting. Such causes include acute myopathies, periodic paralysis, polymyositis or dermatomyositis, or Guillain-Barré syndrome. Rhabdomyolysis associated with strenuous exercise or fasting or repeat episodes of rhabdomyolysis suggest an inherited metabolic myopathy.[3]

TREATMENT

PREHOSPITAL CARE

For victims of **crush injury**, patients strongly suspected of having rhabdomyolysis, or accident victims with prolonged extrication and transport times, early and vigorous IV fluid resuscitation is the most important treatment to prevent acute renal failure.[9,10] Once a limb is extricated, IV normal saline should be initiated at 1 L/h. After extrication, IV normal saline should be continued at 500 mL, alternating with 5% dextrose in normal saline at 1 L/h. **Avoid potassium- or lactate-containing solutions.** There is no evidence that the administration of sodium bicarbonate is beneficial.

ED CARE

Once the patient is in the ED, continue aggressive IV rehydration for the next 24 to 72 hours. One method is rapid correction of the fluid deficit with IV crystalloids followed by infusion of 2.5 mL/kg/h, with the goal of maintaining a minimum urine output of 2 mL/kg/h.[11] Another method is a goal of 200 to 300 mL of urine output each hour.[12]

No prospective controlled studies have demonstrated benefit from alkalinization of the urine with sodium bicarbonate or forced diuresis with mannitol or loop diuretics.[12-14] Bicarbonate is widely recommended but without an evidence base. If bicarbonate is given, maintain an isotonic solution and avoid metabolic alkalosis or hypokalemia.[12] Mannitol may be harmful because it may cause osmotic diuresis in hypovolemic patients.

Place a urinary catheter in patients in critical condition and those with acute renal failure to monitor urine output. Institute cardiac monitoring because electrolyte and metabolic complications can cause dysrhythmias. For patients with heart disease, comorbid conditions, or preexisting renal disease or for elderly patients, hemodynamic monitoring may be necessary to avoid fluid overload. Serial measurements of urine pH, electrolytes, creatine kinase, calcium, phosphorus, BUN, and creatinine are needed.

Hypocalcemia observed early in rhabdomyolysis usually requires no treatment. Calcium should be given only to treat hyperkalemia-induced cardiotoxicity or profound signs and symptoms of hypocalcemia. If hypercalcemia is symptomatic, continue saline diuresis. Treat hyperphosphatemia with oral phosphate binders when serum levels are >7 milligrams/dL. Treat hypophosphatemia when the serum level is <1 milligram/dL. Hyperkalemia, which is usually most severe in the first 12 to 36 hours after muscle injury, can be significant and prolonged. Traditional insulin and glucose therapy, although recommended, may not be as effective in rhabdomyolysis-induced hyperkalemia. The use of ion-exchange resins (e.g., sodium polystyrene sulfonate) is effective. Dialysis may be needed (see chapter 17, Fluids and Electrolytes).

Avoid prostaglandin inhibitors such as nonsteroidal anti-inflammatory drugs because of their vasoconstrictive effects on the kidney. Finally, treat the underlying cause.

DISEASE COMPLICATIONS

The complications of rhabdomyolysis include acute renal failure, metabolic derangements, disseminated intravascular coagulation, and mechanical complications (e.g., compartment syndrome or peripheral neuropathy)[15] (**Table 89-2**). Factors that contribute to rhabdomyolysis-induced acute renal failure include hypovolemia, acidosis or aciduria, tubular obstruction, and the nephrotoxic effects of myoglobin.[3,12] In exertional rhabdomyolysis, acute renal failure is rare without the presence of factors like dehydration, heat stress, trauma, or underlying disease such as sickle cell anemia.[6] Renal tubular obstruction occurs secondary to precipitation of uric acid and myoglobin. Ferrihemate, the breakdown product of myoglobin, is responsible for the direct toxic effect on the kidneys. This effect, however, appears to occur only in the presence of hypovolemia and aciduria (pH <5.6). Renal failure may be oliguric (most common) or nonoliguric. Patients with initially elevated creatinine and BUN and a large base deficit[16,17] have an increased risk for

TABLE 89-2 Complications of Rhabdomyolysis

Complications of Rhabdomyolysis
Acute renal failure
Metabolic derangements
Hypercalcemia (late)
Hyperkalemia
Hyperphosphatemia
Hyperuricemia
Hypocalcemia
Hypophosphatemia (late)
Disseminated intravascular coagulation
Mechanical complications
Compartment syndrome
Peripheral neuropathy

rhabdomyolysis-induced acute renal failure. However, neither the presence of myoglobinuria nor the degree of creatine kinase elevation is predictive of acute renal failure.

Anticipate a rise in the serum potassium level due to release of potassium from injured skeletal muscle. Renal function, however, appears to be the most important determinant of the degree of elevation. Hyperkalemia can be a significant complication of rhabdomyolysis if acute renal failure occurs.

Elevated uric acid levels can occur, especially in crush injures, due to release of muscle adenosine nucleotides and the subsequent conversion to uric acid by the liver. Uric acid levels usually correlate with serum creatine kinase levels.

Serum phosphorus levels initially may be elevated, due to the leakage of phosphorus from injured muscle. Later in the disease course, mild hypophosphatemia may be seen but rarely requires treatment. Hypocalcemia occurs early and is usually asymptomatic. It results from the deposition of calcium salts in necrotic muscle, due to the hyperphosphatemia and decreased levels of 1,25-dihydroxycholecalciferol. Soft tissue calcifications sometimes can be observed on radiographs of the involved limb muscles. Hypocalcemia can occur, however, without elevated levels of phosphorus. Later, as calcium is mobilized from damaged muscle, hypercalcemia may be observed.

Disseminated intravascular coagulation occurs in severe rhabdomyolysis and can result in hemorrhagic complications.

The mechanical complications of rhabdomyolysis consist of compartment syndrome and peripheral nerve injury. The associated muscle swelling may exert pressure on peripheral nerves, resulting in neuronal ischemia and causing paresthesias or paralysis. Nerve injury is often proximal, and multiple nerves may be involved in the same extremity.[15] Compartment syndrome occurs secondary to marked swelling and edema of the involved muscle groups and is discussed in chapter 278, Compartment Syndrome.

DISPOSITION AND FOLLOW-UP

The majority of healthy patients with *exertional rhabdomyolysis* and *without comorbidities* (i.e., heat stress, dehydration, trauma) can usually be treated with oral or IV rehydration, observed in the ED, and then released.[6] Otherwise, patients should be admitted for IV hydration, diuresis, management of complications, and treatment of the underlying cause. For at least the initial 24 to 48 hours, admission should be to a monitored bed to identify dysrhythmias. The nephrology service should be consulted to evaluate the need for dialysis, especially for patients with hyperkalemia unresponsive to therapy.

PRACTICE GUIDELINES

No internationally recognized organization has published validated guidelines for the management of rhabdomyolysis, but the Finnish Medical Society has issued nonvalidated literature-based guidelines that are available on the Internet (see Useful Web Resource).

REFERENCES

The complete reference list is available online at www.TintinalliEM.com.

CHAPTER 90

End-Stage Renal Disease

Mathew Foley
Ninfa Mehta
Richard Sinert

INTRODUCTION AND EPIDEMIOLOGY

End-stage renal disease (ESRD) is the irreversible loss of renal function, resulting in the accumulation of toxins and the loss of internal homeostasis. Uremia, the clinical syndrome resulting from ESRD, is universally fatal without some form of renal replacement therapy. At present, renal replacement therapy consists of two basic modalities: renal transplant and dialytic therapy, either hemodialysis or peritoneal dialysis (PD).

Hemodialysis is the initial therapy in the vast majority of new cases of adult ESRD, with a few starting PD and an even smaller number receiving predialytic renal transplants. The proportions are reversed in children, with most children receiving transplants. More than 90,000 Americans await a renal transplant, with a median time of 2.6 years on a transplant wait list.

Approximately half of hemodialysis and PD patients will be alive 3 years after starting therapy, with cardiac causes accounting for about half of all deaths. Infections trigger death in up to a quarter of patients, with cerebrovascular events and malignancy being other causes.

PATHOPHYSIOLOGY

Uremia, contamination of the blood with urine, differs from azotemia, the buildup of nitrogen in the blood. Renal failure assumes many forms, often co-existing.

Excretory failure leads to elevated levels of >70 chemicals in uremic plasma, which gives rise to the hypothesis that these toxins, individually or in combination, cause uremic organ dysfunction and produce the symptoms of uremia. Urea is not the major toxin, and potential uremic toxins include cyanate, guanidine, polyamines, and β2-microglobulin.[1] If uremia were simply a toxidrome, then dialysis would reverse all its untoward effects; however, it does not, in part because many toxins are highly protein bound and nondialyzable.[2] Because many uremia-related organ dysfunctions persist after dialysis, other processes are clearly important.

Biosynthetic failure refers to the aspects of uremia caused by loss of the renal hormones 1,25$(OH)_2$-vitamin D_3 and erythropoietin. The kidneys are primarily responsible for the secretion of erythropoietin and 1α-hydroxylase, which is necessary to produce the active form of vitamin D_3. Because 85% of erythropoietin is produced in the kidneys, ESRD patients have depressed levels of erythropoietin, which contributes to anemia. Vitamin D_3 deficiency results in decreased GI calcium absorption, inducing secondary hyperparathyroidism, leading to renal bone disease.

Regulatory failure results in an oversecretion of hormones, leading to uremia by disruption of normal feedback mechanisms. The uremic state produces excess free oxygen radicals, which react with carbohydrates, lipids, and amino acids to create advanced glycation end products, linked to atherosclerosis and amyloidosis in ESRD patients.[3] This may explain the progressive nature of the atherosclerosis and amyloidosis seen in ESRD patients.[4]

TABLE 90-1 Clinical Features of Uremia and Dialysis

Neurologic
Uremic encephalopathy: cognitive defects, memory loss, decreased attentiveness, slurred speech, reversal of sleep-wake cycle, asterixis, seizure, coma, symptomatic improvement with dialysis
Dialysis dementia: progressive neurologic decline, failure to improve with dialysis, fatal
Subdural hematoma: headache, focal neurologic deficits, seizure, coma
Peripheral neuropathy: singultus (hiccups), restless leg syndrome, sensorimotor neuropathy, autonomic neuropathy
Cardiovascular
Coronary artery disease
Hypertension: essential hypertension, glomerulonephritis, renal artery stenosis, fluid overload
Heart failure: fluid overload, uremic cardiomyopathy, high-output arteriovenous fistula
Pericarditis: uremic, dialysis related, pericardial tamponade
Hematologic
Anemia, decreased red blood cell survival, decreased erythropoietin levels
Bleeding diathesis
Immunodeficiency (humoral and cellular)
GI
Anorexia, metallic taste, nausea, vomiting
GI bleeding
Diverticulosis, diverticulitis
Ascites
Renal bone disease
Metastatic calcification (calciphylaxis)
Hyperparathyroidism (osteitis fibrosa cystica)
Vitamin D_3 deficiency and aluminum intoxication (osteomalacia)

CLINICAL FEATURES OF UREMIA

Uremia is a clinical syndrome, and no single symptom, sign, or laboratory test result reflects all aspects of uremia. Although a correlation exists between the symptoms of uremia and low glomerular filtration rate (8 to 10 mL/min/1.73 m^2), BUN and serum creatinine levels are inaccurate markers of the clinical syndrome of uremia. The decision to start long-term dialysis is based on the severity of the patient's symptoms related to uremia (**Table 90-1**). The most common reasons for emergency dialysis are hyperkalemia, severe acid-base disturbances, and pulmonary edema resistant to usual therapy.

NEUROLOGIC COMPLICATIONS

Stroke occurs in approximately 6% of hemodialysis patients, with about half being hemorrhagic and half ischemic. Subdural hematomas occur 10 times more frequently in dialysis patients than in the general population.

Uremic encephalopathy is a constellation of nonspecific central neurologic symptoms associated with renal failure. Uremic encephalopathy is best diagnosed after eliminating structural, vascular, infectious, toxic, and metabolic causes of neurologic dysfunction. Neurologic findings of uremic encephalopathy improve with dialysis.

Dialysis dementia is nonspecific in presentation from other encephalopathies. This manifestation of ESRD and treatment is progressive, with the 2- to 4-year survival for these patients being 24%. This disorder usually becomes evident after at least 2 years of dialysis therapy and fails to respond to increases in dialysis frequency or renal transplantation.

Peripheral neuropathy is one of the most frequent neurologic manifestations of ESRD, with greater lower than upper limb involvement. The most frequent clinical features reflect large-fiber involvement, with paresthesias, reduction in deep tendon reflexes, impaired vibration sense, muscle wasting, and weakness. Autonomic dysfunction results in impotence, postural dizziness, gastric fullness, bowel dysfunction, and reduced sweating. Reduced heart rate variability and baroreceptor control impairment occur.

Nerve conduction studies demonstrate findings consistent with a generalized neuropathy of the axonal type. No single pathologic correlate has been identified for peripheral uremic neuropathy. Conventional hemodialysis does not seem to improve autonomic dysfunction; however, daily short hemodialysis and long nocturnal hemodialysis may reduce the elevated sympathetic activity.

CARDIOVASCULAR COMPLICATIONS

The mortality from cardiovascular disease is 10 to 30 times higher in dialysis patients than in the general population. Coronary artery disease, left ventricular hypertrophy, and congestive heart failure are common. The etiology of cardiovascular disease in ESRD patients is multifactorial, related to preexisting conditions (e.g., hypertension, diabetes), uremia (e.g., uremic toxins, hyperlipidemias, homocysteine level, hyperparathyroidism), and dialysis-related conditions (e.g., hypotension, dialysis membrane reactions, hypoalbuminemia).[5]

The diagnosis of ischemic cardiovascular disease in ESRD patients often has been clouded by the misconception that the traditional serum protein markers of myocardial damage (troponins I and T) are unreliable in dialysis patients. Elevated levels of **troponin I and T** are common even in asymptomatic hemodialysis patients and probably reflect left ventricular hypertrophy and microvascular disease. Asymptomatic elevations of cardiac biomarkers are, however, associated with long-term risks of coronary artery disease.[6] To account for higher baseline levels of troponin T and I, many define myocardial infarction only by a 20% or more dynamic rise and with at least one value above the 99th percentile (see chapter 48, "Chest Pain").

Hypertension is present in most patients starting dialysis. Maintenance of hypertension depends mostly on increased total peripheral resistance. Increases in blood volume, decreased vascular compliance, the vasopressor effects of native kidneys, the renin-angiotensin system, and the sympathetic nervous system also play roles in ESRD hypertension.[7]

Management of hypertension in ESRD patients begins with control of blood volume. If that is unsuccessful, most cases can be controlled with adrenergic blocking agents, angiotensin-converting enzyme inhibitors, or vasodilating agents, such as hydralazine or minoxidil. Bilateral nephrectomy is rarely necessary for blood pressure control.

Heart failure most commonly results from hypertension, followed by coronary artery disease and valvular defects. Causes unique to ESRD include uremic cardiomyopathy, fluid overload, and arteriovenous fistula–related high-output failure (see section "Complications of Vascular Access" later in the chapter). **Natriuretic peptide levels** are elevated in hemodialysis patients, often from concomitant left ventricular hypertrophy and systolic dysfunction. Elevation of natriuretic peptides in hemodialysis patients correlates with higher short-term mortality rates, but there are no reliable thresholds to identify fluid overload.

Uremic cardiomyopathy is a diagnosis of exclusion when all other causes of congestive heart failure have been excluded. In most uremic patients, left ventricular dysfunction is related to ischemic heart disease, hypertension, and hypoalbuminemia. Dialysis rarely improves left ventricular function in uremic patients with congestive heart failure.

Pulmonary edema in ESRD patients is commonly ascribed to fluid overload, but acute myocardial ischemia can also trigger depressed left ventricular function. Cornerstones of therapy are supplemental oxygen if needed, bilevel positive airway pressure, nitrates, and angiotensin-converting enzyme inhibitors. Loop diuretics, such as furosemide (60 to 100 milligrams IV), may aid even in those with minimal urine output from their short-lived vasodilatory actions. **Hemodialysis is the ultimate treatment for fluid overload** in ESRD patients. Preload reduction by inducing diarrhea with sorbitol or by phlebotomy may help in low-resource situations. Removing as little as 150 mL of blood is safe and effective in some with pulmonary edema. Improved oxygenation produced by phlebotomy offsets the decrease in oxygen-carrying capacity due to the decrease in hemoglobin. Blood withdrawn during phlebotomy should be collected in transfusion bags, so plasma can be extracted by the blood bank and the red blood cells transfused back to the patient later during dialysis. PD does not remove volume fast enough to have a significant impact on pulmonary edema.

Cardiac tamponade is a concern in any critically ill ESRD patient, often presenting without classic findings. Instead, signs of cardiac tamponade in these patients include changes in mental status, hypotension, or shortness of breath. Increased interdialytic weight gain, increased edema, and intradialytic hypotension are other warning signs suggesting the diagnosis of tamponade. In addition to hypotension, an increased heart size on chest radiograph suggest effusion and potential tamponade. Bedside US is the best method to detect pericardial effusion and tamponade. Hemodynamically significant pericardial effusions require pericardiocentesis under fluoroscopic or US guidance. Bedside pericardiocentesis (see chapter 34, "Pericardiocentesis") is used only in hemodynamically unstable patients because of its high complication rate.

Pericarditis is usually due to uremia. Uremic pericarditis is linked to fluid overload, abnormal platelet function, and increased fibrinolysis and inflammation. Pericardial contents are sterile unless infected and are abundant with fibrin and inflammatory cells.

Uremic pericarditis causes pericardial friction rubs, which are louder than in most other forms of pericarditis, often palpable, and frequently persist for some time after metabolic abnormalities have been corrected. BUN level is nearly always >60 milligrams/dL. One of the unique features of uninfected uremic pericarditis is that the inflammatory cells do not penetrate into the myocardium, so typical ECG changes of acute pericarditis are absent. Most often, the ECG demonstrates associated abnormalities, such as left ventricular hypertrophy, ischemia, and metabolic abnormalities (e.g., hyperkalemia and hypocalcemia). When the ECG has features typical of acute pericarditis, infection should be suspected.

Dialysis-related pericarditis is most common during periods of increased catabolism (trauma and sepsis) or inadequate dialysis due to missed sessions or vascular access problems. The pathophysiology of dialysis-related pericarditis is the buildup of middle molecules and hyperparathyroidism. Dialysis-related pericarditis is more common during hemodialysis than during PD, although now somewhat less frequent because of improved dialysis techniques. Fever and malaise are more common and severe than in uremic pericarditis. Pericardial effusion is the most important complication and tends to be recurrent. Due to the recurrent nature of dialysis pericarditis, adhesions and fluid loculations are common, which complicates the interpretation of echocardiographic scans and images obtained using other modalities.

Management of uremic and dialysis-related pericarditis in patients in hemodynamically stable condition is intensive dialysis. Hemodialysis is preferred over PD because of the higher clearance rates of the former, recognizing the risks of tamponade from heparin and rapid fluid shifts. Hemodialysis is effective in the majority of cases of dialysis-related pericarditis, usually after 10 to 14 days. Indomethacin, colchicine, and steroids are not useful for ESRD pericarditis. If pericardial effusion persists for longer than 10 to 14 days with intensive dialysis, anterior pericardiectomy is often used, with total pericardiectomy reserved for constrictive pericarditis.

HEMATOLOGIC COMPLICATIONS

Anemia is multifactorial, caused by decreased erythropoietin, blood loss from dialysis, frequent phlebotomy, and decreased red blood cell survival times. In addition, the wide fluctuations in plasma blood volume seen in dialysis patients often cause factitious anemia. Without treatment, the hematocrit should stabilize at 15% to 20%, with normocytic and normochromic red blood cells. Bone marrow shows erythroid hypoplasia, with little effect on leukopoiesis or megakaryocytopoiesis. Anemia is treated with regular infusions of human recombinant erythropoietin. Erythropoietin replacement therapy improves the quality of life for ESRD patients by increasing exercise capacity and tolerance.

The **bleeding diathesis** of ESRD patients increases the risks of GI tract bleeding, subdural hematomas, subcapsular liver hematomas, and intraocular bleeding. Several mechanisms, including decreased platelet function, abnormal platelet-vessel wall interactions, altered von Willebrand factor, anemia, and abnormal guanidinosuccinic acid–dependent production of nitric oxide, create uremic bleeding. The skin bleeding test is the best predictor of clinically important defects in hemostasis. Patients receiving aspirin or warfarin are at greater risk of major bleeding. **Improvement in bleeding times with infusions of desmopressin (benefit in 1 h), cryoprecipitate (benefit in 4 h), or conjugated estrogens (benefit in 6 h) is an option** (see chapter 233, "Acquired Bleeding Disorders" for further discussion).

Immunologic deficiency in ESRD patients results in high morbidity and mortality from infectious diseases. Depressed leukocyte chemotaxis and phagocytosis from many causes is the key feature, along with abnormal T-cell activation. Dialysis does not improve the immune function and may exacerbate immunodeficiency by complement activation after exposure to the hemodialysis filter membrane.

GI COMPLICATIONS

Anorexia, nausea, and vomiting are common symptoms of uremia and used to initiate and monitor dialysis adequacy. There is an increased incidence of gastritis and upper GI bleeding in ESRD patients, but the incidence of gastric and duodenal ulcers is similar in ESRD patients and the general population.

Chronic constipation is common secondary to decreased fluid intake and the use of phosphate-bonding gels. ESRD patients have an increased incidence of diverticular disease and colonic perforation, especially patients with polycystic kidney disease.

Dialysis-related ascites is secondary to fluid overload, portal hypertension from polycystic liver disease, and osmotic disequilibrium. Treatment of refractory ascites is possible with peritoneovenous shunts.

RENAL BONE DISEASE

As the glomerular filtration rate falls, phosphate excretion decreases, which results in increased serum phosphate levels. When the calcium-phosphate product [Ca^{2+} (milligrams/dL) × PO_4 (milligrams/dL)] is higher than 70 to 80, **metastatic calcification** can ensue. Joint pain from **pseudogout** develops from calcification of synovial membrane–lined joints. Metastatic calcification in small vessels results in skin and finger necrosis, and life-threatening calcifications can occur in the cardiac and pulmonary systems. Short-term mortality rate is higher in ESRD patients with a calcium-phosphate product of >72. Treatment consists of the use of low-calcium dialysate and phosphate-binding gels.

As ESRD progresses, the combination of calciphylaxis and vitamin D_3 deficiency results in depressed ionized calcium levels and stimulation of the parathyroid gland, causing **hyperparathyroidism**. The increased production of parathyroid hormone results in high bone turnover and weakened bones susceptible to fracture. Bone pain and muscle weakness are other symptoms. High alkaline phosphatase and parathyroid hormone levels make the diagnosis. Treatment consists of control of serum phosphate levels with binding gels, vitamin D_3 replacement, and, if necessary, subtotal parathyroidectomy.

A subset of ESRD patients develops **osteomalacia**, a defect in bone calcification. The signs and symptoms are weakened bones, bone pain, and muscle weakness, similar to those of hyperparathyroidism. Osteomalacia is characterized by low to normal alkaline phosphatase levels and low parathyroid hormone levels. Elevated serum aluminum and bone aluminum levels are useful for confirming the diagnosis. Treatment with desferrioxamine helps aluminum bone disease.

β_2-MICROGLOBULIN AMYLOIDOSIS

Dialysis-related amyloidosis (β_2-microglobulin amyloidosis) can occur in dialysis patients >50 years of age and on dialysis for >10 years. Advanced glycation end products appear central to the chronic inflammatory condition, leading to amyloidosis. Amyloid deposits are found in the GI tract, bones, and joints. Complications include GI perforation, bone cysts with pathologic fractures, and arthropathies, including carpal tunnel syndrome and rotator cuff tears. Patients with amyloidosis have higher mortality rates than do those without this disorder.

HEMODIALYSIS

TECHNICAL ASPECTS OF HEMODIALYSIS

Hemodialysis substitutes a filter for the glomerulus to produce an ultrafiltrate of plasma. Small amounts of IV heparin, 1000 to 2000 units, are used to prevent thrombosis at the vascular access site. Hemodialysis sessions typically take 3 to 4 hours. Adjustment of the pressure gradient across the hemodialyzer filter during hemodialysis controls the amount of fluid removal (ultrafiltration). Solute removal (clearance) during hemodialysis depends on the filter pore size, the amount of ultrafiltration (solute drag), and the concentration gradient across the filter (diffusion). During hemodialysis, blood is removed from the vascular access site by large-bore needles (typically 15 gauge), circulated through the dialysis machine at rates of 300 to 500 mL/min, and returned to the patient. The dialysate usually flows at a rate of 500 to 800 mL/min through the dialysis filter in the direction opposite to blood flow.

COMPLICATIONS OF VASCULAR ACCESS

In cases in which a native artery or vein is not suitable for arteriovenous fistula creation, an interposing vascular graft made of an autologous vein, polytetrafluoroethylene, or bovine carotid artery must be used for vascular access. Such grafts generally are associated with a higher complication rate and shorter functional life expectancies than are natural arteriovenous fistulas. The third form of vascular access for hemodialysis is the use of tunneled-cuffed catheters. The most common site for tunneled-cuffed catheter placement is the right internal jugular vein. Because of the cuff, tunneled-cuffed catheters should not be removed by pulling.

Complications of vascular access account for more inpatient hospital days than any other complication of hemodialysis. The most common complications of hemodialysis vascular access are failure to provide adequate flow (300 mL/min) and infection.[8] If referred to the ED for inadequate access flow that impairs dialysis, missing a single session should not result in uremic encephalopathy, allowing emergency dialysis for those with hyperkalemia and fluid overload in the ED (see chapter 88, "Acute Kidney Injury").

Thrombosis and stenosis of the vascular access are the most common causes of inadequate dialysis flow. Grafts generally have a higher rate of stenosis than do fistulas. Stenosis or thrombosis presents with loss of bruit and thrill over the access. Stenosis and thrombosis can be treated within 24 hours by angiographic clot removal or angioplasty. Thrombosis of vascular access can also be treated with direct injection of alteplase, usually in conjunction with a vascular surgeon.[9]

Vascular access infections occur in 2% to 5% of arteriovenous fistulas and approximately 10% of grafts over their functional lifetimes. Patients with an infected access often present with fever, hypotension, or an elevated WBC count. The classic signs of infection of pain, erythema, swelling, and discharge from an infected vascular access are often missing. Dialysis catheter–related bacteremia is a very common and potentially life-threatening. After 6 months with a dialysis catheter, approximately half of patients develop bacteremia, with a serious complication (death, endocarditis, osteomyelitis, septic arthritis, epidural abscess) occurring in 5% to 10% of patients with bacteremia. Most authorities prefer a trial of IV antibiotics in an attempt to maintain the dialysis access before removal, the latter often done if there is ongoing fever after 2 to 3 days of antibiotics. To narrow the potential source of bacteremia, peripheral and catheter blood samples for culture are drawn simultaneously. A four-fold higher colony count in the catheter blood culture than in the peripheral blood culture suggests the catheter as the source of bacteremia.

The most common infecting organism is *Staphylococcus aureus*, followed by gram-negative bacteria. Patients with access infections usually require hospital admission, and vancomycin is the drug of choice (15 milligrams/kg or 1 gram IV) because of its effectiveness against methicillin-resistant organisms and long half-life (5 to 7 days) in dialysis patients. An aminoglycoside (gentamicin 100 milligrams IV initially and after each dialysis treatment) is added if gram-negative organisms are suspected, but the patient is monitored closely because of toxicity. Alternatives or adjuncts to IV antibiotics include removal and delayed replacement of the catheter, catheter exchange over a guidewire, and the use of antimicrobial/citrate lock solutions, although limited controlled data exist.

TABLE 90-2 Treatment Options for Control of Vascular Access Hemorrhage

Technique	Comments
Direct pressure to hemorrhage site using gloved finger initially	Hold for 5–10 min minimum, longer if needed.
Absorbable gelatin sponges soaked in reconstituted thrombin, or chemical thrombotic [HemCon® (chitosan; HemCon Medical Technologies, Inc., Portland, OR) or QuikClot (1% zeolite; Z-Medica Corp., Wallingford, CT; with water, thermal injury may occur; see package directions)], placed directly on hemorrhage site	Apply pressure after application for 10 min minimum.
Protamine given at a dose of 0.01 milligram per unit of heparin dispensed during dialysis	If the dose of heparin is unknown, protamine, 10 to 20 milligrams, will be sufficient to reverse the typical 1000 to 2000 units of heparin given at dialysis.
Desmopressin acetate, 0.3 microgram/kg IV	Use as an adjunct; consult nephrologist or vascular surgeon as needed.
Tourniquet proximal to vascular access	Temporizing measure only while awaiting urgent vascular surgery consultation.

Hemorrhage from a vascular access is a rare but life-threatening complication. Hemorrhage can result from aneurysms, anastomosis rupture, or overanticoagulation. Control bleeding immediately with manual pressure applied to the puncture sites for 5 to 10 minutes, and observe the patient for 1 to 2 hours if ceased. **Table 90-2** lists further options for control of hemorrhage. Consult a vascular surgeon when simple methods fail to control hemorrhage or large-volume bleeding occurs.

Vascular access aneurysms result from repeated punctures; true aneurysms are very rare. Most aneurysms are asymptomatic, with patients occasionally complaining of pain or an associated peripheral impingement neuropathy. Aneurysms rarely rupture.

Vascular access pseudoaneurysms result from subcutaneous extravasation of blood from puncture sites. Signs are bleeding and infection at the access site. Arterial Doppler US studies identify any aneurysm or pseudoaneurysm, and if detected, a vascular surgeon should be consulted.

Vascular insufficiency of the extremity distal to the vascular access occurs in approximately 1% of all patients. This "steal syndrome" is the result of preferential shunting of arterial blood to the venous side of the access. Signs and symptoms are exercise pain, nonhealing ulcers, and cool, pulseless digits. Doppler US or angiography is the best diagnostic approach, and treatment is surgical.

High-output heart failure can occur when >20% of the cardiac output is diverted through the access. The Branham sign, a drop in heart rate after temporary access occlusion, is useful for detecting this complication. Doppler US can accurately measure access flow rate and establish the diagnosis. Surgical banding of the access is the treatment of choice to decrease flow and treat heart failure.

COMPLICATIONS DURING HEMODIALYSIS

Hypotension is the most frequent complication of hemodialysis, occurring during 50% of treatments (**Table 90-3**). Fluid removal during hemodialysis averages 1 to 3 L over a 4-hour session, but removal of up to 2 L/h is possible. Maintenance of a normal blood pressure during ultrafiltration depends on cardiovascular compensatory mechanisms and refilling of the vascular space by fluid shifts from the interstitial and intracellular compartments. Excessive ultrafiltration due to underestimation of the patient's ideal blood volume (dry weight) is the most common cause of intradialytic hypotension. Optimal dry weight is often clinically defined when hypotension prevents further fluid removal.

TABLE 90-3 Differential Diagnosis of Peridialytic Hypotension

Excessive ultrafiltration
Predialytic volume loss (GI losses, decreased oral intake)
Intradialytic volume loss (tube and hemodialyzer blood losses)
Postdialytic volume loss (vascular access blood loss)
Medication effects (antihypertensives, opiates)
Decreased vascular tone (sepsis, food, dialysate temperature >37°C or 98.6°F)
Cardiac dysfunction (left ventricular hypertrophy, ischemia, hypoxia, arrhythmia, pericardial tamponade)
Pericardial disease (effusion, tamponade)

Myocardial dysfunction from ischemia, hypoxia, arrhythmias, and early pericardial tamponade are in the differential diagnosis of intradialytic hypotension. Abnormalities of vascular tone from sepsis or antihypertensive medications also contribute to hypotension. Vascular refilling can be enhanced by improving nutrition, performing ultrafiltration before dialysis, and increasing the sodium concentration of the dialysate solution.

The timing of intradialytic hypotension is often helpful in formulating a differential diagnosis. **Hypotension early in the dialysis session** is usually due to preexisting hypovolemia. Predialysis losses should be suspected when the patient starts hemodialysis at a weight below his or her dry weight; consider GI bleeding, sepsis, vomiting, diarrhea, or decreased intake of salt and water. Intradialytic blood loss can occur from blood tubing or hemodialyzer filter leaks. Hypotension near the end of dialysis is usually the result of excessive ultrafiltration, but pericardial or cardiac disease is possible.

Intradialytic hypotension produces nausea, vomiting, and anxiety. Orthostatic hypotension, tachycardia, dizziness, and syncope may occur. Treatment of intradialytic hypotension includes halting hemodialysis and placing the patient in the Trendelenburg position. If hypotension persists, the patient is given salt by mouth (broth) or normal saline, 100 to 200 mL IV. If these conservative measures fail, a more extensive evaluation is the next step.

When the patient is transferred to the ED for further evaluation, assess for adequacy of volume status, impairment of cardiac function, pericardial disease, infection, and GI bleeding. Further volume expansion or the administration of vasopressors to support blood pressure may require invasive hemodynamic monitoring in an intensive care setting.

Dialysis disequilibrium is a clinical syndrome occurring at the end of dialysis and is characterized by nausea, vomiting, and hypertension, which can progress to seizure, coma, and death. Dialysis disequilibrium occurs when large solute clearances occur during hemodialysis, as during the patient's first dialysis session or during hypercatabolic states. The cause of dialysis disequilibrium is believed to be cerebral edema from an osmolar imbalance between the brain and the blood. During high solute removal, the blood has a transiently lower osmolality than the brain, which favors water movement into the brain and causes cerebral edema. This condition can be prevented by limiting solute clearance when initiating hemodialysis. Treatment is stopping dialysis and administering mannitol IV to increase serum osmolality.

Air embolism is always a risk when blood is pumped through an extracorporeal circuit. The clinical presentation depends on the patient's body position at the time of the incident. If the patient was sitting, air passes retrograde through the internal jugular vein to the cerebral circulation, causing increased intracranial pressure and neurologic symptoms. In a recumbent position, air goes into the right ventricle and pulmonary circulation, causing pulmonary hypertension and systemic hypotension. The passage of air through a right-to-left shunt (e.g., patent foramen ovale) creates an arterial air embolism, which can lodge in the coronary or cerebral circulation, causing myocardial infarction or stroke.

Symptoms of an air embolism are acute dyspnea, chest tightness, and loss of consciousness, and sometimes full cardiac arrest. Signs include cyanosis and a churning sound in the heart from air bubbles in the blood. If air embolism is suspected, **clamp the venous blood line and place the patient supine.** Give 100% oxygen to aid reabsorption of the air. Other therapies for vascular air embolism include percutaneous aspiration of air from the right ventricle, IV administration of steroids, full heparinization, and hyperbaric oxygen treatment.

TABLE 90-4 Key Historical Elements for Hemodialysis Patients

Cause of end-stage renal disease
Dialysis schedule: any missed dialysis sessions?
Recent complications of hemodialysis
Dry weight, baseline laboratory values, and vital sign values
Average intradialytic weight gain
Does patient usually make dry weight by end of hemodialysis?
Does patient experience intradialysis hypotension? (Timing of hypotension?)
Which vascular access is currently functioning?
Symptoms of uremia
Retention of native kidneys?
Still producing urine?

Electrolyte abnormalities can occur due to errors in mixing the dialysate concentrate with water, which results in rapid osmolar shifts and hemolysis. In some communities, water contains high concentrations of calcium and magnesium and produces a final dialysate high in these minerals. Use of this dialysate can result in the "hard water syndrome," characterized by significant hypercalcemia and hypermagnesemia. Patients develop nausea, vomiting, headaches, burning skin, muscle weakness, lethargy, and hypertension. Treatment consists of properly filtering the dialysis water to lower calcium and magnesium concentrations.

Hypoglycemia occurs in diabetic and nondiabetic ESRD patients. In addition to drugs, malnutrition and sepsis are important causes of hypoglycemia.

ED EVALUATION OF HEMODIALYSIS PATIENTS

Patients treated with hemodialysis may develop complications related to ESRD or hemodialysis, or these conditions may be incidental to the reason for the ED visit. The medical history is very important, because many of the same diseases that caused ESRD (e.g., hypertension, diabetes) persist after the patient's kidneys have failed. The patient should be asked about the ESRD and hemodialysis (**Table 90-4**). Repeated episodes of intradialytic hypotension may provide important early clues to pericardial tamponade or myocardial ischemia. Repeated access infections may represent a worsening immunologic status.

Identify the hemodialysis schedule; most patients in the United States are on an every-other-day schedule (Monday, Wednesday, and Friday or Tuesday, Thursday, and Saturday), with each session lasting approximately 4 hours. Certain centers use high-flux hemodialysis machines with higher blood flows, allowing shorter sessions. Note all missed sessions and reasons, allowing identification about medical or social issues that need to be addressed.

Dialysis patients are often knowledgeable about their dry weights and baseline laboratory test results. If not, the center the patient uses should be contacted and asked about the dry weight, average interdialytic weight gains, and any recent complications. Ask about uremic symptoms as markers of inadequate hemodialysis, and ask if the native kidneys are retained since these can be sources of hypertension, infection, and nephrolithiasis.

Examine the access site (**Table 90-5**), looking for the presence of flow by identifying a bruit and thrill. The classic signs of infection—erythema, swelling, tenderness, and purulent discharge—are often

TABLE 90-5 Key Elements of Physical Examination of Hemodialysis Patients

Vital signs
Vascular access: bruit, thrill, erythema, warmth, swelling, tenderness, discharge, bleeding, Branham sign
Cardiac: signs of heart failure, murmurs, muffled (distant) heart sounds
Neurologic: mental status changes, peripheral neuropathy, asterixis

limited until the infection is far advanced. Look for congestive heart failure, effusion, or high-output fistula-related heart failure; peripheral edema, hepatojugular reflux, and jugular venous distention can be present in both fluid overload and pericardial tamponade. A loud cardiac murmur may just represent increased flow secondary to anemia or the arteriovenous access. Neurologic dysfunction in hemodialysis patients is generally diffuse and nonfocal. Any focal neurologic findings require neuroimaging. Seek GI bleeding with rectal examination and occult blood testing, and obtain Doppler US examination if any question about vascular insufficiency, aneurysm, or pseudoaneurysm exists.

PERITONEAL DIALYSIS

TECHNICAL ASPECTS OF PERITONEAL DIALYSIS

In PD, the peritoneal membrane is the blood–dialysate interface. The amount of ultrafiltration is determined by osmotic pressure differences between the blood and dialysate, which are manipulated by changing the dialysate glucose concentration. Similarly to hemodialysis, PD relies on the separate processes of clearance (solute removal) and ultrafiltration (fluid removal) to replace the functions of the nephron. Most solute removal occurs via diffusion down chemical gradients established by altering dialysate electrolyte concentrations. Dialysate is supplied in 1.5% and 4.25% glucose formulations, which can be alternated to increase or decrease ultrafiltration.

Typical PD regimens use four exchanges daily, with 2 L of dialysate infused and left in place for several hours before draining. During the day, approximately 8 L is infused and about 10 L is drained, for a removal of approximately 2 L/d of fluid. PD can be accomplished in an acute setting, over the long term via exchanges of solution throughout the day (continuous ambulatory PD), or through multiple exchanges at night while the patient sleeps (continuous cyclic PD).

COMPLICATIONS OF CONTINUOUS AMBULATORY PERITONEAL DIALYSIS

Peritonitis is the most common complication of PD, with an incidence of about one episode every 15 to 18 patient care-months. Mortality rates from peritonitis range between 2.5% and 12.5%. Symptoms and signs of peritonitis in PD patients are fever, abdominal pain, and rebound tenderness. Cloudy effluent suggests peritonitis, confirmed by Gram stain, cell count, and culture. **The cell count in PD-related peritonitis is usually >100 leukocytes/mm,^{3} with >50% neutrophils.** Results of the Gram staining are positive in only 10% to 40% of cases of culture-proven PD-related peritonitis. Organisms isolated in PD-related peritonitis are *Staphylococcus epidermidis* (approximately 40% of cases), *S. aureus* (10%), *Streptococcus* species (15% to 20%), gram-negative bacteria (15% to 20%), anaerobic bacteria (5%), and fungi (5%).[10]

Empiric therapy begins with a few rapid exchanges of fluid lavaged to decrease the number of inflammatory cells in the peritoneum, with added heparin (500 to 1000 units/L dialysate) to decrease fibrin clot formation. A first-generation cephalosporin (e.g., cephalothin) can be mixed with the dialysate, 500 milligrams/L with the first exchange and 200 milligrams/L with subsequent exchanges. In penicillin-allergic patients, use vancomycin 500 milligrams/L and maintenance doses of 50 milligrams/L per exchange. If seeking gram-negative coverage, add gentamicin 100 milligrams/L and maintenance doses of 4 to 8 milligrams/L per exchange. Most recommend treating for 7 days after the first negative culture results, usually resulting in a total of 10 days of therapy. Admission decisions are based on the patient's clinical appearance. Parenteral antibiotics are not used.

Infections around a PD catheter present with pain, erythema, swelling, and discharge around the catheter exit site. The most common causative bacteria are *S. aureus* and *Pseudomonas aeruginosa*. Empiric therapy consists of an oral first-generation cephalosporin or ciprofloxacin for outpatient therapy. Refer patients to their continuous ambulatory PD centers for follow-up the next day.

TABLE 90-6 Key Historical Elements for Peritoneal Dialysis Patients

Cause of end-stage renal disease
Type of peritoneal dialysis (continuous ambulatory peritoneal dialysis vs continuous cyclic peritoneal dialysis)
Peritoneal dialysis parameters: concentration, number of exchanges per day
Recent complications of peritoneal dialysis
Baseline weight, laboratory values, and vital sign values
Symptoms of uremia
Retention of native kidneys?
Still producing urine?

TABLE 90-7 Key Elements of Physical Examination of Peritoneal Dialysis Patients

Abdominal examination: inspection for hernia, auscultation of bowel sounds, test for rebound tenderness
Peritoneal catheter: examination of surrounding skin, palpation of tunnel

Abdominal wall hernias occur in 10% to 15% of PD patients. Immediate surgical repair of pericatheter hernias is common because of the high risk of incarceration.

ED EVALUATION OF PERITONEAL DIALYSIS PATIENTS

Table 90-6 lists important elements of patient history for PD patients. As with hemodialysis patients, the disease that caused the renal failure frequently persists.

The physical examination focuses on the abdomen: signs of infection of the peritoneum, tunnel, and exit site should be identified (**Table 90-7**).

REFERENCES

The complete reference list is available online at www.TintinalliEM.com.

CHAPTER 91 Urinary Tract Infections and Hematuria

Kim Askew

URINARY TRACT INFECTIONS

In 2010, urinary tract infection (UTI) was the sixth most common diagnosis in women age 15 to 64 years and the fourth most common diagnosis in women age 65 years and older presenting to the ED.[1] The self-reported annual incidence of UTI in women is 12%, and by the age of 32 years, half of all women report having had at least one UTI. Although younger women are more likely to be affected than men by a ratio of 35:1, the gender gap decreases to 2:1 by age 66, most likely due to prostatic hypertrophy and need for instrumentation in elderly men.[2] All age groups from neonates to the elderly are affected, carrying risks in special populations.[3] (See chapters 132, "Urinary Tract Infection in Infants and Children" and 99, "Comorbid Diseases in Pregnancy").

PATHOPHYSIOLOGY AND DEFINITIONS

UTIs can be grouped based on the anatomic site involved as well as patient characteristics. These classifications are important when determining treatment modalities.

ASYMPTOMATIC BACTERIURIA

Asymptomatic bacteriuria is the presence of >100,000 (>10^5) colony-forming units (CFU)/mL of a single pathogen on two successive urine cultures in a patient without symptoms.[4]

Prevalence of asymptomatic bacteriuria is up to 10% in pregnant woman, 40% in male and 50% in female residents of nursing homes, and up to 100% in patients with indwelling catheters for more than 1 month. There is evidence to suggest that asymptomatic bacteriuria may provide some protection against symptomatic infection with invasive organisms in patients with indwelling catheters[5] and in patients with recurrent UTIs.[6] Treatment of asymptomatic bacteriuria is recommended only in pregnant woman (see chapter 99) and in patients immediately prior to invasive urinary procedures.[4]

URETHRITIS AND CYSTITIS

Infections of the lower urinary tract include urethritis and cystitis. *Acute cystitis* is an infection isolated to the bladder. Acute cystitis without coexisting pyelonephritis in otherwise healthy, nonpregnant young females with no obstruction is a benign illness with a 24% spontaneous cure rate; less than 1% of patients go on to develop pyelonephritis.[7] Competent ureteral valves prevent ascent of the bacteria into the kidneys in most cases. The diagnostic criterion in acutely symptomatic patients is a positive urine culture of ≥10^2 to >10^3 CFU/mL.[8] *Urethritis,* commonly associated with sexually transmitted diseases, presents with similar symptoms but typically is associated with a vaginal discharge or irritation.

PYELONEPHRITIS

Pyelonephritis is an infection of the upper urinary tract. *Acute pyelonephritis* involves the renal parenchymal and pelvicalyceal system. Pyelonephritis is differentiated from cystitis primarily by clinical findings: a syndrome of flank pain or costovertebral angle tenderness, with or without fever, in the setting of a positive urine culture of 10^5 CFU/mL, and frequently other systemic symptoms such as nausea or vomiting. Infections of the upper urinary tract can progress into three patterns of renal infection not commonly considered part of the UTI spectrum: acute bacterial nephritis, renal abscess, and emphysematous pyelonephritis. These diagnoses are made based on imaging studies performed in patients who have an inadequate or atypical response to treatment for presumed acute pyelonephritis.

UNCOMPLICATED URINARY TRACT INFECTION

***Uncomplicated UTI* is a UTI in a patient without structural or functional abnormalities within the urinary tract or kidney parenchyma, without relevant comorbidities that place the patient at risk for more serious adverse outcome, and not associated with GU tract instrumentation.**[9,10] This classification is thus limited to young, healthy, nonpregnant women with normal anatomic and functioning urinary tracts. Women are more susceptible than men to UTI due to a shorter urethra for uropathogenic bacteria to ascend. The traditional diagnostic criterion dating from 1960 had been a positive urine culture of 10^5 CFU/mL; however, in symptomatic patients, low-colony-count infections with ≥10^2 to 10^3 CFU/mL are clinically valid.[8-10]

COMPLICATED URINARY TRACT INFECTION

***Complicated UTI* is infection involving a functional or anatomically abnormal urinary tract or infection in the presence of comorbidities that place the patient at risk for more serious adverse outcomes.**[11] Risk factors for complicated UTI, including UTI in males, are listed in **Table 91-1**.[9] The diagnostic criterion is the isolation of 10^5 CFU/mL of urine culture. Unfortunately, patients with complicated UTIs are a very heterogeneous group, and few clinical trials have been conducted to guide management. In general, patients in this group are more likely to be infected with resistant organisms.[11] Although older literature categorized pyelonephritis as a complicated UTI, current guidelines do not.[10-12] *Uncomplicated pyelonephritis* refers to the clinical syndrome of fever and flank pain or tenderness with or without vomiting in a patient with an anatomically normal urinary tract without comorbidities. However, the recommended management of patients with uncomplicated pyelonephritis is similar to recommendations for patients with complicated UTI and differs from the management of patients with uncomplicated cystitis (see "Treatment" later in the chapter).

TABLE 91-1 Risk Factors for Complicated Urinary Tract Infection (UTI)

Risk Factor	Comments
Male sex	In young males, dysuria is more commonly secondary to sexually transmitted disease; suspect underlying anatomic abnormality in men with culture-proven UTI.
Anatomic abnormality of the urinary tract or external drainage system	Indwelling urinary catheter, ureteral stent, nephrolithiasis, neurogenic bladder, polycystic renal disease, or recent urinary tract instrumentation.
Recurrent UTI plus additional risk factor(s)	Recurrent UTI is common in patients with anatomic or functional abnormalities of the urinary tract; however, recurrent infection alone is not a criterion for complicated UTI.
Advanced age in men	Presence of prostatic hyperplasia, recent instrumentation, or recent prostatic biopsy.
Nursing home residency	With or without indwelling bladder catheter.
Neonatal state	See chapter 132.
Comorbidities	Diabetes mellitus, sickle cell disease, others.
Pregnancy	See chapter 99.
Immunosuppression	Active chemotherapy, acquired immunodeficiency syndrome, immunosuppressive drugs.
Advanced neurologic disease	Spinal cord injuries, stroke with disability, others.
Known or suspected atypical pathogens	Non–*Escherichia coli* infections.
Known or suspected resistance to typical antimicrobial agents for UTI	Resistance to ciprofloxacin predicts multidrug resistance.

RECURRENT URINARY TRACT INFECTION

Recurrent UTI is defined as two uncomplicated UTIs in 6 months or three or more uncomplicated UTIs in the preceding 12 months.[13,14] Recurrent UTIs can be classified into two different categories that affect treatment decisions: relapse and reinfection. **Relapse of UTI is a recurrence of a UTI within 2 weeks of treatment completion caused by the same organism** from a focus within the urinary system, and represents treatment failure. **Reinfection is a recurrent UTI caused by a different bacterial isolate** or by the previously isolated bacteria after a negative intervening culture or a period of 2 weeks between infections.[13] Reinfection is more common than relapse. Behavioral factors can lead to increased risk for uncomplicated UTIs. The concentration of bacteria in the female bladder may increase 10-fold after sexual intercourse, whereas the use of a diaphragm and spermicide is also associated with recurrent UTI, probably because the spermicide enhances vaginal colonization with *Escherichia coli.*[15]

MICROBIOLOGY

UTIs typically arise from ascending infection from the urethra to the bladder, although hematogenous and lymphatic spread can occur. Uropathogenic organisms often have adhesins, fibrillae, or pili that allow the bacteria to adhere to and invade the uroepithelium.[15,16] *E. coli* remains the most common pathogen by a large margin (**Table 91-2**).

First reported in 1983, but with an increase since 2000,[17] community-acquired extended-spectrum β-lactamase–producing *E. coli* has emerged as a small but growing source of antibiotic resistance, affecting approximately 4% to 6% of outpatients with UTI.[17,18] Emergence of this resistant isolate of *E. coli* has important implications for treatment (see

TABLE 91-2 Etiologic Agents in Uncomplicated Urinary Tract Infection

Organism	Incidence (%)
Escherichia coli	>80
Klebsiella species	5–20
Proteus species	
Enterobacter species	
Pseudomonas species	
*Chlamydia trachomatis**	<5
*Staphylococcus saprophyticus**	
Mycobacterium tuberculosis (in human immunodeficiency virus infection)	

*Much more common in the "dysuria-pyuria" syndrome in which sterile or low-colony-count culture results are obtained. *S. saprophyticus* may account for up to 15% of acute lower tract infections in young, sexually active females, but rarely progresses to involve the upper tract.

"Treatment" later in the chapter)[19] and can increase mortality in those affected.[20]

Several anatomic, genetic, and age-related factors increase risks for bacterial invasion of the urinary tract. Select women have specific uroepithelial cell *E. coli*–binding glycolipids that promote fecal coliform colonization of the vagina.[2] In postmenopausal women, decreased estrogen has been associated with a conversion of vaginal flora from lactobacillus to *E. coli* and other Enterobacteriaceae.[2] Incomplete bladder emptying disrupts the bladder's ability to eradicate bacteria from its mucosal surface, increasing its susceptibility to infection, especially in patients with neurogenic bladder, women with uterine prolapse, and men with prostate hypertrophy.

CLINICAL FEATURES

Clinical features of UTI vary by anatomic site involved and the patient's risks for complicated UTI. Asymptomatic bacteriuria is a laboratory-based diagnosis (see "Pathophysiology and Definitions" discussed earlier).

URETHRITIS

In males, dysuria with a urethral discharge indicates urethritis (see chapter 149, "Sexually Transmitted Infections"). UTI is uncommon in healthy young adult males, but if the clinical diagnosis does not suggest urethritis or prostatitis in a male with dysuria, bacteriuria is likely due to UTI. In women, *Chlamydia* infection should be suspected in the following settings: a new sexual partner, a partner with urethritis, examination findings of cervicitis, or low-grade pyuria with no bacteria seen on urinalysis. Concurrent gonorrhea is common with *Chlamydia* infections.

CYSTITIS

Symptoms and signs of cystitis are frequency, urgency, hesitancy, suprapubic pain, visible (gross) hematuria, and/or suprapubic tenderness. The nature and severity of symptoms are determined by the etiologic organism(s), the portions of the urinary tract involved, and the patient's ability to mount an immune and inflammatory response.[12] **A history of vaginal discharge or irritation is more often associated with vaginitis, cervicitis, or pelvic inflammatory disease than with UTI.** Fever is uncommon with simple cystitis.

PYELONEPHRITIS

Flank pain, costovertebral angle tenderness, or specific renal tenderness to deep palpation may be associated with cystitis because of referred pain. However, when these findings occur, especially in association with fever, chills, nausea, vomiting, or prostration, the clinical diagnosis is *acute pyelonephritis*. Patients with pyelonephritis may or may not have coexistent symptoms of cystitis. The presentation of pyelonephritis may be subtle, and it might be difficult to distinguish lower from upper UTI, especially in patients who do not experience pain normally (those with spinal cord injury), immunocompromised patients, and the aged. A missed diagnosis of cystitis is unlikely to lead to patient deterioration[7,9]; in contrast, missed pyelonephritis could lead to untreated sepsis.

UROSEPSIS

Patients with urosepsis may or may not exhibit the symptoms listed above for cystitis or pyelonephritis. As graded by the European Section for Infections in Urology,[10,21] simple urosepsis presents with temperature change (>38°C or <36°C), rising heart rate (>90 beats/min), elevated respiratory rate (>20 breaths/min), and commonly leukocytosis. Severe urosepsis includes hypotension, and/or organ dysfunction, and/or hypoperfusion as evidenced by lactic acidosis, oliguria, or acute altered mental status. Uroseptic shock adds the criteria of hypotension or ongoing evidence of hypoperfusion despite adequate fluid resuscitation (see chapter 150, "Toxic Shock Syndromes").

COMPLICATED URINARY TRACT INFECTION

For patients at risk for complicated UTI (Table 91-1), the clinical features and the classic presenting signs and symptoms of UTI may vary widely or be entirely absent. Fever, pain, and an inflammatory response may be absent. Suspect UTI in more complicated cases involving patients with atypical and diverse signs and symptoms, including weakness, malaise, altered mental status, fever, and flank or abdominal pain. Guidelines suggest the following criteria be used to define symptomatic catheter-associated UTI: new onset or worsening of fever, rigors, altered mental status, malaise, or lethargy with no other identified cause; flank pain; costovertebral angle tenderness; acute hematuria; pelvic discomfort; and in those whose catheters have been removed, dysuria, urgent or frequent urination, or suprapubic pain or tenderness.[22,23] In patients with spinal cord injury, increased spasticity, autonomic dysreflexia, and sense of unease are also compatible with catheter-associated UTI.[22]

DIAGNOSIS

A definitive diagnosis of UTI combines appropriate historical findings with laboratory confirmation.[9,24] However, a clinical diagnosis of acute uncomplicated cystitis can be made with a moderate probability based on a history of dysuria, frequency, and urgency, in the absence of vaginal discharge or irritation, in women who have no other risk factors for complicated UTIs.[10] However, the false-positive rate for the diagnosis of UTI based on history alone has been reported to be 33% in outpatients[24,25] and as high as 43% in ED patients. Although empiric treatment of uncomplicated cystitis based on history alone in select women continues to be advocated by some experts,[10] three systematic reviews do not recommend history-based diagnosis due to inaccuracy,[26-28] and other authors advocate laboratory confirmation to reduce the growing problem of antibiotic resistance.[19,29,30]

URINALYSIS

The *clean-catch, midstream voiding specimen* is as accurate as urine obtained by catheterization if the patient follows instructions carefully. If the sample is properly collected, it should contain no or few epithelial cells. **Bacteria in urine double each hour at room temperature, so urine should be refrigerated if not sent directly to the laboratory.** Catheterization is indicated if the patient cannot void spontaneously, is too ill or immobilized, or is extremely obese. **Avoid unnecessary catheterization, because 1% to 2% of patients develop a UTI after a single catheter insertion.**

Visual inspection or assessment of the odor of the urine is generally not helpful in determining infection because cloudiness and odor are caused by noninfectious etiologies. **Table 91-3** lists normal reference values for urinalysis. UTI often results in positive dipstick test for protein in the urine, but this finding is not specific enough to be useful in diagnostic decision making to rule in infection.

Values for individual laboratories may differ from the listed norms in Table 91-3. Dipstick testing is performed on a fresh uncentrifuged urine specimen and is quick and easy to perform at the bedside. Urine for

TABLE 91-3 Normal Urinalysis Results

Value	Normal Range	Specimen Type
RBCs, female	0–5/HPF	Centrifuged specimen
RBCs, male	0–3/HPF	Centrifuged specimen
WBCs	0–4/HPF	Centrifuged specimen
Bacteria	None/HPF	Centrifuged specimen
Leukocyte esterase	None—dipstick test	Fresh urine
Nitrite	None—dipstick test	Fresh urine

Abbreviations: HPF = high-power field; RBCs = red blood cells.

microscopic analysis is routinely centrifuged prior to analysis. If examination of uncentrifuged urine is desired, make a specific request to the laboratory to account for different normal values between centrifuged and uncentrifuged specimens.

NITRITE REACTION BY DIPSTICK TEST

The urine nitrite reaction has a very high specificity (>90%), and a positive result is very useful in confirming the diagnosis of a UTI caused by bacteria that convert nitrates to nitrite, primarily the coliform bacteria, including *E. coli*. ***Enterococcus*, *Pseudomonas*, and *Acinetobacter* species do not convert nitrates to nitrites in the urine and therefore are not detected by the nitrite test.** Unfortunately the urine nitrite reaction has a low sensitivity (~50%), so it is not always useful as a screening examination because a negative result does not exclude the diagnosis of UTI.

LEUKOCYTE ESTERASE REACTION BY DIPSTICK TEST

Using positive culture results as the criterion standard, the leukocyte esterase urine dipstick test has an overall sensitivity of 48% to 86% and a specificity of 17% to 93% for identifying infection. Performance varies by clinical setting. In the ED, using culture findings of 10^5 CFU/mL as the criterion, a positive leukocyte esterase reaction result has a sensitivity of 77% and a specificity of 54%. The sensitivity of positive leukocyte esterase reaction result for detecting infection decreases for specimens with less bacterial growth at culture, ranging from a sensitivity of 79.5% when culture growth is $>10^5$ CFU/mL to 50.4% when culture growth is 10^3 CFU/mL. Therefore, if the clinician uses a lower culture threshold to define infection, the leukocyte esterase test performs with lower sensitivity to detect infection. **In summary, a positive urinary dipstick nitrite or leukocyte esterase test result supports the diagnosis of UTI, but a negative test result does not exclude it.**

URINE WBC COUNT OR PYURIA BY MICROSCOPY

The assessment of pyuria using standard centrifuged urine is imperfect due to variable specimen preparation techniques. A WBC count of >5 cells/high-power field (HPF) in a centrifuged specimen from a symptomatic patient is abnormal. Although the combination of pyuria and bacteriuria is likely to be found with typical coliform infection, lower degrees of pyuria with or without bacteriuria may be clinically significant, especially in the presence of UTI symptoms.

In a symptomatic patient who has <5 WBCs/HPF in a centrifuged specimen, other causes of false-negative pyuria should be considered such as dilute precentrifuged urine, systemic leukopenia, or patient self-treatment with leftover antibiotics. Pyuria may be intermittent or absent if the patient has an obstructed and infected kidney. **In men, >1 or 2 WBCs/HPF in a centrifuged specimen can be significant when bacteria are present.** Urethritis and prostatitis are far more likely causes of pyuria in young males who are sexually active and complain of dysuria, regardless of the presence or absence of urethral discharge.

BACTERIURIA BY MICROSCOPY

Bacteriuria is a sensitive tool for detection of UTI in the symptomatic patient. **The presence of any bacteria on a Gram-stained specimen of uncentrifuged urine (>1 bacterium/HPF or 1000×) is significant and highly correlates with culture results of $>10^5$ CFU/mL.** For Gram-stained centrifuged specimens, >1 bacterium/HPF (1000×) is 95% sensitive and >60% specific to predict a culture with 10^4 CFU/mL. Both of these methods of looking for bacteria under the microscope fail to detect low-colony-count UTI or infection caused by *Chlamydia*. False-positive results can occur when vaginal or fecal contamination is present. Female patients with symptoms suggestive of UTI *and* vaginal discharge or dyspareunia should have a pelvic examination to investigate for pelvic inflammatory disease.

COMBINED RESULTS OF DIPSTICK TESTING, URINE CELL COUNTS, AND HISTORICAL INFORMATION

Two meta-analyses found that classic historical findings of cystitis were weak predictors of positive culture or failed to predict cystitis.[27,28] Vaginal discharge weakly decreased the likelihood of cystitis; however, in both studies, diagnostic accuracy was significantly improved using dipstick testing, particularly a positive test for nitrites.[27,28] A 2013 systematic review of four ED-based studies pooled 948 patients using a reference culture threshold of 10^4 to 10^5 CFU/mL and found that no single historical variable of cystitis could rule in or rule out infection, but a dipstick test positive for nitrates, moderate pyuria, and/or bacteriuria were accurate predictors of a UTI,[26] effectively ruling in the diagnosis of UTI. However, **no single test or combination of testing results can effectively rule out UTI in women presenting to the ED with symptoms of cystitis.** Therefore, there will be a subset of women for whom test results are equivocal who should either be treated empirically or receive phone-in treatment based on culture, if follow-up cannot be assured in 2 to 3 days.

URINE AND BLOOD CULTURE

For the patient with typical symptoms of *cystitis* or an *uncomplicated UTI* and "positive" findings on urinalysis—pyuria on microscopic examination, bacteria in a Gram-stained specimen, positive leukocyte esterase test result, and/or positive urine nitrite test result—urine culture is not required. The vast majority of patients respond to empiric therapy. Urine culture should be performed for the following patients: those with complicated UTI, pregnant women, adult males, patients with relapse or reinfection, and septic patients. If the patient is symptomatic, a single positive culture result is significant.

Results of blood cultures in patients admitted for clinical pyelonephritis are positive in 25% to 29% of cases; organisms in blood culture match those in urine culture in 97% of cases, and blood culture results usually do not alter management. The primary indication for blood cultures in patients with suspected UTI is clinical sepsis.

IMAGING

Renal imaging studies are not indicated in otherwise healthy patients with acute pyelonephritis who can be managed as outpatients. Male, elderly, diabetic, or severely ill patients with acute pyelonephritis should be considered for imaging, particularly if there is a renal stone or a poor initial response to antibiotic therapy. The kidneys can be imaged with bedside US to evaluate for obstruction and focal parenchymal abnormalities. Plain film radiography and US have poor sensitivity for detection of intrarenal gas formation in emphysematous pyelonephritis. If kidney or ureteral stones or emphysematous pyelonephritis are suspected, CT is the best imaging modality.[9]

Table 91-4 lists the differential diagnoses for dysuria.

TREATMENT

ACUTE CYSTITIS AND UNCOMPLICATED URINARY TRACT INFECTION

Selection of antibiotics depends on the organism suspected of causing the infection, the patient's ability to adhere to the treatment regimen, local resistance patterns, potential drug toxicity, and cost. The Infectious Disease Society of America and the European Society for Microbiology

TABLE 91-4 Differential Diagnosis for Dysuria

Disorder	Comments
Urinary tract infection	Cystitis and pyelonephritis
Vaginitis/cervicitis	Infections (STD), atrophy, allergy
Urethritis	Infections (STD), allergy
Trauma	Trauma involving vagina, urethra, or bladder
Allergy	Typically a reaction to a hygienic product or spermicide
Bladder/urethral cancer	—
Nephrolithiasis	—
Urethral stricture or obstruction	—
Uterine/bladder/vaginal prolapse	—
Fistulas	Ileovesicular, urethral, urethrorectal, bladder
Urethral foreign body	Includes urethral stone disease
Urethral diverticulum	—
Cystocele	—
Chemical irritation	Spermicides, cleansing douches, feminine hygiene products
Behavioral symptom without detectable pathology	Consider previous rape, sexual abuse
Chronic disorders	Chronic cystitis, chronic urethritis

Abbreviation: STD = sexually transmitted disease.

and Infectious Disease published updated recommendations on antibiotics for uncomplicated UTI in 2010 (**Table 91-5**).[12] Other guidelines have been incorporated.[10]

Table 91-5 contains treatment recommendations for three separate groups of patients with UTI: (1) uncomplicated lower tract disease, (2) complicated UTI or pyelonephritis, and (3) women with UTI symptoms in whom coexistent urethritis cannot be excluded.[10,12]

Three-day regimens are recommended for uncomplicated infections in nonpregnant women.[12] A total of 3 to 6 days of therapy is sufficient for treating uncomplicated UTIs in elderly women; however, patient selection guidelines must be strictly adhered to because most elderly women have comorbidities that exclude them from the classification of "uncomplicated UTI."[31] Trimethoprim-sulfamethoxazole continues to be recommended because it is inexpensive and has limited side effects. Rates of resistance to trimethoprim-sulfamethoxazole are reported to be over the 20% threshold for treatment exclusion in the western and southern United States;[32] however, hospital culture data primarily reflect complicated UTI, and trimethoprim-sulfamethoxazole treatment may be successful for uncomplicated UTI.[33] Fosfomycin has less efficacy than short courses of other regimens. Within regions, local resistance patterns vary widely and change rapidly. Currently, recommendations are to avoid trimethoprim-sulfamethoxazole as the first-line empiric agent of choice when local resistance rate exceeds 20%, unless treating based on the results of urine culture with sensitivity testing.

Nitrofurantoin is indicated for treatment of UTI in pregnancy, although it is not effective against *Staphylococcus saprophyticus*. A 5-day course of extended-release nitrofurantoin is as effective as 3 days of trimethoprim-sulfamethoxazole therapy.[34] A single 3-gram dose of **fosfomycin** is a first-line choice for uncomplicated UTI[12] because the resistance rate is only 2%.[35] Both nitrofurantoin and fosfomycin are recommended oral agents in the event of extended-spectrum β-lactamase–producing *E. coli* infection, because resistance is reported to be only 6% and 3%, respectively.[36]

Because of bacterial resistance to traditional antibiotics used for UTI, use local sensitivities to guide the substitution of alternative agents such as cephalosporins. Third-generation cephalosporins are highly effective against enterobacteria, whereas first-generation cephalosporins are more effective against staphylococci. Amoxicillin-clavulanate is less effective than fluoroquinolones or oral cephalosporins for UTI due to enterobacteria. It also often leads to selection of *Klebsiella*. Aminopenicillins are therefore not recommended as first-line therapy in uncomplicated UTI.

If the patient has UTI symptoms and there is also suspicion of *Chlamydia* or *Neisseria gonorrhoeae* infection (cervicitis and/or salpingitis), antibiotic treatment is more complex. The patient should be tested[37]

TABLE 91-5 Guidelines for Outpatient Management of Urinary Tract Infection (UTI) Including Pyelonephritis

Patient	UTI Type	Antimicrobial Regimens	Culture/Treatment Comments
Adult female	Lower (cystitis) Uncomplicated	Nitrofurantoin monohydrate/macrocrystals, 100 milligrams twice a day × 5 d or TMP-SMX DS (160/800 milligrams), 1 tab twice a day × 3 d or Fosfomycin, 3 grams in single dose *or* (where available) Pivmecillinam, 400 milligrams bid × 5 days (lower efficacy than some other recommended agents; avoid if early pyelonephritis suspected)	No initial culture is required. Consider community resistance; if >20%, use another agent. Amoxicillin-clavulanate, cefpodoxime-proxetil, cefdinir, and cefaclor, in 3- to 7-d regimens are appropriate choices for therapy when other recommended agents cannot be used. The fluoroquinolones should be reserved for important uses other than acute uncomplicated cystitis.
Adult female or male	Lower (cystitis), upper (pyelonephritis) Complicated	Ciprofloxacin, 500 milligrams twice a day × 7 d *or* Levofloxacin, 750 milligrams once a day × 5 d *or* Cefpodoxime, 400 milligrams twice a day × 7–14 d *or* Only if susceptibilities are known, consider: TMP-SMX DS (160/800 milligrams), 1 tab twice a day, 14 d minimum *or* Amoxicillin-clavulanate, 875/125 milligrams twice a day	Urine culture is advised. Consider community resistance; if >20%, use another agent. Coliforms are common. Treat for at least 7 d (mild symptoms) or 14 d (more severe symptoms, clear pyelonephritis). Admit if patient is significantly ill, unable to retain fluids or medications, or pregnant. Consider IV dose of ceftriaxone if sensitivity uncertain.
Adult female	Lower (urethritis)	Ceftriaxone, 250 milligrams IM *plus* Azithromycin, 1 gram single dose *or* Doxycycline, 100 milligrams twice a day × 7 d	Culture for *Chlamydia*, and *Neisseria gonorrhoeae*. Fluoroquinolones no longer recommended for treatment of *N. gonorrhoeae* and *Chlamydia*. Consider adding a regimen listed above for cystitis if coexistent infections are strongly suspected.

Abbreviations: DS = double strength; TMP-SMX = trimethoprim-sulfamethoxazole.

TABLE 91-6 Empiric Initial Treatment for Inpatient Management of Pyelonephritis and Complicated Urinary Tract Infection

Ciprofloxacin, 400 milligrams IV every 12 h
Ceftriaxone, 1–2 grams IV once daily
Cefotaxime, 1–2 grams IV every 8 h
Gentamicin or tobramycin, 3 milligrams/kg/d divided every 8 h, ± ampicillin, 1–2 grams every 4 h
Piperacillin-tazobactam, 3.375 grams IV every 6 h
Cefepime, 1–2 grams IV every 8 h
Ertapenem, 1 gram IV every day
Imipenem, 500 milligrams IV every 8 h
Meropenem, 1 gram IV every 8 h

Note: Alternatives include ceftazidime, 1–2 grams IV every 8–12 h; amikacin, 7.5 milligrams/kg IV loading dose, then 15 milligrams/kg/d or divided dose every 8 h; and others based on local resistance and sensitivity patterns.

and empirically treated[38] for *Chlamydia* and *N. gonorrhoeae* (see Table 91-5; also see chapter 149. Fluoroquinolones were formerly recommended in this setting as a treatment for both cystitis and urethritis, but the Centers for Disease Control and Prevention no longer recommend them due to *N. gonorrhoeae* resistance. If coexistent cystitis is suspected in a patient with clinical urethritis, add a recommended treatment for cystitis (Table 91-5) to the treatment for urethritis; alternatively, culture the urine and treat for cystitis pending results.

ACUTE PYELONEPHRITIS AND COMPLICATED URINARY TRACT INFECTION

Recommendations for antibiotic therapy and cultures for patients whose condition is stable enough for outpatient treatment are listed in Table 91-5. Antibiotics for inpatient management are listed in **Table 91-6.**[10,12,] For patients whose vital signs are unstable, see chapter 150, "Toxic Shock Syndromes." After clinical improvement has been achieved with parenteral antibiotics, treatment should be changed to oral agents as listed in Table 91-5. Patients may require fluid resuscitation with crystalloids to replace fluid losses due to vomiting or sweating. Although treatment courses as short as 5 days have been studied in patients with pyelonephritis and catheter-associated infections,[9,10] guidelines recommend a total of 7 to 14 days of therapy for the majority, regardless of whether or not parenteral therapy is used.[10] Men with UTI without immunocompromise may have improved outcomes with therapy for 7 days, rather than 14 days.[39,40] For patients with sepsis syndrome, a total of 21 days of treatment may be required to eradicate bacteriuria.[10]

RECURRENT INFECTION

Women presenting to the ED with an acute UTI and a history of greater than two UTIs in 6 months or greater than three UTIs in 12 months should be cultured, treated empirically, and referred to a primary care physician in 1 to 2 weeks for repeat culture and possible prophylaxis.[41-43] The patient can be treated with recommended treatments for uncomplicated cystitis from Table 91-5 including 3-day regimins,[41] unless the recurrence is a relapse (see "Pathophysiology and Definitions" discussed earlier). Treat relapse with an alternative agent, such as one of those recommended for complicated UTI (Table 91-5).[41] Prophylaxis may take the form of continuous, postcoital, or intermittent self-treatment during symptomatic episodes.[41-43] Woman with recurrent UTI using spermicide with contraception should be encouraged to inquire about an alternative method of contraception.[41-43]

DISPOSITION AND FOLLOW-UP

The decision to admit a patient with UTI is based on age, host factors, and response to initial ED interventions. Admit patients who are unable to retain fluids and medication or those with systemic signs of UTI and a stone (see chapter 94, "Urologic Stone Disease"), and choose antibiotics as listed in Table 91-6. Eighty-four percent of patients are discharged.[44] Healthy females tolerating fluids and medication with uncomplicated pyelonephritis are candidates for outpatient management.[45] Adjunctive therapies at discharge include increased fluids and frequent voiding to diminish tissue contact with bacteria. An oral bladder analgesic, such as phenazopyridine (200 milligrams PO three times daily), reduces dysuria. Cranberry juice appears to be mildly effective in reducing the incidence of recurrent infection. There is no conclusive evidence that postcoital voiding prevents cystitis.[43] Ask patients to return to the ED if they experience increasing pain, fever, or vomiting. Consider systemic analgesics and antiemetics for patients with pyelonephritis.

Overall, approximately 1% to 3% of patients with acute pyelonephritis die from the infection, with younger patients experiencing the fewest complications. Factors associated with an unfavorable prognosis are advanced age and general debility, renal calculi or obstruction, a history of recent hospitalization or instrumentation, diabetes mellitus, evidence of chronic nephropathy, sickle cell anemia, underlying carcinoma, and immunocompromised state (e.g., chemotherapy, human immunodeficiency virus infection/acquired immunodeficiency syndrome [HIV/AIDS]).

Dangerous complications of acute pyelonephritis include acute papillary necrosis with possible ureter obstruction, septic shock, perinephric abscesses, and emphysematous pyelonephritis.

SPECIAL POPULATIONS

PREGNANCY

See chapter 99 for a detailed discussion.

PATIENTS WITH HUMAN IMMUNODEFICIENCY VIRUS INFECTION/ ACQUIRED IMMUNODEFICIENCY SYNDROME

In HIV/AIDS patients, resistance to TMP-SMX is increased due largely to its use in *Pneumocystis jiroveci* prophylaxis. Fluoroquinolones should be the initial antibiotic used for UTI in these patients unless urine culture and sensitivity test results are available to guide therapy. Most UTIs in HIV/AIDS patients are caused by typical pathogens or common sexually transmitted disease organisms. *Mycobacterium tuberculosis* is an infrequent cause of UTI in the HIV/AIDS population. Close outpatient follow-up (recheck in 1 week) and possible infectious disease consultation are warranted when treating UTI in this population (see chapter 154, "Human Immunodeficiency Virus Infection").

PRACTICE GUIDELINES

The European Association of Urology updates its "Guidelines on Urogenital Infections" yearly.[10] The Infectious Diseases Society of America and the European Society for Microbiology and Infectious Diseases updated its "International Clinical Guidelines for the Treatment of Acute Uncomplicated Cystitis and Pyelonephritis in Women" in 2010.[12] "Complicated Urinary Tract Infection in Adults" guidelines were published by the Canadian Association of Medical Microbiology and Infectious Diseases in 2005.[11]

HEMATURIA

INTRODUCTION AND EPIDEMIOLOGY

Gross hematuria is visible to the eye, whereas microscopic hematuria is a laboratory diagnosis. Other pigments, particularly myoglobin, may discolor the urine and simulate gross hematuria. UTI is the most common cause of hematuria associated with urgency, dysuria, and nocturia[26,27]; however, these symptoms are also common in the much smaller group of patients who ultimately are diagnosed with cancer of the urinary tract.[46,47] Painless hematuria is more often due to neoplastic, hyperplastic, and vascular causes.

It takes approximately 1 mL of whole blood per liter of urine to result in visible hematuria. Gross hematuria may also result in false proteinuria.

The incidence of gross hematuria in the general population and in patients presenting to the ED is unknown. However, gross hematuria is more common in premenopausal women due to UTIs and contamination with menstrual blood.[48] The incidence of bladder cancer associated with gross hematuria rises with increasing age.

The American Urological Association recently redefined *microscopic hematuria* as ≥3 red blood cells (RBCs)/HPF (400×) on a properly collected and centrifuged urinary specimen in the absence of an obvious benign cause,[48] removing the prior American Urological Association requirement for a positive repeat specimen (one of the next two) as part of the definition. Hematuria from malignant causes is frequently intermittent.[48] Normal urine contains a small number of RBCs, usually too few to be detected by routine chemical dipstick testing or microscopic urinalysis. Population-based studies have found at least one episode of transient microscopic hematuria in 4% to 13% of individuals.

PATHOPHYSIOLOGY

Any process that results in infection, inflammation, or injury to the kidneys, ureters, bladder, prostate, male genitalia, or urethra may result in hematuria (**Tables 91-7 and 91-8**).[49]

In men >50 years old, tumors of the prostate or elsewhere in the ejaculatory system and benign prostatic hypertrophy are considerations when hematuria is present. In patients <40 years, common causes are infections and inflammatory conditions, including prostatitis, urethritis, sexually transmitted diseases, epididymo-orchitis, calculi with inflammation, and tuberculosis. Testicular tumors may occur in men younger than 50 years old.

False hematuria occurs when the urine appears bloody but dipstick test results are negative for blood and there are no RBCs on microscopic evaluation, or blood has been added to a previously blood-free specimen by the patient (**Table 91-9**). Free hemoglobin, myoglobin, or porphyrins in the urine result in a positive urine test strip reaction for blood.

CLINICAL FEATURES

A careful history, including information regarding sexual activity, recent urologic procedures, medications used, and HIV and tuberculosis risk factors, should be obtained. The patient's general health and condition, vital signs, abdomen, external genitalia, and prostate in males should be evaluated.

Initial hematuria is the appearance of blood at the beginning of micturition, with subsequent clearing, and suggests urethral disease including cancer. Gross hematuria more often indicates a lower tract cause.[26] In younger patients, microscopic hematuria is most often caused by nephrolithiasis or UTI.[26] In older patients, infections and nephrolithiasis remain common causes of hematuria; however, hematuria in patients >50 years old warrants follow-up because renal, bladder, and prostate cancer increase in frequency and may coexist with UTI or kidney stones.[46,48] Risk factors for uroepithelial cancer are age >50 years, male sex, smoking, family history of bladder cancer, occupational exposures in the chemical, rubber, or leather industries (e.g., exposure to dyes, benzenes, or aromatic amines), and excessive analgesic use.[46] Hematuria in a patient taking oral anticoagulants should not be attributed to the anticoagulant alone, because the incidence of underlying disease is up to 80% in patients referred to urology for evaluation.[46] Expanding abdominal aortic aneurysms may erode into the urogenital tract or cause inflammation or obstruction from direct pressure.

TABLE 91-7 Most Common Causes of Hematuria

Cause	Associated Age
Urinary tract infections	Any age
Nephrolithiasis	Usually >20 years
Neoplasms	Typically >50 years (except Wilms')
Benign prostatic hypertrophy	Males >40 years
Glomerulonephritis*	Mostly young patients and children
Schistosomiasis†	Any—underdeveloped country inhabitant

*See chapter 134, "Renal Emergencies in Children."

†See chapter 161, "Global Travelers."

TABLE 91-8 Differential Diagnosis of Hematuria

Urologic (lower tract)
- **Any location**
  - Iatrogenic/postprocedure
  - Trauma
  - Infection
  - Stones/calculi
  - Erosion or mechanical obstruction by tumor
- **Ureter(s)**
  - Dilatation of stricture
- **Bladder**
  - Transitional cell carcinoma
  - Vascular lesions or malformations
  - Chemical or radiation cystitis
- **Prostate**
  - Benign prostatic hypertrophy
  - Prostatitis
- **Urethra**
  - Stricture
  - Diverticulosis
  - Foreign body
  - Endometriosis (cyclic hematuria with menstrual pain)

Renal (upper tract)
- **Glomerular**
  - Glomerulonephritis
  - Immunoglobulin A nephropathy (Berger's disease)
  - Lupus nephritis
  - Hereditary nephritis (Alport's syndrome)
  - Toxemia of pregnancy
  - Serum sickness
  - Erythema multiforme
- **Nonglomerular**
  - Interstitial nephritis
  - Pyelonephritis
  - Papillary necrosis: sickle cell disease, diabetes, NSAID use
  - Vascular: arteriovenous malformations, emboli, aortocaval fistula
  - Malignancy
  - Polycystic kidney disease
  - Medullary sponge disease
  - Tuberculosis
  - Renal trauma

Hematologic
- Primary coagulopathy (e.g., hemophilia)
- Pharmacologic anticoagulation
- Sickle cell disease

Miscellaneous
- Eroding abdominal aortic aneurysm
- Malignant hypertension
- Loin pain–hematuria syndrome
- Renal vein thrombosis
- Exercise-induced hematuria
- Cantharidin (Spanish fly) poisoning
- Bites or stings by insects and reptiles having venom with anticoagulant properties

Abbreviation: NSAID = nonsteroidal anti-inflammatory drug.

TABLE 91-9 Causes of False Hematuria on Visual Inspection

Munchausen's syndrome, malingering, drug seeking
Patients may add blood to voided urine for secondary gain
Medications
NSAIDs, phenytoin, phenothiazines, quinine, rifampin, sulfasalazine, others
Foods and dyes
Beets, berries, rhubarb
Serratia marcescens infection
Amorphous urates
Hemoglobinuria, myoglobinuria, porphyrins

Abbreviation: NSAID = nonsteroidal anti-inflammatory drug.

Malignant hypertension, embolic renal infarction, and renal vein thrombosis are other serious diagnoses that can cause hematuria. In pregnancy, hematuria can be associated with UTI, nephrolithiasis, or pre-eclampsia. Recent instrumentation of the urinary tract may produce hematuria.

The reported incidence of hematuria in HIV-infected patients is 18% to 50%. Causes include UTI, chlamydial and gonococcal urethritis, glomerulonephritis, neurogenic bladder, thrombocytopenia, subclinical uroepithelial Kaposi's sarcoma, and urethral trauma. However, in up to 80% of patients, no specific cause is found.

The physical examination should note the vital signs and the patient's appearance. Hypertension and edema imply nephrotic syndrome. A new heart murmur (endocarditis) or atrial fibrillation increases the likelihood of embolic disease and renal infarction. A full genital-urinary examination is essential for both males and females. Systemic signs need to be correlated to potential diseases that cause hematuria (Table 91-8).

DIAGNOSIS

Potential causes of hematuria are often suggested by considering the patient's age, sex, demographic characteristics, habits, potential risk factors, history of recent GU instrumentation, and comorbidities.[48]

LABORATORY TESTING

A clean-catch midstream urine collection is appropriate for most patients. Catheter-collected specimens are recommended for women with a vaginal discharge or menstrual or vaginal bleeding; however, urethral catheterization induces hematuria in 15% of patients. Brown or smoke-colored urine, along with dysmorphic RBCs, cellular casts, and proteinuria, suggests a glomerular source.[48] Red, clotted blood in the urine indicates a source below the kidneys.

A urine dipstick test for blood can detect as little as 150 micrograms/L of free hemoglobin, corresponding to 5 to 20 intact RBCs/mL on microscopic analysis. False-negative results may be obtained with urine dipstick tests for blood if the urine has a high concentration of ascorbic acid (>5 milligrams/dL) or a high specific gravity. False-positive results occur in the presence of free hemoglobin, myoglobin, or porphyrins.

For patients with a clinical picture that does not provide a clear cause of hematuria on dipstick analysis (or indication for an urgent evaluation), urinalysis with microscopy should be performed to confirm hematuria before further work-up.[48] Hemorrhagic cystitis with invasive infection of the bladder wall by bacteria resulting in shedding and bleeding is a common cause of hematuria and resolves with appropriate antibiotic treatment.

For patients taking anticoagulants, obtain appropriate coagulation studies in the ED, with imaging at follow-up for older patients to exclude malignancy.

The finding of normal RBCs on microscopic examination of the urine together with bacteriuria and leukocytes in a young healthy patient supports UTI as the probable cause of hematuria. Additional laboratory studies may be needed depending on the results of the history, physical examination, and presumptive differential diagnosis. The presence of normal RBCs without evidence of infection should prompt further urologic evaluation to determine the site of bleeding; however, in stable patients without an urgent cause suggested by history and physical examination, an outpatient evaluation is appropriate.

TABLE 91-10 Risk Factors for Significant Disease in Patients with Microscopic Hematuria

Age >50 y
Male sex
History of gross hematuria
Smoking history
Occupational exposure to chemicals or dyes (benzenes or aromatic amines)
Analgesic abuse
History of pelvic irradiation
Cyclophosphamide use
Pregnancy
Known malignancy
Sickle cell disease
Renal insufficiency

IMAGING

Initial upper and lower urinary tract imaging for hematuria is now typically done with noncontrast helical CT or renal US.[48,50] Helical CT clearly delineates most renal tumors, obstructions, or stones and their precise location.[48,50]

Renal US is useful when screening for obstruction, hydronephrosis, or abdominal aortic aneurysm. It is the study of choice in pregnant patients with suspected nephrolithiasis. However, renal US rarely identifies or locates stones in the ureters that are not large enough to give findings of obstruction. Renal US also does not provide any assessment of renal function—normal enhancement and excretion of contrast by both kidneys. Helical CT with contrast provides this important information.

Gross hematuria in patients with blunt or penetrating trauma to the abdomen, flank, or back warrants an aggressive approach to identify the source of bleeding and to guide management (see chapter 265, "Genitourinary Trauma").[48]

TREATMENT, DISPOSITION, AND FOLLOW-UP

Treatment of hematuria is directed at the cause (Tables 91-7 and 91-8). Outpatient management and referral for follow-up are appropriate for patients in hemodynamically stable condition without an apparent life-threatening cause of the hematuria. The urgency for follow-up depends on the presence of gross hematuria or risk factors for significant disease (**Table 91-10**).[48,50] Patients with gross hematuria or listed significant risk factors should ideally be reevaluated at follow-up within 2 weeks.

The American Urological Association guideline recommends referral to urology to assess for urinary tract malignancy in all patients with microscopic hematuria without an obvious benign cause.[48] Follow-up within 1 month is acceptable for patients with microscopic hematuria without significant risk factors.

Gross hematuria may lead to intravesical clot formation and bladder outlet obstruction. See chapter 92, "Acute Urinary Retention" for management.

Patients with intractable pain, intolerance of oral fluids and medications, significant comorbid illness, bladder outlet obstruction, evidence of hemodynamic instability, or possible life-threatening causes of hematuria should be admitted, and the appropriate specialist should be consulted.

PRACTICE GUIDELINES

Practice guidelines include those from the American Urological Association.[48]

REFERENCES

The complete reference list is available online at www.TintinalliEM.com.

CHAPTER 92

Acute Urinary Retention

David Hung-Tsang Yen
Chen-Hsen Lee

INTRODUCTION AND EPIDEMIOLOGY

Acute urinary retention is a common painful urologic emergency characterized by a sudden inability to pass urine, with lower abdominal distention or pain. Most patients with urinary retention are elderly men with benign prostatic hyperplasia.[1,2] The incidence and risk increase with age. There is a 20% recurrence within 6 months after an episode of urinary retention.[2] Few data are available for women. In men with spontaneous urinary retention, the mortality rate at 1 year increases from 4.1% in patients age 45 to 54 years to 32.8% in those age 85 years and older.[3]

PATHOPHYSIOLOGY

The voiding process, or micturition, involves the complex integration and coordination of high cortical neurologic (sympathetic, parasympathetic, and somatic) and muscular (detrusor and sphincter smooth muscle) functions. As the sensory impulse of bladder distention transmits to cortical centers, these areas of the brain smoothly coordinate voluntary urination. Continent urine storage in the bladder requires both relaxation of the detrusor muscle (through β-adrenergic stimulation and parasympathetic inhibition) and contraction of the bladder neck and internal sphincter (through α-adrenergic stimulation). The contraction of bladder detrusor muscle (by cholinergic muscarinic receptors) and relaxation of both the internal sphincter of bladder neck and the urethral sphincter (through α-adrenergic inhibition) contribute to smooth urination.[6]

Any causes that interfere with the neurologic control of the voiding process can result in voiding dysfunction. Urinary retention is the inability to void voluntarily despite a distended bladder and results from the dysfunction of the detrusor muscle and its coordination with the control of the bladder outlet. As bladder outlet obstruction progressively increases, the urine stream decreases in strength and size despite forceful and prolonged detrusor contraction. In chronic decompensation of urination, diminished detrusor muscle contractility is more pronounced, with a large amount of residual urine volume, compared to acute decompensation.

CLINICAL FEATURES

The causes of urinary retention (**Tables 92-1** to **92-3**) are categorized into several domains: obstructive, neurogenic, traumatic, infectious, operative, psychogenic, childhood, extraurinary, and pharmacologic.[4-7] A detailed history of the present illness and physical examination, especially the neurologic examination, supported by imaging and urodynamic studies, reveal the cause in the majority of patients.

The most common presentation is an elderly male with inability to void for several hours and lower abdominal distention or pain, secondary to benign prostatic hyperplasia.

TABLE 92-1 Gender-Specific Causes of Acute Urinary Obstruction

Men	Women
Obstructive Causes	**Obstructive Causes**
Benign prostatic hypertrophy*	Cystocele
Prostate cancer	Ovarian tumor
Phimosis	Uterine tumor
Paraphimosis	**Operative Causes**
Meatal stenosis	Incontinence surgery
Urethral strangulation	**Infectious Causes**
Infectious Causes	Pelvic inflammatory disease
Prostatitis	

*Most common cause.

TABLE 92-2 Causes of Acute Urinary Retention in Both Sexes

Obstructive Causes	**Extraurinary Causes**
Urethral stricture	Perirectal or pelvic abscesses
Bladder calculi	Rectal or retroperitoneal masses
Bladder neoplasm	Fecal impaction
Foreign body, urethral or bladder	Abdominal aortic aneurysm
Neurogenic Causes	**Psychogenic Causes**
Multiple sclerosis	Psychosexual stress
Parkinson's disease	Acute anxiety
Shy-Drager syndrome	**Infectious Causes**
Brain tumors	Cystitis
Cerebral vascular disease	Herpes simplex (genital)
Cauda equina syndrome	Herpes zoster involving pelvic region
Metastatic spinal cord lesions	Local abscess
Intervertebral disk herniation	**Operative Causes**
Neuropathy (diabetes, other causes)	Postoperative bleeding (clots)
Nerve injury from pelvic surgery	Epidural anesthesia
Postoperative retention	**Childhood Causes**
Traumatic Causes	Posterior urethral valves
Urethral injury	Rhabdomyosarcoma of the bladder
Bladder injury	Urethral atresia
Spinal cord injury	**Pharmacologic Agents (Table 92-3)**

Collect past medical history to look for a history of prostatism, prostate or urinary bladder cancer, bladder calculi, indwelling urethral catheter or injury to urethra, prostate surgery, or pelvic radiation therapy. Ask about history of urinary urgency, frequency, or hesitancy; decreased force and caliber of stream; terminal dribbling; nocturia; and incontinence (typically due to overflow phenomena). Gross hematuria may indicate infection, bladder calculi, or urinary tract neoplasm. A patient with urethral stricture may have a history of Foley catheter insertion, cystoscopy, trauma, or previous radiation therapy or infection. Collect any history of new medications, including common cold preparations, anticholinergics (including bronchodilators), sympathomimetic agents, and psychogenic and other potential agents (Table 92-3). Obtain a detailed neurologic history, looking for a causative lesion from high cortical function down to peripheral nerves that determine end-organ function. Identify possible spinal cord injury by determining recent activities including any remote trauma.

Fever, tachycardia, tachypnea, and hypotension suggest infection or sepsis. Hypertension or tachycardia may be transient and may resolve after bladder decompression. Consider urinary retention in patients complaining of lower abdominal pain, even if they do not offer urinary complaints. On abdominal examination, palpitate or percuss from the epigastric area to the lower abdomen to identify a painful mass (distended

TABLE 92-3 Pharmacologic Agents Associated with Urinary Retention

α-Adrenergic agents	Carbamazepine
Amphetamines	Decongestants
Androgens	Estrogens
Anesthesia agents	Hydralazine
Anticholinergics	Muscle relaxants
Antihistamines	Nonsteroidal anti-inflammatory drugs
Antiparkinsonian agents	Opiates
Antipsychotic agents	Progesterones
Antispasmodics	Selective serotonin reuptake inhibitors
Benzodiazepines	Tetracyclic antidepressants
β-Adrenergic agents	Tricyclic antidepressants
Calcium channel blockers	

bladder) in the lean patient. Examine the external genitalia to identify phimosis, paraphimosis, meatal stenosis or stricture, or evidence of urethral or penile trauma.

Perform digital rectal examination (either before or after relief of obstruction, depending on patient comfort) to evaluate the anal-rectal area and prostate, assessing anal tone, perineal sensation, prostate enlargement, stool impaction, and any possibility of malignancy. A nodular or rock-hard prostate may suggest prostate cancer, which must be confirmed at a later date. Women with urinary retention should receive a pelvic examination to detect possible inflammatory lesions or pelvic or adnexal masses. Perform a neurologic examination to determine any neurogenic cause. After successful drainage of the distended bladder, a repeat physical examination of the lower abdomen is indicated to help exclude an unresolved extraurinary bladder problem (e.g., appendicitis) needing further management.

DIAGNOSIS

Bedside US can easily identify urinary retention. However, the need for further diagnostic tests will depend on the nature of the clinical presentation, precipitating factors, and the patient's comorbidities. Obtain a urine culture to identify urinary tract infection. Hematuria secondary to the physical trauma of catheter insertion that clears over time is common (see chapter 91, "Urinary Tract Infections and Hematuria"). A CBC should be checked for patients with suspected severe infection, massive hematuria with possible hypovolemia, or hematologic diseases. Prolonged obstruction may result in impaired renal function and electrolyte imbalance, so obtain renal function studies and serum electrolytes. Formal abdominal US or CT may be indicated to identify pelvic or abdominal masses, bladder stones, or hydronephrosis, but are not routinely needed if symptoms resolve after catheter placement. Neuroimaging or spinal imaging is needed if examination identifies neurologic deficits. Cystourethrography may be required eventually to evaluate the pathology in the lower urinary tract; however, this is not an ED procedure.

TREATMENT

The goal of ED management is outlined in **Table 92-4**. Bladder decompression is by urethral or suprapubic catheterization. Difficult catheterization in males can result from urethral stricture, prostatic enlargement, or postsurgical bladder neck contractures. **If the patient recently underwent urologic surgery (e.g., radical prostatectomy or complex urethral reconstruction), consult the urologist before attempts at catheter placement.**

TABLE 92-4 Steps in Evaluation and Management of Acute Urinary Retention

Recognition	Recognize a patient with possible acute urinary retention.
Initial assessment	Obtain complete history and physical examination to identify underlying diseases and precipitating factors: obstructive, pharmacologic, infectious, neurogenic, traumatic, childhood, or psychogenic causes. Assess bladder volume with bedside US.
Initial stabilization	Place a urethral or suprapubic catheter.
Risk assessment	Assess for risk of recurrence, need for surgical intervention, and morbidity: age, severity of clinical presentation, causes, comorbidity, prostate size, postvoid residual, and maximum urine flow rate.
Need for inpatient care	Admit for treatment of significant underlying medical illness or precipitating factors. Consider malignancy, spinal cord compression or injury, unresolved hematuria, or urinary tract infection with possible sepsis.
Need for urologic consultation	Discuss with urology consultant in the event of urethral stricture, meatal stenosis, urethral injury, suspected prostate cancer, acute prostatitis, or urologic postoperative complications.
Outpatient management	Acute urinary retention without significant comorbidities and without evidence of complications, such as bleeding, infection, or renal function impairment: discharge with Foley catheter, leg bag, α-adrenergic receptor blocker, (i.e., alfuzosin, 10 milligrams daily, or tamsulosin, 0.4 milligram daily) and follow up with urology in 3–7 d.

URETHRAL CATHETERIZATION TECHNIQUE

Most catheters are made of latex, but silicone catheters are available for patients with latex allergy. The retrograde injection of 10 to 15 mL of water-soluble anesthetic lubricant (e.g., 2% lidocaine jelly) 5 to 10 minutes before inserting the catheter can alleviate patient discomfort (**Figure 92-1**). Retract the foreskin when inserting the catheter, and remember to reduce the foreskin once the catheter is in place. The catheter is in place when urine is freely draining. Do not inflate the retention balloon until urine begins to flow through the catheter into the clear extension tube. **The urethra can be injured from inflation of the retention balloon within the urethra.** If the catheter balloon is inflated in the prostatic urethra and not the bladder, urine may or may not drain freely, and balloon inflation causes extreme pain[8] (**Figure 92-2**). Forceful attempts at catheter removal with the balloon still inflated can cause edema and tears to the urethra.

If attempts at passage of a straight 14- to 18-French Foley catheter fail, use a firm angulated coudé catheter, positioned so the tip points anteriorly. The curved tip adjusts to the course of the prostatic urethra. A modification of the standard catheterization technique was reported in a small convenience sample, using US guidance while applying transrectal pressure to help smooth out the course of the prostatic urethra and simultaneously gently advancing the catheter.[9] Applying this technique requires two healthcare providers—one using US and applying rectal pressure, and another advancing the catheter.

During insertion, a false lumen can be created, or the catheter may kink in the urethra, especially in patients with underlying urethral strictures or prostate enlargement. Consult urology for management. If catheterization produces gross blood, deflate the balloon, remove the catheter, and do not attempt reinsertion because a false passage (through the penile soft tissue instead of the urethra) may have been produced. Management may require urology consultation for the use of a guidewire, flexible filiforms, and dilation followers for progressive dilation of the urethra to place a catheter.

SUPRAPUBIC CATHETERIZATION TECHNIQUE

Suprapubic catheterization can be performed in patients after failure of several attempts of urethral catheterization and as long as there is no obvious pelvic trauma or abnormal anatomy in the lower abdomen. This may be the only option to decompress an extremely painful, distended bladder when urethral catheterization is not possible. US-guided suprapubic catheterization has a low complication rate.[10] Prepare the suprapubic area with betadine and local anesthesia. Visualize the distended bladder with US. While monitoring with US, advance a 22-gauge spinal needle with 10-mL syringe posteriorly and caudally at a 30-degree angle from the true vertical and 60 degrees from the horizontal plane of the abdomen, 3 to 4 cm above the pubic symphysis in the midline. Advance the needle while withdrawing on the syringe. US visualization of the needle in the bladder and urine return indicates correct placement. Use the depth and position of this attempt to direct the placement of the obturator. Make a small skin incision in the midline at the point of prior needle removal. The cystostomy catheter and obturator assembly are then placed in similar manner as the spinal needle, again aspirating for urine (**Figures 92-3** and **92-4**).

After inflating the retention balloon, withdraw the obturator and leave the catheter in the bladder. Secure the catheter with a suture. If a guidewire is used for catheter insertion, remove the pull-apart sheath after successful bladder placement.

POSTCATHETERIZATION CARE

Patients with long-standing obstruction are at risk for postobstructive diuresis and postobstructive renal failure. Monitor for 4 hours minimum for significant hourly urinary output (>200 mL/h over input)

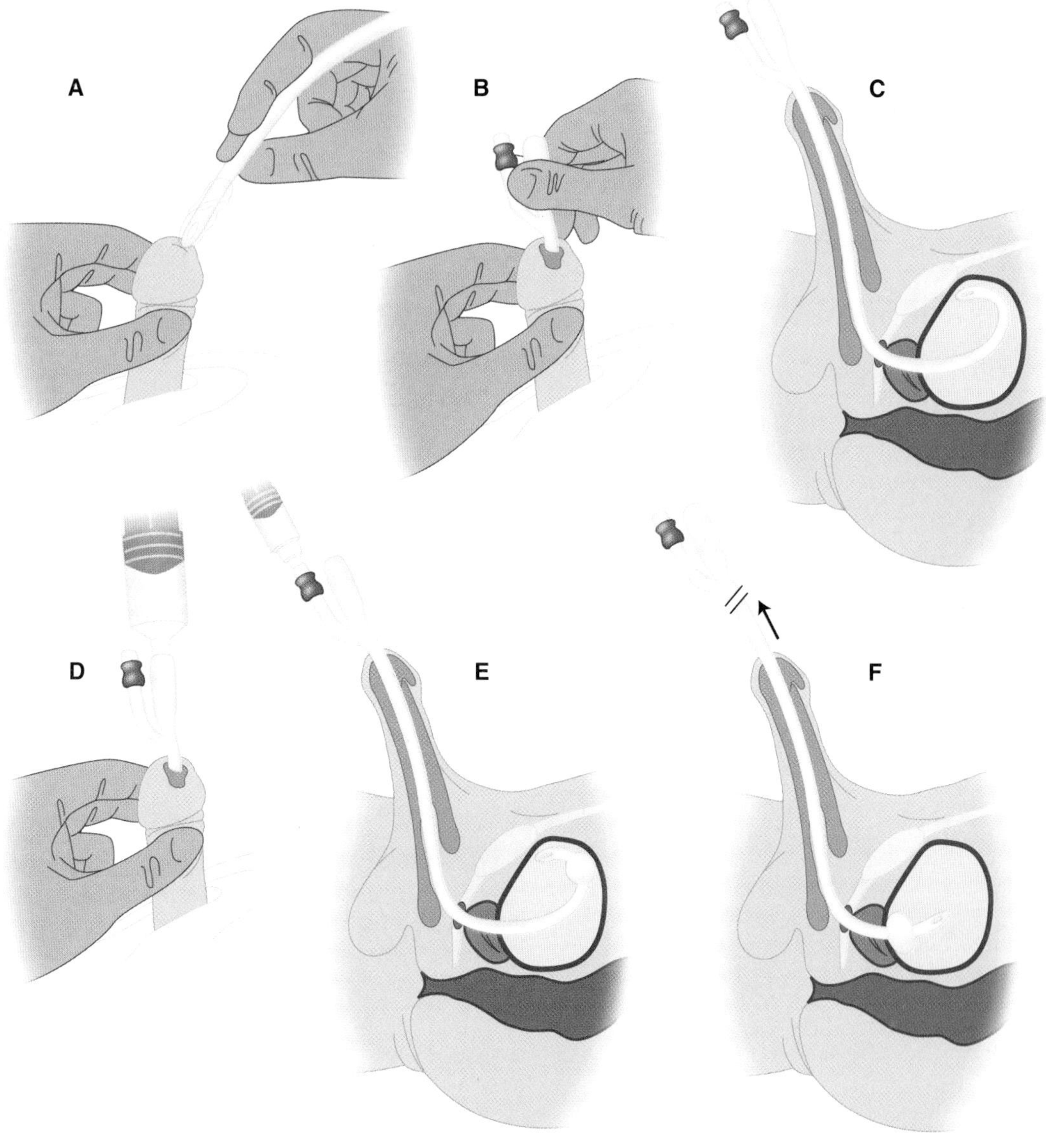

FIGURE 92-1. Urethral catheter insertion. **A.** Insert the lubricated catheter into the urethra. **B.** Advance the catheter until the ports are at the meatus. **C.** Cross-section of the male pelvis showing the distal catheter and cuff positioned within the bladder. **D.** Urine aspiration confirms proper placement of the catheter. **E.** If urine is flowing freely, inflate the balloon at the tip of the catheter. **F.** Gently withdraw the catheter to lodge the cuff against the bladder neck. [Reproduced with permission from Reichman EF, Simon RR: *Emergency Medicine Procedures*. © 2004, Eric F. Reichman, PhD, MD, and Robert R. Simon, MD.]

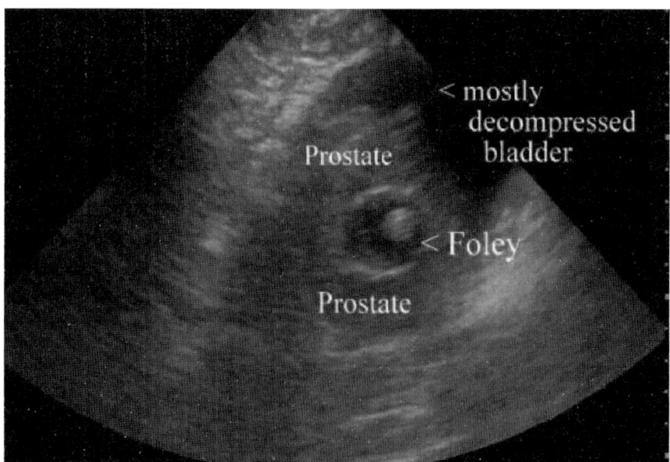

FIGURE 92-2. Foley catheter balloon inflated within the prostatic urethra. [Used with permission of Brady Pregerson MD & EMresource.org.]

after initial return. If this degree of output continues, admit the patient with volume replacement adjusted hourly according to urine output. Patients with significant elevations of BUN or creatinine should be admitted. Patients should be reassessed after Foley insertion for resolution of symptoms.

Routine use of antibiotics for the prevention of bacteriuria or for the treatment of asymptomatic bacteriuria is not suggested. Antibiotics are reserved for symptomatic urinary tract infection[4] (see chapter 95, "Complications of Urologic Procedures and Devices").

Pharmacologic therapy with an α-adrenergic receptor blocker, which exerts its effects on the bladder neck and prostate, may relax bladder smooth muscle, reducing outlet resistance to urinary flow (**Table 92-4**). α-Adrenergic blockers such as alfuzosin, 10 milligrams daily, or tamsulosin, 0.4 milligram daily, increase the success of spontaneous voiding after the catheter is removed.[11] Warn patients, especially the elderly, about possible postural hypotension. α-Adrenergic blockers may also shorten the interval of time before a successful voiding trial and prevent recurrent episodes.[12]

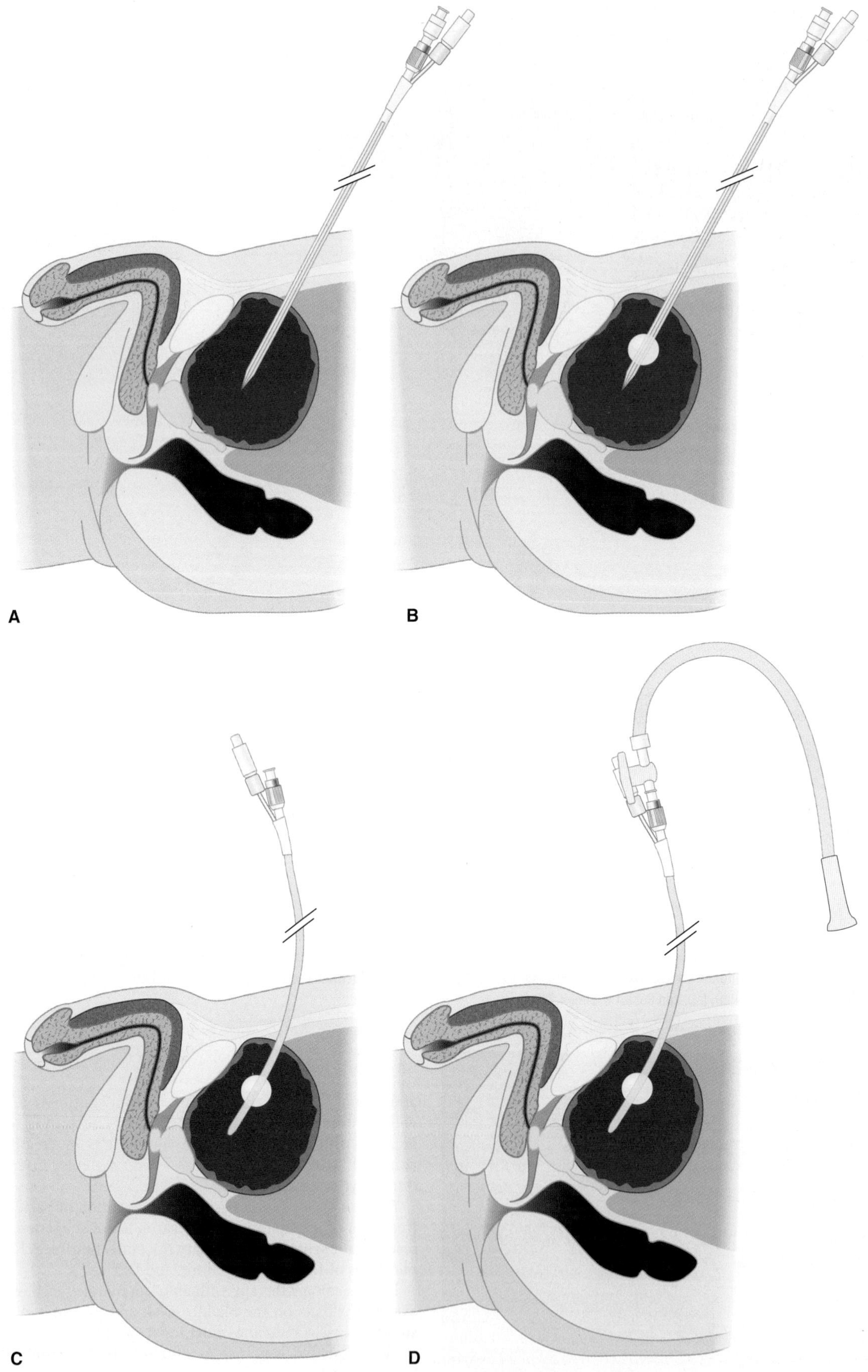

FIGURE 92-3. The obturator technique. **A.** The obturator is within the catheter. The system is inserted 60 degrees to the skin and advanced into the bladder. **B.** The balloon is inflated. **C.** The obturator is removed while the catheter remains within the bladder. **D.** The collecting tube is attached to the catheter. [Reproduced with permission from Reichman EF, Simon RR (eds): *Emergency Medicine Procedures.* © 2004, Eric F. Reichman, PhD, MD, and Robert R. Simon, MD.]

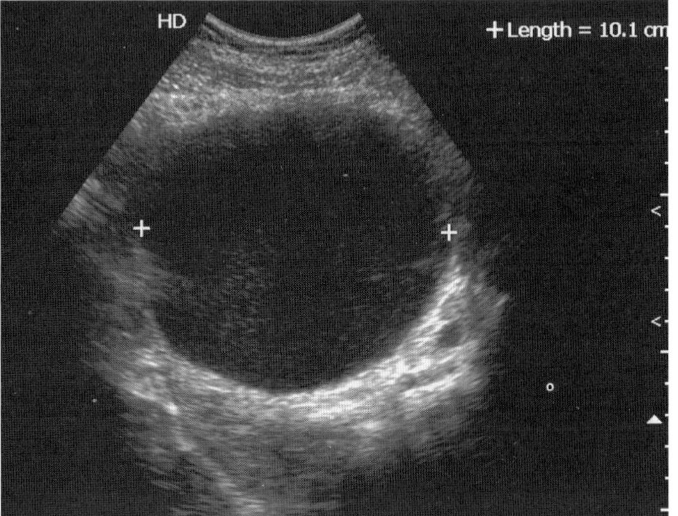

FIGURE 92-4. US visualization of distended bladder. Make sure bladder measurement is at least 2 cm in two planes before attempting suprapubic aspiration. Visualize the needle in the bladder before inserting the catheter. [Reproduced with permission from Ma OJ, Mateer JR, Blavais M: *Emergency Ultrasound, 2nd ed.* © 2008, McGraw-Hill, New York, NY.]

DISPOSITION AND FOLLOW-UP

The majority of patients with urinary retention are discharged home with a catheter connected to a leg bag and wait for further surgical intervention after the urology clinic visit. Patients should be educated in Foley catheter care and bag drainage and given a list of alarm symptoms that should prompt return to the ED. These include fever, return of symptoms, repeated vomiting, abdominal pain, catheter blockage, or penile pain. Penile pain suggests migration of the balloon into the proximal urethra. Feelings of urgency or bladder spasm can be treated with oxybutynin, 2.5 milligrams PO two or three times a day. Oxybutynin has anticholinergic properties and can cause the same adverse effects as any anticholinergic agent. There is no satisfactory treatment for urinary leakage around the catheter. Placement of a larger catheter is not typically effective.

α-Adrenergic blockers can be prescribed as needed (Table 92-4). Recommend urology follow-up within 3 to 7 days. A longer period of Foley drainage is encouraged in patients with retention volumes >1.3 L to improve chances of successful voiding. The serum prostate-specific antigen assay and long-term use of a 5α-reductase inhibitor could be evaluated at urology follow-up.

For precipitated urinary retention, remove the catheter in the ED and allow a voiding trial. Discontinue offending medications. Patients with clot retention, hematuria and coagulopathy, sepsis, possible neurologic cause of urinary retention, or other significant comorbidities should be admitted.[12]

SPECIAL CONSIDERATIONS

FEMALES WITH URINARY RETENTION

Urinary retention in women is uncommon. The obstructive causes of urinary retention in women are usually related to gynecologic problems (Table 93-1), but neurogenic causes can develop in both men and women.[13]

The management of urinary retention in females involves catheterization and attending to any treatable cause. The ideal selection of catheterization method, including in and out catheterization, short-term indwelling urethral catheter followed by a trial of voiding, or clean intermittent self-catheterization, depends on the clinical assessment of precipitating factors and underlying conditions. α-Adrenergic blockers do not appear to be helpful in women with urinary retention. If there is no apparent cause, refer to a gynecologic urologist for urodynamic studies.[13]

GROSS HEMATURIA AND CLOT RETENTION

Gross hematuria can lead to clot retention, resulting in pain and hypertension and tachycardia from acute bladder distention. Management of gross hematuria is placement of a 20- to 24-French triple-lumen catheter (one port for urine drainage, one port for balloon inflation, one port for bladder irrigation) and irrigation with saline until clear to evacuate clots.[14] Patients with clot retention may require admission, because clot retention may reoccur and may require cystoscopic clot removal. Patients with gross hematuria from coagulopathy (i.e., warfarin) should have clotting parameters corrected as appropriate and be admitted.

POSTOPERATIVE URINARY RETENTION

Treatment is discussed in chapter 87, "Complications of General Surgical Procedures." For patients with retention after GU or pelvic procedures, consult with the operating surgeon. Otherwise, for patients with normal renal function and no obstruction, bladder catheterization to relieve symptoms and then removal of the catheter and a trial of voiding are usually all that is necessary.

REFERENCES

The complete reference list is available online at www.TintinalliEM.com.

Male Genital Problems

Jonathan E. Davis

INTRODUCTION

This chapter reviews the common acute infectious and structural or anatomic GU disorders. There are five GU emergencies: testicular torsion, Fournier's gangrene, paraphimosis, priapism, and significant GU trauma (see chapter 265, "Genitourinary Trauma"). Related emergencies include strangulated inguinal hernia (see chapter 84, "Hernias") and ruptured abdominal aortic aneurysm (see chapter 60, "Aneurysmal Disease"), which may present with scrotal pain.

ANATOMY

PENIS

Three cylindrical bodies—the corpus spongiosum, which surrounds the urethra, and the paired corpora cavernosa—form the shaft of the penis (**Figure 93-1**). The corpora cavernosa are the major erectile bodies,

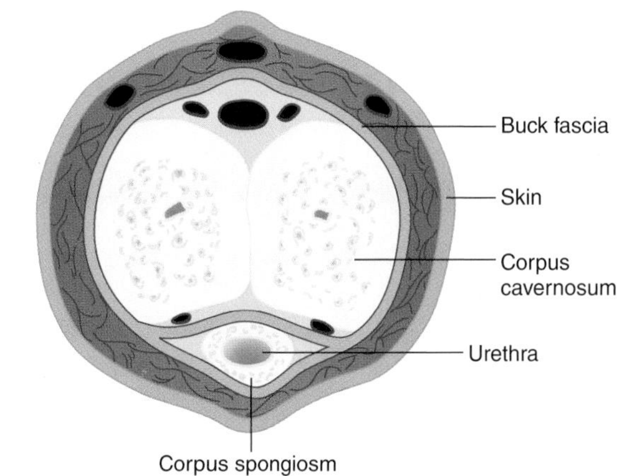

FIGURE 93-1. Cross-section of the penis.

extending distally from the pubic rami and capped by the glans penis. These cylindrical structures are encased in a thick tunic of dense connective tissue, the tunica albuginea. External to the tunica albuginea is Buck's fascia, which fuses with Colles' fascia at the level of the urogenital diaphragm. The internal pudendal artery provides the blood supply, which branches to form the deep and superficial penile arteries. Lymphatics drain from the penis into the deep and superficial inguinal nodes.

SCROTUM

The prepubertal scrotal skin is thin and thickens with subsequent hormonal stimulation during puberty. Immediately beneath the skin are the smooth muscle and elastic tissue layers of Dartos' fascia, similar to the superficial fatty layer (Camper's fascia) of the abdominal wall. The deep membranous layer (Scarpa's fascia) of the abdominal wall extends into the perineum, where it is referred to as *Colles' fascia*, and forms part of the scrotal wall (**Figure 93-2**). The blood supply is derived primarily from branches of the femoral and internal pudendal arteries. Lymphatics from the scrotum drain into the inguinal and femoral nodes.

TESTES

The testes average in size between 4 and 5 cm in length and 3 cm in width and depth, and usually lie in an upright position, with the superior portion tipped slightly forward and outward. Each testis is encased in a thick fibrous tunica albuginea except posterolaterally, where it is in tight apposition with the epididymis. The enveloping tunica vaginalis covers the anterior and lateral aspects of the testes and attaches to the posterior scrotal wall. Superiorly, the testes are suspended from the spermatic cord; inferiorly, the testis is anchored to the scrotum by the scrotal ligament (gubernaculum). Maldevelopment with lack of firm posterior fixation of the tunica vaginalis leaves the testes and epididymis at risk for torsion about the spermatic cord. The posterior (visceral) leaf of the tunica vaginalis is adherent with the tunica albuginea of the anterior testicular surface. A potential space exists between this visceral leaf and the anterior (parietal) tunica vaginalis. Any traumatic or inflammatory event can impede the normal parietal tunica vaginalis from absorbing viscerally secreted fluid, resulting in hydrocele formation anterior to the testes (**Figure 93-3**). Hematocele results from accumulation of blood in the potential space.

The internal spermatic and external spermatic arteries provide the blood supply, traveling together in the spermatic cord. Venous return is primarily by the internal spermatic, epigastric, internal circumflex, and scrotal veins. The lymphatics drain toward the external, common iliac, and periaortic nodes.

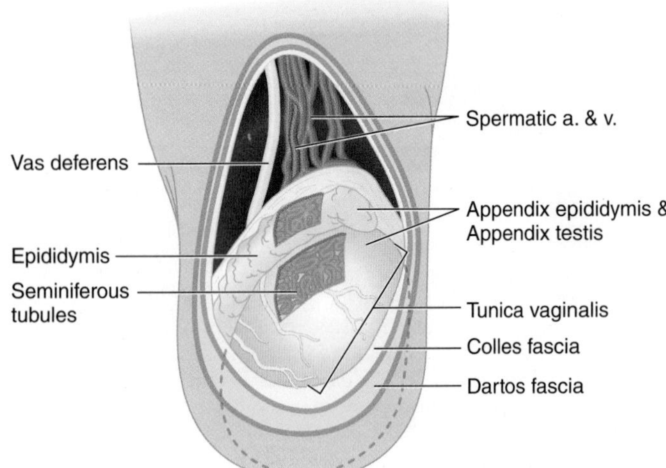

FIGURE 93-2. Anatomy of the scrotum and the testis. a. = artery; v. = vein.

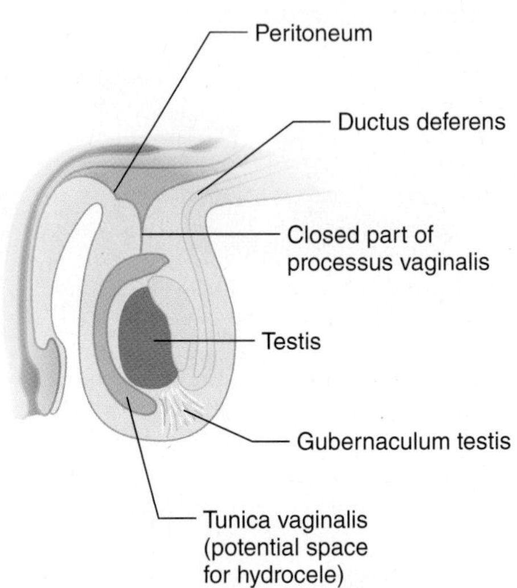

FIGURE 93-3. Embryonic retroperitoneal testis descends into the scrotum and invaginates into the tunica vaginalis, which anchors it to the posterior scrotal wall. Note the potential space in the tunica vaginalis for development of a hydrocele.

EPIDIDYMIS AND VAS DEFERENS

The epididymis is a single, fine, tubular structure approximately 4 to 5 m long compressed into an area of about 5 cm. It serves to promote sperm maturation and motility. Vestigial embryonic structures, the appendix epididymis and the appendix testis, which have no known physiologic function, are often associated with the testes and epididymis. The appendix epididymis is found attached to the head of the epididymis, or globus major. The appendix testis, a pear-shaped structure, is usually situated on the uppermost portion of the testis at the junction of the testis and the globus major of the epididymis, although anatomic variation exists.

The vas deferens is a distinct muscular tube that is easily palpable within the scrotal sac. It extends cephalad in the spermatic cord from the tail of the epididymis (globus minor), traverses the inguinal canal, and crosses medially behind the bladder over the ureters to form the ampullae of the vas, where it joins with the seminal vesicles to form the paired ejaculatory ducts in the prostatic urethra.

PROSTATE

The prostate originates from the urogenital sinus at approximately the third month of embryonic life. It is continually enlarging and, in the young male, is often not definable on rectal examination. As a man matures, the prostate may enlarge dramatically, resulting in significant bladder outlet obstruction. The anterior, median, posterior, and lateral lobes define the divisions of the prostate.

PHYSICAL EXAMINATION

The GU examination should be performed with the male patient in both the supine and upright positions in a well-illuminated, warm room if feasible. In uncircumcised males, fully retract the foreskin to inspect the glans, coronal sulcus, and preputial (foreskin) areas for ulceration or lesions. Note the location of the urethral meatus and presence of discharge. Replace the foreskin to its native position following examination to prevent iatrogenic paraphimosis. Carefully palpate the penile shaft for skin or subcutaneous lesions.

Testicular nodularity or firmness should be considered carcinoma until proven otherwise. The epididymis usually lies on the posterolateral aspect of the testis and has a soft, fleshy feel similar to that of the earlobe. Many males experience pain and tenderness with palpation of a normal globus major (head), body, and globus minor (tail) of the epididymis. Males experience some discomfort during palpation of a normal prostate, and a lateral supine position helps prevent an infrequent vasovagal response.

The prostate has a heart-shaped contour, with its apex located more distally, abutting the urogenital diaphragm. The consistency of the normal prostate has the same resiliency as the cartilaginous tip of the nose, whereas suspicious carcinogenic areas feel more like the bony prominence of the chin. The posterior lobe is small and thin, allowing palpation of the median raphe that distinguishes the two lateral lobes. A rectal prostate examination cannot assess the anterior or median lobes. The seminal vesicles, lying just superior to the prostate, cannot normally be distinguished unless there is inflammation, induration, or enlargement.

Examination of the inguinal canals for hernias and the scrotal spermatic cords for varicoceles is best done in the upright position, with the patient straining at the designated time. When the patient is upright, it should be determined whether the testes are aligned along a vertical or horizontal axis. Horizontally aligned testes are at greater risk for torsion. Likewise, an elevated, horizontally aligned testis may be the result of torsion.

DISORDERS OF THE SCROTUM

An acute scrotum is defined as acute pain or painful swelling of the scrotum or its contents, accompanied by local signs or general symptoms. Testicular torsion and Fournier's gangrene are the most time-sensitive diagnoses of the acute scrotum; the first priority in the evaluation of patients with scrotal pain is differentiation these life- or testicular-threatening disorders from other entities.

SCROTAL EDEMA

Insect bites, human bites, and contact dermatitis may cause scrotal edema, or it may be idiopathic in young boys.[1] In the setting of hypoalbuminemia, or anasarca from any cause, contiguous scrotal and penile edema may occur. Idiopathic scrotal edema presents as unilateral or bilateral pain with scrotal, perineal, and inguinal swelling and erythema in boys between 3 and 9 years of age. US findings include an easily compressible thickened scrotal wall (mean 11.2 mm), increased peritesticular blood flow, and in some cases, a reactive hydrocele.[2,3] Episodes resolve in 1 to 4 days with scrotal elevation, rest, and nonsteroidal anti-inflammatory drugs, although recurrences occur.[4] Antibiotics are sometimes used, but are not typically needed unless fever, increased warmth, or purulence is noted.

SCROTAL ABSCESS

Management of a scrotal abscess depends on its depth. In the case of a simple hair follicle abscess, the phlegmon is localized to the scrotal wall. A superficial abscess should be differentiated from a deeper abscess involving or originating from infection in one of the primary intrascrotal organs (i.e., testis, epididymis, or bulbous urethra). This distinction is difficult late in the course of the infection when a general scrotal mass may be the only physical finding. US can determine contiguous involvement of an inflammatory mass in the testis or epididymis with the scrotal skin. When in question, a retrograde urethrogram will delineate the integrity of the urethra.

A simple hair follicle scrotal wall abscess is managed by incision and drainage. Frequently, wound care can be simplified by circumferential excision of the entire roof of the abscess. This allows access for wound care and sitz baths and assures healing from the base outward.[1] Antibiotics are rarely needed in an immunocompetent male unless there are signs of cellulitis or systemic involvement. Definitive care of deep-seated or complex abscesses require consultation with urology.

FOURNIER'S GANGRENE

Fournier's gangrene is a polymicrobial, synergistic, infective necrotizing fasciitis of the perineal, genital, or perianal anatomy. This process typically begins as a benign infection or simple abscess that quickly becomes virulent, especially in an immunocompromised host, and results in microthrombosis of the small subcutaneous vessels, leading to the development of gangrene of the overlying skin. (**Figure 93-4**).[5]

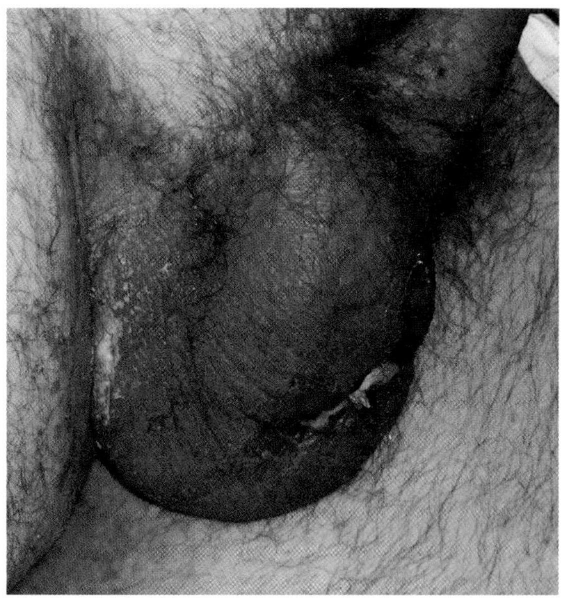

FIGURE 93-4. A patient with Fournier's gangrene of the scrotum. Note the sharp demarcation of gangrenous changes (black portion) and the marked edema of the scrotum and the penis.

Patients with diabetes and alcohol abuse are disproportionately affected with Fournier's gangrene.[6] Mortality rates have varied from 3% to 67%,[7] but contemporary estimates range from 20% to 40%.[8-13] Age over 60 and complications during treatment are the most important predictors of death.[12,13]

In advanced Fournier's gangrene, the local signs and symptoms are usually dramatic, with marked pain and swelling. Crepitus and ecchymosis of the inflamed tissues are common features. Prompt recognition of Fournier's gangrene in its early stages may prevent extensive tissue loss that accompanies delayed diagnosis or treatment. Treat with aggressive fluid resuscitation, gram-positive, gram-negative, and anaerobic antibiotic coverage (see also chapter 151, "Sepsis"). Recommended agents include piperacillin-tazobactam, 3.375 to 4.5 grams IV every 6 hours, or imipenem, 1 gram IV every 24 hours, or meropenem, 500 milligrams to 1 gram IV every 8 hours, plus vancomycin.[7-9] Urgent urologic consultation is required for wide surgical debridement.[7] The addition of clindamycin, 600 to 900 milligrams IV every 8 hours, or metronidazole, 1 gram IV, then 500 milligrams IV every 8 hours, to the antimicrobial regimen may be of benefit.[7] Hyperbaric oxygen therapy in the pre- and postoperative setting is a treatment option but does not improve mortality.[14] Admission to the intensive care unit postoperatively is typically required.[7]

DISORDERS OF THE PENIS

Ischemic priapism, paraphimosis, and entrapment injuries are priority diagnoses that, if left untreated, can result in necrosis of the penis.

BALANOPOSTHITIS

Balanitis (inflammation of the glans penis), posthitis (inflammation of the foreskin), and balanoposthitis (inflammation of the glans and the foreskin) are primarily caused by inadequate hygiene or external irritation with subsequent colonization with *Candida* species, *Staphylococcus* species, *Streptococcus* species,[15] and less commonly, *Mycoplasma genialium*.[16] Infections are frequently mixed flora.[15] On examination, when foreskin retraction is attempted, the glans and apposing prepuce appear purulent, excoriated, malodorous, and tender. **Balanoposthitis can be the sole presenting sign of diabetes.**[17] Consider *Candida*, *Gardnerella*, and anaerobes as potential causes.[15] Treatment consists of cleansing the area with saline, ensuring adequate dryness after cleaning, application of antifungal creams (nystatin or clotrimazole), treatment with an oral

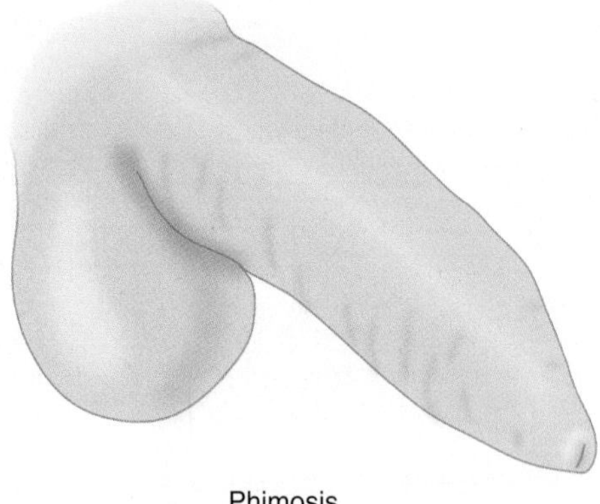

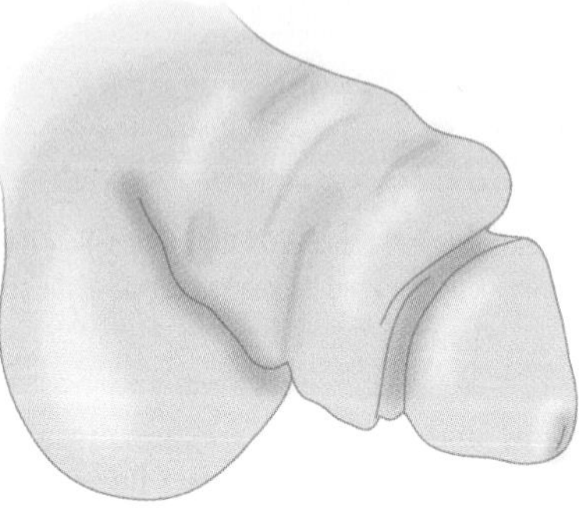

FIGURE 93-5. Phimosis and paraphimosis.

azole in severe cases (fluconazole 150 milligrams orally), and circumcision for recurrent cases.[15] Soap may increase inflammation during the acute phase, but routine hygiene is essential to prevent reoccurrence. Bacterial infection is suggested by warmth, erythema, and edema of the glans, foreskin, and penile shaft; anaerobic organism is suggested by foul smell.[15] If these signs are present, oral clindamycin, 300 milligrams three times per day for 7 days, or metronidazole, 500 milligrams two time per day for 7 days, is recommended.[15,18] Cases that persist warrant culture for potential infective causes or biopsy and follow-up with urology.

PHIMOSIS

Phimosis is the inability to retract the foreskin proximally and posterior to the glans penis (**Figure 93-5**). Physiologic phimosis occurs naturally in uncircumcised newborns. By 3 years of age, fewer than 10% of foreskins remain nonretractile, with nearly all becoming retractile by late adolescence. Infection, poor hygiene, and previous preputial injuries with scarring are common causes of pathologic phimosis. Scarring at the tip of the foreskin can occlude the preputial meatus, infrequently causing urinary retention. Hemostatic dilation of the preputial ostium will temporarily relieve the urinary retention. Circumcision is curative. Alternatively, topical steroid treatment (such as betamethasone, 0.05% to 0.10% twice daily) applied from the tip of the foreskin to the glandis corona for 1 to 2 months, along with daily manual preputial retraction, has been shown to be an effective nonsurgical management option for phimosis.[19]

PARAPHIMOSIS

Paraphimosis, a true urologic emergency, is the inability to reduce the proximal edematous foreskin distally over the glans penis into its natural position (Figure 93-5). The resulting glans edema and venous engorgement can progress to arterial compromise and gangrene.

Paraphimosis can often be reduced by compression of the glans for several minutes to reduce edema and allow for successful reduction of the now smaller glans through the foreskin. **Tightly wrapping the glans with a 2-inch elastic bandage for 5 minutes will reduce edema.** A local anesthetic block of the penis can help the patient tolerate the pain of compression but also adds fluid to an already swollen penis. The patient may require an anxiolytic before the injection of a "ring" of local anesthetic at the base of the penis. If these methods are unsuccessful, local infiltration of the constricting band with 1% lidocaine without epinephrine followed by superficial dorsal incision of the band will allow foreskin reduction.[20] Use of an iris scissor may help prevent damage to underlying tissue. The examining provider should perform this procedure in cases of impaired perfusion to the glans, unless a urologist is immediately available.

ENTRAPMENT INJURIES

Circumferential objects surrounding the penis can occlude the veins and, subsequently, the arterial blood supply. Hair, string, metal rings, and wire have been wrapped around the penis for accidental, experimental, or sexual reasons. Removing the offending object requires care and ingenuity.[21] Removal techniques include compression and cooling the penis, cutting the object, and urologic surgical removal.[21] Lubrication with petroleum jelly may assist. Ice packs can help decrease inflammation and edema, but take care to avoid cooling injury. The compression technique uses the same modified string method recommended for removing finger rings, with the addition of inserting an 18-gauge needle into the end of one of the two corpora cavernosa through the glans to allow edema and blood to be pushed out by the proximal to distal compression of the penis. Start by inserting the short end of the tape under the constriction device to be left proximally, while the long end is used to compress the penis winding in a proximal to distal direction.[21] Cutting devices can remove penile rings. Protect underlying skin with a hard object, preferably metal. Also avoid overheating the surrounding tissues. Urologic consultation may be required depending on the entrapment complexity and physiologic concerns.[21]

The **penile hair-tourniquet syndrome** (**Figure 93-6**) seen in young males presents with swelling of the glans. The offending hair may be

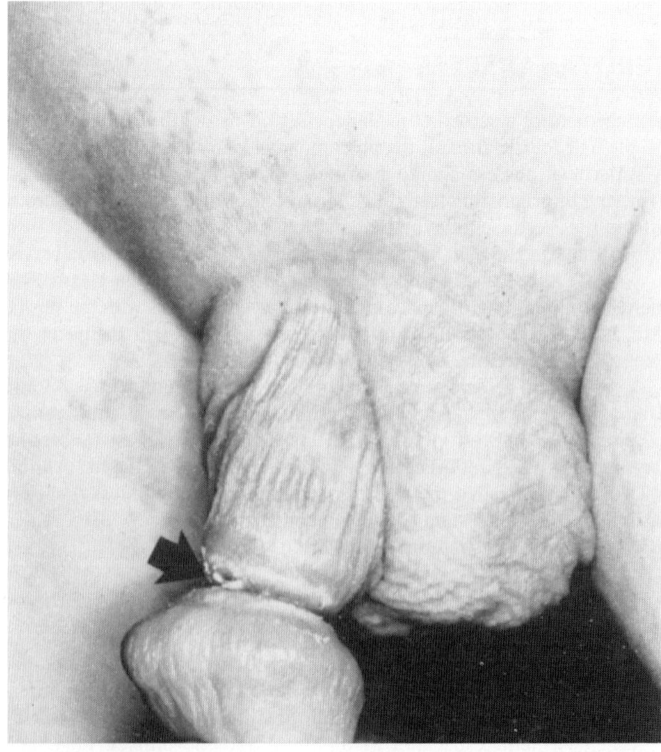

FIGURE 93-6. Hair is entrapped behind the coronal sulcus (*arrow*), constricting and progressively amputating the glans.

invisible within the edematous coronal sulcus. Several common techniques for removal consist of unwinding the hair, lancing the hair when easily accessible, or surgical removal when circumferential edema prevents access to the constricting source.[22]

Another common entrapment injury is penile or scrotal entrapment in a zipper. The reported interventions include dismantling the zipper with wire cutters or trauma shears and surgical interventions like circumcision. First, cleanse the affected area with povidone-iodine and provide local anesthesia with 1% to 2% lidocaine. Next, try coating the zipper and affected area with mineral oil or other nontoxic lubricant. If this does not free the zipper, cut the zipper away from clothing to make the zipper easier to handle. Next, try cutting the sliding bar of the zipper and the zipper teeth.[23] The bottom bar of the zipper apparatus can also be cut and then unzipped from below.

FRACTURE OF THE PENIS

A penile fracture occurs when the tunica albuginea of one or both corpus cavernosa ruptures due to direct trauma to the erect penis.[24] It can be associated with partial or complete urethral rupture (18%) or deep dorsal vein injury.[24] The most common cause is sexual intercourse, but other causes include animal bites, stabbing, bullet wounds, and self-mutilation.[24,25] On examination, the penis is acutely swollen but flaccid, discolored, and tender. A retrograde urethrogram may be necessary to assure urethral integrity, but radiologic evaluation rarely influences surgical managment.[25] Surgical treatment consists of hematoma evacuation and suture apposition of the disrupted tunica albuginea.

PEYRONIE'S DISEASE

Peyronie's disease produces progressive penile deformity, typically curvature with erections, that is painful and may result in erectile dysfunction or preclude successful vaginal penetration during intercourse.[26] Examination of the penile shaft will disclose a thickened plaque, typically on the dorsum, involving the tunica albuginea of the corpora bodies. Urologic referral is warranted. Peyronie's disease of the penis has been noted in association with Dupuytren's contractures of the hand.

PRIAPISM

Priapism is a urologic emergency that is characterized by persistent, usually painful, pathologic erection in which both corpora cavernosa are engorged with stagnant blood.[27] Even though the glans penis and the corpus spongiosum are characteristically soft and uninvolved, urinary retention may develop. Impotence can result in 35% of cases with sustained erections for prolonged periods, so emergency urologic consultation is needed.

Many cases of priapism in adults are pharmacologically related to intracavernosal injection of vasoactive substances for impotence (papaverine, prostaglandin E_1), use of oral agents for hypertension (hydralazine, prazosin, calcium channel blockers), neuroleptic medications (chlorpromazine, trazodone, thioridazine), or oral agents related to erectile dysfunction.[27] Most cases of priapism in children are due to hematologic disorders, usually sickle cell disease.

Priapism is classified into high-flow (nonischemic) priapism and low-flow (ischemic) priapism. High-flow (nonischemic) priapism is rare, most often painless, and usually results from traumatic fistulae between the cavernosal artery and the corpus cavernosum. Blood gas analysis of the first corporal aspirate is recommended to differentiate arterial (high-flow) from ischemic priapism.[27] High-flow priapism may be further delineated by color Doppler US and is treated by embolization. Low-flow (ischemic) priapism is more common, is usually quite painful, and is diagnosed by the aspiration of dark acidic intracavernosal blood from the corpus cavernosum.

Provide adequate narcotic analgesia. Corporal aspiration followed by irrigation (with plain saline or α-adrenergic agonists [i.e., phenylephrine]) is the primary treatment method for persistent priapism. The urologic consultant usually performs this procedure, but if one is not readily available, the examining provider may need to intervene. On each lateral side of the proximal penis, raise a wheal with 1% lidocaine using a 27-gauge needle. After local anesthesia, insert a 19-gauge butterfly needle into the corpora cavernosa on each side, approximately 0.5 cm deep. The needle must penetrate the skin, subcutaneous tissue, and the tunica albuginea in order to enter the corpus cavernosum. The needles can be supported in place by using a combination of small gauze pads on either side of the "butterfly wings" and roller gauze around the penis to secure its position. Aspirate blood from each side.[27] If medical treatment or phenylephrine irrigation fails to produce detumescence, surgery may be required.[27] If priapism due to sickle cell crisis fails to respond to adequate analgesia and hydration, consult both urology and hematology. The role of exchange transfusion has been reexamined; penile aspiration and irrigation, with or without instillation of α- or β-adrenergic agonists, is recommended for acute ischemic episodes in sickle cell patients.[28]

PENILE CARCINOMA

Carcinoma of the penis is rare, usually appearing in the fifth or sixth decade in an uncircumcised male. Carcinoma may appear as a nontender ulcer or warty growth beneath the foreskin in the area of the coronal sulcus or glans penis and is often hidden by an inflamed phimotic foreskin.

DISORDERS OF THE TESTES AND EPIDIDYMIS

TESTICULAR TORSION

The differential diagnosis of acute scrotal pain includes testicular torsion, torsion of the testicular appendages, epididymitis, incarcerated hernia, and trauma, among others. Frequent causes of acute scrotal pain include testicular torsion or epididymitis in adults, with the added possibility of appendage torsion in children (**Table 93-1**). Because of the potential for infarction and infertility, testicular torsion must be the primary consideration in acute scrotal pain. The annual incidence of testicular torsion is 3.8 in 100,00 males under the age of 18.[29] Testicular torsion presents in a bimodal age distribution, with extravaginal torsion occurring in the perinatal period and intravaginal torsion peaking during puberty,[29] although this may occur at any age.

Torsion of the testis or spermatic cord results from abnormal fixation of the testis within the tunica vaginalis. This allows the testis to twist, especially after episodes of minor trauma and during periods of testicular growth such as puberty. Torsion usually occurs in the absence of a preceding event; only a small percentage occurs due to associated trauma. Torsion may occur during sleep, when unilateral cremasteric muscle contraction results in twisting of the testis. Inadequate fixation of the tunica vaginalis to the posterior scrotal wall (bell-clapper deformity) places the testis at risk for torsion. A testis aligned along a horizontal rather than a vertical axis is at particular risk.

Patients usually complain of acute severe pain, usually felt in the lower abdominal quadrant, the inguinal canal, or the testis. Although the pain may be constant or intermittent, it is not positional in nature, because testicular torsion is primarily an ischemic event that becomes inflammatory only after the testis has infarcted. The presence of vomiting makes the diagnosis of testicular torsion more likely.[30]

When examined early, the involved testis is firm, tender, and often higher than the contralateral testis and frequently with a transverse lie.[31] The epididymis may be displaced and not found in its normal posterolateral position. The most sensitive finding in excluding testicular torsion is the unilateral presence of the cremasteric reflex. Testicular torsion has, however, been reported in the setting of an intact cremasteric reflex. Although commonly associated with testicular torsion, the absence of an ipsilateral cremasteric reflex is a nonspecific finding and may be associated with scrotal inflammation from any cause. In addition, some healthy young males may have an underdeveloped reflex, particularly in the first few years of life. Relief of pain with elevation of the affected testicle (Prehn sign–positive for epididymitis) does not reliably distinguish torsion from epididymitis.

TABLE 93-1 Differential Diagnosis of Acute Scrotal Pain

	Testicular Torsion	Epididymitis	Appendage Torsion
Historical Features			
Peak incidence	Neonates, adolescents	Adolescents, young adults	Prepubertal
Risk factors	Undescended testicle (neonate), rapid increase in testicular size (adolescent), failure of prior orchiopexy	Sexual activity/promiscuity, GU anomalies, GU instrumentation	Presence of appendages
Pain onset	**Sudden**	Gradual, progressive	Variable
Nausea/vomiting	**More likely**	Less likely	Less likely
Dysuria	Less likely	**More likely**	Less likely
Physical Findings			
Fever	Less likely	**More likely**, particularly in advanced disease (epididymo-orchitis)	Less likely
Location of swelling/tenderness (early)	Testicle, progressing to diffuse hemiscrotal involvement	Epididymis, progressing to diffuse hemiscrotal involvement	Localized to head of affected testicle or epididymis
Cremasteric reflex	Testicular torsion less likely if present	May be present or absent	May be present or absent
Testicle position	High riding, transverse alignment	Normal position, vertical alignment	Normal position, vertical alignment

In obvious cases of testicular torsion, emergent urologic consultation and surgical exploration are essential. With acute torsion, testicular salvage is related to the duration of symptoms before surgical detorsion. Excellent salvage rates are expected with <6 hours of symptoms, but salvage declines rapidly thereafter. There are no readily available clinical or laboratory parameters to judge the degree or duration of testicular ischemia. Therefore, no matter how long the patient has been symptomatic, a rapid evaluation, including emergency scrotal exploration if necessary, should be performed. Doppler US and radionuclide scintigraphy are two imaging modalities used to evaluate patients with equivocal clinical presentations. Both may be useful, but their routine clinical use is limited by timely availability and operator experience in interpreting the images, particularly for radionuclide scintigraphy. These studies are considered "positive" for testicular torsion when they demonstrate absent or clearly reduced ipsilateral intratesticular blood flow, and "negative" when flow is normal or increased. Older duplex US studies report sensitivities ranging from 69% to 90% and specificities ranging from 98% to 99% for testicular torsion[1]; however, a 2013 prospective study found a sensitively of only 83%.[32] Importantly, partial torsion may reveal falsely reassuring blood flow in an ischemic testicle. Likewise, normal or increased flow may be seen in a high-risk testicle following spontaneous detorsion. Gray-scale US imaging of the spermatic cord itself assessing for coils or kinks may aid in diagnosis. US findings need to be interpreted with caution in the context of the overall clinical picture. US has the advantage of demonstrating scrotal anatomy, which may indicate an alternative diagnosis. Within these limitations, testicular imaging modalities, when used in equivocal cases, can be very helpful tools.[1]

For emergency or preoperative treatment, consider manual detorsion of the affected testis. Explain to the patient that detorsion is a painful procedure but successful detorsion will help to relieve the presenting pain. Most testes twist in a lateral to medial fashion (two thirds of cases); therefore, detorsion initially should be done in a medial to lateral motion.[33] **Detorsion is typically done in a manner similar to opening a book (Figure 93-7A).** If one were to stand at the patient's feet, the patient's right testis would be rotated in a counterclockwise fashion and the patient's left testis in a clockwise fashion (**Figure 93-7B**). The initial attempt should include one and one-half rotations (540 degrees). Any relief of pain is a positive end point, and the success of the maneuver can be assessed with Doppler US, demonstrating restoration of blood flow. An occasional patient will require manipulation beyond the initial one and one-half rotations. A worsening of the patient's pain suggests that detorsion should then be done in the opposite direction (one third of cases). Successful detorsion converts an emergent procedure to an elective one. The timing of the elective surgical correction should depend on the patient's compliance and responsibility.

Young boys may present to the ED with nonspecific abdominal pain suggestive of gastroenteritis only to return 1 to 2 days later with a diagnosis of testicular torsion. Whether these patients had undisclosed testicular torsion at their initial evaluation is not known, but **consider testicular torsion in the differential diagnosis of any male presenting with abdominal pain or vomiting.**

APPENDAGEAL TORSION

The four testicular appendages—appendix testis, appendix epididymis, paradidymis (organ of Giraldes), and vas aberrans—have no known physiologic function. These pedunculated structures are capable of torsion and, in prepubertal boys, probably twist more often than the testes, with the appendix epididymis and appendix testes accounting for approximately 8% and 90% of appendage torsion, respectively. Presenting symptoms, although similar to testicular torsion, classically lack the

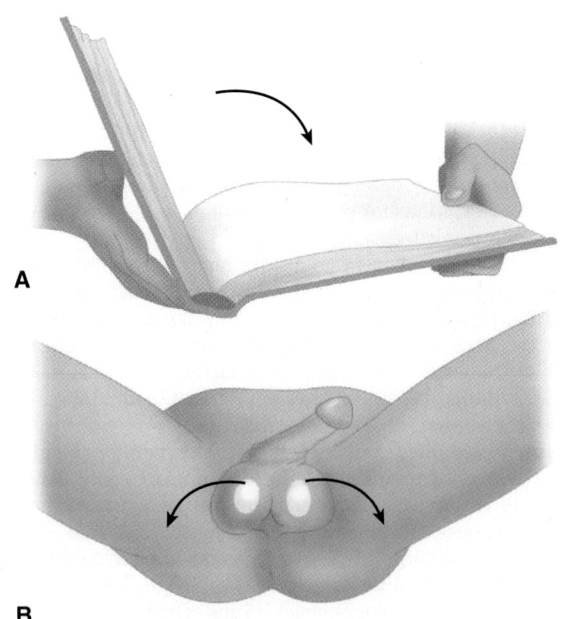

FIGURE 93-7. Testicular detorsion. This procedure is best done standing at the foot of or on the right side of the patient's bed. **A.** The torsed testis is de-torsed in a fashion similar to opening a book. **B.** The patient's right testis is rotated counterclockwise, and the left testis is rotated clockwise. [Reproduced with permission from Strange GR, Ahrens WR, Schafermeyer RW, et al: *Pediatric Emergency Medicine*, 3rd ed. © 2009, McGraw-Hill, Inc., New York, NY, p. 679.]

systemic symptoms of nausea and vomiting. If the patient is seen early, with the pain localized to the upper pole of the testis or epididymis, a blue spot may be observed through the scrotal skin—the "blue dot sign." This "sign" is pathognomonic for torsion of the appendix testis or epididymis. If the diagnosis can be assured and normal intratesticular blood flow to the involved testis is confirmed by color Doppler US, surgical exploration is not necessary. Torsion of an appendage is usually self-limiting and best managed with analgesics, bed rest, supportive underwear, and reassurance, with the expected symptom resolution within 3 to 5 days. If late in the process and testicular swelling is present, or if the color Doppler US is equivocal, then urologic consultation and surgical exploration are needed to exclude testicular torsion.[1]

EPIDIDYMITIS

The onset of pain in epididymitis or epididymo-orchitis is usually gradual. Bacterial infection is the most common cause, and the type of infection tends to depend on age. In young boys, epididymitis or epididymo-orchitis is commonly associated with sterile reflux of urine, but may be due to coliform bacteria, often associated with congenital anomalies of the lower urinary tract. Other considerations include increases in abdominal pressure from lifting or straining, which promote urinary reflux into the tail of the epididymis and subsequent inflammation. In young men <35 years old, epididymitis is due primarily to sexually transmitted diseases or associated complications (i.e., urethral stricture). Consider fungal or coliform infection of the lower urinary tract in addition to the more common sexually transmitted disease organisms in the setting of anal insertive intercourse. In men >35 years old, epididymitis is more commonly caused by common urinary pathogens, such as *Escherichia coli* and *Klebsiella*, or sexually transmitted diseases. In elderly men with epididymitis and urinary tract infection, consider associated benign prostatic hypertrophy or urethral stricture. Large residual urine volume (>50 to 100 mL urine) suggests outlet obstruction as the cause of the patient's infection (see chapter 92, "Acute Urinary Retention"). Chemical epididymitis can occur due to reflux of sterile urine and should be considered as a cause of prolonged symptoms despite appropriate antibiotic treatment.

CLINICAL FEATURES

Epididymitis may cause lower abdominal, inguinal canal, scrotal, or testicular pain alone or in combination. The retrograde progression of infection from the prostatic urethra to the epididymis explains the location and progression of pain. Epididymitis represents a more advanced GU tract infection when compared with urethritis. Patients with epididymitis are more prone to lower urinary tract voiding discomfort and may note transient pain relief in the recumbent position with scrotal elevation. Initially, isolated firmness and nodularity of the affected globus minor are noted on examination. As the disease progresses, the sulcus between the epididymis and testis becomes obliterated, and the inflammatory epididymal mass may become contiguous with the testis, producing a large, tender scrotal mass (epididymo-orchitis) that may be difficult to differentiate from testicular torsion or abscess.

Urinalysis may show pyuria in about half of patients. Obtain a specimen for gonorrhea and *Chlamydia* if urethral discharge is present, or in patients <35 years old. Obtain urine culture in children and elderly men. Adjunctive diagnostic modalities, such as color flow duplex Doppler sonography or radionuclide scintigraphy, will demonstrate increased or preserved blood flow to the testes. A reactive hydrocele may be seen on US.

TREATMENT

Most cases of epididymitis can be managed with oral antibiotics (**Table 93-2**).[34] Admission criteria for epididymitis include fever and clinical toxicity, which can be indicative of epididymal or testicular abscess formation. The ambulatory patient should wear a scrotal supporter, being careful not to lift heavy objects or strain when having a bowel movement, both of which will increase intra-abdominal pressure and exacerbate the inflammatory cycle. A urologist will need to reevaluate the patient in 5 to 7 days and then ultimately decide when the patient may return to work based on his job description (i.e., a sedentary worker would be able to return sooner than a laborer).

TABLE 93-2 Empiric Outpatient Treatment of Epididymitis and Epididymo-Orchitis

Age <35 y
Treat for gonorrhea and *Chlamydia**
Ceftriaxone, 250 milligrams IM single dose, plus doxycycline, 100 milligrams PO twice a day for 10 d
Age >35 y
Treat for gram-negative bacilli*
Ofloxacin, 300 milligrams PO twice a day for 10 d
Levofloxacin, 500 milligrams PO every day for 10 d

*Antibiotic treatment should be adjusted depending on patient risk factors for sexually transmitted disease (STD) and culture results. If age >35 y with risk factors for STD, consider ceftriaxone, 250 milligrams IM single dose, in addition to ofloxacin or levofloxacin orally.

ORCHITIS

Isolated orchitis, or inflammation of the testicle, is quite rare and usually occurs in conjunction with other systemic infections, such as mumps or other viral illnesses (coxsackie virus, Epstein-Barr virus, varicella, or echovirus). Mumps orchitis presents with unilateral involvement in 70% of cases, followed by contralateral involvement in 1 to 9 days. Bacterial orchitis is almost always associated with epididymitis. Orchitis in immunocompromised patients can be due to mycobacteriosis, cryptococcosis, toxoplasmosis, or candidiasis. Patients with orchitis usually present with testicular tenderness and swelling over a few days in duration. The diagnosis is primarily clinical using history and physical examination, but US can exclude testicular torsion or abscess. Treatment for acute episodes starts with antibiotic coverage as listed above for epididymitis; IV antibiotics should be considered for patients with abnormal vital signs.[34] Immunocompromised patients or patients with risks for tuberculosis (exposure, uncontrolled human immunodeficiency virus, or diabetes) require admission if they have abnormal vital signs or, if not, referral to urology and/or infectious disease for further management.

TESTICULAR MALIGNANCY

The hallmark of testicular carcinoma is an asymptomatic testicular mass with firmness or induration. Ten percent of tumors will present with pain secondary to acute hemorrhage within the tumor. Metastatic testicular tumors can be insidious and must be suspected in any male with unexplained supraclavicular lymphadenopathy, abdominal mass, or chronic nonproductive cough from a lung metastasis. Testicular examination may disclose a primary tumor. Any unexplained testicular mass must be approached as a possible tumor with urgent urologic referral.

ACUTE PROSTATITIS

Acute prostatitis is bacterial inflammation of the prostate gland. Patient complaints can include low back pain; perineal, suprapubic, or genital discomfort; obstructive lower urinary tract voiding symptoms; frequency or dysuria; perineal pain with ejaculation; and fever or chills. Risk factors include anatomic or neurophysiologic lower urinary tract obstruction, acute epididymitis or urethritis, anal receptive intercourse, phimosis, intraprostatic ductal reflux, and indwelling urethral catheter or condom drainage. The causative organism is *E. coli* in most cases, with other uropathogens such as *Pseudomonas*, *Klebsiella*, *Enterobacter*, *Serratia*, or *Staphylococcus* causing the remainder. In contrast to acute prostatitis, chronic bacterial prostatitis is characterized by prolonged or recurrent symptoms and relapsing bacteriuria.

Clinical findings include perineal tenderness, rectal sphincter spasm, and prostatic tenderness or bogginess. The diagnosis is clinical, because urinalysis and urine culture may both be negative. Prostatic massage is not necessary to make the diagnosis. Obtain urethral cultures or first-void urine for gonorrhea and chlamydia testing.

Initial treatment is fluoroquinolone antimicrobial therapy for 2 to 4 weeks,[35] such as ciprofloxacin, 500 milligrams orally for 14 days, with plan for primary care revelation at 2 weeks for possible continued therapy as needed. If drug cost is an issue, trimethoprim-sulfamethoxazole double-strength, one tablet PO twice a day, is an alternative, although cure rates are lower than for the fluoroquinolones. Consider treating for sexually transmitted disease organisms in younger patients or older patients with sexually transmitted disease risk factors; give ceftriaxone, 250 milligrams IM as a single dose, plus doxycycline, 100 milligrams PO twice a day for 14 days. Provide adequate narcotic analgesia.

Most patients can be treated as outpatients. Patients with abnormal vital signs should be admitted and given a broad-spectrum antibiotic such as piperacillin-tazobactam, 3.375 to 4.5 grams IV, or cefotaxime combined with an aminoglycoside.[35] If associated with urinary retention, urology consultation is needed. Urologic follow-up should be provided for discharged patients to ensure eradication of infection and to provide continuity of care in case of relapse. Chronic prostatitis is managed with urine cultures after prostatic massage, long-term antibiotics based on culture for chronic bacterial infections, anti-inflammatory medicines plus α-blockers for nonbacterial chronic prostatitis, and urology follow-up.

DISORDERS OF THE URETHRA

URETHRITIS

Urethritis is characterized by purulent or mucopurulent urethral discharge. Diagnosis is clinical, although it can be confirmed by evidence of pyuria or bacteriuria in a first-void urine specimen. Most cases are due to *Neisseria gonorrhoeae* or *Chlamydia trachomatis*. Herpes simplex virus, *Ureaplasma urealyticum*, or *Trichomonas vaginalis* are less frequent causes. Physical examination should exclude other disorders such as epididymitis, disseminated gonococcemia, or Reiter's syndrome. Treatment for urethritis is ceftriaxone, 250 milligrams IM, and azithromycin, 1 gram PO, or doxycycline, 100 milligrams PO twice a day, for 7 days. Failure to respond suggests reinfection or reexposure or infection with *T. vaginalis* or doxycycline-resistant *U. urealyticum*. Treatment with metronidazole or azithromycin should be considered depending on the infectious etiology. See chapter 149, "Sexually Transmitted Infections" for further discussion of sexually transmitted diseases.

URETHRAL STRICTURES

In decades past, sexually transmitted diseases caused the largest percentage of urethral strictures; however, trauma (such as pelvic fractures) and urinary instrumentation have been shown to cause the majority of strictures in recent assessment (**Figure 93-8**).[36]

If a patient requires measurement of his residual urine volume, simple bedside US can be performed. Most urologists agree that postvoid volumes of 50 to 100 mL may signify an abnormal residual urine volume. If the patient has difficulty voiding or is in urinary retention and a 14- or 16-F Foley or Coudé catheter cannot be easily placed into the bladder, the differential diagnostic possibilities include urethral stricture, voluntary external sphincter spasm, bladder neck contracture, or benign prostatic hypertrophy. If time permits, retrograde urethrography can be done, which will define the location and extent of a urethral stricture. Only cystoscopy can confirm a bladder neck contracture or the extent of an obstructing prostate gland. Suspected voluntary external sphincter spasm can be overcome by holding the penis upright and encouraging the patient to relax his perineum and breathe slowly during urinary catheter insertion. Liberal preapplication of intraurethral anesthetic lubricant jelly for male urinary catheterization is prudent.

When a urethral stricture is encountered, copious anesthetic lubrication is placed intraurethrally after the foreskin has been controlled with folded 4 × 4 gauze. This latter maneuver is especially important in uncircumcised patients. A 12- or 14-F Coudé catheter may negotiate the strictured area, because this catheter has an angled bend near its tip. If there are previous false passages from attempts at dilation or unsuccessful instrumentation, passage of the Coudé catheter may be difficult. Further urethral manipulation may create new false passages, leading to unnecessary hemorrhage and possible gram-negative bacteremia. If two or three gentle attempts to pass the catheter fail, urologic consultation is indicated. A catheter guide or urethral sound should be used only by a urologist.

For emergency bladder decompression, consider a suprapubic cystostomy using the Seldinger technique (see chapter 92, "Acute Urinary Retention").

URETHRAL FOREIGN BODIES

Patients of all ages, but especially young children, may be victims of innocent urethral exploration or attempts to heighten sexual experiences by using a variety of foreign bodies such as bobby pins; long, thin paint brushes; or ball point pens.[37] Bloody urine combined with infection and slow, painful urination should suggest a possible foreign body in the lower urinary tract. An x-ray of the bladder and urethral areas may disclose the presence of a radiopaque foreign body.

Foreign bodies often require cystoscopic removal or even open cystotomy. Occasionally a gentle milking action of the proximal end of the urethral foreign body by an experienced examiner will allow its retrieval from the distal urethral meatus. Even then, retrograde urethrography or endoscopic confirmation of an intact urethra is indicated.

HEMATOSPERMIA

Hemospermia, or hematospermia, is a disturbing symptom that produces extreme anxiety in sexually active males. The incidence and prevalence of this condition are not known. For all practical purposes, hematospermia can be regarded as gross hematospermia—that is, visually apparent to the patient—as microscopic analysis of semen is rarely performed. Most symptomatic men seek medical attention after one or two occurrences. Any process that results in trauma or other injury (e.g., tumor with erosion), inflammation, or infection of the male ejaculatory

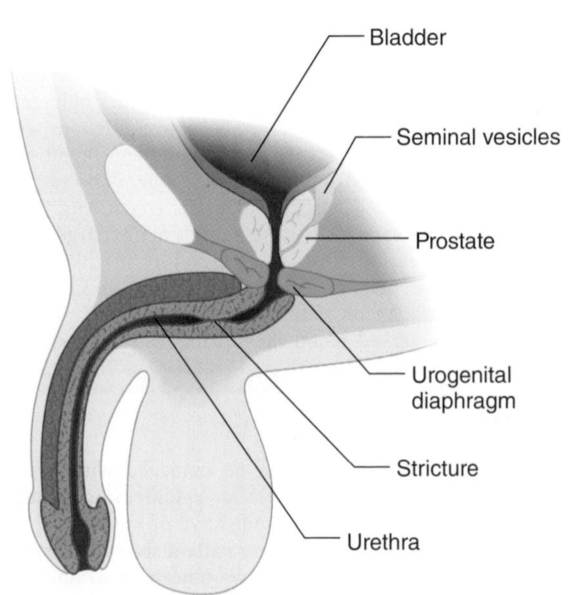

FIGURE 93-8. Stricture of the bulbous urethra.

system may result in bloody semen.[38] It is not uncommon after vigorous sexual activity. Unless the cause can be determined on physical exam, the diagnosis cannot be completed in the ED. Seventy percent of cases are diagnosed as idiopathic hematospermia after a complete outpatient urologic workup. Hematospermia should be differentiated from hematuria based on a clean catch urinalysis (see chapter 91, "Urinary Tract Infections and Hematuria"). Infection, including sexually transmitted disease, should be considered, and if suspected based on history and physical, the patient should be cultured and treated appropriately. Although all patients with hematospermia should be referred to a urologist, those >40 years are at higher risk for cancer and should be strongly advised to seek further evaluation by a urologist even when there is spontaneous resolution of hematospermia.

REFERENCES

The complete reference list is available online at www.TintinalliEM.com.

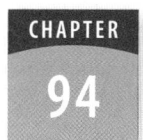

Urologic Stone Disease

David E. Manthey
Bret A. Nicks

INTRODUCTION AND EPIDEMIOLOGY

Emergency medicine management is directed at relieving pain, assessing kidney function, and determining the likelihood of spontaneous stone passage. This chapter discusses renal and ureteral stones. Bladder stones are discussed in chapter 92, "Acute Urinary Retention."

The prevalence of kidney stones in the United States has risen from 5.2% in 1994[1] to 8.8% in 2010.[2] The prevalence is 10.6% in men and 7.1% in women.[2] Increasing prevalence is documented in Europe and Southeast Asia.[3] Obesity and diabetes are strongly associated with kidney stones.[2] The lifetime risk is approximated at 10% to 15% in the United States and other developed countries. Urinary calculi recur in 37% of patients in the first year, 50% of patients within 10 years, and 75% of patients in 20 years.[4] Children <16 years old constitute about 7% of all renal stone cases.[5] Unique to children is a 1:1 sex distribution.[4] The most common causes in children involve metabolic abnormalities (50%), urologic anomalies (20%), infection (15%), immobilization syndrome (5%), and idiopathic causes (10%).[5] Ethnically, whites develop stones more frequently than blacks.[2]

PATHOPHYSIOLOGY

Stone formation requires supersaturation of dissolved salts in the urine, which condense into a solid phase. Increasing the amount of solvent (urine) and decreasing the amount of solute presented to the kidney (i.e., calcium, oxalate, uric acid) can aid in prevention. Inhibitory substances, such as citrate, and magnesium can prevent crystal precipitation and stone formation.

About 80% of calculi are composed of calcium oxalate, calcium phosphate, or a combination of both. Calcium excretion is elevated in conditions that include hyperparathyroidism, absorptive and renal hypercalciuria, and immobilization syndrome. Randall's plaque, a collection of interstitial suburothelial calcium phosphate particles on the surface of the renal papillae, serves as a nucleation surface for calcium oxalate stones.[6,7] Complex interactions between the gut, kidney, and bones contribute to calcium oxalate stone formation. A diet restricting calcium paradoxically increases calcium stone formation because there is less calcium to bind oxalate in the intestinal lumen, leading to increased absorption of oxalate from the gut, recruitment of calcium from bones, osteoporosis, and symptomatic stone disease in predisposed patients.

About 10% of stones are struvite (magnesium-ammonium-phosphate). These stones are associated with infection by urea-splitting bacteria (*Proteus*, *Klebsiella*, *Staphylococcus* species, *Providencia*, and *Corynebacterium*) and are the most common cause of staghorn calculi, which are large stones that form a cast of the renal pelvis. Antibiotic penetration into staghorn calculi is poor, and the potential for urosepsis exists as long as the stones remain.

Uric acid causes about 10% of urolithiasis. Twenty-five percent of patients with gout will develop kidney stones, and they occur at a rate of approximately 1% per year after the first gout attack. Urate stones are radiolucent, and the urine is typically acidic. Cystine stones are rare, account for approximately 1% of all stones, and occur in patients with cystinuria, an autosomal recessive genetic disorder affecting amino acid transport (COLA: *c*ysteine, *o*rnithine, *l*ysine, *a*rginine). Stones can be made of many other miscellaneous substances, including indinavir, triamterene, xanthene, and silicate.

Some medications predispose to stone disease. The protease inhibitor indinavir sulfate, used to treat the human immunodeficiency virus, is associated with a 4% to 10% incidence of symptomatic urolithiasis. Pure indinavir stones are radiolucent on plain abdominal x-ray and CT scan. Carbonic anhydrase inhibitors, triamterene, and laxative abuse also increase the prevalence of renal stones.[8] With appropriate evaluation, 90% of patients will have a cause identified, and over 50% of calcium oxalate stone recurrences can be prevented.[9] **Table 94-1** lists risk factors associated with kidney stones.[2,3,10]

Pain associated with kidney stones is due to obstruction of a hollow viscus organ (ureter) and subsequent hydronephrosis creating pressure against Gerota's fascia, causing flank pain. Isolated small renal pelvis stones (not staghorn) do not cause pain unless they cause intermittent obstruction of the entrance to the ureter. A migrating but nonobstructive stone also causes pain. **During acute obstruction, most patients have no rise in serum creatinine because the unobstructed kidney functions at up to 185% of its baseline capacity.** A rise in serum creatinine in acute obstruction suggests a solitary kidney or preexisting renal disease such that the unobstructed kidney is unable to compensate completely. Fortunately, most patients have incomplete ureteral obstruction, and many patients can be safely observed over weeks. Irreversible renal damage from an obstructive kidney stone is rare if obstruction has been present for ≤1 month.[11]

The probability of spontaneous passage of stones is determined by multiple factors, including size, shape, location, and degree of ureteral obstruction. Bizarre or irregularly shaped stones with spicules or sharp edges have a lower spontaneous passage rate. With complete obstruction, there is a lower rate of spontaneous passage than if the blockage is partial. **The most common sites of obstruction include the ureteropelvic junction, where the 1-cm pelvis constricts into the 2- to 3-mm ureter; the pelvic brim, where the ureter courses over both the pelvis and the iliac vessels; and finally, the ureterovesical junction, because this is the most constricted site of the ureter due to the muscular coat of the bladder.** Based on stone size alone, 98% of stones <5 mm will pass within 4 weeks

TABLE 94-1 Kidney Stone Risk Factors

Risk Factor	Mechanisms
Obesity	May promote hypercalciuria
Low urine volume	Allows solute to supersaturate
Excess dietary meat (purine)	Creates acidic urinary milieu; depletes available citrate (inhibitor); promotes hyperuricosuria
Excess dietary sodium	Promotes hypercalciuria
Insulin resistance, metabolic syndrome	Ammonia mishandling; alters pH of urine
Family history	Genetic predisposition
Gout	Promotes hyperuricosuria
Bowel surgery, inflammatory bowel disease	Promotes low urine volume; acidic urine depletes available citrate (inhibitor); hyperoxaluria
Primary hyperparathyroidism	Creates persistent hypercalciuria
Prolonged immobilization	Bone turnover creates hypercalciuria

without intervention. Sixty percent of stones 5 to 7 mm and 39% of stones >7 mm will pass within 4 weeks. **Stone size on plain radiographs is magnified by up to 20%, and a measured stone on CT is 88% of actual stone size.**[12]

CLINICAL FEATURES

The classic symptom complex for nephrolithiasis is the acute onset of a crampy intermittent flank pain that radiates toward the groin. As pain originates from a hollow viscus (ureter), the pain is visceral in nature without associated peritoneal irritation. Patients writhe in pain, unable to find a position of comfort. However, patients with renal colic may demonstrate rebound tenderness (29%), guarding (61%), and rigidity (8%).[13] Pain is commonly accompanied by nausea and vomiting (50%). The adrenergic response to pain can result in tachycardia, hypertension, and diaphoresis. **Hematuria is present in only 85%** of patients with renal colic, and 30% have gross hematuria.

The location of the pain correlates somewhat with the location of the stone. Stones in the upper ureter refer pain to the flank, whereas those in the mid-ureter radiate to the lower anterior quadrant of the abdomen. A distal ureter stone, which is where 75% of stones are diagnosed, refers pain to the groin. Stones positioned at the ureterovesical junction can mimic a urinary tract infection by causing frequency, urgency, and dysuria in 3% to 24% of patients.[13] Extracorporeal shock wave lithotripsy fractures stones into small particles with the use of focused sound waves. The resulting "sludge" is passed in the urine. When there are large fragments, an acute episode of renal colic occurs.

In children, symptoms vary with age. Older children are more likely to present with typical adult symptoms. Younger children may complain of nonspecific abdominal or pelvic pain. Although renal colic is rare in infants, symptoms may be mistakenly attributed to intestinal colic. Overall, 20% to 30% of children may have only painless hematuria with urologic stone disease.

During the patient interview, elucidate three important items of history: assess risk factors for stone development (Table 94-1), prior stone-related outcome, and important mimickers. The risk factors for a poor outcome with stones include three categories: renal function at risk, history of difficulty with stones, and infection (**Table 94-2**). Two mimickers that are very important to exclude are abdominal aortic aneurysm and renal artery infarction. **Nephrolithiasis is the most common misdiagnosis given to patients with a rupturing or expanding abdominal aortic aneurysm.** Recall that stones do not usually present in men older than age 60 and do not cause hypotension, even transiently. Renal artery thrombosis can mimic stone symptoms due to swelling of the infarcted kidney and can also be associated with hematuria. However, early in the course, noncontrast CT will not necessarily show inflammation around the kidney, and because no contrast is used, the function of the kidney is not assessed.

TABLE 94-2 Risk Factors for Poor Outcome with Stones

Renal function at risk
Diabetes
Hypertension
Renal insufficiency
Single kidney
Horseshoe kidney
Transplanted kidney
History of difficulty with stones
Extractions
Stents
Ureterostomy tubes
Lithotripsy
Symptoms of infection
Fever
Hypotension
Systemic illness
Urinary tract infection

DIAGNOSIS

The diagnosis of urologic stone disease is clinically suspected and supported by the presence of hematuria; imaging confirms the diagnosis with certainty.

Many diagnoses can be confused with renal colic (**Table 94-3**). History and physical examination can be difficult because the patient's discomfort may interfere with adequate information collection. The most critical diagnoses to consider are aortic dissection and ruptured abdominal aortic aneurysm. Renal colic and abdominal aortic aneurysm may have similar presentations.

LABORATORY EVALUATION

The laboratory evaluation centers on evaluating for infection, kidney dysfunction, and possibility of pregnancy. **Test all females of childbearing potential for pregnancy when considering renal colic.** With pregnancy, consider ectopic pregnancy in the differential diagnosis while minimizing radiation exposure to the fetus.

TABLE 94-3 Differential Diagnoses for Ureterolithiasis

Vascular	Aortic dissection
	Abdominal aortic aneurysm
	Renal artery embolism
	Renal vein thrombosis
	Mesenteric ischemia
Renal	Pyelonephritis
	Papillary necrosis
	Renal cell carcinoma
	Renal infarct
	Renal hemorrhage
Ureter	Blood clot
	Stricture
	Tumor (primary or metastatic)
Bladder	Tumor
	Varicose vein
	Cystitis
GI	Biliary colic
	Pancreatitis
	Perforated peptic ulcer disease
	Appendicitis
	Inguinal hernia
	Diverticulitis
	Cancer
	Bowel obstruction
Gynecologic	Ectopic pregnancy
	Pelvic inflammatory disease/tubo-ovarian abscess
	Ovarian cyst
	Ovarian torsion
	Endometriosis
GU	Testicular torsion
	Epididymitis
Other	Drug-seeking behavior
	Shingles
	Retroperitoneal hematoma/abscess/tumor

Urinalysis is needed to rule out infection. If infection is found, obtain urine culture and sensitivities to guide antibiotic therapy.[14] In suspected pediatric nephrolithiasis, a culture is often sent regardless, because identification of a urinary tract infection in children can be more difficult (see chapter 132, "Urinary Tract Infection in Infants and Children").

Hematuria (three or more red blood cells per high-power field), or even its absence, can mislead the physician. Although 10% to 15% of patients with nephrolithiasis will have no hematuria, approximately **24% of patients with flank pain and hematuria have no radiographic evidence of ureterolithiasis.**[15] Therefore, although hematuria may contribute to diagnostic decision making, it should not be used alone to exclude or confirm the diagnosis of ureterolithiasis[15] (see chapter 91, "Urinary Tract Infections and Hematuria").

Check renal function because the overwhelming majority of patients who form stones have reduced creatinine clearance.[16] Unless febrile or systemically ill, a WBC count does not aid in the evaluation; many patients will have an elevated WBC count due to stress demargination. Other laboratory studies, such as serum calcium or uric acid, are not useful in the initial evaluation or treatment but help determine stone type and long-term therapy.

IMAGING

Imaging confirms the presence of a ureteral stone, rules out other diagnoses, identifies complications, defines stone location, and assists with management if the stone fails to pass spontaneously.[17] Imaging is recommended by the American Urological Association in patients with suspected first-time stones.[18] For young, healthy, stable patients with a history of kidney stones in whom the diagnosis is clinically clear, imaging may be deferred until the follow-up visit provided that a reliable follow-up mechanism exists.[19] However, clinicians are frequently incorrect in their clinical impression in 20% to 70% of cases.[20] CT scanning reveals an alternative diagnosis in 33% of the patients.[20] Thus, the physician should determine the need for confirmation of the diagnosis based on the patient's past medical history, dangers of accumulated radiation exposure, clarity of the clinical diagnosis, and ease of follow-up and ability to return for worsening symptoms.

CT The noncontrast helical CT scan is sensitive and specific, with "diagnostic" positive and negative likelihood ratios for detection of renal stones (**Table 94-4**).[21] Images are obtained from the top of the kidney to the bladder base. Secondary signs of ureteral obstruction, such as ureteral dilatation, stranding of perinephric fat, dilatation of the collecting system, and renal enlargement, can be helpful in making the diagnosis. In combination, unilateral ureteral dilatation and perinephric stranding have a positive predictive value of 96% for stone disease.[22] If both are absent, the negative predictive value is 93% to 97%[22] (**Figures 94-1** and **94-2**).

Noncontrast helical CT has advantages over other imaging modalities, including superior speed, the avoidance of radiocontrast media, and greater ability to identify other pathologies. However, because radiocontrast is not used, the specificity and sensitivity for other diagnoses (e.g., abdominal aortic aneurysm, appendicitis, renal infarct, or perinephric abscess) are not as great as with imaging protocols using contrast, and renal function is not assessed.

Low-dose CT has been studied in small numbers. Low-dose CT is as sensitive as standard CT in detecting stones >3 mm in patients with a body mass index <30. However, it was not as sensitive for smaller stones or at higher body mass indices.[23]

IV Urography IV urography (or IV pyelogram) is rarely used, but yields information on renal function and anatomy. It detects calculi with modest sensitivity but excellent specificity[21] (Table 94-4). IV urography can be an adjunct to CT if functional information and knowledge of the degree of obstruction are required.

Plain Abdominal Radiographs Approximately 90% of urinary calculi are radiopaque because calcium phosphate and calcium oxalate stones have a density similar to that of bone. Magnesium-ammonium-phosphate (struvite) is slightly less radiodense, followed by cystine, which is only partly radiopaque. Uric acid and matrix stones are essentially radiolucent, as are most stones associated with medications such as indinavir. Unfortunately, because of small size and overlapping soft tissue and bone shadows, urinary stones are visible much less frequently on plain films. A plain kidney-ureter-bladder film is neither sensitive nor specific enough to rule in or rule out stone. However, once the location of a stone is identified on CT scan, the progression of the stone can be followed by a kidney-ureter-bladder film assuming the stone is visible.

US If patients are not candidates for CT due to concerns about radiation (e.g., during pregnancy or in children), US can assist in the diagnosis. Although useful in the detection of larger stones (**Figure 94-3**), US may miss smaller (<5 mm in diameter) ureteral stones.[24] US is helpful in diagnosing stones in the proximal and distal ureters but is insensitive for mid-ureteral stones. Overall, US has only modest sensitivity and specificity for detecting renal stones (Table 94-4) but is 78% sensitive for detecting hydronephrosis. This sensitivity for hydronephrosis goes up from 75% for stones <6 mm to 90% for stones >6 mm. However, of hydronephrosis diagnosed by US, up to 22% of studies do not represent obstruction; but rather, normal anatomic variation, full bladder, and renal cysts. Rapid bolus infusion of crystalloid can result in a false-positive finding of hydroureter.

US provides information on renal size and, with Doppler scanning, renal blood and urine flow. Obesity may interfere with obtaining good-quality scans, and US can miss early obstructive signs. Accuracy of the US study is dependent on the skill and experience of the operator.

Bedside US Although not quite as accurate as a screening examination would need to be, compared with CT, bedside US by ED physicians had a sensitivity of 80% (95% confidence interval [CI], 65% to 89%), specificity of 83% (95% CI, 61% to 94%), and overall accuracy of 81% (95% CI, 69% to 89%) in the detection of hydronephrosis.[25-27] Bedside US may be useful to detect larger stones unlikely to respond to conservative measures.

TREATMENT

PAIN AND NAUSEA

Treatment for symptomatic nephrolithiasis in the ED includes pain and nausea/vomiting control as needed, antibiotics for those with evidence of infection, and medical expulsion therapy. Forced IV hydration results in no difference in pain control or stone passage rates when compared

TABLE 94-4 Ancillary Tests in Urologic Stone Disease

Test	Sensitivity (%)	Specificity (%)	LR+	LR–	Comments
Noncontrast CT	94–97	96–99	24–∞	0.02–0.04	Advantages: speed, no RCM, detects other diagnoses Disadvantages: radiation, no evaluation of renal function
IV urogram	64–90	94–100	15–∞	0.11–0.15	Advantage: evaluates renal function Disadvantage: RCM (allergy, nephrotoxicity, metformin related acidosis)
US	63–85	79–100	10–∞	0.10–0.34	Advantages: pregnancy, no RCM, no radiation, no known side effects Disadvantages: insensitive in middle third of the ureter, may miss smaller stones (<5 mm)
Plain abdominal radiograph	29–58	69–74	1.9–2.0	0.58–0.64	Advantage: may be used to follow stones Disadvantage: poor sensitivity and specificity

Abbreviations: LR = likelihood ratio; RCM = radiocontrast media.

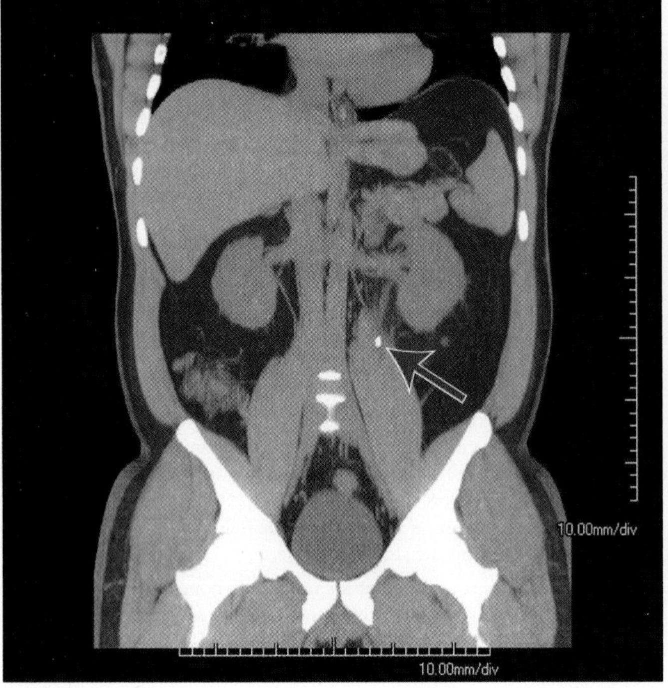

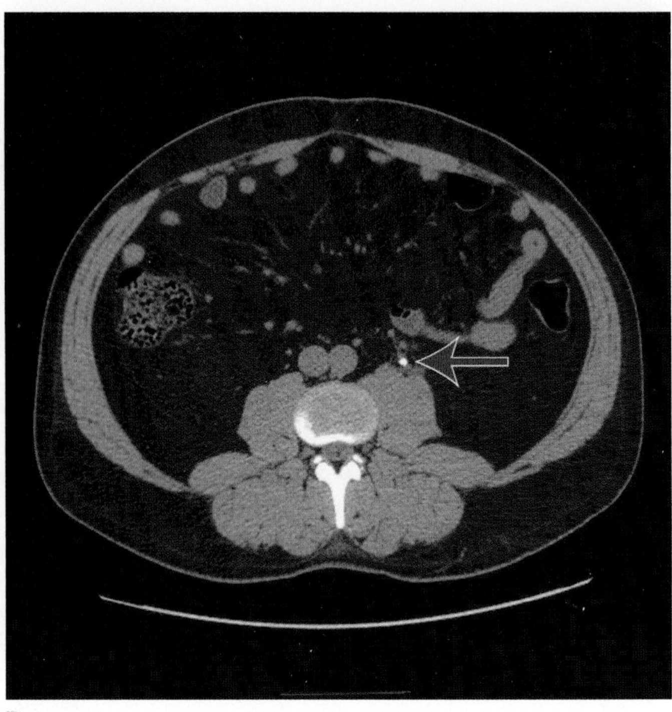

A B

FIGURE 94-1. **A.** *Red arrow* shows 6-mm stone within the proximal third of the left ureter on noncontrast CT reformatted image of upright abdomen. **B.** From same patient as in **A**, note 6-mm stone (*arrow*) within the proximal third of the left ureter on noncontrast CT.

to minimal IV hydration.[28] Fluids should be given to correct any fluid deficit due to vomiting or limited oral intake.

Nonsteroidal anti-inflammatory drugs (NSAIDs) are the primary choice of analgesics in the treatment of stone disease, because they have a direct action on the ureter by inhibiting prostaglandin synthesis.[29,30] IV administration achieves more rapid relief than IM or PO dosing[31] (e.g., ketorolac, 30 milligrams IV). There are several U.S. Food and Drug Administration boxed warnings regarding NSAID use: do not give NSAIDS in those with aspirin or NSAID hypersensitivity; avoid in coagulopathy or patients at risk for bleeding; NSAIDS increase risk of GI bleeding at any time during therapy and without warning; and avoid in renal impairment. Urology may delay the use of lithotripsy on patients who receive any drugs affecting platelet function for 3 to 10 days. Narcotics (e.g., hydromorphone, 0.5 to 2.0 milligrams IV) are good analgesics but do not affect the cause of pain. Because both the pain of the stone and narcotics can cause nausea and vomiting, address these symptoms as well.

FIGURE 94-2. CT image shows 5-mm stone (*arrow*) at left ureterovesical junction. Other calcifications are seen in the pelvis, unrelated to the urinary outflow system.

Metoclopramide is the only antiemetic that has been specifically studied in the treatment of renal colic. In two double-blinded studies, metoclopramide provided pain relief equivalent to narcotic analgesics in addition to relieving nausea. Metoclopramide works by blocking dopaminergic receptors in the CNS but is less sedating than other centrally acting dopamine antagonists.[32]

URINARY TRACT INFECTION

Patients with fever, renal insufficiency, and systemic signs of infection are treated with IV antibiotics and admitted. Options include gentamicin or tobramycin, 3.0 milligrams/kg/d divided every 8 hours, plus ampicillin, 1 to 2 grams every 4 hours; piperacillin-tazobactam, 3.375 grams IV every 6 hours; cefepime, 2 grams IV every 8 hours; ticarcillin-clavulanic acid,

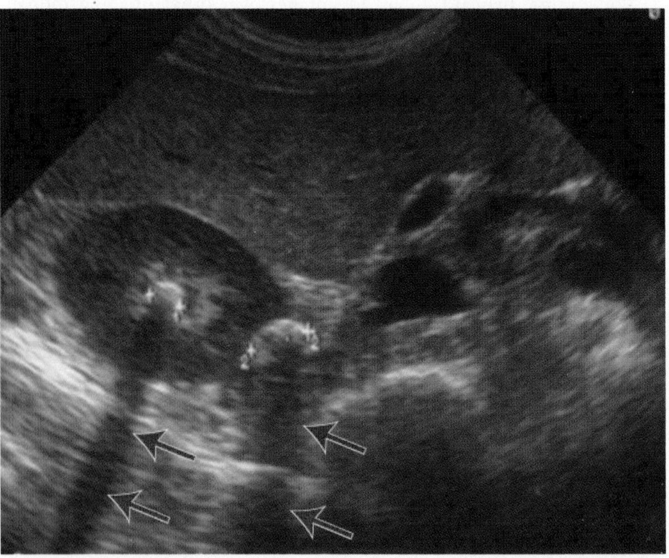

FIGURE 94-3. US of renal pelvis showing stones (marked with 1+ and 2+) with shadowing effects (*arrows*).

3.1 grams every 6 hours; or ciprofloxacin, 400 milligrams every 12 hours, if local sensitivities do not predict treatment failure.

Patients who have a ureteral stone with an associated urinary tract infection but no evidence of significant obstruction, fever, or systemic illness can be treated as outpatients, provided follow-up in 48 to 72 hours can be accomplished (see section "Disposition and Follow-Up" later in the chapter). The choice of antibiotic should cover gram-negative rods and be appropriate for antibiotic sensitivity at your institution. Resistance rates of >10% to 20% should preclude use of that antibiotic. Choices include ciprofloxacin, 500 milligrams PO twice a day for 10 to 14 days; levofloxacin, 500 milligrams PO once a day for 10 to 14 days; cefpodoxime, 200 milligrams PO twice a day for 10 to 14 days; or others predicted to be successful based on local sensitivities.

MEDICAL EXPULSION THERAPY

Medical expulsion therapy is commonly used in clinical practice and is recommended by the urologic societies.[33,34] α-Blockers are associated with increased rate of expulsion, decreased time to expulsion, and decreased pain, with a number needed to treat of 3.3 and a 2- to 6-day improvement in time to expulsion.[33,35] The benefit shown is attributable to stones in the distal third of the ureter because these were the ones most commonly included in the studies. The most commonly used agent is tamsulosin (0.4 milligram PO daily for up to 4 weeks), but terazosin (5 to 10 milligrams daily) and doxazosin (4 milligrams daily) are also as effective.[33,35] Renal colic is an off-label use of these agents; 4% of patients develop side effects including hypotension, but the drugs generally appear to be well tolerated. Calcium channel blockers, specifically nifedipine (30 milligrams PO daily up to 8 weeks), have adverse effects in approximately 15% of patients, a number needed to treat of 3.9, and time to stone expulsion reported as <28 days.[33] Some studies, including one that involved primarily ED patients, have called into question the benefit of this therapy.[36,37] One double-blinded study showed that there was no benefit in stones <6 mm.[38] Steroids are not currently recommended.[34]

DISPOSITION AND FOLLOW-UP

Most patients with stones are discharged with urologic or primary care follow-up, at which time preventive therapy may be considered based on stone type.[18] Because of lower rates of spontaneous passage, discuss disposition of patients with large (>5 mm), irregular, or proximal stones (**Table 94-5**). Also discuss with urology the disposition of patients with renal insufficiency, severe underlying comorbidities, complete obstruction, multiple ED visits associated with the stone, or associated urinary tract infection without sepsis.

Discharge is appropriate in patients with smaller stones, in the absence of infection, and when pain is controlled by oral analgesics. Give patients a urinary strainer with instructions to save any stones they pass for pathologic evaluation. **Average time for stone passage varies according to size and location but may range up to 7 to 30 days for stones 5 to 6 mm in diameter.** Patients should be counseled to return promptly for fever, vomiting, or uncontrolled pain. A prescription for an oral opiate and NSAIDs should be provided, as well as for medical expulsive therapy if used. Follow-up with a urologist within 7 days should be recommended.

TABLE 94-5 Indications for Admission in Patients with Nephrolithiasis

Absolute Indications for Admission	Relative Indications for Admission
Intractable pain or vomiting	Fever
Urosepsis*	Solitary kidney or transplanted kidney without obstruction
Single or transplanted kidney with obstruction*	Obstructing stone with signs of urinary infection
Acute renal failure	Urinary extravasation
Hypercalcemic crisis	Significant medical comorbidities
Severe medical comorbidities/advanced age	Stone unlikely to pass—large stone above the pelvic brim

*Indication for urgent decompression.

If the stone passes in the ED, no further treatment is required. Elective urologic consultation is recommended so that the etiology of the stone is evaluated and a prophylactic strategy can be arranged. **Patients with hematuria, negative imaging studies, and no other source require outpatient urologic follow-up to determine the cause of hematuria.**

SPECIAL POPULATIONS/CONSIDERATIONS

PREGNANCY

Stones occur in 1 in 1500 pregnancies, and 80% to 90% present in the second or third trimester. The presentation is the same as in non-pregnant patients with flank pain (89%) and hematuria (95%). The study of choice in pregnancy is US to identify hydronephrosis. Unfortunately, up to 90% of pregnant patients display physiologic hydronephrosis. US techniques recommended to improve sensitivity and diagnostic accuracy include endovaginal approach and looking for ureteral jets and calculating resistive indices for the kidneys.[39] If US does not provide the information necessary for management, low-dose CT[40,41] or MRI[42] should be considered in consultation with a urologist and obstetrician. **The radiation doses for various imaging modalities for stones are as follows: kidney-ureter-bladder, 0.05 to 0.15 cGy; three-film IV pyelogram, 0.15 to 0.20 cGy; and CT scan, 2.2 to 2.5 cGy.**[42] The American College of Obstetrics recognizes the use of CT scan in the evaluation of emergent conditions in pregnancy, including nephrolithiasis.[43]

With regard to treatment of pregnant patients, NSAIDS are not recommended, so narcotic pain control is most commonly used. Medical expulsive therapy with α-blockers, which are category B drugs in pregnancy, is acceptable.[41]

CHILDREN

Children with stones need investigation for metabolic disease and anatomic abnormality. Up to 30% of children with kidney stones have urinary tract anomalies. CT scans are most commonly used to identify stones in the pediatric ED, although radiation exposure remains a concern. US evaluation should be considered, especially in patients with a history of stones. Treatment includes pain and nausea control. Medical expulsive therapy is not recommended in children.

PRACTICE GUIDELINES

Practice guidelines have been issued by the European Association of Urology[34] (www.uroweb.org/gls/pdf/21_Urolithiasis_LR.pdf) and the American Urological Association (http://www.auanet.org/education/clinical-practice-guidelines.cfm).

REFERENCES

The complete reference list is available online at www.TintinalliEM.com.

Complications of Urologic Procedures and Devices

Elaine B. Josephson

COMPLICATIONS OF URINARY CATHETERS

Urinary catheters should be used sparingly. Indwelling urethral catheters are the most common; suprapubic catheters require a surgical procedure but have fewer infectious complications (see chapter 92, "Acute Urinary Retention"). **Most catheters are made of latex; however, silicone catheters are available for patients with latex allergy.**[1] **Table 95-1** lists the complications of urinary catheters.

TABLE 95-1 Complications of Urinary Catheters

Indwelling Urethral Catheters	Suprapubic Urethral Catheter
Infection	Local complications
Asymptomatic bacteriuria	Hematoma formation
Urinary tract infection (UTI)	Persistent leakage
Pyelonephritis	Insertion failure
Prostatitis	Infection
Epididymitis	Asymptomatic bacteriuria
Scrotal abscess	UTI
Gross and microscopic hematuria	Pyelonephritis
Creation of false lumen	Abdominal wall cellulitis
Urethral disruption	
Bladder perforation	
Mechanical obstruction	
Nondeflating catheter balloon	
Intraluminal encrustation	

INFECTION

Catheter-associated urinary tract infections (UTIs) are one of the most common causes of nosocomial infections. The risk of infection is approximately 1% to 2% with a catheter in place for <24 hours, with the prevalence of bacteriuria reaching almost 100% for long-term catheterization (by 30 days).[2] Comorbidities that increase the risk of catheter-associated UTI include female sex, prostatic hypertrophy, creatinine >2 milligrams/dL, diabetes, advanced age, nonsurgical disease, and debilitation.[3] Microbial factors associated with an incidence of catheter-associated UTI include the source of the organisms, the specific bacteria, the route of invasion, and the duration of catheterization.

Pathophysiology In the noncatheterized urinary tract, bacteria are efficiently eliminated. In contrast, most bacterial strains that are introduced into the catheterized urinary tract are able to multiply to high concentrations in 24 hours. Bacteria may be able to gain access to the urinary tract through the catheter lumen (intraluminal) or along the catheter surface (extraluminal). The drainage tube of a urinary catheter must be opened periodically to drain the accumulated urine. If the drainage tube lumen is colonized, bacteria may ascend the collection bag and catheter, causing an infection. An infection from the catheter lumen route begins with the formation of a biofilm on the catheter's inner surface. This biofilm extends from the uroepithelium through catheters to the drainage bag and allows adherence of bacteria to a catheter or mucosal surface. Organisms become embedded within the biofilm and gain protection from the mechanical flow of urine, host defenses, and antibiotics.[2] The microbiology of catheter-associated UTI varies according to the duration of catheter placement. During short-term catheterization, infections are usually due to single organisms, most commonly *Escherichia coli*, followed by *Klebsiella*, *Pseudomonas*, *Enterobacter*, and gram-positive cocci such as staphylococci. With long-term catheterization (≤30 days), catheter-associated UTIs are usually polymicrobial from *E. coli*, *Proteus mirabilis*, *Pseudomonas*, *Morganella morganii*, and *Candida* species. These infections are usually difficult to treat due to antibiotic resistance by the infecting bacteria.[2]

Asymptomatic bacteriuria usually occurs with short-term catheterization, and removal of the catheter clears the bacteriuria. **Antibiotic treatment of asymptomatic bacteriuria in a patient with a short-term indwelling urinary catheter is not recommended[2-5] (unless the patient is pregnant or immediately pending a urologic procedure).** Guidelines and reviews recommend antibiotics for symptomatic catheter-associated UTI only.[2-4]

Clinical Features Signs and symptoms include fever, rigors, altered mental status, malaise, or lethargy with no other identified cause; flank pain; costovertebral angle tenderness; acute hematuria; pelvic discomfort; and in those whose catheters have been removed, dysuria, urgent or frequent urination, or suprapubic pain or tenderness. In patients with spinal cord injury, increased spasticity, autonomic dysreflexia, and sense of unease are also compatible with catheter-associated UTI.[4]

TABLE 95-2 Infectious Complications of Indwelling Urethral Catheters

Symptomatic Urinary Tract Infection Type	Diagnosis Requires Symptoms
Cystitis	New onset or worsening of fever, rigors, suprapubic pain or tenderness , altered mental status, malaise, acute hematuria (compare to prior assessment); pelvic discomfort or lethargy with no other identified cause.
Pyelonephritis	Syndrome, including fever, rigors, flank pain, or costovertebral angle tenderness.
Symptomatic urinary tract infection in patients with spinal cord injury	Fever, rigors, increased spasticity, autonomic dysreflexia, or sense of unease.
Bacteremia	Diagnosis supported by correlation between blood and urine cultures.
Sepsis syndrome	See chapter 151, "Sepsis"
Suppurative Complications	
Urethritis	See chapter 93, "Male Genital Problems."
Epididymitis	See chapter 93.
Prostatitis	See chapter 93.
Abscess, scrotal, urethral	See chapter 93.

Diagnosis Diagnoses of catheter-associated UTI symptoms are listed in **Table 95-2**.[4] **Pyuria is universal for patients with long-term (>1 month) indwelling catheters; in the absence of clinical symptoms, pyuria should not be used in the diagnosis of symptomatic infection.**[2-4] Hematuria is a better indicator of infection and also may suggest urinary obstruction. Bedside US can identify urinary obstruction.[4]

Pyelonephritis (complicated UTI; see chapter 91, "Urinary Tract Infections and Hematuria") is the most common complication of catheter-associated UTI with fever. Other related infections include prostatitis, epididymitis, and scrotal abscess. Obtain urine cultures prior to empiric antibiotic therapy, and obtain blood cultures if the patient is septic or immunocompromised.[2]

Treatment Remove the catheter if clinically feasible, or replace the catheter if it has been in place for >7 days.[2,4] Empiric antibiotics should be instituted promptly in most cases[4] unless the fever is low grade and the clinical condition allows for time to perform cultures and continued observation.[2] Assess local resistance patterns if available before instituting therapy. Treatment for complicated UTI is reviewed in Table 91-6. Outpatient treatment for patients without clinical toxicity is presented in Table 91-5 in chapter titled "Urinary Tract Infections and Hematuria". A total of 7 total days is the recommended duration of antimicrobial treatment for patients with catheter-associated UTI who have prompt resolution of symptoms, and a total of 10 to 14 days of treatment is recommended for those with a delayed response.[4] Alter drug regimens for renal insufficiency. If candiduria exists, remove the catheter, and consider antifungal agents in symptomatic patients.[2,4]

CATHETER OBSTRUCTION AND LEAKAGE

Urethral catheters can become obstructed for many reasons, most commonly from the formation of intraluminal encrustations during long-term placement. These concretions are composed of compounds, such as ammonium magnesium sulfate (struvite) and calcium phosphate (apatite), often with urease-splitting organisms, such as *Protease* and *Morganella*. Such encrustations can increase the risk of formation of infectious stones and cause bladder trauma, leading to blood clots. A catheter obstruction may lead to urinary leakage around the catheter and acute urinary retention. Management options include repeated bladder irrigations, methenamine treatment, and removal of the catheter if the other methods fail.

NONDEFLATION OF FOLEY RETENTION BALLOON

The Foley balloon is typically inflated with 10 mL of sterile water after successful insertion. Nondeflation of the retention balloon on the catheter can be caused by a faulty valve mechanism or crystallization of balloon fluid, yielding entrapment of the Foley catheter.[6] One noninvasive method is introduction of a flexible guidewire into the balloon inflation channel after cutting off the plastic cylindrical valve from the catheter just below its head. The guidewire dilates the channel and may allow the balloon to deflate. If unsuccessful, try step 2; a 22-gauge central venous catheter can be passed over the guidewire. When the catheter tip is into the balloon, the wire can be removed, and the balloon may drain. If step 2 is unsuccessful, instill 10 mL of mineral oil and leave for 15 minutes in an attempt to dissolve the balloon. Repeat once (10 more mL of mineral oil) if unsuccessful. If simple methods do not work, urologic consultation for intervention and potential cystoscopy is recommended.[7] Another alternative is US-guided percutaneous rupture of the balloon using a needle, typically done by the radiologist in the US suite with input from urology.

COMPLICATIONS OF PERCUTANEOUS NEPHROSTOMY

Percutaneous nephrostomy is a urinary drainage procedure used for supravesical or ureteral obstruction secondary to malignancy, pyonephrosis, GU stones, and ureteral strictures. It is also adjunctive to lithotripsy and ureteral stents. Nephrostomy tubes are also used for urinary diversion associated with vesical fistula, ureteral transection, and trauma. The percutaneous procedure to remove renal calculi is known as *percutaneous nephrolithotomy*. Nephrostomy tubes or stents are commonly left in place, but the tubeless percutaneous nephrolithotomy technique may have less risk of morbidity.[8] Patients develop postoperative complications days or months after the percutaneous nephrostomy. In general, the risk of complications is low and includes bleeding, infection, mechanical complications related to the catheter (dislodgement or obstruction), and accidental punctures of adjacent organs.[8]

During insertion, injury can occur to the renal collecting system (subintimal dissection), lungs (pneumothorax), liver, spleen, and bowel (perforation).[9] This complication usually is clinically apparent during or immediately after the procedure, but recognition may be delayed a few days.[9]

Bleeding and hemorrhage can occur, especially if the patient has a coagulopathy. Check hemoglobin, hematocrit, and renal function. Obtain coagulation studies (prothrombin time, partial thromboplastin time, and platelet count) and type and cross-match if bleeding is excessive or if coagulopathy is suspected. Most bleeding episodes are mild and can be managed with irrigation to clear nephrostomy tube blood clots. More severe bleeding can be handled by catheter tamponade, a procedure undertaken by the urologist and radiologist. Severe hemorrhage occurs from vascular injury, such as laceration of an artery, formation of an arteriovenous fistula, or bleeding from a pseudoaneurysm, and may occur in the retroperitoneal space or perirenal areas. In such cases, fluid resuscitation and blood transfusion, in addition to more definitive interventions, are required. Angiographic studies with possible embolization may be needed to ascertain the site of bleeding and effect treatment.[9] Infectious complications from nephrostomy tubes include simple bacteriuria, pyelonephritis, renal abscess, bacteremia, and urosepsis. Signs and symptoms are fever, chills, rigors, pain, and purulent drainage at the site or from the tube. Obtain urine and wound drainage (if present) cultures, and give antibiotics after consultation with the urologist.

Mechanical complications, such as catheter dislodgement, tube blockage, and residual stone fragments, can occur with these devices. CT scan may be helpful for specific diagnosis. The risk of catheter dislodgement increases with increasing duration of the nephrostomy. Dislodgement occurring in the early postoperative period usually requires creation of a new tract at a different site. Dislodgement occurring after some period may be treated by recannulation under fluoroscopic guidance. Tube blockage can occur secondary to encrustations and kinking. The urologist has several techniques available to reestablish access to an obstructed nephrostomy tube.[8,9]

URINARY DIVERSION AND ORTHOTOPIC BLADDER SUBSTITUTION

The most common method of urinary diversion in the United States is the ileal conduit. With this procedure, a section of small bowel is isolated, and the free ends of the remaining small bowel are reunited, allowing for normal bowel function. The ureters are reimplanted to the isolated section of small bowel, most commonly at the base of the conduit. A stoma is created, typically on the anterior abdominal wall, where a collecting bag is attached. Postoperative complications include bowel obstruction, pyelonephritis, skin breakdown surrounding the stoma, stenosis of the stoma, and inflammatory changes of the upper tract due to reflux of urine back into the ureters. Complications occur in 66% of patients, including deterioration in kidney function (27%), stoma stenosis or infection (24%), bowel obstruction or symptoms (24%), symptomatic UTI/pyelonephritis (23%), conduit/ureteral anastomosis dysfunction (14%), and urolithiasis (9%).[10]

There are multiple newer methods of creating a neobladder for orthotopic bladder substitution. These methods all have a goal of creating a continent reservoir for urine without reflux of the urine into the reimplanted ureters, which predisposes the patient to pyelonephritis. Options include other means of isolating portions of the small bowel (Kock pouch, T pouch, "W" shape neobladder) or large bowel (ileocecal segment). An evidenced-based evaluation of multiple methods has failed to identify a superior procedure.[11] Bacteriuria is common after the procedure (85%) and mostly involves skin flora but may occasionally include uropathogenic strains (gram-negative Enterobacteriaceae species like *E. coli*, *Proteus*, *Pseudomonas*, and *Enterococcus faecalis*).[2,3,12] Clean intermittent catheterization, frequently required after procedure, is associated with increased bacteriuria and pyuria. **Diagnosis of infection should be made on evidence of symptomatic infection based on fever, flank pain, a change in chronic symptoms, or culture of pathologic organisms.** A threshold of at least 10^4 colony-forming units/mL should be used as the criterion for a positive culture.[13] Consultation with urology may be required for optimal management.

LITHOTRIPSY

Extracorporeal shock wave lithotripsy is the application of repetitive high-intensity sound waves to fragment GU calculi so they can pass down the ureter more easily.[14] Common complications include colicky pain in 15% to 40%, gross hematuria in 32%, skin bruising in up to 26%, and steinstrasse ("street of stone," aggregate of stone fragments lining and/or impacting the ureter) in up to 24%.[15-17] Uncommon complications include spleen rupture, kidney rupture, pyelonephritis/sepsis, bowel injury, ureteric perforations, psoas abscess, vascular injury, and pancreatitis (a small rise in lipase is common).[15-18] Postlithotripsy patients may present with abdominal and flank pain, nausea, vomiting (especially 48 hours after procedure), skin ecchymosis, gross hematuria, or fever in up to 30%. Uncommonly, patient may be unstable with hypotension or sepsis. Hematuria is generally self-limited (<24 hours); however, UTI may be coexistent. Diagnosis of minor complications usually requires blood counts, basic chemistries, urinalysis, and renal US if obstruction is suspected. CT scan or MRI (only if stable) is indicated if the serious complications are suspected (consider with flank hematoma, fall in hematocrit, hypotension, syncope, or significant pain). Acute management may include IV fluid hydration, antiemetics, analgesics, monitoring, fluid resuscitation, blood transfusions, and antibiotics. Most patients are managed conservatively with close monitoring of hemodynamic status, urine output, and laboratory studies to assess for decreasing hematocrit and renal function. Consult urology early on, because specific treatments, such as embolization and nephrectomy, may be required.[14]

COMPLICATIONS OF URETERAL STENTS

Ureteral stents are used primarily in patients to relieve ureteral obstruction and maintain ureteral lumen patency. Obstruction to the ureter may result from causes such as stones, strictures, trauma, malignancies, or

TABLE 95-3 Complications of Ureteral Stents

Complication	Management
Fever with pyelonephritis or sepsis	Admission, IV antibiotics, consult urology
Simple urinary tract infection (UTI)	Oral antibiotics
Microscopic hematuria/gross hematuria	Microscopic hematuria is expected, consult urology for gross hematuria
Pyuria	Treat if coexistent bacteriuria
Irritative bladder symptoms	Analgesics, anticholinergics, rule out UTI
Dysuria/urgency/frequency	Analgesics, anticholinergics, rule out UTI
Flank pain/abdominal pain	Analgesics, anticholinergics, rule out UTI
Pain with voiding	Analgesics, anticholinergics, rule out UTI
Incontinence	Analgesics, anticholinergics, rule out UTI
Obstruction	Consult urology
Stent migration/stent fragmentation	Consult urology
Encrustation	Consult urology if obstructed
Erosion of the urinary tract	Consult urology
Vascular-ureter fistula	Consult urology, resuscitation
Malposition	Consult urology
Stent malfunction	Consult urology

retroperitoneal fibrosis. Stents can be placed during ureteroscopy, by the percutaneous nephrostomy route, during surgery involving the GU tract to maintain urinary patency and drainage, and in very specific cases as an adjunct to lithotripsy in the management of nephrolithiasis. **Table 95-3** lists the complications of ureteral stents.

Many factors contribute to stent-related UTIs. Stents induce a foreign body reaction, which increases the risk for infections. Encrustation of stents in the presence of infection with urea-splitting organisms also promotes infection. More serious infections, such as pyelonephritis and sepsis, can occur but are less common.

Most minor infections can be managed with outpatient antibiotics and do not require stent removal (see antibiotic recommendations for catheter-associated UTI in the "Infection" section above). If pyelonephritis or a systemic infection is suspected, IV antibiotics, radiologic studies to determine the position of the stent, and urologic consultation are required. Stents usually can be visualized by plain abdominal x-rays due to the presence of radiodense marking embedded within the catheters. US imaging can detect hydronephrosis, along with confirmatory CT studies if obstruction or pyelonephritis is present.[19,20]

Symptoms, such as mild flank pain, and signs suggestive of an irritative bladder, such as dysuria, urgency, frequency, incontinence, and pain during voiding, occur commonly in patients with ureteral stents. Treatment options for these symptoms can include analgesics and anticholinergic medications and obtaining urine specimen to exclude UTI. New complaints and symptoms, such as severe flank pain, require evaluation for stent migration, infection, or obstruction. Asymptomatic microscopic hematuria is usually of no clinical significance, but gross hematuria may indicate stent migration or ureteral erosion. Imaging studies are needed to identify stent position.[19,20]

Serious problems, such as stent migration and stent fragmentation—or even rarer, ureteral-arterial fistulization due to stent erosion into a nearby vessel—are usually late complications seen with long-term stent placements. Stent migration can occur upward above the ureteropelvic junction or downward below this junction. See **Figure 95-1** for a radiographic demonstration of ureteral stent migration. Such migration can lead to obstruction and infections. Stent migration results in symptoms of new-onset abdominal pain, fever, and irritative bladder symptoms and hematuria.[19,20] For new anemia without hematuria, obtain a CT without contrast to rule out a stent-caused retroperitoneal hematoma.[21] In the presence of severe gross hematuria and syncope or hypotension, assume vascular fistulization from an eroding stent exists until proven otherwise.[21] Resuscitate with IV fluids, and conduct lab studies, bladder irrigation as indicated, and possible blood transfusion. Serious complications require immediate consultation with the urologist, and depending on the case, a surgeon and radiologist may need to be consulted.

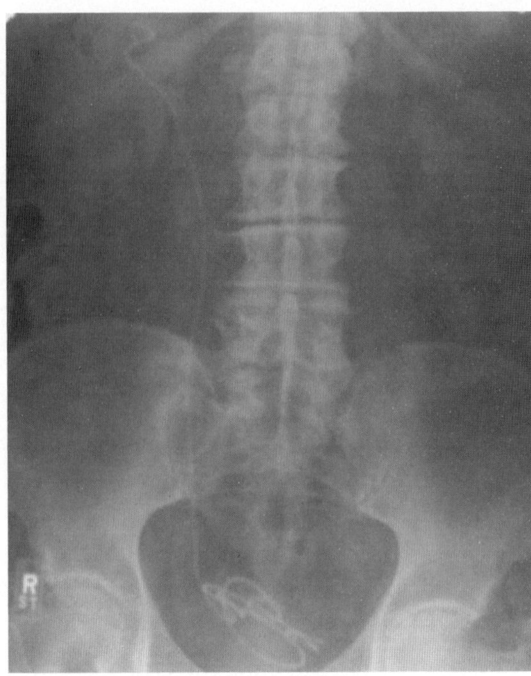

FIGURE 95-1. Ureteral stent migration. This abdominal plain film demonstrates stent migration with the distal portion of the stent coiled within the bladder. [Reproduced with permission from Cline D, Stead L: *Abdominal Emergencies*. © 2008, McGraw-Hill Inc., New York.]

PROSTATE SURGICAL PROCEDURES

Prostate surgery is commonly performed for symptomatic benign prostatic hyperplasia or prostate cancer. Surgical techniques include prostate needle biopsy, transurethral resection of the prostate, transurethral electrovaporization of the prostate, transurethral microwave thermotherapy of the prostate, transurethral needle ablation of the prostate, and visually assisted laser prostatectomy.[22,23] Complications include urinary retention (3%), clot retention (2%), UTI (1.7%), and bleeding requiring transfusion (0.4%). Less common complications include blood per rectum, urethral strictures, and urosepsis.[22,23] Patients may also experience obstructive or irritative voiding symptoms, including incontinence, dysuria, hesitancy, dribbling, urgency, and frequency.

Depending on severity of illness, appropriate laboratory studies may include urinalysis, CBC, blood type and screen, blood chemistries, and renal function. Assess for hemodynamic instability and treat with IV fluids or blood for life-threatening bleeding. Patients with outflow obstruction should be treated with a three-way Foley catheter. Start with manual irrigation to remove clots, and then initiate continuous irrigation with normal saline until clear or slight pink return.[6] If bleeding does not clear, consult urology. **Prolonged irrigation requires monitoring of serum electrolytes to assess for hyponatremia.**[6] If infection is suspected, obtain urine cultures, administer antibiotics, and consult with the urologist.

COMPLICATIONS OF ARTIFICIAL URINARY SPHINCTERS

The artificial urinary sphincter is used for urinary incontinence secondary to sphincter disturbance, postsurgical incontinence, neurogenic bladder with incontinence, trauma to the urethra, and congenital conditions associated with bladder dysfunction, such as exstrophy and epispadias. There are many different models of sphincter devices. The basic principle of the artificial sphincter is to increase the resistance around the urethra and, thus, provide urinary continence.[24,25] Mechanical parts of the artificial sphincter include a pump, an inflatable cuff that encircles the urethra, and a pressure-regulating reservoir balloon

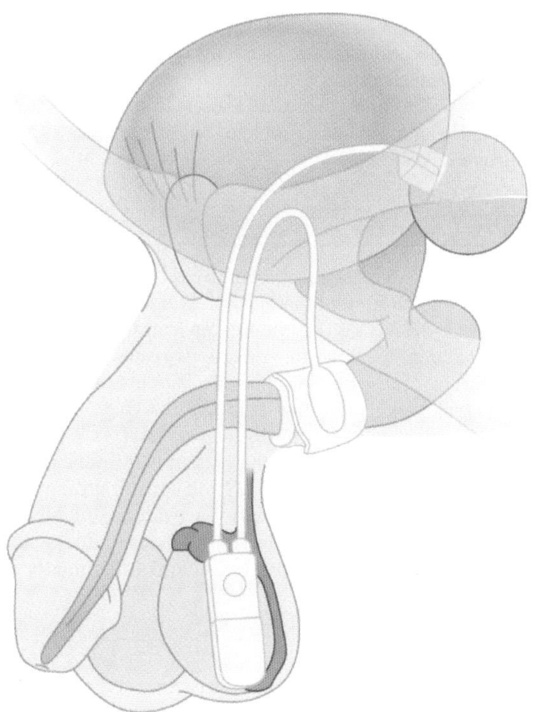

FIGURE 95-2. Diagram of artificial urinary sphincter. [Adapted with permission from James MH, McCammon KA: Artificial urinary sphincter for post-prostatectomy incontinence: a review. *Int J Urol* 21: 536, 2014. Copyright John Wiley & Sons.]

(**Figure 95-2**). These are connected by a set of two tubes. Continence occurs when fluid is moved from the balloon to the cuff. To allow urination, the cuff is emptied, and fluid moves to the reservoir. Both activities are controlled by the pump, which is implanted in the scrotum of males or the pelvis of females.[25]

Postoperative complications can include bleeding (including hematoma), infection, and malfunctions. Hematomas usually occur in the scrotum or the labia, and most resolve spontaneously. Larger hematomas may need to be drained to aid with the healing process (consult the surgeon).[24,25]

Infections are the most serious complication of the artificial sphincter. Periprosthetic infection can present early or late after surgical implantation. Infections occurring early after implantation are usually due to skin flora. Later infections are usually due to gram-negative organisms of the urinary tract. Symptoms and signs of infection can range from pain, swelling, and induration of the site to localized erythema of the pump or cuff site. More serious infections can present with fever, cellulitis, local abscess formation, drainage from incision sites, and erosion of the pump or the cuff. Infections can cause the components (e.g., cuff) to externalize out onto the skin or erode the urethra.[26] Treatment of periprosthetic infection requires antibiotics and removal of the sphincter. Patients with an artificial sphincter in place should receive antibiotic prophylaxis when undergoing procedures that may cause hematogenous seeding of the device, such as dental procedures.[26]

Retained air bubbles, tube kinking, fluid leaks, and perforation of the cuff are some of the mechanical complications that can occur with the artificial sphincter. Air bubbles can cause blockage of the pump, leading to filling defects and, thus, incontinence. Ineffective device functioning secondary to fluid leakage also can lead to sudden onset of incontinence. Tube kinking, a rare complication, can result in fluid blockage, thereby leading to urinary retention. A careful history may provide clues to malfunction. A pump that is difficult to squeeze implies blockage due to any cause, whereas a pump that remains compressed after squeezing signifies pressure loss or fluid leakage. Incorrect urinary catheterization and damage to the device components during other nonurologic surgeries may account for iatrogenic malfunction of the artificial sphincter. Plain radiographs of the pelvis and other imaging studies are used to assess continuity of the mechanical components.[24,25]

Urethral erosion secondary to infection or excessive cuff pressure around the urethra is another serious complication and one that is seen most commonly within several months after the implantation. Signs and symptoms include pain, swelling along the urethra and in the perineum, urinary incontinence, bloody urethral discharge, and infection. Cystourethroscopy and cuff removal are necessary for management of erosions.[24-26]

Recurrent incontinence after artificial sphincter placement can have many causes—infection, cuff erosion, fistulas due to surgical injuries, or mechanical failure. Evaluation requires urodynamic studies to accurately define the cause. Acute urinary retention in a patient with an artificial sphincter implant may occur as a result of bladder neck contractures, urethral strictures, or cuff erosion. Evaluation usually requires cystourethrography or cystourethral endoscopy.

Evaluation in the ED of complications related to the artificial sphincter requires a thorough history noting the model type and make; symptom assessment; a detailed physical examination; urinalysis; appropriate labs, cultures, and imaging studies; and consideration for IV antibiotics as indicated. **Never introduce a urethral urinary drainage catheter through an artificial urinary sphincter.** Consult the urologist for further evaluation and management.

COMPLICATIONS OF DEVICES FOR ERECTILE DYSFUNCTION

The most common causes of erectile dysfunction are diabetes, priapism, vascular disease, Peyronie's disease (deformity especially seen on erection due to nodules/fibrous plaques in penile tissue), pelvic trauma or surgery, spinal cord injury, and psychogenic reasons. Although oral medication and penile injectable device treatment currently exist for erectile dysfunction, some patients with erectile dysfunction fail pharmacologic therapy and are treated with nonpharmacologic interventions such as vacuum therapy, external splint devices, and the surgically implantable prostheses.[27] Two forms of injection therapy for erectile dysfunction are available: intracavernosal and intraurethral.

INTRACAVERNOSAL INJECTIONS

The intracavernosal injections are given along the lateral aspect of the penis, directly into the corpora cavernosa. The basic mechanism involves vasodilatation of arteries and veins leading to corporal smooth muscle relaxation and penile erection. Drugs used are papaverine, phentolamine, and alprostadil, a prostaglandin E_1 analog, singly or in combination. Side effects include penile pain, prolonged erections (4 to 6 hours), priapism (painful erection for longer than 6 hours), and localized hematoma. Of these, priapism is the most critical complication. Management of priapism includes emergent urology consultation for direct injection of terbutaline or α-adrenergic agonists, such as phenylephrine, and corporal aspiration of blood (see chapter 93).[28]

INTRAURETHRAL INJECTION

Intraurethral injections of alprostadil are successful in producing penile engorgement. One marketed product, the MUSE® (medicated transurethral system for erection), uses a medicated pellet via an applicator that allows insertion of the drug into the urethra. The basic mechanism of intraurethral administration is similar to intracavernosal injections. The drug is absorbed from the urethra and through the local communicating vessels and exerts its actions on the corpora. Side effects are few and can include penile pain, urethral bleeding, laceration of the cavernosal artery, and dizziness. Very rarely, priapism can occur. Intraurethral administration is usually free of any major systemic side effects, but syncope secondary to a vasovagal reaction due to the anxiety of the injection and the vasodilatory effects of the drug can occur.[29]

VACUUM DEVICES AND PENILE SPLINTS

Vacuum devices work by use of negative pressure and the use of a constriction ring to cause venous and arterial congestion, thus causing penile engorgement. The most common complaint reported is pain during application of the device and during ejaculation secondary to inappropriate pressure rise. Both symptoms can be resolved with proper education on use of the device. Local skin cyanosis secondary to a drop in penile blood flow from the negative pressure may also be seen. Serious complications from the use of a vacuum device include penile skin necrosis, urethral bleeding, ischemia, and subcutaneous hemorrhage with ecchymosis. Peyronie's disease and Fournier's gangrene have also been reported.[30]

The external penile splint consists of two steel support rods in a silicone cover that have a support loop at the distal end, to loop around the subcoronal sulcus, and support rings at the proximal end, to position around the base of the penis. Aside from occasional dislodgement during sexual intercourse, these splints are relatively free of side effects.[27]

PENILE PROSTHESES

Surgical implantation of a penile prosthesis is reserved for men who fail pharmacologic treatment. Several different kinds of implantable penile prostheses are used: the malleable or semirigid devices, and inflatable types that contain fluid to give a more natural erection. The malleable or semirigid device consists of implanted semirigid rods and is always somewhat firm. The penis may be positioned away from the body to achieve penetration. There are self-contained and three-piece inflatable devices. The self-contained device consists of a pair of inflatable cylinders inserted in the cavernosa and a scrotal pump. The three-piece device is composed of a pair of inflatable cylinders, a scrotal pump, and an abdominal fluid reservoir. Postoperative urinary retention, penoscrotal hematoma formation, and superficial wound infections have been reported. Infection is the most devastating of all penile prosthesis complications and usually occurs soon after the primary surgery for implantation. Late infections can occur years after the procedure secondary to seeding through the bloodstream. Organisms causing penile prosthesis infection are typically *Staphylococcus epidermidis*, *Staphylococcus aureus*, and gram-negative bacilli. Infections present as pain along the device (e.g., in the scrotum or along the penis), erosion, and purulent urethral discharge. Treatment requires antibiotics and removal of the entire device by the urologist.[29,30]

Erosion of the prosthesis can occur into penile tissue and often is accompanied by an infection in the same area. Migration of the device may occur proximally or distally, presenting as extrusion through the urethral meatus. Erosion problems and device migration require consultation with the urologist for removal of the prosthesis. Penile ischemia and necrosis are rare but serious complications occurring mainly in patients with predisposing factors such as diabetes and vascular disease. Mechanical failures may occur, such as pump autoinflation or fluid leakage from tubing, cylinder, or reservoir. Evaluation of mechanical problems requires an assessment of the device by a urologist.[27,29]

VASECTOMY

With few exceptions, vasectomies are completed in the urologist's office. Complications of infection, symptomatic hematoma, and chronic scrotal pain occur in 1% to 3%.[31] Less common complications include bleeding and scrotal hematoma, local wound infections (cellulitis and abscess), epididymitis, and painful sperm granulomas. Patients may develop persistent testicular pain or congestive epididymitis (pain and testicular tenderness on the affected side) months to years later.[31]

Evaluate for infection especially if the patient is immunosuppressed, and treat accordingly; consider scrotal US and consult urology for deep abcess (see chapter 93). When there is no evidence of bleeding or wound infection, treat postvasectomy epididymitis with ice packs, scrotal support, and analgesia with nonsteroidal anti-inflammatory drugs or opiates.

ADULT CIRCUMCISION

Circumcision, or foreskin resection, is usually performed on infant males. However, the procedure is also performed in adolescents and adults.[32] Complications after circumcision include bleeding and infection (most common), pain, hematomas, swelling, suture tears, and wound dehiscence due to premature erection before completion of healing. Treat minor bleeding with direct pressure, or a topical thrombostatic agent as needed. Administer oral antibiotics (trimethoprim-sulfamethoxazole or ciprofloxacin) with local wound care for minor infections. Give analgesia as indicated. Consult urology for significant bleeding or infection.

REFERENCES

The complete reference list is available online at www.TintinalliEM.com.

SECTION 11

Obstetrics and Gynecology

CHAPTER 96 Abnormal Uterine Bleeding

Bophal Sarha Hang

INTRODUCTION

Abnormal uterine bleeding is an overarching term that is defined as bleeding from the uterine corpus that is irregular in volume, frequency, or duration in absence of pregnancy (**Table 96-1**).[1] Vaginal bleeding is a common complaint in the ED, and differential diagnoses include pregnancy, structural abnormalities (e.g., polyps, fibroids), endometritis, coagulopathies, trauma, and various other causes. The prevalence of abnormal bleeding is estimated at 9% to 14% in the general population. Although vaginal bleeding may present as an acute or chronic problem, this chapter will focus on the ED evaluation and management of abnormal uterine bleeding.

MENSTRUAL CYCLE

In North America, average age of menarche is 12.5 years of age, approximately 2 years after the development of thelarche (breast budding). Early cycles are often anovulatory and irregular due to the immaturity of the hypothalamic-pituitary axis. Regular ovulatory cycles develop on average 2 years after the start of menarche.

The normal menstrual cycle is 28 days and is divided into four phases: menses, follicular, ovulation, and luteal or secretory. **Figure 96-1** depicts hormonal and endometrial changes associated with a normal menstrual cycle.

In response to the rising estrogen levels, the pituitary gland secretes follicle-stimulating hormone and luteinizing hormone, which stimulates the release of the mature oocyte. The residual follicular capsule forms the corpus luteum. During the luteal phase, the corpus luteum secretes estrogen and progesterone, which maintains the integrity of the endometrium and makes it more receptive to implantation. If fertilization and implantation occur, the developing embryo secretes human chorionic gonadotropin into the bloodstream, signaling the corpus luteum to continue the production of progesterone and estrogen necessary to support early pregnancy. In the absence of human chorionic gonadotropin, the corpus luteum involutes, and estrogen and progesterone levels fall. Hormonal withdrawal causes vasoconstriction in the spiral arterioles of the endometrium. As a consequence, the ischemic endometrial lining becomes necrotic and sloughs, which leads to menses. The vaginal effluvium contains blood, endometrial tissue, and fluid. The average amount of menstrual blood loss ranges from 25 to 60 mL.

The average tampon or pad absorbs 20 to 30 mL of vaginal effluent. However, judging the amount of blood loss by usage may be unreliable because personal habits vary greatly among women. In women with heavy bleeding, there may be insufficient time for fibrinolysis, so blood clots form.

TABLE 96-1 FIGO Terminology for Bleeding*

Type	Definition
Abnormal uterine bleeding	Bleeding that is abnormal in regularity, volume, frequency, or duration. Bleeding may be acute or chronic and is present for at least 6 months.
Heavy menstrual bleeding *(heavy uterine bleeding [HUB] replaces menorrhagia)*	Excessive menstrual bleeding that interferes with a woman's physical, emotional, social, and quality of life. Note that the definition is menstrual bleeding deemed excessive by the patient regardless of duration, frequency, or timing.
Amenorrhea	Bleeding that is absent for >6 months.
Prolonged menstrual bleeding	Menstrual bleeding that is absent for >6 months.
Intermenstrual bleeding *(replaces metrorrhagia)*	Bleeding episodes between normally timed menstrual periods.
Irregular menstrual bleeding	Unpredictable onset of menses, with cycle variations >20 days over a period of 1 year.
Postmenopausal bleeding	Any bleeding that occurs >12 months after cessation of menstruation.

Abbreviation: FIGO = International Federation of Gynecology and Obstetrics.

*Discarded terms include dysfunctional uterine bleeding, menorrhagia, functional uterine bleeding, hypermenorrhea, hypomenorrhea, menometrorrhagia, metrorrhagia, oliogomenorrhea, polymenorrhea, and uterine hemorrhage.[2]

CLINICAL FEATURES

HISTORY

Obtaining a focused medical history should include details of current bleeding episode, associated symptoms, and past medical history including reproductive and sexual history (**Table 96-2**). Pregnancy-related bleeding should always be considered and ruled out in reproductive-age patients. Patients may describe heavy bleeding as soaking of more than one pad or tampon within 1 hour or passing large clots. **Up to 20% of women with heavy uterine bleeding have an underlying coagulation disorder, with von Willebrand's disease being the most common.** Screening for history of heavy menstrual bleeding since menarche, postpartum hemorrhage, surgery- or dental-related bleeding, and family history may help guide further evaluation for bleeding disorders. It is also important to ask about oral contraceptive use because missed doses are a frequent cause of bleeding. Questions about drug interactions and smoking are also important in determining the cause of bleeding.

To obtain an accurate sexual history from an adolescent patient, assure physician confidentiality and maintain a nonjudgmental attitude. If a female physician is requested, try to honor the request if at all possible. Always ask the parents for an opportunity to interview the patient without the parent present. Furthermore, all states allow minors to consent to diagnosis and treatment of sexually transmitted diseases and drug abuse without parental consent.

PHYSICAL EXAMINATION

The initial assessment includes evaluation of vital signs and hemodynamic status. However, significant signs of volume depletion may not be present until bleeding is profuse. Perform a focused physical examination including pelvic (speculum and bimanual) and abdominal exam to determine the cause of bleeding and to exclude life-threatening blood loss requiring emergent surgical intervention. Look for signs of other illnesses, including hyper- and hypothyroidism, galactorrhea, obesity associated with hirsutism, and liver disease. Petechiae, purpura, and mucosal bleeding require hematologic investigation.

For pelvic examinations in the ED, both male and female physicians are equally advised to have a chaperone present. Decisions regarding parent or guardian presence during examination of adolescents depend

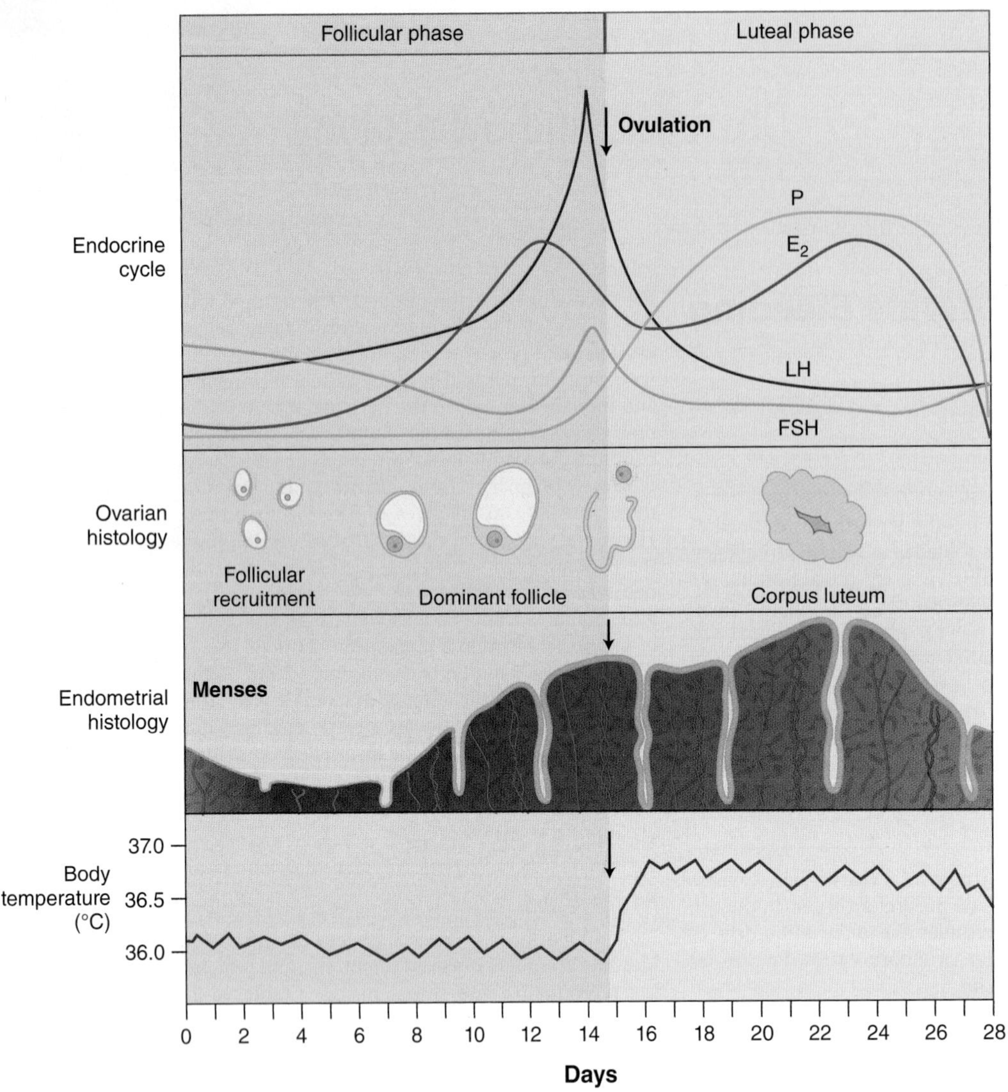

FIGURE 96-1. The hormonal, ovarian, endometrial, and basal body temperature changes and relationships throughout the normal menstrual cycle. E_2 = prostaglandin E_2; FSH = follicle-stimulating hormone; LH = luteinizing hormone; P = progesterone. [Reproduced with permission from Patel DR, Greydanus DE, Baker RJ: *Pediatric Practice Sports Medicine.* © 2009, McGraw-Hill, New York, NY.]

on the patient's age and maturity level. Inspect the perineum, vulva, urethra, and perianal region before internal speculum exam. Evaluate the vaginal canal and cervix for lacerations, fissures, lesions, infection, tumors, and foreign bodies. On bimanual examination, determine the softness and patency of the cervical os, and ask about pain on cervical movement. Palpate the uterus and adnexa for size, consistency, tenderness, and masses.

In a virginal patient, a rectovaginal digital examination is generally sufficient. In the case of trauma, concern for sexual abuse, or vaginal foreign body, a vaginal examination is necessary. Adolescents with intact hymen can generally tolerate a speculum examination if a narrow Pederson-type adolescent or Huffman pediatric speculum is used. Conscious sedation or full anesthesia may be required, depending on the psychological response of the patient, the circumstances, and the extent of the injury or disease.

Several techniques may help facilitate performing a pelvic examination in elderly women, including using a smaller speculum with generous lubrication and proper positioning. Age, immobility, and degenerative joint disease may make it difficulty to place the patient in the dorsal lithotomy position. Patients may be positioned supine, with the head supported with a pillow, and with knees flexed and with hips externally rotated (frog-leg position). The pelvis may be elevated using padding or an upside-down bedpan. If vaginal bimanual examination cannot be performed due to vaginal atrophy, a recto-abdominal approach may be attempted. Abnormalities such as irregular nodules, masses, or thickened rectovaginal septum may suggest malignancy.

CAUSES OF VAGINAL BLEEDING

The causes of abnormal vaginal or uterine bleeding in nonpregnant females are classified into structural and nonstructural causes, using the acronym: PALM-COEIN: **P**olyp, **A**denomyosis, **L**eiomyoma, **M**alignancy and hyperplasia, **C**oagulopathy, **O**vulatory dysfunction, **E**ndometrial, **I**atrogenic, and **N**ot otherwise classified.[2] Causes of bleeding based on age are shown in **Table 96-3**. The term *abnormal uterine bleeding* encompasses all causes of abnormal bleeding in nonpregnant women, and the most likely causes are largely determined by patient age. Because the first clinical signs of heavy menstrual bleeding (heavy uterine bleeding) are noted after the onset of menses during early adolescence, structural causes are uncommon. Anovulatory and bleeding disorders are most common during this time period (ages 13 to 19). **Pregnancy-related complications become the most common cause of abnormal vaginal bleeding during the reproductive years.** Issues regarding pregnancy are covered in chapters 98, "Ectopic Pregnancy and Emergencies in the First 20 Weeks of Pregnancy" and 100, "Maternal Emergencies after 20 Weeks of Pregnancy and in the Postpartum Period."

Abnormal uterine bleeding as a result of local structural pathology such as polyps and fibroids is not typically seen until women reach their

TABLE 96-2 Important Historical Elements in Uterine Bleeding

Category	Details
Reproductive history	Age of menarche Menstrual history Date of the last menstrual period Pattern of normal and abnormal bleeding or discharge Presence of dysmenorrhea
Sexual history	Current sexual activity Contraception Use of barrier protection Pregnant—yes/no? Gravida and para Previous abortion or recent termination History of ectopic pregnancy History of pelvic inflammatory disease, sexually transmitted diseases, human immunodeficiency virus, and hepatitis status
History of trauma	—
Possibility of retained foreign body	—
Medications, including alternative and complementary medicine	—
Past medical history	Signs and symptoms of coagulopathy, including nosebleeds, petechiae, and ecchymoses Endocrine disorders, including diabetes, pituitary tumors, polycystic ovary disease, hyperthyroidism, and hypothyroidism Liver disease
Associated symptoms	Urinary, GI, musculoskeletal symptoms; fever or syncope

mid 30s. Perimenopausal anovulatory bleeding is typically seen in the mid to late 40s. Postmenopausal bleeding is often related to atrophic vaginitis, exogenous hormones, and malignancy. A summary of the causes by age is provided in **Table 96-3**.

STRUCTURAL CAUSES OF VAGINAL BLEEDING

POLYPS

Endometrial and endocervical polyps are epithelial proliferations that most often are benign. Although most polyps are asymptomatic, polyps can be a cause of abnormal uterine bleeding in women older than 35 years. A common symptom is intermenstrual bleeding, and diagnosis is made on hysteroscopy.

ADENOMYOSIS

Adenomyosis is the presence of endometrial glands and stroma within the myometrium. The histopathology is often diffuse within the uterus, but localized areas of growth are called adenomyomas. Symptoms include painful, heavy periods most commonly seen in the fourth and fifth decade of life. ED management is aimed at symptomatic treatment, analgesics, and evaluation for anemia. Leuprolide acetate (Lupron), a gonadotropin-releasing hormone analog plus add-back therapy, or a levonorgestrel intrauterine device (Mirena) for 6 months may be initiated as an oupatient.[3] MRI is the imaging modality of choice, but US is a good alternative. Patients with severe bleeding unresponsive to medical management often require surgical management.

LEIOMYOMAS

Uterine fibroids (also called leiomyoma or myoma) are the most common benign tumors of the pelvis in women; an estimated 25% of white women and 50% of black women have fibroids in their reproductive years. This number increases with age. The cause is unclear, but fibroid growth is dependent on genetic factors and hormones: gonadotropin-releasing hormone, estrogen, and progestin. Leiomyomas decrease in size during menopause. In some cases, fibroids will enlarge early in pregnancy and with oral contraceptive pill use. Most fibroids are asymptomatic, but up to 30% of patients with leiomyomas experience pelvic pain and abnormal bleeding. Acute pain is rare, but severe pain may be experienced with torsion or degeneration. Degeneration results from rapid growth and loss of blood supply, often seen during early pregnancy. A rare case of spontaneous fibroid rupture causing massive intra-abdominal hemorrhage has been reported in the literature.[4]

Signs and symptoms of fibroids vary depending on fibroid size and location. Large fibroids may be palpated on abdominal or rectal exam. Symptoms of acute degeneration include tenderness, rebound guarding, fever, and elevated WBC count. Pedunculated subserosal leiomyomas may undergo torsion or cause uterine cramping. Rapid growth at any age or growth after menopause is highly suspicious for malignant transformation. The best diagnostic test is ultrasonography and is as sensitive as MRI.

The management of uterine fibroids depends on the severity and duration of symptoms. In the ED, management is focused on treating complications associated with fibroids. Iron deficiency anemia is often long-standing and may require a blood transfusion. Other complications are rarer, but constipation, urinary retention, vaginal or intraperitoneal hemorrhage, deep vein thrombosis, and mesenteric thrombosis have been reported.[5] Nonsteroidal anti-inflammatory drugs (NSAIDs) are the mainstays for analgesia in the ED. Medical management with hormonal agents may be initiated in the ED with gynecologic consultation. Intrauterine fibroids are treated surgically with hysteroscopy. Surgical removal is associated with a 25% to 30% rate of recurrence and significant bleeding complications. Uterine artery embolization is an effective treatment for symptomatic fibroids, resulting in decreased fibroid volume and alleviation of symptoms.[6-8]

MALIGNANCY

Any malignancy of the genital tract, in particular endometrial or cervical cancer, may produce bleeding. **Consider endometrial hyperplasia or endometrial cancer in women >45 years old or in younger women**

TABLE 96-3 Causes of Bleeding by Age Group*

Adolescent	Reproductive	Perimenopausal	Postmenopausal
Anovulation (hypothalamic-pituitary-ovarian immaturity)	Pregnancy	Anovulation	Atrophic vaginitis (30%)
Pregnancy	Anovulation (PCOS)	Uterine leiomyomas	Exogenous hormone use (30%)
Exogenous hormones or OCP	Exogenous hormone use or OCP	Cervical and endometrial polyps	Endometrial lesions, including cancer (30%)
Coagulopathy	Uterine leiomyomas	Thyroid dysfunction	Other tumor—vulvar, vaginal, cervical (10%)
Pelvic infections	Cervical and endometrial polyps		
	Thyroid dysfunction		

Abbreviations: OCP = oral contraceptive pill; PCOS = polycystic ovary syndrome.

*Prepubertal bleeding is discussed in chapter 133, "Pediatric Urologic and Gynecologic Disorders."

TABLE 96-4 Factors Frequently Used to Determine the Cause of Abnormal Bleeding in Perimenopausal Women

	Cause of Bleeding					
Distinguishing Features	Perimenopause	Neoplasia	Fibroid	Adenomyosis	Polyp	Pregnancy Related
History						
Associated hot flashes	Yes	No	No	No	No	No
Increased cramping	No	Sometimes	Sometimes	Yes	No	Sometimes
Bleeding pattern						
Skips and misses	Yes	Possible	No	No	No	—
Amenorrhea	Yes	No	No	No	No	Yes
Regular but shorter interval	Yes	No	No	No	No	No
Regular but heavy	No	No	Yes	Yes	Yes	No
Irregular	Yes	Possible	No	No	Yes	Yes
Physical examination						
Enlarged uterus	No	Sometimes	Yes	Yes	No	Yes
Enlarged and tender uterus	No	No	No	Yes	No	Possible
Ultrasonography						
Enlarged uterus	No	No	Yes	Yes	No	No
Enlarged uterus with intrauterine mass	No	Yes	Sometimes	No	Yes	Yes
Laboratory tests						
Follicle-stimulating hormone	Elevated	Normal	Normal	Normal	Normal	Normal
Complete blood count	Usually normal	Normal/low	Normal/low	Normal/low	Normal/low	Normal/low
Human chorionic gonadotropin	Negative	Negative	Negative	Negative	Negative	Positive

with other risk factors.[1,9,10] The amount of bleeding does not correlate with the severity of disease. Elderly patients may not be able to accurately describe the location of pain or bleeding in the proximity of the bladder, uterus, or rectosigmoid. Therefore, make sure to adequately visualize the vagina and cervix on pelvic examination.

All patients with postmenopausal bleeding warrant prompt referral for evaluation. Outpatient US and endometrial biopsy should be arranged for stable patients.

Vaginal bleeding, especially when seen in conjunction with atrophic vaginitis, may be associated with the use of pessaries and douche solutions, which can irritate the mucosa. Cervical polyps can also cause vaginal bleeding. However, an endometrial biopsy is ultimately required to rule out other serious causes of bleeding (**Table 96-4**).

NONSTRUCTURAL CAUSES OF VAGINAL BLEEDING

Consider these causes in the differential diagnosis by methodical history and physical examination. Pursue as needed with further investigations and consultations.

COAGULOPATHIES

Primary coagulation disorders account for 5% to 20% of acute uterine bleeding in adolescents.[11,12] von Willebrand's disease is the most common cause, but myeloproliferative disorders and immune thrombocytopenia also may be diagnosed. In adults, bleeding may result from anticoagulation agents or acquired bleeding disorders. Cirrhosis may lead to bleeding secondary to reduced capacity of the liver to metabolize estrogens.

OVULATORY DYSFUNCTION

Acute uterine bleeding secondary to anovulation is seen in 10% to 15% of gynecologic patients. Signs include irregular and/or heavy menstruation. Ovulatory dysfunction is common in perimenarchal and perimenopausal women, as well as in patients with endocrine disorders, polycystic ovary syndrome, exogenous hormone use, and liver or renal disease.

Anovulatory uterine bleeding in adolescence is due to the immature hypothalamic-pituitary-ovarian axis. In this situation, the amount of bleeding is usually minimal and painless. Dilatation and curettage (D&C) is rarely required. Severe anemia from heavy menstrual bleeding in early adolescence should prompt evaluation for bleeding disorders (e.g., von Willebrand's disease, factor VIII deficiency). **Table 96-5** outlines the medical management of acute uterine bleeding from ovulatory dysfunction in the ED.

Anovulatory bleeding in the reproductive-age female may be regular in timing but more often is irregular because of fluctuating estrogen levels below the critical level required to maintain endometrial growth. The level of estrogen depends on the age, number, and activity of ovarian follicles. As some follicles degenerate, others resume the production of estrogen, and the endometrium continues to proliferate for weeks to

TABLE 96-5 Treatment of Acute Uterine Bleeding from Ovulatory Dysfunction

Drug	Suggested dose	Dose Schedule	Potential Contraindications
Conjugated equine estrogen (Premarin)	25 milligrams IV	Every 4–6 h for 24 h	Breast cancer, liver disease, VTE*
Combined oral contraceptives (e.g., Sprintec®, 0.25 milligram of norgestimate and 0.035 milligram of ethinyl estradiol)	Monophasic† combined OCP that contains at least 35 micrograms of ethinyl estradiol	Three times per day for 7 d	Smokers >35 y, HTN, VTE, CVA, breast cancer, liver disease, thromboembolic disorders, diabetes with vascular disease, heart disease, major surgery with immobilization
Medroxyprogesterone acetate (Provera)	20 milligrams orally	Three times per day for 7 d	VTE, liver disease, breast cancer

Abbreviations: CVA = cerebrovascular accident; HTN = hypertension; OCP = oral contraceptive pill; VTE = venous thromboembolism (including deep venous thrombosis and pulmonary embolism).

*Caution in patients with cardiovascular or thromboembolic risk factors.

†Monophasic delivers the same amount of estrogen and progestin every day.

months, which may cause glandular hyperplasia ("Swiss cheese" hyperplasia). The estrogen steady-state is insufficient to meet the growing needs of the endometrium and produces a relative estrogen insufficiency, and uterine bleeding ensues. Alternatively, when follicle degeneration and stimulation are not balanced, absolute estrogen levels fall, and withdrawal bleeding occurs. Characteristically, anovulatory cycles present as prolonged amenorrhea with periodic menorrhagia. Because of the lack of progesterone-mediated myometrial contractions and arteriolar vasospasm, anovulatory cycles are rarely associated with cramping. This pattern of bleeding increases the risk of endometrial hyperplasia and adenocarcinoma.

Hypothyroidism may be associated with heavy uterine bleeding or intermenstrual bleeding from ovulatory dysfunction, with an estimated incidence of 0.3% to 2.5%.[13] Eating disorders, excessive weight loss, stress, and exercise can also cause abnormal uterine bleeding. Obtain levels of thyroid-stimulating hormone in women with uterine bleeding of undetermined origin or in those with thyroid nodule or goiter.

ENDOMETRIAL CAUSES

Acute uterine bleeding that occurs in the context of normal ovulation and with a structurally normal endometrial cavity is attributed to endometrial causes. Normal ovulation is based on a history of predictable, cyclical menstrual periods. Bleeding may be preceded by breast tenderness, abdominal bloating, and pelvic pain. The diagnosis is made when patients have heavy menstrual bleeding with no other identifiable abnormalities.

Ovulatory bleeding is generally treated with oral contraceptives, NSAIDs, or progestins. Endometrial ablation may be useful for those who do not respond to medical therapy; hysterectomy is reserved for those who fail medical management and have excessive blood loss.

IATROGENIC CAUSES

Oral contraceptive pill (OCP) use remains the most common cause of intermenstrual bleeding. Additionally, medications (e.g., antiseizure medications) that increase the P450 system of the liver may increase the metabolism of endogenous hormonal glucocorticoids and may cause withdrawal bleeding.

Hormone replacement therapy, which can relieve symptoms associated with menopause, may also be associated with vaginal bleeding. Hormone replacement therapy for this purpose has been called into question, as there is no clear benefit for primary and secondary prevention of cardiovascular disease, and excessive risk of endometrial, breast, and colorectal cancer and thromboembolism has been noted.[14-16]

Forty percent of women receiving continuous OCP therapy will experience abnormal bleeding in the initial 4 to 6 months. Bleeding after 6 months of continuous combined hormone replacement therapy, unexpected bleeding with cyclic hormone replacement therapy, or bleeding that recurs after amenorrhea is established should prompt referral for evaluation. There are no acceptable criteria for "abnormal bleeding" on these therapies. The most common etiologies for bleeding while on hormone replacement therapy are poor compliance, poor GI absorption, drug interactions, failure to synchronize therapy with endogenous ovarian activity, and coagulation disorders.

OTHER CAUSES OF VAGINAL BLEEDING

Pelvic inflammatory disease or infections that cause endometritis can cause abnormal vaginal bleeding. Cervical erosions, polyps, and cervicitis may cause bleeding from the cervix. Vaginal infections, trauma, and foreign bodies may also present with abnormal bleeding. Emergency therapy should be directed at investigating and treating obvious causes of bleeding. For further details, see chapters 103, "Pelvic Inflammatory Disease" and 102, "Vulvovaginitis."

LABORATORY EVALUATION AND IMAGING

Obtain a pregnancy test in women of childbearing age (except those with hysterectomy) to rule out pregnancy as a cause of bleeding. A CBC identifies anemia. Obtain coagulation studies only when indicated by history or physical examination. In individuals with suspected endocrine disorders, determination of thyroid-stimulating hormone and prolactin levels may be helpful, but the levels may not be available for ED evaluation.

Ultrasonography is the first-line imaging modality for gynecologic conditions such as vaginal bleeding, adnexal or uterine masses, or pelvic pain. US can determine uterine size and endometrial characteristics and can identify the presence of leiomyoma, ovarian cysts, hydrosalpinx, pelvic adhesions, tubo-ovarian abscesses, endometriosis, and tumors. Transvaginal ultrasonography further delineates ovarian cysts and fluid in the cul-de-sac. Depending on the degree of pain and findings on physical examination, US can be done on an emergency basis or deferred for outpatient evaluation.

CT is used primarily in the ED for the evaluation of acute abdominal or pelvic pain (see chapter 97, "Abdominal and Pelvic Pain in the Nonpregnant Female"). MRI is used primarily for cancer staging and is rarely indicated during ED evaluation. The National Guideline Clearinghouse has published guidelines for radiology for abnormal vaginal bleeding.[17]

TREATMENT

ACUTE UTERINE BLEEDING

Patients who are hemodynamically unstable need immediate resuscitation and emergent gynecologic consultation (**Figure 96-2**). Do not attempt vaginal packing, because it increases the risk of infection and may hide ongoing blood loss. In addition to fluid resuscitation, blood transfusion, and correction of underlying coagulopathies, assess for other potential causes of bleeding including trauma, bleeding dyscrasia, infection, and retained foreign bodies. The options for management of acute hemorrhage include hormonal, surgical, and hemostatic interventions.

Perimenopausal women with abnormal uterine bleeding should have an endometrial biopsy *before* the initiation of hormone replacement therapy. Otherwise, hormonal agents are first-line medical management for acute uterine bleeding in patients without an underlying bleeding disorder.[18,19] Short-term hormonal treatment allows the endometrium to stabilize and slows acute bleeding. Acute treatment options include intravenous estrogen and oral progestins (**Table 96-5**). For severe hemorrhage, give conjugated estrogen (Premarin) at a dose of 25 milligrams IV every 4 to 6 hours until bleeding stops, with ED observation, followed by an oral contraceptive. In women with a history of blood clot or cardiovascular disease, high-dose estrogen therapy is contraindicated. Progestin is used when there is concern for underlying endometrial pathology or hyperplasia. US finding may reveal a thickened endometrial strip, fibroids, or polyps.

Tranexamic acid, a lysine derivative that prevents fibrin degradation, is used primarily for intraoperative gynecologic bleeding.[20,21] Use depends on geography and institution, so obtain gynecologic consultation if administration is considered, especially to discuss risks and benefits. Clinical studies on the effectiveness of tranexamic acid have excluded patients with potential for thrombosis.

HEAVY MENSTRUAL BLEEDING

Heavy menstrual bleeding is treated with NSAIDs and combined or progestin-only oral contraceptives. Progesterone works by decreases the number of available estrogen receptors and stabilizing the endometrium. Common side effects of this regimen include nausea and vomiting. One recent report recommended IM depot-medroxyprogesterone combined with a short 3-day oral course of an oral contraceptive; the mean time for bleeding cessation was 2.6 days, and all patients stopped bleeding within 5 days.[22] Simplified ED regimens for combined OCPs and progestin-only pills are outlined in Table 96-5. The median time to stop bleeding for either regimen (combined OCP or progestin-only regimen) is 3 days. However, multiple different hormonal doses and schedules are also effective. In general, for young healthy women where bleeding is often related to anovulation and there is no concern for endometrial pathology, then OCPs are favored. For older patients, or obese/perimenopausal patients where there could be concern for endometrial pathology, then progestin-only is preferred.

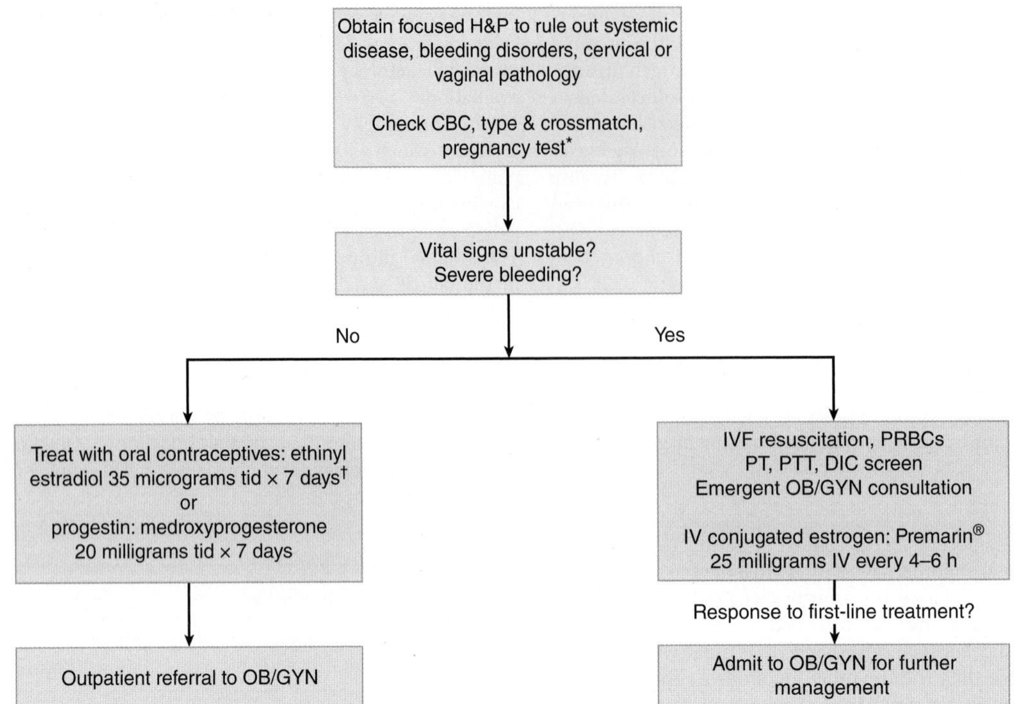

FIGURE 96-2. Algorithm for ED evaluation and treatment of acute vaginal bleeding (**Also see Table 96-5 for more detail.**). *Consider other laboratory tests if positive screen for suspected bleeding disorders based on history and physical (H&P). †Contraindications to hormonal agents need to be considered before administration. Other oral contraceptive and progestin formulations and dose schedules may be equally effective. DIC = disseminated intravascular coagulation; IVF = IV fluid; OB/GYN = obstetrician/gynecologist; PRBCs = packed red blood cells; PT = prothrombin time; PTT = partial thromboplastin time.

DISPOSITION AND FOLLOW-UP

Stable patients can be discharged home with arrangements for prompt follow-up within 1 week.

The need for surgical management is based on clinical stability. If medical management fails or if there is a contraindication (e.g., thromboembolic disease), then surgical management is the next step. Surgical options are directed by suspected etiology and include dilatation and curettage, hysteroscopy, endometrial balloon tamponade, and uterine artery embolization. Hysterectomy is used as a last resort in patients with acute life-threatening bleeding unresponsive to other treatment measures.

Provide referral for endometrial biopsy for patients at risk for endometrial cancer and all women >45 years old. Perimenopausal bleeding is associated with malignancy in 10% of women. Risk factors include obesity, nulliparity, history of anovulation, tamoxifen use, infertility, and a family history of endometrial or colon cancer. Other diagnostic procedures performed at follow-up may include sonohysterography, hysterosalpingography, and hysteroscopy with directed biopsy and dilatation and curettage.[23]

LONG-TERM MANAGEMENT

It is essential to establish a definitive diagnosis before initiating long-term management. Expectant management is appropriate if episodes of heavy or irregular bleeding are infrequent. Several choices for long-term medical management of heavy menstrual bleeding exist. Overall, there is insufficient evidence to define an optimal medical management strategy.[24,25]

OCPs have long been an excellent choice for adolescents and women requiring contraception. Heavy menstrual bleeding is decreased by 50%, with a similar reduction in the degree of pain associated with bleeding. However, a recent systemic review found levonorgestrel intrauterine device (71% to 95% reduction) superior to combined OCPs (35% to 69% reduction) and NSAIDs (10% to 52% reduction).[26]

NSAIDs are effective in reducing pain and blood loss in 20% to 50% of women with abnormal uterine bleeding secondary to ovulatory dysfunction.[27] NSAIDs should be started on the first day of the period and continued until bleeding stops and pain resolves.

All NSAIDs inhibit cyclooxygenase in the arachidonic acid cascade. Prostaglandin inhibitors alter the ratio of prostaglandin $F_2\alpha$, which causes vasoconstriction, to prostaglandin E_2, which causes vasodilation. NSAIDs also increase levels of thromboxane A_2, which causes vasoconstriction and increases platelet aggregation. NSAIDs have a mild side effect profile and are inexpensive. Treatment choices include mefenamic acid, 500 milligrams three times a day PO, naproxen, 500 milligrams twice per day PO, and ibuprofen, 400 milligrams every 6 hours. Any of these may be administered to reduce bleeding and pain associated with use of an intrauterine device.[28] NSAIDs are less useful in patients with uterine leiomyomas.

Additional long-term treatment options that may be prescribed at follow-up include clomiphene citrate, medroxyprogesterone acetate, gonadotropin-releasing hormone agonists, and tranexamic acid. Clomiphene citrate may be used to decrease bleeding as well as to induce ovulation if pregnancy is desired. If there is no contraindication to progestin usage, medroxyprogesterone acetate, 10 milligrams daily PO for 10 days, can be used to produce scheduled bleeding. Intrauterine progesterone release is a highly effective treatment option. Patients may still ovulate when using this medication. Gonadotropin-releasing hormone agonists may be used to induce amenorrhea, but women on this therapy become menopausal. Other drawbacks include medication expense and bone loss when used for >6 months. Tranexamic acid, a fibrinolytic, reduces vaginal bleeding with minimal side effects. An improved quality of life in patients using tranexamic acid when compared with hormone therapy and NSAIDS has been reported.[29]

Nonmedical invasive management strategies may be required if medical treatment fails. These include hysteroscopy, endometrial ablation, or myomectomy. Hysteroscopy can be used to sample the endometrium and resect polyps and myoma. Endometrial ablation may be performed in patients who do not desire fertility, have no pathologic diagnosis, and for whom medical therapy has failed.[30] Myomectomy may be useful in patients with symptomatic fibroids. Hysterectomy is reserved for selected patient populations. Uterine artery embolization is an effective nonsurgical option for the management of bleeding caused by fibroids.[31]

SPECIAL POPULATIONS

GENITAL TRAUMA

Vaginal injuries after intercourse are not uncommon. The majority of coital injuries result from vigorous voluntary sexual activity, although violent involuntary sexual activity should be considered. The most common site of injury is the posterior vaginal fornix. Misdiagnosis of coital injuries occurs frequently because either the physician fails to take an adequate history or the patient does not admit to antecedent sexual activity. Most coital injuries are minor, but severe injuries may lead to hemorrhagic shock.

BLOOD DYSCRASIAS

Bleeding disorders may become apparent with an initial presentation of abnormal menstrual bleeding. Uterine hemostasis is not well understood, and any disorder of blood vessels, platelet abnormalities, and coagulation disorders, including von Willebrand's disease, may result in excessive menstrual bleeding. Of historical interest, the first described case of von Willebrand's disease was in a 13-year-old who died as a result of uncontrollable uterine bleeding.[32] Abnormal uterine bleeding is present in the majority of women with von Willebrand's disease or factor XI deficiency and in carriers of hemophilia.

A multidisciplinary approach is recommended. Initial treatment options are similar to those without bleeding disorder: antifibrinolytics, OCPs, and levonorgestrel intrauterine device. Hormonal agents raise factor VIII and von Willebrand factor levels and are an effective and popular form of therapy. Antifibrinolytics, such as tranexamic acid, reduce both plasminogen activator activity and plasmin activity. Desmopressin acetate (DDAVP) stimulates endogenous release of factor VIII and von Willebrand factor and may be used prophylactically for minor procedures or treatment of bleeding episodes and heavy menstrual bleeding. Desmopressin acetate is administered intranasally, parenterally, or by SC injection. The blood of patients with von Willebrand's disease must be typed and screened for antibodies before instituting desmopressin acetate because it may induce thrombocytopenia in certain subgroups. NSAIDs are ineffective in decreasing uterine bleeding and may increase blood loss in this population.

POLYCYSTIC OVARY SYNDROME

Polycystic ovary syndrome, one of the most common endocrine disorders, is the association of hyperandrogenism and anovulation without underlying disease of the adrenal or pituitary glands.[33] A triad of obesity, hirsutism, and oligomenorrhea is classically described, although obesity is not universally seen. When menses occurs, it is heavy and prolonged. The syndrome is further characterized by acne, androgen-dependent alopecia, elevated serum concentrations of androgens, hyperinsulinemia, and hypersecretion of luteinizing hormone with a normal or low follicle-stimulating hormone level. Typical ovarian morphology, which may be seen by US, is not necessary for the diagnosis and may, in fact, represent a response of the ovary to chronic anovulation. The differential diagnosis includes hyperprolactinemia, acromegaly, congenital adrenal hyperplasia, and androgen-secreting tumors of the ovary or adrenal gland. Management of menorrhagia in women who do not desire fertility includes low-dose oral contraceptives or cyclic progestin administration.

HUMAN IMMUNODEFICIENCY VIRUS

In general, there is no need to change the approach to vaginal bleeding in human immunodeficiency virus–positive women. Look for associated infections and complications of chronic illness. The rate of vaginal and pelvic infections and cervical dysplasia is high in this cohort of patients. In a cross-sectional survey of 386 women <50 years old, with and without human immunodeficiency virus, neither infection nor immunosuppression affected menstruation or the rate of abnormal vaginal bleeding.[34] This was also seen in a study of 85 seropositive women, although the power of the study was low.[35]

STRESS, ILLNESS, AND RAPID WEIGHT CHANGE

Periods of physical or psychological stress, illness, malnutrition, rapid weight gain or loss, and intense physical regimens affect the hypothalamus and disrupt the normal pattern of gonadotropin release. This usually causes amenorrhea but may result in irregular, heavy bleeding. In obese women, menorrhagia may be a result of increased circulating levels of estrogen from peripheral conversion of androstenedione to estrone in fatty tissue. Patients with liver and renal disease may also develop irregular bleeding.

REFERENCES

The complete reference list is available online at www.TintinalliEM.com.

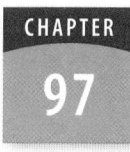

CHAPTER 97 Abdominal and Pelvic Pain in the Nonpregnant Female

Melanie Heniff
Heather R.B. Fleming

INTRODUCTION AND EPIDEMIOLOGY

This chapter reviews diagnosis and treatment of abdominal and pelvic pain in nonpregnant women. Even after the possibility of pregnancy is eliminated, abdominal pain in women remains a challenging diagnosis because of physical proximity and overlapping spinal segment innervation and similar symptoms of GI, urologic, and gynecologic organ systems. Discussion of the pregnant woman with abdominal/pelvic pain is found in chapters 100, "Maternal Emergencies after 20 Weeks of Pregnancy and in the Postpartum Period," 103, "Pelvic Inflammatory Disease," and 71, "Acute Abdominal Pain."

CLINICAL FEATURES

HISTORY

Define characteristics of the pain including onset, duration, location, quality, radiation, and exacerbating and alleviating factors. History should include questions about GI symptoms (nausea, vomiting, diarrhea, and constipation), urologic symptoms (dysuria, hematuria, frequency, and urgency), and gynecologic symptoms (vaginal bleeding, discharge, dyspareunia, and menstrual history). **History of sexual activity and menstrual history should never be relied upon to exclude pregnancy.** Obtain past medical, surgical, and family history, as well as details of prior pregnancies and outcomes. Active lactation and medication use, including specific methods of birth control, should be part of the history. Ask about infertility treatments because ovulation-inducing treatments increase risk of ovarian torsion, cysts, and ovarian hyperstimulation syndrome. When obtaining a sexual history and social history, it is wise to interview the patient alone, which may help patients feel more comfortable discussing potentially sensitive or embarrassing topics. Ask about pelvic inflammatory disease risk factors including unprotected intercourse, prior sexually transmitted infections, and multiple sexual partners. While the patient is alone, ask her about safety at home, and assess for any potential abusive situations. Patients with history of physical and sexual abuse may develop a variety of somatic complaints including abdominal and pelvic pain, and this pain is often chronic in nature. Social history should include living situation, occupation, and personal habits (use of tobacco, alcohol, and drugs).

PHYSICAL EXAMINATION

A standard head-to-toe systematic approach beginning with vital signs is essential. The patient should be adequately undressed for a careful examination. In focusing on the examination of the abdomen, it is helpful to determine in what quadrant(s) of the abdomen the pain is located; this may help to narrow the differential diagnosis (**Figure 97-1**).

In addition to palpating for tenderness or masses, evaluate for surgical scars, rashes, bruising, or ascites. Peritoneal signs may be less obvious in

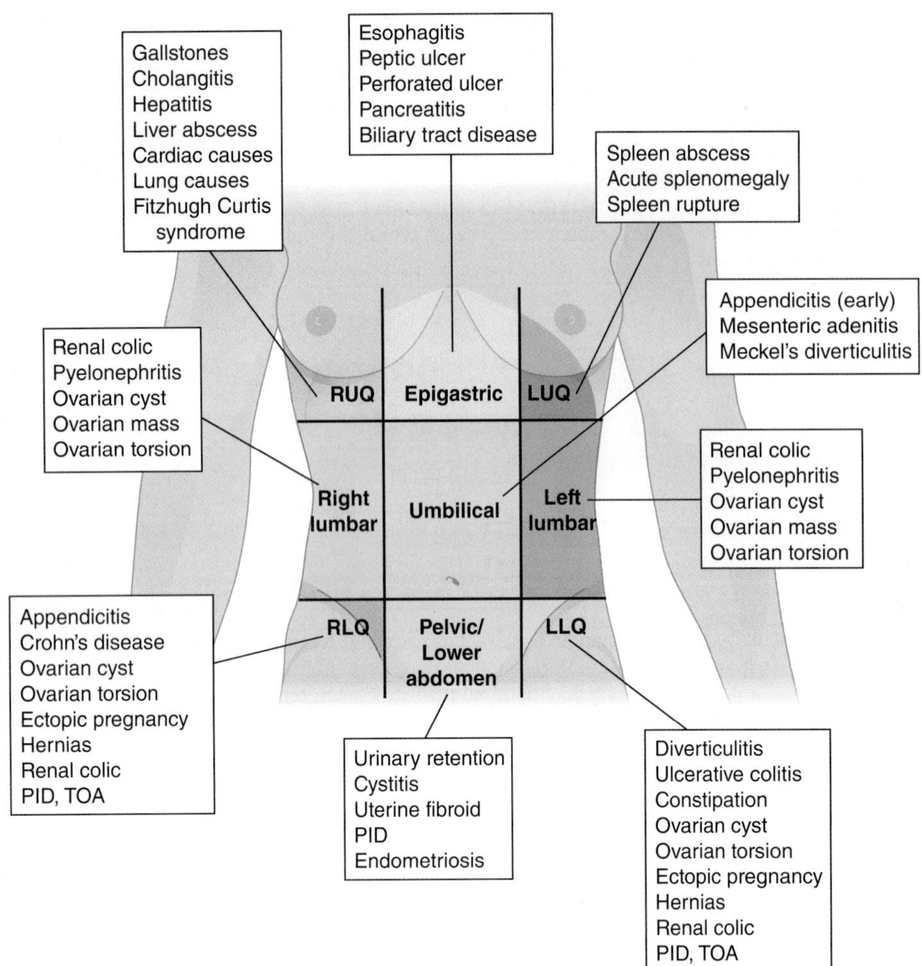

FIGURE 97-1. Differential diagnosis of abdominal pain based on location.

patients who are elderly, are obese, or have altered neurologic status. A digital rectal exam is helpful, if indicated, to evaluate complaints of rectal pain or bleeding.

A pelvic examination is usually a routine component of the exam of women with lower abdominal pain, but studies report a lack of accuracy and reproducibility of pelvic examination findings.[1,2] Pelvic examination is useful for obtaining lab specimens for sexually transmitted infections, palpation for tenderness or mass, and to check for vaginal bleeding, discharge, or foreign body.

DIAGNOSIS

In a nonpregnant female with abdominal pain, ED testing beyond a thorough history and exam is not always mandatory. For example, in a patient with multiple prior similar presentations and recent normal imaging studies, it is unnecessary, rarely helpful, and potentially harmful to repeat imaging.[3] In cases where further ED testing is determined to be unnecessary, the physician must still pay careful attention to symptom control, careful reassessment, and disposition. At the time of discharge, providers should review with the patient arrangements for close follow-up, often in 12 to 24 hours, as well as indications for return to the ED. **When benign causes are not clear from the initial evaluation and concerns for serious pathology remain, lab and/or imaging tests are necessary.**

LABORATORY EVALUATION

Obtain a pregnancy test in all women of childbearing age who still have a uterus and ovaries. See chapter 98, "Ectopic Pregnancy and Emergencies in the First 20 Weeks of Pregnancy" for a detailed discussion of pregnancy testing. A CBC is often obtained, but the WBC count is not reliable to rule in or exclude serious disease.[5] Obtain a urinalysis, and add a urine culture in pediatric patients, pregnant women, and patients at risk for complicated urinary tract infections. See chapter 91, "Urinary Tract Infections and Hematuria" for detailed discussion of urinalysis. **Be cautious in making a definitive diagnosis of urinary tract infection as the sole cause of a patient's symptoms.** For further discussion, see chapter 71.

IMAGING

US is the imaging modality of choice for genital tract pathology (ovarian cyst, ectopic pregnancy, uterine or ovarian mass, or tubo-ovarian abcess). CT is preferred when GI or GU pathology (appendicitis, diverticulitis, bowel obstruction, or renal stones) is highest in the differential diagnosis.

Bedside US can facilitate rapid diagnosis and treatment. For example, a positive focused assessment with sonography for trauma exam could help diagnose a ruptured ectopic pregnancy or significant hemorrhage from an ovarian cyst.[5] ED US can quickly identify a normal intrauterine pregnancy. Pelvic US is the primary imaging modality for evaluation of lower abdominal pain in the female patient in whom a gynecologic diagnosis is considered most likely. US is useful in diagnosis of pelvic inflammatory disease, tubo-ovarian abcess, leiomyoma, and ovarian cysts. In evaluation of possible ovarian torsion, pelvic US should include Doppler flow. Transabdominal and intravaginal probes are used for imaging of pelvic organs. In transabdominal imaging alone, a full bladder aids visualization of pelvic organs. In transvaginal imaging, an empty bladder aids visualization. US studies should never be delayed waiting for a full bladder, particularly when there is concern for a serious diagnosis such as ovarian torsion. US may be useful to evaluate for appendicitis, but it is less sensitive than CT and is operator dependent.

CT of the abdomen and pelvis is sensitive for evaluation of most abdominal and pelvic conditions. Usually IV contrast alone is sufficiently sensitive for evaluation of possible appendicitis.[6] If there is concern for pelvic abscess, or the patient weighs less than 70 kg, oral contrast may enhance accuracy of evaluation. MRI is accurate in diagnosis of many abdominal and pelvic conditions, but cost and limited availability limit its use in most EDs.

TREATMENT

Specific treatment depends on diagnosis (see below), but because the diagnostic process can be time consuming, control of pain and nausea and fluid resuscitation take priority. There is no evidence that judicious use of opiates obscures abdominal exam findings or negatively impacts outcomes. Opiates can be titrated to control pain, without causing excessive somnolence or respiratory depression. Antiemetics including ondansetron, metoclopramide, promethazine, and prochlorperazine are safe and effective. Antibiotics should be given in the ED for suspected severe intra-abdominal infection or sepsis. Choice of antibiotics depends on severity of infection and factors relevant to patients' individual risk, such as comorbid conditions and possibility of hospital-acquired infections.[7,8] See chapters 71 and 103 for further discussion of antibiotic selection.

DISPOSITION AND FOLLOW-UP

When a serious or potentially surgical diagnosis is considered likely, early consultation with the appropriate specialist (general surgery, urology, or obstetrics/gynecology) is indicated. If there is persistent concern for serious pathology, admission or observation is appropriate. This applies even if the diagnosis is unclear. Patients with abnormal vitals, poorly controlled pain, and/or vomiting are best served by inpatient treatment. In many cases, diagnosis is clear after a period of observation and serial exams. Many patients seen in the ED have significant symptoms, but a specific condition may not be diagnosable in the relatively brief period of time a patient spends in the ED. Significant comorbid conditions (immunocompromised, unstable medical problems, inability to care for oneself at home) should prompt strong consideration for observation or admission.

In most patients with abdominal/pelvic pain in the ED, hospitalization is not necessary. **It is common and appropriate to discharge patients with a diagnosis of undifferentiated abdominal pain. In patients who are discharged, instructions for follow-up and indications for return to the ED should be very specific. Instructions should specify a time course during which patients should be seen for repeat exam.** Re-evaluation in 12 to 24 hours is appropriate for patients with acute abdominal pain and diagnostic uncertainty. In more chronic abdominal/pelvic pain, follow-up with a primary care provider is still important, but timing of follow-up should be specified according to individual patient needs.

OVARIAN CYSTS

Ovarian cysts, when symptomatic, usually present with sudden-onset unilateral pain that is more common on the right than left. Cervical motion tenderness and mild vaginal bleeding are sometimes present. Pain often starts during physical activity such as exercise or sexual intercourse. Functional (benign) cysts are fluid-filled sacs that develop during a normal menstrual cycle. **Follicular cysts** contain a maturing ovum and rupture at ovulation. **Corpus luteum cysts** are present after the ovum is released. If no conception occurs, the corpus luteum involutes. If fertilization takes place, the corpus luteum cyst enlarges and secretes estrogen and progesterone. **Hemorrhagic cysts** occur if a blood vessel in the cyst wall ruptures (**Figure 97-2**).

Mittelschmerz (German for middle pain) is midcycle pain at the time of ovulation caused by normal follicular enlargement prior to ovulation or follicular bleeding at ovulation. Pain is usually mild and lasts a few hours up to a few days.

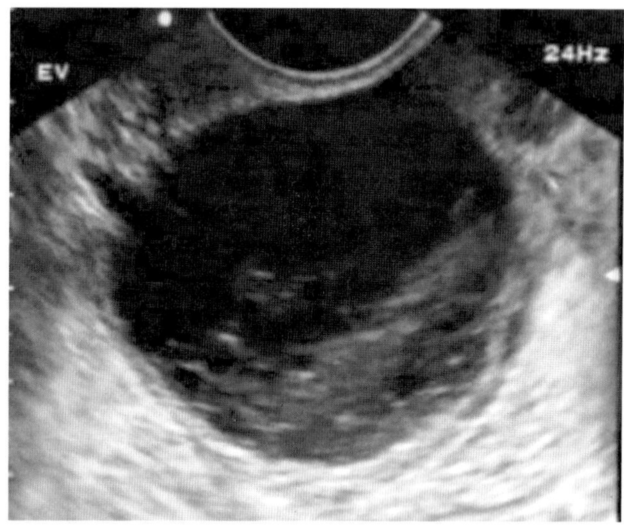

FIGURE 97-2. A 4-cm hemorrhagic ovarian cyst demonstrated by endovaginal US. [Reproduced with permission from Ma OJ, Mateer JR, Blaivas M: *Emergency Ultrasound*, 2nd ed. © 2008, McGraw-Hill, New York. Fig. 14-10, p. 362.]

Complicated cyst rupture is characterized by abnormal vital signs and an acute abdomen. Hospitalization or observation is needed for serial examinations and hematocrits. Surgery may be necessary to control hemorrhage.

A **dermoid cyst** is an ovarian germ cell neoplasm that presents as a multicystic mass that contains various types of tissue including fat, skin, hair, and teeth. These cysts usually occur between age 10 and 30 years. Most are benign, but risk factors for malignant teratomas include age over 45, diameter greater than 8 cm, and rapid growth. Most uncomplicated cyst ruptures are from follicular and corpus luteum cysts. Vital signs are stable, and symptoms only last a few days.

Ovarian cysts that are <8 cm, unilocular, and unilateral are generally observed and typically resolve within two menstrual cycles. **Cysts that are large (>8 cm), solid, and multiloculated are worrisome for neoplasm, dermoid cysts, or endometriomas**. Patients with ovarian cysts, regardless of size, should be referred to the gynecologist or primary care physician for follow-up.

ENDOMETRIOMAS

Endometriomas are called "chocolate cysts" because they usually contain thick brown fluid. They present as a pelvic mass caused by growth of ectopic endometrial tissue within an ovary. Endometriomas may rupture, and patients can present with peritoneal signs/symptoms. Endometriomas may also present similar to endometriosis (pelvic pain, dysmenorrhea, and dyspareunia).

OVARIAN NEOPLASM

An ovarian mass in a postmenopausal woman is malignant until proven otherwise. The mean age at diagnosis is 50 to 60 years. Patients present with nonspecific signs/symptoms, including anorexia, dyspepsia, early satiety, constipation, bloating, and ascites. Cancers of the endometrium, breast, and GI tract may metastasize to ovaries and fallopian tubes.

OVARIAN HYPERSTIMULATION SYNDROME

Ovarian hyperstimulation syndrome is a complication of ovulation induction treatments, with a clinical spectrum of severity. The syndrome can occur early, 5 to 7 days after ovulation, or later, due to rising human chorionic gonadotropin levels.

The severe syndrome is characterized by massive transudation of albumin and fluid from the vascular compartment to the peritoneal, pleural, and sometimes, pericardial cavities.[9] Venous and arterial thrombosis are the most dreaded complications. Reports include thrombosis of the jugular, subclavian, retinal, and extremity veins and cerebral venous thrombosis. Stroke, ST-segment elevation myocardial infarction, and pulmonary embolism are also reported.[9]

ENDOMETRIOSIS AND ADENOMYOSIS

Endometriosis occurs when endometrium-like tissue outside the uterus induces a chronic inflammatory reaction. This is a common cause of pelvic pain and infertility. When endometrial tissue is in the uterine wall, it is termed adenomyosis. Both conditions cause chronic, recurrent, and cyclic pain. Dysmenorrhea and dyspareunia are often reported. US may show cystic or solid masses. Laparoscopy is the definitive method of diagnosis. Primary diagnosis is usually not made in the ED. If suspected, pain control and outpatient referral are appropriate.

FOREIGN BODY/TRAUMA

Vaginal foreign bodies (such as a retained tampon) may cause pelvic pain and vaginal discharge or bleeding. Trauma or foreign body should be considered in the differential diagnosis. Patients are not always immediately forthcoming with history due to fear or embarrassment. Complications such as abscess or perforation are rare.

OVARIAN TORSION

Ovarian torsion is a surgical emergency that requires prompt diagnosis to preserve ovarian function. Adnexal torsion is an ischemic condition almost always associated with ovarian enlargement, generally due to ovarian cysts or masses. The enlargement causes the ovary to twist, creating a fulcrum around which the oviduct revolves. Initial blockage of venous return causes congestion, leading to decreased distal arterial blood flow, which produces ischemia and necrosis of the ovary. Although the process may involve the ovary alone, torsion of both the ovary and the oviduct (adnexal torsion) is more common. Nearly 70% of torsions occur on the right side, due to the increased length of the utero-ovarian ligament on the right and the sigmoid on the left, limiting space for movement.[10]

Risk factors for torsion are pregnancy due to enlarged corpus luteum, presence of large ovarian cysts or tumors, chemical induction of ovulation (ovarian hyperstimulation syndrome), and tubal ligation. Classically, patients present with sudden-onset, severe, unilateral, lower abdominal pain that may develop after episodes of exertion. Unfortunately, atypical presentations are common, with half of patients reporting gradual onset of pain that is intermittent in nature. Nausea and vomiting is present in 70% of cases.[11]

Clinical findings classically consist of unilateral lower abdominal tenderness with guarding, unilateral adnexal tenderness on bimanual examination, and presence of a latero-uterine mass. Conversely, nearly 30% of patients have bilateral adnexal tenderness on bimanual examination, and a minority of patients may have no tenderness at all. Fifty percent of patients are initially misdiagnosed.[12]

Transvaginal US with Doppler is the primary diagnostic modality for suspected torsion. An ovary greater than 4 cm in size due to cyst, tumor, or edema is the most common ultrasonographic finding associated with torsion.[13] Conversely, given the dynamic nature of the torsion process, up to 26% of US studies reveal normal adnexa. Up to 60% of cases of torsion can be missed on arterial Doppler alone, given that arterial disruption of flow is a late clinical finding.[14] However, a positive Doppler study has a 100% positive predictive value for adnexal torsion. Recent improvements in US technology have led to assessment of venous Doppler flow, which may be the only abnormality identified in early ovarian torsion.[15] Given the dynamic nature of the torsion process, there is no one finding that conveys certainty of the absence of torsion. Thus, clinical suspicion based on history and physical exam remains important in involving gynecologic consultation if US is negative, but clinical concern remains high.[16]

Acknowledgment: We wish to gratefully acknowledge the support and assistance of our colleagues in the Department of Emergency Medicine at Indiana University who made this chapter possible.

REFERENCES

The complete reference list is available online at www.TintinalliEM.com.

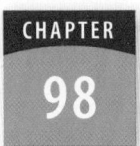

Ectopic Pregnancy and Emergencies in the First 20 Weeks of Pregnancy

Heather A. Heaton

GENERAL APPROACH TO WOMEN OF CHILDBEARING AGE

The differential diagnosis for women of childbearing potential who present with abdominal or pelvic symptoms or abnormal vaginal bleeding is broad (**Table 98-1**). The major clinical goals are, first, diagnosis of pregnancy, and then if pregnant, differentiating ectopic pregnancy from threatened abortion. Consider ectopic pregnancy in women of childbearing age who report abdominal or pelvic pain or discomfort, vaginal spotting or a cycle of amenorrhea, or unexplained signs or symptoms of hypovolemia. There are rare case reports of ectopic pregnancy in patients with ovaries but without a uterus. No combination of signs or symptoms is sufficient to exclude ectopic pregnancy. **If pregnancy is detected, ectopic pregnancy remains in the differential diagnosis until it can be either confirmed or excluded with conviction.**

PREGNANCY TESTING

The diagnosis of pregnancy is central to the diagnosis of ectopic pregnancy. Pregnancy tests currently in use rely on the detection of the β subunit of human chorionic gonadotropin (β-hCG) in the urine or serum. hCG is a hormone produced by the trophoblast. Intact hCG consists of the α and β subunits. Tests based on detection of the intact molecule or the α subunit can cross-react on immunologic assays with hormones found in the nonpregnant individual and are thus less specific than tests for the β-hCG subunit.

hCG preparations are currently standardized in relation to the Third International Reference Preparation. Other standard preparations are not equivalent. A preparation often referred to in earlier literature is the Second International Standard. The Third International Reference Preparation is

TABLE 98-1 Differential Diagnosis of Ectopic Pregnancy

All Patients	Pregnant Patients
Appendicitis	Normal (intrauterine pregnancy)
Inflammatory bowel disease	Threatened abortion
Ovarian pathology	Inevitable abortion
Cyst	Molar pregnancy
Torsion	Heterotopic pregnancy*
Pelvic inflammatory disease	Implantation bleeding
Endometriosis	Corpus luteum cyst
Sexual assault/trauma	
Urinary tract infection	
Ureteral colic	

*Heterotopic pregnancy = combined intrauterine pregnancy and ectopic pregnancy.

TABLE 98-2 Estimated β-Human Chorionic Gonadotropin (β-hCG) Levels After Conception[4]

Postconception Week	β-hCG Levels (mIU/mL)
<1 week	5–50
1–2 weeks	50–500
2–3 weeks	100–5000
3–4 weeks	500–10,000
4–5 weeks	1000–50,000
5–6 weeks	10,000–100,000
6–8 weeks	15,000–200,000
8–12 weeks	10,000–100,000

roughly equal to 1.7 times the Second International Standard. To avoid confusion when interpreting the literature, pay attention to the standard used. In this chapter, hCG and β-hCG concentrations refer to the Third International Reference Preparation unless otherwise noted.

Very early in either an intrauterine pregnancy (IUP) or an ectopic pregnancy, detectable amounts of β-hCG are released into the serum and filtered into the urine. The concentration of β-hCG is fairly closely correlated in the urine and serum, with urinary concentration also depending on urine specific gravity. Qualitative urine and serum tests for pregnancy usually use the enzyme-linked immunosorbent assay methodology. In the laboratory setting, enzyme-linked immunosorbent assay tests can detect β-hCG at concentrations <1 mIU/mL.

Qualitative tests in clinical use are typically reported as "positive" when the β-hCG concentration is ≥20 mIU/mL in urine and ≥10 mIU/mL in serum. A positive qualitative test therefore implies that β-hCG is present in at least this concentration. At this level of detection, the false-negative rate for detection of pregnancy will not be >1% for urine and 0.5% for serum. In clinical use, the performance of urine qualitative testing is 95% to 100% sensitive and specific compared with serum tests.

Urine tests can be performed rapidly at the bedside, and kits from some manufacturers may be used for either urine or serum. **Dilute urine may cause a false-negative urine pregnancy test**, particularly early in pregnancy when β-hCG levels are low (<50 mIU/mL). Additionally, when hCG levels are present in large amounts (generally with concentrations of 1,000,000 mIU/mL), a **"hook effect phenomenon"** can occur, giving false-negative results. This is thought to be related to excess hCG saturating both the fixed, solid-phase antibody and the labeled, soluble antibody of the assay, causing an absence of signal. The resultant false-negative test can be mitigated by diluting the sample.[1] Point-of-care hCG whole-blood assay shows promising results, with 95.8% sensitivity (negative predictive value, 97.9%) when compared with standard urine testing.[2]

When a bedside urine test is negative and ectopic pregnancy is still being considered, perform a quantitative serum test. **The sensitivity of quantitative serum testing for the diagnosis of pregnancy is virtually 100% when an assay capable of detecting ≥5 mIU/mL of β-hCG is used.**[3] Estimated β-hCG levels after conception are listed in **Table 98-2**.

ECTOPIC PREGNANCY

INTRODUCTION AND EPIDEMIOLOGY

Ectopic pregnancy occurs when a conceptus implants outside of the uterine cavity and is a leading cause of maternal death in the first trimester of pregnancy.[5]

The current incidence of ectopic pregnancy is difficult to determine but is probably increasing. Reasons include the increased incidence of sexually transmitted tubal infections, unsuccessful tubal sterilizations, assisted reproductive techniques, previous pelvic surgery, and more sensitive and earlier diagnostic techniques. Major risk factors are shown in **Table 98-3**, but a significant number of ectopic pregnancies occur in women in whom no risk factors are identified.[6,7]

TABLE 98-3 Major Risk Factors for Ectopic Pregnancy

Pelvic inflammatory disease, history of sexually transmitted infections
History of tubal surgery or tubal sterilization
Conception with intrauterine device in place
Maternal age 35–44 (age-related change in tubal function)
Assisted reproduction techniques (cause unknown, as tube is bypassed in implantation)
Previous ectopic pregnancy
Cigarette smoking (may alter embryo tubal transport)
Prior pharmacologically induced abortion

PATHOPHYSIOLOGY

Fertilization of the oocyte usually occurs in the ampullary segment of the fallopian tube. In normal pregnancy, after fertilization, the zygote passes along the fallopian tube and implants into the endometrium of the uterus. An ectopic pregnancy occurs when the zygote implants in any location other than the uterus—the fallopian tube or extratubal sites (the abdominal cavity, cervix, or ovary). Death results from maternal exsanguination after tubal rupture.

The vast majority of ectopic pregnancies implant in the ampullary portion of the **fallopian tube**. The underlying cause is most often damage to the tubal mucosa from previous infection, preventing transport of the ovum to the uterus. Other causes include tubal surgery, defects in the ovum resulting in premature implantation, and elevated estradiol or progesterone levels, which inhibit tubal migration.

Tubal implantation results in the penetration of the ovum into the muscular wall of the tube, and maternal blood seeps into tubal tissue. Intermittent distention of the fallopian tube with blood can occur, with leakage of blood from the fimbriated end of the fallopian tube into the peritoneal cavity. The aborting ectopic pregnancy and associated hematoma can be completely or partially extruded out of the end of the fallopian tube or through a rupture site in the tubal wall.

Abdominal ectopic pregnancies (~1% of ectopic pregnancies) most commonly derive from early rupture or abortion of a tubal pregnancy, with subsequent reimplantation in the peritoneal cavity.

Cervical ectopic pregnancies occur in <1% of ectopic pregnancies, with predisposing factors similar to those associated with ectopic pregnancies (previous dilatation and curettage, previous cesarean delivery, in vitro fertilization, adhesions or fibrosis of the endometrium, prior instrumentation, infertility, previous ectopic pregnancy). Patients develop profuse vaginal bleeding. Bimanual exam reveals a soft, large cervix when compared to the uterus or an hourglass-shaped uterus, and diagnosis is confirmed with US.[8,9]

Cesarean scar pregnancy is rare but can cause massive maternal hemorrhage. Diagnosis is difficult and is based on US demonstrating an empty uterine sac and cervical canal and a gestational sac in the uterine isthmus.

HISTORY

Determine the timing and characteristics of the last few periods. The menstrual history is often, but not always, abnormal. The classic sign of amenorrhea from 4 to 12 weeks after the last normal period is reported in 70% of ectopic pregnancy cases. **No missed menses are reported in 15% of ectopic pregnancy cases.** Although vaginal bleeding is often scant, heavy bleeding does not exclude an ectopic pregnancy.

Ask about previous pregnancies, pregnancy problems, and miscarriages. Typical early pregnancy symptoms may occur and may not differ from symptoms of previous normal IUPs. Discuss previous medical and surgical history, and ask about substance abuse and smoking. Ask about sexual activity and contraception. Identify risk factors for ectopic pregnancy or spontaneous abortion. Determine current medications, including over-the-counter drugs.

Pregnancy in a patient with prior tubal surgery for sterilization is assumed to be an ectopic pregnancy until proven otherwise. Patients are at particularly high risk if they have undergone laparoscopic partial salpingectomy or electrodestruction tubal ligation at a young age (age <28 years), especially 5 to 15 years after the procedure.[10]

In a woman of childbearing age, hysterectomy with oophorectomy excludes ectopic pregnancy. In the situation of hysterectomy without oophorectomy, ectopic pregnancy is exceedingly rare. A literature review identified only 27 such case reports since 1918, after both vaginal and abdominal hysterectomies. The theory is that a fistulous tract after hysterectomy enables embryo implantation in the tube or adnexae.[11]

Abdominal pain or discomfort is the most common symptom of ectopic pregnancy and is reported in 90% of ectopic pregnancies.[12] Pain is due to tubal distention or rupture. The classic pain of rupture is lateralized, sudden, sharp, and severe. Shoulder pain due to diaphragmatic irritation from a ruptured ectopic pregnancy can also occur. Any lateral or bilateral abdominal discomfort or tenderness in a woman of childbearing age requires consideration of ectopic pregnancy. **Lack of pain in a woman with vaginal spotting or bleeding does not exclude ectopic pregnancy.**

PHYSICAL EXAMINATION

Obtain vital signs and focus on the abdominal and pelvic examination. The physical examination in ectopic pregnancy is highly variable, and ectopic pregnancy is difficult to diagnose or exclude based on physical examination. In cases of ruptured ectopic pregnancy, patients may present in shock, with no findings on pelvic examination, or with peritoneal signs and an adnexal mass and tenderness. Cervical motion tenderness can be elicited on pelvic exam in some cases. Relative bradycardia may occur as a consequence of vagal stimulation. There is poor correlation between the volume of hemoperitoneum and vital signs in ruptured ectopic pregnancy.[13] In cases of rupture without hemodynamically significant bleeding, a more benign abdominal exam may be present without significant alteration of vital signs. Fever is rare. In the more common situation of an unruptured ectopic pregnancy, the vital signs are likely to be normal.

If an adnexal mass or fullness with tenderness is detected, it may be due to ectopic pregnancy or to a **corpus luteum cyst,** a 3- to 11-cm, thin-walled, unilocular cyst seen after ovulation that can cause pain and tenderness on exam as well as menstrual irregularities, mimicking an ectopic pregnancy. Cervical motion tenderness may be seen, and blood is often present in the vaginal vault; however, the pelvic exam may be completely normal. The cervix may have a blue coloration, as in a normal pregnancy. Uterine size for estimated gestational age is most often normal. Vaginal examinations in stable women presenting with first-trimester bleeding may add little to the clinical diagnosis; some providers are moving away from routine use of vaginal examinations in initial patient assessment as long as a transvaginal US is obtained.[14]

DIAGNOSIS

The definitive diagnosis of ectopic pregnancy is made by US, by direct visualization by laparoscopy, or at surgery. No single or combination of laboratory tests has a sufficient negative or positive predictive value to completely exclude ectopic pregnancy or to definitively establish the diagnosis.

Serum β-hCG Differences in the dynamics of β-hCG production in normal and pathologic pregnancy are useful in the diagnosis of ectopic pregnancy. Early in normal pregnancy, β-hCG levels rise rapidly until 9 to 10 weeks of pregnancy and then plateau. Expected postconception ranges of β-hCG are listed in Table 98-2. β-hCG levels decline in nonviable pregnancies and in successfully treated ectopic pregnancy. Absolute levels of β-hCG tend to be lower in pathologic pregnancies than in IUPs, but there is much overlap. Due to the variability in absolute levels and the overlap between normal and pathologic pregnancies, **no single β-hCG level can reliably distinguish between a normal and a pathologic pregnancy**. *Doubling time* refers to the time needed for β-hCG concentration in the serum to double. Absolute levels of β-hCG are lower and doubling times longer in ectopic pregnancy and other abnormal pregnancies. This and many other observations have led to the widely used rule of thumb stating that the serum concentration of β-hCG approximately doubles every 2 days early in a normal pregnancy and that longer doubling times indicate pathologic pregnancy. Varying degrees of sensitivity (36% to 75%) and specificity (63% to 93%) are obtained using different criteria for evaluating the rate of increase of β-hCG levels for the diagnosis of ectopic pregnancy. The minimum hCG rise in normal pregnancy may be as low as 53% in 48 hours,[15] and the median rise in β-hCG level was 53% in 1 day and 124% in 2 days. Conversely, in spontaneous abortion, hCG is expected to fall by 21% to 35% in 2 days.[16] Thus, hCG levels that fail to increase by 53% or more in 2 days are suggestive but not diagnostic of ectopic pregnancy or an abnormal IUP. However, **an increase of >53% does not rule out ectopic pregnancy**.

In stable patients, serial measurements of β-hCG are used to either heighten or lower the suspicion for ectopic pregnancy, but are not diagnostic. Repeat serum β-hCG measurement made at least 2 days after the initial presentation is useful in characterizing the risk of ectopic pregnancy and the probability of a viable IUP.[17] Although rates of decline vary depending on the initial hCG value, a decrease of less than 21% at 2 days or 60% at 7 days suggests retained trophoblasts or an ectopic pregnancy; additional testing should be performed.[15] **Table 98-4** describes the American College of Emergency Physicians' clinical policy regarding women with early pregnancies.[17]

Progesterone Progesterone is a steroid hormone secreted by the ovaries, adrenal glands, and placenta during pregnancy. During the first 8 to 10 weeks of pregnancy, ovarian production of progesterone predominates, and serum levels remain relatively constant. After the tenth week of pregnancy, placental production increases and serum levels rise. Absolute levels of progesterone are lower in pathologic pregnancies and fall when a pregnancy fails. This observation has led multiple authors to propose various progesterone levels as a diagnostic aid in differentiating an early normal from a pathologic pregnancy. Most pathologic pregnancies have progesterone levels of ≤10 nanograms/mL. With progesterone ≤5 nanograms/mL, nearly 100% of pregnancies will be pathologic; there are no normal pregnancies reported with progesterone ≤2.5 nanograms/mL. Progesterone levels >25 nanograms/mL have 97% sensitivity for viable IUP. An empty uterus or nonspecific fluid collection on US associated

TABLE 98-4 ED Management of Early Pregnancy[17]

Clinical Issue	Recommendation	Level of Recommendation*
Use of transvaginal US to detect IUP, ectopic pregnancies when serum β-hCG <1000 mIU/mL	Perform or obtain a transvaginal US for symptomatic pregnant patients with β-hCG below the discriminatory threshold.	Level C
Use of β-hCG for predicting ectopic pregnancy in women with indeterminate transvaginal US	β-hCG values do not exclude the diagnosis of an ectopic pregnancy in patients with indeterminate transvaginal US.	Level B
Implications for ED management of women receiving methotrexate for confirmed or suspected ectopic pregnancy	Consider ruptured ectopic pregnancy for persistent abdominal pain or vaginal bleeding.	Level B
Anti-Rh_0 (D) immunoglobulin for ectopic pregnancy	50 micrograms of RhoGAM for all Rh-negative women with threatened loss or loss of established first-trimester pregnancy (full dose of 300 micrograms is not needed when the patient is at <12 weeks of gestation due to the small volume of red cells in the feto-placental circulation).	Level B

Abbreviations: β-hCG = β-human chorionic gonadotropin; IUP = intrauterine pregnancy.

*Level A: reflects high degree of clinical certainty; Level B: reflects moderate clinical certainty; Level C: reflects preliminary or conflicting evidence or based on consensus.

with progesterone ≤5.0 nanograms/mL is highly predictive of abnormal IUP or ectopic pregnancy.[18]

There is considerable overlap between progesterone levels in normal and pathologic pregnancy. Thus, very low values for serum progesterone should increase the clinical suspicion for ectopic pregnancy or abnormal IUP, but as with β-hCG levels, no value is diagnostic or can completely exclude or definitively diagnose ectopic pregnancy. Progesterone levels may not be routinely available on an urgent basis, and as noted, many patients have intermediate values, thus limiting the usefulness of the test. Consequently, the role of serum progesterone assays is currently unclear.

Numerous other serum markers for the diagnosis of ectopic pregnancy have been investigated. These include secretory endometrial protein, estradiol, the pregnancy-associated proteins A to D, and others, as well as routine laboratory tests such as amylase, creatine kinase, erythrocyte sedimentation rate, and others. None has been accepted as equal or superior to β-hCG measurements at this time.

US and Ectopic Pregnancy **The primary goal of US in early pregnancy is determination of a viable IUP and exclusion of ectopic pregnancy (Figure 98-1).**

US findings may also be useful in planning therapy when an ectopic pregnancy is discovered. Additionally, US provides information regarding fetal age and viability when an IUP is present.

It has previously been assumed that if an IUP exists, the diagnosis of ectopic pregnancy has been excluded. This assumption is based on the historical incidence of heterotopic pregnancy (combined IUP and ectopic pregnancy), reported to occur in 1 in 30,000 pregnancies. This is no longer a completely safe assumption, with heterotopic pregnancy now occurring in up to 1 in 3000 pregnancies in the general population. **In vitro fertilization and other efforts to enhance fertility with the use of ovulation-inducing drugs have resulted in a higher incidence of heterotopic pregnancy.** A study of 725 in vitro fertilization pregnancies found 4% to be ectopic pregnancies with 2 of 29 heterotopic gestations.[18] Heterotopic pregnancy should be considered even when US demonstrates an IUP in the assisted reproduction population. For other patients, demonstrating an IUP still provides a high degree of confidence in ruling out ectopic pregnancy. This confidence should be somewhat tempered when a patient has risk factors for ectopic pregnancy.

Advances in sonographic imaging and the use of transvaginal US scanning allow earlier detection of an IUP or an ectopic pregnancy. These advances have contributed to increasing use of real-time, bedside US in the ED performed by emergency physicians. ED US has the further advantage of allowing a potentially unstable patient to remain under continuous observation in the ED. When performed by trained individuals, bedside ED US in the first trimester of pregnancy is accurate and contributes to earlier diagnosis and treatment of ectopic pregnancy. However, US is operator-dependent, and there is limited validation in the community setting of the positive results obtained in academic teaching hospitals. Therefore, keep in mind the limitations of the procedure, equipment, and operator experience.[19]

The sequencing of transabdominal versus transvaginal US is situation- and operator-dependent. Usually, transabdominal scanning is performed first. Among other differences, transabdominal scanning is less invasive and offers a wider field of view and easier orientation to the pelvic organs. A full bladder is required for an appropriate acoustic window.

When transabdominal US is not diagnostic, transvaginal scanning should be performed. A full bladder is not required. The shallower depth of field and higher frequencies made possible by the lack of interposed abdominal fat allow better visualization of early pregnancies. There are reports of negative transvaginal but positive transabdominal US in cases of ectopic pregnancy, so both studies should be performed if the study performed first is not diagnostic. However, in one study of >5000 women with early pregnancy, pregnancy location was accurately diagnosed in >90% with a single transvaginal scan.[20]

When US reveals an unequivocal IUP and no other abnormalities, ectopic pregnancy is effectively excluded unless the patient is at high risk for heterotopic pregnancy. An embryo with cardiac activity seen within the uterine cavity is referred to as a *viable IUP*. When an embryo without cardiac activity is visualized within the uterus, the diagnosis of fetal demise can be entertained, provided that the crown–rump length is at least 5 mm. Briefly, transvaginal scanning can usually visualize the early sonographic signs of pregnancy, the gestational sac, yolk sac, and fetal pole, at 4.5, 5.5, and 6.0 weeks, respectively. Visualization by transabdominal scanning can be done approximately 1 week later.

No further diagnostic testing is needed when sonographic findings confirm or are highly suggestive of ectopic pregnancy. An empty uterus with embryonic cardiac activity visualized outside the uterus is diagnostic of ectopic pregnancy. This is seen in <10% of ectopic pregnancies using transabdominal scanning, but in up to 25% of cases when the transvaginal approach is used. When a pelvic mass or free pelvic fluid is seen in conjunction with an empty uterus, ectopic pregnancy is considered highly likely (**Figure 98-2**). The combination of an echogenic adnexal mass with free fluid in the setting of an empty uterus confers a risk of ectopic pregnancy near 100%, whereas a large amount of free

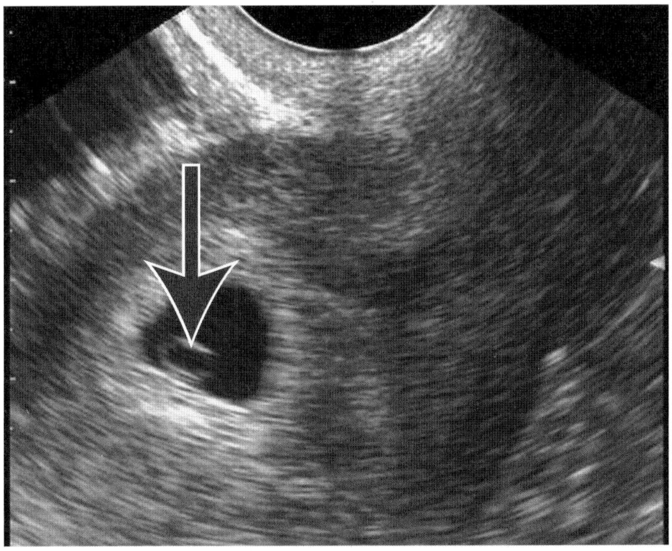

FIGURE 98-1. Yolk sac (*arrow*) within an intrauterine gestational sac. Normal early pregnancy. Transvaginal image. [Reproduced with permission from Ma OJ, Mateer JR, Reardon RF, Joing SA: *Ma & Mateer's Emergency Ultrasound*, 3rd ed. © 2014, McGraw-Hill Inc., New York.]

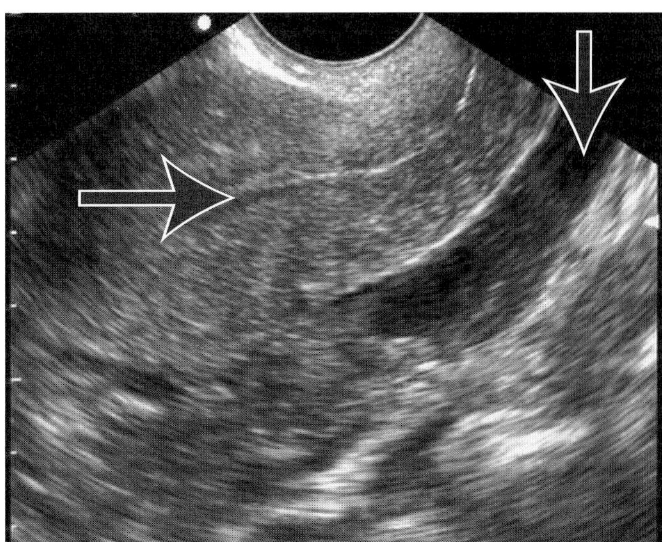

FIGURE 98-2. Ectopic pregnancy: empty uterus and free fluid in the posterior cul-de-sac. Transvaginal sagittal image. *Horizontal arrow* points to empty uterus (uterine stripe), and *vertical arrow* points to fluid in the cul-de-sac. [Reproduced with permission from Ma OJ, Mateer JR, Reardon RF, Joing SA: *Ma & Mateer's Emergency Ultrasound*, 3rd ed. © 2014, McGraw-Hill Inc., New York.]

TABLE 98-5 Ancillary US Findings Suggestive of Ectopic Pregnancy in High-Risk Patients

Ancillary Findings	Risk of Ectopic Pregnancy (%)
Any free pelvic fluid	52
Complex pelvic mass	72
Moderate/large amount of free pelvic fluid	86
Tubal ring	>95
Mass and free fluid	97
Hepatorenal free fluid	~100

Source: Reproduced with permission from Ma OJ, Mateer JR, Reardon RF, Joing SA: *Ma & Mateer's Emergency Ultrasound*, 3rd ed. New York: McGraw-Hill Inc., 2014; Table 14-2, p. 404.

fluid alone has a 86% risk (**Table 98-5**). In addition to a living extrauterine pregnancy, an extrauterine gestational sac is highly predictive of ectopic pregnancy (**Figure 98-3**). Any adnexal mass (other than a simple cyst) seen with US also has high positive predictive value for the diagnosis of ectopic pregnancy.[21,22] It has also been suggested that increased thickness of the endometrial stripe is predictive of ectopic pregnancy when no other diagnostic findings are noted on US. However, the wide overlap between endometrial stripe thickness in normal and ectopic pregnancy limits the usefulness of this observation.[23]

The Discriminatory Zone If US fails to reveal a definite IUP or fails to show findings strongly suggestive or diagnostic of an ectopic pregnancy, the test should be considered indeterminate and interpreted in light of quantitative serum β-hCG levels. The concept of the "discriminatory zone" was developed to relate β-hCG levels and US findings in a clinically useful way.[22] The discriminatory zone is the level of β-hCG at which findings of an IUP are expected on US. A β-hCG level higher than the discriminatory zone and an empty uterus on US suggest an ectopic pregnancy. An empty uterus with a β-hCG level below the discriminatory zone is indeterminate, neither confirming nor negating the diagnosis of ectopic pregnancy. The actual level of β-hCG representing the discriminatory zone is operator- and technique-dependent. With

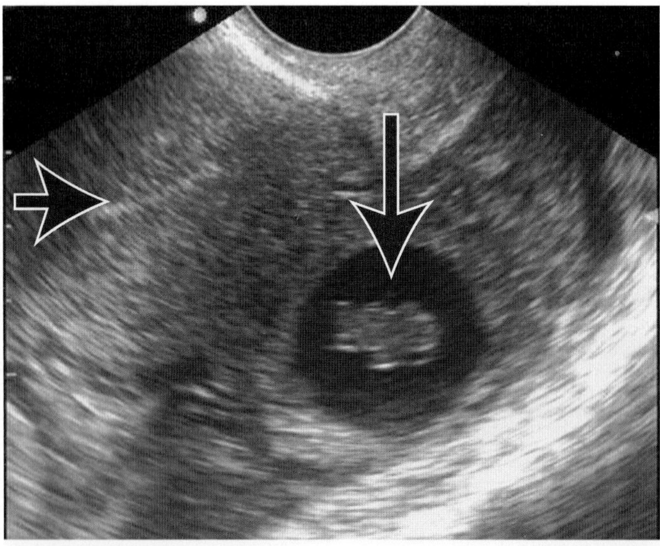

FIGURE 98-3. US of ectopic pregnancy. A living embryo in the adnexa and empty uterus is seen in this ectopic pregnancy (endometrial echo is visible in the left upper portion of the image). Embryonic cardiac activity was present on real-time imaging. Transvaginal image. *Horizontal arrow* points to empty uterus (uterine stripe), and *vertical arrow* points to ectopic pregnancy in the adnexa. [Reproduced with permission from Ma OJ, Mateer JR, Reardon RF, Joing SA: *Ma & Mateer's Emergency Ultrasound*, 3rd ed. © 2014, McGraw-Hill Inc., New York.]

transvaginal scanning, the discriminatory zone is often considered to be 1500 mIU/mL. For transabdominal scanning, an IUP should be detectable when the β-hCG level reaches about 6000 mIU/mL. Clinicians should understand this concept and collaborate closely with imaging specialists in equivocal cases to avoid confusion. **When ectopic pregnancy is suspected, US should be performed even in patients with low β-hCG levels**, because ectopic pregnancy can occur even at very low (<500 mIU/mL) β-hCG levels.[24] Further, decision to intervene on a pregnancy should not be made solely on a single hCG level; if the patient is hemodynamically stable with a β-hCG greater than the discriminatory zone and no visible intrauterine or extrauterine pregnancy, watchful waiting is an appropriate management strategy with close follow-up and strict return precautions.[25]

Other Diagnostic Modalities **MRI** has high sensitivity and specificity for the diagnosis of ectopic pregnancy, but cost, availability, and the time to perform the study make the use of MRI of only theoretical interest at the present time.

Culdocentesis has been supplanted by tests for β-hCG in combination with US, but it may have use when US is unavailable. A positive test facilitates an appropriate, rapid surgical intervention. Possible results include a dry aspiration, which has no diagnostic value. If clear, nonbloody peritoneal fluid is aspirated, the tap is considered negative. Aspiration of nonclotting blood constitutes a positive tap and is considered indicative of an ectopic pregnancy. However, there is no consensus regarding the criteria for a positive test. Various authors have proposed volumes between 0.3 and 10 mL, with hematocrit from 3% to 15%. The pathophysiologic basis for culdocentesis is that a ruptured ectopic pregnancy will bleed into the pelvic peritoneal cavity. Some 85% to 90% of patients with a ruptured ectopic pregnancy will have a positive culdocentesis. Surprisingly, up to 70% of patients with an unruptured ectopic pregnancy will also have a positive result. A basic limitation of the technique is that it is less sensitive in the diagnosis of unruptured than ruptured ectopic pregnancy. Another cause of false-negative results is that, in cases of rapid bleeding, intraperitoneal blood may clot due to the lack of sufficient dwell time to produce defibrination. False-positive results occur because of technical errors (entering a vein or other vascular structure with the needle) or a ruptured corpus luteum cyst. Aspiration of purulent material may indicate another diagnosis, such as pelvic inflammatory disease.

Laparoscopy may be both diagnostic and therapeutic. Laparoscopy is primarily useful in patients with suspected ectopic pregnancy and a nondiagnostic US. It may provide an earlier diagnosis and a possible route for definitive treatment when compared with serial β-hCG measurements and US. As with other invasive techniques, results vary with the skill of the operator and the quality of the available equipment.

Dilatation and curettage may provide a definitive diagnosis of IUP, thus excluding ectopic pregnancy except in cases of heterotopic pregnancy. Dilatation and curettage diagnoses an IUP when chorionic villi are obtained from the uterine cavity. The procedure terminates an IUP and is applicable only when termination of pregnancy is desired or when a nonviable pregnancy has been documented.

TREATMENT

The treatment of ectopic pregnancy can be divided into surgical and medical approaches. If laparoscopy is needed for diagnosis, a surgical approach is most appropriate. For unruptured ectopic pregnancy, the most frequently used surgical approach is laparoscopic salpingostomy; the most frequently used medical approach is systemic methotrexate treatment. There is no difference in success rates between methotrexate, salpingotomy, and salpingectomy in appropriately selected women with unruptured ectopic pregnancies.[26,27] Laparotomy is the treatment of choice in hemodynamically unstable patients. Laparoscopy is preferred in a hemodynamically stable patient.

Methotrexate **Methotrexate** is the only drug currently recommended as a medical alternative to surgical treatment of ectopic pregnancy and is ideally used in patients with hemodynamic stability, minimal abdominal pain, the ability to follow up reliably, and normal baseline liver and renal function tests. Contraindications to methotrexate use are listed in

TABLE 98-6 Contraindications to Methotrexate Administration[28]

Absolute Contraindications	Relative Contraindications
Intrauterine pregnancy	Embryonic cardiac activity detected by transvaginal US
Evidence of immunodeficiency	Human chorionic gonadotropin concentrations >5000 mIU/mL
Moderate to severe anemia, leukopenia, or thrombocytopenia	Ectopic pregnancy >4 cm in size as imaged by transvaginal US
Sensitivity to methotrexate	Refusal to accept blood transfusion
Active pulmonary disease	Inability to reliably return for follow-up
Active peptic ulcer disease	
Clinically important hepatic or renal dysfunction	
Breastfeeding	
Hemodynamic instability	

Table 98-6.[28] Methotrexate is a folic acid antagonist that inhibits dihydrofolate reductase, causing depletion of cofactors needed for DNA and RNA synthesis. Different methotrexate regimens have been used, including both systemic IM injections and direct injection into the ectopic gestational sac. IM methotrexate is the most commonly used approach, eliminating the need for laparoscopy or US guidance. The failure rate is 14.3% or higher with single-dose methotrexate when pretreatment β-hCG levels are >5000 mIU/mL, compared with 3.7% for levels <5000 mIU/mL.[29] If β-hCG levels are higher than 5000 mIU/mL, multiple doses may be appropriate.[30] The success rate of the multiple-dose regimen was statistically significantly higher than that seen with a single dose of methotrexate (92.7% vs 88.1%).[31]

The most common side effects associated with methotrexate include abdominal pain after treatment (up to 75% of patients) followed by flatulence and then stomatitis. Lower abdominal pain lasting up to 12 hours is common 3 to 7 days after methotrexate treatment and is thought to be secondary to methotrexate-induced tubal abortion or tubal distention due to hematoma formation ("separation pain").[32] The pain is usually self-limited and may respond to nonsteroidal anti-inflammatory drugs.

Abdominal pain after methotrexate treatment represents a clinical dilemma. It is difficult to differentiate expected pain from therapeutic tubal abortion and hematoma formation with fallopian tube distension (separation pain) from pain associated with rupturing persistent ectopic pregnancy.[32] Suggested evaluation of patients presenting with abdominal pain in this time frame after methotrexate administration includes a CBC and abdominopelvic US to rule out tubal rupture and hemoperitoneum and consideration of other causes of abdominal pain.[3] Such patients may need admission to the hospital for observation. Hemodynamic instability and/or falling hematocrit require consideration for surgical intervention. Many centers will proceed to surgical intervention in patients with moderate to severe pain, free fluid in the cul-de-sac, or rebound tenderness, although conservative treatment has proven successful in stable patients after methotrexate therapy.[32] Prognostic factors associated with a higher failure rate for methotrexate treatment include larger tubal diameter, higher initial β-hCG levels, severe abdominal pain, and fetal cardiac activity.[33]

Methotrexate administration in properly selected patients with ectopic pregnancy may be initiated in the ED, clinic, or obstetrician/gynecologist's office. Treatment initiated in the ED should be in close conjunction with an obstetrician/gynecologist or other physician capable of providing follow-up care. Keep pelvic examinations after methotrexate treatment to a minimum to decrease the risk of tubal rupture. Patient instruction on discharge should include the following points:[34]

- Treatment failure occurs in up to 36% of cases.
- Elective or emergency surgical treatment may be necessary if medical therapy fails or tubal rupture occurs (~5% of cases).
- Vaginal bleeding, abdominal pain, weakness, dizziness, or syncope after treatment should be evaluated immediately as possible signs of tubal rupture.[16]
- Patients should refrain from sexual intercourse for 14 to 21 days after treatment (until β-hCG levels are undetectable), because it may increase the risk of tubal rupture.

Rh Seroconversion and Indications for Anti-D Immunoglobulin

Rh_0 (D) antigen can be detected as early as 5.5 weeks and certainly by 6 weeks of gestation. Alloimmunization can occur with as little as 0.1 mL of fetal blood admixing with the mother's. Alloimmunization can occur from ectopic pregnancy. Circulating blood volume of the fetus is <5 mL in the first trimester. **Both the American College of Emergency Physicians and the American College of Obstetricians and Gynecologists recommend treatment with 50 micrograms of RhoGAM for Rh-negative women with ectopic pregnancy when diagnosed prior to 12 weeks of gestation due to the small volume of red cells in the fetoplacental circulation, although administration of a full dose of 300 micrograms is acceptable as well.**

DISPOSITION AND FOLLOW-UP

When a patient with signs or symptoms suggestive of ectopic pregnancy is found to be pregnant, determine if the pregnancy is intrauterine (**Figure 98-4**). The nature and timing of additional diagnostic measures depend on the clinical condition of the patient. Unstable patients with suspected ectopic pregnancy should receive resuscitation, urgent consultation, and operative intervention. Surgery may be both diagnostic and therapeutic if an ectopic pregnancy is found or may reveal another cause for the patient's condition. When bedside ED US is available, it may be valuable even in unstable patients, as it should not interfere with resuscitation, consultation, and rapid transfer to the operating room.

Ideally, all pregnant patients with suspected ectopic pregnancy should receive immediate US. However, issues of availability during off hours may make this impractical. Stable patients who are judged to be at low risk for ectopic pregnancy can be considered for discharge and outpatient follow-up. Such patients should have a quantitative β-hCG level obtained to facilitate subsequent management. Culdocentesis remains an option where US is unavailable, but currently is used rarely due to its limitations and the unfamiliarity of many emergency physicians with the technique.

Stable patients with β-hCG levels above the discriminatory zone and an empty uterus on US, with or without other US findings of an ectopic pregnancy, are presumed to have an ectopic pregnancy. These patients should receive consultation in the ED.

Management options for stable patients with a β-hCG level below the discriminatory zone and indeterminate US include consultation in the ED or discharge for follow-up in 2 days for reexamination and repeat β-hCG levels. Culdocentesis, dilatation and curettage, and laparoscopy are also options in this circumstance; however, the decision is normally left to the obstetrician's discretion. Figure 98-4 illustrates a suggested diagnostic approach.

OTHER CAUSES OF BLEEDING IN THE FIRST 20 WEEKS OF PREGNANCY

Common causes of bleeding during early pregnancy are listed in **Table 98-7**.

SPONTANEOUS ABORTION

The World Health Organization defines spontaneous abortion as loss of pregnancy before 20 weeks or loss of a fetus weighing <500 grams. Estimates of pregnancies that abort spontaneously range from 20% to 40%. Approximately 75% of spontaneous abortions occur before 8 weeks of gestation (**Table 98-8**).

The most common cause of fetal loss is chromosomal abnormalities. Other associations include advanced maternal age, prior poor obstetric history, concurrent medical disorders, previous abortion, infection (including syphilis and human immunodeficiency virus), and some anatomic abnormalities of the upper genital tract. Exposure to some agents, such as certain anesthetic agents, certain heavy metals, and tobacco, may also contribute to the incidence of abortion.

Bleeding with or without abdominal pain is the most common presenting complaint.

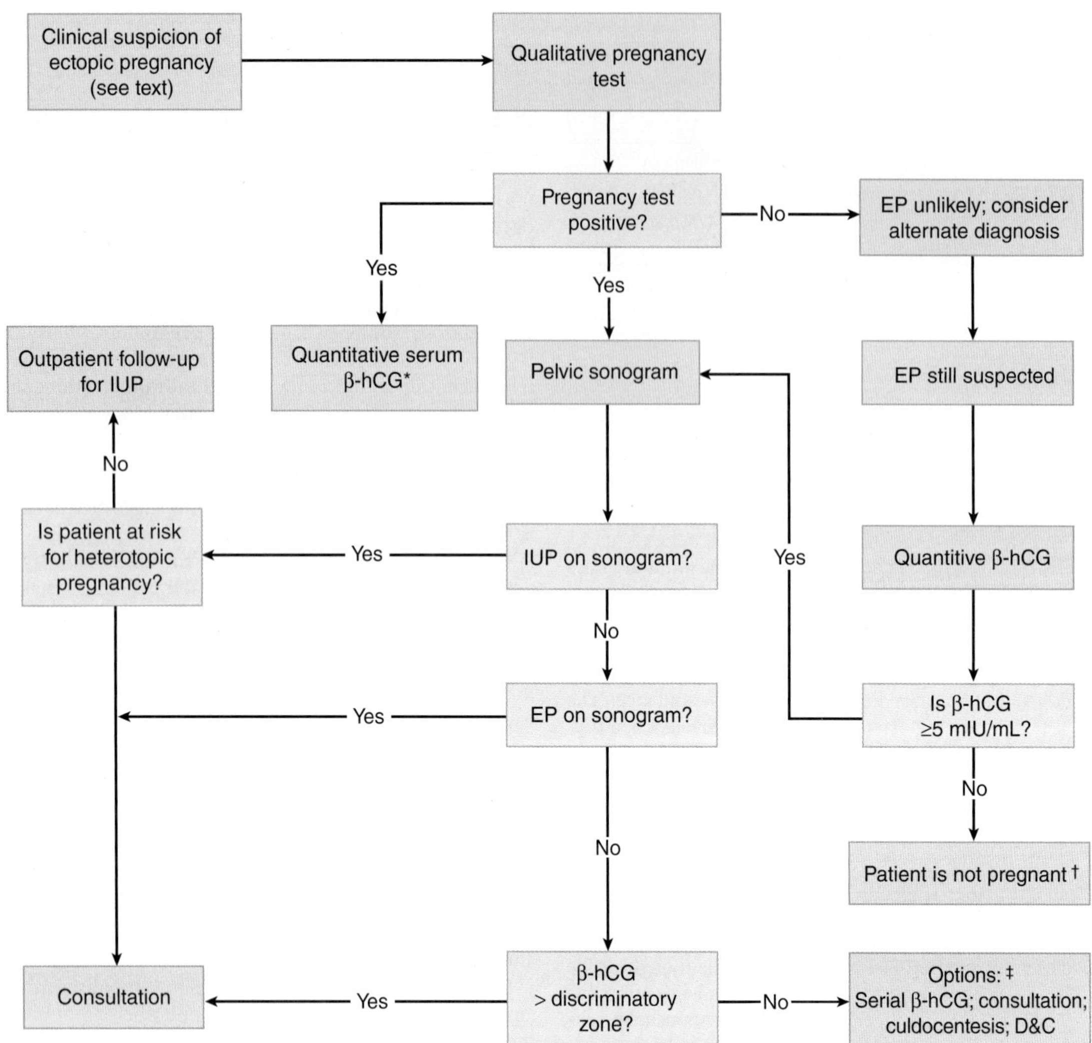

FIGURE 98-4. Diagnostic algorithm for suspected ectopic pregnancy. *Quantitative measurement of β subunit of human chorionic gonadotropin (β-hCG) before US may facilitate rapid patient disposition by saving time. †There have been extremely rare reports of pregnancy with β-hCG <5 mIU/mL. ‡Serial outpatient β-hCG measurements are recommended only for stable patients judged to be at low risk for ruptured ectopic pregnancy. D&C = dilatation and curettage; EP = ectopic pregnancy; IUP = intrauterine pregnancy.

TABLE 98-7 Common Causes of Vaginal Bleeding During the First Trimester of Pregnancy

Abortion
Ectopic pregnancy
Gestational trophoblastic disease
Implantation bleeding (physiologic)

TABLE 98-8 Spontaneous Abortion Terminology

Terminology	Definition
Threatened abortion	Pregnancy-related bloody vaginal discharge or frank bleeding during the first half of pregnancy without cervical dilatation
Inevitable abortion	Vaginal bleeding and dilatation of the cervix
Incomplete abortion	Passage of only parts of the products of conception
	More likely to occur between 6 and 14 weeks of pregnancy
Complete abortion	Passage of all fetal tissue, including trophoblast and all products of conception, before 20 weeks of conception
Missed abortion	Fetal death at <20 weeks without passage of any fetal tissue for 4 weeks after fetal death
Septic abortion	Evidence of infection during any stage of abortion

DIAGNOSIS

In addition to the standard medical history, determine the amount of bleeding as pads used per hour to anticipate blood loss, last menstrual period, and past obstetric history. A pelvic examination is needed to define the type of abortion and to determine the amount and site of bleeding, whether the cervix has dilated, and whether any tissue has been passed.

The diagnosis of pregnancy is central to the diagnosis of abortion. Obtain a quantitative serum β-hCG level, CBC to evaluate for blood loss, blood type, Rh factor and antibody screen, and urinalysis (urinary tract infection has been associated with increased fetal wastage). US can help rule out ectopic pregnancy, aid as a prognostic tool for fetal viability, and diagnose retained products of conception. US studies combined with determinations of β-hCG levels can be both diagnostic and prognostic. Although a β-hCG of 1500 IU/mL is a somewhat arbitrary value when evaluating pregnancy, it is still useful when comparing with US findings. Although institution-dependent, an IUP should be visible on transvaginal US at this concentration. **Table 98-9** describes expected US findings at certain gestational ages and β-hCG values.[35]

TREATMENT

Patients with threatened abortion can be discharged safely if follow-up is ensured. Although a low level of activity and even bed rest are

TABLE 98-9 Comparison of Gestational Age, β-hCG, and US Findings

Gestational Age	β-hCG (mIU/mL)	Transvaginal US Findings	Transabdominal US Findings
4–5 weeks	<1000	Intradecidual sac	N/A
5 weeks	>2000	Yolk sac (± embryo)	Gestational sac
6 weeks	10,000–20,000	Embryo with cardiac activity	Yolk sac (± embryo)
7 weeks	>20,000	Embryonic torso/head	Embryo with cardiac activity

Source: Reproduced with permission from Ma OJ, Mateer JR, Reardon RF, Joing SA: *Ma & Mateer's Emergency Ultrasound*, 3rd ed. New York: McGraw-Hill Inc., 2014; Table 14-1, p. 400.

sometimes advised, there is no proven effectiveness of this practice. Generally speaking, a miscarriage cannot be avoided. Patients should avoid intercourse and tampons to minimize risk of infection.

Patients with a diagnosis of incomplete abortion should have the uterus evacuated. The decision to proceed with medical treatment, such as PO misoprostol, 600 micrograms, or surgical treatment, such as dilatation and curettage, should be made in consultation with the patient and an obstetrician.[36]

Patients with a complete abortion, as shown by US and complete passage of products of conception, can be discharged safely, with follow-up ensured. If there is any doubt, obtain obstetrics consultation for possible dilatation and curettage.

Patients with a nonviable fetus can be either admitted or discharged to be followed up within 1 week, depending on the comfort level of the patient and physician with this decision. Patients should return immediately if there is heavy bleeding (more than one pad per hour for 6 hours), pain, or fever.

Pregnant women with vaginal bleeding who are Rh-negative should be treated with Rh_0 (D) immunoglobulin (RhoGAM). RhoGAM should be administered before discharge, if possible, but it also can be administered within 72 hours by the primary care physician or obstetrician when the woman presents several days or weeks after vaginal bleeding has begun.

SEPTIC ABORTION

A septic abortion is a spontaneous or other abortion complicated by a pelvic infection. Presenting complaints include fever, abdominal pain, vaginal discharge, vaginal bleeding, and history of recent pregnancy. The most common causes are retained products of conception due to incomplete spontaneous or therapeutic abortion and introduction of either normal or pathologic vaginal bacteria by instrumentation.

Perform a history and physical examination, including a pelvic examination. Obtain a quantitative serum β-hCG level, CBC to evaluate for anemia due to blood loss, blood type, Rh factor and antibody screen, urinalysis, and blood cultures. An US will help identify retained products of conception in the uterus, adnexal masses, and free fluid in the cul-de-sac. Treatment consists of fluid resuscitation, broad-spectrum IV antibiotics, and early obstetric consultation for evacuation of the uterus. Antibiotics, such as ampicillin/sulbactam, 3 grams IV, or clindamycin, 600 milligrams, plus gentamicin, 1 to 2 milligrams/kg IV, should cover both normal vaginal flora and those causing sexually transmitted disease.

GESTATIONAL TROPHOBLASTIC DISEASE

Gestational trophoblastic disease consists of a broad spectrum of conditions ranging from an uncomplicated partial hydatidiform molar pregnancy to stage IV choriocarcinoma with cerebral metastases.[37] It is a neoplasm that arises in the trophoblastic cells of the placenta. It complicates 1 in 1700 pregnancies in North America and is more common in Asian women. The noninvasive form of the disease is the hydatidiform mole, which is either complete or partial. Complete moles are more common, and in this form, there is no actual fetus, whereas in the partial mole, a deformed, nonviable fetus is present. Both moles and invasive forms are composed of trophoblasts that produce β-hCG. Patients with a history of hydatidiform molar pregnancy are at increased risk of future molar pregnancies, with a risk of 1% in subsequent gestations after one molar pregnancy and a risk as high as 23% after two molar gestations.

Symptoms include vaginal bleeding in the first or second trimester (75% to 95% of cases) and hyperemesis (26%). Gestational trophoblastic disease, or molar pregnancies that persist into the second trimester, are associated with pre-eclampsia. **When pregnancy-induced hypertension is seen before 24 weeks of gestation, consider the possibility of a molar pregnancy.** The uterus is excessive in size for gestational age and shows a placenta with many lucent areas interspersed with brighter areas on US study. Because not all molar pregnancies are found on US, all tissue extracted from the uterus on suction curettage or during pelvic examination should be sent for histologic examination. If trophoblastic disease is suspected because of abnormally high β-hCG levels, a uterine size either larger or smaller than expected, and US findings suggestive of the diagnosis, obtain obstetric consultation. Treatment is by suction curettage in the hospital setting because of risk of hemorrhage. β-hCG levels that fail to decrease after evaluation are evidence of persistent or invasive disease necessitating chemotherapy. Metastasis to lung, liver, and brain may occur, but the prognosis for most patients is very good. Trophoblastic embolization, although extremely rare, may occur, with resulting rapid onset of respiratory distress resembling amniotic fluid embolus.

IMPLANTATION BLEEDING

Implantation bleeding can occur as the embryo implants into the vascular uterine decidual tissue. Bleeding can be scant or like menstrual bleeding and usually occurs at 5 or 6 weeks after the last period. Pelvic examination is normal. Implantation bleeding is diagnosed only after excluding ectopic pregnancy.

NAUSEA AND VOMITING OF PREGNANCY AND HYPEREMESIS GRAVIDARUM

EPIDEMIOLOGY

Nausea and vomiting of pregnancy generally are seen in the first 12 weeks. The etiology is unknown. Severe nausea and vomiting of pregnancy is known as hyperemesis gravidarum and is defined as intractable vomiting with weight loss, volume depletion, and laboratory values showing hypokalemia or ketonemia. It occurs in up to 2% of all pregnancies. Patients with gestational trophoblastic disease also may present with intractable vomiting for unknown reasons.

CLINICAL FEATURES

Findings on physical examination in nausea and vomiting of pregnancy are usually normal except for signs of volume depletion. Laboratory tests to consider include CBC, serum electrolytes, BUN, creatinine, and urinalysis. The finding of ketonuria is important because it is an early sign of starvation. However, there is no evidence that ketosis per se is harmful to the fetus. Serial measurements of urinary ketones can be used to determine success of therapy.

The presence of abdominal pain in nausea and vomiting of pregnancy or hyperemesis gravidarum is highly unusual and should suggest another diagnosis. Ruptured ectopic pregnancies occasionally present with nausea and vomiting, as well as diarrhea and abdominal pain. Gallbladder dilatation and biliary sludge increase in pregnancy, predisposing to stone formation. Cholelithiasis and cholecystitis are more common in pregnant women than in women of comparable age and health status who are not pregnant. Differential diagnosis of vomiting or vomiting with abdominal pain should include cholecystitis, cholelithiasis, gastroenteritis, pancreatitis, appendicitis, hepatitis,

TABLE 98-10 Antiemetics

Antiemetic	Brand Name	U.S. Food and Drug Administration Category	PO	PR	IV
Promethazine	Phenergan	C	12.5–25 milligrams every 4 h	12.5–25 milligrams every 4 h	IV administration is generally recommended against; 12.5–25 milligrams IM every 4 h
Prochlorperazine	Compazine	—	10 milligrams every 6–8 h	25 milligrams every 12 h	10 milligrams over 2 min Maximum of 40 milligrams every 24 h
Chlorpromazine	Thorazine	C	10–25 milligrams every 4–6 h	100 milligrams every 6–8 h	25 milligrams in 500 mL NS at 250 mL/h
Ondansetron	Zofran	B	4–8 milligrams every 8 h	—	8 milligrams IV over 5 min
Metoclopramide	Reglan	B	10 milligrams orally every 6–8 h	—	10 milligrams over 1–2 min every 6–8 h
Maintenance Therapy for Nausea and Vomiting					
Doxylamine with pyridoxine	Diclegis/ Diclectin	A	2 tablets every evening	—	—
Vitamin B_6	—	—	25 milligrams every 8 h	—	—
Ginger	—	—	500–1000 milligrams daily	—	—
Diphenhydramine	Benadryl	B	25–50 milligrams every 6 h	—	—

Abbreviation: NS = normal saline.

Source: Adapted with permission from Pearlman M, Tintinalli JE (eds): *Emergency Care of the Woman*. New York: McGraw-Hill, 1998.

peptic ulcer, pyelonephritis, ectopic pregnancy, fatty liver of pregnancy, and the syndrome of *h*emolysis, *e*levated *l*iver enzymes, and *l*ow *p*latelets (HELLP syndrome).

TREATMENT

Treatment consists of IV fluids containing 5% glucose in either lactated Ringer's solution or normal saline to replete volume and reverse ketonuria. A number of antiemetic drugs can be used (**Table 98-10**) for patients who remain nauseated or continue to vomit. Initially, the patient should be given nothing by mouth. Oral fluids should be started after the nausea and vomiting are controlled but before discharge.

DISPOSITION AND FOLLOW-UP

The patient may be discharged after reversal of ketonuria, correction of electrolyte imbalance, and a successful trial of oral fluids. Discharge with antiemetic medication is usually necessary. There is no clear drug of choice.

Phenothiazines can cause drowsiness or dystonic reactions in some patients. Ondansetron (Zofran®), 8 milligrams IV or 4 milligrams PO three times daily, can cause headache, constipation, diarrhea, or lightheadedness. It does not cause dystonia. Its chief disadvantage is cost. It is apparently no more effective than promethazine.[15] Doxylamine and pyridoxine (Bendectin®), a mainstay of therapy in the past, was discontinued due to fears of teratogenicity, but with new information, it does not represent an increase in fetal risk and has been reintroduced on the North America market as Diclegis/Diclectin (also put in trademark sign after Diclegis/Diclectin).[16,38]

Admission guidelines include uncertain diagnosis, intractable vomiting, persistent ketone or electrolyte abnormalities after volume repletion, and weight loss of >10% of prepregnancy weight.

REFERENCES

The complete reference list is available online at www.TintinalliEM.com.

Comorbid Disorders in Pregnancy

Lori J. Whelan

INTRODUCTION

This chapter reviews the most common comorbid conditions encountered in pregnant women in the ED environment: diabetes and hypoglycemia; thyroid disorders; hypertensive disorders; cardiac arrhythmias; thromboembolism; asthma; renal disease; urinary tract infections; sickle cell disease; headache; seizures; substance abuse; and intimate partner violence. Drug risk during pregnancy, lactation, and fetal effects of radiation are summarized based on currently available data. Resuscitation is covered in chapter 25, "Resuscitation in Pregnancy."

DIABETES IN PREGNANCY

Maternal diabetes affects >8% of the 4 million live births annually in the United States.[1] Three fourths of pregnant patients with diabetes have either gestational diabetes or type 2 diabetes diagnosed through prenatal screening. Of the remaining 25%, 1% have preexisting type 1 diabetes, and the remaining are type 2 diabetics. Pregnant diabetic women are at increased risk for spontaneous abortion, particularly patients with poor glycemic control early in pregnancy, preexisting vascular disease, and pre-eclampsia. Pregnant diabetics are also at increased risk for several pregnancy complications, including pregnancy-induced hypertension, preterm labor, spontaneous abortion, pyelonephritis, and diabetic ketoacidosis (DKA). The goal of treatment during pregnancy is to prevent spontaneous abortions, hyperglycemia-induced congenital abnormalities and ketoacidosis, and hypoglycemia.

Oral hypoglycemic agents, such as metformin and glyburide, are occasionally used in select patients with gestational diabetes.[2] A significant portion of gestational diabetics can be managed with diet alone if they can maintain glycemic goals with frequent glucose monitoring.

The American College of Obstetricians and Gynecologists recommends the following goals for maintaining euglycemia in pregnant diabetic patients: a fasting blood glucose concentration of ≤95 milligrams/dL and a 2-hour postprandial glucose concentration

≤120 milligrams/dL.[3] Patients with gestational diabetes who are managed by diet alone rarely develop acute hyperglycemic complications because glucose values rarely reach levels consistent with DKA. Among patients with preexisting type 1 and type 2 diabetes, the need for insulin increases throughout the course of pregnancy. Historically, all type 2 diabetics were switched to insulin as soon as possible (even prior to conception) to ensure appropriate glycemic control and due to concerns over the safety of oral hypoglycemic agents in pregnancy. Recent studies in gestational diabetes have not shown metformin or glyburide to have any harmful fetal effects, but long-term studies are needed. Although metformin may be continued in select patients, there is no consensus on the use of these oral agents alone in the pregnant patient with type 2 diabetes.[2-5]

In general, during the first trimester, the initial insulin requirement is 0.7 units/kg/day. By late pregnancy, patients generally require 1 unit/kg/day.[6]

Neutral protamine Hagedorn (NPH)/regular insulin combinations are still first-line insulin therapy, but the long-acting analog insulin detemir (Levemir) is approved by the U.S. Food and Drug Administration for use in pregnancy and is category B. Compared to NPH, insulin detemir improves fasting plasma glucose and decreases hypoglycemic events. There is a strong evidence base to recommend insulin detemir in pregnancy, but the lack of definitive fetal benefit means that there is no pressing need to switch a woman whose diabetes is well controlled by NPH insulin to insulin detemir.

Insulin glargine (Lantus) is still category C. It is generally not initiated during pregnancy. However, it seems reasonable to continue insulin glargine when it was successful maintaining excellent glycemic control in a woman who is now pregnant.[7]

HYPOGLYCEMIA

Women with type 1 diabetes have three to five times more hypoglycemic episodes than the period prior to pregnancy.[8] Risk factors for severe hypoglycemia during pregnancy include a history of severe hypoglycemia in the year preceding pregnancy, impaired hypoglycemia awareness, long duration of diabetes, low HbA_{1c} in early pregnancy, fluctuating plasma glucose levels, and excessive use of insulin injections between meals.[8] Hypoglycemia generally presents as sweating, tremors, blurred or double vision, weakness, hunger, confusion, paraesthesias, anxiety, palpitations, nausea, headache, or stupor. Moderate and infrequent hypoglycemic episodes are generally well tolerated by the fetus.[4] Pregnant diabetic women should be educated about the symptoms and treatment of hypoglycemia. Treat mild hypoglycemia (i.e., a glucose level of <70 milligrams/dL in patients who are able to follow commands) by giving juice, glucose, or food by mouth. Provide standard treatment for more severe hypoglycemia, with IV glucose or PO glucose or glucagon 1 to 2 milligrams SC or IV (see chapters 223, "Type 1 Diabetes Mellitus" and 224, "Type 2 Diabetes Mellitus").

DIABETIC KETOACIDOSIS IN PREGNANCY

A pregnant diabetic who is ill appearing, has persistent nausea and vomiting, and/or has a blood glucose level ≥180 milligrams/dL should be screened for DKA with serum or urine ketones and a serum chemistry panel. Management guidelines for pregnant women with DKA are the same as for nonpregnant patients[9] (see chapter 225, "Diabetic Ketoacidosis"). In addition to the usual care, obtain fetal heart tones, administer oxygen, and for third-trimester patients, place in the left lateral decubitus position to displace the uterus and improve uterine blood flow. Most fetal heart rate abnormalities subside after correction of maternal hypovolemia and acidosis. Consult with the patient's physician, and admit the patient to the hospital.

The incidence of DKA in pregnancy decreases with early diagnosis of insulin-dependent diabetes, improved prenatal counseling, and care with an identifiable primary care provider.[10,11] DKA most commonly affects women in the second or third trimester or pregnant women with new-onset type 1 diabetes.[10,12]

Women who use continuous SC insulin infusions (the insulin pump) can develop DKA whether they are pregnant or not. DKA can develop very quickly and unexpectedly, especially in patients who have recently started using the pump.[13,14] Use of continuous insulin pumps during pregnancy is equivalent, but not superior, to scheduled injections. Management of DKA in a pregnant woman with an insulin pump is the same as the nonpregnant patient.

DKA is not an indication for delivery. Although fetal heart rate monitoring in maternal DKA may initially demonstrate a nonreassuring pattern, patterns usually improve as maternal ketoacidosis is corrected, and mother will tolerate delivery or cesarean section better once acidosis resolves.[10,15]

THYROID DISORDERS

TRANSIENT HYPERTHYROIDISM OF HYPEREMESIS GRAVIDARUM

Women in the first trimester with weight loss, tachycardia, and vomiting consistent with hyperemesis gravidarum may also demonstrate laboratory evidence of hyperthyroidism, or biochemical or transient hyperthyroidism. The most likely cause is thyrotropin receptor stimulation from high human chorionic gonadotropin serum concentrations. Women with transient hyperthyroidism have no previous history of thyroid disease, no palpable goiter, and except for tachycardia, no other symptoms or signs of hyperthyroidism. Test results for thyroid antibodies are negative. With transient hyperthyroidism of hyperemesis gravidarum, thyroid-stimulating hormone (TSH) may be suppressed and free thyroxine (T_4) elevated, but triiodothyronine (T_3) is **lower** than in true hyperthyroidism. With true hyperthyroidism, both free T_4 and T_3 are usually **elevated**. Only symptomatic treatment is suggested for transient hyperthyroidism, and antithyroid medication is not recommended.[16]

HYPERTHYROIDISM

True hyperthyroidism in pregnancy increases the risk of pre-eclampsia, low birth weight, and possibly congenital malformations. Symptoms of hyperthyroidism can mimic symptoms of normal pregnancy and may consist of nervousness, palpitations, heat intolerance, and inability to gain weight despite a good appetite. Methimazole and propylthiouracil (PTU) are equally efficacious in the treatment of pregnant women. However, methimazole has a possible association with congenital abnormalities during first-trimester organogenesis, and PTU can cause hepatotoxicity. Therefore, during the first trimester, hyperthyroidism in pregnancy is treated with PTU followed by methimazole during the second and third trimesters.[17-19] Agranulocytosis and aplastic anemia are rare but serious complications in patients treated with antithyroid drugs. If this occurs, immediately discontinue the medication and obtain obstetrical consultation.

THYROID STORM

Patients with thyroid storm develop fever, volume depletion, or high-output heart failure. Labor, cesarean section, and infection all may precipitate thyroid storm in a woman with a history of hyperthyroidism. Thyroid storm has been associated with a mortality rate of up to 25%. The principles of treatment are summarized in **Table 99-1** and are similar to those for nonpregnant patients (see chapter 229, "Hyperthyroidism").

HYPERTENSION

Hypertensive disorders are the most common medical complication of pregnancy. Hypertension in pregnancy can be divided into five categories: chronic hypertension in pregnancy, gestational hypertension, pre-eclampsia, HELLP syndrome, and eclampsia. Chronic hypertension is discussed below, and the other disorders are discussed in detail in chapter 100, "Emergencies after 20 Weeks of Pregnancy and the Postpartum Period."

TABLE 99-1 Principles of Treatment of Thyroid Storm during Pregnancy

Principle	Comment
Inhibit thyroid hormone release with thionamides (PTU is preferred over methimazole; also blocks conversion of T_4 to T_3)	**Propylthiouracil** (PTU) 600–1000 milligrams PO loading dose followed by 200–250 milligrams PO every 4 h (first trimester) or **Methimazole** 40 milligrams PO loading dose followed by 25 milligrams PO every 4 h (second and third trimesters)
Inhibit new thyroid hormone production (give at least 1 h after above step)	**Lugol solution** 8–10 drops every 6–8 h or **Potassium iodine** 5 drops PO every 6 h or **Iopanoic acid** 1 gram IV every 8 h **Do not use radioactive iodine because the fetus will concentrate iodine-131 after the 10th to 12th week of gestation, resulting in congenital hypothyroidism**
Block peripheral thyroid hormone effects	**Propranolol** 1–2 milligrams IV every 10–15 min and start **Propranolol** 40 milligrams PO every 6 h or **Esmolol** 500 micrograms/kg IV bolus, then 50 micrograms/kg/min maintenance Hold if evidence of heart failure is present
Prevent conversion of T_4 to T_3	**Hydrocortisone** 100 milligrams IV every 8 h or **Dexamethasone** 2 milligrams IV every 6 h
Supportive care	Left lateral decubitus position Oxygen Cooling blankets IV fluids Acetaminophen 650 milligrams PO every 4 h[20]

CHRONIC HYPERTENSION IN PREGNANCY

Chronic hypertension is sustained elevation of blood pressure to >140/90 mm Hg, measured on two separate occasions before 20 weeks of gestation or persistent beyond 12 weeks postpartum.[21,22] Patients with mild hypertension (140/90 mm Hg) and no evidence of renal disease should be counseled on lifestyle modifications and observed. Because there is no consensus that antihypertensives can reduce the risk of fetal death, growth restriction, abruption, or eclampsia, treatment with antihypertensive medication is **not** usually necessary unless renal disease develops.[23] Despite the lack of evidence supporting the benefit of antihypertensive therapy in women with blood pressure <180/110 mm Hg, there is a general consensus that pregnant women with hypertension in the blood pressure range of 150 to 160/100 to 110 mm Hg should be treated with antihypertensive therapy.[22-24] There is insufficient evidence to support or refute the theory that bed rest, either in the hospital or at home, improves outcomes.[25]

Maternal mortality in patients with chronic hypertension results from **severe** hypertension and associated congestive heart failure or stroke. Fetal perinatal outcome is associated most closely with pre-eclampsia or placental abruption.

Commonly used agents for the treatment of chronic hypertension in pregnancy are listed in **Table 99-2** and include labetalol, α-methyldopa (Aldomet), clonidine, and nifedipine. Based on the overall low rate of adverse effects and good efficacy, labetalol is a good option for first-line treatment of chronic hypertension in pregnancy.[22] Thiazide diuretics can be continued during pregnancy.[22] **Angiotensin-converting enzyme inhibitors and angiotensin receptor blockers are the only class of antihypertensive medications contraindicated in pregnancy.**[22]

CARDIAC ARRHYTHMIAS

Pregnancy can precipitate cardiac arrhythmias not previously present in seemingly well individuals. The risk of arrhythmias rises during labor and delivery. Factors that promote arrhythmias in pregnancy include the direct cardiac electrophysiologic effects of hormones, changes in hemodynamics or autonomic tone, hypokalemia, and underlying heart disease. Reduction of uterine blood flow during prolonged tachyarrhythmic episodes may adversely affect the fetus. The incidence of arrhythmias in pregnancy is rising due to increasing maternal age and pregnancies in women successfully treated for congenital heart disease.[26] **Just as in a nonpregnant patient, treat any hemodynamically unstable arrhythmia in pregnancy with direct-current cardioversion (50–200 J).**[27,28] Treat hemodynamically stable arrhythmias medically. The chronic use of β-blockers in pregnancy can influence fetal and newborn size, but only atenolol is singled out as being a Food and Drug Administration class D drug in this regard (some evidence for harm to the fetus). Other β-blockers are Food and Drug Administration class B (sotalol) or C. Digoxin, verapamil, diltiazem, and adenosine have their usual efficacy without adverse fetal affects.[26]

CARDIAC ARRHYTHMIA TREATMENT

Paroxysmal supraventricular tachycardia is the most common nonsinus tachycardia in women of childbearing age. The treatment of supraventricular tachycardia in pregnant women is the same as for nonpregnant women.[26] If vagal maneuvers are ineffective, give adenosine. Case reports show both efficacy and a lack of any direct adverse or teratogenic side effects to the fetus.[29] Additionally, acute treatment with β-blockers, verapamil, and diltiazem is safe in pregnancy when used in standard dosage.

The goal of management of **atrial fibrillation** in pregnancy is rate control or conversion to sinus rhythm. Use diltiazem, β-blockers, and/or digoxin, all of which are safe in pregnancy and with unchanged dosages.[29] Anticoagulation with unfractionated or low-molecular-weight heparin is safe in pregnancy and should be used if the patient meets criteria for anticoagulation described for nonpregnant patients.

Ventricular arrhythmias may occur during pregnancy, particularly in patients with congenital heart disease, cardiomyopathy, or valvular disease. **Amiodarone is categorized as class D** because its main metabolite (desethylamiodarone) and iodine cross the placenta. Chronic fetal exposure to amiodarone and its subsequent iodine overload are associated with neurotoxicity, fetal/neonatal hypothyroidism, and less frequently, goiter. Therefore, the use of amiodarone in pregnancy is limited to maternal/fetal tachyarrhythmias that are resistant to other drugs or are life threatening, because short-term use has not been linked to any harmful effects.[29]

The presence of an artificial pacemaker or implantable cardiac defibrillator does not affect the course of pregnancy.[30]

THROMBOEMBOLISM

A detailed discussion of clinical features, diagnosis, and treatment of thromboembolism in pregnancy is found in chapter 100.

The pregnancy-related changes that increase the risk of thromboembolism include physiologic alterations in coagulation and reduced venous return from the legs, with venous pooling and endothelial injury. The clinical assessment is difficult because many of the typical clinical signs and symptoms are seen in normal pregnancy, including leg edema, shortness of breath, and tachycardia. The Wells Score for deep venous thrombosis (see Table 56-4), the most validated clinical decision rule in the diagnosis of deep vein thrombosis, has not been validated in pregnant women.[31,32]

Obtain Doppler compression ultrasonography for diagnosis.[33] D-Dimer levels normally increase throughout pregnancy, and thromboembolism has been reported with normal D-dimer levels.[34,35] Imaging modalities for diagnosis are provided in Table 100-1.

Treatment is low-molecular-weight heparin (Table 100-2).[36] Do not use warfarin in pregnancy because it crosses the placenta and is

TABLE 99-2 Treatment of Hypertension in Pregnancy

Agent	For Existing Hypertension	Adjunct to Existing Treatment	Urgent Control of Acute Hypertension	Potential Adverse Effects (Maternal)
Hydralazine	N/A	50–300 milligrams daily in 2–4 divided doses; use with methyldopa or labetalol to prevent reflex tachycardia*	Loading dose of 5 milligrams IV or IM, maintenance dose thereafter of 5–10 milligrams every 20–40 min up to 300 milligrams; *or* constant infusion of 0.5–10 milligrams/h	Delayed hypotension
Hydrochlorothiazide	N/A	12.5–50 milligrams daily	N/A	Volume depletion and electrolyte disorders
Labetalol	200–2400 milligrams daily in 2–3 divided doses	N/A	Loading dose of 20 milligrams IV; maintenance dose of 20–80 milligrams up to 300 milligrams; *or* constant infusion of 1–2 milligrams/min	Headache
Nifedipine	30–120 milligrams daily as slow-release preparation	N/A	10–30 milligrams orally, repeated after 45 min if needed	Headache, interference with labor
Methyldopa	0.5–3.0 grams daily in 2–3 divided doses	N/A	N/A	Sedation, elevated liver function tests, depression

Abbreviation: N/A = not applicable.

*Risk of fetal bradycardia and neonatal thrombocytopenia.

associated with embryopathy in the first trimester; in the second and third trimesters, it may lead to CNS and ophthalmologic abnormalities. Protamine sulfate may be used safely in pregnancy for patients who require rapid reversal of heparin anticoagulation. Thrombolytics are not contraindicated and have been used successfully in multiple cases. Reported rates of maternal bleeding complications are between 1% and 6% with no maternal deaths, and rates of fetal loss are between 2% and 5%.[37-40]

ACUTE ASTHMA

Asthma is the most common medical disease in pregnancy and complicates between 3.7% and 8.4% of all pregnancies.[41] The clinical course may improve, remain unchanged, or worsen during pregnancy. Women with asthma have higher odds of pre-eclampsia, gestational diabetes, placental abruption, placenta previa, preterm delivery, low birth weight, maternal hemorrhage, pulmonary embolism, and intensive care unit admission.[42]

Symptoms of cough, wheezing, and dyspnea are the same as in nonpregnant patients. Initial assessment should include history of asthma exacerbations and intubation, peak expiratory flow rate measurements or forced expiratory volume in 1 second, physical examination, assessment of oxygen saturation, and a fetal assessment (if >20 weeks' gestation). Peak expiratory flow rate is not altered in pregnancy, with normal rates ranging between 380 and 550 L/min. Use peak expiratory flow rate as a guide to therapy. If the pregnancy has reached viability, apply continuous electronic fetal monitoring.

Treat rapidly and aggressively to reduce re-admission rates and improve fetal outcomes.[43] The principles of management are the same as in nonpregnant patients. Maintain oxygen saturation >95%, administer repetitive or continuous inhaled β_2-agonist (albuterol/salbutamol); give inhaled ipratropium and systemic corticosteroids; monitor maternal response to therapy; and monitor the fetus for signs of distress.[44] Terbutaline sulfate, 0.25 milligrams every 20 minutes, administered SC, may be used if needed. Avoid epinephrine because concerns exist about epinephrine vasoconstriction of the uteroplacental circulation.

Admission and discharge criteria are the same as in the nonasthmatic patient. For discharged women, prescribe oral prednisone, 40 to 60 milligrams per day (or equivalent), for 5 to 10 days, and a short-acting rescue β-agonist. Inhaled corticosteroids reduce recurrence during pregnancy and decrease re-admission rates following a hospitalization for asthma.[45] Anticipate maternal hyperglycemia when systemic corticosteroids are given.

CHRONIC RENAL DISEASE

Maternal risks associated with renal disease are linked to the patient's degree of renal compromise. Patients with mild renal insufficiency and no hypertension tend to have good outcomes and preserved renal function. Patients with moderate or severe renal insufficiency are more prone to further decline in renal function and pre-eclampsia and preterm delivery. Patients with lupus nephropathy are at greatly increased risk for disease exacerbation and superimposed pre-eclampsia.

Angiotensin-converting enzyme inhibitors and angiotensin II receptor blockers, which are frequently used in patients with chronic renal failure, are teratogenic and should be stopped at the first indication of pregnancy.

ASYMPTOMATIC BACTERIURIA, CYSTITIS, AND PYELONEPHRITIS

Hormonal and mechanical changes of pregnancy increase the risk of urinary stasis and subsequent urinary tract infection. After mid-pregnancy, mild right-sided hydronephrosis is found in 75% of women, and mild left-sided hydronephrosis is found in 33%.

Asymptomatic bacteriuria is diagnosed by urine culture, demonstrating the presence of bacteria in the urine in the absence of maternal symptoms of urinary tract infection. Reagent strips have limited sensitivity, and use in screening depends on resources available, but in general, a positive leukocyte esterase or urinary nitrite should be treated and a negative specimen should be cultured.[46,47] Treatment reduces the incidence of pyelonephritis and low birth weight.[48]

Causative organisms of symptomatic cystitis and pyelonephritis are similar to those in the general population and include *Escherichia coli* (75%), *Klebsiella pneumoniae*, *Proteus*, and gram-positive organisms such as group B *Streptococcus*. Obtain a urinalysis and culture with drug sensitivities in pregnant women with urinary tract symptoms and also in those with hyperemesis. Urinary tract infections need prompt treatment because acute pyelonephritis can precipitate preterm labor, bacteremia, or septic shock.

Recurrent infections can occur as a result of bacteriuria, glycosuria, and mechanical compression of the ureter in the third trimester. Reflux nephropathy increases the risk of sudden escalating hypertension and worsening renal function.[49] Urolithiasis is associated with recurrent urinary tract infections.

Treat asymptomatic bacteriuria and simple cystitis with oral nitrofurantoin, 100 milligrams PO two times per day, or an oral cephalosporin. Recommendations on the length of treatment vary from 3 to 10 days. Trimethoprim-sulfamethoxazole is not a good choice in pregnancy.

Trimethoprim, a folate antagonist, can be used **after the first trimester**; sulfonamides can be taken during the first and second trimesters **but not during the third trimester** because sulfonamides can cause kernicterus in the infant. Do not use fluoroquinolones and tetracyclines during pregnancy because of possible toxic effects on the fetus.

Pregnant women with pyelonephritis are generally hospitalized, aggressively hydrated, and treated with parenteral antibiotics. The antibiotic of choice is a second- or third-generation cephalosporin. Continue IV antibiotics until the patient is afebrile for at least 48 hours and costovertebral angle tenderness has resolved. The most common reason for treatment failure is antibiotic resistance. Patients discharged after hospitalization need to complete a 10-day course of therapy. Many providers choose to continue women with an episode of pyelonephritis on antibiotic suppression for the remainder of pregnancy. Nitrofurantoin, 50 to 100 milligrams PO once per day, is a common treatment.

SICKLE CELL DISEASE

Women with sickle cell disease, including sickle cell trait, are at increased risk for miscarriage, preterm labor, and other complications due to impaired oxygen supply and sickling infarcts in the placental circulation. Maternal complications are more common in the third trimester and postpartum period and include cerebral vein thrombosis, pneumonia, sepsis, and pyelonephritis.

Presentation and treatment of painful crises in pregnancy are similar in pregnant women and nonpregnant patients (see chapter 237, "Acquired Hemolytic Anemia"). Cornerstones of management are oxygen, aggressive hydration, PO or IV narcotics, and evaluation and treatment of the precipitating cause. Place the woman in the left lateral decubitus position, if in the third trimester. Avoid nonsteroidal anti-inflammatory drugs, particularly after 32 weeks of gestation, because these drugs cross the placenta. In early pregnancy, nonsteroidal anti-inflammatory drugs are associated with miscarriage and neonatal defects. In later pregnancy, nonsteroidal anti-inflammatory drugs are associated with risk of oligohydramnios and premature closure of the fetal ductus arteriosus. Blood transfusions are reserved for sickle cell crises when conservative measures have not improved maternal or fetal status.[50] Indications for transfusion include severe anemia with a hemoglobin level <5 milligrams/dL, pre-eclampsia, hypoxemia, acute chest syndrome, new-onset neurologic event, or anticipation of surgical intervention or angiographic dye load.[51]

Institute fetal monitoring and consult with an obstetrician if the fetus is potentially viable. Fetal heart rate patterns should normalize as the crisis resolves. Consult with an obstetrician for emergency delivery in the face of ongoing fetal distress.

HEADACHE AND STROKE SYNDROMES IN PREGNANCY

In pregnant women, headaches can be a symptom of a variety of neurologic or systemic disorders. **Table 99-3** lists the differential diagnosis of headaches in pregnancy (see chapter 165, "Headache").

TABLE 99-3 Causes of Headaches in Pregnancy
Life threatening
Subarachnoid hemorrhage
Intraparenchymal hemorrhage
Central venous thrombosis
Ischemic stroke
CNS tumor or infection
Pre-eclampsia/eclampsia
Non–life threatening
Tension headache
Migraine
Sinus headache
Benign intracranial hypertension (pseudotumor cerebri)

TABLE 99-4 Warning Symptoms and Signs of Headaches
New-onset headaches in pregnancy
Postpartum headaches
Need to exclude cerebral vein thrombosis
Headaches with different characteristics from previous headaches
Worst headache of life
Focal neurologic deficit
Meningismus
Fever
Altered consciousness
Papilledema or other signs of increased intracranial pressure
Retinal hemorrhages
Increased blood pressure (may herald pre-eclampsia or eclampsia)

Warning symptoms and signs of a potentially life-threatening disease are important to elicit during the initial evaluation and are listed in **Table 99-4**.

Obtain imaging studies if concerning signs or symptoms are encountered. CT scan of the brain can be safely performed with appropriate shielding of the fetus. CT scan is best to evaluate acute intracranial or subarachnoid hemorrhage, whereas MRI is superior for evaluation of cerebral infarct, tumor, infection, or cerebral vein thrombosis.

INTRACEREBRAL HEMORRHAGE

In pregnancy, the incidence of intracerebral hemorrhage ranges from 0.01% to 0.05 % but is the cause for 5% to 12% of all maternal deaths.[52] The risk of cerebral hemorrhage extends from pregnancy through the **6-week postpartum period**.[52] Risk factors include older maternal age, African American race, and alcohol or cocaine use. The most common cause for spontaneous intracerebral hemorrhage is **hypertension**. If there is no history of hypertension, then consider other causes such as neoplasm, hemorrhagic disorder, and vascular malformation.

Presenting symptoms vary with the location and extent of hemorrhage, so consider cerebral hemorrhage in a woman with an abrupt neurologic change. For diagnosis, obtain CT/MRI and consult the neurosurgeon. Treatment is blood pressure control and correction of coagulopathy.

SUBARACHNOID HEMORRHAGE

Subarachnoid hemorrhage during pregnancy is the third most common cause of nonobstetric maternal death, and more than half of cases occur **postpartum.**[52] Causes include hypertension,[53] aneurysm, vascular malformation, tumors, and venous thrombosis.

Independent risk factors for subarachnoid hemorrhage from all etiologies include advancing age; African American race; Hispanic ethnicity; hypertensive disorders; coagulopathy; tobacco, drug, or alcohol abuse; intracranial venous thrombosis; sickle cell disease; and hypercoagulability.

Suspect subarachnoid hemorrhage in a woman with severe headache, nausea, vomiting, decreased level of consciousness, or seizure. Diagnosis is by CT/MRI and/or lumbar puncture. In general, pregnant women should be treated the same as nonpregnant patients with bed rest, analgesia, sedation, neurologic monitoring, and control of blood pressure.[52]

STROKE

Pregnancy is associated with an increased risk of ischemic and hemorrhagic stroke, and stroke contributes to more than 12% of all maternal deaths, with the majority occurring in the **third trimester or puerperium.**[54] Arterial occlusion is the most common cause of pregnancy-related stroke.[54] Risk factors include hypertension, heart disease, smoking, diabetes, lupus, sickle cell disease, African American heritage, substance abuse, and cesarean delivery. Consider stroke in women with neurologic deterioration or new focal neurologic deficits.

Once hemorrhage and eclampsia are excluded, consider thrombolytic therapy after consultation with neurology and obstetrics. To date, there are no randomized controlled trials of thrombolytics for stroke in pregnancy; however, recombinant tissue plasminogen activator (risk category C) does not cross the placenta, and there is no evidence of teratogenicity in animal studies.[55] There are more than 200 reports in the literature of pregnant women who have received thrombolytic therapy for various indications including myocardial infarction, pulmonary embolism, superior vena cava syndrome, and ischemic stroke.[54] Use of thrombolytics in pregnancy is not without its risks, although the overall maternal mortality and fetal loss is relatively low at 1% and 6%, respectively.[54]

CENTRAL VENOUS THROMBOSIS

Central venous thrombosis usually presents in the second and third trimesters and may occur up to 4 weeks postpartum. Symptoms include severe headache, focal neurologic deficit, vomiting, or seizure, depending on which veins are occluded. Venous thrombosis increases venous pressure and cerebral blood volume, elevating dural sinus pressure and leading to rupture of small cortical veins.[56] Treatment is low-molecular-weight heparin, unless there is associated intracranial hemorrhage. Once the patient has been stabilized and hemorrhage from an aneurysm is excluded, the mainstay of treatment for the underlying thrombosis is still anticoagulation for the duration of the pregnancy.[56]

MIGRAINE HEADACHE

Although the ergot alkaloids are contraindicated in pregnancy, acute migraine headaches can be successfully treated in pregnancy with the same first-line antiemetics that are used in nonpregnant patients. Metoclopramide (Reglan) is class B, and prochlorperazine (Compazine), promethazine (Phenergan), and droperidol (Inapsine) are all class C. Avoid nonsteroidal anti-inflammatory drugs. Sumatriptans (class C) do not appear to increase fetal malformations, and if already prescribed by the obstetrician or primary physician during pregnancy, sumatriptans can be continued as an outpatient.[57]

GI DISORDERS IN PREGNANCY

GASTROESOPHAGEAL REFLUX DISEASE

Gastroesophageal reflux disease (GERD) is extremely common in pregnancy and is characterized by epigastric pain or burning radiating into the chest and neck, pain with recumbency, and pain exacerbated by acidic foods. Symptoms increase in the second trimester and peak in the third trimester due to loosening of the lower esophageal sphincter and delayed gastric emptying from pregnancy-related hormones. Treat mild symptoms with H_2 antagonists such as cimetidine or ranitidine. Moderate to severe symptoms can be treated with sucralfate and proton pump inhibitors. Both H_2 antagonists and proton pump inhibitors have been extensively studied for teratogenic effects, and no significant abnormal findings have been associated with their use in pregnancy.[58,59]

HEMORRHOIDS

Hemorrhoids are common during pregnancy and are caused by a combination of constipation due to slowed bowel transit from progesterone effects in the last trimester and elevated pressure in the veins below the level of the enlarged uterus. Most symptoms are mild and can be treated with prevention of constipation with increased fluids and high-fiber intake and topical medications including witch hazel compresses, suppositories, corticosteroids, or topically applied anesthetics.[60] Do not use agents containing epinephrine or phenylephrine. Proctofoam has specifically been studied and is safe.[61] Consider surgical or obstetric referral for prolapsed, bleeding, or incarcerated hemorrhoids or when conservative measures fail. There are no studies of the risks/benefits of ED excision of a thrombosed clot in pregnancy. Risks include hemorrhage and recurrence.

CHOLECYSTITIS

During pregnancy, approximately 1 in 1000 women will develop cholecystitis. Pregnancy-related hormones affect gallbladder contractility and increase residual gallbladder volume and sludge, which in turn can lead to gallstone formation. Many women ultimately require cholecystectomy during pregnancy for persistent symptoms. It is preferable to wait until the second trimester if the patient's condition allows, as surgery during the first trimester carries a risk of spontaneous miscarriage, and cholecystectomy in the third trimester is technically difficult and can result in preterm labor.[62]

APPENDICITIS

Appendicitis occurs about once in every 500 to 2000 pregnancies and is the most common extrauterine condition requiring abdominal operation in pregnancy. The diagnosis is often missed or delayed because mild abdominal discomfort, nausea, and vomiting occur frequently in normal pregnancies. Additionally, the appendix shifts in location from the right lower quadrant to the right upper quadrant during the second and third trimesters. The diagnosis is best made with US, which is 80% accurate with experienced technicians. However, if perforation has occurred, US accuracy decreases to 30%.[63,64] Adequate visualization of the appendix is more difficult later in pregnancy. If US is not available or is inadequate, obtain an MRI.[65] If CT is used to make the diagnosis, focal appendiceal CT provides less radiation to the fetus than full abdominopelvic CT. However, focal abdominal imaging may limit discovery of an alternate diagnosis. An abdomen/pelvis CT confers about 30 mGy of radiation, and 50 mGy of radiation is generally accepted to be safe in pregnancy.[66]

OVARIAN TORSION

Torsion of the ovary is a true gynecologic emergency, and up to one fifth of ovarian torsion occurs during pregnancy. Torsion can occur in any trimester, although it is most common in the first trimester.[67] Infertility treatment is a risk factor. Ovarian torsion can recur in the same pregnancy, in particular in enlarged multicystic ovaries.[68] The corpus luteal cyst and enlarged ovaries stemming from the pregnancy hormones are thought to increase the risk. Tissue necrosis can occur rapidly, so timely diagnosis is essential to preserve ovarian function and the pregnancy. The diagnosis is often missed due to the vague clinical presentation of moderate unilateral lower abdominal pain, which may also be intermittent or constant. US may show an enlarged or edematous ovary with absent or decreased blood flow. **However, the presence of ovarian blood flow does not exclude the diagnosis of torsion if symptoms are suggestive.**[69] Therefore, consult an obstetrician/gynecologist as soon as the diagnosis is clinically suspected.

SEIZURE DISORDERS

Seizure frequency can increase in pregnancy because of the increased volume of distribution and plasma clearance of antiepileptic drugs in pregnancy or because of poor medication compliance.

Most of the antiepileptic drugs can cause a range of birth defects.[70] **Valproic acid, carbamazepine, and phenytoin are all class D and are teratogenic.** Yet, discontinuing these drugs can increase morbidity and mortality for both the mother and fetus.[71] Therefore, the risks and benefits of chronic treatment should be discussed and managed by the primary physician. Medication doses may need to be increased in pregnancy. Therapeutic serum target levels remain unchanged. **Monotherapy with levetiracetam or lamotrigine (both class C) should be used whenever possible.**[72]

Acute treatment of seizures in the pregnant woman is similar to that in the nonpregnant patient (see chapter 171, "Seizures"). Even though lorazepam and diazepam are class D medications, they are so categorized based on long-term use. **Use of benzodiazepines for an acute seizure outweighs any potential risk to the fetus.**[73]

If the seizure if self-limited, administer oxygen and position the patient in the left lateral decubitus position and provide supportive care. Fetal bradycardia lasting for up to 20 minutes may follow a single brief maternal seizure. **Status epilepticus** poses a real threat to both mother and the fetus, with a significant maternal and fetal mortality. Provide aggressive management, including intubation and ventilation, early in the management of pregnant women with status epilepticus (see chapter 171).

HUMAN IMMUNODEFICIENCY VIRUS INFECTION

Pregnancy does not appear to alter the natural course of human immunodeficiency virus (HIV) disease, nor do uninfected babies born to HIV-positive women appear to be at increased risk for neonatal complications when compared with appropriate control patients.

Some women may choose to delay initiation of antiretroviral therapy until after the first trimester, when the fetus is less susceptible to the potential teratogenic effects of medications. However, all pregnant HIV-infected patients beyond 12 weeks' gestation should be on a highly active antiretroviral therapy three-drug regimen that includes zidovudine. Use of zidovudine has reduced the vertical transmission rate of HIV to <2% in the United States.[74] There are many combinations of three-drug regimens that can be used in pregnancy. However, several of the medications used in the highly active antiretroviral therapy regimen are potentially harmful when used during pregnancy. For example, the combination of didanosine and stavudine can cause a potentially fatal lactic acidosis in pregnant women. Nevirapine can cause severe hepatotoxicity.[75]

Recommended regimens as of this writing are as follows: **for a treatment-naïve HIV-infected pregnant female,** zidovudine *plus* lamivudine *plus* lopinavir/ritonavir *or* atazanavir/ritonavir; **for a treatment-naïve HIV-infected pregnant female with hepatitis B coinfection:** tenofovir *plus* lamivudine *or* emtricitabine *plus* lopinavir/ritonavir *or* atazanavir/ritonavir.[76]

Prophylaxis for opportunistic infections is similar to that for nonpregnant patients. Patients with CD4+ T-cell counts of <200/μL should be maintained on prophylaxis for *Pneumocystis jiroveci* pneumonia using trimethoprim-sulfamethoxazole. Weigh the risks and benefits of trimethoprim-sulfamethoxazole therapy during the first trimester. Folate supplementation may be added, but it is unclear whether folate supplementation lowers risk. Alternatively, aerosolized pentamidine may be used in the first trimester, as it is minimally systemically absorbed.[77]

Treatment of overt opportunistic infections in HIV-infected pregnant women is addressed in the same way as in nonpregnant women. Early intubation to reverse hypoxemia may be necessary to improve maternal-fetal outcome in women with respiratory infections.

SUBSTANCE ABUSE DURING PREGNANCY

Substance abuse in pregnancy results in approximately 225,000 infants yearly with prenatal exposure.[78] Refer pregnant women identified in the ED as substance abusers to a high-risk obstetrics clinic and offer them substance abuse counseling.

COCAINE

Cocaine use is associated with placental abruption, fetal death in utero, intrauterine growth restriction, preterm labor, premature rupture of membranes, spontaneous abortion, and cerebral infarcts in the fetus. Maternal complications of cocaine use include myocardial infarction, hypertension (which can result in aortic dissection), pulmonary edema, and cardiac dysrhythmias. Subarachnoid hemorrhage, ruptured aneurysms, and strokes are reported in cocaine users and are most likely related to transient hypertension. Treatment of the pregnant woman with acute cocaine intoxication is handled in the same manner as in the nonpregnant patient (see chapter 187, "Cocaine and Amphetamines").

OPIOIDS

Although acute opioid withdrawal poses minimal maternal risk, there is significant risk to the fetus, including meconium, hypoxia, preterm labor, and fetal demise.[79] Illicit opioid use can cause intermittent fetal withdrawal when there is maternal lack of access to the drug.

Therefore, it is standard to refer opioid-addicted pregnant patients for supervised methadone or buprenorphine therapy for the duration of the pregnancy. Even though methadone/buprenorphine will cause neonatal abstinence syndrome (opioid withdrawal) after birth, this is a treatable condition and carries less harm to the infant than acute opioid withdrawal in utero. Maternal detoxification from opioids should be done in a supervised inpatient setting, and only for select patients, as the relapse rate is very high.[79]

Maternal mild opioid withdrawal can be treated with clonidine 0.1 to 0.2 milligrams every hour until the signs of withdrawal resolve. Severe maternal opioid withdrawal may require administration of an opioid agonist and admission for fetal monitoring and induction of methadone therapy.[79,80]

ALCOHOL

Alcohol consumption during pregnancy is a risk factor for fetal alcohol syndrome, birth defects, and low birth weight. Binge drinking is particularly harmful to fetal neurodevelopment.

In the United States, the prevalence of fetal alcohol syndrome is estimated at 0.5 to 2.0 cases per 1000 births, but other fetal alcohol spectrum disorders are believed to occur approximately three times as often as fetal alcohol syndrome.[81]

Pregnant women who present in coma due to acute alcohol intoxication or in alcohol withdrawal are managed in the same way as nonpregnant patients. **Disulfiram (Antabuse) is a potential teratogen. Do not prescribe in pregnancy.**

INTIMATE PARTNER VIOLENCE

Between 4% and 20% of pregnant women are victims of intimate partner violence.[82] Factors associated with intimate partner violence during pregnancy are late entry into prenatal care, unintended pregnancy, drug and alcohol use, depression, and housing problems. Violence increases the risk for preterm labor, placental abruption, fetal fractures, uterine rupture, chorioamnionitis, delivering a low-birth-weight infant, and homicide. The American College of Obstetricians and Gynecologists recommends routine screening for intimate partner violence during pregnancy.[83]

Pregnant women with injuries should be treated according to usual trauma protocols. Institute fetal monitoring for direct or indirect blunt abdominal trauma and major multiple trauma. Administer Rh immunoglobulin to Rh-negative women with blunt abdominal trauma (see chapter 25, "Resuscitation in Pregnancy").

MEDICATIONS IN PREGNANCY AND LACTATION

The classic teratogenic period is 2 to 15 weeks of gestation. During this critical time, organs are forming, and teratogens may cause malformation. Administration of drugs early in the period of organogenesis affects the organs developing at that specific time, such as the heart or neural tube. Teratogens given closer to the end of the classic teratogenic period will affect the ear and palate. Before week 2, exposure to a teratogen produces an all-or-none effect (i.e., the conceptus either does not survive or survives without anomalies). If the organism remains viable after exposure before week 2, organ-specific anomalies do not develop because repair or replacement permits normal development. A similar insult at a later stage of development may produce organ-specific defects.

The U.S. Food and Drug Administration lists five categories of labeling for drug use in pregnancy (**Table 99-5**).

Some therapeutic agents that should not be used during pregnancy are listed in **Table 99-6**. The National Library of Medicine provides a detailed reference list in the Developmental and Reproductive Toxicology Database (see Useful Web Resources below).

Table 99-7 lists some general cautions for using drugs during lactation. When prescribing, check each drug individually. Because information can change, we recommend referring to the following sources for information about drug safety in lactation:

- Drugs and Lactation Database (LactMed), U.S. National Library of Medicine—http://toxnet.nlm.nih.gov/cgi-bin/sis/htmlgen?LACT (accessed December 31, 2013)
- World Health Organization, Breastfeeding and Maternal Medication (last updated 2003)—http://whqlibdoc.who.int/hq/2002/55732.pdf (accessed December 31, 2013)
- Hale Thomas, Medications and Mothers' Milk, ISBN-13 (978-0984774630), Hale Publishing, May, 2012, 15th ed.

TABLE 99-5 U.S. Food and Drug Administration Categorization of Drug Risk in Pregnancy

Drug Category	Risk during Pregnancy
A	Controlled studies show no fetal risk in any trimester, and so the possibility of fetal harm is remote.
B	Animal studies show no fetal risk, but there are no controlled human studies. Or Animal studies have shown an adverse effect that was not confirmed in controlled human studies in women in the first trimester (and there is no evidence of risk in later trimesters).
C	Animal studies have shown adverse fetal effects (teratogenic or embryocidal), and there are no controlled studies in humans. Or No human or animal studies are available. Drugs should only be used if the potential benefit justifies the potential fetal risk.
D	Evidence of human fetal risk exists, but the benefits of use in pregnant women may be acceptable despite the risk.
X	Studies in animals or humans have shown fetal risk, or there is evidence of fetal risk based on human experience. The risk of use in pregnancy clearly outweighs any possible benefit. Drugs are contraindicated for use in women who are or may become pregnant.

FETAL RADIATION EFFECTS

For radiation imaging during pregnancy, weigh the risks of exposure and subsequent fetal adverse effects against the risk of incorrect maternal diagnosis. The major factor determining the degree of risk to the fetus is the quantity of ionizing radiation exposure during imaging. **Fetal exposure to low-dose radiation, defined as <5 rads (<50 mGy), does not increase the risk of fetal or infant death, mental defects, or growth retardation.** More than 5 rads (>50 mGy) is considered the threshold for human teratogenesis.[66] The fetus is most vulnerable to teratogenicity between 3 and 15 weeks of gestation at doses >10 rads (>100 mGy) (**Table 99-8**). The risk and incidence of carcinogenesis are not known.[66]

The estimated radiation doses involved in procedures commonly used for ED diagnosis are listed in **Table 99-9**.[66,84-86]

TABLE 99-6 Drugs Used in Emergency Settings with Known Adverse Effects in Human Pregnancy

Drug	Effect
Angiotensin-converting enzyme inhibitors and angiotensin receptor blockers	Renal failure, oligohydramnios
Aminoglycosides	Ototoxicity (gentamicin class D, Black Box Warning)
Androgenic steroids	Masculinize female fetus
Anticonvulsants (carbamazepine, hydantoins, valproate)	Dysmorphic syndrome, anomalies, neural tube defects
Antithyroid agents	Fetal goiter
Aspirin (high doses)	Bleeding, antepartum and postpartum
Cytotoxic agents (e.g., methotrexate)	Multiple anomalies
Erythromycin estolate	Maternal hepatotoxicity
Fluoroquinolones	Fetal cartilage abnormality
Isotretinoin	Hydrocephalus, deafness, anomalies
Lithium	Congenital heart disease (Ebstein's anomaly)
Nonsteroidal anti-inflammatory drugs (prolonged use after 32 wk)	Oligohydramnios, constriction of fetal ductus arteriosus
Streptomycin	Fetal cranial nerve VIII damage
Sulfonamides	Fetal hemolysis, neonatal kernicterus (near term)
Tetracyclines	Fetal teeth and bone abnormalities
Trimethoprim, methotrexate	Folate antagonist (first trimester)
Thalidomide	Phocomelia
Warfarin	Embryopathy—nasal hypoplasia, optic atrophy

TABLE 99-7 World Health Organization General Cautions for Drugs and Breastfeeding

Guideline	Drugs
Breastfeeding contraindicated	Anticancer drugs, radioactive substances, nitrofurantoin (for <1 mo old, and for those with glucose-6-phosphate dehydrogenase deficiency)
Avoid unless absolutely necessary	Chloramphenicol, tetracyclines, metronidazole, fluoroquinolones
Monitor infant for drowsiness	Selected psychiatric and anticonvulsant agents
Monitor infant for jaundice	Sulfonamides, dapsone, sulfadoxine/pyrimethamine (Fansidar), mefloquine
May inhibit lactation; use alternative drug	Estrogens, thiazides

TABLE 99-8 Teratogenic Radiation Effects

Gestational Age	Effect of 5–10 rads (50–100 mGy)	Effect of >10 rads (>100 mGy)
0–2 wk	Probably none	Possible spontaneous abortion
3–8 wk	Unknown; probably none detectable	Possible malformations with increasing dose
9–15 wk	Unknown; probably none detectable	Possible mental development defects with increasing dose
≥16 wk	None	None detectable or none

TABLE 99-9 Radiation Exposure to the Uterus/Fetus

Procedure	Dosage in mGy
Threshold for human teratogenesis	100
Accepted as safe in pregnancy	**50**
Abdominal/pelvis CT	25–35
CT, kidney-ureter-bladder protocol (reduced radiation dose)	10
Lumbosacral spine series (three view)	1.6–3.5
Ventilation–perfusion scan (total)	2.1
Abdominal series (two view)	2
Lung **perfusion** scan with technetium	1.7
Normal background radiation over 9 months	**1**
Head CT	<0.5
Lung **ventilation** scan with xenon	0.4
Anteroposterior pelvis x-ray	0.4
Chest CT (10-mm slices, 10 slices), for standard or pulmonary embolism protocol	0.2
Cerebral angiography	0.1
Mammography—diagnostic for suspected breast cancers	0.07–0.2
Chest radiography (two view) with shielding of the maternal abdomen	<0.001
Cervical spine (two view)	<0.001

Note: 1 rad = 10 mGy = 10 mSv.

REFERENCES

The complete reference list is available online at www.TintinalliEM.com.

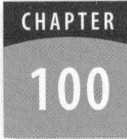

Maternal Emergencies After 20 Weeks of Pregnancy and in the Postpartum Period

Janet Simmons Young

INTRODUCTION

This chapter examines the diagnosis and treatment of the most important maternal emergencies occurring after 20 weeks of pregnancy and during the postpartum period. The second half of pregnancy is often characterized as ≥20 weeks of gestation for simplicity, but until 24 weeks, the chances of fetal survival are less than 50%. The postpartum period is generally accepted as the 6 weeks after delivery. Vast physiologic shifts in maternal cardiovascular tone occur as pregnancy progresses, highlighting the need for maternal blood pressure recordings and fetal heart tones during any ED visit. Conditions discussed are thromboembolic disease; chest pain; disorders associated with elevated blood pressure (hypertension, preeclampsia and HELLP syndrome [hemolysis, elevated liver enzymes, and low platelet count], and eclampsia); vaginal bleeding in the second half of pregnancy; premature rupture of membranes; postpartum hemorrhage; amniotic fluid embolus; peripartum cardiomyopathy; and endometritis.

THROMBOEMBOLIC DISEASE OF PREGNANCY

Venous thromboembolism includes deep venous thrombosis (DVT) and pulmonary embolism (PE) and is the leading cause of maternal morbidity and mortality in industrialized nations. Compared with nonpregnant women, the risk of venous thromboembolism increases fivefold during pregnancy and is increased by 60-fold in the first 3 months after delivery.[1,2]

PATHOPHYSIOLOGY

Pregnancy-related hypercoagulability is due to increased levels of clotting factors, increased platelet and fibrin activation, and decreased fibrinolytic activity, all of which are adaptations to prevent maternal hemorrhage. Physiologic changes include venous stasis, decreased venous outflow, and uterine compression of the inferior vena cava and iliac veins (particularly the left common iliac and left leg veins). Clots tend to develop in the deep venous system of the legs and pelvis, which includes the internal iliac, femoral, greater saphenous, and popliteal veins. Up to 24% of DVTs are complicated by PE, so early DVT diagnosis is important.[1-6]

RISK FACTORS AND CLINICAL FEATURES

Physiologic signs and symptoms of thromboembolic disease, such as tachycardia, tachypnea, lower extremity edema, and dyspnea are nonspecific and also occur during normal pregnancy. Predictive scoring criteria, such as Wells criteria, have not been validated in pregnant women, but left leg symptoms, calf circumference difference ≥2 cm, and leg symptoms in the first trimester are associated with DVT. Iliac vein thrombosis often presents with unilateral swelling of the entire leg and groin or back pain.

A personal or family history of thrombosis is an important risk factor. Other major risk factors include thrombophilias (not identifiable at the first presentation), obesity, maternal age >35, smoking, sickle cell disease, diabetes, hypertension, immobility, in vitro fertilization (greater risk for twins than for singleton), and preeclampsia. Cesarean delivery and postpartum complications further increase the risk.[1,4,5]

DIAGNOSIS OF DEEP VENOUS THROMBOSIS

Compression or duplex US is the test of choice, with a reported sensitivity and specificity for detecting proximal DVT in nonpregnant patients of 89% to 96% and 94% to 99%, respectively.[7] Compression US is less accurate for isolated calf and iliac vein thrombosis. MRI, either with or without contrast venography, is highly sensitive and specific for the diagnosis of pelvic and iliac vein thrombosis. MRI without contrast is preferred with the addition of contrast only if absolutely needed.[8,9] Impedance plethysmography and CT scan of the pelvis are alternatives to diagnose iliac vein thrombosis if MRI is not available. Impedance plethysmography is not widely available and requires operator expertise. CT exposes the fetus to radiation, and iodinated contrast media may affect fetal thyroid tissue.[1] If imaging resources are limited, venography with pelvic shielding is another option.[10]

D-dimers are not useful to include or exclude DVT or PE because levels progressively increase throughout pregnancy, and venous thromboembolism has been reported with negative D-dimers.[11] See chapter 56, Venous Thromboembolism, for a detailed discussion of D-dimers.

DIAGNOSIS OF PULMONARY EMBOLISM

Pregnant women with symptoms suggestive of PE and compression US results positive for DVT should receive anticoagulation without waiting for further confirmatory diagnostic studies.

Women with normal findings on US with suspicion of PE require further diagnostic imaging. The major options for definitive imaging are chest CT–pulmonary angiography and pulmonary perfusion scanning. **As of this writing, the fetal and maternal radiation dose with either modality is felt to be within acceptable limits.[1,12]** Typically, in most institutions, a consensus is obtained between emergency physicians, obstetricians, and radiologists in deciding the imaging steps. **Table 100-1** lists advantages and disadvantages of different imaging modalities.

TABLE 100-1 Imaging Modalities for Diagnosis of Pulmonary Embolism in Pregnancy

	Radiation	Limitations	Disadvantages	Advantages	Lactation
Chest Radiograph	Minimal	Nonspecific and nonsensitive	Results determine next imaging study, requiring more time to diagnosis	May identify another cause of pulmonary symptoms	No change
CT-PA	High maternal breast radiation; lower fetal radiation than V/Q scan	Contrast allergy and renal insufficiency	Hyperdynamic state in pregnancy can affect interpretation	High sensitivity and specificity; needed if abnormal chest radiograph	No need to discard breast milk
V/Q scan	Low breast radiation but higher fetal radiation than CT-PA	Not useful if abnormal chest radiograph, asthma, COPD, underlying pulmonary disease	If negative or inconclusive and suspicion for PE remains, will need a CT-PA; limited availability and time for isotope preparation, which delays diagnosis	Negative perfusion study effectively rules out PE	Discard breast milk for 12 h
MRI/MRV	No radiation	Gadolinium safety for fetus is unknown; do not use in maternal renal insufficiency	Limited availability	Can detect pelvic and iliac thrombosis	No need to discard breast milk

Abbreviations: COPD = chronic obstructive pulmonary disease; CT-PA = chest CT–pulmonary angiography; V/Q scan = ventilation-perfusion scan; MRV = magnetic resonance venography.

Consensus documents based on expert opinions of pulmonologists and radiologists recommend a plain chest radiograph first.[13] If the chest radiograph is abnormal, or the patient has chronic pulmonary disease, asthma, or chronic obstructive pulmonary disease, chest CT–pulmonary angiography is preferred.[13] If the chest radiograph is normal, a negative perfusion scan can be relied upon to exclude the diagnosis of PE, but an inconclusive perfusion scan will then require a chest CT.[1,12-14]

Magnetic resonance angiography (MRA) can detect PE, but its use in pregnancy has not been well studied. Institutions in which MRA of the pulmonary vasculature is performed routinely have demonstrated a sensitivity of 78% and specificity of 99% when the study is qualified as technically adequate.[15]

TREATMENT OF DEEP VENOUS THROMBOSIS AND PULMONARY EMBOLISM

Venous thromboembolism during pregnancy is treated with either unfractionated heparin (UFH) or low-molecular-weight heparin (LMWH) (**Table 100-2**).[1,16,17] UFH and LMWH do not cross the placental barrier. UFH is preferred over LMWH in patients in a hemodynamically unstable condition with PE, patients who are likely to bleed, patients with renal insufficiency, patients in labor, those receiving regional anesthesia, and patients undergoing cesarean delivery. Monitor activated partial thromboplastin times when using UFH.[11] Dosing requirements of UFH and LMWH increase due to the physiologic changes of pregnancy. Adverse effects of UFH include uteroplacental hemorrhage, heparin-induced thrombocytopenia, and heparin-induced osteopenia. LMWH has fewer adverse effects and fewer bleeding episodes than UFH, and monitoring with anti–factor Xa levels is needed only in special circumstances. See chapter 239, Thrombotics and Antithrombotics, for further discussion of heparins.

Fondaparinux is used in the United States for the prevention and treatment of venous thromboembolism in heparin-allergic or heparin-intolerant pregnant patients.[1] However, fondaparinux is transported across the placenta in low concentrations, and minimal data exist on maternal-fetal safety.[1,17]

Do not prescribe warfarin (Coumadin®) in pregnancy because it crosses the placental barrier, causes CNS abnormalities, and causes warfarin embryopathy (bone and cartilage abnormalities and nasal and limb hypoplasia). Warfarin increases the risk of maternal and fetal hemorrhage, especially during delivery. Warfarin is only considered for women with mechanical heart valves who demonstrate a continued risk of venous thromboembolism despite treatment with UFH or LMWH.[1]

An inferior vena cava filter is indicated when anticoagulation is contraindicated, when an acute embolic event occurs despite anticoagulation, or when acute venous thromboembolism occurs with impending delivery of the fetus.[18]

Treatment of Life-Threatening Pulmonary Embolism Treatment options include systemic thrombolysis, catheter-guided thrombolysis, and surgical or catheter-guided embolectomy.[19-22] Data regarding maternal-fetal outcomes in conditions of maternal extremis are limited to case reports, and catheter-guided thrombolysis and embolectomy require precious time for preparation. **Recombinant tissue plasminogen activator** (10-milligram bolus, 90-milligram infusion over 2 hours) does not cross the placenta and has a lower rate of hemorrhagic complications and lower mortality rate than do streptokinase and urokinase in the nonpregnant population. **Streptokinase** (250,000-unit bolus, 100,000 units/h infusion for 24 hours) is also used but with a higher rate of subchorionic hemorrhage, allergic complications, and longer infusion duration than recombinant tissue plasminogen activator. Catheter-directed thrombolysis allows for earlier reperfusion and likely improves long-term pulmonary function compared with systemic therapy.[1,19] Fetal loss subsequent to surgical embolectomy is higher than with thrombolysis.[20,22]

CHEST PAIN

The differential diagnosis of chest pain in pregnant women is similar to that of nonpregnant women, but disorders such as aortic dissection and cardiomyopathy are associated with pregnancy. Advances in reproductive technology resulting in pregnancies in older women may result in an increase in **coronary artery disease** in this population. **Coronary artery dissection** and **coronary vasospasm** are more likely in women who smoke and those with migraine. Coronary artery disease is more likely in those >35 years old, diabetics, and hypertensives.[23] Treat **acute myocardial infarction** with low-dose aspirin, heparin, and percutaneous coronary intervention rather than with thrombolytics.[24,25] **Aortic dissection**, although rare, is usually encountered in the third trimester and the postpartum period. Risk factors are pregnancy, bicuspid aortic valve, connective tissue disorders (e.g., Marfan's syndrome), syncope, hypertension, and a family history of aneurysm.[26] Chest radiograph may not demonstrate a widened mediastinum, and diagnosis is made by MRI or CT scan.[23]

Peripartum cardiomyopathy is a dilated cardiomyopathy that can occur at any stage of gestation, but is classically defined as occurring in the last month of gestation or within the first 5 months after delivery, without an apparent cause or preexisting history of cardiac disease. The cause is unknown. Risk factors include cardiomyopathy during prior pregnancies, multiparity, maternal age >40 years old, chronic hypertension before pregnancy, gestational hypertension, preeclampsia, and HELLP syndrome. Symptoms and signs of peripartum cardiomyopathy are dyspnea, orthopnea, cough, palpitations, chest pain, edema, rales, and jugular venous distention. Diagnose and treat congestive heart failure and pulmonary edema with standard modalities (see chapter 53, Acute Heart Failure) **except that nitroprusside is relatively contraindicated in pregnancy because it can cause thiocyanate and cyanide accumulation in the fetus**. In the postpartum patient, angiotensin-converting enzyme inhibitors may be given. Anticoagulate with heparins because of increased risk of thromboembolism. **Do not use warfarin during pregnancy. Warfarin can be given in the postpartum period.**[27,28]

TABLE 100-2 Initial Treatment for Venous Thromboembolism during pregnancy[(1,16,17)]

Antithrombotic Agent	Initial Dose
Recommended: LOW MOLECULAR WEIGHT HEPARINS (LMWH)	
Enoxaparin (Lovenox®)	1 milligram/kg SC every 12 h
Dalteparin (Fragmin®)	100 units/kg SC every 12 h
Tinzaparin (Innohep®)	175 units/kg SC every 24 h
UNFRACTIONATED HEPARIN (LMWH)	10,000 units SC every 8-12 h to achieve aPTT 2-2.5 times base 6 hrs after dose
For heparin allergy or heparin-induced thrombocytopenia	
Fondaparinux (Arixtra®)	50-100 kg, 7.5 milligrams SC every 24 h; > 100 kg, 10 milligrams SC every 24 h
Danaparoid	removed from US market

DISORDERS ASSOCIATED WITH ELEVATED BLOOD PRESSURE: HYPERTENSION, PREECLAMPSIA AND HELLP SYNDROME, AND ECLAMPSIA

CHRONIC AND GESTATIONAL HYPERTENSION

The decrease in systemic vascular resistance results in a decrease in maternal blood pressure, and blood pressure reaches its nadir at 16 to 18 weeks of pregnancy. Blood pressure returns to prepregnancy values near the end of the second trimester.

Chronic hypertension in pregnancy is defined as a systolic blood pressure of ≥140 mm Hg or a diastolic blood pressure of ≥90 mm Hg that existed prior to pregnancy, is diagnosed before the 20th week of gestation, or persists longer than 12 weeks after delivery. Severe chronic hypertension is systolic blood pressure >160 mm Hg or diastolic pressure >110 mm Hg. Women with chronic hypertension are at increased risk for placental abruption, preeclampsia, low birth weight, cesarean delivery, premature birth, and fetal demise.[29]

Gestational hypertension is hypertension present only after the 20th week of pregnancy or in the immediate postpartum period but without proteinuria.

Safe treatment options for hypertensive women who are pregnant are labetalol and methyldopa.[30] **All antihypertensive drugs cross the placenta.** Labetalol is the first-line agent for chronic hypertension in pregnancy.[29] The starting dose is 100 milligrams PO twice a day, and the usual maintenance dose is 200 to 400 milligrams PO twice a day. Methyldopa, used safely in pregnancy for decades, is started at 250 milligrams every 6 hours PO and titrated to achieve the desired blood pressure. The usual daily dose is 500 milligrams to 3 grams divided in two to four doses per day, with a maximum of 3 grams per day.

Long-acting nifedipine may be added if blood pressure is not controlled with methyldopa or labetalol. Long-acting nifedipine is started at 30 milligrams PO once a day and can be increased up to 120 milligrams per day slowly if needed. For acute management of **hypertensive emergencies**, hydralazine 5 milligrams IV or IM, labetalol 20 milligrams IV, or nifedipine 10 to 30 milligrams PO (not a Food and Drug Administration–approved indication) may be used during pregnancy.[29-31] **Angiotensin-converting enzyme inhibitors and angiotensin receptor blockers are contraindicated because of their teratogenic effects on fetal scalp, lungs, and kidneys.**[29]

PREECLAMPSIA

Preeclampsia, or gestational hypertension with proteinuria, is characterized by hypertension before 20 weeks of gestation with either new-onset proteinuria, sudden increase in proteinuria, or development of **HELLP syndrome.**

The cause of preeclampsia is unknown. The histologic hallmark lesion of preeclampsia is acute atherosis of decidual arteries. Atherosis and thrombosis are thought to lead to placental ischemia and infarctions. Poor placental perfusion is presumed to lead to the formation of free radicals, to oxidative stress, and to inflammatory responses that may influence the mechanistic development of preeclampsia.[30]

Preeclampsia is associated with intrauterine growth retardation, premature labor, low birth weight, abruptio placentae, and future risk of maternal cardiovascular disease.[30,32]

Preeclampsia during an initial pregnancy increases the chances of recurrence in future pregnancies. Other important risk factors for preeclampsia include maternal age >40 years old, hypertension, diabetes, renal disease, collagen vascular disease, and multiple gestation. Low-dose aspirin therapy can prevent preeclampsia and its complications.[33,34]

Diagnosis of Preeclampsia Diagnostic criteria for preeclampsia are listed in **Table 100-3**, and laboratory evaluation is outlined in **Table 100-4.**[35]

TABLE 100-3 Diagnostic Criteria for Preeclampsia

Criteria for *mild* preeclampsia
Systolic blood pressure ≥140 mm Hg OR diastolic blood pressure ≥90 mm Hg
AND
Proteinuria >0.3 grams in a 24-h collection
AND
>20-wk gestation
AND
No other systemic signs or symptoms
Criteria for *severe* preeclampsia
Blood pressure ≥160 mm Hg systolic or ≥110 mm Hg diastolic measured on two occasions at least 6 h apart with the patient at rest
AND
Visual disturbances or mental status disturbances
OR
Pulmonary edema or cyanosis
OR
Epigastric or right upper quadrant pain; abnormal liver function studies
OR
Thrombocytopenia
OR
Oliguria (<500 mL in 24 h)
OR
Proteinuria of ≥5 grams in a 24-h collection or ≥3+ on two random urine samples collected at least 4 h apart
Impaired fetal growth

HELLP Syndrome The **HELLP syndrome (Table 100-5)** is an important clinical variant of preeclampsia. HELLP is more common in the multigravid patient than in the primigravida. Hypertension may not be present initially or at all. This fact, combined with the usual complaint of epigastric or right upper quadrant pain, makes it easy to misdiagnose HELLP syndrome for other causes of abdominal pain, such as gastroenteritis, cholecystitis, hepatitis, pancreatitis, or pyelonephritis. **A pregnant woman at >20 weeks gestation or up to 7 days postpartum with abdominal pain should be evaluated for HELLP syndrome.**

Complications of severe preeclampsia, HELLP syndrome, and eclampsia include disseminated intravascular coagulopathy, spontaneous hepatic and splenic hemorrhage, end-organ failure, abruptio placentae, intracranial bleeding, maternal death, and fetal death.[35]

Treatment of Preeclampsia For **mild eclampsia**, outpatient management is an option after consultation with the obstetrician, as long as arrangements are made for frequent clinical and laboratory evaluation and close fetal surveillance.[35] Headache, scintillating scotomata or other visual changes, abdominal pain, vaginal bleeding, and decreased fetal movement require immediate reevaluation. Treat **severe preeclampsia** (blood pressure >160 mm Hg) with antihypertensive agents **(Table 100-6)**

TABLE 100-4 Laboratory Evaluation for Preeclampsia

Test	Comments
CBC with differential	May see hemoconcentration or falling hematocrit. Thrombocytopenia suggests severe disease.
Creatinine	Elevation suggests severe disease.
Alanine and aspartate aminotransferase concentrations	Elevation suggests severe disease.
Lactate dehydrogenase level	Elevation suggests microangiopathic hemolysis.
Protein in urine	3+ proteinuria; 24-h collection may be done by obstetric service. >5 grams/24 h suggests severe disease.
Protein/creatinine ratio	0.1–0.3 indicates need for 24-h collection[29]
Uric acid level	Level ≥5.5 milligrams/dL may suggest superimposed preeclampsia on chronic hypertension[29]

TABLE 100-5 Laboratory Abnormalities in HELLP Syndrome

Test	Findings
CBC and test of peripheral smear	Schistocytes
Platelet count	<100,000/μL <150,000/μL suspicious for syndrome
Liver function tests (alanine aminotransferase, aspartate aminotransferase levels)	Elevated but below levels usually seen in viral hepatitis (<500 U/L)
Renal function tests	Normal or elevated blood urea nitrogen and creatinine levels
Coagulation profile	Abnormal
Lactate dehydrogenase	>600 U/L suspicious for hemolytic anemia
Total bilirubin	>1.2 milligrams/dL

and IV magnesium sulfate.[35-37] Consult with the obstetrician for admission or transfer to a center that manages high-risk pregnancy especially in the presence of HELLP syndrome. **The only *definitive* resolution for preeclampsia is delivery.**

The initial management of **HELLP syndrome** is similar to that of **severe preeclampsia** or **eclampsia**: IV magnesium, blood pressure control, and hospital admission for stabilization. Correct coagulopathy. If HELLP syndrome is suspected and obstetric care is not available locally, stabilize the patient as best as possible and transfer to a tertiary care center with high-risk obstetrics facilities. The definitive treatment is delivery, especially if the patient is ≥34 weeks of gestation. Corticosteroid administration can help delay delivery and improve fetal outcome in pregnancies <34 weeks of gestation.

ECLAMPSIA

Eclampsia is the development of new-onset seizures, superimposed upon preeclampsia, in a woman between 20 weeks of gestation and 4 weeks postpartum.

Eclampsia should be suspected and treated in any pregnant woman who is at >20 weeks of gestation or <4 weeks postpartum who develops seizures, coma, or encephalopathy. Occasionally, eclampsia can present with seizure in the absence of blood pressure elevation and proteinuria.[30] **Management of eclampsia includes treatment of seizures, treatment of hypertension, and emergent obstetric consultation to facilitate urgent delivery of the fetus.** Treat seizures with **magnesium sulfate**, 4 to 6 grams IV in 100-mL aliquot given over 20 to 30 minutes followed by an infusion of 2 grams per hour for at least 24 hours.[35-37] Magnesium is renally excreted, and in women with renal insufficiency, reduce the dose to 2 grams IV bolus and obtain a serum magnesium level before increasing the dose. The main side effects of high levels of magnesium are flushing, diaphoresis, hypothermia, hypotension, flaccid paralysis, and respiratory depression. When levels approach toxicity, patellar reflexes diminish and respiratory rate slows. Administer antihypertensives as suggested in Table 100-6. Replace coagulation factors if there is coagulopathy. Obtain emergency obstetric consultation for prompt delivery. If obstetric services are not available, stabilize the patient as best as possible and transfer to a center with facilities for advanced obstetric care.

VAGINAL BLEEDING IN THE SECOND HALF OF PREGNANCY

The causes of serious vaginal bleeding in the second half of pregnancy include abruptio placentae, placenta previa, and vasa previa. All can cause severe hemorrhage. **Do not perform a digital or speculum pelvic examination to assess vaginal bleeding until a transvaginal US is performed to determine the location of the placenta. Mechanical disruption of the placenta by speculum or digital examination may precipitate catastrophic hemorrhage.** When transvaginal US is properly and carefully performed by those experienced in transvaginal US (vaginal probe is angled against the anterior lip of the cervix, probe is not advanced to contact the placenta, probe is not inserted into the cervix), the technique does not cause hemorrhage.[40] If there is no evidence of placenta previa or vasa previa, then a sterile speculum examination may be performed to determine if premature rupture of membranes or abruption is present.

ABRUPTIO PLACENTAE

Abruptio placentae is the premature separation of a normally implanted placenta from the uterine lining (**Figure 100-1**). The incidence of spontaneous abruption is highest between 24 and 28 weeks of gestation.[41] Abruption can cause uteroplacental insufficiency and fetal distress or demise. Maternal complications include coagulopathy, hemorrhagic shock, uterine rupture, and multiple organ failure. Abruption usually occurs spontaneously but is also associated with trauma, even minor trauma. See chapter 256, Trauma in Pregnancy. Risk factors for abruption include abdominal trauma, cocaine use, oligohydramnios, chorioamnionitis, advanced maternal age or parity, eclampsia, and chronic or acute hypertension.

Clinical features depend on the degree of placental abruption. Mild abruption is characterized by mild uterine tenderness, no or mild vaginal bleeding, normal maternal vital signs, no coagulopathy, and fetal distress. Signs and symptoms of severe abruption are no or heavy vaginal bleeding, fetal distress, coagulopathy, severe uterine pain or tenderness, continuous or repetitive uterine contractions, and maternal hypotension or shock. Nausea, vomiting, and back pain may also be present. **Consider placental abruption in pregnant women with acute, painful vaginal bleeding or with acute abdominal/uterine pain.**

Diagnosis is made by the clinical features. Electronic fetal monitoring (cardiotocodynamometry) is very sensitive for identifying fetal distress as a sign of placental abruption and has a 100% negative predictive value for adverse outcomes when monitoring is reassuring.[42] Transvaginal US is fairly specific for the diagnosis, but is not sensitive for the detection of

TABLE 100-6 Antihypertensive Drugs for Treatment of Acute, Severe Hypertension in Preeclampsia and Eclampsia[38,39]

Generic Name	Mechanism of Action	Onset of Action	Dosage	Comment
Labetalol	Selective α and nonselective β antagonist	5 min	20 milligrams IV, then 40–80 milligrams IV every 10 min as needed (maximum, 300 milligrams); IV infusion 1–2 milligrams/min titrated	Less hypotension and reflex tachycardia than hydralazine. Higher doses cause neonatal hypoglycemia. Longer use associated with fetal growth restriction.
Hydralazine	Arterial vasodilator	20 min	5 milligrams IV or 10 milligrams IM, repeat at 20-min intervals; consider other drug if no response at maximum of 20 milligrams IV or 30 milligrams IM	Maternal hypotension, fetal distress; must wait 20 min for response between IV doses.
Nifedipine	Calcium channel antagonist	10–20 min	10 milligrams PO, repeat in 30 min if necessary	Food and Drug Administration does not approve short-acting nifedipine for treatment of hypertension.

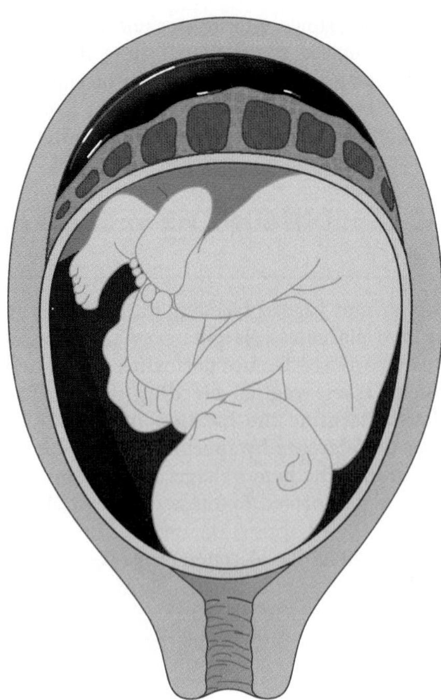

FIGURE 100-1. Abruptio placentae. The placenta has separated from the superior pole of the uterus.

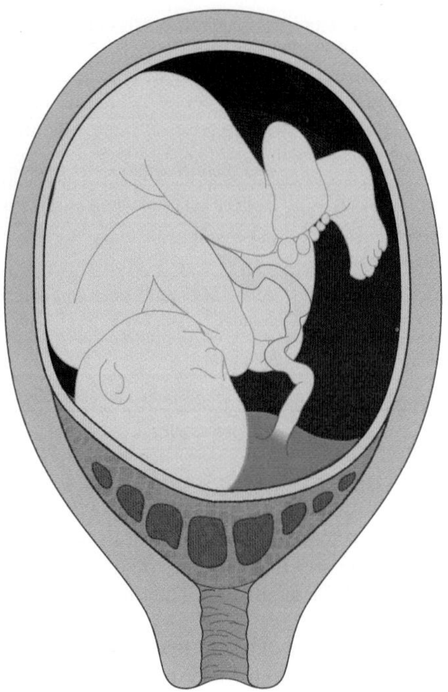

FIGURE 100-2. Complete placenta previa. Placenta overlies the internal os.

retroplacental clot because the appearance of clotted blood evolves in echotexture over time.[41] MRI is diagnostic but requires the transport of a potentially unstable patient out of the ED or intensive care unit for imaging.

Treatment consists of maternal stabilization, cardiotocographic monitoring to detect fetal distress, and emergency obstetric consultation. Place two large-bore IVs; obtain a CBC, metabolic panel, coagulation panel, fibrin degradation product, and fibrinogen levels; and type and cross-match maternal blood. Administer RhoGAM® if the mother is Rh negative. For disseminated intravascular coagulation, replace coagulation factors. Immediate delivery is indicated for severe abruption.

PLACENTA PREVIA

Placenta previa is a placenta that extends near, partially over, or beyond the internal cervical os. Normal placental implantation is in the corpus or fundal region, whereas in placenta previa, implantation is lower in the uterus. The cause is unknown. Although low-lying or partial placenta previa is not uncommon early in pregnancy, the placenta usually migrates to a normal position as the pregnancy nears term.

Risk factors for placenta previa include cesarean delivery, multiple uterine surgeries, advanced maternal age, minority group status, cigarette smoking, and cocaine use. Patients with symptomatic placenta previa present with painless bright-red vaginal bleeding, which should be differentiated from the normal passage of blood-stained mucus that occurs near the onset of labor. There are three subclasses of placenta previa: marginal placenta previa, which reaches the internal os but does not cover it; partial placenta previa, where the placenta partially covers the internal os; and complete placenta previa, which completely covers the internal os (**Figure 100-2**).

While proceeding with further patient assessment, place two large-bore IVs for fluid resuscitation; obtain CBC and coagulation parameters; and type and cross-match blood. **Do not perform a digital or speculum vaginal examination until normal placental position is confirmed by US, as disruption of the cervical-placental junction could precipitate catastrophic hemorrhage.** Carefully perform transvaginal US (see earlier). Once placenta previa is identified, consult obstetrics for management options. A double setup, in which two teams of staff are available in the operating room during a vaginal examination, may be indicated in cases where the placenta lies within 1 to 2 cm of the cervical os and labor is imminent. Otherwise, women in the second half of pregnancy with placenta previa are usually admitted to the hospital for observation and fetal monitoring

VASA PREVIA

Vasa previa is a rare cause of late-pregnancy bleeding. In vasa previa, umbilical vessels course in the amniotic membrane at the level of the cervical os, so that when the cervix begins to dilate in labor with membrane rupture, the blood vessels tear. Fetal distress or fetal demise may result from fetal exsanguination or vessel compression. Risk factors associated with vasa previa are placenta previa, in vitro fertilization, velamentous insertion of the umbilical cord, and bilobed placenta. Vasa previa can sometimes be diagnosed by Doppler color US performed early in pregnancy. Otherwise, it is seldom recognized prior to catastrophic vessel disruption during labor. Treatment is rapid operative delivery.

PREMATURE RUPTURE OF MEMBRANES, PRETERM LABOR, AND PRETERM BIRTH

Premature rupture of membranes is rupture of membranes prior to onset of contractions. **Membrane rupture before 37 weeks of gestation is known as preterm premature rupture of membranes.** The time from membrane rupture to delivery, known as the latent period, is usually inversely proportional to the gestational age when preterm premature rupture of membranes occurs. For pregnancies between 25 and 32 weeks, 33% had latent periods longer than 3 days. For pregnancies at 33 to 34 weeks and 35 to 36 weeks, 16% and 4.5% had latencies greater than 3 days, respectively.[43] The latent period allows for pharmacologic intervention to improve fetal lung maturity and increase fetal survival.

Preterm (premature) labor is labor prior to 37 weeks of gestation and is often preceded by premature rupture of membranes. Preterm labor is thought to be a syndrome initiated by multiple mechanisms, including infection, inflammation, uteroplacental ischemia or hemorrhage, uterine overdistention secondary to multiple gestation, stress, and other immunologically mediated processes.[44] Several non–genital tract infections, including pyelonephritis, asymptomatic bacteriuria, pneumonia, appendicitis, and periodontal disease, are also implicated in preterm labor.

Untreated *Chlamydia*, gonorrhea, *Trichomonas vaginalis*, and bacterial vaginosis infections increase the risk of preterm premature rupture of membranes and preterm labor. With appropriate patient selection, vaginal progesterone gel or suppository or IM progesterone can reduce the likelihood of preterm delivery.[45]

Preterm birth is birth before 37 weeks of gestation, and may occur spontaneously or as a result of premature rupture of membranes or placental abruption or may be induced for medical reasons. Surviving preterm neonates are at risk for sepsis, neurologic defects, feeding problems, blindness, deafness, and respiratory distress. Infants weighing <1500 grams or born at <32 weeks of gestation are at greatest risk for these problems, but even infants born at between 34 0/6 and 36 6/7 weeks gestation (late preterm infants) may require intensive care admission for IV fluids, sepsis, hyperbilirubinemia, and mechanical ventilation.[41,43]

DIAGNOSIS OF PREMATURE RUPTURE OF MEMBRANES

Details of the history taking and physical examination that aid in the diagnosis of premature rupture of membranes are listed in **Table 100-7. Avoid digital cervical examination because it decreases the latent period and may increase the likelihood of infection. Perform speculum examination and visually examine the cervix to identify dilation and test vaginal fluid (Table 100-7).** The combination of history, nitrazine paper, and fern testing (**Figure 100-3**) are reported to diagnose 90% of cases of premature rupture of membranes.[46] US assessment of amniotic fluid volume correctly identifies premature rupture of membranes when a low amniotic fluid index (≤10 cm) is present.[47]

Premature labor or premature rupture of membranes requires obstetric consultation. If obstetric services are unavailable, transfer the patient to a center where such services are available. Obstetric treatment includes corticosteroids and antibiotics to treat group B *Streptococcus*.

Corticosteroids given at <34 weeks of gestation speed fetal lung maturity, decrease the incidence of intraventricular hemorrhage, reduce the duration of mechanical ventilation, and reduce the incidence of necrotizing enterocolitis without increasing maternal or fetal infection. Betamethasone (12 milligrams IM every 24 hours for 2 days) or dexamethasone (6 milligrams IM every 12 hours for 2 days) can be used for gestations between 24 and 34 weeks.[48]

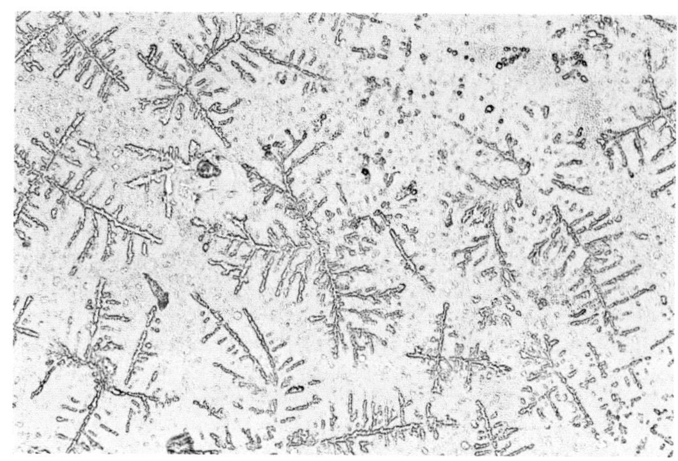

FIGURE 100-3. Ferning of amniotic fluid. [Photo contributed by Robert Buckley, MD.]

Antibiotics can decrease neonatal infection, prolong latency, and reduce the incidence of postpartum endometritis, chorioamnionitis, neonatal infections, and intraventricular hemorrhage. Antibiotic choices are penicillin G (5 million units IV then 2.5 to 3 million units every 4 hours until delivery), ampicillin (2 grams IV then 1 gram every 4 hours until delivery), and cefazolin (2 grams IV). Clindamycin or vancomycin

TABLE 100-7 Keys to Diagnosis of Premature Rupture of Membranes

Information Obtained	Comments
History	
Gush of fluid and continued leakage of fluid	Ask patient to perform a Valsalva maneuver while speculum is in place to look for gush of fluid, or apply fundal pressure.
Details of contractions	Determine if active labor is in process.
Date of last menstrual period	Use to calculate estimated date of delivery and gestational age. Gestational age is number of weeks from first day of last menstrual period.
Vaginal bleeding	Raises concern for placenta previa.
Recent intercourse	
Fever	Infection raises fetal and maternal risk.
Physical Examination	
Measurement of fundal height	
Auscultation of fetal heart tones	
Sterile speculum examination	Check for: Cervical dilatation and effacement. Pooling in vagina of fluid leaking from cervix. If no fluid is noted, apply fundal pressure or ask patient to perform a Valsalva maneuver or cough.
Laboratory Evaluation	
Vaginal fluid	Test with nitrazine paper. **Blue color indicates pH >6.5, signaling presence of amniotic fluid.** Note: Blood, semen, bacterial vaginosis, trichomoniasis, soap, and antiseptics may cause false positive; false negative, about 7%.[46]
Swab of vaginal walls or posterior fornix; do not swab cervical mucus; cervical mucus produces thick, dark, wide arborization pattern, not delicate ferning	Examine glass slide preparation for ferning. **Ferning indicates presence of amniotic fluid.** Blood may obscure ferning. Mucus results in a false-positive fern test finding. Test for *Chlamydia*, *Neisseria gonorrhoeae*, group B streptococci, and bacterial vaginosis.

are alternatives for those allergic to penicillins. Macrolides are not recommended.[49] Do not give amoxicillin-clavulanate because it is associated with necrotizing enterocolitis. There is no need for prophylactic antibiotics if membranes are intact.[50]

Tocolytic therapy using magnesium sulfate, β-mimetics, indomethacin, or calcium channel blockers is controversial and is relatively contraindicated in the patient with preterm premature rupture of membranes. Tocolysis may allow time for antenatal administration of corticosteroids and antibiotics and transfer of the patient to an appropriate neonatal center. Because there are no widely accepted protocols for tocolytic management, consult the obstetrician, who can explain the pharmacologic risks, benefits, and alternatives to the patient. Magnesium sulfate may reduce the risk and severity of cerebral palsy in infants when birth is anticipated before 32 weeks of gestation.[51]

Management guidelines for expedited delivery in the near-term gestation vary. Expedited delivery was historically recommended in patients with preterm premature rupture of membranes at >34 weeks of gestation to avoid the complications of chorioamnionitis and neonatal sepsis, but recent trials suggest that induction of labor does not reduce the risk of neonatal sepsis.[52]

MATERNAL EMERGENCIES DURING LABOR AND DELIVERY

The most important maternal emergencies of labor and delivery are postpartum hemorrhage, uterine rupture, and amniotic fluid embolism. Difficult deliveries are discussed in chapter 101, Emergency Delivery.

POSTPARTUM HEMORRHAGE

Postpartum hemorrhage usually occurs within the first 24 hours of delivery and is referred to as **primary postpartum hemorrhage**. The main causes of primary postpartum hemorrhage are **uterine atony, retained placental fragments, lower genital tract lacerations, uterine rupture, uterine inversion**, and **hereditary coagulopathy. Table 100-8** lists the most common risk factors. **Secondary postpartum hemorrhage** occurs after the first 24 hours and up to 6 weeks postpartum. The most common causes of secondary postpartum hemorrhage are failure of the uterine lining to subinvolute at the former placental site, retained placental tissue, genital tract wounds, and uterogenital infection.[53,54]

Excessive blood loss in the postpartum period is defined as a 10% drop in the hematocrit, a need for transfusion of packed red blood cells, or volume loss that causes symptoms of hypovolemia. Normally, plasma volume increases by 40% and red blood cell volume by 25% at the end of the third trimester. The hematologic changes of pregnancy can mask the typical symptoms of hemorrhage, and the first sign may be only a mild increase in pulse rate. Up to a 30% loss in total blood volume may be required before blood pressure drops.

Most cases of postpartum hemorrhage are due to uterine atony. Another 20% result from cervical, vaginal, or perineal lacerations. Retention of placental tissue may account for another 10%, and underlying coagulopathy is uncommon but potentially treatable.[55] **The initial steps are to begin aggressive fluid and blood resuscitation while simultaneously identifying and treating the underlying cause (Tables 100-9 and 100-10).** Nonpneumatic antishock garments can be applied in combination with fluid resuscitation and uterotonics, resulting in reduced blood loss and increased maternal survival in remote settings or with delayed transport.[56]

TABLE 100-8 Risk Factors for Postpartum Hemorrhage
Primiparity or grand multiparity
Previous postpartum hemorrhage
Preeclampsia
Prior cesarean section
Placenta previa or low-lying placenta
Marginal umbilical cord insertion
Transverse fetal lie
Labor induction or augmentation
Cervical or uterine trauma
Fetal age <32 weeks of gestation
Fetal birth weight >4500 grams
Prolonged third stage of labor

Uterine atony is the most common cause of postpartum hemorrhage. Risk factors include preeclampsia, prolonged use of uterotonics or tocolytics, prolonged labor, multifetal gestation or fetal macrosomia, multiparity, retained placenta, and uterine infection. Initiate bimanual uterine massage; place a fist in the anterior fornix and compress the uterine fundus against the hand in a suprapubic location (**Figure 100-4**).

Uterine inversion mostly results from previous cesarean section or overzealous attempts to remove the placenta to manage the third stage of labor.[53] Inversion can also occur in patients with connective tissue disorders and uterine structural anomalies. It can be a difficult diagnosis to make, especially if the fundus remains cephalad to the cervix. The diagnosis can be made with transvaginal or transabdominal ultrasound. Uterine inversion requires immediate manual replacement of the uterus. A Rüsch balloon catheter can be applied to correct uterine inversion.[57] Whatever technique is used, correction of uterine inversion is a very painful and difficult procedure that may require general anesthesia and tocolytic agents.

Retention of placental fragments or **abnormal placental implantation** (placenta accreta) may cause severe hemorrhage and may require emergency pelvic embolectomy, hemostatic brace sutures (B-Lynch sutures), or peripartum hysterectomy.

Uterine rupture is a rare complication but carries high maternal and fetal mortality. Previous cesarean section is the primary risk factor for uterine rupture, and single-layer surgical closure of the uterus, fetal size >3500 grams, and labor augmentation increase the rate of rupture during a trial of labor. Anatomic abnormalities such as a bicornuate uterus, grand multiparity, history of connective tissue disorders, and abnormal placentation are also associated with rupture. Clinical signs of uterine rupture are persistent abdominal pain, severe vaginal bleeding, loss of fetal station, and palpable uterine defect. Fetal monitors may show fetal distress and bradycardia. The diagnosis of uterine rupture must be made clinically and rapidly. Treatment is aggressive fluid and blood resuscitation and surgical delivery of the fetus.

AMNIOTIC FLUID EMBOLUS

Amniotic fluid embolus is a rare and often catastrophic complication of pregnancy that occurs when amniotic fluid and cells of fetal origin enter the maternal circulation during labor or delivery. Most cases occur before delivery. Fetal and maternal mortality rates are high. Amniotic fluid embolism is difficult to diagnose and is usually a diagnosis of exclusion. The onset of symptoms until cardiovascular collapse can range from seconds to over 4 hours. Presenting signs include respiratory distress, hypoxia, pulmonary edema, altered mental status, seizures, sudden maternal cardiovascular collapse, disseminated intravascular coagulation, and sudden onset of fetal distress.[58]

Postulated causes are antigenic stimuli or activation of the clotting cascade when amniotic fluid enters the maternal circulation. Physiologically, the hemodynamic changes shown on echocardiogram during confirmed cases of amniotic fluid embolism are due to the acute onset of severe pulmonary hypertension, right ventricular failure with leftward deviation of the septum, and the absence of pulmonary edema. Secondarily, left ventricular filling becomes impaired due to profound right heart failure, eventually resulting in myocardial ischemia.[58]

Death can occur rapidly. Treatment is supportive, and there are no specific interventions currently available; prevent and/or treat hypoxia, hypotension, and hypoperfusion. Place the woman in the left lateral decubitus position to minimize vena cava compression; give oxygen by nonrebreather mask or endotracheal tube; resuscitate with fluid and blood; and administer pressors to support maternofetal circulation until emergency delivery of the fetus is performed. Obtain emergency obstetric consultation. If the gravid patient cannot be resuscitated, perimortem cesarean delivery within 5 minutes of cardiac arrest increases the chances of neonatal survival.

TABLE 100-9 Drug Regimens for Postpartum Hemorrhage

Drug	Comments
Oxytocin (Pitocin®) 10 units IM *or* 20-40 units in 1 L NS; give 500 mL over 10 min, then 250 mL/h	First-line treatment. Uterotonic agent. Rapid administration may cause transient hypotension.
Carboprost (Hemabate®) 0.25 mg IM, repeat as needed every 15-90 minutes for a total dose of 2 milligrams	Prostaglandin. Side effects: nausea, vomiting, diarrhea, hypertension, bronchospasm. Avoid in patients with hypertension or asthma.
Misoprostol (Cytotec®, Apo-Misoprostol®) 1000 micrograms rectally	Prostaglandin. Side effects: nausea, vomiting, diarrhea. Not FDA approved for this indication; widely used internationally due to heat stability.
Methylergonovine (Methergine®) or Ergonovine® 0.2 milligrams IM, repeat as needed every 2-4 h to maximum of 5 doses	Ergot. Contraindicated in patients with hypertension or preeclampsia.

Abbreviations: FDA = Food and Drug Administration; NS = normal saline; SL = sublingual.

TABLE 100-10 Common Causes and Treatment of Postpartum Hemorrhage

Tone	Perform bimanual uterine massage. Give drugs to improve uterine tone as outlined in Table 100-9.
Trauma	Examine for cervical, vaginal, or perineal lacerations or hematomas. Repair lacerations. Incise, drain, and appropriately ligate bleeding vessels causing a hematoma. Correct uterine inversion with manual replacement. Uterine rupture requires surgery.
Tissue	Inspect the placenta for missing fragments; if a portion is absent, manually evacuate the uterine cavity. Invasive placentation may require hysterectomy. Perform transvaginal or transabdominal US to identify abnormal fluid-filled uterus. Consider a balloon tamponade with either uterine-specific balloon device (Bakri or Rüsch) or an adaptation of a Foley catheter or condom as a temporizing measure.
Thrombin	Consider DIC in the setting of severe preeclampsia, sepsis, placental abruption, shock, or intrauterine fetal demise, although undiagnosed coagulopathies may rarely present in nulliparas. Replace coagulation factors.

Abbreviation: DIC = disseminated intravascular coagulation.

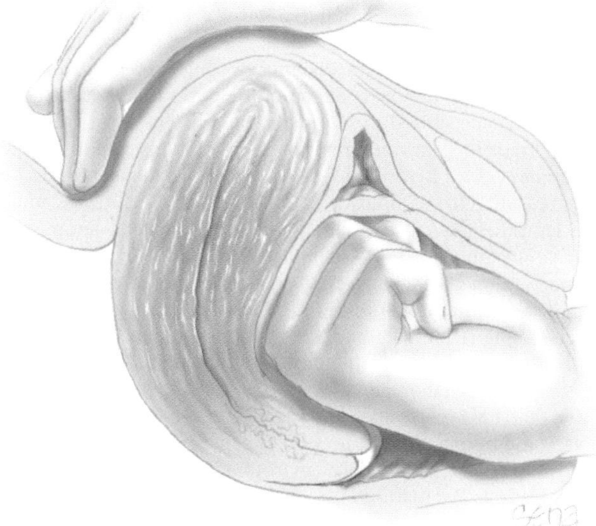

FIGURE 100-4. Bimanual method for uterine massage. [Reproduced, with permission, from Cunningham G, Leveno KL, Bloom SL, Hauth JC, Rouse DJ, Spong CY (eds): *Williams Obstetrics*, 23rd ed. © 2010. The McGraw-Hill Companies, Inc. New York, Figure 35-17.]

POSTPARTUM ENDOMETRITIS

Most postpartum infections are identified after hospital discharge. **In a postpartum woman with fever, assume pelvic infection until proven otherwise. Also consider respiratory tract infection, pyelonephritis, mastitis, thrombophlebitis, and appendicitis.**[59] Risk factors for postpartum endometritis are listed in **Table 100-11**.

The most common pathogens are gram-positive and gram-negative aerobes, anaerobes, *Mycoplasma hominis*, *Chlamydia trachomatis*, and *Neisseria gonorrhoeae*. *Gardnerella vaginalis* is isolated more often in younger women. Many infections are polymicrobial. Group A streptococcal infections are less common, but are increasing causes of postpartum endometritis.[60]

Symptoms of postpartum endometritis are fever, foul-smelling lochia, leukocytosis, tachycardia, pelvic pain, and uterine tenderness. Only scant vaginal discharge may be present, especially in patients infected with group B streptococci. In patients who are status post cesarean section, there may be surgical wound tenderness and purulent exudate.

Vaginal samples are of little value because of contamination with local flora. Blood cultures are rarely positive. Culture any purulent material from surgical incisions. Creatine phosphokinase levels may be elevated in group B streptococcal endometritis. Consult the obstetrician for disposition decisions. Admission is needed for patients who appear ill, have had cesarean section, or have underlying comorbidities. Treatment consists of antibiotics (**Table 100-12**), abscess drainage, and debridement of necrotic tissue.

After consultation with and recommendation by the obstetrician, patients with mild illness and those for whom follow-up in 24 hours is assured can be treated as outpatients with oral antibiotics, such as clindamycin, 300 milligrams three times per day PO for 10 days, or doxycycline, 100 milligrams twice per day for 10 days. **Do not give doxycycline to women who are breastfeeding**.

Complications of endometritis include parametrial phlegmons; surgical, incisional, and pelvic abscesses; infected hematomas; septic pelvic thrombophlebitis; necrotizing fasciitis; and peritonitis.

TABLE 100-11 Risk Factors for Postpartum Endometritis

Cesarean section*
Multiple gestation
Younger maternal age
Long duration of labor and membrane rupture
Internal fetal monitoring
Low socioeconomic level
Digital examination after 37 wk of gestation
Maternal human immunodeficiency virus infection

*Most significant risk factor.

TABLE 100-12 Inpatient Treatment of Postpartum Endometritis*
Cefoxitin (2 grams IV every 6 h) and vancomycin 1 gram IV every 12 h
OR
Cefotetan (2 grams IV every 12 h) and vancomycin 1 gram IV every 12 h
OR
Cefotaxime (2 grams IV every 6 h) and vancomycin 1 gram IV every 12 h
OR
Clindamycin (500 milligrams IV every 6 h) *plus* gentamicin (4.2 milligrams/kg IV daily) and vancomycin 1 gram IV every 12 h
OR
Ampicillin (2 grams IV every 4 h) *plus* gentamicin (4.2 milligrams/kg IV daily) and vancomycin 1 gram IV every 12 h
OR
Metronidazole (500 milligrams IV every 8 h) *plus* ampicillin (2 grams IV every 4 h) *plus* an aminoglycoside and vancomycin 1 gram IV every 12 h

*Consult the hospital pharmacist to determine if the antibiotic regimen selected is appropriate for breastfeeding.

TRANSFER OF THE PREGNANT PATIENT AND THE EMERGENCY MEDICAL TREATMENT IN ACTIVE LABOR ACT

There are times when a pregnant woman must be transferred to another hospital. Emergency physicians who work in a hospital that does not provide obstetric services should be familiar with the protocols in place for transfer and inpatient care of such patients. The **Emergency Medical Treatment and Active Labor Act** specifically addresses the care of pregnant women before and during transfer (see chapter 303, Legal Issues in Emergency Medicine).

A woman having contractions is considered to have an emergency medical condition if there is insufficient time for transfer before delivery or if the transfer may pose a threat to the health or safety of the child. In such a situation, the patient should not be transferred prior to delivery unless the patient requests transfer. If contractions are not present, an emergency medical condition is not automatically present, and the regular rules of providing medical care and determining the need for transfer of patients apply.

Acknowledgment: The authors gratefully acknowledge the previous authors, Michelle A. Echvarria and Gloria J. Kuhn, and the contributions of Antonio F. Didonato, who provided the illustrations for this chapter.

REFERENCES

The complete reference list is available online at www.TintinalliEM.com.

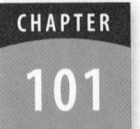

CHAPTER 101 Emergency Delivery

Sarah Elisabeth Frasure

INTRODUCTION AND EPIDEMIOLOGY

The thought of a woman presenting to the ED in active labor is justifiably a cause for anxiety—the emergency physician must contend not only with the often rusty recollection of the stages of normal delivery, but also with the knowledge that there are serious and even fatal complications associated with labor. Maternal and fetal survival may depend on the ability to successfully manage pre-eclampsia, eclampsia, hemorrhage, shoulder dystocia, malpresentation, cord prolapse, breech delivery, or fetal distress. Every ED should be prepared to take care of a woman in active labor. Tools include a basic delivery kit, an infant warmer or isolate, and medical supplies and equipment for neonatal resuscitation (see chapter 108, "Resuscitation of Neonates" and **Tables 101-1** and **101-2**).

TABLE 101-1 Equipment and Supplies for Emergency Delivery
Sterile gloves
Sterile towels and drapes
Povidone-iodine (Betadine) to cleanse the perineum
Sterile lubricant gel
Sterile scissors
Kelly clamps
Cord clamps
Rubber suction bulb
Towel or blanket for the infant
Gauze sponges (4×4)
Syringes (10 mL) and needles (22–24 gauge)
Placenta basin
Suture (3-0 chromic and 2-0 Vicryl) and needle driver

Note: List excludes standard adult and neonatal resuscitation equipment.

Out-of-hospital births occurred in 1.36% of births in 2012, and out-of-hospital births in the United States had a lower risk profile than in-hospital births, so that fewer teen, preterm, low-birth-weight, and multiple births occurred out of hospital.[1] Occasionally, planned home deliveries experience medical complications and require rapid transport to the ED to assist with labor and delivery. In a prospective study of home births in the United States and Canada, nearly 12% of 5400 women who had planned a home delivery ultimately required urgent transfer to a hospital during the course of labor. The majority of *intrapartum* transfers were performed for failure to progress, need for pain management, and maternal exhaustion. *Postpartum* transfers encompassed a variety of obstetric and/or neonatal complications such as maternal hemorrhage, retained placenta, or newborn respiratory distress.[2]

Out-of-hospital deliveries may also occur due to inadequate or nonexistent prenatal care, transportation difficulties, remote setting, or the onset of premature labor. Occasionally, a woman may also attempt to avoid the hospital/physician fees associated with pregnancy until the delivery of her child, presenting to a hospital for the first time when in active labor.

The development of obstetric centers for high-risk pregnancy has led to a significant decline in neonatal mortality in the United States, and transports to specialized units have increased. The most common reasons for transport include preterm labor (41%), premature rupture of membranes (21%), hypertensive disease (16%), and antepartum hemorrhage (13%).[3] Other indications for transport include eclampsia or pre-eclampsia, fetal distress, multiple gestation, fetal anomalies, and maternal health problems, including traumatic injuries. EMS units transporting an actively laboring patient should carry sterile delivery packs, relevant medical supplies (Table 101-1), and appropriate medications (Table 101-2). The transport team should be trained to assist in the precipitous delivery of an infant. Prehospital protocols regarding the complications of labor and delivery should be reviewed regularly to ensure that EMS personnel are adequately prepared for both normal delivery and potentially catastrophic pregnancy-related events.

For deliveries in an austere environment or in a disaster zone, the United Nations Population Fund provides a vaginal delivery kit for use during disaster relief, which includes a plastic sheet to lay on the ground, soap for washing hands and the perineum, string and a razor blade to tie and cut the umbilical cord, and a blanket to protect the newborn baby.[4]

TABLE 101-2 Medications for Emergency Delivery and Indications for Use

Classification	Medication	Dosage	Indication/Use	Contraindications
Uterotonic	Oxytocin	10–40 units/1000 mL normal saline or 10 units IM	Stimulation of uterine contraction or as uterotonic for PPH	Hypersensitivity
	Misoprostol	1000 micrograms PR once	Unlabeled use for PPH	Hypersensitivity
	Methylergonovine	0.2 milligram IM or IV or PO; may repeat at 2–4 h intervals	PPH	Hypersensitivity, hypertension
	Carboprost	250 micrograms IM every 15–90 min (total dose 2 milligrams)	PPH	Asthma
Antihypertensive	Hydralazine	5 milligrams IV, followed by 5- to 10-milligram boluses every 20 min	Pre-eclampsia/eclampsia, hypertensive emergency	Hypersensitivity
	Labetalol	20 milligrams IV, followed by doubled doses up to 80 milligrams (20–40–80–80) every 10 min; maximum total dose, 220 milligrams	Pre-eclampsia/eclampsia, hypertensive emergency	Hypersensitivity, sinus bradycardia
Anticonvulsant	Magnesium sulfate	Loading dose of 4–6 grams IV over 15 min, followed by 2 grams/h infusion; can also give 5 grams IM in each buttock	Seizure prophylaxis in pre-eclampsia/eclampsia	Myasthenia gravis
Electrolyte supplement toxicity	Calcium gluconate	1 gram IV over 5–10 min	Magnesium toxicity	Hypersensitivity, cardiac arrhythmia
Analgesic	Lidocaine 1%	1–10 mL injected locally	Local anesthetic	Hypersensitivity
	Fentanyl, 50 micrograms/mL	50 micrograms/mL	Short-acting opiate analgesic	Hypersensitivity
Opiate antagonist	Naloxone	0.4–2.0 milligrams IV every 2–3 min as need up to 10 milligrams cumulative dose	Narcotic overdose	Hypersensitivity
Antiemetic	Ondansetron	4 milligrams IV	Nausea, vomiting	Hypersensitivity

Abbreviation: PPH = postpartum hemorrhage.

PHYSIOLOGY

RUPTURE OF MEMBRANES

Determining rupture of membranes predicts not only the likelihood of imminent labor, but also the potential for complications, such as infection or cord prolapse. Spontaneous rupture of membranes occurs during the course of active labor in the majority of patients, although it also happens *prior* to onset of labor in approximately 8% of third-trimester patients.[5] Fifty percent of women who experience premature rupture of membranes deliver within 5 hours, and 95% give birth within 28 hours of this event.[6] The history of spontaneous rupture of membranes typically involves report of a gush of clear or blood-tinged fluid. Occasionally, patients recount continued leaking or dampening of their underwear on standing or with a Valsalva maneuver. Thick greenish brown fluid suggests the presence of meconium in amniotic fluid.

Rupture of membranes may be confirmed by using nitrazine paper to test residual fluid in the fornix or vaginal vault while performing a sterile speculum examination. **Amniotic fluid has a pH of 7.0 to 7.4 and will turn nitrazine paper a dark blue.** Vaginal fluid, on the other hand, typically has a pH of 4.5 to 5.5; the nitrazine strip, thus, remains yellow. False-positive results may occur, however, in the presence of blood, lubricant, *Trichomonas vaginalis*, semen, or even cervical mucus. **Another test that confirms rupture of membranes is ferning, which is the observation of sodium chloride crystals on a microscope slide as amniotic fluid dries (Figure 101-1).**

Premature Rupture of Membranes Rupture of the amnion and chorion *prior* to the onset of labor is called *premature* or *prelabor rupture of membranes.* If rupture of membranes occurs prior to 37 weeks of gestation, it is termed *preterm premature rupture of membranes.* Prolonged rupture of membranes transpires if delivery does not take place within 18 hours of rupture of membranes. It is important to understand the difference between and management of premature and preterm premature rupture of membrane as these patients may present to an ED for an initial evaluation.[7] Risk factors related to both premature rupture of membranes and preterm premature rupture of membranes include infection, history of trauma, multiple gestation, fetal anomalies, abruptio placentae, and placenta previa. Obtain emergency obstetrics consultation for preterm premature rupture of membranes.

CERVICAL DILATATION

Cervical dilatation describes the diameter of the internal cervical os and indicates the progression of labor. The index and middle fingers of the examining hand are used to estimate the diameter, which is expressed in centimeters (from closed to 10 cm). **Ten centimeters indicates full dilatation.** As labor progresses, the cervix also undergoes thinning, known as **effacement**, which is described in terms of a percentage (%) of normal cervical length. Unfortunately, this estimate is poorly reproducible among examiners. **Station** indicates the level that the fetus occupies in the pelvis. The maternal ischial spines serve as the reference point and are palpable on either side of the vaginal canal (located at 4 and 8 o'clock). If the presenting fetal part remains above the ischial spines, the station is described as negative. Once the presenting

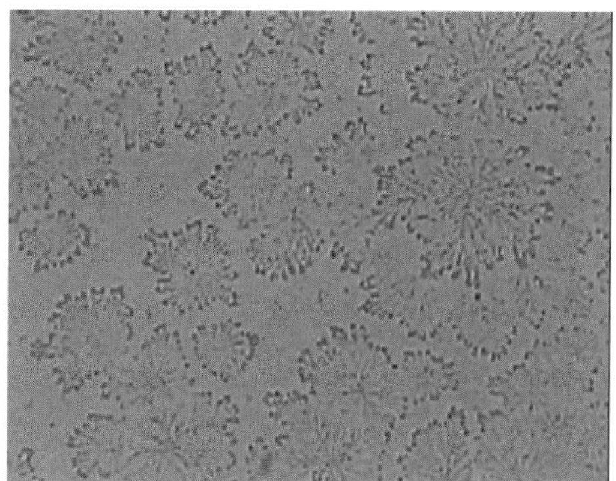

FIGURE 101-1. Typical ferning of dried amniotic fluid.

TABLE 101-3 True Versus False Labor

	True Labor	False Labor
Contractions		
Rhythm	Regular	Irregular
Intervals	Gradually shorten	Unchanged
Intensity	Gradually increases	Unchanged
Discomfort		
Location	Back and abdomen	Lower abdomen
Sedation	No effect	Usually relieved
Cervical dilatation	Yes	No

Source: Reproduced with permission from Cunningham FG, Leveno KJ, Bloom SL, Hauth JC, Rouse DJ, Spong CY (eds): *Williams Obstetrics*, 23rd ed. McGraw-Hill, Inc., 2010. Table 17-4 on AccessMedicine.com.

fetal part has reached the level of the ischial spines, the station is 0, with further descent into the pelvis described as +1 or +2. Therefore, a +3 station corresponds to visible scalp at the introitus, indicating a fetal position consistent with impending delivery.

TRUE VERSUS FALSE LABOR

Distinguishing **true from false labor** is an important initial step in the management of the pregnant patient (**Table 101-3**). **False labor** is defined as uterine contractions that do not produce cervical changes and is characterized by irregular, brief contractions that are usually confined to the lower abdomen. Commonly known as **Braxton Hicks contractions**, they are irregular in both intensity and duration. False labor may persist for several days and is commonly treated with hydration and rest.

True labor, on the other hand, is characterized by painful, repetitive uterine contractions that increase steadily in both intensity and duration and result in cervical effacement and dilatation. Specifically, true labor pains typically commence in the fundal region and upper abdomen and radiate into the pelvis and lower back. True labor leads not only to cervical dilatation and effacement, but also to the progressive descent of the fetus into the pelvis, in preparation for delivery.

STAGES OF LABOR

There are three **stages of labor** (**Table 101-4**). The first stage commences with the onset of regular uterine contractions and ends with full cervical dilatation. The first stage can be subdivided into two phases: latent and active. The latent phase is characterized by moderately uncomfortable uterine contractions that are infrequent and irregular, resulting in gradual cervical changes. In this preparatory phase the uterus orients to contractions and the cervix undergoes both effacement and softening. The active phase is typically noted to arise once the cervix has dilated to 3 to 4 cm, and results in cervical dilatation at an average rate of 1.2 cm/h in nulliparous and 1.5 cm/h in multiparous women. The second stage of labor commences at full dilatation and ends with the delivery of the infant.[8] The mean length of the second stage of labor is 20 minutes for multiparous women and 54 minutes for nulliparous women.[9] The third stage of labor starts after the delivery of the infant and ends with the delivery of the placenta. The third stage usually lasts less than 10 minutes, and active intervention is usually not required until after 30 minutes, unless hemorrhage occurs.

TABLE 101-4 Stages of Labor

Stage	Definition	Comments
First stage	From onset of regular uterine contractions to full cervical dilatation	—
Latent phase	Irregular, infrequent contractions	Preparatory phase, cervix softens and effaces
Active phase	Begins once cervix has dilated to 3–4 cm	Nulliparas: cervix dilates at 1.2 cm/h Multiparas: cervix dilates at 1.5 cm/h
Second stage	From full dilatation to delivery	Nulliparas: mean duration 54 min Multiparas: mean duration 20 min
Third stage	From delivery of infant to delivery of placenta	10 min; intervention not needed until >30 min

FETAL DISTRESS

Fetal distress may occur during active labor. Thus, evaluate for signs of fetal status frequently. Indicators of fetal distress include fetal bradycardia or tachycardia, or late decelerations in fetal heart rate, which are defined as persistent drops in fetal heart rate both during and more than 30 seconds after a contraction. A physician or nurse trained in fetal monitoring can identify fetal distress (**Figure 101-2**). Doppler measurement of fetal heart tones is not reliable to detect decelerations. If decelerations are suspected, obtain emergency obstetrics consultation, and try to increase maternal blood flow by positioning the patient in the left lateral position, provide IV hydration, and administer oxygen. Further information is provided in the Advanced Life Support Course for Obstetrics (see later section "Useful Web Resources").

CLINICAL EVALUATION

When a patient >20 weeks' gestation presents to the ED with signs of labor, immediately obtain both maternal vital signs (blood pressure, heart rate, respiratory rate, oxygen saturation, temperature) and the fetal heart rate. Doppler US can be used to measure fetal heart rate; a **normal fetal heart rate is generally 120 to 160 beats/min, bradycardia is defined as less than 110 beats/min, and tachycardia is greater than 160 beats/min.**[10] A persistently slow fetal heart rate indicates fetal distress and requires emergency obstetric consultation. As part of the initial evaluation, obtain IV access, procure baseline laboratory studies including blood type, and send a urinalysis.

HISTORY

Ask about the onset and frequency of uterine contractions, fetal membrane status, presence or absence of vaginal bleeding, and presence or absence of fetal movement. The obstetric history should include parity, history of complications with prior deliveries, history of precipitous deliveries, prenatal care during this pregnancy, and estimated date of delivery. Obtain a medical and surgical history, a list of current medications, and allergies, and ask the patient about substance abuse. Inquire about symptoms of infection, such as fevers, chills, or foul-smelling vaginal discharge.

Gestational Age If the patient knows the first day of her last menstrual period, the estimated date of delivery can be calculated by adding 9 months and 7 days to that date (**Nägele's rule**). Fundal height also provides a rapid estimate of gestational age and is measured in centimeters (cm) from the pubic symphysis to the top of the fundus (cm = weeks of gestation ± 2 weeks). Fundal height may be falsely overestimated in the obese patient. Bedside US also provides a useful assessment of gestational age in the third trimester, but estimated age can vary by ± 3 weeks.

PHYSICAL EXAMINATION

Monitor vital signs for evidence of maternal fever, tachycardia, or elevated blood pressure. Assess fetal heart tones for bradycardia or tachycardia. Do not keep the pregnant woman flat on her back for a prolonged time period; compression of venous return by the gravid uterus can lead to hypotension in the mother, which in turn results in decreased blood supply to the fetus. So, place the **patient in the left lateral position following the physical examination**. On abdominal examination, determine fundal height, abdominal or uterine tenderness to palpation, and presence of uterine contractions. Examine the perineum for perineal lesions, such as those caused by herpes simplex virus, which might be a contraindication for a vaginal delivery.

PELVIC EXAMINATION

Patients with vaginal bleeding should be evaluated with bedside US prior to speculum or bimanual examination, in order to rule out

placenta previa. Patients without vaginal bleeding should be evaluated first with a sterile speculum examination to determine if membranes have been ruptured, to note cervical dilatation and effacement, and to determine fetal station and presentation.

If rupture of membranes is suspected, perform a sterile speculum examination (do not use lubricant because lubricant may produce a false-positive nitrazine test), but do not perform a digital examination because even one digital examination increases the risk of infection.[11] **Also avoid digital examinations in the preterm patient in whom the prolongation of gestation is desired.**

Using sterile vaginal examination, examine the cervix for dilatation, effacement, and station.

Bedside US is the simplest method to verify presentation. Vertex presentation and lie can also be confirmed through palpation of the cranial sutures on digital examination. Palpation of small parts, such as feet or hands, often indicates malpresentation. If meconium is present on the examining finger, be prepared for neonatal resuscitation (see chapter 108).

EMERGENCY DELIVERY

The first steps in the management of a woman in active labor are to measure vital signs and initiate supportive therapy. Obtain venous access, provide IV hydration, and initiate maternal and fetal monitoring (if available). Delivery is imminent if the pelvic examination reveals complete cervical effacement and the fetus is at the introitus. Labor can progress very rapidly, particularly in multiparous patients. Both the stage of labor and the parity of the patient should be taken into account when considering whether to transport a laboring patient to the labor and delivery suite or to another facility. **If the cervix is fully effaced and dilated or the fetal head is visible during contractions, the obstetrician**

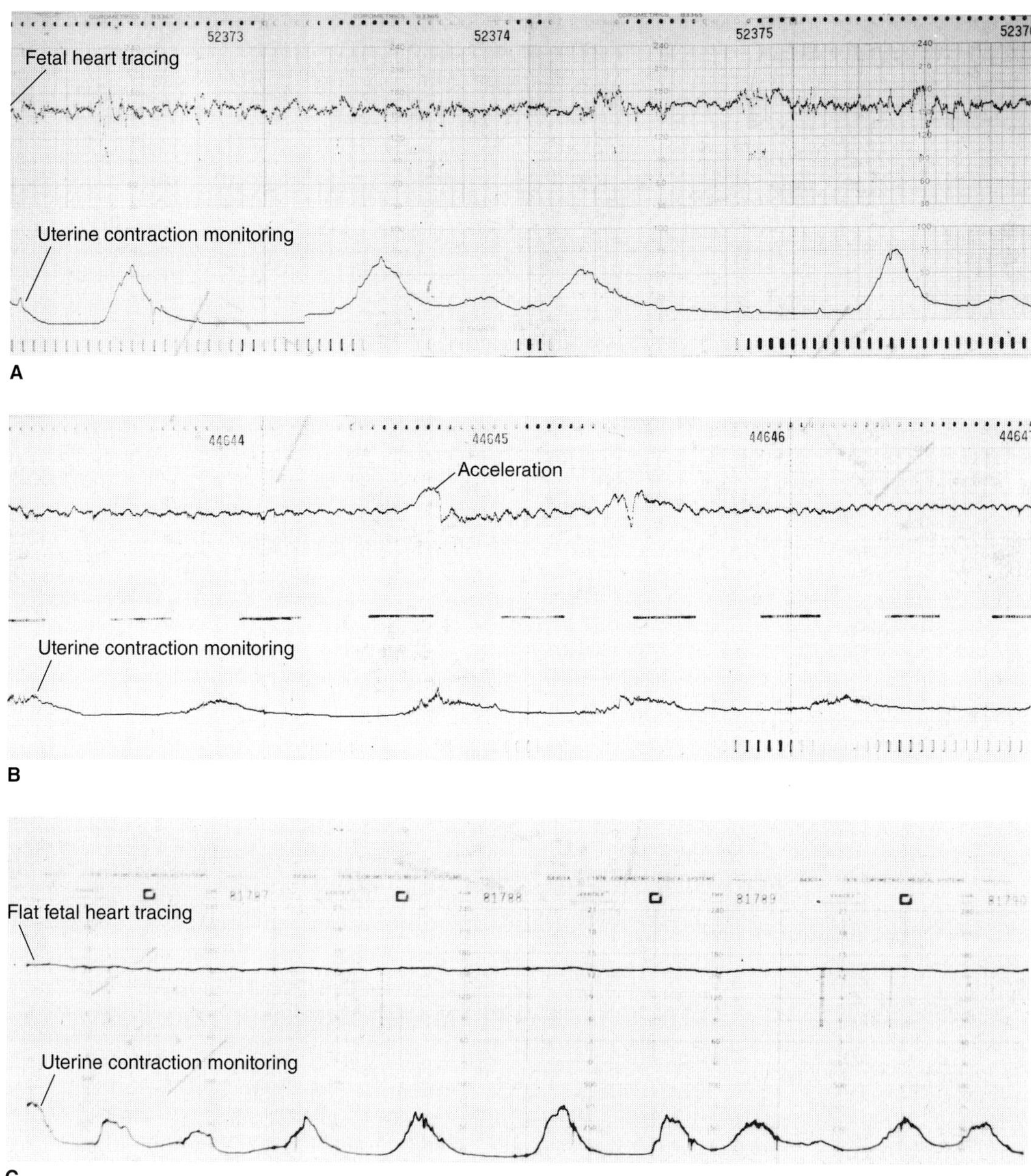

FIGURE 101-2. Fetal heart rate variability and uterine contraction patterns. **A.** Good variability. **B.** Good variability with brief accelerations. Fetal heart rises above baseline and quickly returns to normal. A reassuring pattern. **C.** Poor variability. May be due to fetal hypoxia. **D.** Variable decelerations. No relationship to uterine contractions. May represent cord compression. **E.** Late deceleration. Occurs at onset of contraction and slow return to baseline after contraction ends. Signifies uteroplacental insufficiency and fetal hypoxia. [Reproduced with permission from Pearlman MD, Tintinalli JE, Dyne PL (eds): *Obstetric and Gynecologic Emergencies: Diagnosis and Management.* McGraw-Hill, Inc., 2003. Figs. 10-9 and 10-10, pp. 131 and 132.]

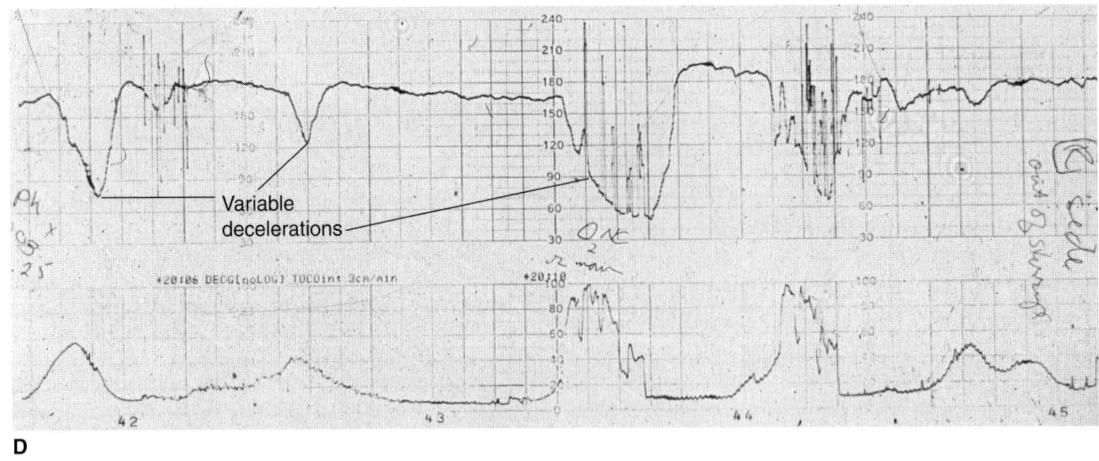

D

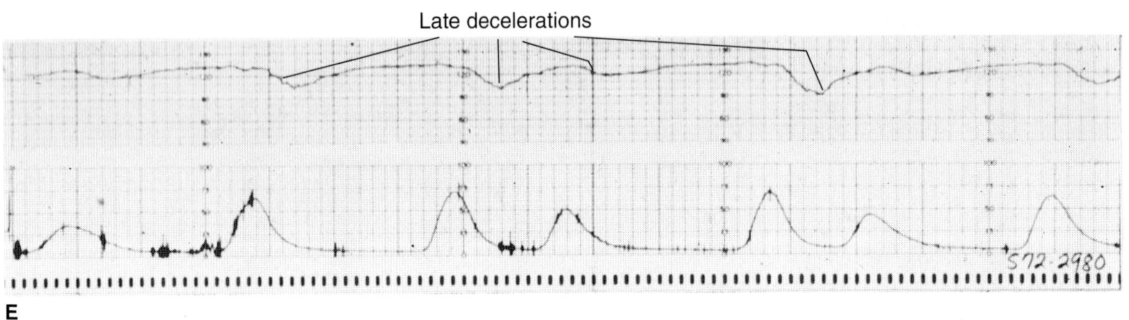

E

FIGURE 101-2. *(Continued)*

(if available) should come to the ED rather than risk a precipitous delivery during transport to the delivery suite.

As the cervix fully dilates, effacement becomes complete, the fetus descends into the pelvis, and the patient will experience the urge to push. The cervix should be fully dilated before the patient begins to push in order to avoid cervical lacerations. Determine fetal presentation by palpating skull sutures and fontanelle or the buttock or extremity. Bedside US can confirm presentation.

If time allows, prepare the perineum by washing it with mild soap and water and swabbing with povidone-iodine. Place drapes over the patient. Medical personnel attending to the patient should don gowns, masks, and gloves. Call for obstetric support.

Six cardinal movements describe the process of fetal descent during labor and delivery: (1) engagement, (2) flexion, (3) descent, (4) internal rotation, (5) extension, and (6) external rotation (**Figure 101-3**). *The following discussion describes delivery in the cephalic, occiput anterior position.* As the fetus descends through the birth canal and reaches the introitus, the perineum bulges in order to accommodate the fetal head. Gentle digital stretching of the inferior portion of the perineum can aid delivery. The perineum undergoes gradual thinning and stretching to enable passage of the newborn.

EPISIOTOMY

Routine **episiotomy** for a normal spontaneous vaginal delivery varies with practitioner, institution, and country. Episiotomy may be necessary to expedite a delivery in cases of fetal distress or shoulder dystocia or if forceps or vacuum devices are used (**Figure 101-4**).[12] The episiotomy can be performed in the midline or mediolaterally (45 degrees from the midline). Median episiotomy is easy to perform, but mediolateral episiotomy has a lower risk of extension to the anal sphincter (third-degree extension) or to the rectum (fourth-degree extension) than median episiotomy. If an episiotomy is clinically necessary, first inject 5 to 10 mL of 1% lidocaine solution with a small-gauge needle into the posterior fourchette and perineum. While protecting the infant's head, make a 2- to 3-cm incision with scissors in order to extend the vaginal opening, either at the midline or 45 degrees from the midline. A median incision must be supported with manual pressure from below. Take care to prevent extension of the incision into the rectum.

COMPLETION OF DELIVERY

Do not drop the baby. The combination of amniotic fluid, blood, and vernix generates a very slippery infant. Before delivering the rest of the body, place your posterior hand underneath the axilla of the infant. Use the anterior hand to grasp the ankles of the infant with a firm grip. Following delivery, keep the infant warm and provide gentle stimulation. Do not routinely aspirate the nose and mouth. Gently bulb aspirate only if there are obvious obstructions from secretions. If delivery is uncomplicated, and the infant has responded well to initial stimulation with a clear airway and good respiratory effort, the mother may hold the child immediately while the cord is cut.

Apgar scores are calculated at 1 and 5 minutes after delivery. Scoring parameters include general color, tone, heart rate, respiratory effort, and reflexes (**Table 101-5**).

For an APGAR score of <7 refer to the chapter 108. Provide positive-pressure ventilation for all newborns with a heart rate <100 beats/min or who are gasping or apneic after 30 seconds.

CLAMPING THE UMBILICAL CORD

Do not clamp the umbilical cord of term or preterm infants for at least 1 to 3 minutes after birth. Delayed cord clamping increases neonatal iron stores. **Double-clamp the umbilical cord 3 cm distal to its insertion at the umbilicus and transect with sterile scissors.** In delivery settings where aseptic care is routine, there is no clear benefit to any additional topical care of the umbilicus. When aseptic care is *not* available, however, antiseptic topical care of the umbilicus with chlorhexidine reduces the risk of omphalitis and neonatal mortality.[16] Once the umbilical cord is cut, dry the infant and either give the infant to the mother or place it in a warming unit.

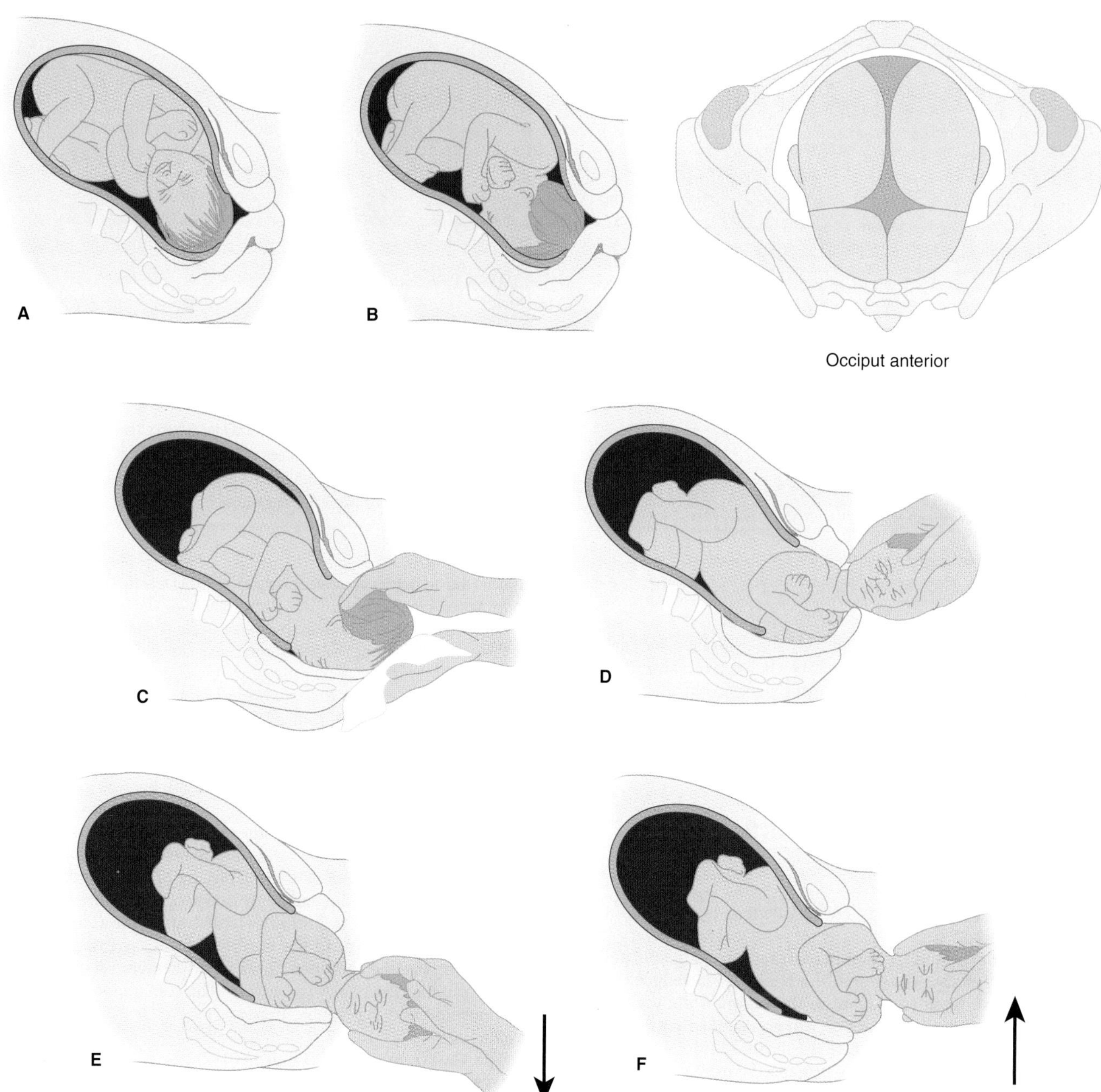

FIGURE 101-3. The movements of normal delivery for a vertex presentation. **A.** Engagement, flexion, and descent with vertex anterior. **B.** Internal rotation with occiput becoming anterior. **C.** Extension and delivery of the head. As the infant's head emerges from the introitus, support the perineum by placing a sterile towel along the inferior part of the perineum with one hand, and support the fetal head with the other hand. Ask the mother to breathe through contractions (rather than bear down) in order to deter rapid expulsion of the baby. Provide mild counterpressure for controlled extension of the fetal head. As the infant's head presents, use the inferior hand to control the fetal chin and keep the superior hand on the crown of the head, supporting the delivery. **D.** External rotation, bringing the thorax into the anteroposterior diameter of the pelvis. As the head delivers, palpate the infant's neck to assess for the presence of a nuchal cord. Nuchal cord is noted in approximately 25% to 35% of all term deliveries.[13] If the cord is loose, move it over the infant's head, and allow delivery to proceed as usual. If the cord is wound tightly around the neck, however, apply two close clamps in the most accessible area, and then cut the cord. **E.** Delivery of the anterior shoulder. Once the head is delivered, it will turn to one side or the other. Grasp the sides of the head with both hands, and apply **gentle** downward traction (go with gravity) until the anterior shoulder is delivered. Jerky or aggressive traction may injure the brachial plexus. If you have not checked for a nuchal cord, do so now. As the head rotates, place the hands on either side of the head, providing gentle downward traction. This maneuver allows for the delivery of the anterior shoulder. **F.** Delivery of the posterior shoulder. Use an upward movement to deliver the upward shoulder. Do not apply traction. If meconium is present or the newborn is limp or poorly responsive, stimulate the baby and be prepared to begin the steps of neonatal resuscitation with ventilation and oxygenation[14,15] (see chapter 108).

DELIVERY OF THE PLACENTA

The placenta usually delivers approximately 10 to 30 minutes after delivery of the infant. Allow the placenta to separate spontaneously and provide only *gentle* traction. Aggressive traction on the cord can lead to uterine inversion, tearing of the cord, or even disruption of the placenta, all of which can result in severe vaginal bleeding. After the placenta has been removed, gently massage the abdomen at the level of the fundus to promote contraction. Give oxytocin (10 to 40 units in 1 L normal saline at 250 mL/h or 10 units IM) to sustain uterine contraction.

The estimated blood loss during a vaginal delivery is usually less than 500 mL. Uterine atony, however, which occasionally follows a precipitous

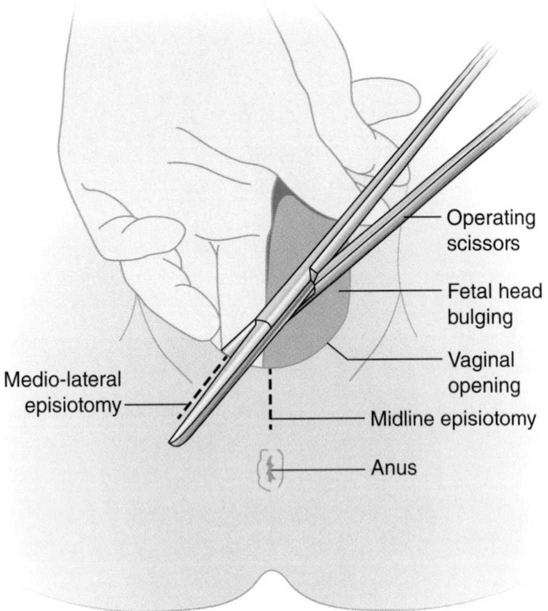

FIGURE 101-4. Methods for episiotomy.

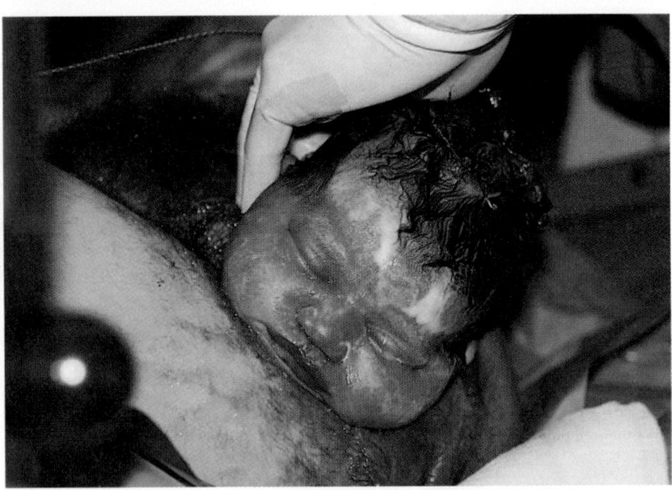

FIGURE 101-5. Clinical appearance of shoulder dystocia. The infant's head is impacted against the perineum. [Reprinted with permission from Buckley RG, Knoop KJ: Gynecologic and obstetric conditions, in Knoop KJ, Stack LB, Storrow AB (eds): *Atlas of Emergency Medicine*, 2nd ed. New York, McGraw-Hill, 2002, Figure 10.46.]

delivery, can lead to excessive vaginal bleeding. In that case, give additional oxytocin or another uterotonic of choice (see Table 101-2). As contractile agents are administered, provide vigorous bimanual massage.[17] Delay episiotomy or laceration repair until an experienced obstetrician is available to close the laceration and inspect for fourth-degree perineal lacerations.

COMPLICATIONS OF LABOR AND DELIVERY

UMBILICAL CORD PROLAPSE

Umbilical cord compression is life threatening to the fetus. Obtain immediate obstetric assistance, as emergent cesarean delivery is indicated. **Should the bimanual examination reveal a palpable, pulsating umbilical cord, elevate the presenting fetal part to reduce compression on the cord. Keep your hand in the vagina while the patient is transported and prepared for surgery to prevent further compression of the cord by the fetal head. Place the mother in the Trendelenburg position. Do not try to reduce the prolapsed cord.**[18]

SHOULDER DYSTOCIA

Shoulder dystocia is the impaction of fetal shoulders at the pelvic outlet after delivery of the head. Typically, the anterior shoulder is trapped behind the pubic symphysis and prevents delivery of the rest of the infant.[19,20] Complications of shoulder dystocia include fetal brachial plexus injury (due to overaggressive traction), clavicle fracture, fetal hypoxia (due to impaired respirations and/or compression of the umbilical cord), postpartum hemorrhage, and fourth-degree perineal lacerations.

Prior to delivery of the head, the head may retract between contractions. Shoulder dystocia then becomes evident when routine downward traction fails to deliver the anterior shoulder once the head has been delivered. After the infant's head is delivered, the head retracts tightly against the perineum (turtle sign; **Figure 101-5**).[21] Several steps can be used to relieve shoulder dystocia (**Table 101-6**). Immediately place the mother in the extreme lithotomy position, with her legs sharply flexed up to the abdomen and the knees held as widely apart as possible (**McRoberts maneuver; Figure 101-6**). Either the mother or an assistant should keep the legs held widely apart. **Simultaneously apply suprapubic pressure. If a second assistant is available, he or she should place their hands in a CPR position, and apply downward pressure just above the pubic symphysis for 1 to 2 minutes to disimpact the anterior shoulder. Do not apply pressure to the uterine fundus, as this maneuver can further impact the shoulder.** Suprapubic pressure serves to rotate the shoulder under the pubic symphysis.[21] The combination of the McRoberts position and suprapubic pressure relieves about 50% of shoulder dystocias.

The **Gaskin maneuver** (**Figure 101-7**) can also be employed. It is a simple maneuver, but with IVs and monitors in place or with an exhausted mother, it can be difficult to achieve. Place the patient on all fours. Exert gentle downward traction on the infant's head. In order to remember the direction of traction, remember to "go with gravity."

TABLE 101-5 Apgar Scoring for Newborns

	Sign	0 Points	1 Point	2 Points
A	Activity (muscle tone)	Absent	Arms and legs flexed	Active movement
P	Pulse	Absent	Below 100 beats/min	Above 100 beats/min
G	Grimace (reflex irritability)	No response	Grimace	Sneezing, coughing, pulling away
A	Appearance (skin color)	Blue-gray, pale	Normal, except extremities	Normal over entire body
R	Respiration	Absent	Slow, irregular	Good, crying

TABLE 101-6 Steps to Relieve Shoulder Dystocia

Steps	Comments
Flex thighs and keep knees apart as much as possible	McRoberts maneuver
Apply suprapubic pressure	Keep patient in McRoberts position. Place one hand with wrist clenched, immediately above the pubic symphysis; if an assistant is available, place two clenched wrists in CPR position just above pubic symphysis. Compress for 1 min. Do not compress uterine fundus. This worsens impaction.
Move patient to all- fours position	Gaskin maneuver. Deliver with gentle downward traction on the infant's head.
Corkscrew maneuvers	Typically require episiotomy. See text.

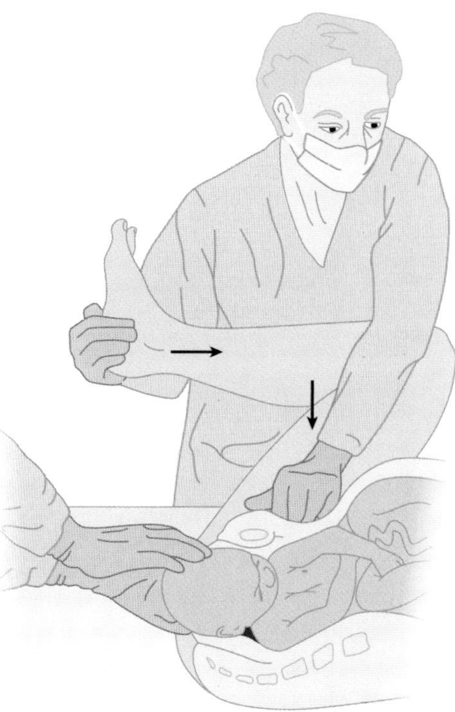

FIGURE 101-6. McRoberts maneuver. Sharply flex the thighs up onto the abdomen, as shown by the *horizontal arrow*, and keep the knees spread widely. Simultaneously provide suprapubic pressure (*vertical arrow*). [Adapted with permission from Cunningham FG, Leveno KL, Bloom SL, et al: *Williams Obstetrics*, 22nd ed. New York, McGraw-Hill, 2005, Figure 20-14.]

In 80% of cases, this maneuver allows the posterior shoulder to successfully deliver.[22]

Should the previous maneuvers fail, rotational maneuvers, which move the shoulders into an oblique position, can be performed. Allow 2 minutes for these maneuvers. The maneuvers typically require an episiotomy. For the Rubin maneuver, place fingers behind the anterior fetal shoulder, and push the shoulder with your fingertips toward the baby's chest. This may reduce the dimension of the shoulder girdle and allow for delivery. For the **Woods corkscrew maneuver** (**Figure 101-8**), keep fingertips behind the anterior shoulder, and with the opposite hand, apply pressure to the back of the posterior shoulder, and rotate the shoulder girdle clockwise into an oblique position, allowing delivery. The **reverse corkscrew maneuver** is in the opposite direction. Place your fingers in front of the posterior shoulder and behind the anterior shoulder, and apply pressure counterclockwise.[23]

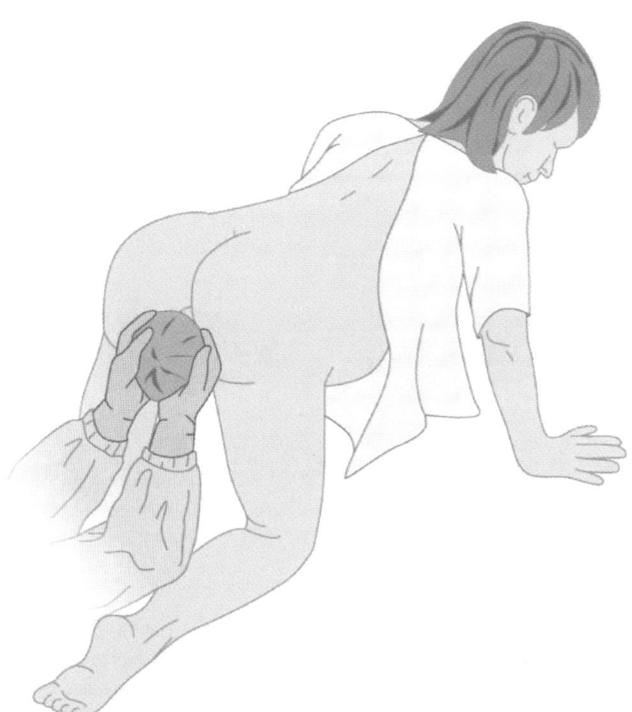

FIGURE 101-7. Gaskin maneuver for shoulder dystocia.

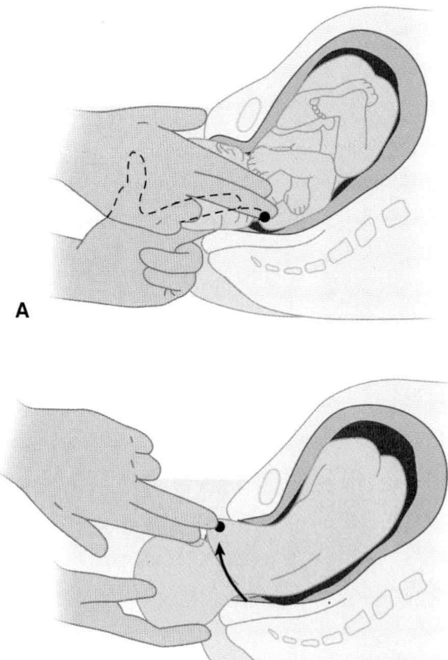

FIGURE 101-8. Corkscrew maneuver. **A.** Place fingertips behind anterior shoulder and in back of posterior shoulder. **B.** Then gently rotate clockwise until shoulder delivers.

BREECH PRESENTATION

Breech presentations occur in 3% to 4% of term pregnancies. Risks of breech presentations include umbilical cord prolapse, trauma, hypoxia, and fetal distress. Breech presentations occur most frequently in the delivery of *premature* infants; approximately 25% to 30% of all preterm infants (<28 weeks' gestation) present in breech position.[24] Given the increased perinatal/neonatal morbidity and mortality associated with vaginal breech deliveries, cesarean section is recommended in breech presentations.[24]

Head entrapment is a major concern in a breech delivery. In a normal cephalic delivery, the larger head dilates the cervical canal, which ensures that the rest of the infant's body can follow. In a breech delivery, however, the head emerges last and may become stuck in an incompletely dilated cervix.

In frank and complete breech deliveries, the buttocks dilate the cervix almost as effectively as the fetal head; therefore, delivery may proceed in an uncomplicated fashion. **In these cases, allow the delivery to proceed spontaneously** (**Figure 101-9**). The emergency physician subsequently places the index and middle fingers over the infant's maxillary bones (not in the infant's mouth) to help keep the head flexed, allowing the mother to expel the infant. It is important to refrain from pulling on the fetus, because this may impact the head in the pelvis or even entrap the extended fetal arm. **Footling and incomplete breech positions are not safe for vaginal delivery due to the risk of cord prolapse or incomplete dilatation of the cervix.** In any breech delivery, obstetric consultation should be obtained immediately.

PRETERM DELIVERY

The incidence of preterm delivery is approximately 12% and contributes substantially to perinatal morbidity and mortality.[25] Preterm labor is also

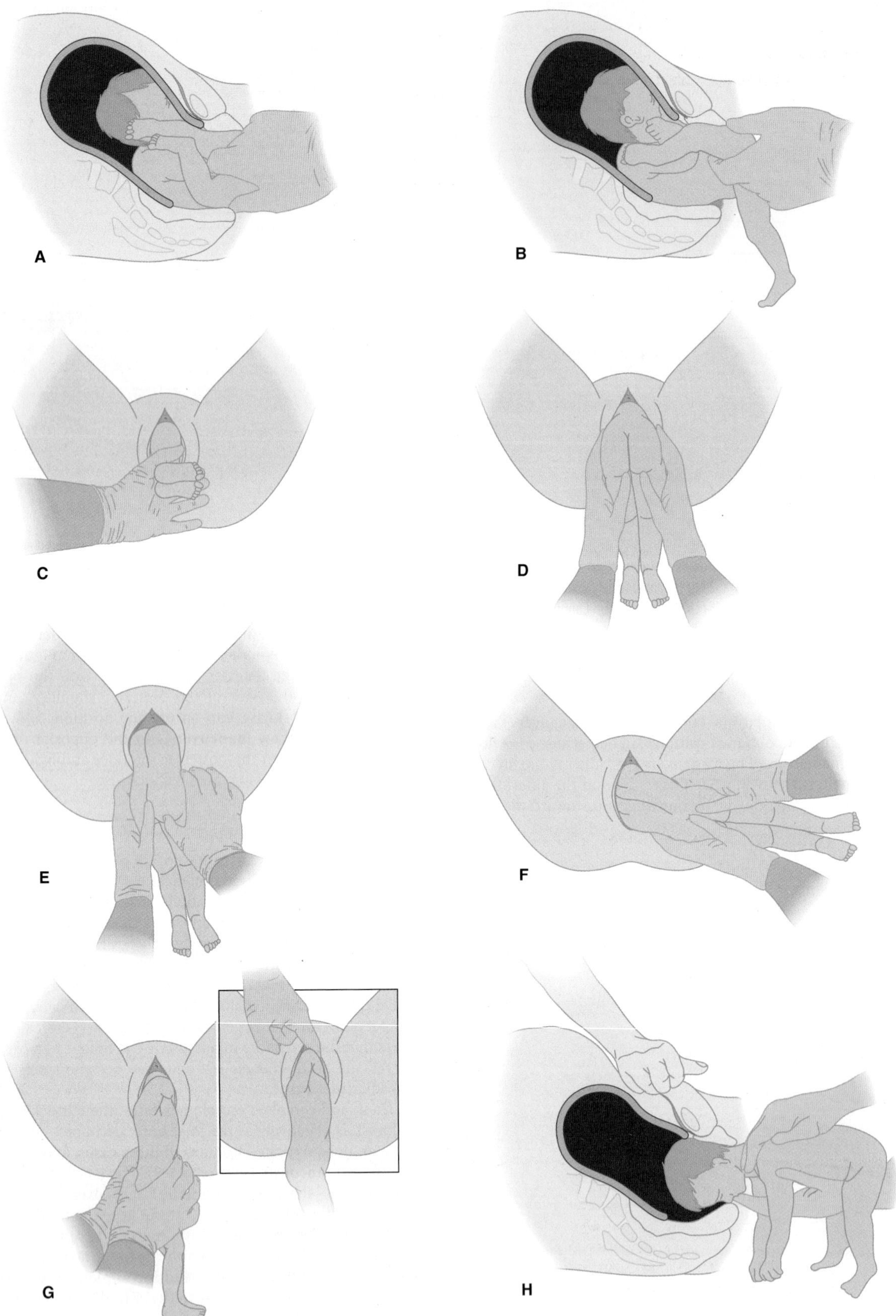

FIGURE 101-9. Breech delivery. **A.** Grasp the thigh to allow delivery of the leg. **B.** Grasp the other leg to allow its delivery. **C.** Grasp the feet at the ankles and rotate the sacrum anteriorly. **D.** The sacrum is rotated anteriorly. Maternal efforts deliver the baby to the level of the umbilicus. Wrap the trunk and legs in a towel. **E.** Maternal efforts further deliver to the level of the scapulae. Apply steady, gentle traction until scapulae come into view. **F.** Once the axilla is visible, the shoulder can be delivered. Rotate counterclockwise to deliver the anterior shoulder. (It does not matter which shoulder is delivered first.) **G.** Delivery of the anterior arm. When the scapulae appear, gently rotate the baby until one humerus can be followed down, rotated across the chest, and swept out. Then turn the baby clockwise to allow delivery of the other arm. **H.** Deliver the vertex of the skull by placing fingers at the maxillary process, and keep body parallel to the horizontal. Do not pull. Do not lift above the parallel to avoid neck hyperextension. Apply suprapubic pressure to aid delivery of the head.

a major cause of precipitous delivery in EDs. Preterm infants present more frequently in the breech position. The delivery maneuvers are similar to those described above. Be prepared to initiate neonatal resuscitation. The decision as to whether to initiate resuscitative efforts in the ED is often difficult because patients may deliver an extremely premature fetus of unknown gestational age. **Survival of the newborn increases significantly for each completed week from 21 weeks of gestation (0% survival) to 25 weeks of gestation (75% survival).**[26] When gestational age is known, initiate resuscitation of newborns 22 weeks of gestation or older. It is justified to cease resuscitative efforts after 10 minutes, and certainly, after 15 minutes of asystole.

Acknowledgment The author gratefully acknowledges the contributions of Michael J. VanRooyen, Jennifer A. Scott, and Kimberly B. Fortner, coauthors of this chapter in the previous editions.

REFERENCES

The complete reference list is available online at www.TintinalliEM.com.

CHAPTER 102

Vulvovaginitis

Ciara J. Barclay-Buchanan
Melissa A. Barton

INTRODUCTION

Vaginal discharge is caused by a wide variety of disorders, including vaginitis, cervicitis, and pelvic inflammatory disease.[1] Vaginitis is a spectrum of diseases that cause vulvovaginal symptoms including burning, irritation, itching, odor, and abnormal discharge. The factors associated with acute vaginitis are listed in **Table 102-1**. **The most common infectious causes of vaginitis in symptomatic premenopausal women are bacterial vaginosis (40% to 45%), vulvovaginal candidiasis (20% to 25%), and trichomoniasis (15% to 20%).** Vulvovaginal candidiasis, contact vaginitis, and atrophic vaginitis may occur in virgins and postmenopausal women; however, the other forms of infectious vulvovaginitis are generally found in sexually active women. In approximately 30% of women with vaginal complaints, the disorder remains undiagnosed even after comprehensive testing.[2-4]

The clinical diagnosis may be challenging, because women may have more than one disease, and signs and symptoms are frequently not specific to a particular cause. Polymicrobial infection is not uncommon.

Although infectious vaginitis rarely requires hospitalization, it may have serious sequelae. Both bacterial vaginosis and trichomoniasis have been shown to be associated with premature rupture of membranes, preterm labor, and low infant birth weight.[5,6] Trichomoniasis is associated with pelvic inflammatory disease in patients infected with human immunodeficiency virus and increases risk of human immunodeficiency virus acquisition and transmission.[7,8] When overgrowth of certain bacteria occurs, the protective effect of vaginal lactobacilli strains, which inhibit the growth of bacteria and destroy human immunodeficiency virus in vitro, is lost.[1]

TABLE 102-1 Factors Associated with Acute Vulvovaginitis
Infections
Irritant or allergic contact
Local response to a vaginal foreign body
Lack of estrogen in perimenopausal and postmenopausal women (atrophic vaginitis)
Postirradiation changes

PHYSIOLOGY

In females of childbearing age, estrogen causes the development of a thick vaginal epithelium with a large number of superficial glycogen-containing cells and serves a protective function. Glycogen is used by the normal flora, such as lactobacilli and acidogenic corynebacteria, to form lactic and acetic acids. The resulting acidic environment favors the normal flora and discourages the growth of pathogenic bacteria. Lack of estrogen or a dominance of progesterone results in an atrophic condition, with loss of the protective superficial cells and their contained glycogen, and subsequent loss of the acidic environment.

Normal vaginal secretions vary in consistency from thin and watery to thick, white, and opaque. The quantity may also vary from a scant to a rather copious amount. Secretions are odorless and produce no symptoms. The normal vaginal pH varies between 3.8 and 4.5. Alkaline secretions from the cervix before and during menstruation, as well as alkaline semen, reduce acidity and predispose to infection. Before menarche and after menopause, the vaginal pH varies between 6 and 7. Because of scant nerve endings in the vagina, the patient usually does not have symptoms until both the vagina and vulva are involved in an inflammatory or irritant process.

Vulvovaginal inflammation is the most common gynecologic disorder in prepubertal girls and includes both infectious causes (e.g., bacterial, fungal, pinworm) and noninfectious causes (e.g., contact/irritant, lichen sclerosis, foreign body). Factors thought to contribute to vaginitis in prepubertal females include less protective covering of the vestibule by the labia minora, low estrogen concentration resulting in a thinner epithelium, exposure to chemical irritants such as bubble bath, poor hygiene, front-to-back wiping and the short distance between the vagina and anus, foreign bodies, chronic medical conditions (eczema, seborrhea, and other chronic diseases), and sexual abuse. Infectious causes include respiratory and enteric bacterial organisms such as *Haemophilus influenzae*, *Staphylococcus aureus*, group A streptococci and *Streptococcus pneumoniae*, *Escherichia coli*, *Shigella flexneri*, *Neisseria gonorrhoeae*, and *Chlamydia*, as well as *Candida* and pinworms. Infectious causes may be more common in adolescents, especially those who are sexually active.[4]

GENERAL APPROACH

Obtain a detailed gynecologic history and perform a pelvic examination. History should include details of vaginal discharge, odor, irritation, itching, burning, bleeding, dysuria, and dyspareunia. Inquire about associated abdominal pain, new sexual partners, use of barrier protection during intercourse, relationship of symptoms to menses, use of antibiotics and contraceptives, and hygiene practices. Note the presence of vulvar edema or erythema, vaginal discharge, cervical inflammation, and abdominal and cervical motion tenderness.

During speculum examination, obtain a swab of the discharge and test for gonorrhea and chlamydial infection. If a patient refuses pelvic examination or it is not feasible, the patient may submit a self-swab of vaginal secretions or a urine sample.[9]

Microscopic examination of secretions and evaluation of pH are useful diagnostic tools. However, microscopes and reagents are not available in all EDs, microscopic examination is time consuming and tedious, and results depend on operator skill. To test pH, obtain a sample from the mid portion of the vaginal sidewall to avoid false elevations in pH caused by mucus. **Sampling from the posterior fornix may yield inaccurate results because cervical mucus, blood, semen, douches, and vaginal medications can elevate the pH.** Microscopic evaluation of fresh vaginal secretions using both normal saline solution and 10% potassium hydroxide slide preparation and fishy odor on whiff test help provide evidence for a diagnosis[10] (**Tables 102-2 and 102-3**). Signs of vulvar inflammation and minimal discharge suggest the possibility of mechanical, chemical, allergic, or other noninfectious causes of vulvovaginitis.

BACTERIAL VAGINOSIS

Bacterial vaginosis is the most common cause of vaginitis and accounts for up to 50% of cases in acutely symptomatic women.

TABLE 102-2 Diagnosis of Vaginitis Based on Vaginal Secretions

Test	Finding	Diagnosis	Comments[13]
pH	4.0–4.5	Normal	—
	4.0–4.5	Candidiasis	If undiagnosed after pelvic examination and evaluation of wet mount, treatment with a single dose of fluconazole is cost effective, but also test for *Neisseria* and *Chlamydia*.
	>4.5	Bacterial vaginosis	If undiagnosed after pelvic examination and evaluation of wet mount, treatment with 2 grams of metronidazole ± a single dose of fluconazole is cost effective, but also test for *Neisseria* and *Chlamydia*.
	>4.5	Trichomoniasis	If undiagnosed after pelvic examination and evaluation of wet mount, treatment with 2 grams of metronidazole ± a single dose of fluconazole is cost effective, but also test for *Neisseria* and *Chlamydia*.
Microscopy of specimen prepared with normal saline solution	Clue cells	Bacterial vaginosis	—
	Motile trichomonads	Trichomoniasis	—
	Pseudohyphae and/or buds	Candidiasis	—
Whiff test of swab specimen prepared with potassium hydroxide	Fishy odor	Bacterial vaginosis	—
Microscopy of specimen prepared with potassium hydroxide	Pseudohyphae and/or buds	Candidiasis	—

However, up to 50% of women who meet clinical criteria for this diagnosis are asymptomatic.

Bacterial vaginosis is a polymicrobial infection that occurs when the normal hydrogen peroxide–producing lactobacilli are replaced by other species including *Gardnerella vaginalis, Ureaplasma, Mycoplasma*, and various anaerobes. Risk factors include multiple sexual partners, intercourse with an uncircumcised male partner, vaginal intercourse immediately after receptive anal intercourse, lack of condom use, douching, and absence of peroxide-producing lactobacilli in the vaginal flora.[1,11] Women who have never been sexually active are less commonly affected. Bacterial vaginosis is not classified as a sexually transmitted infection, but it is generally agreed upon that sexual activity plays a role in transmission and may promote infection.[12]

DIAGNOSIS

The most common clinical presentation of women with bacterial vaginosis is vaginal discharge and odor. Classically, a thin, whitish-gray discharge is present, generally with an increase in discharge volume. The absence of discharge or the presence of only a mild discharge makes the diagnosis less likely. When an odor is present, it may be described as a fishy smell. Introital or vaginal irritation, such as redness, tissue fissures, excoriations, or edema, is not common with bacterial vaginosis.

The diagnosis is based on history, speculum vaginal examination, microscopic evaluation of vaginal secretions, and point-of-care testing. Obtain secretions from the mid sidewall of the vagina, and mix with one to two drops of 0.9% normal saline. Cover with a coverslip for microscopic evaluation for clue cells; to check for fishy or amine odor, add one drop of 10% potassium hydroxide and assess vapors for fishy (amine) smell (see additional methods for amine testing below). To check pH, apply a small amount of secretions directly onto pH paper. The presence of three of the following four criteria makes the diagnosis:

1. A thin, homogeneous vaginal discharge
2. More than 20% clue cells on a wet mount (**Figure 102-1**)
3. Positive results on test for amine release, or whiff test
4. A vaginal pH level >4.5

The criterion with the highest sensitivity (89%) is vaginal pH, whereas that with the highest specificity (93%) is the amine odor, or positive result on whiff test. If vaginal pH is >4.5 and there is an amine odor, the diagnosis of bacterial vaginosis can be made with confidence.[14] A colorimetric card test for bacterial vaginosis detects a vaginal pH of ≥4.7 and volatile vaginal fluid amines. Commercially available tests that might be useful for the diagnosis of bacterial vaginosis include card tests for proline aminopeptidase (Pip Activity TestCard; Quidel, San Diego, CA), a

TABLE 102-3 Vaginitis Signs and Symptoms

Causative Organism	Sign or Symptom
Candida	Thick, curdy discharge
	Itching
Gardnerella or other bacteria	Fishy odor
	Whitish-gray, thin discharge
Trichomonas	Frothy odorous discharge
	Vaginal erythema or edema

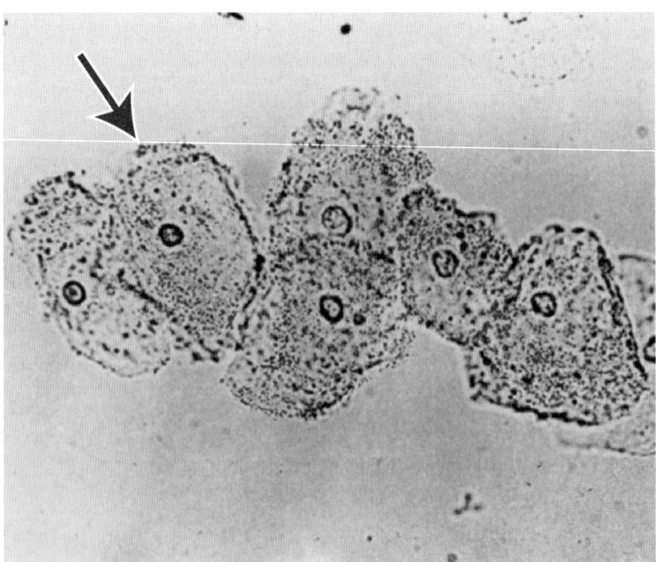

FIGURE 102-1. Bacterial vaginosis. Saline wet mount with clue cells (*arrow*). [Reproduced with permission from DeCherney AH, Nathan L, Laufer N, Roman AS (eds): *Current Diagnosis & Treatment: Obstetrics & Gynecology*, 11th ed. McGraw-Hill, Inc., 2013. Fig. 39-9.]

DNA probe–based test for high concentrations of *G. vaginalis* (Affirm VP III; Becton Dickinson, Sparks, MD), and the OSOM BVBlue test (Sekisui Diagnostics, Lexington, MA), all of which have performance characteristics that are comparable to Gram stain. Cards are available for the detection of elevated pH and trimethylamine; however, they have a low sensitivity and specificity and thus are no longer recommended. Cultures of vaginal discharge are not beneficial, because *Gardnerella* organisms are part of the normal vaginal flora. Polymerase chain reaction for various organisms is being used in research but is not clinically relevant at this time.[1]

The combination of bacterial vaginosis and leukorrhea (more WBCs than epithelial cells seen on a wet mount) is associated with a positive test result for *Chlamydia* (odds ratio = 3.8).[15] For this reason, women who complain of vaginal discharge should be screened for and, depending on clinical suspicion, treated presumptively for *N. gonorrhoeae* and *Chlamydia* infection at the initial visit (Table 102-2). The Centers for Disease Control and Prevention also recommends syphilis testing for women engaged in high-risk sexual behavior, such as those having multiple sexual partners or a new sexual partner or engaging in unprotected intercourse. Finally, women of childbearing age should be screened for pregnancy, because this may impact medical treatment.

TREATMENT

Recommended treatment regimens are listed in **Table 102-4**. The use of *Lactobacillus* intravaginal suppositories and probiotics to restore the normal vaginal flora is an ongoing area of research. Treating male sexual partners is not beneficial for preventing recurrence, but consider treating female partners, particularly with frequent recurrences, because bacterial vaginosis can spread between female partners.[2] Counsel patients receiving metronidazole against consuming alcoholic beverages during the treatment period and for the following 24 hours to avoid a disulfiram-like reaction. Advise patients to refrain from intercourse or to use condoms during treatment.[1]

Overall cure rates 4 weeks after treatment do not differ significantly for a 7-day regimen of oral metronidazole, metronidazole vaginal gel, and clindamycin vaginal cream. Metronidazole vaginal gel has fewer side effects (i.e., GI disturbance and unpleasant taste) but should not be used in women who are allergic to the oral preparation.

Recurrence of symptoms is seen within 3 months in 30% of treated patients who initially show a response. The reasons for this are unclear but could be from sexual transmission.[15] Metronidazole gel 0.75% twice weekly for 4 to 6 months prevents recurrence.[1]

TABLE 102-4 Treatment Regimens for Bacterial Vaginosis

Agent	Dosage
Recommended Regimens	
Metronidazole*	500 milligrams PO twice a day for 7 d
Clindamycin cream 2%	One full applicator intravaginally every night for 7 d
Metronidazole gel 0.75%	One full applicator intravaginally once a day for 5 d
Alternative Regimens	
Clindamycin	300 milligrams PO twice a day for 7 d
Clindamycin ovules	100 milligrams intravaginally every night for 3 d
Tinidazole	2 grams PO daily for 2 d
Tinidazole	1 gram PO daily for 5 d
Regimens for Pregnant Women	
Metronidazole*	250 milligrams PO three times a day for 7 d
Metronidazole*	500 milligrams PO twice a day for 7 d
Clindamycin	300 milligrams PO twice a day for 7 d

*Avoid alcohol during and 24 h after treatment. Metronidazole is a pregnancy category B drug.

BACTERIAL VAGINOSIS COMPLICATIONS

Bacterial vaginosis has been associated with several adverse health outcomes, including facilitation of co-infection with sexually transmitted infections such as human immunodeficiency virus, herpes simplex virus-2, *Chlamydia trachomatis*, and *N. gonorrhoeae* by decreasing local secretory leukocyte protease inhibitor levels.[1,12] Bacterial vaginosis is also linked to complications related to pregnancy and surgical procedures, such as spontaneous abortion, premature rupture of membranes, amniotic fluid infection, chorioamnionitis, preterm delivery, postpartum endometritis, pelvic inflammatory disease, postoperative wound infection, and infection after vaginal and abdominal hysterectomy.[16]

PREGNANT WOMEN

The Centers for Disease Control and Prevention recommends treating all symptomatic pregnant women. Recommended treatment regimens are listed in Table 102-4. The Centers for Disease Control and Prevention no longer recommends routine screening of asymptomatic pregnant women.[1] Pregnant women who are at high risk for preterm labor should be considered for treatment to avoid preterm labor and other adverse outcomes of pregnancy.[5] However, studies have not been able to demonstrate clear benefit in preventing adverse outcomes of pregnancy.[1,17-19] **Topical clindamycin preparations should not be used in the second half of pregnancy** because of an increased association of adverse events, including low infant birth weight and neonatal infections.

CANDIDA VAGINITIS

***Candida* species are the second most common cause of infectious vaginitis.**[20] Prevalence data for vulvovaginal candidiasis vary because the disease is not reportable, many women self-medicate with over-the-counter preparations, and as many as half the women in whom candidiasis is diagnosed also have other conditions.[20] The Centers for Disease Control and Prevention estimates that 75% of women will have at least one episode of vulvovaginal candidiasis in their lifetime.[1]

The organism is isolated in up to 20% of asymptomatic, healthy women of childbearing age, some of whom are celibate. Some women remain entirely asymptomatic despite being heavily colonized with *Candida* species.

Vulvovaginal candidiasis is rare in nonestrogenized premenarchal girls but does occur and is common under 2 years of age. Consider undiagnosed juvenile diabetes or other forms of immunosuppression if *Candida* is diagnosed in a toilet-trained child.[4] Incidence decreases after menopause unless replacement estrogen is being used, which further emphasizes the hormonal dependence of the infection.

Candidiasis can be classified as either an uncomplicated or complicated infection. Uncomplicated infections are sporadic, produce mild to moderate symptoms, are the result of *Candida albicans*, and occur in the nonpregnant, immunocompetent host. Complicated infections are recurrent (four or more infections per year), produce severe symptoms or findings, are the result of suspected or proven non-*albicans* candidiasis, and occur in an abnormal host (women who have uncontrolled diabetes, debilitation, or immunosuppression, or are pregnant). Approximately 10% to 20% of women have complicated disease. Recurrent vulvovaginal candidiasis occurs in <5% of women.[1,21]

C. albicans strains account for 85% to 92% of *Candida* organisms isolated from the vagina. *Candida glabrata* and *Candida tropicalis* are the most common non-*albicans* strains and are often more resistant to conventional therapy.

Candidal organisms gain access to the vaginal lumen and secretions predominantly from the adjacent perianal area. Candidal organisms must first adhere to the vaginal epithelial cells for colonization to take place, and *C. albicans* adheres in greater numbers than other species.

The growth of *Candida* is held in check by the normal vaginal flora, and symptoms of vaginitis usually occur only when the normal balance is upset. Increased colonization by *Candida* resulting in subsequent symptomatic infection may be caused by conditions that (1) inhibit the growth of normal vaginal flora, particularly *Lactobacillus* species (e.g., systemic antibiotics); (2) diminish the glycogen stores in vaginal epithelial cells (e.g., diabetes mellitus, pregnancy, oral contraceptive use, and hormonal replacement therapy); or (3) increase the pH of vaginal secretions (e.g., menstrual blood or semen). Factors that favor increased rates of vaginal colonization include pregnancy, oral contraceptive use, uncontrolled diabetes mellitus, and frequent visits to sexually transmitted infection clinics (perhaps as a result of antimicrobial therapy). This infection is not considered a sexually transmitted infection, although it can be transmitted by sexual intercourse. The wearing of tight-fitting, particularly synthetic, undergarments may also contribute to the problem because of increased temperature. Although all of these factors are thought to be associated with symptomatic disease, there is poor evidence to prove that any of them is causative.[20] Evidence supporting an association between antibiotic use and vulvovaginal candidiasis is limited. However, antibiotics are thought to increase the risk of vulvovaginal candidiasis by killing endogenous normal flora.

DIAGNOSIS

Clinical symptoms include leukorrhea, severe vaginal pruritus, external dysuria, and dyspareunia. **Vaginal pruritus is the most common and specific symptom.** Complaints of discharge vary from little to copious white vaginal discharge. Symptoms vary in severity, but exacerbation is frequently seen in the week prior to menses or with coitus, perhaps because these factors cause the pH to become more alkaline. Odor is unusual and, if present, favors a diagnosis of bacterial vaginosis rather than candidiasis.

Gynecologic examination may reveal vulvar erythema and edema, vaginal erythema, and discharge. Discharge varies from none to watery to homogeneously thick and "cottage cheese–like." Discharge often adheres to the vaginal walls.

The diagnosis is confirmed with a normal vaginal pH (4.0 to 4.5) and visualization of budding yeast and pseudohyphae on slide preparation of vaginal secretions (**Figure 102-2**). The sensitivity of microscopic examination using a sample prepared with normal saline is only 40% to 60%. Adding two drops of 10% potassium hydroxide to the vaginal secretions dissolves the vaginal epithelial cells while leaving yeast buds and pseudohyphae intact. This increases the sensitivity of microscopic examination to 80% and yields almost 100% specificity. Empiric treatment is suggested for symptomatic patients with negative findings on microscopic examination if *Candida* cultures cannot be obtained.[1]

TREATMENT

Recommended treatment regimens are listed in **Table 102-5**. Therapy regimens are effective in treating over 80% of cases of uncomplicated vaginal candidiasis. Topically applied azole drugs are more effective than nystatin, with relief of symptoms in 80% to 90% of patients who complete treatment. Consider patient preference because creams, lotions, sprays, vaginal tablets, suppositories, and coated tampons are all equally efficacious.[22]

The azole drugs are all available over the counter in treatment regimens of 1, 3, or 7 days. Uncomplicated vulvovaginal candidiasis responds to all azoles, including single-dose therapy.[23] Other than initial burning and irritation, side effects of topical agents are unusual.

Single-dose treatment with oral fluconazole is as effective as topical therapy in the treatment of uncomplicated vulvovaginal candidiasis. Patient preference should be considered, because oral therapy is often more convenient, although insurance and cultural variables can influence preference.[24] Oral treatment may occasionally cause GI symptoms, headache, and rash.[25] Ketoconazole can cause liver toxicity, and therefore, it as been removed from many formularies. The oral azoles can interact with a variety of other medications, including astemizole, calcium channel antagonists, cisapride, warfarin, cyclosporine A, oral hypoglycemic agents, phenytoin, protease inhibitors, tacrolimus, terfenadine, theophylline, trimetrexate, and rifampin.

Sexual partners should not be treated unless the woman has frequent recurrences.

Self-medication is sometimes advised in women with recurrence of previously diagnosed vulvovaginal candidiasis; however, studies demonstrate poor ability to accurately self-diagnose candidiasis even with a

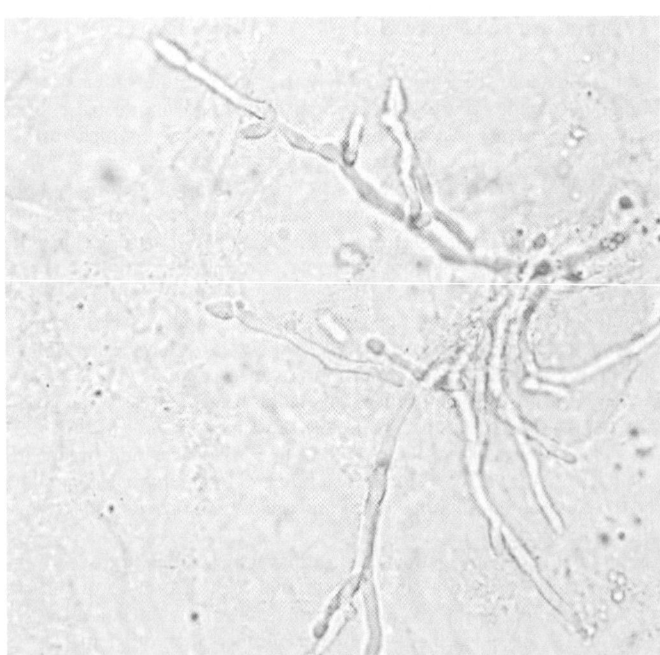

FIGURE 102-2. Hyphae of *Candida albicans,* potassium hydroxide wet mount. [Reproduced with permission from Knoop et al: *The Atlas of Emergency Medicine*, 3rd ed. © 2010 McGraw-Hill Inc. Fig 25-16. Photo contributor: H. Hunter Handsfield: *Atlas of Sexually Transmitted Diseases.* New York, NY: McGraw-Hill; 1992.)

TABLE 102-5 Treatment Regimens for Vulvovaginal Candidiasis*

Agent	Formulation	Dosage
Uncomplicated Vulvovaginal Candidiasis		
Butoconazole†	2% cream	1 applicator intravaginally QHS × 3 d
Clotrimazole	1% cream	1 applicator intravaginally QHS × 7 d
	2% cream	1 applicator intravaginally QHS × 3 d
	100-milligram suppository	1 suppository intravaginally QHS × 7 d
	200-milligram suppository	1 suppository intravaginally QHS × 3 d
	500-milligram suppository	1 suppository intravaginally QHS × 1 dose
Miconazole	2% cream	1 applicator intravaginally QHS × 7 d
	4% cream	1 applicator intravaginally QHS × 3 d
	100-milligram suppository	1 suppository intravaginally QHS × 7 d
	200-milligram suppository	1 suppository intravaginally QHS × 3 d
	1200-milligram suppository	1 suppository intravaginally QHS × 1 dose
Nystatin	100,000-unit vaginal tablet	1 tablet QHS × 14 d
Terconazole	0.4% cream	1 applicator intravaginally QHS × 7 d
	0.8% cream	1 applicator intravaginally QHS × 3 d
	80-milligram suppository	1 suppository intravaginally QHS × 3 d
Tioconazole	6.5% ointment	1 applicator intravaginally QHS × 1 dose
Fluconazole†	150 mg oral tablet	1 tablet PO × 1 dose

*Not all possible regimens listed.

†Not recommended in pregnancy. **Pregnant patient should be treated with topical azoles for 7 days. Oral fluconazole is a Category C medication and thus should be avoided in pregnancy.**

Abbreviation: QHS = every night at bedtime.

prior history of the disease.[5,26] Therefore women who fail to respond to over-the-counter therapy or have recurrence within 2 months should be evaluated by a physician.

The treatment of **complicated vulvovaginal candidiasis** (both severe and recurrent cases) requires longer duration of therapy with topical and oral azoles or alternative therapies. In severe cases, consider treating with a topical azole for 7 to 14 days or treatment with oral fluconazole, 150 milligrams on days 1 and 3 for a total of two doses. In cases of recurrence, consider treating with a topical azole for 7 to 14 days or fluconazole, 100, 150, or 200 milligrams on days 1, 4, and 7 for a total of three doses.[1,25,26]

CANDIDIASIS COMPLICATIONS

Vaginal and microscopic examinations should be performed if symptoms persist or recur within 2 months, and precipitating factors, such as high blood glucose levels, should be controlled. However, most women with recurrences do not have obvious precipitating causes. Vaginal cultures should be obtained to confirm clinical diagnosis but also to indentify any unusual species such as *C. glabrata*. Azoles are not very effective in treating vaginitis caused by *C. glabrata*.

Management of women with frequent recurrence is aimed at control with a long-term suppressive prophylactic regimen, rather than cure. The reason that some women, many of whom have no underlying pathology, experience frequent recurrences of infection with resulting morbidity is not fully understood. Current views suggest that local vaginal immune mechanisms may be responsible for frequent relapses. Maintenance regimens with oral fluconazole (100-, 150-, or 200-milligram doses weekly for 6 months) are the first line of treatment.[1]

TRICHOMONAS VAGINITIS

Trichomonas vaginalis **is the most common nonviral sexually transmitted infection and accounts for 15% to 20% of cases of acute vaginitis.** There are an estimated 3.7 million Americans infected with *T. vaginalis*, more than *N. gonorrhoeae* and *Chlamydia* combined.[27] Both men and women can be infected, and it is spread through sexual contact. Infection is more common in certain racial and ethnic groups. Incidence is highest among black women at 13.3%, compared with 1.8% of Hispanic women and 1.3% of white women.[28] The prevalence of *T. vaginalis* infection increases with age,[1] unlike other sexually transmitted infections, such as *Chlamydia* and *N. gonorrhoeae*, for which the prevalence is highest among adolescents and young adults. Risk of *T. vaginalis* infection is associated with increasing numbers of sexual partners (recent or remote), early initiation of sexual activity, lower educational levels (high school or below), and poverty.

Trichomoniasis is a parasitic infection with the single-celled protozoan *T. vaginalis*, a flagellated organism (**Figure 102-3**). Infection can produce local inflammation when the organism attaches to the vaginal mucosa. As many as 50% of women are asymptomatic. Clinically symptomatic women with *Trichomonas* vaginitis present with vaginal discharge, pruritus, and irritation. The classic discharge is described as frothy and malodorous. Symptoms generally develop within 5 to 28 days; however, untreated infections can last for months to years and produce symptoms at any time.[29]

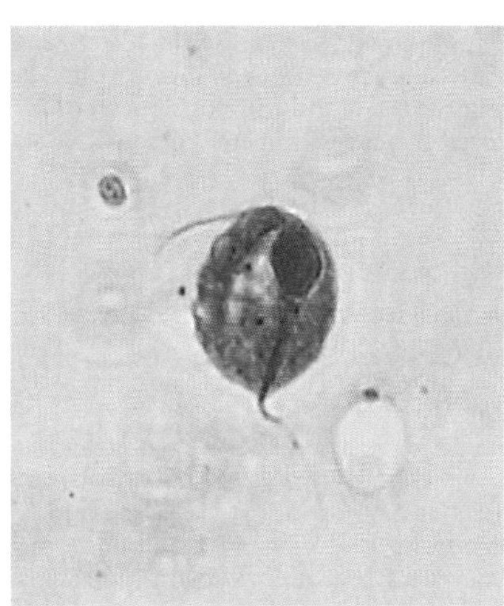

FIGURE 102-3. Trichomonad. [Reprinted with permission of Piotr Rotkiewicz.]

DIAGNOSIS

Clinical diagnosis of *Trichomonas* vaginitis traditionally relies on microscopic examination of the vaginal secretions and visualization of motile trichomonads (Figure 102-3). Microscopy should be performed immediately following sample collection or the organism will lose motility. The sensitivity of microscopic identification of trichomonads is 60% to 70%.[1] Although associated with low cost and immediate results, there are several disadvantages to this method, including operator error and overall poor sensitivity. Culture is 95% sensitive and considered the gold standard in diagnosis. However, results may not be available for 2 to 5 days. There are several newer testing options, including two different point-of-care diagnostic tests. Results of the immunochromatographic capillary flow dipstick technology test, OSOM Trichomonas Rapid Test (Genzyme Diagnostics, Cambridge, MA), and the nucleic acid probe test, Affirm VP III (Becton Dickinson, San Jose, CA), are available in 10 minutes and 45 minutes, respectively. Both have a sensitivity of >83% and specificity of >97%.[1,30,31] The U.S. Food and Drug Administration–cleared polymerase chain reaction assay for *N. gonorrhoeae* and *Chlamydia* infection, Amplicor (Roche Diagnostics, Indianapolis, IN), has been modified for *T. vaginalis* detection in both vaginal and endocervical swabs, as well as urine. The sensitivity ranges from 88% to 97%, and the specificity ranges from 98% to 99%. APTIMA *T. vaginalis* Analyte Specific Reagents are available for RNA-mediated amplification testing using the instrumentation platform APTIMA Combo2 (Gen-Probe, Bedford, MA) currently used to diagnose *N. gonorrhoeae* and *Chlamydia* infections. The sensitivity ranges from 74% to 98%, and the specificity ranges from 87% to 98%.[1]

TREATMENT

Treatment regimens for acute *Trichomonas* vaginitis are listed in **Table 102-6**. The nitroimidazoles, metronidazole and tinidazole, are the only medications effective in treating trichomoniasis. Metronidazole gel is considerably less effective (<50%) than oral metronidazole preparations, and so the gel is not recommended. Single-dose treatment is preferable because of lower cost, fewer side effects, and greater patient adherence to the regimen. However, patients whose infection is not responsive to single-dose therapy may require a 7-day course of therapy. There is a 90% cure rate with either the single- or multiple-dose regimen. Cure rates increase to >90% when sexual partners are treated simultaneously. Patients with a true allergy can undergo desensitization in consultation with a specialist.[1]

TABLE 102-6 Treatment Regimens for Trichomoniasis

Agent	Dosage
Recommended Regimen	
Metronidazole*	2 grams PO in a single dose
Tinidazole†	2 grams PO in a single dose
Alternative Regimen	
Metronidazole*	500 milligrams PO twice a day for 7 d

*Metronidazole is a pregnancy Category B drug.

†Tinidazole is a pregnancy Category C drug.

Counsel patients to abstain from sexual intercourse until drug therapy has been completed and the patient and their partner(s) are asymptomatic and to avoid alcohol use during therapy and for 24 hours after completion of drug therapy with metronidazole to avoid a disulfiram-like reaction.

TRICHOMONIASIS COMPLICATIONS

The spread of *Trichomonas* infection is difficult to control, because up to 50% to 75% of those infected are asymptomatic and reinfection is common. Recurrence of disease is frequent and may necessitate multiple courses of treatment.

T. vaginalis infection is associated with several adverse health outcomes, including preterm birth, delivery of low-birth-weight infants, and pelvic inflammatory disease. It has also been associated with increased transmission of several other infections, including human immunodeficiency virus, herpes simplex virus, and human papillomavirus infection. Not only does *Trichomonas* infection increase the likelihood of human immunodeficiency virus acquisition, but it also promotes human immunodeficiency virus transmission and viral shedding.[32,33]

SPECIAL POPULATIONS

Human immunodeficiency virus–positive individuals are more likely to become infected with *T. vaginalis* and have higher complication rates. Consider 7-day therapy for human immunodeficiency virus–positive individuals because studies have indicated that single-dose therapy is less effective.[1]

Due to the potential adverse outcomes, pregnant women should receive treatment with oral metronidazole. Women can be safely treated with single-dose metronidazole therapy at any stage of pregnancy. Tinidazole safety in pregnancy is not well studied. Breastfeeding mothers should withhold nursing during treatment with metronidazole and for 12 to 24 hours after the last dose. If treated with tinidazole, patients should hold breastfeeding for 3 days after the last dose.

CONTACT VULVOVAGINITIS

Contact dermatitis results from the exposure of the vulvar epithelium and vaginal mucosa to a primary chemical irritant or an allergen. Irritant dermatitis is more common than allergic dermatitis.[34] Common irritants and/or allergens include chemically scented douches, soaps, bubble baths, and deodorants; perfumes, dyes, and scents in toilet paper, tampons, pads, and feminine hygiene products; topical vaginal antibiotics; laundry detergents, dryer sheets, and fabric softeners; and tight slacks, pantyhose, and synthetic underwear. Benzocaine, used by women to control vulvar discomfort, can also cause a particularly severe contact dermatitis.

DIAGNOSIS AND TREATMENT

Diagnosis may be difficult due to variation in severity of symptoms and presence of other preexisting conditions. Clinically, patients report local swelling and itching or a burning sensation. Physical findings range from local erythema and edema to excoriation, ulceration, and secondary infection. Local vesiculation and ulceration are more common with allergens or with primary irritants used in strong concentrations. Also consider herpes infections if vesicles are present. Vaginal pH changes may promote colonization and infection with *C. albicans*, which can obscure the primary cause.

Diagnosis of contact vulvovaginitis is made by ruling out an infectious cause and identifying the offending agent. Most cases of mild vulvovaginal contact dermatitis resolve spontaneously when the causative agent is withdrawn. Cool sitz baths and application of wet compresses of dilute boric acid or Burow's solution may afford relief for patients with severe painful reactions. A few days of therapy with topical corticosteroids, such as hydrocortisone acetate (0.5% to 2.5%), fluocinolone acetonide (0.01% to 0.2%), or triamcinolone acetonide (0.025%), applied two or three times daily, provide symptomatic relief and promote healing. Oral antihistamines may be helpful if a true allergic reaction is present. Superinfection with *C. albicans* should be treated as previously described in the section on *Candida* vaginitis.

ATROPHIC VAGINITIS

Vaginal atrophy, present in 60% of women 4 years after menopause, can result in atrophic vaginitis.[35] Decreases in ovarian steroid production that occur in the menopausal woman lead to profound changes in the vulva, vagina, cervix, urethra, and bladder. The changes vary widely from one patient to another. The vagina loses its normal rugae, and the vaginal mucosa becomes attenuated, pale, and almost transparent as a result of decreased vascularity. The squamous epithelium atrophies, the glycogen content of the cells decreases, and the vaginal pH ranges from 5.5 to 7.0. The upper one third of the vagina constricts, and the entire vagina becomes shorter in length and loses its elasticity. The mucosa is only three or four cells thick and is less resistant to minor trauma and infection. The cervix atrophies and retracts and may become flush with the apex of the vault.

DIAGNOSIS AND TREATMENT

Symptoms include vaginal dryness, soreness, itching, dyspareunia, and occasional spotting or discharge. Discharge is thin, scant, and yellowish or pink. The vaginal epithelium appears thin, inflamed, and even ulcerated.

A clinical vaginal infection with copious purulent discharge may develop due to increased vaginal pH, which permits growth of nonacidophilic coliform organisms and the disappearance of *Lactobacillus* species. *Candida* and *Trichomonas* infections are rare in the postmenopausal woman unless estrogenic replacement therapy is used.

Wet preparations demonstrate erythrocytes, increased polymorphonuclear neutrophils, and small, round epithelial cells, which are immature squamous cells that have not been exposed to sufficient estrogen.

Treatment of atrophic vaginitis consists primarily of topical vaginal estrogen. Creams, pessaries, tablets, and the estradiol vaginal ring are all effective in treating the symptoms.[35] Side effects of treatment may include uterine bleeding, breast pain, perineal pain, and endometrial hyperstimulation. Estrogen should not be prescribed to patients with a history of cancer of any of the reproductive organs. Atrophic vaginitis is usually not seen in patients who are already taking systemic estrogen replacement therapy.

Patients should be referred to their own doctors or a clinic for treatment and follow-up to monitor therapy, because all formulations of estrogen, even at low dosages, show systemic absorption and have potentially harmful side effects.[36] In addition, any patient with postmenopausal bleeding, either by history or physical examination, should be referred to a gynecologist to rule out carcinoma.

BARTHOLIN GLAND CYST AND ABSCESS

Bartholin glands are located in the labia minora. The ducts of the glands drain into the posterior vestibule at the 4 o'clock and 8 o'clock positions. Normally the glands are pea sized, but may form a cyst or abscess. The glands begin to function at puberty to provide moisture for the vestibule and involute as women age. Obstruction of the duct may result in a cyst or abscess. A cyst does not need to be present for an abscess to develop. Abscesses may become quite large and cause extreme pain. Bartholin gland abscesses tend to be polymicrobial, although *N. gonorrhoeae* and *C. trachomatis* have been implicated.[37]

DIAGNOSIS AND TREATMENT

Bartholin gland abscess is characterized as a mass in the posterior introitus near the 4 o'clock or 8 o'clock position that has developed over several days. If the abscess was preceded by a cyst, the abscess may develop over a longer period of time. Pain, induration, and fluctuance are usually present. Systemic symptoms such as fever and chills are rarely present.

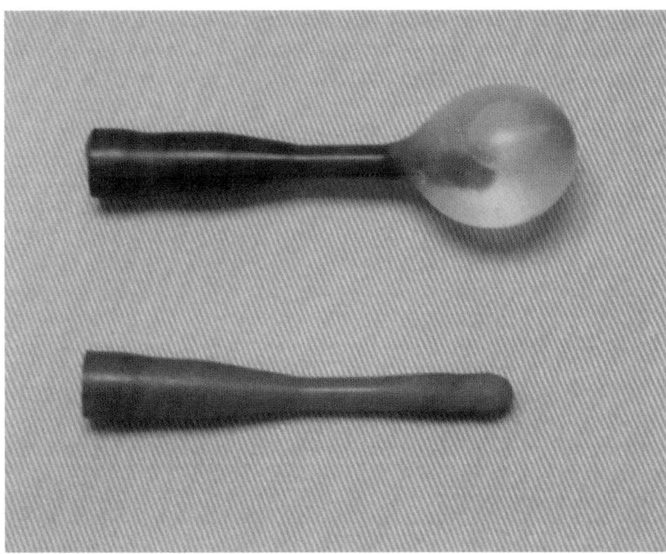

FIGURE 102-4. Word catheter. [Reproduced with permission from Reichman EF: *Emergency Medicine Procedures,* 2nd ed. McGraw-Hill, Inc., 2013. Figure 138-2, p. 932.]

Incision and drainage of an abscess is usually necessary but should not be performed until the abscess is a well-defined, walled-off structure. If the abscess is not ready for incision and drainage, give the patient broad-spectrum antibiotics and analgesics, and advise warm sitz baths. Most patients present with an exquisitely tender, hyperemic, fluctuant mass that needs drainage.

Provide analgesia with a local injection of 2 to 4 mL of 1% lidocaine. To drain the abscess, make a stab incision with a #11 scalpel on the mucosal surface of the vestibule, just lateral to the hymenal ring in the region of the Bartholin gland, where the abscess cavity is closest to the mucosal surface. Extend the stab incision only for a few millimeters—an incision that is too large will result in displacement of the Word catheter. A Word catheter (**Figure 102-4**) is the size of a #10 Foley catheter with a 1-in (2.5-cm) stem and an inflatable balloon. Insert the Word catheter into the incision site, and inflate the balloon with 2 to 4 mL of water. Tuck the end of the catheter into the vagina. The catheter should remain in place for 4 to 6 weeks to avoid recurrence.[38] Case reports describe using plastic tubing (**Figure 102-5**) and pediatric Foley catheters for abscess drainage when a Word catheter is not available.[39,40] Prescribe analgesics and broad-spectrum antibiotics, and give instructions for follow-up care. If *N. gonorrhoeae* and *C. trachomatis* infection are possible, direct antibiotic coverage accordingly (Table 102-2). Patients with recurrent abscess may require definitive surgical care and should be provided with specialty referral.

VAGINAL FOREIGN BODIES

Consider a vaginal foreign body in patients with chronic vaginal discharge. Objects removed in the ED include retained tampons and toilet tissue, items used for sexual stimulation, packets of illegal drugs, and various other items.

Premenarchal children presenting with vaginal discharge, especially if bloody or brown, should be evaluated for a vaginal foreign body, which is found in 4% to 10% of such cases. The discharge associated with a foreign body occurs daily and is often malodorous.[4] Potential foreign bodies include small pieces of toilet paper or cloth and small toys/objects.

Vaginal irrigation with 0.9% normal saline can be attempted to visualize and remove a foreign body in cooperative children >7 years of age. Vaginoscopy under anesthesia in the operating room may be necessary in younger children.

The use of imaging modalities is limited by the composition of the foreign body. Radiolucent foreign bodies are not seen on plain radiographs and may not be detected by pelvic ultrasound. MRI may aid in the localization of nonmetallic objects but is not always available and is not necessarily conclusive.

Treatment of vaginal foreign bodies is removal either manually or by irrigation.

PINWORMS

Patients with pinworms (*Enterobius vermicularis*) complain of anal and/or vaginal pruritus, which is more intense at night (when the gravid female pinworms pass out from the intestinal tract to lay eggs on the

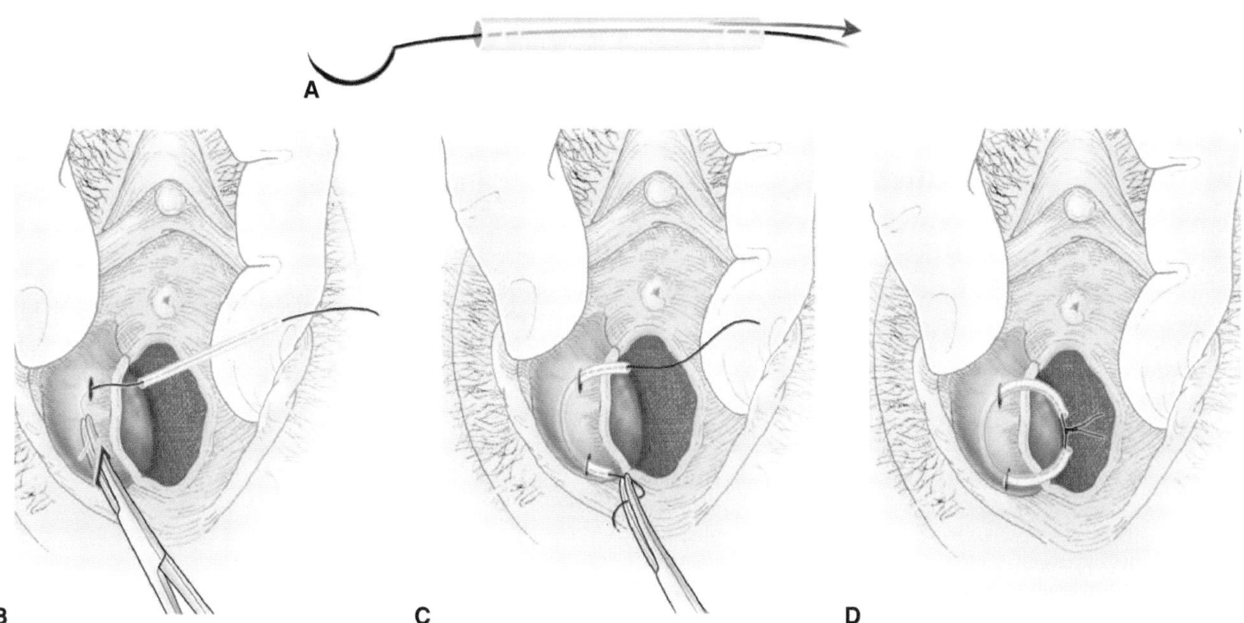

FIGURE 102-5. A. Obtain 7 cm of narrow tubing, and insert silk suture through tubing. B. After drainage, make a second stab incision into the abscess cavity and insert the threaded tubing. C. Use a hemostat to grasp the threaded tubing through both stab sites. D. Suture the threads so they are secure. [Reproduced with permission from Reichman EF: *Emergency Medicine Procedures,* 2nd ed. McGraw-Hill, Inc., 2013. Figure 138-5, Parts A, E, F, G, p. 934.]

TABLE 102-7 Treatment Regimens for Trichomoniasis

Agent and Dosage	Comments
Mebendazole 100 milligrams PO × 1 Repeated in 1 wk	Use with caution in pregnancy
Albendazole 400 milligrams PO × 1 Repeated in 2 wk	Contraindicated in pregnancy
Pyrantel pamoate 11 milligrams/kg PO × 1 (maximum single dose, 1 gram) Repeat dose every 2 wk × 2	Available without prescription

perineal skin). The worms may migrate from the anus to the vagina in children.

The diagnosis is made by visualization of 1-cm-long, thin white worms exiting the anus. Alternately, a sample can be obtained on cellophane tape and used for identification of ova, which are large and double-walled in appearance, on microscopy.

Treat the child and all family members with an antiparasitic agent (**Table 102-7**). Treatments are repeated, because mature worms are more vulnerable to treatment than young worms.[4]

VULVAR TRAUMA

Nonobstetric vulvar trauma is uncommon; however, it is associated with significant physical and psychological consequences. Various types of trauma can be seen including injuries sustained during consensual and nonconsensual sexual activity, accidental injuries including straddle-type injuries, other forms of physical assault, and self-mutilation. Patients may present with abrasions, tears, lacerations, hematomas, burns, and bite wounds. Depending on the situation, gynecologic consultation and examination under anesthesia may be necessary.

Evaluate patients with vulvar trauma for associated vaginal, urethral, anal, and bony pelvis injuries, and treat accordingly.[41]

Acknowledgement: The authors wish to thank Drs. Gloria Kuhn and Robert Wahl who contributed to this chapter in the previous edition.

REFERENCES

The complete reference list is available online at www.TintinalliEM.com.

CHAPTER 103 Pelvic Inflammatory Disease

Suzanne M. Shepherd
Brian Weiss
William H. Shoff

INTRODUCTION AND EPIDEMIOLOGY

The term pelvic inflammatory disease (PID) comprises a spectrum of infections of the female upper reproductive tract. It is a common and serious disease initiated by ascending infection from the vagina and cervix. PID includes salpingitis, endometritis, myometritis, parametritis, oophoritis, and tubo-ovarian abscess and may extend to produce periappendicitis, pelvic peritonitis, and perihepatitis (Fitz-Hugh–Curtis syndrome). PID is the most common serious infection in sexually active women age 16 to 25 years.[1]

Long-term sequelae, including tubal factor infertility, implantation failure after in vitro fertilization, ectopic pregnancy, and chronic pain, may ultimately affect 11% of reproductive-aged women.[2] The most common cause of death is rupture of a tubo-ovarian abscess, and the mortality associated with rupture remains at 5% to 10%, even with current treatment methods.

PATHOPHYSIOLOGY

ORGANISMS ASSOCIATED WITH PID

Neisseria gonorrhoeae and *Chlamydia trachomatis* can be isolated in many cases of PID, and therapy is directed primarily against these organisms. However, polymicrobial infection, including infection with anaerobic and aerobic vaginal flora, is evident from cultured material from the upper reproductive tract.[3] **Table 103-1** lists common pathogenic organisms associated with PID. *N. gonorrhoeae* and *C. trachomatis* are often instrumental in initial infection of the upper genital tract, whereas anaerobes, facultative anaerobes, and other bacteria are isolated increasingly as inflammation increases and abscesses form.

Bacterial vaginosis (BV) is frequently identified in women with PID, and the type of BV-associated microorganism (*Gardnerella vaginalis, Mycoplasma hominis, Ureaplasma urealyticum*, pigmented or nonpigmented anaerobic gram-negative rods) may make a difference in the likelihood of developing PID.[4,5]

Infection with ***Trichomonas vaginalis*** is associated with a fourfold increase in the incidence of acute endometritis. Co-infection with **herpes simplex virus 2** and ***C. trachomatis, N. gonorrhoeae,*** or bacteria causing vaginosis is also associated with acute endometritis. Infection with herpes simplex virus 2 causes fallopian tube inflammation and lower tract ulceration that may disrupt the endocervical canal mucous barrier.[6] **Human immunodeficiency virus 1 (HIV-1)** infection is associated with an increased incidence of *C. trachomatis* infection, increased incidence of co-infection with *Candida* and human papillomavirus, and increased risk of progression to PID.[7]

PID may result from ***Mycobacterium tuberculosis*** infection in endemic areas.[8] **Schistosomes** can cause genital infection, including a PID-like tubal infection, infertility, and chronic abortion, and a recent report links schistosomiasis to HIV transmission in Africa. ***Actinomyces*** species have been identified almost exclusively in patients with intrauterine devices (IUDs).[9]

ASCENDING INFECTION

Most cases of PID are presumed to originate with sexually transmitted infections (STIs) of the lower genital tract, followed by ascending infection of the upper tract. The original STI may be asymptomatic. The precise mechanisms by which upper genital tract infection and inflammation are initiated and propagated are not well known. Although the cervical mucus serves as a functional barrier to ascending infection much of the time, its efficacy may be decreased by hormonal changes during menstruation and ovulation and by retrograde menstruation. Intercourse may contribute to the ascent of infection due to rhythmic

TABLE 103-1 Organisms Associated with Pelvic Inflammatory Disease

Sexually Transmitted Organisms
Chlamydia trachomatis
Neisseria gonorrhoeae
Herpes simplex virus (types 1 and 2)
Trichomonas vaginalis
Endogenous Genital Tract *Mycoplasma*
Mycoplasma genitalium, Mycoplasma hominis, Ureaplasma urealyticum
Anaerobic Bacteria
Bacteroides species, Peptostreptococcus, Prevotella bivia, Leptotrichia sanguinegens/amnionii, Atopobium vaginae
Aerobic Bacteria
Gardnerella vaginalis, Haemophilus influenzae, Streptococcus agalactiae, Escherichia coli, and other gram-negative rods, *Actinomyces israelii, Campylobacter fetus*

TABLE 103-2 Risk Factors Associated with Pelvic Inflammatory Disease[11-17]

Multiple sexual partners
History of sexually transmitted infection or pelvic inflammatory disease
History of sexual abuse
Frequent vaginal douching
Intrauterine device insertion within previous month
Adolescence, younger adulthood
Lower socioeconomic status
Postabortal

mechanical uterine contractions. Bacteria also may be carried by, or along with, sperm into the uterus and tubes. Uterine infection usually is limited to the endometrium but can be more invasive in a gravid or postpartum uterus. Tubal infection initially affects only the mucosa, but acute, complement-mediated transmural inflammation may develop rapidly and increase in intensity with repeated infection. Inflammation may extend to uninfected parametrial structures, including the appendix and bowel. Infection may spread by direct extension of purulent material from the fallopian tubes or via lymphatic spread beyond the pelvis to involve the hepatic capsule with acute perihepatitis (Fitz-Hugh–Curtis syndrome) and produce acute peritonitis.

RISK FACTORS FOR PID

Multiple risk factors are associated with development of PID (**Table 103-2**).[4,10-17]

IUD use has been associated with an increased risk for PID. Although the majority of risk occurs within 21 days of insertion, the presence of an IUD is associated with complicated PID irrespective of the duration of use.[9,13-15] The risk of PID in IUD users is more related to the development of STI than the IUD,[18,19] and STI screening and treatment at the time of insertion can significantly decrease the likelihood that PID will develop.[20]

Pregnancy decreases the risk of PID because the cervical os is protected by the mucous plug. However, PID can occur during the first trimester and is associated with substantial fetal loss and preterm delivery.

COMPLICATIONS OF PID

PID is associated with a number of serious clinical sequelae. Tubo-ovarian abscess is reported in up to one third of women hospitalized for PID. Infection and inflammation can lead to scarring and adhesions within tubal lumens. **Ectopic pregnancy is more frequent in women who have had PID than in those who have never had an ectopic pregnancy.** Tubal factor infertility is increased by 12% to 50% in women with a past diagnosis of PID, and the incidence increases with the number and severity of past PID episodes.[21] Asymptomatic or silent PID appears to be associated with tubal factor infertility as well. Sequelae of PID include recurrence of PID, chronic pelvic pain, menstrual disturbances, and chronic dyspareunia. Recurrence of PID may occur because of inadequately treated infection, nontreatment of partner(s), or reinfection from another sexual contact. In follow-up to the Pelvic Inflammatory Disease Evaluation and Clinical Health trial, those with recurrence of PID were five times more likely to experience chronic pelvic pain.[22] PID may also be associated with an increased risk of ovarian borderline tumors.[23]

CLINICAL FEATURES

The clinical presentation of PID is variable. The most common presenting complaint is lower abdominal pain, most frequently described as bilateral and dull or crampy. Pain may be exacerbated by movement or by sexual activity. Other symptoms include abnormal vaginal discharge (75% of individuals), vaginal and postcoital bleeding (more than one third of patients), irritative voiding symptoms, fever, malaise, nausea, and vomiting.[24] Symptoms occur most commonly early in the menstrual cycle or at the end of the menses and are attributed to low progesterone levels and coincident thinning of the cervical mucosal barrier.

The physical examination is usually notable for lower abdominal tenderness, cervical motion tenderness, and uterine or adnexal tenderness. Involuntary guarding and rebound tenderness may be present and may indicate associated peritonitis. The positive predictive value of these findings varies depending on the prevalence of PID in a given clinical population. Adnexal tenderness appears to have a sensitivity of 95%.[25] Mucopurulent cervicitis is a common finding, and its absence should raise consideration of another diagnosis. In women who are suspected of having PID and for whom there is no likely alternative diagnosis for abdominal pain, the presence of fever, adnexal tenderness, and an elevated erythrocyte sedimentation rate are significant independent predictors of endometritis and correctly classify 65% of patients with laparoscopically proven PID (95% confidence interval, 61% to 99%).[25,26]

Right upper quadrant tenderness, particularly with jaundice, may indicate perihepatic inflammation. **Fitz-Hugh–Curtis syndrome** is perihepatitis, demonstrated by right upper quadrant pain in a woman with a clinical diagnosis of PID and no other cause for this pain. It is an uncommon complication and responds to standard antibiotic treatment for PID.[27]

The differential diagnosis of PID is broad and includes cervicitis, ectopic pregnancy, endometriosis, ovarian cyst, ovarian torsion, spontaneous abortion, septic abortion, cholecystitis, gastroenteritis, appendicitis, diverticulitis, pyelonephritis, and renal colic. Look for signs of other STIs, such as herpes simplex, syphilis, and human papillomavirus infection.

DIAGNOSIS

The diagnosis is based on history and clinical findings. No single piece of historical, physical, or laboratory information is sensitive and specific for the disease. **Laboratory evaluation of any woman of childbearing age in the ED always should include a pregnancy test.** Consider the possibility of ectopic pregnancy or septic abortion; the most common alternative diagnosis in missed ectopic pregnancy is PID. Concurrent pregnancy also influences patient treatment and disposition.

Current Centers for Disease Control and Prevention guidelines encourage initiation of empiric treatment in women at risk for PID who exhibit lower abdominal pain, adnexal tenderness, and cervical motion tenderness. Guidelines stratify diagnostic criteria into the three groups shown in **Table 103-3**.

TABLE 103-3 Diagnostic Criteria for Pelvic Inflammatory Disease (PID)

Group 1: Minimum criteria. Empiric treatment if no other cause to explain findings.
Uterine or adnexal tenderness
Cervical motion tenderness
Group 2: Additional criteria improving diagnostic specificity.
Oral temperature >101°F (38.3°C)
Abnormal cervical or vaginal mucopurulent secretions
Elevated erythrocyte sedimentation rate
Elevated C-reactive protein level
Laboratory evidence of cervical infection with *Neisseria gonorrhoeae* or *Chlamydia trachomatis* (i.e., culture or DNA probe techniques)
Group 3: Specific criteria for PID based on procedures that may be appropriate for some patients.
Laparoscopic confirmation
Transvaginal US (or MRI) showing thickened, fluid-filled tubes with or without free pelvic fluid or tubo-ovarian complex
Endometrial biopsy results showing endometritis

Source: Reproduced with permission from Centers for Disease Control and Prevention, Workowski KA, Berman SM: Sexually transmitted diseases treatment guidelines, 2010. *MMWR Recomm Rep* 59(RR-12): 12, 2010.

LABORATORY TESTING

Obtain saline- and potassium hydroxide–treated wet preparations of vaginal secretions to identify leukorrhea (more than one polymorphonuclear leukocyte per epithelial cell) and trichomonads, and to test for BV, including clue cells, pH, and a whiff test. Leukorrhea is sensitive but not specific for upper tract infection,[28] and the absence of leukorrhea is a negative predictor for PID. Although endocervical swab specimens may be sent for culture and can be gram stained for gonococci, nucleic acid amplification tests and DNA probes for *N. gonorrhoeae* and *Chlamydia* have replaced culture and gram staining in many settings. Unfortunately, these results are not available to the ED at the time of initial evaluation. Several sensitive and specific diagnostic tests are currently available for *Trichomonas* testing, including a nucleic acid amplification test (Aptima®; GenProbe, San Diego, CA), approved in 2013, that is performed on the same clinical samples as those for *Chlamydia* and gonorrhea testing.[29,30]

If PID is clinically suspected, an elevated WBC count, erythrocyte sedimentation rate, or C-reactive protein level supports the diagnosis.[28] Because a patient may have multiple STIs, also obtain a rapid plasma regain test for syphilis. Test for HIV and hepatitis. Urinalysis can exclude urinary tract infection, but a positive urinalysis does not exclude PID, because any inflammatory process in the contiguous pelvis can produce WBCs in the urine. Blood cultures do not aid in diagnosis or treatment.

IMAGING

Transvaginal pelvic US may demonstrate thickened (>5 mm), fluid-filled fallopian tubes or free pelvic fluid in acute severe PID. Pelvic or tubo-ovarian abscesses appear as complex adnexal masses with multiple internal echoes. Pelvic US can demonstrate as many as 70% of adnexal masses missed on physical examination. US also may be helpful in ruling in or out other causes in the differential diagnosis of pelvic pain, including ectopic pregnancy, ovarian torsion, hemorrhagic ovarian cyst, and possibly appendicitis or endometriosis.[31]

Abdominopelvic CT and MRI may also be used in the diagnosis of PID and the exclusion of other important causes of pelvic pain. If appendicitis or other surgical or GI diagnoses cannot be excluded, obtain an abdominopelvic CT. For further discussion, see chapter 97, "Abdominal and Pelvic Pain in the Nonpregnant Female." CT findings in PID include obscuration of the pelvic fascial planes, cervicitis, oophoritis, salpingitis, thickening of the uterosacral ligaments, and the presence of simple or complex pelvic fluid or abscess collections. MRI is especially helpful in characterizing complicated soft tissue masses, including dilated fallopian tubes and abscesses. MRI imaging is more specific and accurate than US to assess PID, with a sensitivity of 95% and a specificity of 89%.[32,33]

TREATMENT

Treatment is aimed at relieving acute symptoms, eradicating current infection, and minimizing the risk of long-term sequelae. From a public health perspective, another objective of treatment is to reduce the risk of transmission of infection to other new partners and to identify and treat past and current sexual partners to prevent disease spread. Early diagnosis and treatment are critical because duration of symptoms is an independent risk factor for infertility.

Due to the difficulty of diagnosis and the potential for serious sequelae, the Centers for Disease Control and Prevention recommend a low threshold for empiric treatment, with overtreatment preferred to a missed diagnosis with resultant delayed or no treatment.

Provide adequate analgesia, control of emesis and fever, and fluid replacement in those with nausea, vomiting, and dehydration and in those who appear toxic. Nonsteroidal anti-inflammatory drugs are very useful for the management of pain of pelvic origin. ED treatment should include empiric broad-spectrum antibiotic therapy to cover the full range of likely organisms. Screen for BV and treat when screening is positive. Treatment regimens should follow both national guidelines from the Centers for Disease Control and Prevention and local health department surveillance reports.

The Pelvic Inflammatory Disease Evaluation and Clinical Health trial, which included 654 females age 14 to 37 years old and excluded those who had been treated with antibiotics during the preceding 7 days, had experienced an abortion, delivery, or gynecologic surgery during the preceding 14 days, were homeless, or had an allergy to study medications, demonstrated no differences between oral and parenteral regimens in women with mild to moderately severe acute PID uncomplicated by pregnancy or the presence of a tubo-ovarian abscess.[34,35]

Currently accepted inpatient and outpatient treatment regimens are summarized in **Tables 103-4 and 103-5**. Current geographic patterns of drug resistance may change recommendations. Patients with PID who require IV antibiotics initially can be switched to oral antibiotics after clinical improvement.

TABLE 103-4 Parenteral Treatment Regimens for Pelvic Inflammatory Disease

Cefotetan, 2 grams IV every 12 h, or cefoxitin, 2 grams IV every 6 h
plus
Doxycycline, 100 milligrams PO or IV every 12 h*
or
Clindamycin, 900 milligrams IV every 8 h
plus
Gentamicin, 2 milligrams/kg IV or IM loading dose, followed by gentamicin, 1.5 milligrams/kg every 8 h maintenance dose†
Alternative Parenteral Regimen (limited data on effectiveness)
Ampicillin/sulbactam, 3 grams IV every 6 h
plus
Doxycycline, 100 milligrams PO or IV every 12 h*

*PO doxycycline has the same bioavailability as IV doxycycline and avoids painful infusion.

†Gentamicin dosing may be 3–5 milligrams/kg every 24 h.

Source: Reproduced with permission from Centers for Disease Control and Prevention, Workowski KA, Berman SM: Sexually transmitted diseases treatment guidelines, 2010. *MMWR Recomm Rep 59*(RR-12): 12, 2010.

TABLE 103-5 Oral and Outpatient Treatment Regimens for Pelvic Inflammatory Disease

Ceftriaxone, 250 milligrams IM once, *or* cefoxitin, 2 grams IM once, *and* probenecid, 1 gram PO once administered concurrently
or
Other parenteral third-generation cephalosporin (e.g., ceftizoxime or cefotaxime)
plus
Doxycycline, 100 milligrams PO twice a day for 14 d
with or without
Metronidazole, 500 milligrams PO twice a day for 14 d
If parenteral cephalosporin therapy is not feasible and community prevalence of fluoroquinolone resistance is low:
Levofloxacin, 500 milligrams PO, *or* ofloxacin, 400 milligrams twice daily every day for 14 d
with or without
Metronidazole, 500 milligrams PO twice a day for 14 d

Note: Other parenteral third-generation cephalosporins can be substituted for ceftriaxone or cefoxitin. Since the Centers for Disease Control and Prevention guidelines were published in 2006, clinically significant resistance to the fluoroquinolones (6.7% of infections in heterosexual men, an 11-fold increase from 0.6% in 2001) has emerged in the United States. Fluoroquinolone antibiotics are no longer recommended to treat gonorrhea in the United States.[27] Fluoroquinolones may be an alternative treatment option for disseminated gonococcal infection if antimicrobial susceptibility can be documented.

Source: Reproduced with permission from Centers for Disease Control and Prevention, Workowski KA, Berman SM: Sexually transmitted diseases treatment guidelines, 2010. *MMWR Recomm Rep* 59(RR-12): 12, 2010.

TREATMENT WITH IUD IN PLACE

In the past, IUDs were generally removed, based on the belief that because it is a foreign body, removal of the IUD would allow treatment to be more effective. There is a low risk of PID from IUD insertion, especially when STI testing is done concomitantly and immediate treatment is initiated.[70] **Current Centers for Disease Control and Prevention guidelines suggest that there is insufficient evidence to recommend IUD removal before treatment for PID, because the device is usually not the source of infection.** For individuals using IUD for birth control who develop PID, there are no data to support the use of one treatment regimen over another. Close clinical follow-up is prudent. If there is a concern regarding PID in a patient with an IUD placed in the last 3 weeks, it is reasonable to consult a gynecologist regarding removal.

TREATMENT IN HIV INFECTION

Microbiologically, HIV-positive women are more likely to have concomitant *Candida*, *Mycoplasma hominis*, HPV, and streptococcal infection. HIV-positive women with PID may experience more severe symptoms irrespective of CD4 count and are more likely to have sonographically diagnosed tubo-ovarian abcess. However, they appear to respond similarly to treatment for uncomplicated PID as do women who are not infected with HIV.[36-38] HIV-positive status alone is not a criterion for hospitalization.[36,39] Although HIV status has been removed from specific admission considerations, the 2010 Centers for Disease Control and Prevention STI guidelines note that "whether the management of immunodeficient HIV-infected women with PID requires more aggressive interventions (e.g. hospitalization or parenteral antimicrobial regimens) has not been determined."[40]

TREATMENT OF ADOLESCENTS

Several studies have raised additional concerns about the outpatient management of early adolescents. Early and mid-adolescents were not well represented in the Pelvic Inflammatory Disease Evaluation and Clinical Health study, and of those enrolled, adolescents had increased risk of recurrent PID and a shorter time to pregnancy after an acute episode compared with adult enrollees. Adolescents hospitalized in pediatric centers often receive services beyond IV antibiotics, including education on risk reduction, emotional support, social work intervention, assistance with communicating the nature of their illness with parents, and assistance to arrange close follow-up.[41,42]

ALTERNATIVE ANTIBIOTICS

For those with severe cephalosporin allergy, **spectinomycin** is recommended in Canada and Europe but is not currently available in the United States. For more information, see the Centers for Disease Control and Prevention Web pages on antibiotic-resistant gonorrhea at http://www.cdc.gov/std/Gonorrhea/arg/default.htm.[28]

Multiple studies have demonstrated poor compliance with doxycycline therapy (25%; 50% with partial compliance), and 20% to 25% of patients never fill their prescriptions.[43-45] Recently, generic doxycycline has been difficult to find due to manufacturing shortages and, when available, may be quite expensive, resulting in patient noncompliance with treatment. For PID treatment, **azithromycin** is an alternative, with dosing as either 250 milligrams PO once a day for 7 days or 1 gram once a week for 2 weeks.[43] The long half-life of azithromycin requires significantly fewer doses, which is thought to improve the likelihood of patient compliance. Azithromycin also provides intrinsic anti-inflammatory effects and may reduce local tissue damage. Weigh these potential benefits against the lack of large-scale or long-term studies comparing the effectiveness of azithromycin to doxycycline in the treatment of PID and the possibility of emerging resistance to azithromycin.[43,46-49]

TUBO-OVARIAN ABSCESS

Disproportionate unilateral adnexal tenderness or adnexal mass or fullness may indicate a tubo-ovarian abscess. In women with clinical toxicity and asymmetric pelvic findings, obtain a pelvic US. Most tubo-ovarian abscesses (60% to 80%) resolve with antibiotic administration alone.[50-52] In the setting of tubo-ovarian abscess, oral therapy should be continued with clindamycin (450 milligrams PO four times per day) or metronidazole with doxycycline for better anaerobe coverage for 14 days. Patients who do not improve after 72 hours of treatment should be reevaluated for possible CT- or US-guided percutaneous drainage, laparoscopic drainage, posterior colpotomy with drainage, surgical intervention, or reconsideration of other possible diagnoses. Abscesses 9 cm or larger on imaging appear to have a higher likelihood of requiring surgical therapy. An enlarging pelvic mass may indicate bleeding secondary to vessel erosion or a ruptured abscess.

DISPOSITION AND FOLLOW-UP

Guidelines for admission (**Table 103-6**) and inpatient treatment (Table 103-4) have evolved over the past decade. There are no data demonstrating that inpatient treatment is more effective than outpatient treatment. Among the problems encountered with outpatient care are the provision of adequate guideline-driven treatment, patient adherence to the prescribed therapeutic regimen, difficulty in arranging outpatient administration of parenteral medications, and coordination of 72-hour follow-up evaluation, all of which have been implicated as causes of treatment failure. Consider these and other constraints when determining the patient's ability to follow or tolerate an outpatient regimen.

Institutions should consider adoption of protocolized treatment guidelines to help to ensure fidelity to standards of care. **Admission decisions in the ED are based on severity of illness, likelihood of adherence to outpatient medication regimen, likelihood of major anaerobic infection (IUD, suspected pelvic or tubo-ovarian abscess, or history of recent uterine instrumentation), certainty of diagnosis, coexisting illness and immunosuppression, pregnancy, patient age, and other major fertility issues.**

If the patient is discharged, arrange reevaluation within 72 hours for clinical improvement and adherence to the prescribed regimen. Encourage partner evaluation and treatment. Test and treat for other STIs if not already done. Educate patients about the use of barrier contraceptives and other "safe sex" techniques to lessen the risk of reinfection. Counsel the patient to remain abstinent from sexual activity until 1 week after treatment is finished for both the patient and partner and symptoms have abated.

Partner treatment is crucial to preventing repeated episodes of PID. This can be difficult to ensure. If the current partner has accompanied the patient to the ED, and the patient is willing to tell this partner about her infection, she can be asked to suggest immediate ED evaluation to her partner. If not, the patient should be instructed to notify partners with whom she has had sexual contact in the 60 days preceding the onset of her symptoms to go to the local public health department or STI clinic for empiric treatment of *N. gonorrhoeae* and *C. trachomatis*. A 6-minute PID outreach video has been developed and was found in one randomized controlled trial to improve partner treatment.[53]

Acknowledgement: The authors gratefully acknowledge the contributions of Amy Behrman, a coauthor of this chapter in the previous edition.

TABLE 103-6 Admission Considerations
Inability to exclude surgical emergency from the differential diagnosis
Pregnancy
Failure to respond to outpatient treatment
Inability to tolerate or comply with outpatient treatment
Severe toxicity, high fever, nausea, vomiting
Tubo-ovarian abscess

Source: Reproduced with permission from Centers for Disease Control and Prevention, Workowski KA, Berman SM: Sexually transmitted diseases treatment guidelines, 2010. MMWR Recomm Rep 59(RR-12): 12, 2010.

REFERENCES

The complete reference list is available online at www.TintinalliEM.com.

Breast Disorders

Bophal Sarha Hang

INTRODUCTION

The most common breast complaints in the ED involve breast pain, breast mass, nipple discharge, infection, or postoperative complications. Approximately 30% of women will present to a physician with a chief complaint related to the breasts.[1] Although the problems are rarely emergent except when systemic symptoms such as fever are present, concerns about the potential for breast cancer contribute to patient anxiety.

PATHOPHYSIOLOGY

Adult breast is composed of approximately 20% glandular tissue, and the remaining breast volume consists of fat and connective tissue that give the breast its characteristic texture and shape. Glandular lobules drain into lactiferous ducts, which converge and open at the nipple. In nonpendulous breast, the nipple is an important landmark located over the fourth intercostal space.

Normal breast tissue extends from the sternocostal junction medially to the midaxillary line laterally and from the second to the sixth ribs in the midclavicular line. An axillary tail of breast tissue often extends into the axilla. Blood supply arises from the internal mammary, lateral thoracic, thoracodorsal, and subscapular arteries, whereas venous drainage starts in the subareolar plexus and empties into the intercostals, internal mammary, and axillary veins. Lymphatic drainage of the breast is primarily to the axilla, with a small portion going to internal mammary lymph nodes.

Cyclic variances in estrogens, progesterone, follicle-stimulating hormone, and luteinizing hormone signal stromal and glandular changes in breast physiology.

CLINICAL FEATURES

HISTORY

Ask the patient about onset of any mass or pain, location of the affected area, and duration of the symptoms. Complaints that vary with menses suggest a benign cause, whereas cancers are often asymptomatic. Radiation of the pain to any other body site is particularly important when a malignancy is suspected. The presence of symptoms in the contralateral breast parenchyma is also more reassuring for a benign diagnosis. Assess the color and consistency of any nipple discharge, although the color of the discharge does not differentiate a benign from a malignant process. Changes that the patient notes on breast self-examination may be significant and should be correlated with the menstrual cycle. Ask about family history, specifically about first-degree relatives with breast cancer and other risk factors (delay of childbearing to after age 30 years, biopsy confirmation of atypical hyperplasia, or history of chest irradiation). However, most women who develop breast cancer have no obvious risk factors beyond the two strongest factors, namely, female gender and age. More than 50% of breast cancers are diagnosed in women ≥65 years of age, and women <30 years of age are diagnosed with <1% of all breast cancers.[2]

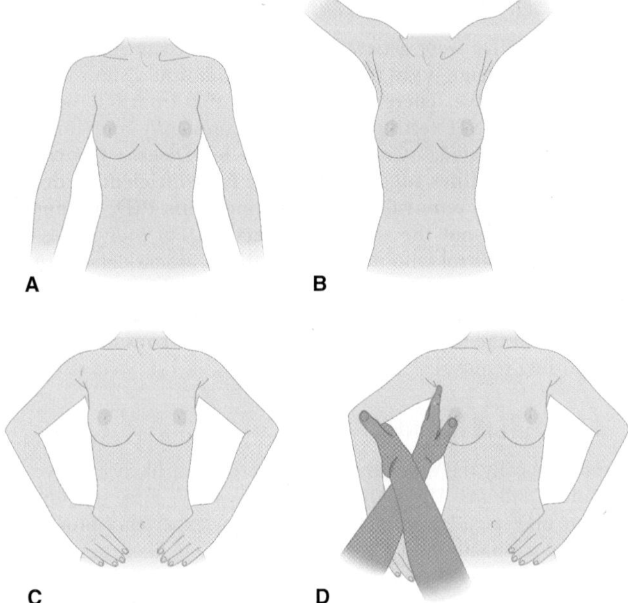

FIGURE 104-1. A through D. Positioning for the examination of the breasts.

PHYSICAL EXAMINATION

The breast examination (**Figure 104-1**) includes both inspection and palpation. Compare the breasts with the patient sitting upright, and note any breast asymmetry or skin dimpling. Subtle abnormalities in the lower quadrants may be accentuated by having the patient raise her arms above her head. Also examine the axillae, including the mammary tail and lymph nodes, in the sitting position. Perform the rest of the examination with the patient supine and ipsilateral hand behind the head. Examine the upper outer quadrant of each breast with extra care, because about half of breast carcinomas originate in that area, with a higher propensity for left-sided involvement.[2,3] Examine the nipple-areola complex with gentle manipulation to detect subareolar masses and latent nipple discharge. Women with breast augmentation may be challenging to examine, but give attention to tissue changes or deviation of the implant.

DISORDERS OF THE LACTATING BREAST

ABNORMAL LACTATION

Any inappropriate secretion of milky discharge from the breast is called *galactorrhea*. Galactorrhea often results from abnormally elevated levels of prolactin, although some women have normal prolactin levels on testing. Hyperprolactinemia may be caused by inadequate inhibition of secretion or increased production of prolactin. Causes of elevated prolactin levels are listed in **Table 104-1**.

Prolactinomas, benign anterior pituitary neoplasms, are distinguished by symptoms of galactorrhea, amenorrhea, hirsutism, facial acne, visual field deficits, and headaches. Chronic renal failure results in a diminished capacity to clear circulating prolactin. Hypothyroidism causes increased levels of thyrotropin-releasing hormone, which result in increased pituitary secretion of prolactin. Hypercortisolism (Cushing's disease) and acromegaly due to elevated growth hormone levels are both associated with galactorrhea.

Evaluation of the patient with galactorrhea focuses on any history of associated menstrual abnormalities and the presence of acne, hirsutism, infertility, or libido changes. Symptoms of increased intracranial pressure and hypothyroidism should be investigated. All medications and dietary supplements should be reviewed.

The physical examination includes evaluations of the visual fields, breasts, skin, and thyroid gland. ED studies include a urine or serum pregnancy test and may include neuroimaging (CT or MRI) and

TABLE 104-1 Causes of Elevated Prolactin Levels

Physiologic causes	Sleep, stress, exercise, volume depletion, intercourse or orgasm, pregnancy, breast stimulation, seizures
Abnormal stimulation of the chest wall	Surgery, trauma, herpetic infection
Damage to or disruption of the pituitary stalk	—
Endogenous hypothalamic-pituitary signaling	—
Neoplasms	Prolactinomas, renal cell carcinoma, lymphoma, craniopharyngioma, bronchogenic carcinoma, hydatidiform mole
Medications	Antidepressants (monoamine oxidase inhibitors, selective serotonin reuptake inhibitors, tricyclic antidepressants), antihypertensives (atenolol, methyldopa, reserpine, verapamil), antipsychotic phenothiazines, antihistamines, herbs and vitamin supplements (anise, fennel, nettle, clover, thistle, fenugreek seed), amphetamines, cocaine, opioids, marijuana
Systemic disease	Chronic renal failure, hypothyroidism, hypercortisolism (Cushing's disease), acromegaly

neurosurgical consultation if there is concern for an intracranial mass. Treatment for galactorrhea, other than the discontinuation of a medication suspected to be causative, is deferred to the primary care physician or the follow-up specialist.

COMPLICATIONS OF LACTATION

Breast engorgement usually presents on the third to fifth postpartum day, with symptoms of painful, hard, and enlarged breasts. The pain may be accompanied by nausea and low-grade fever. Engorgement results from inadequate removal of milk from the breast. This may be due to infant separation, sore nipples, or improper breastfeeding techniques.[4] Ensuring proper latch-on while breastfeeding or pumping usually alleviates the pain and allows for decompression of the nipple-areola complex. Warm showers or manual massage may also help facilitate milk letdown and relieve pain due to engorgement.

Nipple irritation or soreness is common and usually caused by poor positioning or latch-on techniques. Other causes include trauma, plugged ducts, candidiasis, and inflammatory skin disorders. Purified lanolin cream, analgesics, and breast shields may help facilitate healing. There may be some benefit to applying expressed breast milk to nipples.[4,5] There is controversy regarding the role of antifungals for treatment of breast and nipple pain associated with breastfeeding.[6] Reynaud's phenomenon can cause nipple pain in some women and may respond to topical nefedipine.[7]

Puerperal mastitis, or endemic mastitis, presents with severe pain, tenderness, swelling, and redness. Patients may also develop fever, chills, and myalgias. Mastitis is more common in primiparous women in the first few weeks to months of breastfeeding. There is often an associated history of nipple pain or breakdown and inadequate milk drainage that leads to bacterial colonization and infection. Differentials include marked breast engorgement, clogged milk duct, and inflammatory carcinoma, a rare condition.

Mastitis, like other inflammatory processes, has the US appearance of hypoechoic fluid surrounding subcutaneous fat lobules without a discrete fluid collection (**Figure 104-2**), in contrast to abscess (**Figure 104-3**), which presents as a hypoechoic (dark) fluid collection in the tissue with the absence of vascular signals.

Puerperal mastitis is caused by *Staphylococcus aureus* in 40% of cases, although *Escherichia coli* and *Streptococcus* species are also known pathogens. Mastitis can be associated with *S. aureus* nasal carriage in the breastfeeding infant.[8] Consider community-acquired methicillin-resistant *S. aureus* and methicillin-resistant *S. aureus* infections associated with puerperal mastitis and abscess.[5] **There is no need to interrupt breastfeeding.** Treatment requires frequent analgesia, breast emptying, and early antibiotics with antistaphylococcal penicillins or cephalosporins (**Table 104-2**). **Sulfamethoxazole-trimethoprim cannot be given to lactating mothers with infants <2 months old.** If the infection fails to respond rapidly to antibiotics, suspect abscess and broaden antibiotic coverage.

Breast abscess complicates mastitis in approximately 3% of cases. An abscess may present with the signs and symptoms of mastitis or may demonstrate only minimal focal induration, making clinical differentiation difficult. If US examination identifies a subcutaneous fluid collection, US-guided drainage is an initial first-line treatment (Figures 104-2 and 104-3). **Breastfeeding should be continued throughout the course of treatment unless the antibiotic regimen is contraindicated with newborns.**[4,6,9] Surgical drainage may be necessary for large multiloculated fluid collections but is reserved as a last resort in lactating patients to avoid the potential for milk fistulas.[10] Management also includes antibiotic coverage for possible drug-resistant *Staphylococcus* such as oral cephalosporins or clindamycin. Intravenous vancomycin is a good choice for septic patients requiring inpatient hospitalization. In a subset of patients with recurrent

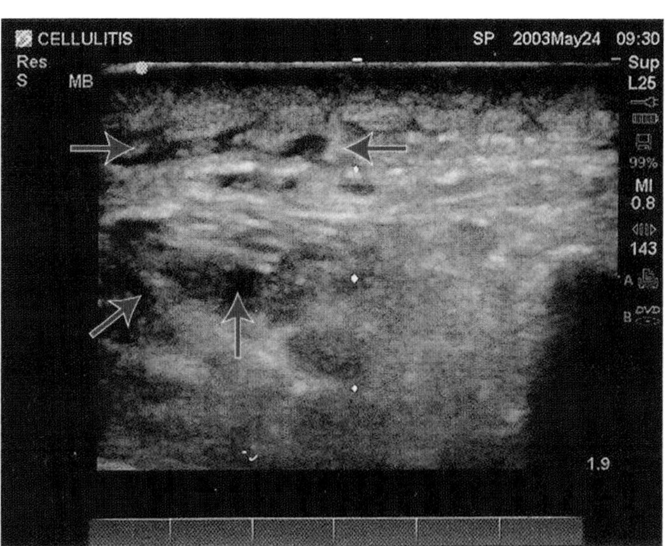

FIGURE 104-2. Mastitis, like other inflammatory processes, has the US appearance of hypoechoic fluid surrounding subcutaneous fat lobules without a discrete fluid collection (*arrows*).

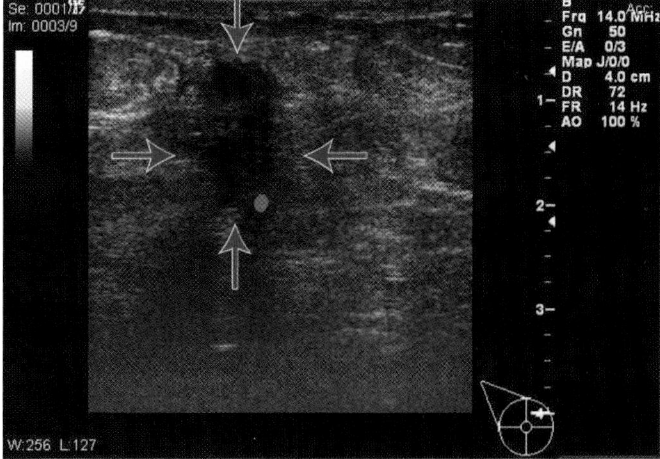

FIGURE 104-3. Breast abscess presents as a hypoechoic (dark) fluid collection in the tissue (*arrows*) with the absence of vascular signals.

TABLE 104-2 Mastitis, Abscess, and Hidradenitis

	Signs and Symptoms	Treatment	Comments
Puerperal mastitis	Erythematous area on breast with area of well-localized pain Fever, chills, myalgias, flulike symptoms	Frequent breast emptying Routine hand washing prior to breast manipulation Analgesia Antibiotics: Dicloxacillin, 500 milligrams four times a day for 10–14 d or Cephalexin, 500 milligrams four times a day for 10–14 d or Clindamycin, 300 milligrams four times a day for 10–14 d	Occurs during first few month or weeks postpartum. Breastfeeding may continue. Early antibiotics and milk drainage are cornerstone of treatment. Must rule out abscess if rapid response to antibiotics does not occur. Cover for MRSA. US to differentiate mastitis from abscess. Follow up with obstetrician.
Nonpuerperal mastitis	Erythematous area on breast with area of well-localized pain Fever, chills, myalgias, flulike symptoms	Analgesia Antibiotics: Dicloxacillin, 500 milligrams four times a day for 10–14 d or Cephalexin, 500 milligrams four times a day for 10–14 d or Clindamycin, 300 milligrams four times a day for 10–14 d or TMP-SMX, 160/800 milligrams twice a day	Must rule out abscess if rapid response to antibiotics does not occur. US helps differentiate between mastitis and abscess. Follow up with surgeon.
Breast abscess	Erythematous area on breast with area of well-localized pain Fever, chills, myalgias, flulike symptoms	US-guided needle aspiration for abscess Analgesia Antibiotics: Dicloxacillin, 500 milligrams four times a day for 10–14 d or Cephalexin, 500 milligrams four times a day for 10–14 d or Clindamycin, 300 milligrams four times a day for 10–14 d or TMP-SMX, 160/800 milligrams twice a day	Needle aspiration is first-line treatment. Obtain surgical consultation for treatment failure and multiloculated abscesses. Immunocompromised patients and those with signs of systemic illness require IV antibiotics, surgical consultation, and admission. Follow up with surgeon.
Periductal mastitis	Varies with age: Younger women—cellulitis or recurrent subareolar abscesses Perimenopausal and postmenopausal women—nipple discharge, nipple retraction, or subareolar mass	Analgesia Antibiotics: Dicloxacillin, 500 milligrams four times a day for 10–14 d or Cephalexin, 500 milligrams four times a day for 10–14 d or Clindamycin, 300 milligrams four times a day for 10–14 d or TMP-SMX, 160/800 milligrams twice a day	Dilated or ectatic ducts with retained secretions. Follow up with surgeon.
Hidradenitis suppurativa	Painful superficial cutaneous abscesses along inferior, pendulous surface of breast	Incision and drainage	Chronic inflammatory disease involving the obstruction of sweat glands. Antibiotics may be indicated in immunocompromised patients.

Abbreviation: MRSA = methicillin-resistant *Staphylococcus aureus*; TMP-SMX = trimethoprim-sulfamethoxazole.

infections, the surgeon may need to perform an excisional biopsy of tissue to rule out an associated inflammatory carcinoma.[11]

INFLAMMATORY BREAST CONDITIONS

The differential diagnosis of an inflamed breast includes infectious mastitis, breast abscess, periductal mastitis, ruptured breast cyst, inflammatory neoplasm, metastatic cancer from a primary lesion, tuberculosis, and Paget's disease. Each entity can mimic the other, more benign conditions. Although the classic *peau d'orange* (orange peel) appearance is highly suggestive of cancer, other clinical signs such as erythematous demarcation, amount of tissue involvement, and the presence of ulceration are not pathognomonic for any specific diagnosis. **A failure of the condition to improve with antibiotic therapy indicates the need for urgent surgical consultation and possible biopsy to exclude the presence of an inflammatory cancer.**[11]

CELLULITIS, ACUTE MASTITIS, AND BREAST ABSCESS IN NONLACTATING WOMEN

Cellulitis, mastitis, and breast abscesses exist along a continuum, with similar clinical presentation of pain, redness, swelling, fever, and malaise. **Cellulitis** can be identified on US as diffuse thickened and hyperechoic skin and increased echogenicity of subcutaneous tissue. However, breast cellulitis is uncommon and requires referral to a breast surgeon for imaging and possibly biopsies. Initial treatment includes dicloxacillin, amoxicillin–clavulanic acid, or a first-generation cephalosporin. However, the increasing incidence of infection with methicillin-resistant *S. aureus* may necessitate the use of trimethoprim-sulfamethoxazole, clindamycin, or tetracycline depending on the patient's history of infections and the local prevalence of methicillin-resistant *S. aureus*.[12] Cellulitis requires follow-up with a breast surgeon.

Acute mastitis and abscesses in nonlactating women (Figures 104-2 and 104-3) are categorized by location as either periareolar or peripheral. They can be difficult to treat and may recur. All require follow-up with a breast surgeon. Either mastitis or abscess may cause systemic toxicity. General indications for admission and immediate surgical consultation are obvious sepsis or hemodynamic compromise, immunosuppression or immunocompromise (e.g., diabetes), rapidly progressive infection, and failure of outpatient antibiotic therapy. Initial recommended empiric parenteral antibiotics are third-generation cephalosporins (e.g., ceftazidime), clindamycin, vancomycin, fluoroquinolones, or linezolid with consideration of the addition of metronidazole for deeper abscesses. Polymicrobial infections account for a significant number of nonpuerperal breast abscesses, and coagulase-negative *Staphylococcal* species and *Pseudomonas* are frequently isolated as well. The prevalence of methicillin-resistant *S. aureus* infections continues to increase and has been reported in up to 20% of cases of breast abscess.[12]

Patients without systemic toxicity can be treated as outpatients. Antibiotics should provide anaerobic coverage. Infections should respond to antibiotics within 48 hours. Refer the patient to a breast surgeon for US-guided needle aspiration and therapy.[13-16]

HIDRADENITIS SUPPURATIVA

Hidradenitis suppurativa frequently presents with recurrent multiple cutaneous abscesses, sinus tracts, and scarring of the breast folds, axillae, and groin and perineum. It is a chronic inflammatory disease involving the obstruction of sweat glands and polymicrobial colonization, usually with *Staphylococcus* and *Streptococcus* species. Frequently, patients present with painful superficial cutaneous abscesses along the inferior, pendulous surface of the breast and require surgical drainage for pain relief. Incision and drainage usually are adequate therapy for a limited area of abscess formation. Antibiotics are rarely used for outpatient management of hidradenitis abscesses in immunocompetent patients, although clindamycin or rifampin may be used by dermatologists or surgeons to decrease the frequency and severity of the disease. There is no cure, and the disease often requires extensive surgical excision of the apocrine tissue.

INFLAMMATORY BREAST CANCER

Of all the potential presentations of a breast malignancy, inflammatory breast cancer is the entity associated with the highest mortality and longest delay from initial presentation to definitive diagnosis. The clinical presentation is characterized by symptoms of mastalgia and breast inflammation due to tumor infiltration of dermal lymphatics and inflammation of the breast stroma. The combination of erythema and edema results in the classic *peau d'orange* appearance of the overlying skin and ultimately nipple retraction as the edema progresses. Initially, the patient presents with a clinical syndrome of breast enlargement, breast warmth, tenderness, edema, erythema, and sometimes discoloration of the overlying skin. The absence of a palpable underlying mass or axillary lymphadenopathy does not rule out the diagnosis. **The signs of inflammatory breast cancer are often indistinguishable clinically from infection.** Prompt mammography and biopsy of the skin and any palpable or radiographic breast lesions will be required by the follow-up physician. **Similarly, the diagnosis of *inflammatory breast cancer* must be considered promptly if there is not an initial good response to antibiotics or if breast cellulitis or abscess fails to completely resolve.**

NONINFLAMMATORY PAINFUL BREAST DISORDERS

MASTODYNIA

Breast pain is also termed *mastodynia* or *mastalgia*. Irritation to the intercostal nerves at T3-T5 can cause pain in the breast or nipple. The pain is bilateral and usually most severe in the upper outer quadrants of the breast. Pain may be referred to the axilla or scapula. Diagnosis relies on findings of the history and physical examination to confirm that the pain actually originates from the breast. Breast pain is an uncommon symptom of breast cancer.[17] Cyclic mastodynia is usually most severe in the immediate premenstrual phase and decreases or resolves completely following menstruation. At times, the examination reveals tender, nodular breasts, which suggests a diagnosis of fibrocystic changes, although breast cancer must remain in the differential diagnosis. For most patients, reassurance and use of a supportive bra provide adequate initial treatment. Refer to a primary care physician for follow-up treatment and consideration of imaging.[18,19]

SKIN AND NIPPLE ABNORMALITIES

NIPPLE DISCHARGE

Table 104-3 lists some common causes of nipple discharge. In general, nipple discharge that is bilateral, occurs with nipple manipulation, and can be expressed from several ducts is not suggestive of cancer. Nipple discharge that originates in a single breast, emanates from a single duct, and is clear, pink, bloody, or serosanguineous is associated with an increased risk of carcinoma.[20] Follow-up with the patient's primary care physician for mammography and possible fluid analysis of the discharge is always needed.

Intraductal papillomas usually present with a unilateral bloody nipple discharge in women from 20 to 40 years of age. Bleeding is secondary to increased tissue vascularity. A mass may not be palpable on examination. Other causes of bloody nipple discharge include mammary duct ectasia and breast cancer. Ductal ectasia involves the stasis or plugging of lactiferous ducts, which then progresses to an infiltrative inflammatory process. The cause of mammary duct ectasia is unknown.

Bilateral spontaneous milky nipple discharge can indicate an elevated serum prolactin level (see earlier discussion under "Abnormal Lactation"). Any postmenopausal nipple discharges are significant, so refer to a breast specialist.

MONDOR'S DISEASE

Thrombophlebitis of the superficial thoracoepigastric vein, or Mondor's disease, results in a cordlike mass in the breast, sometimes associated with skin changes such as dimpling. Although no identifiable cause is found in most cases, localized trauma or an inflammatory process has been associated with Mondor's disease. Breast pain is the usual presenting complaint, with examination findings of a characteristic cordlike mass in the superficial subcutaneous tissue of the breast, most commonly in the lower quadrants. Mondor's disease, which can be mistaken for an inflammatory cancer, is benign and self-limited. US can establish the diagnosis of superficial thrombophlebitis. Past treatment was

TABLE 104-3 Possible Causes of Different Types of Nipple Discharge

Type of Discharge	Cause
Purulent	Infection
	Periductal mastitis
Milky (galactorrhea)	Pregnancy
	Prolactinoma
	Pituitary adenoma or intracranial mass
	Drugs: hormones, psychotropics (phenothiazines), histamine-2 receptor antagonists, antiemetics (metoclopramide), antihypertensives (methyldopa, verapamil)
Serous or serosanguineous	Intraductal papilloma
	Ductal ectasia
	Cancer
Watery	Papilloma
	Cancer
Green, gray, black, or tan	Duct ectasia or periductal mastitis

nonsteroidal anti-inflammatory medication. Consider thrombophilic evaluation and treatment with low-molecular-weight heparins after hematology consultation.[21] Refer for appropriate follow-up.

NIPPLE IRRITATION

Nipple irritation may be caused by repeated friction from clothing or sunburn. The nipples are easily protected from chronic abrasion by application of a small dab of petroleum jelly or use of protective pads inserted into the cups of a support bra. Nipple irritation, however, also may be indicative of atopic dermatitis, erosive adenomatosis, or Paget's disease. Erosive adenomatosis is a benign proliferation of the lactiferous ducts presenting with eczema or an erosion of the nipple. Referral to a breast specialist is needed for the latter condition because the treatment is surgical excision. Paget's disease is often heralded by the appearance of a weeping, eczematoid lesion of the nipple. Paget's disease is almost always associated with an underlying breast carcinoma and usually is diagnosed in postmenopausal women. Paget's disease may present with an associated palpable breast mass, often correlating with the presence of an intraductal carcinoma. Because skin edema and inflammatory changes may respond transiently to incorrectly prescribed topical treatments, there is usually a delay of 6 to 12 months in diagnosis. Provide urgent referral for bilateral mammography and follow up with a breast specialist.

FIBROCYSTIC DISEASE AND THE EVALUATION OF A BREAST MASS

Fibrocystic breast disease is a constellation of symptoms linked by the pathognomonic finding of breast cysts. Breast nodularity and tenderness, which occur as a result of breast tissue responses to hormonal cycling, are referred to as *fibrocystic breast disease* or *fibrocystic changes of the breast*. Fibrocystic changes **do not include** skin thickening, edema, discoloration, nipple retraction, or discharge. If the history and physical examination findings in the ED are normal, then outpatient mammography and follow-up with a specialist should occur, regardless of patient age. Further imaging, including additional mammography and MRI, may also be indicated. Women with recurrent or severe symptoms, skin changes, solid masses, nipple abnormalities, or anxiety about the possibility of cancer should be referred to a breast specialist.

Breast cancer is rare in patients <20 years of age and uncommon in women <30 years of age. Risk factors for young women include inheritance of the *BRCA1* or *BRCA2* gene, a history of childhood malignancy, or a history of chest irradiation. A family history of a first-degree relative with breast cancer, increased exposure to endogenous estrogens (nulliparity or delay of childbearing until after age 30), or biopsy-confirmed atypical breast hyperplasia increases the risk for women ≥30 years old. However, most patients diagnosed with breast cancer have only two risk factors: age >50 years and female gender.[22]

Physical signs that should prompt urgent surgical referral include a palpable mass with or without the following: lymphadenopathy, skin ulceration, mass fixation to the chest wall, fixed axillary nodes, and the presence of ipsilateral arm edema.

Characteristics associated with a delayed diagnosis and poorer survival of breast cancer are black race, lower socioeconomic status, unmarried state, normal or false-negative mammogram results, presentation with nipple lesions or axillary mass, and younger age at time of diagnosis.[23-27]

BREAST TRAUMA

Blunt trauma to the breast is usually seen in association with multiple thoracic injuries and is often accompanied by extensive chest wall ecchymoses, commonly referred to as the "seat belt sign." Traumatic breast injuries rarely need specific therapy unless there is significant avulsion of breast tissue or an expanding hematoma, which should prompt emergent surgical evaluation and management. The presence of a significant isolated breast injury should raise the possibility of abuse or cancer. Long-term sequelae of breast trauma include inflammatory and architectural distortions of the breast, as well as persistent microcalcification observed on mammography. Fat necrosis is the most common type of inflammatory response to breast injury, but few patients actually remember a discrete breast injury. Fat necrosis can be confused easily with carcinoma because it may present with a palpable mass and even skin dimpling and retraction. Although no specific treatment is required for fat necrosis, the presence of cancer must be excluded. Any persistent mass after trauma must raise the question of underlying pathology or malignancy, and referral to a breast specialist for evaluation is required.

PERIOPERATIVE AND POSTOPERATIVE COMPLICATIONS

BREAST HEMATOMA

Immediately postoperative hemorrhage or expanding hematoma formation is best evaluated and treated by the operating surgeon. Up to 1.5 L of blood can extravasate into traumatized breast parenchyma. Emergent evaluation requires determination of whether the hematoma is expanding, tensely distended, or stable. Expanding hematomas, especially those occurring within the first few postoperative days, may signify the presence of continued bleeding and usually require surgical evaluation for evacuation of the hematoma or ligation of bleeding vessels. Later presentations of breast hematoma are usually managed conservatively, with analgesics, a compressive bra, and the correction of any coagulopathy. Aspiration of the hematoma generally is not effective in the ED. The presence of an infected hematoma requires inpatient management with US-guided percutaneous drainage or open surgical drainage; parenteral antibiotics generally are indicated.

WOUND INFECTION

Postoperative wound infections may be treated with an oral first-generation cephalosporin on an outpatient basis if there is no evidence of abscess, systemic signs of toxicity, or immunocompromise. Worsening signs of cellulitis or systemic response to infection, development of purulent drainage, or failure to improve after 48 hours of treatment requires inpatient management. Infections of postoperative drains generally require drain removal and antibiotic therapy. Any fluid collections that develop subsequently usually require drainage either by repeated aspiration or by incision. The operating surgeon should be consulted regarding any postoperative complications.

REFERENCES

The complete reference list is available online at www.TintinalliEM.com.

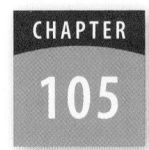

Complications of Gynecologic Procedures

Nikki Waller

INTRODUCTION AND EPIDEMIOLOGY

Advancements in minimally invasive gynecologic surgical techniques, such as laparoscopy and hysteroscopy, have allowed more outpatient procedures for patients. Postoperative complications among inpatients are now seen out of the hospital. The prevalence of all postoperative complications after gynecologic procedures is reported to be 9%, whereas 3.7% are considered major complications.[1] The most common reasons for ED visits during the postoperative period after gynecologic procedures are pain, fever, and vaginal bleeding.

CLINICAL FEATURES

HISTORY

Patient risk factors for postoperative complications include age >80 years, medical comorbidities, dependent functional status, and obesity or unintentional weight loss.[1] Key historical questions are listed in **Table 105-1**. The interval between surgery and the onset of symptoms is very important in determining the cause of symptoms. For example, most cases of early postoperative fevers (<24 hours) are not infectious but rather result from pulmonary atelectasis, hypersensitivity reactions to antibiotics, pyogenic reactions to tissue trauma, or hematoma formation. Fever occurring on postoperative days 3 to 5 may be due to a urinary tract infection. On postoperative days 4 to 6, consider venous thromboembolism, and ≥7 days after surgery, consider a surgical site infection.[2]

PHYSICAL EXAMINATION

Examine all appropriate body systems. Do not assume that complaint is gynecologic, and investigate other potential explanations of symptom. Postoperative pain and tenderness can be difficult to assess. After laparoscopy, patients may have shoulder or upper abdominal pain because of carbon dioxide bubbles trapped between the liver and diaphragm after insufflation for the procedure, with 50% to 70% of patients still being affected 48 hours after surgery.[3] Postoperative pain and tenderness are concerning if associated with fever, nausea and vomiting, and a change in bowel sounds.

Examine the surgical wound and perform a pelvic examination, including both a sterile speculum and a bimanual examination. **In patients undergoing fertility treatment, defer the pelvic examination until consulting with the gynecologist, due to the possibility of rupturing enlarged ovarian follicles.** During sterile speculum examination, the cervix or vaginal cuff must be visualized. After vaginal hysterectomy, no special precautions are needed for a speculum examination. Note any evidence of bleeding, discharge, erythema, and cuff or labial cellulitis. After a vaginal or abdominal hysterectomy, record the presence of tenderness, masses, and an intact cuff. After hysteroscopy or dilatation and curettage, evaluate cervical motion, uterine, and adnexal tenderness. Perform a rectal examination to assess for tenderness, masses, or fecal impaction.

LABORATORY TESTING

Laboratory studies should be directed toward the patient's complaints. A CBC with a manual differential count is almost always indicated. Obtain a serum β-human chorionic gonadotropin level for all women with childbearing potential. A clean-catch or catheterized urine specimen along with urine, blood, wound, and cervical (if present) cultures should be obtained if the patient is febrile. A complete chemistry panel may be necessary to evaluate hepatic and renal function.

Imaging is often necessary. A chest radiograph can confirm pneumonia or inappropriate air under the diaphragm. **Air or insufflated carbon dioxide should be completely absorbed by the third postoperative day.**

TABLE 105-1 Key Historical Questions to Assess Postoperative Complications

Surgical procedure performed
Route of procedure
Abdominal
Vaginal
Laparoscopic
Reason for procedure
Time of symptom onset
Proximity of symptom to the surgery
Complications already experienced
Other postsurgical history
Medications prescribed

Supine and erect abdominal series help confirm bowel obstruction. Although pelvic sonogram is helpful for visualizing the pelvic structures, CT is the gold standard for diagnosing most postoperative abdominal complications, with a sensitivity and specificity of >90%.[4] MRI may be indicated in the evaluation of septic pelvic thrombophlebitis.

COMPLICATIONS OF ENDOSCOPIC PROCEDURES

LAPAROSCOPY

Gynecologic laparoscopy is used for diagnosis and treatment. Indications for laparoscopy are listed in **Table 105-2**. Laparoscopy is almost always an ambulatory surgical procedure and is performed under general anesthesia with endotracheal intubation.

After cesarean sections, abortion, cholecystectomy, and coronary angioplasty, tubal sterilization is the next most common operation in the United States, with a rate of 12.2 procedures per 1000 unsterilized women.[5-7] When not performed postpartum with cesarean sections, the procedure is almost always performed laparoscopically.[6] Laparoscopic hysterectomy is another common procedure.

Reported overall laparoscopic complication rates range from 0.2% to 10.3%.[8] Major laparoscopic procedures are associated with a higher rate of complications compared with minor procedures (0.6% to 18% vs 0.06% to 7.0%, respectively).[8]

Both diagnostic and therapeutic gynecologic laparoscopy are accomplished by passing a rigid endoscope through a trocar that is inserted bluntly through a small infraumbilical incision into the abdominal cavity after a Veress needle has been used to insufflate the abdomen with carbon dioxide. The pneumoperitoneum must be sufficient to displace the bowel and is maintained throughout the surgery. Additional trocars may be placed so that other accessories can be used during the surgery. The majority of complications occur during entry of these instruments.

All laparoscopic procedures entail the same potential complications (**Table 105-3**), but more complex surgeries carry considerably more risk.

Bowel injury is uncommon, but may not be noted at the time of surgery. **Patients with greater than expected pain after laparoscopy should be considered to have a bowel injury until proven otherwise.** Signs and symptoms include abdominal pain and distention, fever, nausea, vomiting, and an elevated WBC count. Plain radiographs may show an ileus or free air under the diaphragm. Complications include peritonitis, abscess, enterocutaneous fistula, and septic shock. There are three major types of bowel injury: traumatic, thermal, and vascular.

Although many significant complications of laparoscopy are recognized in the operating room under direct visualization, **thermal injury** can easily be missed. Patients may not develop symptoms for several days or weeks postoperatively.[9-11] Early gynecologic consult is critical if a thermal injury is suspected, because damage is usually more extensive than may be apparent.

Vascular injury is uncommon[9-11] and is usually recognized during the operation. Patients may later present with a postoperative hematoma, which requires wound exploration by the gynecologist.

The rate of **urinary tract injuries** is about 4%.[12] Injuries can occur from mechanical or thermal trauma. Trocar or dissection injuries to the bladder are typically recognized intraoperatively. Thermal injuries, however, may not be initially apparent and may present later as peritonitis or fistula. The diagnosis of a ureteral injury is usually delayed. Thermal

TABLE 105-2 Common Indications for Laparoscopy

Sterilization
Lysis of adhesions
Carbon dioxide laser ablation of endometriosis
Uterine surgery (including myomectomy)
Tubal surgeries (including salpingectomy)
Ovarian surgery (including oophorectomy and oophorocystectomy)
Paraovarian cyst excision
Hysterectomy

TABLE 105-3	Major Complications Associated with Laparoscopy
Bowel injury	
Thermal injury	
Vascular injury	
Urinary tract injuries	
Incisional hernia	
Wound dehiscence	

injury may present up to 14 days postoperatively with abdominal or flank pain, fever, and peritonitis. An abdominopelvic CT with IV contrast shows extravasation of urine or a urinoma. Mechanical obstruction of the ureter from sutures or staples may be recognized intraoperatively by direct visualization but may also present up to 1 week postoperatively with fever and flank pain. An IV pyelogram or CT helps define the site and degree of obstruction.

Incisional hernias and dehiscence are rare complications after laparoscopy. Incisional hernias are more common when defects >10 mm are made and can develop within the first postoperative week. Patients may be asymptomatic or may note pain, mass, evisceration, or signs and symptoms of a mechanical bowel obstruction. Fever may present if the bowel is incarcerated, and peritonitis may develop after bowel perforation. Dehiscence usually involves protrusion of the omentum and, in rare cases, the small bowel. Immediate incisional repair by a gynecologist is usually sufficient; however, a laparotomy is needed for bowel incarceration or perforation.

Wound infection after laparoscopy is uncommon and rarely a serious complication. Most infections are minor skin infections that can be managed with oral antibiotics and possible drainage. Antibiotics should cover against staphylococci, including methicillin-resistant *Staphylococcus aureus* and streptococci. Excluding minor skin infections, pelvic infection is quite rare and includes pelvic cellulitis, abscess, and necrotizing fasciitis.

HYSTEROSCOPY

Hysteroscopy is the direct visualization of the cervical canal and endometrial cavity using a rigid or flexible fiberoptic instrument. Hysteroscopy can be done as an office procedure under IV sedation or in an operating room. Complications (**Table 105-4**) are uncommon and occur more frequently as a result of operative hysteroscopy than diagnostic hysteroscopy.[13]

The most common indication for hysteroscopy is abnormal vaginal bleeding. Other indications include uterine leiomyomata, intrauterine adhesions, proximal tubal obstruction, removal of intrauterine devices, müllerian anomalies, and infertility evaluation. Therapeutic applications include directed biopsies, removal of small myomata or polyps, and endometrial ablation for menorrhagia. Also, hysteroscopic sterilization is growing in popularity. The Essure® microinsert system is currently the only method available in the United States. The device is deployed in the fallopian tube and stimulates surrounding tissue growth, resulting in fallopian tube occlusion and permanent sterilization.

Uterine perforation is rare and usually noted at surgery. Infection is very rare and most commonly occurs in patients with concurrent genital tract infections. Postoperative bleeding can be uterine or cervical in origin. Cervical lacerations are caused by forceful dilation or tears from the tenaculum. Uterine bleeding can result from resection procedures. Gas embolism is the most feared complication of using carbon dioxide gas as a distention medium for laparoscopy.[14] This complication is likely to occur during or shortly after insufflation.

TABLE 105-4	Complications Associated with Hysteroscopy
Fluid overload	
Uterine perforation	
Postoperative bleeding	
Gas embolism	
Infection	

COMPLICATIONS OF MAJOR ABDOMINAL SURGERY

Complications from major abdominal procedures that lead to ED visits usually occur at least 3 days postoperatively (**Table 105-5**).

Hysterectomy remains one of the most common major surgical procedures in the United States, with the abdominal approach composing 60% of cases (14% laparoscopic and 26% vaginal).[2,15] A total hysterectomy is removal of the uterus and part or all of the cervix and is unrelated to removal of the ovaries. A subtotal hysterectomy involves removal of the uterus without removal of the cervix. Patients may be unsure of the type of hysterectomy that was performed.

The risk of postoperative infection after hysterectomy is 3% to 10%, with higher rates in the abdominal versus the vaginal approach.[16] Risk factors for postoperative infections include obesity, diabetes, and long operative time.[16]

WOUND INFECTION

Most wound infections occur within the first 2 postoperative weeks; however, they can present several months after surgery. Symptoms include fever and increased pain at the incision site. Examination reveals wound tenderness, skin erythema, induration, purulent discharge from the incision, and possible dehiscence.

Empiric antibiotics should provide coverage against staphylococci, including methicillin-resistant *S. aureus*, and streptococci. If an **incisional abscess** is diagnosed, first open and drain the wound. Probe the wound with a sterile cotton swab to confirm an intact fascia. Then, irrigate the wound copiously with normal saline and pack with saline-soaked wet-to-dry dressings. If staples have been placed, they should be removed. Obtain aerobic and anaerobic cultures to tailor antibiotic therapy.

For invasive infections, consult with the operating gynecologist. Give parenteral antibiotics and, usually, admit to the hospital.

WOUND SEROMA AND HEMATOMA

Wound seromas and hematomas are characterized by drainage, rather than fever or pain, and can be visualized by bedside US. Small seromas and hematomas can be managed by observation and will usually resolve spontaneously. Large seromas can be aspirated. If there are any signs of infection, the wound should be opened and drained and then packed with wet-to-dry dressings.

VAGINAL CUFF CELLULITIS AND PELVIC ABSCESS

The vaginal cuff formed during hysterectomy is composed of the contiguous retroperitoneal space immediately above the vaginal apex and the surrounding soft tissue. Vaginal cuff cellulitis usually occurs early

TABLE 105-5	Common Complications Related to Major Abdominal Gynecologic Surgery
Wound infection	
Infected vaginal cuff hematoma, cellulites, or abscess	
Ovarian abscess	
Dehiscence and evisceration	
Bleeding	
Phlebitis	
Urinary tract infection/urinary retention	
Bladder and ureteral injury	
Ileus, bowel injury, and bowel obstruction	
Pneumonia and atelectasis	

after surgery. Patients complain of fever; purulent vaginal discharge; and pelvic, back, or abdominal pain. Pelvic examination reveals tenderness and induration of the vaginal cuff and purulent discharge.

Vaginal cuff and pelvic abscesses and infected hematomas are rare and usually present 10 to 14 days postoperatively. Symptoms include fever, chills, tachycardia, pelvic pain, and rectal pressure. Examination findings include lower abdominal and vaginal cuff tenderness, a tender or fluctuant mass near the cuff, and bloody or purulent drainage from the cuff. US or CT can define the size and location of an abscess or hematoma.

Admit patients for parenteral antibiotics and possible drainage by interventional radiology or colpotomy. Give broad-spectrum antibiotics, such as imipenem-cilastatin, gentamicin and clindamycin, or ciprofloxacin and metronidazole, to cover gram-negative and gram-positive bacteria and anaerobic organisms.[17]

DEHISCENCE AND EVISCERATION

Wound dehiscence is the failure of normal healing and the disruption of fascia and peritoneum. Evisceration occurs when omentum or bowel presents through the incision. The classic sign of impending dehiscence is the sudden outpouring of serosanguineous blood from the incision. The patient may describe a "pop" or tearing sensation. Most often, dehiscence occurs between postoperative days 5 and 8 for abdominal surgeries.[18]

Vaginal cuff dehiscence usually occurs 1.5 to 3.5 months after hysterectomy.[19] Patients complain of postcoital bleeding, watery discharge, and pelvic pain. If bowel evisceration has occurred, patients note vaginal and pelvic pressure or a bulge.

When abdominal evisceration has occurred, cover the abdomen with moist sterile towels and support the dressing with tape to prevent further gut extrusion. The patient should be taken directly to the operating room for closure. In cases in which there is a sudden appearance of blood but no bowel, it is best to follow the same procedure because evisceration usually is imminent. Vaginal cuff dehiscence can be managed conservatively if small or partial, whereas large or complete vaginal cuff dehiscence usually requires surgical closure.

GENITOURINARY INJURY

Genitourinary injury occurs more often during the performance of abdominal hysterectomy than during any other pelvic surgery. Most **bladder injuries** are apparent at the time of surgery, but some ureteral injuries go unrecognized. Ureteral injury occurs less frequently than bladder injury but is generally underestimated. Operative injury to the ureter results from one of three types of trauma: crushing, transection, or ligation. Each type of injury can be either partial or complete.

Suspect **ureteral injury** in women who develop flank pain shortly after surgery. Fever, hematuria, and costovertebral angle tenderness may also be present. Obtain a urinalysis and abdominopelvic CT with IV contrast. Admit to the hospital for ureteral catheterization under cystoscopic guidance and possibly exploratory laparotomy. Percutaneous nephrostomy with delayed repair may also be considered. Provide parenteral antibiotics if infection is suspected.

Vesicovaginal fistulas can become evident 10 to 14 days after surgery with a watery vaginal discharge. The diagnosis can be confirmed by inserting a cotton tampon into the vagina and then instilling methylene blue or indigo carmine dye via a transurethral catheter. If the tampon stains blue, a vesicovaginal fistula is present. If no staining occurs, a ureterovaginal fistula must be ruled out by injecting 5 mL of indigo carmine dye IV. If a ureterovaginal fistula is present, the tampon should stain blue within 20 minutes.

Gynecologic consultation is necessary. Patients with a vesicovaginal fistula require prolonged urinary drainage with a Foley catheter. Although some fistulas close spontaneously, most require surgical repair.

OTHER COMPLICATIONS

Urinary tract infection is a common complication.[2] For detailed discussion, see chapter 91, "Urinary Tract Infections and Hematuria." Urinary retention in a healthy female after gynecologic surgery is uncommon. **Urinary retention** is usually a temporary result of pain or bladder atony resulting from anesthesia. However, many women experience either an inability to void or incomplete emptying of the bladder during the postoperative period, most frequently after radical hysterectomy or surgeries that involve the urethra and bladder neck (i.e., anterior repair or any modification of the retropubic urethropexy). Retention is initially relieved with insertion of a Foley catheter for 12 to 24 hours. Most patients are able to void after this period. For further discussion, see chapter 92, "Acute Urinary Retention."

Pulmonary emboli account for nearly 40% of all deaths after gynecologic surgery.[2] The prevalence of postoperative deep venous thromboembolism is 11% to 25%.[2] Fifty percent of venous thromboembolic events occur in the first 24 hours after surgery, and 75% occur in the first 3 postoperative days. There is no difference in the incidence of venous thromboembolism between abdominal, vaginal, or laparoscopic hysterectomy, but risk factors include age >60 years, cancer, and other comorbidities.[20] For complete discussion of diagnosis and treatment, see chapter 56, "Venous Thromboembolism."

Septic pelvic thrombophlebitis complicates 0.1% to 0.5% of gynecologic procedures, more commonly after cesarean delivery than hysterectomy.[21] The two forms of septic pelvic thrombophlebitis, ovarian vein thrombosis and deep septic pelvic thrombophlebitis, often occur together. Signs include abdominal pain and fever. The diagnosis may be aided by CT and MRI, but a negative study does not exclude disease.[21,22] Treatment is heparin and parenteral antibiotics. Long-term anticoagulation is not needed unless septic pulmonary emboli develop.

POSTCONIZATION BLEEDING

High-grade squamous intraepithelial lesions of the cervix are treated by loop electrocautery, laser ablation, or cold-knife conization. The most common complication of conization procedures is bleeding, which can be rapid and severe. Delayed hemorrhage may occur 7 to 14 days postoperatively.

Visualization of the cervix is the key to controlling bleeding. Application of **Monsel solution** (a commercially available ferrous subsulfate solution) is a reasonable first step if it is readily available. Monsel solution should be available from the hospital pharmacy. Direct pressure for 5 minutes with a large cotton-tipped swab may also be effective. Alternatively, cauterization with silver nitrate may be attempted. If these maneuvers are unsuccessful, consult the gynecologist for suturing or cauterization of the bleeding arteriole. The vagina can be packed with gauze if the bleeding is severe while waiting for definitive therapy. Often the patient must be taken to the operating room for repair because adequate visualization is difficult in the ED.

INDUCED ABORTION

There are three major methods for termination of pregnancy: instrumental evacuation by vaginal route, stimulation of uterine contraction, and major surgical procedures. Overall, less than 1% of women have complications.[23] Complications can be categorized by time after procedure: immediate, delayed, or late (**Table 105-6**).

Due to the approval of mifepristone in 2000, medical abortions now account for 23% to 37% of all nonhospital abortions.[24,25] Mifepristone is

TABLE 105-6 Complications Associated with Induced Abortion

Timing	Complication	Possible Etiologies
Immediate complications: within 24 h after procedure	Bleeding, pain	Uterine perforation, cervical lacerations
Delayed complications: between 24 h and 4 wk after procedure	Bleeding	Retained products of conception, postabortive endometritis
Late complications: >4 wk after procedure	Amenorrhea, psychological problems, Rh isoimmunization	—

usually followed by misoprostol, a regimen with a 92% efficacy rate.[26] Common side effects include nausea, vomiting, diarrhea, headaches, dizziness, and fatigue. Methotrexate, in combination with misoprostol, is an alternative therapy.

Uterine perforation occurs in approximately 0.1 to 3 per 1000 abortion procedures.[27] Most perforations are noted at the time of surgery; however, small perforations may go unnoticed. Patients can present with pain and/or bleeding and, possibly, signs of shock.

If a **cervical laceration** is noted, treatment includes pressure, followed by application of Monsel solution or use of silver nitrate sticks. Suturing may be necessary if there is no resolution of bleeding.

Incomplete abortion and **retained products of conception** occur in 0.5% of medical abortions and 0.29% to 1.96% of all abortions.[25] Women present with abdominal pain, bleeding, and possibly fever. On physical examination, the cervical os is usually open, and the uterus is boggy, enlarged, and tender. A pelvic US is the diagnostic test of choice and can identify a thickened endometrium and retained echogenic contents. Treatment consists of dilatation and curettage or medical management with misoprostol. If coexistent endometritis is present, treatment with broad-spectrum antibiotics is required for at least 10 to 14 days.

Postabortal **endometritis** not associated with retained products of conception presents with a closed cervical os and a firm yet tender uterus. Uncomplicated endometritis is treated with antibiotics.

Women who are Rh negative require Rh0 (D) immunoglobulin, 300 micrograms IM, after spontaneous or induced abortion. If it is not prescribed within 72 hours, the overall risk of sensitization in the second pregnancy is approximately 3%.

Obtain gynecologic consultation for all patients with complications after induced abortion.

INTRAUTERINE DEVICES

Serious complications from intrauterine devices are rare, occurring in less than 1% of patients, and include pelvic inflammatory disease, ectopic pregnancy, and uterine perforation.[28] The only possible indication for removal of an intrauterine device in the ED is infection (salpingitis, endometritis, pyosalpinx, or pelvic peritonitis). The risk of pelvic inflammatory disease in intrauterine device users is more related to preexisting sexually transmitted infections rather than the intrauterine device itself.[29,30] Patients may present to the ED for intrauterine device removal for other reasons, such as irregular menses or pain; however, patients should be referred to their gynecologist for removal.

If referral is impractical, grasp the string of the intrauterine device with a Kelly clamp or long forceps and pull with steady, gentle force until the intrauterine device emerges from the uterus. Do not jerk the string because it may detach from the intrauterine device, making removal more difficult. If the string cannot be visualized, a lost intrauterine device may be located with ultrasonography. If the intrauterine device is extrauterine or fractured, surgical removal will be necessary.

ENDOMETRIAL ABLATION

Endometrial ablation is used to treat abnormal uterine bleeding. Although there are numerous technologies, they share similar postoperative complications, including pregnancy after ablation, pain-related obstructed menses, and infection. Pregnancy incidence after endometrial ablation is 0.7%.[31] There is a much greater risk of complications during these pregnancies, including preterm birth, intrauterine scarring, and postpartum hemorrhage. Also, the ectopic rate is 6.5%, almost three times the baseline risk. Persistent endometrium is common after ablation, as are uterine contracture and scarring. This results in obstructed egress of menses, causing cyclic cramping and pain. The incidence of infectious complications ranges from 1% to 2%, including endometritis, myometritis, pelvic inflammatory disease, and pelvic abscess.[31] Patients present with fever, uterine and/or adnexal tenderness, and vaginal discharge usually within 3 days of surgery.

PELVIC ORGAN PROLAPSE SURGERY AND SYNTHETIC MESH

Surgery using transvaginal mesh can be used to treat pelvic organ prolapse. Associated complications include bladder perforation, mesh erosion and vaginal exposure, chronic pelvic pain, dyspareunia, infection, and fistula formation.[32] This has prompted the U.S. Food and Drug Administration to release several public notifications on the safety and effectiveness of transvaginal mesh for treatment of prolapse.

ASSISTED REPRODUCTIVE TECHNOLOGY

Transvaginal US-guided aspiration of oocytes is used during in vitro fertilization. Complications related to US-guided retrieval and preparation for retrieval of oocytes are rare and include **ovarian hyperstimulation syndrome**, pelvic infection, intraperitoneal bleeding, and adnexal torsion. Occasionally, complications develop hours to weeks after the procedure and require prompt surgical intervention.

Ovarian hyperstimulation syndrome occurs in 1 in 10 women going through in vitro fertilization. Rarely, it can be a life-threatening complication. Symptoms of mild disease include abdominal distention, ovarian enlargement, and weight gain. Patients with severe disease have rapid weight gain, tense ascites due to third spacing of fluid into the abdominal cavity, pleural effusions, tachypnea, orthostatic hypotension due to hypovolemia, tachycardia, progressive oliguria, and electrolyte abnormalities. Increased coagulability and decreased renal perfusion are also noted. The moderate-to-severe form is seen in 1% to 2% of patients undergoing assisted reproduction.

Bimanual pelvic examination is contraindicated due to extremely fragile ovaries that are at high risk of rupture or hemorrhage. Defer examination until after discussion with the gynecologist. Laboratory evaluation includes a CBC, chemistry panel, coagulation studies, and blood for type and cross-match. An ECG to evaluate hyperkalemia should also be obtained.

Treatment in the ED consists of IV volume repletion. Consult the gynecologist for admission. Patients with suspected adnexal torsion should undergo evaluation with Doppler US.

POSTEMBOLIZATION SYNDROME

Uterine artery embolization is a safe, effective approach for treating symptomatic uterine fibroids that may help patients avoid myomectomy and hysterectomy. It is an outpatient procedure performed by interventional radiologists in collaboration with the gynecologist. Compared to hysterectomy, uterine artery embolization is less expensive, results in a move favorable short-term quality of life, and has a significantly lower rate of major complications.[33]

Postembolization syndrome is characterized by abdominal pain, fever, and leukocytosis after embolization and occurs in 2.8% of patients.[33] It is likely caused by an inflammatory response to myometrial and fibroid ischemia and necrotic tissue. Symptoms begin 1 to 2 days after the procedure and can last up to 7 days. In the ED, control pain and consider other possible causes for symptoms, particularly infection such as endometritis. Evaluation may include a CBC and a CT scan. Vaginal discharge and fibroid expulsion may be seen on pelvic exam. Approximately 1% of patients require hysterectomy due to infection. Some patients may require admission for pain control and IV antibiotics.

Acknowledgment: The author gratefully acknowledges the contributions of Michael A. Silverman, contributing author of this chapter in the previous edition.

REFERENCES

The complete reference list is available online at www.TintinalliEM.com.

CHAPTER 106 Emergency Care of Children

Garth Meckler

INTRODUCTION

Children are not just small adults. This standard mantra is heard in EDs around the world. About one third of all ED visits are by children. Anatomic, physiologic, and developmental differences between children and adults give rise to a unique epidemiology, pathophysiology, and differential diagnosis. Key elements of the medical history must often be elicited from caretakers, not from the child. It may be difficult to perform a physical examination on a child, and cardinal signs of disease are different in children compared to adults. Diagnostic testing can cause pain or potentially long-term harm. Drugs require weight-based dosing, and equipment selection must be tailored to the child's size. Disposition may require transfer to a specialized children's hospital. Finally, even though the child is the primary patient, management must be family centered and often involves addressing the fears and stresses of family members.

ANATOMY AND PATHOPHYSIOLOGY

Pediatric age groups are divided into *neonates* (birth to 1 month), *infants* (1 month to 1 year), *toddlers* (1 to 3 years), *school-aged children* (3 to 12 years), and *adolescents* (12 to 18 years). Significant developmental and physiologic changes occur across these age groups; **Table 106-1** summarizes the developmental milestones as they relate to the ED evaluation and approach, and **Table 106-2** lists the age-dependent vital signs.

Neonates undergo the most profound changes as they transition from metabolic and respiratory dependence on the placenta to independence as air-breathing beings. The cardiovascular and respiratory systems switch from near complete shunting of blood flow away from the lungs to typical adult circuitry and dependence on the lungs for oxygenation as the ductus arteriosus closes (see chapter 126, "Congenital and Acquired Pediatric Heart Disease"). Oxygen-avid fetal hemoglobin changes to adult hemoglobin with predictable changes in hemoglobin levels throughout the first years of life. The neonatal and infant immune systems depend on passive maternal humoral protection transferred through the placenta and breast milk until cellular and humoral defenses mature. Immunologic immaturity predisposes to bacterial and viral systemic infections early in life. The neurologic system is characterized by rapid growth, differentiation, and myelination and changes in the balance of excitatory and inhibitory neurotransmitters, which account for susceptibility to seizures.

Anatomically, growth and development of every organ system characterizes infancy and childhood and affects emergency care across the life span. A relatively large occiput, small jaw, high and anterior larynx, narrow cricoid cartilage, and large tongue require unique considerations in airway management (see chapter 111, Intubation and Ventilation in Infants and Children). A soft, compliant chest wall, obligate nose breathing, and gastric inflation from swallowed air alter the mechanics, symptoms, and signs of respiratory distress in young children. **Neonates, infants, and children increase cardiac output through an increase in heart rate rather than stroke volume.** Tachypnea, an increased rate of breathing, not hyperpnea, an increased depth of respiration, is the primary respiratory compensatory mechanism. The musculoskeletal system of young children differs from that of older children and adults not only in its proportions (e.g., relatively large head), but also because **ligaments are stronger than bones, predisposing to fractures rather than sprains**. Linear growth of long bones occurs from specialized cartilaginous end plates (physes), which results in unique fracture patterns (see chapter 140, "Musculoskeletal Disorders in Children").

EPIDEMIOLOGY

Table 106-3 lists the top five causes of pediatric mortality in the United States and worldwide. In the United States, consider congenital anomalies, inherited disorders (see chapter 144, "Metabolic Emergencies in Infants and Children"), complications of prematurity and pregnancy, and accidental and nonaccidental trauma in the first year of life. Injuries, malignancy, and congenital heart disease are the predominant causes of death among children after the first year of life, with injury, suicide, and homicide becoming leading killers in adolescents. Worldwide, infectious diseases, including diarrheal illness, respiratory infections, and preventable or treatable conditions such as measles, malaria, and human immunodeficiency virus infection, predominate.

CLINICAL FEATURES

HISTORY

For preverbal children, obtain the medical history from caregivers. The reliability and quality of historical information are variable. Astute caregivers know their children well and often infer symptoms and complaints from subtle changes in behavior that may not be apparent to the ED physician; this is particularly true for children with special healthcare needs whose medical history and technology may be complex. The expression of some cardinal symptoms of disease varies by age group. For example, vomiting and crying are both common and nonspecific in younger children and may signal serious disease including infection, heart disease, metabolic disease, and surgical abdominal disease.

For neonates and infants, carefully review maternal complications during this and previous pregnancies: a history of spontaneous abortions or maternal liver disease, for example, may indicate inherited metabolic disease, and maternal infections may be congenitally acquired by the neonate. The birth history is important, because gestational age, complications of labor and delivery, and immediate perinatal events alter the differential diagnosis.

Review growth and development and childhood immunizations (**Table 106-4**) to assess overall health. For older children and adolescents, the history should be obtained from both the child and caregiver. Social history becomes important, including questions about risk taking.

PHYSICAL EXAMINATION

The examination is different for children in each developmental stage. Infants are easily separated from parents, whereas children 1 to 3 years of age have stranger anxiety and must be examined in a parent's lap. Crying may make evaluation of the heart, lungs, and abdomen difficult. The sequence of examination should progress from the least to most invasive aspects. Adolescents require special considerations for privacy and autonomy.

TABLE 106-1 Pediatric Developmental Stages and ED Assessment

Stage	Milestone	Strategy
Early infancy (0–6 mo)	Motor: lifts head, reaches	Observation
	Verbal: cooing	Examine in parent's arms
	Social: responsive smile	Direct approach
Late infancy (6–18 mo)	Motor: reaches/obtains, sits, walks	Observation
	Verbal: jargon, few words	Examine in parent's arms
	Social: stranger anxiety/ dependence	Indirect approach
Toddler (18–36 mo)	Motor: walks well, scribbles	Observation
	Verbal: speaks in phrases	Indirect approach
	Social: stranger anxiety/ autonomy	
Preschool (3–5 y)	Motor: runs well, colors	Indirect or direct approach
	Verbal: speaks in sentences	Explain briefly just before procedures
	Social: magical thinking	
School age (5–12 y)	Motor: schoolwork, sports	Direct approach
	Verbal: concrete reasoning	Explain in detail before procedures
	Social: task oriented	
Adolescence (12–17 y)	Motor: adult	Direct approach
	Verbal: abstract reasoning	Confidentiality
	Social: autonomy, rebellion	Treat as adult

Vital signs are age dependent (Table 106-2). For best precision, obtain rectal temperature in infants and young children. Measure blood pressure in all four extremities when considering congenital heart disease. Calculate weight and growth percentiles. Observe skin color, capillary refill, and respiratory effort. For infants and children, note the response to stimulation and check motor tone to identify listlessness or lethargy. Meningismus is present in <15% of infants with bacterial meningitis. Focal abdominal tenderness is difficult to appreciate in the younger child, which leads to delay in the diagnosis of conditions like appendicitis. Skin temperature, color, and capillary refill are affected by ambient temperature, fear, and pain. The inability of the infant to take a deep breath on command makes chest auscultation less reliable for the diagnosis of pneumonia in young infants compared with older children.

DIAGNOSIS

LABORATORY EVALUATION

The pretest probability of disease varies by the child's age and the potential differential diagnosis. The sensitivity and specificity of many common laboratory tests may be unique for children compared with adults. Urinalysis, for example, is less sensitive for detecting infection in young infants who do not store urine long enough to allow accumulation of inflammatory or metabolic markers (e.g., leukocyte esterase and nitrites). Conversely, noninvasive collection of urine by perineal bag or "clean catch" in young infants, although sensitive, lacks specificity in infants due to perineal contamination with bacteria. Other common laboratory screening tests, such as the basic metabolic panel and CBC, have little specificity and predictive power for most childhood conditions (see chapter 128, "Vomiting, Diarrhea, and Dehydration in Infants and Children"; chapter 129, "Fluid and Electrolyte Therapy in Infants and Children"; and chapter 116, "Fever and Serious Bacterial Illness in Infants and Children"). Unless specifically directed by the history and examination, screening labs that are commonly used in adults add little value to the routine evaluation of common pediatric emergencies such as dehydration, febrile seizures, and chest pain. Carefully consider the need for blood tests in children, because of the technical difficulties and the anxiety and pain caused by venipuncture.

IMAGING

Weigh the potential risks and benefits of diagnostic imaging in children. The lifetime risk of a fatal malignancy from a single CT scan may be as high as 1 in 2000 in infants and 1 in 5000 for older children.[1] Early exposure to ionizing radiation from radiologic imaging may result in harmful long-term neurologic outcomes, such as decreased intelligence.[2] If infants and young children require sedation for imaging, the risks of sedation are added to the risk of ionizing radiation. Radiographs can be avoided for a number of childhood respiratory conditions (see chapter 124, "Wheezing in Infants and Children"). US is the imaging modality of choice for a number of disease conditions in children, such as pyloric stenosis, appendicitis, and **intussusception**. Bedside US (e.g., focused abdominal sonography in trauma), although standard in adults, is less reliable in children.

TREATMENT

Many treatment parameters are age specific. Resuscitation principles differ for neonates, children, and adults (see chapter 108, "Resuscitation of Neonates" and chapter 109, "Resuscitation of Children"). Neonatal resuscitation focuses primarily on respiratory assistance with effective positive-pressure ventilation. **Children maintain normal blood**

TABLE 106-2 Pediatric Vital Signs by Age (Awake and Resting)

Age	Heart Rate, Upper Limit (beats/min)	Respiratory Rate, Upper Limit (breaths/min)	Blood Pressure,* Lower Limit (mm Hg)	Weight,† (kg)
0–1 mo	180	60	60/40	3–4
2–12 mo	160	50	70/45	5–10
12–24 mo	140	40	75/50	10–12
2–6 y	120	30	80/55	13–25
6–12 y	110	20	90/60	25–40
>12 y	100	20	90/60	140–60

*May be estimated by:

Systolic blood pressure (5th percentile) = 70 + [2 × (age in years)]

†May be estimated by:

12 mo: weight (kg) = 4 + (age in months/2)

1–12 y: weight (kg) = 10 + [2 × (age in years)]

TABLE 106-3 Leading Causes of Mortality in the United States and Worldwide by Age in Years

	United States*					Worldwide†				
Rank	<1 y	1–4 y	5–9 y	10–14 y	15–24 y	<1 y‡	1–4 y	5–9 y	10–14 y	15–19 y
1	Congenital anomalies	Unintentional injuries	Unintentional injuries	Unintentional injuries	Unintentional injuries	Malaria	Malaria	Malaria	Human immunodeficiency virus	Suicide
2	Short gestation	Congenital defects	Malignancy	Malignancy	Suicide	Pneumonia	Malnutrition	Human immunodeficiency virus	Malaria	Road traffic injuries
3	Sudden infant death syndrome	Homicide	Congenital anomalies	Suicide	Homicide	Malnutrition	Human immunodeficiency virus	Typhoid/paratyphoid	Drowning	Malaria
4	Maternal complications of pregnancy	Malignancy	Homicide	Homicide	Malignancy	Diarrheal illness	Measles	Drowning	Typhoid/paratyphoid	Drowning
5	Unintentional injury	Heart disease	Heart disease	Congenital defects	Heart disease	Congenital anomalies	Pneumonia	Diarrheal illness	Environmental exposure	Fire

*Ten leading causes of death and injury. Centers for Disease Control and Prevention, 2010–11. Available at: http://www.cdc.gov/nchs/data/nvsr/nvsr61/nvsr61_06.pdf. Accessed March 15, 2014.

†Global Burden of Disease Study 2010. Results by Cause. Available at: http://healthintelligence.drupalgardens.com/content/causes-death-world-1990-2005-2010. Accessed March 15, 2014.

‡Data excluding the neonatal period.

pressure until very late in critical illness, so compensated shock and respiratory distress require early and aggressive intervention; **cardiac arrest is most commonly secondary to respiratory failure in children**, rather than primary as in adults. Try to include parents and caretakers in the room during pediatric resuscitation.

Children require special medication dosage calculations based on weight or body surface area due to age-dependent metabolic pathways and differing body composition, volumes of drug distribution, and organ development. Most prescription medications have not been formally tested in children and do not have specific U.S. Food and Drug Administration approval for use in children due to the ethical and practical difficulties of performing drug trials in children. Common medications can have adverse effects in children, such as dental staining from tetracycline antibiotics and life-threatening complications from antimotility drugs commonly used for adult diarrheal disease.

Children generally do not understand the transient nature of painful procedures or of their relative risks and benefits. Such comprehension allows adults to consent to and cooperate with common emergency procedures. Chapter 113, "Pain Management and Procedural Sedation in Infants and Children," discusses the pharmacologic and nonpharmacologic approach to this important topic.

Caretakers make legal decisions on behalf of their children. Consent for treatment and procedures must be obtained from legal guardians for all minors except in cases of emergency medical necessity. A variable exception is the confidential provision of care to adolescents with regard to their reproductive and mental health.

DISPOSITION AND FOLLOW-UP

Disposition decisions in children require consideration of caretaker abilities and indications for transfer to another institution. Discharge to reliable caretakers is an important part of practice guidelines for many common pediatric conditions, including minor head injury (see

TABLE 106-4 Recommended Childhood Immunizations

	Vaccine*												
Age	DTaP (Tdap >6 y)	Hib	Hep B	Polio	Pneumococcal (conjugate)	Rotavirus	HPV	MMR	VZV	Hep A	Meningococcus (conjugate)	Influenza†	BCG
Birth			C, U, W				C						W
2 mo	C, U, W	C, U, W	C, U, W	C, U, W	C, U, W	C, U, W	C				C		
4 mo	C, U, W	C, U, W		C, U, W	C, U, W	C, U, W					C		
6 mo	C, U, W	C, U, W	C, U, W	C, U, W	U, W	C, U, W	C				C	C, U, W	
12–15 mo		U			C, U			C, U, W	C, U	U, W			
15–23 mo	C, U	C								U			
2–4 y											W	U	
4–6 y	U			C, U				C, U	C, U			C	
10–12 y	U						U, W				C, U		
14–17 y	C										U		

Abbreviations: BCG = bacillus Calmette-Guérin; C = Canada (Public Health Agency of Canada); DTaP = diphtheria, tetanus, acellular pertussis; Hep A = hepatitis A; Hep B = hepatitis B; Hib = *Haemophilus influenzae* type b conjugate; HPV = human papilloma virus; MMR = measles, mumps, rubella; U = United States (Centers for Disease Control and Prevention); W = World Health Organization.

*The exact sequence varies according to manufactured brand of vaccine, and many combination vaccines and conjugate vaccines with variable serotypes exist. Schedule is approximate. World Health Organization (W) guidelines recommend additional vaccination of high-risk patients for the following: Japanese encephalitis, yellow fever, tick-borne encephalitis, typhoid, cholera, and rabies. See http://www.who.int/immunization/documents/positionpapers for more information.

†Given annually beginning as early as 6 months of life; requires two-vaccine series for children under 9 years of age; avoid live vaccine in children <2 years of age and those with asthma or who are immunocompromised.

chapter 138, "Head Injury in Infants and Children") and fever without source in the infant (see chapter 116, "Fever and Serious Bacterial Illness in Infants and Children"). Children requiring hospitalization may require transfer to a tertiary-care pediatric hospital. The emergency physician has responsibility for determining the need, risks, and benefits of transfer, and the mode of transporting children to a higher level of care. Ultimately, the disposition requires close communication with receiving facilities and with the child's family.

REFERENCES

The complete reference list is available online at www.TintinalliEM.com.

CHAPTER 107

Neonatal and Pediatric Transport

Samuel J. Prater
Manish Shah

INTRODUCTION

Regionalized intensive care for neonatology and pediatric care[1] focuses expensive, high-technology, labor-intensive therapies to a few regional centers. This model is based on the reduction of morbidity and mortality for trauma patients at designated trauma centers.[2,3] Because patients in need of specialized services often present to other hospitals, interfacility transport is an important complement to regionalized intensive care.[4] Specialized pediatric transport services improve safety, decrease unplanned adverse events (especially airway events), and lower mortality.[4-6] This chapter reviews the general and pediatric considerations for the interfacility transport of critically ill neonates and children.

THE TRANSPORT TEAM

Caring for critically ill children is best accomplished with at least two patient care providers on each team in addition to the driver or pilot. One of the patient care members should be a registered nurse with a minimum of 5 years of experience, typically at least 3 years of neonatal or pediatric critical care or ED training.[4] Additional member(s) may include a respiratory therapist, physician, or paramedic. The condition of the child and local resources determine the exact composition of the specialized transport team.

TRANSPORT ENVIRONMENT

Transporting critically ill patients adds to the risks of the illness or injury because of the hazards associated with the transport environment, particularly for neonates and children.[7] The features of transport that distinguish the transport environment from the ED setting and the effects of these features on patients and caretakers are outlined in **Table 107-1**.

PRECAUTIONS

Suggested guidelines to minimize the impact of the limitations inherent in a transport environment are

1. *Prepare the transport vehicle.* Transport vehicles should be prepared to meet the special needs of children (e.g., accessory lighting, controlled thermal environment) and should be stocked with the necessary

TABLE 107-1 Features of Transport versus Inpatient Setting and Effects

Feature	Effects	Solutions
Noise	Reach levels 90–110 dB[8,9] Arterial desaturation in infants Inability to auscultate	Ear plugs Monitors to allow visual cues
Vibration	Autonomic/central nervous system motion-induced illness (sopite, nausea syndromes) Equipment motion artifact	Accommodation Ondansetron, gastric decompression Alternative monitoring
Inadequate lighting	Poor visual cues Complications with procedures	Compartmental lighting 400 lux Task lighting 1000–1500 lux
Temperature	Gradient-dependent heat loss by convection and radiation	Limiting time in transport Thermal regulation of vehicles and surfaces Double-walled isolettes for neonates and infants
Humidity	Nonhumidification of respiratory gases causes dehydration, secretion tenacity	Humidify gases for long (>2 h) transports
Altitude	Decreased Po_2 Expansion of gases in closed spaces Significant for nonpressurized aircraft above 5000 ft (1500 m)	Pressurize aircraft Ventilate closed-space gas to atmosphere Orogastric tube, decompress pneumothorax
Confined space	Limits crew, workspace, equipment Typical sizes: 47 sq. ft (ambulance) 22–36 sq. ft (helicopter) 150 sq. ft (neonatal intensive care unit patient space)	Efficient use of patient care space in vehicle Experience
Limited support	Hospital-based radiographic and laboratory services unavailable No onsite additional clinical expertise	Portable blood analyzer (i-STAT®) Thoughtful planning of radiographic needs Consultants via telecommunications
Equipment failure	Exhaustion of respiratory gases, supplies, medications Monitor deterioration secondary to vibration	Backup equipment Thorough supply checks Routine accelerated maintenance schedule

Abbreviation: Po_2 = partial pressure of oxygen.

equipment. A list of the minimum necessary equipment for ambulances, which can serve as a guide for EMS agencies, has been published by the Emergency Medical Services for Children program.[10]

2. *Stabilize the patient before transport.* Unless the immediate needs of the patient can only be met in the receiving hospital (e.g., emergent surgery), ample time should be devoted to stabilizing the patient in the referring hospital. Time spent undertaking goal-directed intensive care interventions early in the course of the patient illness at the referring hospital does not worsen patient outcomes.[11]
3. *Monitor as many physiologic parameters as possible electronically.* Because physical examination is difficult during transport, and because children often are transported during dynamic changes in their physiologic condition, electronic monitoring is essential. Important monitoring equipment commonly used during transport includes cardiorespiratory monitor (selected based on its size, weight, battery life, and resistance to motion artifact); continuous pulse oximetry with a plethysmographic waveform to assist in identifying motion artifact; temperature monitor (of infants and incubator air temperature); carbon dioxide monitor using continuous inline infrared analysis (or transcutaneous carbon dioxide monitoring or arterial blood analysis), which can aid in early identification of unplanned extubation[12]; invasive or noninvasive blood pressure monitoring; and portable blood gas analyzer.
4. *Anticipate deterioration.* Preparation of the patient should include not only care for the identified problems but also anticipation of problems that may arise during transport. The application of this principle may lead to performance of procedures or therapies before transport such as gastric decompression, placement of a chest tube for pneumothorax, or transfusion.

PREPARATION OF A PATIENT FOR TRANSPORT

DECISION TO TRANSPORT

Children require transfer to a regional center if the current or anticipated medical care needs of the patient exceed the resources of the local hospital. Arranging transfer to the regional center can occur simultaneously with assessment, resuscitation, and stabilization at the local hospital. Discussion with the receiving hospital and specialists can aid in decisions regarding the mode of transport and composition of the transport team.

ASSESSMENT

Proper assessment is the cornerstone of neonatal and pediatric critical care, as management cannot begin until the critical patient is correctly identified. An important tool in pediatric assessment is the **Pediatric Assessment Triangle** (**Figure 107-1**). Each face of the triangle represents a critical feature in neonatal and pediatric assessment: **Appearance**, **Work of Breathing**, and **Circulation**. This method can be applied quickly to reliably and accurately assess a potentially critically ill patient and determine the need for life-saving interventions.

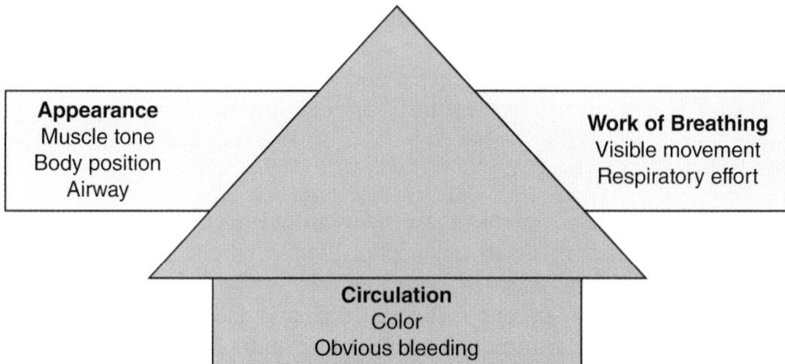

FIGURE 107-1. The Pediatric Assessment Triangle. [Reproduced with permission from Strange GR, Ahrens WR, Schafermeyer RW, Wiebe RA: *Pediatric Emergency Medicine*, 3rd ed. © 2009. The McGraw-Hill Companies, Inc. New York, Figure 150-2.]

BASIC ASSESSMENT

Stabilization is the responsibility of the referring hospital personnel, to the limits of their abilities and resources. Because dealing with a sick neonate is an infrequent occurrence for people working outside of neonatal intensive care units, the **S**ugar/Safe care, **T**emperature, **A**irway, **B**lood pressure, **Lab** evaluation, **E**motional support (STABLE) mnemonic was created by the developers of the **S.T.A.B.L.E.® course** (http://www.stableprogram.org) to aid recall of the steps for managing infants prior to transport.[13] The principles of **STABLE** include maintaining blood glucose at 50 milligrams/dL for transport; sustaining a neutral thermal environment with a core temperature range for a neonate of 36.5°C to 37.5°C (97.7°F to 99.5°F); assuring airway patency and respiratory support necessary for optimal ventilation and oxygenation; maintaining adequate blood pressure to provide oxygen delivery to the tissues (normal blood pressure for preterm infants is 45 to 60/25 to 35 mm Hg); laboratory evaluation directed by the underlying condition; and emotional support for the family in crisis.

AIRWAY MANAGEMENT

Intubation and mechanical ventilation are performed to (1) protect the airway from obstruction, (2) ensure adequate ventilation, or (3) provide adequate oxygenation. While this principle applies to both inpatients and those being prepared for transport, the threshold for intervention is lowered for patients requiring transport.[14] For example, an infant with an elevated partial pressure of arterial carbon dioxide level might be observed without ventilatory support in the inpatient setting but may need to be intubated and ventilated in preparation for transport. In addition, children without respiratory failure but in whom deterioration is anticipated should be intubated in preparation for transport. This more aggressive approach to airway management is justified because the ability to identify respiratory failure and to intubate is impaired during transport.

Principles of infant and pediatric airway management including appropriate airway equipment and sizes are reviewed in chapter 111, "Intubation and Ventilation in Infants and Children."

Some airway problems specific to transport are worthy of mention. Even if the child is already intubated at the transferring institution, or if intubated by the transport team confirm or reconfirm tube placement by several methods: direct visualization, auscultation, end-tidal carbon dioxide detection, or chest radiograph for positioning.[15] Make sure the endotracheal tube is well secured, and stabilize the tube by hand when moving the child to make sure movement doesn't dislodge the tube from the trachea into the esophagus. Right mainstem intubation is common in neonates. Prolonged right mainstem intubation increases the likelihood of pneumothorax and is particularly hazardous in premature infants, many of whom will later receive surfactant through the endotracheal tube. Before departure, and soon after the initiation of mechanical ventilation, obtain an arterial blood gas analysis to ensure appropriate oxygenation and ventilation.

Ventilators for transport should accommodate the needs of all pediatric age groups. Neonates are most often ventilated with time-cycled, pressure-limited ventilators using intermittent mandatory ventilation. Older infants and children typically require volume-assisted ventilation using synchronized intermittent mandatory ventilation. Causes of acute decompensation in the mechanically ventilated patient can be remembered using the **DOPE mnemonic**: (1) **d**islodgement or obstruction of the endotracheal tube; (2) faulty **o**xygen source; (3) **p**neumothorax; and (4) **e**quipment failure.

Initial Ventilator Settings Neonates are most often ventilated with time-cycled, pressure-limited ventilators using intermittent mandatory ventilation. The goals of mechanical ventilation are to maintain adequate tissue oxygenation while minimizing pressure-induced trauma to the lungs. This is best achieved utilizing a strategy of effective lung recruitment with positive end-expiratory pressure combined with permissive hypercapnia.[16]

Preset peak inspiratory pressure, a positive end-expiratory pressure, and an inspiratory time determine the volume of each breath. Suggested initial peak inspiratory pressure for term neonates is 20 to 25 cm of water depending on the severity of respiratory disease, while positive end-expiratory pressure is usually set at 5 cm of water, with an inspiratory time of 0.3 to 0.35 seconds and a rate of 20 to 40 breaths per minute.

Older infants and children typically require volume-assisted ventilations using synchronized intermittent mandatory ventilation, with a volume of 8 to 10 mL/kg, positive end-expiratory pressure of 5 cm of water, pressure support of 10 cm of water, fraction of inspired oxygen >60%, and variable rate depending on normal rate for age and underlying disease process. Obtain an arterial blood gas after initiation of mechanical ventilation to guide future changes. Increases in oxygenation can be achieved by increasing positive end-expiratory pressure and fraction of inspired oxygen, whereas increases in ventilation can be achieved by increasing rate and pressure support.

Ventilator Troubleshooting Causes of acute decompensation in the mechanically ventilated patient can be remembered using the **DOPE mnemonic**, discussed earlier: (1) **d**islodgement or obstruction of the endotracheal tube; (2) faulty **o**xygen source; (3) **p**neumothorax; and (4) **e**quipment failure.

The Difficult Airway Success rates for pediatric direct laryngoscopic intubation are lower than those for adults, and providers must be familiar with advanced airway techniques (see chapter 111, "Intubation and Ventilation in Infants and Children").[17] Supraglottic devices like the laryngeal mask airway and esophageal-tracheal combination tubes can serve as potential rescue devices, and video-assisted laryngoscopy devices may help indirectly visualize the difficult airway.

VASCULAR ACCESS

Nearly all patients should have intravascular access during transport. Critically ill children should have at least two lines of vascular access in case one becomes dislodged or several medications need to be administered simultaneously. For newborns, consider using umbilical vessels for vascular access. Intraosseous cannulation is an alternative technique for fluid and drug administration when intravascular lines cannot be placed or the severity of illness demands immediate access (see chapter 112, Intravenous and Intraosseous Access in Infants and Children).

In small children, IV lines should be infused with the use of pumps. Open "drips" should not be used, even with volumetric drip chambers, because of the risk of fluid overload from inadvertent administration of large boluses. The amount of fluid administered before and during transport should be monitored and carefully recorded.

A small subset of children may do better without IV placement, because IV placement can agitate the child and further compromise the airway. This is particularly true for children with a partial airway obstruction from croup, a foreign body, or epiglottitis. The best measure in the situation of partial airway obstruction may be to keep the child as calm as possible, allow the child to sit in the caregiver's lap during transport, and refrain from IV placement.

CONDUCT OF A TRANSPORT

Pre-established transfer protocols should provide information about each regional center to which a patient might be referred, including (1) special services available; (2) criteria for referral; (3) telephone numbers for consultation, referral, and transport; (4) distance and usual response time; (5) type of transport personnel and their capabilities; (6) type of transport vehicles; and (7) protocols for preparation of patients. Establish formal agreements with regional centers that outline the circumstances under which patients can be transported without prior administrative approval. Clinical approval of transfers is always physician to physician.

Once the decision has been made to transport a child, the referring hospital has certain legal obligations to the patient in addition to provision of medical care.[18] In the United States, the referring physician is responsible for arranging an appropriate mode of transport to a hospital capable of providing the services needed by the patient and stabilizing the patient as best as possible before transport. The referring physician should inform caregivers of the need for transfer and the risks and benefits, and discuss the transport modality. Written consent for transport should be obtained from a parent or other legal guardian. Important documentation to provide for the receiving facility and care team includes a copy of the current medical record, laboratory data, radiographs, and old medical records, if available.

Clear communication between the referring and receiving physicians is essential. Standardized techniques can help mitigate communication errors, such as the **ISBARQ (introduction, situation, background, assessment, recommendation, questions) model** developed by Children's Hospital of Philadelphia: During the *introduction*, the referring physician and patient are identified; the *situation* is conveyed by the working diagnosis and current medical condition; *background* includes what is known about the patient, such as past medical history and past tests or treatments; *assessment* communicates what is happening at the time of transport (current findings, patient needs, treatments, new test results); *recommendations* are made by receiving physicians regarding further stabilization of the patient, sometimes at the request of the referring doctor (although referring physicians are not obligated to follow these recommendations if they are considered to be medically inappropriate or beyond the capabilities of the referring hospital); and the process concludes with mutual *questions* that allow for further clarification.[18,19]

For most critically ill children, ideal care is provided when the ED of the referring hospital devotes its energy to providing emergent short-term medical care, and the responsibility for transport is left to a regional center. This is particularly true for neonates because of the special equipment and expertise required for transport. When transport services are not provided by the regional center or when time is critical, the only option may be for the referring hospital to provide transport. In these circumstances, it is the responsibility of the referring center to ensure the adequacy of care, as best as possible given available resources and personnel, during transport.

In many areas, physicians have a choice between air and ground transportation. This decision should be made collaboratively between the referring and accepting physicians.[20] The risks and benefits of air transport are discussed in chapter 3, Air Medical Transport. Time, distance, traffic, weather, geographic constraints, and availability all factor into the decision regarding mode of transport. When the transport team arrives, the referring physician and local ED staff should be available to coordinate the transition of care and communicate the patient history, recent events, and the care already provided.

Referring providers should provide the family members with written directions to the receiving institution when they are not able to accompany their child in the transport vehicle. Additional helpful information includes parking information, nearby accommodations, and visiting policies of the receiving institution, if known. Allowing a family member to accompany the child during ground transport is valued by the patient and family and does not interfere with the delivery of care.[21,22] Clear communication with family members about the medical needs of the patient, appropriate parental behavior, and logistics involved may help alleviate disruptions during transport. Ultimately, if it is anticipated that family member involvement will diminish the quality of care, it will be necessary to encourage them to meet their child at the receiving institution.

SPECIAL PROBLEMS OF THE NEONATE

Critically ill neonates depend on extrinsic factors to maintain homeostasis. This is particularly true when birth occurs before term; the complexity of care is often inversely related to birth weight and gestational age. Aspects of clinical care that deserve special consideration when preparing neonates for transport can be remembered using the **STABLE mnemonic** described earlier.[13] Common neonatal emergencies are discussed in chapter 114, Neonatal Emergencies and Common Neonatal Problems, and specific considerations for transport are summarized in the following.

HYPOGLYCEMIA

The most common metabolic abnormality in newborns is hypoglycemia, which is discussed in detail in chapter 144, Metabolic Emergencies in Infants and Children. At birth, blood glucose in the neonate is approximately 60% to 70% of the maternal level and falls to approximately 40 milligrams/dL (2.22 mmol/L) within 1 to 2 hours. This decline may be accentuated in premature or small-for-gestational-age infants, acutely ill infants with increased glucose utilization, and certain other high-risk infants (e.g., infants of diabetic mothers, large-for-gestational-age infants). Because of the risk of hypoglycemia, **all neonates should receive**

glucose-containing fluids in preparation for and during transport. An initial glucose infusion rate of 4 to 6 milligrams/kg/min should be targeted, and this can be achieved with 10% dextrose in water infused at a rate of 80 mL/kg/d. Sometimes a bolus of dextrose may be necessary, which can be achieved with 4 to 5 mL/kg of 10% dextrose solution. Repeat measurement of blood sugar at 15- to 30-minute intervals, with a goal to maintain serum glucose at 50 milligrams/dL (2.7 mmol/L).

HYPOTHERMIA

The normal core temperature range for a neonate is 36.5°C to 37.5°C (97.7°F to 99.5°F). A neutral thermal environment is provided when the infant's body temperature is normal and there is a minimal gradient between the core and the skin temperature.

Newborns attempt to conserve heat by several mechanisms: (1) peripheral vasoconstriction, (2) increasing voluntary muscle activity, (3) flexion to conserve exposed surface area, and (4) nonshivering thermogenesis. All of these mechanisms, except nonshivering thermogenesis, are less effective in the neonate than in older infants and children. Unintentional hypothermia in the neonate and young infant can lead to apnea, multisystem organ failure, inability to resuscitate, or intracranial hemorrhages in those most susceptible. The transport vehicle should be equipped with a closed heated incubator with an automatic temperature regulator. If the transport vehicle does not have a closed incubator, an overhead radiant heat source and increasing the heat inside the transport vehicle are other options. During transport, it is necessary to monitor the patient's body temperature frequently to avoid hyper- or hypothermia.

INDUCED HYPOTHERMIA

Therapeutic hypothermia is now a standard of care for neonates with perinatal asphyxia. Guidelines from the International Liaison Committee on Resuscitation recommend therapeutic hypothermia for term or near-term infants with evolving moderate to severe hypoxic-ischemic encephalopathy. Hypothermia lowers mortality rates and improves neurodevelopmental outcomes (number needed to treat = 9).[23] Initiate cooling to a temperature of 33.5°C within the first 6 hours of life using the whole-body method or selective head cooling, and continue cooling throughout transport.

HYPOXEMIA

Recommendations from the 2010 international consensus on neonatal resuscitation[23] state that **resuscitation of term babies should begin with room air rather than 100% oxygen and that administration of supplemental oxygen should be regulated by blending oxygen and room air, to a concentration guided by pulse oximetry**. A normal newborn would not be expected to achieve normal oxygen saturation during the first 10 minutes. Begin resuscitation of neonates <32 weeks of gestation with 30% to 90% oxygen and titrate according to pulse oximetry (**Table 107-2**); if blended oxygen and air is not available, use room air (see chapter 108, Resuscitation of Neonates).

For mechanically ventilated patients, arterial blood gas is the gold standard for assessing the efficacy of ventilation and oxygenation and modifying ventilator settings; however, capillary or venous blood is acceptable for measurement of the partial pressure of carbon dioxide and pH in the absence of access to arterial blood. The target ranges for oxygenation and ventilation of neonates differ according to the disease process and gestational age (**Table 107-2**). No clear relationship has been established between specific partial pressure of arterial oxygen values and adequate tissue oxygenation. It is acceptable to use pulse oximetry alone to guide fraction of inspired oxygen. The overall goal during transport should be to deliver the minimum required fraction of inspired oxygen to maintain adequate tissue oxygenation. The blending of oxygen and air to deliver the minimum fraction of inspired oxygen required to achieve adequate oxygenation is essential in premature infants because of the known retinal and pulmonary toxicities of oxygen.[24,25]

TABLE 107-2 Target Ranges for Oxygenation and Ventilation of Neonates

Oxygenation	Arterial Blood Gas	Pulse Oximetry
Premature infant with RDS*	Pao_2 50–70 mm Hg	Sao_2 85%–94%
Term infant (no lung disease)	Pao_2 60–90 mm Hg	Sao_2 >95%
Infant with persistent pulmonary hypertension of the newborn	Pao_2 60–90 mm Hg	Sao_2 >95%
Infant with CHD	Pao_2 35–50 mm Hg	Sao_2 75%–85%
Ventilation		
Premature infant with respiratory distress syndrome	$Paco_2$ 50–55 mm Hg	
Term infant (no lung disease)	$Paco_2$ 35–50 mm Hg	
Infant with persistent pulmonary hypertension	$Paco_2$ 30–40 mm Hg	
Infant with CHD	$Paco_2$ 35–50 mm Hg	

Abbreviations: CHD = cyanotic heart disease; $Paco_2$ = partial pressure of arterial carbon dioxide; Pao_2 = partial pressure of arterial oxygen; RDS = respiratory distress syndrome; Sao_2= arterial oxygen saturation.

*Gestational age dependent.

RESPIRATORY DISTRESS SYNDROME

Premature infants with respiratory distress syndrome present with progressively worsening retractions, tachypnea, and oxygen requirements because their lungs are too immature to synthesize surfactant. This disease has a characteristic radiographic pattern that includes "ground glass" opacities in the lung parenchyma and prominent air bronchograms (**Figure 107-2**). Initial therapy for respiratory distress syndrome involves **continuous positive airway pressure** to stent open airways, thereby reducing collapse of alveoli and limiting further damage. Continuous positive airway pressure can be administered during transport through specially designed nasal cannula–type devices (with a continuous pressure of 4 to 6 cm of water) in the nonintubated patient with mild respiratory distress. A similar strategy should be used in the intubated patient by adjusting the ventilator to provide a positive end-expiratory pressure of 4 or 5 cm of water such that there is never a period of negative pressure during passive exhalation. For intubated infants with respiratory

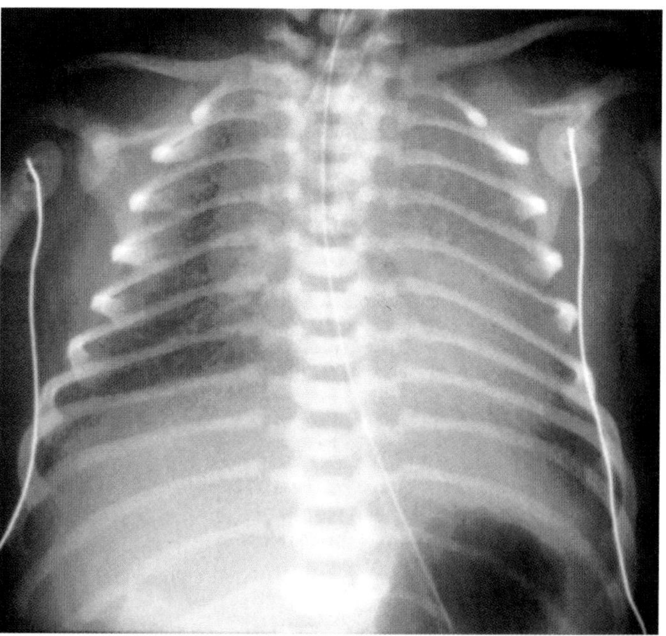

FIGURE 107-2. Chest radiograph of intubated infant illustrating classic findings of respiratory distress syndrome. Note the granular or "ground glass" appearance of the lung parenchyma, the poor inflation, the lack of focal opacities, and the prominent air bronchograms.

distress syndrome, administer surfactant through the endotracheal tube. This procedure can result in rapid changes in pulmonary compliance, can cause transient airway obstruction, and can be associated with pulmonary hemorrhage. For these reasons, only experienced personnel should administer surfactant. **When an infant needs surfactant but the referring institution is unable to administer it, transport personnel to administer surfactant as soon as they arrive on site, thereby minimizing further treatment delay.**

PERSISTENT PULMONARY HYPERTENSION

Pulmonary circulation is attenuated in the fetus by high intrinsic vascular resistance in the pulmonary arterioles and bypass shunting around the lungs via the ductus arteriosus. The rapid transition from fetal to newborn circulation includes a precipitous drop in pulmonary vascular resistance concomitant with lung expansion, followed by increased pulmonary blood flow in the first minutes of life and a gradual closing of the ductus arteriosus over the next 48 hours. Unfortunately, there are several common conditions that can disrupt this progression, including meconium aspiration, hypothermia, sepsis, and birth depression. Early diagnosis of persistent pulmonary hypertension is essential to prevent patient morbidity.

Infants with persistent pulmonary hypertension demonstrate labile oxygenation despite adequate ventilation due to right-to-left shunting of blood through the ductus arteriosus (**Figure 107-3**) or patent foramen ovale. This usually can be detected by placing a pulse oximetry probe on the right hand (preductal) and a second probe on a foot (postductal). Shunting is suggested by a preductal saturation greater than postductal by >10% in a newborn. With shunting exclusively at the atrial level, saturations are low, but the preductal to postductal saturation difference will not be observed.

Initial management of severe persistent pulmonary hypertension includes intubation, administration of 100% oxygen (a pulmonary vasodilator), optimization of ventilation to promote lung recruitment (**Table 107-2**), correction of acidosis, maintenance of high-normal blood pressures (with fluid boluses and inotropic agents if necessary), maintenance of a normal hematocrit, correction of metabolic abnormalities (hypocalcemia, hypoglycemia), sedation, and sometimes paralysis (to minimize intrathoracic pressure). These therapies may transiently stabilize critically ill infants with persistent pulmonary hypertension but are damaging in the long term. Inhaled nitric oxide is a potent pulmonary vasodilator that can be used after conventional therapies are optimized. Some neonatal transport teams carry portable inhaled nitric oxide tanks. When possible, transport of a neonate with persistent pulmonary hypertension should be performed by a team that can administer inhaled nitric oxide, thus minimizing the time to treatment. Infants who do not respond to conventional therapy or inhaled nitric oxide are likely to require extracorporeal membrane oxygenation for survival. For this reason, infants with severe persistent pulmonary hypertension should be transported preferentially to extracorporeal membrane oxygenation centers.

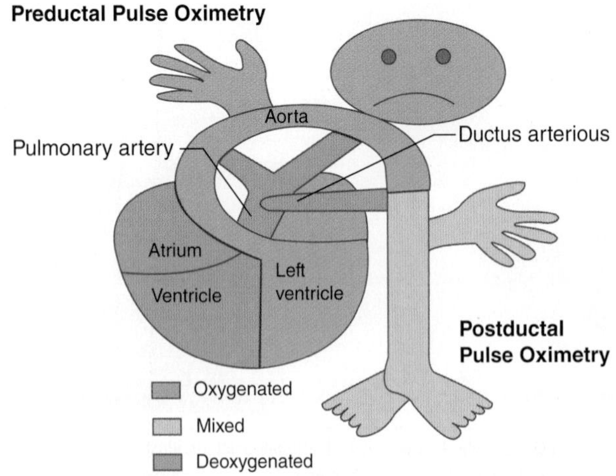

FIGURE 107-3. Homunculus illustrating right-to-left shunting through the ductus arteriosus due to persistent pulmonary hypertension of the newborn.

CONGENITAL HEART DISEASE

Because fetal oxygenation occurs through the placenta, cyanotic heart lesions usually are asymptomatic in the fetus, and a number of cyanotic heart lesions dependent on the ductus arteriosus for pulmonary blood flow at birth remain clinically silent until the time of ductal closure. This sequence of events can result in delayed diagnosis of cyanotic heart disease and a subsequent need for emergency management. The presentation and management of congenital heart disease is discussed in chapter 126, Congenital and Acquired Pediatric Heart Disease, and includes (1) supportive interim management and (2) reopening and maintaining ductus arteriosus patency with a prostaglandin E_1 infusion. Prostaglandin E_1 typically is started by the transport team at 0.05 microgram/kg/min and titrated according to oxygen saturation up to 0.1 microgram/kg/min when trying to reopen the ductus in a severely ill patient. Patients with previously undiagnosed cyanotic heart lesions should be transferred to a tertiary facility that can perform pediatric cardiovascular surgery.

HYPOTENSION

Neonatal hypotension is defined as a systolic blood pressure less than 60 mm Hg. In newborns, hypotension occurs secondary to hypovolemia (intrapartum or postpartum hemorrhage), cardiogenic failure, sepsis, or a combination of these conditions. Physical examination findings of hypotension include weak peripheral pulses, cyanosis, poor perfusion (represented as a capillary refill time >3 seconds), pallor, and cool and mottled skin. Treatment for neonates with hypovolemic shock relies on volume resuscitation initially with normal saline at 10 mL/kg, as larger volumes may be associated with increased risk for intraventricular hemorrhage. In the presence of hypovolemic shock and anemia, administer cross-matched packed red blood cells. Treat cardiogenic failure with inotropic agents (dopamine at 2.5 micrograms/kg/min titrated to desired blood pressure up to 20 micrograms/kg/min).[16] In septic shock, capillary leak and the ongoing third space losses will require volume replacement, and the cardiac effects will require inotropic support. Requiring large amounts of volume replacement is not uncommon for infants in septic shock.

To provide volume and inotropes, peripheral venous access must be obtained, and this may be technically challenging. Consider emergent cannulation of the umbilical vessels or use of intraosseous lines (see chapter 112, Intravenous and Intraosseous Access in Infants and Children).

INFECTION

Signs and symptoms of infection in a neonate are often nonspecific and may be indistinguishable from those associated with other diseases. See chapter 116, Fever and Serious Bacterial Illness in Infants and Children, for details on the evaluation and management of neonates and infants with fever, and consider empiric administration of broad-spectrum antibiotics including meningitic dosages of ampicillin (50 milligrams/kg) and gentamicin (2.5 milligrams/kg).[26] A third-generation cephalosporin should be added or substituted for gentamicin when gram-negative meningitis is suspected or confirmed on a cerebrospinal fluid gram stain.[27] Sick neonates require stabilization and rapid administration of empiric antibiotics, which should not wait for diagnostic studies such as lumbar puncture.

INBORN ERRORS OF METABOLISM

Inborn errors of metabolism encompass a complicated set of diseases involved with the metabolism of carbohydrates, fats, or proteins and are discussed in detail in chapter 144, Metabolic Emergencies in Infants and Children. Regardless of which defect is involved, the end result is depletion of ATP stores and the accumulation of toxic metabolites. Common presentation includes nonspecific symptoms such as vomiting, lethargy, and poor feeding. Fortunately, the principles of management for all emergent presentations of metabolic disease are the same: stop feedings, provide dextrose, and facilitate removal of the toxic metabolites. **Stabilization therapy is 10% dextrose in normal saline at 5 mL/kg/h.**

Additional therapies are discussed in chapter 144, Hypoglycemia and Metabolic Emergencies in Infants and Children.

VIABILITY

Delivery of premature infants who are at the limits of viability is not an uncommon occurrence in the ED. The first priority of the physician caring for the infant is to determine whether resuscitation is justified. **In the United States, an infant born at a gestational age of <23 weeks, weighing <400 grams, and with gelatinous/translucent skin generally should not be resuscitated or transported.** According to the 2010 guidelines,[23] when congenital anomalies are associated with almost certain death or an unacceptable high morbidity is likely among survivors, resuscitation is not indicated. Infants born after 23 weeks of completed gestation and without a congenital anomaly associated with a high rate of mortality or unacceptable morbidity are capable of relatively good outcomes and should be supported aggressively after birth. The decision to initiate support must be made immediately because any delay can have a deleterious effect on the infant's prognosis. If the decision is not clear or there is a condition associated with borderline survival and a high rate of morbidity, medical control should be contacted for further directions. The parents' views on resuscitation should be sought and supported. In a newly born baby with no detectable heart rate after 10 minutes of resuscitation, it is acceptable and appropriate to consider stopping resuscitation at that point.[23]

The death of a newborn judged to be nonviable often does not occur rapidly, even in the absence of spontaneous respiration. After a decision has been made to withhold interventional care, it is important that the staff remain supportive and available to the parents. Additional support, such as family members, friends, or members of the clergy, should be identified and contacted. If the parents desire, the child can be held in a quiet place with a physician checking periodically to determine the time of death. This period, around the time of death, may be emotionally difficult for the staff as well as for the family. Futile efforts at resuscitation or interfacility transport should not be a substitute for compassionate support without medical intervention.

SPECIAL PROBLEMS ASSOCIATED WITH PEDIATRIC TRANSPORT

CONSENT FOR TRANSPORT

In most of the United States, the legal age of majority is 18 years old. However, in most states, mothers of younger ages have authority to consent for medical therapies for their children unless specifically prohibited by court order. Likewise, in many states, medical care for minors can be given without parental consent when it is emergent or involves reproductive health. Thus, the definition of the age of majority is situational and must be addressed on an individual basis within the confines of both federal and state law. In situations in which transport of a minor patient is advisable and a parent or guardian is not available (often the case with pediatric traumas), the minor patient can be transported under the principle of beneficence. In these cases, legal authorization for interfacility transport requires documentation from the referring physician stating that failure to transport would endanger the patient's well-being.

ANXIOLYSIS, ANALGESIA, AND SEDATION

Pediatric pain management is often overlooked but important, especially in anticipation of prolonged interfacility transport. In addition to comfort, adequate sedation may increase transport safety and help to prevent complications such as labile oxygenation and accidental extubation. Chapter 113, Pain Management and Procedural Sedation in Infants and Children, details the approach to assessment and treatment of pediatric anxiety, pain, and sedation.

SURGICAL ABDOMEN

Pediatric patients with surgical abdominal processes often require transfer to a pediatric center for definitive care. Common surgical conditions in the neonate and child are discussed in chapter 130, Acute Abdominal Pain in Infants and Children. Pretransport stabilization of these patients includes correction of hypovolemia, provision of adequate analgesia, decompression of the stomach with nasogastric or orogastric tubes (particularly for patients with obstruction who require unpressurized air transport), and maintenance of nothing by mouth status.

REFERENCES

The complete reference list is available online at www.TintinalliEM.com.

Resuscitation of Neonates

Marc F. Collin

INTRODUCTION AND EPIDEMIOLOGY

Resuscitation of the newborn is required to some extent in nearly 10% of all births. Extensive resuscitation is required in about 1%. Delivery room resuscitation is required for >50% of the high-risk population of very-low-birth-weight (<1500 grams) newborns. Worldwide, nearly 25% of neonatal deaths result from birth asphyxia.[1] With proper antenatal and intrapartum surveillance, the potential need for active resuscitation at birth can often be identified before birth. Unfortunately, the arrival of a newborn to the ED is never planned. This chapter reviews the principles of emergency resuscitation of neonates.

PATHOPHYSIOLOGY

The transition from intrauterine to extrauterine life is a treacherous time. Even the normal laboring process places significant stress on the placental-fetal unit. Blood flow and, therefore, oxygen delivery are transiently impaired during uterine contractions. Compression of the umbilical cord, when it occurs, further impairs circulatory flow. Although antenatal/intrapartum US imaging and fetal heart tone monitoring have permitted better surveillance of fetal well-being, prediction of fetal status at birth remains inexact. Maternal complications of pregnancy can predispose newborns to complications and include infections, chronic or gestational disease (e.g., diabetes, lupus), and illicit or prescribed medication use. Complications of labor, such as preterm delivery and/or prolonged rupture of membranes, maternal fever, breech or transverse fetal position, placental abruption, and umbilical cord problems such as a nuchal cord (cord wrapped around the neck) or true knots in the cord, can significantly heighten the risk to the fetus.

Once delivery occurs, the newborn still faces a variety of risks as the transition to extrauterine life unfolds. Requirements of this transition include the onset of respiration, absorption of lung fluid, reduction of pulmonary vasculature resistance to allow flow to the pulmonary vascular circuit, and closure of the ductus arteriosus and foramen ovale. Premature infants and infants who are small for gestational age are at risk for additional challenges in transitioning from fetal to infant physiology including insufficient pulmonary surfactant, fragile germinal matrices within the cerebral ventricles, and thin skin that impairs thermoregulation. The transition from the sterile intrauterine environment to the extrauterine world teeming with bacteria places yet another burden on the newborn.

CLINICAL FEATURES

HISTORY

Obtain a brief history from the mother, including the date of last menstrual period/estimation of gestational age, number of fetuses, number of previous pregnancies and living children, history of diabetes, hypertension or pregnancy-related problems, prenatal care (including known congenital anomalies), prolonged rupture of membranes, fever, and meconium-stained amniotic fluid.

PHYSICAL EXAMINATION

The need for resuscitation or routine newborn care (see "Treatment" below) is determined by the initial physical examination. For the term infant who is crying or breathing and who has good muscle tone at delivery, provide routine newborn care with the infant skin-to-skin on the mother. A slightly more detailed examination using the Apgar scoring system has been used for generations to assist medical personnel in assessing newborns both for the need for resuscitation and the response to resuscitation. Evaluate the newborn at 1 and 5 minutes after delivery for ***heart rate*** (absent = 0, <100/min = 1, >100/min = 2), ***respiratory effort*** (absent = 0, weak = 1, crying or normal = 2), ***muscle tone*** (limp = 0; some flexion = 1; active, fully flexed = 2), ***reflex irritability*** (no response = 0, grimace = 1, crying or active = 2), and ***color*** (blue or pale = 0, acrocyanosis = 1, completely pink = 2). If the 5-minute Apgar score is <7, continue Apgar scoring at 5-minute intervals until a score of 7 or more is reached. The expanded Apgar scoring system includes a section to document resuscitative measures.[2] For infants requiring resuscitation, monitor pulse oximetry with the probe placed on the newborn's right hand (preductal) (see targets for resuscitation below).

LABORATORY EVALUATION

Routine laboratory studies are not required for most term or preterm deliveries. However, obtain point-of-care glucose testing in infants born to diabetic mothers, infants who are small or large for gestational age, or depressed or irritable infants, or if there is poor response to the initial steps of resuscitation. Obtain a type and screen or crossmatch of blood in infants requiring significant resuscitation in the setting of suspected blood loss.

IMAGING

Routine imaging is not required for most deliveries. In rare circumstances, an x-ray of the chest and abdomen may be useful to confirm endotracheal tube placement, suspected pneumothorax, and some congenital defects (e.g., diaphragmatic hernia).

TABLE 108-1 Neonatal Resuscitation Equipment

Neonatal Resuscitation Equipment
Radiant warmer with servocontrol temperature sensor
Prewarmed towels/receiving blankets
Wall suction, suction catheters, bulb syringes
Heated, humidified oxygen source
Compressed air source and oxygen blender
Cardiorespiratory monitor/monitor leads
Pulse oximeter
Bag (flow-inflating or self-inflating) *with* manometer
Masks (sizes 1, 2, 3, 4)
Laryngoscope (0, 1 blade)
Endotracheal tubes (2.5, 3.0, 3.5, 4.0)
Meconium aspirator
CO_2 detector
Nasogastric tubes (5F, 8F)
IV infusion equipment
IV fluids (10% dextrose in water, normal saline)
Umbilical catheter tray
Curved hemostat
Two iris curved forceps, no teeth
Scalpel handle/blade
Needle holder
Scissors
Syringes
2 × 2 gauze sponges
3.5F, 5F umbilical catheters
Three-way stopcock
Suture material
Umbilical tape
Povidone-iodine solution

PREPARATION AND EQUIPMENT

EQUIPMENT

Table 108-1 lists equipment that may be needed during neonatal resuscitation. A compressed air source, an oxygen blender with flow meter, pulse oximetry for neonatal use, and laryngeal mask airways are standard resuscitation equipment.

UMBILICAL CORD CLAMPING

Do not clamp the umbilical cord of newborns (term or preterm) who do not require positive-pressure ventilation or immediate resuscitation for at least 1 to 3 minutes after birth. Delayed cord clamping reduces the need for blood transfusion, increases neonatal iron stores, and may decrease the risk of requiring treatment for hyperbilirubinemia.[1] For newborns requiring positive-pressure ventilation, the cord may be clamped and cut to allow effective ventilations to be performed.

ROUTINE NEWBORN CARE

Provide routine newborn care to term infants who are breathing or crying with good tone. Leave the newborn with the mother, provide warmth (skin-to-skin or blankets), clear the nose and mouth with bulb suction only if signs of obstructed breathing are noted, dry the baby, and provide ongoing assessment of respiratory effort and tone. Even before initiation of the ABCs (airway, breathing, circulation) of resuscitation, provide a neutral thermal environment for the newborn. Although vigorous term infants may be placed skin-to-skin with their mother for warmth, preterm or depressed newborns should be placed under a preheated radiant heat source. Place the infant on his or her back in the warmer. Then, gently dry the newborn with a warm towel while preparing to initiate resuscitation. Very-low-birth-weight newborns and those <29 weeks of estimated gestational age should be placed in polyethylene bags that have been developed for that purpose (plastic food wrap or a food-grade 1-gallon plastic bag may also be used). Avoid hyperthermia, which may precipitate apnea and worsen hypoxic-ischemic injury.

RESUSCITATION

Newborn resuscitation almost exclusively involves care of primary respiratory compromise (**Table 108-2**). Consensus guidelines[3] recommend a timed sequence of steps (30, 60, and >60 seconds). Most important is the rapid establishment of effective ventilation and determining the heart rate before initiating CPR.[4,5]

INITIAL STEPS (FIRST 30 SECONDS)

Within the first 30 seconds of birth, provide warmth, and dry and stimulate the baby. Current guidelines[3] no longer advise the routine suctioning of the newborn nose and mouth. **Infants who are spontaneously breathing, whether delivered through clear or meconium-stained amniotic fluid, do not require tracheal suctioning because tracheal suctioning can cause reflex bradycardia and apnea.** If the infant is not breathing initially, dry and provide stimulation by rubbing the back two to three times; if there is no response, open the airway using jaw thrust and towels beneath the shoulders to provide a sniffing position. If there appears to be obstruction from amniotic fluid, gently suction the nose and throat with a bulb or 8F catheter.

After these initial steps, assess the respiratory effort and heart rate.

ONGOING RESUSCITATION (30 TO 60 SECONDS)

After warming, drying, and stimulating, reassess the respiratory effort and the heart rate. If the infant begins breathing without significant

TABLE 108-2 Steps in Neonatal Resuscitation

Newborn Appearance	Management	Comments
Infant breathing, crying, good tone	Routine care: warm, dry, delay cord clamping 1–3 min, observe	Vigorous term babies may be warmed skin-to-skin with mother. Stimulate nonvigorous babies after drying by rubbing back vigorously several times.
Poor tone/respiratory effort *or* respiratory distress	Warm, open airway and clear nose and mouth if obstructed, dry, stimulate	
Labored breathing or persistent cyanosis with HR >100 beats/min	Clear nose and mouth, monitor O_2 saturation; provide O_2 only to maintain levels in Table 108-3. Consider CPAP.	Oxygen monitor should be placed on right upper extremity (preductal).
Apnea, gasping, or HR <100 beats/min	PPV Continue PPV for 30 s, taking corrective steps for ventilation if no improvement in HR	Provide PPV with BVM at a rate of 40–60 breaths/min using room air. Provide 30 cm H_2O pressure for term infants and 20–25 for preterm infants.
HR <60 beats/min	Initiate CPR:3:1 compression-to-ventilation ratio 90:30 compressions and ventilations per minute	Use thumb-encircling technique to provide chest compressions to lower one third of sternum.
HR <60 beats/min after appropriate ventilation and CPR	Administer epinephrine	May be given IO, IV, or through a UV or ETT
	Consider volume expansion if blood loss; treat hypoglycemia	

Abbreviations: BVM = bag-valve mask; CPAP = continuous positive airway pressure; ETT = endotracheal tube; HR = heart rate; IO = intraosseous; O_2 = oxygen; PPV = positive-pressure ventilation; UV = umbilical vein.

effort and with good color, return to the mother for routine care. If the heart rate is >100 beats/min but there is persistent cyanosis or labored breathing, open the airway and suction the nose and mouth if there is a visible obstruction; attach pulse oximetry to the right hand or wrist (preductal) and apply supplemental oxygen to achieve targeted preductal oxygen saturation goals as per **Table 108-3**.

Apneic or depressed newborns delivered through meconium are at risk for meconium aspiration syndrome, but current evidence indicates that tracheal suctioning does not reduce morbidity or mortality.[3] Naloxone is not recommended for treatment of neonatal respiratory depression, even after maternal opioid exposure or use.[3] Provide usual respiratory support and ventilation.

Initiate positive-pressure ventilation using a bag and mask for infants with a heart rate of <100 beats/min or who are gasping or remain apneic after the initial steps of newborn resuscitation. Begin resuscitation using room air because newborn blood oxygen levels, even in healthy newborns, take time to reach extrauterine values and excessive oxygenation is associated with increased mortality.[6] Table 108-3 provides subsequent oxygen saturation goals throughout neonatal resuscitation.

POSITIVE-PRESSURE VENTILATION

Provide positive-pressure ventilation with a self-inflating or flow-inflating infant bag or a T-piece resuscitator for all newborns with an HR <100 beats/min or who are gasping or apneic after 30 seconds. Bradycardia, even extreme, is typically the result of respiratory failure, and chest compressions or medications should not be initiated until effective ventilations have been provided. Administer positive-pressure ventilation if available. Use a manometer to monitor peak inspiratory pressures: a peak inspiratory pressure of 20 cm H_2O is usually sufficient, although initial peak inspiratory pressures as high as 30 to 40 cm H_2O may be required. Generally, flow-inflating bags are preferred, because they allow better control of inflation pressures. Self-inflating bags are superior if supplemental air or oxygen is unavailable. Be careful when using a self-inflating bag, because pop-off valve pressures, usually set at 30 to 40 cm H_2O, can be exceeded if excessive pressure is applied. T-piece resuscitators have the advantage of delivering a consistent pressure with each artificial breath. **Excessive inflation pressures can cause pneumothorax and compromise resuscitation. Provide 40 to 60 breaths/min.** Good chest rise and an increase in heart rate (usually within 5 to 10 breaths) are the best indicators of effective ventilation.

TABLE 108-3 Targeted Pulse Oxygen Levels During Newborn Resuscitation

Time After Birth	Target Oxygen Saturation (preductal)
1 min	60%–65%
2 min	65%–70%
3 min	70%–75%
4 min	75%–80%
5 min	80%–85%
10 min	85%–90%

Most infants will respond to initial positive-pressure ventilation as outlined above. The most likely reason for a poor response to positive-pressure ventilation is inadequate positive-pressure ventilation, and corrective steps should be taken to assure effective ventilation prior to further resuscitation measures. The American Heart Association recommends use of the pneumonic "MR SOPA," which stands for **M**ask (adjust to improve the seal), **R**eposition the head to open the airway, **S**uction the mouth then nose, **O**pen the mouth with a jaw thrust, and increase the **P**ressure until chest rise is noted (maximum peak inspiratory pressure 40 cm H_2O), and if none of these is effective, proceed to definitive **A**irway control (endotracheal intubation).

Infants with significant labored breathing may benefit from **continuous positive airway pressure ventilation** if the necessary equipment and expertise are available.

ENDOTRACHEAL INTUBATION

In the absence of improvement with bag-mask ventilation, endotracheal tube insertion and ventilation are indicated. Other potential indications for endotracheal intubation in the newborn include (1) concomitant need for chest compressions, (2) administration of endotracheal medications, (3) known or suspected congenital diaphragmatic hernia (to avoid inflating stomach/bowel situated in the chest), and (4) extremely low birth weight (<1000 grams).[7]

The technique for endotracheal intubation is discussed in detail in chapter 111, Intubation and Ventilation in Infants and Children. **Tables 108-4 and 106-5** provide recommended equipment sizes for neonatal resuscitation. **If time allows, precut the endotracheal tube proximally at the 13-cm mark at the endotracheal tube adapter site.** This may eliminate the need to do so later, after the newborn has already been intubated. Uncut tubes allow for excessive "dead space" and are prone to kinking. A stylet is not essential but may allow for easier intubation by providing both greater rigidity and better concave curvature to the relatively soft endotracheal tube.

Confirm tube placement by direct visualization, observation, and auscultation of bilateral chest rise and breath sounds and by confirmation of end-tidal carbon dioxide detection. A rule of thumb for proper

TABLE 108-4 Selection of Endotracheal Tube Size

Tube Size (mm)	Weight (grams)	Gestational Age (wk)
2.5	<1000	<28
3.0	1000–2000	28–34
3.5	2000–3000	34–38
4.0	>3000	>38

tube insertion depth is **6 + weight in kg at the lips** (e.g., 3-kg infant would be 6 + 3 = 9 cm at the lip).

ADVANCED RESUSCITATION: CIRCULATION (>60 TO 90 SECONDS)

If, despite assisted ventilation for 30 seconds, the newborn remains severely bradycardic with an HR <60 beats/min, start chest compressions. Deliver chest compressions to the lower one third of the sternum to a depth of about one third of the anteroposterior diameter of the chest. The compression phase should be slightly shorter than the relaxation phase to allow for cardiac filling. Avoid simultaneous compressions and ventilation. Deliver chest compressions and ventilations in a ratio of **three chest compressions to one breath for** a total of **90 compressions and 30 breaths/min**.

There are two techniques to perform chest compressions.[7] In the "two-thumb" technique, the chest is compressed with both thumbs with the fingers encircling the newborn's back. In the "two-finger" technique, the operator's second and third digits compress the lower one third of the sternum, often with the other hand supporting the newborn's back. The "two-thumb" technique seems to be superior in generating greater peak systolic pressures. The "two-finger" technique may be more practical if a colleague is simultaneously attempting umbilical vessel catheterization.

Stop chest compressions when the HR exceeds 60 beats/min. Once chest compressions have been discontinued, increase the ventilation rate to 40 to 60 breaths/min, because interference from the chest compressions is no longer an issue. Slowly wean positive-pressure ventilation when the HR exceeds 100 beats/min and the newborn has begun to breathe spontaneously.

Medications and Volume Expansion **If bradycardia continues despite bag-mask ventilation followed by endotracheal intubation, adequate ventilation with 100% oxygen, and chest compressions for 45 to 60 seconds, then give epinephrine. Epinephrine is the primary drug used for neonatal resuscitation and should be administered IV or IO, although it can be given intracheally (use larger dose below) if vascular access cannot be obtained (see "Vascular Access" below for umbilical venous catheter placement). The dose of epinephrine is 0.01 to 0.03 milligram/kg IV/IO** (0.1 to 0.3 mL/kg of 1:10,000 solution). Intratracheal dosing is 0.05 to 0.1 milligram/kg or 0.5 to 1 mL/kg of 1:10,000. Naloxone and sodium bicarbonate are no longer recommended for routine use in neonatal resuscitation. **Naloxone is contraindicated in the newborn when maternal narcotic addiction is suspected, because neonatal seizures may result. Sodium bicarbonate may worsen intracellular acidosis.**[8,9]

Consider **volume expansion** when there is known or suspected blood loss (pallor, poor perfusion, or weak pulses). Administer 10 mL/kg of 0.9% saline solution (normal saline) or O-negative blood. Volume should be given slowly (3 to 5 minutes), especially to premature infants who are at risk for intraventricular hemorrhage.

Hypoglycemia in neonates is associated with adverse outcomes following birth asphyxia, whereas hyperglycemia is not. Although there is no evidence-based target for serum glucose in newborns, administer 2 mL/kg of 10% dextrose in water IV/IO for glucose <25 milligrams/dL (1.38 mmol/L) in the first few hours of life (see "Hypoglycemia," under "Special Problems in the Newborn," below).

Postresuscitation Care Newborns with any degree of asphyxia, even those who respond to resuscitative efforts, require a period of close observation. Transfer or admission to a special care nursery or neonatal intensive care unit will depend on the degree of resuscitation required.

Several large trials have demonstrated significant decrease in mortality and improved 18-month neurologic outcomes among term (≥36 weeks of gestational age) newborns with moderate to severe hypoxic-ischemic encephalopathy treated with hypothermia.[7,10-12] Consider inducing hypothermia between 33.5°C and 34.5°C for term neonates requiring extensive resuscitative care,[13] and obtain emergency neonatologist consultation whenever possible.

TABLE 108-5 Selection of Laryngoscopy Equipment

Tube Size/Gestational Age (wk)	Laryngoscope Blade Size	Suction Catheter Size
2.5/<28	Miller 0	5F or 6F
3.0/28–34	Miller 0	6F or 8F
3.5/34–38	Miller 0	8F
3.5–4.0/>38	Miller 0–1	8F or 10F

VASCULAR ACCESS

Peripheral venous access is often difficult in the newborn, so intraosseous access is a good alternative (see "Vascular and Intraosseous Access"). The most readily available site for venous access in the newborn is the umbilical vein. The umbilical vein is easily differentiated from the two umbilical arteries by its larger orifice and thin wall versus the smaller, thicker-walled arteries (**Figure 108-1**).

PREPARATION

Using sterile technique, snugly tie the umbilical cord at its base. The tie can be tightened as needed to avoid oozing through the umbilical vessels once the cord has been cut with a scalpel. Then, cut the cord below the umbilical clamp that was placed at the time of birth, leaving a residual umbilical stump of 1 to 2 cm.[14]

TECHNIQUE

Flush a 3.5F or 5F umbilical catheter with normal saline. Next, attach the preflushed catheter to a 3-mL syringe with a three-way stopcock. Advance the catheter into the umbilical vein until a free flow of blood is seen—this site will be below the level of the liver. At this point, the catheter can be used for volume expansion and medication administration.

Ultimately, the ideal position for the umbilical venous catheter is in the inferior vena cava above the liver and diaphragm, but below the heart, at the T7 to T8 level (Figure 108-1). To achieve this position, either measure the length from the xiphoid to the umbilicus and add 1 to 2 cm, *or* measure total body length, divide by 6, and add 1 to 2 cm. Positioning of the catheter can be confirmed with an x-ray after the patient has been resuscitated.

If placing an umbilical arterial catheter for monitoring purposes, the ideal final catheter positions are either between T6 and T10 (high line) or L2 and L4 (low line). To place a high line, measure total body length (cm), divide by 3, and add 1 to 2 cm *or* measure the shoulder to umbilicus length (cm) and add 1 to 2 cm.

WITHHOLDING AND DISCONTINUING NEONATAL RESUSCITATION

The ED is typically the site of precipitous, unplanned deliveries. If there is uncertainty about gestational age, infant weight, or viability, it is best to err on the side of resuscitation.

A fetus at <22 weeks of gestation and weighing <400 grams is not viable. At 22 weeks of gestation, survival is about 10%; at 23 weeks of gestation, survival is 35% to 40%; and at 24 weeks of gestation, survival is 60% to 65%.[19] **Resuscitation should be initiated on newborns**

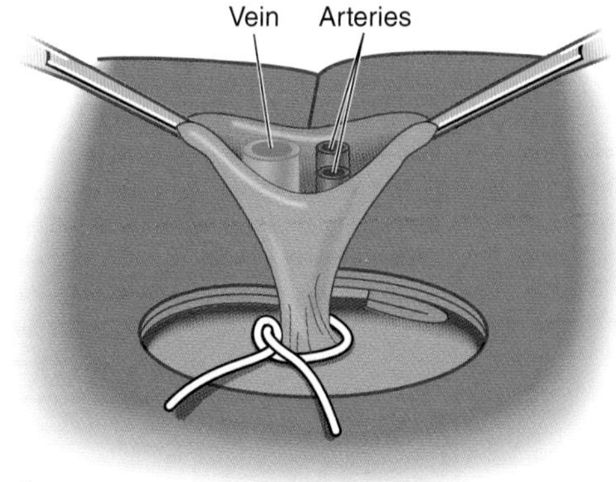

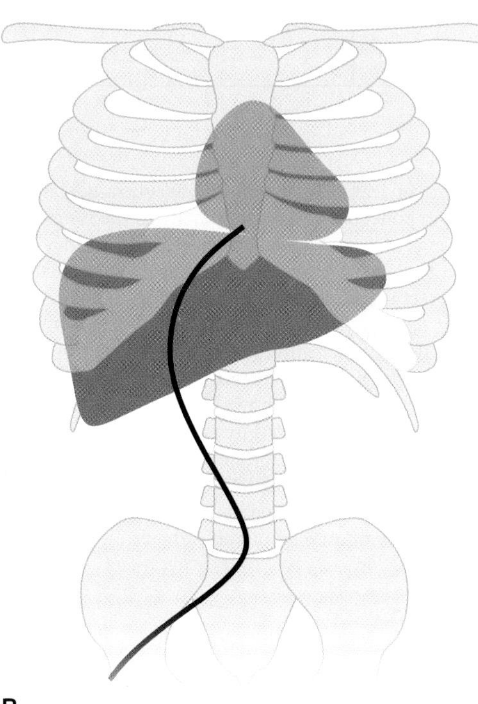

FIGURE 108-1. **A.** Inserting an umbilical catheter. **B.** Correct location of umbilical venous catheterization. When the results of the x-ray are known, reposition the catheter if necessary.

who are 23 weeks of gestation or older. Some centers are now routinely attempting resuscitation of newborns beginning at 22 weeks of gestation. It is difficult to identify with precision the week of gestation at borderline viability based exclusively on anatomic features.

DISCONTINUING NEONATAL RESUSCITATION

Newborns with no sign of life after 10 minutes of continuous and active resuscitation are virtually certain to suffer severe morbidity and/or mortality if continued resuscitation is successful in restoring vital signs. **Therefore, it is justified to cease resuscitative efforts after 10 minutes and, certainly, after 15 minutes of asystole.**[7]

SPECIAL PROBLEMS IN THE NEWBORN

NEONATAL CYANOSIS

Cyanosis is a common finding in the newborn. The first step is differentiating central cyanosis from peripheral cyanosis.

Clinical Features Peripheral cyanosis, or acrocyanosis, is a normal finding in the first few days of life secondary to vasomotor instability and requires no specific evaluation or intervention. Central cyanosis is cyanosis involving the mucous membranes/lips, tongue, and skin. It indicates the presence of at least 4 to 5 grams/dL of unsaturated hemoglobin. The very anemic newborn may present as pale but not cyanotic if the level of unsaturated hemoglobin is below the 4 to 5 grams/dL threshold.

The breathing pattern often provides valuable clues to the cause of cyanosis (**Table 108-6**). On auscultation, unilaterally decreased breath sounds with retractions are associated with a pneumothorax or a space-occupying lesion of the chest. Bilaterally decreased breath sounds with retractions may suggest upper airway obstruction. Stridor also suggests an upper airway cause. Rales and rhonchi may be heard with pneumonia, respiratory distress syndrome, or meconium aspiration syndrome.

A thorough knowledge of the differential diagnosis for cyanosis allows for quick, organized assessment, diagnosis, and treatment (Table 108-6).

Obtain simultaneous preductal (e.g., right radial) and postductal (e.g., lower extremity) or arterial blood gases to help diagnose persistent pulmonary hypertension of the newborn: the postductal Pao_2 is significantly lower than the preductal Pao_2. Using pre- and postductal pulse oximetry may serve the same purpose.

A discrepancy between upper and lower limb blood pressures or reduced femoral pulses may suggest coarctation of the aorta. Babies with coarctation of the aorta often develop new-onset tachypnea and absent femoral pulses later in the first day of life or into the second day of life. Femoral pulses are palpable at birth but disappear after the ductus arteriosus has closed with coarctation of the aorta.

Patients with hypoplastic left heart syndrome may present with poor pulses in all four limbs, poor perfusion, and tachypnea after the immediate newborn period once the ductus arteriosus has closed (see chapter 126, "Congenital and Acquired Pediatric Heart Disease").

Stepped Evaluation and Treatment See **Table 108-7.**

Evaluation The **hyperoxia test** is a quick method to help differentiate a cardiac from a noncardiac cause for cyanosis. Place the newborn in a 100% hood for 5 to 10 minutes. Cyanotic newborns with a pulmonary disorder can increase their oxygen saturation >20% and their Pao_2 to >100 mm Hg. Those with a fixed shunt secondary to congenital cyanotic heart disease or the right-to-left shunting of persistent pulmonary hypertension of the newborn cannot do so.

Obtain a chest x-ray to identify pulmonary disease, abnormalities of pulmonary blood flow, and abnormalities of heart size. If physical examination and chest x-ray have not pointed to a particular diagnosis, an echocardiogram will be needed later on. An echocardiogram is not necessary in the ED during the initial resuscitation.

Treatment **Although oxygen therapy is the mainstay of treatment for cyanosis, treat the underlying cause.** Provide positive-pressure ventilation (continuous positive airway pressure or endotracheal intubation and mechanical ventilation) to the cyanotic newborn with significant respiratory symptoms. Monitor blood gas and pulse oximetry. Establish vascular access, and initiate 10% dextrose in water at 3.3 mL/kg/h (80 mL/kg/24 h) if in the first 24 hours of life. Check serum glucose every 30 to 60 minutes until stable (see "Hypoglycemia" below). Administer empiric antibiotics for sepsis while obtaining appropriate labs (CBC with differential count and platelets, blood culture, chest x-ray, and, possibly, urine culture and C-reactive protein).

If, after initial examination and testing, cyanotic heart disease cannot be ruled out, begin an infusion of **prostaglandin E_1 starting at 0.05 microgram/kg/min, and titrate to the lowest effective dose** to maintain ductal patency.

PNEUMOTHORAX

Pulmonary air leaks are seen more commonly in newborns with respiratory distress syndrome, meconium aspiration syndrome, pneumonia, pulmonary hypoplasia, and congenital diaphragmatic hernia. Pneumothoraces may occur in the otherwise normal newborn in the first few minutes after birth due to increased intrathoracic pressure created with the onset of respiration in the fluid-filled newborn lungs. Air can also dissect into the pulmonary interstitium, mediastinum, pericardium, peritoneum, and subcutaneous space. Pneumothoraces may also be

TABLE 108-6 Causes of Neonatal Central Cyanosis

Airway Obstruction (retractions and/or grunting respirations; stridor)	Cardiac Disorders (tachypnea*, no grunting or retractions)	Pulmonary Disorders (tachypnea* with grunting and/or retractions; rales or rhonchi)	CNS and Metabolic Disorders (slow, shallow respirations without retractions)
Choanal atresia	Transposition of great arteries	Respiratory distress syndrome	Intracranial hemorrhage
Laryngeal web/cyst	Tricuspid atresia	Meconium aspiration syndrome	Brain anomalies (Dandy-Walker malformation, congenital hydrocephalus)
Tracheal stenosis	Truncus arteriosus	Pneumonia	Central hypoventilation syndrome
Pierre Robin sequence	Total anomalous pulmonary venous return	Congenital diaphragmatic hernia	Polycythemia
Cystic hygroma/goiter	Pulmonary atresia	Pulmonary hypoplasia	Hypoglycemia
	Coarctation of aorta	Congenital lobar emphysema	Sepsis/shock
	Hypoplastic left heart syndrome	Congenital cystic adenomatoid malformation	Methemoglobinemia
	Primary pulmonary hypertension of the newborn		

*Tachypnea defined as >60 breaths/min.

iatrogenic secondary to overexuberant bagging during resuscitation, especially with already compromised lungs. Unfortunately, the disorders that most commonly lead to pneumothoraces are also associated with respiratory distress and cyanosis, which may delay the suspicion and diagnosis of the pneumothorax.

Clinical Features and Diagnosis Tension pneumothorax requires rapid treatment to avoid severe respiratory compromise, cardiovascular collapse from impaired venous return to the heart, and, possibly, death. In the preterm newborn, tension pneumothoraces are also highly related to subsequent intracranial hemorrhage, presumably secondary to venous backup into the cerebral circulation.

Tachycardia, tachypnea, and retractions are noted. On auscultation, breath sounds are decreased on the side of the pneumothorax. If there is a tension pneumothorax, heart sounds and point of maximum impulse may be displaced in the direction away from the pneumothorax. Transillumination of the chest with a bright light is another method to help rapidly establish pneumothorax, by "lighting up" the pleural air. Bedside US can also identify pneumothorax. Chest x-ray will confirm the diagnosis.

Treatment The management of a pneumothorax depends on pneumothorax size and the tension it creates in the pulmonary space. A small, nontension pneumothorax can be observed without evacuation. In a term or near-term newborn, the nitrogen washout technique, placing the baby in a 100% oxygen hood for 6 to 12 hours, will usually accelerate clearance of the air leak. This technique is contraindicated in preterm newborns due to concerns of oxygen toxicity to the lungs and retinas.

Emergency evacuation of a tension pneumothorax may be performed with an 18- or 20-gauge 1-inch percutaneous catheter. Instill local anesthetic at the insertion site before the procedure if the patient is not in extremis. After elevating the neonate's affected side with towels under the back, insert the catheter into the fourth intercostal space at the anterior axillary line, which should correlate with the nipple line. Once the pleural space is penetrated, withdraw the needle, and attach the catheter to a three-way stopcock connected to a 10- or 20-mL syringe. Open the stopcock to the syringe, and aspirate the pleural air. More than one syringe of air may be evacuated if a large pneumothorax is present. Clinical improvement should occur after removal of the pleural air. A 10F or 12F chest tube or an 8.5F pigtail catheter can then be placed.

TABLE 108-7 Steps to Evaluate and Treat Neonatal Central Cyanosis

1. Identify breathing pattern to characterize infant into airway obstruction, cardiac pulmonary, or CNS/metabolic pattern.
2. Obtain peripheral oxygen saturation pre- and postductal, check pulses in all 4 extremities, and obtain ABG.
3. Perform hyperoxia test. Deliver 100% oxygen for 5–10 min. Congenital cyanotic heart disease cannot increase oxygen saturation >20% or raise Pa_{O_2} to 100 mm Hg.
4. Obtain stat chest x-ray to identify pneumothorax, congenital diaphragmatic hernia, or pulmonary infiltrates, and assess cardiac size and shape and pulmonary vasculature for clues to congenital heart disease.
5. Establish vascular access in umbilical or peripheral vein, obtain POC glucose, CBC, and metabolic panel. Treat hypoglycemia (glucose <25 milligrams/dL [1.38 mmol/L]) with 10% dextrose in water, 2 mL/kg IV bolus, or 3.3 mL/kg/h (see "Hypoglycemia" section below).
6. Institute continuous positive airway pressure or intubate and ventilate if O_2 saturation does not improve with standard methods for oxygen delivery.
7. If oxygenation still does not improve, treat as presumptive congenital cardiac disease with prostaglandin E_1 starting at 0.05 microgram/kg/min and titrate to the minimum effective dose.

Abbreviations: ABG, arterial blood gas; POC, point of care.

HYPOGLYCEMIA

In the first four hours after birth, asymptomatic hypoglycemia requiring IV therapy is defined as <25 milligrams/dL. Levels of 25 to 44 milligrams/dL (1.38 to 2.4 mmol/L) require feeding and repeat evaluation in 1 hour. After 4 hours of age, serum glucose levels should be ≥45 milligrams/dL (2.4 mmol/L), with levels of 35 to 44 milligrams/dL (1.94 to 2.4 mmol/L) requiring feeding and 1-hour postprandial glucose checks. Risk factors for hypoglycemia in the newborn include prematurity, low birth weight (<2.5 kg), small for gestational age, large for gestational age (>4 kg), infant of a diabetic mother, hypothermia, sepsis, and intrapartum stress.

Clinical Features Symptoms of hypoglycemia are quite varied and include tremors, irritability, lethargy, hypotonia, apnea, tachypnea, tachycardia, cyanosis, high-pitched cry, and seizures. Hypoglycemic newborns may be asymptomatic despite very low glucose levels.

Treatment Treat mild hypoglycemia (25 to 44 milligrams/dL [1.38 to 2.4 mmol/L]) in an otherwise well newborn by feeding. Treat significant hypoglycemia (<25 milligrams/dL [1.38 mmol/L]) immediately with a bolus of dextrose (10% dextrose in water, 2 mL/kg IV/IO), and then administer continuous IV therapy with 10% dextrose in water at 100 mL/kg/24 h and adjust based on serum glucose levels every 30 to 60 minutes until stable and ≥45 milligrams/dL (2.4 mmol/L).

CONGENITAL DIAPHRAGMATIC HERNIA

Congenital diaphragmatic hernias are frequently diagnosed prenatally with US, which expedites proper initial newborn resuscitation.

Anatomically, congenital diaphragmatic hernia is a diaphragmatic defect, either posterolaterally through the foramen of Bochdalek or, less commonly, through the retrosternal foramen of Morgagni. Most are left-sided.[16-19] The diaphragmatic defect allows intra-abdominal contents, including stomach, bowel, and, occasionally, liver, to enter the chest during the second trimester of gestation, leading to pulmonary hypoplasia.

The lung ipsilateral to the diaphragmatic defect is hypoplastic, although the degree of hypoplasia may vary. Ultimate morbidity and mortality are determined both by the extent of hypoplasia of the contralateral lung secondary to compression from the abdominal contents in the thoracic space and whether or not the liver is located in the thorax.[17] Total lung volumes >45% of normal are predictive of survival.[18] Significant associated malformations, especially cardiac defects, are seen in one fourth to one half of patients with congenital diaphragmatic hernia.

Clinical Features The clinical hallmark is persistent respiratory distress at birth, often with a characteristic "seesaw" side-to-side respiratory pattern due to the severely hypoplastic ipsilateral lung. A halting, gasping type of respiratory pattern along with persistent cyanosis is frequently noted. The abdomen appears scaphoid, because abdominal contents are partially situated in the thoracic space. Auscultation of bowel sounds in the chest strongly suggests the presence of congenital diaphragmatic hernia. Radiographic examination is confirmatory.

Treatment Rapid endotracheal intubation is the treatment of choice for respiratory distress. **Bag-mask ventilation will inflate the GI contents in the chest and will further compromise ventilation.** Endotracheal intubation followed by ventilation with a rate of 40 to 50 breaths/min and lowest peak inspiratory pressures that allow for normal chest rise will help avoid pneumothoraces due to barotrauma to the hypoplastic lungs. Gentle hyperventilation to a P_{CO_2} between 30 and 35 mm Hg may help lower pulmonary vasculature resistance and allow for an easier stabilization phase before surgical correction of the diaphragmatic defect. Place a large-bore (10F) orogastric tube set to low continuous suction to minimize further lung compression from overaerated GI contents.

Obtain chest and abdominal x-rays and blood gas analysis to confirm the initial diagnosis and guide stabilization and management. After initial stabilization, emergent referral to a pediatric specialty center is essential.

Despite the advent of antenatal diagnosis, alternate ventilatory strategies (high-frequency oscillatory ventilation), a larger armamentarium to treat pulmonary hypertension (inhaled nitric oxide therapy, sildenafil, and extracorporeal membrane oxygenation), and changing surgical strategies (delayed repair to allow more time for resolution of pulmonary hypertension), mortality from congenital diaphragmatic hernia remains quite high at 30% to 60%.[19-21]

GASTROSCHISIS AND OMPHALOCELE

A gastroschisis is a defect located to the right of the umbilicus from which uncovered intestine is extruded. An omphalocele is a large, centrally located defect of the abdominal wall containing stomach, intestine, and, frequently, liver that is covered by the mesentery. The umbilical cord inserts directly into the omphalocele sac. Rarely, an omphalocele may be ruptured either before delivery or during delivery. Associated anomalies are seen in 10% to 21% of patients with gastroschisis and 40% to 75% of patients with omphalocele.[22-24] Associated defects include cardiac defects (such as tetralogy of Fallot), syndromes (Beckwith-Wiedemann), and chromosomal abnormalities (trisomy 13, trisomy 18), in addition to associated intestinal atresias.

Treatment The initial management of gastroschisis and omphalocele is similar: handle the covered sac and free intestine with care. Place the newborn on a radiant warmer to help prevent hypothermia due to increased heat loss from the exposed abdominal contents. The ABCs of stabilization should be performed as needed.

If an omphalocele is present, note its size and contents. Cover the sac with warmed saline gauze wrapped gently around the baby with Kerlix, and then place an additional cover with plastic wrap to help minimize evaporative losses. Start IV 10% dextrose in water at 1.5× maintenance (i.e., 5 to 6 mL/kg/h or 120 to 150 mL/kg/24 h) to compensate for the additional insensible water loss. Monitor urine output and electrolytes closely to determine ongoing fluid needs.

If a gastroschisis is present, immediately check for dusky or cyanotic intestine, which indicates reduced flow to the affected bowel due to torsion and vascular occlusion. Gently rotate the bowel to relieve torsion if necessary to prevent bowel infarction. Emergency pediatric surgical consultation is essential. If the intestine appears pink, cover with warmed saline gauze, wrap with Kerlix, and further cover with plastic wrap. **Be careful not to compress the intestine, which could result in obstruction of blood flow to the bowel.** Insensible water loss is much greater in the newborn with gastroschisis due to the open defect with large amounts of extruded bowel. Therefore, IV 10% dextrose in water should be started at 6 to 7 mL/kg/h (at least 150 mL/kg/24 h).

Check glucose periodically. Antibiotics, usually ampicillin, 50 to 100 milligrams/kg IV, and gentamicin, 4 to 5 milligrams/kg IV, should be given.

Immediate consultation with a neonatologist and pediatric surgeon is necessary. The overall outcome for gastroschisis is quite good, with survival exceeding 90%.[25,26] Survival with omphalocele is somewhat less at 73% to 88%, depending largely on the presence of associated anomalies.[25]

TRACHEOESOPHAGEAL FISTULA

Tracheoesophageal fistula develops secondary to a failure of separation of the developing foregut structures, the trachea and esophagus, during the embryologic stage of development. There are five types of tracheoesophageal fistula: (1) esophageal atresia with a distal tracheoesophageal fistula (88% of cases), (2) isolated esophageal atresia without tracheoesophageal fistula (7%), (3) esophageal atresia with proximal tracheoesophageal fistula (1%), (4) esophageal atresia with proximal and distal tracheoesophageal fistulas (1%), and (5) H-type fistula without esophageal atresia (3%). Tracheoesophageal fistula is highly associated with several other malformations, designated as the acronyms VATER or VACTERL association: *v*ertebral anomalies, *a*nal atresia, *c*ardiac anomalies, *t*racheo*e*sophageal fistula, *r*adial anomaly/*r*enal anomalies, and *l*imb anomalies.

Diagnosis The diagnosis of tracheoesophageal fistula can be missed during prenatal US examination. When esophageal atresia is present, polyhydramnios is usually noted before or at delivery. Newborns with tracheoesophageal fistula/esophageal atresia will usually have excessive oral secretions noted shortly after birth. When attempting to pass a nasogastric tube, the tube coils in the esophageal pouch and often comes back out of the mouth. No air passage will be heard when a 5-mL air bolus is injected into the nasogastric tube. A chest x-ray with a nasogastric tube in place will demonstrate the esophageal pouch. Confirmatory contrast studies are not indicated and may actually be contraindicated because the esophageal contents can be aspirated into the lungs.

Treatment Management of tracheoesophageal fistula includes placing the child in head-up (reverse Trendelenburg) positioning to help prevent passage of gastric contents through the tracheoesophageal fistula into the lungs, placing the nasogastric tube into the esophageal pouch on low intermittent suction to prevent buildup and possible aspiration of oral secretions, and giving the newborn nothing by mouth. Initially, standard 10% dextrose in water IV fluids are best. Immediate referral to a center with neonatologists and pediatric surgeons is essential.

REFERENCES

The complete reference list is available online at www.TintinalliEM.com.

Resuscitation of Children

William E. Hauda, II

INTRODUCTION AND EPIDEMIOLOGY

The resuscitation of children differs from that of adults in a number of important ways. For example, the most common cause of primary cardiac arrest in adults is coronary artery disease, whereas respiratory failure and shock are more common causes among children and infants; hypoxemia, hypercapnia, and acidosis subsequently lead to bradycardia,

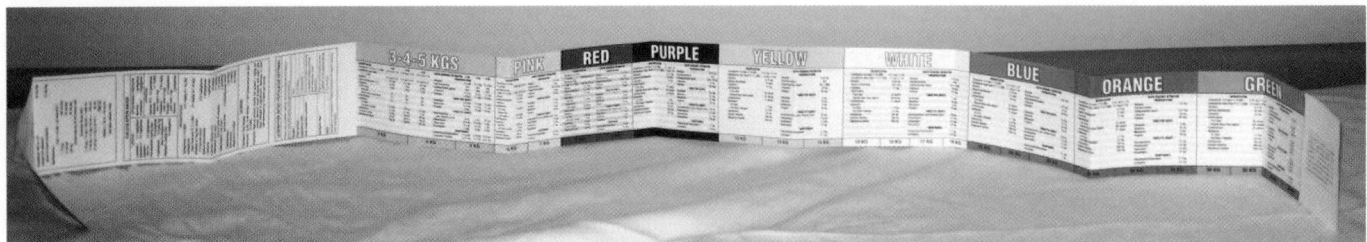

FIGURE 109-1. The Broselow resuscitation tape. [Broselow® tape; Armstrong Medical Industries, Inc., Lincolnshire, IL.]

hypotension, and secondary cardiac arrest in children. After resuscitation, survival to discharge may be greater among children and adolescents than in infants or adults.[1-4] The survival rate without devastating neurologic sequelae in children varies by age, ranging from 1% to 2% in infants and young children to 11% for adolescents in whom a shockable rhythm is more common; survival rates as high as 30% have been seen after sudden out-of-hospital witnessed ventricular fibrillation.[5-7] The best chance for a good outcome is to recognize impending respiratory failure or shock and intervene to prevent the development of cardiopulmonary arrest.

Age-related differences are important considerations when treating children. An appropriate drug dose for a 6-month-old infant may be excessive for a 1-month-old newborn but inadequate for a 5-year-old child. Other aspects of resuscitation, such as endotracheal tube size, tidal volumes, cardiac compression rates, and respiratory rates, vary with a child's age. Equipment selection and medication dosing are based on age and body weight. Valuable time can be lost in weight estimation, dosage calculations, and equipment selection. Emergency personnel must be able to find the proper equipment rapidly. Equipment can be stored on shelves or in drawers labeled by age and weight, or a system of color codes can be used in which color-coded shelves, carts, or equipment organizers correspond to specific length categories as illustrated in **Figure 109-1**.

BASIC LIFE SUPPORT

The American Heart Association Guidelines[8] use the following age group delineations: *newborn*, 1 month or less in age; *infant*, 1 month to 1 year of age; and *child*, 1 year of age to the onset of puberty. As in adults, the priorities of resuscitation are airway, oxygenation, ventilation, and shock management. An important change in the 2010 American Heart Association Guidelines is the order of basic life support assessment. Instead of using ABC (airway, breathing, circulation) as a mnemonic, the American Heart Association recommends CAB, emphasizing the importance of chest compressions beginning as rapidly as possible (**Figure 109-2**). Reasons for this change in approach include the following: (1) starting with chest compressions reduces the delay to the start of the first compression; (2) all rescuers can start chest compressions immediately, because airway management requires manipulation and positioning of the patient; and (3) simplifying the basic life support resuscitation approach is consistent for all patients regardless of the arrest cause.[8,9] Cardiopulmonary arrest should be prevented whenever possible with prompt recognition of and intervention for compromised physiology.[10] International consensus guidelines for basic life support procedures are listed in **Table 109-1**.[8,11]

AIRWAY

ANATOMY

A child's airway is much smaller than an adult's, and airway size varies by age. Anatomic and functional differences are more pronounced in infants and young children. **The airway is higher and more anterior in a child's neck than in an adult's.** The tongue and epiglottis are relatively larger, and, thus, more likely to obstruct the airway. Infants <6 months are primarily nasal breathers, so keeping the nasal passages clear is vital if spontaneous ventilation is present. Infants >6 months are able to breathe through their mouths. During CPR, ventilation by the oral route is sufficient to maintain adequate ventilation.

POSITIONING

When a child is supine, the prominent occiput causes flexion of the neck on the chest and occludes the airway. Correct airway occlusion by mild extension of the neck to the sniffing position. Overextension or hyperextension of the neck, acceptable for adults, causes obstruction and may kink the trachea, because the cartilaginous support is poor.

Maintain the sniffing position by placing a towel or other object beneath the shoulders. Despite good head position, a child's hypotonic mandibular tissues may still allow the relatively large tongue to occlude the airway posteriorly. This condition can be relieved by a chin lift or jaw thrust that elevates the mandible anteriorly and separates the tongue from the posterior pharyngeal wall. Use the jaw thrust technique in a child with a possible cervical spine injury because it minimizes the movement of the neck and allows maintenance of a neutral position of the cervical spine. The jaw thrust may be superior to the standard chin lift and is also useful in maintaining an open airway during bag-valve mask ventilation.[12] If these maneuvers are unsuccessful, consider an oral airway device or endotracheal tube.

BASIC AIRWAY ADJUNCTS

Nasopharyngeal airways can be useful adjuncts for maintaining airway patency during resuscitation, particularly in the awake child; however, nasopharyngeal airway insertion can cause nasal trauma or bleeding due to small nasal passages and hypertrophic adenoid tissue in the posterior nasopharynx. Oral airways should be used only in unconscious children. Oral airways are most useful in children who need a continuous jaw thrust or chin lift to maintain airway patency. Oral airways are inserted with a tongue depressor to push the tongue down into the mandible so that the airway can be inserted under direct vision.

Advanced airway management in neonates and infants and the difficult pediatric airway are discussed in chapter 111.

CHOKING AND FOREIGN-BODY MANAGEMENT

The back blow and chest thrust are recommended maneuvers to clear an infant's airway. The American Heart Association specifically discourages two common maneuvers used with adult patients: (1) **do not use the "Heimlich maneuver" for patients <1 year old**, because of the potential for injury to abdominal organs; and (2) **do not use blind finger sweeps**, because of the possibility of pushing the foreign body farther into the airway.[8,11]

CONSCIOUS CHILDREN

A child who is choking but is able to maintain some ventilation or vocalization should be allowed to clear the airway by coughing. Once a child cannot cough, vocalize, or breathe, a sequence of steps must be instituted immediately. ***Choking infants are treated with an alternating sequence of five back blows and five chest thrusts.***[11] With the infant's torso positioned prone and head down along the rescuer's arm, or the older child draped prone and head down across the rescuer's knees, deliver five blows to the interscapular area. Then reposition the

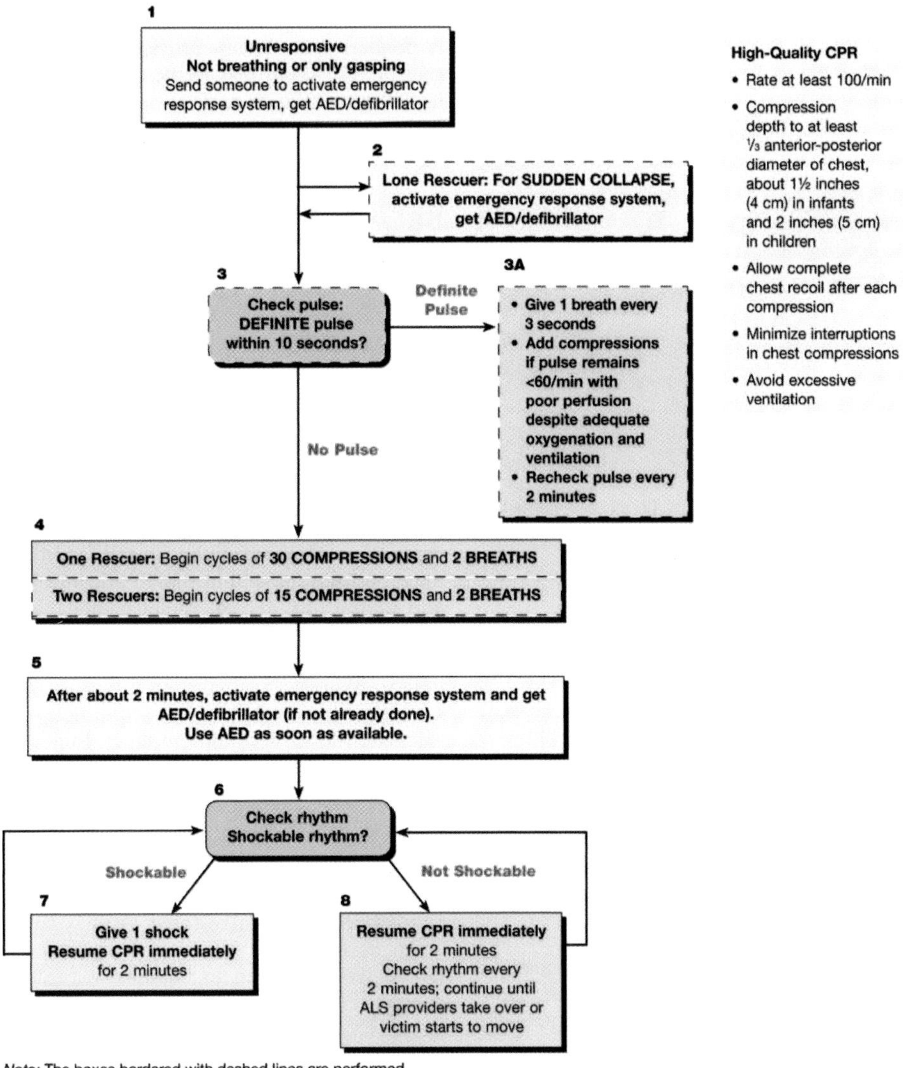

Pediatric BLS Healthcare Providers
1
Unresponsive
Not breathing or only gasping
Send someone to activate emergency response system, get AED/defibrillator
2
Lone Rescuer: For SUDDEN COLLAPSE, activate emergency response system, get AED/defibrillator
3
Check pulse: DEFINITE pulse within 10 seconds?
Definite Pulse
3A
• Give 1 breath every 3 seconds
• Add compressions if pulse remains <60/min with poor perfusion despite adequate oxygenation and ventilation
• Recheck pulse every 2 minutes
No Pulse
High-Quality CPR
• Rate at least 100/min
• Compression depth to at least ⅓ anterior-posterior diameter of chest, about 1½ inches (4 cm) in infants and 2 inches (5 cm) in children
• Allow complete chest recoil after each compression
• Minimize interruptions in chest compressions
• Avoid excessive ventilation
4
One Rescuer: Begin cycles of 30 COMPRESSIONS and 2 BREATHS
Two Rescuers: Begin cycles of 15 COMPRESSIONS and 2 BREATHS
5
After about 2 minutes, activate emergency response system and get AED/defibrillator (if not already done).
Use AED as soon as available.
6
Check rhythm
Shockable rhythm?
Shockable
Not Shockable
7
Give 1 shock
Resume CPR immediately for 2 minutes
8
Resume CPR immediately for 2 minutes
Check rhythm every 2 minutes; continue until ALS providers take over or victim starts to move
Note: The boxes bordered with dashed lines are performed by healthcare providers and not by lay rescuers
© 2010 American Heart Association

FIGURE 109-2. Pediatric basic life support (BLS) algorithm. For both single and multiple rescuers, the sequence of approach follows CAB (circulation, airway, breathing): chest compressions are initiated immediately upon recognition of the arrest. AED = automated external defibrillator. [Reprinted with permission 2010 American Heart Association Guidelines For CPR and ECC Part 13: Pediatric Basic Life Support *Circulation.2010;122[suppl 3]:S862-S875* © 2010, American Heart Association, Inc.]

TABLE 109-1 Guidelines for Pediatric Basic Life Support[8]

Maneuver	Newborn	Infant <1 Y	Child 1 Y to Puberty	Onset of Puberty to Adult
Airway	Head tilt/chin lift	Head tilt/chin lift	Head tilt/chin lift	Head tilt/chin lift
If trauma	Jaw thrust	Jaw thrust	Jaw thrust	Jaw thrust
If foreign body–conscious	Suction	Back blows and chest thrusts	Abdominal thrusts	Abdominal thrusts
If foreign body–unconscious	Suction	Chest compressions	Abdominal thrusts	Abdominal thrusts
Breathing rate	30–60/min (every 1–2 s)	12–20/min (every 3 s)	12–20/min (every 3 s)	10–12/min (every 5 s)
Circulation				
Pulse check	Umbilical	Brachial	Carotid or femoral	Carotid or femoral
Compression				
Location	One finger below intermammary line	One finger below intermammary line or lower half of sternum	Lower half of sternum	Lower half of sternum
Method	Two fingers or two thumbs	Two fingers or two thumbs	Heel of one hand or two hands	Two hands
Depth	One third of chest	One third to one half of chest	One third to one half of chest	One third of chest
Rate	120/min	100/min	100/min	100/min
Compression-to-ventilation ratio	3:1	15:2 (single rescuer–30:2)	15:2 (single rescuer–30:2)	30:2

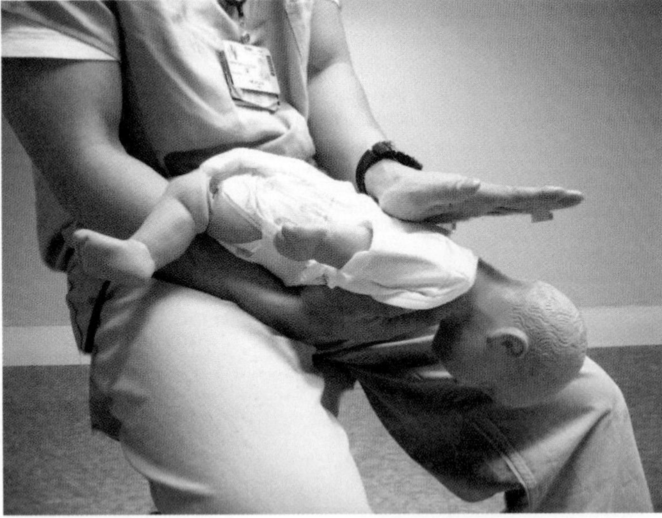

FIGURE 109-3. Back blows to clear airway of choking infant. [Image used with permission of Rita K. Cydulka, MD, MS, MetroHealth Medical Center.]

infant supinely along the rescuer's arm, or place the larger infant on the floor, as for external cardiac compression, and deliver five chest thrusts (cardiac compressions) (**Figures 109-3 and 109-4**). Continue this sequence until the airway obstruction is relieved or the child becomes unconscious. In older children, use the obstructed airway ("Heimlich") maneuver, with the rescuer kneeling or standing behind the child. Place the rescuer's clenched fist at the level of the umbilicus, and deliver firm upward thrusts until the obstruction is cleared or the child becomes unconscious.

UNCONSCIOUS CHILDREN

If a child loses consciousness due to a presumed airway obstruction, begin chest compressions immediately. After 30 compressions, open the airway and look for a foreign body in the mouth. Attempt to deliver two rescue breaths. If successful, then check for a pulse. If the obstruction is still present, then continue with alternating cycles of compressions and attempted rescue breaths until the obstruction is relieved. Chest compressions will circulate blood if there is a loss of perfusion (unconsciousness) and may relieve the obstruction. After each cycle and before each attempt at ventilation (lone rescuer: 30 to 2; two rescuers: 15 to 2), inspect the airway to see if an object is present and remove visible objects. **Do not perform blind finger sweeps.**

The foregoing recommendations are directed primarily at first responders or healthcare providers who have neither access to nor the skills to use airway management equipment. For unconscious children in EDs, direct laryngoscopy, visualization, and removal of the foreign body with McGill forceps can be attempted. Until this equipment is ready, use basic life support techniques.

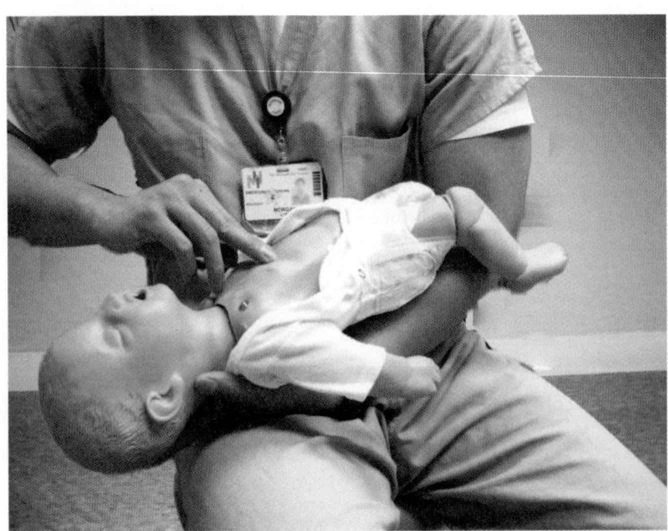

FIGURE 109-4. Chest thrusts to clear airway of choking infant. [Image used with permission of Rita K. Cydulka, MD, MS, MetroHealth Medical Center.]

BREATHING

MOUTH TO MOUTH

The size of the child dictates whether to use mouth-to-mouth or mouth-to-mouth-and-nose ventilation. The rate of ventilation is shown in Table 109-1. Perform ventilations slowly to avoid the generation of high airway pressures, which can impede venous return, cause barotrauma, and result in gastric distention and regurgitation.[11]

BAG-VALVE MASK

The self-inflating bag-valve mask system is most commonly used for ventilation. **Ventilation bags used for infants and children should have a minimum volume of 450 mL, and 1000 mL for older children and adolescents.**[11] Pediatric lung compliance is very good, and children can tolerate relatively high pressures. **Pneumothoraces usually result from the administration of excessive tidal volume rather than from high pressures.** The tidal volume necessary to ventilate children is the same as that for adults: 10 to 15 mL/kg. Because it is impractical to calculate the tidal volume in emergency situations, start ventilation with the smallest volume that causes adequate chest rise. Carefully monitor the rate of ventilation to **avoid excessive hyperventilation.**

OXYGEN

It is reasonable to provide 100% oxygen during CPR; however, once circulation has been restored, studies suggest improved outcomes when normal arterial oxygen and carbon dioxide levels are maintained. Wean oxygen to maintain saturations of >93% and assure eucapnia.[11,13,14]

CIRCULATION

Monitor the brachial pulse in infants <1 year old; for older children, the femoral or carotid pulse is most easily accessible.[11] Begin cardiac compression in the absence of pulse or with poor perfusion (heart rate ≤60 beats/min). Perform compressions over the lower sternum, not the midsternum.[8] The depth of compressions should be about one third of the anteroposterior chest diameter.

Place patients on a hard surface to improve the effectiveness of compressions. Palpate pulses during compression to assess the adequacy of the compression depth and rate. With bag-valve mask ventilation, pause chest compressions only long enough to deliver effective ventilations; however, once an advanced airway is established, chest compressions do not need to be paused for ventilations. See chapter 111 for further discussion.

INFANTS

Use the two-thumb technique when two healthcare providers are present. Compress at a rate of at least 100 per minute. The compression-to-ventilation ratio is 15:2 for two healthcare providers performing CPR on an infant.[8] If the patient is intubated, then compressions and ventilations may be performed without synchronization, but the rate of compressions should be maintained at 100 per minute.

CHILDREN 1 YEAR OLD TO THE ONSET OF PUBERTY

Compress the lower half of the sternum with the heel of one hand. If unable to adequately depress the sternum with one hand, then use the two-hand technique. The rate of compression is at least 100 compressions per minute. If there are two healthcare providers, then perform compressions in a series of 15:2 compressions to ventilations. If there is only one healthcare provider, perform 30 compressions for every 2 ventilations. If the patient is intubated, then compressions and ventilations may be performed without synchronization, but keep the rate of compressions at 100 per minute.

CHILDREN AFTER PUBERTY (ADOLESCENTS)

Children who are of pubertal age or older are treated as adults with respect to basic life support.[8] Use the two-hand technique of chest compressions. The compression-to-ventilation ratio and rate of compressions are the same as with children, 15:2 for two-person CPR and 30:2 for one-person CPR with a rate of 100 compressions per minute.

VASCULAR ACCESS

Difficulty in obtaining rapid IV access is certainly one of the major differences between adult and pediatric resuscitation. Keep several important facts in mind. First, a significant portion of children respond to airway management alone because most cardiac arrests in children are secondary to hypoxia from respiratory arrest. Do not waste time securing vascular access in children at the expense of airway management. Intraosseous infusion and fluid administration are quick, safe routes for resuscitation drugs (see chapter 112, "Intravenous and Intraosseous Access in Infants and Children"). If vascular access is needed rapidly, establish an intraosseous site until venous access is obtained. Once the child is intubated, use the tracheal route to administer drugs, such as *l*idocaine, *e*pinephrine, *a*tropine, and *n*aloxone (mnemonic: LEAN). **Although the ideal endotracheal doses for drugs other than epinephrine have never been studied in children, current recommendations support the use of two to three times the respective IV dose.**[8,10]

The most frequently used peripheral sites are the scalp, arm, hand, antecubital veins, and external jugular vein. If central venous access is needed, then the femoral vein is the most familiar and least complicated site. The general order of peripheral venous attempts during resuscitation should be antecubital, then hand or foot.

FLUIDS

If hypotension is due to volume depletion, give isotonic fluid boluses of 20 mL/kg as rapidly as possible and repeat as needed.[10] Use a syringe attached to a three-way stopcock and extension tubing to rapidly deliver aliquots of fluid, until the entire bolus is administered. This method is far superior to the use of gravity or pressure bags.

Deliver the bolus in <20 minutes and more rapidly, if possible. Reassess the child's condition after each bolus. If blood pressure normalizes, maintain fluid administration at the minimum rate to keep the vein open or at a rate to compensate for ongoing fluid losses. Adjust fluids and electrolytes based on calculations or laboratory results after emergency stabilization. If volume depletion is corrected with three to four fluid boluses but hypotension persists, consider a pressor agent.

Always use a pediatric microdrip assembly when resuscitating children to prevent accidental overhydration and for easy monitoring of the total volume given. It is easy to overhydrate infants and children, even when IV lines are set to keep the vein open, if adult equipment is used for children.

WEIGHT ESTIMATION AND MEDICATION CALCULATIONS

Proper dosage of medications in children requires knowledge of the patient's weight, knowledge of the dose (usually given in milligrams per kg), and error-free calculation and delivery. Use a chart with precalculated drug doses to reduce dosage errors (**Tables 109-2 and 109-3**).

Reformulating drug preparations so that all children receive 0.1 mL/kg regardless of the medication results in a 50% reduction in time to administration and a significant reduction in dosing errors even compared with the use of a length-based drug calculation device.[17]

To calculate the proper drug dosage from the table, accurately determine the child's weight. Because it is not possible to weigh a child during resuscitation, several alternative methods are available for estimating a child's weight, but each of these has inherent challenges and problems (**Table 109-4**).

LENGTH-BASED ESTIMATION

Systems based on a direct measurement of a patient's length have been developed for estimating weight, dosages, and selecting equipment in pediatric emergencies (**Table 109-5**).[18] The use of a length-based system is currently included in the American Heart Association Pediatric Advanced Life Support Course.[10] These systems use a tape measuring device (**Broselow® tape**; Armstrong Medical Industries, Inc., Lincolnshire, IL) to assist in making appropriate selections. Most tapes are two-sided and display emergency resuscitation drug dosage and equipment selection based on length (Figure 109-1). Fluid volumes for resuscitation and appropriate basic life support techniques are often also displayed.

The length-based systems many not be accurate in all populations of children.[19-21] Forty-three percent of children 10 to 12 years of age are longer than the tape used for the weight estimation.[22] The Broselow® tape underestimates some weights, resulting in underdosing medications.[20,23] Although there are limitations in using the length-based systems for weight estimation, their use in EDs provides a very rapid tool during a critical resuscitation. Length-based systems also help provide accurate selection of appropriately sized equipment.[24]

AGE-BASED ESTIMATION

There are several formulas based on a child's age to assist in estimating a child's weight. The commonly used estimates of weights based on age noted in **Table 109-6** have never been formally validated. The original Advanced Pediatric Life Support formula, (years + 4) × 2, underestimates weights of 1-year-old children by 9.7% and underestimates weights of 12-year-olds by 34.2%[25] and has, therefore, been updated to be more accurate, but at the cost of increased complexity (Table 109-4). Luscombe and colleagues suggest that the formula (years × 3) + 7 bears a more consistent relationship to a child's true weight. A large study comparing various formulas to estimate weights in Australian children found the Best Guess and updated Advanced Pediatric Life Support formulas were most accurate overall.[23] No formulas are perfect. The Argall formula was within 10% of actual weight in only 37% of Australian children studied.[26] It also correlates poorly with the weight estimates of the Broselow® tape in whites.[27] Both the Nelson formula and the Best Guess formula would be challenging to apply rapidly from memory in the ED but are accurate when used for white children.[28]

HEALTHCARE PROVIDER ESTIMATION

Estimations by healthcare providers without using a specific tool are quite variable.[29] Healthcare providers should not rely on a visual estimation of the child's weight, but must use some tool in estimating a child's weight for all resuscitation medications.

PARENTAL ESTIMATION

Parental estimations of a child's weight are often the most accurate estimation compared with formulas and length-based devices.[27] One author has suggested that parental estimations should be used, if available; if not, then use length-based weight estimations.[29]

PHARMACOLOGIC AGENTS

The pharmacology of resuscitation drugs has been well described in other chapters (see chapter 19, "Pharmacology of Antiarrhythmics and

TABLE 109-2 Drugs for Pediatric Resuscitation[15,16]

Drug	Pediatric Dosage	Remarks
Adenosine	IV/IO: 0.1 milligram/kg, followed by 2–5 mL NS bolus Double dose and repeat once, if needed	Maximum single dose: 6 milligrams first dose, 12 milligrams second dose.
Amiodarone	IV/IO: 5 milligrams/kg over 20–60 min; then 5–15 micrograms/kg/min infusion	Maximum bolus repetition to 15 milligrams/kg/d. Use lowest effective dose. Bolus may be given more rapidly in shock states.
Atropine	IV/IO: 0.02 milligram/kg, repeat in 5 min (minimum single dose is 0.1 milligram) Endotracheal: 0.04–0.06 milligram/kg diluted with NS to 3–5 mL	Maximum single dose: 0.5 milligram (child) and 1.0 milligram (adolescent). Maximum cumulative dose: 1.0 milligram (child) and 2.0 milligrams (adolescent).
Calcium chloride (10%)	IV/IO: 20 milligrams/kg (maximum dose 2 grams)	*Not routinely recommended.* Use in documented hypocalcemia, calcium channel blocker overdose, hypermagnesemia, or hyperkalemia. Administer slowly.
Epinephrine	Bradycardia: IV/IO: 0.01 milligram/kg (0.1 mL/kg of 1:10,000) Endotracheal: 0.1 milligram/kg (0.1 mL/kg of 1:1000) Pulseless arrest: IV/IO: 0.01 milligram/kg (0.1 mL/kg of 1:10,000) Endotracheal: 0.1 milligram/kg (0.1 mL/kg of 1:1000)	Maximum dose: 1 milligram IV/IO; 2.5 milligrams ETT. Unlike other agents, epinephrine per endotracheal tube is 10× the IV dose. Follow endotracheal dose with several positive pressure ventilations. Maximum dose: 1 milligram IV/IO; 2.5 milligrams ETT. No evidence for high-dose parenteral epinephrine (may worsen outcomes).
Glucose	IV/IO: Newborn: 5 mL/kg $D_{10}W$ Infants and children: 2 mL/kg $D_{25}W$ Adolescents: 1 mL/kg $D_{50}W$	
Lidocaine	IV/IO: 1.0 milligram/kg bolus Endotracheal: double IV dose and dilute with NS to 3–5 mL	
Naloxone	IV/IO: If <5 y or ≤20 kg: 0.1 milligram/kg If >5 y and >20 kg: 2.0 milligrams	Titrate to desired effect.
Sodium bicarbonate	IV/IO: 1 mEq/kg (1 mEq/mL)	*Not routinely recommended.* Infuse slowly and use only if ventilation is adequate for tricyclic antidepressant overdose and hyperkalemia.

Abbreviation: $D_{10}W$ = 10% dextrose in water; $D_{25}W$ = 25% dextrose in water; $D_{50}W$ = 50% dextrose in water; ETT = endotracheal tube; NS = normal saline.

TABLE 109-3 Calculation for Dosage of Medications Delivered by Constant Infusion Using the Rule of 6

Drug	Continuous Infusion Dose	Conversion Factor	Delivery
Epinephrine	0.1–1.0 microgram/kg/min	0.6 milligram × wt (kg)	1 mL/h = 0.1 microgram/kg/min
Dobutamine	2–20 micrograms/kg/min	6 milligrams × wt (kg)	1 mL/h = 1.0 microgram/kg/min
Dopamine	2–20 micrograms/kg/min	6 milligrams × wt (kg)	1 mL/h = 1.0 microgram/kg/min
Norepinephrine	0.1–2.0 micrograms/kg/min	0.6 milligram × wt (kg)	1 mL/h = 0.1 microgram/kg/min
Lidocaine	20–50 micrograms/kg/min	60 milligrams × wt (kg)	1 mL/h = 10 micrograms/kg/min
Nitroprusside	0.5–8 micrograms/kg/min	6 milligrams × wt (kg)	1 mL/h = 1 microgram/kg/min
Isoproterenol	0.1–1.0 microgram/kg/min	0.6 milligram × wt (kg)	1 mL/h = 0.1 microgram/kg/min
Dosage of medications delivered by constant infusions is calculated in terms of micrograms per kg per minute. Actual calculation can be confusing and a source of lethal decimal errors. The rule of 6 can be used for dopamine and dobutamine to simplify dosage calculation:			
The medication is mixed in an IV set with a measured chamber and a microdrip (1 drop/min = 1 mL/h). Rate of administration is best set by an electric pump.	6 milligrams × wt (kg), fill to 100 mL with D_5W		
Example: For a 10-kg infant requiring dopamine	6 milligrams × 10 = 60 milligrams dopamine		
In a measured chamber, fill to 100 mL with D_5W. Weight is now factored in so that:	1 mL/h = 1 microgram/kg/min 5 mL/h = 5 micrograms/kg/min 10 mL/h = 10 micrograms/kg/min		
For epinephrine and isoproterenol, the rule of 6 is:	0.6 milligram × wt (kg), fill to 100 mL with D_5W 1 mL/h = 0.1 microgram/kg/min 5 mL/h = 0.5 microgram/kg/min		

Abbreviations: D_5W = 5% dextrose in water; wt = weight.

TABLE 109-4 Estimating Weight in Infants and Children

Formulas by name	Argall	(Years + 2) × 3
	Luscombe	(Years × 3) + 7
	Advanced Pediatric Life Support	Infants: (age in months × 0.5) + 4 Children 1–5 y: (2 × age in years) + 8 Children 6–12 y: (3 × age in years) + 7
	Nelson	<12 mo: (months + 9)/2 1–6 y: (years × 2) + 8 7–12 y: (years × 7) − 5
	Best Guess	<12 mo: (months + 9)/2 1–4 y: (years + 5) × 2 5–14 y: (years × 4)
Formulas by age	Infants	(months + 9)/2
	1 to 5 or 6 y	(years × 2) + (7, 8, or 10)
		Or
		(years × 3) + 7
	6 or 7 to 12 or 14 y	(years × 2) + 8
		Or
		(years × 3) + 7
		Or
		Years × 4
		Or
		(years × 5) − 5

Antihypertensives," and chapter 20, "Pharmacology of Vasopressors and Inotropes"), but a few peculiarities pertain to pediatric resuscitation drug use.

EPINEPHRINE

Epinephrine is the one drug universally used in cardiac arrest; however, its beneficial effect on survival remains questionable. It is specifically indicated for hypoxia- or ischemia-induced slow rates that fail to respond to adequate oxygenation and ventilation and for pulseless arrest situations (i.e., asystole, pulseless electrical activity, and ventricular fibrillation). If the initial dose of epinephrine is not effective, give subsequent doses at the same dose. High-dose epinephrine (0.1 milligram/kg of the 1:1000 concentration) for resuscitation in infants and children does not increase survival. The American Heart Association currently recommends that subsequent doses of epinephrine be at the standard dose.[8] High-dose epinephrine may be useful in catecholamine-resistant states, such as anaphylaxis, α- or β-blocker overdose, or severe sepsis. Adverse effects associated with the use of high-dose epinephrine include intracranial hypertension, myocardial hemorrhage, myocardial necrosis, and a postresuscitation hyperadrenergic state.[30]

Epinephrine, rather than dopamine, is the vasopressor infusion of choice in children (Table 109-3), because dopamine requires release of endogenous norepinephrine. In children with cardiac arrest, norepinephrine stores may be low. There is no evidence to recommend use of vasopressin over epinephrine in children.

TABLE 109-6 Body Weight Estimation by Age

Age	Weight (kg)	Estimation
Term infant	3.5	Birthweight
6 mo	7	2 × birthweight
1 y	10	3 × birthweight
4 y	16	One-fourth adult weight of 70 kg
10 y	35	One-half adult weight

AMIODARONE

Amiodarone can treat atrial and ventricular arrhythmias and is currently included in the algorithm for ventricular fibrillation and pulseless ventricular tachycardia, although a single study of children found higher rates of return of spontaneous circulation among those treated with lidocaine compared to amiodarone.[31] Amiodarone is a potent vasodilator and a potential proarrhythmic agent. Dosage for pediatric patients is 5 milligrams/kg over 20 to 60 minutes and may be repeated to a maximum of 15 milligrams/kg/d. Administer amiodarone rapidly for ventricular tachycardia or ventricular fibrillation resistant to electrical cardioversion. If the patient has a perfusing rhythm, then consultation with a pediatric

TABLE 109-5 Length-Based Equipment Chart (Length = Centimeters)*

Item	54–70	70–85	85–95	95–107	107–124	124–138	138–155
Endotracheal tube size (mm)	3.5	4.0	4.5	5.0	5.5	6.0	6.5
Lip–tip length (mm)	10.5	12.0	13.5	15.0	16.5	18.0	19.5
Laryngoscope	1 straight	1 straight	2 straight	2 straight or curved	2 straight or curved	2–3 straight or curved	3 straight or curved
Suction catheter	8F	8F–10F	10F	10F	10F	10F	12F
Stylet	6F	6F	6F	6F	14F	14F	14F
Oral airway	Infant/small child	Small child	Child	Child	Child/small adult	Child/adult	Medium adult
Bag-valve mask	Infant	Child	Child	Child	Child	Child/adult	Adult
Oxygen mask	Newborn	Pediatric	Pediatric	Pediatric	Pediatric	Adult	Adult
Vascular access (gauge)							
Catheter	22–24	20–22	18–22	18–22	18–20	18–20	16–20
Butterfly	23–25	23–25	21–23	21–23	21–23	21–22	18–21
Nasogastric tube	5F–8F	8F–10F	10F	10F–12F	12F–14F	14F–18F	18F
Urinary catheter	5F–8F	8F–10F	10F	10F–12F	10F–12F	12F	12F
Chest tube	10F–12F	16F–20F	20F–24F	20F–24F	24F–32F	28F–32F	32F–40F
Blood pressure cuff	Newborn/infant	Infant/child	Child	Child	Child	Child/adult	Adult

*Directions for use: (1) measure patient length with centimeter tape; (2) using measured length in centimeters, access appropriate equipment column.

Source: Reproduced with permission from Luten RC, Wears RL, Broselow J, et al: Length-based endotracheal tube sizing and emergency equipment for pediatric resuscitation. *Ann Emerg Med* 21: 900, 1992, ©1992, Elsevier, Philadelphia, PA. Copyright Elsevier.

a pediatric cardiologist or critical care specialist is strongly recommended prior to amiodarone administration.[8]

Avoid amiodarone if there is the potential for a long QT syndrome either due to a primary cardiac dysrhythmia or medication administration or overdose, because amiodarone prolongs the QT interval and its administration may cause irreversible dysrhythmias in these circumstances.

ATROPINE

Atropine is the first-line drug for treatment of symptomatic bradycardias **in the absence of reversible causes** (Class IIa). In children, hypoxia and shock are the primary causes of symptomatic bradycardia. Although primary cardiac causes of slow rates are rare in children, atropine is recommended if slow rates persist after adequate oxygenation and ventilation. The recommended dose of atropine is 0.02 milligram/kg IV. The minimum dose is 0.1 milligram, with maximum single doses of 0.5 milligram for children and 1.0 milligram for adolescents. The dose may be repeated once, with maximum total doses of 1.0 milligram for children and 2.0 milligrams for adolescents. There is no particular proscription against additional doses, but the maximum recommended dose is considered fully vagolytic. If no response to atropine is seen, then dosing beyond the vagolytic amount is unlikely to be effective. If an effect is seen but not maintained, give additional doses. **Large doses of atropine are needed to treat exposure to organophosphates or nerve agents.**

SODIUM BICARBONATE

Bicarbonate therapy has a primary role in treating overdoses of sodium channel blocking agents, such as procainamide, flecainide, and tricyclic antidepressants (Class IIa). It has an uncertain utility in calcium channel blocker overdoses (Class Indeterminate). Because other resuscitation drugs are less effective in the face of severe acidosis, sodium bicarbonate may be useful during prolonged resuscitations. Adverse effects of bicarbonate include reducing systemic vascular resistance (thereby lowering coronary perfusion pressure), inhibition of oxygen release (by shifting the oxyhemoglobin dissociation curve), inducing hypernatremia and hyperosmolality, inactivation of simultaneously administered catecholamines, and paradoxical worsening of intracellular acidosis (by the production of carbon dioxide, which diffuses rapidly through cell walls). **An initial dose of 1 mEq/kg IV is given only after adequate ventilation has been established.** Without adequate ventilation, the child cannot compensate for the release of carbon dioxide by buffering the hydrogen ions, and the adverse effects of bicarbonate therapy surpass any beneficial effects. **In neonates or premature infants, dilute sodium bicarbonate 1:1 with sterile water, not saline, to reduce the hyperosmolarity of the solution.**

CALCIUM

Routine calcium administration is not recommended during resuscitation because of lack of proven efficacy and because of possible harmful effects. Calcium should be used for documented and symptomatic hyperkalemia, hypocalcemia, and calcium channel blocker overdose. Whenever possible, follow ionized calcium levels to direct calcium administration (total calcium levels do not correlate with the need for calcium therapy in critically ill patients).[32] Calcium may be given as calcium chloride, 20 milligrams/kg (0.2 mL/kg of a 10% solution), or calcium gluconate, 60 to 100 milligrams/kg (0.6 to 1.0 mL/kg of a 10% solution) via the IV or intraosseous route.

DYSRHYTHMIAS

Dysrhythmia management plays only a small role in the resuscitation of children. **Because rhythm disturbances are usually secondary to hypoxia and not primary cardiac events, first provide ventilation and oxygenation, and correct hypoxia, acidosis, and fluid balance.**

A child with an abnormal cardiac rhythm or rate, coupled with evidence of poor end-organ perfusion (cyanosis, mottled skin, lethargy, etc.) is unstable and requires immediate intervention. The parameters of clinical assessment and expression of instability vary with a child's age. In infants and children, variations in heart rate may be well tolerated clinically, and a blood pressure of 70 plus (age in years) divided by 2 mm Hg or less, coupled with evidence of poor end-organ perfusion, may be used to define instability. **Figures 109-5, 107-6, and 109-7** summarize the approach to unstable cardiac rhythms in children, and **Table 109-7** lists the weight-based electrical dose when cardioversion or defibrillation is indicated.[8] American Heart Association guidelines for pediatric ALS are available at: http://circ.ahajournals.org/content/122/18_suppl_3.toc.

The most common rhythms seen in pediatric arrest are the bradycardias, which lead to asystole if untreated. **Again, treatment consists of maximizing oxygenation and ventilation.** Begin chest compression in children with a heart rate <60 beats/min and signs of poor perfusion.

Paroxysmal atrial tachycardia (supraventricular tachycardia) is seen most commonly in infants and most often presents as a narrow complex tachycardia with rates usually between 250 and 350 beats/min. Treatment of unstable patients consists of rapid synchronized cardioversion. Treatment of stable patients varies. Adenosine, vagal maneuvers, and cardioversion are used to treat stable supraventricular tachycardia. **Adenosine (0.1 milligram/kg) is the current recommended drug for supraventricular tachycardia in children; administer via rapid IV push using a three-way-stopcock setup and normal saline flush in a proximal vein or intraosseous line.** This dose can be doubled if the first dose is unsuccessful.

Differentiating a rapid secondary sinus tachycardia from a rapid primary cardiac tachycardia can be difficult but is critical to patient management. Although heart rates of 150 to 200 beats/min in adults are usually cardiac in origin, small infants and young children not uncommonly have compensatory sinus tachycardias as fast as 200 to 220 beats/min. **A rate of >220 beats/min in an infant or >180 beats/min in a child is likely supraventricular tachycardia.** ECG may not be very helpful, because identifiable P waves may not be readily apparent at very fast rates. History compatible with volume loss suggests sinus tachycardia. Congestive heart failure is more likely associated with a pathologic rhythm than a compensatory sinus tachycardia. Children can tolerate primary cardiac tachydysrhythmias for long periods before congestive heart failure or lethal dysrhythmias develop.

CARDIOVERSION, DEFIBRILLATION, AND PACING

Electric conversion is used on an emergency basis to treat ventricular fibrillation (defibrillation) and symptomatic tachydysrhythmia (cardioversion). Ventricular fibrillation is an unusual presenting rhythm in infants and children, but more common with advancing age, and may be present at some point in up to 27% of children with in-hospital cardiac arrest.[7,8,33] Energy requirements for defibrillation and cardioversion are listed in Table 109-7.

Paddle Size Paddle size is 4.5 cm for infants (who weigh <10 kg) and 8 cm for children. The paddle should be in contact with the chest wall over its entire surface area. The larger, 8-cm paddles can be used for infants in the anteroposterior position.

Paddle Interface Electrode cream, electrode paste, and saline-soaked gauze pads are acceptable. Alcohol pads should not be used because serious burns may occur. Make sure that the interface substance from one paddle does not come in contact with the substance from the other paddle. Contact creates a short circuit, and insufficient energy may be delivered to the heart. Many defibrillation devices use cables with integrated adhesive pads for delivery of energy. Adhesive pads are used with the same general guidelines as metal paddles, including the recommendations on sizing and positioning.

Electrode Position Place one paddle to the right of the sternum at the second intercostal space. Place the other paddle at the left midclavicular line at the level of the xiphoid. The anteroposterior approach also can be used, although improved success with anteroposterior positioning has not been documented.[8]

Defibrillation Defibrillate as quickly as possible for pulseless ventricular tachycardia or ventricular fibrillation. The first shock success rate during cardiac arrest due to ventricular arrhythmia is 18% to 50%.[8] Initially, use 2 J/kg. Immediately after defibrillation, and before additional attempts at

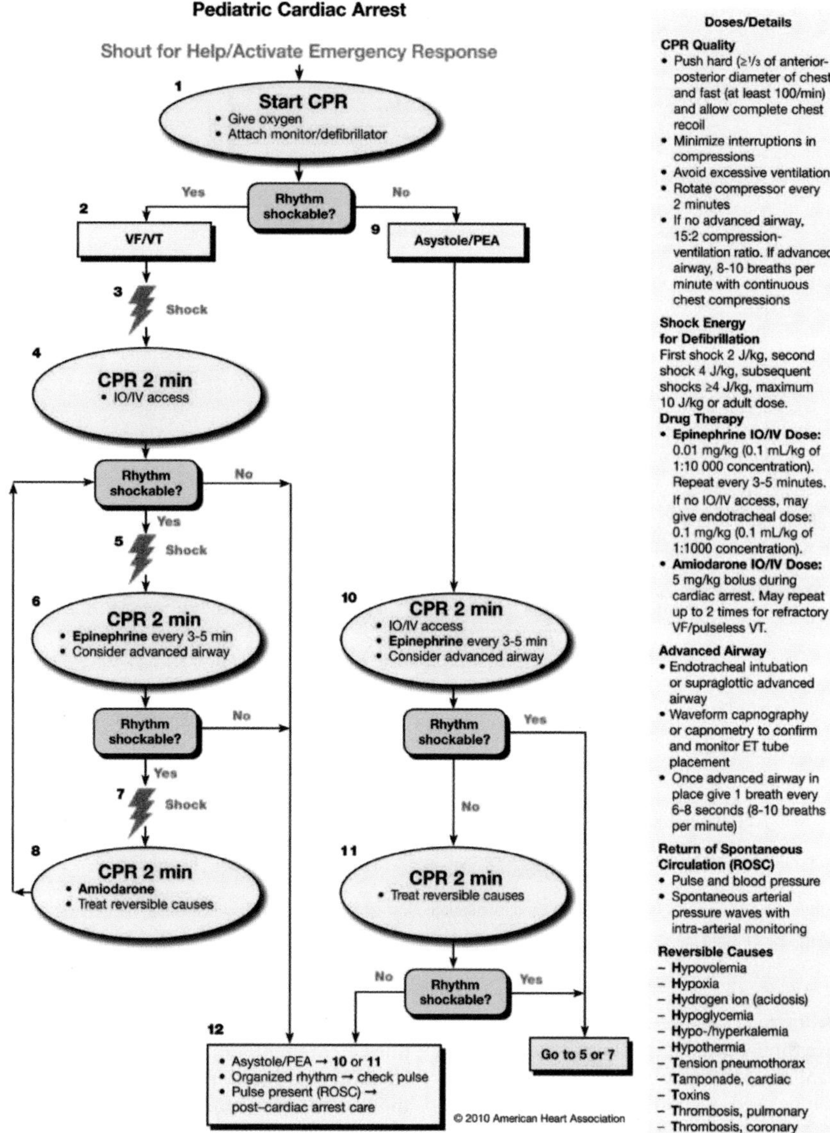

FIGURE 109-5. Pediatric pulseless arrest decision tree. PEA = pulseless electrical activity; VF = ventricular fibrillation; VT = ventricular tachycardia. [Reprinted with permission 2010 American Heart Association Guidelines For CPR and ECC Part 14: Pediatric Advanced Life Support *Circulation. 2010;122[suppl 3]:S876-S908* © 2010, American Heart Association, Inc.]

defibrillation, provide 2 minutes of high-quality uninterrupted CPR to restore coronary perfusion and improve delivery of oxygen to the myocardium. If the first defibrillation attempt is unsuccessful, double the defibrillation energy to 4 J/kg, and use this higher energy level for all additional defibrillation attempts; refractory ventricular fibrillation may require higher energy to a maximum of 10 J/kg or the maximum adult dose.[8]

Provide 2 minutes of chest compressions with ventilations after each defibrillation attempt, regardless of the postdefibrillation rhythm. Nearly all patients will be in a low-perfusion state after defibrillation, and external chest compressions (with ventilations) will improve the perfusion of the vital organs.

If medications such as epinephrine are administered, they are probably most effective when given 1 to 2 minutes before repeating a defibrillation attempt.

Cardioversion Tachydysrhythmias are generally very sensitive to electric conversion. **The initial dose is 0.5 J/kg, in the synchronized mode** (Table 109-7). Double the energy level if the first attempt is unsuccessful. If the device has only a few energy settings available, choose the one closest to the desired energy setting. If the device does not provide the synchronized mode, then obviously the unsynchronized mode must be used.

Transcutaneous Pacing Severe bradycardia or asystole due to an intrinsic myocardial block may respond to transcutaneous pacing. Oxygenation, chest compressions, and medications should precede attempts at pacing in children with severe symptomatic bradycardia due to heart block or sinus node dysfunction. Pacing is not indicated if the bradycardia is due to hypoxic or ischemic myocardial injury or if due to respiratory failure.

Use adult pacing patches in children who weigh >15 kg.[34] Anterior-posterior positioning does not appear to have an advantage over the standard anterior positioning. If using the anterior-posterior positioning, place the negative electrode patch on the anterior chest at V_3, and place the positive electrode patch on the posterior chest between the shoulder blades at the T4 vertebral level. Ventricular capture is determined by the palpation of a pulse or the appearance of an arterial waveform, if an arterial pressure catheter is present. Maximal energy output is used until ventricular capture occurs, then the energy setting is decreased progressively until the lowest setting is found that allows ventricular capture. Set the pacing rate slightly higher than the normal rate for age.

Transcutaneous pacing has not been associated with greatly improved survival rates, but may be advantageous in a child with sudden asystole or bradycardia due to intrinsic atrioventricular node or sinus node dysfunction and with congenital or acquired heart disease.

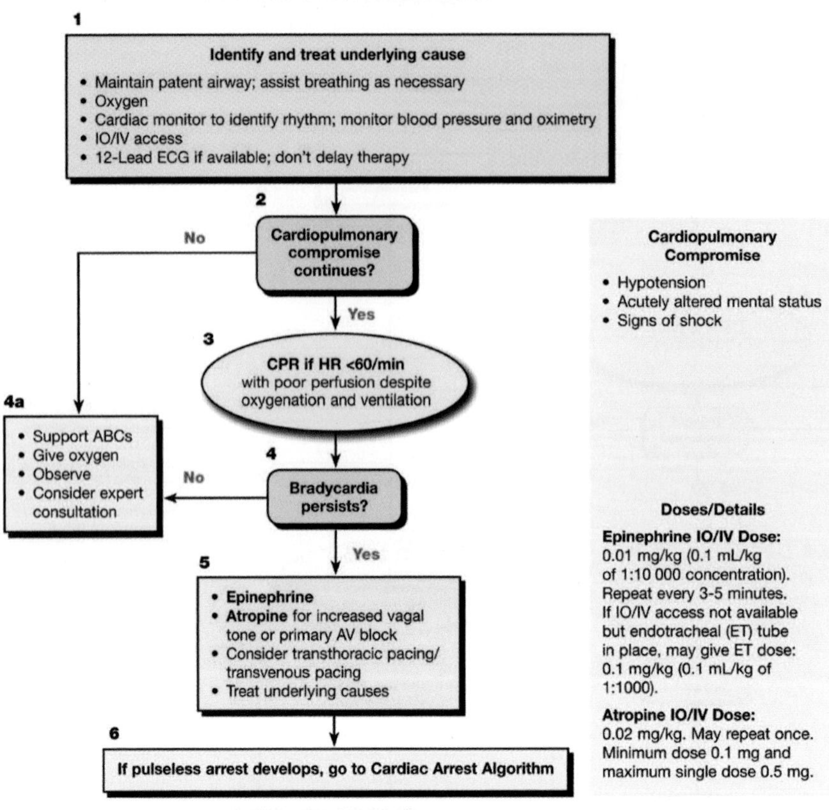
Pediatric Bradycardia
With a Pulse and Poor Perfusion
1
Identify and treat underlying cause
• Maintain patent airway; assist breathing as necessary
• Oxygen
• Cardiac monitor to identify rhythm; monitor blood pressure and oximetry
• IO/IV access
• 12-Lead ECG if available; don't delay therapy
2
Cardiopulmonary compromise continues?
No
Yes
3
CPR if HR <60/min with poor perfusion despite oxygenation and ventilation
4a
• Support ABCs
• Give oxygen
• Observe
• Consider expert consultation
4
Bradycardia persists?
No
Yes
5
• Epinephrine
• Atropine for increased vagal tone or primary AV block
• Consider transthoracic pacing/ transvenous pacing
• Treat underlying causes
6
If pulseless arrest develops, go to Cardiac Arrest Algorithm
Cardiopulmonary Compromise
• Hypotension
• Acutely altered mental status
• Signs of shock
Doses/Details
Epinephrine IO/IV Dose:
0.01 mg/kg (0.1 mL/kg of 1:10 000 concentration). Repeat every 3-5 minutes. If IO/IV access not available but endotracheal (ET) tube in place, may give ET dose: 0.1 mg/kg (0.1 mL/kg of 1:1000).
Atropine IO/IV Dose:
0.02 mg/kg. May repeat once. Minimum dose 0.1 mg and maximum single dose 0.5 mg.
© 2010 American Heart Association

FIGURE 109-6. Pediatric bradycardia decision tree. ABC = airway, breathing, circulation; AV = atrioventricular; HR = heart rate; ICP = intracranial pressure. [Reprinted with permission 2010 American Heart Association Guidelines For CPR and ECC Part 14: Pediatric Advanced Life Support *Circulation. 2010;122[suppl 3]:S876-S908* ©2010, American Heart Association, Inc.]

Automated External Defibrillators Because children ≥8 years old may have life-threatening arrhythmias similar to those in adults and because their body weights approach those of adults, an automated external defibrillator (AED) can be used. A child ≥8 years and weighing >25 kg with sudden collapse should have an AED applied as soon as possible. An AED with a pediatric dose attenuator is ideal for a child 1 to 8 years of age because this feature allows the delivery of a lower dose of energy in pediatric patients. More AEDs are available that allow changing the cardioversion energy levels. If an AED with a pediatric dose attenuator is not available, then use a standard AED. AEDs may be used in infants, but a manual defibrillator is preferred.

Because ventricular fibrillation is an uncommon presentation in children, it is uncertain whether there is greater benefit from providing five cycles of CPR before application of the AED or withholding CPR until the AED has completed its analysis of the heart rhythm. Guidelines for adults recommend 2 minutes of chest compressions before allowing the AED to analyze the rhythm in unwitnessed arrests or when the time since collapse is >5 minutes.[10] For witnessed arrests and arrests in the hospital, the AED should be applied and allowed to analyze as soon as possible. Start chest compressions the instant cardiac arrest is confirmed, and continue compressions until the moment the AED is in place and ready to analyze the rhythm. Realistically, with more than one rescuer, a cycle or two of chest compressions can be provided before the AED is able to analyze the rhythm. If the AED does not recommend defibrillation, then continue CPR. Keep the AED applied until other means of cardiac monitoring become available.

TERMINATION OF EFFORTS

Pediatric cardiopulmonary arrest lasting >20 minutes or with no response to two doses of epinephrine and good CPR is associated with a poor outcome.[1] If hypothermia is thought to be responsible for the arrest, and cardiac electrical activity is present, continue resuscitation until a core temperature of 30°C (86°F) is reached. The likelihood of survival and intact neurologic function diminish as the duration of the resuscitation attempt increases. Unfortunately, no single factor is predictive of outcome, so integrate all the circumstances of the arrest and the patient's premorbid condition before terminating resuscitative efforts. Neurologically intact survival can occur after very prolonged ED resuscitations with high-quality CPR,[8] so developing a strict time for termination of resuscitation efforts is not possible.

FAMILY PRESENCE DURING RESUSCITATION

Family presence during resuscitation efforts continues to increase in acceptance. ED staff may worry about the family's critique of the resuscitation or the family's unwillingness to terminate efforts. Some family members may become distressed or exceedingly emotional while care is being given to a loved one. Positive and negative family responses can occur during resuscitation.[35] Most family members wish to be present during resuscitation.[35] Having family members present during resuscitation is a holistic approach to patient care, with the family's and the patient's needs addressed simultaneously. The current 2010 American Heart Association Guidelines consider family presence during the resuscitation to be a Class I recommendation.[8] A social worker, chaplain, or nurse can assist the family during resuscitative efforts.

COPING WITH THE DEATH OF A CHILD

Both family members and members of the resuscitation team mourn the death of a child.[36] Several *tasks of mourning* have been described that must occur for successful resolution of grieving (**Table 109-8**).[37]

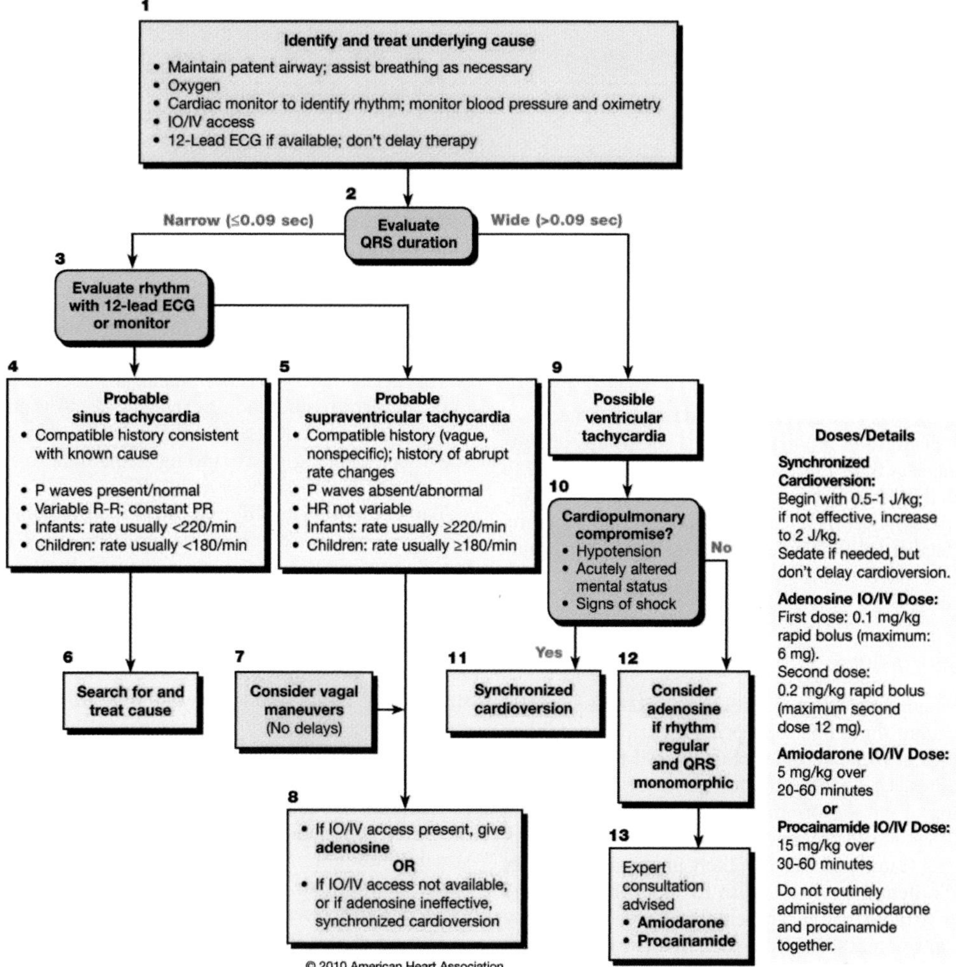

FIGURE 109-7. Pediatric tachycardia decision tree for infants and children with rapid rhythm and poor perfusion. ABC = airway, breathing, circulation; bpm = beats per minute; HR = heart rate. [Reprinted with permission 2010 American Heart Association Guidelines For CPR and ECC Part 14: Pediatric Advanced Life Support *Circulation.2010;122[suppl 3]:S876-S908* ©2010, American Heart Association, Inc.]

TABLE 109-7 Energy Requirements for Defibrillation and Cardioversion

Rhythm	Type of Shock	Initial Dose	Subsequent Doses
Ventricular fibrillation or pulseless ventricular tachycardia	Defibrillation (unsynchronized)	2 J/kg	4 J/kg to maximum of 10 J/kg or adult dose
Unstable supraventricular tachycardia or ventricular tachycardia with pulse but poor perfusion	Synchronized cardioversion	0.5–1 J/kg	2 J/kg

Physicians and other healthcare providers can shape the way families remember the death of a child. Guidelines for communicating with parents are listed in **Table 109-9**.[38] Parents remember how compassionately the bad news is given, but most families still want the "bottom line" when they are first told of their child's death. They are waiting for it.

TABLE 109-8 Tasks of Family Mourning a Lost Child

Accept the reality of the loss.
Work through painful grieving.
Adjust to life without the child.
Emotional resolution and return to normal activities.

TABLE 109-9 Giving Bad News Effectively

Use support staff such as chaplains and social workers.
Early in your delivery of the news, let the family know the child has died.
Use simple, direct, understandable language.
Speak with compassion and caring.
Answer questions from any family members honestly.

Saying, "I am very sorry, we did everything we could, but Sally died" is compassionate and direct. Most families do not want all the technical details about the resuscitation efforts. After delivering the bad news, have a chaplain or social worker stay with the family to allow the family time to deal initially with the shocking news. The physician should remain quietly in the room or return after a few minutes (or later, if other duties require) to answer questions. This is also the time to ask whether the family would like to see the child and to prepare them for what they will see. Although parents do not regret organ donation, donation is not associated with a higher likelihood of successful grieving.[38]

REFERENCES

The complete reference list is available online at www.TintinalliEM.com.

CHAPTER 110 Pediatric Trauma

Camilo E. Gutiérrez

INTRODUCTION AND EPIDEMIOLOGY

Pediatric trauma is a leading cause of morbidity, mortality, and disability for children. More than 9143 children died in the United States due to trauma-related injuries in 2010.[1] For each childhood death associated with injury, more than 1000 children received medical attention for nonfatal injuries.[2] According to the American College of Surgeons National Databank 2013 Pediatric Report, 152,884 patients younger than 19 years of age were admitted to 803 facilities across the United States and Canada with 2834 fatalities. Trauma is the leading cause of death in children over age 1 and exceeds all other causes of death combined.[3]

Unintentional injury death rates are high in some subgroups including newborns and infants less than 1 year of age and teenagers age 15 to 19 years old.[4] Gun-related injuries in this population lead to 8.87 hospitalizations per 100,000 persons <20 years of age in 2009, with 6.1% dying in the hospital (35.1% fatality from suicide).[5] In 2010, gun-related injuries accounted for 6570 deaths of children and young people (1 to 24 years of age).[6]

BEHAVIORAL CONSIDERATIONS

In general, a child's developmental stage dictates the expected behavioral response to injury. An infant should be appropriately curious and interactive or afraid of strangers, while an older child should respond with fear to invasive procedures. Understanding normal child development helps identify alterations of the sensorium, which may be the result of traumatic brain injury, hypoperfusion, or hypoxemia.

Family presence during trauma care is extremely important, not only to help assess the child's mental status, but also to support the injured child. Studies repeatedly demonstrate that parental presence is beneficial for both the patient's and parent's psychological well-being, does not interfere with medical efforts or increase stress in the healthcare team for the most part, and does not result in increased medicolegal issues. **Family presence during resuscitation is an important standard practice in pediatric care.**[7-9]

ED PREPAREDNESS

Children require age- and size-based medication and equipment, so EDs should prepare an appropriate pediatric resuscitation area, provide personnel with adequate training in the care of children, and stock appropriately sized pediatric resuscitation equipment.[10] In 2013, the American Academy of Pediatrics, the American College of Emergency Physicians, the Emergency Nurses Association, and the Emergency Medical Services for Children developed the Pediatric Readiness Project[11] to improve care for children in the ED, to provide a quality improvement process following the Guidelines for Care of Children in the Emergency Department,[12] and to measure ED improvements over time. Approximately 5000 EDs with a response rate of over 80% were involved, resulting in one of the most successful assessments to date.[13]

PEDIATRIC ANATOMY

The pediatric head has a larger surface area that is prone to significant bleeding either from open scalp wounds with brisk arterial bleeding or in the form of cephalohematomas or subgaleal hematomas that can cause hypovolemic shock in small infants. The cranium is thinner, transmits energy easily, and predisposes to skull fractures.[14] Open sutures in infants can accommodate increases in intracranial pressure and delay the recognition of serious intracranial injuries. Infants have prominent extra-axial intracranial spaces through which bridging cortical vessels traverse and are prone to sheer and acceleration-deceleration forces such as those sustained in aggressive shaking; this accounts for classic findings such as subdural hemorrhages in inflicted injury victims.[15] Finally, the size of the head in young children is larger compared to the body, which predisposes to closed head injury when children fall and will also occlude the airway when placed supine without back support.

The facets in the pediatric cervical spine are more horizontal than in adults, with less calcified vertebral bodies, increased laxity of spinal ligaments, and weaker supporting musculature, all of which allow translational forces to cause spine injuries without bony abnormalities. Due to the weaker neck musculature and larger cranium, the fulcrum of force is more cephalad, predisposing children to higher cervical spine injuries compared to adults (see chapter 139, "Cervical Spine Injury in Infants and Children").[16,17]

Significant anatomic differences between pediatric and adult airways are discussed in chapter 111, "Intubation and Ventilation in Infants and Children," as they relate to advanced airway management. The pediatric laryngeal cartilages are more pliable and therefore less prone to fracture than the firm ossified adult cartilages.[18,19] Although the larynx is relatively protected, children have higher risk for airway compromise due to soft tissue swelling or expanding hematoma in relation to the smaller size of the pediatric airway and neck.

The chest wall in children is more compliant, its tracheobronchial structures are more vulnerable, and the heart is more anterior with mobile mediastinal structures, all of which predispose to intrathoracic injury such as pulmonary contusions with minimal thoracic wall injury. Delicate tracheobronchial structures are susceptible to barotrauma especially in situations of excessive volume ventilations during resuscitation generating iatrogenic pneumothorax. The diameter of the respiratory structures is much smaller than adults, and a change in the inner diameter (from aspirated fluids or secretions) has a four-fold impact on the resistance to air flow as stated by the Hagen-Poiseuille equation, predisposing to airway obstruction.

The child's abdomen is relatively larger in size compared with the rest of the trunk, has underdeveloped musculature, and has relatively larger size intra-abdominal organs, which predisposes to solid organ injuries in blunt abdominal trauma and hollow viscus injuries in certain acceleration-deceleration mechanisms such as seat belt injuries.

The skeleton is incompletely calcified, which renders bones more pliable and leads to bowing and greenstick injuries; multiple active growth centers and weaker epiphysis explain certain fracture types specific to children such as supracondylar fractures of the elbow and epiphyseal injuries such as the ones described by the Salter-Harris classification (see chapter 140, "Musculoskeletal Disorders in Children").[20]

The higher body surface area to overall body mass in children and thin epidermal and dermal layers of the skin along with a paucity of subcutaneous fat and immature thermoregulatory mechanisms lead to increased propensity for hypothermia in cold environments which must be considered when assessing an exposed child in the trauma bay.[21]

PHYSIOLOGY

Table 110-1 shows the expected vital signs according to age. Be alert to abnormalities in heart rate, respiratory rate, and peripheral perfusion that can indicate acute deterioration in the setting of trauma.[22]

TABLE 110-1 Normal Pediatric Vital Signs

	Pulse (beats/min)	Systolic BP (mm Hg)	Diastolic BP (mm Hg)
Newborn	95–145	60–90	30–45
Infant	125–170	75–100	30–70
Toddler	100–160	80–110	40–90
Preschool	70–110	80–110	45–85
School age	70–110	85–120	45–88
Adolescent	55–100	95–120	60–90

Abbreviation: BP = blood pressure.

Source: Reproduced with permission from Iserson, *Improvised Medicine* © 2012, McGraw-Hill Education, New York, NY.

Cardiac output is mediated primarily by heart rate in children as opposed to stroke volume in adults. Children with significant blood loss develop tachycardia, which can be sustained for a variable period of time before cardiac output is compromised. In addition, the vasculature is quite sensitive to endogenous catecholamines, allowing children to modify vascular tone in response to hemodynamic changes and regulate perfusion to the core organs. These two parameters, capacity to increase heart rate and modulate peripheral vascular resistance, help children maintain normal blood and perfusion pressures in the face of significant hemorrhage (25% to 30%), and **hypotension is a very late and ominous sign of cardiovascular compromise in children.**[23]

In children, pulmonary tidal volume is relatively fixed, so minute ventilation is maintained primarily by respiratory rate (tachypnea) rather than depth (hyperpnea). Small residual volumes contribute to atelectasis, and a smaller functional residual capacity contributes to rapid desaturation during apnea.[24]

Finally, the metabolic demands in children are higher than adults. Children have a much higher energy expenditure and caloric requirement at baseline. Although stress-induced **hyperglycemia** is common in the setting of polytrauma, **hypoglycemia** can occur and should be treated promptly.

THE PRIMARY SURVEY

AIRWAY

The most important step in trauma care for children is assessment and stabilization of the airway. Children experience desaturation sooner than adults, and desaturation is quickly followed by respiratory arrest, which can lead to full cardiac arrest. For this reason, the most experienced clinician should be in charge of airway management.

Assess the **patency** of the airway first; note a hoarse or muffled cry or voice, stridor or sonorous respirations, increased work of breathing, or poor chest rise with bag-valve mask ventilation. Evaluate the **maintainability of a protected airway** in the presence of facial or neck trauma or facial burns, or in patients with neurologic compromise that precludes them from having an organized breathing pattern.

Perform basic airway maneuvers such as jaw thrust and oropharyngeal suctioning and maintain a sniffing position to align the airway axes, often by placing a towel roll under the shoulders. Consider use of airway adjuncts such as nasal trumpets, oral airways, or supraglottic devices until a definitive airway through endotracheal intubation can be achieved (see chapter 111).

Maintain in-line cervical spine stabilization at all times. Rapid sequence intubation is the safest method of intubating a trauma patient with a full stomach. When possible, limit positive-pressure ventilation before intubation to avoid gastric insufflation and vomiting. Indications for endotracheal intubation in the trauma patient include:

1. Glasgow coma score <8 or inability to maintain or protect the airway
2. Inadequate oxygenation or ventilation
3. Inability to ventilate or oxygenate with bag-valve mask
4. Potential for clinical deterioration (e.g., facial burns, inhalation injury)
5. Flail chest
6. Decompensated shock resistant to fluid resuscitation
7. Anticipated surgical intervention or need for radiologic investigation outside of the ED in an unstable patient

BREATHING

Assess the adequacy of breathing, ventilation, and oxygenation through careful observation of the rate, depth, pattern, and work of breathing, including tracheal position and symmetry of chest wall rise and fall. Note that alterations in the mental status might signify hypoxia (agitation) or hypercarbia (somnolence) from inadequate breathing.

Remember that small children are predominantly diaphragmatic breathers, are highly sensitive to increased intra-abdominal pressure, and have mobile mediastinal structures that predispose to pneumothorax, hemothorax, or flail chest that can rapidly compromise respiration and ventilation.

When there is concern for tension pneumothorax, perform needle thoracostomy by placing a 14- to 18-gauge IV catheter in the midclavicular line at the second intercostal space attached via a three-way stopcock to a 10- to 20-mL syringe; do not wait for radiologic confirmation in the hemodynamically unstable child.

CIRCULATION

Recognize early signs of circulatory shock including tachycardia, mental status, and color and perfusion abnormalities, because hypotension is typically a terminal event in children. **Estimate normal systolic blood pressure in children 1 to 10 years of age using the following formula: 90 + (2 × age) mm Hg; hypotension can be estimated as systolic blood pressure less than 70 + (2 × age) mm Hg.**[25]

Evaluate the heart rate, peripheral pulses, capillary refill time, skin color, body temperature, and mental status, which is an important surrogate for perfusion. Control external hemorrhage by applying direct pressure to limit ongoing blood loss; perform additional maneuvers such as scalp suturing, fracture reduction, and pelvic binding to limit ongoing hemorrhage.

Vascular access can be challenging in small children and is more difficult in shock. Ideally, place two proximal large-bore IV catheters, but limit attempts in the unstable child and proceed to intraosseous access if unsuccessful after 90 seconds (see chapter 112, "Intravenous and Intraosseous Access in Infants and Children").

For compensated or uncompensated shock, give a rapid infusion of crystalloid (20 mL/kg of normal saline or lactated Ringer's solution). Give two to three boluses rapidly as needed, ideally within 5 minutes each using an automated "rapid infuser," a frequently monitored pressure bag, or the "hand push and pull method."[26] After two to three crystalloid boluses, consider 10 mL/kg boluses of warmed O-negative blood.

Although techniques such as permissive hypotension and "damage control resuscitation" with goals to limit hemorrhage, hemodilution, and the disruption of the clotting process have been widely studied and practiced in adult trauma care,[27] there are insufficient data to recommend routine use in pediatric trauma patients. Children may tolerate relative hypotensive states better than adults, but the current standard of care is to maintain tissue perfusion with crystalloid boluses and blood component replacement until definitive surgical control of hemorrhage is achieved.[10]

Pediatric rapid or massive transfusion protocols, on the other hand, have been widely studied and used in pediatric trauma centers. Implement a massive transfusion protocol, if available, when the need for transfusion is anticipated to equal one or more blood volumes within a 24-hour time frame or half of a blood volume in 12 hours is suspected. Massive transfusion protocols replace red blood cells, plasma, and platelets in specific amounts (usually 1:1:1) with the goal of minimizing the coagulopathy associated with significant hemorrhage and minimizing the effects of hypothermia and acidosis.[28]

DISABILITY

Assess mental status and neurologic deficits as part of the primary survey. Mental status can be assessed using the **modified pediatric Glasgow coma scale**, which mirrors the familiar adult Glasgow coma scale in assigning points for eye opening and motor response using the same scale, but defines verbal response in an age-appropriate way (**Table 110-2**).

TABLE 110-2 Modified Pediatric Glasgow Coma Scale

Coos or babbles = 5
Irritable cry = 4
Cries to pain = 3
Moans to pain = 2
No response = 1

TABLE 110-3 AVPU Score

A = Awake
V = Responds to verbal stimuli
P = Responds to pain
U = Unresponsive

However, the Glasgow coma scale lacks good interobserver reliability and reproducibility and does not accurately predict outcomes in individual patients.[29] A simpler and validated method to assess mental status in children is by using the AVPU score, which is currently recommended by the pediatric advanced life support guidelines[25] (**Table 110-3**).

In addition to assessing mental status, perform a pupillary examination and focused assessment of tone and strength.

EXPOSURE

To identify all potential injuries and perform life-saving procedures, disrobe and expose the child; however, children are particularly susceptible to hypothermia when exposed to cold environments or receiving room temperature fluids.[30] To avoid iatrogenic hypothermia, maintain a warm resuscitation environment, remove wet clothing, and place warm blankets underneath the child. Additional measures to maintain euthermia include use of radiant warmers and infusion of warmed intravenous fluids. Monitor and record temperature carefully throughout assessment and resuscitation.

THE SECONDARY SURVEY

Begin the secondary survey after the primary survey is complete and resuscitative measures have been initiated. For the secondary survey, perform a complete head-to-toe physical examination, cervical spine evaluation, and clearance. Ancillary tools such as pulse oximetry, blood gas measurement, and quantitative end-tidal carbon dioxide (CO_2) monitoring help guide therapy. Initiate laboratory evaluation, bedside ultrasonography, and radiographic imaging. During the secondary survey, perform nonemergent procedures such as placing a nasogastric or orogastric tube and Foley catheter (minimum urine output should be 0.5 mL/kg/h). A nasogastric tube will decompress the stomach, as a full stomach can restrict functional residual capacity.

In this phase, stabilize the child's condition sufficiently to allow transfer to the radiology suite or inpatient unit or a facility that can provide a higher level of care. **Reassess the airway, breathing, circulation, and neurologic status continually because some injuries may manifest over time and complications from therapeutic interventions can occur**. Consider endotracheal tube dislodgment, equipment failure, pneumothorax, regurgitation and aspiration of stomach contents, occult hemorrhage, and progression of intracranial hypertension as causes for deterioration. Carefully monitor fluid administration to prevent inadvertent overhydration. **Provide appropriate analgesics and sedatives because pain treatment is often neglected in children**.

REFERRAL TO A PEDIATRIC CENTER

Pediatric trauma center designation in the United States is conferred by governmental authority, and requirements vary from state to state. Guidelines have been created by American College of Emergency Physicians and American College of Surgeons to delineate the capabilities of a pediatric trauma center.[18] The receiving institution should have a dedicated pediatric trauma service; comprehensive pediatric services should be available from scene care to rehabilitation and reintegration into the family and society. The trauma team should be immediately available at all times and capable of treating at least two patients simultaneously. Additional pediatric specialists should be on site or immediately available, including specialists in pediatric emergency medicine, anesthesiology, neurosurgery, radiology, orthopedics, critical care, and nursing. A pediatric intensive care unit is an essential component of a designated pediatric trauma center.

TABLE 110-4 Pediatric Trauma Score*

	−1	+1	+2
Size (kg)	<10	10–20	>20
Airway	Unmaintained	Maintained	Normal
Systolic blood pressure (mm Hg)	<50	50–90	>90
Level of consciousness	Comatose	Altered	Awake
Wounds	Major open	Minor open	None
Skeletal trauma	Open/multiple	Closed	None

*Total score is calculated by adding the score corresponding to the appropriate value from each column.

Use of trauma triage scores can help identify a child with more severe injuries, increase awareness of the need for higher level of care and monitoring, and predict outcomes. Two of the most commonly used systems are the Pediatric Trauma Score (**Table 110-4**) and the Revised Trauma Score (**Table 110-5**). Their advantages over other systems include use of physiologic variables instead of reliance solely on anatomic factors. Lower scores are associated with greater mortality and thus a need for pediatric trauma center care: **a Revised Trauma Score of <12 or a Pediatric Trauma Score of <8 should prompt transfer to a pediatric trauma center.**[31]

Additional indications for transfer to a pediatric trauma center are listed in **Table 110-6**.[32] Anatomic and physiologic parameters are most useful in determining which children should be transported to a trauma center.

Care of seriously injured children at a pediatric trauma center is associated with improved survival. In a study of 53,702 pediatric traumas comparing children treated at adult or pediatric trauma centers, the adjusted odds of mortality was 20% lower for children seen at trauma centers with pediatric qualifications.[33] If not available, transport to a designated trauma center, adult or pediatric, is still associated with improved outcomes.[34,35] Interfacility transfer of critically injured children is best done by a specialized pediatric transport team or a critical care transport team with pediatric experience when available (see chapter 107, "Neonatal and Pediatric Transport").

GENERAL ASSESSMENT

The goals of evaluation in a trauma victim are to determine the extent and severity of injury, what interventions, if any, are needed, and the level of monitoring required if admission is indicated. The mechanism of injury, history, and initial physical examination influence the degree of suspicion for intra-abdominal injury and guide subsequent radiographic and laboratory evaluation. Persistent emesis (especially bilious or bloody), abdominal distention, abdominal pain or any signs of peritoneal irritation, gross hematuria, and blood on rectal examination are indications for further investigation.

Carefully inspect the abdomen for signs of trauma including distention, abrasions, seat belt marks, or ecchymosis. Palpate for abdominal tenderness, which has a has a high positive predictive value for intra-abdominal injury. In high-mechanism injuries, maintain a high index of suspicion because pancreatic and hollow viscus injuries can present with delayed symptoms such as pain or emesis. Clinical evaluation of patients with altered mental status or distracting or associated injuries is difficult, and in this setting, a normal abdominal examination does not rule out the possibility of injury.

TABLE 110-5 Revised Trauma Score*

Number	Glasgow Coma Scale Score	Systolic Blood Pressure (mm Hg)	Respiratory Rate (breaths/min)
4	13–15	>89	10–29
3	9–12	76–89	>29
2	6–8	50–75	6–9
1	4–5	1–49	1–5
0	3	0	0

*Total score is calculated by adding the score corresponding to the appropriate value from each column.

TABLE 110-6 Indications for Transfer to a Pediatric Trauma Center

Mechanism of injury	Ejection from motor vehicle
	Fall from a significant height
	Motor vehicle collision with prolonged extrication
	Motor vehicle collision with death of another vehicle occupant
Anatomic injury	Multiple severe trauma
	More than three long-bone fractures
	Spinal fractures or spinal cord injury
	Amputations
	Severe head or facial trauma
	Penetrating head, chest, or abdominal trauma

Source: Reproduced with permission from Harris BH, Barlow BA, Ballantine TV, et al: American Pediatric Surgical Association principles of pediatric trauma care. *J Pediatr Surg* 27: 423, 1992. Copyright Elsevier.

LABORATORY INVESTIGATION

Routine laboratory "trauma panels" are frequently obtained in the evaluation of injured children, but individual laboratory abnormalities, while common, are seldom useful to dictate therapy, and no single laboratory test has acceptable sensitivity or negative predictive value to safely and effectively screen patients with abdominal trauma when used alone.[36] Even organ-specific chemistries predicted injury poorly in children, are of little value, and alter acute management in only 5% to 6% of trauma patients.[37] Although elevated liver function tests, particularly alanine aminotransferase, are suggestive of liver injury, no consensus exists as to the cut point for determining risk. Alanine aminotransferase levels >80 to 125 units/L have a sensitivity of 77%, specificity of 82%, but a positive predictive value of only 16%.[38,39] An exception to the generally poor utility of liver function tests is in the setting of suspected inflicted injury in infants and young children, for whom liver function tests are recommended as a screening tool to detect occult blunt intra-abdominal injury.[40]

Amylase is not sensitive for acute pancreatic or other intra-abdominal organ injury, but lipase levels are fairly specific for pancreatic injury and can be used to serially monitor children for the development of complications such as pseudocyst formation or small bowel injury.[41] In the seriously injured child, a base deficit >8 on blood gas analysis and lactate >4.0 mg/dL correlate with severe intra-abdominal injury and prognosis.[42-44]

Urinalysis is frequently obtained in trauma patients, but microhematuria alone is poorly predictive of either genitourinary or intra-abdominal injury across a range of cut points for number of red blood cells per high-power field; gross hematuria and mechanism of injury, rather than microhematuria, should guide imaging studies.[45]

IMAGING

Plain Radiography Plain radiography is still advocated as part of the trauma series in which the cervical spine, chest, and pelvis are imaged. Plain radiography has a low sensitivity for detecting intra-abdominal injury.

US Bedside ultrasonography is an extension of the physical examination of adult trauma patients. The FAST and extended FAST are used to evaluate for fluid in the peritoneal, pericardial, or pleural spaces. The utility of FAST is predicated upon its ability to identify free fluid (hemoperitoneum) and the assumption that the presence of free fluid is an indication of serious intra-abdominal injury requiring further evaluation. FAST is an appealing test due to its rapid bedside acquisition, relatively low cost, and lack of radiation, but there are a number of limitations in pediatric use. **Due to anatomic and physiologic differences between children and adults, up to 30% of children with solid organ injury have no demonstrable free fluid on FAST, decreasing the sensitivity of this exam for solid organ injuries and limiting its negative predictive value, particularly in hemodynamically stable patients.** Moreover, unlike adults in whom free fluid (hemoperitoneum) usually requires laparotomy, the vast majority of children with hemoperitoneum are successfully managed nonoperatively, so a positive FAST does not always change management. On the other hand, in the hemodynamically unstable patient with multiple trauma, FAST can provide valuable information as to the source of instability and help to focus resuscitative and surgical efforts when positive.[46-48] As in adults, FAST poorly detects retroperitoneal and hollow viscus injury.

CT CT scan is the study of choice for the evaluation of blunt pediatric abdominal trauma. Advantages of CT include its speed, excellent depiction of solid organs, and widespread availability. Reformatted images in the coronal and sagittal planes allow good depiction of anatomy, and CT angiography can provide additional detail. Disadvantages include the need to remove the patient from the controlled and monitored setting of the trauma bay, radiation exposure, and potential complications related to the use of contrast materials. The main limitation to CT use is persistent hemodynamic instability despite adequate fluid resuscitation.

Common indications for CT include intubated children with multisystem trauma; altered mental status in the setting of trauma; spinal cord injuries resulting in loss of abdominal sensation; gross hematuria; abdominal pain and tenderness on examination; free fluid on FAST examination; abdominal or flank bruising or seat belt mark above the iliac crests; suspected inflicted trauma to the abdomen with elevated liver function tests; and direct blow to the abdomen from bicycle handlebars.[49,50]

PEDIATRIC HEAD TRAUMA

Minor head injury (Glasgow coma scale >13) and concussion, including pathophysiology and clinical decision rules to decide which children require neuroimaging, is discussed in chapter 138, "Head Injury in Infants and Children." Inflicted head injuries are discussed in more detail in chapter 148, "Child Abuse and Neglect". This section focuses on more severe traumatic brain injury (Glasgow coma scale <14).

IMAGING

Plain Films Plain films of the skull have limited use in the evaluation of pediatric head trauma except in children less than 2 years old in whom they are an acceptable screening tool for fractures when there is a large, usually boggy scalp hematoma noted on physical examination. However, if a skull fracture is identified by plain film, obtain a CT scan to rule out an intracranial injury, as there is a four- to six-fold risk of intracranial pathology associated with skull fracture.[51] A four-view series is recommended and consists of anteroposterior, right and left lateral, and Towne (30-degree caudal angulation) views.[52] Plain films can be difficult to interpret due to normal cranial sutures and may miss as many as 25% of skull fractures, and plain films have a low sensitivity for intracranial injuries.[53,54]

US A number of studies suggest an emerging role for bedside ultrasonography to detect skull fractures in children, with a sensitivity ranging from 94% to 100% and a specificity up to 96%,[55,56] and US may be more sensitive than plain films for certain types of fractures.[57] Brain US can be used in infants with open anterior fontanel to assess for intraventricular hemorrhage and is commonly used in preterm neonates, but its use has not been validated in trauma, and there is a risk that it might miss peripheral or extra-axial hemorrhages. US interpretation is highly dependent of sonographer skill, however, and when compared to CT scan, has limited ability to detect traumatic brain injury in the absence of skull fractures. US is not yet a reliable tool to determine if CT can be avoided in children with a single isolated risk factor for intracranial injury and no evidence of fracture by US.

CT CT is the gold standard in the diagnosis of traumatic brain injury and has 100% sensitivity and 100% specificity for significant intracranial lesions.[58] In the setting of significant trauma, CT of the head is typically performed without contrast, and sedation is rarely required. See chapter 138 for further discussion of CT imaging decision rules in pediatric head injury.

MRI MRI is not widely available, scan times are lengthy, and MRI is not appropriate in unstable patients. MRI is an option once the patient has been stabilized and additional information is needed regarding extent of injury and prognosis. MRI may be useful when there are inconsistencies between the clinical picture and the CT findings, for dating of extra-axial hemorrhage, and for detecting diffuse axonal injury.

TREATMENT

Emergent treatment for serious traumatic brain injury is listed in **Table 110-7**.

PALATAL INJURIES

Children commonly place objects in their mouth and may trip and fall leading to penetrating injuries of the oropharynx. It is estimated that around 1% of children suffer such injuries.[59] Such injuries present a diagnostic challenge for several reasons: soft palate injuries can heal rapidly leaving few visible clues; the size of the lacerations does not relate to the depth of the wound; most of these injuries are caused by long, thin, sharp objects (i.e., pencils) that can penetrate deeply; and the potential for severe complications related to vascular injury is high. Well-known complications based on observational studies[60] include compression, thrombosis or laceration of the carotid artery, deep soft tissue infections and mediastinitis, and stroke.[61,62]

Wounds longer than 2 cm or with evidence of flaps require repair, while smaller ones usually heal by primary intention.[63] The location of the wound is most important, as lateral wounds (over tonsillar pillars) have a greater risk of vascular injury than wounds near the midline where the hard palate is located. Obtain CT when a foreign body is noted or suspected.

The imaging modality of choice for lateral palatal injuries or those associated with focal neurologic injury, the presence of a bruit, persistent bleeding, or concern for significant mechanism of injury is CT or MRI angiography or digital subtraction carotid angiography. There are differences in the sensitivity and specificity of the various imaging modalities, and a balance needs to be established between radiation exposure, the need for sedation, and the length of time required to complete the study.[64] Admit patients with lateral palatal penetrating injury for observation and serial neurologic exams unless vascular injury has been excluded by angiography. In patients with midline hard palate lacerations, minor trauma, or trivial injuries, no imaging is necessary. Provide clear discharge instructions with signs and symptoms of complications for which to seek prompt medical care, including fever, dysphagia, persistent bleeding, or symptoms of stroke. The use of empiric antibiotics such as clindamycin, ampicillin, or amoxicillin with clavulanic acid is recommended, although evidence is lacking. Provide tetanus prophylaxis as appropriate.

NECK TRAUMA

Although adult penetrating neck trauma accounts for 5% to 10% of trauma visits and carries an overall mortality of 3% to 10%,[65] penetrating neck trauma is rare in children, comprising only 0.5% of trauma admissions.[66] Blunt neck injuries are more common than penetrating injuries in children and are a result of falls into stationary objects, direct impact during sports, "clothesline injuries," and intentional hanging injuries. Hanging can result in laryngeal fractures or separation injuries.[67] For a complete discussion of neck injuries, see chapter 260, "Trauma to the Neck" in the adult section.

An approach to the evaluation of pediatric blunt neck trauma is shown in **Figure 110-1**. Assess children with neck injuries in a position of comfort to avoid airway compromise; avoid forcing a patient into recumbence when the physiology dictates tripoding and neck hyperextension in order to maintain airway patency.

TABLE 110-7 Management of Serious Traumatic Brain Injury in Children

Considerations	Primary Goal	Comments
Cervical spine	Maintain spinal precautions	
Airway	Maintain airway, intubate for GCS <8 or as needed for oxygenation and ventilation	
Oxygenation and ventilation	Oxygen saturation >90%; Pco_2 35–40 mm Hg	No prophylactic hyperventilation
Blood pressure	SBP > 70 + (2 × age)	No permissive hypotension
Cerebral perfusion pressure (CPP)	CPP = 40–65 mm Hg (ref)	
Intracranial pressure (ICP) monitoring	ICP ≤20 mm Hg	Consultation with neurosurgeon
GCS	GCS before paralytics if possible	Serial GCS to document changes
Sedation and pain management	Midazolam Fentanyl	Consider paralytics once thorough neurologic examination is completed
Neuroimaging (noncontrast head CT and cervical spine CT when indicated)	Identify intracranial injury and signs of increased intracranial pressure or herniation	Transcranial Doppler[108] may be useful in infants with open fontanelles but requires an experienced pediatric radiologist
Glucose	Treat hypoglycemia and hyperglycemia	Maintain normal blood glucose
Increased ICP/impending herniation	Elevate head of bed 30 degrees	3% normal saline 5 mL/kg bolus over 10 minutes followed by infusion of 0.1 mL/kg/h to maintain serum Na within 155–165 mEq/L *or* Mannitol 0.5–1 gram/kg if normotensive (response is not dose-dependent)
Core temperature	Maintain temperature 36–38°C	Hypothermia in children not recommended[109]; avoid hyperthermia
Seizure prophylaxis	Optional: consider for children with witnessed posttraumatic seizures and intracranial blood	Phenytoin 20 milligrams/kg (or fosphenytoin 20 PE/kg) *or* Levetiracetam 10–20 milligrams/kg (maximum, 500 milligrams/dose)[111] for first week following severe traumatic brain injury
Anemia	Transfuse for hemoglobin <7 grams/dL[110]	
Neurosurgery/transfer	ICP monitoring, evacuation of intracranial blood, or cerebrospinal fluid shunt for refractory intracranial hypertension	

Abbreviations: GCS = Glasgow coma scale; Pco_2 = partial pressure of carbon dioxide; PE = phenytoin equivalent; SBP = systolic blood pressure.

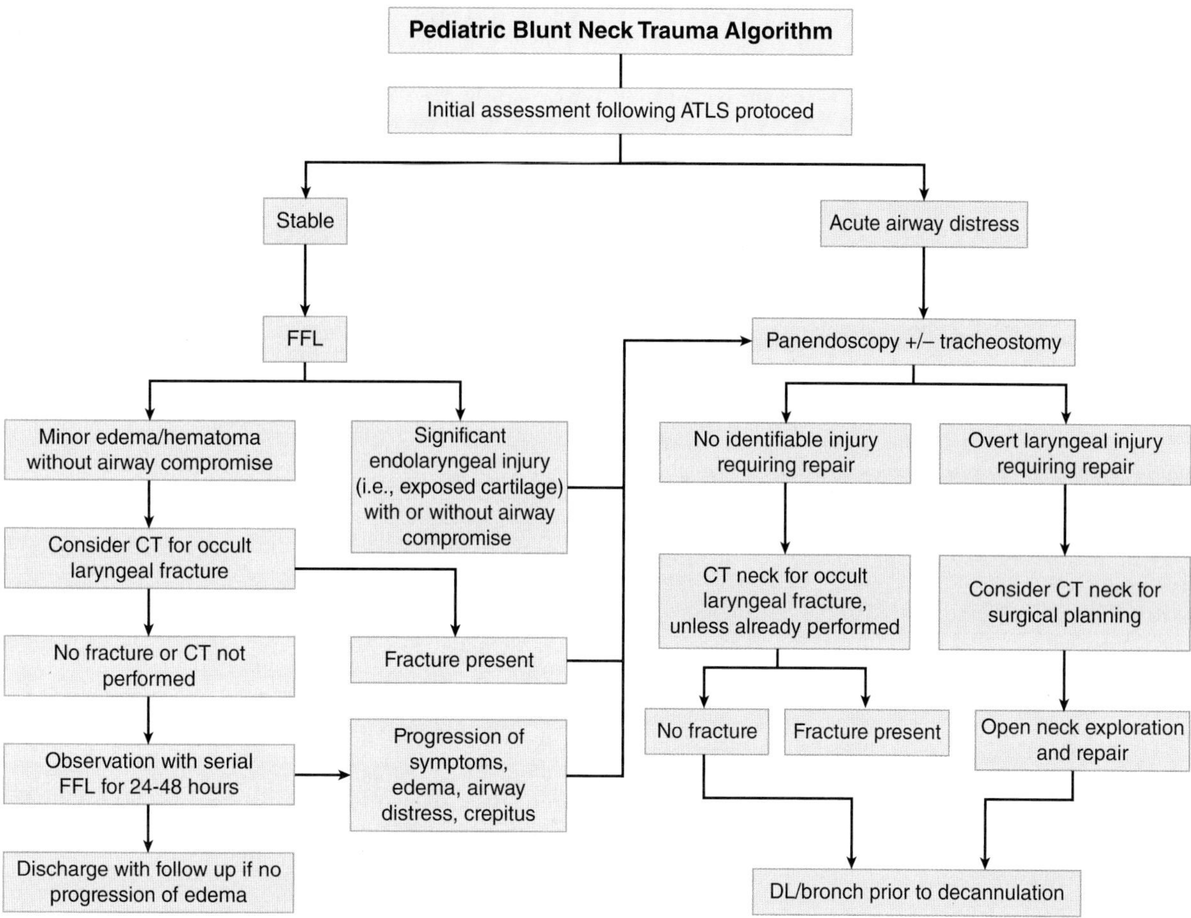

FIGURE 110-1. Algorithm for the evaluation of pediatric blunt neck trauma. ATLS = advanced trauma life support; DL/Bronch = direct laryngoscopy bronchoscopy; FFL = flexible fiberoptic laryngoscopy. [*Source:* Hernandez, et al: Emergency airway management for pediatric blunt neck trauma. *Clin Pediatr Emerg Med* 15: 1522, 2014. © 2014 Elsevier Inc. All Rights Reserved.]

THORACIC TRAUMA

Thoracic injuries occur infrequently in children, accounting for 5% to 12% of pediatric trauma admissions, but are the second leading cause of death from trauma after closed head injury. Isolated chest trauma in children carries a 4% to 12% mortality rate in isolation, but when associated with closed head injuries and abdominal trauma, mortality increases to 40%.[68]

Blunt forces account for 80% to 85% of pediatric thoracic injuries. Motor vehicle crashes, pedestrian accidents, and inflicted injury are more common in younger children, whereas falls, sports-related injuries, and high-speed crashes are more common in older children and teenagers.[69] Penetrating trauma is rare in children and most commonly the result of impaling injuries; accidental gunshot wounds in younger children have become increasingly common as the number of firearm injuries steadily increases in the United States.

Pulmonary contusions are the most common injury in blunt chest trauma in children and may present with minimal or no external signs of trauma.[70] Anatomic changes in pulmonary contusion include interstitial edema and alveolar hemorrhage with subsequent consolidation. Areas of ventilation/perfusion mismatch reflect poor lung compliance and are associated with disordered ventilation and oxygenation.[71]

Pneumothoraces are common and present in up to 33% of trauma victims; they should alert the clinician to the possibility of associated injuries. Tension pneumothorax is of special concern in younger children due to the relatively easier compromise of cardiopulmonary physiology and detrimental effect on right side heart-filling pressures. Signs like jugular venous distention are less prominent in children than in adults, and their absence can be falsely reassuring. Treat tension pneumothorax emergently with needle decompression and closed chest thoracostomy without waiting for confirmatory chest x-ray in the child with unstable vital signs and asymmetric breath sounds.

Hemothorax is relatively less common in children than adults. No clear guidelines exist with regard to initial output volume or continuous blood drainage from a closed chest thoracostomy to indicate the need for surgical intervention. A child's hemithorax can contain up to 40% of the effective blood volume, and intrathoracic bleeding can lead to hemorrhagic shock. Hemothorax is associated with morbidity from infection, lung scarring, and chronic atelectasis.[72]

Rib fractures are uncommon in children as a result of the elasticity of the rib cage. When present, however, rib fractures are often associated with severe injuries due to the high force required to cause them, and mortality increases with an increasing number of ribs fractured.[73] In the absence of a witnessed high-energy mechanism, rib fractures, especially posterior, are highly suggestive of inflicted injury in infants. Obtain a chest x-ray to assess for acute or healing rib fractures when abuse is suspected.

Cardiac contusions are uncommon in infants and children but may be seen in sports-related blunt chest trauma in school-age children and teenagers. They can manifest as sudden death, commotio cordis, or arrhythmias with ECG changes and elevation of cardiac enzymes.[74]

ASSESSMENT

Begin the evaluation of the thorax with careful inspection for bruising or laceration. Observe chest rise and fall, noting paradoxical chest movement suggestive of flail chest or pneumothorax. Palpate for bony defects and crepitus associated with subcutaneous emphysema, and auscultate for symmetry of breath sounds.

Plain chest x-ray can identify rib fractures and most pneumothoraces (a small pneumothorax can layer anteriorly in the supine patient and be missed by an anteroposterior view of the chest). Point-of-care US has better specificity and sensitivity to detect small pneumothoraces than x-ray. Pulmonary contusions may not be visible on initial radiographs, and serial imaging may be required to reliably determine the progression of parenchymal lung injuries. Evolving contusions can be exacerbated by overhydration and might not be present until well into the first hours of the hospital course.

Plain radiography is a screening tool for significant injury in children, and CT scan is an adjunct to the clinical evaluation and initial plain radiography.[75,76] Although thoracic CT is more sensitive than chest x-ray at recognizing intrathoracic injuries, CT seldom results in significant changes in patient management and is not routinely indicated for the emergent evaluation of chest trauma.[77,78] CT is indicated in blunt thoracic injury when suspicion of aortic disruption is high and has a sensitivity of 95% to 100% and negative predictive value of 99% to 100% for this aortic injury. Surgical intervention is the standard of care for these patients.[79,80]

Tracheobronchial injuries are difficult to detect with radiography and are best evaluated by bronchoscopy. Consider tracheobronchial disruption in the setting of persistent air leak, pneumothorax, or pneumomediastinum, although presentation can be subtle.[81]

TREATMENT

The management of injuries such as flail chest, pneumothorax, hemothorax, and pulmonary contusions is similar to that in adults (see chapters 261, "Pulmonary Trauma" and 262, "Cardiac Trauma" in the adult section). Emergency thoracotomy is rarely indicated in pediatric patients and has no role in blunt traumatic arrest in children. Thoracotomy should be considered for children with penetrating chest injuries who lose vital signs during transport or in the trauma bay. Overall, emergency thoracotomy yields minimal improvement in patient survival, poses substantial risk of injury to staff, and carries significant financial impact.[82,83]

ABDOMINAL TRAUMA

Abdominal trauma is the third most commonly injured anatomic region in children but the most common site of initially unrecognized fatal injury and the third leading cause of injury-related mortality in the pediatric population of all ages in the United States after head injuries and thoracic trauma.[1,84,85] Blunt abdominal trauma accounts for approximately 10% of all trauma admissions to pediatric hospitals and usually results from motor vehicle collisions, pedestrian injuries, falls, or direct trauma (bicycle handlebar), although blunt abdominal trauma is also common in inflicted injuries (see chapter 148).[86] Penetrating abdominal injuries are less common in children and account for 10% of abdominal injuries, mostly from firearms in adolescents (87% of all pediatric firearm injuries),[2] although children of all ages suffer firearm-related injuries.[87] The abdomen is injured in 25% of children with gunshot wounds, and 14% of these injuries are fatal.[2] Other causes of penetrating injuries in this age group include impalement, animal bites, and stab wounds.

Pediatric anatomy differs from adults and accounts for the different response to abdominal trauma: the abdominal wall and ribs in children are more compliant than in adults, providing less effective protection of intra-abdominal and thoracic structures. The relative size of solid organs is comparatively larger in the child than in the adult, which further increases the potential risk for injury, and a thick capsule limits hemoperitoneum in solid organ injury in children, decreasing the sensitivity of FAST to detect significant injury. The lower intra-abdominal fat content and elastic ligamentous attachments in children (i.e., perinephric fat, sigmoid and ascending colon peritoneal attachments) contribute to increased vulnerability to injury from acceleration-deceleration or abdominal compression. In infants and younger children, the bladder boundaries extend cephalad to just below the umbilicus and the bladder is vulnerable to direct blows to the lower abdomen.

Blunt abdominal trauma can be divided according to the different structures that are involved. Abdominal wall contusions are frequent in children secondary to minor accidents, often sports related. Solid organs are more commonly injured in high-energy mechanisms. The spleen is the most commonly injured solid organ (25% to 39%), followed by the liver (15% to 37%) and kidney (19% to 25%). Hollow viscous injuries involve the jejunum, duodenum, colon, and stomach (15%) in decreasing order of frequency. Pancreas injuries are less commonly seen in pediatric abdominal trauma (7%).[88]

CLINICAL DECISION RULES FOR BLUNT ABDOMINAL TRAUMA

A number of clinical decision rules have been developed to risk stratify children with blunt abdominal trauma. The largest study to date was conducted by the Pediatric Emergency Care Applied Research Network group, in which 20 EDs enrolled 12,044 children with blunt abdominal trauma in a prospective observational study, and an algorithm was used to identify patients at very low risk for intra-abdominal injury requiring intervention (surgery, embolization, transfusion for abdominal bleeding, IV fluid requirement >48 hours). Children are classified as very low risk if they meet the following criteria:

1. No evidence of abdominal wall trauma/seat belt sign or Glasgow coma scale <14 with blunt abdominal trauma
2. No abdominal tenderness on examination
3. No thoracic wall trauma, and no complaints of abdominal pain, decreased bowel sounds, or vomiting

Forty-two percent of the study population met these very low risk criteria, among whom the risk of intra-abdominal injury requiring intervention was 0.1%. The Pediatric Emergency Care Applied Research Network rule has a sensitivity of 97% and negative predictive value of 99.9%.[89]

SPLEEN INJURIES

Splenic injury may present with diffuse abdominal pain or localized tenderness in the left upper quadrant. Pain can be referred to the left shoulder from accumulation of blood in subphrenic spaces. Concomitant injuries include left lower rib fractures and pulmonary contusion. The American Association for the Surgery of Trauma grades splenic injuries from 1 to 5 according to the size of the subcapsular hematoma and degree of parenchymal or vascular involvement on CT.[90]

The management of acute splenic injury in children is often nonoperative and is based on observation with serial abdominal examinations and laboratory values (hemoglobin/hematocrit) or imaging; this conservative approach has led to a decreased incidence of postsplenectomy sepsis syndrome.[91,92] Prognosis is excellent, with full recovery from splenic injury in 90% to 98% of children. Emergent laparotomy is indicated for splenic injury causing hemodynamic instability, massive organ disruption, or continuing transfusion requirements.[93] Surgical options include partial or total splenectomy or splenic autotransplantation (revascularization of splenic tissue in other intra-abdominal locations such as the omental pocket). Children who require splenectomy should receive vaccination against encapsulated bacteria (meningococcal and streptococcal pneumonia) as well as common antibiotic prophylaxis.[112]

HEPATIC INJURY

Blunt hepatic trauma is the most common cause of fatal intra-abdominal injury in children. Localized tenderness to the right upper quadrant and diffuse abdominal tenderness are the most common physical findings. The American Association for the Surgery of Trauma classifies hepatic injuries as grades 1 to 6 according to the size of the subcapsular hematoma and degree of parenchymal and vascular injury.[113] As with splenic injury, conservative management is the rule, dictated by the hemodynamic stability of the patient, and can be achieved in over 90% of traumas.[94] Close monitoring, serial exams, and occasional follow-up imaging are the cornerstones of management. Success rates for nonoperative management are between 85% and 90%.[114]

KIDNEY INJURY

Renal injury is seen with high-energy mechanisms such as motor vehicle and pedestrian collisions, falls, and occasionally sport injuries. Urologic injuries usually accompany other injuries and rarely are the cause of death. The Organ Injury Scaling Committee of the American Association for the Surgery of Trauma grades renal injury from 1 to 5 based on degree of contusion, laceration, subcapsular or retroperitoneal hematomas, and involvement of the vascular hilar structures or collecting system. Contusions and hematomas comprise 60% to 90% of renal injuries, whereas lacerations comprise only 10% of injuries.

Clinical findings include localized flank tenderness, ecchymosis, or a palpable flank mass. **Microscopic hematuria is common after blunt trauma and does not require further investigation as an isolated finding; the pediatric trauma victim with microscopic hematuria can be followed clinically and with serial urinalysis and does not require imaging unless indicated for other injuries.** Although gross hematuria indicates potential serious injury, up to 50% of patients with vascular hilar injuries have no hematuria. Obtain imaging in patients with history of significant force trauma or with gross hematuria. Approximately 95% of renal injuries can be treated conservatively, although surgical or radiologic intervention is indicated for expanding retroperitoneal hematoma, vascular pedicle injury, or urinomas, and total nephrectomy may be required for major renal vascular injury.

PANCREATIC INJURY

Pancreatic injury is uncommon in children and usually due to focal upper abdomen trauma, often from bicycle handlebar injuries. Pancreatic injuries are difficult to diagnose due to their nonspecific and indolent clinical presentation. When present, the combination of epigastric pain, a palpable abdominal mass, and elevated liver and pancreatic enzymes suggests pancreatic pseudocyst, although this classic triad is rarely seen in children. Pancreatic enzymes are neither sensitive nor specific for pancreatic injury in pediatric blunt abdominal trauma: they can be elevated without otherwise demonstrable pancreatic injury, and are normal in up to 30% of patients with complete pancreatic transection.

Most patients with pancreatic injury respond to conservative supportive management. Severe injuries with parenchymal disruption may lead to pancreatitis and pancreatic pseudocyst formation. Treat traumatic pancreatitis conservatively with close monitoring, often initially in an intensive care setting. Pseudocysts often require surgical or percutaneous drainage, although spontaneous resolution occurs in up to one fourth of children specially with cysts <5 cm. Patients with pancreatic duct injury or transaction more often require surgical exploration and repair.[114]

HOLLOW VISCUS INJURY

Intestinal trauma is less common than solid organ injury and is usually associated with motor vehicle versus pedestrian trauma, seat belt injuries, or inflicted injury. Injury can result from a direct blow producing visceral compression or acceleration-deceleration forces at anatomic points of fixation, resulting in visceral and mesenteric tears. Visceral injuries include bowel perforation, bowel wall hematoma, and mesenteric tears. Acute symptoms are nonspecific and sometimes mild, making the diagnosis difficult. Imaging is less reliable than with solid organ injury due the minimal and often nonspecific findings. Persistent or worsening abdominal pain, vomiting (particularly bilious), or the development of peritonitis or fever should alert the clinician to the possibility of hollow viscus injury. Surgical exploration is often required for definitive diagnosis.

Duodenal injuries are often associated with handlebar injuries and classically present in a delayed manner 48 to 72 hours after the injury, as expansion of the hematoma causes partial or complete obstruction. Abdominal pain and bilious vomiting are the most common symptoms.[95]

The **seat belt injury complex** is a pattern of blunt abdominal injury seen in children who are inappropriately restrained with a lap belt positioned over the abdomen instead of the pelvic girdle. Acceleration-deceleration forces crush the bowel between the seat belt and the spine. Classic findings include a "seat belt sign" (abdominal wall contusion in the distribution of the lap belt), with small bowel injury and Chance fractures of the lumbar spine. Seat belt sign may be present in up to 10% of motor vehicle collisions and, when present, confers a risk of intra-abdominal injury around 80%; the presence of a Chance fracture is associated with a 50% incidence of associated intra-abdominal injury.[96-98] Small bowel injuries are difficult to diagnose with CT and require a high index of suspicion and serial physical examination and monitoring of labs (lipase, lactate, complete blood cell count).[99]

PEDIATRIC SPINE AND SPINAL CORD INJURY

PEDIATRIC CERVICAL SPINE TRAUMA

Any pediatric patient involved in significant trauma has the potential for a cervical spine injury; therefore, immobilize the patient until injury is ruled out either clinically or radiologically to avoid significant morbidity and mortality.[100] Guidelines for immobilization and imaging as well as specific injuries are discussed in chapter 139, "Cervical Spine Injury in Infants and Children."

PEDIATRIC THORACIC AND LUMBAR SPINE TRAUMA

Children account for only 2% to 5% of all spine injuries, and only 5% of pediatric fractures occur in the spine.[101] Twenty to 60% of pediatric spine fractures occur in the thoracic or lumbar spine, with older children experiencing more lumbar fractures and younger children more prone to cervical and thoracic fractures.[102] There is a bimodal age distribution in pediatric spine injuries, with one peak in children <5 and another in children >10 years of age. Falls and motor vehicle accidents account for the first peak; motor vehicle accidents account for the majority of spine injuries in older children; and sports-related mechanisms account for the majority of injuries in adolescents.[102]

The pediatric spine differs from that of adults in that children have greater ligamentous elasticity and flexibility, more horizontal facets, and relatively weak musculature, particularly before the age of 8, with a transition toward adult anatomy and physiology after this age. Distraction forces can result in Salter-type fractures of the thoracolumbar spine in children, and anatomic differences make multilevel injuries more common in children than adults in the setting of compression forces.[101]

Evaluate the pediatric spine during the secondary survey with careful palpation of the entire spine and paraspinous region for tenderness, step-offs, crepitus, bruising, or open injuries. Physical examination is 87% sensitive and 75% specific for thoracolumbar injuries.[101] In one prospective study, the sensation of "breath arrest" (a feeling of breathlessness in the few seconds immediately following the injury) had a sensitivity of 87%, specificity of 67%, positive predictive value of 69%, and negative predictive value of 86% for predicting thoracolumbar spine fractures.[103]

Obtain anteroposterior and lateral x-rays of the entire spine in all children with symptoms or signs of spinal injury during physical exam, because up to one third of children with spine injury have multilevel imaging. CT scan, although commonly used in adults, exposes children to significant ionizing radiation and should be limited to those with neurologic deficits or significant concern for intra-abdominal or intrathoracic injuries requiring cross-sectional imaging for other reasons. Stable children with thoracolumbar spine injury associated with neurologic deficits should be imaged with MRI.

Thoracolumbar injuries can be classified using the Thoracolumbar Injury Classification and Severity Score System, which appears to be valid in children as well as adults.[102] This scoring system, based on morphology (compression, burst, rotation/translation, or distraction), integrity of posterior ligaments (intact, suspected disruption, confirmed disruption), and neurologic status (intact, nerve root deficits, cord and conus medullaris, and cauda equina function), helps to guide surgical versus nonsurgical management. Generally speaking, most stable fractures are treated conservatively with the use of braces such as the thoracolumbosacral orthosis.

Compression fractures are the most common fracture in the thoracolumbar spine and are usually stable and managed with bracing. Fractures of the spinous or transverse processes are often associated with blunt trauma and carry low risk for associated visceral injury; most of these fractures are managed with analgesics and rest, often without immobilization. The flexion-distraction injury known as the Chance fracture (see Table 258-1) deserves special consideration. This injury typically results from inappropriate restraint of children with a lap belt and is a high-energy flexion injury; this fracture is associated with intra-abdominal injury in up to 40% of children and should prompt a thorough search for such injuries.

PEDIATRIC SPINAL CORD INJURY AND SPINAL CORD INJURY WITHOUT RADIOGRAPHIC ABNORMALITY

Pediatric spinal cord injury is uncommon, occurring in 1.99 of 100,000 children. Children <15 years old account for only 10% of spinal cord injuries, which are often related to motor vehicle accidents and involve the cervical spine in 60% to 80% of identified injuries in this age group.[104] Adolescent spine injuries are more often caused by sports-related mechanisms. The mortality rate for children <5 years of age is 18.5%, and most deaths were associated with injuries to the upper cervical spine.[105]

Overall, neurologic recovery is better among children than adults with traumatic spinal cord injury, with incomplete injuries associated with better outcomes. A unique pediatric feature of spinal cord injury is **spinal cord injury without radiographic abnormality**, which is reported to occur in 4.5% to 35% of children with spinal cord injury and 0.2% of all pediatric traumas.[105] Scoliosis can be a sequel to spinal cord injury, particularly among younger children.[105] Spinal injuries are often associated with other injuries, with rates ranging from 42% to 65% and most commonly involving thoracic structures (pulmonary contusion, pneumothorax, rib fractures) or other contiguous or noncontiguous fractures of the appendicular skeleton or spine.[106]

The clinical evaluation and presentation of spinal cord injury and syndromes as well as the principles of physical examination and stabilization are similar to that of adults (see chapter 258, "Spine Trauma"). As with adults, hypotension with relative bradycardia and flaccid paralysis suggests spinal shock that may require administration of vasopressors, because aggressive fluid administration may worsen spinal cord edema. **Corticosteroids are not recommended to treat acute spinal cord injury in children. Steroids increase the risk of infection and do not result in significant neurologic improvements in children.**[107]

REFERENCES

The complete reference list is available online at www.TintinalliEM.com.

CHAPTER 111

Intubation and Ventilation in Infants and Children

Robert J. Vissers
Nathan W. Mick

INTRODUCTION

There are significant physiologic, anatomic, and equipment differences between children and adults that must be considered when planning the approach to the emergent pediatric airway. The presentation of a critically ill child requiring intubation is relatively uncommon compared to adults.[1-3] This chapter presents the physiologic and anatomic characteristics of the pediatric airway, strategies for effective airway management, and organization methods for equipment to minimize errors in equipment sizing and medication dose calculation.[4]

PHYSIOLOGIC CHARACTERISTICS

Due to a higher metabolic rate, oxygen consumption is increased in children, especially in infants. Infants and children have an increased relative cardiac output and minute ventilation to match the increased metabolic demand. However, children are vulnerable to rapid desaturation when oxygenation or ventilation is reduced. Children have relatively small-volume lungs with small functional residual capacities. This translates into a reduced oxygen reservoir, which decreases the effectiveness of preoxygenation and makes optimal preoxygenation more difficult. Therefore, be prepared to support oxygenation with bag-mask ventilation, often before an intubation attempt, while awaiting the onset of induction and paralysis. Attempts at intubation may need to stop once oxygen saturation drops below 90% to allow for bag-mask ventilation before the next attempt. Below an oxygen saturation of 90%, desaturation is particularly rapid.[5] The vast majority of children are easily bag ventilated when the proper technique is used, even when partial obstruction is present. **The key is anticipation and early use of good bag-mask ventilation.**

Children can develop gastric distention from air swallowing during distress as well as insufflation during bag-mask ventilation. Gastric distention can further compromise functional residual capacity, tidal volume, and ventilation. Early placement of an orogastric or nasogastric tube may remedy this. Gastric tubes have also been recommended to minimize the risk of reflux from an incompetent gastroesophageal junction, but the incidence of aspiration in children appears to be quite low, even in emergent intubation.

Children have a proportionally larger extracellular fluid compartment than adults. This results in a quicker onset and shorter duration of action of drugs and may require higher doses per kilogram for many of the drugs used to facilitate rapid-sequence intubation.

ANATOMIC CHARACTERISTICS

There are a number of anatomic characteristics of children that must be appreciated to optimize the success of endotracheal intubation (**Table 111-1**). Most of the unique anatomic characteristics are present

TABLE 111-1 Anatomic Considerations in the Pediatric Airway

Pediatric Anatomy	Potential Implications	Airway Maneuvers
Large head and occiput	May push head forward, occluding airway	Shoulder roll should be used to align airway axes
Large tongue	May occlude upper airway in obtunded or paralyzed patient	Jaw thrust, oral or nasopharyngeal airway, Miller (straight) laryngoscope blade
Superior larynx and anterior cords	May make visualization of cords difficult	Shoulder roll may be required to align airway axes, straight laryngoscope blade to lift epiglottis
Cricoid narrowing	Subglottic space is narrowest portion of the pediatric airway, prone to inflammation and upper airway obstruction	Monitor cuff insufflation pressures in small children
Large adenoids and tonsils	May cause upper airway obstruction; may bleed with nasal intubation	Avoid blind nasal intubation in young children
Small cricoid cartilage	Makes open cricothyrotomy technically difficult	Needle cricothyrotomy preferred in young children
Large stomach, low gastroesophageal sphincter tone, relatively small lungs	Insufflation of stomach with bag-valve mask ventilation or swallowed air can compromise respiratory status; children are prone to vomiting	Consider early placement of orogastric or nasogastric tube to deflate stomach when using positive-pressure ventilation or in the obtunded patient

in the first few years of life. From 2 to 8 years of age, there is a transition to a smaller but similarly proportioned anatomy compared to adults. Most children do not have the many acquired anatomic challenges present in older adults, and the differences in children are predictable. With good technique and anticipation of these differences, the majority of pediatric airways are successfully managed.

Alignment of the oral, pharyngeal, and tracheal axes, to allow visualization of the glottis, is affected by several features most pronounced in the infant: (1) a relatively large head and occiput, (2) a disproportionately large tongue and small mandible, and (3) a larynx that is more superior and anterior than in adults. **This acute angle can be overcome by extending the neck (unless cervical injury is suspected) and, in some cases, placing a small roll under the shoulders (Figure 111-1).**

The use of a straight laryngoscope blade is helpful in the presence of a large tongue and redundant soft tissues. The infant glottic opening, epiglottis, and aryepiglottic folds are more prominent, soft, and mobile than in an adult or older child. This redundant tissue can obscure the view and make it hard to identify the trachea. Under tension from a laryngoscope blade, the esophageal inlet can appear similar to the cords, because it can form a triangle and the edges appear white when stretched.

The narrow trachea, combined with the redundant, mobile periglottic tissues, predisposes the young child to airway obstruction.[6] **The narrowest point of the child's trachea is at the cricoid ring**, which is also the site of mucosal swelling associated with croup. Airway resistance increases disproportionately with any reduction in diameter and dramatically increases when airflow becomes turbulent rather than laminar. A 25% reduction in diameter from swelling (e.g., 4 mm to 3 mm) reduces the cross-sectional area by 50% and increases resistance by 200%. The swollen, mobile tissues create a dynamic obstruction, and, in the agitated, crying, young child with subsequent turbulent airflow, the work of breathing can increase 32-fold.[7] This can lead to complete obstruction and respiratory arrest. **This principle underscores the need to keep children with partial airway obstructions as calm as possible in a quiet, comforting environment.** Because the obstruction is dynamic, children with airway edema usually respond well to positive-pressure bag-mask ventilation. Also, croup—by far the most common infectious cause of pediatric upper airway obstruction—causes inflammation below the glottic opening, and laryngoscopy usually provides normal visualization of the cords.

Some procedures are not indicated in children because of anatomic differences. **Blind nasotracheal intubation is relatively contraindicated in children <10 years old**, because the prominent adenoidal and tonsillar lymphoid tissue is likely to bleed and the acute airway angles described earlier make success less likely. Also, **surgical cricothyrotomy is contraindicated in children <10 years old because the cricothyroid membrane is too small. Therefore, in children <10 years of age, needle cricothyrotomy is the subglottic, invasive airway of choice.**[8]

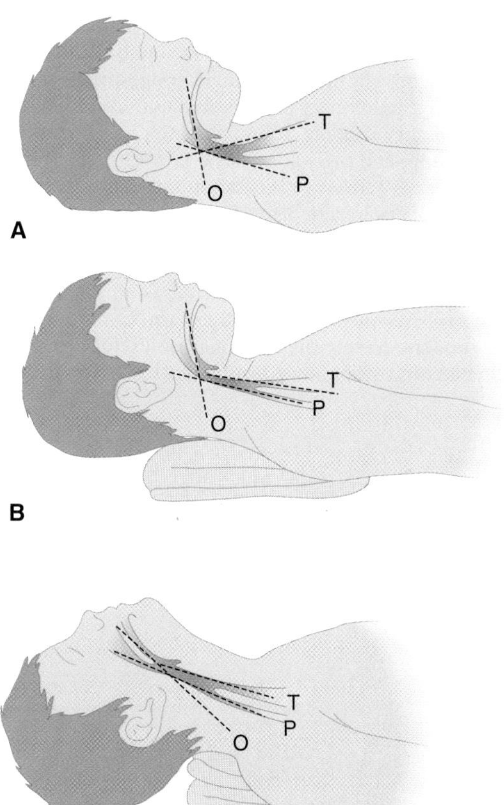

FIGURE 111-1. Alignment of axes. **A.** Large occiput and anterior airway make alignment of airway axes difficult. **B.** Shoulder roll aligns tracheal and pharyngeal axes, but (**C**) neck extension may be needed to align all three airway axes. O = oral; P = pharyngeal; T = tracheal.

EQUIPMENT

The principal challenge with children is selecting the appropriate-size equipment. Although there are formulas that can assist in the estimation of equipment sizing, all EDs should have pediatric airway equipment stocked and organized by age or size and easily accessible. Equipment restocking must also be reliable, so that all sizes are immediately available when needed. The Broselow® tape represents a system that uses length-based estimates of equipment and medications, organized by color.[7] Airway carts can be similarly color-coded. Regardless of the system used, the goal is to eliminate reliance on memory to determine the best equipment size and medication dose.

ENDOTRACHEAL TUBES

Endotracheal tube size can be estimated by using the Broselow® length-based system noted earlier. The following formulas can also reasonably estimate the size, as measured by internal diameter in children >1 year of age:

$$(\text{age} + 4) \div 4 \text{ for uncuffed tubes}$$

$$(\text{age} + 4) \div 3.5 \text{ for cuffed tubes}$$

Endotracheal tubes with <5.5-mm internal diameter are traditionally recommended to be uncuffed. This is because the cricoid ring represents the narrowest point of a pediatric airway and serves as a physiologic cuff. More recent data suggest that the use of cuffed tubes in younger children is safe; however, cuff inflation pressures must be closely monitored (**Tables 111-2** and **111-3**). Cuffed tubes may be beneficial in cases where high airway pressures or changing compliance are anticipated (e.g., asthma, pneumonia, acute respiratory distress syndrome).

TABLE 111-2 Age-Based Airway Equipment Size

Age	Internal Diameter (mm)	Blade Size
Premature	2.5 Uncuffed*	0 Straight
Newborn	3.0 Uncuffed*	1.0 Straight
1–6 mo	3.5 Uncuffed*	1.0–1.5 Straight
6–12 mo	4.0 Uncuffed*	1.5 Straight
1–2 y	4.5 Uncuffed*	1.5 Straight
3–4 y	5.0 Uncuffed*	1.5–2.0 Straight or curved
5–6 y	5.5 Uncuffed*	2.0 Straight or curved
7–8 y	6.0 Cuffed	2.0 Straight or curved
9–10 y	6.5 Cuffed	2.0 Straight or curved
≥11 y	7.0 Cuffed	3.0 Straight or curved

*Cuffed tubes also acceptable as long as cuff pressures can be monitored.

TABLE 111-3 Length-Based Equipment Chart (length)*

Item	54–70 cm	70–85 cm	85–95 cm	95–107 cm	107–124 cm	124–138 cm	138–155 cm
Endotracheal tube size (mm)	3.5	4.0	4.5	5.0	5.5	6.0	6.5
Lip–tip length (mm)	10.5	12.0	13.5	15.0	16.5	18.0	19.5
Laryngoscope	1 Straight	1 Straight	2 Straight	2 Straight or curved	2 Straight or curved	2–3 Straight or curved	3 Straight or curved
Suction catheter	8F	8F–10F	10F	10F	10F	10F	12F
Stylet	6F	6F	6F	6F	14F	14F	14F
Oral airway	Infant/small child	Small child	Child	Child	Child/small adult	Child/adult	Medium adult
Bag-valve mask	Infant	Child	Child	Child	Child	Child/adult	Adult
Oxygen mask	Newborn	Pediatric	Pediatric	Pediatric	Pediatric	Adult	Adult
Vascular access (gauge)							
Catheter	22–24	20–22	18–22	18–22	18–20	18–20	16–20
Butterfly	23–25	23–25	21–23	21–23	21–23	21–22	18–21
Nasogastric tube	5F–8F	8F–10F	10F	10F–12F	12F–14F	14F–18F	18F
Urinary catheter	5F–8F	8F–10F	10F	10F–12F	10F–12F	12F	12F
Chest tube	10F–12F	16F–20F	20F–24F	20F–24F	24F–32F	28F–32F	32F–40F
Blood pressure cuff	Newborn/infant	Infant/child	Child	Child	Child	Child/adult	Adult

*Directions for use: (1) measure patient length with centimeter tape; (2) using measured length in centimeters, access appropriate equipment column.

LARYNGOSCOPE BLADES

Straight laryngoscope blades (Miller) are preferred to curved blades in young children because the large epiglottis can be lifted directly and the large tongue is more easily displaced to provide direct visualization. A blade that is too small or short is potentially more difficult to use than one that is too large, because a short blade may not reach the supraglottic area. To determine proper blade length, place the blade handle joint at the child's upper incisors and the tip at the angle of the mandible. The length of the blade from its tip to the handle joint should be within 1 cm proximal or distal of the angle of the mandible.[9] The #0 straight (Miller) blade or #1 curved (MacIntosh) blades are only used for the small or premature newborn (**Figure 111-2**).

AIRWAY ADJUNCTS

Oversized masks do not allow a proper seal. Proper mask size is shown in **Figure 111-3**. Correct sizing is also needed for stylets, bag-mask ventilators, oxygen masks, and suction. Undersized bag-mask ventilators (250 mL) do not provide adequate tidal volume for most children.

The selection of alternative airway techniques or rescue devices for children is limited. However, most children can be bag-mask ventilated should laryngoscopy fail. Intubating stylets, or bougies, are available in pediatric sizes small enough to accept a 3.0-mm internal diameter endotracheal tube. **The Combitube is not recommended for patients <48 inches tall.**

As noted in the earlier section "Anatomic Characteristics," emergency subglottic, surgical airways in children <10 years of age are restricted to needle cricothyrotomy. The indications for these alternative airway options are discussed in more detail below.

APPROACH TO AIRWAY MANAGEMENT IN NEONATES, INFANTS, AND CHILDREN

NONINVASIVE VENTILATION

Noninvasive ventilation has been used in adult patients as a technique for respiratory support in order to stave off intubation. Its application has been most rigorously studied in adult congestive heart failure and chronic obstructive pulmonary disease. Studies in children have focused mostly on respiratory support in bronchiolitis. Nasal continuous positive airway pressure and high-flow (i.e., 6 L/min) nasal cannula, where humidified oxygen is delivered via nasal cannula, have been evaluated in the literature as means to support respiratory effort in infants and children with bronchiolitis.[10-13] Use of this technique has been shown to improve ventilation and, in some children, obviate the need for subsequent intubation and should be considered as an adjunct in cases of moderate to severe bronchiolitis. Another form of noninvasive ventilation, bilevel positive airway pressure, may be useful in chronic conditions associated with respiratory insufficiency such as neuromuscular

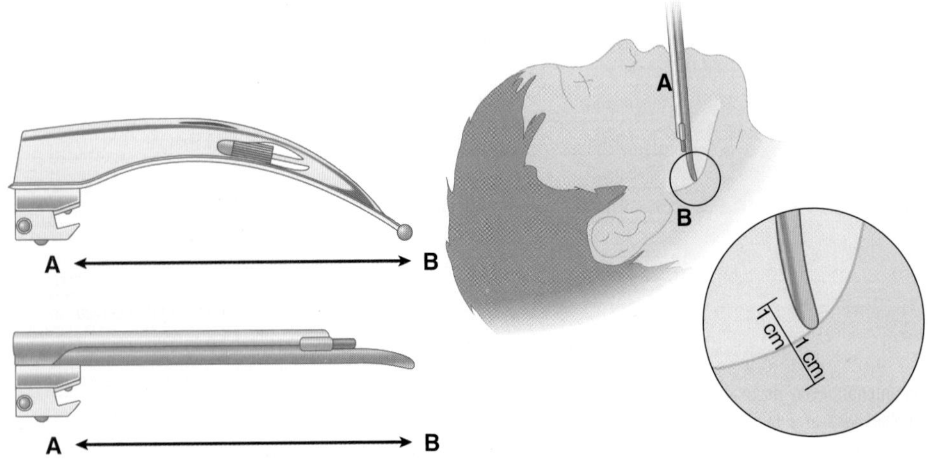

FIGURE 111-2. Measurement of proper laryngoscope length for curved and straight blades. [Instruments on left: Reproduced with permission from Mellick LB, Edholm T, Corbett SW: Pediatric laryngoscope blade size selection using facial landmarks. *Pediatr Emerg Care* Apr;22(4):226-229, 2006. Copyright Wolters Kluwer Health.]

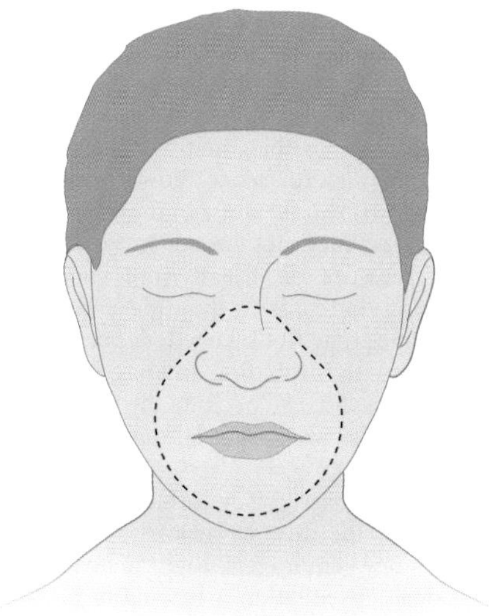

FIGURE 111-3. Proper facemask size.

disorders or syndromes associated with anatomic upper airway obstruction (e.g., craniofacial syndromes, Down's syndrome with macroglossia), as well as acute conditions including asthma.[14,15]

PREPARATION FOR INTUBATION

Begin preparation for endotracheal intubation when noninvasive means of ventilatory support and oxygenation are insufficient. Initiate preoxygenation, even if oxygen saturation is 100%. Maximize preoxygenation through elevation of the head of the bed when possible and high-flow oxygen through a non-rebreathing mask. Prepare appropriately sized equipment before initiating rapid-sequence intubation. Prepare different sized blades and at least one size smaller endotracheal tube. Make sure that oral and endotracheal suction catheters are functioning and of proper size. Assess airway difficulty (see later section "The Difficult Pediatric Airway") and have rescue devices at hand. In some situations, such as partial airway obstruction, the best strategy may include anesthesia or otolaryngology consultation and consideration of intubation in the operating room. Even if the plan is to defer final management to another setting or a consultant, have equipment at the bedside in case of clinical deterioration requiring immediate action. Specialty equipment, such as a pediatric Magill forceps for foreign body obstruction, should also be at the bedside.

Ensure reliable IV access. In cases of urgency and no IV access, an IO line may be needed. Finally, a fluid bolus (20 mL/kg normal saline) is often beneficial before initiation of rapid-sequence intubation. Many children require intubation for respiratory failure, which is often associated with dehydration from reduced oral intake and increased insensible losses. In addition, **positive pressure resulting from ventilation after intubation may decrease preload, making preintubation fluid resuscitation important**.

BAG-MASK VENTILATION

Bag-mask ventilation is frequently required in children, and good technique is important. Rapid oxygen desaturation in children requires bag-mask ventilation before any laryngoscopic attempt, and bag-mask ventilation is the principal rescue technique in children when intubation attempts fail. Correctly sized bags and masks are essential to good ventilation, regardless of the provider's skill.

A common error in pediatric bag-mask ventilation is the tendency to bag too rapidly, rather than match the rate and volume appropriate for the child's age. On occasion, the rate or volume will need to be adjusted for the disease state. For example, lower volumes and longer expiratory times are often needed in asthma, but one must first understand the normal ventilatory parameters before adjustments can be made (**Table 111-4**).

TABLE 111-4 Initial Ventilation Parameters in Children

Patient weight (kg)	3–9	10–18	19–36
Patient length (cm)	46–75	76–109	110–146
Tidal volume (mL/kg)	8–10	8–10	8–10
Rate (breaths/min)	20–25	15–25	12–20

Another common error is pressing the mask into the face in an attempt to achieve a good seal, which causes flexion of the neck and subsequent airway obstruction.

Because of the relatively large occiput, elevation of the head is usually not required, and in infants, a supine position may cause flexion of the neck, occasionally requiring a roll under the shoulders to prevent flexion. Optimal alignment of the oral, pharyngeal, and tracheal axes (Figure 111-1) can then be achieved with extension at the atlanto-occipital junction, known as the *sniffing position*. In a well-positioned airway, a horizontal line extending from the external auditory canal will lie just anterior to the shoulder.

A mask seal can be obtained using a one-handed "C-grip" or "E-C clamp" technique in smaller children, with the thumb and index finger positioned on the mask and the remaining fingers pulling the mandible up into the mask, while maintaining extension at the atlanto-occipital junction (**Figure 111-4A**). In larger children, a two-handed technique can be used (**Figure 111-4B**). With either technique, it is important

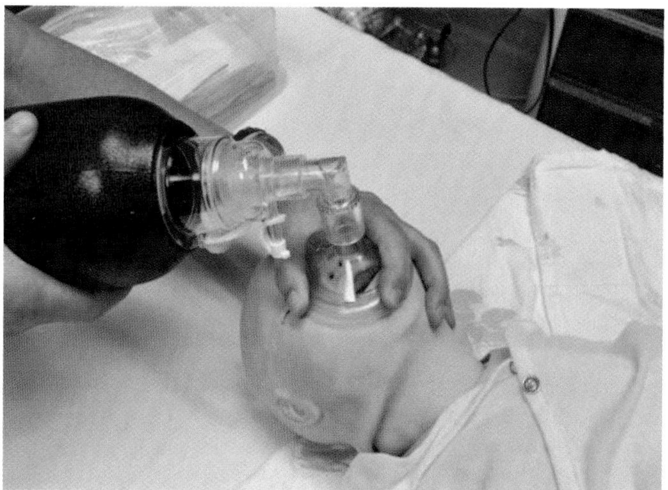

A

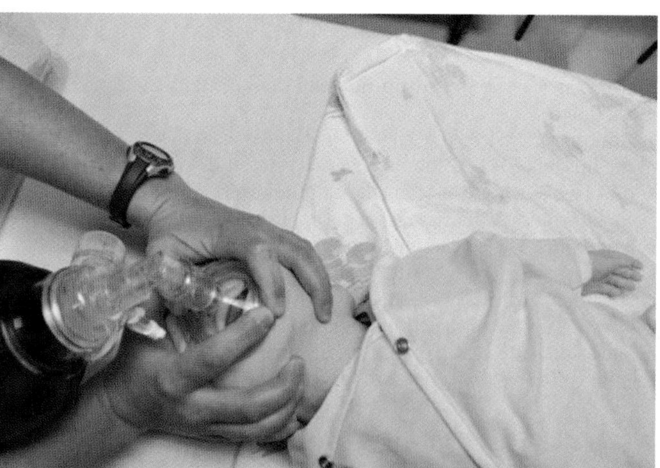

B

FIGURE 111-4. Bag-mask ventilation using (**A**) the "C-grip" or "E-C clamp" technique for small children, pulling the face into the mask, and (**B**) the two-person, two-handed technique.

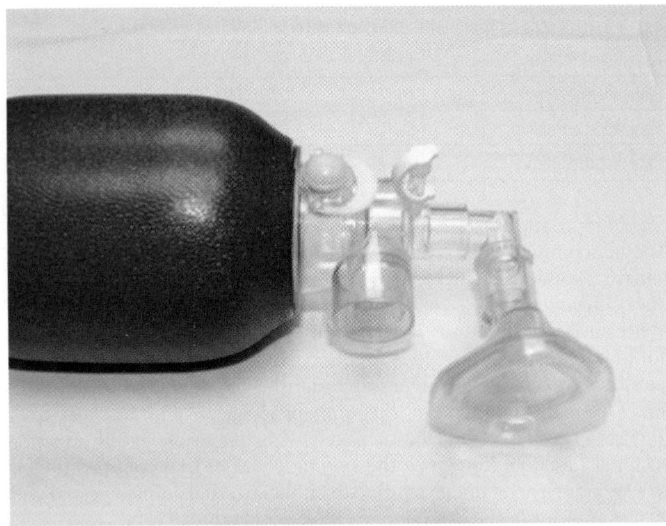

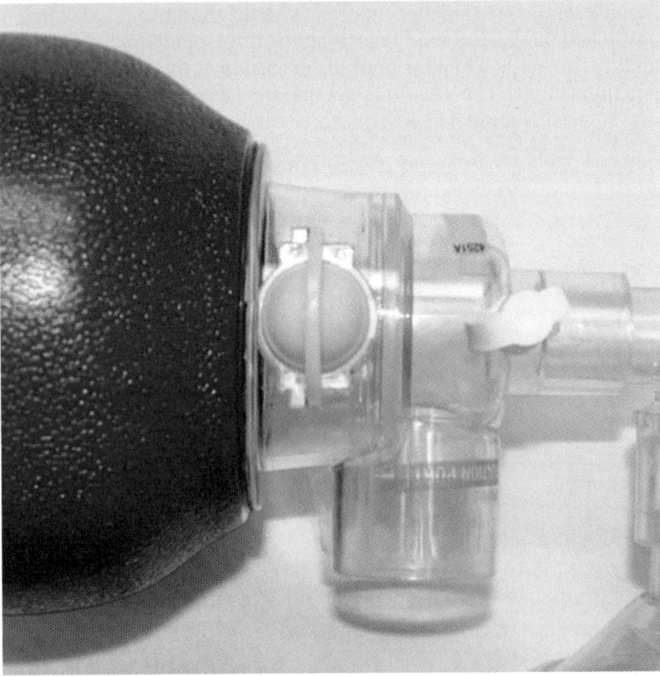

FIGURE 111-5. The pop-off valve on a pediatric bag-valve mask, designed to prevent barotraumas, may need to be occluded when higher pressures are required, such as in patients with asthma.

that the airway be pulled up into the mask, rather than pushing the mask down.

Appropriately sized oral airways (measured from the mandibular angle to the lip; Table 111-3) should always be placed in the unconscious child and can assist with displacement of the relatively large pediatric tongue.

Finally, most pediatric bags incorporate a pop-off, or pressure-relief, valve (**Figure 111-5**). Designed to avoid barotrauma, the valve will open at a preset peak pressure (usually 35 to 40 cm H_2O of pressure). However, in some diseases associated with high airway pressures, such as asthma or airway obstruction, higher peak pressures may be needed to achieve adequate ventilation. In these circumstances, disable or occlude the pop-off valve manually.

LARYNGOSCOPY AND TRACHEAL INTUBATION

The technique for laryngoscopy is similar between children and adults and is described in detail in chapter 29 "Intubation and Mechanical Ventilation." Proper positioning is critical, and optimal alignment of the airway axes for laryngoscopy is the same as described in the previous section for bag-mask ventilation (Figure 111-1). If using a straight blade, the large epiglottis overlies the vocal cords. Pick up the epiglottis with the straight blade to see the cords below. In younger children, there is a tendency to place the blade too deeply, into the esophagus. If identification of structures is impossible, the tip of the blade is usually in the upper esophagus, or retroglottic space. Slowly withdraw the blade, and the cords or the epiglottis should come into view.

Visualization may or may not be enhanced by use of *b*ackward-*u*pward-*r*ightward *p*ressure on the thyroid cartilage (the "**BURP**" **maneuver**), displacing the cords to the right and posterior into better view.[16] **Cricoid pressure may not be needed, because it has been associated with difficulty with intubation and bag-mask ventilation,**[17] **and in children, cricoid pressure can occlude the pliable trachea.** If cricoid pressure is applied, release pressure if laryngoscopy and intubation are difficult.

There is a tendency to insert the endotracheal tube too far in the very young child, in whom the distance from laryngeal cords to tracheal carina may just be a few centimeters. Right mainstem intubation is not always appreciated on auscultation, particularly in the infant, because breath sounds may be transmitted throughout the chest. Therefore, predetermine endotracheal tube depth and adhere to that depth during intubation. Depth can be estimated using the formula below:

$$\text{Tube internal diameter} \times 3 = \text{tube depth at lips}$$

For example, a 4.0-mm internal diameter tube should be 12 cm at the lips. Length-based systems can also be used (Table 111-3).

RAPID-SEQUENCE INTUBATION

Rapid-sequence intubation remains the preferred method of intubation in children and is associated with the highest success and lowest complication rates, compared to other methods.[18] Specific induction and paralytic agents for children are presented in **Table 111-5**. The indications and

TABLE 111-5 Common Rapid-Sequence Intubation Medications in Children*

Medication	Dose†	Comments
Induction agents		
Etomidate	0.3 milligram/kg	Preserves hemodynamic stability; may suppress adrenal axis even in a single dose; short acting, requires anxiolysis or analgesia after intubation
Ketamine	1–2 milligrams/kg	Bronchodilator, preserves respiratory drive, cardiovascular stimulant; drug of choice for intubation for asthma and sepsis
Propofol	1–2 milligrams/kg	Rapid push, higher dose in infants, may cause hypotension; short acting, requires ongoing anxiolysis or analgesia after intubation
Paralytics		
Rocuronium	1 milligram/kg	Nondepolarizing agent; longer duration than succinylcholine
Succinylcholine	<10 kg: 1.5–2.0 milligrams/kg >10 kg: 1.0–1.5 milligrams/kg	Shorter duration than rocuronium; better intubating conditions at 60 s; may cause bradycardia in children and hyperkalemic cardiac arrest in children with undiagnosed neuromuscular disease
Sedatives		
Midazolam	0.1 milligram/kg	Short-acting sedative
Lorazepam	0.1 milligram/kg	Longer-acting sedative
Analgesics		
Fentanyl	1–2 micrograms/kg	Short-acting analgesic; preserves hemodynamic stability
Morphine	0.1–0.2 milligram/kg	Longer-acting analgesic; may cause histamine release

*Premedication is no longer routinely recommended in children due to a lack of supporting evidence.

†Rapid-sequence intubation medications can be given IO when IV access cannot be obtained.

TABLE 111-6 Complications and Contraindications of Succinylcholine

Hyperkalemia
Burns >5 d old
Denervation injury >5 d old
Significant crush injuries >5 d old
Severe infection >5 d old
Neuromuscular diseases, myopathies
Preexisting hyperkalemia
Masseter spasm
Increased intragastric, intraocular, and possibly intracranial pressure
Malignant hyperthermia
Bradycardia
Prolonged apnea with pseudocholinesterase deficiency
Fasciculations

contraindications are the same as for adults. A detailed review of the pharmacology of rapid-sequence intubation is beyond the scope of this chapter.

Succinylcholine or rocuronium are both commonly used neuromuscular blocking agents for paralysis during pediatric rapid-sequence intubation.[19,20] There are no comparative studies in children demonstrating benefit of one agent over another. Succinylcholine may have a more rapid onset, has a shorter duration of action (8 minutes for succinylcholine vs 45 minutes for rocuronium), and is associated with better glottic visualization at 1 minute in adult comparative studies.[21] Succinylcholine can cause fatal hyperkalemia in a number of conditions (**Table 111-6**), usually apparent on patient presentation (see Table 29-4); however, its specific association with cardiac arrest in children with undiagnosed neuromuscular disease has caused some practitioners to prefer the use of rocuronium in children.[19] Many clinicians prefer succinylcholine in the absence of contraindications due to their familiarity with the agent.

In children, there is an absence of literature to support the use of pretreatment agents in rapid-sequence intubation. The administration of weight-based medications, particularly in critically ill pediatric patients, can create delays and the potential for drug error. The rationale for the administration of pretreatment agents is to attenuate the pathophysiologic responses to laryngoscopy and intubation that may be harmful in certain clinical circumstances. The reflex sympathetic response can cause hypertension and tachycardia. Laryngeal stimulation also can have respiratory effects, including laryngospasm, cough, and bronchospasm. In children, the vagal response predominates and can result in significant bradycardia, even in the absence of succinylcholine.

Lidocaine may be considered in children with possible elevation of intracranial pressure; however, most data on its use are extrapolated from the adult experience.[19] There is no evidence that lidocaine improves outcomes in children with reactive airways undergoing intubation. **A pretreatment dose of a nondepolarizing neuromuscular blocking agent is no longer recommended as a pretreatment agent in rapid-sequence intubation.**

The routine use of atropine in children to prevent reflex bradycardia from airway manipulation and succinylcholine is not necessary.[22] Pretreatment with atropine does not consistently prevent bradycardia in children. **Give atropine if symptomatic bradycardia occurs.**

POSTINTUBATION MANAGEMENT

Immediately after intubation, confirm endotracheal tube placement using a capnograph or a colorimetric end-tidal carbon dioxide detector.[23] A small-sized colorimetric end-tidal carbon dioxide detector should be used for children weighing <15 kg. For larger children, weighing >15 kg, use the adult-sized carbon dioxide detector, because there can be a resistance to flow when using the smaller device with larger tidal volumes (**Figure 111-6**). Continuous waveform capnography is now considered standard of care for postintubation monitoring.

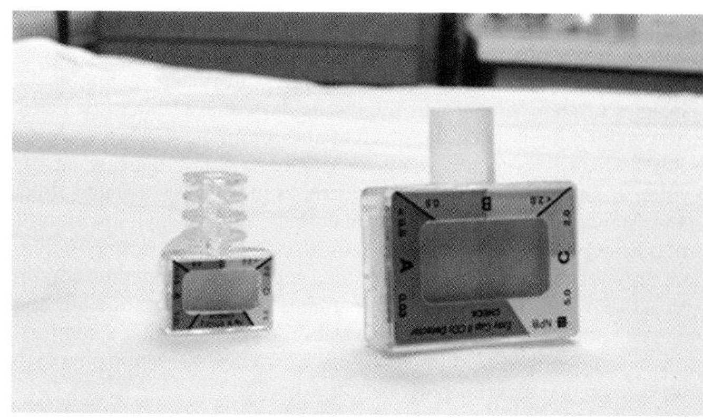

FIGURE 111-6. Examples of a pediatric colorimetric end-tidal carbon dioxide detector for children <15 kg and a standard one for larger children.

Visualization of the tube through the cords or fogging of the tube is not adequate confirmation of tube placement in the trachea. Likewise, equal breath sounds do not preclude right mainstem bronchus intubation, and a chest x-ray should be obtained shortly after intubation to confirm appropriate depth.

Carefully secure the tube at the mouth, using either tape adhered to the maxilla with skin adhesive or available commercial devices.[24] Because of the short distance between the glottic opening and the end of the endotracheal tube, infants are prone to displacement of the tube into the oral pharynx with head extension and into the right mainstem bronchus with head flexion. **Immobilize the head and neck in a neutral position in intubated young children.**

Most children will be placed on a volume-limited ventilator. However, in children <10 kg, try to use pressure-limited ventilator settings. **Initial rates of 20 to 25 breaths/min, with peak inspiratory pressures between 15 and 20 cm H_2O, will usually give a tidal volume of 8 to 12 mL/kg.**[25] An initial inspiration-to-expiration ratio of 1:2 is suggested but may need to be adjusted, particularly in the presence of reactive airways, which will require a longer expiratory phase. A small amount of positive end-expiratory pressure (3 to 5 cm H_2O) can also be added. In volume-limited ventilation, base initial respiratory rates on age, with starting volumes of 6 to 10 mL/kg. Regardless of the initial settings, frequent reevaluation, monitoring, and the use of arterial blood gases should guide ongoing ventilation parameters.

Provide adequate sedation and analgesia before the effects of induction and paralysis agents wear off. This is particularly important when rocuronium or other longer-acting muscle relaxants are used, because their duration is often much longer than most induction agents used in rapid-sequence intubation.

THE DIFFICULT PEDIATRIC AIRWAY

IDENTIFICATION

A difficult airway as defined by the American Society of Anesthesiologists is difficulty with bag-mask ventilation, difficulty with tracheal intubation, or both.[26,27] **Other characteristics of the difficult airway include (1) more than two attempts at intubation with the same laryngoscopic blade, (2) need for a change in blade or use of intubation stylet, and (3) need for an alternative intubation technique or rescue.** The incidence of difficult pediatric airways in the emergency setting is not known, although the child who cannot be intubated and cannot be ventilated appears to be less common than the adult.[18]

Three questions will help guide management decisions:

1. Will I be able to bag-mask ventilate to maintain oxygenation?
2. Are laryngoscopy and intubation likely to be successful?
3. What rescue device, if needed, is most appropriate for this patient?

Difficult pediatric airways fall into three categories: acute upper airway infections, such as croup and retropharyngeal abscesses; acute airway obstructions, such as foreign bodies, trauma, or burns; and congenital anatomic airway abnormalities.[7] An approach to each potential difficulty is beyond the scope of this chapter. However, an understanding of the principles of management and the rescue devices available in pediatric airway management will usually lead to an appropriate strategy.

Small changes in airway diameter can significantly increase airway resistance, and when airflow is turbulent, as in a crying, agitated child, the resistance to flow increases exponentially. This is why most significant *partial* pediatric airway obstructions, potentially requiring intubation, are best managed in the controlled setting of the operating room with assistance from appropriate consultants, such as anesthesiology and otolaryngology. Until that time, maintain the child in a quiet, comforting environment, with minimal stimulation. The emergency physician must remain prepared for potential deterioration.

UPPER AIRWAY INFECTION

See chapter 123, "Stridor and Drooling in Children in Infants and Children" for a detailed discussion of infectious causes of upper airway obstruction in children. Acute upper airway infections, such as croup, are usually gradual in onset and may respond to medical intervention. Supraglottic infections, such as epiglottitis or pharyngeal abscesses, may make laryngoscopic visualization difficult, and rescue devices (see later section "Supraglottic Devices"), such as a laryngeal mask airway, should be readily available. If respiratory failure should occur before intervention, bag-mask ventilation is usually successful because positive-pressure stents open the mobile soft tissues.

FOREIGN BODY OBSTRUCTION

Patients with partial obstruction from a foreign body are another category in which expectant management is advised until care is transferred to a consultant skilled in fiberoptic or endoscopic removal. Should complete obstruction occur before intervention, perform the Heimlich maneuver for children >1 year of age (see chapter 109, "Resuscitation of Children"). For infants, perform five back blows followed by five chest thrusts and repeat these maneuvers and intersperse them with attempts at ventilation if the child remains conscious. If the child becomes unconscious, perform direct laryngoscopy. If the foreign body is supraglottic, it can possibly be removed using Magill forceps during laryngoscopy. If the obstruction is subglottic, intubation or bag-mask ventilation may push the foreign body into a mainstem bronchus, allowing temporary ventilation of the other lung until removal with bronchoscopy. Subglottic surgical approaches, such as needle cricothyrotomy and supraglottic rescue devices, are rarely helpful in this setting because the obstruction usually lies within the trachea, below the level of the cricothyroid membrane.

Partial obstruction may require intervention in the ED, due to rapid progression of the occlusion and the anticipated difficulty of laryngoscopy and bag-mask ventilation should complete obstruction occur. Early subspecialty consultation may be needed before any transfer out of the emergency setting. Burn patients, caustic ingestions, expanding hematomas, and anaphylactic reactions not responding to medical therapy fall into this category. Preparation for possible needle cricothyrotomy should be considered in these cases.

CONGENITAL AIRWAY ANOMALIES

Children with congenital abnormalities associated with difficult laryngoscopy and bag-mask ventilation, such as Pierre Robin syndrome, are uncommon but challenging. The ideal management is aggressive medical treatment of the underlying disease, in hopes of obviating the need for intubation. Early subspecialty involvement is also needed in most cases. The most common issue is micrognathia, pushing the tongue posterior and superior, and obscuring attempts at laryngoscopy. A subtly recessed mandible may not be appreciated unless specifically looked for. This can be assessed by drawing a line from the forehead to the anterior maxilla, and the extension of this line should touch on the anterior chin in a normal-size mandible.[4] **Most pediatric patients with micrognathia respond to bag-mask ventilation or ventilation through a laryngeal mask airway.**[25]

AIRWAY RESCUE DEVICES FOR CHILDREN

SUPRAGLOTTIC DEVICES

Consider supraglottic airway devices when ventilation with bag-mask is inadequate and attempts at endotracheal intubation fail. Supraglottic devices provide oxygenation by creating a seal between the oropharynx and the glottic opening and ventilating through a port placed between. A wide range of supraglottic devices are available for use in children including infants and newborns.[14]

One of the first supraglottic devices available for use in children is the laryngeal mask airway, which consists of a large-bore tube terminating in an ovoid, fenestrated cup with an inflatable rim that, when properly placed, forms a seal over the laryngeal orifice (**Figure 111-7**). The result is an airway that is superior to a facemask in that it prevents supraglottic obstruction and greatly reduces the likelihood of gastric insufflation, but it is less reliable at preventing aspiration than an endotracheal tube. Because the laryngeal mask airway is placed blindly, it avoids the complications of endotracheal intubation that arise from the need to visualize and penetrate the glottic opening.

The laryngeal mask airway has been described as a successful rescue device in the pediatric difficult airway.[28,29] The device recommended in children is the standard laryngeal mask airway, which comes in sizes small enough to be used in premature newborns and remains the supraglottic device best supported by the literature[29-33] (**Figure 111-8**).

Table 111-7 presents a guideline of sizes according to weight.

The insertion technique is described in chapter 29. Placement is rapid, and the ability to successfully ventilate is very high, even in the presence of distorted anatomy. Approximately 5% to 10% of insertions are associated with an initial failure to ventilate. Occasionally this is caused when the tip of the laryngeal mask airway pushes the epiglottis over the glottic opening, a complication that is more common in children due to the larger epiglottis.[34] If ventilation is difficult, manifest by poor chest rise or high peak pressures, the clinician should attempt to reposition the laryngeal mask airway by deflating the cuff and partially or completely removing and reinserting. The laryngeal mask airway does not represent a definitive airway, because it does not prevent aspiration, but it is an excellent means of ventilation and oxygenation when laryngoscopic attempts have failed.

Intubating laryngeal airways can be used as a conduit for subsequent endotracheal intubation.[29,32] The **laryngeal mask airway Fastrach™** is an intubating laryngeal airway, but only comes in one pediatric size, designed for children 30 to 50 kg. By contrast, the **air-Q®** intubating laryngeal airway has been successfully used to pass cuffed tubes in infants as small as 4 kg.[29] Another recent supraglottic device with high success rates is the i-gel®, which uses a noninflatable cuff with a gastric access port and comes

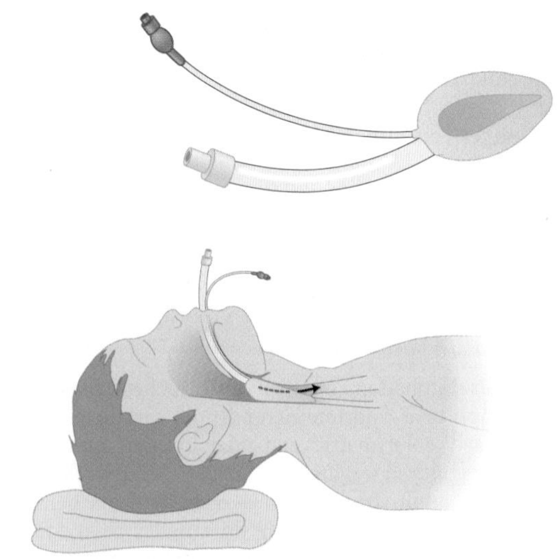

FIGURE 111-7. Pediatric laryngeal mask inserted into airway.

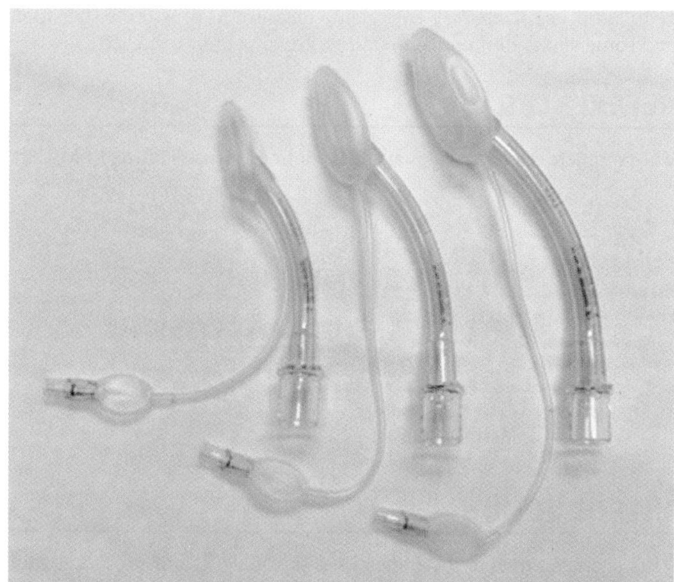

FIGURE 111-8. Pediatric-sized laryngeal mask airways.

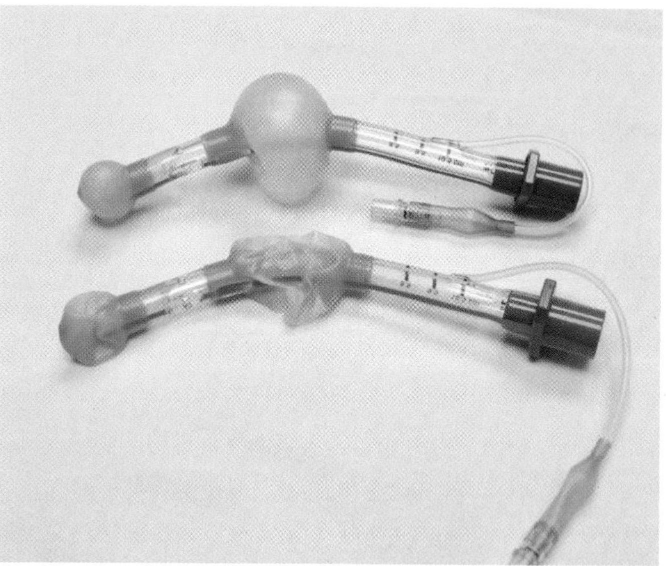

FIGURE 111-9. Pediatric-sized King LT® (King Systems, Noblesville, IN) inflated and deflated.

in sizes ranging from neonates to adults. Studies suggest that the clinical performance of i-gel is similar to the laryngeal mask airway.[35]

There are a number of double-balloon devices in which the tip is placed into the upper esophagus, and ventilation occurs between one balloon occluding the proximal esophagus and another occluding the airway above the glottis. The most studied device is the Combitube, which can only be used in patients >48 inches tall. The King LT® (King Systems, Noblesville, IN) (**Figure 111-9**) is a newer device that comes in pediatric sizes and shows promise in early adult studies; however, experience in pediatrics is lacking at this time.[36]

OTHER RESCUE AND DIFFICULT AIRWAY DEVICES

There are a limited number of rescue devices available for children. Even fewer rescue devices have any significant literature to support their use in the ED. This is likely due to the high success rate associated with good technique in bag-mask ventilation in pediatrics, the subsequent rare need for a rescue device, and the issue of multiple sizes needed in any product development.

The **flexible fiberoptic scope** is available in pediatric sizes and can be useful to evaluate airway difficulty and facilitate intubation. Experience and practice are needed to obtain facility with these devices, and the occasion to use them is rare, which makes it a challenge to ED application. Furthermore, most instances require an awake, cooperative patient, which is unlikely in the distressed young child, even with good topical anesthesia. Therefore, consultation with experienced subspecialists is often needed, with performance of the procedure in the operating room.

Fiberoptic stylets allow direct visualization through an eyepiece mounted on the proximal end of a rigid or malleable stylet, which incorporates a fiberoptic bundle. The Shikani Optical Stylet® (Clarus Medical LLC, Minneapolis, MN) and the Bonfils Retromolar Intubation Scope® (Karl Storz Endoscopy, Culver City, CA) are two such devices that are available in pediatric sizes. There are small case series describing the Shikani scope's successful use in dysmorphic pediatric cases.[37]

Video laryngoscopy displays the laryngeal view on an external monitor from a microvideo camera located at the tip of the laryngoscope blade. Although the blade and handle have the familiarity of a traditional laryngoscope, the operator performs the intubation watching a video screen rather than looking directly into the oropharynx. A growing literature on these devices suggests that, in most cases, video laryngoscopy provides equivalent or better views of the glottic opening than direct laryngoscopy.[38] Some devices, such as the GlideScope® (Verathon, Bothell, WA) and CMAC® (Karl Storz Endoscopy, Culver City, CA), provide blades small enough for the newborn. There is a growing body of research demonstrating successful use of videolaryngoscopy in children, although most of the published literature is from the operating room setting.[39-41] Given the benefits of videolaryngoscopy in adults and demonstrated safety and feasibility in children, use of these devices in the ED is becoming more common.

TABLE 111-7 Laryngeal Mask Airway (LMA) Sizes by Patient Weight

Weight, kg	LMA Size
<5	1
5–10	1.5
10–20	2
20–30	2.5
30–50	3
50–70	4
>70	5

SURGICAL AIRWAY

Subglottic surgical cricothyrotomy is the final airway solution when traditional laryngoscopy and rescue airways have failed or are impossible and the patient cannot be oxygenated. The most common indication is the "can't intubate, can't ventilate" scenario, which is extremely rare in emergency pediatric airway management.[8] **Open surgical cricothyrotomy is not an option in children <10 years old, due to the small cricothyroid membrane. Needle cricothyrotomy is therefore recommended in children <10 years old.** Actual experience in the ED is limited, but success has been described in case reports, animal studies, and the operating room. The procedure involves placing a large-gauge, over-the-needle catheter (usually 14 gauge) through the cricothyroid membrane or upper trachea. Nonkinking catheters are available for this purpose and are preferred, but a standard 14-gauge over-the-needle catheter can be used. **Jet ventilation, through high-pressure oxygen tubing attached directly to 50-psi wall-mounted oxygen and the catheter, should only be used for children >5 years old due to the potential for barotrauma.** If jet ventilation is used in children, the pressure should be reduced using a pressure gauge or air leak available in commercial transtracheal jet ventilation devices designed for this purpose. In children <5 years old, ventilate through the catheter with a bag ventilator. This method can be used in older children also. Use the adapter from a 3.0-mm internal diameter endotracheal tube to connect a standard catheter to the bag (**Figure 111-10**). Transtracheal jet

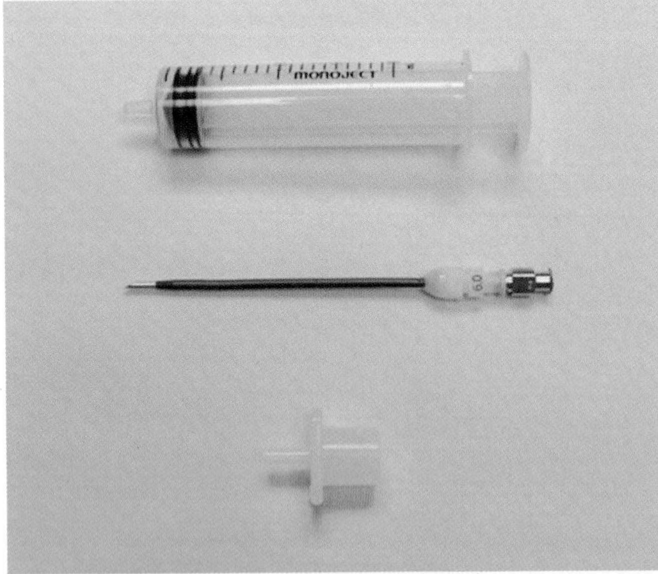

A

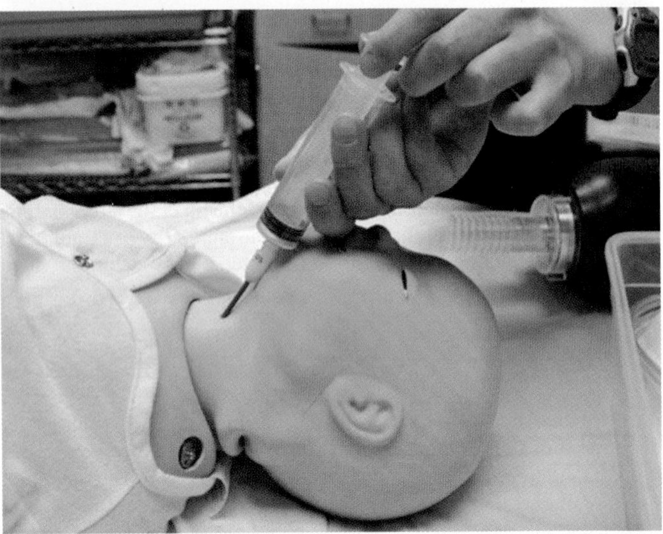

B

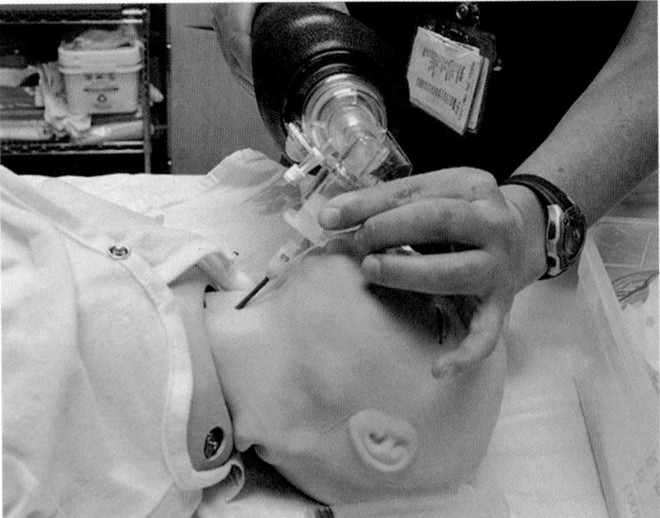

C

FIGURE 111-10. Technique for needle cricothyrotomy. **A.** Equipment required for a needle cricothyrotomy: a 14-gauge over-the-needle catheter (ideally nonkinking), a 3.0-mm internal diameter endotracheal tube adapter, and a 10-mL syringe. **B.** Placement of catheter into trachea. **C.** Ventilation through the catheter using a 3.0-mm endotracheal tube adapter.

ventilation is a *temporary* emergency measure to provide oxygenation and some ventilation until a definitive airway can be achieved.

REFERENCES

The complete reference list is available online at www.TintinalliEM.com.

CHAPTER 112

Intravenous and Intraosseous Access in Infants and Children

Matthew Hansen

INTRODUCTION

This chapter presents the indications, advantages, and procedures for vascular access techniques in children: intraosseous, central venous, US-guided peripheral venous, and umbilical venous access in the newborn.

INTRAOSSEOUS ACCESS

Intraosseous access has the advantage of cannulating a noncollapsible structure that connects to the central circulation. The intraosseous approach is particularly useful for children as a result of their high percentage of red bone marrow and relatively thin bony cortex.

Intraosseous access is indicated when there is an emergent need for vascular access and other sites are difficult, high risk, or excessively time-consuming. Mechanical intraosseous insertion devices have insertion times of only seconds with consistently >90% success rates.[1-6] Insertion devices include simple hand-twist needles, hand-held power drills, and spring-loaded devices.

There are few contraindications to intraosseous placement (**Table 112-1**), and the rate of serious complications from intraosseous insertion is ≤1%. The most common complication is extravasation at the insertion site. By comparison, central venous catheters have complication rates of at least 3.4%.[7,8]

MEDICATIONS AND FLUIDS ADMINISTERED BY THE INTRAOSSEOUS ROUTE

Any medication or fluid that can be given through an IV can be administered by the intraosseous route. Paralytics, anticonvulsants, analgesics, benzodiazepines, and vasopressors such as epinephrine have comparable intraosseous and IV infusion rates. Blood and blood products can be given by the intraosseous route.[9] Medications for rapid-sequence intubation can be administered by the intraosseous route, although the time to effect may be delayed.[10] In a study of sheep given IV or intraosseous succinylcholine, the IV route induced respiratory arrest in a mean of 30.8 seconds, whereas the intraosseous route took 57.5 seconds.[11]

The principal limitation of intraosseous access is a relatively low maximum flow rate. Resistance to flow within the bone marrow cavity limits the flow rate of intraosseous needles, and flow rates per kilogram tend to be higher in young patients who have a greater percentage of low-resistance red marrow compared to adults. The speed of administration of intraosseous infusions can be improved with pressure devices.

TABLE 112-1 Contraindications to Intraosseous Placement
Overlying infection
Exposed bone
Underlying fracture
Structural bone disorders (e.g., osteogenesis imperfecta)

TABLE 112-2 Intraosseous Laboratory Findings Compared with Phlebotomy

	Equivalent	Use Caution in Interpretation
Hematologic	Hemoglobin	Leukocytes, hematocrit, platelets
Chemistries	Sodium, chloride, glucose, bilirubin, bicarbonate, urea, and creatinine	Potassium, aspartate aminotransferase, alanine aminotransferase, alkaline phosphatase
Venous gas	pH	Pco_2, Po_2
Transfusion	ABO, Rh typing, and leukocyte activity	—

Abbreviations: Pco_2 = partial pressure of carbon dioxide; Po_2 = partial pressure of oxygen.

LABORATORY TESTING OF BONE MARROW ASPIRATE

The comparison of marrow aspirate with peripheral blood has been explored in small trials of hematology and oncology patients undergoing routine marrow sampling (**Table 112-2**). Two of these human studies have shown a close correlation of marrow aspirate to venous blood in regard to hemoglobin, sodium, chloride, bilirubin, pH, bicarbonate, urea, and creatinine concentrations.[12,13] In another study, bone marrow taken for medical diagnosis correlated with the peripheral blood for ABO, Rh typing, and leukocyte activity.[14] Correlation between bone marrow and peripheral blood is less reliable for leukocytes, platelets, glucose, potassium, aspartate aminotransferase, alanine aminotransferase, alkaline phosphatase, partial pressure of carbon dioxide, and partial pressure of oxygen; however, the degree of discrepancy likely has minimal clinical significance. Aspirates obtained from the marrow after prolonged CPR may be considerably different from serum levels.[15]

INTRAOSSEOUS CANNULATION DEVICES

There are several devices available for intraosseous insertion. The two most common manual insertion devices include the Cook® intraosseous needle (Cook Medical, Bloomington, IN) and the Jamshidi® style intraosseous needles. Powered devices are also available for intraosseous needle insertion; two examples are the EZ-IO® (Vidacare Corp., San Antonio, TX) and the Bone Injection Gun (BIG®) (Waismed, Ltd., Hertzliya, Israel). There is one prospective randomized study comparing manual to powered insertion devices in pediatrics in the prehospital setting, which compared the Jamshidi needle to the BIG. There were only 22 children in the cohort, which was primarily comprised of adults. There were no significant differences in time to insertion, which was less than 1 minute for both devices, or success rate, which was approximately 80% for both devices.[4] Several studies have demonstrated rapid insertion and high success rates (>90%) using the EZ-IO in children, even among providers with minimal training.[4,16] Small randomized studies in adults comparing the EZ-IO to the BIG suggest faster time to insertion and a higher first-time insertion success rate for the EZ-IO.[5,6] The EZ-IO is a battery-powered cordless drill with a specialized needle (**Figure 112-1**). The needle is chosen based on the patient's weight and the distance from the skin to the bone (**Figure 112-2**). This device is intended for use in the proximal tibia, distal tibia, or proximal humerus. The BIG is a spring-loaded device that can be used in the proximal tibia; the pediatric device allows adjustable depths of insertion based on the patient's age. The BIG has the potential to cause injury to patient or provider if fired at the wrong time.

PLACEMENT AND INSERTION OF INTRAOSSEOUS NEEDLE

Placement Sites The ideal location for intraosseous access is a large bone with easily palpable landmarks, a thin cortex, and limited proximity to vital structures. The proximal or distal tibia, distal femur, and sternum are the sites most commonly described. The flat surface of the anteromedial proximal tibia is easily accessible given the paucity of overlying tissue, making it the most commonly accessed site (**Figure 112-3**).[16] Insert the needle 2 cm inferior (distal) to the tibial tuberosity to avoid the physeal plate in children (**Figure 112-4**). When accessing the distal tibia, enter just superior to the medial malleolus, avoiding the saphenous vein (**Figure 112-5**), which is located 2 cm anterior and 2 cm superior to the malleolus. In adults, the distal tibia has thinner cortex than that of the proximal tibia. The anterior distal femur is an alternate site for children when the proximal tibia cannot be used or has failed (**Figure 112-6**). Insert the needle two fingerbreadths superior (proximal) to the distal end of the femur in the midline.

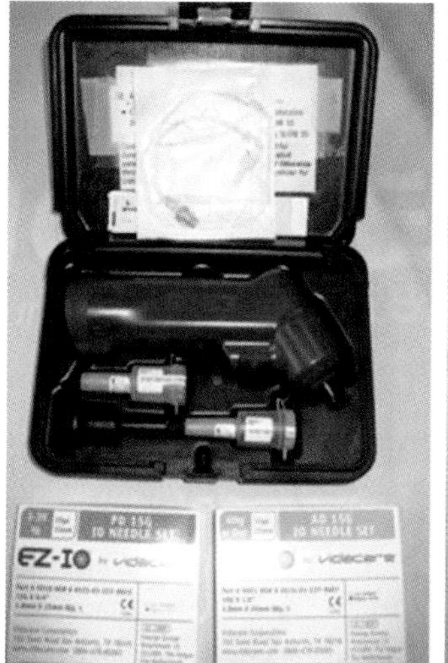

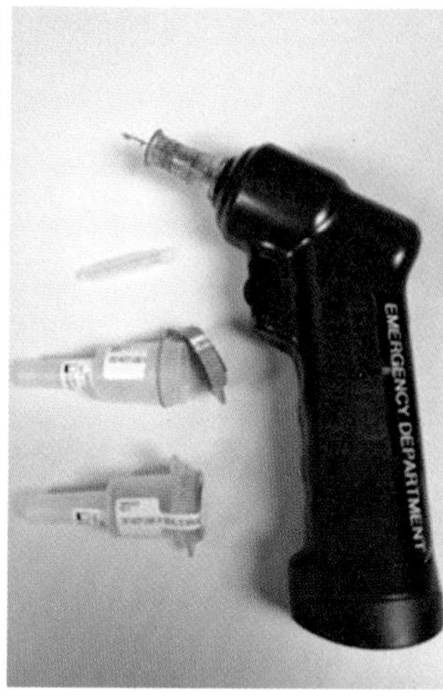

FIGURE 112-1. EZ-IO® device and needles. [Reproduced with permission from Vidacare Corp., San Antonio, TX. For updates see http://www.vidacare.com/ez-io/index.html.]

Steps for Insertion Once the appropriate insertion site has been selected, place the intraosseous needle perpendicular to the bone against the skin. Manual needles are pushed into the bone using steady pressure and slow rotation of the needle back and forth. If using an intraosseous drill, depress the trigger while applying gentle pressure on the needle. The drill significantly reduces the amount of pressure needed to penetrate the bone. Keep the trigger depressed during insertion, as the skin can twist and cause significant pain if the drill is repeatedly started and stopped. Once the cortex is penetrated, there will be a sudden decrease in resistance. At that point, release the trigger and detach the drill from the needle, which, in the EZ-IO, is secured with a magnetic chuck. Unscrew the stylet from the needle and attach a 5- or 10-cc luer lock syringe to the intraosseous needle and aspirate. Return of blood or bone marrow confirms placement, but return does not always occur, even when the needle is properly placed. Flush the intraosseous needle with 5 to 10 cc of normal saline, which should flow easily and further confirm placement. If the intraosseous needle has penetrated the posterior cortex or if the tip is not in the medullary cavity for another reason, fluids will extravasate into the soft tissues. This could include spaces posterior to the bone being cannulated, such as the gastrocnemius in a proximal tibial attempt. **Palpate the area carefully to ensure that no**

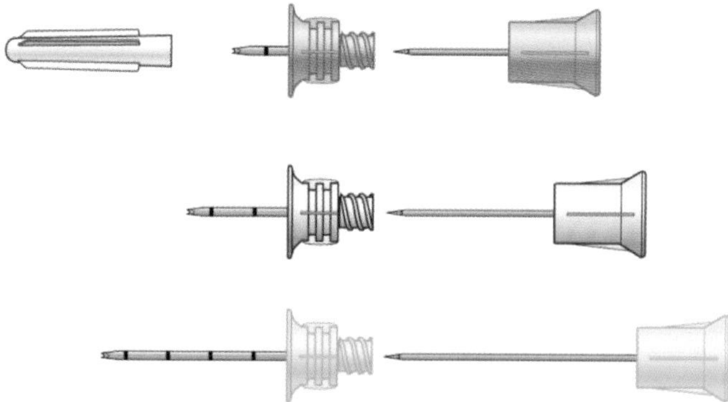

FIGURE 112-2. EZ-IO® needle sizes. The pink needle set is 15 mm in length (EZ-IO PD). This size is used in most children. The blue needle set is adult sized at 25 mm in length (EZ-IO AD), and the yellow needle set is for larger adults and is 45 mm in length (EZ-IO LD). The length and color are the only differences between needle sets. [Reproduced with permission from Vidacare Corp., San Antonio, TX. For updates see http://www.vidacare.com/ez-io/index.html.]

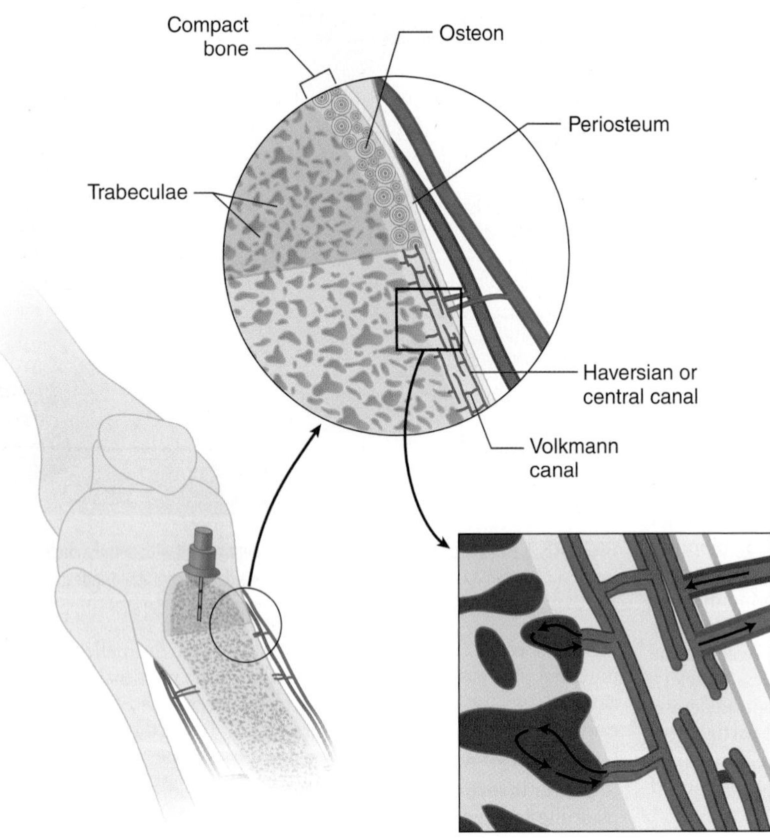

FIGURE 112-3. Anatomy of the proximal tibia. [Reproduced with permission from Vidacare Corp., San Antonio, TX. For updates see http://www.vidacare.com/ez-io/index.html.]

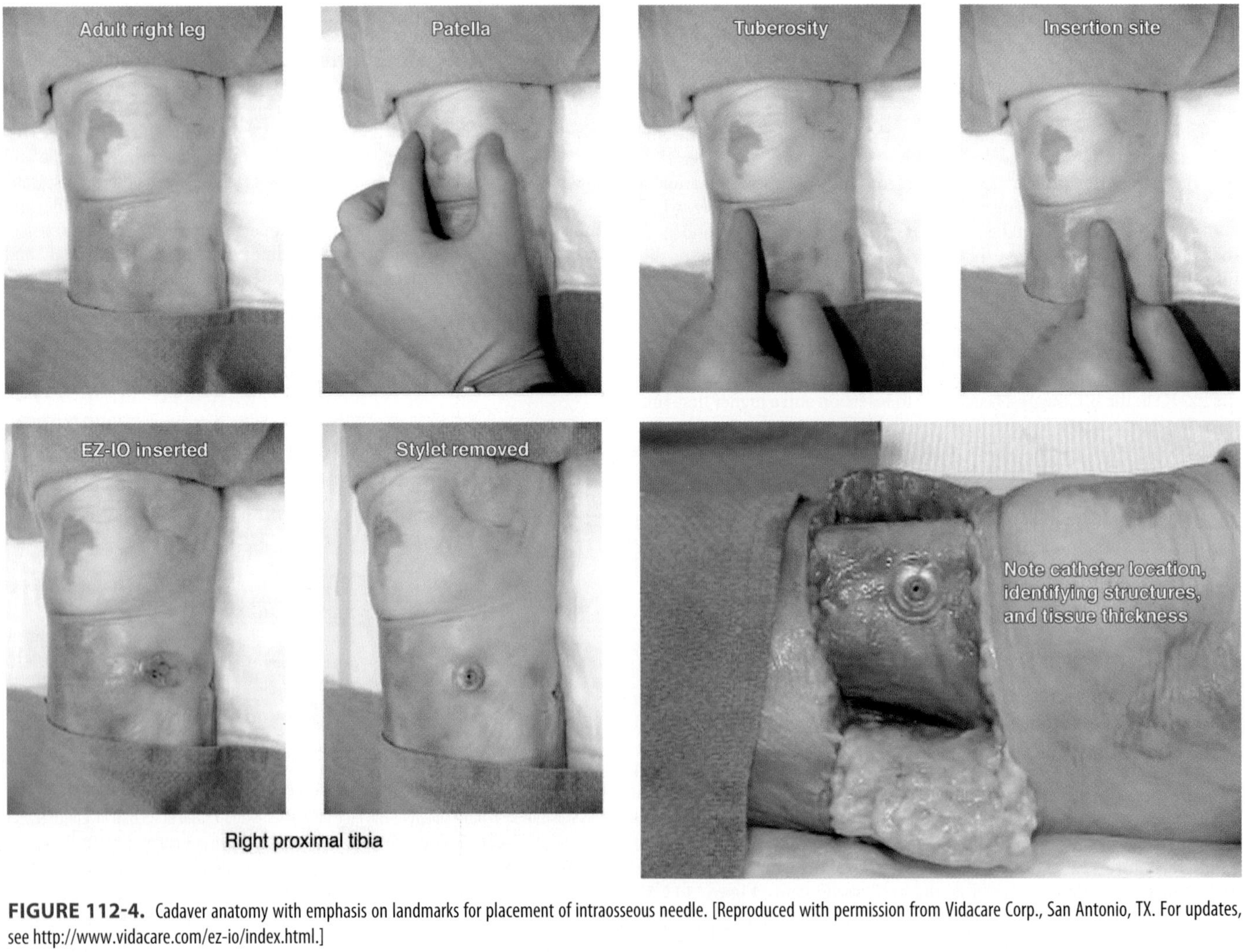

FIGURE 112-4. Cadaver anatomy with emphasis on landmarks for placement of intraosseous needle. [Reproduced with permission from Vidacare Corp., San Antonio, TX. For updates, see http://www.vidacare.com/ez-io/index.html.]

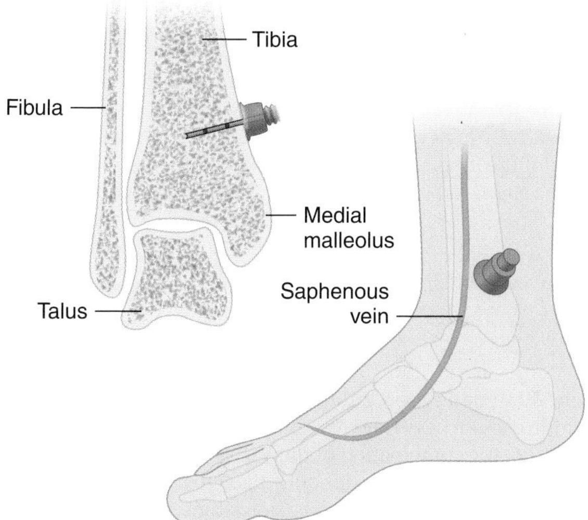

FIGURE 112-5. Anatomy of the distal tibia site for intraosseous placement.

extravasation is present. If the needle is misplaced, remove it and select a different bone for subsequent attempts. Frequently, automated gravity-based infusions and even automated pumps may not provide adequate pressure for infusion, and pneumatic pressure bags may be required. Secure the needle with bulky gauze dressing, but leave the dressing loose enough to check the site for signs of extravasation as infusions continue.

COMPLICATIONS OF INTRAOSSEOUS PLACEMENT

The complication rate is low. The most common complication is pain during insertion and infusion. Discomfort during infusion is thought to be due to pressure within the marrow cavity and can be reduced with the administration of lidocaine. The manufacturer of the EZ-IO recommends giving a 0.5 milligram/kg dose of 2% lidocaine without epinephrine (20 to 40 milligrams in adults) followed by a 10-mL normal saline flush after the intraosseous route is established.

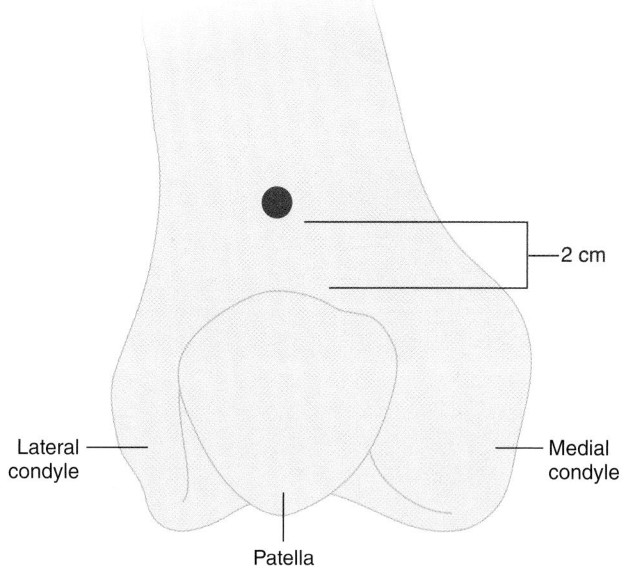

FIGURE 112-6. Distal femur. The distal femur is an alternative site for intraosseous access. The red circle represents the site of insertion of the intraosseous needle. [Reproduced with permission from Hoffman ME, Ma OJ: Intraosseous infusion, in Reichman E, Simon RR (eds): *Emergency Medicine Procedures*. Figure 44-4, http://www.accessemergencymedicine.com/content.aspx?aID=50506.]

In a prospective cohort of 95 patients who had intraosseous placement in the field or in the ED, no complications were noted other than difficulty removing the needle.[3] A retrospective series of 42 patients with intraosseous placement had one serious complication of tibial fracture in a 10-day-old.[17] A case series of 58 insertions in pediatric critical care transport team noted a 12% complication rate, all of which were minor local tissue edema or infiltration.[16] A population-based study found no serious complications in 281 intraosseous insertions using administrative data.[18] Case reports have described serious complications including compartment syndrome, osteomyelitis, fat embolism, cerebral air embolism, and skin necrosis from extravasation of caustic medications.[18] Soft tissue fluid accumulation may be more likely in the setting of multiple attempts at intraosseous placement in the same bone. As a result, **no more than one attempt per bone is recommended.**[19] Growth plate injuries are possible if not inserted at the proper site.[20] Tibial fracture is a rare complication that is more likely in children with underlying bone disorders. In general, radiographs are not needed following intraosseous removal unless there is suspicion of a complication.

INTRAOSSEOUS REMOVAL

Each device has specific instructions for removal. The EZ-IO is removed by attaching a luer lock syringe then applying traction while twisting in a *clockwise* direction. If the syringe is twisted counterclockwise, it will unscrew from the short hub, which can be difficult to grasp. Other needles can be removed with traction and a back-and-forth twisting motion. Remove intraosseous needles as soon as another stable route of vascular access is established.

US-GUIDED PERIPHERAL VENOUS ACCESS IN INFANTS AND CHILDREN

Peripheral venous access with US guidance is an additional option when blind peripheral attempts fail. Both arm and leg veins can be accessed using either a transverse or longitudinal approach to localize the vein and directly guide cannulation. One randomized trial demonstrated significantly reduced time to peripheral venous access with fewer total attempts when US was used compared to traditional techniques in pediatric patients with difficult IV access.[21] The saphenous vein has also been described as a reliable site for US-guided IV placement. Another study showed no improvement in success when using US after one failed IV attempt among practitioners with little experience using US, which suggests that operator experience likely plays a significant role in success with this technique.[22]

CENTRAL VENOUS ACCESS IN INFANTS AND CHILDREN

Central venous access is safe in all age groups as long as proper techniques are followed. In older children, complications are similar to those encountered in adults. Insertion of central venous catheters >6-French size in children <1 year old, <10 kg in weight, or <75 cm in height is associated with higher complication rates.[23] Typically, a 5-French catheter is used for term neonates and infants, and a 3-French catheter for preterm (<36 weeks) neonates.

Indications for pediatric central venous access in the ED are listed in **Table 112-3**.

Rapid large-volume resuscitation is not always an indication for central access. The rate of flow through a catheter is inversely related to the length of the cannula; thus central lines have slower flow rates than peripheral catheters of the same diameter. However, large-bore central catheters,

TABLE 112-3 Indications for Pediatric Central Venous Access
Inability to obtain peripheral access
Need for invasive hemodynamic monitoring
Administration of caustic or hypertonic solutions
Need for long-term vascular access
Need for transvenous pacemaker placement

TABLE 112-4 Complications of Pediatric Central Venous Access

Complications
Pneumothorax (subclavian and internal jugular vein sites)
Thoracic duct injury (left-sided internal jugular vein)
Arterial puncture
Cardiac tamponade
Air embolism
Arrhythmia
Incorrect position
Hemothorax (subclavian and internal jugular vein sites)
Subcutaneous hematoma (subclavian vein cannulation in coagulopathy)
Neuropathies
Death
Infection

which are shorter than common multi-lumen catheters, allow extremely rapid infusion. The choice of central venous catheter size in children should be predicated on the primary disease and intended use as well as the child's age, weight, and height.

PLACEMENT OF CENTRAL VENOUS CATHETERS

The three most common anatomic locations for obtaining central access in children are the subclavian vein, the internal jugular vein, and the femoral vein (see chapter 31, Vascular Access, for descriptions of these procedures). The anatomical landmarks and insertion techniques are the same in adults and children, although key differences are described below. The choice of location depends on patient factors as well as practitioner experience with a particular site. Complications of central venous access are listed in **Table 112-4**. Multiple attempts (more than two) and the subclavian approach are associated with higher complication rates.[24]

SUBCLAVIAN VEIN

The anatomy of the subclavian vein and technique for line placement are similar in children and adults. The primary disadvantage is a higher rate of mechanical complications of insertion compared to other sites including the relatively high potential for pneumothorax in children given the extension of the lung apices above the clavicles.

Place the child's head in a neutral position, without the use of a shoulder roll, as this maximizes vein diameter.[25] For a detailed explanation of technique, see chapter 31.

INTERNAL JUGULAR VEIN

The anatomy of the internal jugular vein is similar in adults and children. As in adults, US guidance is recommended in children and likely improves success rates.[26]

In children, the combination of the Valsalva maneuver, liver compression, and Trendelenburg positioning maximizes the distention of the internal jugular vein. The effect is significant in young children, but negligible in infants.[27] For further discussion, see chapter 31.

FEMORAL VEIN

The anatomic location of the femoral vein in children is similar to that in adults. In adults, femoral lines have high rates of infection and are generally avoided. In children, the femoral site may not be associated with higher infection rates and is easier to place in a responsive child, and mechanical complications are less likely to be severe (e.g., pneumothorax and pericardial tamponade).

The femoral artery overlaps the femoral vein at least partially in up to 15% to 20% of children.[28,29] US studies have demonstrated that the optimal position to reduce overlap is to place the leg in 30 to 60 degrees of abduction.[30] In addition, US guidance lowers the rate of arterial puncture.[31] For further demonstration of the technique, see chapter 31.

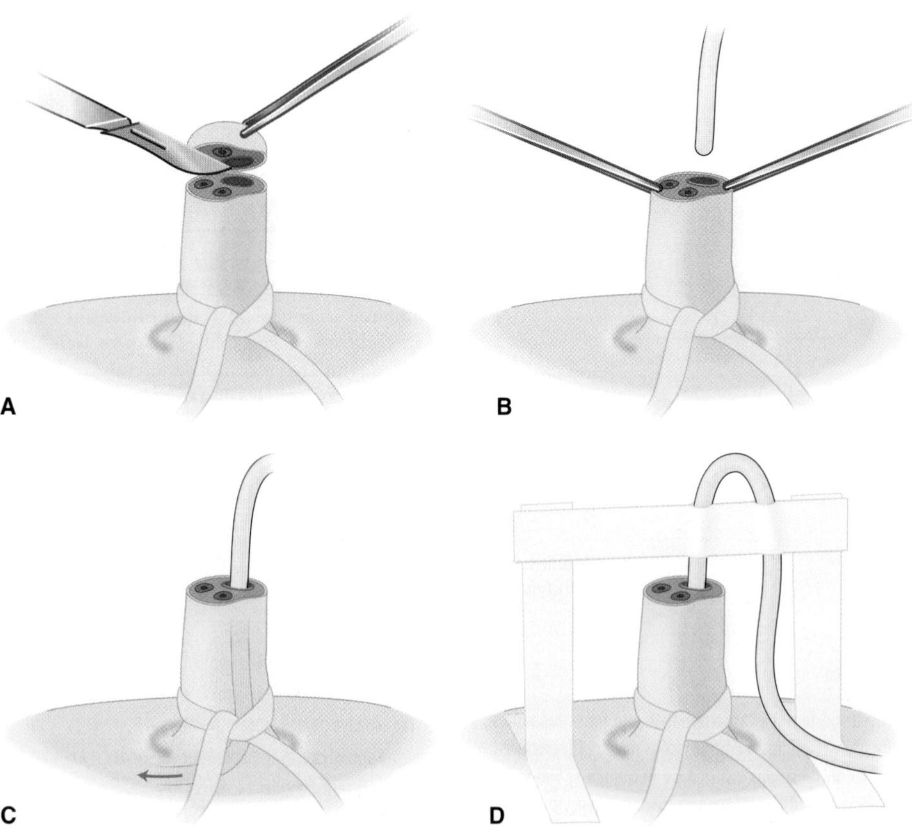

FIGURE 112-7. **A through D.** Umbilical vein access.

UMBILICAL VEIN ACCESS

In general, umbilical venous catheterization is limited to the first week of life. The umbilical vein is continuous with the portal vein. An alternative to umbilical access for neonatal resuscitation is intraosseous placement, which may be preferable for those not trained in umbilical access.

UMBILICAL CANNULATION PROCEDURE

Use a 5.0-French catheter for term infants and a 3.5-French catheter for preterm infants. For emergency access, insert the catheter only 4 to 5 cm in depth. Preflush the catheter and attach it to a closed stopcock connected to a syringe. Use standard iodine-based sterile preparation of the umbilicus and sterile drapes. Tie a string loosely around the skin at the base of the umbilicus; this can be tightened in case of bleeding (**Figure 112-7**).

Cut the cord with a scalpel approximately 2 cm from the abdominal wall and identify the vein and two arteries. The vein is larger, thin walled, and usually at the 12 o'clock position. The arteries are smaller with a thicker muscular layer and located roughly at 4 and 8 o'clock. The vein may need to be dilated or thrombus cleared from the lumen with small forceps. Holding the catheter near the tip, insert it into the vein, checking every centimeter for blood return by drawing on the syringe. If resistance is met at the base of the stump, loosen the umbilical tie. In emergency situations, advance the catheter only 1 to 2 cm beyond the point of good blood return; this is typically 4 to 5 cm from the end of the umbilical stump in a term infant. If there is free return of blood, the line can be used. In this technique, the catheter extends only a few centimeters into the abdomen so radiographic confirmation is not necessary. At that point, tighten the purse string or umbilical tie and tie it off. A suture may be placed through the stump and tied around the catheter or the catheter can be held in place manually.

COMPLICATIONS OF UMBILICAL VEIN CANNULATION

Umbilical vein cannulation carries serious risks, which are similar to those for standard central venous catheters but also include hepatic necrosis if a line is placed in the hepatic vein.[32] However, many of these risks apply only to longer lines placed in the intensive care unit, and the umbilical vein should be considered a viable bridge to other access. Monitor for tachycardia or signs of increasing abdominal distention, which suggests vessel or bowel perforation.[33]

REFERENCES

The complete reference list is available online at www.TintinalliEM.com.

CHAPTER 113 Pain Management and Procedural Sedation in Infants and Children

Peter S. Auerbach

INTRODUCTION

Pain and anxiety are very common experiences for patients of all ages in the ED, and both are frequently undertreated. This is particularly true for children. There are many reasons for this, including the idea that very young children do not experience true pain or will not remember, the perceived difficulty in measuring pain and anxiety in children, fear of masking the signs and symptoms of serious disease processes, concerns that addressing pain takes too much time or effort, and lack of familiarity and comfort with medication dosing in children. These concerns should not stand in the way of providing adequate analgesia, anxiolysis, and sedation for children, however, and addressing these concerns is the primary goal of this chapter.

Caring for children in the ED requires constant attention to pain and anxiety. Common situations include fractures, lacerations, abdominal pain, lumbar puncture, incision and drainage of abscesses, and IV placement. Full procedural sedation may be necessary for invasive procedures in children. This chapter discusses pain management goals (**Table 113-1**) and pharmacologic and nonpharmacologic measures to minimize pain and anxiety experienced by children in the ED, with an emphasis on both basic concepts and newer developments in this topic of daily relevance to ED care providers.

TABLE 113-1 General Goals of Pediatric Analgesia, Anxiolysis, & Sedation
Minimize physical pain and discomfort
Alleviate anxiety
Maximize amnesia
Minimize negative psychological responses to treatment
Control behavior/motion to expedite performance of procedures
Maintain safety and minimize risk to patient

ASSESSMENT OF PAIN AND ANXIETY BY AGE

The first step in the treatment of pain and anxiety in children is to quantify the severity of symptoms. The level of pain or distress may be obvious to the care provider, such as when a child has a visibly displaced fracture. Other scenarios are not as straightforward, however, such as the common complaint of abdominal pain. Preverbal and young children are especially challenging. As a result, specific pain scales have been developed for children at different developmental stages (**Table 113-2**). Familiarity with and application of these pain scales greatly reduces uncertainty in treating pain and anxiety in children of all ages. In addition, measuring and addressing pain is one of the Centers for Medicare & Medicaid Quality Measures.

Children with cognitive developmental delay may compound the challenges of assessing and treating pain and anxiety by combining the physical size and strength of an older child with the cognitive and behavioral attributes of the young. Furthermore, many of the patients in whom this "cognitive-physical mismatch" exists are medically complex and have already experienced a large number of medical encounters, including painful procedures, so baseline anxiety is high. Relying on parental pain assessment and providing empiric analgesia for procedures that are expected to be painful is the most prudent approach to these children.

INFANTS AND TODDLERS

A variety of pain scales have been developed for use in infants and young children, before they are able to self-report and quantify pain. These scales are based on physiologic parameters such as heart rate and observations of behavioral reactions such as crying, facial expressions, and activity level. In the United States, the FLACC Scale© (Face, Legs, Activity, Cry, Consolability) is most commonly used.

PRESCHOOL CHILDREN

Beginning at about 3 years of age, many children are able to describe and rate pain, and pain scales utilizing self-report become possible and are the preferred means of assessing pain. The most commonly used is the

TABLE 113-2 Assessment of Pain by Age: Pain Scales	
Infants & toddlers	FLACC© (Face, Legs, Activity, Cry, Consolability) scale
Young children (preschool)	Wong-Baker FACES© pain scale
Older children & adolescents	Verbal Numeric Scale or Visual Analog Scale

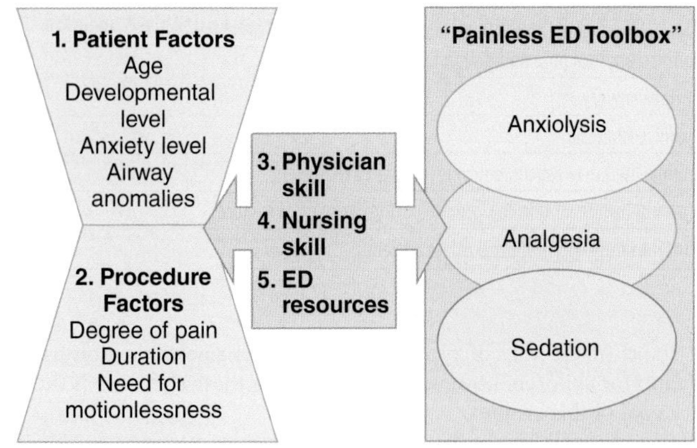

FIGURE 113-1. Elements for anxiolysis, analgesia, and sedation in children.

Wong-Baker FACES© pain scale: the child points to one of six face drawings ranging from very happy (0; no pain) to very sad (5; worst pain). Similar scales include the Faces Pain Scale-Revised© (which uses a 0 to 10 scale) and the Oucher Scale© (which incorporates photographs of children instead of simple drawings and offers a variety of ethnic versions). Samples of these scales are readily available online.

OLDER CHILDREN AND ADOLESCENTS

Older children are able to self-report pain and can use numeric pain scales. The Verbal Numeric Scale©, also called the Numeric Rating Scale, rates pain from 0 (no pain) to 10 (worst pain) and is validated in children aged 8 to 17 years.[1] The experience of pain itself is subjective, and self-reported pain assessment is based on prior experiences and varies widely from individual to individual. Nevertheless, assigning a numeric score to pre- and post-treatment pain provides the most objective method available for assessing pain and anxiety.

ELEMENTS OF PAIN MANAGEMENT

The approach to analgesia, anxiolysis, and sedation in children consists of five general elements (**Figure 113-1**). The variables affecting the choices and outcome of pediatric analgesia, anxiolysis, and sedation can also be thought of as four interfacing "domains"—patient, procedure, medications, and setting (**Table 113-3**).

To choose the best option(s) in any given scenario, assess the child and his/her physical and psychological development, along with the procedure and its level of pain and associated anxiety, and whether the procedure requires complete stillness (such as CT with IV contrast). Synthesize these characteristics to apply the modalities available in the "tool box" (Figure 113-1).

ANXIOLYSIS

Anxiety potentiates pain, and anxiety itself is unpleasant for children and their families. Common examples of anxiety-provoking procedures are laceration repair and lumbar puncture. Although theoretically both procedures should be nearly painless, particularly with the use of topical anesthetics such as LET® (lidocaine, epinephrine, and tetracaine, for lacerations) and LMX® (liposomal lidocaine cream, applied before lumbar puncture), both the waiting period and the procedure itself can be highly anxiety provoking. Anxiety can be addressed in a variety of ways, both pharmacologic and nonpharmacologic.

TABLE 113-3 Domains Related to Pediatric Analgesia & Sedation

Patient Factors	Procedural Factors	Medication Factors	Setting Factors
Age	Urgency	Route of administration	Provider skill and experience
Weight	Duration	Pharmacokinetics	Institutional policies
Comorbidities	Requirement for emotionlessness	Properties (anxiolytic, hypnotic, analgesic, amnestic)	Resources
Medication	Anxiety	Side effects	Equipment
Allergies	Pain		Time constraints
NPO status			

Abbreviation: NPO = nil per os.

NONPHARMACOLOGIC ANXIOLYSIS

Parental presence (and sometimes involvement) is a fundamental technique to reduce anxiety that is both cost-free and highly effective. The form of parental presence used may vary by age of the child, but generally, for painful procedures, a well-prepared parent can "coach" the child and reduce anxiety. Allowing the parent on the stretcher with the child is particularly helpful with toddlers and school-aged children.

Distraction for younger children can take the form of picture books, stories read aloud, bubbles, light wands, songs, or music. Guided imagery and hypnosis are both effective but require specific provider training. Education and advance preparation are also useful. Procedures should be explained in a developmentally appropriate context. Child life specialists, if available, are extremely effective in reducing anxiety and acting as patient advocates.

PHARMACOLOGIC ANXIOLYSIS

Benzodiazepines are widely used for their anxiolytic, sedative, amnestic, and hypnotic properties. In the ED, midazolam is almost universally preferred over other agents in this class because of its relatively short duration of action. Midazolam can be given by the intranasal route, which avoids the need for IV access and affords a more rapid onset of action than the oral route. However, benzodiazepines do not have analgesic properties and should be combined with other agents if pain is also an issue. Luckily, fentanyl can also be given by the intranasal route (**Table 113-4**). Midazolam can cause paradoxical agitation, particularly at lower doses, and can cause respiratory depression and hypotension, particularly in hypovolemic patients. Adjunctive depressant medications can potentiate these effects.

The main advantage of intranasal administration is a more rapid onset of action than the oral route, higher blood levels (by avoiding "first pass effects" of the GI system), and no need for IV placement. High-concentration solutions must be used because the maximum volume that can be delivered to each nostril is limited to approximately 1 mL. Because the medication particles must be within a specific size range (approximately 10 to 50 microns) to be absorbed by the nasal mucosa, commercially available (and inexpensive) "mucosal atomizer devices" are used for intranasal delivery.

Regardless of the route of administration, midazolam is more effective when dosed at the higher end of the range (e.g., 0.4 milligrams/kg for the intranasal route). Oral midazolam (which avoids the nasal irritation of intranasal administration) may be appropriately paired with topical lidocaine-epinephrine-tetracaine suspension for wound repair, as both take 20 to 30 minutes to be effective. Oral midazolam has a longer duration of effect than intranasal or IV preparations, so warn parents to protect the child from falls due to incoordination for several hours after discharge.

When IV access has already been obtained, midazolam may be used IV for anxiolysis, which has the advantage of rapid onset and is easier to titrate than other routes of administration. A lower dose (0.05 to 0.1 milligram/kg IV) is usually sufficient and should be considered, for example, in children and teens requiring lumbar puncture. Higher doses of IV midazolam can cause respiratory depression, and a few children can exhibit a paradoxical reaction to midazolam, with agitation, confusion, or crying. These reactions are self-limited and can occur with PO and intranasal administration. Both paradoxical agitation and respiratory depression may be treated with flumazenil, although this is rarely necessary.

ANALGESIA

NONPHARMACOLOGIC STRATEGIES

There are a wide variety of nonpharmacologic techniques to reduce pain. Some of them, such as proper immobilization, application of ice, and elevation of fractures, may make a larger difference for the patient

TABLE 113-4 Intranasal Medications Commonly Used for Children in the ED

Drug	Concentration	IN Dose	Onset	Duration	Side Effects/Warnings
Midazolam	5 milligrams/mL	0.2–0.4 milligram/kg; max 10 milligrams	5–15 min	0.5–2 h	Excitation/paradoxical reaction Somnolence Nasal irritation Bitter taste
Fentanyl	50 micrograms/mL	2 micrograms/kg; max 100 micrograms	5–10 min	20–60 min	Nausea Respiratory depression (*outlasts analgesic effect*) Dizziness

than medications. Although techniques such as immobilization are widely known, they are often overlooked, delayed, or omitted. Other techniques include distraction, massage, breathing techniques, acupressure, and emotional support.

PHARMACOLOGIC STRATEGIES

Oral Sucrose for Neonates Neonates must often undergo unpleasant and painful procedures, and when their pain is not addressed, it can have long-lasting effects on future response to pain. Examples of painful ED procedures include urinary catheterization, venipuncture, heel sticks, IM injections, and lumbar puncture. Oral sucrose is an effective analgesic for brief, painful procedures[2] and is thought to work by activating endogenous opioids through taste receptors. It is given orally as a concentrated solution by a syringe (e.g., 2 mL of a 24% sucrose solution) or applied to a pacifier. Sucrose solution comes in a variety of commercially available formulations (such as Sweet-Ease®, a premixed 24% sucrose and water solution). Regardless of the formulation used, oral sucrose reduces physiologic measures of pain (e.g., heart rate), behavioral measures (e.g., time crying), and newborn pain scale scores.

Topical Anesthetics for Intact Skin Topical anesthetics reduce the pain of minor procedures, such as phlebotomy, Mediport access, and lumbar puncture, and are appropriate for children of all ages. Two commercially available products are EMLA® and LMX®. EMLA® (eutectic mixture of 2.5% prilocaine and 2.5% lidocaine) and LMX® (4% liposomal lidocaine) are both fat-absorbable creams that anesthetize the skin. The time to maximal effect is up to 60 minutes for EMLA® and 30 minutes for LMX®. The use of topical anesthetics may result in a delay in the time to IV access or other procedures, but it is usually appropriate to wait the additional time for the benefit of patient comfort.

Topical Anesthetics for Open Wounds LET® (lidocaine 4%, epinephrine 0.1%, and tetracaine 0.5%) is a topical anesthetic mixture for open wounds and is safe and effective for almost all laceration repairs in children. It can be applied to fingers, toes, lips, and other end-organ tissues despite the vasoconstriction effects of the epinephrine.

LET® is most effective for wounds that are not deeper than the subcutaneous tissues. LET® should be applied half into the wound and half on a saturated piece of sterile cotton (rather than gauze) at a maximum dose of 0.2 mL/kg. The adequacy of anesthesia from LET® is highly dependent on proper application technique. LET® is prepared by hospital pharmacies as a liquid, but is also available commercially as a gel. LET® should be left in place for at least 20 to 30 minutes for satisfactory wound anesthesia, with longer times (up to 45 minutes or more) generally leading to more complete anesthesia (though highly vascular tissues such as lips require less time). Blanching of the skin from the vasoconstriction effects of epinephrine is a good sign that topical anesthesia has been achieved.

Another option for topical anesthesia prior to procedures such as venipuncture and lumbar puncture is the use of a needle-free injection system. This is a highly effective alternative to EMLA® or LMX®, with the major advantage that it is nearly instantaneous.[3] Needle-free injection systems deliver lidocaine into the dermis using a self-contained high-pressure delivery system such as a carbon dioxide gas cartridge. The J-tip® (National Medical Products, Irvine, CA) is currently the most widely used needle-free injection system for local anesthesia.

Local Anesthetic Injection Slow injection with a small-gauge needle decreases the discomfort of injection. The addition of sodium bicarbonate (typically in a 1:9 ratio) buffers the acidity of lidocaine and further reduces the pain of injection, but must be added immediately before use or precipitation of the solution may result. When possible, regional nerve blocks should be used because they produce a greater area of anesthesia with less medication and can avoid distortion of local tissues in cosmetically important areas such as the lip (see chapter 36, Local and Regional Anesthesia). The onset of action of bupivacaine is slightly longer than that of lidocaine, but it provides much longer lasting anesthesia.

Systemic Analgesia • *Oral Agents* Oral acetaminophen and ibuprofen are the mainstays of treatment for mild to moderate pain in children. Unless a specific contraindication to one of these exists, they should be used whenever oral systemic analgesia is required. Codeine has been widely used as an analgesic for many years in children, both alone and in combination with acetaminophen, probably because it is widely available and thought to have a favorable side effect profile. However, the combination of acetaminophen and codeine is no more effective than ibuprofen alone.[4,5] In addition, codeine is poorly efficacious as an analgesic and much less safe than previously believed. **As a result, ibuprofen should be considered the first-line oral agent in the treatment of mild to moderate pain in children, particularly for acute musculoskeletal injuries, and is preferred over the use of codeine (with or without acetaminophen).** Although laboratory studies in tissue culture demonstrate inhibition of osteoblasts by nonsteroidal anti-inflammatory drugs, no human studies have demonstrated clinically significant delay in fracture healing from their use.[5,6] Oral opioid analgesics such as hydrocodone and oxycodone provide superior analgesia when compared with codeine.[7] Consider these agents instead of codeine when ibuprofen alone is insufficient. A convenient liquid formulation of hydrocodone plus acetaminophen (7.5 milligrams/500 milligrams per 15 mL) is available both generically and under the brand name Lortab®, and dosing is simplified by the use of a chart such as that shown in **Table 113-5**. The liquid opioid/acetaminophen combination should replace the use of codeine/acetaminophen in pediatric practice.

Intranasal Fentanyl Intranasal fentanyl is an alternative to oral or IV opioids when acute pain management is necessary, the time required for absorption of oral mediations is too long, and IV placement is not otherwise necessary. Intranasal fentanyl at doses of 1.5 to 2 micrograms/kg provides adequate and rapid analgesia comparable to that of IV morphine.[8] The time to administration of analgesia is reduced when intranasal fentanyl

TABLE 113-5 Hydrocodone/Acetaminophen (7.5 milligrams/500 milligrams/15 mL dosage)

Body Weight	Approximate Age	Dose (every 4 hours as needed)	Maximum in 24 Hours (6 doses)
12–15 kg	2–3 years	3.75 mL	22.5 mL
16–22 kg	4–6 years	5 mL	30 mL
23–31 kg	7–9 years	7.5 mL	45 mL
32–45 kg	10–13 years	10 mL	60 mL
>45 kg	>14 years	15 mL	90 mL

TABLE 113-6 Pediatric Parenteral Opiates

Drug	IV Dose	Onset	Duration	Side Effects/Warnings
Morphine	0.1–0.2 milligram/kg	5–10 min	1–4 h	Histamine release/pruritus Seizures in neonates Nausea Hypotension
Hydromorphone	0.015–0.020 milligram/kg	5–10 min	1–4 h	Nausea Pruritus
Fentanyl	1–2 micrograms/kg	1–2 min	30–60 min	Bradycardia Respiratory depression (*outlasts analgesic effect*) Chest wall rigidity (risk increases with larger doses, rapid push)

is compared with IV analgesics such as morphine.[9] Intranasal medications (specifically fentanyl and midazolam) are also useful in the prehospital setting.

IV Nonsteroidal Anti-inflammatory Agents IV access provides additional options for the acute treatment of pain. IV ketorolac is particularly effective for musculoskeletal pain, the pain of cholelithiasis and ureterolithiasis, and gynecologic pain. It is approved by the U.S. Food and Drug Administration for use in children as young as 24 months. The dose is 1 milligram/kg IM (maximum 30 milligrams) or 0.5 milligram/kg IV (maximum 15 milligrams). Ketorolac is *not* more effective than ibuprofen or other nonsteroidal anti-inflammatory drugs when given orally and is not approved by the U.S. Food and Drug Administration for use in children.

IV Opiates Children require more opiates proportionate to their weight than adults. Undertreatment of pediatric pain out of fear of adverse effects of opiates or due to lack of recognition of pain is a common problem in the ED. Morphine, for example, should be administered in doses of 0.1 to 0.2 milligram/kg and can then be repeated at 10- to 15-minute intervals until adequate analgesia is accomplished. For example, an 18-kg 3-year-old might receive 2 to 3 milligrams as an initial dose—nearly the same as the typical 4-milligram "starting dose" for an adult weighing five times as much.

The specific choice of parenteral opiates is determined by the individual characteristics of the drug, the clinical indication, and the patient's prior experience with opiates. Fentanyl, for example, is associated with less histamine release than the nonsynthetic opioids and has a relatively short duration of action, which makes it useful for short, painful procedures. Hydromorphone has a much higher potency than morphine and may be useful for ongoing pain in children (e.g., sickle cell pain crisis) and in children with extensive prior use of opiates.

Table 113-6 lists pediatric parenteral opiates and their individual considerations. If fentanyl is given as a rapid IV bolus or in high doses to younger patients, it can cause the "rigid chest phenomenon," which may require emergency reversal with naloxone or neuromuscular blockade.

PROCEDURAL SEDATION

Benzodiazepines, ketamine, etomidate, propofol, and nitrous oxide are all well studied agents for ED procedural sedation. Most of these agents have the potential to cause a loss of respiratory drive and airway protective reflexes, and their use is typically limited to physicians specifically credentialed to provide deep sedation who are trained in advanced airway management. Although there are numerous sedative agents that may be used for procedural sedation, it is best to become knowledgeable about and comfortable with only a few agents, to use those agents regularly, and to choose the proper agent or combination of agents most appropriate to the goals of the specific clinical scenario. The traditional continuum of sedation is thought of as starting with moderate sedation (previously called "conscious sedation"), progressing to deep sedation, and then general anesthesia. These terms are fairly arbitrary, however, with considerable overlap. Ketamine is sometimes placed in its own category, "dissociative sedation," because although ketamine causes depressed response to verbal or painful stimuli, it is not expected to have effects on respiratory drive or protective airway reflexes.

In general, procedural sedation can be broken down into five distinct steps:

1. **Determine the indications for sedation and obtain informed consent.**
2. **Assess the patient** to assure that the child is an appropriate candidate for sedation.
3. **Select the appropriate sedative agents.**
4. **Monitor** the patient throughout the procedure.
5. **Provide postsedation monitoring until recovery.**

INDICATIONS FOR SEDATION AND INFORMED CONSENT

Procedural sedation is commonly used for painful procedures and for those requiring motionlessness in the ED (**Table 113-7**). Conversely, there are many common ED procedures that do not routinely need sedation (**Table 113-8**). These are only general guidelines, however, and there is room for individual judgment. Once the decision is made to proceed with sedation, consideration then turns to choosing the proper medication or combination of medications. Obtain informed consent from the responsible adult (see chapter 303, Legal Issues in Emergency Medicine), which involves explaining the anticipated effects and potential adverse effects specific to the medications and procedure.

ASSESS THE PATIENT AND SELECT THE AGENT(S)

Perform a thorough history and physical examination to identify the risk of complications during sedation. Consider contraindications to specific agents at this time. For example, a significant upper respiratory infection or a history of psychosis may make ketamine a poor choice for sedation.

Presedation assessment usually incorporates the American Society of Anesthesiologists classification: (1) normal healthy patient; (2) mild systemic disease; (3) severe systemic disease; (4) severe systemic disease that is a threat to life; (5) moribund patient; (6) brain-dead patient undergoing organ harvest. Children who are in American Society of Anesthesiologists category 3 or higher may not be candidates for elective procedural sedation in the ED, and sedation or general anesthesia in the operating room may be safer. Examples might be children with significant

TABLE 113-7 Indications for Procedural Sedation in Children

Indications for Procedural Sedation in the ED	Examples
Very painful procedures of any length	Reduction of fracture
Moderately painful protracted procedures	Incision and drainage of subcutaneous abscess
Extreme anxiety or developmental barriers when attempts at anxiolysis have failed	Developmentally delayed 14-year-old with simple arm laceration
Need for complete motionlessness	Repair of complex facial laceration in a toddler

TABLE 113-8 Common Procedures Not Usually Requiring Routine Procedural Sedation

Procedures That Do Not Generally Warrant Sedation in the ED	Examples
Short, painless diagnostic procedures	CT scans (other than when IV contrast is given)
Ultra-short painful procedures	Reduction of nursemaid's elbow or subluxed patella
Painful procedures for which adequate analgesia can be provided without sedation	Simple laceration repair, lumbar puncture

congenital heart disease or children who require multiple pharmacologic agents to maintain hemodynamic stability.

Next, perform a focused airway assessment in order to predict a difficult airway *before* problems arise. The **Mallampati grading system** (**Figure 113-2**) is one commonly used means to predict the technical ease of intubation. High Mallampati scores may also predict difficult bag-mask ventilation and airway obstruction if neuromuscular paralytics are given. Pediatric patients with congenital conditions may present challenging airway abnormalities, including trisomy 21 patients with relatively large tongues and cervical spine instability and patients with Pierre Robin's syndrome with micrognathia. If the clinical scenario allows, consider sedation or anesthesia in the operating room for these children.

Determining nil per os (NPO) status is also traditionally emphasized as an important part of the presedation assessment, but **there is no correlation between fasting status and the incidence of aspiration or other untoward outcomes in procedural sedation**. This is particularly true for ketamine, which is the most widely used sedative agent in children. The Pediatric Sedation Research Consortium documented only a single aspiration in 30,037 pediatric sedations outside the operating room, and this single case occurred in a patient who had fasted >8 hours.[10] **There is therefore no evidence to support specific fasting requirements before procedural sedation in the ED.** The American College of Emergency Physicians Clinical Policy on sedation of pediatric patients in the ED states: "Procedural Sedation may be safely administered to pediatric patients in the ED who have had recent oral intake" (Level B recommendation), although clinical judgment in each specific case is still advised.[11]

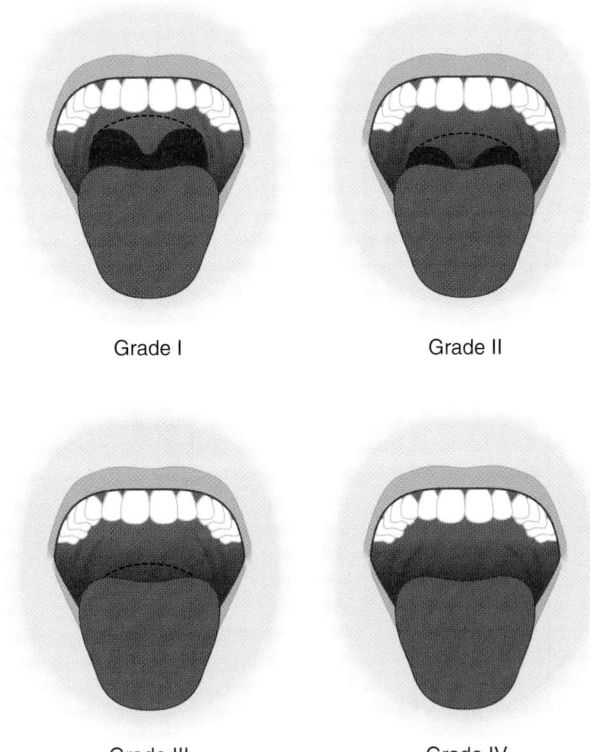

FIGURE 113-2. Mallampati grading scale for airways.

Postoperative vomiting has no relationship to fasting, but vomiting is relatively common after procedural sedation, typically in the recovery phase, and does not usually result in aspiration or other significant adverse outcomes.[10] Depending on the medications used, the risk of vomiting may decrease with pretreatment using ondansetron. For example, the incidence of vomiting decreases if children sedated with ketamine are pretreated with ondansetron. Therefore, **consider routine use of ondansetron with ketamine**, especially in younger adolescents.[12,13]

High-flow oxygen use during ED procedural sedation with propofol reduces the incidence of hypoxemia, but the clinical significance of this remains unclear.[14]

Select Medications for Procedural Sedation Common medications used in procedural sedation in the ED are listed in **Table 113-9**.

Ketamine **Ketamine** is a dissociative anesthetic and is the most commonly used medication for procedural sedation of children in the ED in the United States. It is safe and effective in children of all ages and has anesthetic, analgesic, and amnestic effects. It is relatively short acting, poses little risk of respiratory or cardiovascular depression, and has bronchodilatory effects. However, **it is emetogenic, particularly in adolescents,** and may increase intraocular pressure as well as salivation. Ondansetron administered before sedation with ketamine may reduce the associated nausea and vomiting, which may be particularly true for adolescents and adults.[12] A clinical practice guideline for the ED use of ketamine for procedural sedation has been published and updated in 2011.[15] Specific changes in the 2011 update include the following: (1) expansion of the guideline to include adults; (2) reduction in minimum recommended age to 3 months; (3) removal of minor oropharyngeal procedures and head trauma as contraindications to ketamine sedation; (4) emphasis on IV over IM route when feasible; (5) removal of recommendation for prophylactic anticholinergic medications or benzodiazepines in children; (6) addition of prophylactic ondansetron to prevent vomiting.

Ketamine does not have a typical dose-response continuum with progressive titration. At doses lower than a threshold, analgesia and sedation occur. Once a critical dosing threshold is exceeded (about 1.0 to 1.5 milligrams/kg IV or 3 to 4 milligrams/kg IM), the characteristic dissociative state abruptly appears.[16] This dissociation has no observable levels of depth. The only value of additional ketamine is to prolong the dissociative state for extended procedures.

Sub-dissociative doses (e.g., <1 milligram/kg IV) do have analgesic and amnestic effects despite the lack of a dissociative state. Greater than 90% of children are adequately sedated by a ketamine dose of 1.5 milligrams/kg IV, which is currently the recommended starting dose (1 milligram/kg for adults). Ketamine may also be administered IM at a dose of 4 to 5 milligrams/kg, but IM administration may cause more vomiting and has a prolonged recovery time compared with the IV route. IM ketamine, however, may be advantageous in children in whom IV access is difficult or traumatic (e.g., developmental delay).

Midazolam has often been given along with ketamine to minimize emergence reactions, but research does not support the utility of this practice.[17] The use of anticholinergics such as atropine or glycopyrrolate to reduce salivation as adjuncts to ketamine sedation is also unnecessary and no longer recommended in the current clinical practice guideline.[18]

Opiates are commonly given to children before procedural sedation with ketamine. For example, a painful fracture may be treated with morphine or fentanyl before imaging, with subsequent administration of ketamine for sedation during reduction and splinting. There is no increased incidence of adverse events with the addition of opiates to ketamine.

Propofol **Propofol** is attractive for use in children because of its ultra-short duration of action (shorter than ketamine) and, to a lesser extent, its mildly antiemetic properties. However, propofol provides no analgesia

TABLE 113-9 Medications for Procedural Sedation

Class	Drug	Route	Dose	Onset	Duration	Advantages	Disadvantages	Examples	Comments
Anxiolytic	Midazolam	PO, PR, IV, IM, IN	PO/PR 0.5 milligram/kg IV/IM 0.05–0.1 milligram/kg IN 0.2–0.4 milligram/kg	PO/PR 20–30 min IV 3–5 min IM 10–20 min IN 5–10 min	1–4 h	Flexible route of administration	No analgesia, paradoxical reaction	Premedication for IV start, laceration repair using local anesthetic	Acidic, nasal administration stings, may cause increased secretions; oral/rectal slow onset, less predictable
Hypnotic/sedative	Propofol	IV	1–2 milligrams/kg, followed by 0.5 milligram/kg repeat doses as needed	Seconds	Minutes	Rapid onset and short duration, motionlessness, muscle relaxant	No analgesia, respiratory and cardiovascular depressant	CT scan, LP with topical analgesic, laceration repair, reduction of dislocation	Non-analgesic, increased requirement for younger patients, painful injection
	Etomidate	IV	0.2–0.3 milligram/kg	Seconds	Minutes	Rapid onset, short duration	No analgesia, myoclonus, respiratory depressant	CT scan, short procedures requiring motionlessness	Avoid in patients with increased tone (e.g., CP) due to myoclonic jerks, painful injection
	Pentobarbital	IV	1–2 milligrams/kg, repeated every 3–5 min as needed	<1 min	15–45 min	Well studied, motionlessness, neuroprotective	No analgesia, respiratory and cardiovascular depressant	CT scan, no reversal agent	Variable dosing, long recovery times
	Methohexital	IV	0.5–1 milligram/kg	Seconds	10–60 min	Rapid onset	No analgesia, respiratory and cardiovascular depressant	CT scan, no reversal agent	—
Dissociative	Ketamine	IV, IM	IV 1–1.5 milligrams/kg IM 4–5 milligrams/kg	IV 1–2 min IM 3–5 min	IV 15 min IM 30–45 min	Analgesic, anesthetic, motionlessness, respiratory and cardiovascular stimulant, bronchodilator	Increased intraocular pressure, intracranial pressure, salivation; emetogenic; laryngospasm	Painful procedures requiring motionlessness (complex lacerations, fracture reductions, I & D), no reversal agent	Consider pretreatment with ondansetron; atropine and midazolam co-administration unnecessary
Combinations	Fentanyl + midazolam	IV	Fentanyl 1–2 micrograms/kg, midazolam 0.05–0.1 milligram/kg	1–2 min	1–3 h	Analgesic and anxiolytic	Respiratory depressant	Fracture reduction, reduction of dislocation, laceration repair	Reversal with flumazenil and naloxone
	Propofol + ketamine	IV	Propofol 1 milligram/kg, ketamine 0.5 milligram/kg	1 min	Propofol (minutes); ketamine 15–45 min	Decreased dosing for both agents, complementary side effects (lessens respiratory and cardiovascular depression, emesis)	—	Fracture reduction, I & D, complex laceration	Consider ondansetron pretreatment
Other	Nitrous oxide	Inhaled	Titrate to effect	Minutes	Minutes	Self-dosing	Not readily available	Adjunct to anesthetics	—

Abbreviations: CP = cerebral palsy; I & D = incision and drainage; IN = intranasally.

when used alone, so parenteral, local, or regional analgesics/anesthetics must be co-administered with propofol. Because of its short duration of action and recovery time, overall ED length of stay is decreased when propofol is used compared with ketamine. Propofol may cause hypotension and may cause respiratory depression or apnea. These effects are short-lived and not usually clinically significant.[19] Hypotension from propofol results from a combination of vasodilation and direct cardiac effects and may be exacerbated in hypovolemic patients; administration of crystalloids before sedation with propofol may be prudent in these patients, though the evidence of benefit is mixed.[20,21] Do not administer propofol to children with mitochondrial disorders.[22]

Propofol is ideal for short procedures requiring complete stillness such as neuroimaging and can be given as a single IV bolus (2 milligrams/kg for infants, 1 milligram/kg for older children). It is particularly useful for ultra-short procedures requiring muscle relaxation such as reduction of dislocations. Propofol can be administered as repeated IV boluses in combination with local, regional, or systemic analgesics for longer procedures (e.g., facial laceration repair) or as a bolus followed by continuous infusion at 100 to 200 micrograms/kg/minute. IV administration may cause local burning at the injection site, which can be mitigated with 0.5 milligrams/kg lidocaine either prior to or mixed with propofol.[19]

Propofol and Ketamine The combination of ketamine and propofol is safe and effective, and the use of both agents together had advantages over either agent used alone.[23,24] The two medications have complementary side effect profiles. For example, propofol can cause hypotension and respiratory depression and is an antiemetic, whereas ketamine may cause hypertension and vomiting and has little effect on respiratory drive. When used in combination, lower doses of each agent are used. This results in shorter overall sedation times compared with ketamine alone. In addition, the two medications are pharmacologically compatible and can be given combined in a single syringe (sometimes referred to as "**ketofol**"). The most common practice is to give a bolus dose of combined ketamine and propofol, followed by repeated doses of propofol as needed to maintain the desired level of sedation (ketamine is longer acting, and does not require titration).

Midazolam and Fentanyl Before the widespread use of ketamine and propofol, **midazolam plus opiates—most often short-acting fentanyl**—was the combination of choice for pediatric sedation. This combination provides somewhat less predictable sedation and analgesia, requires careful titration (as opposed to ketamine), and carries the same risks of hypotension and respiratory depression seen with propofol. Although some practitioners still use this combination, ketamine and propofol, with or without adjunct medications, are superior in their effectiveness and safety profile.[25]

Barbiturates **Barbiturates** are useful medications when motionlessness is required, such as for imaging, although propofol is largely replacing their use for this indication. Ketamine is not as useful for imaging due to the fact that it does not reliably induce stillness. Both pentobarbital and methohexital have been used for many years for sedation during radiologic procedures and are particularly useful for imaging in the setting of potential intracranial hypertension.[26,27] The main drawbacks to these agents include hypotension, respiratory depression, and long recovery times (although methohexital is shorter acting than pentobarbital).

Etomidate **Etomidate** is thought to work at the γ-aminobutyric acid receptor to produce hypnosis without analgesia. Most emergency physicians are familiar with etomidate for its use as a sedative during rapid-sequence intubation. When administered for intubation, etomidate provides brief deep sedation with minimal cardiovascular effects, minimal respiratory depression, and maintained or increased cerebral perfusion. Etomidate may be useful for brief, painless procedures requiring stillness, such as neuroimaging. However, etomidate is similar to propofol in that the protective airway reflexes may be briefly reduced or lost, and providers should be prepared to manage the airway when using etomidate for procedural sedation.

Nitrous Oxide Inhaled nitrous oxide is a mild dissociative anesthetic gas that produces anxiolysis, sedation, and analgesia. It is useful for minor procedures such as IV placement and Mediport access. It is commonly administered in up to a 70%/30% mixture with oxygen, has maximal effect within a minute, and wears off quickly upon discontinuation. It does not typically affect hemodynamics, respiratory drive, or protective airway reflexes. It has an excellent and well-documented safety record when used for pediatric procedural sedation in the ED.[28] Nitrous oxide does not reliably produce effective sedation for painful procedures such as fracture reduction, however, which limits its utility as a single agent in the ED. As a result, it must often be combined with other agents such as opioids for efficacy. A good combination, which does not require IV access, is intranasal fentanyl with inhaled nitrous oxide. For laceration repair, nitrous oxide can be combined with topical LET® and/or injected local anesthetics.

A disadvantage of nitrous oxide is that it requires patient cooperation, limiting usefulness in young children. In older patients it can be administered using a self-administered demand valve, which limits the degree of sedation, but in young children it must be given by a continuous flow device. In either case, a gas scavenging system is necessary to prevent inhalation by healthcare personnel. The most common adverse reactions are dizziness and vomiting. Hypoxemia is rare, likely because nitrous oxide is administered in combination with oxygen.

Monitoring During Sedation Some hospital policies require that two physicians must be present throughout the sedation and recovery, but most do not. In an ideal setting, one physician would be responsible for sedation and airway management, and the second would perform the procedure. An experienced pediatric respiratory therapist can sometimes fulfill the role of the second physician.

In instances in which the child may require side or prone positioning (e.g., incision and drainage of buttocks abscess), or when the procedures involve the mouth or airway (dental procedures, intraoral lacerations), establish a plan among all providers for abandoning the procedure and repositioning the patient to open the airway in case of a complication. Suction should be available in the rare event of vomiting during sedation, and providers should be prepared to turn the patient's head in order to avoid aspiration should this occur.

Monitor the child for the entire duration of sedation. Monitored parameters include heart rate, respiratory rate, blood pressure, oxygen saturation, capnography, and electrocardiogram recordings.

Capnography is a noninvasive means to assess baseline end-tidal carbon dioxide at the initiation of sedation and to continuously assess for real-time changes during sedation such as hypoventilation, apnea, or upper airway obstruction. In spontaneously breathing patients, capnography is done with a nasal cannula device, which continuously measures exhaled carbon dioxide, while simultaneously delivering low-flow oxygen (if desired). Capnography can alert the clinician to respiratory depression before it is clinically apparent.[29] It is particularly helpful in situations in which clinical observation is difficult, such as in the radiology suite or when patient positioning makes direct assessment of respiratory effort challenging.

The use of supplemental oxygen during sedation, in the absence of oxygen desaturation, is currently considered optional. The administration of supplemental oxygen during sedation may delay or mask the recognition of hypoventilation. If oxygen is administered, it should be in combination with continuous capnography.

Postsedation Monitoring and Recovery After the procedure, monitor patients until recovery is complete and the child has resumed presedation baseline mental status. Immediately after the procedure, with the cessation of painful stimuli, oversedation and respiratory depression can develop. If using ketamine, even with the addition of ondansetron, nausea and vomiting may occur and should be anticipated. Discharge criteria include the following: normal serial vital signs, including blood pressure and pulse oximetry; return to presedation mental status (if sleeping, the ED staff should be able to easily awaken the patient to presedation mental status); and ability to sit unaided (except when not a baseline skill developmentally). Because nausea and vomiting are common but relatively benign side effects of many sedative agents, a PO trial is not routinely indicated before discharge, although caregivers should be warned that vomiting might occur. Parents should review and understand written postsedation discharge instructions, which warn them to closely observe their child for abnormal somnolence and to restrict activities that require coordination until all medication effects have worn off.

REFERENCES

The complete reference list is available online at www.TintinalliEM.com.

Neonatal Emergencies and Common Neonatal Problems

Quynh H. Doan
Niranjan Kissoon

INTRODUCTION AND EPIDEMIOLOGY

Neonates are infants ≤1 month old, or preterm infants within 30 days of their term due date. Symptoms that precipitate ED visits in neonates are often vague and nonspecific. Signs are usually subtle and may not point to a specific diagnosis. For example, respiratory distress can be caused by pulmonary or cardiac disease, generalized sepsis, abdominal pathology, or metabolic disorders. Many visits occur because of caregiver concerns about normal variants of newborn vegetative functions. Such concerns must be distinguished from potentially life-threatening congenital and acquired conditions that can present in the first month of life. This chapter reviews normal neonatal vegetative patterns, life-threatening neonatal emergencies, and common neonatal problems.

NORMAL NEONATAL VEGETATIVE FUNCTIONS

FEEDING PATTERNS

In the first few weeks of life, expect variation in times between feedings, but by the end of the first month, the vast majority of newborns establish a regular feeding schedule. Most healthy, bottle-fed infants eat 2 to 4 ounces every 2 to 4 hours (six to nine feedings in 24 hours) by the end of the first week of life; breastfed infants prefer shorter intervals—feeding every 1 to 3 hours. Intake is adequate if the neonate gains weight appropriately and appears content between feedings. Feedings are progressing well if the infant is no longer losing weight by 5 to 7 days of age and is gaining weight by 12 to 14 days of age.

WEIGHT GAIN

Weigh neonates completely undressed. Normal newborns may lose up to 12% of their birth weight during the first 3 to 7 days of life, with earlier and slightly more accentuated weight loss in exclusively breastfed newborns. A weight loss of up to 10% is acceptable if the infant's examination, stooling, and voiding frequency and behavior are normal. On average, infants gain between 20 and 30 grams per day in the first 3 months of life and between 15 and 20 grams per day for the next several months.

STOOL PATTERNS

The number, color, and consistency of bowel movements can vary greatly in the same infant and between infants, regardless of diet or environment (**Table 114-1**).

An excessive intake of human milk or maternal use of laxatives increases the water content of the infant's stool. Overfeeding or use of formula that is too concentrated or too high in sugar content also can produce loose stools.

Stool color has no significance unless it is acholic or bloody. The first stool, which consists of meconium, is usually passed within the first 24 hours after birth and is thick, sticky, and black. Transitional stools, which are greenish brown, appear after initiation of milk feeding and are replaced by typical yellow, seedy milk stools 3 to 4 days later. Infrequent bowel movements do not necessarily mean constipation, because breastfed infants may occasionally go 5 to 7 days without a bowel movement. **Failure to pass meconium in the first 48 hours of life may suggest Hirschsprung's disease or cystic fibrosis.**

BREATHING PATTERNS

The normal respiratory rate in neonates is 30 to 60 breaths/min. Newborn breathing is almost entirely diaphragmatic, and the soft front of the thorax is usually drawn inward during inspiration while the abdomen protrudes. Count the respiratory rate for a full minute with the infant resting or preferably asleep. **Neonates increase minute ventilation almost entirely through an increase in respiratory rate rather than inspiratory volume; a neonate with a resting respiratory rate of >60 breaths/min during periods of regular, quiet breathing requires evaluation for the causes of tachypnea.** Observe respirations to determine if breathing is thoracic or abdominal. Thoracic breathing or tachypnea usually signifies intrathoracic or intra-abdominal pathology. Check the nares and upper airway, as neonates are obligate nose breathers, and nasal congestion, or choanal stenosis or atresia, can cause respiratory distress.

Newborn infants, especially those born prematurely, may exhibit **periodic breathing** that is characterized by alternating periods of a normal or fast rate and periods of a markedly slow rate of respiration, with pauses of 3 to 10 seconds between breaths. Irregular respiratory patterns are seen in many premature babies during sleep, but are less common in term infants. **Periods of apnea >20 seconds or apnea accompanied by bradycardia, cyanosis, or a change in muscle tone is abnormal and requires evaluation** (see chapter 115, Sudden Infant Death Syndrome and Apparent Life-Threatening Event).

SLEEPING AND FEEDING PATTERNS

Infants are not born with the ability to sleep through the night. Instead, they awaken every 20 minutes to 6 hours, and sleep periods are spread evenly across the day and night. By 3 months of age, most sleep occurs at night, and by 6 months, most infants are sleeping through the night. Night waking is defined as waking and crying once or more between midnight and 5 A.M. for ≥4 nights per week, for ≥4 consecutive weeks. Night waking occurs in about 25% of bottle-fed infants and about 50% of breastfed infants <12 months old. When the child cries during the night, parents should make sure that there is no physical reason for crying. If there is no physical problem, parents may ignore the crying so that the child learns to fall asleep on his or her own. If parents usually feed the child at that time and the child is about ≥6 months old, the volume of the night feedings should be progressively tapered and then discontinued, so all nourishment is given during the daytime.

TABLE 114-1 Stool Frequency Ranges in Neonates and Infants

Authors	Number	Age	Feed	Mean Number of Stools/d	Range (number of stools/d)
Hyams et al. (1995)[1]	283	1 mo	Breastfed	4.2	0.3–9.6
			Cow's milk formula	2.3	0.4–6.7
			Cow's milk formula with iron	2.1	0.9–4.1
			Soy formula	2.2	0.7–4.1
			Extensively hydrolyzed cow's milk formula	3.6	1.1–8.6
Tham et al. (1996)[2]	140	0–24 mo	Breastfed	4.4	0.3–8.0
			Formula fed	1.6	0.6–3.9

TABLE 114-2 Conditions Associated with Uncontrollable Crying, Irritability, and/or Lethargy in Neonates

System	Emergent	Less Serious
CNS	Intracranial hemorrhage (neonatal alloimmune thrombocytopenia, birth trauma, nonaccidental trauma, vitamin K deficiency)	—
	Meningitis	
	Elevated intracranial pressure	
Eye, ear, nose, throat	Nasal obstruction (choanal atresia or stenosis)	Corneal abrasion, ocular foreign body
		Otitis media
		Nasal congestion (upper respiratory infection)
		Oral thrush
		Stomatitis
Pulmonary	Pneumonia	—
Cardiac	Supraventricular tachycardia	—
	Heart failure	
GI	Volvulus	Gastroesophageal reflux disease (reflux)
	Intussusception	
	Incarcerated hernia	Gastroenteritis
		Anal fissure
		Colic
GU	Testicular torsion	Urinary tract infection
	Genital hair tourniquets	Diaper rash
	Paraphimosis	
Musculoskeletal	Hair tourniquet of finger/toe	Injuries (diaper pin, sharp or irritating objects from clothing)
	Nonaccidental trauma	
Infectious	Sepsis	Upper respiratory infection
	Pneumonia	
	Meningitis	
Metabolic	Inborn errors of metabolism	—
	Hypoglycemia	
	Congenital adrenal hyperplasia	

CRYING

The symptom complex of crying or irritability is fairly common yet difficult to treat, even in the presence of an identifiable cause. Most neonates exhibit varying degrees and periods of crying during a 24-hour period. Total crying time increases after birth, peaking at 3 to 5 months of age. Infants who present with an episode of acute, **inconsolable crying**, however, require careful evaluation for an underlying cause (**Table 114-2**).

THE CRITICALLY ILL NEONATE

Principles of basic life support, pediatric advanced life support, and the Neonatal Resuscitation Program are reviewed in chapter 108, Resuscitation of Neonates. A brief discussion of critical neonatal illness is presented here (**Table 114-3**), with further discussion of specific complaint-based differential diagnosis and management to follow.

For the neonate with respiratory and/or cardiovascular distress, pay primary attention to adequacy of the airway and breathing. There are more stresses and fewer compensatory responses available to the neonate. The neonate has a compliant chest wall and cannot increase inspiratory force; the neonatal airway is small; neonatal metabolism is characterized by high oxygen consumption; and abdominal distention can further impair ventilation. Consider the early use of positive-pressure ventilation or endotracheal intubation for respiratory insufficiency and nasogastric tube placement for gastric distention. **Bradycardia in the neonate is almost always due to respiratory failure and hypoxia and usually corrects with restoration of adequate airway and breathing.**

TABLE 114-3 Causes of Critical Illness in Neonates

Sepsis (bacteremia, urinary tract infection, meningitis)
Congenital heart disease (ductal-dependent lesions)
Pneumonia (bacterial, viral, chlamydia, aspiration)
Bronchiolitis
Congenital anatomic airway anomalies (cleft palate, laryngeal or tracheomalacia, laryngotracheal cleft, tracheal webs, tracheoesophageal fistula, tracheal hemangiomas, and vascular rings)
Neuromuscular disease (infant botulism, muscle weakness)
Inborn errors of metabolism
Congenital adrenal hyperplasia
Intracranial hemorrhage (vitamin K deficiency, nonaccidental trauma)
Abdominal catastrophe (malrotation, volvulus, necrotizing enterocolitis)

Tachypnea can be caused by minor problems, such as gaseous abdominal distention, or life-threatening illnesses, such as sepsis. **True tachypnea (respiratory rate >60 breaths/min) or grunting is an emergency**; admit for further investigations, monitoring, and therapy in all but the mildest cases.

Cardiorespiratory symptoms in neonates are nonspecific and may be due to cardiovascular or respiratory failure or to systemic diseases. Search for pathologic conditions in all organ systems. For example, sepsis, meningitis, gastroenteritis, and metabolic acidosis may cause respiratory distress as the predominant symptom. Regardless of the cause, assess and stabilize the cardiac and respiratory systems before, or simultaneously with, further diagnostic evaluation.

When a specific cause cannot be identified, initiate a full sepsis evaluation (see chapter 116, Fever and Serious Bacterial Illness in Infants and Children) and begin broad-spectrum antibiotics, and add IV acyclovir if there are any findings consistent with or suggestive of exposure to herpes simplex virus.

Conditions discussed in the following sections include common and uncommon symptom complexes in the critically ill neonate: neonatal sepsis; congenital heart disease; pneumonia; bronchiolitis; anatomic airway lesions; inborn errors of metabolism; congenital adrenal hyperplasia; neuromuscular disorders; intracranial hemorrhage; and abdominal catastrophe.

NEONATAL SEPSIS

Overwhelming neonatal sepsis is the most common cause of neonatal cardiorespiratory distress. **Fever or hypothermia** signals serious infection in the neonate. **Fever in the first month of life is a rectal temperature ≥38°C (100.4°F), and hypothermia is a rectal temperature <36.5°C (97.7°F).** Neonates have about twice the risk of serious bacterial infection as do infants 4 to 8 weeks of age. Neonatal sepsis tends to appear as an "**early-onset**" or a "**late-onset**" syndrome, with some overlap. **Early-onset disease** is seen in the first few days of life, tends to be fulminant, and is usually associated with maternal or perinatal risk factors, such as maternal fever, prolonged rupture of membranes, and fetal distress. **Late-onset disease** usually occurs after 1 week of age, tends to develop more gradually, and is less likely to be associated with risk factors. Septic shock and neutropenia are more common with early-onset syndrome, and meningitis is more common in late-onset disease.

Clinical signs of early- or late-onset sepsis are not specific. Septic infants may exhibit any of a variety of symptoms as described in **Table 114-4**. Tachypnea and respiratory distress may be a sign of sepsis, meningitis, or urinary tract infection. Localizing signs may be absent—for instance, nuchal rigidity and Kernig and Brudzinski signs are present in a small minority of neonates with meningitis.

Bacterial causes of neonatal sepsis reflect organisms that colonize the female genital tract and nasal mucosa of caregivers. In general, the two groups of pathogens most frequently encountered are gram-positive cocci,

TABLE 114-4 Signs and Symptoms of Neonatal Sepsis
Temperature instability (fever, hypothermia)
CNS dysfunction (lethargy, irritability, seizures)
Respiratory distress (apnea, tachypnea, grunting)
Feeding disturbance (vomiting, poor feeding, gastric distention, diarrhea)
Jaundice
Rashes

such as β-hemolytic streptococci, and enteric organisms, such as *Escherichia coli* and *Klebsiella* species, and *Haemophilus influenzae. Listeria monocytogenes* also causes sepsis and meningitis in neonates. **Viral infections** are another cause of fever and are most likely due to enteroviruses (coxsackievirus and echovirus) acquired at the time of delivery or respiratory syncytial virus and influenza A virus acquired postnatally. The height of the temperature does not distinguish a viral versus bacterial cause in neonates.

The clinical investigation for neonatal sepsis is similar to that of an older infant except that the threshold for a full sepsis workup, including cerebrospinal fluid analyses, is lower. Admit all neonates to the hospital and initiate treatment with empiric IV antibiotics. Initial treatment of a neonate with suspected bacterial septicemia or meningitis usually includes **ampicillin (50 milligrams/kg to cover group B *Streptococcus* and *Listeria*)** and an **aminoglycoside (gentamicin, 2.5 milligrams/kg) to cover *E. coli* and other gram-negative organisms and possible gram-negative meningitis. Avoid ceftriaxone in neonates as it can cause kernicterus. When gram-negative meningitis is strongly suspected, replace gentamicin with cefotaxime or ceftazidime (50 milligrams/kg)**, which have better CNS penetration. Add **IV acyclovir** for neonates with a maternal history of herpes or suspicious cerebrospinal fluid findings (predominance of lymphocytes and erythrocytes in a nontraumatic lumbar puncture) and all neonates who are ill appearing.[3] For further detailed discussion, see chapter 116.

CONGENITAL HEART DISEASE

Suspect **congenital heart disease** in a well-developed neonate who presents with unexplained cardiorespiratory collapse, cyanosis, and or tachypnea, especially without chest retractions or use of accessory muscles for breathing (see chapter 126, Congenital and Acquired Pediatric Heart Disease). Undiagnosed **congenital heart disease** may be first identified *after* discharge from the newborn nursery and typically becomes symptomatic at one of two distinct time frames: in the first week of life or after the second week of life (see also chapter 126, Congenital and Acquired Pediatric Heart Disease). In the first week of life, lesions dependent on pulmonary or systemic blood flow through the ductus arteriosus (e.g., hypoplastic left heart syndrome, critical coarctation of the aorta) present with shock and acidosis as the duct begins to close. Lesions that involve left-to-right shunting of blood (ventricular and atrial septal defects) typically present after the second week of life with congestive heart failure as pulmonary vascular resistance falls, allowing pulmonary overcirculation and the onset of congestive heart failure.

PNEUMONIA

The lungs are the most common site of infection in neonates. Neonatal pneumonia contributes to significant mortality in developing countries, whereas the incidence of neonatal pneumonia in full-term infants in developed countries is lower. **Table 114-5** displays the various causes, the associated clinical picture, and suggested management of neonatal pneumonia.[4] Chapter 125, Pneumonia in Infants and Children, further addresses pneumonia after the neonatal period.

BRONCHIOLITIS

A detailed discussion of bronchiolitis can be found in chapter 124, Wheezing in Infants and Children. Neonates are at particularly high risk for serious complications from bronchiolitis, because of obligate nose breathing and respiratory mechanics. **Factors that predispose to complications of bronchiolitis include prematurity, underlying pulmonary or congenital heart disease, initial oxygen saturation <92%, and bronchiolitis caused by respiratory syncytial virus.**

Acute bronchiolitis is a clinical diagnosis, and neonates present with nasal discharge and sneezing followed by diminished appetite, difficulty with feeds, cough, dyspnea, irritability, and, occasionally, periods of apnea. Respiratory symptoms include hypoxia, wheezing, retractions, and possibly palpable liver and spleen due to pulmonary hyperinflation. **Bronchiolitis caused by respiratory syncytial virus is associated with apnea, especially in neonates and preterm infants delivered at <34 weeks of gestational age.** While apnea usually presents within the first 3 days of illness, it may develop even if the neonate displays only minimal respiratory distress, and **there are no reliable predictors for the development of apnea.**

Perform a nasal wash for rapid respiratory syncytial virus testing in all neonates and admit those who test positive. Obtain a chest radiograph in critically ill neonates and in those in whom the diagnosis is not clear, although bacterial pulmonary infection is not likely in confirmed viral bronchiolitis. **Obtain a urinalysis in febrile neonates (temperature >38.0°C [100.4°F]), as up to 4% of febrile infants with bronchiolitis have concomitant urinary tract infection.**[5,6] The risk of bacteremia and meningitis associated with bronchiolitis is quite low, and full sepsis evaluation is not needed unless the neonate appears ill.[5,6]

Administer a trial of nebulized racemic epinephrine for treatment of wheezing and evaluate response with respiratory rate and oxygen saturation. Continue racemic epinephrine treatment only if the neonate shows improvement with the first dose. Inhaled β-adrenergic bronchodilators provide no clinical benefits. There is conflicting evidence surrounding the use of corticosteroids. There is no role for antibiotics.

ANATOMIC AIRWAY LESIONS

The anatomically correctable causes of respiratory distress in newborns are less common and include anomalies of the upper respiratory tract (e.g., choanal atresia, laryngomalacia, tracheomalacia, micrognathia, macroglossia, tracheoesophageal fistula, vascular slings) or lower respiratory tract (e.g., congenital lobar emphysema, sequestration, cystic adenomatous malformation, congenital diaphragmatic hernia). Most of these anomalies are identified in the newborn nursery, but in the ED, these diagnoses should be considered in any infant with respiratory distress. Admission is needed for diagnosis.

NEUROMUSCULAR DISORDERS

Any form of muscle weakness may be associated with shallow breathing and a compensatory increase in respiratory rate. **Infantile botulism** is one possible acquired cause and is usually preceded by constipation, followed by a weak cry and feeding difficulties. Ocular palsies, apnea, weakness or hypotonia, and lethargy are late symptoms of botulism. Other causes of hypotonia that may cause respiratory symptoms include Down's syndrome; hypoxic-ischemic encephalopathy; spinal cord lesions, such as myelomeningocele; spinal muscular atrophy; myasthenia gravis; metabolic disorders; and myotonic dystrophy.

INBORN ERRORS OF METABOLISM

Inborn errors of metabolism may manifest as lethargy or respiratory and/or cardiovascular collapse in the neonate. Although the differential diagnosis of inborn errors of metabolism is extensive, the ED evaluation necessitates only a few tests, including bedside glucose, electrolytes, blood gas analysis, serum ammonia, and urine for ketones. More specific testing can wait until after resuscitation. Administer dextrose-containing IV fluids for suspected metabolic disease until specialty consultation can be obtained. For further discussion, see chapter 144, Metabolic Emergencies in Infants and Children.

CONGENITAL ADRENAL HYPERPLASIA

Congenital adrenal hyperplasia is one of the few acute life-threatening endocrine emergencies that present in the neonatal period (see chapter 144,

TABLE 114-5 Neonatal Pneumonia

Etiology	Clinical Presentation	Management Approach
Common bacterial [group B *Streptococcus* (most common), *Escherichia coli*, *Listeria monocytogenes*, *Haemophilus influenzae* B, *S. pneumoniae*, *Klebsiella* species, *Enterobacter aerogenes*]	Fulminant illness with onset within 48 h of birth, with infection likely acquired in utero from contaminated amniotic fluid environment.	Full evaluation for sepsis (blood and urine cultures, chest radiographs, and CBC). Blood culture results are typically negative. Two culture samples may increase diagnostic yield fourfold.
	Respiratory distress, unstable temperature (high or low), irritability or lethargy, tachycardia, and poor feeding may be present.	A lumbar puncture should be done if there are no contraindications.
		Hospitalization, supportive care (oxygen), and parenteral antibiotics (ampicillin and gentamicin; adjust as per culture and sensitivities when available).
Chlamydia	Develops in 3%–16% of exposed neonates (in colonized mothers).	Sepsis evaluation as indicated.
		CXR may show hyperinflation with interstitial infiltrates.
	Usually occurs after 3 wk of age, accompanied by conjunctivitis in one half of cases. Often afebrile, tachypneic, with prominent "staccato" cough. Wheezing uncommon.	Definitive diagnosis by nasopharyngeal swab PCR or cultures.
		Eosinophilia may be seen on peripheral blood count.
		Treatment: macrolide (erythromycin, clarithromycin, or azithromycin).
Bordetella pertussis	In addition to pneumonia, may cause paroxysms of cough ± cyanosis and posttussive emesis in otherwise well-looking infant. Characteristic whoop is not present in neonates. Apnea may be the only symptom. Suspect when adult caregiver also has persistent cough.	Sepsis evaluation as indicated.
		Diagnosis via nasopharyngeal swab for PCR and/or culture.
		Lymphocytosis in peripheral blood count is nonspecific but supports the diagnosis.
		Macrolides are effective against *B. pertussis* but are not approved by the U.S. Food and Drug Administration for infants <6 mo.
		No available data on efficacy of azithromycin or clarithromycin in infants <1 mo old, but case series show less adverse effects with azithromycin.
		Neonates should be admitted during treatment and monitored for adverse effects.
Mycobacterium tuberculosis	Half of infants born to actively infected mothers develop TB if not immunized or treated.	Sepsis evaluation as for bacterial pneumonia.
		CXR, culture of urine, gastric and tracheal aspirates.
	May be acquired by transplacental means, aspiration/ingestion of infected amniotic fluid, or postnatal airborne transmission.	Skin testing not sensitive in neonates.
		Routine anti-TB treatment.
	Often presents with nonspecific systemic symptoms with multiorgan involvement (fever, failure to thrive, respiratory distress, organomegaly).	Supportive treatment as needed.
Viral pneumonia/pneumonitis (herpes simplex virus, respiratory syncytial virus, adenovirus, human metapneumovirus, influenza, parainfluenza)	Initial upper respiratory illness progressing to respiratory distress and feeding difficulty.	Sepsis evaluation as indicated and intravenous acyclovir if HSV is suspected.
	Hypoxia, apnea, and bradycardia (with HSV) may be present.	Viral testing (direct antigen detection/PCR/cultures) of nasopharyngeal washings (swab).
	Often indistinguishable from bronchiolitis.	Rate of concurrent bacterial infections in confirmed viral infection is low.
		CXR for significant respiratory distress.
		Supportive therapy; monitoring for apnea in young and premature infants.

Abbreviations: CXR = chest roentgenogram; HSV = herpes simplex virus; PCR = polymerase chain reaction; TB = tuberculosis.

Metabolic Emergencies in Infants and Children). Although many state newborn screens test for this disorder, infants may present in shock before screening results are known, typically in the first or second week of life. On examination, look for virilization, ambiguous genitalia, and hyperpigmentation. Hyponatremia and hyperkalemia occur in the salt-wasting form of congenital adrenal hyperplasia. Administer hydrocortisone (12.5 to 25.0 milligrams IV/IM/IO) promptly, while undertaking other resuscitative measures. Treat hyperkalemia with standard measurements only if associated with electrocardiogram changes.

INTRACRANIAL HEMORRHAGE

Intracranial hemorrhage, either as a result of birth trauma or nonaccidental trauma, is another consideration in the critically ill neonate. Risk factors include home delivery without administration of vitamin K (associated with hemorrhagic disease of the newborn) or traumatic vaginal delivery. Consider head CT after initial resuscitation if a diagnosis is not apparent or intracranial pathology is suspected.

ABDOMINAL CATASTROPHE

Consider **abdominal catastrophe** in the critically ill neonate with abdominal symptoms. Congenital malrotation can lead to midgut volvulus and intestinal infarction, with bilious vomiting, a distended rigid abdomen, sepsis, and circulatory collapse. Necrotizing enterocolitis, while typically a disease of premature infants, can present in the term neonate with poor feeding; abdominal distension, tenderness, and discoloration; lethargy or irritability; vomiting or diarrhea; temperature instability; apnea; and circulatory collapse. These and other abdominal considerations are discussed in chapter 130, Acute Abdominal Pain in Children, and are reviewed briefly later (see "GI Symptoms").

SYMPTOM-BASED NEONATAL PROBLEMS

Common symptom-based neonatal problems that may result in ED visits include irritability, colic, upper airway complaints, apnea and periodic breathing, GI symptoms, eye complaints, and abnormal movements.

IRRITABILITY

Normal crying was discussed earlier (see "Normal Neonatal Vegetative Functions"), and Table 114-2 lists the important causes of irritability in the neonate. Obtain a thorough history focusing on symptoms other than crying, such as changes in feeding, temperature instability, and vomiting, and perform a systematic head-to-toe examination. Palpate the fontanelles for signs of dehydration (sunken) or infection or intracranial hemorrhage (bulging). If corneal abrasion is possible, examine the eyes with fluorescein staining.[7] Inspect the mouth for oral thrush and check diaper area and groin for rashes, hair tourniquets (also check fingers and toes), and hernias or testicular torsion. Auscultate the heart to appreciate dysrhythmias or murmurs, and observe respiratory effort that may point to a pulmonary or metabolic cause of irritability. Obtain a bedside glucose in all neonates with altered mental status, vomiting, or a history of poor oral intake. Examine the abdomen for tenderness, distension, or discoloration suggestive of intra-abdominal pathology and the extremities for signs of trauma.

If a careful history and complete physical examination reveal no source for the crying and the infant quiets during the ED visit, further testing is unnecessary and parents can be reassured and advised to follow up with their primary care physician.

INTESTINAL COLIC

Colic is a symptom complex consisting of the sudden onset of paroxysmal crying, a flushed face, circumoral pallor, tense abdomen, drawn up legs, cold feet, and clenched fists. The cause is not known. **Colic is defined as a paroxysm of crying for ≥3 hours per day for ≥3 days per week over a 3-week period.** It may begin as early as the first week of life but seldom lasts beyond 3 to 4 months of age. **Infant colic is a diagnosis of exclusion.** Physical examination is normal, and laboratory tests are not required. However, when the diagnosis is unclear, a careful history, physical examination, and appropriate laboratory investigations are necessary to rule out conditions listed in Table 114-2.

There is no specific treatment for colic. Overfeeding without adequate burping during feedings may result in an irritable, crying infant. Improved feeding practices may decrease symptoms.

Administration of drugs or sedatives is contraindicated. A 1-week trial of hypoallergenic formula (non–cow's milk protein) may help. Infant colic can create significant caregiver stress and fatigue and is a risk factor for nonaccidental neonatal trauma. Carefully assess the caretaker's mental health and explore strategies to provide respite if needed.

UPPER AIRWAY COMPLAINTS

Cough and Nasal Congestion Cough associated with sneezing and nasal congestion is usually due to viral upper respiratory infection. Neonates with underlying pulmonary or heart disease such as bronchopulmonary dysplasia or hypoplastic left heart may develop respiratory failure with even mild upper respiratory infections. Inquire about sick siblings and perinatal infectious risk factors. Pay attention to the relation between respiratory symptoms and feeding that might suggest reflux and aspiration, or even congenital tracheoesophageal fistula, as a cause. Respiratory difficulty when quiet and improvement during crying suggest **choanal atresia**. Treat the underlying condition: cough is the infant's primary protective reflex; do not give cough suppressants to neonates. **Over-the-counter cold medications are not effective, may be dangerous in infants, and are contraindicated for children <24 months old.** Treat nasal congestion with instillation of saline drops and bulb suctioning.

Noisy Breathing and Stridor Noisy breathing is a common presenting complaint in neonates and is usually benign, but consider serious underlying pathology. Distinguish between inspiratory and expiratory sounds through careful listening in order to distinguish stertor, stridor, and wheezing. **Stertor** is an inspiratory sound like snoring or snorting that localizes to the nose or nasopharynx and is usually benign, but can be a symptom of choanal stenosis. Inability to pass a small nasogastric tube through the affected nostril is diagnostic of this condition. **Stridor** is a sign of upper airway obstruction and may be evident on both inspiration and expiration. The most common cause of stridor in neonates is **laryngomalacia**, which is characterized by noisy, crowing, inspiratory sounds, usually present from birth, that usually decrease during the first year of life. Nasal pharyngoscopy by an otolaryngologist confirms the diagnosis.

Stridor may also be a symptom of congenital anomalies causing a fixed obstruction anywhere from the nose to the trachea and bronchi, such as webs, cysts, atresia, stenosis, clefts, and hemangiomas. Stridor from fixed lesions is often biphasic, although it may be predominant in either inspiration or expiration. Stridor worsening with cry or increased activity suggests laryngomalacia, tracheomalacia, or subglottic hemangioma (which often become symptomatic after the first few weeks of life). Stridor accompanied by feeding difficulties suggests a vascular ring, laryngeal cleft, or tracheoesophageal fistula. Occasionally an **H-type tracheoesophageal fistula** may present in the first month of life or later with recurrent pneumonia, respiratory distress after feedings, and problems clearing mucus. **Tracheal stenosis** may present initially with noisy breathing or a high-pitched cry and disproportionate respiratory distress with mild upper respiratory infections. Stridor with hoarseness or weak cry suggests **vocal cord paralysis**, which is typically present at birth. Infants who were intubated in the neonatal period may develop **subglottic stenosis** causing stridor. Infection (e.g., croup, epiglottitis, and abscess) as a cause of stridor in neonates is rare and is associated with fever. When the diagnosis is in doubt, admit the neonate for further evaluation, which may include pharyngoscopy, bronchoscopy, radiographs, or even ultrasonography.

APNEA AND PERIODIC BREATHING

Periodic breathing, which occurs in normal neonates, must be differentiated from apnea; however, periodic breathing may precede apnea, and both may occur in the same patient. **Periodic breathing** is alternating periods of a normal or fast respiratory rate with periods of a slow rate of respiration, with pauses of 3 to 10 seconds between breaths. **Apnea is cessation of breathing for ≥20 seconds, or cessation of breathing for a period <20 seconds accompanied by bradycardia, cyanosis, or a change in muscle tone.** It signifies critical illness and warrants investigation and admission for monitoring and therapy. Apnea may be precipitated by any of the disease conditions listed in Table 114-4 and usually indicates respiratory muscle fatigue and impending respiratory arrest. Provide airway and ventilatory support, and search for the cause. If no obvious cause is found, presume sepsis, obtain cultures, and initiate broad-spectrum antibiotics and acyclovir if there is concern for herpes simplex virus. Chapter 115, Sudden Infant Death Syndrome and Apparent Life-Threatening Event, covers conditions associated with apnea in detail.

GI SYMPTOMS

Common GI symptoms that bring neonates to the ED include feeding difficulties, gastroesophageal reflux, vomiting, blood in the diaper, diarrhea and dehydration, abdominal distension, and constipation.

Feeding Difficulties Most visits for feeding difficulties occur because parents perceive that the infant's food intake is inadequate; normal feeding and benign feeding problems are discussed earlier (see "Normal Neonatal Vegetative Functions"). Rarely, anatomic abnormalities may cause difficulty in feeding and swallowing. A careful history usually pinpoints such difficulties as having started at birth, and these infants appear malnourished and dehydrated. Potential causes include upper GI abnormalities (e.g., stenoses, strictures, laryngeal clefts, or cleft palate) and compression of the esophagus or trachea by a double aortic arch. Infants with a recent decrease in intake usually have acute illness, most often infectious, and should be evaluated urgently.

Regurgitation and Gastroesophageal Reflux Regurgitation of small amounts of milk or formula is common in neonates due to reduced lower esophageal sphincter pressure and relatively increased intragastric pressure. **Regurgitation** is independent of effort or muscular contraction and likely represents the ultimate degree of GI reflux. Parents may confuse regurgitation with vomiting. As long as the neonate is gaining weight, parents can be reassured that regurgitation is of no clinical significance and will decrease as the infant grows. Strategies to reduce reflux include thickening of feeds and upright feeding positioning. Infants who are not thriving or have respiratory symptoms related to feeding should be investigated for anatomic causes of regurgitation or chronic aspiration.

Regurgitation rarely results from pathologic processes, such as intrinsic compression of the esophagus or, occasionally, compression of the trachea, in which case it is usually accompanied by stridor and cough.

Dysphagia, irritability, feeding aversion, anemia, and malnutrition are sequelae of chronic regurgitation with esophagitis, but this condition is rare. Investigations such as pH monitoring, endoscopy, and biopsy confirm the diagnosis of reflux esophagitis.

Vomiting **Vomiting** results from forceful contraction of the diaphragm and abdominal muscles. A detailed discussion of vomiting in childhood is provided in chapter 128, Vomiting, Diarrhea, and Dehydration in Children, while surgical conditions that present with vomiting are discussed in chapter 130, Acute Abdominal Pain in Children; those specific to the neonatal period are briefly discussed here.

Vomiting beginning at birth is most likely due to an anatomic abnormality, such as tracheoesophageal fistula (with esophageal atresia), upper GI obstruction (e.g., duodenal atresia, which has a higher incidence among Down's infants), or midgut malrotation. Vomiting may be a symptom unrelated to the GI tract, such as increased intracranial pressure, metabolic disorders, or infections (e.g., sepsis, urinary tract infections, and gastroenteritis).

Pyloric Stenosis **Projectile vomiting** is usually seen in infants with pyloric stenosis and may assume its characteristic pattern, projectile vomiting at the end of feeding or shortly thereafter, after the second and third weeks of life. **Pyloric stenosis classically presents between 6 weeks and 6 months of age and is the most common surgically correctible cause of vomiting in newborns.** The vomitus does not contain bile or blood, and typically the infant appears well with an increased appetite. Perform an abdominal examination with the infant relaxed and the stomach empty. Observe for prominent gastric waves progressing from left to right. Palpate for a firm olive-shaped mass under the liver edge. Observe the neonate feeding to confirm projectile vomiting and distinguish this from regurgitation. Definitive diagnosis is most commonly made with ultrasound examination of the pyloric length and diameter, although barium studies may also make the diagnosis.[8]

The well-appearing infant without dehydration, malnutrition, or electrolyte abnormalities can be discharged with a plan for outpatient surgical correction. Admit ill-appearing or dehydrated infants.

Other Surgical Causes of GI Complaints Emergent surgical causes of vomiting in the neonate include malrotation with volvulus, intussusception, necrotizing enterocolitis, and incarcerated hernia, all of which are discussed in chapter 130.[8]

Blood in the Diaper Parents may come to the ED complaining of blood in the neonate's diaper. Several important distinctions must be made: first, confirm that the discoloration is blood by testing with a guaiac card if possible; it is not uncommon in the neonatal period to find urinary crystals that may cause an orange or red discoloration in the diaper that can be mistaken for blood. If blood is confirmed, the next important distinction is whether the origin is the GI tract or, in girls, the vagina. Bloody or mucous discharge is common and normal in female neonates due to withdrawal from placental estrogen. Physical examination may reveal a small anal fissure as the source of bleeding. **In the first 2 to 3 days of life, blood in the diaper is most commonly due to maternal blood that is swallowed during delivery.** This possibility may be confirmed by the Kleihauer-Betke or Apt-Downey test, performed on a stool sample or scraped from the diaper if possible, which differentiates fetal from maternal hemoglobin in the stool. **After the first few days of life, most causes of blood in the diaper are idiopathic, but consider coagulopathies, necrotizing enterocolitis, allergic or infectious colitis, and congenital defects.** Cow's milk allergy is an immunoglobulin E–mediated disorder, but most infants have cow's milk protein intolerance rather than true allergy. Both conditions cause changes in the bowel mucosa that result in gassy, bloody, and mucous bowel movements; painful feeds; and worsened reflux. Eosinophils may be present in the stool, and the diagnosis may be confirmed by resolution of the problem after cow's milk is removed from the diet. For unresponsive or severe cases, endoscopy and biopsy may be needed for diagnosis. A newborn with a single event of hematochezia and no concerning findings may be observed as an outpatient. Persistent symptoms or concerning exam findings should be further evaluated, and depending on the infant's condition (hydration status and weight gain), admission with appropriate subspecialty care may be necessary (see chapter 131, Gastrointestinal Bleeding in Infants and Children).

Diarrhea and Dehydration Diarrhea and dehydration are discussed in detail in chapter 128, and fluid and electrolyte therapy in chapter 129, Fluid and Electrolyte Therapy in Infants and Children. *Diarrhea* is abnormally frequent and liquid stools (Table 114-1). The modifier *abnormal* is critical because stools can normally be frequent and liquid in young children. Consider infection in addition to feeding-related causes, although infectious diarrhea is predominantly seen in older infants in the United States. Neonates are particularly susceptible to dehydration and electrolyte abnormalities associated with severe diarrhea. In an infant, the normal extracellular fluid volume is 25% of body weight; therefore, a loss of 8% of body weight as extracellular fluid results in severe dehydration.

Weigh all neonates with diarrhea unclothed to allow comparison with previous weights and to provide a baseline for monitoring subsequent weights during the course of the disease. Start the physical examination with a general assessment of mental status and hydration (see Table 129-2).[9] Document rectal temperature, pulse, and blood pressure, which provide additional information concerning the degree of illness. Consider rectal examination to look for anal fissures as a potential source of blood, and obtain a stool sample for detection of occult blood, culture, examination for leukocytes, measurement of pH, and detection of reducing substances.

Obtain serum electrolytes, particularly sodium and glucose, in all neonates with diarrhea and dehydration. Markedly elevated serum urea nitrogen with a relatively normal creatinine may indicate recent or rapid dehydration. Serum creatinine values tend to be low in infants and young children, and a creatinine value of 1 milligram/dL may represent a doubling in the normal value. In addition to stool testing as above, obtain a urine sample in the setting of fever to evaluate for urinary tract infection.

Admit most newborns with ongoing GI losses to the hospital for rehydration, since the loss of even seemingly small volumes of stool may cause severe dehydration in the neonate. Diarrhea, particularly when bloody or containing mucus, may be a symptom of a more severe surgical abdominal process, such as volvulus, intussusception, or necrotizing enterocolitis, although all three of these conditions typically present with vomiting as well.

Abdominal Distention Abdominal distention may be normal in neonates and is usually due to lax abdominal musculature, relatively large intra-abdominal organs, and distension from swallowed air. If the infant is comfortable and feeding well and the abdomen is soft, there is no need for concern. Abdominal distention may also occur in association with bowel obstruction, constipation, necrotizing enterocolitis, or ileus due to sepsis or gastroenteritis. Congenital organomegaly (e.g., hepatomegaly, splenomegaly, or renal enlargement) undetected in the perinatal period also may cause abdominal distention.

Constipation Infrequent bowel movements in neonates do not necessarily mean that the infant is constipated. Infants occasionally may go without a bowel movement for 5 to 7 days and then pass a normal stool. However, if the neonate has never passed stools, especially if there has not been a stool in the first 48 hours of life, consider intestinal stenosis, Hirschsprung's disease, or meconium ileus associated with cystic fibrosis. Constipation occurring after birth but within the first month of life suggests Hirschsprung's disease, hypothyroidism, anal stenosis, or an anteriorly displaced anus. Correct anatomic positioning of the anus is determined by measuring the distance between the gluteal cleft and the posterior fourchette in girls or the median raphe in boys. The anus should be no more anterior than two thirds of this distance. Neonates with constipation should have a careful evaluation of the lumbosacral spine for evidence of occult dysraphism, which may be associated with neurogenic bowel or bladder. The diagnosis of Hirschsprung's disease is supported by absence of feces on rectal examination, a tonic or tight sphincter tone, and an abrupt change in bowel luminal size on barium enema, and is confirmed by a rectal biopsy demonstrating absence of ganglion cells. Infants with hypothyroidism present with constipation, feeding problems, a weak or hoarse cry, a large anterior fontanelle, hypothermia, hypotonia, and peripheral edema. Thyroid testing as part of the routine newborn metabolic screen varies from state to state in the United States.

JAUNDICE (HYPERBILIRUBINEMIA)

Jaundice signifies hyperbilirubinemia and can represent normal newborn physiology or a pathologic process. Bilirubin is a breakdown product of hemoglobin that is conjugated in the liver by glucuronyl transferase before it is excreted with bile into the GI tract. Once bilirubin reaches the intestinal lumen, brush border enzymes deconjugate some of the bilirubin, which is then reabsorbed through enterohepatic circulation. The remainder of the bilirubin is either oxidized by intestinal bacteria to urobilinogen (which is excreted in the urine) or passed in the feces, creating the normal yellow color of neonatal stool. **Physiologic jaundice is characterized by a slow rise in bilirubin (<5 milligrams/dL per 24 hours), with a peak of 5 to 6 milligrams/dL during the second to the fourth days of life and a decrease to <2 milligrams/dL by 5 to 7 days.** Decreased neonatal hepatic glucuronyl transferase activity, a shortened life span of neonatal red blood cells and relative polycythemia, and decreased intestinal bacterial colonization all lead to an increase in enterohepatic circulation that produces the normal rise in bilirubin seen in physiologic jaundice. Other processes, both benign and pathologic, often cause bilirubin levels that are significantly higher than 6 milligrams/dL, and excessive hyperbilirubinemia can lead to permanent brain injury—**kernicterus**. Practice parameters for the evaluation and treatment of neonatal jaundice are summarized in **Table 114-6.**[10]

Distinguishing between physiologic and pathologic neonatal jaundice is important, and the timing of the onset of jaundice in the newborn provides useful clues. **Table 114-7** lists various causes of hyperbilirubinemia in the neonate and their timing.

The evaluation of the jaundiced neonate begins with a thorough history, including maternal infections during pregnancy; maternal blood type and RhoGAM® administration; estimated gestational age (i.e., term or preterm); feeding patterns, including formula or breast milk, frequency, duration, and whether maternal milk supply is adequate and latching successful; stool history, including timing of first stool and transitional stools, color (yellow, acholic), and frequency; regurgitation or vomiting; urine output; and documented fever. A family history of hemolytic anemia or prior neonatal jaundice might indicate an inherited disorder. Review maternal and fetal medications. When possible, obtain results of the infant's blood type and maternal antibody screen.

On physical examination, note the degree of jaundice, which progresses in a cephalocaudal direction, although the level of jaundice does not reproducibly correlate with serum bilirubin levels. Scleral icterus is typically noted with serum bilirubin >5 milligrams/dL. Examine the head for cephalohematoma and assess the fontanelles for signs of dehydration or possible infection. Palpate the abdomen for organomegaly that might signify congenital infection or liver disease.

It is important to distinguish unconjugated hyperbilirubinemia from conjugated hyperbilirubinemia. Unconjugated hyperbilirubinemia is much more common, presents earlier in the neonatal period, and is related to the normal or abnormal breakdown of hemoglobin, although inherited enzyme deficiencies or infection may be pathologic causes. Conjugated hyperbilirubinemia results from the inability to excrete bilirubin into the bile and intestines and is usually the result of primary hepatic or biliary disease such as biliary atresia or hepatitis. Conjugated hyperbilirubinemia is always pathologic and often presents later in the neonatal period with jaundice, acholic stools, and dark urine.

TABLE 114-7 Causes of Jaundice in Neonates

<24 h	Hemolysis due to ABO, Rh incompatibility
	Congenital infection (rubella, toxoplasmosis, cytomegalovirus infection)
	Excessive bruising from birth trauma (cephalohematoma or intramuscular hematoma)
	Acquired infection (e.g., sepsis, pneumonia)
2–3 d	Physiologic
3 d–1 wk	Acquired infection (e.g., sepsis, urinary tract infection, pneumonia)
	Congenital decrease in glucuronyl transferase (e.g., Crigler-Najjar syndrome, Gilbert's syndrome)
	Congenital infections (syphilis, toxoplasmosis, cytomegalovirus infection)
>1 wk	Breast milk jaundice
	Acquired infection (e.g., sepsis, urinary tract infection, pneumonia)
	Biliary atresia
	Congenital and acquired hepatitis
	Red cell membrane defects (e.g., sickle cell anemia, spherocytosis, elliptocytosis)
	Red cell enzyme defects (e.g., glucose-6-phosphate dehydrogenase deficiency)
	Hemolysis due to drugs
	Endocrine disorders (hypothyroidism)
	Metabolic disorders (galactosemia, fructosemia)
	Pyloric stenosis

At a minimum, laboratory studies for the jaundiced neonate should include a direct and indirect bilirubin. Transcutaneous bilirubin measurement correlates fairly well with total serum levels but does not distinguish conjugated and unconjugated bilirubin. Transcutaneous measurement is thus limited to very low-risk neonates with a normal physical examination.[11,12] When other pathologic conditions are suspected, the evaluation should be determined by the differential diagnosis and may include a CBC for anemia and red cell indices, a blood smear for hemolysis, reticulocyte count, and liver function tests. When infection is a concern, obtain appropriate cultures and Gram stains (urine, cerebrospinal fluid).

Septic infants with hyperbilirubinemia may have an increase in bilirubin by greater than the acceptable 5 milligrams/dL per 24-hour period and have other features of sepsis, such as vomiting, abdominal distention, respiratory distress, and poor feeding. **Breast milk jaundice** is thought to be due to the presence of substances that inhibit glucuronyl transferase in the breast milk; it may start as early as the third to fourth day and reaches a peak of 10 to 27 milligrams/dL by the third week of life. Although cessation of breastfeeding will result in a rapid decline of bilirubin over 2 to 3 days, it is not routinely recommended. **Breast milk jaundice is unlikely to cause kernicterus and usually can be treated with phototherapy, when necessary.** This should be distinguished from *breastfeeding jaundice*, or *starvation jaundice*, which can occur when a

TABLE 114-6 Neonatal Risk and Bilirubin Treatment Threshold for Hyperbilirubinemia

	Age of Neonate						
Bilirubin Treatment Threshold (milligrams/dL)	24 h	48 h	72 h	96 h	5 d	6 d	7 d
Low-risk neonates*	12	16	19	21	22	23	23
Intermediate-risk neonates†	9	13	15	16	17	17	17
High-risk neonates‡	8	11	13	14.5	15	15	15

*Full-term, well-appearing, and no risk factors (isoimmune hemolytic disease, glucose-6-phosphate dehydrogenase deficiency, asphyxia, lethargy, temperature instability, sepsis, acidosis, hypoalbuminemia [<3.0 grams/dL if measured]).

†Thirty-five to 37 6/7 weeks estimated gestational age without risk factors, or term with risk factors.

‡Thirty-five to 37 6/7 weeks estimated gestational age with risk factors.

newborn is exclusively breastfed and the mother's milk supply is still inadequate. *Poor oral intake* resulting in reduced bowel movement and bilirubin excretion through the GI tract, coupled with relative dehydration, may accentuate physiologic jaundice. Optimizing the neonate's feeding pattern with controlled supplementation, whether with expressed breast milk, donated breast milk, or formula, usually resolves the problem, but severe hyperbilirubinemia may require treatment.

The treatment of hyperbilirubinemia depends on the cause, but for most cases of unconjugated hyperbilirubinemia, phototherapy is sufficient. **Phototherapy** causes a configurational change in the bilirubin structure that allows it to be excreted in the urine. There is no additional benefit to IV fluids coupled with phototherapy, so enteral feeding should always be encouraged, although the dehydrated infant may require fluid resuscitation. Extreme levels of hyperbilirubinemia are treated emergently with exchange transfusion and require admission to hospital.

Risk factors include hemolysis risks (e.g., isoimmune hemolytic disease, glucose-6-phosphate dehydrogenase deficiency, ABO incompatibility), sepsis (lethargy, temperature instability, irritability), asphyxia, hypoalbuminemia, and acidosis. In the first 24 hours of life, response to phototherapy is less predictable, and specific exchange transfusion indications are less certain during this period.

EYE COMPLAINTS

Watery Eyes Clear eye discharge, and occasionally crusting over of the eyelashes without associated conjunctival redness or irritation, is commonly seen in neonates and infants and results from narrow or obstructed nasolacrimal ducts. This condition usually resolves spontaneously and requires antibiotics only when complicated by conjunctival erythema and inflammation (conjunctivitis or dacryocystitis). Ophthalmologic consultation for nasolacrimal duct probing is appropriate if this problem persists past 12 months of age or earlier if complicated by recurrent infection.

Red Eye and Irritation Corneal irritation or abrasion can result from an eyelash or scratch from a fingernail. Perform fluorescein staining and evaluate with a Wood's lamp or a hand-held slit lamp to identify **corneal abrasions**. **Acute glaucoma**, although rare, also presents as a red, teary eye. The cornea is cloudy, the anterior chamber is shallow, and the intraocular pressure may be increased. Promptly consult pediatric ophthalmology for all suspected cases of glaucoma.

Red Eye and Discharge Conjunctivitis is described in detail in chapter 119, Eye Emergencies in Infants and Children. The most common causes of neonatal conjunctivitis are chemical irritation, bacterial or chlamydial infection, and herpes simplex infection. **Chemical conjunctivitis** due to ocular prophylaxis usually occurs on the first day of life and requires no treatment.

Gonococcal conjunctivitis generally has its peak time of onset between 3 and 5 days after birth. Despite antibiotic prophylaxis at delivery, the failure rate of prophylaxis is about 1%. *Neisseria gonorrhoeae* invades superficial layers of the conjunctiva and, if untreated, causes corneal ulceration and can result in permanent loss of vision. For diagnosis, obtain a Gram stain and culture for *N. gonorrhoeae*. Treat gonococcal conjunctivitis with cefotaxime (50 milligrams/kg IV or IM). **Cefotaxime is recommended for neonates, as ceftriaxone can displace bound bilirubin and precipitate kernicterus.** Perform septic workup including lumbar puncture. Disseminated disease should be suspected until CSF cultures are negative. Supportive care includes ocular irrigation with normal saline as soon as diagnosis is suspected, with frequent irrigation until the discharge is eliminated. Admit the neonate and obtain ophthalmology consultation. Topical antibiotic treatment alone is inadequate and unnecessary when systemic antibiotic treatment is given.

Chlamydial conjunctivitis becomes evident by the end of the first week throughout the first month after birth. The disorder varies in severity, from mild to severe hyperemia with a thick, profuse mucopurulent discharge and pseudomembrane formation. There often is severe edema of both lids. Because isolation of *Chlamydia trachomatis* requires specialized tissue cultures, assure proper technique in collecting culture specimens (e.g., Dacron swabs) and specimens for antigen detection.

Treat chlamydial conjunctivitis and pneumonia in neonates with oral erythromycin (50 milligrams/kg PO per day in four divided doses, for 14 days). Oral sulfonamides may be used after the immediate neonatal period for infants who do not tolerate erythromycin. Topical treatment is unnecessary. Because the efficacy of erythromycin therapy is approximately 80%, a second course is sometimes required. A specific diagnosis of *C. trachomatis* infection in an infant should prompt the treatment of the mother and her sexual partners.

The finding of vesicles anywhere on the skin or mucous membranes in association with neonatal conjunctivitis suggests **herpes simplex infection** and warrants a full sepsis evaluation with cerebrospinal fluid evaluation for herpes simplex virus and treatment with acyclovir, 20 milligrams/kg/dose three times a day.

ABNORMAL MOVEMENTS AND SEIZURES

Seizures are covered in detail in chapter 135, Seizures in Infants and Children. It is important to distinguish benign sleep myoclonus in infancy and the **normal startle reflex** from actual seizures. **Sleep myoclonus** consists of rhythmic myoclonic jerks observed when the infant is drowsy or in quiet sleep and can be suppressed upon touching and/or waking the infant; the startle reflex is a single myoclonic jerk with extension of the arms and legs triggered by noise or tactile stimulation. Tetany due to **hypocalcemia** is associated with congenital syndromes, such as DiGeorge's syndrome, and must also be distinguished from **seizure** activity. Recognition of seizures in the newborn period is important, because seizure management and outcome are different than at any other age. Neonatal seizures are likely to present with subtle manifestations, such as eye deviation, tongue thrusting, eyelid fluttering, apnea, pedaling movements, or arching, rather than generalized activity. Neonatal seizures usually indicate a severe underlying structural or metabolic problem and are rarely idiopathic.

Acknowledgment: The authors gratefully acknowledge the contributions of Tonia J. Brousseau, the lead author of this chapter in the previous edition.

REFERENCES

The complete reference list is available online at www.TintinalliEM.com.

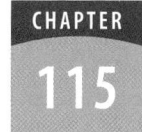

Sudden Infant Death Syndrome and Apparent Life-Threatening Event

Ilene Claudius
Joel S. Tieder

SUDDEN INFANT DEATH SYNDROME

Sudden infant death syndrome (SIDS) is the unexpected death of infants <1 year old for which no pathologic cause can be determined by a thorough history, physical examination, postmortem examination, and environmental investigation. **SIDS is a diagnosis of exclusion.** The syndrome has been a leading cause of death of infants between 1 month and 1 year of age. In the past, between 5000 and 10,000 infants (1 to 2 per 1000 live births) succumbed yearly to SIDS. With recent changes in infant sleep position, the number of deaths has decreased to about 2200, or 0.57 deaths per 1000 infants.[1] Certain autopsy features seem relatively consistent among infants succumbing to SIDS, including intrathoracic petechial hemorrhages, thyromegaly, encephalomegaly, microcardia, unclotted blood in the heart, kidney growth restriction, and an empty bladder and rectum.[2] *Sudden unexplained infant death* is a broader term that includes all unexpected deaths, including cases of SIDS as well as deaths for which a cause is found, such as channelopathies and disorders of fatty acid oxidation.[3]

EPIDEMIOLOGY

The peak incidence is between 2 and 4 months of age. SIDS is rare in the first month of life, probably because neonates have a better anaerobic capacity for survival and may be able to raise their Pa_{O_2} over 20 mm Hg with a gasp. There are a disproportionate number of SIDS deaths in lower socioeconomic groups, although this is true for deaths in infancy from all causes. There is ethnic variation, with Asian Americans at lower risk and African Americans and Native Americans at higher risk. It is more common for mothers of SIDS victims to be <20 years old, unwed, smoke, use drugs, and have made few prenatal and postpartum visits. Prenatal and postnatal maternal smoking increases the incidence of SIDS. SIDS is more likely to occur during the winter months and when the infant is asleep. Thirty percent to 50% of SIDS patients have some acute infection, usually an upper respiratory tract infection, at the time of the event. Otitis media and gastroenteritis also have been associated with SIDS.

Sleep position has received a great deal of attention as a modifiable SIDS risk factor. The prone sleep position is associated with an increased odds ratio of 4.92. In clinical trials, prone infants were found to rebreathe expired air and experience hypercarbia.[4] In addition, infants normally dissipate heat through their head, and prone sleeping may inhibit heat loss, thereby exacerbating hyperthermia, another noted risk factor for SIDS.[5] A disproportionate number of infants succumb to SIDS while with a babysitter.[6] Many of these infants are found in the prone position. For some infants, this is the first time they have been placed in the prone position, and investigators have proposed that these infants have poor strength and tone in their neck muscles. Side-sleeping is also considered a risk factor for SIDS and discouraged. Because of these observations related to the prone position, the American Academy of Pediatrics has recommended a supine sleeping position for normal infants since 1992 and issued a useful statement in 2011 addressing specific issues related to sleep. Among the recommendations is an acknowledgement that the supine sleeping position does not increase aspiration risk in infants with gastrointestinal reflux and should apply to premature infants as well, even in neonatal intensive care units, as soon as they are medically stable. Infants should be placed on a firm mattress in a crib, bassinet, or portable crib (rather than adult bed), and protected from overheating. Bed sharing is discouraged, particularly in situations where the infant is <3 months of age; if the parent is a smoker, excessively tired, or on sedative substances; or on soft surfaces such as couches or beds with soft bedding.[7] Prone sleeping, bed sharing, or sleeping in a location other than a crib or bassinet was associated with 92.2% of SIDS deaths.[8] A recent paper found sofas to be a particularly hazardous sleep environment, accounting for 12.9% of sleep-related infant deaths.[9]

Other risk factors include pre- or postnatal smoke exposure, prenatal drug exposure, overweight status of infant or mother, low birth weight, and prematurity.[2] Use of a pacifier,[10] breastfeeding,[11] and immunizations[12] are protective against SIDS. Home monitoring has not been shown to prevent SIDS.[13] Although a recognized case of abuse would not meet the criteria for SIDS, 1% to 5% of cases of sudden unexplained death in infancy are attributable to infanticide.[14] Familial cases of "SIDS" raise the possibility of abuse. The presence of traumatic head injury, bruises, long-bone fractures, rib fractures, internal hemorrhages, evidence of physical neglect, or blood around the nares suggests abuse.[15] A history inconsistent with the usual events surrounding a SIDS death also may raise the suspicion of abuse. Some infants with abusive head trauma may present with nonspecific symptoms, including apparent life-threatening events.[16]

PATHOPHYSIOLOGY

The etiology and pathophysiology of SIDS remain unclear despite continued investigation. Over the years, >70 different theories have been proposed to explain SIDS, including suffocation from sleeping with a parent (overlaying), milk allergy, and thymic enlargement. Because most SIDS victims are found dead in their cribs, early theories emphasized the role of apnea and ventilatory control, as well as possible cardiac etiologies. Although cardiac dysfunction related to prolonged QT interval or Wolff-Parkinson-White syndrome has been reported,[17] prospective studies monitoring infants failed to show antecedent dysrhythmia in infants who subsequently succumbed to SIDS. More recent studies on the brains of infants who have died from SIDS demonstrate the presence of medullary serotonergic (5-hydroxytryptamine) pathology, including abnormal firing, synthesis, release, and clearance,[18,19] and morphologic differences in the brainstem.[20] Autonomic dysfunction has recently been postulated to play a role.[21] Currently, emphasis is placed on the interplay between developmental factors related to autoregulation, arousal, and environmental stressors. The triple-risk model for SIDS[22] hypothesizes a "perfect storm" of underlying vulnerability, a critical period of development, and exogenous stressors. Factors contributing to underlying vulnerability can include age <6 months, genetic factors, male gender, race, poverty, or prenatal exposure to cigarettes, alcohol, and illicit drugs. Although no single genetic locus for SIDS has been identified, the 10-fold increased risk among the siblings of SIDS victims suggests a genetic component. Recently, polymorphism in the interleukin-10 gene promoter has been associated with SIDS and sudden unexpected death associated with infection.

CLINICAL FEATURES AND MANAGEMENT

Generally, SIDS victims present in one of two ways: not amenable to resuscitation or potentially responsive to resuscitation measures. **Infants with rigor mortis, livedo reticularis, pH <6, and a significantly reduced core temperature in the absence of a history of environmental hypothermia should not be resuscitated.** On the other hand, the warm infant with apnea and no pulse may benefit from attempts at resuscitation. Regardless of the presentation of SIDS, obtain a thorough history and perform a complete physical examination. Important questions include complete description of the circumstances, caretakers, recent illness, prenatal and birth history, maternal and family history of miscarriages or other infant deaths, and family history of metabolic disease. For epidemiologic information, documentation of sleep position, sleep location, when and by whom the infant was last seen alive, when and in what position the infant was found, and whether or not bed sharing was involved is helpful to the coroner. Examination of the infant may be unrevealing or may show subtle though relevant signs of trauma, such as facial bruising, petechiae, or a torn frenulum, raising suspicion of inflicted trauma. Physical data, including rectal temperature, blood in the nose or the mouth, presence of petechiae on the face or conjunctiva, apparent injuries, and presence of rigor mortis or lividity, will help the coroner in determining an approximate time of death and the likelihood of suffocation or abuse.

The management of a nonresuscitative SIDS infant and the infant's family is challenging for the entire team. The emergency provider is confronted by a distraught caregiver who often has found the baby cold, blue, and lifeless only hours after having fed the infant. Frequently, valiant, albeit unsuccessful, efforts are carried out in the ED, or the infant is revived briefly, only to succumb after several hours in the intensive care unit. The major responsibility of the physician is then to notify, counsel, and educate the family. Frequently, the family wants to spend time with the deceased infant. **In general, the infant's body should not be manipulated or photographed after death has been declared unless permission is granted by the coroner.** If the family wants a hand or footprint, inkless pads must be used, and this must be documented in the medical record. Do not remove any lines or tubes placed during attempted resuscitation. If the presence of tubing is disconcerting to the family, tubes may be cut at the skin to appear less obvious. Unless directed otherwise by the coroner, the family should be allowed to hold the deceased infant in a private setting that allows discrete monitoring of the family.

In most jurisdictions, victims of sudden and unexplained deaths must be reported as soon as possible to the coroner's office. **As treating physician, complete the form reporting the death, but do not sign the official death certificate, as the cause of death will not be evident until the coroner's investigation is finished.** SIDS is technically a postmortem diagnosis, and *sudden unexpected death in infancy* is a more appropriate term for an ED record. If blood samples were drawn, put the samples on hold in the laboratory for later access by the coroner. Once death has been pronounced, the physician does not have jurisdiction to perform postmortem sampling or radiography unless directed to do so by the coroner.

A home scene investigation is often conducted. Some jurisdictions have infant death teams that fully evaluate the circumstances surrounding the unexpected death of young infants. If the physician believes the infant is a victim of SIDS, the family should be so advised but told that the final confirmation awaits the autopsy report. Involving the primary care provider, who may follow up on the autopsy and remain in contact with the family, is of paramount importance. The hospital chaplain or social worker may provide additional support, and a chaplain consult may be especially needed in cases in which the laws regarding autopsy before burial are at odds with the family's religious doctrine. For infants requiring a perimortem baptism, this is ideally done by a chaplain but can be performed by a medical provider if no chaplain is available. Most communities have organizations for parents of SIDS victims, and information about these organizations can be obtained from First Candle (1-800-221-SIDS, www.firstcandle.org). Parents also may be referred to Web sites such as http://www.sidsfamilies.com. Some states also require notification of organ procurement agencies.

APPARENT LIFE-THREATENING EVENT

An apparent life-threatening event (ALTE) is an episode that is frightening to a caregiver and involves some combination of apnea, color change (cyanosis, pallor, or plethora), change in muscle tone (limp or stiff), choking, or gagging.[23] An ALTE is a description of a constellation of symptoms, not a diagnosis. The term *ALTE* is defined by subjective symptoms, and often clinicians must interpret historical information from nonmedical caregivers. For example, without a respiratory monitor, quantifying change in color or change in respiratory effort is challenging, even for medical providers. Currently, the American Academy of Pediatrics is developing a practice guideline with recommendations for the definition, diagnosis, and management of ALTEs.

EPIDEMIOLOGY

The true incidence of ALTE is difficult to ascertain but likely ranges from 0.05% to 6.0%, depending on the population studied.[24] Between 0.2% and 0.9% of infants have an ALTE resulting in admission, yielding an incidence of 200 per 10,000 admits per year for this diagnosis. However, when parents are questioned regarding periods of prolonged apnea, 4% to 6% recall such an event.[24] The peak incidence is between 1 week and 2 months of age, with the majority of ALTEs occurring before 10 weeks of age.[25] The male-to-female ratio is 2:1.[26] Known risk factors for ALTE include respiratory syncytial virus infection, prematurity, recent anesthesia, gastroesophageal reflux, and airway/maxillofacial anomalies.

PATHOPHYSIOLOGY

Apnea is typically characterized as central, obstructive, or mixed. **Apneic pauses of >20 seconds or those associated with changes in color, tone, or heart rate are considered pathologic.** *Central apnea* implies a disruption in the central respiratory centers resulting in a cessation of respiratory effort. There is no attempt to breathe. *Normal periodic breathing* is characterized by pauses of several seconds in respiration between normal to rapid periods of breathing. Infants with *obstructive apnea* appear to be attempting to breathe through an occluded airway, with paradoxical movements of the chest and abdomen and a dip of 3% or greater in oxygen saturation.[27] Many parents describe components of both central and obstructive apnea, indicating a *mixed picture*. *Apnea of prematurity* is a disorder in the control of breathing in premature infants, occurring in up to 25% of this group.[28] Its frequency decreases with increasing maturity, and it is usually outgrown by 37 weeks of postconceptual age but occasionally persists a few weeks past term.[29] **An ALTE occurring in a premature infant who has reached 37 weeks of postconceptual age and is without a recent history of apnea of prematurity should be investigated with the assumption that there is a new underlying etiology.**

Changes in infant skin color are often difficult for caretakers to characterize and may represent cyanosis, plethora, or pallor. The color change may be a manifestation of normal infant physiology (e.g., acrocyanosis) or may indicate more serious problems with perfusion or oxygenation (e.g., central cyanosis). Cyanosis becomes apparent when at least 5 grams/100 mL of blood is deoxygenated. Because young infants are often polycythemic, this threshold is more easily met in this age group, and cyanosis may be observed in normal newborns, typically seen in the dense perioral veins or in the distal extremities (acrocyanosis), due to vasomotor instability. Both of these entities are benign. Normal infant polycythemia can also lead to a ruddy appearance (plethoric), which, in the crying infant, may be misinterpreted by lay caregivers as cyanosis or "purple" coloring. Pallor is characteristic of the vasovagal response and can be seen in association with a gastroesophageal reflux event.

In neonates, changes in muscle tone are difficult to classify, because baseline neurologic status is variable due to immaturity. Seizures in infants uncommonly present as stereotypical tonic-clonic activity and are more likely to present with altered consciousness or intermittent high and low tone. In addition, infants may exhibit changes in tone (either decreased or increased) in the postictal state. Changes in tone may also be secondary to hypoxia resulting from apnea. Stiffening and arching behavior have been well described in infants with gastroesophageal reflux events (Sandifer's syndrome).

Choking, gagging, and coughing are also common symptoms in infants and may be due to gastroesophageal reflux, overfeeding, or incoordination of the normal suck-swallow-breath sequence. The latter can be exacerbated by congestion from an upper respiratory infection. Rarely, congenital anatomic malformations, such as tracheoesophageal fistula, may lead to choking, gagging, or coughing with feeds. Some respiratory infections, such as pertussis and respiratory syncytial virus, may be associated with a number of observed changes that are part of the ALTE diagnostic criteria: coughing (which may be staccato in pertussis), gagging (from thick mucus secretions in respiratory syncytial virus), color changes (including true cyanosis), and stiffening or loss of tone are well described. Apnea has also been described in the setting of both pertussis and respiratory syncytial virus, and may occur in the absence of significant congestion, nasal discharge, cough, or work of breathing, particularly in neonates.

DIFFERENTIAL DIAGNOSIS

In the case of an ALTE for which no cause is identified after a reasonable workup, the term *idiopathic ALTE* is applied. A large literature review on this topic indicated that 26% of 643 patients studied were termed idiopathic,[30] whereas the European Society for the Study and Prevention of Infant Death found that number to be as high as 50%.[31] Assigning a specific diagnosis in the ED is not unreasonable, but in a study of patients admitted through the ED, the final diagnosis was changed by the time of ward discharge in 51% of cases. Therefore, initial diagnoses may be viewed with some uncertainty. **Table 115-1** lists common, uncommon, and rare diagnoses assigned to patients presenting with ALTE. More common processes are discussed independently below.

GASTROESOPHAGEAL REFLUX

As a final diagnosis, gastroesophageal reflux is among the most common and the most controversial of the potential sources for ALTE. Gastroesophageal reflux is the involuntary passage of gastric contents into the esophagus, and it occurs daily in children during the first year of life. This form of reflux, commonly characterized by frequent "spitting up," is entirely normal and should be considered physiologic. Pathologic gastroesophageal reflux disease, however, is defined as regurgitation of gastric contents into the esophagus with accompanying symptoms and complications such as failure to thrive. If ALTEs are recurrent and appear to be related to gastroesophageal reflux disease, then empiric treatment is indicated, including small, frequent, and upright feedings. Medications used to alter the acidity of the gastric contents are indicated.[32]

Given the temporal correlation between peak age for ALTE and that of gastroesophageal reflux, and the fact that reflux of gastric contents into the hypopharynx can trigger laryngospasm, a diagnosis of gastroesophageal reflux disease provides an easy explanation for an ALTE.

TABLE 115-1 Reported Final Diagnoses for Patients Presenting with Apparent Life-Threatening Event

Common Diagnoses	Less Common Diagnoses	Rare Reported Diagnoses
Seizure/febrile seizure	Pertussis	Arrhythmia or other cardiac process
Gastroesophageal reflux	Inflicted injury	
Respiratory tract infection (upper or lower tract)	Poisoning	Anemia
	Serious bacterial infection	Breath-holding spell
Misinterpretation of benign process such as periodic breathing	Electrolyte abnormality (including glucose)	Metabolic disease
Vomiting/choking episode		Anatomic maxillofacial obstruction

However, researchers have been unable to demonstrate a temporal relationship between episodes of gastroesophageal reflux on pH probe and ALTEs or apneic events,[33,34] and the literature on the topic is mixed. Some studies have shown a decrease in repeated brief apneas after initiating appropriate medications in patients with gastroesophageal reflux disease.[35] Other studies demonstrate that reflux events may be unrelated,[36] secondary to apnea,[33] or even protective in stimulating a patient out of succumbing to an apneic episode.[37] Moreover, the risk of a recurrent ALTE among patients diagnosed with gastroesophageal reflux disease is not significantly different than with a negative pH probe (relative risk 1.26).[38]

BRONCHIOLITIS

A number of studies have reported an increased risk of both central and obstructive apnea during respiratory infections in infants, especially respiratory syncytial virus bronchiolitis. Dysregulation of mucosal immune responses and sensorineural stimulation have been postulated.[39,40] Obstructive apnea commonly occurs when infants choke on respiratory secretions. Episodes of central apnea have also been demonstrated during sleep in infants with bronchiolitis.[41] Diagnosis can be difficult, because **apnea may be the first presenting symptom of bronchiolitis**. Apnea on presentation is a risk factor for recurrent apnea with bronchiolitis, as is younger age, lower temperature, higher $P{CO_2}$, or radiographic signs of atelectasis.[42,43] Most studies have been performed on clinical or respiratory syncytial virus–proven bronchiolitis, but recently, the same association was found with metapneumovirus-associated bronchiolitis.[44] A recent paper by Wilwerth et al[43] found a 2.7% rate of apnea among infants admitted with bronchiolitis. All patients with apnea in this study were <1 month of age if full-term or 48 weeks of postconceptual age if premature or had a history of apnea upon presentation to the ED.[43] Use of over-the-counter cough and cold medications may contribute to the increased risk of apnea during a respiratory illness, and these medications have been withdrawn from the market. However, these medications can often be obtained by prescription or as adult medications, and it is prudent to counsel parents not to use them.

SEIZURES

Seizures have been identified in 4% to 7% of infants with ALTE and may be obvious or subtle when associated with apnea. In younger infants, apnea may be the sole manifestation of a seizure.[45] Interictal electroencephalograms may be normal, making the diagnosis challenging. Rarely, seizures are secondary to underlying causes such as congenital brain malformation, metabolic disorders, electrolyte abnormalities, perinatally acquired brain injury, or intracranial bleeding (including abusive head injury), and these possibilities must be considered. One study of infants presenting with an ALTE caused by a seizure found that 11% were eventually diagnosed as child abuse, 3.6% developed chronic epilepsy, and 3% developed developmental delay. This paper concluded that, although an inpatient workup is not mandatory, close follow-up must be ensured.[46]

CHILD ABUSE/POISONING

Child abuse is reported in 1.4% to 2.5% of infants presenting with ALTE.[47-49] **Suffocation, abusive head injury, and poisoning are among the most concerning possible causes of an ALTE.** Truman and Ayoub[50] reported a high risk of future death or recurrent ALTEs among children presenting with fresh blood from the nose/mouth, and an increased risk of moderate to high suspicion for nonaccidental trauma in infants >6 months of age with ALTE. Southall et al[51] performed covert video surveillance in a highly selective population of recurrent ALTE patients considered suspicious for abuse, which confirmed abusive behavior in 33 of 39 cases. Interestingly, 29% of the siblings of this group had died unexpectedly. Southall's group also found an association between intentional suffocation and bleeding from the nose and mouth, as well as high rates of marital dissatisfaction and personality disorders among the parents.[51] One study (with small numbers) found subsequent abuse-related death to occur in 9% of patients followed for 12 months after an ALTE due to abuse.[52] Poisoning as a cause of an ALTE is also a concern and may be intentional or unintentional. Intentional poisonings frequently involve narcotics, benzodiazepines, or phenothiazines in an attempt to quiet or sedate a fussy infant.[53] Unintentional poisonings may involve inappropriate dosing of medications or mixing of over-the-counter cough and cold preparations containing ingredients with similar activity. Homeopathic medications, such as colic preparations, have also been linked to ALTE.[54]

PERTUSSIS

Bordetella pertussis, or "whooping cough," causes a respiratory infection that persists despite vaccination due to waning immunity in older individuals, vaccine failures, and vaccine refusal. Infants <6 months old are particularly susceptible because the initial immunization series begins at 2 months old and is only partially effective, particularly until the series is completed at 6 months old. Classically, the disease starts with upper respiratory infection symptoms (catarrhal phase) and progresses to paroxysmal coughing (paroxysmal phase) over 3 to 6 weeks. However, the textbook presentation is often absent or blunted in infants, in whom **the disease may present with isolated apnea**. In children <2 years of age, apnea occurs in 0.5% to 12.0% of cases[55,56] and is most common in those <3 months of age. Complications of pertussis include respiratory failure, pneumonia, airway obstruction, seizures, encephalitis, and apnea. Infants <12 months old have the highest complication rates, and most infant mortality occurs in patients <2 months old.[57]

SERIOUS BACTERIAL INFECTIONS

Serious bacterial infections (SBIs) must be considered in all febrile infants with an ALTE (see chapter 116, "Fever and Serious Bacterial Illness in Infants and Children"). Reported rates range from 0% to 8.2%, and even in the infant presenting with an afebrile ALTE, the risk of bacteremia, meningitis, or urinary tract infection should be considered, particularly in a patient who continues to look ill in the ED. Concern is greatest in the infant <60 days old, who may manifest few other symptoms to indicate the possibility of SBI. A study of 112 infants <60 days old with ALTE who underwent testing for SBI identified three cases of bacteremia and one urinary tract infection, as well as one case of pertussis. This constituted 2.7% of the sample, and prematurity and hypothermia were found to confer additional risk.[58] Other studies that include infants over 2 months of age have shown that urinary tract infections can rarely present as an ALTE (3.1%), but rates of meningitis and bacteremia were negligible.[59]

Although many providers will perform a full "rule out sepsis" or SBI evaluation for the afebrile infant <2 months old presenting with ALTE (CBC, urinalysis, and cultures of blood, urine, and cerebrospinal fluid), in term infants without infectious risk factor and who are asymptomatic and afebrile, this approach will rarely identify an occult infection. One study identified one urinary tract infection, three cases of bacteremia, one case of pertussis, and four pneumonias among 112 infants <60 days old presenting with ALTE who had a complete or partial workup for SBI. The study was not sufficiently powered to evaluate meningitis. Prematurity was found to be a risk factor for an occult infection.[58] Another population of 198 ALTE patients <12 months old were assessed by either testing or a 4-week follow-up phone call. None was found to have an SBI, and two were diagnosed with enteroviral meningitis.[60] A third study examined 243 febrile and afebrile ALTE patients <12 months of age, 95 of whom received an infectious diagnosis. Of these, 30 were bacterial, accounting for 12% of the overall ALTE group. Fourteen patients had pneumonia (age range, 1 to 5 months old), with all but one patient having clinical signs of respiratory illness. Two had pertussis, one had *Chlamydophila pneumoniae*, five had urinary tract infections (aged 1 to 5 months old), three had bacteremia (all with toxic appearance), three had bacterial meningitis (all with signs), and one had aseptic meningitis.[61] These multiple single-center studies with variability in case definitions and patient populations reported sufficiently conflicted outcomes, making it difficult to calculate the diagnostic yield of routine testing for SBI in patients with ALTE. **Clearly, toxic- or ill-appearing infants and those with localizing symptoms and signs of infection should receive appropriate SBI testing.** Urine testing may be considered in all ALTE patients, even in the absence of a fever, but should be strongly considered in those less than 2 months of age unless an alternative diagnosis is likely. Chest radiograph may be similarly contemplated, although in absence of any respiratory findings, false positives can be common.

BREATH-HOLDING SPELLS

Breath-holding spells occur in 4% to 5% of children <8 years of age and entail a cessation of respiration at the end of expiration, usually in response to pain, anger, or fear. Spells typically last <1 minute and may be accompanied by cyanosis, pallor, syncope, and seizures. Cyanotic breath-holding spells have not been associated with any underlying medical condition; there is some literature supporting the finding that pallid spells are associated with pronounced QT dispersion and may have a cardiac etiology. Breath-holding spells are generally easily recognized in older children, but they may be diagnosed in infants as young as 6 months of age: one study found that in 15% of children with breath-holding spells, the age of onset was <6 months.[62] Although breath-holding should be a diagnosis of exclusion in younger patients, it is likely that some ALTEs are early manifestations of breath-holding spells.

OTHER CAUSES

Anatomic anomalies of the airway such as laryngomalacia have been linked to ALTE. Parents of these patients will usually report breathing difficulties or noisy breathing present since birth. Approximately 0.6% of ALTE patients will ultimately require an otolaryngologic intervention.[63]

ED APPROACH TO AN APPARENT LIFE-THREATENING EVENT

Typically, ALTE patients can easily be categorized into one of three discrete groups. The *first group* consists of those for whom a proximate cause for the ALTE is clear from the history or physical examination. Fever in a neonate with signs suggestive of sepsis, a cough classic for pertussis or bronchiolitis, or a seizure witnessed by a member of the healthcare team and confirmed as similar to the presenting complaint by the caretaker are examples of this type of patient. The *second group* comprises infants for whom the diagnosis is not immediately clear but who appear unstable. The *third and largest group* consists of well-appearing infants and a physical examination that is either normal or noncontributory.

STABLE PATIENTS WITH A CLEAR DIAGNOSIS

Manage stable infants with a clear diagnosis according to the identified disease, and consider that a history of apnea may confer higher risk of subsequent events. For example, one episode of apnea is a risk factor for further apneic events in bronchiolitis. Even a single episode of apnea in an infant with pertussis is concerning, so consider hospitalization. Conversely, obstructive apnea after a gastroesophageal reflux event may be managed by conservative measures such as small, frequent, and upright feedings. In general, the disposition should be dictated by the physician's concern that a life-threatening event will recur, the underlying illness, the duration and severity of the ALTE, the resuscitation required, single versus multiple events, the severity of other symptoms, and the follow-up available to the child.

STABLE PATIENTS WITHOUT A CLEAR DIAGNOSIS

Stable and asymptomatic patients lacking a clear diagnosis represent the largest group of ALTE patients and the greatest diagnostic conundrum. In the vast majority, the ALTE is associated with a benign self-limiting condition. However, a small minority will have a condition that if left undiagnosed may lead to a poor outcome. This group includes infants who, by history, have had an ALTE but appear well in the ED. They may have upper respiratory infection symptoms or nonspecific examination findings, but nothing to render them unstable or suggest an obvious diagnosis. Specific information that should be obtained in the history is outlined in **Table 115-2**.

UNSTABLE PATIENTS

For unstable patients without a clear diagnosis, the priority is stabilization, which may require assisted ventilation for the infant with persistent ventilatory compromise. In such a situation, head injury, sepsis, metabolic or electrolyte disorder, poisoning, pertussis with complications, and bronchiolitis (in the neonate or ex-preemie) are the most likely possibilities. The disposition of this group is clearly hospitalization, and persistently unstable infants may require an intensive care setting.

DIAGNOSTIC TESTING

A careful history and physical examination, resulting in a categorization into one of the three discrete groups identified above, should indicate which patients require additional evaluation, diagnostic imaging, or monitoring in the vast majority of cases. Maintain a high index of suspicion for an occult condition in children <2 months old.

Several experts have offered algorithms to guide management decisions, but there is not a clear, evidence-based pathway that works for all patients. **It is clear, however, that a routine battery of tests for all ALTE patients is unnecessary and inappropriate. Testing and hospitalization should be reserved for higher-risk groups.**[64]

Many ALTE patients seen in the ED undergo extensive laboratory testing, including 55% who are checked for electrolyte abnormalities and 77% who receive a CBC.[65] One study at a single hospital in New York of 243 ALTE patients found a low rate of abnormal tests, and fewer still that contributed to the diagnosis: WBC count contributed to the identification of infection in 6 of 223 tests performed, whereas hemoglobin was useful in 2 of 223 cases (abusive head injury), sodium in 3 of 215 cases (afebrile seizure), calcium in 2 of 215 cases (afebrile seizure), and metabolic screen in 1 of 44 cases. Platelets, carbon dioxide, potassium, chloride, glucose, blood gas, and coagulation profile were not helpful in any case. Of these tests, only one (an elevated WBC count) was identified in a child without signs or symptoms to point toward a specific abnormality. Based on this, the authors recommend that a careful history and physical examination be performed and that laboratory testing be directed by specific signs and symptoms in the well-appearing child with ALTE.[66] Urinary toxicology screens were not studied in this paper, but other literature points to a positive rate as high as 8.4%, and this test should be considered in all ALTE infants in whom another diagnosis is not strongly likely.[67]

The study by Brand et al[66] also evaluated the utility of imaging and monitoring. Of 459 tests performed in patients based on signs and symptoms, 106 (23%) were abnormal. Thirty-two (11%) of 291 tests performed in patients with a noncontributory history were abnormal, but 29 of 32 of the tests were positive for GI reflux,[66] a common diagnosis in all infants

TABLE 115-2 Important Historical Questions in the Apparent Life-Threatening Event (ALTE) Patient

Past medical history	Prematurity (before 37 wk) Prior hospitalization, surgery, ED visits History of prior apnea or ALTE Prior respiratory difficulties (snoring, stridor) Prior feeding difficulties (choking, gagging, coughing with feeds) Immunization status (pertussis) Prior history of urinary tract infection or risk factors for bacterial infection (chorioamnionitis or Guillain-Barré syndrome)
Family history	History of sudden infant death syndrome or sudden death Cardiac arrhythmias or congenital heart disease Seizure disorder Metabolic disease
Event history	Duration of event Resuscitation required (e.g., stimulation, mouth-to-mouth, chest compressions) Temporal relationship with feeding, sleep, crying, vomiting, choking, gagging Color (cyanosis, pallor, plethora) Change in tone (including seizure activity) Central vs obstructive pattern of apnea (i.e., apparent respiratory effort) Number of ALTEs experienced within 24 h of presentation Episodic vs sustained change in mental status (syncope, postictal phase, irritability, obtundation, loss of consciousness)
Review of systems	Respiratory symptoms or other intercurrent illness Period of fasting (e.g., recent onset of sleeping through the night) Medication use, medications in the home or used by breastfeeding parent Possible trauma
Social history	Possibility of follow-up (an identified physician, transportation, proximity) Comfort level of parents Concern for abuse Parental psychiatric issues or marital stress (e.g., absentee parent) Infectious exposure (pertussis, respiratory syncytial virus, upper respiratory tract infection, lower respiratory tract infection)

that may or may not be the proximate cause of an ALTE. This number is similar to the population prevalence (12%) of GI reflux in infants <2 years of age.[68] GI reflux is a common diagnosis in all infants that may or may not be the proximate cause of an ALTE. ECGs are performed in 43% of cases[69] but uncommonly identify contributory information.

DISPOSITION AND FOLLOW-UP

It is common to admit patients to the hospital for workup and monitoring.[70] However, this is not without cost: the mean adjusted charge for children's hospitals in the United States is $15,567 per admission (average length of stay, 4.4 days).[71] The financial burden is compounded by the frequency of iatrogenic complications, including medical errors and nosocomial infections, and the social implications from unnecessary admission and added anxiety. In response, several authors have attempted to identify high- and low-risk subsets of infants based on the likelihood of a subsequent ALTE or adverse outcome.[72-74] Prematurity, postconceptual age <43 weeks,[72] multiple events at the time of ED presentation,[73,74] significant past medical history,[74] and upper respiratory tract infection symptoms increase the risk of a serious event. Age is somewhat controversial, with some investigators reporting a higher risk in older infants, whereas others report a higher risk in neonates in the first month of life.[65,73] A conservative but rational approach (presented in **Table 115-3**) would be to admit for monitoring and further workup all patients <48 weeks of postconceptual age, as well as those who are ill appearing or have concerning findings on physical examination and those with bronchiolitis or pertussis and apnea, suspicion of nonaccidental trauma, more than one event within 24 hours of presentation, a past medical history that places them at risk for poor outcomes, prolonged central apnea, ALTE requiring significant resuscitation, or poor follow-up. Any history of prematurity, family history of SIDS, or patient history of multiple ALTEs may warrant overnight observation (Table 115-3).

Routine use of empiric histamine-2 blockers or proton pump inhibitors for gastroesophageal reflux is not recommended. If the events persist or there is continued evidence of gastroesophageal reflux disease, then referral to a gastroenterologist may be indicated. Cough and cold preparations are contraindicated in infancy even when it appears that an infant has choked on mucus. Reassure the family that the ALTE is not a precursor or related to SIDS. CPR instruction, if feasible, may provide additional reassurance to caregivers. Finally, communicate with the primary care provider regarding the event and discuss recommendations for further evaluation and subspecialist referral. Children with a family history of SIDS or recurrent ALTE may need referral to a pulmonologist for a sleep evaluation or home monitoring. Infants with a concern for an airway abnormality should be evaluated by an otolaryngologist. Infants presenting with seizure in the first year of life will

TABLE 115-3 Reasons for Admission for Apparent Life-Threatening Event (ALTE)

<38 wk postconceptual age (prematurity)
Ill appearing
Reason for admission identified in the ED (e.g., hypoxemia)
Concerning findings on physical examination
Bronchiolitis or pertussis with apnea
Nonaccidental trauma or child abuse suspected
More than one event in past 24 h
Abnormalities in past medical history
Concern for prolonged central apnea, >20 s
ALTE requiring resuscitation
Inadequate follow-up
Family history of sudden infant death syndrome or sudden unexplained death

certainly need neurologic consultation; the advantage of an inpatient versus outpatient workup is controversial (see chapter 135, "Seizures in Infants and Children").

LONG-TERM OUTCOME

The greatest fear for the ED physician is to discharge home an infant who subsequently succumbs to SIDS or occult illness. Although ALTE is not considered a risk factor for SIDS, a very small portion of ALTE patients may still be at risk. One small study found a subsequent mortality rate of 10% among patients requiring cardiopulmonary resuscitation for ALTE and a 28% rate in such infants after multiple ALTE episodes.[75] Another study reported a 1.9% death rate in infants with ALTE requiring CPR, much higher than the population risk of 0.8%.[76] Identification of a cardiac illness as the cause of ALTE is a risk factor for subsequent death.[77] Focusing on the immediate postdischarge period, Kant et al[78] identified 2 of 176 children who died within 2 weeks of hospitalization for ALTE, both of pneumonia not present at the time of hospital admission, stressing the need for follow-up. Currently, monitors are only recommended for infants with one or more severe ALTEs, symptomatic preterm infants, siblings of two or more SIDS victims, and infants with certain diseases such as central hypoventilation.

Acknowledgment: The authors would like to thank Denise Bertone, RN, and James Ribe, MD, of the Los Angeles Coroner's Office for their assistance in preparing this chapter and Carol Berkowitz for her authorship in past editions of this chapter and inspiring work in this field.

REFERENCES

The complete reference list is available online at www.TintinalliEM.com.

Fever and Serious Bacterial Illness in Infants and Children

Vincent F. Wang

INTRODUCTION AND EPIDEMIOLOGY

Fever is the most common chief complaint of children presenting to the ED, accounting for ~30% of pediatric outpatient visits. It is critical to differentiate mildly ill from seriously ill children with fever, especially in the neonate and infant. This challenge is compounded by the nonspecific symptoms and lack of a focus of infection in most children with fever. Many factors influence evaluation and management, including clinical assessment, physical examination findings, patient age, immunization status, and height of the fever.

This chapter focuses on the management of a neonate, infant, or child with acute fever at risk for serious bacterial illness, because morbidity and mortality are high if not properly treated. Neonates are infants <1 month old. For preterm neonates, the age should be calculated from the date of term birth, rather than from the actual preterm birth date. The significance of age groups is discussed in the subsequent sections.

FEVER

Any elevation in temperature above normal is considered a fever, but the threshold for clinically important fever varies with the age group and is related to the ability of signs and symptoms to identify the underlying cause of fever. **In the neonate or infant <2 to 3 months of age, the threshold for concerning fever is 38°C (100.4°F); in infants and children 3 to 36 months old, the threshold has traditionally been 39°C (102.2°F).**[1] In children >36 months old, the definition of significant fever is not fixed because concern for serious bacterial illness in this age group should be directed by other signs or symptoms of the underlying cause. In children with developmental delay, with limited ability to demonstrate specific signs and symptoms, the cause of fever may be difficult to determine, and more testing is often necessary.

Axillary temperatures are 0.6°C (1°F) lower than oral temperatures, which are 0.6°C (1°F) lower than rectal temperatures. Temperatures taken with infrared thermometers that scan the tympanic membrane are of variable reliability and reproducibility.[2]

Fever is treated with acetaminophen or ibuprofen. The dosage of acetaminophen is 15 milligrams/kg/dose (maximum daily dose, 80 milligrams/kg) every 4 to 6 hours, up to five times per day. Acetaminophen can be given PO or PR. The dosage of ibuprofen is 10 milligrams/kg/dose (maximum daily dose, 40 milligrams/kg) every 6 to 8 hours. Ibuprofen can be given PO or IV and is recommended for children older than 1 year of age.

SERIOUS BACTERIAL ILLNESS

Infants ≤3 months of age, and especially neonates, are relatively immunodeficient. Neonates and young infants demonstrate decreased opsonin activity, decreased macrophage and neutrophil function, and bone marrow insufficiency.[3] Infants and children demonstrate a poor immunoglobulin G antibody response to encapsulated bacteria until 24 months of age. Immune development is a continuum and improves as the child matures. Therefore, the age of the patient and the virulence of the bacteria are considerations for the evaluation of fever in children and the identification of serious bacterial illness. The most common manifestations of serious bacterial illness in children are discussed: urinary tract infection (UTI), bacteremia and sepsis, pneumonia and sinusitis, and meningitis. Of note, the following discussion applies primarily to Western countries.

URINARY TRACT INFECTION

Pathophysiology Overall, the most common serious bacterial illness is UTI with or without pyelonephritis (see chapter 132, Urinary Tract Infection in Infants and Children). Among young children presenting to EDs with fever and no obvious source of infection, between 3% and 8% have UTI.[4] The overall incidence of UTI is 5% in children between 2 months and 2 years old.[5] Uncircumcised boys have a rate of UTI 5 to 20 times greater than circumcised boys. The presence of a fever of 39°C (102.2°F) and a urine suggestive of infection indicate renal parenchymal involvement, or **pyelonephritis**. Additional risk factors in boys include history of previous UTI, ill appearance, age less than 12 months, fever for at least 2 days, absence of another source for fever, and nonblack race.[6] After 2 years of age, UTI remains a frequent bacterial cause of fever in girls but is more commonly associated with urinary symptoms. UTI is uncommon in boys older than 1 to 2 years of age, unless underlying risk factors exist.

Escherichia coli and other gram-negative bacteria are the most common causative organisms, although gram-positive organisms comprise a significant minority in older boys and in children with underlying medical conditions such as neurogenic bladder. **UTIs may not produce symptoms other than fever, so routinely obtain a urinalysis and culture in the evaluation of the febrile neonate or infant without other source.**

Diagnosis The ideally obtained urine specimen for a child in diapers has traditionally been by urethral catheterization or suprapubic aspiration. In children with labial adhesions or phimosis, a bag collection specimen may be preferred as a screening test. However, if the urinalysis is positive from a bagged specimen, obtain a urine specimen for culture by suprapubic aspiration or clean-catch midstream method before initiating antibiotic therapy, because bag collection methods produce frequent false-positive cultures (up to 88%) from skin contamination.[5]

The initial diagnosis of UTI is made with chemical strip testing or a microscope urinalysis (see Table 132-4). Chemical testing detects leukocyte esterase or nitrites. **A positive test for leukocyte esterase has a sensitivity of 67% to 85% for UTI, whereas a positive test for nitrites has a specificity of 95% to 99% for UTI.** A positive test for leukocytes on microscope urinalysis testing is a urine WBC count of 5 to 10/high-power field and has a sensitivity of 51% to 91%. The identification of bacteria on Gram stain has a sensitivity and specificity of 80% to 97% and 87% to 99%, respectively. When Gram stain is not readily available, chemical and microscopy testing compares favorably with gram stain.

Before beginning antibiotic treatment, obtain an appropriate urine sample for culture and susceptibility testing. Consider blood and cerebrospinal fluid testing in young infants suspected to have a UTI. Approximately 5% to 10% of febrile infants with UTI will have **bacteremia.**[7,8] UTIs can be associated with bacteremia in up to 30% of infants between 4 and 8 weeks of age.[9]

One study reported that 13% of infants (15 of 117 infants) <3 months of age with a febrile UTI admitted to the hospital had a sterile pleocytosis of the cerebrospinal fluid thought to be due to systemic release of inflammatory mediators or low bacterial virulence in the subarachnoid space.[7-12] Less than 1% of febrile infants with UTI will have a bacterial meningitis, but concomitant infection of the urine and cerebrospinal fluid has been reported.

A recent American Academy of Pediatrics practice parameter on UTI suggested that patients with a negative microscope urinalysis or chemical strip testing in association with a positive urine culture are likely to have asymptomatic bacteriuria, rather than a true UTI.[5] Based on this reasoning, they suggested that negative urine microscope urinalysis or chemical strip testing does not warrant ordering urine culture. However, the recommendations are Level C, based on previous studies not directly relevant to the infant or child presenting to the emergency department with fever.[13,14] **Therefore, if a patient is at risk for UTI, obtain a urine culture even if the initial urinalysis is negative.**

BACTEREMIA AND SEPSIS

Most studies of febrile infants ≤3 months old cite a bacteremia/sepsis incidence of 2% to 3%. The most common causes of bacteremia and meningitis in this age group are *E. coli*, group B *Streptococcus*, and *Listeria monocytogenes*. Ill-appearing neonates or those identified at high risk because of laboratory testing have an incidence of serious bacterial illness of 13% to 21%.[15] Overall, however, viral infections are the most frequent cause of fever in infants.

Before the widespread use of the pneumococcal conjugate vaccine, in febrile infants and children between 3 and 36 months old, high fever, WBC >15,000/mm^3, and absolute neutrophil count >10,000/mm^3 were independent predictors of occult bacteremia. The presence of any of these factors increased the incidence of bacteremia to 8% to 17%.

Administration of the *Haemophilus influenzae* type b vaccine and the heptavalent pneumococcal conjugate vaccine has decreased the occult bacteremia rate of well-appearing, febrile children 3 to 36 months of age from approximately 2% to 3% to 0.5% to 0.7%.[16] The Centers for Disease Control and Prevention reports a 76% reduction in invasive infections from *Streptococcus pneumoniae* when comparing 2005 with 1998 data in the United States. The incidence of serious bacterial illness in children 2 to 6 months old, who were incompletely or not immunized, decreased because the widespread use of the vaccine resulted in herd immunity.[17] In 2009, a decavalent pneumococcal conjugate vaccine was released in Europe, and in 2010, the 13-valent pneumococcal conjugate vaccine was introduced in the United States, both of which are expected to further decrease the incidence of pneumococcal disease.[18] Ongoing Centers for Disease Control and Prevention Active Bacterial Core Surveillance cites declining national estimates of invasive disease.[19] Given these declines and the fact that 80% of pneumococcal bacteremia resolves spontaneously, the traditional standards for routine evaluation of the febrile infant 3 to 36 months old will be changing as the prevalence of occult bacteremia decreases.[20]

PNEUMONIA AND SINUSITIS

Pneumonia and sinusitis are common bacterial infections of childhood, frequently associated with or following upper respiratory tract symptoms (see chapter 120, Nose and Sinus Disorders in Infants and Children; chapter 121, Mouth and Throat Disorders in Infants and Children; and chapter 125, Pneumonia in Infants and Children). Pneumonia occurs in all age groups, with the most common causative agents being the same as those for bacteremia or meningitis in each age group. The incidence of pneumococcal pneumonia in all ages has decreased since the introduction of the pneumococcal conjugate vaccine.[21-23] Sinusitis is uncommon in children <3 years of age because sinus formation is incomplete.

Plain chest radiographs remain the gold standard for diagnosis of pneumonia. In neonates and young infants, routine chest radiographs are not necessary unless the patient has specific physical examination findings suggestive of pneumonia, such as respiratory distress, rales, grunting, significant tachypnea, or hypoxemia.[7,24] In older children with chronic medical problems, such as cystic fibrosis, congenital heart disease, or malignancy, consider pneumonia in the differential diagnosis of fever and upper respiratory tract symptoms, even if there are no signs of lower tract infection. In one study performed before the widespread use of the pneumococcal conjugate vaccine, a WBC count of 20,000/mm^3 was associated with occult pneumonia in 19% of patients without focal findings.[25] Without predisposing conditions or abnormal test results, the decision to obtain a chest radiograph can otherwise be made clinically. Pneumonia in a febrile but otherwise asymptomatic child is unlikely.

MENINGITIS

In Western countries, most studies of febrile infants <3 months old cite a bacterial meningitis incidence of 1%. The most common organisms are the same as those for bacteremia/sepsis: *E. coli*, group B streptococci, and *L. monocytogenes*. For children >3 months old, the most common organisms are *S. pneumoniae, Neisseria meningitidis*, and *Staphylococcus aureus*, with a lower incidence of *S. pneumoniae* meningitis since routine vaccinations with the conjugate vaccine.

Outside of North America, the epidemiology of meningitis is more complex, depending on the region of the world in which the patient has been living or traveling. *N. meningitidis* and *Mycobacterium tuberculosis* are the more common causes. Although *N. meningitidis* rarely occurs in North America (groups B, C, W135, X, and Y), different serogroups exist elsewhere, especially group A in sub-Saharan Africa. **In patients with symptoms of meningitis and recent travel to Africa, meningococcal meningitis should be considered as a diagnosis.** Treatment is similar to other causes of bacterial meningitis. Tuberculosis meningitis is discussed in chapter 174, Central Nervous System and Spinal Infections.

The diagnosis of meningitis is made by obtaining cerebrospinal fluid by lumbar puncture (see later section, Procedures in Children: Lumbar Puncture). It is often difficult to distinguish between viral and bacterial meningitis because there is a wide overlap in cerebrospinal fluid and peripheral blood findings. **Cerebrospinal fluid WBC >30 cells/mm^3 in the neonate and >10 cells/mm^3 in children >1 month old have been traditional markers to suggest meningitis.** Risk factors for bacterial meningitis in children 29 days to 18 years old are listed in **Table 116-1.**[26] Each risk factor counts as a single point added toward the bacterial

TABLE 116-1 Bacterial Meningitis Score for Infants >2 Months Old and Well Appearing

Risk Factor*	
CSF ANC	≥1000 cells/mm^3
CSF protein	≥80 milligrams/dL
Peripheral blood ANC	≥10,000 cells/mm^3
CSF:serum glucose	Not reliable for decision making because infrequently drawn
Seizure	Before or after presentation
CSF Gram stain	Positive Gram stain 61% sensitive, 99% specific for bacterial meningitis

Abbreviations: ANC = absolute neutrophil count; CSF = cerebrospinal fluid.

*Any one factor (one point) = high risk for bacterial meningitis. Very low risk of bacterial meningitis if infant lacks all high-risk criteria (negative predictive value = 100%; any one factor positive has sensitivity and specificity of 98.3% and 61.5%, respectively, for bacterial meningitis).

meningitis score. A negative bacterial meningitis score does not exclude some treatable causes of meningitis/encephalitis such as herpes virus or Lyme disease.

Because of the serious morbidity of missed meningitis, it is best to admit any ill-appearing patient or patients <2 months old with any degree of pleocytosis and administer appropriate antibiotics in the ED.

The pathogenesis of bacterial meningitis suggests that steroids may attenuate the inflammatory response associated with meningitis. However, the use of steroids has been associated with decreased bactericidal activity by some antibiotics and decreased antimicrobial penetration into the cerebrospinal fluid. Studies are conflicting. However, a recent Cochrane review found no difference in mortality among studies of children (162/1229 in the steroid group vs. 166/1202 in the placebo group), but did suggest a positive effect in the prevention of hearing loss among pediatric patients (relative risk, 0.74; 95% confidence interval, 0.62 to 0.89) with the strongest effect seen in cases of *H. influenzae*. Subgroup analysis showed possible survival benefit from steroids in meningitis caused by *S. pneumoniae* when adults and children were combined.[27] If given, administer steroids before or during antibiotic administration.

Infants with aseptic meningitis generally should be hospitalized and ensured adequate long-term follow-up because they are at greater risk for dehydration and subsequent neurologic and learning disabilities.

For those with cerebrospinal fluid pleocytosis and likelihood of viral meningitis, if the child is to be discharged from the ED, it is wise to administer a long-acting parenteral antibiotic (ceftriaxone, 100 milligrams/kg IM or IV) and ensure follow-up in 24 hours.[26]

GENERAL TREATMENT AND DISPOSITION PRINCIPLES BASED ON AGE

The clinical challenge is to distinguish the cause of fever: a benign viral infection, serious bacterial illness, or a noninfectious illness. Most causes are due to viral infections, but bacterial infections are not infrequent. The significance of fever depends on multiple factors. If the physical examination identifies the source of infection, evaluation, testing, and treatment are dictated by the presumptive diagnosis. If the physical examination does not identify a source of infection causing fever, decision making is based first on age and then by height of fever. There are no absolute rules in the evaluation and management of fever, but the guidelines in **Table 116-2** are suggested for the management of neonates, infants, and children who are well appearing, have had all relevant immunizations, and have no obvious cause for the fever. Again, this discussion should be applied judiciously to non-Western countries or patients recently emigrated from non-Western countries, because the epidemiology of fever may be more diverse in international settings and is beyond the scope of this chapter. Detailed discussion of evidence-based information is provided later in the section, Decision Rules for Assessment of Fever in Neonates and Young Infants. Any ill-appearing infant or child should have a complete sepsis evaluation performed and should be admitted for parenteral antibiotic therapy.

Meningismus is unreliable in infants <6 months of age, and its absence does not exclude meningitis. **Because of the declining prevalence of meningitis in the United States with age, we recommend routine lumbar puncture in infants <2 months of age, but selective lumbar puncture in infants 2–6 months of age.** Peripheral WBC count does not predict the risk for meningitis, and the decision to perform a lumbar puncture should be made independently of the peripheral WBC count.

FEVER EVALUATION IN NEONATES AND INFANTS ≤3 MONTHS OF AGE

CLINICAL FEATURES

In infants <3 months of age, review the birth history, including the length of the gestation, the use of peripartum antibiotics in the mother or infant during labor or delivery, and the presence of neonatal complications, such as fever, tachypnea, or jaundice. Signs and symptoms of serious bacterial illness are typically nonspecific in this age group. For example, vomiting and diarrhea accompany many problems, including gastroenteritis, otitis media, UTI, and meningitis. Alternatively, crying may be either a manifestation of serious bacterial illness or a benign condition of infancy (colic or hunger).

Undress infants completely. Assess age-appropriate normal vital signs. Tachypnea or hypoxemia may be a clue to lower respiratory tract infection. Inconsolable crying or increased irritability when handled is frequently seen in infants with meningitis. Although fullness of the anterior fontanelle may be noted in some infants with meningitis, other signs of meningeal irritation, such as nuchal rigidity, are usually absent. Perform a head-to-toe evaluation to identify a focus of infection, such as an inflamed tympanic membrane or evidence of cellulitis.

Treatment of neonates and infants <3 months old with a focal source for fever is controversial. In a small study of tympanocentesis-confirmed acute otitis media, there were no cases of bacteremia or meningitis, but UTI was found in 9%.[28] The sample size of this study was not adequate to determine that blood testing or lumbar puncture was not necessary. As of this writing, there are no other studies that have identified the incidence of bacteremia, meningitis, or UTI in children <3 months old who have a focal source such as cellulitis, otitis media, or other identified bacterial infections. Therefore, even with an identified source, caution is urged, especially in children <3 months old, and laboratory testing is recommended to detect occult infection.

DECISION RULES FOR ASSESSMENT OF FEVER IN NEONATES AND YOUNG INFANTS

Clinical assessment of the severity of illness in neonates and young infants is difficult. The three most commonly applied outpatient criteria for the management of fever in well-appearing neonates and young infants are the **Rochester Criteria**, the **Philadelphia Protocol**, and the **Boston Criteria** (**Table 116-3**). All three have limitations for clinical decision making. A comparison of these decision rules is difficult because of differences in inclusion criteria, laboratory testing, and clinical implications for decision making. In addition, the routine administration of antibiotics to pregnant women who test positive for group B *Streptococcus* on vaginal cultures and improved immunization practices have decreased the incidence of serious bacterial illness, making it difficult to extrapolate these three decision rules to current practice.

The **Rochester Criteria** state that in well-appearing neonates and infants ≤60 days old, without prior or peripartum illness and with a normal CBC, a negative urinalysis and negative chest radiograph (if indicated) are sufficient to exclude serious bacterial illness.[29] However, the Rochester Criteria miss 1% of patients with serious bacterial illness and do not include lumbar puncture as one of the diagnostic tests. The Rochester Criteria are the least sensitive of the three guidelines.

In the largest validation study of the Rochester Criteria, the cohort of 1057 patients included 511 who met low-risk criteria (Table 116-3). Five patients, or 1% of patients identified as "low risk," had serious bacterial illness that was missed. Lumbar puncture was not included in the rules, so the criteria do not provide the ability to exclude meningitis. Of note, the incidence of meningitis was 0.3% of the entire cohort of 1057 patients, which is lower than the 1% meningitis incidence cited in most other studies. In summary, the Rochester Criteria miss 1% of patients with SBI and do not exclude meningitis.

The **Philadelphia Protocol** (Table 116-3) includes the results of lumbar puncture in clinical decision making and includes young infants 29 to 56 days old.[30] The sensitivity of the low-risk criteria for excluding serious bacterial illness (neonatal bacteremia, UTI, or meningitis) is 98%; specificity is 44%; positive predictive value is 14%; and negative predictive value is 99.7%. The temperature criterion for fever was 38.2°C (100.8°F), not 38°C (100.4°F). The incidence of meningitis in this cohort was 1.2%. Using the Philadelphia Protocol, all patients with meningitis were identified. One of 288 patients, who had otherwise met low-risk criteria, was identified by an elevated cerebrospinal fluid WBC alone. In addition, all cases of bacteremia and UTI were identified by the Philadelphia Protocol.

TABLE 116-2 Suggested Guidelines for the Evaluation and Management of Neonates, Infants, and Children with Fever Who Are Well Appearing, Have Had All Relevant Immunizations, and Have No Clinical Source for Fever

Age Group	Evaluation	Treatment
Neonate, 0–28 d* of age, ≥38°C (100.4°F) SBI incidence of ill appearing: 13%–21%; if not ill appearing: <5%	CBC and blood culture *and* Urinalysis and urine culture *and* CSF cell count, Gram stain, and culture. Chest x-ray is optional, if no respiratory symptoms. Stool culture if diarrhea is present.	*Admit and treat with:* Parenteral antibiotic therapy with ampicillin, 50 milligrams/kg, and either cefotaxime, 50 milligrams/kg, or gentamicin, 2.5 milligrams/kg.
Infant 29–56 d* of age, ≥38.2°C (100.8°F) (Philadelphia Protocol) SBI incidence of ill appearing: 13%–21%; if not ill appearing: <5%	Same as for neonates.	*Discharge if:* WBC ≤15,000/mm^3 and ≥5000/mm^3 and < 20% band forms. Urinalysis negative. CSF WBC <10 cells/mm^3. Negative chest x-ray or fecal leukocytes if applicable. *Admit if:* Any of above criteria are not met and treat with parenteral ceftriaxone, 50 milligrams/kg with normal CSF, 100 milligrams/kg with signs of meningitis.
Infants 57 d* to 6 mo* of age, ≥38°C (100.4°F) Non-UTI SBI incidence is estimated to be negligible UTI is 3%–8%.	Urinalysis and urine culture alone. *or* For conservative management, treat infants 57–90 d using Philadelphia Protocol above.	*Discharge if negative.* *Treat for UTI* with cefixime, 8 milligrams/kg/dose daily, or cefpodoxime, 5 milligrams/kg/dose twice a day, or cefdinir, 7 milligrams/kg/dose twice daily for 10 d as outpatient. *Admit and treat* with parenteral ceftriaxone if fails conservative criteria for discharge.
Infants 57 d to 6 mo* of age ≥39°C (102.2°F) SBI incidence is estimated as <1%; non-UTI SBI incidence is estimated to be negligible. UTI is 3%–8%.	Urinalysis and urine culture alone. *or* Urinalysis and urine culture in addition to CBC and blood culture.	*Discharge if negative.* *Treat for UTI as above.* If WBC ≥15,000/mm^3, consider treatment with ceftriaxone, 50 milligrams/kg IV/IM, and follow-up in 24 h. If WBC ≥20,000/mm^3, consider chest x-ray and CSF testing.†
Infants/children 6–36 mo of age Non-UTI SBI incidence is <0.4% UTI in girls ≤8% UTI in boys (<12 mo) ≤2% Uncircumcised boys (1–2 y) remains 2%	Urinalysis and urine culture. Girls 6–24 mo Boys 6–12 mo Uncircumcised boys 12–24 mo	*Discharge if negative.* *Treat for UTI* as above as outpatient.
Children >36 mo and older	No workup is routinely necessary.	*Discharge and treat with antipyretics:* acetaminophen, 15 milligrams/kg PO/PR every 4 h, or ibuprofen, 10 milligrams/kg PO every 6 h as needed.

Abbreviations: CSF = cerebrospinal fluid; SBI = serious bacterial illness; UTI = urinary tract infection.

*For preterm infants, count age by estimated postconception date and not by actual delivery date for the first 90 days of life.

†Meningismus is difficult to discern in infants <6 months of age, and especially in infants <2 months of age. Therefore, we recommend routine CSF testing in infants <2 months of age, but selective CSF testing in infants 2–6 months of age. There is no absolute cutoff point for prediction of meningitis with a peripheral WBC count.

The **Boston Criteria** (Table 116-3) attempted to identify young infants at lower risk of SBI and safely treat them as outpatients with empiric ceftriaxone.[31] The Boston Criteria included infants 28 to 89 days of age and accepted a peripheral WBC up to 20,000/mm^3 as normal. Lumbar puncture was performed in all patients, and all patients with meningitis were excluded. In those who met low-risk criteria, <1% of patients had a missed serious bacterial illness, and none had complications after empiric treatment with ceftriaxone. By using the Boston Criteria, a greater number of patients are discharged.

Subsequent studies applying the Rochester, Philadelphia, and Boston decision rules missed serious bacterial illness in neonates 0 to 30 days old.[10,30,32,33] The safest course for 0- to 30-day-old infants is sepsis testing, admission, and empiric antibiotic treatment (Table 116-2).

The recognition of occult serious bacterial illness in well-appearing neonates and infants <3 months of age is difficult. No single clinical variable or diagnostic test can correctly or reliably identify it in this age group. In addition, as noted earlier with the Rochester, Philadelphia, and Boston decision rules, these rules differ in their inclusion criteria. Combinations of variables can be helpful. A study from Boston chose statistically significant cutoff points for predictive variables for SBI.[34] In order of greatest statistical significance for prediction were positive urinalysis, WBC >20,000/mm^3, temperature >39.6°C (103.3°F), WBC <4100/mm^3, and age <13 days old. No variable or cutoff point was 100% sensitive or specific, and the number of meningitis cases was too small to lead to the inclusion of results of lumbar puncture in the decision rule. This study challenges the previous study protocols by introducing clinical and diagnostic test variables that were determined to be statistically significant. Although this is not standard of care, this added information may help determine different thresholds for fever evaluation in the neonate or for admission and antibiotic therapy.

TABLE 116-3 Comparison of Low-Risk Rochester Criteria, Philadelphia Protocol, and Boston Criteria for Assessment of Fever in Well-Appearing Neonates and Infants*

Low-Risk Criteria for Serious Bacterial Infection*	Rochester Criteria	Philadelphia Protocol	Boston Criteria
Fever	T ≥38°C (100.4°F)	T ≥38.2°C (100.8°F)	T ≥38°C (100.4°F)
Age	≤60 d	29–56 d	28–89 d
Past medical history	Term infant ≥37 wk gestation	No immunodeficiency syndrome	No immunizations within 48 h
	No perinatal or postnatal antibiotics		No recent antibiotics
	No treatment for jaundice		
	No chronic illnesses or admissions		
	Not hospitalized longer than mother		
Physical examination	Well appearing	Same	Same
	Unremarkable examination		
Laboratory values			
Blood count	WBC ≥5000, ≤15,000/mm³	WBC ≤15,000/mm³	WBC ≤20,000/mm³
	Absolute band count ≤1500/mm³	Band-to-neutrophil ratio ≤0.2	
Urinalysis	WBC ≤10 per high-power field	WBC ≤10 per high-power field	WBC ≤10 per high-power field
Stool	WBC ≤5 per high-power field	—	—
Lumbar puncture and cerebrospinal fluid findings	None	WBC ≤8 per high-power field	WBC ≤10 per high power field
			Negative Gram stain
Chest radiograph	None	Negative	Negative if obtained
Comments	Excluded lumbar puncture, so number of missed meningitis cases is unknown. UTIs missed in those with negative urinalysis. The least sensitive of the low-risk criteria.	Sensitivity of low-risk criteria for SBI 98%; specificity 44%; PPV 14%; NPV 99.7%	5 of low-risk neonates and infants had SBI (8 bacteremia, 8 UTI, 10 bacterial gastroenteritis); 96% sensitive to ceftriaxone

Abbreviations: NPV = negative predictive value; PPV = positive predictive value; SBI = serious bacterial illness; T = temperature; UTI = urinary tract infection.

*Any single deviation from the criteria is interpreted as failure of low-risk criteria.

TREATMENT, DISPOSITION, AND FOLLOW-UP

There is no "community standard of practice" regarding the need for hospitalization of infants 3 months of age and younger. Some physicians hospitalize all febrile infants <3 months old, and others hospitalize selectively. Some have attributed this difference in management to a difference in bias, with physicians in private practice having a bias toward wellness (the infant is basically healthy) and emergency physicians having a bias toward illness (worst-case scenario approach).[35] Because the differentiation between sick and well infants <28 days of age is difficult, with varying reports of missed serious bacterial illness, all such febrile infants should have sepsis evaluations, including CBC, blood culture, urinalysis, urine culture, cerebrospinal fluid cell count, Gram stain and culture, and admission for parenteral antibiotics. Infants who are ill appearing or fail to meet the low-risk criteria (Table 116-3) should be admitted and administered parenteral antibiotics. Ampicillin (50 milligrams/kg/dose every 8 hours) and a cefotaxime (50 milligrams/kg/dose every 8 hours) is a common antibiotic regimen (or ampicillin and gentamicin, 2.5 milligrams/kg/dose), but choose antibiotics based on regional susceptibility patterns for group B *Streptococcus*, *E. coli*, and *L. monocytogenes*. **Do not give ceftriaxone to infants <1 month old because it may displace bilirubin and worsen hyperbilirubinemia.**

The decision to discharge a febrile infant home must be made after careful clinical and appropriate laboratory assessment and after ensuring the reliability of follow-up. Utilization of the Rochester Criteria, the Philadelphia Protocol, or the Boston Criteria may be considered. No missed cases of meningitis have been described with the Philadelphia Protocol and the Boston Criteria. The Philadelphia Protocol is recommended due to its high sensitivity.

If low-risk criteria are met for the Philadelphia Protocol, the patient may be discharged home without antibiotic administration, with evaluation in 24 hours. Additional factors for outpatient management are a reliable caretaker with a telephone and an infant who can maintain hydration. Any child who is ill appearing should be admitted and given parenteral antibiotics, regardless of the age.

Baskin et al[36] proposed parenteral ceftriaxone and 24-hour observation (with negative cultures at 24 hours) for febrile neonates between 2 and 4 weeks of age who were low risk for serious bacterial illness by the Boston Criteria. Utilization of the data from viral testing may also influence the decision to discharge to home or admit for observation.

In a large, multicenter, retrospective study, Schnadower et al[37] proposed that febrile infants 29 to 60 days old who demonstrate evidence of UTI, but meet low-risk criteria, may be safely discharged with antibiotic therapy. Significant adverse events, such as meningitis and sepsis, requiring critical care intervention occurred in 2.8% of patients. Bacteremia occurred in 6.5% of patients. Low-risk criteria for both adverse events and bacteremia were lack of ill appearance in the ED and lack of high-risk past medical history. Additional low-risk criteria for bacteremia included peripheral band count of <1250 cells/mm³ and peripheral neutrophil count of ≥1500 cells/mm³[37].

Antibiotics are administered for clinically evident bacterial disease, such as pneumonia, meningitis, otitis media, cellulitis, and septic arthritis. Specific management is outlined in chapter 118, Ear and Mastoid Disorders in Infants and Children; chapter 125, Pneumonia in Infants and Children; chapter 140, Musculoskeletal Disorders in Children; and chapter 141, Rashes in Infants and Children.

SPECIAL SITUATIONS: NEONATES AND INFANTS <3 MONTHS OF AGE WITH FEVER AND RECOGNIZABLE VIRAL ILLNESS

Neonates and infants with bronchiolitis have a significant incidence of UTI.[38] Similarly, neonates and infants with enterovirus and parainfluenza virus also have a significant incidence of serious bacterial illness (UTI and bacteremia).[15] ED evaluation should therefore also include a minimum of a urinalysis and urine culture in patients with bronchiolitis and a urinalysis, urine culture, CBC, and blood culture in patients with suspected or proven enterovirus or parainfluenza infection.

SERUM BIOMARKERS

Although the serum WBC count, absolute neutrophil count, or band-to-neutrophil ratio remain the standard biomarkers for serious bacterial illness in young infants (see previous section on decision rules), the value of several other potential biomarkers deserves mention. The most widely available and best studied of the emerging serum biomarkers is **C-reactive protein**. A systematic review of the accuracy of C-reactive protein to detect bacterial infections in febrile infants and children found limited value of the test among seven studies conducted in the ED.[39] Cutoff values ranged from 2 to 7 milligrams/dL and yielded a positive predictive value of 22% and a negative predictive value of 2% given an estimated prevalence of serious bacterial illness of 7%. The pooled sensitivity for C-reactive protein in discriminating between serious bacterial illness and nonbacterial infection was 77%, and the specificity was 79%.

Using a cut point of 0.12 nanograms/mL, Maniaci et al[40] found that **procalcitonin** had a sensitivity of 95.2%, specificity of 25.5%, and negative predictive value of 96.1% for serious bacterial illness among febrile infants in the first 3 months of life.

Manzano et al[41] compared the test characteristics of **WBC, absolute neutrophil count, C-reactive protein, and procalcitonin** for distinguishing serious bacterial illness among febrile infants and children 1 to 36 months of age with no identifiable source for fever. The sensitivity and specificity of procalcitonin and C-reactive protein were 87.5% and approximately 70% using cut points of 0.2 nanograms/mL and 17.7 milligrams/L, respectively; using a cut point of 14,000/mm^3 for WBC and 5200/mm^3 for absolute neutrophil count, the sensitivity was only 75%. The authors concluded that serum biomarkers were superior to clinical impression for the detection of serious bacterial illness in children with fever and no source, but insufficiently sensitive or specific for clinical decision making.

INFANTS 3 TO 36 MONTHS OLD

CLINICAL FEATURES

Clinical assessment is more reliable for older infants and young children than for young infants. Viral illnesses, including respiratory infections and gastroenteritis, account for most febrile illnesses and usually have system-specific symptoms, such as vomiting, diarrhea, rhinorrhea, cough, or rash. Characteristics to note are willingness of patients to make eye contact, playfulness and positive response to interactions, negative response to noxious stimuli, alertness, and ease of consolation. Toxic infants will not respond appropriately.

Otitis media is generally caused by ***S. pneumoniae*** or nontypeable ***H. influenzae***. Although pneumonia is commonly viral, it is difficult to distinguish bacterial from viral causes. In older infants or young children with UTI, fever is usually the only presenting sign, but a history of foul-smelling urine or crying with urination may be noted. Cellulitis is clinically apparent. Abscess may be associated with these patients as well. Bacterial pharyngitis is unlikely under the age of 3 years old.

Nuchal rigidity and Kernig or Brudzinski signs may be absent in children with meningitis even up to the age of 2 years old. A bulging fontanelle, vomiting, irritability that increases when the infant is held, inconsolability, or a complex febrile seizure may be the only signs suggestive of meningitis. Infants with aseptic meningitis generally should be hospitalized and provided with long-term follow-up because they are at greater risk for dehydration and subsequent neurologic and learning disabilities.

Petechiae noted on physical examination are concerning for infection by *N. meningitidis*. However, most children with fever and petechiae will have a viral cause, such as adenovirus, whereas **purpura fulminans** (see Figure 249-19), hypotension, lethargy, and meningismus predict meningococcemia. For the well-appearing child with fever and petechiae, there are no good predictors for SBI. Ultimately, time may be the best diagnostic test, with a brief observation period or admission warranted for cases that are indeterminate.

DIAGNOSIS

The American Academy of Pediatrics practice guidelines that advocate testing for UTI in children 2 months to 2 years of age may be broken down into guidelines for girls and boys.[5] *Ill appearance and history of UTI exclude patients from these guidelines.* For girls, testing should be done if they have two or more of the following risk factors: (1) white race; (2) age <12 months; (3) temperature ≥39°C; (4) fever ≥2 days; and (5) absence of another source of infection. Uncircumcised boys should be tested if no apparent focus of infection is present.[5] Circumcised boys should be tested if two or more of the following risk factors exist: (1) nonblack race; (2) temperature ≥39°C; (3) fever >24 hours; and (4) absence of another source of infection.

Many would advocate that empiric blood testing and treatment for these patients is no longer necessary. Although reports of decreased bacteremia incidence have been published, as of this writing no studies to determine predictors of bacteremia, outcome of empiric antibiotic use, reduction of complications, or outcome of nontreatment protocols have been published since the introduction of the pneumococcal conjugate vaccine. In addition, no practice parameters have established a current standard of care, and the American Academy of Pediatrics has not renewed its practice guideline since 1993. The physician is therefore left with evidence of decreased incidence of bacteremia but no studies or practice parameters supporting a selective testing or nontesting protocol.

Given the decrease in invasive pneumococcal disease[42] and the limited predictive value of an elevated WBC for bacteremia,[43] three options exist. The *first option* is following the previous practice parameters and obtaining a CBC and blood culture on all children between 3 and 36 months old with a fever >39°C (102.2°F), and then treating with ceftriaxone only if the WBC is >15,000/mm^3. Because of the low positive predictive value of an elevated WBC, the *second option* is obtaining a blood culture and waiting for results before beginning empiric treatment. The *third option* is to assume that the incidence of pneumococcal disease has decreased so substantially that laboratory evaluation in a well-appearing child is unnecessary, so discharge with primary care follow-up is reasonable. Variants on the first and second options may be to evaluate children between 2 and 6 months of age because these children have not received the first three vaccine series.

TREATMENT, DISPOSITION, AND FOLLOW-UP

Any child who appears ill or toxic, is unable to maintain oral hydration, or has inadequate follow-up after discharge should be admitted for IV hydration and/or parenteral antibiotic therapy. Choices for antibiotics depend on the organism and the regional susceptibilities.

For recognized **bacterial infections**, use appropriate antibiotics based on the type of infection and regional and national standards. Treatment with high-dose amoxicillin (30 milligrams/kg/dose given three times daily, to a maximum adult dose) is recommended for otitis media, pneumonia, and sinusitis. Alternatives include amoxicillin/clavulanic acid, basing the dosing on high-dose amoxicillin, or azithromycin (10 milligrams/kg daily for 3 days) for penicillin-allergic patients.

Patients with **cellulitis** should be treated with appropriate antistreptococcal and antistaphylococcal antibiotic therapy. Cephalexin (20 to 25 milligrams/kg per dose four times a day for 10 days) or amoxicillin/clavulanic acid (22.5 milligrams/kg/d twice daily) are appropriate choices. Given the increase in methicillin-resistant *S. aureus*, consider using an antibiotic regimen effective against this organism: clindamycin (10 milligrams/kg per dose three times a day for 10 days) or a combination of cephalexin and trimethoprim-sulfamethoxazole (trimethoprim, 4 milligrams/kg per dose twice a day for 10 days). The choice of antibiotic therapy for UTIs should be based on regional antibiotic susceptibility testing. UTI isolates are increasingly resistant to trimethoprim-sulfamethoxazole. Therefore, cefixime (8 milligrams/kg daily for 7 days), cefpodoxime (5 milligrams/kg/d twice a day), or cefdinir (7 milligrams/kg/d twice a day) is a reasonable choice.

Approximately 80% of patients with *S. pneumoniae* bacteremia will have spontaneous resolution, but in 20% of patients, complications will arise, such as meningitis, pneumonia, or sinusitis. Each of these factors may be considered if occult bacteremia is suspected. If treatment is indicated, obtain a blood culture before administration of ceftriaxone at a single dose of 50 milligrams/kg. Ceftriaxone reduces the risk of complications from bacteremia.[44] While reducing the incidence of infectious sequelae, the difficulty with empiric antibiotic treatment arises when the blood culture returns as positive but no cerebrospinal fluid studies were sent.

POSITIVE BLOOD CULTURES IN CHILDREN 3 TO 36 MONTHS OLD

Recall all children with positive blood cultures. In the case of positive *S. pneumoniae* cultures: If the child is receiving appropriate antibiotics, is clinically well, and is afebrile, the child should complete the course of therapy. If the child is afebrile and clinically well but not receiving antibiotics, opinions differ regarding the need for additional blood cultures and antibiotic therapy. In general, neither is necessary unless the child has developed a specific focus of infection.

The febrile child with a positive blood culture should receive a complete sepsis evaluation (CBC, urinalysis, and lumbar puncture). For the persistently febrile patient who is well appearing and has a normal evaluation, admission is usual, although empiric treatment with ceftriaxone and follow-up as an outpatient may be considered.

For any patient who is ill appearing, obtain the sepsis evaluation and admit for parenteral antibiotics.

Children with cultures positive for *N. meningitidis* or methicillin-resistant *S. aureus* should be admitted for parenteral antibiotic therapy. For organisms other than *S. pneumoniae, N. meningitidis,* or methicillin-resistant *S. aureus*, more conservative management may be warranted.

Any child who appears ill or toxic should be admitted to the hospital. Likewise, children who are thought to be at risk for serious bacterial illness and do not have reliable follow-up or the ability to return to the hospital should also be admitted for inpatient management.

FEVER IN CHILDREN >36 MONTHS OF AGE

Children >36 months old are easier to evaluate, and their complaints are usually more specific. Children with infections such as UTI, meningitis, pneumonia, pharyngitis, and otitis media are more likely to complain of symptoms typical for these diagnoses. **Pharyngitis** due to group A *Streptococcus* becomes more common in this age group, especially in the school-aged child. However, **infectious mononucleosis** also becomes more prevalent in this age group and may mimic the signs and symptoms of group A streptococcal pharyngitis. Treatment for group A streptococcal infection is amoxicillin (25 milligrams/kg twice daily for 10 days), penicillin G benzathine (50,000 units/kg IM single dose, up to 900,000 units IM for older pediatric patients), or azithromycin (10 milligrams/kg daily for 3 days) for penicillin-allergic patients.

Kawasaki's disease (see chapter 126, Congenital and Acquired Pediatric Heart Disease) is the most common cause of acquired cardiac disease in children and typically presents in children <5 years of age. Patients usually have high fevers for 5 days, strawberry-appearing tongue, conjunctivitis and iritis, red mucous membranes in the mouth and dry cracked lips, and swollen lymph nodes. Peeling of the skin in the hands, feet, and genital area may also occur in the later phases. Variants of Kawasaki's disease also occur, with fewer of these classic signs. Untreated patients with Kawasaki's disease may develop life-threatening coronary aneurysms. Treatment for Kawasaki's disease involves aspirin and IV immunoglobulin.

PROCEDURES IN CHILDREN: LUMBAR PUNCTURE

The usual goal of lumbar puncture (LP) in children is to obtain CSF to test for markers of infection. Measuring opening pressure is not necessary, and therefore the procedure is straightforward. The condition of children with hypoxemia, respiratory distress, hypotension, and tachycardia may deteriorate when they are positioned for LP, so resuscitation and empiric administration of IV antibiotics is needed prior to LP. **In children with thrombocytopenia or factor deficiencies, replace platelets or factor before attempting LP.**

PATIENT PREPARATION

Anticipate the procedure and its difficulties. Assemble a needle of the correct size, the appropriate specimen containers and preprinted labels, and ensure a quiet environment without interruptions. Explain the procedure to the caregivers. In some institutions, written informed consent for LP is required. Describe the process of procedural sedation if it is needed and obtain consent.

Apply a topical anesthetic cream or spray prior to needle insertion to reduce pain and improve the success rate of the LP.[45,46] For infants, sucking on a pacifier dipped in sucrose solution is analgesic and calming and decreases crying. Prepare the skin using sterile technique.

POSITION

Have an experienced health care provider, the "holder," restrain the infant or child. Wrapping the child in sheets may help limit leg movement. Flexing the hips is more important than flexing the neck. In addition, flexing the neck may lead to respiratory difficulty. Whether to choose the lateral recumbent position or the sitting position depends upon the preference of the physician. In one study using US to measure the width of the spinous processes, the sitting position was found to be better than the lateral decubitus position.[47] Although the sitting position may improve flexion of the hips, this position may be more difficult for the holder to maintain.

LUMBAR PUNCTURE TECHNIQUE

Most LPs are performed with a 22-gauge LP needle, usually 1½ in. in length for infants, 2½ in. for children 2 years to 8 years, and 3½ in. for older children. In obese patients, choosing an LP needle may be more difficult. One study calculated that an LP needle length (in centimeters) of 1 + [17 × (weight in kilograms/height in centimeters)] was most accurate.[48] LP depth was measured on abdominal CT scans to derive this formula. Lumbar needles with a clear hub show CSF flow sooner than those with metal or opaque hubs.

Insert the LP needle between the L4 and L5 spinous processes in the intervertebral space in the midline of the back, and direct the needle toward the umbilicus. This interspace is easily located because it lies in line between the iliac crests. Introduce the needle with the bevel of the needle up. Insert the needle until the characteristic "pop" identifies introduction into the subarachnoid space. An alternative method is to remove the stylet from the needle[49] after the needle pierces the skin. Advance the needle, without the stylet, incrementally until CSF flows. Occasionally rotating the lumbar needle clockwise or counterclockwise up to 360 degrees may help improve flow if the bevel of the needle is sideways. When removing the lumbar needle, replace the stylet.

Bonadio originally reported early stylet removal as the "Cincinnati method" in 1992.[49] Early experience with hollow-bore needles without a stylet associated this technique with the development of epidermoid tumors after the procedure. However, by puncturing the epidermis with the stylet in place and removing the stylet after introduction through the epidermis, this complication should be eliminated. Two separate reports found that the use of this Cincinnati method and the administration of topical anesthetics were associated with improved success rates.[45,46]

After successful entry into the subarachnoid space, collect three tubes of CSF, each with at least 0.5 mL of fluid. Send the first tube for cell count, which includes white blood cell and red blood cell counts; send the second tube for protein and glucose measurement; and send the third tube for routine bacterial culture and Gram staining (**Table 116-4**). Additional tubes may be collected for polymerase chain reaction testing for bacteria and viruses as needed (e.g., enterovirus, herpes simplex virus). If the child has been pretreated with antibiotics, latex agglutination testing may be performed for *Haemophilus influenzae* type b, *Streptococcus pneumoniae*, group B streptococci, *Escherichia coli*, and *Neisseria meningitidis*

TABLE 116-4 Normal Cerebrospinal Fluid Values in Children

Parameter	Preterm Infant	Term Neonate	Child
Cell count (WBCs/mm^3)	9 (0–25) WBCs (>30 cells/mm^3 suggests meningitis)	8 (0–22) WBCs (>30 cells/mm^3 suggests meningitis)	0–7 WBCs (>10 cells/mm^3 in children >1 mo suggests meningitis)
Polymorphonuclear neutrophils (%)	57	61	0
Glucose (milligrams/deciliter)	52 (24–63)	52 (34–119)	40–80
Protein (milligrams/deciliter)	115 (65–150)	90 (20–170)	5–40
Red blood cells	0	0	0

Abbreviation: WBCs = white blood cells.

Reproduced with permission from Strange GR, Ahrens W, Lelyveld S, et al: *Pediatric Emergency Medicine: A Comprehensive Study Guide,* 2nd ed. New York, McGraw-Hill, 2002.

serogroups A, B, C, Y, and W135. However, latex agglutination testing does have poor sensitivity for bacterial infection.

FAILED ATTEMPTS

After a failed attempt, obtain a new needle and restart the procedure. Insertion into the L3-L4 intervertebral space or the L5-S1 intervertebral space may be successful. US- or fluoroscopy-guided lumbar needle insertion may be necessary when all else fails.

REFERENCES

The complete reference list is available online at www.TintinalliEM.com.

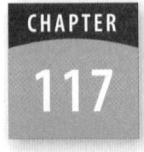

CHAPTER 117 Meningitis in Infants and Children

Amy Levine

INTRODUCTION AND EPIDEMIOLOGY

Meningitis is an inflammation of the leptomeninges, tissues that cover the brain and spinal cord. Untreated **bacterial meningitis** has a mortality of nearly 100%, so treat suspected bacterial meningitis promptly. Unfortunately, even with rapid antibiotic treatment, long-term neurologic sequelae occur. **Viral meningitis** has a range of severity. Mild cases resolve without sequelae. However, some viruses, such as herpes virus, can cause severe infections. **Meningoencephalitis** is an inflammation of the brain as well as the meninges. It is less common than meningitis but can be devastating.

The most common causes of bacterial meningitis vary with the child's age. In neonates, important organisms are group B *Streptococcus*, *Escherichia coli*, and *Listeria monocytogenes*. Other gram-negative bacteria can be occasional causes of meningitis as well. In infants >1 month old and children, the leading organisms are *Neisseria meningitides*, *Streptococcus pneumoniae*, and *Haemophilus influenzae* type b. Vaccination programs have had a huge impact on the epidemiology of bacterial meningitis in developed countries. Prior to the widespread use of ***H. influenzae*** **type b (Hib)** conjugate vaccines, *H. influenzae* type b was the most common cause of bacterial meningitis in children in the United States. Since the introduction of Hib vaccines, the incidence of *H. influenzae* type b meningitis has decreased by 99% in the United States.[1] Similar dramatic decreases have occurred in other developed countries. Immunization has also had a big impact on the incidence of meningitis from *S. pneumoniae* in the United States and other developed countries. At present, the primary cause of bacterial meningitis in the United States is *N. meningitides*.[2] Other important causes of bacterial meningitis in children include *Mycobacterium tuberculosis* and *Borrelia burgdorferi*, the causative agent of Lyme disease.

Viral meningitis is fairly common. **Enteroviruses** are the most frequent cause. Meningoencephalitis can be caused by enteroviruses, arboviruses (including West Nile virus), and herpes viruses. Herpes simplex virus type 1 (HSV-1) infection occurs sporadically and causes a severe meningoencephalitis in children and adults. Herpes simplex virus type 2 (HSV-2) develops in neonates born to infected mothers. Varicella-zoster virus can cause CNS infections including acute cerebellar ataxia. Many other viruses can cause CNS infections, including cytomegalovirus, Ebstein-Barr virus, mumps virus, adenovirus, influenza virus, parainfluenza virus, rubeola virus, rubella virus, and rabies virus.

Fungal meningitis can occur in both normal and immunocompromised hosts. Important causes include *Cryptococcus neoformans*, *Coccidioides immitis*, and *Candida albicans*.

Parasite infections can cause eosinophilic meningitis, defined as meningitis with at least 10 eosinophils/mm^3 of cerebrospinal fluid (CSF).[3] The most frequent cause of eosinophilic meningitis throughout the world is helminth infection.

PATHOPHYSIOLOGY

Bacterial meningitis in children usually results from bacteremia, arising from organisms colonizing the nasopharynx. Less commonly, meningitis is caused by direct spread of bacteria from a contiguous site of infection, such as sinusitis, or from penetration of the CSF space from trauma, dermal sinus tracts, or open neural tube defects. Viral respiratory infections can increase the likelihood of meningitis if the nasopharynx is colonized by bacteria.

Meningitis starts with breakdown of the blood–brain barrier. Then organisms enter the subarachnoid space. Once there, they can multiply quickly because the CSF has low levels of complement, antibodies, and other host defenses. Bacterial cell wall components and toxins produce an inflammatory response that increases vascular permeability and attracts leukocytes. The inflammatory response is responsible for much of the damage that ensues. Viral pathogens also produce damage by direct tissue destruction as well inflammation.

CLINICAL FEATURES

HISTORY

Infants ≤30 days old are at risk for meningitis due to an immature immune response. Symptoms in this age group are variable and nonspecific and include both fever and hypothermia. Neonates can present with a history of lethargy, poor feeding, fussiness, bulging fontanelle, vomiting, diarrhea, seizures, grunting, or respiratory distress. Elements in the birth history that increase the likelihood of bacterial meningitis include prematurity, low birth weight, delivery complications, maternal infection, and maternal colonization with group B streptococci or herpes simplex. Some neonates present with few symptoms early in the course of their illness, so maintain a high degree of suspicion for early meningitis when confronted with a potentially sick newborn.

SIGNS AND SYMPTOMS

Bacterial Meningitis Certain signs and symptoms are especially helpful for diagnosing bacterial meningitis in infants and children. Caregiver reports of bulging fontanelle (likelihood ratio [LR] 8, 95% CI 2.4–26), *or* neck stiffness (LR 7.7, 95% CI 3.2–19), *or* seizures (outside of the febrile seizure range of 6 months to 6 years; LR 4.4, 95% CI 3.0–6.4), *or* reduced feeds (LR 2, 95% CI 1.2–3.4) are concerning for meningitis.[4] Children with meningitis can present with the rapid onset of shock and altered mental status or with more gradual symptoms including fever, headaches, photophobia, upper respiratory symptoms, GI symptoms, irritability, and rash.

The World Health Organization's *Pocket Book of Hospital Care for Children* reported the performance of signs and symptoms for bacterial meningitis in infants and children and did not find any single clinical feature distinctive enough to make a "robust diagnosis of bacterial meningitis."[5] However, the combination of fever, seizures, meningeal signs, and altered consciousness was consistently associated with bacterial meningitis.[6]

Viral Meningitis Infants with viral meningitis typically present with irritability and decreased activity. Headache and fever are the usual complaints in children. Other symptoms include photophobia, rashes, nausea, vomiting, and pain in the neck, back, and legs. Most children with West Nile virus will be asymptomatic or have mild illness. Severe neurologic illness from West Nile virus is more common in adults than in children.[7] Arboviruses can cause viral meningitis, encephalitis or acute flaccid paralysis.

Herpes simplex virus can cause devastating infection in neonates. Infection can present in three ways: (1) as disseminated disease with involvement of the CNS in 60% to 75% of cases; (2) as primary CNS disease; or (3) as disease localized to the skin, eyes, and/or mouth. About two thirds of infants with disseminated or CNS disease will have skin lesions, but these may not be present at the time of diagnosis. Neonatal herpes infections, including herpes simplex meningitis, can occur at up to 6 weeks of age.[8] Herpes infection can be transmitted through an infected maternal genital tract but may also be transmitted from a nongenital maternal infection, for example, if a mother with oral herpes kisses the baby. Herpes simplex encephalitis (HSV-1) beyond the neonatal period presents with fever, altered mental status, seizures, and focal neurologic findings. It occurs sporadically.

PHYSICAL EXAMINATION

Neonates and infants <90 days old may have fever, normal temperature, or hypothermia. A normal temperature does exclude meningitis. Toxic appearance, lethargy, mottling, bulging fontanelle, abnormal cry, grunting, respiratory distress, and increased or decreased tone are all supportive of the diagnosis, but these signs can be absent. Jaundice or rash may occasionally be seen. Infants in the first months of life are unlikely to have a stiff neck. **Fever in neonates (rectal temperature of 100.5°F or higher) should always prompt suspicion for meningitis.** In the absence of fever, a clinician should be concerned about infants who are ill appearing, have the signs or symptoms listed earlier, or are just not "acting right" according to their caregivers.

Older infants (>90 days old) with meningitis may also have fever, hypothermia, toxic appearance, lethargy, mottling, bulging fontanelle, abnormal cry, grunting, and respiratory distress at presentation. **Children (>36 months of age)** may have fever and nuchal rigidity. The **Kernig sign** (with the patient lying supine and the hip flexed at 90 degrees, the patient cannot extend the knee fully without pain) and **Brudzinski sign** (with the patient lying supine, there is involuntary flexion of the legs with passive neck flexion) may be present. Children may have altered mental status, shock, focal neurologic signs, or signs of increased intracranial pressure. Rash or another focal sign of infection may be present. Consider bacterial meningitis in the child with seizures, outside the range of 6 months to 6 years.

DIAGNOSIS

DIFFERENTIAL DIAGNOSIS

In neonates, the most common causes of meningitis in the United States are group B *Streptococcus*, *E. coli*, and *L. monocytogenes*. Other organisms that cause meningitis include *S. pneumoniae*, other streptococci, nontypeable *H. influenzae*, *Staphylococcus* species, *Klebsiella*, *Enterobacter*, *Pseudomonas*, *Treponema pallidum*, and *M. tuberculosis*.[9] Neonates can develop meningitis from primary viral infection with HSV or enteroviruses. The differential diagnosis of neonatal sepsis and meningitis includes infection from fungi (*Candida*) and protozoa (malaria crosses the placenta, and maternal malaria can infect the neonate). Noninfectious illnesses that can appear similar to sepsis and meningitis include cardiac disease, necrotizing enterocolitis, congenital adrenal hyperplasia, inborn errors of metabolism, and intracranial hemorrhage.

TABLE 117-1 ED Treatment of Bacterial Meningitis by Age Group[10]

Neonatal Meningitis Treatment	Meningitis Treatment in Older Infants and Children
Ampicillin* 50 milligrams/kg every 6 h AND	Cefotaxime† 75 milligrams/kg every 6 h OR Ceftriaxone† 100 milligrams/kg every 24 h
Gentamicin 2.5 milligrams/kg every 12 h for 0–7 days old; every 8 h for >7 days old OR Cefotaxime* 100 milligrams/kg every 8 h	
AND if herpes suspected	AND if herpes suspected
Acyclovir 20 milligrams/kg every 8 h	Acyclovir 20 milligrams/kg every 8 h

*For penicillin/β-lactam allergy, substitute chloramphenicol 50 milligrams/kg every 12 hours.[11]

†For penicillin/β-lactam allergy, substitute chloramphenicol 25 milligrams/kg every 6 hours.[11]

In older infants and children, the usual dilemma is differentiating acute viral and bacterial meningitis. The typical bacterial causes are *N. meningitides*, *S. pneumoniae*, and *H. influenzae* type b. Less common organisms include *M. tuberculosis*, *Nocardia* species, *T. pallidum*, and *B. burgdorferi*.[2] Fungal infections and parasitic infections can produce infection of the CNS. Infections around the brain and spinal cord may appear similar to meningitis. Collagen vascular disease, malignancy, and certain drugs and toxins should also be included in the differential diagnosis.

LABORATORY TESTING

All children suspected of having meningitis should undergo a lumbar puncture when they are clinically stable. Although establishing a diagnosis is important, patients who are unstable but suspected of having bacterial meningitis should receive antibiotics as quickly as possible (see **Table 117-1**). Defer lumbar puncture until the child is stabilized and can tolerate the procedure. Positioning an infant or child for lumbar puncture before stabilization can result in hypoxia and hypotension. There are a few contraindications to lumbar puncture in children besides hypoxia and clinical instability. These include focal neurologic findings, thrombocytopenia, local infection at the lumbar site, and vertebral abnormalities. See chapter 116, Fever and Serious Bacterial Illness in Infants and Children, for details of pediatric lumbar puncture.

Children with focal neurologic signs should undergo a head CT scan prior to lumbar puncture and should receive antibiotics promptly without waiting for the results of the scan or lumbar puncture. CSF abnormalities of meningitis, such as neutrophilic pleocytosis, low glucose, and high protein, will persist for days despite antibiotic treatment. Bacteria are generally not evident on Gram stain after antibiotics have penetrated the CSF (time intervals for clearance of bacteria in the CSF range from 15 minutes to several hours; see later section, "The Child Pretreated with Antibiotics").

Spinal fluid should be sent for cell count, protein, glucose, Gram stain, and culture. In the event of a traumatic tap, send fluid for culture and use clinical judgment in the interpretation of other results. **Decision rules correcting the WBC count based on the number of red cells may not be reliable.**

The CSF of patients with bacterial meningitis tends to have lower glucose, higher protein, higher WBC counts, and a more frequent predominance of neutrophils relative to the CSF of patients with viral meningitis, but there is considerable overlap between the two groups.[12-14] Data for the development of the Bacterial Meningitis Score were collected on children from 20 U.S. EDs from 2001 to 2004, and *any one* of the following risk factors was associated with bacterial meningitis: CSF protein >80 micrograms/L; positive CSF Gram stain; peripheral absolute neutrophil count ≥10,000 cells/μL; CSF absolute neutrophil count ≥1000 cells/μL; or a seizure before or after presentation.[15] The Bacterial Meningitis Score predicted a very low risk of bacterial meningitis for those children with none of the above risk factors (sensitivity, 98.3%; negative predictive value, 99.9%). Two children, both <2 months old, had bacterial meningitis despite a negative Bacterial Meningitis Score. The overall worldwide generalizability of the score, or its stability in view of a country's vaccination practices, is not known. The biomarkers of erythrocyte sedimentation rate, C-reactive protein, interleukin-6, and procalcitonin do not perform robustly enough to serve as proxies for lumbar puncture and examination and culture of CSF.

Polymerase chain reaction is especially helpful in diagnosing viral meningitis. Polymerase chain reaction is available for HSV, Epstein-Barr virus, enterovirus, and cytomegalovirus, as well as others. Polymerase chain reaction is useful for the diagnosis of meningitis due to tuberculosis and is sensitive for acute neurosyphilis as well.[16]

Latex agglutination testing has been proposed for the rapid diagnosis of bacterial meningitis, particularly when the patient has already received antibiotics. However, testing is only available for certain bacteria. Furthermore, sensitivity varies depending on the organism. A negative test does not rule out bacterial meningitis. Although latex agglutination testing may be helpful in certain situations, it is not recommended for routine use.[17,18] Counterimmunoelectrophoresis can also be used for identifying bacterial causes of meningitis. It requires special equipment and is cumbersome to perform.[19] Counterimmunoelectrophoresis has relatively poor specificity, creating a number of false positives.

ED TREATMENT

ANTIBIOTICS

Antibiotics may have difficulty penetrating the blood–brain barrier. Therefore, doses used to treat meningitis are frequently higher than the doses used for other pediatric infections (Table 117-1).

For neonates, presumptive therapy for meningitis is generally ampicillin and cefotaxime or gentamicin. For older infants and children, Table 117-1 lists empiric treatment that will cover the three major bacterial causes of meningitis in the United States (*N. meningitides*, *S. pneumoniae*, and *H. influenzae* type b).

Patients with viral meningitis and meningoencephalitis generally receive supportive treatment, although acyclovir should be used when HSV infection is suspected. Lyme disease, tuberculous meningitis, fungal meningitis, and parasitic infections of the CNS all require specific therapy.

STEROIDS

Much of the damage caused by bacterial meningitis results from the inflammatory response in the CNS. In particular, labyrinthitis can result from bacterial meningitis, producing sensorineural hearing loss. For that reason, **dexamethasone** therapy to reduce CNS inflammation has been studied as a possible adjunct to antibiotic therapy.

Data supporting the benefits of dexamethasone treatment have not been robust in children. Dexamethasone does appear to reduce the likelihood of hearing loss in children with meningitis due to *H. influenzae* type b. Reviews have not shown a consistent benefit of steroid treatment for other bacterial causes of infection, including *S. pneumoniae*.[11,20]

The American Academy of Pediatrics states that dexamethasone *may be* considered for treatment of infants and children with meningitis due to *H. influenzae* type b[21] but does not recommend steroid use in other bacterial forms of meningitis. If it is used for bacterial meningitis, dexamethasone needs to be given before or with the first dose of antibiotics to be most effective. The dose of dexamethasone is 0.15 milligrams/kg IV every 6 hours. Steroids such as prednisolone are recommended for parasitic eosinophilic meningitis.[22]

The opportunity for giving steroids for bacterial meningitis in the ED is very limited. The diagnosis of *H. influenzae* type b meningitis is not clinical but depends on the Gram stain and other analyses—studies that return after the time frame for steroid administration. Thus, the ED circumstances for administering dexamethasone for meningitis are rare.

In children with bacterial meningitis, the risks of dexamethasone therapy have been minor. A small number of patients have had GI bleeding. Recurrence of fever after dexamethasone has been stopped has also been seen. Theoretically, dexamethasone could decrease the concentration of vancomycin in the CSF, but there are no specific vancomycin dosing changes when dexamethasone is given.[23]

DISEASE COMPLICATIONS

Mortality from bacterial meningitis has been reduced to <10% with antibiotics and supportive care.[2] However, survivors can experience sensorineural hearing loss, visual impairment, seizures, hydrocephalus, cognitive impairment, learning disabilities, and emotional problems.[24] Factors predicting hearing loss include *S. pneumoniae* as the etiologic agent and low glucose levels in CSF. Factors predicting mortality include coma, seizures, shock, respiratory distress, neutropenia, and a high protein level in CSF. Factors predicting adverse neurologic consequences in general include coma, seizures, fever for at least 7 days, and a low WBC count in CSF. Additional, although less robust, predictors include symptoms for more than 48 hours, male gender, fever, and absence of petechiae.[25]

In the ED, physicians may see respiratory compromise, shock, seizures, hypoglycemia, and hyponatremia in children with meningitis. Hypoglycemia results from sepsis and physiologic stress and is treated with administration of dextrose. Hyponatremia most commonly results from the syndrome of inappropriate antidiuretic hormone secretion due to brain inflammation. If syndrome of inappropriate antidiuretic hormone secretion is suspected, initiate fluid restriction to 75% of maintenance requirements after treating shock and dehydration. Low sodium can also be due to home therapy: oral rehydration with hypotonic liquids. Seizures can be due to brain inflammation, hypoglycemia, or hyponatremia, so correct glucose and sodium before administering antiepileptic medications.

Children with meningitis can also develop subdural effusions, empyemas, and strokes during treatment for bacterial meningitis, but these are not usually present at the time of ED presentation.

Viral meningitis and meningoencephalitis can range from mild illness to a fulminating course leading to death or permanent neurologic disability. Some lasting effects can be subtle, such as learning disorders. Fungal meningitis can cause death or severe disability, particularly in immunocompromised hosts. Eosinophilic meningitis from helminth infection is generally self-limited and does not require antifungal therapy.

DISPOSITION AND FOLLOW-UP

In almost all circumstances, admit children with suspected bacterial or viral meningitis for definitive diagnosis, treatment, and supportive care. After discharge, children need long-term monitoring for neurodevelopmental problems and hearing loss.

SPECIAL CONSIDERATIONS AND SPECIAL PATIENTS

THE CHILD WITH A VENTRICULOPERITONEAL SHUNT

One of the most common causes of shunt failure in patients with shunted hydrocephalus is shunt infection. Most infections occur soon after shunt placement. The predominant organism is *Staphylococcus epidermis*, suggesting that the infecting organism is likely introduced at the time of surgery. Other infecting agents include *Staphylococcus aureus*, gram-negative rods, *Enterococcus faecalis*, and *Propionibacterium* species. Predictors of shunt infection include premature birth, use of a neuroendoscope during shunt placement, and replacement of an infected shunt.[26] Only about 10% of shunt infections occur more than 1 year after shunt surgery. Patients with late infections frequently develop peritonitis, often from appendicitis.[27] Shunt infections can present with symptoms of increased intracranial pressure, fever, redness or swelling along the shunt, or abdominal pain. Treatment should include vancomycin and a third-generation cephalosporin. Add an aminoglycoside if the Gram stain shows gram-negative rods.

THE UNVACCINATED CHILD

Widespread immunization against Hib and *S. pneumoniae* has drastically reduced the rate of serious bacterial illness or meningitis from these two organisms. Children who are not immunized benefit from herd immunity. Nevertheless, when unvaccinated neonates or children develop fever, consider meningitis. Prior to the age of 18 months, children are less likely to develop meningismus, and it is difficult to exclude meningitis on clinical grounds alone. The septic-appearing infant or child with no immunizations should be managed conservatively with a lumbar puncture to exclude meningitis.

The real question is what to do with the unimmunized child with a fever who is not toxic appearing and has no obvious source for fever on physical examination. In children who have not been immunized, obtain a WBC count and blood culture and give ceftriaxone if the WBC count is ≥15,000/mm^3. Arrange 24-hour follow-up either in the ED or with the child's primary provider. See chapter 116, for further discussion.

THE CHILD PRETREATED WITH ANTIBIOTICS

Children who have signs or symptoms of meningitis but who have been pretreated with antibiotics present an important challenge. In one study, after receiving ≥50 milligrams/kg of a third-generation cephalosporin, sterilization of the CSF occurred as early as 15 minutes in meningococcal meningitis, about 4 hours in pneumococcal meningitis, and about 8 hours in group B streptococcal meningitis. Blood cultures obtained prior to antibiotic treatment were positive in 74% of cases.[28] Antibiotic pretreatment was examined in another study, which showed that CSF WBC count and absolute neutrophil count were unaffected by antibiotic administration, but patients had higher CSF glucose levels and lower protein levels after about 12 hours of antibiotic administration.[29] In the situation where a child has been pretreated, CSF assays with polymerase chain reaction, latex agglutination, or counterimmunoelectrophoresis may be helpful for the diagnosis of meningitis. In differentiating bacterial from viral meningitis, erythrocyte sedimentation rate and C-reactive protein have not performed well, but serum procalcitonin may be helpful. Using 0.5 nanograms/mL as the cut-off point (<0.5 for viral infection and >0.5 for bacterial infection), the sensitivity of procalcitonin is reported as 99% and specificity as 83%.[30]

THE CHILD WITH CSF LEAK

Children with CSF rhinorrhea or otorrhea are most likely to develop meningitis from *S. pneumoniae*. The signs and symptoms of meningitis tend to be milder in this group than in children with pneumococcal meningitis from bacteremia. Therefore, this is a situation in which meningitis is still a possibility despite a somewhat well-appearing child. Recommended treatment is with a third-generation cephalosporin and vancomycin.[31]

THE CHILD WITH PENETRATING HEAD TRAUMA

Children who have experienced penetrating head trauma can get meningitis from *S. aureus*, coagulase-negative staphylococci such as *S. epidermidis*, and gram-negative rods. Initial therapy should consist of a combination of drugs including vancomycin; cefepime, ceftazidime, or meropenem; plus an aminoglycoside such as gentamicin or amikacin.[32]

THE CHILD WITH A COCHLEAR IMPLANT

A cochlear implant increases the risk of meningitis in children. In most cases, the initial event is an acute episode of otitis media in the side with the implant, followed by the development of meningitis. In the first 2 months after cochlear implant surgery, treat otitis media with parenteral antibiotics. After 2 months, treat nontoxic children with otitis media with oral antibiotics.[33] *S. pneumoniae* is the most common cause of meningitis in children with implants. Obtain cultures of middle ear fluid and CSF in children with suspected meningitis.

Children with meningitis in the first 2 weeks after implantation are at risk of a greater range of pathogens than patients presenting later and should receive broad-spectrum antibiotics, such as meropenem and vancomycin. Children with symptoms of meningitis developing later than 2 weeks after implantation should receive the standard empiric treatment for meningitis (Table 117-1). Consult ear, nose, and throat specialists for imaging recommendations and possible surgical management.[33]

THE CHILD WITH A FEBRILE SEIZURE

Children with meningitis can present with seizures. However, simple febrile seizures are more common. Simple febrile seizures occur in up to 5% of children between 6 and 60 months of age. About one third of children will experience a recurrence. The American Academy of Pediatrics defines simple febrile seizures as seizures that are generalized, last less than 15 minutes, and do not recur within 24 hours. Per the guidelines, a lumbar puncture should be performed if the child has an examination consistent with meningitis.[34] Children between 6 and 12 months of age should be considered for a lumbar puncture if they are missing immunizations against Hib or *S. pneumoniae* or if their immunization status is not known. Clinicians should be able to recognize meningitis clinically after 12 months of age. A lumbar puncture should also be considered in children pretreated with antibiotics because antibiotics can mask the development of meningitis. Routine blood work, imaging, and electroencephalogram are not recommended.[34]

REFERENCES

The complete reference list is available online at www.TintinalliEM.com.

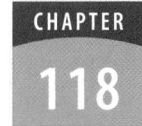

CHAPTER 118 Ear and Mastoid Disorders in Infants and Children

Carmen Coombs

INTRODUCTION

Ear pain, or otalgia, is one of the most common pediatric outpatient chief complaints. The differential diagnosis is listed in **Table 118-1**. This chapter discusses acute otitis media, otitis media with effusion, otitis externa, acute mastoiditis, and foreign body. Anatomically, the ear is divided into three major parts: (1) the outer ear, which includes the auricle and the external auditory canal; (2) the middle ear, which is bound by the tympanic membrane laterally, contains the auditory ossicles, and is connected to the nasopharynx via the eustachian tube; and (3) the inner ear, which includes the semicircular canals, the cochlea, and the auditory nerve (**Figure 118-1**).

ACUTE OTITIS MEDIA

EPIDEMIOLOGY

Otitis media is a general term used to describe inflammation within the middle ear, and acute otitis media (AOM) specifically refers to the acute onset of signs and symptoms of middle ear inflammation. Otitis media is one of the two most common diagnoses for outpatient sick visits in children under 15 years old, accounting for 7.4% of all ED visits,[1] and is second only to acute upper respiratory infection.[2] However, visits appear to be decreasing due to a combination of increased financial barriers to care, improved public education regarding the viral nature of most infectious diseases, and the administration of contemporary pneumococcal and influenza vaccines.[3]

The peak incidence of AOM is between 6 and 18 months of age.[4] In the United States, up to 50% of children will have had at least one episode of AOM by the age of 1 year.[5] The incidence is higher in children who are Native Americans, Eskimos, males, day care attendees, exposed to tobacco smoke, born with craniofacial anomalies, prone position sleepers, pacifier users, or born with immunodeficiency syndromes.[4,5] The incidence is also higher in infants who are diagnosed with their first episode of AOM before 6 months of age. Breastfed infants have a lower incidence of AOM compared to infants who are formula-fed.[5]

TABLE 118-1 Differential Diagnosis of Acute Ear Pain

Common
Acute otitis media
Otitis externa
Foreign body in the external ear canal
Otitis media with effusion
Impacted cerumen
Less common
Cholesteatoma
Referred pain from oral cavity pathology (e.g., dental caries and infections, pharyngitis)
Cellulitis of the auricle/pinna
Contact dermatitis (e.g., earrings)
Trauma to the auricle/pinna (e.g., hematoma and subsequent pressure necrosis of cartilage)
Physical trauma or barotrauma to the tympanic membrane and middle ear
Rare
Mastoiditis
Herpes zoster oticus (Ramsay Hunt syndrome)
Hemotympanum due to basilar skull fracture
Rhabdomyosarcoma of the ear or temporal bone

PATHOPHYSIOLOGY

The middle ear is a laterally compressed cavity within the temporal bone bounded by the tympanic membrane laterally and the eustachian tube medially (Figure 118-1). In the healthy state, this space is aerated and contains the auditory bones, which transmit sound to the inner ear. Compared with adults, the eustachian tube in children is shorter and more horizontally oriented. This orientation is the anatomic rationale for the increased incidence of middle ear disease seen in children. An upper respiratory tract infection can obstruct the eustachian tube and disrupt its function of aerating the middle ear, creating conditions favorable to the development of sterile or purulent effusions.

Microorganisms responsible for AOM originate from the nasopharynx, enter the middle ear space via the eustachian tube, and include both bacteria and viruses. Both bacteria and viruses can be isolated in 66% of cases of AOM, bacteria alone in 27%, and viruses alone in 4%, and cultures are negative for both in 4%.[6] The most common bacterial pathogens are *Streptococcus pneumoniae* (49%), nontypeable *Haemophilus influenzae* (29%), and *Moraxella catarrhalis* (28%). Common viruses identified in cases of AOM include picornaviruses such as rhinovirus and enterovirus, respiratory syncytial virus, and parainfluenza virus.[6]

CLINICAL FEATURES

The classic symptom is rapid-onset ear pain. Young or nonverbal children may hold, tug, or rub the ear or be fussy and irritable. Fever is present in many but not all, although fever ≥40.5°C (104.9°F) is rare.[7] Older children may complain of decreased hearing due to conductive hearing loss of middle ear effusion. An antecedent history of rhinorrhea, congestion, and/or cough is common because an upper respiratory tract infection creates conditions favorable to the development of AOM.

The most common acute complication is tympanic membrane perforation. More serious acute complications are rare and include mastoiditis, spread to the intracranial cavity (meningitis, encephalitis, abscess, sinus thrombosis, otitis hydrocephalus, facial or abducens nerve palsy), and involvement of the inner ear (labyrinthitis). Acquired sensorineural hearing loss can result from chronic or recurrent AOM and secondary inflammatory changes in the inner ear.

DIAGNOSIS

The diagnosis is clinical. Although tympanocentesis is the gold standard for diagnosis, it is outside the scope of most pediatricians and emergency physicians. Guidelines for clinical diagnosis are listed in Table 118-2.[3] **Erythema of the tympanic membrane alone is insufficient for the diagnosis of AOM because erythema can be caused by middle ear inflammation, crying, or fever.**

For proper otoscopic examination, use a bright light source, clean otoscope head, and properly fitting speculum. To immobilize the child's head, have the caregiver hold the child's head against the caregiver's shoulder or chest. Or place the child supine with the examiner controlling the head of the child and the parents holding the child's arms. Remove impacted cerumen with a soft speculum or by gently irrigating

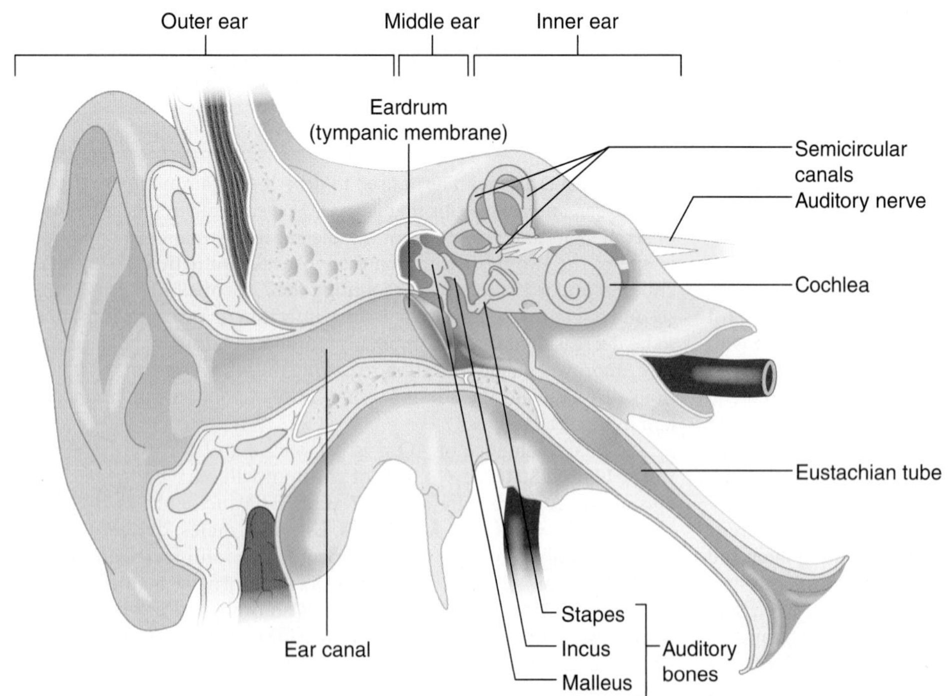

FIGURE 118-1. Anatomy of the outer, middle, and inner ear.

TABLE 118-2 Clinical Criteria for the Diagnosis of Acute Otitis Media (AOM)

Scenario 1	Moderate to severe bulging of the tympanic membrane
Scenario 2	Mild bulging of the tympanic membrane and at least 1 of the following: Acute onset of ear pain (<48 h) Intense erythema of the tympanic membrane
Scenario 3	New onset of otorrhea not due to otitis externa or foreign body (indicating perforation of the tympanic membrane or AOM in a child with tympanostomy tubes)

the canal with warm water. Both procedures can cause pain and/or traumatic perforation of the tympanic membrane and must be done carefully. Adjunctive use of a topical ceruminolytic agent such as docusate may be helpful in some cases.[8]

Assess for the presence or absence of discharge in the ear canal and the tympanic membrane's position, color, degree of translucency, and mobility in response to positive and negative pressures created by the pneumatoscope. **Table 118-3** and **Figures 118-2** and **118-3** compare normal and abnormal tympanic membrane findings of effusion.

TREATMENT

Most cases of AOM resolve spontaneously and without complications. Tympanic membrane perforation typically heals spontaneously after AOM resolution, but persistent perforations require ear, nose, and throat referral.

Antibiotics are recommended for some but not all cases of AOM.[3] **Pain control, however, is an essential treatment modality and should be provided whether or not antibiotics are prescribed.**

PAIN CONTROL

The medications most commonly used to treat ear pain are shown in **Table 118-4**. Ibuprofen and acetaminophen are analgesic and antipyretics. Opioids medications such as oxycodone and hydrocodone may be considered for severe ear pain but should be reserved as second-line agents and used cautiously. Topical otic analgesic drops may be used in combination with systemic analgesics because they have a rapid onset and may provide temporary relief of ear pain but have a short duration of action.[9-11] **Topical analgesics are contraindicated in patients with perforation of the tympanic membrane and those with tympanostomy tubes.**

ANTIBIOTICS OR OBSERVATION

Consensus guidelines from the American Academy of Pediatrics and American Academy of Family Physicians recommend an initial observation option (defined as withholding immediate antibiotics) for **select children** with AOM.[3,12] An observational approach for AOM has been used successfully in areas of Europe with similar rates of mastoiditis (the primary suppurative complication of AOM) compared to the United States,[13] and this approach is now supported by several randomized controlled trials, systemic reviews, and observational studies.[3] **Tables 118-5** and **118-6** describe which children require initial antibiotics and which children can initially be observed without antibiotics.

TABLE 118-3 Tympanic Membrane (TM) Characteristics: Normal versus Middle Ear Effusion

TM Finding	Normal	Middle Ear Effusion
Position*	Flat	Bulging
Color	Pearly gray	Erythematous or hemorrhagic
Translucency	Translucent with easily discernable bony landmarks	Opaque without easily discernable bony landmarks
Mobility	Freely mobile	Decreased or absent

*The TM may also be in the retracted position, which is usually a normal variant or reflective of otitis media with effusion rather than acute otitis media.

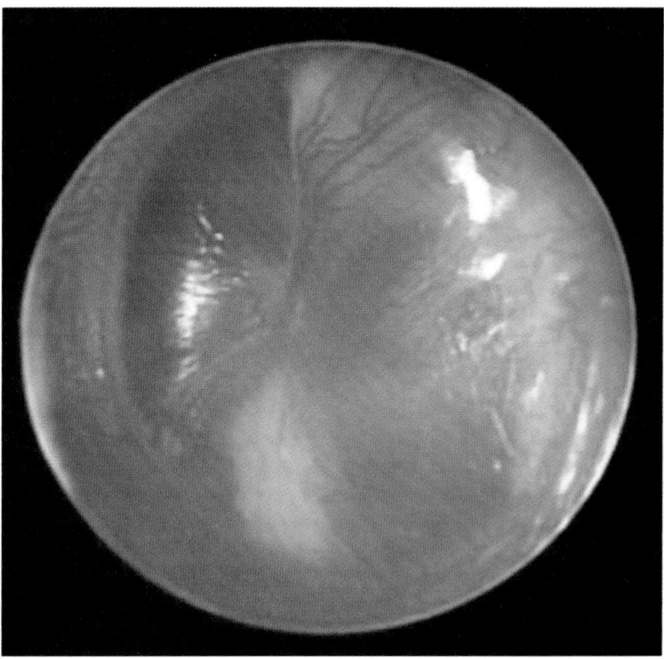

FIGURE 118-2. Normal right tympanic membrane (TM). TM is flat, pearly gray, and translucent. [Image used with permission of Dr. Shelagh Cofer, Department of Otolaryngology, Mayo Clinic.]

If acceptable to both the provider and caregivers, initial observation with close follow-up and initiation of antibiotics only if the child develops worsening symptoms or fails to improve within 48 to 72 hours of onset of symptoms is appropriate for children who do not fall into one of the categories listed in Table 118-5. This group consists of healthy children with uncomplicated AOM who are 6 to 23 months old with **unilateral** AOM without severe signs or symptoms and children ≥24 months old with **bilateral or unilateral** AOM without severe signs or symptoms.[3] When observation is used, a mechanism must be in place to ensure follow-up and initiation of antibiotics if the child worsens or fails to improve. A wait-and-see antibiotic prescription can be provided at the initial visit with instructions for the caregiver to initiate antibiotics if the child worsens or fails to improve.

CHOICE OF INITIAL ANTIBIOTICS

Initial antibiotic treatment for AOM in which antibiotics are prescribed is shown in **Table 118-7**. High-dose amoxicillin (45 milligrams/kg/dose PO twice daily) for 5 to 10 days is the first-line treatment.[3] The higher dose achieves concentrations in the middle ear that exceed the minimum inhibitory concentration for highly resistant forms of *S. pneumoniae*, the most common bacteria found in AOM.

With initiation of appropriate antibiotics, fever and ear pain should be expected to persist for 24 to 48 hours. If symptoms persist 72 hours after antibiotic therapy has been initiated, however, reevaluation is needed and antibiotics may need to be adjusted. Management of AOM after failure of initial antibiotic is shown in **Table 118-8**. If high-dose amoxicillin fails, change to amoxicillin-clavulanate or ceftriaxone to provide coverage against β-lactamase–producing *M. catarrhalis* and nontypeable *H. influenzae*. If the second antibiotic regimen fails, treat with clindamycin and a third-general cephalosporin, or consult ear, nose, and throat for tympanocentesis and culture (Table 118-8).

A suggested algorithm for treatment of AOM is illustrated in **Figure 118-4**.

OTITIS MEDIA WITH EFFUSION

Otitis media with effusion (OME) is fluid in the middle ear space without clinical signs of inflammation or acute symptoms of illness. OME can occur spontaneously as a result of poor eustachian tube function but

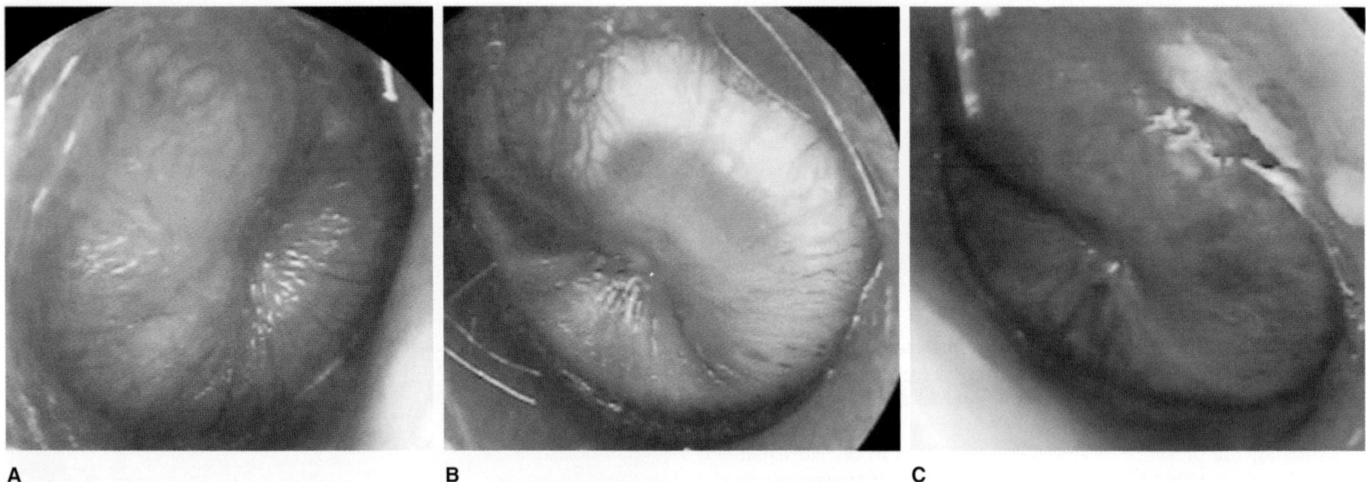

FIGURE 118-3. Tympanic membrane findings consistent with acute otitis media. **A.** Severe bulging and opaque. **B.** Moderate bulging and opaque with intense erythema. **C.** Mild bulging with intense erythema. [Photos used with permission of Alejandro Hoberman, Department of Pediatrics, Children's Hospital of Pittsburgh.]

more commonly results from an inflammatory response after an episode of AOM. Approximately 2 million episodes of OME are diagnosed annually in the United States, with an estimated annual cost of $4 billion.[14] The peak incidence is between 6 months and 4 years of age, and 90% of children will be affected at some time before school age.[14]

Many children with OME are asymptomatic. In some children, however, the effusion can cause mild intermittent ear pain, fullness, or a popping sensation. Because the effusion can impair the mobility of the tympanic membrane, mild to moderate conductive hearing loss in the range of 10 to 20 dB can occur and can have adverse effects on speech, language, and learning in the developing child.

DIAGNOSIS

Diagnosis is by pneumatic otoscopy. A cloudy tympanic membrane often with a visible effusion (visualized as either an air-fluid level or bubbles) and with significantly impaired mobility is the classic otoscopic finding of OME (**Figure 118-5**). Although there is overlap of some of the otoscopic findings of OME and AOM, it is important to remember that the disorders are separate entities and distinguishing between the two is essential. The critical distinguishing feature is that AOM has acute signs and symptoms and OME does not.

TABLE 118-4 Treatment of Ear Pain from Acute Otitis Media

Medication	Comments
Systemic	
Ibuprofen (10 milligrams/kg PO every 6 h PRN)	First-line agents Also work as an antipyretic
Acetaminophen (15 milligrams/kg PO/PR every 4 h PRN)	
Oxycodone (0.1 milligram/kg PO every 4 h PRN)	Second-line agents Consider for severe otalgia Use cautiously due to side effects
Hydrocodone (0.2 milligram/kg PO every 6 h PRN)	
Topical	
Antipyrine/benzocaine (2–3 drops every 1–2 h PRN)	Apply drops to a small piece of cotton and place in external ear canal
Lidocaine (2% aqueous) (2–3 drops every 1–2 h PRN)	Provide rapid but short-term relief Contraindicated with perforation or tympanostomy tubes

Abbreviation: PRN = as needed.

TREATMENT

Close to 90% of episodes of OME resolve spontaneously and without complications.[15] Watchful waiting is appropriate for children with OME who are not at risk for complications.[15] Long-term benefits of antihistamines, decongestants, corticosteroids, and antibiotics are unproven and not routinely recommended. Reexamine children at 3- to 6-month intervals until the effusion is no longer present, significant hearing loss is identified, or structural abnormalities of the eardrum or middle ear are suspected. Hearing and language testing is recommended if OME lasts >3 months or at any time that hearing loss or language delay is suspected in a child with OME.[15]

For children with underlying sensory, physical, cognitive, or behavior factors, OME can compound the risk for speech, language, and learning delays.[15] Children with autism, Down's syndrome, or blindness are examples of at-risk children.

Management of at-risk children with OME should include hearing and language testing and may include speech and language therapy, hearing aids, and/or more aggressive medical and/or surgical management of OME. Refer to an otolaryngologist. Although long-term benefit of antimicrobial therapy with or without steroids has not been demonstrated, a single trial of therapy for 10 to 14 days can be tried in select high-risk cases.[15]

Candidates for surgery include children with OME lasting 4 months or longer with persistent hearing loss or other signs and symptoms, recurrent or persistent OME in children at risk regardless of hearing status, and OME with structural damage to the tympanic membrane or

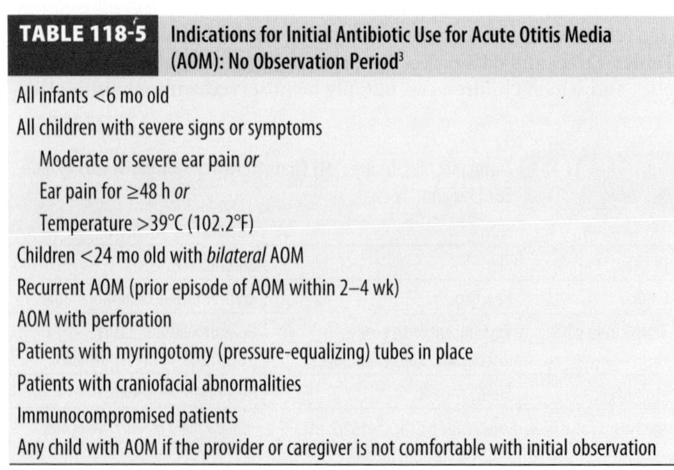

TABLE 118-5 Indications for Initial Antibiotic Use for Acute Otitis Media (AOM): No Observation Period[3]

All infants <6 mo old
All children with severe signs or symptoms
Moderate or severe ear pain *or*
Ear pain for ≥48 h *or*
Temperature >39°C (102.2°F)
Children <24 mo old with *bilateral* AOM
Recurrent AOM (prior episode of AOM within 2–4 wk)
AOM with perforation
Patients with myringotomy (pressure-equalizing) tubes in place
Patients with craniofacial abnormalities
Immunocompromised patients
Any child with AOM if the provider or caregiver is not comfortable with initial observation

TABLE 118-6 Indications for Consideration of Initial Observation for Acute Otitis Media (AOM)*

Children 6–23 mo old with *unilateral* AOM without severe signs or symptoms Mild ear pain for <48 h Temperature <39°C (102.2°F)
Children ≥24 mo old with *unilateral or bilateral* AOM without severe signs or symptoms Mild ear pain for <48 h Temperature <39°C (102.2°F)

*When observation is used, a mechanism must be in place to ensure follow-up and initiation of antibiotics if the child worsens or fails to improve within 48 to 72 hours of onset of symptoms.

TABLE 118-7 Initial Antibiotic Treatment for Uncomplicated Acute Otitis Media (AOM)[3]

	Antibiotic	Dosing
First-Line Treatment		
AOM (with or without tympanic membrane perforation)	Amoxicillin	40–45 milligrams/kg/dose PO 2 times daily for 5–10 d
Special Situations		
Penicillin allergy	Cefdinir	7 milligrams/kg/dose PO 2 times daily for 5–10 d
	Cefuroxime	15 milligrams/kg/dose PO 2 times daily for 5–10 d
	Cefpodoxime	5 milligrams/kg/dose PO 2 times daily for 5–10 d
	Clindamycin	10 milligrams/kg/d PO 3 times daily for 5–10 d
Amoxicillin received in past 30 days *or* Concurrent purulent conjunctivitis *or* History of recurrent AOM unresponsive to amoxicillin	Amoxicillin-clavulanate	45 milligrams/kg/d PO of amoxicillin with 3.2 milligrams/kg/d of clavulanate 2 times daily for 5–10 d
Myringotomy tubes	Ofloxacin otic drops	5 gtts in affected ear twice daily for 5–10 d
Unable to tolerate PO antibiotics	Ceftriaxone	50 milligrams/kg/d IM or IV for 1–3 days

TABLE 118-8 Management of Acute Otitis Media after Failure of Antibiotic Regimen

	Management	Dosing
Failure of Initial Antibiotic		
First-line treatment	Amoxicillin-clavulanate	45 milligrams/kg/d of amoxicillin with 3.2 milligrams/kg/d of clavulanate 2 times daily
	Ceftriaxone	50 milligrams/kg/d IM or IV for 3 d
Penicillin allergy	Clindamycin	10–12 milligrams/kg/dose PO 3 times daily
Failure of Second Antibiotic		
Treatment options	Clindamycin + third-generation cephalosporin	10–12 milligrams/kg/dose PO 3 times daily
	Consult an otolaryngologist for tympanocentesis and culture	

middle ear.[15] The decision to pursue surgery must always take into consideration the risks and benefits of the procedure for the specific child. When surgery is indicated, tympanostomy tube insertion is the preferred initial procedure.

ACUTE OTITIS EXTERNA

Acute otitis externa is diffuse inflammation of the external ear canal with or without inflammation of the auricle and/or tympanic membrane. The peak prevalence occurs between 7 and 12 years of age, and it is rarely diagnosed before the age of 3 years.[16] Acute otitis externa results almost exclusively from colonization of the external ear canal by invasive organisms, the most common of which are *Pseudomonas aeruginosa* (20% to 60%) and *Staphylococcus aureus* (10% to 70%), which often coexist.[17,18] Fungal infection is rare in primary acute otitis externa and is more commonly associated with chronic otitis externa. Otitis externa is most likely to occur when protective features of the ear canal are compromised. The most common risk factor is hyperhydration and maceration of the epithelial tissue, often induced when a child is submerged during swimming ("swimmer's ear"). Occasionally, otitis externa can occur from mechanical debridement of the epithelial layer, as by a cotton swab inserted in the external canal.

CLINICAL FEATURES

The early stages of otitis externa are often characterized by a sense of ear fullness and/or itching. As the disease progresses, pain becomes prominent and is often exacerbated by manipulation of the auricle as well as by any range of motion of the temporomandibular joint. A purulent and sometimes foul-smelling discharge can develop and fill the canal. Because the discharge as well as canal edema can obstruct sound waves, temporary hearing loss may be present. In the severe form of otitis externa, further anterior spread can cause tenderness and inflammation of the surrounding lymphoid and subcutaneous tissue. Rarely, posterior spread can involve the mastoid or can cause osteomyelitis of the skull. Malignant otitis externa is osteomyelitis of the ear canal and should be suspected with the presence of fever >38.9°C (102°F), severe otalgia, and/or facial paralysis or meningeal signs.

DIAGNOSIS

Diagnosis is clinical. According to the American Academy of Otolaryngology–Head and Neck Surgery Foundation, a diagnosis of otitis externa requires the rapid onset (within 48 hours) in the past 3 weeks of at least one primary symptom (otalgia, itching, or fullness) and one primary sign (tenderness of the tragus/pinna or diffuse ear canal edema/erythema) of otitis externa (**Table 118-9**).[18]

Acute otitis externa must be distinguished from other causes of ear pain, otorrhea, and inflammation such as foreign body and AOM with perforation of the tympanic membrane. Placing the speculum of the otoscope into the external ear canal may induce pain and should be done gently.

TREATMENT

Treatment is pain relief and eradication of infection. Provide oral analgesics, such as ibuprofen, to reduce pain. Clean and dry the external ear canal. Dry mopping with a cotton-tipped wire applicator may be sufficient and curative in mild cases.

Topical fluoroquinolone drops, such as ofloxacin or ciprofloxacin, instilled into the ear canal two to four times daily, are the standard treatment. Ciprofloxacin drops are also available in preparations that include hydrocortisone or dexamethasone. Polymyxin B/neomycin/hydrocortisone preparations have been also been traditionally recommended as first-line therapy, but neomycin hypersensitivity is common so fluoroquinolone drops may be preferable. Acidifying agents,

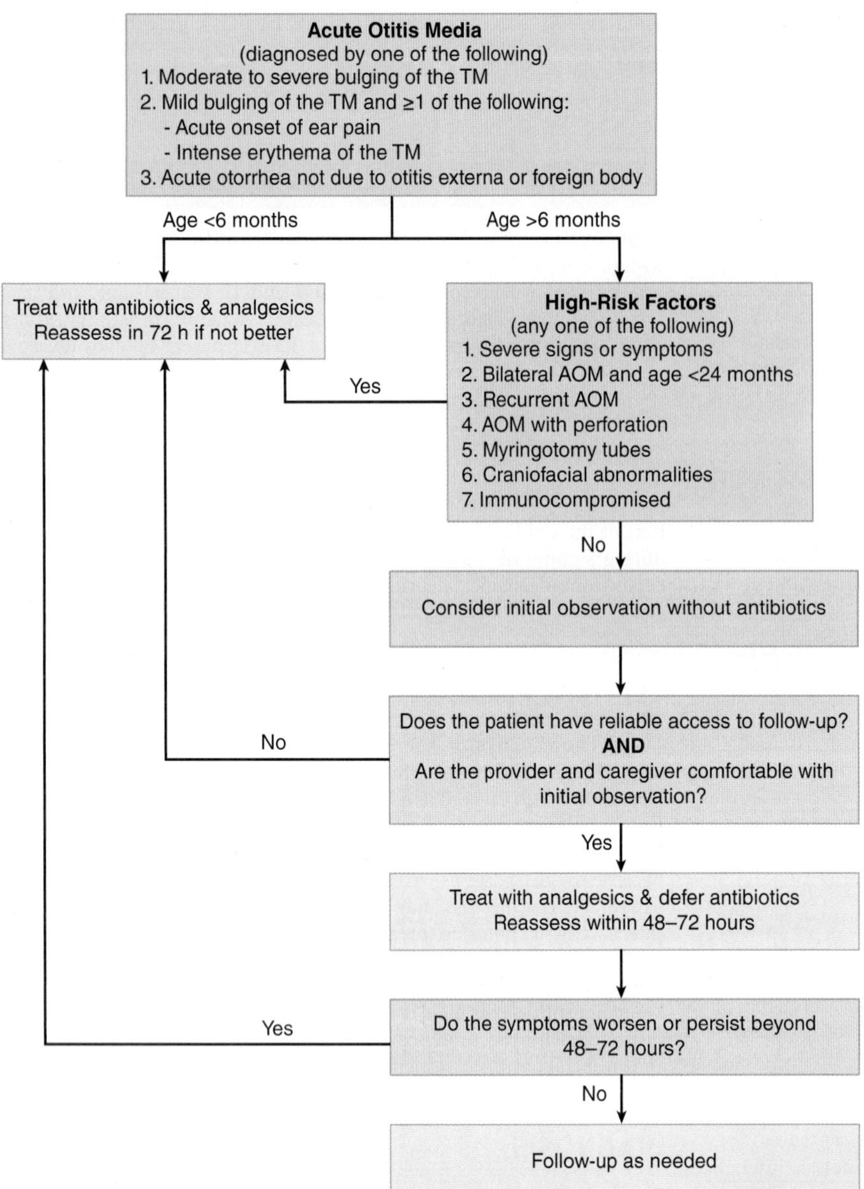
Acute Otitis Media
(diagnosed by one of the following)
1. Moderate to severe bulging of the TM
2. Mild bulging of the TM and ≥1 of the following:
- Acute onset of ear pain
- Intense erythema of the TM
3. Acute otorrhea not due to otitis externa or foreign body
Age <6 months
Age >6 months
Treat with antibiotics & analgesics
Reassess in 72 h if not better
High-Risk Factors
(any one of the following)
1. Severe signs or symptoms
2. Bilateral AOM and age <24 months
3. Recurrent AOM
4. AOM with perforation
5. Myringotomy tubes
6. Craniofacial abnormalities
7. Immunocompromised
Yes
No
Consider initial observation without antibiotics
Does the patient have reliable access to follow-up?
AND
Are the provider and caregiver comfortable with initial observation?
No
Yes
Treat with analgesics & defer antibiotics
Reassess within 48–72 hours
Do the symptoms worsen or persist beyond 48–72 hours?
Yes
No
Follow-up as needed

FIGURE 118-4. Algorithm for management of acute otitis media (AOM). TM = tympanic membrane.

such as 2% acetic acid drops, are painful upon application and are contraindicated in the presence of a suspected tympanic membrane perforation or tympanostomy tubes. When instilling antibiotic drops, lie the child down with the affected ear upward. When filling the ear with the topical agent, move the pinna gently moved back and forth to improve delivery throughout the entire external canal. Have the child remain in this position for 5 minutes after application. If the external canal is extremely edematous, place an ear wick to improve delivery of topical treatments. Remove the wick in 3 days if it has not fallen out on its own as edema improves. Children who fail initial therapy should be reexamined in 48 to 72 hours, and the clinician should consider other diagnoses. Avoid swimming until the canal heals.

Systemic antibiotics should not be given for uncomplicated cases of acute otitis externa. Systemic antimicrobial therapy should only be considered if there is extension of the disease outside of the ear canal and/or there are specific host factors (e.g., immunocompromised) that indicate a need for systemic therapy. Cultures of the external canal may be useful in these cases and should be obtained if possible. Parenteral therapy may be required in severe cases and should include coverage against *Pseudomonas* (e.g., ceftazidime, 50 milligrams/kg IV every 8 hours) and penicillinase-producing organisms (e.g., methicillin, 50 milligrams/kg/dose every 6 hours).

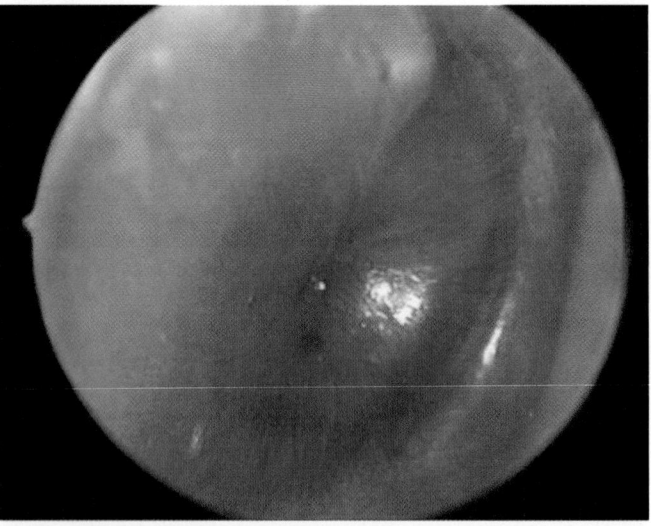

FIGURE 118-5. Well-appearing toddler with middle ear effusion. Note slight bulging of tympanic membrane and visible fluid level. [Image used with permission of Dr. Shelagh Cofer, Department of Otolaryngology, Mayo Clinic.]

TABLE 118-9 Diagnostic Criteria for Acute Otitis Externa: Rapid Onset (within 48 hours) in the Past 3 Weeks of at Least One Primary Sign and One Primary Symptom[14]

Symptoms of Otitis Externa		Signs of Otitis Externa	
Primary (at least 1)	Secondary	Primary (at least 1)	Secondary
Otalgia (often severe) Itching Sense of ear fullness	Hearing loss Jaw pain (pain in the ear canal and TMJ region intensified by jaw motion)	Tenderness of the tragus and/or pinna Diffuse ear canal edema and/or erythema	Otorrhea Regional lymphadenitis Tympanic membrane erythema Cellulitis of the pinna and adjacent skin

Abbreviation: TMJ = temporomandibular joint.

PREVENTION

With repeated infections in children who swim, recommend earplugs while swimming. Cotton swabs applied to the external canal may cause further trauma to the lining of the canal wall. During at-risk periods such as swimming season, daily prophylaxis with acidifying and drying drops (e.g., vinegar and isopropyl alcohol as 1:1 solution) may prevent infection.

ACUTE MASTOIDITIS

Acute mastoiditis is a bacterial infection of the mastoid and almost always develops as a complication of AOM. At birth, the mastoid consists of a single cell called the *antrum,* but air cells quickly develop during the first few years of life, and most children have well-developed mastoids by 3 years of age. The incidence of mastoiditis is highest in children 12 to 36 months of age. The incidence rate of mastoiditis in the United States ranges from 1.2 to 2.0 cases per 100,000 person-years.[13] This incidence is similar in the Netherlands, which has a low rate of antibiotic prescriptions for AOM.[13] There is no evidence that the incidence in the United States has increased since 2004 when an initial observation option without antibiotic therapy was recommended for some children with AOM. Risk factors for acute mastoiditis include recurrent AOM, immunocompromise, or the presence of a cholesteatoma. Cholesteatomas are destructive, expanding growths in the middle ear consisting of keratinizing epithelial cells and can be congenital or acquired (**Figure 118-6**).

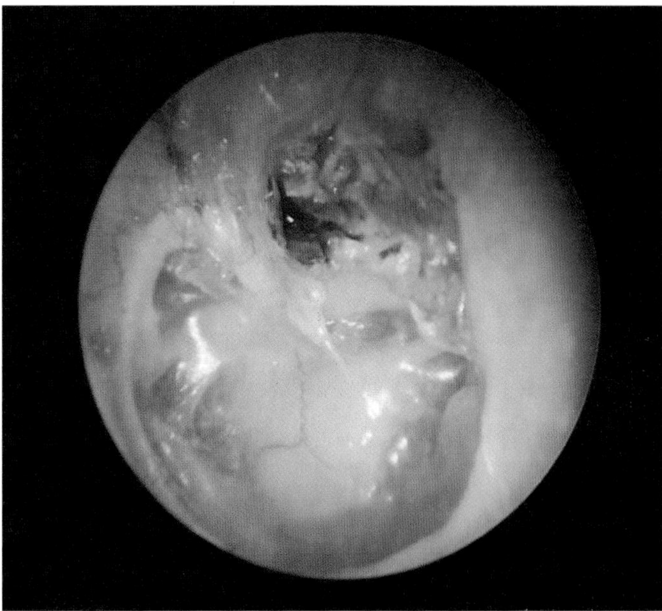

FIGURE 118-6. Cholesteatoma. Cholesteatomas are destructive, expanding growths in the middle ear and/or mastoid that consist of keratinizing squamous epithelial cells. Note the yellow epithelial debris and distortion of anatomy. Cholesteatomas can be congenital or acquired. [Image used with permission of C. Bruce Macdonald, MD; reproduced with permission from Knoop et al: *Atlas Of Emergency Medicine*, 2nd ed. Jauch et al: Chapter 5, Ear, Nose, and Throat Conditions, Figure 5-9.]

PATHOPHYSIOLOGY AND MICROBIOLOGY

Acute mastoiditis develops when inflammation of the middle ear spreads into the cells of the mastoid through the aditus ad antrum. This happens when bacteria in the middle ear space cannot be resorbed properly or when the eustachian tube is obstructed. This process can induce destruction of the mastoid bone and periosteum.

The same three bacterial organisms most commonly associated with AOM (*S. pneumoniae*, nontypeable *H. influenzae*, and *M. catarrhalis*) are common causes of acute mastoiditis, but other important bacteria implicated include *S. aureus*, *Streptococcus pyogenes*, and *P. aeruginosa*. A review of 86 children in Israel with acute mastoiditis found that *S. pneumoniae* and *P. aeruginosa* were the two most common organisms identified.[19]

CLINICAL FEATURES

Fever and ear pain are the classic symptoms of uncomplicated AOM and are also usually present in children with AOM complicated by acute mastoiditis. AOM is evident in >80%, and mastoiditis is unlikely if middle ear examination is normal. Clinical features that distinguish acute mastoiditis from uncomplicated AOM include erythema, edema, and/or tenderness of the mastoid area posterior to the auricle. This process eventually leads to outward protrusion of the auricle (**Figure 118-7**). Advanced disease may cause palsies of the VI (abducens) or VII (facial) nerves.

Complications include direct extension into the intracranial cavity (e.g., intracranial abscess, meningitis), hematogenous spread of infection to separate sites, and otitic hydrocephalus. Otitic hydrocephalus is due to thrombosis of the transverse sinus of the dura and should be

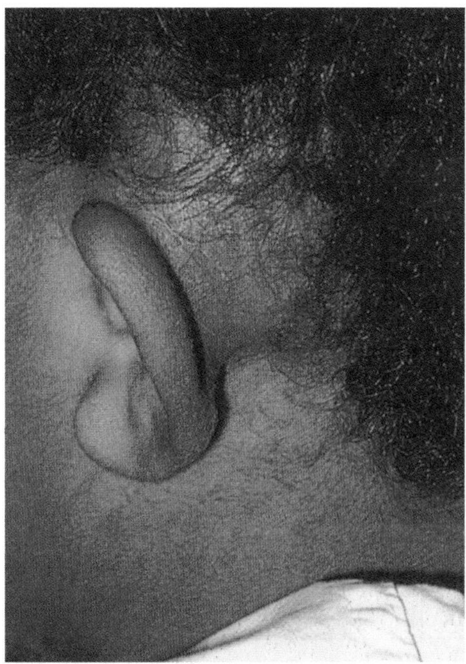

FIGURE 118-7. Acute mastoiditis with postauricular erythema and edema and outward protrusion of the auricle. [Image used with permission of Dr. Shelagh Cofer, Department of Otolaryngology, Mayo Clinic.]

suspected in children with mastoiditis with signs and symptoms of elevated intracranial pressure.

DIAGNOSIS

The diagnosis is clinical. Confirmation is by CT of the mastoid. CT has a high sensitivity (>90%) to confirm the diagnosis and can also evaluate for spread of the disease into the intracranial space. Laboratory tests rarely change outcome. Consider blood cultures in children with fever. Aspiration and culture of middle ear fluid by tympanocentesis are useful to identify the specific organism.

TREATMENT

Broad-spectrum IV antibiotics and inpatient admission are indicated for the vast majority of cases of acute mastoiditis. Initial antibiotic therapy should be directed toward the most common bacteria (*S. pneumoniae*, nontypeable *H. influenzae*, *M. catarrhalis*, *S. aureus*, *S. pyogenes*, and *P. aeruginosa*). Piperacillin-tazobactam plus vancomycin is an example of an appropriate regimen. Antibiotic therapy should be narrowed once a specific organism is identified and continued for 2 weeks after hospital discharge.

Consult pediatric ear, nose, and throat for myringotomy with or without placement of tympanostomy tubes. Mastoidectomy is typically reserved for cases in which there is not significant clinical improvement within 48 hours of initiation of treatment and for cases of mastoiditis associated with extramastoid spread of disease.

FOREIGN BODY IN THE EAR

The foreign body can be anything from a bead to a small toy to a corn kernel to a piece of paper to a button battery. On occasion, a live insect will crawl into the ear during sleep.

Some children will report putting something in their ear and come to medical attention before symptoms are present. Others will develop ear pain and/or discharge as the ear canal becomes inflamed and may also complain of hearing loss. In the case of an insect, acute onset of extreme pain often with the sensation of something moving in the ear is classic.

Diagnosis is confirmed by direct visualization with otoscopy.

Most foreign bodies can be easily removed at the bedside. Young children may first require an anxiolytic medication such as intranasal midazolam. Kill live insects by instilling mineral oil into the ear canal. Foreign bodies that are irregularly shaped can be grasped and extracted with alligator forceps.[20] Consult ear, nose, and throat if the foreign object is a hazardous material such as a button battery. Foreign bodies that do not have easily graspable parts but are not deeply embedded can be removed with an ear curette, suctioning, or irrigation with warm water.[20] For irrigation, thread a thin catheter attached to a syringe filled with warm water into the ear canal posterior to the foreign body, so that irrigation pushes the foreign body out of the canal rather deeper into it. If inflammation is noted after foreign body removal, a short course of topical antibiotic-hydrocortisone otic drops (e.g., ciprofloxacin 0.3% and dexamethasone 0.1%) is indicated.[20] If the above techniques are unsuccessful or there is ear trauma, ear, nose, and throat consultation is needed.

Acknowledgment: We are grateful to Dr. Shelagh Cofer for her otoscopic pictures and photographs of mastoiditis and Dr. Alejandro Hoberman for his otoscopic pictures.

REFERENCES

The complete reference list is available online at www.TintinalliEM.com.

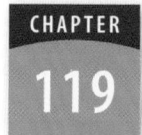

CHAPTER 119 Eye Emergencies in Infants and Children

Janeva Kircher
Andrew Dixon

INTRODUCTION

Pediatric ophthalmologic problems are a common yet challenging issue for all emergency physicians. The history often comes from the parents, particularly in preverbal children, and it may even be difficult for older children to fully articulate their symptoms. The child and the parents need to be calmed and reassured sufficiently to allow for a complete and thorough examination. This chapter includes a review of eye examination techniques and illnesses specific to the care of children. Because the care of pediatric and adult trauma to the eye and its surrounding structures is similar, only those areas of difference are discussed in this chapter. Further discussion of eye emergencies is provided in chapter 241, "Eye Emergencies."

EYE ANATOMY

Eye anatomy is presented in **Figures 119-1**, **119-2**, **119-3**, and **119-4**.

EYE EXAMINATION IN A CHILD

If a history of chemical exposure is obtained, triage as highest priority, and immediately irrigate the eye with 1 to 2 L of saline.

A complete eye exam includes gross examination, assessment of visual acuity, extraocular movements, and ophthalmoscopic exam of the eye. A slit lamp exam of the eye should be performed whenever possible.

Begin by performing a general survey, adopting an outside-in approach, to note any obvious abnormalities such as rash, soft tissue changes, matter on the lashes, ptosis, misalignment of the eyes, injection of the conjunctiva, drainage from the eye, or corneal/lens opacities. Newborns may appear cross-eyed during the first 2 months of life as ocular fixation develops.

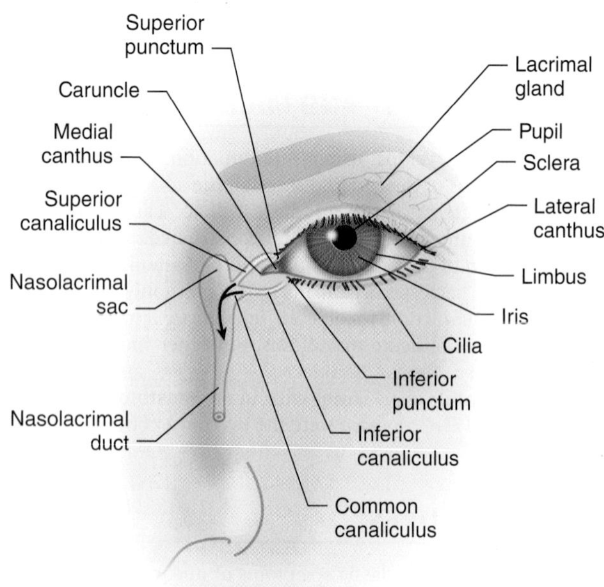

FIGURE 119-1. Anatomic diagram of the eye and the adnexa.

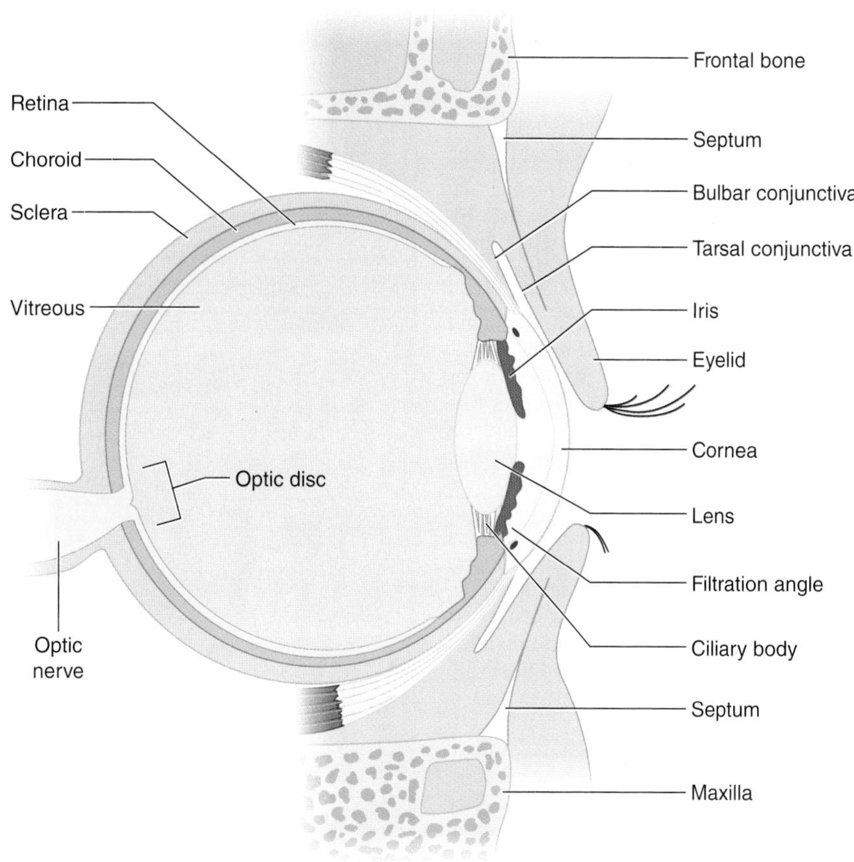

FIGURE 119-2. Horizontal cross-sectional diagram of the eye.

VISUAL ACUITY AND EXTRAOCULAR MOVEMENTS

Visual acuity (V_A) is the vital sign of the eye, and it should be the first objective measurement obtained after the history. Obtaining V_A in a child will depend on the child's age and level of development. A child 6 months to 3 years old should be able to fix and follow a face, toy, or light; a child 3 to 5 years old should have a V_A of 20/40 or better with one line acuity difference between eyes; and a child >5 years old should have a V_A of 20/25 or better with no acuity difference between eyes.[1]

Several different eye charts can be used to check distance V_A in children, including the Snellen, Allen picture, and tumbling E charts. There is no consensus on the best eye chart for use in young children, but if the child knows letters of the alphabet (typically 4 to 6 years of age), the standard Snellen eye chart should be used. Consider using the tumbling E chart if the child is illiterate or has a cognitive disability. Generally, if the child can identify the letters or objects when standing beside the chart, then it is appropriate to formally test the child's vision. To use the Snellen chart,

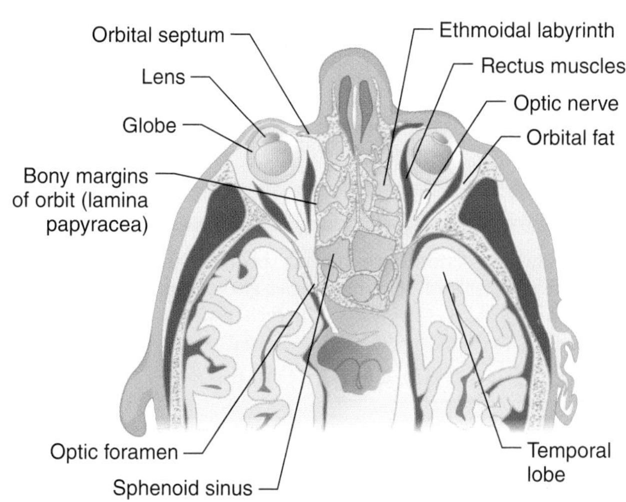

FIGURE 119-3. Orbital anatomy. [Reproduced with permission from Shah BR, Lucchesi M: *Atlas of Pediatric Emergency Medicine*. © 2006, McGraw-Hill, New York, Figure 8-13.]

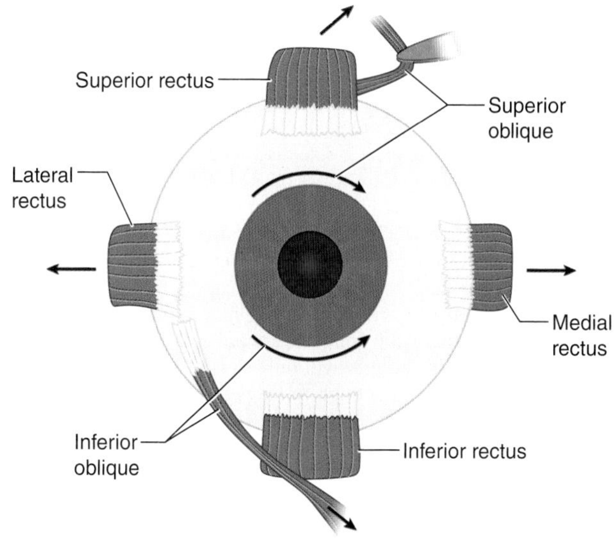

FIGURE 119-4. Extraocular muscles of the eye.

check acuity at a distance of 20 ft. Document V_A for the lowest line on which four or more characters were correctly identified. One can also chart "20/30 minus 3," which indicates the patient incorrectly identified three characters in the 20/30 line. When using the Allen picture or tumbling E chart, acuity should be assessed at a distance of 10 ft. from the patient.

If the child cannot stand, use the Rosenbaum near vision card or the Allen reduced picture cards, held at 14 in. (36 cm) from the eyes to check V_A. Record which chart was used and the distance at which it was tested.

Check acuity in the nonaffected eye first to establish baseline function. If the child holds his or her hand to cover the eye not being tested, make sure to use the palm and not the fingers, so as not to "peek" or put pressure on the globe. A solid occluding device is preferred. V_A should be assessed with the patient wearing corrective lenses. If not available, then use a commercial pinhole occluder or a card with five to six holes created with an 18-gauge needle. If the child is unable to read the top line of an eye chart, then hold up one or more fingers at 3 ft. (1 m) and ask how many fingers are visible. If the child is unable to count fingers, then move your hand from side to side at 1 to 2 ft. (30 to 60 cm) and ask if the child sees motion. Document these responses with the distance your hand is from the patient (i.e., "count fingers at 3 ft." or "hand motion at 2 ft."). If the child is unable to see motion, then shine a bright light into the eye and document the presence or absence of light perception.

For V_A in children from approximately 3 months to 3 years of age, use a brightly colored object, light source, or moving toy to attract the child's attention. See if the child is able to follow it with both eyes and then with each eye individually with the opposite eye occluded.

Extraocular movements can be assessed after V_A. In cooperative children, have the child follow your finger or an object through the cardinal directions of gaze, often in an "H" pattern, as you would in an adult. In younger children, try using a toy or brightly colored object to direct gaze while the head is held stationary. If this is not possible, the examiner can move the head gently while the child stares at a stationary object to watch the eyes move passively in the orbit.

Relieving pain will make your exam much easier, especially in a child unwilling to open his or her eye. With the patient supine, analgesic drops can be applied to the space between the medial canthus and the nose. The drops will flow into the eye when the child eventually opens his or her eye.[2]

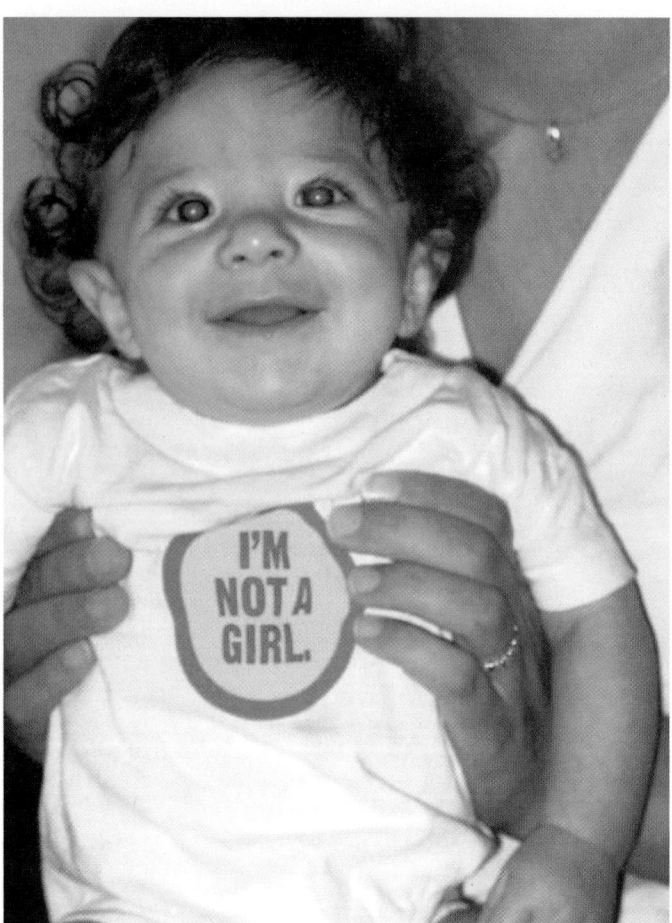

FIGURE 119-5. Normal red reflexes. [Reproduced with permission from Shah BR, Lucchesi M: *Atlas of Pediatric Emergency Medicine*. © 2006, McGraw-Hill, New York, Figure 8-18.]

EXAMINATION OF PUPILS AND FUNDUS

Older and more cooperative children can be examined sitting independently or on a parent's lap. Infants, toddlers, developmentally delayed children, and uncooperative children may need to be swaddled in a sheet. Some patients require an eyelid retractor to examine the eye. One can use a standard Desmarres retractor or an eyelid speculum. If neither of these is available, an eyelid retractor can be made from a bent paper clip cleaned with an alcohol swab.

First, document pupil diameter in ambient light. When checking pupil size, have the child focus on a distant object to exclude accommodative miosis and record whether the size was obtained in bright, ambient, or dark illumination. If the difference between pupils is 0.5 mm or greater, then anisocoria exists. A greater size discrepancy in a dark room when compared with a light room indicates physiologic anisocoria, which is of no clinical significance. It is also important to look for leukocoria (white appearance of pupil), which may be indicative of problems with the cornea, lens, or anterior or posterior chamber. Leukocoria is discussed later in the chapter.

Next, check the direct and consensual light reflexes. A bright light source is recommended for children around age 5 years or older. In younger children, a bright light will only cause the child to shut his or her eyes. If the child is old enough to cooperate, have him or her focus on a distant object in the room, such as a brightly colored picture attached to a wall, or have a parent hold up two fingers while standing at the end of the room and direct the child's attention to the parent. Assess the direct light reflex by shining a light source into the pupil and watching for the pupil to constrict. Then assess the consensual light reflex by shining light into one eye and watching for the pupil of the *other eye* to constrict. Finally, assess for a relative afferent pupillary defect, a sign of unilateral optic neuropathy. First, shine a light source into one eye, and then swing it to the consensual eye. The consensual pupil should remain constricted in response to the now direct light exposure. If the pupil dilates in response to direct light, a positive relative afferent pupillary defect is present. Repeat the procedure with the other eye and document your observations. Some children will have a small amount of pupillary movement (dilation and contraction) in the consensual eye when the light is swung from the direct to the consensual eye. This is pupillary escape and can be a normal response.

Continue with examination of the red reflex, which should be performed in children of all ages.[3] In a dimly lit room, look at the pupils through the direct ophthalmoscope or panoptic scope; position yourself at the patient's eye level about 1 to 2 ft. away. Document the presence or absence of the red reflex for each eye (**Figure 119-5**). With older children, perform the same funduscopic examination that you would in an adult.

SPECIFIC PEDIATRIC EYE PROBLEMS

In the following sections, specific eye problems in children are discussed. Eye injuries and eye emergencies also commonly seen in adults are discussed in chapter 241, "Eye Emergencies."

STRABISMUS AND AMBLYOPIA

Strabismus is ocular misalignment. Knowledge of preexisting strabismus helps differentiate between congenital/childhood strabismus and acquired emergent causes of strabismus. Terminology used to describe strabismus is listed in **Table 119-1**. Normal newborns may have transient misalignment that usually improves by 3 to 4 months of age as the strength of extraocular muscles improves.[4]

TABLE 119-1 Strabismus Terminology

Term	Description
Esotropia	Inward eye deviation
Exotropia	Outward eye deviation
Hypertropia	Upward eye deviation
Hypotropia	Downward eye deviation
Esophoria	Inward eye deviation when other eye is covered
Exophoria	Outward eye deviation when other eye is covered

Amblyopia is a loss of V_A not correctable by glasses in an otherwise healthy eye. If children have unilateral visual impairment, their brain will "choose" the image presented by the eye with better vision. If amblyopia is not corrected by about age 10 years old, the brain eventually suppresses visual information presented by the impaired eye, leading to permanent vision loss.

CAUSES OF STRABISMUS

Emergent causes of strabismus include cranial nerve palsy and muscle restriction or entrapment that may be associated with trauma, stroke, tumor, aneurysm, thyroid-associated orbitopathy or other infiltrative process, increased intracranial pressure, or infection. The innervation of the extraocular muscles defines which cranial nerve is involved. Cranial nerve VI innervates the ipsilateral lateral rectus muscle, and palsy will lead to esotropia. Cranial nerve IV innervates the ipsilateral superior oblique muscle, and palsy will cause hypertropia. Cranial nerve III innervates all other extraocular muscles, and palsy will lead to exotropia, hypertropia or hypotropia (depending on which branch is affected), and ptosis (Figure 119-4).

DIAGNOSIS AND MANAGEMENT

Strabismus is usually suspected after general inspection. Some children have epicanthal folds that lead to pseudostrabismus, or the appearance of ocular misalignment, when the eyes are in fact in proper alignment (**Figure 119-6**). To identify true strabismus, two simple tests must be performed.

Begin with the **Hirschberg test** by holding a penlight several feet from the child and observe the reflection of the light on each cornea. In normal ocular alignment, the light reflection will appear on the same position of each eye. Then, a cover test can be performed. Have the child fixate on a distant object and then cover one of the child's eyes. If the uncovered eye then moves, it can be assumed that it was not properly fixated on the object and strabismus is present. When the eyes are uncovered, they will revert to their original misalignment. Misalignment can further be described as a "tropia," or constant misalignment, or a "phoria," or intermittent misalignment, such as when the patient is tired or fusion is broken (Table 119-1). With a "phoria," the eyes will revert to normal (equal) alignment when both eyes are uncovered.

Historical clues to an emergent cause of strabismus include trauma, diplopia, report of abnormal extraocular movements, sunsetting of the eyes (upgaze deficit), nausea, vomiting, and lethargy. If an emergent cause of strabismus is suspected, obtain imaging directed at the suspected condition.

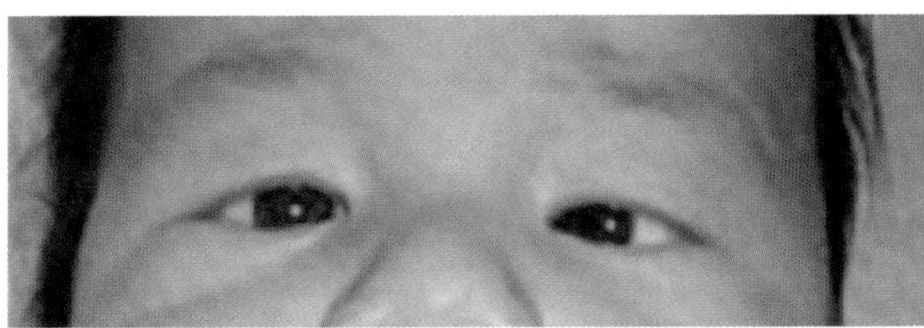

FIGURE 119-6. Pseudostrabismus.

Congenital strabismus caused by extraocular muscle weakness usually self-resolves in infancy. Stable strabismus that persists into childhood should be referred nonemergently to an ophthalmologist. Strabismus caused by amblyopia often resolves with glasses that equalize the vision, although a patch over the "good" eye or surgical correction may be required.

LACRIMAL SYSTEM PROBLEMS

Tears are produced in the lacrimal gland and drain at the medial aspect of the eye through the nasolacrimal duct and lacrimal sac through the canalicular system to the Hasner valve and finally into the nose. Several common problems seen in pediatrics can arise in the gland and canalicular system.

DACRYOSTENOSIS

Dacryostenosis, or nasolacrimal duct obstruction, is a narrowing or obstruction of the nasolacrimal duct. It occurs in 6% of all newborns and usually resolves with conservative management.[5] Dacryostenosis is a common condition presenting to the ED, and infants may present with epiphoria, eyelash matting, and tears that appear thicker and yellowish in color, which may be mistaken by parents as infection. Fluorescein applied to the eye and left for 5 minutes will accumulate, whereas it normally would be cleared by the lacrimal system. An important clinical feature is the lack of accompanying signs or symptoms, such as fever, irritability, or conjunctivitis. If the conjunctiva are not inflamed, the cause is dacryostenosis with evaporation of the aqueous layer of poorly draining tears, which leaves the yellow mucus layer behind and mimics conjunctivitis.

Treatment of dacryostenosis is supportive and does not require antibiotics. Parents should be taught gentle massage with a downward motion to the nasolacrimal duct three to four times a day. If still present after 12 months of age, ophthalmology referral is indicated for possible dilation of the duct.

DACRYOCYSTITIS

Inflammation and bacterial superinfection of the lacrimal sac will cause dacryocystitis. Common pathogens are *Streptococcus pneumoniae*, staphylococci, and *Haemophilus influenzae*.[5,6] Patients develop a chronic mucopurulent discharge followed by erythema and swelling inframedially to the eye (**Figure 119-7**).

In children of all ages, dacryocystitis is usually a secondary bacterial infection following a viral upper respiratory infection. The diagnosis is made when gentle pressure with a finger or cotton swab applied to the

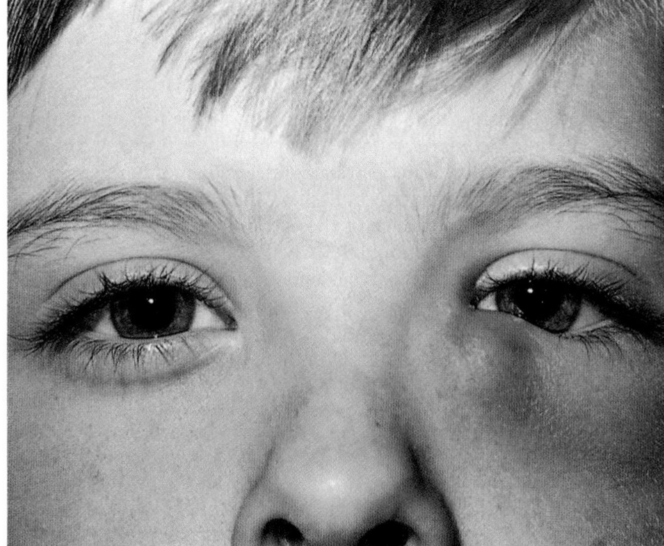

FIGURE 119-7. Dacryocystitis. [Reproduced with permission from Knoop K, Stack L, Storrow A: *Atlas of Emergency Medicine*, 2nd ed. © 2002, McGraw-Hill, New York, Figure 2-10.]

nasolacrimal sac causes a reflux of mucopurulent material. The discharge should be cultured to identify the causative agent.

Improperly treated dacryocystitis may lead to periorbital and orbital cellulitis. Children are often quite ill and require hospital admission with parenteral antibiotics until the infection begins to improve.[7,8] A cephalosporin, such as cefuroxime (50 milligrams/kg IV every 8 hours) or cefazolin (33 milligrams/kg IV every 8 hours), may be used, or clindamycin (10 milligrams/kg IV every 6 hours) may be used for penicillin-allergic patients. If methicillin-resistant *Staphylococcus aureus* is suspected, vancomycin (10 to 13 milligrams/kg IV every 6 to 8 hours) is indicated.[7,9]

DACRYOCELE

A dacryocele is a small, bluish-hued, palpable mass in the location of the nasolacrimal duct (inferior and medial to the eye) without conjunctival erythema, discharge, or other pathologic findings. It is caused by an obstruction at the valve of Hasner and the common canaliculus.[5] Due to possible need for marsupialization, patients should be urgently referred to a pediatric otolaryngologist or ophthalmologist.[4]

DACRYOADENITIS

Dacryoadenitis is inflammation of the lacrimal gland and can be acute or chronic. Chronic dacryoadenitis is caused by noninfectious inflammatory disorders such as Sjögren's syndrome, sarcoidosis, or thyroid disease. Acute dacryoadenitis is usually infectious. In both acute and chronic disease, children will have soft tissue swelling, especially in the region of the lateral upper lid. With infectious causes, systemic symptoms such as malaise and fever may also be present.

Viral dacryoadenitis causes less intense discomfort and erythema than bacterial dacryoadenitis. Causative viral pathogens include Epstein-Barr virus, mumps virus, coxsackievirus, cytomegalovirus, and varicella-zoster virus. Bacterial dacryoadenitis is associated with intense eye discomfort, tenderness, and erythema. The most common causative bacterial pathogen causing dacryoadenitis is *S. aureus*, but streptococci, *Neisseria gonorrhea*, *Chlamydia trachomatis*, and *Brucella melitensis* have also been implicated.[7]

The first-line treatment of bacterial dacryoadenitis is oral or parenteral antibiotics against *S. aureus*. For mild infections, an oral first-generation cephalosporin, such as cephalexin (25 milligrams/kg PO every 6 hours), until the infection has resolved is appropriate. If methicillin-resistant *S. aureus* is suspected, sulfamethoxazole-trimethoprim (20 milligrams/kg PO [or IV] every 12 hours) or linezolid (10 milligrams/kg PO [or IV] every 12 hours) may be used. For more severe infections, parenteral antibiotic therapy is indicated. Nafcillin (37.5 milligrams/kg IV every 6 hours) is appropriate when methicillin-resistant *S. aureus* is not suspected. Vancomycin (10 to 13 milligrams/kg IV every 6 to 8 hours) is indicated for severe dacryoadenitis caused by methicillin-resistant *S. aureus*.[7]

BLEPHARITIS

Blepharitis is inflammation of the eyelid that may present with eye redness, tearing, photophobia, crusting of the lid margin, swelling, or pruritus. Anterior blepharitis is usually infectious in nature (staphylococci) and affects the base of the eyelashes, whereas posterior blepharitis affects the conjunctival surface of the eyelid and is usually caused by meibomian gland dysfunction.[9] Both types of blepharitis are treated with warm compresses and baby shampoo scrubs once to twice daily. Have caregivers apply shampoo to a washcloth and then gently scrub the eyelids. This should be continued until symptoms have resolved completely, which usually requires prolonged treatment. In addition, staphylococcal blepharitis should be treated with erythromycin or bacitracin-polymyxin ointment one to three times a day for 7 days, with the length of treatment depending on severity.[9]

PERIORBITAL AND ORBITAL CELLULITIS

The orbital septum is a connective tissue extension of the orbital periosteum that extends into the upper and lower eyelids and acts as a barrier to the spread of infection. However, infection can be facilitated by the valveless drainage system of the midface region that permits bacteria to travel hematogenously in an anterograde fashion (i.e., away from the heart) despite a retrograde venous system.[10] Periorbital, or preseptal, cellulitis must be distinguished from orbital, or postseptal, cellulitis. The diagnosis may be difficult clinically, and imaging is often required to make the appropriate diagnosis.

PERIORBITAL CELLULITIS

The average age of presentation with periorbital cellulitis is 2 years old. Periorbital cellulitis can be caused by local infection, hematogenous spread, and extension of sinusitis.

Local infection, such as conjunctivitis, dacryoadenitis, dacryocystitis, hordeolum, or even a minor traumatic cellulitis after an insect bite or small scratch, can spread to the periorbital area (**Figure 119-8**).

Hematogenous spread of nasopharyngeal pathogens can also lead to periorbital cellulitis. Affected children tend to be younger (often <18 months old) and have a history of a viral upper respiratory infection followed by abrupt onset of fever and eyelid swelling. The most common pathogens are *S. pneumoniae* and *Streptococcus pyogenes*.[11]

Finally, periorbital cellulitis may be the result of acute sinusitis. Sinusitis can be associated with reactive edema and mild inflammation of the eyelids noted upon awakening that regresses during the day as dependent edema resolves. Unilateral periorbital edema that does not regress may indicate cellulitis. Bacteria that cause sinusitis, such as *S. pneumoniae*, nontypeable *H. influenzae*, and *Moraxella catarrhalis*, are the most common pathogens for this type of periorbital cellulitis.[4]

Clinical Features and Diagnosis Periorbital cellulitis is characterized by an erythematous, tender, indurated, swollen, and warm eyelid and periorbital area. **There is no associated decrease in V_A, conjunctival injection, impairment of extraocular movements, proptosis, pain with eye movement, or other intraorbital pathology.** It may not be possible to always differentiate clinically between an insect bite near the eye, a mild allergic reaction, and early periorbital cellulitis. Children with moderate to severe periorbital cellulitis may have difficulty opening their eyelids for the examiner, so eyelid retractors may be required to fully examine the eye and its movements. A CT scan of the orbits may be required to differentiate between periorbital cellulitis and the often more severe but less common orbital cellulitis.

Treatment, Disposition, and Follow-Up Children who are well appearing and are afebrile are candidates for outpatient oral antibiotic therapy. Amoxicillin-clavulanate (20 milligrams/kg PO twice a day) is appropriate oral therapy. Those with more severe periorbital cellulitis

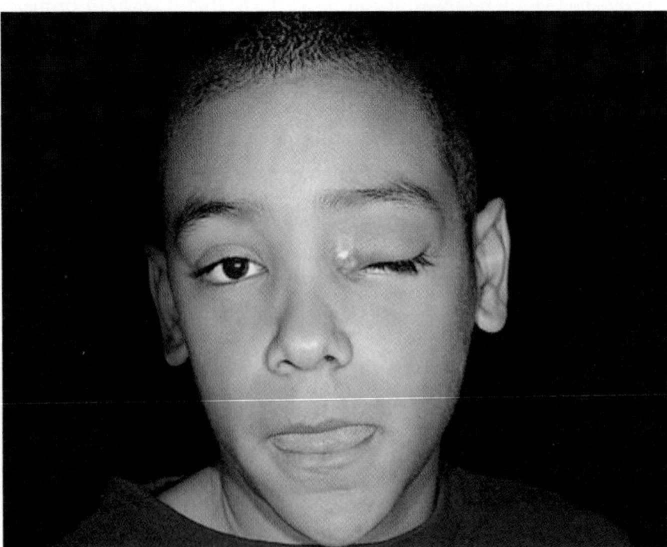

FIGURE 119-8. Hordeolum with preseptal cellulitis. [Reproduced with permission from Shah BR, Lucchesi M: *Atlas of Pediatric Emergency Medicine*. © 2006, McGraw-Hill, New York, Figure 8-10.]

or in whom hematogenous spread is suspected require parenteral therapy and hospitalization. Cefuroxime (50 milligrams/kg IV every 8 hours), ceftriaxone (50 milligrams/kg IV every 12 hours), or ampicillin-sulbactam (50 milligrams/kg IV every 6 hours) are appropriate choices. Add vancomycin if methicillin-resistant *S. aureus* is suspected.[4,7]

ORBITAL CELLULITIS

Orbital cellulitis is usually an extension of a sinus infection into the orbit behind the septum, but may also be spread hematogenously or from traumatic inoculation (**Figure 119-9**). The average age of presentation is 12 years old. Complications include subperiosteal abscess, orbital abscess, cavernous sinus thrombosis, panophthalmitis, or endophthalmitis. The most common bacterial pathogens are *S. pneumoniae*, *H. influenzae*, *M. catarrhalis*, *S. aureus*, *S. pyogenes*, and anaerobic upper respiratory flora such as *Bacteroides* and *Fusobacterium* species.[7]

Clinical Features and Diagnosis Orbital cellulitis is characterized by erythema and swelling around the eye. **Suspect orbital cellulitis if the eyelid or periorbital inflammation is accompanied by any of the following: proptosis, impaired extraocular movements, pain with eye movement, decreased V_A, chemosis, or an afferent pupillary defect** (**Figure 119-10**). Fever may or may not be present.[12]

Diagnosis of orbital cellulitis is primarily clinical, but an orbital and sinus CT can differentiate between periorbital and orbital cellulitis as well as delineate any concomitant abscess or other pathology. Culture of the blood, nares, and conjunctiva may be obtained to help identify the bacterial source. After neuroimaging, consider lumbar puncture for symptoms such as headache, lethargy, neurologic symptoms, or toxic appearance to exclude associated meningitis.

Treatment, Disposition, and Follow-Up Orbital cellulitis requires inpatient management. Consult otolaryngology and ophthalmology for evaluation and possible surgical drainage of abscesses. Parenteral therapy is indicated until significant clinical improvement is noted, followed by oral antibiotics to complete a 3-week course. Cefuroxime (50 milligrams/kg IV every 8 hours) and ampicillin-sulbactam (50 milligrams/kg IV every 6 hours) are appropriate first-line antibiotics. If cefuroxime is used or if an anaerobic infection is strongly suspected, add clindamycin (10 milligrams/kg IV every 6 hours) or metronidazole (15 milligrams/kg IV every 12 hours). Also add vancomycin for life-threatening infections or suspected methicillin-resistant *S. aureus*.[4,7]

THE RED EYE

There are many problems that may produce a red eye in a child. In this section, we focus on the most common pediatric complaints, corneal abrasion and conjunctivitis, and then discuss other pertinent pediatric problems, including Kawasaki's disease and pediculosis. Inflammatory conditions including scleritis, episcleritis, uveitis, and iritis are covered in chapter 241.

CORNEAL ABRASION

CLINICAL FEATURES

Corneal abrasions in older children are characterized by a foreign body sensation, pain, photophobia, injection, and a history of direct trauma, ultraviolet light exposure, or pain from windblown particulate matter in the eye. Smaller children and infants often lack a history of trauma to the eye and may present with a chief complaint of inconsolable crying and an otherwise normal physical examination. If instillation of an anesthetic drop such as tetracaine 0.5% onto the surface of the eye calms the child, it strongly suggests that injury to the surface of the eye may be the source of the child's distress.

DIAGNOSIS AND TREATMENT

A thorough eye examination with instillation of fluorescein confirms the diagnosis of corneal abrasion. An abrasion will fluoresce to a yellow-green color under the cobalt blue filter in the slit lamp or handheld Wood's lamp. The presence of a vertical linear abrasion suggests the presence of a retained foreign body, and the upper eyelid should be everted and the superior conjunctiva examined. If details on the iris are not visible due to corneal opacification, this may indicate a corneal ulcer, and the patient should be seen by an ophthalmologist the same day.[13]

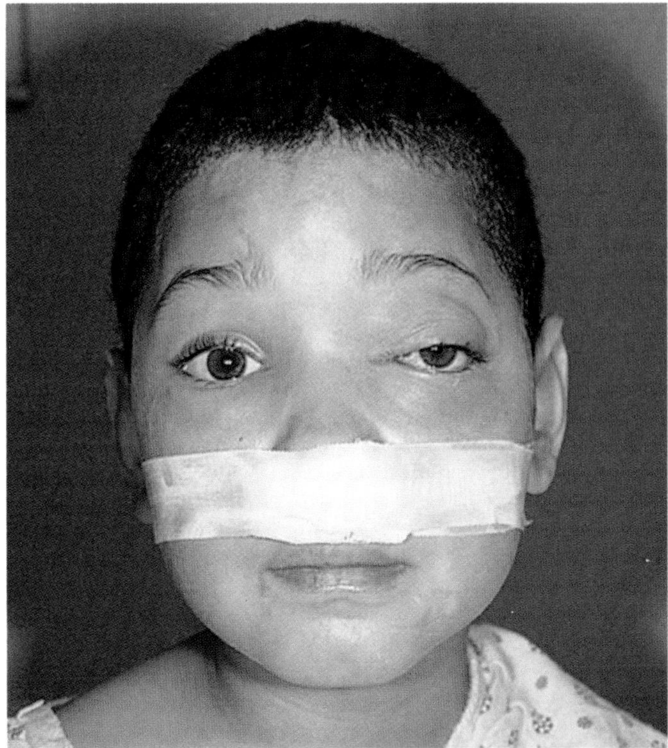

A

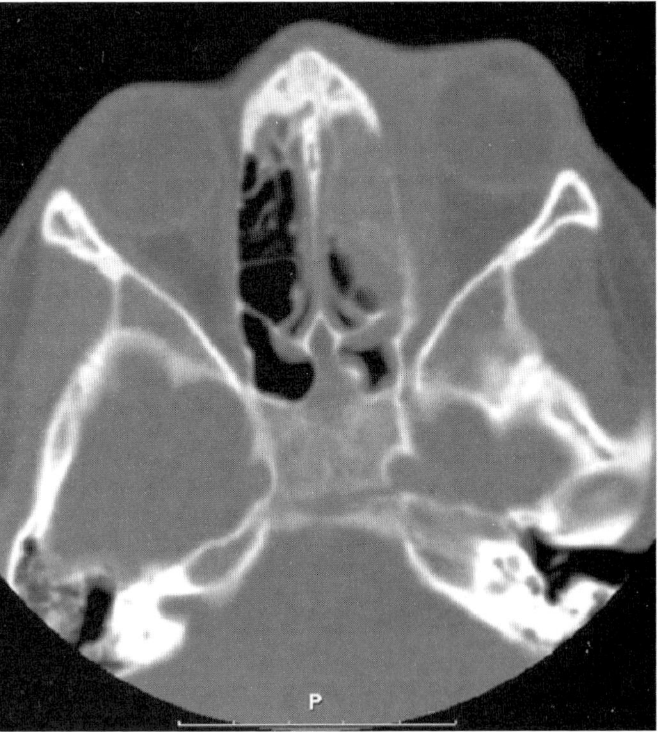

B

FIGURE 119-9. A and B. Sinusitis with orbital cellulitis. [Reproduced with permission from Shah BR, Lucchesi M: *Atlas of Pediatric Emergency Medicine*. © 2006, McGraw-Hill, New York, Figure 8-15.]

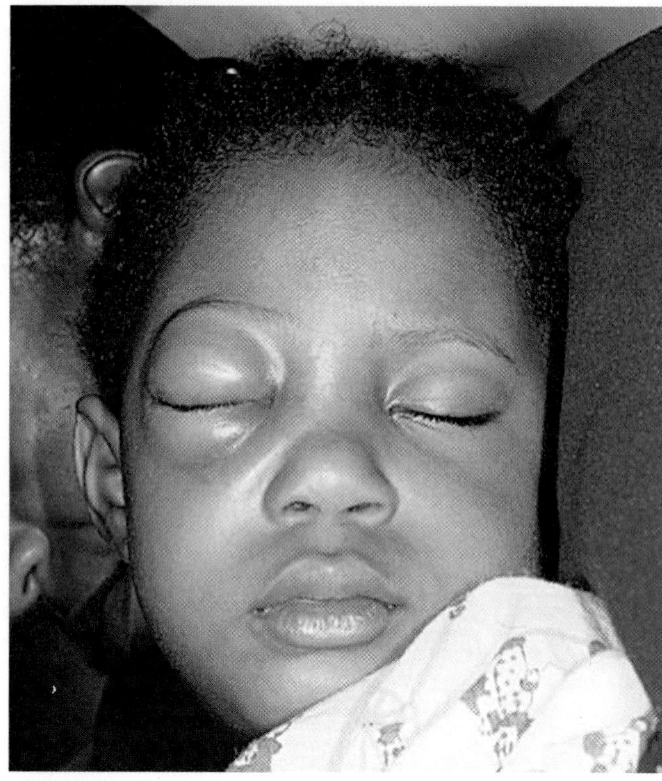

A

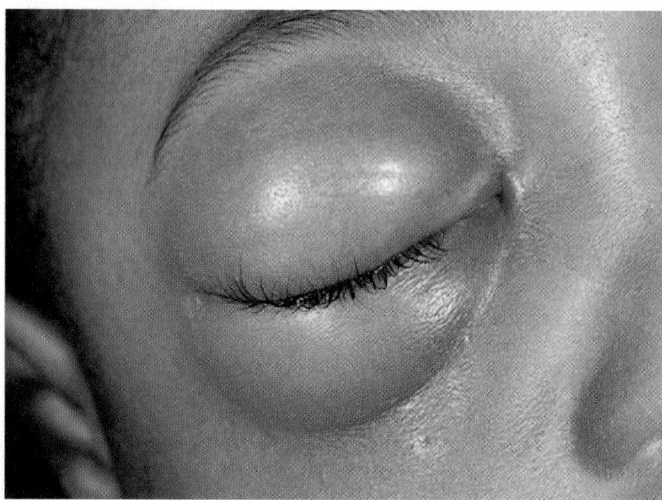

B

FIGURE 119-10. **A and B.** Orbital cellulitis. [Reproduced with permission from Shah BR, Lucchesi M: *Atlas of Pediatric Emergency Medicine*. © 2006, McGraw-Hill, New York, Figure 8-14.]

Treatment of a corneal abrasion is erythromycin or bacitracin-polymyxin ophthalmic ointment to help avoid superinfection and provide lubrication.[13] Avoid ointments containing neomycin due to hypersensitivity reactions.[14] Cyclopentolate 0.5% drops may alleviate pain by reducing ciliary spasm. Occasionally nonsteroidal anti-inflammatory drops are also used (such as ketorolac), but the evidence is not robust.[15] Eye patching is not routinely recommended but may be useful for any child who frequently attempts to scratch or rub the injured eye. Although the need for tetanus prophylaxis of a corneal abrasion is debatable, the ED visit should be used to remind the caregiver to check the child's tetanus status with the primary care provider. In a tetanus-prone injury, using the same criteria as a standard skin abrasion, updating unknown tetanus status is recommended.[16]

For uncomplicated and simple corneal abrasions, recommend follow-up in 48 hours with the pediatrician or other primary care provider. Children with involvement of the visual axis should follow up the next day with ophthalmology. Children or adolescents who use contact lenses, have a history of herpes, or may have a retained foreign body should also be evaluated by an ophthalmologist. Contact lenses should not be worn until all symptoms have resolved. Corneal abrasions heal quickly, and patients who continue to have a foreign body sensation 2 to 3 days after initial presentation require urgent ophthalmologic reevaluation.

OPHTHALMIA NEONATORUM

Ophthalmia neonatorum is conjunctivitis in neonates up to 30 days old. The five primary categories of neonatal conjunctivitis are chemical, gonococcal, chlamydial, other bacterial, and viral (**Table 119-2**). Gonococcal, chlamydial, and viral neonatal conjunctivitis can all lead to severe morbidity. Although specific diagnoses and treatments are discussed in the following sections, in the ED, it may not be possible to determine the specific etiology. A rapid Gram stain of discharge should be obtained in all cases and will aid in management.

CHEMICAL OPHTHALMIA NEONATORUM

Chemical conjunctivitis occurs in the first 24 hours of life following erythromycin ointment prophylaxis.[13] Infants present with bilateral conjunctivitis, inflamed eyelids, and watery discharge. Gram stain of the discharge would reveal the absence of pathologic bacteria and only a few WBCs. Treatment of neonatal chemical conjunctivitis is watchful waiting. Symptoms should resolve within 48 hours.

GONOCOCCAL OPHTHALMIA NEONATORUM

Erythromycin ophthalmic ointment prophylaxis is used at birth in all babies to diminish the risk of conjunctivitis caused by *Neisseria gonorrhoeae*. **Gonococcal conjunctivitis usually presents at 2 to 7 days of life with intense bilateral bulbar conjunctival erythema, chemosis, and a copious purulent discharge** (**Figure 119-11**). The diagnosis is made by Gram stain, revealing gram-negative diplococci, and culture using chocolate agar. **Admit all infants with gonococcal conjunctivitis and**

TABLE 119-2 Ophthalmia Neonatorum

Type	Cause	Age of Presentation	Key Findings	Treatment
Chemical	Erythromycin ointment prophylaxis	24 h	Bilateral, watery discharge, negative Gram stain	Watchful waiting
Gonococcal	*Neisseria gonorrhoeae*	2–7 d	Intense chemosis, copious discharge, gram-negative diplococci on Gram stain	Admission, IV antibiotics
Chlamydial	*Chlamydia trachomatis*	7–14 d	Intense erythema, purulent discharge	Admission, PO and topical antibiotics
Other bacterial	*Staphylococcus aureus*, nontypeable *Haemophilus influenzae, Staphylococcus epidermidis, Escherichia coli, Pseudomonas*	7–14 d	Identify etiology on Gram stain	Topical antibiotics
Viral	HSV-2, less commonly HSV-1	14–28 d	Dendrites on fluorescein exam	Admission, IV and topical antivirals

Abbreviation: HSV = herpes simplex virus.

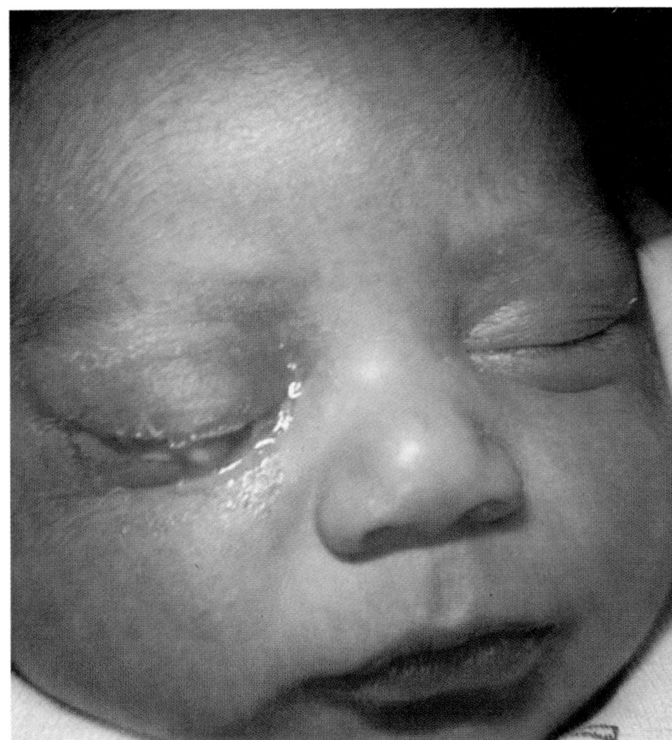

FIGURE 119-11. Gonococcal ophthalmia. [Reproduced with permission from Shah BR, Lucchesi M: *Atlas of Pediatric Emergency Medicine.* © 2006, McGraw-Hill, New York, Figure 8-1.]

obtain ophthalmology consultation, and evaluate for disseminated disease.[17] Test blood, urine, cerebrospinal fluid, and any other sites with suspected infection. Therapy for isolated conjunctivitis in a neonate without hyperbilirubinemia is a single dose of parenteral ceftriaxone (50 milligrams/kg IV; maximum, 125 milligrams). To avoid exacerbation of hyperbilirubinemia or if disseminated infection is suspected and longer-term antibiotics are required, use cefotaxime (50 milligrams/kg IV every 8 hours). Irrigate the infant's eyes with normal saline frequently to eliminate the purulent discharge. Gonococcal ophthalmia neonatorum may progress to ulceration and perforation of the cornea if improperly treated.

CHLAMYDIAL OPHTHALMIA NEONATORUM

Symptoms of chlamydial conjunctivitis present slightly later than those caused by gonorrhea, typically around 7 to 14 days of age. Signs are unilateral or bilateral purulent discharge with intense erythema of the palpebral conjunctiva (**Figure 119-12**). Chlamydial ophthalmia may be associated with chlamydial pneumonia. Diagnosis is confirmed with Giemsa stain, culture, or nucleic acid amplification of conjunctival scrapings. Treat chlamydial conjunctivitis with or without associated pneumonia with a 14-day course of oral erythromycin (12.5 milligrams/kg PO every 6 hours) and erythromycin ophthalmic ointment.[13] Ophthalmology consultation is recommended. Patients with isolated chlamydial ophthalmia who do not have respiratory symptoms or evidence of pneumonia may be safely discharged to home with follow-up in 24 hours.

OTHER BACTERIAL OPHTHALMIA NEONATORUM

Bacterial conjunctivitis due to bacteria other than chlamydia and gonorrhea is also less common when erythromycin topical prophylaxis has been given.[17] The most common bacterial pathogens are *S. aureus*, nontypeable *H. influenzae*, *Staphylococcus epidermidis*, *Escherichia coli*, and *Pseudomonas*.[4] Symptoms are variable and usually begin within 2 weeks of birth with hyperemia, purulent discharge, and edema. Gram stain and culture will identify the cause. Parenteral or oral therapy is not necessary in almost all cases, except nontypeable *H. influenzae*, and topical therapy with bacitracin-polymyxin ointment is sufficient.[4] Nontypeable *H. influenzae* requires admission to the hospital, a full septic workup, and parenteral antibiotics.

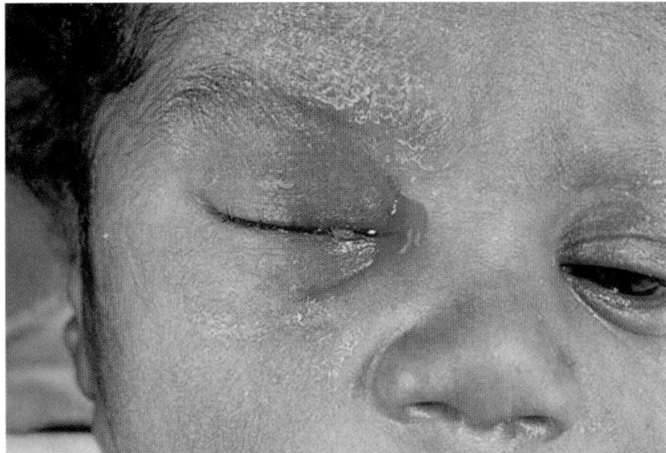

A

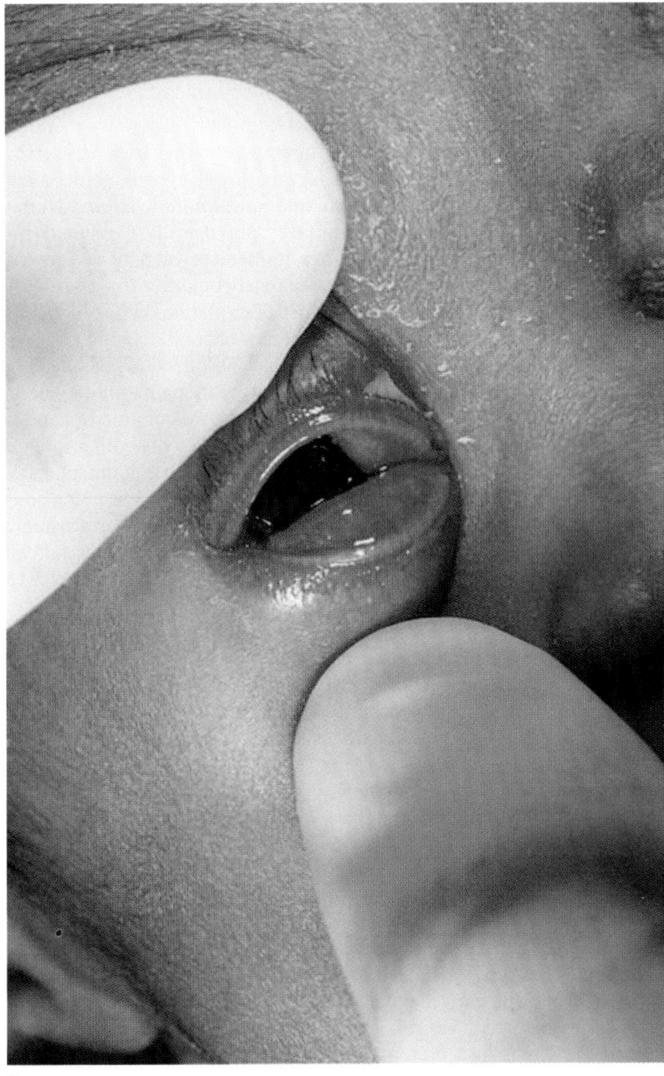

B

FIGURE 119-12. **A and B.** Chlamydial ophthalmia. [Reproduced with permission from Shah BR, Lucchesi M: *Atlas of Pediatric Emergency Medicine.* © 2006, McGraw-Hill, New York, Figure 8-2.]

VIRAL OPHTHALMIA NEONATORUM

Viral neonatal ophthalmia, caused by herpes simplex virus types 1 and 2, is a rare cause of neonatal conjunctivitis. Because there is a significant risk of keratitis and devastating disseminated infection, early identification and treatment are critical. Symptoms develop at 14 to 28 days of life with bilateral lid edema and conjunctival erythema. Suspect herpes infection in a neonate with associated mucocutaneous lesions and a maternal history of herpes; however, a history of maternal infection is not necessary for the diagnosis. Herpes conjunctivitis is confirmed with the presence of keratitis or corneal dendrites on fluorescein examination and viral culture or nucleic amplification tests. Neonates with suspected herpetic ophthalmia require hospital admission, full septic evaluation (including lumbar puncture with herpes polymerase chain reaction testing of cerebrospinal fluid), IV acyclovir (20 milligrams/kg IV every 8 hours for 14 to 21 days), and topical antivirals (1% trifluridine, 0.1% iododeoxyuridine, or 3% vidarabine).[17] **Steroid drops should be strictly avoided in herpes conjunctivitis.**

CHILDHOOD CONJUNCTIVITIS

Conjunctivitis, or inflammation of the conjunctiva, is very common in children and may be caused by viruses, bacteria, or allergy; less commonly, it may be a symptom of a systemic disease. Each type of conjunctivitis is discussed in the following sections.

VIRAL CONJUNCTIVITIS

Viral conjunctivitis in childhood is most frequently caused by adenovirus. Less frequent pathogens are rhinovirus, enteroviruses, influenza, and Epstein-Barr virus.[4] Measles virus can also cause conjunctivitis but is an unlikely diagnosis with proper childhood immunization. Measles outbreaks can occur among unimmunized populations. Conjunctivitis caused by the herpes viruses requires immediate therapy to prevent permanent vision loss and is covered separately below.

Viral conjunctivitis has several distinct presentations. **Pharyngoconjunctival fever** presents with fever, acute onset of conjunctivitis, pharyngitis, and preauricular adenopathy, and may be unilateral or bilateral. **Epidemic keratoconjunctivitis** can present with pain, photophobia, subepithelial defects, and pseudomembranes over the conjunctiva, and is usually bilateral. **Follicular conjunctivitis** often presents with a foreign body sensation and erythema of the conjunctiva. On examination, an aggregation of lymphocytes around networks of blood vessels in the conjunctiva will give the appearance of follicles. Finally, **acute hemorrhagic conjunctivitis** presents with hyperemic conjunctiva, subconjunctival hemorrhages, chemosis, swelling, photophobia, and pain. **Figure 119-13** shows a child with adenoviral conjunctivitis.

The treatment of these categories of viral conjunctivitis is supportive only. Cool compresses may offer patients symptomatic relief. Artificial tears and topical vasoconstrictors may improve redness and the sensation of dryness. **Topical antibiotics should not be prescribed because there is no evidence of protection against secondary infections and there is suspicion of harm.**[18] Symptoms may last 2 to 3 weeks, and patients should be referred to ophthalmology if conjunctivitis is persistent or worsening. Viral conjunctivitis is very contagious, and families should not share face cloths, towels, or pillows.

CONJUNCTIVITIS CAUSED BY HERPES VIRUSES

Conjunctivitis caused by **varicella** most often occurs during primary infections. However, it can also occur with herpes zoster ophthalmicus, which is when the varicella virus lies dormant in the trigeminal nerve and causes recurrent vesicles in the V_1 distribution. **Herpes simplex virus type 1** may also present similarly with unilateral vesicles in the same distribution. A typical dendritic pattern will be seen on the cornea with fluorescein examination.

Treat both primary and secondary varicella conjunctivitis presenting in the first 72 hours of symptoms with oral acyclovir (for age >2 years old: 20 milligrams/kg PO every 6 hours for 5 days; maximum dose, 3200 milligrams/d) and obtain ophthalmology consultation.[19] Similarly, herpes simplex infections of the eye in children also require ophthalmology consultation but may be treated with topical antivirals such as trifluridine, iododeoxyuridine, or vidarabine.[17] Topical steroids may be prescribed by an ophthalmologist for both varicella and herpes simplex infections of the eye but should not be prescribed by the emergency physician.

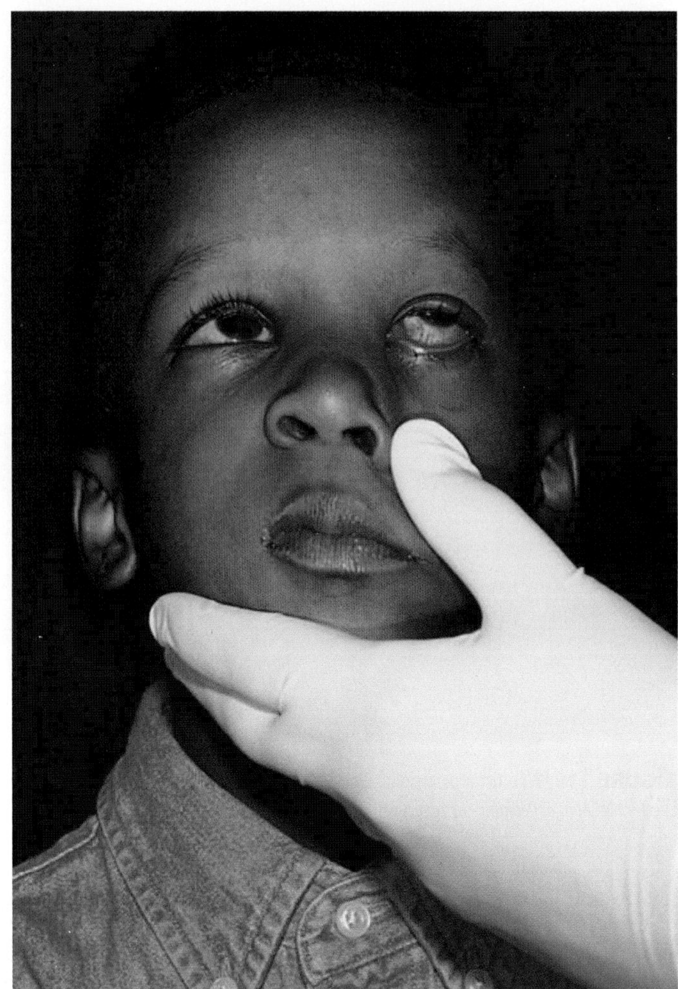

A

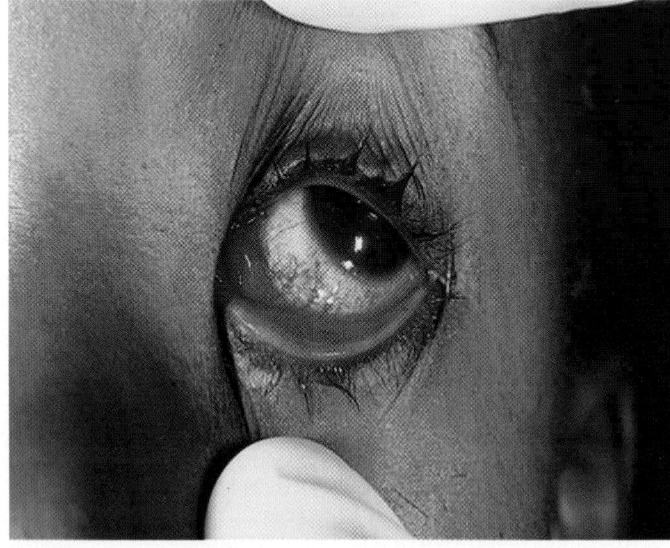

B

FIGURE 119-13. A and B. Adenoviral conjunctivitis. [Reproduced with permission from Shah BR, Lucchesi M: *Atlas of Pediatric Emergency Medicine.* © 2006, McGraw-Hill, New York, Figure 8-3.]

CHILDHOOD BACTERIAL CONJUNCTIVITIS

Bacterial conjunctivitis in childhood is most frequently caused by *Haemophilus* species, *S. pneumoniae*, *M. catarrhalis*, and *S. aureus*.[4] Less common pathogens include *Pseudomonas aeruginosa*, group B

Streptococcus, E. coli, and Neisseria meningitidis. Oculoglandular syndrome is a rare infection often caused by *Bartonella henselae* (**cat-scratch disease**) or **tularemia**, which causes ipsilateral conjunctivitis and lymphadenopathy, often axillary. Physical exam findings include normal vision, mucopurulent matting of the lashes (especially after sleep), and eyelid edema. Photophobia and eye pain are not present, although patients will have some discomfort. Consider **chlamydial and gonococcal conjunctivitis** in the differential diagnosis, especially in sexually active adolescents and neonates, as mentioned above.

The diagnosis of bacterial conjunctivitis is primarily clinical. If patients have concomitant otitis media, the diagnosis is most likely conjunctivitis-otitis syndrome caused by nontypeable *H. influenzae*, and oral antibiotics should be prescribed. Otherwise, treat with a broad-spectrum topical antibiotic such as a fluoroquinolone (ciprofloxacin or ofloxacin ophthalmic, which, due to limited absorption, are acceptable for use in children), bacitracin-polymyxin, or trimethoprim-polymyxin.[4] An ointment is preferable to eye drops. Although erythromycin ointment is inexpensive, it does not provide adequate coverage for *H. influenzae* or *M. catarrhalis*. Therefore, if erythromycin ointment has been prescribed and the patient is not clinically improving, change the topical antibiotic ointment.

Patients with isolated bacterial conjunctivitis or conjunctivitis-otitis syndrome may be safely discharged to home. Symptoms that do not improve after 7 days of therapy merit ophthalmology referral.

It may be difficult in the ED to differentiate bacterial from viral conjunctivitis. In addition to the earlier noted differences, clues to bacterial etiology include history of discharge causing eyelash matting and mucoid or mucopurulent discharge on exam. Viral conjunctivitis is likely in the presence of preauricular lymphadenopathy, recent respiratory illness, and conjunctivitis that spreads among close contacts.[9] Consider a swab of the conjunctiva for severe or recurrent cases.

ALLERGIC CONJUNCTIVITIS

Children with a history of atopy are most likely to suffer allergic conjunctivitis, but almost any child can be affected. Children with allergic conjunctivitis may have bilateral itchy eyes, tearing, thin mucoid discharge, mild redness, and eyelid edema, as well as chemosis. In severe cases, patients may have mild photophobia. Treat allergic conjunctivitis with allergen avoidance, topical antihistamines, and mast cell stabilizers. Ketotifen (one drop to each eye every 8 to 12 hours) and olopatadine (one to two drops to each eye daily), which are both antihistamines and mast cell stabilizers, are very effective.[20,21] Topical nonsteroidal anti-inflammatory drugs, vasoconstrictors, and lubricants may provide symptomatic relief. Cool compresses may also be beneficial. Oral antihistamines are discouraged because they can cause eye dryness, exacerbating symptoms.

OTHER CAUSES OF CHILDHOOD CONJUNCTIVITIS

Although almost all pediatric conjunctivitis is due to bacterial, viral, or allergic causes, a differential diagnosis of the red eye includes iritis, keratitis, uveitis, glaucoma, corneal abrasion, Kawasaki's disease, and pediculosis. Kawasaki's disease, glaucoma, and pediculosis of the eyelashes are discussed in the following sections.

KAWASAKI'S DISEASE

Kawasaki's disease, a severe medium-sized vessel vasculitis that can cause coronary artery aneurysms, predominantly presents in children 1 to 8 years of age (see chapter 141, "Rashes in Infants and Children"). Nonpurulent bilateral conjunctivitis is a key diagnostic feature of Kawasaki's disease. In typical cases, patients have a fever (>5 days), dry and erythematous lips and oropharynx, enlarged cervical lymph node (>1.5 cm), nonvesicular rash, edema, or peeling of the hands and feet. A diagnosis of Kawasaki's disease requires inpatient admission, IV γ-globulin, aspirin therapy, cardiology consult, and, in most institutions, either infectious disease or rheumatology consultations.

PEDICULOSIS

Lice can infest the eyelashes of a child of any age, leading to itching and scratching, with a mild conjunctivitis caused by the louse's saliva. Occasionally by scratching, children can cause a secondary bacterial infection or corneal abrasion.

Do not use pediculicide shampoos to treat pediculosis of the eyelashes because the shampoo is toxic to the eyes. Rather, attempt to remove nits (eggs) and then smother the lice with petroleum jelly or other ophthalmic ointment three times a day. Although the head and body louse may frequently involve the eyelashes of children, if *Pthirus pubis* (pubic louse) is identified, consider sexual abuse.

PEDIATRIC GLAUCOMA

Pediatric glaucoma is an important worldwide cause of visual impairment. It is the result of an abnormality of the trabecular network of the eye and can be classified as either primary or secondary. Primary pediatric glaucoma is the result of dysgenesis of the chamber angle leading to decreased outflow of aqueous humor and increased intraocular pressure. In secondary glaucoma, aqueous outflow is diminished by systemic disease, scarring, trauma, inflammation, or infection. Primary pediatric glaucoma is more common than secondary glaucoma in children and is often familial. Estimates of incidence range from 1 in 10,000 to 1 in 18,500 births.[22,23] Approximately 75% of cases are bilateral, and 80% of cases will present before 1 year of age. Pediatric syndromes associated with glaucoma include Sturge-Weber syndrome, Lowe's syndrome, Down's syndrome, neurofibromatosis, and maternal rubella syndrome. It is important to be familiar with the presenting signs of pediatric glaucoma so that proper ophthalmologic consultation and referral may be made.

Children with pediatric glaucoma will have a number of pathologic ocular signs and symptoms. Intraocular pressure will be elevated (≥20 mm Hg), and the cornea will appear enlarged and often cloudy and edematous (**Figure 119-14**). A full-term newborn cornea is nearly adult sized, with a horizontal diameter range of 9.0 to 10.5 mm versus 10.5 to 13.0 mm in an adult.[4] **Children <1 year of age should not have a corneal diameter >12 mm, and no child should have a corneal diameter >13 mm.**[24] There is associated blepharospasm, conjunctival

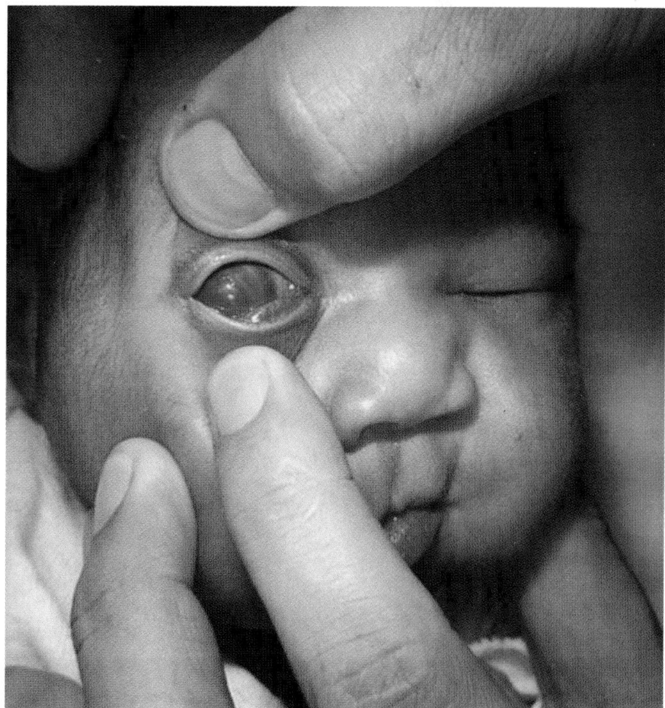

FIGURE 119-14. Infantile glaucoma. [Reproduced with permission from Shah BR, Lucchesi M: *Atlas of Pediatric Emergency Medicine*. © 2006, McGraw-Hill, New York, Figure 8-32.]

injection, and myopia. The globe may appear enlarged. If the optic disc can be visualized, abnormal cupping or asymmetry may be found.

In consultation with ophthalmology, initiate medical therapy of pediatric glaucoma to temporarily decrease intraocular pressure while awaiting definitive surgical repair. Therapies include oral and topical carbonic anhydrase inhibitors and topical β-blockers.[25] Acetazolamide (3 milligrams/kg PO every 6 hours) can be used for short periods of time, and pediatric doses are prepared by crushing the tablets used for adults. Topical carbonic anhydrase inhibitors such as dorzolamide or brinzolamide may also be used with fewer systemic side effects. Topical β-blockers such as timolol 0.25% are recommended at a starting dose of one drop daily. Surgery is required for definitive treatment.

LEUKOCORIA

Leukocoria is a white-appearing pupil (**Figure 119-15**). Normally when a bright light is directed at the pupil, a "red reflex" appears as the light is reflected off the retina. With leukocoria, the red reflection is blocked. Despite routine screening during pediatric well-child examinations, leukocoria is frequently discovered by parents after a photograph with flash photography is noticed to have unequal "red eye."[26]

Leukocoria has many causes, as listed in **Table 119-3**. Of patients age 0 to 10 years old presenting with leukocoria, up to 60% will have congenital cataracts and 18% will have retinoblastoma.[27] Leukocoria requires prompt emergency evaluation by an ophthalmologist to avoid loss of vision or life.

TABLE 119-3 Causes of Leukocoria in Children

Causes of Leukocoria in Children
Congenital cataracts
Retinoblastoma
Retinal detachment
Retinoschisis
Retinopathy of prematurity
Falciform retinal fold
Persistent hyperplastic primary vitreous
Coats' disease
Retinal coloboma
Endophthalmitis or panophthalmitis
Posterior uveitis
Vitreous hemorrhage
High myopia
Sarcoma
Corneal opacity
Phakomatosis
Other tumors
Ocular larva migrans

CATARACTS

Cataracts are one of the most common causes of childhood visual impairment and the most frequent nonmalignant cause of leukocoria.[28] Although cataracts are not treated in the ED, it is important for the ED physician to recognize and refer children with cataracts promptly to avoid permanent visual loss.

Pediatric cataracts can be unilateral or bilateral. Unilateral cataracts have a higher association with other ocular abnormalities and may be idiopathic (92%), hereditary (6%), or secondary to infection or other perinatal injury (2%). Bilateral cataracts, on the other hand, are more frequently hereditary (56%) and less commonly idiopathic (38%) or from infection or other perinatal injury (6%).[29] Hereditary cataracts can be inherited in an autosomal dominant or recessive pattern. Cataracts recognized in the neonatal period are most frequently from the TORCH infections (toxoplasmosis, syphilis, rubella, cytomegalovirus, and herpes simplex). Cataracts may also be associated with a variety of systemic illnesses and syndromes such as trisomy 21, galactosemia, Lowe's syndrome, Alport's syndrome, homocystinuria, Wilson's disease, and many more.

Children with cataracts present with any one of the following: leukocoria (**Figure 119-16**), strabismus, and/or nystagmus. On direct or slit lamp examination, lens opacities will be seen that can have partial or complete lens involvement, obscuring the retina.

Cataracts require referral to an ophthalmologist. Although there are a wide variety of surgical techniques used, generally central cataracts that are >3 mm warrant surgical removal. Children older than 2 years old may benefit from intraocular lens placement. Patients may also require surgery to repair concomitant strabismus.

RETINOBLASTOMA

The most common presenting signs of retinoblastoma are leukocoria and strabismus, and most children are identified by 2 years of age (Figure 119-15). Leukocoria in children with retinoblastoma is most

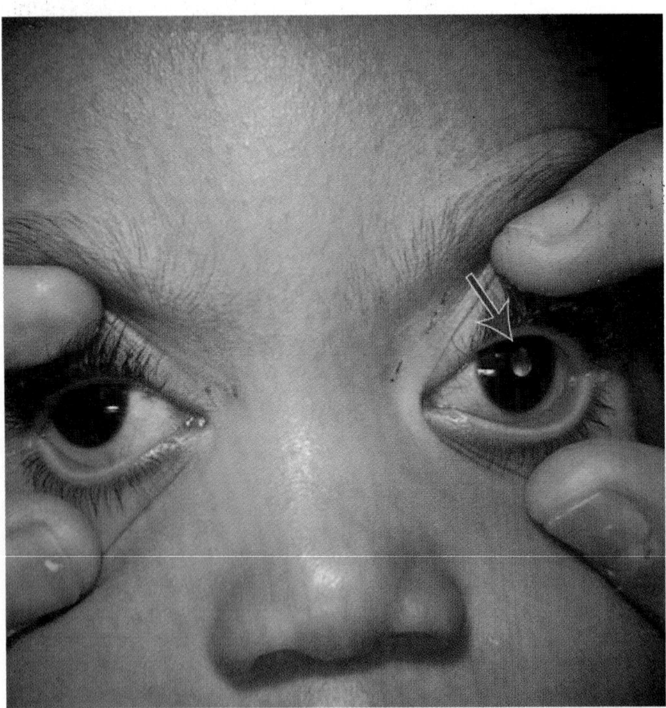

FIGURE 119-15. Leukocoria (*arrow*) due to retinoblastoma. [Reproduced with permission from Shah BR, Lucchesi M: *Atlas of Pediatric Emergency Medicine.* © 2006, McGraw-Hill, New York, Figure 8-19.]

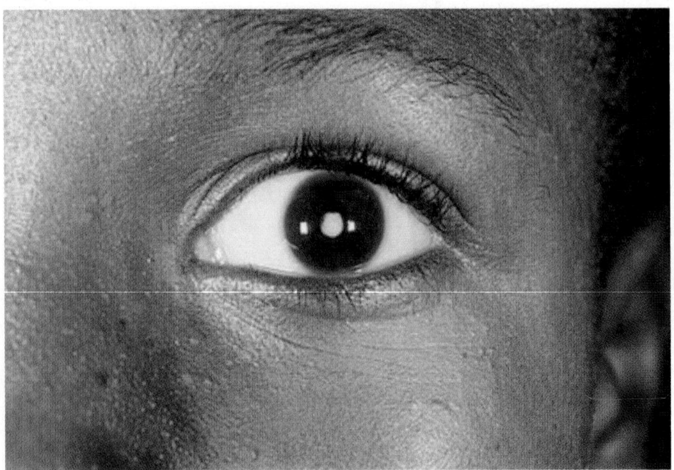

FIGURE 119-16. Cataract. [Reproduced with permission from Shah BR, Lucchesi M: *Atlas of Pediatric Emergency Medicine.* © 2006, McGraw-Hill, New York, Figure 8-21.]

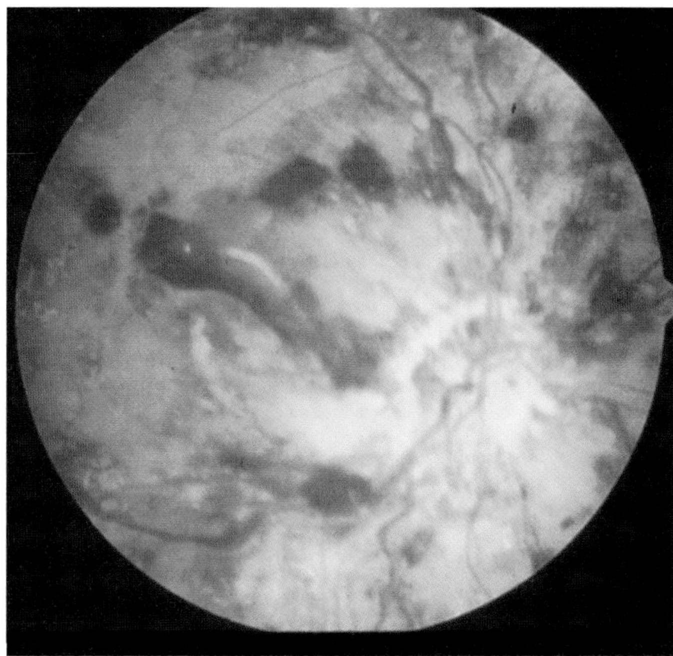

FIGURE 119-17. Retinal hemorrhage. [Reproduced with permission from Knoop K, Stack L, Storrow A: *Atlas of Emergency Medicine*, 2nd ed. © 2002, McGraw-Hill, New York, Figure 15-33.]

often detected by family and friends (80% of cases), and less commonly by ophthalmologists (10%) and pediatricians (8%).[26] Children may also present with proptosis, retinal detachment, glaucoma, hyphema, vitreous hemorrhage, and a red, painful eye due to ocular inflammation that may be confused with orbital cellulitis. Retinoblastoma is further discussed in chapter 143, "Oncologic and Hematologic Emergencies in Children."

RETINAL HEMORRHAGES

The incidence of shaken baby syndrome is approximately 29.7 per 100,000 infants.[30] Shaken baby victims have subdural hemorrhages and encephalopathy, as well as extensive retinal hemorrhages in 83% of cases (**Figure 119-17**).[31] Because child abuse is discussed elsewhere (see chapter 148, "Child Abuse and Neglect"), this section focuses on ocular pathology.

Retinal hemorrhages appear to be caused by shaking of the infant's head and are not sequelae of intracranial injury. One theory suggests that retinal hemorrhages are the result of an abrupt increase in venous pressure from elevated intracranial pressure or elevated thoracic pressure, whereas a second theory postulates that the injury is the result of vitreoretinal traction and shearing sustained during the violent acceleration and deceleration of the child's head.[32] Although retinal hemorrhages are pathognomonic of shaken baby syndrome in most settings, rarely, victims of a severe head crush injury have similar findings.[33] Although children may suffer vision loss from ocular pathology, the most common cause of blindness in shaken baby syndrome is cortical blindness, rather than retinal hemorrhage.

Obtain ophthalmologic consultation to detect retinal hemorrhage if child abuse is suspected.

PREVENTION OF EYE INJURIES AND PROTECTION FROM ULTRAVIOLET RADIATION

A visit to the ED is an opportunity to educate the patient and family about prevention of ocular injury. The annual incidence of eye trauma is 8 to 15.2 per 100,000 children, and most events are thought to be preventable.[34] Protective eyewear and adequate supervision during recreational and competitive sports should be available and may prevent injuries.[34] Advise parents that frame-only safety glasses without lenses are insufficient.

An ED visit is also an excellent opportunity to discuss the use of sunscreen and sunglasses before going outdoors for any sustained period of time. Emphasize the importance of using sunglasses with both ultraviolet A and ultraviolet B protection. Sun exposure is cumulative, and there is some research that it has an effect on development of cataracts and macular degeneration.[35] Ultraviolet B rays may also increase the risk of developing pterygia and pinguecula (yellowish-white vascular conjunctival lesions) later in life.

Acknowledgments: The authors would like to thank Thomas A. Mayer, Katherine Fullerton, and Bill Bosley, authors of this chapter in the previous edition.

REFERENCES

The complete reference list is available online at www.TintinalliEM.com.

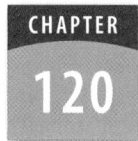

CHAPTER 120 Nose and Sinus Disorders in Infants and Children

Joanna S. Cohen
Dewesh Agrawal

ACUTE BACTERIAL SINUSITIS

Acute bacterial sinusitis is bacterial infection of one or more of the paranasal sinuses lasting <30 days.[1] The most common predisposing factor is a viral upper respiratory infection (URI). The incidence of viral URIs in children age 6 months to 35 months is approximately six episodes per patient-year, with approximately 8% of those becoming complicated by acute bacterial sinusitis. Bacterial sinusitis in children is most common in the 12 to 23 months age group, probably because these children are most likely to be in daycare, predisposing them to URIs.[2] The cost of acute pediatric bacterial sinusitis in the United States is approximately $20,000 per hospitalized patient, and a large geographic variation in healthcare utilization exists.[3] In 1996, total healthcare costs in the United States incurred from treating sinusitis in children <12 years of age had been estimated at $1.8 billion a year.[4]

PATHOPHYSIOLOGY

The sinuses are air cavities lined with ciliated columnar epithelium that helps mucus clearance by pushing mucus and debris out of the sinus ostia into the nasal cavity. Blockage of the ostia by mucus and inflammation predisposes to bacterial sinusitis. The ethmoid and maxillary sinuses are present at birth and are most commonly involved in sinusitis in children. The sphenoid sinuses form at 3 to 5 years of age. The frontal sinuses do not appear until 7 to 8 years of age and remain incompletely pneumatized until late adolescence. The most common predisposing factors for acute bacterial sinusitis are diffuse mucositis secondary to viral rhinosinusitis in about 80% and allergic inflammation in about 20%.[5] Less common predisposing factors include nonallergic rhinitis, cystic fibrosis, dysfunctional or insufficient immunoglobulins, ciliary dyskinesia, and anatomic abnormalities.[6]

The most common pathogen of acute bacterial sinusitis is *Streptococcus pneumoniae*, recovered in 30% of children with acute sinusitis. Nontypeable *Haemophilus influenzae* and *Moraxella catarrhalis* are each recovered in 20%.[6,7]

CLINICAL FEATURES

Children with acute bacterial sinusitis typically present with high fever and purulent nasal discharge. Headache, particularly behind the eye, is variable. Complaints of facial pain in children are rare.[2] The physical examination findings of acute bacterial sinusitis are often similar to those of uncomplicated viral sinusitis, with swollen and erythematous

TABLE 120-1 Clinical Features of Acute Bacterial Sinusitis[9]

Persistent symptoms lasting >10 d without improvement	Nasal or postnasal discharge and/or Daytime cough
Worsening course	Worse or new onset of nasal discharge, daytime cough, or fever after initial improvement
Severe onset	Fever ≥39°C (102.2°F) Purulent nasal discharge for ≥3 d

turbinates and mucopurulent discharge. However, reproducible unilateral tenderness to percussion or direct pressure of the frontal or maxillary sinus may indicate acute bacterial infection, and periorbital edema might indicate ethmoid sinusitis.[2] Transillumination of the maxillary sinuses is unreliable in children <10 years of age.[8]

DIAGNOSIS

Although the gold standard for diagnosis of acute bacterial sinusitis is the recovery of ≥10^4 colony-forming units/mL of bacteria from the paranasal sinuses, sinus aspiration is painful and impractical in the ED.[6] Therefore, diagnosis is often based on clinical criteria that help to distinguish acute bacterial sinusitis from an uncomplicated viral URI in an ill-appearing child (**Table 120-1**).[1]

Imaging studies should not be obtained to differentiate acute bacterial sinusitis from viral URI because of the high incidence of sinus mucosal abnormalities in patients with simple upper respiratory symptoms or no clinical symptoms at all.[1] In one study, mucosal sinus changes were evident in 97% of infants who had a URI in the 2 weeks preceding a cranial CT done for unrelated reasons.[10] Plain films have limited utility because they require correct positioning that is technically difficult in young children, and there is only a 70% to 75% correlation of culture confirmation with abnormal-appearing sinus radiographs.[11] A paranasal sinus CT with contrast or an MRI with contrast is, however, recommended for suspected orbital or CNS complications of bacterial sinusitis, including preseptal or postseptal cellulitis, subperiosteal abscess, cavernous sinus thrombosis, osteomyelitis of the frontal bone (Pott's puffy tumor), subdural empyema, epidural or brain abscess, and meningitis.[1,11]

TREATMENT

Patients with mild symptoms suggestive of a viral infection can be observed for 7 to 10 days, with no antibiotics prescribed. However, if symptoms persist or are severe (Table 120-1), suspect acute bacterial sinusitis and prescribe antibiotics to speed recovery, prevent suppurative complications, and minimize asthma exacerbations in susceptible children (**Figure 120-1**).[1]

Antibiotic treatment for acute sinusitis is outlined in **Table 120-2**.

Decongestants, antihistamines, and nasal irrigation are not effective for children with acute bacterial sinusitis.[12] Adjunctive therapy with intranasal steroids (e.g., fluticasone propionate, one to two sprays per nostril daily, or beclomethasone, one to two sprays per nostril twice a day) has modest benefits and may be considered.[1,13,14]

Complications of acute bacterial sinusitis are rare but usually involve the orbit or CNS. If suspected, obtain a contrast-enhanced CT scan or an MRI if possible.[15] Proptosis or impairment of extraocular muscle movement suggests orbital inflammation, usually from extension of an ethmoidal infection (**Figure 120-2**). Frontal and sphenoidal inflammation can lead to intracranial extension, causing frontal lobe and subdural abscesses as well as meningitis and empyema. IV antibiotics are needed, and surgical management may be necessary. Consult an ophthalmologist and/or neurosurgeon promptly for complications.1 For further discussion of the management of periorbital and orbital sinusitis, see chapter 119, "Eye Emergencies in Infants and Children."

CHRONIC BACTERIAL SINUSITIS

Chronic rhinosinusitis is an inflammatory process involving the mucosa of the nose and sinuses that lasts >3 months.[16] Factors associated with chronic sinusitis include older age, allergic rhinitis, recurrent viral URIs, immunodeficiency, ciliary dyskinesia, anatomic abnormalities, and fungal colonization of the sinuses.[17] The most common organisms identified are α-hemolytic *Streptococcus, H. influenzae*, and *S. pneumoniae*.[18] Chronic sinusitis has been linked to asthma, and treatment of chronic sinusitis reduces asthma symptoms.[19]

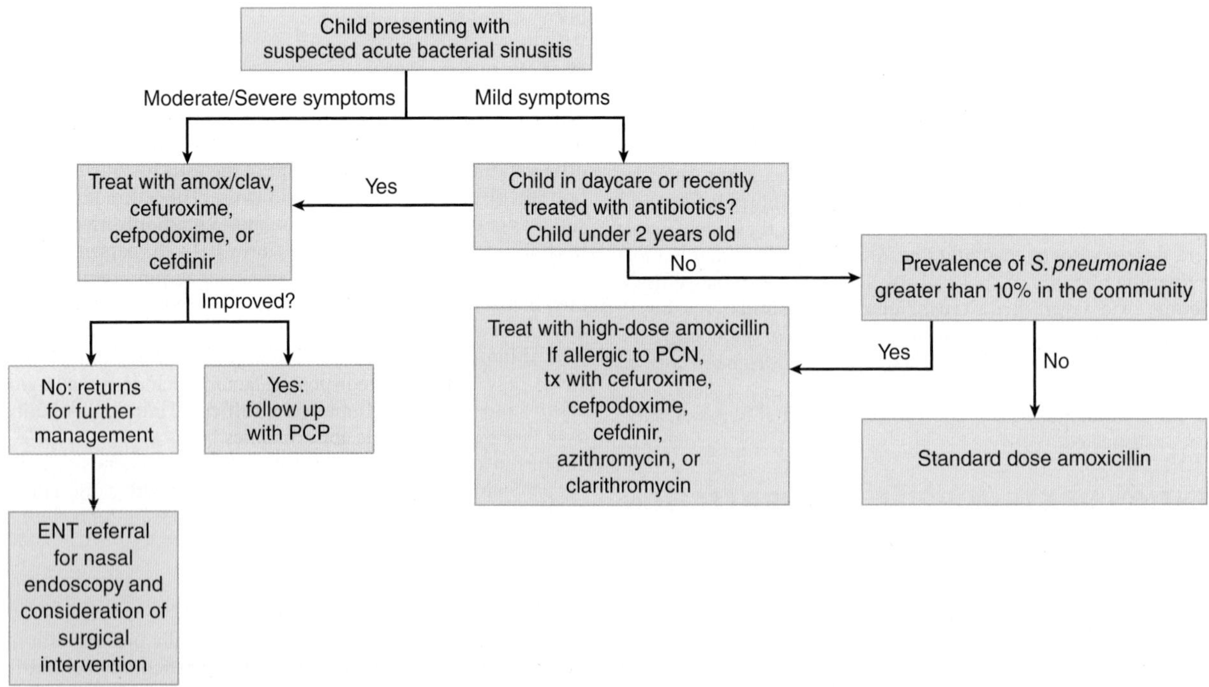

FIGURE 120-1. Management of uncomplicated acute bacterial sinusitis in children. amox = amoxicillin; clav = clavulanate; ENT = ear, nose, and throat; PCN = penicillin; PCP = primary care provider; tx = treat.

TABLE 120-2 Antibiotic Treatment for Bacterial Sinusitis

Clinical Scenario	Additional Factors	Treatment	Duration of Treatment
Mild symptoms or age >2 y	Not in daycare, no antibiotics in past 4 wk	Amoxicillin 22.5 milligrams/kg PO twice daily	10–28 d
	>10% *Streptococcus pneumoniae* prevalence	Amoxicillin 40–45 milligrams/kg PO twice daily	*or*
Moderate-severe symptoms or age <2 y	Attending daycare or recent amoxicillin administration	Amoxicillin 40–45 milligrams/kg with clavulanate 3.2 milligrams/kg PO twice daily	7 d beyond resolution of symptoms
	Vomiting, noncompliant	Ceftriaxone 50 milligrams/kg IV/IM once a day	Substitute PO agent when tolerable
Penicillin allergic		Cefdinir 7 milligrams/kg PO twice daily *or* Cefuroxime 15 milligrams/kg PO twice daily *or* Cefpodoxime 5 milligrams/kg PO twice daily	10–28 d *or* 7 d beyond resolution of symptoms

In addition to the more common pathogens seen in acute bacterial sinusitis, chronic sinusitis may also be caused by *Staphylococcus aureus*, anaerobes, and, rarely in children, fungi, including *Aspergillus*, *Fusarium*, *Bipolaris*, *Curvularia lunata*, and *Pseudallescheria boydii*.[17] Antibiotics for chronic sinusitis should cover the usual pathogens of acute sinusitis as well as aerobic and anaerobic β-lactamase–producing bacteria. Commonly used oral antimicrobial agents include amoxicillin-clavulanate (22.5 milligrams/kg PO twice daily), clindamycin (8 milligrams/kg PO three times daily), and the quinolones (moxifloxacin, 400 milligrams PO daily) for adolescents.[20] Chronic bacterial sinusitis is treated with prolonged antibiotics, typically for at least 4 weeks.[21]

For patients with chronic sinusitis who have failed antibiotic trials and nasal saline irrigation, otolaryngology referral is recommended for complete evaluation with nasal endoscopy and consideration of surgical options.[22] Definitive therapies may involve adenoidectomy or, in select cases, endoscopic sinus surgery, in which the ostiomeatal area is opened, antrostomies are created, and ethmoid partitions are removed.[22] This has an estimated success rate of 83% in a combined pediatric and adult study.[23] In the pediatric population, however, a less invasive approach known as a **functional endoscopic sinus surgery**, which is essentially a drainage procedure, has good efficacy, with 90% of patients showing marked reduction in symptoms.[24]

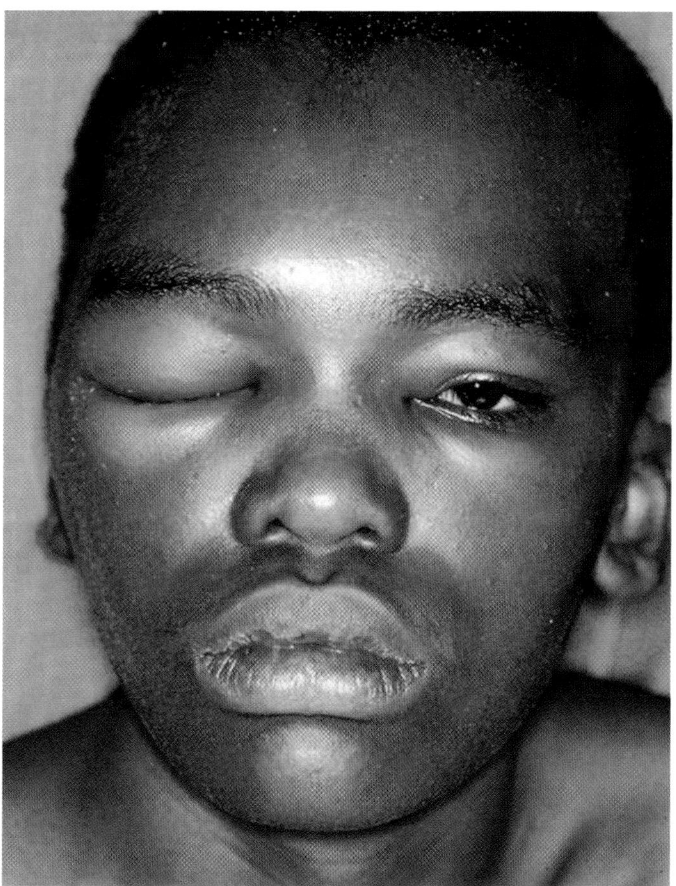

FIGURE 120-2. Sinusitis. Adolescent with pansinusitis complicated by periorbital cellulitis. The patient was also found to have osteomyelitis of the frontal bone (Pott's puffy tumor). [Reproduced with permission from Knoop K, Stack L, Storrow A: *Atlas of Emergency Medicine*, 2nd ed. © 2002, McGraw-Hill, New York.]

SPECIAL POPULATIONS

Children with recurrent or refractory sinusitis should be evaluated for immune deficiencies with quantitative immunoglobulin levels, immunoglobulin G subclasses, immunoglobulin A, and T- and B-cell counts. The most commonly diagnosed immune deficiencies in patients presenting with recurrent or refractory sinusitis are selective immunoglobulin A deficiency, common variable immunodeficiency, and immunoglobulin G subclass deficiency.[25] Children with **cystic fibrosis** have thick mucus that predisposes them to sinusitis. Cystic fibrosis is diagnosed through sweat chloride testing. Suspect cystic fibrosis in a child who presents with nasal polyps or chronic sinusitis, particularly in conjunction with failure to thrive and chronic cough.[5]

ALLERGIC RHINITIS

Allergic rhinitis is an IgE-mediated chronic or recurrent inflammatory response of the nasal mucosa that is induced by an allergen and typically affects children >2 years old. The worldwide prevalence of symptoms of allergic rhinoconjunctivitis is 2.2% to 14.6% in children age 6 to 7 years old and 4.5% to 45.5% in adolescents age 13 to 14 years old.[26] Approximately 80% of children with asthma have allergic rhinitis, and allergic rhinitis makes it more difficult to control asthma, making it an important topic for the emergency medicine physician caring for children.[26]

PATHOPHYSIOLOGY

Seasonal allergic rhinitis (commonly known as hay fever) is usually caused by airborne allergens such as pollen, whereas perennial allergic rhinitis is usually caused by dust mites, animal dander, and mold. Allergic rhinitis is an immunoglobulin E–mediated inflammatory response in the nasal mucosa that occurs after sensitization with a specific allergen. Immunoglobulin E binding triggers mast cell degranulation and subsequent histamine release. The binding of histamine to the histamine-1 receptor on nasal neurons and nasal vasculature is the ultimate mechanism responsible for the nasal itch, sneeze, rhinorrhea, and nasal obstruction of allergic rhinitis.

CLINICAL FEATURES

Allergic rhinitis presents with clear rhinorrhea, nasal pruritus, and sneezing. Ocular symptoms, such as conjunctival hyperemia and pruritus, may coexist. Symptoms can lead to sleep disturbance, limitations in activity, and poor school performance.[27]

DIAGNOSIS

Patients with allergic rhinitis report symptoms of paroxysmal sneezing, nasal pruritus, rhinorrhea, oropharyngeal pruritus, hyperemia, and ocular pruritus. On physical examination, there may be hypertrophy of the nasal turbinates and clear secretion from the nares. Concomitant wheezing suggests an association with asthma. A patient with severe symptoms who does not respond to treatment may warrant a referral to an allergist for skin testing to detect immediate hypersensitivity reactions to allergens. Total IgE levels are neither sensitive nor specific for atopic disease.[28]

TREATMENT

Treatment involves recommending environmental controls such as avoidance of allergens and irritants, including pollutants and cigarette smoke. Nasal saline irrigation with a syringe or spray reduces the use of antibiotics and other medications.[29]

Intranasal steroids, such as fluticasone furoate nasal spray, are effective for treatment of allergic rhinitis.[30] Intranasal corticosteroids reduce inflammation of the nasal mucosa. Daily morning dosing minimizes the impact on the hypothalamic-pituitary-adrenal axis. Oral antihistamines are also commonly used to treat allergic rhinitis, but there is a lack of evidence for the benefit of oral antihistamine therapy in addition to topical nasal steroids for children with allergic rhinitis.[31] Second-generation antihistamines, such as loratadine (5 milligrams daily for age 2 to 6 years; 10 milligrams daily for >6 years of age) and cetirizine (2.5 to 5.0 milligrams daily age 2 to 6 years; 5 to 10 milligrams daily for >6 years of age), are preferable because they are less likely to cross the blood–brain barrier and therefore cause less sedation than first-generation antihistamines such as diphenhydramine and hydroxyzine. Other therapies target the immune system directly. Montelukast, a leukotriene receptor antagonist, and disodium cromoglycate, a mast cell stabilizer, have been used with success for symptom reduction.[32,33] Sublingual and subcutaneous immunotherapy has also been shown to be effective in improving symptoms of allergic rhinitis in children.[34,35]

NASAL FOREIGN BODIES

Foreign body insertion is a common pediatric complaint in the ED. Foreign bodies in the external ear canal predominate, followed by nasal foreign bodies. Children who insert objects into their nose are, in general, younger than patients with auditory foreign body insertion.[36] Although pharyngeal foreign bodies can present in adults, nasal foreign bodies are almost exclusively a pediatric problem. Common objects include beads, paper, rocks, toy parts, and organic material such as peas, corn, seeds, nuts, and legumes.

CLINICAL FEATURES

The child with a nasal foreign body may present with local pain (23% to 55%), nasal discharge (7% to 36%), epistaxis, or admission by the child. Alternatively, the parent may witness the child placing something in the nose, or the object may be found during routine childcare. Most children with nasal foreign bodies are asymptomatic.[36,37]

DIAGNOSIS

Most nasal foreign bodies can be directly visualized. Have a high index of suspicion for a nasal foreign body in an appropriately aged child who presents with persistent, unilateral, purulent, foul-smelling nasal discharge (**Figure 120-3**).

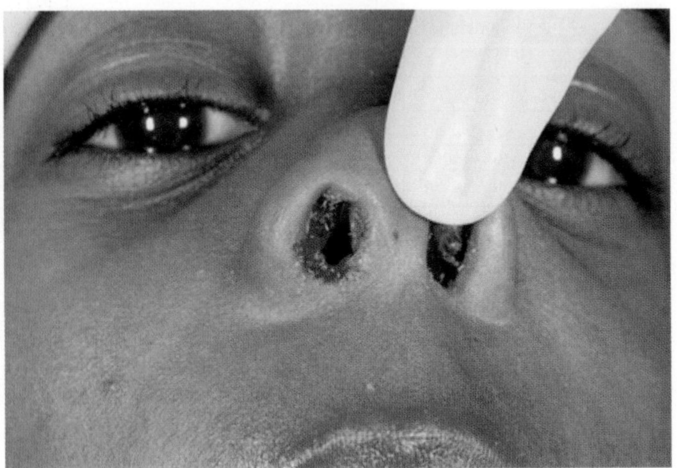

FIGURE 120-3. A 6-year-old child was brought to the ED with a complaint of a foul-smelling serosanguineous discharge from the right nostril. He confessed to putting a button in his nostril about 1 week before this visit. [Reproduced with permission from Shah BR, Lucchesi M: *Atlas of Pediatric Emergency Medicine*. © 2006, McGraw-Hill, New York, Figure 9-9.]

TREATMENT

The key to successful removal is immobilization. Approximately 20% of patients undergoing nasal foreign body removal in the ED are given procedural sedation, most commonly with ketamine.[38] Place the child in a supine position, and pretreat the nasal mucosa with topical 1% lidocaine and 0.5% phenylephrine.[36] Phenylephrine shrinks inflamed nasal mucosa, allowing for easier removal of entrapped foreign bodies, and also reduces the likelihood of procedural epistaxis. The most common methods for removal include forceps, the Foley catheter technique, applied positive pressure via an anesthesia bag, and the use of a suction catheter. All have varying degrees of success and failure. Alligator forceps work best if the object is close to the anterior nares and can be easily grasped. If the object is friable, there is a risk of pulling it apart and leaving pieces in the nose. Other techniques include the advancement of a lubricated 5- or 6-French Foley balloon catheter past the object, inflating the balloon with air and withdrawing the catheter to gently remove the foreign body; positive pressure applied to the mouth while occluding the contralateral naris; or use of a suction catheter to remove the object.[36] A particularly deep nasal foreign body may need to be removed by an otolaryngologist. Although it is possible to aspirate a nasal foreign body, this is rare, and most complications of nasal foreign bodies occur during attempted removal.[36,37] Complications of nasal foreign body removal include failure to remove the object, epistaxis, laceration, and, rarely, septal perforation. If irrigation is attempted and the object is expandable, such as rice, vegetable matter, or sponge, the foreign body can swell, impeding its extraction.

SPECIAL CONSIDERATIONS

Button batteries pose an important risk to children, particularly those less than 5 years old.[39] A button battery in the nasal cavity can cause liquefactive necrosis and septal perforation in as little as 7 hours.[40] For this reason, remove button batteries as quickly as possible. Do not instill any type of nasal drops before removal because the electrical charge of the battery will produce electrolysis with any electrolyte-rich fluid. This results in a severe alkaline burn. Button batteries are often not directly visualized in the ED because of extensive mucopurulent discharge and mucosal edema. For this reason, consider a plain radiograph to characterize a nonvisible foreign body or unilateral foul-smelling nasal discharge.[41]

Although more common in the external ear, live foreign bodies in the nose also require special mention. Cockroaches, mosquitoes, and beetles are all uncommon foreign bodies. They are often related to sleeping on the floor or poor hygiene. The recommended approach is to first kill the insect with 2% lidocaine or mineral oil and then attempt removal.

EPISTAXIS

Epistaxis usually occurs in children age 2 to 10 years old. It is rare in infants and older children.[42] Nose bleeds in children are most often secondary to digital trauma (nose picking) or rhinitis sicca. Rhinitis sicca is more common in northern latitudes during the winter when the humidity is low and dry air heating systems can cause nasal mucosa desiccation and frequent bleeding.

Other causes of epistaxis include facial trauma, foreign bodies, sinusitis, or increased vascular pressure secondary to excessive coughing. Less commonly, epistaxis can be the presenting complaint of a coagulopathy, leukemia, or nasal tumor. Most pediatric epistaxis originates from Kiesselbach plexus, a venous vascular plexus on the anterior nasal septum. Although anterior bleeds usually ooze, posterior bleeds tend to be more profuse because they originate from the sphenopalatine artery. This type of bleeding, while rare, carries a higher risk of airway compromise, aspiration of blood, and life-threatening hemorrhage.

TREATMENT

Most epistaxis can be controlled with conservative methods, such as pinching the nostrils together for 5 to 10 minutes with the patient slightly bent forward at the waist so as to avoid aspirating or swallowing blood. Ice or phenylephrine can also be applied to the nose to promote vasoconstriction. Application of cotton gauze under the upper lip can be used to compress the labial artery. Cautery with silver nitrate can be used if the bleeding site can be identified. If all else fails, the nares can be packed with absorbable gelatin foam, oxidized cellulose, or preformed devices (Rhino Rocket Child®, Shippert Medical Technologies Corporation, Centennial, CO). See chapter 244, "Nose and Sinuses" for the procedure and related information.

DISPOSITION AND FOLLOW-UP

Most children with simple epistaxis can be sent home with instructions to avoid digital trauma and apply petroleum jelly to the nares at night to help lubricate the mucosa. Children with recurrent or severe epistaxis and a family history of a bleeding disorder or abnormal screening prothrombin time or activated partial thromboplastin time should be referred to a hematologist for a complete coagulopathy evaluation. Approximately one third will have a diagnosable coagulopathy, most often von Willebrand's disease type 1.[42] If bleeding is recurrent, unilateral, and associated with nasal obstruction, a neoplasm may be suspected, and an otolaryngology consult is warranted. In an adolescent male with profuse unilateral epistaxis requiring packing, juvenile nasal angiofibroma should be suspected, and the patient should be evaluated with a CT scan.

Acknowledgments: We gratefully acknowledge the contributions of Kimberly S. Quayle, Susan Fuchs, and David M. Jaffe, the authors of this chapter in a previous edition.

REFERENCES

The complete reference list is available online at www.TintinalliEM.com.

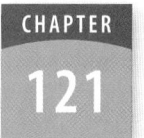

Mouth and Throat Disorders in Infants and Children

Derya Caglar
Richard Kwun
Abigail Schuh

INTRODUCTION

Lesions of the mouth and throat are common in children and can range from benign conditions that require no intervention to significant systemic illness requiring extensive treatment and support (**Table 121-1**).

TABLE 121-1 Common Causes of Oral Lesions in Children

Anterior	Posterior	Diffuse
Aphthous ulcers	Adenovirus pharyngitis	Autoimmune disease
Contact stomatitis	Coxsackie virus	Candidiasis (thrush)
Herpes simplex gingivostomatitis	Cytomegalovirus Epstein-Barr virus	Chemotherapy-related mucositis
Trauma	Streptococcal pharyngitis	Medication-related (phenytoin [Dilantin])
Vincent's angina		
		Stevens-Johnson syndrome Varicella-zoster

Making the distinction between these conditions can be difficult. Mouth pain secondary to viral infections of the oropharynx is one of the most common presenting complaints of pediatric patients; however, most patients require no treatment beyond supportive care and pain control. Bacterial infections of the mouth and throat, such as pharyngitis and uvulitis, cause local and systemic illness and rarely can lead to life-threatening complications. The management of dental injuries, whether from neglect or trauma, differs for primary and permanent teeth.

NORMAL VARIANTS

Epstein pearls are remnants of embryonic development that present as white, slightly raised nodules seen most commonly midline at the junction of the soft and hard palates of neonates. They are often seen incidentally during feeding and do not cause the child any pain or discomfort. Most resolve spontaneously.

Geographic tongue or migratory glossitis (**Figure 121-1**) can be a source of great parental concern. It is a benign, asymptomatic condition and is often incidentally noticed by parents during another illness. Findings are an area of erythema and atrophy of the papillae of the tongue surrounded by a serpiginous, elevated white or yellow border usually located in the anterior two thirds. The lesions will improve and disappear gradually over time but tend to recur in other areas of the tongue. There is no known cause, although it has been associated with childhood allergies and atopy. No treatment other than reassurance is necessary.

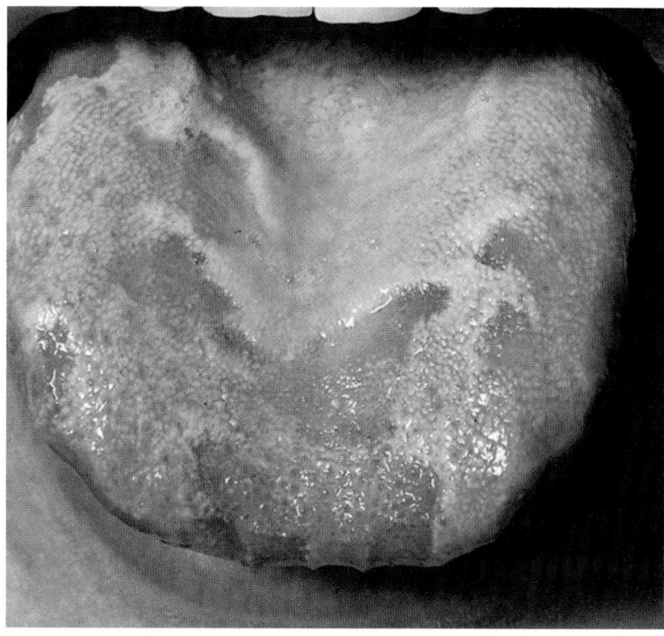

FIGURE 121-1. Geographic tongue. [Reproduced with permission from Wolff K, Johnson RA, Saavedra AO: *Fitzpatrick's Color Atlas and Synopsis of Clinical Dermatology*, 7th ed. © 2013 by McGraw-Hill, New York, Figure 33-4.]

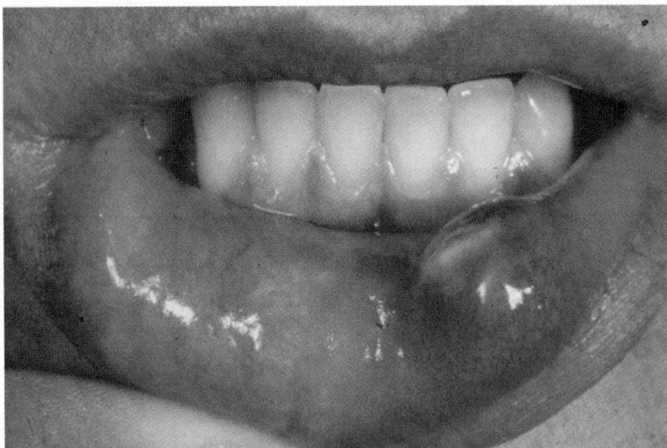

FIGURE 121-2. Mucocele. [Reproduced with permission from Wolff KL, Johnson R, Suurmond R: *Fitzpatrick's Color Atlas & Synopsis of Clinical Dermatology*, 6th ed. © 2009, McGraw-Hill, New York, Figure 34-14.]

Mucoceles (**Figure 121-2**) and **ranulas** are lesions of the oral mucosa that present as small, bluish, discrete, mucosal swellings on the lower lip or sublingual areas.[1] These are most often caused by minor trauma such as biting the lip.[2] Intervention is needed only with disruption of feeding or development of speech. Adjacent salivary glands are usually removed in addition to the lesion to prevent recurrence.

Eruption cysts are smooth, painless bluish-black areas of swelling found over an erupting tooth that usually resolve with the eruption of the underlying tooth. Although these findings are frightening to the parent, they are benign in nature, often asymptomatic, and require no intervention.

APHTHOUS ULCERS

Aphthous ulcers, also known as *canker sores*, are the most common form of recurrent oral ulcers, occurring in 5% to 25% of the general population.[3] They present in children and adolescents as painful, shallow ulcers on the oral mucosa (**Figures 121-3** and **121-4**). The etiology of canker sores is unknown, but genetic factors, food allergies, local trauma, endocrine changes, stress, and anxiety are all thought to contribute to recurrence.[4] They are found most frequently on the buccal and lingual mucosa. Spontaneous resolution after 7 to 10 days is the norm. Topical medications, such as antimicrobial mouthwashes and topical analgesics, can achieve the primary goal of reducing pain but do not hasten healing or improve recurrence or remission rates.

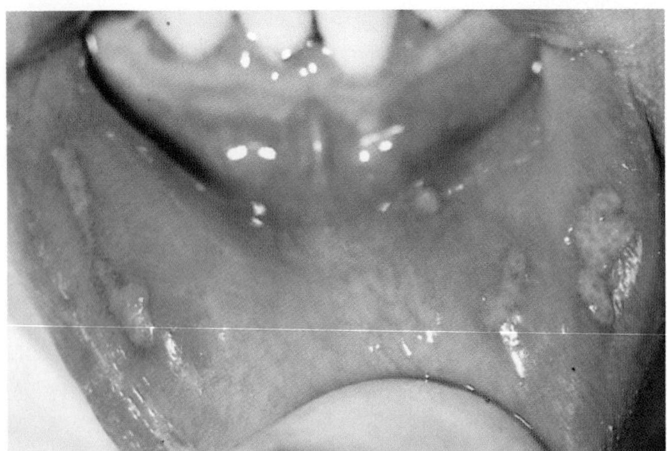

FIGURE 121-3. Aphthous ulcers: Note the multiple ulcers of various sizes located on the lip and gingival mucosa. These lesions rarely occur on the immobile oral mucosa of the gingiva or hard palate. [Reproduced with permission from Knoop K, Stack L, Storrow A: *Atlas of Emergency Medicine*, 2nd ed. © 2002, McGraw-Hill, New York, Figure 6-33.]

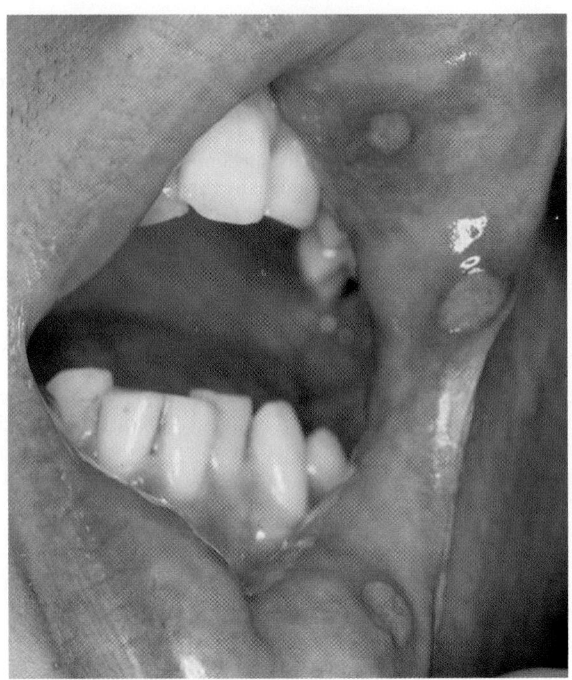

FIGURE 121-4. Aphthous ulcers: minor, multiple, very painful, gray-based ulcers with erythematous halos on the labial mucosa. [Reproduced with permission from Wolff KL, Johnson R, Suurmond R: *Fitzpatrick's Color Atlas & Synopsis of Clinical Dermatology*, 6th ed. © 2009, McGraw-Hill, New York, Figure 31-1.]

Less commonly, periodic fever, aphthous stomatitis, pharyngitis, and cervical adenitis syndrome (**PFAPA**) can cause aphthous ulcers in children 2 to 6 years of age. Patients present with fever, malaise, exudative pharyngitis, cervical lymphadenopathy, and multiple oral ulcers lasting 4 to 6 days, often recurring multiple times a year. **Recurrence is the key to diagnosis,** as this constellation of symptoms is difficult to distinguish from viral infection, particularly in the ED where patient care is cross-sectional rather than longitudinal. The cause of PFAPA remains unknown, but most patients respond well to oral steroids, with resolution of symptoms within 24 hours. Some studies have also shown that tonsillectomy leads to complete resolution of symptoms and that vitamin D supplementation reduces number and duration of PFAPA episodes.[5,6]

STOMATITIS

The majority of infectious mouth and throat lesions are viral. Enteroviral infections commonly cause oral lesions with or without other physical findings such as fever, rash, abdominal pain, or diarrhea. Herpes viruses can cause oropharyngeal lesions that are extremely painful, may be recurrent, and are usually associated with high fever during primary infection. Adenovirus can cause acute pharyngitis in association with fever and tonsillar erythema. Exudative pharyngitis in association with fevers, fatigue, and malaise is frequent in infections with Epstein-Barr virus and cytomegalovirus.

HERPANGINA

Herpangina is an enteroviral infection that causes a vesicular enanthem (**Figure 121-5**) of the tonsils and soft palate, affecting children 6 months to 10 years of age during late summer and early fall. It is primarily caused by Coxsackie virus A16 and human enterovirus 71, although other Coxsackie A and B genotypes are also common etiologic agents.[7] These vesicles are often very painful and are accompanied by fever, difficulty swallowing, and dysphagia. Patients may complain of headache, vomiting, and abdominal pain. Diagnosis is primarily clinical. Viral culture is the gold standard for confirmation of infection; however, enteroviral

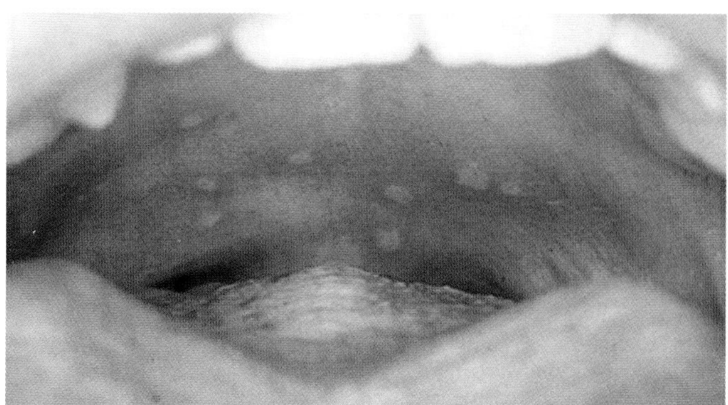

FIGURE 121-5. Herpangina: Typical elliptical or oval-shaped papulovesicular lesions with erythematous rims are seen on the posterior soft palate. [Reproduced with permission from Shah BR, Lucchesi M: *Atlas of Pediatric Emergency Medicine*. © 2006, McGraw-Hill, New York, Figure 3-67.]

polymerase chain reaction can detect enteroviral RNA from nasopharyngeal secretions, blood, urine, or feces much sooner and with higher sensitivity (87% to 100%; 95% from throat culture).[8]

Treatment is palliative because the symptoms are usually mild and lesions heal spontaneously after 3 to 5 days. Antipyretics and systemic analgesics aid with supportive care. **Viscous lidocaine is generally not recommended for pain relief** because it has no benefit over placebo in improving oral intake in affected children and also carries a risk of toxicity from lidocaine ingestion, with associated seizures.[9,10] A mixture of **diphenhydramine and Maalox** applied orally in a swish-and-swallow fashion can provide local pain relief. When topical treatment does not suffice, systemic analgesics, including narcotics, may be necessary. Pay close attention to hydration status, because children can quickly become dehydrated, requiring admission for IV fluid replacement.

HAND, FOOT, AND MOUTH DISEASE

Hand, foot, and mouth disease is also seen with enteroviral infections.[11] Coxsackie virus A16 is the most common cause, but A5, A9, A10, B2, B5, and enterovirus 71 subtypes have also been implicated.[12,13] The disease is typically seen in children <5 years old but is most common in infants and toddlers. The infection has a seasonal distribution and primarily occurs in the spring and summer months.

The illness generally follows a mild course, starting with a low-grade temperature lasting 2 to 3 days and associated with decreased appetite, malaise, vague abdominal pain, and mild upper respiratory symptoms. Children will then develop an enanthem of vesicles, followed by the exanthema, although both can occur simultaneously.

Oral lesions usually begin as erythematous macules and evolve into vesicles and ulcers over the course of 1 to 3 days, with new lesions appearing throughout the duration of illness. Lesions typically involve the palate, buccal mucosa, gingiva, and tongue. Pain from these ulcerations often leads to decreased oral intake and mild dehydration.

The associated rash appears on the palms of the hands, soles of the feet, and buttocks (**Figure 121-6**). Lesions begin as erythematous macules that later may develop into small nontender vesicles. The oral and skin lesions tend to resolve over 4 to 7 days.

Diagnosis is primarily clinical, although the virus can be isolated by viral culture or polymerase chain reaction from swabs of the vesicles and from stool specimens. Treatment involves supportive and symptomatic care with antipyretics, topical and oral analgesics, and oral rehydration. In rare cases, pain may lead to inadequate oral intake. Analgesics and IV fluids may be needed to treat dehydration. Rare complications of these infections include viral meningitis, meningoencephalitis, myocarditis, and sepsis.[14,15] Diligent hand washing among children and caregivers is key to preventing spread.[16]

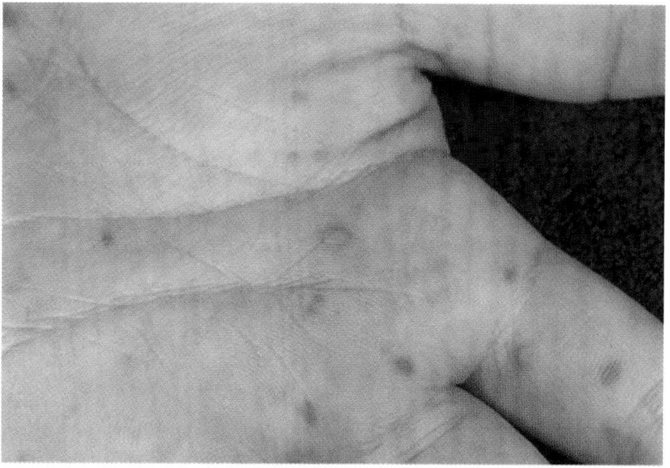

A

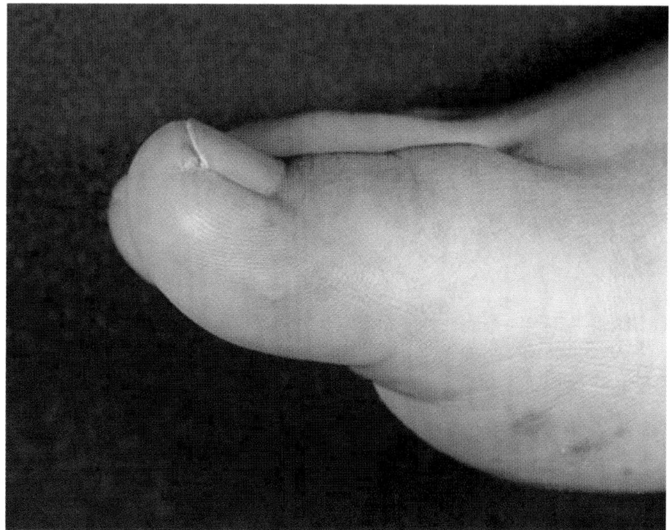

B

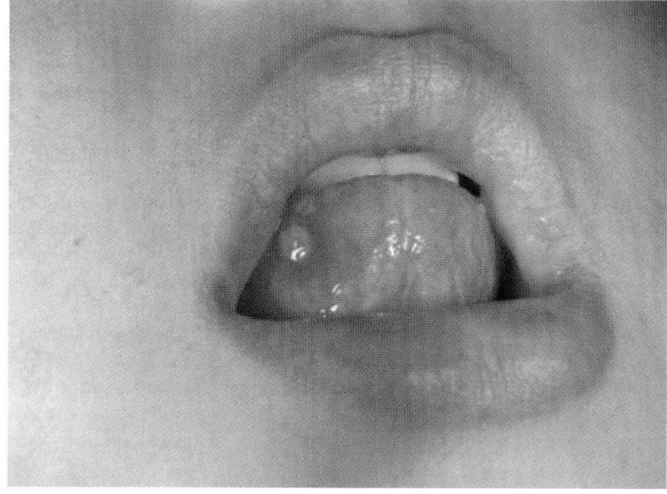

C

FIGURE 121-6. Hand, foot, and mouth disease: typical erythematous macules on the palms or soles. [Reproduced with permission from Shah BR, Lucchesi M: *Atlas of Pediatric Emergency Medicine*. © 2006, McGraw-Hill, New York, Figure 3-65.]

HERPES SIMPLEX GINGIVOSTOMATITIS

Herpes simplex virus can cause a variety of symptoms in the pediatric population. Infants and toddlers will often present with high fever, pharyngitis, and gingivostomatitis during their primary infection.[17] Initial infection is often very difficult to distinguish from other viral etiologies. Most children go undiagnosed with herpes simplex virus until they later present with a more classic painful labial reactivation lesion.

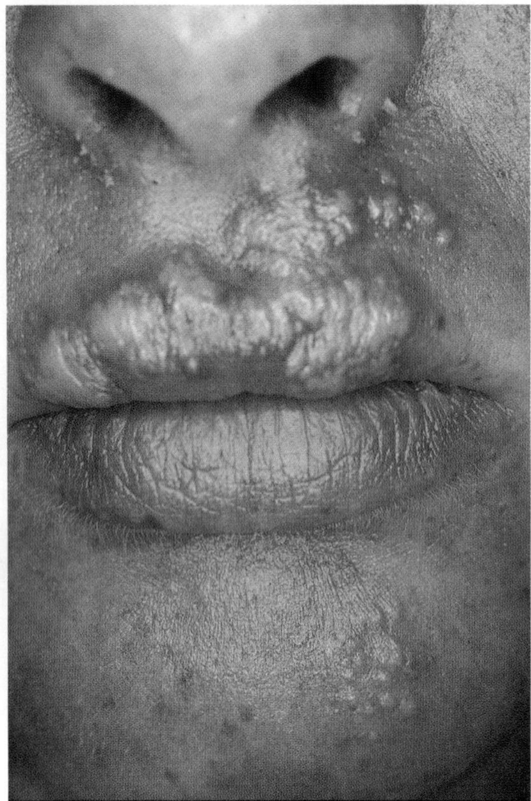

FIGURE 121-7. Herpes simplex virus (HSV): Extensive vesicular lesions along the vermilion border and surrounding tissues are consistent with HSV infection. [Reproduced with permission from Knoop K, Stack L, Storrow A: *Atlas of Emergency Medicine*, 2nd ed. © 2002, McGraw-Hill, New York, Figure 6-31.]

Acute herpetic gingivostomatitis is the most common presentation of primary herpes infection in children[18,19] (**Figure 121-7**). It usually presents at 6 months to 5 years of age, although primary herpes simplex virus infection may occur in older children and adults. Ninety percent of cases are due to herpes simplex virus type 1; however, herpes simplex virus type 2 has also been found to cause disease.[20] Herpes transmission occurs via contact with infectious saliva, typically from caregivers who may be unaware of their infectious risk. The incubation period is 2 to 12 days, with a mean of 4 days.

Clinically, the disease presents with abrupt onset of high fever, irritability, decreased oral intake and drooling, and swollen, erythematous, friable gingiva. Physical findings include vesicular lesions in the oral cavity, ulcerations, and tender cervical lymphadenopathy. Symptoms may persist for up to 3 weeks, but more commonly last <1 week.[21]

Diagnosis is primarily clinical. Viral culture has been the gold standard of laboratory testing for years. However, the recovery of virus from lesions is low (7% to 25%). Herpes simplex virus polymerase chain reaction is a newer, more accurate assay with improved sensitivity in detecting infection from any lesions that are present.[22] Tzanck smear of fluid from unroofed lesions 24 to 48 hours old showing multinucleated cells can also confirm the diagnosis but cannot differentiate infection between viruses within the herpesvirus family.

Treatment consists of supportive care with oral analgesics/antipyretics (acetaminophen or ibuprofen), topical analgesics, and systemic antiviral therapy for severe disease (acyclovir, 15 milligrams/kg PO divided five times a day for 7 days).[23] Immunocompromised patients are at significantly higher risk for systemic dissemination, and hospitalization and treatment with IV acyclovir are recommended.

Prognosis of a primary herpes simplex virus infection beyond the fetal/neonatal period is usually very good. As the primary infection resolves, a lifelong latent residency of the virus within the trigeminal ganglion occurs, which may lead to less severe recurrences at the same site in the future.

TABLE 121-2 Causes of Viral Pharyngitis in Children
Adenovirus
Coronavirus
Enterovirus (coxsackievirus)
Respiratory syncytial virus
Rhinovirus
Measles
Herpes simplex virus types 1 and 2
Parainfluenza virus
Epstein-Barr virus
Cytomegalovirus virus
Human immunodeficiency virus
Influenza virus A and B

PHARYNGITIS

It is important to distinguish between superficial and deep space infections of the mouth and throat. Deep space infections are discussed in chapter 123, "Stridor and Drooling in Infants and Children," and are typically associated with toxic appearance, high fever, drooling, stridor, or changes in phonation, trismus, or torticollis. Simple pharyngitis, on the other hand, accounts for 1% to 2% of all visits to outpatient clinics and EDs, resulting in 7.3 million annual visits for children.[24] Viral etiologies predominate in children with acute pharyngitis (**Table 121-2**).

Symptoms associated with acute pharyngitis include sore throat, odynophagia, fever, headache, abdominal pain, nausea and vomiting, cough, hoarseness, coryza, diarrhea, arthralgias, myalgias, and lethargy. Physical examination may reveal tonsillopharyngeal erythema and/or exudates, soft palate petechiae, uvulitis, anterior cervical lymphadenitis, rash, conjunctivitis, anterior stomatitis, and discrete ulcerative lesions. It is often difficult to distinguish between viral and bacterial causes of pharyngitis based on physical examination alone,[25] and *tonsillar exudate does not imply bacterial etiology*. This often results in overdiagnosis of bacterial etiology and unnecessary antibiotic treatment. Most viral infections are self-limited and require only symptomatic treatment. Interestingly, patient satisfaction appears to be greatest when a physician shows concern and provides reassurance and is not related to whether or not antibiotics are prescribed.[26]

VIRAL PHARYNGITIS

Pharyngitis is the best known acute clinical manifestation of **Epstein-Barr virus** infection (**Figure 121-8**). It often begins with malaise, headache, and fevers before development of the more specific signs of exudative

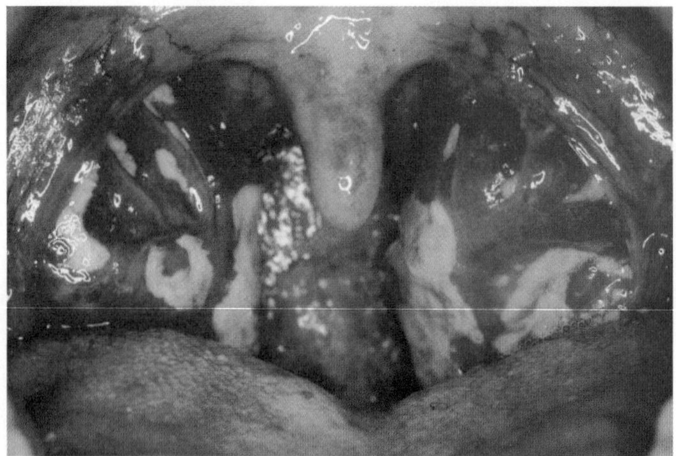

FIGURE 121-8. Marked white exudates on the tonsils of a child with Epstein-Barr virus infection. [Reproduced with permission from Kane KSM, Lio P, Stratigos A, Johnson R: *Color Atlas & Synopsis of Pediatric Dermatology*, 2nd ed. New York, McGraw-Hill, 2010.]

pharyngitis and posterior cervical lymph node enlargement. Splenomegaly and hepatomegaly can also occur. Patients mistakenly treated for a bacterial pharyngitis with amoxicillin or ampicillin often develop a characteristic pruritic maculopapular rash that aids in diagnosis.

Diagnosis is often clinical, although a heterophile test (monospot) can aid in diagnosis. It is important to remember that this test relies on cross-reactivity of patient antibodies and is relatively insensitive in pediatric patients (25% positive in 10 to 24 months vs 75% in 24 to 28 months). Furthermore, the monospot test typically does not turn positive in cases of Epstein-Barr virus until symptoms have been present for 1 week or more. A negative test, therefore, does not exclude the diagnosis of Epstein-Barr virus; when necessary, testing for Epstein-Barr virus immunoglobulin M and immunoglobulin G is both sensitive and specific, although results are not immediately available. Atypical lymphocytes may be present on the CBC, if obtained. Epstein-Barr virus infection may be associated with other organ involvement, including hepatitis. Patients with right upper quadrant tenderness should have liver enzymes evaluated.

Treatment is largely supportive; however, some patients may require IV fluids and pain medication. Although there is no evidence of efficacy, a dose of oral or parenteral steroid can be considered to reduce tonsillar enlargement when swallowing or respiratory symptoms are attributed to enlarged tonsils. When splenomegaly is noted, proper counseling regarding risk factors and symptoms of splenic rupture should be given (avoid contact sports until splenomegaly has resolved as determined by the primary care physician).

Cytomegalovirus infection can very closely mimic Epstein-Barr virus mononucleosis. Symptoms and signs of the two infections are almost identical. Indeed, patients presenting with classic infectious mononucleosis who are heterophile-negative are often infected with cytomegalovirus. Fever, malaise, and systemic complaints predominate in the clinical picture of cytomegalovirus, with less prominent cervical lymphadenopathy or splenic enlargement than Epstein-Barr virus. Distinguishing between the two etiologies is difficult, and often, the diagnosis is confirmed with laboratory testing for cytomegalovirus immunoglobulins M and G. Treatment is again supportive.

Acute retroviral syndrome, or acute infection with **human immunodeficiency virus,** may present similarly to Epstein-Barr virus pharyngitis in 50% to 70% of patients. Differences implicating human immunodeficiency virus from other viral illnesses may include presence of high-risk behaviors in the social history, the acuity of onset, the absence of exudate and prominent tonsillar hypertrophy, presence of a rash, and mucocutaneous ulceration.

Acute infection with human immunodeficiency virus is uncommon in the pediatric patient, although it must be considered in adolescents in whom high-risk behaviors are identified. In addition to the usual causes of pharyngitis, opportunistic infections, such as *Candida albicans* and *Mycobacterium avium*, should be considered in the immunocompromised patient.[27]

BACTERIAL INFECTIONS

Group A β-Hemolytic *Streptococcus* **Group A β-hemolytic *Streptococcus* (GABHS) pharyngitis** is the most commonly occurring form of acute bacterial pharyngitis for which antibiotic therapy is indicated.[28] It typically occurs in the winter and early spring, is rare in children <2 years of age,[29] and primarily affects children age 5 to 15 years old.[30] Although GABHS accounts for only 15% to 30% of pharyngitis in children, approximately 53% of children with pharyngitis receive antibiotics.[31] Additionally, a substantial proportion of patients treated for GABHS pharyngitis receive an inappropriate antibiotic. Clinical trials are under way to evaluate the safety and efficacy of a multivalent group A *Streptococcus* vaccine.[32]

Several clinical prediction rules have been created to identify cases of GABHS pharyngitis, and most are modifications of the original Centor criteria[33] (**Table 121-3**). These can be useful in determining which patients require testing for GABHS. With zero or one criterion, GABHS is unlikely, and testing and treatment for GABHS are not indicated. With two or more criteria, testing should be performed using a rapid antigen detection test and/or culture.[34]

Although bacterial culture remains the gold standard, with a sensitivity of 90% to 95%, the 18- to 48-hour wait time for definitive diagnosis is often impractical, and the use of rapid antigen detection has become popular. The sensitivity of rapid antigen detection varies from 80% to 90%. As a result, current guidelines recommend confirmatory throat culture for all patients with a negative antigen test.[35] Back-up cultures are not necessary for patients with a positive antigen test because the test is highly specific.

TABLE 121-3 Centor Criteria for Likelihood of Group A β-Hemolytic *Streptococcus* Pharyngitis
Tonsillar exudates
Tender anterior cervical lymphadenopathy
Absence of cough
History of fever

The antibiotic treatment of GABHS pharyngitis is effective to: (1) shorten the duration of illness, (2) prevent transmission, (3) prevent suppurative complications (acute otitis media, acute sinusitis, and peritonsillar abscess), and (4) prevent systemic illness such as rheumatic fever, rheumatic heart disease, and poststreptococcal glomerulonephritis. Antibiotics for the treatment of GABHS pharyngitis should be reserved, however, for patients with a positive antigen test or culture, or those meeting clinical criteria for diagnosis. GABHS pharyngitis is typically a self-limited disease, with fever and constitutional symptoms diminishing markedly at days 3 and 4 after symptom onset, and antibiotics only decrease the duration of symptoms by approximately 16 hours.[36]

Treatment Treatment can be delayed safely for up to 9 days after symptom onset and still prevent major nonsuppurative sequelae; thus, waiting for confirmatory cultures and providing a wait-and-see-prescription for antibiotics are safe. There is no definitive evidence that antibiotic use can prevent acute glomerulonephritis. Further confounding the decision to treat is the possibility that a percentage of patients may be GABHS carriers and that acute infection with another organism may be causing disease rather than GABHS pharyngitis.

Penicillin remains the treatment of choice, based on its efficacy, safety, narrow spectrum, ease of dosing (twice-daily dosing), compliance, and cost (**Table 121-4**).[35] No clinical isolate of GABHS has been documented to be penicillin resistant. Treatment failures may be attributable to viral pharyngitis with GABHS carriage, medication noncompliance, or reinfection of patients successfully treated for GABHS. A course of 10 days of oral therapy with twice-a-day dosing is recommended for complete pharyngeal eradication; similar efficacy is achieved with once-daily dosing of amoxicillin for 10 days or with a single IM dose of benzathine penicillin.

Several alternative therapy options exist for those unable to take penicillin. The efficacy of amoxicillin appears to be comparable to that of penicillin and is acceptable in children who more easily tolerate the taste of the suspension. Clarithromycin and first-generation cephalosporins are suitable alternatives in penicillin-allergic patients. Clindamycin may be required for macrolide-resistant GABHS in the penicillin-allergic patient. Macrolide resistance is increasing worldwide. Currently, 6% to 7% of GABHS isolates in the United States appear to be macrolide resistant, but this is expected to increase given higher resistance patterns in other parts of the world and the widespread use of macrolides for the treatment of upper and lower respiratory tract infections.[37]

Routine antibiotic prophylaxis is not recommended for household members exposed to GABHS, because the risk of developing subsequent pharyngitis is approximately 10%.[38] Although tonsillectomy is clearly indicated for recurrent tonsillitis in children, there is only modest evidence to support tonsillectomy for recurrent pharyngitis. Patients undergoing tonsillectomy have been shown to have a modest reduction in frequency of GABHS infections for up to 2 years after surgery.[39]

Benefits of antibiotic treatment for other bacterial pharyngitides are unclear at this time. There have been no cases of acute rheumatic fever due to non-GABHS, such as groups C and G *Streptococcus*. If treated, antibiotics used in the treatment of GABHS are appropriate for pharyngitis due to groups C and G *Streptococcus*.

Several other bacterial etiologies must be considered in patients with pharyngitis. These include *Neisseria gonorrhoeae*, *Corynebacterium diphtheriae*, *Arcanobacterium haemolyticum*, *Yersinia enterocolitica*, *Yersinia*

TABLE 121-4 Antibiotics for the Treatment of Streptococcal Pharyngitis

Medication	Dosage	Route	Duration
Penicillin V (first line)	Child: 250 milligrams *two times daily* Adolescent/adult: 500 milligrams twice a day	PO	10 d
Amoxicillin (first line)	50 milligrams/kg once daily; maximum dose, 1000 milligrams or 25 milligrams/kg/dose twice daily; maximum dose, 500 milligrams	PO	10 d
Benzathine penicillin G	<27 kg: 600,000 units ≥27 kg: 1,200,000 units	IM	One dose
Cephalexin (alternative for penicillin-allergic patients without anaphylaxis)	20 milligrams/kg/dose twice daily; maximum dose, 500 milligrams	PO	10 d
Clindamycin (alternative for penicillin-allergic patients)	7 milligrams/kg three times daily; maximum dose, 300 milligrams	PO	10 d
Azithromycin (alternative for penicillin-allergic patients)	Child: 12 milligrams/kg once daily Adolescent/adult: 500 milligrams on day 1, then 250 milligrams on days 2–5	PO	5 d
Clarithromycin (alternative for penicillin-allergic patients)	7.5 milligrams/kg/dose twice daily; maximum dose, 250 milligrams	PO	10 d

pestis, *Francisella tularensis*, *Mycoplasma pneumoniae*, and *Chlamydia* species.

Gonococcal Pharyngitis Gonococcal pharyngitis is difficult to distinguish from other bacterial causes of pharyngitis. A careful sexual history, including exposure to partners with known sexually transmitted diseases and oral sex practices, should be elicited in all adolescent patients presenting with pharyngitis. Gonococcal infection of the throat may be associated with infection elsewhere, including proctitis, vaginitis, and/or urethritis. The diagnosis requires special culture on Thayer-Martin medium, although nucleic acid amplification testing is also available. A positive culture in a prepubertal child is highly suspicious for sexual abuse, and further investigation is warranted with involvement of the appropriate child protection agencies. IM ceftriaxone (250 milligrams) is the only therapy recommended by the Centers for Disease Control and Prevention for the treatment of uncomplicated pharyngeal gonorrhea. Empiric treatment for concomitant chlamydia with the addition of 1 gram of azithromycin should be given unless it has specifically been ruled out.

Diphtheria Although occurrence is rare in developed countries due to vaccination, *C. diphtheriae* should be considered in patients who are under- or unimmunized. Toxigenic strains of this bacterium produce an exotoxin that causes localized necrosis of the respiratory mucosa and can lead to both cardiac and neurologic complications. Pseudomembrane formation in the respiratory tract can result in airway obstruction. Identification of the causative organism is made using Loeffler or tellurite selective medium. Treatment of pharyngeal diphtheria is aimed at bacterial eradication and exotoxin neutralization. Penicillin and erythromycin are the antibiotics of choice, along with equine diphtheria antitoxin. Serious sequelae can be prevented with prompt antibiotic administration, and treatment should be started when diphtheria is clinically suspected.

***Arcanobacterium* Pharyngitis** *A. haemolyticum* closely mimics GABHS pharyngitis and may also produce a scarlatiniform rash in teenagers; rarely, it produces a membranous pharyngitis similar to that of diphtheria. It may be missed on routine cultures and may be more readily detected on human-blood agar plates. Both macrolide and β-lactam antimicrobial agents are effective treatments.

UVULITIS

Isolated inflammation of the uvula is unusual and has infectious and noninfectious causes. When associated with pharyngitis, the most common bacterial etiology is GABHS.[40] In the unimmunized patient, *Haemophilus influenzae* type b is the next most common cause and may occur with epiglottitis. Other bacterial causes are *Fusobacterium nucleatum*, *Prevotella intermedia*, *Streptococcus pneumoniae*, and *C. albicans*. Noninfectious causes include trauma from instrumentation, irritant inhalation, vasculitis, allergic reaction, and angioedema.[41]

The inflamed uvula appears erythematous, enlarged, and edematous (**Figure 121-9**). Patients may present with fever, sore throat, difficulty swallowing, odynophagia, drooling, and/or respiratory distress.

Uvulitis is a clinical diagnosis. When there is associated pharyngitis, test for GABHS. *H. influenzae* diagnosis requires culture on Loeffler or tellurite selective medium.

Antibiotics to cover GABHS should be based on antigen testing or throat culture results. Acute airway obstruction is unusual with isolated uvulitis; however, when epiglottitis is also present, intubation may be required. When allergic reaction or angioedema is suspected, treatment may include epinephrine, antihistamines, and steroids. Precipitants, such as inhaled irritants and allergens, and responsible medications, such as an angiotensin-converting enzyme inhibitor, should be discontinued.

ORAL PROBLEMS

DENTAL TRAUMA

The evaluation and management of pediatric dental trauma, including subluxation, luxation, intrusion, extrusion, avulsion, and fracture, differ between primary and secondary (permanent) teeth (**Figure 121-10**).

Most dental injuries occur in the toddler years, when children are learning to walk; although in all children, nonaccidental trauma must be considered.[42,43] Up to 75% of abused children may have orofacial injuries, and a high index of suspicion must be maintained. Two other significant periods of trauma include school-aged children, from play injuries, and adolescents, mainly due to sports. The most commonly injured teeth are the maxillary central incisors.

Primary tooth eruption begins at approximately 6 months of age and is usually complete by 3 years of age. Secondary teeth may begin to erupt

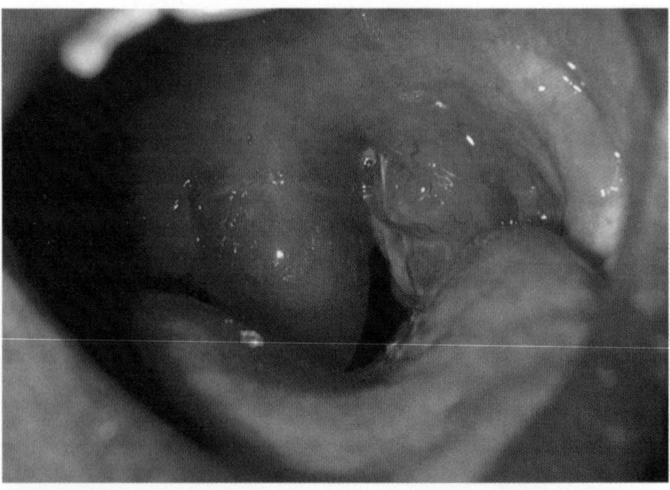

FIGURE 121-9. Uvulitis: Edematous, erythematous uvula. [Reproduced with permission from Knoop K, Stack L, Storrow A: *Atlas of Emergency Medicine*, 2nd ed. © 2002, McGraw-Hill, New York, Figure 5-28.]

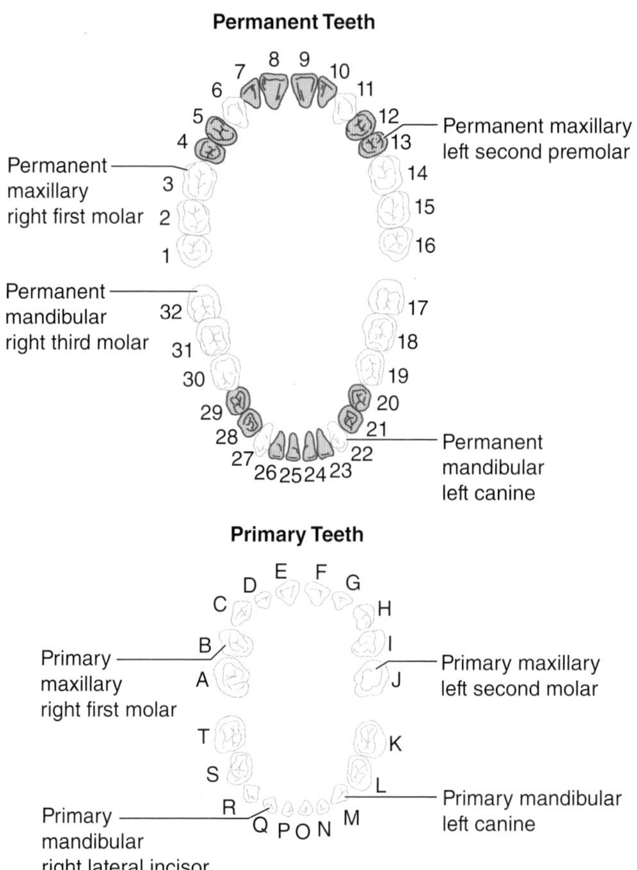

FIGURE 121-10. Primary and secondary dentition.

at 6 years of age and can continue past adolescence if the wisdom teeth are not extracted.

Subluxation refers to loosening of the tooth without displacement and is due to periodontal ligament damage (**Figure 121-11**). On examination, the tooth is mobile, and sulcal bleeding may be present. When subluxation is noted in a primary tooth, no intervention is required; however, permanent teeth may require splinting. Dental follow-up is recommended in either case, as pulpal necrosis may occur.[44]

Luxation is a loosening and displacement of a tooth from its normal anatomic position and occurs when the periodontal ligament is torn. The tooth is often nontender and immobile, and may be fixed in its new position. Primary teeth may be allowed to passively reposition, although dental consultation is recommended. Permanent teeth require active repositioning and splinting as soon as possible.

Intrusion occurs when a tooth is driven apically into the socket, displacing into the alveolar bone. The tooth appears shortened, or even absent, and, when visible, is not mobile or tender. Ninety percent of intruded teeth will re-erupt spontaneously in 2 to 6 months. Extraction of primary teeth is indicated when the apex is displaced toward the permanent tooth germ, as determined by radiography. Permanent teeth with immature root formation may be allowed to re-erupt; mature teeth require orthodontic or surgical extrusion.

Extrusion occurs when a tooth is displaced from its socket. The tooth appears elongated and is mobile, due to tearing of the periodontal ligament. Both primary and permanent teeth should be repositioned and splinted as soon as possible. If the injury is severe enough, primary teeth may require extraction in the ED.

Avulsed primary teeth should not be replanted, because this may damage the permanent tooth germ. Permanent teeth, by contrast, require urgent reimplantation, because success is time dependent. There is 85% to 97% survival of permanent teeth when replaced within 5 minutes, and near-zero survival at 1 hour. Avulsed teeth should be handled by the crown to avoid damaging the periodontal ligament. Debris should be removed with gentle rinsing in saline or water; scrubbing should be avoided because it may cause further damage. If the tooth cannot be replanted within 5 minutes, it should be stored, in order of preference, in ViaSpan, Hanks' Balanced Salt Solution, cold milk, saliva, physiologic saline, or water.

Fracture of the tooth enamel alone (a type 1 fracture using the Ellis classification system) or of the enamel and dentin (Ellis type 2 fracture) may be managed conservatively (**Figures 121-12** and **121-13**). Treatment of an Ellis type 3 fracture, involving the pulp (**Figure 121-14**), includes pulp capping and partial and complete pulpectomy. A root fracture, or Ellis type 4 fracture, involves the dentin, pulp, and cementum. In both primary and permanent teeth, the coronal fragment should be repositioned and stabilized in its anatomically correct position. In primary teeth, alternatively, the coronal fragment may be extracted, allowing the periodontal ligament and neurovascular supply to heal.

Radiographs may be obtained to confirm any of the diagnoses above or to confirm a tooth avulsion when there is question of an intrusion into the alveolar bone.

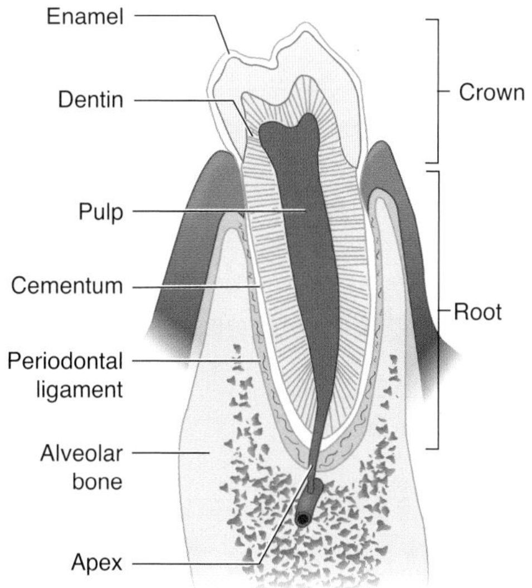

Enamel
Dentin
Crown
Pulp
Cementum
Root
Periodontal ligament
Alveolar bone
Apex

FIGURE 121-11. Normal anatomy of the tooth.

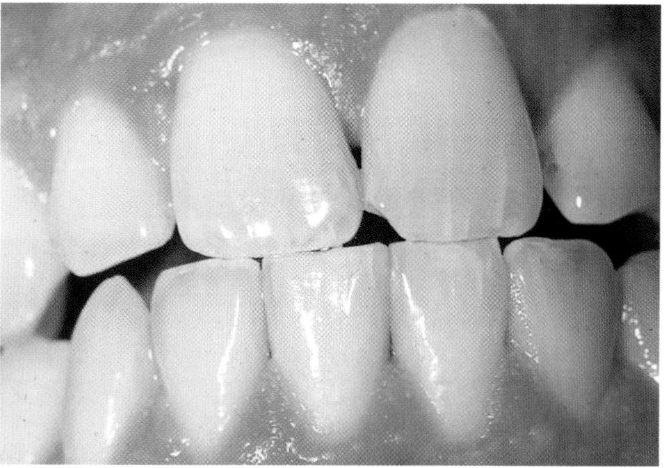

FIGURE 121-12. Ellis type 1 fracture: Note the fracture of the left upper central incisor. The sole involvement of the enamel is consistent with an Ellis type 1 injury. [Reproduced with permission from Knoop K, Stack L, Storrow A: *Atlas of Emergency Medicine*, 2nd ed. © 2002, McGraw-Hill, New York, Figure 6-5.]

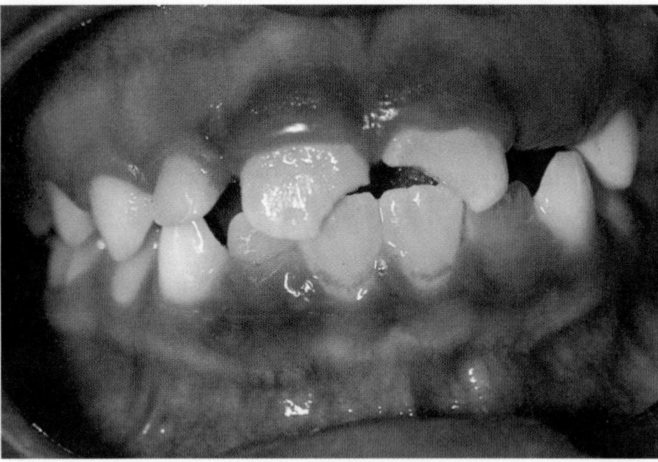

FIGURE 121-13. Ellis type 2 fracture: Bilateral maxillary central incisor injuries with exposed enamel and dentin consistent with an Ellis class 2 fracture. [Reproduced with permission from Knoop K, Stack L, Storrow A: *Atlas of Emergency Medicine*, 2nd ed. © 2002, McGraw-Hill, New York, Figure 6-6.]

SOFT TISSUE INJURIES OF THE MOUTH

Repair large lacerations of the gingiva with absorbable sutures. Wounds can allow entry of foreign bodies, such as food particles, dental fillings, and tooth fragments, leading to infection. Frenulum lacerations of the maxilla usually heal well without intervention. By contrast, the vascularity around the mandibular frenulum often requires primary closure. Tongue lacerations can usually be treated conservatively, especially if the wound is <1 cm in length, is in the central portion of the tongue, and does not gape, and bleeding is controlled.[45] Tongue lacerations greater than one third of the total diameter and those at the tip causing forking that may affect speech require suturing.

In general, lacerations limited to the inner mucosal surface heal well on their own and do not require primary repair. By contrast, full-thickness lacerations and those that disrupt the vermillion border require suturing.

CARIES

Children are particularly susceptible to developing caries soon after the initial eruption of teeth if care is not taken to properly examine and clean the new teeth. "Baby bottle" caries occur in 24% to 28% of all children age 2 to 5 years old.[46] Risk factors include prolonged breast or bottle feeding (beyond 12 months), prolonged pacifier use, frequent consumption of beverages high in sugar, and use of a bottle at bed time.

Encourage parents to minimize beverage choices high in sugar content. Teeth should be cleaned daily from time of eruption to 24 months of age with a soft toothbrush and increased to twice a day thereafter. Transition to a training cup by 1 year of age and removal of the bottle can also significantly reduce the occurrence of caries. Additionally, an initial screening dental examination between 12 and 18 months of age is recommended to look for signs of decay or a need for fluoride supplementation. In communities without fluoridated water, supplemental fluoride should be prescribed by the primary care provider.

Dental neglect is a form of child abuse probably underreported or unrecognized by medical providers. It is defined as the "willful failure of parent or guardian to seek and follow through with treatment necessary to ensure a level of oral health essential for adequate function and freedom from pain and infection." Poor oral hygiene may be secondary to family isolation, lack of finances, parental ignorance, unfluoridated water, bottle-propping, or lack of perceived value of oral health, and clinicians should determine whether one or more of these situations are contributing factors.[47]

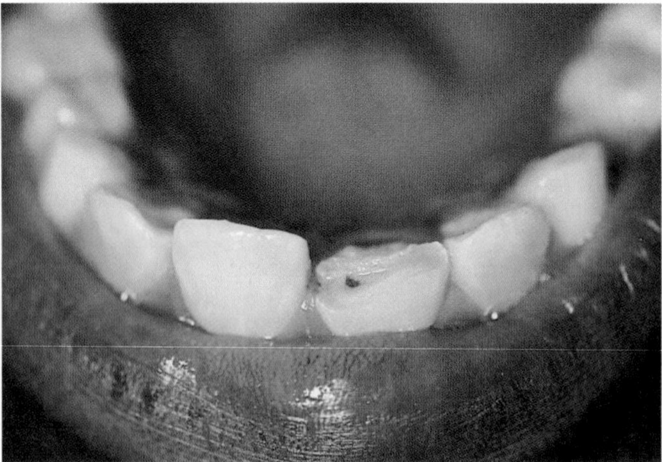

FIGURE 121-14. Ellis type 3 fracture: A fracture demonstrating blood at the exposed dental pulp. This sign is pathognomonic for an Ellis class 3 fracture. [Reproduced with permission from Knoop K, Stack L, Storrow A: *Atlas of Emergency Medicine*, 2nd ed. © 2002, McGraw-Hill, New York, Figure 6-7.]

GINGIVITIS

Gingivitis is inflammation of the gums that presents as tender, erythematous, often ulcerated or vesiculated areas of tissue. It is seen mainly in the setting of poor dental hygiene but can occur with viral and bacterial infections, certain medications (e.g., phenytoin [Dilantin]), or even as a presentation of leukemia. Although there are many causes of gingivostomatitis, viral infections are particularly common in children.

Acute necrotizing ulcerative gingivitis is a progressive infection of the gingiva, leading to pain, significant edema, and ulceration. The incidence typically peaks in the teens to early 20s but may be seen in younger children in developing countries due to poor access to adequate dental care or malnutrition. Other factors that may predispose patients to acute necrotizing ulcerative gingivitis include smoking, immunosuppression, viral infections, stress, and sleep deprivation. Patients present with fever, halitosis, decreased appetite, and generalized malaise. Acute necrotizing ulcerative gingivitis is a mixed infection that includes spirochetes, specifically, *Prevotella intermedia*. Untreated, acute necrotizing ulcerative gingivitis can spread beyond the gingiva to involve deeper tissues or the tissues of the mouth floor (Ludwig's angina) or face. Treatment consists of analgesia to facilitate better oral hygiene and antimicrobial oral rinses. Patients with more extensive disease or systemic symptoms may require admission for local debridement and parenteral antibiotic therapy with penicillin or metronidazole. The patient should be referred to a dentist for close follow-up care.

REFERENCES

The complete reference list is available online at www.TintinalliEM.com.

CHAPTER 122 Neck Masses in Infants and Children

Charles E. A. Stringer
Vikram Sabhaney

INTRODUCTION AND EPIDEMIOLOGY

Neck masses are common in childhood, and although most are benign, malignancy is always a primary consideration. Correct diagnosis is challenging, but differentiating neck masses into inflammatory, congenital, or neoplastic categories is the first step toward diagnosis.

In patients referred to tertiary centers for surgical excision of a cervical lesion, 90% to 96% of lesions are benign and are predominantly congenital.[1,2]

GENERAL APPROACH

CLINICAL FEATURES

A thorough history and physical examination will narrow the broad differential for cervical lymphadenopathy. The acuity and laterality of node swelling are helpful for diagnosis. Typically, acute bilateral lymph nodes are due to a viral cause, acute unilateral nodes are due to a bacterial cause, and subacute/chronic nodes (>4 to 6 weeks) are due to granulomatous bacteria or noninfectious causes. This framework is most effective for diagnosis when combined with the general and specific features of different causes (**Tables 122-1** and **122-2**). Carefully record the features of all head and neck masses for future comparison. Lymph node location and characteristics give clues based on lymphatic drainage patterns. Look for systemic disease by assessing for generalized lymphadenopathy, hepatosplenomegaly, testicular masses and/or enlargement in males, and the child's overall condition.

GENERAL MANAGEMENT

Ideally, the treatment of a childhood neck mass is directed at the specific cause; however, due to the many etiologies, this is not always obvious at first presentation. The majority of presentations are benign; however, the priority of childhood neck masses is to correctly identify those that are neoplastic. The algorithm in Figure 122-1 provides an approach to management based on suspected etiology and should be adapted to the individual patient. Follow-up of patients who are treated with antibiotics is necessary at 48 to 72 hours; if improvement of symptoms is not seen, then expanded coverage to include periodontal flora or MRSA is encouraged, and aspiration of fluctuant nodes for culture may be considered. Most lymphadenopathy will improve after 2 weeks of observation or antibiotics; however, all cases require 6-week follow-up to ensure resolution.

TABLE 122-1 Key Features from History

Historical Feature	Associated Etiology
Duration >4-6 weeks	Granulomatous lymphadenitis, congenital lesions, malignancies
Rate of growth	Fluctuating → inflammatory Progressive → malignancy
Pain	Infectious, or infected congenital lesion
Recent illness	Viral URTI → Reactive lymphadenopathy Pharyngitis → EBV, GAS
Neonatal period	Group B *Streptococcus*
Pain with meals	Sialoadenitis
Tuberculosis exposure (travel or sick contacts)	Tuberculosis mycobacteria
Undercooked meat or unpasteurized milk exposure	Toxoplasmosis
Cat exposure	Cat-scratch disease or toxoplasmosis
Animal exposure (including rabbits)	Tularemia, cat-scratch disease, toxoplasmosis
Mass since birth	Congenital
Birth trauma, forceps delivery	Fibromatosis colli
Constitutional symptoms (fever, weight loss, night sweats)	Tuberculosis mycobacteria, malignancy
Recent blood transfusions	EBV, CMV, HIV
Recent immunizations (DPT, polio, typhoid)	Reactive lymphadenopathy
Medications	Phenytoin, carbamazepine, isoniazid, hydralazine, and others

Abbreviations: CMV = cytomegalovirus; DPT = diphtheria, pertussis, and tetanus; EBV = Epstein-Barr virus; GAS = group A *Streptococcus*; HIV = human immunodeficiency virus; URTI = upper respiratory tract infection.

TABLE 122-2 Key Features on Examination

Physical Examination Finding	Associated Etiology
Laterality	Bilateral → viral Unilateral → bacterial
Size	>3 cm more likely congenital or malignant; fluctuations in size more likely infectious
Location	Depends on lymph drainage pattern (**Figure 122-2**)
Hard, rubbery, fixed, matted nodes	Possibly malignant
Signs of inflammation (tenderness, erythema, warmth)	Bacterial lymphadenitis or infected congenital lesion
Fluctuance	Abscess, often due to *Staphylococcus aureus*, or GAS
Difficulty swallowing or drooling	Deep space infection—retropharyngeal abscess
Viral URTI (cough, rhinorrhea, conjunctivitis)	Reactive lymphadenopathy
Pharyngitis	EBV mononucleosis, GAS
Periodontal disease	Anaerobic bacteria
Purulent salivary duct drainage	Sialoadenitis
Crossing jaw—suggests parotid involvement	Sialoadenitis, mumps, salivary gland malignancy
Violaceous skin change	Granulomatous lymphadenitis (TbM, NTM, CSD, tularemia)
Cold node	Granulomatous lymphadenitis or malignancy
Midline, moves with swallowing or tongue protrusion	Thyroglossal duct cyst
Transillumination	Lymphangioma (cystic hygroma)
Torticollis, laterally mobile, vertically immobile	Fibromatosis colli
Supraclavicular mass	Lymphoma, or less likely metastatic node
Midline mass	Thyroid cancer, thyroglossal duct cyst, dermoid cyst
Posterior mass	Rubella, toxoplasmosis, nasopharyngeal cancer
Hepatosplenomegaly	Malignancy, mononucleosis, systemic disease
Wasting or cachexia	Malignancy

Abbreviations: CSD = cat-scratch disease; EBV = Epstein-Barr virus; GAS = group A *Streptococcus*; NTM = nontuberculous mycobacteria; TbM = tuberculous mycobacteria; URTI = upper respiratory tract infection.

INFLAMMATORY NECK MASSES

The most common pediatric neck mass is an enlarged lymph node caused by infection. Be careful to consider masquerading lesions such as salivary gland infections, acutely infected congenital lesions, and, most importantly, malignancies.

Cervical lymph nodes drain the skin of the head and neck as well as the entire nasal, oral, and pharyngeal mucosa (Figure 122-2). Submandibular and cervical nodes are most common because they drain much of the oropharynx, including the adenoids and tonsils.[3,4] Supraclavicular lymphadenopathy is suspicious for metastasis because it drains the abdomen and thorax.[4]

Palpable cervical lymph nodes are found in about 28% to 44% of healthy infants and children, with the incidence peaking in early childhood.[3,5,6] Lymph nodes ≤1 cm in children <12 years old are considered normal.[7,8] Most lymphadenopathy represents nonspecific reactive hyperplasia, often due to a viral upper respiratory tract infection.[9]

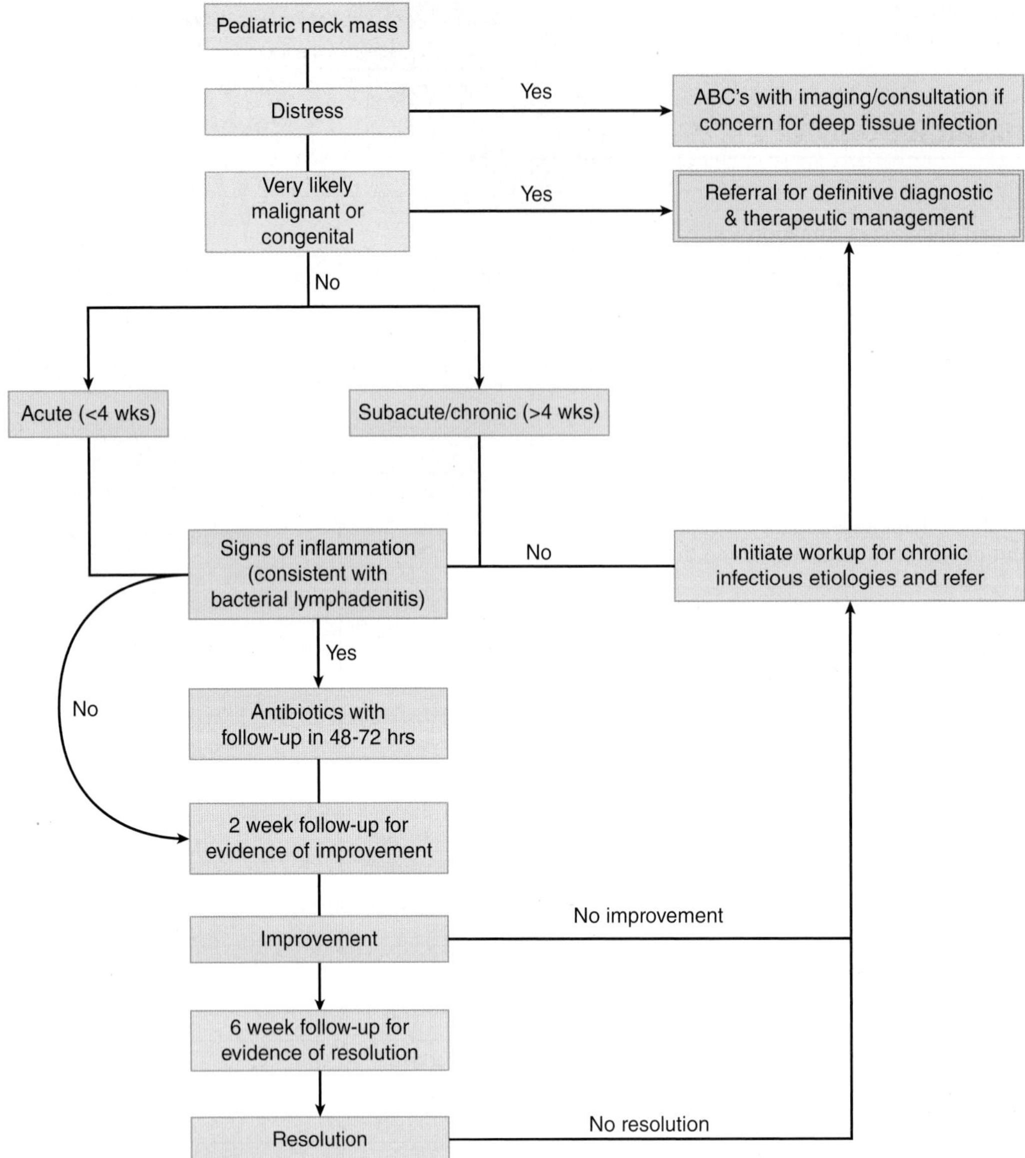

FIGURE 122-1. Approach to the pediatric neck mass in the ED. ABC = airway, breathing, circulation.

Lymphadenitis is lymph node inflammation (swelling, tenderness, warmth, erythema) and is most commonly due to viral or bacterial causes. Infection with a pyogenic organism may lead to liquefactive necrosis (suppuration) and abscess formation (**Figure 122-3**). If the immune system is unable to eradicate a particular organism, macrophages will attempt to contain it, forming a chronic granulomatous lymphadenitis.

ACUTE BILATERAL LYMPHADENOPATHY

Acute bilateral lymphadenopathy is usually due to viral infection and is self-limited. Common viruses include rhinovirus, parainfluenza, influenza, respiratory syncytial virus, coronavirus, reovirus, and adenovirus.[10] Treatment is symptomatic and expectant.

Alternative viral causes include **infectious mononucleosis**, characterized by fever, exudative pharyngitis, and significant lymphadenopathy (**Figure 122-4**). Heterophile antibodies or Epstein-Barr virus–specific immunoglobulin M confirms the diagnosis, and in immunocompetent patients, treatment is symptomatic. The classic viral exanthems associated with lymphadenopathy are **measles** (Koplik spots, conjunctivitis, and a descending rash) and **rubella** (associated with Forchheimer spots, rash, and polyarthritis). Acute bilateral lymphadenopathy and oral lesions may also be due to **herpes simplex virus** (gingivostomatitis) or **coxsackie virus** (herpangina). Pharyngitis caused by group A *Streptococcus* is accompanied by cervical lymphadenopathy.[11] Bilateral swelling that extends over the jaw suggests **parotid gland** involvement due to mumps and may be associated with orchitis and a rash.

ACUTE UNILATERAL LYMPHADENOPATHY

Acute unilateral lymphadenopathy is most often due to bacterial lymphadenitis (**Figure 122-5**) caused by *Staphylococcus aureus* and group A *Streptococcus*.[12] Lymph nodes will likely have signs of inflammation, and if an abscess has developed, fluctuance may be appreciated. Often the source of group A *Streptococcus* is the pharynx, whereas *S. aureus* originates from a break in the skin. Careful examination of the head, neck, throat, skin, and ears may identify a source that can be cultured.

Generally, lymph nodes <1 cm are normal and do not need treatment. If lymphadenitis measures between 1 and 3 cm, appropriate antibiotics treating group A *Streptococcus* and *Staphylococcus* for up to 2 weeks should lead to complete resolution.[13] Nodes >3 cm raise suspicion for malignancy, but if the nodes are acute and inflammatory, a course of antibiotics and observation is reasonable.

Due to increasing β-lactamase–resistant *Staphylococcus*, first-line oral antibiotic choices are first-generation cephalosporins, cloxacillin/

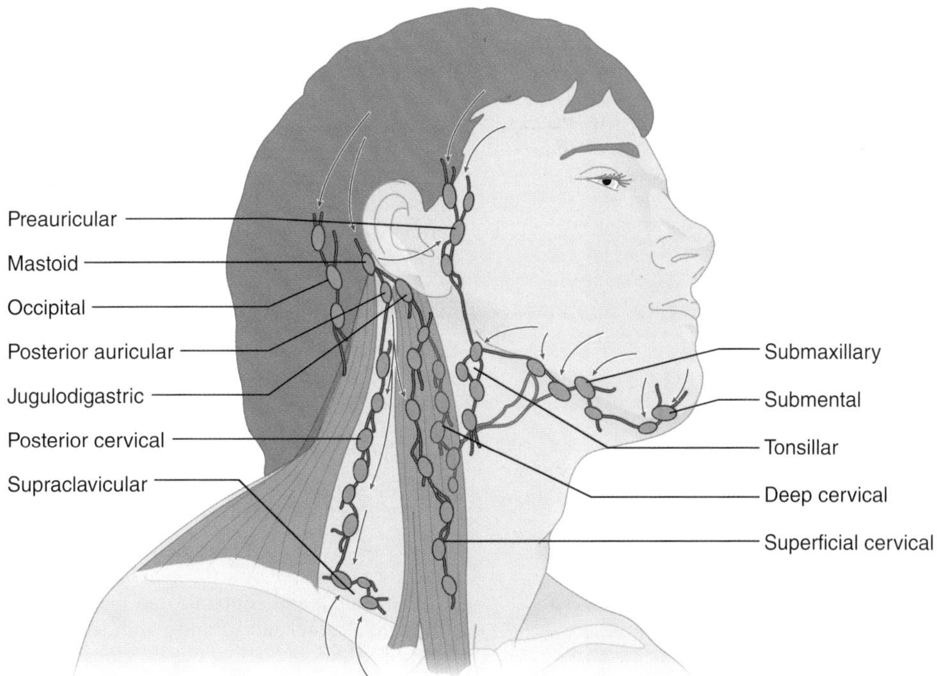

FIGURE 122-2. Cervical lymph node drainage.

dicloxacillin/oxacillin, or clindamycin.[12,14,15] If the child is unwell or immunocompromised, treat with IV cefazolin, nafcillin, or clindamycin. Reassess in 48 hours, and if no improvement is appreciated, consider changing antibiotics to treat methicillin-resistant *S. aureus*.[16,17]

Fluctuance of the node suggests abscess formation due to pyogenic bacteria, with the source often from the tonsils.[15] Fluctuant nodes typically respond to antibiotics alone, but needle aspiration after local anesthesia may be helpful to avoid incision in cosmetically important areas.[15] If a superficial abscess is pointing or not resolving within 2 weeks of antibiotics, then evaluation by US and incision and drainage may be necessary.[18] When associated with torticollis or trismus, suspect a retropharyngeal abscess, and obtain imaging and/or surgical consultation (see chapter 123, "Stridor and Drooling in Infants and Children").

Infants have a higher incidence of infection with group B *Streptococcus* rather than *S. aureus* or group A *Streptococcus*. Group B streptococcal

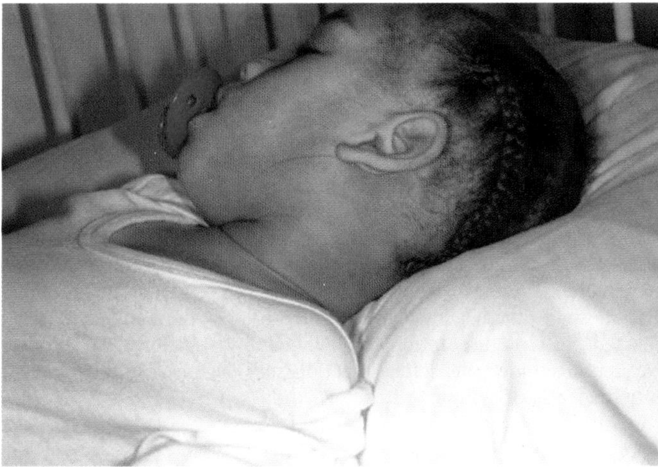

FIGURE 122-3. Suppurative lymphadenitis. [Reproduced with permission from Shah BR, Lucchesi M, Amodio J (eds): *Atlas of Pediatric Emergency Medicine*, 2nd ed. © 2013, McGraw-Hill Education, New York, NY, Figure 3-2.]

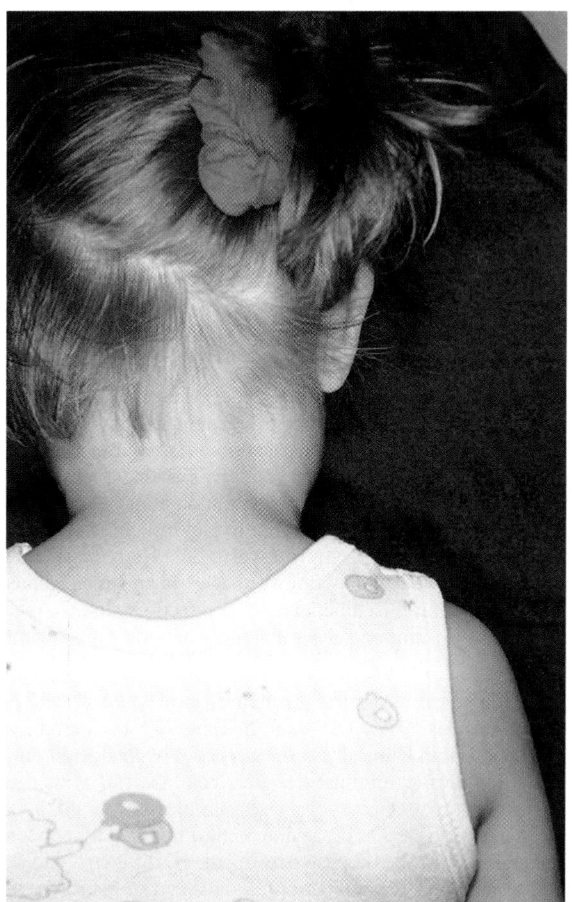

FIGURE 122-4. Infectious mononucleosis typically presents with bilateral lymphadenopathy. A 6-year-old girl demonstrating bilateral lymphadenopathy. [Reproduced with permission from Shah BR, Lucchesi M: *Atlas of Pediatric Emergency Medicine*. © 2006, McGraw-Hill Education, New York, NY, Figure 11-14.]

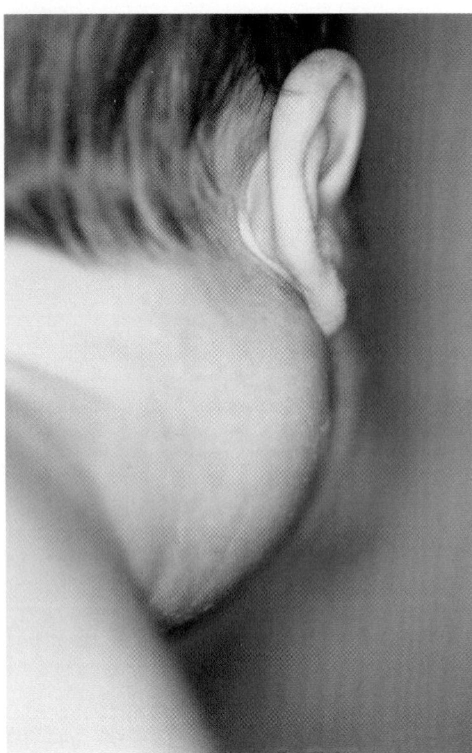

FIGURE 122-5. An infant with unilateral lymphadenitis due to *Staphylococcus aureus* infection. [Photo Contributed by Dr. J. P. Ludemann, BC Children's Hospital, Vancouver, British Columbia, Canada.]

infection can be associated with bacteremia, pneumonia, and meningitis.[19,20] Infections originating from the oral mucosa, seen most commonly in children age 5 to 15 years with periodontal disease, are more likely to contain anaerobic bacteria requiring coverage with penicillin V, amoxicillin-clavulanic acid, or clindamycin.[14] Sialoadenitis is characterized by unilateral swelling crossing the jaw and tenderness after meals, and can be associated with purulent discharge from Wharton's and Stensen's ducts (**Figure 122-6**). Sialolithiasis can cause recurrent infections due to outflow obstruction of the gland.

SUBACUTE/CHRONIC LYMPHADENOPATHY

Chronic lymphadenopathy is defined as persistence for 6 weeks without resolution. Persistent lymphadenopathy, generalized lymphadenopathy, or failure to respond to 2 to 4 weeks of antibiotics requires evaluation for uncommon infectious, congenital, and neoplastic causes. Persistent infectious agents evade eradication by granuloma formation. Generally, the course of evolution is slower than a typical inflammatory lymphadenitis and may be characterized by a violaceous overlying skin change. Refer to otolaryngology for definitive diagnosis and management.[21-23] Refer immunocompromised patients to an infectious disease specialist. Some of the more common causes of granulomatous lymphadenitis are covered below.

Mycobacterial Lymphadenitis Chronic cervical lymphadenitis may be due to tuberculous (*Mycobacterium tuberculosis*) or nontuberculous mycobacterial strains. Clinically, both varieties of lymphadenitis are characterized by a chronic, minimally tender, "cold abscess," with overlying violaceous skin. Spontaneous drainage can transform into a chronic draining sinus.[22] It is important to differentiate between tuberculous and nontuberculous strains because treatment is different. Differential Mantoux testing with a combination of antigens can identify strains in about 93% of patients.[24] Consider *M. tuberculosis* lymphadenitis in children with risk of tuberculosis exposure, in those exhibiting constitutional signs, and in those with an abnormal chest x-ray and with a strongly reactive purified protein derivative skin test,[25] and treat for 8 to 12 months. Treatment for nontuberculous lymphadenitis is surgical excision.[26]

Cat-Scratch Disease Cat-scratch disease is caused by *Bartonella henselae*, with inoculation by a scratch or a bite from a kitten. The inoculation site develops into a painless, erythematous vesicle or pustule after 3 to 10 days, which may disappear before other symptoms develop. After 1 to 3 weeks, regional lymphadenopathy typically develops. Suppuration is uncommon. Diagnosis involves serologic testing, but because antibody development may be delayed and the primary lesion may have resolved, rely on a strong history of cat exposure and an inoculating lesion. No treatment is needed. Serious complications (encephalitis) can develop in immunodeficient patients, with treatment options based primarily on case reports.

Toxoplasmosis *Toxoplasma gondii* is a protozoan parasite with a complex life cycle that can infect humans through ingestion of undercooked meat, exposure to oocysts in cat feces, or through maternal-fetal transmission (congenital toxoplasmosis). Infection is widespread; an estimated 22.5% of children in the United States are infected by the age of 12 years old; in some countries, up to 95% of the population has been infected. The lymphatic system is the most common organ system involved. Diagnosis is usually made serologically with antibody titers. Treatment is not typically needed in healthy children.

Tularemia Tularemia is caused by the bacteria *Francisella tularensis*, which is transmitted by arthropod bites, handling infected animals (classically rabbits), and contaminated food and water. The most common forms are ulceroglandular and glandular tularemia. In the ulceroglandular form, the inoculation site develops from an erythematous tender papule into an exudative ulcer within days. Regionally draining lymphadenopathy subsequently develops that may spontaneously suppurate and drain if not treated. Tularemia is diagnosed serologically with microagglutination testing. Gentamicin is the treatment of choice.

Other Causes Other causes of cervical lymphadenopathy include recent immunizations (diphtheria, pertussis, and tetanus; polio; typhoid), blood transfusions (causing Epstein-Barr virus, cytomegalovirus, or human immunodeficiency virus exposure), various medications (including phenytoin, carbamazepine, isoniazid, and hydralazine) and systemic disease (Kawasaki's disease; sarcoid; periodic fever, aphthous stomatitis, pharyngitis, and adenitis; and autoimmune) (Tables 122-1 and 122-2).

CONGENITAL NECK MASSES

In patients referred to tertiary centers for surgical excision of a cervical lesion, 90% to 96% of lesions are benign, and most are congenital.[1,2] Congenital lesions are the most common cause of noninflammatory pediatric neck masses,[1] but a mass may not be recognized until infection develops. The sternocleidomastoid muscle divides the neck into anterior and posterior triangles, and congenital neck masses can be organized into midline, anterior, and posterior groups (**Table 122-3**). The most common congenital neck masses and their characteristic features are discussed below.

THYROGLOSSAL DUCT CYSTS

Thyroglossal duct cysts (**Figure 122-7A**) account for approximately 70% of the congenital neck masses and are the second most common benign neck mass after lymphadenopathy.[27] Thyroglossal duct cysts result from the persistence of any segment of the thyroglossal duct along its course from the foramen cecum of the tongue to the pyramidal lobe of the thyroid and are located in the midline of the neck within the anterior triangle.[28] Most of the lesions are infrahyoid (65%), whereas suprahyoid cysts account for 20%, and another 15% of lesions are at the level of the hyoid bone.[29,30] The pathognomonic feature is a painless fluctuant mass that moves with swallowing or protrusion of the tongue. Acutely infected cysts require antibiotics. Further investigations and surgical excision are undertaken after infection subsides because they carry a very small risk of malignant transformation.[31]

DERMOID CYSTS

Dermoid cysts are developmental anomalies involving pluripotent embryonal stem cells and occur most often in children <3 years old. Dermoid cysts are usually suprahyoid[32] and midline and are often misdiagnosed as

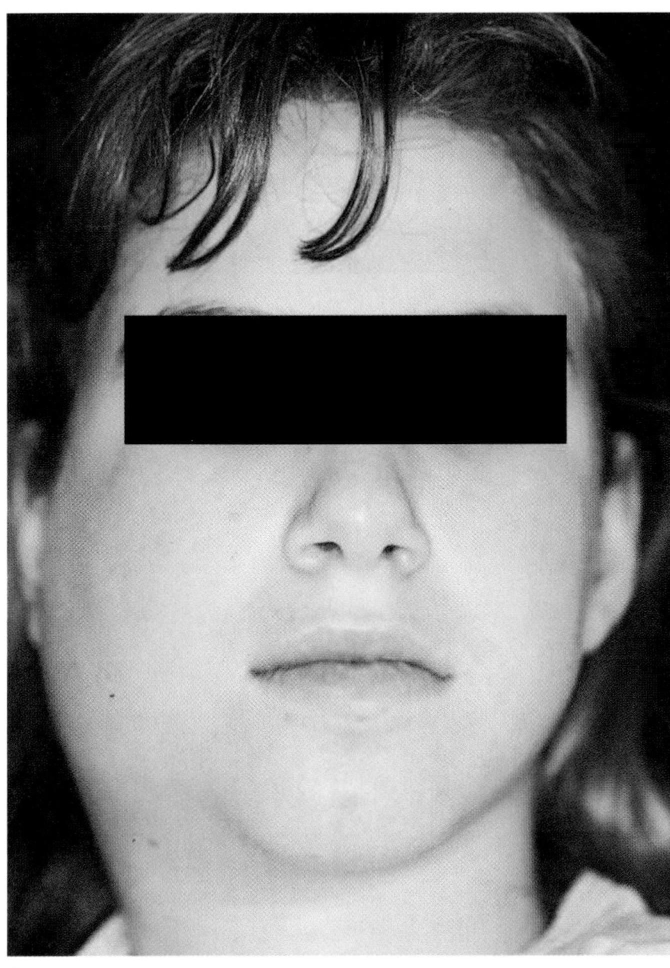

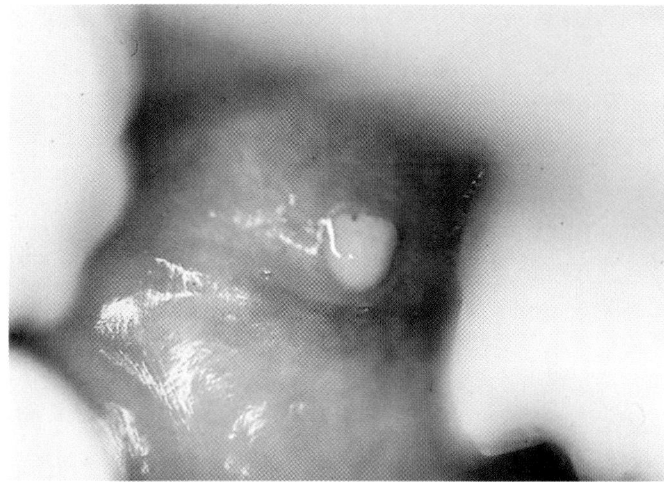

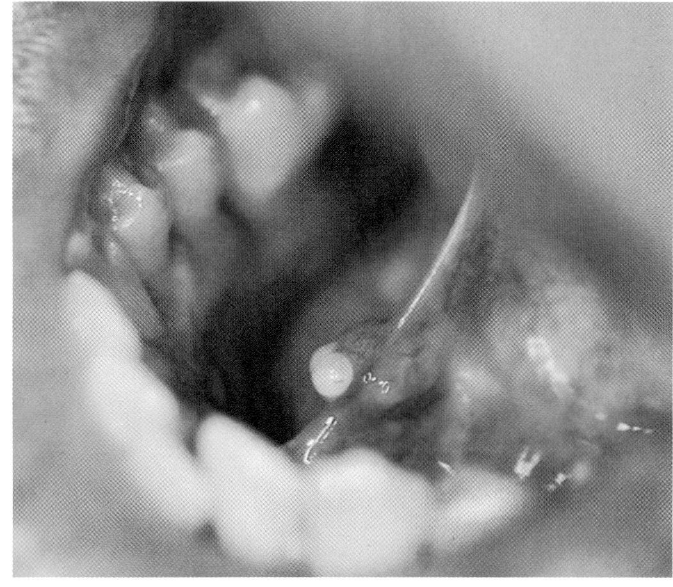

FIGURE 122-6. Sialoadenitis. **A.** Unilateral swelling crossing the angle of the mandible. **B** and **C.** Purulent drainage from Stensen's and Wharton's salivary ducts, respectively. [Reproduced with permission from Knoop KJ, Stack LB, Storrow AB: *Atlas of Emergency Medicine,* 2nd ed. © 2002, McGraw-Hill, New York, Figures 5-32 and 5-33.]

TABLE 122-3 Common Congenital Neck Cysts by Location, Signs, and Typical Age of Onset

Type	Location	Signs	Age
Thyroglossal duct	Midline (infrahyoid mostly)	Cyst moves with swallowing or tongue protrusion.	Birth–elderly
Dermoid/ epidermoid	Midline (suprahyoid)	Cyst may move with swallowing.	Birth–adult
Branchial	Anterior triangle anterior to sternocleidomastoid muscle near angle of the mandible	May be associated with draining sinus.	Childhood–adult
Lymphangioma (cystic hygroma)	Posterior triangle	Soft; enlarges in first few weeks of life. Transilluminates.	Birth–infancy

thyroglossal duct cysts.[33,34] Dermoid cysts are mobile, but they do not move with tongue protrusion. Management is surgical excision.

BRANCHIAL CLEFT CYSTS

Incomplete obliteration of the branchial apparatus, predominately the cleft, leads to branchial cleft anomalies: cysts, sinuses, or fistulae.[28] Up to 95% of branchial cleft cysts arise from remnants of the second branchial cleft,[35] which are most often anterior to the sternocleidomastoid muscle near the angle of the mandible (**Figure 122-7B**). The cysts are round, smooth, and mobile, but are not tender unless they become infected. There may be a history of recurrent swelling or infection in the same area. Cysts may spontaneously rupture, forming an external sinus or fistula. Oral antibiotics are indicated for infected cysts prior to definitive surgery.

LYMPHANGIOMAS

Lymphangiomas (also known as cystic hygromas) result from sequestration of lymphatic channels that fail to communicate with the internal jugular vein leading to a blockage of the lymphatic system.[36] They can occur anywhere in the body, but nearly 75% arise within the neck, most

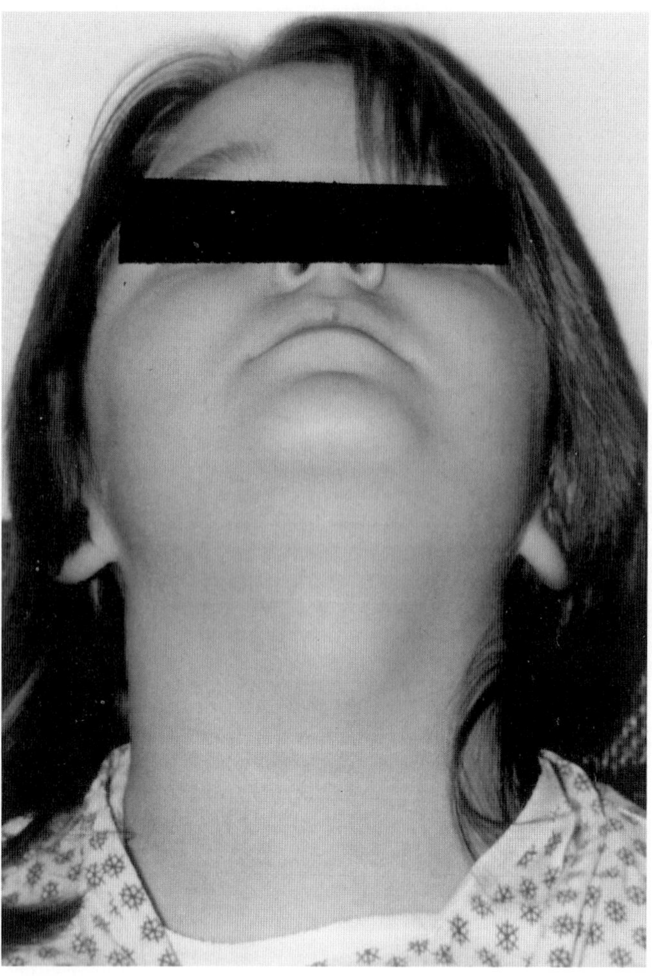
A

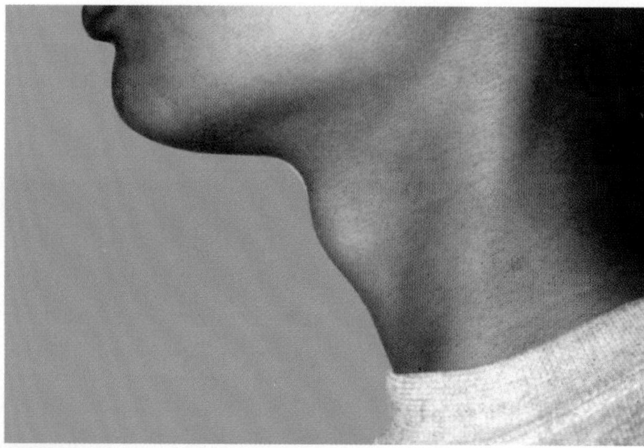
B

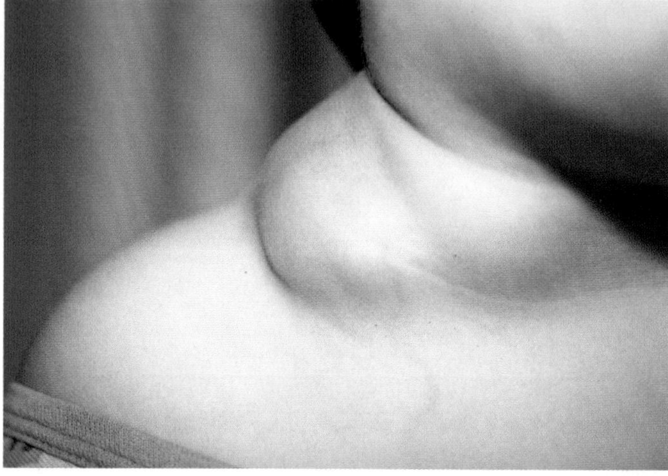
C

FIGURE 122-7. Congenital lesions. **A.** Large thyroglossal duct cyst. **B.** Second arch branchial cleft cyst. **C.** Lymphangioma. [**B:** Photo contributor: Scott Manning, MD. Reproduced with permission from Knoop KJ, Stack LB, Storrow AB, Thurman RJ: *Atlas of Emergency Medicine*, 3rd ed. © 2010, McGraw-Hill, New York, Figure 14-48. **C:** Reproduced with permission from Knoop KJ , Stack LB, Storrow AB, Thurman RJ: *Atlas of Emergency Medicine*, 2nd ed. © 2002, McGraw-Hill, New York, Figure 14-35.]

commonly along the jugular chain of lymphatics. Cervical lymphangiomas are soft, painless, and compressible, and can be very large (**Figure 122-7C**). Morbidity is usually secondary to compression of surrounding structures, and large neck lesions may cause serious airway and feeding problems. Sixty-five percent present at birth, and 90% are clinically detected by the end of the second year.[29,36] Sudden enlargement can occur from infection or hemorrhage into the lesion. Careful inspection of the oral cavity and palpation of the trachea for deviation are important in assessing the airway of patients with large cystic hygromas. Injection of sclerosing agents can be used in some lesions, although surgical excision is the definitive treatment.[36]

NEOPLASTIC NECK MASSES

Malignancy should always be considered as a potential etiology in the evaluation of a child with a neck mass. Of childhood malignancies, 5% to 12% present as a head or neck mass, of which 99% are primary tumors.[1,37-40] Diagnosing malignancies is made challenging by their rarity; only 1% of pediatric superficial lumps are malignant;[41] accordingly, a high index of suspicion and attention to worrisome features from history and physical examination are required (**Table 122-4**).[12,25,39-43] One review demonstrated that in 80% of superficial masses, malignancy can be ruled out with 99.7% accuracy based on the absence of five clinical features (Table 122-4).[41] The presence of any worrying features should prompt urgent referral for further diagnostic workup that may include fine-needle aspiration cytology, imaging, or excisional biopsy.

BENIGN NEOPLASMS

Benign noninflammatory pediatric neck masses comprise 5% of presentations.[44] An exhaustive review is not included in this chapter; instead, benign masses with specific identifying features are highlighted.

Hemangiomas Hemangiomas are congenital vascular tumors that present at 2 to 4 weeks, usually grow rapidly until 9 to 10 months of age, and typically regress thereafter. When palpable, they are soft, mobile, and frequently have a bluish hue.[45] Almost 90% of hemangiomas resolve spontaneously without the need for therapy. Lesions showing unusually rapid growth, hemorrhage, recurrent infection, or compression of adjacent

TABLE 122-4 Worrisome Features of Head and Neck Masses

Worrisome Features of Head and Neck Masses
Constitutional symptoms (fever, weight loss, night sweats, fatigue)
History of malignancy
Mass features (onset in the neonatal period*; size >3 cm; duration >4–6 weeks; supraclavicular, posterior, or midline location; rapid and progressive enlargement*; hard or rubbery consistency; fixation to skin or deep fascia*; associated skin ulceration*)
Generalized lymphadenopathy
Inflammatory mass >3 cm persistent for >6 wk, despite treatment
Mass greater than 3 cm with firm or hard consistency*

*If these five features are absent, then there is 99.7% accuracy that superficial lump is not malignant in 80% of cases.[41]

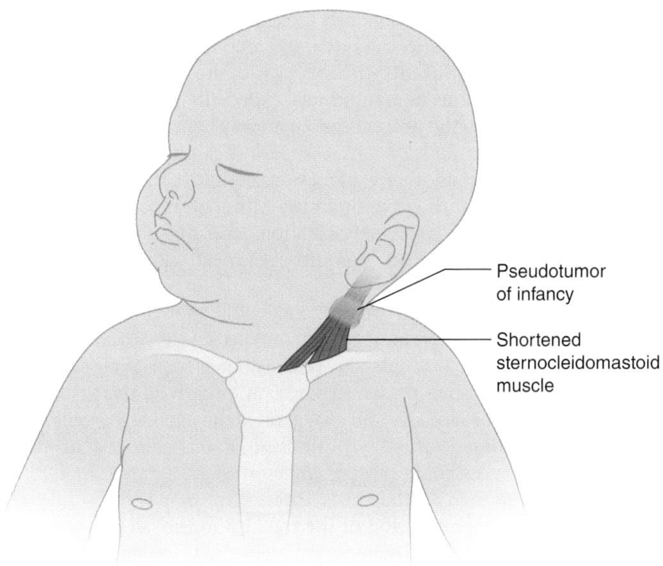

FIGURE 122-8. Schematic of fibramoatosis colli or pseudotumor of infancy.

structures may require treatment by a specialist, including β-blockers, steroids, and laser or surgical excision.[46] Hemangiomas compromising the airway result in biphasic stridor not responsive to nebulized epinephrine and may be associated with cutaneous lesions in a beard distribution.

Neurofibromas and Schwannomas Neurofibromas and schwannomas are rare usually large tumors often involving the orbits, the skull base, or the parotid region, and are frequently associated with neurofibromatosis type I, which may present with café-au-lait spots and other classic features.[44]

Fibromatosis Colli Fibromatosis colli (also known as pseudotumor of infancy) presents in the neonatal period as a mass in the sternocleidomastoid muscle (**Figure 122-8**). Often due to birth trauma with forceps delivery, part of the involved muscle is replaced by dense fibrous tissue.[44,47] Parents will often notice a mass or limited range of motion of the neonate's neck in the first weeks of life. Physical examination reveals a firm, solid, immobile mass located within the sternocleidomastoid muscle that is horizontally mobile, vertically fixed, and moves with the muscle when the head is turned. It is often associated with some degree of sternocleidomastoid contracture (torticollis). The diagnosis can often be made clinically, and imaging is not necessary. Treatment involves stretching and physical therapy, resulting in spontaneous resolution over a period of 4 to 8 months.[30,44,47]

MALIGNANT NEOPLASMS

Malignant head and neck masses are rare, accounting for approximately 1% of all etiologies. However, assessment for worrying features is important in the ED (Table 122-4); management of a suspected malignant lesion should include urgent referral for definitive treatment. The more common childhood malignancies presenting as a neck mass are highlighted briefly (see also chapter 143, "Oncologic and Hematologic Emergencies in Children").

Lymphoma Lymphoma is the most common childhood malignancy of the head and neck.[28,39,44] Most lymphomas present as a large, firm mass that is often mobile but can be fixed and is commonly located in the anterior triangle or the supraclavicular area.[1,37,39,48,49] One study found that 35% of childhood head and neck lymphomas presented as a supraclavicular mass.[1] Hodgkin's lymphoma is more likely nodal, found in the supraclavicular area, and seen more often in teenagers, whereas non-Hodgkin's lymphoma is primarily extranodal and has increasing incidence with age. Diagnosis requires excisional biopsy. Do not give steroids before biopsy because steroids interfere with staging.

Rhabdomyosarcoma Rhabdomyosarcoma is a frequent malignancy of the head and neck in children.[44] This tumor presents in the neck in 40% of cases, often as a large painless mass, rarely causing compression or infiltration of adjacent structures, most notably the airway.[37,38] Peak incidence is at 2 to 5 years old and again at 15 to 19 years old. Neck tumors may present with brachial plexus palsy.

Neuroblastoma Neuroblastoma is a malignancy of the sympathetic chain, and the adrenal glands are the most common primary site.[30,50] Most present before the age of 5 years, and those arising in the neck (5%) have a better prognosis than tumors of adrenal origin.[28,51] Neuroblastoma may present with local compressive signs such as hoarseness, dysphagia, airway obstruction, Horner's syndrome, or cranial nerve palsies.

Thyroid Cancer Thyroid cancer accounts for 21% of pediatric head and neck cancers; however, its incidence is decreasing due to declining radiation exposure.[40] Childhood thyroid cancer is usually papillary, presenting at a more advanced stage, with node, muscle, and metastatic involvement in 90% of cases; despite its advanced presentation, the prognosis is better than adult thyroid cancer.[52] Benign causes of diffuse thyroid enlargement include symptomatic thyrotoxicosis or Hashimoto's thyroiditis,[53] although goiter is seen in some parts of the world.

Metastatic Disease Metastatic disease may also present as cervical lymphadenopathy, accounting for 1% of childhood head and neck cancers. Tumors that metastasize to the neck include nasopharyngeal carcinoma and some thoracic/GI tumors. The location of the metastasis may give a hint to the origin of the primary tumor: posterior triangle nodes are often seen in nasopharyngeal carcinoma, whereas isolated supraclavicular nodes suggest a mediastinal or abdominal mass.

REFERENCES

The complete reference list is available online at www.TintinalliEM.com.

CHAPTER 123 Stridor and Drooling in Infants and Children

Elisa Mapelli
Vikram Sabhaney

INTRODUCTION

Stridor is a high-pitched, harsh sound produced by turbulent airflow through a partially obstructed airway. Both inspiratory and expiratory stridor are associated with airway obstruction. As air is forced through a narrow tube, it undergoes a decrease in pressure (the Venturi effect). The decrease in lateral pressure causes the airway walls to collapse and vibrate, generating stridor. Airway resistance is inversely proportional to the fourth power of the airway radius. This translates into a 16-fold increase in resistance when the radius is reduced by half. **Even 1 mm of edema in the normal pediatric subglottis reduces its cross-sectional area by >50%. A small amount of inflammation can result in significant airway obstruction in children.**

Immediately assess the child with stridor, because stridor indicates a difficult airway, and advanced airway management may be necessary (see chapter 111, "Intubation and Ventilation in Infants and Children"). A thorough history and examination will often lead to a "working diagnosis." If time permits, ask about the time and events surrounding the onset of stridor, the presence of fever, known congenital anomalies, perinatal problems, prematurity, and previous endotracheal intubation.

The level of obstruction can often be identified on examination. Partial obstruction of the upper airway at the nasopharynx and oropharyngeal levels produces sonorous snoring sounds, called *stertor*. Obstruction of the supraglottic region may cause inspiratory stridor or stertor.

TABLE 123-1 Causes of Stridor

Children <6 mo of age
Laryngotracheomalacia
Vocal cord paralysis
Subglottic stenosis
Airway hemangioma
Vascular ring/sling
Children >6 mo of age
Croup
Epiglottitis
Bacterial tracheitis
Foreign body aspiration
Retropharyngeal abscess

Obstruction of the glottis and subglottic and tracheal areas often cause both inspiratory and expiratory stridor. **Consider airway foreign body until proven otherwise if there is marked variation in the pattern of stridor.** The noise made by a child with stridor is often interpreted as wheezing by parents unfamiliar with stridor. Clarify what the parent means when the word "wheezing" is used—whether the sound occurs when the child breathes in or breathes out. The provider can imitate a stridor sound to help ED diagnosis. The differential diagnosis of stridor depends on the child's age (**Table 123-1**).

STRIDOR IN CHILDREN <6 MONTHS OLD

An infant <6 months old with a long duration of symptoms typically has a congenital cause of stridor. The major causes are laryngomalacia, tracheomalacia, vocal cord paralysis, and subglottic stenosis. Less common but important considerations include airway hemangiomas and vascular rings and slings. Stridor presenting in the first 6 months of life will often require direct visualization of the airway through endoscopy or advanced imaging. The timing of this evaluation (emergent or outpatient) is dictated by the severity of symptoms and clinical suspicion.

Laryngomalacia accounts for 60% of all neonatal laryngeal problems and results from a developmentally weak larynx. Collapse occurs with each inspiration at the epiglottis, aryepiglottic folds, and arytenoids. Generally, stridor worsens with crying and agitation but often improves with neck extension and when the child is prone. **Laryngomalacia usually manifests shortly after birth**, which is a key diagnostic feature, and generally resolves by age 18 months old. In many cases, the tracheal support structures are similarly affected, resulting in laryngotracheomalacia. Symptom exacerbations may occur with upper respiratory infections or increased work of breathing from any cause. Definitive diagnosis can often be made with flexible fiberoptic laryngoscopy. Surgery may be required if a child suffers from failure to thrive, apnea, or pulmonary hypertension.

Vocal cord paralysis can be congenital or acquired. Unilateral vocal cord paralysis is more common than bilateral cord paralysis and presents with feeding problems, stridor, hoarse voice, and cry changes. Children with bilateral cord paralysis often have a normal voice associated with stridor and dyspnea, and symptoms include cyanosis and apneic episodes. Diagnosis is by flexible nasolaryngoscopy. Endotracheal intubation can be difficult with bilateral cord paralysis, and needle cricothyroidotomy and subsequent tracheotomy may be required to secure the airway.

Subglottic stenosis may be acquired or congenital and is diagnosed when there is a narrowing of the laryngeal lumen. Congenital stenosis is usually diagnosed in the first few months of life when the child is noted to have persistent inspiratory stridor. Mild cases may present later in childhood as recurrent or persistent croup. Prolonged endotracheal intubation in premature babies is the most common cause of acquired subglottic stenosis. Treatment is based on the severity of the stenosis, but symptoms typically resolve by a few years of age.

Hemangiomas are benign congenital tumors of endothelial cells or vascular malformations that can occur anywhere on the body (80% are located above the clavicles), including the airway where they can cause obstruction and stridor. Hemangiomas typically enlarge throughout the first year of life, may not be noticed at birth, and tend to spontaneously regress by age 5 years old. **For infants <6 months old, thoroughly examine the skin, because cutaneous hemangiomas, especially in a beard distribution, may be a clue to the presence of an airway hemangioma.** Consider airway hemangioma in new-onset stridor beginning after the first month of life without another explanation; definitive diagnosis requires airway visualization through endoscopy. Although most hemangiomas spontaneously regress, large malformations and those causing significant respiratory symptoms may require treatment with β-blockers, steroids, laser, or surgery.[1-3]

Vascular rings and slings are rare congenital anomalies of the aortic arch and pulmonary artery in which anomalous vessels can compress the trachea or esophagus. Examples include a double- or right-sided aortic arch. Symptoms are often present from birth or early in the first month of life, and may be progressive and exaggerated during intercurrent upper respiratory infections; difficulty with feeding may also occur if the esophagus is compressed. Because these anomalies are rare, a high index of suspicion is required for diagnosis. Chest x-ray may reveal subtle narrowing or anterior compression of the trachea on the lateral view or an abnormal (e.g., right-sided) aortic arch. Further evaluation includes bronchoscopy, CT angiography, and echocardiography to evaluate for associated congenital heart anomalies. Definitive treatment is surgical.

STRIDOR IN CHILDREN >6 MONTHS OLD

The child >6 months old with a relatively short duration of symptoms (hours to days) characteristically has an acquired cause of stridor. Causes are either inflammatory/infectious, such as croup or epiglottitis, or noninflammatory, such as a foreign body aspiration (**Table 123-2**).

CROUP

Croup (viral laryngotracheobronchitis) is the most common cause of stridor outside the neonatal period, commonly affecting children 6 months to 3 years old, with a peak in the second year of life. The incidence is highest in the fall and the early winter months, and more cases occur during odd-numbered years.[4] Croup is acquired through inhalation of the virus. The most common viruses are parainfluenza virus and rhinovirus, followed by enterovirus and respiratory syncytial virus, influenza virus, human metapneumovirus, and human bocavirus. Co-infection by more than one virus is common.[5-7]

CLINICAL FEATURES

The clinical course of croup varies, but symptoms typically begin after 1 to 3 days of nasal congestion, rhinorrhea, cough, and low-grade fever. Classic symptoms are a harsh barking cough, hoarse voice, and stridor. Symptoms may be worse at night. The severity of symptoms is related to the amount of edema and inflammation of the airway. Assess for tachypnea, stridor at rest, nasal flaring, retractions, lethargy or agitation, and oxygen desaturation. The "typical" duration of symptoms ranges from 3 to 7 days. **Symptoms are most severe on the third and fourth days of illness and then improve.**

DIAGNOSIS

Diagnosis is clinical. Laboratory studies, viral tests, or radiographs are needed only in children who fail to respond to conventional therapy or if considering another diagnosis such as epiglottitis, retropharyngeal abscess, or aspirated foreign body.[8] If radiographs are ordered, provide physician monitoring during the procedure, because agitation may worsen existing airway obstruction.[5] Radiographs may demonstrate subglottic narrowing (**"steeple sign"**) (**Figure 123-1**). However, the steeple sign may be present in normal children and can be absent in up to 50% of those with croup.

TREATMENT

Croup is often classified as mild, moderate, or severe (**Table 123-3**), and treatment is directed primarily at decreasing airway obstruction. Croup

TABLE 123-2 Common Acquired Causes of Stridor

	Viral Croup	Bacterial Tracheitis	Epiglottitis	Peritonsillar Abscess	Retropharyngeal Abscess	Foreign Body Aspiration
Etiology	Parainfluenza viruses (occasionally respiratory syncytial virus and rhinovirus)	*Staphylococcus aureus* (most)	*Streptococcus pneumoniae*	Polymicrobial	Polymicrobial	Variable
				Streptococcus pyogenes	*S. pyogenes*	Foods
		S. pneumoniae	*S. aureus*	*S. aureus*	*S. aureus*	Peanuts
		Haemophilus influenzae	*H. influenzae*	Oral anaerobes	Gram-negative rods	Seeds
		Moraxella catarrhalis			Oral anaerobes	Balloons/other toys
Age	6 mo–3 y old	3 mo–13 y old	All ages	10–18 y old (most)	6 mo–4 y old	Any
	Peak 1–2 y old	Mean, 5–8 y old	Classically 1–7 y old	6 mo–5 y old (rare)	Rare >4 y old	6 mo–5 y old most common
						80% <3 y old
Onset	1–3 d	2–7 d viral upper respiratory infection	Rapid, hours	Antecedent pharyngitis	Insidious over 2–3 d after an upper respiratory infection or local trauma	Immediate or delayed possible
		Suddenly worse over 8–12 h				
Effect of positioning on symptoms	None	None	Worse supine	Worse supine	Neck stiffness and hyperextension	Usually none
			Prefer erect, chin forward			Location-dependent
Stridor	Inspiratory and expiratory	Inspiratory and expiratory	Inspiratory	Uncommon	Inspiratory when severe	Location-dependent
Cough	Seal-like bark	Usually	No	No	No	Often transient or positional
		Possible thick sputum				
Voice	Hoarse	Usually normal	Muffled	Muffled	Often muffled	Location-dependent
	Not muffled	Possibly raspy	"Hot potato"	"Hot potato"	"Hot potato"	Primarily if at or above glottis
Drooling	No	Rare	Yes	Often	Yes	Rare—often if esophageal
Dysphagia	Occasional	No	Yes	Yes	Yes	Rare—typically if esophageal
Radiologic appearance	Subglottic narrowing "steeple sign" (no diagnostic value)	Subglottic narrowing	Enlarged epiglottis "thumbprint sign"	May see enlarged tonsillar soft tissue	Thickened bulging retropharyngeal soft tissue	Often normal
		Irregular tracheal margins	Thickened aryepiglottic folds			Possible radiopaque density
		Stranding across trachea				Ball-valve effect
						Segmented atelectasis

scoring systems are more useful as research tools than for clinical practice. The score, if calculated, should only be used as one piece of data in the decision-making process.

Place children in a position of comfort, often in the lap of the caretaker. Assess respiratory distress through observation, without disturbing the child. Agitation and crying increase oxygen demand and may worsen airway compromise. Humidified air or cool mist do not appear to improve clinical symptoms.[9,10] However, anecdotally, exposing children with croup to cold air at home reduces the intensity of symptoms.[5]

Current standard treatment is nebulized epinephrine for moderate to severe croup and corticosteroids for all (**Table 123-4**).

Epinephrine Mild croup generally does not require epinephrine. Give nebulized epinephrine for moderate to severe croup. For those with moderate or severe croup who receive nebulized epinephrine, observe in the ED for 3 hours before considering discharge.[11]

Epinephrine decreases airway edema through vasoconstrictive alpha effects. Clinical effects of epinephrine are seen in as few as 10 minutes and last for more than 1 hour.[12,13] Use of epinephrine decreases the number of children with croup requiring intubation, intensive care unit admission, and admission to the hospital in general. Studies comparing L-epinephrine with racemic epinephrine show no significant difference in response initially; however, at 2 hours after administration, patients receiving L-epinephrine have lower croup scores.[14,15] Administration of nebulized intermittent positive-pressure breathing has no benefit over simple nebulization.[16]

ED observation for about 3 hours is recommended because an increase in croup scores can occur between the second and third hours after epinephrine nebulization in those patients ultimately requiring admission.[17,18]

Corticosteroids All patients with croup, whether mild, moderate, or severe, benefit from the administration of oral steroids as a one-time dose. Steroids reduce the severity and duration of symptoms[19,20] and result in a decrease in return visits and ED or hospital length of stay. **Dexamethasone is equally effective if given parenterally or orally.** Currently, a single dose of 0.6 milligram/kg PO of the oral dexamethasone preparation is recommended, but doses as low as 0.15 milligram/kg of dexamethasone may be considered.[19-23] Traditionally, onset of action for oral dexamethasone is considered to be 4 to 6 hours after oral administration, but effects can be seen within 1 hour of oral administration.[21] Most clinicians initially prescribe oral corticosteroids because of ease of administration. The volume of a PO dose of IV dexamethasone is smaller than the volume of the PO dexamethasone preparation and may be associated with less vomiting. Nebulized budesonide and IM dexamethasone are alternatives to PO dexamethasone in children who are vomiting.

Agents with No Benefit in Croup Heliox, in a 70% helium/30% oxygen ratio, has theoretical treatment benefits for severe, refractory croup. Replacing nitrogen with the less dense helium decreases airway resistance and improves gas flow through a compromised airway.

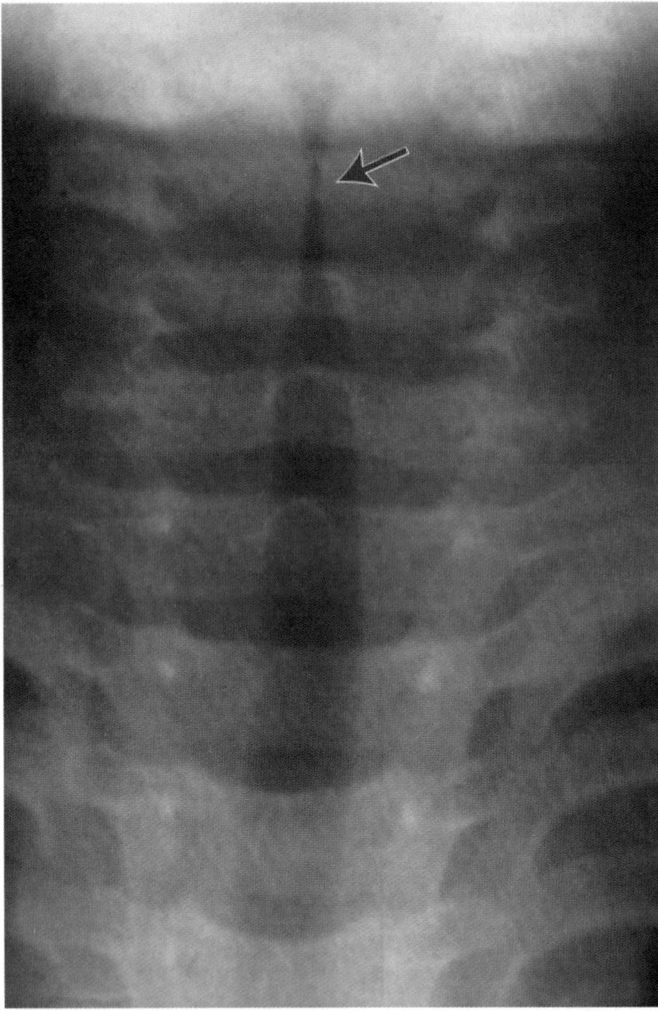

FIGURE 123-1. Anteroposterior neck radiograph in patient with croup; note presence of the "steeple sign" (*arrow*). [Photo used with permission of W. McAlister, MD, Washington University School of Medicine, St. Louis, MO.]

An important limitation is the low fractional concentration of inspired oxygen in the gas mixture. Despite its theoretical benefits, studies show no definitive advantage of heliox over conventional treatment.[24-28]

Although historically used in children with mild to moderate croup, the use of **humidified air** is likely ineffective.[29]

There are insufficient data to determine whether nebulized **β_2-agonists** are beneficial in children with croup.[27] In addition, there is theoretical risk of worsening upper airway obstruction with β-agonists in croup: β-receptors on the vasculature cause vasodilation (as compared to the vasoconstrictive α effects of epinephrine), which might worsen upper airway edema in croup, and there is no smooth muscle in the upper airway. **Therefore, β-agonists are not recommended for treatment of croup.**

TABLE 123-3 Assessment of Croup Severity

Mild	Moderate	Severe
Occasional barking cough	Frequent barking cough	Frequent barking cough
No audible stridor at rest	Easily audible stridor at rest	Prominent inspiratory and occasionally expiratory stridor
Mild or no chest wall/subcostal retractions	Chest wall/subcostal retractions at rest	Marked sternal retractions
No agitation and distress	Little or no agitation and distress	Agitation and distress

TABLE 123-4 Croup Pharmacotherapy

Medication	Dose	Notes
Dexamethasone	0.15–0.6 milligrams/kg PO/IM (10 milligrams maximum)	Give for mild, moderate, or severe croup. May crush pills and mix in juice or applesauce or administer the IV formulation orally.
Budesonide	2 milligrams nebulized	Consider if PO steroids vomited.
L-Epinephrine (1:1000)	0.5 mL/kg nebulized (5 mL maximum)	Use for moderate or severe croup; may need repeat dose if severe.
Racemic epinephrine (2.25%)	0.05 mL/kg/dose nebulized (maximum 0.5 mL)	Use for moderate or severe croup; may need repeat dose if severe.

DISPOSITION AND FOLLOW-UP

Most children with croup can be safely discharged to home (**Table 123-5**). Children who have received nebulized epinephrine should be observed in the ED for 3 hours after administration. **Children with persistent stridor at rest, tachypnea, retractions, and hypoxia or those who require more than two treatments of epinephrine should be admitted to the hospital.**[5,17,18] Intubation is reserved for cases of severe croup not responding to medical treatment. When intubation is necessary, use endotracheal tubes smaller than recommended for patient size and age to avoid traumatizing the inflamed mucosa.

EPIGLOTTITIS

Epiglottitis, or supraglottitis, is an acute inflammatory condition of the epiglottis that may progress rapidly to life-threatening airway obstruction. Widespread administration of *Haemophilus influenzae* type B vaccine has significantly reduced the number of cases of childhood epiglottitis. In the postvaccine era, most cases of infectious epiglottitis are caused by streptococcal and staphylococcal species. *Candida* species can cause epiglottitis in the immunocompromised patient. Noninfectious causes, such as thermal injury, caustic burns, and direct trauma, may cause swelling and inflammation of the epiglottis with a clinical picture identical to that of infectious epiglottitis in the absence of fever.

CLINICAL FEATURES

Infection typically presents with the abrupt onset of fever, drooling, and sore throat. Symptoms may progress rapidly, with inability to handle oral secretions followed by stridor and respiratory distress. Cough is often absent, but the voice may be muffled. Most children appear toxic and anxious and may assume a tripod or sniffing position with the neck hyperextended and the chin forward to maintain the airway.[30]

DIAGNOSIS

The ideal approach to the diagnosis of epiglottitis varies, depending on the practice and the environment. Each institution should have a written "suspected epiglottitis management protocol." Important components of all protocols are listed in **Table 123-6**.

In older children and those with mild respiratory distress, gentle direct visualization of the epiglottis may be attempted. Despite concerns that such maneuvers could trigger worsening distress, no documented reports show this to be unsafe. Patients with suspected epiglottitis who

TABLE 123-5 Criteria for Discharge from ED in Patients with Croup

3 h since last epinephrine
Nontoxic appearance
Able to take fluids well
Caretaker able to recognize change in child's condition and has adequate transportation to return if necessary
Parents have a phone and no social issues for concern

TABLE 123-6 Suspected Epiglottitis Management Protocol

Immediate recognition and triage to a resuscitation area
Continuous monitoring by someone trained in the management of a difficult airway
Rapid consultation with appropriate colleagues from otolaryngology and anesthesiology
Consideration and risk-benefit analysis of patient transfer with appropriate personnel present during the transfer
Bedside radiology without disturbing the patient or, if moved to the x-ray suite, constant monitoring by a physician with appropriate airway equipment and skills

are initially seen in an office or clinic without pediatric or otolaryngologic subspecialty support should be transported to a referral center accompanied by personnel who can manage the airway.

Lateral neck radiographs are usually unnecessary in patients with the classic presentation of epiglottitis. When the diagnosis is uncertain, obtain soft tissue neck radiographs with the neck extended during inspiration. Affected children typically hold their heads in a sniffing position and have prolonged inspiration already, making it quite simple to obtain radiographs. Lateral neck radiographs may show an enlarged epiglottis protruding from the anterior wall of the hypopharynx (often called the "**thumb sign**") and thickened aryepiglottic folds (**Figure 123-2**). If suspicion for the diagnosis still exists despite normal-appearing radiographs, direct visualization of the epiglottis is necessary to exclude the diagnosis (**Figure 123-3**).

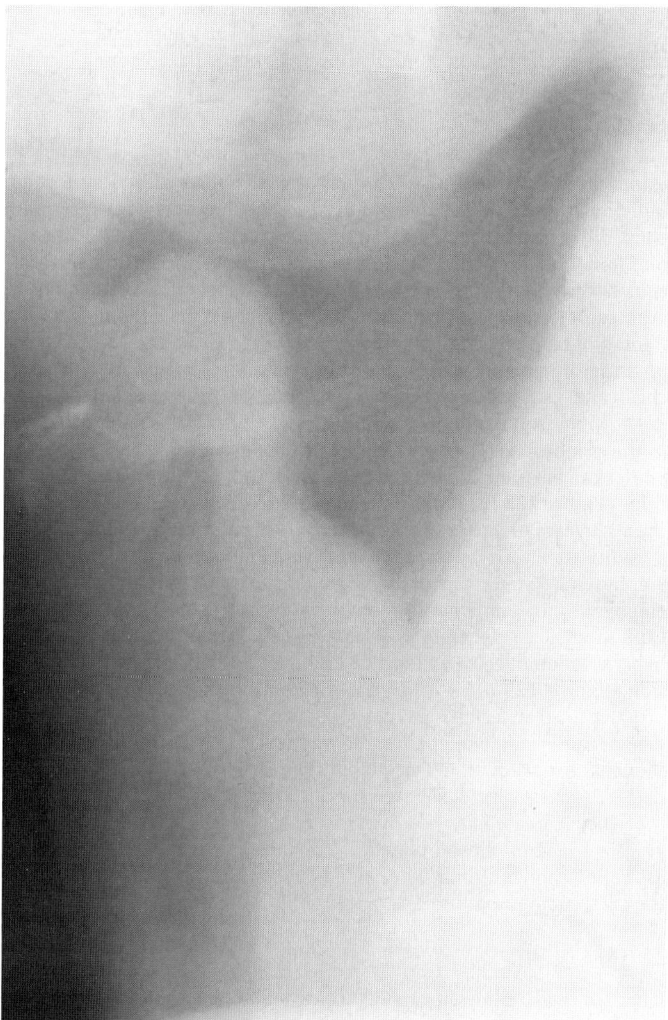

FIGURE 123-2. Lateral neck view of a child with epiglottitis. [Photo used with permission of W. McAlister, MD, Washington University School of Medicine, St. Louis, MO.]

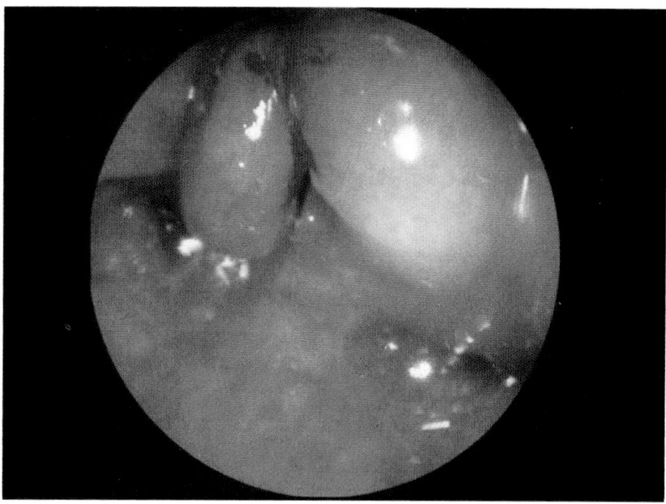

FIGURE 123-3. Epiglottitis at laryngoscopy. [Reproduced with permission from Knoop K, Stack L, Storrow A: *Atlas of Emergency Medicine,* 3rd ed. McGraw-Hill, New York. Part 2 Specialty Areas, Chapter 14, Pediatric Conditions, Figure 14-38.]

TREATMENT

Keep the child seated and upright in a position of comfort. Provide oxygen. Administer nebulized racemic or L-epinephrine to decrease airway edema. Alert the referral center or pediatric otolaryngologist as soon as possible so decisions concerning intubation or tracheotomy can be made in concert with consultants and support personnel can be mobilized. The most skilled individual available should perform intubation as soon as the diagnosis is made. Use sedation, paralytics, and vagolytics as needed. For a child who is able to maintain an airway, the decision to administer paralytics must be accompanied by absolute certainty that intubation will be successful. Have multiple endotracheal tube sizes immediately available. If endotracheal intubation is unsuccessful, an emergent surgical airway is required. Administer a second- or third-generation cephalosporin, such as cefuroxime (50 milligrams/kg IV) or ceftriaxone (50 milligrams/kg IV), to ensure adequate coverage of the most common infectious pathogens. With the increasing incidence of *Staphylococcus aureus* and highly resistant *Streptococcus pneumoniae* as a cause of epiglottitis, one may also empirically add vancomycin (10 milligrams/kg IV) to the antibiotic regimen. Antibiotics are typically continued for 7 to 10 days. Steroids are often employed to decrease mucosal edema of the epiglottis.

BACTERIAL TRACHEITIS

Bacterial tracheitis, also known as *membranous laryngotracheobronchitis* or *bacterial croup*, is an uncommon infection that can cause life-threatening upper airway obstruction. It can be a primary or secondary infection. The mean age of presentation is now 5 to 8 years of age compared with the 4 years of age that has been classically described.[31,32]

Bacterial tracheitis often develops secondarily after a viral upper respiratory tract infection. A history of upper respiratory infection symptoms followed by sudden worsening with high fever, stridor, and cough (which may be productive of thick sputum) and a toxic appearance suggest the diagnosis. Thick mucopurulent secretions of the trachea result in upper airway obstruction. Children with tracheitis often complain of sore throat and will point to their trachea when asked where it hurts; there is often tenderness with palpation of the trachea. Management is similar to that of epiglottitis, with patients ideally going to the operating room for sedation, intubation, and bronchoscopy. Cultures and Gram stain of the mucopurulent secretions should be obtained at this time, because Gram stain findings may help guide the antibiotic therapy. Bronchoscopy may be therapeutic, because the removal of purulent pseudomembranes improves tracheal toilet and may lessen

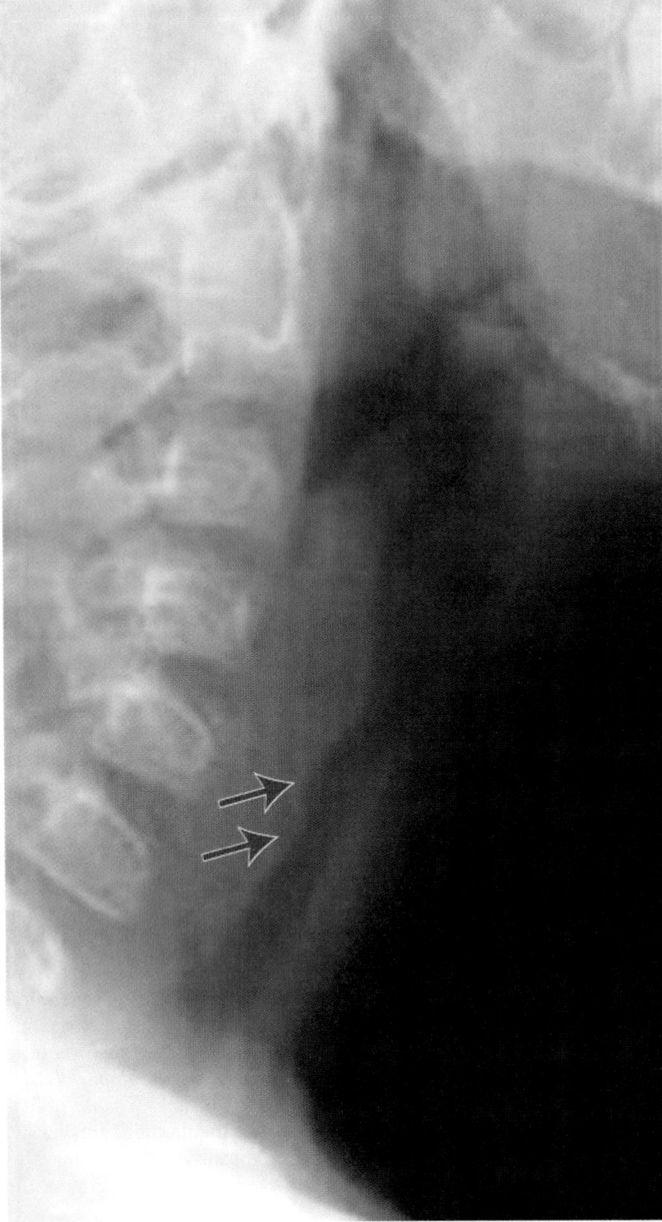

FIGURE 123-4. Lateral neck view of patient with bacterial tracheitis. Note presence of irregular tracheal margins (*arrows*). [Photo used with permission of W. McAlister, MD, Washington University School of Medicine, St. Louis, MO.]

upper airway obstruction. For continued management, most patients with bacterial tracheitis require intubation and ventilatory support.

The most commonly isolated pathogen obtained from culture at bronchoscopy is *S. aureus*. Other organisms implicated in bacterial tracheitis include *S. pneumoniae*, *Streptococcus pyogenes*, *Moraxella catarrhalis*, *H. influenzae*, and anaerobes.[33-36] Initial antibiotic choices include ampicillin/sulbactam or the combination of a third-generation cephalosporin and clindamycin. Add vancomycin for methicillin-resistant *S. aureus*. Laboratory studies other than tracheal cultures are of limited use in the diagnosis. Neck radiographs are not needed to make the diagnosis. When obtained to evaluate for other potential diagnostic entities, neck films may show subglottic narrowing of the trachea and irregular tracheal margins in patients with tracheitis (**Figure 123-4**). Because no single clinical or radiographic feature can definitively make a diagnosis, bronchoscopy is the diagnostic method of choice in bacterial tracheitis.

AIRWAY FOREIGN BODY

Airway foreign body aspiration occurs most commonly in children between 1 and 3 years old as a result of increasing mobility and oral exploration. Foreign body aspiration in children <6 months old often involves a well-meaning sibling who places an object in the infant's mouth. The most common objects aspirated fall into two groups: food and toys. Commonly aspirated foods include peanuts, sunflower seeds, carrots, raisins, grapes, and hot dogs.

A high index of suspicion is needed for diagnosis. **Consider foreign body aspiration in a young child with respiratory symptoms, regardless of the duration of symptoms, because many children may present >24 hours after foreign body aspiration.** If the clinical scenario clearly indicates the presence of a foreign body or airway obstruction, immediately implement a protocol for obstructed airway management. **Suspect foreign body aspiration with a history of sudden coughing and choking in the child; this is the most predictive of all signs and symptoms in foreign body aspiration.**[37,38] In many cases, the choking episode is not witnessed by a caregiver.

CLINICAL FEATURES

Although the location of the aspirated foreign body plays a role in determining the symptoms and signs on presentation, there is great overlap between groups, and some children may be asymptomatic on presentation. "Classic dogma" is that laryngotracheal foreign bodies cause stridor and hoarseness, whereas bronchial foreign bodies cause unilateral wheezing and decreased breath sounds. Eighty percent to 90% of airway foreign bodies are found in the bronchi. Children may develop severe immediate-onset stridor or even cardiopulmonary arrest, but a significant proportion will have no cough, wheeze, or stridor. The most important factor in reducing mortality from an airway foreign body is the recognition of the child in acute airway distress.

DIAGNOSIS

Radiographs are helpful to *confirm* the diagnosis of airway foreign body but should not be used to *exclude* the diagnosis, because plain chest radiographs are normal in >50% of tracheal foreign bodies and one fourth of bronchial foreign bodies.[39] Laryngeal and tracheal foreign bodies often constitute an acute emergency, and radiography is omitted. If performed, posteroanterior and lateral neck radiographs are the radiographic examinations of choice. Foreign bodies lodged in the proximal esophagus may also present with airway compression. Tracheal and esophageal foreign bodies can be differentiated on neck radiographs: foreign bodies typically lodge in the trachea in profile and in the esophagus en face (see Figure 77-2). Suspected bronchial foreign bodies can be evaluated with the use of posteroanterior and lateral chest films (**Figure 123-5**). **More than 75% of airway foreign bodies in children <3 years of age are radiolucent.**[37,40-42] Indirect radiologic signs of a radiolucent airway foreign body include unilateral obstructive emphysema, atelectasis, and consolidation. Unilateral obstructive emphysema is seen when a foreign body obstructs airflow, mainly on expiration. This generates a check-valve obstruction that results in hyperinflation of the affected side and mediastinal shift to the opposite side (**Figure 123-6**). A foreign body that obstructs a bronchus may produce focal atelectasis and consolidation visible on chest films. Inspiratory and expiratory chest radiographs can aid in the diagnosis by showing hyperinflation (air trapping) on expiratory films. Bilateral decubitus chest films have been used to demonstrate air trapping; however, they increase false positives without increasing true positives, suggesting a lack of clinical benefit.[43] A clinically suspected foreign body aspiration should ultimately be ruled out by bronchoscopy, regardless of the chest radiograph findings.[44-47]

TREATMENT

Children with complete airway obstruction are typically unable to breathe or speak and require emergency basic life support measures to relieve airway obstruction. For detailed discussion, see chapters 108,

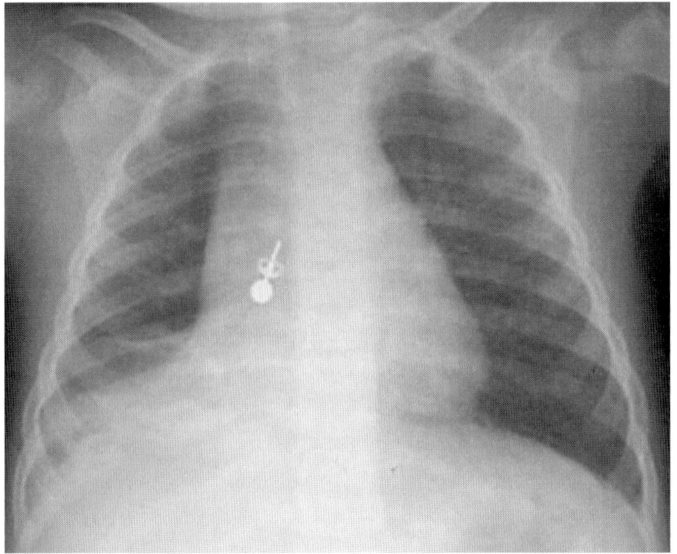

A

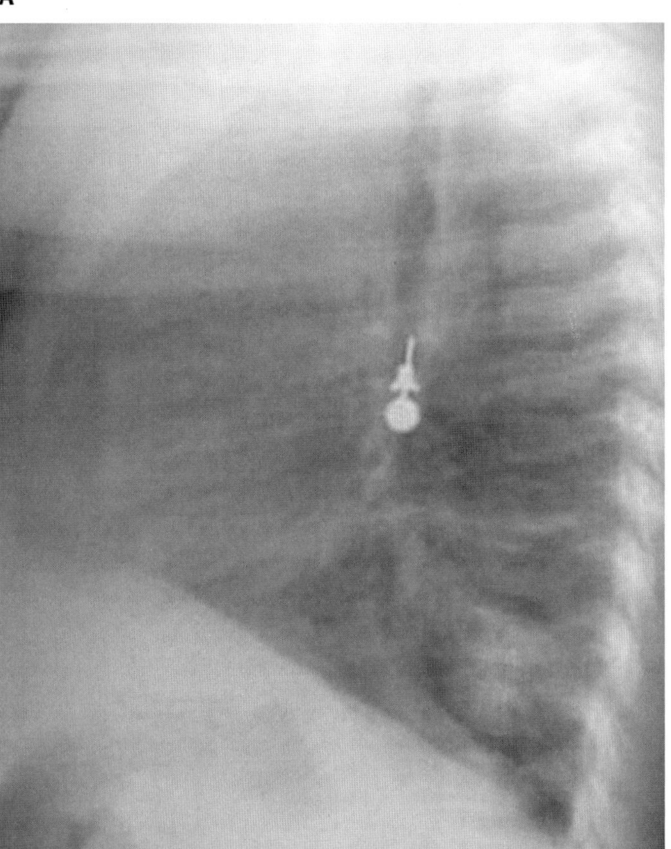

B

FIGURE 123-5. (**A**) Posteroanterior and (**B**) lateral chest radiographs showing radiopaque bronchial foreign body. [Photos used with permission of W. McAlister, MD, Washington University School of Medicine, St. Louis, MO.]

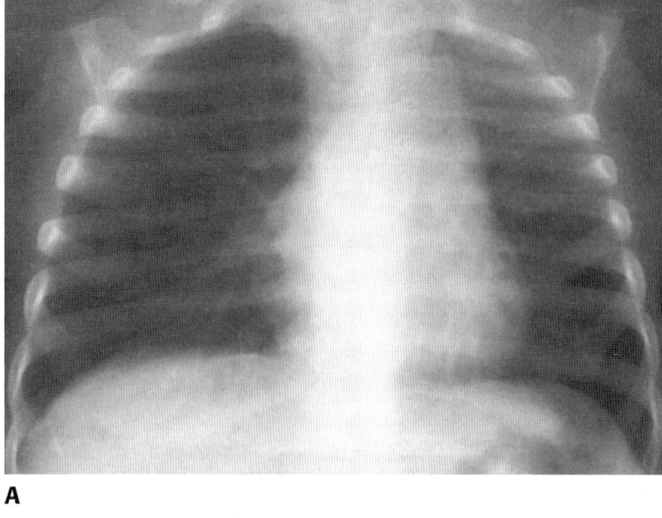

A

B

FIGURE 123-6. (**A**) Inspiratory and (**B**) expiratory chest radiographs showing air trapping on the left with shift of the mediastinum to the right caused by a peanut in the left mainstem bronchus. [Photos used with permission of W. McAlister, MD, Washington University School of Medicine, St. Louis, MO.]

"Resuscitation of Neonates" and 109, "Resuscitation of Children." If basic life support maneuvers fail, direct laryngoscopy and foreign body extraction with Magill forceps should be attempted. When the foreign body is not visible or able to be removed, orotracheal intubation with dislodgment of the foreign body more distally (often into the right mainstem bronchus) can relieve the complete obstruction and may be life-saving. If the foreign body cannot be removed and ventilation cannot be provided through an endotracheal tube, needle cricothyroidotomy or emergency tracheostomy should be performed. Those patients who do not have complete airway obstruction should have their respiratory status closely monitored while preparations are made for bronchoscopic removal under general anesthesia.

RETROPHARYNGEAL ABSCESS

The retropharyngeal space occupies the space between the posterior pharyngeal wall and the prevertebral fascia and extends from the base of the skull to approximately the level of the second thoracic vertebrae. This space is fused down the midline and contains two chains of lymph nodes extending down each side. These lymph nodes tend to regress by age 4 years old, obliterating this potential space, which explains the decreasing frequency of retropharyngeal abscess in older children. The formation of a retropharyngeal abscess is believed to be secondary to suppuration of these lymph nodes that have been seeded from a distant infection. Localized penetrating trauma with subsequent invasion of this space by bacteria is another cause of retropharyngeal infection. This most commonly occurs in children who fall with a stick or other similar object in their mouth. Infection can also occur from traumatic esophageal instrumentation or ventral extension of vertebral osteomyelitis. Retropharyngeal infection typically progresses from an organized phlegmon to a mature abscess.

CLINICAL FEATURES

Most cases of retropharyngeal abscess evolve insidiously over a few days after a relatively minor upper respiratory infection. Fever is typically present but may be absent in >10% of patients.[48-51] Signs and symptoms include neck pain, fever, dysphagia, excessive drooling, and neck swelling. The child may maintain the neck in an unusual position, with stiffness, torticollis, and hyperextension. A unique finding is bulging of the posterior oropharynx. Abscess progression can lead to stridor and respiratory distress. Pleuritic chest pain is an ominous sign, indicating extension of the infection into the mediastinum.

DIAGNOSIS

Initial imaging includes a soft tissue lateral neck radiograph. The radiograph should be taken during inspiration with the neck extended to limit false-positive results. **The diagnosis of retropharyngeal abscess/cellulitis is suggested when the retropharyngeal space at C2 is twice the diameter of the vertebral body or greater than one half the width of the C4 vertebral body (Figure 123-7).** Rarely, gas may be seen within the mass. Contrast-enhanced CT scan may demonstrate necrotic nodes, inflammatory phlegmon, or fluid collection within a ring-enhancing abscess (**Figure 123-8**). CT is helpful for diagnosing and defining the extent of the infection and planning a surgical procedure. However, CT scans are limited in their ability to differentiate between abscess and cellulitis/phlegmon. Therefore, imaging results should be correlated to clinical findings when guiding the decision of conservative versus surgical treatment.[52-57] Unstable patients should be intubated before going to the radiology suite for CT scan. Patients requiring sedation to obtain a scan may require presedation intubation if airway obstruction is present. A physician accustomed to managing the difficult pediatric airway should escort patients without airway compromise to radiology, and appropriate equipment should accompany the patient.

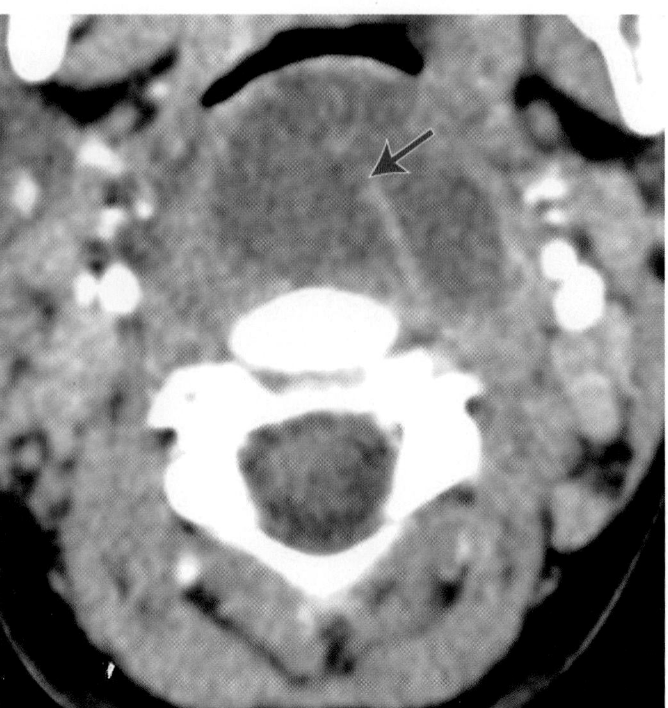

FIGURE 123-8. Contrast-enhanced neck CT showing a retropharyngeal fluid collection (*arrow*).

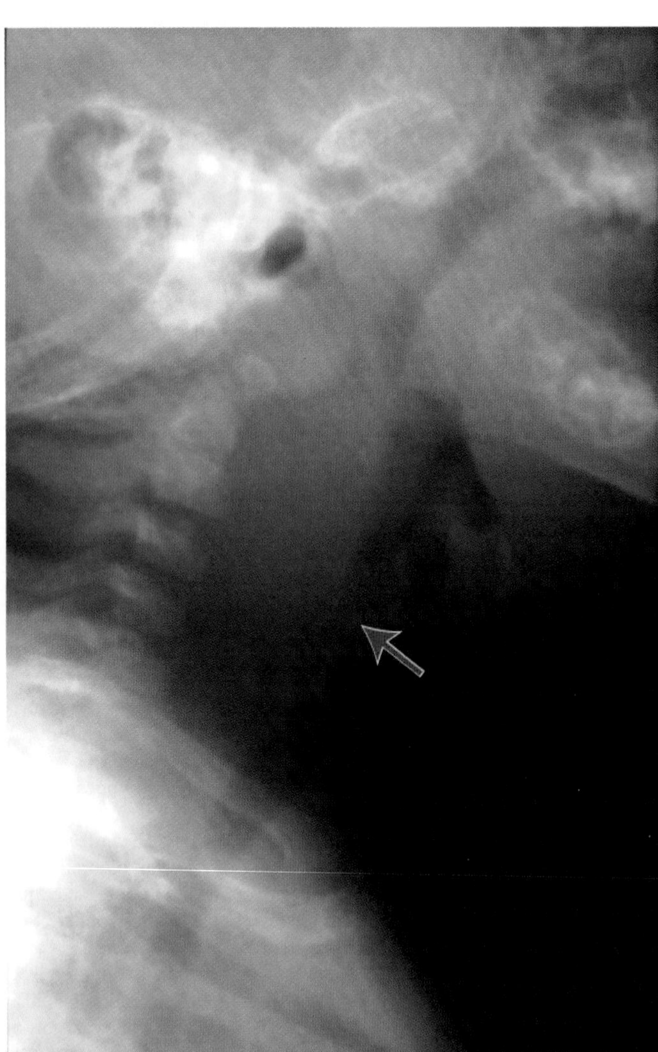

FIGURE 123-7. Lateral soft tissue neck radiograph demonstrating retropharyngeal swelling (*arrow*).

TREATMENT

Carefully monitor and stabilize the airway. Obtain IV or IO access to administer fluids, antibiotics, and CT contrast. Retropharyngeal cellulitis and small, localized abscesses may be treated successfully with antibiotic therapy alone. All other cases should undergo operative incision and drainage, usually by an otolaryngologist. Steroids can reduce airway edema, inflammation, and the progression of cellulitis into an abscess. Most retropharyngeal abscesses are found to contain mixed flora when cultured.[31] Common organisms include *S. aureus*, *S. pyogenes*, *Streptococcus viridans*, and β-lactamase–producing gram-negative rods. Oral anaerobes are also frequently seen. Single-agent antimicrobial therapy includes ampicillin/sulbactam or clindamycin. Unusual complications of retropharyngeal abscess include airway obstruction, spontaneous abscess perforation, mediastinitis, sepsis, aspiration, and jugular venous thrombosis.

PERITONSILLAR ABSCESS

Peritonsillar abscess is a deep oropharyngeal infection. It can occur in patients of any age, but most commonly occurs in adolescents and young adults. The disease typically begins as a superficial infection that progresses to an accumulation of pus in a space between the tonsillar capsule and the superior constrictor muscle. Most are unilateral, and <10% are bilateral at the time of diagnosis.

CLINICAL FEATURES AND DIAGNOSIS

Patients with peritonsillar abscess typically present with sore throat, fever, chills, trismus, and voice change ("hot potato voice"). Patients will often complain of "the worst sore throat" of their life and may drool due to difficulty swallowing their saliva. Ipsilateral ear pain and

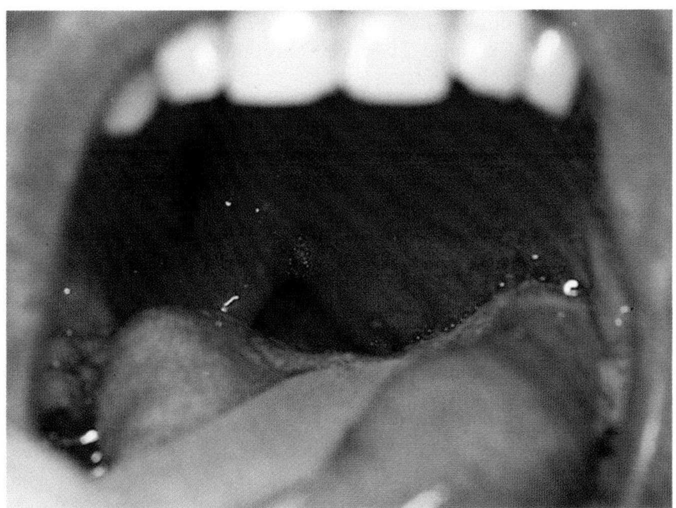

FIGURE 123-9. Peritonsillar abscess. [Reproduced with permission from Knoop K, Stack L, Storrow A: *Atlas of Emergency Medicine, 3rd ed.* McGraw-Hill, New York. Part 1 Regional Anatomy, Chapter 5, Ear, Nose & Throat Conditions, Figure 5-27.]

torticollis may be present. On examination, bulging of the affected tonsil and deviation of the uvula away from the involved tonsil are evident (**Figure 123-9**).

Differentiating peritonsillar cellulitis from peritonsillar abscess can be difficult. If the child is toxic, consider a peritonsillar abscess until proven otherwise. Imaging with CT scan or US can differentiate between the two.

TREATMENT

In nontoxic-appearing adolescents with good follow-up and with findings most consistent with peritonsillar cellulitis, a trial of oral antibiotics (e.g., penicillin) may be the best choice for treatment. Most cases of peritonsillar abscess are managed as outpatients with prompt aspiration or incision and drainage using local anesthetics in the ED. Young and uncooperative children may require procedural sedation to facilitate adequate evaluation and drainage. Complications of needle aspiration and incision and drainage include hemorrhage, puncture of the carotid artery, and airway aspiration of purulent material. CT with IV contrast is the imaging modality of choice for assessment of suspected infection in patients who have failed incision and drainage and in whom trismus or lack of cooperation prevents a thorough intraoral examination.

Most peritonsillar abscesses are polymicrobial infections. Predominant organisms include anaerobes, group A β-hemolytic streptococci, *S. aureus*, and *H. influenzae*.[58] The fluid obtained from needle aspiration should be sent for Gram stain and culture. IV antimicrobial therapy may include ampicillin/sulbactam or clindamycin. Outpatient management antibiotic choices include penicillin, clindamycin, and amoxicillin/clavulanate. Single high-dose steroid administration may improve symptoms in patients with peritonsillar abscess.[59]

LUDWIG'S ANGINA

Ludwig's angina is a potentially life-threatening, rapidly expanding infection of the submandibular space. The submandibular space is composed of two spaces subdivided by the mylohyoid muscle into the sublingual and submylohyoid space (submaxillary space) and extends from the floor of the mouth to muscular attachments at the hyoid bone. Infectious expansion into this space spreads superiorly and posteriorly and often involves the entire submandibular space (**Figure 123-10**). **Most cases arise from an odontogenic source, often from the spread of periapical abscesses of mandibular molars.**

CLINICAL FEATURES

Ludwig's angina usually begins with a mild infection that progresses rapidly to severe mouth pain, drooling, trismus, tongue protrusion, and

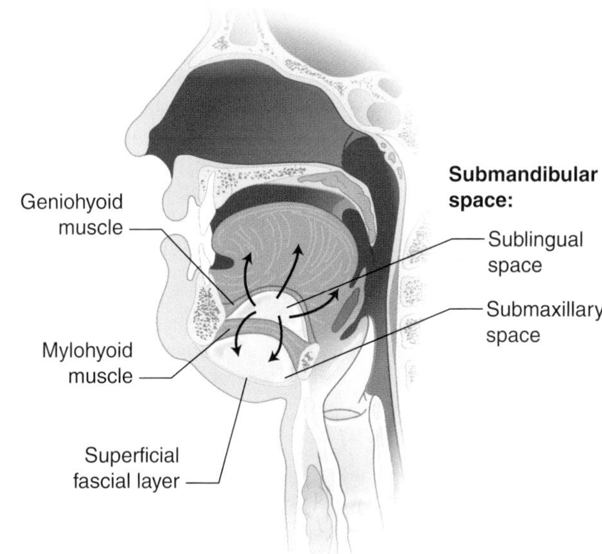

FIGURE 123-10. Spread of infection within the submandibular space of the neck.

brawny neck swelling. The child may lean forward to maximize airway diameter. Stridor may develop with subsequent progressive airway obstruction. Control the airway early, because intubation can be extremely difficult late in the clinical course of the disease. One case series reports that 11 of 20 patients had an unsuccessful attempt at intubation resulting in emergent tracheotomy.[60] Treatment is antibiotics and oral surgery to remove the dental abscess that is the source of the infection. IV antibiotics should cover β-lactamase–producing aerobic or anaerobic gram-positive cocci and gram-negative bacilli. Consideration must be given to including coverage of community-acquired methicillin-resistant *S. aureus* as well.

DIPHTHERIA

Diphtheria is an acute toxin-mediated disease caused by *Corynebacterium diphtheria* and has largely been eradicated in developed nations through widespread vaccination. It is transmitted from person to person through respiratory secretions or skin lesions. In cases of pharyngeal diphtheria, symptoms include sore throat, malaise, dysphagia, and low-grade fever. Characteristic thick gray membranes (pseudomembranes) can develop over the tonsils and soft palate and potentially cause respiratory obstruction and death. Laryngeal diphtheria is characterized by a classic "barking" cough, stridor, hoarseness, and difficulty breathing, accompanied by marked edema of the neck referred to as "bull neck."

Complications include myocarditis and neuritis potentially leading to diaphragmatic paralysis and death from respiratory failure. Diagnosis is confirmed by isolation of *C. diphtheria* by cultures of a nasopharyngeal swab. Treatment includes antitoxin and antibiotics (erythromycin or penicillin G) and respiratory support as needed.

OROPHARYNGEAL TRAUMA

Traumatic oropharyngeal injuries in children typically occur during a fall with an object in the mouth. Such injuries are often referred to as "pencil injuries" and most commonly occur in patients between 2 and 4 years of age. When evaluating these injuries, ask if a foreign body was removed intact or if part of the object may have broken off into the soft tissue. If there is suspicion of retained foreign body, imaging is required.

CLINICAL FEATURES

Children with oropharyngeal trauma may present with bleeding, drooling, or dysphagia. Most wounds do not require surgical intervention and closure, but large gaping wounds and those with persistent bleeding may require closure under sedation or anesthesia. Prophylactic antibiotics play an inconclusive role in the treatment of intraoral wounds.[61] There are rare but well-known complications of penetrating pharyngeal injury. Entrance of free air into the neck or chest can result in stridor and acute airway obstruction. Subsequent retropharyngeal infection from introduction of bacteria into the penetrating wound can occur. A more severe complication of oropharyngeal trauma is **carotid artery injury**. The carotid artery is closely associated with the lateral oropharynx and is at risk of injury from penetrating and blunt impact forces. Penetrating injury results in massive hemorrhage, whereas blunt injuries can cause compression of the carotid artery between the object and upper cervical vertebrae. The resultant shearing effect can cause an intimal tear in the vessel with subsequent thrombosis formation. Symptoms may evolve over hours to days and can result in significant neurologic sequelae (stroke in the distribution of the common carotid territory).

DIAGNOSIS AND TREATMENT

Neither mechanism nor degree of injury is helpful in determining the possibility of neurovascular compromise. Soft tissue lateral neck films can assist in the evaluation of air in soft tissues, radiopaque foreign bodies, and evaluating for abscess. Normal retropharyngeal soft tissue in airway films is no more than one half of the width of the adjacent vertebral body. An increase in the width and the presence of air in the retropharyngeal space indicate pharyngeal injury and may warrant further investigation. CT is superior to plain radiographs for the detection of free air, inflammation, or abscess. CT angiography is needed if carotid injury is suspected and should be considered for patients who are unstable, who cannot be adequately assessed, and for whom lateral pharyngeal trauma raises concern for vascular injury.[62] Treatment is specific for the complication and involves consultation with surgery or otolaryngology.

REFERENCES

The complete reference list is available online at www.TintinalliEM.com.

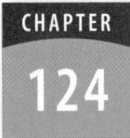

CHAPTER 124 Wheezing in Infants and Children

Allan Shefrin
Alia Busuttil
Roger Zemek

INTRODUCTION

Wheezing is a high-pitched sound that occurs when there is an elevation of airway resistance due to an obstructive process. The clinician must differentiate between stridor and wheeze because this determines location of the airway obstruction. Stridor is a sign of upper airway obstruction (above the thoracic inlet) that is more marked during inspiration, whereas wheeze signifies lower airway obstruction distal to the thoracic inlet that is more marked during expiration (see chapter 123, "Stridor and Drooling in Infants and Children").[1-4] Wheezing implies a generalized obstructive airway disease when diffuse and focal obstruction when localized. However, severe flow limitation may exist without wheezing, for example, the silent chest in a severe asthma exacerbation. Bronchiolitis is the most frequent cause of wheezing in infants, and asthma is the most frequent cause in children and adolescents.

RESPIRATORY PHYSIOLOGY

The nasal passages account for 50% of total airway resistance. Nasal resistance increases in the presence of nasal mucus or edema and may be clinically important in the infant with bronchiolitis. The conducting airways extend from the trachea to the terminal bronchioles and do not participate in gas exchange. The distal transitional and respiratory zones are the gas-exchanging units.

Lung tissue has elastic properties; functional residual capacity is the resting balance of stretch and recoil forces. Normally, at functional residual capacity, the tissue is relaxed at end expiration, and inspiration begins with minimal effort at the onset of inspiratory muscle contraction. Inspiration is an active process generated by the diaphragm and external intercostal muscles. During exertion, inspiration is aided by the use of accessory muscles including scalene and sternocleidomastoid muscles.[5] Expiration is normally a passive process, facilitated by elastic recoil of the stretched lung.

In the presence of diffuse (e.g., asthma, bronchiolitis) or focal (e.g., foreign body) intrathoracic airway obstruction, the normally passive process of expiration becomes active in an attempt to overcome airway resistance. Abdominal and internal intercostal muscles are recruited. Positive intrapleural pressure is generated, and increasing external pressure is applied to the airways. This leads to progressively increasing airway obstruction as expiration proceeds, a phenomenon referred to as *dynamic airway compression* (**Figure 124-1**).[6]

Dynamic airway compression results in prolonged expiratory time. The net result is failure of alveoli and distal airways to fully empty at end expiration, resulting in air trapping and increased functional residual capacity. Before subsequent inspiratory flow can begin, inspiratory muscles must overcome this increased elastic recoil, which substantially increases the work of breathing, a phenomenon referred to as *auto-positive end-expiratory pressure*. Finally, air trapping and subsequent atelectasis result in areas with ventilation–perfusion mismatch and hypoxemia.

Infants have smaller airways, highly compliant bronchial and bronchiolar cartilage, and more peripheral airway smooth muscle than older children and adults. These factors result in an even greater tendency toward airway collapse during expiration, air trapping, and auto-positive end-expiratory pressure. Thus, infants not only are more likely to experience wheezing illnesses, but are also more likely to suffer the physiologic consequences of airway obstruction.

WHEEZING

Approximately 25% to 30% of infants will have one episode of wheezing, and nearly 50% of children will have a history of wheezing by 6 years of age.[2,7,8] Obtain a thorough history for any child with wheezing (**Table 124-1**). Consider age, family history, onset, pattern, seasonality, positional changes, and associated symptoms.[2] Identify possible triggers. A recurrent and episodic pattern, history of cough, association with identifiable triggers, and documented response to bronchodilators are highly suggestive of asthma in a child >2 years old.[9-11] A prior history of hospitalization, particularly to a critical care unit, and prior endotracheal intubation are important risk factors for severe disease. An exposure to sick contacts during a viral season, nasal congestion, poor feeding, and age <1 year suggest bronchiolitis.[2] Choking or gagging indicates possible foreign body aspiration.

CLINICAL FEATURES

On physical examination, use the pediatric assessment triangle to assess **appearance, work of breathing, and circulation.**[12] Assess the general appearance of the child using the **TICLS** mnemonic (**tone, interactivity, consolability, look, and speech**). Assess work of breathing by observing the child's position (e.g., sniffing, tripod), accessory muscle use (e.g., nasal flaring, tracheal tug, scalene retraction, intercostal muscle use, abdominal breathing), and presence of stridor or wheeze. Assess circulation rapidly by observing the patient's color, especially noting cyanosis. Determine respiratory rate (see **Table 124-2** for age-related ranges).

Monitor oxygen saturation by either intermittent or continuous pulse oximetry. It is common for some infants and children with asthma or bronchiolitis to develop ventilation–perfusion mismatch, which may result in mild hypoxemia (92% to 94%) that is correctable with minimum supplemental oxygen (1 to 2 L/min). **More severe hypoxemia** (<91%) **suggests moderate to severe disease.** Hypoxemia refractory to

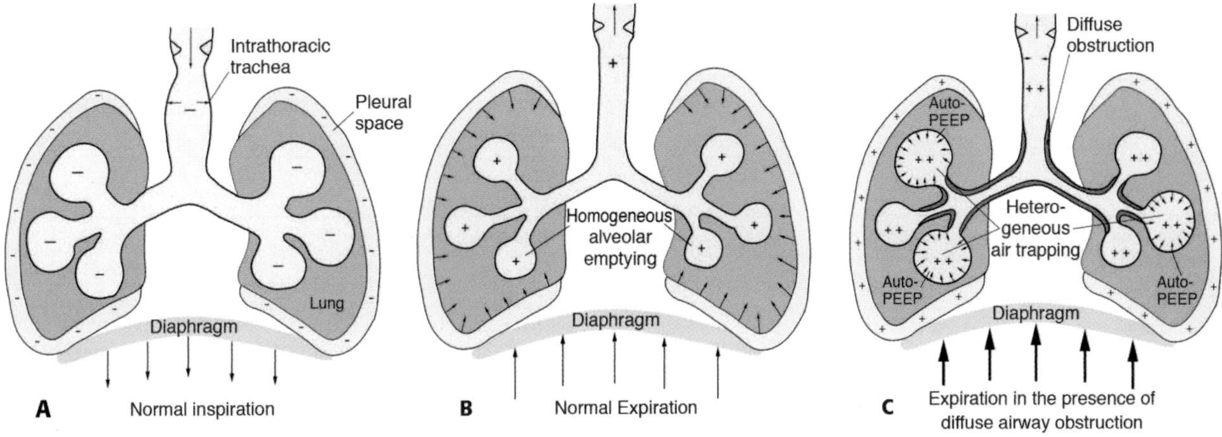

FIGURE 124-1. Normal inspiration and expiration (**A, B**) and dynamic airway compression (**C**) with development of auto–positive end-expiratory pressure (Auto-PEEP).

bronchodilators and supplemental oxygen may suggest alternate diagnoses such as pneumonia, pneumothorax, pulmonary shunt, or congenital cardiac lesion (especially in the hypoxemic neonate). **Diaphoresis, confusion, and drowsiness are ominous signs indicating imminent respiratory failure.** Check for audibility and symmetry of breath sounds to assess adequacy of ventilation. Inspiratory-to-expiratory ratios of less than the normal 2:1 (e.g., 1:2 or 1:3) reflect the prolonged expiratory times seen with obstructive airway disease. **Perhaps more important than the initial physical examination findings are the changes in these findings in response to bronchodilators and other treatments.**

DIAGNOSIS

Table 124-3 lists the differential diagnosis of wheezing.

Asthma and bronchiolitis account for the majority of wheezing episodes in children, although a broader differential diagnosis must always be considered and ruled out on history, on physical exam, or with ancillary investigations. This is particularly important when the patient's history or physical findings are not consistent with a diagnosis of asthma or bronchiolitis or when the illness does not respond to interventions appropriate to these disease processes. **Table 124-3 outlines the signs, symptoms, context, and ancillary testing for the different causes of wheezing.**

Stridor is not associated with lower airway obstruction and suggests an upper airway obstructive process (see chapter 123). The association of wheezing with feedings suggests gastroesophageal reflux or tracheoesophageal fistula with aspiration. **Grunting**, a physiologic response to generate positive end-expiratory pressure in an attempt to maintain alveolar inflation, suggests pneumonia, loss of surfactant, or other alveolar disease, although it may also result from extrapulmonary disease including GI emergencies. Inspiratory crackles or rales may result from atelectasis associated with bronchiolitis and asthma, although pneumonia should be considered, especially if these findings persist after initial bronchodilator therapy. **Consider the possibility of foreign body aspiration and congestive heart failure because these disorders frequently cause wheezing.**

TABLE 124-1 Important Historical Features and Their Significance in Infants and Children with Wheezing

Feature	Significance
Age	<1 y: bronchiolitis more common 1–2 y: mixed >2 y: asthma more common
Family history	Positive family history of wheeze suggests atopy, making asthma more likely
Pattern	Single episode: any etiology possible Recurrent: asthma Chronic illness: asthma, cystic fibrosis, congestive heart failure, anatomic abnormality
Onset	Sudden onset: foreign body aspiration, allergic reaction, asthma
Identifiable trigger	Concurrent viral illness: bronchiolitis, asthma Pollens, pets, dust, smoke and other irritants: asthma Choking episode: foreign body aspiration
Response to bronchodilators	Improvement with β_2-agonist treatment is diagnostic for asthma Bronchiolitis may improve with inhaled epinephrine
Previous hospitalization	More severe disease, inability to care for child at home
Previous critical care unit admission ± intubation	More severe or life-threatening disease

BRONCHIOLITIS

Bronchiolitis is the most common lower respiratory tract infection in infants and children ≤2 years of age and is the leading cause for hospitalization in children <1 year of age.[13] The most common cause is **respiratory syncytial virus**, although bronchiolitis may be caused by other viruses including, but not limited to, human metapneumovirus, adenovirus, influenza, rhinovirus, and parainfluenza viruses.[14]

PATHOPHYSIOLOGY

The viral infection in bronchiolitis causes inflammation of the lower respiratory tract, with resultant edema, epithelial cell necrosis, bronchospasm, and increased mucus production within the bronchioles.[15] These features result in variable degrees of air trapping, atelectasis, and hyperinflation of the lower airways. The increase in airway resistance

TABLE 124-2 Age-Specific Respiratory Rate Ranges

Age	Respiratory Rate (breaths/min)
<1 y	30–60
1–2 y	24–40
2–5 y	22–34
6–12 y	18–30
>12 y	12–16

TABLE 124-3 Differential Diagnosis for Wheezing in Infants and Children

Potential Diagnosis	Typical Age of Onset	Cardinal Symptoms and Signs	Confirmatory Tests
Asthma	>2 y	Recurrent episodes of wheeze and/or nighttime cough, identifiable triggers such as seasonality, allergens, exercise Responsive to bronchodilators	Trial of β-agonist Pulmonary function tests Allergy testing
Bronchiolitis	<2 y	URI symptoms, seasonal (winter months), nasal flaring and congestion, wheezes, rales, rhonchi	(Viral antigen testing)
Gastroesophageal reflux Tracheoesophageal fistula	Present from birth	Cough, gagging, emesis related to feeding	Esophageal pH probe Barium swallow
Vascular ring, sling, malformation, or airway hemangioma or polyp Laryngomalacia Tracheomalacia	Early infancy Present from birth, improves during first year of life	Stridor that changes with position of the neck, exacerbations with URI	CXR, CT angiography, bronchoscopy, barium swallow Laryngoscopy
Congenital heart disease with left-to-right shunting and congestive failure Myocarditis	2–6 mo Any age	Diffuse or basilar rales, tachycardia, hepatomegaly, cardiac murmur/gallop	CXR, ECG, echocardiography ECG, CXR, troponin, echocardiography
Foreign body aspiration Vocal cord dysfunction (paradoxical vocal cord motion)	Usually >6 mo From birth (paralysis) Late school age/adolescents	History of choking episode with subsequent acute onset of stridor and/or wheezing. Stridor and/or wheezing, poor response to β-agonists	Right and left lateral decubitus CXRs* Flexible fiberoptic laryngoscopy
Epiglottitis	School age or adolescent	Stridor and high fever, toxic appearance, drooling and tripod positioning	Soft tissue radiographs of the neck*
Pneumonia	Any age	Fever, cough, tachypnea, rales, grunting	CXR
Cystic fibrosis Ciliary dyskinesia Immunodeficiency	Present from birth	Recurrent lower respiratory tract infections, failure to thrive	Sweat chloride concentration Ciliary biopsy Immunoglobulin assays

*Consider portable x-rays because patients with possible foreign body aspiration or epiglottitis outside of the ED may experience sudden and complete airway obstruction.

Abbreviations: CXR = chest x-ray; URI = upper respiratory infection.

and development of lower airway obstruction result in increased work of breathing. Because the nasal passages account for 50% of total airway resistance, increased nasal mucus production may cause upper airway obstruction due to the small nasal passages of infants. This in itself can cause modest respiratory distress, particularly in young infants, who are obligate nasal breathers.

Respiratory syncytial virus is transmitted by direct contact with contaminated secretions, including large droplets into the mucosa of the eyes and nose. Infected secretions found on fomites remain contagious for several hours. Because respiratory syncytial virus is highly infectious, self-contamination and nosocomial spread are common. Hand washing and contact precautions are important to limit the spread of disease. The incubation period for respiratory syncytial virus ranges from 2 to 8 days.

CLINICAL FEATURES

Although bronchiolitis can be seen throughout the year, its peak occurrence in North America is from November to March. Typical symptoms are rhinorrhea, tachypnea, wheezing, and coughing. Use of accessory muscles, nasal flaring, and fever may also occur. **These symptoms last on average 7 to 21 days and are often the worst in the first week of the illness.**[16] The peak of symptoms is often between the third and fifth day after onset. Associated symptoms include irritability, cyanosis, and poor feeding.

A subset of infants with bronchiolitis will develop severe disease and apnea. **Apneic episodes** may be brief and self-limited or progress to more frequent and prolonged episodes that lead to hypoxia and the need for endotracheal intubation. Some infants presenting with apnea have minimal other symptoms. Several factors associated with a greater risk of severe disease and apnea are listed in **Table 124-4.**[15,17] Infants with bronchiolitis and these risk factors may have prolonged hospital stays, greater need for mechanical ventilation, and higher mortality rates. Consider bronchiolitis in infants with apparent life-threatening events and monitor such infants closely (see chapter 115, "Sudden Infant Death Syndrome and Apparent Life-Threatening Event").

On chest examination, wheezing and crackles are heard diffusely throughout both lung fields. Respiratory rates should be measured for 1 full minute and may vary from normal to profound tachypnea (Table 124-1). Accessory muscle use and intercostal or subcostal retractions develop as respiratory distress worsens. Patients with bronchiolitis are at risk for dehydration as blocked nasal passages inhibit feeding while increased work of breathing and a higher metabolic rate contribute to increased insensible losses. Assess for signs of dehydration including dry mucous membranes, tachycardia, lethargy, delayed capillary refill, inadequate urine output, and a sunken fontanelle.

DIAGNOSIS

Bronchiolitis is a clinical diagnosis based on the findings of the history and physical examination, which include typical symptoms of rhinorrhea, tachypnea, crackles, and/or wheezing in a child <2 years of age. There are several published scoring systems for assessing the severity of illness and change over time used for research purposes, although none has been validated or gained wide acceptance in clinical application. Obtain pulse oximetry readings at presentation to detect

TABLE 124-4 Risk Factors for Severe Disease and Apnea in Infants with Bronchiolitis

Prematurity (<37 wk gestational age, especially if <32 wk gestational age)
Age <12 wk
Previous episode of apnea
Underlying cardiopulmonary disease
Immunodeficiency
Chronic lung disease

hypoxemia that may not be readily suspected on physical examination, and repeat readings during the course of the ED visit. Obtain intermittent oxygen saturation monitoring for children with mild disease and continuous monitoring for those with moderate or severe disease.

Rapid viral antigen detection tests may be useful. Sensitivity of the rapid tests generally ranges from 80% to 90% and specificity from 90% to 99%. Test results remain positive as long as virus is being shed. For respiratory syncytial virus, this may be up to 2 weeks after the onset of symptoms. The use of reverse transcriptase polymerase chain reaction testing to detect nucleic acid offers greater sensitivity. Results of viral culture are not available for several days and are not useful for guiding ED treatment.

Ancillary tests, such as blood work and radiographs, are not routinely needed unless other diagnoses need to be excluded.[15] The incidence of serious bacterial infections in infants <28 days of age with bronchiolitis and fever is 3% to 10%, similar to that in other neonates with fever, so the standard testing of blood, urine, and cerebrospinal fluid is indicated. In infants >30 days of age, the incidence of serious bacterial infection in association with bronchiolitis remains 3% to 5%, with the most common infection being a urinary tract infection.[18] **Chest radiographs are not routinely indicated but may be considered when the illness is severe or associated with hypoxia, or when the course is atypical.**[19] Although the chest radiograph in bronchiolitis may demonstrate atelectasis, bacterial pneumonia is unusual.

TREATMENT

Figure 124-2 outlines an ED algorithm for bronchiolitis treatment based on severity of illness. **In 2014, the American Academy of Pediatrics published an updated clinical practice guideline for the treatment of bronchiolitis in children age 1 to 23 months that highlights some of the challenges clinicians encounter in the inpatient and ED settings.**[15]

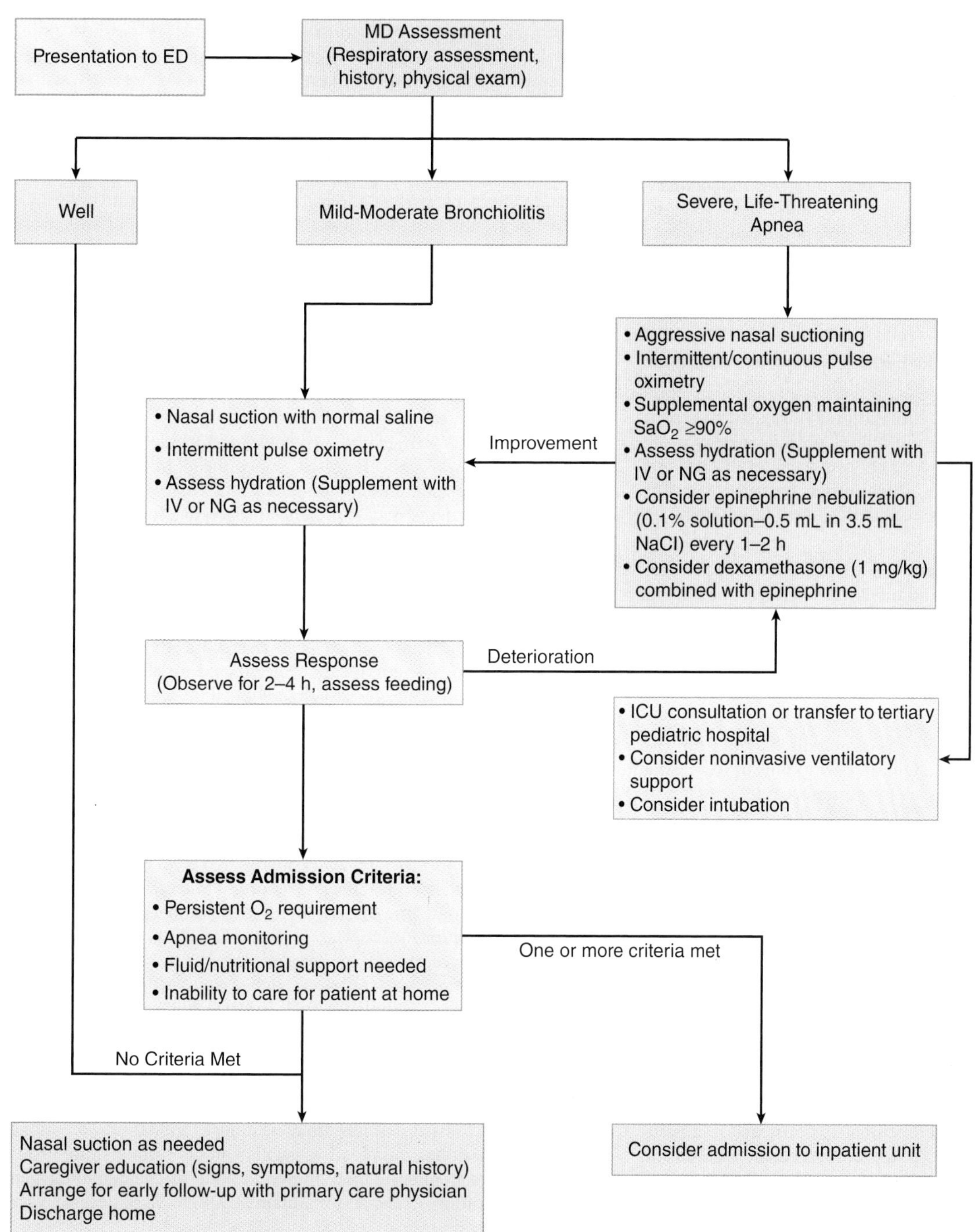

FIGURE 124-2. ED algorithm for the treatment and disposition of a patient with bronchiolitis. ICU = intensive care unit; MD = physician; NG = nasogastric.

Infants with bronchiolitis who do not meet criteria for admission can be managed as outpatients, and few need hospital admission. **The most important treatment is frequent instillation of saline into the nares followed by suctioning.** Support for feeding includes more frequent and smaller feeds and the use of prefeed suctioning. Caretakers should use frequent hand washing to minimize contagion.

Bronchodilators **No benefits have been shown on oxygen saturation, hospitalization rates, or duration of hospitalization by using β_2-agonists (including salbutamol/albuterol, ipratropium bromide, and terbutaline),**[20,21] and they should not be given routinely. Inhaled epinephrine has not been shown to affect rates of admission from the ED or hospital length of stay among patients admitted for bronchiolitis; however, there may be a role in children with severe or acutely deteriorating bronchiolitis.[15,21,22]

Corticosteroids The combined use of dexamethasone and epinephrine decreased admission rates in a large, multicenter, Canadian study that examined the effects of dexamethasone (1 milligram/kg) given in the ED with or without inhaled epinephrine followed by 5 days of dexamethasone (0.6 milligram/kg/d) at home.[23] Infants in the dexamethasone-only and epinephrine-only groups did not show any benefits. Therefore, there is insufficient evidence to support stand-alone use of systemic or inhaled corticosteroids for bronchiolitis. **Current guidelines advocate consideration for steroid use in combination with epinephrine in the treatment of bronchiolitis.**[24]

Nebulized Hypertonic Saline The effect of hypertonic saline in bronchiolitis is mixed. Hypertonic saline may improve mucociliary clearance by loosening mucous plugs through osmotic draw of fluid from submucosal and adventitial spaces. The preponderance of evidence suggests no meaningful clinical benefit from nebulized hypertonic saline (3% or 7%) in the ED, and the 2014 American Academy of Pediatrics clinical practice guideline recommends against its routine use.[15,25-28]

Oxygen **The American Academy of Pediatrics recommends maintaining an oxygen saturation of >90%.**[15]

Ventilatory Support Noninvasive ventilation measures, such as nasal continuous positive airway pressure and bilevel positive airway pressure, may help avoid or delay the need for endotracheal intubation and mechanical ventilation.[29,30] However, when other measures do not work, endotracheal intubation with mechanical ventilation may be necessary.

Heliox Heliox does not affect the rates of intubation or mechanical ventilation or length of intensive care admission.[31] There may be a small benefit on hospital length of stay by using heliox via tight-fitting facemask or nasal continuous positive airway pressure.[32]

DISPOSITION AND FOLLOW-UP

The majority of children with bronchiolitis can be discharged from the ED. Educate caregivers regarding the signs and symptoms of increasing respiratory distress, including an increase in respiratory rate, presence of retractions, and inability to feed, and tell them to bring the child for immediate reevaluation if any of these develop. Demonstrate proper nasal suctioning techniques to caregivers. Counsel parents that symptoms may persist for up to 3 weeks to help avoid unnecessary ED returns for persistent mild symptoms.[16]

Factors that contribute to the need for admission include prematurity, corrected age <1 month old, persistent tachypnea or work of breathing despite therapy, dehydration, and oxygen requirement (arterial oxygen saturation [Sa_{O_2}] <90% on room air). **Admit infants with witnessed episodes of apnea and those with risk factors for apnea, even when they are clinically well appearing.** Factors such as sex, race, duration of symptoms, parental history of asthma, and prior ED visits are not related to safety for discharge.[33]

More detailed information about bronchiolitis is provided in a practice guideline available at the American Academy of Pediatrics Web site (http://pediatrics.aappublications.org/content/early/2014/10/21/peds.2014-2742.full.pdf+html).

ASTHMA

Asthma is a chronic disease characterized by episodic and reversible airflow obstruction due to bronchial smooth muscle hyperreactivity and inflammation, that is responsive to bronchodilator and corticosteroid treatments.[9,10,34]

More than 95% of children age 2 to 18 years presenting to the ED with asthma exacerbations exhibit wheezing, shortness of breath, cough, and/or dyspnea secondary to decreased expiratory airflow.[35] Milder cases of acute asthma exacerbations may present with only wheezing or mild dyspnea, whereas severe exacerbations present with dyspnea at rest, inability to speak, and marked increased work of breathing and may be associated with peak expiratory flow of <40% of predicted value.[10] Severe exacerbations may progress to status asthmaticus and respiratory failure, which may be life-threatening.[36,37]

PATHOPHYSIOLOGY

The three pathophysiologic processes of asthma are inflammation, bronchospasm, and airway obstruction. The inflammatory cascade either directly leads to or contributes to the severity of bronchospasm and airway obstruction. Multiple inflammatory pathways are activated in asthma and involve a complex interplay of cytokines, chemokines, immunoglobulin E (IgE), lymphocytes, mast cells, and eosinophils.

Bronchospasm results in decreased airflow and symptoms during exacerbations and may be precipitated by triggers such as infection, irritants, or allergens. Irritant-induced bronchospasm may involve non–IgE-dependent pathways (e.g., aspirin, nonsteroidal anti-inflammatory drugs), and may also involve as yet undefined mechanisms (e.g., exercise, emotional stress). Allergens precipitate bronchospasm as a result of IgE-dependent release of histamine, leukotrienes, and other mediators from mast cells.

The third primary pathophysiologic process in acute asthma is airway obstruction. Inflammation causes airway mucosal edema and contributes to airway obstruction indirectly as a result of mucus hypersecretion, formation of mucous plugs, and structural airway changes. These changes, in a process termed *airway remodeling,* include hyperplasia and hypertrophy of airway smooth muscle, subepithelial fibrosis, and thickening of the sub-basement membrane. As a result of airway remodeling, some asthmatic patients may experience progressive loss of lung function that may not be reversible.[10]

CLINICAL FEATURES AND INITIAL ASSESSMENT AND TREATMENT

Obtain a thorough, detailed history to determine the progression of illness and ability for ongoing care at home and for disposition planning. Identify possible triggers, such as viral illnesses, pneumonia, or allergens[38]; progression of symptoms at home; and home treatments. Ask about past ED visits, hospitalizations, prior intensive care admission, and any invasive and noninvasive airway support. Obtain any family history of asthma or eczema.

Assess airway and breathing immediately; the degree of respiratory distress and impaired ventilation dictate the tempo of the evaluation and intensity of interventions. Serial assessments are key to ED management because changes in clinical status and response to treatment are usually more relevant to outcome and need for admission than the level of severity at presentation.

Physical signs are useful in determining the severity of airway obstruction. Mental status changes such as agitation may indicate hypoxemia, whereas somnolence may indicate hypercarbia. Respiratory rate (Table 124-2) and air entry indicate the adequacy of gas exchange and ventilation.

Determine oxygen saturation at presentation. Perform continuous pulse oximetry for patients who are hypoxemic or moderately to severely ill. Intermittent oximetry may be done in milder exacerbations or once the patient has improved, is stable, and does not require bronchodilators more frequently than hourly. Provide supplemental oxygen for oxygen saturation <92%, and maintain at 93% to 98%, because very high saturations of oxygen may decrease minute ventilation and result in elevations of pulmonary end tidal carbon dioxide ($ETCO_2$).[39,40]

Mild hypoxemia (>92% at sea level) does not directly provide information regarding ventilation and airflow obstruction.[41-43] Oxygen and β_2-agonists are pulmonary vasodilators and may contribute to ventilation–perfusion mismatch by augmenting perfusion of underventilated lung units. This phenomenon may worsen hypoxemia, but hypoxia generally resolves by 1 to 2 hours as pulmonary autoregulation corrects mismatch. If oxygen saturation remains <92% after initial treatment, consider worsening asthma, pneumothorax, or pneumonia.

Consider $ETCO_2$ monitoring in all children with severe or life-threatening asthma exacerbations, because a rising $ETCO_2$ is a marker of fatigue or worsening of the disease. Levels of $ETCO_2$ are normally 3 to 5 mm Hg lower than capillary or arterial partial pressure of arterial carbon dioxide ($Paco_2$).[44,45] $Paco_2$ should be lower than normal in children with asthma exacerbations due to increased minute ventilation (normal range, 35 to 40 mm Hg).[46,47]

Accessory muscle use reflects the work of breathing necessary to overcome auto-positive end-expiratory pressure and airway resistance. Heart rate, respiratory rate, and accessory muscle use are associated with diminished percentage of predicted forced expiratory volume in 1 second.[48,49] Accessory muscle recruitment progresses in a caudal to cephalad direction. Subcostal and intercostal muscle use occurs with mild to moderate obstruction, whereas neck muscle use suggests severe obstruction. Wheezing is pathognomonic for airway obstruction and typically occurs more during expiration than during inspiration; **however, the quiet chest is an ominous sign of severely compromised ventilation and indicates insufficient airflow to generate wheezing.**

The severity of an acute asthma exacerbation may be assessed based on signs and symptoms, without assigning a numeric score, and classified as **mild, moderate, severe, or imminent respiratory failure**. However, asthma scoring systems are a means to assess severity and response to treatment and to communicate among providers. The Pediatric Respiratory Assessment Measure (PRAM; **Figure 124-3**) has been validated in patients 2 to 17 years old with asthma and is responsive to changes in a patient's respiratory status.[50-52]

TABLE 124-5 Indications for Chest Radiography in Acute Asthma

Fever not explained by apparent viral illness
Chest pain, cardiovascular instability, or absent breath sounds (rule out pneumothorax)
Poor response to treatment (consider congestive heart failure or foreign body aspiration)
Life-threatening exacerbation (consider alternate diagnoses, comorbidities)

DIAGNOSIS

There are three essential diagnostic questions for the child with signs and symptoms suggestive of an acute asthma exacerbation: (1) Does this patient have asthma? (2) What is the severity of airway exacerbation? (3) Is there a treatable trigger for this exacerbation?

For children >2 years old who do not have a history of health professional–diagnosed asthma, a provisional diagnosis of asthma is made when there are signs and symptoms of wheezing, shortness of breath, cough, dyspnea, diminished air entry, or retractions **and** demonstration of reversibility with β_2-agonist bronchodilators (e.g., salbutamol/albuterol). Children 1 to 2 years old with viral-induced wheeze may be treated as having either asthma or bronchiolitis. Children <1 year old with first episode of wheeze should be treated as having bronchiolitis.

Although spirometry may be a useful adjunct to clinical assessment, spirometry cannot be performed in children <6 years old, is challenging to perform in severe respiratory distress, and must be performed by qualified and trained personnel.

Atelectasis is common in children with acute asthma exacerbations, whereas bacterial pneumonia is much less common. A chest radiograph for a child with acute asthma and fever is likely to demonstrate atelectasis, especially if done early during treatment, and the question arises whether this finding represents pneumonia. A reasoned approach to chest radiography is presented in **Table 124-5**.[53,54]

TREATMENT

Acute asthma exacerbations often require multiple medications (**Table 124-6**), review of current medication use, and an individualized

Paediatric Respiratory Assessment Measure (PRAM)

SIGNS/SCORING	0	1	2	3	PATIENT'S SCORE
Suprasternal retractions	Absent		Present		(max 2)
Scalene muscle contraction	Absent		Present		(max 2)
Air entry*	Normal	Decreased at bases	Widespread decrease	Absent/minimal	(max 3)
Wheezing*	Absent	Expiratory only	Inspiratory and expiratory	Audible without stethoscope/silent chest with minimal air entry	(max 3)
O_2 Saturation in room air	≥95%	92%–94%	<92%		(max 2)
*If asymmetric findings between the right and left lungs, the most severe is rated **PRAM SCORE TOTAL**					**(MAX 12)**

PRAM Score 0–3 **MILD** Asthma
PRAM Score 4–7 **MODERATE** Asthma
PRAM Score 8–12 **SEVERE** Asthma

IMPENDING RESPIRATORY FAILURE
is based on clinical presentation

[1]Chalut, D. S., Ducharme, F. M., & Davis, G.M. (2000). The Preschool Respiratory Assessment Measure (PRAM): A responsive index of acute asthma severity. The Journal of Pediatrics, 137 (6), 762-768.

[2]Ducharme, F., Chalut, D., Plotnick, L., Savdie, C., Kudirka, D., Zhang, X., et al. (2008). The Pediatric Respiratory Assessment Measure: A Valid Clinical Score for Assessing Acute Asthma Severity from Toddlers to Teenagers. *The Journal of Pediatrics, 152*(4), 476-480.e1.

FIGURE 124-3. The Pediatric Respiratory Assessment Measure (PRAM).

TABLE 124-6 Treatment for Acute Asthma Exacerbations

Treatment	Comments
Short-acting β_2-agonist bronchodilators	For all patients with acute asthma exacerbations in the ED. **Add ipratropium bromide for severe or life-threatening exacerbations.**
Systemic steroids	For all patients with moderate or worse exacerbations as early as possible in course. May be given orally or parenterally.
Oxygen	In patients with arterial oxygen saturation ≤92%.
Magnesium sulfate	Intravenous or nebulized smooth muscle–relaxing bronchodilator for severe exacerbations not responding to initial therapy.
Inhaled corticosteroids	No role in acute ED management, but prescribe inhaled corticosteroids for home use.

discharge plan. The PRAM helps identify the severity of exacerbations and may be incorporated into treatment algorithms such as the Ontario Lung Association Pediatric Asthma Care Pathway (**Figure 124-4**). Dosages of drugs for acute exacerbations are listed in **Table 124-7**, and treatment recommendations for acute exacerbations by severity are provided in **Table 124-8**.

Short-Acting β_2-Receptor Agonists β_2-Agonists are the mainstay of acute asthma therapy. They act specifically on β_2-receptors to relax bronchial wall smooth muscles and are the most effective agents for relieving acute bronchospasm. **Salbutamol/albuterol** is the most widely available and used β_2-agonist. After inhalation, the onset of action is within 3 to 5 minutes, the peak effect is seen within 30 to 120 minutes, and the duration of action is 2 to 5 hours.[55]

Levosalbutamol (levalbuterol), the R-enantiomer of salbutamol, is not any more effective or safer than salbutamol and is much more expensive.[56]

β_2-Agonists are frequently delivered by metered-dose inhalers **with an age-appropriate valved holding chamber or via wet nebulization.** Metered-dose inhalers are as effective as nebulizers for mild to moderate exacerbations and decrease length of ED stay while causing less side effects such as nausea, tachycardia, and tremor.[57] A primarily metered-dose inhaler–based algorithm may also confer benefits for infection control and may be more cost effective than a nebulizer-based algorithm[58]

There is no therapeutic advantage of β_2-agonist administration by the IV route versus the inhaled route in the child who is ventilating reasonably well. However, for the patient with significantly diminished air entry, the IV route may allow for critical initial bronchodilation that permits subsequent inhaled medications to reach distal airways.[59,60]

Oral albuterol is not recommended due to the delayed onset and prominent tachycardia, tremulousness, and behavioral changes accompanying this form.

Epinephrine has α- and β-agonist properties that facilitate vasoconstriction and rapid resolution of mucosal edema. However, it causes more side effects, because it is not as selective for lower airways as β_2-agonists.

Corticosteroids Systemic corticosteroids inhibit the inflammatory cascade and enhance β-receptor expression, sensitivity, and function. They provide rapid beneficial physiologic effects, usually within 4 hours, which reduces both the need for hospitalization and the likelihood of relapse.[61,62] **Most patients should be treated immediately with systemic corticosteroids and discharged on a 3- to 5-day course of the drugs to prevent early relapse.**[63,64] Early administration of corticosteroids by a triage nurse can decrease ED length of stay and admission rates.[65]

Prednisone should be given orally at a dose of 2 milligrams/kg or equivalent within the first hour of ED presentation followed by 1 milligram/kg/d (maximum 60 milligrams/d) for the subsequent 4 days upon discharge to complete a 5-day total course. A taper is not required for short treatments. Prednisolone suspension, at the same dose, is palatable; unpalatable agents lead to poor compliance (50% to 60% fill rates).[66] When the patient is severely ill or not responding to therapy, IV methylprednisone (1 milligram/kg/dose) may be given every 6 hours. Dexamethasone is palatable and, in addition to the oral route, may be given intramuscularly or intravenously. There are different dosing regimens for dexamethasone that are therapeutically equivalent to 5 days of prednisone including a single dose (0.6 milligram/kg) or a 2-day course at 0.6 milligram/kg/d or a 3- to 5-day course at 0.2 to 0.3 milligram/kg/d.[67-70]

Inhaled corticosteroids have no role in the acute ED management but are an essential part of maintenance therapy and should be prescribed to all patients with persistent asthma at discharge (see "Disposition and Follow-Up" section for further discussion).[71]

Anticholinergic Agents Anticholinergic agents such as ipratropium bromide relieve bronchiole obstruction by blocking muscarinic receptors in the bronchiole wall, leading to bronchodilation and decreased mucus secretion. However, they are not as potent or rapid as β_2-agonists.[72] When used in combination with short-acting β_2-agonists, anticholinergics decrease hospitalization rates versus anticholinergic use alone.[73,74] Addition of multiple high doses of ipratropium (0.5 milligram) to nebulized albuterol treatments has additive benefit and results in reduced hospitalization in children with severe exacerbations.[65,75]

Magnesium Magnesium sulfate acts as a bronchodilator by inhibiting smooth muscle contraction[76,77] and may reduce the need for hospitalization or intensive care admission.[77-80] It is given IV. Nebulized magnesium is not effective.[81-83]

Ketamine Ketamine is a dissociative sedative agent that is commonly used for both procedural sedation and as an induction agent for endotracheal intubation. The sympathomimetic properties of ketamine and its bronchodilation effect make it the ideal induction agent for the patient with respiratory failure due to asthma. One case series found that ketamine alleviated the need to intubate when given as part of induction in children,[84] but there are few data about dosing and indications other than for induction during intubation.[85,86] Low ketamine doses, 0.2 milligram/kg followed by a 2-hour infusion of 0.5 milligram/kg, are ineffective.[87]

Heliox Heliox, a mixture of helium and oxygen, is less dense than air, leading to laminar instead of turbulent airflow in obstructed airways.[88] It may be a better vehicle for medication delivery and improves gas exchange. It has no direct pharmacologic or biologic effect and has an extremely low risk profile.[86,89-92] The evidence for routine heliox use is conflicted, and the equipment required to use it makes this treatment difficult in the ED setting.

Methylxanthines Methylxanthines (theophylline and aminophylline) have been replaced by safer and more effective short-acting β_2-agonists. Adverse effects include tachycardia, vomiting, and CNS excitation, including seizures.[93,94] Current treatment guidelines recommend against its use primarily due to its side effect profile and narrow therapeutic window.[95]

TREATMENT OF NEAR-FATAL ASTHMA

Patients with acute severe asthma who do not respond adequately to maximal medical therapy and who continue to manifest severe airway obstruction and hyperinflation are at risk for fatal asthma. One third of pediatric deaths from asthma are in children who previously had only mild asthma. Clinical signs of this progression include worsening hypoxemia, increasing respiratory rate, diaphoresis, inability to speak, somnolence, and fatigue. The decision to undertake advanced airway management for near-fatal asthma is based on clinical judgment.

One must weigh the need for intubation against the potential adverse outcomes, including worsening bronchospasm, laryngospasm, pneumothorax, ventilator-associated pneumonia, and hemodynamic instability.[96,97]

Noninvasive Positive-Pressure Ventilation Bilevel positive airway pressure is the preferred noninvasive modality in the care of the patient with severe, nonresponsive asthma. It delivers different pressures during inspiration and expiration to decrease the work of breathing, stent the airways open, and improve gas exchange. It also appears to have a bronchodilator effect.[98] The largest study of bilevel positive airway pressure use in children found that 88% tolerated the intervention and demonstrated

Indications to start Paediatric Asthma Clinical Pathway

- Age 1-17 years with wheeze and/or cough

AND

- asthma diagnosis and/or past history of wheeze

Physician assessment required prior to starting on clinical pathway if:

- any active chronic condition other than asthma OR
- prior serious adverse reaction to albuterol/salbutamol, ipratropium bromide, or oral corticosteriods OR
- active chickenpox or suspected incubation of chickenpox OR
- heart rate greater than or equal to 200 beats/min

**PRAM 0 - 3 (Mild)

***FEV_1 greater than 70% of predicted or personal best, if known

- **MD** to assess within 60 min
- Albuterol/salbutamol now and q 60 min prn (via MDI† + spacer)
- Vital Signs + PRAM q 60 min

**PRAM 4 - 7 (Moderate)

***FEV_1 50 -70% of predicted or personal best, if known

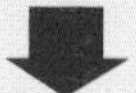

- **MD** to assess within 30 min
- Administer oxygen to keep SpO_2 greater than or equal to 92%
- Albuterol/salbutamol now and q 30 - 60 min prn (via MDI† and spacer)
- **Give oral corticosteroid AS SOON AS POSSIBLE** after 1st albuterol/salbutamol dose (within 60 min of triage)
- Vital Signs + PRAM q 30 - 60 min if not improving (PRAM unchanged or less than 3 point improvement), consider: ipratropium bromide

**PRAM 8 - 12 (Severe)

***FEV_1 less than 50% of predicted or personal best, if known

- **MD** to assess within 15 min
- Administer oxygen to keep SpO_2 greater than or equal to 92%
- Albuterol/salbutamol + ipratropium NOW, + q 20 min x 3 doses (via MDI† + spacer or nebulizer), then q 20-60 min prn
- **Give systemic corticosteroid AS SOON AS POSSIBLE** after 1st albuterol/salbutamol/ipratropium dose (within 20 min of triage)
- Vital Signs + PRAM q 20 - 60 min
- Consider IV access and blood gases

Complete all of above within 60 min of triage.

Impending Respiratory Failure

lethargy, cyanosis, decreasing respiratory effort, and/or rising pCO_2

- **MD** to assess STAT and remain in attendance until patient stabilized
- Administer 100% oxygen
- Support ventilation if required (bag & mask); do not over-ventilate as this will increase air trapping
- Continuous cardiopulmonary monitoring
- Continuous nebulized albuterol/salbutamoll with ipratropium
- **Systemic corticosteroid AS SOON AS POSSIBLE** after 1st albuterol/salbutamol/ipratropium dose:
- Obtain IV access

MD to consider:

- IV magnesium sulfate (caution: can cause low BP)
- IV fluids
- CXR + blood gas measurement
- Contact ICU or Regional Tertiary Centre regarding management & transport

CritiCall Ontario
1-800-668-HELP (4357)

Mild: Reassess Vital Signs + PRAM q 60 min

If PRAM greater than or equal to 4 or ***FEV_1 less than 70% of predicted:

- MD to reassess and move to top of '**Moderate**' pathway

If PRAM remains less than or equal to 3 or ***FEV_1 greater than or equal to 70% of predicted:

- MD to consider discharge
- Provide asthma teaching
- Provide discharge instructions

Moderate: Reassess Vital Signs + PRAM q 30-60 min

If at any time PRAM is greater than or equal to 8 or ***FEV_1 is less than 50% of predicted, or if PRAM is unchanged or has improved less than 3 points:

- MD to reassess and move to top of '**Severe**' pathway

If 6-8 hrs post corticosteroid, PRAM is greater than or equal to 4 or ***FEV_1 is less than 70% of predicted:

- MD to reassess and consider admission

If PRAM less than or equal to 3 or ***FEV_1 greater than or equal to 70% of predicted:

- MD to consider discharge; provide asthma teaching and discharge instructions

Severe: Reassess Vital Signs + PRAM q 20-60 min

If poor response (PRAM unchanged or less than 3 point improvement) or signs of impending respiratory failure at any time:

- MD to reassess STAT and move to top of '**Impending Respiratory Failure**' pathway

If 4 hrs post corticosteroid, PRAM is greater than or equal to 4 or ***FEV_1 is less than 70% of predicted:

- MD to reassess and consider admission

If PRAM improving, move to 'Moderate' pathway

†Inhaled medication delivery by metered dose inhaler (MDI) and age appropriate valved spacer is preferred unless continuous oxygen is required. Small volume nebulizer is an acceptable alternate.
**See below for PRAM scoring.
***FEV_1 (or as second choice, PEF) should only be used in children aged 6 years and older with demonstrated reproducibility within 10% and when performed by health care personnel trained in spirometry.
NOTE: FEV_1 results may be discordant with the severity level indicated by the PRAM (as clinical signs and lung function are different parameters); in case of discordance, the physician is invited to use his/her best judgment to decide which parameter to use to manage the child. **Do not delay treatment to obtain FEV_1 and/or peak flow.**

Medication Guidelines

BRONCHODILATORS

Metered Dose Inhaler (MDI)† via age appropriate spacer, allow 30 sec between puffs

albuterol/salbutamol salbutamol (100 mcg/puff)
1 - 3 yrs: 4 puffs/dose 4 - 6 yrs: 6 puffs/dose
7 years and older: 8 puffs/dose

ipratropium bromide (20 mcg/puff)
3 puffs/dose, alternate each puff with albuterol/salbutamol

Wet Nebulization† driven by oxygen flow of 6-8 L/min via well-fitting mask

albuterol/salbutamol (5mg/mL solution or unit dose nebule)
less than 10 kg: dose = 1.25 mg; use 1.25 mg nebule OR 0.25 mL of 5 mg/mL sol'n in 3 mL NaCl
10 to 20 kg: dose = 2.5 mg; use 2.5 mg nebule OR 0.5 mL of 5mg/mL sol'n in 3 mL NaCl
greater than 20 kg: dose = 5 mg; use 2 x 2.5 mg nebule OR 5 mg nebule OR 1 mL of 5 mg/mL sol'n in 3 mL NaCl

ipratropium bromide
all patients: 250 mcg, mixed with albuterol/salbutamol

CORTICOSTEROIDS

Oral route
prednisone/prednisolone 2 mg/kg x 1 (max 50 mg/dose)

Parenteral route
methylprednisolone 1 mg/kg/dose IV or IM (max 125 mg/dose) x 1; could be repeated q 6h

MAGNESIUM SULFATE

magnesium sulfate (requires cardiorespiratory monitoring and frequent BP checks)
50 mg/kg/dose IV x 1 (max 2 g/dose), give over 20-30 min

†Inhaled medication delivery by MDI and age-appropriate valved spacer is preferred unless continuous oxygen is required. Small volume nebulizer is an acceptable alternate.

PRAM scoring table

O_2 Saturation	≥ 95%	0
	92-94%	1
	< 92%	2
Suprasternal retraction	Absent	0
	Present	2
Scalene muscle contraction	Absent	0
	Present	2
Air entry*	Normal	0
	↓ at the base	1
	↓ at the apex and the base	2
	Minimal or absent	3
Wheezing§	Absent	0
	Expiratory only	1
	Inspiratory (± expiratory)	2
	Audible without stethoscope or silent chest (minimal or no air entry)	3
	PRAM score : (max. 12)	

Score	0-3	4-7	8-12
Severity	Mild	Moderate	Severe

* In case of asymmetry, the most severely affected (apex-base) lung field (right or left, anterior or posterior) will determine the rating of the criterion.
§ In case of asymmetry, the two most severely affected auscultation zones, irrespective of their location (RUL, RML, RLL, LUL, LLL), will determine the rating of the criterion.

Disclaimer:
This Clinical Pathway is not intended to set the standard of care applicable in any particular clinical situation. It is merely prepared as a guide to assist physicians, nurses, respiratory therapists and other healthcare providers, in deciding on the appropriate care required for a particular patient. At all times, physicians, nurses, respiratory therapists and other healthcare providers must exercise their independent clinical judgment, based on their knowledge, training and experience, taking into account the specific facts and circumstances of each patient, when deciding on the appropriate course of investigation and/or treatment to recommend in a particular clinical situation. Any reference throughout the document to specific pharmaceutical products as examples does not imply endorsement of any of these products.

The views expressed are the views of the authors and do not necessarily reflect those of the Government of Ontario.

This clinical pathway was developed with input from and endorsed by:

FIGURE 124-4. The Ontario Lung Association Pediatric Asthma Care Pathway. [Reproduced with permission from The Ontario Lung Association. In: *Paediatric Emergency Department Asthma Care Pathway: Information Package March 2014*. The Lung Association Ontario; 2014:4. Available at: http://machealth.ca/programs/paediatric-emergency-department-asthma-care-pathway/m/mediagallery/1921/download.aspx]

TABLE 124-7 Dosages of Medications for Asthma Exacerbations

Medication	American Pediatric Dosages[55]	Alternate Pediatric Dosages
Bronchodilators		
Salbutamol/albuterol (aerosol or nebulized)	MDI (90 micrograms/puff); *delivered via valved holding chamber*: ≤1 y: 2 puffs/dose 1–3 y: 4 puffs/dose ≥4 y: 8 puffs/dose	MDI (100 micrograms/puff); *delivered via valved holding chamber*: ≤1 y: 2 puffs/dose 1–3 y: 4 puffs/dose 4–6 y: 6 puffs/dose ≥7 y: 8 puffs/dose
	Nebulization (unit dose nebule or 5 milligrams/mL solution): 0.15–0.3 milligrams/kg/dose (minimum 2.5 milligrams)	Nebulization (unit dose nebule or 5 milligrams/mL solution): <10 kg: 1.25-milligram nebule or 0.25 mL of 5-milligram/mL solution* 10–20 kg: 2.5-milligram nebule or 0.5 mL of 5-milligram/mL solution* >20 kg: 5-milligram nebule or 1 mL of 5-milligram/mL solution*
	IV: *Not available*	IV: 0.5–3 milligrams/kg/h continuous infusion (maximum 15 milligrams/h)
	PO: *Not recommended*	PO: *Not recommended*
Ipratropium bromide (aerosol or nebulized)	MDI (20 micrograms/puff); *delivered via valved holding chamber:* 4–8 puffs/dose PRN, alternated with salbutamol	MDI (20 micrograms/puff); *delivered via valved holding chamber:* 3 puffs/dose for all patients, alternated with salbutamol
	Nebulization: 250–500 micrograms for all patients, mixed with salbutamol	Nebulization: 250 micrograms for all patients, mixed with salbutamol
Systemic corticosteroids		
Prednisone (PO)	1–2 milligrams/kg/dose (maximum 60 milligrams) for 3–10 d	2 milligrams/kg (maximum 50 milligrams) in ED, then 1 milligram/kg/d for 4 d
Methylprednisolone (IV, IM)	2 milligrams/kg/dose load, then 0.5–1 milligram/kg/dose every 6 h	1 milligram/kg/dose (maximum 125 milligrams/dose), repeated every 6 h or change to oral regimen
Dexamethasone (PO, IV, IM)	0.6 milligram/kg/dose (maximum 16 milligrams) for 1–2 d	Multiple dosing regimens: 0.6 milligram/kg/d for 1–2 d 0.3 milligram/kg/d for 3–5 d
Other medications		
Magnesium sulfate (IV)	25–75 milligrams/kg/dose (maximum 2 grams) × 1	50 milligrams/kg/dose × 1 (*monitor blood pressure*)
Ketamine (IV)†	1–2 milligrams/kg/dose × 1	2 milligrams/kg/dose × 1 (*may alleviate need for intubation, given as induction agent for intubation*)

*Mixed in 3 mL of normal saline solution.

†Consider only if standard therapies have failed in order to prevent intubation.

Abbreviation: MDI = metered-dose inhaler.

clinically significant improvements in respiratory rate and oxygenation without adverse effects.[99] Bilevel positive airway pressure may be effective in preventing the need for endotracheal intubation even if applied for only several hours.

Use of a well-fitting facemask and close attention to patient comfort are essential. Most patients tolerate bilevel positive airway pressure well, but sedation is frequently required with low doses of benzodiazepines (0.05 to 0.1 milligram/kg of midazolam or lorazepam) or ketamine (0.5 to 1 milligram/kg followed by 0.25 milligram/kg/h). Reasonable initial applied bilevel positive airway pressures for severe asthma are an inspiratory positive airway pressure of 12 cm H_2O and expiratory positive airway pressure of 6 cm H_2O, with ranges of 12 to 18 cm H_2O and 6 to 12 cm H_2O, respectively.[98-100] Aerosolized medications can be administered through the bilevel positive airway pressure airway circuit.

TABLE 124-8 Summary of Treatment Recommendations by Severity for Acute Asthma Exacerbations

	$β_2$-Agonist	Systemic Corticosteroid	Anticholinergic
Mild	+	–	–
Moderate	++	+	–
Severe*	+++	+	+

*Severe patients not responding to full therapy should be considered for IV magnesium and/or other adjuvant therapies.

Endotracheal Intubation and Assisted Ventilation An extremely small number of children will require intubation despite aggressive management. It is best to try to avoid the need to intubate due to challenges in ventilatory management and potential for adverse effects due to air trapping, and noninvasive ventilation strategies such as bilevel positive airway pressure may prevent the need for intubation. Select the largest appropriate cuffed endotracheal tube. Preoxygenate with 100% oxygen. If reasonable, give a normal saline fluid bolus (20 mL/kg) prior to intubation to minimize hypotension.

Drugs for rapid-sequence intubation in severe asthma are listed in **Table 124-9** and should be administered with the patient sitting up or in another comfortable position to maximize preoxygenation. **Ketamine is the preferred induction agent because it provides bronchodilation and does not directly cause hypotension.** Give it immediately before the paralytic agent. Atropine is only indicated to treat symptomatic bradycardia. For full discussion of pediatric intubation, refer to chapter 111, "Intubation and Ventilation in Infants and Children." Once the endotracheal tube is in place, an appropriate tidal volume and a sufficiently low respiratory rate to allow for expiratory emptying and avoid hyperinflation should be provided manually.

The key pulmonary mechanics of the disease process are hyperinflation, auto–positive end-expiratory pressure, and markedly prolonged expiratory time constants that result in failure of the airways to empty. Mechanical ventilation must be tailored to these features. The principles of ventilator management are thus to use low respiratory rates and tidal volumes, long expiratory times, and high flow rates (**Table 124-10**).[101,102]

TABLE 124-9 Drugs for Rapid-Sequence Intubation of a Child with Near-Fatal Asthma

Drug	Dose
Intubation Induction	
Ketamine*	2 milligrams/kg
Short-term paralysis during intubation	
(*Use caution with paralysis*)	
Succinylcholine	<10 kg: 2 milligrams/kg; >10 kg: 1 milligram/kg
Or	
Rocuronium	1 milligram/kg
Postintubation paralysis†	
Vecuronium	0.1 milligram/kg/h
Postintubation sedation	
Ketamine†	2–3 milligrams/kg/h
or	
Fentanyl	1–2 micrograms/kg bolus then 1 microgram/kg/h
and	
Midazolam	0.1 milligram/kg/h

*Immediately prior to paralytic agent.

†Patient-ventilator dyssynchrony may necessitate postintubation paralysis. The use of ketamine for sedation may also obviate the need for paralysis.

TABLE 124-10 Initial Ventilator Settings for the Intubated Pediatric Patient with Asthma

Ventilator Parameter	Setting
Mode	Synchronized intermittent mandatory ventilation/ pressure-regulated volume control
Tidal volume	6–10 mL/kg
Peak pressure	45 cm H_2O
Respiratory rate	8–15/min
Inspiratory time	0.5–1.0 s
Expiratory time	4–8 s

The practice of controlled hypercapnic hypoventilation is a recommended ventilator strategy.[10] The aim is to minimize hyperinflation and airway pressures while providing adequate oxygenation.[103] This mode of ventilation may be key to allowing for the prolonged expiratory times necessary to minimize auto-positive end-expiratory pressure and hyperinflation. Provide adequate sedation to avoid ventilator dyssynchrony, tachypnea, and breath stacking. Ketamine, benzodiazepines, and opiates, or a combination of these, are appropriate, and paralysis is usually necessary.

DISPOSITION AND FOLLOW-UP

The decision regarding hospital admission or discharge of the child with asthma must consider both the adequacy of response to treatment and the ability of the patient and caretaker to provide necessary ongoing care. **The ED relapse rate of 7% to 15% reflects the potential uncertainty of disposition decisions.**[41,104,105] Clinical improvement so that only minimal symptoms remain is a useful guide for discharge. Most patients should be observed for at least 60 minutes after the most recent bronchodilator dose. A PRAM score of 8 or higher at 3 hours after ED presentation strongly predicts the need for admission.[106] If more aggressive therapies have failed, consider early admission.

Dischargeable patients should be prescribed an inhaled short-acting β_2-agonist on discharge from the ED. An age-appropriate valved holding chamber (e.g., AeroChamber®) must be prescribed with the metered-dose inhaler and proper instructions for inhaler technique reviewed. Patients treated with systemic corticosteroids should be prescribed a 5-day oral course. Inhaled corticosteroids should be prescribed at discharge for all classes of asthma severity except mild intermittent asthma.[107] (See **Table 124-11** for dosing guidelines.)

Partner with the primary care physician to ensure appropriate follow-up, symptom and trigger management, monitoring of anti-inflammatory therapy, and implementation of other elements of the National Asthma Education and Prevention Program guidelines.[108]

National and international guidelines recommend treatment with long-term controller medications in all children with persistent asthma.[10] However, primary care physician adherence to these guidelines has been suboptimal. Despite published guidelines stating that inhaled steroids should be prescribed at discharge, fewer than 50% of children with persistent asthma treated by pediatric emergency physicians receive them.[107]

A visit to the ED is an indication of inadequate long-term asthma management and insufficient understanding of how to manage an exacerbation. The goal upon discharge should be to prevent future exacerbations requiring ED visits. A written asthma action plan focused on patient symptoms is superior to action plans based on peak flows.[109,110] The provision of a combined asthma action plan plus prescription increases patient adherence to medications and improves asthma control.[111] One of the proposed benefits of a combined plan with prescription may be the reinforcement of the medical recommendations by the family physician as well as by the pharmacists filling the prescription.[111] At the time of discharge, the physician, nurse, and/or respiratory therapist should review the appropriate use, technique, and timing of all prescribed medications and review early symptom identification and management. A symptom checklist such as the "Asthma Quiz for Kidz" may help self-monitoring of asthma control.[112] Provide clear plans for follow-up appointments and instructions for managing relapse or future exacerbations (**Figure 124-5**).

TABLE 124-11 Recommended Dose Ranges for Inhaled Corticosteroids*

Drug	Dosage	Alternate Formulations
Budesonide (Pulmicort®) dry powder inhaler (90 or 180 micrograms/spray)	180–360 micrograms twice daily	
Budesonide nebulizer suspension (Pulmicort® Respules) (0.25, 0.5, 1 milligram/2 mL units)	0.5–1 milligram divided once or twice daily	
Fluticasone MDI (Flovent®) (44, 120, or 220 micrograms/spray)	88–440 micrograms twice daily For children <5 y: 1 puff of 120 micrograms twice daily	50, 125, or 250 micrograms/spray MDI: 50–250 micrograms twice daily
Beclomethasone (QVAR®) MDI (40, 80 micrograms/spray)	40–80 micrograms twice daily	50, 100 micrograms/spray MDI: 50–100 micrograms twice daily
Ciclesonide MDI (Alvesco®) (80, 160 micrograms/spray)	80–320 micrograms twice daily	100, 200 micrograms/spray MDI: 100 micrograms once daily to 200 micrograms twice daily

*Prescribers should use the lowest effective doses to prevent side effects including adrenal suppression.

Abbreviation: MDI = metered-dose inhaler.

Emergency Department
Asthma Clinical Pathway
Paediatric: 1 to 17 years
Discharge Instructions

ADDRESSOGRAPH

PHYSICIAN: Complete and initial beside selected orders.
PHARMACIST: Label short-acting (relief) inhaler as "Take as directed as per EDACP Discharge Instructions". Fill other medications as directed by physician.

Weight: _______ kg

GREEN ZONE

Asthma **under control**

Breathing is good.
Run & play normally.
Cough or wheeze less than 4 times a week.

CONTROLLER Medicine: ☐ ____________ (specify name)
____ mcg/inhalation, take ____ inhalations ____ times per day, for 3 months, Refill 3
☐ metered dose inhaler (puffer) **OR** ☐ dry powder inhaler
☐ Other ____________

QUICK RELIEF Medicine: ☐ ____________ (specify name)
(usually a blue inhaler)
___mcg/inhalation, take ___inhalations every 4 to 6 hours as needed, 1 inhaler, Refill 1
☐ metered dose inhaler (puffer) **OR** ☐ dry powder inhaler

SPACER DEVICE: ☐ (specify name) ____________
☐ Infant with mask ☐ Paediatric with mask ☐ Adult with mouthpiece

YELLOW ZONE

Asthma **not well controlled**

Signs of a cold.
Mild to moderate cough or wheezing.
Waking up because of asthma.

Continue GREEN ZONE CONTROLLER medicine.
Take QUICK RELIEF medicine every 4 hours until better.
____

If the effect of the QUICK RELIEF medicine does not last 4 hours, or if the child's symptoms are getting worse, see a doctor.

Today, your child was seen in the Emergency Department for a significant asthma exacerbation. To treat this attack, in addition to your Controller and Quick Relief medicines, also give:
☐ prednisolone liquid ____ mg daily for ___ days, Refill **0** **OR** ☐ prednisone tablet ____ mg daily for ___ days, Refill **0**
Additional discharge instructions: ____________

RED ZONE

Asthma **out of control**

Very short of breath.
Severe wheezing.
"Pulling in" of skin between ribs.
Cannot do usual activities.
Severe trouble breathing, walking or talking.
Blueness of lips or skin.
Tired because of effort of breathing.

Take QUICK RELIEF medicine (usually a blue inhaler) every 4 hours.

If the effect of the QUICK RELIEF medicine does not last 4 hours, or if the child's symptoms are getting worse, seek medical attention NOW.

If still in Red Zone after 15 minutes or you have not reached your doctor, call 911 or go to nearest emergency department NOW.

Take QUICK RELIEF medicine as needed (even every 10 or 20 minutes if not improving) on way to hospital.

Schedule appointment with: ☐ family doctor ☐ asthma educator ☐ specialist ____________ within _____ weeks.
If you have any questions about asthma, call The Lung Association **Lung Health Information Line: 1-888-344-LUNG (5864).**

Physician: ____________ (print name) **License #** ________ **Signature:** ____________ **Date:** ________ (dd/mm/yyyy)

ORIGINAL – PHARMACY, COPY 1– MEDICAL CHART, COPY 2 – FAMILY PHYSICIAN, COPY 3 – PATIENT

Created by the Children's Hospital of Eastern Ontario. Adapted with permission for use in the Ontario Lung Association ED Asthma Care Pathways

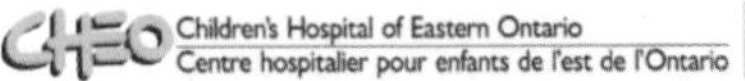

FIGURE 124-5. The Ontario Lung Association Pediatric Asthma Action Plan Pathway. [Reproduced with permission from The Ontario Lung Association. In: *Paediatric Emergency Department Asthma Care Pathway: Information Package March 2014*. The Lung Association Ontario; 2014:4. Available at: http://machealth.ca/programs/paediatric-emergency-department-asthma-care-pathway/m/mediagallery/1921/download.aspx] (*Continued*)

ASTHMA QUIZ FOR KIDZ*

* Adapted from Canadian Respiratory Journal 2004; 11(8):541-6.

	YES	NO
1. Did you **cough, wheeze**, or **have a hard time breathing** 4 or more days out of the last 7 days?	☐	☐
2. Did you wake up at night because you were coughing, or wheezing, or having a hard time breathing 1 or more times in the last 7 days?	☐	☐
3. Did you use your blue puffer 4 or more times in the last 7 days?	☐	☐
4. In the last 7 days, did you do less exercise or sports because it was making you cough, wheeze, or you were having a hard time breathing?	☐	☐
5. In the last 30 days, did you miss school or regular activities because you were coughing, wheezing, or having a hard time breathing?	☐	☐
6. In the last 30 days, did you go to a clinic or a hospital without an appointment because you were coughing, wheezing, or having a hard time breathing?	☐	☐

- How many times did you answer YES? _____
- If you said YES 2 or more times, your asthma is not well controlled. Talk to your mom and dad about seeing a doctor. Let your doctor be your asthma coach!

TRIGGERS

Follow these steps to avoid these common triggers:

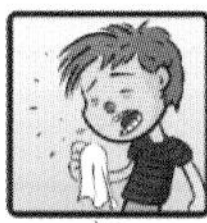

COLDS: Most common trigger. Wash hands before touching your mouth or nose to prevent colds. Follow Yellow Zone at first sign of a cold.

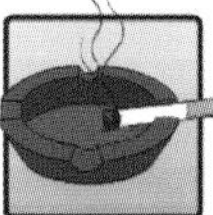

SMOKE: Don't smoke! Do not allow others to smoke in your home or car. Encourage your parents to STOP smoking. Even if they smoke outside, the smoke in their clothes and hair can trigger your asthma.

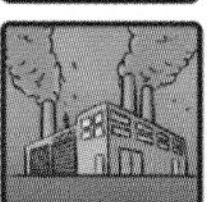

AIR POLLUTION: Avoid fumes and chemicals.

Follow these steps if you have any of the following allergies:

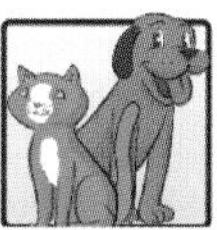

PETS: Avoid pets with fur or feathers. If you have pets, wash them often.

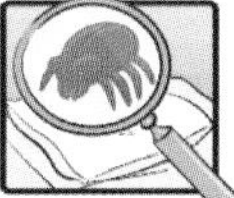

DUST MITES: Wash bed sheets in hot water. Vacuum and dust often. Cover pillows and mattresses with dust mite-resistant covers.

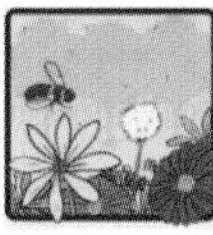

POLLEN: Close windows during pollen season (Spring and Fall). Air conditioning helps. Avoid freshly cut grass.

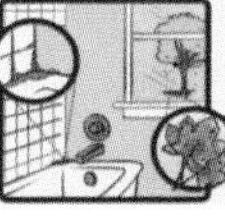

MOLD: Keep bathroom and basement dry. Keep away from decomposing leaves and garden waste.

Controlling your asthma

1. **Avoid your triggers.**
2. **Know your medication and how and when to take it. Take controller medications regularly.**
3. **Follow your action plan.**
4. **After any emergency room visit, you must schedule a follow-up appointment with a doctor in the next 2 weeks.**
5. **Always have spare quick relief medication (blue inhaler) available.**

FIGURE 124-5. *(Continued)*

Acknowledgment: The authors gratefully acknowledge the contributions of Donald H. Arnold, David M. Spiro, and Melissa L. Langhan, the authors of this chapter in the previous edition. We also appreciate the assistance of Avery Ross in the editing of this chapter.

REFERENCES

The complete reference list is available online at www.TintinalliEM.com.

CHAPTER 125 Pneumonia in Infants and Children

Joseph E. Copeland

INTRODUCTION AND EPIDEMIOLOGY

Pneumonia is an infection of the lung and lower respiratory tract, below the level of the larynx. Globally, pneumonia is a leading cause of morbidity and mortality, with an estimated 120 million cases annually resulting in nearly 1.3 million deaths.[1] The greatest burden of disease and mortality occurs in the developing world, and young children under the age of 2 account for 81% of pediatric deaths from pneumonia. Although survival in industrialized countries is better than in the developing world, the burden of disease remains high, with an estimated 2 to 2.6 million cases annually, resulting in nearly a million hospitalizations.[2] This chapter addresses the clinical and radiographic diagnosis of pneumonia, common viral and bacterial causes, evidence-based treatments, and appropriate disposition and follow-up for children seen in the ED. Wherever possible, you will see special mention of unusual microbes, changing patterns of immunization and resistance, and special considerations for children with underlying medical conditions. If you have limited pediatric experience, you may find the section on the use and interpretation of chest radiographs in children helpful.

PATHOPHYSIOLOGY

Pneumonia occurs through invasion of the lower respiratory tract by pathogens. Anatomic and mechanical barriers to infection include the nasal hairs and turbinates, cilia, epiglottis, and cough reflex. Humoral immunity is largely mediated by secretory immunoglobulin A, whereas cellular immunity and phagocytic cells (e.g., alveolar macrophages) further protect against infection. Infectious agents may be inhaled or aspirated directly into the lungs, invade respiratory epithelium and spread contiguously, or, less commonly, reach the lungs hematogenously. Viral inoculation is typically by droplet or fomite (e.g., influenza, respiratory syncytial virus), whereas bacterial pneumonia often follows colonization of the nasopharynx. Infection can result in injury or death of the respiratory epithelium, interstitial inflammation, or alveolar injury. The air space fills with exudate and WBCs, which disrupt oxygenation and cause air space collapse, with eventual ventilation-perfusion mismatch.

In most cases, the causative agent is never known. Definitive microbiologic diagnosis requires invasive procedures such as bronchial lavage or sampling of pleural effusion for culture, which are unavailable or impractical in the ED.

Overall, viruses predominate in younger children, although bacterial, atypical, fungal, parasitic, and opportunistic organisms can also cause disease. Infection with *Mycobacterium tuberculosis* can occur in areas where it is endemic and among children with immunodeficiency, so one should take into account local and regional epidemiology, individual immunization status, and underlying health problems that may influence which pathogens are likely. The types and causes of pneumonia vary considerably according to the age of the child; a few general rules and specific exceptions are described below.[3,4]

CLINICAL FEATURES AND ETIOLOGY

The cardinal symptoms of lower respiratory tract infection include cough, fever, tachypnea, and respiratory distress. However, signs and symptoms vary by age and specific causative agents. Both age-based etiology and pathogen-specific clinical patterns of disease are described below.

AGE-SPECIFIC CAUSES OF PNEUMONIA

Neonates Neonates (0 to 30 days of age) require special consideration because they are at risk from bacterial pathogens acquired from the birth canal at or around the time of delivery. Specific organisms of concern include group B streptococci, gram-negative enteric bacteria such as *Klebsiella* and *Escherichia coli*, and *Listeria monocytogenes*. Late-onset neonatal pneumonia may be caused by *Staphylococcus aureus*, *Streptococcus pneumoniae*, or *Streptococcus pyogenes*. Pneumonia due to maternal genital *Chlamydia trachomatis* has been largely eliminated in developed countries through the systematic screening and treatment of pregnant women[5] but is still a consideration if the mother has had little or no prenatal care. Any neonate with pneumonia is also at risk of sepsis, and **between birth and 3 months, infants with pneumonia should be evaluated for sepsis.**

Infants and Children between 30 Days and 2 Years of Age **Pneumonia in older infants and toddlers is usually viral rather than bacterial.**[6] Common causes include respiratory syncytial virus, influenza virus, parainfluenza virus, human metapneumovirus, and adenovirus. In this age group, the most common **bacterial** cause of community-acquired pneumonia remains *S. pneumoniae*. Other agents include *Haemophilus influenzae* type b in nonimmunized children and nontypeable *H. influenzae* in all children. Less common but important pathogens include *S. aureus* and *Bordetella pertussis*.

Children 2 to 5 Years Old As children get older and attend day care or school, they come into contact with many pathogens, particularly respiratory viruses.

In children between 2 and 5 years of age, most community-acquired pneumonia is caused by respiratory viruses, followed by *S. pneumoniae*, *H. influenzae* type b, or nontypeable *H. influenzae*.[4,7] *Mycoplasma* and *Chlamydophila pneumoniae* are thought to be less common in children <5 years old.[4,7,8] Pneumonias due to varicella-zoster virus, measles, *H. influenzae* type b, *B. pertussis*, and some strains of *Pneumococcus* are increasingly rare in areas of widespread vaccination and herd immunity.

Children 5 to 13 Years Old In children from age 5 to adolescence, *Mycoplasma pneumoniae* is thought to be a chief cause of community-acquired pneumonia, with *C. pneumoniae* and *S. pneumoniae* still important considerations.[7,9] Less common bacterial causes include *S. aureus* and *Legionella*.[6] *M. tuberculosis* is a rare but important agent to consider. Pertussis immunity from the newer acellular vaccine appears to wane (in the 5 years after vaccination), so consider *Bordetella* even in the immunized child if clinical symptoms are **strongly** suggestive.[10]

Adolescents By adolescence, most patients are assumed to have the same infectious risks as healthy adults. The prevalence of specific pathogens may vary according to region, season, and cyclical epidemics in the population. In North America, the role of atypical agents, especially mycoplasma and *C. pneumoniae*, is estimated to be significant, but data and guidelines from other parts of the industrialized world (e.g., Europe) suggest regional differences.[11]

UNIQUE AND HIGH-RISK GROUPS

Tuberculosis remains a consideration for children with known exposures and those from endemic areas such as Native reserves, Alaska, northern Canada, and some inner-city settings. Consider tuberculosis in immigrants from high-prevalence areas of the world, including Africa, Asia, and parts of Eastern Europe.

Children with underlying disease are at risk for specific infections. For example, younger children with cystic fibrosis are often infected with *S. aureus* in the first years of life, and later with *Pseudomonas*. Children with sickle cell disease are particularly susceptible to infection with encapsulated bacteria (e.g., pneumococcus, *Salmonella*, *Klebsiella*), which can cause acute chest syndrome and sepsis. Children with congenital or acquired immune deficiencies such as human immunodeficiency virus infection, malignancy, and congenital immunodeficiencies are at risk for opportunistic infections with agents such as *Pneumocystis jirovecii*, cytomegalovirus, and fungi.[1]

Unvaccinated children and those with incomplete immunization are at risk of serious morbidity and mortality from a variety of vaccine-preventable pathogens. They should be managed accordingly.

PATHOGEN-SPECIFIC PATTERNS OF DISEASE

"**Typical pneumonias**" classically present with high fever, chills, pleuritic chest pain, and productive cough and suggest a bacterial cause, especially *S. pneumoniae.* In contrast, "**atypical pneumonias**" are characterized by gradual onset over days to weeks, low-grade fever, nonproductive cough, and malaise, and suggest infection with agents like mycoplasma or *C. pneumoniae.* Unfortunately, there is significant overlap in the agents causing these symptoms, and it is not possible to pinpoint specific causative organisms by clinical findings alone.[4,12] If definitive identification of the pathogen is important, perform laboratory testing.

Despite these limitations, some patterns of disease do suggest certain etiologies (**Table 125-1**). **Staphylococcal pneumonia,** which may follow influenza, is notorious for rapidly progressing symptoms, high fever, toxicity, and presence of pulmonary abscesses. ***C. trachomatis*** infection in infants (which is rare where there is prenatal screening and treatment) often presents with a staccato cough, diffuse rales, and lack of fever, so-called *afebrile pneumonitis.* Scattered rales, rare wheezes, and bilateral interstitial infiltrates are all possible findings. Older children may complain of sore throat and dysphagia. *B. pertussis* and respiratory viruses are also implicated as possible causes.[13] ***Mycoplasma*** infection typically produces a hacking, dry cough and may be associated with extrapulmonary manifestations including arthralgias, rash, and even CNS symptoms.[14] An upper respiratory tract prodrome followed by paroxysmal cough, gasping respirations, and color change is characteristic of ***B. pertussis*** infection (whooping cough); the postinfection cough may persist for months. Consider **tuberculosis** with prolonged cough in the setting of identified risk factors and characteristic radiographic findings. Note that classic signs and symptoms of tuberculosis such as hemoptysis or tuberculosis-positive sputum may be absent in children, especially those with immune deficiencies.[15] Tuberculosis in infants and young children tends to progress more rapidly from infection to clinical disease than it does in older children and adults, and hematogenous spread to extrapulmonary sites is also possible.[16,17]

Wheezing in a young infant with respiratory infection typically points to **bronchiolitis** of viral origin. In older, school-age children, wheezing may suggest viral infection or *Mycoplasma* pneumonia.[5] Distinguishing between viral and bacterial causes of pneumonia is often difficult, and radiographs may not provide a specific diagnostic pattern.

TABLE 125-1 Patterns of Disease by Specific Pathogen

Infective Agent	Disease Characteristics	Comments
Staphylococcus aureus	Rapid onset, high fever, toxicity, pulmonary abscesses	Infection with influenza may predispose to secondary *Staphylococcus* pneumonia
Chlamydia trachomatis	Staccato cough, diffuse rales, "afebrile pneumonitis," possible wheeze; bilateral infiltrates	Primarily seen in neonates and young infants but rare with prenatal maternal screening and treatment
Mycoplasma pneumoniae	Hacking dry cough, headache, sore throat; may cause wheezing in school-age children	Extrapulmonary symptoms: arthralgias, rash, CNS involvement
Bordetella pertussis	Upper respiratory prodrome followed by paroxysmal cough, gasping, stridor, color change	Cough may persist for months
Mycobacterium tuberculosis	Prolonged cough and/or fever, extrapulmonary spread	Consider in children from endemic areas and those with known exposure; classic symptoms seen in adults (e.g., hemoptysis) may be absent in children
Respiratory syncytial virus	Upper respiratory symptoms, cough, wheezing, rales, rhonchi	Clinical diagnosis of classic symptoms in child <2 years old; seasonal epidemics

TABLE 125-2 Differential Diagnosis of Pneumonia

Infectious Causes	Noninfectious Causes	Extrapulmonary Causes
Upper respiratory tract infection ("cold"), otitis media	Foreign body aspiration	Sepsis
Bronchiolitis	Inhalation pneumonitis (e.g., hydrocarbon inhalation, chronic gastroesophageal reflux disease)	Cardiac anomalies (cyanotic heart disease, congestive heart failure, myocarditis)
	Intoxication (e.g., salicylate poisoning, carbon monoxide exposure)	Endocrinopathies (e.g., diabetic ketoacidosis)
	Congenital disorders (e.g., cystic fibrosis, sickle cell disease with chest crisis)	Neuromuscular disorders
	Anatomic abnormalities (e.g., congenital lobar emphysema, pulmonary sequestration, tracheoesophageal fistula, congenital cystic adenomatous malformation)	Inborn errors of metabolism
		GI emergencies (e.g., appendicitis with grunting)
	Neoplasm, metastasis	
	Pulmonary embolism	

SEVERE DISEASE

The British Thoracic Society Guidelines for community-acquired pneumonia in children defines severe disease in infants as a fever >38.5°C, respiratory rate >70 breaths/min, nasal flaring, grunting, cyanosis, apnea, and poor feeding. Severe disease in older children is similarly defined by fever >38.5°C, signs of respiratory distress (respiratory rate >50 breaths/min, cyanosis, grunting), and signs of dehydration.[3]

DIFFERENTIAL DIAGNOSIS

The differential diagnosis of pneumonia includes both infectious and noninfectious conditions as well as extrapulmonary disorders that may mimic or complicate lower respiratory tract infection (**Table 125-2**). Formulating a differential diagnosis is especially important for infants and very young children, who may have undiagnosed congenital anomalies.

For children with respiratory distress but *no* fever, look for causes other than pneumonia. Congenital heart disease may present with cyanosis, quiet tachypnea, or respiratory distress related to congestive heart failure (see chapter 126, "Congenital and Acquired Pediatric Heart Disease"). Kussmaul breathing suggests diabetic ketoacidosis or other metabolic disease. Toddlers are particularly at risk for foreign body aspiration and ingestion of toxins. Adolescents may intentionally or unintentionally take drug overdoses that speed or slow breathing.

DIAGNOSIS

HISTORY

Relevant history depends on age of the patient and the underlying health of the child. Many complaints are nonspecific (e.g., cough and fever) and are common to both upper and lower respiratory tract disease. The predictive value of specific signs and symptoms is discussed below (see "Physical Examination" section).

Ask about the presence, timing, and duration of cough, fever, rapid breathing, and difficult breathing. Ask about specific exposures, sick contacts, travel, and pets, when relevant.

Choking or persistent or recurrent lower respiratory tract symptoms suggest foreign body aspiration. Recurrent pneumonias may signify underlying disease such as cystic fibrosis, immune disorders, or anatomic abnormalities.

In young children, abdominal pain may be a clue to lower lobe pneumonia or effusion.

Fever is a common but nonspecific sign of both upper and lower respiratory tract infections.

Birth History Because neonates may acquire infections perinatally, be sure to ask questions about the mother's prenatal and perinatal health, including maternal infections (e.g., chlamydia, gonorrhea, group B streptococci, genital herpes, and human immunodeficiency virus status), intrapartum or postpartum fever, and any specific antibiotic or antiviral therapy received during labor and delivery. Other perinatal risk factors include prolonged rupture of membranes, prematurity, and immediate peripartum complications. Meconium aspiration may cause chemical or bacterial pneumonia in the first 24 to 72 hours of life. Neonatal stays in hospital suggest an underlying health problem and also increase the risk of nosocomial infection.

Medical History Ask about the child's hospitalizations since birth and major illnesses, especially chronic respiratory problems (e.g., asthma, recurrent wheezing). In the young child, consider an undiagnosed respiratory, cardiac, renal, or immune dysfunction. Children with congenital respiratory problems (e.g., cystic fibrosis, neuromuscular disorders, immune compromise) are at increased risk of infection with common and rare agents, respiratory failure, and treatment failure. Adjust treatment and disposition accordingly (see Table 125-4).

Social History Take a brief, focused social history, because it may influence both diagnosis and treatment. For example, children from the far north, Native reserves, or countries with high rates of tuberculosis may be exposed to this uncommon but serious infection. A travel history may also be relevant. Children born to human immunodeficiency virus–positive mothers are at risk of vertical transmission and immunocompromise. Social history may also influence treatment decisions. For outpatient management, make sure that caregivers understand instructions, can afford medication, and can provide the required care (see "Disposition and Follow-Up" section below).

Immunization History Always inquire about childhood immunizations, and review records for confirmation when possible. Table 106-4 in chapter titled Emergency Care of Children provides a typical childhood immunization schedule. Ensure that enough time has elapsed to develop protective antibodies—typically 4 to 6 weeks for primary vaccination and 1 week for a booster. An *unvaccinated* child is at risk of serious morbidity, and even death, from vaccine-preventable illness.

Annual immunization against influenza is recommended for children ≥6 months of age and for those at high risk due to underlying health conditions. Influenza vaccine must be given annually to account for seasonal antigenic changes (see "Special Considerations" section below). Priority is given to children with asthma, cystic fibrosis, and other pulmonary diseases; those with significant cardiac, renal, and immune disorders; and those with diabetes. Caregivers and healthcare providers should also be immunized to avoid transmission to these at-risk children.[18]

Around the globe, immunization against polio, pertussis, measles, and *H. influenzae* type b infection has significantly lowered the risk of pneumonias and respiratory failure associated with these diseases. In some cases, simple herd immunity has decreased the chances that a child will come into contact with these once-feared diseases, but sporadic outbreaks exist in nonimmunized populations.

Immunization against varicella (chickenpox) should protect against the secondary pneumonias associated with this virus, although use of the vaccine is not yet universal. Similarly, the administration of the bacillus Calmette-Guérin vaccine to provide partial protection against certain forms of tuberculosis varies by state, province, and country.

The introduction of a seven-strain pneumococcal conjugate vaccine (Prevnar®, PCV-7) in 2000 to 2001 led to dramatic decreases in invasive disease and modest but promising trends in the reduction of pneumococcal pneumonias, especially in children <2 years old.[19,20] Early reports suggested a somewhat diminished impact in human immunodeficiency virus–positive children.[21] Vaccine-specific serotypes are being replaced globally by nonvaccine strains, although newer PCV-10 and PCV-13 vaccines are expected to counteract some of this serotype substitution. Children who received the initial PCV-7 series should receive a booster with PCV-13 to gain additional immunity.[19] Vaccine coverage is universal in Canada but varies by state and private insurance provider in the United States.

TABLE 125-3 Tachypnea as an Indicator for Pneumonia*

Age	Tachypnea	Comments
<60 d old	>60 breaths/min	>70 breaths/min indicates severe disease
2–12 mo old	>50 breaths/min	
>1–5 y old	>40 breaths/min	>50 breaths/min indicates severe disease
>5 y old	>20 breaths/min[22]	>50 breaths/min indicates severe disease

*Determine rate before examination and when child is calm or sleeping; count respiratory rate for a full minute[23]; fever may increase the rate by up to 10 breaths/min for every 1°C (1.8°F) rise in patient temperature.[24]

The older 23-valent polysaccharide vaccine (Pneumovax®) is effective in children ≥2 years of age, and it should be confirmed that the vaccine has been given to children with sickle cell disease, those who have undergone splenectomy, and others at high risk for pneumococcal disease. A booster may be required.

PHYSICAL EXAMINATION

In the developing world where imaging equipment and laboratory tests are limited, the World Health Organization has proposed a diagnostic algorithm based *entirely* on the presence or absence of tachypnea, respiratory distress, and lower chest retractions or indrawing. Although physicians in industrialized nations have many tools at their disposal, the diagnosis of pneumonia can still be made clinically.

Rapid respiratory rate is a simple, standardized screening tool for pneumonia[4] (**Table 125-3**).

Children at very high altitudes may have a resting respiratory rate higher than children at sea level do, so oxygen saturation may be a more useful measure. Note that children who are severely malnourished or dehydrated or have impending respiratory failure may not be capable of generating rapid respiratory rates.

Markers of respiratory distress include nasal flaring, tracheal tug, and intercostal indrawing. Lower chest or "abdominal" indrawing or retractions and grunting suggest more severe pneumonia.[25] **In infants, intermittent apnea, grunting, and an inability to feed are surrogate markers of dyspnea.** Cough is less common in neonates or very young children, and productive cough is rarely seen before late childhood.

Document oxygen saturation, because **hypoxia on room air (arterial oxygen saturation <93% at sea level) increases the risk of oral amoxicillin treatment failure in severe pneumonia,**[26] and oxygen saturation <93% is a strong independent predictor of radiographic pneumonia.[27]

Auscultate the chest using an appropriately sized stethoscope with the chest fully exposed, assessing all lung zones. Localized fine crackles (rales), coarse breath sounds (rhonchi), or diminished breath sounds suggest pneumonia, but sound recognition may not be consistent across observers[23]; a toxic appearance and overall impression of illness as judged by the clinician show better diagnostic sensitivity than focal auscultatory findings.[4]

CLINICAL DIAGNOSIS

No single physical finding in isolation is diagnostic of pneumonia, and constellations of signs are more useful. For example, the combination of fever plus either tachypnea, decreased breath sounds, or fine crackles predicts x-ray–positive pneumonia with a sensitivity of 93% to 96%. **The presence of fever plus *all three* of the other variables raises sensitivity to 98%,** so much so that a radiograph is not required to make the diagnosis.[28]

Conversely, a small but frequently cited study confirms that the child without tachypnea, respiratory distress, rales, and decreased breath sounds does not have pneumonia; a radiograph is not indicated.[29]

Presumptive diagnosis of the causative organism and empiric treatment are made by considering historical and social factors (see above), immunization status (see above), and age of the child. See Table 125-4 for the most common causes of pneumonia by age as well as their treatment. Use care when assessing children with incomplete or no immunizations. Such children may be partially or fully susceptible to pneumonia associated with *B. pertussis*, *H. influenzae* type b, and all strains of pneumococcus, as well as measles, influenza, and varicella-zoster viruses.

LABORATORY EVALUATION

Because the results of most laboratory investigations are not known in the ED, tests are usually initiated to guide *future* treatment, except for rapid bedside tests for specific respiratory viruses. **Nasopharyngeal assays for respiratory syncytial virus, influenza, and human metapneumovirus can be valuable, because they are quick and specific and results may negate the need for imaging, invasive testing, and antibiotic therapy.** One may also defer imaging and antibiotic treatment for nontoxic children with clinical bronchiolitis or influenza, especially those with a positive nasopharyngeal swab finding.[3,22]

Bacterial cultures of nasopharyngeal samples are generally *not* helpful, because results are delayed and oral flora correspond poorly with the organisms causing disease in the lung. The majority of newer serologic and polymerase chain reaction techniques to detect organisms such as *H. influenzae* or *C. pneumoniae* have not been validated in children and have produced variable results.[3,5,22]

The routine collection of blood cultures *is not* recommended in healthy children with mild community-acquired pneumonia.[22] For toxic-appearing children and those with severe disease requiring hospitalization, obtain blood for culture, CBC, electrolytes, and renal and hepatic function. Currently, the literature does not support the routine use of inflammatory markers (C-reactive protein or erythrocyte sedimentation rate), acute-phase reactants, or procalcitonin to distinguish bacterial from viral pneumonia in children.[22]

When tuberculosis is suspected, obtain induced sputum samples from older children or gastric aspirates from infants for microscopy and confirmatory culture.[30] These tests require equipment and expertise beyond the scope of the ED.

IMAGING

Guidelines on the use of routine chest radiography are inconsistent.[3,22,31] Consider chest radiographs only when the results are likely to alter diagnosis, treatment, or outcome.

Benefits of radiography include diagnosis or confirmation of pneumonia and occasionally the discovery of a significant congenital abnormality. Risks and disadvantages include cost, delay, repeated exposure to ionizing radiation, and overdiagnosis of bacterial pneumonia.[32] Several studies and major guidelines state that imaging should *not* be performed routinely in children with mild, uncomplicated acute lower respiratory tract infections.[3,22,33,34] Most of these studies and guidelines reference outpatient settings, in which children with prolonged cough, severe symptoms, and other "red flag" features were excluded, so these recommendations may not apply to the ED setting.

The chest radiograph is *not* the gold standard of diagnosis, because it is neither 100% sensitive nor 100% specific[35] and may be falsely negative (e.g., when clinical disease precedes radiographic changes) or falsely positive (e.g., poor inspiration or rotation; **Figures 125-1 and 125-2**). Chest radiographs do not reliably distinguish between bacterial and viral causes.[36,37] Young children with straightforward viral bronchiolitis may show radiographic areas of atelectasis or patchy collapse, resulting in a temptation to initiate antibiotic therapy for viral disease.

Although routine radiographs are not usually necessary, potential indications for chest radiography are listed below:[8,38-40]

1. Infants and children with a toxic appearance and respiratory findings
2. Age of 0 to 3 months with fever, as part of a full sepsis evaluation
3. Child <5 years old, with a temperature of >39°C (102.2°F), WBC of ≥20,000/mm^3, and no clear source of infection
4. Suspicion of a complication, such as pleural effusion or pneumothorax
5. Pneumonia that is prolonged or unresponsive to treatment
6. Children with biphasic illness (typical symptoms of upper respiratory tract infection followed by acute worsening of [respiratory] symptoms and high fever)
7. Suspected foreign body aspiration

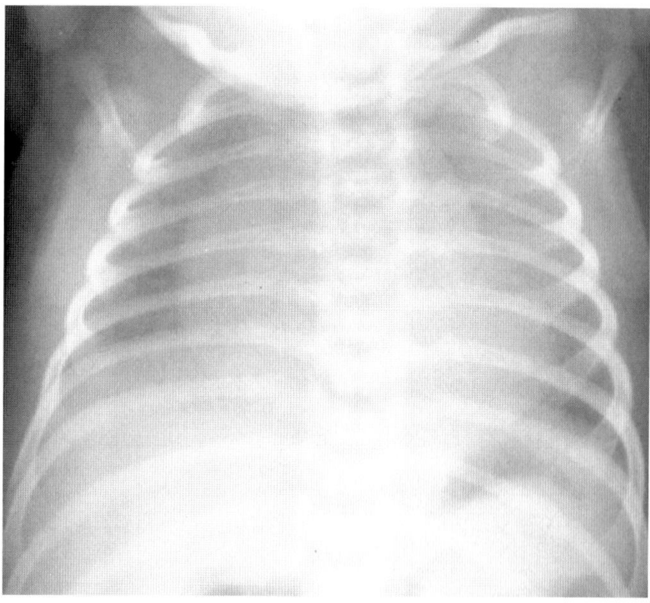

FIGURE 125-1. Poor inspiration results in the appearance of pulmonary infiltrates and cardiomegaly in this normal 4-month-old infant. [Photo contributed by BC Children's Hospital, Vancouver, British Columbia, Canada.]

8. Suspected congenital lung malformation (e.g., sequestration or congenital cystic adenomatous malformation)
9. Follow-up of "round pneumonia" (see Figure 125-5) to exclude an underlying mass

For a brief overview of important normal and abnormal radiographic findings unique to children, see the "The Pediatric Chest Radiograph" section at the end of this chapter.

TREATMENT

Treatment is based on the presumptive pathogen using information from history, immunizations, and age group (**Tables 125-4 to 125-6**).

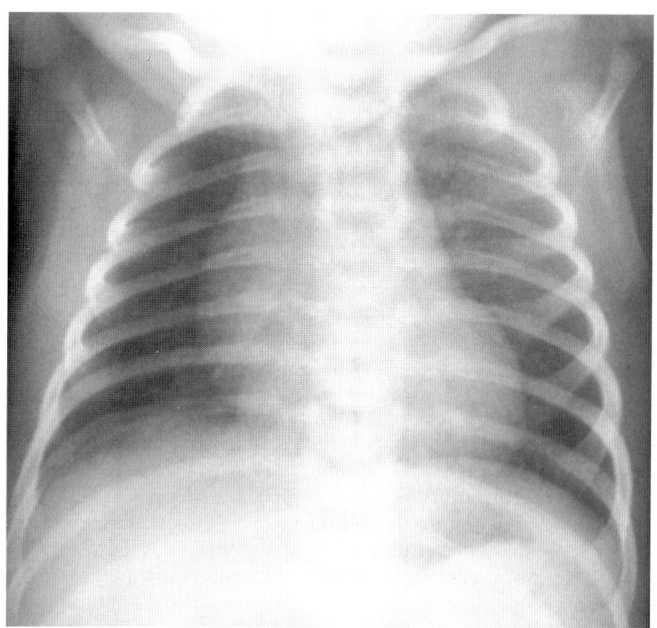

FIGURE 125-2. The same child as in Figure 125-1, with adequate inspiration. Note that persistent rotation (see clavicles) causes a false difference in left and right lung density. [Photo contributed by BC Children's Hospital, Vancouver, British Columbia, Canada.]

TABLE 125-4 Bacterial Organisms and Empiric Treatment for Pneumonia in Otherwise Healthy Children

Age Group	Bacterial Pathogens	Outpatient Treatment	Inpatient Treatment
Neonates	Group B *Streptococcus* Gram-negative bacilli *Listeria monocytogenes*	Initial outpatient management not recommended	Ampicillin + Gentamicin or cefotaxime
1–3 mo	*Streptococcus pneumoniae* *Chlamydia trachomatis* *Haemophilus influenzae* *Bordetella pertussis* *Staphylococcus aureus*	Initial outpatient management not recommended	Ampicillin or Ceftriaxone or Cefotaxime or Cefazolin or vancomycin[*] ± Macrolide[†]
3 mo–5 y[‡]	*S. pneumoniae* *H. influenzae* type b[#] Nontypeable *H. influenzae* *S. aureus*	Amoxicillin ± Clavulanate or Cefuroxime axetil	Ampicillin or Ceftriaxone or Cefotaxime or Cefazolin or vancomycin[*] ± Macrolide[†]
5–18 y	*Mycoplasma pneumoniae* *S. pneumoniae* *Chlamydophila pneumoniae* *H. influenzae* type b[#] *S. aureus*	Macrolide[*] or Amoxicillin ± Clavulanate or Doxycycline[ƒ] or Cefuroxime axetil	Ampicillin or Ceftriaxone or Cefotaxime or Cefazolin or vancomycin[*] ± Macrolide[†]

[*]For suspected *S. aureus:* cefazolin suggested if methicillin sensitive; vancomycin when methicillin-resistant *S. aureus* is suspected

[†]Macrolide should be used for suspected atypical infections (e.g., *M. pneumoniae, C. trachomatis, C. pneumoniae, B. pertussis*), and options include clarithromycin, erythromycin, or azithromycin.

[‡]The majority of pneumonias in preschool-age children are viral, not bacterial, and do not require antibiotics.[22]

[#]Uncommon where vaccination against *H. influenzae* type b is universal.

[ƒ]Do not use doxycycline for children <8 years of age to avoid staining permanent teeth.

SUPPORTIVE AND SYMPTOMATIC TREATMENT

General supportive measures include supplemental oxygen to maintain oxygen saturation >92%; antipyretics; oral, nasogastric, or intravenous fluids to offset respiratory losses; and bronchodilators for wheezing. Because children depend on cough to clear mucus, cough suppressants are not generally indicated. Over-the-counter cough suppressants are not effective and have been withdrawn from the market in several countries for children <5 years of age. Narcotic-based cough suppressants are occasionally prescribed in older children, but data on their effectiveness and proper dosage are lacking. Codeine in particular is discouraged due to the risk of respiratory suppression in some children.[41]

Treat noninfectious pneumonitis (e.g., chemical inhalation, aspiration) and likely viral pneumonia (e.g., age 3 months to 5 years, audible wheezing, positive bedside test for respiratory syncytial virus, or influenza) with supportive measures as outlined above. **Antibiotics are not indicated for viral pneumonia.** Febrile infants (even those <3 months of age) with bronchiolitis (clinical and respiratory syncytial virus–positive) are at low risk for concurrent bacterial pneumonia, bacteremia, and meningitis and do not require radiographs, blood or cerebrospinal fluid testing, or empiric antibiotic therapy for their respiratory infection. **The exception is infants less than 90 days old, who still have a small risk of concurrent urinary tract infection and should have their urine tested as part of a partial septic workup.**[33]

TABLE 125-5 Antibiotic Dosages for Bacterial Pneumonia

Antibiotic	Dosage[*]
Oral	
Amoxicillin ± clavulanate	80–100 milligrams/kg/d (amoxicillin component) in 3 divided doses
Azithromycin	10 milligrams/kg on day 1, then 5 milligrams/kg/d every 24 h for 4 doses
Clarithromycin	15 milligrams/kg/d in 2 divided doses
Erythromycin	30–50 milligrams/kg/d in 4 divided doses
Doxycycline[†]	2–4 milligrams/kg/d in 2 divided doses
Cefuroxime axetil	30 milligrams/kg/d in 2 divided doses
Parenteral	
Ampicillin	200 milligrams/kg/d every 6 h IV, IM
Cefotaxime	150 milligrams/kg/d every 8 h IV
Ceftriaxone	100 milligrams/kg/d every 12–24 h IV, IM
Gentamicin	7.5 milligrams/kg/d once daily IV, IM
Vancomycin[‡]	40–60 milligrams/kg/d every 6–8 h IV
Cefazolin	150 milligrams/kg/d every 8 h IV
Erythromycin lactobionate	20 milligrams/kg/d every 6 h
Azithromycin	10 milligrams/kg/d on days 1 and 2 of therapy and then transition to oral

[*]Weight-based amounts should not exceed maximum adult doses.

[†]Do not use doxycycline in children <8 y to avoid staining adult teeth.

[‡]Consult infectious disease or pediatric specialist for severely ill children with suspected methicillin-resistant *Staphylococcus aureus* pneumonia.

EMPIRIC ANTIBIOTIC TREATMENT

Treat all children with suspected *bacterial* pneumonia with prompt administration of empiric antibiotics.[4,6,8,38] Table 125-4 summarizes empiric treatment by age group, and Table 125-5 lists recommended antibiotic dosing.

Neonates In **neonates**, who are at risk of sepsis, administer ampicillin to cover *Listeria* and group B *Streptococcus* in conjunction with an aminoglycoside (e.g., gentamicin) or a third-generation cephalosporin (e.g., cefotaxime) for expanded coverage of gram-negative organisms such as *E. coli*. **Ceftriaxone is contraindicated in neonates because it can displace bound bilirubin.**

TABLE 125-6 Special Cases

Condition	Drug
Varicella pneumonia	Acyclovir
Respiratory syncytial virus pneumonia	Ribavirin, if high-risk patient
Interstitial pneumonia in a patient with human immunodeficiency virus	Trimethoprim-sulfamethoxazole ± prednisone[*]
Cytomegalovirus pneumonia	Ganciclovir and γ-globulin
Gram-negative pneumonia	Ceftazidime
Pneumonia in a patient with sickle cell disease	Cefotaxime ± macrolide ± vancomycin (in severely ill)
Pneumonia in a patient with cystic fibrosis[†]	Piperacillin + tobramycin *or* ceftazidime + tobramycin
Methicillin-resistant *Staphylococcus aureus* pneumonia	Clindamycin or vancomycin

[*]Empiric treatment for *Pneumocystis* infection.[15] World Health Organization recommends additional antibiotic therapy in severe cases.[42]

[†]Where possible, base selection on patient's most recent culture and sensitivity reports. Consult infectious disease specialist.

Young Infants 1 to 3 Months Old The syndrome of **afebrile** pneumonitis described in infants 1 to 3 months old (staccato cough, tachypnea, with or without progressive respiratory distress and diffuse pulmonary infiltrates) may be viral in origin but has also been associated with atypical bacteria, so authors have suggested empiric treatment with erythromycin or clarithromycin in this group.[4] **Note that azithromycin is not included in the treatment of patients this young, because it has not been approved by the U.S. Food and Drug Administration.**

Infants and Children ≥3 Months Old For children ≥3 months old, the choice of treatment remains largely empiric. There are notable differences between some North American and European recommendations,[3,11] but all presume the most frequent cause of bacterial pneumonia to be *S. pneumoniae*. For this reason, **high-dose oral amoxicillin (80 to 100 milligrams/kg/d) or another β-lactam antibiotic remains the drug of choice.** For children >5 years old, some North American guidelines assume that atypical agents such as *Mycoplasma* and *C. pneumoniae* play a more important role, so macrolides are often listed as first choice. This recommendation presumes that macrolides will treat both atypical pathogens *and* pneumococci. High rates of pneumococcal resistance to macrolides in vitro are a growing concern in many areas of the world, and several major guidelines now recommend amoxicillin with or without clavulanate as initial therapy for *all* children ≥3 months of age with simple community-acquired pneumonia.[3,22] **In cases where resistant pathogens or multiple pathogens are suspected, all guidelines make provisions for double coverage with β-lactams or cephalosporins *plus* macrolides.** With these considerations in mind, typical choices for primary or secondary bacterial pneumonia are listed in Tables 125-4 and 125-6.

For a child with significant underlying illness or fulminant viral pneumonia, special agents and antimicrobials may be indicated, and consultation is strongly advised. Specific cases and treatment suggestions are listed in Table 125-6.

These guidelines may need to be adapted according to formulary, familiarity, and local patterns of antibiotic resistance. Antibiotic choices for children with allergies, unusual exposures, or specific risk factors should be tailored in consultation with a specialist.

The choice of oral versus parenteral antibiotics depends on the clinical picture. Oral antibiotics provide adequate coverage for most mild-to-moderate cases of bacterial pneumonia. Parenteral therapy is usually limited to neonates and those with severe pneumonia requiring hospitalization.[4] Even for children who are admitted, oral treatment can be sufficient within the monitored setting of the hospital.[43]

The recommended duration of outpatient treatment is typically 7 to 10 days (5 days in cases in which azithromycin is used). This is based on historical precedent, although some literature suggests equivalent outcomes in mild pneumonia with as few as 3 to 5 days of outpatient treatment.[44-46] There are theoretical concerns, however, that shorter courses of treatment and poor adherence may drive bacterial resistance.

In pediatrics, the choice of antibiotic may also be influenced by important nonmicrobial factors, such as taste, cost, frequency of administration, availability of a liquid formulation, and the child's ability to swallow.

CONTROVERSIES OF TREATMENT

The use of macrolides (erythromycin, clarithromycin, azithromycin) as first-line agents in young children is an area of controversy.[5,47] Macrolides are generally effective against atypical and intracellular agents, which are more common in children after the age of 5 years, but they may be ineffective against common *S. pneumoniae*. **Pneumococcal resistance to macrolides in Europe and North America ranges from 7.5% to >50.0%.**[11] The indiscriminate use of azithromycin in treating upper respiratory tract infections appears to be driving streptococcal resistance in some populations.[48] The liquid suspension of azithromycin is not approved for children <6 months of age by the U.S. Food and Drug Administration. Some suggest that children who have fever of <2 days in duration and who are <3 years of age have a very low risk of community-acquired *Mycoplasma* infection and that macrolides can be safely excluded as first-line antibiotics.[49] If a preschool child fails to improve when taking amoxicillin or an equivalent β-lactam, consider adding a macrolide.

Pneumococcal resistance to penicillin and other β-lactams is another area of concern around the globe. To date, most antibiotic resistance in community-acquired streptococci has been documented in vitro, rather than in vivo, and clinical response is still satisfactory when clinicians use an increased dosage, as noted in Table 125-4.[50] The safety and efficacy of fluoroquinolones for respiratory infections in children is not established, and their use is generally restricted due to theoretical risks of arthropathy. Doxycycline, a much older and less expensive agent, has activity against atypical pathogens as well as streptococci but is restricted to use in adolescents and adults, because use in young children may cause permanent staining of the adult teeth. As resistance to amoxicillin, macrolides, and other antibiotics grows, the importance of *prevention* using pneumococcal conjugate vaccines is likely to increase.

DISEASE COMPLICATIONS

Most **viral** pneumonias resolve spontaneously without specific therapy. Complications are similar to those for bronchiolitis and include dehydration, bronchiolitis obliterans, and apnea. Apnea is a potential complication of infection with respiratory syncytial virus, *Chlamydia*, or *B. pertussis* infection in very young infants. Pleural effusions can occur with viral pneumonias but are not common.

Uncomplicated bacterial pneumonia usually responds within 72 hours to antibiotic therapy. Failure to respond or worsening of disease suggests a complication. These include pleural effusion, empyema, pneumothorax, or pneumatocele. Although effusions can occur in a small number of pneumococcal and mycoplasmal pneumonias, they are more commonly associated with *H. influenzae* type b infections; *S. aureus* is associated with empyema, abscess, and pneumatoceles. *Mycoplasma* pneumonia may cause extrapulmonary complications such as arthritis and meningitis, whereas local and hematogenous spread of tuberculosis can result in myriad manifestations both inside and outside the lung. Systemic complications of pneumonia include dehydration, sepsis, and hemolytic-uremic syndrome.

The child with pneumonia who returns to the ED with a worsening clinical picture should always cause concern. If the initial treatment was supportive care for a presumed viral pneumonia, consider secondary bacterial pneumonia or an alternative diagnosis (e.g., cardiac disease, congenital anomaly, foreign body).[51] Similarly, a child receiving antibiotics who returns with diminished breath sounds, dullness to percussion, or worsening respiratory distress should prompt you to look for complications, such as empyema, effusion, or pneumothorax. If you suspect antibiotic-resistant pneumonia, you may need to get blood or pleural fluid cultures because clinical findings cannot reliably differentiate between drug-resistant and drug-sensitive pathogens.[52,53]

DISPOSITION AND FOLLOW-UP

Recommendations for outpatient, inpatient, and intensive care treatment of pneumonia are presented in **Table 125-7**.[3] In addition to these clinically based criteria, neonates and infants up to 90 days old require hospital admission, as do infants and children with significant comorbid disease (e.g., cystic fibrosis, sickle cell disease, underlying immunodeficiency or malignancy). Social indications for admission include the inability of parents or caregivers to afford, understand, or ensure outpatient treatment.[3] If there is a risk that adults cannot bring a child back for follow-up with a healthcare provider in 24 to 48 hours, also consider admission.

Infants with suspected *B. pertussis* infection (whooping cough) are at risk for apnea and should be admitted under respiratory isolation. Indications for hospitalizing patients with respiratory syncytial virus pneumonia are the same as those for patients with respiratory syncytial virus bronchiolitis (see chapter 124, "Wheezing in Infants and Children"). Admit children of any age with suspected active pulmonary tuberculosis, under respiratory isolation. Patients who fail a trial of oral antibiotics and those with complications of pneumonia require admission for further diagnosis and therapy. The finding of a pleural effusion or pneumatocele or findings suggestive of a bacterial infection in a child <1 year of age suggest a pathogen other than *S. pneumoniae* (in particular *H. influenzae* type b or *S. aureus*); hospitalize these children.

TABLE 125-7 Disposition of Infants and Children with Pneumonia

Age	Outpatient Management	Inpatient Management	Intensive Care Management
Infants	Mild-to-moderate symptoms (no cyanosis, grunting, significant retractions), oxygen saturation >92%, respiratory rate (RR) <70 breaths/min, feeding well and well hydrated, reliable caretakers and outpatient follow-up	Oxygen saturation <93%, RR >70 breaths/min, respiratory distress (retractions, grunting, apnea), poor feeding, dehydration, family unable to provide appropriate home observation or assure follow-up	Inability to maintain oxygen saturation >92% with fraction of inspired oxygen >0.6, severe respiratory distress or recurrent apnea, respiratory fatigue, signs of shock
Children	Mild-to-moderate symptoms (no cyanosis, grunting, significant retractions), oxygen saturation >92%, RR <50 breaths/min, feeding well and well hydrated, reliable caretakers and outpatient follow-up	Oxygen saturation >93%, RR >50 breaths/min, respiratory distress (retractions, grunting, apnea), poor feeding, dehydration, family unable to provide appropriate home observation or assure follow-up	

DISCHARGE INSTRUCTIONS

Provide all children and families with specific instructions on the dosage and scheduling of medications and the signs of worsening respiratory distress. Encourage return to medical care for children who cannot take prescribed antibiotics or adequate amounts of fluid. Ensure that all children discharged with the diagnosis of pneumonia have follow-up within a day or two with a primary care provider. Younger children require closer follow-up.

Many factors predispose children to pneumonia. Quickly review the following topics with parents and caregivers:

1. Hand washing and general hygiene to prevent transmission
2. Breastfeeding of infants, which is known to be protective
3. Avoidance of smoking (by teens) and second-hand smoke
4. Vaccination, including pneumococcal conjugate vaccine (Prevnar®, Synflorix®), as well as polysaccharide vaccine (Pneumovax®) for at-risk children older than 2 years

SPECIAL CONSIDERATIONS

For a child with significant underlying illness or fulminant viral pneumonia, special agents and antimicrobials may be indicated, and consultation is strongly advised. Specific cases and treatment suggestions are listed in Table 125-6.

INFLUENZA

Influenza is a common cause of respiratory infections worldwide. Classic symptoms include fever, cough, runny nose, headache, and myalgias, lasting up to 7 days.

Complications of influenza include secondary bacterial pneumonia and occasionally a pneumonia from the virus itself.[54] Apnea is a rare but serious complication in young infants.

Point-of-care and other rapid testing may be helpful in pinpointing influenza as the source of fever in children and avoiding a search for additional causes. Sensitivities are moderate (40% to 70%), but specificities are high (85% to 100%), if performed within the first 4 days of symptoms.[55] If a false-negative result is suspected, you can perform confirmatory polymerase chain reaction or viral culture.

Treatment of influenza is largely supportive, with fluids, rest, and fever control. Note that acetylsalicylic acid should not be used for fever control, due to the risk of Reye's syndrome.

The role for antivirals is unclear. A 2012 Cochrane meta-analysis of the older medications amantadine and rimantadine showed a limited role in prevention and amelioration of influenza A in children. The number needed to treat was high (n = 12), and the quality of evidence was low.[56]

The newer neuraminidase inhibitors oseltamivir (Tamiflu®) and zanamivir (Relenza®) showed initial promise, but subsequent reviews of the data have cast serious doubts on the utility of these drugs to shorten symptoms or prevent serious complications such as pneumonia.[57]

With few treatments available, the best defense against influenza and its associated pneumonias remains annual vaccination, frequent hand washing, and droplet precautions.

The U.S. Centers for Disease Control and Preventions and the American Academy of Pediatrics recommend routine annual influenza vaccination for children 6 months and older. Special emphasis is placed on children 4 years and under, because they are most at risk for complications and most likely to transmit disease in the community.

Children generally require a single dose of the vaccine annually, to account for antigenic changes in the virus from year to year. Those being vaccinated for the very first time may require a second dose at least 28 days later.

A nasal form of the vaccine containing live, attenuated virus is approved for children 2 years of age and older and may improve compliance. However, there is an increased risk of wheezing when used in children with a prior history of wheeze. Those with asthma or immune suppression should use the standard, injectable vaccine, which contains no live virus.

TUBERCULOSIS

Children of all ages are susceptible to tuberculosis, and most have *primary* disease, rather than secondary reactivation. Both upper lobe infiltrates and hilar lymphadenopathy on chest radiograph suggest the diagnosis, but classic findings can be absent in children, especially those with immune deficiencies.[15] Infants and young children tend to progress rapidly from infection to clinical disease, and hematogenous spread can lead to the radiographic "snowstorm" appearance of miliary tuberculosis.[16] Secondary tuberculosis has a predilection for the upper segments of the lung, as in adults, and may yield a cavitary lesion in some cases. *Mycobacterium avium* lesions may be indistinguishable from those of secondary tuberculosis.

OPPORTUNISTIC INFECTIONS

Nodular findings in the lungs may alert the astute clinician to the presence of other, rare infectious agents, such as *Histoplasma*, *Aspergillus*, and *Pneumocystis*. Pediatric patients with human immunodeficiency virus/acquired immunodeficiency syndrome may be susceptible to all of these, as well as cytomegalovirus, lymphomas, and lymphocytic interstitial pneumonia.

CYSTIC FIBROSIS

Children with cystic fibrosis have decreased mucus clearance, which leads to small-airway obstruction. More advanced disease results in chest radiograph findings such as peribronchial thickening and mucous plugging, with subsequent cystic or bullous lung lesions, segmental atelectasis, and hilar adenopathy. Air trapping may be seen on expiratory views. Patients with cystic fibrosis are also at risk for pneumothorax.

ASPIRATION PNEUMONIA

Patchy atelectasis and air space consolidation in the dependent zones of the lung should raise suspicion of aspiration pneumonia or pneumonitis. Recurrent aspiration pneumonias may occur in children with chronic gastroesophageal reflux disease, tracheoesophageal fistula, developmental delay, immobility, or neuromuscular disorders.

THE PEDIATRIC CHEST RADIOGRAPH

NORMAL NEONATAL ANATOMY

The chest of a neonate (<1 month of age) has a more pyramidal or trapezoidal shape than the long, rectangular form of the adult. The cardiac silhouette may occupy up to 60% or 65% of the chest width on

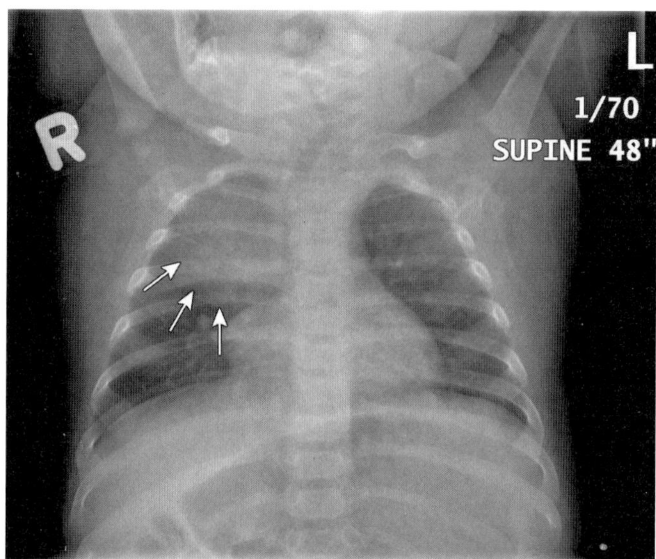

FIGURE 125-3. *Arrows* indicate a normal thymus. Rotation, apparent from the location of the heart, trachea, and clavicles, makes this thymus appear to be far right of midline. [Photo contributed by BC Children's Hospital, Vancouver, British Columbia, Canada.]

the frontal view and still be considered normal. In infants, bronchial branching may be visible beyond the level of the carina, giving the false impression of pathologic air bronchograms. The thymus appears as a large, dense, anterior mediastinal "sail," until involution occurs around age 6. A normal thymus can often be recognized by the sharp inferior edge of its silhouette and occasionally by a "wave" or "sail" sign at the lateral edge, where the adjacent ribs indent this soft, solid organ. Occasionally the thymus may be confused with a lobar pneumonia, mediastinal mass, or hilar lymphadenopathy (**Figure 125-3**). A lateral view can help to confirm the **anterior** location of the thymus (**Figure 125-4**). A silhouette that extends behind the heart shadow or posterior to the vertical lucency of the trachea should be investigated.

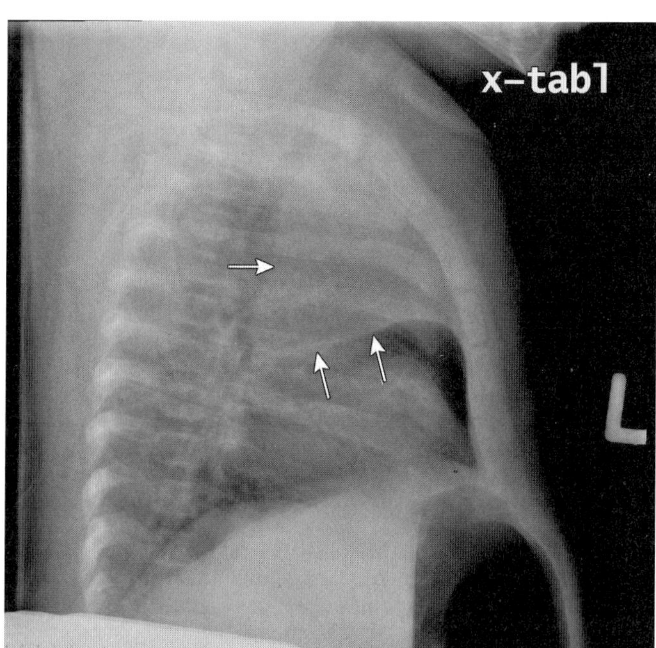

FIGURE 125-4. Lateral view confirms thymic density fully confined to the anterior mediastinum (*arrows*). [Photo contributed by BC Children's Hospital, Vancouver, British Columbia, Canada.]

TRANSIENT TACHYPNEA OF THE NEWBORN AND MECONIUM PNEUMONITIS

Occasionally parents may bring a very young newborn to the ED because of real or perceived breathing difficulties. Noninfectious causes of tachypnea and respiratory distress in the first few days of life include transient tachypnea of the newborn, or "wet lung," and chemical pneumonitis from meconium aspiration. The former may cause increased vascular markings, linear interstitial opacities, and even pleural effusions on radiographs due to interstitial edema. Meconium aspiration can block small airways, leading to hyperinflation and bilateral air space opacities

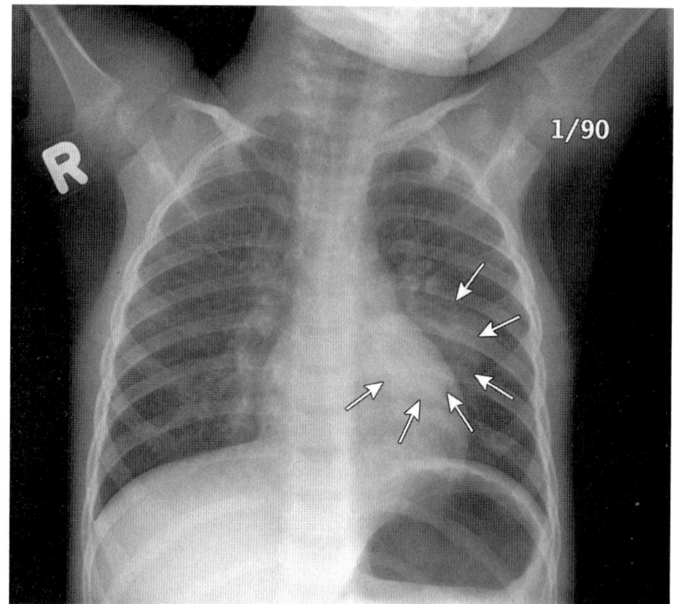

A

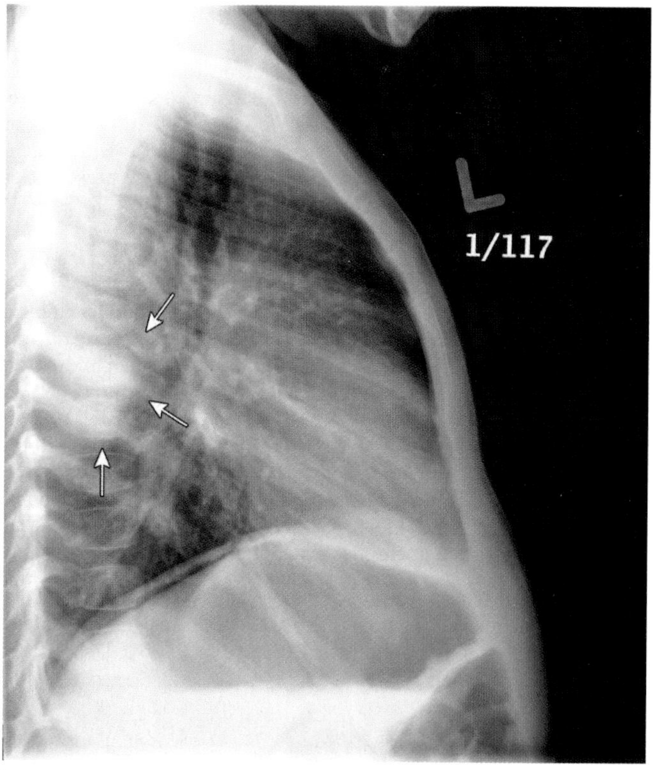

B

FIGURE 125-5. Anterior-posterior (**A**) and lateral views (**B**) show lower lobe consolidation (*arrows*). [Photos contributed by BC Children's Hospital, Vancouver, British Columbia, Canada.]

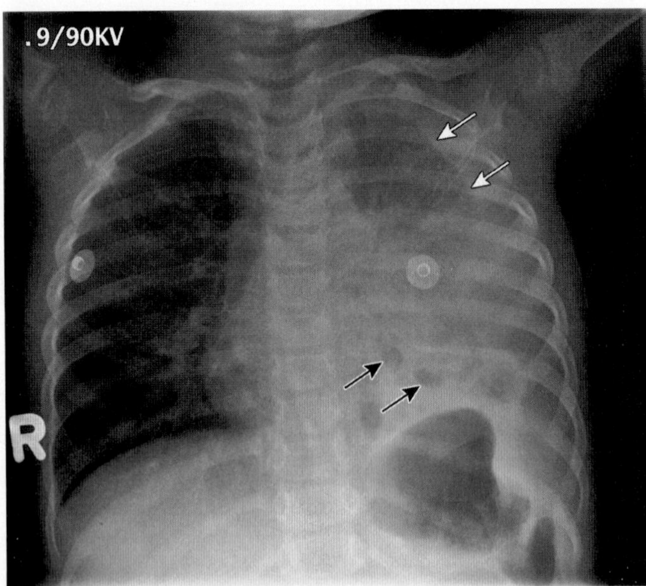

FIGURE 125-6. Complicated left-sided pneumonia. Note the pleural effusion (*white arrows*) and cavitation (*black arrows*). [Photo contributed by BC Children's Hospital, Vancouver, British Columbia, Canada.]

on plain radiographs. Signs of interstitial opacities or edema should prompt observation and/or consultation with a specialist.

FOREIGN BODY OR HYDROCARBON ASPIRATION

In addition to pneumonias from the infectious causes, toddlers are susceptible to choking and foreign body aspiration from objects they can reach. These may include organic materials (e.g., food) or inorganic objects (coins, buttons, batteries), as well as volatile toxins such as cleaning products, gasoline, or other hydrocarbons. Retained foreign bodies can lead to respiratory distress and febrile aspiration pneumonia. Radiopaque foreign bodies will appear on the chest radiograph; signs of *radiolucent* foreign bodies include asymmetric air trapping or segmental collapse past an obstructed bronchus. By contrast, inhaled hydrocarbons and irritants may yield a pneumonitis with patchy lower air space opacities and even pneumatoceles if the presentation is delayed.

PNEUMONIA IN THE OLDER CHILD

By school age, the radiographic signs of chest infection in children become more like the typical findings in adults. There may be obvious lobar consolidation or patchy, multifocal findings. Younger children can also present with "round pneumonia" (**Figure 125-5**), a sharply defined consolidation often found in the posterior lower lobe, classically from pneumococcal infection. **Children with round pneumonias should have radiographic follow-up** to confirm resolution and ensure that this finding is not actually a mass. Cavitation and pleural effusions should arouse suspicion of infection with *S. aureus* or *S. pneumoniae*, particularly penicillin-resistant pneumococcus (**Figure 125-6**).

Acknowledgments: The author would like to thank Dr. Gordon Culham, Department of Radiology, BC Children's Hospital, Vancouver, British Columbia, and Dr. James McCormack of the BC Therapeutics Initiative for their input.

REFERENCES

The complete reference list is available online at www.TintinalliEM.com.

CHAPTER 126 Congenital and Acquired Pediatric Heart Disease

Esther L. Yue
Garth D. Meckler

INTRODUCTION

This chapter reviews congenital and acquired heart disease in children. The section on congenital heart defects begins with a review of fetal and neonatal cardiac physiology, followed by a discussion of specific lesions and their diagnosis and management organized by clinical presentation. A brief discussion of pediatric murmurs follows, and the section concludes with a discussion of common surgical procedures for repairing congenital heart defects and associated complications.

The section on acquired heart disease in children reviews inflammatory and infectious disorders and cardiomyopathies, of which the most important is hypertrophic cardiomyopathy.

PEDIATRIC CARDIAC PHYSIOLOGY

FETAL CIRCULATION

Fetal circulation involves a number of shunts to bypass the liquid-filled lungs, which are incapable of providing oxygen to circulating blood. Blood oxygenated by the maternal lungs passes through the placenta via the umbilical vein to the fetus. Roughly half of the blood flow passes through the liver and half through the ductus venosus to the inferior vena cava, where it mixes with deoxygenated fetal blood returning from the lower body. The inferior vena cava enters the right atrium, where deoxygenated blood returning from the upper body and head via the superior vena cava mixes with that from the inferior vena cava. Blood from the right atrium travels in one of three routes: A portion passes through the foramen ovale into the left atrium, where it subsequently travels to the left ventricle, through the aorta, and into the vessels supplying the fetal head and upper extremities; most of the remainder enters the right ventricle and passes into the pulmonary artery, where the majority is shunted away from the lungs through the ductus arteriosus connecting the pulmonary artery with the aorta; and a small amount of blood travels to the lungs to provide oxygen and nutrients to support fetal lung growth.[1]

TRANSITIONAL CIRCULATION

The newborn's lungs expand and become air filled with gradual reabsorption of fetal lung fluid. This increases the partial pressure of arterial oxygen (Pa_{O_2}) of blood flowing through the newborn lung, which in turn mediates a cascade of events that completes the transition to adult circulatory patterns. Flow through the umbilical arteries ceases, and the venous flow through the cord slows and then stops. Pulmonary vascular resistance falls, and pulmonary blood flow increases (pulmonary vascular resistance continues to fall with increases in blood flow over the first 30 to 45 days of extrauterine life). The ductus venosus and ductus arteriosus close, and decreased pulmonary arterial resistance coupled with increased systemic resistance create increased blood flow through the atria. Left atrial pressure exceeds right atrial pressure, which leads to closure of the foramen ovale.

NEONATAL CARDIAC PHYSIOLOGY

Because neonates and small children have relatively noncompliant ventricular walls, they cannot increase stroke volume but rely on changes in heart rate to adjust cardiac output. Thus, sinus tachycardia is usually the first response to stress in infants and young children. The neonatal myocardium requires more oxygen than the infant's or child's heart and has a lower systolic reserve, which predisposes to congestive heart failure. Although the ductus arteriosus and foramen ovale are usually functionally closed by 15 hours of life and 3 months of age, respectively, shunting may still occur through these pathways during times of stress.[2] Finally, the neonatal right ventricle is still predominant, whereas the left ventricle is predominant in older infants and children, and pulmonary vascular resistance is relatively high and oxygen responsive.

Preload is the amount of blood that the heart receives to distribute to the body. Decreasing the amount of blood flowing into the heart lowers cardiac output. Similarly, increasing the amount of blood into the heart increases cardiac output in accordance with Starling forces, to the point of maximum compliance of the ventricular wall. When the ventricular wall compliance is exceeded, cardiac output decreases dramatically and congestive heart failure occurs.

Afterload is the resistance to blood flow out of the heart and is determined in neonates by the size and compliance of the ventricles, peripheral vascular resistance (which is largely mediated by catecholamines), and, when present, anatomic obstructions such as aortic stenosis or critical coarctation of the aorta.

Contractility or *inotropy*, which is the ability of the cardiac muscle to pump blood out of the heart, refers to the force or power of cardiac contraction and determines the amount of work that the heart can perform. Increasing the cardiac contractility increases the stroke volume and hence the cardiac output. Cardiac contractility is normally regulated by neural or humoral mechanisms. The ability of the neonatal heart to increase contractility is limited, as previously mentioned, and stroke volume is primarily increased through increases in rate.

Cardiac rate or *chronotropy* is the ability of the heart muscle to pump blood out of the heart per fixed unit of contraction. In the typical circumstance, chronotropy and inotropy cannot be differentiated with regard to therapeutic maneuvers. Typically, both the cardiac rate and the relatively fixed contractility of the neonatal heart contribute to the overall cardiac output, with the former contributing more of the output. In the hearts of children older than 4 or 5 years, there is a more balanced contribution to cardiac output, with the contractility playing a much more prominent role.

CONGENITAL HEART DISEASE

INTRODUCTION AND EPIDEMIOLOGY

Congenital heart defects can present at different ages with clinical signs and symptoms ranging from cyanosis to cardiovascular collapse or congestive heart failure depending on the anatomy and physiology of the lesion. Long-term survivors are at risk for a number of postoperative complications.

Congenital heart defects occur in approximately eight in 1000 births and range from benign to life threatening. About 10% of congenital heart defects are associated with genetic syndromes such as trisomy 21, Turner's syndrome, and Noonan's syndrome, and heart defects may accompany other organ malformations in conditions such as VACTERL association (*v*ertebral anomalies, *a*nal atresia, *c*ardiac anomalies, *t*racheoesophageal fistulas, *e*sophageal atresia, *r*enal and *l*imb anomalies, and single umbilical artery). The remaining 90% of congenital heart defects result from isolated embryologic malformation or as yet undefined genetic lesions.

Congenital heart disease is usually classified based on physiology (presence or absence of cyanosis, with or without persistent fetal circulation) or on the nature of the anatomic defect (shunt, obstruction, transposition, or complex defect). Most textbooks separate cyanotic from acyanotic lesions.

Cyanotic lesions result in mixing of deoxygenated and oxygenated blood or right-to-left shunting; cyanotic lesions include the **"five Ts"**: **tetralogy of Fallot**, tricuspid anomalies including **tricuspid atresia** and **Ebstein's anomaly**, **truncus arteriosus**, **total anomalous pulmonary venous return**, and **transposition of the great arteries**. **Acyanotic lesions** include those that result in pulmonary overcirculation such as **ventricular septal defect**, **atrial septal defect**, **patent ductus arteriosus**, and **atrioventricular canal** as well as those with restricted pulmonary or systemic blood flow such as pulmonary stenosis, aortic stenosis, and aortic coarctation.

It is often more useful to organize congenital heart disease by clinical presentation (**Table 126-1**). Distinct clinical presentations are discussed further in later sections, including the pathophysiology, clinical features and treatment, and individual defects within each group. Discussion of murmurs and arrhythmias included in this chapter is limited to those related to congenital heart disease. Rhythm disturbances are discussed in greater detail in the later section, "Acquired Heart Disease," and syncope and sudden death are discussed in chapter 127, Syncope, Dysrhythmias, and ECG Interpretation in Children.

TABLE 126-1 Clinical Presentations of Congenital Heart Disease

Clinical Presentation	Causative Conditions in Neonates	Causative Conditions in Infants and Children
Cyanosis	Transposition of the great arteries, TOF, tricuspid atresia, truncus arteriosus, total anomalous pulmonary venous return	TOF, Eisenmenger's complex
Cardiovascular shock	Critical AS, coarctation of the aorta, HLHS	Coarctation of the aorta (infants)
Congestive heart failure	Rare: PDA, HLHS	PDA, VSD, ASD, atrioventricular canal
Murmur	PDA, valvular defects (AS, PS)	VSD, ASD, PDA, outflow obstructions, valvular defects (AS, PS)
Syncope	—	AS, PS, Eisenmenger's complex
Hypertension	—	Coarctation of the aorta
Arrhythmias	—	ASD, Ebstein's anomaly, postsurgical complication after repair of congenital heart defect

Abbreviations: AS = aortic stenosis; ASD = atrial septal defect; HLHS = hypoplastic left heart syndrome; PDA = patent ductus arteriosus; PS = pulmonic stenosis; TOF = tetralogy of Fallot; VSD = ventricular septal defect.

CYANOSIS IN CONGENITAL HEART DISEASE

Cyanosis is the bluish discoloration of the skin that occurs from the presence of deoxygenated hemoglobin (which is blue) in capillary beds. For cyanosis to be clinically apparent, 3 to 5 milligrams/dL of deoxyhemoglobin must be present, corresponding to an oxygen saturation of 70% to 80% on room air.[3-5] Compression of the placenta during birth typically leads to polycythemia in term newborns, and, as a result, clinical cyanosis develops more readily in newborns because a smaller percentage of circulating hemoglobin must be desaturated to manifest this sign.

Congenital heart defects that present with cyanosis include transposition of the great arteries, tetralogy of Fallot, tricuspid atresia, truncus arteriosus, and total anomalous pulmonary venous return. These lesions have in common the mixing of oxygenated and deoxygenated blood, circulation of desaturated hemoglobin, and a cardinal manifestation as cyanotic heart disease. Another condition resulting in cyanosis is **persistent fetal circulation**, which can be caused by structural heart disease or noncardiac disease, including meconium aspiration, pneumonia, sepsis, and pulmonary hypertension. Lesions that restrict pulmonary blood flow, such as critical pulmonary stenosis, do not typically cause cyanosis without the presence of associated defects (atrial septal defect, ventricular septal defect) that allow for right-to-left shunting.

Congenital heart defects can lead to cyanosis in the first weeks of life or, for some lesions, episodically throughout childhood if uncorrected. Lesions such as transposition of the great arteries are associated with mixing of oxygenated and deoxygenated blood, usually through an associated ventricular septal defect or atrial septal defect, and produce cyanosis in the period immediately after birth. Conditions associated with persistent pulmonary hypertension allow blood to shunt right to left through a patent foramen ovale or through a septal defect. Tetralogy of Fallot (see the next section, "Tetralogy of Fallot") can produce cyanosis at birth through mixing, but is also associated with episodic cyanosis ("**tet spells**"; see the later section, "Treatment of Tet Spells") throughout infancy and childhood if uncorrected. Large uncorrected septal defects (e.g., ventricular septal defect) can cause cyanosis in adolescents and young adults in a condition termed Eisenmenger's complex. Chronic left-to-right shunting across a nonrestrictive defect leads to hypertrophy of pulmonary arteriolar musculature that causes a gradual and irreversible rise in pulmonary vascular resistance and right-sided heart pressures until supersystemic pressures develop and shunting switches to right to left, which produces cyanosis.

Noncardiac causes of cyanosis range from benign peripheral vasoconstriction in response to cold or crying, causing peripheral cyanosis, to sepsis with poor perfusion or even effects of toxins such as methemoglobin.[6] The most common congenital heart defects that must be considered in the cyanotic neonate are briefly reviewed in the sections below before returning to a general approach to the evaluation and management of cyanotic congenital heart disease.

Tetralogy of Fallot Tetralogy of Fallot is the most common cyanotic congenital heart disease manifesting in the postinfancy period and comprises as much as 10% of all congenital heart disease.[7-10] There are four primary components of tetralogy of Fallot: a large ventricular septal defect, right ventricular outflow obstruction (created by valvular or supravalvular pulmonic stenosis), an overriding aorta, and right ventricular hypertrophy.

The intensity of cyanosis depends on the amount of obstruction of the right ventricular outflow tract. A nonrestrictive ventricular septal defect balances the systolic pressures in the right and left ventricles. The amount of right ventricular outflow obstruction determines whether shunting is left to right, bidirectional, or right to left. Severe pulmonic stenosis creates a right-to-left shunt, resulting in cyanosis and decreased pulmonary blood flow. The acyanotic form of tetralogy of Fallot is characterized by mild pulmonic stenosis with a left-to-right shunt. In addition to cyanosis, examination findings can include a systolic thrill at the lower and middle left sternal border. A loud single S_2, an aortic ejection click, a loud systolic ejection murmur (heard best at the middle to lower left sternal border), and a continuous patent ductus arteriosus murmur may also be apparent on examination.

Transposition of the Great Arteries Comprising about 5% to 8% of all congenital heart disease, transposition of the great arteries is the most common cyanotic heart lesion manifesting in the newborn period. Compared to other congenital heart defects, extracardiac anomalies occur less often in babies with transposition of the great arteries (<10%).[11] There are many variations in transposition of the great arteries, but the underlying elements are that the aorta arises from the right ventricle and the main pulmonary artery originates from the left ventricle. This arrangement gives rise to two distinct circulatory systems. Because the main pulmonary artery has higher oxygen saturation than the aorta, hyperoxic blood goes through the pulmonary system and hypoxic blood flows through the systemic system. Mixing of the two circulatory systems is the only manner in which oxygenated blood enters the systemic blood flow. A ventricular septal defect, atrial septal defect, or patent ductus arteriosus must exist in order for the infant to survive. In 20% to 40% of patients, a ventricular septal defect is present. The physical examination is notable for a loud and single S_2, and if a ventricular septal defect exists, a systolic murmur may be heard.

Total Anomalous Pulmonary Venous Return Total anomalous pulmonary venous return represents 1% of congenital heart disease.[12] The pulmonary veins empty into the right atrium instead of returning blood from the lungs into the left atrium. Total anomalous pulmonary venous return is usually separated into four groups depending on where the pulmonary veins empty. In the supracardiac type (50% of all total anomalous pulmonary venous return cases), the common pulmonary vein is attached to the superior vena cava. In the cardiac type (20%), the common pulmonary vein drains into the coronary sinus. In the infracardiac/subdiaphragmatic type (20%), the common pulmonary vein empties into the portal vein, ductus venosus, hepatic vein, or inferior vena cava. Mixed lesions comprise the remaining 10%. Survival depends on the mixing of blood, so an atrial septal defect or a patent foramen ovale must be present.

When pulmonary venous return arrives in the right atrium, there is mixing of the pulmonary and systemic circulations. In the right atrium, blood crosses the atrial septal defect to the left atrium or crosses the tricuspid valve to the right ventricle. Systemic arterial blood becomes desaturated because of the mixing of pulmonary and systemic arterial flow. Pulmonary blood flow determines the degree of desaturation of systemic arterial blood. If there is no obstruction to pulmonary venous return, systemic blood is minimally desaturated. Obstruction to pulmonary venous return results in severe cyanosis. Because of the extra volume returning to the right side of the heart, right ventricular and atrial enlargement can develop.

Although total anomalous pulmonary venous return more commonly presents with signs and symptoms of congestive heart failure (see later section, "Congestive Heart Failure in Congenital Heart Disease"), tachypnea, tachycardia, hepatomegaly, and cyanosis are commonly seen. Children with pulmonary venous obstruction often have a history of frequent pneumonias and growth retardation. The physical examination reveals a right ventricular heave and fixed split S_2. A grade 2/6 to 3/6 systolic ejection murmur heard at the left upper sternal border and a mid-diastolic rumble at the left lower sternal border are also heard. Total anomalous pulmonary venous return with pulmonary venous obstruction leads to respiratory distress and cyanosis with a loud and single S_2 and a gallop but, on most occasions, no murmur.

Tricuspid Atresia Tricuspid atresia represents 1% to 2% of congenital heart disease.[13] There is no tricuspid valve, and the development of the right ventricle and pulmonary artery is interrupted. Pulmonary blood flow is decreased. With no flow existing between the right atrium and right ventricle, an atrial septal defect, ventricular septal defect, or patent ductus arteriosus is necessary for survival because the right atrium requires a right-to-left shunt in order to empty. The great arteries are transposed, with a ventricular septal defect and pulmonic stenosis in 30% of cases. Artery anatomy is normal, with a small ventricular septal defect and pulmonic stenosis in half of cases.

With all of the systemic venous return shunted from the right atrium to the left atrium, right atrial dilatation and hypertrophy occur. Increased volume from the systemic and pulmonary circulations causes enlargement of the left atrium and left ventricle. The extent of cyanosis and the amount of pulmonary blood flow are inversely related.

Usually patients have marked cyanosis, tachypnea, and poor feeding. A single S_2 is evident, as well as a grade 2/6 or 3/6 regurgitant systolic murmur heard best at the left lower sternal border. The continuous murmur of a patent ductus arteriosus may also exist. Hepatomegaly is present if there is congestive heart failure.

Truncus Arteriosus (Common Arterial Trunk) In truncus arteriosus, all of the pulmonary, systemic, and coronary circulations originate from a single arterial trunk. The defect comprises <1% of all congenital heart disease.[14] Associated with truncus arteriosus are a large ventricular septal defect, coronary artery irregularities, and DiGeorge's syndrome (hypocalcemia, hypoparathyroidism, absent or hypoplastic thymus, and chromosomal abnormalities). Pulmonary blood flow is determined by the type of truncus, and flow can be normal, increased, or decreased. There is a direct relationship between the amount of pulmonary blood flow and systemic arterial oxygen saturation. Decreased pulmonary blood flow creates marked cyanosis, whereas increased pulmonary blood flow produces minimal cyanosis but is associated with congestive heart failure from left ventricular volume overload.

Congestive heart failure and cyanosis typically develop within the first few weeks of life. A loud regurgitant 2/6 to 4/6 systolic murmur at the left sternal border may be accompanied by a high-pitched diastolic decrescendo murmur or diastolic rumble. A single S_2 is prominent.

Clinical Features of Cyanosis in Congenital Heart Disease • ***History*** The cardinal clinical presentation of cyanotic congenital heart defects is cyanosis. The history taking should elicit details of the pregnancy, gestational age, fetal US results if applicable, and complications of labor and delivery, including cyanosis in the period immediately after birth. For older infants and children with known congenital heart defects, details of the anatomy and surgical procedures and current medications should be obtained. Baseline oxygen saturations may be known by caretakers and are helpful when intercurrent illness leads to an ED visit. A careful

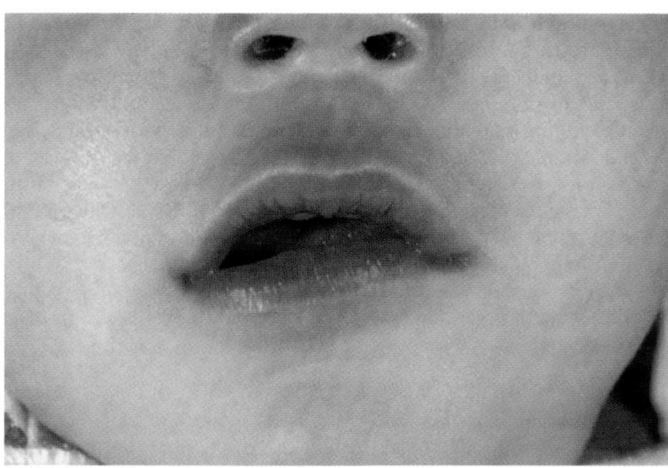

A

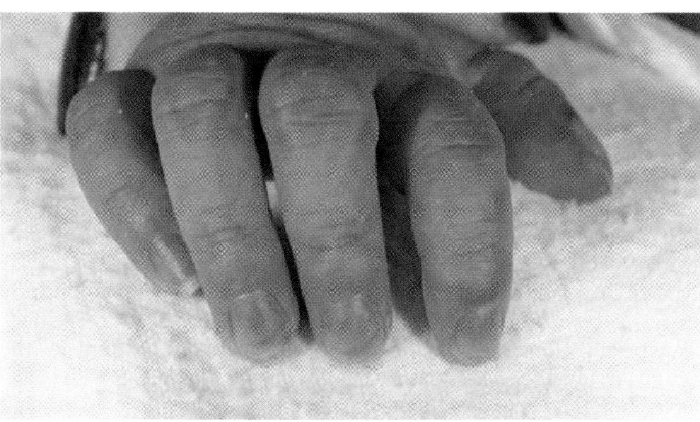

B

FIGURE 126-1. Cyanosis of the mucous membranes (**A**) and nail beds (**B**). [Reproduced with permission from Shah BR, Lucchesi M (eds): *Atlas of Pediatric Emergency Medicine*. New York: McGraw-Hill; 2006.]

feeding history should be obtained, focusing on changes in oral intake, slow or difficult feeding, sweating with feeds, and growth, and a complete review of systems should be performed.

Physical Examination Measure all vital signs, including blood pressure in the upper and lower extremities. A difference in upper and lower extremity blood pressures may signal an obstructive lesion such as coarctation of the aorta (see later section, "Coarctation of the Aorta"). Document weight and growth parameters. Note if cyanosis is **central** (mucosal) or **peripheral** (acral, involving digits) (**Figure 126-1**). Listen for cardiac murmurs, noting location, timing, and loudness (see later section, Pediatric Murmurs), and a gallop or fixed splitting of S_2 (characteristic of atrial septal defect). Palpate the chest for heaves, lifts, and thrills, and note surgical scars. Observations of the strength, quality, and symmetry of pulses help in the assessment of cardiac output. Hepatomegaly and splenomegaly suggest right-sided heart failure. Observe for signs of increased work of breathing, and auscultate for rales, which suggest congestive heart failure. **Neonates with cyanosis secondary to congenital heart disease rarely have respiratory symptoms other than tachypnea.** Neonates with lung disease producing cyanosis show respiratory distress, grunting, tachypnea, and retractions. Cyanotic infants with CNS disturbances or sepsis have apnea, bradycardia, lethargy, and seizures. Neonates with **methemoglobinemia** show minimal distress despite their cyanotic appearance. The neurologic examination includes observation and examination of muscle tone and mental status—irritability may be a symptom of hypoxemia. Performing a complete head-to-toe examination is important in the cyanotic patient without a known history of congenital heart defects to exclude noncardiac causes.

Diagnosis in Cyanotic Heart Disease Laboratory tests are not typically helpful in the evaluation of cyanotic congenital heart defects, although they help exclude other causes of cyanosis. Results of the **"hyperoxia test" (Pao_2 in response to breathing 100% oxygen)** may help distinguish heart disease from other causes of cyanosis. **Neonates with cyanotic heart disease do not demonstrate an increase in Pao_2 >20 mm Hg, because of the right-to-left shunting of the circulation.** Most neonates with lung disease or sepsis, however, demonstrate an increase in Pao_2 after breathing 100% oxygen for 20 minutes. Infants with persistent pulmonary hypertension may or may not demonstrate a significant rise in Pao_2. There is no response to oxygen in the neonate with methemoglobinemia. **When a blood specimen is exposed to air, it turns pink in all the conditions described above except in methemoglobinemia, in which the blood remains chocolate colored.** In an infant without known congenital heart defects, results of arterial blood gas analysis with the infant breathing room air and 100% oxygen can be compared: Failure of the Pao_2 to rise significantly with 100% oxygen suggests cardiac mixing or right-to-left shunting, whereas improvement in the Pao_2 in response to oxygen suggests a pulmonary cause.

The primary diagnostic tests for the patient with suspected cyanotic congenital heart defects are chest radiography and electrocardiogram (**Table 126-2**). Chest radiographic studies are essential in assessing the size and shape of the heart and in evaluating pulmonary blood flow. The chest radiograph also provides some information about the position of the aortic arch, which should be normally left sided. In the normal left-sided aortic arch, there is rightward displacement of the esophagus and trachea. An abnormal position of the aortic arch may be a clue to the diagnosis of the congenital cardiac lesion. Right-sided aortic arches are seen in truncus arteriosus, transposition of the great arteries, tetralogy of Fallot, tricuspid atresia, and total anomalous pulmonary venous return. The chest radiograph is critical to the assessment of pulmonary vascularity. With small left-to-right shunts, the pulmonary vascularity is normal. Pulmonary vascularity can also be normal in conditions that cause pulmonary stenosis, such as valvular pulmonic stenosis or functional pulmonic stenosis associated with tetralogy of Fallot. Increased pulmonary vascularity may be seen with any cause of left-to-right shunting or in any cause of left-sided failure, such as outflow obstruction.

The electrocardiogram is useful to evaluate chamber size, electrical axis, and cardiac conduction. Age-related normal values should be used as a reference to determine axis deviation, atrial enlargement, or ventricular hypertrophy.[15,16] The electrical axis most often defines abnormal

TABLE 126-2 Cyanotic Congenital Cardiac Lesions: Typical Chest Radiograph and Electrocardiogram Findings

Cardiac Lesion	Chest Radiograph	Electrocardiogram
Tetralogy of Fallot	Boot-shaped heart, normal-sized heart, decreased pulmonary vascular markings	Right axis deviation, right ventricular hypertrophy
Transposition of the great arteries	Egg-shaped heart, narrow mediastinum, increased pulmonary vascular marking	Right axis deviation, right ventricular hypertrophy
Total anomalous pulmonary venous return	Snowman sign, significant cardiomegaly, increased pulmonary vascular markings	Right axis deviation, right ventricular hypertrophy, right atrial enlargement
Tricuspid atresia	Heart of normal to slightly increased size, decreased pulmonary vascular markings	Superior QRS axis with right atrial hypertrophy, left atrial hypertrophy, left ventricular hypertrophy
Truncus arteriosus	Cardiomegaly, increased pulmonary vascular markings	Biventricular hypertrophy

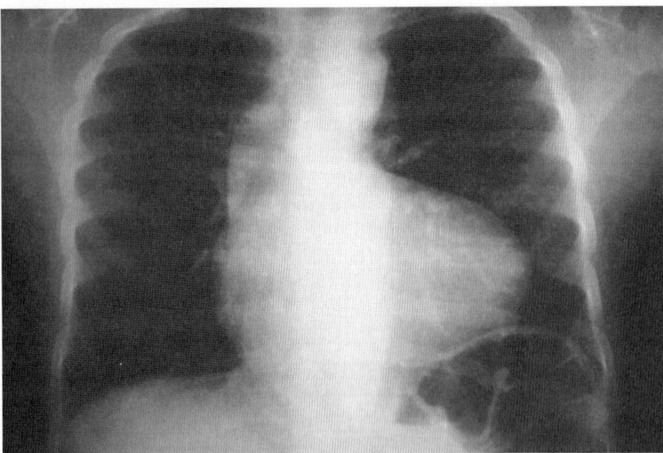

FIGURE 126-2. Chest radiograph revealing the classic "boot-shaped heart" of tetralogy of Fallot. [Reproduced with permission from Shah BR, Lucchesi M (eds): *Atlas of Pediatric Emergency Medicine*. New York, NY: McGraw-Hill; 2006.]

chamber diameters and usually does not suggest cardiac ischemia as in the adult population. Table 126-2 lists characteristic chest radiograph and electrocardiogram findings of cyanotic congenital heart defects. **Figure 126-2** depicts the typical "boot-shaped heart" of tetralogy of Fallot.

When available, bedside echocardiography may delineate structural heart disease, although adequate imaging depends on the availability of an ultrasonographer with pediatric cardiac experience.

Treatment in Cyanotic Heart Disease The management of cyanotic congenital heart defects depends on the age of the patient, hemodynamic stability, and prior diagnosis and medical management. Most cyanotic congenital heart defects are hemodynamically stable. With obstructive lesions, in contrast, adequate circulation often depends on systemic or pulmonary blood flow through a patent ductus arteriosus, and such lesions can be fatal if patency is not maintained with prostaglandins (see later section, "Shock in Congenital Heart Disease"). Although central cyanosis and low oxygen saturation are alarming and may tempt one to administer oxygen immediately, **neonates have significant amounts of oxygen-avid fetal hemoglobin and tolerate oxygen saturation percentages in the 70s (characteristically seen in most mixing lesions) without tissue or brain hypoxemia.** Moreover, oxygen is a potent pulmonary vasodilator. **Oxygen administration and pulmonary vasodilation are helpful in treating cyanotic congenital heart defects associated with pulmonary hypertension or vasoconstriction, but may actually lead to pulmonary vascular overcirculation or even "steal" of systemic blood flow in patients with a patent ductus arteriosus and ductal-dependent systemic blood flow. Oxygen administration should be reserved for patients with signs and symptoms of inadequate tissue perfusion, those without known heart disease in whom it may be diagnostic as well as therapeutic, and patients with known congenital heart defects with oxygen saturation significantly below known baseline values.**

The primary management objective in the cyanotic neonate or infant is the treatment of intercurrent illness, exclusion of noncardiac causes of cyanosis, and diagnosis of cyanotic congenital heart defects in those who do not have a previous diagnosis. Treatment thereafter involves consultation with a pediatric cardiologist and transfer to a tertiary pediatric hospital or clinic.

Treatment of Tet Spells **A tet spell is caused by right-sided outflow tract obstruction leading to right-to-left shunting through a ventricular septal defect. Hypoxia and acidosis cause pulmonary arterial vasoconstriction, thus increasing pulmonary resistance and exacerbating shunting.** The management goals for tet spells are to increase pulmonary blood flow by increasing preload, provide pulmonary vasodilation, and increase afterload in order to reverse right-to-left shunting and promote pulmonary blood flow. **This is often achieved through simple maneuvers such as administering 100% oxygen via a non-rebreathing face mask, calming the child by minimizing stimulation and placing the child in a parent's arms, and flexing the child's knees to the chest in order to increase venous return to the heart and increase systemic vascular resistance to mitigate right-to-left shunting.** Second-line intervention includes administration of morphine, 0.1 to 0.2 milligram/kg IM, SC, or IV, and isotonic fluid (normal saline 20 mL/kg bolus) to increase preload. If these measures are unsuccessful, next options include administration of sodium bicarbonate 2 mEq/kg as an IV bolus to treat acidosis and promote pulmonary vasodilation; propranolol 0.2 milligram/kg IV to relieve infundibular spasm; or phenylephrine 2 to 10 micrograms/kg/min to increase systemic vascular resistance. Refractory spells may require neuromuscular blockade and rapid-sequence intubation.

SHOCK IN CONGENITAL HEART DISEASE

The presentation of congenital heart defects as shock or cardiovascular collapse is dramatic. Cardiogenic shock can be the final common pathway for a wide variety of disease processes, both noncardiac and cardiac. Sepsis, hypovolemic shock, metabolic disease, adrenal insufficiency, respiratory failure, trauma, and poisonings can all lead to cardiogenic shock and are discussed in other chapters. Consider noncardiac causes of shock and low cardiac output states, and treat the patient accordingly while contemplating the possibility of congenital heart disease.

Congenital heart defects that present as shock or cardiovascular collapse include lesions that depend on flow through the ductus arteriosus to provide systemic or pulmonary perfusion. The classic examples are severe coarctation of the aorta and hypoplastic left heart syndrome. In both of these conditions, systemic blood flow is restricted by the underlying defect but maintained by flow through a patent ductus arteriosus that bypasses the coarctation in the former and allows blood pumped by the functional right ventricle to perfuse the aorta in the latter. The ductus typically closes and becomes the ligamentum arteriosum by the second or third week of life, and as it constricts, patients with duct-dependent flow manifest poor peripheral perfusion with increasing acidosis and eventual cardiovascular collapse.

Once the ductus arteriosus begins to close, some cardiac lesions become incompatible with life, because blood can no longer reach the lungs or distal circulation. Both cyanotic and acyanotic lesions may present in this fashion.

Acyanotic lesions include severe coarctation of the aorta, critical aortic stenosis, and a hypoplastic left ventricle. Transposition of the great arteries, pulmonary atresia, and hypoplastic right heart syndrome are examples of the cyanotic lesions that may present with shock.

Nonstructural cardiac causes of shock include dysfunctional myocardium, which may mimic the signs and symptoms seen with shunt-dependent anatomic lesions. Such cardiomyopathies are uncommon in pediatric patients but can easily be confused with anatomic lesions. Cardiomyopathies in children are discussed later in the "Acquired Heart Disease" section.

Patent duct arteriosis–dependent acyanotic congenital lesions are briefly reviewed in the following sections.

Coarctation of the Aorta Coarctation of the aorta represents 8% to 10% of congenital heart disease and has a 2:1 male predominance. Congenital narrowing of the aorta takes place around the ductus arteriosus in the upper thoracic aorta. Factors determining the severity and clinical manifestations of disease include the degree of narrowing, the length of narrowing, and the presence of associated defects. Infants who present early have a right ventricle that supplies the descending aorta through a patent ductus arteriosus in fetal life. A ventricular septal defect, patent ductus arteriosus, aortic hypoplasia, and underdeveloped collateral circulation can also be seen.

A patent ductus arteriosus delays the obstructive effects of coarctation by allowing blood to flow distal to the obstruction. With closure of the patent ductus arteriosus, pulmonary hypertension occurs, leading to pulmonary venous congestion and congestive heart failure. Blood flow distal to the aortic obstruction is compromised. Shock, metabolic acidosis, tachypnea, and feeding difficulty are common; when congestive heart failure occurs, a loud gallop and weak pulses with or without a murmur can usually be appreciated.

Finding decreased pulses in the lower extremities is essential to diagnosing a coarctation. Comparing right upper extremity blood pressures and pulse oximeter readings with those of the lower extremities aids in diagnosis unless the patient is in shock, in which case pulses may be decreased all over.

Hypoplastic Left Heart Syndrome Hypoplastic left heart syndrome consists of hypoplasia of the left ventricle and ascending aorta and aortic arch. Atresia or marked stenosis of the mitral and aortic valves and regressed development of the left atrium are also common. These combined lesions lead to minimal left ventricular outflow. In utero pulmonary vascular resistance remains higher than systemic vascular resistance. The right ventricle is able to maintain normal perfusion of the body through right-to-left shunting through the patent ductus arteriosus as a result of elevated pulmonary resistance. Systemic blood flow is based entirely on the ductus arteriosus. After birth, major problems occur as reversal of the fetal pulmonary-systemic pressure gradient takes place and the ductus arteriosus closes. Cardiac output collapses and aortic pressure falls, which results in circulatory shock and metabolic acidosis. Pulmonary edema also develops because of increased pulmonary blood flow and increased left atrial pressure. Signs at presentation include an ashen gray color, tachypnea, and listlessness, and a single heart sound, systolic ejection murmur, and decreased pulses are noted.[17,18]

Aortic Stenosis Aortic stenosis comprises 6% of congenital heart disease and has a 4:1 male predominance. Stenosis can occur at the valvular, supravalvular, or subvalvular levels. Infants with severe obstruction (10% to 15%) present with congestive heart failure and poor distal perfusion or shock. Left ventricular hypertrophy typically develops in severe stenosis. Patients with aortic stenosis who are asymptomatic in infancy can present in childhood with syncope and hypertension.[19-21]

A bicuspid aortic valve is the most common form of aortic stenosis. Supravalvular aortic stenosis, elfin facies, mental retardation, and pulmonary artery stenosis comprise Williams' syndrome. A systolic thrill may be noticed at the right upper sternal border, suprasternal notch, or carotid arteries along with an ejection click. There can also be a rough or harsh grade 2/6 to 4/6 systolic murmur at the right or left sternal border with transmission to the neck.

Clinical Features of Shock in Congenital Heart Disease • *History* The typical history of the neonate with duct-dependent congenital heart defects is one of a day or two of poor feeding, irritability, or lethargy followed by decreasing responsiveness, typically in the second or third week of life. By the time the neonate arrives in the ED, he or she is often in severe shock. A complete history of the pregnancy, labor and delivery, and immediate perinatal period should be obtained and symptoms should be reviewed to rule out noncardiac causes of shock such as vomiting, diarrhea, fever, and respiratory distress.

Physical Examination Assessment of vital signs should include four-extremity blood pressure measurement to identify a gradient between upper and lower extremities characteristic of coarctation of the aorta. **Pulse oximetry measurements in the right (preductal) and left (postductal) upper extremities may also reveal a difference suggesting duct-dependent flow.** Tachycardia is usually severe, and tachypnea may reflect profound metabolic acidosis or may be a manifestation of heart failure. Hypoxemia and cyanosis may accompany cyanotic lesions with duct-dependent flow. An ashen or gray color is characteristic of the infant with left-sided outflow obstruction in systemic shock, and extremities may be cold and mottled with severely delayed capillary refill. A single heart sound is characteristic of hypoplastic left heart syndrome, and a harsh systolic murmur transmitted to the neck may be heard in patients with aortic stenosis. A gallop rhythm may be appreciated when congestive heart failure accompanies shock. Pulses are typically thready and may be absent in the lower extremities with significant delay between right brachial and femoral pulses. The lung examination may reveal rales, tachypnea, and retractions or grunting in neonates with both shock and congestive heart failure. The infant may be limp and lethargic.

Diagnosis in Congenital Heart Disease with Shock Laboratory studies that may aid in the diagnosis and management of duct-dependent congenital heart defects include arterial blood gas analysis, which often demonstrates profound metabolic acidosis. Other electrolyte abnormalities are rare, although renal insufficiency from hypoperfusion may accompany severe shock. A CBC is not routinely helpful but may be obtained to rule out noncardiac causes of shock, such as sepsis.

TABLE 126-3 Duct-Dependent Acyanotic Congenital Cardiac Lesions: Typical Chest Radiograph and Electrocardiogram Findings

Cardiac Lesion	Chest Radiograph	Electrocardiogram
Coarctation of the aorta	Cardiomegaly with pulmonary edema (neonate)	RVH, right bundle-branch block (neonate)
	Rib notching and collateral vascularity (child)	LVH (child)
Hypoplastic left heart syndrome	Cardiomegaly	Right atrial enlargement, RVH, peaked P waves
Aortic stenosis	Cardiomegaly	LVH in severe cases

Abbreviations: LVH = left ventricular hypertrophy; RVH = right ventricular hypertrophy.

Electrocardiogram and chest radiography are typically performed and may be useful in narrowing the differential diagnosis of suspected congenital heart defects. **Table 126-3** lists the characteristic findings in duct-dependent acyanotic lesions.

Radiographs are less helpful in duct-dependent acyanotic congenital heart defects than in cyanotic heart disease, but may be useful when clinical symptoms and signs of congestive heart failure exist. Signs of aortic stenosis outside of infancy are cardiomegaly and posterior rib notching of the third to eighth ribs from collateral vessels. Bedside echocardiography requires an ultrasonographer experienced in examining for pediatric heart disease.

Treatment of Shock in Congenital Heart Disease Although oxygen is typically administered to patients in shock in order to increase the dissolved oxygen content of blood and enhance tissue oxygenation, **oxygen is a potent pulmonary vasodilator and decreases right-to-left flow through the ductus arteriosus, potentially worsening systemic perfusion. Oxygen is also a vasoconstrictor of the ductus arteriosus, which further worsens perfusion.** Infants requiring rapid-sequence intubation are at high risk for complications, and pretreatment with atropine is recommended (0.02 milligram/kg IV 2 minutes prior to sedation and paralysis).[22]

The single most important therapeutic intervention for duct-dependent lesions is the infusion of **IV prostaglandin E_1** to restore ductal patency and improve left-to-right shunting and systemic blood flow. **The initial dose of prostaglandin E_1 is 0.1 microgram/kg/min, and improvement in peripheral perfusion typically occurs in minutes.** Subsequent titration to the lowest effective dosage is recommended, typically 0.05 microgram/kg/min. **Prostaglandin E_1 can be administered through an umbilical venous catheter, central line, intraosseous line, or peripheral IV line with equal efficacy. Side effects include vasodilation and flushing, hyperthermia, hypotension (although blood pressure typically improves), and apnea.** Continuous monitoring of infants receiving prostaglandin E_1 is therefore advised. In certain obstructive variants of total anomalous pulmonary venous return, administration of prostaglandin E_1 can exacerbate the patient's condition because it increases pulmonary flow and decreases pulmonary resistance, thereby increasing pulmonary venous congestion.

Give a bolus of 10 mL/kg of normal saline with careful reassessment after each bolus to increase preload and improve cardiac output. Infants with severe congestive heart failure may not tolerate much volume. Sodium bicarbonate, 1 to 2 mEq/kg, can be considered for severe metabolic acidosis (pH <7.0), but may cause paradoxical intracellular worsening of acidosis and myocardial dysfunction, and adequate ventilation must be ensured. Occasionally, pressors such as dopamine or dobutamine may be helpful after prostaglandin E_1 infusion has been initiated.

Sepsis cannot be excluded on clinical grounds, so also give ampicillin, 50 milligrams/kg, and gentamicin, 2.5 to 5 milligrams/kg, or cefotaxime, 50 milligrams/kg, should be given.

Consultation with a pediatric cardiologist and pediatric critical care specialist is of great importance. Although many practitioners routinely intubate infants receiving prostaglandin E_1 prior to transport to tertiary hospitals, infants in stable condition may safely be transported unintubated.[23]

CONGESTIVE HEART FAILURE IN CONGENITAL HEART DISEASE

Congenital heart defects can lead to congestive heart failure because of left-sided outflow obstruction resulting in elevated left atrial pressure (e.g., aortic stenosis) or pulmonary overcirculation through a patent ductus arteriosus or septal defect. Such lesions typically present later in infancy, often in the second through fourth months of life, with failure to thrive, feeding difficulties, sweating with feeds, and gradually increasing respiratory distress that may worsen with respiratory infection. A number of acquired heart conditions, including myocarditis, cardiomyopathy, and arrhythmias, as well as noncardiac conditions such as sepsis, metabolic disease, or severe anemia can also cause congestive heart failure in infants and children (see later section, "Acquired Heart Disease").

Important factors in the development of congestive heart failure include increased afterload from left-sided obstructive lesions (e.g., coarctation or stenosis of the aorta), increased preload or pulmonary circulation from left-to-right shunts (e.g., large ventricular septal defect, atrial septal defect, patent ductus arteriosus), decreased inotropic function (e.g., cardiomyopathy), and rhythm abnormalities (e.g., sustained tachyarrhythmias).

In addition to congenital structural heart disease, noncardiac disorders and acquired heart disease should be considered as causes of congestive heart failure. Congenital structural causes of congestive heart failure not already discussed are described further in the following sections.

Atrial Septal Defects Atrial septal defects comprise 10% of congenital heart disease.[24] Only 10% of infants with an atrial septal defect develop clinical symptoms. Large or multiple defects can cause significant left-to-right shunting with overloading of the pulmonary circulation. Surgical intervention is needed for larger atrial septal defects, whereas smaller ones may close spontaneously. Difficulty feeding and trouble gaining weight are common with larger lesions.

Ostium secundum defects represent the majority of atrial septal defects and result from the incomplete adhesion of the foramen ovale and septum secundum. Ostium primum atrial septal defects result from the insufficient merging of the septum primum and endocardial cushion with associated abnormalities of the mitral and tricuspid valves. Sinus venosus atrial septal defects occur when the atrium does not merge with the sinus venosus. In these lesions, a widely split and fixed S_2 with a grade 2/6 to 3/6 systolic ejection murmur at the left sternal border can often be appreciated, along with a mid-diastolic rumble.

Ventricular Septal Defects Ventricular septal defects are the most common congenital heart defect, comprising over 25% of all such defects.[25,26] Ventricular septal defects allow blood to mix in the ventricles. The size of the ventricular septal defect determines the clinical extent of disease, with small defects having little or no effect and large defects contributing to pulmonary hypertension and congestive heart failure. Large ventricular septal defects create volume and pressure overload in the right ventricle and volume overload in the left atrium and left ventricle. This results in congestive heart failure and poor weight gain and may lead to developmental delay. A grade 2/6 to 5/6 holosystolic, harsh murmur can often best be heard at the left lower sternal border and may have an associated systolic thrill or diastolic rumble with a narrowly split S_2.

Patent Ductus Arteriosus A patent ductus arteriosus is present in 10% of cases of congenital heart disease and occurs when the ductus arteriosus fails to close spontaneously.[27] The degree of shunting through the ductus arteriosus depends on the length and diameter of the lesion and the pulmonary vascular resistance. Symptomatic patients have large left-to-right shunts. Normally, the ductus arteriosus closes within 15 hours of birth and seals completely at 3 weeks of age, becoming the ligamentum arteriosum. Prematurity and hypoxia can delay closure of the ductus arteriosus. As with all left-to-right shunts, a large patent ductus arteriosus presents as congestive heart failure. A grade 1/6 to 4/6 continuous "machinery" or "to-and-fro" murmur may be appreciated and is loudest at the left upper sternal border. A diastolic rumble and bounding pulses can also be present.

Endocardial Cushion Defect (Common Atrioventricular Canal) Incorrect development of the endocardial cushion causes defects in the atrial septum, ventricular septum, and atrioventricular valves. Complete defects involve the entire endocardial cushion and involve the atrial and ventricular septum as well as the common atrioventricular valve. Incomplete or partial defects have atrial involvement with an intact ventricular septum. Endocardial cushion defects represent 3% of congenital heart disease cases, with two thirds manifesting as complete defects.[27] **Down's syndrome and endocardial cushion defects are strongly associated.**

Typical presentations include failure to thrive and frequent respiratory infections. There is a direct relationship between left-to-right shunting and the magnitude of the defects, and complete lesions often lead to congestive heart failure from volume overload of both ventricles early in life.

Usually there is a hyperactive precordium, a systolic thrill, a loud holosystolic regurgitant murmur, and a loud and widely split S_2. The electrocardiogram is important and demonstrates a pathognomonic superior QRS axis with right ventricular hypertrophy, right bundle-branch block, left ventricular hypertrophy, and a prolonged PR interval.

Anomalous Left Coronary Artery Arising from Pulmonary Artery Anomalous left coronary artery arising from pulmonary artery is very rare and occurs when the left coronary artery branches from the pulmonary artery instead of the aorta. The decreased pressure in the pulmonary artery causes significantly lower flow in the anomalous left coronary artery and actually reverses blood flow ("coronary steal"), resulting in left ventricular insufficiency. This is one of the most common causes of myocardial ischemia and infarction, mostly anterolateral infarct; unfortunately, 90% of untreated children die within 1 year of life.

Presenting symptoms of infants include irritability (angina) and diaphoresis with feeds. There may be a murmur present consistent with mitral regurgitation. Mitral regurgitation results from infarction of the papillary muscle or from annular dilation.[28]

Clinical Features of Heart Failure in Congenital Heart Disease • *History* The typical history of congenital heart defects presenting with congestive heart failure depends on the pathophysiology of the underlying lesion. **Cyanotic lesions often present early in the neonatal period, whereas obstructive duct-dependent lesions typically present in the second week of life with feeding difficulties and shock, as previously discussed.** Patients with pulmonary overcirculation from truncus arteriosus, patent ductus arteriosus, and large ventricular septal defect or atrial septal defect lesions usually present after the neonatal period with poor or prolonged feeding, diaphoresis, and respiratory distress associated with feeds, and poor weight gain, sometimes associated with developmental delay. Parents may notice increased work of breathing, cyanosis, or frequent respiratory infections or wheezing. Tachyarrhythmias and anemia can also lead to congestive heart failure.

Physical Examination Assessment of vital signs may reveal tachycardia and tachypnea with or without associated hypoxemia, depending on the underlying defect. Upper and lower extremity blood pressure differences may signal left outflow tract obstruction. Wide pulse pressure suggests a shunting lesion such as patent ductus arteriosus, whereas a narrow pulse pressure may indicate cardiomyopathy or carditis. Weight should be recorded and compared with birth and previous weights as an indicator of overall growth. Careful palpation of the chest wall may reveal a hyperdynamic precordium or thrill; palpation of the pulses may uncover a delay between upper and lower extremities or weak distal pulses or may reveal bounding pulses characteristic of patent ductus arteriosus. Murmurs may be noted with nearly all congenital heart defects resulting in congestive heart failure and may be characteristic (e.g., continuous murmur of patent ductus arteriosus); the presence of a diastolic rumble suggests significant pulmonary overcirculation as seen with a large unrestrictive ventricular septal defect. A fixed split S_2 is suggestive of an atrial septal defect. Gallops may be present, especially with cardiomyopathy, and occasionally a friction rub may be appreciated in pericarditis.

TABLE 126-4 Acyanotic Congenital Cardiac Lesions Resulting in Congestive Heart Failure: Typical Chest Radiograph and Electrocardiogram Findings

Cardiac Lesion	Chest Radiograph	Electrocardiogram
Atrial septal defect	Cardiomegaly with increased vascular markings	Right axis deviation, RVH, RBBB
VSD	Cardiomegaly with increased vascular markings	LAH, LVH (RVH with larger VSDs)
PDA	Cardiomegaly with increased vascular markings	LVH, RVH with larger PDAs
Endocardial cushion defect	Cardiomegaly with increased vascular markings	Superior QRS axis with RVH, RBBB, LVH, prolonged PR interval
Anomalous origin of the left coronary artery	Cardiomegaly	Abnormally deep and wide Q waves with precordial ST-segment changes

Abbreviations: LAH = left atrial hypertrophy; LVH = left ventricular hypertrophy; PDA = patent ductus arteriosus; RBBB = right bundle-branch block; RVH = right ventricular hypertrophy; VSD = ventricular septal defect.

The hallmarks of congestive heart failure with elevated left-sided pressure are pulmonary rales and increased work of breathing, although rales are less often detected in infants and young children as compared to older children. Hepatomegaly, with or without splenomegaly, and peripheral or generalized edema suggest right-sided heart failure. Jugular venous distention is often difficult to appreciate in neonates and infants and may not be present.

Diagnosis of Heart Failure in Congenital Heart Disease The laboratory evaluation of congestive heart failure includes measurement of electrolytes and renal function tests, which may be helpful in determining volume status. A CBC may reveal anemia, and determination of red cell indices may point to a cause.

Chest radiograph may reveal a cardiac silhouette suggestive of a particular congenital defect, cardiomegaly, and pulmonary edema or pleural effusion. **Table 126-4** outlines characteristic chest radiograph and electrocardiogram findings in congenital heart defects presenting as congestive heart failure. Echocardiography provides a definitive diagnosis.

Treatment of Congestive Heart Failure Administer oxygen cautiously. Oxygen saturation of >95% may cause pulmonary vasodilation and worsen congestive heart failure in overcirculating lesions such as ventricular septal defect and patent ductus arteriosus. Elevate the head of the infant's bed. Provide volume expansion cautiously if at all. **A bolus of 5 to 10 mL/kg of normal saline may improve cardiac output in some circumstances, but may worsen failure in others.**

The mainstays of congestive heart failure treatment are **furosemide (1 to 2 milligrams/kg IV)** for diuresis and inotropic support. Adjustments to preload (end-diastolic volume is roughly equivalent to intravascular volume), afterload, contractility, and heart rate can be attempted.

Dopamine and dobutamine should be considered in the acutely ill patient with congestive heart failure. Dopamine increases heart rate, blood pressure, and urine output. Dopamine is given as a continuous infusion at 5 to 15 micrograms/kg/min. Dobutamine reduces afterload through peripheral vasodilation and improves cardiac output without increasing blood pressure. Dobutamine is given as a continuous infusion at 2.5 to 15 micrograms/kg/min, but in infants <1 year of age, tachycardia can result, and the dose may need to be lowered. Congestive heart failure associated with hypotension may require treatment with dopamine and dobutamine.[29,30]

Milrinone has inotropic effects, improves diastolic relaxation, and causes vasodilation but does not augment heart rate and does not increase myocardial oxygen demand.

The dose of amrinone is 0.5 milligram/kg IV administered over 3 minutes. Milrinone is given as a loading dose of 50 micrograms/kg IV administered over 10 to 60 minutes followed by a continuous infusion of 0.25 to 0.75 microgram/kg/min. Adjuvant agents such as synthetic brain natriuretic peptide and calcium sensitizers are being investigated in the pediatric population.[31]

Afterload reduction may be useful for conditions unresponsive to standard measures and in consultation with a cardiologist. Nitroprusside is a mixed vasodilator and can be administered as an infusion of 1 to 10 micrograms/kg/min. Calcium channel blockers may be more effective in cases of diastolic dysfunction and include diltiazem (0.2 to 0.5 milligram/kg/dose PO or sublingual) and nifedipine (0.25 to 1.0 milligram/kg PO), but are contraindicated in infants <1 year of age.

A pediatric cardiologist should be consulted to help guide diagnosis and management. Transfer to a tertiary care pediatric facility may be necessary.

For patients in stable condition, **digoxin** is the inotrope of choice and improves cardiac contractility and output. The *total digitalizing dose* is 20 to 30 micrograms/kg for term neonates of >2 kg and 30 to 50 micrograms/kg for infants and children between 1 month and 2 years of age. **The total digitalizing dose is administered over 16 to 24 hours as follows: half the total dose is given as an initial IV bolus; one fourth of the total dose is given 6 to 12 hours after the initial dose; and the remaining one fourth is given 6 to 12 hours later.** Digoxin is less helpful in the acute setting as it takes time to reach therapeutic levels. If digoxin is given, check and recheck doses before administration to avoid dosing errors.

PEDIATRIC MURMURS

Common benign pediatric murmurs need to be distinguished from murmurs that represent congenital heart defects. The characteristic murmurs of specific cyanotic and acyanotic congenital heart defects were described in the preceding brief overviews of each lesion. **Usually, innocent flow murmurs are of low intensity and do not radiate, are brief murmurs, and are most often systolic.**[32,33] **Table 126-5** lists the most common benign pediatric murmurs and their characteristics.

INTERVENTIONAL AND SURGICAL REPAIR OF CONGENITAL HEART DEFECTS

In many infants, heart defects can be definitively corrected through surgical repair or the use of devices delivered through catheterization. This section provides a brief review of commonly used techniques for the correction of congenital heart defects. **Table 126-6** lists common surgical procedures used in the treatment or palliation of congenital heart defects.

COMPLICATIONS OF CONGENITAL HEART DEFECTS

This section discusses complications of medical management, common complications related to surgery for repair of congenital heart defects, and infectious complications in children with congenital heart defects. Diagnosis and management typically require pediatric cardiology consultation and transfer to a tertiary care center.

Arrhythmias Arrhythmias may be caused by the underlying lesion, the surgical repair, or digitalis toxicity. Supraventricular tachycardia is common with procedures that employ atriotomy (Senning operation, Mustard operation, Fontan procedure, atrial septal defect repair, total anomalous pulmonary venous return repair). Bradycardia may occur in patients who have undergone the Fontan procedure, and atrioventricular block is not uncommon after atrioventricular canal repair.

Some lesions recur after surgery. This is most commonly seen with coarctation of the aorta, which recurs in 10% of cases. Pulmonary stenosis and aortic stenosis balloon dilation may also be complicated by restenosis or valvular incompetence.

Surgical Shunt Dysfunction When palliative shunt procedures are performed in the neonatal period prior to definitive operative repair of complex congenital heart disease, shunts can malfunction. Typically, infants with surgical shunt failure develop acute distress with increasing cyanosis when the shunt flow narrows to <50% of usual. Ordinarily, a continuous murmur should be heard over the shunt. Diminution or disappearance of the murmur suggests occlusion of the shunt. Typically, emergency physicians can do nothing for these infants. Palliative therapy with 100% oxygen is used, and transfer to a tertiary center is expedited.

TABLE 126-5 Benign Cardiac Murmurs

Murmur	Age	Character	Positioning	Cause	Differential Diagnosis
Still's vibratory murmur	Most common benign murmur in children 2–6 y; can occur in infancy to adolescence	Grade 1/6–3/6 early systolic ejection murmur, left lower sternal border to apex, vibratory musical quality	Louder when patient is supine	Postulated to be from flow across valvular cordi	Ventricular septal defect murmur is harsher.
Pulmonary flow murmur	Childhood to young adulthood	Grade 2/6–3/6 crescendo-decrescendo, early to midsystolic, left upper sternal border, second intercostal space	Louder when patient is supine, increased on full expiration	Turbulent flow in the pulmonary outflow tract	Atrial septal defect has fixed split S_2; pulmonic stenosis has higher-pitched, longer murmur, ejection click.
Peripheral pulmonic stenosis murmur	Birth to 1 y	Grade 1/6–2/6 low pitched, early to midsystolic ejection murmur in pulmonic area and radiating to axillae and back	Increased with viral respiratory infections, lower heart rate, decreased with tachycardia	Turbulence at peripheral pulmonary artery branches due to acute angles in infants	Significant branch pulmonary artery stenosis in Williams' syndrome; congenital rubella has higher-pitched murmur, extends beyond S_2, older child.
Supraclavicular or brachiocephalic murmur	Childhood to young adulthood	Crescendo-decrescendo, systolic, low pitched, above the clavicles, radiating to neck, abrupt onset and brief	Decreases with hyperextension of shoulders and reclining position	Turbulent flow through major brachiocephalic vessels arising from aorta	Idiopathic hypertrophic subaortic stenosis: louder with Valsalva maneuver and softer with rapid squatting. Aortic stenosis: higher pitched, ejection click.
Venous hum	Childhood	Faint to grade 6, continuous, humming, low anterior neck to lateral sternocleidomastoid muscle to anterior chest below clavicle	Louder when sitting, looking away from murmur; softer when lying, with compressed jugular vein or head turned toward murmur	Turbulence from internal jugular and subclavian veins entering superior vena cava	Patent ductus arteriosus has machinery murmur, not compressible, bounding pulses.
Mammary soufflé	Pregnancy or lactation, rarely adolescence	High pitched, systole into diastole, anterior chest over breast, varies day to day	—	Plethora of vessels over chest wall	Patent ductus arteriosus has machinery murmur, does not vary day to day.

Reproduced with permission from Strange GR, Ahrens WF, Schafermeyer RW, et al (eds): *Pediatric Emergency Medicine, 3rd ed.* New York: McGraw-Hill Professional; 2009, Table 47-2.

The use of thrombolytic therapy has been attempted, but thrombolytic agents should be administered by a pediatric cardiologist either directly into the shunt or systemically. In all cases, definitive treatment consists of surgical repair.

Pulmonary Hypertensive Crisis Many children with congenital heart disease have increased pulmonary artery pressure, particularly those with large ventricular septal defects. Pulmonary vasospasm can develop in response to painful procedures. In such conditions, cyanosis and lethargy can develop and can mimic the hypercyanotic episodes of tetralogy of Fallot. Treatment is administration of 100% oxygen to facilitate pulmonary vasodilation and consideration of alkalinization with IV sodium bicarbonate, 1 mEq/kg. Anxiolysis and analgesia are useful.

Diuretic Complications Because dosing of diuretic medications is weight based, normal infant growth may lead to inadequate diuretic therapy that presents as congestive heart failure. Conversely, during times of excess fluid losses, such as from diarrhea or vomiting, dehydration can occur with hemoconcentration that can compromise cardiac function or shunt integrity. Electrolyte imbalances are a common side effect of many diuretics and can be exacerbated during intercurrent illness, so potassium levels should always be checked.

Digoxin Toxicity Because of digoxin's narrow therapeutic window, digoxin toxicity can easily develop. In infants, toxicity often presents with bradycardia or other dysrhythmias. The usual adult patterns of atrial and ventricular tachycardia are not seen in younger children,

TABLE 126-6 Surgical Procedures for the Treatment of Congenital Heart Defects

Procedure	Cardiac Lesion	Objective
Rashkind balloon atrial septostomy	Transposition of the great arteries	Palliative procedure creates an atrial communication to allow for the mixing of oxygenated and deoxygenated blood.
Blalock-Taussig shunt, modified Blalock-Taussig shunt (Gore-Tex® shunt involving less dissection)	Pulmonary stenosis, pulmonary atresia, tetralogy of Fallot	Connects the subclavian artery to the ipsilateral pulmonary artery, allowing for improved pulmonary blood flow.
Fontan procedure	Hypoplastic left heart syndrome, tricuspid atresia, hypoplastic right heart syndrome, single right ventricle lesions	Cavocaval baffle to pulmonary artery anastomosis allows all systemic venous return to be directed to the pulmonary arteries.
Arterial switch operation	Transposition of the great arteries	Aortic trunk is connected to the left ventricle; pulmonic trunk is connected to the right ventricle.
Glenn operation	Hypoplastic left heart syndrome, hypoplastic right heart syndrome	Cavopulmonary shunt connects the superior vena cava to the right pulmonary artery.
Norwood operation, Norwood operation with Sano modification	Hypoplastic left heart syndrome, single ventricle lesions with aortic atresia or hypoplasia	Aortic arch reconstruction using the main pulmonary artery and ascending aorta, atrial septectomy, and modified Blalock-Taussig shunt provides unobstructed systemic blood flow and adequate coronary artery perfusion.

although they may occur in adolescents. It is always good practice to monitor digoxin concentrations expectantly during any visit at which blood is drawn. Usually, increased serum concentrations can be managed by withholding dosages of digoxin. Rarely, pharmacologic intervention is required for bradycardia. Ventricular dysrhythmias are managed medically with lidocaine or phenytoin. For severely intoxicated children, the use of digoxin immune globulin (Digibind®) is indicated and reverses toxicity rapidly. Usually, the dosage can be calculated readily based on the amount of digoxin elevation in nanograms above the normal level (see chapter 193, Digitalis Glycosides).

Anticoagulation Problems Some children with congenital heart disease require lifelong anticoagulant therapy to prevent shunt occlusion or thrombosis of surgically implanted valves or grafts. The risk of serious bleeding is small, but must be considered in any elective repair of fractures or lacerations. Prothrombin time and the INR should be monitored. **Reversal of anticoagulation with vitamin K or fresh frozen plasma should be undertaken only after consultation with a pediatric cardiologist.**

Anemia and Polycythemia Children with cyanotic congenital heart defects develop an increase in hemoglobin concentration to compensate for hypoxemia. When hemoglobin concentrations fall to normal, these infants can become symptomatic, with tachycardia, feeding difficulty, or congestive heart failure. Conversely, polycythemia causes increased blood viscosity and the potential for stroke. Iron supplementation is important for the prevention of anemia. When polycythemia occurs, therapeutic phlebotomy may be warranted.

Viral Infections in Congenital Heart Disease Children with congenital heart disease are at high risk for serious complications from infection with viruses such as influenza virus, parainfluenza virus, or respiratory syncytial virus, and mortality and morbidity are dramatically higher than in normal infants. Children with lesions that increase pulmonary blood flow are at greater risk because of pooling of alveolar secretions. Pooled secretions allow for stasis and secondary bacterial overgrowth. Treat acute influenza according to standard current guidelines. Prophylactic treatment after exposure to influenza virus is recommended only if the patient is not vaccinated against the influenza virus strains circulating at the time of exposure.[34] Annual influenza immunization is recommended for all infants with congenital heart defects. Antiviral therapy for respiratory syncytial virus infection is controversial, but prevention with virus-specific immune globulin is recommended for most infants with congenital heart defects. No effective therapy is available for parainfluenza virus infection.

Serious Bacterial Illness and Subacute Bacterial Endocarditis Although occult bacteremia has the same probability of occurrence in a child with congenital heart disease as in a child without congenital heart defects (see chapter 116, Fever and Serious Bacterial Illness in Infants and Children), bacterial endocarditis is always a concern in a child with congenital heart defects and fever, and parenteral antibiotics (ceftriaxone, 50 milligrams/kg) should be administered presumptively after appropriate specimens for culture are obtained. A follow-up visit in 12 to 24 hours is mandatory for those discharged home from the ED.

Children with congenital heart disease are at risk of developing endocarditis. Uncorrected congenital heart defects carry a 0.1% to 0.2% annual risk of endocarditis, which falls to 0.02% after correction of most lesions. The highest risk is seen for uncorrected complex lesions and may be as high as 1.5% per year in these cases, whereas atrial septal defect, ventricular septal defect, patent ductus arteriosus, coarctation, and pulmonary stenosis carry low risk. Transient iatrogenic bacteremia produced by procedures such as dental work or respiratory manipulation can lead to localized colonization and infection. Although the focus of most primary care providers is toward prevention of this disease, cases still occur. The usual presentation is unexplained fever in children with known congenital heart disease. Appropriate evaluation includes multiple blood cultures, urine culture and analysis, and CBC. Parenteral or oral antibiotics should be administered in consultation with a pediatric cardiologist familiar with the child's history. In cases with a known source of infection, such as otitis media or pneumonia, multiple blood cultures should be performed, and appropriate therapy should be directed at the site of primary infection. Acutely ill children with high fever require hospitalization, multiple blood cultures, and echocardiographic study of the heart. Usually, treatment is instituted after culture specimens are obtained and is directed toward the most common pathogens. Establishment of a diagnosis is followed by 4 to 6 weeks of IV antibiotic therapy.[35] Endocarditis is discussed further in the later section, Endocarditis, under Acquired Heart Disease.

Prophylactic treatment is recommended for patients who have congenital heart malformations or who have had rheumatic fever with valvular disease and who are undergoing surgical or dental procedures or instrumentation involving mucosal surfaces. The latest prophylaxis guidelines are reviewed in the later section, "Endocarditis," under "Acquired Heart Disease."

ACQUIRED HEART DISEASE

INFLAMMATORY DISEASES

Myocarditis Myocarditis is an inflammatory disorder of the myocardium, affecting children of all ages, and is the leading cause of dilated cardiomyopathy requiring transplantation. This inflammatory disease of the heart frequently results from common viral infections as well as post-viral immune-mediated responses. Viral causes include parvovirus B19, human herpesvirus 6, and adenovirus and enteroviruses (e.g., coxsackie viruses). Additional causes are influenza (subtypes A and H1N1), human immunodeficiency virus–associated myocarditis, and chronic Epstein-Barr myocarditis. Many bacterial species have been associated with myopericarditis but not myocarditis alone. Noninfectious causes include conditions such as **Kawasaki's disease** (see later section, "Kawasaki's Disease"), juvenile idiopathic arthritis, and lupus erythematosus.[35-37]

Clinical Features Myocarditis is often preceded by a viral respiratory illness. Presenting signs and symptoms are often respiratory distress, fever, tachypnea, tachycardia, generalized malaise, and myalgias. Vomiting, decreased activity, and poor feeding are present. Arrhythmias may complicate myocarditis and give rise to symptoms of palpitation or syncope in older children. Chest pain may be a symptom of concurrent pericarditis.[35,37]

The physical examination reveals signs of decreased cardiac output and compensatory response: tachycardia, weak pulses, cool extremities with delayed capillary refill, skin mottling, or cyanotic skin. Auscultation of the heart may reveal distant heart sounds, an S_3 or S_4 gallop, and a regurgitant murmur. There may be signs of congestive heart failure.

Diagnosis Diagnostic evaluation includes CBC, serum chemistries, and blood cultures to identify bacterial infection. Inflammatory markers, such as erythrocyte sedimentation rate and C-reactive protein, are nonspecific but may be elevated. Respiratory viral cultures or viral titers may help to identify a specific infectious cause. Troponin T or I may be elevated.

Electrocardiogram changes are nonspecific, with sinus tachycardia, low QRS voltages (<5 mm in limb leads), flattened or inverted T waves with ST- and T-wave changes, and prolongation of the QT interval. A prolonged QRS duration of >120 milliseconds is associated with poor clinical outcome. Left ventricular hypertrophy or strain can be seen. Arrhythmias include premature ventricular contractions, atrial tachycardias, junctional tachycardia or, occasionally, heart block or ventricular tachycardia.[35,37]

Chest radiograph may reveal cardiomegaly and pulmonary edema. Echocardiography is useful to define cardiac function as well as to rule out other causes of heart failure such as valvular disease, hypertrophic cardiomyopathy, or restrictive cardiomyopathy. Emerging modalities such as cardiovascular magnetic resonance are being studied.[2] Endomyocardial biopsy is the diagnostic gold standard.

Treatment Treatment of myocarditis depends on the cause, with the initial goal of managing heart failure and arrhythmias. Therapeutic agents consist of afterload reduction, preload reduction in the case of true volume overload, or inotropic support. Diuretics will worsen the condition if cardiac output is dependent on preload. Children with heart failure should be admitted to a pediatric tertiary care facility where care can be guided by a pediatric cardiologist. Since much of the myocyte damage in myocarditis is caused by the host's immune response, treatments targeting the host's immune system have been studied, namely IV immunoglobulin. However, a systematic review of pediatric and adult literature determined that there is insufficient evidence to support the use of IV immunoglobulin in the treatment of acute myocarditis.[38]

Pericarditis Pericarditis is inflammation of the pericardium and has many causes. Infectious causes are common and can be bacterial, viral, fungal, parasitic, or tubercular. Viral etiologies predominate in the infant. Pericarditis is often associated with myocarditis, with myocarditis being the predominant entity. *Staphylococcus aureus, Streptococcus pneumoniae, Haemophilus influenzae, Neisseria meningitidis,* and streptococci species are causes of bacterial pericarditis. Noninfectious inflammatory causes include acute rheumatic fever, collagen vascular disease, Kawasaki's disease, and uremia. Rarely, pericarditis may be caused by malignant disease, including leukemia, lymphoma, and cardiac rhabdosarcoma.[39]

Clinical Features Pericarditis often follows or accompanies upper respiratory infection. Chest pain may be a symptom of pericardial inflammation and is classically positional, with worsening in the supine position and improvement leaning forward. Pain can worsen with respirations and may be referred to the upper abdomen.[37,40]

Vital signs may reflect tachycardia, tachypnea, and hypotension with a narrow pulse pressure. Pulsus paradoxus is the sine qua non of pericardial effusion with cardiac tamponade and is defined by a 20–mm Hg fall in systolic blood pressure with inspiration. Auscultation of the heart may reveal a friction rub and muffled or distant heart sounds. Peripheral pulses may be decreased, with cool extremities, mottled skin, and sluggish capillary refill.

Diagnosis Routine blood tests are not typically helpful for diagnosis, but specific testing may identify the cause: A positive purified protein derivative or **Mantoux screening test** suggests tuberculosis, circulating blasts indicate hematologic malignancy, and positive blood cultures may occasionally be seen in bacterial pericarditis.

Electrocardiogram findings include decreased precordial voltage in the setting of large pericardial effusions. Diffuse ST elevations and T-wave inversion are also common and indicate myocardial involvement. Sinus tachycardia is usually present.

The chest radiograph may demonstrate cardiomegaly with a water bottle–shaped heart or a pleural effusion. Echocardiography is best to detect pericardial effusion or tamponade associated with pericarditis but may be normal if there is minimal fluid accumulation or the fluid is loculated. If a tamponade is present, there will be collapse of the right atrial wall or right ventricular wall during diastole.

Treatment Treatment depends on the underlying cause. Tamponade requires emergency pericardiocentesis (see chapter 55, Cardiomyopathies and Pericardial Disease, and chapter 34, Pericardiocentesis). Empiric antibiotic therapy for bacterial pericarditis includes oxacillin, 50 milligrams/kg, or vancomycin, 10 milligrams/kg, for methicillin-sensitive *S. aureus* and methicillin-resistant *S. aureus*, with the addition of gentamicin, 5 to 7.5 milligrams/kg, in immunocompromised patients.[5] The treatment of pericarditis without effusion or tamponade includes outpatient treatment with nonsteroidal anti-inflammatory drugs such as naproxen, 5 to 10 milligrams/kg/dose every 12 hours. Patients should be followed for complications such as myocarditis, pericardial effusion, or cardiac tamponade.

Kawasaki's Disease Kawasaki's disease (mucocutaneous lymph node syndrome) is a generalized systemic vasculitis of unknown cause. Along with Henoch-Schönlein purpura (see chapter 130, Acute Abdominal Pain in Infants and Children; chapter 141, Rashes in Infants and Children; and Chapter 134, Renal Emergencies in Children), **Kawasaki's disease is one of the principal pediatric systemic vascular diseases and is the leading cause of acquired heart disease in North American and Japanese children.** It affects infants and young children and can occur in endemic and community-wide epidemic forms. There is seasonal variation, with more cases in the late fall through early spring, both in North America and in northeast Asia. Male-to-female ratio is about 1.5:1.[41,42]

Clinical Features The diagnosis is clinical. Criteria for the diagnosis are outlined in **Table 126-7**, and these criteria can be applied after excluding diseases of similar findings such as viral illnesses (measles, adenovirus, enterovirus), bacterial illnesses (cervical adenitis, scarlet fever, staphylococcal scalded skin syndrome), or immune-mediated syndromes (serum sickness, Stevens-Johnson syndrome, toxic shock syndrome).

Cardiac complications are the most severe manifestations of Kawasaki's disease and include coronary artery aneurysms, myocarditis, pericarditis, pericardial effusion, valvular dysfunction, left ventricular dysfunction, and arrhythmias. Coronary artery aneurysms or ectasia occur in 15% to 25% of untreated children and can lead to myocardial infarction, sudden death, or ischemic heart disease.[42] Left ventricular dysfunction is seen in almost half of patients.

Noncardiac findings of Kawasaki's disease include arthritis or arthralgia, vomiting and abdominal pain, hydrops of gallbladder, extreme irritability due to systemic inflammation, aseptic meningitis, urethritis, and desquamating rash in the groin (as compared to desquamation of fingers and toes in weeks 2 and 3 of illness).

Kawasaki's disease is divided into three phases: The acute febrile phase typically lasts for the first 2 weeks of illness; the subacute phase lasts from 2 to 4 weeks; and the convalescent phase lasts from 4 to 6 weeks. Laboratory results are nonspecific in the acute phase, but for those children who do not fulfill diagnostic clinical criteria, the following findings lend support to the diagnosis: (1) elevated erythrocyte sedimentation rate, (2) elevated C-reactive protein, and (3) leukocytosis with neutrophil predominance. Anemia from prolonged inflammation, hypoalbuminemia, hyponatremia, increased alanine aminotransferase, and sterile pyuria may be seen. Additionally, there may be elevated plasma lipid and elevated serum gamma-glutamyl transpeptidase. Thrombocytosis is not usually noted until the second week of illness.[41]

Patients <1 year old and those >9 years old tend to present with incomplete Kawasaki's disease, leading to delayed diagnosis and higher risk of coronary artery abnormalities.[41-44] Due to the importance of identifying patients at risk of developing coronary artery abnormalities, cardiovascular biomarkers will become important for diagnosis in the future. One biomarker, N-terminal pro-B-type natriuretic peptide, is increased in patients with Kawasaki's disease and incomplete Kawasaki's disease compared with febrile controls.[45]

Cardiac complications vary depending on the stage of disease and are presented in **Table 126-8**. A number of demographic, clinical, and laboratory findings have been identified as conferring higher risk for the development of coronary artery aneurysms and are listed in **Table 126-9**.

The acute phase of disease results in myocarditis and pericarditis, which typically resolve without treatment. The most common cardiac findings include tachycardia out of proportion to fever and a gallop rhythm. Inflammation of aortic and mitral valves can lead to murmurs of valvular incompetence, usually during the acute phase of disease.

Pericardial effusions are rarely large or life threatening. Reduced left ventricular function and arrhythmias are more common in the acute phase of illness than in later phases.

Although coronary arteritis begins during the acute phase and aneurysms can be seen as early as 6 days after the fever starts, **most coronary artery aneurysms develop during the third and fourth weeks of illness.** Aneurysms of arteries other than the coronaries (subclavian, brachial, iliac, femoral) can also develop but are rare. Myocardial infarction is a complication of coronary artery aneurysm and is the leading cause of death in Kawasaki's disease. The majority of infarcts occurs in the first 6 months of the disease but may present later.

Echocardiography should be performed during the acute stage of disease and repeated in the subacute and convalescent stages and beyond. Findings include pericardial effusion, poor left ventricular function, aortic or mitral valve regurgitation, perivascular brightness of the coronary arteries (acute phase), and coronary artery aneurysms.[41,42,46,47]

Treatment Treatment is directed at reducing inflammation and preventing cardiac complications. **Administration of IV immunoglobulin (2 grams/kg over 12 hours) results in rapid and dramatic symptomatic improvement in 90% of patients and prevents aneurysm formation in 95%.** In addition to IV immunoglobulin, treat with high-dose aspirin (20 to 25 milligrams/kg/dose every 6 hours). High-dose aspirin and IV immunoglobulin have a synergistic anti-inflammatory effect. The dose is later reduced to 3 to 5 milligrams/kg once daily for 6 to 8 weeks. A second dose of IV immunoglobulin may be given (same dosage) if the patient remains febrile 48 hours after the initial dose, because refractory fever may be a risk factor for coronary artery abnormalities. As many as 12% to 38% of patients require a second dose of IV immunoglobulin, and despite

TABLE 126-7 Diagnostic Criteria and Definitions of Kawasaki's Disease

Classic or Complete Kawasaki's Disease

Fever for ≥5 d and ≥4 of the 5 following clinical criteria:

- Bilateral, nonpurulent, bulbar conjunctivitis (not palpebral conjunctivitis)
- Oropharyngeal erythema; any of the following:
  - Strawberry tongue
  - Nonexudative erythematous oropharynx
  - Fissured, cracked, erythematous lips
- Polymorphous rash (diffuse and nonspecific, not bullous or vesicular lesions)
- Peripheral extremity changes; any of the following:
  - Erythema of palms and soles
  - Edema of palms and soles (sausage digits)
  - Periungal desquamation during subacute phase
- Cervical lymphadenopathy (>1.5 cm, usually unilateral, nonfluctuant)

Fever for ≥5 d with <4 diagnostic criteria with coronary artery abnormalities on two-dimensional echocardiography or on angiography

Incomplete Kawasaki's disease

Fever for ≥5 d with only 2 or 3 of the above clinical criteria:

- CRP level ≥3.0 milligrams/dL or ESR ≥40 mm/h
- ≥3 of the following supporting laboratory findings:
  - WBC count ≥15,000 cells/mm^3
  - Anemia for age
  - Platelet count ≥450 × 10^3 cells/mm^3 if ≥7 d of fever at presentation
  - Albumin level of ≤3.0 grams/dL
  - Alanine aminotransferase level elevation
  - Urinary WBC count of >10 cells per high-power field

Fever for ≥5 days with only 2 or 3 of the above clinical criteria

- CRP level ≥3.0 mg/dL or ESR ≥40 mm/h
- <3 of the above supportive laboratory findings with coronary artery abnormalities on two-dimensional echocardiography

Infants <6 months of age with 7 d of fever without other explanation, even if no clinical criteria met, should undergo laboratory testing and, if indicated, two-dimensional echocardiography

Atypical Kawasaki's Disease

Patient who meets all the clinical criteria for complete Kawasaki's disease but who also have additional clinical features not typical of Kawasaki's disease (e.g., child with Kawasaki's disease and nephrotic syndrome)

Abbreviations: CRP = C-reactive protein; ESR = erythrocyte sedimentation rate.

retreatment with IV immunoglobulin, 3% to 4% of patients may still not respond. A single dose of corticosteroids administered before IV immunoglobulin does *not* improve coronary outcome. However, for patients with persistent treatment resistance, rescue dosing of corticosteroids is being studied. The use of infliximab, cyclosporine A, methotrexate, and cyclophosphamide remains to be elucidated in future prospective trials.[41,42,47]

INFECTIONS

Endocarditis Infective endocarditis is closely associated with congenital heart disease. Only 20% of pediatric patients with endocarditis have normal cardiac anatomy.[39] Clinical manifestations are often subtle and may be protracted. Definitive diagnosis is often difficult. Although mortality has declined, it remains high at 10% to 15%. Significant complications, such as septic emboli, valvular dysfunction, and congestive heart failure, occur in 20% to 30% of patients. A high index of suspicion is therefore important to prevent, diagnose, and treat patients with risk factors for endocarditis.[39,48]

Infectious endocarditis occurs when damaged endocardium is exposed to circulating bacteria, and both conditions are necessary for vegetations to develop. Congenital heart defects predispose to infection through turbulent blood flow that creates endothelial damage and promotes thrombus formation. The risk for endocarditis is enhanced by the presence of prosthetic heart valves or graft material within the heart.

Invasive medical procedures are associated with transient bacteremia, and complex dental procedures confer the highest risk (**Table 126-10**). *Streptococcus viridans*, *S. aureus*, coagulase-negative *Staphylococcus*, *S. pneumoniae*, enterococci, and the **HACEK organisms** are common

TABLE 126-8 Cardiac Complications of Kawasaki's Disease

Phase of Illness	Cardiac Complications
Acute (0–2 wk)	Myocarditis, pericarditis, coronary arteritis, arrhythmias
Subacute (2–4 wk)	Coronary artery abnormalities
Convalescent (4–6 wk)	Coronary artery abnormalities

TABLE 126-9 Risk Factors for Coronary Artery Abnormalities

Patient Characteristics	Clinical Course	Laboratory Values
Age <1 y old	Prolonged fever (>16 d)	Hematocrit <35%
Male	Recurrent fever after 48 h afebrile Cardiomegaly on presentation Delayed time to diagnosis	WBC count >12,000/mm^3 Platelets >350,000/mm^3 C-reactive protein >3 milligrams/dL Albumin <3.5 grams/dL

TABLE 126-10 Risk Stratification for Antibiotic Prophylaxis for Endocarditis

High-Risk Patients/Conditions	High-Risk Procedures
Prosthetic valve or material used for repair Unrepaired CHD, including palliative shunts and conduits	Dental procedures that involve manipulation of gingival tissue or periapical region of the teeth, or perforation of oral mucosa
Repaired CHD using prosthetic material or device, during the first 6 months after the procedure	Procedures on the respiratory tract, infected skin, skin structures, and musculoskeletal tissue
Repaired CHD with residual defects	
Cardiac transplant recipients with valvulopathy	
Low risk—no prophylaxis recommended	Low risk—no prophylaxis recommended
All other CHD	GI and GU procedures
Repaired CHD with prosthetic material after 6 months postrepair	Minimally invasive dental procedures: injection of anesthetic, radiographs, removable prosthodontic or orthodontic appliances, shedding of deciduous teeth, bleeding from trauma to the lips or oral mucosa

Abbreviation: CHD = cyanotic heart disease.

agents associated with endocarditis. A HACEK organism is a slow-growing gram-negative bacterium that is part of normal human flora. **The term *HACEK* is derived from the first letter of the bacteria in the group (*Haemophilus*, *Actinobacillus*, *Cardiobacterium*, *Eikenella*, and *Kingella*).**[39,48-50]

Fungal infections can also cause endocarditis, and 12% of endocarditis is culture negative.

Clinical Features The symptoms of endocarditis are vague and often difficult to distinguish from common childhood illness. Unexplained or persistent fever is the most common complaint. In the patient with cyanotic heart disease, pneumonia, new neurologic deficits, hematuria, or skin rashes prompt consideration of infective endocarditis. Other symptoms include malaise, fatigue, chills, diaphoresis, headache, myalgias, and weight loss.

Fever, tachycardia, and a new murmur may be noted. CNS embolization can cause focal neurologic deficits. Rales or decreased breath sounds accompany septic pulmonary emboli. Examine the skin for evidence of cutaneous emboli that appear as splinter hemorrhages of the nail beds, painless erythematous macules on the palms or soles (**Janeway lesions**), and tender subcutaneous nodules on the fingers (**Osler nodes**). Although these skin findings are typical for infectious endocarditis, they can be seen in other conditions such as lupus or typhoid fever. Retinal emboli are difficult to visualize in young children. Splenomegaly may be appreciated.

Diagnosis The diagnosis is made through a combination of clinical features, laboratory investigations, and echocardiography. Blood cultures may be negative and require multiple, large-volume samples (1 to 3 mL in infants, 3 to 5 mL for toddlers and preschool-aged children, and 10 mL for school-aged children and adolescents). The CBC may reveal anemia of chronic disease, but leukocytosis may be absent. Nonspecific inflammatory markers, such as erythrocyte sedimentation rate and C-reactive protein, are usually elevated. The mean erythrocyte sedimentation rate in endocarditis is 55 mm/h. Subacute or chronic endocarditis may produce a positive rheumatoid factor. Urinalysis demonstrates proteinuria and microscopic hematuria in roughly half of patients.[48,50]

An echocardiogram is not 100% sensitive or specific, and a negative echocardiogram does not rule out endocarditis. Transthoracic echocardiography is more sensitive in infants and children than adults and may reveal vegetations, abscess, or valvular regurgitation. Histologic confirmation of disease from a vegetation or abscess is sometimes required for definitive diagnosis.

The modified Duke criteria for endocarditis use a combination of diagnostic and echocardiographic findings (**Table 126-11**). Clinical diagnosis requires two major criteria, *or* one major and three minor criteria, *or* five minor criteria.

TABLE 126-11 Modified Duke Criteria for Infective Endocarditis

Major Criteria	Minor Criteria
Two positive blood cultures for a typical microorganism for endocarditis *or* Persistently positive blood culture—two or more positive blood cultures for the same organism over 12 h or three or more positive blood cultures for the same organism with 1 h between first and last culture *or* Single culture for *Coxiella burnetii* Endocardial involvement demonstrated by echocardiography	Fever ≥38°C (100.4°F) Predisposing heart condition or injection drug use Vascular emboli Immunologic phenomena such as elevated rheumatoid factor, immune complex glomerulonephritis, Osler nodes Positive blood culture but not meeting major criterion or serologic evidence of endocarditis

Treatment The ultimate goal of treatment is complete eradication of the infecting organisms, which often requires a prolonged course of parenteral antibiotics. The clinical condition at the time of presentation determines the initial ED management. After proper blood and urine cultures are obtained, if the child is septic or toxic, administer penicillin G (50,000 to 100,000 units/kg IV every 6 hours), ceftriaxone (50 milligrams/kg IV daily), or nafcillin (25 to 50 milligrams/kg IV every 4 hours) plus gentamicin (5 to 7.5 milligrams/kg IV every 24 hours) for synergistic bactericidal effect.[39,48-50]

Hospitalization and consultation with a pediatric cardiologist are indicated. Patients with hemodynamic instability may require assessment by a pediatric cardiac surgeon for emergent intervention.

Endocarditis Prophylaxis The 2007 American Heart Association guidelines[49] recognize that bacteremia from daily activities is a much more common event than bacteremia from specific medical procedures and that only a small number of cases of bacterial endocarditis can be prevented with antibiotic prophylaxis. Indications for prophylaxis are listed in Table 126-10; **administer prophylactic antibiotics 30 to 60 minutes before the procedure:**

- Oral: amoxicillin (50 milligrams/kg)
- Parenteral: ampicillin (50 milligrams/kg) *or* cefazolin (50 milligrams/kg) *or* ceftriaxone (50 milligrams/kg)
- Penicillin allergic: cephalexin (50 milligrams/kg PO) *or* clindamycin (20 milligrams/kg PO/IV) *or* azithromycin (15 milligrams/kg PO) *or* cefazolin (50 milligrams/kg IM/IV) *or* ceftriaxone (50 milligram/kg IM/IV)

CARDIOMYOPATHIES

Cardiomyopathies are uncommon but significant because of the high mortality and severe disability that they produce. They are the most common cause of heart transplantation in children older than 1 year of age. *Cardiomyopathy* refers to a heterogeneous group of disorders involving abnormalities of the myocardial muscle fibers. They may be inherited or acquired and are usually classified into distinct groups: dilated, hypertrophic, and restrictive. Clinical and therapeutic features differ according to subtypes, which are discussed separately below. The overall annual incidence of pediatric cardiomyopathy in the United States is 1.13 per 100,000.[51] The incidence is highest among infants in the first year of life, with a second peak in children 12 to 18 years of age, and is higher among boys than girls. Ethnic and regional variation also exists. Dilated cardiomyopathies comprise 51% of cases, followed by hypertrophic (42%) and restrictive (3%).[51]

Dilated Cardiomyopathy Dilated cardiomyopathy is characterized by dilation of all four cardiac chambers and may be accompanied by some degree of hypertrophy. Typically, the left side is more involved than the right, and systolic dysfunction predominates. The cause is unknown in most cases, and thus the term *idiopathic dilated cardiomyopathy* is applied. Known causes include myocarditis from infections (coxsackieviruses, echovirus, Epstein-Barr virus, cytomegalovirus, rickettsia, parasites, and fungus), neuromuscular disease (muscular dystrophies, Friedreich's ataxia), collagen vascular disease, anemias, nutritional deficiencies, medications (anthracyclines, cyclophosphamide), metabolic disorders (mitochondrial disorders, glycogen storage disease, fatty acid oxidation defects, mucopolysaccharidoses), and chromosomal deletions.

Dilated cardiomyopathy is the most common form of cardiomyopathy in children, with an annual incidence of roughly 1 per 100,000 in children in the United States, and the average age at diagnosis is 18 months old. Boys are more often affected than girls. There is a genetic component in roughly 20% to 30% of patients who have affected relatives. Patterns of inheritance are varied, with autosomal dominant being the most common.[51-53]

The symptoms are usually insidious and vague, although dramatic acute heart failure may occur. Poor feeding, irritability, sweating, failure to thrive, and malaise are typical nonspecific symptoms. Cough, wheezing, and orthopnea are easily confused with upper respiratory infection or reactive airway disease. Older children may complain of chest pain, palpitations, decreased exercise tolerance, or syncope. Some children are asymptomatic, and cardiomegaly or electrocardiogram changes may be incidental findings. A careful family history should be obtained given the frequency of inherited disease.

The physical examination may reveal signs of congestive heart failure: tachycardia, tachypnea, rales, or decreased breath sounds. Peripheral pulses may be weak and the skin pale, cool, or mottled with poor capillary refill. Dependent edema and hepatomegaly may be present. The heart examination may reveal a gallop rhythm (S_3/S_4), regurgitant murmurs, and an accentuated P_2.

The diagnosis is often suggested by cardiomegaly noted on chest radiograph, which may also demonstrate a prominent left ventricular apex and elevation of the left mainstem bronchus by left atrial enlargement. Pulmonary congestion or effusions may be present. Echocardiography is the diagnostic study of choice and can evaluate the degree of chamber dilation and cardiac dysfunction. Electrocardiogram changes are typically nonspecific. The diagnosis is further refined by cardiac catheterization, angiography, and biopsy.

The treatment in the ED is supportive. Administer oxygen and generally avoid IV fluids. Admission and pediatric cardiology consultation are required.

Hypertrophic Cardiomyopathy Hypertrophic cardiomyopathy is a term used for a diverse group of myocardial disorders characterized by hypertrophy of one or more of the cardiac chambers. The left ventricle is most commonly involved, although all chambers can be affected. Systolic function is often preserved, and diastolic dysfunction predominates. Hypertrophic cardiomyopathy is usually genetic in origin, specifically in sarcomeric and other cardiac genetic abnormalities, and is inherited as an autosomal dominant trait in many cases. The disorder may also result from inborn errors of metabolism, neuromuscular disorders, malformation syndromes (e.g., Noonan's syndrome), and glycogen storage disease.

Hypertrophic cardiomyopathy is the second most common form of pediatric cardiomyopathy, comprising 35% to 40% of cardiomyopathies, with an annual incidence of five per million. Males are more commonly affected than females, and the median age of diagnosis is 7 years of age, with peaks in both infancy and adolescence. Hypertrophic cardiomyopathy is more common in adults, and children under the age of 12 years old account for <10% of cases. First-degree relatives of affected children can be shown to have echocardiographic evidence of disease in 25% of cases.[53-55]

The pathophysiology depends on the underlying genetic defect. Most familial cases result from defects in genes encoding myosin and actin, which result in disorganized myofibrils, fibrosis, and, ultimately, hypertrophy. Coronary artery abnormalities may be associated with thickened intima predisposing to ischemia. Contractile function of the ventricles is normal, but relaxation (diastolic function) is impaired, leading to increased end-diastolic pressures. Some forms involve asymmetric hypertrophy of the ventricular septum, which may lead to left ventricular outflow tract obstruction. Typically, this obstruction is dynamic and worsened by increased left-sided volume.

The symptoms are variable. Infants typically present with vague symptoms associated with heart failure: poor feeding, irritability or lethargy, sweating with feeds, and increased work of breathing. Older children may complain of chest pain, exercise intolerance, dizziness, syncope or near-syncope (particularly with exercise), or palpitations. **Sudden cardiac death** may be the first indication of disease, is most common in adolescents, and is often associated with exercise.

The physical examination can be normal or with signs of heart failure. The precordial impulse may be laterally displaced and forceful, and the second heart sound may be paradoxically split. Left ventricular outflow obstruction results in a systolic ejection murmur, loudest between the apex and left sternal border, and radiating to the suprasternal notch. **Maneuvers that increase preload (e.g., Valsalva, squatting) or increase afterload (e.g., hand grip) will *decrease* the murmur, whereas standing (which decreases preload) will *increase* the murmur.** In advanced disease associated with mitral regurgitation, a holosystolic murmur is heard radiating to the axilla.

Chest radiograph is nonspecific but may demonstrate cardiac hypertrophy with left atrial enlargement. Echocardiography is the study of choice and will reveal a thickened septal wall and ventricular hypertrophy. Systolic anterior motion of the mitral valve is commonly seen with obstructive disease. Systolic function is typically normal. Electrocardiogram findings are nonspecific but may include left ventricular hypertrophy, ST-T wave abnormalities, axis deviation, and conduction abnormalities.

Cardiac catheterization and myocardial biopsy are needed for definitive diagnosis.

Treatment Treatment is typically directed by a pediatric cardiologist. The primary role of the emergency physician is to make the diagnosis, exclude secondary causes (e.g., metabolic disease), and reduce the risk of sudden cardiac death that includes exclusion of vigorous exercise until cleared by a cardiologist. Hospitalization is recommended for patients with heart failure, arrhythmias, syncope or near-syncope, or other significant symptoms. Outpatient management with exercise restriction may be appropriate for asymptomatic patients.

Pharmacologic therapy includes β-blockers and calcium channel blockers that may decrease outflow obstruction and improve diastolic relaxation.[54] Propranolol can be initiated at 0.01 to 0.1 milligram/kg IV over 10 minutes or prescribed at 0.5 milligram/kg PO every 6 to 8 hours. Verapamil should be used in children >1 year of age (increased mortality in infants) and can be administered at 0.1 milligram/kg IV over 2 minutes and repeated every 10 to 30 minutes as needed. Maintenance dosing is 1 to 2 milligrams/kg four times a day.

Acknowledgment: The authors gratefully acknowledge the contributions of C. James Corrall and Linton Yee, the authors of this chapter in the previous editions.

REFERENCES

The complete reference list is available online at www.TintinalliEM.com.

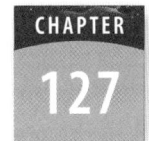

Syncope, Dysrhythmias, and ECG Interpretation in Children

Andrew C. Dixon

SYNCOPE

INTRODUCTION

Syncope, or fainting, is the abrupt loss of consciousness and postural tone resulting from transient global cerebral hypoperfusion, followed by complete spontaneous recovery.[1] In children, this process is usually benign, but it can be a symptom of serious cardiac, neurologic, or metabolic pathology. Assessing syncope in children is complicated by the variability of symptoms and lack of a gold standard for diagnosis. The primary goal of the emergency physician is to differentiate children with benign syncope from those with serious disease.

EPIDEMIOLOGY

Syncope is a presenting symptom in 1% to 3% of pediatric emergency visits[2,3] and 6% of hospital admissions[4] and is more common in adolescents than in younger children. Between 15% and 25% of adolescents experience at least one episode of syncope.[5] Only 10% to 15% of patients evaluated in the pediatric ED for syncope are ultimately diagnosed with a serious illness.[6] About 80% of pediatric fainting is neurocardiogenic (previously known as vasovagal) syncope. Neurologic disorders, mostly seizures, account for about 10% of episodes, and 2% to 3% are due to cardiac pathology.[6,7]

PATHOPHYSIOLOGY

Neurocardiogenic syncope, or neurally mediated syncope, is a mix of vasodepressor syncope (due to vasodilation) and cardioinhibitory syncope (due to vagal stimulation). Neurocardiogenic syncope can be triggered by a variety of conditions in which a reduction in venous return enhances vagal tone causing hypotension, bradycardia, and reduced cerebral perfusion. Recovery of consciousness occurs over 1 to 5 minutes, but symptoms of nausea and fatigue can last for several hours.

Cardiac syncope occurs when there is an interruption of cardiac output due to an intrinsic cardiac abnormality. These causes are divided into tachydysrhythmia, bradydysrhythmia, outflow obstruction, and myocardial dysfunction.

Any event that causes sufficient cerebral hypoperfusion can lead to sudden death. The most common causes are seizures, cardiac diseases, and metabolic diseases. Little is known about the most common dysrhythmias that cause sudden death in children, because such cardiopulmonary arrests are unwitnessed. In children, bradycardic or asystolic arrests are thought to be most common, especially in infants <1 year, but ventricular fibrillation is also seen in older children, although at much lower rates than in adults.[8]

CLINICAL FEATURES

Syncope is characterized by the sudden onset of falling with a brief episode of loss of consciousness. Other associated symptoms or signs are usually related to the cause for the syncopal event. Two thirds of children experience a prodrome of light-headedness or dizziness before the event,[5] and vertigo is uncommon. Involuntary motor movements, related to cerebral hypoxia, occur with all types of syncopal events but are more common with seizures. A careful history can usually differentiate tonic-clonic movements associated with seizures from the myoclonus of cerebral hypoxia, by their onset after loss of consciousness, less rhythmic nature, and shorter duration.

RISK FACTORS FOR A SERIOUS CAUSE OF SYNCOPE

Risk factors are outlined in **Table 127-1**. Events that may mimic syncope in children are listed in **Table 127-2**.

Exertion before a syncopal event increases the suspicion of structural heart disease, specifically cardiac outflow obstruction. Conditions such as aortic stenosis, hypertrophic obstructive cardiomyopathy, and other vascular or valvular anomalies may cause cardiac outflow obstruction.

Prior to age 6, syncope is much more likely to be associated with seizures, breath-holding spells, and cardiac arrhythmia.[1] Preexisting cardiac disease heightens suspicion of ventricular arrhythmias as a cause of syncope. Bradyarrhythmias secondary to ischemia, overmedication, or pacemaker malfunction also cause syncope. A history of heart murmur, or discovery of one on exam, may indicate undiagnosed congenital heart disease.

TABLE 127-1 Risk Factors for a Serious Cause of Syncope
Exertion preceding the event
Age <6 years
History of cardiac disease or heart murmur in the patient
Family history of sudden death, long QT syndrome, sensorineural hearing loss, or cardiac disease
Recurrent episodes
Recumbent episode
Prolonged loss of consciousness
Associated chest pain or palpitations
Absence of premonitory symptoms or physical precipitating factors
Use of medications that can alter cardiac conduction

Several familial inherited syndromes are associated with syncope and sudden death. Romano-Ward syndrome is an autosomal dominant syndrome associated with prolonged QT interval and ventricular arrhythmias; Jervell and Lange-Nielsen syndrome is an autosomal recessive syndrome associated with prolonged QT interval, deafness, and ventricular arrhythmias. The presence of a family history of dysrhythmias should prompt a more thorough investigation.

When more than one episode of syncope has occurred, the presence of ongoing cardiac disease producing a low-flow state must be considered. Illnesses associated with valvular insufficiency, congestive heart failure and diastolic dysfunction, or recurrent supraventricular tachycardia or atrial fibrillation causing rate-dependent hypoperfusion should be considered, even in children. Recurrence also raises the probability of a neurologic cause (i.e., seizures).

Episodes that occur when the patient is supine can suggest ventricular arrhythmias or seizures, which are unrelated to activity.

An extended period of loss of consciousness is worrisome and can be a sign of hypotension resulting from cardiac disease that causes prolonged cerebral hypoperfusion. Alternatively, prolonged loss of consciousness, lasting for hours, is often seen with pseudosyncope or pseudoseizures in adolescent females.[9] Syncope in association with chest pain may result from acute myocardial infarction or aortic dissection, whereas preceding palpitations should raise suspicion for possible arrhythmia.

Antidysrhythmic medications, blood pressure agents, tricyclic antidepressants, amphetamines, and cocaine are all agents that can precipitate electrical conduction disturbances. Many common medications can prolong QT interval and predispose to syncope (see Table 127-5).

No clinical or historical features can reliably exclude all serious causes of syncope.[7] Certain elements in the history increase the likelihood of a potentially serious cause (Table 127-1), and a careful history taking and physical examination are necessary. Many of the diseases that cause syncope also cause sudden death in children. A syncopal event can be the presenting symptom of these more serious illnesses. Up to 25% of children who die suddenly have a history of at least one prior syncopal event.[10] Syncope is a very common event, however, and a syncopal event by itself is not associated with an increased risk of sudden death unless certain features are present (Table 127-1).[5]

TABLE 127-2 Events Easily Mistaken for Cardiovascular Syncope

Condition	Distinguishing Characteristics
Basilar migraine	Headache, rarely loss of consciousness, other neurologic symptoms
Seizure	Loss of consciousness simultaneous with motor event, prolonged postictal phase
Vertigo	Rotation or spinning sensation, no loss of consciousness
Hyperventilation	Inciting event, paresthesias or carpopedal spasm, tachypnea
Hysteria	No loss of consciousness, indifference to event
Hypoglycemia	Confusion progressing to loss of consciousness, requires glucose administration to terminate

HISTORY

Obtain a history focused on hydration status, last meal, environmental conditions, activity preceding the syncopal event, and the use of drugs and medications. Note the position the child was in when syncope occurred, because recumbent positioning is less consistent with neurocardiogenic syncope. Be sure to include interviews with any family members, friends, or witnesses who were with the child just before the event. **A history of syncope during exertion or exercise increases the likelihood of a serious cause.** A prodrome of warmth, nausea, lightheadedness, and a visual gray-out or tunneling of vision is indicative of benign neurocardiogenic syncope. The sequence and timing of motor movements and postural positioning help to differentiate primary seizures from syncope. **Loss of consciousness occurs *with* the onset of movements in seizures, but loss of consciousness *precedes* movements in most cases of true syncope.** Inquire about past history such as previous syncopal events, cardiac disease, diabetes, seizures, medication or drug use, and psychiatric or psychological problems. Ask about a family history of structural cardiac disease, dysrhythmias, sudden death, migraines, or seizures. Take statements by the witnesses that the patient appeared dead and required CPR seriously and characterize the duration of pulselessness and the degree of intervention required. Whenever CPR has been performed, even if by an inexperienced layperson, consider the event resuscitation from sudden death and evaluate comprehensively.

PHYSICAL EXAMINATION

Complete cardiovascular, neurologic, and pulmonary examinations are crucial, but the findings are normal in the vast majority of children with syncope, regardless of the seriousness of the cause. Perform a neurologic examination including deep tendon reflex, gait, and coordination testing. Examine the cardiovascular system including blood pressure, resting heart rate, oxygen saturation, and respiratory rate. Assess pulse quality in all extremities. Measure blood pressure and heart rate with positional changes (orthostatic vital signs), especially if syncope occurred during positional change. Auscultate the heart to identify any murmurs, abnormalities in rhythm, and variations or abnormalities in heart sounds. Any abnormal findings in the cardiovascular assessment require an in-depth cardiac evaluation.

LABORATORY EVALUATION

Obtain an ECG in all children with syncope.[11] However, abnormalities on the ECG may not correlate with the syncopal event, and some patients with an arrhythmic cause of syncope have normal ECGs.[3] See the section "ECG Interpretation in Infants and Children" at the end of chapter for detailed discussion.

A detailed history, physical exam, and ECG have a 96% sensitivity for detecting cardiac syncope.[12] Selection of other laboratory tests should be guided by clinical suspicion (e.g., a hemoglobin measurement for a patient with possible anemia or a glucose measurement for a patient with diabetes). **Routine laboratory studies are not needed in a child with a clear episode of vasovagal syncope.** For patients with an atypical presentation or worrisome associated symptoms, a serum chemistry panel, hematocrit, thyroid function tests, and chest radiograph may be performed in the ED if indicated by history. For example, hyperthryroidism predisposes children to supraventricular tachycardia, so thyroid function tests are appropriate when supraventricular tachycardia is considered. In adolescents, consider serum alcohol level and a urine drug screen to rule out illicit drug use (most commonly cocaine and amphetamines).

Obtain an echocardiogram for those with known cardiac disease, abnormal heart sounds, abnormal cardiac murmurs, evidence of cardiac chamber enlargement, or repolarization abnormalities on ECG, or other features that suggest myocardial dysfunction. If an echocardiogram cannot be obtained in the ED, then consider admission for inpatient evaluation.

EEG has very low diagnostic yield in syncope and is not needed routinely.[13] The clinical utility of other tests, such as stress tests, tilt-table tests, electrophysiologic studies, and cardiac catheterization, usually is determined by the pediatric cardiologist and is beyond the scope of this chapter.

Children resuscitated from sudden death must undergo a complete evaluation unless a clear cause for the arrest is apparent. The diagnostic possibilities are extensive, so laboratory and radiographic studies should be directed by clinical and historical information. For all such patients, obtain a serum chemistry panel, cardiac enzymes, a CBC, serum alcohol level, urine drug screen, thyroid function tests, chest radiograph, and ECG. Look for complications resulting from the arrest, such as hypothermia, acidosis, rhabdomyolysis, and cerebral edema or hypoxia. Inpatient evaluation can include an echocardiogram, cardiac catheterization, stress test, and electrophysiologic testing as directed by the pediatric cardiologist.

TREATMENT

Most children experiencing syncope have recovered fully by the time they arrive at the ED.[5,6] Continued altered level of consciousness should prompt an evaluation for continued neurologic, cardiovascular, or psychological derangements. Treatment should be tailored to current symptoms. Correct compromised oxygenation, ventilation, or circulation. Apply a cardiac monitor to document any transient dysrhythmias while gathering the history and physical findings. Manage ongoing cardiac dysrhythmias or seizures as appropriate (see chapters 109, "Resuscitation of Children" and 135, "Seizures in Infants and Children"). Most patients, however, have no treatable dysrhythmias in the ED.

Treatment is targeted to specific identified causes of the syncopal event; 80% of the time, this will be neurocardiogenic syncope, and treatment for these patients includes reassurance, increasing water (1.5 to 2.5 L/d or until urine consistently clear) and salt intake (2 to 5 g/d), and isometric counter-pressure maneuvers. There is little evidence to support the use of compression devices.

DISPOSITION AND FOLLOW-UP

A child who had a syncopal event can present a challenging disposition decision, although in the majority of patients, the condition is benign.

Admit any child with a dysrhythmia documented by prehospital providers or on the ECG in the ED. Children who have any of the risk factors listed in Table 127-1 should be seen by a pediatric cardiologist, either in the ED or in follow-up. Patients with a normal ECG but a history suspicious for dysrhythmia are candidates for outpatient ambulatory cardiac monitoring. Identified causes of syncope should be treated as appropriate in the ED, and admission to the hospital should be directed by the need for further evaluation or therapy. All children admitted for an evaluation of syncope should be placed on a cardiorespiratory monitor.

If, after appropriately thorough history taking, physical examination, and ECG, no concerning features are elicited, the child may be discharged to home with close follow-up by the child's primary physician. Because neurally mediated syncope accounts for up to 80% of the cases of syncope in children, most children without cardiac risk factors or exercise-induced symptoms may be safely evaluated as outpatients.

SPECIFIC CONDITIONS

SUDDEN DEATH

Sudden unexpected death includes many causes, such as a seizure, asthma, or toxic ingestion, whereas sudden cardiac death includes just those events that directly relate to cardiovascular dysfunction. Sudden unexpected death in children occurs in 7.5 cases per 100,000 children overall with a much higher rate of 96 per 100,000 in children less than 1 year old.[14] Sudden cardiac death rates range from 0.8 to 6.2 per 100,000.[10,15] These numbers are approximate because there is no centralized registry of these cases. Excluding trauma, sudden cardiac death is the most common cause of sports-related death in young athletes, accounting for about 100 deaths per year in the United States.[16] The greatest risk for sudden cardiac death is in patients with congenital or acquired structural cardiac disease, including those with congenital heart disease who have undergone corrective surgery. The most frequent causes of sudden cardiac death in children are listed in **Table 127-3.**[17] Hypertrophic cardiomyopathy and congenital artery anomalies are the most common causes of sudden cardiac death in adolescents without known cardiac disease.[16]

TABLE 127-3 Predisposing Factors for Sudden Cardiac Death in Children

Structural/functional cardiac disease	Hypertrophic cardiomyopathy
	Coronary artery anomalies
	Dilated or restrictive cardiomyopathy
	Acute myocarditis
	Congenital heart disease
	Arrhythmogenic ventricular cardiomyopathy
Rhythm disturbances	Long QT syndrome
	Wolff-Parkinson-White syndrome
	Brugada syndrome
	Complete heart block
Systemic disease	Marfan's syndrome (aortic rupture)

Sudden cardiac death is usually an unexpected, unwitnessed, terminal event.

Survival from an out-of-hospital cardiac arrest is very unlikely, with reported rates from 2.5% to 5%.[18,19] Any surviving patients must undergo rapid stabilization, and any identified conditions must be quickly treated, following the principles of pediatric advanced life support (see chapter 109). Avoid use of class Ia agents such as procainamide and quinidine for the treatment of wide QRS complex tachydysrhythmias if long QT syndrome is suspected, because these medications act by prolonging the QT interval; use class Ib drugs, such as phenytoin or amiodarone, instead (see chapter 109).

After stabilization, children who have experienced a sudden cardiac arrest should be transferred to a pediatric intensive care unit that is capable of managing cardiac disorders. A crew capable of treating cardiac arrest from any dysrhythmia must perform any transfers. In general, this should be done by a dedicated pediatric critical care transport team and in consultation with the receiving pediatric intensivist.

NEUROCARDIOGENIC SYNCOPE

The majority of neurally mediated syncope is a mixed pattern of vasodepressor syncope (due to vasodilation) and cardioinhibitory syncope (due to vagal stimulation). **Neurocardiogenic syncope is the most common type of syncope in children[1] and usually is preceded by a sensation of warmth, nausea, light-headedness, and a visual gray-out or tunneling of vision.[5]** This type of syncope frequently lasts <1 minute.[4] Common precipitating factors include prolonged recumbence just before standing or prolonged standing, sight of blood or disfiguring injury (e.g., fractures or soft tissue injuries), emotional upset, mild physical trauma or pain, physical exertion, and hot or crowded conditions. Other contributing factors that are less common include hypovolemia, anemia, dehydration, and pregnancy. **Breath-holding spells are a variant of this form of syncope.** Medications that alter vascular tone or heart rate may contribute to the development of syncope, including β-blockers, calcium channel blockers, and diuretics. Hypovolemia can result from diuretic use in young athletes, such as wrestlers, who must comply with weight restrictions.

Diagnosing neurocardiogenic syncope in the ED can be challenging, because there is no specific diagnostic test. A history of position change, prodromal symptoms, an absence of previously noted red flags, a normal physical exam, and normal ECG fairly reliably confirm that the syncopal event is benign in nature.

BREATH-HOLDING SPELLS

Breath-holding spells are a form of neurally mediated syncope. Typical occurrence is in a 6- to 18-month-old, and an intense emotional trigger that causes crying precipitates the spell and then breath-holding during expiration.[20] The child may become cyanotic or pale and lose consciousness from progressive cerebral hypoperfusion. Myoclonic activity or seizure activity may occur. The episode is usually short, requires no specific intervention, and rapidly resolves with gasping respirations and progressive loss of cyanosis or pallor. Up to 20% of children who have breath-holding spells develop neurocardiogenic syncope in later life.[20]

ORTHOSTATIC SYNCOPE AND POSTURAL ORTHOSTATIC TACHYCARDIA SYNDROME

Factors that predispose children to orthostatic syncope include anemia, dehydration, and use of certain medications, especially calcium channel blockers and angiotensin-converting enzyme inhibitors.[5] A drop of >20 mm Hg in blood pressure with an increase in heart rate of >20 beats/min when the child changes from a supine position to a standing position is often considered diagnostic of orthostatic hypotension. Postural orthostatic tachycardia syndrome is a form of chronic orthostatic intolerance, defined by elevation in heart rate of >35 to 40 beats/min, with stable or increased blood pressure on tilt-table testing combined with symptoms of orthostatic intolerance and sympathetic overactivation.[21]

SITUATIONAL SYNCOPE

Urination, defecation, coughing, and swallowing have been described as causing syncope. The pathophysiology probably is related to an exaggerated Valsalva response causing cardioinhibitory syncope. Stretching, neck extension, external neck pressure, and hair grooming also have been described as causing syncope, presumably due to carotid sinus hypersensitivity or abnormal Valsalva responses.

PEDIATRIC AUTONOMIC DISORDERS

Abnormalities in heart rate and blood pressure control can be inherited as a primary disorder. These disorders are associated with general autonomic dysfunction and present with many more symptoms than syncope. The most common is familial dysautonomia (Riley-Day syndrome). This disorder results from abnormal development of the sensory and autonomic ganglia, due to a genetic defect that inhibits neurotransmitter production. Manifestations include failure to thrive, developmental delay, temperature instability, abnormal sweating, absent lacrimation, breath-holding spells, and seizures.

HYPERTROPHIC CARDIOMYOPATHY

Hypertrophic cardiomyopathy, also known as *idiopathic hypertrophic subaortic stenosis*, results in a dynamic and a fixed subvalvular obstruction (see chapter 126, "Congenital and Acquired Pediatric Heart Disease"). Exertional syncope is a common presentation, but infants may present with congestive heart failure and cyanosis. This diagnosis must be considered in any child with exertion-related syncope. A typical loud crescendo-decrescendo murmur may be heard at the left sternal border, which is accentuated by standing or Valsalva (decreased left ventricular preload). The ECG is abnormal in >75% of patients, usually with findings of left ventricular hypertrophy.[16] Onset of symptoms in early childhood is associated with a greater risk of mortality—the 10-year mortality rate is 50% for children diagnosed before 14 years of age.[22] Syncopal events appear to be related to myocardial ischemia and/or ventricular tachycardia, probably secondary to the long QT syndrome. Echocardiography is necessary to exclude or confirm this diagnosis and should be performed in the ED or on the inpatient ward. Patients with hypertrophic cardiomyopathy should be advised against playing competitive sports to reduce risk of sudden death. Implanted cardiac defibrillators are controversial benefit in pediatric hypertrophic cardiomyopathy and should be considered in consultation with a pediatric cardiologist.

DILATED CARDIOMYOPATHY

Dilated cardiomyopathy is unusual in children but can occur by three general mechanisms: idiopathic, with congenital heart disease, or after myocarditis (see chapter 126). Syncope and death are thought to be caused by ventricular dysrhythmias or severe myocardial dysfunction.

ARRHYTHMOGENIC VENTRICULAR CARDIOMYOPATHY (FORMERLY ARRHYTHMOGENIC RIGHT VENTRICULAR DYSPLASIA)

Arrhythmogenic ventricular cardiomyopathy has a general prevalence of 1:2000; however, it is a common cause of adolescent death in certain countries such as Italy and parts of Greece.[23] The disorder is more common in older adolescents and adults. Once thought to only affect the right ventricle, this has been shown to be a biventricular disease with a right-sided predominance. Patients usually present with congestive heart failure, cardiomegaly, and syncope or sudden death from a dysrhythmia. ECG abnormalities include left bundle-branch block and T-wave inversion, but some patients may have normal ECG findings. Even the echocardiogram, cardiac catheterization, and myocardial biopsy results can be nondiagnostic, which makes exclusion of this disorder by the ED physician problematic.

CONGENITAL CYANOTIC AND NONCYANOTIC HEART DISEASE

Hypercyanotic spells may progress to syncope in tetralogy of Fallot, tricuspid atresia, transposition of the great arteries, and Eisenmenger's syndrome. Children with structural heart disease are also prone to ventricular dysrhythmias and atrioventricular block (see chapter 126).

VALVULAR DISEASES

Several valvular lesions are associated with syncope and sudden death. In general, the degree of valve dysfunction correlates with the risk of sudden death. *Aortic stenosis* is usually due to a congenital defect and is often associated with a bicuspid valve. Other associated cardiac anomalies, in particular coarctation of the aorta, also may present as syncope. Most patients with valvular disease are identified by the presence of a murmur. Exertional syncope is caused by reduced cerebral blood flow and is commonly associated with chest pain, dyspnea on exertion, and poor exercise tolerance. *Mitral valve prolapse* itself is probably not associated with an increased risk of sudden death, but children with the disorder do appear to have a higher frequency of syncope and arrhythmias.[24] A child with mitral valve prolapse and syncope requires a more intensive diagnostic workup. *Ebstein's malformation of the tricuspid valve* is an uncommon disorder (see chapter 126). Sudden death in patients with this anomaly is thought to be due to the development of supraventricular or ventricular dysrhythmias.

PULMONARY HYPERTENSION

Primary pulmonary hypertension (without structural heart disease) is uncommon but can present in adolescence. It is often associated with dyspnea on exertion, shortness of breath, exercise intolerance, and syncope. Eisenmenger's syndrome is acquired pulmonary hypertension due to a cardiac shunt. High blood flow to the pulmonary circulation from a left-to-right shunt leads to a reactive increase in pulmonary resistance. After months to years, the development of pulmonary hypertension causes the shunt to reverse to a right-to-left shunt, and cyanosis becomes apparent. One half of patients with pulmonary hypertension develop syncope. Physical findings include an increased ventricular impulse, a loud second heart sound, and cyanosis, which is particularly prominent in patients with Eisenmenger's syndrome. Syncope and sudden death usually are related to a dysrhythmia.

CORONARY ARTERY ABNORMALITIES

Coronary artery abnormalities can cause sudden death during exercise or exercise-induced syncope. Abnormalities of coronary artery origin include the origination of the left main artery from the right sinus of Valsalva and, less frequently, the origination of the right artery from the left sinus. In both cases, the aberrant artery often passes between the aorta and the pulmonary artery, which thus places it at risk for extrinsic compression, especially during physical exertion. The ECG in abnormal left coronary arteries shows evidence of anterolateral myocardial infarction and abnormal R-wave progression. Other coronary abnormalities include myocardial overbridging, coronary artery fistulas, coronary artery spasm, coronary ostial stenosis, coronary artery aneurysms, and stenosis from Kawasaki's disease.

NONCARDIOVASCULAR CAUSES OF SYNCOPE

Noncardiovascular causes of syncope are listed in Table 127-2.

DYSRHYTHMIAS IN CHILDREN

Outpatient continuous portable ECG monitoring (Holter monitoring) identifies the cause of syncope in <1% of cases.[7,11] Case series indicate value in implantable loop recorders in cases of recurrent syncope with a history concerning for cardiac dysrhythmia. A cardiac dysrhythmia should be suspected if syncope is associated with an intense sympathetic stimulus, such as fright, anger, surprise, or physical exertion. The event usually starts and ends abruptly and may be associated with palpitations, irregularities of heartbeat, or chest pain.

A number of variations in rhythm can occur in normal children that are not considered pathologic. Significant P-P interval variation is common in children and represents an exaggerated respiratory reflex (slowing during expiration) leading to this benign sinus arrhythmia. Infants in particular may demonstrate sudden prolongation of the P-P interval (up to 1.9 seconds), which is normal. Other common and benign variations include isolated ventricular premature beats (up to 40% of adolescents), which are typically of uniform morphology. Isolated supraventricular premature beats are also common in children of all ages. First-degree atrioventricular block, Mobitz type 1 second-degree atrioventricular block, and junctional rhythms can also be seen in normal children.[25]

Dysrhythmias occur as a result of altered cardiac impulse formation, conduction, or both, and may be related to congenital structural disease (e.g., Ebstein's anomaly, mitral valve prolapse, mitral stenosis), operative repair of congenital heart defect (e.g., corrected transposition of the great arteries, tetralogy of Fallot, atrial septal defect, or Fontan procedure), systemic disease (e.g., electrolyte abnormalities, neuromuscular disorders, metabolic or endocrine disease), acquired heart disease (e.g., myocarditis, endocarditis, Kawasaki's disease), or isolated electrical abnormalities.[26,27]

In general, children are able to tolerate higher rates without the usual ischemic phenomenon often present in adults. Dysrhythmias can occur in the absence of underlying structural heart disease or metabolic condition. Many conditions that occur in the adult population—such as hypoxia, electrolyte imbalance, collagen vascular diseases, and overzealous use of sympathomimetic agents—rarely occur in children. Because much of the prognosis with regard to the reoccurrence of a dysrhythmia depends on the nature of underlying structural cardiac defects, cardiologic evaluation is needed for all first-time occurrences of dysrhythmias.

The symptoms of true dysrhythmias can be subtle and nonspecific, particularly in neonates and infants in whom poor feeding and irritability may be the only signs of early tachyarrhythmia. Sustained tachyarrhythmia may progress to signs of poor cardiac output and the development of congestive heart failure, edema, and poor capillary refill. Older children, on the other hand, may verbalize more classic adult symptoms of palpitations or tachycardia. Symptoms related to decreased cerebral blood flow that may suggest arrhythmia include syncope or dizziness, whereas those related to decreased coronary blood flow include chest pain. Detailed discussion of dysrhythmias is provided in "Cardiac Rhythm Disturbances." Some dysrhythmias with features or treatments unique to children are discussed below.

ATRIOVENTRICULAR BLOCK

Atrioventricular block is most common in children with congenital heart disease after heart surgery but also occurs as a rare congenital disorder. Congenital atrioventricular block is associated with death in infancy, but children may be asymptomatic into adolescence.[28] Congenital atrioventricular block is more prevalent with connective tissue disease in the mother. Atrioventricular block also occurs with acquired heart diseases, such as hypertrophic cardiomyopathy, myocarditis, and muscular dystrophy, and in 87% of children with carditis associated with

Lyme disease.[29] **Syncope from a high-degree atrioventricular block warrants urgent referral to cardiology.**

The treatment of sinus bradycardia or complete heart block in symptomatic patients begins with atropine (0.02 milligrams/kg IV) as a temporizing measure. The minimum dose is 0.1 milligram, with maximum single doses of 0.5 milligrams for children and 1.0 milligram for adolescents. The maximum total dose (which is fully vagolytic) is 1.0 milligram for children and 2.0 milligrams for adolescents. Isoproterenol infusion (0.1 to 2 micrograms/kg/min) or epinephrine infusion (0.1 to 2 micrograms/kg/min of 1:10,000 dilution) can also be used, although definitive treatment usually requires pacing. Transthoracic pacing in children is discussed in detail in chapter 109, "Resuscitation in Children."

Prophylactic pacemaker insertion is routinely performed in children with acquired or congenital atrioventricular block.

SUPRAVENTRICULAR TACHYCARDIA

Supraventricular tachycardia can lead to syncope while the patient is recumbent if the heart rate is high enough to inhibit cardiac filling or if coincident vasomotor abnormalities occur.[30] Wolff-Parkinson-White syndrome (see next section) and atrial fibrillation are the most common causes, but primary supraventricular tachycardia can also occur. Episodes of supraventricular tachycardia are associated with congenital heart disease, including Ebstein's anomaly and corrected transposition of the great arteries.

The differentiation of sinus tachycardia from supraventricular tachycardia can be difficult in young children. **A rate of greater than 220 beats/min in an infant or greater than 180 beats/min in a child, with a rate out of proportion to clinical status, is likely supraventricular tachycardia.** Causes of sustained high-rate sinus tachycardia important to exclude are severe dehydration, fever, pain, hemorrhage, hyperthyroidism, sepsis, and drug toxicity from ingestion or iatrogenic medication administration. If vagal maneuvers can slow the heart rate and P waves become visible, the diagnosis is sinus tachycardia.[26,27] Treatment of supraventricular tachycardia is described in chapter 109.

WOLFF-PARKINSON-WHITE SYNDROME

Accessory pathways are common in infants and children with supraventricular tachydysrhythmias. They consist of thin strands of subendocardial tissue with conductive properties that create a "bypass" tract around the atrioventricular node, allowing direct conduction of atrial impulses to the ventricular myocardium. Accessory pathways often carry impulses faster than the normal atrioventricular conduction system and are not subject to the normal conduction delay of the atrioventricular node. Some accessory pathways carry impulses bidirectionally, whereas others may conduct in only one direction. Those that conduct in a retrograde-only direction are known as "concealed" because they are not visible on ECG during sinus rhythm, but can lead to atrial preexcitation and fibrillation. Those that conduct in an antegrade-only fashion can cause atrioventricular reentrant tachycardia that is conducted in the retrograde direction through the atrioventricular node, resulting in wide complex tachycardia.

Wolf-Parkinson-White syndrome is the most common form of ventricular preexcitation in children and was first described in 1930. It has a prevalence of 0.1 to 3.1 per 1000 and is more common in boys than girls. Although most cases of Wolf-Parkinson-White syndrome are sporadic, familial autosomal dominant inheritance has been described. As many as one in five patients with Wolf-Parkinson-White syndrome have associated cardiac anomalies including Ebstein's, hypertrophic obstructive cardiomyopathy, atrial septal defect, ventricular septal defect, transposition of the great arteries, and coarctation. Wolf-Parkinson-White syndrome is characterized by an accessory pathway that may be asymptomatic or can lead to recurrent episodes of tachydysrhythmia through ventricular preexcitation.[31]

The diagnosis of Wolf-Parkinson-White syndrome is typically made electrocardiographically through signs of preexcitation: a short PR interval (<0.12 seconds), a prolonged QRS complex (>0.12 seconds), and the "delta wave," which represents a slurred upstroke of the QRS complex (**Figure 127-1**). These findings may be subtle during normal sinus rhythm or absent during paroxysmal supraventricular tachycardia, but may be enhanced with vagal maneuvers or immediately after conversion of a tachydysrhythmia.[31]

The clinical presentation of Wolf-Parkinson-White syndrome ranges from asymptomatic discovery on ECG to symptoms of dysrhythmia including palpitations, dizziness, shortness of breath, chest pain, or syncope. Arrhythmias occur in approximately 50% of patients with Wolf-Parkinson-White syndrome and are usually characterized by narrow complex tachycardia through atrioventricular reentrance (antegrade conduction through the atrioventricular node with retrograde conduction through the accessory pathway—"orthodromic"); atrial fibrillation

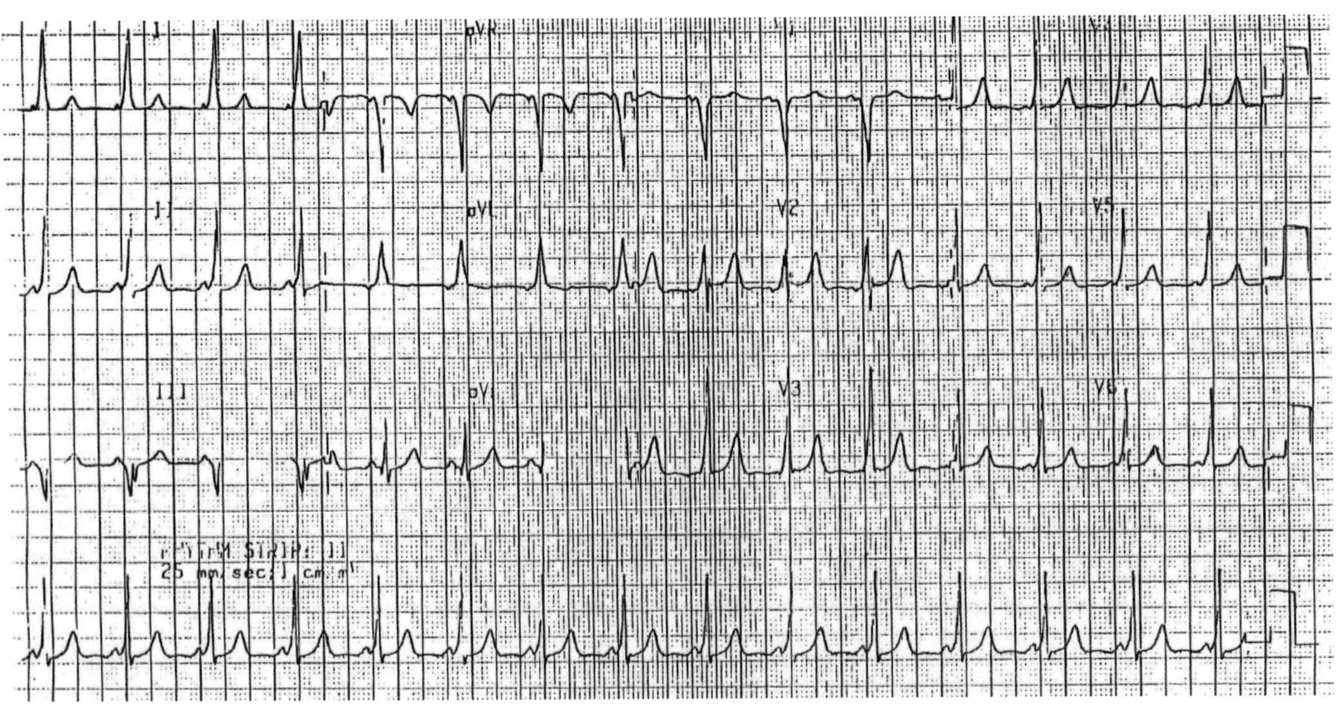

FIGURE 127-1. Wolf-Parkinson-White syndrome. Note the short PR interval and widened QRS with delta waves.

TABLE 127-4 Management of Patients with Accessory Pathways (Wolf-Parkinson-White Syndrome)

Clinical Situation	Treatment	Comments
Supraventricular tachycardia	Pharmacologic: Treat as per Figure 109-7 Definitive treatment: radiofrequency catheter ablation	Adenosine may induce atrial fibrillation/flutter with rapid ventricular response; avoid digoxin and flecainide, which can lead to lethal arrhythmias.
Atrial fibrillation		
Stable	Procainamide 3–6 milligrams/kg/dose over 5 min *or* 12–15 milligrams/kg over 30 min (maximum dose, 100 milligrams)	Avoid nodal blocking agents such as verapamil, diltiazem, adenosine, β-blockers, and digoxin because these may precipitate ventricular fibrillation.
Unstable	Synchronized cardioversion 0.5–2 J/kg	
Prevention of recurrence	Pharmacologic: propranolol 1 milligram/kg/dose 2 to 3 times a day *or* sotalol 0.5–2 milligrams/kg/dose 2 times a day Definitive treatment: radiofrequency catheter ablation	

is common in patients with orthodromic accessory pathways with Wolf-Parkinson-White syndrome. Occasionally, antidromic tachycardia (antegrade conduction through the accessory pathway with retrograde conduction through the atrioventricular node) can lead to ventricular fibrillation and death.[31]

The acute management of supraventricular tachycardia in patients with Wolf-Parkinson-White syndrome is similar to that of supraventricular tachycardia from other causes: in stable patients, vagal maneuvers or adenosine may be useful; unstable patients are treated with immediate synchronized cardioversion. Two important caveats, however, should be noted in the pharmacologic management of supraventricular tachycardia with accessory pathways: verapamil and digoxin should not be used in this setting because they may precipitate lethal arrhythmias; similarly, flecainide should be avoided in patients with Wolf-Parkinson-White syndrome. Because of the risk of recurrence of arrhythmias in Wolf-Parkinson-White syndrome, definitive treatment usually consists of radiofrequency catheter ablation.[31] Pharmacologic options for the treatment of atrial fibrillation associated with Wolf-Parkinson-White syndrome and the prevention of recurrent arrhythmias are listed in **Table 127-4**.

LONG QT SYNDROME

Long QT syndrome is an inherited or acquired channelopathy and is characterized by a prolonged QT interval on the ECG. Inherited long QT syndrome is relatively rare, occurring at a rate of 1 in 2000 to 5000 births. It is associated with an increased risk of polymorphic ventricular tachyarrhythmias and sudden cardiac death in young individuals with normal cardiac morphology.[32] Classically, a patient with long QT syndrome should have a corrected QT interval that is >0.44 seconds on the ECG; however, registry evidence indicates that the risk of cardiac events increases only with corrected QT of >0.50 seconds in children and >0.53 seconds in adolescents.[32] Therefore, patients with corrected QT <0.5 and no history of syncope are considered at low risk of cardiac events. Other abnormalities on the ECG associated with long QT syndrome include torsade de pointes, T-wave alternans, notched T waves in three leads, and prominent U waves. Children with long QT syndrome may have a normal ECG in the ED. The disorder may then be diagnosed by discovery of a history of long QT syndrome in a family member (familial), stress testing (exertional), or Holter monitoring (intermittent). On history, review any recent use of medications that can prolong the QT interval (**Table 127-5**). Appropriate treatment can reduce the

TABLE 127-5 Common Medications That Prolong QTc

Drug Class	Examples	Comments
Antiarrhythmics	Class 1 (flecainide, procainamide, quinidine) Class 3 (amiodarone, sotalol, bretylium)	
Antihistamines	Diphenhydramine, hydroxyzine, terfenadine, astemizole	
Antimicrobials	Macrolides (azithromycin, erythromycin, clarithromycin) Quinolones (ciprofloxacin, ofloxacin, moxifloxacin) Antifungals (cotrimoxazole, fluconazole, ketoconazole, voriconazole) Other (trimethoprim sulfa, pentamidine)	
Psychiatric drugs	Tricyclics Phenothiazines Others (citalopram, clozapine, fluoxetine, haloperidol, lithium, methadone, risperidone, quetiapine, sertraline, trazodone, venlafaxine, ziprasidone)	
GI agents	Cisapride, ondansetron	
Anticonvulsants	Fosphenytoin, felbamate	
Immunosuppressives	Tacrolimus	
Migraine medications	Sumatriptan, zolmitriptan	
Stimulants	Albuterol, epinephrine, dopamine, dobutamine, isoproterenol, methylphenidate, phenylephrine, terbutaline	
Other	Antimalarials, chloral hydrate, octreotide, vasopressin	
OTC/illicit drugs	Phenylephrine, pseudoephedrine, Cocaine, amphetamine	

risk of aborted cardiac arrest and sudden cardiac death approximately 50%.[32] β-Blockers are the mainstay of treatment, but they are ineffective for some long QT variants. Therapy should be started in consultation with a cardiologist. Genetic studies to date have identified 13 genetic loci associated with long QT syndrome, all of which encode proteins involved in sodium, calcium, and potassium transport.[33]

SICK SINUS SYNDROME

Sick sinus syndrome is also known as *tachycardia-bradycardia syndrome*. Isolated sinus node dysfunction rarely causes syncope, and syncope associated with sick sinus syndrome is more likely to be due to a reentrant atrial tachycardia. Most commonly, these dysrhythmias are associated with prior heart surgery, especially the Mustard or Senning operation for transposition of the great vessels and the Fontan procedure. **Syncope and sudden death can occur after pacemaker placement, because the pacemaker prevents bradycardia but not tachycardia.**

PACEMAKER MALFUNCTION

Although pacemaker use is not common in childhood, any child with a pacemaker who develops syncope or presyncope should be presumed to have a pacemaker malfunction.

ECG INTERPRETATION IN INFANTS AND CHILDREN

The pediatric ECG is characterized by age-related variations and, as a result, can be very difficult to interpret. The age-related variations reflect the maturation of the pediatric myocardium and vascular system from the neonate to adult. Developmental changes in the pediatric ECG from birth to adolescence include a gradual shift from right to left ventricular

TABLE 127-6 Normal Pediatric Heart Rates[36]

Age	Heart Rate
Birth–4 weeks	130–190
1–3 months	125–185
3–6 months	110–165
6–12 months	105–195
1–3 years	100–155
3–5 years	70–120
5–8 years	60–110
8–12 years	55–100
12–16 years	50–100

TABLE 127-8 Age-Specific ECG Intervals[36]

Age	PR (seconds)	QRS (seconds)	QTc (seconds)
Birth–4 weeks	0.08–0.12	0.05–0.09	0.38–0.46
1–3 months	0.08–0.13	0.05–0.08	0.38–0.46
3–6 months	0.08–0.14	0.05–0.09	0.39–0.45
6–12 months	0.08–0.14	0.05–0.09	0.38–0.45
1–3 years	0.08–0.15	0.05–0.09	0.38–0.45
3–5 years	0.1–0.15	0.06–0.09	0.38–0.45
5–8 years	0.09–0.16	0.06–0.1	0.37–0.45
8–12 years	0.1–0.17	0.07–0.1	0.37–0.45
12–16 years	0.1–0.18	0.7–0.11	0.36–0.46

dominance, decrease in the resting heart rate, a lengthening of the PR and QRS intervals, and a change from inverted to upright T waves in the precordial leads.[25,34,35] Use a systematic approach to ECG interpretation, checking rate, rhythm, axis, hypertrophy of the atria and ventricles, and repolarization changes. Reference tables with age-specific values are necessary to deal with the progressive changes in heart rate, axis, interval duration, and morphology. The most important changes are described below.

NORMAL ECG INTERVALS

Heart Rate The normal heart rate is age dependent (**Table 127-6**). The neonatal and infant heart has a limited capacity to increase stroke volume, and cardiac output is therefore dependent largely on rate, which is relatively high in the young infant to meet increased metabolic demands. Significant state-dependent and beat-to-beat variability in resting heart rate is characteristic of the normal neonatal and infant heart. Sinus tachycardia in the neonate can often reach 200 to 220 beats/min and is common in the setting of fever or pain. In general, bradycardia with normal perfusion and without evidence of heart block (discussed below) rarely requires treatment or investigation.

P and QRS Axes Because blood is shunted away from fetal lungs and the right ventricle provides the majority of systemic blood flow in utero, the right ventricle predominates in the neonate. In the first few months of life, this is characterized by right ventricular dominance and right axis deviation. P waves should be upright in leads I and aVF with the P axis between 0 and +90 degrees. The precordial leads have increased R wave amplitude in V_1 and V_2 and decreased amplitude in V_5 and V_6. With a subsequent increase in left ventricular size during infancy and early childhood, the QRS axis shifts leftward, so that R wave amplitude decreases in V_1 and V_2 and increases in V_5 and V_6 (**Table 127-7**).

PR, QRS, and QT Intervals The PR interval varies with age, gradually lengthening from 0.08 to 0.12 seconds in neonates to 0.11 to 0.18 seconds in adolescents.[36] The QRS interval also lengthens over time from 0.05 to 0.09 seconds in the neonate to 0.07 to 0.11 seconds in the adolescent.[36]

TABLE 127-7 Age-Specific QRS Axis[36]

Age	Mean Axis in Degrees	Range in Degrees
Birth–4 weeks	105	60–160
1–3 months	85	40–140
3–6 months	68	0–110
6–12 months	68	0–120
1–3 years	66	0–120
3–5 years	70	0–115
5–8 years	72	−10 to 120
8–12 years	68	−20 to 120
12–16 years	65	−10 to 110

TABLE 127-9 Voltage Criteria for Left and Right Ventricular Hypertrophy by Age[34,37]

	Age				
LVH	0–7 days	7 days–1 year	1–3 years	3–5 years	> 5 years
RV_6	> 12 mm	> 23 mm	> 21–23 mm	> 24–25 mm	> 25–27 mm
SV_1	> 23 mm	> 15–18 mm	> 21 mm	> 22 mm	> 26 mm
$SV_1 + RV_6$	> 28 mm	> 35 mm	> 38 mm	> 42 mm	> 47 mm
RVH					
RV_1	> 26 mm	> 20–22 mm	> 18 mm	> 14–18 mm	> 13 mm
SV_6	> 10 mm	> 7–10 mm	> 7 mm	> 6 mm	> 4 mm
$RV_1 + SV_6$	> 37 mm	> 43 mm	> 30 mm	> 24 mm	> 17 mm

The QT interval (measured from the onset of the QRS complex to the end of the T wave) is subject to variations in heart rate, and a correction for heart rate is calculated using Bazett's formula: QTc = QT/the square root of the RR interval. The QTc should be <0.49 seconds in the first 6 months of life and <0.44 seconds thereafter, although different definitions for prolonged QTc have been suggested.[34] Age-specific normal intervals are listed in **Table 127-8**.

T Waves Pediatric T-wave changes are typically nonspecific. Flat or inverted T waves are usually normal in the newborn. T-wave inversion in the right precordial leads is common in the first years of life and may persist into adolescence or revert in early childhood to the typical upright pattern seen in adults.[34] T-wave changes are common in infants and children and rarely reflect ischemia.

Chamber Size Evaluating the ECG for signs of chamber size is important when considering congenital or acquired heart disease in the pediatric patient. P-wave amplitude is relatively age-independent and best measured in lead II. P waves >0.25 mV should be considered abnormal and may indicate right atrial enlargement.[36] Left atrial enlargement is suggested by prolonged P-wave duration, which should not be >0.08 seconds in infants or >0.12 seconds in adolescents.[34] Voltage criteria for left ventricular hypertrophy and right ventricular hypertrophy depend on age and are listed in **Table 127-9**.[34,37] Left ventricular hypertrophy is also suggested by a q-wave amplitude >4 mm in V_5 or V_6 or inverted T wave in V_6, whereas right ventricular hypertrophy is suggested by an RSR′ pattern in V_1 with an R′ >15 mm in infants or >10 mm in children after the first year of life, or with a q wave in lead V_1.[25,34,37]

REFERENCES

The complete reference list is available online at www.TintinalliEM.com.

CHAPTER 128

Vomiting, Diarrhea, and Dehydration in Infants and Children

Stephen B. Freedman
Jennifer D. Thull-Freedman

INTRODUCTION

Acute viral gastroenteritis is the most common cause of vomiting and diarrhea in children and continues to cause approximately 800,000 deaths globally each year in children <5 years old.[1]

Transmission of GI infections can be reduced by attention to good hand hygiene. Hand washing can reduce the incidence of diarrheal disease by approximately 30% in both high- and low-income countries.[2] The provision of alcohol-based hand sanitizer and educational materials can reduce GI illnesses in child care centers,[3] and a multifactorial intervention including hand sanitizer and surface disinfection similarly reduces illness due to enteric pathogens in elementary school students.[4]

Rotavirus accounts for a large majority of severe cases and contributes significantly to hospitalizations in developed countries. Two live oral rotavirus vaccines, marketed as RotaTeq® and Rotarix®, are currently licensed for use in the United States and numerous other countries. These vaccines are recommended by the World Health Organization for immunization of children worldwide. They have been introduced into the immunization programs of >50 countries. Routine rotavirus vaccination, which began in the United States in 2006, has resulted in an approximately 80% reduction in rotavirus-related hospitalizations and ED visits for rotavirus among immunized children.[5,6] Although a prospective postlicensure study of more than 200,000 doses identified an increase in the rate of intussusception after vaccination (attributable risk ~5.3 per 100,000 infants vaccinated); this increased risk must be weighed against the benefits of preventing rotavirus-associated illness.[7]

Although the clinical diagnosis of gastroenteritis requires the presence of diarrhea, many infants present with isolated vomiting. This chapter focuses on one of the most frequent and important causes of vomiting and diarrhea in children, gastroenteritis, and will also review other important causes of these symptoms.

VOMITING

Vomiting is the forceful act of expelling gastric contents through the mouth. It is controlled by the vomiting center in the reticular formation of the medulla and the chemoreceptor trigger zone underlying the floor of the fourth ventricle. Trigger areas that excite the CNS vomiting centers are found in the pharynx, cardiac vessels, peritoneum, bile ducts, and stomach. Vomiting results when the stomach relaxes, the gastric pylorus constricts, and the contractions of surrounding muscles cause expulsion of the gastric contents. Acute vomiting is usually caused by a self-limited viral illness. Nonetheless, serious diagnoses that need to be considered include infections, metabolic abnormalities, neurologic processes, acute surgical/GI diseases, or other major organ system dysfunction. The differential diagnosis of vomiting is age specific (**Table 128-1**). **Bilious or bloody vomitus, hematochezia, or significant abdominal pain should trigger concerns of a disease process other than simple viral gastroenteritis or a potential complication of viral gastroenteritis (Tables 128-2 and 128-3).**

Bilious vomiting suggests an obstructive lesion distal to the ampulla of Vater and portends a surgical emergency. From one third to half of newborns with bilious vomiting have a surgical lesion, often malrotation with volvulus or Hirschsprung's disease.[8,9] For further discussion, see chapter 130, "Acute Abdominal Pain in Infants and Children." For discussion of hematemesis, see chapter 131, "Gastrointestinal Bleeding in Infants and Children."

TABLE 128-1 Causes of Vomiting, by Age

Newborn	
Obstructive intestinal anomalies	Esophageal stenosis/atresia, pyloric stenosis, intestinal stenosis/atresia, malrotation ± volvulus, incarcerated hernia, meconium ileus/plug, Hirschsprung's disease, imperforate anus, enteric duplications
Neurologic	Intracranial bleed/mass, hydrocephalus, cerebral edema, kernicterus
Renal	Urinary tract infection, obstructive uropathy, renal insufficiency
Infectious	Viral illness, gastroenteritis, meningitis, sepsis
Metabolic/endocrine	Inborn errors of metabolism (urea cycle, amino/organic acid, carbohydrate), congenital adrenal hyperplasia
Miscellaneous	Ileus, gastroesophageal reflux, necrotizing enterocolitis, GI perforation
Infant (<12 mo)	
Obstructive intestinal anomalies	Pyloric stenosis, malrotation ± volvulus, incarcerated hernia, Hirschsprung's disease, enteric duplications, intussusception, foreign body, bezoars, Meckel's diverticulum
Neurologic	Intracranial bleed/mass, hydrocephalus, cerebral edema
Renal	Urinary tract infection, obstructive uropathy, renal insufficiency
Infectious	Viral illness, gastroenteritis, meningitis, sepsis, otitis media, pneumonia, pertussis, hepatitis
Metabolic/endocrine	Inborn errors of metabolism, adrenal insufficiency, renal tubular acidosis
Miscellaneous	Ileus, gastroesophageal reflux, posttussive, peritonitis, drug overdose, food allergy
Child (>12 mo)	
Obstructive intestinal anomalies	Malrotation ± volvulus, incarcerated hernia, Hirschsprung's disease, intussusception, foreign body, bezoars, Meckel's diverticulum, acquired esophageal stricture, peptic ulcer disease, adhesions, superior mesenteric artery syndrome
Neurologic	Intracranial bleed/mass, cerebral edema, postconcussive, migraine
Renal	Urinary tract infection, obstructive uropathy, renal insufficiency
Infectious	Viral illness, gastroenteritis, meningitis, sepsis, otitis media, pneumonia, hepatitis, streptococcal pharyngitis
Metabolic/endocrine	Inborn errors of metabolism, adrenal insufficiency, renal tubular acidosis, diabetes mellitus, Reye's syndrome, porphyria
Miscellaneous	Ileus, gastroesophageal reflux, posttussive, peritonitis, drug overdose, food allergy, appendicitis, pancreatitis, gastritis, Crohn's disease, pregnancy, psychogenic, cyclic vomiting syndrome

Diagnostically, it is important to consider children with **isolated vomiting** separately from those who present with *vomiting and diarrhea*. The differential diagnosis of vomiting is vast and age specific (Table 128-1). Gastroesophageal reflux, intussusception, pyloric stenosis, and malrotation are discussed briefly below and more fully in chapter 130.

GASTROESOPHAGEAL REFLUX

Gastroesophageal reflux is the spontaneous regurgitation of gastric contents into the esophagus. Reflux is physiologic in young infants and usually resolves by the end of the first year of life. It is considered pathologic only in the small subset that experiences complications. The typical infant with uncomplicated gastroesophageal reflux effortlessly brings up small amounts of milk after feeding but

TABLE 128-2 Causes of Vomiting with Significant Morbidity

Newborn Period (birth–2 wk)	
Obstructive intestinal anomaly	Esophageal or intestinal stenosis/atresia, bowel malrotation ± midgut volvulus, meconium ileus/plug, Hirschsprung's disease, imperforate anus, enteric duplications
Other GI disease processes	Necrotizing enterocolitis, perforation with secondary peritonitis
Neurologic	Mass lesion, hydrocephalus, cerebral edema, kernicterus
Renal	Obstructive anomaly, uremia
Infectious	Sepsis, meningitis
Metabolic	Inborn errors of metabolism, congenital adrenal hyperplasia
Infant (2 wk–12 mo)	
Acquired esophageal disorders	Foreign body, retropharyngeal abscess
GI obstruction	Bezoar, foreign body, pyloric stenosis, malrotation ± volvulus, enteric duplications, complications of Meckel's diverticulum, intussusception, incarcerated hernia, Hirschsprung's disease
Other GI disease processes	Gastroenteritis with dehydration, peritonitis
Neurologic	Mass lesion, hydrocephalus
Renal	Obstruction, uremia
Infectious	Sepsis, meningitis, pertussis
Metabolic	Inborn errors of metabolism
Toxic ingestions	—
Child (>12 mo)	
GI obstruction	Bezoar, foreign body, posttraumatic intramural hematoma, malrotation ± volvulus, complications of Meckel's diverticulum, intussusception, incarcerated hernia, Hirschsprung's disease
Other GI disease processes	Appendicitis, peptic ulcer disease, pancreatitis, peritonitis
Neurologic	Mass lesions
Renal	Uremia
Infectious	Sepsis, meningitis
Metabolic	Diabetic ketoacidosis, adrenal insufficiency, inborn errors of metabolism
Toxic ingestion	—

continues to grow well. Symptoms may begin as early as the first week of life and often resolve around the time of solid food introduction and the assumption of the sitting position. In infants with significant vomiting, pathologic conditions should be considered. Complications that can occur include esophagitis, **failure to thrive/weight loss**, respiratory disease, refractory asthma, recurrent pneumonia, apnea, and acute life-threatening events. In most infants, the diagnosis can be made based on clinical findings. The gold standard diagnostic test is continuous esophageal pH monitoring to detect the presence of gastric acid in the distal esophagus. Semi-supine positioning (e.g., infant carrier or car seat) may exacerbate gastroesophageal reflux and should be avoided, especially after feeding.[10] Although severe cases may require a histamine-2 receptor antagonist or a proton pump inhibitor, the overuse of medications in the "happy spitter" should be avoided.[11]

TABLE 128-3 Causes of Diarrhea with Significant Morbidity

Infection: *Salmonella* gastroenteritis with bacteremia, *Shigella*, *Clostridium difficile* (pseudomembranous colitis)
Anatomic abnormalities
Intussusception
Hirschsprung's disease with toxic megacolon
Partial obstruction
Appendicitis
Inflammatory bowel disease with toxic megacolon
Verotoxigenic *Escherichia coli* infection with the secondary development of hemolytic-uremic syndrome

INTUSSUSCEPTION

Intussusception occurs when one segment of bowel invaginates into a more distal segment. It is the leading cause of acute intestinal obstruction in infants and occurs most commonly between 3 and 12 months of age. The most common location is ileocolic, and the lead point usually is a hypertrophied Peyer patch. However, in children >2 years of age, a specific pathologic lead point should be considered. The primary manifestation is colicky abdominal pain followed by the onset of vomiting. The "classic" triad of colicky abdominal pain, vomiting, and bloody stools is present in only 20% of cases. For further discussion of intussusception, see chapter 130.

PYLORIC STENOSIS

Pyloric stenosis results from pyloric muscle hypertrophy that obstructs gastric outflow. The incidence is 1 in 250 live births, and >80% of cases occur in males[12]; other risk factors include white race, first born birth order, and a positive family history. Over 90% of cases are diagnosed by 10 weeks of life, with a sharp increase in the incidence after the second week of life, peaking at the fifth week and then steadily declining until the tenth week.[12] Children typically present with nonbilious projectile vomiting associated with weight loss and dehydration. Initially, the vomiting is mild and often mistaken for regurgitation. However, vomiting progresses and becomes more severe over several days. ED treatment includes the correction of fluid and electrolyte abnormalities. The pathognomonic electrolyte abnormalities are a hyponatremic, hypokalemic, and hypochloremic metabolic alkalosis. At present, the diagnosis is usually confirmed by US.

MALROTATION

Malrotation occurs when incomplete rotation of the gut in utero places the cecum in the right upper quadrant and fixes the dorsal mesentery on a narrow base instead of the broad fixation that usually extends from the ligament of Treitz to the ileocecal junction. These anomalies place the small bowel at risk for twisting on the narrow pedicle of mesentery, resulting in a volvulus that subsequently impairs blood flow to the bowel. Although malrotation can present at any age, roughly one third of patients present in the first month of life.[12] Symptoms may include bilious vomiting, pain, abdominal distention, and, ultimately, shock due to intestinal ischemia. Bilious emesis, particularly in a young infant, should immediately raise a concern for possible malrotation and volvulus. In some children, the volvulus can be intermittent, resulting in episodic vomiting and pain. Prompt diagnosis and surgical repair are needed to minimize the risk of bowel necrosis and death.

DIARRHEA

Diarrhea is loose or liquid stools and/or an increase in the frequency of evacuations with at least three stools in 24 hours. The child's age and diet affect stool consistency and frequency. For example, in the first month of life, a change in stool consistency is more specific for diarrhea than absolute stool number. Breastfed infants typically have several poorly formed, yellow-green stools per day. Recognition of diarrhea in infants is important, because given their small size, they have limited fluid reserves and are at high risk for developing dehydration.

Most children with diarrhea have an acute viral infection, but diarrhea may be a presenting symptom of many conditions (**Tables 128-4** and **128-5**). Preexisting conditions may contribute to the clinical presentation or predispose the patient to an unusual cause of diarrhea, so it is

TABLE 128-4 Causes of Diarrhea

Infection
Viral: rotavirus, norovirus, enteric adenoviruses, sapoviruses, astroviruses
Bacterial: *Salmonella, Shigella, Yersinia, Campylobacter, Escherichia coli, Aeromonas hydrophila, Vibrio species, Clostridium difficile*
Parasitic: *Giardia lamblia, Entamoeba histolytica, Cryptosporidium*
Dietary disturbances
Overfeeding, food allergy, starvation stools
Anatomic abnormalities
Intussusception, Hirschsprung's disease, partial obstruction, appendicitis, blind loop syndrome, intestinal lymphangiectasia, short bowel syndrome
Inflammatory bowel disease
Malabsorption or secretory diseases
Cystic fibrosis, celiac disease, disaccharidase deficiency, acrodermatitis enteropathica, secretory neoplasms
Systemic diseases
Immunodeficiency, endocrinopathy (hyperthyroidism, hypoparathyroidism, congenital adrenal hyperplasia)
Miscellaneous
Antibiotic-associated diarrhea, secondary lactase deficiency, irritable colon syndrome, neonatal drug withdrawal, toxins, hemolytic-uremic syndrome

important to inquire about previous GI surgery or chronic illnesses such as inflammatory bowel disease and immunodeficiency states. Bacterial and parasitic infections are more likely in institutionalized children and those returning from travel in low- and middle-income countries. Other causes of diarrhea include food allergies, antibiotic-associated diarrhea, and secondary lactase deficiency.

Acute onset of **bloody diarrhea** suggests a bacterial cause and a need to perform stool cultures. **If there is a known outbreak of *Escherichia coli* O157:H7 or clinical features of hemolytic-uremic syndrome, obtain further testing to exclude renal failure, thrombocytopenia, and hemolytic anemia** and provide early volume expansion.[13] An infant with intermittent, crampy abdominal pain, vomiting, and bloody stools raises concern for intussusception, pseudomembranous colitis, parasitic infection, or inflammatory bowel disease.

DEHYDRATION

Regardless of the cause of vomiting and diarrhea, the end result is fluid loss. Parental reports of dehydration, although highly sensitive, have a high false-positive rate. However, a history of *normal fluid intake* and *normal urine output* drastically reduces the likelihood of significant dehydration.[14] Thus, for the majority of children, the physical examination remains crucial and should begin by assessing the child's overall appearance, level of activity, responsiveness, respiratory pattern, and vital signs. Although the American Academy of Pediatrics, Centers for Disease Control and Prevention, World Health Organization, and European Society for Paediatric Gastroenterology, Hepatology, and Nutrition have developed treatment guidelines based on the degree of dehydration, no single variable in isolation is sufficiently accurate to determine the severity of dehydration.[15] The percentage of body weight lost remains the gold standard measurement of dehydration, but it is infrequently available in the ED. Thus, physicians need to continue to rely on the presence of a combination of clinical findings as well as historical features to determine the degree of dehydration (see Table 129-2).

Three clinical signs have significant positive likelihood ratios for 5% dehydration: prolonged capillary refill time, abnormal skin turgor, and abnormal respiratory pattern.[15] Well appearance, moist mucous membranes, and the absence of sunken eyes can help exclude dehydration.[15]

TABLE 128-5 Mechanisms of Infectious Diarrheal Disease

Pathogen Type	Characteristic Examples	Mechanism	Pathologic Impact	Clinical Impact
Viral enteropathogens	Rotaviruses Adenoviruses	Invade small intestinal mucosa villous epithelium	Loss of mature absorptive cells, producing a proliferative response, resulting in repopulation of intestinal epithelial lining with poorly differentiated cells.	Salt and water absorption is decreased Carbohydrate malabsorption and osmotic diarrhea
Bacterial enteropathogens	**Invasive** *Shigella* *Salmonella* *Yersinia enterocolitica* *Campylobacter jejuni* *Vibrio parahaemolyticus*	Adhere to mucosal cells followed by invasion and multiplication, primarily in large intestine	Intramucosal multiplication elicits an acute mucosal inflammatory reaction, resulting in ulceration and synthesis of a variety of secretagogues.	Salt and water absorption is decreased (secretory diarrhea)
	Cytotoxic *Shigella* Enteropathogenic *Escherichia coli* Enterohemorrhagic *E. coli* *Clostridium difficile*	Elaboration of cytotoxins	Cause cell damage and death by inhibiting protein synthesis or by inducing the secretion of one or more inflammatory mediator substances.	Decreased intestinal absorptive surface
	Toxigenic *Shigella* Enterotoxigenic *E. coli* *Y. enterocolitica* *Aeromonas* *Vibrio cholerae*	Colonize small intestine and secrete enterotoxins	Enterotoxin binds to specific mucosal receptors, increasing the concentration of an intracellular mediator (adenosine 3′:5′-cyclic phosphate or cyclic guanosine monophosphate).	Alter intestinal salt and water transport without affecting mucosal morphology
	Adherent Enteropathogenic *E. coli* Enterohemorrhagic *E. coli*	Colonization and adherence to intestinal surface of small and large intestine	Binding to epithelial cells indents the surface and causes glycocalyx dissolution and microvilli flattening.	Decreased intestinal absorptive surface

TABLE 128-6 Clinical Dehydration Score

Score	General Appearance	Eyes	Oral Mucosa (Tongue)	Tears
0	Normal	Normal	Moist	Normal
1	Thirsty, restless, lethargic but irritable	Mildly sunken	Sticky	Decreased
2	Drowsy/nonresponsive, limp, cold, diaphoretic	Very sunken	Dry	None

Score >0 = some dehydration; score >5 = moderate-severe dehydration.

A validated dehydration score (**Table 128-6**) derived from several clinical studies[16-20] correlates with length of stay and need for IV rehydration.[20]

GASTROENTERITIS

EPIDEMIOLOGY

Diarrheal diseases are the second leading cause of death worldwide in children. Rotavirus is the most common pathogen in areas without a vaccination program,[21] and in areas with widespread rotavirus vaccination,[22] norovirus is the most common pathogen.

PATHOPHYSIOLOGY

To cause diarrhea, an infectious agent must overcome numerous host defense factors, including gastric acidity, intestinal immunity, motility, mucus, and the resident microflora. The interaction between these factors and the infecting agent's virulence mechanisms determines the subsequent clinical course (Table 128-5). No matter what the mechanism is, acute gastroenteritis is associated with fluid shifts and has the potential to cause dehydration, shock, and even death. The common final pathway results in fluid output exceeding the absorptive capacity of the GI tract. Fasting, which sometimes occurs with gastroenteritis, actually worsens the capacity of the bowel to absorb fluids. Continued feeding not only slows the progression of dehydration by increasing the volume of fluid available to the intravascular space, but the presence of nutrients in the bowel lumen also promotes mucosal recovery and improves fluid absorption.[23]

CLINICAL FEATURES

Diarrhea associated with acute **viral gastroenteritis** typically lasts <7 days and not longer than 14 days, and it may be accompanied by vomiting or fever. Clinical features associated with the most important causes of **bacterial gastroenteritis** are listed in **Table 128-7. Isolated vomiting should not be diagnosed as acute gastroenteritis.** The differential diagnosis for isolated vomiting in the absence of diarrhea is broad.

Abdominal pain is often associated with gastroenteritis, but pain is typically poorly localized and crampy with no peritoneal signs on examination. If peritoneal signs are present, consider an alternative diagnosis, such as acute appendicitis. **Although appendicitis typically manifests with abdominal pain followed by vomiting associated with constipation, it may also cause diarrhea, particularly once the appendix has perforated. This is presumed to occur because the inflammation irritates the colon, resulting in diarrhea.** Stools tend to be frequent, mucus-containing, and small in volume. For further discussion, see chapter 130, "Acute Abdominal Pain in Infants and Children."

LABORATORY TESTING

Obtain a CBC only if the child is ill appearing or has bloody diarrhea (mainly to identify bacterial enterocolitis or hemolytic-uremic syndrome). The WBC count and C-reactive protein are not reliable for distinguishing viral from bacterial gastroenteritis.[25-27] The C-reactive protein is only helpful for following activity of inflammatory bowel disease. **Given that the reported prevalence of hypoglycemia may be as high as 9% in pediatric gastroenteritis,[28] measuring serum glucose in infants and young children is essential.**

Obtain serum electrolytes only in specific circumstances.[29,30] Table 128-8 lists the European Society for Paediatric Gastroenterology, Hepatology, and Nutrition recommendations for measuring electrolytes in children with gastroenteritis.

In a study assessing the utility of routinely obtaining electrolytes in 182 children receiving IV rehydration,[31] an electrolyte abnormality was present in nearly half, and management changed in 10% of children. **All interventions were related to the administration of fluids and glucose or potassium.**

Although BUN is elevated in severe dehydration, it does not identify lesser degrees of dehydration very well. Serum bicarbonate>15 mEq/L makes dehydration unlikely.[32] Last, urinary indices have been demonstrated to correlate poorly with severity of dehydration.[33]

RAPID STOOL TESTS

Classic gastroenteritis of bacterial origin arises in the distal small bowel or colon to cause dysentery, with fecal blood, pus, and mucus. Most viral, parasitic, and toxin-mediated etiologies do not cause significant inflammation. Thus, tests for inflammatory markers might help differentiate between viral and bacterial gastroenteritis. Identifying fecal leukocytes has technical limitations, including the need for an experienced technician and a fresh stool sample to provide an accurate identification. More than five WBCs per high-power field has a sensitivity of 73% (95% confidence interval, 0.33% to 0.94%) and specificity of 84% (95% confidence interval, 0.50% to 0.96%) and is moderately useful for identifying bacterial gastroenteritis.[34] A marker for fecal leukocytes, **fecal lactoferrin**, is increased during bacterial infection and in children with clinically more severe disease, and thus it may be a good marker for predicting and monitoring intestinal inflammation in children with infectious diarrhea.[35]

STOOL CULTURES

With a diagnostic yield as low as 2% and a high cost per positive result, **routine stool cultures are not necessary in acute gastroenteritis.** In select instances, however, stool culture is warranted. Several high-risk factors have been identified: >10 stools in the previous 24 hours,[36,37] travel to high-risk country,[36] fever,[36] older age child,[36] blood or mucus in stool,[37,38] and abdominal pain/tenderness.[37] Obtain stool cultures in cases of persistent diarrhea, when a specific antimicrobial treatment is being considered, or when infection must be excluded to support another diagnosis, such as inflammatory bowel disease.

Five bacterial pathogens commonly produce gastroenteritis in North America (Table 128-7): *Salmonella*, *Shigella*, *Yersinia*, *Campylobacter*, and pathogenic *E. coli*. All but *E. coli* do not normally inhabit the alimentary tract, so their identification in stool specimens diagnoses bacterial gastroenteritis. *E. coli*, however, is part of the usual gut flora and is rarely pathogenic; therefore, serotyping is useful for detecting *E. coli* O157, which causes hemolytic-uremic syndrome. In some parts of the world, *Vibrio cholerae* is a common bacterial cause of gastroenteritis.

IMAGING

In general, radiologic investigations play a very limited role in assessment of pediatric acute gastroenteritis. Imaging is valuable when the diagnosis is uncertain, such as may occur in children with isolated vomiting. Although plain films of the abdomen are usually nonspecific and have low sensitivity, they may be a useful starting point when looking for bowel obstructions, foreign bodies, and bowel perforation. On the other hand, in a group of neonates with bilious vomiting in the first 72 hours of life, 56% of lesions requiring surgical repair were not detected with the use of plain abdominal x-rays, reinforcing the need for further imaging when clinically indicated.[39] A history of abdominal surgery or foreign body ingestion or evidence on exam of abnormal bowel sounds, abdominal distension, or peritonitis has 93% sensitivity and 40% specificity in detecting diagnostic or suggestive radiographs in patients with major diseases potentially requiring procedural intervention.[40] Abdominal ultrasonography has an

TABLE 128-7 Clinical Features and Treatment of Bacterial Gastroenteritis[24]

Organism	Typical Clinical Features	Risk Factors	Complications	Antimicrobial Therapy
Shigella	Ranges from watery stools without constitutional symptoms to fever, abdominal pain, tenesmus, mucoid stools, hematochezia; *Shigella dysenteriae* serotype 1 causes more severe symptoms	Contact with infected host or fomite, poor sanitation, crowded living conditions, day care	Pseudomembranous colitis, toxic megacolon, intestinal perforation, bacteremia, Reiter's syndrome, hemolytic-uremic syndrome, encephalopathy, seizures, hemolysis	Typically self-limited Treat if: immunocompromised, severe disease, dysentery or systemic symptoms If susceptibility unknown: azithromycin, ceftriaxone, ciprofloxacin; if susceptible, ampicillin or trimethoprim-sulfamethoxazole
Salmonella	Nontyphoidal: May be asymptomatic or cause watery diarrhea, mild fever, abdominal cramps Enterica serotypes: "enteric fever" may include high fever, constitutional symptoms, headache, abdominal pain, dactylitis, hepatosplenomegaly, rose spots, altered mental status	Direct contact with animals: poultry, livestock, reptiles, pets; consuming food contaminated by human carrier: beef, poultry, eggs, dairy, water	Meningitis, brain abscess, osteomyelitis, bacteremia, dehydration, endocarditis, enteric (typhoid or paratyphoid) fever	Typically self-limited Treat if: <3 mo of age, hemoglobinopathy, immunodeficiency, chronic GI tract disease, malignancy, severe colitis, bacteremia, sepsis Options: ampicillin, amoxicillin, trimethoprim-sulfamethoxazole; if resistant, azithromycin, fluoroquinolone Invasive disease: cefotaxime, ceftriaxone
Campylobacter	Diarrhea, hematochezia, abdominal pain, fever, malaise	Contamination from poultry feces or undercooked poultry, untreated water, unpasteurized milk, pets (dogs, cats, hamsters, birds); person-to-person transmission possible	Acute: dehydration, bacteremia, focal infections, febrile seizures Convalescence: reactive arthritis, Reiter's syndrome, erythema nodosum, acute idiopathic polyneuritis, Miller Fisher syndrome, myocarditis, pericarditis	Often self-limited; 20% have relapse or prolonged symptoms Treat if: moderate-severe symptoms, relapse, immunocompromised, day care and institutions Options: erythromycin, azithromycin, ciprofloxacin
Escherichia coli–Shiga toxin producing	Initially nonbloody diarrhea, often becoming bloody; severe abdominal pain	Food or water contaminated with human or cattle feces, undercooked beef, unpasteurized milk	Hemorrhagic colitis, hemolytic-uremic syndrome	None indicated; debated risk of increased incidence of hemolytic-uremic syndrome with treatment
E. coli–enteropathogenic	Severe watery diarrhea, usually children <2 years in resource-limited countries	Food or water contaminated with feces	Dehydration	Treat if severe Options: trimethoprim-sulfamethoxazole, azithromycin, ciprofloxacin
E. coli–enterotoxigenic	Moderate watery diarrhea, abdominal cramps; traveler's diarrhea	Food or water contaminated with feces	Dehydration	Treat if severe Options: trimethoprim-sulfamethoxazole, azithromycin, ciprofloxacin
E. coli–enteroinvasive	Fever, bloody or nonbloody diarrhea, dysentery	Food or water contaminated with feces	Dehydration	Treat if severe Options: trimethoprim-sulfamethoxazole, azithromycin, ciprofloxacin
E. coli–enteroaggregative	Watery diarrhea, may be prolonged	Food or water contaminated with feces	Dehydration	Treat if severe Options: trimethoprim-sulfamethoxazole, azithromycin, ciprofloxacin
Yersinia	Bloody diarrhea with mucus, fever, abdominal pain; pseudoappendicitis syndrome: fever, right lower quadrant pain, leukocytosis; *Yersinia* pseudotuberculosis causes fever, scarlatiniform rash, abdominal pain	Contaminated food: improperly cooked pork, unpasteurized milk, untreated water; contact with animals (ungulates, rodents, rabbits, birds)	Acute: bacteremia, pharyngitis, meningitis, osteomyelitis, pyomyositis, conjunctivitis, pneumonia, empyema, endocarditis, acute peritonitis, liver/spleen abscess; convalescence: erythema nodosum, glomerulonephritis, reactive arthritis	Typically self-limited; if severe, treat with trimethoprim-sulfamethoxazole, aminoglycosides, cefotaxime, fluoroquinolones, tetracycline, doxycycline, chloramphenicol
Vibrio cholerae	Voluminous watery diarrhea, usually without cramps or fever, classically described as "rice water" stools	Travel to affected areas, consumption of contaminated water or food (particularly undercooked seafood)	May rapidly lead to hypovolemic shock, hypoglycemia, hypokalemia, metabolic acidosis, seizures	Treat if moderate or severe: azithromycin, doxycycline; ciprofloxacin or trimethoprim-sulfamethoxazole if resistant

important diagnostic role in pediatric centers; however, technical expertise is required to obtain optimal sensitivity and specificity.

TREATMENT

Oral Rehydration Therapy Treatment is directed at (1) preventing or treating dehydration, (2) replacing ongoing fluid losses, and (3) meeting nutritional needs. The worldwide adoption of oral rehydration therapy has revolutionized the treatment of dehydration. Oral rehydration therapy has reduced mortality in developing nations and is a safe and effective treatment for dehydrated children in developed nations.

The physiologic effectiveness of oral rehydration therapy is based on the coupled transport of sodium and glucose molecules at the brush border of intestinal epithelial cells, which provides a gradient for the passive absorption of water. This mechanism remains relatively intact, even in severe diarrheal disease, and functions optimally when the sodium-to-glucose ratio is 1:1.[30] The World Health Organization recommends an oral rehydration solution with a sodium concentration of

TABLE 128-8 Recommendations for Measuring Glucose and Serum Electrolytes

Moderately dehydrated children whose history and physical examination findings are inconsistent with acute gastroenteritis
All severely dehydrated children
All children requiring IV rehydration[31]

Source: Reproduced with permission from Guarino A, Albano F, Ashkenazi S, et al: European Society for Paediatric Gastroenterology, Hepatology, and Nutrition/European Society for Paediatric Infectious Diseases evidence based guidelines for the management of acute gastroenteritis in children in Europe. *J Paediatr Gastroenterol Nutr* 46: S81, 2008. Copyright Lippincott Williams & Wilkins.

75 mmol/L, and it is effective for children with noncholera diarrhea as measured by reduced stool output, reduced vomiting, and a reduced need for supplemental IV therapy.[29] Most commercially available oral rehydration solution formulations in North America and Europe contain 45 to 60 mmol/L of sodium (**Table 128-9**). **Many other beverages traditionally suggested for children with vomiting and diarrhea, such as tea, juice, or sports drinks, are deficient in sodium and may provide excessive sugar, amplifying fluid losses.** These beverages are not suitable for use as rehydration solutions but may be appropriate in nondehydrated children. For children who are not dehydrated and have only mild symptoms, there is currently no evidence to determine whether oral rehydration solution has advantages over a child's usual beverage of choice. Many potential oral rehydration solution additives have been studied for the purpose of enhancing clinical efficacy. Examples include alternative carbohydrates, such as rice starch, and although these may be of benefit in patients with cholera diarrhea, they are not routinely indicated in children with noncholera diarrhea.

Although oral rehydration therapy should be the first-line treatment for most children with acute gastroenteritis, it is often underused by healthcare providers in industrialized countries, who too often elect to administer IV rehydration. This may be due to misperceptions about the effectiveness of IV rehydration or unfamiliarity with published guidelines.[29,30] **IV rehydration is appropriate and necessary in children with severe dehydration or hemodynamic compromise or when altered mental status precludes safe oral administration of fluid.**[30] **Children with mild to moderate dehydration are candidates for oral rehydration therapy and should not receive IV rehydration as first-line therapy.** When comparing oral rehydration therapy with IV therapy, a Cochrane review concluded that there is no difference in failure to rehydrate, weight gain, or total fluid intake; oral rehydration therapy is associated with a shorter hospital stay. For every 25 children treated with oral rehydration therapy, one child would fail and require IV rehydration.[41] A sample ED algorithm incorporating oral rehydration therapy is provided in **Figure 128-1**.

In children with moderate dehydration undergoing oral rehydration therapy, the fluid deficit should be corrected rapidly (over 4 hours). **Give 50 to 100 mL of oral rehydration solution per kilogram of body weight, plus additional oral rehydration solution to compensate for ongoing losses (approximately 10 mL/kg per stool and 2 mL/kg per emesis).** Offer small volumes initially, such as 5 mL every 2 to 5 minutes, and increase as tolerated. **A general rule is to aim for about 1 ounce (30 mL) of oral rehydration solution per kilogram of body weight per hour.** Do not limit breastfeeding during any phase of oral rehydration therapy, both for the nutritional support of the infant and to avoid a decrease in the mother's milk supply. If necessary, oral rehydration solution may be provided as a supplement. **When oral rehydration is not feasible, enteral rehydration by the nasogastric route provides an effective alternative to IV rehydration.** This method allows for rehydration at a steady rate and is as successful as, and more cost effective than, IV rehydration.[42] Children with severe dehydration requiring IV rehydration can begin oral rehydration therapy when perfusion and mental status return to normal. Caregivers should understand the technique and rationale of oral rehydration therapy and should be provided with helpful equipment such as a clock and a syringe or dropper. Recognizing caregiver expectations and addressing potential obstacles, such as misconceptions about oral rehydration therapy or exhaustion, may also contribute to a successful outcome.

IV Hydration Parenteral therapy is discussed in chapter 129, "Fluid and Electrolyte Therapy in Infants and Children."

Antiemetics Although vomiting is not a contraindication to oral rehydration therapy and does not usually preclude successful oral rehydration, the presence of ongoing vomiting may be an obstacle to initiating or continuing oral rehydration therapy. **Ondansetron, a 5-hydroxytryptamine (serotonin) receptor antagonist, may be used as an adjunct to oral rehydration therapy in children with persistent vomiting at a dose of 0.15 mg/kg/dose PO. The use of intravenous ondansetron and multiple dose therapy is not supported by the evidence which associates both such approaches with increased side effects and no additional benefit beyond a single oral dose.**[43]

Do not use dopamine receptor agonists (such as promethazine, prochlorperazine, metoclopramide, and droperidol) to treat vomiting in children because of the potential for respiratory depression and extrapyramidal reactions.[44] **In addition, they lack evidence of efficacy.** The U.S. Food and Drug Administration issued an alert in 2006 indicating that promethazine (marketed as Phenergan®) should not be used in children <2 years of age because of the potential for fatal respiratory depression.

Maintenance Phase and Diet For children with minimal or no dehydration and those who have been successfully rehydrated, the priority is to prevent dehydration by providing maintenance fluid needs and replacing losses. Fluid needs may be met with oral rehydration solution or regular diet. Children undergoing oral rehydration therapy should resume feedings with an age-appropriate, palatable, and nutritionally complete diet as soon as the initial fluid deficit has been replaced. **Do not withhold feedings for >4 hours in a dehydrated child or for any length of time in a child who is not dehydrated.** Early refeeding during oral rehydration therapy has clinical and nutritional benefits and is supported in major guidelines.[29,30] The introduction of full-strength formula or regular diet immediately after rehydration is associated with increased weight gain and does not limit the success of oral rehydration therapy. **Most young children can continue to receive lactose-containing milk or formula.** However, there does appear to be a slight reduction in the duration of diarrhea and the treatment failure rate among inpatients administered lactose-free products, and this approach may be considered in this patient population.[45]

The banana, rice, applesauce, and toast diet is unnecessarily restrictive and may not provide enough nutrition, so it is no longer recommended.[30] Because fats are an important source of calories, low-fat diets are discouraged. Although yogurt has been shown in some studies to lead to an improvement in symptoms, it is not a standardized food and would not be expected to provide consistent effects. Beverages with high sugar content can increase intestinal fluid losses and are not recommended.[29]

Antidiarrheal Medications Antidiarrheal medications are not recommended either due to safety concerns or a lack of data to support effectiveness. Potential risks outweigh benefits. Loperamide, a peripheral opiate receptor agonist that can

TABLE 128-9 Composition of Standard ORS, Reduced-Osmolarity WHO ORS, and Other Commonly Consumed Beverages

	Carbohydrate (mmol/L)	Sodium (mmol/L)	Potassium (mmol/L)	Chloride (mmol/L)	Base (mmol/L)	Osmolarity (mOsm/L)
WHO reduced osmolarity (2002)	75	75	20	65	10	245
Pedialyte®	139	45	20	35	20	250
Enfalyte® (formerly Ricelyte)	167	50	25	45	34	200
Apple juice	666	0.4	44	45	N/A	730
Coca-Cola Classic®	622	1.6	N/A	N/A	13.4	650
Ginger ale	500	3.5	0.1	N/A	3.6	565
Gatorade®	322	20	3	N/A	3	350
Chicken broth	44	260	0.5	260	N/A	450

Abbreviations: N/A = not available; ORS = oral rehydration solution; WHO = World Health Organization.

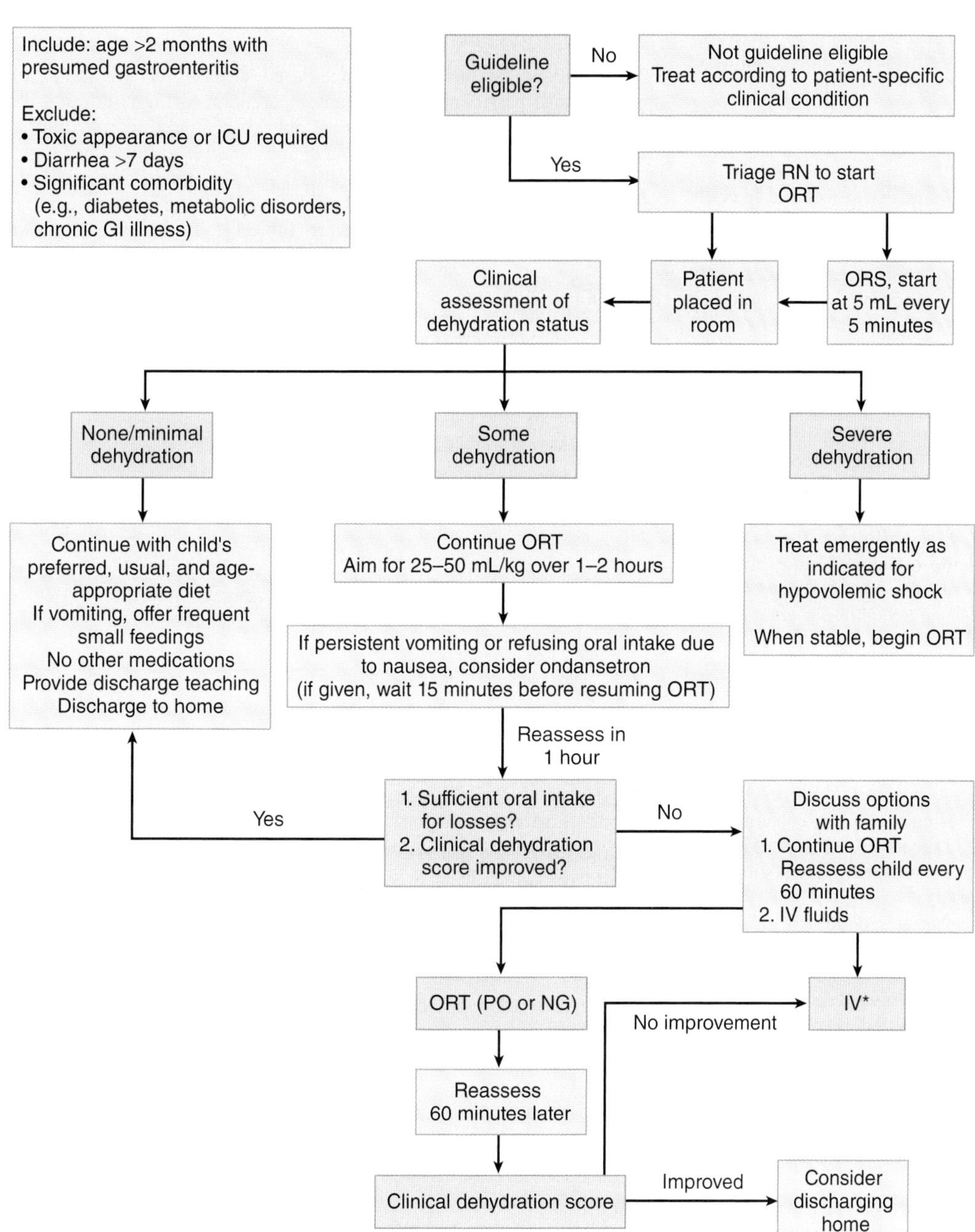
Include: age >2 months with presumed gastroenteritis
Exclude:
• Toxic appearance or ICU required
• Diarrhea >7 days
• Significant comorbidity (e.g., diabetes, metabolic disorders, chronic GI illness)
Guideline eligible?
No
Not guideline eligible
Treat according to patient-specific clinical condition
Yes
Triage RN to start ORT
Clinical assessment of dehydration status
Patient placed in room
ORS, start at 5 mL every 5 minutes
None/minimal dehydration
Some dehydration
Severe dehydration
Continue with child's preferred, usual, and age-appropriate diet
If vomiting, offer frequent small feedings
No other medications
Provide discharge teaching
Discharge to home
Continue ORT
Aim for 25–50 mL/kg over 1–2 hours
Treat emergently as indicated for hypovolemic shock
When stable, begin ORT
If persistent vomiting or refusing oral intake due to nausea, consider ondansetron
(if given, wait 15 minutes before resuming ORT)
Reassess in 1 hour
Yes
1. Sufficient oral intake for losses?
2. Clinical dehydration score improved?
No
Discuss options with family
1. Continue ORT
Reassess child every 60 minutes
2. IV fluids
ORT (PO or NG)
IV*
No improvement
Reassess 60 minutes later
Clinical dehydration score
Improved
Consider discharging home

FIGURE 128-1. Algorithm for evaluation and management of acute gastroenteritis in children >2 months of age based on clinical assessment of dehydration status. *If IV access is difficult, consider nasogastric (NG) oral rehydration solution (50 mL/kg) over 3 hours instead. Continue oral rehydration therapy (ORT) during IV therapy. RN = registered nurse.

reduce diarrhea, is absolutely contraindicated in children <2 years old and for those with bloody stools or suspected bacterial gastroenteritis from *Salmonella*, *Shigella*, or *Campylobacter*. The drug can cause lethargy and paralytic ileus. Additionally, loperamide may be associated with a possible increased risk of hemolytic-uremic syndrome when used in the setting of enterohemorrhagic *E. coli* infection. Although older children with viral gastroenteritis who take an age-appropriate dose are unlikely to experience serious events, potential risks likely outweigh benefits in most children.

Adsorbents and Antisecretory Agents Smectite is an aluminomagnesium silicate that binds some toxins, bacteria, and viruses and is used in several European countries as an antidiarrheal agent. Although some trials and a recent meta-analysis have reported effectiveness in reducing diarrhea, the limitations of the studies prevent any firm conclusions from being drawn. Bismuth subsalicylate is an antisecretory agent that is commonly found in over-the-counter diarrhea medications. **Although bismuth has a modest effect on reducing severity of diarrhea, it can cause elevated salicylate levels in children.[46] Consequently, products containing bismuth subsalicylate (e.g., Kaopectate) in the United States are now labeled for use only in adults and children 12 years of age and older.** Racecadotril is a prodrug that must be hydrolyzed to its active metabolite (thiorphan), which then acts as an enkephalinase inhibitor that decreases intestinal secretion by preventing the breakdown of endogenous GI opioids. It is available in Europe and Southeast Asia, but not in the United States. In a systematic review including nine trials and 1,384 children, twice as many patients had diarrhea resolution at any time point when administered racecadotril relative to placebo.[47] Although it has also been shown to reduce stool frequency (stool ratio of racecadotril to placebo = 0.63), it has not demonstrated an improvement in major clinical outcomes such as hospitalization.[48]

Probiotics Probiotics are living organisms that, when ingested, can modulate mucosal and systemic immunity by altering microbial balance in the intestinal tract. Data from several meta-analyses show a moderate clinical benefit of certain probiotic strains in reducing the duration and/or volume of diarrhea in hospitalized children. However, more data are needed to determine the optimal organism, dosing, and duration of treatment.[49] The only pediatric ED study to date, which evaluated *Lactobacillus rhamnosus* GG, reported no reduction in the time to normal stool or the number of diarrheal stools.[50] Prebiotics, which are nondigestible food components believed to improve microbial balance in the intestinal tract, have not been extensively studied and are not recommended. There is no high-quality published evidence regarding the use of homeopathic or herbal medications for the management of gastroenteritis.

Zinc Zinc is necessary for intestinal mucosal healing, and its deficiency has been associated with increased diarrhea severity. Malnourished children >6 months old benefit the most from zinc therapy (27-hour reduction in diarrhea duration), and its use should likely be limited to such groups of children.[51] Because zinc is an effective therapy for diarrhea and reduces morbidity and mortality in the setting of low-income countries,[52] the United Nations Children's Fund and the World Health Organization recommend zinc supplementation as a universal treatment for children with diarrhea in low-income countries at a dose of 20 milligrams/d of any zinc salt orally for 10 to 14 days (10 milligrams/d for infants <6 months old).

Antibiotics for Acute Gastroenteritis Because the cause of gastroenteritis is rarely known upon presentation, treatment decisions must be made before the identification of a pathogen is possible. Because the vast majority of episodes of pediatric gastroenteritis are of viral origin, **do not routinely give antibiotics.** See recommendations for specific pathogens and clinical settings in Table 128-7. **Give antibiotics for symptoms of inflammatory infection such as acute onset of bloody diarrhea with mucus and high fever.** The most common bacterial causes of this presentation are *Shigella*, *Campylobacter*, and *Salmonella enterica* species. The choice of antimicrobial agent depends on local prevalence and resistance patterns. Parenteral rather than oral antibiotic therapy is appropriate for patients unable to take oral medications, patients with toxic appearance or underlying immunodeficiency, and febrile infants <3 months of age. **Children with watery diarrhea generally should not receive empiric antibiotics unless they have been exposed to cholera.**

Antibiotics are effective in reducing the symptoms and infectivity of *Shigella* gastroenteritis. Because of increasing resistance, use ampicillin or trimethoprim-sulfamethoxazole only if the strain is susceptible. Otherwise, azithromycin is an appropriate first-line agent. Ceftriaxone is the treatment of choice for parenteral therapy.

Do not use antibiotics to treat *Salmonella* gastroenteritis unless specific risk factors are present. A Cochrane review (12 trials, 767 patients) demonstrated no evidence of benefit from antibiotic therapy in otherwise healthy individuals with nontyphoidal *Salmonella* gastroenteritis.[53] Although the number of young children studied was small, adverse events were more common in participants who received antibiotic treatment. Thus, antibiotics should only be administered to high-risk children to reduce the risk of *Salmonella* bacteremia and extraintestinal infections. High-risk children include those with underlying immune deficiencies, sickle cell disease, immunosuppressive therapy, or inflammatory bowel disease and infants <3 months old.

Antibiotic therapy for *Campylobacter* gastroenteritis has a modest effect on symptoms and is most effective if treatment is started within 3 days of disease onset.[54] Antibiotics reduce the duration of fecal excretion of organisms and are recommended to reduce transmission in day care centers and institutions.

Antibiotics for Shiga toxin–producing *E. coli* do not significantly affect the clinical course. Additionally, an increased risk of hemolytic-uremic syndrome after antibiotic treatment has been reported, but results are conflicting, and a meta-analysis concluded that the risk is unclear.[55] **Therefore, children with *E. coli* O157:H7 should not receive antibiotics.** Intravenous volume expansion is an underused intervention that may decrease the frequency of oligoanuric renal failure in children with diarrhea-associated hemolytic-uremic syndrome (hematocrit <30% with evidence of intravascular erythrocyte destruction), thrombocytopenia (platelet count $<150 \times 10^3/mm^3$), and impaired renal function.[13] **Antibiotics may be useful for severe forms of enteroinvasive, enteropathogenic, or enterotoxigenic E. coli infection.** Azithromycin and trimethoprim-sulfamethoxazole are treatment options.

Antibiotics reduce the severity of *V. cholerae* diarrhea. Treatment options include doxycycline, azithromycin, or trimethoprim-sulfamethoxazole.

Antimicrobial treatment of *Yersinia* species is appropriate if severe disease, bacteremia, or extraintestinal infection is suspected. Options include trimethoprim-sulfamethoxazole, aminoglycosides, cefotaxime, fluoroquinolones, tetracycline, doxycycline, and chloramphenicol.

DISPOSITION AND FOLLOW-UP

There are no established evidence-based criteria for admission of patients with gastroenteritis. In general, well-appearing children with minimal or no dehydration who are able to receive oral rehydration therapy at home should be discharged, and caregivers should be taught how to administer oral rehydration therapy and recognize signs of dehydration. Discharge instructions should be verbal and written. Sample discharge instructions are presented in **Table 128-10**. Ideally, caregivers

TABLE 128-10 Sample Gastroenteritis Discharge Instructions

Your child has been diagnosed with gastroenteritis. Gastroenteritis is an illness that consists of vomiting and diarrhea. It is often caused by viruses and usually can be treated without medications. Preventing dehydration is the most important goal in caring for children with gastroenteritis.

How will I know if my child is becoming dehydrated?

Dry lips and mouth.

Decreased activity level.

Sunken eyes.

Sunken fontanelle (soft spot) in babies <1 y.

Not urinating as often as usual or dark urine.

Reduced tears when crying.

What should I give my child to eat and drink?

Children who do not have signs of dehydration can drink what is usual for them. You do not need to stop giving milk. Drinks with a lot of sugar, such as fruit juices, can make diarrhea worse.

Your child should return to his or her normal diet as soon as possible. A special diet is not necessary. Good nutrition is important, even if there is still vomiting or diarrhea.

If you are breastfeeding, continue breastfeeding. Babies taking formula can continue to receive their usual formula.

Children who are showing some signs of dehydration should receive oral rehydration solutions (see below).

What types of fluids are acceptable for oral rehydration?

Over-the-counter rehydration solutions are ideal for rehydration. Some brands include Pedialyte and Enfalyte. Generic solutions are also available. Flavored solutions are usually preferred by children.

Sports drinks are not the same as oral rehydration solutions and should not be used in infants or children who are dehydrated. They may be acceptable in older children with minimal dehydration.

Plain water and tea do not have sugar or salt and can cause electrolyte changes, especially if given to small babies.

Soda/pop and juices have too much sugar and not enough salt to be used for oral rehydration.

Children who are not dehydrated do not need a special oral rehydration solution.

How do I give oral rehydration?

If your child is vomiting, start with small amounts of oral rehydration fluid, such as one teaspoon (5 mL) every 5 min. Increase the amount gradually, as tolerated.

If your child is breastfed, continue breastfeeding. Oral rehydration solutions can supplement breast milk after or between breast feedings, but should never take the place of breast milk.

When should I call my child's doctor or seek help?

Call your doctor immediately or go to the nearest emergency department if:

- Your child seems dehydrated and is not able to drink.
- Your child's vomit is green or bloody.
- Your child has severe abdominal pain.
- Your child appears to be very sick.
- Your child has blood in the diarrhea.
- Your child has a fever and is <3 mo of age.

When should I follow up with my child's doctor?

If your child is <6 mo of age, follow up within 24–48 h.

If your child is >6 mo of age, call your doctor's office and schedule a follow-up if symptoms continue.

will have had the opportunity to practice oral rehydration therapy and ask questions while in the ED. Children with moderate or severe dehydration, intractable or bilious vomiting, a suspected surgical condition, or significant laboratory or neurologic abnormalities, including lethargy or seizures, require further testing and should be observed in the ED or admitted. Patients not likely to succeed with home oral rehydration therapy, such as those with large ongoing losses or inadequate support, should also be observed or admitted. Many patients with dehydration who require ongoing treatment can be successfully managed in an observation unit.[56] Young infants are at risk for more rapid and severe dehydration, so the threshold for admission should be low, and follow-up in 24 hours should be ensured if discharge is considered. Families who are discharged should be instructed to return to seek further care if their child becomes unable to receive oral rehydration therapy, has persistent or bilious emesis, or shows increasing evidence of dehydration, or if symptoms are worsening.

SPECIAL SITUATIONS

DIARRHEA WITH OR WITHOUT VOMITING

Adverse Food Reactions Adverse food reactions can be due to either an adverse immunologic response, otherwise known as an allergy, or an adverse physiologic response, often referred to as food intolerance.[57] The National Institute of Allergy and Infectious Diseases recognizes four categories of immune-mediated adverse food reactions: immunoglobin E (IgE)-mediated, non–IgE-mediated, mixed, and cell-mediated.[58] IgE-mediated GI allergic symptoms may consist of nausea, abdominal pain, cramping, vomiting, or diarrhea developing within minutes to 2 hours of the ingestion of a food allergen. GI symptoms are often accompanied by symptoms involving the mouth or skin and may also include respiratory and systemic manifestations. Eosinophilic gastroenteritis is an example of a mixed IgE and non-IgE food allergy, with T-cell–mediated responses playing a significant role in pathogenesis.[59] Patients may present at any age, and many will have other allergic or atopic conditions. The portion of the GI track involved determines symptoms. Because symptoms tend to be delayed, identifying the offending food(s) may be challenging. Infants often present with feeding difficulties, gastroesophageal reflux, vomiting, and failure to thrive. Older children may present with vomiting, abdominal pain, or symptoms similar to irritable bowel syndrome. A history of dysphagia or food impactions suggests eosinophilic esophagitis.

Non–IgE-mediated food allergies are primarily T-cell–mediated and tend to result in delayed symptoms. Examples include food protein–induced enterocolitis syndrome, food protein–induced allergic proctocolitis, and celiac disease.[59] Food protein–induced enterocolitis syndrome is a potentially severe condition with a peak incidence in infants between 0 and 9 months old. Proteins in cow's milk or soy formulas are the most common triggers in infants, and symptoms consist of profuse vomiting and diarrhea for several hours after exposure, at times resulting in shock. Many other foods have been implicated in food protein–induced enterocolitis syndrome, and children regularly exposed to the allergenic food may develop chronic vomiting, diarrhea, anemia, or failure to thrive. Food protein–induced allergic proctocolitis most often presents in breastfed infants in the first 2 months of life. Infants generally appear healthy but have stools characterized by the presence of blood and mucus. Cow's milk in the maternal diet is the most common trigger, and symptoms begin to improve within a few days of dietary modification. The condition generally resolves between the ages of 6 months and 2 years. Diagnostic tests used for IgE allergies such as skin prick testing are not useful in identifying the offending agents in non-IgE–mediated food allergies; therefore, the diagnosis is based on clinical suspicion. Dietary avoidance is the mainstay of management.

Celiac disease is a T-cell–mediated inflammatory response triggered by the ingestion of gluten in genetically predisposed individuals. GI presentations are common in children and include chronic or intermittent diarrhea, abdominal pain, abdominal distension, and failure to thrive. Whereas young children most often have a "typical" presentation, extraintestinal symptoms such as fatigue, osteopenia, iron deficiency anemia, and short stature become more common as age increases. Treatment consists of lifelong adherence to a gluten-free diet.[60]

Antibiotic-Associated Diarrhea Antibiotic-associated diarrhea is otherwise unexplained diarrhea that occurs in association with the administration of antibiotics. The frequency of this complication varies, with diarrhea occurring in 5% to 10% of children treated with ampicillin, 10% to 25% treated with amoxicillin-clavulanate, and 15% to 20% treated with cefixime. The spectrum of findings in antibiotic-associated diarrhea ranges from mild diarrhea to severe colitis that may include abdominal cramping, fever, leukocytosis, fecal leukocytes, hypoalbuminemia and colonic thickening with characteristic changes visible on endoscopy and biopsy. Although infection with *Clostridium difficile* accounts for only 10% to 20% of the cases of antibiotic-associated diarrhea, it accounts for most cases of colitis associated with antibiotic therapy. Nonclostridial antibiotic–associated diarrhea may be caused by other enteric pathogens, by the direct effects of antimicrobial agents on the intestinal mucosa, or by the metabolic consequences of reduced concentrations of fecal flora. **Clindamycin, cephalosporins, and penicillins are the antibiotics most frequently implicated in *C. difficile* diarrhea.**

C. difficile disease can only be firmly diagnosed once its toxin is identified. However, because children can be asymptomatic hosts of toxin-producing strains, testing for *C. difficile* should only be performed on diarrheal stools. When identified in the stool of children < 2 years of age (even if diarrheal), it most commonly is not the etiology of the diarrhea and usually does not require treatment. The following two-step testing strategy has been proposed: screening should be performed through the conduct of an enzyme immunoassay for glutamate dehydrogenase, which is present in almost all strains of *C. difficile*, including those that do not produce toxin.[61,62] If positive, this should be followed by a confirmatory enzyme immunoassay test for toxins A and B or preferably, by a cell cytotoxin assay that demonstrates cytotoxicity of stool for human fibroblast cells. Polymerase chain reaction testing is a rapid, sensitive, and specific test that appears promising. However, significant variations exist in testing methodologies and kits and thus further evaluation of its utility is warranted before widespread adoption.[63,64] Indications for treatment include positive assays for *C. difficile* toxin, plus one of the following: evidence of colitis, moderate to severe diarrhea, persistent diarrhea despite the discontinuation of the implicated agent, or the need to continue treating the original infection. Oral metronidazole is the treatment of choice in most cases of pediatric *C. difficile* colitis. In the most severe cases, vancomycin (oral or rectal) may be used in conjunction with IV metronidazole. The anticipated response to treatment is resolution of fever within 1 day and resolution of diarrhea in 4 to 5 days. Treatment does not eradicate *C. difficile*, and asymptomatic patients should not be retested or treated based on a positive stool test. **Metronidazole is preferred because it is less expensive than vancomycin and avoids the potential risk of promoting vancomycin-resistant enterococci.**

Secondary Lactase Deficiency Secondary lactase deficiency implies that a pathophysiologic condition has resulted in an acquired lactase deficiency and lactose malabsorption. The most common etiology is acute GI infection resulting in small intestinal injury with loss of lactase-containing epithelial cells at the tips of the villi. The immature epithelial cells that replace these are often lactase deficient, leading to secondary lactase deficiency and lactose malabsorption. Despite this, children with infectious diarrheal illnesses who have no or only mild dehydration can continue consuming human milk or standard formula without a significant effect on clinical course. Secondary lactase deficiency with clinical signs of lactose intolerance can be seen in celiac disease, Crohn's disease, and immune-related and other enteropathies, and should be considered as a possible etiology for diarrhea in children with these conditions. Diagnostic evaluation should be performed when secondary lactase deficiency is suspected and infection is not the cause.

Parasitic Infection Parasites are uncommon causes of diarrhea but may be the source of waterborne outbreaks and are more severe in immunocompromised children. *Cryptosporidium* and *Giardia* are the parasites most likely to cause diarrhea. Nitazoxanide is the drug of choice for *Cryptosporidium* infections, and either metronidazole, tinidazole, or nitazoxanide may be used in the treatment of *Giardia* infections. For further discussion of parasitic diseases, see the chapters 159, "Food and Waterborne Illnesses," and 161, "Global Travelers."

TRAVELER'S DIARRHEA

Limited data suggest that diarrhea is common in children traveling to high-risk regions. Although many cases of traveler's diarrhea are self-limited, antibiotic therapy is appropriate for children with a history of travel to a high-risk region who have severe or prolonged symptoms (>5 days). Macrolides such as azithromycin are the first-line antibiotic therapy, and trimethoprim-sulfamethoxazole may also be considered.

PRACTICE GUIDELINES AND SOCIETY POSITION STATEMENTS

King CK, Glass R, Bresee JS, Duggan C, Centers for Disease Control and Prevention: Managing acute gastroenteritis among children: oral rehydration, maintenance, and nutritional therapy. *MMWR Recomm Rep* 52:(RR16): 1, 2003.

National Collaborating Centre for Women's and Children's Health: *Diarrhoea and Vomiting Caused by Gastroenteritis: Diagnosis, Assessment and Management in Children Younger Than 5 Years.* London: National Institute for Health and Clinical Excellence; April 2009.

REFERENCES

The complete reference list is available online at www.TintinalliEM.com.

TABLE 129-1 Causes of Dehydration in Children

Decreased Intake:
- Voluntary or involuntary
  - Anatomic or pathologic diseases (pharyngitis, stomatitis, cleft lip/palate, facial dysmorphism, airway obstruction)
  - Neurologic diseases (meningitis, encephalitis, brain tumor, seizures)
  - Febrile illnesses

Increased Output:
- Insensible losses (fever, heat, respiratory diseases, diaphoresis, thyroid disease, cystic fibrosis)
- GI losses (vomiting, diarrhea)
- Renal losses:
  - Osmotic (DKA, acute tubular necrosis)
  - Nonosmotic (renal diseases, electrolyte disturbance, diabetes insipidus)

Sodium losing (adrenal disease, diuretics, kidney disease, pseudohypoaldosteronism)

Systemic Diseases:
- Moderate to severe burns
- Ascites
- Respiratory disease
- Peritonitis: medical or surgical with third spacing
- Anaphylaxis

Abbreviation: DKA = diabetic ketoacidosis.

CHAPTER 129 Fluid and Electrolyte Therapy in Infants and Children

Melissa Chan
Paul Enarson

INTRODUCTION

This chapter provides a basic a guide to parenteral rehydration, maintenance fluids, and management of common electrolyte abnormalities in children.

The most common cause of fluid and electrolyte abnormalities in children is dehydration.[1] Dehydration results from a negative fluid balance due to decreased intake, increased output (renal, GI, or insensible losses from the skin or respiratory tract), or disease states such as burns, sepsis, or diabetes. Negative fluid balance can occur in the intracellular fluid or extracellular fluid compartments and may be accompanied by derangements in electrolytes. **Table 129-1** lists some of the common causes of dehydration. Common signs of dehydration are listed in **Table 129-2**, and a validated clinical scoring system predicting the need for parenteral rehydration is provided in Table 129-7 of chapter 128, "Vomiting, Diarrhea, and Dehydration in Infants and Children."

PATHOPHYSIOLOGY

Infants and children are particularly susceptible to dehydration for a number of developmental and physiologic reasons. They are dependent on caretakers to provide oral fluids and therefore cannot regulate their intake. In addition, young children and infants have increased fluid requirements and are at risk of increased fluid losses compared to adults and older children. Basal metabolic rates are highest in young children, peaking at 12 months of age and gradually decreasing starting at 3 years of age.[2] Infants also have a higher turnover rate for water. Total body water as a percentage of body weight decreases from 75% in a term infant to 60% at 1 year of age, remaining at this percentage until puberty.[3] The high percentage of total body water, coupled with a decreased ability to control water loss (e.g., insensible losses from larger surface area–to–body ratio and faster respiratory rate) and a decreased ability to concentrate the urine, predispose infants to dehydration. Furthermore, young children are more prone to hypermetabolic states, such as high fever, which also increase the need for free water. Fever increases the basal metabolic rate by 13% for each degree above 37.8°C.[4]

Because sodium and water are tightly regulated together, dehydration is often described in relation to serum sodium concentrations. Children can develop isonatremic (isotonic) dehydration (sodium level of 135 to

TABLE 129-2 Clinical Guidelines for Assessing Dehydration in Children

	None to Minimal Dehydration (<3% loss of body weight)	Some (mild to moderate) Dehydration (3% to 9% loss of body weight)	Severe Dehydration (>9% loss of body weight)
Mental status	Well, alert	Fatigued, restless, irritable	Apathetic, lethargic, unconscious
Thirst	Normal, slight increase, or refusing fluids	Increased, eager to drink	Very thirsty or too lethargic to indicate
Heart rate	Normal	Normal to increased	Tachycardic with bradycardia in severe cases
Blood pressure	Normal	Normal	Normal to reduced
Pulse quality	Normal	Normal to reduced	Weak, thready
Breathing	Normal	Normal to tachypneic	Deep
Eyes	Normal	Slightly sunken orbits	Deeply sunken orbits
Tears	Present	Decreased	Absent
Mucous membranes	Moist	Dry	Parched
Anterior fontanelle	Normal	Sunken	Sunken
Skin turgor	Instant recoil	Recoil in <2 s	Recoil in >2 s
Capillary refill	Normal	Prolonged 1–2 s	Prolonged >2 s
Extremities	Warm	Cool	Cold, mottled, cyanotic
Urine output	Normal to decreased	Decreased (<1 mL/kg/h)	Minimal (<0.5 mL/kg/h)

Courtesy of Stephen Freedman, MD, and Jennifer Thull-Freedman, MD.

145 mEq/L), hyponatremic (hypotonic) dehydration (sodium level of <135 mEq/L), or hypernatremic (hypertonic) dehydration (sodium level of >145 mEq/L). Isonatremic dehydration is the most common form of dehydration. Isonatremic (isotonic) dehydration occurs when the fluid sodium losses are proportionate in the intracellular fluid and extracellular fluid compartments. Hyponatremic (hypotonic) dehydration occurs when fluid that is lost contains proportionately more sodium than blood, which leads to osmotic shifts of free water from the intracellular fluid to the extracellular fluid compartments. Hypernatremic (hypertonic) dehydration occurs when the fluid lost contains less sodium than the blood, which causes extracellular fluid free water to move into the intracellular fluid space.

CLINICAL FEATURES

HISTORY

Suspicion of fluid or electrolyte disorders can often be raised through a properly taken history. Questions to be asked on history include symptoms (what they are, when they started, where they started; e.g., was the child in a hot environment), whether fever is present, whether the child is tachypneic, and prior treatment. Prior treatment is of utmost importance beause this will demonstrate if intake has matched output and if appropriate (or more importantly, inappropriate) fluid replacement has occurred. For breastfeeding infants, inquire about frequency of feeds, whether the mother feels she has a good milk production, and whether the infant is feeding or engaged in nonnutrient sucking for comfort. If not breastfeeding, ask what type of fluid has been given, because hypotonic fluids (e.g., water or other hypotonic solutions) that increase the risk of hyponatremia are often used during illnesses. If the infant is bottle-fed, ask whether the formula is premixed or made from powder; hypernatremia or hyponatremia can result from inappropriately prepared formula. Questions surrounding output aid in assessing whether replacement of losses has been adequate; excess output results from vomiting or diarrhea (quantify the frequency and volume if possible). Assess urine output by asking how often the child is urinating or the number of wet diapers if the child is not yet toilet trained. Inquire about volume status by asking about tear production, the presence or absence of sweat, and the child's general appearance and mental status: Is the child increasingly irritable or lethargic? Has the parent noticed a change in the skin (cyanotic, pale, mottled)? **Most important, if known, is a change in weight, because weight loss is the gold standard for assessment of volume status.**[5] In addition to the specific questions, ask about signs or symptoms of infection, recent travel, sick contacts, and underlying chronic disease, which may point to a specific cause of dehydration. Children are at risk for accidental ingestion of toxins or plants, many of which can cause vomiting and lead to electrolyte disturbances, so such exposure should be specifically assessed.

PHYSICAL EXAMINATION

Physical findings related to individual electrolyte disorders are discussed in relation to specific electrolyte disorder below. In general, children with dehydration demonstrate a spectrum of physical findings ranging from a normal exam if dehydration is mild, to hypovolemic shock if dehydration is severe. Table 129-2 lists common signs and symptoms, and Table 128-6 presents a simplified clinical scoring system for dehydration. Tachycardia is an early sign of dehydration as the body compensates for a decreased circulatory volume. Tachycardia can present with normal blood pressure with or without signs of shock (compensated shock), but may be accompanied by hypotension (uncompensated shock) in severe dehydration. Tachypnea may also be noted as metabolic acidosis develops in moderate to severe dehydration. Note the mental status and the presence of lethargy or hypotonia, because these suggest severe dehydration or electrolyte abnormalities. In infants, the quality of the fontanelle (flat or sunken) may aid in assessment of hydration status, along with the presence or absence of tears when crying; assess the mucous membranes for cracked, dry lips, or decreased saliva in mouth, and the temperature, color, and turgor of the skin (cool, mottled, cyanotic, decreased elasticity), as well as capillary refill time, which should be <2 seconds when normal. Finally, note the character of the pulses because diminished pulses may also reflect significant dehydration.

LABORATORY EVALUATION

Laboratory testing for individual electrolyte disorders is discussed individually below. **Routine laboratory testing for assessing dehydration alone is generally not required**, because numerous studies have found a lack of correlation between laboratory values and degree of dehydration based on percent weight lost. Measure serum electrolytes if IV insertion is required for rehydration and signs of electrolyte disturbance are present,[5,6] or if electrolyte abnormalities are expected due to certain underlying medical condition (e.g., diabetic ketoacidosis or congenital adrenal hyperplasia). **Perform a bedside glucose test in any child presenting with altered sensorium, and rapidly correct hypoglycemia** (see chapter 144, "Metabolic Emergencies in Infants and Children").

INITIAL TREATMENT OF DEHYDRATION

Three main modalities exist for rehydration in children: oral, nasogastric, and parenteral. Treatment at each level of dehydration is discussed below and summarized in **Table 129-3**.

MILD TO MODERATE DEHYDRATION

Mild and moderate dehydration can be successfully managed with oral or nasogastric rehydration. Oral rehydration therapy and the role of antiemetics for vomiting patients are discussed in detail in chapter 128. Nasogastric hydration is effective, even in vomiting patients.[7,8] In a large study comparing nasogastric hydration versus IV hydration over 3 hours, subjects in the nasogastric-treated group had fewer complications, achieved resolution of ketonuria more often, and had greater reduction in specific gravity than IV-treated subjects. Nasogastric treatment is more cost effective than IV treatment.[8]

MODERATE AND SEVERE DEHYDRATION

The child unable to tolerate oral/nasogastric rehydration therapy or with severe dehydration requires prompt fluid resuscitation with large volumes of fluid over a short period of time[9,10] (**Table 129-4**). Give 20 mL/kg boluses

TABLE 129-3 Treatment for Mild, Moderate, and Severe Dehydration

	Mild	Moderate	Severe
Primary phase	PO*	PO*	IV†, IO, NG
Secondary phase (if primary phase fails)	NG/IV	NG/IV‡	IO Central line
Tertiary phase (after rehydration to ensure ability to maintain oral intake—optional)	PO*	PO*	± PO* after initial IV/IO rehydration
Laboratory studies	None	Optional#	Electrolytes, BUN, creatinine, calcium, glucose levels; urinalysis
Discharge criteria	Appears clinically well, alert, and orientated Vital signs within normal limits for age Urine output during hydrating period Intake is equal or greater to ongoing losses		
Treatment failure	Admit or place in observation unit		

*PO: Use commercial rehydration solution such as Pedialyte® or Enfalyte® or WHO reduced-osmolality ORS. Rehydrate with 5 mL (1 tsp) every 2–3 min. Increase based on patient tolerance; aim for 50–100 mL/kg replacement plus 10 mL/kg per stool and 2 mL/kg per emesis episode.

†IV (severe dehydration): 20 mL/kg over 5–30 min (NS or lactated Ringer's solution). Aim for 60–100 mL/kg in the first hour. Contraindications include some forms of cardiac disease (e.g., cardiomyopathy).

‡IV NS 20 mL/kg over 20-30 min, repeat as needed; NG oral rehydration solution at a rate of 10-20 mL/kg/hour.

#Perform laboratory testing based on dietary history or disease state.

Abbreviations: NG = nasogastric; NS = normal saline; ORS = oral rehydration salts; WHO = World Health Organization.

TABLE 129-4 IV Rehydration for Moderate to Severe Dehydration

Degree of Dehydration	IV Rehydration	Replacement of Ongoing Losses after Initial Rehydration
Severe with uncompensated shock	20 mL/kg 0.9% saline bolus over 5 min, repeated until hemodynamically stable	5–10 mL/kg 0.9% saline or 5% dextrose in 0.9% saline for each watery diarrheal stool *and* 2 mL/kg 0.9% saline or 5% dextrose in 0.9% saline for each emesis
Moderate to severe without signs of shock	20 mL/kg 0.9% saline bolus over 1 h followed by 5% dextrose in 0.9% saline at 1–2× maintenance rate for 1 h	

over 5 to 10 minutes repetitively until hemodynamics stabilize. Up to 60 mL/kg or more may be required in the first hour, unless contraindicated based on underlying disease.[11] Use an isotonic solution such as 0.9% saline or a lactated Ringer's solution during this resuscitation phase.[12]

For patients with moderate dehydration requiring parenteral fluids, there is no advantage of rapid or ultrarapid (50 to 60 mL/kg in 1 hour) hydration over standard hydration with 20 mL/kg over 1 hour, and a blinded randomized trial found increased hospitalization rates among those receiving ultrarapid hydration.[13] Furthermore, a study of fluid resuscitation among dehydrated children in Africa found that aggressive bolus fluid resuscitation was associated with increased mortality.[14]

After initial volume expansion, continue replacement with either normal saline or 5% dextrose in 0.9% normal saline. Use clinical judgment, because there is no strong evidence to recommend one fluid over the other, although dextrose-containing fluids help clear ketones in the patient who has not been eating or drinking.[15,16]

MAINTENANCE TREATMENT

Caloric expenditure and therefore fluid requirements can be estimated from body surface area, which is relatively large in infants in comparison with older children and adults. However, in the ED, weight is a sufficiently accurate value for calculating fluid requirements. The primary formula for daily fluid requirements is calculated as follows:

For the first 10 kg: 100 mL/kg/d (4 mL/kg/h)

For the second 10 kg: 50 mL/kg/d (2 mL/kg/h)

For each kg >20 kg: 20 mL/kg/d (1 mL/kg/h)

For example:

A 10-kg baby requires: 100 mL × 10 kg, or a total of 1000 mL/d.

A 20-kg child requires: (100 mL × 10 kg) + (50 mL × 10 kg) = 1500 mL/d.

A 40-kg child requires: (100 mL × 10 kg) + (50 mL × 10 kg) + (20 mL × 20 kg) = 1900 mL/d.

Electrolyte requirements remain constant throughout childhood and can be estimated by body weight. All infant formulas contain sufficient electrolytes to satisfy these requirements, as do the commercially available oral rehydration solutions such as Pedialyte®. The requirement is 2 to 3 mEq/kg/d for sodium and 2 mEq/kg/d for potassium.

Because hyponatremia is the most common intragenic complication of IV fluid therapy, it is important that isotonic solutions be used as maintenance fluid, such as normal saline with 5% dextrose.[17,18] An exception is during the neonatal period (**Table 129-5**). Although there is little evidence as to which maintenance fluids should be used early in life, neonates have immature kidneys and higher glucose requirements compared to older infants and children, and do not require sodium or chloride during their first day of life, but do require higher dextrose concentrations (e.g., dextrose 10% in water). Between days 2 and 7 of life, sodium can be added but at lower concentrations than for older children (e.g., dextrose 5% in 0.45% saline). After the first week of life, increasing sodium concentration should be used, with a transition to isotonic fluids as mentioned above.

TABLE 129-5 Maintenance Fluids in Neonates

Age	Recommended Maintenance Fluid Based on Age
Day 1 of life	Dextrose 10% with no electrolytes (i.e., dextrose 10% in water)
Days 2–7 of life	Dextrose 5% in 0.45% sodium chloride
>1 week of life	Dextrose 5% in 0.9% sodium chloride

DISORDERS OF SODIUM

Table 129-6 outlines disease states associated with disruption in serum sodium levels and total body water (volume).

HYPONATREMIA

Hyponatremia is a serum sodium level <135 mEq/L. First determine if a low sodium value is a true value by relating the sodium value to the osmolarity. If hyponatremia occurs in a hyperosmolar state (i.e., >290 mOsm/kg), this suggests an osmotically active solute in the plasma such as excess glucose or alcohol. If hyponatremia occurs in the presence of normal osmolarity (275 to 290 mOsm/kg), this is likely due to hyperlipidemia

TABLE 129-6 Conditions Altering Serum Sodium and Total Body Water Balance

Total Body Water (volume)	Hypernatremia	Hyponatremia
Increased	Excessive saline infusion	Congestive heart failure Cirrhosis Nephrotic syndrome Advanced renal failure
Normal	Hypertonic saline infusion Bicarbonate intoxication Salt poisoning Hyperaldosteronism	SIADH Primary polydipsia Exercise-induced Low solute intake Renal osmostat Hypothyroidism Glucocorticoid deficiency Nephrogenic SIADH
Decreased	Cutaneous losses Sweating Radiant warmers Phototherapy Burns Inadequate intake Improperly prepared formula GI losses Vomiting Nasogastric suctioning Diarrhea Osmotic stool softeners	Diuretics Renal losses Interstitial nephritis Mineralocorticoid deficiency Burns, heat illnesses (exhaustion/stroke) Ascites Cystic fibrosis
	Renal free water losses Diabetes insipidus Increased osmoles (diabetes mellitus, mannitol) Chronic kidney disease ATN (if polyuric) Postobstructive diuresis	

Abbreviations: ATN = acute tubular necrosis; SIADH = syndrome of inappropriate secretion of antidiuretic hormone.

TABLE 129-7 Treatment of Hyponatremia

Symptoms	Treatment*
If hypovolemic and hemodynamically unstable	Correct instability with NS boluses (20 mL/kg over 5 min followed by reassessment after each bolus)
Asymptomatic	Correct deficit to normal over 48 h mEq Na required = [(Na$^+$ desired) − (measured Na$^+$)] × (0.6 × weight in kg)
Neurologic symptoms (altered mental status, seizures)	1–2 mL/kg/h of 3% sodium chloride until asymptomatic or Na level >120 mEq/mL, then increase Na level 0.5 mEq/mL/h (not to exceed increase of 12 mEq/mL in first 24 h or 18 mEq/mL in first 48 h)

*Does not include maintenance requirements and ongoing losses.

0.9% NS = 0.15 mEq Na/L; 3% saline = 0.5 mEq Na/L

Abbreviation: NS = normal saline.

TABLE 129-8 Treatment of Hypovolemic or Euvolemic Hypernatremia

Condition	Treatment*
If hypovolemic and hemodynamically unstable	Correct instability with NS boluses (20 mL/kg boluses followed by reassessment after each bolus)
Once hemodynamically stable and hypovolemic or euvolemic hypernatremia	Correct deficit to normal over 24 h Free water deficit (mL) = 4 mL × body weight (kg) × [desired change in serum sodium mEq/L (mmol/L)] Subtract bolus fluids given from deficit; correct remaining deficit giving half of deficit over first 8 h and remainder over the next 16 h (see text for monitoring criteria)†

*Does not include maintenance requirements and ongoing losses.

†Tonicity of fluid used for correction will depend on initial severity of hypernatremia.

Abbreviation: NS = normal saline.

or hyperproteinemia.[19] In such cases, correct the underlying disorder rather than the serum sodium level. When hyponatremia occurs in a hypo-osmolar state (<275 mOsm/kg), this is likely due to gain of free water or loss of sodium. The most common causes of hyponatremia seen in the ED are GI losses and water intoxication caused by ingestion of hypotonic replacement fluids, especially during infancy.

Signs and symptoms of hyponatremia depend on the serum sodium level and the speed at which sodium level falls. Symptoms primarily involve the CNS, as free water moves from the extracellular to intracellular space, and the musculoskeletal system. Neurologic symptoms include nausea, vomiting, headache, mental status changes, altered consciousness, diminished reflexes, hypothermia, pseudobulbar palsy, and seizures. Musculoskeletal symptoms include weakness, muscle cramps, and lethargy.

Although patients may be only mildly symptomatic with sodium levels as low as 120 mEq/L, if the low level is chronic (>48 hours), symptoms usually occur with an acute drop in serum sodium level below 120 mEq/L. Without appropriate treatment, complications include respiratory failure, seizures, and death.

Treatment depends on the stability of the patient and associated symptoms. General guidelines are presented in **Table 129-7**. **Take special care to avoid rapid shifts in sodium levels.** Although hyponatremia itself can have dire consequences, rapid correction can cause severe demyelination of brainstem neurons.[20] Therefore, correct hyponatremia slowly and in a controlled manner (Table 129-7). The exception to this is in the setting of severe neurologic symptoms, such as confusion, altered level of consciousness, or seizures, typically with sodium level <120 mmol/L. When this occurs, a rapid, controlled increase in sodium level is required until neurologic symptoms resolve or a sodium level of 120 mmol/L is achieved.[21]

For euvolemic hyponatremia, after correction of serum sodium level, institute water restriction and treat the underlying disorder. For hypervolemic hyponatremia (edema), institute sodium and water restriction, and administer diuretics if needed to treat the clinical condition (e.g., congestive heart failure).

HYPERNATREMIA

Hypernatremia is a serum sodium level >145 mEq/L. Hypernatremia generally indicates a lack of total body water in relation to total body solute and often occurs as a result of dehydration (loss of water through the GI tract, kidney, or insensible losses), but may also occur secondary to excessive sodium intake (e.g., inadequate water intake or hypertonic solution intake) (**Table 129-8**).[22] Diarrhea is the most common cause in children. Other diseases to consider include renal disease and diabetes insipidus. Children are at risk for hypernatremia if free water is limited or if formula is mixed improperly. Mild hypernatremia is commonly found in ill children, particularly infants with gastroenteritis. If mild, it is usually asymptomatic and corrects with treatment of the underlying cause. Serum sodium levels of >160 mEq/L require immediate attention due to the potential for serious complications and permanent neurologic sequelae, including intellectual deficits, seizure disorder, or other neurologic impairments. Conversely, patients who have a sodium level of <160 mEq/L and receive treatment typically have symptoms that are relatively mild and self-limited.

Signs and symptoms of hypernatremia result from cellular dehydration as free water moves from the intracellular to extracellular space and include mental status changes, muscular weakness, ataxia, tremors, hyperreflexia, seizures, unresponsiveness, intracerebral hemorrhage, permanent neurologic dysfunction, and death. In addition, when extracellular fluid hypertonicity develops, brain intracellular osmolar contents increase to prevent or minimize cell shrinkage. In severe hypernatremic dehydration, neurologic findings may include any of the following: increased peripheral tone with brisk reflexes, muscle weakness, high-pitched cry, nuchal rigidity, myoclonus, asterixis, chorea, altered level of consciousness, or seizures.[22,23]

Treatment is the restoration of intravascular volume while decreasing the serum sodium level. **Correct serum sodium gradually to avoid cerebral edema and associated central pontine myelinolysis** (Table 129-8). Closely monitor serum sodium levels every hour initially to ensure that the level is reduced no faster than 1 mEq/L/h and no more than 15 mEq/L in the first 24 hours. This may require more than 48 hours for complete correction. Monitor urine output given the risk of acute tubular necrosis.[22] Correct underlying causes. Hypervolemic hypernatremia may require dialysis if sodium levels cannot be decreased without volume overload. Dialysis may also be required for hypernatremia of any type if the initial serum sodium is >180 mmol/L.

DISORDERS OF POTASSIUM

HYPOKALEMIA

Hypokalemia occurs when the serum potassium level falls to <3.4 mEq/L and most commonly occurs secondary to profuse vomiting and/or diarrhea. Other common causes include therapy with loop or thiazide diuretics, mineralocorticoids, or laxatives and diabetic ketoacidosis. In diabetic ketoacidosis, profound hypokalemia can result from osmotic diuresis, although in the face of the hydrogen–potassium shift that accompanies acidemia, serum levels may be normal or falsely elevated. Uncommon causes of hypokalemia include renal tubular acidosis, Bartter's or Gitelman's syndrome, Cushing's syndrome, and familial hypokalemia-induced paralysis.

In most cases, hypokalemia occurs slowly, and thus patients are asymptomatic. Clinical signs tend to reflect the rate of fall of serum potassium rather than the absolute level. However, severe potassium depletion can result in skeletal muscle weakness, ileus, and cardiac conduction disturbances. A prominent ECG manifestation is the U wave.

Treatment is generally with oral replacement with potassium, 2 to 5 mEq/kg/d in two or three divided doses (maximum 40 mEq/dose). However, dehydration and magnesium abnormalities must also be corrected to maintain normal potassium levels. If IV therapy is necessary, potassium 0.2 to 0.3 mEq/kg/h is generally adequate. In extremely urgent situations, such as hypokalemia-induced respiratory insufficiency or cardiac manifestations, potassium 0.5 mEq/kg/h can be administered (maximum 20 mEq/dose), with continuous ECG monitoring.[24] If potassium chloride infusion concentration exceeds 60 mEq/L, the infusion will need to run through a central line, because potassium is a vein irritant. In diabetic ketoacidosis, potassium repletion should begin early in the course of therapy, because diuresis-induced depletion can result in profound hypokalemia as acidosis is corrected and serum potassium shifts into cells (see chapter 145, "Diabetes in Children").

HYPERKALEMIA

Hyperkalemia is a serum potassium level of >5.5 mEq/L. In infants and children, a laboratory finding of hyperkalemia is most commonly due to hemolysis from phlebotomy and does not reflect serum levels. However, do not assume hyperkalemia is false; repeat the potassium level, reexamine the patient, obtain an ECG, and place the child on a cardiac monitor. Some common causes of true hyperkalemia include renal failure, rhabdomyolysis, burns, heat stroke, trauma, tumor lysis syndrome, hemolytic anemia, use of potassium-sparing diuretics, and adrenal corticoid insufficiency (e.g., Addison's disease, salt wasting congenital adrenal hyperplasia). Metabolic acidosis can result in hyperkalemia due to hydrogen–potassium shifts.

Cardiac conduction delay is the most common manifestation of hyperkalemia and is potentially life threatening. Peaked T waves are the first manifestation, followed by prolonged PR interval and then widening of the QRS complex, an ominous finding that can precede the characteristic "sine wave" pattern leading to ventricular dysrhythmias and asystole. Any patient with ECG changes requires emergent therapy to reverse cardiac conduction toxicity.

Treatment is detailed in **Table 129-9**. Asymptomatic patients with normal ECG findings usually do well with therapy to enhance potassium excretion. In patients with renal failure with a gradual rise in serum potassium levels, sodium polystyrene sulfonate can be given. It is a resin that exchanges sodium for potassium at a 1:1 ratio and therefore enhances potassium excretion and can be administered orally or by enema. A dose of 1 gram/kg lowers the serum potassium level by up to 1.2 mEq/L. When administered orally, it is usually given with a cathartic to speed transit time through the GI tract. Hypernatremia and volume overload are potential complications. In patients with severe hyperkalemia from renal failure, dialysis is usually necessary, but emergency correction of potassium must be done first (Table 129-9). In patients with hyperkalemia secondary to metabolic acidosis, normalization of serum pH usually restores serum potassium to normal levels.[24]

TABLE 129-9 Treatment of Hyperkalemia

Purpose	Agent	Dose
Increase cardiac stability	Calcium gluconate 10% (10% calcium gluconate contains 100 milligrams/mL)	100 milligrams/kg (1 mL/kg/dose) IV at rate not to exceed 100 milligrams/min; maximum 3 grams/dose. Can be administered peripherally or centrally. May be repeated in 5 min if necessary.
	Calcium chloride 10% (10% calcium chloride contains 100 milligrams/mL)	20 milligrams/kg (0.2 mL/kg/dose) IV at rate not to exceed 100 milligrams/min; maximum 1 gram/dose. Calcium chloride must be given via central line or IO due to vein sclerosis. May be repeated in 5 min if necessary.
Decrease potassium	Albuterol (Ventolin) 0.5% solution	2.5–5 milligrams via nebulization; every 20 min as needed.
	Sodium bicarbonate	If acidotic (pH <7.3), 1–2 mEq/kg IV/IO; typical adult dose 50–100 mEq. Onset of action is in minutes. May be repeated every 5–10 min as needed.
	Regular insulin	0.1 unit/kg IV in 5 mL/kg 10% dextrose in water, 0.5 gram/kg IV over 30 min; check glucose level every 30 min; onset of action, 30 min. May be repeated every 30–60 min.
	Furosemide	If renal function normal and patient is not hypovolemic, 0.5–1 milligram/kg/dose IV to a maximum of 40 milligrams/dose. Peak effect seen at 30 min.
	Sodium polystyrene sulfonate	1 gram/kg to a maximum of 60 grams orally, via nasogastric tube, or rectally. Onset of action, 1–2 h orally, <30 min rectally.

DISORDERS OF CALCIUM

HYPOCALCEMIA

Hypocalcemia is a serum calcium level <8 milligrams/dL (2 mmol/L) or ionized calcium level <4.4 milligrams/dL (1.1 mmol/L); however, levels must be adjusted for albumin levels and pH of the blood. Low calcium levels tend to result from hypoparathyroidism or end-organ resistance to parathyroid hormone. True hypoparathyroidism can be idiopathic, be associated with DiGeorge's syndrome, occur after thyroid surgery, and/or be associated with magnesium deficiency. End-organ resistance to parathyroid hormone is most commonly associated with vitamin D deficiency. The most common causes are dietary deficiency and chronic renal failure. Young infants fed cow's milk, which is high in phosphate, can develop severe hypocalcemia. Another common cause of hypocalcemia is hyperventilation: the decreased partial pressure of carbon dioxide results in an acute respiratory alkalosis that rapidly decreases levels of ionized calcium.

Clinical manifestations of hypocalcemia include muscle weakness, vomiting, and irritability. Infants may simply appear "jittery." In severe cases, tetany, laryngospasm, carpopedal spasm, and seizures can occur. Carpopedal spasm is especially common in children with hyperventilation syndrome. The most characteristic ECG abnormality is a prolonged QT interval. Investigation of hypocalcemia includes laboratory measurement of total serum and ionized calcium, phosphate, total protein and albumin, parathyroid hormone, BUN, and creatinine levels. Urine calcium level should also be collected. If a neonate is seen with hypocalcemia, a chest x-ray should be done to look for a thymic shadow in infants and young children. If the thymus is not present, consider DiGeorge's syndrome.

Treatment is the administration of IV calcium (**Table 129-10**). Give calcium gluconate 10% in a dose of 100 milligrams/kg at a rate not to exceed 100 milligrams/min, with continuous ECG monitoring. Following initial correction, a calcium infusion may be required to maintain calcium levels. Further management depends on the cause.[25]

HYPERCALCEMIA

Hypercalcemia is a serum calcium level of >11 milligrams/dL and most often results from increased bone resorption. Probably the most

TABLE 129-10 Treatment of Disorders of Calcium and Magnesium

	Treatment	Comments
Calcium		
Hypocalcemia	10% calcium gluconate IV, 100 milligrams/kg, at a rate <100 milligrams/min	Continuous ECG monitoring
Hypercalcemia	Hydrate with twice maintenance fluids, furosemide 1–2 milligrams/kg IV to a maximum of 40 milligrams	Treat underlying cause
Magnesium		
Hypomagnesemia	10% magnesium sulfate, 25–50 milligrams/kg over 30 min	
Hypermagnesemia	Hydration, diuresis 1–2 milligrams/kg IV furosemide to a maximum of 40 milligrams; or 10% calcium gluconate IV, 0.5 mL/kg	

common cause in children is malignancy involving the lymphoreticular system. Less common causes include vitamin A or D intoxication, hyperparathyroid syndromes, hyperthyroidism, adrenal insufficiency, and pheochromocytoma.

Clinical manifestations include hypotonia, fatigue, irritability, anorexia, vomiting, and constipation. Affected children may be clinically dehydrated and complain of polyuria and/or polydipsia. An ECG may reveal bradycardia and a shortened QT interval.

The laboratory evaluation of hypercalcemia includes measurement of total serum and ionized calcium levels, a CBC, and evaluation of total protein and albumin and alkaline phosphatase levels. An evaluation of the vitamin D level may also be indicated, depending on the patient's medical history.

Treatment (Table 129-10) depends on the cause. Acutely, patients with functioning kidneys can be treated with aggressive IV hydration (e.g., twice maintenance),[26] with or without furosemide, 1 to 2 milligrams/kg IV, to a maximum of 40 milligrams. Then, treat the underlying cause.

DISORDERS OF MAGNESIUM

HYPOMAGNESEMIA

Serum magnesium levels are age independent and range from 1.5 to 2.2 mEq/L. Dietary magnesium is absorbed in the intestine and reabsorbed in the urine, particularly in states of decreased intake. Serum levels of <1.5 mEq/L are considered low and usually result from GI or renal losses as well as some endocrine disturbances. Diarrhea, malabsorption, short gut, and fistulas are potential mechanisms of GI magnesium loss, but iatrogenic causes of renal loss (osmotic diuretics, parenteral fluids, antibiotics, and chemotherapeutics) predominate. Hypercalcemia may cause magnesium loss as well as hypophosphatemia. Hypomagnesemia may also occur in diabetes, disorders of the parathyroid glands, and primary hyperaldosteronism.

Clinical manifestations are similar to those seen with hypocalcemia: muscle spasms, weakness, or even atrophy may occur; CNS symptoms include ataxia, abnormal movements, nystagmus, and seizures and occur with very low magnesium levels. Cardiac changes include prolonged PR and QT intervals and may predispose to arrhythmias such as torsade de points.

Treatment (Table 129-10) depends on the underlying cause. Include magnesium in parenteral or enteral nutritional liquids in chronically ill children. In symptomatic patients (e.g., those with seizures, arrhythmias), give IV magnesium sulfate, 25 to 50 milligrams/kg administered as a 10% solution over 30 minutes, and repeat every 4 to 6 hours as needed.

HYPERMAGNESEMIA

Hypermagnesemia is rare, and serum levels of >2.2 mEq/L are considered elevated. The most common cause is ingestion of exogenous magnesium, typically found in antacids and laxatives. Patients with renal dysfunction are at increased risk. Clinical manifestations include hypotension, loss of deep tendon reflexes, and respiratory failure. Cardiac manifestations include widening of the QRS, PR, and QT intervals.

Treatment (Table 129-10) is removal of exogenous sources and hydration accompanied by diuresis. Severe symptoms may be mitigated with IV calcium, 0.5 mL/kg as calcium gluconate. Dialysis is effective in patients with renal failure.

REFERENCES

The complete reference list is available online at www.TintinalliEM.com.

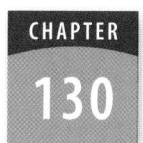

CHAPTER 130 Acute Abdominal Pain in Infants and Children

Ross J. Fleischman

INTRODUCTION

The diagnoses discussed in this chapter are challenging, since emergent surgical conditions in children may present with predominant symptoms other than pain, including vomiting, fever, irritability, or lethargy. **Table 130-1** classifies conditions by age, although many conditions cross categories.

The pathophysiology of abdominal pain is discussed in chapter 71, Acute Abdominal Pain and gynecologic causes are discussed in chapter 97, Abdominal and Pelvic Pain in the Nonpregnant Female.

PHYSICAL EXAMINATION

The assessment of young children depends on careful observation for subtle clues. Stillness suggests conditions that irritate the peritoneum, such as appendicitis. Writhing for a position of comfort suggests obstruction, such as intussusception or renal colic.

Inspect, auscultate, and then palpate the abdomen, starting away from the expected area of maximal tenderness. Bringing the knees up relaxes the abdominal muscles. Move the hips to test for hip pathology or irritation caused by appendicitis or a psoas abscess. **Thoroughly examine the diaper area to identify testicular torsion, paraphimosis, hair tourniquet, hernia, and imperforate hymen, as the young child may be unable to articulate problems in that area and the older child may be embarrassed to do so.** Rectal exam may identify gross or occult blood, constipation, abnormalities of anogenital anatomy, and inflammatory processes. Evaluate for extra-abdominal causes of abdominal pain such as pharyngitis or pneumonia.

TABLE 130-1 Causes of Abdominal Pain by Age Group

Age	Emergent	Nonemergent
0–3 months old	Necrotizing enterocolitis Volvulus Incarcerated hernia Testicular torsion Nonaccidental trauma Hirschsprung's enterocolitis	Constipation Acute gastroenteritis Colic
3 months–3 years old	Intussusception Volvulus Testicular torsion Appendicitis Vaso-occlusive crisis	Urinary tract infections Constipation Henoch-Schönlein purpura Acute gastroenteritis
3 years old–adolescence	Appendicitis Diabetic ketoacidosis Vaso-occlusive crisis Ectopic pregnancy Ovarian torsion Testicular torsion Cholecystitis Pancreatitis Urinary tract infections Tumor Pneumonia	*Streptococcus* pharyngitis Inflammatory bowel disease Pregnancy Renal stones Peptic ulcer disease/gastritis Ovarian cysts Henoch-Schönlein purpura Constipation Acute gastroenteritis Nonspecific viral syndromes

SPECIAL CONSIDERATIONS BY AGE GROUP

NEONATES AND YOUNG INFANTS (0 TO 3 MONTHS)

The major life-threatening diagnoses in young infants are necrotizing enterocolitis, malrotation with midgut volvulus, incarcerated hernias, and nonaccidental trauma. Young infants typically eat every 2 hours, so inconsolability and lethargy with poor feeding are signs of serious disease. **The maxim that bilious vomiting portends a surgical emergency until proven otherwise is well supported, since between 27% and 51% of children with bilious vomiting require surgery.**[1]

Intermittent, paroxysmal pain is often associated with intussusception, colic, and gastroenteritis. Necrotizing enterocolitis and volvulus are associated with constant pain. Pain after feeding may be caused by gastroesophageal reflux. **Pyloric stenosis causes progressive painless projectile vomiting followed by renewed interest in feeding.**

Past medical history includes the complications of pregnancy and delivery. Constipation, with a history of not passing meconium within the first 24 to 48 hours of life, suggests Hirschsprung's disease. Hirschsprung's enterocolitis is a serious complication that presents with explosive diarrhea, fever, vomiting, abdominal pain, and distension. It is common in the first 2 years after resection of the aganglionic segment, but also occurs in patients with undiagnosed disease.

Fever in this age group requires thorough investigation (see chapter 116, Fever and Serious Bacterial Illness in Infants and Children).

OLDER INFANTS AND TODDLERS (3 MONTHS TO 3 YEARS OLD)

Intussusception, urinary tract infections, testicular torsion, and accidental and nonaccidental trauma are serious causes of abdominal pain in older infants and toddlers. Malrotation with midgut volvulus and appendicitis are less common but remain considerations. Constipation is a common cause of abdominal pain that can be severe and often begins around the time of toilet training. Parents may not offer a bowel history unless asked.

Stranger anxiety is prevalent at this age. Take a few moments to gain the confidence of the child before any examination or procedures. It may be helpful to ask a parent to palpate the child's abdomen while you observe, before palpating yourself or with the toddler's assistance. **Observe the child while coughing, walking, or jumping as a test for peritoneal irritation.** Toddlers may not be able to differentiate pain from nausea.

CHILDREN (3 TO 15 YEARS OF AGE)

Diagnoses in this age group include problems that are common in adults. **Appendicitis is the most common surgical emergency.**

Other important etiologies are diabetic ketoacidosis (chapter 145, Diabetes in Children), urinary tract infection (chapter 132, Urinary Tract Infection in Infants and Children), testicular torsion, ectopic pregnancy, pelvic inflammatory disease (chapter 133, Pediatric Urologic and Gynecologic Disorders), pancreatitis, inflammatory bowel disease, cholelithiasis (chapter 130, Acute Abdominal Pain in Infants and Children), sickle cell anemia (chapter 142, Sickle Cell Disease in Children), Henoch-Schönlein purpura, and renal colic (chapter 134, Renal Emergencies in Children). Upper respiratory symptoms may be associated with mesenteric adenitis, which may mimic appendicitis.

An examination of the testicles is required. If two testicles cannot be identified, consider torsion of an undescended testis. Perform a pelvic examination in sexually active girls. Adolescents may offer additional information if some of the history is taken with parents out of the room.

LABORATORY STUDIES

Bedside glucose measurement is a first step in the evaluation of any ill-appearing child or in cases of persistent vomiting or poor oral intake. Obtain a chemistry panel if there is suspicion for electrolyte or renal abnormalities in ill-appearing children and in the first 6 months of life, in which sodium or metabolic abnormalities are more common. Urinalysis identifies urinary tract infection, microscopic hematuria, and pregnancy. **The WBC count is a poor screening test for undifferentiated abdominal pain.**

DIAGNOSTIC IMAGING

US is the first-line test for appendicitis, pyloric stenosis, intussusception, testicular torsion, and biliary and gynecologic pathology. CT scan is the most sensitive study for appendicitis, urolithiasis, and intra-abdominal abscesses and may uncover a wide variety of pathology. Current thinking is that one fatal cancer will be induced by every 1000 CT scans performed on young children.[2] IV contrast has a significant risk of allergic reactions and contrast nephropathy; therefore, reducing unnecessary CT use should be a goal of emergency physicians.

Plain radiographs give a much lower radiation dose (1/600th the dose for a chest radiograph compared with an abdominal CT).[3] Radiography should be used selectively to exclude or support specific diagnoses, not for undirected screening. Free air from a perforation can be seen on upright or left lateral decubitus views, although these are insensitive tests. Barium oral or rectal contrast should never be given if perforation is suspected; instead, use water-soluble contrast.

PAIN MANAGEMENT

Contrary to fears that analgesics may mask surgical conditions, analgesia improves the physician's ability to assess pain and does not worsen outcomes. See chapter 113, Pain Management and Procedural Sedation in Infants and Children.

SPECIFIC CONDITIONS

NECROTIZING ENTEROCOLITIS

Necrotizing enterocolitis is a neonatal disease thought to be caused by an immune overreaction to an insult to the intestine followed by inflammation, bacterial translocation, and coagulation necrosis of the intestine. Overall mortality is 15% to 30%, with many survivors left with short bowel syndrome and growth retardation.[4] While necrotizing enterocolitis is largely a disease of prematurity, 10% of cases occur in term infants.[5] Predisposing conditions include congenital heart disease, sepsis, neonatal asphyxia, polycythemia, and hypotension.[6] The range of mean ages at onset of disease is between 2 and 9 days of age. **Therefore, although the disease rarely presents outside of the neonatal intensive care unit, its severity makes it an important consideration in near-term infants or those with comorbidities in the first 3 weeks of life.**

Clinical Features and Imaging Presenting signs and symptoms are poor feeding, lethargy, abdominal distension, bilious vomiting, temperature instability, apnea, and abdominal tenderness. Gross or occult blood in the stool increases the likelihood of necrotizing enterocolitis but is neither sensitive nor specific.[7]

Obtain antero-posterior and lateral decubitus abdominal radiographs. Inclusion of the chest will screen for cardiopulmonary abnormalities. Early in the disease, abdominal radiographs may show signs of ileus or obstruction. **Pneumatosis intestinalis (air in the bowel wall) and portal venous gas are both pathognomonic (Figure 130-1),**[8] but normal abdominal radiographs do not exclude the disorder.

Treatment **Evaluation must include a search for underlying causes, especially sepsis.** Management includes nothing by mouth status, gastric tube decompression, aggressive IV hydration, broad-spectrum antibiotics, and surgical consultation. Consider ampicillin to cover gram-positive organisms, gentamicin or cefotaxime for gram-negative organisms, and metronidazole or clindamycin for anaerobes.[9] Although necrotizing enterocolitis is first managed medically, many cases require resection of necrotic bowel. Admit to intensive care.

MALROTATION AND VOLVULUS

Volvulus is a life-threatening complication of malrotation. **Eighty percent of malrotation presents within the first month of life and 90% within the first year, but it can present at any time in life.**[10] At approximately 10 weeks of gestation, the growing intestines return to the abdomen from the yolk sac, and the midgut undergoes a 270-degree counterclockwise turn around the superior mesenteric artery. Abnormal rotation can

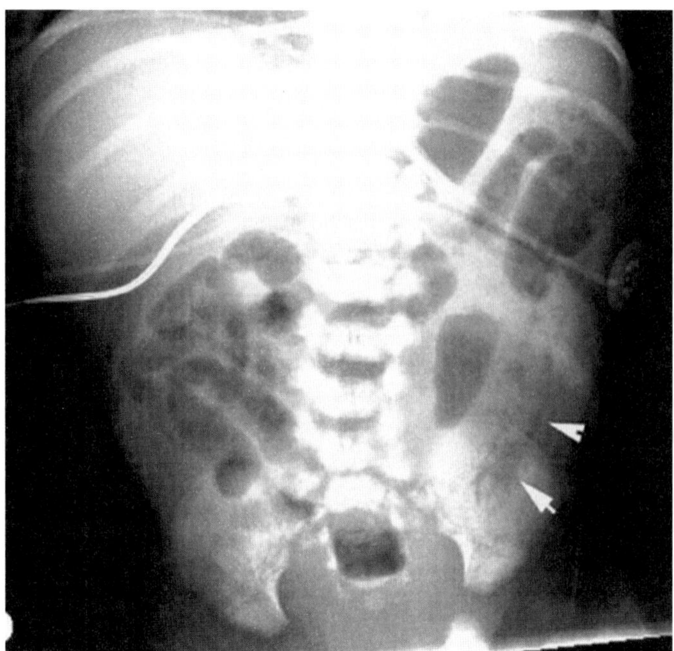

FIGURE 130-1. Plain abdominal film demonstrating air in the intestinal wall (*arrows*), which is pathognomonic of necrotizing enterocolitis. [Reproduced with permission from Strange GR, Ahrens WR, Schafermeyer RW, Wiebe RA: *Pediatric Emergency Medicine*, 3rd ed. © 2009. The McGraw-Hill Companies, Inc. New York, Figure 9-12.]

leave the cecum high in the abdomen, with its peritoneal attachments (Ladd's bands) crossing the duodenum. Down's syndrome, heterotaxy, and duodenal atresia are associated with malrotation.

Clinical Features The child may be well until the malrotated gut twists (volvulus) or becomes obstructed by Ladd's bands, causing ischemia.

Volvulus is a surgical emergency as it can result in gangrene of the entire midgut within hours. The infant with volvulus often has no significant past medical history and presents with the abrupt onset of constant abdominal pain, bilious vomiting, abdominal distention, and irritability. Patients with volvulus are typically ill appearing and may have signs of shock. The abdomen is diffusely tender and distended and may be rigid. Intermittent volvulus may present with stable vital signs and focal tenderness on abdominal examination. The absence of fever can be helpful in distinguishing volvulus from sepsis.

Imaging and Treatment Imaging studies should not delay surgical consultation, as rapid detorsion of the volvulized bowel is necessary to prevent loss of the entire small intestine. Upper GI series with contrast remains the test of choice for diagnosing malrotation with sensitivities of 93% to 100% for malrotation and 54% to 79% for volvulus.[11] The normal location of the duodenojejunal junction is at the level of the duodenal bulb and to the left of the spine. In malrotation, the junction is commonly located low and to the right of the spine. If midgut volvulus is present at the time of the study, there may be an abruptly tapered cutoff of contrast in the duodenum (bird's beak) or a corkscrew appearance of the bowel. If concern persists after a negative study and surgical consultation, options for additional evaluation include repeat upper GI series to exclude intermittent volvulus, abdominal CT, US, and contrast enema.

Plain abdominal radiographs are neither sensitive nor specific for malrotation. The most common findings on plain abdominal x-ray are an air-filled stomach with little distal gas, which may show a distal obstruction, nonspecific, or even normal gas pattern.[12]

Treatment consists of resuscitation and immediate surgical consultation. Electrolytes, CBC, coagulation studies, and a type and cross-match for packed red blood cells are helpful to guide resuscitation and operative management.

INTUSSUSCEPTION

Intussusception is the most common cause of intestinal obstruction in children under 2 years of age. It is rare before 2 months. The male:female ratio is 2:1.[13,14]

Intussusception occurs when one segment of the intestine telescopes into another, usually the ileum into the colon. Constriction of the mesentery results in engorgement of the intussusceptum and bowel ischemia. In infants, lymphoid hyperplasia from viral illness may cause a "lead point," which drags one portion of bowel into another. In older children, causes of intussusception include Meckel's diverticulum, intestinal polyps, congenital duplications, lymphoma, and Henoch-Schönlein purpura, and possibly exposure to antibiotics.[15]

Clinical Features Intussusception is notoriously difficult to diagnose because its two common presentations, intermittent pain and lethargy, are insensitive signs of intussusception. The classic presentation of the "intermittentsception" is an infant aged 5 to 12 months who suddenly develops a few minutes of severe abdominal pain with the legs drawn to the chest and who then appears well until the next episode of pain. An alternate presentation is an infant with unexplained lethargy, which may divert the provider to an evaluation for altered mental status. Vomiting is not usually present at first but develops over 6 to 12 hours and may be bilious.

The physical examination between attacks may be normal, although a sausage-shaped mass may be palpated in the right upper quadrant. **Occult blood is found in 70% of stools and gross blood in about 50%, although it rarely resembles the classic "currant" jelly.**[16,17]

Diagnosis and Treatment A history consistent with the intermittent symptoms of intussusception should prompt further evaluation or observation even if the patient is asymptomatic at the time.

US should be the first study when the diagnosis is ambiguous. In research settings, the accuracy of US for intussusception is nearly 100% (**Figure 130-2**).

Children with a high suspicion of intussusception should undergo immediate air-contrast enema, which is both diagnostic and therapeutic.[17] Prepare the child for reduction with boluses of normal saline, as volume loss due to intestinal edema, decreased intake, and vomiting is a common comorbidity. A surgeon should be notified prior to air-contrast enema in case the reduction is unsuccessful or perforation occurs. **Children with peritonitis, with free air on plain radiographs, or who are in shock should not undergo air-contrast enema and require emergent surgical reduction.**

Plain abdominal radiographs are not highly useful unless needed to rule out perforation, but they may show a mass or paucity of bowel gas in the right abdomen, a "crescent sign" where the curved edge of one segment of bowel visibly protrudes into another, or an obstructive pattern (**Figure 130-3**).[16]

Children have traditionally been admitted after enema reduction because of a 10% recurrence rate, usually within the first 24 to 48 hours.[17] However, discharge after a few hours of observation to exclude complications may be appropriate in children with a normal WBC count, who can tolerate oral intake, and who can easily return should they have a recurrence.[18] A recurrence should prompt a second enema reduction. Further recurrences may require surgery.

APPENDICITIS

Appendicitis is the most common surgical emergency in children. The peak ages for appendicitis are between 9 and 12 years, with a male predominance.[19]

The appendix is a diverticulum that arises from the cecum. Appendicitis usually begins with obstruction of the appendiceal lumen by fecaliths, lymphoid hyperplasia, or less commonly parasites, tumors, or foreign bodies. Multiplying bacteria and mucus secretion increase pressure on the wall, leading to dilation, ischemia, and perforation.

Clinical Features The classic progression of periumbilical pain that migrates to the right lower quadrant followed by vomiting and fever is seen in less than 50% of children with appendicitis.[20] Many of the

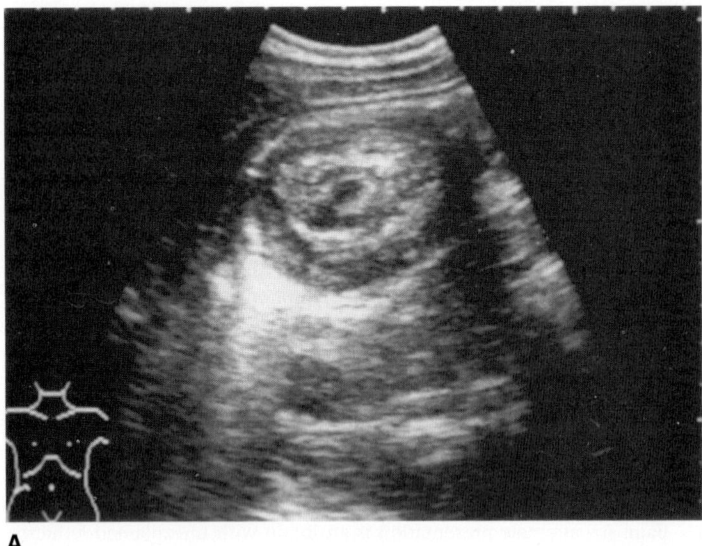

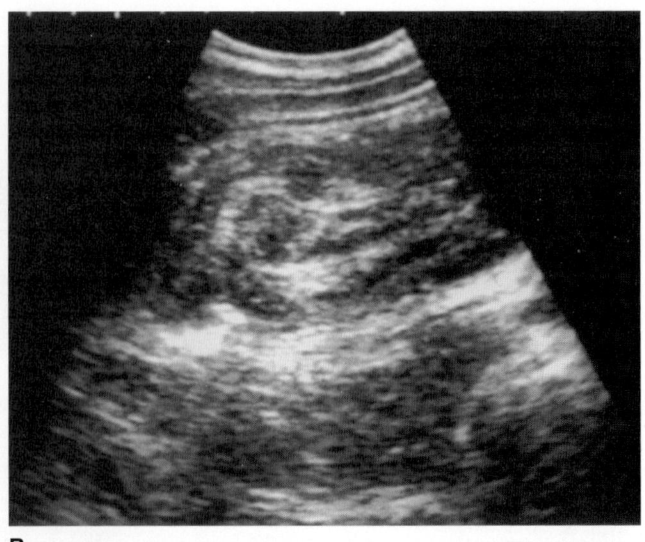

FIGURE 130-2. **A** and **B.** US image of intussusception showing the classic target appearance of bowel-within-bowel. [Reproduced with permission from Ma OJ, Mateer JR, Blaivas M: *Emergency Ultrasound,* 2nd ed. © 2008, McGraw-Hill, New York, Figure 9-15.]

classic symptoms are seen with only moderate frequency: pain of <48 hours in duration (82%), nausea or emesis (71%), anorexia (60%), and migration of pain to the right lower quadrant (50%). Constipation is seen in 9% to 33% of cases and diarrhea in 10% to 33%.[21] **Perforation rates approach 90% in children <4 years old, so younger children are more likely to present with vomiting, fever, peritonitis, or sepsis.**[22]

FIGURE 130-3. The crescent-shaped head of the intussusceptum is seen as an intraluminal mass in the gas-filled transverse colon (*asterisk*). [Reproduced with permission from Schwartz: *Emergency Radiology Cases Studies* © 2008, The McGraw-Hill Companies, Inc. New York. Figure II-4-6 Part A.]

Children with appendicitis may perforate early in the course of the disease. One study of children aged 3 to 18 found no perforation before 12 hours, but a 10% perforation rate at 18 hours and 44% by 36 hours.[23] Perforation may cause a brief remission in pain prior to the development of peritonitis and worsening symptoms.

Tenderness may be localized to the right lower quadrant (68% of cases) or McBurney's point (two thirds of the way from the umbilicus to the anterior-superior iliac spine), or may involve the entire abdomen. Assessing pain when the child coughs, walks, and jumps is a useful tool to assess for peritoneal inflammation. Rebound tenderness and guarding are more common with perforation and may be absent early. Assess for hernias and perform a testicular examination in boys. A pelvic examination may be needed in adolescent females to compare the tenderness of McBurney's point to the adnexa. Rectal tenderness had a positive likelihood ratio of 2.3 and negative ratio of 0.7 in a summary of three studies.[22]

Diagnosis There is a high potential for missing the diagnosis of appendicitis in children. The Alvarado and Samuel scores have been widely cited but have insufficient positive predictive values to safely identify the need for surgery for appendicitis in children, and other decision rules may or may not be generalizable[24-26] (**Table 130-2**). Problems with interrater reliability make it difficult to apply decision rules in the clinical prediction of appendicitis[15] (**Table 130-3**).

WBC count has insufficient sensitivity or specificity to confirm the diagnosis of appendicitis; however, a normal WBC is strongly correlated

TABLE 130-2 A Clinical Decision Rule to Identify Children at Low Risk of Appendicitis[*] (rule has poor positive predictive value)

Criterion	Points
Absolute neutrophil count $>6.75 \times 10^3/\mu L$	6
Rebound pain or pain with percussion	2
Unable to walk or walks with limp	1
Nausea	2
History of migration of pain to right lower quadrant	1
History of focal right lower quadrant pain	2

Note: A score of ≤5 indicates low risk for appendicitis (sensitivity, 96.3%; 99% confidence interval, 87.5%–99.0%). If appendicitis is still suspected, repeat examination during ED observation, repeat examination within 12 hours, or US examination should be considered.

[*]*Caution:* Interrater reliability is only fair to moderate for some of these variables.

TABLE 130-3 Interrater Reliability of Selected Historical and Clinical Variables Used in the Clinical Assessment of Appendicitis

Sign or Symptom	Agreement, %	Kappa (95% CI)
Focal RLQ pain	84.9	0.48 (0.39–0.58)
Migration of pain to RLQ	68.4	0.37 (0.29–0.45)
Nausea	72	0.44 (0.37–0.52)
Rebound	68.4	0.32 (0.24–0.40)
Abdominal pain with walking, jumping, or coughing	83.6	0.54 (0.45–0.63)

Abbreviations: CI = confidence interval; RLQ = right lower quadrant.

with a decreased likelihood of appendicitis.[24] A WBC <10,000/mm^3 is a strong negative predictor for appendicitis (negative likelihood ratio = 0.26). C-reactive protein is a nonspecific later marker of inflammation and correlates with severity of appendicitis and may be helpful for distinguishing ruptured or gangrenous appendicitis from early disease. No single cut-point for C-reactive protein has been established, however, as a sensitive or specific marker of acute surgical appendicitis; some studies suggest that C-reactive protein in conjunction with WBC and clinical signs and symptoms may add to the diagnostic evaluation of children with abdominal pain.[27-33] Sterile pyuria can be seen with acute appendicitis as the inflamed appendix irritates the nearby ureters.

Imaging Patients with a history and examination compelling for acute appendicitis should have surgical consultation without diagnostic imaging. **When the diagnosis is uncertain, US is often the preferred initial imaging exam.** Appendiceal findings include a maximal diameter >6 mm, wall thickness ≥3 mm, lack of compressibility, hyperemia on color Doppler US, surrounding edema or fat stranding, and an appendicolith (**Figure 130-4**).[25] If done by experienced technicians, US is highly sensitive and specific (88% and 94%).[26] However, studies of the performance of US outside of controlled research settings have been less optimistic, and one study reported visualizing the appendix in only 24% of children.[34] US is useful to exclude gynecologic processes such as ovarian torsion and ruptured cysts. A US with findings of appendicitis in a patient with a consistent clinical picture is sufficiently specific to warrant surgery. When the appendix is visualized and normal, US is sufficiently sensitive to exclude appendicitis in many cases. If clinical suspicion for appendicitis is very high, visualization of a normal appendix should not exclude the diagnosis, and additional evaluation should be undertaken. This may include surgical consultation, CT scan, admission for observation, or repeat US.

Abdominal CT scanning has superior test characteristics to US, with a sensitivity and specificity of 94% and 95%, respectively (**Figure 130-5**). Abdominal CT is useful for identifying perforation and abscess formation, which may require percutaneous drainage and antibiotics rather than immediate appendectomy, and therefore may be the preferred imaging modality in children with prolonged pain or diffuse peritoneal signs suggestive of rupture. CT may also identify alternative diagnoses such as mesenteric adenitis, epiploic appendagitis, inflammatory bowel disease, renal stones, and tumors. Disadvantages of CT are the radiation exposure, the time required for oral and/or rectal contrast when requested, and the possibility of allergic reactions and IV contrast nephropathy. One study suggests that a single CT scan may triple the risk of malignancy, although the absolute risk remains small and the authors caution that radiation doses from CT scans be kept as low as possible.[35] Institutional protocols often determine whether IV contrast CT or both oral and IV contrast CT is the preferred CT modality.

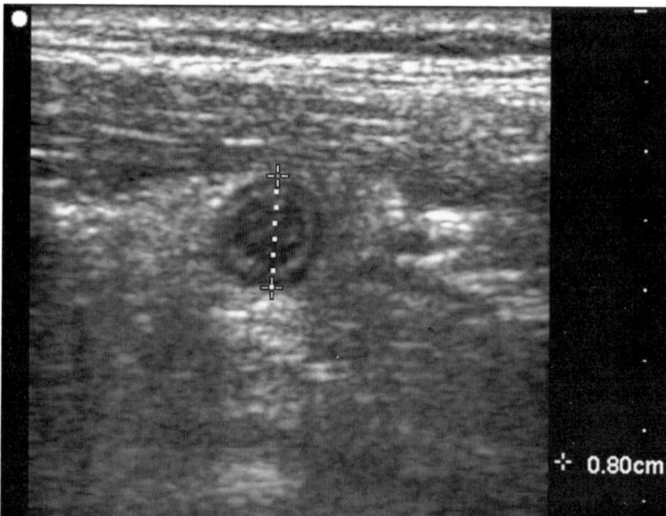

FIGURE 130-4. US of acute appendicitis with a diameter of 8 mm in short-axis view. [Reproduced with permission from Ma OJ, Mateer JR, Blaivas M: *Emergency Ultrasound*, 2nd ed. © 2008, McGraw-Hill, New York, Figure 18-23.]

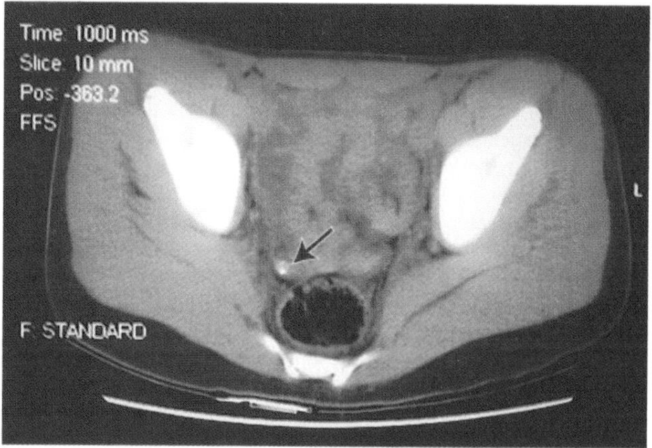

A

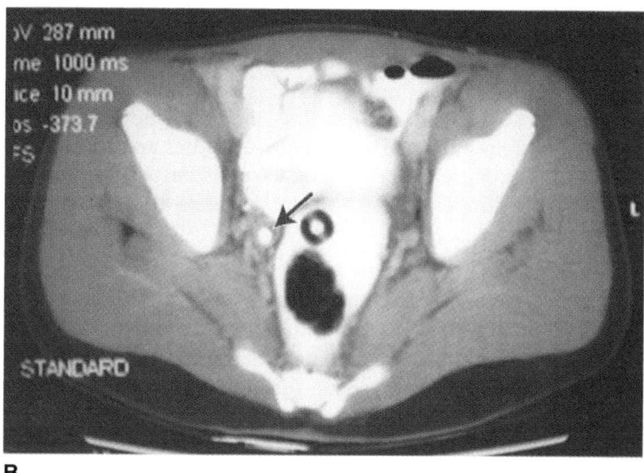

B

FIGURE 130-5. Acute appendicitis. **A.** A non–contrast-enhanced axial CT scan through the pelvis reveals a calcific appendicolith (*arrow*) in a pelvic appendix. Inspissated, sometimes calcified fecal material leads to obstruction followed by secondary bacterial invasion. Radiographic evidence of a fecalith is seen in 20% of cases. The presence of an appendicolith along with inflammation is indicative either of acute appendicitis or of impending appendicitis. **B.** Contrast-enhanced CT scan of the pelvis reveals the previously described appendicolith (*arrow*) in a dilated fluid-filled and thick-walled appendix. Enhancement of the appendiceal wall is also noted. [Reproduced with permission from Shah BR, Lucchesi M: *Atlas of Pediatric Emergency Medicine*. © 2006, McGraw-Hill, New York, Figure 10-8.]

Treatment Once the diagnosis of appendicitis is highly suspected or confirmed, obtain surgical consultation and admit to the hospital for appendectomy. Antibiotics for nonperforated appendicitis include cefoxitin or ampicillin/sulbactam; for perforated appendicitis, monotherapy with piperacillin/tazobactam is as effective as multidrug therapy.[36] Percutaneous drainage may be done if an abscess is present, followed by delayed appendectomy to prevent recurrence. In ambiguous cases, admission for serial abdominal examination by a surgeon is reasonable.

HENOCH-SCHÖNLEIN PURPURA

Henoch-Schönlein purpura is a vasculitis of children between 2 and 11 years of age with slight peaks in the fall and winter months. The cause is unknown, although a viral pathogen or group A *Streptococcus* may trigger the condition. Immunoglobulin A deposits are seen in the glomeruli and vessel walls.

Clinical Features The typical clinical presentation of Henoch-Schönlein purpura is **a triad of palpable purpuric rash, acute abdominal pain, and arthritis**. The rash occurs in all cases and is the presenting sign in 50% of cases (see chapter 141, Rashes in Infants and Children). The rash may initially be urticarial or macular-papular. The lesions typically appear first on the extensor surfaces of the lower extremities and buttocks; they may involve the arms and ears. The face, palms, and soles are usually spared.

GI symptoms including abdominal pain and GI bleeding occur in 50% to 75% of cases.[37] The pain is usually diffuse and colicky in nature and may be associated with vomiting. Abdominal pain usually presents after the rash, but can precede the rash in 30% to 43% of patients. **Intussusception occurs in 3.5%.**[38] Arthralgia or arthritis occurs in 80% of cases and is the presenting sign in 25%. Joint symptoms are migratory and usually involve the knees and ankles with periarticular swelling and tenderness.

Renal involvement including hematuria, edema, and proteinuria is the most significant long-term consequence (see chapter 134, Renal Emergencies in Children). Obtain a urinalysis on all patients to detect hematuria. When hematuria is present, obtain renal function tests. Although microscopic hematuria is relatively common in patients with Henoch-Schönlein purpura, proteinuria and gross hematuria represent more extensive renal involvement. Perform a rectal examination to assess for gross and occult blood. Stool guaiac may be positive in nearly half of cases and, in the absence of intussusception symptoms, does not require further evaluation. Additional laboratory studies, including CBC and coagulation studies, are not routinely indicated in the patient with a characteristic presentation of Henoch-Schönlein purpura, because these studies are normal in this condition. **If the patient has a history consistent with accompanying intussusception, obtain an abdominal US or air-contrast enema to assess for this.**

Treatment Treatment is mainly supportive. If the child is ill appearing, unable to tolerate oral fluids, or dehydrated, begin IV fluid hydration and arrange for admission. Nonsteroidal anti-inflammatory drugs, such as ibuprofen and ketorolac, are used for management of arthritis, painful edema, and abdominal pain if renal function is normal based on urinalysis. Oral corticosteroids reduce symptoms of severe abdominal and joint pain. Care of patients with gross hematuria, more than small proteinuria, abnormal renal function, hypertension, or nephritic syndrome should be discussed with a pediatric nephrologist. Patients without these findings do not need steroids for prophylaxis of renal disease.[39] Arrange for repeat urinalysis and blood pressure measurements within 7 days, continuing for 6 months.[40]

INGUINAL HERNIA

Inguinal hernias occur in up to 45% of children and are more common in those born prematurely.[41] Incarceration refers to a hernia that cannot easily be reduced and is the presenting sign of the hernia in up to 65% of cases.[42] **Incarceration is most common in the first year of life.**

Clinical Features A simple inguinal hernia is often asymptomatic and is noted as a scrotal or inguinal mass. Symptoms of incarcerated hernia may include irritability, poor feeding, and vomiting. **The differential diagnosis includes torsion of the testicle** or testicular appendage, hydrocele of the cord or the scrotum, undescended testicle, inguinal lymphadenopathy, inguinal node abscess, orchitis, and trauma. The incarcerated sac may contain omentum, bowel, or ovary. Because it can be difficult to differentiate an incarcerated hernia from testicular torsion if significant swelling is present, it may be necessary to proceed with consultation and evaluation for both of these time-dependent emergencies simultaneously.

Treatment An incarcerated hernia may progress to strangulation and is therefore a surgical emergency. Attempt reduction as soon as possible. Place the patient in the Trendelenburg position. Apply pressure to the hernia sac with one hand while the other guides the contents through the inguinal ring. Reduction may take minutes of steady pressure. Sedation and analgesia can be quite helpful. **One third of children redevelop incarceration, so patients should either be admitted for repair or expedited outpatient care should be arranged within 24 hours.** If manual reduction is unsuccessful, request immediate surgical consultation. **Unlike adults, even inguinal hernias in children that have not become incarcerated require referral for early repair because of the high risk of incarceration.**

INFLAMMATORY BOWEL DISEASE

Children account for 20% to 25% of new diagnoses of inflammatory bowel disease.[43] In one series, **95% of those <10 years old with Crohn's disease initially presented with abdominal pain, 77% with diarrhea, and 60% with bloody stools.**[44] The pain in Crohn's disease is often colicky and either diffuse or in the right lower quadrant, mimicking appendicitis. Weight loss is seen in 80% of patients with Crohn's disease. Growth failure may be the only symptom in 5%. Up to 25% of children with inflammatory bowel disease have a positive family history.

Tachycardia and hypotension may be present secondary to dehydration or anemia from chronic blood loss. Inspect the anal area for fistulas, fissures, and skin tags suggestive of Crohn's disease. Extraintestinal signs, including arthritis, ankylosing spondylitis, and erythema nodosum, occur in 20%.

Most children with moderate to severe disease will have anemia and an elevated erythrocyte sedimentation rate. Measure electrolytes in cases of severe diarrhea. If a new diagnosis is being considered, obtain stool culture, ova and parasite examination, and *Clostridium difficile* toxin to assess for infectious causes. An abdominal CT is commonly obtained to evaluate for thickening of the terminal ileum and complications of Crohn's disease such as intra-abdominal abscesses and fistula. Definitive diagnosis requires endoscopy and biopsy, and a pediatric GI specialist should be consulted for further management, which may include oral or IV corticosteroids. Toxic megacolon is a complication of severe ulcerative colitis in which large bowel dilation is present on abdominal radiograph or CT in the setting of fever, abdominal pain, and laboratory markers of systemic inflammation.[45] Treatment requires hospital admission for steroids.[46]

RENAL STONES

Calcium-containing renal stones are the most common type in children. Predisposing factors include immobilization, hyperparathyroidism, corticosteroids, diuretics, and neoplasms. Both ketogenic diets and antiepileptic drugs used to treat seizure disorders can predispose to stone formation.

Clinical Features and Diagnosis Children with renal stones present with abdominal pain only 50% of the time. Microscopic or gross hematuria is present in 85% of children with urolithiasis.[47,48] **The ED workup should include imaging to exclude severe obstruction (CT or US) and urinalysis to exclude infection, as both of these potentially require immediate intervention. If the patient has never had imaging to confirm the presence of two normal kidneys and labs to confirm baseline normal renal function, these should be obtained.** If these studies are abnormal, contact a pediatric nephrologist or urologist.

The imaging evaluation of urolithiasis in children may begin with either US or CT. See chapter 94, Urologic Stone Disease, for a discussion of imaging in adults. In children, US has good specificity but limited sensitivity for urolithiasis (90% for stones within the kidneys, but only 38% for ureteral stones, which are more likely to cause pain). Therefore, US is a sufficient first study if positive, but should be followed by noncontrast CT if negative and urolithiasis is highly suspected. A negative US alone is sufficient if the goal of testing is not to confirm urolithiasis but to rule out obstruction. Plain radiographs have poor sensitivity for stones.

Because of the high rate of underlying metabolic abnormalities in children with urolithiasis (38% to 90%), all children with a new diagnosis require a metabolic evaluation, although this need not be done in the ED.[49] Workup may include a basic metabolic panel, serum calcium, phosphorus, parathyroid hormone, and a 24-hour urine collection.[50] Anatomic abnormalities including vesicoureteral reflux, ureteropelvic and ureterovesicular junction obstruction, and neurogenic bladder were found in 11% of children with urolithiasis, so plans should be made for subsequent imaging.[51] **Parents should be instructed to strain the urine so the stone can be analyzed.**

Treatment ED management is centered on pain and nausea control. If IV placement is indicated for dehydration, pain control, or blood draws, provide aggressive rehydration. Indications for admission include urinary tract infection with obstruction, abnormal renal anatomy or function, uncontrolled pain or nausea, and dehydration. **Most stones in the distal ureters smaller than 3 mm will pass spontaneously, while those larger than 4 mm will likely require intervention.**[52] Discuss patients with larger stones or mild to moderate obstruction with a urologist to plan follow-up. One study of doxazosin 0.03 milligram/kg up to 2 milligrams daily failed to show a benefit for stone passage in children.[53] Interventional therapy includes extracorporeal shock wave lithotripsy and urethral or transcutaneous endoscopy to extract the stone.

Dehydration contributes to stone formation; so encourage oral fluids for all children discharged. Those with known metabolic causes for their stones may benefit from dietary modification, diuretics, or other medications specific to their condition.

PANCREATITIS

Pancreatitis is extremely rare in infants and is most commonly a secondary process in children and adolescents. See chapter 79, Pancreatitis and Cholecystitis, for a discussion of its pathophysiology. **Table 130-4** lists causes of acute pancreatitis in children.[54]

Clinical Features The typical history is an acute onset of epigastric or periumbilical abdominal pain associated with anorexia, nausea, and vomiting. Although 62% to 89% of children with pancreatitis complain of epigastric pain, <10% describe back pain or radiation of the pain to the back; nausea and vomiting are present in 40% to 80% of older children, but only 28% of children <2 years of age.[55] Older children may be able to describe dull, constant epigastric pain that is made worse by eating or lying supine. Physical examination reveals guarding or distension in fewer than half of children with pancreatitis, and Grey Turner sign is present in 2%.[55,56] The child may be lying quietly on his or her side with knees flexed.

TABLE 130-4 Causes of acute pancreatitis in children

Cause	Frequency
Biliary: gallstones and sludge, pancreas divisum	10%–30%
Medications: valproic acid, L-asparaginase, 6-mercaptopurine	<25%
Idiopathic	13%–34%
Multisystem disease: sepsis, shock, systemic lupus erythematosus	33%
Trauma	10%–40%
Infectious: mumps, hepatitis, other viral infection, *Mycoplasma*	<10%
Metabolic: diabetic ketoacidosis, hypertriglyceridemia, hypercalcemia	2%–7%
Hereditary: cystic fibrosis	5%–8%

Diagnosis and Treatment **Acute pancreatitis is defined by an elevation of either lipase or amylase of three times the upper limit of normal, or imaging consistent with pancreatitis.** Lipase is between 73% and 100% sensitive in children.[57] Lipase rises within hours and remains elevated for up to 14 days. Also testing for amylase will identify some cases of pancreatitis with normal lipase values.[55] The level of enzyme elevation does not correlate with the severity of the disease. Obtain electrolytes, including calcium, and liver enzymes, which may suggest hepatic disease or biliary obstruction.

Obtain a US or CT scan to assess for biliary causes (gallstones or sludge) or anatomic abnormalities of the pancreas. US has greater sensitivity for gallstones and gives no ionizing radiation. CT is better at identifying complications of severe pancreatitis including necrosis, fluid collections, and hemorrhage, although these complications are more likely to present a few days into the disease. CT should be ordered if trauma is suspected.

Because intra-abdominal third spacing, shock, and multiorgan system failure are potential complications of acute pancreatitis, aggressively administer normal saline or lactated Ringer's solution. Treat pain and admit the patient to the hospital.

CHOLECYSTITIS

Acute cholecystitis is very rare in children as compared to adults, with only 0.1% to 0.2% of gallstone disease being diagnosed in patients under age 15.[58] **Bile stones from hemolytic disease, such as sickle cell disease, and total parenteral nutrition are the most common type in children, comprising 9% to 50% in case series.** Acute or chronic illness with dehydration, fasting, or mechanical ventilation can cause gallbladder sludge and obstruction in the absence of stones (acalculous cholecystitis). When complicated by bacterial infection of the common bile duct, cholangitis results and is associated with a high risk of sepsis and shock. Children who have undergone surgical Roux-en-Y procedures (e.g., Kasai procedure for biliary atresia) are at risk for ascending cholangitis.

Clinical Features and Diagnosis Children with biliary pain are typically restless and unable to lie still. **Jaundice is more common in children than adults and may occur in the absence of common bile duct obstruction.** Right upper quadrant tenderness and a positive Murphy sign may be elicited in older children and adolescents.

Obtain liver function tests and lipase, which may be normal even in cases of acute cholecystitis. US is the first-line test for evaluation of biliary disease. CT scan may demonstrate acute cholecystitis but misses 20% of gallstones.

Treatment A child with biliary colic (cholelithiasis without acute cholecystitis, whose pain has resolved) may be discharged with outpatient follow-up. Children with cholecystitis or cholangitis should be admitted. Administer antibiotics for findings of gallbladder infection including fever and elevated WBC count: One common regimen is ampicillin, gentamicin, and clindamycin.[59] Cholangitis, with Charcot's triad of right upper quadrant pain, fever, and jaundice, is a medical emergency and requires immediate intervention.

PNEUMONIA

Although a child with pneumonia will often present with respiratory signs and symptoms and fever, the predominant complaint may be abdominal pain. The diagnosis and management of pneumonia in children is discussed in chapter 125, Pneumonia in Infants and Children.

STREPTOCOCCUS PHARYNGITIS

***Streptococcus* pharyngitis can cause abdominal pain with or without vomiting and without sore throat.** Examine the oropharynx of any child ≥3 years of age with abdominal pain. If signs of pharyngitis are present, test for group A *Streptococcus*. If the rapid strep test is negative, send a throat culture because of the rapid antigen test's good specificity but poor sensitivity.[60] See chapter 121, Mouth and Throat Disorders in Infants and Children.

COLIC

Colic is excessive, unexplained paroxysms of crying in a healthy infant from 2 weeks to 4 months of age, peaking at 6 weeks. Wessel's "rule of threes" is a mnemonic for colic: **crying >3 hours per day for >3 days per week for >3 weeks.** Sufferers will flex their legs, turn red, and pass large amounts of gas. Colic is a diagnosis of exclusion made by the chronicity of episodes and exclusion of dangerous alternative diagnoses. See chapter 114, Neonatal Emergencies and Common Neonatal Problems.

CONSTIPATION

Constipation is defined as stools that are hard, infrequent, or painful to pass. **Constipation may cause significant abdominal pain, prompting extensive evaluation.** Normal infants may occasionally go up to 7 days without a bowel movement. As long as the child is not symptomatic and the stool is not hard, no evaluation is necessary.

Hirschsprung's disease is a pathologic cause of constipation in infants. Hirschsprung's disease is caused by a failure of colonic ganglion cells to migrate during gestation and is more common in trisomy 21. A history of failing to pass meconium in the first 24 to 48 hours of life is suggestive of Hirschsprung's disease or cystic fibrosis. Symptoms include infrequent, explosive bowel movements, poor growth and feeding, and progressive abdominal distension.

Constipation may be seen in older children with chronic medical conditions such as anorexia nervosa, cerebral palsy, neuromuscular disease, depression, or hypothyroidism. Acute causes include dehydration, electrolyte abnormalities (hypercalcemia or hypokalemia), or drug ingestions.

Constipation may still be present with a recent, watery bowel movement if the child is passing soft stool around a mass of hard stool. Pencil-like stools suggest a stricture. Spasticity or delayed motor milestones may be signs of occult spinal dysraphism. Toilet training is a common inciting event for functional constipation.

While constipation may be very painful, it should not cause an ill or toxic appearance. The abdomen may be distended, and firm columns of stool may be felt in the descending and ascending colons. A rectal exam with an empty vault and increased sphincter tone that emits a burst of gas on insertion of a finger suggests Hirschsprung's disease. Examine the anal and sacral area for tufts of hair, dimples, and lipomas, which may suggest neurologic malformations including spina bifida and tethered cord.[61] An anteriorly displaced anus (more than two thirds the distance from the coccyx to the scrotal-perineal junction in males and the posterior fourchette in females) should prompt outpatient surgical referral. Fissures may cause painful defecation, leading to a cycle of retention and functional constipation. Check lower extremity tone, reflexes, and gait for signs of spasticity. Botulism from contaminated honey may present as a hypotonic child with constipation.

Treatment If the constipation is presumed to be causing acute pain, the physician may wish to treat in the ED with response guiding further evaluation (**Table 130-5**).[62,63] Oral polyethylene glycol is as effective as enemas for outpatient treatment. Children with constipation refractory to ED management may require hospitalization for polyethylene glycol by nasogastric tube.

TABLE 130-5 Treatment of Constipation in Children

Dietary management: Fruits, vegetables, avoidance of processed foods, water or nonsugar fluids to avoid dehydration.
Glycerin suppositories: ED treatment of constipation in infants <2 years; 1 suppository × 2.
Normal saline enemas: ED treatment of acute constipation; 0–6 months, 120–150 mL; 6–18 months, 150–250 mL; 18 months–5 years, 300 mL. Enemas are most effective when held as long as possible.
Sodium phosphate enemas: ED treatment of acute constipation in children 2–11 years, 2.25-oz pediatric enema. Children >11 years, 4.5-oz adult enema. May repeat.
Polyethylene glycol (PEG): Initial treatment 1–1.5 grams/kg/d divided to two to four times per day for 3 days. Then decrease to 0.78 gram/kg/d divided daily or twice daily for maintenance therapy. Inpatient treatment for cleanout by nasogastric tube with PEG + electrolyte solution is 14–40 mL/h.

ACUTE GASTROENTERITIS

Gastroenteritis is the most common cause of abdominal pain in children of all ages (see chapter 128, Vomiting, Diarrhea, and Dehydration in Children).

NONSPECIFIC ABDOMINAL PAIN

The largest single group of children will have no definite diagnosis and will receive the *diagnosis of exclusion* of nonspecific abdominal pain. **Patients should not be given unsubstantiated diagnoses such as gastroenteritis, gastritis, or constipation without strong support for these diagnoses.** Patients discharged without a clear diagnosis should have a planned reexamination.

Acknowledgment: The authors gratefully acknowledge the contributions of Anupam B. Kharbanda and Rasha D. Sawaya, the authors of this chapter in the previous edition.

REFERENCES

The complete reference list is available online at www.TintinalliEM.com.

CHAPTER 131 Gastrointestinal Bleeding in Infants and Children

Sarah M. Reid

INTRODUCTION AND EPIDEMIOLOGY

GI bleeding varies in its epidemiology and presentation depending on whether it originates from the upper or lower GI tract. Upper GI (UGI) bleeding is bleeding proximal to the ligament of Treitz, whereas lower GI (LGI) bleeding originates distal to this ligament. UGI bleeding is a relatively uncommon presentation in pediatrics, with one population-based survey reporting an incidence of 1 to 2 per 10,000 children/year.[1] LGI bleeding is more common, but most cases are benign and self-limited.[2] In one study, LGI bleeding constituted the chief complaint of 0.3% of children presenting to a pediatric ED, but only 4.2% of these patients had bleeding considered to be life-threatening.[3]

The signs and symptoms of GI bleeding in children vary: bright red blood in small strands or clots in emesis or bowel movements, vomiting of gross blood (hematemesis), black tarry stools (melena), or the passage of bright red or maroon-colored blood from the rectum (hematochezia). Occult bleeding may result in unexplained pallor, fatigue, and anemia. Severity is assessed by vital signs, physical appearance, and the hemodynamic status of the patient, all of which lead to an estimation of the volume of blood loss. Worrisome symptoms and signs include pallor, diaphoresis, lethargy, abdominal pain, tachycardia, hypotension, and altered mental status. GI bleeding can be life threatening. Advances in endoscopy, radiology, and newer therapeutic modalities have helped identify the causes of bleeding more accurately and have provided more treatment options.

CLINICAL APPROACH

Assess bleeding and institute resuscitation if the child has signs of hemorrhagic shock. Next, obtain a history and perform a physical examination, and try to establish the level of bleeding as UGI or LGI, because the subsequent diagnostic and treatment steps differ. Then, narrow the differential diagnosis based on history, physical examination, laboratory studies, and the categorization of age-related causes of UGI and LGI bleeding. The presence of any one of melena, hematochezia, unwell appearance, or moderate to large volume of fresh blood in the vomitus was associated with a clinically significant UGI bleed (defined as a hemoglobin drop of >20 g/L, need for blood transfusion, need for emergent endoscopy, or need for surgical procedure).[4]

ASSESS BLEEDING AND BEGIN RESUSCITATION

There are several important questions to consider. Is the patient stable or unstable? Is this really blood, and is it coming from the GI tract? Is it a small amount of blood or a large volume? Has the child had prior episodes of bleeding, and if so, do the parents know the cause and prior treatment?[5]

IS THE PATIENT STABLE OR UNSTABLE?

The presence of tachycardia, pallor, tachypnea, prolonged capillary refill time, altered mental status, metabolic acidosis, and/or hypotension indicates significant GI bleeding. Tachycardia and tachypnea are the first clinical signs, followed by delayed capillary refill, decreased urine output, altered mental status, metabolic acidosis, and pallor. Orthostatic changes in heart rate and blood pressure indicate that significant bleeding has occurred. Hypotension is a late sign and indicates uncompensated hemorrhagic shock. Any signs of hemorrhagic shock require simultaneous resuscitation, diagnosis, and treatment. Maintain the airway, monitor oxygen saturation and provide oxygen, place two large-bore IVs (20 gauge or larger), and administer boluses of crystalloid and, if necessary, blood products.

IS THIS REALLY BLOOD?

Determine whether or not the vomit or stool really contains blood. Beets, food coloring, and fruit juices can look like blood. Black and tarry stools can result from vitamins with iron, bismuth (Pepto-Bismol®), spinach, cranberries, blueberries, or licorice. Urinary (urate) crystals in the neonatal diaper are often orange in color and may be interpreted by a caregiver as blood. The Gastroccult® and Hemoccult® tests (Beckman Coulter, Brea, CA) can be used to document the presence of blood in gastric contents or stool, respectively. These guaiac-based tests rely on the peroxidase activity of the heme portion of hemoglobin. False-positive results are associated with foods that have peroxidase activity such as red meat, melons, grapes, radishes, turnips, cauliflower, and broccoli. False-negative results can result from the ingestion of vitamin C due to its antioxidant properties.

IS BLOOD COMING FROM THE GI TRACT?

Evaluate the child for epistaxis, recent dental work, or gingival bleeding, because swallowed blood may lead to hematemesis. The neonate can swallow maternal blood during delivery or from breastfeeding if the mother has fissures on her nipples. In the toddler, blood could come from an injury to the oropharynx or nose. Make sure that blood does not originate from the throat or lungs. Distinguish whether the blood in the diaper is from a GU or GI source. Examine the perineum and urethra. Neonatal girls may develop some vaginal bleeding from maternal hormone withdrawal.

IS IT A SMALL OR LARGE AMOUNT OF BLOOD?

It is difficult to gauge the amount of bleeding from caretaker descriptions, because even small amounts of blood can appear alarmingly large. Assess the clinical status of the patient, vital signs, results of laboratory studies, and results of serial clinical examinations to determine the amount of bleeding. The hemoglobin and hematocrit are unreliable indicators of blood loss in the early stages.

See **Tables 131-1, 131-2,** and **131-3,** for potential recurrent causes of GI bleeding organized by age and symptoms.[2,5]

HISTORY

Ask whether the child had prior episodes of bleeding. If so, ask whether the caregivers know the cause and prior treatments. There are many causes of UGI and LGI bleeding in children, and the causes vary significantly by age (Tables 131-1 and 131-2). In addition to the age-based approach to the differential diagnosis of GI bleeding, the clinical presentation and constellation of associated symptoms are often useful in narrowing the differential diagnosis for a particular child. Table 131-3 describes symptom complexes along with the differential diagnosis of GI bleeding.

The type and implications of questioning differ depending on the age of the child (Tables 131-1 and 131-2). If the child is verbal, obtain the history from both the child and the parent or caregiver. Elicit an accurate chronology of events, and ask questions to help frame the differential diagnosis (**Table 131-4**). Vomiting of bright red blood or coffee-ground emesis is the classic presentation of UGI bleeding. Bloody diarrhea and bright red blood mixed with or coating normal stool are the classic presentations of LGI bleeding. Hematochezia, melena, or occult GI blood loss could represent UGI or LGI bleeding.[6]

PHYSICAL EXAMINATION

Obtain vital signs and pulse oximetry. Assess the airway, breathing, and circulation of the patient. Perform a complete physical examination. Gain the confidence of the child before any painful examination or procedures are performed. Examine the nose for any signs of epistaxis and the oral pharynx for any signs of injury, infection, bleeding, or ulcers. Examine the skin for bruises or petechiae (a sign of coagulopathy), jaundice and abnormal venous pattern on the abdomen that would point toward liver disease, cutaneous vascular malformations that may signal lesions of the GI tract, or the palpable purpura associated with Henoch-Schönlein purpura. Allow the young child to rest on the caregiver's lap while examining the abdomen. Start with visual inspection, then auscultate for bowel sounds, and finally, palpate the abdomen for tenderness, guarding, rebound, rigidity, organomegaly, ascites, or masses. External examination of the anus and digital rectal examination are necessary to identify fissures, skin tags, fistulae, hemorrhoids, polyps, and impacted stool and to test for fecal blood.

DIAGNOSIS

Try to determine if the source of bleeding is UGI or LGI. In cases where it is unclear if UGI bleeding is occurring, consider nasogastric lavage. Nasogastric lavage is performed with **a 12-French nasogastric tube in small children and a 14- to 16-French tube in older children.** Instill 50 mL of saline for infants and 100 to 200 mL for older children while keeping the child's head elevated to 30 degrees to reduce the risk of aspiration. After 2 to 3 minutes, gently aspirate gastric contents. Blood-flecked or coffee-ground aspirate suggests a slow rate of UGI bleeding, whereas bright red blood suggests serious hemorrhage. The usefulness of nasogastric lavage is limited, because clear aspirate does not exclude major bleeding from the UGI tract. For example, a duodenal ulcer distal to the pylorus may not reflux blood into the stomach and could yield a negative gastric aspirate.

Laboratory studies are guided by the results obtained from the history and physical examination, the child's appearance (ill or not), and the differential diagnosis (see chapter 130, "Acute Abdominal Pain in Infants and Children" and chapter 128, "Vomiting, Diarrhea, and Dehydration in Infants and Children").

The stable child with minimal or self-limited bleeding may require no further diagnostic evaluation. A CBC, type and screen or cross-match of blood, serum electrolytes, renal function tests, liver function tests, coagulation panel, urinalysis, and stool testing for enteric pathogens or *Clostridium difficile* toxin should be obtained, as needed.

For minimal or moderate GI bleeding, it may be difficult to determine the exact cause in the ED. Diagnosis may require ultrasonography, radiographic imaging, endoscopic evaluation, or a technetium-99m (Meckel) scan.[2]

DIFFERENTIAL DIAGNOSIS FOR UPPER GI BLEEDING BY AGE GROUP

Although the differential diagnosis is guided by the results of history and physical examination and age-related causes, there is considerable overlap among age groups (Table 131-1). Mucosal lesions such as gastritis, esophagitis, ulcer disease, and Mallory-Weiss tears can be seen in

TABLE 131-1 Age-Based Causes of Upper and Lower GI Bleeding

Upper GI Bleeding

Neonate	Infant/Toddler	Child/Adolescent
Common	*Common*	*Common*
Swallowed maternal blood	Non-GI source (e.g., epistaxis)	Mallory-Weiss tear
Milk/soy protein allergy	Mallory-Weiss tear	Gastritis (especially *Helicobacter pylori* gastritis)
Trauma (nasogastric tube in NICU)	Esophagitis	Esophagitis
Uncommon	Gastritis	Peptic ulcer disease
Stress ulcer/gastritis	*Uncommon*	*Uncommon*
Esophagitis	Stress gastritis or ulcer	Esophageal varices
Vascular malformation	Peptic ulcer disease	Toxic/caustic ingestion
Hemorrhagic disease of newborn (vitamin K deficiency)	Vascular malformation	Foreign body
Coagulopathy/bleeding diathesis	GI duplication	Vasculitis
Coagulopathy associated with infection	Gastric/esophageal varices	Vascular malformation
	Bowel obstruction	Bowel obstruction
	Toxic/caustic ingestion	Crohn's disease
	Coagulopathy/bleeding diathesis	Coagulopathy/bleeding diathesis
	Foreign body	GI stromal tumors
		Dieulafoy's lesion

Lower GI Bleeding

Neonate	Infant/Toddler	Child/Adolescent
Common	*Common*	*Common*
Swallowed maternal blood	Anal fissure	Anal fissure
Anal fissure	Milk/soy protein allergy	Infectious gastroenteritis
Milk/soy protein allergy	Infectious gastroenteritis	Polyps; benign, familial
Infectious gastroenteritis	*Uncommon*	*Uncommon*
Uncommon	Intussusception	Henoch-Schönlein purpura
Meckel's diverticulum*	Meckel's diverticulum*	Hemorrhoids
Necrotizing enterocolitis	GI duplication	Inflammatory bowel disease
Vascular malformation	Hemolytic-uremic syndrome	Meckel's diverticulum*
Hemorrhagic disease of newborn (vitamin K deficiency)	Henoch-Schönlein purpura	Hemolytic-uremic syndrome
Intussusception	Malrotation with volvulus	Vascular malformation
Malrotation with volvulus	Polyps; benign, familial	Celiac disease
Hirschsprung's-associated enterocolitis (toxic megacolon)	Coagulopathy/bleeding diathesis	
GI duplication	Vascular malformation	

Abbreviation: NICU = neonatal intensive care unit.

*Most common cause of severe LGI bleeding in all ages.

children of any age. Massive bleeding can occur from esophageal varices, ulcer disease, vascular malformations, Meckel's diverticulum, and GI duplication.

Neonates **Hematemesis in the newborn** is most likely the result of swallowed maternal blood at delivery or during breastfeeding from cracked nipples. The **Apt test** is a qualitative test that distinguishes fetal from maternal hemoglobin. The blood in question is mixed with alkali to detect conversion of oxyhemoglobin to hematin. Fetal hemoglobin is more resistant to denaturation than adult hemoglobin. If the supernatant stays pink after the addition of alkali, the blood is fetal in origin (reported as a positive test). If it turns brown, it is maternal blood. Hemorrhagic disease of the newborn is rare, but if there was failure to administer vitamin K in the immediate postpartum period (e.g., home birth), a prolonged prothrombin time can result in neonatal bleeding.

Infants and Children Children with severe **gastroesophageal reflux** may develop esophagitis and hematemesis. Mallory-Weiss tears after acute forceful vomiting or retching can also cause hematemesis. Any child with significant illness or injury (shock, polytrauma, respiratory failure, burns, head injury, renal failure, or vasculitis) can develop stress-related peptic ulcer disease.

Ingestion of a sharp foreign body or **button battery** can occasionally cause GI bleeding. Removal by endoscopy is indicated. See chapter 77, "Esophageal Emergencies" for further discussion of button battery ingestions.

Preschool and older children can develop idiopathic ulcer disease. **Peptic ulcer disease** in the child is similar to that in adults, and there may be a positive family history. Young children may have poorly localized abdominal pain, bleeding, or even signs of obstruction or perforation. The adolescent will describe epigastric burning pain in a pattern more typical of the adult. If the bleeding is low grade, chronic symptoms of weakness and fatigue may develop. *Helicobacter pylori* is a leading cause of secondary gastritis and peptic ulcer disease in older children. Diagnosis should be made using endoscopy and is based on both positive histopathology and either a positive rapid urease test or positive culture.[7] *H. pylori* eradication is confirmed using either a stool antigen immunoassay or the ^{14}C-Urea Breath Test (Kimberly-Clark Corp., Roswell, GA).[7]

TABLE 131-2 Causes of GI Bleeding by Type

Hematemesis	
Infant	Swallowed maternal blood
	Vitamin K deficiency
	Vascular malformation
Child/adolescent	Swallowed blood from epistaxis, dental work, oral trauma
	Mallory-Weiss tear
	Esophagitis/gastritis
	Peptic ulcer disease
	Esophageal varices
	Vascular malformation
	Toxic ingestion
	Foreign body
	Coagulopathy/bleeding diathesis
Hematochezia and melena	
Infant	Upper GI sources
	Anal fissure
	Milk/soy protein allergy
	Infectious gastroenteritis
	Meckel's diverticulum
	Intussusception
	Malrotation with volvulus
	Ischemic bowel
Child/adolescent	Upper GI sources
	Anal fissure
	Infectious gastroenteritis
	Polyps
	Henoch-Schönlein purpura
	Hemorrhoids
	Inflammatory bowel disease
	Intussusception
	Meckel's diverticulum
	Malrotation with volvulus
	Ischemic bowel
	Hemolytic-uremic syndrome
	Celiac disease
	Vascular malformation

Variceal bleeding is the most common cause of severe UGI bleeding in children.[5] Consider esophageal variceal bleeding in older children and those with underlying chronic hepatic or vascular disease resulting in portal hypertension. Primary diseases of the liver that may lead to portal hypertension include biliary atresia, cystic fibrosis, hepatitis, α_1-antitrypsin deficiency, or congenital hepatic fibrosis. Portal hypertension may occur following liver transplant or operative repair of liver diseases such as biliary atresia. Other predisposing factors to portal hypertension include neonatal omphalitis, umbilical venous cannulation, abdominal sepsis, and abdominal/surgical trauma, although many cases remain idiopathic.[8]

Reactive gastritis can occur due to anti-inflammatory drugs, alcohol, cocaine ingestion, iron ingestion, *H. pylori*, Crohn's disease, Henoch-Schönlein purpura, or foreign bodies. GI stromal tumors can arise from the wall of the GI tract mesentery or omentum. Most of these are found in the stomach and are associated with genetic disorders such as neurofibromatosis.

An unusual cause of UGI bleeding in children is **Dieulafoy's lesion**. Symptomatic lesions result when an abnormal submucosal artery erodes through a tiny mucosal defect, typically in the fundus of the stomach, causing massive bleeding. The characteristic history is recurrent massive

TABLE 131-3 Symptom Complexes and Differential Diagnosis for GI Bleeding

Symptom Complex	Differential Diagnosis
Painless hematemesis	Swallowed blood (non-GI source)
	Coagulopathy/bleeding diathesis
Hematemesis and abdominal, epigastric, or chest pain	Peptic ulcer disease
	Helicobacter pylori–associated gastritis
	Esophagitis/gastritis
Hematemesis, hematochezia, or melena with underlying systemic disease	Esophageal varices
	Inflammatory bowel disease
Vomiting, hematochezia, or melena with abdominal pain	Intussusception
	Malrotation with volvulus
	Ischemic bowel
	Henoch-Schönlein purpura
	Necrotizing enterocolitis
Vomiting, hematochezia, or melena with fever	Infectious gastroenteritis
	Inflammatory bowel disease
Painless rectal bleeding	Polyp
	Meckel's diverticulum
	GI duplication
	Vascular malformation

hematemesis without any prodromal symptoms. Definitive diagnosis is usually made during endoscopy.[9]

DIFFERENTIAL DIAGNOSIS FOR LOWER GI BLEEDING BY AGE GROUP

The presence of melena, hematochezia, or bright red blood per rectum can help to differentiate causes of LGI in children (**Figure 131-1**). The differential diagnosis for LGI bleeding is also age dependent (Table 131-1).

TABLE 131-4 Focused Historical Questions

Chief complaint	Frequency and volume of vomiting
	Blood-streaked, coffee-ground, or bloody vomitus
	Frequency and volume of diarrhea
	Bloody diarrhea
	Constipation with blood-streaked stool
	Blood on toilet paper or blood in toilet bowl
	Abdominal pain along with bloody vomitus or stool
	Dyspepsia; heartburn; dysphagia
	Fever
Review of systems	Rashes; joint pain; oral ulcers; perianal lesions; ocular symptoms; weight loss; fatigue; delayed puberty; failure to thrive; abnormal bleeding; dehydration
Medications	Iron; aspirin; nonsteroidal anti-inflammatory drugs; steroids; alcohol; recent antibiotics
Environment	Foreign body ingestion; foreign travel; sick contacts; raw meat/poultry; unpasteurized milk/cheese; animal contacts; water source
Trauma	Injury to abdomen (especially epigastrium or right upper quadrant) or significant body surface area burns
Past medical history	Term or premature; umbilical artery catheter; postpartum care; abdominal surgery; sepsis; liver disease; GI disease (enterocolitis, intussusception, congenital anomalies); coagulopathy/bleeding diathesis
Family history	GI bleeding; polyps; vascular anomalies; coagulopathy/bleeding diathesis; inflammatory bowel disease

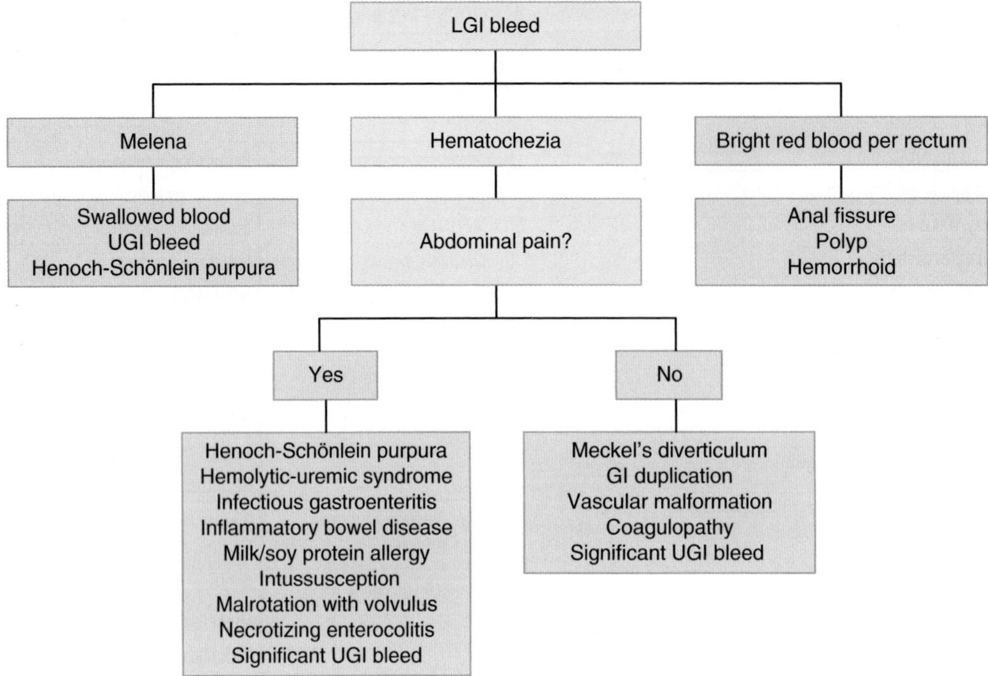

FIGURE 131-1. Diagnostic algorithm for lower GI (LGI) bleeding in children. UGI = upper GI.

The approach to LGI bleeding in the neonate can be organized based on whether the baby appears well or unwell (**Figure 131-2**).

Neonates and Infants The neonate with dark, tarry stools likely has swallowed maternal blood from delivery or breastfeeding. Birth history is important because failure to replace vitamin K can lead to coagulopathy and massive bleeding.

As the infant ages, other disorders become important. **Anal fissures** are a common cause of bright red rectal blood on the surface of well-formed stools or toilet paper in children of all ages and highlight the importance of a careful rectal examination and spreading of anal skin folds. **Milk protein allergy** has a prevalence of 2% to 3% in infants, and cross-reactivity with soy protein exists in at least 10% of cases. Approximately 60% of cases are immunoglobulin E–mediated; both humoral and cell-mediated mechanisms lead to a range of clinical symptoms. Protein-induced allergic enterocolitis/proctitis/proctocolitis may lead to blood-streaked, mucousy, loose stools. Food protein-induced enterocolitis is a rare, delayed non–immunoglobulin E–mediated reaction typically presenting with profuse vomiting and diarrhea 2 to 3 hours after ingestion of the offending allergen. The diarrhea may be frankly bloody, and the infant may develop profound dehydration and lethargy. The basis of therapy in milk/soy protein allergy is removal of the offending protein using hydrolyzed or elemental formula. Breastfed infants whose mothers ingest dairy or soy may also suffer from this condition, and the offending protein must be eliminated from the maternal diet.[10]

Necrotizing enterocolitis is most commonly seen in preterm infants in the neonatal intensive care unit, but may rarely be seen in

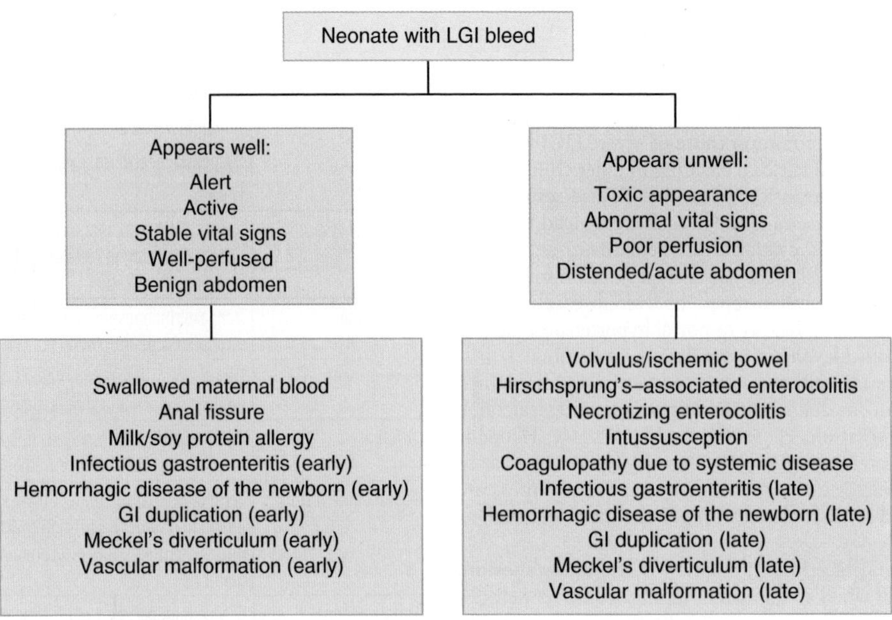

FIGURE 131-2. Approach to lower GI (LGI) bleeding in a neonate.

term infants. Infants will be systemically unwell and present with abdominal distension and hematochezia. Plain radiographs reveal ileus and the pathognomonic *pneumatosis intestinalis* diagnostic of this condition. Infants with **Hirschsprung's disease** (congenital aganglionic megacolon) may develop Hirschsprung's-associated enterocolitis or toxic megacolon, also characterized by abdominal distension and hematochezia.

In older infants who develop sudden painless hematochezia, congenital malformations such as **Meckel's diverticulum** and **GI duplication** must be considered. Meckel's diverticula are remnants of the omphalomesenteric duct in the distal ileum and are present in approximately 2% of the population. They may be lined with ectopic gastric mucosa and typically present with painless rectal bleeding in the 2-month to 2-year-old age group.[11] Diagnosis is made using a Meckel scan. **Intussusception** is another important consideration in children under 2 years with a peak incidence between 5 and 10 months of age.[12] Intussusception is associated with episodes of colicky abdominal pain and vomiting. As the intussusception progresses, painful episodes may alternate with periods of lethargy, and gross blood ("currant jelly") may be noted in the stool. Diagnosis is made using US or contrast/air enema. Painful LGI bleeding in the infant can also be a symptom of **malrotation with volvulus**. Volvulus most commonly presents with abdominal pain, distension, and bilious vomiting, but may lead to bowel ischemia and subsequent LGI bleeding as the condition progresses. Both intussusception and volvulus represent true surgical emergencies and are further discussed in chapters 128 and 130.

Children Age 2 to 5 Years Old Children in the 2- to 5-year-old age range have a different spectrum of disorders causing LGI bleeding: juvenile polyps, infectious gastroenteritis, hemolytic-uremic syndrome, and Henoch-Schönlein purpura. A review of recent literature suggests an estimated detected prevalence of colorectal polyps in 12% of all children with LGI bleeding undergoing colonoscopy.[13] Manifestations of **polyps** range from chronic heme-positive stools to acute hematochezia from autoamputation of the polyp at its stalk. Juvenile polyps are usually benign hamartomas, and most have no malignant potential. Multiple adenomatous polyps should suggest diagnoses such as familial adenomatous polyposis.

Infectious gastroenteritis should be evident by history and physical examination (**Table 131-5**).[14] Also see chapter 128. Patients with typical diarrhea-associated hemolytic-uremic syndrome caused by Shiga toxin–producing strains of *Escherichia coli* have an antecedent episode of hemorrhagic enterocolitis within 2 to 12 days before the onset of thrombotic microangiopathy.[15] Children who have recently been exposed to antibiotics may develop bloody diarrhea from pseudomembranous colitis associated with ***C. difficile* infection**. In **Henoch-Schönlein purpura**, 50% to 75% of patients have episodic abdominal pain and/or blood in their stool from intestinal vasculitis. One-third of Henoch-Schönlein purpura patients develop acute intestinal bleeding manifested as gross or occult blood per rectum.[16] Intussusception develops in 1% to 5% of children with Henoch-Schönlein purpura.[17] Henoch-Schönlein purpura is further discussed in chapter 130.

Children >5 Years Old In children >5 years of age, juvenile polyps and infectious gastroenteritis remain common causes of LGI bleeding. Both **Crohn's disease** and **ulcerative colitis** also become evident in this age group, and the incidence of these diseases is increasing.[18] Symptoms are varied and involve multiple systems: skin lesions such as erythema nodosum and pyoderma gangrenosum; extraintestinal GI problems such as nonspecific hepatitis, cholelithiasis, sclerosing cholangitis, and

TABLE 131-5 Infectious Causes of Bloody Diarrhea in Children

Infectious Agent	Historical Facts	Symptoms	Diagnosis	Treatment
Salmonella	1–4 y Foodborne Reptiles	Fever Abdominal pain	Stool culture	Supportive; antibiotics if typhoid fever, septic, <3 months old, or immunosuppressed
Shigella	<5 y Child care center Travelers	Fever Abdominal pain	Stool WBC count (nonspecific) Shiga toxin Stool culture	Antibiotics unless very mild disease
Yersinia	Uncommon Livestock transmission	Abdominal pain (pseudoappendicitis) Fever Scarlatiniform rash	Stool culture	Antibiotics for systemically ill patients; otherwise unclear
Campylobacter jejuni	Unpasteurized milk, improperly cooked chicken	Often self-limited No fever Abdominal pain 10%–20% have severe, prolonged, or relapsing illness	Stool culture	Antibiotics
Escherichia coli (Shiga toxin)	Ground beef Petting zoos Contaminated raw fruits	—	Stool culture for 0157:H7 Produces Shiga toxin	Antibiotics not proven beneficial
E. coli (enteroinvasive)		Fever Vomiting	Stool cultures not helpful (normal flora)	Antibiotics
Entamoeba histolytica	Southeast United States Low socioeconomic class Travelers from endemic areas	Increasing severity of diarrhea Lower abdominal pain Tenesmus	Stool for ova and parasites may be negative (serial testing may be necessary) Serology with enzyme immunoassay kit	Antibiotics followed by luminal amebicide
Aeromonas hydrophila	Warm weather Waterborne	Chronic diarrhea	Stool culture (requires special media)	Antibiotics only in special populations
Clostridium difficile	Recent antibiotic usage	Pseudomembranous colitis Toxic megacolon (rare)	Stool culture not helpful *C. difficile* toxin studies on diarrheal stool	Antibiotics if symptomatic

pancreatitis; skeletal involvement including aseptic necrosis of bone, arthralgias, and arthritis; ocular problems with uveitis and scleritis; renal disorders such as stones and nephritis; hematologic abnormalities such as anemia, thrombocytopenia, and hypercoagulability; and general failure to thrive. Crohn's disease is twice as common as ulcerative colitis and is characterized by abdominal pain, weight loss, growth failure, and anemia.[18] Ulcerative colitis often presents with rectal bleeding, bloody diarrhea, urgency/tenesmus, and abdominal pain.[18] In the acutely ill patient, diagnosis can be made with a combination of laboratory studies (blood count, erythrocyte sedimentation rate, C-reactive protein, albumin, liver function tests) and CT or MRI enterography.[18] Imaging can show areas of inflammation and can identify complications such as abscess or perforation.[19] Definitive diagnosis requires upper endoscopy, colonoscopy, and biopsy.

TREATMENT

Severe bleeding requires acute resuscitation and teamwork with the pediatric surgeon and/or gastroenterologist, depending on the suspected cause of bleeding. Treatment goals for UGI and LGI bleeding are: (1) resuscitation from hemorrhagic shock and restoring the intravascular volume; (2) restoring normal oxygen-carrying capacity by transfusion with packed red blood cells; (3) identifying the source of bleeding; and (4) stopping ongoing blood loss.

Management begins with an assessment of the airway, breathing, and circulation, followed by the rapid administration of serial 20 mL/kg crystalloid fluid boluses. If three boluses of crystalloid do not restore volume, administer 10 mL/kg of packed red blood cells.

Avoid overexpansion of intravascular volume, particularly if the bleeding is from varices. Correct for shock and restore urine flow, but then titrate additional fluid volume or blood administration based on estimated blood loss and response of the vital signs (**Figure 131-3**).

TABLE 131-6 Pantoprazole Dosing

Patient Weight	Bolus	Infusion
5–15 kg	2 milligrams/kg/dose IV	0.2 milligram/kg/h IV
15–40 kg	1.8 milligrams/kg/dose IV	0.18 milligram/kg/h IV
>40 kg	80 milligrams/dose IV	8 milligrams/h IV

UPPER GI BLEEDING

Emergency endoscopy is needed for children with moderate to severe, persistent or recurrent bleeding, and may be both diagnostic and therapeutic (e.g., coagulation, sclerotherapy, banding).

Variceal Bleeding For unstable patients in whom endoscopy cannot be performed, **octreotide** is the drug of choice for esophageal variceal bleeding. Administer octreotide at 1 to 2 micrograms/kg bolus up to 50 micrograms, and follow with a continuous infusion of 1 to 2 micrograms/kg/h, which may be increased hourly by 1 microgram/kg up to 4 micrograms/kg/h.[6,20] The major adverse effect of octreotide is hyperglycemia, which requires monitoring of serum glucose.

If octreotide is unavailable, consult with a pediatric gastroenterologist regarding the use of **vasopressin**. The dose of vasopressin is 0.002 to 0.005 unit/kg/min titrated as needed (maximum 0.01 unit/kg/min). If bleeding stops for 12 hours, then vasopressin is tapered off over 24 to 48 hours.[21] Intensive care unit admission is needed. Vasopressin use is limited by the side effects of peripheral and central vasoconstriction.

Nonvariceal Bleeding Medical treatment of bleeding from mucosal lesions, such as peptic ulcers, can include proton pump inhibitors, histamine-2 receptor antagonists, antacids, and sucralfate. **Proton pump inhibitors** are more efficacious than histamine-2 receptor antagonists.[6] Intravenous pantoprazole, given as a bolus dose followed by an infusion, is used for control of active bleeding (**Table 131-6**).[21]

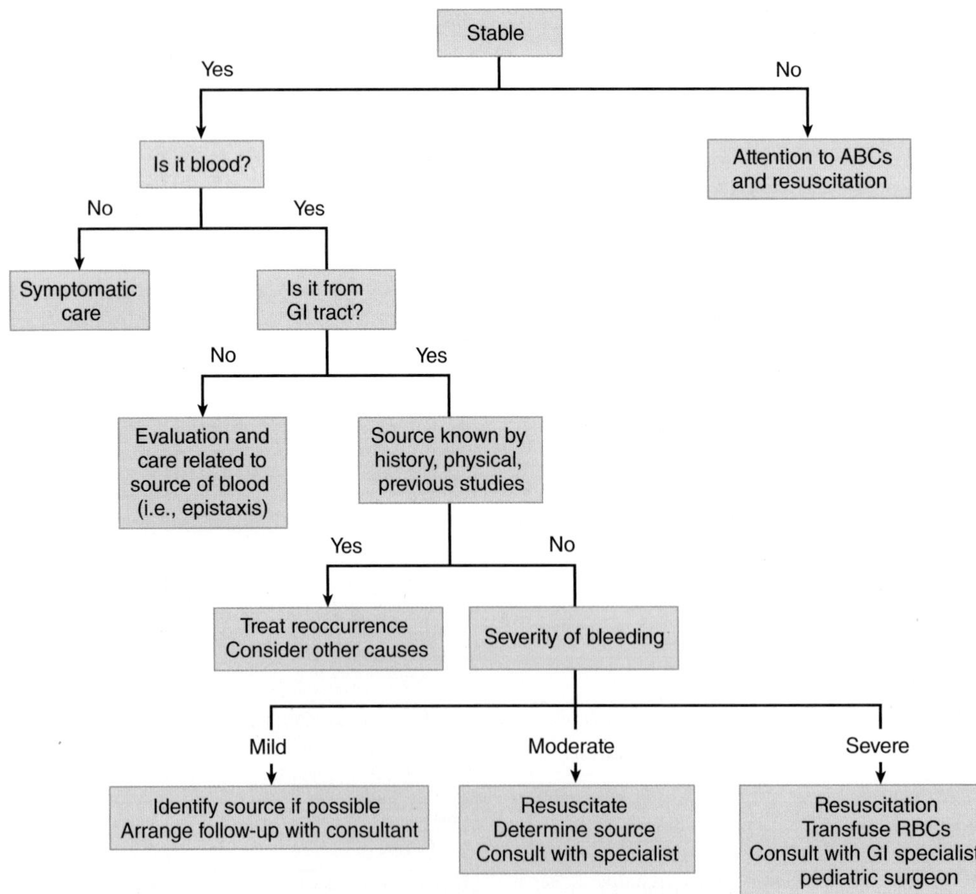

FIGURE 131-3. Initial management of GI bleeding. ABCs = airway, breathing, and circulation; RBCs = red blood cells

If bleeding is persistent and endoscopy fails to identify a bleeding site, angiography may be indicated, although it is technically difficult in young children and a minimum rate of bleeding of 1 to 2 mL/min is required for diagnosis using this modality.

LOWER GI BLEEDING

Hemorrhagic shock is not common as a result of LGI bleeding. There are some important exceptions, however. Meckel's diverticulum may result in significant blood loss in children of any age and requires surgical excision. Painless hematochezia should point to this diagnosis, and a Meckel scan is diagnostic. Definitive treatment is surgical resection. Bleeding associated with Henoch-Schönlein purpura can be severe, but resuscitation and stabilization are the mainstays of treatment. GI duplications and vascular malformations may also cause significant bleeding.

DISPOSITION AND FOLLOW-UP

The management of potential surgical abdominal emergencies such as intussusception and volvulus are discussed in chapter 130. Children with LGI bleeding associated with abdominal pain should not be discharged from the ED until symptoms have resolved or definitive diagnosis has been made. Small amounts of bright red blood per rectum in an otherwise healthy child or signs of chronic blood loss in well-compensated patients can be referred to a gastroenterologist for outpatient colonoscopy. Infants with suspected milk/soy protein allergy who appear well and in whom close follow-up can be arranged do not require specific therapy in the ED; dietary changes are best left to the primary care physician who will follow these patients longitudinally.

When follow-up in 24 to 72 hours can be ensured, the majority of children with mild GI bleeding can be discharged from the ED without a definitive diagnosis. Hemodynamically stable children without systemic symptoms or significant abdominal pain do not require inpatient treatment or evaluation. Conditions that can generally be diagnosed simply or presumptively in the ED and managed safely in the outpatient setting include swallowed maternal blood in the infant, Mallory-Weiss tears, gastritis, peptic ulcer disease, anal fissures, juvenile polyps, milk/soy protein allergy, and infectious gastroenteritis effectively treated with oral rehydration therapy. Stable patients with suspected inflammatory bowel disease can often have definitive diagnosis made in the outpatient setting as well.

Patients with large-volume blood loss, even with a normal hematocrit on initial evaluation, and those with associated abdominal pain in whom surgical or serious causes cannot be excluded require admission to the hospital for continued evaluation and treatment.

Acknowledgment: Special thanks to Dr. Areej Shahbaz for her help in the preparation of this chapter.

REFERENCES

The complete reference list is available online at www.TintinalliEM.com.

Urinary Tract Infection in Infants and Children

Justin W. Sales

INTRODUCTION AND EPIDEMIOLOGY

Pediatric urinary tract infections (UTIs) are now the most common serious bacterial infection in young children, since the introduction of successful immunizations and the resultant decrease in pediatric sepsis, meningitis, and occult bacteremia. UTIs should be considered as a possible diagnosis in all febrile infants and young children presenting to EDs and in all older children with abdominal or urinary symptoms whether or not there is fever.

TABLE 132-1 Risk Factors for Pediatric UTI

Factor	Risk
Gender	3 times higher risk in females
Age	Variably increased risk in infants and younger children
Circumcision status	4–20 times higher risk in uncircumcised males
Race/ethnicity	Half the risk in African American children compared with nonblack children
Fever	Increased risk with fever > 39°C for both boys and girls, and with fever duration > 24 h in boys or > 48 h in girls
History of UTI	2-fold increased risk
Genital sexual activity	Increased risk
Previous urinary tract infection	Increased risk

Estimates of UTI prevalence are highly variable depending on the population. Pediatric UTI occurs in up to 8% of febrile children presenting to the ED with no obvious source of infection.[1-3] Approximately 1% of boys and 3% of girls are diagnosed with a UTI before puberty.[4] The highest incidence occurs during the first year of life for both genders.[3] Some of the baseline characteristics that increase the risk of UTI are listed in **Table 132-1**.[1,2,5-11] It is unclear why African American children have a lower risk of UTI, but this difference is consistently noted.[11]

PATHOPHYSIOLOGY

Bacteria most commonly cause UTIs, although viruses and other infectious agents can also be urinary pathogens. The vast majority of UTIs in all age groups typically occur from retrograde contamination of the lower urinary tract with organisms from the perineum and periurethral area. In neonates, however, UTIs typically develop after seeding of the renal parenchyma from hematogenous spread.

Escherichia coli is the most common cause of UTI in children, and this is likely because of its ubiquitous presence in stool combined with bacterial virulence factors that improve adhesion to and ascent of the urethra.[4] Additional pathogens include *Klebsiella*, *Proteus*, and *Enterobacter* species. *Enterococcus* species, *Staphylococcus aureus*, and group B streptococci are the most common gram-positive organisms and are more common in neonates. *Staphylococcus saprophyticus* can cause UTI in adolescents, and *Chlamydia trachomatis* may be present in adolescents with urinary tract symptoms and microhematuria. Adenovirus may cause culture-negative acute cystitis in young boys.

Mechanical defenses in humans, such as normal urinary outflow, clear most bacteria that are introduced into the bladder. Anatomic abnormalities can make bacterial proliferation or persistence in the bladder more likely. Additional factors influencing the development of UTI include virulence of the pathogen, vesicoureteral reflux, urolithiasis, poor hygiene, voluntary urinary retention, and abnormal bladder function due to constipation. There are occasionally patients, usually preschool- or school-aged females, who have recurrent UTI without a clear anatomic abnormality or identifiable risk factors. Genetic investigation may allow identification of these at-risk individuals.[12] Rare causes of UTI in children include indwelling urinary catheters or UTI from embolism or secondary to infection of other body areas.

CLINICAL FEATURES

HISTORY AND COMORBIDITIES

Clinical features vary markedly by age. The initial history should focus on the acute illness, including the presence of fever, vomiting, or abdominal pain, and questioning about symptoms that might suggest another source of fever such as rhinorrhea, cough, or diarrhea. Neonates with UTIs may appear septic, with fever, jaundice, poor feeding, irritability, and lethargy.[13] Older infants and young children typically develop GI complaints, with fever, abdominal pain, vomiting, and change in appetite. GU symptoms in a verbal child should always trigger consideration of a UTI. In school-aged children and adolescents, cystitis and urethritis (lower tract disease) typically present with urinary frequency, urgency, hesitancy, and dysuria. Pyelonephritis (upper tract disease) typically presents with fever, chills, back pain, vomiting, and dehydration. **In nonverbal children, a history of high (>40°C [104°F]) or prolonged fever appears to be one of the most predictive symptoms of UTI.**[11] A parental report of "smelly" urine does not appear to be helpful.[14]

Medical history should include a prenatal history and ascertainment of whether a late-term prenatal US was obtained. A normal late-term US decreases the likelihood of some GU abnormalities that increase the risk of UTI. Additionally, a previous history of UTI and family history of UTI is important to guide subsequent evaluation.

PHYSICAL EXAMINATION

Assess the child's health and degree of acute illness. If the child is lethargic, dehydrated, or in respiratory distress, then institute appropriate therapy. Examine the genitalia for anatomic abnormalities (e.g., labial adhesions, phimosis) or other causes of GU symptoms. Note circumcision status in male infants. Perform a careful abdominal and groin examination to evaluate for suprapubic tenderness,[11] costovertebral angle tenderness, hernias, and any abnormal masses. A complete physical examination helps to exclude other causes of illness. **Although the presence of another source of fever lowers the risk of UTI, it does not eliminate it, and UTI can coexist with common viral syndromes such as respiratory syncytial virus bronchiolitis.**[11,15,16]

DIAGNOSIS AND DIFFERENTIAL DIAGNOSIS

In infants and young children, the only cardinal feature of UTI is a febrile illness without other definitive source. The approach to neonates and infants <3 months of age with fever and no identifiable source is discussed in detail in chapter 116, Fever and Serious Bacterial Illness in Infants and Children. Urine testing (including urine chemical strip testing, microscopy, and culture) is an important part of a more comprehensive evaluation in this age group. As mentioned earlier, UTI should be considered in infants with bronchiolitis, particularly in the presence of high fever (temperature of 40°C [104°F]).[16,17] In verbal children, dysuria combined with suprapubic tenderness on examination is the classic constellation of symptoms and signs.

There are no clinical criteria that confirm the diagnosis of UTI in children without urinary testing and culture.[18] Evidence-based clinical practice guidelines for the evaluation and treatment of pediatric UTI from the American Academy of Pediatrics are limited to infants and young children 2 to 24 months of age and require *both* pyuria and bacteriuria with ≥50,000 colonies/mL of a single uropathogenic organism (in a properly collected specimen, <1 hour old at room temperature and <4 hours old refrigerated) for definitive diagnosis of UTI.[19] Positive urine cultures in the absence of pyuria/bacteriuria may represent asymptomatic bacteriuria. For infants <2 months old, a positive urine culture is the gold standard for diagnosis.

In adolescents, symptoms of dysuria without vaginal or urethral discharge, or an examination consistent with UTI/pyelonephritis, such as suprapubic or costovertebral angle tenderness, in the presence of a positive urine chemical strip for pyuria and/or nitrites, allow a *presumptive* diagnosis of UTI. A careful sexual history (with assurance of confidentiality and respect for privacy) is important in this age group, because urethral symptoms (such as dysuria) may predominate in both UTI and sexually transmitted infections. Urine culture remains important for definitive diagnosis, and pyuria without uropathogenic culture growth may suggest sexually transmitted infection. Consider pelvic examination for sexually active girls and appropriate testing in both boys and girls with dysuria who are sexually active (see chapter 149, Sexually Transmitted Infections).

TABLE 132-2 Causes of Culture-Negative Dysuria and Pyuria in Children

Culture-Negative Dysuria
Viral urethritis/cystitis
May be hemorrhagic in some viral infections such as adenovirus
Meatitis/urethritis
Often in young boys due to irritation from clothes or self-stimulation
Can be from vaginitis in the vaginal vault in girls. The common causes of vaginitis in young girls include irritant vaginitis from poor hygiene and residual urine that is persistently not cleaned after voiding or irritant vaginitis from soaps or other chemicals. Occasionally, premenarchal girls have bacterial vaginitis. Candidal vaginitis generally does not occur in prepubertal girls.
Balanitis
Culture-Negative Pyuria
Kawasaki's disease (from urethritis)
Pelvic abscess or infection
Appendicitis, pelvic inflammatory disease, colitis, etc.
Sexually transmitted diseases (e.g., *Chlamydia*, gonorrhea*)
In sexually active adolescents, strongly consider these if there is pyuria with a negative culture.
Intrinsic renal disease (e.g., glomerulonephritis)
Allergic bladder or renal disease (e.g., interstitial nephritis)

*Sexually transmitted disease can cause both dysuria and pyuria.

DIFFERENTIAL DIAGNOSIS

UTI is a possible diagnosis in all infants with fever. In children with dysuria but no fever, the most common concerns are listed in **Table 132-2**.

LABORATORY EVALUATION

Urine Sample Collection If children can *void on command*, then attempt collection of a spontaneously voided specimen. Perineal cleaning before voiding reduces the rate of false-positive urinary dipstick tests and the rate of contaminated culture results.[20]

In infants and children who are not able to void on command, bladder catheterization is the preferred method for urine collection. Suprapubic aspiration, although invasive, is also acceptable. The value of perineal bag specimens is limited by the high false-positive results and low specificity. Although the sensitivity of perineal bag specimens for UTI is generally similar to that collected from catheterized or suprapubic specimens, the specificity is low, and a positive culture result from a perineal bag specimen has a high likelihood of significant contamination with perineal bacterial flora. The only (rare) circumstance where a perineal bag specimen may be used is to *exclude disease* when the pretest probability of UTI is very low, in which case a negative test rules out disease; if the results from a perineal bag specimen are positive, confirmation *before giving antibiotics* requires culture of a specimen collected in a sterile manner. Due to this diagnostic delay, many clinicians prefer obtaining a definitive specimen initially.

Urine Culture **The definitive test for UTI is a urine culture**, and colony counts indicating infection are based on the type of sample collection (**Table 132-3**). **Do not give antibiotics until a urine culture is obtained using a sterile method** (bladder catheterization or suprapubic aspiration; see Procedures later). Based on the clinical scenario, length of illness, and urinalysis results, lower colony counts or mixed-growth cultures cannot necessarily be dismissed. Gram-negative urine culture results are usually available within 24 hours of the time that the culture plate is prepared.

Colorimetric or Chemical Test Strip Testing and Microscopic Analysis Urine culture results are not available at the first ED visit, so chemical test strips that can detect leukocyte esterase and urinary nitrites, in conjunction with microscopic urinalysis, help predict the results of the urine culture. Leukocyte esterase is an enzyme found in some white blood cells, and its presence on testing suggests pyuria.

TABLE 132-3 Urine Culture Results Indicating UTI

Sample Collection	Positive Culture*
Clean catch	≥50,000 cfu/mL
Catheterization	≥50,000 cfu/mL
Suprapubic catheterization	Any single species bacterial growth if combined with acute symptoms or signs of urinary tract infection

Abbreviation: cfu = colony-forming unit.

*Urine culture results listed here should be considered indicative of urinary tract infection only in the setting of pyuria.

Nitrite in the urine depends on coagulase-splitting bacteria that can reduce urinary nitrate to nitrite. **Enterobacteria generally reduce nitrate to nitrite if the urine has been in the bladder long enough (about 4 hours), but most gram-positive bacteria do not reduce nitrate to nitrite, so nitrite testing has insufficient sensitivity for detection of UTI (53%; range, 15% to 82%).**[19] Urinary nitrites and leukocyte esterase alone are not sensitive markers for children who empty their bladders frequently. Urinary nitrites are highly specific (98%; range, 90% to 100%)[19] and are therefore helpful when positive.[21] Microscopy of spun or unspun urine for leukocytes and bacteria and/or Gram stain of unspun urine are also helpful for immediate diagnosis; urine Gram stain performs as well as a chemical test strip for urine infection.[22] Gram stain can also identify the bacterial morphology and help guide appropriate initial antibiotic therapy. **Table 132-4** summarizes the test characteristics of the urinalysis.

Regardless of the results from chemical testing strip or microscopic analysis, send the sample for a urine culture. There are two situations where one might not send urine for culture: (1) in low-risk patients with a completely normal urinalysis and another explanation for the symptoms; and (2) in older adolescent females with a very high posttest probability of UTI, without severe illness or complicating medical problems, and in an area with a predictable antibiotic resistance pattern. Because pyuria alone does not confirm a UTI, refer to Table 132-2 for some causes of culture-negative pyuria.

Imaging Acute imaging of the urinary tract is rarely necessary in UTI assessment or treatment. If children have persistent fever or are worsening despite appropriate therapy or symptoms are unusually severe, then renal US is indicated to rule out abscess, stone, or obstruction. A renal US and bladder US are recommended for children 2 to 24 months old after the first UTI.[19] Routine urethrocystography after first UTI is not recommended.[19] Voiding cystourethrography is indicated if renal-bladder US reveals hydronephrosis, scarring, or other findings that would suggest either high-grade vesicourethral reflux or obstructive uropathy. This testing is arranged on an outpatient basis or is performed during hospitalization and is not typically facilitated from the ED. Some expert groups recommend against imaging after the first UTI, if the infection follows a typical clinical course. In Britain, US is recommended in the setting of atypical response to therapy or recurrent infection.[23,24]

Other Suggested Testing Testing beyond urinalysis and culture is not necessary for afebrile children with isolated UTI before initiating treatment. Children with atypical presentations or significant comorbidities may require further investigation as directed by the clinical picture. Febrile neonates and young infants (<2 months of age) require further evaluation prior to initiating antibiotics. Approximately 10% of young infants with febrile UTI admitted to the hospital demonstrate a sterile cerebrospinal fluid pleocytosis thought to be due to systemic release of inflammatory mediators.[27,28] Less than 1% of febrile infants with UTI will also have bacterial meningitis. **Perform lumbar puncture and obtain blood cultures in febrile infants <1 month old with UTI before starting empiric antibiotics (see chapter 116).** Lumbar puncture is not needed in febrile older infants and children with UTI unless there are signs or symptoms suggestive of meningitis, or if the child is clinically ill or the illness does not respond to treatment.[29]

Most febrile infants with UTI have upper tract involvement, and laboratory tests are unlikely to differentiate those with bacteremia from those without bacteremia.[30] About 5% to 10% of febrile infants with UTI

TABLE 132-4 Characteristics of Urinary Diagnostic Tests, Alone and in Combination

	Test Characteristic Ranges				Post-test Probability (%) of UTI in Different Patients				
	Sensitivity (%)	Specificity (%)	Test Result	Likelihood Ratio*	Patient A	Patient B	Patient C	Patient D	Patient E
Individual Tests[19]									
Leukocyte esterase	67–94 (83)	64–92 (78)	+	3.8	22.2	3.7	19.5	20.9	27.3
			–	0.2	1.5	0.2	1.3	1.4	1.9
Nitrite†	15–82 (53)	90–100 (98)	+	26.5	66.6	21.1	62.8	64.8	72.4
			–	0.5	3.6	0.5	3.1	3.4	4.7
Leukocytes on microscopy	32–100 (73)	45–98 (81)	+	3.8	22.2	18.3	58.6	60.7	68.7
			–	0.3	2.2	2.2	12.3	13.3	17.9
Bacteria on microscopy	16–99 (81)	11–100 (83)	+	4.8	26.5	21.1	62.8	64.8	72.4
			–	0.2	1.5	1.5	8.7	9.4	12.9
Combined Tests[19,25]									
Leukocyte esterase and nitrite	27–48 (37)	92–97 (95)	+	7.4	35.8	7	32.1	34	42.3
			–	0.7	5.0	0.7	4.3	4.6	6.5
Leukocyte esterase, nitrite, and blood	33–55 (44)	94–99 (97)	+	14.7	52.5	12.9	48.4	50.5	59.2
			+	0.6	4.3	0.6	3.7	4	5.6
Any positive test on dipstick	99–100 (99.8)	60–92 (70)	+	3.3	19.9	3.2	17.4	18.7	24.6
			–	<0.1	0.2	<0.1	0.1	0.1	0.2

Note: Patient A: female patient in ED, <1 year old, fever with no definitive source on examination, pretest probability of UTI 7%[1,2]; Patient B: male patient in ED, <1 year old, circumcised, fever with no definitive source on examination, pretest probability of UTI 1%[26]; Patient C: male patient in ED, <1 year old, uncircumcised, fever with no definitive source on examination, pretest probability of UTI 6%[26]; Patient D: female patient in ED, 2–6 years old, no fever but GU symptoms, pretest probability of UTI 6.5%[2]; Patient E: female patient in ED, adolescent age range, no fever but urinary symptoms, pretest probability of UTI 9%.[2]

*Positive and negative likelihood ratio calculated from mean sensitivity and specificity.

†Test characteristics are for all subjects. However, test likely has no use if urine infection is due to gram-positive organism or if urine has not stayed in the bladder.

TABLE 132-5 Treatment of First UTI in Children*

Age	Comment
≤1 mo old	Hospital admission and IV antibiotics for 3–5 d followed by variable course of oral antibiotics for 14 d.
>1 mo old–2 y old	If toxic, admit to hospital. If nontoxic, not vomiting, and well hydrated, may give ceftriaxone, 50 milligrams/kg in ED; follow with oral antibiotic (Table 132-6) for 7–14 d. Follow up in 24 h.
>2 y old	Select an oral antibiotic from Table 132-6 based on local resistance patterns. Children >2 y old to age 13 y, treat for 7 d. Follow up with pediatrician in 2–3 d. Adolescent girls (≥13 y old), option to treat for 3 d.

*In children with normal GU anatomy.

have bacteremia.[27] There is low risk of bacteremia and adverse events in well-appearing infants and children with febrile UTI.[29,31,32] For older patients being sent home for UTI treatment who have been initially committed to oral antibiotics, a blood culture is not likely to be helpful.

TREATMENT

Do not give antibiotics to children until a urine culture is obtained, because typical choices for antibiotics will likely sterilize the urinary tract and make bacteriologic diagnosis impossible.[19] Treatment and disposition depend on the age of the patient and severity of the illness. Most children can be treated orally.[33-35] Goals of therapy are to reduce symptoms/eliminate the acute infection, prevent complications and septicemia, and decrease the risk of renal scarring. Pyelonephritis can be demonstrated by renal scan in up to 61% of children <2 years old with febrile UTI, so children <2 years old with UTI have presumptive pyelonephritis.[30] Renal scarring is associated with adverse long-term outcomes such as hypertension, proteinuria, risk of preeclampsia in pregnant women, and eventual renal insufficiency. Treatment guidelines for first UTI are listed in **Table 132-5**, and **Table 132-6** lists suggested parenteral and oral antibiotics. For children with relapsing or recurrent UTI or with underlying GU anatomic abnormalities, treat according to culture and sensitivity reports.

E. coli is the most common etiologic agent causing UTI, so antibiotics should be directed toward its eradication. *Due to regional variation in antimicrobial susceptibility, physicians should be familiar with the local susceptibilities of the common urinary pathogens in their geographic region.* Medications listed in Table 132-6 are generally acceptable, but emerging resistance is a continuing problem. Local sensitivities should guide antibiotic selection. Typical effective first-line agents to treat *E. coli* include cephalosporins, aminoglycosides, and extended-spectrum penicillins. Many strains of *E. coli* are now resistant to amoxicillin and trimethoprim-sulfamethoxazole, limiting the use of these two agents for empiric UTI treatment. A fluoroquinolone should be used in children *only* if sensitivities indicate that this is the only effective agent. Agents that do not achieve therapeutic concentrations in the bloodstream, such as nalidixic acid or nitrofurantoin, should not be used for UTI in febrile children. Once culture results with sensitivities for the infection are known, antimicrobial therapy should be tailored and simplified, based on the actual bacteria isolated. **Children with anatomic urinary tract abnormalities need individualized treatment.**

***Enterococcus faecalis* is a gram-positive organism that can cause UTI in children approximately 5% of the time,**[37] **and *S. saprophyticus* can cause UTI in adolescents.** When *Enterococcus* is suspected because of prior infections with that organism, or gram-positive bacteria are identified on urine Gram stain, add ampicillin/amoxicillin or vancomycin to other therapy. The presence of *Enterococcus* increases the likelihood of an underlying urinary tract abnormality in a patient.[36] *S. saprophyticus* is typically sensitive to standard treatments.

TABLE 132-6 Antibiotic Treatment of Pediatric UTI[36]

Parenteral Antibiotics	
Antimicrobial	**Dosage in Normal Renal Function**
Ceftriaxone	50 milligrams/kg every 24 h
Cefotaxime	150 milligrams/kg/d divided every 8 h
Ceftazidime	150 milligrams/kg/d divided every 8 h
Cefazolin	50 milligrams/kg/d divided every 8 h
Gentamicin	7.5 milligrams/kg/d divided every 8–24 h
Tobramycin	5 milligrams/kg/d divided every 8 h
Ticarcillin	300 milligrams/kg/d divided every 6 h
Ampicillin	100 milligrams/kg/d divided every 6 h
Oral Antibiotics	
Antimicrobial	**Dosage in Normal Renal Function**
Amoxicillin	40–80 milligrams/kg/d in 2–3 doses
TMP in combination with SMX	6–12 milligrams TMP, 30–60 milligrams SMX per kg per d in 2 doses
Sulfisoxazole	120–150 milligrams/kg/d in 4 doses
Cefixime	8 milligrams/kg/d in 1 or 2 doses
Cefpodoxime	10 milligrams/kg/d in 2 doses
Cefprozil	30 milligrams/kg/d in 2 doses
Cephalexin	50–100 milligrams/kg/d in 3 doses

Abbreviations: SMX = sulfamethoxazole; TMP = trimethoprim.

DISPOSITION AND FOLLOW-UP

All neonates (<1 month old) and children with UTI who appear ill or septic should be hospitalized for parenteral antibiotics and fluid resuscitation and to guard against worsening of shock when endotoxins are released after antibiotics lyse gram-negative bacteria. Children over 1 month of age with uncomplicated UTI may be appropriate for outpatient care with oral antibiotics if they appear well, can tolerate oral medication, are not dehydrated, and are not immunocompromised. They may receive a single dose of IM or IV ceftriaxone (50 milligrams/kg) in the ED and start on outpatient oral antibiotics. Length of antimicrobial therapy should be 7 to 14 days with close pediatric follow-up to ensure appropriate antibiotic use and to consider the need for imaging. Adolescent girls (>13 years old) with UTI may be treated like adults with the option for a 3-day oral antibiotic regimen.

SPECIAL SITUATIONS

PEDIATRIC UTI WITH UROLITHIASIS

Although uncommon, urolithiasis occurs in children, and the incidence is increasing and may be associated with the increasing prevalence of childhood obesity.[38-40] **Children with symptoms suggestive of urolithiasis (colicky abdominal or flank pain, often radiating to the groin, and gross or microscopic hematuria) require imaging to evaluate for the possibility of stones. While noncontrast enhanced CT is the imaging modality of choice in adults, consideration of the potential long-term effects of radiation exposure must be weighed carefully, and renal US or MRI should be considered as alternatives.**[41] **In the setting of fever, pyuria, and an obstructing stone, initial treatment should be parenteral with inpatient management and consultation with pediatric urology. Additional urine studies may be obtained to identify predisposing factors and chemical composition of stones, which may guide future management.**

PRACTICE GUIDELINES

Practice parameters for the diagnosis, treatment, and evaluation of an initial UTI in febrile infants and young children are available from the American Academy of Pediatrics[19] and the Royal College of Obstetrics and Gynaecology.[23]

REFERENCES

The complete reference list is available online at www.TintinalliEM.com.

Pediatric Urologic and Gynecologic Disorders

Deborah R. Liu

SCROTUM

Scrotal pain is one of the most common urologic emergencies seen in boys. Although many causes of scrotal pain may not require an immediate organ-preserving procedure, some causes can lead to rapid and permanent loss of testicular function without timely intervention. Thus, the clinician must identify patients who need emergent diagnostic and/or therapeutic procedures and those who need observation and reassurance.

TESTICULAR TORSION

Consider testicular torsion in males with acute scrotal pain, because torsion is a urologic emergency. The estimated incidence of torsion in U.S. males younger than 18 years is 3.8 per 100,000 children.[1] Testicular torsion has a bimodal age presentation, with one peak in the immediate neonatal period and another peak during early puberty. Because the testicle of neonates with prenatal torsion is not salvageable, many urologists agree that neonates can be taken to the operating room on a semi-elective basis when the infant is a few months of age to decrease the anesthesia risk. However, in perinatal torsion, the contralateral side may also be torsed, even without abnormal physical examination findings or an abnormal US.[2]

Most boys with testicular torsion present between 12 and 18 years of age. Classically, the pain is abrupt in onset and severe and is usually associated with nausea or vomiting. The testicle is extremely painful, and often the patient will walk with a wide-based gait to minimize the contact of the scrotum to the thigh. There may be a preceding history of a sports activity or even minor trauma to the area, which may lead the clinician to a misdiagnosis of traumatic injury. In some cases, the patient may recall episodes of previous scrotal pain that rapidly resolved without intervention, which may represent intermittent torsion with spontaneous detorsion. Episodes of intermittent torsion may predispose a patient to acute complete testicular torsion.[3]

Classic physical examination findings of acute testicular torsion include a swollen, tender, high-riding testis, with an abnormal transverse lie. There are often scrotal skin changes. Ipsilateral loss of the cremaster reflex is almost always noted but is not 100% sensitive, especially in young boys.[4,5]

Doppler US is the diagnostic imaging study of choice,[6] with radionuclide imaging a distant second. If the time to obtain diagnostic imaging may lead to delay of surgical intervention, advocate for emergent surgical exploration by a urologist, rather than waiting for an imaging study to be completed. Time is especially critical if the duration of symptoms is <6 hours, as the salvage rate is excellent in such cases. Beyond 6 hours, the salvage rate becomes progressively worse, and after 48 hours of symptoms, the salvage rate is near zero. Patients presenting with equivocal signs of torsion or who have had pain for >6 hours may benefit from a Doppler US, which can visualize blood flow to the testis. In acute torsion, Doppler demonstrates an enlarged testis with decreased or absent flow compared with the unaffected side. In patients with suspected intermittent torsion who have a normal Doppler US and resolution of pain, counsel the patient and family to seek medical attention immediately should the pain recur, and recommend urologic follow-up as an outpatient.

Manual detorsion may be indicated for patients with torsion when there is no urologist immediately available and when the duration of symptoms is too long for surgical salvage. Administer parenteral opioid analgesia, local anesthesia (infiltrating the spermatic cord near the external ring with lidocaine), or procedural sedation. Because the testis tends to torse in the medial direction, manual detorsion is accomplished by holding the testis between the thumb and index finger and rotating the testis in an outward direction toward the thigh (as if opening a book). However, the spermatic cord may be twisted >180 degrees, making it difficult to recognize how many times the testis should be outwardly rotated. Also, a very swollen hemiscrotum may make isolating the testis between two fingers challenging. The unsedated, older, verbal patient may be able to describe relatively immediate relief upon successful detorsion. Bedside or formal Doppler US may be useful in determining improvement of flow. The success rate of manual detorsion is quite variable and is not definitive therapy. Even after manual detorsion, patients need emergent surgical exploration to confirm complete detorsion and to perform bilateral orchidopexy.

TORSION OF TESTICULAR APPENDAGE

The appendix testis and appendix epididymis are testicular embryologic remnants that can twist, resulting in venous congestion and subsequent infarction of the appendage. Torsion of a testicular appendage is most common in males between 7 and 12 years of age, although it can occur at any age. Typically, the patient's symptoms are more insidious than true testicular torsion, with less severe pain and lack of systemic symptoms. Early in the course before scrotal edema and erythema develop, it may be possible to localize the point of tenderness to the upper pole of the testis or epididymis. In addition, one may observe the infarcted appendage through the scrotal skin (**"blue dot sign"**). If Doppler US is obtained, there should be normal testicular flow with a small hyperechoic region adjacent to the testis. Management consists of scrotal support, limitation of activity, and oral analgesics (e.g., nonsteroidal anti-inflammatory drugs). If torsion of the testicular appendage is diagnosed early in its course, the pain may worsen before ultimate improvement due to ongoing inflammation, and this is an important point of counseling to prevent return to the ED.

EPIDIDYMITIS

Epididymitis, or inflammation of the epididymis, is a common cause of scrotal pain in pre- and postpubertal boys that does not require surgical intervention. In a 2014 study of 252 patients with epididymitis presenting to an outpatient pediatric urology referral practice, the mean age at first presentation was 10.92 years, with the majority of cases occurring between 10 and 14 years.[7] In sexually active males, acute epididymitis may result from ascending urethral infection due to *Chlamydia trachomatis* or *Neisseria gonorrhoeae*. Epididymitis may also result from enterovirus or adenovirus infection.[8] Symptoms are insidious in onset, with dysuria, frequency, or fever. Prehn's sign (relief of pain by elevating the scrotum) is not consistently reproducible in boys. Typically, the affected testis is mildly enlarged and tender with hemiscrotal erythema and swelling (**Figure 133-1**). Urinalysis may demonstrate pyuria and bacteriuria. Obtain urine culture and sensitivity, and in suspected sexual transmission, obtain urethral cultures for *C. trachomatis* and *N. gonorrhoeae* and treat with empiric antibiotics pending culture results.

Doppler US, if the diagnosis is in doubt, shows an enlarged epididymis with increased blood flow, and normal blood flow to the testis. It is often difficult to differentiate torsion of a testicular appendage from epididymitis by US, but neither disorder requires surgical intervention. Treatment of epididymitis is somewhat controversial, with some advocating analgesics and limited activity only and others supporting treatment with antibiotics, even in the non–sexually active male.

HYDROCELE

Hydrocele (**Figure 133-2**), the accumulation of fluid around the testis, is the most common cause of painless scrotal swelling in children. Parents often note intermittent swelling of one or both sides of the scrotum. This painless swelling may resolve when supine or sleeping and become more prominent when awake or crying. Hydrocele is termed *noncommunicating* if there is residual but static swelling after the processus vaginalis has

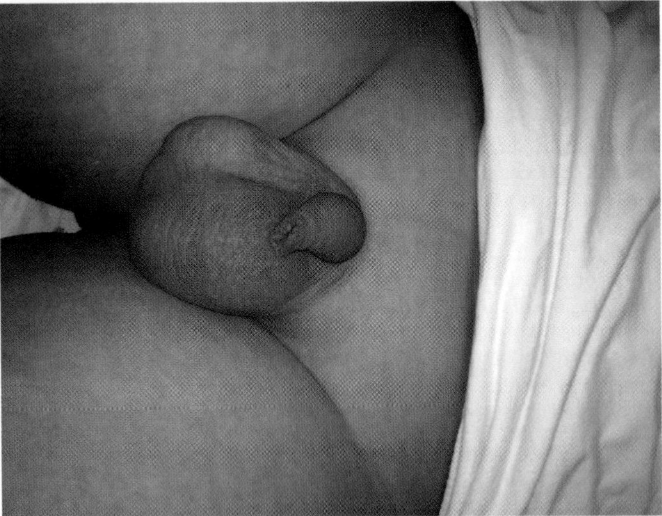

FIGURE 133-1. Epididymo-orchitis. A 5-year-old boy with 1 day of left testicular pain and swelling, consistent with epididymo-orchitis.

closed, or *communicating* if swelling increases and decreases through a patent processus vaginalis. The diagnosis is confirmed by transillumination, whereby an otoscope or other light source is placed on the affected hemiscrotum and the hydrocele fluid is illuminated like a lantern; by contrast, a thickened scrotal wall or pure testicular enlargement will not transilluminate.

Most simple hydroceles resorb by 18 to 24 months of age. A communicating hydrocele is often associated with inguinal hernia, and as long as the hernia is reducible, it does not require emergent surgical repair. Management of most hydroceles includes outpatient scrotal US with referral to urology.

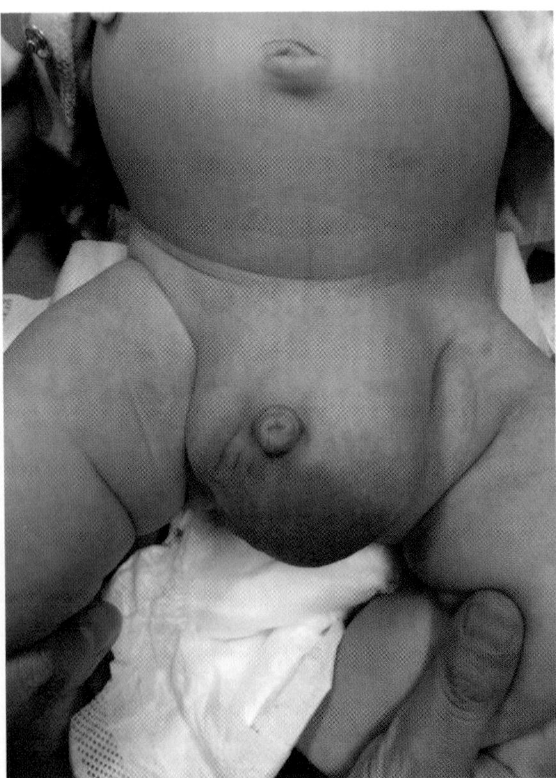

FIGURE 133-2. Hydrocele. A 3-month-old boy with bilateral hydroceles (left greater than right).

VARICOCELE

Varicocele is another cause of painless scrotal swelling and typically presents at the onset of puberty. It is due to abnormal dilation of spermatic cord veins, also known as the *pampiniform plexus*, due to faulty valvular venous return. Most varicoceles occur on the left, possibly due in part to the acute angle of confluence with the left renal vein and resulting higher venous pressure. Classically the mass of enlarged veins can be palpated superior and posterior to the testis ("bag of worms") and is more prominent when standing or with the Valsalva maneuver; even large varicoceles may be missed in the supine position. Varicoceles are managed on an outpatient basis by urology. The implications of possible subfertility should be discussed in the urologist's office.

INTRASCROTAL TUMORS

Intrascrotal tumors are uncommon in young children; however, testicular tumors are the most common solid tumor among adolescent males.[9] The testicular or paratesticular tumor usually presents as a painless, firm, unilateral scrotal mass. Evaluation includes serum α-fetoprotein and tumor β-human chorionic gonadotropin levels, scrotal US, and urgent urologic consultation.

DISORDERS OF THE PENIS

A swollen, red, or painful penis can usually be categorized as a disorder of the foreskin or of the shaft of the penis. The most common abnormalities of the foreskin are phimosis, paraphimosis, and balanoposthitis. Penile shaft disorders occur less commonly and include priapism, tourniquet syndrome, and zipper injury.

PHIMOSIS

Phimosis is caused by stenosis of the distal aspect of the foreskin, preventing retraction of the foreskin over the glans. There may be a history of ballooning of the foreskin during urination, with dribbling of entrapped urine after voiding is complete (**Figure 133-3**). Most uncircumcised infants have normal, physiologic phimosis. Nearly all cases of physiologic phimosis spontaneously resolve by 5 years of age and rarely require treatment other than daily cleaning while bathing. If a patient has persistent phimosis beyond school age and the parent desires treatment, topical steroid cream can be effective.[10,11] Acquired cases of phimosis may be secondary to recurrent balanoposthitis, poor hygiene, or forcible retraction of the foreskin. Acquired cases are often refractory to medical management and may ultimately require circumcision. One of the few true emergencies related to phimosis occurs when the foreskin

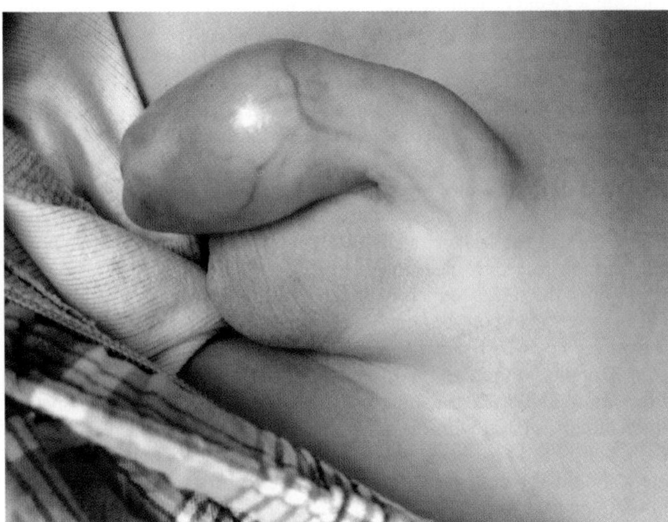

FIGURE 133-3. Phimosis in a toddler leading to ballooning of foreskin caused by entrapped urine.

is nearly completely sealed off, causing acute urinary retention. Such cases may require dilation of the foreskin under procedural sedation or dorsal penile block to place a Foley catheter.

PARAPHIMOSIS

Paraphimosis is a true urologic emergency. This occurs when a tight ring of phimotic foreskin is retracted proximal to the glans and becomes trapped in that position. Subsequent impairment of venous and lymphatic drainage causes progressive swelling of the glans and foreskin. If the paraphimosis is not promptly reduced, arterial blood supply becomes compromised, and the glans may necrose.

Symptoms of paraphimosis are pain, erythema, and swelling of the shaft and glans, distal to the constricting ring of foreskin (**Figure 133-4**). The area of the shaft proximal to the constriction appears normal. Because delay in reduction will lead to worsening edema resulting in a more difficult manual reduction, paraphimosis should be reduced as soon as possible. Mild paraphimosis may be manually reduced without the need for sedation or analgesia. More difficult cases will require either a dorsal penile nerve block or procedural sedation, depending on the age and degree of cooperativeness of the patient.

The dorsal penile nerve provides most of the somatosensory innervation to the shaft and glans penis. The dorsal penile block (**Figure 133-5**) is useful for minor painful procedures of the penis, such as paraphimosis reduction, dorsal slit procedure, or zipper entrapment release. Using a 25- or 27-gauge needle, inject lidocaine hydrochloride *without* epinephrine into the base of penis, at the junction between the penis and the suprapubic skin, off the midline to avoid the superficial dorsal vein. Inject the lidocaine just deep to the Buck fascia, which is located 3 to 5 mm beneath the skin.

A slight "pop" is usually felt as the needle passes through the fascial layer. Aspirate before injecting the lidocaine, because the dorsal arteries and veins are within close proximity to the nerve. Depending on the size of the child, between 1 and 5 mL of lidocaine should be used. Half of the volume is injected at the 10 o'clock position, with the other half injected at the 2 o'clock position. Another technique involves injecting only once at the midline through the Buck fascia, with injection of the full volume

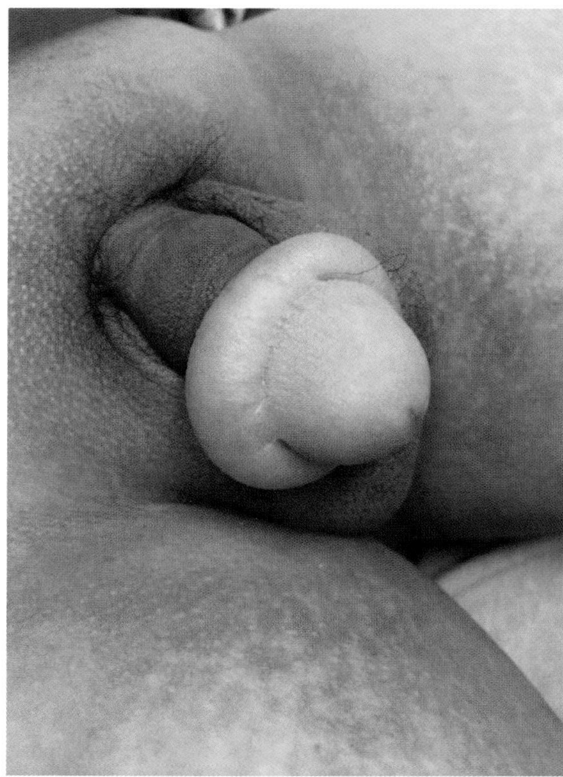

FIGURE 133-4. A 12-year-old boy with paraphimosis for more than 24 hours.

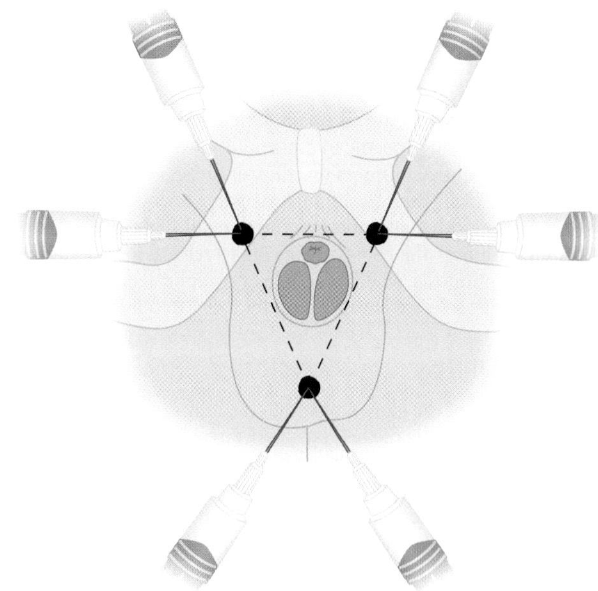

FIGURE 133-5. Dorsal penile block. Local anesthesia infiltration around the base of the penis. *Black dots* represent the locations of the skin wheals. [Reproduced with permission from Reichman EF, Simon RR: *Emergency Medicine Procedures,* Copyright © 2004, The McGraw-Hill Companies, Inc., all rights reserved. Section 10. Genitourinary Procedures, Chapter 125, Anesthesia of the Penis, Testicle, and Epididymis, Figure 125-3.]

directed toward each direction after negative aspiration of blood. Like most nerve blocks, optimal analgesia is achieved after 5 minutes.

Once analgesia is achieved either by dorsal nerve block or procedural sedation, manual reduction of the paraphimosis may be attempted. To decrease penile edema, it is often helpful to use a bag of ice (for 3-minute increments to avoid cold injury) or manual compression before attempting reduction. Squeezing the glans and swollen foreskin using one's palm or a compression dressing for 5 minutes usually decreases the edema to allow successful manual reduction. The most common technique for manual reduction involves placing both thumbs over the glans, with both index fingers and long fingers surrounding the trapped foreskin. One pushes the glans back into the foreskin while pulling the foreskin back into normal position. This may require a few minutes of constant pressure before the glans slips through the paraphimotic ring (**Figure 133-6**).

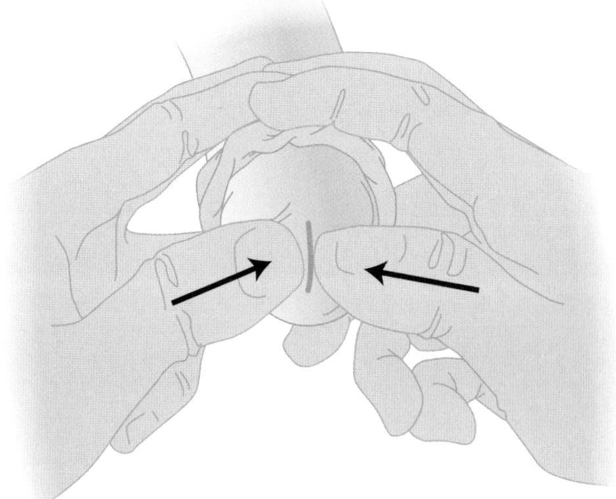

FIGURE 133-6. Manual reduction of paraphimosis. After appropriate analgesia is administered, place both thumbs over the glans, with both index and long fingers surrounding the trapped foreskin. The foreskin can then be reduced by placing pressure on the glans. [Reproduced with permission from Reichman EF, Simon RR: *Emergency Medicine Procedures,* Copyright © 2004, The McGraw-Hill Companies, Inc., Figure 129-4.]

Manual reduction may fail if there is extreme swelling of the foreskin and glans from prolonged paraphimosis. Emergent urologic consultation is necessary for such cases. Although more invasive procedures are ideally done by a surgeon, the emergency physician may need to perform such procedures if necrosis is imminent. One commonly used technique involves using a 21-gauge needle to make multiple punctures in the foreskin followed by gentle compression, thus draining some of the edema. Manual reduction can then be attempted again. A dorsal slit procedure may be necessary if other attempts at reduction fail. This involves making a vertical incision over the constricting ring to release the paraphimosis. All cases of paraphimosis, whether simple or complicated, require follow-up with a urologist to assess healing and the need for circumcision.

BALANOPOSTHITIS

Balanitis (cellulitis of the glans), posthitis (cellulitis of the foreskin), and balanoposthitis (cellulitis of the glans and foreskin) are common diagnoses in young males. Poor hygiene and phimosis predispose children to such infections (**Figure 133-7**). On examination, the glans, the foreskin, or both the glans and foreskin are swollen, tender, and edematous. In most cases, empiric treatment with oral antibiotics with a first-generation cephalosporin and warm soaks are sufficient. In cases in which there is an associated erythematous papular rash with satellite lesions, antifungal cream may also be indicated.

PRIAPISM

Priapism is a prolonged, unwanted erection not associated with sexual stimulation. Low-flow (venous) and high-flow (arterial) priapism are managed differently.

High-flow (nonischemic) priapism is generally due to an arteriovenous fistula from trauma (i.e., lacerated cavernous artery shunting blood into the cavernous bodies). This can lead to a persistent partial or full erection for days to weeks, but is generally not painful. Because of the continuous inflow of arterial blood, ischemia or impotence does not occur. Therefore, high-flow priapism is not a true urologic emergency. Most cases are treated conservatively, and only a few cases require angioembolization of the lacerated artery.

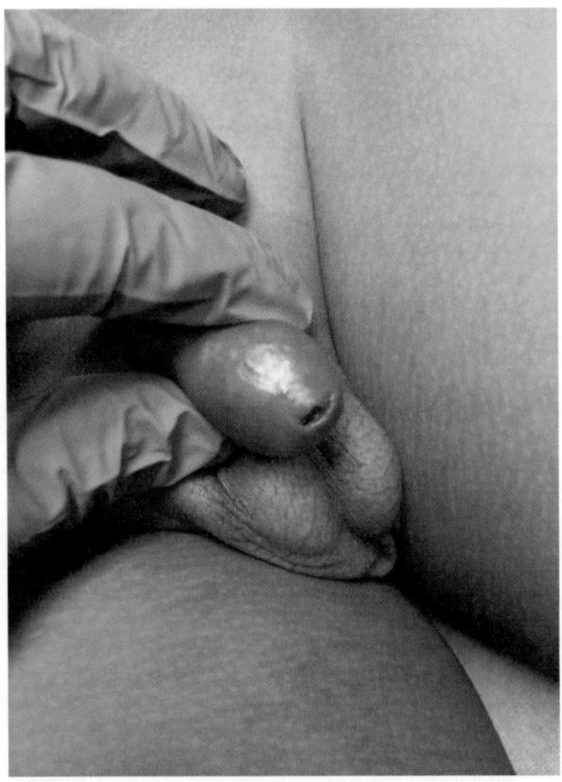

FIGURE 133-7. A 4-year-old boy with posthitis and phimosis.

Low-flow (ischemic) priapism is caused by sludging of red blood cells, leading to impaired venous drainage, venous congestion, and ischemia. In children, the most common cause of low-flow priapism is sickle cell disease.[12] Other less common causes in children include illicit drugs (cocaine and cannabis), antidepressants, antipsychotics, and leukemia (presenting with extreme hyperleukocytosis).[13] Low-flow priapism causes a very rigid and extremely painful erection.

The type of priapism can usually be identified by history and physical examination. Doppler US can distinguish the type of priapism, with low-flow priapism showing decreased or no blood flow in the cavernosal arteries. The most reliable method, however, involves testing aspirated blood from the corpus cavernosum for blood gas analysis. Aspiration of the corpus cavernosum should be done only by an experienced urologist. Blood from low-flow priapism will be dark in color, with a partial pressures of oxygen (Po_2) <30 mm Hg, a partial pressure of carbon dioxide (Pco_2) >60 mm Hg, and a pH <7.25. Cavernous blood gas from high-flow priapism is bright red in color with numeric values similar to normal arterial blood.

Without a history of pelvic, genital, or perineal trauma, nearly all priapism is low flow and usually secondary to sickle cell crisis. Priapism can occur in all forms of sickle cell disease, including sickle hemoglobin C and the sickle thalassemias. Among patients with sickle cell disease, a single episode of priapism was reported by 31% to 64% of patients, with approximately 50% reporting recurrent episodes.[12] Such recurrent episodes are termed *"stuttering" priapism* and are unpredictable and of variable duration.

Obtain a history including the duration of symptoms and any precipitating events (i.e., medications or illicit drugs). When low-flow priapism lasts for >4 hours, the risk for permanent damage leading to impotence is significant and requires emergency urology consultation. While waiting for the urologist, administer IV fluids, opioid analgesics, and supplemental oxygen, and maintain the patient as NPO (nothing by mouth) for possible procedural sedation or operative management. If sickle cell disease is the underlying cause, treat with IV venous hydration at 1.5 times maintenance rates and consider red blood cell exchange transfusion (see chapter 142, "Sickle Cell Disease in Children"). Prolonged priapism requires concurrent aggressive urologic management with corporeal aspiration and irrigation, intracavernous injection of a sympathomimetic drug (such as phenylephrine or epinephrine), or, potentially, surgical shunting as a last resort.[14] Opioids may actually prevent detumescence, whereas **ketamine is an established detumescent**.[15] Ketamine should be preferentially considered for patients requiring procedural sedation prior to corporeal aspiration or irrigation.

TOURNIQUET SYNDROME OF THE PENIS

First reported in the literature in 1832, Reinisch and colleagues coined the term *hair-thread tourniquet syndrome* in 1988, when they described six cases of young infants with digit strangulation.[16] In a 2004 review, among the 90 cases of tourniquet syndrome found in the literature, toes were affected in 47%, penis in 25%, fingers in 20%, clitoris in 6%, and labia in 2%.[17]

Tourniquet syndrome of the penis presents with penile redness, swelling, and pain. Occasionally, the presenting sign is irritability of unknown cause, so a thorough history and physical are crucial to identify a tourniquet syndrome. On physical examination, the area of the penis distal to the strangulation is erythematous, edematous, and tender. Edema often obscures the hair or thread itself. Treatment includes cutting the hair or thread if visualized, or using a depilatory agent, such as Nair®. **Depilatory creams will not work on synthetic fibers**, however, and if unable to remove the constriction, urologic consultation is necessary. Damage from the tourniquet can range from mild penile edema, to glandular disfigurement, urethral transaction, and even penile amputation.[18] Although most cases are unintentional, they can also result from abuse.

ZIPPER INJURY

Penile zipper entrapment is most often seen in school-age boys, most commonly when not wearing underpants. The patient's shaft, foreskin, or glans becomes entrapped between the locked teeth of the zipper or

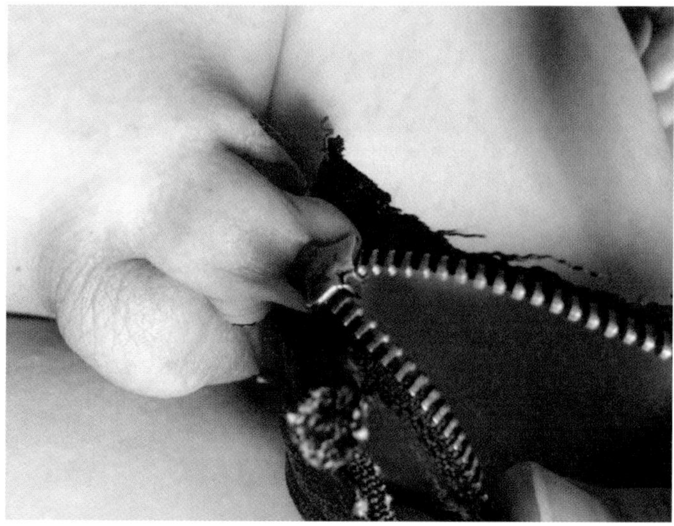

A

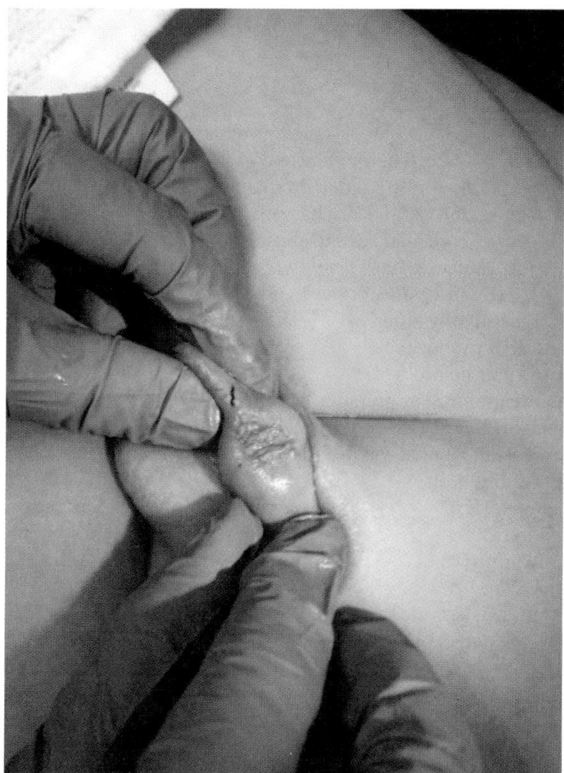

B

FIGURE 133-8. A 4-year-old boy with (**A**) penile zipper entrapment and (**B**) post-zipper removal after cutting the median bar.

within the fastener itself (**Figure 133-8**). If the skin is trapped between the teeth of the zipper, cut the cloth between the locked teeth, and separate the teeth of the zipper. However, if the skin is caught within the fastener of the zipper, releasing the skin is more difficult.

There are several methods described in the literature for zipper release. The most commonly used method is to use sturdy wire cutters or bone cutters to cut the median bar of the zipper (**Figure 133-9**). This requires a special tool, which may not be available, and in some cases the angle of the zipper and type of zipper preclude easy access to the median bar. Other methods include using a mini hacksaw to cut the median bar,[19] dousing the area with liberal amounts of mineral oil and then freeing the entrapped skin with gentle traction,[20] and twisting a small flathead screwdriver between the two faceplates of the zipper to widen the gap and allow release of the tissue.[21]

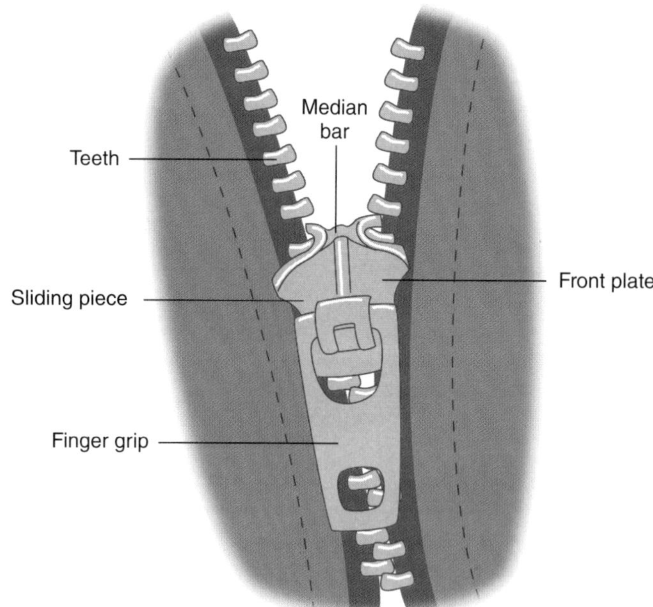

FIGURE 133-9. Parts of zipper are identified for penile zipper release. The most common method is to cut the median bar, thus releasing the entrapped skin. [Reproduced with permission from Reichman EF, Simon RR: *Emergency Medicine Procedures,* Copyright © 2004, McGraw-Hill, New York, Figure 131-1.]

The age and degree of cooperativeness of the patient will determine type of analgesia and/or sedation needed. The patient may need oral analgesics, IV analgesics, or a dorsal penile block with or without procedural sedation. If all attempts fail at bedside zipper release, consult the urologist for removal under general anesthesia in the operating room.

FEMALE GYNECOLOGIC PROBLEMS

One of the most challenging physical examinations to perform is the gynecologic examination of the young female. Provide extra care and attention to create a nonthreatening environment to obtain a thorough, less anxiety-provoking examination. Tell the child that the parent approves the examination and that he or she will remain in the room. Tell the child why the examination is necessary and that everything will be explained to her beforehand. It is helpful to have the parent stand near the head of the bed while holding the child's hand. Never forcibly restrain a child for a gynecologic examination. If the examination is difficult, procedural sedation or an examination under general anesthesia is an alternative approach. Regardless of practitioner gender, obtain third-party assistance (such as a nurse or social worker).

The first position in which to examine the young female external genitalia is the frog-legged position (**Figure 133-10**), with the child lying supine (or near-supine on a parent's lap). Spread the child's knees apart. Sometimes, this position can be aided with the soles of the feet brought together. The vestibule and hymen can be seen by gently pressing the labia majora laterally and posteriorly. Examine the child in the knee-chest position (**Figure 133-11**) for visualization of the perianal area and the outer vaginal vault. Ask the child to position herself on the examination table on her hands and knees, like a baby crawling. With her parent standing at the head of the bed, ask the child to put her head down onto her hands, with her elbows resting on the examination table. Apply gentle lateral and upward traction over the buttocks and labia majora to inspect the vaginal vault.

LABIAL ADHESIONS

Labial adhesions (**Figure 133-12**) are a fusion of the labia minora, most commonly seen in infant and preschool-aged girls. The exact cause is unknown, although they are thought to be related to a girl's low level of

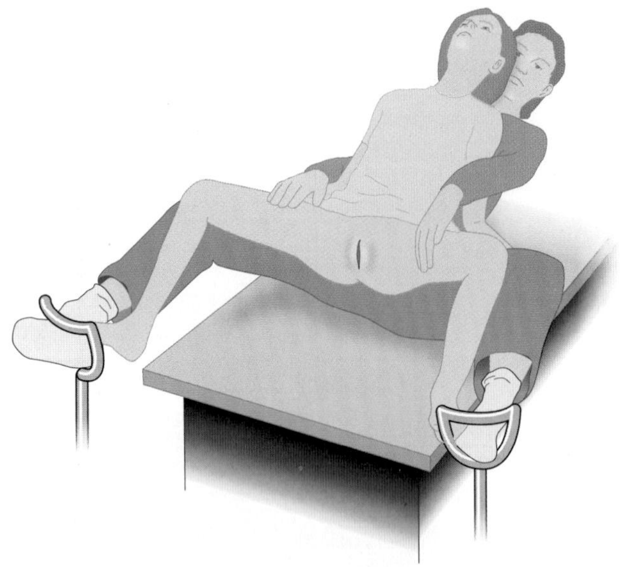

FIGURE 133-10. Girl lying in frog-legged position with knees spread apart and feet together. This position is best for examining the vestibule and hymen.

estrogen, which predisposes the epithelium to irritation. Irritation may be due to poor hygiene, harsh soaps, bubble baths, or minor trauma. Re-epithelialization occurs as a response to irritation, forming the labial adhesions.

The adhesions appear as a flat, connected surface, inferior to the clitoris, with a thin, vertical raphe. Adhesions may extend from the clitoris over the entire introitus, or they can be partial with some perforations.

Labial adhesions are often asymptomatic and may be discovered on routine examination or when obtaining a catheterized urine specimen, although occasionally the child may complain of dysuria. Most labial adhesions resolve spontaneously during puberty, or topical estrogen cream can be applied over the area twice a day for 2 to 4 weeks. Topical estrogen may cause transient hyperpigmentation of the area, and prolonged use may induce reversible secondary sexual characteristics. Once lysis of the adhesions occurs, the parent should apply petroleum jelly to the area for another 2 to 3 weeks to maintain labial separation. Do not manually separate adhesions, as they will likely recur.

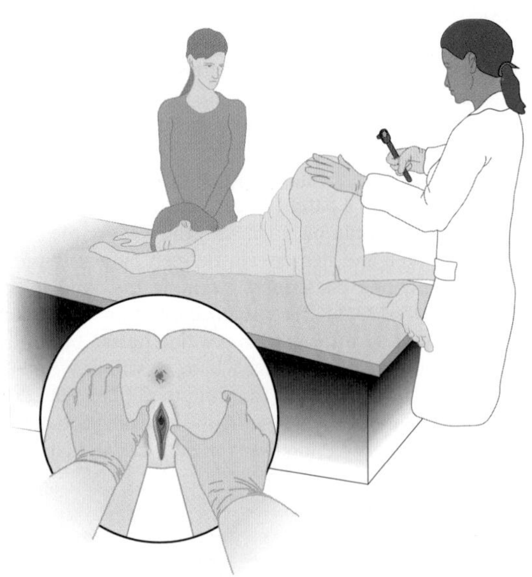

FIGURE 133-11. Girl in knee-chest position with elbows resting on examination table. This position is best for examining the perianal area and the vaginal vault.

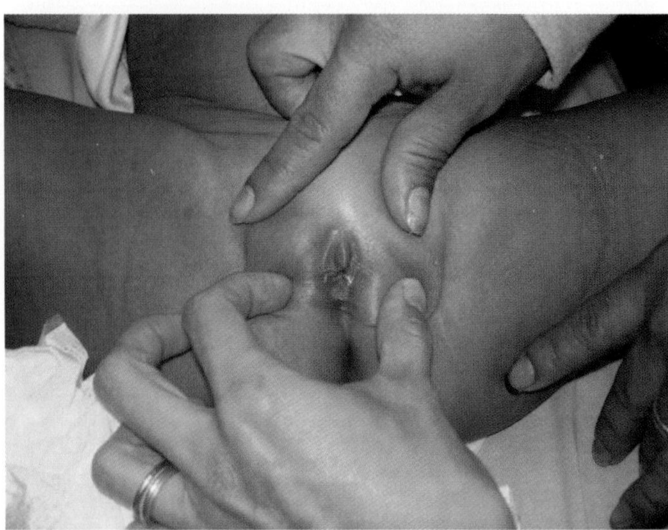

FIGURE 133-12. Eight-month-old girl who was noted to have labial adhesions when a catheterized urine specimen was ordered in the ED for a fever workup.

VAGINAL DISCHARGE

During the first 2 to 3 weeks of life, many infant girls have normal physiologic vaginal discharge. The leukorrhea is thin, slippery, and clear or white in color. Among older infants and young girls, there are two common causes of vaginal discharge: vaginal foreign body and vulvovaginitis. Also, consider sexual abuse with infection from *N. gonorrhoeae*, *C. trachomatis*, or *Trichomonas* as a possibility.

Vaginal foreign bodies present with foul-smelling vaginal discharge, which can be slightly bloody. The patient may complain of voiding symptoms secondary to local irritation. Symptoms are often present for a long period of time before presentation to a physician. The most common vaginal foreign body in prepubertal females is toilet paper. Examination of the patient in knee-chest position (Figure 133-11) is the best method to visualize the vaginal vault and possible foreign body. If the foreign body is readily seen, it can be removed using forceps or warm water vaginal lavage. If bedside removal is not possible, the patient may require examination and removal under procedural or general anesthesia.

Vulvovaginitis is a very common cause of vaginal discharge, pain, and pruritus. Most cases are not associated with any specific organism, but irritation is secondary to poor hygiene, wiping back to front after urination or defecation, bubble baths, tight clothing or underwear, or perfumed bathing products. Treatment for such cases includes proper hygiene habits and eliminating offending agents. Among bacterial causes of vaginitis in the prepubertal female, the most common are group A β-hemolytic *Streptococcus*, *Staphylococcus aureus*, *Escherichia coli*, and *Shigella*. *Candida* vaginitis is not common among prepubertal females because of the alkaline pH of the vagina.

Vaginal bleeding is another common complaint in the pediatric ED. In the first 2 to 3 weeks of life, as maternal hormonal levels wane, the newborn female may experience sloughing of her endometrium with subsequent vaginal bleeding. This form of nonpathologic bleeding is always self-limited and requires no treatment other than reassurance to the parents.

In children, **urethral prolapse** occurs predominantly in prepubertal black females between the ages of 2 and 10 years old. The complaint is usually painless blood spotting on the underwear, although some patients may also experience mild irritation with voiding. The mucosa of the distal urethra prolapses outward beyond the meatus, causing venous congestion of the prolapsed tissue. Prolapse appears as a red-purple, doughnut-shaped mass with a central dimple. If the diagnosis is in doubt, pass a urinary catheter through the central opening for confirmation. The treatment of choice is sitz baths and topical estrogen cream for 2 weeks. Constipation may exacerbate the prolapse if the child strains with defecation, so providing a stool softener is often helpful. If conservative medical management fails, or if the prolapsed tissue becomes necrotic, the tissue may have to be surgically reduced and/or removed.

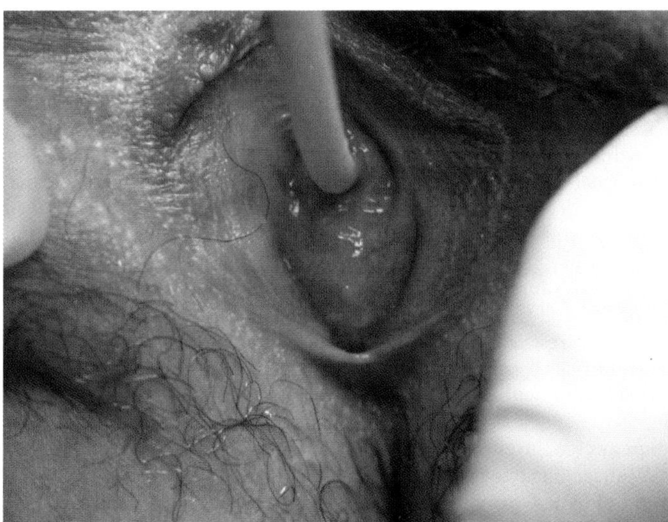

FIGURE 133-13. Teenage female with imperforate hymen (with Foley catheter in place).

Fortunately, most **straddle injuries** cause only minor superficial abrasions, lacerations, or hematomas of the perineum. Such cases can be treated with supportive care and sitz baths. Pain with voiding can be relieved by allowing the child to urinate in a bathtub of warm water. More significant injuries, such as an expanding hematoma, a laceration beyond the superficial layers, a wound that continues to actively bleed, any rectal bleeding, or inability to urinate, require immediate gynecologic evaluation. In addition, sexual abuse or assault should always be considered as a possible cause of genital injury and should be reported to the appropriate state agency as mandated by law.

The vast majority of vaginal bleeding in adolescents is caused by **dysfunctional uterine bleeding**. Irregular menses with or without prolonged bleeding is especially common in females during the first year after menarche, due to the high number of anovulatory cycles. Dysfunctional uterine bleeding is best managed initially with a trial of a combined estrogen-progestin pill. The estrogen stops the bleeding, and the progestin stabilizes the endometrium. There are multiple forms of oral contraceptive pills that would be appropriate as first-line therapy. For further discussion, see chapter 96, "Abnormal Uterine Bleeding."

IMPERFORATE HYMEN

Cases of imperforate hymen (**Figure 133-13**) typically present to the ED as a teenage female with chronic, vague abdominal pain, who has secondary sexual characteristics, yet is still "premenarchal." Physical examination reveals a bluish bulging membrane covering the introitus, representing accumulated menstrual blood and hematocolpos. If the hematocolpos is large, the patient may have symptoms of urinary urgency, frequency, or dysuria. Treatment in adolescents is urgent surgical repair, but in asymptomatic infants and young girls, surgery is performed on an elective basis.

REFERENCES

The complete reference list is available online at www.TintinalliEM.com.

CHAPTER 134 Renal Emergencies in Children

Andrew Dixon
Brandy Stauffer

ACUTE KIDNEY INJURY

Acute kidney injury (AKI; previously called acute renal failure) is the sudden loss of renal function necessary to maintain normal fluid and electrolyte balance and clear metabolic waste.[1,2] AKI is typically manifested by an increase in serum creatinine, although the increase will not necessarily cause the creatinine to be outside the normal range. Use of serum creatinine alone to define AKI, however, is problematic because creatinine is an inaccurate estimate of glomerular filtration rate (GFR) and can be removed by dialysis, and variable cut-off values for creatinine have been used in AKI. Therefore, the international classification system, Kidney Disease: Improving Global Outcomes (KDIGO) (**Table 134-1**), is preferred. The system uses creatinine and urine output criteria and can be applied to both children and adults, minimizing practice variation.[3]

PATHOPHYSIOLOGY

AKI is the result of nephrotoxic and/or hypoxic injury to the glomeruli and renal tubules.[1] Reduced blood flow causes hypoxic injury and damages the proximal tubular cells. Common nephrotoxins include aminoglycosides, contrast agents, calcineurin inhibitors, amphotericin B, and nonsteroidal anti-inflammatory drugs.[4] Inflammatory mediators intensify renal tubular damage.[2]

AKI is frequently classified based on three major anatomic locations of injury: prerenal, renal, and postrenal disease. Prerenal disease is typically caused by inadequate renal perfusion and is the most common class of AKI. Prerenal AKI is typically due to hypovolemia (e.g., bleeding or GI losses such as vomiting and diarrhea), decreased renal artery blood flow, or reduction in effective circulation (e.g., heart failure, cardiogenic shock, third spacing in septic shock). Renal disease or intrinsic renal disease occurs when there is structural damage to the renal parenchyma. Common causes of renal disease include glomerular diseases (e.g., pyelonephritis, nephrotic syndrome, glomerulonephritis, Henoch-Schönlein purpura), vascular diseases (e.g., hemolytic-uremic syndrome, thrombosis, vasculitides), interstitial diseases (e.g., interstitial nephritis, infections), and tubular injuries (e.g., ischemia, nephrotoxins, hypotension). Lastly, postrenal disease is typically due to an obstruction caused by congenital or acquired anomalies to the lower urinary tract. Examples include nephrolithiasis, renal vein thrombosis, pelvic masses (e.g., lymphoma, rhabdomyosarcoma), and urethral obstruction (posterior ureteral valves).

TABLE 134-1 KDIGO Classification of Renal Injury

Stage*	Lab Criteria	Urine Output Criteria	Other Criteria
I	Serum creatinine 1.5–1.9 times baseline *or* increase of ≥ 0.3 mg/dL	Urine output <0.5 mL/kg/h for 6 h	
II	Serum creatinine 2–2.9 times baseline	Urine output <0.5 mL/kg/h for 12 h	
III	Serum creatinine 3 times baseline *or* increase in serum creatinine to ≥4 mg/dL	Urine output <0.3 mL/kg/h for 24 h *or* anuria for ≥12 h	Initiation or renal replacement therapy

Abbreviation: KDIGO = Kidney Disease: Improving Global Outcomes.

*Stage is determined by meeting any criterion (lab or urine output or other) in that row.

CLINICAL FEATURES

HISTORY

Direct the initial history to determine risk factors or causes for AKI. Many symptoms and signs relate to the underlying disorder, although patients can also be asymptomatic. Vomiting and diarrhea may suggest intravascular depletion and a prerenal cause of AKI. Other important historical features include history of streptococcal infection (suggests poststreptococcal glomerulonephritis), bloody diarrhea (hemolytic-uremic syndrome), and joint symptoms, rash, or purpura (Henoch-Schönlein purpura). Signs of obstruction include complete anuria or poor urinary stream. Symptoms of renal failure itself include nausea, anorexia (secondary to uremia), changes in urine output or color, edema (may be dependent, periorbital, scrotal/labial, or generalized), and headache from hypertension. Perform a full review of systems and obtain the medical history and pertinent family history.[1,2] Identify all medications used, including prescription and nonprescription drugs, herbals, and sport supplements.

PHYSICAL EXAMINATION

The physical examination should be thorough, with special emphasis on vital signs (especially blood pressure), weight, hydration status, and joint and skin findings.[1] Note the presence or absence of edema. Auscultate the lungs for rales, which suggest fluid overload, and the heart for uremic rubs. Palpate the abdomen for masses and organomegaly, which may indicate fluid overload in young children.

DIAGNOSIS

LABORATORY EVALUATION

Acute renal failure laboratory findings include alterations of renal function, such as elevated creatinine and BUN or an abnormal urinalysis.

Analysis of the urine can distinguish between prerenal, renal, and postrenal causes of acute renal failure. In children who are not toilet trained, it may be necessary to obtain a urine specimen by catheterization. In prerenal AKI, urinalysis may be normal. Hematuria, presence of casts, and proteinuria characterize the "active sediment" of glomerulonephritis. Proteinuria alone suggests nephrotic syndrome. WBCs and bacteria suggest infection. A urine dipstick test positive for blood in the absence of observed red blood cells (RBCs) suggests myoglobinuria or hemoglobinuria. Hyaline casts may be seen in acute tubular necrosis. Urine specific gravity is often high (>1.025) in prerenal acute renal failure and may be normal to low in acute tubular necrosis.

Obtain serum electrolyte levels when acute renal failure is suspected because hyperkalemia and other electrolyte abnormalities may require emergent treatment. Hyperkalemia may result from a combination of factors including reduced GFR, decreased tubular secretion of potassium, tissue breakdown with release of intracellular potassium, and metabolic acidosis resulting in transcellular movement of potassium. Other electrolyte abnormalities may include hyponatremia secondary to fluid retention or hypernatremia from dehydration in prerenal failure. Hyperphosphatemia from impaired renal excretion may lead to secondary hypocalcemia. A blood gas may show an anion gap metabolic acidosis secondary to impaired renal excretion of acid and reabsorption and regeneration of bicarbonate. A CBC is useful to identify anemia, hemolysis, and thrombocytopenia (characteristic of hemolytic-uremic syndrome), signs of systemic infection, or eosinophilia (interstitial nephritis). Additional studies are dictated by the clinical picture.

An ECG will identify cardiac arrhythmias and hyperkalemia. Renal biopsy is the definitive study for most cases of intrinsic renal disease and may be done on an outpatient or inpatient basis.[1,2]

IMAGING

A chest radiograph can identify an increase in heart size or pulmonary edema. US identifies anatomic abnormalities, hydronephrosis, and/or hydroureter. Voiding cystourethrogram is obtained in boys with suspected posterior urethral valves. Additional imaging depends on the differential diagnosis.

TREATMENT

Treatment of acute renal failure is different for prerenal, renal, and postrenal failure. In all cases, careful monitoring of vital signs, including baseline weight and urine output, is necessary. In prerenal failure, treat dehydration and hypovolemia with a 10- to 20-mL/kg crystalloid bolus of normal saline. If hemorrhagic shock is the cause for hypovolemia, initiate a crystalloid bolus until blood products are available. Packed RBCs are transfused at a volume of 10 mL/kg. Fresh frozen plasma and platelets may be necessary in massive hemorrhage.

In renal failure from intrinsic renal disease, the specific cause must be identified and treated. Depending on the clinical state, manage oliguria with fluid restriction, limiting replacements to insensible losses only. Discontinue all nephrotoxic medications or adjust dose for GFR. Treat hypertension with antihypertensive agents (avoid angiotensin-converting enzyme [ACE] inhibitors and angiotensin receptor blockers) or diuretics (see "Hypertension" below).

Manage oliguria of postrenal failure with fluid restriction and treatment of hypertension. A Foley catheter may be necessary to relieve the obstruction. In all types of AKI, electrolyte management is important. The management of life-threatening hyperkalemia and hyponatremia is discussed in chapter 129, "Fluid and Electrolyte Therapy in Infants and Children."

When conservative management fails, consider acute renal replacement therapy (dialysis). Indications for acute renal replacement therapy are severe electrolyte abnormalities, fluid overload not relieved by administration of loop diuretics, and intractable metabolic acidosis not responding to bicarbonate therapy. Peritoneal dialysis is the preferred method of acute dialysis for children because it is inexpensive and requires less expertise to perform than hemodialysis.[1,2]

DISPOSITION AND FOLLOW-UP

Although the primary care physician can manage mild renal insufficiency caused by dehydration, pyelonephritis, postinfectious glomerulonephritis, or Henoch-Schönlein purpura on an outpatient basis, consult a pediatric nephrologist for the management of more significant renal insufficiency, which often requires inpatient therapy. Children with hypertension with or without other findings require inpatient evaluation and management. Pediatric urology consultation is needed for postrenal failure.[1] Admit children with severe electrolyte abnormalities and fluid overload to a pediatric intensive care unit.

NEPHROTIC SYNDROME

Nephrotic syndrome is a chronic disease in children that alters permeability at the glomerular capillary wall, which causes a urinary loss of protein. The disease is classically characterized by proteinuria (>40 milligrams/m^2 in 24 hours), hypoalbuminemia (serum albumin <30 grams/L), hyperlipidemia, and edema. However, hyperlipidemia and edema are not consistently present. Nephrotic syndrome can be primary (involving only the kidney) or secondary (multisystem). The cause is unknown.

PATHOPHYSIOLOGY

The glomerular membrane is damaged, resulting in increased permeability of the glomerulus to proteins normally not able to pass through the glomerular capillary wall. Increased permeability results in the two diagnostic hallmarks of nephrotic syndrome: proteinuria and hypoproteinemia. Nephrotic syndrome also leads to salt and water retention. The combination of low intravascular oncotic pressure from the loss of proteins, coupled with the retention of salt and water, gives rise to the clinical feature of edema. As fluids shift to the extracellular space, the kidney is stimulated through the renin-angiotensin-aldosterone system to increase distal sodium reabsorption, which exacerbates the cycle.[5]

Although viral upper respiratory tract infection often precedes symptomatic nephrotic syndrome, a causal link has not been established. The classification of primary nephrotic syndromes includes minimal change disease, focal segmental sclerosis, membranous nephropathy, membranoproliferative nephritis, and proliferative nephritis (diffuse, focal, or mesangial). Causes of secondary nephrotic syndrome include systemic diseases such as lupus, Henoch-Schönlein purpura, sickle cell anemia, and systemic infections, as well as potential drug or toxin exposure (e.g., heavy metals). TORCH (toxoplasmosis, syphilis, varicella, rubella, cytomegalovirus, and herpes simplex virus) infections may cause a congenital nephrotic syndrome in neonates.

CLINICAL FEATURES

HISTORY AND COMPLICATIONS

Edema is the most common complaint. Focus the history on the duration and location of edema. Anasarca consists of marked peripheral edema, ascites, scrotal or vulvar edema, and severe periorbital edema. Shortness of breath, cough, and orthopnea suggests a pleural effusion. Ask about urine output, because oliguria is often associated with more severe edema. Nausea, vomiting, and anorexia suggest ascites or edema of the bowel wall. Review of systems should note fever, fatigue, and headache as well as the character of the urine (foamy, bloody, and tea colored).[2] The presence of hematuria, hypertension, or reduced renal function, age at onset, medical and family history of disease, and biopsy findings are all important predictors of disease outcome.

The main life-threatening complications of nephrotic syndrome are severe infection and thromboembolic events (venous and arterial). Serum complements, antibodies, and coagulation factors are lost as protein in the urine, leading to relative immunocompromise. Steroid therapy for nephrotic syndrome increases the risk of infection. Hyperlipidemia may lead to hyperviscosity, and increased levels of fibrinolytic inhibitors increase thrombotic risks.

PHYSICAL EXAMINATION

Rebound abdominal tenderness, ascites, and scrotal or labial swelling are potential findings.[5] Perform a full cardiopulmonary and abdominal exam. Auscultate for findings of pleural effusion and pulmonary edema. Be careful not to confuse facial swelling due to nephrotic syndrome with swelling secondary to allergic reaction.

DIAGNOSIS

The four diagnostic criteria of nephrotic syndrome are as follows:

1. Hypoproteinemia with disproportionately low albumin level (<3 grams/dL)
2. Urine protein (milligrams/deciliter) to urine creatinine (milligrams/deciliter) ratio >2 in a first morning void or a 24-hour urine protein loss that exceeds 50 milligrams/kg or 40 milligrams/m^2
3. Hypercholesterolemia (>200 milligrams/dL)[2]
4. Generalized edema

Renal biopsy is not indicated during the initial episode of acute nephrotic syndrome. Renal biopsy may be done when there is a definitive need to make a specific diagnosis for therapeutic reasons or to provide a diagnosis.[2,5]

LABORATORY EVALUATION

In general, blood and urine samples are sent for study to confirm the diagnosis of nephrotic syndrome (tests for proteinuria, hypoproteinemia, and hyperlipidemia), distinguish primary from secondary causes (tests for hematuria, serum immunoglobulin and complement levels, and antinuclear antibody level; hepatitis serologic testing), and aid in management (CBC, serum electrolyte levels, and renal function test). Serum creatinine may be normal for age and height. Total serum calcium is often low, although ionized calcium is usually normal. Serum sodium level is low secondary to increased triglycerides. Imaging studies are rarely indicated unless there is clinical concern for pulmonary edema or effusions. Symptoms or signs suggestive of potential thrombotic complications of nephrotic syndrome should prompt the appropriate evaluation (e.g., duplex US of renal vessels, CT angiography).

TREATMENT

ED MANAGEMENT

The goal is to treat acute symptoms, make the diagnosis of nephrotic syndrome, and arrange for appropriate follow-up. Treat hypovolemic shock with isotonic fluid, even if edema is severe. For the mildly to moderately dehydrated patient, provide oral rehydration with small, frequent aliquots of sodium-deficient solutions. Treat volume overload with furosemide, 1 to 2 milligrams/kg. Diuretics may not be effective when there is profound hypoalbuminemia, and in that situation, infusion of albumin (0.5 to 1.0 gram/kg) followed by furosemide may be effective, but intensive care monitoring is required. Treat infection or thrombotic complications as clinically indicated.

SPECIFIC TREATMENT OF NEPHROTIC SYNDROME

The mainstay of the treatment of nephrotic syndrome is oral corticosteroids, but the response to steroids varies with the cause. Minimal change disease and mesangial proliferative nephritis are often steroid responsive; membranous nephropathy may respond to steroids; focal segmental sclerosis and membranoproliferative nephritis are typically steroid resistant.[2,5] When indicated, prednisone is often started at 2 milligrams/kg/d in two or three divided doses, or 60 milligrams/m^2 for the initial dose and 40 to 60 milligrams/m^2 for the subsequent doses, given daily for 6 weeks with an additional 6 weeks of alternate-day administration. No steroid taper is required for this initial therapy.[6] In patients with known steroid-responsive disease who experience relapse, the ED physician may restart steroids as above in consultation with a pediatric nephrologist. In steroid-resistant nephrotic syndrome, the nephrologist must be consulted for initiation of medications. There are three types of medications that can be used for steroid-resistant nephrotic syndrome (5% of cases): immunosuppressive, immunostimulatory, and nonimmunosuppressive medications. Examples include cyclosporine, cyclophosphamide, chlorambucil, and levamisole.[6]

DISPOSITION AND FOLLOW-UP

Admit patients with severe edema, pulmonary effusions or respiratory symptoms, or signs and symptoms suggestive of systemic infection or thrombotic complications to the hospital. Children with mild or moderate edema can often be treated as outpatients with a low-salt (<2 grams/d) diet and close follow-up with their primary care physician or pediatric nephrologist.[2]

Children with nephrotic syndrome are at high risk for bacterial peritonitis from *Streptococcus pneumoniae* and should receive the pneumococcal (23-valent) vaccine to avoid peritonitis. The varicella vaccine should also be administered to children with nephrotic syndrome once they are in remission and no longer receiving steroid therapy.[5]

GLOMERULONEPHRITIS

Glomerulonephritis is a spectrum of inflammatory disorders characterized by hematuria and proteinuria. Signs of glomerulonephritis vary from asymptomatic proteinuria and microscopic hematuria to gross hematuria, nephrotic syndrome, hypertension, and impaired renal functioning requiring renal replacement therapy.[2] Glomerulonephritis is caused by several disorders, all of which cause inflammation leading to glomerular injury. Examples of hereditary glomerular diseases include systemic lupus erythematosus nephritis, thin glomerular basement membrane disease, and Alport's syndrome.[2,7] Poststreptococcal glomerulonephritis, immunoglobulin A (IgA) nephropathy, and Henoch-Schönlein purpura will be discussed in this section.

PATHOPHYSIOLOGY

Glomerulonephritis is an inflammatory process affecting the glomerulus. It can be caused by immune-mediated disorders, inherited disorders, or postinfection sequelae. Glomerulonephritis usually results from deposition of immune complexes within the glomeruli. These immune complexes activate a number of processes including complement activation, leukocyte recruitment, and release of growth factors and cytokines. This leads to inflammation and injury. Sclerosis occurs within the glomeruli, and fibrosis occurs in the tubulointerstitial cells.[2,7]

Glomerulonephritis may be classified as primary (isolated to the kidney) or secondary (a result of a systemic disorder). There are four main presentations: acute glomerulonephritis, rapidly progressive glomerulonephritis, recurrent macroscopic hematuria, and chronic glomerulonephritis. Although glomerulonephritis caused by streptococcal disease or Henoch-Schönlein purpura usually resolves completely and without sequelae, glomerulonephritis from other causes can progress to renal damage and ultimately end-stage renal failure.[2]

CLINICAL FEATURES

Glomerulonephritis is often associated with hypertension, which may cause headaches when severe. Symptoms related to hypertension may be the chief complaint of a child with undiagnosed glomerulonephritis.[2,7] Patients may complain of bloody or foamy urine (a result of proteinuria), oliguria, fatigue, and lethargy.[2,7] In glomerulonephritis, the urinalysis demonstrates macroscopic or microscopic hematuria, RBC casts, and proteinuria. Microscopic examination of urinary sediment shows dysmorphic RBCs and RBC casts. The physical examination is often normal. The blood pressure may be elevated. Other examination findings depend on the underlying disorder.

LABORATORY EVALUATION

The microscopic urinalysis demonstrates dysmorphic RBCs and RBC casts. Send urine for culture, because proteinuria and hematuria may represent urinary tract infection, although RBC casts are not typical of infection.[7] Other useful studies include a CBC, creatinine level, and electrolytes. Serum albumin level is often reduced. Send serum complement levels (C3 and C4), because complement proteins (C3) are decreased in >90% of patients with poststreptococcal glomerulonephritis, whereas levels are usually normal in patients with IgA nephropathy. Consider streptococcal serologic tests (antistreptolysin-I and streptozyme).[7] More specific tests may be needed to make a clear diagnosis in illnesses with systemic manifestations such as Henoch-Schönlein purpura and systemic lupus erythematosus. A renal biopsy is often required for definitive diagnosis in glomerulonephritic disorders.[7]

POSTSTREPTOCOCCAL GLOMERULONEPHRITIS

Poststreptococcal glomerulonephritis is caused by prior infection with group A β-hemolytic streptococci. Only certain strains of this group are "nephritogenic," and infection of the pharynx is the most common type of infection leading to acute glomerulonephritis, which occurs on average 7 to 14 days after infection. Group A β-hemolytic streptococci stimulate immune complex formation secondary to deposition of streptococcal nephritogenic antigens within the glomerulus. Other infections such as *Staphylococcus aureus* and *S. epidermidis* may also lead to renal disease, usually with a longer latency period.

Clinically, poststreptococcal glomerulonephritis consists of microscopic or gross hematuria, proteinuria, hypertension, and edema. Children may give a history of a recent upper respiratory tract or skin infection or have tea-colored urine. The most common serologic markers include an anti-streptolysin O titer, which is typically elevated, and a serum C3 level, which is typically decreased.[8] The recovery phase, where proteinuria and gross hematuria begin to resolve, starts after resolution of the patient's fluid overload.[8]

Treatment is largely supportive. Symptoms of poststreptococcal glomerulonephritis usually resolve in a few weeks. Hypertension rarely requires long-term treatment and tends to resolve within 1 to 2 weeks.[8] Renal biopsy is not indicated for diagnosis, unless atypical clinical features are present.[8] Asymptomatic patients with probable poststreptococcal disease and normal vital signs are eligible for discharge after consultation, and arrangement for follow-up, with a nephrologist.

IGA NEPHROPATHY

IgA nephropathy, also known as Berger's disease, is an autoimmune disease that is responsible for up to 10% of acute glomerulonephritis in the United States. Initially, IgA is deposited on the mesangial cells of the kidney. This alone is not enough to cause IgA nephropathy. In addition, there needs to be reduced IgA clearance, development of glomerular injury, and complement activation, all resulting from dysregulation of mucosal-type IgA immune responses. The cause is unknown.

Clinically, IgA nephropathy may present one of three ways: macroscopic hematuria, microscopic hematuria with mild proteinuria, or acute rapidly progressive glomerulonephritis with edema, hypertension, and renal insufficiency. Macroscopic hematuria is often concurrent with an upper respiratory tract infection and is called synpharyngitic hematuria. The diagnosis is typically based on the clinical history and laboratory data (including urinalysis). Renal biopsy is confirmatory.

Treatment is symptomatic. Immunosuppressant therapy may be initiated to treat underlying inflammation, depending on disease severity. ACE inhibitors or angiotensin receptor blockers may be used to control blood pressure, particularly in patients with proteinuria.[9] IgA nephropathy can either completely resolve or progress to end-stage renal disease.[9] Concern for a IgA nephropathy in the ED warrants an outpatient referral to nephrology. Rapidly progressive glomerulonephritis requires admission.

HENOCH-SCHÖNLEIN PURPURA

Henoch-Schönlein purpura, also known as IgA vasculitis, is a form of systemic vasculitis associated with IgA deposition in the small vessels of the body. Palpable purpura, arthritis/arthralgias, abdominal pain, and renal disease make up the classic presentation tetrad. Henoch-Schönlein purpura nephritis is often asymptomatic, and it is extremely important to follow up to detect persistent renal inflammation.[10] Full discussion of Henoch-Schönlein purpura is in chapter 130, "Acute Abdominal Pain in Infants and Children," and we focus on the renal manifestations here.

Renal complications occur in 20% to 54% of patients with Henoch-Schönlein purpura and include gross or microscopic hematuria, proteinuria, or nephritic syndrome.[11] Of the children diagnosed with Henoch-Schönlein purpura, 40% have mild nephritis, manifested only by microscopic hematuria or low-grade proteinuria.[12] Renal complications may develop any time over a period of 28 days, and 2% of children may develop long-term renal impairment.[13] Obtain a urinalysis to identify RBCs, casts, and protein. Treatment focuses on hydration, rest, and analgesics. Treatment with corticosteroids in Henoch-Schönlein purpura with renal involvement is controversial and may lead to increased recurrence of disease. Nephrology consultation is recommended.

HEMOLYTIC-UREMIC SYNDROME

Hemolytic-uremic syndrome is a multisystem disorder resulting in acute renal failure, thrombocytopenia, and microangiopathic hemolytic anemia. Hemolytic-uremic syndrome is one of the most common causes of AKI in children and typically occurs in those <10 years old. It is classified as typical (diarrhea associated) or atypical. In children, Shiga toxin–producing *Escherichia coli* causes 90% of hemolytic-uremic syndrome cases, presenting with a prodrome of diarrhea.[14] Other causes of hemolytic-uremic syndrome are *S. pneumoniae* infection, genetic disorders, oral contraceptive use, pregnancy, and malignancy.

PATHOPHYSIOLOGY

Epidemic hemolytic-uremic syndrome is usually caused by infection with *E. coli* O157:H7, an organism associated with ingestion of undercooked meat, unpasteurized milk, and contaminated fruits and vegetables. *E. coli*

O157:H7 produces a Shiga toxin, which is absorbed from the intestines into the circulation, causing microangiopathic intravascular thrombosis, RBC hemolysis, thrombocytopenia (due to platelet consumption), and decreased glomerular perfusion.[14] Microthrombi are deposited in kidney parenchyma, causing hypertension, oliguria, and anuria.[15] Renal involvement ranges from mild renal insufficiency to acute renal failure requiring dialysis.

In atypical hemolytic-uremic syndrome associated with *S. pneumoniae*, pathogenesis is initiated by the pneumococcal enzyme neuraminidase. This enzyme cleaves *N*-acetylneuraminic acid from the surface of RBCs and endothelial cells, uncovering the T antigen on the surface of endothelial cells. This in turn leads to an immune response, initiating the cascade leading to hemolytic-uremic syndrome.[16]

CLINICAL FEATURES

The majority of hemolytic-uremic syndrome is associated with *E. coli* enteritis, and the disease starts with nausea, vomiting, and bloody diarrhea with or without fever. Within a week, anemia, oliguria, and seizures or encephalopathy develop. Other complications include hypertension, heart failure, intussusception, diabetes mellitus, acidosis, and colitis.[15] A careful dietary and travel history may identify a potential source of infection to aid public health officials assess epidemic outbreaks.

The differential diagnosis of diarrhea-associated hemolytic-uremic syndrome includes acute gastroenteritis, appendicitis, colitis, intussusception, inflammatory bowel disease, and perforation. Petechiae, hemolysis, and thrombocytopenia are seen in disseminated intravascular coagulation, thrombotic thrombocytopenia purpura, and systemic lupus erythematosus. Some of the symptoms of hemolytic-uremic syndrome may also be seen in malignant hypertension and renal vein thrombosis.

LABORATORY EVALUATION

Microangiopathic hemolytic anemia, one of the cardinal features of hemolytic-uremic syndrome, may be profound with a hemoglobin level between 5 and 9 grams/dL. A peripheral smear demonstrates schistocytes, helmet cells, and burr cells. The Coombs test is negative. The platelet count is <150 000/mm^3. The WBC count may be elevated.

Hyponatremia and hyperkalemia develop as a result of metabolic acidosis from renal failure, and hyperbilirubinemia results from acute hemolysis.

Obtain a stool specimen to test for Shiga toxin, and specifically test for *E. coli* O157:H7. Urinalysis demonstrates gross or microscopic hematuria with granular and hyaline casts and variable proteinuria and leukocyturia.

TREATMENT

ED management is supportive. Correct life-threatening electrolyte disturbances, and treat hypovolemia with IV fluid boluses (10 to 20 mL/kg normal saline). Exercise cautious use of fluids to prevent fluid overload, particularly in patients with oliguria/anuria.[14] **Antibiotics are contraindicated in pediatric diarrheal illness and may increase the risk hemolytic-uremic syndrome.[15] Antiperistaltic agents increase the risk for systemic complications associated with *E. coli* infection and are also contraindicated.[14]** Blood transfusions may be needed for severe anemia. Platelet transfusion is not recommended because it could worsen the thrombotic process. For atypical hemolytic-uremic syndrome, consult with hematology for possible plasma exchange therapy.

All patients with hemolytic-uremic syndrome require hospitalization. Patients with neurologic symptoms and oliguric renal failure should be admitted to the intensive care unit.[15] Renal replacement therapy is required in 15% to 70% of cases of acute hemolytic-uremic syndrome.[14] Most children (90%) survive the acute phase of the illness, and most regain normal renal function.

RENAL TUBULAR ACIDOSIS

Renal tubular acidosis is rare. In the absence of diarrhea, it is defined as hyperchloremic metabolic acidosis with a normal anion gap and a normal to near-normal GFR.[12,17]

TABLE 134-2 Laboratory Findings in Renal Tubular Acidosis (RTA)

Type of RTA	Anion Gap	Urinary Anion Gap	Serum Potassium Level	Additional Laboratory Tests
Distal or type I RTA	Normal	Elevated	Low or normal	Arterial blood gas concentrations, urine pH (>5.5), urine to blood CO_2
Proximal or type II RTA	Normal	Normal	Normal	Arterial blood gas concentrations, urine pH (>5.5, except in severe metabolic acidosis), serum K level, fractional excretion of HCO
Type IV RTA	Normal	Elevated	High	Arterial blood gas concentrations, urine pH (<5.5 with severe metabolic acidosis), urine to blood CO_2, creatinine clearance

In children, renal tubular acidosis is typically secondary to an inherited or acquired defect that affects the kidney's ability to manage bicarbonate, acid, and ammonia. Renal tubular acidosis develops because of failure of reabsorption of bicarbonate in the proximal tubule (type I), failure of excretion of hydrogen ions in the distal nephron (type II), or inability to acidify the urine in the setting of low serum aldosterone level or aldosterone resistance (type IV). For example, Fanconi's syndrome causes a type II renal tubular acidosis and may be associated with hypophosphatemia and rickets. Types I and II renal tubular acidosis result in hyperchloremic metabolic acidosis. Type IV renal tubular acidosis results in hyperkalemia, acidemia, and a low urinary pH.[12,17]

There is no single symptom complex that brings children with renal tubular acidosis to medical attention. Chronic acidosis is associated with failure to thrive, and this may result in an ED visit. Depending on the type of renal tubular acidosis, symptomatic hypokalemia or hyperkalemia (weakness, nausea, constipation), rickets, or nephrolithiasis may prompt an ED visit. Often the diagnosis of renal tubular acidosis is suggested by abnormal results on serum chemistry and urine studies that are incidentally discovered in the process of evaluation for unrelated complaints. **Table 134-2** describes the typical laboratory findings in each type of renal tubular acidosis.

Acute treatment consists of correcting the underlying electrolyte and acid-base abnormalities (see chapter 129). Maintenance treatment includes oral bicarbonate therapy and monitoring of serum potassium for all types of renal tubular acidosis, vitamin D and sodium phosphate for type II renal tubular acidosis, and loop diuretics and fludrocortisone for mineralocorticoid deficiency in type IV renal tubular acidosis.

HYPERTENSION

Pediatric hypertension is increasing in incidence, with a prevalence of 2.5% to 5%.[18] This increase is related to higher rates of childhood obesity, greater salt intake, hyperlipidemia, and decreased physical activity.[18] **Hypertension** is defined as average systolic blood pressure and/or diastolic blood pressure greater than the 95th percentile or higher for sex, age, and height on three or more occasions.[19]

Hypertensive urgency is a severely elevated blood pressure without evidence of target organ damage that, left untreated, may cause end-organ damage.

Hypertensive crisis is defined as blood pressures exceeding the 99th percentile for age and sex with acute end-organ damage and requires immediate treatment.[20] Generally, the CNS, kidneys, and cardiovascular system are the organs most likely to be damaged secondary to hypertension. Hypertensive crises in younger children are usually secondary to an underlying disease.

Essential hypertension is uncommon in younger children and is more prevalent in adolescents.[21] Renal disease (glomerulonephritis, hemolytic-uremic syndrome, chronic infections, obstructive lesions,

TABLE 134-3 Common Causes of Hypertension in Children

Age Group	Cause
Newborn	Renal: thrombosis, stenosis, polycystic kidney disease
	Heart: coarctation of the aorta
	Endocrine: pheochromocytoma, Cushing's disease
Preschool/kindergarten (<6 y)	Renal: parenchymal disease, vascular disease
	Heart: coarctation of the aorta
	Endocrine: pheochromocytoma, Cushing's disease
School age (6–10 y)	Endocrine: pheochromocytoma, Cushing's disease
Adolescence	Essential hypertension
	Renal: parenchymal, vascular
	Endocrine: pheochromocytoma, Cushing's disease
	Drugs of abuse (e.g., cocaine, amphetamines), nonsteroidal anti-inflammatory drugs, monoamine oxidase inhibitors

and renal vascular disease) is the most common cause of secondary hypertension in children. Endocrine causes of hypertension include tumors that secrete vasoactive peptides (pheochromocytoma), abnormal levels of endogenous steroid hormones (Cushing's syndrome), adrenocortical steroid therapy, and hyperthyroidism. Hypertension may also result from congenital heart disease such as coarctation of the aorta. Elevated intracranial pressure may also lead to hypertension in an attempt by the body to maintain cerebral perfusion pressure and can be caused by space-occupying lesions, acute hemorrhage, infection, or obstruction to cerebrospinal fluid flow. Exogenous medications or toxins may also cause hypertension. **Table 134-3** outlines the common causes of hypertension by age group.

CLINICAL FEATURES

HISTORY AND COMORBIDITIES

Focus on signs of hypertension and determine if end-organ damage is present.[20] The most common signs suggesting primary hypertension in children are headache, sleep disturbances (falling asleep, daytime tiredness), chest pain, and abdominal pain.[18] Identify any medications or substances associated with blood pressure elevation, such as oral contraceptives, steroids, and illicit drugs (e.g., cocaine, amphetamines). Inquire about visual changes, headache, epistaxis, chest pain, urine output, hematuria, fever, and changes in mental status. Palpitations, weight loss, flushing, and diarrhea may suggest an endocrine cause. Ask about a family history of essential hypertension, diabetes, obesity, renal disease, hyperlipidemia, stroke, or endocrinopathy.[19,20] For those with an established diagnosis of hypertension, ask about medication adherence.

PHYSICAL EXAMINATION

Obtain an accurate height and weight, and determine percentiles for age.[19] Obtain four-limb blood pressures (a lower blood pressure in the lower extremities compared to the upper extremities or left versus right arms may indicate aortic coarctation), respiratory rate, heart rate, and oxygen saturation. Perform a comprehensive physical examination, including a funduscopic examination (for retinal hemorrhages, papilledema, infarcts) and a neurologic examination.[20] Assess the heart and lungs for signs of congestive heart failure or structural disease (gallops, murmurs, rales). Palpate the abdomen to exclude masses or pregnancy. Auscultation of an abdominal bruit may suggest renovascular disease.

LABORATORY EVALUATION

Assess renal function with a serum BUN, creatinine, electrolytes, glucose, plasma rennin activity, aldosterone levels, and microscopic urinalysis.[18] Obtain a CBC and reticulocyte count to look for rheumatic disorders, appropriate marrow response, and signs of anemia.[18] Perform a urine pregnancy test in pubertal girls. Urine drug screening is indicated if intoxication is suspected. Ordering of more esoteric tests for endocrine abnormalities should be left to subspecialists.

IMAGING

Obtain a chest radiograph and ECG. Obtain a head CT if neurologic findings are present.[20] Renal US is indicated to rule out structural kidney abnormalities. If suspicion for renovascular disease is high, then obtain a CT or MRI. Obtain an echocardiogram to look for left ventricular hypertrophy and to rule out cardiac causes of hypertension.

TREATMENT

Most patients with mild to moderate elevation of blood pressure in the ED are discharged with instructions for follow-up for outpatient evaluation and treatment.

Hypertensive urgency may be treated with oral antihypertensives.[18] Treatment of **hypertensive emergency** begins with evaluation and stabilization of the airway, breathing, and circulation. Obtain IV or IO access and start cardiac monitoring; consider placement of a Foley catheter and arterial line. The goal is to reduce the mean arterial pressure by ≤25% over the first 8 hours, followed by a gradual reduction to normal values over the next 26 to 48 hours.[22] Reducing the blood pressure too aggressively can lead to ischemic complications such as acute neurologic issues, blindness, and renal failure.[18]

Recommendations regarding the most useful drugs for treating severe hypertensive emergency and urgency in children are listed in **Table 134-4** and **Table 134-5**.[22,23] Medications should be chosen according to their side effect profile, availability, and physician familiarity.[20]

TABLE 134-4 Treatment of Hypertensive Emergency in Children 1 to 17 Years Old

Drug	Class	Dosage	Route	Onset of Action	Duration of Action	Comments
Labetalol	α- and β-blocker	Bolus: 0.2–1.0 milligram/kg/dose to a maximum of 40 milligrams/dose, then infusion: 0.25–3.0 milligrams/kg/h	IV bolus or infusion	2–5 min	2–6 h	Contraindications include asthma, chronic lung disease, and evident heart failure. May mask hypoglycemic symptoms.
Nicardipine	Calcium channel blocker	0.5–3.0 micrograms/kg/min IV infusion	IV infusion	2–5 min	30 min–4 h	May cause increased intracranial pressure, headache, nausea, and hypotension.
Hydralazine	Vasodilator	0.1–0.5 milligram/kg/dose; maximum, 20 milligrams/dose	IV, IM	5–30 min	4–12 h	Administer every 4 h when given as IV bolus. Not as strong as other agents. Recommended dose is less than U.S. Food and Drug Administration–approved label.
Sodium nitroprusside	Vasodilator	0.3–8.0 micrograms/kg/min IV infusion	IV infusion	Seconds	Only during infusion	May increase intracranial pressure. Monitor cyanide and thiocyanate levels for patients with renal and liver disease when administering for >24–48 h.
Esmolol	β-Blocker	100–500 micrograms/kg/min (initial dose), then 50–300 micrograms/kg/min	IV infusion	Immediate	10–30 min	May cause bronchospasm, congestive heart failure, and profound bradycardia.

TABLE 134-5 Treatment of Hypertensive Urgency in Children 1 to 17 Years Old

Drug	Class	Dosage	Route	Onset of Action	Duration of Action	Comments
Nifedipine	Calcium channel blocker	0.1–0.25 milligram/kg/dose	PO, sublingual	Immediate release, 20–30 min Extended release, 2.5–5 h	Immediate release, 4–8 h Extended release, 24 h	Precipitous drop in blood pressure, tachycardia, headache
Minoxidil	Vasodilator	0.1–2 milligrams/kg/dose	PO	Within 30 min	Up to 2–5 d	Pericardial effusion
Isradipine	Calcium channel blocker	0.05–0.1 milligram/kg/dose up to 5mg/dose	PO	2–3 h	>12 h	Tachycardia, headache
Clonidine	Central α-agonist	0.05–0.3 milligram	PO	30–60 min	6–10 h	Rebound hypertension, sedation

Many nephrologists administer short-acting nifedipine to treat moderate to severe hypertension in the setting of primary renal disease. Although it is generally safe and effective,[24] there are reports of adverse neurologic events due to rebound hypertension.

DISPOSITION AND FOLLOW-UP

Mild hypertension should be managed on an outpatient basis by the primary care provider or subspecialist. Hypertensive urgencies and emergencies require ED stabilization and initial pharmacologic treatment in the ED with subsequent admission to the intensive care unit or medical ward depending on the degree of end-organ damage and the response to initial interventions.

HEMATURIA

Hematuria is the presence of an increased number of RBCs (≥5 RBCs/μL of urine). Hematuria may be macroscopic (apparent to the naked eye) or microscopic (apparent only on urinalysis). It is frequently asymptomatic.

Hematuria can be divided into three types: macrohematuria, transient hematuria, and persistent microhematuria. Macroscopic hematuria is most frequently caused by urinary tract infections or blunt abdominal trauma. Other causes include nephrolithiasis, poststreptococcal glomerulonephritis, IgA nephropathy, and malignancy. Transient hematuria may be caused by strenuous exercise, trauma, menstruation, bladder catheterization, and fever. Persistent microhematuria can be seen in benign familial hematuria, idiopathic hypercalciuria, IgA nephropathy, Alport's syndrome, and sickle cell trait or anemia or with drugs/toxins.

CLINICAL FEATURES

HISTORY AND COMORBIDITIES

Obtain a complete history, because the differential diagnosis is broad. Distinguish between transient, persistent, and recurrent hematuria.[2,25] Associated dysuria, urinary frequency and urgency, fever, and abdominal or flank pain suggest infection or urolithiasis (see chapter 94, "Urologic Stone Disease" in the adult section). A history of an upper respiratory tract infection, sore throat, or skin infection may suggest postinfectious glomerulonephritis. A current infectious process is suspicious for IgA nephropathy. For transient hematuria, ask about blunt abdominal trauma, recent catheterization, or menstruation.[25] The color of the urine (pink, red, or tea colored) and the timing during micturition—at the beginning (associated with pathology of the urethra), throughout micturition (associated with bleeding above the bladder neck), or at the end of micturition (associated with pathology of the bladder neck, posterior urethra, or prostate)—provides useful diagnostic information.[2,25] Ask about joint pain and rash (Henoch-Schönlein purpura[25,26] or lupus[2]). Some drugs associated with hematuria are nonsteroidal anti-inflammatory drugs, anticonvulsants, warfarin, diuretics, penicillin, and chlorpromazine.[13] Recent vigorous exercise can cause hematuria, which resolves after a period of rest.[2] Obtain a family history carefully, because many causes of hematuria in children are inherited. Questions about family history should be directed to information regarding deafness, hematuria, hypertension, coagulopathy, hemoglobinopathy, calculi, renal failure, dialysis, and transplant.[2,13] Staining reported as "blood on the diaper" of an infant without other symptoms may represent benign urinary crystals, extra–urinary tract blood (e.g., vaginal bleeding in female neonates), or blood from the GI tract. The presence of amorphous crystals in the urine is a common and benign finding in neonates, and because these crystals are often pink or orange, they may be interpreted as blood by parents. Dipstick testing is negative for blood in this situation.

PHYSICAL EXAMINATION

The physical examination findings vary depending on the cause of hematuria suggested by historical information.[2,25] Obtain vital signs to identify hypertension or a fever. Assess for signs of respiratory infection, joint swelling, and skin rashes. Perform a careful GU examination to identify a source of external bleeding such as a periurethral tear.

DIAGNOSIS

LABORATORY EVALUATION

The laboratory evaluation begins with confirmation of hematuria. Medications such as chloroquine, isoniazid, malin, and nitrofurantoin may cause a red-brown discoloration of the urine.[27] Similarly, foods such as beets, rhubarb, or blackberries may also cause discoloration. Because such urinary discoloration may be misinterpreted by parents as blood, screen with a urine dipstick test, which can exclude hematuria. A positive dipstick test result, however, must be followed by microscopic evaluation. Microscopic examination of the urine helps narrow the differential diagnosis: dysmorphic RBCs and casts suggest glomerulonephritis; WBCs and bacteria suggest infection; eosinophils may be seen in interstitial nephritis; and intact RBCs suggest lower tract causes of hematuria. Urinary crystals or stones may be seen in urolithiasis. A dipstick test result positive for blood without evidence of RBCs on microscopy suggests hemoglobinuria or myoglobinuria. Further evaluation of the urine includes rapid or quantitative evaluation for proteinuria, which can be seen in nephritis, nephrotic syndrome, and orthostatic proteinuria.[13] Obtain other laboratory studies to identify serious causes of hematuria, such as hemolytic-uremic syndrome, acute poststreptococcal glomerulonephritis, or renal insufficiency.

IMAGING

US is the imaging method of choice for macroscopic hematuria without proteinuria or RBC casts in the urine and is done to rule out malignancy or structural defects. For patients with trauma, macroscopic hematuria, or >20 RBCs/high-power field a more complete anatomic evaluation is needed, including CT, angiography, or retrograde urethrography depending on the history and clinical suspicion.

TREATMENT

The treatment of hematuria, like its evaluation, depends on the suspected cause. Most children without signs of major or life-threatening etiologies can be managed as outpatients. Children with isolated microscopic hematuria do not require an extensive evaluation if the blood pressure and urine output are normal. Hematuria requires a more rigorous evaluation when the blood pressure is elevated or there is significant proteinuria, so consult with a nephrologist. Refer to a urologist if there is suspicion of a urogenital tract anatomic abnormality, obstructing calculi, tumor, or recurrent nonglomerular macroscopic hematuria.[13]

CHRONIC RENAL FAILURE AND END-STAGE RENAL DISEASE

Chronic kidney disease is defined as the presence of kidney damage as manifested by abnormalities in blood or urine tests, imaging tests, or kidney biopsy or a GFR >60 mL/min/1.73 m^2 for 3 months or more, regardless of the diagnosis.[19] End-stage renal disease occurs when the GFR is <10% of normal for age.[28] Mortality in end-stage renal disease usually results from cardiovascular causes (40% to 50%) and infection (20%).[29] The only definitive treatment for end-stage renal disease is transplantation; however, the morbidity and mortality associated with chronic renal replacement therapy have decreased.

The National Kidney Foundation classifies chronic kidney disease into five separate stages.[30] The recommended method for determination of GFR is with spot urine and serum creatinine using either the Schwartz or Counahan calculation. Twenty-four–hour urine collections for creatinine are no longer recommended.

Stage 1: GFR ≥90 mL/min/1.73 m^2 (kidney damage with normal or increased GFR)

Stage 2: GFR 60 to 89 mL/min/1.73 m^2 (kidney damage with mild reduction of GFR)

Stage 3: GFR 20 to 59 mL/min/1.73 m^2 (moderate reduction of GFR)

Stage 4: GFR 15 to 29 mL/min/1.73 m^2 (severe reduction of GFR)

Stage 5: GFR <15 mL/min/1.73 m^2 or dialysis (kidney failure)

At stage 5, when end-stage renal disease develops, conservative management of chronic renal failure has been exhausted, and dialysis and transplantation become the next options for medical management.[31]

ETIOLOGY AND DIFFERENTIAL DIAGNOSIS

Congenital renal disease is the most common cause of chronic renal failure in young children, whereas glomerulonephritis and reflux nephropathy predominate in older children.[32] Congenital structural lesions include dysplasias and cystic malformations (e.g., polycystic kidney disease). Obstructive uropathy leading to end-stage renal disease may be caused by posterior urethral valves in boys, severe vesicoureteral reflux with recurrent infection, and ureteropelvic junction obstruction. End-stage renal disease in children can be caused by hereditary nephritis or acquired nephropathies such as hemolytic-uremic syndrome, glomerulonephritis, and cortical necrosis (more common in children with sickle cell disease).

CLINICAL FEATURES

Take a complete history to obtain information about changes in urination, fatigue, swelling, anorexia, emesis, bone pain, muscle cramps, headache, and change in mental status. Ask about signs and symptoms related to potential complications from chronic kidney disease.

Complications associated with chronic kidney disease include disorders of fluids, electrolytes, and mineral metabolism. Anemia, hypertension, dyslipidemia, and endocrine abnormalities, including growth impairment, are present. End-stage renal disease is associated with cardiovascular problems and cerebrovascular events from malignant hypertension. Skeletal, hematologic, and intestinal abnormalities accompany renal failure. Renal failure predisposes to non-Hodgkin's lymphoma and skin cancer.[29,32]

Pertinent physical findings in patients with end-stage renal disease include short stature, CNS problems, peripheral neuropathies, and rickets. Fever should prompt an aggressive search for a source. Fluid overload is suggested by peripheral edema and pulmonary congestion. Pericarditis is less common in children with end-stage renal disease than in adults. Abdominal pain and tenderness in children receiving peritoneal dialysis suggests peritonitis.

TREATMENT

The standard of treatment for most patients with end-stage renal disease is hemodialysis. Children <2 years of age are often treated with peritoneal dialysis because it is associated with fewer complications than hemodialysis in young children. Renal transplantation is the ultimate goal.[28,29,32]

In dialysis patients presenting to the ED with fever, an aggressive search for infection must ensue. Use of empiric antibiotics is directed by the source of the infection (e.g., *S. aureus, S. epidermidis*), after cultures are drawn. If a patient on peritoneal dialysis presents with abdominal pain, suspect bacterial peritonitis. In patients presenting with severe electrolyte abnormalities, fluid overload, severe hypertension, or uremic pericarditis, urgent dialysis is indicated. Dialysis patients presenting with syncope should be evaluated for electrolyte abnormalities, hypovolemia, and cardiac dysrhythmias. See chapter 90, "End Stage Renal Disease" in the adult section for detailed discussion.

REFERENCES

The complete reference list is available online at www.TintinalliEM.com.

CHAPTER 135 Seizures in Infants and Children

Maija Holsti

INTRODUCTION AND EPIDEMIOLOGY

Unusual movements and changes in behavior in children often lead to an ED visit. Most seizure activity stops before the child is seen in an ED; therefore, history is key to the correct diagnosis. Although seizures account for many of these events, as many as 30% or more of paroxysmal events may be misdiagnosed as seizures.[1]

There are many different causes of pediatric seizures. The goal is to identify and treat the underlying cause. Some seizures require emergency management and extensive evaluation (e.g., status epilepticus, neonatal seizures), whereas others are common, benign, and need little or no ED evaluation (e.g., febrile seizures, first-time seizure in an otherwise well child). This chapter focuses on the diagnosis and management of ongoing seizures first, and the approach to febrile seizures, neonatal seizures, and seizures in special populations (e.g., children with epilepsy, neurologic shunts, and trauma) are discussed under Special Considerations/Populations.

The incidence of new-onset pediatric seizure in the United States is approximately 120,000 cases per year and is highest in children <2 years and in certain high-risk groups.[2] **Febrile seizures are the most common type of pediatric seizure, affecting 2% to 5% of all children between 6 months and 5 years of age.**[3] Epilepsy is diagnosed when a patient has one or more unprovoked seizures.[4,5] Roughly 326,000 children <15 years have epilepsy, and 1% of the population can be expected to have epilepsy by the age of 20.[2] The incidence of status epilepticus in developed countries is between 17 and 23 cases per 100,000 and is higher for younger children.[6]

PATHOPHYSIOLOGY

Seizures represent abnormal, excessive, paroxysmal neuronal activity in the brain, primarily the cortex. Glutamate released from firing neurons activates N-methyl-d-aspartic acid receptors that subsequently initiate and propagate seizure activity.[7] Seizures are inhibited by gamma-aminobutyric-acid, and failure of this inhibition facilitates seizure spread.[7] Incomplete myelination of the brain may limit secondary generalization of seizure activity in young infants, and a relative imbalance between glutamate and gamma-aminobutyric-acid with paradoxical excitation from gamma-aminobutyric-acid makes younger children more susceptible to seizure activity.

Seizures can be primary (intrinsic) or secondary (the result of another process). Primary seizures are often idiopathic or may be caused by congenital developmental abnormalities, in utero central nervous system insult (e.g., infection, infarct), or genetic factors. Secondary seizures may result from trauma or injury, infection, metabolic abnormalities (e.g., hypoglycemia, electrolyte abnormalities, inborn errors of metabolism), toxins, or systemic illness.

CLINICAL FEATURES

TYPES OF SEIZURE

The clinical manifestation of seizures depends on the area(s) of the brain that are affected and whether the seizure activity is localized (focal) or widespread (generalized). Generalized seizures involve both hemispheres of the brain and lead to loss of consciousness, usually followed by a period of postictal drowsiness. In **convulsive generalized seizures or grand mal seizures**, rhythmic motor activity affects both sides of the body. **Nonconvulsive generalized seizures produce loss of consciousness without motor activity and can only be recognized on electroencephalogram.** In one study, nonconvulsive status epilepticus appeared in 51 of 117 critically ill patients, with 75% of these patients showing no clinical evidence of seizure activity.[8] Other examples of generalized seizures in children include **absence seizures** (brief episode of staring without a postictal state), **atonic seizures** (sudden loss of muscle tone with a sudden "drop" to the floor), and **myoclonic seizures**.

Partial seizures represent focal neuronal activity, and clinical features correlate with the affected area. In simple partial seizures, the patient remains awake, whereas complex partial seizures are focal but produce alterations of consciousness. Partial seizures may secondarily spread and become generalized. Young children with new-onset focal seizures are at increased risk for structural anatomic abnormalities, and neuroimaging is more likely to be abnormal in these children.[9]

Although status epilepticus was originally defined as a seizure lasting longer than 30 minutes, today **any "prolonged" seizure, or recurrent seizures lasting >5 minutes without return to full consciousness, is considered status epilepticus.**[10,11] Status epilepticus is a medical emergency, and rapid termination is important to prevent irreversible neuronal damage.[7,12] Refractory status epilepticus is a prolonged seizure that cannot be controlled with two or more doses of standard treatment.[7,12] **Nonconvulsive status epilepticus may present as a prolonged postictal state**[8] **and must be considered in any patient with altered mental status**; morbidity and mortality increase when nonconvulsive status epilepticus is untreated, though less so than with untreated convulsive status epilepticus.[8,13]

HISTORY

Obtain a detailed history of the event from a reliable observer. **Table 135-1** lists historical clues that may help identify a cause for seizures. Important details include the events surrounding the seizure (e.g., emotional upset and crying that may indicate breath holding in a toddler), the nature of the seizure activity (e.g., tonic stiffening, clonic jerks, generalized or focal characteristics), the duration of the event (often difficult for frightened parents to accurately report), and postictal observations and duration. Ask about recent illness, possible trauma, ingestions, and medications (both over-the-counter and prescribed). Inquire about past medical history (especially epilepsy) and recent changes or missed doses of medication. A developmental history is important, as children with underlying developmental delay are at increased risk for epilepsy. A family history of febrile seizures, epilepsy, or neurologic disease is also important for prognosis. Patient age alone is an important consideration in the potential cause of seizures, as depicted in **Figure 135-1**.

PHYSICAL EXAMINATION

Perform a complete head-to-toe examination with the patient undressed. The physical examination should be focused on whether the patient is actively seizing and identify potential causative factors (e.g., head trauma, rash indicative of infection, neurocutaneous lesions). **Table 135-2** outlines a number of clinical signs and symptoms of seizures. Rhythmic repetitive movement, incontinence of bowel or bladder, postictal state after a seizure, and tongue biting are strong clues to a seizure. Lateral tongue biting was found to have a specificity of 100% and a sensitivity of 24% for the occurrence of a seizure.[14]

TABLE 135-1 History Relevant to the Child Presenting With Seizure
Age of child
Seizure duration and description of seizure activity prior to arrival
History of trauma
History of possible ingestion
History of fever
History of associated illness (vomiting or diarrhea)
Feeding problems (especially in an infant)
Changes in behavior
History of seizures and type of seizures
History of developmental delay
Other medical history
Medications
Anticonvulsants with milligrams per kilogram dose and recent changes or missed doses
Recent new medications (may alter metabolism of antiepileptic drugs)
Allergies
Developmental history
Family history of seizures

DIAGNOSIS

DIFFERENTIAL DIAGNOSIS & CONDITIONS MASQUERADING AS SEIZURES

A number of benign conditions may masquerade as seizures, leading to an ED visit; up to 30% of new-onset paroxysmal events may be misdiagnosed as epileptic.[1] **Syncope is the most common condition that may be mistaken for seizures**; however, there are many differentiating features. Syncope is commonly preceded by dizziness, weakness, tunnel vision, pallor, and diaphoresis (presyncopal aura). It is also associated with a brief loss of consciousness and a quick recovery with no postictal state. Seizures, on the other hand, may be preceded by an aura but usually do not have a provoking factor noted before the event. Seizures are associated with tongue biting, rhythmic motor activity, incontinence, and a slow recovery and postictal state. **Table 135-3** lists nonepileptic causes of syncope and abnormal movements that can mimic seizures. In infants, myoclonic jerks, sleep myoclonus, shudder attacks, and Sandifer's syndrome (gastroesophageal reflux) are common. In toddlers, breath-holding spells become more prevalent. Self-stimulation and night terrors should be considered in preschool and young school-age children, whereas tic disorders typically begin in older children.

LABORATORY TESTING

Check bedside glucose on all seizing or postictal patients. Additional laboratory evaluation is directed by the history and is not routinely indicated for febrile seizures or first-time afebrile seizures that are nonfocal in a child with a normal examination (see Special Considerations/Populations, later). If indicated by the history and examination, labs that may be helpful include electrolytes (including calcium), serum antiepileptic medication levels, toxicologic testing, and spinal fluid for evaluation of possible central nervous system infection in the appropriate setting. Urine culture and analysis is indicated in the evaluation of febrile seizures in the child with fever and no identifiable source.

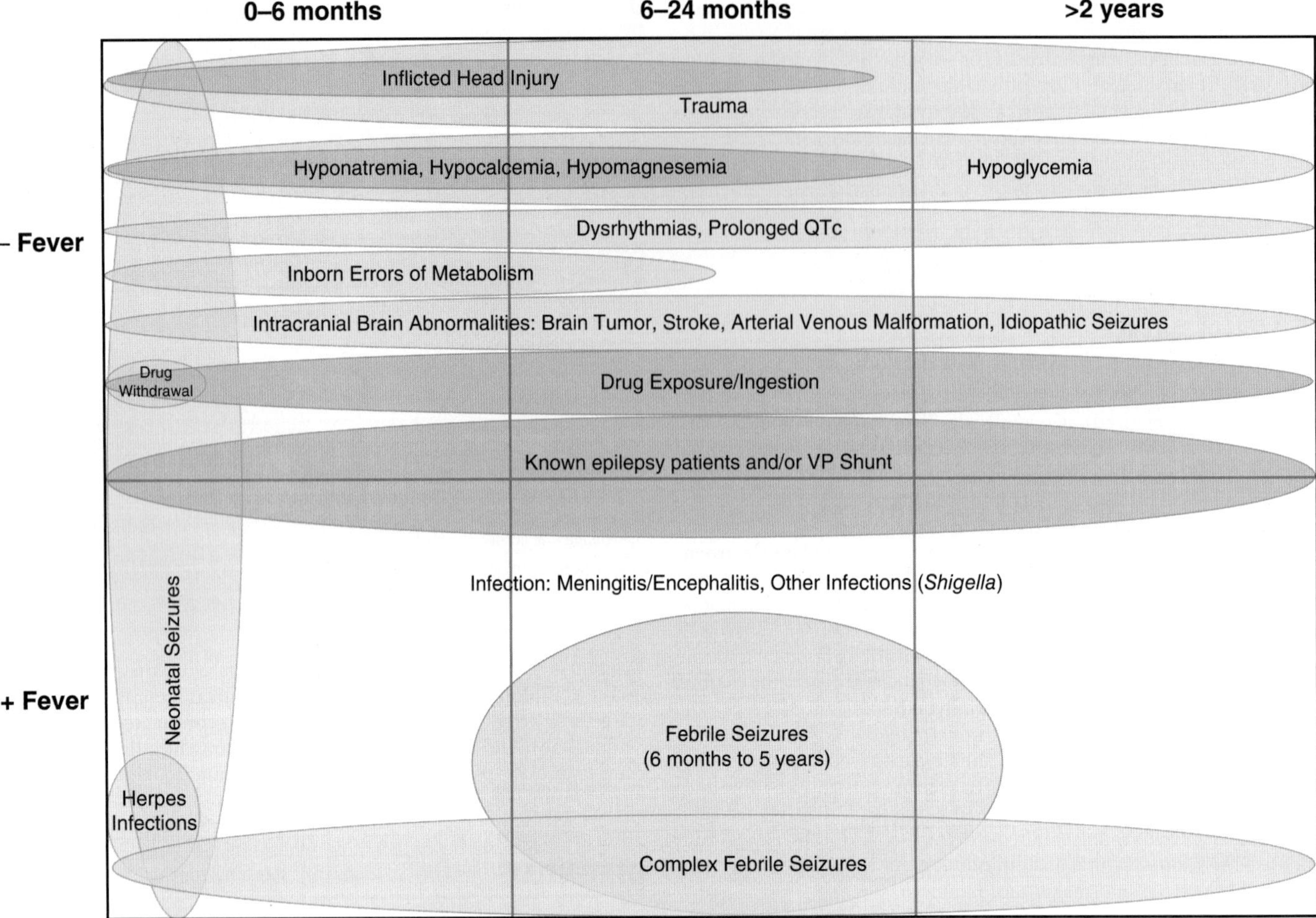

FIGURE 135-1. Age-based approach to the evaluation of pediatric seizures. VP = ventriculoperitoneal.

IMAGING

Similar to laboratory testing, imaging should be directed by the history and examination. Routine neuroimaging is rarely indicated or helpful. When trauma is suspected or in the setting of focal deficits, obtain a head CT. Todd's paralysis is a temporary condition characterized by a focal deficit of unknown etiology that can last up to 36 hours after a seizure.[15] The paralysis is usually unilateral and lasts on average 15 hours[15]; however, it can be bilateral and involve a patient's speech or vision.[13] It may be impossible to distinguish Todd's paralysis from stroke or hemorrhage, and emergent imaging should be considered.[15] Most first-time seizures in the well-appearing child with a normal examination are best evaluated with outpatient MRI, which avoids ionizing radiation and provides better anatomic detail.

TABLE 135-2 Signs and Symptoms Associated With Seizures

Signs and Symptoms
Head deviation
Eye deviation
Rhythmic or repetitive arm or leg movement
Posturing
Stiffening
Jerking
Change in breathing pattern
Increase in heart rate
Increase in blood pressure
Cyanosis or apnea
Eye dilatation
Vomiting
Lip smacking
Tongue biting
Incontinence of bowel or bladder
Postictal or sleepy period after a seizure
Mood or behavior changes before a seizure
Subjective aura before seizure (noted in older patients)

ANCILLARY TESTS

Consider obtaining an electrocardiogram for evaluation of syncope with seizure activity to rule out arrhythmia. Emergent electroencephalogram monitoring may be required for patients with refractory status epilepticus (especially those requiring rapid sequence intubation with a paralytic) or concern for nonconvulsive status epilepticus; otherwise, outpatient electroencephalogram may help identify specific epilepsy syndromes and guide future treatment.

SUMMARY OF APPROACH TO EVALUATION

Figure 135-2 summarizes the approach to the evaluation of pediatric seizures.

TREATMENT

PREHOSPITAL

Children may have been treated at home or by EMS personnel. Take this into consideration when treating refractory status epilepticus.

TABLE 135-3 Events Masquerading as Seizures

Syncope
Breath-holding spells
Cataplexy
Narcolepsy
Vasovagal event
Standing for long periods of time
Standing quickly from lying or sitting
Hair-grooming syncope
Earring-changing syncope
Micturition syncope
Emotional distress or pain
Hypoglycemia
Hypovolemia
Sandifer's syndrome (gastroesophageal reflux)
Acute life-threatening event
Acute dystonic reactions/drug reactions (i.e., promethazine [Phenergan®])
Movement disorders
Tics
Myoclonic jerks
Chills or rigors
Shudder attacks
Mannerisms
Self-stimulation
Choreoathetosis
Night terrors, sleep walking
Migraine variants
Benign paroxysmal vertigo
Nonepileptic paroxysmal event (pseudoseizures)

Note: Events in bold are more common.

Benzodiazepines (**Table 135-4**) are the first-line treatment for prolonged seizures because of their rapid onset and effectiveness; however, not all benzodiazepines or routes are available in the prehospital setting, and establishing IV access can be difficult in a child who is having a seizure.[7,10,15] Benzodiazepines may be given by the intranasal, buccal, rectal, or intraosseous route when an IV is difficult to place.[11,16-25]

Rectal diazepam is one "rescue" medication commonly used at home and by EMS personnel. The advantage is that no refrigeration or IV line is needed. The disadvantage is its short half-life and the need for rectal administration. Midazolam, also an effective rescue medication, can be given safely via the intranasal route using a mucosal atomization device (MAD®, Wolfe Tory Medical, Inc., Salt Lake City, UT).[20,21,26] Midazolam can also be given buccally.[1,12,14-24] Lorazepam is not generally used in the prehospital setting because of its need for refrigeration and recommendations that it only be administered through an IV line. There is new evidence that intranasal lorazepam using a MAD® may be as effective as IV lorazepam in the treatment of status epilepticus.[25,27]

ED TREATMENT

Most seizures stop within 5 minutes and do not require medical treatment.[10] Status epilepticus is a medical emergency, however, and is more responsive to medications when treated early, and treatment becomes less effective with time.[11,17,28] An overview of one treatment algorithm for status epilepticus is depicted in **Figure 135-3**.

Administer oxygen by facemask and institute continuous pulse oximetry and cardiac monitoring. Establish IV or intraosseus (IO) access, but administer medication early via alternate routes (intranasal, IM, PR, buccal) if there is delay.[6] Obtain bedside glucose testing and electrolyte levels when available.[4,7,11] Consider additional laboratory studies and imaging as directed by the history and examination. Subtherapeutic antiepileptic drug levels are found in almost one third of children with epilepsy presenting in status epilepticus.[29] Consider central nervous system infection in the child with fever and status epilepticus.

The decision to intubate is clinical. Intubate for apnea and persistent hypoxia. Blood gas concentrations are not needed to guide the decision to intubate, because the seizure itself causes a metabolic and respiratory acidosis. **The use of a paralytic with intubation obscures the ability to assess ongoing seizure activity, so arrange continuous electroencephalogram monitoring for intubated patients with status epilepticus.**

Administer a **benzodiazepine** (Table 135-4) as the initial treatment for status epilepticus.[11,16,17] Benzodiazepines are effective in terminating seizure activity and act by binding to gamma-aminobutyric-acid receptors[7]; they are preferred over other medications because of their rapid onset of action.[11,16] Lorazepam is generally preferred over other benzodiazepines because of its longer duration of action and some evidence that it has fewer side effects (including respiratory depression) than the other benzodiazepines.[30,31]

Generally, if two doses of benzodiazepines are administered without effect, additional doses are unlikely to be successful and increase the risk for respiratory depression.[32] Because there is no standard treatment for refractory status epilepticus, approaches to treatment and order of medication administration vary,[11,33,34] and Figure 135-3 represents one approach to refractory status epilepticus.

If a seizure persists after two doses of a benzodiazepine have been given, fosphenytoin, levetiracetam, phenobarbital, or valproic acid are preferred second-line treatment choices.[11,33,34] Currently, there are no randomized controlled trials that compare these four treatment options, but a number of small studies have shown the efficacy of each. A provider should generally choose two of the four medications for refractory status epilepticus and then move on to a fourth-line treatment option if a seizure persists. **Table 135-5** summarizes the medications used for refractory status epilepticus.

Second- and Third-Line Treatments Phenytoin and its prodrug, fosphenytoin, inhibit neuronal firing by stabilizing sodium channels and reducing neuronal calcium uptake. **Fosphenytoin** is safe and effective[11,33,34]; it can be administered more rapidly with fewer cardiac effects than phenytoin, which can precipitate in an IV line and cause significant tissue injury with extravasation.[31] Fosphenytoin is preferred as second-line treatment over phenobarbital except in neonates, mainly because it has a different mechanism of action from benzodiazepines and phenobarbital, which both bind gamma-aminobutyric-acid receptors.[11,31] Monitor serum levels in patients with renal or hepatic dysfunction.[31]

Levetiracetam is also safe and effective for treatment of status epilepticus, although it has not been prospectively compared with other anticonvulsants.[11,33-42] Levetiracetam is eliminated solely via renal excretion and has no hepatic metabolism, and it has few adverse effects and essentially no drug and food interactions.[11,33-43] Another advantage of levetiracetam over fosphenytoin (phenytoin) and phenobarbital is that it is commonly used for maintenance therapy for multiple seizure types.[39]

Phenobarbital is most commonly used in neonates who are often maintained on daily phenobarbital for subsequent seizure control.[44] Side effects include sedation and cardiorespiratory depression, which may be amplified by benzodiazepines.[4,11,33,34]

Valproic acid is approved by the U.S. Food and Drug Administration for treatment of status epilepticus and is also effective for partial and generalized seizures.[45] Consider valproic acid for treatment of children already taking this medication who are suspected of having subtherapeutic levels. Twenty to 40 milligrams/kg of IV valproic acid effectively terminates seizure activity with few side effects or less sedation.[11,33,34,45-47] Use with caution in children at risk for metabolic disease, because in rare cases it may cause hepatic failure[11,33,34] and has rarely been associated with thrombocytopenia.[33]

Fourth-Line Treatment **Propofol** is an IV anesthetic agent that acts on gamma-aminobutyric-acid receptors differently from benzodiazepines or barbiturates[34] and has been shown to effectively treat refractory status epilepticus better than pentobarbital.[34,48,49] Propofol has a rapid onset of action, but it is quickly metabolized and should be followed by continuous

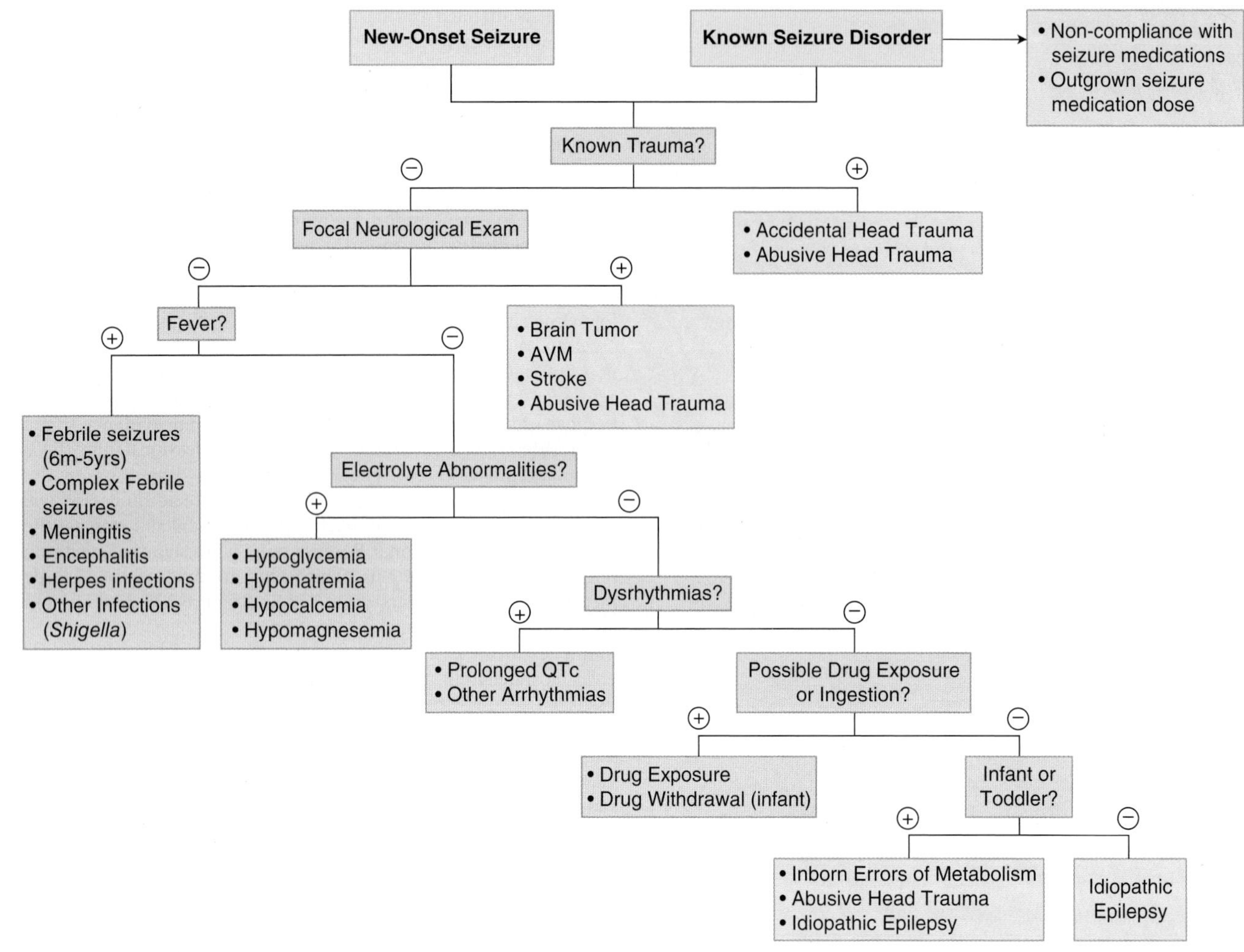

FIGURE 135-2. General approach to the evaluation of pediatric seizures. AVM = arteriovenous malformation.

infusion if seizure activity persists and must be infused slowly because of the potential for serious side effects, including bradycardia, apnea, and hypotension.[34,48] Prepare for intubation and provide continuous cardiopulmonary when administering propofol for seizures.[34,48,49] Patients receiving sustained propofol administration (>24 hours) should be monitored for development of "**propofol infusion syndrome**" (metabolic acidosis, rhabdomyolysis, renal failure, and cardiac failure).[34,50]

TABLE 135-4 Benzodiazepines for Initial Treatment of Prolonged Seizures

Drug	Route	Dose*	Maximum	Onset of Action	Duration of Action
Lorazepam	IV, IO, IN	0.1 milligram/kg	4 milligrams	1–5 min	12–24 h
	IM	0.1 milligram/kg	4 milligrams	15–30 min	12–24 h
Diazepam	IV, IO	0.1–0.3 milligram/kg	10 milligrams	1–5 min	15–60 min
	PR	0.5 milligram/kg	20 milligrams	3–5 min	15–60 min
Midazolam	IV, IO	0.1–0.2 milligram/kg	4 milligrams	1–5 min	1–6 h
	IM	0.2 milligram/kg	10 milligrams	5–15 min	1–6 h
	IN	0.2 milligram/kg	10 milligrams	1–5 min	1–6 h
	Buccal	0.5 milligram/kg	10 milligrams	3–5 min	1–6 h

Abbreviation: IN = intranasal.

*Initial and repeat dose is the same.

A "**pentobarbital coma**," or continuous infusion, has been used for refractory status epilepticus not responsive to multiple anticonvulsant treatments with reported efficacy between 74% and 100%.[34] Side effects include respiratory depression, hypotension, and decreased cardiac contractility, and most patients require intubation and inotropic support.[34]

Midazolam infusion has a low rate of adverse effects; however, compared with propofol and pentobarbital, midazolam has a higher rate of seizure recurrence.[34]

Treatment of Glucose and Electrolyte Abnormalities Most laboratory results are not immediately available when treating status epilepticus. Abnormal glucose, sodium, calcium, and magnesium, especially low levels, can cause seizures. Seizures caused by abnormal electrolytes respond poorly to conventional medication but do respond to replacement electrolyte therapy.

Hypoglycemia Hypoglycemia can be the cause or an effect of prolonged seizures, and bedside testing is essential in seizing patients. Treat hypoglycemia with a rapid infusion of 2 mL/kg of 25% dextrose in water or 5 mL/kg of 10% dextrose in water.[7]

Hyponatremia Hyponatremia (serum sodium <135 mEq/L) is most commonly seen in infants <6 months of age and sometimes in athletes and can cause seizures, especially if the serum sodium is <120 mEq/L. The goal of therapy is to correct the level to >120 mEq/L quickly and then correct to normal levels over the next 24 hours (see chapter 129, Fluid and Electrolyte Therapy in Infants and Children). Treat the seizing patient with hyponatremia with 3% NaCl 4 to 6 mL/kg over 20 minutes, or

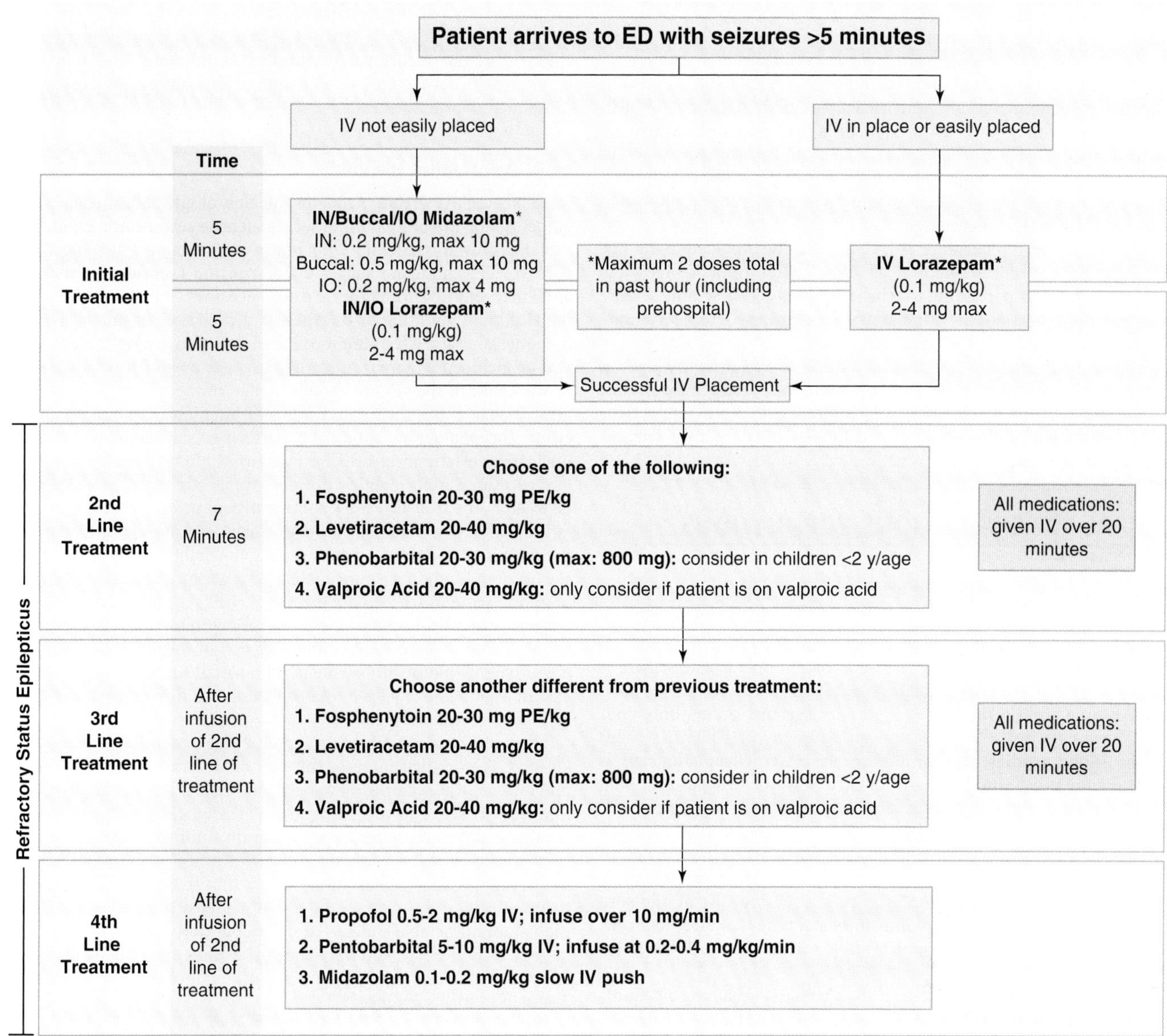

FIGURE 135-3. Initial treatment of status epilepticus: an example of one approach. IN = intranasal; PE = phenytoin sodium equivalents.

begin an infusion of 20 mL/kg of 0.9% NaCl if 3% NaCl is not immediately available. The sodium level should be rechecked after the bolus to determine whether a second bolus is necessary.[6]

Hypocalcemia Hypocalcemia is more common in neonates and young infants and may be associated with congenital anomalies such as DiGeorge's syndrome. Calcium gluconate 0.3 mL/kg over 5 to 10 minutes is preferred over calcium chloride when infusing through a small peripheral IV, as calcium chloride can cause local irritation.[6]

Hypomagnesemia Treat hypomagnesemia (serum magnesium <1.5 mEq/L) with magnesium sulfate 50 milligrams/kg IV infused over 20 minutes.

DISPOSITION AND FOLLOW-UP

Infants >6 months of age with febrile seizures (see later) and children with single seizures lasting <15 minutes who return to baseline mental status and have no focal neurologic deficits or secondary cause of seizure requiring

TABLE 135-5 Medications for Refractory Status Epilepticus

Drug	Route	Loading Dose	Repeat Dose	Maximum	IV Infusion
Fosphenytoin	IV, IM	20–30 milligrams/kg PE	5–10 milligrams/kg PE	30 milligrams/kg PE	3 milligrams/kg/min PE
Phenobarbital	IV	20–30 milligrams/kg	5–10 milligrams/kg	40 milligrams/kg	1–30 milligrams/min
Valproic acid	IV	20–40 milligrams/kg	15–20 milligrams/kg	40 milligrams/kg	5 milligrams/kg/h
Levetiracetam	IV	20–60 milligrams/kg	—	3 grams	—
Pentobarbital	IV	5–10 milligrams/kg	1–2 milligrams/kg	15 milligrams/kg	0.5–5.0 milligrams/kg/h
Propofol	IV	0.5–2.0 milligrams/kg	0.5–1.0 milligram/kg	5 milligrams/kg	1.5–4.0 milligrams/kg/h
Midazolam	IV	0.1–0.2 milligram/kg	0.1–0.2 milligram/kg	10 milligrams	0.05–0.4 milligram/kg/h

Abbreviation: PE = phenytoin sodium equivalents.

ongoing treatment are candidates for discharge and outpatient follow-up with their primary care provider or a pediatric neurologist (in the case of new-onset seizures or breakthrough seizures in children with epilepsy).

Parents of discharged children should be given guidance to prevent injury in association with subsequent seizures: children should not be in a position where they could drown, fall, or injure someone else during a seizure. Caregivers should never allow their children to bathe or swim alone. If they are old enough to take a shower, children should not lock the bathroom door. Those old enough to drive should not be allowed to do so until cleared by a neurologist.

Information about recurrence risk should also be provided in the ED. Although the recurrence risk for a particular child cannot be predicted, population statistics pertaining to febrile seizures and first-time seizure recurrence can be shared with parents (see Special Considerations/Populations, next).

Children with prolonged seizures requiring ED treatment who stop seizing should be observed for 24 hours and monitored for recurrence or side effects from medication. All children with status epilepticus require admission to the hospital, and those with refractory seizures require intensive care.

SPECIAL CONSIDERATIONS/POPULATIONS

FEBRILE SEIZURES

Febrile seizures are common in the general pediatric population, with an incidence of 2% to 5%.

Simple Febrile Seizures The definition of a simple febrile seizure is a generalized tonic-clonic seizure lasting <15 minutes with a fever 38°C (100.4°F) in a child 6 months to 5 years of age that occurs only once in a 24-hour period.[51,52] The American Academy of Pediatrics holds that **no blood studies, neuroimaging, or electroencephalogram is necessary for most simple febrile seizures** and the evaluation should focus on identifying the source of fever (e.g., urinalysis and culture).[51-54] The American Academy of Pediatrics does recommend that a lumbar puncture be strongly considered in these children when there are clinical signs or symptoms that suggest meningitis or intracranial infection. **Consider lumbar puncture for infants 6 to 12 months of age who are unimmunized for *Haemophilus influenza* type B or streptococcus pneumonia and those taking antibiotics, which can mask the signs and symptoms of meningitis.**[51,52]

Parents of children experiencing a simple febrile seizure need education regarding the natural history of febrile seizures. Only 50% of children <12 months and 30% of children >12 months will have another simple febrile seizure.[54] Having a febrile seizure does not mean that a child will develop epilepsy. In fact, children who experience a simple febrile seizure have roughly the same 1% risk as the general population of developing epilepsy by the age of 7 years. Factors that increase that risk to 2% to 4% include a family history of seizures, multiple febrile seizures, and first febrile seizure before 12 months of age. Other factors that increase the risk of recurrence include developmental delay, focal seizures, Todd's paralysis, focal neurologic findings on examination, and abnormal findings on electroencephalogram, CT, or MRI.[54]

Complex Febrile Seizures Complex febrile seizures are defined as seizures with fever that last >15 minutes, that recur within a 24-hour period, are focal, or occur in children <6 months or >5 years of age without any signs of serious infection.[51,54] **Routine blood tests and imaging are not indicated, even in the setting of complex febrile seizure, if the child returns to baseline in the ED.** Consider lumbar puncture for prolonged febrile seizures: one study noted that children with fever and seizures lasting >30 minutes had a significantly higher incidence of bacterial meningitis (15% to 18%) than children with simple febrile seizures (0.4% to 1.2%)[55]; another study, however, found only two patients with meningitis among 526 complex febrile seizures, and both had clinical signs and symptoms of meningitis.[56]

Children with a prolonged seizure associated with a fever who appear ill should undergo evaluation to rule out serious bacterial infection in the blood and cerebrospinal fluid,[29,56] although parenteral antibiotics should not be delayed while sick children are being evaluated.[55]

Treatment of Febrile Seizure Anticonvulsant therapy is not recommended for simple febrile seizures since side effects outweigh the minor risks of seizure recurrence.[54] Although antipyretics are indicated in children with fever, there is no evidence that antipyretics can prevent subsequent febrile seizures.[54,57]

FIRST AFEBRILE SEIZURE

In 2000, the American Academy of Neurology published a practice guideline for the evaluation of a first afebrile seizure in a child, which pertains only to the child who returns to baseline following the seizure.[58,59] The guideline suggests that **routine laboratory evaluations and emergent neuroimaging are not necessary**. If there is evidence that the child had vomiting or diarrhea, is dehydrated, or fails to return to baseline, laboratory tests are recommended. A toxicology screen should also be included if there is concern for drug exposure or substance abuse or the cause of the seizure cannot be determined. Lumbar puncture is unnecessary unless there is a concern for meningitis or encephalitis. An electroencephalogram should be performed, although the timing is unclear: an electroencephalogram within 24 hours of the seizure is most likely to show abnormalities; however, an electroencephalogram within 24 to 48 hours may also show some transient postictal slowing.

Indications for emergent head CT include children with a condition predisposing them to intracranial abnormalities, those with focal seizures, and children younger than 33 months of age with new-onset seizures.[9] Patients who do not meet the criteria for high risk and are well appearing may be discharged with outpatient follow-up. Outpatient MRI should be considered in any child with any of the following: significant cognitive or motor impairment, abnormal findings on neurologic examination, abnormal electroencephalogram findings, partial seizure, or infants <1 year of age.[58,59]

The overall risk of recurrence after a single afebrile seizure is about 40%.[58-60] Factors that increase this risk are a family history of seizures, previous febrile seizures, developmental delay, abnormal CT or MRI findings, presence of focal deficits on neurologic examination, Todd's paralysis, abnormal electroencephalogram findings, and seizure occurring during sleep.[58,59] Most neurologists do not recommend initiating daily anticonvulsant medications after a first seizure.[59] Noninitiation of treatment does not increase the risk of epilepsy, prognosis, or increase the risk of intractable epilepsy or death, but does allow the physician to better clarify the type and frequency of seizures and also avoids the side effects of unnecessary daily anticonvulsant medications in those not destined to for recurrence.[58-60]

NEONATAL SEIZURES

Neonates do not have a fully developed neurologic system, and seizures in this age group can be subtle, are more likely to be focal, and often carry a poor prognosis.[44] Seizures occur in 1.4% of full-term infants and 20% of premature infants.

Identifying seizure activity in the neonate and distinguishing it from normal newborn myoclonus and jitters can be challenging. Subtle focal movements or stereotyped activities (e.g., lip smacking, eye deviation, or bicycling) may represent seizure activity; neonates less often have generalized tonic-clonic seizures.[44] Apparent life-threatening events with pallor or cyanosis and a change in muscle tone may be a manifestation of seizure activity.

A birth and maternal history may identify risks for congenital or neonatal infection (e.g., herpes simplex virus, cytomegalovirus, or group B streptococci) or potential withdrawal from maternal narcotics.[44] Complications with labor and delivery may suggest birth asphyxia with subsequent seizures. Regardless of the history or presence of fever, neonates with witnessed seizures require extensive evaluation. Obtain cultures of blood, urine, and cerebrospinal fluid and test for herpes simplex virus and begin empiric parenteral antibiotics and acyclovir. Toxicologic evaluation may provide the physician with evidence of withdrawal or overdose of abused substances. Neonates with seizures are more likely to have electrolyte abnormalities than older children, and electrolytes including calcium and glucose should be measured. Consider head CT for concerns of nonaccidental trauma, intracranial hemorrhage, infarction,

TABLE 135-6 List of Anticonvulsants Commonly Used in Children

Standard seizure medications used in children
Phenobarbital
Phenytoin (Dilantin®)
Carbamazepine (Tegretol®, Carbatrol®)
Valproic acid (Depakote®, Depakene®)
Newer seizure medications used in children (blood levels not obtainable in ED setting)
Gabapentin (Neurontin®), 1993
Lamotrigine (Lamictal®), 1994
Topiramate (Topamax®), 1996
Levetiracetam (Keppra®), 1999
Oxcarbazepine (Trileptal®), 2000
Zonisamide (Zonegran®), 2000

or mass (even without external signs of injury). Finally, if inborn errors of metabolism are suspected, obtain serum levels of lactate and ammonia, as well as serum amino acids and urine organic acids (see chapter 144, Metabolic Emergencies in Infants and Children).[38] All neonates with witnessed seizure require admission to the hospital.

Treat the actively seizing neonate with benzodiazepines as with older children; consider phenobarbital for second-line therapy. Identify and treat hypoglycemia and electrolyte abnormalities.

SEIZURES IN CHILDREN WITH EPILEPSY

Parents, old records, and pediatric neurologists can be very helpful in identifying past causes of seizures, successful (and unsuccessful) treatments, and other issues that can help direct the care of patients with epilepsy presenting to the ED with seizure. **Table 135-6** lists common anticonvulsants prescribed for children with epilepsy. Subtherapeutic drug levels may result when a child outgrows a previously prescribed dose, vomits medications due to an intercurrent illness, starts a new medication (due to changes in drug pharmacokinetics from drug interactions), or does not adhere to the original drug regimen. Subtherapeutic drug levels are a common cause of breakthrough seizures, and serum levels of home antiepileptic medications should be checked as part of the routine ED evaluation of these patients, although results may not be readily available for some newer agents. When low levels are identified, the cause should be determined so that proper adjustments in daily anticonvulsant dosing can be made with advice from the patient's neurologist.

Children with epilepsy may have a lower seizure threshold with febrile illness, even with therapeutic anticonvulsant levels, and the ED evaluation in these situations may be limited to determining the source of fever. Lumbar puncture is unnecessary unless there are clinical signs or symptoms of meningitis.

SEIZURES IN CHILDREN WITH VENTRICULOPERITONEAL SHUNTS

Many children with ventriculoperitoneal shunts also have a medical history of seizures. Considerations include underlying epilepsy, shunt malfunction, and central nervous system infection. The standard approach to the evaluation for a shunt malfunction consists of a radiographic ventriculoperitoneal shunt series and a head CT or "quick brain MRI" to evaluate for increased ventricular size. If central nervous system infection is a concern, a pediatric neurosurgeon should be consulted and the shunt tapped for cerebrospinal fluid analysis and culture. Seizures in children with ventriculoperitoneal shunts are more likely to be related to shunt infection than to mechanical shunt malfunction, especially if associated with fever,[61] and the risk of infection increases in children with a history of a prior shunt infections.[62] In most cases, consulting past medical records, parents, and the neurosurgeon who placed the shunt is needed for prudent decision making.

SEIZURES IN TRAUMA

"Impact seizures" (seizures that occur within minutes of head trauma) do not, by themselves, increase the risk of having an intracranial injury; seizures that occur in a more delayed fashion, however, are more indicative of severe injuries. Guidelines for the ED evaluation and management of head injury increasingly focus on strategies for risk stratification in order to avoid the potential long-term effects of ionizing radiation and are discussed in detail in chapter 138, Head Injury in Infants and Children. Children with identified intracranial injury and a witnessed seizure should be treated with a loading dose of antiepileptic medication, typically fosphenytoin 20 milligrams/kg IV, to prevent short-term recurrence that can worsen traumatic brain injury and increase intracranial pressure; benzodiazepines remain first-line treatment for active seizures in the setting of trauma.

Abusive Head Trauma Infants and toddlers presenting with vague complaints and seizures may be the victims of abusive head trauma (see chapter 110, Pediatric Trauma), which can present without external signs of injury. Most children with abusive head trauma are <2 years of age, and the majority occur in the first year of life (shaken baby syndrome).[63,64] Subdural hematoma is the most often identified inflicted intracranial injury in these infants. **Maintain a high index of suspicion for trauma in the setting of afebrile seizures in infants.** If intracranial injury is identified, a more complete evaluation for other abusive injuries is necessary, including skeletal survey, retinal examination by an ophthalmologist, screening for blunt abdominal trauma (liver and pancreatic enzymes), and bleeding studies.[63]

Acknowledgments: The author gratefully acknowledges the contributions of Michael A. Nigro, MD, the author of this chapter in the previous edition; Dr. Nanette Dudley, MD (Pediatric Emergency Medicine, University of Utah), Dr. Jeff Schunk, MD (Pediatric Emergency Medicine, University of Utah), Dr. Kim Statler, MD (Pediatric Intensive Care, University of Utah), and Pamela Carpenter, graphic design specialist.

REFERENCES

The complete reference list is available online at www.TintinalliEM.com.

Headache in Children

David C. Sheridan
Garth Meckler

INTRODUCTION AND EPIDEMIOLOGY

Headache is pain in the scalp and cranium. Headaches in children can be mild, refractory, or life threatening, and can represent an acute, subacute, or chronic process. Sustained or recurrent headaches can greatly impact school performance and may even induce behavioral disturbances.[1] Headache accounts for approximately 1% of all pediatric ED visits.[2,3] Headaches increase in prevalence as a child ages; 30% to 60% of children through adolescence experience headaches.[4,5] The most common causes of headache are viral and respiratory illnesses (28.5%),[2,6] posttraumatic headache (20%), possible ventriculoperitoneal shunt malfunction (11.5%), and migraine (8.5%).[3] Serious causes of headache are reported in 4% to 6.9% of children and include subdural hematoma, epidural hematoma, proven ventriculoperitoneal shunt malfunction, brain abscess, pseudotumor cerebri, and aseptic meningitis.[2,3] Factors correlated with dangerous conditions include preschool age, recent onset of pain, occipital location, and the child's inability to describe the quality of the headache. Emergent neurosurgical conditions in children with headache are generally predicted by the presence of focal neurologic signs.[7]

PATHOPHYSIOLOGY

The pathophysiology of headaches is complex and varies according to cause. The cranium, most of the overlying meninges, brain, ependymal lining, and choroid plexus do not possess pain receptors.[6,8,9] Extracranial pain may arise from cervical nerve roots, cranial nerves, or extracranial arteries, and intracranial pain may arise from intracranial venous, arterial, or dural structures. Cranial nerve or root pain can radiate to the occiput, ear, retroauricular areas, or throat.[9,10]

HEADACHE CLASSIFICATION

Headaches are classified as primary or secondary based on the underlying cause. **Primary headaches** are physiologic or functional and are typically self-limited. They are often recurrent and are usually associated with normal findings on physical examination. Their diagnosis is typically based on recurrent symptoms, and they include migraine, tension, cluster, and chronic daily headaches. Migraine headaches are common and account for about 75% of primary pediatric headache disorders seen in the ED.[7]

Specific underlying causes are identifiable for **secondary headaches** (**Table 136-1**), which are usually, but not always, anatomic in nature. Causes include brain tumors, vascular malformations, and intracranial abscesses; craniofacial problems, such as sinusitis, dental abscesses, or otitis; systemic disorders, such as lupus cerebritis; and exposure to toxic substances, such as carbon monoxide, lead, or cocaine. Although primary headaches can be disabling, secondary headaches result in morbidity and mortality if not treated.

The International Headache Society provides one method for headache classification (http://ihs-classification.org/en/). **Table 136-2** associates temporal patterns of headache with possible diagnoses.

HISTORICAL FEATURES

Obtain a thorough history from all possible sources (child, parents, and other caretakers available) in order to help identify or exclude more worrisome secondary causes of headache (Table 136-1). Enquire about the child's personal and family medical histories. Elicit characteristic features of the headache. Obtain details as to whether the child or family has a history of headaches and whether the current headache is similar to past attacks.

TABLE 136-1 Features Suggesting Secondary Headache

Historical Description	Physical Findings
Abrupt onset	Altered mental status
First or worst ever	Septic or toxic appearance
Posttraumatic	External evidence of head trauma
Awakens from sleep	Bradycardia, hypertension, or irregular respirations
Present with fever or a stiff neck	
Aggravated by sneezing, coughing, Valsalva maneuver, lying down	Diaphoresis
	Facial herpes zoster
Vomiting and/or worsening pain in the morning	Petechiae
	Café au lait or ash-leaf spots
Altered mental status or focal neurologic symptoms	Asymmetry of pupillary response
	Ptosis
Change in behavior	Visual field defect
Change in pattern (if chronic) or worsening over time	Retinal hemorrhage or optic disc distortion
Toxic exposure	Asymmetry of motor or sensory responses
Family history of subarachnoid hemorrhage	Thyromegaly
	Nuchal rigidity
	Head tilt

TABLE 136-2 Temporal Patterns of Headache in Children

Type	Temporal Pattern	Causes
Acute headache	Single episode of head pain without history of previous events	Upper respiratory tract infection, sinusitis, first migraine, medication use, trauma
Acute recurrent headache	Pattern of head pain separated by symptom-free intervals	Migraine
Chronic progressive headache	Gradual increase in frequency and severity; may be worse in the morning or awaken at night	Space-occupying lesion, hematoma, pseudotumor cerebri
Chronic nonprogressive headache (chronic daily)	Frequent or constant headache	Tension headache, cluster headache
Mixed headache	Acute recurrent headache superimposed on chronic daily background pattern; variant of chronic daily headache	Typically migraine (acute recurrent headache) superimposed on chronic daily headache

AGE OF FIRST OCCURRENCE OR PATTERN OF PREVIOUS OCCURRENCES

The prevalence of migraine headaches increases with the child's age, and a pattern of prior occurrences suggests primary headache.[3,4,11] Although migraine headaches are unusual in preschool-age or younger children (<5 years old), they are becoming increasingly recognized in this young age group.[12] Complex migraines (hemiplegic, confusional, or basilar type) may have their onset at a young age as well; however, *incapacitating headache* in a young child, especially when associated with vomiting or gait changes, suggests an intracranial mass with an infratentorial location being the most common location.[13] **Predictors of a surgical space-occupying lesion include headache of <6 months' duration, sleep-related headache, vomiting, confusion, absence of visual symptoms, absence of family history of migraine, and abnormal findings on neurologic examination.**[14]

HEADACHE PRECIPITANTS

Viral illnesses and fever are among the most common causes of headache in children, and the associated headaches are most frequently frontal or temporal.[2,6,8] A history of trauma may suggest posttraumatic headache or traumatic brain injury. Posttraumatic headaches may be chronic as well.[15] Migraines, more common and better studied in adults and adolescents, may be accompanied by premonitory symptoms (prodromes such as fatigue, mood changes, or GI symptoms) and have identifiable triggers.[16] Children with prodromes tend to have more characteristic triggers as a whole, which may include specific foods (e.g., chocolate or monosodium glutamate), stress, light, specific odors, and weather changes.[8,12] Headaches are among the most commonly reported symptoms in toxic exposures such as carbon monoxide poisoning.[17] Additional precipitants include medications (e.g., methylphenidate, steroids, oral contraceptives, and anticonvulsants), infection (e.g., sinusitis, pharyngitis, or meningitis), hypertension, anemia, and substance abuse (e.g., cocaine).[18]

TIME AND MODE OF ONSET

Headache coinciding with the onset of fever suggests inflammation of some sort, typically infectious (e.g., sinusitis, pharyngitis, otitis, or meningitis), or may be associated with a more general viral syndrome. **Abrupt occurrence of severe headache due to a serious underlying condition, such as a brain tumor or intracranial hemorrhage, is typically associated with one or more objective findings on neurologic examination (e.g., altered mental status, ataxia, nuchal rigidity, papilledema, or hemiparesis).**[7,8] Cluster headaches also tend to develop acutely, whereas tension headaches have a more subacute onset. Hormonal cycles can trigger migraine headaches in adolescent females. **Migraine headaches in children typically start relatively abruptly,**

intensify over several minutes, and then reach full intensity in about an hour.[19] Young children often have headaches that begin in the late afternoon.

LOCATION OF HEADACHE

In a cohort of children with headaches presenting to a pediatric ED, only 27.5% of patients could identify a precise location of the pain. Among children with intracranial diseases, most either were unable to indicate the location of the pain or had an occipital headache.[7,20] Medications, hypertension, and basilar-type migraines can also cause headaches in the occipital region. Pain at the vertex can be seen with sphenoid sinusitis. Ethmoid, maxillary, and frontal sinus infections tend to cause retro-orbital pain, as does meningitis (along with fever and neck stiffness) and dural sinus thrombosis. Pain seemingly in, around, or in front of the ear (or entire temporal region) is often seen with temporomandibular joint dysfunction and can be reproducible on exam. **Migraine headaches are usually unilateral and involve the frontal or temporal region in adolescents. However, in younger children, they are usually bifrontal or generalized. Only about a third of children have unilateral migraines.**[19] Tension headaches tend to have the greatest variability in location. They may be generalized, frontal, or even occipital/posterior cervical. **Occipital location in children is a red flag that should be investigated further before attributing to a primary headache disorder.**

QUALITY OF HEADACHE

Younger children and many developmentally normal, otherwise healthy children may have a difficult time describing the quality of their headaches. An ability to describe pain quality or a description of the headache as having a pulsating quality is more frequently associated with benign headaches. An inability to describe the pain or a description of the headache as constrictive indicates a greater likelihood of a more serious cause.[7,8,20] Many different qualities of pain can be identified: stabbing or hyperesthetic pain has been associated with herpes zoster; aching pain with tension headaches, meningitis, or encephalitis; and constant pain with sinusitis in all locations. A pulsating quality is one of the diagnostic criteria for migraine headache set forth by the International Headache Society but can also be seen with headaches caused by hypertension or intracerebral hemorrhage.[21] The International Headache Society criteria for migraine were developed for the adult population, but children present differently. In particular children, may have shorter headaches and in different locations. Diagnostic criteria for pediatric migraine are presented in **Tables 136-3 and 136-4.**[22] **Although these diagnostic criteria rely on recurrent attacks, in an ED, a child may present with a first migraine headache due to intractable pain.** One study investigated the utility of applying the International Headache Society criteria in the ED without the "recurrent" requirement ("Irma Criteria") and found the criteria to be quite sensitive in diagnosing first-time migraines when followed long term using the original International Headache Society criteria as the gold standard.[23]

TABLE 136-3 Diagnostic Criteria for Pediatric Migraine Headache without Aura

I	At least 5 attacks with features (II–IV) below
II	Headache between 1 and 48 h
III	At least 2 of the following: Bilateral or unilateral location (not to include posterior location) Pulsating Moderate-to-severe pain Made worse with activity
IV	At least one associated symptom: Nausea/vomiting Photophobia/phonophobia

TABLE 136-4 Diagnostic Criteria for Pediatric Migraine Headache with Aura

I	At least 2 attacks with features below
II	At least 3 of the following: Gradual development of autonomic aura Aura that is fully reversible Aura is present less than 1 h Headache within 1 h of aura

SEVERITY OF HEADACHE

The severity of a headache is neither a sensitive nor a specific characteristic in determining cause. Patients with tension headaches can complain of terrible pain, whereas a child with a brain tumor may complain of mild to moderate pain. Nonetheless, complaints of very intense pain should be taken seriously and assessed in context with other historical elements.[7] Ask about and document presenting pain assessments in children with primary headache disorders because treatment end points will be dictated by improved pain scores in the ED.

DURATION OF HEADACHE

Although the duration of a headache is not particularly useful in assessing the majority of headaches, the International Headache Society definition of migraines requires a duration of symptoms of 4 to 72 hours[21] in adults, but the duration may be less (1 to 48 hours)[22] in children (Tables 136-3 and 136-4). A migraine that lasts >72 hours is known as *status migrainosus*. Children can sometimes come to the ED with this condition and should be treated appropriately.

ALLEVIATING AND EXACERBATING FACTORS

Patients with a sense of restlessness or agitation are more likely to have cluster headaches (more rare in children; **Table 136-5**).[21] They may pace about the room or rock back and forth in a chair. In contrast, patients with migraines typically prefer silence and darkness because the lack of stimulation provides some relief, and photophobia/phonophobia are part of the diagnostic criteria for migraine headache (Table 136-3).[21,22] Tension headaches can be frequent and frustrating but tend *not* to be aggravated by routine physical activity (**Table 136-6**).[21] Positional preferences (such as a head tilt) may be noted in children with space-occupying lesions, in order to avoid positions that increase intracranial pressure or exacerbate diplopia caused by cranial nerve dysfunction. In addition, children with increased intracranial pressure may be unable to look up or may avoid the Valsalva maneuver (e.g., defecation or coughing). Analgesic rebound headaches worsen when the patient goes a certain period of time without taking long-term pain medication or overuses analgesics.

TABLE 136-5 International Headache Society Diagnostic Criteria for Cluster Headache[24]

At least five attacks of headache fulfilling the following criteria:

1. Severe or very severe unilateral orbital, supraorbital, and/or temporal pain lasting 15–180 min if untreated
2. Headache is accompanied by at least one of the following:
   a. Ipsilateral conjunctival injection and/or lacrimation
   b. Ipsilateral nasal congestion and/or rhinorrhea
   c. Ipsilateral eyelid edema
   d. Ipsilateral forehead and facial sweating
   e. Ipsilateral miosis and/or ptosis
   f. A sense of restlessness or agitation
3. Attacks have a frequency from one every other day to eight per day
4. Not attributed to another disorder

TABLE 136-6 International Headache Society Diagnostic Criteria for Tension Headache[24]

Infrequent episodic—at least 10 episodes occurring on <1 d per month on average (<12 d per year) fulfilling criteria 1–4

Or

Frequent episodic—at least 10 episodes occurring on ≥1 but <15 d per month for at least 3 mo (≥12 and <180 d per year) fulfilling criteria 1–4

1. Headache lasting from 30 min to 7 d
2. Headache has at least two of the following characteristics:
   a. Bilateral location
   b. Pressure or tightening (nonpulsating quality)
   c. Mild or moderate intensity
   d. Not aggravated by routine physical activity such as walking or climbing stairs
3. Both of the following:
   a. No nausea or vomiting (anorexia may occur)
   b. No more than one of photophobia or phonophobia
4. Not attributed to another disorder

ASSOCIATED SYMPTOMS

Eliciting associated symptoms can help narrow the differential diagnosis. Migraine headache with aura, by definition, is associated with visual, sensory, or speech disturbances (all fully reversible; Table 136-4).[22] Specific symptomatology may distinguish between types of migraines such as confusional (e.g., distortions of visual size, space, or time) and hemiplegic (e.g., transient hemiparesis or aphasia). Hemiplegic migraines are uncommon, so think carefully about other causes of neurologic deficits when contemplating the differential diagnosis. Abdominal pain, nausea, or vomiting may occur along with migraine headache.[10] Cluster headaches can be associated with multiple ipsilateral symptoms (Table 136-5).[21] Headache with effortless vomiting but no GI complaints is characteristic of elevated intracranial pressure.[7] Irreversible and progressive defects in visual acuity and diplopia are more suggestive of pseudotumor cerebri. Seizures and headache may indicate traumatic brain injury, concussion, arteriovenous malformation, subarachnoid hemorrhage, or tumor. A headache with fever and focal neurologic signs (with or without seizure) may suggest an intracranial abscess, encephalitis, or meningitis (especially with neck stiffness). Children who present with headache, altered mental status, and seizures must be evaluated for meningoencephalitis from herpes simplex virus.[25]

MEDICAL HISTORY

Headaches should be considered both independently and within the context of the child's medical history because secondary headaches can occur even when there is a history of primary headaches. It is helpful if a child has a history of similar headaches, but a first-time headache does not preclude a primary headache disorder as described previously.[23] Concurrent chronic illness may predispose the patient to unique headaches (e.g., those associated with ventriculoperitoneal shunt malfunction or infection), headaches from infection (e.g., related to anatomic defects predisposing to meningitis or acute illness with sinusitis leading to brain abscess), or headaches caused by intracranial hemorrhage (e.g., due to hemophilia or anatomic arteriovenous anomalies). Although the ED is a location for acute care, taking a history regarding psychological factors can be important, because children have been shown to have psychosomatic headaches as well.[26]

FAMILY HISTORY

Headaches occur more often in children who have a family history of headaches in either first- or second-degree relatives.[27] This association is particularly true for children with migraines (family history of migraines in up to 90% of cases). Children with cluster headaches rarely have a family history of similar headaches (about 7%). Children with a parent who experienced a subarachnoid hemorrhage are at a four times greater risk of this type of intracranial bleed than the general population. Predisposing genetic disorders may provide some clue to a familial link in headaches (e.g., bleeding diathesis, familial dyslipidemias, or atherosclerotic events).

TABLE 136-7 Factors Associated with the Occurrence of Benign or Life-Threatening Headache

Factor	Benign	Life-Threatening
Age	School	Preschool
Location of pain	Unilateral/bilateral, frontal, or temporal region	Cannot be described or occipital region
Quality of pain	Can be described or pulsating	Cannot be described or constrictive
Intensity of pain	From slight to intense	Very intense
Associated neurologic signs	None	Focal neurologic deficits, papilledema, ataxia, altered mental status

PHYSICAL EXAMINATION

The physical examination and history will help to distinguish benign from life-threatening headaches (**Table 136-7**). However, examination findings may be normal even if the history suggests a secondary headache. A careful neurologic examination with attention to cranial nerves, gait, strength, and mental status is essential to exclude secondary headache (**Table 136-8**). Focal neurologic findings or gait instability are associated with secondary causes of headache. Additional examination clues to secondary headache are listed in Table 136-8.

DIAGNOSIS

No specific laboratory testing or radiologic imaging is needed for primary headache because the diagnosis is clinical and made by history. **Imaging studies are not needed for primary headache when the findings of the neurologic examination are normal.** Despite the importance of history and examination, one study reported that almost 40% of all children with headache who were evaluated in the ED underwent head imaging with radiation.[28]

If secondary headache is a consideration, obtain laboratory evaluation and imaging dictated by results of the history and physical examination. Blood tests that may be useful in specific clinical situations include CBC, serum glucose level, electrolyte levels, renal function tests, liver function tests, blood culture, and drug screen. Perform a lumbar puncture if meningitis or encephalitis is suspected, and send cerebrospinal fluid for Gram stain, culture, appropriate viral studies, glucose, protein, and cell count. If pseudotumor cerebri is suspected, perform a lumbar puncture with the patient in the lateral decubitus position and measure the opening pressure. A lumbar puncture may also be needed to rule out a subarachnoid hemorrhage if there is a high level of suspicion but the findings of a CT scan of the brain are normal.[29,30] Focal neurologic deficits or signs of increased intracranial pressure warrant a CT scan prior to lumbar puncture; however, clinical signs of probable impending herniation are the best indicators of when to delay a lumbar puncture, even in the setting of normal CT scan results.[31]

IMAGING

Consider imaging in children with abnormal findings on neurologic examination, altered mental status, or concurrent seizures, or if medical history indicates the recent onset of severe (worst) headache,

TABLE 136-8 Physical Examination Findings Associated with Potential Secondary Causes of Headache

Examination Component	Finding	Potential Causes
Growth parameters	Abnormal height, weight, head circumference for age	Failure to thrive indicative of systemic disease; enlarged head circumference suggestive of increased intracranial pressure
Vital signs	Abnormal heart rate, blood pressure, respiratory rate, temperature	Bradycardia, hypertension, and irregular respirations (Cushing's triad) indicative of intracranial hypertension and impending herniation; severe hypertension associated with headache in hypertensive crisis; tachypnea possibly indicative of metabolic acidosis (e.g., diabetic ketoacidosis); fever possibly indicative of CNS or systemic infection (meningitis, encephalitis, viral syndrome)
Head and neck	Cranial or carotid bruits	Arteriovenous malformation
	Bulging fontanelle	Hydrocephalus
	Signs of trauma	Accidental or nonaccidental trauma
Eyes	Papilledema	Increased intracranial pressure (pseudotumor, tumor, shunt failure, intracranial bleeding, hydrocephalus)
	Inability to look up: "sunset eyes"	Hydrocephalus
	Unilateral conjunctival injection, tearing, eyelid edema without tenderness	Cluster headache
	Retinal hemorrhage	Nonaccidental trauma
	Bilateral periorbital edema, facial tenderness, nasal discharge	Sinusitis
Ear, nose, throat	Signs of infection	Otitis media, mastoiditis, sinusitis, pharyngitis (including streptococcal pharyngitis), dental abscess or caries
	Malocclusion, TMJ tenderness	TMJ dysfunction
Heart	Murmurs	Potential shunting lesion with risk of embolic event or cerebral abscess
Skin	Café au lait spots, ash-leaf spots, vascular malformations	Neurofibromatosis, tuberous sclerosis, congenital vascular malformations (risk for CNS hemorrhage)

Abbreviation: TMJ = temporomandibular joint.

a change in the type of headache, or associated features that suggest neurologic dysfunction.[10,32-34] There is a very low incidence of positive findings on neuroimaging studies in children with headache who have normal findings on physical examination.[35-39] Imaging is not indicated in children with recurrent headaches and normal findings on neurologic examination.

CT Scan Reserve CT scans for instances in which there is a highly suspicious history, neurologic findings on examination are abnormal, or an intracranial hemorrhage or a space-occupying lesion is suspected. Noncontrast head CT is sensitive for detecting skull fracture and brain injury from trauma and may identify supratentorial tumors and stroke; give IV contrast if considering intracranial abscess.

MRI A normal head CT does not exclude an intracranial mass because the posterior fossa is not well visualized. The posterior fossa is the most common location of brain tumors in children, and MRI of the brain provides better visualization of the posterior fossa. Magnetic resonance angiography and venography are useful when vascular malformations or dural sinus thrombosis is suspected. MRI may require sedation based on the patient's age. The decision to admit a child for MRI or to obtain outpatient imaging depends on the practice location and deserves a discussion with an inpatient team as well as primary care provider.

TREATMENT

Treatment recommendations vary greatly because few evidence-based data on treatment efficacy are available.[40,41] Treat the underlying cause of secondary headache and provide analgesia for pain. Almost 30% of children presenting with headache to the ED receive opioid medications in the United States.[28] **Do not use narcotics for primary headaches.** Long-term use of narcotics can change the pain-modulatory system in the brainstem and can lead to more intense pain.

PHARMACOLOGIC TREATMENT OF PRIMARY HEADACHES

Table 136-9 lists treatment options for migraine and cluster headache treatment in the ED. Both are initially treated in the same fashion. A recent review of the available evidence in pediatric migraine suggests a treatment algorithm with dopamine antagonists and nonsteroidal anti-inflammatory agents (**Table 136-10**).[41]

The most widely studied abortive medications are the dopamine antagonists, prochlorperazine and metoclopramide. These drugs can cause dystonic or extrapyramidal reactions, which are relieved by diphenhydramine.[42,43] A second class of medications that are well studied are nonsteroidal anti-inflammatory agents, including ketorolac. Ketorolac may not be used if the patient has acutely taken a nonsteroidal anti-inflammatory agent within 6 hours. When compared to dopamine antagonists, ketorolac appears to be less effective than prochlorperazine.[44]

Other options for abortive migraine therapy include the triptans, which may be given orally, intranasally, and subcutaneously. As with most pediatric migraine medications, treatment is "off-label," but a limited number of triptan agents have received Food and Drug Administration approval in adolescents. Dihydroergotamine is effective in the inpatient setting, but no studies exist on ED treatment.[45] Data are lacking in children on dexamethasone for prevention of headache recurrence.[46,47] Many emergency medicine providers use a "cocktail" of medications for migraine treatment that includes ketorolac, prochlorperazine or metoclopramide, and diphenhydramine. This combination is effective and safe.[48] In addition to administering abortive medications in the emergency department, counsel patients to identify and eliminate potential precipitating factors.

Table 136-11 lists additional treatment for cluster headaches, which includes triptans and high-flow oxygen. Consider pediatric neurology consultation to help guide the management of recalcitrant headaches.

TABLE 136-9 Treatment of Migraine and Cluster and Tension Headaches

Medication	Migraine and Cluster Headache Treatment, Dose: Route	Tension Headache Treatment, Dose: Route
NSAIDs		
Ibuprofen	10 milligrams/kg: PO (max: 800 milligrams/dose or 2400 milligrams/d)	10 milligrams/kg: PO (max: 800 milligrams/dose or 2400 milligrams/d)
Ketorolac	0.5 milligram/kg: IV (max: 30 milligrams/dose)	0.5 milligram/kg: IV (max: 30 milligrams/dose)
Analgesics		
Acetaminophen	15 milligrams/kg: orally (max: 1 gram/dose or 4 grams/d)	15 milligrams/kg: PO (max: 1 gram/dose or 4 grams/d)
Dopamine antagonist		
Prochlorperazine	0.15 milligram/kg: IV (max: 10 milligrams/dose)	
Metoclopramide	0.1 milligram/kg: IV (max: 10 milligrams/dose)	
Other antiemetic		
Diphenhydramine	1 milligram/kg: IV (max: 50 milligrams/dose)	
Promethazine	0.25–1 milligram/kg: IV (max: 25 milligrams/dose)	
Triptans (more available than listed below)		
Sumatriptan	Multiple routes: →5–20 milligrams: IN →50–100 milligrams: PO →3–6 milligrams: SC	
Rizatriptan	5–10 milligrams: PO	
Sumatriptan/naproxen combination	Multiple combinations →85 milligrams/500 milligrams: PO (sumatriptan/naproxen) →30 milligrams/180 milligrams: PO →10 milligrams/60 milligrams: PO	

Abbreviation: NSAID, nonsteroidal anti-inflammatory drug.

Source: Adapted with permission from Sheridan DC, Spiro DM, Meckler GD: Pediatric migraine: abortive management in the emergency department. *Headache* 54: 235, 2014. Copyright John Wiley & Sons.

PROPHYLACTIC TREATMENT

Children with chronic headaches that disrupt activities of daily living or school performance may benefit from prophylactic treatment. Medications for the prevention of migraines are summarized in **Table 136-12**. The decision to start prophylaxis should be made by the primary care physician or pediatric neurologist, in consultation with the child and the family, and should include a careful weighing of the risks and benefits of daily medication.

TABLE 136-10 Suggested ED Treatment Algorithm for Primary Headaches*

Migraine and Cluster Headache	Tension Headache
Normal saline bolus (20 mL/kg IV; max of 1 L) + Ketorolac (0.5 milligram/kg IV; max 30 milligrams)† + Prochlorperazine (0.15 milligram/kg IV; max 10 milligrams) OR Metoclopramide (0.1 milligram/kg IV; max 10 milligrams) + Diphenhydramine (1 milligram/kg IV; max 50 milligrams)‡ ↓ If no significant relief, consider neurology consultation prior to other therapies such as dexamethasone	Ketorolac (0.5 milligram/kg IV; max 30 milligrams)† + Acetaminophen PO (15 milligrams/kg; max 1000 milligrams)

*For patients who have failed first-line therapy with oral ibuprofen or acetaminophen.

†Do not give ketorolac if ibuprofen taken within 6 h.

‡Diphenhydramine may be given prophylactically as part of a "cocktail" or used only to treat extrapyramidal side effects of dopamine antagonists.

NONPHARMACOLOGIC TREATMENT

For tension-type headaches, biofeedback and relaxation techniques can be effective.[49] In general, 8 to 10 sessions are necessary to teach these techniques in the outpatient setting. Although acupuncture has been used to treat chronic migraine headaches in both children and adults, several randomized controlled studies failed to show benefit over placebo.

DISPOSITION AND FOLLOW-UP

Admit children with emergent, life-threatening causes of headache to the hospital for definitive treatment and pain control. Consider admission for intractable pain. Arrange close follow-up for any child with headache discharged from the ED. Thoroughly discuss reasons for immediate return to the ED.

TABLE 136-11 Additional Treatment of Cluster Headaches

Headache Type	Treatment	Comment
Cluster	100% oxygen via non-rebreather mask at onset of headache	Most useful at onset of symptoms, less effective later in course of headache
	Various triptans	Refer to Table 136-9 for routes and doses
	Lidocaine, 1% solution in ipsilateral nostril	Effective for mild to moderate pain; can instill via atomizer and syringe
	Prednisone, 1–2 milligrams/kg for 10 d with subsequent 7-d taper	Effective at terminating prolonged cluster headaches and preventing recurrence

TABLE 136-12 Prophylaxis for Migraine Headaches in Children

Class	Medication	Dosage
Calcium channel blocker	Flunarizine	10 milligrams/d
	Nimodipine	10 milligrams/d (<40 kg), 16 milligrams/d (40–50 kg), 20 milligrams/d (>50 kg)
β-Blocker	Propranolol	10 milligrams PO twice a day up to 20 milligrams three times a day as tolerated for age <14 y; 20 milligrams twice a day to 120 milligrams twice a day as tolerated for age >14 y
Nitrogen alkaloid	Papaverine	5 milligrams/kg/d in divided doses twice a day
Tricyclic antidepressant	Amitriptyline	10 milligrams PO at bedtime to maximum of 50 milligrams PO at bedtime for age <12 y and 100 milligrams PO at bedtime for age >12 y
Antiepileptic	Topiramate	50 milligrams/d titrated to 200 milligrams/d in divided doses three times a day
	Divalproex sodium	125–250 milligrams PO at bedtime to twice a day for age >10 y
Vitamin	Riboflavin	400 milligrams/d
Antihistamine	Cyproheptadine	4 milligrams PO at bedtime to maximum of 12 milligrams at bedtime for age >6 y

REFERENCES

The complete reference list is available online at www.TintinalliEM.com.

CHAPTER 137 Altered Mental Status in Children

Sarah Mellion
Kathleen Adelgais

INTRODUCTION

Altered mental status in children is characterized by the failure to respond to verbal or physical stimulation in a manner appropriate to the child's developmental level. The ED incidence of altered mental status in children varies widely depending on the type of institution reporting, the patient population served, and the specific definition of altered mental status used.[1,2] Children with altered mental status require simultaneous stabilization, diagnosis, and treatment. The objectives of treatment are to sustain life and prevent irreversible CNS damage. Once the patient is resuscitated, the goal is to determine the cause and stop disease progression.

PATHOPHYSIOLOGY

Altered mental status is caused by abnormalities of the ascending reticular activating system or the cerebral cortex. The ascending reticular activating system is located in the brainstem and modulates wakefulness in response to the environment, as well as homeostasis and cardiovascular and respiratory functions. Neural pathways from the ascending reticular activating system project to the cerebral cortices, producing awareness. Altered mental status occurs through dysfunction of the neurons or bilateral cerebral cortices.[3,4]

There are many factors that can cause dysfunction in the ascending reticular activating system and cerebral hemispheres, including inadequate substrate for metabolic demand, insufficient blood flow, presence of toxins or metabolic waste products, or alterations of body temperature.[4] Typical causes of bilateral cortical impairment are toxic and metabolic states that deprive the brain of normal substrates.

The pathologic conditions that affect awareness and arousal can be divided into three broad pathologic categories: supratentorial mass lesions, subtentorial mass lesions, and metabolic encephalopathy.[5]

Supratentorial mass lesions compress the brainstem and/or diencephalon. Signs and symptoms of this type of lesion include focal motor abnormalities, which are often present from the onset of the altered level of consciousness. The progression of neurologic dysfunction is from rostral to caudal, with sequential failure of midbrain, pontine, and medullary functions. When compromise due to supratentorial lesions is present, the fast component of nystagmus is in a direction **away from** a cold stimulus during caloric testing.

Subtentorial mass lesions lead to reticular activating system dysfunction, in which prompt loss of consciousness is generally the rule. Cranial nerve abnormalities are frequent, and abnormal respiratory patterns, such as Cheyne-Stokes respiration, neurogenic hyperventilation, and ataxic breathing, are common. With brainstem injury, asymmetric and/or fixed pupils are found. No eye movements occur despite cold water irrigation of both auditory canals.

Metabolic encephalopathy usually causes depressed consciousness before motor signs become depressed. Motor signs are typically symmetric. Respiratory abnormalities are usually secondary to acid-base imbalance. Pupillary reflexes are generally preserved. Pupils may be sluggish, but pupil responses are intact and symmetric, except in the case of profound anoxia or poisoning with cholinergics, anticholinergics, opiates, or barbiturates.

CLINICAL FEATURES

The spectrum of alteration of mental status ranges from confusion or delirium (disorders in perception) to lethargy, stupor, and coma (states of decreased awareness). A lethargic child has decreased awareness of self and the environment. Patients may be aroused from an apparent deep sleep, but they immediately relapse into a state of minimal responsiveness. A stuporous child has decreased eye contact, decreased motor activity, and unintelligible vocalization. Stuporous patients can be aroused with vigorous noxious stimulation. Comatose patients are unresponsive and cannot be aroused by verbal or physical stimulation, such as phlebotomy, arterial catheterization, or lumbar puncture.[6]

Take a methodical and comprehensive history (**Table 137-1**). Ask about the prodromal events before the change in consciousness as well as recent illnesses or infectious exposures, and determine the likelihood of trauma, abuse, or ingestion. Inquire about antecedent fever, headache, head tilt, abdominal pain, vomiting, diarrhea, gait disturbance, seizures, drug ingestion, palpitations, weakness, hematuria, weight loss, and rash. For infants and young children, review developmental

TABLE 137-1 Important Historical Elements for Evaluating Altered Mental Status in Children

Prodromal events	Recent illnesses or infectious exposures
	History of recent trauma
Risk factors	Medications in the home
	Social environment
	Vaccinations
	Family history
	Developmental milestones
Associated symptoms	
Constitutional	Fever, weight loss
GI	Vomiting, diarrhea, abdominal pain
Neurologic	Headache, gait changes, seizure activity, weakness
Cardiac	Palpitations
Musculoskeletal	Head tilt
Dermatologic	Rash

milestones. The medical, immunization, and family histories are important in children of all ages. Be alert for any inappropriate responses, inconsistencies, or delays in seeking care that may arouse the suspicion of child abuse.[6,7]

Proceed with a general examination only after respiratory, cardiac, and cerebral stabilization. The objectives of the examination are to identify occult infection, trauma, toxicity, or metabolic disease. The neurologic examination should document the child's response to sensory input, motor activity, pupillary reactivity, oculovestibular reflexes, and respiratory pattern. Although several coma scales have been published, such as the Modified Pediatric Glasgow Coma Scale (GCS) (**Table 137-2**), the most simplified and functional in an emergency setting is the AVPU scale (**Table 137-3**).

The Glasgow coma scale lacks good interobserver reliability and reproducibility and does not accurately predict outcomes in individual patients.[8] A simpler and validated method to assess mental status in children is using the AVPU score, which has been validated and currently recommended by the Pediatric Advanced Life Support guidelines[9] (Table 137-3).

The A, V, P, and U values correspond to Glasgow coma scale scores of 15, 13, 8, and 3, respectively.[10]

After obtaining a comprehensive history and performing a complete physical examination, anticipate and carefully observe improvement or deterioration.[11]

TABLE 137-2 Modified Pediatric Glasgow Coma Scale

Coos or babbles = 5
Irritable cry = 4
Cries to pain = 3
Moans to pain = 2
No response = 1

TABLE 137-3 AVPU Score

A = Awake
V = Responds to verbal stimuli
P = Responds to pain
U = Unresponsive

DIAGNOSIS

The familiar mnemonic **AEIOU TIPS** (***a**lcohol, **e**ncephalopathy, **i**nsulin, **o**piates, **u**remia, **t**rauma, **i**nfection, **p**oisoning, and **s**eizure*) is a useful tool for organizing the diagnostic possibilities of altered mental status in children (**Table 137-4**).

TABLE 137-4 AEIOU TIPS: A Mnemonic for Pediatric Altered Mental Status

A	**Alcohol.** Ethanol. Isopropyl alcohol. Methanol. Concurrent hypoglycemia is common. **Acid-base and metabolic.** Hypotonic and hypertonic dehydration. Hepatic dysfunction, inborn errors of metabolism. **Arrhythmia/cardiogenic.** Stokes-Adams, supraventricular tachycardia, aortic stenosis, heart block, pericardial tamponade, hypertensive encephalopathy.
E	**Encephalopathy.** Reye's syndrome. Parainfectious encephalomyelitis. Autoimmune encephalitis. **Endocrinopathy.** Addison's disease can present with AMS or psychosis. Thyrotoxicosis can present with ventricular dysrhythmias. Pheochromocytoma can present with hypertensive encephalopathy. **Electrolytes.** Hypo-/hypernatremia and disorders of calcium, magnesium, and phosphorus can produce AMS.
I	**Insulin.** AMS from hyperglycemia is rare in children, but diabetic ketoacidosis is the most common cause. Hypoglycemia can be the result of many disorders. Irritability, confusion, seizures, and coma can occur with blood glucose levels <40 milligrams/dL. **Intussusception.** AMS may be the initial presenting symptom.
O	**Opiates.** Common household exposures are to Lomotil, Imodium, diphenoxylate, and dextromethorphan. Clonidine, an α-agonist, can also produce similar symptoms. **Oxygen.** Disorders of airway, breathing, or circulation may adversely affect oxygen delivery to the brain; hypercapnia from primary lung disease or neurologic dysfunction also may result in altered mental status.
U	**Uremia.** Encephalopathy occurs in over one-third of patients with chronic renal failure. Hemolytic-uremic syndrome can produce AMS in addition to abdominal pain. Thrombocytopenic purpura and hemolytic anemia also can cause AMS. In children with chronic renal failure, neurologic dysfunction may develop secondary to stroke, hypertension, or metabolic derangements.
T	**Trauma.** Hypovolemia or hemorrhage from multisystem trauma may lead to insufficient cerebral perfusion and result in altered mental status. Consider concussion, hemorrhage or contusion, or epidural or subdural hematoma. Remember to look for signs of child abuse, particularly shaken baby syndrome with retinal hemorrhages. **Tumor.** Primary, metastatic, or meningeal leukemic infiltration. Intracerebral tumors commonly produce focal neurologic signs, and posterior fossa tumors typically block the ventricular system and create signs and symptoms suggestive of hydrocephalus. Supratentorial and infratentorial tumors may present abruptly with altered mental status, fever, or meningismus after an intratumor hemorrhage.[12] **Thermal.** Hypo- or hyperthermia. Progressive hypothermia leads to insidious altered mental status. Temperatures >41°C (105.8°F) result in headache, weakness, and dizziness followed by confusion, euphoria, combativeness, and altered mental status.
I	**Infection.** Bacterial meningitis, encephalitis,[13] and brain abscess[14] are the most important causes of AMS in children, especially AMS with fever. Brain abscess is characterized by fever and headache before AMS changes. Presenting symptoms also include generalized or focal seizures. Any systemic infection associated with vasculitis or shock may lead to altered mental status secondary to cerebral hypoperfusion. **Intracerebral vascular disorders.** Subarachnoid, intracerebral, or intraventricular hemorrhages can be seen with trauma, ruptured aneurysm, or arteriovenous malformations. Venous thrombosis can follow severe dehydration or pyogenic infection of the mastoid, orbit, middle ear, or sinuses. Arterial thrombosis is uncommon in children, except in those with homocystinuria. Intracerebral and intraventricular hemorrhages may follow birth asphyxia or trauma in neonates, but in older children, they may signify a congenital or acquired coagulopathy. Cerebral emboli from bacterial endocarditis may cause altered mental status. Acute confusional migraine may be associated with profound alterations in consciousness. Children with sickle cell anemia can develop cerebral thrombosis, status epilepticus, and coma.
P	**Psychogenic.** Rare in children, characterized by decreased responsiveness with normal neurologic examination including oculovestibular reflexes. Psychogenic unresponsiveness may be a conversion reaction, an adjustment reaction, a panic state, or malingering. **Poisoning/ingestion.** Drugs, toxins, or illicit substances can be ingested by accident, through neglect or abuse, or in a suicidal gesture.
S	**Seizure.** Generalized motor seizures and absence status epilepticus are often associated with prolonged unresponsiveness in children.[15] In a child with a history of seizures who presents with AMS, consider nonconvulsive status epilepticus. Seizures in a febrile child suggest intracranial infection. Shunt malfunction should be considered among patients with a ventriculoperitoneal shunt for hydrocephalus.

Abbreviation: AMS = altered mental status.

TABLE 137-5 General Treatment of Altered Mental Status

Assess airway, breathing, and circulation.
Immobilize cervical spine for suspected trauma.
Initiate continuous pulse oximetry; consider capnometry; administer oxygen.
Give dextrose for hypoglycemia; for children, give 25% dextrose in water 2 mL/kg IV; for newborns, give 5 mL/kg of 10% dextrose in water.
Provide fluid resuscitation, 20 mL/kg of isotonic crystalloid, and repeat to total of 60 mL/kg as needed.
Administer broad-spectrum antibiotics for suspected sepsis or meningitis.
Give naloxone for suspected opiate or clonidine overdose, 0.01 to 0.1 milligram/kg IV every 2 min.
Administer flumazenil for suspected pure benzodiazepine overdose, 0.01 milligram/kg IV.
Control seizures with benzodiazepines (lorazepam, 0.1 milligram/kg IV; diazepam, 0.1 milligram/kg IV; or midazolam, 0.1 milligram/kg IV).
Prevent hypothermia with heat lamps during resuscitation; treat hyperthermia.

TREATMENT

Treatment principles are outlined in **Table 137-5**. Begin with airway, breathing, and circulation and administer 100% oxygen until adequate oxygenation is confirmed. Establish an IV, and give normal saline to restore and/or maintain perfusion. **Obtain a stat point-of-care glucose and treat hypoglycemia.** If the history or the exam suggests opiate toxicity, give naloxone.[6]

Once the child is stabilized, the history and physical should suggest either a medical disorder or structural lesion. If a medical cause is suspected, obtain serum electrolyte levels, renal and hepatic function studies, serum ammonia, and coagulation studies. If the history or examination suggests a toxic ingestion, obtain serum levels of suspected agents and a urine toxicology screen. For serious bacterial infection, obtain blood and urine cultures. For suspected meningitis, give antibiotics and/or acyclovir. Correct shock, hypotension, and hypoxia before attempting lumbar puncture (see chapter 116, "Fever and Serious Bacterial Illness in Infants and Children").

Obtain arterial blood gas analysis and pulse oximetry in cases of trauma, respiratory distress, or suspected acid-base imbalance. Obtain a 12-lead ECG and provide continuous cardiac monitoring if there are pathologic auscultatory findings, rhythm disturbance, or suspected overdose.

The clinical scenario directs imaging. Immobilize the cervical spine and x-ray the cervical spine if spine injury is suspected or in the case of multiple system trauma. If an intracranial lesion or vascular disorder is suspected or if there are focal neurologic signs, obtain a noncontrast CT scan of the head. For suspected increased intracranial pressure, also elevate the head of the bed to 30 degrees. A chest radiograph confirms or clarifies examination findings and documents endotracheal tube placement. Abdominal radiographs are indicated to assess for acute ingestion of radiopaque material. Abdominal US may be useful to screen for cases of intussusception.[16]

Other studies that may be useful in specific cases are serum osmolality, blood alcohol level, thyroid function tests, blood lead level, and skeletal survey for suspected abuse. Electroencephalogram will diagnose nonconvulsive status epilepticus.

DISPOSITION AND FOLLOW-UP

Once the patient is stabilized, the child should be observed until his or her mental status improves. The patient's clinical condition and specific disorder dictate whether further management can occur on the inpatient unit or in an intensive care unit.[6] Only patients with transient, reversible causes may be treated, monitored in the ED, and discharged after observation and a return to their baseline mental status. Patients who are discharged (e.g., those with a closed head injury or simple febrile seizure) should receive disease-specific discharge instructions. Children who are evaluated for altered mental status and discharged home should have a repeat evaluation within 24 hours of discharge.

Acknowledgments: The authors gratefully acknowledge the contributions of Jonathan Singer, the author of this chapter in the previous edition.

REFERENCES

The complete reference list is available online at www.TintinalliEM.com.

Head Injury in Infants and Children

Alessandra Conforto
Ilene Claudius

INTRODUCTION AND EPIDEMIOLOGY

Minor head injury in children is responsible for almost 400,000 ED visits each year,[1] with children 0 to 4 years of age most commonly affected. Of all children with minor head injury coming to the ED, it is estimated that about 5% have intracranial injury,[2] and <1% of those with intracranial injury require neurosurgical intervention.[3,4]

Given the rarity with which head-injured children require intervention, the diagnostic challenge is to distinguish the small subset of seriously injured children, while minimizing evaluation of those at low risk of significant intracranial injury. Therefore, careful risk stratification of children with minor head injury is important for safe and efficient medical care.

This chapter focuses on evaluation of children with minor head injury and concussion, as well as the treatment of children in whom significant intracranial injuries are identified.

DEFINITION

The definition of minor head injury varies in the literature. **The American Academy of Pediatrics defines children with minor head injury as "those who have normal mental status at the initial examination, who have no abnormal or focal findings on neurologic (including funduscopic) examination, and who have no physical evidence of skull fracture."**[5] The Glasgow Coma Scale (GCS; **Table 138-1**), or its derivative for younger, preverbal infants and toddlers, is often used

TABLE 138-1 Glasgow Coma Scale Score for Adults and Infants

Response	Adults	Infants	Score
Eye opening	Spontaneous	Spontaneous	4
	To voice	To voice	3
	To pain	To pain	2
	No response	No response	1
Verbal response	Oriented	Coos, babbles	5
	Disoriented	Irritable	4
	Inappropriate words	Cries to pain	3
	Incomprehensible	Moans to pain	2
	No response	No response	1
Motor response	Obeys commands	Makes normal spontaneous movements	6
	Localizes pain	Withdraws to touch	5
	Withdraws to pain	Withdraws to pain	4
	Decorticate posture	Decorticate posture	3
	Decerebrate posture	Decerebrate posture	2
	No response	No response	1

to determine the severity of head injury. **Head injuries resulting in a GCS score of ≤8 are severe, those with scores of 9 to 13 are moderate, and those with scores of 14 or 15 are mild.**

PATHOPHYSIOLOGY

Head trauma is classified as blunt or penetrating based on the mechanism of injury. In children, the vast majority of head trauma is caused by blunt force with the underlying mechanism varying according to the age of the patient. In younger children, the most common causes of head trauma are falls and assaults/child abuse.[6] In fact, in children under 2 years of age, nonaccidental trauma is the leading cause of death due to head trauma. In older children, falls, sports and recreation, assault, and, increasingly, motor vehicle collisions are more common. Penetrating injuries are most frequently related to dog bites in infants or gunshot wounds in older children. In the largest study of pediatric minor head injury to date, including over 42,000 patients, radiographically documented intracranial injuries were found in approximately 1.8% of children with minor head injury who presented to the ED for evaluation, and only 0.9% required intervention.[4] This is a lower number than cited in prior studies, likely due to the inclusion and clinical follow-up of lower-risk children not undergoing CT. The true incidence of intracranial injuries is probably even lower, because many children with mild injuries do not present to the ED.

The pattern of injury is different in children compared to adults. In children, diffuse injuries are proportionally more common, and in adults, focal injuries such as epidural and subdural hematomas and cerebral contusions are more common.[6]

The differences in brain development and pediatric anatomy explain the specific pattern of childhood injuries compared to adults. In blunt head injury, rotation of the brain around its center of gravity leads to more diffuse injuries (diffuse axonal injury and subdural hematoma), whereas linear forces are generally less damaging to the brain and cause local (coup and contrecoup injury) rather than diffuse injury. The type and severity of the injury are determined both by the type of deceleration and its magnitude.[7] Younger age is a significant risk factor for intracranial injury. Even among infants, the greatest risk for intracranial injury is in children under 3 months of age.[2]

More details of physiology are discussed in chapter 257, "Head Trauma."

SKULL FRACTURES

Skull fractures can involve the calvarium or the base of the skull. The presence of skull fractures is a risk factor for underlying brain injury in infants under 2 years of age (**Figures 138-1 and 138-2**).[4]

However, significant brain injury can occur in the absence of skull fractures in 50% of cases.[8] Plain films of the skull should therefore not be obtained as a replacement for CT to evaluate for underlying brain injury.[9] Depressed skull fractures occur in response to the application of significant force and require neurosurgical consultation, as surgical elevation is often required. Compared to adults, skull fractures in children are more common but less frequently associated with underlying brain injury.[6]

A growing fracture can occur when the leptomeninges are torn beneath the fracture, allowing for the formation of a cerebrospinal fluid leptomeningeal cyst that forces apart the fracture edges and leads to nonunion. **Growing skull fractures** typically present weeks to months following an injury resulting in skull fracture. This rare complication is unique to infants and requires neurosurgical repair.

INTRACRANIAL INJURIES

An **epidural hematoma** (**Figure 138-3**) is a collection of blood between the inner skull and the dura and can occur from rapid arterial bleeding from the middle meningeal artery or the dural or diploic vasculature.

The classic presentation is a lucid interval after head trauma followed by rapid deterioration. The presence of a bi-convex hyperdense extra-axial lesion that does not cross the suture lines is indicative of an epidural hematoma on CT.[10] The long-term prognosis depends on the preoperative GCS and the extent of other underlying brain injury,[11] but is generally good if surgical evacuation can be undertaken in a timely manner.

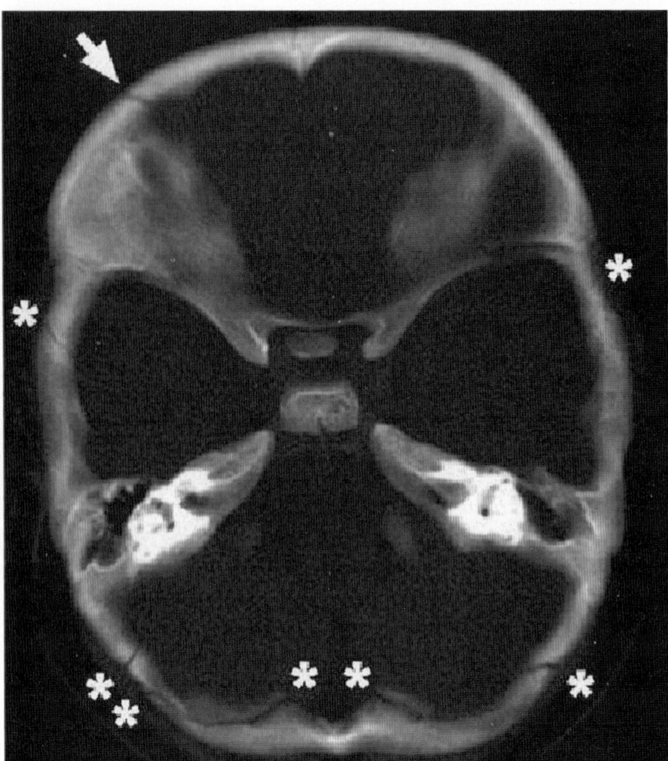

FIGURE 138-1. Linear fracture seen on CT. *Arrow* indicates skull fracture, and *asterisks* indicate normal cranial suture lines. [Image used with permission of Joseph Piatt, Jr., MD, Division of Neurosurgery, A. I. duPont Hospital for Children, Wilmington, Delaware; Departments of Neurological Surgery and Pediatrics, Thomas Jefferson University, Philadelphia, Pennsylvania.]

Subdural hematomas (**Figure 138-4**), located between the arachnoid and the internal dural layer, are more common than epidural hematomas, particularly in infants and younger children. Subdural hematomas are caused by tearing of the subdural veins, are often extensive and bilateral (80% of cases), are frequently associated with underlying brain injury, and have a worse prognosis than epidural hematomas.

Radiographically, a subdural hematoma appears as a crescent-shaped fluid collection with the concavity facing the brain surface. Immediately after the injury, the subdural hematoma appears more dense (brighter white) than adjacent brain tissue. Due to the metabolism of blood products within the hematoma, its radiographic appearance changes over time. In the subacute phase (1 to 3 weeks after injury), the hematoma progressively assumes the same density of the brain tissue and can thus be difficult to recognize. Flattening of the sulci and the presence of a mass effect are indirect evidence of the presence of a subdural hematoma. Subsequently, in the chronic phase, the hematoma appears as a hypodense fluid collection, with a density similar to cerebrospinal fluid.[10] In infants, loss of gray-white matter differentiation and diffuse hypodensity has been described with subdural hematoma.[7]

Cerebral contusions (**Figure 138-5**) are located in the cortex underlying the area of direct impact of a significant force (coup lesions) or on the opposite side (contrecoup lesions) where the brain has struck the cranial surface.

The severity ranges from minor CT findings in an asymptomatic patient to severe brain edema. On CT, the presence of ill-defined hyperdense areas within the cortex of the frontal and temporal lobe represent parenchymal contusions.

Traumatic subarachnoid hemorrhage is often associated with significant trauma and diffuse axonal injury (**Figures 138-6 and 138-7**). Infants more commonly present with diffuse injury and cerebral edema compared to adults because developmental differences render them susceptible to rotational and deceleration forces. Clinically, the child with diffuse axonal injury presents with a profoundly depressed level of consciousness. Radiographic findings on CT may be minimal in the acute

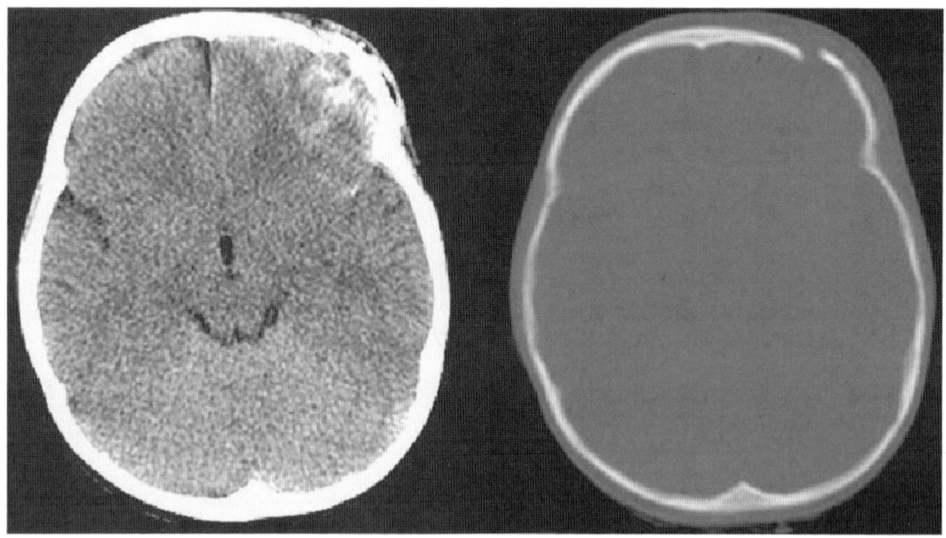

FIGURE 138-2. Open skull fracture with underlying cerebral contusion. This injury was sustained from a fall of two stories. [Image used with permission of Joseph Piatt, Jr., MD, Division of Neurosurgery, A. I. duPont Hospital for Children, Wilmington, Delaware; Departments of Neurological Surgery and Pediatrics, Thomas Jefferson University, Philadelphia, Pennsylvania.]

setting. MRI is more sensitive in the detection of diffuse axonal injury, which can be both hemorrhagic and nonhemorrhagic.[10]

Figure 138-8 provides noncontrast head CT images of a variety of cerebral injuries.

CONCUSSION

The pathophysiology of concussion is complex. Although cerebral blood flow is increased in some children immediately following a concussion, the predominant pattern is transiently decreased blood flow. This is followed by a period of hyperemia from days 1 to 3, followed by return of the low-flow state.[12] In more than one third of concussed children, this phenomenon continues for a month or more.[13] Concussions do not cause gross structural changes, making them difficult to diagnose by conventional radiography. However, animal models indicate that the acceleration-deceleration forces of a concussion initiate a neurochemical cascade that results in neuronal membrane disruption and axonal stretching. This in turn leads to significant ion flux, initially coupled with a transient increase in the cerebral glucose metabolism, followed by hypometabolism lasting days to weeks. Cytokine-mediated inflammation, stretch-mediated axonal disconnection, and neurotransmitter-mediated oxidative dysfunction also contribute to concussion-related impairments.[12]

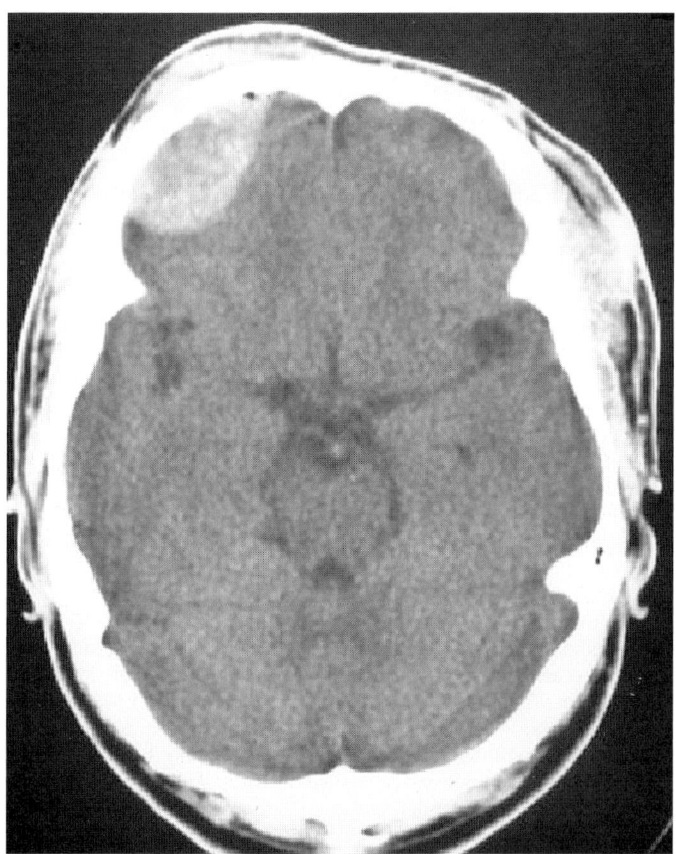

FIGURE 138-3. Epidural hematoma. Note the convex shape and focal location. [Image used with permission of Jack Fountain, Jr., MD, Emory University and Grady Memorial Hospital.]

CLINICAL FEATURES

HISTORY

Obtain the history from adult caregivers, witnesses, and EMS personnel and focus on the mechanism and time of the accident, and whether the child has experienced loss of consciousness, seizure, changes in behavior, or vomiting. Loss of consciousness itself is difficult to correlate with pathophysiology: the absence of loss of consciousness alone is not necessarily reassuring, particularly in children under 2 years of age,[14] nor does loss of consciousness alone predict a significant intracranial injury. Some authors report that falls from <1.5 m (5 ft), result in death only in extremely rare cases (<0.48 deaths per 1 million young children per year); however, head injury requiring neurosurgical intervention has been reported with this mechanism.[2,14,15]

A history that is incompatible with the child's age or situation (e.g., a report that a 1-month-old rolled off of the changing table or that a 6-month-old crawled out of the crib) raises a suspicion of nonaccidental injury.

Although the mechanism of injury contributes to an understanding of forces involved, symptoms such as headache, vomiting, and changes in behavior (e.g., irritability, lethargy) and their progression or resolution guide most decision rules. If possible, ask the child directly. For preverbal children, caregivers who know the child's normal behavior can identify behaviors suggesting headache or pain. Particularly in the young child, symptoms of neurologic injury may be subtle. Lethargy, irritability, seizures, and alterations in muscle tone or level of consciousness, as well as vomiting, poor feeding, breathing abnormalities and apnea, raise the suspicion of significant head injury.[7] Worsening of symptoms suggests intracranial injury. The persistence of symptoms such as headache, confusion, and amnesia suggests either an intracranial injury or a concussion.

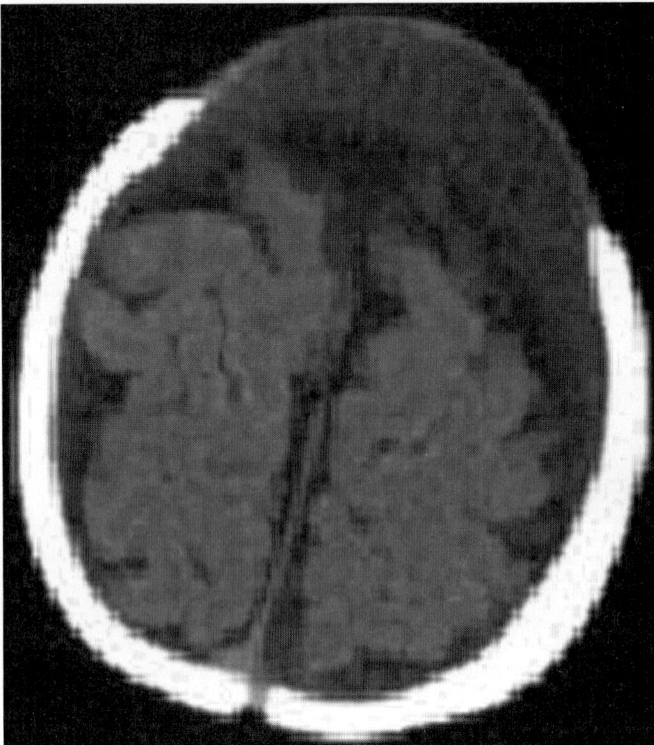

A

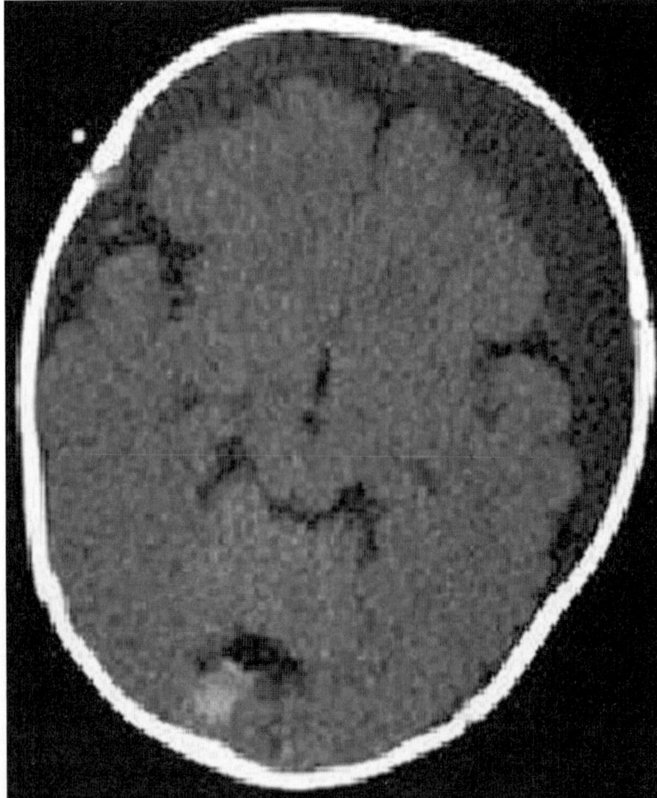

B

FIGURE 138-4. **A.** Bifrontal chronic subdural hematoma extending through the anterior fontanelle in a 1-month old-child. **B.** Second image in the same child showing bifrontal chronic subdural hematoma as well as small, acute intraparenchymal hemorrhage in the posterior fossa.

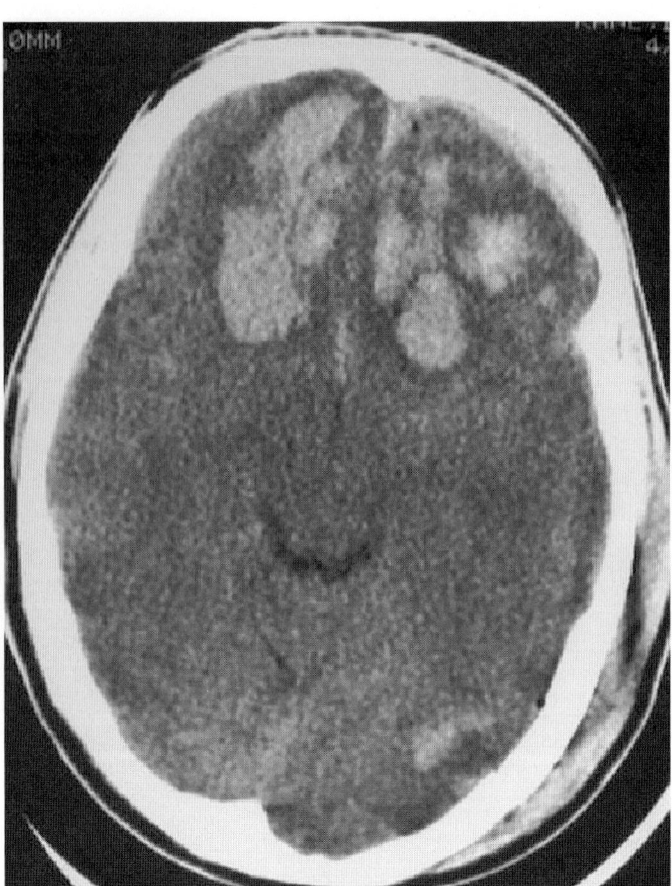

FIGURE 138-5. CT scan demonstrating delayed intraparenchymal hemorrhages from a traumatic contusion. [Image used with permission of Jack Fountain, Jr., MD, Emory University and Grady Memorial Hospital.]

PHYSICAL EXAMINATION

Focus the initial assessment on the immediate evaluation of airway, breathing, circulation, level of consciousness, and GCS (Table 138-1). Protect the cervical spine with a *properly sized* cervical collar. Most children with minor head injury have stable vital signs and are alert, active, and appropriately interactive, and often the cervical spine can be clinically cleared after a thorough evaluation (see discussion on cervical spine injury later in this chapter).

If the child is sleeping on ED arrival, gently arouse the child to assess the level of consciousness or irritability. If the child is upset, allow time for the child to become comfortable with the environment before continuing with the examination. A knowledge of appropriate developmental milestones (e.g., stranger anxiety) and consideration of the child's normal nap time are important factors in assessing the mental status of the head-injured child.

Perform a thorough head-to-toe assessment for trauma, including an age-appropriate complete neurologic examination, musculoskeletal examination, and funduscopic examination. Note any evidence of trauma to the skull and examine the fontanelle in the calm upright child for signs of increased intracranial pressure. **A scalp hematoma in a child <2 years old is associated with an increased risk of skull fracture and intracranial hemorrhage.**[2,10] Hemotympanum or cerebrospinal fluid otorrhea and rhinorrhea may signify basilar skull fracture. Periorbital ecchymoses ("raccoon eyes") and bruising behind the ears ("Battle's sign"), although rare, also suggest basilar skull fracture. Evaluate the cervical spine for tenderness to palpation and evidence of injury. When nonaccidental trauma is suspected in an infant, consult with an ophthalmologist to identify retinal hemorrhages. Anisocoria, hypertension, and bradycardia are clinical signs of impending herniation and are preterminal events.

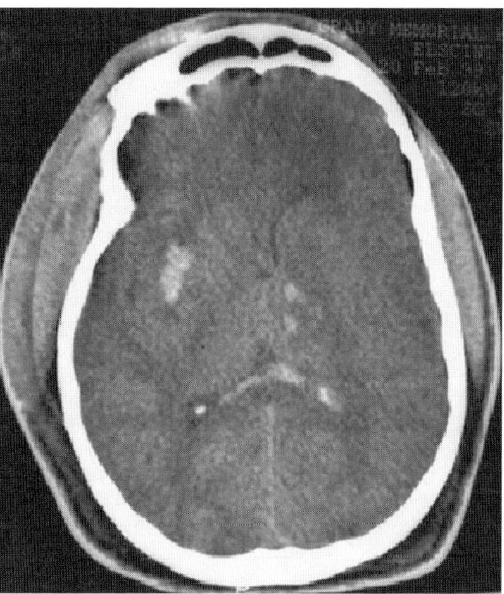

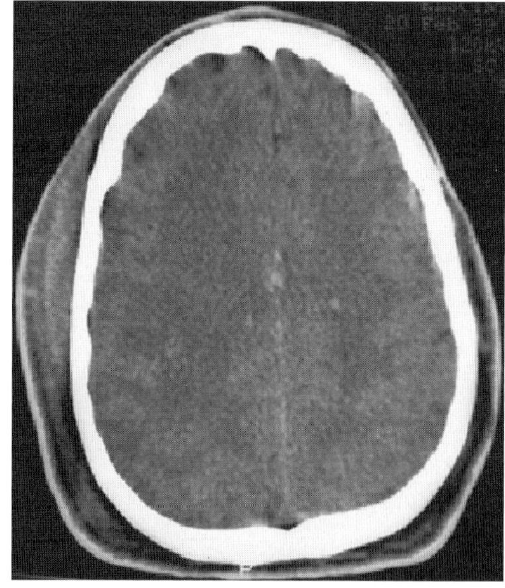

FIGURE 138-6. Diffuse axonal injury with intraventricular blood. [Image used with permission of Jack Fountain, Jr., MD, Emory University and Grady Memorial Hospital.]

DIAGNOSIS

Several factors have led to a disparity in practice patterns and more frequent use of CT scan (12.8% of pediatric head trauma victims in 1995 to 22.4% in 2003) in the evaluation of minor head trauma in children.[16] Significant intracranial injury after a minor head injury is a relatively rare but potentially preventable cause of death and disability in the young. No single clinical finding is pathognomonic for intracranial hemorrhage; therefore, clinical practice has come to rely on CT evaluation. However, ionizing radiation is a long-term carcinogenic risk and should be used only when clinically indicated.[17] Thus, several clinical decisions rules have been developed to guide imaging. Three large studies demonstrate high sensitivity and specificity and include **CHALICE**[18] (Children's Head Injury Algorithm for the Prediction of Important Clinical Events), **CATCH**[19] (Canadian Assessment of Tomography for Childhood Head Injury), and **PECARN** (Pediatric Emergency Care Applied Research Network). PECARN is considered the "best for children and infants, with the largest cohort, highest sensitivity and acceptable specificity of clinically significant ICI (intracranial injury)."[20]

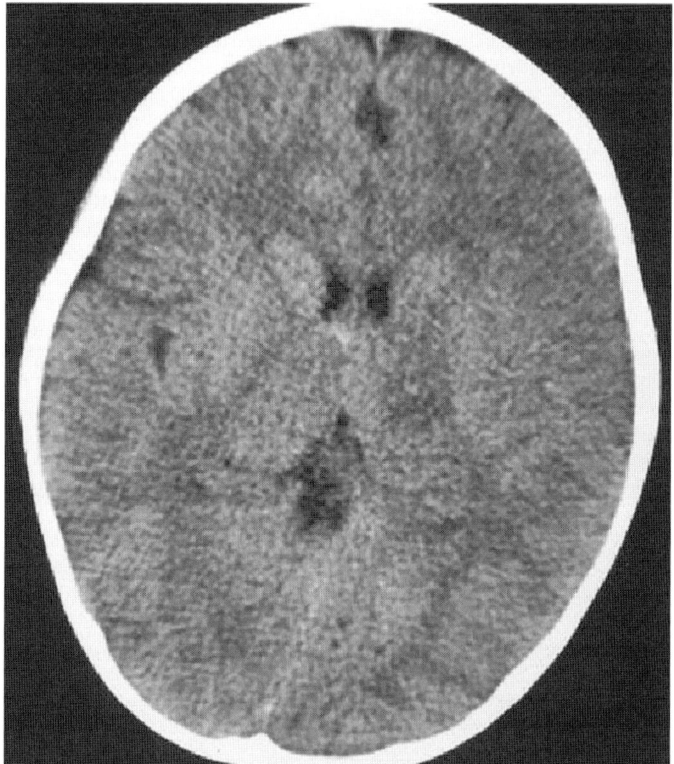

FIGURE 138-7. Diffuse axonal injury with loss of the grey matter–white matter interface. [Image used with permission of Daniel Curry, MD, PhD, Texas Children's Hospital and Baylor College of Medicine.]

In 2009, PECARN derived and validated a novel prediction rule to identify children with minor head injury who are at very low risk of clinically significant intracranial injury. To address concerns of applicability to children of all ages, two prediction rules (**Tables 138-2 and 138-3**)[4] were developed and validated: one for children <2 years old and one for children >2 years old. Among enrolled children <2 years of age, there were 8502 patients in the derivation group and 2216 patients in the validation group; among enrolled children >2 years old, there were 25,283 patients in the derivation group and 6411 patients in the validation group.

The strengths of this study are the presence of both a derivation and a validation population, the strong statistical power provided by the large number of enrolled patients, and the inclusion of a separate study population of preverbal children age <2 years (25% of the study population). **The authors conclude that a CT scan is not indicated in patients meeting all low-risk criteria for age.** Of the clinical criteria suggesting intracranial injury in both age groups, the presence of altered mental status (or GCS of 14) or the presence of skull fracture most strongly correlated with intracranial injury (4.4% risk of clinically significant traumatic brain injury). Of note, the authors explicitly underscore that the findings in the study apply only to patients with a GCS of 14 or 15, because patients with a lower GCS have a higher risk of traumatic brain injury on CT.[4]

By comparison, the **CATCH** study identifies factors associated with high risk for significant intracranial injury requiring neurosurgical intervention among 3866 children <16 years of age presenting to the ED within 24 hours of minor head injury defined as GCS of 13 to 15 with witnessed loss of consciousness, vomiting, amnesia, and disorientation or irritability. High-risk children were those with GCS <15 2 hours after injury, suspected open or depressed skull fracture, worsening headache, or irritability. Medium-risk children were defined as those with signs of basilar skull fracture, a large, boggy scalp hematoma, or a dangerous mechanism of injury (fall >1 meter or five stairs, motor vehicle collision, or fall from a bicycle without a helmet). Using these criteria, the CATCH rule had a sensitivity of 100% and specificity of 70% for identifying high-risk patients who require surgical intervention and 98% and 50% for

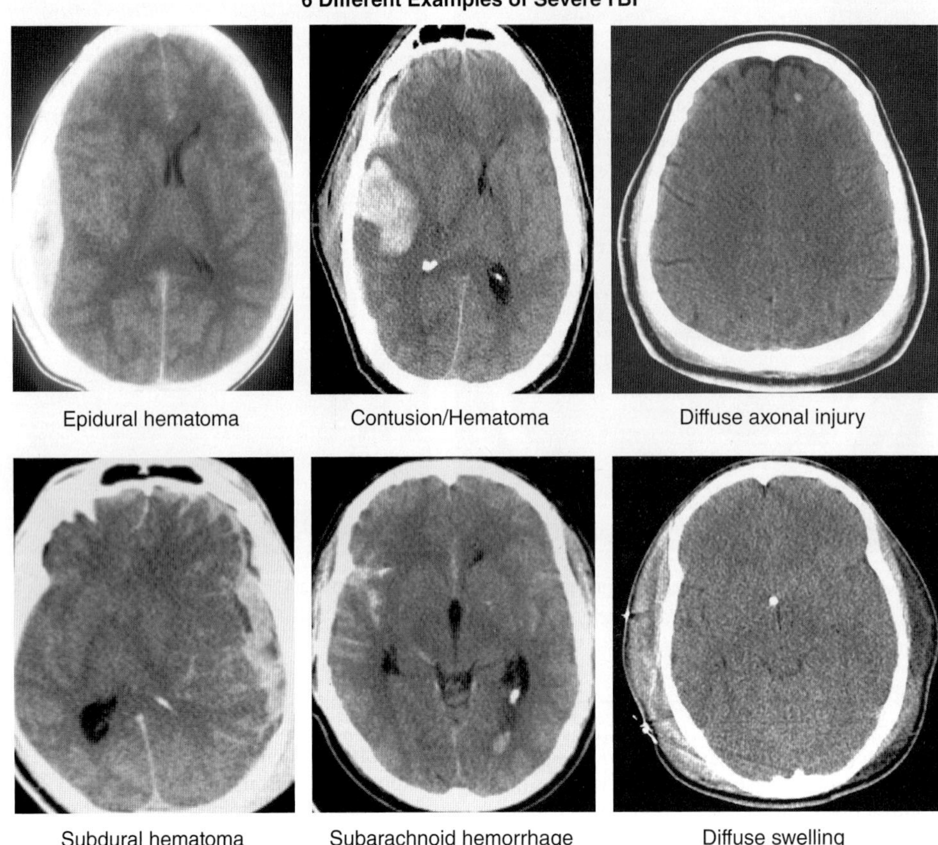

FIGURE 138-8. Six different examples of severe traumatic brain injury (TBI). [Image used with permission of Alisa Green, MD, University of California, San Francisco.]

identifying a CT abnormality among medium-risk patients. Compared to the PECARN rule, implementation of CATCH would lead to significantly lower rates of CT.[19]

The **CHALICE** study included patients with a range of injury severity and without a specific time of evaluation after injury. Conducted in the United Kingdom, 22,722 children <16 years of age were analyzed for factors associated with high risk of clinically significant intracranial injury (death, need for neurosurgical intervention, or significant CT abnormality). Identified risk factors included a witnessed loss of consciousness >5 minutes, amnesia >5 minutes, abnormal drowsiness, more than three episodes of emesis, seizure, suspicion of nonaccidental trauma, GCS <15 in children under 1 year of age or <14 in older children, penetrating or depressed skull injury or signs of basilar skull fracture, bulging fontanelle, scalp swelling, bruising or laceration >5 cm in children <1 year of age, abnormal neurologic exam, and significant mechanism of injury (high-speed motor vehicle collision, fall >3 m, or

TABLE 138-2 PECARN Low-Risk Criteria for Infants and Children with Minor Head Injury*

Age Group	Clinical Criteria
<2 years	Normal mental status
	No scalp hematoma except frontal
	Loss of consciousness <5 s
	Nonsevere mechanism†
	No palpable skull fracture
	Normal behavior per parents
>2 years	Normal mental status
	No loss of consciousness
	No vomiting
	Nonsevere mechanism†
	No signs of basilar skull fracture
	No severe headache

*Minor head injury was defined as a Glasgow Coma Scale score of 14 or 15 in this study.
†Severe mechanism: motor vehicle collision with ejection, rollover, or death of passenger; pedestrian or bicyclist without helmet struck by motorized vehicle; fall >2 m or 5 ft (age >2 y) or >1 m or 3 ft (age <2 y); head struck by high-impact object.
Source: Reproduced with permission from Kupperman N, Holmes JF, Dayan PS, et al: Identification of children at very low risk of clinically-important brain injuries after head trauma: a prospective cohort study. *Lancet* 374: 1160, 2009. Copyright Elsevier.

TABLE 138-3 Pediatric Emergency Care Applied Research Network Low-Risk Criteria for Infants and Children with Minor Head Injury*

Age Group	Population	Sensitivity (95% CI)	Specificity (95% CI)	Negative Predictive Value (95% CI)
<2 years	Derivation (N = 8502)	98.6% (92.6–99.97)	53.7% (52.6–54.8)	99.9% (99.88–99.999)
	Validation (N = 2216)	100.0% (86.3–100.0)	53.7% (51.6–55.8)	100% (99.7–100.00)
>2 years	Derivation (N = 25,283)	96.7% (93.4–98.7)	58.5% (57.9–59.1)	99.95% (99.9–99.98)
	Validation (N = 6411)	96.8% (89.0–99.6)	59.8% (58.6–61.0)	99.95% (99.81–99.99)

*Minor head injury was defined as a Glasgow Coma Scale score of 14 or 15 in this study.
Source: Reproduced with permission from Kupperman N, Holmes JF, Dayan PS, et al: Identification of children at very low risk of clinically-important brain injuries after head trauma: a prospective cohort study. *Lancet* 374: 1160, 2009. Copyright Elsevier.

TABLE 138-4 Treatment of Serious Head Injury

Cervical spine	Maintain spinal precautions	
Airway	Maintain airway, intubate for GCS < 8 or as needed for oxygenation and ventilation	
Oxygenation and ventilation	Oxygen saturation > 90; P_{CO_2} 35–40	No prophylactic hyperventilation
Blood pressure	SBP >70 + (2 × age)	No permissive hypotension Consider sedation and neuromuscular blockade
GCS	GCS before paralytics if possible	Serial GCS to document changes
Stat neuroimaging (noncontrast head CT and cervical spine CT)	Look for signs of increased ICP and identify mass lesions	Transcranial Doppler may be useful in infants with open fontanelles and experienced pediatric radiologists
Glucose	Treat hypoglycemia and hyperglycemia	Maintain normal blood glucose
Increased ICP/impending herniation	Keep head of bed at 30 degrees	3% NS 5 mL/kg over 10 min *or* Mannitol 0.5 milligram/kg if normotensive (response is not dose-dependent)
Core temperature	Maintain temperature 36–38°C	Hypothermia in children not recommended; avoid hyperthermia
Seizure prophylaxis	Optional for children with witnessed seizures	Fosphenytoin or levetiracetam for first week following severe TBI
Neurosurgery/transfer	ICP monitoring and CSF diversion for ICP	
Anemia	Transfuse for Hgb <7 grams/dL	

Abbreviations: CSF = craniospinal fluid; GCS = Glasgow Coma Scale; Hgb = hemoglobin; ICP = intracranial pressure; NS = normal saline; P_{CO_2} = partial pressure of carbon dioxide; SBP = systolic blood pressure; TBI = traumatic brain injury.

struck by high-velocity object). Using these high-risk factors, the CHALICE rule had a sensitivity of 98% and specificity of 87% and resulted in the lowest CT scan rate of the three studies.[18]

TREATMENT OF SERIOUS INTRACRANIAL INJURY

Treatment for children follows the same treatment principles as for adults (see chapter 254, "Trauma in Adults"). Treatment is outlined in **Table 138-4**.

SPECIAL CONSIDERATIONS: CONCUSSION

Approximately 1.6 to 3.8 million athletes suffer a concussion annually in the United States,[12] with the majority affecting children.[21] Eight- to 13-year olds account for 40% of pediatric concussions.[22] Concussion is defined as a "complex pathophysiological process, involving the brain, induced by traumatic biomechanical forces." Common features include a direct blow or transmitted force, rapid-onset but short-lived neurologic impairment, characteristic symptoms that may or may not include loss of consciousness, and lack of structural abnormalities on standard imaging. Grading systems and the use of the terms *simple* and *complex* have been abandoned in lieu of a more symptom-focused approach.[23]

Sideline management involves attention to first aid and cervical spine protection in the appropriate clinical setting. Child and teen athletes suspected of having a concussion should not be returned to play the same day and should be observed for deterioration through the first few hours following the injury, because symptoms can progress over a 6- to 24-hour period. Standardized concussion assessment tools have been published and include the Sport Concussion Assessment Tool–Third Edition and the Child Sport Concussion Assessment Tool–Third Edition.[24] These tools are comprehensive, but impractical in the ED. In addition to assessment for serious head injury, focused tests of cognition and balance (designed for sideline use) are useful for the ED evaluation of the concussed patient, and two such exams, the Maddox questions and the Balance Error Scoring System, are detailed in **Table 138-5** and **Figure 138-9.**[25] Difficulty with definitive diagnosis on the sideline has led to the use of the phrase, "When in doubt, sit them out." Symptoms and signs of a concussion include somatic complaints (headache, dizziness, nausea or vomiting, blurred vision, balance problems, photophobia, phonophobia, fatigue), cognitive complaints (feeling of being in a fog,

TABLE 138-5 Maddox Questions for Sideline Evaluation of Concussion (any incorrect answer is suggestive of concussion)

Where are we at today?
Which half is it now?
Who scored last in the game?
What team did you play last week/last game?
Did your team win the last game?

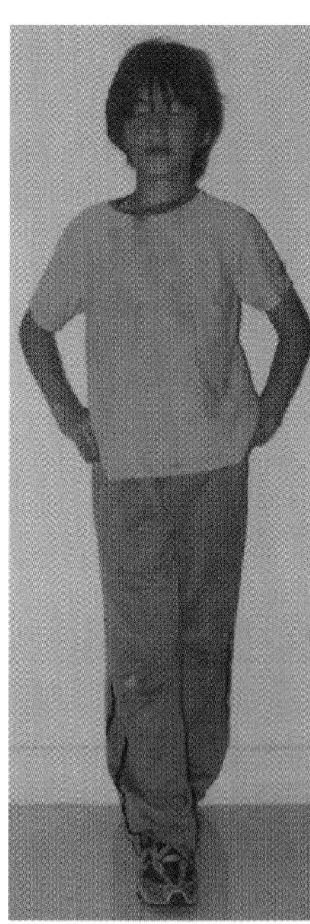

FIGURE 138-9. The athlete stands heel-to-toe with the dominant foot forward, eyes closed, and hands on hips for 20 seconds. More than five errors (lifting hands, opening eyes, stumbling, lifting forefoot or heel, or remaining out of the start position for >5 seconds) may suggest concussion. Note that shoes should not be worn during this test.

delayed reaction time, difficulty concentrating, confusion), emotional lability (irritability, depression, anxiety, apathy), loss of consciousness or amnesia, behavioral changes, and sleep disturbance (insomnia or sleepiness).[26]

In the ED, neuroimaging for diagnosis of a concussion is not recommended, but CT should be performed on children in whom an intracranial injury is suspected. Advanced imaging with certain MRI sequences, magnetic resonance spectroscopy, and positron emission tomography may be abnormal and predictive of outcomes[27] but does not guide management and, thus, is currently used as a research tool. Computerized neurocognitive testing, such as ImPACT, is rarely available in the ED, but should be performed by the primary care physician, particularly if preseason testing of an athlete was done and a comparative baseline is available. In clinically equivocal cases, neurocognitive tests are >90% sensitive to diagnose concussion.[28] Scores may be useful in verifying readiness to return to play, and the 72-hour score is prognostic of recovery time.

Adults typically require 3 to 5 days to return to baseline neurocognitive testing scores, college students 5 to 7 days, and high school students 10 to 14 days. Premorbid conditions such as mental health disorders, migraines, or attention deficit/hyperactivity disorder predict a slower recovery.[29] Fourteen percent of children and adolescents will have persistence of symptoms beyond 3 months, or "postconcussive syndrome."[30] Concerns regarding return to play prior to symptom resolution include second impact syndrome and recurrent concussions. **Second impact syndrome** is a rare entity characterized by loss of vascular autoregulation and cerebral edema in response to a second head injury prior to recovery from the first. It is exclusive to pediatrics, and mortality is high.[25] **Recurrent concussions** are more common in athletes who return quickly to play, and 80% of same-season concussions occur within 10 days of each other.[29]

Physical and cognitive rest are the cornerstones of concussion management. **Return to play should follow a six-step protocol of activity, provided that the child remains asymptomatic for at least 24 hours in between each step:**

1. No activity; complete rest
2. Light aerobic exercise (e.g., walking)
3. Sport-specific exercise, progressive addition of resistance training
4. Noncontact training drills
5. Full-contact training after medical clearance
6. Game play

Children who have recurrence of their symptoms upon progression should return to the previous level until they have been asymptomatic for 24 hours at that level.[28] Advise cognitive rest until the child is minimally symptomatic or asymptomatic. Cognitive rest includes rest from texting and video games and accommodations with schoolwork such as extra time for tests and assistance with note-taking.

Symptomatic treatment of concussive symptoms remains unproven, but described options include nonsteroidal anti-inflammatory medications, simple analgesics, and triptans for headache[31] and ondansetron for nausea and vomiting.[32] Prophylaxis with β-blockers or antiseizure medications can be considered in the outpatient setting.[31,33]

DISPOSITION AND FOLLOW-UP

Asymptomatic infants and children (e.g., not vomiting, normal neurologic and mental status examinations) who are at least 2 to 4 hours post-injury can safely be discharged to reliable caregivers without imaging. Provide careful instructions regarding signs and symptoms for which to **seek immediate care: lethargy, irritability, focal deficits, or intractable vomiting.**

Infants and children thought to be at *intermediate risk* can be observed for 3 to 6 hours, or a head CT scan can be obtained. If the CT is normal or they remain in stable condition on observation, they may safely be discharged to reliable caretakers with primary care follow-up.

Patients for whom a CT scan has been obtained and shows normal findings may safely be discharged to reliable caretakers. **The incidence of delayed deterioration requiring intervention after normal findings on CT is near zero.**[34,35] If a concussion is considered likely, parents should be informed of the specific return to activity guidelines, and encouraged to seek primary care or neurology follow-up.

Children with complex, depressed, or basilar skull fractures should be managed in conjunction with the pediatric neurosurgeon and typically require admission. Stable, asymptomatic infants and children with linear, nondisplaced skull fractures and no intracranial injury are safe for discharge with primary care or neurosurgical outpatient follow-up.[36] Parents should be warned that infants are at risk for "growing fractures" over the weeks to months following a skull fracture.

Patients with intracranial injury and those thought to be at risk of nonaccidental trauma may require transfer to a hospital with appropriate services if admission to an appropriately monitored setting is not available at the presenting institution.

REFERENCES

The complete reference list is available online at www.TintinalliEM.com.

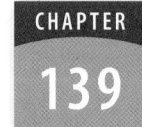

CHAPTER 139 Cervical Spine Injury in Infants and Children

Solomon Behar

CERVICAL SPINE INJURIES IN INFANTS AND CHILDREN

INTRODUCTION AND EPIDEMIOLOGY

Cervical spine injuries occur in 1% to 2% of all pediatric trauma patients. While the incidence of cervical spine injuries in children with trauma is lower than adults, children have higher rates of mortality (~18%) compared to adults (~10%).[1] In children <8 years old, almost three quarters of all spinal injuries occur in the cervical spine,[2] and nearly two thirds of these children have associated neurologic deficits and head or other major organ injury.[3] In addition, spinal cord injury without radiographic abnormality (SCIWORA) may occur in children and typically involves the cervical spine. The incidence of SCIWORA among pediatric trauma patients ranges from 0.15% to 0.2%, compromising 4.5% to 35% of pediatric spine injuries.[4-6] Motor vehicle crashes are the most common mechanism of cervical spine injuries, followed by falls, and in teenagers, diving and sports injuries. Boys are affected more often than girls. Child abuse can result in cervical spine injuries in younger patients via a shaking mechanism, although this is a rare manifestation of nonaccidental trauma.[7]

PATHOPHYSIOLOGY

A number of anatomic differences between the pediatric and adult cervical spine predispose children to different patterns of injury (**Table 139-1**). In particular, the relatively larger head-to-body ratio in

TABLE 139-1 Anatomic Considerations in the Pediatric Cervical Spine
Larger head
Ligamentous laxity
Absent cervical lordosis
Weaker neck muscles
Anterior wedging of vertebrae
Shallow and horizontal vertebral facets
Ossification centers and synchondroses

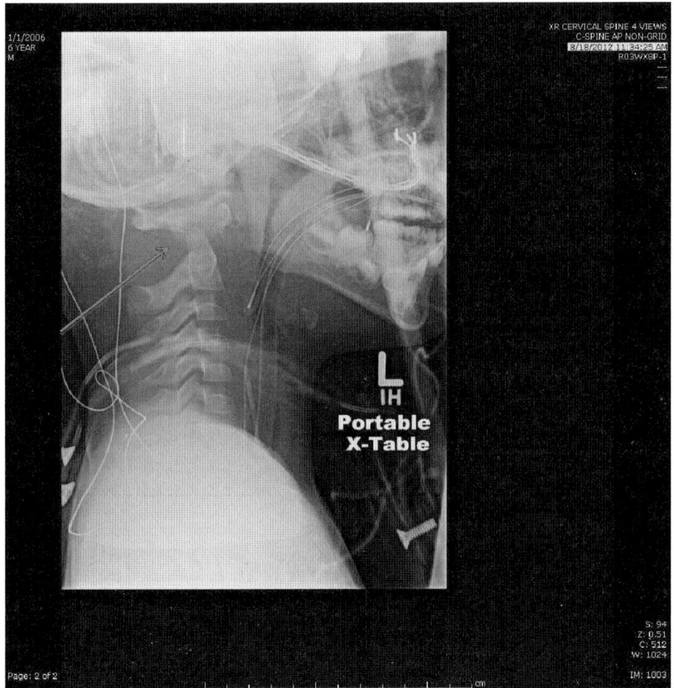

A

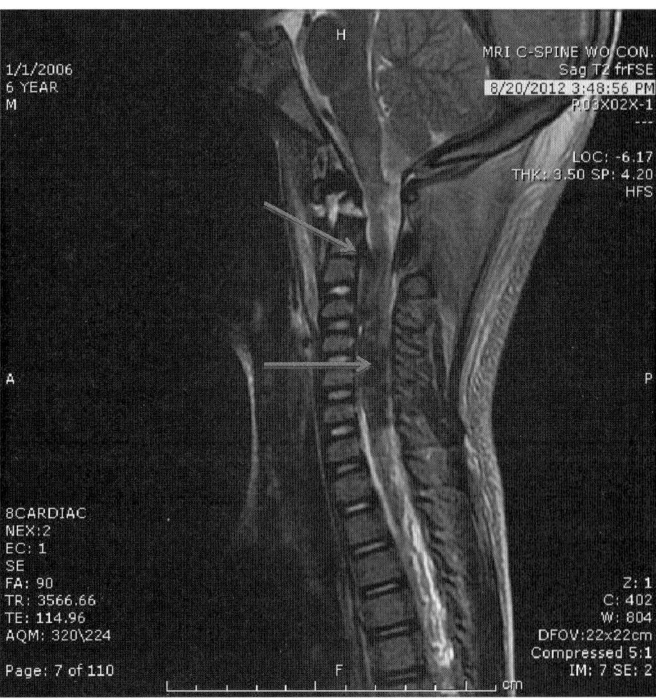

B

FIGURE 139-1. Atlantoaxial dislocation in a 6-year-old boy involved in a motor vehicle crash. **A.** Lateral plain radiograph reveals atlantoaxial dislocation (blue arrow). **B.** MRI of the same patient reveals a near-complete transection of the brain stem at the level of the distal medulla, extensive ligamentous injury with resulting atlantoaxial dissociation, extensive intrathecal hematoma and hemorrhage, C1-C2 interspinous ligament tear, and prevertebral soft tissue swelling and edema around the nuchal ligament (blue arrows).

young children creates a fulcrum at C2-C3 (compared to C5-C6 in adults) that accounts for higher rates of cervical spine injury above C3 in children. Weaker muscles and ligaments combined with anterior wedging and shallow facets connecting cervical vertebrae and immature growth centers together allow for easier anterior-posterior slipping of the vertebrae than in adults.

Patients younger than 8 years of age incur high ligamentous injuries more often than older children and adults. Fractures tend to occur at the weak points in the bones—synchondroses and ossification centers. Dens fractures occur most commonly along the synchondrosis, especially in children younger than age 7 years. The mechanism of injury is usually a forward facing child in a high-speed motor vehicle crash with rapid forward flexion. Atlanto-occipital and atlantoaxial dislocation injuries are devastating vertical distraction injuries that occur in the very young child, most commonly from a motor vehicle crash, and usually result in rapid death (**Figure 139-1**).

IMMOBILIZATION AND NECK STABILIZATION IN INFANTS AND CHILDREN

Proper immobilization of the cervical spine is of primary concern in the ED. Immobilization may be difficult in young children who are frightened or agitated, and placement of a cervical collar in children <7 years old while on a flat surface (e.g., spine board) may cause unwanted flexion of the cervical spine with further harm. A number of untoward effects have been associated with immobilization on a long backboard and cervical spine immobilization, including development of decubitus ulcers, flexion of the neck causing respiratory compromise, worsening of atlanto-occipital distraction injury, increased intracranial pressure, and musculoskeletal pain that may mimic injury and lead to increased radiologic investigation.[8-20]

For those at significant risk for cervical spine injury, neutral positioning of the neck is important; consider elevating the torso 2.5 cm (or more for children <4 years of age) from the spine board in order to alleviate neck flexion caused by the large occiput, and place padding beneath the child. **Neutral position is achieved by aligning the external auditory meatus with the shoulders.** Proper sizing of pediatric cervical collars is equally important and varies depending on the device used. If the proper-size collar is not available, use towel rolls or foam blocks placed on both sides of the child's head and secured to the backboard with tape across the forehead.

CLINICAL FEATURES

HISTORY

Ask parents, witnesses, or prehospital personnel about the mechanism of injury: children with cervical spine injury will usually have a history of high-force acceleration/deceleration (as seen in motor vehicle crashes) or axial loading trauma (falls, diving injuries). Trivial mechanisms such as a ground-level fall usually do not lead to serious spine injury unless the patient has a condition associated with cervical spine instability (see "Special Considerations" later in the chapter). In the cooperative, verbal child, ask about symptoms such as neck pain, sensory deficits, or weakness. One large multicenter case-control study looking at 521 children with blunt trauma and cervical spine injury identified eight factors associated with cervical spine injury after blunt trauma (**Table 139-2**).[21] Absence of these eight factors had a 98% sensitivity and 26% specificity for cervical spine injury. Prospective studies for validation of these risk factors are forthcoming.

TABLE 139-2 Risk Factors for Pediatric Cervical Spine Injury
Altered mental status
Focal neurologic examination
Neck pain
Torticollis
High-risk motor vehicle crash
Substantial torso injury
Predisposing condition associated with cervical spine injury
Diving

PHYSICAL EXAMINATION

Examine the child with a primary survey of airway, breathing, and circulation, followed by a complete head-to-toe examination to identify major and potentially distracting injuries that may complicate the specific evaluation of the cervical spine.

Pay careful attention to breathing, because damage to C3-C5 can injure the phrenic nerve, impairing innervation to the diaphragm, compromising respiratory mechanics, and leading to apnea. Injury to the high cervical spine can affect hemodynamic stability from spinal shock. Intubated or obtunded trauma patients should have a cervical collar remain in place, and imaging should be performed.

In children who are cooperative and alert, assess for midline neck tenderness, the presence of torticollis, and neurologic deficits while maintaining inline stabilization of the neck. Sensory symptoms such as numbness or tingling are the most common neurologic deficits among pediatric cervical spine injury patients, and persistent sensory deficits may help localize the level of the injury.

Test for motor function in the cooperative child: shoulder shrug is controlled by C5, elbow flexion and wrist extension by C6, elbow extension and wrist flexion by C7, and finger flexion by C8. Also check deep tendon reflexes: the biceps reflex tests C5, the brachioradialis reflex tests C6, and the triceps reflex tests C7.

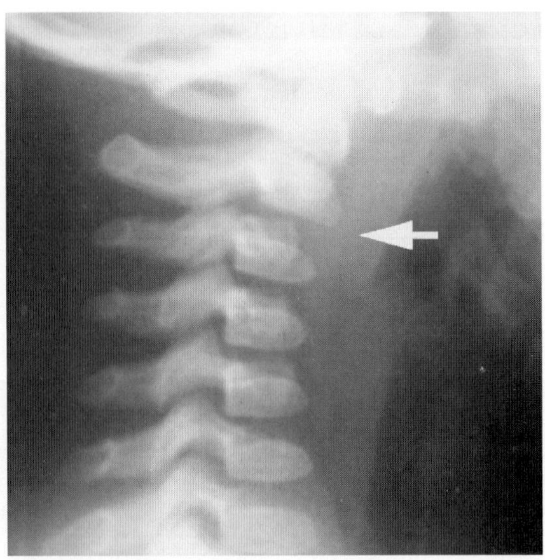

FIGURE 139-2. Pseudosubluxation of C2 on C3. [Reprinted, with permission, from Yamamoto LG: Cervical spine malalignment—true or pseudosubluxation? In: Yamamoto LG, Inaba AS, DiMauro R (eds): *Radiology Cases in Pediatric Emergency Medicine,* Vol. 1, Case 5. Honolulu, HI: University of Hawaii John A. Burns School of Medicine, Department of Pediatrics, 1994. http://www.hawaii.edu/medicine/pediatrics/pemxray/v1c05.html.]

DIAGNOSIS

DIFFERENTIAL DIAGNOSIS

Distinguishing between bony cervical spine injury, **SCIWORA**, and peripheral nerve injury (brachial plexus) from sports-related accidents can be challenging. Transient burning sensation of the hands and fingers has been described with hyperextension injuries among young football players and may indicate central cord contusion. Muscular torticollis causes neck pain in children but typically lacks a history of trauma. Infectious causes of neck pain in children include cervical adenitis and deep space infections such as retropharyngeal and peritonsillar abscess. These conditions are associated with fever and toxic appearance and do not include a history of injury.

LABORATORY TESTING

Routine laboratory testing is not helpful in the general evaluation of cervical spine injury in children but may be useful in the context of multisystem trauma.

IMAGING

Because the history and physical examination can be difficult, particularly in young children or those with multiple injuries, imaging is often considered, and clinical decision rules have been developed to help identify patients who require radiologic investigation.

Adult decision rules such as NEXUS and the Canadian Cervical Spine Rule (CCR) (see Tables 258-4 and 258-5) for cervical spine clearance can safely be applied to children **over 8 years old**, the same age that patient anatomy starts to resemble that of an adult. NEXUS should be used with caution in children under 9 years old, because the cohort examined in the study of NEXUS included no patients with cervical spine injury under the age of 2 years and only four patients under the age of 9 years.[22] A prospective study applying NEXUS in children showed that NEXUS did in fact miss two fractures, both in children under 2 years of age, highlighting the difficulty of ruling out cervical spine injury in the very young patient.[23] Additional clinical algorithms have been published by the Trauma Association of Canada's Pediatric Subcommittee (see Figures 139-4 and 139-5 later).

Plain Radiographs For patients in whom a cervical spine injury is suspected, plain radiographs should be considered first. The sensitivity of plain radiographs for identifying fractures, dislocations, and subluxations in children varies across the literature, ranging from 74% to 98%, with sensitivity increasing with the number of views taken.[24-30] Combining the cross-table lateral and anterior-posterior views identifies 87% of significant cervical spine injury in children younger than 8 years of age.[30] Consider the addition of an odontoid (open mouth) view in cooperative older children, although the added value in children younger than age 8 years has been questioned.[30]

Interpreting pediatric cervical spine radiographs can be challenging as a result of the anatomic differences across the spectrum of age. The principles of evaluation are similar to adults: assess the anterior and posterior vertebral lines, the spinolaminal line, and the spinous processes for alignment; and carefully examine the soft tissue spaces for swelling that might indicate subtle fracture. Widening of the soft tissue space >7 mm in the retropharyngeal space and >14 mm in the retrotracheal space on lateral x-ray may be an indirect sign of cervical spine injury. In addition, assess the pediatric cervical spine for atlantoaxial instability. Useful measurements include Wackenheim's clivus line

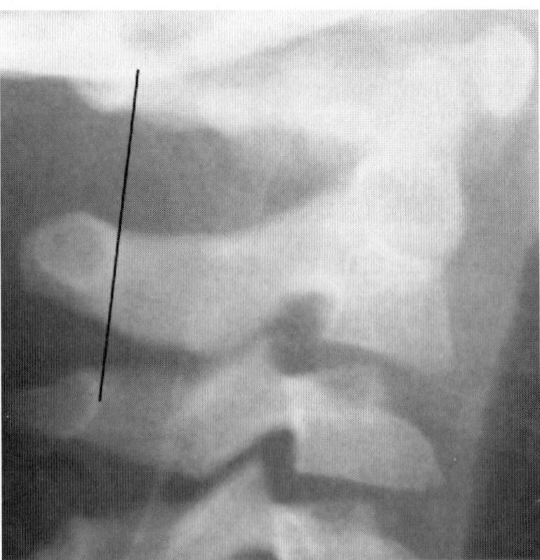

FIGURE 139-3. Posterior cervical line of Swischuk. [Reprinted, with permission, from Yamamoto L: Cervical spine malalignment—true or pseudosubluxation? In: Yamamoto LG, Inaba AS, DiMauro R (eds): *Radiology Cases in Pediatric Emergency Medicine,* Vol. 1, Case 5. Honolulu, HI: University of Hawaii John A. Burns School of Medicine, Department of Pediatrics, 1994. http://www.hawaii.edu/medicine/pediatrics/pemxray/v1c05.html.]

TABLE 139-3 Predispositions to Cervical Spine Injury in Children

Down syndrome: 15% atlantoaxial instability
Connective tissue disorders (e.g., Marfan's syndrome and Ehlers-Danlos syndrome): ligamentous laxity
Klippel-Feil syndrome: cervical vertebral defects
Morquio's syndrome (type IV mucopolysaccharidosis): odontoid hypoplasia
Previous cervical spine surgeries or arthritis

(a line along the posterior edge of the clivus should intersect the odontoid) and the rule of thirds (the dens, cord, and empty space should each occupy one third of the spinal space). Craniocervical dislocation is suggested by a C1-C2:C2-C3 ratio >2.5. Important differences between pediatric and adult cervical spine radiographs include:

1. Normal cervical lordosis may be absent in children.
2. The posterior arch of C1 fuses by age 3 years and the anterior arch by age 10 years.
3. Anterior wedging of the vertebrae caused by secondary growth centers may be mistaken for compression fractures in children under 7 years old.
4. Posterior laminar fusion lines may be mistaken for fractures in children under 7 years old.
5. Children younger than 8 years old may demonstrate pseudosubluxation (up to 46%) on lateral x-ray, usually at the C2-C3 level (**Figure 139-2**).[31]

Swischuk developed a method for distinguishing between true subluxation and pseudosubluxation: draw a line connecting the posterior cortex of the spinous process of C1 to the cortex of the spinous process of C3 (**Figure 139-3**). If this line is more than 2 mm anterior to the spinous process of C2, suspect cervical pathology, such as a

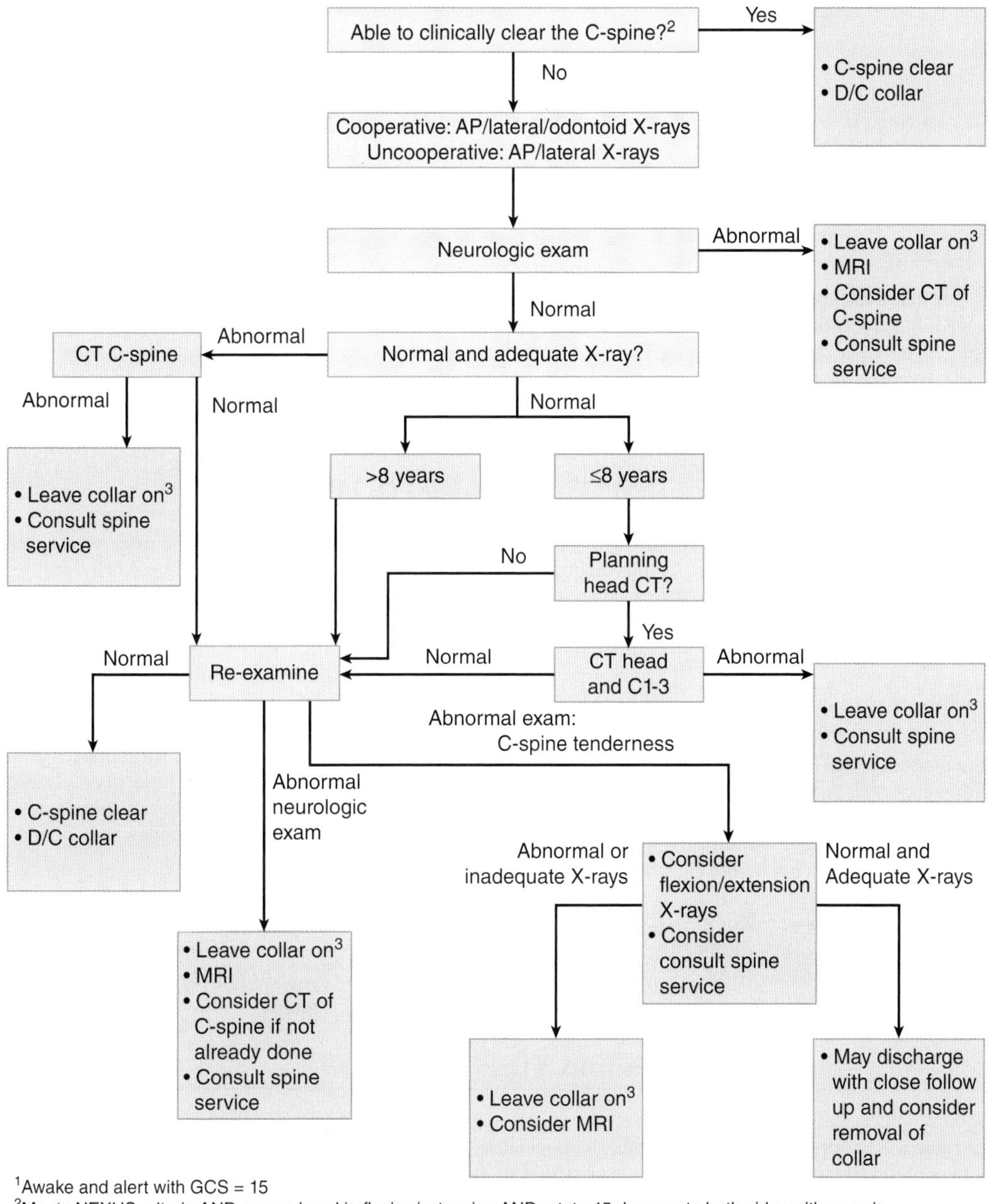

FIGURE 139-4. Algorithm for evaluation of the pediatric cervical spine (C-spine) in the patient with a reliable clinical exam. AP = anteroposterior; GCS = Glasgow Coma Scale. [Reproduced with permission from Chung S, Mikrogianakis A, Wales PW, et al: Trauma Association of Canada Pediatric Subcommittee National Pediatric Cervical Spine Evaluation Pathway: consensus guidelines. *J Trauma*. 2011 Apr;70(4):873-884. Copyright Wolters Kluwer Health.]

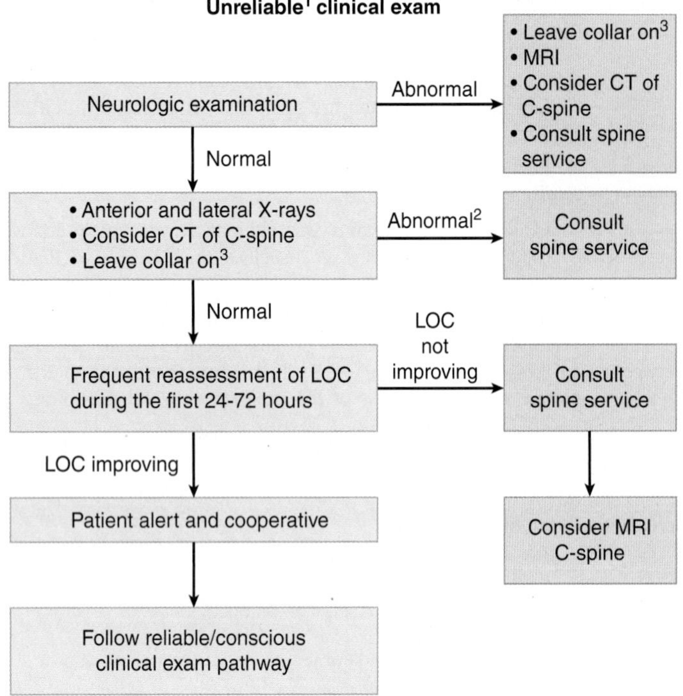

FIGURE 139-5. Algorithm for evaluation of the pediatric cervical spine (C-spine) in the patient with an unreliable clinical exam. GCS = Glasgow Coma Scale; LOC = level of consciousness; T/L = thoracic/lumbar. [Reproduced with permission from Chung S, Mikrogianakis A, Wales PW, et al: Trauma Association of Canada Pediatric Subcommittee National Pediatric Cervical Spine Evaluation Pathway: consensus guidelines. *J Trauma.* 2011 Apr;70(4):873-884. Copyright Wolters Kluwer Health.]

hangman's fracture. There is little role for flexion/extension plain x-rays in the ED for children. Obtain an MRI if ligamentous instability is suspected.

CT Scan Although CT has been advocated as the most cost-effective modality for imaging the cervical spine in adults, it is unclear if this is true for children, in whom radiation exposure is of particular concern. CT scanning exposes a child to 10 to 90 times the radiation of plain films, with an estimated 18-fold increase in thyroid malignancy in a theoretical model if all plain films are replaced by CT scans.[32,33] Given the potential risks and unclear advantages of CT in children, this modality should be reserved for children with inadequate visualization of the cervical spine on plain radiographs, those with abnormal or suspicious plain radiographs, and those with significant mechanism of injury who are obtunded or intubated and undergoing CT evaluation for other injuries. Some experts advocate scanning up to C3 in young children and stopping there if no injury is detected, avoiding irradiation to radiosensitive thyroid tissues.

MRI MRI is the modality of choice for the diagnosis and evaluation of SCIWORA and can be helpful in determining prognosis as well. Patients with normal MRI examinations and SCIWORA have very favorable prognoses; those with minor findings such as cord edema or a minor hemorrhage have good prognoses, whereas those with major hemorrhage or cord transections have poor prognoses for recovery.[34] MRI should be reserved for children who have an obvious neurologic deficit, those with a persistently unreliable clinical examination, the very young with a dangerous mechanism of injury, or those with persistent symptoms and negative plain films and CT scan.[4]

TREATMENT

The ED management of the child with potential cervical spine injury should follow the principles of advanced trauma life support with primary attention to assessment and management of the airway and breathing (especially with a high cervical spine injury, which may compromise respiratory effort) and circulation (particularly in spinal shock).

In adult cervical spine injury, steroids are no longer favored (see chapter 258, "Spine Trauma"), and no large studies have examined the efficacy of steroids in pediatric spine injury, so steroids are not standard of care for children.

Definitive management of cervical spine injury is primarily surgical, through consultation with pediatric neurosurgery or orthopedics.

DISPOSITION AND FOLLOW-UP

Unstable patients and those with radiographic evidence of cervical spine injury require admission, usually to intensive care; a minority require immediate surgical intervention. Children with normal plain radiographs or CT imaging who have persistent neurologic complaints need MRI evaluation. Children with persistent neck pain but without focal neurologic signs or symptoms and normal x-rays or CT imaging will usually be evaluated with an MRI. If imaging is normal and the mechanism of injury is mild, the child may be discharged with an appropriately sized cervical collar and close outpatient medical follow-up. Children without neck pain or neurologic symptoms or deficits and those who have been cleared radiographically may be discharged with instructions to return for symptoms of numbness, tingling, or weakness in the arms, hands, legs, or feet.

THORACIC, LUMBAR AND SACRAL SPINE INJURIES

Injuries to the spine and spinal cord outside of the cervical spine are discussed in chapter 110, "Pediatric Trauma."

SPECIAL CONSIDERATIONS

Certain conditions predispose patients to cervical spine injury as a result of associated abnormalities causing cervical spine instability. These are listed in **Table 139-3**. Children with these conditions should be considered at high risk for cervical spine injury and undergo conservative evaluation.

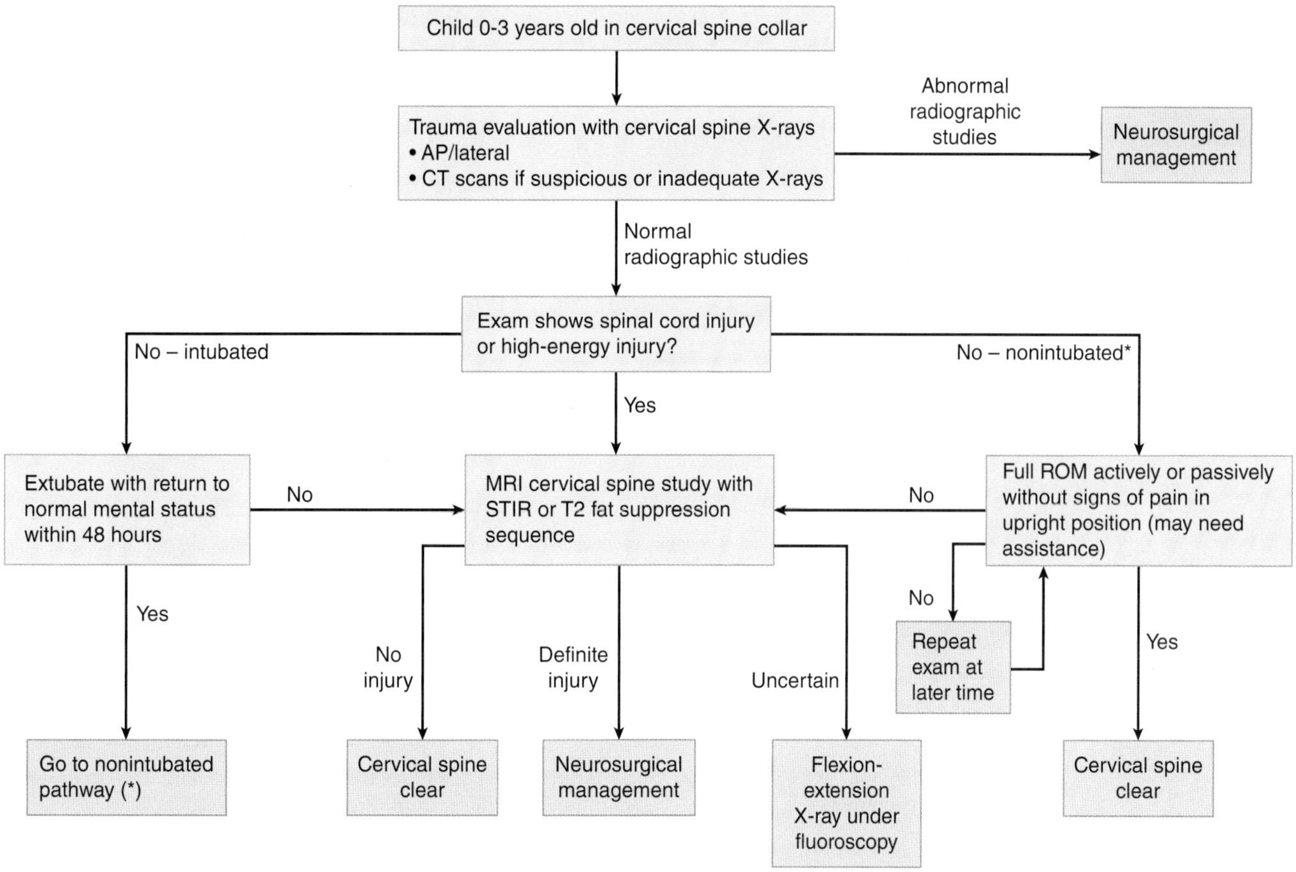

Child 0-3 years old in cervical spine collar

Trauma evaluation with cervical spine X-rays
• AP/lateral
• CT scans if suspicious or inadequate X-rays

Abnormal radiographic studies

Neurosurgical management

Normal radiographic studies

Exam shows spinal cord injury or high-energy injury?

No – intubated

No – nonintubated*

Yes

Extubate with return to normal mental status within 48 hours

No

MRI cervical spine study with STIR or T2 fat suppression sequence

No

Full ROM actively or passively without signs of pain in upright position (may need assistance)

No

Repeat exam at later time

Yes

Yes

No injury

Definite injury

Uncertain

Go to nonintubated pathway (*)

Cervical spine clear

Neurosurgical management

Flexion-extension X-ray under fluoroscopy

Cervical spine clear

FIGURE 139-6. Algorithm for evaluation of the pediatric cervical spine in the patient age 0 to 3 years. AP = anteroposterior; ROM = range of motion; STIR = short T1 inversion recovery. [Reproduced with permission from Anderson RC, Kan P, Vanaman M, et al: Utility of a cervical spine clearance protocol after trauma in children between 0 and 3 years of age. *J Neurosurg Pediatr.* 2010 Mar;5(3):292-296.]

CLINICAL ALGORITHMS

In 2011, the Trauma Association of Canada's Pediatric Subcommittee National Pediatric Cervical Spine Evaluation Pathway released a consensus guideline for evaluation of the pediatric cervical spine summarized in **Figures 139-4, 139-5,** and **139-6.**[35] They divided their algorithms into two parts: the reliable patient (Figure 139-4) and the unreliable patient (Figure 139-5). These algorithms have not been prospectively studied, but represent a reasonable, expert-driven tool to evaluate the pediatric cervical spine. For the youngest victims of cervical spine trauma (age 0 to 3 years), a clinically challenging population, an algorithm for cervical spine evaluation has been developed and prospectively studied on a small scale (Figure 139-6). In a moderate-sized, two-center study, no injury was missed using this protocol.[36]

REFERENCES

The complete reference list is available online at www.TintinalliEM.com.

Musculoskeletal Disorders in Children

Karen J.L. Black
Catherine Duffy
Courtney Hopkins-Mann
Demilola Ogunnaiki-Joseph
Donna Moro-Sutherland

GENERAL PRINCIPLES

The anatomy of the pediatric musculoskeletal system is unique and reflects the active growth and development that occurs during childhood. Fracture classification, treatment approach, and types of complications are directly related to this unique anatomy. In general, both injury patterns and treatment approaches in children in whom closure of the physes (growth plates) has already occurred is similar to those of the adult. Therefore, the major focus of this chapter is directed at injuries occurring in the prepubescent child with open physes. In addition, diseases specific to children that cause nontraumatic musculoskeletal complaints are covered.

The long bones of children consist of discrete anatomic areas. The physis is an area of growth cartilage and may occur at one (e.g., the phalanges) or both (e.g., the tibia and the femur) ends of a long bone. The area of bone between a physis and the adjacent joint is termed the *epiphysis*. An *apophysis* is an outgrowth of bone, usually with its own ossification center in childhood that often serves as a point for muscle or ligament attachment. The midshaft of a long bone is referred to as the

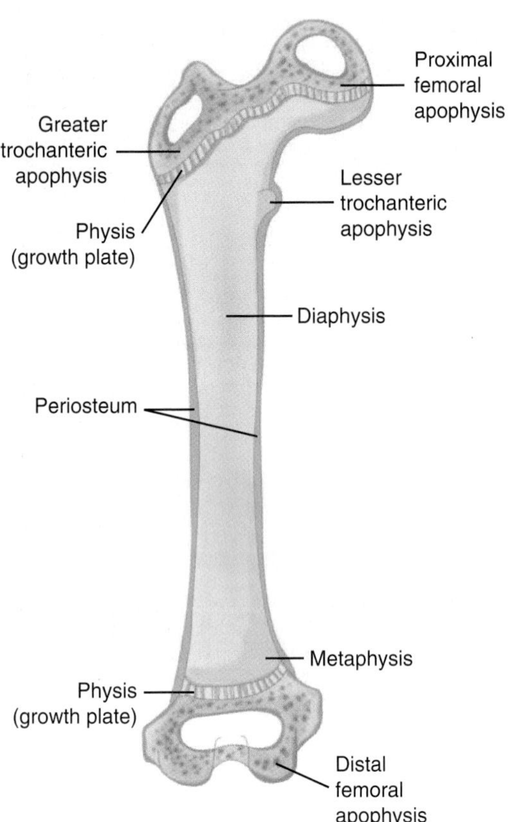

FIGURE 140-1. The anatomy of the pediatric long bone as demonstrated by the femur. Longitudinal growth occurs at the physes (growth plates) located at either end. Bony prominences that serve as sites of muscular or ligamentous attachment are known as apophyses (e.g., greater trochanteric apophysis).

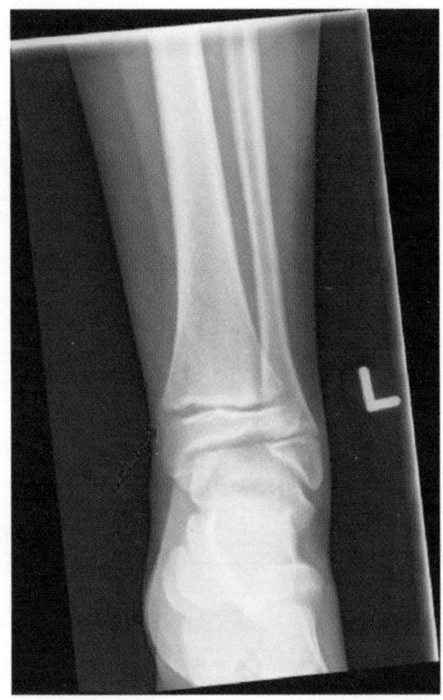

FIGURE 140-2. Salter-Harris type I fracture of distal tibia. Anteroposterior radiograph showing widened physeal line of distal tibia with malalignment of epiphysis with metaphysis (*arrow*). [Photo used with permission of Karen Black, BC Children's Hospital, Vancouver.]

diaphysis. The *metaphysis* of a long bone represents the area between the diaphysis and the physis (**Figure 140-1**; see chapter 267, "Initial Evaluation and Management of Orthopedic Injuries").

The long bones of children are less dense and more porous than the long bones of adults. Pediatric long bones respond to mechanical stress by bowing and buckling rather than fracturing through and through, as in adults. The periosteum of the diaphysis and the metaphysis is thick in children and is continuous from the metaphysis to the epiphysis, surrounding and protecting the mechanically weaker physis. The weakness of the physis is in part related to the reduced oxygen tension found in the hypertrophic zone of the physis. This hypertrophic zone is the location of frequent fractures within the physis. The physis is also sensitive to alterations in the blood supply, and physeal injuries can result in growth disturbance. Compression forces alone may also affect bone growth. This is particularly true when compression forces are applied to the epiphyseal side of the physis. The injury to bone growth caused by compression results from interruption of the epiphyseal circulation to the reproductive cells of the physis.

The growth of the musculoskeletal system and its response to injury are influenced by the growth of muscle and connective tissue. The ligaments of children are stronger and more compliant than in adults, and ligaments tolerate mechanical forces better than the weaker physes. Therefore, apophyseal detachments or epiphyseal fractures are much more common than ligamentous injuries during childhood.

FRACTURE PATTERNS

FRACTURES INVOLVING THE PHYSIS

The Salter and Harris classification system (see Figure 267-7) is based on the relationship of the fracture line to the physis and the prognosis for growth disturbance.

Salter-Harris Type I Fractures Type I physeal injuries occur when the epiphysis separates from the metaphysis. The cleavage is through the hypertrophic cell zone of the physis, with the reproductive cells of the physis remaining with the epiphysis. There are no associated fragments of bone, as the thick periosteal attachments surrounding the physis remain intact. The epiphysis may, however, displace from the metaphysis. **Type I injuries have a low incidence of growth disturbances.**

Suspect a Salter-Harris type I injury when there is point tenderness over a physis. Radiographic findings are typically subtle or absent, and soft tissue swelling or a joint effusion may be the only abnormality. Epiphyseal displacement can usually be appreciated on x-rays in one or more views (**Figure 140-2**); however, in the absence of epiphyseal displacement, the diagnosis is a clinical one.

Treatment of most type I fractures consists of immobilization of the suspected fracture using an appropriate splint, cold compresses, and elevation to limit swelling. Refer to an orthopedic surgeon for monitoring of bone growth disturbances. **Type I fractures of the distal fibula (which happens to be the most common fracture site for type I) are exceptions because they are not associated with growth arrest and can be followed by a primary care physician after splinting.**

Salter-Harris Type II Fractures In a type II injury, the fracture line extends a variable distance along the hypertrophic cell zone of the physis and then out through a piece of metaphyseal bone. The periosteum overlying the metaphyseal fragment remains intact, whereas the periosteum on the opposite side of the fracture is torn away from the diaphysis while remaining adherent to the epiphysis. Growth is preserved because the reproductive layers of the physis maintain their position with the epiphysis and the epiphyseal circulation. Diagnosis is made radiographically by noting a triangular-shaped fragment of metaphysis that is not associated with discernible injury to the epiphysis (**Figures 140-3** and **140-4**).

Treatment of a type II fracture consists of closed reduction of any displacement followed by immobilization in a splint or cast, ice, elevation, analgesia, and orthopedic follow-up.

Salter-Harris Type III Fractures Type III physeal injuries are intra-articular. The fracture line extends intra-articularly from the epiphysis, through the hypertrophic zone of the physis, with the cleavage plane continuing along the physis to the periphery. The prognosis for subsequent bone growth relates to the preservation of circulation to the epiphyseal bone fragment; however, the prognosis is usually quite favorable.

The diagnosis of a type III injury is made radiographically and is based on the appearance of an epiphyseal fragment not associated with an

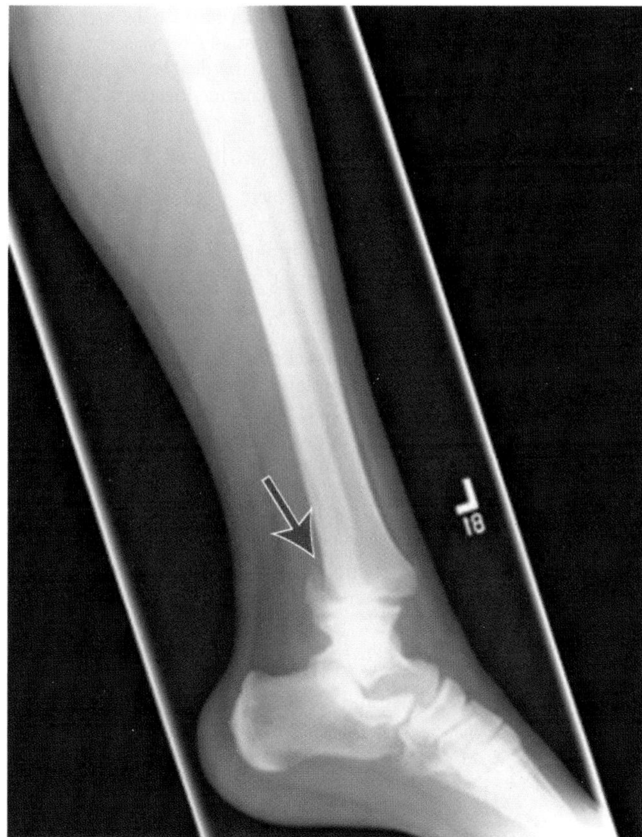

FIGURE 140-3. Salter-Harris type II fracture of distal tibia. Lateral radiograph illustrating fracture extending through physeal growth plate and metaphysis with dorsal displacement of epiphysis requiring reduction. [Photo used with permission of Wake Medical Center, Raleigh, NC.]

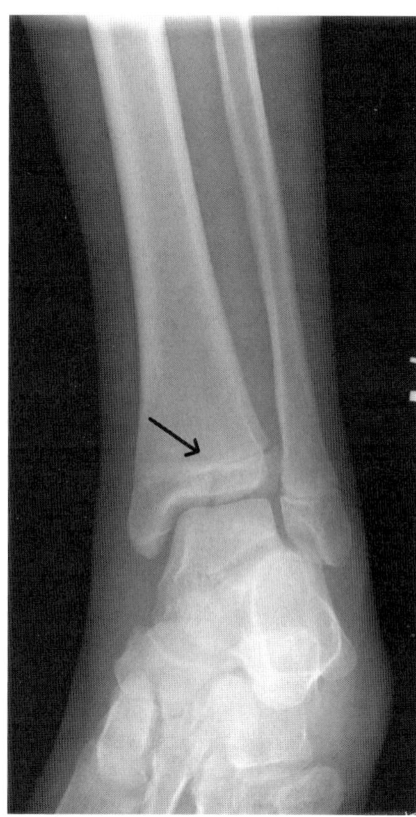

FIGURE 140-5. An x-ray of a Salter-Harris type III fracture of the distal tibia, also known as Tillaux's fracture. Note the intra-articular component extending through the growth plate and the medial epiphysis of the tibia. [Reproduced with permission from Strange GR, Ahrens WR, Schafermeyer RW, Wiebe RA: *Pediatric Emergency Medicine,* 3rd ed. McGraw-Hill, Inc., 2009. Fig 38-8.]

apparent metaphyseal fracture. There may or may not be an associated periosteal injury (**Figure 140-5**). Occasionally, additional imaging with CT or MRI is used to better evaluate the extent of fracture and articular surface involvement. Treatment requires orthopedic consultation and follow-up, as open reduction may be required in some cases to ensure proper alignment of the articular surface.

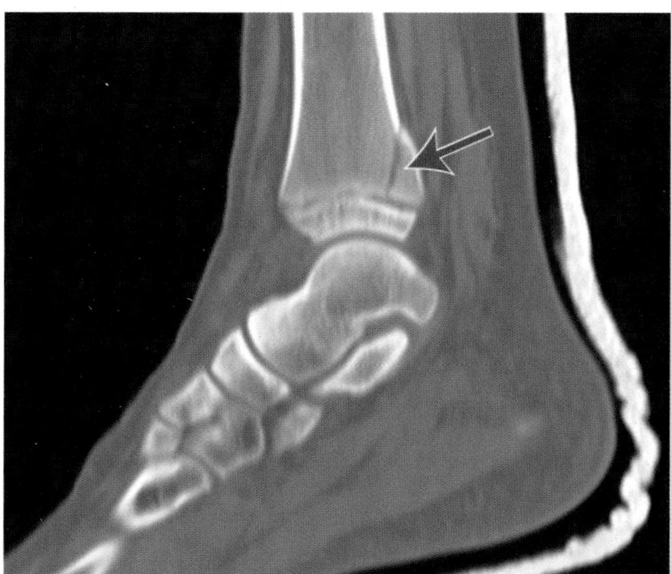

FIGURE 140-4. Salter-Harris type II fracture of distal tibia. CT image illustrating fracture extending through physeal growth plate and metaphysis (*arrow*). [Image used with permission of Wake Medical Center, Raleigh, NC.]

Salter-Harris Type IV Fractures In type IV injuries, the fracture line originates at the articular surface and extends through the epiphysis, the entire thickness of the physis, and continues through the metaphysis (**Figure 140-6**). The risk of growth disturbance with this type of fracture is significant, and reduction must be precise.

The diagnosis of a type IV injury is made radiographically upon identification of epiphyseal and metaphyseal fragments. Treatment is typically open surgical reduction and internal fixation.

Salter-Harris Type V Fractures Type V injuries typically involve the knee or ankle and are the result of a profound compressive force transmitted to the physis, resulting in crushing of the chondrocytes in both the reserve and proliferative zones. Displacement of the epiphysis is usually only minimal despite the significant damage to the physis.

The diagnosis of a type V injury may be difficult initially, leading to a lack of appreciation of the severity of the injury. An initial diagnosis of a sprain or a type I physeal fracture may prove incorrect in view of subsequent development of premature growth arrest during follow-up. Radiographs may appear normal or may demonstrate focal narrowing of the physeal plate. There is also typically a joint effusion. The history, however, should point to a type V injury, as these injuries are typically associated with a significant mechanism. Treatment consists of casting and orthopedic monitoring in anticipation of bone growth arrest.

TORUS FRACTURES

Compressive forces often result in a bulging or buckling of the periosteum rather than a more complete fracture line. Cortical, or *torus,* fractures are so named to describe prominence or bulging of the bony cortex, usually involving the metaphysis. These are also called *buckle fractures.*

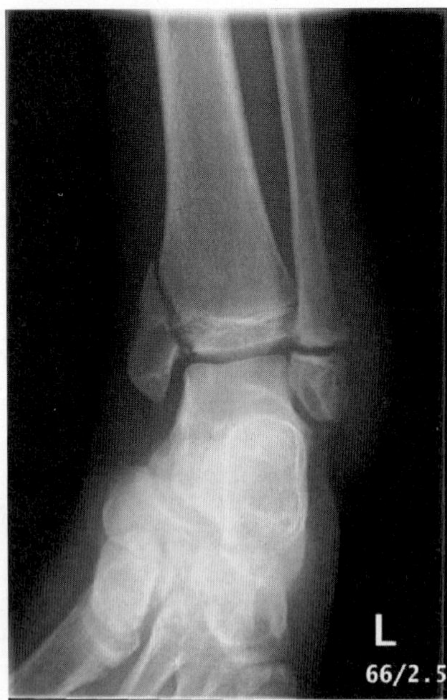

FIGURE 140-6. X-ray of a Salter-Harris type IV fracture of distal tibia with a Salter I fracture of the fibula. [Photo used with permission of Karen Black, BC Children's Hospital, Vancouver.]

A simple torus fracture will not produce a visible deformity to the shape of the extremity; however, there is typically soft tissue swelling and point tenderness over the bony injury. In children who are not obese, the torus fracture is occasionally palpable as a ridge over the metaphyseal area of the long bone.

Radiographically, the torus fracture may be subtle. Carefully inspect the contour of the metaphyseal flare. Any asymmetry, bulging, or deviation of the cortical margin indicates a torus fracture. Soft tissue swelling is also usually evident (**Figure 140-7**). Torus fractures are not associated with angulation, displacement, or rotational abnormalities, so reduction is not necessary. Treat by splinting in a position of function with primary care or orthopedic follow-up within 1 week. Simple torus fractures of the distal radius can need splinting, but orthopedic follow-up is not necessary.

GREENSTICK FRACTURES

A *greenstick* fracture is characterized by cortical disruption and periosteal tearing on the convex side of the bone, with an intact periosteum on the concave side of the fracture. Greenstick fractures are more stable and somewhat less painful than complete fractures because the area of intact periosteum limits bony displacement (**Figure 140-8**).

The need for reduction is determined by the degree of angulation of the fracture, the age of the child, and the anatomic location of the injury.

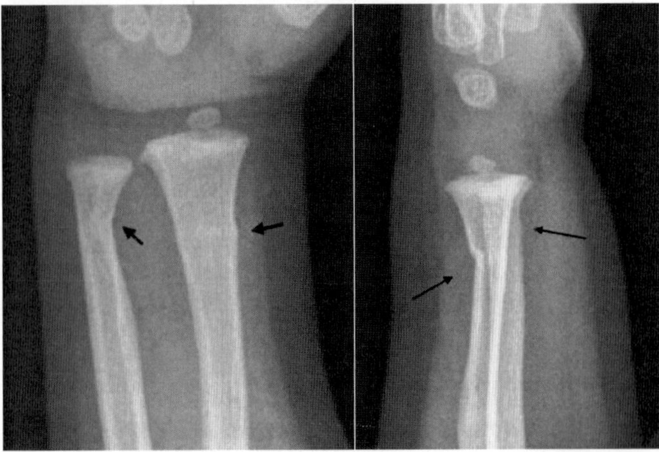

FIGURE 140-7. Torus fractures of the distal radius and ulna. [Figures used with permission of Karen Black, BC Children's Hospital, Vancouver.]

PLASTIC DEFORMITIES (BOWING OR BENDING FRACTURES)

Plastic deformities, also referred to as *bowing* or *bending fractures*, are almost exclusively limited to the forearm and lower leg long bones. Usually, a bowing injury is noted in combination with a complete fracture of the other bone of the forearm or lower leg. The cortex of the diaphysis of the long bone is deformed, but the periosteum along the entire diaphysis is preserved.

Plastic deformity is usually obvious clinically, which should guide the inexperienced clinician who may think that in the absence of an obvious fracture the x-ray appearances are normal.

Proper interpretation of the radiographs requires an awareness of the normal shape of the long bones involved because fracture lines and disruptions in the periosteum are absent. Comparison films of the uninvolved extremity are not typically necessary. Prompt orthopedic consultation is required for any plastic deformities, as proper reduction and realignment are essential. Reduction usually requires completion of the fracture and restoration of proper alignment.

FRACTURES FROM CHILD ABUSE

See chapter 148, "Child Abuse and Neglect" for a complete discussion of child abuse.

UPPER EXTREMITY INJURIES

CLAVICLE FRACTURES

Clavicle fractures occur during two distinct time frames: the newborn period and childhood. Fractures of the clavicle in the newborn usually result from birth injury (**Figure 140-9**). Risk factors include high birth weight and shoulder dystocia. The infant may demonstrate upper extremity palsy secondary to a brachial plexus injury or may have "pseudoparalysis" of the extremity secondary to pain. Although many clavicle fractures are detected at birth, the diagnosis may be delayed, especially if the fracture is nondisplaced. An ED visit may be made when the newborn is not moving one arm during the first week of life, or when a parent notices a small "lump" or callus at the clavicle during the first 2 to 3 weeks of life. Clavicle fractures in the newborn do not need specific treatment. Pain control and careful handling of the baby are usually all that are required.

Clavicle fractures outside of the newborn period usually result from accidental injury in a mobile child. However, **clavicle fractures in the nonambulatory child should raise the possibility of abuse**. The most common mechanism of injury is either a fall onto an outstretched hand or onto the lateral side of the shoulder. The clavicle may fracture in three general sites: the diaphysis, medial end, or lateral end.

FRACTURES OF THE MIDDLE THIRD OF THE CLAVICLE

Fractures of the diaphysis usually occur in the middle third of the clavicle and are the most common of all clavicle fractures. Treatment is an arm sling/shoulder immobilizer or collar and cuff, as tolerated by the child. Even displaced and overlapping fractures tend to heal well with simple immobilization for 3 to 4 weeks. Complete healing and remodeling can take >1 year, and a small callus will become palpable in most cases if the fracture was displaced. Routine follow-up with the primary care physician is typically sufficient.

FRACTURES OF THE MEDIAL CLAVICLE

Fractures at the medial end of the clavicle are uncommon. Given the strong ligamentous attachment of the clavicle to the sternum, injuries to this area are usually epiphyseal disruptions. Orthopedic consultation is recommended for displaced fractures of the medial clavicle.

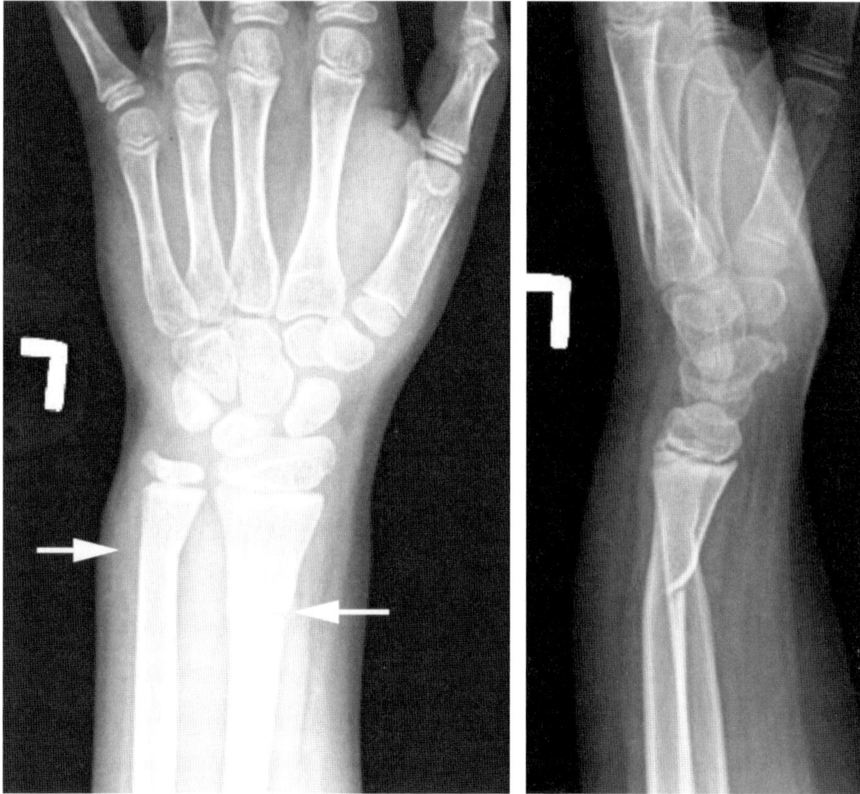

FIGURE 140-8. Anteroposterior and lateral radiographs demonstrating greenstick fractures of the distal radius and ulna in a child. [Reproduced with permission from Sherman SC: *Simon's Emergency Orthopedics,* 7th ed. © 2015, McGraw-Hill, New York. Fig 13-15.]

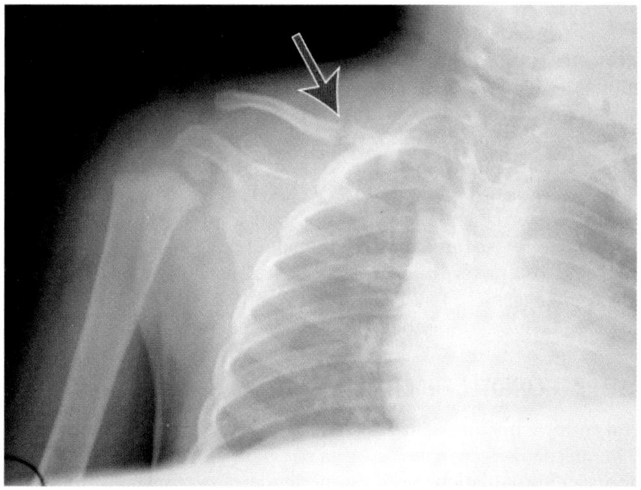

FIGURE 140-9. Nondisplaced clavicle fracture in an infant (*arrow*).

FRACTURES OF THE DISTAL CLAVICLE

Fractures of the distal end of the clavicle are also uncommon in children and again more likely to be epiphyseal disruptions. Minimally displaced distal clavicle fractures only need immobilization with a sling or equivalent. Surgical reduction may be needed for more displaced fractures.

FRACTURES OF THE HUMERUS

Fractures of the humerus are divided into three groups: fractures of the proximal humerus, fractures of the humeral diaphysis, and fractures of the condyles and supracondylar area. Supracondylar and condylar fractures are discussed as part of "The Pediatric Elbow" section below.

FRACTURES OF THE PROXIMAL HUMERUS

Fractures of the proximal humerus may occur at the physis or the proximal humeral metaphysis, and they have an extraordinary ability to repair themselves. Proximal humeral physeal fractures occur more commonly in adolescence because this area becomes relatively weak during this time due to rapid growth. Fractures of the proximal humeral metaphysis are more common in preadolescents. Treatment depends on the age of the child and degree of displacement and/or angulation. Orthopedic consultation is needed to determine the best approach. In general, the younger child can tolerate a greater degree of displacement. For slightly displaced fractures, treatment is conservative, with immobilization in a sling and orthopedic follow-up. Significantly displaced fractures of the proximal humerus in young teens (e.g., off-ended Salter-Harris type II fracture) may need fixation; however, most angulated fractures otherwise will remodel. Brachial plexus injuries can rarely occur when the distal fragment is displaced into the axilla.[1]

FRACTURES OF THE HUMERAL DIAPHYSIS

Fractures of the humeral diaphysis are uncommon in children. Direct trauma can cause a transverse fracture, and violent rotation can cause a spiral fracture. The fracture fragment may injure the radial nerve as it runs in the radial groove. Potential for healing is good, and treatment is usually immobilization in a long arm plaster splint and orthopedic follow-up. Closed reduction (or even open reduction and internal fixation) by orthopedics may be required for displaced fractures in the teenager. Transverse fractures tend to be more unstable than spiral fractures. **Assess radial nerve function on initial examination and following any splinting** (wrist extensors and supinators, sensation of dorsoradial hand, thumb, and second digits). Consider abuse in small children with fractures of the diaphysis of the humerus because of the significant force required to produce fractures in this area.

THE PEDIATRIC ELBOW

Compared with other fractures, elbow fractures in children are commonly missed in the ED. The radiologic diagnosis of elbow fractures is challenging because of the large cartilaginous component of the elbow.

ELBOW RADIOGRAPHS

True lateral and anteroposterior radiographs of the elbow are essential to diagnose fractures (**Figure 140-10**).

If the capitellum falls posterior to the anterior humeral line, an extension-type supracondylar fracture is a possible diagnosis. Other diagnoses to consider include lateral condyle fractures or, rarely, a transphyseal fracture. Additionally, the radius should point to the capitellum in all radiographic views (the radiocapitellar line) (**Figure 140-11**). If not, consider lateral condyle fracture, radial neck fracture, Monteggia's fracture, or elbow dislocation.[2,3]

Lateral radiographs are also used to evaluate for subtle effusions when an occult fracture is suspected. An anterior fat pad may be normal and appears as a small drop of oil hugging the distal anterior humerus. An anterior fat pad that seems to protrude like a sail from the distal humerus may be pathologic ("sail sign"). A posterior fat pad is always pathologic and is evidence of a hemarthrosis from intra-articular injury.

Oblique views or CT scan can be obtained if there is clinical suspicion of fracture without clear radiographic findings on standard anteroposterior and lateral views.

ELBOW OSSIFICATION CENTERS

It is important to identify the ossification centers around the elbow to avoid confusion with fracture. There are six ossification centers appearing at varying ages in the pediatric elbow. The mnemonic used over the years is **CRITOE** (*c*apitellum, *r*adial head, *i*nternal [medial] epicondyle, *t*rochlea, *o*lecranon, external [lateral] *e*picondyle). All of the ossification centers may be seen on the anteroposterior view of the elbow in the appropriately aged child, although the olecranon may be difficult to identify. On the lateral view, all are seen but the trochlea and external (lateral) epicondyle (**CRIO**).

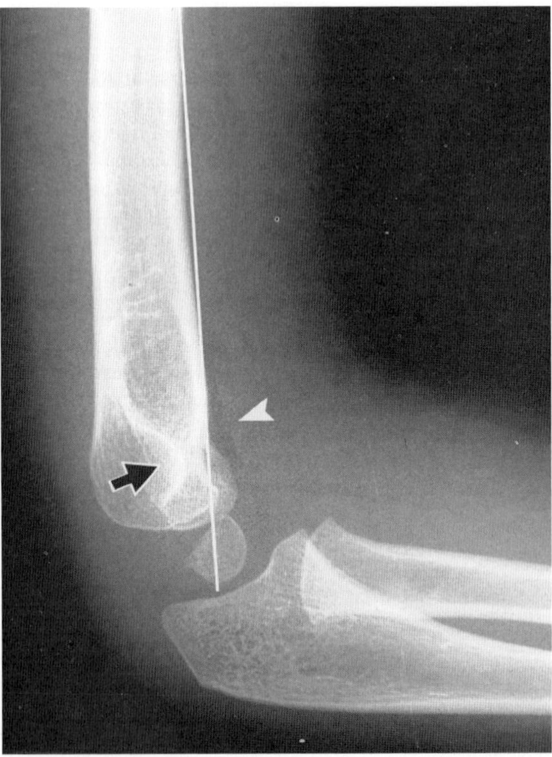

FIGURE 140-10. Anterior humeral line. A line drawn along the anterior cortex of the humeral shaft normally intersects the middle third of the capitellum. A normal radiographic teardrop is seen where the cortices of the olecranon and coronoid fossae come together (*black arrow*). A small normal anterior fat pad is visible (*arrowhead*). [Reproduced with permission from Schwartz D: *Emergency Radiology Case Studies,* © 2008, McGraw-Hill, New York.]

SUPRACONDYLAR FRACTURES

Supracondylar fractures are the most common fractures in children <8 years old. The majority of supracondylar fractures occur in children from 3 to 10 years of age, with the peak incidence occurring between ages 5 and 7 years old. The extension type is by far the most common, accounting for 90% to 98% of cases. An extension-type supracondylar fracture is caused by a fall on an outstretched hand with the elbow hyperextended. A flexion-type fracture results from falling on a flexed elbow and is rare. The complications of a supracondylar fracture, although uncommon, range from transient neurapraxia to Volkmann's ischemic contracture, with the most common being injury to the anterior interosseous nerve resulting in the "pointing finger sign."

Classification of Supracondylar Fractures Classification of supracondylar fractures is based on the extent of fracture fragment displacement. Type I fractures have no displacement or angulation and may have an anterior or posterior fat pad sign as the only radiographic finding (**Figure 140-12**). Confirmation of a supracondylar fracture will be seen on later x-rays done at 2 to 4 weeks that will demonstrate periosteal reaction of the humerus (**Figure 140-13**). Type II fractures are angulated to varying degrees, but the posterior cortex of the humerus is intact (**Figure 140-14**). Type III fractures are completely displaced with no cortical contact (**Figure 140-15**). The distal fragment may be posteromedially (type IIIa) rotated and, as such, can impinge against the radial nerve or be posterolaterally (type IIIb) rotated. **In posterolaterally displaced fractures, the brachial artery and median nerve are at risk for injury, and compartment syndrome can develop.**[1,4] If compartment syndrome is suspected (see chapter 278, "Compartment Syndrome"), emergency orthopedic consultation is needed. Traction and reduction are indicated if the hand is cool, pale, and pulseless. The simple absence of a pulse in an otherwise viable hand is a contraindication to manipulation in the ED.

Treatment The level of displacement and the prereduction physical examination dictate treatment of pediatric supracondylar fractures. Type I supracondylar fractures are inherently stable. The goal of therapy is comfort and immobilization. Apply a double sugar tong splint or a long-arm posterior splint with the elbow at 90 degrees and the forearm in pronation or neutral rotation for 3 weeks. Arrange orthopedic follow-up within 2 to 7 days. While collar and cuff immobilization is used in some centers, it does not offer as good pain management as splinting.[5,6] Type II and III fractures need orthopedic consultation in the ED for definitive management that typically includes operative pinning.[7] Keep these patients fasting for anticipation of surgical intervention.

LATERAL CONDYLE FRACTURES

Lateral condyle fractures can be Salter-Harris type II (most common) or IV. The mechanism of injury is varus stress on an extended elbow with the forearm in supination. Swelling and tenderness are usually limited to the lateral elbow, and neurovascular injury is uncommon. Diagnosis can be made with standard anteroposterior and lateral views, but obtain an oblique view if clinical suspicion is high. Treatment is based on amount of displacement and articular congruence, but often requires open reduction and internal fixation as these fractures are transphyseal and intra-articular. Nonunion, malunion, osteonecrosis, cubitus valgus, and tardy ulnar nerve palsy are well-described complications, so orthopedic consultation is needed to determine the best treatment approach. Displacement can occur even within a cast or splint due to the pull of the forearm extensor tendons (**Figure 140-16**).

MEDIAL EPICONDYLE FRACTURES

Fractures of the medial epicondyle tend to occur in older children, between the ages of 10 and 14 years old. They are not true Salter-Harris injuries, because the apophysis rather than the physis is involved. Simple

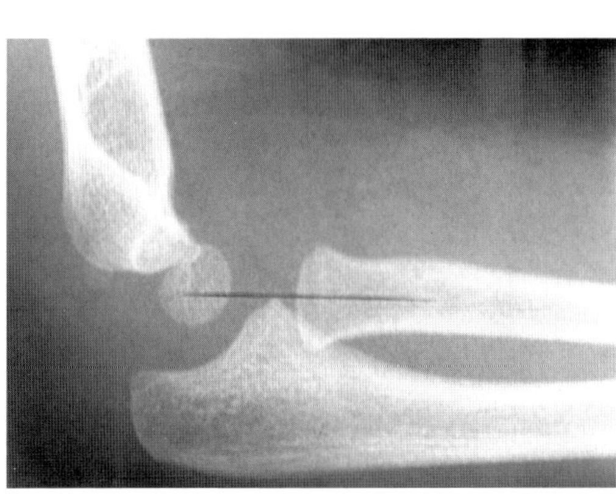

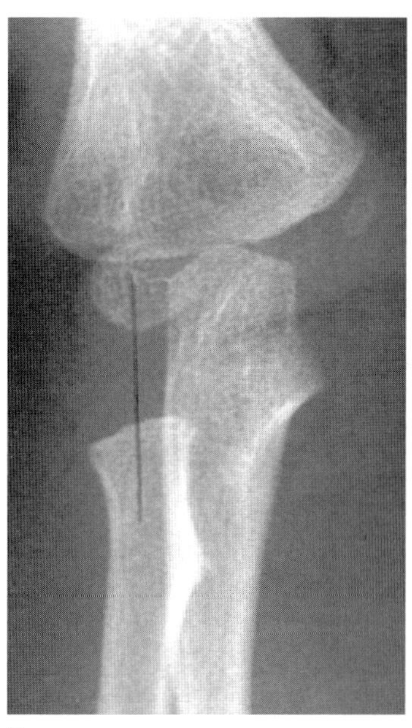

A B

FIGURE 140-11. Radiocapitellar line. **A and B.** A line drawn along the long axis of the radial shaft should intersect the middle of the capitellum on each view. [Reproduced with permission from Schwartz D: *Emergency Radiology Case Studies,* © 2008, McGraw-Hill, New York.]

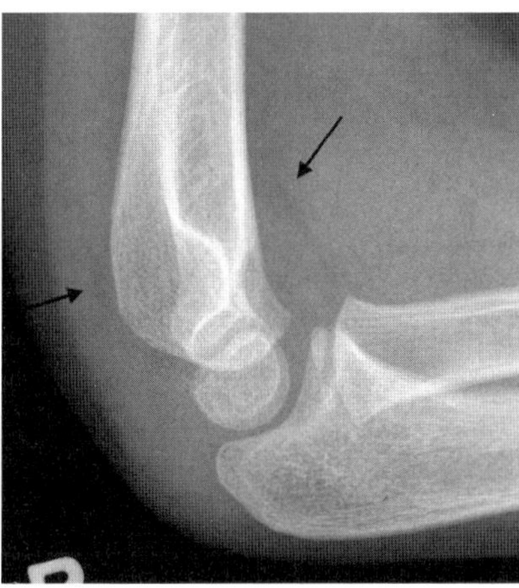

FIGURE 140-12. Type I supracondylar fracture. Note the anterior and posterior fat pad signs suggestive of fracture without displacement of the distal fragment. [Photo used with permission of Karen Black, BC Children's Hospital, Vancouver.]

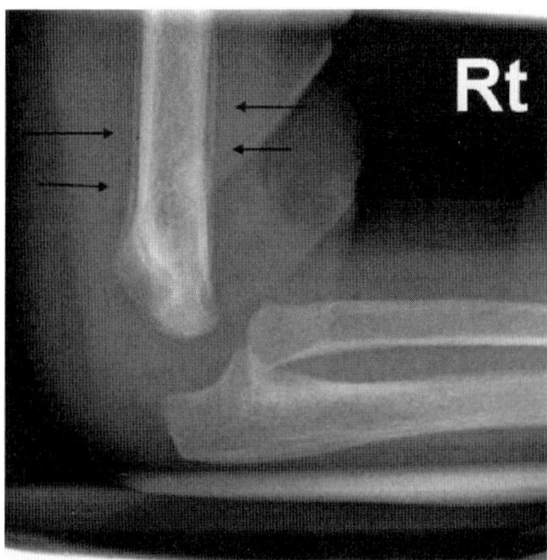

FIGURE 140-13. Healing type I supracondylar fracture with periosteal reaction in a toddler. [Photo used with permission of Karen Black, BC Children's Hospital, Vancouver.]

fractures of the medial epicondyle are extra-articular injuries with limited soft tissue involvement, but nearly half of injuries are associated with elbow dislocation; in such injuries, the epicondyle can become entrapped in the joint.[8,9] Fractures are classified by the amount of displacement and associated extremity injuries, and orthopedic consultation is needed to determine the best approach (**Figure 140-17**).

DISTAL HUMERAL TRANSPHYSEAL FRACTURES

Most distal humeral transphyseal fracture injuries occur in children <2.5 years old. Recognition is both difficult and important, especially in infants, in whom this particular injury is often the result of child abuse. This injury is thought to result from a twisting mechanism that shears off the distal epiphysis and **is an intentional injury (child abuse) until proven otherwise**.

OLECRANON FRACTURES

Olecranon fractures generally result from a fall on the elbow. Orthopedic consultation is best to guide treatment. If the fracture is displaced <5 mm, it should be immobilized in the most stable position, usually 45 degrees of elbow flexion, for 3 to 6 weeks. Open reduction and internal fixation are indicated for unstable fractures. Olecranon fractures occur in association with fractures of the radial head and neck. A "simple" olecranon fracture may be part of Monteggia's lesion, so radial head position should be evaluated carefully.

RADIAL HEAD AND NECK FRACTURES

Fractures of the radial head and neck are uncommon in children (**Figures 140-18 and 140-19**). The radial neck is fractured more frequently than the radial head, and most radial neck fractures occur through the metaphysis. The most common mechanism is a fall. Obtain orthopedic consultation to guide treatment. Reduction is often necessary when angulation is >35 degrees or displacement is >60%.[10]

ELBOW DISLOCATION

Elbow dislocations occur most frequently in males (70%), usually from a fall on the outstretched hand. The most common type of dislocation is posterior, usually accompanied by some lateral displacement (**Figure 140-20**). Carefully examine the radiographs for associated fractures, particularly of

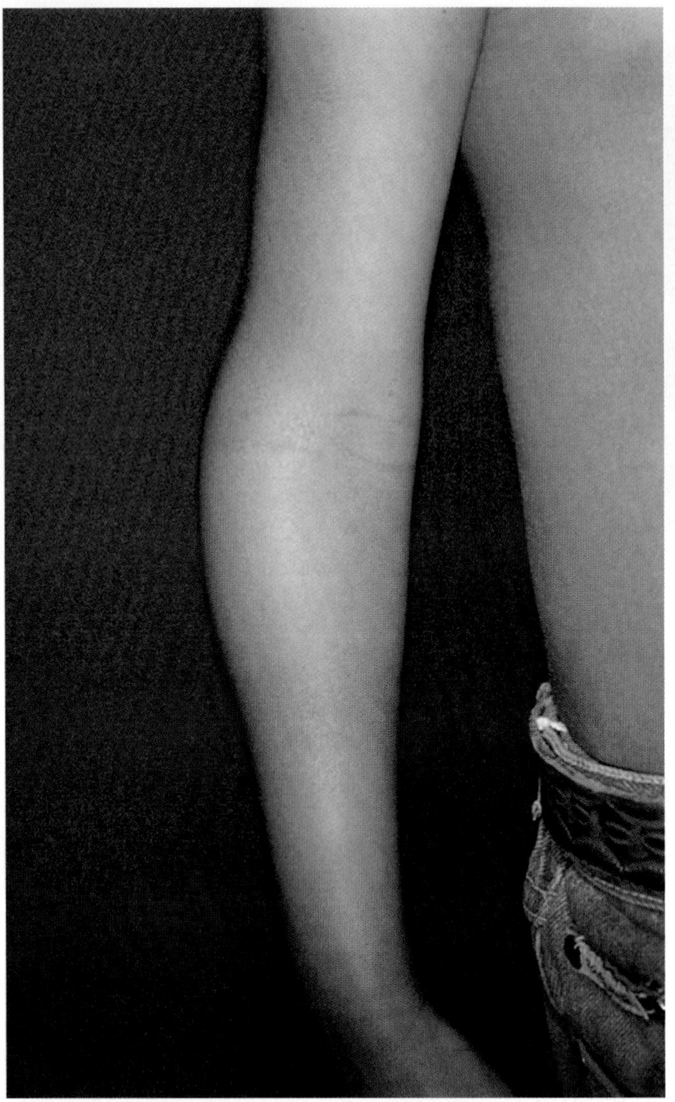

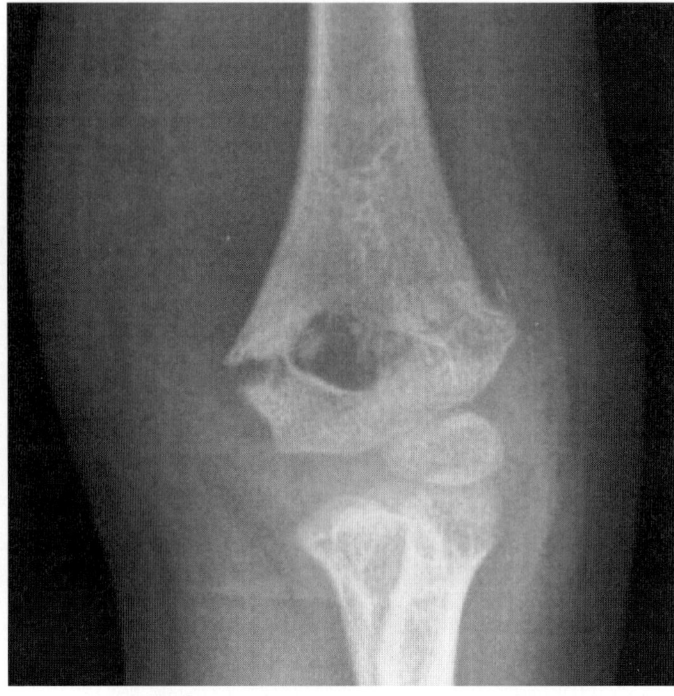

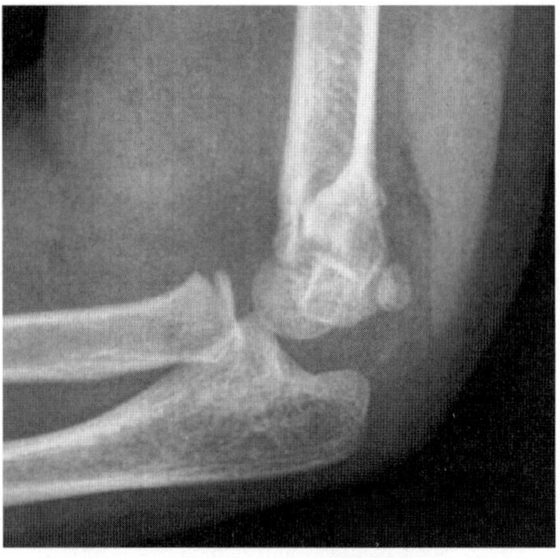

FIGURE 140-14. **A.** Clinical picture of a type II supracondylar fracture with marked soft tissue swelling in a child with a history of falling on an outstretched arm. **B and C.** Anteroposterior (AP) and lateral views of the elbow, demonstrating a supracondylar fracture with medial opening seen on the AP view and posterior displacement of the distal fragment identified on the lateral view. [**A:** Reproduced with permission from Shah BR, Lucchesi M, Amodio J, Silverberg M: *Atlas of Pediatric Emergency Medicine,* 2nd ed. © 2013, McGraw-Hill, New York. Fig. 19-33A. **B and C:** Image used with permission of Karen Black, BC Children's Hospital, Vancouver.]

the medial and lateral epicondyle and radial neck. Neurologic injury is associated with approximately 10% of elbow dislocations. Ulnar neuropathy is the most common and is usually associated with medial epicondyle entrapment. Median nerve injury may be caused by entrapment of the nerve inside the joint, behind the medial epicondyle, or in an epicondyle fracture. Radial nerve and arterial injury are both rare. Consult orthopedics emergently if neurovascular injury is suspected (see chapter 270, "Elbow and Forearm Injuries"). After reduction and review of postreduction x-rays, immobilize the reduced elbow in a posterior mold and refer for orthopedic follow-up within 1 week. The major long-term complication is elbow stiffness.

FOREARM INJURIES

TORUS FRACTURES

Torus or buckle-type fractures (Figure 140-7) of the distal forearm are extremely common and can be radiographically subtle. There is point tenderness over the distal radius and/or ulna, occasionally with associated localized swelling. Manage with application of a volar splint and follow-up with family physician in 1 to 3 weeks.

PHYSEAL FRACTURES

Salter-Harris fractures of the distal radial physis are also very common. Even if radiographs are negative, assume a Salter-Harris I fracture if there is point tenderness or swelling over the distal physis. Immobilize with a sugar tong or volar splint and arrange primary care or orthopedic follow-up in 1 week. Salter-Harris type II injuries require reduction if there is physeal displacement (**Figure 140-21**). For Salter-Harris types III, IV, and V injuries, orthopedic consultation is necessary.

FRACTURES OF THE RADIAL AND ULNAR SHAFTS

Metaphyseal Fractures

Clinical and radiographic assessment should include the forearm and the joints above and below the primary injury to assess for the presence

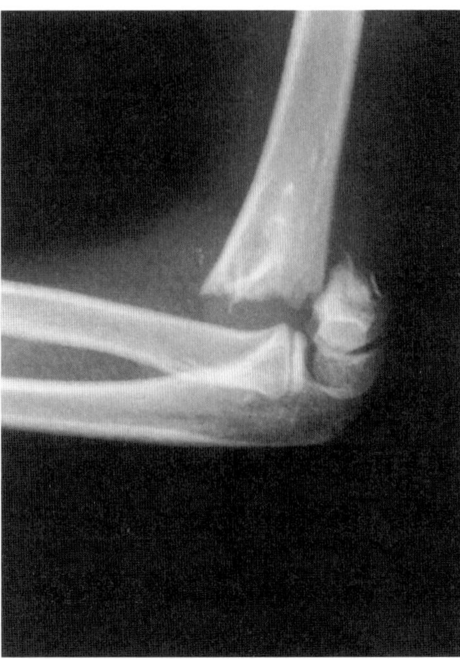

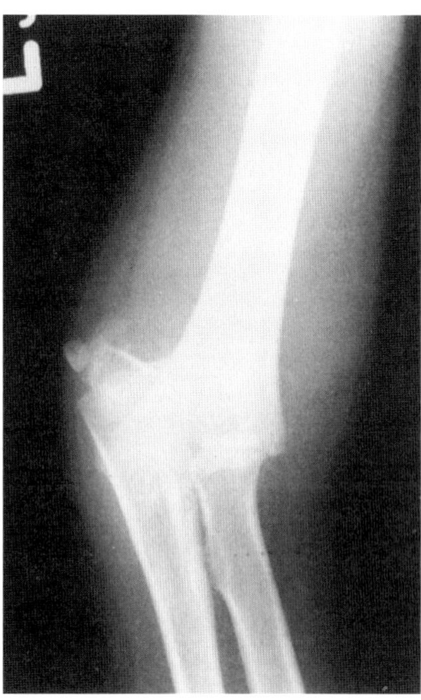

FIGURE 140-15. Type III displaced supracondylar fracture. The distal fragment is displaced posteriorly, proximally, and medially.

of associated fractures or dislocations at those joints. The potential for remodeling is better the younger the child and the more distal the injury. The vast majority of shaft fractures involve the distal third of the forearm. Clinically, there is typically point tenderness, swelling, and obvious deformity. Although all forearm fractures need orthopedic follow-up, the patient's age and degree of deformity determine the need for immediate referral and reduction. **Any fracture with rotational deformity or >10 degrees of angulation in children >8 years of age, or >15 to 20 degrees in younger children, requires consultation with an orthopedist to determine the need for reduction. Otherwise, immobilization in a splint with follow-up within 1 week is adequate treatment.** Greenstick and complete fractures of the distal radius and ulna have a tendency to become further displaced if they are not appropriately immobilized, so use of sugar tong splint or circumferential cast rather than a simple volar splint.

Diaphyseal Fractures Injuries of the midshaft can remain unstable despite attempts at closed reduction and occasionally require open fixation. Failure to correct bowing (which tends to be along the whole bone) may lead to permanent deformity and disability. As with incomplete yet angulated greenstick fractures, bowing fractures may require completion of the break to establish proper realignment.

Isolated Ulnar Fracture Isolated fractures of the ulna (nightstick fractures) are rare and are caused by a direct blow. If caused by an indirect force, typically, there is an associated fracture or dislocation of the radius. **The combination of an ulnar fracture with a dislocation of the radial head is called *Monteggia's fracture* (Figure 140-22).** Clinically, there may be tenderness about the elbow; however, even without significant clinical findings, films of the elbow are essential with fractures of the ulna to evaluate for possible dislocations. Any suspected Monteggia's fracture-dislocation requires immediate evaluation by an

FIGURE 140-16. Lateral condyle fracture (*arrow*) can be subtle in some views but displaces easily in the first week if not fixed operatively. [Photo used with permission of Karen Black, BC Children's Hospital, Vancouver.]

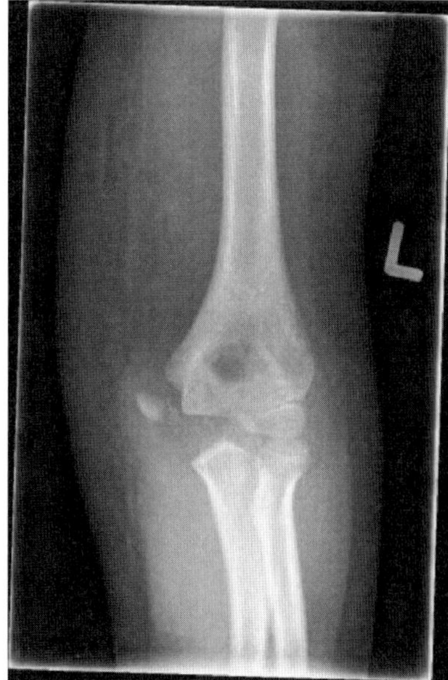

FIGURE 140-17. Medial epicondyle avulsion. Note a flake of the medial condyle has fractured off as well. [Photo used with permission of Karen Black, BC Children's Hospital, Vancouver.]

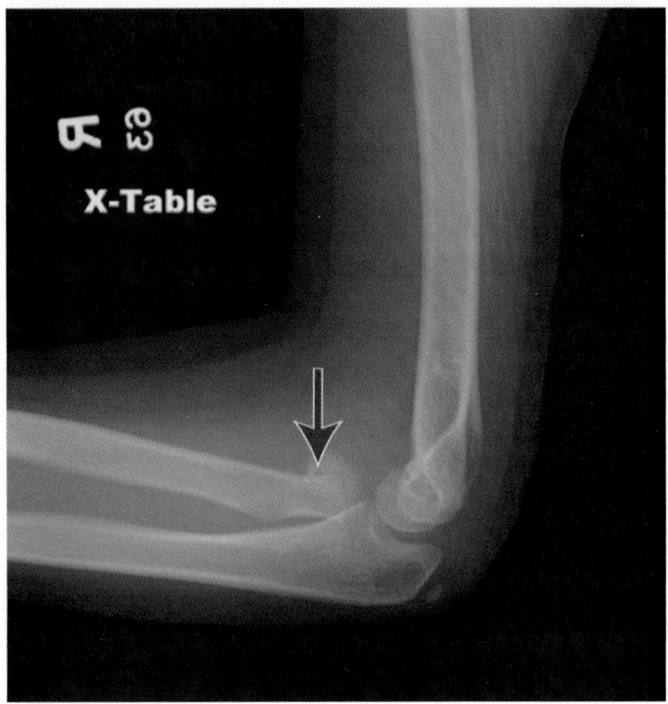

FIGURE 140-18. Lateral radiograph illustrating radial head fracture (*arrow*). [Photo used with permission of Wake Medical Center, Raleigh, NC.]

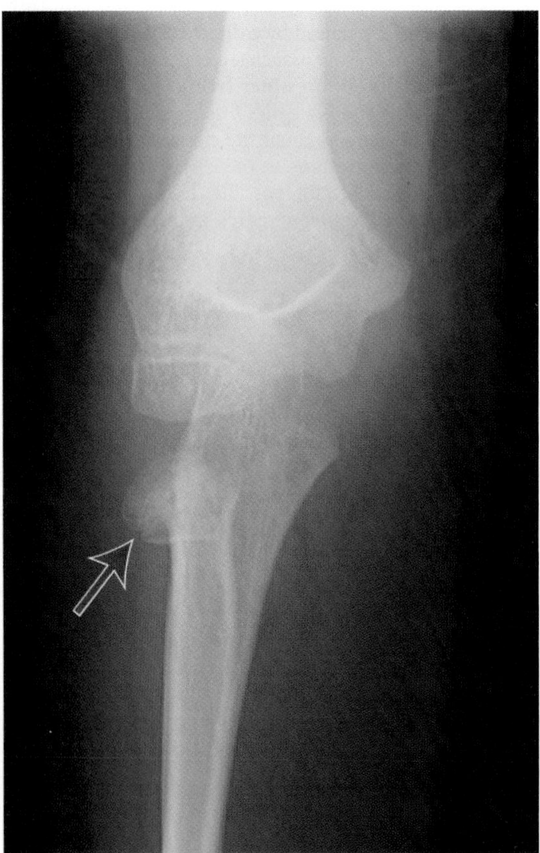

FIGURE 140-19. Anteroposterior radiograph illustrating radial head fracture (*arrow*). [Photo used with permission of Wake Medical Center, Raleigh, NC.]

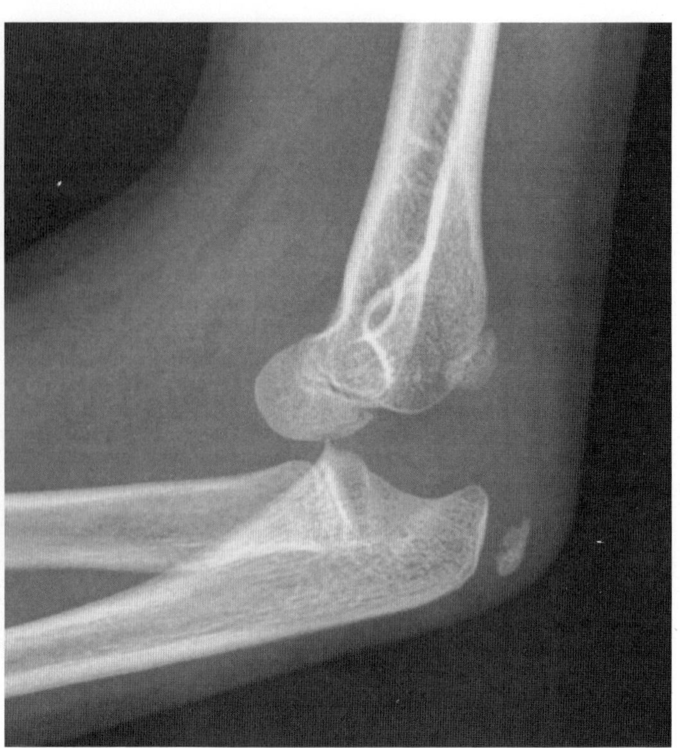

FIGURE 140-20. Radiograph demonstrating elbow dislocation with displacement of both radius and ulna. [Photo used with permission of Karen Black, BC Children's Hospital, Vancouver.]

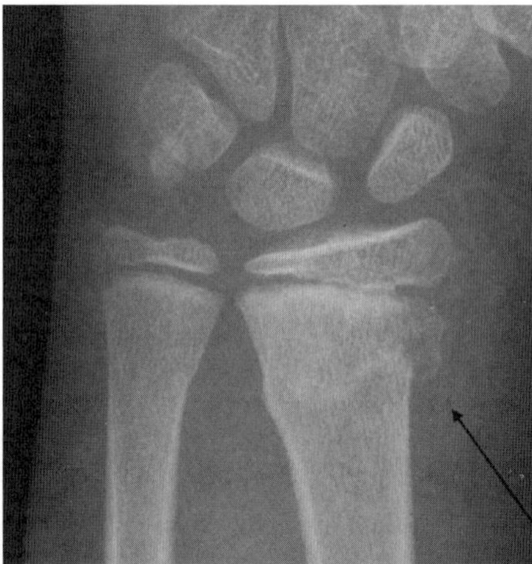

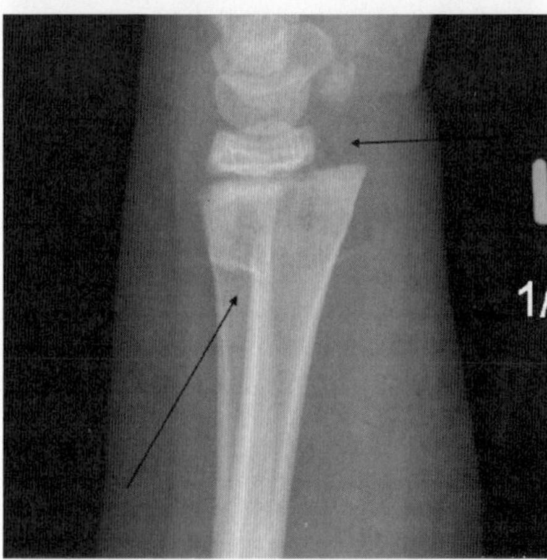

FIGURE 140-21. Anteroposterior and lateral radiographs illustrating Salter-Harris type II fracture of the distal radius requiring reduction for dorsal displacement of distal fragment (*arrows*). [Photo used with permission of Karen Black, BC Children's Hospital, Vancouver.]

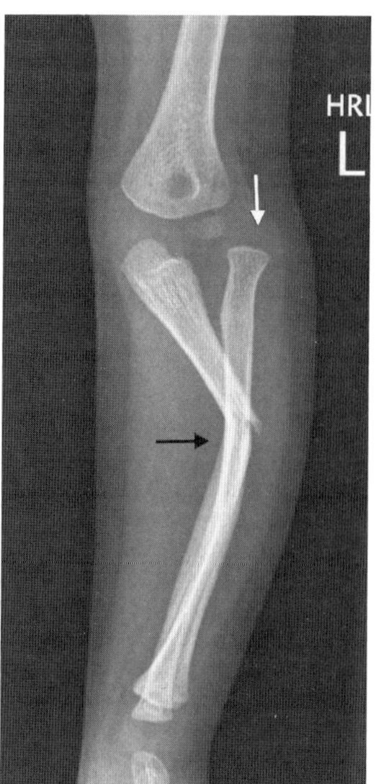

FIGURE 140-22. Type III Monteggia's fracture-dislocation. The angulation of the greenstick fracture of the ulna (*arrow*) points in the direction of the radial head dislocation (*arrowhead*). [Photo used with permission of Karen Black, BC Children's Hospital, Vancouver.]

orthopedist. ***Galeazzi's fracture* is a radial shaft fracture with an associated dislocation of the distal radioulnar joint (Figure 140-23).** Although this injury is uncommon, immediate orthopedic consultation is again warranted.

WRIST INJURIES

Fractures of the carpal bones are quite rare in the skeletally immature child. However, these injuries increase in frequency in the skeletally mature adolescent population. Most are sports-related injuries. Fracture patterns and presentation are similar to the adult. For example, the scaphoid may be fractured in older adolescents with the typical mechanism being that of a fall on an outstretched hand. There is typically the classically expected snuffbox tenderness and pain with longitudinal compression of the thumb. However, unlike adults, nonunion is less common in children. A high index of suspicion for this type of injury is required. Immobilize any suspected fracture of carpal bone in a thumb spica splint and arrange early orthopedic follow-up, even in the absence of radiographic findings. Repeat plain radiographs, CT, or MRI may be used at follow-up for further assessment of the injury.

PHALANGEAL FRACTURES

The most common injury is that to the distal phalanx resulting from a crush injury, typically seen when the child catches his or her hand in a door. Immobilize a distal phalanx "tuft" fracture with a finger splint. If there is associated nail bed injury, the fracture is considered "open," and orthopedic or plastic surgery follow-up in 1 week or less must be arranged. The role of prophylactic antibiotics in open fractures of the distal tuft remains controversial, with no clear evidence of benefit.

Fractures of the phalangeal shaft should be examined for displacement, rotational deformity, and tendon disruption. Significantly displaced or rotated fractures or those with tendon disruption need orthopedic/plastic surgery consultation for reduction and repair.

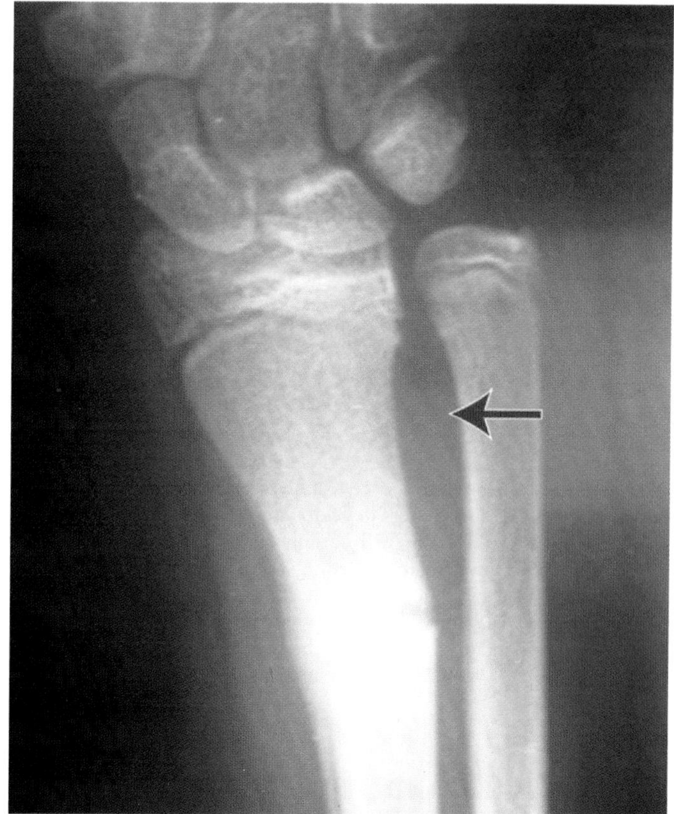

A

B

FIGURE 140-23. Galeazzi's fracture. Note the widening of the distal radial ulnar joint space on the anteroposterior view (**A**) and dislocation of the distal radius relative to the ulna on the lateral projection (**B**) (*arrows*). [Reproduced with permission from Simon RR, Sherman SC, Koenigsknecht SJ: *Emergency Orthopedics: The Extremities,* 5th ed, © 2007, McGraw-Hill, New York.]

LOWER EXTREMITY INJURIES

PELVIC FRACTURES

The immature, relatively cartilaginous pediatric pelvis is somewhat pliable. Therefore, pediatric pelvic fractures usually result from a tremendous force.[11] The exception is the avulsion-type injury, which usually results from sudden muscle contractions associated with athletic injuries.

The most common mechanism for nonavulsion-type pelvic fractures is pedestrian versus motor vehicle collisions. Assume multisystem injury in a child with a pelvic fracture, and transfer to a facility equipped to manage pediatric multiple trauma. In children, life-threatening hemorrhage usually results from injury to other body areas rather than from injury to the pelvic vessels.

Avulsion-type injuries of the pelvis result from sudden contraction of musculature attached to the pelvis and typically occur during athletic activities. These injuries are usually seen in the adolescent after secondary ossification centers develop and are unusual before 8 years of age. Clinically the child will complain of sudden pain and have point tenderness and possibly swelling over the fracture site (usually the anterior-superior iliac spine, but can occur at anterior-inferior iliac spine also). MRI or CT may be needed to confirm the diagnosis, but nearly all avulsion fractures can be managed conservatively with rest, limitation of activity until symptoms resolve, and orthopedic follow-up.

HIP FRACTURES AND DISLOCATIONS

Trauma can result in an epiphyseal disruption or a fracture of the head, neck, trochanteric, or subtrochanteric region of the femur. Proximal fractures involving the femoral head or neck have a high risk of complications such as avascular necrosis and growth arrest. Treatment is almost always urgent operative repair.

Traumatic dislocations of the hip are also rare in the pediatric population and are best divided into those occurring in the older adolescent and those occurring in the skeletally immature child. Most hip dislocations in adolescents are posterior and result from significant trauma. Dislocations in children <10 years old can occur with low-energy trauma. Treatment for pediatric hip dislocations is urgent closed reduction. Immediate orthopedic consultation is indicated, as any significant delay in reduction is associated with a higher incidence of complications including sciatic nerve injury. Pathologic fractures are possible through bone cysts or lesions.

FRACTURES OF THE FEMORAL SHAFT

The femur is the second bone to ossify in the fetus and the largest of the long bones in the body. The strength of the femur continues to increase in later childhood, and therefore significant force is usually required to fracture the femoral shaft. Pediatric femur fractures occur more commonly in boys and seem to follow a bimodal distribution with peaks during late toddler age and mid-teenage years.

The most common mechanisms of injury are falls, pedestrian versus automobile incidents, motor vehicle collisions, and sports-related injuries. **Consider child abuse in a child with a femur fracture who is not yet walking.**[12]

The clinical findings of a femur fracture are obvious. There is typically tenderness and swelling over the fracture site. The child may hold the leg externally rotated and will likely refuse to bear weight. The leg may be shortened. Given the high degree of force needed to fracture the femur, perform a thorough evaluation for multisystem trauma. **Hypotension is usually not related to an isolated femur fracture in a young child and should prompt a search for other injuries.**[13]

All femoral shaft fractures require immediate orthopedic consultation. Treatment depends on the child's age, size, degree of malalignment, and reliability of follow-up.[14]

SLIPPED CAPITAL FEMORAL EPIPHYSIS

Slipped capital femoral epiphysis (also known as slipped upper femoral epiphysis) is a disorder of childhood characterized by slipping of the femoral epiphysis of the hip. Complications include avascular necrosis of the hip and premature closure of the physis. Slipped capital femoral epiphysis is the most common cause of hip disability in adolescents. Etiology is multifactorial, and any child may develop slipped capital femoral epiphysis during a growth spurt; however, many affected children are obese adolescents whose hips are exposed to repetitive minimal trauma, but some are tall, athletic children. Boys with slipped capital femoral epiphysis present at an average age of 14 to 16 years old. Girls typically present earlier, at approximately 11 to 13 years of age, with occurrence after menarche being rare. Hormonal and genetic factors also appear to play a role in the development of slipped capital femoral epiphysis. Atypical slipped capital femoral epiphysis occurs in children in whom obesity is not a risk factor and can be seen in children with juvenile chronic arthritis, certain human leukocyte antigen types, endocrinopathies, renal failure, and previous radiation or chemotherapy (**Figure 140-24**).

The slippage may be chronic, acute, or acute-on-chronic. Acute slipped upper femoral epiphyses are rare but quite dramatic. The child cannot bear weight, and surgery for reduction and fixation is done on an urgent basis. Acute worsening of mild chronic displacement may occur after minimal or no trauma. In cases of chronic slip, clinically, the child may develop hip (groin) pain, or pain is referred to the thigh or, much more commonly, the knee. The pain may be vague and chronic in nature. If you watch the child walk you will observe that the foot on the affected side has a much more external progression angle, and when you examine the hip you will note that the hip flexes into obligate external rotation. **Obtain bilateral hip radiographs in any adolescent with chronic pain in the groin, hip, thigh, or knee to evaluate for slipped capital femoral epiphysis because delay in diagnosis can lead to significant disability.** Adequate radiographs include both anteroposterior and lateral hip x-rays (Lowenstein view). Both hips should be imaged given the high incidence of bilateral disease. The use of frog leg views is controversial given the potential for further epiphyseal displacement in this position.

Radiographically, epiphyseal slippage may be detected by examining the anatomic relationship of the femoral neck to the femoral head (**Figure 140-25**). Several techniques of measuring the presence or degree of slip have been suggested, but subtle cases can be challenging to find on x-ray. Therefore, obtain orthopedic consultation for any child with pain suspicious for slipped capital femoral epiphysis in the ED. Additional imaging with MRI to detect early slips may be recommended. Once the diagnosis is made, the goal of treatment is to prevent further slippage: management includes strict non–weight bearing and definitive operative management. Prophylactic pinning of the contralateral hip, even if apparently unaffected, is also recommended by some authors.[15]

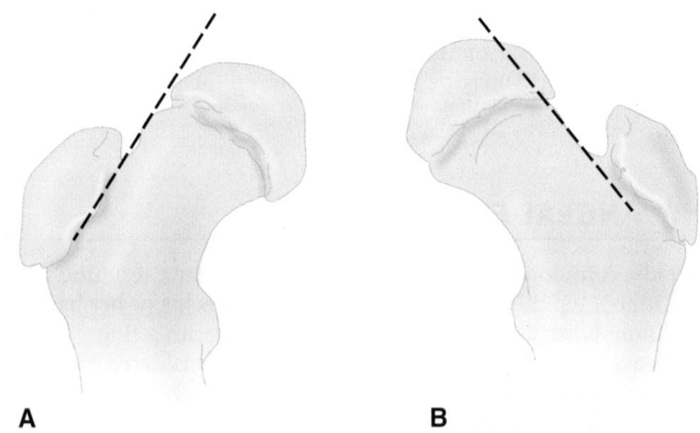

FIGURE 140-24. A line (Klein's line) drawn along the lateral (superior) aspect of the femoral neck fails to transect the lateral quarter of the femoral head in slipped capital femoral epiphysis, seen in **A** (Trethowan's sign). The normal anatomic relationship is illustrated in **B**.

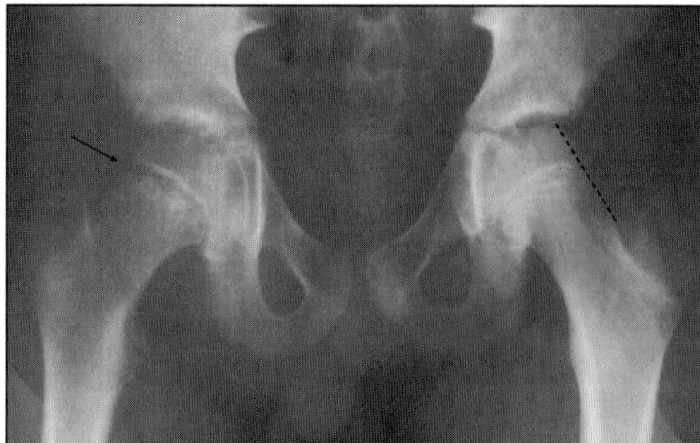

FIGURE 140-25. Anteroposterior radiograph illustrating an early slipped capital femoral epiphysis requiring surgical management in right hip (*arrow*). *Dotted line* represents the Klein's line on the unaffected side. Note that the epiphysis on the affected side would not be intersected by a similar line. [Photo used with permission of Karen Black, BC Children's Hospital, Vancouver.]

Prognosis depends on the degree of displacement; however, even in the best of cases, many patients are left with residual limited range of motion and an increased risk for the development of osteoarthritis.

The differential diagnosis includes a traumatic transphyseal fracture of the proximal femur; however, it is difficult to differentiate between the two acutely in the typical age group because an acute slipped capital femoral epiphysis can be associated with falls. Chronic slipped capital femoral epiphysis has a typically insidious onset and a history of preceding intermittent groin or, more commonly, knee pain, and precipitating trauma is minimal or absent. There can be gait changes and metaphyseal remodeling demonstrated on x-ray. In contrast, significant and acute trauma is necessary to fracture the femoral physis in a healthy hip.

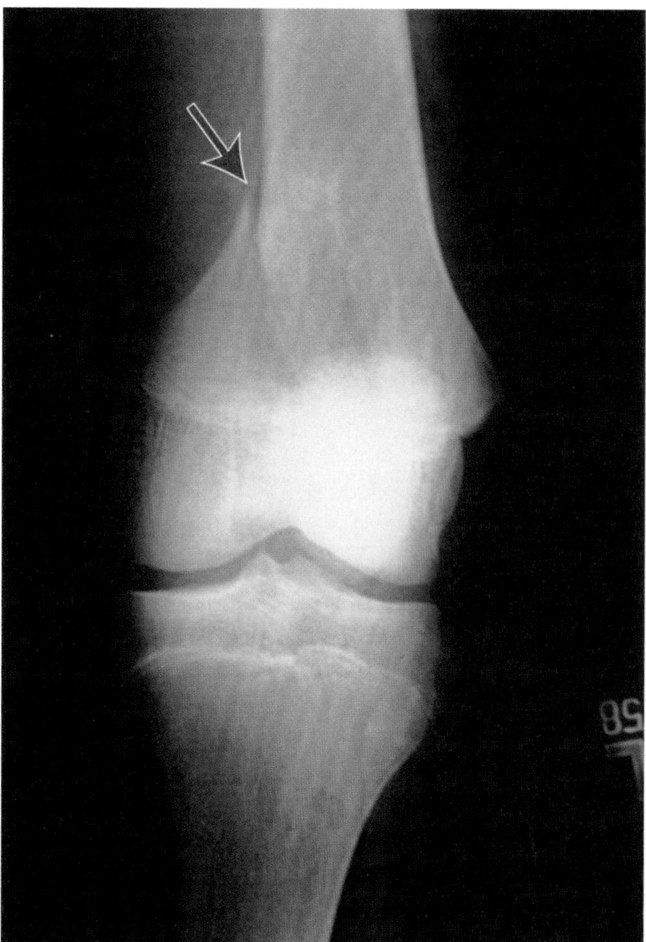

FIGURE 140-26. Distal femur Salter-Harris type II fracture. [Photo used with permission of Wake Medical Center, Raleigh, NC.]

KNEE INJURIES

Compared with the adult, ligamentous injuries to the pediatric knee are much less common than are fractures. **The Ottawa knee rules (see chapter 274, "Knee Injuries") have been validated for children ≥2 years of age** and can help determine the need for radiographs.[16]

FRACTURES OF THE DISTAL FEMORAL PHYSIS

Fractures through the distal femoral physis are uncommon yet carry a significant complication rate. **The popliteal artery lies close to the distal femoral metaphysis and may be injured along with the peroneal nerve.** Growth arrest may also occur secondary to permanent physeal damage. Although Salter-Harris type I injuries may not be appreciated on x-rays, any child suspected of having a significant injury should receive orthopedic follow-up. Any displaced distal femoral physeal disruption needs immediate orthopedic evaluation for reduction (**Figure 140-26**).

PATELLAR DISLOCATIONS

Patellar injuries in children are usually dislocations. In fact, patellar dislocation is one of the most common causes of a traumatic hemarthrosis in children. The typical mechanism is one of pivoting the knee on a fixed lower leg. Often reduction has already occurred at the scene, although a history of the "knee popped out of place" can usually be obtained. If the patient remains dislocated at the ED visit, the displaced patella usually sits laterally and the knee is held in flexion. Reduction need not be delayed for x-rays and is easily accomplished by gently extending the knee while another provider helps "lift" the patella into place. Although the patella does not actually need to be moved into place, the second provider can help prevent a traumatic reduction, resulting in additional fractures. Obtain x-rays after the reduction to assess for fractures, which are most typically seen at either the lateral femoral condyle or the medial margin of the patella. Provide a knee immobilizer and orthopedic follow-up. Most patients improve with conservative management and rehabilitation; however, some children are predisposed to chronic dislocations and may eventually need realignment of their extensor mechanism.

PATELLAR FRACTURE

Fractures of the patella are uncommon in children and usually occur from direct blunt force. The "sleeve" fracture of the patella, in which the distal patellar "sleeve" is avulsed from the body of the patella, is a patellar fracture unique to children. The typical mechanism of an avulsion "sleeve" fracture is forceful contraction of the quadriceps against a fixed lower leg. Consultation with an orthopedist is advised to determine the appropriate treatment.

PROXIMAL TIBIA FRACTURES

FRACTURES OF THE TIBIAL SPINE

Mechanically speaking, an avulsion fracture of the tibial spine is the equivalent of an anterior cruciate ligament rupture in an adult. The anterior cruciate ligament inserts on the tibial eminence, also known as the anterior tibial spine, and this ligament and its insertion are much stronger than the epiphyseal bone in children. Nondisplaced fractures may be managed conservatively with immobilization in extension and orthopedic follow-up. However, any displaced fractures need reduction and immediate orthopedic consultation (**Figure 140-27**).

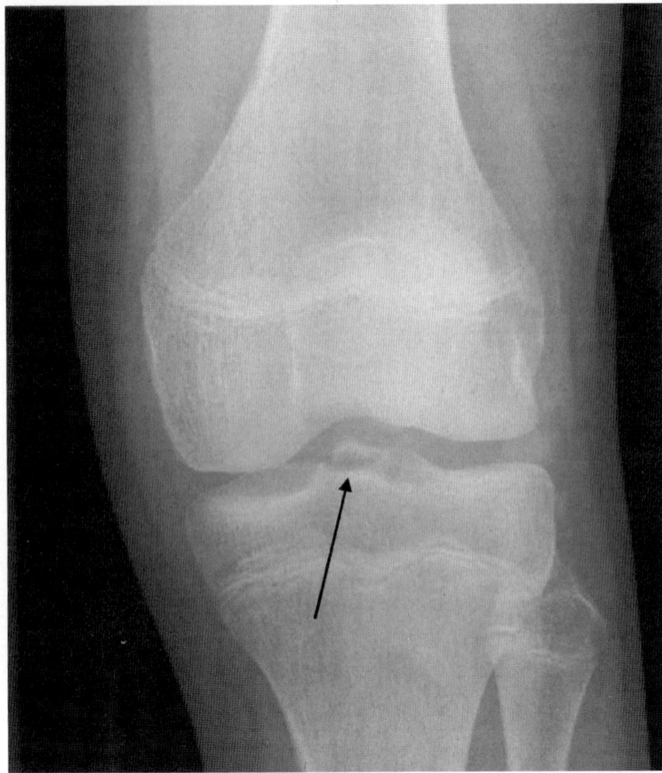

FIGURE 140-27. Anterior tibial spine fracture. Sometimes the "tunnel" view (flexed) is needed to demonstrate this fracture. [Photo used with permission of Karen Black, BC Children's Hospital, Vancouver.]

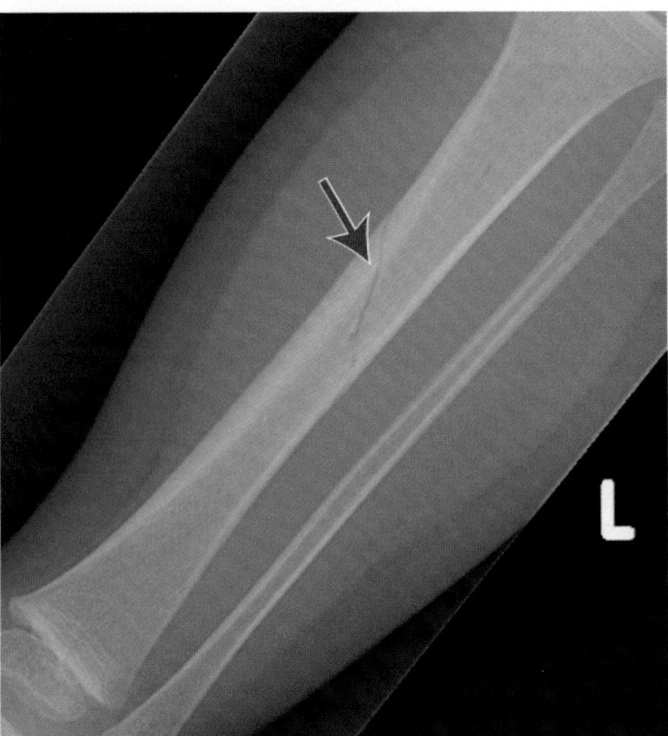

FIGURE 140-28. Anteroposterior radiograph illustrating toddler fracture of tibial shaft (*arrow*). [Photo used with permission of Wake Medical Center, Raleigh, NC.]

TIBIAL TUBEROSITY FRACTURES

Tibial tuberosity fractures are typically avulsion type and occur most commonly from strong contraction of the quadriceps against a fixed leg. Such injuries are usually sports related. Tibial tuberosity fractures are classified as type I, II, or III, depending on the location of the fracture line. Type I injuries are characterized by a fracture through the small distal portion of the tibial tuberosity. Type II fractures occur after the coalescence of the secondary ossification centers of the tuberosity to the metaphysis. The fracture splits the epiphysis of the tuberosity from the epiphysis of the proximal tibia. **Type III injuries involve a fracture into the joint and are at risk for compartment syndrome.** Types I and II fractures are usually treated with immobilization. Displaced type II and type III injuries need reduction and fixation and require immediate orthopedic consultation.

PROXIMAL TIBIAL PHYSIS FRACTURES

Fractures of the proximal tibial physis are relatively uncommon, and most are Salter-Harris type I. Vascular injury to the popliteal artery is a concern, and documentation of intact pulses is important.

PROXIMAL TIBIAL METAPHYSIS FRACTURES

There is a high risk of drift through healing and growth into a valgus deformity of the knee (Cozen's phenomenon) with proximal tibial metaphyseal fractures, even with proper alignment and immobilization. Arrange orthopedic follow-up for these fractures.

FRACTURES OF THE TIBIA AND FIBULA DIAPHYSES

Most fractures of the tibia and fibula occur at the shaft. If the fracture is minimally displaced and there is no evidence of compartment syndrome, immobilize in a long leg posterior splint and arrange orthopedic follow-up. However, if there is >10 degrees of angulation in any plane, orthopedic consultation and reduction are indicated. These are very painful injuries and may require admission for pain relief. The mechanism of injury and the nature of the injury need to be considered when assessing the risk of compartment syndrome. Where there is high-energy injury, if the limb was in highly metabolic state at the time of injury (e.g., taking part in sports), or if there is any element of crush, then there is a risk of compartment syndrome, and the patient should be admitted for observation.

TODDLER'S FRACTURE

The *toddler's fracture* is an isolated spiral fracture of the distal tibia in a toddler (i.e., once learning to walk). The typical mechanism is external rotation of the foot with the knee flexed. Parents report that the child is limping or refusing to bear weight for no evident reason or after seemingly insignificant trauma. Clinically, there is usually pain with palpation and rotation of the distal tibia, although swelling may be minimal or absent and occasionally there is no tenderness. Obtain radiographs of the leg in the limping toddler, even in the absence of physical examination finding. Radiographically, a fracture line may be noticed at the distal third of the tibial shaft (**Figure 140-28**). At times, initial standard x-rays may be normal. Oblique views may show a fracture line when standard views are negative. If a toddler's fracture is clinically suspected and initial radiographs are negative, immobilization and no immobilization are both management options with follow-up in 1 week for repeat x-rays and/or bone scan or MRI.[17,18] The leg should not be in a circumferential cast if the diagnosis is not clear. For radiologically evident fractures, immobilize the leg in a long leg splint or above knee cast with adequate flexion for car seat use and provide orthopedic follow-up within 72 hours for definitive casting if not done in the ED.

ANKLE INJURIES

Ankle injuries in children include both ligamentous disruptions as well as fractures. Ligamentous injuries are uncommon before physeal closure because of the generally stronger nature of ligaments when compared with open physes. Ankle sprains in older children with closed physes are graded and treated as they are in adults.

Fractures of the pediatric ankle may involve the distal tibia, the fibula, or both. A thorough evaluation and appropriate treatment are extremely important because any articular surface disruption in this joint can result in long-term complications despite a seemingly benign initial presentation. Additional imaging techniques such as CT and MRI are frequently used to help define the extent of fracture involvement.

DISTAL FIBULA FRACTURES

The most common fractures of the distal fibula are Salter-Harris types I and II, which account for approximately 90% of isolated distal fibula fractures. Clinically, findings with a Salter-Harris I fracture may be subtle; however, typically there is tenderness at the growth plate, and soft tissue swelling is common. Isolated Salter-Harris I fractures of the distal fibula are distinguished from a lateral ligamentous ankle sprain by the presence of point tenderness over the physis in a fracture. Plain radiographs only show soft tissue swelling at the lateral fibula. In general, any type I or II fracture that is nondisplaced may be managed by immobilization in a weight-bearing cast or commercial immobilizer, and orthopedic follow-up is usually not necessary.[19]

DISTAL TIBIA FRACTURES

The most common fractures of the distal tibia are also Salter-Harris types I and II. In general, these fractures may be managed with closed reduction if any displacement is present, followed by immobilization. Often, open reduction in Salter-Harris II fractures is required due to infolding of the periosteum. Salter-Harris III fractures account for approximately 25% of distal tibia fractures and typically require open reduction of any displacement. Tillaux's fracture is a Salter-Harris type III fracture of the anterolateral portion of the distal tibia (Figure 140-5). The location of Tillaux's fracture is a result of the order in which the distal tibial physis closes. Physeal closure occurs centrally, then medially, and finally, laterally, making the anterolateral portion most vulnerable. Therefore, this type of fracture is typically seen in a child who is nearing skeletal maturity. Treatment is surgical reduction in most cases.

Salter-Harris IV fractures include the triplane fracture, which involves fractures in the sagittal, coronal, and transverse planes, resulting in multiple fracture fragments. CT scan is helpful in delineating the extent of the joint surface injury in both Salter-Harris type III and IV ankle fractures (**Figure 140-29**). The management is surgical reduction.

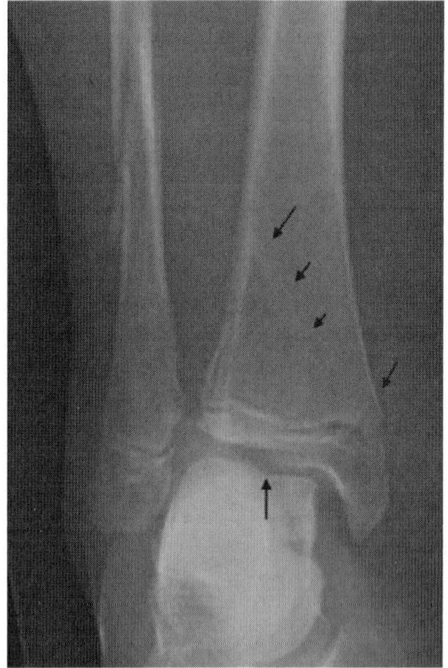

FIGURE 140-29. **A.** Mortise view of the ankle demonstrating a Salter-Harris type IV fracture of the tibia known as the triplane fracture with an associated fibular shaft fracture. **B.** CT lateral projection showing the fracture lines through the metaphysis (coronal plane), physis (transverse plane), and epiphysis (sagittal plane). [Photos used with permission of Karen Black, BC Children's Hospital, Vancouver.]

FOOT AND TOE INJURIES

In early childhood, the pliability and lack of ossification of the foot make fractures in this area rare. As ossification increases with age, fractures become more common, but significant injuries are still unusual. The foot is divided into the hindfoot (calcaneus and talus), the midfoot (navicular, cuboid, second and third cuneiforms), and the metatarsals and phalanges. Fractures of the mid- and hindfoot are rare; however, when they occur, they usually result from a fall. Recognition of fractures in these areas may be difficult, and CT or MRI may be necessary to identify and define these fractures. Fractures of the metatarsals and phalanges are relatively common in children and typically result from a direct blow from a falling object. They typically heal without sequelae. Crush injury to the foot may cause vascular compromise and compartment syndrome; these patients should be admitted for foot elevation and observation even if no fracture is detected.

Most nondisplaced fractures of the metatarsals and phalanges can be managed by immobilization in a posterior short-leg splint and follow-up with an orthopedist. Significantly displaced fractures of the metatarsals and phalanges as well as those of the great toe that have intra-articular involvement may require fixation, although this can typically be done on an outpatient basis.

Fractures of the base of the fifth metatarsal are common with inversion injuries of the ankle as in adults. The evaluation of ankle injuries should therefore include radiographs of the foot when there is tenderness over the fifth metatarsal. The immature skeleton includes an ossification center lateral to the base of the fifth metatarsal to which the peroneus brevis tendon attaches. This ossification center may be confused with a fracture, although an avulsion fracture at this site can also occur and presents with point tenderness and displacement of the ossification center (**Figure 140-30**). Immobilization and orthopedic follow-up are recommended.

SELECTED NONTRAUMATIC MUSCULOSKELETAL DISORDERS OF CHILDHOOD

ACUTE SEPTIC ARTHRITIS

Septic arthritis occurs in all age groups, but especially in children <3 years of age. The reported incidence of septic arthritis varies from 2 to 5 per 100,000 per year in the general population to 28 to 38 per 100,000 per year in patients with rheumatoid arthritis. Although any joint can be infected and multiple joints can be involved, the hip and the knee account for nearly 80% of cases.

Bacteria are the usual pathogens in acute skeletal and joint infections. Bacteria may access the joint hematogenously, by direct extension from adjacent osteomyelitis, or from inoculation, as in arthrocentesis or femoral venipuncture. Hematogenous spread is the most common.

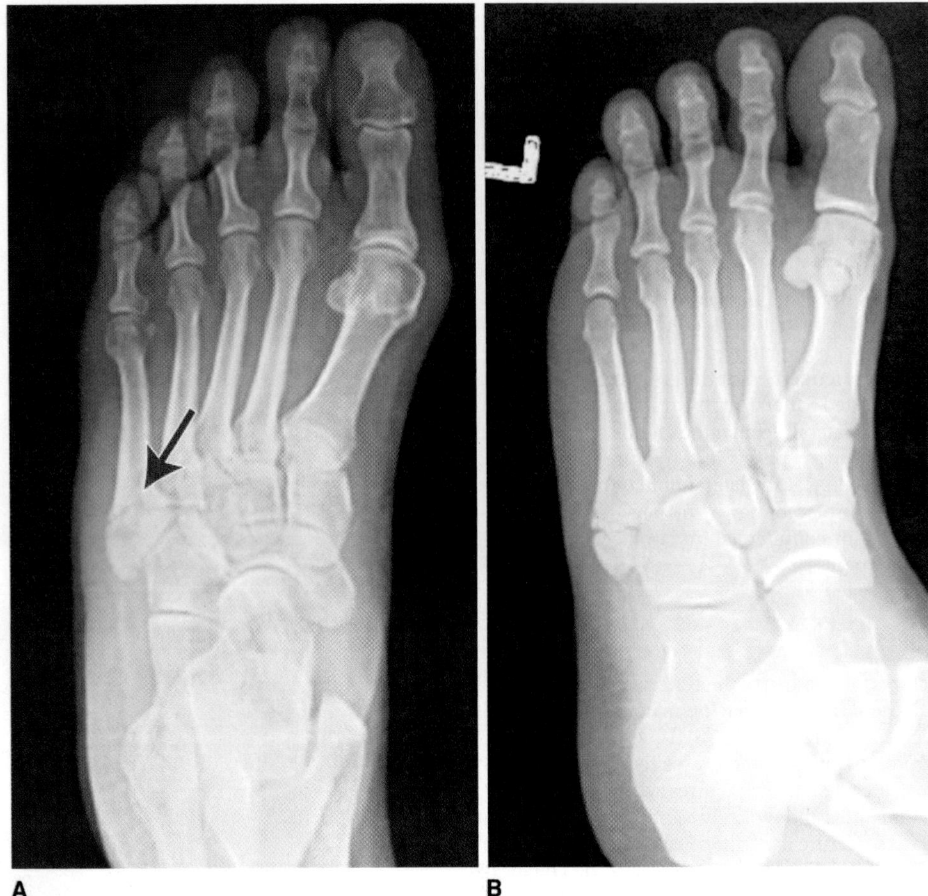

A B

FIGURE 140-30. Fracture of the base of the fifth metatarsal. **A.** Jones' fracture (*arrow*). **B.** Avulsion fracture of the tuberosity. [Reproduced with permission from Sherman SC: *Simon's Emergency Orthopedics*, 7th ed. © 2015, McGraw-Hill, New York. Fig 23-33A&B.]

Although *Staphylococcus aureus* is still the most common pathogen in osteoarticular infections, infection with community-acquired methicillin-resistant *S. aureus* and other multidrug-resistant organisms is increasing. In Europe, *Kingella kingae* (gram-negative coccobacilli) is reported to cause bone and joint infections, with only sporadic case reports of outbreaks in the United States.[20] Widespread vaccination has decreased the prevalence of *Haemophilus influenzae* type B, reducing invasive disease. Common etiologic organisms also vary with the age of the child (**Table 140-1**).

Even though septic infections of joints in children are uncommon, they are important because of their potential to cause permanent disability.

TABLE 140-1 Causes of Suppurative Arthritis in Children in Order of Decreasing Incidence

Newborn (0–2 mo)	Infant (2–36 mo)	Child (>36 mo)
Methicillin-sensitive *Staphylococcus aureus* (MSSA)	MSSA	MSSA
Methicillin-resistant *S. aureus* (MRSA)	MRSA	MRSA
Group B *Streptococcus*	*Streptococcus* species	*Streptococcus* species
Gram-negative bacilli	Gram-negative bacilli	Gram-negative bacilli
Neisseria gonorrhoeae	*Haemophilus influenzae*	*N. gonorrhoeae*
H. influenzae	Unknown or unidentified	
*Candida albicans**		

*Hospital acquired.

CLINICAL FEATURES AND DIAGNOSTIC IMAGING

The earliest signs and symptoms of septic arthritis are subtle. Neonates do not characteristically appear ill and, in half of cases, do not have fever. Older infants, toddlers, and children usually have fever and localizing signs. Infants may have only pseudoparalysis (absence of spontaneous movement) of an extremity or apparent pain on movement of the affected extremity. The child with hip or knee septic arthritis will limp or not walk at all. The child maintains the infected hip in flexion, abduction, or internal rotation. On physical examination of the septic knee, the manifestations are those of any localized infection (i.e., erythema, swelling, tenderness, and pain); these signs are not easily detected in the hip. Older children will appear ill, often with high fever (40.0 to 40.5°C [104 to 105°F]), with apprehension and irritability.

Children at special risk for septic infections of the bone and joint include those with underlying immune deficiency or systemic disease, including recent chickenpox, sickle cell anemia, rheumatoid arthritis, and inflammatory bowel disease. Maintain a high index of suspicion for septic arthritis in such children.

Plain film radiographs are nondiagnostic early in the course of infection but should be obtained to help identify osteomyelitis, fracture, or another process in the differential diagnosis.

Widening of the joint space with joint effusion and distention are late findings. Fat lines are displaced early in septic arthritis because of capsular distention. Views of the contralateral side may be useful for comparison. Ultrasonography is useful to document the presence of a joint effusion and aids in needle aspiration. CT and MRI provide improved soft tissue resolution and can aid in the diagnosis. The differential diagnosis is listed in **Table 140-2**.

TABLE 140-2 Differential Considerations for the Acutely Inflamed Pediatric Joint

Reactive or toxic synovitis
Trauma
Septic arthritis
Acute rheumatic fever
Poststreptococcal reactive arthritis
Gonococcal arthritis
Lyme disease
Sickle cell crisis
Henoch-Schönlein purpura
Legg-Calvé-Perthes disease
Slipped capital femoral epiphysis
Osteomyelitis
Juvenile rheumatic arthritis
Transient synovitis
Hemophilia
Osgood-Schlatter disease

DIAGNOSIS

If septic arthritis is suspected, obtain a CBC, blood cultures, erythrocyte sedimentation rate, C-reactive protein, and throat cultures; call orthopedics; and keep the child fasted/nothing by mouth. Arthrocentesis provides definitive diagnosis and should not be delayed while awaiting laboratory studies (see chapter 284, "Joints and Bursae"). Administer empiric antibiotics immediately if septic arthritis is suspected and orthopedic care is not available within 24 hours. **Patients at risk for septic arthritis usually have temperature >38.5°C (101.3°F), a C-reactive protein >20 milligrams/L (usually high), leukocytosis (>12,000 cells/mm3), severe pain, tenderness on palpation, spasm, and refusal to walk.**

Obtain joint fluid and send fluid for cell count, Gram stain, glucose, and culture and polymerase chain reaction testing.[21] Isolation of an organism from the joint fluid does not occur in approximately one third of cases, but purulent fluid confirms the diagnosis when the clinical exam is suggestive. Fastidious or slow-growing organisms may not grow in culture. Likewise, the bacteriostatic effect of synovial fluid or prior empiric antibiotic therapy may decrease the sensitivity of joint aspirate cultures. When blood cultures are obtained, they are positive in less than half of cases, but they are the only source from which the causative agent is isolated in about 10%. Polymerase chain reaction studies of joint fluid improve organism detection.[21,22]

Concurrent infections at other sites may be associated with septic arthritis, and culture of those sites may help define the pathogen (e.g., urine gram-negative bacilli; skin/wound *S. aureus*; urethra, cervix, rectum, and pharynx *Neisseria gonorrhea*).

TREATMENT

Treatment is prompt joint drainage and wash-out (open, in the operating room) followed immediately by IV antibiotic administration. If orthopedic care will be delayed, then IV antibiotics should be started. **Table 140-3** lists possible choices for initial antibiotic therapy, including empiric treatment. The prognosis depends on the length of time between symptom onset and treatment. A treatment delay of more than 4 days increases the likelihood of orthopedic complications, and infants have less favorable outcomes.

JUVENILE IDIOPATHIC ARTHRITIS

Juvenile idiopathic arthritis is an umbrella term that has replaced the term *juvenile rheumatoid arthritis*. Juvenile idiopathic arthritis includes a heterogeneous group of arthritides of unknown cause that develop in children <16 years old. A detailed presentation of each type of arthritis is beyond the scope of this chapter. Systemic juvenile idiopathic arthritis is discussed in the following paragraphs.

Systemic juvenile idiopathic arthritis is associated with high fevers and chills, characteristically with spikes to at least 39°C (102.2°F) for a minimum of 2 weeks. There is also an accompanying characteristic faint erythematous macular coalescing rash that can involve the trunk, palms,

TABLE 140-3 Initial Antibiotic Therapy of Acute Suppurative Arthritis in Children

Age	Suspected Organism	Antibiotics
Newborn (0–2 mo)	*Staphylococcus aureus*	Vancomycin, 10 milligrams/kg every 6–8 h
		or
		Clindamycin, 10 milligrams/kg every 6–8 h
	Group B *Streptococcus*	Ampicillin, 50–100 milligrams/kg every 6 h
		and
		Cefotaxime, 50 milligrams/kg every 6–8 h
		or
		Ceftriaxone, 50 milligrams/kg every 12 h
	Gram-negative bacilli	Cefotaxime, 50 milligrams/kg every 8 h
	Neisseria gonorrhoeae	Cefotaxime, 50 milligrams/kg every 8 h
	Unknown	Vancomycin or clindamycin and cefotaxime or ceftriaxone (dosing as above)
Infant (2–36 mo)	*S. aureus*	Vancomycin or clindamycin (dosing as above)
	Streptococcus species	Clindamycin/cefotaxime/ceftriaxone (dosing as above)
	Gram-negative bacilli	Cefotaxime or ceftriaxone (dosing as above)
	Haemophilus influenzae	Cefotaxime or ceftriaxone (dosing as above)
	Unknown	Vancomycin or clindamycin and cefotaxime or ceftriaxone
Child (>36 mo)	*S. aureus*	Vancomycin or clindamycin
	Streptococcus species	Clindamycin/cefotaxime/ceftriaxone
	Gram-negative bacilli	Cefotaxime or ceftriaxone
	N. gonorrhoeae	Cefotaxime or ceftriaxone
	Unknown	Vancomycin or clindamycin and cefotaxime or ceftriaxone

and soles. The arthritis is usually polyarticular. Associated findings are hepatosplenomegaly, lymphadenopathy, and pleuritis or pericardial effusion. Laboratory evaluation is not highly specific but can be significant for anemia, leukocytosis, thrombocytosis, elevated acute phase reactants (erythrocyte sedimentation rate and C-reactive protein), and elevated serum immunoglobulins. Arthrocentesis may be necessary to exclude acute septic arthritis, especially in oligoarticular disease. Early in the course, radiographs demonstrate only soft tissue swelling and, possibly, synovial effusions. Bone and cartilage destruction occurs later.

One of the most life-threatening complications is an entity called *macrophage activating syndrome* caused by macrophage and T-lymphocyte proliferation and is characterized by multi-organ system failure. Clinical findings can include high fever, purpura, spontaneous mucosal bleeding, altered mental status, and hepatosplenomegaly. Laboratory evaluation can reveal pancytopenia, liver dysfunction, disseminated intravascular coagulopathy, hyperferritinemia, hypertriglyceridemia, and low fibrinogen. Treatment may include symptomatic care in addition to pulse corticosteroids and cyclosporine A or a biologic.[23]

Hospital admission is needed to establish the diagnosis and to treat suspected acute suppurative arthritis while synovial fluid cultures are pending.

The initial therapy for patients with an established diagnosis includes a short-term trial of nonsteroidal anti-inflammatory drugs, following which, if disease activity is still present, methotrexate is usually started. Corticosteroids are used less commonly than in the past, but can still be useful in overwhelming systemic illness, including pericarditis, myocarditis, or iridocyclitis unresponsive to other therapy. A pediatric rheumatologist should direct management strategies, including intra-articular glucocorticoid injections and use of methotrexate (current first-line agent) and other biologic or nonbiologic disease-modifying antirheumatic drugs.[24]

LEGG-CALVÉ-PERTHES DISEASE

Legg-Calvé-Perthes disease is a hip disorder that generally has an onset between the ages of 4 and 9 years old in 80% of patients, with a range of occurrence from 2 to 13 years. It is the best known form of avascular necrosis or osteochondrosis, occurs in the femoral head, and should be considered in the differential diagnosis of the limping child in this age range. Males outnumber females by a ratio of 4:1, and it is bilateral in 10% of cases. Most children with the disorder are small for their age, with delayed skeletal maturation. Any primary or secondary ossification center can undergo changes as described below with necrosis and alteration of bone growth, with more common sites being the navicular (Koehler's disease), second metatarsal (Freiberg's disease), capitellum (Panner's disease), and lunate (Kienbock's disease), as well as the apophyses of the patella (Sinding-Larsen-Johanssen disease), tibia (Osgood-Schlatter disease), and calcaneus (Sever's disease).[25]

CLINICAL FEATURES

Legg-Calvé-Perthes disease begins with repeated episodes of ischemia of the femoral head, leading to infarction and necrosis. Avascular necrosis is then complicated by a subchondral stress fracture. Reossification and remodeling (resorption) occur over 2 to 4 years. The femoral head flattens and collapses and is prone to subluxation. The outcome ranges from complete recovery of the joint to a painful hip joint with a restricted range of motion, muscle spasms, and soft tissue contractures, and depends largely on the age of onset and the potential of the femoral head to remodel.

The onset of disease is usually insidious. Mild hip pain and limp have been present for weeks to months before making the diagnosis. Initially, pain is mild to none and is often referred to the anteromedial thigh or knee. Physical findings include decreased hip abduction and internal rotation. Sometimes the initial presentation is associated with trauma. Proximal thigh atrophy, and in advanced cases, limb shortening may also be noted.

Radiographically, in the initial stage of the disease (1 to 3 months), the capital femoral epiphysis fails to grow because of the lack of blood supply. The hip radiograph demonstrates widening of the cartilage space of the affected hip and a small-size ossific nucleus of the femoral head

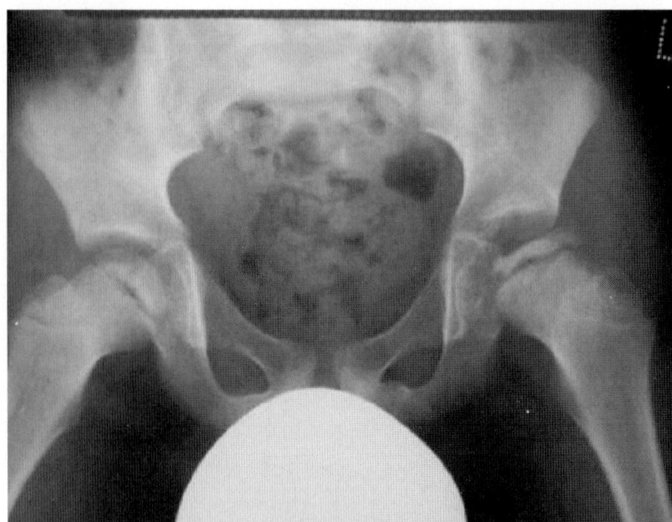

FIGURE 140-31. Legg-Calvé-Perthes disease: note the flattened and radiopaque left femoral epiphysis.

(**Figure 140-31**). Next, a subchondral stress fracture line in the femoral head is evident (Caffey's sign). As the disease progresses, new bone is deposited on avascular trabeculae. Subsequently, calcification of the more radiopaque necrotic marrow occurs, with resultant crushing of the avascular trabeculae in the dome of the epiphysis. Further distortion of the femoral head progresses (although this is not inevitable), along with subluxation and extrusion of the femoral head from the acetabulum.

DIAGNOSIS AND TREATMENT

Diagnosis of Legg-Calvé-Perthes disease demands a high index of suspicion, because initial radiographs sometimes are normal. Bone scan and MRI can detect disease before plain film abnormalities are evident. The differential diagnosis includes toxic synovitis, slipped capital femoral epiphysis, acute rheumatic fever, tuberculosis arthritis, tumors such as eosinophilic granuloma, osteoid osteoma, osteoblastoma, and lymphoma. Initial management is non–weight bearing and referral to a pediatric orthopedist for definitive care.

OSGOOD-SCHLATTER DISEASE

Osgood-Schlatter disease is an apophysitis of the tibial tubercle resulting from repeated normal stresses or overuse. These repetitive stresses imposed by the patellar tendon on its site of insertion result in a series of microavulsions of the ossification center and the underlying cartilage. Inflammation causes patellar tendonitis and the development of a remarkable prominence, induration, and tenderness of the tibial tuberosity. There is no avascular necrosis of the tibial tubercle. Children are usually between 10 and 15 years of age at time of onset; it more commonly occurs in running or jumping athletes. Boys are affected more often than girls, and most cases are bilateral, although symptoms are commonly asymmetric.

CLINICAL FEATURES

Signs and symptoms of Osgood-Schlatter disease are chronic, intermittent pain and tenderness over the anterior aspect of the knee and the tibial tuberosity. Pain is aggravated by activities such as running, kneeling, squatting, and climbing stairs; pain improves with rest. On examination, there is a prominence and soft tissue swelling over the tibial tubercle. The patellar tendon is tender and thick. The remainder of the knee examination usually is normal, and there is no knee effusion.

Radiographs are not essential, but are usually obtained. Radiographic findings of soft tissue swelling and irregularities of the tibial tubercle are nonspecific (**Figure 140-32**). The irregularity of the ossification of the tibial tubercle is normal in this age group. A lateral knee

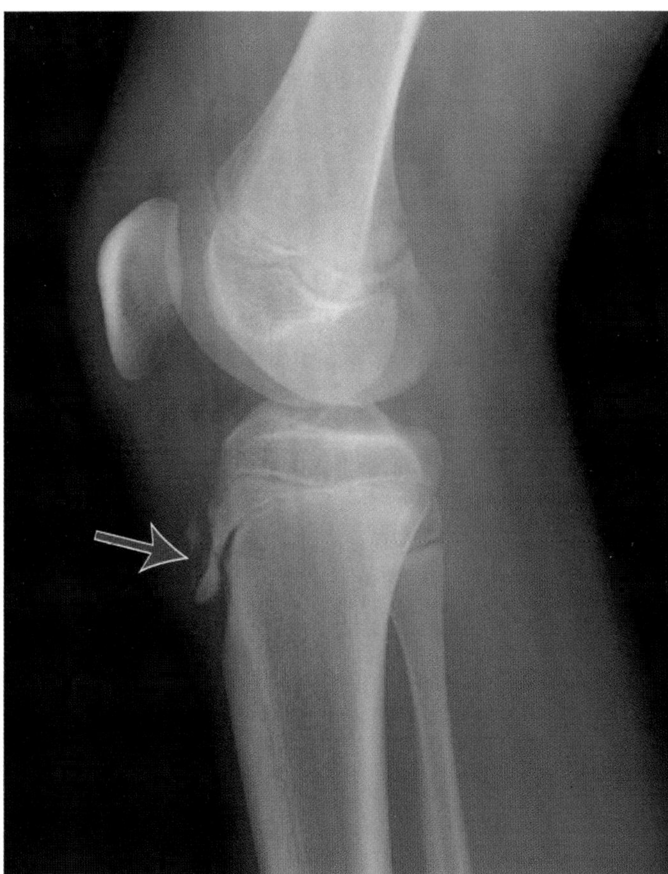

FIGURE 140-32. Lateral radiograph illustrating Osgood-Schlatter disease with prominence of the tibial tuberosity in addition to ossicles separate from the anterior border of the tubercle (*arrow*). [Photo used with permission of Wake Medical Center, Raleigh, NC.]

radiograph may show prominence of the tibial tuberosity, calcification in the tibial tubercle region, or separate ossicles from the anterior border of the tubercle.

TREATMENT

The disease is self-limited, and most patients' symptoms respond to rest and temporary avoidance of the offending activity. However, complete avoidance of activity or sports is not essential. Immobilization is actually contraindicated and can lead to rapid atrophy of the quadriceps muscle. Physical therapy and flexibility exercises to stretch and strengthen the quadriceps and hamstring muscles may help to alleviate stress on the tubercle and avoid recurrences. Applying ice after activity may decrease swelling, and pain can be controlled with nonsteroidal anti-inflammatory drugs. Corticosteroids should not be injected into the patellar tendon or para-apophyseal soft tissues. Parents should be provided reassurance that the condition is benign and self-limited and will resolve after closure of the proximal tibial growth plate. Rarely, an ossicle may persist after skeletal maturity that causes pain and may require excision.

ACUTE RHEUMATIC FEVER

Acute rheumatic fever primarily affects children of school age. The incidence of acute rheumatic fever has steadily fallen in developed countries over the past 50 years. However, sporadic cases of invasive group A β-hemolytic streptococcal infections with presumably more virulent strains means that outbreaks of acute rheumatic fever continue to be regularly reported in North America. It is preceded by infection with certain strains of group A β-hemolytic *Streptococcus* (mucoid types 3, 5, and 18). The connective tissue of the heart, joints, CNS, and subcutaneous tissues and skin are targeted by host antibodies that develop

TABLE 140-4 Revised Jones Criteria for the Diagnosis of Acute Rheumatic Fever

Major Criteria	Minor Criteria
Carditis	Fever
New or changing murmurs	Arthralgia
Cardiomegaly, congestive heart failure	History of previous attack of acute rheumatic fever
Pericarditis	Elevated erythrocyte sedimentation rate, C-reactive protein
Migratory polyarthritis	
Chorea	Prolonged PR interval on ECG
Erythema marginatum	Rising titer of antistreptococcal antibodies
Subcutaneous nodules	

Note: Diagnosis is likely when two major criteria or one major and two minor criteria are met. Group A *Streptococcus* may be documented by a history of scarlet fever, isolation of group A *Streptococcus* from throat culture, or rising titers of antistreptococcal antibodies.

secondary to streptococcal infection. The carditis is an endomyocarditis, with valvulitis primarily involving the mitral and aortic valves. The arthritis is characterized by synovial edema and periarticular swelling with joint effusions.

CLINICAL FEATURES

The child develops the disorder 2 to 6 weeks following streptococcal pharyngitis. Although nonspecific symptoms of systemic illness predominate early on, physical examination eventually reveals evidence of arthritis, carditis, choreiform movements, erythema marginatum, or subcutaneous nodules, individually or in combination. **Table 140-4** lists the Jones criteria for establishing a diagnosis of acute rheumatic fever. Either two major criteria or one major and two minor criteria plus evidence of an antecedent streptococcal infection are necessary to establish the diagnosis.

Arthritis occurs in 60% to 75% of initial attacks and is characterized as a migratory, fleeting polyarticular arthritis primarily affecting the large joints. Carditis occurs in one third of new cases and may be mild or severe. Its presence is heralded by any combination of a new cardiac murmur, tachycardia, a gallop rhythm, a pericardial friction rub, congestive heart failure, or a hyperactive precordium. Sydenham chorea occurs in 10% of cases and may have its initial appearance months following a streptococcal infection. Chorea may be the sole manifestation of acute rheumatic fever. The skin rash of acute rheumatic fever (erythema marginatum) is described as serpiginous and persists only for several days. It usually coexists with the presence of carditis in some form. Subcutaneous nodules are rarer and are located on the extensor surfaces of the wrists, elbows, and knees. The greatest morbidity and mortality are due to carditis.

DIAGNOSIS

Diagnostic studies are used to clarify the associated antecedent infection by group A *Streptococcus* (a pharyngeal swab for culture, antistreptolysin titers, or streptozyme titers) or are used to identify and assess the presence and extent of carditis. Obtain an ECG to identify conduction delays or hypertrophy. A chest x-ray serves to identify cardiac dilatation or pulmonary vascular congestion or edema. Echocardiography identifies valvulitis or valvular insufficiency (see chapter 126, "Congenital and Acquired Pediatric Heart Disease").

The differential diagnosis includes juvenile idiopathic arthritis, septic arthritis, Kawasaki's disease, viral or other forms of cardiomyopathy, leukemias, and other forms of vasculitis, including Henoch-Schönlein purpura, and drug reactions. Rarely, tumors of the CNS require differentiation from acute rheumatic fever when the child's sole clinical manifestation is chorea.

TREATMENT

ED treatment is directed primarily toward the management of complicating features of carditis. In the absence of cardiac or hemodynamic instability (and such is the rule), early consultation with a pediatric cardiologist is recommended, and **admission to the hospital is generally advised in the early stages until the diagnosis is confirmed**. Arthritis is managed with high-dose aspirin therapy (75 to 100 milligrams/kg/d) to achieve a serum salicylate level of 20 to 30 milligrams/dL. Reduce the aspirin dose after approximately 1 week to 50 milligrams/kg/d for an additional 4 to 6 weeks. Weigh the benefits and risks of aspirin therapy during influenza season (i.e., association with Reye's syndrome) carefully. Carditis or congestive heart failure is treated with prednisone, 1 to 2 milligrams/kg/d. Continue prednisone for 2 weeks after the resolution of symptoms and the return of the erythrocyte sedimentation rate to normal, and then taper steroids over 4 to 6 weeks. Chorea can be treated with haloperidol, 0.01 to 0.03 milligram/kg/d in four divided doses. All children with acute rheumatic fever are treated with penicillin, even if the cultures for group A *Streptococcus* are negative. The dose of benzathine penicillin is 600,000 units IM if <27 kg, and 1.2 million units IM if >27 kg. Benzathine penicillin G can be administered in a single dose of 1.2 million units. Penicillin V administered PO is also effective. Erythromycin is substituted for the penicillin-allergic patient. Therapy is administered for 10 days.

Administration of prophylactic antibiotics for 5 years is recommended for children without cardiac involvement; patients with carditis need lifelong prophylaxis. Prophylactic regimens include benzathine penicillin G, 1.2 million units administered IM every month, or daily oral penicillin V potassium or sulfadiazine.

POSTSTREPTOCOCCAL REACTIVE ARTHRITIS

Poststreptococcal reactive arthritis is a poorly understood clinical syndrome in which arthritis of one or more joints occurs after group A streptococcal infection of the pharynx. It is not certain whether poststreptococcal reactive arthritis represents a mild or early form of acute rheumatic fever or whether it is an entirely separate entity. It falls into a group of postinfectious reactive arthritides with multiple etiologies.[26]

Poststreptococcal reactive arthritis is not associated with carditis or other major Jones criteria and is a milder illness. Poststreptococcal reactive arthritis also begins sooner (approximately 10 days) after streptococcal infection than does acute rheumatic fever (approximately 21 days). The arthritis in poststreptococcal reactive arthritis is generally more severe and prolonged and unusually resistant to treatment with salicylates, in contrast to the migratory salicylate-sensitive arthritis generally associated with acute rheumatic fever.

The differentiation between acute rheumatic fever and poststreptococcal reactive arthritis is clinical. The arthritis of acute rheumatic fever is classically a migratory polyarthritis, whereas the arthritis of poststreptococcal reactive arthritis is a nonmigratory mono- or oligoarthritis. Acute rheumatic fever poststreptococcal nonsuppurative sequelae are more commonly observed in younger patients (mean age, 12 ± 4 years). The typical patient with reactive arthritis is older, but it may occur in children as young as 4 years of age. Erythema nodosum and erythema multiforme are frequently associated with poststreptococcal reactive arthritis, whereas they are encountered only infrequently in cases of acute rheumatic fever.

To establish the diagnosis of poststreptococcal reactive arthritis, establish antecedent infection with group A *Streptococcus*. If group A *Streptococcus* is recovered from the throat, treat with antibiotics. The diagnosis of poststreptococcal reactive arthritis should be made only after careful historical and clinical evaluation for nonsuppurative complications or other causes of polyarthritis. Antibiotic prophylaxis may be considered on a short-term basis. If, after further evaluation, there is no evidence of carditis or chorea, prophylaxis may be discontinued. Treatment of poststreptococcal reactive arthritis is nonsteroidal anti-inflammatory drug analgesia.

TRANSIENT SYNOVITIS OF THE HIP

Toxic or transient synovitis is a benign, self-limiting inflammatory process of the hip. It afflicts males more than females and is the most common cause of acute hip pain in children <10 years of age. The peak incidence is between ages 3 and 6 years old, but it is reported from 9 months of age to adolescence. It is eight times more frequent than septic arthritis of any joint. The cause is unknown, but it is most often believed to be a postviral illness sequela, but trauma, bacterial infection, and postvaccine or drug-mediated reactions have also been cited as possible causes. Arthralgia and arthritis are secondary to a transient inflammation and hypertrophy of the synovial membrane.

CLINICAL FEATURES

Symptoms are characterized by an abrupt onset of unilateral hip pain, limp, and restricted hip motion (preferentially held in abduction and external rotation). The child may complain of pain in the anteromedial or anterolateral thigh and knee. Although children complain of discomfort with movement of the limb, it generally remains possible to put the hip through a full range of motion. This is in contrast to the septic hip in which pain and spasms are more severe and range of motion is decreased. The child is nontoxic appearing, and other signs of systemic illness are absent. There can be either no fever or a low-grade temperature elevation. **The mean WBC count and erythrocyte sedimentation rate are significantly lower than in septic arthritis, but they cannot be used to distinguish between transient synovitis and septic arthritis in individual patients** (see discussion of acute septic arthritis above).

Radiographs of the hip may be normal or may demonstrate an effusion. There are no bone changes associated with transient synovitis. US is more sensitive than plain films at detecting joint effusions, although accuracy is decreased in patients <1 year of age. Reports of an effusion of the hip by US in toxic synovitis vary from 50% to 95%.

The differential diagnosis includes Legg-Calvé-Perthes disease and septic arthritis of the hip. Less common causes include acute rheumatic fever, juvenile idiopathic arthritis, and, rarely, tuberculosis of the hip.

DIAGNOSIS

If the peripheral WBC count and erythrocyte sedimentation rate are substantially elevated and a hip effusion is noted on radiograph or US, perform a diagnostic arthrocentesis and obtain orthopedic consultation to exclude a septic joint. Send synovial fluid for Gram stain, aerobic and anaerobic cultures, and acid-fast bacilli with culture. Synovial fluid is sterile and clearly transudative with no organisms on Gram stain.

TREATMENT

Treatment is with rest until the pain resolves, usually 3 to 7 days, followed by limited activity for 1 to 2 weeks. Nonsteroidal anti-inflammatory drugs are the first-line therapy for pain. There are no sequelae from transient synovitis. As long as the diagnosis is certain, reevaluation by the primary care physician can be arranged within 2 weeks.

REFERENCES

The complete reference list is available online at www.TintinalliEM.com.

Rashes in Infants and Children

Gary Bonfante
Amy Dunn

INTRODUCTION

This chapter describes disease processes in children for which dermatologic symptoms are diagnostic and serves as a reference for the presenting complaint of "rash" in children and young adults. Additional detailed descriptions of important skin diseases are provided in chapters in Section 20, "Dermatology," with chapter 248, "Initial Evaluation and Management of Skin Disorders" specifically outlining principles of evaluation of rashes in both children and adults. Several important disease entities presenting with rashes are covered extensively elsewhere within this text (e.g., Lyme disease, Rocky Mountain spotted fever). In addition to the discussion below, chapters in Section 20, "Dermatology," discuss diagnosis based on anatomic location of the rash.

GENERAL APPROACH

Ask about fever and systemic symptoms, prior immunizations, potential human or animal contacts, recent bites or stings, travel, recent prescription or over-the-counter drug administration, and recent food and environmental exposure. Ask about the initial location of rash, the pattern and time frame of rash development, initial morphology, and whether any topical or systemic medications have been applied.

Most exanthems present as an isolated episode in a single child, but outbreaks can also develop in groups of children. When evaluating only a single child with a rash, the diagnosis can usually be made by routine history and physical examination. When several children develop similar-appearing skin lesions, obtain detailed contact and exposure history, and consider the need to involve specialty services or notify local public health authorities.

Perform a complete physical exam and obtain a full set of vital signs. Completely disrobe all patients and place in a gown; examine patients in a room with good lighting to avoid missing important findings. Most rashes are self-limited and benign in children, but some rashes may be the harbinger of serious illness. An ill-appearing child or a child with a nonblanching rash raises suspicion for a serious condition. Check the scalp, ears, neck, mucous membranes, all skinfolds, digits and web interspaces, palms, and soles. Look for ticks that may be adherent in hair-bearing areas or skinfolds. Identify the morphology and determine the location and distribution of the rash.

VIRUSES

ENTEROVIRUSES

Enteroviruses are a very common cause of illness and rash in young children. Enteroviruses are small, single-stranded RNA viruses belonging to the picornavirus group and include polioviruses, coxsackievirus, and echovirus.[1] The enterovirus family has been associated with a wide variety of illnesses, including polio. Enterovirus infections usually occur in epidemics, with a peak prevalence in the summer and early fall. Transmission usually occurs by the fecal–oral route and sometimes by respiratory or oral–oral transmission.[2]

The clinical signs and symptoms of infection with coxsackieviruses and echoviruses vary and can include nonspecific febrile illnesses, upper and lower respiratory infections, GI infections and inflammations, aseptic meningitis, or myocarditis. Similarly, the associated skin manifestations include an array of exanthems. Diffuse macular eruptions, morbilliform erythema, vesicular lesions, petechial and purpuric eruptions, rubelliform rash, roseola-like rash, and scarlatiniform eruptions have all been reported.[2] Strict clinical–virologic associations are difficult to demonstrate, unlikely to be practical in the ED, and equally unlikely to change the course of management.

Infection due to **echovirus 9** or **coxsackievirus A9** is common and produces typical examples of exanthems secondary to enteroviral illness. Both viruses may produce a maculopapular rash beginning on the face and neck and then extending to the trunk and feet. The palms and soles are also sometimes affected. Clinical manifestations include fever that may be accompanied by headache, GI complaints, and upper respiratory symptoms. With echovirus 9, occasionally, there are lesions on the buccal mucosa and soft palate that resemble Koplik spots. Petechiae may develop, raising concern for meningococcemia, although the petechiae due to enterovirus do not typically coalesce or progress to purpura. The exanthem persists for approximately 5 days. The exanthem of coxsackievirus A9, by contrast, may be vesicular or urticarial. Aseptic meningitis may be present.

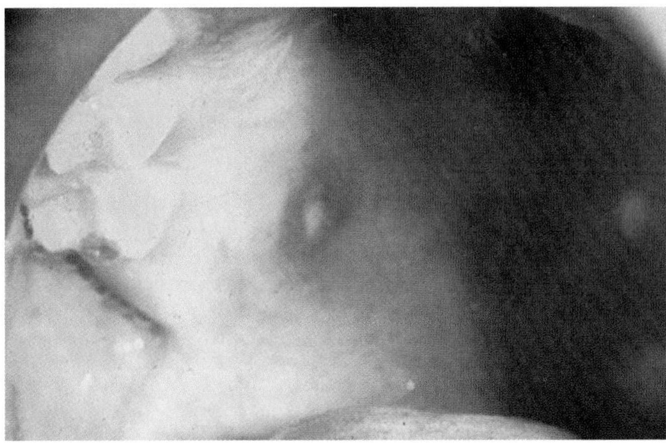

FIGURE 141-1. Oral lesions of hand-foot-and-mouth disease. [Photo contributed by James F. Steiner, DDS. Reproduced with permission from Knoop K, Stack L, Storrow A, Thurman RJ: *Atlas of Emergency Medicine*, 3rd ed. © 2010, McGraw-Hill, New York.]

Another common rash caused by an enterovirus is **hand-foot-and-mouth disease**. Initial signs and symptoms include fever, anorexia, malaise, and sore mouth. Oral lesions appear 1 to 2 days later, and cutaneous lesions appear shortly thereafter (**Figure 141-1**). The oral lesions begin as vesicles on an erythematous base, which subsequently ulcerate. The vesicles are usually 4 to 8 mm in size and are very painful. They are located on the buccal mucosa, tongue, soft palate, and gingiva. The exanthem starts as red papules that change to gray vesicles approximately 3 to 7 mm in size. They are found on the palms and soles but may occur on the dorsum of the feet and hands and on the buttocks as well (**Figure 141-2**). They may be oval, linear, or crescentic and may run parallel to skin lines. They heal in 7 to 10 days.

A particularly severe form of hand-foot-and-mouth disease, attributed to enterovirus 71, has been identified in Southeast Asia and has been associated with serious illness including encephalitis and death. Clinicians caring for patients from this region or those having traveled to that area should be mindful of potential deterioration of these patients.

A similar syndrome of fever, mouth pain, and oral ulcers is caused by other subtypes of the coxsackievirus group A and is known as **herpangina**. Like hand-foot-and-mouth disease, the diagnostic finding is small whitish ulcers, typically located on the soft palate and posterior pharynx, without accompanying skin lesions (**Figure 141-3**).

The clinical differentiation of enteroviral disease is difficult, but because there is no specific therapy for enteroviral infection, it is more important to consider bacterial diseases in the differential diagnosis to

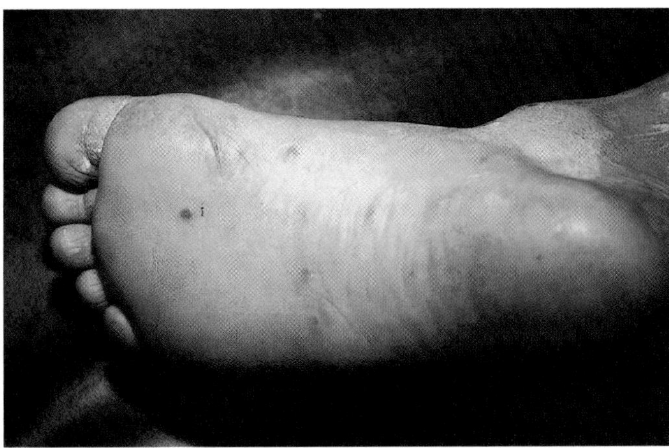

FIGURE 141-2. Hand-foot-and-mouth disease. [Photo contributed by Raymond C. Baker, MD. Reproduced with permission from Knoop K, Stack L, Storrow A, Thurman RJ: *Atlas of Emergency Medicine*, 3rd ed. © 2010, McGraw-Hill, New York.]

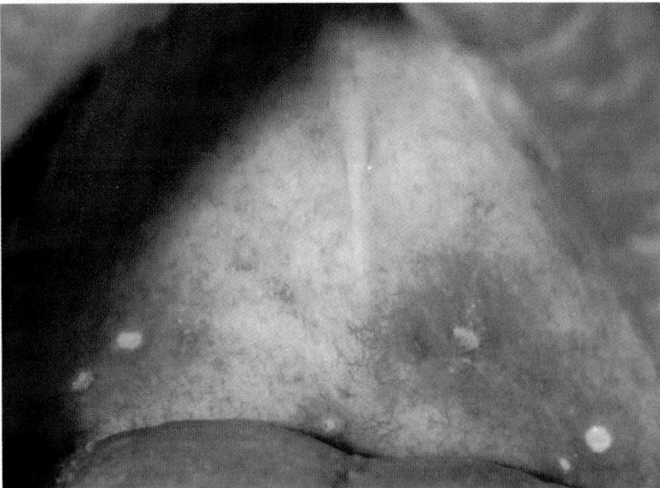

FIGURE 141-3. Herpangina. [Reproduced with permission from Wolff KL, Johnson R, Suurmond R: *Fitzpatrick's Color Atlas & Synopsis of Clinical Dermatology*, 6th ed. © 2009, McGraw-Hill, New York.]

exclude treatable causes of sepsis, meningitis, myocarditis, and pneumonia. Enteroviral polymerase chain reaction testing is commonly available and may be useful in cases of meningitis in which viral testing may decrease length of hospital stay and use of antibiotics. Symptomatic therapy for enteroviral infections includes hydration, antipyretics, and topical oral pain relief preparations. Combinations of Maalox® (or similar) and diphenhydramine liquids applied with a cotton swab to the painful oral lesions may be useful. **Viscus lidocaine should not be used.** A recent U.S. Food and Drug Administration drug safety communication advises that viscus lidocaine 2% solution should not be used in infants and children.[3] In 2014, 22 serious adverse events, including deaths, in children age 5 months to 3.5 years were attributed to the use of oral topical viscus lidocaine. Rarely, analgesia with oral narcotics is needed to prevent dehydration. Hospitalization in patients requiring this level of pain relief may be considered.

MEASLES

The number of measles cases in the United States in 2013 to 2014 is the highest since 2000. Recent outbreaks among adults and children in many states have been attributed to international travel and unvaccinated populations here in the United States. Thimerosal was taken out of childhood vaccines in 2001, and multiple, large, well-designed epidemiologic studies and systematic reviews have found no evidence of an association between thimerosal and autism or other developmental disorders. In fact, autism rates have continued to rise, which is the opposite of what would be expected if thimerosal caused autism.[4]

Serious complications of measles have been reported including encephalitis, bacterial infections such as pneumonia, and death. These complications are more common in children under the age of 5 years than school-age and adolescent patients. All medical care providers must be able to identify the exanthem and enanthem typical of measles in any patient presenting with the undifferentiated rash.

Measles virus (rubeola) is a member of the family Paramyxoviridae, genus *Morbillivirus*. After exposure, the incubation period for measles is approximately 10 days (range, 7 to 21 days). The prodromal period lasts approximately 3 days and is characterized by fever, malaise, and anorexia, followed by conjunctivitis, coryza, and cough. The severity of conjunctivitis is variable and may also be accompanied by lacrimation or photophobia but is typically not exudative. The exanthem develops approximately 14 days following exposure. The rash first appears behind the ears and at the hairline of the forehead and then spreads cephalocaudally and centrifugally to involve the neck, upper trunk, lower trunk, and extremities sparing the palms and soles. It initially consists of erythematous blanching maculopapular lesions but rapidly coalesces, especially where the first lesions appeared on the face (**Figure 141-4, A–C**). In general, the extent and degree of confluence of the rash correlate with the severity of the illness in children. Other rash-causing diseases often confused with measles include roseola (roseola infantum) (see Figure 141-12) and rubella (German measles) (see Figure 141-6).

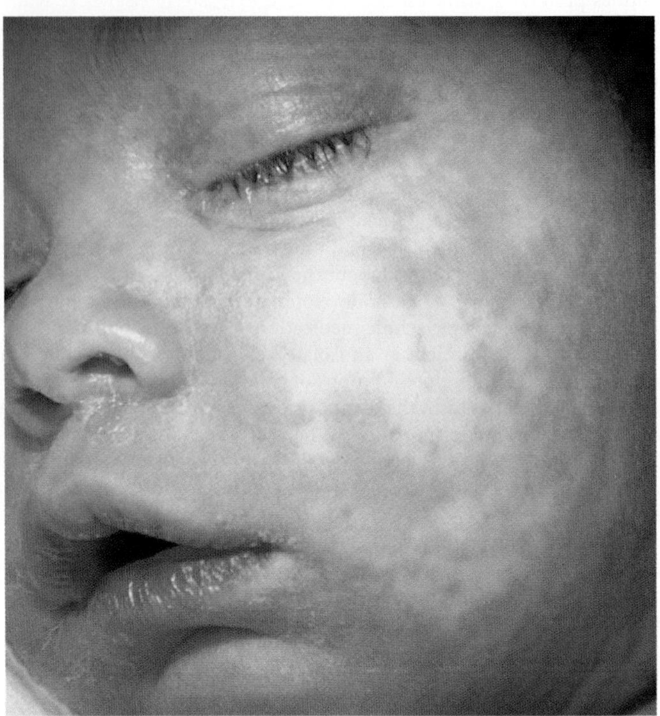

A

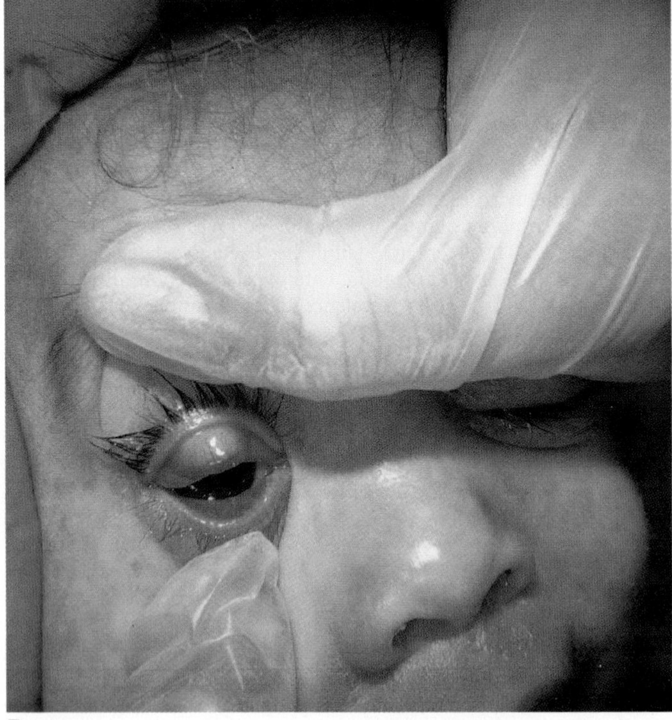

B

FIGURE 141-4. **A–C.** Measles. An 8-month-old child presented with fever, coryza, and marked conjunctivitis associated with intense photophobia. Confluent, erythematous, and maculopapular rash on the face developed on the fourth day of fever. He developed measles during the measles outbreak seen in New York City in 1993. [For A and B: Used with permission of Binita R. Shah, MD. Reproduced with permission from Shah BR, Lucchesi M, Amodio J (Eds). *Atlas of Pediatric Emergency Medicine*, 2d ed. McGraw-Hill, Inc., 2013. Fig 3.54 A&B, Pg 100. For part C: Reproduced with permission from: Shah BR and Laude TL: *Atlas of Pediatric Clinical Diagnosis*. WB Saunders, Philadelphia, 2000.]

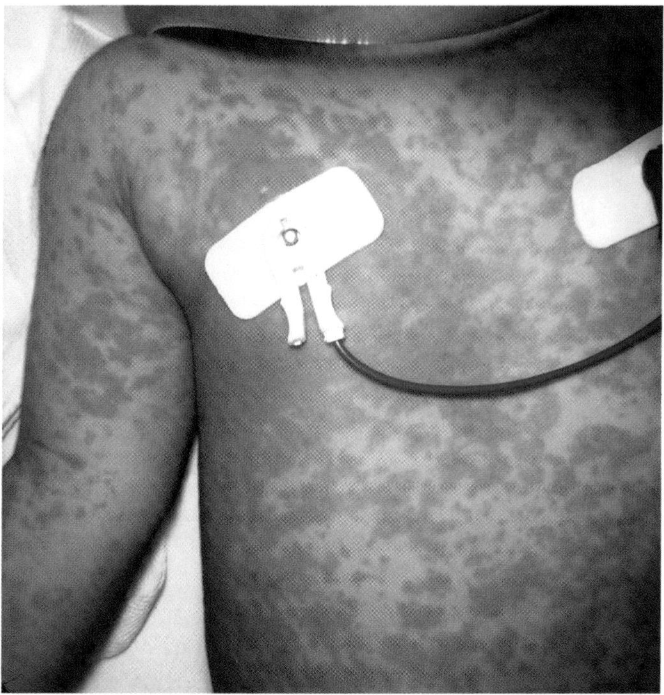

C

FIGURE 141-4. *(Continued)*

Search carefully for Koplik spots (**Figure 141-5**) in patients with suspected measles, because they are pathognomonic for measles infection and occur about 48 hours before the characteristic exanthem. However, they do not appear in all patients.

Treatment is supportive. Recognition is of the utmost importance in preventing the spread of the disease and associated morbidity and mortality. Immunization remains the most important preventative measure. About 1 in 20 children who receive the measles, mumps, rubella, and varicella vaccine will develop a rash following vaccination, which may prompt a trip to the ED. The rash usually involves the trunk and face, is macular and blanching, does not involve systemic symptoms, and is self-resolving. The only treatment is reassurance.[4]

RUBELLA

Rubella, "**German measles**," or "**Third disease**" was once a common childhood disease that had its highest incidence during the spring. The incubation period is 12 to 25 days following exposure, with a 1- to 5-day prodrome of fever, malaise, headache, and sore throat.

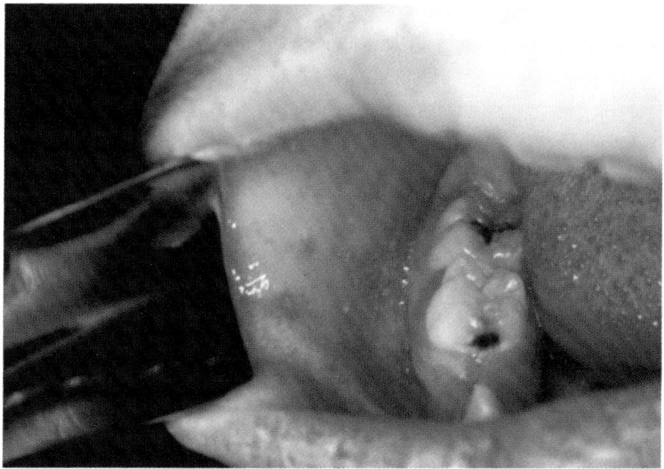

FIGURE 141-5. Koplik spots. [Image used with permission of the Centers for Disease Control and Prevention.]

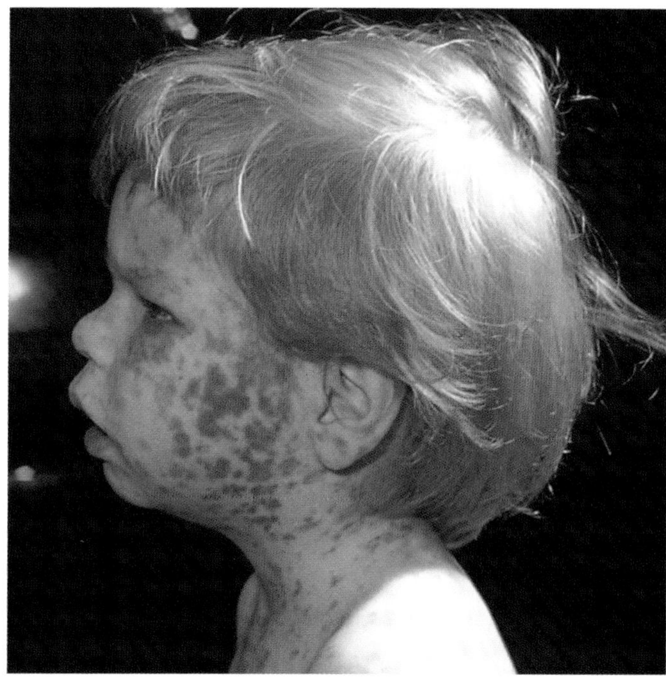

FIGURE 141-6. Rubella. [Image used with permission of the Centers for Disease Control and Prevention.]

The exanthem varies and is sometimes difficult to identify. It may be a short-lived blush, or it may have a more typical and protracted 2- to 3-day course. The exanthem begins as irregular pink macules and papules on the face, spreading to the neck, trunk, and arms in a centrifugal distribution (**Figure 141-6**). The rash coalesces on the face as the eruption reaches the lower extremities and then clears in the same fashion. Forchheimer spots are pinpoint petechiae involving the soft palate that coalesce and may accompany the rash but are nonspecific.

Lymphadenopathy is a clinical manifestation of rubella, with characteristic enlargement of suboccipital and posterior auricular nodes. The clinical diagnosis in an individual case is often difficult, but the epidemic nature of the illness, along with the seasonal variation and high expression rate of the exanthem, help in establishing the diagnosis. A history of inadequate immunizations may assist in the diagnosis. There is no specific therapy.

ERYTHEMA INFECTIOSUM

Fifth disease, or erythema infectiosum, is an acute, febrile illness with a unique exanthem. Outbreaks of erythema infectiosum occur primarily in the spring. During epidemics, the attack rate is highest in children 5 to 15 years of age, but all age groups can be affected. The illness is caused by infection with human parvovirus B19, a single-stranded DNA virus.

The abrupt appearance of the rash is frequently the first manifestation of erythema infectiosum. It begins with a characteristic fiery red rash on the cheeks (**Figure 141-7**). The rash is a diffuse erythema of closely grouped tiny papules on an erythematous base. The edges are slightly raised. The erythema is most intense below the eyes and extends over the cheeks in a pattern reminiscent of butterfly wings; it is sometimes referred to as a slapped-cheek appearance. There is circumoral pallor as well as sparing of the eyelids and chin. The facial rash fades after 4 to 5 days.

Approximately 1 to 2 days after the appearance of the facial rash, a nonpruritic macular erythema or erythematous maculopapular rash occurs on the trunk and limbs. It is at first localized to the deltoid areas, trunk, and forearms, but usually extends to involve a large area. This stage of the exanthem may last 1 week. A distinctive aspect of the rash is that it fades with central clearing, giving a reticulated or lacy appearance (**Figure 141-8**). The palms and soles are rarely affected.

The exanthem may recur in the ensuing 3 weeks, sometimes briefly. The intensity of the recurrent exanthem varies and may be related to

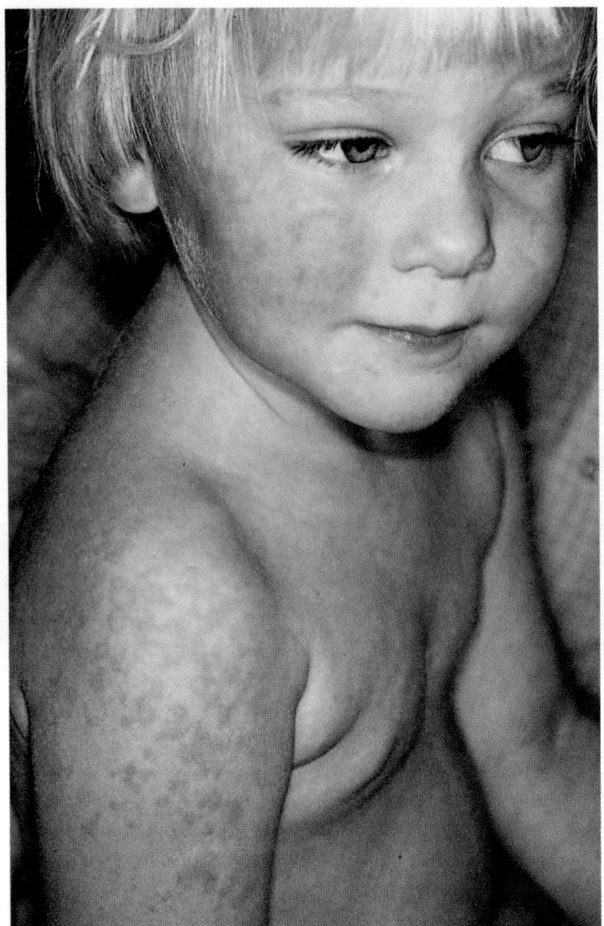

FIGURE 141-7. Erythema infectiosum (fifth disease). [Photo contributed by Anne W. Lucky, MD. Reproduced with permission from Knoop K, Stack L, Storrow A, Thurman RJ: *Atlas of Emergency Medicine*, 3rd ed. © 2010, McGraw-Hill, New York.]

exposure to environmental factors such as sunlight, hot baths, and, perhaps, physical exertion or emotional upset. Associated symptoms frequently occur and may include fever, malaise, headache, sore throat, cough, coryza, nausea, vomiting, diarrhea, and myalgia. Arthralgia and arthritis can occur but are more common in adolescents and adults in whom symptoms can be severe. **Parvovirus infection may also be severe in patients with sickle cell disease, in whom it may precipitate aplastic crisis.** Fetal anemia and hydrops may also occur with acute infection in pregnant women in the first half of pregnancy, and those who have been exposed should be counseled appropriately. In general, parvovirus infection requires only symptomatic therapy, and recovery is usually complete.

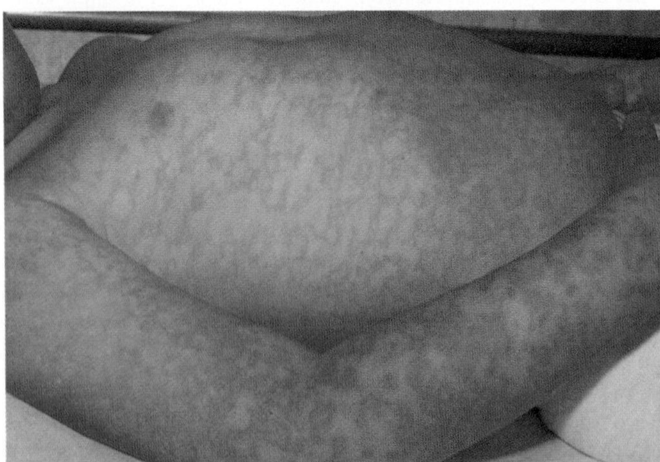

FIGURE 141-8. Erythema infectiosum. Lacy, reticulated rash on the body of a child with erythema infectiosum. [Reproduced with permission from Shah BR, Laude TL: Erythema infectiosum, in: *Atlas of Pediatric Clinical Diagnosis*. Philadelphia, WB Saunders, 2000]

HERPES VIRUS

The two serotypes of herpes simplex virus (HSV) are HSV-1 and HSV-2, which are double-stranded DNA viruses that can present variably based on the organ systems involved and the competency of the host's immune system. Infections may be disseminated, localized to the CNS, or mucocutaneous. In the infant, HSV-2 is usually contracted during childbirth through vaginal secretions. HSV-1 is typically spread through oral secretions. The incubation period for herpes is from 2 to 14 days. With both serotypes, viral shedding may occur from an asymptomatic source. HSV-1 is the most common type identified in lesions of the skin and oral mucosa, but HSV-2 has also been identified. Autoinoculation may also occur. The clinical appearance of both serotypes is indistinguishable, and this point is important when there is concern for sexual abuse. HSV persists for life in a latent form, with the possibility of both symptomatic and asymptomatic reactivation.[5] Visually identifiable lesions presenting to the ED may include oral lesions, skin lesions primarily of the hand or genitalia, or ocular lesions.

Herpes labialis ("cold sores") and gingivostomatitis are two common mucocutaneous presentations of herpes in children and young adults (**Figure 141-9**). A lesion may be single, or lesions may be clustered or, in the case of gingivostomatitis, may be evident diffusely throughout the oral cavity. The clinical appearance of most herpetic infections is of umbilicated vesicles that are extremely painful. They eventually unroof and crust over. Labialis is typically localized to the vermillion border. Gingivostomatitis may make eating painful. As stated earlier, viscus lidocaine preparations should not be used.

Eczema herpeticum (**Figure 141-10**) is the development of vesicular eruptions in the areas of the epidermis previously affected by eczema and may be life threatening. Although fever may present with other forms of HSV infections of children, fever is described more frequently with eczema herpeticum. Treatment includes oral antibiotics to treat *Staphylococcus* and *Streptococcus* (see Table 141-4 regarding antibiotics

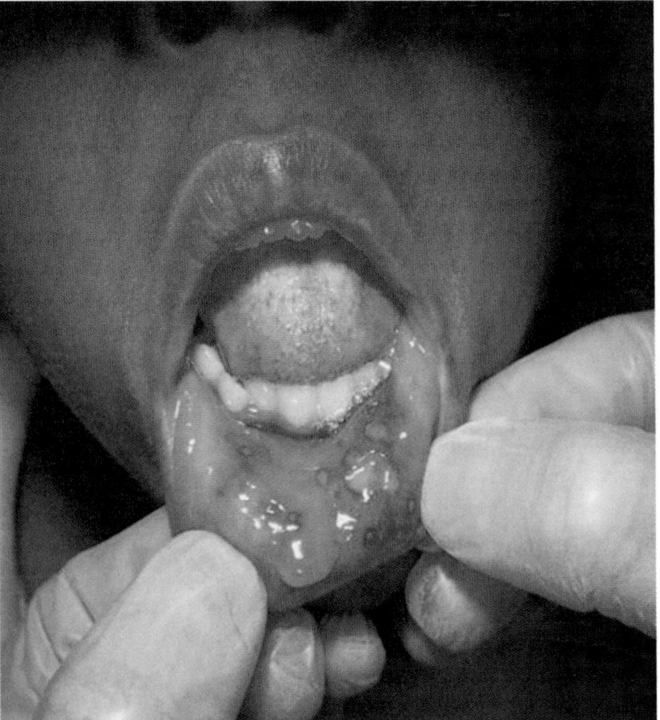

FIGURE 141-9. Primary herpetic gingivostomatitis. Typical lesions of herpes gingivostomatitis on the buccal mucosa. [Reproduced with permission from Shah BR, Lucchesi M: *Atlas of Pediatric Emergency Medicine*, © 2006 by McGraw-Hill, Inc., New York.]

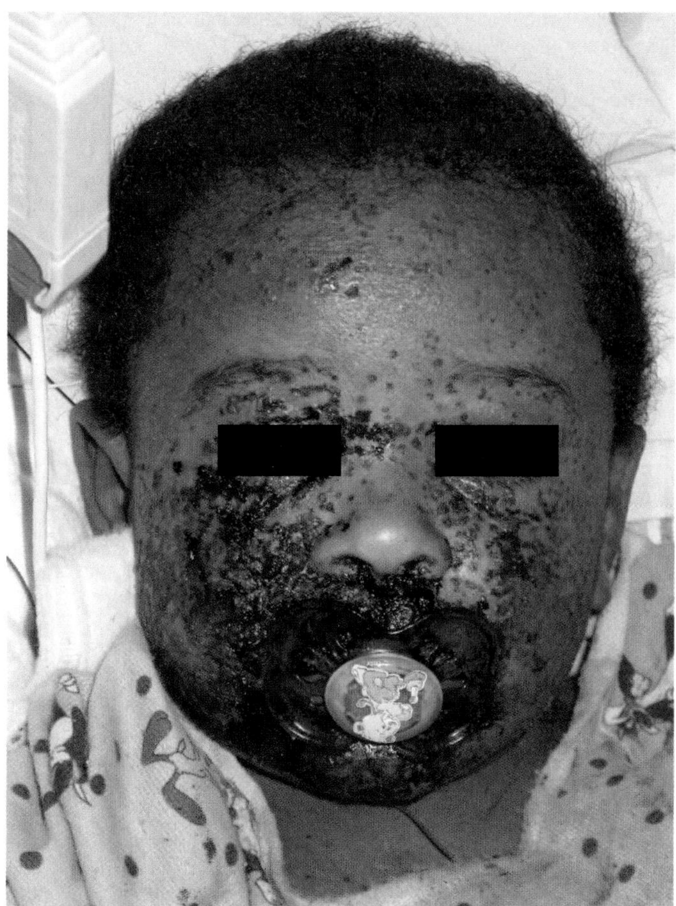

FIGURE 141-10. Eczema herpeticum in areas of atopic dermatitis. [Photo contributed by University of North Carolina Department of Dermatology.]

for cellulitis), as well as antiviral therapy with acyclovir, 80 milligrams/kg/d every 6 hours for 10 days.

Another herpetic skin manifestation is **herpetic whitlow**. This infection of the distal fingers is usually the result of inoculation from an oral infection. Carefully examine the child's eyes to ensure that no herpetic lesions are present on the cornea secondary to direct contact.

Herpetic infections of the ears, thorax, and extremities have also been reported as a result of close contact sports (wrestling). Genital infections are most commonly the result of sexual transmission (consensual or abuse). Diagnosis is usually based on the clinical appearance, but viral cultures should be obtained for confirmation, particularly when sexual abuse is a consideration; obtain cultures from the fluid of an unroofed vesicle. Culture, enzyme-linked immunosorbent assay, direct fluorescent antibody testing, polymerase chain reaction, and Tzanck smear are acceptable forms of testing. Providers should confirm with their laboratories the preferred method of sampling at their institution.[6]

Treatment in the case of oral lesions is symptomatic. Oral antivirals may shorten the course of an acute outbreak and viral shedding when provided early in the disease (first 48 hours). Topical acyclovir is ineffective. The dosing of oral acyclovir is variable based on age and location of the lesions, but is typically 80 milligrams/kg/d divided every 6 hours for 5 days. When initiating antiviral medication in children <2 years old or in immunocompromised children, dosing is more variable, and consultation with a pediatric or infectious disease specialist is appropriate. Ophthalmology should be consulted when herpetic lesions are suspected of having invaded the cornea. This may be evidenced by dendritic-appearing lesions with fluorescein staining.

VARICELLA

Varicella, or chickenpox, is a result of infection with varicella-zoster virus, a herpes virus. In normal children, it is characterized by a pruritic generalized vesicular exanthem with mild systemic manifestations. Cases generally occur in late winter and early spring. It is highly contagious in the prodromal and vesicular stage. Varicella most frequently occurs in children <10 years old but may occur at any age. The rates of varicella and associated hospital admissions and deaths have declined dramatically in surveillance areas with significant vaccine coverage, but cases do occur in vaccinated children, although they are typically mild and more limited than in unvaccinated children.[7] Severe side effects from the vaccine are rare.[8]

Varicella starts on the trunk, and most lesions are clustered in this body region. Lesions are of different stages presenting simultaneously. Within 24 hours, the rash acquires the typical vesicular appearance of varicella. The rash consists of teardrop vesicles on an erythematous base, which then dry and crust over. Successive fresh crops may appear for a few days. The extent of the rash may be minimal, but usually it will spread centrifugally and become widespread (**Figure 141-11**). Palms and soles are spared. Vesicles may occur on mucous membranes and go on to rupture and form shallow ulcers. Atypical and limited cutaneous involvement may occur among immunized children infected with varicella virus. Low-grade fever, malaise, and headache are frequently present but are usually mild. The diagnosis of varicella is usually made clinically based on its distinctive rash. A Tzanck smear of the vesicle contents may demonstrate varicella giant cells with inclusion bodies; polymerase chain reaction may also be performed on skin scrapings. Fluorescent antibody to membrane antigen testing is regarded as the gold standard for identification of varicella-zoster virus antibodies but is not readily available.[8]

Complications of varicella include encephalitis, pneumonia, hepatitis, and bacterial superinfection of the ruptured vesicles with staphylococci or streptococci. Neonates born to mothers with perinatal varicella infection may develop serious illness.

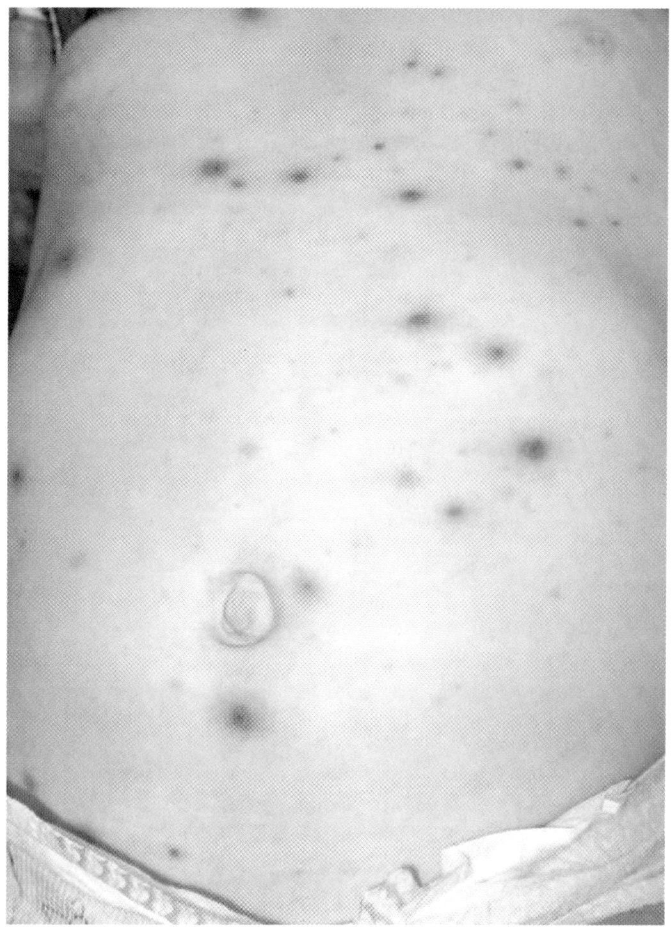

FIGURE 141-11. Varicella. [Photo contributed by University of North Carolina Department of Dermatology.]

Uncomplicated varicella requires no specific therapy. Acetaminophen may be used as needed. **Do not give aspirin because it may predispose to the development of Reye's syndrome**. Oral antihistamines may be useful to reduce itching. Over-the-counter oatmeal-based baths may provide temporary symptomatic relief. Clean lesions regularly to prevent secondary infection. In the absence of CNS complications, the prognosis is excellent. **Routine use of antiviral therapy for uncomplicated varicella infections in immunocompetent children is not commonly recommended.**[9] Acyclovir (80 milligrams/kg/d divided every 6 hours for children >3 months old) may be considered if started within 24 hours of onset but generally only results in a 1-day reduction of fever and a 15% to 30% reduction in other signs and symptoms.[8]

Infants and immunocompromised children with varicella require aggressive treatment with acyclovir. Those less than 1 year of age are treated with 10 milligrams/kg every 8 hours, whereas children older than 1 year receive 500 milligrams/m^2 every 8 hours. Administration of varicella-zoster prophylaxis should be considered for patients exposed to individuals with varicella if provided within 3 days of exposure.[10]

ROSEOLA INFANTUM

Roseola infantum, or **exanthem subitum**, was previously called **sixth disease**. There is no seasonal association. The most likely cause is the human herpesvirus 6, although other viruses have been associated with a roseola-like illness.

Roseola is characterized by a febrile period of 3 to 5 days, defervescence, and the appearance of a rash for 1 or 2 days (**Figure 141-12**). The appearance of the rash immediately following a nonspecific febrile illness is characteristic and aids in the diagnosis. Primarily, young children are affected, with most patients being between 6 months and 3 years of age. The illness begins abruptly with high fever, sometimes as high as 40.6°C (105°F). The child is usually alert and active but may be irritable, especially with very high fever. Associated symptoms are usually mild and may include cough, coryza, anorexia, and abdominal discomfort. Lymphadenopathy may be present. The fever persists for 3 to 5 days, and the child rapidly becomes well.

Although the exanthem in roseola usually coincides with defervescence, the rash may follow a short afebrile interlude. The rash is an erythematous macular or maculopapular eruption that consists of discrete, rose or pale-pink lesions 2 to 5 mm in size. It is most prominent on the neck, trunk, and buttocks, but the face and proximal extremities may also be involved. The lesions blanch with pressure. There is no mucous membrane involvement. The rash lasts 1 to 2 days but may fade rapidly, usually without desquamation.

There is no specific treatment for roseola. Acetaminophen is useful for fever control. Because of the abrupt nature of the fever, febrile seizures may occur and are treated as any febrile seizure.

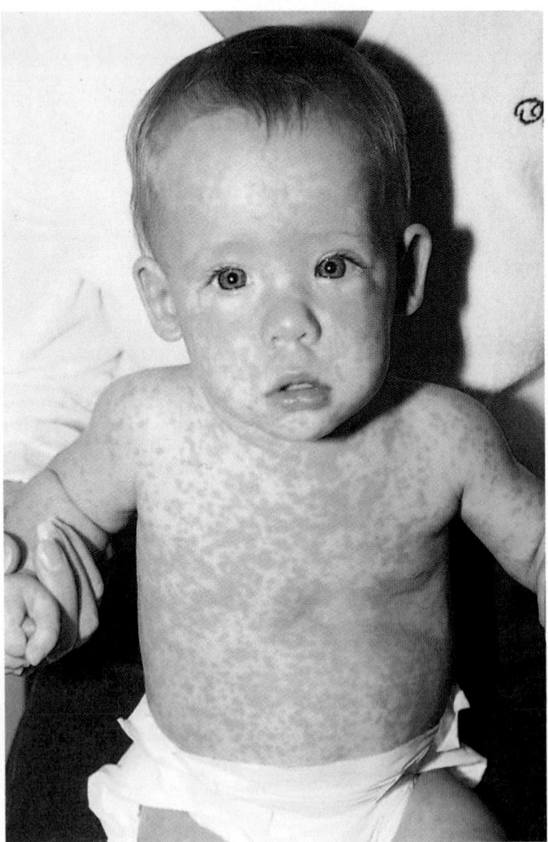

FIGURE 141-12. Roseola infantum. [Photo contributed by Raymond C. Baker, MD. Reproduced with permission from Knoop K, Stack L, Storrow A, Thurman RJ: *Atlas of Emergency Medicine*, 3rd ed. © 2010, McGraw-Hill, New York.]

FUNGAL INFECTIONS

Tinea refers to a broad spectrum of skin infections caused by dermatophytes. These spore-forming organisms invade the stratum corneum and proliferate by feeding on keratin. These superficial infections can affect the nails, skin, scalp, and hair and are named for the area of the body infected. Tinea capitis (scalp) and corporis (skin) are the two most common infections in younger children.[11] Capitis is most common in children <10 years of age with a peak of 3 to 7 years old. Corporis is also common and may be seen in adolescents participating in contact sports. Tinea pedis (foot) and tinea cruris (groin) also occur in children.

The affected areas are typically scaly and vary with a degree of pruritus from intense (as with cruris) to barely present (corporis). Tinea corporis commonly has a ring appearance with central clearing. Tinea capitis causes patchy alopecia as the hair follicles are invaded and lose their structure, causing them to break at the base (**Figure 141-13**). A more severe form of capitis, known as kerion, may occur when there is an exaggerated inflammatory response producing a painful, boggy mass (**Figure 141-14**). The differential diagnosis of a tinea infection includes pityriasis rosea, lichen planus, psoriasis, eczema, and contact dermatitis. Diagnosis can be aided by direct microscopic observation for hyphae. Culturing with Sabouraud dextrose agar may prove useful in cases of capitis or treatment failures.[11] Wood lamp evaluation is not very useful, because many dermatophytes do not fluoresce.

Treatment is typically topical, with the exception of tinea capitis. Some forms of tinea that do not respond to topical treatment may also require oral therapy. For topical treatment, therapy is usually continued for 7 to 10 days beyond resolution of the lesions, which may take 2 to 3 weeks to fade. Multiple topical therapies are available by prescription or over the counter (**Table 141-1**). The treatment of choice for tinea

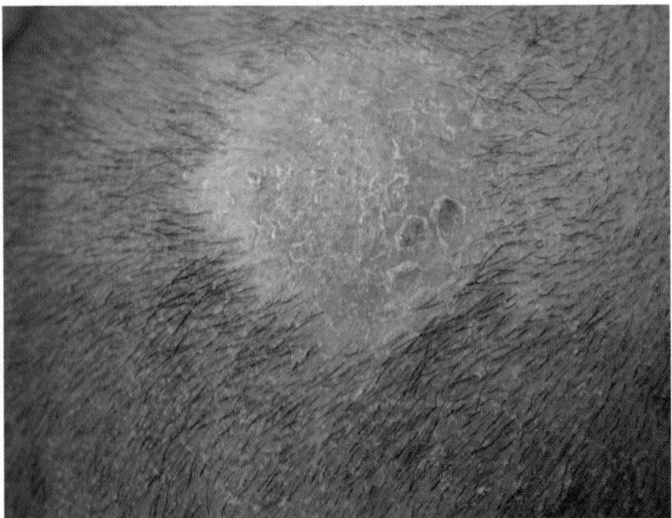

FIGURE 141-13. Tinea capitis. [Photo contributed by University of North Carolina Department of Dermatology.]

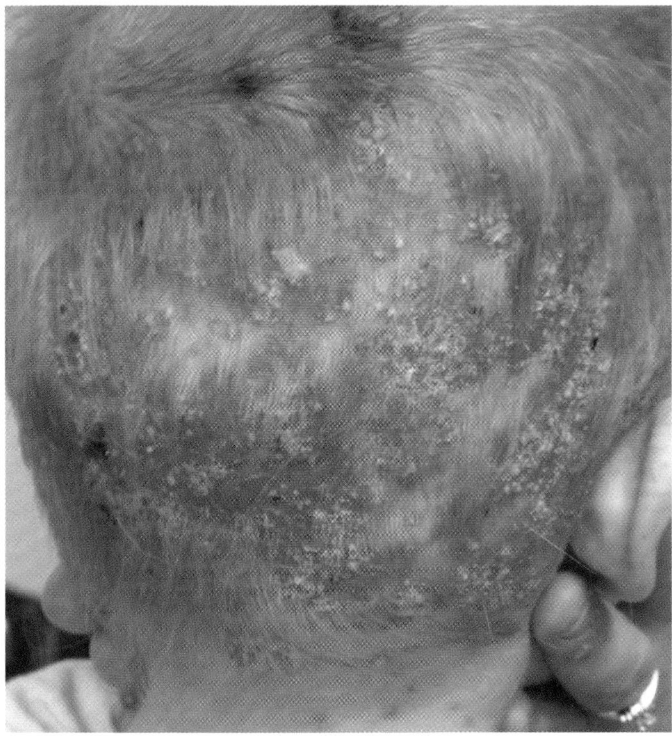

FIGURE 141-14. Tinea capitis with kerion. [Photo contributed by University of North Carolina Department of Dermatology.]

TABLE 141-1 Topical Antifungal Treatment for Tinea Corporis, Pedis, and Cruris

Medication	Dosing	Comments
Clotrimazole 1% cream*	Twice per day × 2–3 wk	None
Miconazole*	Twice per day × 2–4 wk	Not recommended <2 y old
Tolnaftate*	Twice per day × 2–3 wk	Longer treatments in hyperkeratotic patients usually needed
Ketoconazole	Once or twice per day × 2–3 wk	Pedis treated for 4–6 wk; safety in children not established
Oxiconazole 1% cream	Once or twice per day × 2–3 wk	Pedis treated for 4 wk

*Available over the counter without prescription in the United States.

capitis is **griseofulvin** (age >2 years old; microsize 20 to 25 milligrams/kg/d divided every 12 hours or ultramicrosize 10 to 15 milligrams/kg/d also divided every 12 hours). Treat for 6 to 12 weeks with frequent follow-up for testing of liver function and to ensure improvement. Terbinafine (less effective than griseofulvin for *Microsporum* species), itraconazole, and fluconazole[12,13] are also effective, with shorter courses of treatment, but are expensive. Selenium sulfide 2.5% and ketoconazole shampoos are excellent adjunct therapy. Both should be left on the scalp for approximately 5 minutes to improve effectiveness. There is no recommendation for exclusion from school, because there is a high incidence of asymptomatic carriers and spores may be spread for months. Children with painful kerion should be treated with cephalexin (25 to 50 milligrams/kg/d divided every 6 to 8 hours) in addition to systemic antifungal therapy. Acute inflammation may also respond to oral steroids.

BACTERIAL INFECTIONS

IMPETIGO

Impetigo is a superficial infection caused by either *Staphylococcus aureus* or β-hemolytic streptococci (**Figure 141-15**). Impetigo can arise at the site of insect bites or superficial cutaneous trauma; sometimes, there is no apparent predisposing skin lesion. Lesions occur most frequently on the face, neck, and extremities. Fever and systemic signs are uncommon. Diagnosis is made on clinical appearance that takes two forms. In nonbullous impetigo (more common), skin lesions start as small erythematous macules and papules that develop into discrete, thin-walled vesicles, which become pustular and quickly rupture. As the vesicles rupture, a yellow fluid forms an exudate, which dries to form a stratified golden yellow crust that can spread the infection to other parts of the body. The crusts can be readily removed, leaving a smooth, red surface. Initially the lesions are discrete, but they may enlarge and become confluent. Local adenopathy may be present. Cultures are only necessary in patients who fail to respond to standard therapy. Treatment is aimed at preventing spread and eradicating the offending agent. Appropriate cleansing and general hygiene are mandatory. Mupirocin ointment (2% applied three times a day for 7 to 14 days) is the topical antibiotic of choice for localized areas of infection. Cephalexin or clindamycin is given when large areas are affected or topical coverage is impractical (**Table 141-2**).

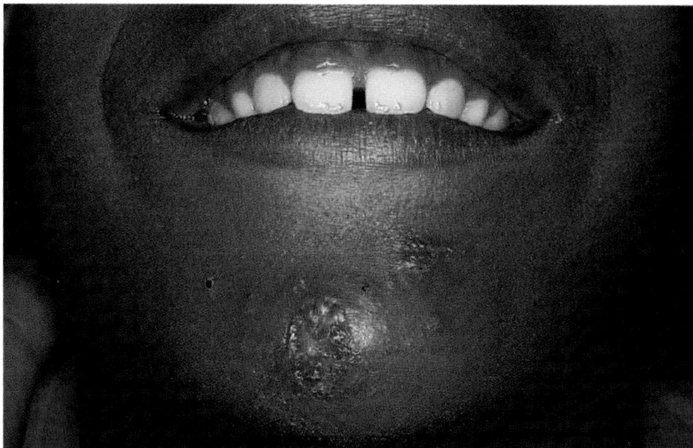

FIGURE 141-15. Impetigo. [Photo contributed by Michael J. Nowicki, MD. Reproduced with permission from Knoop K, Stack L, Storrow A, Thurman RJ: *Atlas of Emergency Medicine*, 3rd ed. © 2010, McGraw-Hill, New York.]

TABLE 141-2 Treatment Options for Impetigo

Medication	Dosing and Duration	Comments
Mupirocin 2%	Three times a day for 7–14 d	For localized infection in patients >2 mo old
Cephalexin	25–50 milligrams/kg/d divided every 6–12 h for 5–7 d	Extensive lesions, suspected *Streptococcus* or methicillin-sensitive *Staphylococcus aureus*
Clindamycin	Generally 10–25 milligrams/kg/d divided every 6–8 h for children >1–2 mo old	Suspected MRSA, good strep coverage, liquid formulation tastes terrible, not routinely covered by insurance; for neonates, see Table 141-3
Trimethoprim-sulfamethoxazole	8–10 milligrams/kg/d every 12 h	Poor strep coverage, some resistance of MRSA; dose based on trimethoprim
Dicloxacillin	<40 kg: 25 milligrams/kg/d divided every 6 h >40 kg: 500 milligrams/kg/d divided every 6 h	Maximum of 2 grams/d; give 1 h before or 2 h after meals
Doxycycline	2.2–4.4 milligrams/kg/d every 12 h	For >8 y old; poor strep coverage; useful for MRSA
Vancomycin	40 milligrams/kg/d every 6–8 h	Parental for widespread/severe infections; for neonates, see Table 141-3

Abbreviation: MRSA = methicillin-resistant *Staphylococcus aureus*; strep = *Streptococcus*.

BULLOUS IMPETIGO AND STAPHYLOCOCCAL SCALDED SKIN SYNDROME

Toxin-mediated erythrodermas, including bullous impetigo and staphylococcal scalded skin syndrome, are part of the spectrum of the same disease. Although the lesions of bullous impetigo are local at the site of infection, those of staphylococcal scalded skin syndrome are distant and widespread. Toxin serotypes A and B produced by *Staphylococcus* are the causative agents for the exfoliative presentation.[14] In bullous impetigo, the epidermolytic toxin acts locally to cause separation of the skin at the granular layer, giving rise to bullae. The infection occurs primarily in newborn infants and young children. The characteristic skin lesions of bullous impetigo are superficial, flaccid, thin-walled bullae that occur most often on the extremities but can occur anywhere. Bullae range in size from 0.5 to 3.0 cm. They can arise from normal skin or may have a thin, red halo. The bullae are filled with a clear, pale-to-yellow fluid and rupture easily, leaving a moist, denuded base that dries rapidly with a shiny coating (**Figure 141-16**). Extensive areas of skin may be involved if left untreated. The clinical appearance of the lesions usually makes diagnosis less complicated. However, single lesions or extensive involvement may not be as typical. Staphylococci cultured from the fluid of aspirated bullae will establish the diagnosis.

Community-acquired methicillin-resistant *S. aureus* may be present in a fair number of these infections, so be aware of the local community epidemiology. In most cases, bullous impetigo may be treated locally and as an outpatient. Topical or oral agents directed at both methicillin-sensitive *S. aureus* and *Streptococcus* are recommended (Table 141-2).

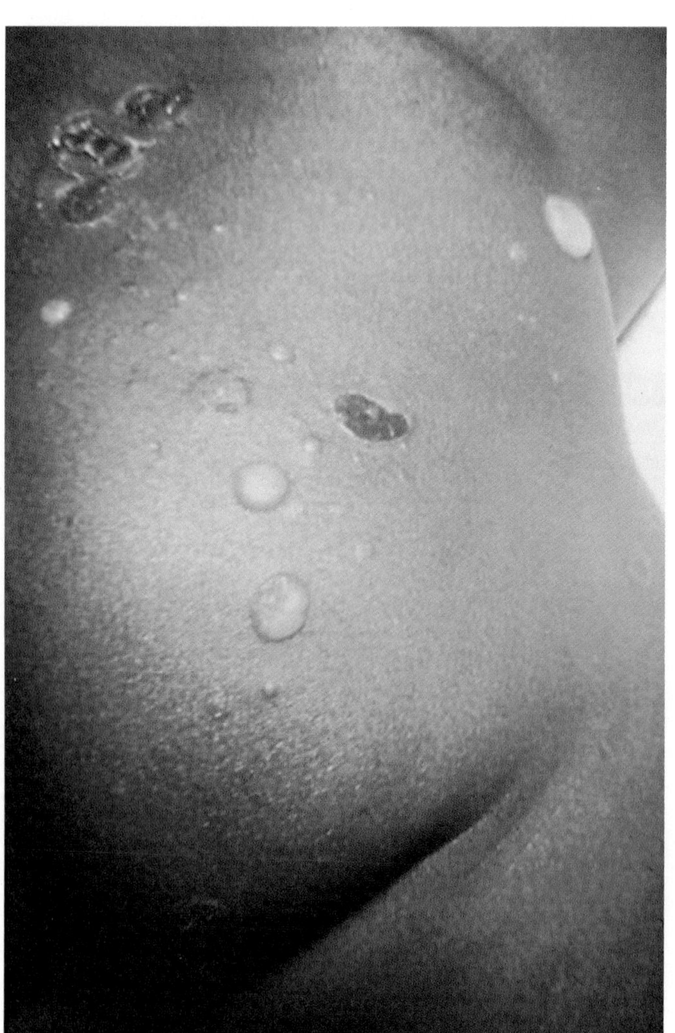

FIGURE 141-16. Bullous impetigo. [Image used with permission of the Centers for Disease Control and Prevention.]

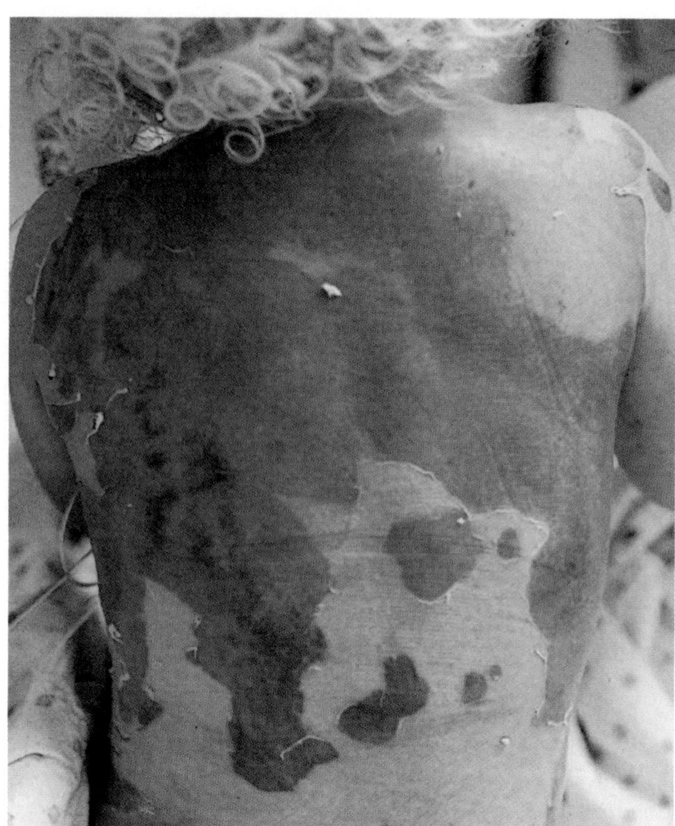

FIGURE 141-17. Staphylococcal scaled skin syndrome. [Photo contributed by Judith C. Bausher, MD. Reproduced with permission from Knoop K, Stack L, Storrow A, Thurman RJ: *Atlas of Emergency Medicine*, 3rd ed. © 2010, McGraw-Hill, New York.]

Some cases will require coverage for methicillin-resistant *S. aureus*. Severe cases require parental antibiotics.

Most children affected by staphylococcal scalded skin syndrome are <2 years old, and nearly all are <6 years old. Outbreaks in nurseries have been reported. Systemic symptoms such as malaise, fever, irritability, and tenderness of the skin are often present. The rash progresses from erythroderma to extensive areas of exfoliation (**Figure 141-17**). Nikolsky sign (separation of the epidermis when pressure is applied) is present with staphylococcal scalded skin syndrome.

Obtain cultures of blood, urine, nasopharynx, and cutaneous lesions; treatment often requires inpatient therapy, fluid resuscitation, and parenteral antibiotics. Patients with diffuse disease should be admitted to a burn unit for further care. Patients with localized infection may be discharged to home with appropriate follow-up. Parental nafcillin, oral dicloxacillin, penicillin G procaine, amoxicillin-clavulanate, cefazolin, and cephalexin are all acceptable therapies. For methicillin-resistant *S. aureus*, options include clindamycin, trimethoprim-sulfamethoxazole, or vancomycin. Coverage is often provided for both methicillin-sensitive and methicillin-resistant *S. aureus*. Linezolid may also be considered first- or second-line therapy in cases of suspected methicillin-resistant *S. aureus* (**Table 141-3**). It has ease of dosing and similar bioavailability in both the PO and IV route.[15] Reports of increased morbidity with the use of linezolid have been related to its off-label use in treating catheter-related infections.

SCARLET FEVER

Second disease, or scarlet fever, is an acute febrile illness, primarily affecting young children, caused by group A β-hemolytic streptococci. Group C *Streptococcus* has been implicated as well. Clinical manifestations include acute onset with fever, sore throat, headache, vomiting, and abdominal pain followed by a distinctive exanthem in 1 to 2 days.

There is both an enanthem and an exanthem associated with scarlet fever, caused by an erythrogenic toxin elaborated by the streptococcal organism. The tonsils and pharynx are red and covered with exudate,

TABLE 141-3 Antibiotics for Staphylococcal Scaled Skin Syndrome

Drug	Dosing
Nafcillin IV	<7 d old, <2 kg or >7 d old, <1.2 kg: 50 milligrams/kg/d divided every 12 h <7 d old, >2 kg or >7 d old, 1.2–2 kg: 75 milligrams/kg/d divided every 8 h All others: 100 milligrams/kg/d divided every 6 h
Dicloxacillin PO	<40 kg: 25 milligrams/kg/d divided every 6 h >40 kg: 500 milligrams/kg/d divided every 6 h Give 1 h before or 2 h after meals
Amoxicillin-clavulanate	<40 kg, <3 mo: 30 milligrams/kg/d divided every 12 h <40 kg, >3 mo: 25-45 milligrams/kg/d divided every 12 h >40 kg: 500 milligrams/kg/d divided every 12 h All doses based on amoxicillin
Cefazolin	<7 d old or >7 d old, <2 kg: 40 milligrams/kg/d divided every 12 h >7 d old, >2 kg: 60 milligrams/kg/d divided every 8 h All others: 50–100 milligrams/kg/d divided every 6–8 h
Cephalexin	25–50 milligrams/kg/d divided every 6–12 h
Clindamycin	<7 d old, <2 kg or >7 d old, <1.2 kg: 10 milligrams/kg/d divided every 12 h <7 d old, >2 kg or >7 d old, 1.2–2 kg: 15 mg/kg/d divided every 8 h All others: 10–40 milligrams/kg/d divided every 8 h
Trimethoprim-sulfamethoxazole	8 milligrams/kg/d divided every 12 h
Vancomycin	<1.2 kg: 15 milligrams/kg once a day <7 d old, 1.2–2 kg: 10–15 milligrams/kg/d divided every 12–18 h <7 d old, >2 kg or >7 d old, 1.2–2 kg: 10–15 milligrams/kg/d divided every 8–12 h All others: 40–60 milligrams/kg/d divided every 8 h
Linezolid	<12 y old: 30 milligrams/kg/d divided every 8 h >12 y old: 600 milligrams every 12 h

although, occasionally, pharyngeal findings are minimal. The tongue may develop a white coating through which red and hypertrophied papillae project, creating the appearance of a "white strawberry tongue." The white coating disappears by day 4 or 5, and the tongue acquires a bright-red appearance, the "red strawberry tongue" (**Figure 141-18**). Bright-red or hemorrhagic spots may be seen on the soft palate or anterior pillars of the tonsillar fossa.

The exanthem of scarlet fever begins 1 or 2 days after the onset of the illness. It starts on the neck, axillae, and groin, and spreads to the trunk and extremities (**Figure 141-19**). The rash is red and finely punctate, consisting of 1- to 2-mm papules that blanch and have a characteristic rough, sandpaper feel. It is sometimes easier to identify the rash by palpation. Linear petechial eruptions, Pastia lines, are often present in the antecubital and axillary folds. There is facial flushing with circumoral pallor. A brawny desquamation occurs at 2 weeks, yielding fine flakes of dry skin.

The diagnosis of scarlet fever is readily made on clinical grounds. Throat swabs usually culture group A β-hemolytic streptococci, although group C may be cultured as well. Treatment with antibiotics is necessary to reduce the incidence of rheumatic fever and may ameliorate the clinical course of the disease, although the effect on other complications such as nephritis remains unclear. Penicillin or amoxicillin are antibiotics of choice. For penicillin-allergic patients, alternatives include cephalexin and clindamycin; macrolide antibiotics remain an option, although resistance of group A streptococci to macrolides is increasing.[16]

ERYSIPELAS AND CELLULITIS

Erysipelas, or St. Anthony fire, is cellulitis and lymphangitis of the skin caused by group A β-hemolytic streptococci. Infection is frequently accompanied by fever, chills, malaise, headache, and vomiting.

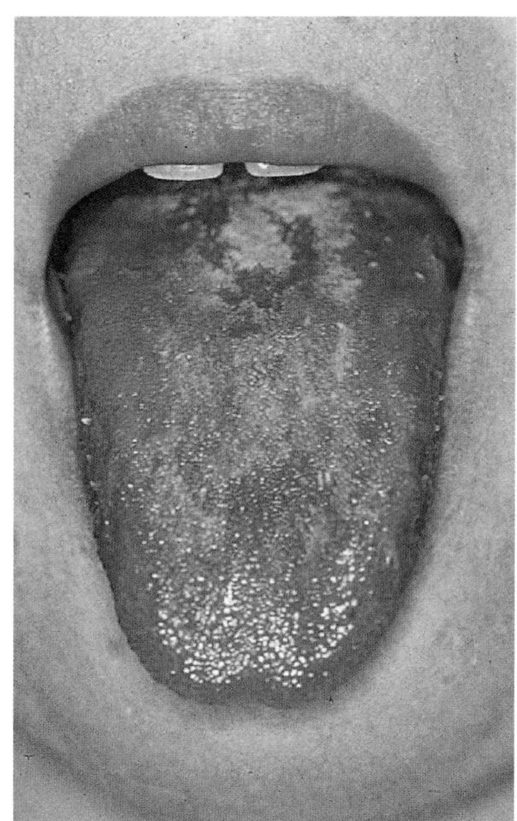

FIGURE 141-18. Scarlet fever: white and red strawberry tongue. [Reproduced with permission from Wolff K, Johnson RA, Saavedra AP (eds): *Fitzpatrick's Color Atlas and Synopsis of Clinical Dermatology*, 7th ed. McGraw-Hill, Inc., 2013, Fig. 25-42.]

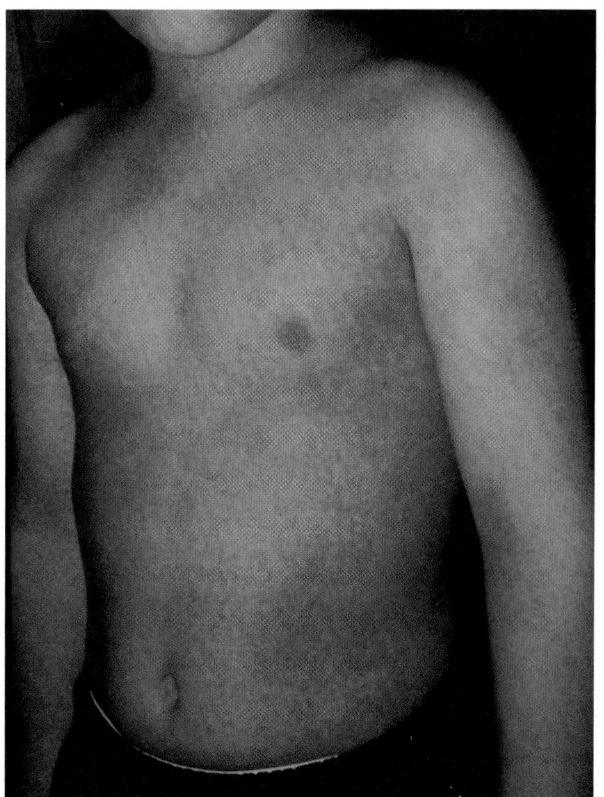

FIGURE 141-19. Sandpaper-like rash of scarlet fever. [Photo contributed by Lawrence B. Stack, MD. Reproduced with permission from Knoop K, Stack L, Storrow A, Thurman RJ: *Atlas of Emergency Medicine*, 3rd ed. © 2010, McGraw-Hill, New York.]

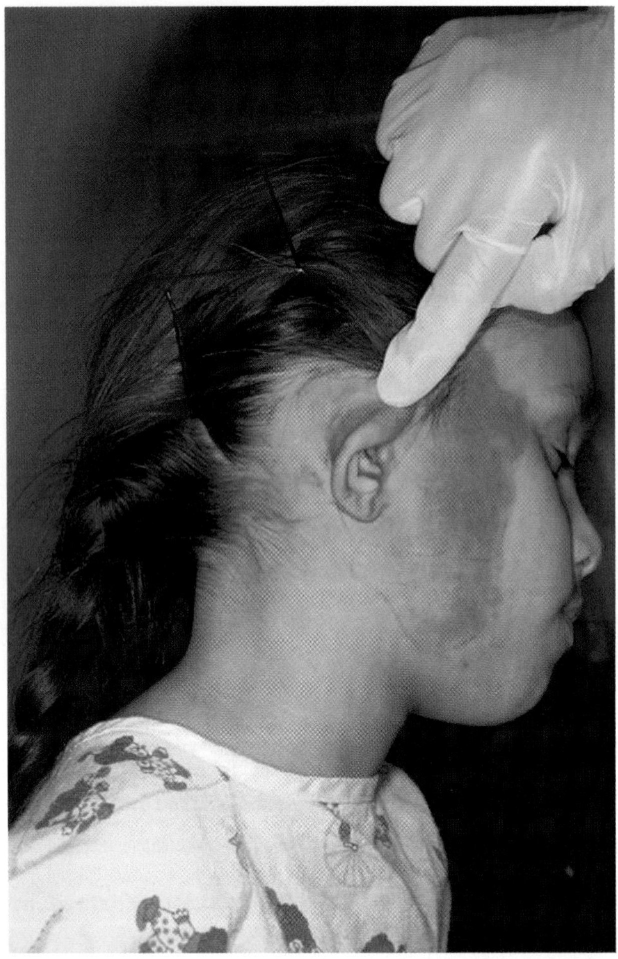

FIGURE 141-20. Erysipelas. [Reproduced with permission from Shah BR, Lucchesi M: *Atlas of Pediatric Emergency Medicine*, © 2006, McGraw-Hill, New York.]

The rash is characterized by local redness, heat, swelling, and a raised, indurated border. There is marked involvement of the superficial dermal lymphatics. The rash starts as an erythematous plaque that rapidly enlarges by peripheral extension. At first, it is scarlet, hot, brawny, swollen, and tender. The edge is raised and sharply demarcated. The rash can vary in appearance from a transient hyperemia to intense inflammation, vesiculation, and bulla formation. The rash may have the appearance of an orange peel. The face was commonly the most frequent site (**Figure 141-20**) of infection, but more recently, infections in children have been more common on the extremities.[17] A skin wound, fissure, or ulcer may act as a portal of entry.

The diagnosis is clinical, and cultures of the blood or from aspiration of the leading edge of the lesion are rarely helpful.[18,19] A brief course of parenteral penicillin G procaine is usually warranted because of the rapid advancement of the infection, the acutely toxic state of the patient, and the possibility of suppurative complications. Rapid clinical response is usually obtained. Cephalosporins, clindamycin, or trimethoprim-sulfamethoxazole may be used in patients unable to take penicillin; macrolides may be considered but are limited by increasing resistance. Other forms of cellulitis are treated in a similar fashion with parenteral or oral antibiotics as listed in **Table 141-4**.

Cellulitis is most commonly caused by *S. aureus*. The affected area is usually erythematous, warm to palpation, and tender. Lymphangitis or regional lymphadenopathy may be seen. Once a mostly institutional issue, methicillin-resistant *S. aureus* has become increasingly prevalent as a community-acquired skin infection. Maintain a high suspicion for community-acquired methicillin-resistant *S. aureus* and be aware of local antibiotic sensitivities. If abscesses are present, they should be drained and cultures obtained. Small (<5 cm) pus collections can typically be treated with incision and drainage alone.[17] Bedside US can localize the abscess and differentiate cellulitis from abscess when the clinical presentation is less clear (**Figure 141-21, A** and **B**).

TABLE 141-4 Antibiotics for the Treatment of Cellulitis

Medication	Dosing	Comments
Cephalexin	25–50 milligrams/kg/d divided every 6–12 h	Use for suspected strep or methicillin-sensitive *Staphylococcus aureus*
Clindamycin	See Table 141-3	Good strep and *Staphylococcus* coverage (MRSA variable); poor taste and insurance coverage for liquid form
TMP-SMX	8–20* milligrams/kg/d divided twice a day	Poor strep coverage; some resistance in MRSA
Doxycycline	4 milligrams/kg/d twice a day	For >8 y of age; poor strep coverage
Azithromycin	10 milligrams/kg on day 1 and then 5 milligrams/kg every day for 4 d	PCN-allergic patients Emerging macrolide resistance
Erythromycin	30 milligrams/kg/d three or four times a day	PCN-allergic patients Emerging macrolide resistance
Clarithromycin	15 milligrams/kg/d twice a day	PCN-allergic patients Emerging macrolide resistance
Linezolid	See Table 141-3	MRSA resistant to clindamycin and TMP-SMX
Cefazolin		Strep, methicillin-sensitive *S. aureus*
Nafcillin		Strep, methicillin-sensitive *S. aureus*
Clindamycin		Strep, MRSA; well absorbed orally; no clear advantage over PO dosing unless unable to tolerate PO
Vancomycin		MRSA coverage

Abbreviations: MRSA = methicillin-resistant *Staphylococcus aureus*; PCN = penicillin; strep = *Streptococcus*; TMP/SMX = trimethoprim-sulfamethoxazole.

*Use 20 milligrams/kg/d when MRSA is suspected.

MENINGOCOCCEMIA

A petechial rash may be the presenting symptom of many viral infections or bleeding disorders or an indication of a very serious life-threatening disease due to bacterial infections such as *Neisseria meningitidis* (**Figure 141-22**). *N. meningitidis* is a gram-negative diplococcus and the causative agent of invasive meningococcal disease. Since the introduction in the United States of *Haemophilus influenzae* type b and pneumococcal polysaccharide-protein conjugate vaccines for infants, *N. meningitidis* has become the leading cause of bacterial meningitis in children and remains an important cause of septicemia. Disease most often occurs in children 2 years of age or younger; the peak incidence occurs in children younger than 1 year of age. Another peak occurs in adolescents and young adults age 16 to 21 years. Outbreaks continue to occur in communities and institutions, including child care centers, schools, colleges, and military recruit camps. However, most cases of meningococcal disease are endemic, with fewer than 5% associated with outbreaks.[20]

The incubation period is 1 to 10 days but usually less than 4 days. Because of the rapid progression from initial symptoms to death, it is important to recognize the first specific clinical symptoms, which can be early indicators of sepsis such as leg pain, cold hands and feet, and abnormal skin color (pallor, mottling). In approximately half of children, the first classic symptom of meningococcal disease is rash, which sometimes evolves from nonspecific to petechial to hemorrhagic over several hours. The petechial rash appears as discrete lesions 1 to 2 mm in diameter, most frequently on the trunk and lower portions of the body. The mucous membranes of the soft palate, ocular, and palpebral conjunctiva should also be examined for signs of hemorrhage. Petechiae may coalesce into larger purpuric and ecchymotic lesions (**Figure 141-23**).

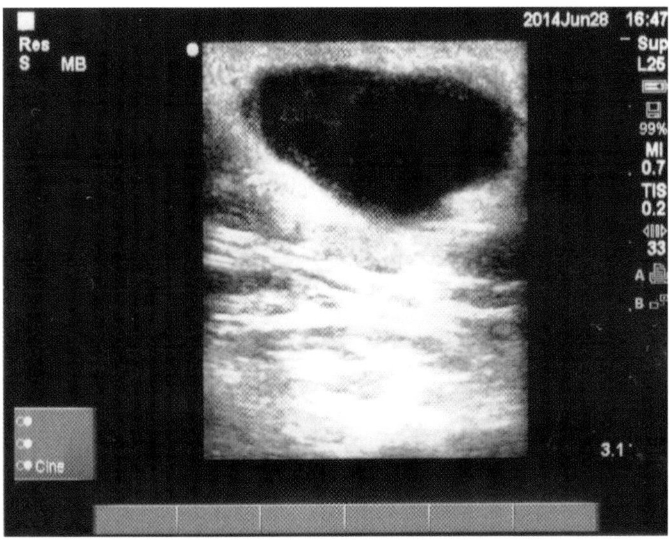

A

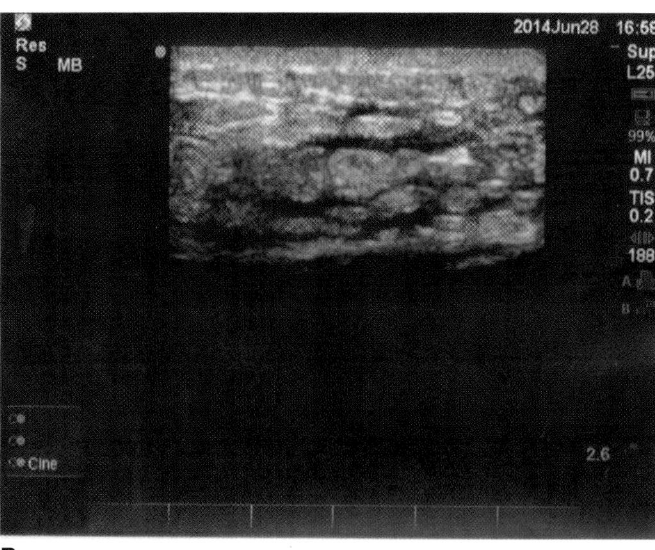

B

FIGURE 141-21. **A.** Abscess as visualized on US. Essentially anechoic area within the surrounding soft tissue. **B.** Cellulitis. Relatively hypoechoic fluid between hyperechoic soft tissue structures. This classic appearance is referred to as "cobblestones." In some cases, the abscess contents may appear hyperechoic and mimic cellulitis. [Photos contributed by Gary Bonfante, DO, FACOEP, FACEP.]

The petechiae correlate with the degree of thrombocytopenia and clinically are important as an indicator of the potential for bleeding complications secondary to disseminated intravascular coagulopathy.

Early identification of a petechial rash is essential to allow for rapid intervention to prevent further progression to fulminant disseminated intravascular coagulopathy, meningitis, and sepsis. It is very important to perform a thorough physical exam as well as a close review of a full set of vital signs to look for early indicators of sepsis such as tachycardia or hypotension. The overall case-fatality rate for meningococcal disease is 10% and is higher in adolescents.

Children with a transient petechial rash who are well appearing do not need extensive testing. But the presence of petechiae in a febrile and ill-appearing child requires testing, especially a CBC to detect thrombocytopenia and leukocytosis. Cultures of blood and cerebrospinal fluid are indicated for patients with suspected invasive meningococcal disease. Cultures of a petechial or purpuric lesion scraping, synovial fluid, and other usually sterile body fluid specimens yield the organism in some patients.[21]

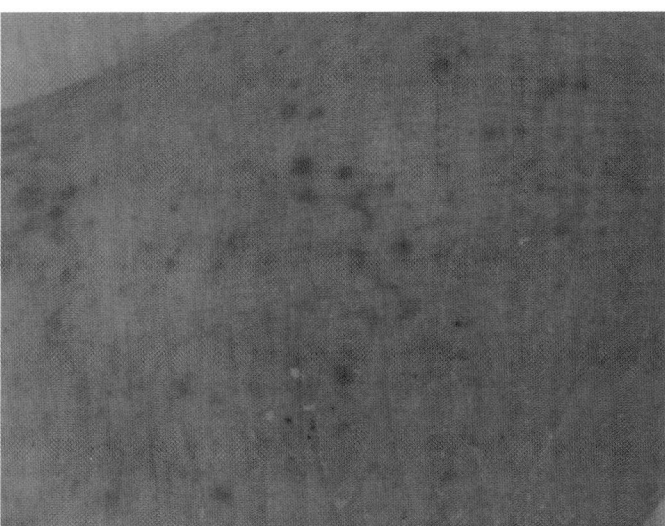

FIGURE 141-22. Petechial rash seen in meningococcemia. [Reproduced with permission from McKean S, Ross JJ, Dressler DD, Brotman DJ, Ginsber JS (eds): *Principles and Practice of Hospital Medicine*. The McGraw-Hill Companies, Inc., 2012, Fig. 147-22.]

Treatment The priority in management of meningococcal disease is treatment of shock in meningococcemia and of raised intracranial pressure in severe cases of meningitis. Empiric therapy for suspected meningococcal disease is an extended-spectrum cephalosporin, such as cefotaxime or ceftriaxone. Once the microbiologic diagnosis is established, definitive treatment with penicillin G (300,000 units/kg/d; maximum, 12 million units/d, divided every 4 to 6 hours), ampicillin, or an extended-spectrum cephalosporin (cefotaxime or ceftriaxone) is recommended.[21]

Chemoprophylaxis is warranted for people who have been exposed directly to a patient's oral secretions through close social contact, such as kissing or sharing of toothbrushes or eating utensils, as well as for child care and preschool contacts during the 7 days before onset of disease in the index case. Rifampin and ceftriaxone are the drugs of choice in children, and ciprofloxacin can be used for adult contacts.[20]

INFESTATIONS

Infestations with mites are common in children and readily spread through families, day care, and school settings where close contact with index cases can occur. Both scabies and lice are common causes of pruritic skin rash that can affect children, and scabies, in particular, may present atypically in young infants.

SCABIES

Scabies is caused by infestation with the *Sarcoptes scabiei* mite. The female burrows into the skin, where eggs are deposited and larvae hatch, resulting in the severe pruritus that characterizes the disease. There is typically a 4- to 6-week incubation period after exposure, which may occur at day care, school, or within the home, and infestation occurs across all socioeconomic levels and is not a reflection of poor hygiene. The classic skin findings in older children and adults include a generalized eruption with linear burrows, papules, pustules, and even vesicles. Lesions show a proclivity for the hands, feet, and groin (**Figure 141-24**). In infants, lesions may be widespread, with involvement of the palms and soles, and hyperpigmented nodules may be noted in the axilla and diaper areas (**Figure 141-25**). Excoriations are common from scratching. The differential diagnosis includes impetigo, atopic dermatitis, insect bites, and drug reactions. A careful history evaluating for other family members or close contacts with similar symptoms should be sought and may provide a clue to the diagnosis, although, occasionally, even co-sleeping parents will deny symptoms. Testing is usually not necessary, because the diagnosis is made on history and physical alone,

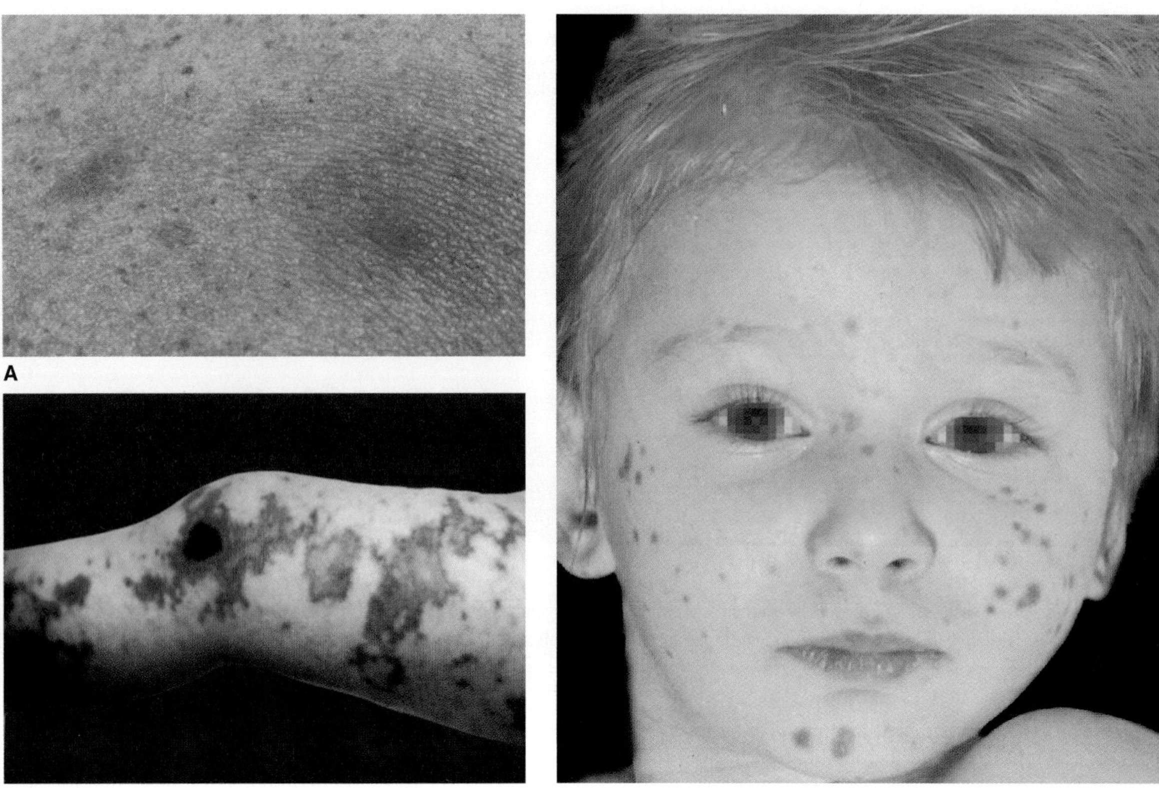

FIGURE 141-23. A–C. Petechial rash can progress to purpuric lesions. [Reproduced with permission from Goldsmith LA, Katz SI, Gilchrest BA, Paller AS, Leffell DJ, Wolff K (eds): *Fitzpatrick's Dermatology in General Medicine*, 8th ed. McGraw-Hill, Inc., 2012, Fig. 180-1 A-C, p. 2180.]

although scrapings of pustules may reveal mites on microscopy. Treatment consists of topical **permethrin cream** applied from the neck down (infants may require application to the scalp and face, avoiding the mucous membranes) and left on for 8 to 12 hours before washing off. **Lindane is contraindicated in young children due to neurotoxicity.** For severe infestations, oral treatment with a single dose of **ivermectin**, 200 micrograms/kg, may be necessary. All linens and clothes should be washed in hot water. Treatment should include all family members to prevent recurrence of infestation. Antipruritics such as diphenhydramine may be useful. Families should be counseled that pruritus may continue for weeks despite successful elimination of infestation.

LICE

As with scabies, infestations with the common head louse, *Pediculus humanus capitis*, are common among children in school and day care. Parents may bring children to the ED as a result of a diagnosis made at school or reports of an outbreak at day care. Spread is by close contact, and hats and combs may act as fomites for transmission. The mites are more commonly found in long, straight hair and, therefore, are more common among girls than boys and less common among children with dark skin tones. Infestations may be asymptomatic and noticed by a caretaker or may present with scratching as a result of pruritus. The diagnosis is confirmed by direct observation of live mites, although the presence of nits (egg sacks) may be considered a presumptive diagnosis. Nits are small (0.3 to 0.8 mm), oval, white or yellow sacks that are found on hair shafts close to the scalp and often concentrated around the ears or nape of the neck (**Figure 141-26**).

Treatment involves the use of pediculicides, careful grooming, hot water washing of linens and clothing, and co-treatment of close contacts. Several over-the-counter and prescription pediculicides are available. Permethrin, 1% lotion, is the most commonly used (Nix®, available without a prescription), although pyrethrins are also available over the counter (e.g., Rid®). Topical benzyl alcohol (5% lotion) is also effective and safe for children as young as 6 months of age.[22] The organophosphate malathion is available by prescription as a 0.5% lotion. Malathion is approved for children >6 years of age and is applied to the hair and scalp (dry hair), left on for 8 to 12 hours, and washed out. Re-treat in 7 to 9 days. **Lindane shampoo is contraindicated in young children and pregnant women due to neurotoxicity.** Retreatment after 7 to 10 days may be necessary with all of these agents, because none is completely effective. Careful removal of the nits with a fine comb (often supplied in over-the-counter products) is an important aspect of successful treatment. Shaving of the head is not necessary.

COMMON NEONATAL RASHES

A number of common rashes affecting neonates and infants are worth noting due to their commonality or unique presentation in this age group and because they are of frequent concern to parents, who often present with their child to the ED for evaluation. These include erythema toxicum neonatorum, neonatal acne, seborrheic dermatitis, atopic dermatitis, and diaper rash.

ERYTHEMA TOXICUM

Despite the name, erythema toxicum is a benign, self-limited rash that occurs in up to 50% of all newborns, typically in the first week of life. The etiology is unknown, and the rash spontaneously resolves over approximately 1 week, although new lesions may develop in the second week of life as well. Characteristic erythematous macules, 2 to 3 cm, develop on the face, trunk, and extremities, and may have central 1- to 3-mm pustules (**Figure 141-27**). The diagnosis is clinical, although Wright-stained scrapings of the pustules will reveal eosinophils if performed to differentiate erythema toxicum from impetigo or HSV. No treatment other than reassurance is necessary.

TRANSIENT NEONATAL PUSTULAR MELANOSIS

Transient neonatal pustular melanosis is less common than erythema toxicum. It is most common in black infants. Transient neonatal pustular melanosis consists of three types of lesions: small pustules on a

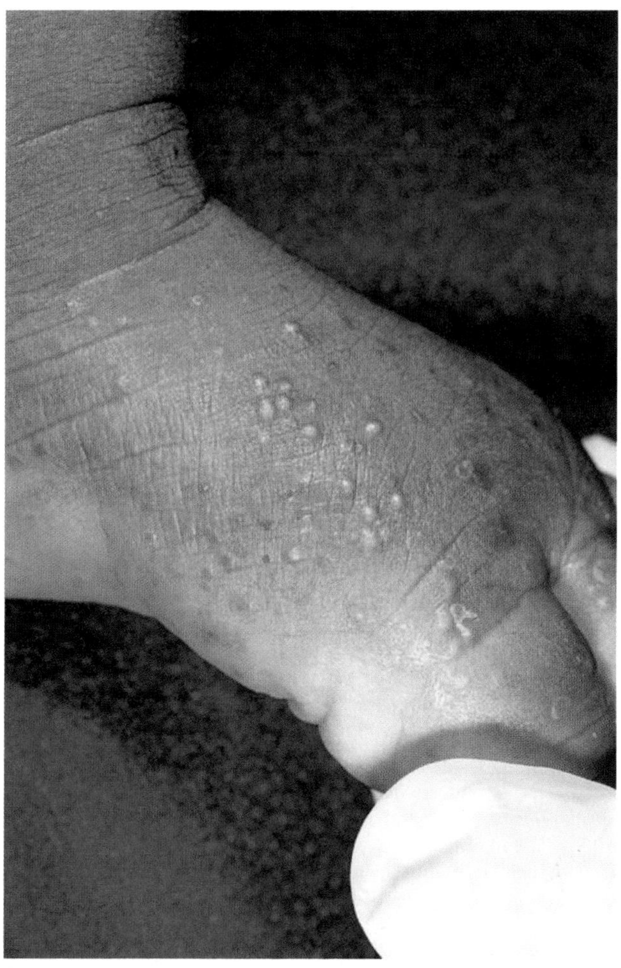

A

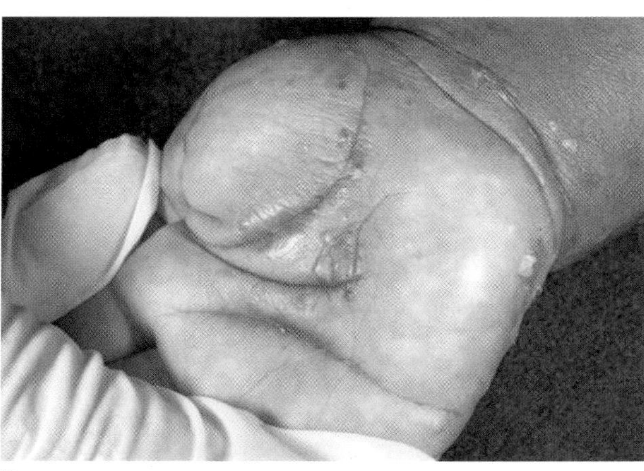

B

FIGURE 141-24. A and B. Scabies on the foot of an infant. [Reproduced with permission from Shah BR, Lucchesi M: *Atlas of Pediatric Emergency Medicine*, © 2006, McGraw-Hill, New York.]

nonerythematous base that may be present at birth, erythematous macules with a surrounding scale that develop as the pustules rupture and may persist for weeks to months, and hyperpigmented brown macules that gradually fade over several weeks to months (**Figure 141-28**).

The diagnosis of transient neonatal pustular melanosis is usually based on the clinical appearance. Microscopic examination of a Wright-stained smear of the contents of a pustule may demonstrate numerous neutrophils and rare eosinophils. This can help differentiate it from the lesions of erythema toxicum, which contain mostly eosinophils. However, this is usually not necessary. Treatment is supportive, and full resolution is expected.

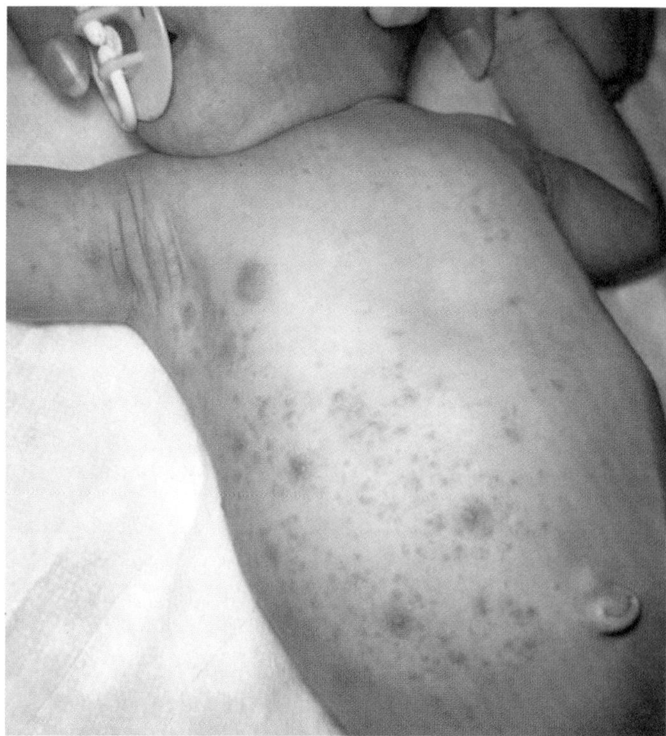

FIGURE 141-25. Infantile scabies. [Reproduced with permission from Shah BR, Lucchesi M: *Atlas of Pediatric Emergency Medicine*, © 2006, McGraw-Hill, New York.]

NEONATAL ACNE

Neonatal or baby acne affects up to 20% of infants and typically appears around the third week of life. It results from stimulation of sebaceous glands by maternal hormones, and males are more commonly affected than females. Erythematous papules and pustules are commonly found on the face, although they may also occur on the trunk (**Figure 141-29**). The diagnosis is clinical, and no testing is necessary. Lesions spontaneously resolve, usually by the third month of life, and reassurance is all that is needed.

SEBORRHEIC DERMATITIS

Seborrheic dermatitis affects neonates and infants as well as adolescents and is an inflammatory condition of unknown etiology, although genetic and environmental factors are thought to play a role. In newborns, the rash typically starts between 2 and 6 weeks of life and improves by 6 months of life. Lesions are greasy yellow or red scales and

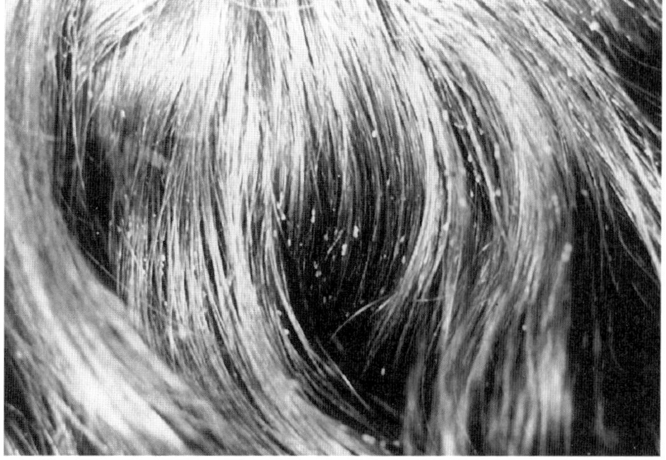

FIGURE 141-26. Head lice.

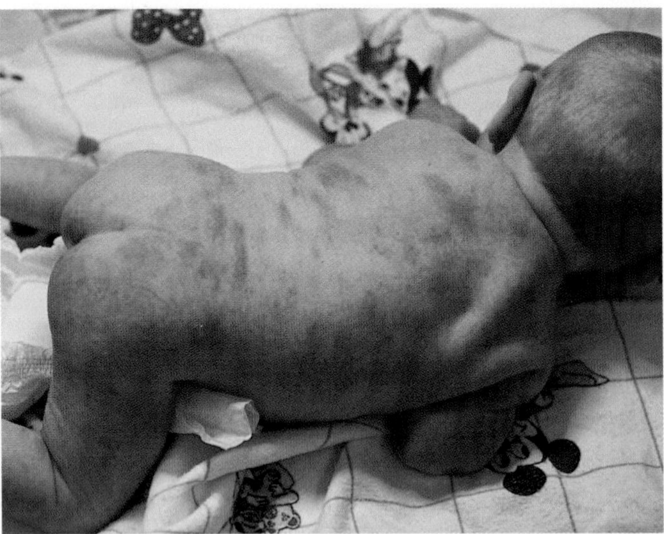

FIGURE 141-27. Erythema toxicum neonatorum. [Photo contributed by Kevin J. Knoop, MD. Reproduced with permission from Knoop K, Stack L, Storrow A, Thurman RJ: *Atlas of Emergency Medicine*, 3rd ed. © 2010, McGraw-Hill, New York.]

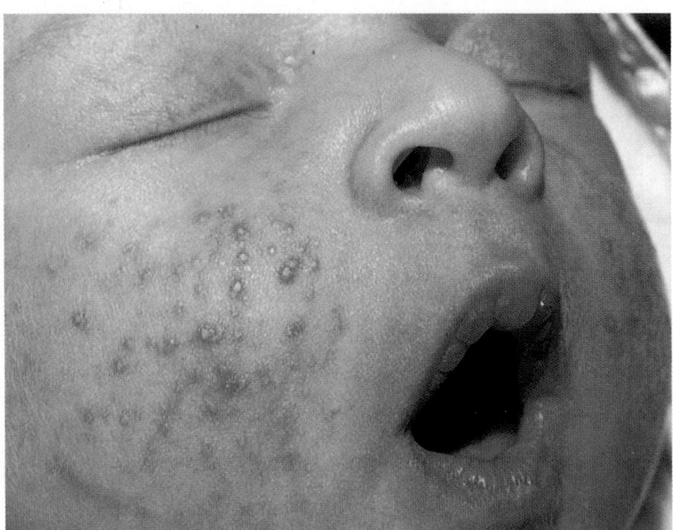

FIGURE 141-29. Neonatal acne. [Reproduced with permission from Wolff K, Goldsmith LA, Katz SI, et al: *Fitzpatrick's Dermatology in General Medicine*, 7th ed. © 2008, McGraw-Hill, Inc., New York.]

have a proclivity for the scalp (cradle cap; **Figure 141-30**), but may appear around the eyebrows, ears, cheeks, or neck and intertriginous areas of the body and diaper area. Unlike atopic dermatitis (see "Atopic Dermatitis"), seborrhea is not usually pruritic. The differential diagnosis includes atopic dermatitis (which should be considered when the onset occurs in the second or third month of life, when lesions are found to be weeping and pruritic, or with a strong family history of atopy), tinea capitis, and psoriasis. The diagnosis is clinical, and testing is usually not necessary. Treatment for cradle cap includes salicylic acid–containing shampoo (Sebulex®) or the application of oils (mineral or olive) followed by washing and removal of scales with a fine-tooth comb.

ATOPIC DERMATITIS

Infantile atopic dermatitis or infantile eczema is a chronic, recurrent inflammatory disorder of the dermis and epidermis of unclear etiology but with a strong genetic component. A complete discussion of the disorder is beyond the scope of this chapter, but atopic dermatitis is common throughout childhood and often presents in the first months of life. Triggers include excessive bathing or desiccation, heat, contact irritants, and allergens (foods and environmental). The disorder is associated with food allergies, asthma, and allergic rhinitis later in life. The infantile form typically manifests between 2 and 6 months of life, somewhat later than seborrheic dermatitis, from which it must be distinguished. Characteristic findings include xerosis (dry skin) and erythematous papular or papulovesicular lesions and plaques that may become excoriated or weep. The classic flexural distribution seen in older children (**Figure 141-31**) is less common in infants in whom the face is most commonly involved, although diffuse involvement is possible (**Figure 141-32**). The nose and diaper areas are typically spared. Lesions are usually pruritic, which, in infants, may manifest as fussiness. **The differential diagnosis includes scabies and seborrheic dermatitis.** A careful history, including affected caretakers and a family history of atopy, and the clinical appearance are usually all that are needed to make the diagnosis.

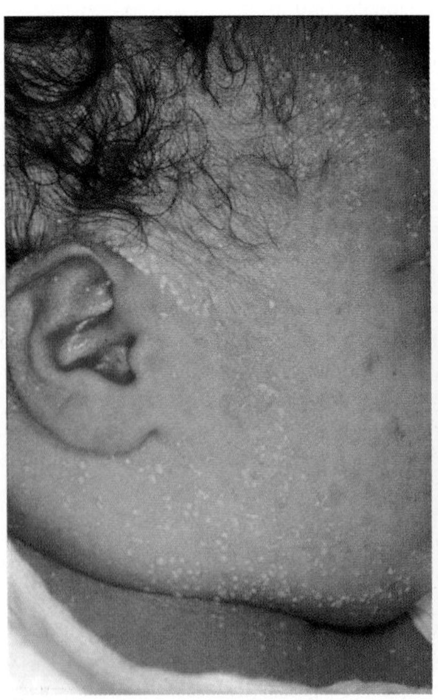

A

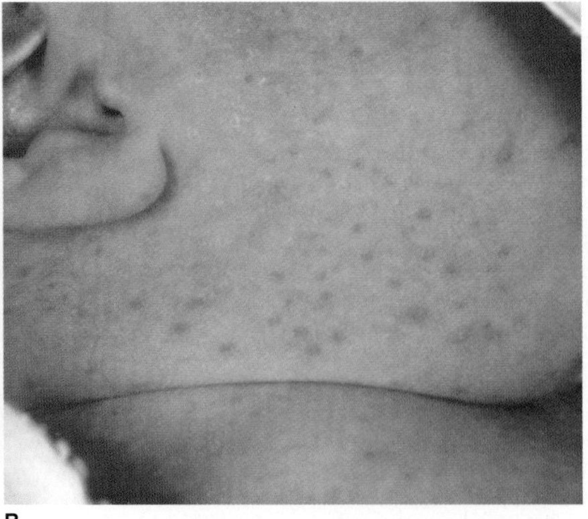

B

FIGURE 141-28. A and B. Transient neonatal pustular melanosis. [Reproduced with permission from Goldsmith LA, Katz SI, Gilchrest BA, Paller AS, Leffell DJ, Wolff K: *Fitzpatrick's Dermatology in General Medicine*, 8th ed. McGraw-Hill, Inc., 2012, Fig. 107-4A&B, p. 1189.]

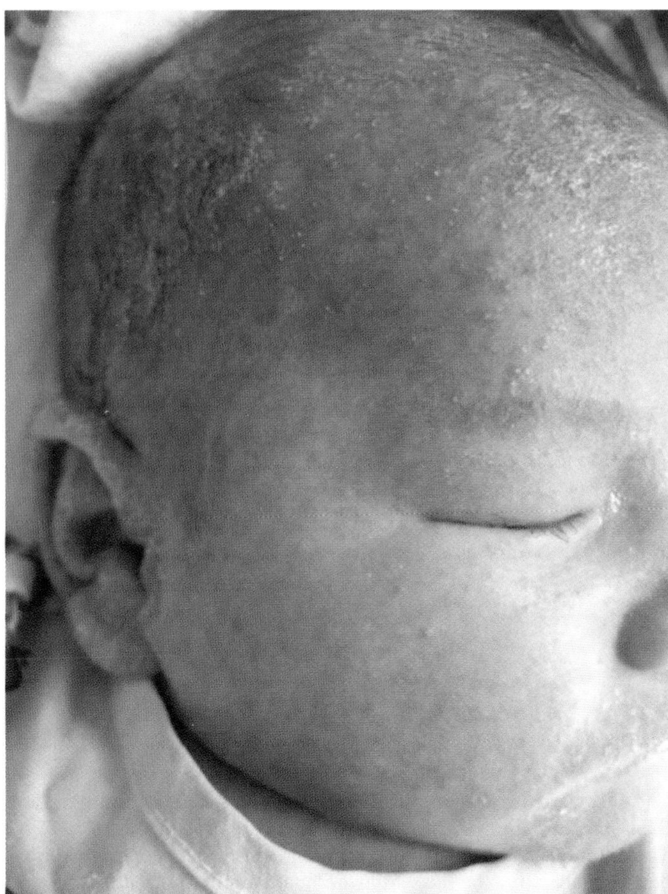

FIGURE 141-30. Cradle cap or infantile seborrheic dermatitis. [Photo contributed by University of North Carolina Department of Dermatology.]

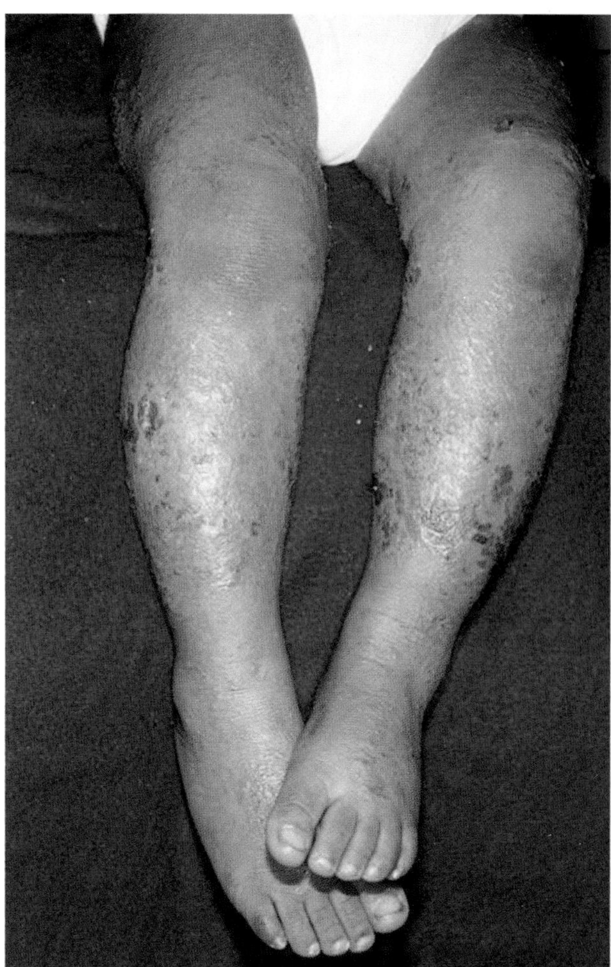

FIGURE 141-31. Atopic dermatitis. [Reproduced with permission from Shah BR, Lucchesi M: *Atlas of Pediatric Emergency Medicine*, © 2006, McGraw-Hill, New York.]

Treatment involves counseling of parents to establish realistic expectations of probable recurrences. Therapy is aimed at identifying and eliminating triggers, reducing drying of skin (including limiting exposure to water with brief and infrequent bathing and minimal use of drying soaps), liberal application of emollients (e.g., Vaseline®), symptomatic treatment of pruritus (e.g., diphenhydramine), and topical steroids for active inflammation. In general, ointments are more effective than creams, and low-potency steroids (see chapter 248, "Initial Evaluation and Management of Skin Disorders") should be used on the face and urogenital area, with medium-potency agents reserved for the trunk and extremities. Immunomodulators, such as tacrolimus ointment, are approved for children >2 years of age but should not be used in infants unless prescribed by a dermatologist. Occasionally, oral antibiotics or antivirals may be indicated for superinfected areas (e.g., impetigo, eczema, herpeticum).

DIAPER DERMATITIS

Diaper rash is a common ED complaint that is specific to neonates and infants. Although rare disorders such as psoriasis, immunodeficiencies, and dietary insufficiencies (e.g., zinc, biotin) may present with diaper rash, for all practical purposes, two forms of diaper rash comprise the vast majority: contact (irritant) dermatitis and candidal dermatitis. Reducing substances in stool and irritants in the urine can cause a contact dermatitis when left in contact with the skin for prolonged periods of time or during diarrheal illness. The characteristic rash is erythematous, macular, or papular, and has well-demarcated borders. The differential diagnosis includes perianal streptococcal infection, which is usually warm, macular, and may be associated with desquamation. Treatment of contact diaper dermatitis includes good hygiene, air-drying, and the use of barrier creams or ointments such as zinc oxide. Candidal diaper dermatitis results from superficial infection with *Candida* species that are ubiquitous in the infant GI tract. Typical lesions are erythematous with papular and pustular lesions and scaling around margins (**Figure 141-33**).

The classic finding is "satellite lesions," which are small pustules beyond the margins of the main rash. The differential diagnosis includes atopic dermatitis, psoriasis, and contact dermatitis, although the diagnosis is usually made by clinical examination alone based on the characteristic scale and satellite lesions. Treatment is with topical application of antifungal agents, most commonly nystatin cream (100,000 units/gram as a cream, powder, or ointment applied three times a day for 10 to 14 days), which may be applied in combination with barrier ointments (zinc oxide applied after nystatin) and topical steroids (1% to 2% hydrocortisone cream or ointment applied after nystatin, but before zinc oxide if used) for severely inflamed lesions. Infants with candidal diaper dermatitis should be carefully examined for concomitant oral thrush. If oral disease is present, it should be treated with oral nystatin in mixtures of 100,000 units/mL. Use 2 mL four times a day in infants and 4 to 6 mL four times a day in children. Administer for up to 48 hours after resolution of oral lesions.

CUTANEOUS DRUG REACTIONS

Many medications commonly used by children can cause a significant exanthem for which parents will seek medical care. Often, the parents suspect an allergic reaction to the medication. There are a number of medications that are known to cause rash including antibiotics and anti-inflammatory and antiepileptic medications. One study found that

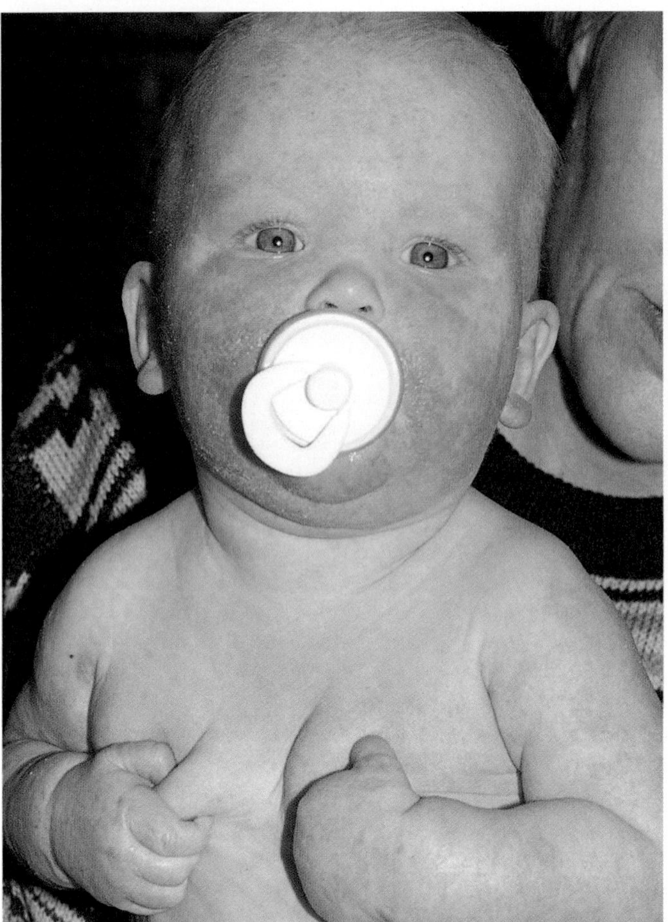

FIGURE 141-32. Infantile atopic dermatitis. [Reproduced with permission from Wolff KL, Johnson R, Suurmond R: *Fitzpatrick's Color Atlas & Synopsis of Clinical Dermatology*, 5th ed. © 2005, McGraw-Hill, New York.]

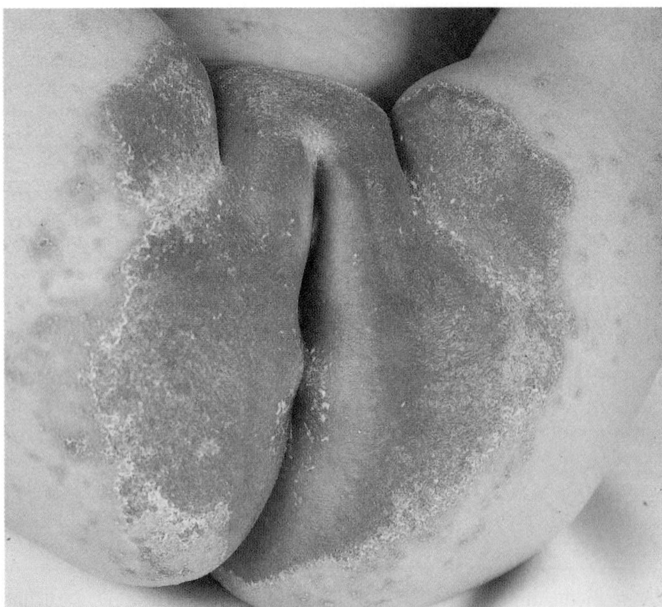

FIGURE 141-33. Diaper rash (*Candida*). [Reproduced with permission from Wolff KL, Johnson R, Suurmond R: *Fitzpatrick's Color Atlas & Synopsis of Clinical Dermatology*, 6th ed. © 2009, McGraw-Hill, New York.]

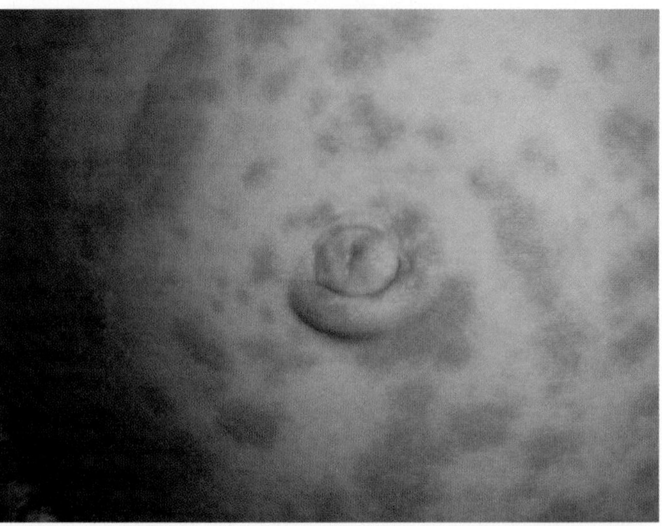

FIGURE 141-34. Coalescing papular lesions of a drug eruption. [Reproduced with permission from Strange GR, Ahrens WR, Schafermeyer RW, Wiebe RA: *Pediatric Emergency Medicine*, 3rd ed. © 2009. The McGraw-Hill Companies, Inc., New York, Fig. 16-1.]

45% of drug reactions were manifested in the skin.[23] Most commonly the rash appears as red macules with papules and can occur any time after drug therapy is initiated (often 7 to 10 days). The rash can take longer to appear, especially with antiepileptic medications, and last 1 to 2 weeks. The reaction usually starts on the upper trunk or head and neck and then spreads symmetrically downward to the limbs (**Figure 141-34**). The eruptions may become confluent in a symmetric, generalized distribution that spares the face. Mild desquamation is normal as the rash resolves. These rashes can sometimes be more morbilliform or even appear as the targetoid lesions of erythema multiforme. Occasionally these rashes can progress to Stevens-Johnson syndrome, toxic epidermal necrolysis (**Table 141-5**), serum sickness, or drug-induced hypersensitivity syndrome. Drug-induced hypersensitivity syndrome involves a distinct triad of fever, rash, and systemic involvement of any internal organ. This should always be discussed with caregivers of children being discharged to home with a diagnosis of cutaneous drug rash as warning signs of worsening illness. Often management just includes discontinuation of the offending drug. Children with more severe skin findings or evidence of systemic involvement may require hospital admission. Treatment is mostly supportive with topical skin care, hydration, topical steroids if necessary, and oral antihistamines as needed.[24]

ERYTHEMA MULTIFORME

Until the early 1990s, erythema multiforme, Stevens-Johnson syndrome, and toxic epidermal necrolysis were classified as a continuum of a spectrum of disease; it is now appreciated that erythema multiforme is distinct from the more serious or even life-threatening Stevens-Johnson syndrome and toxic epidermal necrolysis (see chapter 249, "Generalized Skin Disorders"). Although all may be induced by the use of medications, such as barbiturates, penicillins, sulfonamides, nonsteroidal anti-inflammatory drugs, and phenothiazines, **erythema multiforme in children is most commonly caused by infection, particularly herpes viruses and *Mycoplasma pneumoniae*.**[25] HSV-1 and HSV-2 account for 70% to 90% of all erythema multiforme cases. Erythema multiforme is rare under the age of 3 years old, affects boys more than girls, and does not favor a particular race or ethnicity.

Erythema multiforme typically presents with an abrupt onset of rash, sometimes preceded by a burning sensation. Pruritus is usually absent. The characteristic lesions are described as "target" with two to three zones consisting of a dark, ruddy-appearing center and a lighter colored area surrounding the center (**Figure 141-35**). A red-appearing outer ring is sometimes present. Lesions typically present as plaques and coalesce and frequently involve the palms and soles.

TABLE 141-5 Clinical Distinctions among Common and Serious Skin Infections

Disease	Image Reference	Age	Skin Findings	Mucosal Involvement	Nikolsky	Mortality (normal immune)	Prognosis
Bullous impetigo	Figure 141-16	Newborn and young	Localized bullae. Easily ruptured.	None	Present	None	Excellent.
Staphylococcal scalded skin syndrome	Figure 141-17	<6 y of age	Bullae, easily ruptured. More extensive involvement.	None	Present	Rare	Good.
Erythema multiforme	Figure 141-35	>3 y of age	Target lesions, atypical raised lesions. Blisters less common.	Usually limited to oral mucosa when involved	Usually absent	Possible	Good. May have reoccurrence.
SJS	Figure 245-4	Usually beyond childhood	Widespread blisters, purple macules. Usually <10% TBSA.	Extensive and may involve more than one mucosal surface	Present	5%–10%	Usually good.
Toxic epidermal necrolysis	Figure 245-4	Usually beyond childhood	Same as SJS. >30% TBSA. May involve nails.	Extensive and may involve more than one mucosal surface	Present	30%	Variable.
Cutaneous drug rashes	Figure 141-34	Child through adult	Diffuse maculopapular; become confluent.	Minimal to no mucosal involvement	Absent	Rare	Excellent.

Abbreviations: SJS = Stevens-Johnson syndrome; TBSA = total body surface area.

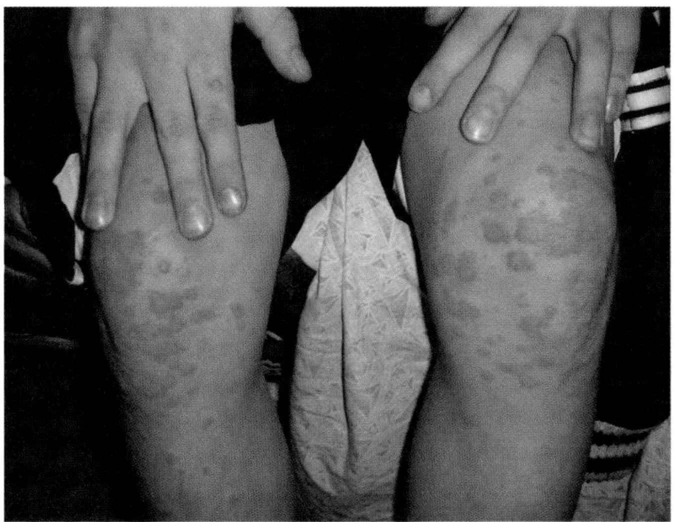

FIGURE 141-35. Symmetric distribution seen with erythema multiforme. [Reproduced with permission from Strange GR, Ahrens WR, Schafermeyer RW, Wiebe RA: *Pediatric Emergency Medicine*, 3rd ed. © 2009. The McGraw-Hill Companies, Inc., New York, Fig. 16-3.]

When limited in distribution, the term erythema multiforme minor is often applied; rarely there is involvement of the oral mucosa, in which case it is termed erythema multiforme major. Lesions last 1 to 3 weeks and may recur.

Differential diagnosis includes urticaria, viral exanthem, hypersensitivity reaction, cutaneous drug eruptions, Stevens-Johnson syndrome, toxic epidermal necrolysis, and vasculitis. Treatment for erythema multiforme is supportive and includes reassurance, although recurrent disease associated with herpes virus has been treated with oral antivirals.[25]

KAWASAKI'S DISEASE

Kawasaki's disease, or mucocutaneous lymph node syndrome, remains a vasculitis of unknown etiology. Infectious processes, toxin-mediated processes, and processes triggering a common inflammatory pathway are all postulated theories of the disease. The most devastating complication is sudden cardiac death in a child as a result of coronary artery aneurysms. However, mortality is less than 0.5% and is most common in the first year following the illness in patients with large aneurysms.[26] Kawasaki's disease peaks at age 18 to 24 months, with most cases occurring by age 10 years and the majority of patients being seen by age 5 years.[27] Children younger than 6 months or older than 9 years tend to have poorer outcomes.[28] Because of the potentially devastating sequelae and the potential for incomplete or atypical presentation of the disease, maintain a high index of suspicion for the diagnosis. Younger infants have increased risk for long-term sequelae and sudden death and are more likely to present with incomplete clinical manifestations. Kawasaki's disease is the leading cause of acquired heart disease in children (see chapter 126, "Congenital and Acquired Pediatric Heart Disease").

Kawasaki's disease is recognized as complete or classic disease and incomplete disease. The criteria for classic and incomplete disease are listed in **Table 141-6. Criteria for classic disease are fever of at least 5 days in duration and the presence of four other findings, which may include bilateral nonexudative conjunctivitis, cervical lymphadenopathy, erythema of the lips and oral mucosa, various skin changes of the extremities, and rash.** The fever is usually high and abrupt. The course of illness spans from acute to subacute to

TABLE 141-6 Diagnostic Criteria for Kawasaki's Disease[29]

Classic Kawasaki's Disease	Incomplete Kawasaki's Disease
Fever for 5 days or more plus four of the following symptoms:	Fever for 5 days and two to three clinical criteria of classic Kawasaki's disease
1. Bilateral nonexudative conjunctivitis	*plus*
2. Mucous membrane changes (erythema, peeling, cracking of lips, "strawberry tongue," or diffuse oropharyngeal mucosae)	C-reactive protein ≥3.0 milligrams/L and/or erythrocyte sedimentation rate ≥40 mm/h plus three or more of the following supplemental labs or positive echo:
3. Changes of the extremities (erythema or swelling of hands/feet, peeling of finger tips/toes in the convalescent stage) 4. Rash	1. Albumin <3 grams/dL 2. Anemia for age 3. Elevated alanine aminotransferase 4. Platelets >450,000/mm^3 after 7 d of fever onset
5. Cervical adenopathy (more than one node >1.5 cm unusually unilateral anterior cervical)	5. WBC count >12,000/mm^3 6. Presence of pyuria

convalescent and occurs over several weeks. Infants and children are typically very irritable. Cervical lymphadenopathy is the least common finding of the case definition. The type of rash is variable, although vesicles have not been described. Its appearance usually accompanies the onset of fever and has a predilection for the perineum. Desquamation in this area as well as the fingers and toes may be seen at various times during the disease, but desquamation in the extremities is more common later in the disease course. Erythema and associated edema in the extremities may cause arthralgia and fussiness. The child may refuse to bear weight. In most cases, all external clinical manifestations have resolved by 6 weeks. Cardiac complications develop early on in the illness, but coronary artery aneurysm development is most prevalent as the fever begins to lessen (see chapter 126, "Congenital and Acquired Pediatric Heart Disease").

Incomplete Kawasaki's disease is suggested by fever for at least 5 days and two of the clinical symptoms of classic disease but with supportive laboratory findings detailed in Table 141-6. Recognition and close follow-up are required in cases of incomplete Kawasaki's disease because the risk for the development of coronary artery aneurysms is greater in incomplete disease than in classic disease. There are no evidenced-based studies upon which to develop strict criteria for incomplete disease.[29] In the presence of fever for 5 days and at least two clinical criteria consistent with the disease, the patient should undergo laboratory evaluation, including C-reactive protein and erythrocyte sedimentation rate. If C-reactive protein is <3.0 milligrams/dL and the erythrocyte sedimentation rate is <40 mm/h, the child is followed daily until resolution or typical peeling occurs. With desquamation, an echocardiogram should be performed. If either C-reactive protein or erythrocyte sedimentation rate is elevated, perform additional laboratory testing. Obtain the specimen tubes for these tests at the time of initial evaluation to avoid additional venipuncture. If less than three criteria are present, the patient should undergo an echocardiogram, and if positive, treatment should be started. If the fever persists after a negative echocardiogram, a repeat study is suggested. If three or more criteria are present, obtain an echocardiogram and begin treatment for the disease.

Once the presence of incomplete Kawasaki's disease is suspected or the disease is thought to be classic, admission and specialty referral are indicated. High-dose aspirin (80 to 100 milligrams/kg/d in four doses for 14 days, then 3 to 5 milligrams/kg/d for 6 to 8 weeks in the absence of coronary aneurysms, and indefinitely in those with aneurysms) with concomitant IV immunoglobulin infusion (2 grams/kg in a single infusion over 8 to 12 hours) is recommended. Aspirin alone does not appear to lessen the appearance of coronary artery aneurysms. IV immunoglobulin should be administered within the first 7 to 10 days of illness. Steroids are not routinely indicated but may be useful in those who do not improve with IVIG. There is practice variability with both the duration of aspirin and the use of steroids.[26] Infliximab and cyclosporine A have been studied as possible therapies. Patients who develop aneurysms or coronary sequelae are referred to a pediatric cardiologist and/or cardiothoracic surgeon.

HENOCH-SCHÖNLEIN PURPURA

Henoch-Schönlein purpura is the most common vasculitis in childhood and presents with the tetrad of a palpable purpura, renal disease, abdominal pain, and polyarthralgias. Episodes of Henoch-Schönlein purpura may be preceded by or associated with upper respiratory infections, streptococcal infections, or medications.[30] Henoch-Schönlein purpura is characterized by deposition of immunoglobulin A, immunoglobulin C3, and other immune complexes in the walls of the smaller vascular supply to multiple organs throughout the body. The kidneys and the GI tract are the two most commonly affected organ systems. Renal involvement occurs in approximately half the cases. Children presenting between the age of 3 and 15 years is typical, with a peak incidence between 5 and 7 years.[31] Males are affected twice as often as females. Adult cases have been reported.[32]

The rash occurs in nearly all patients. It is predominately seen on the buttocks, legs, and arms. Failure to fully undress the child for examination would lead the clinician to miss the diagnosis. The rash is a nonblanching palpable purpura (**Figure 141-36**). It is not pruritic. Lesions range from 2 to 10 mm in size. Colicky abdominal pain is present in about half of patients, and GI bleeding may occur. Nausea, vomiting, and diarrhea may be present and may be the only presenting chief complaint. Arthralgias and painful subcutaneous edema are also typically present, are usually localized to the lower extremities, and occur in 70% to 85% of patients. The patient may refuse to bear weight. The diagnosis may be distinguished from septic arthritis, because Henoch-Schönlein purpura typically presents with bilateral joint pain and fever is usually absent. Bloody stools have also been reported.

The diagnosis is usually readily made by bedside evaluation, and laboratory testing is unnecessary other than evaluation of urine for hematuria and proteinuria, which suggests renal disease. Blood tests may reveal abnormal renal function and mild leukocytosis with elevated eosinophils. Laboratory tests do not alter the course of treatment.

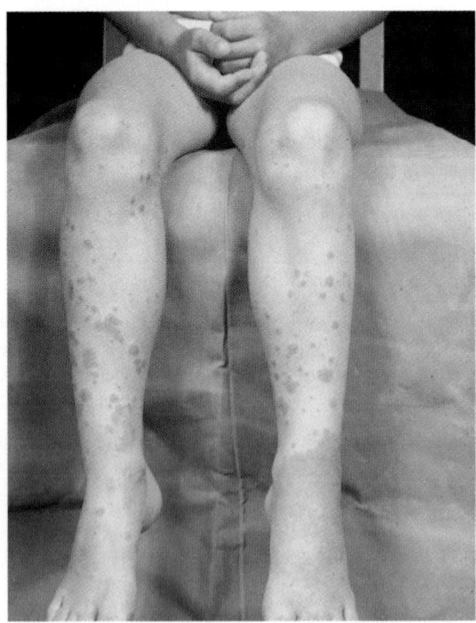

A

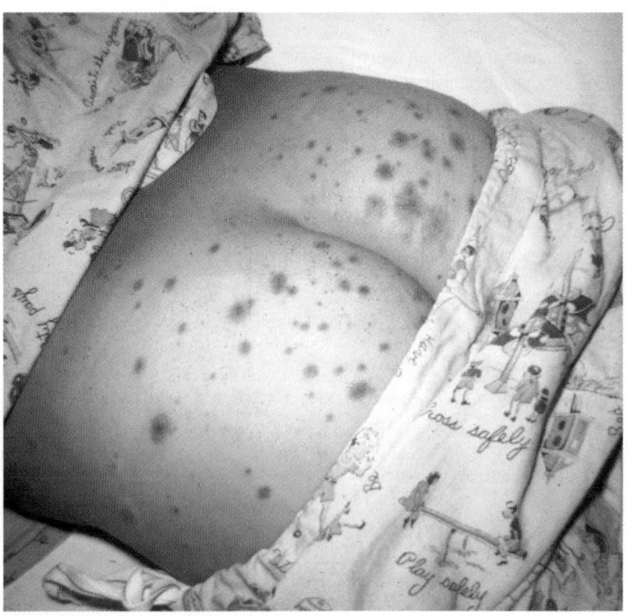

B

FIGURE 141-36. A. Henoch-Schönlein purpura on lower extremities. B. Henoch-Schönlein purpura on buttocks. [Reproduced with permission from Strange GR, Ahrens WR, Schafermeyer RW, Wiebe RA: *Pediatric Emergency Medicine*, 3rd ed. © 2009. The McGraw-Hill Companies, Inc., New York, Fig. 85-3 A&B.]

Streptococcus testing and antistreptolysin O titers have been reported as elevated in approximately 50% of patients. Additional laboratory studies and imaging are only useful to help eliminate other disease processes such as pancreatitis, idiopathic thrombocytopenic purpura, thrombotic thrombocytopenic purpura, and intussusception.

Henoch-Schönlein purpura is typically self-limited and resolves over the course of 3 to 4 weeks. Recurrent disease occurs in approximately one third of patients. Although some patients may have urinary abnormalities for years, only a very small percentage will progress to end-stage renal disease (see chapter 134, "Renal Emergencies in Children"), and most patients can be discharged to home from the ED with follow-up within 1 week for repeat urinalysis. Although there is no demonstrated impact on preventing the development of nephritis, the use of prednisone, 1.0 milligram/kg/d for 2 weeks followed by a 2-week taper, can attenuate joint and GI symptoms. Nonsteroidal anti-inflammatory drugs are effective treatment for pain associated with arthralgias and edema. The treatment of severe nephritis is more controversial, and high-dose steroids, cyclophosphamide, azathioprine, and cyclosporine have all been advocated (see chapter 134).

REFERENCES

The complete reference list is available online at www.TintinalliEM.com.

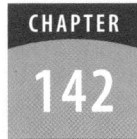

CHAPTER 142 Sickle Cell Disease In Children

John Marshall

INTRODUCTION AND PATHOPHYSIOLOGY

Sickle cell disease is a spectrum of blood disorders of which sickle cell anemia (SCA) is the most serious. SCA is found primarily in children of African, Arab, or Mediterranean descent. It is caused by a single amino acid substitution in the sixth position of the β-globulin chain of normal adult hemoglobin (HbA), which creates the abnormal sickle hemoglobin (HbS). The HbS chain found in patients with SCA creates a hydrophobic region of the hemoglobin tetramer when it is deoxygenated.[1] In this state, noncovalent polymerization of the hemoglobin molecules creates chains that distort the shape of the membrane, causing the characteristic sickle appearance. The altered red blood cell shape and its associated rigidity and decreased deformability cause sickle cells to impede blood flow. This is responsible for most of the clinical manifestations of SCA through two primary mechanisms: hemolytic anemia and vaso-occlusion with subsequent ischemia-reperfusion injury. Interruption of blood flow created by the abnormal cells leads to poor tissue perfusion, acidosis, and hypoxia, which cause further sickling. The need to reverse these conditions is central to the management of SCA-related complications.

Children homozygous for this genetic abnormality have two genetic copies of the HbS mutation and are described as having classic hemoglobin SS (HbSS) disease, whereas heterozygotes for HbS with a second β-globulin chain that is normal (HbA) are considered to have sickle cell trait. These patients have enough HbA to prevent polymerization of the hemoglobin chains and subsequently avoid the more severe complications of the disease. Other patients may be heterozygous for HbS coupled with a second hemoglobin abnormality such as HbC, HbO, or β-thalassemia. Although some of these combinations can cause the severe pathology of SCA, patients with HbSC and the 90% of HbS/β-thalassemia patients with some normal β chains have fewer ischemic and infectious complications than patients with HbSS.

Because fetal hemoglobin (HbF) is unaffected by these genetic mutations, symptoms of SCA do not appear until HbF is replaced by the abnormal HbA. HbF predominates until 4 months of age, after which it rapidly declines, reaching baseline low levels just before 1 year of age. One of the first organs affected by the emerging sickle cells is the spleen. Recurrent splenic infarcts lead to a gradual decline in splenic function between 4 and 12 months of age, resulting in susceptibility to serious infections with encapsulated bacteria.

In the United States, all neonates are screened for SCA using highly sensitive and specific tests, so the diagnosis is rarely made in the ED. The clinical manifestations and potential complications of SCA, however, include symptoms that overlap considerably with diseases not related to SCA. Therefore, the diagnostic portion of this chapter is organized in a symptom-based fashion, and the treatment portion is grouped by disease physiology.

SICKLE CELL ANEMIA SYMPTOMS

EXTREMITY PAIN

Vaso-occlusive crises causing severe extremity pain are the most common manifestation of SCA, accounting for 79% to 91% of ED visits.[2] Common triggers include stress, cold, dehydration, altitude, hypoxia, or illness. Pain preferentially affects the long bones and lower back. Individual patients tend to manifest their pain crises in characteristic locations, but the frequency of vaso-occlusive pain crisis is variable, even among SS homozygotes. Five percent of children with SCA account for 33% of total episodes, averaging between 3 and 10 pain crises per year.[3] Children display variable degrees of tenderness over affected sites and may have slight temperature elevations without true fever. Because anemia can precipitate a crisis, assess patients for an acute drop in hemoglobin; experienced families may know the patient's baseline values.

Severe vaso-occlusive crises can lead to **bony infarction**. Pain episodes caused by bony infarcts typically cause more debilitating and refractory pain than past episodes, and there is often significant localized bone tenderness and an elevated peripheral WBC count. Fat embolism can be a complication. Signs and symptoms of **fat embolism** include acute respiratory distress, hypoxia, and systemic symptoms of petechiae, altered mental status, liver damage, and renal failure. Fat embolism can occur without acute extremity pain, and the aforementioned symptoms should prompt consideration of fat embolization.

When vaso-occlusive crises affect the nutrient arteries of the metacarpals and/or metatarsals, dactylitis results, and children develop tender, painful, swollen hands and feet, which may be accompanied by a low-grade fever (**Figure 142-1**). **Dactylitis** occurs in children <2 years old

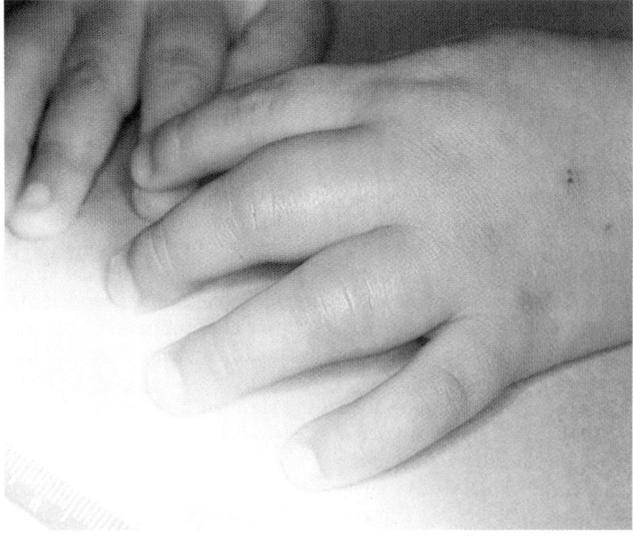

FIGURE 142-1. Acute sickle dactylitis. Bilateral cylindrical swelling of soft tissue of the fingers in sickle cell anemia consistent with vaso-occlusive crisis of the hands. [Photo contributed by Donald L. Rucknagel, MD, PhD. Reproduced with permission from Knoop K, Stack L, Storrow A, Thurman RJ: *Atlas of Emergency Medicine*, 3rd ed. © 2009, McGraw-Hill, Inc., New York.]

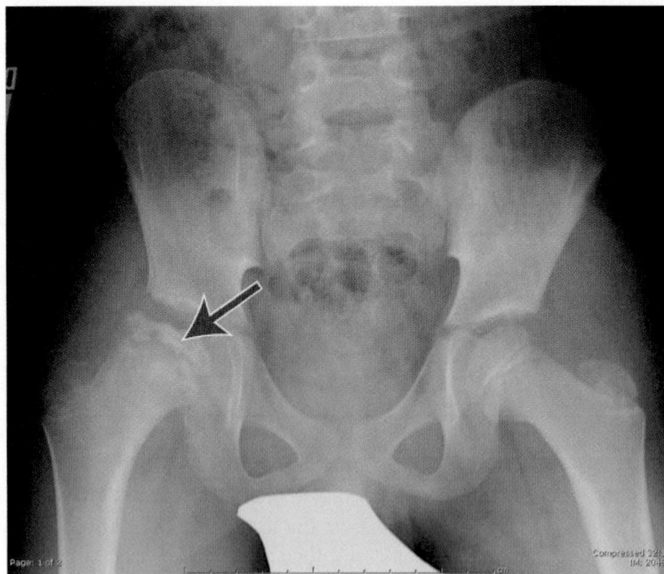

FIGURE 142-2. Avascular necrosis. Note the flattening of the femoral head (*arrow*). [Image used with permission of Dr. Hollie Jackson, MD.]

and may be the initial clinical presentation of SCA, but dactylitis is extremely rare beyond 5 years of age. Any number of extremities can be affected, and symptoms can last from days to 2 weeks. Recurrences are common.

Avascular necrosis of the femoral head occurs in 30% of patients by age 30 years old. Children present with afebrile inguinal pain with weight bearing. Radiographs may demonstrate flattening and collapse of the femoral head (**Figure 142-2**). Less commonly, ischemia can cause similar pain in the humeral head.

Bone and joint infections affect patients with SCA at higher rates than the general population. Infections are often difficult to distinguish from bony infarcts. Symptoms of tenderness, warmth, and swelling may be indistinguishable from those of a vaso-occlusive crisis, although a high fever is more typical of infection. **Limited range of motion of a joint is unusual in vaso-occlusive crisis and should prompt evaluation for a septic joint.** Although leukocytosis occurs with vaso-occlusive crisis, a left shift is unique to infection. **Erythrocyte sedimentation rates are unreliable in patients with SCA.** Radionuclide imaging or MRI may distinguish infection from infarct.

ABDOMINAL PAIN

Abdominal pain is a difficult symptom to assess in any child and is complicated by the potential abdominal manifestations of SCA. Any acute abdominal condition, such as appendicitis, pancreatitis, and hepatitis, must be considered. However, **the abdomen is the next most common site of pain from a vaso-occlusive crisis after the extremities and back**. Abdominal vaso-occlusive crises are due to mesenteric, splenic, and hepatic ischemia and present as sudden onset of poorly localized abdominal pain. Physical examination may reveal tenderness and guarding but typically should not demonstrate rebound or rigidity.

Gallstones are common due to the elevated bilirubin levels from hemolysis in SCA and can occur as early as 2 to 4 years of age. Diagnosis is by US. Although symptoms in children may resolve with time, occasionally, cholecystitis can be severe, and infection can progress rapidly (see chapters 79, "Pancreatitis and Cholecystitis," and 131, "Gastrointestinal Bleeding in Infants and Children"). Right upper quadrant syndrome due to intrahepatic cholestasis is not common. Signs and symptoms include sudden right upper quadrant pain, jaundice, anorexia, tender hepatomegaly, and, often, fever. Bilirubin levels can be as high as 50 milligrams/dL. Although patients with SCA often have bilirubin levels above baseline, bilirubin levels rarely exceed 4 milligrams/dL and are predominantly unconjugated bilirubin. Confirm the diagnosis by US. **Acute hepatic sequestration** is another cause of abdominal pain, and the liver enlarges rapidly. Laboratories are variable, except for low hemoglobin. US or CT scan shows diffuse hepatomegaly in hepatic sequestration.

RESPIRATORY DISTRESS AND CHEST PAIN

Acute chest crisis, due to pulmonary ischemia and infarction, is frequently a complication of pneumonia (Figure 142-3). The incidence of acute chest crisis in children is higher than in adults (21 per 100 person-years in patients with HbSS), but is associated with better outcomes. Children develop any combination of pleuritic chest pain, cough, fever, and dyspnea. Examination findings include retractions, hypoxia, tachypnea, rhonchi, or rales, although dehydration can minimize the presence of rales on examination. An elevated WBC count is often present in both infarct and pneumonia, and thrombocytopenia may accompany severe crises. **Chest radiograph is indicated in any patient with chest symptoms or hypoxia, although findings may be minimal early on and should not dissuade treatment of a patient with potential chest crisis on clinical grounds only**. Radiography demonstrates a new alveolar pulmonary infiltrate, which is typically located in the upper or middle lobe in children, although adults often have multilobar disease. The cause of pneumonia is typically *Chlamydia*, *Mycoplasma*, viral, *Streptococcus pneumoniae*, *Staphylococcus aureus*, or *Haemophilus influenzae*. Sputum or blood cultures are rarely positive and not generally recommended, except in patients ill enough to require mechanical ventilation. Multilobe involvement, history of cardiac disease, and low platelets predict poor outcomes.[4] Chest crisis can result in decreased lung function,[5] poor integrity of the pulmonary vessels, and a propensity to pulmonary edema. Asthma is common in patients with SCA, occurring in 17% to 53%. **Asthma not only complicates the diagnosis of acute chest crisis but also increases the likelihood of chest syndrome by four- to six-fold.**[5]

Pulmonary hypertension develops in 16% to 35% of children with SCA. By adulthood, about one-third have pulmonary hypertension, a

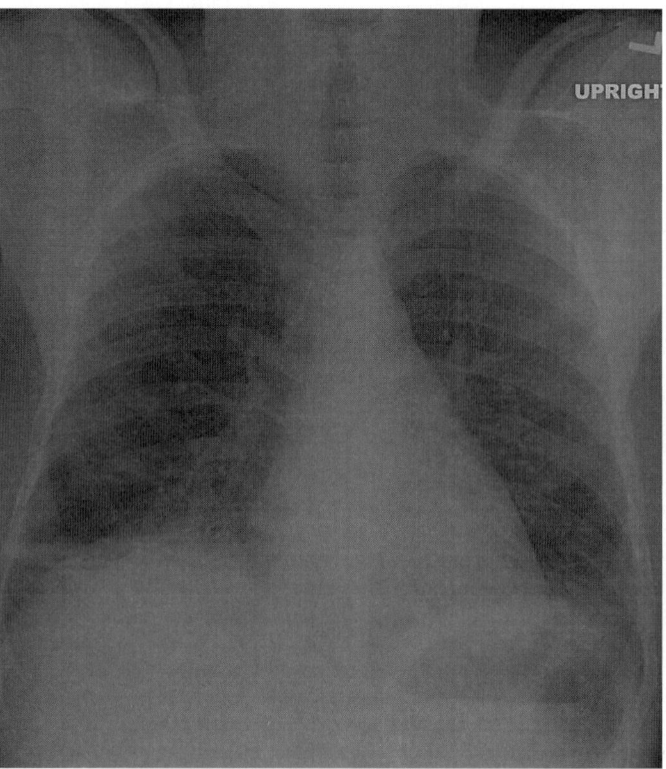

FIGURE 142-3. Acute chest crisis. Note the areas of infiltrate in the right lower lobe and left upper lobe. [Image used with permission of Dr. Hollie Jackson, MD.]

condition that is associated with diastolic dysfunction and increased mortality. Increased intensity of the second heart sound, evidence of right ventricular enlargement, or unexplained desaturation should suggest pulmonary hypertension (see chapters 57 and 58, "Systemic Hypertension" and "Pulmonary Hypertension," respectively, section on pulmonary hypertension). Diagnosis is made by echocardiogram and right heart cardiac catheterization demonstrating a pulmonary artery pressure above 25 mm Hg. Progressive disease can cause chest pain, dyspnea on exertion, resting hypoxia, right-sided heart failure, syncope, and pulmonary thromboembolism.

Cardiomegaly and heart murmurs are common in children with SCA. However, overt heart failure is uncommon in children, except in cases of iatrogenic volume overload associated with transfusion. Heart failure is managed by the usual methods and by correcting anemia.

FEVER

Across all ages, infection is the leading cause of death in patients with SCA.[6] Splenic dysfunction and inability to form immunoglobulin G antibodies to polysaccharide antigens increase susceptibility to infection, particularly with encapsulated organisms. **Children age 6 months to 3 years old are at the greatest risk for sepsis, with *H. influenzae* and *S. pneumoniae* more common in the very young, and *Escherichia coli* and *Salmonella* more frequent in older children.** The rate of bacteremia in children ≤3 years old has been about 8 per 100 patient-years. In children who receive pneumococcal 7-valent conjugate vaccine, invasive pneumococcal disease has decreased by as much as 93.4%.[7] **Table 142-1** reviews risk factors for bacteremia. Workup of potential infection in SCA patients should include a CBC, urinalysis, chest radiograph, oxygen saturation measurement, and cultures of the blood, throat, urine, or other potential source of infection.

Children with SCA also have an increased prevalence of meningitis, pneumonia, arthritis, and osteomyelitis compared to the general population, and have poorer outcomes for these diseases. Similarly, viral infections, including influenza, result in greater morbidity, and **yearly vaccination for influenza is recommended**.

PARVOVIRUS INFECTION

Parvovirus B19 infection is of particular concern. The initial infection is usually asymptomatic or associated with nonspecific upper respiratory symptoms. However, parvovirus can cause several different clinical syndromes. Erythema infectiosum is characterized by fever, headache, nausea, coryza, and slapped cheek appearance with circumoral pallor followed by diffuse maculopapular rash. Gloves and socks syndrome describes well-demarcated painful erythema and edema of the hands and feet that evolves into petechiae, purpura, vesicles, and skin sloughing. Finally, parvovirus can cause symmetric or asymmetric arthropathy of knees and ankles. **Regardless of the clinical presentation, parvovirus can cause a transient aplastic crisis, with the reticulocyte count dropping 5 days after exposure, followed by a decline in hemoglobin (see chapter 143, "Oncologic and Hematologic Emergencies in Children").** Because of the shortened life span of the red cells in SCA, parvovirus can cause serious anemia, which lasts for 2 weeks. Upon recovery, there is an outpouring of nucleated red blood cells from the marrow, and patients late in the illness may have a high reticulocyte count.[8] Infection usually imparts subsequent lifelong immunity to parvovirus.

TABLE 142-1 Risk Factors for Bacteremia in Children with Sickle Cell Anemia

Temperature >40°C (104°F)
WBC count >30,000 or <5000 cells/mm³
Platelet count <100,000/mm³
Hemoglobin <5 grams/dL
Ill appearance, poor perfusion, hypotension
Infiltrate on chest radiograph
History of pneumococcal sepsis

ANEMIA

Splenic sequestration, or intrasplenic trapping of red cells, is a major cause of mortality in children <5 years old. Two types exist, **major** and **minor**. **Major splenic sequestration** causes a rapid drop of more than three points in the hemoglobin, with the development of pallor, left upper quadrant abdominal pain, and splenomegaly. This can progress within hours to altered mental status, hypotension, and cardiovascular collapse. **Minor splenic sequestration** tends to be more insidious, with a smaller change in hemoglobin levels. Often, attacks occur along with bacterial or viral infections. Laboratory studies in either syndrome demonstrate a decline from baseline hemoglobin level, a normal to increased reticulocyte count, and no change in bilirubin, because there is no hemolytic component to this complication. Mild neutropenia or thrombocytopenia may be noted. Patients with HbSS rarely experience this complication beyond 5 years of age (peak, 3 months to 5 years old) due to infarction and scarring of the spleen, but most patients with HbSC and homozygous S/β-thalassemia have a spleen that persists into adulthood, and thus have a risk of splenic sequestration.

As noted earlier, aplastic crisis is an important cause of anemia in SCA patients and can be induced by parvovirus infection or medications. Signs are the gradual onset of pallor without pain or jaundice. Laboratories demonstrate a decline in hemoglobin and a low reticulocyte count. Full recovery is expected within weeks.

NEUROLOGIC COMPLAINTS

Stroke is 250 times more common in children with SCA than in the baseline population[9]: 11% of children with SCA suffer a clinically overt stroke, and another 20% are found to have silent strokes on imaging. The risk of recurrence, untreated, after one stroke is 49% to 90%, and children with HbSS are at four times greater risk than those with HbSC. SCA patients typically have cerebral vasculopathy involving the intima and media of large arteries, usually the middle cerebral artery. Screening transcranial Doppler studies can identify abnormal flow patterns associated with this vasculopathy, which, if untreated, are associated with a 10% risk of stroke within 2 to 3 years of diagnosis.[3] Additionally some children will develop a moyamoya-like syndrome in which clotted vessels induce the development of diffuse small collateral vessels. These weak vessels are prone to aneurysm formation and spontaneous hemorrhage and demonstrate a characteristic "puff of smoke" appearance on cerebral angiography.

Cerebral ischemia can present with fleeting symptoms of transient ischemic attacks, or with hemiparesis, seizure, altered mental status, or coma. Common vascular territories involved include the internal carotid or middle cerebral arteries, but venous sinus thrombosis may cause parieto-occipital or thalamic involvement (**Figure 142-4**).[9] As in adult stroke, the CT scan is less reliable to detect ischemic infarct in the first 36 hours, although CT scan does rule out hemorrhage. Diffusion-weighted MRI demonstrates changes within minutes and T2-weighted MRI within hours of ischemia.

Patients with SCA also have a higher rate of cerebral aneurysms and intracranial hemorrhage than the general population, although hemorrhagic stroke only accounts for 10% of strokes in SCA patients. This complication is rarely seen in children but becomes a concern during late adolescence. Hemorrhagic strokes typically present with headache, vomiting, and alterations in level of consciousness but may present with hemiparesis similar to an ischemic stroke if bleeding is intraparenchymal. There are three potential sites of hemorrhage: subarachnoid from an aneurysm, intraparenchymal from large-vessel vasculopathy or moyamoya, and intraventricular from moyamoya.

Neurologic symptoms are not uncommon in patients with acute chest crisis as well and have been noted in 7% to 10% of cases.[9] Other considerations in the patient with altered mental status and SCA previously mentioned include severe anemia from splenic sequestration and meningitis.

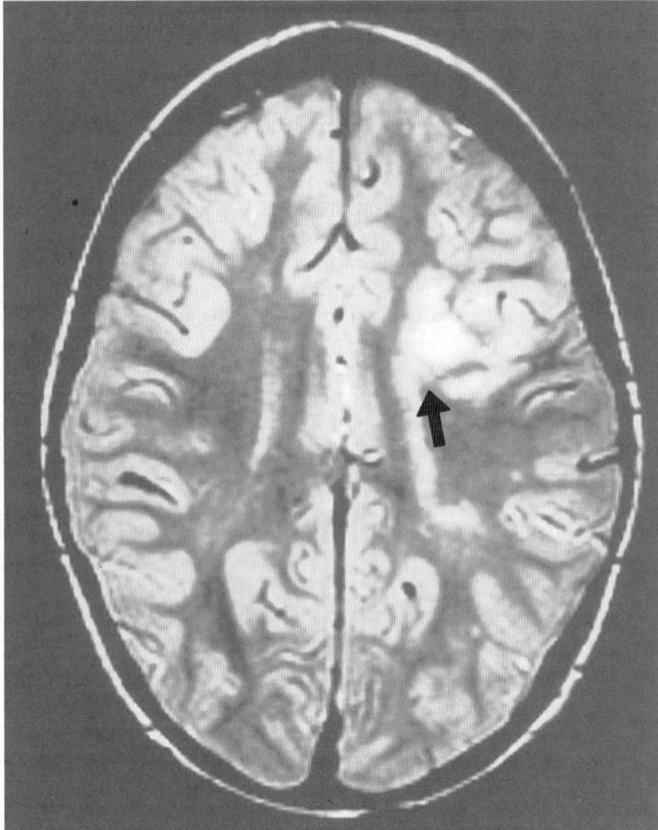

FIGURE 142-4. Acute stroke. T2-weighted MRI scan of the brain shows areas of increased signal intensity (*arrow*) involving the gray and white matter of the left parietal lobe, consistent with an acute infarct. [Reproduced with permission from Shah BR, Laude TL: *Atlas of Pediatric Clinical Diagnosis*, © 2000 WB Saunders, Philadelphia.]

GU COMPLAINTS

Priapism is common in males, with 27% having at least one episode by age 20 years old.[10] There is a bimodal age peak—5 to 13 years old and 21 to 29 years old. Patients present with a painful, swollen, edematous, tender penis, often with difficulty urinating (**Figure 142-5**). The glans itself remains soft. Sickling of the red cells in the sinusoids of the corpus cavernosum cause decreased venous outflow from the penis.[10]

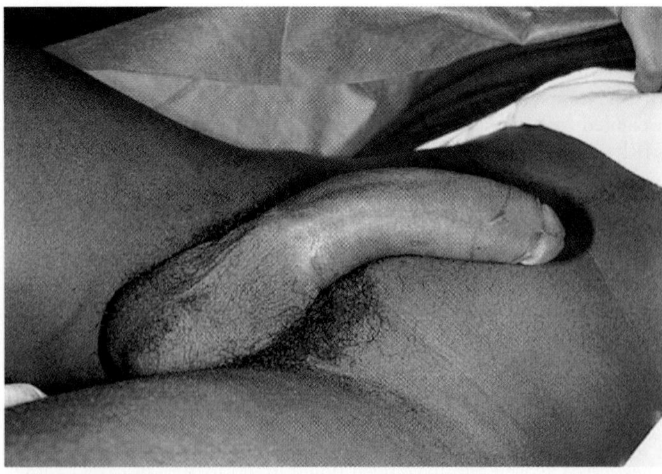

FIGURE 142-5. Priapism in an adolescent male with sickle cell anemia. [Reproduced with permission from Shah BR, Lucchesi M: *Atlas of Pediatric Emergency Medicine*. © 2006, McGraw-Hill, New York.]

The most common renal abnormality is hyposthenuria, the inability to maximally concentrate urine. This may cause enuresis, nocturia, and a propensity for dehydration and hyperkalemia. Renal vaso-occlusive crises are also common and can be asymptomatic or accompanied by colicky intermittent flank pain, costovertebral angle tenderness, gross or microscopic hematuria, and passage of renal tissue. Chronic damage to the kidneys can lead to renal insufficiency at an early age.

Hematuria can also occur with papillary necrosis, a complication seen in both homozygous and sickle trait patients. Urinalysis demonstrates red blood cells without casts or associated pyuria or significant proteinuria.

TREATMENT OF SICKLE CELL ANEMIA SYMPTOMS

ANEMIA

Severe and symptomatic anemia, as well as many of the other complications of SCA, may require transfusion. The general principles of transfusion discussed here are applicable to each of the crises described earlier. **A typical pediatric transfusion of packed red blood cells is 10 mL/kg over a 2-hour period.** In the case of severe anemia, smaller volume transfusions, typically 5 mL/kg, are given more slowly because of the risk of pulmonary edema associated with large fluid shifts. In this case, multiple lower volume transfusions are indicated with reassessment between each infusion. **In general, transfusions are indicated in the case of symptomatic anemia with a hemoglobin <6 grams/dL and an inappropriately low reticulocyte count, or an acute vaso-occlusive crisis with a hemoglobin below 10 grams/dL.** In these cases, a simple transfusion, rather than an exchange transfusion, is the indicated treatment with the goal of treatment being a hemoglobin >10 grams/dL.

Patients requiring transfusion for a specific crisis in which the hemoglobin is >10 grams/dL require an exchange transfusion, with the goal of reducing the proportion of HbS to <30%. Generally, this requires infusion of normal saline followed by removal of 50 to 60 mL/kg of blood prior to the transfusion. This process reduces vaso-occlusion by essentially replacing the patient's diseased erythrocytes with normal red blood cells. Many centers have an automated exchange transfusion machine, but in the event of an extreme emergency, this procedure can be performed manually at the bedside. **All transfusions should be leukoreduced; washed cells are used in patients with a history of allergic reactions; irradiated cells (from an unrelated donor) are indicated for patients who may be candidates for a bone marrow transplantation.**

Anemia secondary to an aplastic crisis is often treated with simple transfusion and close follow-up. Acute splenic or hepatic sequestration with associated anemia is managed with good hydration, analgesia, simple transfusion, and exchange transfusion in refractory cases. Because the recurrence rate for splenic sequestration is 50%, chronic transfusion therapy and/or splenectomy are often considered.

VASO-OCCLUSIVE CRISES

Vaso-occlusive pain crises, regardless of location, are treated with pain control and *gentle* hydration and, in some cases, oxygen. Provide liberal analgesia with frequent reassessment of pain 15 to 30 minutes after medication, and repeat dosing until the patient is comfortable. Although standard drug dosing is presented here, patients with pain crises who require narcotics frequently may have tolerance to these drugs and may require much larger doses to achieve adequate analgesia. Commonly used analgesics are listed in **Table 142-2**. Ketorolac (Toradol®) can be combined with narcotics. IV is the preferred route of administration of morphine, but IM injection can be a temporizing measure. Due to the histamine release from morphine, a frequent side effect is pruritus, which may require treatment with diphenhydramine (Benadryl®) or use of alternative agents. Hydromorphone (Dilaudid®) is a reasonable alternative to morphine and has a similar pharmacokinetic profile. Subsequent narcotic doses may be reduced to half the initial dose, depending on the response and side effects to the initial dose. **Meperidine and fentanyl are not ideal opioid choices due to the side effect profile in the case of meperidine and the short duration of action of fentanyl.**

TABLE 142-2 Medications for Vaso-Occlusive Crisis in Children

Medication	Route	Dose	Onset	Duration	Common Side Effects
Morphine sulfate	IV	0.1 milligram/kg	10–15 min	1–2 h	Pruritus, nausea, respiratory depression, sedation
	IM	0.1 milligram/kg	15–30 min	3–4 h	
Hydromorphone (Dilaudid®)	IV	0.015 milligram/kg	10–15 min	1–2 h	Nausea, respiratory depression, sedation
	IM	0.015 milligram/kg	15–30 min	3–4 h	
Ketorolac (Toradol®)	IV loading	0.5 milligram/kg	10–30 min	4–6 h	Gastritis, bleeding, allergy
Hydrocodone (Lortab®, Vicodin®)	PO	0.15–0.2 milligram/kg every 3–4 h	10–20 min	3–6 h	Sedation
Ibuprofen (Motrin, Advil)	PO	10 milligrams/kg every 6–8 h	Within 60 min	6–8 h	Gastritis, bleeding, allergy

Ketamine is a possible alternative to narcotics, but its use is not yet widespread.[11]

Provide IV hydration at a rate of 1.5 times maintenance with 5% dextrose in half-normal saline. **Because of the risk of increased permeability of pulmonary vasculature and cardiomyopathy, normal saline boluses are not routinely used except to treat acute dehydration or hypovolemic shock.** Consider transfusion for pain crises accompanied by a significant drop in hemoglobin or a total hemoglobin <5 grams/dL (see chapter 113, "Pain Management and Procedural Sedation in Infants and Children"). Oxygen is not useful in the nonhypoxic patient.[12] The decision to admit or discharge is often difficult and is usually made with input from the patient, family, and hematologist. Children requiring two or more doses of narcotic medications in the ED are likely to require admission. Patients discharged home should be instructed to take nonsteroidal anti-inflammatory drugs if no contraindications exist and may require an oral narcotic as well. Hydrocodone (Lortab®, Vicodin®) at a dose of 0.15 to 0.2 milligram/kg given every 3 to 4 hours is generally an effective choice and comes in a solution (Lortab®) for younger children.

For acute chest crisis, treat pain and provide IV hydration and oxygen. Several papers have noted a possible association between morphine sulfate use and the development of acute chest syndrome,[13] but morphine is still commonly and widely used in the treatment of pain associated with SCA. Because pneumonia is frequently a precipitant or complicating factor, give empiric antibiotic treatment with a third-generation cephalosporin and macrolide. For patients whose clinical status deteriorates despite all of these measures, transfusion (simple for hemoglobin <10 grams/dL, or exchange for hemoglobin >10 grams/dL) is indicated. **Generally a partial pressure of arterial oxygen (Pa_{O_2}) below 70 mm Hg or an oxygen saturation that has fallen >10% from baseline in a chronically hypoxic patient should be a trigger for transfusion.** Steroids are not beneficial. Respiratory distress associated with fat emboli may respond to prompt transfusion and/or exchange transfusion.

Other crises, such as renal infarct and right upper quadrant syndrome and papillary necrosis, are usually treated with hydration, analgesia, and other supportive measures.

PRIAPISM

Treat priapism with the use of hydration, analgesia, and transfusion and/or exchange transfusion depending on the current hemoglobin. Additionally, urologic consultation and aspiration of the corpora with a 23-gauge needle may be necessary, followed by irrigation and administration of a 1:1,000,000 epinephrine solution if the priapism continues for more than 4 to 6 hours. Procedural sedation may be required for children needing corporal aspiration. Patients with repeated episodes of priapism may be candidates for prophylaxis with pseudoephedrine, gonadotropin-releasing hormone analogues, diethylstilbestrol, or hydroxyurea.[10]

STROKE

Alteplase (t-PA®) is not recommended for children and has no role in the management of stroke related to SCA. Interventions are aimed at limiting secondary brain injury through aggressive control of hyperpyrexia, correction of hypoglycemia, hypoxia, and hypovolemia, and **urgent exchange transfusion** to decrease the percentage of HbS below 30%. There is currently no consensus opinion on the management of blood pressure.[14] Children with a history of clinical stroke or transient ischemic attack or with abnormal cerebral blood flow on cranial Doppler are often managed long term with a chronic transfusion protocol or hydroxyurea to decrease the risk of subsequent strokes. Neurosurgical consultation is required for management of hemorrhagic stroke.

FEVER

Well-appearing children >1 year old with isolated fever and no signs of sepsis may be candidates for discharge if they are stable for a 4-hour period of observation, have good follow-up, and do not meet the high-risk criteria detailed in the earlier "Fever" section. **Give a dose of ceftriaxone before discharge pending culture results.** Stable children with an identified source for fever (e.g., strep throat, otitis media) can be discharged with disease-specific treatment. Patients <1 year old or those meeting high-risk criteria or demonstrating signs of sepsis require admission. A third-generation cephalosporin (ceftriaxone, 100 milligrams/kg/d, one dose, not to exceed 4 grams/d) is frequently adequate empiric treatment against encapsulated bacteria pending culture results, but areas with high rates of resistant *S. pneumoniae* may consider the addition of vancomycin (10 milligrams/kg IV every 6 hours) as well. Pulmonary infections require the addition of a macrolide. For specific infections, such as bone and joint infections, treatment should be determined based on available culture results and consultation with appropriate subspecialty services. In the case of meningitis, patients are at increased risk of stroke, and the decision to administer a prophylactic exchange transfusion should be made in conjunction with the hematologist.

OTHER PROCEDURES

SCA patients may be admitted for surgery for reasons related or unrelated to the underlying disease. Before surgery, exchange transfusion can be given to decrease HbS to <30%. This should be considered in consultation with the hematologist for all but the most emergent conditions requiring major surgery.[15] Minor procedures may not require transfusion. Transfusion is not indicated before the administration of nonionic contrast materials.

COMMON OUTPATIENT MEDICATIONS AND TREATMENTS

Due to the risk of bacteremia, children are maintained on **oral penicillin** through age 5 years old. Beyond 5 years of age, there does not seem to be any additional benefit from penicillin.[16] **Folate** supplementation is standard due to the increased turnover of red blood cells.

Hydroxyurea is the only disease-modifying drug available for sickle cell disease and is used in SCA patients to decrease the frequency and severity of complications and to reduce mortality. Hydroxyurea induces the production of HbF in addition to other benefits such as decreasing the number of leukocytes and providing some vasodilation. The additional HbF lowers the percentage of HbS, which decreases hemoglobin polymerization, increases erythrocyte size, and improves cellular deformability, thus decreasing the amount of sickling and consequently reducing vaso-occlusion.[15,17] There is strong evidence that hydroxyurea should be started in all children over 9 months of age regardless of severity of the disease to reduce the risk of complications. Although this medication should be started by a primary care physician or sickle cell disease specialist, emergency physicians caring for SCA patients should counsel patients on the availability of this treatment and refer them appropriately. Side effects can include GI discomfort, modest neutropenia, hyperpigmentation, and renal toxicity.

Hypertransfusion or **chronic transfusion therapy** is an option in patients with severe or frequent crises, with the principle that the transfused red cells will decrease anemia and minimize the patient's own production of abnormal red cells. If the percentage of HbS is kept below 30%, the possibility of a sickle crisis is minimized. Clearly, the known risks of infection and transfusion reaction that pertain to any transfusion apply. Transfusion for sickle cell disease patients more frequently results in alloimmunization (5% to 36% of patients) compared to the general population. Alloimmunization is defined as immunization of the patient by donor RBC antigens. The risk can be minimized by using blood matched for minor red blood cell antigens such as C, E, and Kell. In these cases, patients experience a drop to below pretransfusion levels of hemoglobin, despite a negative direct antibody test, due to hemolytic anemia that can be life threatening. This phenomenon also increases the risk for future transfusion reactions in SCA patients.[15]

Finally, chronic **iron overload** is another complication of frequent transfusions and may contribute to cardiomyopathy. Iron overload is treated with deferoxamine chelation therapy, a treatment that is also associated with risk: deferoxamine may increase the susceptibility for fungal infections (and other infections such as *Yersinia*) and lead to growth failure, allergic reactions, ophthalmic toxicity, or ototoxicity.

Bone marrow or stem cell transplantation has been successfully used to cure SCA. However, due to the risks associated with transplantation, this is generally only considered in patients who have a human leukocyte antigen–matched sibling.

Acknowledgments: The author gratefully acknowledges the contributions of Peter J. Paganussi, Thom Mayer, Maybelle Kou, and Ilene Claudius, the authors of this chapter in previous editions.

REFERENCES

The complete reference list is available online at www.TintinalliEM.com.

CHAPTER 143

Oncologic and Hematologic Emergencies in Children

Megan E. Mickley
Camilo Gutierrez
Michele Carney

ONCOLOGIC EMERGENCIES

Children and adolescents develop different types of cancers than adults. The 5-year survival rate for all childhood (0 to 19 years of age) cancers is now >80%[1]; however, malignant neoplasms remain the second leading cause of death for U.S. children age 5 to 14 years.[2] Globally, the American Cancer Society estimates that less than 40% of children younger than 15 years with cancer are adequately diagnosed and treated.[3] The most common childhood malignancies are discussed below.

LEUKEMIA

EPIDEMIOLOGY

Acute leukemias, including acute lymphoblastic leukemia (ALL) and acute myelogenous leukemia (AML), are the most common cancers in children, accounting for over a quarter of all malignancies.[4-6] Chronic leukemias are rare in children and adolescents. ALL accounts for approximately 75% to 80% of pediatric leukemias and, if diagnosed early, carries a 5-year survival rate of 90% in developed countries.[4-7] The peak incidence of ALL is 3 to 5 years of age, with younger children having the best outcomes.[8,9] In the United States, ALL is more common in boys, and more common in white and Hispanic than in African American children.[2-5,10] A number of inherited risk factors, including trisomy 21, are well documented.

AML accounts for approximately 15% to 20% of childhood and adolescent leukemias in the United States.[4,6,11] Cure rates have improved but remain lower than those for ALL. Current estimates are 60% to 70%, and relapsed AML accounts for greater than half of all childhood leukemia-related deaths.[4,11,12] Incidence of AML peaks in the first 2 years of life.[4,6] Environmental exposures, including chemotherapy agents and radiation received during treatment of other childhood cancers, are known causes of secondary AML. Patients being treated for AML have a higher incidence of complications than those with ALL, especially infections. This is primarily due to the greater intensity of chemotherapeutic regimens necessary to achieve remission.

CLINICAL FEATURES

Most signs and symptoms of acute leukemia are due to bone marrow infiltration by blasts, as well as infiltration of extramedullary sites. A detailed history may reveal nonspecific constitutional symptoms: fever, fatigue, anorexia, and weight loss. **Cytopenias from marrow infiltration can present as pallor, easy bleeding/bruising with petechiae and ecchymoses, infections, or bone pain. The reticuloendothelial system is the most common site of extramedullary infiltration, manifesting as hepatomegaly, splenomegaly, and/or lymphadenopathy.** Other sites include the CNS and testes.

Consider leukemia in cases of recurrent or severe unexplained epistaxis or other mucosal bleeding or unusually extensive or abnormally located bruising. In rare cases of AML, solid nodules of leukemic blasts (chloromas) may be noted, most commonly in the skin (leukemia cutis) or gingiva. Bone and joint pain may result in limping or refusal to walk. Such symptoms can result in a delay in diagnosis if pain is attributed to other conditions. Concerning symptoms include abnormal blood counts, a history of nighttime pain, and recurrent or persistent bony complaints.[13,14] For a subset of patients, diagnosis is made incidentally during an evaluation for infection, lymphadenopathy, priapism, or other presentations.

DIAGNOSIS

Begin with a CBC with differential count, a peripheral smear, a coagulation profile, a type and screen, and serum chemistries including calcium, phosphate, magnesium, uric acid, liver function studies, and lactate dehydrogenase. Obtain a chest x-ray, because some children with T-cell ALL can have an anterior mediastinal mass of leukemic cells. If fever or clinical suspicion of infection is present, obtain a blood and urine culture. **Although almost all children with leukemia have some form of hematologic abnormality including anemia, thrombocytopenia, leukocytosis, or neutropenia, very few have an extremely elevated WBC.** Total WBC counts are often normal or only moderately elevated. Hyperleukocytosis is more likely in patients with AML and in infants with either ALL or AML.[15] Definitive diagnosis requires a bone marrow aspirate.

The differential diagnosis of children with marrow suppression includes aplastic anemia, profound iron deficiency anemia (commonly noted in toddlers with excessive milk intake), viral infections (Epstein-Barr virus [EBV], cytomegalovirus [CMV], parvovirus B19), primary immune thrombocytopenia, and rheumatologic diseases. A good rule of thumb is that leukemias commonly involve abnormalities in more than one cell line, whereas other conditions are often restricted to a single cell line.

TREATMENT

The goal is to induce remission while minimizing treatment toxicity. Taking into consideration age and leukocyte count at the time of diagnosis, as well as other risk factors (e.g., genetic abnormalities of leukemic cells with important prognostic significance), children with ALL are usually stratified into different treatment groups.[16] Children with AML receive intensive multiagent chemotherapy. Molecularly targeted therapeutic approaches are in development.[12,17] Some receive hematopoietic stem cell transplantation. **Table 143-1** lists common chemotherapeutic agents used in pediatric oncology and their most common adverse effects.

DISEASE COMPLICATIONS

Most children suspected of having leukemia are stable and receive an initial diagnostic workup (see "Diagnosis" section) but no acute treatment. Occasionally, acute treatment is needed for cytopenias, hyperleukocytosis, coagulopathy, electrolyte abnormalities, and infection. Select treatment after consultation with a pediatric oncologist.

Anemia Anemia is extremely common and multifactorial, including impaired hematopoiesis due to leukemic marrow infiltration, decreased erythropoietin levels, iron deficiency, hemolysis, occult blood loss, and chronic inflammation. There is no universally recommended threshold for transfusion, and in the ED, the decision to transfuse should depend more on the appearance and clinical condition of the child than on any particular laboratory value.[18] Life-threatening hemorrhage, symptomatic anemia, or rapidly consumptive coagulopathy requires transfusion, with the addition of factor replacement as needed. The general goals of transfusion therapy are to raise the hemoglobin level to >8 to 10 grams/dL, depending on the child's condition.[8] However, in the setting of profound anemia and hyperleukocytosis, transfuse to a much lower level to minimize the effect on blood viscosity. The exact numbers will often depend on institutional protocols (see discussion on transfusion below under "Blood Products").

Thrombocytopenia Mild to moderate bruising, petechiae, and/or mucosal bleeding may occur with platelet counts <20,000/mm^3, but the risk of spontaneous intracranial hemorrhage is extremely low until the platelet count dips to <5000/mm^3. **Most protocols reserve prophylactic platelet transfusions in asymptomatic patients to platelet counts <10,000/mm^3 in the absence of other bleeding risk factors. Invasive procedures require a platelet count >50,000/mm^3[3,8,19] and the platelet count should exceed 50,000 to 100,000/mm^3 for surgeries or procedures with bleeding risks.[20]**

Disseminated Intravascular Coagulation Disseminated intravascular coagulation (DIC) is commonly associated with AML. Some subtypes release a procoagulant tissue factor that can lead to a life-threatening consumptive coagulopathy. ED treatment includes replacement of platelets, depleted coagulation factors, fibrinogen with fresh frozen plasma, and cryoprecipitate.

Blood Products A unit of packed red blood cells has a volume of about 250 mL and a hematocrit of 70% to 80%. The typical volume of packed red blood cells given to a child is 10 to 15 mL/kg. Generally, 10 mL/kg of packed red blood cells is expected to raise the hemoglobin level 3 grams/dL in a patient without active hemorrhage.

A dose of platelets is 0.1 unit/kg random donor equivalent units and is expected to raise the platelet count by 30,000 to 50,000/mm^3.[8,20,21] Some institutions release platelets as single apheresis units versus random donor units. Platelets express ABO antigens, and, even though platelets do not express Rh antigens, Rh-negative donors are used for Rh-negative patients because red blood cell contamination may result in Rh alloimmunization. Rh immunoglobulin can be given if Rh-negative

TABLE 143-1 Common Chemotherapy Agents and Their Side Effects

Chemotherapeutic Agent	Common Indications	Common Adverse Effects
Doxorubicin (Adriamycin)	NHL, HL, ALL, AML, neuroblastoma, sarcomas, Wilms' tumor	Myelosuppression, mucositis, cardiomyopathy (acute and chronic), arrhythmia, radiation dermatitis, red urine (from drug), vomiting
Bleomycin	Testicular cancer, germ cell tumor, HL	Pneumonitis, pulmonary fibrosis, vomiting, mucositis
Carboplatin	Germ cell tumors, sarcomas, neuroblastoma, CNS tumors	Myelosuppression (especially platelets), nephrotoxicity, vomiting
Carmustine (bis-chloronitrosourea)	NHL, HL, CNS tumors	Pulmonary fibrosis, stomatitis, myelosuppression
Cisplatin	Testicular cancer, germ cell tumor, lymphoma, osteosarcoma, CNS tumors	Nephrotoxicity, myelosuppression, peripheral neuropathy, vomiting
Cyclophosphamide	NHL, HL, ALL, neuroblastoma, retinoblastoma, soft tissue sarcoma, Ewing's sarcoma	Hemorrhagic cystitis, myelosuppression, vomiting, nephrotoxicity
Cytarabine (cytosine arabinoside)	ALL, AML, NHL	Myelosuppression, seizure, ataxia/encephalopathy, mucositis, typhlitis, vomiting
Actinomycin-D (dactinomycin)	Testicular cancer, sarcomas, Wilms' tumor	Myelosuppression, veno-occlusive disease, vomiting, mucositis
Daunorubicin	ALL, AML	Red urine, myelosuppression, cardiomyopathy, vomiting, arrhythmias, mucositis
Etoposide	Testicular cancer, ALL, AML, NHL, HL, CNS tumors, neuroblastoma, sarcomas	Myelosuppression, vomiting, mucositis
Ifosfamide	Ewing's sarcoma, various refractory tumors	Hemorrhagic cystitis, myelosuppression, encephalopathy, nephrotoxicity, vomiting
L-Asparaginase; pegaspargase	ALL, AML, lymphoma	Venous thrombosis/cerebrovascular accident, pancreatitis, coagulopathy, platelet dysfunction
6-Mercaptopurine	ALL, NHL	Hepatic dysfunction, myelosuppression, mucositis
Methotrexate	ALL, osteosarcoma, NHL	Myelosuppression, renal toxicity, stroke-like syndrome, hepatitis, photosensitivity, mucositis, vomiting
Thioguanine	ALL, AML	Myelosuppression, mucositis, veno-occlusive disease
Vinblastine	Testicular cancer, HL, histiocytosis	Mucositis, myelosuppression, constipation
Vincristine	AML, ALL, HL, NHL, Wilms' tumor, sarcomas, neuroblastoma	Constipation, peripheral neuropathy, syndrome of inappropriate secretion of antidiuretic hormone/hyponatremia, veno-occlusive disease

Abbreviations: ALL = acute lymphoblastic leukemia; AML = acute myelogenous leukemia; CNS = central nervous system; HL = Hodgkin's lymphoma; NHL = non-Hodgkin's lymphoma.

TABLE 143-2 Transfusion of Blood Products in Children

Blood Product Component	Volume	Dose	Typical Transfusion Goals*
Packed red blood cells	Citrate phosphate dextrose adenine, 1 unit = 250 mL†	10 mL/kg increases Hb by 3 grams/dL	Hb, 8–10 grams/dL
	Adsol, 1 unit = 350 mL†	12.5–15.0 mL/kg increases Hb by 3 grams/dL	
Platelets	One apheresis unit = 200–400 mL‡	0.1 unit/kg increases platelets by 30,000–50,000/mm^3	50,000–100,000/mm^3
Fresh frozen plasma	1 unit = 200–250 mL (centrifuged)	20 mL/kg will replace ~50% of most coagulation factors	
	1 unit = 500 mL (apheresis)		
Cryoprecipitate	1 unit = 15 mL	0.1 unit/kg increases fibrinogen by ~50 milligrams/dL#	Fibrinogen, 100 milligrams/dL
	1 unit = 80–100 units factor VIII		
	1 unit = 150–200 milligrams fibrinogen		

Abbreviation: Hb = hemoglobin.

*Varies by clinical circumstance.

†The volume in a single unit of packed red blood cells depends on the additive/preservative used.

‡The random donor platelet unit is used when there is a shortage of apheresis units. A single random donor unit contains a volume of 50 to 70 mL. One apheresis unit = 6–8 random donor units.

#In the absence of ongoing bleeding.

platelets are unavailable. Institutions vary on the use of type-specific platelets and the need for Rh immunoglobulin (**Table 143-2**).

There are several product choices for packed red blood cells and platelets: irradiated, leukocyte reduced, and CMV seronegative (**Table 143-3**). Irradiation of blood products is recommended for profoundly immunosuppressed individuals (e.g., severe immunodeficiency, high-dose chemotherapy, post–bone marrow transplant). Many pediatric cancer centers will transfuse only irradiated blood to *all* oncology patients. Consult with the pediatric oncologist for specific directions before administering blood products.

Hyperleukocytosis Hyperleukocytosis is a WBC >100,000/mm^3. Leukocytosis can cause leukostasis, tumor lysis syndrome, and DIC.[22] **Leukostasis is a clinical diagnosis.** Intravascular aggregations of leukocytes lead to injury of the lungs and CNS most commonly, but can affect other organs as well. In the cerebral circulation, symptoms and signs include headache, mental status changes, visual changes, seizures, and stroke (ischemic and hemorrhagic), whereas in the pulmonary circulation, leukostasis can cause dyspnea, hypoxemia, and respiratory failure. Chest radiographs may be normal or may show a diffuse, nonspecific interstitial infiltrate. AML patients are especially at risk because their leukemic blasts are larger, "stickier," and more rigid.

ED treatment consists of aggressive IV hydration and treatment of tumor lysis syndrome (see discussion in "Tumor Lysis Syndrome" section and Table 143-5). **Avoid treatments that increase blood viscosity such as diuretics and packed red blood cell transfusions.** Platelets do not increase blood viscosity and should be administered for levels <20,000/mm^3 to decrease the risk of cerebral hemorrhage. Leukapheresis is a temporizing measure until definitive antileukemic therapy can be given.

HODGKIN'S LYMPHOMA

EPIDEMIOLOGY

Hodgkin's lymphoma is a lymphoid neoplasm characterized by progressive enlargement of lymph nodes. Age distribution is bimodal, with peaks in young adulthood and older-aged adults. It is the most common malignancy in adolescents between the ages of 15 and 19 years old.[4] Risk factors include EBV (particularly in developing countries) and human immunodeficiency virus.

CLINICAL FEATURES AND DIAGNOSIS

Hodgkin's lymphoma typically presents with painless, firm, "rubbery" lymph nodes, usually cervical or supraclavicular (**Figure 143-1**). If empiric antibiotics are prescribed for presumptive cervical adenitis, the mass continues to increase in size. The lack of overlying erythema and the absence of pain suggest lymphoma. **Systemic "B" symptoms (fever >38°C [100.4°F], night sweats, and weight loss ≥10% over 6 months) are present in 39% to 50% of children and adolescents.**[23,24] Pulmonary symptoms such as cough, stridor, dysphagia, or dyspnea suggest mediastinal involvement, present in two thirds of pediatric patients at the time of diagnosis.[25] Obtain a chest x-ray. Hepatomegaly or splenomegaly can be found due to hematogenous spread. A CT of the soft tissues of the neck, chest, abdomen, and pelvis will help delineate the extent of disease. Subdiaphragmatic primary disease is uncommon; more than 97% of Hodgkin's lymphoma patients present with a lesion above the diaphragm.[23]

The differential diagnosis of cervical lymphadenopathy is extensive. See chapter 122, "Neck Masses in Infants and Children." Diagnosis is confirmed by lymph node biopsy.

TABLE 143-3 Blood Component Therapy

Treatment	Description	Goal	Target Recipient
Leukodepleted blood	99.9% reduction in donor WBCs	Reduces incidence of febrile nonhemolytic transfusion reactions Decreases sensitization to HLA-1 antigens Significantly reduces transmission of CMV*	Patients likely to receive multiple platelet or packed red blood cell transfusions in future
CMV-seronegative blood	Gold standard for CMV-negative blood	Eliminates transmission of CMV*	Patients at high risk for CMV-related complications now or in the future
Irradiated blood	Destroys donor lymphocytes' ability to multiply	Prevent transfusion-associated graft-versus-host disease from donor WBCs (does not prevent CMV transmission)	Profoundly immunocompromised patients Stem cell transplant patients

Abbreviations: CMV = cytomegalovirus; HLA-1 = human leukocyte antigen 1.

*Patients at high risk for CMV-related complications include patients receiving stem cell or solid organ transplants and the severely immunocompromised.

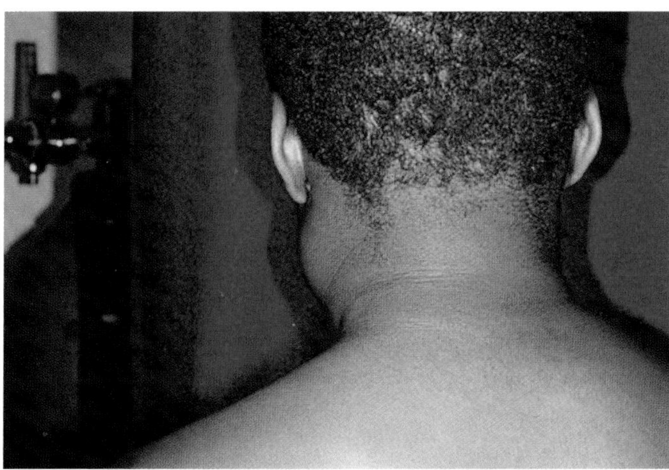

FIGURE 143-1. Hodgkin's lymphoma. A 13-year-old adolescent male presented with a painless, rubbery, firm cervical lymphadenopathy of 4 months' duration. [Reproduced with permission from Shah BR, Lucchesi M: *Atlas of Pediatric Emergency Medicine*, © 2006, McGraw-Hill, New York.]

TREATMENT

ED treatment before confirmatory diagnosis is usually directed at acute complications such as superior vena cava syndrome or upper airway compression (see "Complications of Pediatric Cancer and Oncologic Emergencies" section, below). **Use caution with sedation, given the risk of airway compromise with mediastinal involvement.** The need for admission is individualized. **Do not give steroids to patients with significant lymphadenopathy if lymphoma is in the differential diagnosis.** Following risk categorization, therapeutic management of Hodgkin's lymphoma incorporates chemotherapy and radiotherapy. Significant toxicities, including cardiac, pulmonary, thyroid, and second malignant tumors in long-term survivors, prompted modification of existing protocols to decrease the radiation and chemotherapy exposure while maintaining good outcomes.[25-27]

NON-HODGKIN'S LYMPHOMA

EPIDEMIOLOGY

Non-Hodgkin's lymphoma accounts for 7% of cancer in children and adolescents in the United States, with little variation by age.[28] Non-Hodgkin's lymphoma includes a heterogeneous group of malignant neoplasms that can originate not only in the lymphatic system but in almost any organ in the body, including the skin, cortical bone, GI tract, and CNS. There is a male predominance,[1] and the majority of cases have no known cause. Immunodeficiencies and previous exposure to immunosuppressive agents are known risk factors. In equatorial Africa, non-Hodgkin's lymphoma accounts for almost 50% of childhood cancers and is almost universally associated with EBV.[29] That association exists to a much lesser degree in developed countries.

CLINICAL FEATURES AND DIAGNOSIS

The clinical presentation depends on the site and extent of disease. Constitutional symptoms are not common. Lymphadenopathy, a mass in virtually any location, hepatosplenomegaly, and cytopenias can all be seen. GI manifestations occur with abdominal tumors (usually Burkitt's lymphoma). Mediastinal involvement may lead to pleural or pericardial effusions, upper airway obstruction from mass effect, respiratory symptoms, or superior vena cava syndrome (see "Complications of Pediatric Cancer and Oncologic Emergencies" section, below). Testicular, skin, and CNS or spinal manifestations are seen, but less commonly. The differential diagnosis is broad and includes infectious (tuberculosis, toxoplasmosis, EBV, *Bartonella henselae*, human immunodeficiency virus) and oncologic (Hodgkin's lymphoma, leukemia, rhabdomyosarcoma) processes. Diagnosis is by biopsy.

TREATMENT

Initial workup should include basic laboratory studies and a chest x-ray to evaluate for mediastinal disease. If there is concern for intra-abdominal obstruction (bowel or ureteral), ultrasonography or other imaging (e.g., abdominal and pelvic CT) may be indicated. CT can also further evaluate for chest mass or superior vena cava syndrome. Treatment is multiagent chemotherapy.

CENTRAL NERVOUS SYSTEM TUMORS

EPIDEMIOLOGY

CNS tumors are the second most common pediatric cancer and the most common solid tumor in childhood, accounting for approximately 21% of all pediatric cancers.[4] They are also the leading cause of cancer-related death in children.[30] Survival is worse for infants and young children.[31] For the emergency physician, the specifics of the tumor type are less important than tumor location and clinical effects.

The three most common categories of pediatric CNS tumors are astrocytomas, medulloblastomas, and ependymomas. For most, the cause is unknown.[32] Specific genetic syndromes, including neurofibromatosis, tuberous sclerosis, and Li-Fraumeni syndrome, are predisposing factors. CNS tumors can also be secondary to high-dose cranial radiation for a previously treated childhood cancer.

CLINICAL FEATURES AND DIAGNOSIS

There is heterogeneity in the presentation of CNS neoplasms depending on the location and extent of the tumor and the age of the child. Tumors can be infratentorial or supratentorial but are more often infratentorial in children. Symptoms are often nonspecific (headache, irritability, emesis, behavioral changes), which can delay diagnosis.

The classic presentation of a posterior fossa tumor or other tumors causing obstructive hydrocephalus is **early morning headache** and subsequent vomiting. These symptoms are believed to be due to a rise in intracranial pressure during sleep caused by hypoventilation (hypercarbia causes increased cerebral blood flow) and increased cerebral blood volume in the recumbent position. **Although patients with brain tumors commonly have headaches, children with headaches are *not* statistically likely to have a brain tumor.**[33] Additional clinical signs such as a bulging fontanelle, rapidly increasing head circumference in an infant (from hydrocephalus), sunsetting (preferential downward gaze due to obstructive dilatation of the third ventricle with resultant tectal pressure and paresis of upward gaze), cranial nerve palsies (most commonly the sixth nerve), papilledema, or somnolence also suggest increased intracranial pressure.[34] Infiltration of the brainstem can produce cranial nerve deficits, long tract corticospinal motor weakness, and cerebellar ataxia.

Symptoms of supratentorial neoplasms are dictated by location and include headache, endocrinopathies, declines in school performance, personality changes, motor weakness, and seizures. Craniopharyngiomas arise in the sellar region and produce visual changes due to their proximity to the optic chiasm, as well as significant endocrinologic abnormalities from hypothalamic dysfunction (including diabetes insipidus, stunted growth and sexual development, and hypothyroidism).

TREATMENT

Most CNS malignancies are identifiable on CT, but MRI provides superior visualization of the tumor and the posterior fossa. The most serious threat is increased intracranial pressure leading to herniation. The treatment of increased intracranial pressure is addressed below in "Complications of Pediatric Cancer and Oncologic Emergencies." Treat acute seizures. Give IV dexamethasone to treat vasogenic edema surrounding the tumor (see "Increased Intracranial Pressure" section, below). Consult with neurosurgery and pediatric oncology to arrange definitive treatment.

NEUROBLASTOMA

EPIDEMIOLOGY

Neuroblastoma is a malignant tumor that arises from primitive ganglion cells of the sympathetic nervous system. It accounts for 7% of all childhood cancers and is the most common solid extracranial tumor of childhood and the most common neoplasm in the first year of life.[4,35]

CLINICAL FEATURES

The clinical features are highly variable and depend on tumor size and location. Neuroblastoma may arise anywhere along the sympathetic nervous system; the adrenal gland is the most common primary site, but it may also arise from other intra-abdominal sites, the chest, and the neck. Metastasis is quite common (through circulatory or lymphatic channels) to adjacent lymph nodes, liver, skin, bone, and bone marrow.

The variability in tumor location and extent explains the array of signs and symptoms that may lead to the diagnosis of neuroblastoma. One presentation is a painless abdominal mass. Mass effect from the tumor can lead to compression of the bowel, bladder, venous, or lymphatic structures. Thoracic masses can also lead to compression, causing respiratory distress or superior vena cava syndrome. Paravertebral tumors can invade the spinal canal, causing spinal cord compression. Horner's syndrome (ptosis, miosis, and anhidrosis) may result from disease involving the superior cervical ganglion.

Unique presentations of neuroblastoma that require a high index of suspicion include proptosis and periorbital ecchymoses ("raccoon eyes") or swelling, characteristic of orbital neuroblastoma metastases. Neuroblastoma is the most common primary childhood cancer to metastasize to the orbits, and orbital findings can be the primary manifestation of the tumor.[36] Opsoclonus-myoclonus is a paraneoplastic syndrome also highly associated with occult neuroblastoma.

DIAGNOSIS AND TREATMENT

Obtain basic laboratory studies. Cytopenias suggest bone marrow involvement. X-rays, US, or CT in the ED may detect an intra-abdominal or thoracic mass. Because neuroblastomas often lead to increased levels of catecholamines, the metabolites of which are detectable in the urine, urine homovanillic acid and vanillylmandelic acid can aid in diagnosis. Bone marrow and tumor biopsies confirm the diagnosis.

Treatment includes surgical resection and/or radiation therapy and chemotherapy. Some undergo stem cell transplants.

WILMS' TUMOR (NEPHROBLASTOMA)

EPIDEMIOLOGY

Wilms' tumor, or nephroblastoma, is a malignant embryonal renal tumor that affects children predominantly under the age of 5 years.[4] Overall survival rates are excellent, at approximately 90%.[37]

CLINICAL FEATURES

The classic presentation of Wilms' tumor is an asymptomatic abdominal mass, sometimes noted while dressing or bathing the child. **Vigorous or excessive palpation of the mass can cause tumor rupture.** As opposed to neuroblastoma (given that the age group and abdominal mass at the time of presentation can be similar), children often appear remarkably well with no systemic symptoms. Metastases at the time of diagnosis are uncommon, but can occur to the lungs, liver, or lymph nodes. Hypertension due to increased renin production is present in 25% of cases.[38] Less common symptoms include anorexia, weight loss, emesis, hematuria, or abdominal discomfort. There can be significant mass effect from the tumor, leading to respiratory distress or intra-abdominal obstruction.

DIAGNOSIS AND TREATMENT

The differential diagnosis includes benign hydronephrosis, neuroblastoma, hepatoblastoma, lymphoma, sarcoma, and germ cell tumors.[39] Ultrasonography is appropriate for initial abdominal imaging in the ED.

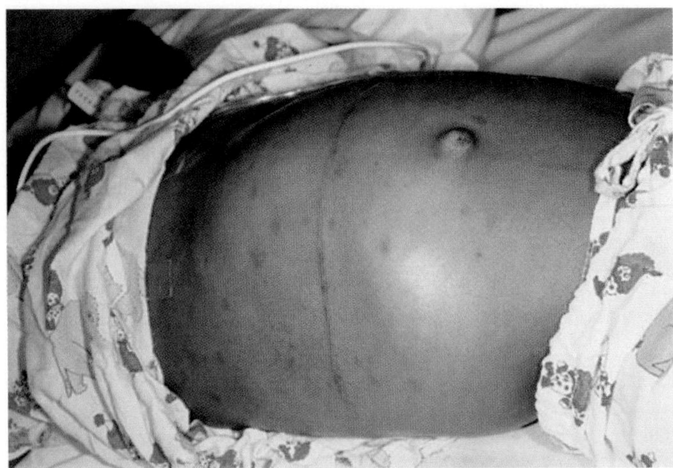

A

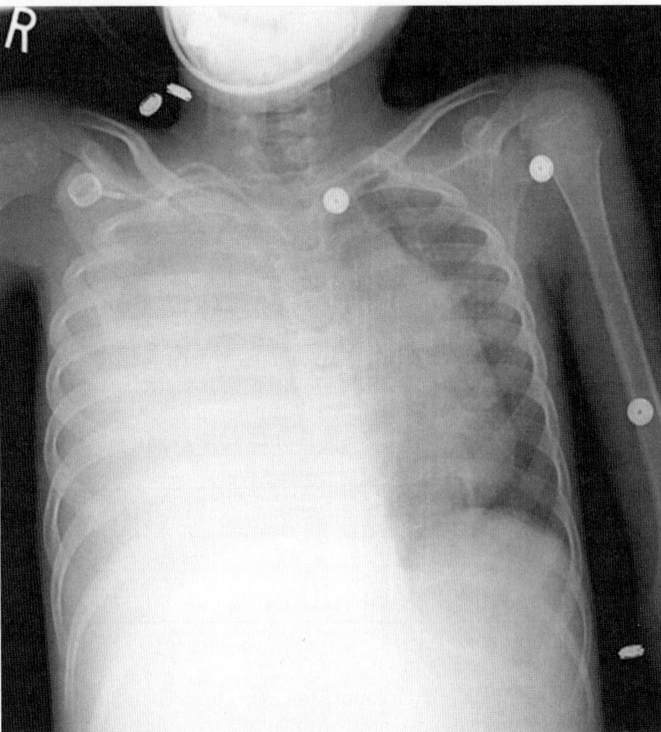

B

FIGURE 143-2. Wilms' tumor. **A.** A 7-year-old child presented with a huge abdominal mass and respiratory distress. Pelvic CT scan followed by laparotomy confirmed the mass as Wilms' tumor. Because of the retroperitoneal location of the kidney, these tumors can be quite large at diagnosis without significant impingement of other vital structures. **B.** Right-sided pleural effusion due to metastatic disease. Almost complete opacification of the right hemithorax with mediastinal shift to the left. [Reproduced with permission from Shah BR, Lucchesi M: *Atlas of Pediatric Emergency Medicine*, © 2006, McGraw-Hill, New York.]

Obtain a chest x-ray to identify pulmonary metastases (**Figure 143-2**). Obtain basic laboratory studies, urine catecholamines to rule out neuroblastoma, and urinalysis. CT or MRI identifies the extent of the disease. Definitive treatment is surgical resection and chemotherapy, with or without radiation therapy.

RETINOBLASTOMA

EPIDEMIOLOGY

Retinoblastoma is the most common pediatric intraocular malignancy.[36] Ninety percent of cases are diagnosed in children younger than 3 years of age.[40] There are both heritable and nonheritable forms, and the majority

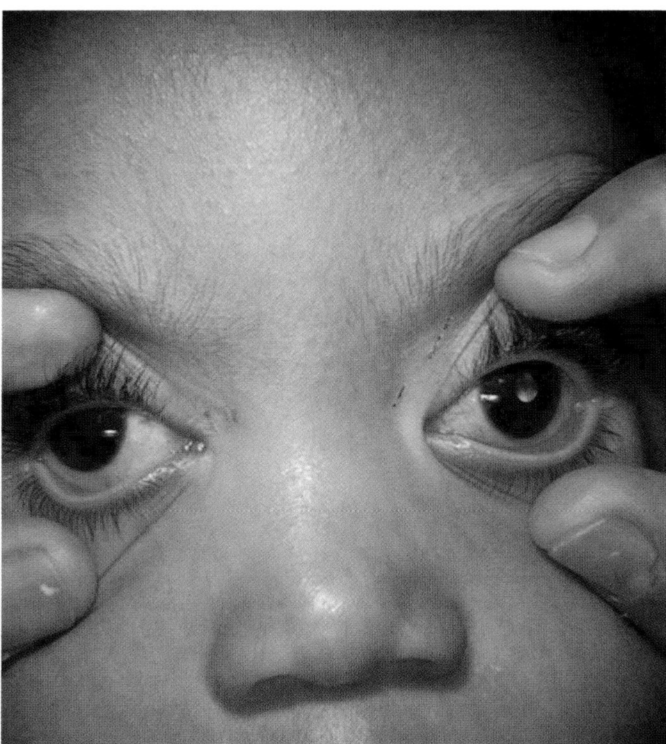

FIGURE 143-3. Leukocoria in retinoblastoma. An 18-month-old child presenting with a left-sided white pupil. [Reproduced with permission from Shah BR, Lucchesi M: *Atlas of Pediatric Emergency Medicine*, © 2006, McGraw-Hill, New York.]

of cases of nonheritable disease are unilateral. The retinoblastoma (*RB*) gene was the first tumor suppressor gene discovered in the human genome.[41] Heritable forms are usually due to a germline mutation in the *RB1* gene and present within the first year of life with bilateral disease.

CLINICAL FEATURES

Leukocoria ("white pupil"), in which the white light reflects off of the tumor instead of red light reflecting off of the retina, is the most common presenting sign (**Figure 143-3**). This may be noted by a primary physician or occasionally by family members when they note the leukocoria in photographs. Other signs may include strabismus, decreased visual acuity, redness, pain, glaucoma, and proptosis (late stage). Young children do not often report visual complaints. The retinoblastoma can spread into the surrounding orbit, as well as metastasize into the CNS and viscera.[36]

DIAGNOSIS AND TREATMENT

If leukocoria or other signs suggestive of an intraocular tumor are noted, consult ophthalmology in the ED. Definitive diagnosis is usually obtained by exam and imaging under anesthesia. Obtain a CT or MRI if there is evidence of orbital inflammation. Treatment options depend on the extent of the disease and include enucleation, chemotherapy, cryotherapy, brachytherapy, thermotherapy, radiotherapy, and laser photocoagulation.[42]

GERM CELL TUMORS

EPIDEMIOLOGY

Germ cell tumors are a heterogenous group of neoplasms that can develop in males and females at any age, although they are more common in adolescents and young adults.[4,43] Extragonadal tumor locations, including sacrococcygeal, mediastinal, and intracranial, are more common in young children, whereas during and after puberty, the primary location is the gonads.[43]

Testicular germ cell tumors are the most common solid tumor in young adult men (**Figure 143-4**).[44] **An undescended testicle increases the risk for testicular cancer 10- to 50-fold.**[45] Prognosis for these tumors is extremely good, even if metastases are present, with an overall cure rate of 85% to 90%.[44] Despite that fact, they remain a significant cause of death in young males. This highlights the importance of encouraging young male patients to perform testicular self-examinations. The median age of diagnosis for ovarian germ cell tumors is 16 to 20 years.[46] Due to the intra-abdominal location, ovarian tumors may go undetected for a longer amount of time than testicular tumors; this increases the potential for rupture.[47]

CLINICAL FEATURES

Testicular tumors typically present with an asymptomatic, nontender testicular mass. Ovarian tumors are most likely to present with abdominal pain (85%).[46] Other ovarian symptoms include abdominal distention, vaginal bleeding, and weight gain. Ten percent of patients with ovarian tumors presenting with abdominal pain from tumor rupture, hemorrhage, or torsion are misdiagnosed.[46] Tumors can metastasize, most commonly to the lymph nodes, liver, lungs, and CNS.

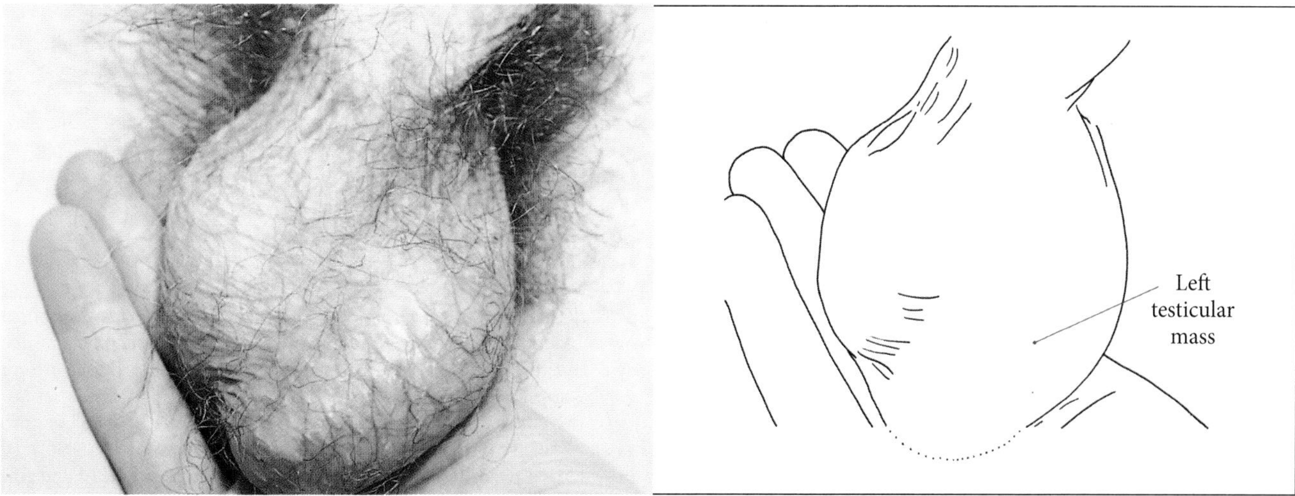

FIGURE 143-4. Testicular tumor. This patient presented with a painless left testicular mass highly suspicious for cancer. [Photo contributed by Patrick McKenna, MD. Reproduced with permission from Knoop K, Stack L, Storrow A, Thurman RJ: *Atlas of Emergency Medicine*, 3rd ed. © 2010, McGraw-Hill, New York.]

DIAGNOSIS AND TREATMENT

A testicular mass or abdominal mass may be palpated upon exam. Ultrasonography identifies an ovarian or scrotal mass. CT delineates the extent of disease. Serum tumor markers can be added to the basic laboratory tests. Treatment includes resection, chemotherapy, and/or radiotherapy. Given that many patients are of reproductive age, treatment attempts to preserve fertility if possible.

BONE AND SOFT TISSUE SARCOMAS

The term *sarcoma* refers to a diverse group of malignant neoplasms derived from mesenchymal cell origin that can arise from virtually any location at any age. Sarcomas are divided into two main types: soft tissue sarcomas and bone sarcomas. There are over 70 recognized subtypes. The most common subtypes diagnosed in pediatrics are rhabdomyosarcoma, osteosarcoma, and Ewing's sarcoma.

RHABDOMYOSARCOMA

Rhabdomyosarcoma accounts for 3% of childhood cancers and 2% of adolescent cancers.[4] Risk factors include a number of inherited cancer predisposition syndromes (e.g., Li-Fraumeni, neurofibromatosis type I). The embryonal subtype (>75% of cases) is most common in children <5 years old, tends to occur in the head and neck, and has a better prognosis. The alveolar subtype can occur at any age, is more aggressive, and is commonly found in the trunk or extremities. Orbital rhabdomyosarcoma accounts for 10% of all rhabdomyosarcoma cases.[36]

Signs and symptoms depend on location, but a painless mass is characteristic. Evaluation in the ED may begin with ultrasonography. More extensive evaluation steps are determined by the oncologist. Treatment includes a combination of surgical excision, chemotherapy, and radiotherapy.

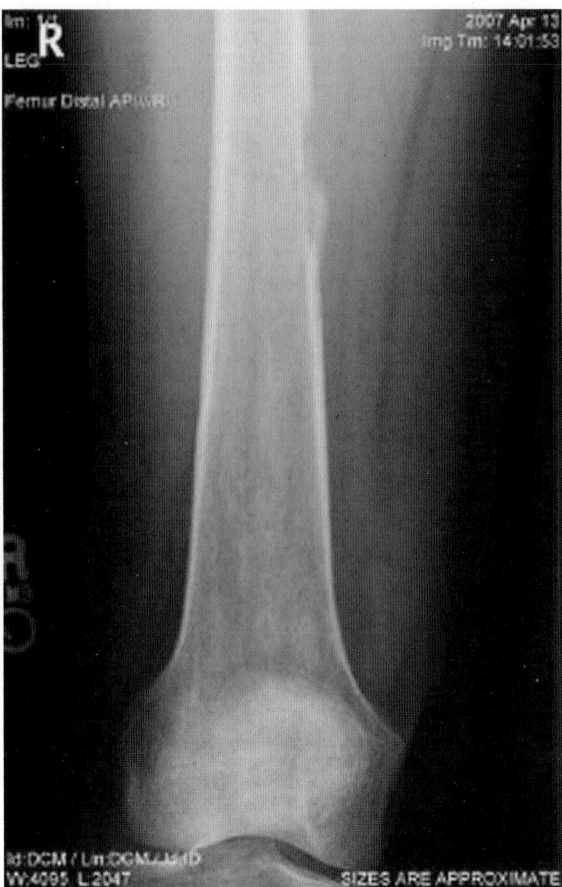

FIGURE 143-5. Osteosarcoma. Note the lytic femoral lesion with cortical destruction.

OSTEOSARCOMA

Osteosarcoma, also called *osteogenic sarcoma*, is the most common primary pediatric bone tumor and is among the most frequent causes of cancer-related death.[48] Incidence peaks in adolescence, particularly during a growth spurt. It can occur in any bone, but the majority of cases arise from the metaphyses of long bones. Over half of cases originate near the knee joint, either at the distal femur or at the proximal tibia.[49] Twenty percent of patients have metastases at the time of diagnosis, most commonly in the lungs, followed by bone.[4] Previous radiation during treatment for a different pediatric neoplasm increases the risk of osteosarcoma, as do several genetic syndromes.

Nonspecific symptoms can lead to a delay in diagnosis. The most common presentation is an adolescent with **persistent bone pain that worsens at night or with activity**. Soft tissue swelling may be noted on exam.

Diagnosis is suggested by plain radiography (**Figure 143-5**). The radiograph may demonstrate a lytic lesion with cortical destruction near the metaphysis. The classic radiographic finding is the "sunburst" appearance of periosteal reaction. Pathologic fracture is an uncommon presentation.[50] The differential diagnosis of radiographically similar lesions includes Ewing's sarcoma as well as more benign lesions. Diagnosis is by biopsy, and treatment includes chemotherapy and limb-sparing surgery. Osteosarcoma is radiation resistant.

EWING'S SARCOMA

Ewing's sarcoma is an aggressive tumor of uncertain origin that can occur in the bone or soft tissues. It is more common in older children and adolescents, but the incidence is half that of osteogenic sarcoma.[51] Hematogenously spread metastases are present in approximately 25% of patients at the time of diagnosis and are most commonly located in the lungs, bone, and bone marrow.[4] Metastatic disease is the most significant prognostic factor.[52]

Ewing's sarcoma typically presents with persistent pain at the tumor site. Tenderness or swelling may be noted on physical exam. The long bones (femur, tibia, humerus) and the axial skeleton (pelvis, ribs, spine) are the most common sites of disease.

Plain radiographs of the primary tumor site may reveal the characteristic "moth-eaten appearance" of the destructive lesion, or the "onion peel" appearance of the periosteal reaction (**Figure 143-6**). Diagnosis is by biopsy, and treatment is multidisciplinary, including chemotherapy and radiotherapy or surgery.

COMPLICATIONS OF PEDIATRIC CANCER AND ONCOLOGIC EMERGENCIES

For the child with cancer, the road to recovery is inevitably interrupted by complications. These complications can be generally classified as **infectious** (e.g., fever and neutropenia), **metabolic** (including tumor lysis syndrome, hypercalcemia, and the syndrome of inappropriate antidiuretic hormone secretion), and **structural** (superior vena cava syndrome, spinal cord compression, and increased intracranial pressure).

INFECTION

Most pediatric cancer patients experience an infectious complication over the course of the illness. Neutropenia is usually seen as an effect of cytotoxic therapy,[53] and many treatment protocols produce profound myelosuppression (Table 143-1).

In the context of a febrile cancer patient, "neutropenia" is defined as an absolute neutrophil count (ANC) <500/mm³ or an ANC <1000/mm³ with a predicted decline. Relative risk of infection is highest at this time. **The ANC nadir typically occurs 5 to 10 days after chemotherapy.**

Fever will occur in up to one third of neutropenic episodes, with a rate of documented infection between 10% and 40%.[54] **Fever in this setting**

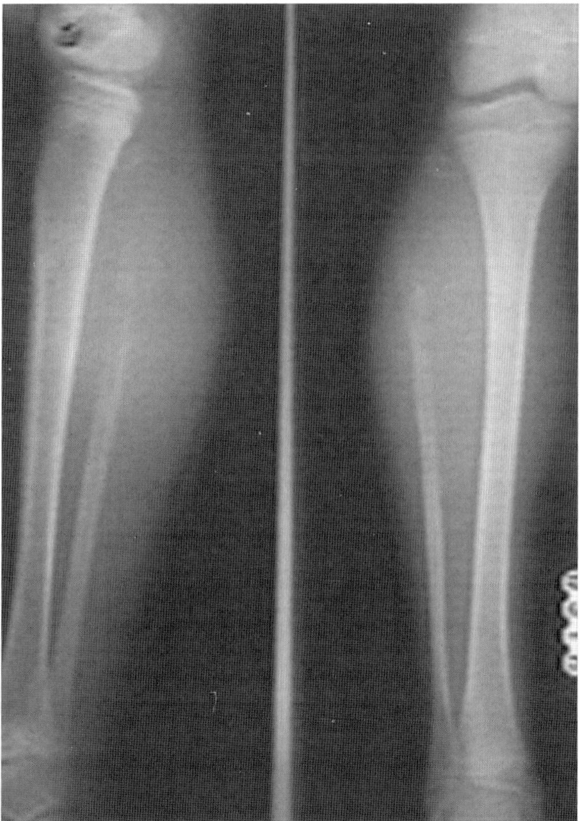

FIGURE 143-6. Ewing's sarcoma. Note the destruction of the proximal fibula.

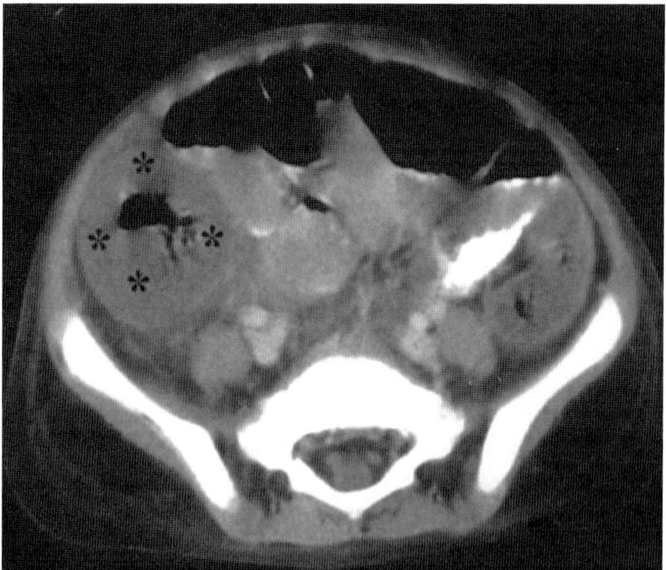

FIGURE 143-7. Neutropenic enterocolitis. *Asterisks* indicate inflamed and thickened bowel wall.

is conservatively defined as a single oral temperature >38.3°C (101°F), or multiple temperatures ≥38.0°C (100.4°F) separated by more than 1 hour.[53] Avoid rectal temperatures due to the risk of bacteremia induced by rectal trauma.

Many patients will not demonstrate a source of fever. Neutropenia, or a decrease in the ability to mount an inflammatory response, limits the development of infectious signs such as abscess, pulmonary infiltrates, or severe abdominal pain. Therefore, perform a meticulous physical examination with close attention to areas of pain, mucosal barriers, and the central line site. Chemotherapeutic regimens that produce profound neutropenia can cause severe mucositis with oral and/or perianal mucosal breakdown.

Typhlitis, or neutropenic enterocolitis, warrants particular attention (**Figure 143-7**). Inflammation usually involves the ileocecal region. The presentation can be as subtle as mild abdominal pain, and **the physical exam may be relatively unrevealing; however, maintain a high index of suspicion for infection**. Bacteremia is common and is often polymicrobial.[55] Other signs and symptoms include fever, nausea, emesis, right lower quadrant pain, abdominal distention, and watery or bloody diarrhea. Due to bowel wall necrosis, bowel perforation with resulting pneumatosis intestinalis is possible.

ED TREATMENT

Children with fever history (even if afebrile upon presentation) and potential for neutropenia require **immediate** clinical evaluation, acquisition of appropriate laboratory studies and cultures, and prompt administration of broad-spectrum antibiotics. **Table 143-4** summarizes management of neutropenic fever, including the 2012 recommendations from the International Pediatric Fever and Neutropenia Guideline Panel.[56] Individual recommendations may differ across institutions. **Administration of antibiotics in patients at high risk of neutropenia should not wait for laboratory confirmation of neutropenia.**

Obtain blood cultures, if at all possible, before administering empiric antibiotics. Anaerobic cultures are very low yield, and many institutions do not require them unless there are specific concerns for an anaerobic infection. Other diagnostic studies are patient specific (e.g., chest radiograph, stool cultures, abdominal imaging, lumbar puncture).

As shown in Table 143-4, empiric therapy for febrile neutropenia begins with broad-spectrum antibiotics directed at the most common pathogens. Antibiotic coverage can be tailored to the specific clinical situation and institutional resistance patterns and then be narrowed as more data become available. Given the high prevalence of central venous lines in this population, greater than 50% of bacteremias in neutropenic patients are caused by gram-positive bacteria.[22] The most common gram-positive organisms are coagulase-negative staphylococci, *Streptococcus viridans*, *Staphylococcus aureus*, and enterococci.[57] Gram-negative organisms, however, are known to be particularly virulent and have an association with sepsis.[58] Intestinal flora provide the source of gram-negative organisms, including *Escherichia coli*, *Klebsiella* species, *Pseudomonas aeruginosa*, and *Enterobacter* species.[57] Special infectious considerations include treatment of *Pneumocystis carinii* in the immunocompromised patient with respiratory signs and symptoms and typhlitis/mucositis warranting broader anaerobic coverage. Although cancer patients are at increased risk for fungal infections, there is little indication for beginning antifungal agents in the ED. Septic patients require immediate, broad-spectrum antipseudomonal antibiotic therapy in addition to vancomycin for coverage of gram-positive organisms. Consider adding a second agent with activity against gram-negative organisms (e.g., gentamicin) in critically ill patients.

Careful monitoring and reevaluation are essential once treatment has begun. There is recent literature regarding risk stratification of pediatric patients to determine who can safely be treated as an outpatient. The majority of patients with febrile neutropenia, however, are admitted to the hospital. The decision to discharge should only be made in consultation with the oncologist.

METABOLIC COMPLICATIONS

TUMOR LYSIS SYNDROME

Tumor lysis syndrome is a constellation of metabolic derangements resulting from the rapid turnover of tumor cells with cell lysis and subsequent release of intracellular potassium, phosphate, and uric acid. Tumor lysis syndrome is associated with rapidly proliferating malignancies, cancers with a high tumor burden, and cancers that are highly sensitive to chemotherapy such as ALL (with hyperleukocytosis), Burkitt's lymphoma, and non-Hodgkin's lymphoma. It is most commonly precipitated

TABLE 143-4 Management of Neutropenic Fever

Definition of neutropenia
Absolute neutrophil count (segs + bands) <500/mm³
Absolute neutrophil count <1000/mm³ and expected to decrease*
Definition of fever†
Oral temperature ≥38.3°C (100.9°F) once
Or
Oral temperature ≥38°C (100.4°F) >2 times, measured 1 h apart
Caveats
Some add 0.5°C (1.0°F) to axillary temperatures for oral equivalent
Confirm with oral temperature when possible
Avoid rectal temperatures
Parental history of objective fever is sufficient
Cultures‡
One culture from each central line lumen (label appropriately)
Peripheral culture in absence of central line, or if recommended by oncologist
Consider urine culture and urinalysis (clean catch or bagged)
Antibiotics#
Well-appearingƒ
Broad-spectrum antipseudomonal monotherapy with β-lactam or carbapenem
Cefepime, 50 milligrams/kg (maximum dose, 2 grams), or ceftazidime, 50 milligrams/kg (maximum dose, 2 grams), or piperacillin-tazobactam, 80 milligrams/kg (maximum dose, 3.375 grams)§
Clinically unstable, suspected resistant infection, or center with high rate of resistant pathogens
Addition of second gram-negative agent and/or glycopeptide:
As above + gentamicin, 2.5 milligrams/kg, and/or vancomycin, 15 milligrams/kg (maximum, 1 gram)
Abdominal/perirectal pain
As above + metronidazole, 7.5 milligrams/kg (maximum, 1 gram)

*Based on serial measurements or history of chemotherapy in the previous 5–10 days.
†Definitions will vary by institution.
‡Most patients will only require aerobic cultures. Consider anaerobic cultures if significant GI symptoms or visible mucositis.
#Do not wait for absolute neutrophil count results if patient is *expected* to be neutropenic.
ƒIndications for the addition of vancomycin include: relapsed acute lymphoblastic leukemia or acute myelogenous leukemia patients, significant mucositis, evidence of skin or soft tissue or line infections, and presence of orthopedic appliances.
§Ceftazidime monotherapy should not be used if there are concerns for gram-positive or resistant gram-negative infections. Use vancomycin + aztreonam for cephalosporin-allergic patients.

TABLE 143-5 Initial Management of Tumor Lysis Syndrome

Labs (repeat every 4–8 h)
CBC
Electrolytes
Renal function studies
Calcium, phosphate, magnesium
Uric acid, lactate dehydrogenase
Urinalysis
ECG
IV fluids, often at >2× maintenance
Specific therapies, if indicated
Hyperuricemia: allopurinol, 100 milligrams/m², or rasburicase,* 0.2 milligram/kg
Symptomatic hypocalcemia: calcium gluconate
Hyperkalemia: calcium/dextrose/insulin/bicarbonate
Poor urine output: Loop diuretic†

*Contraindicated in glucose-6-phosphate dehydrogenase deficiency.
†Patient must be volume replete.

by the induction of chemotherapy, but it can also be present at the time of diagnosis. Symptoms are variable but can be life-threatening, including cardiac dysrhythmias, seizures, and acute renal failure.[53]

The large quantity of intracellular contents released into the circulation can easily overwhelm the excretory capacity of the kidneys. The metabolic derangements, including hyperkalemia, hyperuricemia, hyperphosphatemia, and hypocalcemia, are exacerbated by developing renal failure. **Uric acid** is insoluble at the low pH commonly found in the renal collecting duct, and crystals may precipitate in the collecting tubules, leading to acute kidney injury.[59] **Hyperkalemia** is the most immediate threat to life and should be treated aggressively, even in the absence of overt ECG changes. Lymphoblasts contain four times more phosphate than normal lymphocytes,[60] and the resulting excess phosphate from cell lysis can bind ionized calcium, leading to hypocalcemia. In addition, calcium phosphate crystalluria and obstructive uropathy can worsen acute kidney injury. The signs, symptoms, and treatment of these electrolyte disorders are discussed in chapter 129, "Fluid and Electrolyte Therapy in Infants and Children."

Laboratory studies include CBC, renal function studies, electrolytes, calcium, phosphate, uric acid, lactate dehydrogenase, and urinalysis (**Table 143-5**). Send laboratory studies every 4 hours in high-risk patients who remain in the ED for a prolonged period of time. The ED treatment is directed at the prevention of renal failure, correction of electrolyte derangements, and reduction of uric acid levels. Coordinate management with an oncologist and include aggressive IV hydration, administration of allopurinol or recombinant urate oxidase (rasburicase) for hyperuricemia, and treatment of hyperkalemia and **symptomatic** hypocalcemia (as noted earlier, supplemental calcium can lead to calcium phosphate crystalluria). Allopurinol decreases uric acid production, whereas rasburicase promotes uric acid catabolism to a urine soluble metabolite. Rasburicase is contraindicated in glucose-6-phosphate dehydrogenase deficiency due to its potential to precipitate hemolytic anemia or methemoglobinemia.[22,53,59] Urinary alkalinization is no longer recommended.[22,59] A loop diuretic could be considered in **volume-replete patients**, because volume depletion worsens acute kidney injury. **Avoid rectal Kayexalate**, because rectal administration increases the risk of bacteremia in neutropenic patients. Refractory electrolyte abnormalities or significant acute kidney injury requires dialysis.

HYPERCALCEMIA

Hypercalcemia is uncommon in children (estimated incidence <1%) due in part to the low prevalence of the tumors most commonly responsible for this electrolyte abnormality.[61,62] There are reports of hypercalcemia associated with both hematopoietic malignancies of childhood and solid tumors, usually due to local osteolysis with bone marrow invasion or paraneoplastic secretion of parathyroid hormone–related peptide[62] and to nephropathy secondary to the malignancy or therapeutic measures. Clinical manifestations are reviewed in chapter 129. Obtain a serum ionized calcium in the ED. Treat with hydration. Discontinue predisposing factors, such as vitamin D supplementation.[62] After volume replacement, consider loop diuretics and IV bisphosphonate. Definitive treatment addresses the underlying disease.

SYNDROME OF INAPPROPRIATE ANTIDIURETIC HORMONE AND HYPONATREMIA

Causes of hyponatremia in oncology patients include chemotherapeutic agents, adjunct treatments (e.g., diuretics), clinical conditions (e.g., GI losses), and syndrome of inappropriate antidiuretic hormone secretion. Syndrome of inappropriate antidiuretic hormone secretion is the leading cause of hyponatremia in children undergoing chemotherapy or stem cell transplant.[63] Syndrome of inappropriate antidiuretic hormone secretion can result from CNS disease, infection, drug toxicity (including chemotherapy), surgical intervention for CNS tumors, and the primary malignancy. Cerebral salt wasting is also a possible cause of hyponatremia with CNS disease or following intracranial surgery.[64] **Whereas syndrome of inappropriate antidiuretic hormone secretion is characterized by euvolemia, cerebral salt wasting is characterized by volume**

depletion; this distinction is critical in the ED setting, where inappropriate fluid administration could be catastrophic.

Patients may be asymptomatic, with hyponatremia incidentally noted on routine laboratory studies. Signs and symptoms of profound hyponatremia include fatigue, lethargy, confusion, coma, and seizures. The presentation depends on the rate and severity of the decline in sodium level. **Treatment must be tailored to the patient's underlying cause of hyponatremia.** Guidelines for ED management of hyponatremia are outlined in chapter 129. For syndrome of inappropriate antidiuretic hormone secretion, treatment consists of fluid restriction and slow sodium correction to prevent inducing central pontine myelinolysis. For hypovolemic hyponatremic patients, isotonic fluids are administered. **Treat acutely symptomatic patients with 3% normal saline.**

SUPERIOR VENA CAVA AND SUPERIOR MEDIASTINAL SYNDROMES

Superior vena cava syndrome is the result of compression or obstruction of the superior vena cava causing impaired venous return (**Figure 143-8**). Over 90% of cases are attributable directly to malignancy,[59] but infection and thrombus are additional causes. Superior mediastinal syndrome is superior vena cava syndrome with associated tracheal compression. These two terms are used interchangeably in children, because mediastinal pathology often leads to both.[65] Although these entities are rare, the most common pediatric malignancies presenting with superior mediastinal syndrome are non-Hodgkin's lymphoma, ALL, neuroblastoma, and germ cell tumors.[66]

The signs and symptoms of superior mediastinal syndrome are dictated by the acuity and extent of the underlying process. Some patients are asymptomatic, but young children are at particular risk due to the small size and compliance of the airway.[67] Signs and symptoms include dyspnea, cough, stridor, wheezing, chest discomfort, facial and upper body edema and/or plethora, neck/chest vein dilatation, presence of collateral veins, and syncope (from decreased cardiac output). **The threat of acute cardiorespiratory failure makes this a true medical emergency.** Equally concerning are neurologic symptoms suggestive of cerebral ischemia: headache, confusion, and altered mental status.[68]

ED treatment depends on the clinical acuity. Confirm the diagnosis by chest x-ray or CT scan. Supine positioning for imaging may critically compromise the airway, so a prone position is a preferred alternative for older, cooperative children. **Avoid any intervention, such as sedation, that could potentially compromise the airway. Superior mediastinal syndrome is one of the few conditions in which rapid sequence induction and intubation for respiratory distress may be lethal if the endotracheal tube cannot bypass the site of compression.** Temporizing measures include elevating the head of the bed to maintain an upright posture, high-flow oxygen, bilevel positive airway pressure, and possible consideration of heliox where available. Definitive management is treatment of the underlying malignancy to reduce the amount of compression. In cases where the syndrome is due to thrombotic occlusion, fibrinolytic therapy can be considered. Emergency stents have been placed at centers with appropriate expertise.[68]

NEUROLOGIC EMERGENCIES

SPINAL CORD COMPRESSION

Tumors involving the spine or spinal cord account for only 2% of childhood malignancies, but due to delays in diagnosis and deficits that are not always reversible, they are associated with a disproportionate degree of morbidity.[69] The most common neoplasms involving the spinal cord are CNS tumors, neuroblastoma, sarcomas, lymphoma, and germ cell tumors. Spinal cord compression can present in a child with known malignancy or as an initial presentation of disease. Most commonly, spinal cord compression arises from a hematogenously spread metastasis to vertebral bodies, with subsequent expansion and erosion of the lesion into the epidural space (**Figure 143-9**).[68] However, it can also

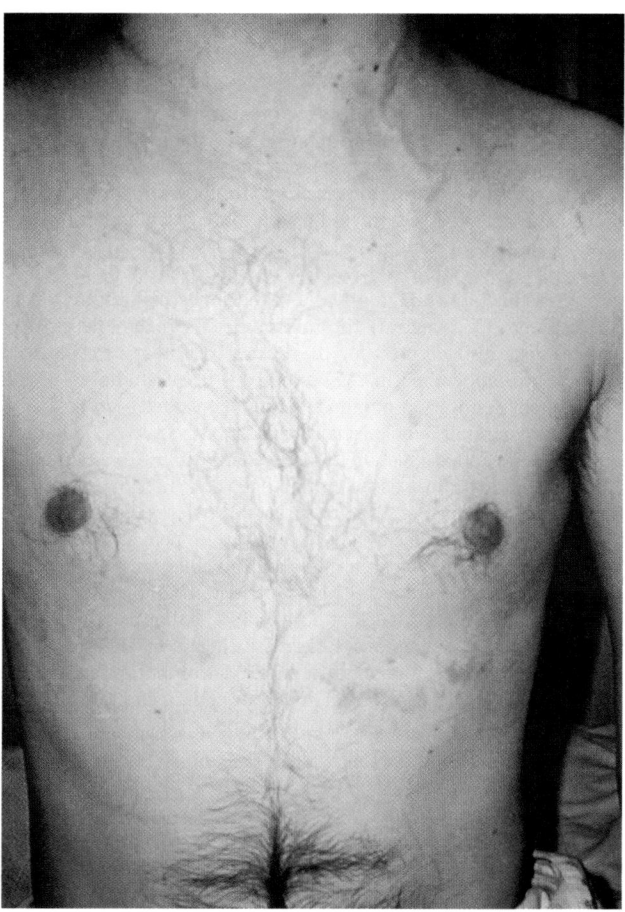

FIGURE 143-8. Superior vena cava syndrome. Note the prominent collateral veins of the chest and neck. [Photo contributed by William K. Mallon, MD. Reproduced with permission from Knoop K, Stack L, Storrow A, Thurman RJ: *Atlas of Emergency Medicine*, 3rd ed. © 2010, McGraw-HIll, New York.]

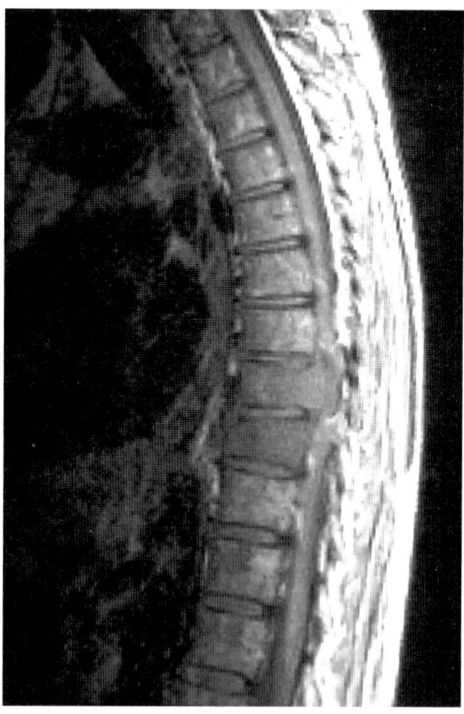

FIGURE 143-9. Spinal cord compression. MRI demonstrating spinal cord compression at T9 due to epidural extension of tumor. T10 vertebral body also has metastasis (decreased signal intensity). [Reproduced with permission from Schwartz D (ed). *Emergency Radiology: Case Studies*. Copyright © 2008 by The McGraw-Hill Companies, Inc., New York, New York.]

result from direct extension of a paravertebral tumor through an intervertebral foramen into the spinal canal.

Back pain is the most common presenting symptom of spinal cord compression in children and adults and often precedes other symptoms, providing an opportunity for early detection and intervention.[59,68,69] If the diagnosis is delayed, progressive symptoms include motor weakness, worsening scoliosis, and gait disturbance. Sensory impairments and sphincter dysfunction are extremely rare in young children. **Consider spinal involvement in any child with a history of cancer presenting with back pain.** Physical exam findings depend on the location of the lesion(s), as well as the degree of spinal cord impingement and the rate at which compression takes place.

MRI is the gold standard for spinal cord imaging and should be obtained emergently.[70] Plain films are ineffective for diagnosis. Given that a significant number of patients present with multiple spinal lesions, image the entire spinal cord.[59,68] Obtain brain imaging if a spinal neoplasm is identified. ED treatment is IV dexamethasone (0.1 milligram/kg to a maximum of 10 milligrams) to decrease vasogenic edema caused by obstruction of the epidural venous plexus and to improve symptoms. **However, if leukemia or lymphoma is in the differential diagnosis for an initial presentation of a spinal tumor, do not administer steroids without consulting the oncologist; steroid administration can mask the tumor and prevent diagnosis and appropriate treatment.** Obtain oncology, neurosurgery, and radiotherapy consultation. The damage is irreversible once ischemia develops and the spinal cord infarcts. Even with aggressive interventions, studies report that 40% to 70% children have residual impairment.[71]

INCREASED INTRACRANIAL PRESSURE

Increased intracranial pressure in children with cancer is usually due to primary CNS tumors. Childhood CNS tumors are often infratentorial, a location where there is potential for cerebrospinal fluid flow obstruction.[72] Nonhematopoietic CNS metastases account for only 2% of all pediatric CNS tumors.[73] Clinical presentation and risk of herniation depend on the location and growth rate of the tumor, as well as the age of the child. Signs and symptoms are often nonspecific. Cushing's triad is rare, but requires emergent intervention.

Brain imaging with MRI or CT can identify a neoplasm, associated vasogenic edema and/or hydrocephalus, and alternative diagnoses; however, CT is the test of choice in the emergency setting. Management is guided by the severity of the presentation. Initial focus in the ED should be a primary survey; in particular, ensure airway protection in a patient with high intracranial pressure and altered mental status. Use of hyperventilation is now debated, because hypercarbia causes cerebral dilation but hypocarbia is an independent predictor of mortality.[74] Mild hyperventilation (pulmonary end tidal carbon dioxide, 30 to 34 mm Hg) is considered appropriate in cases of herniation. Elevate the head of the bed to 30 degrees to improve venous drainage and consult neurosurgery. Administer IV dexamethasone (0.1 milligram/kg to a maximum of 10 milligrams) to reduce tumor-associated vasogenic edema. There are no pediatric data that clearly support antiepileptic administration for seizure prophylaxis,[74,75] but fosphenytoin or another longer-acting antiepileptic can be considered if the patient requires transport. Maintain appropriate electrolyte levels and correct thrombocytopenia or coagulopathy.

STROKE

Stroke, occurring within the first few years of a childhood cancer diagnosis, is rare.[76] Overall prevalence is estimated at 1%.[77] Hemorrhagic strokes and ischemic strokes occur with equal frequency.[76] Risk factors include coagulopathy, thrombocytopenia, hyperleukocytosis, radiation, medications, and primary or metastatic CNS tumors. Stroke can be the sole clinical manifestation from hemorrhage into a previously occult CNS neoplasm.

Treatment depends on the underlying cause. Standard stroke management applies, including brain imaging. Modifiable risk factors should be addressed, including correction of thrombocytopenia to keep platelet levels >100,000/mm^3. Discuss anticoagulant therapy in consultation with neurology and oncology.

SEIZURES

Seizures are common in pediatric oncology patients and may have a number of causes: primary or metastatic CNS lesion, cerebrovascular accident, metabolic derangement (i.e., hyponatremia), infection (e.g., abscess, meningitis), chemotherapeutic agents, and radiation therapy. Fifteen percent of pediatric brain tumor patients experience seizures, and 12% of pediatric brain tumor patients present with seizures.[75]

Initial evaluation of a seizure in a child with cancer should include brain imaging with CT or MRI to identify the cause. If there are no contraindications, perform lumbar puncture to exclude infection. See chapter 135, "Seizures in Infants and Children" for further discussion.

CATHETER-RELATED COMPLICATIONS

The vast majority of pediatric cancer patients undergo central venous line placement for their treatment. These devices include external catheters (e.g., Broviac), totally implantable catheters (e.g., Port), and peripherally inserted central catheters. Rates of catheter-related complications are 40% to 50%,[78,79] and the complications fall primarily into three categories: infectious, mechanical, and thrombotic.

Infection of the central line occurs from contamination of the hub and luminal migration of pathogens within the catheter, from hematogenous seeding of the intravascular portion of the catheter, or from fractures within the catheter itself. The morbidity and mortality attributable to central line–associated bloodstream infections is significant.[80] The incidence of central line infections is three times greater in ambulatory pediatric oncology patients compared to inpatients.[80] Risk factors include frequent access, poor hygiene and sterility, previous infection, and <1 month duration from line insertion. Tunnel infections of the soft tissue surrounding the catheter may also occur shortly after placement, with typical signs of infection. Totally implantable catheters are associated with the least catheter-associated infectious morbidity.[81,82] For further discussion, see "Infection" section, above. Treatment requires IV antibiotics and possible device removal.

A central venous line is the single most important risk factor for developing thromboembolism in any child,[79] **and 50% of children with cancer are reported to have central line–associated thrombosis.**[78] However, common morbidities from thrombosis include infection, embolism to other vessels (including pulmonary embolism), catheter malfunction, loss of venous access, and delay of treatment. Venous Doppler ultrasonography can identify upper extremity or jugular vein thrombosis, but ultrasonography is limited in its inability to visualize more proximal (i.e., central) thrombosis. CT or magnetic resonance venogram may also be used for diagnosis. Treatment of central line–associated thromboembolism may require tissue plasminogen activator (a small alteplase infusion administered to the catheter site if there are concerns for an intraluminal partial occlusion of the catheter), removal of the catheter, and anticoagulation for more significant thromboembolisms. ED staff should not infuse tissue plasminogen activator into a central line without consulting oncology and/or surgery. When anticoagulant therapy is indicated, low-molecular-weight heparin, using pediatric-specific dosing protocols, is usually the preferred choice in children.[83]

Mechanical complications are also quite common in pediatric oncology patients, with a prevalence of 20% to 39%, and are an independent risk factor for poor outcomes.[78] External catheters have increased rates of mechanical complications and failure.[82] Thrombotic occlusions are the most common cause of central line dysfunction, and in turn, central line dysfunction increases the risk of thrombosis.[78] Fracture of the catheter lumen (external to the patient) can occasionally be repaired. Potential nonthrombotic occlusions include intraluminal precipitation of calcium, bicarbonate, or drugs (e.g., phenytoin).

OTHER COMPLICATIONS OF MALIGNANCY

CARDIOPULMONARY COMPLICATIONS

There are a variety of cardiac and pulmonary oncologic complications that are not unique to pediatrics. These include malignant pericardial effusion through direct or metastatic involvement of the pericardium, treatment-induced transudative pericardial effusion, cardiac tamponade, and pleural effusions. These complications and their management are addressed in the adult chapters of this textbook. Chemotherapeutic agents and adjunct therapies can also be associated with cardiomyopathy, hypertension, arrhythmias, and pulmonary fibrosis (Table 143-1).

GASTROINTESTINAL COMPLICATIONS

Mechanical bowel obstruction due to mass effect may occur with any intra-abdominal tumor, most commonly lymphoma. Malignancy should be on the differential for a child presenting with intussusception, because masses can act as lead points for telescoping of the bowel. Postoperatively, patients with oncologic abdominal surgery are at increased risk for developing a bowel obstruction due to adhesions. Patients are also at risk for constipation and ileus due to narcotic administration.

Any component of the GI tract, from mouth to anus, can be affected by mucositis induced by chemotherapeutic agents. Mucosal breakdown can lead to pain, infection, dehydration due to poor oral intake, and bleeding at any location. Herpetic or fungal esophagitis can develop. Typhlitis, or neutropenic enterocolitis, was previously discussed in this chapter (see earlier "Infection" section and Figure 143-7). There are conflicting reports regarding the possibility of increased incidence of appendicitis in pediatric patients with underlying hematologic malignancy. Regardless of incidence, **appendicitis must remain a consideration in the oncology patient with right lower quadrant abdominal pain.** Of note, the typical appendicitis presentation may be blunted in children with neutropenia and/or on corticosteroids.[84] Imaging with CT or US can help to differentiate between appendicitis, typhlitis, and other intra-abdominal processes.

GI bleeding can result from mucositis, high-dose steroids or radiation in the treatment regimen, primary tumor or metastatic invasion, or tumor- or treatment-related cytopenias or coagulopathies. Primary colorectal cancers are extremely rare in children, but those numbers increase when including secondary GI malignancies following a previously treated pediatric cancer. Mallory-Weiss tears can develop from severe chemotherapy-related emesis. Unique GI complications resulting from chemotherapeutic agents are listed in Table 143-1.

GENITOURINARY COMPLICATIONS

Mass effect from abdominal or pelvic tumors can lead to ureteral obstruction and hydronephrosis, necessitating urgent stent placement. Other causes of acute urinary retention include drugs (e.g., narcotics, anticholinergics) or spinal cord compression (see "Neurologic Emergencies," above). Viruses, radiotherapy, and chemotherapeutic agents can all induce hemorrhagic cystitis. Hemorrhagic cystitis treatment requires IV hydration, correction of underlying cytopenia and coagulopathy, and antiviral medications if appropriate. Severe cases warrant urologic consultation for placement of a double-lumen Foley catheter for continuous bladder irrigation or for cystoscopy.[85]

HEMATOLOGIC EMERGENCIES

INTRODUCTION

Bleeding in a child can be a diagnostic dilemma, because the causes range from benign to serious. Children with mild bleeding disorders may not experience an episode of bleeding until faced with a hemostatic challenge, such as an interventional procedure or trauma. On the other hand, children without an underlying bleeding disorder commonly present with complaints of bruising and bleeding such as epistaxis or menorrhagia. **Red flags for a potential bleeding disorder include bleeding or bruising out of proportion to the injury, prolonged and/or recurrent bleeding (particularly with unknown cause or after a small injury or procedure), spontaneous bruising or bleeding, uncommon sites of bleeding (joints, GI) or bruising (proximal extremities, trunk), and a family history of a bleeding disorder.** Consider nonaccidental trauma in the child with unusual bruising patterns (see chapter 148, "Child Abuse and Neglect"). **Figure 143-10** provides a basic approach for the initial ED assessment of a child with bleeding. The most common bleeding disorders presenting in childhood are discussed below.

HEMOPHILIA

A detailed discussion of hemophilias is provided in chapter 235, "Hemophilias and von Willebrand's Disease." **Table 143-6** provides a summary of those bleeding disorders, which are also reviewed below.

EPIDEMIOLOGY

Factor VIII (hemophilia A) and factor IX (hemophilia B) deficiencies are X-linked recessive hematologic disorders and predominantly affect males. One third of cases arise from spontaneous mutations; thus patients may have a negative family history of bleeding disorders.[86] These disorders are clinically indistinguishable but differ in their treatment.

CLINICAL FEATURES

The severity of disease is defined by the factor activity as a percentage of normal (which is defined as 50% to 100%). Risk of bleeding depends on factor activity (see Table 235-1). Patients with mild disease may never spontaneously bleed but have increased bleeding with trauma (**Figure 143-11**), whereas individuals with severe disease have spontaneous bleeding into the joints (hemarthroses; **Figure 143-12**) and soft tissue (hematomas) and may develop life-threatening hemorrhage.

DIAGNOSIS

Most children with hemophilia have already been identified before an ED visit because of a positive family history of bleeding disorder (prenatal testing is possible through chorionic villus sampling or amniocentesis), intracranial hemorrhage, significant hematoma following birth trauma (e.g., traumatic delivery or forceps/vacuum extraction), or prolonged and excessive bleeding after circumcision in infancy. However, some cases, especially mild hemophilia, may escape detection until the child is several years old, when symptoms are provoked by an injury or a small interventional procedure. The event precipitating initial presentation could be as minor as a trip and fall in a newly ambulatory toddler, a common age of diagnosis due to the increased activity level. **Suspect hemophilia in a child who presents with spontaneous bleeding, particularly in unusual locations (e.g., joints, areas not usually injured like the proximal extremities), or with bleeding that is out of proportion to the injury.** Specific bleeding manifestations are listed in Table 235-2. Hemarthroses are the hallmark of hemophilia, accounting for 80% of bleeding episodes in severe hemophiliacs.[87]

Differential diagnosis includes the spectrum of bleeding disorders. The screening test for hemophilia is an activated PTT, which will be prolonged (with the exception of some patients with mild disease). Platelet count, bleeding time, and prothrombin time will be normal. Quantitative factor levels confirm a diagnosis of hemophilia. Mixing studies identify whether factor inhibitors are present.

TREATMENT

The overall treatment goal is to increase levels of the deficient factor. **Early factor replacement is standard of care.** Treatment of hemophilia depends on the specific factor deficiency, the baseline severity of the disease, and the nature and extent of the injury. In severe hemophiliacs, regular scheduled prophylactic administration of clotting factor concentrate is a well-established practice and significantly reduces the incidence of bleeding.[87] Prophylactic therapy is not addressed in detail here.

In patients with known hemophilia, coagulation studies are not necessary upon presentation for a new bleeding episode. However, a level of factor VIII or IX or the presence of a factor inhibitor may be requested by the hematologist to assist in the patient's evaluation and treatment. **Even in the absence of physical findings, promptly order and initiate factor replacement for children with a history that raises concern about high-risk sites for bleeding.** Older children and adolescents describe a burning or tingling sensation preceding signs of hemarthrosis development.[87] A reliable adage in hemophilia is: when in doubt, treat.

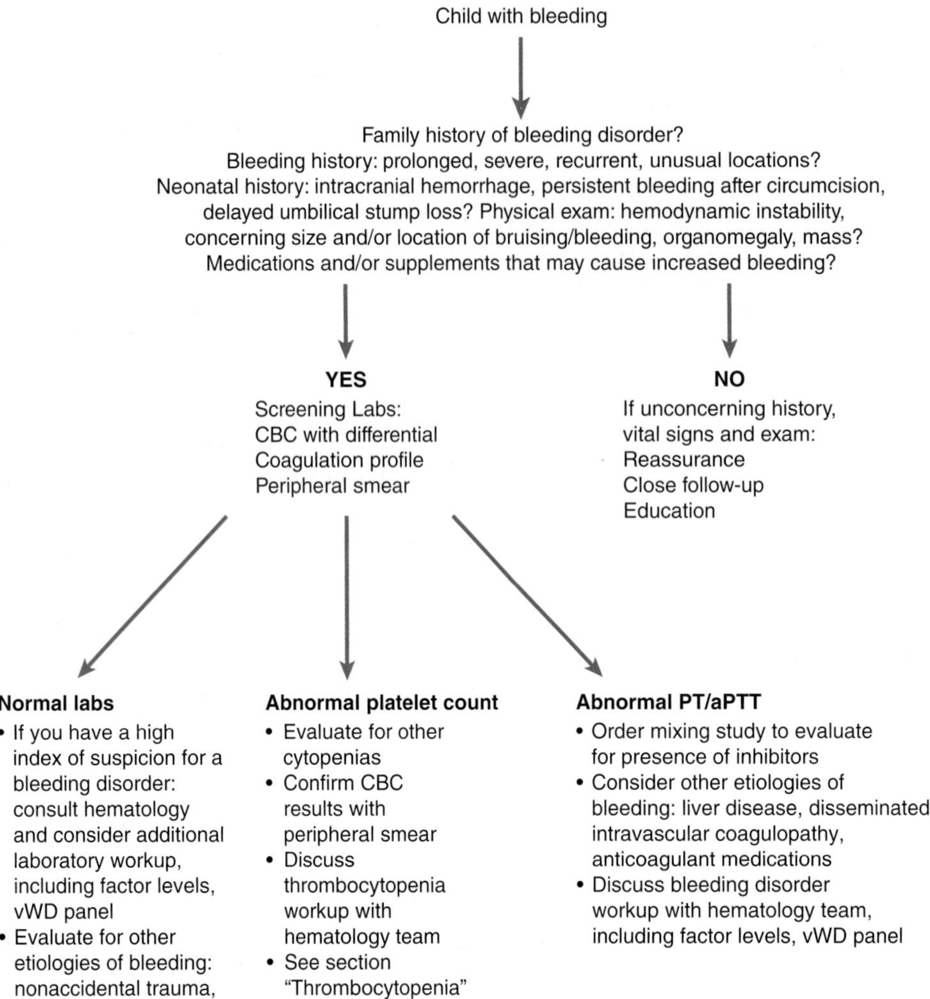
Child with bleeding
Family history of bleeding disorder?
Bleeding history: prolonged, severe, recurrent, unusual locations?
Neonatal history: intracranial hemorrhage, persistent bleeding after circumcision, delayed umbilical stump loss? Physical exam: hemodynamic instability, concerning size and/or location of bruising/bleeding, organomegaly, mass?
Medications and/or supplements that may cause increased bleeding?
YES
Screening Labs:
CBC with differential
Coagulation profile
Peripheral smear
NO
If unconcerning history, vital signs and exam:
Reassurance
Close follow-up
Education
Normal labs
• If you have a high index of suspicion for a bleeding disorder: consult hematology and consider additional laboratory workup, including factor levels, vWD panel
• Evaluate for other etiologies of bleeding: nonaccidental trauma, rheumatologic
Abnormal platelet count
• Evaluate for other cytopenias
• Confirm CBC results with peripheral smear
• Discuss thrombocytopenia workup with hematology team
• See section "Thrombocytopenia"
Abnormal PT/aPTT
• Order mixing study to evaluate for presence of inhibitors
• Consider other etiologies of bleeding: liver disease, disseminated intravascular coagulopathy, anticoagulant medications
• Discuss bleeding disorder workup with hematology team, including factor levels, vWD panel

FIGURE 143-10. Algorithm for the approach to a child with undiagnosed bleeding. vWD = von Willebrand's disease.

The dose of factor replacement and goal level of factor percentage are based on the clinical scenario. **A good rule of thumb is to aim for a desired factor level of approximately 40% to 50% following replacement. For high-risk and/or life-threatening bleeds (CNS, retropharyngeal, ophthalmic, iliopsoas/retroperitoneal, intra-abdominal, intrathoracic, and GI), that goal doubles to 80% to 100%.** Specific factor replacement products are listed in Table 235-3, and factor replacement guidelines are listed in Table 235-4 of that chapter. Recombinant and human plasma-derived factors are available, and efforts should be made to use the patient's home product. Treatment regimens will differ for factor VIII and factor IX products, because they have different dosing requirements and different half-lives. In most patients, 1 unit/kg of factor VIII will increase the clotting activity of treated plasma by 2%; 1 unit/kg of factor IX will only raise factor activity level by **1%**. Given the cost of these products, an effort should be made to use the whole unit dose. In the rare case in which factor replacement products are not immediately available, administer cryoprecipitate for factor VIII deficiency or fresh frozen plasma for factor IX deficiency.

There are a few special clinical situations. Patients with mild hemophilia A who have been pretested to document a response may be treated with **desmopressin** instead of factor replacement. This is particularly advantageous for pediatric patients, because there is an intranasal form. Desmopressin releases stored factor VIII from the subendothelial compartment. See Table 235-5 for desmopressin dosing. Of note, desmopressin is an antidiuretic; patients must be monitored for water retention and hyponatremia. For hemophilia patients requiring surgery and scheduled to go to the operating room from the ED, factor replacement must be given beforehand to optimize factor levels. Minimal oral bleeding (e.g., after dental procedures) may be treated with topical thrombin or aminocaproic acid (Amicar), and minimal anterior epistaxis may respond to conservative therapies, such as direct pressure and phenylephrine, without factor replacement. Patients, usually with severe hemophilia A, who have factor inhibitors (antibodies) may require very high doses of standard factor products to overwhelm the inhibitors present. However, some patients will need to be treated with products that bypass factor VIII and factor IX in the clotting cascade (see Table 235-6). These include activated prothrombin complex concentrates (FEIBA) and recombinant activated factor VIIa (NovoSeven).

COMPLICATIONS

Hemarthrosis is the most common hemorrhagic complication of hemophilia and most commonly affects the knee, ankle, elbow, and shoulder. Minor, often unrecognized, trauma may precipitate spontaneous intra-articular hemorrhage with pain, swelling, and decreased range of motion. Unfortunately, the presence of blood in the joint precipitates a cascade of inflammation and synovial neovascularization. This increases vulnerability to bleeding and leads to synovium fibrosis, irreversible cartilage destruction, and hemophilic arthropathy (**Figure 143-13**).[87] Aggressive measures must be taken to limit the number and extent of these events.

Spontaneous muscle hematomas account for 10% to 25% of hemophilia bleeds and can also present with severe pain and limited range of motion.[88] **Complications from ongoing bleeding include compartment syndrome and nerve compression.** Particularly concerning are iliopsoas

TABLE 143-6 Coagulation Disorders

Disease	Inheritance	Defect	Incidence	Distribution	Subtypes	Inhibitors	Diagnostics	Symptoms	Treatment
Hemophilia A									
Factor VIII deficiency	X-linked recessive	Defect in factor VIII procoagulant activity	1:5000 live male births	Males	Severe: <1% factor VIII activity	30% of those with severe subtype have inhibitors	Platelet count, PT, bleeding time—WNL	Intracranial hemorrhage	Factor VIII replacement
		Quantitative and qualitative			Frequency: 50%–70%		PTT—prolonged	Hemarthroses (large joints)	Desmopressin (in pretested mild hemophiliacs)
					Bleeding spontaneously into joints or soft tissue		Factor VIII assay—low or absent amount	Bleeding after neonatal circumcision	Activated prothrombin complex concentrates (FEIBA)
					Moderate: 1%–5% factor VIII activity			Muscle and soft tissue hematomas	Recombinant activated factor VIIa (NovoSeven)
					Frequency: 10%			Retroperitoneal bleeds	Cryoprecipitate*
					Bleeding with minor trauma or surgery			Epistaxis and mucosal bleeding from oral trauma	
					Mild: >5% factor VIII activity				
					Frequency: 30%–40%			Pharyngeal bleeding (posttussive and after emesis)	
					Bleeding with major trauma or surgery			Hematochezia and melena from GI bleeding	
								Hematuria	
								Menorrhagia	
Hemophilia B (Christmas disease)									
Factor IX deficiency	X-linked recessive	Defect in factor IX procoagulant activity	1:30,000 live male births	Males	Severe: <1% factor IX activity	1%–3% with inhibitors	Platelet count, PT, bleeding time—WNL	Symptoms same as for factor VIII deficiency	Factor IX replacement
		Quantitative and qualitative			Bleeding spontaneously into joints or soft tissue		PTT—prolonged		Activated prothrombin complex concentrates (FEIBA)
					Moderate: <1% factor IX activity		Factor IX assay—low or absent amount		Recombinant activated factor VIIa (NovoSeven)
					Bleeding with minor trauma or surgery				Fresh frozen plasma*
					Mild: >5% factor IX activity				
					Bleeding with major trauma or surgery				

(Continued)

TABLE 143-6 Coagulation Disorders (*Continued*)

Disease	Inheritance	Defect	Incidence	Distribution	Subtypes	Inhibitors	Diagnostics	Symptoms	Treatment
von Willebrand's									
vWF deficiency	Autosomal dominant (type 1 and subtypes of 2); autosomal recessive (subtypes of 2 and type 3)	Defect in vWF	1%–2% of general population	Males = females	Type 1 von Willebrand's (classic) disease	Inhibitors rare	PT—WNL	Types 1 and 2 (mild)	vWF replacement
		Quantitative and qualitative					PTT—prolonged or WNL	Mucocutaneous bleeding	
					Mild quantitative deficiency of vWF			Recurrent or prolonged epistaxis	Desmopressin for type 1 and some type 2
		Variable factor VIII activity			Most common form (80%)		Factor VIII—borderline or decreased		
					Type 2 von Willebrand's disease		vWF activity, antigen and multimer evaluation	Bleeding after surgery or trauma, e.g., dental procedures	Antifibrinolytic agents (ε-aminocaproic acid)
					Variable qualitative abnormalities of vWF			GI bleeding	
								Menorrhagia	
					Type 3 von Willebrand's disease			Type 3	
					Severe quantitative deficiency of vWF			Spontaneous hemarthroses	
					Rare (1–3 per million)			Muscle hematomas	
								Severe bleeding	

Abbreviations: PT = prothrombin time; PTT = partial thromboplastin time; vWF = von Willebrand factor; WNL = within normal limits.

*If concentrated factor products unavailable.

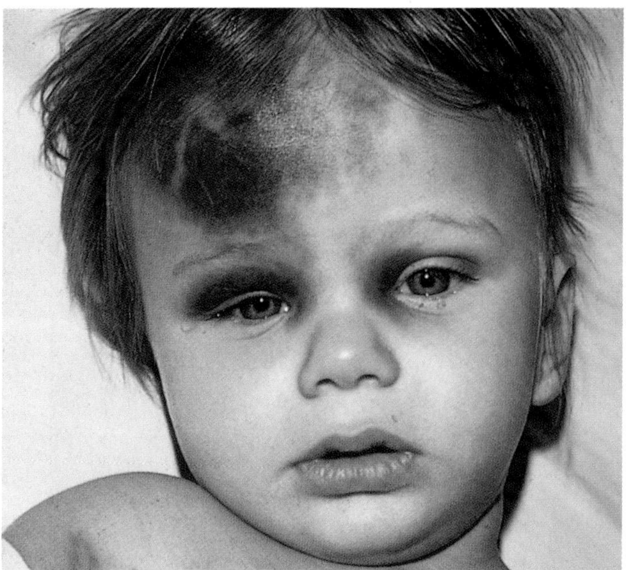

FIGURE 143-11. Hemophilia A. Extensive bruising in a child with factor VIII deficiency. [Photo contributed by Ralph A. Gruppo, MD. Reproduced with permission from Knoop K, Stack L, Storrow A, Thurman RJ: *Atlas of Emergency Medicine*, 3rd ed. © 2010, McGraw-Hill, New York.]

bleeds, which may mimic acute appendicitis or hip pathology, with radiation of pain to the back, groin, and hip. The hip is often held in flexion. Such bleeds can be particularly uncomfortable if there is compression of the femoral nerve or sacral plexus. They require aggressive factor replacement, given the potential for blood accumulation in the retroperitoneal space.

The leading cause of death in children with hemophilia is intracranial hemorrhage, which can be spontaneous or occur after even mild head trauma.[88] Because bleeding can progress slowly, patients may not yet have clinical manifestations of hemorrhage upon presentation. Maintain a high index of suspicion. **Unless directed otherwise by the hematology consultant, treat all reports of head injuries, neurologic symptoms, or visible head trauma presumptively with 100% factor correction.** Obtain immediate head CT imaging to identify intracranial hemorrhage.

Bleeding from the GI tract is rarely severe unless a specific anatomic lesion is present. Gross hematuria may require factor replacement. Obtain urinalysis to rule out infection and renal ultrasonography to identify a serious anatomic lesion. Other uncommon but critical lesions that require aggressive factor replacement (100%) and specialist intervention to avoid massive hemorrhage or permanent injury include tonsillar bleeding, solid organ bleeding from blunt abdominal or thoracic trauma, spinal hematoma, and intraocular hemorrhage.

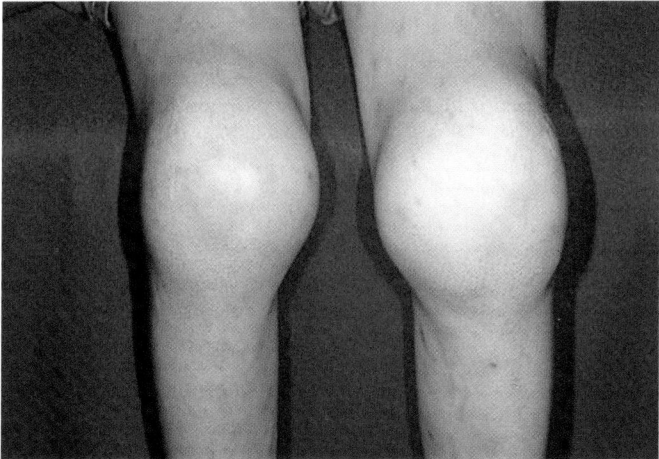

FIGURE 143-12. Hemarthrosis. A child with hemophilia A who presented with bilateral knee hemarthroses. [Reproduced with permission from Shah BR, Lucchesi M: *Atlas of Pediatric Emergency Medicine*, © 2006, McGraw-Hill, New York.]

DISPOSITION

Consult a hematologist for all children with hemophilia and active bleeding prior to disposition. Pediatric hemophilia patients and their families are often comfortable participating in that decision, because they may receive some treatments at home. Children with mild bleeding episodes may be discharged home with careful instructions and a concrete hematology follow-up appointment. Patients with moderate or severe bleeding and those with high-risk bleeds require hospital admission, because close monitoring and documentation of adequate response to factor replacement are necessary, and repeat doses are frequently required.

VON WILLEBRAND'S DISEASE

A detailed discussion of von Willebrand's disease (vWD) is provided in chapter 235; vWD classification and basic treatment are outlined in Table 235-7. There is an extremely rare acquired disorder, "acquired von Willebrand's syndrome," with normal von Willebrand factor (vWF) synthesis but abnormal clearance. This syndrome is not within the scope of this chapter, but is associated with neoplasms, autoimmune diseases, medications, and cardiovascular disease in children.[89]

CLINICAL FEATURES

vWD type 1 is usually associated with mild mucocutaneous bleeding, including easy bruising, recurrent or prolonged epistaxis, and prolonged postprocedural bleeding (e.g., gingival bleeding after dental work). Menorrhagia may be the sole presenting complaint in young women. In type 3 vWD, clinical features can closely resemble those of hemophilia, because significantly reduced amounts of vWF allow increased clearance of factor VIII. In general, the severity of bleeding correlates with the degree of reduction of factor VIII.[90]

DIAGNOSIS

A high index of suspicion is necessary for the diagnosis of vWD because clinical features are mild in most patients, and mucocutaneous bleeding (e.g., bruising, epistaxis) is common in childhood. History should include frequency, duration, severity, and location of bleeding, as well as concurrent medications. Note any family history of "easy" bleeding. ED screening lab work includes a CBC with peripheral smear and a coagulation profile to rule out coagulation factor deficiencies. More specific testing includes vWF antigen, vWF ristocetin cofactor activity, vWF multimers, and factor VIII level.[91,92] Bleeding time, once the gold standard for vWD diagnosis, has difficulties with reproducibility and poor sensitivity and specificity.[92-94] vWD labs usually reveal a normal CBC and prothrombin time, a normal or prolonged activated PTT (if factor VIII is sufficiently reduced), and low vWF levels. vWF multimer helps to distinguish among the different types of vWD. There is an array of more discriminating tests to evaluate for the presence and type of vWD that will not be addressed here. Levels of vWF can be affected by a variety of normal (e.g., stress) and medical (e.g., active bleeding) conditions.[93] Repeat testing should be done if clinical suspicion is high.

TREATMENT

Treatment of active bleeding in a known vWD patient consists initially of localized measures to achieve hemostasis, including direct pressure on bleeding sites, packing dental extraction sites and nasal passages, and the application of topical hemostatic agents. **Amicar, an antifibrinolytic agent, can also be used to treat oral trauma**. Oral contraceptive pills or an intrauterine device help to control menorrhagia. Desmopressin (see earlier section on hemophilia treatment), which releases stored vWF from the endothelium, can be used for treatment and prevention

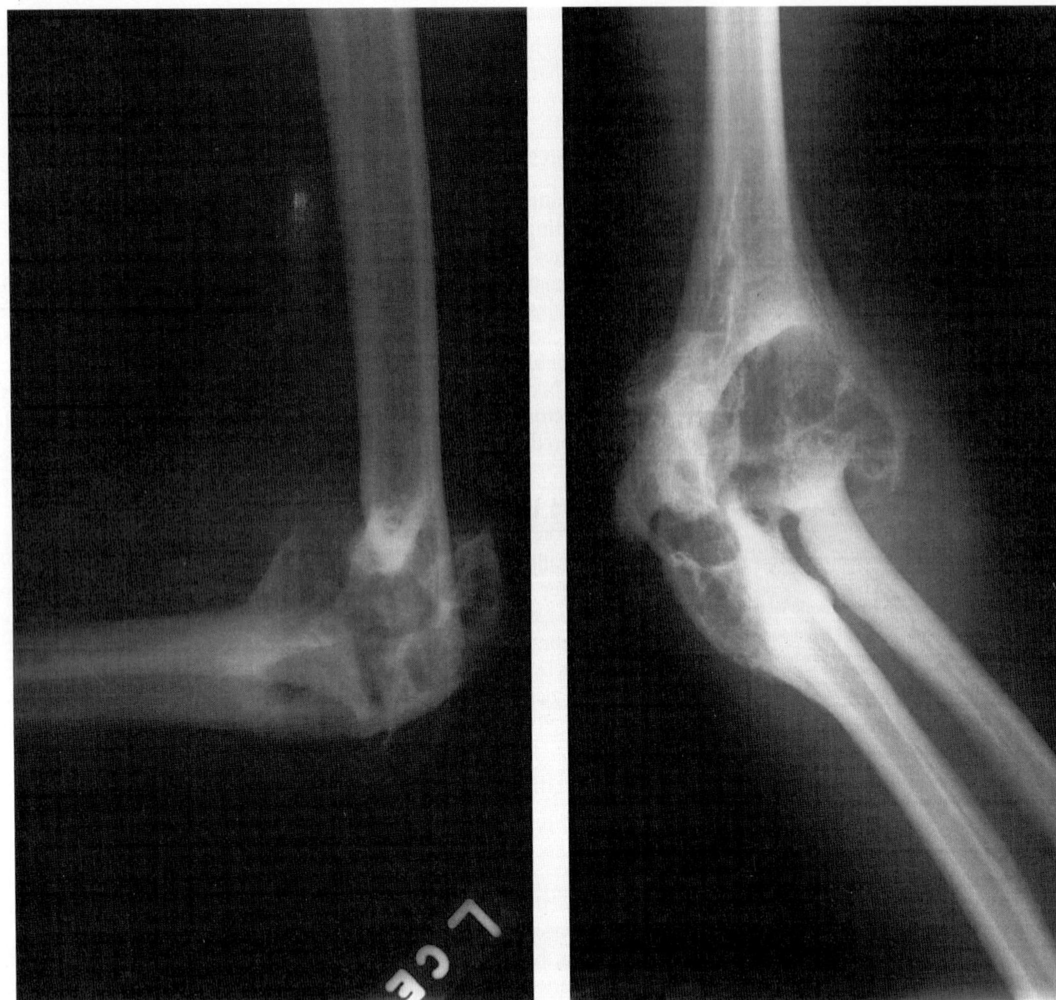

FIGURE 143-13. Hemophilic arthropathy. Note the extensive degenerative changes. [Image used with permission of J. Fitzpatrick, MD, Cook County Hospital. Reproduced with permission from Simon RR, Koenigsknecht SJ: *Emergency Orthopedics: The Extremities*, 5th ed. Copyright © 2007 by The McGraw-Hill Companies, Inc. All rights reserved.]

(e.g., prior to a minimally invasive procedure) of bleeding in patients with type 1 vWD. It has no effect in those with type 3 vWD and variable effect in those with type 2. **Pay attention to the fluid status of patients receiving desmopressin, because dilutional hyponatremia is a rare side effect due to its antidiuretic properties.** For children with an inadequate response to desmopressin or for whom it is ineffective, there are a variety of plasma-derived vWF and factor VIII concentrates available for protein replacement. Such conditions require prophylaxis with concentrate replacement prior to surgical procedures. Dosing of the above medications is reviewed in Tables 235-4 and 235-5. In emergencies, administer cryoprecipitate if no vWF:factor VIII replacement is available. Cryoprecipitate has infectious risks because it does not undergo viral inactivation. Advise all patients with vWD to avoid medications with known antiplatelet effects (e.g., aspirin, nonsteroidal anti-inflammatory drugs).

VITAMIN K DEFICIENCY BLEEDING

Vitamin K deficiency bleeding, formerly known as "hemorrhagic disease of the newborn," is a neonatal bleeding coagulopathy resulting from vitamin K deficiency. Although the American Academy of Pediatrics has recommended intramuscular vitamin K prophylaxis as standard of care in newborns since 1961, there has been an increasing rate of parental refusal in the past few years.[94] Risk factors include breastfed infants (because breast milk contains less vitamin K content than cow's milk formulas), infants with malabsorption or hepatobiliary disorders, and maternal medications (e.g., phenytoin, isoniazid).

In classic cases, bleeding occurs 2 to 14 days after birth; however, there are reports of cases <24 hours after birth and up to 12 weeks after birth.[95] Bleeding can present as mild oozing from the umbilicus or circumcision site or as life-threatening pulmonary and intracranial hemorrhage. Although vitamin K deficiency bleeding is rare in developed countries, 30% to 60% of reported cases are associated with intracranial hemorrhage.[94] Labs reveal a decreased hematocrit, depending upon the severity and duration of the bleed, and prolonged prothrombin time and activated PTT. **Treatment is the immediate administration of 1 milligram of SC, IM, or IV vitamin K (phytonadione). The IM route places the patient at risk for a significant hematoma, whereas the IV route carries a greater risk of an anaphylactoid reaction. Given the risk of intracranial bleeding, do not wait for laboratory results if your clinical suspicion is high.** Life-threatening hemorrhage may require a transfusion of 10 to 20 mL/kg of fresh frozen plasma to increase serum procoagulant levels.

ANEMIA

Children may develop profoundly low hemoglobin levels (e.g., 3 to 4 grams/dL) before coming to medical attention. Patients may be asymptomatic or present with symptoms ranging from pallor and decreased activity to congestive heart failure in an infant. This section reviews the ED diagnosis and management of some important types of anemia in children. The management of anemia due to hemorrhage is discussed in chapters 13, "Fluid and Blood Resuscitation in Traumatic Shock" and 110, "Pediatric Trauma." Hemoglobin levels vary with a child's age, peaking at ~14 to 15 grams/dL in the full-term newborn period and at ~13 grams/dL (females) and ~15 grams/dL (males) in the teenage years. The dramatic increase in oxygen availability after birth briefly shuts down erythropoietin production, resulting in a physiologic nadir, or "physiologic anemia," of about 9 to 11 grams/dL at ~2 months of age. Hemoglobin levels then rise steadily throughout childhood. After the first year of life, the normal reticulocyte count is 1% to 2% of circulating red blood cells, assuming normal red blood cell physiology.[93] Refer to normal hemoglobin and red blood cell values when evaluating pediatric anemia.

ED TREATMENT OF SEVERE ANEMIA

Children with anemia unrelated to acute blood loss rarely require blood transfusion in the ED. Some children with very low hemoglobin levels and a presentation highly consistent with iron deficiency anemia, for example, may be managed as outpatients if close follow-up is assured. Exceptions include hemolytic anemias, bone marrow failure, hemodynamic instability, congestive heart failure, or other symptoms due to severe anemia. Emergency transfusion of patients with nonautoimmune hemolytic anemias poses significantly less risk than transfusion of patients with antibodies. Obtain a hematology consultation to assist with transfusion management.

The decision to transfuse must take into account whether the child has a chronic or acute anemia; those with chronic anemias are at risk for volume overload. For children with hemoglobin ≤8 grams/dL and signs of hemodynamic compromise, active bleeding, or consumptive coagulopathy, consider an initial transfusion of packed red blood cells in 10 to 15 mL/kg aliquots. **With extremely low hemoglobin levels (<5 grams/dL) due to chronic anemia, the transfusion should be small (2 to 3 mL/kg packed red blood cells) and slow (1 mL/kg/h), with continuous monitoring and frequent reassessment.** In cases of volume overload, diuretics can be considered, or an exchange transfusion in severe cases.

CLASSIFICATION OF ANEMIA

As with adults, a differential diagnosis for anemia in childhood can be broken down into microcytic, normocytic, and macrocytic categories (see Figures 231-2, 231-3, and 231-4). The pathologic causes can be classified as those that decrease red blood cell production and those that increase red blood cell destruction, in addition to blood loss and iatrogenic dilutional anemia from fluid administration. To help with those differentiations, a peripheral smear and reticulocyte count should always be sent with the CBC. A more detailed differential diagnosis of anemia is provided in **Table 143-7**. Selected common pediatric anemias are discussed below. For a more thorough discussion of specific etiologies, see chapters 231, 233, "Acquired Bleeding Disorders," 236, "Sickle Cell Disease and Hereditary Hemolytic Anemias," and 237, "Acquired Hemolytic Anemia."

IRON DEFICIENCY ANEMIA

Iron deficiency anemia is the leading cause of anemia in childhood and can be profound. Healthy term infants have adequate iron storage for the first 4 to 6 months of life. After this, iron stores are depleted. Decreased prevalence of iron deficiency anemia may be attributable, in part, to the American Academy of Pediatrics recommendations regarding iron supplementation in breastfed infants, iron-fortified formulas and infant foods, delayed use of cow's milk until after 1 year of age, and universal hemoglobin screening at 1 year of age.[98] However, excessive whole-milk feeding and poor dietary intake of iron make iron deficiency anemia a diagnosis common in the toddler years. Milk proteins may also cause a low-grade colitis with occult GI bleeding. **Nutritional iron deficiency anemia is uncommon in children >3 to 4 years of age and is suspicious for occult bleeding.**[93] Iron deficiency anemia is diagnosed based on clinical suspicion, with labs demonstrating a hypochromic microcytic anemia and low reticulocyte count. Iron studies help to confirm the diagnosis. For hemodynamically stable children, treatment is outpatient oral ferrous sulfate supplementation and primary care follow-up. For children with severe anemia and/or evidence of hemodynamic compromise, inpatient care may be necessary, and hematology should be consulted regarding transfusion guidelines.

TABLE 143-7 Classification of Anemia

Decreased red blood cell (RBC) production
Impaired RBC proliferation
Parvovirus B19 infection
Aplastic anemia (congenital or acquired)
Isolated pure red cell aplasia (Diamond-Blackfan syndrome)
Transient erythroblastopenia of childhood (TEC)
Bone marrow infiltration (e.g., leukemia)
Impaired erythropoietin production
Anemia of chronic disease
Chronic renal disease
Malnutrition
Abnormal hemoglobin synthesis
Lead poisoning
Iron deficiency
Thalassemia
Vitamin B_{12} or folate deficiency
Sideroblastic anemia
Increased RBC destruction
Hemoglobinopathy
Thalassemia
Sickle cell disease
Membrane defect (e.g., hereditary spherocytosis)
Extrinsic disease
Autoimmune hemolytic anemia
Glucose-6-dehydrogenase deficiency
Disseminated intravascular coagulopathy
Microangiopathic process (e.g., hemolytic-uremic syndrome)
Paroxysmal nocturnal hemoglobinuria

SICKLE CELL ANEMIA

This topic is discussed in depth in chapters 236, and 142, "Sickle Cell Disease in Children."

PARVOVIRUS B19 INFECTION

Parvovirus, a common virus in childhood, replicates in erythroid progenitor cells and can cause transient red cell aplasia. In the normal host, parvovirus infection may go unrecognized or be identified by its characteristic reticular rash and slapped cheek appearance (erythema infectiosum, or fifth disease); see "Erythema Infectiosum" in chapter 141, "Rashes in Infants and Children." The red cell aplasia is so short lived that concomitant anemia is usually not discovered. However, in patients with hemoglobinopathy or hemolytic anemias such as sickle cell disease, in whom the life span of a red cell is decreased, even brief periods of red cell aplasia may result in severe anemia and aplastic crisis, often requiring transfusion.

TRANSIENT ERYTHROBLASTOPENIA OF CHILDHOOD

Transient erythroblastopenia of childhood is a gradually developing, self-resolving normocytic anemia caused by a temporary decrease in red blood cell precursors. The cause is unknown. It is most common in the toddlers and preschool age groups but can be diagnosed in children 6 months to 10 years of age.[97] Other cell lines should not be affected, and iron studies are normal. Bone marrow recovery usually occurs in 1 to 2 months, and transfusions are rarely needed.

AUTOIMMUNE HEMOLYTIC ANEMIA

Autoimmune hemolytic anemia is caused by the production of autoantibodies to red blood cells. In primary autoimmune hemolytic anemia (most common in infants and young children), there is no evidence of an underlying disorder; the disease may manifest after a simple viral illness. Older children are more likely to experience autoimmune hemolytic anemia secondary to an underlying systemic illness, such as malignancy, human immunodeficiency virus, or an autoimmune disorder. The clinical presentation may be abrupt and the anemia severe. White cells and platelets are unaffected, and reticulocytes are increased unless the hemolysis is sudden and recent. Labs reveal spherocytes and schistocytes on peripheral blood smear, an indirect hyperbilirubinemia, elevated lactate dehydrogenase, and urine bilirubin metabolites (hemoglobinuria in the absence of red blood cells on urine microscopy). Definitive diagnosis is made by a direct Coombs test. These patients should be hospitalized, and treatment usually begins with corticosteroids. If transfusion is required, the most compatible packed red blood cells are used.

THROMBOCYTOPENIA

A platelet count <150,000/mm^3 should be considered abnormal, and patients with a count <20,000/mm^3 are at high risk for spontaneous bleeding. Consider thrombocytopenia in patients with petechiae (see Figure 233-1A), easy bruising, epistaxis, gingival bleeding, menorrhagia, hematuria, and GI bleeding. Perform a thorough physical exam to assess for signs of systemic disease. Refer to Figure 143-10 for the general approach. The pathophysiology of acquired thrombocytopenia is listed in Table 143-1, and common medications associated with thrombocytopenia are listed in Table 233-2.

IMMUNE THROMBOCYTOPENIA

Immune thrombocytopenia (ITP), previously called "idiopathic thrombocytopenic purpura," is an autoimmune disorder of antiplatelet antibodies leading to platelet destruction and, in some cases, decreased megakaryocyte platelet production. In the childhood form, over 80% of cases are self-limited and resolve within 6 months, and the incidence of life-threatening bleeds is <0.5%.[98] ITP lasting >3 months after diagnosis is termed *persistent*, and the term *chronic* is now used for children with thrombocytopenia >12 months from the time of diagnosis.[98]

The typical presentation is a preschool- or school-age, previously healthy child with acute onset of petechiae and bruising, often following a viral illness. However, 25% of children present with a more insidious course.[98] Additional symptoms and signs are typically absent and, if found, should raise your concern for different diagnoses including hematologic, rheumatologic, oncologic, and infectious diseases. Laboratory studies typically demonstrate isolated thrombocytopenia.

Pharmacologic treatment is controversial and may include corticosteroids, IV immunoglobulin (IVIG), or anti-Rh (D) immunoglobulin (WinRho). There are limited data regarding the use of thrombopoietic agents in children. These treatment options are discussed in further detail in chapter 233. Consult hematology prior to management, activity restrict patients, and avoid all medications with antiplatelet activity. Admission is necessary for any child with a platelet count <20,000/mm^3, with an IV medication regimen, or with spontaneous bleeding, regardless of platelet count.

If steroids are given, there are a variety of effective dosing regimens, including 1–2 milligrams/kg/d of oral prednisone, 30 milligrams/kg (maximum dose, 1 gram) daily of IV methylprednisolone, and 20 milligrams/m^2/d of oral dexamethasone.[99] **Steroids should be started only if the possibility of leukemia or aplastic anemia can be completely excluded on clinical grounds; otherwise, a bone marrow aspirate is necessary to secure the diagnosis before initiating steroid therapy.** IVIG is superior to steroids in improving platelet numbers for ITP patients.[100] The typical IVIG dose is 1 gram/kg/d. Anti-Rh (D) immunoglobulin is only effective in Rh-positive patients and can lead to a 1 to 2 gram/dL drop in the hemoglobin concentration. The anti-Rh (D) dose is 50 to 75 micrograms/kg, and patients require admission due to the risk of severe intravascular hemolysis following infusion. Pretreatment with acetaminophen and diphenhydramine is recommended for both IVIG treatments.

On the rare occasion that a child with ITP develops life-threatening hemorrhage, administer an immediate single-donor platelet transfusion (two to three times normal dose), along with IV methylprednisolone and IVIG or anti-Rh (D). The obvious disadvantage of platelet transfusion in ITP is that platelets will be rapidly consumed by circulating antiplatelet antibodies, and repeat transfusions may be necessary.

HEMOLYTIC-UREMIC SYNDROME

Hemolytic-uremic syndrome is discussed in detail in chapter 134, "Renal Emergencies in Children."

NEUTROPENIA

Isolated neutropenia in childhood is caused by a heterogeneous group of disorders, ranging from transient and benign to chronic and profound immunodeficiency. Neutropenia in the oncology patient is discussed in the "Oncologic Emergencies" section of this chapter.

Neutropenia is an ANC <1500/mm^3. Lower counts can be noted in infants during the first year of life and in individuals of African and Middle Eastern descent, but should not drop below 1000/mm^3.[101,102] Neutropenia can be stratified into categories that are associated with increasing risk of pyogenic infection: mild neutropenia with ANC of 1000 of 1500/mm^3, moderate neutropenia with ANC of 500 to 1000/mm^3, and severe neutropenia with ANC of <500/mm^3. **Severe neutropenia places the patient at risk for life-threatening infections.** Perform a through history and physical examination to identify a nidus of infection. Physical exam should include the oral mucosa, skin, ears, lungs, abdomen, and perineal region. Avoid digital rectal examinations and rectal temperatures, as well as catheter urine sampling, because these maneuvers can result in a portal of infection. Obtain a family history to evaluate for inheritable conditions.

The underlying cause of isolated neutropenia is critical in defining infectious risk. A benign, transient neutropenia is quite common in healthy children and usually arises in the context of a viral infection, resolving within weeks to months. A number of medications, including antiepileptic drugs, antibiotics, antipsychotics, and antithyroid drugs, can cause severe neutropenia and comorbidities, and reports of drug-induced neutropenia quote a 2.5% to 10% mortality rate.[102] Neutropenia due to bone marrow depletion is a known entity in the septic child; therefore, **suspect serious bacterial infection in a critically ill child with neutropenia. Typical symptoms and signs of infection (e.g., purulence) may be absent in a neutropenic patient due to reduced inflammatory response.**

Chronic (>3 months) neutropenia can be idiopathic, autoimmune, nutritional, or associated with congenital or acquired bone marrow failure. Neonates may develop a self-resolving but significant isoimmune neutropenia from maternal/fetal antigen incompatibility or have placental transfer of antibodies from a mother with autoimmune neutropenia.[101] A benign autoimmune neutropenia can also be noted during infancy or early childhood, when repeat CBCs reveal persistent neutropenia. Children with autoimmune neutropenia tend to have more frequent (rather than more severe) infections, and the neutropenia resolves spontaneously within a few years. Lack of resolution should prompt further evaluation. If severe chronic neutropenia is noted in infancy, severe congenital neutropenia and other inherited marrow failure disorders must be excluded. Distinguishing benign neutropenia from worrisome neutropenia often requires a bone marrow examination to distinguish normal versus abnormal myelopoiesis.

Cyclic neutropenia, inherited as an autosomal dominant disorder, is characterized by episodic severe neutropenia on an approximately 21-day cycle. Episodes typically last 4 to 6 days.[102] Affected children are more likely to experience fevers and non–life-threatening infections such as stomatitis, pharyngitis, cellulitis, otitis media, and lymphadenitis. They are also at high risk for more profound infections.

For the otherwise healthy child with acute, asymptomatic neutropenia identified on routine CBC, close outpatient observation and serial blood counts are usually performed. Consult hematology for children with persistent neutropenia, concern for a heritable cause of neutropenia,

neutropenia associated with syndromic features on clinical exam, or serious pyogenic infections associated with neutropenia.

Fever in children with neutropenia, regardless of etiology, must be treated as a medical emergency with broad-spectrum antibiotics.

REFERENCES

The complete reference list is available online at www.TintinalliEM.com.

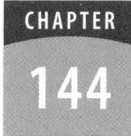

Metabolic Emergencies in Infants and Children

Garth Meckler
Nadeemuddin Quereshi
Mohammed Al-Mogbil
Osama Y. Kentab

INTRODUCTION

Metabolic emergencies are challenging childhood disorders, often presenting with nonspecific signs and symptoms that may mimic more common conditions such as sepsis. Delay in accurate diagnoses can lead to significant morbidity and mortality, whereas early aggressive management based on probable diagnosis can be lifesaving and reduce long-term neurologic sequelae.

In any healthy neonate, sudden acute deterioration should prompt consideration of metabolic disease. **Vomiting, altered mental status, and poor feeding are the most common clinical features of metabolic emergencies.** Appropriate initial management can be started in the ED without definitive diagnosis. This chapter reviews the most common metabolic disorders presenting as acute decompensation in the young infant and the ED treatment. Hypoglycemia is discussed separately. Congenital adrenal insufficiency is included here because of the overlap in presentation with other inherited metabolic disorders and the importance of prompt recognition and treatment in the critically ill neonate. Inherited metabolic disorders that present in later childhood, such as lysosomal storage disease, are often diagnosed and managed outside of the ED, and these disorders are not included here.

HYPOGLYCEMIA

Hypoglycemia is a plasma glucose level of <45 milligrams/dL (2.6 mmol/L) in any symptomatic child or <35 milligrams/dL (<1.9 mmol/L) in an asymptomatic neonate.[1,2] Intellectual performance is poor at 18 months in premature infants with persistent serum glucose <47 milligrams/dL,[3] and MRI of infants with episodes of hypoglycemia demonstrates patterns of brain injury.[4-6] This has led to the recommended treatment threshold of 45 milligrams/dL (2.6 mmol/L) for neonates, who may be at higher risk of poor neurologic outcomes than older infants and children.[7] Hypoglycemia in children requiring resuscitation is associated with increased mortality, and hypoglycemia in the setting of seizures is associated with poor neurologic outcomes.[2,8]

PATHOPHYSIOLOGY

Neonates are born with 60% to 80% of maternal glucose levels. Within 2 to 4 hours, neonates begin to regulate their own serum glucose. Maintenance of serum glucose depends on intake and endogenous gluconeogenesis and glycogenolysis mediated by various hormones. Serum glucose level is affected when there is an imbalance between insulin (hypoglycemic hormone) and its counterregulatory hormones cortisol, growth hormone, glucagon, and epinephrine (hyperglycemic hormones). Insulin stimulates cellular glucose uptake and suppresses lipolysis, whereas hyperglycemic hormones stimulate lipolysis and glycogenolysis. Excess insulin (hyperinsulinemia) results in hypoglycemia with absence of urinary ketones. Hypoglycemia in the neonate or infant may result from inadequate oral intake, excess insulin, deficient hyperglycemic hormones (e.g., growth hormone or adrenal hormone deficiency), disorders of fatty acid oxidation or carbohydrate metabolism, aminoacidopathies and organic acidurias (due to inhibition of gluconeogenesis), or systemic infection (sepsis). Infants of diabetic mothers, postterm infants, and large for gestational age infants are at risk for hypoglycemia due to excess fetal insulin levels in response to elevated maternal serum glucose levels, whereas premature infants or those small for gestational age are at risk due to inadequate glycogen stores.[9-11]

CLINICAL FEATURES

HISTORY

Neonates and infants with hypoglycemia typically present with alterations in mental status. Nonspecific symptoms include poor feeding, an abnormal or high-pitched cry, cyanosis, and hypothermia, and varying degrees of irritability and jitteriness or lethargy.[12] Severe hypoglycemia may result in coma or seizures.

Inquire about maternal complications during pregnancy (including gestational diabetes, growth retardation, and infections) as well as any history of prior spontaneous abortions or early infant deaths, which may signal inherited metabolic disease. Obtain a detailed feeding history, and document duration and progression of symptoms as well as the presence of associated signs and symptoms of vomiting, diarrhea, abnormal urine output, jaundice, and temperature instability.

PHYSICAL EXAMINATION

The classic signs of hypoglycemia seen in older children and adults are a result of the hyperglycemic hormones and include signs of adrenergic stimulation such as tachycardia, diaphoresis, tremor, anxiety, and tachypnea. **Neonates and infants may not manifest these signs, and lethargy, apnea, or seizures may be the prominent finding.** A careful neurologic examination should focus on mental status, tone, and reflexes, and may reveal focal neurologic deficits similar to Todd's paralysis in cases of prolonged, severe hypoglycemia. Seizures may be noted.

A complete physical examination is important to search for primary and secondary causes of hypoglycemia. Document weight and compare with birth weight (if known) in the neonate. Macrosomia or growth retardation may provide a quick clue to potential cause. Dysmorphic features should be documented. Fever or hypothermia suggests infection. The cardiac examination may suggest congenital heart disease (e.g., critical coarctation of the aorta), and the pulmonary examination may reveal tachypnea, apnea, or respiratory distress suggestive of pneumonia or sepsis. The abdominal examination is important in an infant with a history of vomiting to exclude abdominal catastrophe or obstruction (e.g., atresia, volvulus, intussusception, or pyloric stenosis). The GU examination may reveal ambiguous genitalia suggestive of congenital adrenal hyperplasia (discussed later separately in the "Congenital Adrenal Hyperplasia [Adrenal Insufficiency]" section).

DIAGNOSIS

The most important diagnostic test in the ED for the neonate, infant, or child who is critically ill or shows altered mental status is a **rapid bedside screen for serum glucose level**. Confirm abnormal results with a venous sample sent to the laboratory. Although the treatment of hypoglycemia must be prompt and should not be delayed, the first blood sample taken from the hypoglycemic neonate or infant is critical for making a definitive diagnosis, and when possible, a gray-topped sample tube should be filled and placed on ice for additional studies, which may include serum insulin, C-peptide, growth hormone, cortisol, and glucagon levels.[13]

Evaluation of urine for ketones is the second important step. Ketonuria is characteristic of ketotic hypoglycemia, adrenal or growth hormone deficiency, and other inborn errors of metabolism. A lack of urinary ketones suggests hyperinsulinism or fatty acid oxidation defects.[14,15] Serum insulin, C-peptide, and hormone analysis, as described above, can help differentiate among these diagnostic possibilities.

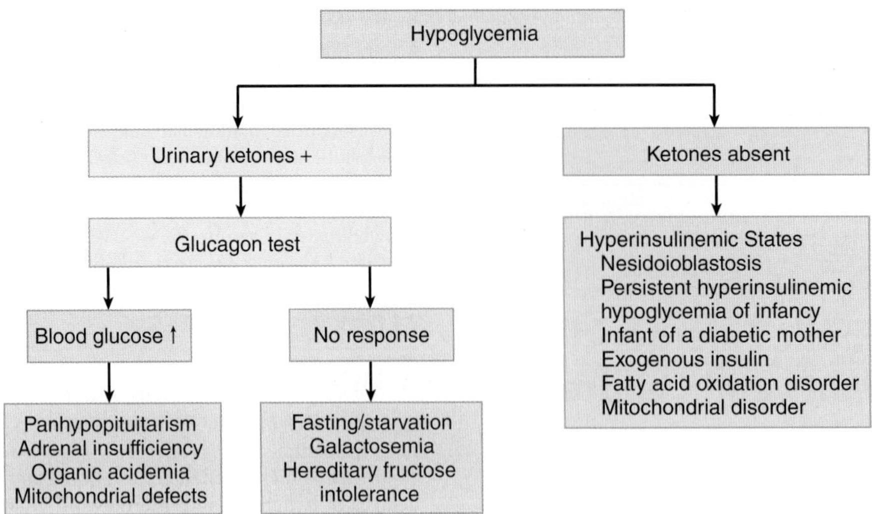

FIGURE 144-1. Evaluation of hypoglycemia in the ED.

The administration of **glucagon** (0.3 milligram/kg IM or IV) in hypoglycemic states can be diagnostic and therapeutic. If glucagon is effective in normalizing serum glucose level, then the presence of hepatic stores is confirmed and the hypoglycemia is likely due to hormonal deficiency (panhypopituitarism or adrenal insufficiency) (**Figure 144-1**). Lack of response to glucagon suggests poor glycogen stores. Among nonresponders to glucagon, fasting is the most common cause, followed by galactosemia and hereditary fructose intolerance, although children with ketotic hypoglycemia often fail to respond to glucagon as well.

Additional laboratory evaluation is directed by the clinical picture and differential diagnosis and may include cultures of the blood, urine, and cerebrospinal fluid when sepsis is suspected. Definitive diagnosis of specific inborn errors of metabolism may require evaluation of levels of urine organic acids and serum amino acids and serum lactate (discussed later in "Inborn Errors of Metabolism"), as well as serum ammonia and lactate.

Routine imaging studies are not required for most cases of hypoglycemia, but may be useful if there are underlying organ anomalies.

TREATMENT

Treat hypoglycemia promptly while awaiting diagnostic results. IV dextrose is the primary treatment and may be given enterally (PO, nasogastric tube) or parenterally (IV or IO). **The dose of dextrose is 0.5 to 1.0 gram/kg regardless of the route of administration. Newborns should receive 5 mL/kg of 10% dextrose, whereas infants and children should receive 1 to 2 mL/kg of 25% dextrose.** With adequate IV access, 1 mL/kg of 50% dextrose may be administered to older children as to adults. Some recommend a 0.2 gram/kg dextrose bolus to minimize hyperglycemia and resultant insulin secretion, which prolongs hypoglycemia. Use of dilute solutions in younger patients is suggested to minimize the vascular injury associated with more concentrated fluids.

Provide maintenance dextrose at a rate of 6 to 8 milligrams/kg/min with 10% dextrose, which is 1.5 times the normal maintenance rate for infants and children. If IV or IO access or nasogastric tube placement cannot readily be initiated, glucagon, 0.3 milligram/kg IM, may be given. Refractory hypoglycemia may be seen in hyperinsulinemic states such as insulin-secreting tumors and is suggested by hypoglycemia requiring administration of more than 6 to 8 milligrams/kg/min. Frequent reevaluation and titration of infused dextrose are necessary in this situation. **If adrenal insufficiency is suspected, give hydrocortisone, 25 grams IV or IM for neonates and infants, 50 grams for toddlers and school-age children, and 100 grams for adolescents.** The management of hypoglycemia is summarized in **Table 144-1**.

Because sepsis is always in the differential diagnosis of the neonate, infant, or child who is critically ill or shows altered mental status, provide prompt broad-spectrum antibiotics as indicated by the clinical

TABLE 144-1 Management of Hypoglycemia in the ED

Patient Age	Dextrose Bolus Dose	Dextrose Maintenance Dosage	Other Treatments to Consider
Neonate	D10 5 mL/kg PO/NG/IV/IO	6 mL/kg/h D10	Glucagon, 0.3 milligram/kg IM Hydrocortisone, 25 grams PO/IM/IV/IO
Infant	D10 5 mL/kg PO/NG/IV/IO *or* D25 2 mL/kg	6 mL/kg/h D10	Glucagon, 0.3 milligram/kg IM Hydrocortisone, 25 grams PO/IM/IV/IO
Child	D25 2 mL/kg PO/NG/IV/IO	6 mL/kg/h D10 for the first 10 kg + 3 mL/kg/h for 11–20 kg + 1.5 mL/kg/h for each additional kg >20 kg	Glucagon, 0.3 milligram/kg/IM Hydrocortisone, 50 grams PO/IM/IV/IO
Adolescent	—	6 mL/kg/h D10 for the first 10 kg + 3 mL/kg/h for 11–20 kg + 1.5 mL/kg/h for each additional kg >20 kg	Glucagon, 0.3 milligram/kg IM Hydrocortisone, 100 grams PO/IM/IV/IO

Abbreviations: D10 = 10% dextrose; D25 = 25% dextrose; NG = (via) nasogastric tube.

picture. This includes ampicillin, 50 milligrams/kg, and gentamicin, 5 to 7.5 milligrams/kg, or cefotaxime, 50 milligrams/kg, for neonates and infants in the first 2 months of life, and ceftriaxone, 50 milligrams/kg (100 milligrams/kg if meningitis is suspected), for older infants and children.

DISPOSITION AND FOLLOW-UP

All neonates and infants with symptomatic hypoglycemia requiring ED resuscitation should be admitted to the hospital for further evaluation and treatment. Patients for whom sepsis is a concern and those requiring dextrose beyond the expected 6 to 8 milligrams/kg/h may require admission to the intensive care unit.

INBORN ERRORS OF METABOLISM

Although the diversity and complexity of inborn errors of metabolism in infants and children may seem overwhelming, keep in mind that making a definitive diagnosis is not as important as maintaining a high suspicion and that acute stabilization and management are relatively simple. As a group, these disorders involve enzyme deficiencies that lead to errors of metabolism resulting in the accumulation of various toxic biochemical products, which can cause dysfunction of multiple organ systems, especially the CNS. Although each **individual** type of inborn error of metabolism is extremely rare, as a group they are relatively common, with an incidence ranging from 1 in 1400 to 1 in 200,000 live births.[13,14]

Clinical manifestations of inborn errors of metabolism are a result of the accumulation of toxic metabolites and their effects on end-organs. Common symptoms and signs of inherited metabolic disorders include acute encephalopathy with or without metabolic acidosis and hypoglycemia (discussed earlier in "Hypoglycemia"). **Because most metabolic toxins cross the placenta and are cleared by maternal enzymes, most newborns are asymptomatic and present after varying delays once enteral feeding begins.** Hypoglycemia may be the primary presentation of some inherited disorders of metabolism and is discussed earlier (see "Hypoglycemia"). Jaundice and hepatic dysfunction can be seen in a number of inherited disorders such as galactosemia.[16] Shock and cardiovascular collapse can occur with congenital adrenal insufficiency, but nonmetabolic conditions such as congenital heart disease and sepsis must be considered in the differential diagnosis of infants presenting in extremis. The discussion here is limited to conditions that typically present in early infancy with the potential for life-threatening consequences.

PATHOPHYSIOLOGY

Most inborn errors of metabolism result from single-gene defects with a variety of inheritance patterns. The defects result in abnormal metabolism of protein, fat, carbohydrates, or other complex molecules. Affected proteins include enzymes, enzyme cofactors, and transport proteins. The result of these varied deficiencies is the accumulation of toxic substrates upstream of the impaired protein or of intermediates derived from alternate metabolic processes downstream. On the basis of metabolic and clinical manifestations, these disorders can often be grouped into those defects resulting in hyperammonemia, metabolic acidosis, hypoglycemia, or hyperbilirubinemia and liver dysfunction.[16]

Urea cycle defects, organic acidemias, and some fatty acid oxidation defects may result in the accumulation of ammonia, leading to encephalopathy.[17] Examples of organic acidemias that present in the first 24 hours of life are glutaric acidemia and pyruvate carboxylase deficiency (which causes lactic acidemia). Urea cycle defects typically present after the first 24 hours of life and often lack associated metabolic acidosis. Examples are ornithine transcarbamylase deficiency, carbamyl phosphate synthetase deficiency, and citrullinemia. Ornithine transcarbamylase deficiency is X-linked in its inheritance, and therefore affects male infants.

Although organic acidemias can also lead to hyperammonemia, they are typically accompanied by metabolic acidosis. Examples are methylmalonic acidemia, propionic acidemia, and isovaleric acidemia. Defects in pyruvate metabolism, defects in enzymes of the respiratory chain, and mitochondrial disorders also result in metabolic acidosis, which is often independent of protein intake. These disorders result in lactic acidosis with normal urine organic acid levels and include pyruvate dehydrogenase deficiency.

Disorders of carbohydrate, lipid, or fatty acid metabolism include glycogen storage diseases and medium-chain acyl coenzyme A dehydrogenase deficiency. These disorders impair the ability to use or produce glucose, which leads to hypoglycemia, often in the setting of fasting or poor oral intake. Glycogen and lipid storage diseases usually present later in infancy or childhood with developmental delay, dysmorphic or progressively coarse features, and hepatomegaly. Fatty acid metabolism defects result in nonketotic hypoglycemia (see "Hypoglycemia" above), which is a distinguishing characteristic. Secondary carnitine deficiency is often seen in medium-chain acyl coenzyme A dehydrogenase deficiency.

Hyperbilirubinemia and liver dysfunction may be the presenting feature of inborn errors of metabolism such as galactosemia, tyrosinemia, or α1-antitrypsin deficiency. Galactosemia results from the deficiency of galactose-1-phosphate uridylyltransferase, which leads to an accumulation of galactose-1-phosphate and other metabolites that are toxic to the liver. In addition to hepatic dysfunction, these infants may develop hypoglycemia, hyperbilirubinemia, hemolysis, or overwhelming infection.

CLINICAL FEATURES

HISTORY

Many inborn errors of metabolism present with nonspecific symptoms, including irritability, lethargy, vomiting, and poor feeding; severe hypoglycemia or metabolic encephalopathy may present with seizures. A careful characterization of these symptoms, however, may point toward a metabolic disorder: poor feeding and lethargy may be more notable in the morning prior to the first feeding as a result of a relative period of fasting. Parents may note aversion to protein or carbohydrates. Diarrhea may accompany carbohydrate metabolism disorders or mitochondrial disease. Parents may report an abnormal body or urinary odor, although this is more commonly noted by clinicians. Abnormal odor is typical of isovaleric acidemia, glutaric acidemia, and maple syrup urine disease, which, as the name suggests, is accompanied by a characteristic sweet smell of the urine.

Obtain a dietary and developmental history. Frequent changes in formula due to vomiting or failure to thrive may indicate undiagnosed metabolic disease. Unexplained developmental delay may also be a clue to diagnosis. Take a thorough medical history. A history of recurrent hospitalizations with a response to IV fluids and glucose may suggest an underlying metabolic disorder. The maternal history taking should include questions about previous spontaneous abortions or miscarriages and the death of previous infants early in life. Maternal complications during pregnancy, such as acute fatty liver or HELLP syndrome (*h*emolysis, *e*levated *l*iver enzymes, *l*ow *p*latelets), may be related to heterozygosity for fatty acid oxidation defects. The family history should include information about relatives with early cardiac disease, sudden infant death syndrome, neurologic disease, and liver disease with onset in childhood, all of which may signal inherited disorders of metabolism.

PHYSICAL EXAMINATION

The physical examination begins with attention to the vital signs. Tachycardia is often present during acute metabolic crisis; congenital adrenal hyperplasia may cause hypotension. Hypothermia may accompany many metabolic diseases, particularly the urea cycle defects and organic acidemias. Tachypnea without increased work of breathing may be noted in patients with metabolic acidosis and may result in a respiratory alkalosis. Although the majority of inborn errors of metabolism that present in early infancy are not associated with other specific findings on physical examination, those that present later in childhood, such as glycogen storage disease, liposomal storage disease, and mucopolysaccharidoses, may manifest with hepatosplenomegaly, growth retardation, poor muscle tone, developmental delay, and coarse features.[18] Some metabolic disorders have ocular findings, including cataracts (e.g., galactosemia) or dislocated lenses (e.g., homocystinuria). The GU

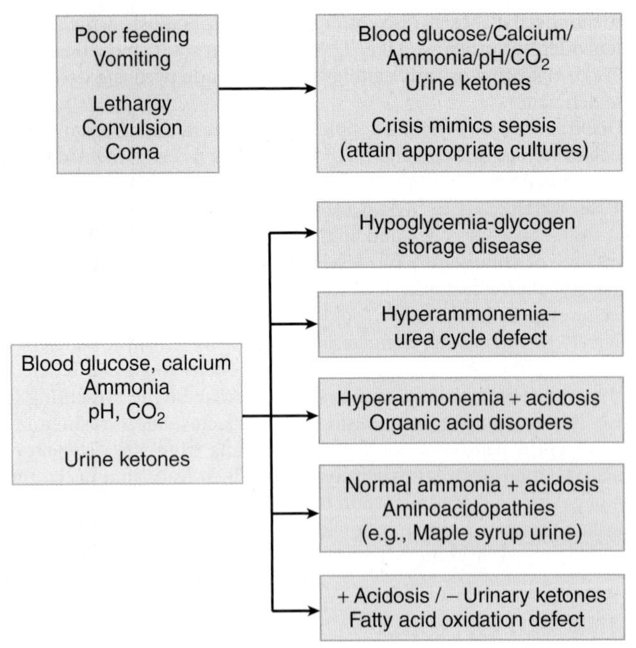

FIGURE 144-2. Approach to suspected metabolic disorders. CO_2 = carbon dioxide.

examination is important when adrenal insufficiency is a consideration, because females with one specific defect may show signs of virilization (see "Congenital Adrenal Hyperplasia [Adrenal Insufficiency]" below). A complete head-to-toe physical examination should be performed, of course, despite the lack of characteristic findings in most inborn errors of metabolism presenting during infancy, in order to exclude alternative diagnoses, including sepsis and congenital heart disease.

DIAGNOSIS

Due to the rarity and diversity of these disorders, the aspects of their acute clinical presentations and management in the ED have yet to be well defined. A simplified, although not exhaustive, approach to inborn errors of metabolism is presented in the following sections and in **Figure 144-2**. The key laboratory studies that are most useful to the emergency physician in directing immediate management and suggesting potential diagnoses include bedside glucose level, urine ketone level, plasma ammonia concentration, basic metabolic screen, blood gas analysis, and plasma lactate level. These are discussed in more detail in the following sections. Additional clues may be provided by a CBC, liver function tests, and muscle function tests (lactate dehydrogenase, creatine kinase, and myoglobin levels) (**Table 144-2**). Definitive diagnosis often depends on plasma or serum levels of amino acids, acylcarnitine profile, and lactate and pyruvate levels, as well as urine test results for organic acids, acylglycines, and orotic acid, and potentially on results of cerebrospinal fluid studies, including tests for lactate, pyruvate, and organic and amino acids.[16,18,19] A summary of laboratory evaluations for suspected metabolic disease and their utility and significance is provided in Table 144-2.

BEDSIDE GLUCOSE AND URINE KETONE LEVELS

Hypoglycemia may be a feature of several inborn errors of metabolism, including glycogen storage disease, fatty acid oxidation disorders, and disorders of gluconeogenesis. Some organic acidemias may also be associated with hypoglycemia. **Hypoglycemia in the absence of urinary ketones suggests a fatty acid oxidation defect, and hypoglycemia with urinary ketones can be seen in organic acidemias.**

PLASMA AMMONIA CONCENTRATION

Ammonia is formed during the deamination of amino acids and excreted as urea in the urine. Urea is produced in the hepatocyte mitochondria and cytosol through the metabolic process known as the *urea cycle*. Normal neonatal ammonia concentrations are <65 micromoles/L, but may be two to three times this in stressed or nonfasting newborns and infants. Levels >200 micromoles/L suggest metabolic disease and are the hallmark of urea cycle disorders. Hyperammonemia detected in the first 24 hours of life may be seen with pyruvate carboxylase deficiency, whereas hyperammonemia associated with urea cycle defects usually presents after protein feeding has begun and may reach ammonia concentrations well above 400 micromoles/L. The severe hyperammonemia of urea cycle disorders may stimulate central hyperventilation, resulting in respiratory alkalosis. Secondary causes of more modest hyperammonemia include mitochondrial, respiratory chain, or fatty acid oxidation defects, which are often associated with metabolic and/or lactic acidosis.

BLOOD GAS ANALYSIS AND BASIC METABOLIC PANEL

Evaluation of acid-base status is best achieved through analysis of blood gas samples and serum electrolyte levels. Serum lactate levels (discussed below in "Plasma Lactate Level") provide additional information. The anion gap (sodium – [chloride + bicarbonate]) is usually <15 mEq/L but increases with excess acid production. **Organic acidemias are associated with significant anion gap acidosis, often higher than 30 to 50 mEq/L.** Other inborn errors of metabolism associated with metabolic acidosis include respiratory chain disorders, disorders of pyruvate metabolism, and some glycogen storage diseases. In comparison with organic acidemias,

TABLE 144-2 Additional Laboratory Tests in the Diagnosis of Metabolic Disease

Test	Result	Diagnostic Implications
Liver function tests	Unconjugated hyperbilirubinemia	Galactosemia
	Hepatic failure	Fatty acid oxidation disorders, mitochondrial disorders, urea cycle disorders
CBC	Pancytopenia	Aminoacidopathy (propionic acidemia, isovaleric acidemia, methylmalonic acidemia)
Creatine kinase	Elevated	Mitochondrial disorders
Aldolase	Elevated	Fatty acid oxidation defects
Serum amino acids	Abnormal quantitative results	Aminoacidopathy, organic aciduria, urea cycle defect, mitochondrial disorder
Serum acylcarnitine	Abnormal profile	Organic acidurias, fatty acid oxidation defects, mitochondrial disorders, carnitine deficiency
Profile		
Urine-reducing substances	Positive test result is always abnormal	Aminoacidopathy (tyrosinemia), carbohydrate intolerance disorders (galactosemia)
Urine organic acids	Abnormal profile	Aminoacidopathy, organic aciduria, fatty acid oxidation defects, mitochondrial disorders, peroxisomal disorders
Urine orotic acid	Elevated	Urea cycle defects (ornithine transcarbamylase deficiency)
Urine acylglycines	Abnormal	Aminoacidopathies, organic acidurias

these conditions typically include significant accumulation of lactic acid, which helps distinguish them from organic acidemia.[15,16,18]

PLASMA LACTATE LEVEL

Lactate is produced from pyruvate, and lactic acidosis is a common feature of severe illnesses ranging from sepsis to hypoxia from pulmonary or cardiac disease or hypovolemic shock. Dehydration often accompanies metabolic disease and may produce some degree of lactic acidosis in any critically ill neonate with a metabolic disorder; however, subtracting the plasma lactate from the anion gap can aid in distinguishing between primary lactic acidosis resulting from mitochondrial disorders, fatty acid oxidation defects, and some glycogen storage disease (normal anion gap after subtraction of lactate), and secondary metabolic causes such as organic acidemias (elevated anion gap after subtraction of lactate).[16]

TREATMENT

Despite the diverse etiology and complexity of inborn errors of metabolism, ED resuscitation and stabilization are relatively simple. **Neonates, infants, and children presenting in metabolic crisis, regardless of cause, show some combination of dehydration, metabolic acidosis, and encephalopathy, which must be immediately addressed.** Therefore, the goals of treatment are to improve circulatory status by restoring circulatory volume, provide energy substrate to halt catabolism, remove the inciting metabolic substrate (formula or breast milk), and help eliminate toxic metabolites.[20-22]

FLUID RESUSCITATION

As with any critically ill patient, attending to the ABCDs (*a*irway, *b*reathing, *c*irculation, *d*isability [neurologic status]) is the first step. Apnea, hypoventilation, and hypoxia are treated with positive-pressure ventilation or endotracheal intubation and administration of oxygen. **Take care when paralyzing the infant in metabolic crisis, because metabolic acidosis can be worsened by respiratory acidosis if insufficient ventilation is provided.** Restore circulation with crystalloid boluses, typically 10 to 20 mL/kg in the neonate and 20 mL/kg in the infant, with frequent reassessment and further fluid administration as clinically indicated. (Because congenital heart disease can present similarly to metabolic crisis, careful reevaluation after each fluid bolus is essential.) Even a patient who is not in shock may benefit from a bolus of normal saline followed by double the usual level of maintenance fluids with dextrose, because aggressive hydration promotes urine output with increased clearing of toxic metabolites (e.g., organic acids, ammonia), whereas dextrose provides a substrate for metabolism. Avoid hypotonic fluids because they may increase the risk of cerebral edema, particularly in hyperammonemic states. Assess neurologic status before definitive airway management. The cause of altered mental status (hypoglycemia or hyperammonemia) must be determined and may be reversible but is difficult to assess in the paralyzed or sedated patient (see below).

Metabolic acidosis during metabolic crisis can arise from dehydration, which may respond to fluid administration, or from the underlying metabolic defect. The ongoing production of acidic metabolites may necessitate the administration of sodium bicarbonate; however, treatment may be associated with side effects, including sodium overload, cerebral edema, and cardiac dysfunction. **A conservative approach is to treat a blood pH of <7.0 with 0.5 mEq/kg/h.**[13,20]

All patients in metabolic crisis should be kept NPO to remove potential inciting metabolic substrates (protein, carbohydrates, fats), and adequate dextrose should be provided for anabolic substrate. Dextrose 10% is usually preferred and should be administered at twice the usual maintenance rates.

ELIMINATE TOXIC METABOLITES

Elimination of toxic metabolites is the next step. Hyperammonemia, as seen in urea cycle defects and some organic acidemias, is the most common cause of metabolic encephalopathy in infants. Ammonia levels of <500 micromoles/L should be treated with a combination of sodium phenylacetate and sodium benzoate (Ammonul®): 250 milligrams/kg in 10% dextrose is administered through a central venous line (or intraosseous line) over 90 minutes followed by 250 milligrams/kg/d as a continuous infusion. Arginine, 210 milligrams/kg IV/IO in 10% dextrose over 90 minutes followed by 210 milligrams/kg/d continuous infusion, should also be provided (**Figure 144-3**). Empiric therapy with arginine with or without sodium benzoate can reduce ammonia levels drastically. Early aggressive treatment may eliminate the need for hemodialysis for excessive ammonia removal. Additional therapy may include empiric carnitine, 400 milligrams IV/IO, which combines with organic acids to form acylcarnitines that are readily excreted from urine (**Figure 144-4**), although no prospective trials have been performed.[23] Reduction in acyl coenzyme A levels eliminates their inhibitory effect on the urea cycle, resulting in reduced serum ammonia levels.[17,21]

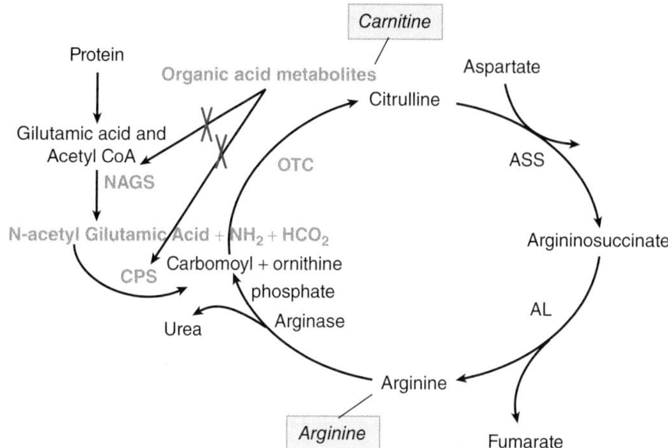

FIGURE 144-3. Combined role of carnitine and arginine in metabolic crisis in inborn errors of metabolism. Acetyl CoA = acetyl coenzyme A; AL = argininosuccinate lyase; ASS = argininosuccinate synthase; CPS = carbamoyl phosphate synthetase; NAGS = *N*-acetylglutamate synthase; OTC = ornithine transcarbamylase.

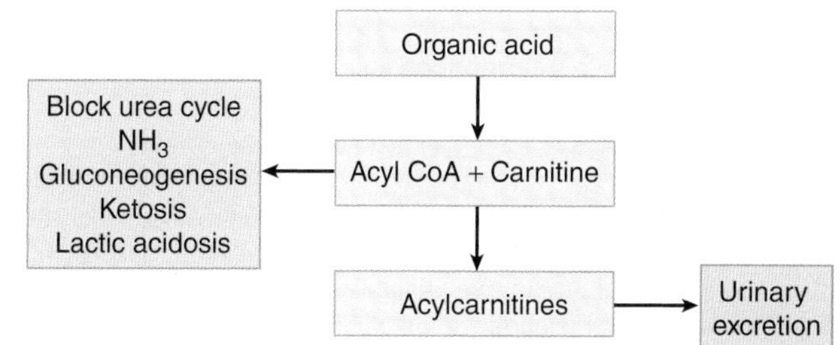

FIGURE 144-4. Role of carnitine in metabolic crisis in inborn errors of metabolism. Acyl CoA = acyl coenzyme A.

ADDITIONAL THERAPIES

For hyperammonemia of >400 to 600 micromoles/L, consider dialysis. For infants with seizures, empiric administration of pyridoxine, 100 milligrams IV/IO, for pyridoxine-dependent metabolic disease can be tried. If this is ineffective, folinic acid, 2.5 milligrams IV/IO, or biotin, 10 milligrams by nasogastric tube, can be considered.[13] A summary of second-tier therapies for specific suspected inborn errors of metabolism is provided in **Table 144-3**.

COMPLICATIONS

During metabolic crisis, the accumulation of various organic acids can suppress granulopoietic stem cells and thereby cause bone marrow suppression of all cell lines. This leads to an immunocompromised state

TABLE 144-3 Specific Therapies for Inborn Errors of Metabolism

Inborn Error of Metabolism	Drug	Dosage
Urea cycle defects	Arginine HCl 10%	210 milligrams/kg IV/IO over 90 min
	Sodium benzoate and/or phenylacetate	250 milligrams/kg IV/IO continuous infusion over 24 h
Organic acidemias	Carnitine	400 milligrams IV/IO or PO
Fatty acid oxidation defects	Biotin	10 milligrams IV/IO or PO
Pyridoxine-dependent seizures	Pyridoxine	100 milligrams IV/IO
Maple syrup urine disease, primary lactic acidosis	Thiamine	25–100 milligrams IV/IO

with an increased incidence of **sepsis** due to unusual organisms. **The incidence is 15% to 30% per 100 episodes.** Therefore it is essential to rule out sepsis in all patients with metabolic crisis. Chronic anemia and thrombocytopenia may accompany a number of inborn errors of metabolism and may be exaggerated during metabolic crisis. Give empiric broad-spectrum antibiotics such as ceftazidime, 50 milligrams/kg IV.

Hyperammonemia is a specific risk factor for **cerebral edema**, especially when hypotonic solutions are administered during therapy. Cerebral edema is a clinical diagnosis and should be suspected when laboratory parameters improve but altered mental status continues. Treatment for cerebral edema is mannitol (0.5 gram/kg IV/IO) and avoidance of hypo-/hyperventilation. **Do not give steroids because steroids exacerbate hyperammonemia.**

DISPOSITION AND FOLLOW-UP

All patients in metabolic crisis should be admitted to the hospital or transferred to a tertiary care children's hospital where metabolic specialists are available to help with definitive diagnosis and dietary management. Patients with severe metabolic abnormalities requiring hemodialysis require intensive care.

CONGENITAL ADRENAL HYPERPLASIA (ADRENAL INSUFFICIENCY)

Congenital adrenal hyperplasia results from deficiency in one of the five enzymes involved in the production of cortisol. Absence of these enzymes leads to decreased conversion of 17-hydroxyprogesterone to 11-desoxycortisol with resultant cortisol deficiency. Most of the enzyme deficiencies also impair conversion to progesterone and 11-desoxycorticosterone in the mineralocorticoid pathway, which leads to decreased aldosterone production. Deficiency of 21-hydroxylase accounts for up to 95% of congenital adrenal hyperplasia cases and occurs in 1 in 10,000 to 15,000 live births.[24] Seventy-five percent of affected newborns manifest the classic salt-losing, virilizing variant in which urinary salt wasting with hyperkalemia and hyponatremia dominate the clinical picture. Twenty-five percent of cases are the non–salt-losing simple virilizing type. Infants with salt-losing forms of congenital adrenal hyperplasia typically present during the second to fifth weeks of life in crisis, sometimes before the results of newborn screening tests for the disease are available.

PATHOPHYSIOLOGY

Congenital adrenal hyperplasia is a group of disorders of adrenal steroid biosynthesis that result from a defect in one of five enzymes (**Figure 144-5**). Depending on the specific enzyme deficiency, cortisol deficiency may be accompanied by mineralocorticoid deficiency, leading to hypoaldosteronism with resultant salt wasting. Because the hypothalamic-pituitary axis is suppressed by cortisol, the deficiency results in increased secretion of adrenocorticotropic hormone without feedback suppression. Uninhibited excess adrenocorticotropic hormone stimulates the adrenal gland, which leads to hypertrophy. Elevated adrenocorticotropic hormone levels can also cause hyperpigmentation of the skin, which is best observed on the labial or scrotal folds and the nipples. Steroid hormone precursors upstream of the enzyme defect build up and are shunted into alternate pathways. Deficiencies in 21-hydroxylase lead to the accumulation of precursors that are metabolized to androgens. This, in turn, causes virilization of affected females, which manifests as clitoromegaly. Affected males may go undetected at birth because their genitalia appear normal.

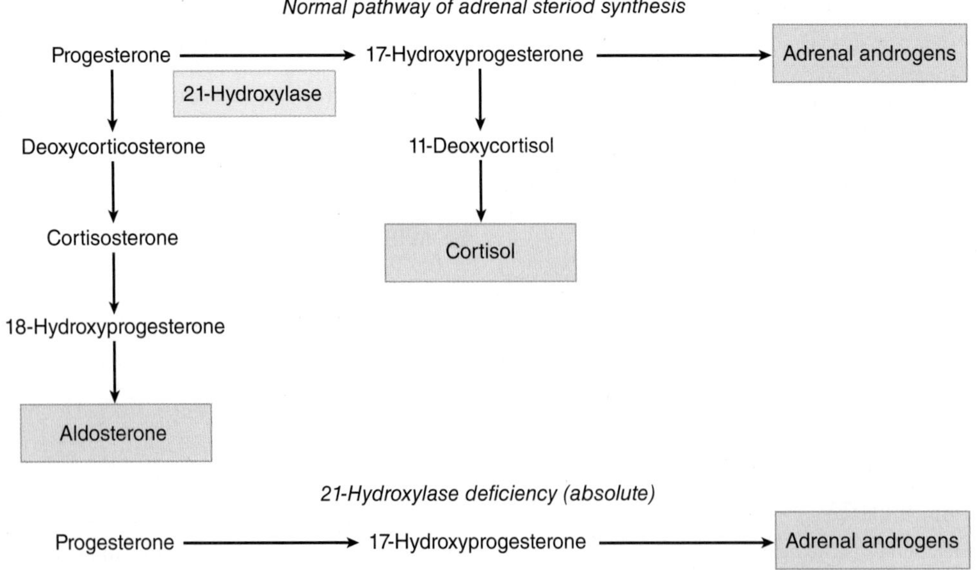

FIGURE 144-5. Normal pathway of adrenal steroid synthesis.

CLINICAL FEATURES

HISTORY

Salt-wasting variants of congenital adrenal hyperplasia typically manifest as acute crisis in the second week of life. Symptoms are vague and include lethargy, irritability, poor feeding, vomiting, and poor weight gain. Depending on the duration and severity of symptoms, infants may present with significant dehydration or even shock. Obtain a complete history of the presenting symptoms, because the differential diagnosis of adrenal salt-wasting crisis includes sepsis, congenital heart disease, and other inborn errors of metabolism. Review gestational age and birth weight as well as maternal history regarding complications of pregnancy, prior pregnancies, miscarriages, spontaneous abortions, and previous infant deaths. Try to obtain results of newborn screening.

PHYSICAL EXAMINATION

Record vital signs and weight, and assess hydration and mental status. In addition to performing a complete head-to-toe examination, carefully examine the genitalia: females may have fusion of the labia and an enlarged clitoris. Males may have normal genitalia or a small phallus or hypospadias. Note any hyperpigmentation, especially in the scrotal or labial folds and around the nipples.

DIAGNOSIS

The most important laboratory studies are a bedside glucose level and serum electrolyte levels. Although hypoglycemia is rare, poor feeding and vomiting may cause secondary hypoglycemia requiring urgent treatment. **The classic electrolyte abnormalities in salt-wasting congenital adrenal hyperplasia are hyponatremia and hyperkalemia.** Serum potassium level may be elevated to between 6 and 12 mEq/L, although changes in cardiac function and ECG are unusual. Metabolic acidosis typically accompanies the classic electrolyte abnormalities as a result of aldosterone deficiency and dehydration.

Definitive diagnosis depends on analysis of blood hormone levels. If possible, obtain results of a steroid profile prior to treatment, but do not delay treatment in the critically ill neonate. Because the presentation of adrenal salt-wasting crisis is nonspecific, consider alternative diagnoses such as sepsis.

Although infants generally tolerate hyperkalemia well, obtain a 12-lead ECG, because hyperkalemic changes may alter emergent therapy and disposition. Imaging studies are not routinely indicated or helpful.

TREATMENT

Circulatory collapse from cortisol deficiency and dehydration is common, so establish IV or IO access rapidly. Administer IV fluids in the form of 10 to 20 mL/kg of normal saline. Fluid loss in congenital adrenal hyperplasia is isotonic, and fluid replacement should be with normal saline. Treat hypoglycemia with 5 mL/kg of 10% dextrose as discussed above in "Hypoglycemia."

Initiate steroid hormone replacement urgently: give hydrocortisone, 25 milligrams IV/IO to neonates, 50 milligrams to toddlers and school-age children, and 100 milligrams to adolescents. Although mineralocorticoid deficiency in congenital adrenal hyperplasia is primarily treated by sodium repletion with normal saline, there is some mineralocorticoid effect at these doses of hydrocortisone.

If hyperkalemia results in ECG changes or arrhythmia, treat with IV calcium gluconate (10%), 100 milligrams/kg (1 mL/kg), and sodium bicarbonate, 1 mEq/kg. **Do not give insulin and glucose for hyperkalemia in infants, because this may result in profound hypoglycemia.** The administration of normal saline and hydrocortisone is usually sufficient to lower serum potassium levels in the absence of cardiac manifestations.

DISPOSITION AND FOLLOW-UP

All infants with salt-wasting crisis require admission to the hospital. Infants with signs of shock or severe hyperkalemia with ECG changes should be admitted to the intensive care unit, with endocrinology consultation.

Acknowledgment: The authors thank Ralph Cordle, author of this chapter in the previous edition.

REFERENCES

The complete reference list is available online at www.TintinalliEM.com.

CHAPTER 145 Diabetes In Children

Adam Vella

INTRODUCTION AND EPIDEMIOLOGY

Diabetes is subclassified into several different forms. Type 1 diabetes, previously referred to as *insulin-dependent diabetes mellitus* or *juvenile-onset diabetes* because of its earlier onset, is characterized by an abrupt and frequently complete decline in insulin production. Type 2 diabetes, formerly referred to as *non–insulin-dependent diabetes mellitus* or *adult-onset diabetes*, is marked by increasing insulin resistance and most commonly occurs in the overweight adult or adolescent; there is a strong genetic tendency toward the disease. The third main form of diabetes affecting children is gestational diabetes, which can affect pregnant teens as well as the infants of diabetic mothers. There has been an increase in the prevalence of type 1 diabetes of 21% between 2001 and 2009, and an increase of 31% in type 2 diabetes in the same time period.[1] While the cause of the increase in type 1 diabetes is unknown, some experts suggest that the increasing prevalence of type 2 diabetes may be a result of minority population growth, obesity, exposure to diabetes in utero, and perhaps endocrine-disrupting chemicals.[1] Diabetes is the most common pediatric endocrine disorder, with an estimated prevalence of 1 in 400. As many as 34% of children with new-onset type 1 diabetes present in diabetic ketoacidosis (DKA).[2] In children with known diabetes, DKA is much less common and tends to be clustered in a small subset of patients, with 5% of children with diabetes accounting for nearly 60% of DKA episodes.[3] DKA is the leading cause of mortality in patients with diabetes <24 years of age, and cerebral edema is the leading cause of mortality in DKA.[4]

PATHOPHYSIOLOGY

The fundamental cause of DKA is an absolute or relative insulin deficiency that results in the inability of cells to take up and use glucose. Levels of counterregulatory hormones (catecholamines, cortisol, growth hormone, and glucagon) are elevated, which drives many of the physiologic disturbances observed in DKA. These hormones increase glucose production by promoting glycogenolysis, gluconeogenesis, lipolysis, and ketogenesis, and further decrease glucose utilization by antagonizing insulin.

As the serum glucose level exceeds the renal absorption threshold, an obligatory osmotic diuresis ensues, which results in the classic symptoms of polyuria and polydipsia. If not recognized early, this can lead to profound dehydration and electrolyte disturbances. Acidosis stems from the complex metabolic derangements induced by insulin deficiency and unopposed glucagon. The cellular milieu of the body is essentially in a state of functional starvation, unable to use the excess serum glucose. Decreased lipid uptake by adipose tissue and increased lipolysis result in an overabundance of circulating free fatty acids, which are converted by the liver into the ketoacids acetoacetate and β-hydroxybutyrate.

Despite this profound shift in substrate production, ketoacid utilization and renal elimination are both impaired, which results in a wide anion gap metabolic acidosis. In certain patients, the acid-base status may be more complex. Persistent vomiting and severe volume depletion may result in a superimposed metabolic alkalosis that may mask the severity of the acidosis by producing a relatively normal pH. Severe dehydration and poor perfusion further lead to lactic acidosis, which results in a superimposed anion gap acidosis. Alternatively, a patient who remains relatively well hydrated will lose sodium with keto anions in the urine while retaining chloride and demonstrate a significant non–anion gap acidosis.

See the chapters 223 and 224, "Type 1 Diabetes Mellitus" and "Type 2 Diabetes Mellitus," respectively, for more discussion of the pathophysiology of diabetes.

CLINICAL FEATURES

Polyuria, polydipsia, and polyphagia are the classic symptom triad of type 1 diabetes. Other common symptoms include weight loss, secondary enuresis, anorexia, vague abdominal discomfort, visual changes, and genital candidiasis in a toilet-trained child. The diagnosis is established by demonstrating hyperglycemia and glucosuria in the absence of other causes such as steroid therapy, Cushing's syndrome, pheochromocytoma, hyperthyroidism, or other rare disorders. Signs of uncontrolled diabetes span the entire spectrum from simple hyperglycemia without ketonuria to diabetic ketosis (hyperglycemia with ketonuria) to full-blown DKA.

DKA

DKA is generally defined as a metabolic acidosis (pH <7.30 or serum bicarbonate level of <15 mEq/L) with hyperglycemia (serum glucose level of >200 milligrams/dL or 11 mmol/L) and ketonemia or ketonuria.[5,6] DKA is much more common in patients with type 1 diabetes than in those with type 2, but it is not uncommon for patients with type 2 to develop acidosis under moderately severe physiologic stress. This acidosis has been referred to as the hyperglycemic hyperosmolar state, which can result in severe total body water, potassium, and phosphorus deficits. Hyperglycemic hyperosmolar state, which is estimated to account for 1% of all diabetic admissions, has a case fatality rate of 5% to 20%.[5,7]

In the patient with known diabetes, the diagnosis of DKA is relatively straightforward. The most common cause of DKA in children and adolescents with known diabetes is poor adherence to the prescribed insulin regimen. Other precipitants include intercurrent viral illness and focal infections such as urinary tract infection or gastroenteritis. Patients complain of polydipsia and polyuria (if not dehydrated), diffuse nonfocal abdominal pain often associated with vomiting, difficulty breathing, and generalized malaise, in addition to any localizing complaints related to a precipitating trigger. Kussmaul breathing may be mistaken for pulmonary pathology or even anxiety with hyperventilation.

Physical findings in DKA are due to dehydration and metabolic acidosis. Children appear dehydrated, are tachycardic, and may be hypotensive. Respiratory compensation for acidosis is noted in the deep Kussmaul respirations, which may be accompanied by paresthesias. Acetoacetate is converted to acetone and is responsible for the classic breath odor of nail polish. The level of consciousness may range from alert to somnolent to comatose. **In a child with DKA and a depressed level of consciousness, consider the development of cerebral edema.**

Abdominal pain and vomiting often accompany DKA. Distinguish nonspecific abdominal pain or gastroenteritis from more serious intra-abdominal disorders such as acute appendicitis. Focal abdominal tenderness, failure of pain to resolve with fluid therapy, and associated fever suggest an underlying intra-abdominal process.

An elevated glucose level in the presence of ketonemia/ketonuria and acidosis almost always indicates DKA. However, other rare conditions possess similar clinical characteristics. Any condition resulting in prolonged vomiting or excessive fasting can result in ketoacidosis, but the glucose level is not elevated. **In adolescent patients without known diabetes, consider toxic ingestions of ethylene glycol, isopropyl alcohol, or salicylates.**

CEREBRAL EDEMA

PATHOPHYSIOLOGY

Cerebral edema, which occurs in approximately 0.5% to 1% of all children presenting with DKA, is the most dreaded complication, accounting for 60% to 90% of all pediatric DKA-associated deaths.[4] Mortality rates range from 21% to 24%, and only 14% to 57% of children who develop the disorder recover neurologically normal.[8] Cerebral edema more commonly develops in children <5 years old and is rare in persons >20 years old (see **Table 145-1**).[8] It is likely that all patients with severe DKA have some degree of subclinical cerebral edema,[9] but the **specific risk factors associated with overt, life-threatening cerebral edema are young age, severe hyperosmolality, persistent hyponatremia, and severe acidosis.**[5,8] Failure of serum sodium level to rise commensurately with the fall in glucose level during therapy may be an important predictor.[8] **Newer studies refute the belief that overaggressive fluid resuscitation per se is a significant risk factor.**[2,10] The incidence of cerebral edema has not changed over the past 15 to 20 years, despite the introduction of gradual rehydration protocols over the same interval.[10] Furthermore, a randomized study of two rehydration protocols in DKA was assessed for the risk of associated MRI-documented subclinical cerebral edema and showed no difference in the rate of cerebral edema between an aggressive and a more judicious rehydration protocol.[11] A vasogenic process has been postulated as the predominant mechanism of cerebral edema formation in DKA rather than osmotic cellular swelling.[9,12] A study using perfusion MRI during DKA treatment in children demonstrated increased cerebral blood flow suggesting a difference in the hemodynamic states of dehydrated and resuscitated children with DKA. The authors further noted that the patients with greater dehydration and more profound hypocapnia had an increased risk of cerebral edema, possibly as a result of cerebral hypoperfusion and ischemia prior to treatment.[12] Regardless of the exact mechanism, caution in fluid administration is prudent, particularly in the extremely hyperosmolal child (i.e., osmolarity of >340 mOsm/L).

TABLE 145-1 Management of Cerebral Edema

Factors indicating high risk
Age <5 y
Severe acidosis
Severe hyperosmolality
Failure of serum sodium level to rise with therapy
Prevention
Avoid high-dose insulin therapy
Judicious fluid management historically, but recent studies refute this as a cause
Early clinical recognition
Avoid administration of sodium bicarbonate
Treatment
Mannitol, 0.5–1 gram/kg IV bolus, or 10 mL/kg of 3% saline over 30 min
Fluid restriction
Appropriate airway management and ventilation

CLINICAL FEATURES

Cerebral edema typically manifests itself 6 to 12 hours after the onset of therapy (**Figure 145-1**).[5] Many children appear to be improving clinically and biochemically prior to deterioration from cerebral edema. **Premonitory symptoms occur in as few as 50% of patients and include severe headache, declining mental status, seizures, and papillary edema.** Unfortunately, respiratory arrest may be the first sign of cerebral edema. Early aggressive intervention based on the clinical evaluation, *often before confirmatory CT findings*, is vital to prevent respiratory arrest, herniation, and death.[8,13] Once respiratory arrest has occurred, meaningful recovery is unlikely.[8]

TREATMENT

Standard treatment for cerebral edema is mannitol (0.25 to 1 gram/kg IV bolus) and endotracheal intubation if necessary. A recent case series reported improvement after infusion of hypertonic saline. Four children given **10 mL/kg of 3% hypertonic saline** infused over 30 minutes had improved findings on neurologic examination with no apparent

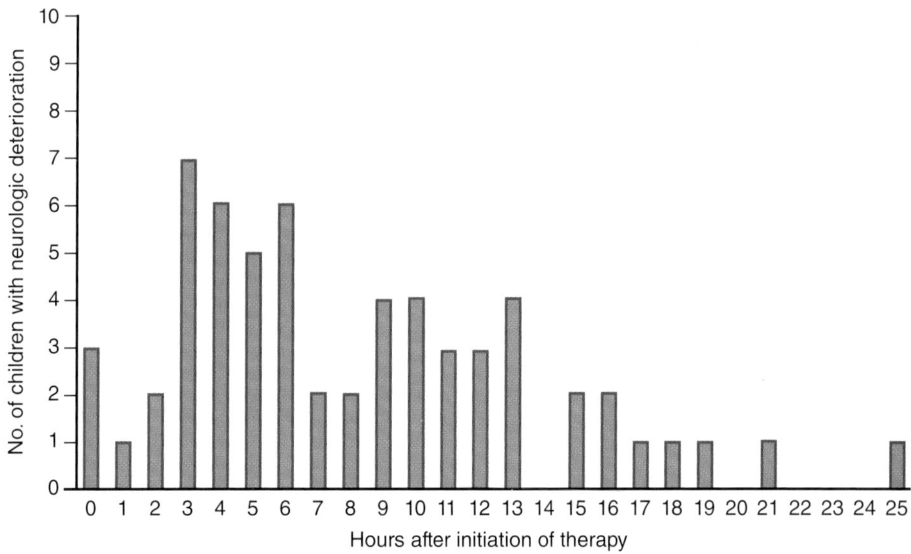

FIGURE 145-1. Time between the initiation of therapy and neurologic deterioration in children with diabetic ketoacidosis and cerebral edema.

complications.[14] Limit additional fluid administration to the minimum possible to retain a functioning IV catheter or use a heparin lock to allow immediate IV access as necessary. If the child appears more clinically stable and is still in the ED, give **half** of normal maintenance fluids until the child reaches the pediatric intensive care unit.

Historically the teaching has been that hyperventilation reduces cerebral blood flow and may worsen cerebral ischemia; however, failure to compensate for the metabolic acidosis through adaptive hyperventilation may lead to hyperemia and worsening of cerebral edema.[15] **Avoidance of a normocapnic state in patients with a severe metabolic imbalance certainly seems prudent.** Consider cerebral venous sinus thrombosis in the child with clinical symptoms of cerebral edema without obvious findings on CT, as this diagnosis may be missed without contrast administration and is better demonstrated on MRI.

LABORATORY EVALUATION IN DKA

Routine blood studies should include serum glucose level, electrolyte panel including calcium and phosphate, venous blood gas analysis, and urinalysis (**Table 145-2**). Hyperglycemia, metabolic acidosis, and ketones in the urine confirm the diagnosis of DKA. Obtain venous blood samples rather than arterial for assessing the degree of acidosis and hypocarbia, which avoids an additional painful procedure (or procedures); **the pH determined by venous blood gas analysis is only 0.03 less than that measured by arterial blood gas analysis and is an accurate reflection of the acid-base status.**[16] Obtain other laboratory studies as clinically indicated.

TABLE 145-2 Laboratory Evaluation in Diabetic Ketoacidosis

Initial Laboratory Studies	
Essential	*Optional*
Glucose level	Magnesium level
Electrolyte panel	Calcium level
Venous blood gas analysis	Serum osmolality
Phosphate level	Serum ketone test
Test for urinary ketones	Complete blood count
	Lactate level
Every Hour	
Bedside serum glucose measurement	
Every 2 Hours	
Electrolyte panel	
Venous blood gas analysis	

Several factitious laboratory abnormalities may be seen in DKA. An increased WBC count is common in DKA and should be interpreted in the context of physical findings and results of diagnostic studies for infection. Elevated salivary amylase level in DKA confounds the diagnosis of pancreatitis, and lipase level is more accurate. **Depending on the type of laboratory analysis used to measure creatinine, serum ketones may result in a factitious elevation in the serum creatinine level.**

The serum glucose level is usually >350 milligrams/dL (19.4 mmol/L), but a glucose level of <300 milligrams/dL (16.6 mmol/L) can be consistent with DKA. Euglycemic DKA may occur in a young, well-hydrated diabetic who is adherent to the insulin regimen but has relative insulin deficiency caused by an intercurrent illness. **Even in the absence of hyperglycemia, insulin is needed when acidosis and ketonemia or ketonuria are present.**

Change in the **serum potassium** level is the most critical electrolyte disturbance in DKA. Hypokalemia can be both profound and present despite relatively normal initial laboratory values due to ion shifts in response to acidosis. The average potassium deficit is 3 to 5 mEq/kg (150- to 250-mEq potassium deficit in a 50-kg adolescent), and the initial serum level is often normal or high. Potassium depletion is a result of insulin deficiency (which normally drives potassium into cells), acidemia (which causes the redistribution of potassium out of the cells in exchange for hydrogen), volume contraction, and tissue catabolism. These processes all provide increased potassium available for urinary excretion. Within this context, initial hypokalemia signifies a severe deficit and a potentially dangerous situation that requires potassium supplementation once urine output is established.

Serum bicarbonate is invariably low, and a wide anion gap acidosis from the ketonemia is usually noted. In simple DKA, the bicarbonate level should fall to the extent that the anion gap increases. A decrease in the bicarbonate level *less* than expected for a given increase in the anion gap in the vomiting patient indicates the presence of an accompanying metabolic alkalosis. Conversely, a fall in the bicarbonate level *greater* than expected for the increase in the anion gap indicates a concomitant non–anion gap acidosis. This is frequently seen in well-hydrated patients who are still able to excrete the keto anions while retaining chloride or in severely dehydrated patients with accompanying lactic acidosis.

The **serum osmolality** is increased in DKA, and its rise correlates with the decrease in the level of consciousness at presentation. Osmolarity of >340 mOsm/L often results in a stuporous or comatose state, whereas a serum osmolarity of <300 mOsm/L should prompt reconsideration of the cause of a decreased level of consciousness. The development of cerebral edema may be correlated with the rate of decline in the serum osmolarity; thus, it is critical that fluid deficits be corrected less rapidly in patients with high serum osmolarity.

Sodium deficits average 5 to 10 mEq/kg, but the serum sodium level may be normal because of excessive free water loss. More typically, the serum sodium level is factitiously low because of hyperglycemia, and a corrected value may be arrived at by using the formula *corrected sodium level = {1.6 × [(serum glucose level – 100)/100]} + measured serum sodium level.*

The major **ketoacid** produced is β-hydroxybutyrate. Unlike acetoacetate, however, it does not react with the nitroprusside used in urine and serum ketone assays, so measured ketone levels may appear low for the degree of acidosis and do not reflect the true extent of ketonemia. This fact also explains the paradoxical rise in measured ketone levels with therapy: β-hydroxybutyrate is converted to acetoacetate, which reacts more strongly with the assay. Using bedside ketone testing to monitor recovery is further complicated by the persistence of urine ketones after clearance of serum ketones.[17]

TREATMENT OF DKA

Intensive monitoring and meticulous care of the patient with DKA improves outcome. **Current consensus statements recommend continuous cardiac monitoring of all children with DKA,[4] and a prolonged QT_c interval occurs frequently during DKA and is correlated with ketosis.[18]** QT_c prolongation can lead to life-threatening arrhythmias such as torsade de pointes. Avoid medications that may further prolong the QT interval such as ondansetron if the ECG demonstrates prolongation.

Direct attention to perfusion, electrolyte disturbances, mental status, hyperglycemia and ketonemia (Table 145-3). Concurrently identify and treat associated infections.

FLUID RESUSCITATION

The average fluid deficit is 10% of body weight, but is often greater. Give an initial 20 mL/kg bolus of normal saline if the child is in shock and repeat if needed. **Once vital signs have stabilized, resist the desire to correct the fluid deficit too rapidly, especially if there is a high calculated osmolarity (i.e., >340 mOsm/L).** Many institutions replace the deficit evenly over 24 to 48 hours; this moderated approach helps to avoid overhydration, pulmonary complications, and possibly cerebral edema. The traditional approach is 50% deficit replacement in the first 8 hours with the rest replaced over the next 16 to 24 hours.

ELECTROLYTE REPLACEMENT

Sodium depletion from vomiting and urinary losses rarely causes a problem by itself and is most often related to the extent of dehydration. The main concern with sodium level lies in its correction: failure of serum sodium level to rise in the treatment of DKA is associated with the development of cerebral edema.[8] Typical protocols historically recommended 0.9% sodium chloride correction at 1.5 times the maintenance level for empiric replacement therapy. But in an attempt to decrease the risk of cerebral edema, some newer protocols advocate sodium concentrations of 0.66% (typically mixed by the pharmacist) to 0.9% sodium chloride and calculate fluid replacements to tighten control over biochemical parameters.[4] This approach is effective in ensuring a steady rise in the sodium concentration.

Withhold **potassium** until hyperkalemia (i.e., potassium level of >6.0 mEq/L) is excluded and the child is urinating. ECG findings may be normal in the face of hyperkalemia, so monitor the serum potassium level. Total body potassium deficits are often large, and both initial rehydration and insulin therapy can cause a precipitous decline in potassium levels due to redistribution.

Initial hypokalemia (i.e., <3.0 mEq/L) indicates a profound deficit, and therapy should be aggressive; insulin will further lower serum potassium, so close monitoring and replacement are essential. **The recommended rates of potassium replacement vary widely, but in general, maintenance fluids should contain between 30 and 40 mEq $[K^+]$ per liter.** Consider higher doses for children with demonstrated hypokalemia, although a central line is needed and intensive care unit monitoring is required at most institutions. Monitor serum potassium at least every 2 hours.

Phosphate depletion in DKA is well described, but the value of IV replacement has never been proven. Many authorities recommend half of the potassium replacement in the form of potassium phosphate. In the absence of replacement, one should monitor for symptomatic hypophosphatemia (serum phosphate level of <1 mmol/L, muscular weakness, rhabdomyolysis, respiratory depression). The same rule applies to **magnesium** replacement. **Hypocalcemia,** when present, is likely secondary to overaggressive phosphate replacement.

TABLE 145-3 Management of DKA in Children

1. 10 mL/kg NS bolus over 1 h unless hypotensive.*
2. Begin NS at 1.5 times maintenance level in the ED.†
3. If $[K^+]$ is 3.5–5.5 mEq/L and patient is urinating, add 30 mEq potassium per liter (1/2 as potassium chloride and 1/2 as potassium phosphate). If initial $[K^+]$ is 2.5–3.5 mEq/L, add 40 mEq $[K^+]$ per liter; consider adding more if the $[K^+]$ is <2.5 mEq/L.
4. Begin regular insulin at 0.1 units/kg/h after IV fluid bolus (if given) is complete. Adjust dose to maintain glucose decline at 50–100 milligrams/dL/h. **Do not decrease insulin infusion to <0.05 units/kg/h because insulin is required to clear ketosis even when glucose has normalized.**
5. Add dextrose to IV fluids when blood glucose level is <200–250 milligrams/dL (11–14 mmol/L).
6. Measure serum electrolyte levels every 2 h; measure serum glucose level every hour.

Abbreviations: K = potassium; NS = normal saline (0.9% sodium chloride).

*In the setting of hypotension, bolus patient with 20 mL/kg NS repeatedly until normotensive.

†Alternatively, calculate fluid deficit and correct 50% over the first 12–16 h. Some authorities recommend a higher calculated sodium concentration of between 0.45% and 0.9% sodium chloride.

INSULIN IN DKA

Fluid resuscitation will reduce serum glucose levels somewhat, but do not correct the underlying metabolic problem or improve ketonemia or acidosis. After the patient is hemodynamically stable, begin a low-dose insulin infusion. High-dose insulin therapy does not improve the rate of recovery and places the patient at greater risk of hypoglycemia and hypokalemia. **A loading *bolus* of 0.1 units/kg is no longer considered beneficial and is considered potentially harmful because it has been associated with an increased risk for cerebral edema.[19]**

The insulin infusion dosage is 0.1 unit of regular insulin per kilogram per hour. As a rule of thumb, serum glucose level should decrease by 50 to 100 milligrams/dL/h (2.8 to 5.6 mmol/L) in a slow, controlled fashion to prevent intracerebral osmolar shifts. If improvement of the pH is too slow (<0.03 pH units per hour), the insulin infusion rate can be doubled. **Generally, glucose level corrects faster than the ketoacidosis, so add dextrose to the IV fluids when the blood glucose level drops to <250 milligrams/dL (14 mmol/L) without stopping the insulin infusion, with the goal of maintaining a serum glucose level of 150 to 300 milligrams/dL (8.3–16.6 mmol/L) until resolution of the ketoacidosis.**

Initiate glucose along with insulin for the patient with **euglycemic DKA**. If the blood glucose level continues to decline, provide additional glucose before considering adjustment of the insulin drip. If the child is receiving the maximum glucose concentration available (or maximum tolerable concentration if through a peripheral line), then the administration of insulin can be temporarily held for 10 to 15 minutes before restarting the insulin drip at a lower rate. **In general, this rate should not be <0.05 units/kg/h.** The short half-life of IV insulin (5 to 10 minutes), along with the continued administration of glucose, will correct transient hypoglycemia. Continued insulin administration is the mainstay of therapy and should be maintained until reversal of ketoacidosis.

Do not transition the insulin infusion to SC administration until the pH is >7.30, bicarbonate level is >15 mEq/L, and serum ketones have disappeared. At that point, taper the IV insulin to 0.02 to 0.05 unit/kg/h and initiate multidose SC insulin using a regular insulin (short-acting) at a dose of 0.1 unit/kg every 2 hours to maintain serum glucose between 150 and 200 mg/dL (8.3 to 13.8 mmol/L); stop the IV insulin infusion

1 to 2 hours after initiating SC therapy. Do not simply discontinue insulin therapy altogether when DKA resolves, because DKA will recur without adequate continued serum insulin. There is institutional variation regarding the preferred SC insulin regimen, so consult with a pediatric endocrinologist about preferred local practices.

INSULIN PUMP AND DKA

Because most episodes of DKA are related to inadequate insulin delivery, this implies malfunctioning of the insulin pump. Alternatively, the pump may be functioning correctly but the child may have an intercurrent illness with increased and unmet insulin needs. **Either way, shut off the pump and treat the child like any other insulin-dependent diabetic patient with DKA.**

BICARBONATE THERAPY FOR ACIDOSIS

The use of bicarbonate in the treatment of DKA is not recommended, because it has never been shown to improve outcome and has been associated with a fourfold increase in the development of cerebral edema.[5] In addition, bicarbonate therapy can lead to volume overload, accelerated hypokalemia, hypernatremia, and paradoxical CNS acidosis.[20] **Bicarbonate administration should be limited to critically ill patients with a pH of <7.0 and hemodynamic compromise (unresponsive to fluid resuscitation) from depressed cardiac contractility and poor perfusion.** If necessary, depending on the pH and the patient's clinical condition, bicarbonate may be administered slowly at 0.5 to 2.0 mEq/kg over 1 to 2 hours. Correction should never exceed a pH of 7.1 or a serum bicarbonate level of 10 mEq/L.

DKA DISPOSITION AND FOLLOW-UP

Most patients with DKA require admission to the intensive care unit, even once stabilized, because of intensive monitoring needs. Furthermore, many hospitals restrict the use of insulin infusions to intensive care settings. Patients with known diabetes who have a pH of >7.35 and a bicarbonate level of >20 mEq/L, have a known and resolving precipitant for DKA and a good clinical appearance, and have a solid social situation and will follow up closely with their primary physicians may be discharged home. In as many as 69% of patients with a starting pH of >7.20 or a serum bicarbonate level of >10 mEq/L, acidosis is corrected within 6 hours.[6]

HYPERGLYCEMIA WITHOUT KETOACIDOSIS

NEW-ONSET HYPERGLYCEMIA

Many children with new-onset diabetes present with classic symptoms of diabetes such as polydipsia, polyuria, and malaise, and are identified before significant ketoacidosis develops. They are frequently sent from the outpatient physician's office to the ED for management and admission. ED management for these children is less intensive and should be done in coordination with an endocrinologist. In general, children with hyperglycemia but no DKA are only mildly dehydrated, urinary ketones may or may not be present, and the serum pH is >7.3. The speed at which such children descend toward actual DKA is largely a function of hydration status and age. Infants and very young children progress more rapidly because of their inability to access fluids independently and their increased metabolic rate. With appropriate hydration and timely insulin administration, DKA is very unlikely to develop in the hospital in the absence of serious underlying illness.

ED management should be restricted to drawing samples for baseline laboratory studies; providing fluids PO or IV, depending on the need; and possibly administering the first dose of insulin. **An acceptable initial dose is 0.1 unit/kg SC of regular insulin.** Whether or not children with new-onset diabetes are particularly sensitive to insulin is a matter of debate. Still, monitor serum glucose levels closely—every hour after insulin is administered. Consider admission for education and to establish daily insulin requirements. **Daily insulin requirements** are generally in the range of 0.5 to 1.0 unit/kg/d in divided doses, two thirds in the morning and one third in the evening.

HYPERGLYCEMIA IN PATIENTS WITH PREDIAGNOSED DIABETES

For a diabetic child with hyperglycemia with or without an intercurrent illness or injury, management should focus on the primary reason for the ED visit. **An additional dose of 10% of the child's normal daily insulin dose can be administered as regular insulin SC for simple hyperglycemia.**

For children with an intercurrent illness, more specific management guidelines may vary among endocrinologists and also may depend on whether or not urinary ketones are present. **An acceptable approach if the child has an intercurrent illness and no urinary ketones is to administer an additional 5% of the daily insulin dose every 4 to 6 hours until the condition resolves. If the child has urinary ketones, administer 10% of the daily dose every 4 to 6 hours until the ketonuria resolves, and then decrease to 5%, as noted above.**

HYPERGLYCEMIA IN PATIENTS TAKING INSULIN GLARGINE

Occasionally, a child will present with hyperglycemia without DKA after missing one or more doses of **insulin glargine (Lantus)**. Glargine is a long-lasting once-daily insulin preparation that has no peak effect. Generally, glargine is given at approximately 50% of the daily insulin requirement, with the rest given as a short-acting preparation, so that missing a single dose of glargine is not equivalent to missing all insulin doses for the day.

If the child is off schedule for insulin glargine and does not have DKA, a single injection of neutral protamine Hagedorn (NPH) insulin can be given, followed by resumption of the regular dosing schedule.

If the child is off schedule for insulin glargine and has DKA, treatment is no different from management of other cases of DKA.

REFERENCES

The complete reference list is available online at www.TintinalliEM.com.

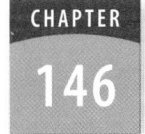

The Child With Special Healthcare Needs

Lila O'Mahony

INTRODUCTION AND EPIDEMIOLOGY

Children with special healthcare needs are children with chronic physical, developmental, behavioral, or emotional conditions that require health and related services beyond what is required by children in general.[1,2] This population accounts for about 16% of children in the United States,[3,4] accounts for 40% to 80% of all pediatric healthcare utilization and costs, and is the fastest-growing group in pediatrics.[3,5-9] Compared to children without chronic conditions, children with chronic conditions tend to be older, male, and from non-Hispanic white racial/ethnic groups.[4,6,10,11] The clinical spectrum of conditions is diverse, and complex medical devices are often required for care (**Tables 146-1 and 146-2**).[6,8-10,12-14]

EMERGENCY CARE PLAN

An emergency care plan provides information and instructions for emergency care. Components of the plan include an information form, special instructions for devices or emergency conditions, and ancillary replacement supplies.

The individualized emergency information form should be provided at the ED visit (http://www.childrensnational.org/files/PDF/EMSC/PubRes/EIForm.pdf). Informational elements of the form include demographic and emergency contact information; names and contact information for

TABLE 146-1 Congenital or Developmental Disorders and Associated Medical Conditions[15,16]

Chromosomal disorders[6,7]

Down syndrome (trisomy 21 syndrome)

Seizure disorder (12%–15%); atlantoaxial instability (14%–22%); cataracts (15%); serous otitis media (50%–70%); deafness (75%); congenital heart disease (50%): ASD, VSD, AV canal, PDA, tetralogy of Fallot, pulmonary hypertension; GI atresias (12%); Hirschsprung's disease (1%); constipation, fecal impaction from medications or hypothyroidism; thyroid disease (15%); diabetes mellitus; leukemia (1%); acquired hip dislocation (6%); and psychiatric disorders (22%)

Fragile X syndrome

Recurrent serous otitis media (60% in males), strabismus (30%–56% in males), seizures (14%–50% in males), autism (16% in males), self-abusive, and mitral valve prolapse (22%–77% in males)

Trisomy 18

Congenital heart disease (99%): VSD, ASD, and PDA

Turner's syndrome (XO syndrome)

Short stature in females, horseshoe kidney, heart disease (bicuspid aortic valve in 30%, coarctation of the aorta in 10%, valvular aortic stenosis, mitral valve prolapse, aortic dissection later in life, and hypertension)

Noonan's syndrome

Webbing of the neck, pectus excavatum, cryptorchidism, and pulmonic stenosis

Disorders with facial defects as major feature

Pierre Robin syndrome

Micrognathia, glossoptosis, and cleft soft palate; primary defect: early mandibular hypoplasia

Waardenburg's syndrome

Lateral displacement of medial canthi, partial albinism, and deafness

Occasional associations: VSD, Hirschsprung's disease, esophageal atresia, and anal atresia

Treacher Collins syndrome

Malar hypoplasia with downward-slanting palpebral fissures, defect of lower lid, and malformation of the external ear

Disorders with limb defects as major feature

Holt-Oram syndrome

Upper limb defect, cardiac anomaly (ASD, VSD, arrhythmia), and narrow shoulders

Fanconi's pancytopenia syndrome

Radial hypoplasia, hyperpigmentation, pancytopenia, and renal anomaly

Radial aplasia thrombocytopenia (TAR syndrome)

Inherited metabolic disorders

Phenylketonuria (autosomal recessive)

Light pigmentation, eczema (33%), poor coordination, seizures (25%), and autistic behavior

Hunter's syndrome (X-linked recessive)

Developmental lag after age 6–12 mo, coarse facies, growth deficiency, stiff joints by age 2–4 y, clear corneas, and hepatosplenomegaly

Hurler's syndrome (autosomal recessive)

Developmental lag after age 6–10 mo, coarse facies, stiff joints, mental deficiency, cloudy corneas by age 1–2 y, hepatosplenomegaly, and rhinitis

Connective tissue disorders

Marfan's syndrome

Arachnodactyly with hyperextensibility, lens subluxation, and aortic dilatation

Ehlers-Danlos syndrome

Hyperextensibility of joints, hyperextensibility of skin, and poor wound healing with thin scar

Osteogenesis imperfecta congenital

Short, broad, long bones; multiple fractures; and blue sclera

Hamartoses

Sturge-Weber sequence

Flat facial hemangiomata and meningeal hemangiomata with seizures

Tuberous sclerosis syndrome

Hamartomatous skin nodules (thumb print macules), seizures, angiomyolipomata (45%–81%), phakomata, and bone lesions

Neurofibromatosis syndrome

Multiple neurofibromata, café-au-lait spots, presence or absence of bone lesions, seizures and/or EEG changes in 20%, cerebrovascular compromise, and headaches

Environmental agents (toxins)

Fetal alcohol syndrome

Vision problems (94%), recurrent serous otitis (93%), hearing loss (66%), heart defects (29%–41%), renal hypoplasia, duplication of the kidney and collecting system, and bladder diverticula (10%)

Other environmental exposures include fetal hydantoin syndrome, fetal trimethadione syndrome, fetal valproate syndrome, fetal warfarin syndrome, and retinoic acid embryopathy

(Continued)

TABLE 146-1 Congenital or Developmental Disorders and Associated Medical Conditions[15,16] (*Continued*)

Trauma
Traumatic brain injury
Visual and hearing disturbances; cranial nerve damage; spasticity, incoordination, ataxia, and feeding disorders; GERD; neuropsychiatric disturbances
Cerebral palsy
Seizures (33%), strabismus (50%), hearing loss (10%), hip dislocation, scoliosis, contractures, gait disorder, GERD (8%–10%), chronic aspiration and recurrent RAD, pulmonary fibrosis and bronchiectasis
Miscellaneous
Angelman's syndrome (happy puppet syndrome)
Puppet-like gait, paroxysms of laughter, and characteristic features; seizures vary from major motor to akinetic, beginning usually at age 18–24 mo
Beckwith-Wiedemann syndrome
Macroglossia, omphalocele, macrosomia, and ear creases; neonatal polycythemia and hypoglycemia in early infancy; associated with Wilms' tumor
CHARGE syndrome
Coloboma, heart disease (tetralogy of Fallot, PDA, double-outlet right ventricle with an atrioventricular canal, VSD, ASD, and right-sided aortic arch), atresia choanae, retarded growth and development and/or CNS anomalies, genital anomalies and/or hypogonadism, and ear anomalies and/or deafness
Prader-Willi syndrome
Mental retardation, hypotonia, hypogonadism, obesity, hyperphagia, gastric perforation, hypoventilation, obstructive sleep apnea, cor pulmonale, NIDDM, scoliosis, strabismus, inability to vomit, decreased sensitivity to pain, seizure disorder, hypoxia, right-sided heart failure, and pulmonary hypertension
Rett's syndrome
Hyperventilation, breath holding, air swallowing, bruxism, ataxia, muscle wasting, poor circulation, scoliosis, seizures, and intermittent flushing
VATER syndrome
Vertebral defects and VSD, imperforate anus, tracheoesophageal fistula, renal anomalies, and single umbilical artery
Williams' syndrome
Elfin-like syndrome, cardiovascular disease, supravalvular aortic stenosis, pulmonic stenosis, coarctation of the aorta, strabismus, joint contractures, hypertension, urethral stenosis, vesicoureteral reflux, constipation, ulcers, and hypercalcemia

Abbreviations: ASD = atrial septal defect; AV = atrioventricular; EEG = electroencephalogram; GERD = gastroesophageal reflux disease; NIDDM = non-insulin-dependent diabetes mellitus; PDA = patent ductus arteriosus; RAD = reactive airway disease; TAR = thrombocytopenia-absent radius; VSD = ventricular septal defect.

the primary and specialty care physicians; diagnoses, past procedures, and baseline examination findings; allergies; immunizations; procedures to avoid; common acute problems and suggested management; and comments on other specific medical issues or special instructions for device malfunction. Information should be regularly updated. Copies of the form should be available at the home, physician's office, and care facilities.

The care plan should include special instructions for EMS personnel, first responders, or family members who may need to provide emergency care for the child.[12,13] A "go-bag" or kit with specialized equipment should accompany the child. Such kits contain extra tracheostomy tubes, appropriate size suction catheters, equipment to change a tracheostomy tube, syringes and adapters to decompress a feeding catheter, a bag-valve mask resuscitator, and needles to access central lines.[17]

GENERAL APPROACH

Optimal emergency care requires access to multiple healthcare resources, including family, primary care physicians, specialists, and home health nurses (**Table 146-3**).[12,13,17] Long-term caregivers know the child's baseline status and are familiar with medications and supportive equipment.

TABLE 146-2 Common Home Medical Devices and Equipment

Apnea monitors
Tracheostomies
Feeding tubes and pumps
Central venous lines or percutaneous IV catheters and pumps
Oxygen/suction
Ventilators
Nebulizers
Colostomies
Internal pacemakers or defibrillators
Ventricular peritoneal shunts
Vagus nerve stimulators

HISTORY AND PHYSICAL EXAMINATION

The child may not be able to communicate directly. Elicit essential elements of the history and subtle symptoms from family or care providers; occasionally, a call to a chronic care facility or review of past medical records is necessary to obtain important details. Inquire about advanced directives, limitations of care, and family goals as well as treatments prior to ED arrival. Carefully review medications including recent changes or missed doses, allergies (e.g., latex), and comorbidities. The physical examination, too, often relies on accompanying family or care providers, particularly with regard to mental status, assessment of pain, and changes from baseline. Obtain vital signs. Baseline vital signs for children with complex medical conditions may be out of the range of normal. Core temperature may be low at baseline, and a "normal" temperature may represent fever; baseline values for heart rate, respiratory rate, and oxygen saturation may be abnormal; vital signs may be controlled by a pacemaker or ventilator. Obtain an accurate weight to calculate weight-based medication dosing. To obtain a current weight, if a conventional floor scale is not appropriate, ask caregivers for the most recent weight, use a bed scale, or consider a length-based tape to estimate weight. When performing a head-to-toe evaluation, pay special attention to medical devices and equipment: palpate ventricular shunts

TABLE 146-3 Checklist for Emergency Care

Fully involve the family and caregivers and use the care plan.
Inquire about advanced directives and family goals of emergency care.
Use family information when assessing child's pain, mental status, and symptoms.
Anticipate latex allergy.
Identify proper equipment sizes (e.g., tracheostomies, gastrostomy tubes, colostomies).
Anticipate difficult intubation in the child with craniofacial or cervical vertebrae anomalies or contractures.
Recognize and treat comorbid states.
Consider physical or sexual abuse in the child with special needs.

for swelling or tenderness; check patency of tracheostomy tubes; assess central or peripherally inserted vascular catheters for patency and signs of infection; and examine gastrostomy sites and feeding tubes.

LABORATORY TESTING AND IMAGING

The specific evaluation depends on the presenting problem and underlying special healthcare needs. Perform bedside glucose testing in all complex patients with altered mental status. Check serum drug levels (e.g., anticonvulsants) as appropriate. Compare plain radiographs and CTs with prior imaging results to distinguish acute from chronic changes.

TREATMENT

Although treatment is tailored to the presenting condition, the universal approach of prioritizing airway, breathing, circulation, and disability remains the same. A general overview of common respiratory, metabolic, neurologic, GI, and musculoskeletal problems and suspected abuse follows. A review of the complications common to children dependent on medical technology is discussed separately later, under "Technology-Dependent Children."

RESPIRATORY DISORDERS

Oral motor dysfunction and gastroesophageal reflux can lead to aspiration, wheezing, pneumonia, and chronic congestion. Scoliosis and neuromuscular disease may compromise pulmonary mechanics and lead to functional restrictive lung disease with limited respiratory reserve. To evaluate acute respiratory complaints, obtain a thorough history of past respiratory function, especially in the situation of prematurity; escalating home therapy including supplemental oxygen use; reactive airway disease; or tracheomalacia. Airway instability can develop in the child with poor head control, and simple head repositioning or jaw thrust may improve airway mechanics and decrease pooling of saliva in the oropharynx. Suction and change tracheostomies as needed. Consider foreign body aspiration in appropriate clinical circumstances. Treatment of respiratory distress in this population may include deep suctioning, replacement of malfunctioning equipment (tracheostomy tubes, ventilators), β-agonists for bronchospasm, antibiotics for pneumonia, and subspecialty consultation for airway foreign bodies. Admission is generally warranted for pneumonia, increased home oxygen requirement, persistent respiratory distress, or removal of a foreign body.

METABOLIC DISORDERS

This diverse category of disorders is due to genetic defects that lead to abnormalities in the metabolic pathways of proteins, carbohydrates, and lipids (see chapter 144, "Metabolic Emergencies in Infants and Children"). Although a detailed understanding of individual biochemical pathways is not necessary for emergency management and evaluation, general familiarity with presenting signs and symptoms is necessary, because recognition in the ED could be lifesaving. Initial laboratory studies should include a CBC, serum glucose, electrolytes with anion gap, blood gas, ammonia, liver function tests, urine ketones, and lactate dehydrogenase, aldolase, and creatine kinase if there are muscular symptoms. After verifying adequate airway, breathing, and circulation, direct care to correct acute metabolic abnormalities such as hypoglycemia (**Table 146-4**).[18]

Consult a biochemical geneticist for further diagnostic evaluation and management guidance.

TABLE 146-4 Emergency Treatment of Inborn Errors of Metabolism

Primary	Airway, breathing, circulation; vascular access, nothing by mouth (NPO)
Fluid resuscitation	Use normal saline boluses 10–20 mL/kg Avoid lactated Ringer's with concerns for worsening lactic acidosis Avoid hypotonic fluid load due to concerns for risk of cerebral edema
Prevent catabolism	Glucose bolus for hypoglycemia 5 mL/kg D10 for neonates and infants or 2 mL/kg D25 for children and adolescents. Maintenance glucose and electrolytes D10 normal saline at 1.5 times maintenance (6 mL/kg/hr for first 10 kg of weight + 3 mL/kg/h for 11–20 kg + 1.5 mL/kgh for each additional kg >20 kg). Insulin 0.2–0.3 U/kg/h to treat hyperglycemia if necessary.

SEIZURES

The prevalence of epilepsy is estimated at 4 to 9 cases per 1000 children but is as high as 35% among children with special needs.[19-21] In general, the nature and complexity of the seizure syndromes differ considerably between patients, but seizure syndromes are generally consistent in the individual. The initial evaluation and management follow the standard approach to seizures (see chapter 135 "Seizures in Infants and Children"), with a few caveats in the child with special healthcare needs: note anomalies or comorbid conditions that might lead to airway or respiratory compromise with the use of respiratory depressant anticonvulsants; obtain a careful history including the baseline frequency and type of seizures and efficacy of past medications (ask the child's family what has and has not worked previously); confirm allergies and potential drug interactions; and consult with the primary neurologist if multiple medications are needed for seizure control and determine if therapeutic adjustments are required. Obtain serum anticonvulsant medication levels as indicated.

Adequate seizure control may require multiple medications. Intractable seizures, those that do not respond to at least two anticonvulsants, affect approximately 1 in 10 children with epilepsy[22] and may be associated with underlying disorders or syndromes. Patients with refractory seizures, including those with epileptic encephalopathies (e.g., Lennox-Gastaut and Dravet's syndromes) may be placed on a ketogenic diet or have an implanted vagus nerve stimulator. **For children on a ketogenic diet, it is critical to avoid sugars and maintain ketosis.** Therefore, ask caregivers about baseline serum glucose levels before administering dextrose, as dextrose may increase seizures previously controlled by therapeutic ketosis. In addition, consider working with a pharmacist to ensure that the vehicle in which a medication is provided is not contraindicated for a ketogenic diet. For example, most chewable and suspension medications and common medications such as acetaminophen and ibuprofen contain sugar.

GI DISORDERS

GI complaints may include dehydration, feeding tube complications, and constipation. Dehydration may result from poor oral intake, oral motor dysfunction, or increased fluid losses from infection. Children with growth retardation (in particular below the fifth percentile) or marginal reserves may dehydrate even from minimal vomiting and diarrhea. In addition to the clinical signs of dry mucous membranes, tachycardia, and oliguria, ask the family about weight loss, changes in baseline function, and ability to orally or enterally hydrate. IV access may be difficult, and the child may require central or intraosseous access (see chapter 112, "Intravenous and Intraosseous Access in Infants and Children"). Constipation may be associated with nonspecific symptoms such as abdominal pain, change in bowel habits, anorexia, or overflow diarrhea. Treat acute constipation with enemas, suppositories, polyethylene glycol, and dietary adjustments. Avoid mineral oil in children with aspiration potential to avoid pulmonary complications and impaired fat-soluble vitamin absorption. Do not recommend chronic use of Fleet enemas because electrolyte abnormalities may result.

MUSCULOSKELETAL/DERMATOLOGIC DISORDERS

Children with disorders that require orthopedic braces, have prolonged periods of immobility, or result in wheelchair dependence may develop painful skeletal or cutaneous complications. The risk of pathologic fractures increases from disuse and nutritionally induced osteopenia. Although fractures may occur from therapy, falls, or accidents, also

TABLE 146-5 Ventilator Troubleshooting

Alarm	Possible Causes	Interventions
High pressure	Plugged or obstructed airway Coughing/bronchospasm	Clear obstruction Suction tracheostomy Administer bronchodilator
Low pressure/apnea	Loose or disconnected circuit Leak in circuit Leak around tracheostomy site	Ensure all circuits are connected Check tracheostomy balloon Ensure tracheostomy is well seated
Low power	Internal battery depleted	Plug the ventilator into a power outlet
Setting error	Settings incorrectly adjusted	Manually ventilate patient Transport ventilator and patient
Power switchover	Unit switched from AC to internal battery	Press "alarm silent" button after ensuring battery is powering ventilator

consider abuse, particularly for comminuted fractures. Assess for orthopedic injuries in the irritable, severely impaired, or nonverbal child by palpating all extremities and checking range of motion. Inspect the skin, especially in dependent areas, for pressure ulcers or skin breakdown. Evaluate wheelchair-dependent children on stretchers and out of their chairs to check the entire body.

NEGLECT AND ABUSE

Children with disabilities are three to four times more likely to be neglected or abused when compared with children without disabilities.[23] They often place higher emotional, physical, economic, and social demands on their families.[24-26] The added attention required, coupled with limited caregiver resources, can result in failure of the child to receive needed medications, medical care, and appropriate educational placement. Maintain a heightened awareness for potential abuse, and work closely with the primary physician who is most familiar with the child and his or her care providers.

TECHNOLOGY-DEPENDENT CHILDREN

A technology-dependent child is one who needs a medical device to compensate for the loss of a vital body function and substantial nursing care to avert death or further disability.[27] Devices include ventilators, pacemakers, tracheostomies, gastrostomy tubes, central venous catheters, ventriculoperitoneal shunts, and vagus nerve stimulators.[27,28] Contact the child's primary physician and home health nurse early in the evaluation process to avoid unnecessary tests, to determine need for inpatient admission, and to simplify care.

TRACHEOSTOMY CARE

There are many types and sizes of tracheostomy tubes, so clarify the exact type and size of tube. Common complications related to tracheostomy tubes include decannulation, bleeding at the cannulation site, obstruction, and tube reinsertion into a false passage, resulting in subcutaneous emphysema, pneumomediastinum, or pneumothorax. Granuloma or stricture formation at the stoma or tracheal wall can cause bleeding with cannula manipulation or by suctioning. Erosion into the innominate artery is rare and is usually related to an inferiorly placed tracheostomy stoma. Consider otolaryngology consultation and urgent bronchoscopy for bleeding.

Infections associated with tracheostomies include tracheitis, bronchitis, and pneumonia. Normal secretions are generally clear to white and thin in consistency. Abnormal secretions are thick and yellow to green in color. Obtain a tracheal aspirate and culture in children with fever, respiratory distress, or a change in secretions or oxygen requirement.

MECHANICAL VENTILATION

Chronic respiratory support is necessary for a variety of conditions: neurologic and neuromuscular disease accounts for about half, and chronic lung disease accounts for only 7%.[29] Ventilator-related complications, such as pneumothorax or machine failure, are managed according to standard principles. Provide bag ventilation for total ventilator failure. **Table 146-5** provides a checklist for ventilator troubleshooting.

FEEDING TUBES

Complications of a nasogastric tube include sinusitis, nasal and esophageal irritation, tube dislodgement or clogging, and pulmonary aspiration. Gastrostomy tubes can be associated with gastroesophageal reflux, tube dislodgement or clogging, peristomal wound infection, abdominal wall abscess, peritonitis, gastric perforation or hemorrhage, gastrocolic fistula, gastric ulceration, and gastric outlet obstruction. The gastrostomy tube may become dislodged or broken and can be difficult to reinsert if left out for any period of time. Insert a small feeding tube or Foley catheter to prevent stoma closure while arranging for the appropriate tube to be reinserted (see chapter 86, "Gastrointestinal Procedures and Devices"). Additional complications of gastrojejunostomy tubes include diarrhea, tube migration, small bowel perforation, and intussusception (see chapter 87, "Complications of General Surgical Procedures").

Stomal complications include dermatitis, allergic hypersensitivity, granulation, cellulitis, and fungal infections. Superficial bleeding due to granulation tissue can be cauterized using silver nitrate sticks.

Complications of parenteral feeding include catheter obstruction or occlusion, air embolism, catheter breakage, catheter displacement, or catheter-related infection. Other complications include cholestasis that may lead to irreversible liver disease or metabolic bone disease.

INDWELLING VENOUS CATHETERS[30]

Indwelling catheters, often tunneled central venous catheters, can be of multiple types but will be accessible through either externalized catheter tubing, such as a Hickman device, or a subcutaneous reservoir, such as a Port-a-Cath device. Complications include occlusion, breakage, dislodgement, air embolism, and infection. Various agents can be used to relieve catheter obstruction in the ED, such as tissue plasminogen activator in the instance of intraluminal coagulated blood, but protocols are typically institution dependent. Surgical or interventional radiology consultation may be necessary if initial attempts at removing the obstruction are unsuccessful. For breakage or dislodgement, clamp externalized catheters proximal to the affected segment and repair with a special kit if available. For nonexternalized catheters, especially when there is concern for dislodgment, seek surgical consultation promptly. Air embolism may be associated with symptoms of respiratory distress and hemodynamic instability. If air embolism is suspected, clamp the catheter and place the child in left-sided Trendelenburg position with supplemental oxygen.[30] For suspected infection, obtain blood cultures and administer antibiotics to cover gram-positive organisms, which are the most common pathogens.

CEREBROSPINAL FLUID SHUNTS

Cerebrospinal shunt placement is the most common neurosurgical procedure performed in children.[30] Complications include separation or disruption of the tubing or device, infection, and overdrainage[31,32] (**Table 146-6**).

TABLE 146-6 Symptoms and Signs of Ventriculoperitoneal Shunt Obstruction or Malfunction

Symptom	Signs
Headache	Shunt site swelling or normal exam
Visual disturbances	Papilledema
Nausea or vomiting	Bulging fontanelle, enlarged head, or normal exam
Lethargy and/or irritability	Engorged head veins
Lack of developmental progress and/or poor school performance	McEwen sign (cracked-pot sound during skull percussion)

Neurologic findings: increased deep tendon reflexes or lower extremity tone, positive Babinski sign, lateral (sixth) or upward (fourth) gaze palsy (sun-setting), and respiratory compromise.

Shunt malfunction occurs most often in the year following placement,[33] with approximately 40% of standard shunts malfunctioning during this time.[34] After the first year, the annual rate of shunt malfunction is about 5%.[35]

Seizures are generally accompanied by other signs and symptoms and are seldom, if ever, the only sign of shunt malfunction. Patients with impending herniation may develop **Cushing's triad**: hypertension, bradycardia, and irregular respirations. This is a late sign of impending herniation and a true neurosurgical emergency. When neurosurgical consultation is not immediately available and the patient is experiencing symptoms of herniation, removing cerebrospinal fluid through the shunt reservoir may be lifesaving.

Shunt infections occur most commonly within a few months of shunt placement, many within the first few weeks, and they generally decrease in frequency with time. Infection rates vary from 1% to 40%, with most in the range of 5% to 15%.[36] Signs and symptoms of shunt infection may be nonspecific, such as fever, behavior change (irritability or lethargy), vomiting, and/or abdominal pain. Infected shunts may be accompanied by mechanical shunt failure. Antibiotics should be selected to treat gram-positive (most commonly, coagulase-negative *Staphylococcus*, *Staphylococcus aureus*, and *Streptococcus*) and gram-negative (*Escherichia coli*, *Enterococcus* species, and *Haemophilus influenzae*) species. Intra-abdominal cerebrospinal fluid loculations or peritoneal pseudocysts can occur at the distal tip of the catheter with or without peritonitis. Less common intra-abdominal complications are bowel obstruction due to adhesions, subphrenic abscess, and cerebrospinal-enteric fistula.[37]

The evaluation for mechanical shunt malfunction includes plain radiographs of the skull, neck, chest, and abdomen to evaluate continuity of shunt hardware, and head CT or quick-brain MRI to assess ventricular size and shunt positioning. Increased cerebral ventricle size, particularly when compared with previous studies, indicates shunt malfunction. However, malfunction may be present with unchanged ventricular size due to a loss of surrounding tissue compliance. A "negative" neuroimaging study does not rule out shunt malfunction or obstruction. Approximately 11% of shunt failures present with small ventricles, and neuroimaging should not be used as the sole or definitive diagnostic modality when evaluating shunt function. If shunt malfunction or infection is suspected, consult neurosurgery for further evaluation, including shunt aspiration, nuclear medicine flow studies, admission, and monitoring. Programmable shunts will need to be reprogrammed after MRI because the magnet alters the set pressure level. Programming requires an on-site, trained provider.

URINARY DIVERSIONS

Urinary diversions include vesicostomies, ureterostomies, ileal loop conduits, and bladder augmentations. Complications include prolapse and stomal stenosis in vesicostomies, stenosis of ureterostomies, pyelonephritis, stricture of the ureteroileal anastomosis, peristomal hernia, or stenosis in ileal loop conduits. Small bowel obstruction can be a complication of constriction of the ileal conduit. Most complications are managed in consultation with the child's urologist.

SPECIAL POPULATIONS

AUTISM SPECTRUM DISORDER

Autism spectrum disorder is a category of disorders characterized by restrictive, repetitive, and stereotyped patterns of behaviors with impaired social interaction and communication.[38] The disorder has a wide variety of clinical expressions, severity, and levels of function. The increase in prevalence over the past few decades may be due to improved and earlier detection.[39] The current prevalence is about 1 in 88 children.[40] The cause is unknown, but there is no relationship with childhood immunizations. In general, most children with autism spectrum disorder do not have associated medical disorders and have medical needs similar to those of age-matched, normally developing children. Sensory defensiveness, unusual social behaviors, and aggressive self-protective responses to medical procedures and examinations can complicate medical interactions. Always ask the parents or primary caregivers about the most effective means of communication for each child, as well as specific "do's and don'ts." Consider reducing auditory, visual, and tactile stimulation, and allow a period of adjustment to the ED environment; if possible, limit the number of medical providers who are unfamiliar to the child. Sedation may be needed for examination and procedures.

INTELLECTUAL DISABILITY AND GLOBAL DEVELOPMENTAL DELAY

Intellectual disability occurs in approximately 1% to 3% of the population[41] and is defined by cognitive impairment and decreased adaptive behaviors resulting from injury, disease, or abnormality occurring before the age of 18. Global developmental delay refers to intellectual disability in children <5 years old and is characterized by significant deficits in learning and adaptive behaviors.[42] Intellectual disability is associated with disorders such as Down's syndrome, Rett's syndrome, Williams' syndrome, fragile X syndrome, and fetal alcohol syndrome, but has no disorder-specific associations in most cases. Children with intellectual disability can be difficult to approach, have impaired social and communication skills, and may become aggressive or combative when confronted by new or painful stimuli. The parent or primary caregiver is the best source of information for effective interaction strategies. The various medical problems found in these patients can be specific to the underlying syndrome, but treatment is generally the same as with developmentally normal children. Review medication profiles to prevent drug interactions and to identify potential drug side effects.[16]

DOWN'S SYNDROME

Down's syndrome is a relatively common genetic disorder, most often resulting from a trisomy of chromosome 21, that occurs in just over 1 in 1000 live births. The syndrome (see Table 146-1) is characterized by developmental delay, intellectual disability, congenital heart defects, GI abnormalities, thyroid dysfunction, insulin-dependent diabetes mellitus, increased risk of upper respiratory and ear infections, atlantoaxial instability, and leukemia. Congenital heart defects affect about half of children and include atrioventricular canal defects, ventricular and atrial septal defects, tetralogy of Fallot, and patent ductus arteriosus. These defects generally are detected in early infancy, but pulmonary hypertension and congestive heart failure can develop over time if treatment is not successful. GI abnormalities occur in about 5% of cases[43] and include esophageal atresia, tracheoesophageal fistula, pyloric stenosis, duodenal atresia, Meckel's diverticulum, Hirschsprung's disease, and imperforate anus. Therefore, feeding difficulties or vomiting in the infant with Down's syndrome requires thorough investigation. Gastroesophageal reflux responds to standard therapy. Midface malformations affect the normal functioning of eustachian tubes, leading to recurrent and chronic infections of the ear, sinuses, and upper respiratory tract. **Asymptomatic atlantoaxial instability is present in about 13% of children with Down's syndrome. Maintain a high index of suspicion for cervical spine injury after trauma.** Specifically, deceleration injuries raise concern for **atlantoaxial subluxation** or dislocation. Children with Down's syndrome, compared

TABLE 146-7 Cerebral Palsy

Motor abnormality	Spastic	Increased tone; muscle stiffness
	Dyskinetic	Involuntary, nonpurposeful, uncoordinated movements
	Ataxic	Wide-spaced, unsteady gait; movement uncoordinated and clumsy
	Hypotonic	Floppy; generalized muscle weakness and flaccidity
Distribution	Diplegia	Paralysis affecting symmetrical parts of the body
	Paraplegia	Paralysis of both legs
	Hemiplegia	Involvement of one half of the body
	Quadriplegia	Four-limb paralysis

to those without, have a 10- to 20-fold increased risk of developing leukemia,[44] most commonly acute lymphoblastic leukemia.

CEREBRAL PALSY

The term cerebral palsy describes a collection of nonprogressive disorders of movement and posture originating from injury sustained by the developing brain within the first 3 to 5 years of life. The prevalence is 2 to 4 cases per 1000 individuals. Although motor deficits are the primary feature, cerebral palsy can also be associated with seizures, cognitive impairments, and sensory, communication, and behavioral abnormalities. There is a wide spectrum of intellectual and physical function, ranging from normal intelligence and mild motor deficits to severe disability. Cerebral palsy is often classified by the type of motor abnormality, its distribution, and the degree of involvement (**Table 146-7**).

Prenatal injury may occur from teratogen exposure, genetic syndromes, intrauterine infections, brain malformations, intrauterine cerebrovascular accidents, or fetal-placental malfunctions. The perinatal period may be affected by pre-eclampsia, complications of labor and delivery, sepsis or CNS infection, asphyxia, or prematurity. Older infants and children can develop cerebral palsy as a result of meningitis, traumatic brain injury, or toxic exposures. About 25% have no obvious cause.[45-47] Children with severe spasticity may have an intrathecal baclofen pump. Baclofen pump complications include malfunction, dislodgement, infection, or acute medication withdrawal. **Life-threatening baclofen withdrawal can occur and may present with malignant hyperthermia, hypotension, myoclonus, seizures, rhabdomyolysis, disseminated intravascular coagulation, multisystem organ failure, cardiac arrest, coma, and death.** In addition to life-saving supportive measures, oral baclofen and benzodiazepines are used to treat symptoms.

NEURAL TUBE DEFECTS

Neural tube defects result from the failure of the neural tube to close during the early embryonic stage of development and account for most congenital abnormalities of the CNS. The cause is multifactorial, but folic acid deficiency is associated with an increased risk, and maternal supplementation is currently recommended as early as possible in pregnancy.[48] The most common and most severe form of neural tube defect is meningomyelocele, which involves the spinal cord, meninges, and vertebral column. Spina bifida and spina bifida occulta are other examples of neural tube defects. Complex medical problems result from the impairment of sensory and motor control of voluntary and autonomic activities at or below the site of the lesion (**Table 146-8**).

Autonomic dysreflexia is a serious, potentially life-threatening complication of neural tube defects. Autonomic dysreflexia consists of paroxysmal sympathetic and parasympathetic hyperactivity initiated by stimuli below the level of the lesion, such as bladder overdistention, fecal impaction, or fracture. The symptoms of autonomic dysreflexia are sweating, flushing, pounding headache, hypertension, bradycardia, and piloerection. The primary intervention is to determine and eliminate the offending stimulus through bladder emptying, disimpaction with local

TABLE 146-8 Neural Tube Defect Complications

Autonomic dysreflexia
Neurogenic bowel and bladder dysfunction
Contractures
Scoliosis
Hydrocephalus
Chiari II malformation
Tethering of the spinal cord
Spinal cord syrinx
Vesicoureteral reflux
Latex allergy
Recurrent urinary tract infections
Constipation
Growth failure
Respiratory compromise
Seizures
Vision impairment
Osteoporosis
Cognitive impairment
Gastroesophageal reflux

anesthesia, discontinuation of painful procedures, or repositioning. If elevated blood pressure does not respond to repositioning or stimulus reduction, institute standard treatment for hypertensive emergencies.

Chiari Malformation Chiari malformation consists of a downward displacement of the cerebellar tonsils through the foramen magnum, frequently causing obstructive hydrocephalus. Although mild tonsillar herniation seen in type I Chiari malformation can be asymptomatic, the more severe Chiari II is common in children with meningomyelocele and consists of malformation of the cerebellum, hindbrain, and brainstem (**Table 146-9**), requiring early ventricular shunt placement. Even minor cervical hyperflexion and extension injuries can cause symptoms in children with Chiari malformation; **any deceleration injury, even mild, requires cervical spine stabilization and assessment for spinal cord injury due to instability of the craniocervical junction.** Consider Chiari II malformation as a possible cause of new-onset stridor in the child with meningomyelocele. Monitor closely for progression to complete airway obstruction. Diagnosis requires emergent MRI of the craniocervical junction. If respiratory function is not severely compromised and the airway remains stable, outpatient disposition may be considered in consultation with subspecialists caring for the child.

URINARY TRACT

Complications of a neurogenic bladder include recurrent urinary tract infection, urinary retention or incontinence, and complications of self-catheterization. Medications or prophylactic antibiotics may be prescribed to enhance continence and minimize damage to the upper urinary tract. Because bacterial colonization of the urine is common, only treat symptomatic infection with antibiotics. Suspect formation of a false passage

TABLE 146-9 Chiari II Malformation Symptoms

Infant	Older child
Apnea	Vision dysfunction
Vocal cord paralysis	Motor incoordination
Stridor	Headache
Oral motor dysfunction	Hand weakness
Vision disturbances	
Upper extremity weakness	
Incoordination	

during self-catheterization with difficult catheter passage, pain, or urethral bleeding. Do not attempt recatheterization in the ED for these symptoms, for fear of compounding the underlying injury, but obtain urologic consultation. Long-term indwelling catheterization predisposes the patient to the development of **latex allergy**.

Acknowledgment The author gratefully acknowledges the contributions of Douglas R. Trocinski and Donna Moro-Sutherland, the lead authors of this chapter in previous editions.

REFERENCES

The complete reference list is available online at www.TintinalliEM.com.

CHAPTER 147 Behavioral Disorders in Children

Quynh Doan
Tyler R. Black

INTRODUCTION

Pediatric mental health emergencies encompass a range of conditions, including psychological disorders such as mood and anxiety disorders (depression, bipolar disorder, suicidal ideation, obsessive compulsive disorders, posttraumatic stress syndrome), exacerbations of behavioral disorders (attention-deficit/hyperactivity disorder, aggressive outbursts, conduct disorders), deteriorating neurodevelopmental disorders (autistic spectrum disorders, tic disorders, intellectual disabilities), addictive disorders, and eating disorders. The psychological and sometimes physical aftermath of child maltreatment, mass casualty incidents and disasters, and exposure to violence and unexpected deaths are also likely causes of mental health emergencies.[1-4]

The role of the emergency physician includes medical stabilization, differentiating physical from mental health issues, performing a psychosocial assessment, and directing patients and families toward appropriate resources for acute and long-term needs. Initial management may include pharmacologic therapy, physical restraint, and referral for inpatient admission.[2,5]

EPIDEMIOLOGY

The mental health crisis involves all socioeconomic and ethnic groups and is not unique to any one geographic area, state, or region. The cause of the dramatic rise in pediatric mental health emergencies is multifactorial and complex. A Centers for Disease Control and Prevention report of a 5-year (2005 to 2011) mental health surveillance among children in the United States cited a prevalence of mental health disorders of 13% to 20% and suicide as the second most common cause of mortality among children 12 to 17 years old in 2010.[6] The National Comorbidity Survey–Adolescent Supplement data found the lifetime a prevalence of any one *Diagnostic and Statistical Manual of Mental Disorders* class disorder among adolescents of 51%.[7] In Canada, 14% to 25% of children and youth are affected by at least one diagnosable mental disorder.[8,9] Factors contributing to high prevalence of mental illnesses among children and youths include family instability or dysfunction, economic crisis or financial hardship, inadequate numbers of mental health professionals (especially those with pediatric expertise), lack of access to care, shortage of funding for mental health services, and failure to seek care due to cultural stigma.[1] In addition, social networking exposes youths to cyberbullying, online harassment, social isolation, and "Facebook depression," adding further risks for developing mental health illnesses.[10]

Multiple economic forces negatively impact the availability and delivery of mental health services[1,4,5,11,12] and have transformed EDs into the safety net for a fragmented mental health infrastructure.[5] Mental health follow-up or aftercare is also a problem. Of patients discharged from psychiatric emergency facilities, 40% to 60% do not receive aftercare, which increases the risk of repeat ED visits.[11]

It is therefore not surprising that ED use for mental health care by children and youth is increasing. In the United States, both the absolute number (from 565,000 to 823,000) and proportion of all ED visits (from 2.0% to 2.8%) by children and youth for a mental health problem are on the rise.[13] The Pediatric Emergency Care Applied Research Network reported that 3.3% of all participating pediatric ED visits were made for psychiatric-related visits. These visits are more frequently arriving by ambulance, are associated with longer length of stays, and result in admission to the hospital more commonly than other causes for ED visits.[14] Pediatric psychiatric emergencies show seasonal variation and are more common during the school year, peaking in May and November, while reaching a nadir in July and August. While the visit distribution over days of the week appears to be even, visits occur more frequently in the evening, coinciding with a time period when most outpatient community mental health resources are not easily reachable.[15]

CLINICAL ASSESSMENT

GENERAL GOALS

The first goal in the assessment of children with mental health emergencies is to identify and treat acute life-threatening medical emergencies. The second goal is to determine whether the child in a medically stable condition poses an imminent threat to his or her own life or the life of others, because this determines the need for hospitalization. Next, exclude organic causes. The general approach to making this determination is outlined here, and individual psychiatric conditions are further detailed below in "Management of Psychiatric Presentations." **Table 147-1** lists medical and psychiatric conditions that may present with agitation, psychosis, or obtundation. **Table 147-2** enumerates some general characteristics that may distinguish organic from psychiatric causes of psychosis.

HISTORY

Focus the history on the chief complaint and details of the presenting symptoms, circumstances, and precipitating events (e.g., social stressors). The timing and sequence of events and associated symptoms may help to distinguish organic from psychiatric conditions, and a thorough review of systems aids in this regard. Auditory hallucinations are associated with psychosis, whereas visual hallucinations may indicate intoxication or organic causes. A history of head injury, chronic or progressive headaches, visual changes, vomiting (especially morning vomiting), and deterioration of motor skills or gait suggests an intracranial process such as a brain tumor or subdural hematoma. Constitutional symptoms that may provide clues to an organic etiology include temperature instability, palpitations, and changes in appetite, stool patterns, hair, or skin.

The past medical history and family history will help identify the pattern and chronicity of the presenting symptoms. Similarly, a review of medications, including adherence to prescribed medication regimens, and their efficacy will guide the treatment plan and disposition. A family history of psychiatric or organic disease may indicate a potential genetic predisposition.

In addition to noting these standard components of history, pay particular attention to the social history. Many psychosocial screening tools exist, and some have been validated, such as the HEADS-ED (**Table 147-3**). The HEADS-ED assesses the degree of acute distress in domains pertaining to the **h**ome, **e**ducation, **a**ctivities and peers, **d**rugs and alcohol, **s**uicidality, **e**motions and behavior, and **d**ischarge resources.[16] In addition to facilitating the assessment, this tool also guides management decisions.

PHYSICAL EXAMINATION

Assess vital signs and the airway, breathing, and circulation status, and perform a detailed neurologic examination. Alterations in vital signs may provide clues to potential intoxication, ingestions, or organic pathology (endocrinologic and metabolic). Tachycardia, hypertension,

TABLE 147-1 Medical and Psychiatric Causes of Altered Mental Status in Children

Medical Conditions	Psychiatric Conditions
CNS disorders	Acute mania
Brain tumor	Bipolar disorder
Temporal lobe epilepsy	Depression
Trauma	Acute psychosis (e.g., schizophrenia)
Infection (abscess, encephalitis, meningitis)	Personality disorder
	Conduct disorder
Metabolic/endocrine disorders	
Hyperglycemia, hypoglycemia	
Thyroid disease	
Uremia	
Hepatic failure	
Porphyria	
Collagen vascular diseases	
Lupus erythematosus	
Vasculitis	
Hyperpyrexia	
Intoxication	
Drugs of abuse (alcohol, stimulants, hallucinogens)	
Medications (antipsychotics, corticosteroids)	
Environmental substances (anticholinergics, heavy metals)	
Withdrawal	
Alcohol	
Barbiturates	
Benzodiazepines	

pyrexia, and tachypnea may suggest intoxication with stimulants such as amphetamines, cocaine, and "ecstasy" (3,4-methylenedioxymethamphetamine). Assessment for toxidromes may help identify anticholinergic symptoms or salicylate toxicity. The pupillary responses, presence or absence of nystagmus, skin temperature and moisture, and condition of the mucous membranes are all helpful in identifying toxidromes.

Focus the neurologic examination on level of consciousness, gait and coordination, and reflexes, and administer the Mini-Mental State Examination. Note the child's affect and general appearance, content and organization of thought, and articulation and expression of speech. Pressured speech with flight of ideas may signal acute mania, whereas echolalia, "word salad," and other disordered thought may indicate acute psychosis.

TABLE 147-2 Differentiation of Organic and Psychiatric Psychosis

Characteristic	Organic Cause	Psychiatric Cause
History: onset and progression	Acute	Gradual/progressive
Vital signs	Often disturbed	Usually normal
Physical examination		
Focal neurologic symptoms	May be present	Usually absent
Mental status	Delirium, visual hallucinations, agitation	Anger, sadness, auditory hallucinations, agitation
Laboratory findings	May be altered	Usually normal

LABORATORY TESTING AND IMAGING

Laboratory tests and imaging are dictated by the history and physical examination. Pubertal girls should have a urine pregnancy test, because many psychiatric medications can affect the fetus. Urine drug screening can be helpful when intoxication from drugs of abuse is suspected. Obtain serum acetaminophen (Tylenol) and aspirin levels in children who have ingested drugs or attempted suicide. Hyperglycemia, hypoglycemia, and hyperammonemia can cause alterations in mental status, and measurement of glucose and ammonia levels may be useful in obtunded patients. A 12-lead ECG is useful in cases of potential ingestion or intoxication to identify interval prolongation or conduction abnormalities. Document normal sinus rhythms at baseline, before initiating psychotropic medications that may accentuate long QT disorders. Screening laboratory tests performed in psychiatric emergencies vary by institution. Many inpatient psychiatric facilities require basic chemistry panels and screening for thyroid disorders. See chapter 137, "Altered Mental Status in Children" for further discussion of altered mental status.

Imaging studies are rarely indicated or helpful except as dictated by the findings of the history and physical examination. Chest radiographs may identify aspiration in the obtunded vomiting patient. Abdominal radiographs may identify radiopaque foreign objects or ingestions. Neuroimaging can exclude intracranial mass lesions in those with suggestive clinical signs and symptoms.

MANAGEMENT OF PSYCHIATRIC PRESENTATIONS

A detailed summary of child and youth mental health issues is beyond the scope of this book. Formal diagnoses of mental health conditions usually occur after the ED presentation. Therefore, this section will focus on the approach to, and treatment of, **psychiatric presentations**. Many care environments use social workers, youth care workers, nurses, and other clinicians to conduct significant portions of the mental health assessment in the ED.

SUICIDAL IDEATION AND ATTEMPTS

Suicide is complex. Although it is one of the most common causes of death in youth (4.9 per 100,000 per year between the ages of 10 and 19, more than neoplasm, respiratory, and cardiovascular deaths combined),[17] the vast majority of youth who have suicidal thinking or behaviors do not go on to complete suicide (**Table 147-4**).[18-20] Risk prediction is currently not possible.[21] Therefore, the standard of care in an approach to suicide is not risk prediction; rather the focus should be on **risk/protective factor identification and acuity assessment, collateral history, clinical synthesis, and safety management.**

A number of **risk factors** are associated with increased suicide risk, and suicide risk is fluid and can change rapidly. Identification of risk factors should be carried out with the goal of separating **chronic** (longstanding and unlikely to change) from **acute** (recent and possible to change) risk factors. Chronic risk factors convey ongoing risk and are important for informing systemic, rather than individual approaches. Acute risk factors allow for individual approaches for suicide safety planning to occur. Protective factors reduce risk overall and should be considered in risk factor identification. A representative, noncomprehensive list of risk and protective factors is presented in **Table 147-5**.[22-26]

Assessment scales and tools for assessment should be used to gather information to contribute to the assessment process rather than rigid structures to guide decision making. In the ED, brief screening questionnaires like the Ask Suicide-Screening Questions can help identify patients with suicidal thinking.[27] The Ask Suicide-Screening Questions consists of four questions: (1) current thoughts of being better off dead; (2) current wish to die; (3) current suicidal ideation; and (4) past suicide attempt. A positive response to any one question identified 97% of those at risk for suicide (sensitivity 96.7%, specificity 87.6%).[27] The Columbia–Suicide Severity Rating Scale (available for download at http://www.cssrs.columbia.edu/scales_practice_cssrs.html) can help guide assessment of suicidal thinking and behaviors and has been validated for use

TABLE 147-3 Proportion of Patients Referred for Psychiatric Consult and Admitted by Level of HEADS-ED

	Score	Total Sample, 313 (100), *n* (%)	Consult, 149 (47.8), *n* (%)	Admitted, 66 (21.1), *n* (%)
Home			*	NS
Supportive	0	142 (45.4)	64 (45.4)	34 (23.9)
Conflicts	1	144 (46.0)	66 (45.8)	24 (16.7)
Chaotic/dysfunctional	2	27 (8.6)	19 (70.4)	8 (29.6)
Education			**	**
On track	0	124 (39.7)	40 (32.3)	13 (10.5)
Grades dropping	1	149 (47.8)	85 (57.4)	40 (26.8)
Failing/not attending school	2	39 (12.5)	23 (59.0)	12 (30.8)
Activities and peers			**	**
No change	0	164 (52.7)	53 (32.3)	11 (6.7)
Reduced	1	116 (37.3)	74 (63.8)	37 (31.9)
Withdrawn	2	31 (10.0)	22 (73.3)	18 (58.1)
Drugs and alcohol			*	*
No or infrequent	0	216 (69.5)	93 (43.3)	36 (16.7)
Occasional	1	52 (16.7)	27 (51.9)	14 (26.9)
Frequent/daily	2	43 (13.8)	28 (65.1)	15 (34.9)
Suicidality			**	**
No thoughts	0	68 (21.7)	15 (22.1)	2 (2.9)
Ideation	1	167 (53.4)	67 (40.1)	15 (9.0)
Plan or gesture	2	78 (24.9)	67 (87.0)	49 (62.8)
Emotions and behavior			**	**
Mildly anxious/sad/acting out	0	39 (12.5)	6 (15.4)	2 (5.1)
Moderately anxious/sad/acting out	1	198 (63.3)	88 (44.7)	27 (13.6)
Significantly distressed/unable to function/out of control	2	76 (24.3)	55 (72.4)	37 (48.7)
Discharge resources			NS	NS
Ongoing/well connected	0	94 (30.3)	48 (51.1)	18 (17.0)
Some/not meeting needs	1	148 (47.7)	66 (44.6)	28 (18.9)
None/on wait list	2	68 (21.9)	32 (47.8)	19 (27.9)

NS, nonsignificant.

*$P < .05$;

**$P < .01$.

Source: Reproduced with permission from Cappelli M, Gray C, Zemek R, et al: The HEADS-ED: a rapid mental health screening tool for pediatric patients in the emergency department. *Pediatrics* 130: e321, 2012. Table 5. Copyright American Academy of Pediatrics.

in multiple settings including the ED for both adolescents and adults.[28,29] Internal validity and usability rate high for such scales. Some more commonly used scales, such as the SADPERSONS, have little evidentiary support, contain many inaccurate assumptions about suicide risk, and do not accurately predict suicide.[30-34]

Clinical interview, impression, and analysis are crucial aspects of suicide risk assessment. Collateral history for the youth (parents, caregivers, clinicians, teachers, etc.) adds to the confidence of the assessment and can significantly affect the quality of the risk assessment. If an interview has poor reliability or rapport, the "collected data" may be inaccurate. The tone of the patient themselves, their family, and the support network around them can alter the impression of hope or despair. The importance of clinical and interpersonal factors cannot be understated and is why a reliance on rigid data, forms, or quantities is perilous.[35]

TABLE 147-4 Relative Frequency of Suicide-Related Thoughts and Behaviors in Adolescents

	1-Year Prevalence	Frequency
Feeling sad or hopeless for 2 weeks*	30.0%	1:3.3
Nonsuicidal self-injury	18.0%	1:5.6
Suicidal ideation*	17.0%	1:5.8
Suicide planning*	13.6%	1:7.4
Suicide attempt (any)*	8.0%	1:12.5
Suicide attempt (potentially lethal)*	2.7%	1:37
Death by suicide†	0.005%	1:21,000

*Females generally twice as likely.

†Males generally four times as likely.

Safety management, following an adequate risk assessment, flows naturally from identified risk and protective factors. By dividing risk factors into acute and chronic categories, targeted interventions for **any acute risk factors** can be made. Creating safety plans for families and youth to use when suicidal ideation occurs can increase compliance with follow-up programming,[36] encourages appropriate re-presentation to the ED, and provides a sense of structure and support to families struggling with suicide concerns. **Figure 147-1** provides an emergency approach to suicidal presentations, and the approach can be done in a multidisciplinary way—a physician is not required for any one step.

Determination of the risk factors will influence the services consulted; social issues require social support services, whereas psychiatric issues require mental health supports. Rigid consultation of all suicidal patients to psychiatric care is neither necessary nor effective; inpatient and involuntary approaches to patients are beneficial when the risk profile is simply too high to manage in the outpatient environment and inpatient services are required to reduce the identified risk factors. Examples of nonpsychiatric

TABLE 147-5 Selection of Common Chronic and Acute Risk Factors and Protective Factors for Suicide

Chronic Risk Factors	
History of suicidal thinking or behavior	Any suicidal factor by history is one of the only consistent predictive measures for suicide risk.
History of mental health disorder	Lifetime risk of suicide is increased in almost all mental health disorders.
Age	Exceedingly rare <10 y of age. Risk starts at approximately age 10 and increases consistently until the age of 24. **Adolescents are less at risk for suicide than adults.**
Sex	Males 4–5 times more likely by adolescence.
Ethnic or cultural risk group	Aboriginal youth, homeless youth, LGBTQ youth.
Chronic illness	Any chronic illness causing pain, disability, or fatigue.
Family history of suicide	Closer-degree relatives infer a greater risk.
History of trauma, abuse, neglect, loss	Duration, frequency, and severity of trauma is additive.
Acute Risk Factors	
Recent suicidal thoughts or behaviors	Ideation < planning < nonlethal attempt < lethal attempt. **New/changing suicidality** should prompt full assessment.
Suicide planning	Passive (nonspecific wish to die) confers less risk than active (specific, formed plan).
Accessibility to lethal means	Unsecured substances, medications, firearms. Feasibility of plan.
High agitation/anxiety presentation	Strong (yet poorly specific) prediction of acute suicide risk.
Current mental health/substance use disorder	Lack of treatment response, noncompliance to treatment, worsening or rapidly changing disorders, should be targets of suicide risk reduction.
Family dysfunction/caregiver unavailable	Chaotic, dysfunctional homes confer suicide risk. A responsible caregiver must be in place to institute safety management measures.
Lack of professional supports	Can include supports that are not effective.
Recent crisis/major life change	Conflicts, relationships, school, failures, losses, etc. *Directly addressing these crises reduces risk.*

Protective Factors		
Parent connectedness	Sport/activity participation	Positive social supports
Safety of environment	Strong professional supports	Future orientation
Good therapeutic connection	Strong cultural identity	Responding to treatment

Abbreviation: LGBTQ, lesbian, gay, bisexual, transgender, queer/questioning.

risk reduction maneuvers include removing lethal means, securing firearms, creating safety plans, referring to social support services, providing family supports, and addressing social and school concerns. Resolution of any triggering crisis severely reduces severity risk.

NONSUICIDAL SELF-INJURY

Nonsuicidal self-injury is "the deliberate, self-inflicted destruction of body tissue without suicidal intent and for purposes not socially sanctioned,"[37] and refers to a wide variety of behaviors including cutting, burning, carving, punching, and picking. Approximately 18% of adolescents have engaged in nonsuicidal self-injury in the past year, and recent studies report that as many as 47% of females have tried it, even briefly. Nonsuicidal self-injury begins in puberty and is twice as common in females, peaking in middle adolescence and declining thereafter. Although it increases suicide risk, over 90% of youth presenting to crisis services with nonsuicidal self-injury have no intent of suicide.[38] Biologic predispositions to self-injury include an absent stress cortisol response, sensitivity of opioid receptors, and genetics.

First, address the sequelae of the injury, and focus on the **distress** and **events** that led to self-injury. Avoid overreaction to superficial injuries; comments such as "you could have killed yourself" or "these injuries look awful" may harm the patient and even increase subsequent behavior. Such comments can confuse the message that self-injury is different from suicide. Second, conduct suicide risk assessment, especially for new or changing self-injury, or in the presence of other developing mental health issues. Explain the difference between nonsuicidal self-injury and suicidal behaviors to caregivers. Finally, provide social and mental health support resources to improve **distress tolerance**, **stress management,** and **family supports**.

AGGRESSION

Aggression can occur prior to ED presentation, before or during assessment, and in subsequent care. Consider patient and environmental safety, potential trauma to the child or family, engagement and deescalation whenever possible, and safe medication and restraint policies.[39]

Pharmacologic interventions require consideration of the *intention* of the intervention. If the underlying issue is psychosis or mania, potent antipsychotic medications are warranted. However, if agitation is behavioral, reactionary, or anxiety-driven in nature, and the goal of intervention is sedation, many less potent and potentially less dangerous approaches can be taken.

An approach to aggression in the ED is outlined in **Table 147-6**, with pharmacologic options in **Table 147-7**.[40,41]

ANXIETY AND DEPRESSION

ED presentations for anxiety and depression are common. For anxiety, this is often in the form of panic, dysregulation, or regressive behavior. In depression, common presentations include irritability, hopelessness, or sadness. Signs and symptoms of anxiety and depression vary with age: younger children exhibit more regressive, agitated, or withdrawn behaviors, whereas adolescents tend to be able to express their emotional state through direct conversation. Both anxiety and depression in youth can also present with impaired concentration, fatigue, and insomnia. Perform suicide risk screening and assessments as appropriate.

Anxiety or irritability can be relieved in the ED through the use of sublingual lorazepam. Most often, treatments of anxiety and depressive disorders are combination approaches;[47] proper treatment includes the use of therapeutic approaches (cognitive behavioral therapy, interpersonal therapy) and medications (selective serotonin reuptake inhibitors) that usually exceed the scope of an ED. Severe, disabling, or suicide-related anxiety or depression concerns should warrant a consultation to psychiatric service; for more mild issues, referral to appropriate mental health supports can be made.

PSYCHOSIS

Psychosis is a generic term that describes a process in which someone's thought or sensory process no longer conforms to reality. Often it is confused as a diagnosis (for example, schizophrenia), when in fact, the presentation of psychosis can be brought about by a variety of conditions,[48] including benign (hypnagogic hallucinations that occur in sleep-wake transition, normal bereavement), medical (CNS tumors, delirium), psychiatric (schizophrenia, bipolar mania), and substance-induced (steroids, drugs of abuse). Psychosis is a syndrome of exclusion; potentially dangerous medical diagnoses must be considered and ruled out prior to psychiatric treatment (see Tables 147-1 and 147-2, above).

Psychiatric causes of psychosis are rare in prepubertal children; in fact, these disorders usually manifest at around 20 years of age. However, many adolescents can have prodromal presentations, and early-onset bipolar disorder, schizophrenia, and other psychiatric causes of psychosis are possible. Predictors of psychosis include a family history (especially first-degree relatives), progressive decline (rather than abrupt), and a history of subclinical psychotic symptoms.[49]

The approach to psychosis varies depending on the cause (**Table 147-8**). In the ED, the antipsychotic medications in Table 147-7 can be tried for agitation or urgent symptom concerns; however, caution must be used, because delirium or substance intoxication as a root cause of the psychosis could be worsened by the addition of psychotropic medications.

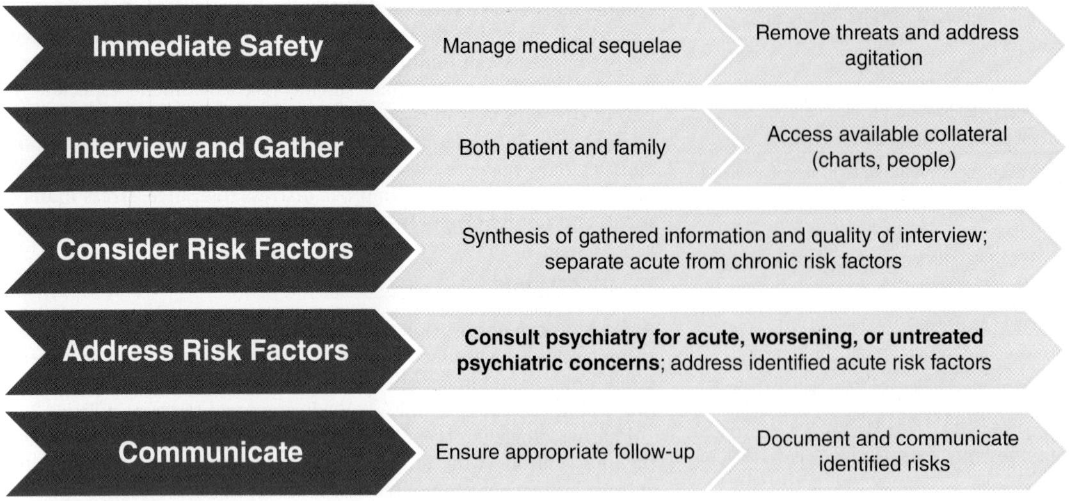

Immediate Safety → Manage medical sequelae → Remove threats and address agitation

Interview and Gather → Both patient and family → Access available collateral (charts, people)

Consider Risk Factors → Synthesis of gathered information and quality of interview; separate acute from chronic risk factors

Address Risk Factors → **Consult psychiatry for acute, worsening, or untreated psychiatric concerns**; address identified acute risk factors

Communicate → Ensure appropriate follow-up → Document and communicate identified risks

FIGURE 147-1. Approach to suicidality in the ED.

BEHAVIORAL DISORDERS

Behavioral disorders is a broad term, generally focused on maladaptive behaviors that have progressed to a point of severe dysfunction, risk, or negative outcome. They are seen as a pathologic extension of normal behavioral issues. **Oppositional defiant disorder** is a persistent pattern of provocative, hostile, and noncompliant behavior, characterized by low temper threshold.[50] **Conduct disorder** is a more severe, antisocial pattern of rule-breaking behavior that includes aggression to people and animals, deceitfulness and theft, serious rule-breaking, and destruction of property.[51] Treatment is largely environmental and familial, and pharmacologic interventions are of mixed benefit. Behavioral disorders have extremely high psychiatric comorbidity, particularly with attention-deficit/hyperactivity disorder, and treatment of comorbid conditions is necessary. Stimulants, nonstimulant ADHD medications, clonidine, guanfacine, antiepileptic medications, and antipsychotic medications have mixed evidence, but trials are often necessary to reduce impulsivity, sometimes induce sedation, and are used off-label.[52]

TABLE 147-6 Approach to the Pediatric Aggressive Patient

Safety	Secure patient and staff safety. Recognize the compromise between security and safety: higher security measures (such as pharmacologic or physical restraint) may also confer greater risk for patient harm. Use these measures when appropriate.
Engagement	Youth often use aggression as their last resort to express or achieve something: expressing anger, being left alone, interfering in treatment, or receiving something desired. Engaging the youth whenever possible to help achieve these goals can reduce the need for further measures. **ALWAYS allow the situation to "step down."** (i.e., reoffer oral medications before injection)
Interventions, in the order they should be attempted when possible:	
1. Environment and engagement	Secure the environment so the patient can safely be agitated and engagement is possible. Environments with safe furniture and objects, full observation abilities, and adequate staffing are required.
2. Pharmacology (voluntary)	**See Table 147-7.** Consider low doses and reengage as necessary.
3. Pharmacology (involuntary)	**See Table 147-7.** Minimize the need for reinjection of medications by choosing dosing appropriately. Physical restraint is often necessary. Offer oral medications immediately before intramuscular medications.
4. Seclusion and restraint	Ensure the facility has appropriate seclusion and restraint policies; both can be fatal if used incorrectly or inappropriately. All seclusion and restraint should mandate 1:1 observation levels. Remove whenever possible. Special consideration should be given to the possibility of rhabdomyolysis with physical restraints and asphyxia with person-to-person holds.

SUBSTANCE MISUSE AND WITHDRAWAL

Alcohol use and misuse have decreased over the past 20 years in youth, with record-low numbers being seen in recent surveys, both in extreme (<13 years) underage drinking and overall alcohol use.[18] However, the 1-year prevalence of being drunk at least once is 20% in adolescence, and 6% of adolescents will drink more than 10 drinks in a row, making acute intoxication a common adolescent event. Marijuana use has remained stable, with 40% of adolescents reporting ever using. However, cocaine, hallucinogen, inhalant, ecstasy, and methamphetamine use **has halved in the past 15 years**.

The management of individual toxidromes is described in the Toxicology section of this book. A very small percentage of adolescents with alcohol misuse experience any withdrawal symptoms, and an even smaller percentage require pharmacologic treatment. Paced alcohol discontinuation is a successful approach to managing alcohol withdrawal in teens, and treatment of severe symptoms can be carried out as in adults, using benzodiazepines such as diazepam and chlordiazepoxide.[53] Refer any youth with a substance use problem to available substance misuse services; the remission rates are low, but a nonjudgmental, continuous, motivational approach reduces rates of misuse.

CHILD ABUSE AND NEGLECT

Worldwide, 1 in 5 female children and 1 in 10 male children are sexually abused.[54] Approximately 25% of children are emotionally abused by their caregivers, and physical abuse affects 18% of children under the age of 18. Neglectful care of a child occurs in 6.5% of children every year.[55] Overall, these numbers are staggering and reflect a dire need for increased assessment, screening, and recognition of child maltreatment. It is *mandatory* to report any suspected child abuse to the legal authorities, and this should be done in any injury for which the mechanism is not explained; any behavior, phrase, or suggestion of abuse must be reported. The psychological, medical, and quality-of-life impacts of child maltreatment are severe, and early recognition and intervention can reverse these impacts. Children and adolescents presenting to the ED with behavioral or psychiatric emergencies should be asked about exposure to violence at home or school. See also chapter 148, "Child Abuse and Neglect."

SPECIAL CONSIDERATIONS IN THE DEVELOPMENTALLY DISABLED PATIENT

Assessing psychiatric emergencies in patients with a developmental disability is tremendously challenging (see chapter 146, "The Child with Special Healthcare Needs"). The following principles can be applied both in children and adults with developmental disabilities:[56]

1. **Establish a baseline.** In developmental disability, age cannot be relied upon to understand normal behavior. Ask caregivers what is normal for the patient, what has changed, and when.

TABLE 147-7 Pharmacologic Management of the Agitated Child

Drug	Child Dosing	Adolescent Dosing	Notes
Appropriate for Sedation in Children			
Diphenhydramine 1 milligram/kg May repeat q30min	25–50 milligrams PO/IM Maximum: 200 milligrams/24 h	50–100 milligrams PO/IM Maximum: 300 milligrams/24 h	Anticholinergic. Directly treats dystonia from antipsychotic treatment. Liquid form available.
Lorazepam 0.05 milligram/kg May repeat q30min	0.5–2 milligrams PO/IM Maximum: Until sedated or ataxic	1–2 milligrams PO/IM Maximum: Until sedated or ataxic	Paradoxical reaction possible. Respiratory depression. Sublingual tablet available.
Appropriate for Sedation and/or Psychosis in Children			
Olanzapine 0.1 milligram/kg May repeat q30min	2.5 milligrams PO/IM Maximum: 5 milligrams/24 h	5–10 milligrams PO/IM Maximum: 20 milligrams/24 h	QTc sparing. Dystonic reaction can occur but unlikely. Warning: IM preparation coadministered with benzodiazepine IM is not recommended because it can cause bradycardia and hypotension. Dissolvable tablet available. Anticholinergic.
Risperidone 0.05 milligram/kg May repeat q60min	0.25–0.5 milligram PO Maximum: 2 milligrams/24 h	0.5–1 milligram PO Maximum: 4 milligrams/24 h	QTc sparing. Dystonic reaction can occur. Dissolvable tablet and liquid form available.
Chlorpromazine 1 milligram/kg PO 0.5 milligram/kg IM May repeat q30min	25 milligrams PO/25 milligrams IM Maximum: 100 milligrams/24 h PO 75 milligrams/24 h IM	50 milligrams PO/12.5 milligrams IM Maximum: 200 milligrams/24 h PO 100 milligrams/24 h IM	Hypotension, QTc prolonging, lowers seizure threshold. Anticholinergic.
Appropriate for Psychosis in Children (when other treatments unavailable or failed)			
Haloperidol 0.05 milligram/kg May repeat q60min	0.5–2 milligrams PO/IM Maximum: 5 milligrams/24 h	2–5 milligrams PO/IM Maximum: 10 milligrams/24 h	QTc prolonging. **Extrapyramidal symptoms very likely in youth,**[42-46] especially dystonia. Consider coadministration of prophylactic anticholinergic (e.g., diphenhydramine as above or benztropine 1–2 milligrams PO/IM).

2. **Use developmentally appropriate approaches.** Use visual scales, toys, language cards, gestures, and simple words as required. Ask the caregiver for advice on interaction.
3. **Consider medical/pain sources.** Especially in patients with limited verbal output, changes in behavior, mood, and aggression can be due to simple issues such as urinary tract infections, dental pain, or headaches.
4. **Be pharmacologically conservative.** Use the minimum doses of medications (e.g., the child dosing in Table 147-7), resist polypharmacy, and make sure the medication has an observable effect prior to long-term prescription.
5. **Consider comorbidities.** Many patients with developmental disabilities have a high rate of psychiatric and medical comorbidities. Treatment of these comorbidities is necessary, and all efforts must be made to diagnose these conditions.

TABLE 147-8 Approach to Psychosis in the ED by Suspected Cause

Unknown	Rule out medical causes after thorough history and physical examination. Treat agitated patients or patients with distressing symptoms with the antipsychotics as per Table 147-7. Consult psychiatry when medically appropriate.
Substances	Use antidote/countering medication if available or necessary. Use environmental controls to reduce stimulation. May need to use medications as per Table 147-7, but cautiously due to interaction with intoxicant. Often clears as substance is metabolized.
Medical	Treat the underlying medical cause. Caution in using Table 147-7 medications that have anticholinergic properties. Consult psychiatry to manage psychiatric comorbidities.
Psychiatric	Primary psychosis (schizophrenia, etc.): use medications as per Table 147-7. Mania/psychotic depression: use antipsychotics as per Table 147-7 with combination of sedative medications as necessary. The goal in mania is to "settle the brain down" first; in psychotic depression, urgent psychiatric treatment is required. When psychiatric causes are suspected, consult psychiatry.

REFERENCES

The complete reference list is available online at www.TintinalliEM.com.

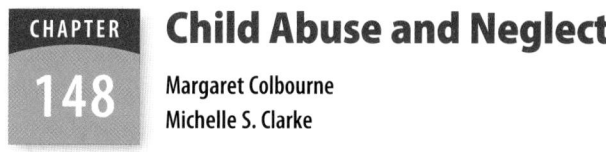

CHAPTER 148 Child Abuse and Neglect

Margaret Colbourne
Michelle S. Clarke

INTRODUCTION AND EPIDEMIOLOGY

Child maltreatment is, unfortunately, a common occurrence. In the United States, over 650,000 children suffer some form of child abuse or neglect each year, and approximately 12% of these children will present to a hospital with injuries.[1] It is estimated that between 2% and 10% of children visiting the ED are victims of child abuse or neglect.[2] Therefore, emergency physicians are in a unique position to identify nonaccidental injuries and potentially prevent further abuse. Child maltreatment takes many forms including neglect (68%), physical abuse (16%), sexual abuse (8%), and emotional abuse and medical child abuse (8%)[1] (previously called Munchausen syndrome by proxy).

NEGLECT

Child neglect is the most common form of child maltreatment and the most difficult to evaluate and manage; it contributes to as many as 50% of fatalities from child maltreatment.[3] Neglect occurs when a caregiver fails to meet a child's basic needs in provision of food, shelter, clothing, health care, education, supervision, and nurturance.[3-5] Further, this failure either results or is very likely to result in serious impairment of a child's health or development. While many types of neglect may occur, seldom does any one form exist on its own. Carefully consider each neglect risk factor individually, identifying whether there is overt

TABLE 148-1 Types of Neglect	
Types of Neglect	Description
Physical	Failure to provide the basic physical necessities of food, shelter, and adequate clothing.
Emotional	Failure to provide necessary nurturing, affection, and stimulation.
Educational	Failure to provide an educational program; this may include chronic truancy.
Medical/dental	Failure to provide basic medical and dental care, which results, or has the potential to result, in harm; this may include noncompliance with healthcare recommendations.
Supervisory	Failure to adequately supervise and ensure safety of a child, given the child's developmental needs.

historical or physical evidence of each subtype of neglect (**Table 148-1**).

Given that neglect is rarely a single act, but is rather an accumulation of harm over time, the often brief, single encounter of an ED assessment cannot provide the comprehensive assessment required. The goals of the ED encounter are to recognize when child neglect may be at issue, to clearly document the presenting concerns, and to trigger the appropriate multidisciplinary team approach for the investigation and management of these complex cases. The recognition of child neglect in the ED requires knowledge of the multiple risk factors associated with neglect (**Table 148-2**).[4-7] Poverty, parental substance abuse, and mental health issues are three of the most common risk factors for child maltreatment and neglect.[4,6] Although not all poor families are neglectful, poverty has an overwhelming effect on the parents' ability to provide basic care for their children and may contribute to social isolation and a lack of supports.[7] Substance abuse may result in a parent who is both physically and emotionally unavailable to the child, and substance abuse may divert funds for basic necessities.

CLINICAL FEATURES

Children and adolescents may be brought to the ED for a variety of reasons when neglect is the underlying problem. Presenting symptoms may include failure to thrive, malnutrition, chronic respiratory or skin infections, repeated injuries, poisonings, behavioral problems, or mental health concerns. Children with chronic disabilities or chronic medical conditions may present repeatedly with clinical deterioration if a parent is noncompliant with healthcare recommendations.

History Review the hospital record prior to obtaining the medical history from the parent. Be alert to chronic health problems, repeated accidents or injuries, and missed medical appointments. The medical history must address both the presenting complaint as well as any past illnesses or injuries. Note whether the parents are able to provide a clear history and are knowledgeable about their child's health and developmental milestones. Document the child's immunization status and any past or current medications. The young infant or child who presents with feeding problems or failure to thrive requires a thorough perinatal history as well as a detailed dietary record. In the case of maternal depression, the history provided by the mother may be vague and difficult to obtain. Inquiries into the family history should specifically address known risk factors for child neglect including parental mental health issues and substance abuse.

Physical Examination The physical examination begins during the process of gathering the history, with observations of the interaction between the parents and child, and notes on the child's clothing and hygiene. Observe for unusual demeanor or extreme behaviors such as flat affect, listlessness, overt fear, or out-of-control behavior. Document objective growth parameters including weight, height, and head circumference, and compare with previously reported measures when possible. In general, weight is the first growth parameter to be adversely affected by inadequate nutrition.

The physical examination is typically focused on the system of chief complaint; however, concern for neglect should prompt special attention to the skin (bruises, scars, infection, diaper rash), hair (alopecia, lice infestation), and teeth (dental caries). Determine if muscular tone is decreased or increased. Ear, nose, throat, and respiratory examinations may reveal evidence of chronic, untreated infection. Abdominal exam should note any distention, organomegaly, or unusual masses. Look for evidence of peripheral edema. Note the presence of adequate subcutaneous fat as well as muscular development, particularly over the suprascapular and buttock regions.

Laboratory Testing and Imaging Investigations vary depending on the severity of illness or injury. For failure to thrive, a comprehensive nutritional and metabolic profile is generally indicated. A complete skeletal survey should be considered in any situation of serious neglect to identify physical abuse and to assess skeletal abnormalities from nutritional deficiency or undiagnosed metabolic disease.

TREATMENT AND DISPOSITION

Focus on initial stabilization of acute medical illness and injury. For severe malnourishment with fluid and electrolyte imbalance, initial management may require intensive care support to manage metabolic complications such as "refeeding syndrome." Most infants with failure to thrive due to environmental neglect will respond rapidly to appropriate feeding.

Educate the parents in a thoughtful, respectful, and culturally sensitive manner on the most urgent problems and need for further investigation and treatment. Early consultation with pediatric specialists or child abuse pediatricians is warranted for all concerns of child neglect, even if hospitalization is not indicated. Comprehensive management of child neglect requires frequent ongoing reevaluation, which goes beyond the routine duties of the emergency physician.

TABLE 148-2 Risk Factors for Child Maltreatment	
Child risk factors	Premature birth Young age Multiple gestation (twin/triplet) births Chronic disability
Parent risk factors	Substance abuse Cognitive impairment Adolescent parents Domestic violence Mental health issues Lack of education/unrealistic expectations
Family/social risk factors	Isolation Single-parent families Unemployment Family illness History of involvement with child welfare services

PHYSICAL ABUSE

CLINICAL FEATURES

Physical abuse accounts for approximately 16% of all cases of child abuse and is perhaps the most easily identified type of maltreatment.[1] Child physical abuse is defined as injury inflicted on a child by a caregiver. Injuries can occur to all parts of the body, but the more commonly injured areas are the skin (bruising, burns), skeleton (fractures), head, and abdomen. Evaluate the child medically and treat injuries. Medical evaluation and treatment of the child always take precedence over the legal investigation. Although the forensic or legal evaluation is best performed by trained investigators or child abuse specialists, data gathered in the ED often guides and informs further investigation.

History Obtain a detailed history from all involved including the child, parents, caregivers, and any witnesses. Document details of the onset and progression of symptoms leading to the ED visit. Especially in young infants, pinpoint the last time the child was completely well. In a critically ill child, provide immediate resuscitation. In most cases of accidental injury, there is a clear and consistent history of an accident with the child presenting for care soon afterward. **Historical features concerning for abuse include no history of trauma, changing important details of the history, explanations inconsistent with the injury or with the developmental stage of the child, discrepancies in the history provided by different caregivers, or a significant delay in seeking care.**[8-10]

Obtain past medical history including the birth history, chronic or congenital conditions, previous injuries, and previous hospitalizations and surgeries. Document any family history of bleeding or bone disorders and any relevant metabolic or genetic conditions. Review the diet and medication history including vitamin K at birth and any subsequent vitamin or nutritional supplementation. Note current developmental status and progress. Important social history should identify the primary caregiver and other caregivers, household composition, any history of past abuse to the child or siblings, and previous child protective services involvement.

Physical Examination Begin with a general assessment of the child's alertness and demeanor. A brief evaluation of the work of breathing, cardiovascular perfusion, and level of alertness will identify a critically ill child in need of resuscitation. Note whether there is spontaneous and symmetric movement of the extremities. Lack of use of an extremity or pain with examination or movement may indicate a fracture. Document the head circumference and examine the scalp, noting any hematomas or step-offs, which may indicate a skull fracture. Funduscopic exam may reveal retinal hemorrhages, although it is often very difficult to perform an undilated exam in a child. Injuries to the mouth, such as a torn frenulum, may be indicative of forced feeding. Fully expose the skin and document the precise location, size, and shape of any bruises, burns, bite marks, or scars. Palpate the chest, abdomen, spine, and extremities for any tenderness. Perform and document a neurologic examination if there is concern for head trauma.

DIAGNOSIS

Bruises Bruising is the most common manifestation of physical abuse and is often overlooked. Up to a third of children with fatal or near-fatal abusive injuries have previous medical assessments in which bruising was noted.[11,12] Because bruising is also very common in nonabused children, distinguishing between nonaccidental and accidental bruising requires careful consideration of the child's age and developmental level, the history, and any other associated injuries. **Accidental bruises occur on the front of the body over bony prominences, on the extremities, and on the forehead.**[13] **Nonaccidental bruises, on the other hand, are more commonly found on the torso, neck, and ears (Figure 148-1) and the soft parts of the body such as the cheeks and the buttocks.** Nonaccidental bruises are also more likely than accidental bruises to be found in clusters, to be on the back of the body, and to be symmetrical. In addition, nonaccidental bruises tend to be larger and more numerous than accidental bruises. Patterned bruises may be evident if a child has been struck with a hand or an implement (**Figure 148-2**). Although the presence of bruises of different colors was previously thought to indicate bruises of different ages, the dating of bruises is highly inaccurate, so document bruise description and do not attempt to date the bruises.[14]

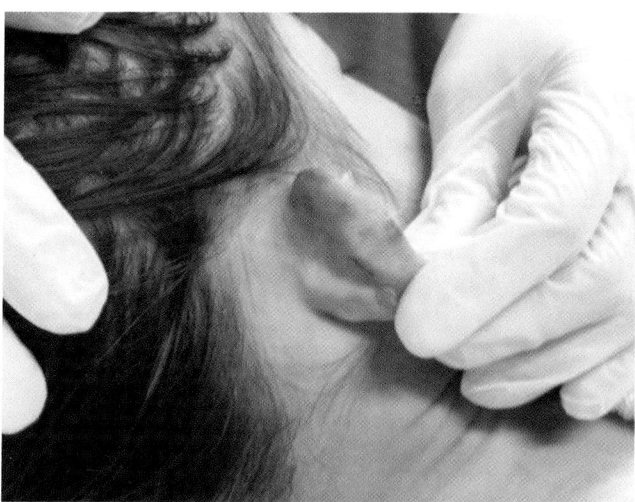

FIGURE 148-1. Bruising and petechiae on the ear from physical abuse.

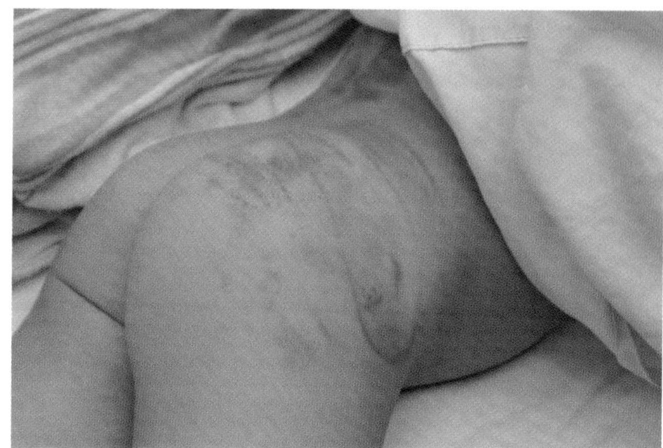

FIGURE 148-2. Multiple bruises to the back and buttock from physical abuse. Note the patterned loop bruising from impact with a cord.

Bruises in young infants deserve special consideration because infants very rarely sustain accidental bruises. The adage *those who don't cruise rarely bruise* is supported by the observation of bruising in only 0.6% of infants less than 6 months of age and in only 2.2% of infants not yet able to walk, while bruising is present in over half of toddlers.[15] Bruising in infants is associated with more serious abusive injuries. Additional injuries are diagnosed in up to one half of infants with isolated bruising.[16] The **TEN-4** bruising clinical decision rule identifies bruises to the thorax, ears, and neck, as well as any bruising in infants less than 4 months, as particularly concerning for abuse (**Figure 148-3**).[17]

The **differential diagnosis of bruises** includes skin conditions such as congenital dermal melanocytosis (Mongolian spots) and cultural practices such as cupping and coining. A number of medical conditions are associated with bruising, the most common of which is idiopathic thrombocytopenic purpura. Inherited factor deficiencies such as hemophilia and von Willebrand's disease predispose children to bruising from

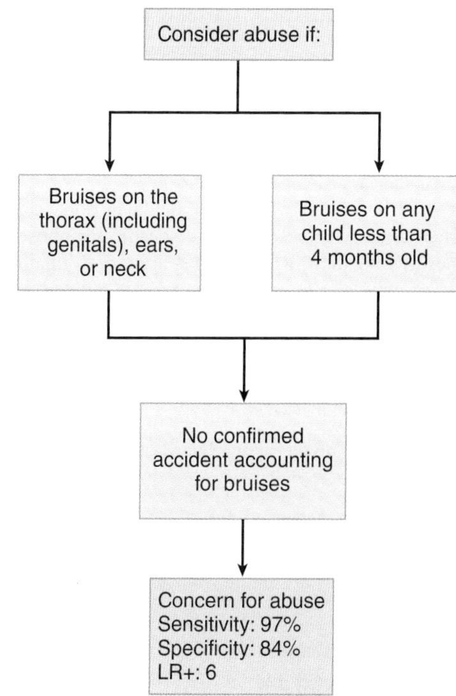

FIGURE 148-3. TEN-4 bruising clinical decisions rule for bruises concerning for abuse. LR+ = positive likelihood ratio.

inconsequential trauma. Other medical conditions include infections (e.g., meningococcemia), leukemia, nutritional deficiencies, and Henoch-Schönlein purpura.

Burns Burns account for 6% to 20% of abusive injuries. Most burns, both accidental and abusive, are scalds and affect children age 1 to 4 years old.[18] Accidental scalds typically occur when young children pull hot beverages off tables or stovetops, spilling the hot liquid onto themselves. The resulting burns are generally asymmetric, have irregular borders, are of varying depth, and are distributed over the face, neck, and upper torso.[18] In contrast, most inflicted burns are caused by immersion in hot tap water.[18] Abusive burns are often in a glove and stocking distribution with a sharp line of demarcation between the burned and uninjured skin. The child may have been held seated in a tub of hot water, resulting in burns to the perineum and feet with doughnut shaped sparing of the buttocks where the skin was in contact with the cooler porcelain of the tub.

When assessing nonscald burns, consider the distribution and extent of the burn. Children usually burn themselves when they reach out and touch a hot object. Most accidental burns, therefore, occur on the palms and the fingers and have an indistinct contour. In contrast, inflicted burns tend to be on the dorsal surface of the hands and on the back of the body. The margins of inflicted burns are often more distinct and may take the shape of the heated object used to inflict the burn.[18]

Burns due to neglect are nine times more common than inflicted burns.[19] Even when a burn itself does not appear inflicted, it is important to consider whether lack of adult supervision or exposure to an unsafe environment or substances played a role in the injury. The **differential diagnosis of burns** includes bullous impetigo, Stevens-Johnson syndrome, and severe diaper dermatitis.

Fractures Fractures are the second most common manifestation of physical abuse. Over 80% of abusive fractures occur in children less than 18 months of age, and 12% to 20% of fractures in infants and toddlers are caused by physical abuse.[20,21] Because fractures are also very common accidental injuries, accounting for between 8% and 12% of all pediatric injuries, distinguishing between accidental and abusive fractures can be challenging, particularly when the caregiver may not provide an accurate history.[8,22] In children <3 years old, up to 20% of abusive fractures were initially attributed to accidents or other causes.[23] Children with abusive fractures may present with nonspecific complaints such as irritability, swelling, not using a limb, or refusal to weight bear. Fractures may also be discovered incidentally during evaluation for other conditions or injuries.

There are a number of historical and clinical factors associated with an increased likelihood of physical abuse; however, **the single most important risk factor for abusive fractures is young age (Table 148-3).**[22] It is very unusual for nonmobile infants to sustain fractures.[21,22] Abuse accounts for one in two femur fractures in children less than 1 year of age, whereas the likelihood of abuse as a cause of femur fractures in 2- to 3-year-olds drops to less than one in five.[22-26]

Any fracture can be caused by either accidental or nonaccidental means; however, certain fracture types are more specific for abuse and should prompt further investigation. **Rib fractures** are rare in infants and young children and are generally only seen in cases of severe trauma such as motor vehicle collisions (**Figure 148-4**). In the absence of severe trauma, a child with rib fractures has a 7 in 10 chance of having been abused.[22] Posterior rib fractures are most highly correlated with physical abuse.[27]

TABLE 148-3 Risk Factors for Physical Abuse in a Young Child with Fracture

Age <1 year old with fracture
No history/inconsistent history of trauma
High-risk fractures:
Rib fractures
Metaphyseal fractures
Humerus fracture in child <15 months old
Femur fracture in nonambulatory child
Multiple fractures or fractures of different ages
Presence of other injuries

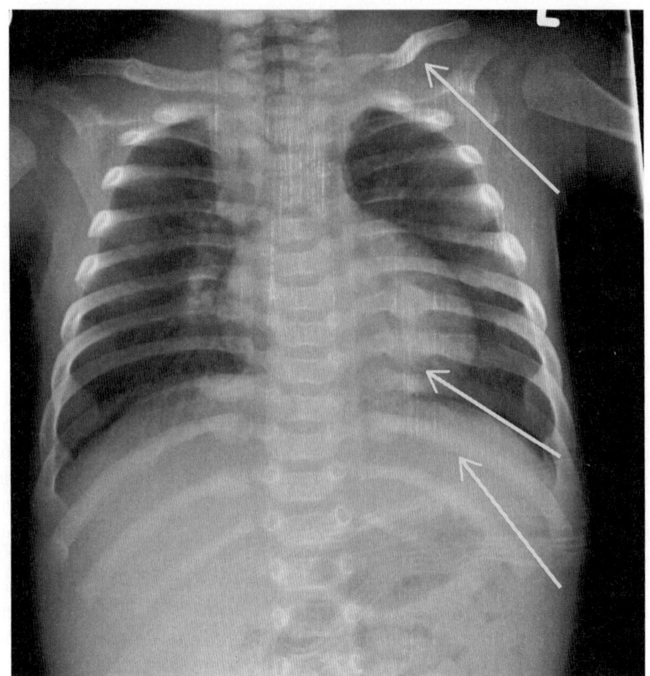

FIGURE 148-4. Acute left clavicle and healing rib fractures in an infant.

Classic **metaphyseal fractures** are shear injuries to the immature ends of growing bones in infants caused by the rapid acceleration and deceleration associated with yanking or shaking (**Figure 148-5**). They are highly specific for child abuse.[28]

Additional injuries, such as linear skull fractures and long bone fractures, are common in both accidental and nonaccidental injuries. Knowledge of possible injury mechanisms resulting in each fracture type guides the clinician in assessing whether the reported history accounts for the injury.

Consider the **differential diagnosis of fractures**. Although the lack of any reported history of trauma should raise concern about abusive injuries, toddler's fractures are an exception to this rule. **Toddler's**

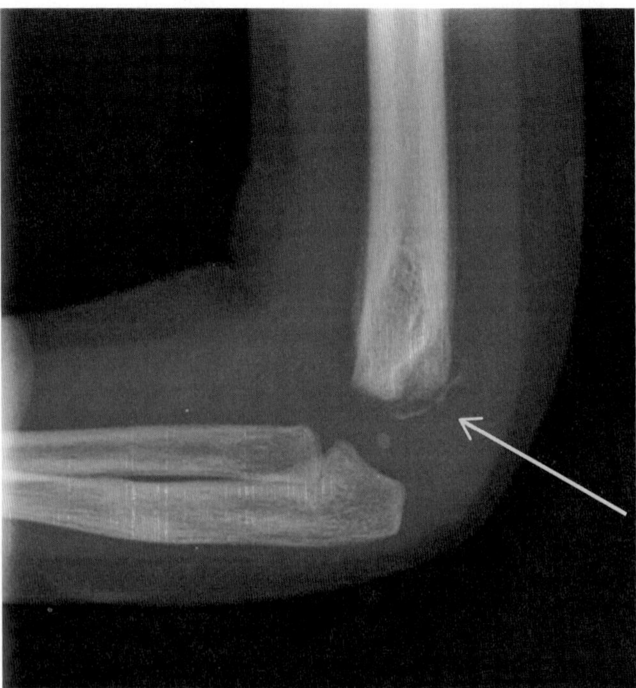

FIGURE 148-5. Classic metaphyseal fracture of the humerus with bucket handle appearance.

fractures are nondisplaced spiral fractures occurring in the distal third of the tibia in ambulatory children between 9 months and 4 years of age. These are accidental fractures that occur when the child twists and falls on a planted foot. Certain medical conditions such as inherited bone diseases (osteogenesis imperfecta), chronic medical conditions (renal osteodystrophy), or nutritional deficiencies result in weaker bones that may fracture with relatively minor trauma. These conditions are far less common than child abuse and are often easily identified by the medical history, the physical exam, and the radiographic appearance of the bones.

Abusive Head Trauma Abusive head trauma is the most common cause of traumatic death and disability in infancy and early childhood.[29-31] Although a number of terms have appeared in the medical literature over the years to describe the spectrum of cranial and ocular injuries that occur due to inflicted head injury in children, the American Academy of Pediatrics currently recommends the term *abusive head trauma* as the appropriate medical diagnostic terminology.[32]

Abusive head trauma demonstrates a distinct pattern of injuries characterized by intracranial injury (hemorrhage, edema, or infarction) and ocular injury (retinal hemorrhage or retinoschisis).[32-36] Skull, rib, or long bone fractures may be present; however, remarkably, there may also be no external evidence of trauma at all. Retinal hemorrhages occur in up to 80% of patients with abusive head trauma and typically are extensive, occurring in multiple layers of the retina and extending out to the ora serrata.[35,36]

Infants and children with abusive head trauma are brought to the ED with a broad spectrum of clinical concerns and findings. Children may present in extremis, with obvious signs of physical trauma, or alternately, they may present with only very subtle suggestions of irritability or feeding problems and no history of trauma at all. Apnea and seizures both have a significantly higher association with abusive head trauma than with accidental trauma.[37] Unfortunately, a substantial number of cases of abusive head trauma go unrecognized due to the mild, nonspecific nature of the presenting symptoms and signs.[11]

The **differential diagnosis of abusive head trauma** includes a number of conditions, but perhaps the two most common are birth-related and accidental trauma. Subdural and retinal hemorrhages secondary to birth are typically asymptomatic, resolving well within the first month of life.[36,38] Accidental falls may cause head injury and, very rarely, sparse retinal hemorrhage usually isolated to the posterior pole. Accidental falls are extremely unlikely to result in severe intracranial injury and typically result in focal damage with clear evidence of blunt impact to the head. Other underlying medical conditions such as coagulopathies or metabolic or congenital abnormalities will very rarely present with features similar to abusive head trauma.

Abdominal Trauma Although abdominal injuries due to child abuse are less common than other types of abusive injuries, abdominal trauma is the second leading cause of death in abused children, after abusive head injury.[9] Injuries to virtually every organ have been reported; however, liver and small bowel injuries are the most commonly seen. While no single feature allows identification of children with intra-abdominal trauma, features associated with a higher likelihood of abusive trauma than of accidental abdominal injuries include young age and small bowel injury.[9] Abdominal injuries due to abuse are much more common in toddlers (median age, 2.6 years), whereas accidental injuries are more common in older children (median age, 7.8 years). Accidental injury to the small intestine is exceedingly rare in children less than 5 years of age. In older children, accidental small bowel injuries most commonly are the result of motor vehicle collisions or handlebar injuries. Duodenal injuries in particular are very concerning for abuse in young children.[9] The mechanism of injury is typically a direct blow to the abdomen compressing the fixed duodenum against the spine.

Because many cases of abdominal trauma are asymptomatic or have other confounding injuries and there is often no history of trauma provided, be alert for any potential sign of injury and have a low threshold for investigation. Although bruising to the abdomen is a clear sign to consider intra-abdominal injury, it is only present in 20% of cases.[39] Signs and symptoms of intra-abdominal injury range from nonspecific irritability, lethargy, vomiting, poor feeding, and abdominal discomfort or distention to shock with frank peritonitis.

The gold standard for diagnosis of intra-abdominal trauma is a CT scan of the abdomen; however, given the difficulty in identifying abdominal injuries due to abuse, some advocate screening for intra-abdominal injuries using **hepatic transaminases** in all young children where there are concerns about physical abuse.[10,39,40] However, hepatic transaminases may not be elevated in cases of small bowel injury, so obtain abdominal CT scan if clinical suspicion warrants.

LABORATORY TESTING AND IMAGING FOR SUSPECTED ABUSE AND NEGLECT

Investigations for any form of injury are guided by the nature and severity of the injury, the age of the child, and the physical examination findings. In general, the more severe the injury and the younger the child, the more extensive the investigations required and the more likely they are to reveal additional injuries. Consultation with a pediatrician or child abuse specialist is recommended.

Laboratory Testing Laboratory investigations include a CBC with differential and coagulation studies, including a platelet count, a prothrombin time, and a partial thromboplastin time. Results may reveal anemia secondary to an intracranial hemorrhage or an abnormal coagulation profile due to the brain injury itself. Further coagulation studies may be indicated in cases of extensive bruising or intracranial hemorrhage. In the child with unexplained fractures, obtain a serum calcium, phosphate, and alkaline phosphatase. Children with severe injuries, including those suspected of abusive head trauma or occult abdominal trauma, should undergo a complete trauma panel including hepatic transaminases.

Imaging **A skeletal survey is a specific series of radiographs of all the long bones, chest, spine, hands, feet, pelvis, and skull that is indicated in all infants and young children in whom there is a concern for inflicted trauma.**[8,10,16] A properly performed skeletal survey frequently reveals previously unsuspected injuries including multiple fractures or fractures at various stages of healing.

Noncontrast head CT is indicated for any child suspected of sustaining acute intracranial trauma. Radiologic features with significant association for abusive head trauma include subdural hemorrhage, particularly if diffuse, interhemispheric, or infratentorial; hypoxic ischemic injury; and cerebral edema.[41] MRI may further delineate the extent of brain injury and may offer some guidance for the timing of injuries. Inclusion of the neck and spine in MRI studies may identify ligament injury or spinal hemorrhage.[42]

Abdominal CT should be included when there is concern for intra-abdominal injury.[10] Although it may be tempting to screen for intra-abdominal injury by US, US is not sensitive enough to identify all clinically significant intra-abdominal injuries in both abusive and accidental injuries.[40,43]

TREATMENT AND DISPOSITION

Rapidly identify and resuscitate life-threatening injuries. Once the child has been stabilized, attention shifts to further medical and legal evaluation. Because the comprehensive investigation of child abuse requires a multidisciplinary approach, most potential victims of serious physical abuse should be admitted to the hospital while the appropriate medical, surgical, and child protection teams complete their respective investigations. Children with head and abdominal injuries due to abuse have both longer hospitalizations and higher mortality compared with children with accidental injury.[31,44]

Older children with minor or superficial injuries may be discharged provided they have been assessed by child protective services and a safe environment can be assured.

CHILD SEXUAL ABUSE

Reports suggest that 26% of girls and 5% of boys have experienced some form of sexual abuse by the age of 17 years.[45] When there is concern for possible sexual abuse, determine the best ED method for evaluation; decide when to refer to other professionals and child protection authorities; and decide how to counsel the parents. The child's ED visit may be triggered by a broad spectrum of issues including anogenital bleeding, vaginal/urethral discharge, dysuria, urinary tract infection, sexualized behaviors, suicidality, or as commonly happens, a recent disclosure of sexual abuse without any specific physical symptoms. The sexual abuse may be either recent or remote relative to the time of presentation and may have involved numerous contacts over a period of time. The offender is typically well known to the child and, indeed, is often a parent or family member.[45-47] As a result, the child's caregivers typically present in emotional crisis, even though the child may not be suffering any physical trauma. The family requires a patient, supportive individual to listen to their concerns and provide appropriate guidance and reassurance.

First begin by assessing the urgency of the situation and determining when and where the full assessment should most appropriately be performed. In some jurisdictions, **sexual assault nurse examiners** or child abuse pediatricians are available. Emergency evaluation with collection of forensic evidence is indicated if the abuse has been recent, the child has genital bleeding or concerns of acute trauma, or there are other concerns for occult trauma. As yet, there is no consensus on the outside limit for the timing of forensic evidence collection in the pediatric patient. Research suggests that physical examination should be performed as soon as possible after an assault, yet evidence collection is unlikely to produce positive results in child victims outside the first 24-hour period.[48] Whether or not forensic evidence is collected, an immediate physical examination is recommended for all children disclosing sexual abuse within 72 hours of the last event.[49,50] Physicians should be aware of the policies for the timing of forensic evidence collection within their own jurisdiction.

CLINICAL FEATURES

There are numerous factors that make conclusive evaluation of alleged child sexual assault challenging:

- **The medical diagnosis of sexual abuse is heavily reliant on the history provided by the child.**[47,51] A proper forensic interview should be conducted by trained child protection investigators.
- **The absence of physical findings does not exclude abuse.**[47,51-54] Many sexually abusive activities leave no physical marks on the child, and in the rare instances where traumatic injuries do occur, they often heal well, with no obvious evidence of prior injury.
- **Forensic evidence is most often lacking in child sexual abuse.**[47-49,55] Forensic evidence may include blood, seminal fluid, sperm, saliva, or other foreign debris. The likelihood of obtaining forensic evidence from the prepubertal child is low, and the majority of evidence will be found on linens or clothing.[47,48,55]

History Obtain the initial historical details from ancillary personnel (parents, guardians, police, or social workers) without the child present. Often the most compelling evidence for criminal prosecution is the detailed, forensic interview of the child performed by child protection investigators. Thus, direct questioning of the child by the emergency physician should be limited to a medical history that addresses acute physical symptoms or concerns only. Record verbatim any spontaneous disclosures or statements of significance that the child makes during the course of the history or physical examination.

Document past medical history including any previous genitourinary trauma, urinary tract or anogenital infections, discharge, or toileting concerns. Note immunization status and any recent medications.

Physical Examination Much emphasis is placed on the importance of the physical examination, even though most pediatric victims of sexual abuse have a normal examination. If the child's disclosure suggests the abuse was remote to the time of presentation, then a straightforward physical examination to ensure that the child is currently physically well may be all that is required in the ED. All children should have a parent or supportive adult who is known to them present during the examination. Explain the procedure for the assessment prior to beginning the examination, addressing any parental concerns in advance. For the child, a simple age-appropriate review of systems generally guides them through the various body parts being evaluated. Do not force the examination. Subtle distraction techniques and frequent gentle reassurance are helpful. If the child remains uncooperative, decide whether the

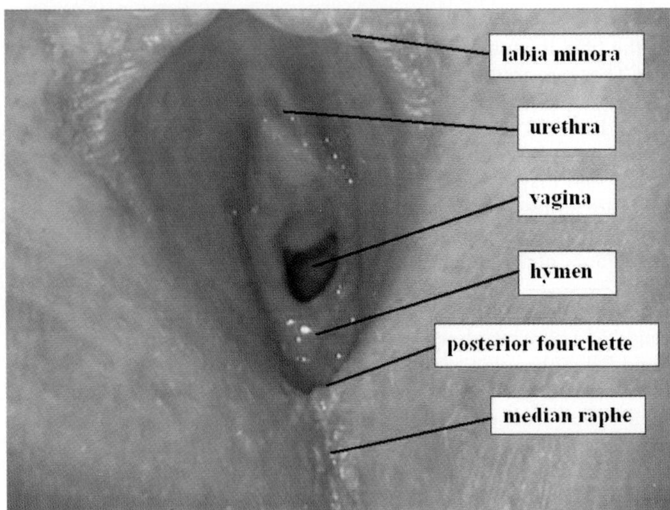

FIGURE 148-6. Normal prepubertal genital anatomy.

examination should continue under procedural sedation or general anesthesia or whether the assessment can be rebooked for a future time.

A complete examination begins with a comment on the child's overall appearance including emotional state and demeanor. Prior to palpation, ask the child about any painful areas. Thoroughly inspect all parts of the skin and hair and document bruises, petechiae, abrasions, areas of swelling, or bite marks. Carefully examine the oropharynx for signs of trauma.

Anogenital Examination Examination of the anogenital area can generally be accomplished with inspection only. The supine, frog-leg position optimizes visualization of the genital structures. Speculum examinations are not required in the prepubescent child. If the hymenal margin is not well visualized while supine, or if abnormalities are suspected, then examine the child in the prone knee-chest position. This position allows gravity to pull the margins of the hymen down into clearer view. Toddler-age children who are reluctant to undergo genital examination may be examined while lying supine in the parent's lap.

A systematic approach to anogenital examination is helpful to ensure complete documentation. Initial inspection details the appearance of the labia majora, labia minora, and the posterior fourchette. With gentle separation and traction of the labia, the clitoris, urethra, hymen, vaginal vault, and fossa navicularis come into view (**Figure 148-6**). Describe relevant findings using a "clock face" orientation, with 12 o'clock being anterior/superior and 6 o'clock being inferior/posterior. Document any evidence of trauma including bruising, bleeding, edema, lacerations, or abrasions. Accidental genital trauma typically results in bruises or abrasions to the labia or posterior fourchette. The hymen is rarely injured with accidental trauma given its more protected, recessed position. Note all nonspecific findings of erythema, ulceration, hypopigmentation, or discharge. Describe the hymen by noting both the shape and the integrity of the hymen margin (**Figure 148-7**). Typically the hymen is thickened and redundant at both infancy and puberty, due to maternal hormonal effect at birth and endogenous hormonal effect later. Small mounds (bumps), tags, or rolled edges are common nonspecific findings contributing to a wide degree of variation in normal genital morphology.[51] Note any deep notches or clefts to the rim of the hymen as well as any transections, either acute or healed, that extend to the base of the hymen. Acute superficial lacerations generally heal well with no intervention; however, deeper lacerations with extension into the vagina are less common and should be assessed by a gynecologist.

Genital examination of young boys is generally more straightforward. Note the presence of past circumcision and document any evidence of acute trauma including bruises, bite marks, or petechiae.

Anal examination of both boys and girls is most often normal or nonspecific; however, make note of any acute physical findings including bruising, abrasions, fissures, or edema. Recent anal trauma may result in either spasm of the anal sphincter or anal dilatation. Minor anal dilatation is a normal finding, particularly if there is stool present in the rectal vault. Anal dilatation of greater than 2 cm is concerning for a

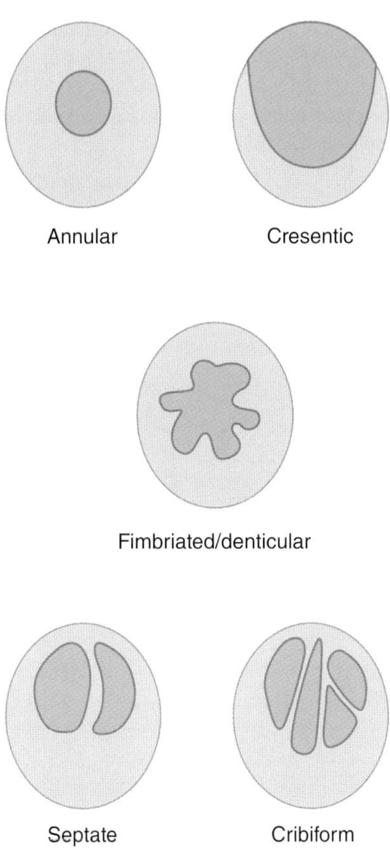

FIGURE 148-7. Normal hymen morphology.

history of trauma but should be interpreted with caution if there has been no disclosure of sexual abuse.[51]

Laboratory and Forensic Investigation Initial investigation is dictated by history and clinical findings. If the child appears stable, laboratory investigations may be limited to assessment for sexually transmitted infections (STIs) and/or forensic evidence collection.

Sexually Transmitted Infections The prevalence of STIs in the pediatric abuse population is exceedingly low, often less than 1% to 4%.[56,57] Current recommendations suggest testing for the presence of STIs in high-risk situations only.[49] High-risk situations include the following: presence of genitourinary symptoms or injury; assailant has or is at high risk for STI; a sibling has an STI; or parents or patient request testing. A non–clean catch urine should be sent for nucleic acid amplification technique testing for gonorrhea and *Chlamydia*. Although urine nucleic acid amplification technique testing is an acceptable standard for vaginal infections, it is not yet approved for rectal or oral swabs. For forensic purposes, positive tests should be confirmed with culture or with a second nucleic acid amplification technique probe. Vesicles or ulcerations are not common in the pediatric patient and, if present, should be swabbed for viral studies. Serologic studies for syphilis and the human immunodeficiency virus are not routinely indicated but may be considered if clinical suspicion warrants or if requested by the patient or parent.

Forensic Specimens Be familiar with the forensic evidence collection kits provided by the criminal investigation units in your area. All forensic specimens must be properly labeled and packaged, with appropriate chain-of-evidence documentation. Place the child's underwear and clothing (if worn at the time of the assault) in a paper bag and then seal the bag. Obtain forensic swabs from any areas suspicious for oral, genital, or ejaculatory fluid contact. Examination with Woods light may help guide collection of specimens.

TREATMENT AND DISPOSITION

Treatment begins at initial contact with the family. A timely assessment performed by a reassuring health professional is often the first step toward a positive therapeutic outcome for both the patient and family. If the history involves significant behavioral or emotional concerns, a referral to mental health professionals may be indicated on either an urgent or elective basis depending on the child's current state.

Pharmacologic treatment should be dictated by the individual's history and physical examination findings. Pregnancy and STI prophylaxis are not routinely recommended in the young pediatric patient following a disclosure of sexual abuse; however, they should be considered for older girls and adolescents.[49,58] Arrange counseling and follow-up in an outpatient setting to ensure appropriate repeat assessment. It is important to ensure resolution of any physical injuries, to assess for any new symptoms, and to inquire as to any emotional or behavioral sequelae.

MEDICAL CHILD ABUSE

Medical child abuse, which has been known in the past as **Munchausen syndrome by proxy** or **pediatric condition falsification**, has also been termed **caregiver fabricated illness.**[59] This condition is an uncommon form of child abuse in which a parent or caregiver induces or fabricates illness or injury in a child. Cases are generally highly complex, often necessitating detailed and comprehensive assessments by multiple subspecialty pediatric teams. Although the role of the emergency physician may seem minor, it is often the detailed emergency documentation of numerous clinical presentations and responses to investigation and intervention that provides objective information needed for eventual diagnosis.

Be alert to the possibility of this condition when presented with a pediatric case that involves persistent or recurrent illness that is not adequately explained and yet results in multiple medical or surgical procedures. Often the medical diagnoses that the caregiver describes do not match the objective findings, and the child tends not to respond to the usual therapies. Hospitalization is often required to coordinate a multidisciplinary evaluation.

REPORTING

Although laws governing the reporting of suspected child maltreatment vary around the world, in all states and provinces in the United States and Canada, **any physician who has reason to believe that a child is at risk of abuse or neglect has a legal obligation to report to local child welfare authorities**. The legal duty to report overrides any duty of patient confidentiality. It is not necessary to be certain of the diagnosis of abuse, but one should have *reasonable suspicion* that abuse or neglect may have occurred. Healthcare providers reporting concerns of suspected maltreatment are protected from civil litigation. Reports must be made in a timely manner because the risk of future maltreatment to other children in the home must be considered.

Informing parents of your obligation to report to child protection services should be respectful and nonaccusatory. Communication should focus on accurately identifying the underlying medical problem, managing the child's injuries, and providing honest, straightforward medical information.

In some cases, particularly when parents are engaged in legal custody disagreements, the history may be quite vague and the physical examination may be entirely normal. If the only concern for abuse or neglect is with the parent or guardian and there is no disclosure from the child and no witnessed abuse or concerning physical findings, then the emergency physician may provide the parent with the appropriate information to make a report on their own. Be familiar with local laws and the methods for reporting. If uncertainty exists about the need to report, consult with a child abuse pediatric specialist.

PRACTICE GUIDELINES

1. Kellogg ND, Committee on Child Abuse and Neglect: Evaluation of suspected child physical abuse. *Pediatrics* 119: 1232, 2007.
2. Flaherty EG, Perez-Rossello JM, Levine MA, et al: Evaluating children with fractures for child physical abuse. *Pediatrics* 133: e477, 2014.

3. Christian CW, Block R, American Academy of Pediatrics Committee on Child Abuse and Neglect: Abusive head trauma in infants in children. *Pediatrics* 123: 1409, 2009.
4. www.cps.ca/english/statements/pp/AHT.pdf. (Bennett S, Agrey N, Anderson L, et al: Canadian Pediatric Society. Multidisciplinary guidelines on the identification, investigation and management of suspected abusive head trauma.) Accessed September 30, 2014.
5. Kellogg N, American Academy of Pediatrics Committee on Child Abuse and Neglect: The evaluation of sexual abuse in children. *Pediatrics* 116: 506, 2005.
6. Adams JA: Medical evaluation of suspected child sexual abuse: 2011 update. *J Child Sex Abus* 20: 588, 2011.
7. Flaherty EG, MacMillan HL, Committee on Child Abuse and Neglect: Caregiver fabricated illness in a child: a manifestation of child maltreatment. *Pediatrics* 132: 590, 2013.

REFERENCES

The complete reference list is available online at www.TintinalliEM.com.

SECTION 13

Infectious Diseases

CHAPTER 149

Sexually Transmitted Infections

Flavia Nobay
Susan B. Promes

INTRODUCTION

Sexually transmitted infections (STIs) are a major public health problem. In 2010, there were 1,307,893 cases of chlamydia infection, 309,341 cases of gonorrhea, and 45,834 cases of syphilis reported in the United States.[1] The World Health Organization estimates that 500 million people are infected each year by a curable STI.[2]

The primary medical goals are identifying and treating STIs, but important secondary goals include preserving future health (including fertility), protection of any sexual contacts, preventive education, and provision of instructions for future screening. Lack of treatment can contribute to infertility, cancer, and urogenital complications. Failure of patients to follow up and adhere to a prescribed medical regimen complicates individual care and public health reduction efforts.

Multiple STIs frequently occur together. Once an STI is diagnosed, further testing for human immunodeficiency virus (HIV) infection and hepatitis B is warranted.[3]

Because of frequent changes in treatment guidelines and resistance patterns, we recommend that the reader access the *Morbidity and Mortality Weekly Report* (http://www.cdc.gov/mmwr) to check any modifications for treatment and also to obtain patient information in several languages.

GENERAL PRINCIPLES FOR DIAGNOSIS AND SCREENING

The signs and symptoms of an STI may be obvious, such as a genital lesion or vaginal discharge, or less specific, such as dysuria, lower abdominal pain, painful intercourse, or spotting and abnormal periods. Less specific signs lead to frequent ED STI underrecognition. Obtain a thorough sexual history in an objective, nonjudgmental manner to determine the risk of STI, HIV infection, or hepatitis. The young (13 to 24 years old), pregnant women, and homosexual men are all at higher risk of STI and subsequent morbidity. The Centers for Disease Control and Prevention have questions that providers can use when obtaining a sexual history and determining a patient's risk for an STI (**Table 149-1**).

Perform a pregnancy test in all females of childbearing potential, because pregnancy can affect treatment options. As appropriate, have chaperones present whenever breast, genital, or rectal examinations are performed. In women, perform a vaginal speculum examination, bimanual examination, and rectal examination. In males, retract the foreskin in uncircumcised patients to fully examine the area. Examine the areas between skinfolds, particularly in obese patients. Obtain directed site test specimens, which may include urine, vaginal, rectal, and urethral samples.

GENERAL RECOMMENDATIONS FOR TREATMENT AND FOLLOW-UP

Based on advice from the Centers for Disease Control and Prevention, we recommend the following[3,5] (**Table 149-2**):

1. When an STI is suspected, especially for gonorrhea and chlamydia infection, treat the patient in the ED with single-dose antibiotic regimens.
2. Obtain a pregnancy test and consult or refer promptly if the patient is pregnant.
3. If one STI is suspected or diagnosed, screen for other STIs (HIV infection, syphilis, and hepatitis) in the ED or through follow-up.
4. Report any notifiable infections such as *Chlamydia trachomatis*, gonorrhea, HIV infection, and syphilis. This is often based on final laboratory testing and can be automated.
5. Counsel all patients with suspected STIs about prevention and co-infection risks (notably HIV and hepatitis) in the ED and ensure follow-up options. Although no method aside from abstinence is 100% effective for STI prevention, male latex condoms and female condoms are useful in preventing STIs.
6. Advise that the partner(s) must seek treatment before any reengagement in sex.
7. Arrange follow-up to ensure relief of symptoms, compliance, and STI cure.

Although the Centers for Disease Control and Prevention recommend that health care providers in all settings routinely screen for HIV infection in all patients aged 13 to 64 years, the ED remains an underused venue for HIV screening.[6] Rapid HIV testing in the ED is not routine but is becoming more prevalent.[7]

SEXUALLY TRANSMITTED INFECTIONS PRESENTING WITH URETHRITIS, CERVICITIS, AND/OR DISCHARGE

CHLAMYDIAL INFECTIONS

Clinical Features In the United States and the United Kingdom, *C. trachomatis* infection is the most frequently reported STI. It is one of the causes of nongonococcal urethritis and commonly coexists with gonorrhea infections. It is most prevalent in people <25 years of age and is frequently asymptomatic, especially in women.[7]

Chlamydial infections in men can cause urethritis, epididymitis, proctitis, or Reiter's syndrome (urethritis, conjunctivitis, and rash). Women generally have asymptomatic cervicitis when infected with *Chlamydia*, although if present, symptoms include vaginal discharge, bleeding between menses, and dysuria. The discharge may be mucopurulent (**Figure 149-1**) when *Neisseria gonorrhoeae* is a co-infectant. **Consider urethral chlamydial infection in the differential diagnosis of sterile pyuria.** Complications in women include pelvic inflammatory disease, ectopic pregnancy, and infertility.

Diagnosis Nonculture methods of detection, such as direct immunofluorescence, enzyme-linked immunosorbent assays, nucleic acid hybridization tests, and nucleic acid amplification testing (NAAT), are preferred tests for diagnosis. NAAT has a high sensitivity (90%) and specificity (99%) for *Chlamydia*. NAAT is approved by the U.S. Food and Drug Administration for urine testing, and some tests are approved for use with vaginal specimens.

Treatment The Centers for Disease Control and Prevention recommend single-dose azithromycin or twice-a-day doxycycline for 7 days.[9] Table 149-2 lists dosages and alternative treatment options.[3] Azithromycin is safe for pregnant women, and pregnant women should undergo a test of cure 3 to 4 weeks after treatment. Amoxicillin is a safe alternative in pregnancy if azithromycin cannot be given.

Refer partners for testing and treatment if there was sexual contact in the last 60 days. Some providers choose to have the patient deliver

TABLE 149-1 Centers for Disease Control and Prevention Recommended Questions for the Five Ps of Sexually Transmitted Infection (STI) Prevention[4]

1. *P*artners
   "Are you currently sexually active?" "If no, have you ever been sexually active?"
   "In recent months, how many sex partners have you had?"
   "Are your sex partners men, women, or both?"
2. *P*revention of pregnancy
   "Are you currently trying to conceive or father a child?"
   "Are you concerned about getting pregnant or getting your partner pregnant?"
   "Are you using contraception or practicing any form of birth control?"
   "Do you need any information on birth control?"
3. *P*rotection from STI
   "Do you and your partner(s) use any protection against STI?" "If not, could you tell me the reason?"
   "If so, what kind of protection do you use?"
   "How often do you use this protection?" "If 'sometimes,' in what situations or with whom do you use protection?"
   "Do you have any other questions, or are there other forms of protection from STI that you would like to discuss today?"
4. *P*ractices
   "What kind of sexual contact do you have or have you had? Genital (penis in the vagina)? Anal (penis in the anus)? Oral (mouth on penis, vagina, or anus)?"
5. *P*ast history of STI
   "Have you ever been diagnosed with an STI?" "When?" "How were you treated?"
   "Have you had any recurring symptoms or diagnoses?"
   "Have you ever been tested for HIV or other STI?" "Would you like to be tested?"
   "Has your current partner or any former partners ever been diagnosed or treated for an STI?"
   "Were you tested for the same STI(s)?" "If yes, when were you tested?" "What was the diagnosis?" "How was it treated?"

Abbreviation: HIV = human immunodeficiency virus.

treatment to their partners—endorsed by the Centers for Disease Control and Prevention—as a way of preventing the spread of this STI. Universal adoption of this method at this time is incomplete because of ethical issues and medicolegal consequences including some state prohibitions.[10]

Counsel patients to avoid sexual contact until 7 days have elapsed after completion of antibiotic treatment and their symptoms have resolved. Encourage women to be retested approximately 3 months after treatment because of the high incidence of recurrence.[3]

GONOCOCCAL INFECTIONS

Gonorrhea is the second most commonly reported STI, caused by *N. gonorrhoeae,* a gram-negative diplococcus.

Clinical Features Most gonococcal infections in women are asymptomatic, and many coexist with chlamydial infection. Subclinical gonorrheal infections result in complications ranging from ectopic pregnancy to chronic pelvic pain to pelvic inflammatory disease.[8,9] Women who are symptomatic from a gonoccal infection tend to present with nonspecific lower abdominal discomfort and mucopurulent cervicitis after a 7- to 14-day incubation period. Eighty percent to 90% of men develop symptoms within 2 weeks of exposure. In men, dysuria and profuse, purulent penile discharge (**Figure 149-2**) are the most common presenting symptoms, but symptoms of acute epididymitis and prostatitis may result in an ED visit. Rectal infection with mucopurulent anal discharge and pain occurs in 30% to 50% of women with gonococcal cervicitis, and the rectum can be the only site of infection in homosexual men. *N. gonorrhoeae* also can be isolated from the pharynx but rarely causes pharyngitis.

Signs and symptoms of **disseminated gonococcemia** are petechial or pustular acral skin lesions on an erythematous base (**Figure 149-3**), asymmetric arthralgias, tenosynovitis or septic arthritis, and fever or general malaise. Infection with *N. gonorrhoeae* and other STIs is associated with increased HIV shedding.[11]

Diagnosis The Centers for Disease Control and Prevention recommend that NAAT be performed on cervical, vaginal, urethral, or urine specimens. Specimens can be self-collected by the patient. Not all NAAT is the same; some tests can be used only on certain specimen types, so know what is available at your institution. Culture and nucleic acid hybridization tests require endocervical or urethral swab specimens.

In men, a Gram-stained specimen with the classic intracellular diplococci and polymorphonuclear leukocytes confirms the diagnosis. This diagnostic method is not recommended as a screening tool for asymptomatic men and is not sufficient for endocervical, pharyngeal, or rectal specimens. Diagnosis of disseminated gonococcal infection is difficult, with only 20% to 50% of cultures of blood, lesion, and joint specimens yielding positive results. Culture of cervical, rectal, and pharyngeal specimens may improve the chance of diagnosis.

Treatment Given emerging resistance patterns, the Centers for Disease Control and Prevention recommend dual therapy with ceftriaxone 250 milligrams IM or cefixime 400 milligrams PO plus either azithromycin 1 gram or doxycycline 100 milligrams PO twice a day for 7 days for the treatment of gonorrhea (Table 149-2).[3,5] Fluoroquinolones are no longer recommended for first-line treatment of gonorrhea because of antibiotic resistance. Pregnant women should be treated with a cephalosporin or, if allergic, with 2 grams of either azithromycin PO or 2 grams of spectinomycin IM (not available in the United States) in a single dose. Instructions to sexual contacts are the same as with chlamydial infections. Treat disseminated disease with higher doses of ceftriaxone (1 gram IM or IV every 24 hours for 1 to 2 days) followed by cefixime 400 milligrams PO twice a day for a minimum of 1 week. Gonococcemia requires hospitalization for IV administration of antibiotics and evaluation for possible endocarditis and meningitis. Patients with gonococcal arthritis rarely require surgical drainage and irrigation of affected joints.

NONGONOCOCCAL URETHRITIS

Nongonococcal urethritis is diagnosed when *N. gonorrhoeae* is absent in someone with clinical symptoms. Although nongonococcal urethritis is usually caused by *C. trachomatis,* other causes of nongonococcal urethritis include *Ureaplasma urealyticum*, *Mycoplasma genitalium*, *Trichomonas vaginalis*, herpes simplex virus, and adenovirus. Alternative pathogens are seen more often in older men, and often no singular pathogen is identified. Specific tests for *U. urealyticum* and *M. genitalium* are not indicated.

If a patient's urethral specimen has five or more white blood cells per oil immersion field or the first-void urine specimen suggests infection, treat empirically as chlamydial urethritis. If the symptoms persist, the patient was noncompliant with their prior treatment regimen, the patient was exposed to a new sexual partner, or the previous partner was not treated, repeat treatment for chlamydial urethritis. Otherwise, obtain a specimen for culture for *T. vaginalis* and treat with metronidazole, 2 grams as a single oral dose, or with a combination of tinidazole, 2 grams PO, plus azithromycin, 1 gram PO as a single dose.

TRICHOMONAL INFECTIONS

T. vaginalis is a flagellated protozoan that causes urogenital infections mostly in women, with a prevalence of approximately 3%. The Centers for Disease Control and Prevention recommend routine screening for *Trichomonas* in women with abnormal vaginal discharge. *T. vaginalis* infection is associated with a high prevalence of coinfection with other STIs, notably HIV.[12,13]

Clinical Features Trichomoniasis can range from asymptomatic carrier states to severe, inflammatory disease, and incubation can be 3 to 28 days. The symptomatic presentation commonly has vulvar irritation and a malodorous, thin watery discharge with associated burning, pruritus, dysuria, urinary frequency, and dyspareunia, and occasionally low abdominal pain. Symptoms can worsen during menstruation. The classic yellow-green, frothy discharge is infrequently found, and many

TABLE 149-2 Treatment of Sexually Transmitted Infections

Sexually Transmitted Infection	First-Line Treatment	Alternative(s)	Pregnancy/Lactation
Bacterial vaginosis	Metronidazole, 500 milligrams PO two times daily × 7 d	Tinidazole, 2 grams PO daily × 3 d	Metronidazole, 500 milligrams PO two times daily × 7 d
	or	or	
	Metronidazole vaginal gel 0.75%, 5 grams intravaginally daily × 5 d	Tinidazole, 1 gram PO daily × 5 d	
	or	or	
	Clindamycin vaginal cream 2%, 5 grams intravaginally at bedtime × 7 d	Clindamycin, 300 milligrams PO twice daily × 7 d	
		or	
		Clindamycin ovule, 100 milligrams intravaginally at bedtime × 3 d	
Chancroid	Azithromycin, 1 gram PO single dose		Azithromycin, 1 gram PO single dose
	or		or
	Ceftriaxone, 250 milligrams IM single dose*		Ceftriaxone, 250 milligrams IM single dose*
	or		
	Ciprofloxacin, 500 milligrams PO, two times daily × 3 d		
	or		
	Erythromycin base, 500 milligrams PO three times daily × 7 d		
Chlamydia (treat for *Neisseria gonorrhoeae* concurrently)	Azithromycin, 1 gram PO single dose	Erythromycin base, 500 milligrams PO four times daily × 7 d	Azithromycin, 1 gram PO single dose
	or	or	or
	Doxycycline, 100 milligrams PO two times daily × 7 d	Erythromycin ethylsuccinate, 800 milligrams PO four times daily × 7 d	Amoxicillin, 500 milligrams PO three times daily × 7 d
		or	or
		Levofloxacin, 500 milligrams PO once daily × 7 d	Erythromycin base, 500 milligrams PO four times a day for 7 d
		or	or
		Ofloxacin, 300 milligrams PO twice daily × 7 d	Erythromycin base, 250 milligrams PO four times a day for 14 d
			or
			Erythromycin ethylsuccinate, 800 mg orally four times a day for 7 d
			or
			Erythromycin ethylsuccinate, 400 mg orally four times a day for 14 d
Gonorrhea (treat for *Chlamydia trachomatis* concurrently)	Ceftriaxone*, 250 milligrams IM single dose AND azithromycin, 1 gram PO single dose	Cefixime, 400 milligrams PO single dose AND azithromycin, 1 gram PO single dose	Ceftriaxone*, 250 milligrams IM single dose AND azithromycin, 1 gram PO single dose
	or	or	or
	Ceftriaxone*, 250 milligrams IM single dose AND doxycycline, 100 milligrams PO twice a day for 7 d	Cefixime, 400 milligrams PO single dose AND doxycycline, 100 milligrams PO twice a day for 7 d	Cefixime, 400 milligrams PO single dose AND azithromycin, 1 gram PO single dose
		or	or
		Azithromycin, 2 grams PO single dose AND test-of-cure in 1 week	Azithromycin, 2 grams PO single dose AND test-of-cure in 1 week
			or
			Spectinomycin 2 grams IM single dose
Granuloma inguinale (donovanosis)	Doxycycline, 100 milligrams PO two times daily for at least 3 weeks until lesions completely healed	Azithromycin, 1 gram PO weekly for at least 3 weeks until lesions completely healed	Erythromycin base, 500 milligrams PO four times daily for at least 3 weeks until lesions completely healed
		or	or

(*Continued*)

TABLE 149-2 Treatment of Sexually Transmitted Infections (*Continued*)

Sexually Transmitted Infection	First-Line Treatment	Alternative(s)	Pregnancy/Lactation
Granuloma inguinale (donovanosis) (*continued*)		Ciprofloxacin, 750 milligrams PO two times daily for at least 3 weeks until lesions completely healed	Azithromycin, 1 gram PO weekly for at least 3 weeks until lesions completely healed
		or	or
		Erythromycin base, 500 milligrams PO four times daily for at least 3 weeks until lesions completely healed	Gentamicin 1 milligram/kg IV every 8 hours (if the above therapy is ineffective)
		or	
		Trimethoprim-sulfamethoxazole, double-strength (160/800 milligrams) PO two times daily for at least 3 weeks until lesions completely healed	
Herpes simplex *First episode*	Acyclovir, 400 milligrams PO three times daily × 7–10 d		Acyclovir, 400 milligrams PO three times daily × 7–10 d
	or		or
	Acyclovir, 200 milligrams PO five times daily × 7–10 d		Acyclovir, 200 milligrams PO five times daily × 7–10 d
	or		or
	Famciclovir, 250 milligrams PO three times daily × 7–10 d		Valacyclovir, 1 gram PO two times daily × 7–10 d
	or		
	Valacyclovir, 1 gram PO two times daily × 7–10 d		
Recurrent or suppressive therapy for patients without HIV	Valacyclovir, 500 milligrams daily if >9 episodes/year		Acyclovir, 400 milligrams orally three times a day for 5 d
	or		or
	Valacyclovir, 1 gram PO daily × 5 d		Valacyclovir 1 PO daily × 5d
Severe	Acyclovir, 5–10 milligrams/kg IV every 8 h × 2–7 d then oral meds for total treatment time of 10 d		Acyclovir, 5–10 milligrams/kg IV every 8 h × 2–7 d then oral meds for total treatment time of 10 d
			or
			Valacyclovir, 500 milligrams PO once per day
Lymphogranuloma venereum	Doxycycline, 100 milligrams PO two times daily × 21 d	Erythromycin base, 500 milligrams PO four times daily × 21 d	Erythromycin base, 500 milligrams PO four times daily × 21 d
Syphilis *Primary, secondary, and early latent*	Benzathine penicillin G, 2.4 million units IM single dose	Doxycycline, 100 milligrams PO two times daily × 14 d	Benzathine penicillin G, 2.4 million units IM single dose
		or	
		Tetracycline, 500 milligrams PO four times daily × 28 d	
		or	
		Ceftriaxone, 250 milligrams IM or IV daily × 10–14 d (early syphilis)	
		or	
		Azithromycin, 1 gram PO single dose (early syphilis)	
Latent	Benzathine penicillin G, 2.4 million units IM one time a week × 3 weeks	Doxycycline, 100 milligrams PO two times daily × 28 d	
		or	
		Tetracycline, 500 milligrams PO four times daily × 28 d	
Trichomoniasis	Metronidazole, 2 grams PO single dose	Metronidazole, 500 milligrams PO two times daily × 7 d	Metronidazole, 2 grams PO single dose (only if symptomatic)
	or		or
	Tinidazole, 2 grams PO single dose		If asymptomatic, deferral of treatment until after 37 weeks
			Consider withholding breastfeeding until 12–24 h after last dose

*Ceftriaxone is painful IM and may be mixed with lidocaine 1% to decrease patient discomfort with administration.

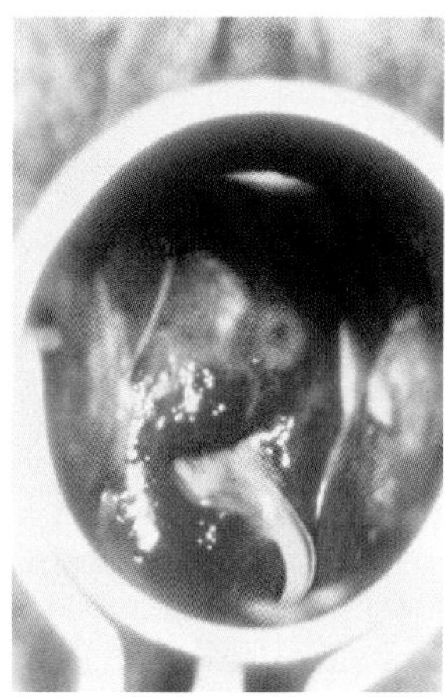

FIGURE 149-1. Viscous, opaque discharge emanating from the cervical os, consistent with mucopurulent cervicitis. The string from an intrauterine device is seen descending through the os in this patient. [Reproduced with permission from Knoop KJ, Stack LB, Storrow AB, Thurman RJ: *The Atlas of Emergency Medicine*, 3rd ed. © 2009 by McGraw-Hill, Inc., New York.]

women have minimal symptoms.[3] Physical examination is consistent with an irritated vulvar region with inflamed vaginal mucosa, and punctate cervical hemorrhages may also be seen. In men, the disease is often asymptomatic but may present as urethritis.

Diagnosis Microscopic confirmation of the classic motile parasites is diagnostic. Protozoan motility is present for 10 to 20 minutes after collection, making wet preparations of cervical smears or spun urine samples not sensitive. Culture is the most sensitive and specific test available, although it may take up to 7 days to obtain results. Because of this delay to diagnosis, commercially available tests using DNA probes and monoclonal antibodies are used in some institutions.

Treatment Patients should avoid intercourse for about 1 week after the last dose of antibiotics. All patients with *Trichomonas* infection should be treated irrespective of symptoms, and sexual partners should be treated to prevent reinfection. Metronidazole, 2 grams PO in a single dose or 500 milligrams PO twice daily for 7 days, cures 90% to 95% of patients.[13] Single-dose regimens are associated with better adherence and less vaginal candidiasis, whereas the lower dose, prolonged course has fewer systemic side effects.[3] Patients must avoid alcohol when taking metronidazole given the disulfiram-like reaction. Metronidazole gel is less effective than oral treatment.[13]

Trichomonas infections are linked to an increase in pregnancy-related complications. Because **metronidazole is a pregnancy category B drug**, it is the drug of choice for treating symptomatic pregnant patients, with no evidence linking metronidazole exposure with teratogenic effects.[14] Despite the Centers for Disease Control and Prevention

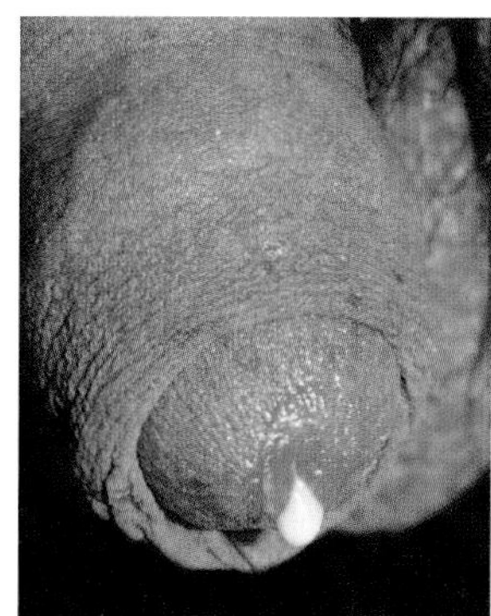

FIGURE 149-2. Gonococcal urethritis in a male. Mucopurulent ureteral discharge is caused by infection with *Neisseria gonorrhoeae*. [Reproduced with permission from Goldsmith LA, Katz SI, Gilchrest BA, et al: *Fitzpatrick's Dermatology in General Medicine*, 8th ed. © 2012 by McGraw-Hill Inc., New York.]

recommendations of a 2-gram singular dose coupled with evidence supporting the safety of metronidazole treatment in symptomatic pregnant women, some clinicians avoid oral treatment in the first trimester. Treatment of partners includes administration of the same medications as for the patient plus an STI clinic referral given the high rate of co-transmission of other STIs.

SEXUALLY TRANSMITTED INFECTIONS PRESENTING WITH GENITAL ULCERS

Genital ulcers are caused by syphilis, herpes virus infection, chancroid, lymphogranuloma venereum, and granuloma inguinale (donovanosis). These infections have high rates of co-infection with HIV. Not all infections associated with genital ulcers are sexually transmitted. Characteristics of the lesions and their accompanying signs and symptoms are provided in **Table 149-3**.

SYPHILIS

Treponema pallidum, a spirochete, is the causative agent of syphilis as well as yaws and pinta. The organism enters the body through mucous membranes or nonintact skin. *T. pallidum* remains very sensitive to penicillin. The incidence of syphilis in the United States was on the rise from 2001 to 2009, possibly because of behavior associated with drug use and male-to-male transmission.[1]

Clinical Features Syphilis consists of three phases: primary, secondary, and tertiary or latent syphilis. The disease may be diagnosed in any of these three stages.

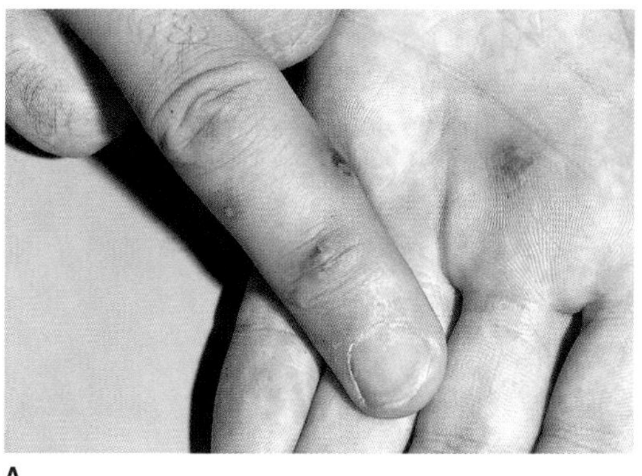

A

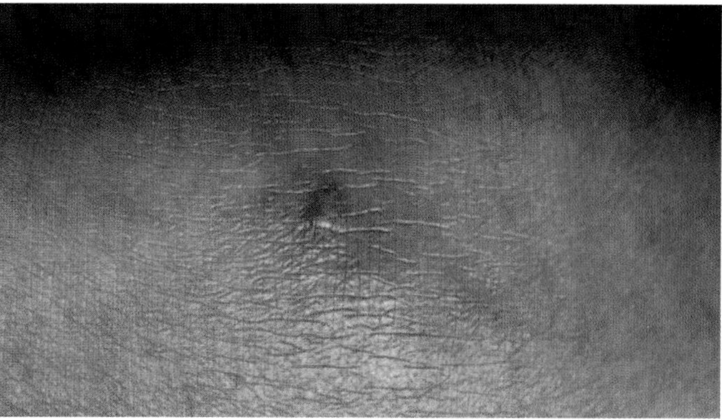

B

FIGURE 149-3. Disseminated gonococcal infection. **A.** Maculopapules on the hands. **B.** Lesion on the extensor surface of the wrist in a sexually active adult female. The macropapule has a petechial component and an erythematous periphery.

TABLE 149-3 Clinical Features of Genital Ulcerative Infections

Disease	Clinical Diagnosis	Presence of Pain	Inguinal Adenopathy	Comment
Syphilis	Indurated, relatively clean base; heals spontaneously	No	Firm, rubbery, discrete nodes; not tender	Primary: chancre Secondary: rash, mucocutaneous lesions, lymphadenopathy Tertiary: cardiac, ophthalmic, auditory, central nervous system lesions
Herpes simplex virus infection	Multiple small, grouped vesicles coalescing and forming shallow ulcers; vulvovaginitis	Yes	Tender bilateral adenopathy	Cytologic detection insensitive; false-negative culture results common; type-specific serologic test
Chancroid (*Haemophilus ducreyi*)	Multiple painful, irregular, purulent ulcers with potential exudative base	Yes	50% painful, suppurative, inguinal lymph nodes potentially requiring drainage	Cofactor for human immunodeficiency virus transmission; 10% have co-infections with herpes simplex virus infection or syphilis
Lymphogranuloma venereum	Small and shallow ulcer, associated proctocolitis with fistulas and strictures	No	Tender lymph nodes	Caused by *Chlamydia trachomatis* L1, L2, L3
Granuloma inguinale (donovanosis)	Painless, beefy red, bleeding ulcers	No	No	Endemic in Africa, Australia, India, New Guinea; rare in United States

Primary syphilis, or the initial stage of infection, is characterized by a painless chancre with indurated borders on the penis (**Figure 149-4**), vulva (**Figure 149-5**), or other areas of sexual contact.

The incubation period is approximately 21 days, with lesions disappearing after 3 to 6 weeks. There are no constitutional symptoms, and a lesion may even be absent with primary disease. The lesion resolves spontaneously.

Secondary syphilis develops 3 to 6 weeks after the end of the primary stage and is characterized by rash and lymphadenopathy. Nonspecific symptoms of sore throat, malaise, fever, and headaches are common. The rash often starts on the trunk (**Figure 149-6**) and flexor surfaces of the extremities, spreading to the palms (**Figure 149-7**) and soles. The rash takes on many forms but is often dull red-pink and papular. Secondary syphilis resolves spontaneously.

Tertiary or latent syphilis develops in about one third of patients after secondary syphilis, occurring 3 to 20 years after the initial infection. Involvement of the nervous and cardiovascular systems is characteristic, with widespread granulomatous lesions (gummata). Specific manifestations include meningitis, dementia, neuropathy (tabes dorsalis), and thoracic aneurysm.

Diagnosis *T. pallidum* cannot be cultured in the laboratory, and there is no single optimal test. The sensitivity and specificity of tests for syphilis depend on the stage of the disease and the type of test. Direct visualization of the organism using darkfield microscopy is diagnostic of primary, secondary, or early congenital syphilis, no matter what the results on serology. However, failure to visualize the organism does not exclude syphilis. Nontreponemal tests (Venereal Disease Research Laboratory

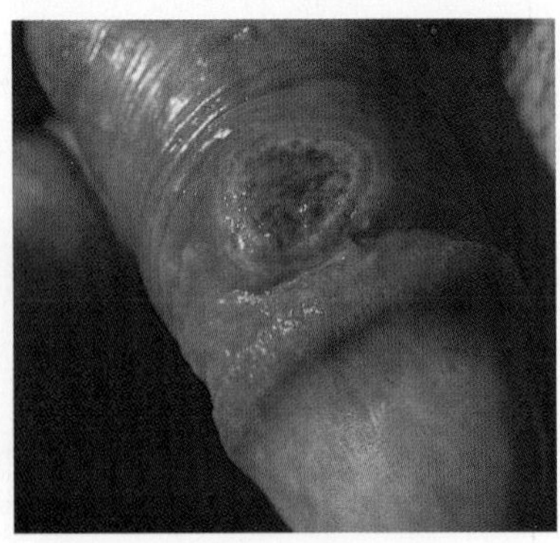

FIGURE 149-4. Painless chancre. [Reproduced with permission from Wolff KL, Johnson R, Suurmond R: *Fitzpatrick's Color Atlas & Synopsis of Clinical Dermatology*, 5th ed. © 2005, McGraw-Hill, New York.]

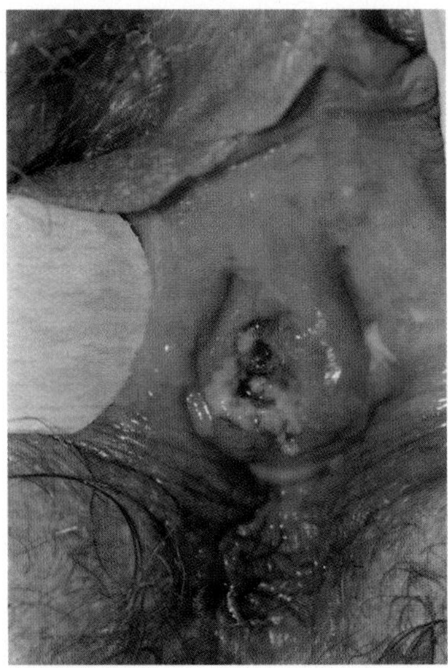

FIGURE 149-5. Syphilis chancre in a female. A painless ulcer is seen on the vulva. [Reproduced with permission from Goldsmith LA, Katz SI, Gilchrest BA, et al: *Fitzpatrick's Dermatology in General Medicine*, 8th ed. © 2012 by McGraw-Hill Inc., New York.]

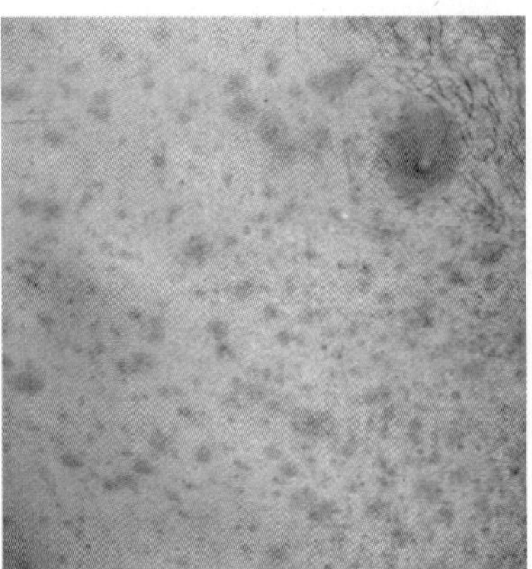

FIGURE 149-6. Disseminated papulosquamous eruption on the right chest wall characteristic for secondary syphilis. [Reproduced with permission from Wolff K, Johnson RA, Saavedra AO: *Fitzpatrick's Color Atlas and Synopsis of Clinical Dermatology*, 7th ed. © 2013 by McGraw-Hill, Inc., New York.]

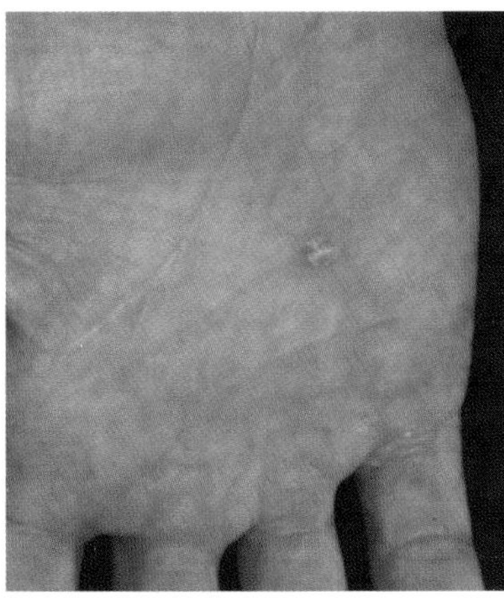
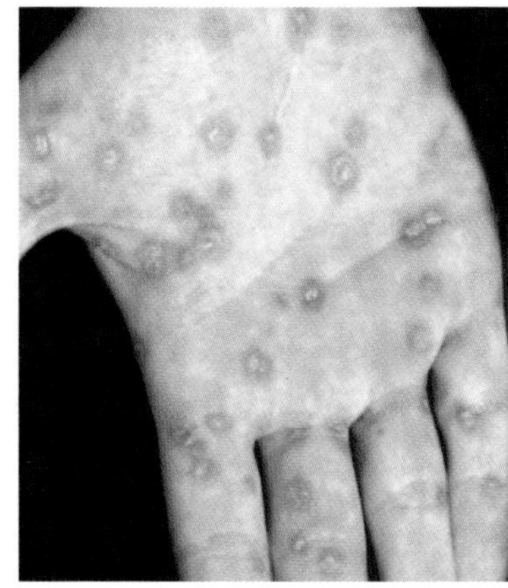

FIGURE 149-7. Papulosquamous eruption on the right palm characteristic for secondary syphilis. [Reproduced with permission from Goldsmith LA, Katz SI, Gilchrest BA, et al: *Fitzpatrick's Dermatology in General Medicine*, 8th ed. © 2012 by McGraw-Hill, Inc., New York.]

[VDRL] test, rapid plasma reagin test) detect nonspecific antibodies to cardiolipins, which are released as a result of infection. The VDRL and rapid plasma reagin tests are used as screening tests and also, once diagnosis is made, to assess disease activity and response to treatment. If used for screening, the VDRL and rapid plasma reagin tests are associated with both false-negative and false-positive results. Tests do not become positive until about 1 to 4 weeks after a chancre appears. Positive results must be confirmed with an immunoassay specific for *T. pallidum* antibodies. Some laboratories now begin the testing sequence with sensitive and specific *Treponema*-specific assays (reverse screening) and follow response to treatment with nontreponemal tests.[15]

For **secondary syphilis**, nontreponemal antibody tests are nearly 100% sensitive with high specificity.[16] The blood of treated patients usually becomes nonreactive on nontreponemal antibody tests. **Patients who develop disease and have a reactive result on a specific treponemal antibody test will have a reactive test result for life regardless of disease activity or treatment.**

A presumptive diagnosis of syphilis is made if a positive result on a nontreponemal antibody test (i.e., rapid plasma reagin or VDRL) is supported by a positive confirmatory result on a treponemal antibody test (i.e., fluorescent treponemal antibody absorption test).[16,17] Treat based on strong clinical grounds while results of confirmatory tests are pending, if follow-up is uncertain. When uncertain about testing interpretation, review the Centers for Disease Control and Prevention Web site (http://www.cdc.gov/STD/syphilis/default.htm) for detailed clarification of laboratory diagnosis or contact the local health department.

Treatment **For primary and secondary syphilis** treat with penicillin G benzathine, 2.4 million units IM in a single dose. Doxycycline twice daily for 2 weeks may be used in penicillin-allergic patients (Table 149-2). Pregnant women should be treated with parenteral penicillin G; if allergic, they must be desensitized and then given this medication. The **Jarisch-Herxheimer reaction** occurs most frequently in treatment of early syphilis and is characterized by an acute febrile reaction associated with headache and myalgias within the first 24 hours after treatment. Inform patients about this possible reaction. Recommend treatment of sexual partner(s) exposed in the previous 90 days. For a more detailed explanation of partner treatment, please refer to the Centers for Disease Control and Prevention Web site: http://www.cdc.gov/std/ept/default.htm.

Treat **tertiary syphilis** with 2.4 million units of penicillin G benzathine IM weekly for 3 weeks. Either a primary care physician or the department of public health should closely follow all patients for repeat serologic testing at 6 and 12 months.

HERPES SIMPLEX INFECTIONS

Herpes simplex virus (HSV) type 1 or type 2 infections are lifelong. Genital herpes is caused by exposure of mucosal surfaces or nonintact skin to the HSV virus. Approximately 25% of the U.S. population has serologic evidence of herpes infection. Most genital infections are caused by the HSV-2 virus; but anogenital infections are also caused by HSV-1.[18] Only 10% to 25% of individuals who are HSV-2 seropositive report a history of genital herpes, which suggests that most infected people have unrecognized symptomatic or completely asymptomatic infections. Viral shedding in persons who are unaware that they are infected is likely responsible for the majority of HSV transmission.[3]

Clinical Features "Classic" outbreaks of primary genital HSV infection begin with a prodrome lasting 2 to 24 hours that is characterized by localized or regional pain, tingling, and burning. Next, constitutional symptoms of headache, fever, painful inguinal lymphadenopathy, anorexia, or malaise are common. Women are more likely to have constitutional symptoms than men. As the disease progresses, papules and vesicles on an erythematous base become evident. The vesicles erode in hours to days. Patterns of HSV-1 and HSV-2 infection appear identical: vesicles usually are uniform in size, and the tense center umbilicates to form a depressed center. Lesions usually crust and then re-epithelialize and heal without scarring.

In men, HSV ulcers often appear on the shaft or glans of the penis (**Figure 149-8**). In women, ulcers can occur on the introitus (**Figure 149-9**), urethral meatus, labia, and perineum. Lesions are exquisitely painful and sometimes are associated with serous discharge. In

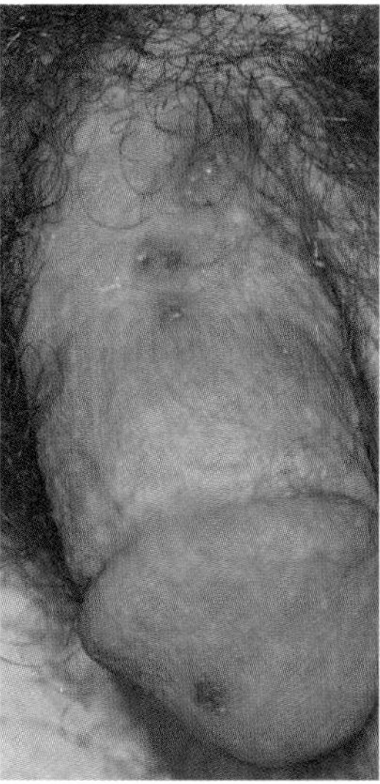

FIGURE 149-8. Genital herpes in a male. These formerly vesicular lesions have crusted over. [Reproduced with permission from Goldsmith LA, Katz SI, Gilchrest BA, et al: *Fitzpatrick's Dermatology in General Medicine*, 8th ed. © 2012 by McGraw-Hill Inc., New York.]

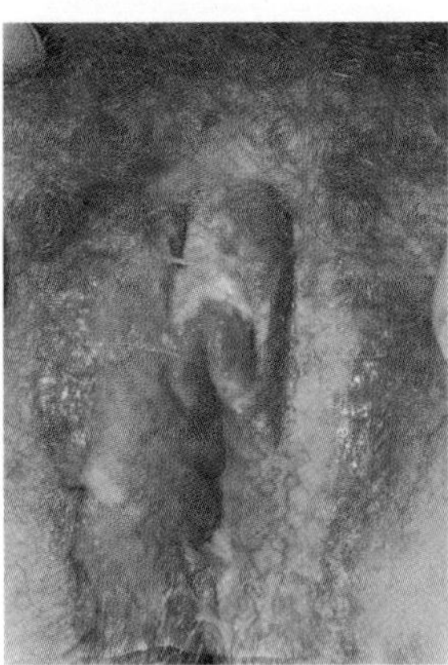

FIGURE 149-9. Genital herpes in a female. These formerly vesicular lesions have crusted over. [Reproduced with permission from Goldsmith LA, Katz SI, Gilchrest BA, et al: *Fitzpatrick's Dermatology in General Medicine*, 8th ed. © 2012 by McGraw-Hill Inc., New York.]

both sexes, lesions may be found on the perianal area, thighs, or buttocks. Dysuria is common in women and may progress to urinary retention secondary to severe pain.

Complete healing usually occurs within 3 weeks, and viral shedding persists for 10 to 12 days after the onset of the rash. Recurrent outbreaks generally are milder than the initial episode. There are typically fewer grouped lesions, and viral shedding occurs at a lower concentration and for a shorter duration (i.e., about 3 days).[19] The disease can be transmitted despite the absence of ulcers.

Diagnosis Diagnosis is usually made on clinical features. If uncertain, a Tzanck test may demonstrate large intranuclear inclusions. Laboratory diagnosis is either by cell culture or polymerase chain reaction. When obtaining a specimen for analysis, puncture the vesicle and swab the fluid. Swab the base of the lesion vigorously, because the virus is cell associated.[3] Lack of HSV detection does not indicate a lack of HSV infection, because viral shedding is intermittent.

Treatment Treatment hastens recovery but does not cure. Antiviral medications decrease the time until all lesions are crusted and healed, decrease pain and constitutional symptoms, and decrease the period of viral shedding by several days.[3]

Treat the first clinical episode with acyclovir, famciclovir, or valacyclovir (Table 149-2). Extend treatment duration if lesions persist. To treat proctitis or oral infections, use higher dosages (acyclovir, 400 milligrams five times a day for 7 to 10 days). For hospitalized patients, give acyclovir, 5 to 10 milligrams/kg IV every 8 hours for 5 to 7 days. Famciclovir and valacyclovir have high oral bioavailability and are alternative oral agents with easier dosing regimens for patients.

Treat episodic recurrent infection for 5 days with acyclovir, famciclovir, or valacyclovir at dosages reduced from primary therapy (Table 149-2). Begin treatment within 1 day. Suppressive therapy is available for individuals who experience more than six episodes per year, which reduces recurrence and shedding but does not eliminate either event. **Treat severe recurrent infections** (seen primarily in immunocompromised patients) with acyclovir, 5 to 10 milligrams/kg every 8 hours IV, for at least 2 days before switching to oral therapy. A primary diagnosis of HSV should prompt the search for other STIs including HIV.

CHANCROID

Haemophilus ducreyi is a pleomorphic gram-negative bacillus that causes chancroid, seen as painful genital ulcers and lymphadenitis. This disease is on the decline in most of the world with sporadic male outbreaks.[20] Chancroid increases HIV transmission and often is accompanied by other infections when chancroid is present; 10% of infected patients in the United States also have HSV or *T. pallidum*.[20]

Clinical Features A painful erythematous papule appears at the site of infection (usually confined to the genital region) after an incubation period of 4 to 10 days. One to 2 days later, the lesion becomes eroded, ulcerated, and often pustular (not vesicular). The ulcers are usually 1 to 2 cm in diameter with sharp, undermined margins and are very painful (**Figure 149-10**). The friable base of the ulcer is covered with yellow-gray necrotic exudates. Multiple lesions are present in up to 50% of patients (more so in women), and "kissing lesions" (infection of adjacent skin areas due to autoinoculation) are frequent. Painful inguinal lymphadenopathy develops 1 to 2 weeks after primary infection (**Figure 149-11**). A bubo will develop if chancroid is untreated, and the lymph nodes become necrotic or pus filled. Constitutional symptoms are rare, and ulcerations are rarely recurrent.

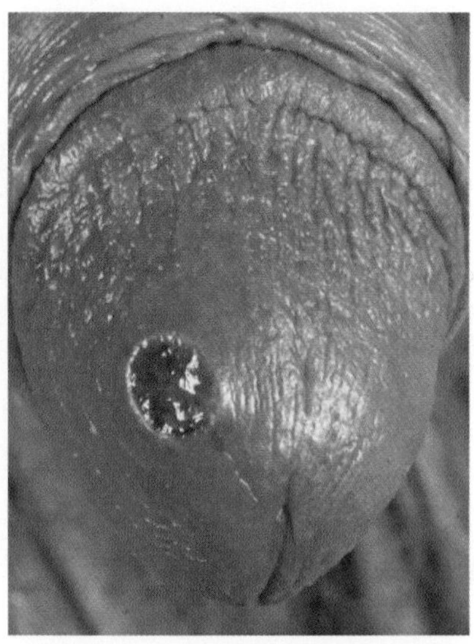

FIGURE 149-10. Painful, punched out ulcer of chancroid. [Reproduced with permission from Fleischer AB Jr, Feldman SR, McConnell CF, et al: *Emergency Dermatology: A Rapid Treatment Guide.* © 2002, McGraw-Hill, New York.]

Diagnosis Diagnosis can generally be made on clinical grounds with a painful ulcer and regional lymphadenopathy, but other infections (such as HSV infection and syphilis) are possible. A swab of a lesion or pus from a suppurative lymph node can be cultured, but a special medium is required that is not widely available, and culturing has a sensitivity of <80%. There is no current Food and Drug Administration–approved polymerase chain reaction test.

Treatment Azithromycin PO in a single dose, ceftriaxone IM in a single dose, ciprofloxacin for 3 days, or erythromycin base for 7 days are all

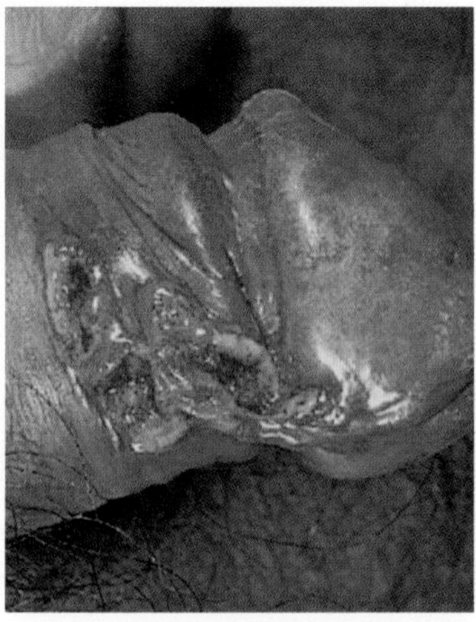

FIGURE 149-11. Chancroid with characteristic penile ulcers and associated left inguinal adenitis. [Photo contributor: H. Hunter Handsfield. Atlas of Sexually Transmitted Diseases. New York: McGraw-Hill; 1992. Reproduced with permission from Knoop K, Stack L, Storrow A, Thurman RJ: *Atlas of Emergency Medicine*, 3rd ed. © 2010, McGraw-Hill, New York. Fig 9-22.]

effective for the treatment of *H. ducreyi* infection (Table 149-2), with the choice based on local antibiotic resistance patterns and patient factors. Generally, azithromycin and ceftriaxone are used in patients without HIV infection, with ciprofloxacin as an alternative. Erythromycin is inexpensive, but the need for multiple doses and GI toxicity make it less desirable. Incision and drainage or aspiration of buboes can be considered for symptomatic relief, prevention of fistulas, and secondary ulcers.

Symptoms improve in about 3 days, and lesions are visibly improved within a week. Larger ulcers may require 2 to 3 weeks to heal. Partners should be treated if they have had sexual contact in the last 10 days, regardless of symptoms.[3] Pregnant women are usually treated with ceftriaxone or erythromycin as an alternative. All patients should be tested for HSV, syphilis, and HIV at or near the time of diagnosis of chancroid and again 3 months later if tests are initially negative.

LYMPHOGRANULOMA VENEREUM

Three specific serotypes (L1, L2, and L3) cause lymphogranuloma venereum, also referred to as struma, tropical bubo, or Durand-Nicolas-Favre disease. Lymphogranuloma venereum is endemic worldwide but is seen only sporadically in the United States. The Netherlands has seen an increased incidence of this STI in homosexuals.[21] The primary lesion can take many forms and be confused with the lesions of other STIs (Table 149-3).

Clinical Features The painless primary chancre is almost never noticed and lasts only 2 to 3 days (**Figure 149-12**). Generally, 1 to 3 weeks after the appearance of the initial lesion, unilateral inguinal lymphadenopathy is noted (60% of cases) (**Figure 149-13**). Often the overlying skin has a purplish hue. The initial lesion progresses to suppurative lymphadenopathy, resulting in either spontaneous abscess rupture or firm inguinal masses. Lymphogranuloma venereum proctitis (rectal ulcers, bleeding, and discharge) is also seen, primarily in homosexual men, and can be confused with new onset of ulcerative colitis. Scarring of these masses may cause linear depressions parallel to the inguinal ligament, forming the so-called *groove sign* (**Figure 149-14**). Lymphogranuloma venereum infections can cause fever, chills, arthralgias, erythema nodosum, or rarely meningoencephalitis. Lymphogranuloma venereum is easily confused with syphilis, chancroid, and HSV, and it also facilitates the transmission and acquisition of HIV.

Diagnosis Chlamydia serologic testing for lymphogranuloma venereum is not standardized and not helpful except to support the diagnosis in the appropriate setting. Culture, direct immunofluorescence testing, and nucleic acid detection of a lesion swab or bubo aspirate are not widely available, nor is genotyping. Given these diagnostic constraints, patients with a clinical picture suggestive of lymphogranuloma venereum and epidemiologic information should simply be treated. The Centers for Disease Control and Prevention may be able to assist with testing.

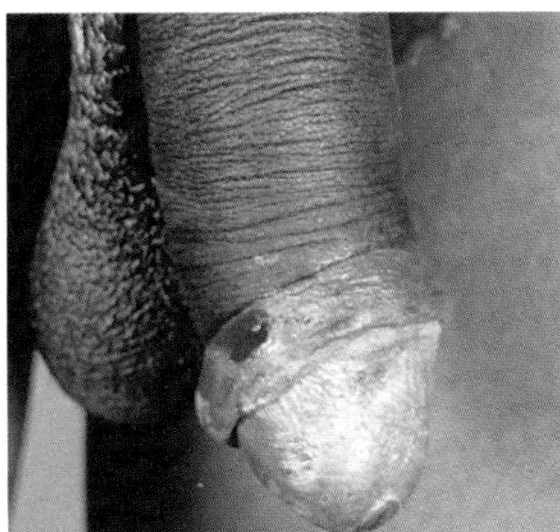

FIGURE 149-12. Lymphogranuloma venereum chancre. This ulceration was painless to the patient. [Reproduced with permission from Goldsmith LA, Katz SI, Gilchrest BA, et al: *Fitzpatrick's Dermatology in General Medicine,* 8th ed. © 2012 by McGraw-Hill Inc., New York.]

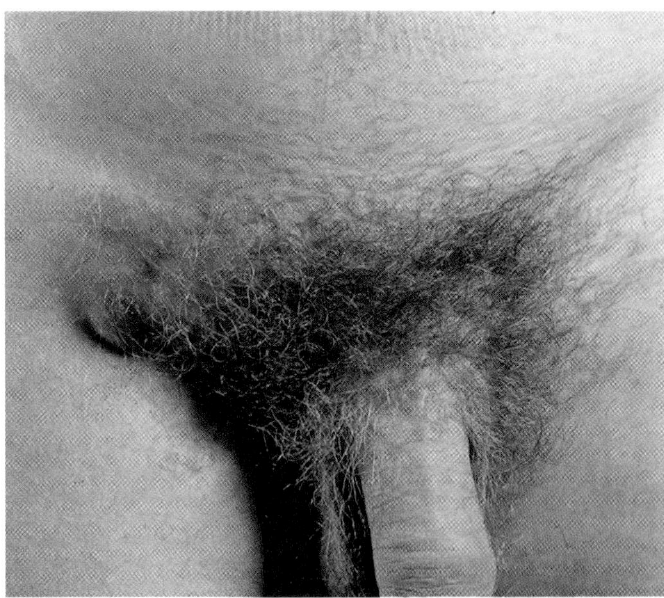

FIGURE 149-13. Lymphogranuloma venereum. Marked lymphadenopathy with small central eschar/ulcer. [Reproduced with permission from Wolff KL, Johnson R, Suurmond R: *Fitzpatrick's Color Atlas & Synopsis of Clinical Dermatology,* 5th ed. © 2005, McGraw-Hill, New York.]

Treatment Doxycycline for 21 days is the usual regimen (Table 149-2). Alternatives include erythromycin, azithromycin, or extended treatment with fluoroquinolones.[3] Mild untreated cases resolve spontaneously in 8 to 12 weeks. Treat pregnant or lactating women with erythromycin or azithromycin. Refer partners with whom the individual has had sexual contact within the past 60 days for treatment. Sexual activity should be avoided until the full course of antibiotic treatment is completed and lymphadenopathy has resolved.[3]

GRANULOMA INGUINALE (DONOVANOSIS)

Granuloma inguinale, also called donovanosis, is caused by *Klebsiella granulomatis*, a gram-negative intracellular bacterium. The disease is rare in the United States but is endemic in India, southern Africa, and central Australia.

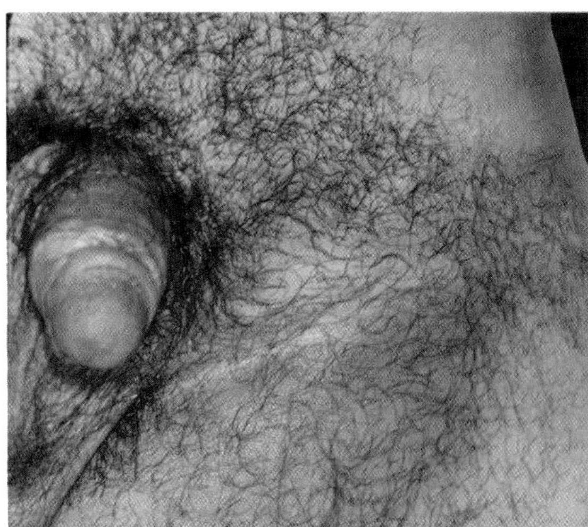

FIGURE 149-14. An example of the linear depression parallel to the inguinal ligament in lymphogranuloma venereum, the groove sign. [Reproduced with permission from Goldsmith LA, Katz SI, Gilchrest BA, et al: *Fitzpatrick's Dermatology in General Medicine,* 8th ed. © 2012 by McGraw-Hill Inc., New York.]

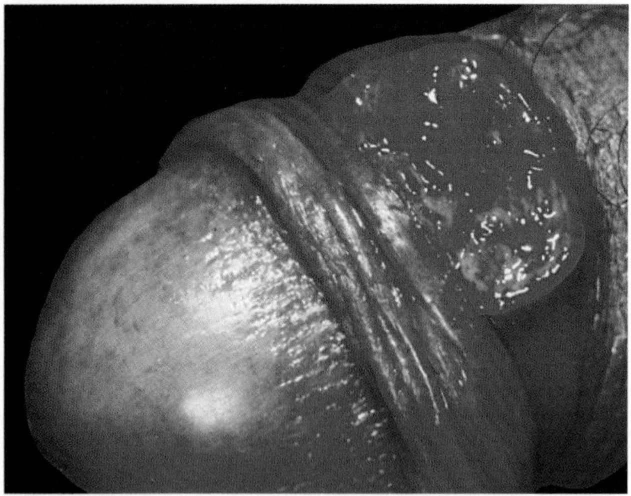

FIGURE 149-15. Granuloma inguinale in a male. The painless, ulcerative lesion is classically beefy red and bleeds easily. [Reproduced with permission from Goldsmith LA, Katz SI, Gilchrest BA, et al: *Fitzpatrick's Dermatology in General Medicine*, 8th ed. © 2012 by McGraw-Hill Inc., New York.]

Clinical Features After a variable incubation period of 2 weeks to 6 months, granuloma inguinale begins as subcutaneous nodules on the penis or labial-vulvar area. The nodules then progress to the more classic painless, ulcerative lesions (**Figure 149-15**). These lesions are highly vascular, which explains both their appearance (beefy red) and their tendency to bleed easily on contact. Lymphadenopathy is not usually present, but subcutaneous granulomas may occur and mimic lymphadenopathy. Superinfection may complicate these open, bleeding lesions and complicate the diagnosis. Granuloma inguinale is not highly contagious, and multiple exposures are required to contract the disease. Autoinoculation can occur, leading to oral and GI tract involvement.

Diagnosis *K. granulomatis* is difficult to culture, and diagnosis often requires visualization of characteristic Donovan bodies on tissue biopsy.

Treatment Doxycycline PO for at least 3 weeks stops progression of the lesions (Table 149-2), although longer treatment may be needed to allow complete healing of the ulcers. Azithromycin, ciprofloxacin, erythromycin base, and trimethoprim-sulfamethoxazole are alternatives for at least 3 weeks and until the lesions heal. Doxycycline, ciprofloxacin, and sulfonamides are contraindicated in pregnancy. Erythromycin base is the recommended treatment for pregnant or lactating women with the potential addition of a parenteral aminoglycoside. Individuals with whom the patient had sexual contact within 60 days of the appearance of the lesions should also be treated if symptomatic.[22]

GENITAL WARTS

Over 40 different genotypes of human papillomavirus (HPV) can infect the human genital tract by direct transmission. It is estimated that just under 25% of the U.S. population is currently infected with genital HPV.[23] As many as half of these infections are in adolescents and young adults, age 15 to 24 years.[23] HPV infection is so common that most sexually active adults become infected at some point in their lives. The significance of genital warts goes beyond their discomforting presence, with many genotypes being oncogenic.

Two Food and Drug Administration–approved vaccines are available against HPV. The quadrivalent vaccine (Gardasil®) works against the two most important oncogenic HPVs (genotypes 16 and 18) and those that cause genital warts (genotypes 6 and 11). The bivalent vaccine (Cervarix®) works against genotypes 16 and 18 only. The three-dose vaccine is routinely recommended for 11- and 12-year-old girls and is given over 6 months. The vaccine series can be started at 9 years of age. Catch-up vaccination is recommended for 13- through 26-year-old females who have not yet received or completed the vaccination series.[24] Gardasil is used in males age 9 to 27 years old to prevent genital warts.

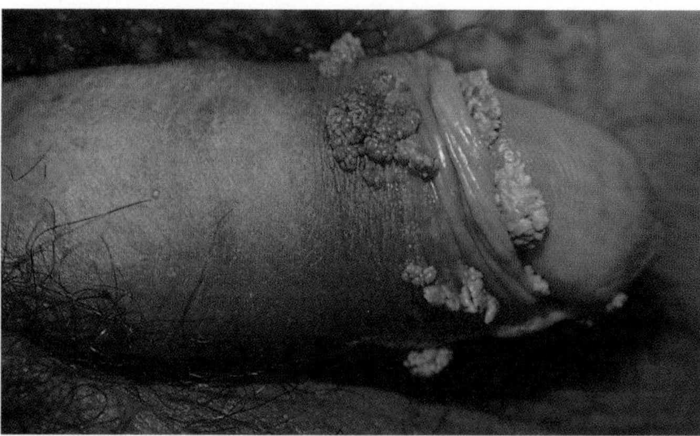

FIGURE 149-16. Condylomata acuminata in a 25-year-old male with a 3-month history of penile lesions. Multiple cauliflower floret–like papules are seen on the penile shaft and foreskin. [Reproduced with permission from Wolff K, Johnson RA: *Fitzpatrick's Color Atlas and Synopsis of Clinical Dermatology*, 6th ed. © 2009 by McGraw-Hill, Inc., New York.]

Clinical Features Genital warts are flesh-colored papules or cauliflower-like projections that usually appear after an incubation period of 1 to 8 months and may coalesce to form condylomata acuminata (**Figure 149-16**). In women, they are seen on the external genitalia (**Figure 149-17**) and in the perianal region. Genital warts are usually painless, but depending on their anatomic location can be friable, painful, or pruritic and often enlarge during pregnancy. Infected males often complain of nonhealing penile lesions, occasionally with pruritus and urethral discharge. Perianal condylomata have been seen in up to 80% of women with vulvar condylomata and are seen frequently in homosexual males.

Diagnosis Diagnosis is clinical.

Treatment Many topical treatments exist that can be used for days to weeks, but these are not usually initiated in the ED. Treatment decisions are based on the size and number of lesions, the amount of discomfort they are causing, and patient preferences. The treatment of external genital warts may help reduce viral load but is not a cure. All treatment options are considered equally effective and chosen based on the discretion of the patient and provider.

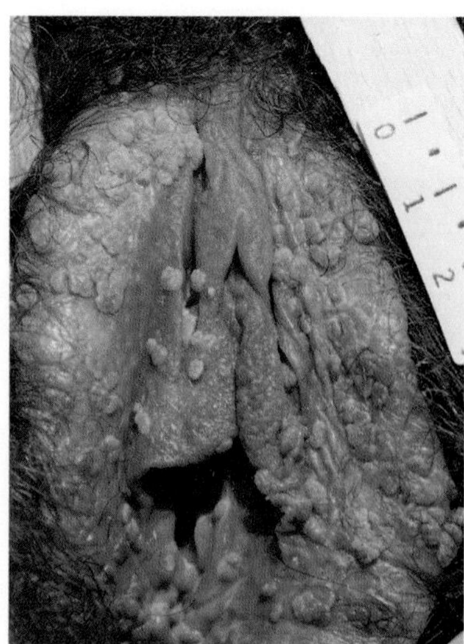

FIGURE 149-17. Condylomata acuminata of the vulva. Multiple pink-brown, soft papules are seen on the labia. [Reproduced with permission from Wolff K, Johnson RA, Saavedra AO: *Fitzpatrick's Color Atlas and Synopsis of Clinical Dermatology*, 7th ed. © 2013 by McGraw-Hill, Inc., New York.]

Patients with HPV infections rarely require emergent management. However, counseling in the ED regarding this distressing condition is relatively common. Emphasize the following: it is common for sexually active people to have HPV at some point in their lives, and most people clear serologic evidence of HPV spontaneously without external evidence of the disease. Condoms are protective with HPV, but they are not preventative, and the only way to decrease exposure is to limit the number of sexual partners. It is an incorrect assumption that having HPV indicates an oncogenic certainty or a change in fertility.

PRACTICE GUIDELINES

The Centers for Disease Control and Prevention publishes guidelines for the diagnosis and treatment of STI every few years. The most recent full publication was issued in 2010 and is available at http://www.cdc.gov/std/treatment/2010/default.htm.

SPECIAL CONSIDERATIONS

TREATMENT OF SEXUALLY TRANSMITTED INFECTIONS DURING PREGNANCY

Refer pregnant patients with STIs to the physician providing their prenatal care. Penicillin, ceftriaxone, azithromycin, cefixime, metronidazole, erythromycin, and acyclovir are thought to be safe for use during pregnancy and can be started pending follow-up.

PROPHYLAXIS AFTER SEXUAL ASSAULT

Sexual assault is discussed in detail in chapter 293, "Female and Male Sexual Assault," but a brief review of prophylactic regimens follows. Once all appropriate forensic investigation and culture specimens have been taken, three-agent prophylaxis with single doses of ceftriaxone, 250 milligrams IM; metronidazole, 2 grams PO; and azithromycin, 1 gram PO, or doxycycline, 100 milligrams PO, twice daily for 7 days should be given, with adjustments as needed for allergy and pregnancy. Hepatitis B vaccine (initial and remaining doses to complete three-shot course) without hepatitis B immune globulin should be given to those who are unimmunized. HIV prophylaxis requires decision making on a case-by-case basis and is discussed in chapter 293. Repeat evaluation for STIs should be done in 1 to 2 weeks to make sure that infection has been eradicated.

REFERENCES

The complete reference list is available online at www.TintinalliEM.com.

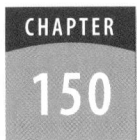

Toxic Shock Syndromes

Stephen Y. Liang

INTRODUCTION

The two classic toxic shock syndromes are attributed to *Staphylococcus aureus* or to group A *Streptococcus* (*Streptococcus pyogenes*). Each is a life-threatening illness stemming from toxin production by gram-positive organisms, creating hemodynamic compromise and fulminant multiorgan dysfunction. This cascade makes diagnosis a challenge, with the features looking like the more common entities of sepsis and septic shock. Characteristic epidemiology, pathophysiology, clinical presentations, and management strategies set these syndromes apart (**Table 150-1**). Early recognition and definitive treatment are the keys to improving patient outcomes.

TABLE 150-1 Distinguishing Characteristics of Toxic Shock Syndrome and Streptococcal Toxic Shock Syndrome

	Toxic Shock Syndrome (TSS)	Streptococcal Toxic Shock Syndrome (STSS)
Organism	*Staphylococcus aureus* (including MRSA)	Group A *Streptococcus* (*Streptococcus pyogenes*)
Toxin	Toxic shock syndrome toxin-1 (TSST-1) Staphylococcal enterotoxins	Streptococcal pyrogenic exotoxins (most commonly A and B)
Risk factors	Retained foreign body (e.g., tampon, female barrier contraceptive) Skin and soft tissue infections Varicella Surgery Trauma Childbirth Influenza	Necrotizing soft tissue infections Varicella Surgery Trauma Childbirth Influenza
Presence of pain	Uncommon	Common
Presence of rash	Common	Uncommon
Blood culture positivity	5%	60%
Mortality	≤5%	20%–45%

Abbreviation: MRSA = methicillin-resistant *Staphylococcus aureus*.

STAPHYLOCOCCAL TOXIC SHOCK SYNDROME

INTRODUCTION AND EPIDEMIOLOGY

Staphylococcal toxic shock syndrome (TSS) was first described in 1978 in a series of seven children presenting with systemic illness punctuated by fever, headache, confusion, vomiting, diarrhea, scarlatiniform rash, desquamation, hypotension, and multiorgan dysfunction.[1] A toxigenic strain of *S. aureus* isolated from mucosal (nasopharyngeal, tracheal, vaginal) and sequestered sites (abscess, empyema) in five of the patients was the causative organism. During the early 1980s, TSS was linked to tampon use in young menstruating women,[2,3] with incidence rates as high as 13.7 per 100,000 menstruating women between the ages of 15 and 24.[4] Education on the proper frequency and duration of use of tampons coupled with the removal of highly absorbent tampons from the market are widely credited with reducing menstrual TSS rates, although tampon use remains an important risk factor for menstrual TSS to this day in the United States, Canada, and Western Europe.

Nonmenstrual TSS is associated with a wide range of skin and soft tissue infections including abscesses, cellulitis, mastitis, and infected surgical and postpartum wounds, including vaginal and cesarean deliveries.[5] Sinusitis and superimposed infections of burns, abrasions, and varicella lesions have been described in other cases, particularly in children. Patients with influenza may develop TSS in the setting of secondary *S. aureus* respiratory tract infections (e.g., pneumonia, tracheitis).[6] Because the vagina and nares are known sites of *S. aureus* colonization, retained foreign bodies, including **female barrier contraceptives** (*e.g.*, diaphragm, contraceptive sponge) and **nasal packing material**, are risk factors for developing nonmenstrual TSS. Nasal packing is not a current common trigger, and routine prescription of antibiotics is not needed to stop this from occurring.[8] Nonmenstrual TSS affects men and women alike, and patients tend to be older and have more comorbid illnesses than those seen with the menstrual form of the disease.

Population-based surveillance shows that TSS incidence has been stable in the United States for the past 30 years.[9,10] Women between the age of 13 and 24 years have a higher incidence of menstrual TSS, at a rate of 1.41 per 100,000 persons.[9] The overall case fatality rate for TSS is 4.1%, with higher rates in nonmenstrual TSS (5%) compared to menstrual TSS (3%).[11]

PATHOPHYSIOLOGY

TSS is a superantigen-mediated disease. Toxigenic *S. aureus* strains produce pyrogenic exotoxins including toxic shock syndrome toxin-1 (TSST-1) and staphylococcal enterotoxins that bind directly to the major histocompatibility complex class II molecule and T-cell receptor on antigen-presenting cells.[12] Massive T-cell and antigen-presenting cell activation leads to enhanced cytokine expression (e.g., interleukin-1, -2, and -6; tumor necrosis factor-α; interferon-γ), establishing a proinflammatory state. Increased vascular permeability, hemodynamic shock, metabolic acidosis, coagulopathy, and multiorgan dysfunction ensue, mirroring that of the cascade triggered by lipopolysaccharide (endotoxin) in gram-negative sepsis.

Almost all menstrual TSS cases are tied to TSST-1.[13,14] Disease starts with colonization of the vagina by a toxigenic strain of *S. aureus* capable of producing TSST-1. Approximately 9% of women are vaginally colonized with *S. aureus*, only 1% of whom are considered toxigenic.[15] TSST-1 must cross the vaginal epithelium for clinical disease to occur, and the host cannot possess neutralizing antibodies to TSST-1 that might confer immunity. One reason why menstrual TSS rates have remained low yet consistent throughout the years may be due to the development of durable immunity to TSST-1,[15] perhaps from either transient or persistent asymptomatic colonization with toxigenic *S. aureus*.[16]

In contrast to menstrual TSS, TSST-1 is implicated in only half of nonmenstrual TSS cases,[17] with the remaining share attributed to staphylococcal enterotoxin B and other members of that family.[18] Vulnerability to nonmenstrual TSS usually starts with infection or colonization involving a toxigenic strain of *S. aureus* at a localized site, notably mucosa, skin, wound, lung, or a foreign body.

CLINICAL FEATURES

A case definition created for the National Notifiable Diseases Surveillance System by the U.S. Centers for Disease Control and Prevention (**Table 150-2**) provides criteria for reporting TSS in its most severe form, although many of these symptoms may not be evident on initial evaluation of the patient presenting to the emergency department and should not be used to exclude the diagnosis of TSS. These definitions are periodically updated at the National Notifiable Diseases Surveillance System Web page (http://wwwn.cdc.gov/nndss).

TABLE 150-2 Case Definition for Toxic Shock Syndrome

Clinical criteria:

- Fever: temperature ≥38.9°C or 102.0°F
- Rash: diffuse macular erythroderma
- Desquamation: 1–2 weeks after onset of rash
- Hypotension: systolic blood pressure ≤90 mm Hg (adult) or <5th percentile by age (children <16 years of age)
- Multiorgan involvement (≥3 organ systems):
  - Gastrointestinal: vomiting and/or diarrhea at onset of illness
  - Muscular: severe myalgia or CPK ≥2 times the upper limit of normal
  - Mucous membrane: vaginal, oropharyngeal, or conjunctival hyperemia
  - Renal: BUN or serum Cr ≥2 times the upper limit of normal for laboratory or urinary sediment with pyuria (≥5 leukocytes per high-power field) in the absence of urinary tract infection
  - Hepatic: total bilirubin, ALT, or AST ≥2 times the upper limit of normal
  - Hematologic: platelet count <100,000/mm^3
  - Central nervous system: disorientation or alterations in consciousness without focal neurologic signs when fever and hypotension are absent

Laboratory criteria: *Negative* results on the following tests, if obtained:

- Blood or cerebrospinal fluid cultures (blood culture may be positive for *Staphylococcus aureus*)
- Serologies for Rocky Mountain spotted fever, leptospirosis, or measles

Case classification:

- Probable: ≥4 clinical criteria + laboratory criteria met
- Confirmed: 5 clinical criteria + laboratory criteria met, including desquamation (unless death occurs prior to desquamation)

Abbreviations: ALT = alanine aminotransferase; AST = aspartate aminotransferase; CPK = creatine phosphokinase; Cr = creatinine.

Time of onset of initial symptoms is highly variable, ranging from as little as 48 hours in postoperative nonmenstrual TSS[5] to several days after the start of menstruation in menstrual TSS.[3] **Patients presenting early on in the disease process may exhibit a nonspecific prodrome** consisting of any combination of fever, chills, malaise, myalgias, headache, sore throat, vomiting, diarrhea, or abdominal pain. The progression of an unexplained febrile illness to include hypotension, erythroderma, and multiorgan dysfunction should raise clinical suspicion for TSS. Hypotension with a systolic blood pressure of ≤90 mm Hg in adults or less than the fifth percentile for children <16 years of age heralds severe disease as a consequence of systemic vasodilation and increased capillary permeability. Decreased urinary output signals acute kidney injury, which may result from renal hypoperfusion, rhabdomyolysis, or other causes. Lethargy, agitation, and confusion can result from shock or be related to cerebral edema. Respiratory failure can occur from acute respiratory distress syndrome or pulmonary edema from toxic cardiomyopathy. Patients with TSS may also present to care with second- or third-degree heart block or, more rarely, ventricular arrhythmias.

The erythroderma of TSS is characterized as a painless, diffuse, red, macular rash resembling "sunburn." The rash can be either patchy or confluent, and it can be modest and evanescent, involving the palms and soles. Desquamation, notably of the hands and feet, begins anywhere from 1 to 3 weeks after the initial onset of symptoms. Mucosal involvement can include conjunctival and scleral hemorrhage as well as vaginal, cervical, or oropharyngeal hyperemia ("strawberry tongue") and ulceration. In the patient at risk for menstrual TSS, pelvic examination gauges mucosal disease and allows a look for retained foreign bodies such as tampons.

Surgical wounds infected or colonized with toxigenic *S. aureus* in nonmenstrual TSS patients may have little or no erythema, induration, or purulent drainage to raise clinical suspicion of infection,[5,19] likely due to unique properties associated with TSST-1 and staphylococcal enterotoxin B. Any wound in a patient presenting with concern for TSS should be considered a potential source for toxigenic *S. aureus*.

DIAGNOSIS

Timely diagnosis of TSS relies on identifying patient risk factors; recognizing an evolving pattern of febrile illness, hemodynamic compromise, and organ injury; and considering the diagnosis before profound illness occurs even if all of the case criteria are not met. **TSS is a clinical diagnosis.**

Laboratory evaluation reveals the adverse sequelae of organ hypoperfusion and dysfunction, but nothing more specific. Usually, a CBC, comprehensive metabolic panel with liver function tests, coagulation studies, creatine phosphokinase level (particularly if myalgias are a primary complaint), urinalysis, chest radiograph, and an ECG are obtained to assess organ function. Leukocytosis, anemia, or thrombocytopenia may be present. Azotemia indicative of acute kidney injury can be accompanied by electrolyte disturbances including hyponatremia, hypocalcemia, and hypophosphatemia.[20] Metabolic acidosis in the presence of hypotension is common. Hypoalbuminemia from capillary leakage and liver function abnormalities with coagulopathy can also be seen. Absent coagulopathy, CT of the brain accompanied by lumbar puncture is often needed in those with altered sensorium.

Obtain blood cultures, but **positive blood cultures are uncommon**: *S. aureus* is grown in less than 5% of TSS cases.[5] In contrast, **cultures from wounds, mucosal sites, and retained foreign materials are frequently positive for *S. aureus***. Get all possible cultures early, optimally before initiating antibiotic therapy, to facilitate identification of a toxin-producing strain of *S. aureus* and to allow antibiotic susceptibility testing.

Differential Diagnosis **Streptococcal toxic shock syndrome** and **myonecrosis** due to *Clostridium perfringens*, both commonly associated with traumatic and surgical wounds, are important considerations in the differential diagnosis of TSS. Toxic shock syndrome due to *Clostridium sordellii*, associated with gynecologic surgery, childbirth, miscarriage, and abortions, can also present similarly, but often without fever. **Staphylococcal scalded skin syndrome**, mediated by exfoliative toxin A or B, can present with fever, lethargy, and desquamation similar to TSS, but is not typically accompanied by hypotension or multiorgan dysfunction. In the absence of erythroderma, TSS is indistinguishable from sepsis or septic shock due to any number of gram-positive or gram-negative bacteria. Other infectious diseases classically associated with fever, rash, and multiorgan dysfunction include **Rocky Mountain spotted fever and leptospirosis.** Also, consider **meningococcemia** if any severe headache or a petechial rash is seen. Noninfectious illnesses including **Stevens-Johnson syndrome**, **toxic epidermal necrolysis**, and **Kawasaki's disease** are occasional alternative diagnoses.

TREATMENT

The initial management of TSS in the ED is based on treating shock and eliminating the source of infection. Start with aggressive isotonic crystalloid fluid resuscitation, and use vasopressors and inotropes as needed if volume alone does not resolve hypotension or organ hypoperfusion. Mechanical ventilation may be necessary for respiratory failure. Drain abscesses and other infected fluid collections, obtain surgical consultation for debridement of potentially infected wounds, and remove retained foreign bodies that might represent a focus for toxigenic *S. aureus* (e.g., tampons, nasal or surgical packing material). Patients suspected of having TSS require hospital admission, usually to the intensive care unit, given the hemodynamic compromise, respiratory failure, and multiorgan dysfunction.

Administer antibiotics to treat infection, eliminate *S. aureus* carriage, and reduce recurrences, although the role of antibiotics in curbing the inflammatory response of TSS is unclear (**Table 150-3**). With the growing prevalence of methicillin-resistant *S. aureus* (MRSA), decisions about empiric antistaphylococcal therapy should hinge on local *S. aureus* antibiotic resistance patterns. Both community- and hospital-acquired MRSA strains have been reported to cause TSS through TSST-1[21] and staphylococcal enterotoxin production, although the exact proportion of TSS cases attributable to MRSA is not known. Empiric therapy should consist of **vancomycin**, 15 milligrams/kg IV every 12 hours (maximum single dose of 2.25 grams), with adjustment of the dosing interval based on creatinine clearance. **Linezolid**, 600 milligrams IV every 12 hours, is an alternative to treat MRSA and may also directly suppress TSST-1 production.[22] If the concern for MRSA is low, an antistaphylococcal penicillin, such as oxacillin, 2 grams IV every 4 hours, or nafcillin, 2 grams IV every 4 hours, is adequate. Clindamycin, 900 milligrams IV every 8 hours, is added as a second agent given its ability to inhibit protein synthesis and toxin production in TSS,[23] but should not be used as monotherapy. The duration of antibiotic therapy is based on the clinical response and typically ranges from 7 to 14 days.

Reserve IV immune globulin for cases where supportive care, source control, and antibiotic therapy fail to elicit improvement within the first 6 hours of care. Although dosing recommendations will vary by patient age and comorbidity, many require higher doses of IV immune globulin to inhibit staphylococcal toxins.[24] Give IV immune globulin only after consultation with infectious disease or critical care specialists. An initial dose of 1 to 2 grams/kg is recommended. Immunoglobulin A deficiency is an absolute contraindication to the use of IV immune globulin. High-dose corticosteroids are not recommended in the treatment of TSS.[25]

TABLE 150-3 Differential Diagnosis and Recommended Antibiotic Regimens for Staphylococcal Toxic Shock Syndrome

Differential diagnosis

Streptococcal toxic shock syndrome
Rocky Mountain spotted fever
Stevens-Johnson syndrome
Clostridial myonecrosis
Leptospirosis
Toxic epidermal necrolysis
Staphylococcal scalded skin syndrome
Meningococcemia
Kawasaki's disease

Recommended Antibiotic Regimen	Organism
Vancomycin, 15 milligrams/kg IV *or* Linezolid, 600 milligrams IV *and* Clindamycin, 900 milligrams IV	MRSA
Oxacillin, 2 grams IV *or* Nafcillin, 2 grams IV *and* Clindamycin, 900 milligrams IV	MSSA

Abbreviations: MRSA = methicillin-resistant *Staphylococcus aureus*, MSSA = methicillin-sensitive *Staphylococcus aureus*.

STREPTOCOCCAL TOXIC SHOCK SYNDROME

INTRODUCTION AND EPIDEMIOLOGY

Streptococcal toxic shock syndrome (STSS) is a complication of invasive infections involving group A *Streptococcus* (*S. pyogenes*), including skin and soft tissue infections, pneumonia, and bloodstream infections. First recognized in 1987, STSS shared many of the same clinical features of TSS seen with *S. aureus*.[26] However, in a case series of 20 patients published just 2 years later, STSS emerged as a disease associated with necrotizing fasciitis and myositis, marked by a significantly higher morbidity and mortality compared with that of TSS.[27] Annual incidence rates for invasive group A *Streptococcus* (GAS) infection have ranged from 3 to 6 cases per 100,000 persons,[28-30] with those age 65 years and older or under the age of 1 greatest affected. In prospective population-based surveillance across 11 European countries in 2003 and 2004, 13% of invasive GAS infections were complicated by STSS, with half of all STSS cases reported in patients with necrotizing fasciitis.[29] More recently, population-based surveillance at sentinel sites in the United States have reported STSS in 3.4% of invasive GAS infections.[31] Mortality rates for STSS are high, ranging from 19% to 44% in recent studies.[28-30,32]

Despite the preponderance of invasive GAS infections at the extremes of age, STSS cases occur in all age groups. Underlying medical conditions including heart, liver, and kidney disease; diabetes mellitus; alcoholism; and drug abuse are more common in patients who develop STSS,[30,33] but many patients are healthy prior to the illness.[27,34] Surgical procedures, traumatic injuries, vaginal or caesarean delivery, varicella infection in children,[35] and influenza are all associated with STSS and other invasive GAS infections. Rare outbreaks of severe GAS infection with some progressing to STSS have occurred in daycare centers,[36] healthcare facilities,[37] and other institutional settings.

In recent years, STSS has been linked to infections involving group B, C, and G streptococci.[38] *Streptococcus suis* (a pathogen in pigs) is another newly identified trigger of invasive soft tissue infections accompanied by an STSS-like syndrome in China.[39]

PATHOPHYSIOLOGY

As with *S. aureus* TSS, STSS is mediated by toxins that function as superantigens. Streptococcal pyrogenic exotoxins, predominantly A and B, are produced by GAS in severe infections. These toxins also bind to the major histocompatibility complex class II molecule and T-cell receptor on antigen-presenting cells, thereby activating T cells and triggering cytokine expression.[12] Fever, increased vascular permeability, hemodynamic compromise, and multiorgan dysfunction are the products of this systemic inflammatory response. Virulence factors including M proteins confer resistance to phagocytosis and may impart other properties that further enhance the severity of disease.

Breaches in skin and mucosal surfaces (e.g., oropharynx, vagina), as well as minor trauma without obvious skin disruption resulting in hematoma, contusion, or muscle injury, are common starting points for severe GAS infections. In many cases, a portal of entry is never identified.

CLINICAL FEATURES

Fulminant STSS, as defined by the Centers for Disease Control and Surveillance case definition (**Table 150-4**), is often preceded by a nonspecific prodrome of fever, chills, sweats, malaise, arthralgias, cough, sore throat, rhinorrhea, anorexia, nausea, vomiting, abdominal pain, and diarrhea in adults and children alike.[27,40] A diffusely erythematous and macular rash is infrequently seen in STSS and may progress to desquamation, although its presence is not required to solidify the diagnosis of STSS. Confusion, somnolence, and agitation may follow. Given the strong association between STSS and necrotizing soft tissue infections, many patients are likely to present initially with **pain out of proportion to physical findings** at a localized site, often an extremity or the abdomen.[27] Progressive violaceous discoloration, skin crepitus and necrosis, and bullae formation at the site are ominous signs of underlying necrotizing fasciitis and myositis. Compartment syndrome can be a complication. Refractory hypotension rapidly ensues from a combination of vasodilation, capillary leakage, and myocardial depression from toxic cardiomyopathy.[34] Acute kidney injury, myocardial and cerebral ischemia, acute respiratory distress syndrome, rhabdomyolysis from muscle destruction, liver dysfunction, and disseminated intravascular coagulation can lead to death within hours to days.

DIAGNOSIS

As with *S. aureus* TSS, the surveillance case definition for STSS may not be fully met on the initial presentation.

Laboratory evaluation has no specific diagnostic role, although it usually includes CBC, comprehensive metabolic panel with liver function tests, coagulation studies, creatine phosphokinase level (particularly if myositis or necrotizing fasciitis is suspected), arterial blood gas analysis, urinalysis, chest radiograph, and an ECG. Athough leukocytosis may be modest, a marked bandemia, sometimes in excess of 40%, can be present.[27] Anemia, thrombocytopenia, and coagulopathy may be evident. Transaminitis, azotemia, metabolic acidosis, hypoalbuminemia, and hypocalcemia are common findings, particularly as hypotension and capillary leakage progress. In necrotizing soft tissue infections, creatine phosphokinase will be elevated.

Obtain blood and wound cultures prior to administering antibiotics when possible to confirm the presence of GAS and guide therapy. **Blood cultures are positive in up to 60% of STSS cases; cultures from infected sites almost always yield GAS.**[27,40]

Consult a surgeon immediately for all patients believed to have a necrotizing soft tissue infection. CT and MRI showing soft tissue destruction establishes this diagnosis but should never delay timely surgical evaluation.

Differential Diagnosis Staphylococcal TSS, myonecrosis associated with *C. perfringens* or *Clostridium septicum*, nonclostridial myonecrosis due to mixed anaerobes and other bacteria, and *C. sordellii* toxic shock syndrome are principal contenders in the differential diagnosis of STSS. Other systemic infections including meningococcemia, Rocky Mountain spotted fever, and leptospirosis are potential candidates as well.

TREATMENT

Management of STSS begins with aggressive isotonic fluid resuscitation to restore volume and tissue perfusion. In light of the profound refractory hypotension and capillary leakage associated with STSS, large volumes of IV crystalloid fluid (10 to 20 L/d) may be required. Vasopressors or inotropic therapy are often necessary. More than half of patients with STSS will develop acute respiratory distress syndrome, often requiring intubation and mechanical ventilation.

Obtain surgical consultation for early and often extensive operative debridement, fasciotomy, and even amputation if a significant burden of infected and necrotic tissue exists. Admit to the intensive care unit.

Given the overlap in clinical presentations between STSS and septic shock and the high mortality associated with both, empiric broad-spectrum antibiotic therapy to cover GAS and other potential pathogens is best until culture data are available (**Table 150-5**). Use a β-lactamase inhibitor (e.g., piperacillin-tazobactam, 4.5 grams IV every 6 hours) or a carbapenem (e.g., meropenem, 1 gram IV every 8 hours) in combination with clindamycin, 900 milligrams IV every 8 hours,[41] the latter for suppression of toxin formation.[42] In areas where MRSA is prevalent, add vancomycin, 15 milligrams/kg IV every 12 hours (maximum single dose of 2.25 grams). Adjust antibiotic dosing for acute kidney injury.

Once the presence of GAS is identified, consider narrowing antibiotic therapy to penicillin G, 4 million units IV every 4 hours (for a total of 24 million units per day), in combination with clindamycin.[43] The duration of antibiotic therapy should be at least 14 days but may be longer based on the extent of the infection and the patient's clinical response.

Although retrospective studies have shown decreased mortality with IV immune globulin,[44,45] a multicenter, randomized controlled trial has failed to find benefit.[46] Obtain consultation before giving IV immune globulin to treat STSS.[47]

Surveillance case definitions for TSS and STSS are available from the Centers for Disease Control and Prevention Web site at http://www.cdc.gov/nndss.

TABLE 150-4 Case Definition for Streptococcal Toxic Shock Syndrome

Clinical criteria:

- Hypotension: systolic blood pressure ≤90 mm Hg (adult) or <5th percentile by age (children <16 years of age)
- Multiorgan involvement (≥2 organ systems):
  - Renal: serum Cr ≥2 milligrams/dL (≥177 μmol/L) for adults or ≥2 times the upper limit of normal for age. In patients with preexisting renal disease, >2-fold elevation above baseline.
  - Coagulopathy: platelet count ≤100,000/mm³ (≤100 × 10⁶/L) or disseminated intravascular coagulation, defined by prolonged clotting times, low fibrinogen level, and presence of fibrin degradation products
  - Hepatic: total bilirubin, ALT, or AST ≥2 times the upper limit of normal for the patient's age. In patients with preexisting liver disease, >2-fold elevation above baseline.
  - Acute respiratory distress syndrome: acute onset of diffuse pulmonary infiltrates and hypoxemia in the absence of cardiac failure or by evidence of diffuse capillary leak manifested by acute onset of generalized edema, or pleural or peritoneal effusions with hypoalbuminemia.
  - Skin: generalized erythematous macular rash that may desquamate
  - Soft tissue necrosis, including necrotizing fasciitis or myositis, or gangrene

Laboratory criteria:

- Isolation of group A *Streptococcus*

Case classification:

- Probable: All clinical criteria met + absence of other identified etiology for illness + isolation of group A *Streptococcus* from a nonsterile site
- Confirmed: All clinical criteria met + isolation of group A *Streptococcus* from a sterile site (e.g., blood, cerebrospinal fluid, synovial fluid, pleural fluid, or pericardial fluid)

Abbreviations: ALT = alanine aminotransferase; AST = aspartate aminotransferase; Cr = creatinine.

TABLE 150-5 Differential Diagnosis and Recommended Antibiotic Regimen for Streptococcal Toxic Shock Syndrome

Differential diagnosis	
Staphylococcal toxic shock syndrome	
Clostridial myonecrosis	
Meningococcemia	
Rocky Mountain spotted fever	
Leptospirosis	
Recommended Antibiotic Regimen	**Organism**
Piperacillin-tazobactam, 4.5 grams IV	Group A *Streptococcus*
or	
Meropenem, 1 gram IV	
and	
Clindamycin, 900 milligrams IV	
and consider	
Vancomycin, 15 milligrams/kg IV	If MRSA cannot be ruled out

Abbreviation: MRSA = methicillin-resistant *Staphylococcus aureus.*

REFERENCES

The complete reference list is available online at www.TintinalliEM.com.

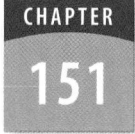

Sepsis

Michael A. Puskarich
Alan E. Jones

INTRODUCTION AND EPIDEMIOLOGY

Sepsis is a heterogeneous syndrome characterized by widespread inflammation and potential organ harm initiated by a microorganism. Although gram-positive and gram-negative bacteria account for the majority of cases, fungi, viruses, mycobacteria, rickettsiae, and protozoans can trigger sepsis. Invasion of the blood is not necessary to develop or identify sepsis, which is determined by the host response to the infectious insult. As sepsis severity increases, a multifactorial series of events lead to impairments in oxygen delivery, secondary to macro- and microvascular malperfusion, as well as direct cellular damage secondary to inflammation. Eventually, multisystem organ failure occurs, and mortality is high.

The varying clinical presentation, differences in coding, and methodologic differences between studies lead to a wide range of estimates of the annual incidence of severe sepsis, ranging from 300 to 1000 cases/100,000 persons per year.[1] Over 500,000 patients each year present to the ED with suspected severe sepsis, the largest group of all sepsis patients hospitalized. The incidence is increasing and is multifactorial in origin; a key component of this increase relates to an aging patient population, which is not surprising given the fact that sepsis incidence increases >100-fold with age (0.2 per 1000 in children age 10 to 14 years to 26.2 per 1000 in those >85 years of age).[2]

The mean ED length of stay of a patient with sepsis is 5 hours. Once admitted, more than half of patients with severe sepsis will require care in an intermediate or intensive care unit,[2] where it represents the leading cause of death. Despite advances in care, mortality rates from severe sepsis remain high, with approximately 20% dying[3] during hospitalization in optimal clinical trial scenarios[4,5]; this rate approaches 50% when considering the sicker subset of those with septic shock.[6] These mortality rates exceed many other high-visibility acute care conditions such as acute myocardial infarction,[7] massive pulmonary embolism,[8] and cerebrovascular accident.[9] Morbidity is high and prolonged, and a long-term deficit in cognition and functioning is common.[10] Finally, sepsis care is costly; estimates from 10 years ago suggest a mean case cost of $22,100 with annual national costs reaching $16.7 billion,[2] figures that have certainly increased in the last decade.

Since 1987, gram-positive bacteria outside of the surgical setting are the predominant pathogens of sepsis.[11] With the rise of antimicrobial resistance, methicillin-resistant *Staphylococcus aureus*, vancomycin-resistant *Enterococcus*, and other multidrug-resistant organisms are more common.[12] Similarly, the incidence of fungi as the source has risen, particularly in immunosuppressed patients. The most likely causative microorganism varies based on the likelihood of exposure to drug-resistant microorganisms (due to recent healthcare exposures) and the anatomic site of infection, with pneumonia, intra-abdominal, urinary, and skin/soft tissue being the most common locations.

DEFINITIONS

Sepsis syndromes are a continuum, with specific definitions regularly updated to include children[13,14] (**Table 151-1**). Although the definitions provide a conceptual and practical framework for recognition of the systemic inflammatory response to infection, definitions often are not sensitive or specific in the real-world clinical setting. In general, sepsis is defined as suspected or confirmed infection with evidence of systemic inflammation (demonstrated either through evidence of the systemic immune response syndrome or laboratory abnormalities), whereas severe sepsis is generally defined as sepsis plus evidence of new organ dysfunction thought to be secondary to tissue hypoperfusion. Septic shock exists when cardiovascular failure occurs, evidenced as persistent hypotension or need for vasopressors despite adequate fluid resuscitation; this latter category has a particularly poor prognosis.

SYSTEMIC INFLAMMATORY RESPONSE SYNDROME PROGNOSIS

Having systemic inflammatory response syndrome criteria does not confirm the presence of infection or sepsis because these features are shared by many other noninfectious conditions such as trauma, pancreatitis, and burns (**Figure 151-1**). **The systemic inflammatory response syndrome response is not a diagnosis or a good indicator of outcome; it is a crude means of stratification of patients with systemic inflammation.** In a prospective study of the epidemiology of patients demonstrating systemic inflammatory response syndrome (infectious and noninfectious), mortality rates were 3% in patients without systemic inflammatory response syndrome, 6% in those meeting two criteria, 10% in those meeting three criteria, and 17% in those meeting all four criteria.[14] Death rates were similar whether or not patients had positive blood cultures.

Complementary methods of classification of sepsis based primarily on physiologic abnormalities include the third Acute Physiology and Chronic Health Evaluation acuity system,[15] the Sequential Organ Failure Assessment score, and the Mortality in Emergency Department Score[16]; each allows for prognostication. These scoring systems are typically limited to research and are not for guiding patient care. Any evidence of septic shock confers the highest mortality risk assessment.

Serum lactate across a wide spectrum[17] provides excellent prognostic data in those with sepsis, but is not a singular test to diagnose or exclude sepsis. Lactate has traditionally been attributed to anaerobic metabolism secondary to tissue hypoperfusion; it also accumulates from changes in *aerobic* metabolism that occur in response to widespread inflammation.[18] As lactate increases, the risk of mortality rises, with the degree of lactate elevation and hypotension being independent predictors of mortality.[19,20] Specifically, 28-day mortality rate associated with modest elevation of serum lactate to 2 to 4 mmol/L approaches 15% even in those patients without hypotension,[21] and the rate continues to rise with increasing lactate levels. In general, venous or arterial lactate levels on either point-of-care bedside devices or measured in a central laboratory are useful if done with good clinical technique[22]; even better are serial levels using the same method of sampling (arterial or venous) to identify improvement that mirrors clinical responses.[22] This is called **lactate clearance** and is defined as a drop over time; lactate clearance provides an independent prognostic value in addition to

TABLE 151-1 Definition of Sepsis in Adults and Children

Systemic Inflammatory Response Syndrome (SIRS) criteria:
1. Fever (temperature >38.3°C) or hypothermia (temperature <36°C)
2. Pulse rate (>90 beats/min or >2 SDs above the normal value for age)
3. Tachypnea (respiratory rate >20 breaths/min)
4. Leukocytosis (WBC >12,000 cells/μL) *or* leukopenia (WBC <4000 cells/μL), *or* normal WBC with >10% immature forms
Sepsis: *Infection (documented **or** suspected), and some of the following:*
General Parameters:
Fever (temperature >38.3°C)
Hypothermia (temperature <36°C)
Pulse rate (>90 beats/min or >2 SDs above the normal value for age)
Tachypnea
Altered mental status
Significant edema or positive fluid balance (>20 mL/kg during 24 h)
Hyperglycemia (plasma glucose >140 milligrams/dL or 7.7 mmol/L) in the absence of diabetes
Inflammatory Parameters:
Leukocytosis (WBC >12,000 cells/μL)
Leukopenia (WBC <4000 cells/μL)
Normal WBC with >10% immature forms
Plasma C-reactive protein (CRP) >2 SDs above the normal value
Plasma procalcitonin >2 SDs above the normal value
Hemodynamic Parameters:
Arterial hypotension (SBP <90 mm Hg, MAP <70 mm Hg, or an SBP decrease >40 mm Hg in adults or <2 SDs below normal for age)
Organ Dysfunction Parameters:
Arterial hypoxemia (P_{a02}/F_{I02} <300)
Acute oliguria (urine output <0.5 mL/kg per hour for at least 2 h despite adequate fluid resuscitation)
Creatinine level increase >0.5 milligrams/dL
Coagulation abnormalities (INR >1.5 or aPTT >60 s)
Ileus (absent bowel sounds)
Thrombocytopenia (platelet count <100,000 cells/μL)
Hyperbilirubinemia (plasma total bilirubin >4 milligrams/dL)
Tissue Perfusion Parameters:
Hyperlactatemia (above upper limits of laboratory normal levels)
Decreased capillary refill or mottling
Severe Sepsis: *Sepsis-induced tissue hypoperfusion or organ dysfunction (any of the following thought to be due to infection)*
Sepsis-induced hypotension
Lactate level above upper limits of laboratory normal levels
Urine output <0.5 mL/kg per hour for at least 2 h despite adequate fluid resuscitation
Acute lung injury with P_{a02}/F_{I02} <250 in the absence of pneumonia as infectious source
Acute lung injury with P_{a02}/F_{I02} <200 in the absence of pneumonia as infectious source
Creatinine level >2.0 milligrams/dL
Bilirubin level >2 milligrams/dL
Platelet count <100,000 cells/μL
Coagulopathy (INR >1.5)

Abbreviations: aPTT = activated partial thromboplastin time; F_{I02} = fraction of inspired oxygen; INR = international normalized ratio; MAP = mean arterial pressure; P_{a02} = arterial partial pressure of oxygen; SBP = systolic blood pressure; SD = standard deviation.

Source: Adapted with permission from Levy et al.[13] Copyright Wolters Kluwer Health.

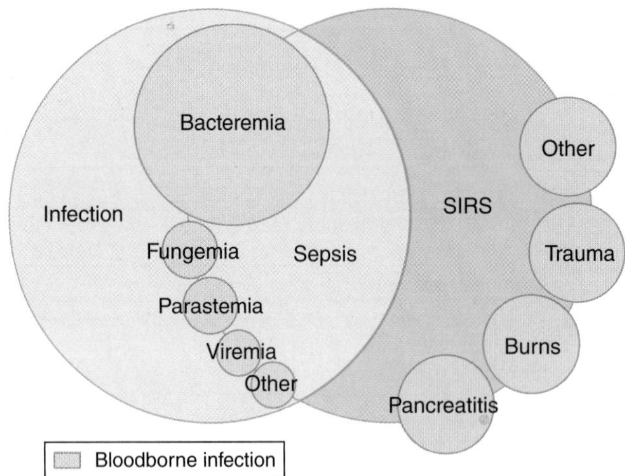

FIGURE 151-1. Interrelationship between systemic inflammatory response syndrome (SIRS), sepsis, and infection.

vital signs and other measurements. Patients with sepsis who do not clear lactate (adequate is at least a 10% drop with therapy over the first few hours) have a higher mortality rate than patients who do clear the lactate.[23,24] The major limitation is that **lactate is nonspecific and can be elevated in a number of conditions, and it must be used together with clinical judgment**.

PATHOPHYSIOLOGY

In sepsis, the host immune response fails to control and/or overreacts to invasive pathogens, leading to two critical events.[25,26] The first event involves marked abnormalities in the inflammatory response in the host. The host response typically varies from a hyperinflammatory response in the early stages of sepsis, to a blunted inflammatory response in the later stages of sepsis, which leads to an increased risk of secondary hospital-acquired infections. The blunted inflammatory response results in programmed death of key immune, epithelial, and endothelial cells, leading to tissue injury and perpetuating multiorgan dysfunction.

The second event is an imbalance in procoagulant and anticoagulant functioning; in the most extreme of situations, this results in the clinical syndrome of disseminated intravascular coagulation. Disseminated intravascular coagulation results in micro- and macrovascular clot formation, impaired microvascular tissue perfusion, and thrombosis of small vessels. Notably, subclinical disseminated intravascular coagulation is often lurking despite relatively normal basic laboratory findings, with impaired microvascular perfusion (detectable in research settings) that is associated with a worse prognosis.[27] Continued microvascular ischemia likely contributes to organ failure, as well as to the release of proinflammatory intracellular contents, which further stimulates the innate immune response and perpetuates the underlying pathology.[28] As these events progress, they intensify the inflammatory response and a destructive cycle ensues, as illustrated in **Figure 151-2**. At this time, there are no specific therapies to remedy microvascular dysfunction.

CLINICAL FEATURES

While some presentations of severe sepsis are immediately clinically apparent, sepsis can present in a subtle or occult manner, particularly early in the course. Given that systemic inflammation produces physiologic changes, vital sign abnormalities—notably fever, hypotension, and/or tachycardia—are a hint to sepsis, recognizing that many patients with these findings may have another cause. In ED patients with undifferentiated hypotension, 40% will ultimately have an infectious cause of symptoms.[29]

Although traditionally sepsis is categorized as an example of distributive shock (peripheral vasodilation evidenced by warm extremities with

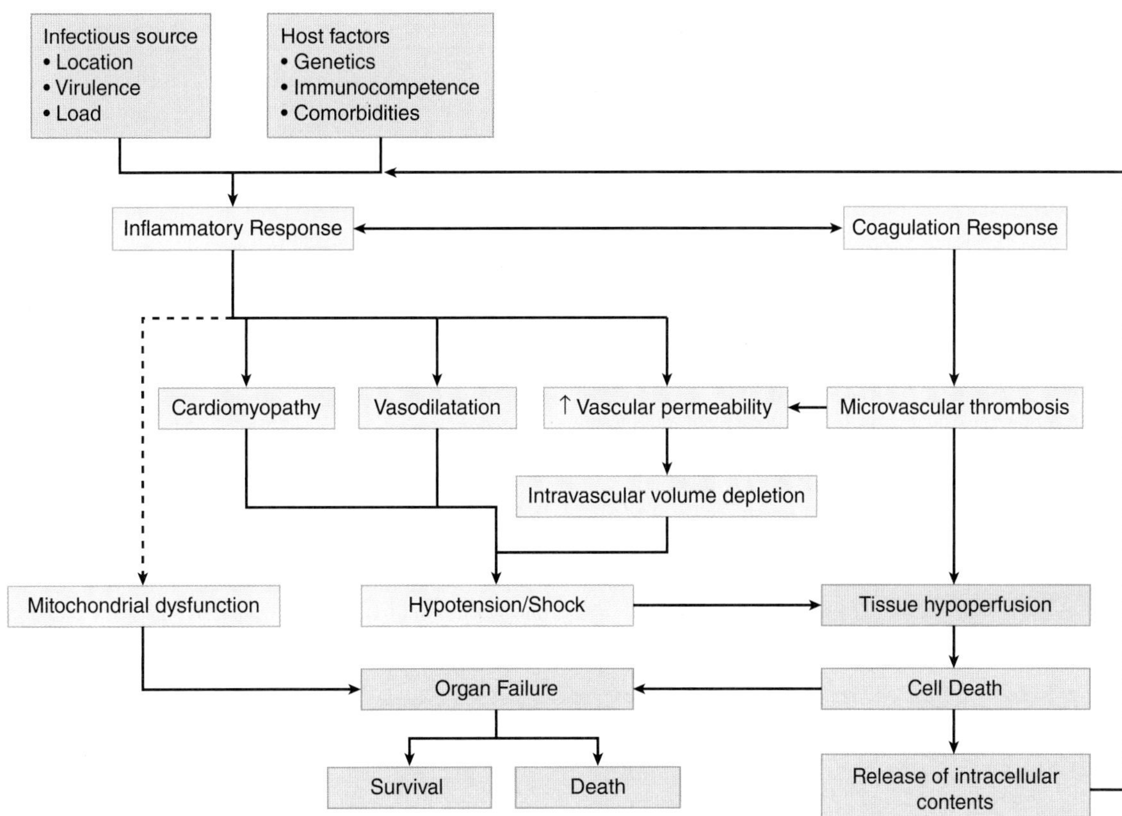

FIGURE 151-2. Pathogenic sequence of events in septic shock.

a compensatory increased cardiac output), this presentation does not accurately describe all patients with sepsis. ED patients with sepsis are often volume depleted from decreased intake and increased fluid losses (from emesis, diarrhea, or insensible losses associated with fever and tachypnea). Intravascular volume depletion directly affects preload, cardiac output, and ultimately peripheral perfusion. Further complicating matters is **septic cardiomyopathy**, a reversible process characterized by impaired systolic function and diastolic relaxation.[30] Finally, the combination of intravascular volume depletion and septic cardiomyopathy may manifest as "cold shock," impaired peripheral perfusion and cool extremities.

PULMONARY INJURY

Widespread inflammation secondary to sepsis commonly affects pulmonary function even in the absence of pneumonia. Acute lung injury is common and may result in acute respiratory distress syndrome, which is characterized by new lung edema from increased alveolar and capillary permeability. Classification of acute respiratory distress syndrome is based primarily on the degree of hypoxemia.[31] The three mutually exclusive categories are mild (P_{aO2} divided by fraction of inspired oxygen [F_{IO2}] of 200 to 300), moderate (P_{aO2}/F_{IO2} of 100 to 200), and severe (P_{aO2}/F_{IO2} <100), within 1 week of a clinical insult or change in respiratory status coupled with new bilateral pulmonary infiltrates on chest radiographs not explained by effusions, lung collapse, or nodules and not fully explained by heart failure or volume overload. Clinically, severe refractory hypoxemia, noncompliant lungs noted on mechanical ventilation, and a chest radiograph showing bilateral pulmonary alveolar infiltrates suggest the diagnosis. Mortality increases from 27% to 45% with increasing severity of acute respiratory distress syndrome.

RENAL INJURY

The kidney is another common sepsis target; acute kidney injury can present with azotemia, oliguria, or anuria. Factors increasing acute kidney injury risk include pre-existing kidney dysfunction or vasculopathy, depth and duration of hypotension, dehydration, and use of nephrotoxic substances (e.g., aminoglycoside antibiotics, nonionic intravenous contrast). Renal ischemic injury from hypoperfusion is a major factor in the pathogenesis of acute kidney injury in sepsis, although toxic products resulting from neutrophil-endothelial interactions, endothelial damage by various mediators, reperfusion injury, and microvascular thrombosis also contribute.

HEPATIC INJURY

The most frequent hepatic abnormality is cholestatic jaundice, although it occurs infrequently. Increased concentrations of transaminase, alkaline phosphatase (one to three times the normal level), and bilirubin (usually not >10 milligrams/dL) may be observed. Marked elevations of transaminases or bilirubin are less common unless septic shock is present; if seen, consider a biliary source of infection. Smaller elevations in liver function tests can result from intermittent or prolonged macro- or microvascular hypoperfusion and ischemia or can be secondary to direct endotoxin, cytokines, or immune complex damage. Red blood cell hemolysis from microvascular coagulation can also rarely cause jaundice.

GI CHANGES

The most common GI manifestation of sepsis is ileus, which may persist for days after shock resolves. Major blood loss secondary to upper GI bleeding is rare in septic patients. Minor GI blood loss within 24 hours of developing severe sepsis can result from painless erosions in the mucosal layer of the stomach or duodenum.

HEMATOLOGIC CHANGES

Multiple abnormalities are possible in the hematologic system in the setting of sepsis, including neutropenia or neutrophilia, thrombocytopenia, or disseminated intravascular coagulation. Neutrophilic leukocytosis with a "left shift" results from demargination and release of newer granulocytes from the marrow storage pools. However, the presence of excessive bands (the immature neutrophil) is neither sensitive nor specific for infection. **Neutropenia** occurs rarely and is associated with an increase in mortality; it results from increased peripheral use of neutrophils, damage to neutrophils by bacterial by-products, or depression of marrow granulocyte production by inflammatory mediators. Functional neutropenia also creates a relative immunosuppression, particularly later in patients' hospital course. Both red cell production and survival decrease during sepsis, but anemia is not expected unless it existed prior to the infection, the infection is extremely prolonged, or there is concomitant bleeding.

Thrombocytopenia may arise as a consequence of disseminated intravascular coagulation but is present in >30% of cases of sepsis even in the absence of overt disseminated intravascular coagulation, and lower platelet levels are associated with worse outcomes.[32,33] Proposed mechanisms of thrombocytopenia include inhibition of thrombopoiesis, increased platelet turnover (due to a consumptive coagulopathy), increased endothelial adherence, and increased destruction secondary to immunologic mechanisms.

Finally, fulminant **disseminated intravascular coagulation** where clinical clotting and bleeding exist is rare but associated with a very poor prognosis.[26] Occult disseminated intravascular coagulation, with microvascular flow abnormalities, subclinical increased activation of the coagulation system, and evidence of increased fibrinogen split products in the absence of overt bleeding and clotting, is much more common. The activation of the hemostatic (clotting) system is due primarily to the activation of the extrinsic pathway of clotting. The fibrinolytic system is also activated in sepsis and plays an important role in limiting fibrin deposition in the microcirculation. The release of tissue plasminogen activator activates the fibrinolytic system, at least initially in sepsis. As sepsis progresses, there is an increased release of plasminogen activator inhibitor 1, which blocks plasmin generation and thus contributes to fibrin deposition in the microcirculation and subsequent multiple-organ failure. Laboratory studies suggesting the presence of disseminated intravascular coagulation include thrombocytopenia, prolonged prothrombin and activated partial thromboplastin values, decreased fibrinogen and antithrombin III levels, and increased fibrin monomer, fibrin split products, and D-dimer levels.

METABOLIC CHANGES

Sepsis induces multiple metabolic changes. Abnormalities in lactate metabolism due to tissue hypoperfusion with resultant anaerobic metabolism as well as increased aerobic production of lactate have been discussed previously (see "Systemic Inflammatory Response Syndrome Prognosis"). Hyperglycemia is seen even in patients without a history of diabetes; in this latter group, it is associated with a worse prognosis, in contrast to less impact of glucose elevations in those with known diabetes.[34] Hypoglycemia with glucose levels as low as 10 to 20 milligrams/dL is reported but uncommon, and may result due to depletion of hepatic glycogen and inhibition of gluconeogenesis and/or adrenal insufficiency. Adrenal insufficiency can occur,[35] caused by hypoperfusion of the adrenal glands, adrenal or pituitary hemorrhage, cytokine dysfunction of the adrenals, drug-induced hypermetabolism, inhibition of steroidogenesis by chemotherapeutics (e.g., ketoconazole), and desensitization of glucocorticoid responsiveness at the cellular level.

SKIN

There are five potential cutaneous manifestations of sepsis: direct bacterial involvement of the skin and underlying soft tissues (cellulitis, erysipelas, and fasciitis); lesions from hematogenous seeding of the skin or the underlying tissue (petechiae, pustules, cellulitis, ecthyma gangrenosum); lesions from hypotension and/or disseminated intravascular coagulation (acrocyanosis and necrosis of peripheral tissues); lesions from intravascular infections (microemboli and/or immune complex vasculitis); and lesions caused by toxins (toxic shock syndrome). Look for any necrotizing or surgical source of sepsis, and recall that the toxic shock syndromes present in an overlapping fashion (see chapter 150, "Toxic Shock Syndromes").

DIAGNOSIS

In the ED, **sepsis is a clinical diagnosis** predicated on suspicion or confirmation of infection, systemic inflammation, and evidence of new organ dysfunction and/or tissue hypoperfusion.[36] Septic shock is present or likely in any individual with the preceding signs (Table 151-1) and a systolic blood pressure of <90 mm Hg (or 2 standard deviations below normal for age in children) after an initial fluid bolus (often cited as 20 to 30 mL/kg crystalloid, generally 1.5 to 3 L in adults), or who displays evidence of inadequate organ perfusion.

Many patients with minor infections can meet consensus criteria for sepsis due to evidence of systemic inflammation. If there is new organ dysfunction or tissue hypoperfusion secondary to sepsis, consider more aggressive assessments and interventions. However, in the absence of new organ failure, the diagnosis of sepsis does not necessarily imply a poor prognosis.

The differential diagnosis of severe sepsis and septic shock includes other causes of shock. This includes cardiogenic, hypovolemic, anaphylactic, neurogenic, or obstructive shock (pulmonary embolism, cardiac tamponade), or endocrine disorders (adrenal insufficiency, thyroid storm) that mimic sepsis. **Given the high frequency of sepsis in ED patients with undifferentiated shock (40%), think of this cause when uncertain.** Children may not have hypotension until very late in the course of the disease process due to an ability to upregulate their heart rate as a compensatory response to tissue hypoperfusion. This means considering compensated shock and occult sepsis in infected children who do not appear well, even with normotension.

Once sepsis is diagnosed, seek the source, but **do not withhold** interventions such as resuscitative measures and antimicrobials. Often the source is clear, as the patient may present with signs and symptoms attributable to a pulmonary, genitourinary, skin and soft tissue, or intra-abdominal source. However, a source of infection may not be readily apparent or may be difficult to detect because of altered mental status.

The most common sepsis trigger is **acute bacterial pneumonia**, although viral and bacterial etiologies are difficult to differentiate initially. The most frequent causative organisms are *Streptococcus pneumoniae*, *S. aureus*, gram-negative bacilli, and *Legionella pneumophila*. A chest radiograph may identify air space changes and pneumonia, although radiograph findings can lag behind the clinical presentation (see also chapter 65, "Pneumonia and Pulmonary Infiltrates").

Acute pyelonephritis, typically due to gram-negative enteric bacteria or enterococci, is another frequent cause of severe sepsis. Other abdominal triggers include **cholecystitis** and **cholangitis**, each rare but particularly devastating sources of septic shock, and both require immediate surgical assessment. If there is abdominal tenderness or peritonitis, the possibilities include perforated viscous, appendicitis, diffuse colitis, or intra-abdominal abscesses. Acute pancreatitis can result in a presentation identical to that of septic shock due to widespread inflammation.[37] If peritonitis or organ ischemia/necrosis exists, early surgical consultation is needed. In women of childbearing age, septic abortion and postpartum endometritis or myometritis are unusual etiologies of septic shock.

The most common skin and soft tissue infection triggering a sepsis syndrome is cellulitis due to *S. aureus* or *Streptococcus pyogenes*. Soft tissue infections caused by gram-negative organisms are indistinguishable from those caused by staphylococci or streptococci. Shock associated with a generalized erythematous macular rash may be a toxic shock syndrome. Necrotizing soft tissue infections are usually seen in immunocompromised patients, diabetic patients, or patients with a history of poor vascular circulation (see chapter 152, "Soft Tissue Infections"). Pay close attention to skin and soft tissue infections, particularly in elderly or obtunded patients. Include an assessment for decubitus ulcers and a genitourinary assessment to look for a necrotizing infection such as Fournier's gangrene.

Individuals without an obvious source of septic shock may have a primary bacteremia or endocarditis. The most prevalent causes of primary bacteremia in outpatients are *S. aureus*, *S. pneumoniae*, and *Neisseria meningitidis*. *Pseudomonas aeruginosa* and other gram-negative bacteria are occasional causes of bacteremia and endocarditis in injection drug users. Secondary bacteremia from indwelling medical devices, including intraperitoneal or intravascular dialysis catheters, chemotherapy ports, peripherally inserted central catheters, ventriculoperitoneal shunts, and pacemaker/defibrillators, is possible. Although bacteremia can be suspected, it takes time for a blood culture to be fully assessed, making ED diagnosis difficult.

Acute bacterial meningitis is a devastating but rare cause of septic shock. Community-acquired meningitis with shock is usually caused by *S. pneumoniae* or *N. meningitidis* (see chapter 174, "Central Nervous System and Spinal Infections"). Brain and spinal abscesses, subdural or epidural empyemas, and viral CNS infections are seldom associated with shock on the initial presentation. Shock is also unusual in neurosurgical patients with *S. aureus* or enteric gram-negative meningitis secondary to neurosurgical procedure or skull fracture.

LABORATORY TESTING AND IMAGING

Tests are useful to assess the general hematologic and metabolic state of the patient and aid in detecting occult bacterial infection, uncovering a specific microbial cause of infection, and identifying occult severe sepsis. Common tests include a CBC with platelet count; serum electrolytes (including calcium and glucose); renal function panel (BUN and creatinine levels); lactic acid level; liver function panel (bilirubin, alkaline phosphate, and aspartate and alanine aminotransferase levels); and urinalysis. An arterial blood gas will aid in assessing the metabolic, ventilatory, and oxygenation adequacy in select patients. Type and screening of red blood cells is wise with any hypotension or anemia. In the setting of active bleeding or suspected disseminated intravascular coagulation, consider prothrombin time, activated partial thromboplastin time, fibrinogen, and D-dimer.

Given the frequency of pneumonia or concomitant acute respiratory distress syndrome, obtain a chest radiograph. Abdominal plain radiographs or CT scans are needed in patients if perforation or diffuse inflammation is suspected as a potential source of intra-abdominal sepsis, and US can identify a biliary source. Soft tissue CT scans to assess for the presence of free air in the tissue or deep space abscesses may assist in making the diagnosis of necrotizing skin and soft tissue infections. Perform head CT and lumbar puncture in any patient with potential meningitis, but do not delay antibiotics pending these tests (see chapter 174). If considering a spinal epidural abscess, an MRI is obtained after resuscitation.

In adults with sepsis, obtain at least two separate sets of specimens for blood culture from different venipuncture sites when possible. Order Gram staining and culture of secretions from any potential site of infection, if possible.

Other tests of interest in the assessment of sepsis include C-reactive protein and procalcitonin, both of which reflect systemic inflammation; neither of these tests can exclude sepsis, and they are not routinely needed in the ED.[37,38] Both of these tests may be better suited to guide the necessity of initiating or continuing antimicrobial therapy outside of sepsis or after a treatment course.[39]

TREATMENT

The cornerstones of the initial treatment and stabilization of severe sepsis are **early recognition, early reversal of hemodynamic compromise, and early infection control**.[36] Base the resuscitation on administering fluids, frequently assessing response, and adding adjunct therapies including vasopressors based on the conditions. The specific method of titrating resuscitation is less important than treating early and aggressively.

The goals of resuscitation are to improve preload, tissue perfusion, and oxygen delivery. There is no "set amount of fluid," although most patients will require a total (bolus plus infusion) of 2 to 5 L of crystalloid in the first 6 hours to achieve optimal outcomes. Similarly, **do not delay vasopressors when blood pressure does not respond to volume or if volume overload seems likely**. Administer appropriate antibiotics, and remove any nidus of infection. Each of these interventions will be discussed in detail below. Once the patient is stabilized, other interventions such as appropriate management of oxygenation and ventilation, fever control to reduce metabolic demand, and control of hyperglycemia may be needed to improve patient outcomes.

EARLY QUANTITATIVE RESUSCITATION

The primary deficit leading to poor outcomes in shock states (typically studied in hemorrhagic shock) is a mismatch between oxygen supply and demand,[40] and after a certain time point, processes initiated by this mismatch are irreversible. In 2001, Rivers et al[41] described the use of an early, structured hemodynamic resuscitation protocol driven by a central venous catheter with continuous oximetric capability to titrate fluids to central venous pressure, vasopressors to mean arterial pressure, and transfusion of blood or inotropes to central venous oxygen saturation (S_{CVO2}). This protocol, termed "early goal-directed therapy," decreased mortality when compared with standard care, although all patients had central venous catheters placed early. Follow-up uncontrolled observational studies confirmed that even partial use of this approach lowered mortality in settings compared with previous times without aggressive early sepsis detection or care.[42-46]

In a second large trial, Jones et al[4] randomized patients to the Rivers early goal-directed therapy protocol or to a protocol that measured lactate clearance of ≥10% rather than S_{CVO2}. The lactate clearance protocol was noninferior to continuous S_{CVO2} monitoring in the setting of ED-based resuscitation of septic shock. Lactate clearance–guided therapy (titrating fluids and vasopressors) became an alternative to invasive S_{CVO2} monitoring and early goal-directed therapy. Although the ideal lactate clearance target remains unclear, a minimum of 10% relative lactate clearance[23,24] and normalization of lactate to <2 mmol/L emerged as goals.[36,47] Still, about one third of patients with severe sepsis have a normal lactate,[47] and up to one half or more have a normal S_{CVO2},[48] limiting either tool in guiding therapy.

The newly released ProCESS trial[49] compared three ED treatment groups after early identification and antibiotics: protocol-based resuscitation using invasive central venous monitoring (the Rivers early goal-directed therapy protocol), protocol-based care using clinical parameters such as blood pressure and shock index (but no catheter-driven care), and nonprotocol usual care chosen by the bedside physician(s). These resuscitative approaches all delivered different care, but all groups received aggressive fluids and pressors in addition to early recognition and antibiotic use; however, **no one approach was superior** in terms of morbidity or mortality. Thus, the ProCESS trial emphasizes that the **early recognition of sepsis, administration of antimicrobials, adequate volume resuscitation, and assessment of the adequacy of circulation are the important elements that improve outcomes, not any specific path of resuscitation**. These observations allow providers or sites the flexibility of crafting the best approach to care but show that mandatory central venous catheterization and monitoring of central venous pressure or S_{CVO2} are not necessary for all patients with sepsis.

VOLUME RESUSCITATION

When resuscitating an ED patient with sepsis, first assess and replenish circulating volume, typically with an initial 20 to 30 milligram/kg crystalloid bolus, preferably through large-bore IVs. This amounts to an approximate 1- to 2-L bolus of saline or lactated Ringer's solution in a 70-kg adult, although some patients require more or less. Saline can produce a hyperchloremic metabolic acidosis if used in large-volume resuscitation, causing some to switch to lactated Ringer's if large volumes are planned. Colloids are not needed in early sepsis care, and hydroxyethyl starch can worsen acute kidney injury.

The most important variable process in volume replacement is determining if a patient is volume responsive. There are several more sophisticated measurements that can be used to make this determination such as cardiac output and stroke volume variation. The latter entails lifting the legs of a supine patient for 60 seconds; improved blood pressure or less variation in the peak blood pressure wave (if an arterial line is present) identifies a volume-responsive patient who will likely benefit from more fluid. If these tools are unavailable, assess the need for further volume expansion with empiric crystalloid boluses until the patient fails to demonstrate a physiologic or hemodynamic response (e.g., rise in systolic or mean pressure, decrease in heart rate, improvement in peripheral pulses or extremity perfusion, increase in urinary output).

VASOPRESSORS

Once the patient fails to respond to further intravenous volume expansion, provide adequate perfusion pressure with vasoactive agents. In general, a mean arterial pressure goal of 65 mm Hg is sought; routine targeting of a higher mean arterial pressure does not aid outcomes, although in some patients, it may be necessary.[50] A mean arterial pressure is preferable to a specific systolic blood pressure goal; however, use of systolic pressure is often preferred by clinicians, who often seek a goal of 90 mm Hg or higher.

Ideally, deliver vasoactive agents through a central venous line to limit extravasation and resultant tissue necrosis. If a central line is unavailable, use a large, secured peripheral IV temporarily for vasopressor administration. In septic shock, **norepinephrine** at a dose of 0.5 to 30 micrograms/min is the best first choice since the dual α- and β-adrenergic effects result in peripheral vasoconstriction and cardiac inotropy. Dopamine has a higher rate of complications, most notably dysrhythmias and failure, compared with norepinephrine and is no longer routinely recommended.[51] **Vasopressin** is a second-line agent and may allow for the down-titration of the norepinephrine dose.[52] Give vasopressin as a constant infusion at a rate of 0.03 or 0.04 U/min. Do not titrate the dose, because higher rates are associated with vasospasm and high morbidity. **Epinephrine** at a dose of 1 to 20 micrograms/min appears safe and equivalent to norepinephrine when dosed appropriately,[53] although the risk of medication dosing errors related to epinephrine concentration may make norepinephrine a superior choice. If tachydysrhythmias are a problem, phenylephrine is an option as a pure α-adrenergic agonist.

CENTRAL VENOUS OXYGENATION

After volume repletion and perfusion pressure optimization, if tissue perfusion appears to continue to be compromised (cool extremities, poor pulses, worsening organ function), one may assess oxygen balance. Although not needed routinely, insertion of a continuous central venous oxygen saturation (S_{CVO2}) measuring catheter can aid additional therapy as outlined in the early goal-directed therapy approach.[41] If S_{CVO2} is less than 70%, it implies a relative oxygen supply and demand mismatch.

LACTATE CLEARANCE

An alternative is to guide therapy through the use of lactate clearance, because a relative decrease in lactate over time suggests a restoration of adequate tissue perfusion. Measure lactate using the same method 1 to 2 hours apart; improvement of 10% or more is associated with improved clinical outcomes.

TREAT INFECTION

Give broad-spectrum antibiotics as early as possible for severe sepsis.[36] Combination antibiotic therapy as opposed to monotherapy leads to improved outcomes, potentially due to higher rates of bactericidal activity.[55] Recommendations for antibiotic regimens are in **Table 151-2.** Therapy can later be tailored based on clinical response and microbiologic data. Given the rising rates of community-acquired methicillin-resistant *S. aureus* (CA-MRSA), ensure this is covered along with gram-negative pathogens and anaerobic organisms. Vancomycin is often underdosed in clinical practice, which can impair recovery[55]; guidelines suggest an initial vancomycin dose of 25 to 30 milligrams/kg in critically ill patients.[56] In immunosuppressed patients, consider antifungal or antiviral agents.

The Surviving Sepsis Campaign recommends giving antibiotics as soon as feasible, ideally within 1 hour of the recognition of severe sepsis and/or within 3 hours of triage. However, these are suggestions, not a standard of care,[36] and these recommendations are often not achievable.[57] Whether antimicrobials are best given initially or only after hemodynamic stabilization of the patient is unclear; given the poor prognosis associated with delays in either resuscitation or infection therapies, we recommend delivering both concurrently. Ideally, sample any organ infectious source and obtain blood cultures *prior* to the initiation of antibiotics, *but do not delay* the initiation of antibiotics to obtain cultures.[36]

Infection control is not confined to antimicrobial administration; it also includes addressing potential surgical sources of infection. Drain any source and remove indwelling vascular lines and other medical devices suspected as infected once the patient is stabilized.

OTHER THERAPIES: VENTILATION, GLYCEMIC CONTROL, ACTIVATED PROTEIN C, AND STEROIDS

Sepsis is the leading cause of acute respiratory distress syndrome. Data from a large study of patients with acute respiratory distress syndrome found that low tidal volume ventilation (6 mL/kg ideal body weight) leads to superior outcomes compared with large (12 mL/kg) volume ventilation,[58] with the latter likely creating barotrauma from overdistension of the alveoli. Thus, low tidal volume ventilation with a positive end expiratory pressure adequate to prevent alveolar collapse is recommended. Although starting at a low tidal volume is recommended,[36] it is unclear whether a fixed volume of 6 mL/kg is best for all; some titration is permissible. To accommodate low tidal volumes, patients may be allowed some hypercapnia as long as the accompanying acidosis does not threaten hemodynamic deterioration.

Multiple trials note a link between hyperglycemia and worsened outcomes in the setting of sepsis, notably in patients without pre-existing diabetes. Although there is evidence of improved outcomes in patients who achieve tight glucose control (target glucose level of 80 to 110 milligrams/dL), the high rate of hypoglycemia occurring with attempts at this targeted glycemia may explain increased harm seen.[59] More modest efforts (seeking blood glucose <180 mg/dL) allow for similar outcomes with less variation.[59] Glucose control is most important after initial care and is best if protocolized, especially for patients receiving extended sepsis care in the ED.

Therapies to manipulate the coagulation cascade are unproven; the most promising candidate to date, activated protein C, failed to improve outcomes and is not used.[60] Systemic corticosteroids are the only anti-inflammatory agent in use in clinical practice but are controversial. Despite early literature suggesting a mortality benefit,[61] recent data failed to confirm these findings.[62] Corticosteroids shorten the time to shock reversal and are adjunctive agents in patients with *refractory* hemodynamic shock (i.e., requiring more than one vasopressor or active upward titration of vasopressors after adequate volume restoration). Stimulation testing using adrenocorticotropic hormone is not clinically helpful. Although even a single dose of etomidate may alter adrenal activity as measured by laboratory tests,[63] there is no clear evidence that the use of etomidate to facilitate endotracheal intubation alters any clinically important outcome.

SPECIAL POPULATIONS

PATIENTS WITH POSITIVE BLOOD CULTURES

There is no consensus for interpretation or management of positive ED blood cultures. Before assessing positive blood culture reports and choosing a plan, you should know local typical pathogens and contaminants along with patient data, including reason for seeking care, past medical history, immune status, and current condition at the time the positive culture was called to the clinician. *Corynebacterium* spp., *Bacillus* spp., and *Propionibacterium acnes* rarely represent true bacteremia or require action. Other pathogens such as viridans group streptococci, enterococci, and coagulase-negative *Staphylococcus* (the most common organism reported on blood culture notifications) may represent a pathogen or require new care in a given patient. In both ambulatory and ED patients, blood cultures are positive in less than 10% of cases, with only one third to two thirds of those cultures representing true bacteremia.[64]

TABLE 151-2 Empiric Antibiotic Selection in Severe Sepsis and Septic Shock

Host	Likely Pathogens	Initial Antibiotic Selection
Adults (nonneutropenic) without an obvious source of infection	*S. aureus,* streptococci, gram-negative bacilli, others	Imipenem, 500 milligrams every 6 h to 1 gram IV every 8 h *or* Meropenem, 1 gram IV every 8 h *or* Doripenem, 500 milligrams IV every 8 h *or* Ertapenem*, 1 gram IV every 24 h *plus* Vancomycin†, 15 milligrams/kg loading dose
Adults (nonneutropenic), suspected biliary source	Aerobic gram-negative bacilli, enterococci	Ampicillin/sulbactam, 3 grams IV every 6 h *or* Piperacillin/tazobactam, 4.5 grams IV every 6 h *or* Ticarcillin/clavulanate, 3.1 grams IV every 4 h
Adults (nonneutropenic), suspected pneumonia	*S. pneumoniae*, methicillin-resistant *S. aureus*, gram-negative bacilli, *Legionella*	Ceftriaxone, 1–2 grams IV every 12 h *plus* Azithromycin, 500 milligrams IV, then 250 milligrams IV every 24 h *plus* Levofloxacin, 750 milligrams IV every 24 h *or* moxifloxacin, 400 milligrams IV every 24 h *plus* Vancomycin†, 15 milligrams/kg loading dose
Adults (nonneutropenic), suspected illicit use of IV drugs	*S. aureus*	Vancomycin†,15 milligrams/kg loading dose
Adults with petechial rash	*N. meningitidis,* RMSF	Ceftriaxone, 2 grams IV every 12 h *or* Cefotaxime, 2 grams IV every 4–6 h *Consider* Addition of doxycycline 100 milligrams IV every 12 h for possible RMSF
Adults (nonneutropenic), suspected intra-abdominal source	Mixture of aerobic and anaerobic gram-negative bacilli	Imipenem, 500 milligrams IV every 6 h to 1 gram IV every 8 h *or* Meropenem, 1 gram IV every 8 h *or* Doripenem, 500 milligrams IV every 8 h *or* Ertapenem, 1 gram IV every 24 h *or* Ampicillin/sulbactam, 3 grams IV every 6 h *or* Piperacillin/tazobactam, 4.5 grams IV every 6 h
Adults (nonneutropenic), suspected urinary source (hospitalized with pyelonephritis)	Aerobic gram-negative bacilli, enterococci	Levofloxacin, 750 milligrams IV every 24 h *or* Moxifloxacin, 400 milligrams IV every 24 h *or* Piperacillin/tazobactam, 4.5 grams IV every 6 h *or* Ceftriaxone, 1–2 grams IV every 12–24 h *or* Ampicillin, 1–2 grams IV every 4–6 h *plus* gentamicin, 1.0–1.5 milligrams/kg every 8 h‡

(*Continued*)

TABLE 151-2 Empiric Antibiotic Selection in Severe Sepsis and Septic Shock (*Continued*)

Host	Likely Pathogens	Initial Antibiotic Selection
Adults (nonneutropenic), suspected urinary source (complicated urinary tract infection/ urinary catheter)	Enterobacteriaceae, *P. aeruginosa*, enterococci, rarely *S. aureus*	Piperacillin/tazobactam, 4.5 grams IV every 6 h *or* Imipenem, 500 milligrams every 6 h to 1 gram IV every 8 h *or* Meropenem, 1 gram IV every 8 h *or* Doripenem, 500 milligrams IV every 8 h *or* Ampicillin, 1–2 grams IV every 4–6 h *plus* gentamicin, 1.0–1.5 milligrams/kg every 8 h‡
Neutropenic adults	Aerobic gram-negative bacilli, especially *P. aeruginosa, S. aureus*	Ceftazidime, 2 grams IV every 8 h *or* Cefepime, 2 grams IV every 8 h *or* Imipenem, 500 milligrams IV every 6 h to 1 gram IV every 8 h *or* Meropenem, 1 gram IV every 8 h *or* Piperacillin/tazobactam, 4.5 grams IV every 6 h *plus* Levofloxacin, 750 milligrams IV every 24 h *or* moxifloxacin, 400 milligrams IV every 24 h *plus* Vancomycin†, 15 milligrams/kg loading dose *and consider* Fluconazole, 400 milligrams IV every 24 h *or* micafungin, 100 milligrams every 24 h
Patients with suspected anaerobic source: intra-abdominal, biliary, female genital tract infection; necrotizing cellulitis; odontogenic infection; or anaerobic soft tissue infection	Anaerobic bacteria plus gram-negative bacilli	Metronidazole, 15 milligrams/kg IV load then 7.5 milligrams/kg every 8 h# *or* Clindamycin, 600–900 milligrams IV every 8 h
Patients with indwelling vascular devices	Coagulase-negative *Staphylococcus*, methicillin-resistant *S. aureus*	Vancomycin†, 15 milligrams/kg loading dose
Patients with potential for *Legionella* species infection		Azithromycin, 500 milligrams IV then 250 milligrams IV every 24 h *or* Erythromycin, 800 milligrams IV every 6 h *should be added to the regimen*
Asplenic patients	*S. pneumoniae, N. meningitidis, Haemophilus influenzae, Capnocytophaga*	Ceftriaxone, 1 gram IV every 24 h up to 2 grams IV every 12 h if meningitis

Abbreviation: RMSF = Rocky Mountain spotted fever.

*Ertapenem has no antipseudomonal coverage and is not recommended in many intensive care units due to concerns of potentiating pseudomonal antimicrobial resistance.

†In most communities in the United States, methicillin-resistant *S. aureus* colonization is extremely high, and consideration should be given to including vancomycin in addition to the antibiotic recommendations given in the table. Although initial vancomycin dosage is typically suggested at 15 milligrams/kg, this results in delayed time to effective antimicrobial activity, and initial dosages of 25 to 30 milligrams/kg have been recommended by some authorities. If the patient has an allergy to vancomycin, linezolid 600 milligrams IV can be substituted.

‡Multiple daily dosing: 2 milligrams/kg load then 1.7 milligrams/kg every 8 h.

#Metronidazole is often prepackaged as 500-milligram bags. Dosing at 500 milligrams IV every 6 or 8 h to approximate the milligram/kg dosing may speed time to antibiotic administration by decreasing pharmacy mixing time.

An important predictor of true-positive first blood culture is persistence of the organism on subsequent culture *if* the latter was done separately (time and location); in a discharged patient, this requires re-evaluation, either in the ED or by another provider. Decisions about antibiotics or admission are guided by the pathogen and clinical grounds: All highly lethal pathogens should receive therapy and admission, whereas some pathogens in blood culture may clear with or without therapy, with a plan made after all current data are assimilated.

POSTSPLENECTOMY PATIENTS

Patients without a spleen are at increased risk for infection with encapsulated species such as *Salmonella* or *Haemophilus influenzae*. Table 151-2 details treatment recommendations of these patients. Although not relevant at the time of initial sepsis care, these patients should have appropriate bacterial immunization following a splenectomy.

NEUTROPENIC FEVER

Due to an impaired immune system, neutropenic patients are at increased risk for developing sepsis and having worse outcomes. Any fever in a neutropenic patient is suspicious for infection, and all patients should have source organ and blood cultures drawn followed by empiric antibiotics. After conferring with an oncologist, some patients may be treated at home with oral broad-spectrum agents (often including a quinolone) *if* they look well and are closely followed; the rest are admitted.

Sepsis Checklist

- In those with signs or symptoms of infection, look for cryptic shock: check vital signs and lactate early and repeat if in doubt. Occult shock is dangerous.
- Give appropriate antimicrobials to patients with suspected sepsis as soon as possible.
- Look hard for the infection source, including getting blood cultures and seeking a surgical or indwelling medical device infection.
- Give at least 1 to 2 L bolus of intravenous crystalloid to hypotensive patients or patients with elevated lactate and monitor the response.
- Recheck resuscitation responses using more than one measure—better vital signs/shock index, improved clinical appearance, decreasing lactate, or improved central venous pressure.
- A central venous catheter is not mandatory to resuscitate most patients, and central venous pressure trends are more important than absolute values.
- Give more fluids if not better and there is no evidence of volume overload. Often, 3 to 5 L are needed in the first 6 hours.
- Administer norepinephrine as the first-line vasopressor to patients with refractory hypotension despite adequate fluid resuscitation.
- Although not mandatory for all, consider central venous pressure and central venous oxygen monitoring to titrate dobutamine and packed red blood cells, and consider corticosteroids in those with refractory shock.

REFERENCES

The complete reference list is available online at www.TintinalliEM.com.

CHAPTER 152

Soft Tissue Infections

Elizabeth W. Kelly
David Magilner

INTRODUCTION

This chapter discusses soft tissue infections in adults; impetigo and other soft tissue infections in children are discussed in chapter 141, "Rashes in Infants and Children."

ANATOMY AND DEFINITIONS

The skin consists of the superficial epidermis, dermis, and deeper subcutaneous tissues including fat (**Figure 152-1**). The lymphatics run parallel with the blood vessels (not shown in the figure). *Cellulitis* is an infection of the dermis and subcutaneous tissues of the skin. Cellulitis is divided clinically as *purulent* or *nonpurulent,* and management of the two types is different.[1,2] Purulent cellulitis is cellulitis with an abscess, or cellulitis with drainage or exudate in the absence of a drainable abscess. Nonpurulent cellulitis has no purulent drainage or exudate and no associated abscess.[1,2] *Erysipelas* traditionally has been defined as a more superficial skin infection involving the upper dermis with clear demarcation between involved and uninvolved skin with prominent lymphatic involvement. However, in many countries, the term *erysipelas* is considered synonymous with *cellulitis.*[2] *Folliculitis* is an infection of the hair follicle, often purulent, but is superficial without involvement of the deeper tissues. *Skin abscesses* are collections of pus within the dermis and deeper skin tissues, potentially involving the subcutaneous tissues. Abscesses should be differentiated from simple cellulitis, because abscesses should be treated with incision and drainage.[1] *Furuncles* (or boils) are single, deep nodules involving the hair follicle that are often suppurative.[2] *Carbuncles* are formed by multiple interconnecting furuncles that drain through several openings in the skin.[2] *Necrotizing soft tissue infections* are necrotizing infections involving any of the soft tissue layers including the dermis, subcutaneous tissues, fascia, and muscle.[3]

CELLULITIS AND ERYSIPELAS

EPIDEMIOLOGY

Cellulitis accounts for approximately 1.3% of all ED visits. General risk factors for cellulitis are listed in **Table 152-1**.[4,5] Risk factors for specific organisms causing cellulitis are listed in **Table 152-2**.[1,4,6-11] Cellulitis is observed more frequently among middle-aged and elderly patients, whereas erysipelas is more common among children and elderly patients.[12] Patient characteristics demonstrate a male predominance (61%) and a mean age of 46 years, and the vast majority of infections involve either the lower or upper extremities (48% and 41%, respectively). Approximately 10% of patients diagnosed with cellulitis are hospitalized, the majority of these patients are over age 64 years.

MICROBIOLOGY

Approximately 80% of cellulitis cases are caused by gram-positive bacteria. Community-acquired Methicillin-resistant *Staphylococcus aureus* (MRSA) is now the most common cause of skin and soft tissue infections presenting to the ED,[6,13] regardless of patient risk factors. The Infectious Diseases Society of America recommends differentiation of purulent from nonpurulent cellulitis (see detailed definitions above) for treatment decisions.[1] MRSA is likely to be the causative agent in purulent cellulitis. For nonpurulent cellulitis, the role of MRSA is unknown, and empirical therapy for β-hemolytic streptococcal infection with β-lactams is recommended.[1,14,15]

Gram-negative aerobic bacilli are the third most common etiology. Other less common pathogens causing cellulitis are listed in Table 152-2 with associated risk factors.

Erysipelas is usually caused by β-hemolytic streptococci.[12] Bullous erysipelas is a more severe form, and can represent synergy with beta-hemolytic streptococci and methicillin-resistant staphylococcal aureus.[16]

PATHOPHYSIOLOGY

Most symptoms of cellulitis are secondary to a complex set of immune and inflammatory reactions triggered by cells within the skin itself. Although bacterial invasion is what triggers the inflammation, the organisms are largely cleared from the site within the first 12 hours, and the infiltration of cells, such as Langerhans cells and keratinocytes, releases the cytokines interleukin-1 and tumor necrosis factor that enhance skin infiltration by lymphocytes and macrophages. The net effect is a rapid clearing of bacteria but with significant inflammatory response.

CLINICAL FEATURES

Cellulitis In cellulitis, the affected skin is tender, warm, erythematous, and swollen, and typically does not exhibit a sharp demarcation from uninvolved skin. Edema can occur around hair follicles that leads to dimpling of the skin, creating an orange peel appearance referred to as "peau d'orange" (**Figure 152-2**). Symptoms develop gradually over a few days. Lymphangitis and lymphadenopathy are seen occasionally in previously healthy patients, but purely local inflammation is much more common. In cases of purulent cellulitis, exudate drains from the wound[1]; an abscess may or may not subsequently form. Systemic signs of fever, leukocytosis, and bacteremia are more typical in the immunosuppressed. Recurrent episodes of cellulitis can lead to impairment of lymphatic drainage, permanent swelling, dermal fibrosis, and epidermal thickening. These chronic changes are known as elephantiasis nostra and predispose patients to further attacks of cellulitis.

Erysipelas In erysipelas, the onset of symptoms is usually abrupt, with fever, chills, malaise, and nausea representing the prodromal phase. Over the next 1 to 2 days, a small area of erythema with a burning sensation develops. As infection progresses, the affected skin becomes indurated with a raised border that is distinctly demarcated from the surrounding normal skin. The "peau d'orange" appearance is also

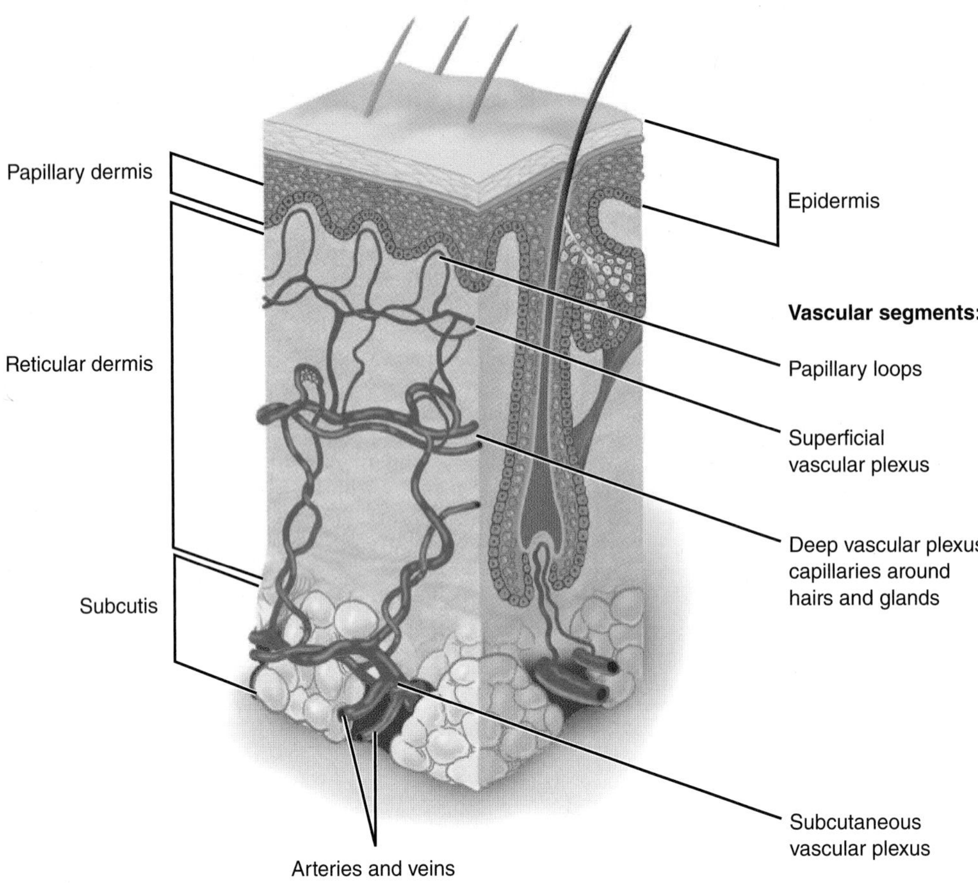

FIGURE 152-1. Schematic diagram of the architecture of the skin. This diagram shows the anatomy of the skin, including the epidermis, dermis, and deeper subcutaneous tissues. Also shown are the blood vessels and a hair follicle. [Reproduced with permission from Wolff et al: *Fitzpatrick's Dermatology in General Medicine*, 7th ed. © 2008, McGraw-Hill, Inc., New York.]

common in erysipelas. A classic description is a "butterfly" pattern over the face (**Figure 152-3**). Complete involvement of the ear is the "Milian ear sign" and is a distinguishing feature of erysipelas because the ear does not contain deeper dermis tissue typically involved in cellulitis. Lymphatic inflammatory changes, known as toxic striations, and local lymphadenopathy are common. Purpura, bullae, and small areas of necrosis warrant a search for possible necrotizing soft tissue infection. On resolution of the infection, desquamation of the site often occurs.

DIAGNOSIS

The diagnosis of cellulitis and erysipelas is clinical. Management should be guided by the clinical differentiation between purulent and nonpurulent soft tissue infections.[1,2] Presence of an abscess defines the soft tissue infection as purulent; purulent cellulitis is defined as cellulitis with drainage or exudate in the absence of a drainable abscess.

Mild disease, for both purulent and nonpurulent forms of cellulitis, is distinguished by the absence of systemic symptoms. In cases of mild infection, blood cultures, needle aspiration, punch biopsy, leukocyte count, or other lab data are of little benefit and are not recommended.[2] Needle aspiration of the leading edge of an area of cellulitis produces organisms in 15.7% of cultures (range, 0% to 40%), and punch biopsy reveals an organism only 18% to 26% of the time.[14] Areas with abscess formation have significantly higher yields; **wound culture** is recommend when the decision has been made to place the patient on antibiotics for purulent cellulitis.[2] Blood cultures are positive in only 5% of cases. For both purulent and nonpurulent cellulitis, in patients with systemic toxicity, extensive skin involvement, underlying comorbidities, immunodeficiency, immersion injuries, failed initial therapy, or recurrent episodes, or in circumstances such as animal bites, cultures of pus, bullae, or blood are recommended.[2,17,18] Routine radiographic evaluation is unnecessary but should be considered if osteomyelitis (see chapter 281, "Hip and Knee Pain") or necrotizing soft tissue infections are suspected (see section below). **Table 152-3** lists differential diagnoses and characteristics that help distinguish cellulitis from the listed disorder.

Bedside US is useful to exclude occult abscess.[19] Doppler studies may be indicated to distinguish lower extremity deep venous thrombosis from cellulitis. The most important diagnosis to exclude is necrotizing soft tissue infection (see section below).

TABLE 152-1 General Risk Factors for Cellulitis and Erysipelas

Risk Factors
Lymphedema
Skin breakdown/site of entry
Venous insufficiency
Leg edema
Obesity
Neutropenia
Immunocompromise
Hypogammaglobulinemia
Chronic renal disease
Cirrhosis

TREATMENT

General Treatment Treatment is elevation of the affected area, incision and drainage of any abscess found (see section below), antibiotics for cellulitis, and treatment of underlying conditions. Elevation helps drainage of edema. Treat skin dryness with topical agents because skin dryness and cracking further exacerbate symptoms. Treat predisposing conditions such as tinea pedis (see chapter 253, "Skin Disorders: Extremities") and refer to primary care for treatment of lymphedema and chronic venous insufficiency.

Treatment for Purulent Cellulitis or Suspected Methicillin-Resistant Staphylococcus aureus See **Table 152-4** for empiric antibiotic recommendations for purulent cellulitis or when MRSA is suspected.[2] Identify

TABLE 152-2 Risk Factors for Specific Organisms Causing Cellulitis

Organism(s)	Risk Factors
Methicillin-resistant *Staphylococcus aureus* (MRSA)	Purulent soft tissue infections Antibiotic use in past month Previous MRSA infection or colonization Patient report of suspected spider bite Previous history of hospitalization or surgery within the past year Residence in a long-term care facility within the past year Hemodialysis Crowded living environments including daycare or homeless shelters, soldiers, prisons Contact sports IV drug users Men who have sex with men Household contacts with MRSA infection Children
β-Hemolytic streptococci	Nonpurulent cellulitis that is culture negative by needle aspiration
Gram-negative bacteria	Elderly patients, cirrhosis, diabetic foot infections, fish bone injury
Aeromonas hydrophila	Fresh water lacerations, contact with wet soil
Vibrio vulnificus, *Vibrio parahaemolyticus*	Salt water lacerations, fish fin or bone injuries, cirrhosis
Pseudomonas aeruginosa	Neutropenia, IV drug use, hot tub exposure
Anaerobic bacteria including clostridia	Bite wounds,* diabetes mellitus, necrotizing infections, gas in tissues
Polymicrobial	Diabetic foot injections, bite wounds*
Pasteurella species	Dog and cat bites*
Capnocytophaga canimorsus	Dog and cat bites*
Mycobacterium marinum	Fish tank exposure
Streptococcus pneumoniae and Haemophilus influenzae	Nonimmunized children and adults

*See chapters 46 and 211-213, "Puncture Wounds and Bites," "Bites and Stings," "Reptile Bites," and "Marine Trauma and Envenomation."

and thoroughly drain an abscess. Bedside US will aid this procedure. Provide empiric therapy for MRSA for patients who have failed initial non-MRSA therapy, those with a previous history of or risks for MRSA, or those who live in an area with a high prevalence of community-associated MRSA infections.[20] For patients with severe infection or systemic toxicity,

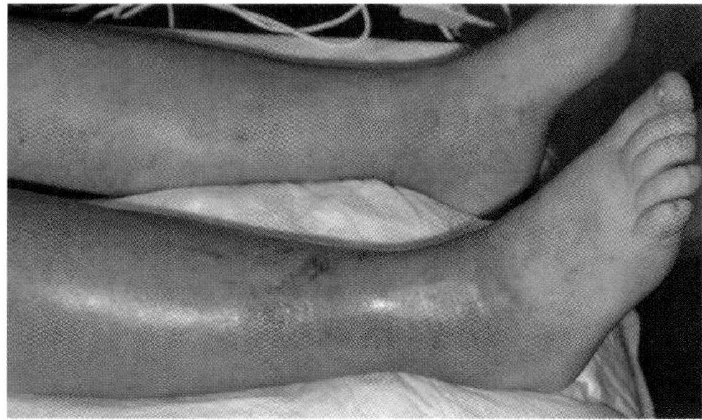

FIGURE 152-2. Cellulitis of the right leg characterized by erythema and mild swelling. [Photo contributed by Lawrence B. Stack, MD. Reproduced with permission from Knoop K, Stack L, Storrow A, Thurman RJ: *Atlas of Emergency Medicine*, 3rd ed. © 2010, McGraw-Hill, New York.]

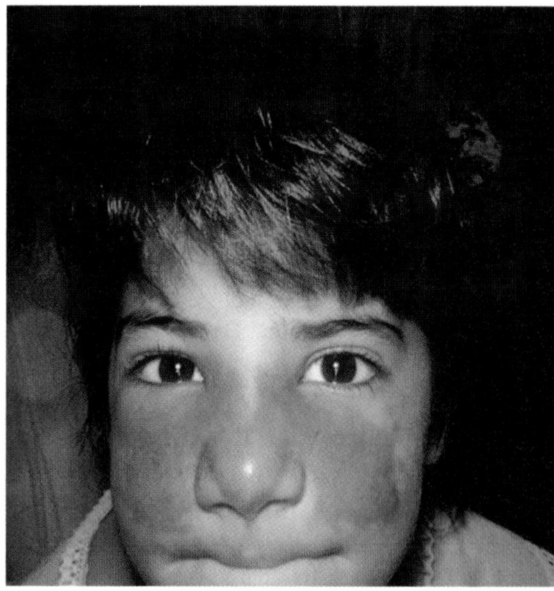

FIGURE 152-3. Butterfly rash of erysipelas. The sharp demarcation between the salmon-red erythema and the normal surrounding skin is evident. [Reproduced with permission from Shah BR, Lucchesi M: *Atlas of Pediatric Emergency Medicine*, © 2006, McGraw-Hill, New York.]

consider necrotizing fasciitis (see later section on necrotizing fasciitis). It may be difficult to clinically distinguish MRSA cellulitis from methicillin-susceptible *S. aureus* cellulitis. Treatment failure rates are similar for both β-lactam antibiotics and MRSA-specific antibiotics such as trimethoprim-sulfamethoxazole.[21,22]

Treatment of Nonpurulent Cellulitis/Erysipelas Guidelines no longer differentiate the treatment of nonpurulent cellulitis from erysipelas.[2] Oral antibiotics are sufficient for simple cellulitis or erysipelas in otherwise healthy adult patients. See **Table 152-5** for guideline-recommended antibiotic options.[2] Consider surgical consultation in patients with bullae, crepitus, pain out of proportion to examination, or rapidly progressive erythema with signs of systemic toxicity, because these signs and symptoms suggest necrotizing infection (see later section on necrotizing fasciitis).

TABLE 152-3 Differential Diagnosis of Cellulitis and Erysipelas

Diagnosis	Distinguishing Clinical Characteristics
Bursitis	Characteristic locations such as suprapatellar or olecranon, may have palpable fluid collection
Contact dermatitis	Pruritus instead of pain, absence of fever, may have bulla, but patient is nontoxic in appearance.
Cutaneous abscess	Abscess may appear similar to cellulitis initially; eventual fluctuance and purulent drainage
Deep vein thrombosis	Typically not associated with skin redness or fever
Drug reactions	Temporal relation to new drug exposure, pruritus instead of pain, absence of fever
Gouty arthritis	Pronounced pain with involved joint movement
Herpes zoster	Characteristic vesicles, dermatomal pattern
Insect stings	Pronounced pain most at onset
Necrotizing soft tissue infection	Rapid progression; triad of severe pain, swelling, and fever; pain out of proportion to exam; severe toxicity; hemorrhagic or bluish bullae; gas or crepitus; skin necrosis or extensive ecchymosis
Osteomyelitis	Deeper involvement, prolonged course, comorbidities
Superficial thrombophlebitis	Typically not associated with fever, limited to venous path
Toxic shock syndrome	Hypotension, multiorgan involvement, severe toxicity

TABLE 152-4 Empiric Antibiotic Treatment of Purulent Cellulitis[*] and/or Soft Tissue Abscess

Guide by Severity of Illness	Antibiotics	Comments
No antibiotics for mild disease: Drainable abscess found with no signs of systemic infection	None required for immunocompetent patients where abscess drainage is complete after procedure	1. Presence of an abscess should be carefully investigated clinically and drained; consider use of US.
Oral antibiotics for moderate disease: Purulent cellulitis* without signs of systemic infection **Or** drainable abscess in the presence of mild to moderate signs of systemic infection ***If*** immunocompromised, see below.	Trimethoprim-sulfamethoxazole double-strength 1–2 tablets twice per day PO for 7–10 d[†] **Or** doxycycline 100 milligrams PO twice per day for 7–10 d[†] **Or** clindamycin, 300–450 milligrams PO four times daily for 7–10 d[†‡]	1. Wound culture is recommended in cases where antibiotics are given. 2. Patients who have failed to improve on outpatient antibiotics or are unable to tolerate oral antibiotics should be admitted to the hospital and receive IV antibiotics; see below.
IV antibiotics for severe disease: Purulent cellulitis* with signs of systemic infection **Or** drainable abscess in the presence of moderate to severe signs of systemic infection[#] or sepsis[ƒ] **Or** an immunocompromised patient	**For MRSA coverage:** Vancomycin 15 milligrams/kg IV every 12 h **Or** linezolid 600 milligrams IV every 12 h[†] **Or** daptomycin 4 milligrams/kg IV every 24 h[†] **Or** telavancin 10 milligrams/kg IV every 24 h[†] **Or** clindamycin 600 milligrams IV every 8 h[†‡]	1. Admit to the hospital. 2. Additional antibiotic coverage is listed below. 3. Consider admission to intensive care unit for patients who meet criteria for sepsis (see also chapter 151, Sepsis). 5. For all patients with severe disease, see later section on necrotizing fasciitis.
Additional coverage for patients with sepsis or for patients with selected indications (see last column to the right)	**For patients with sepsis, or for unclear etiology, add:** Piperacillin-tazobactam, 4.5 grams IV every 6 h[†] **Or** meropenem, 500–1000 milligrams IV every 8 h[†] **Or** imipenem-cilastatin, 500 milligrams IV every 6 h[†]	For **fresh water** exposure (*Aeromonas* species) or for **salt water** exposure (*Vibrio* species) consider adding Doxycycline 100 milligrams IV every 12 hours,[†] plus ceftriaxone 1 gram IV every 24 hours[†]

Abbreviation: MRSA = methicillin-resistant *Staphylococcus aureus*.

[*]Purulent cellulitis is defined as cellulitis with drainage or exudate in the absence of a drainable abscess. In all cases of purulent cellulitis, the presence of an abscess should be carefully investigated clinically and drained. Bedside US can help diagnose occult abscess formation and verify complete drainage after procedure.

[†]Optimal treatment duration has not been established. For mild to moderate disease, 5-day oral treatment regimens have been successful but are recommended only in settings where follow-up at 5 days is feasible.

[‡]Not recommended if local resistance is greater than 10%.

[#]Physicians should use their clinical judgement; there are no validated criteria to differentiate moderate from severe signs for systemic infection.

[ƒ]Criteria for sepsis in the presence of an infection are two or more of the following: temperature >38°C, tachycardia (>90 beats/min), tachypnea (respiratory rate >24 breaths/min), WBC count <400 cells/μL or >12,000 cells/μL), or immunocompromised patients (see chapter 151, Sepsis). Hypotensive patients should be admitted to the ICU.

TABLE 152-5 Empiric Treatment of Nonpurulent Cellulitis[*]/Erysipelas

Guide by Severity of Illness	Antibiotics	Comments
Oral antibiotics for mild disease: Typical cellulitis/erysipelas with no focus of purulence, and no signs of systemic infection	Cephalexin, 500 milligrams PO every 6 h[†] **Or** dicloxacillin, 500 milligrams PO every 6 h[†] **Or** clindamycin, 150–450 milligrams PO every 6 h[†]	Cultures are not recommended because of poor yields.
Monotherapy IV antibiotics for moderate disease: Typical cellulitis/erysipelas with mild to moderate systemic signs of infection‡ ***If*** immunocompromised, see below	Ceftriaxone 1 gram IV every 24 h[†] **Or** cefazolin 1 gram every 8 h[†] **Or** clindamycin 600 milligrams IV every 8 h[†]	Patients who have failed to improve on outpatient antibiotics or are unable to tolerate oral antibiotics should be admitted to the hospital and receive IV antibiotics, with coverage dependant on severity of illness.
Broad-spectrum antibiotics for severe disease (including necrotizing fasciitis): Those with sepsis# or those with clinical signs of deeper infection such as bullae, skin sloughing, hypotension, or evidence of organ dysfunction **Or** an immunocompromised patient	Vancomycin 15 milligrams/kg IV every 12 h[†] **Plus** piperacillin-tazobactam, 4.5 grams IV every 6 h[†] **Or** meropenem, 500–1000 milligrams IV every 8 h[†] **Or** imipenem-cilastatin, 500 milligrams IV every 6 h[†]	1. Consider immediate consultation with surgery for possible debridement (see later section on necrotizing fasciitis for further recommendations). 2. Blood cultures recommended in this treatment group.
Different/additional coverage for patients with selected indications	**Fresh water** exposure (suspected *Aeromonas* species): Doxycycline 100 milligrams IV every 12 h[†] **Plus** ciprofloxacin 500 milligrams IV every 12 h[†] **Salt water** exposure (suspected *Vibrio* species): Doxycycline 100 milligrams IV every 12 h[†] **Plus** ceftriaxone 1 gram every 24 h[†] **Suspected *Clostridium*** species: Clindamycin 600–900 milligrams IV every 8 h[†] **Plus** penicillin 2–4 million units IV every 4 h[†]	1. Consider immediate consultation with surgery for possible debridement (see later section on necrotizing fasciitis below for further recommendations). 2. Blood cultures recommended in this treatment group.

[*]If exudate or abscess is found on exam, the patient should be treated for purulent cellulitis, see Table 152-4 for treatment recommendations

[†]Optimal treatment duration has not been established. For mild to moderate disease, 5-day treatment regimens have been successful but are recommended only in settings where follow-up at 5 days is feasible.

[‡]Physicians should use their clinical judgment; there are no validated criteria to differentiate moderate from severe signs of systemic infection.

[#]Criteria for sepsis in the presence of an infection are two or more of the following: temperature >38°C, tachycardia (>90 beats/min), tachypnea (respiratory rate >24 breaths/min), WBC count <400 or >12,000 cells/mm^3, or immunocompromised state (see chapter 151 "Sepsis"). Hypotensive patients should be admitted to the intensive care unit.

DISPOSITION AND FOLLOW-UP

Admit patients with cellulitis or erysipelas and evidence of systemic toxicity and those with underlying comorbidities such as diabetes mellitus, alcoholism, or immunosuppression (see later section on necrotizing fasciitis). Healthy patients without systemic toxicity can be discharged to home with follow-up and a list of warning signs to prompt return. Follow-up intervals depend on initial presentation, but generally 2 or 3 days are sufficient to evaluate the success of treatment. Mark the patient's skin with an indelible marker along the perimeter of infection so healing can be determined at follow-up; marks also aid the patient in evaluating worsening infection. Reported risk factors for failure of empiric antibiotic therapy include fever, lymphedema or chronic edema, chronic leg ulcers, prior cellulitis in the same area, and cellulitis at a wound site.[23]

CUTANEOUS ABSCESSES, FURUNCLES, AND CARBUNCLES

Furuncles and carbuncles involve the epidermis, and abscesses involve the deeper soft tissue.[2] Skin abscesses, furuncles, and carbuncles can develop in otherwise healthy patients with no risk factors other than skin or nasal carriage of *S. aureus*. Persons in close contact with those who have an active infection with a skin abscess are at increased risk.

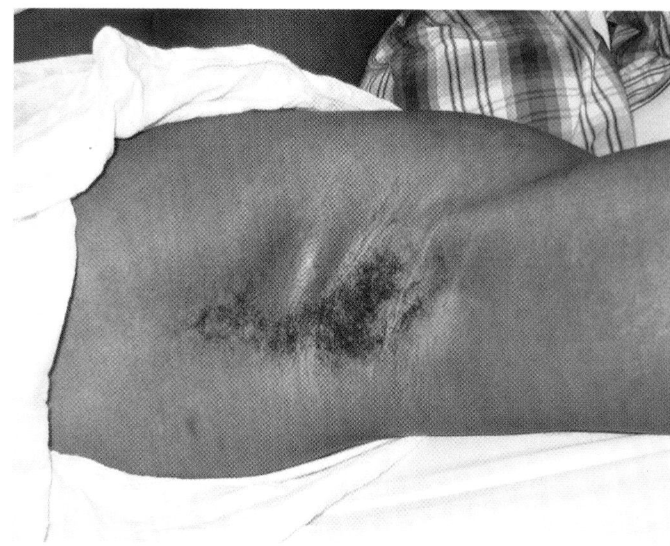

FIGURE 152-4. Subcutaneous abscess is noted in the axilla. [Reproduced with permission from Slaven EM, Stone SC, Lopez FA: *Infectious Diseases: Emergency Department Diagnosis & Management*, © 2006, McGraw-Hill, New York.]

PATHOPHYSIOLOGY

Skin abscesses typically begin as a local superficial cellulitis. Many organisms that colonize normal skin can cause necrosis and liquefaction with subsequent accumulation of leukocytes and cellular debris; however, MRSA causes the majority of skin abscesses presenting to the ED in the United States.[6,13] Loculation and subsequent walling off of these products of infection lead to abscess formation. As the infection progresses and the area of liquefaction increases, the abscess wall thins and ruptures spontaneously, draining either cutaneously or into an adjoining tissue compartment.

Infection can be caused by one or multiple pathogens that typically include skin flora or organisms from adjacent mucous membranes. Pathogens implicated in folliculitis are those that can cause furuncles and carbuncles, namely *Pseudomonas*, *Candida*, and others.

Any process causing a breach in the skin barrier heightens the risk for a skin abscess. Examples include trauma, such as abrasions or shaving; skin foreign bodies; insect bites; and IV drug abuse involving needle injection. Other risk factors for abscess development include diabetes mellitus and immunologic abnormalities. Patients with oral, rectal, or vulvovaginal abscesses are more likely to be infected with multiple organisms, including gram-negative and anaerobic organisms.

CLINICAL FEATURES

Skin abscesses are fluctuant, tender, erythematous nodules, often with surrounding erythema (**Figure 152-4**). Spontaneous drainage of purulent material may occur, and local lymphadenopathy may be present. Signs of systemic toxicity, fever, or chills are rare in the case of simple abscesses. In uncommon cases, skin abscesses may be the result or cause of bacteremia.

Furuncles are clinically very similar to abscesses, and systemic toxicity is rare. Carbuncles are larger infections commonly associated with fever and malaise. Carbuncles are most common on the upper back, chest, buttocks, hips, and axilla but can occur in any hair-bearing region of the body.

DIAGNOSIS

The diagnosis of skin abscesses, furuncles, and carbuncles is clinical; however, physical exam is unreliable for nonsuperficial abscesses.[24] Bedside US is an invaluable tool for distinguishing deep abscess from cellulitis, identifying a foreign body within an abscess, and determining the adequacy of drainage[19,25,26] (**Figure 152-5**).

Radiography is not needed routinely, unless a radiopaque foreign body or underlying osteomyelitis is suspected. Disorders that can mimic abscesses include folliculitis, hidradenitis suppurativa, sporotrichosis, leishmaniasis, tularemia, and blastomycosis, as well as conditions in immunocompromised persons such as *Nocardia* and *Cryptococcus*. Wound cultures are not recommended for simple abscess drainage; however, guidelines recommend cultures when antibiotics are given.[2]

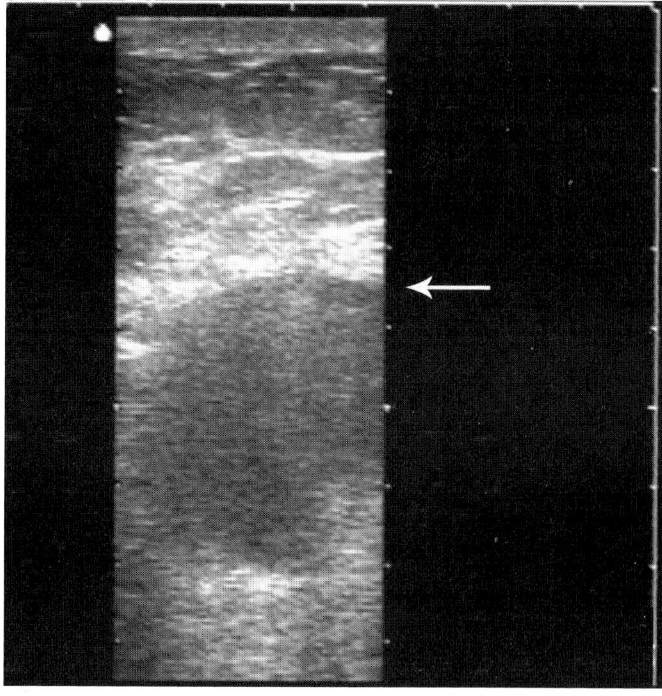

FIGURE 152-5. Long-axis sonogram of a deep midline buttock abscess in the region of the gluteal fold. The skin and immediate subcutaneous tissue exhibit relatively normal echogenicity. The deeper tissues surrounding the rounded abscess cavity appear more hyperechoic and edematous. Note that the superior edge of this large abscess cavity is 3.5 cm from the skin surface (*arrow*). Knowledge of the depth of this abscess cavity was crucial to the individual performing the drainage procedure. [Reproduced with permission from Ma OJ, Mateer JR, Reardon RF, Joing SA: *Ma & Mateer's Emergency Ultrasound*, 3rd ed. 2014, McGraw-Hill Inc., New York. From Chapter 18: Musculoskeletal, Soft Tissue, and Miscellaneous Applications, Figure 18-105, p. 561.]

TREATMENT

It is best to drain extremely large abscesses or those in deep areas in the operating room. Abscesses of the palms, soles, or nasolabial folds can be associated with complications and usually require a specialist.[27] Input from an appropriate specialist is also recommended in areas of the body with cosmetic concerns due to the expected scar formation.[27]

In the case of small furuncles (boils), warm compresses can be used to promote drainage, and no other treatment is needed. Sitz baths are helpful for furuncles in the buttock or perineal regions. Repeat evaluation in 2 to 3 days is best to determine whether suppuration has occurred and surgical drainage is required.

Large furuncles, carbuncles, and skin abscesses require incision and drainage.[28] Simple needle aspiration of abscesses is inadequate to treat abscesses caused by MRSA.[29] Prior recommendations for endocarditis prophylaxis in patients undergoing incision and drainage have changed (see chapter 155, "Endocarditis"). If indicated by the severity of valvular heart disease, the most common regimen is either clindamycin 600 milligrams IV or vancomycin 1 gram IV, 30 to 60 minutes before the procedure.

Incision and Drainage Procedure Before the incision and drainage procedure, obtain consent and explain complications. Use universal precautions, including a face shield with eye protection, because many abscesses are under pressure. There are few complications with superficial abscesses, but these include residual local numbness, the risk of injury to deeper nerves and blood vessels, and poor or delayed wound healing, especially in those with diabetes or peripheral vascular disease. Plan the incision along tension lines to minimize scaring if possible, especially in areas of cosmetic significance.

Position the patient for good access to the abscess. Prepare the area with povidone-iodine solution and drape in a sterile fashion. To provide local anesthesia, approach the abscess from the side and slowly infiltrate the skin over the abscess. Then infiltrate deeper until resistance of the wall of the abscess cavity is overcome. Distend the abscess with several milliliters of lidocaine, taking care to shield the patient and operator from any material forced from the wound due to pressure. The inflamed abscess wall absorbs the lidocaine and lessens pain associated with the procedure.

After appropriate anesthesia, using a No. 11 or 15 scalpel blade, incise the abscess over the area of greatest fluctuance, using the results of preparatory US evaluation to guide the length of the incision. Incisions that are too small or superficial are not likely to provide effective drainage. Express as much pus as possible by gentle compression. Insert a hemostat into the abscess cavity, opening and closing the jaws to break up loculations.

Irrigation of the cavity with saline followed by packing with gauze ribbon to promote drainage is commonly done, but the benefit is uncertain.[30,31] Less painful alternatives to packing include placing a catheter,[32] or tying in a rubber drain after placing two small stab incisions, using a small forceps to reach into one incision, coming out the other, and pulling the drain back through the track before making a knot.[33] Primary closure after abscess drainage shortens healing time for patients treated in the operating room[34] and has been studied in a small randomized controlled trial in the ED;[35] however, recommendations for its use await larger trials.

If placed, maintain packing, catheter, or drain long enough for the cavity to heal from the inside out and to prevent recollection of pus. Patients should apply warm compresses or soaks three times a day. Schedule a follow-up visit in 2 to 3 days for recheck. Maintain catheter or replace packing if the cavity is still draining at the follow-up visit.

Adjuvant Antibiotics Antibiotics are generally unnecessary after incision and drainage of uncomplicated abscesses without significant surrounding cellulitis in healthy patients.[6,36,37] Guidelines recommend antibiotics for patients with multiple lesions, extensive surrounding cellulitis, immunosuppression, or signs of systemic infection; see Table 152-4 for indications and specific antibiotics recommended.[2]

DISPOSITION AND FOLLOW-UP

Most patients with skin abscess, furuncles, and carbuncles are treated as outpatients. Those with systemic toxicity or severe infection may require parenteral treatment and hospital admission. For those discharged to home, remind patients to keep the wound covered and practice frequent hand washing to prevent spread of the infection to household contacts.[28] Patients with open wounds should not participate in activities involving skin-to-skin contacts, such as wrestling or football, until wounds are fully healed. Individuals should not share items such as towels, clothing, soap, razors, or other items that come in contact with a contaminated wound.

NECROTIZING SOFT TISSUE INFECTIONS

Necrotizing soft tissue infections are a spectrum of illnesses characterized by fulminant, extensive soft tissue necrosis, systemic toxicity, and high mortality. Early in their course, these infections can appear deceptively benign.[3,38] Terms used to describe necrotizing soft tissue infections are Fournier's gangrene (see chapter 93, "Male Genital Problems"), necrotizing fasciitis, necrotizing soft tissue infection, or gas gangrene. Risk factors for necrotizing soft tissue infections are advanced age, diabetes mellitus, alcoholism, peripheral vascular disease, heart disease, renal failure, human immunodeficiency virus, cancer, nonsteroidal anti-inflammatory drug use, decubitus ulcers, chronic skin infections, IV drug abuse, and immune system impairment.[39,40] However, infections also occur in young and healthy individuals. The incidence is increasing, but mortality has decreased in the United States from 25% to 10% over the last 20 years.[41] Bacteremia is reported in 25% to 30% of cases and is a strong predictor of mortality. Other patient factors that increase mortality are age <1 year old or >60 years old; IV drug use; comorbid conditions, especially cancer, chronic renal disease, and congestive heart failure; and certain characteristics of the clinical course such as positive blood culture, trunk or perineal involvement, infection related to peripheral vascular disease, and delayed time to diagnosis or treatment.

MICROBIOLOGY

Type I (polymicrobial) infections include 55% to 75% of all necrotizing soft tissue infections, and the causative microbes are a combination of gram-positive cocci, gram-negative rods, and anaerobes. Clostridial infections are now uncommon causes due to improvements in hygiene and sanitation.[38] Type II (monomicrobial) infections are most commonly caused by group A *Streptococcus*. Type II infection is less common (20% to 30%) than type I infection and tends to occur on an extremity in an otherwise healthy host who often has a history of trauma or has had a recent operative procedure at the site of the infection. Community-acquired MRSA is a cause of type II (monomicrobial) infection, particularly in IV drug abusers, athletes, and institutionalized patients.[42,43] Necrotizing infection caused by *Vibrio vulnificus* is classified as a type III infection. This infection is more common in Asia and may occur in patients who have an apparently insignificant break in their skin in a seawater environment. Type IV is associated with fungal infections, primarily in immunocompromised patients.[44]

PATHOPHYSIOLOGY

The rapid necrotizing process typically begins with direct invasion of subcutaneous tissue from external trauma (IV injection, surgical incision, abscess, insect bite, or ulcer) or direct spread from a perforated viscus (usually colon, rectum, or anus). Although spontaneous development is rare, it does occur, and risk factors include diabetes and underlying malignancy. Bacteria proliferate, invade subcutaneous tissue and deep fascia, and release exotoxins that lead to tissue ischemia, liquefaction necrosis, and systemic toxicity.[39]

Skin involvement is secondary to vasculitis and thrombosis of perforating blood vessels. The ischemic tissue environment promotes bacterial growth, propagating the process and resulting in rapid spread of the infection. **Infection can spread as fast as 1 inch/h.** Because thrombosis of large numbers of capillary beds must occur before skin findings develop, early infection has little overlying skin change to indicate the extent of infection.[38] As the disease progresses, widespread gangrene of the skin, subcutaneous fat, fascia, and even skeletal muscle occurs.[39]

In polymicrobial infections, a symbiotic relationship between the different kinds of bacteria seems to promote the necrotizing soft tissue infection. Facultative gram-negative organisms lower the oxygen reduction potential of the tissue and facilitate anaerobic organism growth. Anaerobic organisms impede phagocyte function, favoring aerobic bacterial growth. The alpha-toxin produced by the *Clostridium* species causes tissue necrosis and cardiovascular collapse. *S. aureus* and streptococci produce exotoxins and cause the release of tumor necrosis factor and cytokines that can produce the systemic inflammatory response syndrome and lead to septic shock, organ failure, and death.

The tissue ischemia produced in all such infections impedes immune system destruction of bacteria and prevents adequate delivery of antibiotics.[39] **Thus, antibiotics alone are rarely effective, and immediate surgical intervention remains the cornerstone of successful management.**

CLINICAL FEATURES

Classic symptoms of necrotizing soft tissue infections are severe pain, anxiety, and diaphoresis.[38] Pain is often out of proportion to physical examination findings with tenderness beyond the area of erythema and thus is perhaps the single most important feature to make the diagnosis early. However, some patients may have little pain, and as the condition progresses, the affected areas may become insensate. About 10% to 40% of the time, patients report trauma or a break in the skin roughly 48 hours before onset of symptoms.

On examination, the painful area may demonstrate a brawny edema, and crepitus caused by bacterial gas production may be present. The lack of crepitus does not rule out the diagnosis. Two different studies reported that the only signs present in >50% of patients were erythema, tenderness, or marked edema beyond the area of redness; crepitus was present in only 13% to 31% of patients. Late in the course of the infection, the skin can develop a bronze or brownish discoloration with a malodorous serosanguineous discharge, and bullae may be present (**Figure 152-6**).

Systemic manifestations include a low-grade fever with tachycardia out of proportion to the fever. In fulminant necrotizing infections, particularly from *V. vulnificus*, patients may have cardiovascular collapse due to release of bacterial toxins and release of cytokines, and they may be confused, irritable, or have a rapid deterioration of mental status.

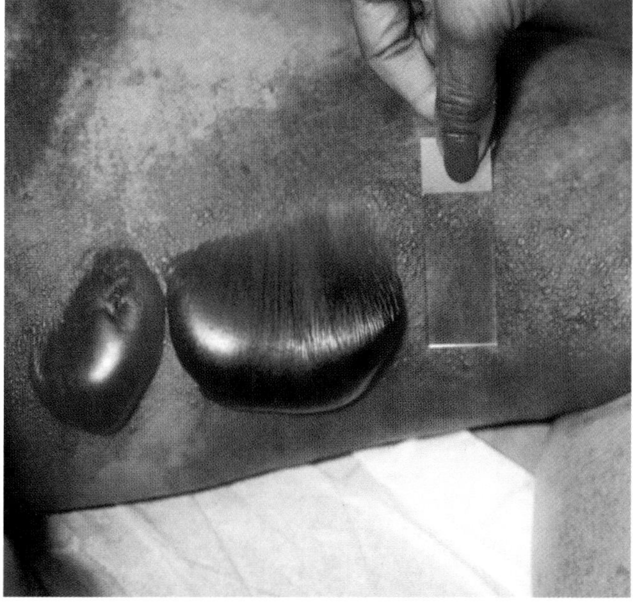

FIGURE 152-6. Necrotizing soft tissue infection. Large cutaneous bullae are seen on the leg of this patient with necrotizing fasciitis. Note the dark purple fluid in the bullae. [Photo contributed by Lawrence B. Stack, MD. Reproduced with permission from Knoop K, Stack L, Storrow A, Thurman RJ: *Atlas of Emergency Medicine*, 3rd ed. © 2010, McGraw-Hill, New York.]

DIAGNOSIS

The diagnosis is based on clinical assessment in combination with laboratory tests and imaging when the clinical picture is unclear. One or more "hard" signs of necrotizing fasciitis—crepitus, skin necrosis, bullae, hypotension, or gas on x-ray—are present in less than half of patients.[45] Many laboratory abnormalities have been investigated to aid in the diagnosis,[46-52] including the laboratory risk indicator for necrotizing fasciitis.[46,47] Since its derivation, the laboratory risk indicator for necrotizing fasciitis has proven to miss many cases of necrotizing fasciitis,[51] especially those cause by *Vibrio* species,[48] and neck infections.[52] **Table 152-6** lists laboratory factors and imaging findings associated with necrotizing fasciitis to help clinicians with medical decision making.[45-55] Clinicians are

TABLE 152-6 Laboratory and Imaging Results Associated with Necrotizing Fasciitis

Laboratory Factors Associated with Necrotizing Fasciitis		
Laboratory Test	**Threshold**	**Comments**
C-reactive protein	>150 milligrams/L	Positive result adds 4 in LRINEC score
WBC count	>15,000 cells/mm³	Positive result adds 1 in LRINEC score, level >25,000 cells/mm³ adds 2
Hemoglobin	<13.5 grams/dL	Positive result adds 1 in LRINEC score,* level <11 grams/dL adds 2 in LRINEC score*
Sodium	<135 mmol/L	Positive result adds 2 in LRINEC score*
Creatinine	>1.6 milligrams/dL	Positive result adds 2 in LRINEC score*
Glucose	>180 milligrams/dL	Positive result adds 1 in LRINEC score*
Potassium	>5.0 mEq/L	Associated with extremity infections
Band count	>7%	Associated with *Vibrio* species
Serum albumin	≤2.0 grams/dL	Associated with *Vibrio* species
Platelets	≤80,000	Associated with *Vibrio* species
Imaging Findings Associated with Necrotizing Fasciitis		
Imaging Test	**Finding**	**Comments**
MRI with contrast	Extensive thickening of the intermuscular fasciae with an appearance suggesting incomplete vascularization	1. Presence of gas is highly specific for necrotizing infection (but not common). 2. Absence of MRI abnormalities of the intermuscular fasciae virtually rules out necrotizing fasciitis.
CT with contrast	1. Fascial thickening of deep facial planes 2. Nonenhancing deep fascia on contrast imaging suggesting necrosis	1. Presence of gas is highly specific, but found in one third of cases or less. 2. Accurate diagnosis requires contrast; acute kidney injury is common in patients with necrotizing fasciitis and may contraindicate IV contrast.
Ultrasonography	1. Fluid collections along the fascial plane 2. Fascia irregularity 3. Subcutaneous air	Radiologists warn that abnormal superficial hyperechogenicity absorbs US and may block diagnostic deeper findings and give false reassurance.
Plain radiographs	Gas in soft tissues	Poor sensitivity

Abbreviation: LRINEC = laboratory risk indicator of necrotizing fasciitis.

*LRINEC score of ≥6 is associated with increased risk of necrotizing fasciitis but misses many cases and therefore should not be used in isolation for the diagnosis and management.

encouraged to consult surgery for possible debridement early when the diagnosis of necrotizing fasciitis is being considered rather than waiting for confirmatory studies that may yield equivocal results. There is no single test or sign that can reliably confirm the diagnosis of necrotizing fasciitis early in the course of this disease process. The finger test has been advocated, which involves making a 2-cm incision over involved tissue down to the fascia after local anesthesia, observing for normal blood flow, and inserting a gloved finger to test for normal tissue firmness.[46] A positive test is lack of normal bleeding, or friable tissue to minimal finger pressure. However, its use has never been studied formally.

Plain x-rays may reveal subcutaneous gas in a minority of patients but may miss deep fascial gas and is therefore a poor screening tool. CT with contrast is more sensitive (80% to 97%) but has a false-positive rate of 19%. The most reliable sign of necrosis on CT is nonenhancing deep tissues, which requires contrast, or gas, seen in only ≤36% of patients.[54] IV contrast is a significant risk in this group of patients who frequently sustain acute renal failure due to sepsis. MRI has better sensitivity (90% to 100%), but false-positive rates are as high as 39%.[55] Finally, MRI imposes significant delays to treatment. Bedside US has been advocated,[53] but radiologists caution against excluding necrotizing fasciitis based its findings.

TREATMENT

Begin aggressive fluid resuscitation immediately. Transfusion of packed red blood cells may be needed to correct anemia from hemolysis. Avoid vasoconstrictors, if at all possible, because vasoconstrictors will decrease perfusion to already ischemic tissue.

Early surgical consultation is indicated for all suspected cases of necrotizing fasciitis. Surgery is the gold standard for diagnosis and treatment. Surgical intervention may include fasciotomy, debridement, and/or amputation. Mortality skyrockets if debridement is delayed >24 hours. See Table 152-5, "Empiric Treatment of Nonpurulent Cellulitis/Erysipelas," the row titled "Broad-spectrum antibiotics for severe disease," for patients with selected indications. Provide tetanus prophylaxis as indicated. Controversial therapies that are typically the decision of the surgical consultant include IV immunoglobulin therapy and hyperbaric oxygen therapy.

OTHER SOFT TISSUE INFECTIONS

FOLLICULITIS

Folliculitis is an inflammation of hair follicles related to infection, chemical irritation, or physical injury to the skin. It typically involves a superficial bacterial infection of the hair follicles with purulent material in the epidermis.

Epidemiology/Microbiology Folliculitis is usually caused by *S. aureus*, and nasal carriage of this organism is a risk factor for folliculitis. "Hot tub folliculitis" or "whirlpool-associated folliculitis" is often attributed to *Pseudomonas* species and occurs in inadequately chlorinated hot tubs, whirlpools, and swimming pools. Symptoms of uncomplicated folliculitis and whirlpool-associated *Pseudomonas* folliculitis are often mild and self-limited, and patients do not seek medical attention.

Individuals exposed to whirlpool footbaths at nail salons are at risk for mycobacterial furunculosis. *Candida* species are implicated in patients receiving broad-spectrum antibiotics or glucocorticoids or who are otherwise immunocompromised.[2]

Clinical Features The most common sites of involvement for folliculitis are the apocrine areas of the upper back, chest, buttocks, hips, and axilla, but folliculitis can develop in any hair-bearing region of the body, especially in areas of repeated shaving. Folliculitis presents with clusters of pruritic, erythematous lesions that are usually <5 mm in diameter, with pustules sometimes present at the centers.[2] Pseudomonal folliculitis can develop over areas exposed to contaminated water, and lesions are often larger (up to 3 cm in diameter).

Pseudofolliculitis is a related noninfectious condition more commonly seen in blacks secondary to shaving. It occurs when the hair follicle becomes trapped and, instead of exiting the follicle, curls and grows into the follicular wall. Such findings in the beard region are called "sycosis barbae" or "folliculitis barbae" and can progress to deep infections that can cause facial scarring (see chapter 250, "Skin Disorders: Face and Scalp").

Diagnosis Folliculitis is diagnosed clinically. It should be differentiated from other disorders, such as acne vulgaris, impetigo, fungal infections, contact dermatitis, scabies, insect bites, and viral disorders such as herpes.

Treatment/Disposition and Follow-Up For simple cases of uncomplicated folliculitis or hot tub folliculitis, stopping exposure or removing the offending agent and twice-daily cleansing with mild hand soap often suffices. Lesions usually resolve spontaneously, but if desired, warm compresses may be applied several times daily, and a topical antibiotic such as bacitracin or polymyxin B can also be used. Shaving should be avoided in the involved areas. Pseudofolliculitis is managed by allowing the hairs to grow 2 to 3 mm above the surface and afterward using commercially available razors designed for this condition. For painful or more extensive cases, oral antibiotics with activity against *Streptococcus* and *Staphylococcus*, such as cephalexin, dicloxacillin, or azithromycin, are recommended.

HIDRADENITIS SUPPURATIVA

Hidradenitis suppurativa is a recurrent, suppurative, and scarring disease of the apocrine glands, most commonly found in the axillae and pubic regions of women and people of African descent. The disorder is neither contagious nor due to poor hygiene. Diagnosis is clinical. Identification and treatment are discussed in chapter 252, "Skin Disorders: Groin and Skinfolds."

PILONIDAL ABSCESS

Pilonidal abscesses are located along the superior gluteal fold. Some think that a pilonidal sinus forms along the gluteal fold possibly at the time of embryogenesis, although others believe it to be an acquired condition secondary to local soft tissue trauma. The sinuses are lined with squamous epithelium and hair, and blockage of the sinus tract with hair and other keratinous material leads to bacterial invasion and infection. The causative organisms typically are normal skin flora, with *Staphylococcus* species being the most common. Contamination with peritoneal and fecal organisms is also possible.

Clinical Features Patients tend to develop symptoms in their late teens and early twenties, and without definitive surgical treatment, they tend to suffer recurrent infections, sometimes developing a chronic draining fistulous tract. Pilonidal abscess is a tender, swollen, and fluctuant nodule located along the superior gluteal fold (**Figure 152-7**).

Treatment ED treatment is incision and drainage, with care taken to remove excess hair and debris from the abscess cavity. See "Incision and Drainage Procedure" given earlier for further recommendations. Antibiotics generally are not needed. Outpatient surgical referral should be recommended for definitive treatment. This typically consists of wide

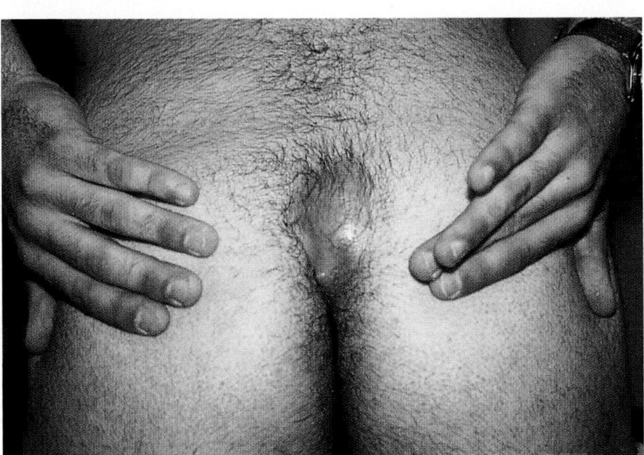

FIGURE 152-7. Pilonidal abscess. Redness, fluctuance, and tenderness in the gluteal cleft are seen with a pilonidal abscess. [Photo contributed by Louis La Vopa, MD. Reproduced with permission from Knoop K, Stack L, Storrow A, Thurman RJ: *Atlas of Emergency Medicine*, 3rd ed. © 2010, McGraw-Hill, New York.]

surgical excision and healing by secondary intention. Surgical treatment, although often successful, may involve difficult wounds and a long healing time. There is a debate in the surgical literature over primary closure versus open healing for pilonidal abscesses. When surgical treatment involves primary closure, wounds heal more quickly but are associated with an increased risk of recurrence.[56] Performing less extensive procedures whenever possible is often in the patient's best interest.

INFECTED EPIDERMOID AND PILAR CYSTS

Epidermoid cysts originate from the epidermis, and pilar cysts originate from hair follicles; both contain a thick, cheesy collection of keratin, not sebum. True sebaceous cysts, as these cysts have erroneously been called in the past, are rare. Sebaceous glands occur diffusely throughout the body. Blockage of the duct of a sebaceous gland may lead to development of a glandular cyst that can exist for a long period without becoming infected. Once bacterial invasion occurs, abscess formation is common. An infected epidermoid or pilar cyst is an erythematous, tender, fluctuant cutaneous nodule. Simple incision and drainage is the appropriate ED treatment. The cyst always contains a capsule that must be removed to prevent further infection. Capsule excision is typically done at follow-up when the initial inflammation has improved or resolved. Occasionally, the wall of the sac can be grasped with a forceps and removed at the time of drainage.

BARTHOLIN GLAND ABSCESS

Bartholin gland abscesses are common in women of reproductive age. An abscess in a perimenopausal woman requires gynecologic follow-up to exclude carcinoma. The Bartholin glands are a pair of pea-sized glands located in the labia minora in the 4 and 8 o'clock positions. They are not palpable if in a noninfected state. Infections are polymicrobial, including vaginal flora, anaerobes, and, in an important minority, *Neisseria gonorrhoeae* and *Chlamydia trachomatis*. Examination of the labia typically reveals a fluctuant 2- to 4-cm mass.

Definitive treatment is marsupialization of the abscess to prevent recurrence. The technique is detailed in **Figure 152-8**. See chapter 102, "Vulvovaginitis" for further discussion.

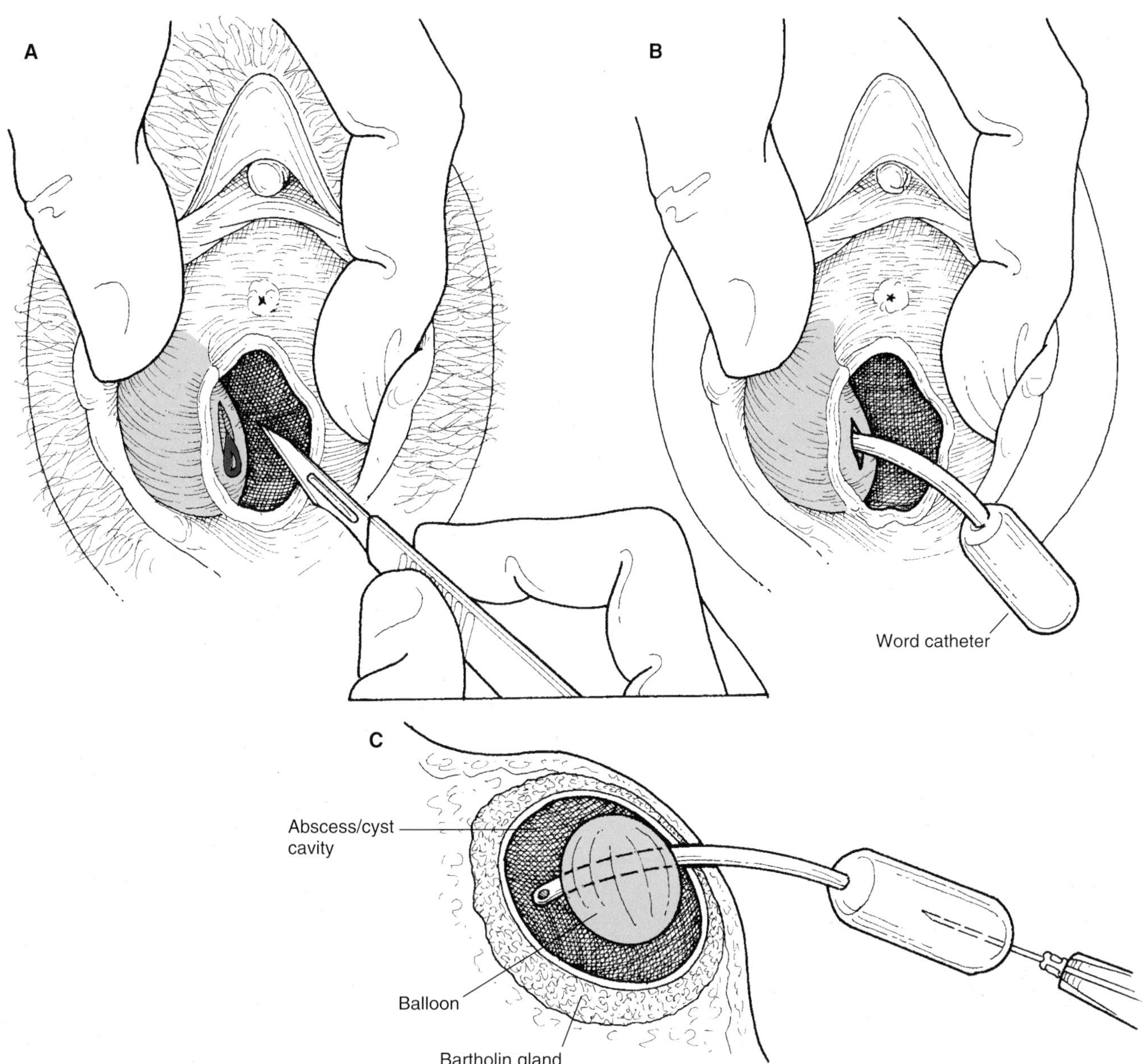

FIGURE 152-8. Incision and insertion of the Word catheter. **A.** Make a 0.5-cm-long stab incision on the mucosal surface of the labia minora. **B.** The cavity has been evacuated and the Word catheter inserted. **C.** The balloon is inflated with saline. [Reproduced with permission from Reichman EF, Simon RR: *Emergency Medicine Procedures*, © 2004, Eric F. Reichman, PhD, MD, and Robert R. Simon, MD.]

PARONYCHIA AND FELONS

Paronychia and felons are discussed in chapter 283, "Nontraumatic Disorders of the Hand."

PERIRECTAL ABSCESSES

Perirectal abscesses are discussed in chapter 85, "Anorectal Disorders."

SPOROTRICHOSIS

Sporotrichosis is a mycotic infection caused by the fungus *Sporothrix schenckii.*

Epidemiology Sporotrichosis occurs worldwide but is most common in tropical and subtropical zones. It is endemic in Central and South America and in Africa. The organism is found most commonly in soil, sphagnum moss, and decaying vegetable matter. It is a common disease among florists, gardeners, and agricultural workers. Inoculation into the host most often occurs when a spine or barb on a plant punctures the skin during handling. Approximately 10% to 62% of patients relate infection to penetrating trauma from plant thorns, wood splinters, or contaminated organic material. The largest outbreak of sporotrichosis in the United States occurred in 1988 and involved 15 states and 84 persons, all of whom handled conifer seedlings shipped in sphagnum moss contaminated with *S. schenckii.*

Transmission from infected animals, especially cats, has been documented. Veterinary workers, animal handlers, and cat owners are therefore at increased risk. The typical patient is a healthy young adult, but the infection can also occur in immunocompromised individuals such as those with alcoholism, diabetes mellitus, hematologic malignancy, organ transplantation, or human immunodeficiency virus infection.

Pathophysiology *S. schenckii* is a thermally dimorphic fungus that changes from its mycelial form to its yeast form on entering a body temperature environment. Disease is usually limited to local cutaneous or lymphocutaneous areas. Osteoarticular involvement, including osteomyelitis, septic arthritis, bursitis, and tenosynovitis, occurs and may extend from a local cutaneous infection or may be secondary to hematogenous spread. Although less common, transmission may occur through inhalation of the fungus through the upper respiratory tract, and subsequent hematogenic dissemination can occur. When inhaled, granulomatous pneumonitis with cavitation may arise.

Clinical Features The incubation period averages 3 weeks following initial inoculation, but varies from a few days to several weeks. After the fungus enters the body through a break in the skin, three types of localized infections may occur. The fixed cutaneous type is characterized by lesions restricted to the site of inoculation and may appear as a crusted ulcer or verrucous plaque (**Figure 152-9**). Local cutaneous type infections also remain local but present as a subcutaneous nodule or pustule. The surrounding skin becomes erythematous and may ulcerate, resulting in a chancre. Local lymphadenitis is common. The lymphocutaneous type is the third and most common type. It is characterized by an initial painless nodule or papule at the site of inoculation that later develops subcutaneous nodules with clear skip areas along local lymphatic channels (**Figure 152-10**). The local reactions in all three types of infections tend to be relatively painless but show no signs of improvement without treatment.

Patients occasionally develop extracutaneous illness from what is most probably hematogenous spread. Most cases of extracutaneous sporotrichosis involve the skeletal system. An indolent form of monoarticular arthritis is the most common symptom. Osteomyelitis, tenosynovitis, and carpal tunnel syndrome are occasionally seen as well. Multiarticular arthritis is usually only seen in patients with immunocompromise. Pulmonary involvement is rare, typically occurring in elderly alcoholic males and clinically resembling tuberculosis. Chronic lymphocytic meningitis can be a delayed complication of sporotrichosis infection and should be considered in patients with chronic meningeal symptoms.

Diagnosis History and physical findings are the keys to diagnosis. Fungal cultures are the best way to isolate the fungus, and tissue biopsy cultures often are diagnostic. Pus, synovial fluid, sputum, blood, or tissue fragment is suitable for culture.

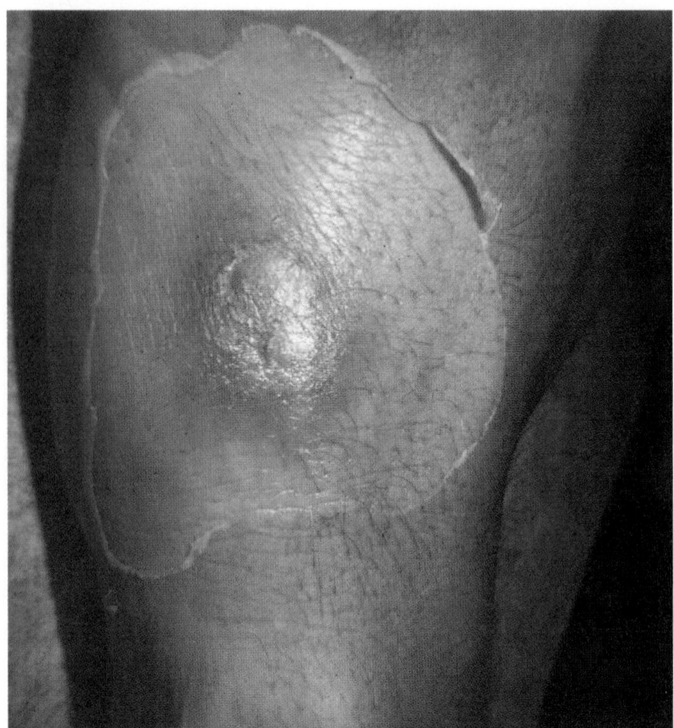

FIGURE 152-9. Fixed sporotrichosis. The ulcer and surrounding erythema of fixed cutaneous sporotrichosis could be confused with a brown recluse spider bite. [Reproduced with permission from Knoop K, Stack L, Storrow A: *Atlas of Emergency Medicine*, 2nd ed. © 2002, McGraw-Hill, New York.]

Routine laboratory tests are nonspecific, but an increased WBC count, eosinophil count, and erythrocyte sedimentation rate may occur. The differential diagnosis includes tuberculosis, subcutaneous abscesses of tularemia, cat-scratch disease, leishmaniasis, staphylococcal lymphangitis, paracoccidioidomycosis, chromoblastomycosis, blastomycosis, bacterial pyoderma, primary syphilis, and infections caused by atypical mycobacteria such as *Mycobacterium marinum.*

Treatment Itraconazole (100 to 200 milligrams daily for 3 to 6 months) is the treatment of choice for localized and systemic infections. Fluconazole is less effective than itraconazole and should be reserved for those few patients not tolerating itraconazole. Ketoconazole has shown even poorer results than fluconazole. IV amphotericin B is effective, but adverse reactions limit its use to disseminated forms of the disease. In endemic regions or in epidemic outbreaks, a saturated solution of potassium iodide is an effective low-cost alternative.

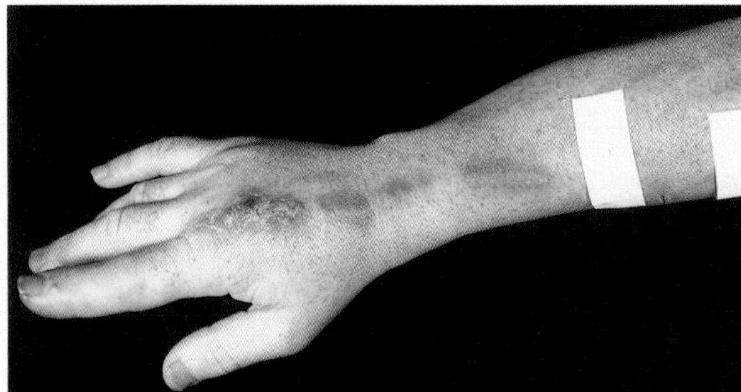

FIGURE 152-10. Sporotrichosis. Chronic lymphocutaneous type—an erythematous papule at the site of inoculation on the index finger with a linear arrangement of erythematous dermal and subcutaneous nodules extending proximally in lymphatic vessels of the dorsum of the hand and arm. [Reproduced with permission from Wolff K, Johnson RA: *Fitzpatrick's Color Atlas and Synopsis of Clinical Dermatology*, 6th ed. © 2009, McGraw-Hill, New York.]

REFERENCES

The complete reference list is available online at www.TintinalliEM.com.

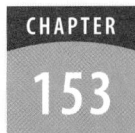

Serious Viral Infections

Sukhjit S. Takhar
Gregory J. Moran

INTRODUCTION

Viral infections are among the most common illnesses encountered in the ED. Although many are self-limited, some are life-threatening, have specific treatments, or have public health implications. We review serious viral infections that cause disseminated illness or have a predilection for the CNS.

INFLUENZA

Human influenza is caused by a large, single-stranded RNA virus from the orthomyxovirus family. Influenza A and Influenza B cause the majority of human infections, with influenza A typically being more serious. Other viruses can cause similar febrile respiratory syndromes, including the coronaviruses linked to severe acute respiratory syndrome and Middle Eastern respiratory syndrome, both emanating from limited geographic areas and associated with high mortality.

EPIDEMIOLOGY

Influenza is highly infectious and is transmitted via aerosolized respiratory secretions, large droplets, or fomites. Seasonal influenza has varying severity, typically striking in the winter months of temperate climates. Seasonal disease causes 250,000 to 500,000 annual deaths worldwide and between 5000 and 50,000 deaths in the United States. Outbreaks spread quickly throughout a community, largely among school-age children. Mortality occurs mostly among the elderly and young infants.

New strains occasionally emerge that can lead to pandemics. The 1918 influenza pandemic killed between 50 and 100 million people worldwide, and the potential for devastation by a novel influenza virus drives anxiety among clinicians and public health personnel. Unlike seasonal influenza, mortality during pandemics occurs mostly among healthy adults. In 2009, a pandemic H1N1 strain emerged in Mexico and followed this pattern, reminding us about the potential danger. A highly pathogenic avian strain of influenza emerged in 1997 in China, which was transmitted from infected chickens to humans. A variety of other animal strains of influenza have since been detected. These remain primarily bird viruses that have not developed the ability for efficient human-to-human transmission.

PATHOPHYSIOLOGY

Influenza is transmitted by respiratory secretions, usually by sneezing or coughing, and via touching hands. The incubation period is typically 1 to 4 days. Influenza viruses undergo minor variations (antigenic drift) in their surface antigens that allow the virus to reinfect individuals and reemerge each winter. Occasionally, there are major antigenic changes (antigenic shift) that increase population susceptibility and lead to a pandemic.

CLINICAL FEATURES

Patients with influenza typically present with an abrupt onset of fevers and respiratory symptoms. Most cases are self-limited; however, some patients, particularly the elderly, the very young, and those with comorbid conditions, require hospitalization or die from complications of influenza. Additionally, influenza can lead to exacerbations of chronic medical conditions, such as congestive heart failure or chronic obstructive lung disease. Delirium is common in the elderly.

TABLE 153-1 Risk Factors for Severe Influenza[3]
Children younger than age 2 years
Adults age 65 years and older
Patients with comorbid conditions
Immunosuppressed
Pregnant patients
Patients younger than 19 years receiving long-term aspirin
American Indians/Alaskan natives
Morbidly obese patients
Residents of nursing homes and long-term care facilities

Pneumonia complicates some influenza infections. Primary influenza pneumonia develops quickly and progresses to acute respiratory distress syndrome, often within 24 hours. Bacterial super-infections also occur. Classically, influenza is associated with secondary *Staphylococcus aureus* pneumonia and, more recently, with community-acquired methicillin-resistant *S. aureus*.

DIAGNOSIS

Most cases of influenza are diagnosed clinically when a patient presents with fever, aches, and cough with influenza virus circulating in the community. However, clinical features of influenza overlap with other respiratory infections; laboratory confirmation can occasionally be helpful in patient care and infection control, especially before influenza has been documented in the community.

Rapid antigen assays identify the surface proteins in influenza A and B. These tests are simple to perform and give results within 15 minutes. However, they can have a low sensitivity, with ranges between 10% and 80% reported in clinical use. Specificity of these tests is between 90% and 95%, so a positive test indicates high likelihood of influenza, especially during an outbreak.

Molecular diagnostic tests, such as polymerase chain reaction for nucleic acids, are available and are more sensitive and specific than antigen tests. They are recommended for patients hospitalized with influenza.[1] Several rapid polymerase chain reaction–based tests return results within the time frame of an ED visit, although they are more costly than rapid antigen tests.

TREATMENT

The majority of patients will have a self-limited, uncomplicated illness requiring only symptomatic care. Patients with more severe influenza may benefit from IV fluids, respiratory support, and occasionally vasopressors. Those with pneumonia should be treated with antibiotics, targeting methicillin-resistant *S. aureus* if severe pneumonia exists.

The benefits of neuraminidase inhibitors for otherwise healthy adults and children are debated;[2] the Centers for Disease Control and Prevention recommend treating higher risk populations. Studies of neuraminidase inhibitors for influenza in uncomplicated cases note benefits limited to patients treated within 48 hours of symptom onset. Antiviral treatment can also benefit patients hospitalized with influenza or bacterial complications of influenza, even if started after 48 hours of illness. Consider empiric antiviral treatment for patients with severe or progressive illness and those with higher risk of complications (**Table 153-1**). Oseltamivir is the most widely used neuraminidase inhibitor (75 milligrams twice daily for 5 days), with longer treatment for critically ill patients. Extracorporeal membrane oxygenation aids those with severe cardiorespiratory dysfunction, especially in pandemic settings where younger patients are afflicted.

HERPES SIMPLEX VIRUS INFECTIONS

Herpes simplex virus type 1 (HSV-1) and herpes simplex virus type 2 (HSV-2) are related double-stranded DNA viruses that cause oral and genital infections; rarely, these create devastating CNS disease. **Herpes simplex infections are treatable with antiviral drugs, making early recognition of serious infection important.**

EPIDEMIOLOGY

HSV is common throughout the world. Transmission occurs when a susceptible individual is exposed to the virus. HSV-1 is usually acquired during childhood through nonsexual contact; HSV-2 is almost always sexually transmitted (see chapter 149, "Sexually Transmitted Infections"). HSV-1 seroprevalence varies by socioeconomic status, age, and geographic location. More than 50% of the U.S. population is seropositive for HSV-1, and 15.7% is seropositive for HSV-2.[4] Rates are higher in developing countries. HSV-1 is one of the most common viral causes of encephalitis in the United States. It occurs most commonly in patients <20 years and >50 years of age.[5] The mortality rate for untreated disease is >70%.

Neonates with HSV infection have a high frequency of both visceral involvement and CNS disease. Encephalitis in neonates is most often caused by HSV-2, which is acquired from the maternal genital tract at the time of delivery. The risk is highest when the mother acquires the infection in the third trimester.

PATHOPHYSIOLOGY

HSVs are transmitted through contact with persons with ulcerative lesions or by those who are shedding the virus by the exchange of saliva, vesicle fluid, semen, and cervical fluid. The virus must come in contact with a mucosal surface or abraded skin, where it replicates and causes localized symptoms before becoming latent in the sensory ganglia. HSV-1 typically resides in the trigeminal ganglia, and HSV-2 is found in the sacral ganglia. Reactivated virus travels to the cutaneous surface and results in localized vesicular eruptions (**Figure 153-1**).

In herpes simplex encephalitis, the virus is thought to gain access to the brain by the olfactory or the trigeminal nerve, with a predilection for the medial and inferior temporal lobes of the brain.

Most healthy hosts are able to control the virus and limit its replication to mucosal surfaces. Rarely during primary infection, the virus can spread beyond the local dorsal root ganglia and cause more widespread involvement. Multiorgan disease is much more common in the immunosuppressed and in neonates.

CLINICAL FEATURES

HSV infections occur year round. Symptoms of HSV depend on multiple factors, including the anatomic site involved, the immune status of the host, virus type, and whether the infection is primary or recurrent. Most HSV infections are subclinical. Symptomatic HSV-1 infection most commonly results in recurrent orolabial lesions, whereas HSV-2 is most often implicated in genital herpes. Primary infections typically produce more extensive lesions involving mucosal and extramucosal sites, often accompanied by systemic signs and symptoms. Gingivostomatitis and pharyngitis are typical manifestations of primary HSV-1 infection (**Figure 153-2**), and recurrence presents as herpes labialis (**Figure 153-3**). Less common skin manifestations include herpetic whitlow and herpes gladiatorum (skin). Eczema herpeticum (see Figure 251-14) can occur in patients with atopic dermatitis. **Bell's palsy** may result from latent HSV-1 in the geniculate ganglia (see chapter 172, "Acute Peripheral Neurologic Disorders"). Herpetic keratitis presents as a painful, red eye, and can be identified by characteristic dendritic lesions on fluorescein slit lamp exam. HSV-1 and HSV-2 can cause identical genital lesions. Genital HSV-2 is more common and has a higher relapse rate, but the proportion of genital disease caused by HSV-1 is increasing.[4] Primary genital infections can present with aseptic meningitis, which is a complication more common in women.

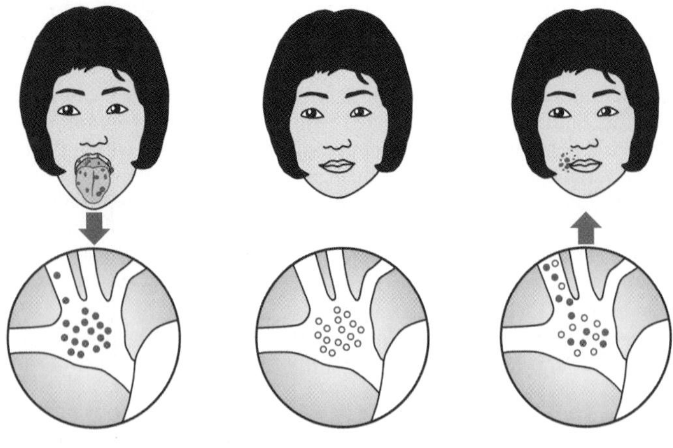

FIGURE 153-1. Herpes simplex virus infection, latency, and recurrence. **A.** Primary infection. **B.** Latent phase. **C.** Recurrence. [Reproduced with permission from Wolff K, Johnson RA: *Fitzpatrick's Color Atlas and Synopsis of Clinical Dermatology*, 6th ed., © 2009 by McGraw-Hill, Inc., New York.]

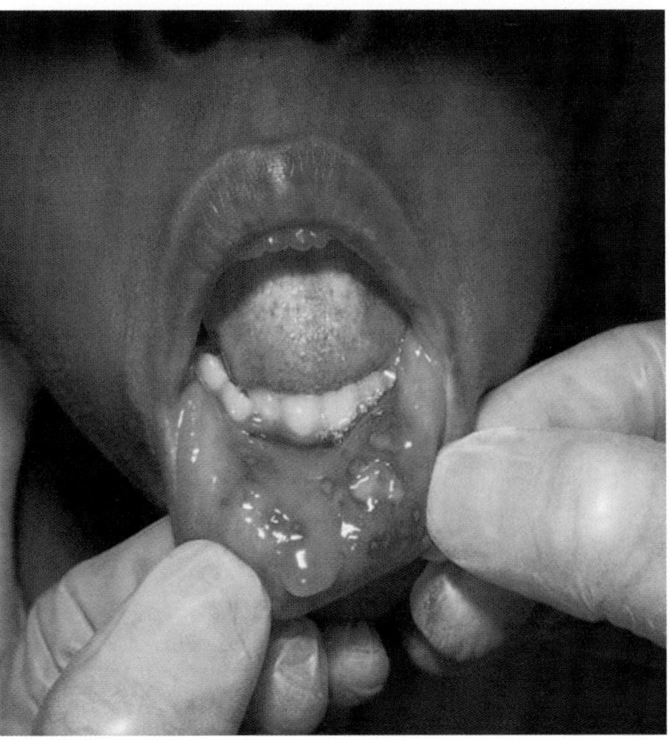

FIGURE 153-2. Primary herpetic gingivostomatitis. Typical lesions of herpes gingivostomatitis on the buccal mucosa. [Reproduced with permission from Shah BR, Lucchesi M: *Atlas of Pediatric Emergency Medicine*, © 2006 by McGraw-Hill, Inc., New York.]

The hallmark of HSV encephalitis is acute onset of fever and neurologic symptoms. Patients can present with hemiparesis, cranial nerve abnormalities, ataxia, focal seizures, and altered mental status or behavioral abnormalities. It can be difficult clinically to distinguish HSV encephalitis from other types of meningoencephalitis. Meningitis occurs in up to 25% of females with primary HSV-2 infections. HSV-2 meningitis, unlike encephalitis, has a benign course, and patients recover uneventfully. Some patients develop recurrent lymphocytic meningitis (Mollaret's syndrome).

HSV infections in immunocompromised hosts can lead to widespread dissemination with multiorgan involvement (**Figure 153-4**). Organ transplant patients may develop esophagitis, hepatitis, colitis, and pneumonia (see chapter 297, "The Transplant Patient"). Severely burned patients are also prone to potentially fatal disease. HSV infections can also cause immune-mediated manifestations such as erythema multiforme, hemolytic anemia, and thrombocytopenia.

DIAGNOSIS

The preferred diagnostic test for confirmation of suspected HSV infection depends on the presentation. Because mucocutaneous infection is lifelong, we recommend laboratory confirmation of the clinical diagnosis. A specimen for viral culture can be obtained from the fluid of an unroofed vesicle. The sensitivity of culture is highest in the early stages

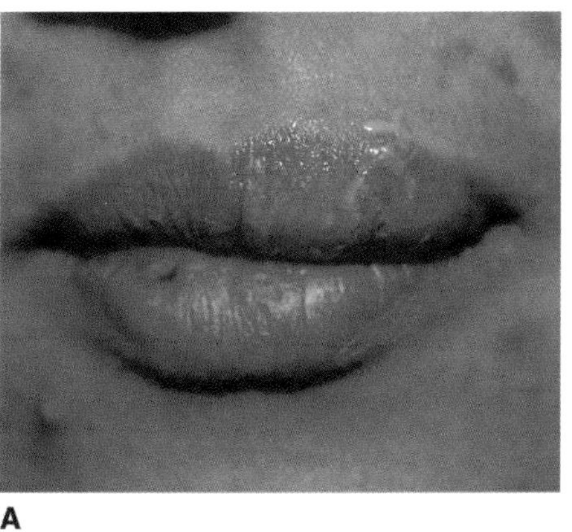
A

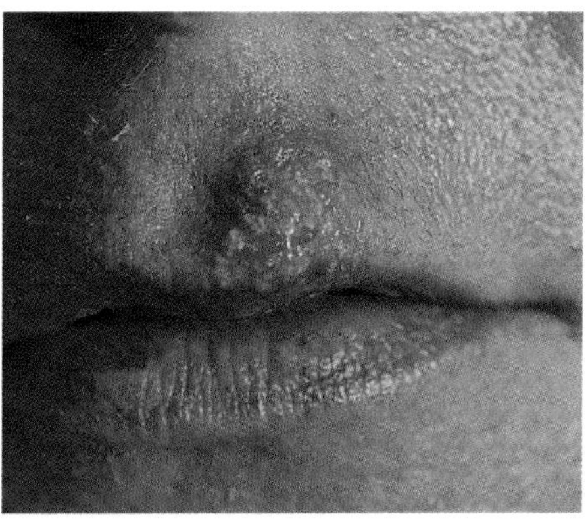
B

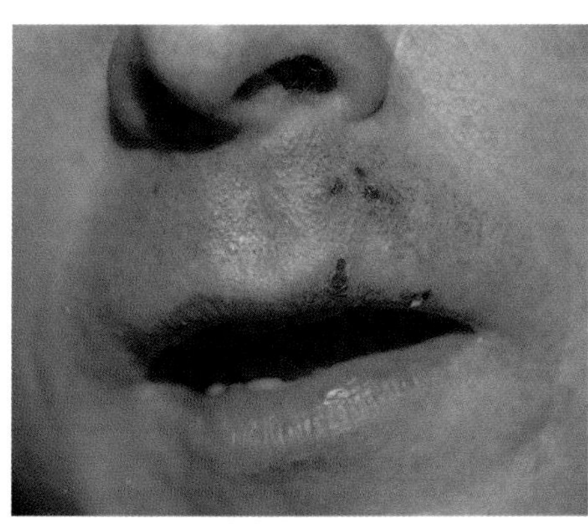
C

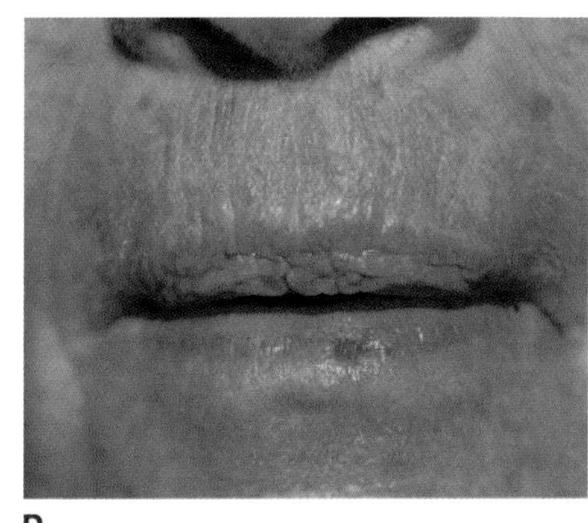
D

FIGURE 153-3. A through D. Herpes labialis. Typical vesicular lesions of the upper and lower lip. [Reproduced with permission from Wolff K, Johnson RA: *Fitzpatrick's Color Atlas and Synopsis of Clinical Dermatology*, 6th ed., © 2009 by McGraw-Hill, Inc., New York.]

and in primary disease. Polymerase chain reaction testing or a direct fluorescent antibody test can be performed on swabbed tissue. A Tzanck test is generally not useful.

Identification of temporal lobe lesions on CT scan or MRI is strongly suggestive of HSV encephalitis (**Figure 153-5**). An electroencephalogram shows typical intermittent, high-amplitude slow waves localized to the temporal lobes.

Cerebrospinal fluid analysis typically shows a lymphocytic pleocytosis with the presence of red blood cells. However, some patients can have normal cerebrospinal fluid parameters. Polymerase chain reaction testing of the cerebrospinal fluid is the testing modality of choice for HSV meningoencephalitis, with high sensitivity and specificity.[5] Viral DNA can be detected within the first 24 hours, and results remain positive for a week or longer. To perform this test, most laboratories need an additional 0.5 to 1.0 mL of fluid beyond that required for standard analysis. Brain biopsy is reserved for difficult cases and for investigation of alternative diagnoses.

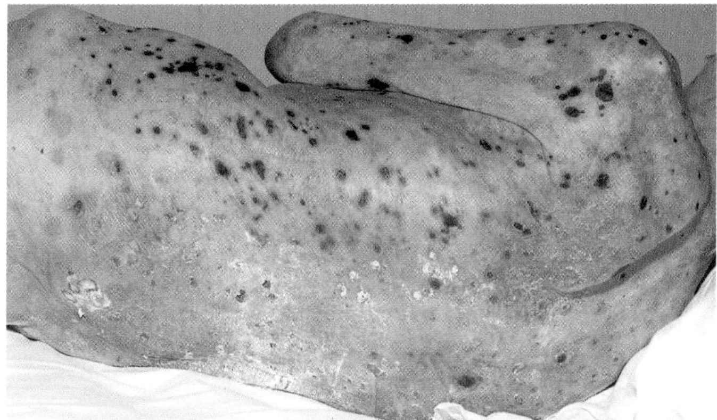

FIGURE 153-4. Disseminated herpes simplex in an immunocompromised host. The rash of disseminated herpes simplex begins as vesicular lesions on an erythematous base, which may umbilicate and may blister and crust over as seen here. [Reproduced with permission from Wolff K, Johnson RA: *Fitzpatrick's Color Atlas and Synopsis of Clinical Dermatology*, 5th ed., © 2005 by McGraw-Hill, Inc., New York.]

TREATMENT

Treatment depends on the severity of the disease and the immune status of the patient (see chapter 149, "Sexually Transmitted Infections"). IV acyclovir is the drug of choice in patients with HSV encephalitis or disseminated disease and in immunocompromised patients with severe mucocutaneous disease (**Table 153-2**). Valacyclovir is a prodrug of acyclovir with higher bioavailability. Famciclovir and valacyclovir require fewer doses per day.

Even with early treatment, patients with HSV encephalitis have a high mortality. Without treatment, mortality is >70%. Survivors are often left with long-term neurologic sequelae. Independent predictors of a poor outcome for patients with HSV encephalitis include a Glasgow Coma Scale score of ≤6, focal CNS lesions on CT scan, increased patient age, and start of antiviral therapy >4 days after onset of symptoms.[5] **Because altered mental status and focal neurologic abnormalities are key features of encephalitis and because it can be clinically difficult to distinguish meningitis from encephalitis, consider adding acyclovir to empiric antibiotic therapy in patients with neurologic findings when the diagnosis of acute bacterial meningitis is also being considered.**[6,7]

Healthy patients with primary HSV-1 or HSV-2 infections can be treated with oral acyclovir, valacyclovir, or famciclovir for 7 to 10 days. Recurrent herpes labialis usually does not require treatment. Those with severe or frequent recurrences may benefit from daily suppressive therapy.

VARICELLA AND HERPES ZOSTER

Varicella-zoster virus is the causative organism of both varicella (chickenpox) and herpes zoster (shingles). It is extremely contagious; prior to routine vaccination, it was usually acquired in childhood.

Varicella occurs year round, but there is a higher incidence during

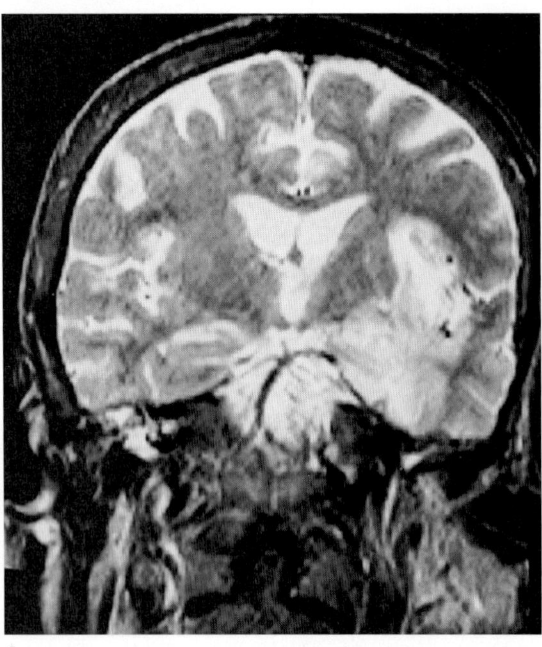

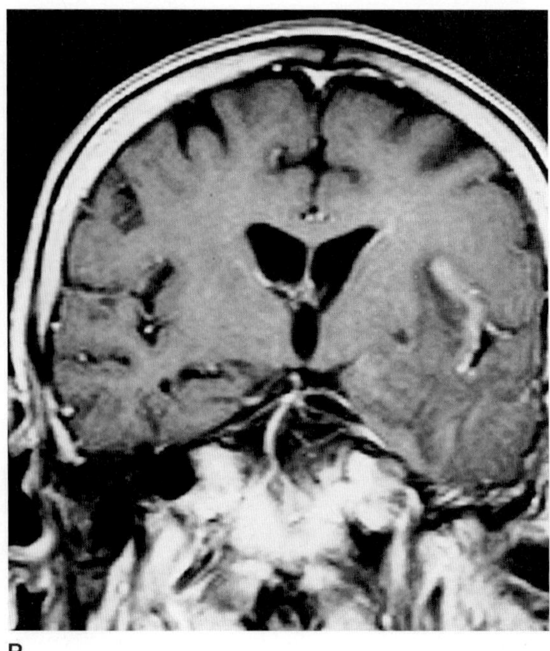

FIGURE 153-5. MRI scans showing hyperintensity involving the left temporal lobe and insular cortex in herpes simplex encephalitis. **A.** T2-weighted coronal MRI scan in the axial plane, taken during the acute stage of the illness. There is increased signal from practically all of the inferior and deep temporal lobe and the insular cortex. **B.** T1-weighted image after gadolinium infusion showing enhancement of the left insular and temporal cortices and early involvement of the right temporal lobe. [Reproduced with permission from Ropper AH, Samuels MA: *Adams and Victor's Principles of Neurology*, 9th ed., © 2009 by McGraw-Hill Inc., New York.]

winter and spring months. The infection rate ranges from 60% to 100% in exposed individuals. The introduction of the varicella vaccine to routine childhood immunizations in 1995 has dramatically reduced the clinical burden of the virus.[8]

Herpes zoster can occur once immune response against the virus wanes, usually with advancing age. Over 90% of adults have serologic evidence of varicella-zoster virus infection, and unvaccinated persons who live to 85 years of age have a 50% risk of herpes zoster.[9] Iatrogenic immune suppression, certain diseases such as lymphoproliferative disorders, human immunodeficiency virus infection, and organ transplantation increase the risk of herpes zoster.

Vaccines are available to prevent both chickenpox and herpes zoster, although neither is 100% effective. Encourage parents to vaccinate their children, and remind those age 60 or older about the availability of a vaccine to prevent herpes zoster. Varicella-zoster immune globulin is available, but its use is generally limited to postexposure prophylaxis for nonimmune pregnant women and the severely immunosuppressed. Healthy individuals who are not immune can be vaccinated after exposure. Exposed individuals should be watched closely, and antivirals should be given to high-risk patients if they develop symptoms.[10]

TABLE 153-2 Antiviral Treatment of Severe Herpes Simplex Virus (HSV) Infection

Infection	Drug	Dosage	Duration
Mucocutaneous HSV infections in immunocompromised patients	Acyclovir	5 milligrams/kg IV every 8 h	7–14 d
	Valacyclovir	500 milligrams–1 gram PO twice per day	
	Famciclovir	500 milligrams PO twice per day	
Herpes simplex encephalitis	Acyclovir	10–15 milligrams/kg IV every 8 h	14–21 d
Neonatal herpes simplex	Acyclovir	10–20 milligrams/kg IV every 8 h	14–21 d
Visceral herpes simplex disease	Acyclovir	10–15 milligrams/kg IV every 8 h	14–21 d

PATHOPHYSIOLOGY

Varicella-zoster virus spreads to the respiratory mucosa of a susceptible host via aerosolized droplets of respiratory secretions of patients with chickenpox. It can also spread from direct contact with vesicle fluid in herpes zoster but is not as highly contagious in this situation. The virus multiplies in regional lymph nodes and then disseminates to the nasopharyngeal surfaces and the skin, causing the characteristic rash. It is contagious until all the lesions have crusted over. Varicella-zoster virus remains latent in the dorsal root ganglion and can later reactivate along dermatomes, resulting in shingles (**Figure 153-6**).

VARICELLA CLINICAL FEATURES

Varicella (chickenpox) is a febrile illness with a vesicular rash. Often it is associated with nonspecific symptoms of headache, malaise, and loss of appetite. The rash is superficial and appears in crops, so patients typically have lesions at varying stages, including papules, vesicles, and crusted lesions (**Figure 153-7**). Lesions are concentrated more on the torso and face and typically crust and slough off after 1 to 2 weeks. Most infections are minor and self-limited. Immunized patients can occasionally develop mild chickenpox.

A range of complications can occur, more often in those at extremes of age or the immunocompromised. Bacterial superinfections of skin lesions, most often with group A streptococci, can cause serious illness including necrotizing fasciitis. Children with lymphoma and leukemia may develop progressive varicella in which vesicles continue to erupt into the second week of illness, sometimes with visceral involvement of the lung, liver, and brain. CNS complications such as cerebellar ataxia, meningitis, meningoencephalitis, and vasculopathy are well described. **Pneumonitis can be severe and is more common in pregnant women.**[8]

HERPES ZOSTER CLINICAL FEATURES

Herpes zoster (shingles) often begins with a prodrome of malaise, headache, and photophobia. The patient notes pain, itching, and paresthesias in one or more dermatomes. These symptoms are followed by the development of a maculopapular rash that becomes vesicular. The eruption does not cross the midline (**Figure 153-8**). Most commonly, herpes

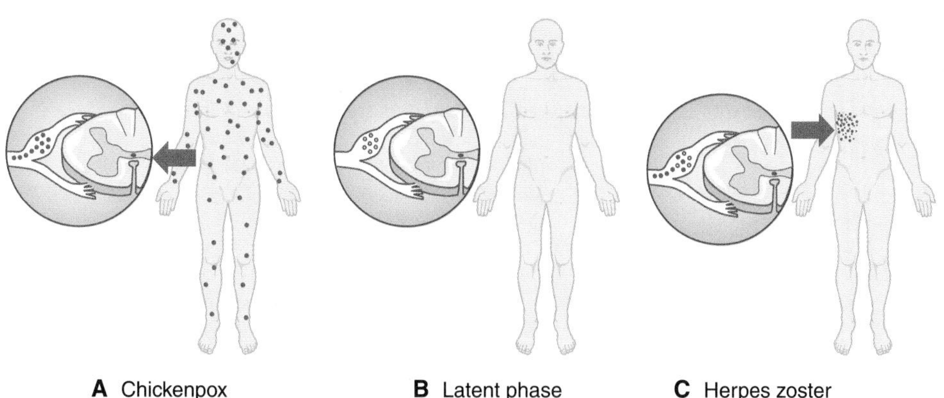

FIGURE 153-6. Primary infection, latency, and reactivation of varicella-zoster virus. **A.** Generalized distribution of primary varicella. **B.** Latent phase. **C.** Reactivation phase of clinical herpes zoster. [Reproduced with permission from Wolff K, Johnson RA: *Fitzpatrick's Color Atlas and Synopsis of Clinical Dermatology,* 6th ed., © 2009 by McGraw-Hill, Inc., New York.]

zoster affects the chest or face, but it can affect any dermatomal level. Herpes zoster ophthalmicus can cause blindness and is the result of reactivation along the ophthalmic distribution of the trigeminal nerve (see chapter 241, "Eye Emergencies"). The seventh cranial nerve can be involved, causing facial nerve paralysis and lesions along the auditory canal (herpes zoster oticus). Postherpetic neuralgia, pain that persists for >30 days, is a feared complication. The incidence increases with advancing age, and pain may last months or years.

Dissemination of varicella-zoster virus can occur in immunocompromised patients. **Herpes zoster involving more than three dermatomes is often a clue to an immunodeficient condition. The presence of herpes zoster in a young, healthy person may be a sign of human immunodeficiency virus infection.** In many cases of disseminated disease, the skin is the only involved structure. However, the virus may spread to the visceral organs and cause pneumonitis, hepatitis, and encephalitis.

DIAGNOSIS

Varicella-zoster virus infections have a characteristic appearance, so a clinical diagnosis is sufficient in most cases. Clinicians should look for the characteristic rash of chickenpox, which involves vesicles that appear in crops in different stages of development. Herpes zoster is diagnosed when clusters of vesicles and papules appear in a dermatomal pattern.

Laboratory diagnosis is needed in patients with atypical illness or severe disease. This is accomplished through viral culture, antigen testing, or polymerase chain reaction testing of vesicle fluid. Although smallpox has been eradicated, it remains a potential threat as a biologic weapon, and the lesions could be confused with those of varicella. The lesions of smallpox are larger and distributed more on the extremities, and all lesions are at the same stage of development.

Obtain a chest radiograph if pneumonitis is suspected. An MRI of the brain, lumbar puncture, and polymerase chain reaction testing for varicella-zoster virus are appropriate for suspected brain involvement.

VARICELLA TREATMENT

Most healthy patients need only supportive care for chickenpox. Acyclovir and similar antiviral agents decrease the number of lesions and shorten the course if therapy is started within 24 hours of rash onset. However, the impact of treatment is modest, so it is not routinely recommended for those who are otherwise healthy. Secondary skin infections are typically caused by group A streptococci and can be treated with a first-generation cephalosporin.

Consider acyclovir for those at higher risk for complications, including adults and children >12 years of age, patients with chronic skin or pulmonary disorders, those receiving long-term salicylate therapy, and immunocompromised patients. Varicella-zoster virus is less sensitive to acyclovir than herpesvirus and requires higher and more frequent dosing. Although chosen by some for dosing simplicity, famciclovir and valacyclovir are not licensed for the treatment of varicella (chickenpox) in the United States.

HERPES ZOSTER TREATMENT

Antiviral agents hasten lesion resolution, reduce new lesions, reduce viral shedding, and decrease acute pain, but **do not reduce the severity of postherpetic neuralgia.**[9] Using antiviral therapy in immunocompromised

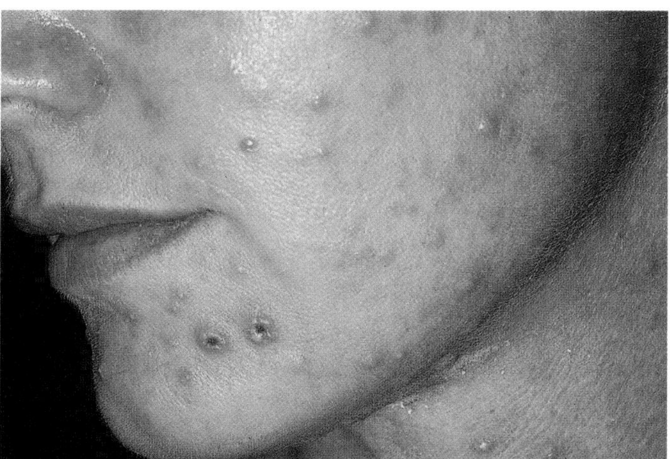

FIGURE 153-7. Rash of primary varicella (chickenpox), demonstrating lesions of multiple stages, including papules, vesicles, and crusted lesions. [Reproduced with permission from Wolff K, Johnson RA: *Fitzpatrick's Color Atlas and Synopsis of Clinical Dermatology,* 6th ed., © 2009 by McGraw-Hill, Inc., New York.]

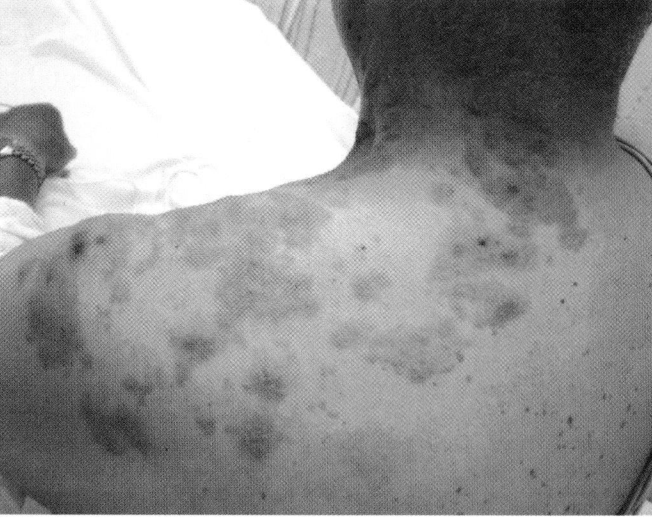

FIGURE 153-8. Dermatome distribution of the classic rash of herpes zoster (shingles).

patients may reduce the risk of severe disseminated disease. **Start antiviral medication within 72 hours of the onset of rash, and consider treatment at >72 hours if new vesicles are still present or developing. Treat immunocompromised patients regardless of the time since rash onset.** Benefits are more pronounced in patients >50 years of age. Therapy is well tolerated, and the risk of adverse events is minimal.

Treat those with disseminated herpes zoster, those with CNS involvement, and severely immunosuppressed patients with herpes zoster with IV acyclovir. Use valacyclovir in those with herpes zoster ophthalmicus, along with ophthalmologist consultation (see chapter 241, "Eye Emergencies").

Herpes zoster can be extremely painful and require opioid analgesia. Corticosteroids in combination with antivirals may provide a modest decrease in acute pain but do not decrease the development of postherpetic neuralgia.[9] **Adjunctive corticosteroids can be considered in older individuals with severe pain who do not have contraindications to their use.**

EPSTEIN-BARR VIRUS INFECTION

Epstein-Barr virus (EBV) is implicated in a variety of human illnesses. It is the causative agent of heterophile-positive infectious mononucleosis. EBV infection is also associated with cancers such as B-cell lymphoma, Hodgkin's disease, Burkitt's lymphoma, and nasopharyngeal carcinoma.

There are two age-related peaks of infection: early childhood and young adulthood. In developing countries, EBV infection is widespread in early childhood and is often asymptomatic. College students and military recruits experience the highest morbidity. EBV requires close contact for transmission. The infection is usually contracted from an asymptomatic individual who sheds the virus.

PATHOPHYSIOLOGY

EBV is transmitted via salivary secretions. After infecting the oropharyngeal epithelium, it disseminates through the bloodstream. The virus infects B lymphocytes and causes an increase in T lymphocytes, which results in enlargement of lymphoid tissue. In immunocompromised patients with decreased T-cell function, the B cells continue to proliferate, and proliferation may lead to neoplastic transformation.

CLINICAL FEATURES

The manifestations of EBV infection depend on age and immune status. Infections in infants and young children are often asymptomatic or have mild pharyngitis. Teenagers and young adults can develop infectious mononucleosis, which presents as fever, lymphadenopathy, and pharyngitis. Tonsillar exudates are frequent and often extensive and may be necrotic appearing (**Figure 153-9**). Splenomegaly occurs in more than half of patients. Symptoms generally resolve over 2 to 3 weeks, and most patients recover uneventfully. Severe fatigue is a prominent feature and can persist for months. **Patients treated with ampicillin or amoxicillin for suspected streptococcal pharyngitis often develop a nonallergic morbilliform rash if they have infection with EBV.**

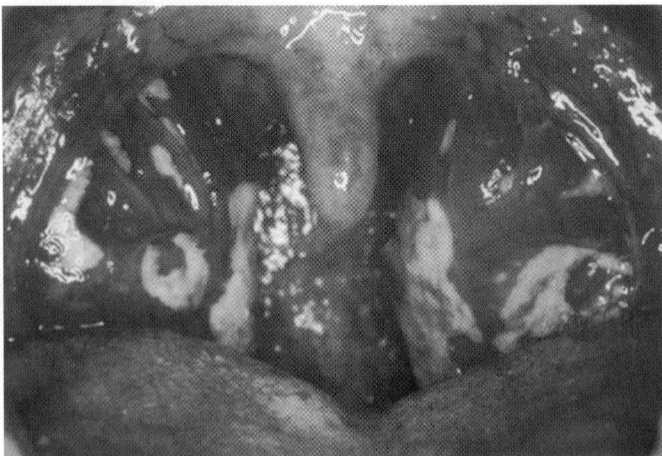

FIGURE 153-9. Classic findings of tonsillopharyngitis associated with infectious mononucleosis caused by Epstein-Barr virus. [Reproduced with permission from Shah BR, Lucchesi M: *Atlas of Pediatric Emergency Medicine,* © 2006 by McGraw-Hill, Inc., New York.]

EBV can affect nearly all organ systems. Neurologic complications such as encephalitis, meningitis, and Guillain-Barré syndrome have been described. Hepatitis, myocarditis, and hematologic disorders are also known complications. Rarely death results from splenic rupture, CNS complications, and airway obstruction. A rare form of chronic EBV infection characterized by a high titer of viral DNA has been reported. Patients are ill for ≥6 months and have histologic evidence of major organ involvement. The prognosis is poor, and treatment is not well defined.

DIAGNOSIS

If infectious mononucleosis is suspected based on the history and physical examination, a CBC and a monospot test can provide confirmation. Typically, there is lymphocytosis with >50% lymphocytes, and atypical lymphocytes are found on examination of the smear. These are reactive cytotoxic T cells that can also be found in other illnesses, including cytomegalovirus infection, human immunodeficiency virus infection, and viral hepatitis. The monospot test identifies heterophile antibodies that agglutinate animal erythrocytes, and a positive result is considered diagnostic of EBV infection in the right clinical setting. The monospot test result may be negative early in the course of disease, requiring a second test later if unclear. The sensitivity of the test is also decreased in infants and the elderly. Testing is particularly important in pregnant patients, because some other causes of heterophile-negative mononucleosis can be teratogenic. Tests for specific antibodies to the EBV viral capsid and nuclear antigen are available but are usually not needed because of the high sensitivity and specificity of the monospot test.

TREATMENT

Rest and analgesia are the mainstays of therapy, with most cases self-limited and not requiring specific therapy. **Use of corticosteroids is associated with increased complications and is recommended only for patients with severe disease, such as upper airway obstruction, neurologic disease, or hemolytic anemia.** Acyclovir is active against EBV but is thought to be effective only for oral hairy leukoplakia associated with human immunodeficiency virus infection. **Advise patients to avoid all contact sports for a minimum of 3 weeks after illness onset to avoid splenic injury.**[11]

CYTOMEGALOVIRUS INFECTION

Cytomegalovirus (CMV) is an important human pathogen that causes a wide variety of diseases, ranging from asymptomatic infections in most to life-threatening pneumonia in transplant patients. Like other herpesviruses, it causes a primary infection and then recedes into lifelong latency.

CMV is not highly contagious, and transmission requires repeated or prolonged exposure. The virus is spread by sexual contact, saliva, breastfeeding, and transplantation, as well as transplacentally and through blood transfusion. Seroprevalence rates approach 100% in Africa and in some Asian countries. In the developed world, it is not unusual for older individuals to acquire a primary infection. This is of particular concern in women of childbearing age because of teratogenic effects. The risk of fetal CMV infection is highest in the first trimester of pregnancy in a previously seronegative mother who acquires a primary infection.

Organ transplant patients can acquire infection, most often between 1 and 4 months after transplant. The risk is highest when a seronegative patient receives a CMV-positive organ.

PATHOPHYSIOLOGY

CMV is usually inoculated on the mucosal surface of the upper respiratory or genital tract, where the virus multiplies and then disseminates. Most infections are only mildly symptomatic. Primary disease in late adolescence and adulthood results in an infectious mononucleosis syndrome. The virus remains latent in most individuals unless immunity is severely suppressed.

CLINICAL FEATURES

Primary infection in healthy individuals is usually asymptomatic. CMV can cause a heterophile-negative infectious mononucleosis syndrome, characterized by prolonged fever, myalgias, and lymphocytosis, but no exudative pharyngitis. Severe disease in the otherwise healthy host includes hepatitis, colitis, Guillain-Barré syndrome, encephalitis, and hemolytic anemia.[12]

Congenital and neonatal infections are associated with some of the most important complications of primary CMV infection. Symptoms in infants can be devastating and include hepatosplenomegaly, jaundice, microcephaly, petechiae, and growth retardation. Severe infections carry a high mortality, and those who survive often have neurologic sequelae.

Infections in immunocompromised patients can be severe and involve any organ. Infection can be primary or the result of reactivation of latent virus. Severe disease can develop in previously healthy CMV-seropositive individuals with an abnormal T-cell response during critical illness. Infections after solid-organ and hematopoietic stem cell transplantation are a leading cause of morbidity (see chapter 297, "The Transplant Patient"). The infection typically begins in the transplanted organ and subsequently may disseminate, causing pneumonia, hepatitis, and CNS involvement. CMV infections can also cause late-onset chronic graft-versus-host disease in stem cell transplant patients. Symptoms often begin with prolonged fever, night sweats, and fatigue.

In human immunodeficiency virus–infected patients with CD4 counts of <50 cells/mm^3, retinitis is the most common manifestation of infection, causing painless loss of vision. Other manifestations associated with human immunodeficiency virus infection include encephalopathy, colitis, and peripheral polyradiculopathy.

DIAGNOSIS

A specific diagnosis is not made in the ED. Body fluids such as urine, saliva, blood, tears, semen, and vaginal fluid can be subjected to antigen testing, polymerase chain reaction testing, antibody testing, histologic analysis, and viral culture. The hallmark of CMV infection on histologic examination is a large cell containing a large basophilic intranuclear "owl's eye" and intracytoplasmic inclusion bodies.

TREATMENT

Several systemic antiviral agents are active against CMV infection, including ganciclovir, valganciclovir, foscarnet, and cidofovir (**Table 153-3**). Illness in the otherwise healthy host is usually self-limited and does not require antiviral therapy. CMV-induced infectious mononucleosis is treated symptomatically.

Transplant recipients with CMV disease are treated more aggressively (see chapter 297). Treatment may include the use of CMV hyperimmune globulin along with ganciclovir or valganciclovir.[13] Ganciclovir implants are available for human immunodeficiency virus patients with CMV retinitis.

TABLE 153-3 Treatment of Cytomegalovirus Disease

Patient Population	Syndrome	Treatment
Healthy host	Heterophile-negative infectious mononucleosis	Symptomatic care
Bone marrow transplant recipient	Pneumonia, GI disease, graft-versus-host disease	IV ganciclovir plus immunoglobulin
Acquired immunodeficiency syndrome patient	Retinitis, GI disease, neurologic disease	IV ganciclovir, valganciclovir
Organ transplant recipient	Pneumonia, GI disorder, infection of transplanted organ, nonspecific febrile illness	IV ganciclovir

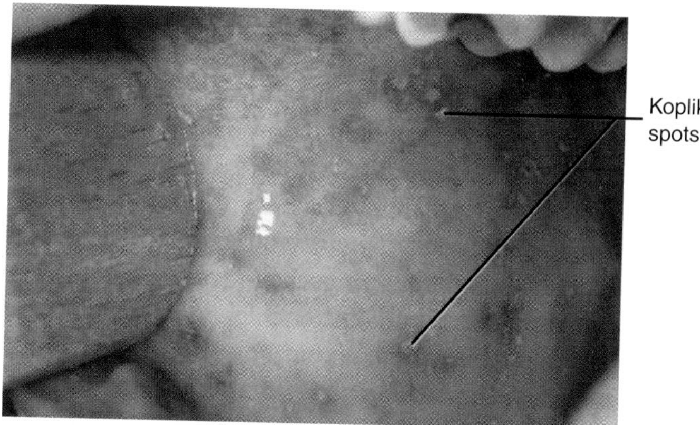

FIGURE 153-10. Oral Koplik's spots on day 3 of measles. [Reproduced with permission from Nester EW, Anderson DG, Roberts CE Jr, Nester MT: *Microbiology: A Human Perspective*, 6th ed. New York: McGraw-Hill, 2008.]

MEASLES

Measles was a common childhood illness before vaccination became routine in the 1960s. Most measles deaths occur among children in developing countries, but developed countries are now seeing occasional outbreaks related to parents choosing not to vaccinate their children, largely due to unfounded fears about vaccine safety. Measles is caused by an RNA virus that is the most infectious virus known to humans and is communicable before symptoms begin. Illness starts with fever, malaise, cough, and runny nose, often with conjunctivitis. Small, white Koplik's spots (**Figure 153-10**) appear on the buccal mucosa early in the illness, followed by a red maculopapular rash that typically starts on the head and spreads throughout the body. **Diagnosis is usually clinical, with pathognomonic Koplik's spots and the characteristic rash.** Measles can be confirmed by detection of immunoglobulin M antibodies, which are present at rash onset. Treatment is supportive, with particular attention to insuring adequate nutrition, especially vitamin A. Mortality in developed countries is less than 1/1000, but can be up to 20% to 30% among infants in developing countries, often from pneumonia.

ARBOVIRAL INFECTIONS

Arboviral infections are infections spread by biting mosquitoes, ticks, and flies. Japanese encephalitis is one of the most common and important causes of encephalitis in the world. The emergence of West Nile virus infection has caused renewed interest in North America regarding epidemic viral encephalitis. This section reviews some of the more important and severe arboviral infections, concentrating on those that occur in North America[14] (**Table 153-4**). Other significant arboviral diseases are discussed in chapter 161, "Global Travelers."

TABLE 153-4 Arboviral Infections in North America

Virus	Geographic Distribution	Groups at Highest Risk
West Nile virus	United States, Canada, Mexico	Elderly adults
St. Louis encephalitis virus	United States, Canada, Mexico	Elderly adults
La Crosse virus	Central, northeastern United States	Children
Eastern equine encephalitis virus	Eastern and Gulf Coast states, eastern Canada	All ages
Western equine encephalitis virus	Western and midwestern United States and western Canada	Infants and elderly adults
Venezuelan equine encephalitis virus	Florida, Texas, Mexico	All ages

EPIDEMIOLOGY

Arboviral infections tend to be seasonal, with increased incidence in warmer months due to the breeding patterns of the arthropod vectors. The major hosts are mammals and birds. When migratory birds are involved, the virus can spread quickly over large distances. Humans are usually an incidental host and acquire the diseases when they venture into areas occupied by the reservoir host.

The age group affected often depends on local prevalence. Japanese encephalitis, which is highly endemic in certain parts of Asia, usually affects children. Most adults have been exposed and are immune. Elderly adults are at risk for St. Louis encephalitis.

Dengue, yellow fever, Rift Valley fever, and chikungunya viruses are among the viruses causing hemorrhagic fever syndromes (see chapter 161). Dengue virus is a common cause of fever and rash (**Figure 153-11**) in tropical areas with large mosquito populations, and transmission has been found in the southern United States. Severe dengue hemorrhagic fever can develop in locals who are exposed to a second infection with a different serotype. Chikungunya fever causes rash, myalgias, arthralgias, and fever. Although fatalities are rare, arthralgias can be debilitating and last for months. The disease is reported in Asia, Africa, and more recently in the Caribbean and southeastern United States. Yellow fever is found in the tropics of Africa and South America. The *Aedes aegypti* mosquito vector for the yellow fever virus was once eradicated in the United States, but it is now starting to reappear. This mosquito can also spread dengue and chikungunya viruses.

Japanese encephalitis virus causes >15,000 deaths yearly, primarily in Asia, and is now spreading to Australia. West Nile virus and the viruses causing La Crosse encephalitis, St. Louis encephalitis, eastern equine encephalitis, and western equine encephalitis are found in North America.[13,14]

PATHOPHYSIOLOGY

A mosquito or other appropriate vector becomes infected after it feeds on the blood of a viremic host. Humans are infected when the arthropod takes a blood meal. The virus replicates near the site of inoculation before it enters the reticuloendothelial system and then disseminates to various target organs.[14,15] There is often a low-grade viremia until the host can produce immunoglobulin M neutralizing antibodies. If the immune system is unable to clear the virus, then the more serious manifestations of hemorrhagic fever or encephalitis may become evident.

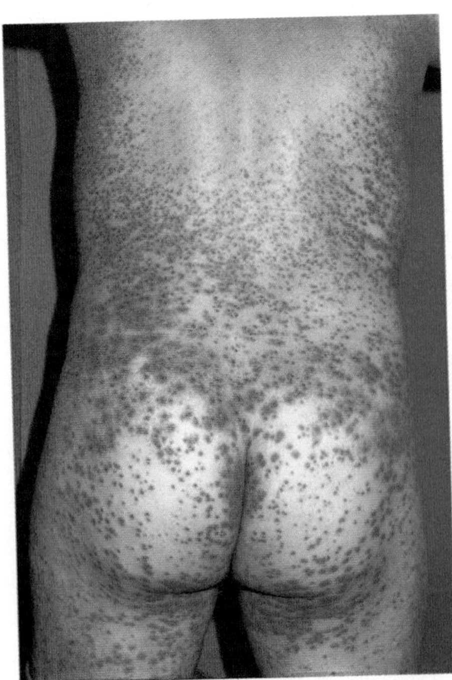

FIGURE 153-11. Maculopapular rash of dengue hemorrhagic fever with areas of dermal hemorrhage, petechiae, and edema. [Reproduced with permission from Wolff K, Johnson RA: *Fitzpatrick's Color Atlas and Synopsis of Clinical Dermatology*, 6th ed., © 2009 by McGraw-Hill, Inc., New York.]

CLINICAL FEATURES

Most arbovirus infections are either asymptomatic or cause a nonspecific mild illness. Only a few individuals develop hemorrhagic fever or encephalitis. **Severe human arboviral diseases most commonly manifest as four syndromes: fever and myalgia, arthritis and rash, encephalitis, and hemorrhagic fever.** These syndromes can overlap; viruses that cause encephalitis and hemorrhagic fever may also cause fever and myalgia. Headache is a common symptom of most arboviral infections and may be quite severe. Hemorrhagic fever presents with bleeding from the gums, petechiae, and GI tract. The classic presentation of viral encephalitis is fever, headache, and altered level of consciousness. Patients can be lethargic and confused and occasionally present with seizures.[14] In general, individuals at extremes of age are more likely to have severe disease.

DIAGNOSIS

Obtaining a detailed travel and exposure history and knowing local epidemiologic patterns help in diagnosing arboviral infections. Patients with encephalitis should undergo CT or MRI of the brain. MRI is more sensitive and may show foci of increased signal intensity in the parenchyma.

Cerebrospinal fluid typically shows a lymphocytic pleocytosis and a slightly elevated protein level, although these findings are nonspecific. When encephalitis is in the differential diagnosis, save an extra vial of cerebrospinal fluid for further testing, because less common infections are often diagnosed only with stepwise testing after more common causes have been ruled out.

Serologic testing is the main method for diagnosis of arboviral infections. Viral cultures are labor intensive and technically demanding. Furthermore, patients are viremic for only a few days after the onset of illness. Generally, immunoglobulin M appears within a few days. Patients who are tested very early in the course of illness may have a false-negative result. A presumptive diagnosis of the suspected arboviral infection can be made based on an elevated immunoglobulin M level, and this can be confirmed with an increase in antibody titers between acute and convalescent samples. Many arboviruses are antigenically similar and cross-react on testing. Arboviral infections are reportable to public health authorities in many areas.[16]

TREATMENT

Symptomatic management is the mainstay of treatment after excluding other serious, treatable causes of meningitis and encephalitis. Antiviral drugs, interferon, and steroids are not useful. Empiric treatment with acyclovir and antibiotics is appropriate until HSV encephalitis and bacterial meningitis are ruled out. Anticonvulsant therapy may be required if seizures occur.

Hemorrhagic fever is also treated with supportive care. Patients with hemorrhagic fever require diligent fluid management to avoid overload.[14,15]

EBOLA VIRUS DISEASE AND OTHER HEMORRHAGIC FEVERS

Viral hemorrhagic fevers are caused by several groups of RNA viruses with varying geographic distributions. These rare diseases elicit tremendous fear among the public and healthcare providers, now exacerbated by the large outbreak in Western Africa. Examples include Hantavirus pulmonary syndromes, Lassa fever, and perhaps the most notorious, Ebola virus disease. Geographic exposure and contact with an infected traveler are the most important clues to suspecting viral hemorrhagic fevers in an individual patient. Clinical presentation varies between viruses, with some causing relatively minor illness and some with high mortality. Symptoms typically begin with fever, myalgia, and malaise, which then progress to GI and other system involvement. Increased vascular permeability results in hypotension, pulmonary edema, and renal failure. Coagulation defects lead to diffuse hemorrhage, which can be worse in patients with thrombocytopenia or platelet dysfunction, sometimes with extensive bleeding, organ damage, and shock. Ebola and most other viral hemorrhagic fevers can be confirmed with acute serology to identify antibodies or, more commonly, reverse transcriptase polymerase chain reaction identification of the virus that is performed at specialized labs such as the Centers for Disease Control and Prevention.

Periodic Ebola virus outbreaks in western Africa have occurred with high mortality. The virus is spread through contact with infected body fluids such as bloody vomit and diarrhea, and the lack of personal protective equipment in developing countries contributes to spread within healthcare facilities.[17] Important aspects of preparing for Ebola and other severe viral hemorrhagic fevers in EDs include screening at triage for illness in travelers returning from areas of current outbreak, and rapid initiation of appropriate isolation. **Ebola and many other viral hemorrhagic fevers require contact and droplet precautions including full gown, gloves, and face mask with eye protection**. Staff should be instructed on proper donning and removal of protective equipment to avoid contamination with body fluids. **It is important to notify the hospital laboratory to take proper precautions and to plan for sending specimens to specialized labs**. Treatment of Ebola and most other VHFs is supportive, with fluids, renal replacement, and respiratory support. Experimental serologic treatments and vaccines are in development.

REFERENCES

The complete reference list is available online at www.TintinalliEM.com.

Human Immunodeficiency Virus Infection

Richard Rothman
Catherine A. Marco
Samuel Yang

EPIDEMIOLOGY

The human immunodeficiency virus (HIV) is the leading cause of infectious disease deaths worldwide. As of 2013, approximately 36 million patients died of HIV-related illnesses, and an estimated 35.3 million people were living with HIV infection/acquired immunodeficiency syndrome (AIDS). Although HIV exists everywhere, the vast majority of new infections (95%) occur in individuals living in low- and middle-income countries. As an example, in sub-Saharan Africa, which is the world's most affected region, nearly 1 in every 20 adults are living with HIV.[1]

Despite the global burden, the number of new HIV infections is falling annually, as are deaths. These improvements result from a global health strategic approach.[2] In 2013, an estimated 1.3 million U.S. citizens had HIV.[3] Despite the overall promising trends, the challenge of reducing new infections persists, with **approximately 50,000 new cases occurring each year in the United States.**

Risks associated with acquiring HIV infection include homosexuality or bisexuality, injection drug use, heterosexual exposure, receipt of a blood transfusion prior to 1985, and maternal HIV infection (risk for vertical and horizontal maternal–neonatal transmission). Rates of HIV attributable to male-to-male sexual contact increased from 55% in 2008 to 62% in 2011. Heterosexual contact accounts for approximately 28% of transmissions, followed by about 8% for injection drug use and 3% for male-to-male sexual contact *and* IV drug use. New HIV infection rates continue to rise among young disadvantaged minority populations (many of whom use the ED for both primary and emergency care). Although African Americans represent only 14% of the total U.S. population, this group accounted for almost half (44%) of new HIV infections in the year 2010. The rate of new infections among black men was the highest of any group by race and sex, notably in men having sex with men. Hispanics also have a higher proportion of new infections (21%) than accounted for by their relative size in the population (14%). Factors associated with the ethnic disparities in HIV include the overall higher prevalence of disease in minority populations, economic barriers that decrease access to testing and treatment, higher rates of incarceration (associated with increased concurrent relationships and higher levels of sexually transmitted infections, both of which increase likelihood of transmissions), and homophobia, which may impede HIV prevention.[4] ED visits by HIV-infected individuals occur at rates higher than the general population[5] due to the characteristics of the populations who use the ED, which are the same groups disproportionately affected by HIV/AIDS.

PATHOPHYSIOLOGY

HIV is a cytopathic retrovirus that kills infected cells. The virus is labile and is neutralized easily by heat and common disinfecting agents such as 50% ethanol, 35% isopropyl alcohol, 0.3% hydrogen peroxide, or a 1:10 solution of household bleach. There are two major subtypes of HIV; HIV-1 is the predominant subtype worldwide and is the cause of AIDS. HIV-2 causes a similar immune syndrome but is restricted primarily to western Africa and is infrequent in the United States, but its incidence is growing.

The HIV virion is a central RNA molecule and a reverse transcriptase protein surrounded by a core protein encased by a lipid-bilayer envelope. After infection, HIV selectively attacks host cells involved in immune function, primarily CD4+ T cells. Within the host cell, HIV-encoded RNA is reverse-transcribed into DNA by the enzyme reverse transcriptase. The viral genome then becomes integrated into the host genome, where it may lie dormant or be actively transcribed and translated to produce virally encoded proteins and new HIV virions. As a result of infection, immunologic abnormalities eventually occur, including lymphopenia, qualitative CD4+ T-cell function defects, and autoimmune phenomena. Defects in cellular immunity ultimately result in development of a variety of opportunistic infections and neoplasms.

HIV exists in saliva, urine, cerebrospinal fluid (CSF), pus, brain, tears, alveolar fluid, synovial fluid, and amniotic fluid. Transmission of HIV occurs through semen, vaginal secretions, blood or blood products, and breast milk, and in utero by transplacental transmission. Transmission does not occur with casual contact. There is only one documented case of transmission from healthcare provider to patient in the United States, which involved an infected dentist in Florida who transmitted the virus to six patients.

NATURAL HISTORY AND CLINICAL STAGES OF HIV INFECTION

Symptoms of acute HIV infection (also called *acute retroviral syndrome*) occur in 50% to 90% of infected patients. The diagnosis is missed in up to 75% of cases due to nonspecific presentation (resemblance to a flulike or mononucleosis-like syndrome) and a lack of suspicion. Symptoms of acute HIV infection usually develop 2 to 4 weeks after exposure and may last for 2 to 10 weeks and include fever (>90%), fatigue (70% to 90%), pharyngitis (>70%), rash (40% to 80%), headache (30% to 70%), and lymphadenopathy (40% to 70%); other reported symptoms are weight loss, headache, and diarrhea.[6]

Seroconversion and detectable antibody response to HIV usually occur 3 to 8 weeks after infection, although delays of up to 11 months have been reported. This phase is followed by a long period of asymptomatic infection, during which patients generally have no findings on physical examination except for possible persistent generalized lymphadenopathy (enlarged lymph nodes in at least two noncontiguous sites other than inguinal nodes). The mean incubation time from exposure to the development of AIDS in untreated patients is estimated at 8.23 years for adults and 1.97 years for children <5 years of age. Virologic studies

TABLE 154-1 Stage 3 AIDS–Defining Opportunistic Illnesses in HIV Infection

Bacterial infections, multiple or recurrent*
Candidiasis of bronchi, trachea, or lungs
Candidiasis of esophagus
Cervical cancer, invasive†
Coccidioidomycosis, disseminated or extrapulmonary
Cryptococcosis, extrapulmonary
Cryptosporidiosis, chronic intestinal (>1 month in duration)
Cytomegalovirus disease (other than liver, spleen, or nodes), onset at age >1 month
Cytomegalovirus retinitis (with loss of vision)
Encephalopathy attributed to HIV
Herpes simplex: chronic ulcers (>1 month in duration) or bronchitis, pneumonitis, or esophagitis (onset at age >1 month)
Histoplasmosis, disseminated or extrapulmonary
Isosporiasis, chronic intestinal (>1 month in duration)
Kaposi's sarcoma
Lymphoma, Burkitt's (or equivalent term)
Lymphoma, immunoblastic (or equivalent term)
Lymphoma, primary, of brain
Mycobacterium avium complex or *Mycobacterium kansasii*, disseminated or extrapulmonary
Mycobacterium tuberculosis of any site, pulmonary†, disseminated, or extrapulmonary
Mycobacterium, other species or unidentified species, disseminated or extrapulmonary
Pneumocystis jirovecii (previously known as *Pneumocystis carinii*) pneumonia
Pneumonia, recurrent†
Progressive multifocal leukoencephalopathy
Salmonella septicemia, recurrent
Toxoplasmosis of brain, onset at age >1 month
Wasting syndrome attributed to HIV

Abbreviations: AIDS = acquired immunodeficiency syndrome; HIV = human immunodeficiency syndrome.

*Only among children aged <13 years. (CDC. 1994 Revised classification system for human immunodeficiency virus infection in children less than 13 years of age. MMWR 1994;43[No. RR-12].)

†Only among adults and adolescents aged >13 years. (CDC. 1993 Revised classification system for HIV infection and expanded surveillance case definition for AIDS among adolescents and adults. MMWR 1992;41[No. RR-17].)

of patients during this period suggest that a steady state of HIV replication and CD4+ T-cell death and replacement exists until increased levels of HIV replication occur. **Variables most predictive of disease stage are viral load and CD4+ T-cell counts,** with a steeper decline in CD4+ T-cell count and a higher viral burden associated with more rapid progression and more outcomes. Other non–HIV-related factors, such as age and malignancy, also impact disease progression.

Early symptomatic infection is characterized by conditions that are more common and more severe in the presence of HIV infection but are not AIDS-indicator conditions. These include thrush, persistent vulvovaginal candidiasis, peripheral neuropathy, cervical dysplasia, recurrent herpes zoster, and idiopathic thrombocytopenic purpura. These conditions occur more often as the CD4+ T-cell count drops below 500 cells/mm^3; if the count drops below 200 cells/mm^3, the frequency of opportunistic infections increases dramatically. HIV infection is classified by the Centers for Disease Control and Prevention as stage 3 (AIDS) by either laboratory evidence or clinical evidence of disease[7] (**Table 154-1**).

DIAGNOSIS

HIV TESTING METHODS

HIV infection is diagnosed using identification of HIV nucleic acid, detection of viral-specific antigen, detection of antibodies to HIV, and isolation of the virus by culture (now rarely used in practice). **The standard and most commonly used testing method for HIV is detection of antibodies to the virus.** Testing involves sequential use of an enzyme-linked immunosorbent assay, followed by a Western blot assay. Enzyme-linked immunosorbent assay is approximately 99% specific and 98.5% sensitive; Western blot testing is nearly 100% sensitive and specific if performed under ideal laboratory conditions. Enzyme-linked immunosorbent assay detects the binding of specific serum antibodies to HIV antigens that are adherent to a microtiter plate. Western blot assay detects HIV antibodies to discrete viral antigens that are electrophoretically separated and transferred to nitrocellulose paper. A positive Western blot result requires detection of at least one gene product, although criteria vary by laboratory. Reasons for indeterminate test results include early seroconversion, cross-reacting antibodies, pregnancy, presence of an autoimmune disease, or technical errors.

Acute HIV is the time from HIV transmission to seroconversion. **Diagnosis of acute HIV infection cannot be made with standard serologic tests** because seroconversion has not yet occurred. Methods for earlier detection of HIV-1 include techniques to detect DNA, RNA, or HIV antigens, although these tests are not always available in the ED. Mean times from transmission to detection are shortest for viral load (17 days), followed by p24 antigen (22 days), enzyme-linked immunosorbent assay positivity (25 days), and Western blot positivity (31 days).[8]

BENEFITS OF EARLY DIAGNOSIS

Although acute HIV infection is not diagnosed in up to 75% of all cases, the benefits of early recognition allow an opportunity to limit risk of further transmission (key in this high viral load period) and to start antiretroviral therapy to potentially reduce symptoms and slow disease progression.[8] For patients in whom acute HIV infection is suspected but not confirmed (i.e., those with a high-risk profile presenting with fever of unknown origin and/or a syndrome suspicious for acute seroconversion), counseling and urgent referral from the ED to an outpatient follow-up setting for appropriate testing are best.

RAPID HIV TESTS

As of 2012, there were eight rapid HIV tests approved for use by the U.S. Food and Drug Administration.[9] The first approved point-of-care rapid HIV test was Orasure HIV-1/2®, and it is the only one that uses oral fluid. Sensitivity and specificity are comparable with those of standard serologic testing, and minimal training is required for administration. Relay any point-of-care results to the patient as *preliminary positive* if reactive, confirming with Western blot testing. Negative test results may miss patients in the window period before seroconversion has occurred; this requires a repeat test at 3 months.

THE NEW HIV TESTING ALGORITHM

In June 2014, the Centers for Disease Control and Prevention released new recommendations regarding laboratory testing practices for HIV.[10] The new algorithm calls for use of automated testing for antibody to HIV-1 and HIV-2 simultaneously with detection of HIV-1 p24 antigen, permitting detection of acute infections. In instances where this set of tests is negative, no further testing is advised, and the patient is counseled that he or she tested negative. For those tests with positive results, follow-up testing differentiates HIV-1 and HIV-2. In cases where the differentiation test is negative, a nucleic acid amplification test confirms acute seroconversion. Turnaround time for the combined assay and HIV-1/2 differentiation assay is about 60 minutes. Turnaround time for confirmatory testing with nucleic acid amplification can take up to a few days. This new algorithm allows better early detection; ED-based studies show this is feasible and will detect new, acutely infected patients.[11,12]

CD4+ T-CELL COUNTS

CD4+ T-cell counts of <200 cells/mm^3 and a viral load of >50,000 copies/mm^3 are associated with increased risk of AIDS-defining illnesses. These indices are also frequently used by the primary care physician or HIV specialist as indicators for initiation of antiretroviral therapy (although the threshold value for initiation of treatment is controversial). When this information is unavailable or the stage of disease is unknown, the total lymphocyte count approximates the CD4+ T-cell count. In a recent ED study, a total lymphocyte count <1700 cells/mm^3 had a sensitivity of 95% for a CD4 count of <200 cells/mm^3.[13]

HIV TESTING PRACTICES IN THE ED

Time limitations, cost, difficulty with follow-up, confidentiality requirements, and questions regarding reimbursement are barriers to HIV testing in the ED. The Centers for Disease Control and Prevention 2006 HIV testing guidelines[14] offer a streamlined approach with decreased requirements for pretest counseling and use of opt-out testing (in which no separate written consent is required). State variability exists for both opt-out versus opt-in approaches and documentation requirements for informed consent. The U.S. Preventive Services Task Force gave a "Grade A" recommendation for routine HIV screening for all people age 15 to 65, as well as younger adolescents and older adults who are at an increased risk for HIV infection and all pregnant women, including those in labor whose HIV status is unknown. The Patient Protection and Affordable Care Act requires new insurance policies to pay for preventive services with "Grade A" recommendation.

American College of Emergency Physicians policy recognizes the need for ED HIV testing based on clinical need and supports screening with caveats. Currently, ED HIV testing in the United States remains relatively low (~0.2% of all ED visits), but programs are increasing, particularly in urban and/or academic centers. Determination of which of several approaches (e.g., nontargeted universal vs targeted) is most rational for ED practice is an area of active research, with local prevalence playing a role in the screening plan chosen.

CLINICAL FEATURES AND TREATMENT

INITIAL CARE: GENERAL CONSIDERATIONS

The spectrum of disease caused by HIV infection varies, from those coming to the ED with asymptomatic infection for symptoms unrelated to HIV disease, to symptomatic patients seeking care from involvement of virtually any organ system and with multiple coexisting symptoms. This makes the ED evaluation and diagnosis of HIV-positive patients challenging.

Maintain confidentiality regarding HIV-related diagnoses in the ED. Begin care without discrimination and without assuming any illness trajectory unless advanced directives, including cardiopulmonary resuscitation, are already in place.

Always use universal precautions (in some hospitals termed *standard precautions*). Healthcare workers are often exposed to the blood and body fluids of HIV-infected patients or patients at high risk of harboring the HIV virus. ED-based studies have demonstrated that substantial numbers of patients continue to have unsuspected HIV infection and that HIV seropositivity cannot be predicted accurately, even after assessment of risk factors.

Occupational exposure is covered in the chapter 162, "Occupational Exposures, Infection Control, and Standard Precautions." Testing, treatment, and follow-up are discussed. Other resources for information on HIV exposures are the Centers for Disease Control and Prevention and the University of California, San Francisco National Clinicians' Post-Exposure Prophylaxis Hotline (888-448-4911, http://www.nccc.ucsf.edu).[15]

Focus the history taking and physical examination on identifying the clinical stage of disease to direct attention to the most likely complications. Obtain a thorough report of past and current medications and previous infections, and ask about the patient's ability to perform activities of daily living. A directed exam seeks findings of organ involvement related to the chief complaint. Physical findings that might specifically assist with staging include the presence of oral candidiasis, skin lesions, temporal wasting, and dementia.

Diagnosis and treatment are directed toward recognition of infection (when not previously diagnosed), assessment of the severity of disease, identifying specific organ(s) involved, and institution of therapy. For the most up-to-date information and details on drug dosing, sources include the Centers for Disease Control and Prevention Web site[16] or the Johns Hopkins University School of Medicine guide to care of the HIV-positive patient.[8]

Consultation with an infectious disease specialist and others with expertise in HIV infection is often necessary to provide proper therapy and disposition. Disposition decisions are based on the need for inpatient evaluation or management and the patient's ability to function as an outpatient, which is often driven by oral intake and ambulation ability and availability of appropriate medical follow-up. Healthcare and family resources can aid decision making about care.

Systemic symptoms such as fever, weight loss, and malaise are common in HIV-infected patients and account for the majority of HIV-related ED presentations.[8] In the ED, look for systemic infection, malignancy, drug toxicity, or metabolic abnormalities. This is done by assessing serum electrolytes with renal function, CBC, liver function studies, blood cultures, urinalysis and urine culture, hepatic function tests, and chest radiograph; serologic testing for syphilis, cryptococcosis, toxoplasmosis, cytomegalovirus infection, and coccidioidomycosis is deployed more selectively. Lumbar puncture is needed after neuroimaging if headache, altered sensorium, visual change, or other focal neurologic symptoms or signs are present.

When treating the febrile ill-appearing HIV patient, provide fluid resuscitation, prompt empiric antibiotics, and admission for further evaluation and management. Outpatient evaluation and treatment are indicated only when all of the following conditions are met: the source of the fever does not dictate admission, the patient is able to function adequately at home (e.g., can maintain sufficient oral intake), and timely medical follow-up can be arranged.

HIV STAGE AND CAUSES OF FEVER

Infections are the most common cause of hospitalization among HIV-infected persons. In HIV-infected persons without obvious localizing signs or symptoms, sources of fever vary by stage of disease. Patients with CD4+ T-cell counts of >500 cells/mm^3 generally have causes of fever similar to those in nonimmunocompromised patients, whereas those with CD4+ T-cell counts between 200 and 500 cells/mm^3 are most likely to have early bacterial respiratory infections. For patients with CD4+ T-cell counts of <200 cells/mm^3, the most common causes of fever without obvious localizing findings are early *Pneumocystis jirovecii pneumonia* (formerly known as *Pneumocystis carinii*); central line infection; infection with *Mycobacterium avium* complex, *Mycobacterium tuberculosis*, or cytomegalovirus; drug fever; and sinusitis. Other causes of fever include endocarditis, lymphoma, and infection with *Histoplasma capsulatum* or *Cryptococcus neoformans*. Fever caused by HIV infection alone tends to occur in the afternoon or evening and generally is responsive to antipyretics.

Disseminated *M. avium* complex infection occurs predominantly in patients with CD4+ T-cell counts of ≤100 cells/mm^3 and not on **antiretroviral therapy** or azithromycin prophylaxis. Persistent fever and night sweats are typical symptoms. Associated symptoms include weight loss, diarrhea, malaise, and anorexia. Dissemination to the bone marrow, liver, and spleen results in anemia and elevated alkaline phosphatase levels. Diagnosis may be made by acid-fast stain of stool or other body fluids or by blood culture. Cultures using the lysis-centrifugation method are more sensitive for *M. avium* complex (and histoplasmosis) and should be ordered for patients with late-stage disease and fever of unknown origin. Treatment for *M. avium* complex reduces bacteremia and improves symptoms but does not eradicate disease; it starts with clarithromycin combined with ethambutol and rifabutin. Azithromycin is an alternative therapy.

Immune reconstitution inflammatory syndrome mimics an autoimmune event, with lymphadenitis, fever, and other symptoms commonly starting weeks to months after beginning antiretroviral therapy, often during tuberculosis therapy. Current treatment guidelines advise continuing antiretroviral therapy; nonsteroidal anti-inflammatory agents are recommended for mild to moderate cases; in severe cases, corticosteroids are advised (prednisone 1 to 2 milligrams/kg or equivalent for 1 to 2 weeks). Add the appropriate antimicrobials if there is a known or suspected infection.

Cytomegalovirus is a common cause of serious opportunistic viral disease in HIV-infected patients. Disseminated disease commonly involves the GI, pulmonary, and central nervous systems. The most important manifestation is retinitis (see "Cytomegalovirus Retinitis" below). Treatment is with foscarnet or ganciclovir. Oral ganciclovir can be used for prophylaxis (**Table 154-2**).

Fever in injection drug users is suspicious for infective endocarditis, which often has a nonspecific presentation in the ED (see chapter 155, "Endocarditis"). Most ED physicians admit febrile injection drug users while awaiting the results of blood cultures and echocardiography given the high morbidity and mortality coupled with the difficulties encountered with outpatient follow-up in the drug user population.

TABLE 154-2 Treatment Recommendations for Common Human Immunodeficiency Virus–Related Infections

Organ System	Infection	Therapy
Systemic	*Mycobacterium avium-intracellulare*	Clarithromycin, 500 milligrams PO twice a day *and* Ethambutol, 15 milligrams/kg PO once a day *and* Rifabutin, 300 milligrams/kg PO once a day
	CMV infection	Ganciclovir, 5 milligrams/kg IV twice a day for 2 wk, then 5 milligrams/kg/d *or* Foscarnet, 90 milligrams/kg every 12 h for 3 wk, then 90 milligrams/kg once a day
Pulmonary	*Pneumocystis jiroveci* (*Pneumocystis carinii*) pneumonia	Trimethoprim-sulfamethoxazole dose using 15–20 milligrams of trimethoprim component per kilogram per day PO or IV in divided doses three times a day for 3 wk If partial pressure of arterial oxygen is <70 mm Hg or alveolar-arterial gradient is >35 mm Hg, then add Prednisone, 40 milligrams twice a day for 5 d, then 40 milligrams once a day for 5 d, then 20 milligrams once a day for 11 d *or* Pentamidine, 4 milligrams/kg/d IV or IM for 3 wk
	Mycobacterium tuberculosis infection*	Isoniazid, 5 milligrams/kg PO once a day *and* Rifampin, 10 milligrams/kg PO once a day *or* rifabutin 5 milligrams/kg PO once a day *and* Pyrazinamide, 15–30 milligrams/kg PO once a day *and* Ethambutol, 15–20 milligrams/kg PO once a day
Central nervous	Toxoplasmosis†	Pyrimethamine, 200-milligram loading dose PO followed by 50–75 milligrams PO once a day for 6–8 wk *and* Sulfadiazine, 1–1.5 grams PO every 6 h for 6–8 wk *and* Leucovorin, 10–25 milligrams once a day
	Cryptococcosis‡	Amphotericin B, 0.7 milligram/kg IV once a day for 2 wk *and* Flucytosine, 25 milligrams/kg IV four times a day for 2 wk *then* Fluconazole, 400 milligrams/d PO for 8–10 wk
Ophthalmologic	CMV infection#	Valganciclovir, 900 milligrams PO twice a day for 14–20 d of induction therapy, then 900 milligrams PO daily for maintenance therapy *and* Ganciclovir, 2 milligrams intravitreal injection 1–4 doses over 7–10 d for patients with immediately sight-threatening lesions *or* Foscarnet, 2.4 milligrams intravitreal injection 1–4 doses over 7–10 d for patients with immediately sight-threatening lesions
GI	Candidiasis (thrush–limited to mouth)	Clotrimazole, 10-milligram troches five times a day *or* Nystatin, 500,000 units five times a day, gargle
	Esophagitis (primarily *Candida*)	Fluconazole, 100–400 milligrams/d PO
	Salmonellosis†	Ciprofloxacin, 500 milligrams PO twice a day for 2–4 wk
	Cryptosporidiosis	No known effective cure; best results with highly active antiretroviral therapy
Cutaneous	Herpes simplex	Acyclovir, 200 milligrams PO five times a day for 7 d *or* Famciclovir, 125 milligrams PO twice a day for 7 d *or* Valacyclovir, 1 gram PO twice a day for 7 d *or* for severe disease Acyclovir, 5–10 milligrams/kg IV every 8 h for 7 d

(*Continued*)

TABLE 154-2 Treatment Recommendations for Common Human Immunodeficiency Virus–Related Infections (*Continued*)

Organ System	Infection	Therapy
	Herpes zoster	Acyclovir, 800 milligrams PO five times a day for 7–10 d *or* Famciclovir, 500 milligrams PO three times a day for 7–10 d *or* Valacyclovir, 1 gram PO three times a day for 7–10 d *or* for ocular or disseminated disease Acyclovir, 5–10 milligrams/kg PO every 8 h for 5–7 d
	Candida or *Trichophyton* infection	Topical clotrimazole two or three times a day for 3 wk *or* Topical miconazole two or three times a day for 3 wk *or* Topical ketoconazole two or three times a day for 3 wk

Abbreviation: CMV = cytomegalovirus.

*Specific drug regimen must be adjusted if patient is receiving highly active antiretroviral therapy.

†Maintenance therapy required.

‡Maintenance therapy required; may be discontinued if CD4+ T-cell count is >150 cells/mm^3 for >16 wk.

#Maintenance therapy required until CD4+ T-cell count is >150 cells/mm^3.

Noninfectious causes of fever in HIV patients include neoplasm and drug fever. Non-Hodgkin's lymphoma is the most frequently occurring neoplasm and is characterized by high-grade, rapidly growing mass lesions. New CNS symptoms, particularly a change in mental status in the presence of fever, require neuroimaging. Definitive diagnosis requires biopsy. Radiotherapy and chemotherapy are effective treatment regimens. Drug fever may be secondary to injection drug abuse or adverse drug reactions (see below).

NEUROLOGIC COMPLICATIONS

Neurologic disease is caused by a variety of opportunistic infections and neoplasms and also by effects of HIV infection or treatment on the CNS. Common presenting symptoms include seizures, altered mental status, headache, meningismus, and focal neurologic deficits. The most common causes of neurologic symptoms include AIDS dementia, *Toxoplasma gondii* infection, and *C. neoformans* infection. Since the widespread use of antiretroviral therapy, rates of CNS infection and malignancy have declined, whereas the rate of AIDS dementia remains unchanged.

ED evaluation should include a complete neurologic examination and CT followed by lumbar puncture, especially when patients have CD4+ T-cell counts of <200 cells/mm^3. Fever, meningismus, altered mental status, and headache are independent predictors of space-occupying lesions. In patients with CD4+ T-cell counts of <200 cells/mm^3, isolated headaches that are protracted or have changed in quality, even in the absence of other neurologic findings, are best evaluated by prompt immediate neuroimaging.

Non-contrast-enhanced CT is the first neuroimaging study in the ED in HIV-infected patients with neurologic symptoms or deficits; if concerned about malignancy or abscess, or the CT scan findings are equivocal or negative, contrast-enhanced CT or MRI is next. Specific CSF studies of value include opening and closing pressures, cell count, glucose level, protein level, Gram staining, India ink staining, bacterial culture, viral culture, fungal culture, toxoplasmosis and cryptococcosis antigen assays, and coccidioidomycosis titer. If possible, save an extra tube (5 mL) of CSF for additional testing if the diagnosis remains unclear. Even if the ED evaluation is unrevealing, all patients with new or changed neurologic signs or symptoms are best admitted to the hospital.

HIV-ASSOCIATED DEMENTIA

HIV-associated dementia (also referred to as *HIV encephalopathy* or *subacute encephalitis*) is a progressive disorder heralded by subtle impairment of recent memory and other cognitive deficits. It occurs in 20% to 40% of HIV-positive patients.[17] In the early stages, HIV-associated dementia is often confused with depression, anxiety disorders, or substance abuse. Later phases of the illness are characterized by obvious changes in mental status or aphasia and motor abnormalities. Patients with an established diagnosis of HIV-associated dementia and progressive neurologic or psychological signs or symptoms warrant further evaluation for systemic or CNS processes. CT images in patients with HIV-associated dementia typically show cortical atrophy and ventricular enlargement. HIV-associated dementia is associated with elevated protein levels in the CSF in 50% to 70% of cases. Antiretroviral therapy is the most effective treatment for HIV-associated dementia.

TOXOPLASMOSIS

Toxoplasmosis is a common cause of focal encephalitis in patients with AIDS. It occurs most commonly in patients with CD4+ cell counts <100 cells/mm^3. Symptoms may include headache, fever, focal neurologic deficits, altered mental status, and seizures. Serologic tests are not useful in making or excluding the diagnosis because antibodies to *T. gondii* are prevalent in the general population. The presence of antibodies to *T. gondii* in the CSF is helpful, although there is a high rate of false-negative results. On unenhanced CT scan, toxoplasmosis typically appears as multiple subcortical lesions with a predilection for the basal ganglia. Contrast-enhanced CT scan typically shows multiple ring-enhancing lesions with surrounding areas of edema. MRI is more sensitive than contrast-enhanced CT scan in detecting toxoplasmosis. Other disorders in the differential diagnosis of ring-enhancing lesions on contrast-enhanced CT include lymphoma, fungal infection, and cerebral tuberculosis.

Patients with suspected toxoplasmosis are admitted and treated with a combination of IV pyrimethamine plus sulfadiazine plus leucovorin (folinic acid); trimethoprim-sulfamethoxazole is an alternative (Table 154-2). Steroids (dexamethasone 4 milligrams IV every 6 hours) are helpful when edema or a mass effect exists. For patients responsive to toxoplasmosis therapy, chronic suppressive therapy with pyrimethamine, sulfadiazine, and folinic acid is usually indicated. Oral sulfamethoxazole-trimethoprim, one double-strength tablet daily, is used as prophylaxis in patients with positive toxoplasmosis serologic test results and CD4+ T-cell counts of <100 cells/mm^3.

CRYPTOCOCCOSIS

Cryptococcal CNS infection produces either focal cerebral lesions or diffuse meningoencephalitis. Cryptococcal infection occurs most commonly in patients with CD4+ counts of <50 cells/mm^3. The most common presenting signs are fever and headache, followed by nausea, altered mentation, and focal neurologic deficits. Presentation may be subtle, and meningismus is uncommon. Neuroimaging studies are usually normal or nondiagnostic.

Diagnosis of CNS cryptococcal infection in HIV patients relies on CSF cryptococcal antigen testing (nearly 100% sensitive and specific), culture (95% to 100% sensitive), or staining with India ink (60% to 80% sensitive). Serum cryptococcal antigen testing helps but has lower sensitivity than CSF testing (~95%). CSF analysis will typically show a pleocytosis with a predominance of lymphocytes. Elevated intracranial pressure is common; if >25 cm H_2O, remove 20 to 30 mL of CSF for therapy.

Patients with CNS cryptococcosis require hospital admission and IV amphotericin B and oral flucytosine for 14 days, followed by fluconazole for 8 weeks to clear the CSF (Table 154-2). Sixty percent of patients respond to therapy, and side effects are frequent, most notably bone marrow suppression. Long-term maintenance therapy with fluconazole (200 milligrams/d) follows initial treatment, although it may be stopped if immune reconstitution occurs.

OTHER NEUROLOGIC DISORDERS

Other less common considerations in the presence of neurologic symptoms include bacterial meningitis, histoplasmosis (usually disseminated), cytomegalovirus infection, progressive multifocal leukoencephalopathy, herpes simplex virus infection, neurosyphilis, and tuberculosis. Noninfectious CNS processes include CNS lymphoma (typically manifested as a subacute neurologic deterioration over several months with a single ring-enhancing lesion on CT), cerebrovascular accidents, and metabolic encephalopathies.

The most common disorder of the peripheral nervous system is HIV neuropathy, characterized by foot pain. Although HIV infection itself is the most common culprit, HIV therapies also are a possible cause, and changing treatment regimens may help. Cyclic antidepressants or membrane-stabilizing drugs may offer pain relief but are not often started in the ED and may cause delirium in patients with concurrent HIV dementia. Short-term opioid analgesia may be needed in severe cases.

OPHTHALMIC COMPLICATIONS

Seventy-five percent of patients with AIDS develop ocular complications, the most common being retinal microvasculopathy characterized by retinal cotton-wool spots identical in appearance to those seen in diabetes or hypertension. Retinal microaneurysms may be seen in the periphery. These lesions are incidental and do not cause visual disturbances. The diagnostic dilemma is to distinguish these findings from early cytomegalovirus infection; prompt ophthalmologic consultation is needed.

CYTOMEGALOVIRUS RETINITIS

Cytomegalovirus retinitis (Figure 154-1) is the most frequent and serious ocular opportunistic infection and is the leading cause of blindness in AIDS patients. In the antiretroviral therapy era, the incidence of cytomegalovirus infection is reduced, due in large part to immune reconstitution associated with the therapy.[18] Retinitis may be asymptomatic early on but later causes changes in visual acuity, visual field cuts, photophobia, and scotoma, and eye redness or eye pain may develop. Findings on indirect ophthalmoscopy are fluffy white perivascular lesions with areas of hemorrhage. First-line therapy is oral valganciclovir; this is often used before intravitreal ganciclovir, IV ganciclovir, IV foscarnet, or IV cidofovir due to its ease of administration, fewer complications, and less toxicity.[19] However, for patients with immediately sight-threatening lesions (lesions <1500 micrometers from the fovea or adjacent to the optic nerve head), intravitreal injection in conjunction with oral valganciclovir is best given promptly to avoid vision loss (Table 154-2). Frequent relapses and progression of disease are common, with 10% of affected patients ultimately going blind.

HERPES ZOSTER OPHTHALMICUS

Herpes zoster ophthalmicus (see chapter 241, "Eye Emergencies") usually presents with paresthesia and discomfort in the distribution of cranial nerve V_1 (ophthalmic branch), followed by the appearance of the typical zoster skin rash. Ocular complications include conjunctivitis, episcleritis, iritis, keratitis, secondary glaucoma, and, rarely, retinitis. Early recognition and treatment can prevent ocular damage.

PULMONARY COMPLICATIONS

The most common causes of pulmonary abnormalities in HIV-infected patients are community-acquired bacterial pneumonia, PCP, tuberculosis, cytomegalovirus infection, cryptococcosis, histoplasmosis, and neoplasms. **The most common cause of pneumonia in HIV-infected patients in the United States and Western Europe is *Streptococcus pneumoniae*.**[20] Pulmonary radiographic findings are helpful in determining likely causes (**Table 154-3**). Admit patients with new-onset or profound pulmonary symptoms, especially in the presence of hypoxemia or any change in sensorium. In patients with known existing pulmonary involvement, disposition and care decisions are based on change from baseline, the effectiveness of ongoing or previous treatment, ability to adhere to therapy, and the ability to obtain outpatient follow-up. The Pneumonia Severity Index and CURB scoring systems are powerful risk assessment tools but not designed for use in those with advanced HIV.

PNEUMOCYSTIS PNEUMONIA

PCP is the most common opportunistic infection among AIDS patients.[21] The causal agent is known as *P. jirovecii* (previously known as

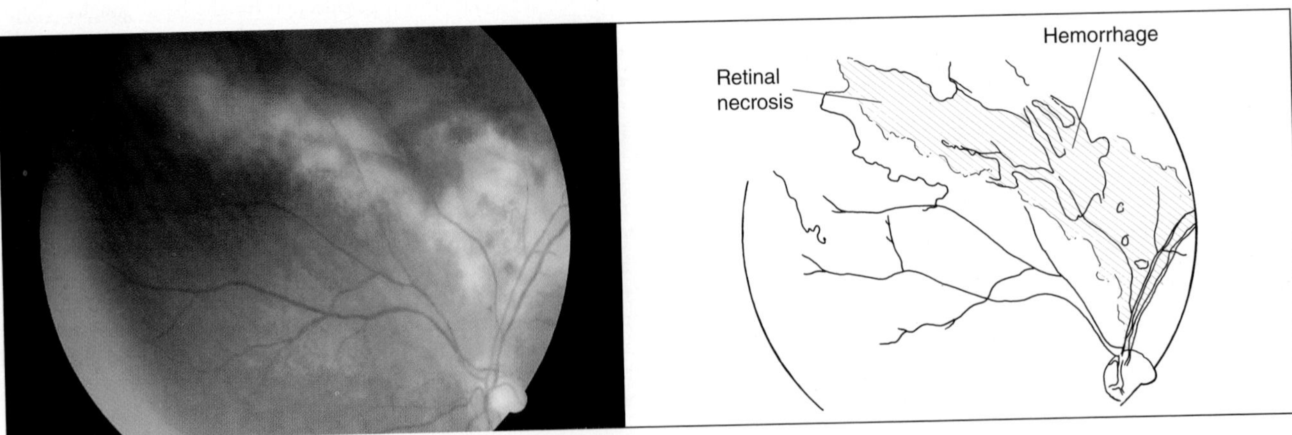

FIGURE 154-1. Cytomegalovirus retinitis. "Pizza pie" or "cheese and ketchup" appearance is demonstrated by hemorrhages and the dirty white granular-appearing retinal necrosis adjacent to major vessels. [Photograph contributed by Richard E. Wyszynski, MD. Reproduced with permission from Knoop KJ, Stack LB, Storrow AB, Thurman RJ: *The Atlas of Emergency Medicine*, 3rd ed, © 2009 by McGraw-Hill Inc., New York.]

TABLE 154-3 Chest Radiographic Abnormalities: Differential Diagnosis in the Patient with Acquired Immunodeficiency Syndrome

Finding	Causes
Diffuse interstitial infiltration	*Pneumocystis jiroveci* (*P. carinii*) infection
	Cytomegalovirus infection
	Mycobacterium tuberculosis infection
	Mycobacterium avium-intracellulare complex infection
	Histoplasmosis
	Coccidioidomycosis
	Lymphoid interstitial pneumonitis
Focal consolidation	Bacterial pneumonia
	Mycoplasma pneumoniae infection
	P. jiroveci infection
	M. tuberculosis infection
	M. avium-intracellulare complex infection
Nodular lesions	Kaposi's sarcoma
	M. tuberculosis infection
	M. avium-intracellulare complex infection
	Fungal lesions
	Toxoplasmosis
Cavitary lesions	*P. jiroveci* infection
	M. tuberculosis infection
	Bacterial infection
	Fungal infection
Adenopathy	Kaposi's sarcoma
	Lymphoma
	M. tuberculosis infection
	Cryptococcosis

P. carinii). Approximately 70% of HIV-infected patients acquire PCP at some time during their illness, and PCP is often the initial opportunistic infection that establishes the diagnosis of AIDS. This infection is the most frequent serious complication of HIV infection in the United States and the most common identifiable cause of death in patients with AIDS. The classic presenting symptoms of PCP are fever, cough (typically nonproductive), and shortness of breath (progressing from being present only with exertion to being present at rest).

Symptoms are often insidious and accompanied by fatigue. Chest radiographs most often show diffuse interstitial infiltrates (Table 154-3), but negative radiographic findings exist in 15% to 25% of patients with PCP.[22] The lactate dehydrogenase level is elevated in patients with PCP, but this test has low sensitivity and specificity, impairing utility. Arterial blood gas analysis usually demonstrates hypoxemia and an increase in the alveolar-arterial gradient. Suspect early PCP if a patient demonstrates a decrease in pulse oximetric values with exercise; even an ED "walk" can detect this exercise desaturation. **Presumptive diagnosis of PCP is often made in the ED if there is hypoxemia without any other explanation.** Inpatient diagnostics include bronchoscopy with specimen analyses.

Initial PCP therapy is trimethoprim-sulfamethoxazole (Table 154-2) PO or IV for 3 weeks (2 double-strength tablets three times daily). Adverse reactions, including rash, fever, and neutropenia, occur in up to 65% of AIDS patients. Pentamidine is an alternative agent (Table 154-2). Give steroids to patients with a partial pressure of arterial oxygen of <70 mm Hg or an alveolar-arterial gradient of >35 mm Hg, usually oral prednisone starting at 40 milligrams twice daily and tapering over 21 days (Table 154-2).

Seventy percent of patients have reinfection within 18 months; thus, prophylactic therapy is key. Oral trimethoprim-sulfamethoxazole, one double-strength tablet daily, is the preferred agent. Prophylaxis for all patients with CD4+ T-cell counts of <200 cells/mm^3 is another common approach to mitigate PCP. Repeat PCP infections are often less responsive to therapy.

TUBERCULOSIS

Approximately 10% of new cases of tuberculosis in the United States occur in HIV-infected persons, varying in regional prevalence based on specific population compositions and public health measures.[23] Clinical manifestations of tuberculosis in HIV-infected patients vary according to the severity of immunosuppression. **Tuberculosis frequently occurs in patients with CD4+ T-cell counts of 200 to 500 cells/mm^3.** Classic manifestations include cough with hemoptysis, night sweats, prolonged fevers, weight loss, and anorexia. With worsening immunosuppression, patient presentation may be more atypical (i.e., fewer of the classic symptoms described above). Classic upper lobe involvement and cavitary lesions are less common as patients become more immunosuppressed, particularly among patients with late-stage AIDS.[24] Negative purified protein derivative skin tuberculosis test results are frequent among AIDS patients due to immunosuppression. Definitive diagnosis of tuberculosis is made by stain and culture of expectorated sputum, although some cases require bronchoscopy. Later stage HIV is also associated with increased frequency of extrapulmonary tuberculosis with clinical manifestation associated with the involved sites of infection. Frequent sites of dissemination are peripheral lymph nodes, bone marrow, CNS, GI, and the urogenital system.

In the ED, think of tuberculosis in any HIV-infected patients with pulmonary symptoms, and begin precautions to avoid transmission. Place the patient in an isolation room and with an appropriate mask immediately and until the diagnosis is excluded, usually after the ED visit. Current treatment guidelines recommend a four-drug initial empirical therapy (Table 154-2; see chapter 67, "Tuberculosis").[19,25-27] Multidrug-resistant tuberculosis remains a concern, increasing the need for suspicion and early isolation. All HIV-infected patients with positive purified protein derivative skin tests should receive isoniazid plus pyridoxine for 9 to 12 months; alternatives include rifampin or rifabutin for 4 months. Also, give empiric treatment to HIV-infected persons in close contact with another patient with active tuberculosis.

BACTERIAL PNEUMONIA

Bacterial pneumonia is the most common pulmonary infection in HIV-infected patients. Common pathogens include *S. pneumoniae*, *Haemophilus influenzae*, and *Staphylococcus aureus*. Productive cough, leukocytosis, and the presence of a focal infiltrate suggest bacterial pneumonia, especially in those with earlier-stage disease. The response to empirical therapy tends to be good; seek a specific pathogen by Gram staining and culture.

FUNGAL PNEUMONIA AND OTHER LUNG DISORDERS

Patients with severe immunosuppression are predisposed to **disseminated fungal infections** such as those caused by *C. neoformans* and *Aspergillus fumigatus*. Other noninfectious disorders of the lung seen in HIV-infected patients include neoplasms (e.g., Kaposi's sarcoma) and lymphocytic interstitial pneumonitis. Cytomegalovirus or *M. avium* complex infections are unlikely unless the CD4+ T-cell count drops to <50 cells/mm^3.

CARDIOVASCULAR COMPLICATIONS

Cardiovascular complications are common in late-stage disease but are difficult to diagnose in the ED. Cardiovascular complications may be related to opportunistic infections, structural defects, or drug toxicity. HIV-associated cardiovascular conditions include cardiomyopathy, infective endocarditis (in injection drug users; see chapter 155, "Endocarditis"), pericardial effusion, congestive heart failure, coronary artery disease, arrhythmias, and HIV-associated pulmonary hypertension. After standard ED evaluation, consultation with a cardiologist and infectious disease specialist is best.

GI COMPLICATIONS

GI complications of HIV infection are common. Approximately 50% of AIDS patients present with GI complaints at some time during their illness. The most frequent presenting symptoms include odynophagia,

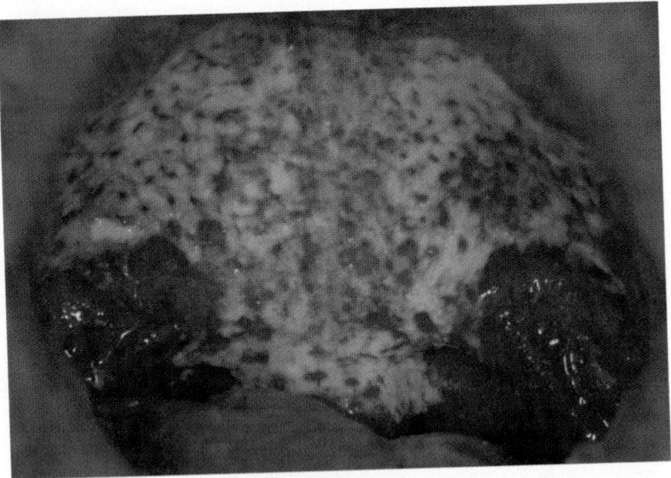

FIGURE 154-2. Oral candidiasis (thrush). Extensive thrush is seen on the hard and soft palate of this immunocompromised patient. [Photograph contributed by Lawrence B. Stack. Reproduced with permission from Knoop KJ, Stack LB, Storrow AB, Thurman RJ: *The Atlas of Emergency Medicine*, 3rd ed, © 2009, McGraw-Hill Inc., New York.]

abdominal pain, bleeding, and diarrhea. ED evaluation seeks to identify the severity of symptoms and perform appropriate initial diagnostic studies. Therapy starts with volume and electrolyte repletion, with anti-infective therapy when appropriate. Disposition is based on the duration of symptoms, the clinical appearance of the patient, and the response to ED therapy.

ORAL AND ESOPHAGEAL COMPLICATIONS

Oral Candidiasis/Thrush Oral lesions are common in HIV-infected patients, frequently contributing to malnutrition. The appearance of oral lesions in HIV patients serves as a potential clinical marker for viral load and degree of immunodeficiency. Oral candidiasis ("thrush"; **Figure 154-2**) affects >80% of AIDS patients. The tongue and buccal mucosa are commonly involved, and the plaques are easily scraped from the erythematous base. Differentiation from hairy leukoplakia (adherent, white, thickened lesion[s] on the lateral tongue border) is challenging, but microscopic examination of a potassium hydroxide smear can confirm the fungal presence. The development of oral candidiasis is a poor prognostic sign and is predictive of progression to AIDS. Most oral lesions can be managed symptomatically on an outpatient basis. Clotrimazole or nystatin suspension or troches (five times daily) is the preferred treatment. Refractory or recurrent disease can be managed with oral fluconazole. Amphotericin B is reserved for severe cases.

Other Oral Lesions Other causes of painful oral and perioral lesions include oral hairy leukoplakia, herpes simplex virus infection, and Kaposi's sarcoma. Herpes simplex virus infection usually can be recognized by the presence of typical vesicular lesions, with diagnosis confirmed by identification of multinucleated giant cells in scrapings or by culture. Both herpes simplex virus infection and hairy leukoplakia are responsive to oral acyclovir. Oral Kaposi's sarcoma appears as a nontender, well-circumscribed, slightly raised violaceous lesion. Diagnosis requires biopsy, and topical treatments are palliative and started outside the ED.

ESOPHAGEAL LESIONS

Esophageal involvement may occur with *Candida*, herpes simplex virus, and cytomegalovirus infection. Complaints of odynophagia or dysphagia are indicative of esophagitis, and these symptoms may be debilitating. Disease typically occurs in patients who have oral thrush and CD4+ T-cell counts of <100 cells/mm^3. Treatment of esophagitis in the ED is presumptive with oral fluconazole (Table 154-2) or oral ketoconazole (200 to 400 milligrams/d for 2 to 3 weeks). IV caspofungin or IV amphotericin B may be used when oral treatment fails. Endoscopy, histologic staining and culture of lesions, and biopsy are reserved for patients who fail to respond to therapy or have atypical presentations. Cytomegalovirus and herpes simplex virus infections discovered by endoscopy are treated with ganciclovir and acyclovir, respectively.

DIARRHEA

Diarrhea is the most frequent GI complaint of those with HIV-related co-infections. Causes include bacteria (*Shigella*, *Salmonella*, enteroadherent *Escherichia coli*, *Entamoeba histolytica*, *Campylobacter*, *M. avium-intracellulare* complex, *Clostridium difficile*, and others), parasites (*Giardia lamblia*, *Cryptosporidium*, *Isospora belli*, and others), viruses (cytomegalovirus, herpes simplex virus, HIV, and others), and fungi (*H. capsulatum*, *C. neoformans*, and others). In many cases, a pathogen is never found. Diarrhea is a side effect of protease inhibitors, most notably nelfinavir and ritonavir.

In the ED, look for stool leukocytes, ova, and parasites; in recalcitrant or severe cases, obtain acid-fast staining and bacterial cultures of stool. Bacterial infections generally follow a more acute and fulminant course, whereas parasitic infections are frequently indolent. If bacterial infection is suspected, treat empirically with ciprofloxacin to cover the common pathogens. *Cryptosporidium* and *Isospora* infections are common parasitic causes and are associated with profuse watery diarrhea. Both organisms can be identified by modified acid-fast staining of a stool specimen. *I. belli* infection is usually responsive to trimethoprim-sulfamethoxazole, but relapse is common. Cryptosporidiosis is difficult to treat, usually starting with an antiretroviral therapy coupled with supportive care, including rehydration and electrolyte repletion. Antimicrobial treatment is not beneficial. Consult with an infectious disease specialist to create a long-term management plan.

In patients with end-stage disease, the most common diarrheal pathogens are cytomegalovirus and *M. avium-intracellulare* complex, each requiring biopsy for diagnosis. Prolonged antimicrobial therapy is indicated, and relapse is frequent for both infections. About 15% of patients with late-stage AIDS experience severe, high-volume watery diarrhea absent a clear pathogen, with the presumed diagnosis of AIDS-related enteropathy. Octreotide may aid some of these patients.

ED management consists of repletion of fluid and electrolytes. Patients who appear nontoxic and can tolerate liquids can be referred for outpatient follow-up to obtain test results. Patients with severe diarrhea who do not require antibiotics may benefit from symptomatic therapy, such as attapulgite (Kaopectate), psyllium (Metamucil), or diphenoxylate hydrochloride with atropine (Lomotil).

OTHER GI COMPLICATIONS

Hepatomegaly occurs in approximately 50% of AIDS patients, often with an elevated alkaline phosphatase level but rarely with jaundice. Co-infection with hepatitis B virus and hepatitis C virus is common, especially among injection drug users. Opportunistic infection with cytomegalovirus, *Cryptosporidium*, *M. avium-intracellulare* complex, and *M. tuberculosis* also may cause hepatitis.

Anorectal disease is common in AIDS patients. **Proctitis** presents with painful defecation, rectal discharge, or tenesmus. Common causative organisms include *Neisseria gonorrhoeae*, *Chlamydia trachomatis*, *Treponema pallidum*, and herpes simplex virus. Proctocolitis includes the same symptoms plus diarrhea, and multiple bacterial organisms may be responsible (most commonly *Shigella*, *Campylobacter*, and *E. histolytica*). Evaluation includes anoscopy with microscopic examination, Gram staining, and culture of pus and/or stool.

RENAL COMPLICATIONS

Renal insufficiency among AIDS patients may be secondary to prerenal azotemia, drug nephrotoxicity, or HIV-associated nephropathy. Renal tubular acidosis is common and explains a finding of hyperchloremic metabolic acidosis. Indinavir therapy is a common cause of nephrolithiasis.

CUTANEOUS COMPLICATIONS

Cutaneous complications occur in approximately 90% of HIV-infected individuals. Generalized cutaneous conditions, such as xerosis (dry skin), seborrheic eczema, and pruritus, are common and may develop before opportunistic infections. Treatment is with emollients and, if necessary, mild topical steroids. Pruritus may respond to oatmeal baths and antihistamines.

CUTANEOUS INFECTIONS

Skin and soft tissue infections occur commonly in the HIV-infected population, including *S. aureus* infection (manifested as bullous impetigo, ecthyma, or folliculitis), *Pseudomonas aeruginosa* infection (which may present with chronic ulcerations and macerations), and syphilis, all treated with standard therapies. Methicillin-resistant *S. aureus* colonization and infection are more prevalent and are associated with low CD4+ cell counts, men who have sex with men, anal intercourse, previous methicillin-resistant *S. aureus* infections, and illicit drug use.[28,29] Human Papillomavirus (HPV) infections manifesting as condyloma acuminata or warts are common; treatment is cosmetic or symptomatic and includes cryotherapy, topical therapy, or laser therapy. Intertriginous infections with *Candida* or *Trichophyton* are frequent in HIV-positive patients; microscopic examination of potassium hydroxide preparations of lesion scrapings aids diagnosis. Treatment is with topical clotrimazole, miconazole, or ketoconazole.

Pruritus is common and related to xerosis, eczema, drug reaction, scabies folliculitis, psoriasis, seborrheic dermatitis, or numerous other cutaneous conditions. ED evaluation includes history, physical examination, removal of offending agents, and treatment of the underlying condition. If no specific diagnosis is found, symptomatic treatment with emollients and antipruritic agents can be effective.[30]

HERPES SIMPLEX VIRUS

Herpes simplex virus infections are common and either localized or systemic. In patients with immunosuppression, infection may become progressive and chronic (see chapter 149, "Sexually Transmitted Infections"). IV acyclovir is the therapy for extensive disease (Table 154-2).

VARICELLA-ZOSTER VIRUS INFECTION

Reactivation of **varicella-zoster virus** is more common in patients with HIV infection and AIDS than in the general population. The clinical course is prolonged, and complications are more frequent. In HIV-positive patients, oral acyclovir, famciclovir, and valacyclovir are options for treatment (Table 154-2). In patients with disseminated disease or ophthalmic herpes zoster, use IV acyclovir.

SCABIES

Scabies occurs in about 20% of HIV-infected patients, but classic intertriginous lesions are less common. Treat any with a scaly, persistent pruritic eruption with permethrin 5% cream, ivermectin, or crotamiton. **Norwegian scabies** occurs in immunosuppressed patients, presenting with extensive hyperkeratosis and crusting of the hands, feet, and scalp. Pruritus is less impressive than is seen in typical scabies. Treatment failures and secondary infection also are common.

KAPOSI'S SARCOMA

Kaposi's sarcoma appears more often in homosexual men than in other risk groups. Clinically, it consists of painless, raised, brown-black or purple papules and nodules that do not blanch. Common sites are the face, chest, genitals, and oral cavity, but widespread dissemination involving internal organs may occur. Treat extensive, painful, or cosmetically disfiguring lesions. Cryotherapy or radiation can be used for localized disease; widespread disease may be responsive to chemotherapy with vincristine, vinblastine, or doxorubicin.

PSYCHIATRIC DISORDERS

HIV infection has a variety of CNS and metabolic disturbances that can produce psychiatric symptoms. HIV infection is also a psychosocial stressor, leading to social isolation, poverty, and hopelessness. In the ED, search for underlying organic causes; delirium suggests an organic disorder or a withdrawal syndrome. Patients with AIDS psychosis develop hallucinations, delusions, or other behavioral changes. Treat as for any psychosis.

Depression occurs in up to 81% of patients.[31] Antidepressant therapy is often started if symptoms of depression continue for >2 weeks and with close monitoring for side effects. Patients with suicidal ideation or profound dysfunction usually require inpatient psychiatric management.

An increased incidence of mania is observed in both the early and late stages of HIV infection. Late-stage mania is closely associated with dementia and carries a poor prognosis. If danger exists, use physical restraints or acute pharmacologic intervention. Neuroleptics and benzodiazepines may be used in combination.

Nearly 50% of those with HIV infection have a history of substance abuse.[32,33] Depression and psychotic symptoms are more prevalent among patients with substance abuse. ED management includes identification and outpatient referral to integrated substance abuse and psychiatric resources.

SEXUALLY TRANSMITTED INFECTIONS

Sexually transmitted infections, HIV, and viral hepatitis share common routes of transmission and may coexist.[34-36] Genital ulcers caused by diseases such as herpes, chancroid, and syphilis are portals of entry for HIV. There is more frequent HIV seropositivity in patients with genital ulcers, gonorrhea, and chlamydial infections. The prevalence of sexually transmitted infections, including syphilis, is increasing and warrants enhanced surveillance.[37] Therapy for sexually transmitted infections is based on current Centers for Disease Control and Prevention guidelines (see chapter 149).

IMMUNIZATION OF HIV-INFECTED PATIENTS

HIV-infected persons should not receive live virus or live bacteria vaccines.[38] The exception to this rule is the measles-mumps-rubella vaccine, which does not have adverse effects in this population.

Killed vaccines pose no danger to immunosuppressed patients.[39] Because symptomatic HIV-infected persons have a suboptimal response to vaccines, all single-dose vaccines are best given as early as possible in the course of HIV infection. **Table 154-4** summarizes the Centers for Disease Control and Prevention recommendations for common immunizations.

ANTIRETROVIRAL THERAPY

After the introduction of antiretroviral therapy, sharp declines in AIDS incidence and mortality occurred,[40] transforming HIV therapeutics into long-term management of a chronic infection. General therapeutic goals include: (1) prolonging and improving the quality of life; (2) reducing

TABLE 154-4 Immunization Recommendations for Adult Human Immunodeficiency Virus–Infected Patients[39]

Vaccine	Adult Recommendation
Tetanus, diphtheria, and pertussis (Tdap)	One booster in adulthood
Tetanus-diphtheria toxoid (Td)	Every 10 years
Measles-mumps-rubella	Avoid in patients with CD4+ T-cell count <200 cells/mm³
Pneumococcal	One dose
Influenza (inactivated)	One dose annually
Hepatitis B	Three doses over a 2-y period
Varicella	Avoid in patients with CD4+ T-cell count <200 cells/mm³

viral load as much as possible to halt disease progression and prevent or reduce the development of resistant variants; (3) promoting immune reconstitution, both quantitative (CD4+ T-cell count) and qualitative (pathogen-specific immune response); and (4) reducing side effects and maintaining therapeutic options. A complete drug list and up-to-date guide for the general classes of antiretroviral drugs, principles for initiating therapy, and common adverse reactions can be found on the Centers for Disease Control and Prevention Web site (http://www.cdc.gov/hiv/pubs/mmwr.htm).

The five main classes of antiretroviral drugs are (1) nucleoside reverse transcriptase inhibitors, which interfere with the action of reverse transcriptase (e.g., zidovudine); (2) nonnucleoside reverse transcriptase inhibitors, which bind to reverse transcriptase and block RNA- and DNA-dependent DNA polymerase activity (e.g., efavirenz); (3) protease inhibitors, which block HIV protease, a key enzyme in establishing HIV infectivity (e.g., indinavir); (4) entry inhibitors, which prevent HIV entry into cells by targeting specific viral surface proteins or their corresponding receptors (e.g., enfuvirtide); and (5) integrase inhibitors, which work by blocking integrase, a protein that HIV needs to insert its viral genetic material into the genetic material of an infected cell (e.g., raltegravir).

Preferred initial treatment regimens include at least three drugs—two nucleoside reverse transcriptase inhibitors *plus* one of the following classes: nonnucleoside reverse transcriptase inhibitor, protease inhibitor (boosted with ritonavir), or integrase strand transfer inhibitor. Currently, all HIV-infected patients with CD4+ cell counts of <350 cells/mm^3 or with a history of AIDS-defining illness receive therapy.[41] Other indications for initiation of antiretroviral therapy regardless of CD4+ count include pregnancy, HIV-associated nephropathy, and hepatitis B virus co-infection requiring treatment.[41] Education and counseling also constitute an integral part of antiretroviral therapy. Decisions regarding initiation of and changes in antiretroviral therapy should be made in consultation with the primary care physician and an infectious disease consultant.

TABLE 154-5 Antiretroviral Medications, Major Adverse Effects, and Interacting Drug Effects[42]

Antiretroviral Medications	Adverse Effects	Interacting Drugs	Effects of Interaction
Nucleoside reverse transcriptase inhibitors			
Abacavir	Stevens-Johnson syndrome, hypersensitivity reaction (fever, rash, myalgia)		
Didanosine	Peripheral neuropathy, lactic acidosis, pancreatitis		
Emtricitabine	Skin hyperpigmentation/discoloration, hepatic steatosis (rare), lactic acidosis		
Lamivudine	Lactic acidosis/hepatic steatosis (rare)		
Stavudine	Pancreatitis, lactic acidosis, peripheral neuropathy, ascending muscle weakness, dyslipidemia		
Tenofovir	Pancreatitis, headache, renal failure, diarrhea, nausea, vomiting		
Zidovudine	Bone marrow suppression		
Nonnucleoside reverse transcriptase inhibitors		Anticonvulsants, rifampin	Decreased concentration of antiretrovirals and increased concentration of anticonvulsants
Delavirdine	Transaminitis rash (blisters), headache		
Efavirenz	Depression, psychosis, suicidal ideation		
Nevirapine	Stevens-Johnson syndrome, hepatic failure		
Protease inhibitors		Antiarrhythmics, anticonvulsants, midazolam, metoprolol, rifampin, warfarin, HMG-CoA reductase inhibitors	Decreased concentration of antiretroviral and increased concentration of the interacting drug; increased risk of rhabdomyolysis with HMG-CoA reductase inhibitors
Amprenavir	Toxicity from propylene glycol diluent		
Atazanavir	Increased indirect bilirubin, prolonged PR interval	Proton pump inhibitors	Decreased absorption of atazanavir; concomitant use contraindicated
		Diltiazem	Increased concentration of diltiazem (decrease diltiazem dose by half)
Darunavir	Headache, nausea, diarrhea, rash		
Fosamprenavir	Hyperlipidemia, rash		
Indinavir	Urolithiasis, nephrotoxicity, indirect hyperbilirubinemia		
Nelfinavir	Secretory diarrhea		
Ritonavir	Hyperlipidemia, nausea, vomiting, hyperglycemia	Digoxin	Increased digoxin concentration (monitor levels)
Saquinavir	Hyperglycemia lipodystrophy		
Tipranavir	Intracerebral hemorrhage, hepatotoxicity		
Entry and fusion inhibitors			
Enfuvirtide	Pneumonia, injection site reaction		
Maraviroc	Abdominal pain, postural hypotension		
Integrase inhibitors			
Raltegravir	Increased creatine phosphokinase, nausea, headache		

Abbreviation: HMG-CoA = 3-hydroxy-3-methylglutaryl-coenzyme A.

DRUG INTERACTIONS AND ADVERSE EFFECTS IN HIV-INFECTED PATIENTS

Current antiretroviral therapy programs include a standard three-drug regimen that may cause a range of changes in metabolic or physiologic functions and be toxic. **Table 154-5** shows the currently available antiretroviral medications, their major adverse effects, and their interacting drug effects. These reactions may be compounded by the effects of antibiotic prophylaxis being taken to fight against opportunistic infections.

Drug interactions are pharmacokinetic (changes in the level of one or more drugs) or pharmacodynamic (changes in effect, therapeutic response, or side effect of one or more drugs).[41] Review of current reference sources and consultation with a hospital pharmacologist and an infectious disease specialist are indicated when drug reactions are suspected.

REFERENCES

The complete reference list is available online at www.TintinalliEM.com.

CHAPTER 155

Endocarditis

Richard Rothman
Catherine A. Marco
Samuel Yang

INTRODUCTION AND EPIDEMIOLOGY

The clinical presentation of endocarditis is often nonspecific and variable, with potential to affect nearly every organ system in an indolent or fulminant course. The vast majority of endocarditis is infective; diagnosis relies on a set of explicit criteria, which include findings from blood culture, echocardiography, and close clinical observation. Unrecognized infective endocarditis has frequent complications and high mortality.

In developed countries, the incidence of infective endocarditis ranges from 2 to 11.6 cases per 100,000 patient-years[1-7] and is higher in urban versus rural settings, likely reflecting the impact of injection drug use. The disease is uncommon among children, where it is associated with structural congenital heart disease, rheumatic heart disease, or nosocomial, catheter-related bacteremia. The disorder affects men more commonly than women, and the hospital mortality rate is up to 18%, varying according to the microorganism involved and presence of complications.[1,2]

Most cases occur either in those with a predisposing identifiable cardiac structural abnormality (congenital or acquired), prosthetic valve, or a recognized risk factor for disease (including injection drug use, intravascular devices, poor dental hygiene, chronic hemodialysis, or infection with the human immunodeficiency virus). The mitral valve is the most commonly affected site, followed in decreasing frequency by the aortic, tricuspid, and pulmonic valves.

For native valve–related infective endocarditis in the developed world, **mitral valve prolapse** is a common predisposing cardiac lesion. Other underlying structural defects include congenital defects (most commonly bicuspid aortic valve), degenerative cardiac lesions (particularly calcific aortic stenosis), and rheumatic heart disease. In developing countries, **rheumatic heart disease** creating valvulopathy remains the leading underlying risk factor. For native valve–related lesions, left-sided disease predominates, and mortality ranges from 16% to 27%. Short-term mortality increases in those with left-sided native valve endocarditis when accompanied by other severe comorbid illnesses, abnormal mental status, congestive heart failure, or a bacterial etiology other than *Streptococcus viridans* and *Staphylococcus aureus*, and when treated with medical therapy absent valve surgery.[8]

The estimated risk in **injection drug users** is 2% to 5% per year, with a mean age of diagnosis being 30 years old. When endocarditis occurs in injection drug users, it has a predilection for the tricuspid valve. Other features include increased susceptibility to recurrence (approximately 40%) and increased mortality in those with concurrent human immunodeficiency virus and evidence of immunosuppression (defined as a CD4+ T-cell count of <200/mm^3). Large vegetation size and fungal organism are predictive of poor outcome in injection drug use–associated right-sided endocarditis.[9]

Indwelling vascular devices create greater risks that microorganisms will attach to valves during bacteremia. Healthcare-associated endocarditis occurs when (1) a diagnosis is made >72 hours after admission in patients with no evidence of endocarditis on admission or in whom the disorder develops within 6 months after hospital discharge; or (2) cardiovascular manipulations have occurred in the ambulatory setting within 6 months before endocarditis develops, including central venous catheter use, arteriovenous fistula for hemodialysis, invasive intravascular techniques, or intracardiac devices (e.g., prosthetic valves, pacemaker, left ventricular assist device).[10,11]

Prosthetic valve endocarditis occurs in 1% to 4% of recipients during the first year following valve replacement and in approximately 1% per year thereafter. There is no difference in risk between mechanical versus bioprosthetic valves. Cases with onset within 60 days after surgery are called *early* prosthetic valve endocarditis and are usually acquired in the hospital. Cases starting beyond 60 days after surgery are called *late* prosthetic valve endocarditis and are usually community acquired. Hospital mortality rates are highest for those with early (30% to 80%) versus late (20% to 40%) prosthetic valve endocarditis, attributable to the greater virulence of the causative organisms involved.

PATHOPHYSIOLOGY

The normal endothelium is resistant to infection and thrombus formation unless it is injured by high-pressure gradients and turbulent flow states. Such abnormal hemodynamic states occur commonly in those with preexisting valvular or congenital cardiac defects. In injection drug use, endothelial damage likely occurs by a different mechanism, such as from repetitive bombardment with particulate matter (i.e., talc) present in injected material or from ischemia brought on by vasospasm from the injected drug. Cocaine use is particularly associated with increased rates of endocarditis. The resultant endothelial damage promotes deposition of platelets and fibrin and the formation of sterile vegetations (nonbacterial thrombotic endocarditis).

Nonbacterial thrombotic endocarditis can also arise as a result of hypercoagulable states, such as in patients with malignancy (marantic endocarditis) or systemic lupus erythematosus (Libman-Sacks endocarditis), and in areas surrounding foreign bodies like vascular catheters or prosthetic valves. In the setting of preexistent nonbacterial thrombotic endocarditis, transient bacteremia may result in colonization of vegetations and conversion to infective endocarditis.

Transient bacteremia can occur from trauma to the skin or mucosal surfaces of the oropharynx or GI or GU tracts (all of which are normally laden with endogenous flora). Even in the absence of trauma, spontaneous bacteremia can occur in patients with periodontal disease or other localized infections. In cases of bacteremia, the bacterial load usually does not exceed 10 organisms per milliliter of blood, and the bloodstream is usually sterilized in <30 minutes. In the presence of nonbacterial thrombotic endocarditis, this time interval is sufficient for bacteria to adhere to the vegetation and transform it into an infected lesion.

The coexistence of bacteremia and nonbacterial thrombotic endocarditis does not uniformly result in infective endocarditis. To cause infective endocarditis, the infecting organism must be able to adhere to the nonbacterial thrombus on the endothelium. Different organisms vary in this ability. Furthermore, although nonbacterial thrombotic endocarditis is often present in those who develop infective endocarditis, it not an absolute prerequisite, and highly invasive organisms (e.g., *S. aureus*) can directly invade the endocardium. Adherent organisms stimulate further deposition of platelets and fibrin, leading to sequestration of organisms into a "protected site" that phagocytic cells cannot easily penetrate. As the disease progresses, the vegetation continuously fragments, shedding surface organisms into the circulation and causing sustained bacteremia.

TABLE 155-1 Microbiology of Infective Endocarditis (IE)

Native Valve IE (% of cases)			Intracardiac Device IE (% cases)		
	Nonaddict	IV Drug Addict		Prosthetic Valve IE	Other Devices*
Staphylococcus aureus	28	68	*S. aureus*	23	35
Coagulase-negative *Staphylococcus*	9	3	Coagulase-negative *Staphylococcus*	17	26
Viridans group streptococci	21	10	*Viridans* group streptococci	12	8
Other streptococci	14	3	*Streptococcus bovis*	10	7
Enterococcus species	11	4	*Enterococcus* species	12	6
HACEK	2	0	HACEK	2	1
Fungus	1	1	Fungus	4	1
Polymicrobial	1	3	Polymicrobial	1	0
Others	4	5	Others	7	6
Culture negative	9	3	Culture negative	12	10

Abbreviation: HACEK = *Haemophilus, Actinobacillus, Cardiobacterium, Eikenella,* and *Kingella group.*

*Including pacemakers and implantable cardioverter-defibrillators.

MICROBIOLOGY

A wide range of bacteria and fungi, as well as *Rickettsia* and *Chlamydophila* species, can cause infective endocarditis. Bacteria are the predominant cause overall, with a small number of species responsible for the majority of cases. Causative microorganisms vary based on the specific conditions (i.e., native vs prosthetic valve) and risk factors (injection drug use or intracardiac devices; **Table 155-1**). Overall, recent reports from the United States and European countries indicate that *Staphylococcus* is the single most common cause, followed by streptococci and enterococci.[1,3,12-14]

The increase in the number of cases caused by staphylococci is likely linked to the observed increase in healthcare-associated endocarditis and also more frequent intravenous drug use. Staphylococcal endocarditis can cause rapid destruction of valves, multiple distal abscesses, myocardial abscesses, conduction defects, and pericarditis. Staphylococcal endocarditis has an increased risk of in-hospital death.[1] In contrast, streptococcal endocarditis tends to be indolent. Patients with enterococcal endocarditis generally have underlying valvular disease and risk factors such as diabetes mellitus or manipulation of the GU or lower GI tract.

Blood cultures are the best initial method for detection but are negative in about 5% of patients; in one third to one half of patients, cultures are negative because of prior antibiotic administration. For those cases associated with negative blood cultures and without prior antibiotic administration, infection is due to fastidious organisms, such as the **HACEK group (*Haemophilus, Actinobacillus, Cardiobacterium, Eikenella,* and *Kingella*), *Bartonella* species, or *Coxiella burnetii*.**

Skin flora and contaminated injection devices are the most frequent sources of microorganisms in injection drug use–associated endocarditis. *S. aureus* accounts for >50% of cases, followed in decreasing frequency by streptococcal species (including enterococci) and coagulase-negative staphylococci. The well-established predilection for *S. aureus* to infect normal heart valves, particularly tricuspid valves, is seen in injection addicts, although streptococci and enterococci often infect abnormal mitral or aortic valves in these patients.

Microorganisms involved in prosthetic valve endocarditis often reflect contamination during the perioperative period, with *Staphylococcus epidermidis* being a commonly isolated organism. *Aspergillus* and *Candida albicans* account for the majority of cases of mycotic prosthetic valve endocarditis and often have large vegetations and emboli.

CLINICAL FEATURES

The clinical manifestations of endocarditis are on a continuum, from acute in onset to insidious and indolent.[12] Common presenting symptoms include fever, chills, weakness, and dyspnea. The most common complications are congestive heart failure (44%), CNS disorder (30%), and peripheral embolization (22%).[14]

FEVER

Early bacteremia produces nonspecific signs and symptoms (**Table 155-2**), usually beginning within 2 weeks of infection. Symptoms include fever, chills, nausea, vomiting, fatigue, and malaise.[15] Fever (>38°C [100.4°F]) is present in almost all patients (>90% overall and >98% in those with injection drug use–associated infective endocarditis).[5,11,12,13] Fever may be absent in the elderly, those with a history of antibiotic or antipyretic use, and those with congestive heart failure, renal failure, or immunosuppression. Clinical symptoms of sepsis may be present.

CARDIAC MANIFESTATIONS

Congestive heart failure occurs in up to 70% of patients from distortion or perforation of valvular leaflets, rupture of the chordae tendineae or papillary muscles, or perforation of cardiac chambers. Heart murmurs are common, heard in 50% to 85% of patients, although less so in cases of right-sided endocarditis (<50%). Valvular abscesses and pericarditis can result from local extension. Other cardiac complications include heart blocks and dysrhythmias that result from extension of infection through the interventricular septum to the conduction system.

NEUROLOGIC MANIFESTATIONS

About 20% to 40% of patients develop neurologic symptoms, notably cerebral ischemic events (often in multiple areas), CNS abscess, intracranial hemorrhage, mycotic aneurysm, meningitis, or seizures.[16] Embolic stroke involving the middle cerebral artery is the most common CNS complication.[15]

ARTERIAL EMBOLIZATION

Friable vegetation fragments can embolize to any artery, resulting in infarction or abscess in remote tissues; finding multiple brain or lung abscesses should trigger a search for endocarditis. Pulmonary complications include pulmonary infarction, pneumonia, empyema, or pleural effusion. Coronary artery emboli usually arise from the aortic valve and

TABLE 155-2 Clinical Features of Infective Endocarditis

Symptoms	%	Signs	%
Fever	80	Fever	90
Chills	40	Heart murmur	85
Weakness	40	New murmur	3–5
Dyspnea	40	Changing murmur	5–10
Anorexia	25	Skin manifestations	18–50
Cough	25	Osler nodes	10–23
Malaise	25	Splinter hemorrhages	15
Skin lesions	20	Petechiae	20–40
Nausea/vomiting	20	Janeway lesions	<10
Headache	20	Splenomegaly	20–57
Stroke	20	Embolic phenomena	>50
Chest pain	15	Septic complications	20
Abdominal pain	15	Mycotic aneurysm	20
Mental status change	10–15	Renal failure	10
Back pain	10	Retinal lesions	2–10

may cause acute myocardial infarction or myocarditis. Embolic splenic infarction causes left upper quadrant abdominal pain with radiation to the left shoulder. Renal emboli result in flank pain and hematuria. Emboli to the mesenteric arteries cause acute abdominal pain and guaiac-positive stool and can lead to bowel ischemia, whereas emboli to arteries of the extremities may produce acute limb ischemia. Rupture of a cerebral mycotic aneurysm results in subarachnoid hemorrhage. Retinal artery embolism may cause acute monocular blindness.

CUTANEOUS FINDINGS

Cutaneous embolic phenomena are less common due to early clinical presentation and treatment. Cutaneous findings may occur in 5% to 10% of cases and may include petechiae, splinter or subungual hemorrhages of the finger or toenails, Osler nodes (small, tender subcutaneous nodules on the pads of the fingers or toes), and Janeway lesions (small hemorrhagic painless plaques on the palms or soles).[17,18] Digital clubbing is infrequent and found only in those with long-standing disease. Cutaneous signs are not specific and may be seen in other disease states characterized by vasculitis or bacteremia.

ADMISSION

Suspicion of endocarditis usually requires hospital admission[19,20] to allow the key diagnostic steps to occur (culture, echocardiography, and clinical observation).[1] Although prediction rules to exclude infective endocarditis exist,[21] none are currently robust enough to permit use in clinical practice. Consider endocarditis in patients with unexplained fever and with risk factors for the disease. Because the prevalence of endocarditis among febrile injection drug users is high (10% to 15%), clinical findings cannot reliably exclude the diagnosis, and follow-up is often a challenge, patients should be admitted to evaluate for bacteremia and endocarditis. Prolonged unexplained fever, malaise, or other constitutional symptoms without another cause are symptoms concerning for endocarditis. Admit all patients with a cardiac prosthetic valve and fever (or persistent malaise, vasculitis, or new murmur) because of the increased risk for endocarditis and the high morbidity and mortality associated with prosthetic valve infections. Look for any new or changed murmur, and seek evidence of vasculitis or embolization. In stable patients for whom there is a low suspicion of endocarditis who were initially discharged, admit immediately once positive blood cultures are found.

DIAGNOSTIC CRITERIA

The **Duke criteria**[22,23] are widely used criteria for diagnosing infective endocarditis (**Tables 155-3 and 155-4**).

TABLE 155-3 Duke Criteria* for Infective Endocarditis

Major Criteria
Positive blood culture for IE
Typical microorganism consistent with IE from two separate blood cultures* as noted below:
Streptococcus bovis, viridans streptococci, HACEK group
or
Community-acquired *Staphylococcus aureus* or *enterococci* in the absence of a primary focus
or
Microorganisms consistent with IE from persistently positive blood cultures defined as:
At least two positive cultures of blood samples drawn >12 h apart
or
All of three or a majority of four or more separate blood cultures (with first and last sample drawn at least 1 h apart)
Single positive blood culture for *Coxiella burnetii* or antiphase I immunoglobulin G antibody titer of >1:800
Evidence of echocardiographic involvement
Positive ECG for IE defined as:
Oscillating intracardiac mass on valve or supporting structures, in the path of regurgitant jets, or on implanted material in the absence of an alternative anatomic explanation
or
Abscess
or
New partial dehiscence of prosthetic valve
New valvular regurgitation (worsening or changing of preexisting murmur not sufficient)
Minor Criteria
Predisposition: predisposing heart condition or injection drug use
Fever: temperature >38°C (100.4°F)
Vascular phenomena: major arterial emboli, septic pulmonary conjunctival hemorrhages, and Janeway lesions
Immunologic phenomena: glomerulonephritis, Osler nodes, Roth spots, and rheumatoid fever
Microbiologic evidence: positive blood culture but does not meet a major criterion as noted in Table 155-4* or serologic evidence of active infection with organism consistent with IE
Echocardiographic minor findings were eliminated in the modified Duke criteria

Abbreviations: HACEK = *Haemophilus, Actinobacillus, Cardiobacterium, Eikenella, and Kingella;* IE = infective endocarditis.

*Excludes single positive cultures for coagulase-negative staphylococci and organisms that do not cause IE.

BLOOD CULTURES

Obtain blood cultures in the ED before beginning antibiotics, drawing three sets from separate sites because fewer collections may not detect bacteremia. Obtain at least 10 mL of blood for each culture bottle. Additional sets of blood cultures may be needed in patients already receiving antibiotics. Ideally, wait at least 1 hour between the first and last blood culture. In patients who are in septic shock or with systemic complications, do not withhold antibiotics to obtain delayed sets of cultures.

For patients who are at risk for culture-negative infective endocarditis, advise the laboratory of the suspected diagnosis to allow initiation of specialized testing to recover fastidious organisms. Polymerase chain reaction techniques aid pathogen detection.

OTHER DIAGNOSTIC TESTS

There are no definitive laboratory tests that diagnose endocarditis in the ED. Common findings are anemia (70% to 90% of cases), hematuria, and elevated erythrocyte sedimentation rate (>90% of cases), C-reactive protein, and procalcitonin.

ECG findings are also nonspecific but can identify conduction abnormalities resulting from infection. Prolonged PR interval, new left bundle-branch block, or new right bundle-branch block with left anterior hemiblock suggests spread of infection from the aortic valve into the conduction system. Junctional tachycardia, Wenckebach block, or complete heart block may indicate likely extension of infection from the mitral annulus into the atrioventricular node or proximal bundle of His.

Chest radiographs may demonstrate other complications, such as pulmonic emboli in patients with right-sided valvular involvement or congestive heart failure in those with left-sided valvular involvement.

ECHOCARDIOGRAPHY

Obtain echocardiography as soon as possible, because (1) echocardiographic abnormalities represent one of the two major criteria required for definitive diagnosis of endocarditis and (2) evaluation of the cardiac valves and surrounding structures provides critical information for management decisions. Bedside ED echocardiography is one tool, in addition to formal inpatient testing.

Two-dimensional transthoracic echocardiography is the first choice for those with native valves. The specificity of transthoracic echocardiography for vegetations is excellent (98%), but sensitivity varies

TABLE 155-4 Modified Duke Criteria for Infective Endocarditis

Definite Infective Endocarditis
Pathologic criteria
Microorganisms demonstrated by culture or histologic examination of a vegetation or in a vegetation that has embolized, or in an intracardiac abscess
or
Pathologic lesions: vegetation or intracardiac abscess present, confirmed by histology showing active endocarditis
Clinical Criteria, Using Specific Definitions Listed in Table 155-3
Two major criteria
or
One major and three minor criteria
or
Five minor criteria
Possible infective endocarditis
One major criterion and one minor criterion
Three minor criteria
Rejected
Firm alternate diagnosis for manifestations of endocarditis
or
Resolution of manifestations of endocarditis with antibiotic therapy for 4 d or less
or
No pathologic evidence of infective endocarditis at surgery or autopsy after antibiotic therapy for 4 d
Does not meet criteria for possible infective endocarditis

according to patient population. Sensitivity of transthoracic echocardiography is highest in injection drug users (88% to 94%), who more often have larger vegetations, a preponderance of right-sided lesions, and a favorable acoustic precordial window characteristic of younger patients. For those with chest wall deformities, obesity, or chronic obstructive pulmonary disease, echocardiography is less sensitive.

Transesophageal echocardiography has greater sensitivity and specificity for valvular abnormalities than transthoracic echocardiography due to improved image resolution, but it can be harder for an awake patient to tolerate. Use transesophageal echocardiography in (1) patients with prosthetic valves or intracardiac devices; (2) those in whom inadequate images are likely to be obtained with transthoracic echocardiography, as described above; and (3) those with intermediate or high clinical probability of endocarditis. Transesophageal echocardiography is of particular value for assessing suspected complications such as myocardial abscess and perivalvular extension.

TREATMENT

INITIAL STABILIZATION

Patients with endocarditis may present with hemodynamic instability, including hypotension, respiratory compromise due to decreased cardiac output and/or pulmonary edema, diminished pulmonary capacity, altered mental status, or acidosis. Emergency stabilization with airway management and hemodynamic monitoring and support are priority interventions. Intra-aortic balloon counterpulsation aids the emergency management of unstable mitral valve rupture but is contraindicated for aortic valve rupture.

Definitive management requires a team approach and may include cardiology, infectious disease, and cardiac surgery. Systemic clot lysis or anticoagulation for treatment of endocarditis-associated stroke is controversial and best decided upon together with a stroke expert.

Anticoagulation for prosthetic valve endocarditis may reduce the risk of thromboembolism without increased risk of intracranial hemorrhage.[24] Patients with prosthetic valves already being treated with anticoagulants may be maintained on established regimens.[25]

EMPIRIC TREATMENT OF SUSPECTED ENDOCARDITIS OF NATIVE VALVES

Antibiotic selection is based on patient characteristics and local resistance patterns. **Table 155-5** lists sample empiric treatment regimens.[25-27] Although some authors recommend awaiting culture results before antibiotic therapy for patients with subacute bacterial endocarditis, we recommend ED initiation of antibiotic therapy for all patients suspected of endocarditis after obtaining appropriate cultures, targeting the most common organisms, *Staphylococcus aureus* and *Streptococcus* species. For patients with suspected native valve infection, empiric antibiotic therapy includes a penicillinase-resistant penicillin or a cephalosporin *and* an aminoglycoside. For patients with complications (including injection drug use, congenital heart disease, nosocomial infections, those who develop endocarditis while taking oral antibiotics, or those with suspected methicillin-resistant *S. aureus*), add vancomycin.

EMPIRIC TREATMENT OF SUSPECTED ENDOCARDITIS OF ARTIFICIAL VALVES

For patients with suspected artificial valve endocarditis, empiric therapy includes vancomycin, an aminoglycoside, and rifampin.

TABLE 155-5 Empiric Therapy of Suspected Bacterial Endocarditis*

Patient Characteristics	Recommended Agents, Initial Dose
Uncomplicated history	Ceftriaxone, 1–2 grams IV *or* Nafcillin, 2 grams IV *or* Oxacillin, 2 grams IV *or* Vancomycin, 15 milligrams/kg *plus* Gentamicin, 1–3 milligrams/kg IV *or* Tobramycin, 1 milligram/kg IV
Injection drug use, congenital heart disease, hospital-acquired, suspected methicillin-resistant *Staphylococcus aureus*, or already on oral antibiotics	Nafcillin, 2 grams IV *plus* Gentamicin, 1–3 milligrams/kg IV *plus* Vancomycin, 15 milligrams/kg IV
Prosthetic heart valve	Vancomycin, 15 milligrams/kg IV *plus* Gentamicin, 1–3 milligrams/kg IV *plus* Rifampin, 300 milligrams PO

*Based on American Heart Association, endorsed by the Infectious Disease Society of America, http://www.idsociety.org/Organ_System/, accessed April 1, 2014. Because of controversy in the literature regarding the optimal regimen for empiric treatment, antibiotic selection should be based on patient characteristics, local resistance patterns, and current authoritative recommendations.

DEFINITIVE TREATMENT OF ENDOCARDITIS

Definitive antibiotic treatment is based on culture and sensitivity results. Most patients will require 4 to 6 weeks of antibiotic therapy. Surgical management is indicated in patients with severe valvular dysfunction, congestive heart failure, relapsing prosthetic valve endocarditis, major embolic complications, fungal endocarditis, new conduction defects or dysrhythmias, or persistent bacteremia after appropriate antibiotic therapy.[28,29] Surgical risk increases in those older than 65 years, on inotropes, with sepsis or with cerebral emboli.[30]

ENDOCARDITIS PROPHYLAXIS

Because everyday dental activities (brushing, flossing, chewing) create bacteremia, good dental care is important. Antibiotic prophylaxis should be given to those at risk **(Table 155-6).**

Prophylaxis is *not* routinely indicated for patients with mitral valve prolapse (with or without regurgitation), pacemakers, hypertrophic cardiomyopathy, physiologic murmurs, prior coronary artery bypass surgery or angioplasty, or previous surgical repair of atrial septal defect, ventricular septal defect, or patent ductus arteriosus.

For highest risk patients, provide antibiotic prophylaxis before dental procedures that involve manipulation of gingival tissue, the periapical region of teeth, or perforation of the oral mucosa. **Prophylaxis is not needed for nondental procedures**, such as local injections, laceration suturing, IV line placement, blood drawing, endotracheal intubation, endoscopy, vaginal delivery, oral trauma and bleeding, urethral catheterization, or uterine dilation and curettage. Some experts recommend prophylaxis for body art, such as tattooing and piercing.

Recommendations for procedures that manipulate infected skin structures or musculoskeletal tissue are Class IIb (may be considered, usefulness is less well established); it is reasonable to administer antibiotics before the procedure for the highest risk groups identified in Table 155-6. The antibiotic should be active against staphylococci and β-hemolytic streptococci. Vancomycin and clindamycin are options for those unable to tolerate a β-lactam or who are known or suspected to have an infection caused by a methicillin-resistant strain of *Staphylococcus*. The incidence of bacteremia with abscess incision and drainage is very low; hence, clear data are lacking.

A simplified strategy for antibiotic prophylaxis is listed in **Table 155-7.**[32] With the endorsement of the National Institute for Health and Clinical Excellence of London,[33] the European College of Cardiology does not recommend prophylaxis before respiratory tract procedures, GI or GU procedures, or uncomplicated dermatologic or musculoskeletal procedures.[34]

With good aseptic technique, prophylactic antibiotics are not recommended prior to invasive procedures such as central lines.[35]

PRACTICE GUIDELINES

The American Heart Association has published guidelines on diagnosis and management (http://circ.ahajournals.org/cgi/reprint/111/23/e394) as well as prophylaxis (www.circ.ahajournals.org/content/lll/23/e394.full [accessed 8/17/2015])for infective endocarditis.

TABLE 155-6 Highest Risk Conditions for Endocarditis[31]

Prosthetic heart valves
Prosthetic material used for valve repair
History of previous infective endocarditis
Unrepaired cyanotic congenital heart disease
Repaired congenital heart defect with prosthetic material or device
Repaired congenital heart disease with residual defects
Cardiac transplant recipients with valve regurgitation due to a structurally abnormal valve

TABLE 155-7 Prophylaxis Against Endocarditis for Highest Risk Patients

Procedure	Patient Characteristics	Antibiotic Agent	Dose
Dental procedures involving manipulation of either gingival tissue or the periapical region of teeth or perforation of the oral mucosa	Able to take oral antibiotics	Amoxicillin	2 grams PO, 30–60 min before procedure
		or	
	Unable to take oral medication	Ampicillin	2 grams IM or IV, 30–60 min before procedure
		or	
		Cefazolin or ceftriaxone	1 gram IM or IV, 30–60 min before procedure
	Allergic to penicillins or ampicillin	Cephalexin	2 grams PO, 30–60 min before procedure
		or	
		Clindamycin	600 milligrams PO, 30–60 min before procedure
		or	
		Azithromycin or clarithromycin	500 milligrams PO, 30–60 min before procedure
	Unable to take oral medication and allergic to penicillins or ampicillin	Cefazolin or ceftriaxone	1 gram IM or IV, 30–60 min before procedure
		or	
		Clindamycin	600 milligrams IM or IV, 30–60 min before procedure
Procedures on infected skin, skin structure, or musculoskeletal tissue	Non–methicillin-resistant strain of *Staphylococcus* or β-hemolytic *Streptococcus* suspected	Dicloxacillin	2 grams PO, 30–60 min before procedure
		or	
		Cephalexin	2 grams PO, 30–60 min before procedure
	Patients unable to tolerate a β-lactam or who are known or suspected to have an infection caused by a methicillin-resistant strain of *Staphylococcus*	Vancomycin	1 gram IV, 30–60 min before procedure
		or	
		Clindamycin	600 milligrams IM or IV, 30–60 min before procedure
Other procedures (respiratory; GI; GU; noninfected dermatologic or musculoskeletal procedures)		Prophylaxis not indicated	

REFERENCES

The complete reference list is available online at www.TintinalliEM.com.

CHAPTER 156 Tetanus

Joel L. Moll
Donna L. Carden

INTRODUCTION AND EPIDEMIOLOGY

Tetanus is uncommon in the United States but continues to have a substantial health impact in developing countries. The worldwide incidence of tetanus is approximately 1 million cases per year, with a mortality rate of 20% to 30%.[1]

The Centers for Disease Control and Prevention defines tetanus as a syndrome of acute onset of hypertonia and/or painful muscular contractions (usually of the muscles of the jaw and neck) and generalized muscle spasms without other apparent medical cause as reported by a health professional.[2] In the United States, tetanus is a reportable disease, aggregated through the National Notifiable Diseases Surveillance System.

Improved childbirth practices, widespread immunization programs for children, decennial tetanus boosters for adults, mechanization of agriculture, and use of chemical fertilizers rather than animal manure have resulted in a >95% decline in the annual incidence of tetanus in the United States since 1947.[2] From 2001 to 2008, 233 tetanus cases were reported in the United States from 45 states, with the majority of cases reported from five states: California (n = 60), Florida (n = 25), Texas (n = 12), New York (n = 12), and Pennsylvania (n = 11).[2] Most patients who develop tetanus have inadequate immunity to the disease. Due to waning immunity and failure to receive routine boosters, only 31% of Americans >70 years old have adequate tetanus immunity.[3] As a result, the average annual incidence of tetanus among those ≥65 years of age is higher (0.23 cases per 1 million population) than among those age 5 to 64 years (0.08 cases per 1 million population). Tetanus among children and neonatal tetanus are uncommon in the United States as well as in other developed countries. The case fatality rate is approximately 13%, with the elderly accounting for the majority of deaths.[2]

Most cases of tetanus in the United States are associated with an acute wound. Puncture, contaminated, infected, or devitalized wounds account for approximately 70% of tetanus cases. Although less common, chronic wounds, ulcers and other wounds in diabetics, and dental abscesses are also associated with the disease. Diabetics and injection drug users have an increased risk of contracting tetanus.[2,4]

Most patients who develop tetanus do not seek medical care for their initial wound. In those who do seek initial treatment and later develop tetanus, up to 95% do not receive appropriate therapy.[2]

PATHOPHYSIOLOGY

Clostridium tetani is a motile, nonencapsulated, anaerobic gram-positive rod, and its toxins cause tetanus. *C. tetani* exists in either a vegetative or a spore-forming state. The spores are ubiquitous in soil and in animal feces and are resistant to destruction, surviving on environmental surfaces for years. In agricultural areas, adults may harbor the organism, and spores have been found on skin or in contaminated heroin.[4,5] *C. tetani* is usually introduced into a wound in the spore-forming, noninvasive state but can germinate into a toxin-producing, vegetative form if tissue oxygen tension is reduced. **Crushed or devitalized tissue, a foreign body, or the development of infection favors the growth of the toxin-producing form of *C. tetani*.**[5,6]

C. tetani produces two exotoxins: tetanolysin, which appears to favor the expansion of the bacterial population, and tetanospasmin, a powerful neurotoxin responsible for all of the clinical manifestations of tetanus. Tetanospasmin reaches the nervous system by hematogenous spread of the exotoxin to peripheral nerves and by retrograde intraneuronal transport. Tetanospasmin does not cross the blood–brain barrier, but retrograde intraneuronal transport of the exotoxin enables tetanospasmin to gain access to the CNS.[6]

Tetanospasmin prevents the release of the inhibitory neurotransmitters glycine and γ-aminobutyric acid from presynaptic nerve terminals, releasing the nervous system from its normal inhibitory control. Loss of inhibition may also affect the preganglionic sympathetic neurons, resulting in sympathetic overactivity and high circulating catecholamine levels.[5-8]

CLINICAL FEATURES

Tetanus results in generalized muscular rigidity, violent muscular contractions, and autonomic nervous system instability.[6] Wounds that become contaminated with toxin-producing *C. tetani* are often puncture wounds, but contaminated wounds range from deep lacerations to minor abrasions.[2] **No wound is identified in up to 10% of patients with tetanus.** Tetanus can also develop after surgical procedures, otitis media, or abortion and can develop in injection drug users from contaminated heroin and in neonates through infection of the umbilical stump.[4,9]

The incubation period for tetanus ranges from <24 hours to >1 month. Short incubation periods are associated with severe disease and a poor prognosis for recovery. Clinical tetanus can be categorized into three forms: generalized, cephalic, and local. **Generalized tetanus** accounts for about 80% of cases. The most frequent presenting complaints of patients with generalized tetanus are pain and stiffness in the masseter muscles (lockjaw). Nerves with short axons are affected initially, so symptoms appear first in the facial muscles, with descending progression to the muscles of the neck, trunk, and extremities. The transition from muscle stiffness to rigidity leads to the development of trismus and the characteristic facial expression: risus sardonicus (sardonic smile). Reflex convulsive spasms and tonic muscle contractions are responsible for the development of dysphagia, opisthotonos flexing of the arms, clenching of the fists, and extension of the lower extremities. Spasms can last for 3 to 4 weeks, and recovery depends on regrowth of axonal nerve terminals and may take months.[6] Complications of tetanus include rhabdomyolysis and long-bone fractures secondary to violent muscle contractions. The mental status is normal, an important consideration in differentiating tetanus from other disorders (**Table 156-1**). Patients remain conscious and alert unless laryngospasm or contraction of respiratory muscles results in respiratory compromise. Other complications of prolonged hospitalization include pulmonary embolus, pneumonia, and sepsis. Aspiration pneumonia is present in 50% to 70% of autopsied cases.[5,6]

Autonomic changes are generally a hypersympathetic state, occurring during the second week of clinical tetanus and including tachycardia, labile hypertension, profuse sweating, hyperpyrexia, and

TABLE 156-1 Differential Diagnosis of Tetanus

Disorder	Comments
Strychnine poisoning	See chapter 201, "Pesticides."
Dystonic reaction (phenothiazines, metoclopramide)	See chapter 180, "Antipsychotics."
Hypocalcemic tetany	See chapter 17, "Fluids and Electrolytes."
Malignant neuroleptic syndrome	See chapter 180, "Antipsychotics."
Serotonin syndrome	See chapter 178, "Atypical and Serotonergic Antidepressants"
Stiff man syndrome	Centrally mediated motor hyperexcitability with persistent and intense spasms, particularly of the proximal lower limbs and lumbar paraspinal muscles.
Peritonsillar abscess	See chapter 246, "Neck and Upper Airway."
Peritonitis	See chapter 71, "Acute Abdominal Pain."
Meningeal irritation (bacterial meningitis, subarachnoid hemorrhage)	See chapters 174, "Central Nervous System and Spinal Infections" and 166, "Spontaneous Subarachnoid and Intracerebral Hemorrhage."
Rabies	See chapter 157, "Rabies."
Temporomandibular joint disease	See chapter 243, "Face and Jaw Emergencies."

increased urinary excretion of catecholamines.[6-8] **Neonatal tetanus**, a form of generalized tetanus, develops in infants born to inadequately immunized mothers, frequently after unsterile treatment of the umbilical cord stump.[9] Infants with neonatal tetanus are weak, irritable, and have an inability to suck. Symptoms are evident by the second week of life.[9]

Cephalic tetanus follows injuries to the head or occasionally otitis media and results in dysfunction of the cranial nerves, most commonly the seventh. It has a poor prognosis.

Local tetanus is manifested by rigidity of muscles in proximity to the site of injury and usually resolves completely after weeks to months. Local tetanus may progress to the generalized form of the disease. Approximately 1% of the cases are fatal.[5,6]

DIAGNOSIS

Tetanus is diagnosed clinically. In the United States, 96% of tetanus cases occur in those with unknown or inadequate immunization history.[2] Certain populations, especially the elderly, those requiring hemodialysis, and the immunocompromised, are more likely to have inadequate immunity.[10,11] There are no laboratory tests to diagnose tetanus, although serum antitoxin titers of >0.01 IU/mL (by mouse neutralization assay) are usually protective. An immunochromatographic dipstick test offers the advantage of rapid assessment of immunity, with an 88% sensitivity and 98% specificity, and may be useful in regions with high disease incidence.[12] However, tetanus has developed in patients with protective levels of antitetanus antibodies.[13] Wound culture is of limited value, because *C. tetani* may be cultured from wounds in the absence of clinical disease and may not be recovered in patients with documented tetanus.

Table 156-1 provides the differential diagnosis of tetanus. **Strychnine poisoning** most closely mimics the clinical picture of generalized tetanus.

TREATMENT

Treatment is summarized in **Table 156-2**. Admit patients with tetanus to the intensive care unit. Respiratory compromise requires immediate neuromuscular blockade and intubation. Minimize environmental stimuli to prevent the precipitation of reflex convulsive spasms.

TETANUS IMMUNOGLOBULIN

Human tetanus immunoglobulin neutralizes circulating tetanospasmin and toxin in the wound but not toxin that is already fixed in the nervous system. Even though tetanus immunoglobulin does not ameliorate the clinical symptoms of tetanus, early reports suggest it reduces mortality.[14] The dose varies depending on the purpose. For postexposure prophylaxis, a single dose of 250 units (4 units/kg in children) IM given in the anterolateral thigh or deltoid is recommended. For the treatment of actual tetanus, the optimal dose of tetanus immunoglobulin is unknown, but 3000 to 6000 units IM is the usual recommended dose, administered in a separate syringe and opposite the site of tetanus toxoid administration. At least a portion of the dose should be administered around the wound itself.[5] **Tetanus immunoglobulin should be given before wound debridement, because exotoxin may be released during wound manipulation.** Repeated doses of tetanus immunoglobulin are unnecessary because of its long half-life of 28 days.

WOUND MANAGEMENT

Identify and debride the wound to improve the oxidation-reduction potential of infected tissue and to prevent further toxin production.

ANTIBIOTICS

Antibiotics are of limited value but are traditionally administered, and **parenteral metronidazole** is the antibiotic of choice.[15,16] **Do not give penicillin because it may potentiate the effects of tetanospasmin.**[6]

MUSCLE RELAXANTS

Tetanospasmin prevents neurotransmitter release at inhibitory interneurons, and therapy of tetanus is aimed at restoring normal inhibition. The benzodiazepines are centrally acting inhibitory agents that have been used extensively for this purpose. However, the large IV doses of benzodiazepines required in tetanus may result in metabolic acidosis secondary to the propylene glycol vehicle in IV lorazepam or diazepam. **Thus, many prefer midazolam, a water-soluble agent, for muscle relaxation.**[6] The effects of baclofen, a specific γ-aminobutyric acid agonist, vary.[6]

NEUROMUSCULAR BLOCKADE

Prolonged neuromuscular blockade aids in control of ventilation, muscular spasms, secondary fractures, and rhabdomyolysis. Succinylcholine can be given early for emergency airway control, whereas vecuronium is a good option for prolonged blockade because of minimal cardiovascular side effects.[15]

TREATMENT OF AUTONOMIC DYSFUNCTION

One randomized controlled trial in 256 patients with severe tetanus demonstrated that magnesium sulfate reduced autonomic instability and muscle spasm in the disease.[7] Furthermore, magnesium sulfate has been shown to reduce urinary catecholamine excretion in patients with severe tetanus.[8] However, a meta-analysis failed to show a benefit of magnesium sulfate on tetanus mortality, and the effect of the drug on duration of intensive care unit and hospital stay and need for ventilatory support was unclear.[17]

Adrenergic blocking agents may treat the autonomic dysfunction of severe tetanus. Choose either a short-acting β-blocker, such as esmolol, or labetalol, a combined α- and β-adrenergic blocking agent, if treating this manifestation of tetanus.

Morphine sulfate reduces sympathetic α-adrenergic tone and central sympathetic efferent discharge and produces peripheral arteriolar and venous dilatation.[6] Clonidine, a central α_2-receptor agonist, may act to reduce the sympathetic hyperactivity that causes autonomic dysfunction and thereby provide better control of crises.[18]

TABLE 156-2 Treatment of Tetanus

Respiratory management	Sedation and neuromuscular blockade with succinylcholine or vecuronium for intubation and ongoing mechanical ventilation
Immunotherapy	Tetanus immunoglobulin, 3000–6000 units IM opposite side of the body from tetanus toxoid, with at least a portion around the wound site *and* Tetanus toxoid (DTaP or Td/Tdap depending on age), 0.5 mL IM at presentation, and 6 wk and 6 mo after presentation
Wound care	Wound debridement
Antibiotic therapy	Metronidazole, 500 milligrams IV every 6 h **No penicillin**
Muscle relaxation	Midazolam preferred
Management of autonomic dysfunction	Magnesium sulfate, 40 milligrams/kg IV loading, then 2 grams/h (1.5 grams/h if ≤45 kg) continuous infusion to maintain blood level of 2.0–4.0 mmol/L *or* Labetalol, 0.25–1.0 milligram/min continuous IV infusion
	Morphine sulfate, 0.5–1.0 milligram/kg/h
	Clonidine, 300 micrograms every 8 h by nasogastric tube

Abbreviations: DTaP = diphtheria and tetanus toxoids and acellular pertussis vaccine; Tdap = tetanus toxoid with lower doses of diphtheria and acellular pertussis than DTaP; Td = tetanus-diphtheria.

IMMUNIZATION

Patients who recover from tetanus must receive active immunization, because infection does not confer immunity and vaccination is the only means of disease prevention. Give adsorbed tetanus toxoid (0.5 mL) IM at the time of presentation and at 6 weeks and 6 months after injury.

In patients with tetanus-prone wounds or those with incomplete vaccinations or greater than 10 years from previous vaccination, use tetanus-diphtheria (Td) if ≥7 years old, and use diphtheria and tetanus toxoids and acellular pertussis vaccine (DTaP) for those under 7 years old.[19] DTaP contains over three times the amount of diphtheria component as Tdap and must be used for primary vaccination series in children. Because of the recent increase in the incidence of pertussis, adolescents and adults should receive a single lifetime dose of Tdap to replace one Td booster.[19] An inadvertent dose of DTaP in an adult would count as the single lifetime dose of Tdap.

The revised Advisory Committee on Immunization Practices guidelines recommend administering a dose of Tdap during each **pregnancy**, irrespective of the patient's prior history of receiving Tdap or interval since last injection, to maximize the maternal antibody response and passive antibody levels in the newborn.[20] Tdap may be given at any point during pregnancy, with optimal timing between 27 and 36 weeks of gestation unless treating a specific wound. For women who have never received Tdap, it should be given to the mother immediately postpartum and to any direct caregivers to reduce the risk of pertussis to the newborn.

Table 156-3 summarizes the guidelines for tetanus immunization and tetanus prophylaxis in wound management.[19] **Only about 60% of patients with an acute injury who seek medical care receive appropriate tetanus wound prophylaxis.**[2] Table 156-2 summarizes the management of tetanus.

Adverse reactions following tetanus immunization include erythema, induration, and pain at the injection site. Local reactions are common and usually self-limited. Exaggerated local reactions (Arthus reactions) occur occasionally after tetanus toxoid and involve extensive pain and swelling of the entire extremity. Arthus reactions occur most often in adults with high serum tetanus antitoxin levels who have received frequent doses of tetanus toxoid, the reason this therapy is limited to 10-year intervals.

Contraindications to Td or Tdap include a history of serious allergic reaction (respiratory compromise or cardiovascular collapse) to vaccine components. History of encephalopathy (e.g., coma or prolonged seizures) not attributable to an identifiable cause within 7 days of administration of a pertussis vaccine is a contraindication to Tdap. Reasons to defer Td or Tdap include Guillain-Barré syndrome ≤6 weeks after a previous dose of tetanus toxoid-containing vaccine, moderate to severe acute illness, unstable neurologic condition, or history of an Arthus hypersensitivity reaction to a tetanus toxoid–containing vaccine administered <10 years previously.[19] If tetanus toxoid is contraindicated, consider passive immunization with tetanus immunoglobulin.

TABLE 156-3 Summary Guide to Tetanus Prophylaxis in Wound Management

	Clean, Minor Wounds		All Other Wounds*	
History of Adsorbed Tetanus Toxoid (doses)	Tdap or Td† IM	TIG, 250 units IM	Tdap or Td†	TIG, 250 units IM
Unknown or less than three	Yes‡	No	Yes	Yes
Three or more#	No^f	No	Yes**	No

*For example, wounds >6 hours old, contaminated with soil, saliva, feces, or dirt; puncture or crush wounds; avulsions; wounds from missiles, burns, or frostbite.

†DTaP for children <7 years of age (DT if pertussis vaccine is contraindicated); Td for persons ≥7 years of age. A single booster dose of Tdap is recommended for adolescents and adults to replace 1 Td booster.

‡The primary immunization series should be completed. Three doses total are required, with the second dose given at least 4 weeks after the first dose and the third dose given 6 months later.

#If only three doses of fluid toxoid have been received, then a fourth dose of *absorbed* toxoid should be given.

^f Yes, if >10 years since last dose.

**Yes, if >5 years since last dose. Boosters more frequent than every 5 years may predispose to side effects.

Abbreviations: DTaP = diphtheria and tetanus toxoids and acellular pertussis vaccine; DT = diphtheria-tetanus toxoids; Td = tetanus-diphtheria; Tdap = tetanus toxoid with lower doses of diphtheria and acellular pertussis than DTaP; TIG = tetanus immunoglobulin.

REFERENCES

The complete reference list is available online at www.TintinalliEM.com.

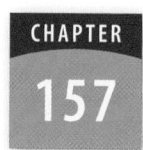

Rabies

David Weber

INTRODUCTION AND EPIDEMIOLOGY

This chapter reviews the epidemiology of rabies, pre- and postexposure rabies prophylaxis, and clinical presentation and treatment of rabies. Current information is available from the Centers for Disease Control and Prevention (http://www.cdc.gov/rabies/).

More than 3 billion people are at risk of rabies in over 100 countries.[1] The World Health Organization estimates that more than 15 million people receive a postexposure preventive regimen with more than 55,000 people dying of rabies annually, despite the availability of effective postexposure prophylaxis.

Rabies is primarily a disease of animals.[2-4] The epidemiology of human rabies reflects both the distribution of the disease in animals and the degree of human contact with these animals. A summary of major rabies vectors is provided in **Table 157-1**.

In the United States, rabies is endemic in many wild animal populations, with more than 6000 rabid animals reported in 2010.[5] Although human rabies is rare in the United States, postexposure rabies prophylaxis is provided to about 40,000 persons each year.[6] From 2001 to 2011, 29 cases of human rabies were reported in the United States, with eight cases contracted in other countries. About 90% of these cases were associated with **bats**. Most cases contracted outside the United States and Canada were from **dog** bites.[5,7,8]

PATHOPHYSIOLOGY

Rabies virus is the prototype member of the genus *Lyssavirus*.[9,10] All lyssaviruses are adapted to replicate in the mammalian CNS, are transmitted by direct contact, and are not associated with transmission by or natural replication in insects.

TABLE 157-1 Major World and U.S. Rabies Vectors

Vector	Region
Dogs	Asia, Latin America, Africa
Foxes	Europe, Arctic, North America
Skunks	Midwest United States, Western Canada
Coyotes	Asia, Africa, North America
Mongooses	Asia, Africa, Caribbean
Bats	North America, Latin America, Europe
No rabies	Hawaii, United Kingdom, Australasia, Antarctica

Viral infection of the salivary glands of the biting animal is responsible for the infectivity of saliva.[2-4,11] After a bite, saliva containing infectious rabies virus is deposited in muscle and subcutaneous tissues. The virus remains close to the site of exposure for the majority of the **long incubation period (typically 20 to 90 days)**. Rabies virus binds to the nicotinic acetylcholine receptor in muscle, which is expressed on the postsynaptic membrane of the neuromuscular junction. Subsequently, the virus spreads across the motor end plate and ascends and replicates along the peripheral nervous axoplasm to the dorsal root ganglia, the spinal cord, and the CNS. Following CNS replication in the gray matter, the virus spreads outward by peripheral nerves to virtually all tissues and organ systems.

Histologically, rabies is an encephalitis, resulting in infiltration of lymphocytes, polymorphonuclear leukocytes, and plasma cells, and focal hemorrhage and demyelination in the gray matter of the CNS, the basal ganglia, and the spinal cord. Negri bodies, in which CNS viral replication occurs, are eosinophilic intracellular lesions found within cerebral neurons and are highly specific for rabies. Negri bodies are found in about 75% of proven cases of animal rabies. Although their presence is pathognomonic for rabies, their absence does not exclude it.

Transmission of rabies virus usually begins when the contaminated saliva of an infected host is passed to a susceptible host, usually by the bite of a rabid animal. Other routes of documented transmission include contamination of mucous membranes (i.e., eyes, nose, mouth), aerosol transmission during spelunking (caving) in bat-infested caves, exposure while working in the laboratory with rabies virus, infected organ transplants (e.g., cornea, liver, kidney, vascular graft, lung), and iatrogenic infection through improperly inactivated vaccine.

PREEXPOSURE PROPHYLAXIS

Preexposure prophylaxis with rabies vaccine is highly recommended for persons whose recreational or occupational activities place them at risk for rabies (**Tables 157-2** and **157-3**).[12] Although the initial rabies preexposure vaccine regimen is similar for all risk groups, the need for booster doses, the timing of booster doses, and the need for and timing of serologic tests to confirm immunity differ based on the degree of individual risk for exposure to rabies. Preexposure prophylaxis may be obtained from the local health department or from a local physician or veterinarian. Preexposure vaccination does not eliminate the need for additional therapy after a rabies exposure, but simplifies postexposure prophylaxis by eliminating the need for human rabies immunoglobulin (HRIG) and by decreasing the number of doses of vaccine required (see later section, Postexposure Prophylaxis in Special Populations).

TABLE 157-3 Rabies Preexposure Prophylaxis Schedule—United States (2008)

Type of Immunization	Route	Regimen
Primary	Intramuscular*	HDCV or PCECV; 1.0 mL (deltoid area), one dose on days 0,† 7, and 21 or 28
Booster‡	Intramuscular*	HDCV or PCECV; 1.0 mL (deltoid area), one dose on day 0† only

Abbreviations: HDCV = human diploid cell vaccine; PCECV = purified chick embryo cell culture vaccine.

*Use deltoid area for adults and older children. For young children, use anterolateral thigh. Do not administer vaccine in the gluteal area.

†Day 0 is the day the first dose of vaccine is administered.

‡Persons in the continuous risk category should have a serum sample tested for rabies neutralizing antibody every 6 months, and persons in the frequent risk category should be tested every 2 years. An IM booster dose of vaccine should be administered if the serum titer falls to maintain the value of at least complete neutralization at a 1:5 serum dilution by rapid fluorescent focus inhibition test. See recommendations by the Centers for Disease Control and Prevention[12] for more details.

POSTEXPOSURE PROPHYLAXIS

RISK ASSESSMENT

The risk of developing rabies following a bite or scratch by a rabid animal depends on whether the wound was a bite, scratch, or nonbite exposure; the number of bites; the depth of the bites; and the location of the wounds (**Table 157-4**).[13]

Risk assessment for postexposure prophylaxis includes determining the epidemiology of animal rabies in the area where the contact occurred; knowing the species of animal involved; understanding the type of exposure (e.g., bite versus nonbite); clarifying the circumstances of the exposure incident; and determining if the animal can be safely captured and tested for rabies (**Table 157-5**). **The distinction between a "provoked" and "nonprovoked" attack should not be used for risk assessment.** Most animal bites are "provoked" from the standpoint of the animal (i.e., interfering with the animal's food, offspring, feeding habits, etc.). In addition, about 15% of animals with rabies do *not* exhibit aggressive behavior but are apathetic ("dumb rabies"). The local health department can provide information about the epidemiology of animal rabies in the area. **Evaluation for postexposure prophylaxis is indicated for persons bitten by, scratched by, or exposed to saliva from a wild or domestic animal that could be rabid (Figure 157-1).**

TABLE 157-2 Rabies Preexposure Risk Assessment and Recommendations

Risk Category	Nature of Risk	Typical Population	Preexposure Recommendations
Continuous	Virus present continuously, often in high concentrations; specific exposures likely to go unrecognized; bite, nonbite, or aerosol exposure	Rabies research laboratory workers,* rabies biologicals production workers	Primary course: serologic testing every 6 months; booster immunization if antibody titer is below acceptable level†
Frequent	Exposure usually episodic with source recognized, but exposure also might be unrecognized; bite, nonbite, or aerosol exposure	Rabies diagnostic laboratory workers,* cavers, veterinarians and staff, and animal-control and wildlife workers in rabies-endemic areas; all persons who regularly handle bats	Primary course: serologic testing every 2 years; booster immunization if antibody titer is below acceptable level†
Infrequent (greater than population at large)	Exposure nearly always episodic with source recognized; bite or nonbite exposure	Veterinarians and animal-control and wildlife workers working with terrestrial animals in areas where rabies is uncommon or rare, veterinary students, travelers visiting areas where rabies is endemic and immediate access to appropriate medical care, including biologicals, is limited	Primary course: no serologic testing or booster immunization
Rare (population at large)	Exposure always episodic with source recognized; bite or nonbite exposure	U.S. population at large, including persons in rabies-endemic areas	No immunization necessary

*Judgment of relative risk and extra monitoring of immunization status of laboratory workers is the responsibility of the laboratory supervisor.

†Minimum acceptable antibody level is complete virus neutralization at 1:5 serum dilution by the rapid fluorescent focus inhibition test. A booster dose should be administered if the titer falls below this level.

TABLE 157-4 Risk of Rabies in the Absence of Postexposure Prophylaxis after Exposure to a Rabid Animal

Multiple severe bites around the face: 80%–100%
Single bite: 15%–40%
Superficial bite(s) on an extremity: 5%
Contamination of a recent wound by saliva: ~0.1%
Contact with rabid saliva on a wound older than 24 hours: 0%
Transmission via fomites (e.g., tree branch): theoretical*
Indirect transmission (e.g., raccoon saliva on a dog): theoretical*

*Literature review revealed no cases due to this theoretical method of transmission.

Give postexposure prophylaxis as soon as possible after exposure to rabies-prone wildlife (**Tables 157-5** and **157-6**).

Bites For the purpose of rabies postexposure prophylaxis, **a bite exposure is defined as any penetration of the skin by the teeth of an animal.**[12] Bites to the face and hands carry the highest risk, but the site of the bite does not influence the decision to begin therapy.

Nonbite Exposures A **nonbite exposure** is contamination of scratches, abrasions, open wounds, or mucous membranes with saliva or brain tissue from a rabid animal. For example, animal licks to nonintact skin have transmitted rabies. Nonbite exposures from animals very rarely cause rabies. If the material containing the virus is dry, the virus can be considered noninfectious. Petting a rabid animal or contact with blood, urine, or feces (e.g., guano) of a rabid animal does not constitute an exposure and is not an indication for prophylaxis.[12]

Exposures to Animals Previously Vaccinated for Rabies A fully vaccinated dog or cat (i.e., two vaccinations) is unlikely to become infected with rabies. No documented vaccine failures have been reported in the United States among dogs or cats that received two vaccinations. Rare cases have been reported among animals that had received only a single dose of vaccine. In the United States, animals other than dogs, cats, and ferrets that can transmit rabies and are the source of an animal bite or scratch to a human should be euthanized and tested for rabies *even if the animals have been vaccinated.*

Exposures to Bats Any direct contact between a human and a bat should be evaluated for a rabies exposure. **Seeing a bat does not constitute an exposure.** Postexposure prophylaxis is not indicated if the person can be *certain* that a bite, scratch, or mucous membrane exposure did not occur or if the bat is available for testing and results are negative for the presence of rabies virus. All bats that might be a source of exposure, if available, should be sent to the public health department and tested for rabies, because approximately 94% of submitted bats in the United States have tested negative for rabies.[8] **The Advisory Committee on Immunization Practices recommends consideration of postexposure prophylaxis for persons who were in the same room as a bat and who were unaware if a bite or direct contact had occurred** (e.g., a sleeping person awakens to find a bat in the room, or an adult witnesses a bat in a room with an unattended child, mentally disabled person, or intoxicated person).[12,14] One article calculated the incidence of rabies following bedroom exposure with contact as 0.6 cases per billion person-years,[8] whereas another article reported that the number needed to treat to prevent a single case of rabies in this context would be 314,000 to 2.7 million persons.[15]

Bites from Healthy-Appearing Animals The Centers for Disease Control and Prevention recommends that a healthy dog, cat, or ferret that bites a person be confined and observed for 10 days.[12,14] At the first sign of illness during confinement, such animals should be evaluated by a veterinarian and a report immediately made to the local health department. If signs suggestive of rabies develop, the animal should be euthanized and its head removed and shipped under refrigeration (not frozen) for examination of the brain by a qualified laboratory designated by the local or state health department.

Bites from Stray Animals Any stray or unwanted dog, cat, or ferret that bites a person may be euthanized immediately and the head submitted for rabies examination. Animals that might have exposed a person to rabies should be reported immediately to the local health department. **An animal other than a dog, cat, or ferret that received prior vaccination** may still require euthanasia and testing if the period of virus shedding is unknown for that species.

Person-to-Person Transmission There are anecdotal reports of person-to-person transmission of rabies. Fluids from the upper and lower respiratory tracts of humans frequently test positive for rabies virus. Despite the lack of proven healthcare-associated transmission, about 30% of healthcare personnel who have had contact with a human diagnosed with rabies have received postexposure prophylaxis. Given the mechanism of disease transmission and concern among healthcare workers, contact isolation precautions should be used for patients with known or suspected rabies, and healthcare workers who care for such patients should wear either masks and eye protection or face shields.[12] **Healthcare personnel with nonintact skin or mucous membrane exposure to infective saliva from patients with rabies should receive postexposure prophylaxis.**

Patients Concerned about Rabies For unusual exposures, the state veterinarian or local public health agency can be contacted for more information. However, for patients who voice concern about rabies exposure even if the risk assessment is virtually nil (**Table 157-6**), vaccination can be offered, along with an explanation of the risks and benefits of vaccination. If the risk of rabies is virtually nil, we discourage the administration of HRIG.

WOUND CARE

First, assess wounds for the presence of a life-threatening condition, such as arterial laceration or pneumothorax.[16] Provide proper wound care, including **tetanus prophylaxis, wound cleansing with soap and water and (if available) a dilute solution of povidone-iodine (1 mL**

TABLE 157-5 Rabies Postexposure Risk Assessment and Recommendations (2012)[14]

Animal Type	Evaluation and Disposition of Animal	Postexposure Prophylaxis Recommendations
Dogs, cats, and ferrets	Healthy and available for 10 d of observations	Persons should not begin vaccination unless animal develops clinical signs of rabies.*
	Rabid or suspected rabid	Immediate immunization.
	Unknown (e.g., escaped)	Consult public health officials.
Skunks, raccoons, foxes, and most other carnivores; bats†	Regard as rabid unless animal proven negative for rabies virus by laboratory tests‡	Consider immediate immunization.
Livestock, horses, rodents, rabbits and hares, and other mammals	Consider individually	Consult public health officials; bites of squirrels, hamsters, guinea pigs, gerbils, chipmunks, mice, rats, rabbits, hares, and other small rodents almost never require rabies postexposure prophylaxis.

*During the 10-day observation period, begin postexposure prophylaxis at the first sign of rabies in a dog, cat, or ferret that has bitten someone. If the animal exhibits clinical signs of rabies, it should be euthanized immediately and tested.

†Provide postexposure prophylaxis immediately.

‡The animal should be euthanized and tested as soon as possible. Holding for observation is not recommended.

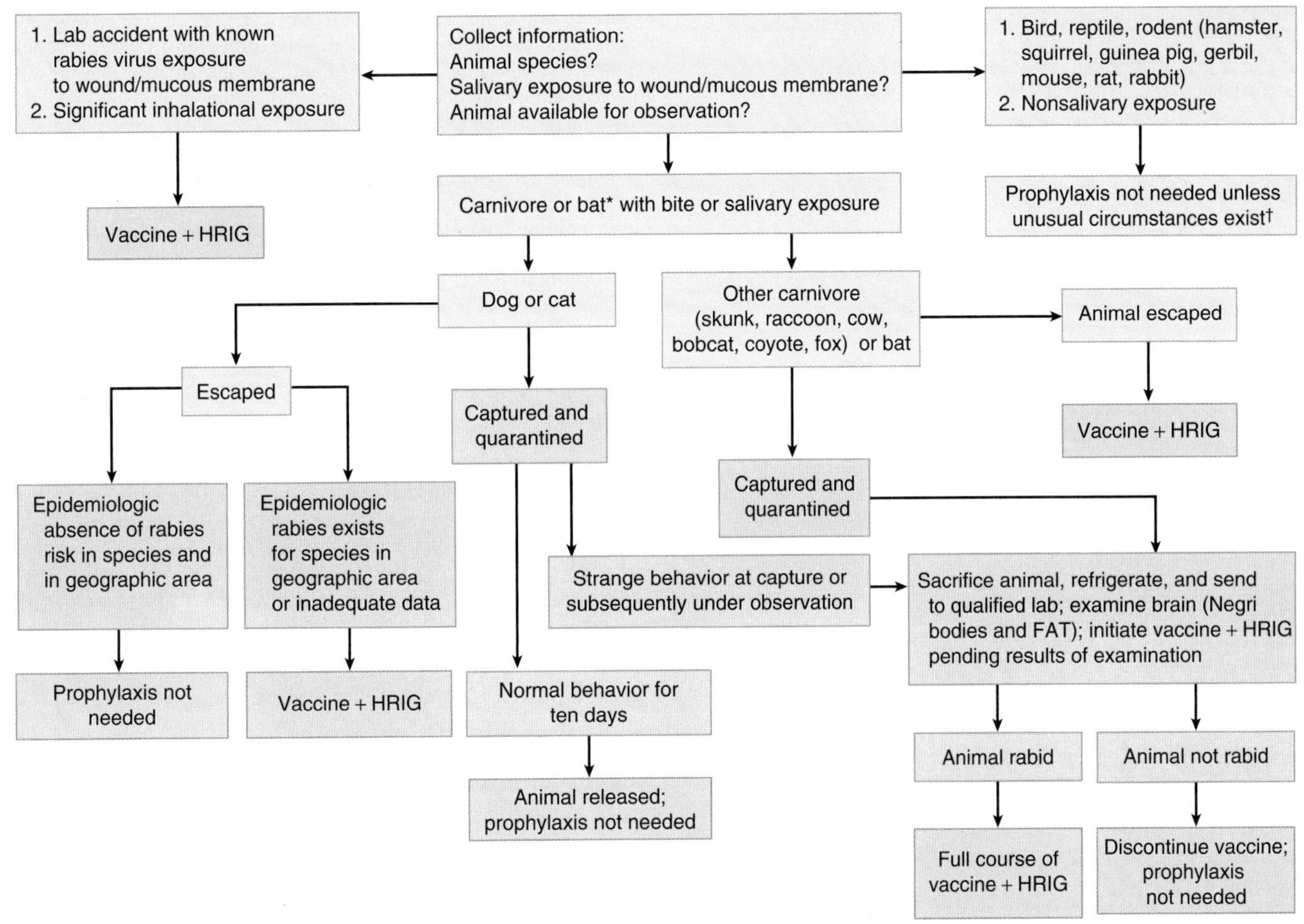

FIGURE 157-1. Clinical guidelines for administration of postexposure prophylaxis. (*) Consider postexposure prophylaxis for persons who were in the same room as a bat and who might be unaware that a bite or direct contact had occurred. (†) The small mammals listed here have never been reported to transmit rabies to humans in the United States, but theoretically, such animals could acquire and transmit rabies. Therefore, postexposure prophylaxis following a bite or scratch from one of these mammals would only be indicated if such an animal had signs typical of rabies or a positive laboratory test for rabies. Consult with local public health officials for reports of rabies in atypical animals. FAT = fluorescent antibody testing; HRIG = human rabies immune globulin.

povidone-iodine in 9 mL of water or normal saline), antibiotics (if indicated) to prevent bacterial infection (see chapter 46, Puncture Wounds and Bites), and **rabies prophylaxis** as indicated.[17]

POSTEXPOSURE PROPHYLAXIS TREATMENT

In the United States, postexposure prophylaxis consists of a regimen of one dose of HRIG and four doses of rabies vaccine over a 14-day period, except for immunocompromised persons, who should receive a five-dose series of vaccine over a 28-day period (**Table 157-7**).[14,17] The shift from a five-dose to a four-dose series of rabies vaccine occurred in 2010 and is based on rabies virus pathogenesis, experimental animal studies, clinical trials, epidemiologic surveillance, and economic analyses.[17] No other aspects of postexposure prophylaxis were altered from the 2008 recommendations (e.g., use of HRIG, site of injection, etc.). HRIG and the first dose of rabies vaccine should be given as soon as possible after exposure, preferably within 24 hours. If HRIG was not administered when vaccination was begun, it can be administered up to 7 days after administration of the first dose of the vaccine.

Follow the Centers for Disease Control and Prevention recommendations for postexposure prophylaxis *exactly* (**Table 157-7**). Although no postexposure prophylaxis vaccine failures have been reported in the United States since the licensing of human diploid cell vaccine in 1980, 13 persons outside the United States have contracted rabies after postexposure prophylaxis with tissue culture–derived vaccine.[2] Each of these cases involved deviation from the recommended protocol; wounds were not cleansed, passive immunization with HRIG was not provided, or rabies vaccine was injected into the gluteal rather than the deltoid area.

Rabies Vaccines Rabies vaccines available in the United States include human diploid cell vaccine (produced in human diploid cells; Imovax®, Sanofi Pasteur, Lyon, France) and purified chick embryo cell culture vaccine (PCECV) (produced in chick embryo cells; RabAvert®, Novartis Vaccines, Emeryville, CA). **The active antibody response requires approximately 7 to 10 days to develop, and detectable rabies virus–neutralizing antibodies generally persist for several years.** All currently used vaccines are produced in cell cultures and are significantly less toxic than older vaccines that were produced in neural tissue. Side effects of human diploid cell vaccine, including mild erythema, swelling, and pain at the injection site, have been reported in 10% to 90% of vaccine recipients. Systemic reactions, such as headache, nausea, abdominal pain, muscle aches, and dizziness, have been reported in 5% to 40% of recipients. Serum sickness–like reactions (type III hypersensitivity) have been noted in approximately 6% of persons receiving booster doses of human diploid cell vaccine and occur 2 to 21 days after administration of the booster dose. Such reactions have not been life threatening and have not been reported with purified chick embryo cell culture vaccine. Anaphylaxis and neurologic symptoms have only rarely been associated with the current rabies vaccines. **Severe egg allergy is a contraindication to the use of purified chick embryo cell culture vaccine.**

Rabies prophylaxis should not be interrupted or discontinued because of local or mild systemic adverse reactions to rabies vaccine.[16] Usually such

TABLE 157-6 Summary of Risk of Acquiring Rabies in the United States

Risk	Exposures
Moderate to high	Bite by skunk, raccoon, fox, and other wild carnivores (unless animal tested negative for rabies)
	Bite or direct contact with bat (unless animal tested negative for rabies)
	Exposure by percutaneous injury, mucous membrane exposure, or inhalation to live rabies virus in a laboratory
	Dog bite in a country with endemic rabies and inadequate immunization of dogs (or bite by feral dog)
Very low to low	Bite by inadequately vaccinated cat or dog that has access to the outdoors (or feral cat or dog)
	Contamination of open wound or abrasion (including scratches) with, or mucous membrane exposure to, saliva or other potentially infectious material (e.g., neural tissue) from a possibly rabid animal (skunk, raccoon, fox, and other wild carnivores, bat)
	Awakening in a room with a bat present
No risk identified	Contact of animal fluids (e.g., saliva, blood, neural tissue) with intact skin
	Indirect contact with saliva from a wild animal (e.g., by cleaning a dog or cat that has had contact with a wild animal)

reactions can be successfully managed with anti-inflammatory and antipyretic agents. When a person with a history of serious hypersensitivity to rabies vaccine must be revaccinated, antihistamines may be given. Epinephrine should be readily available to counteract anaphylactic reactions, and the person should be observed carefully immediately after vaccination (as after any other injection given in a healthcare setting).

Human Rabies Immunoglobulin HRIG is administered only once, at the beginning of antirabies prophylaxis, to provide immediate antibodies until the patient responds to rabies vaccine by producing antibodies. A passive antibody titer is evident in 24 hours. Failure to administer HRIG has led to rabies despite appropriate postexposure prophylaxis with human diploid cell vaccine. If HRIG was not given when vaccination was begun, it can be given through the seventh day after administration of the vaccine.[17] **Beyond the seventh day after vaccination is begun, HRIG is not indicated, because an antibody response is presumed to have occurred.** The Centers for Disease Control and Prevention recommends that as much as possible of the full dose be infiltrated around the wound. HRIG should never be administered in the same syringe or into the same anatomic site as the vaccine. Even if the wound has to be sutured, it should be infiltrated locally with HRIG. This practice is safe and does not create an additional risk of infection. However, caution is needed when injecting into a tissue compartment, such as the finger pulp, because excessive HRIG can increase compartment pressure and lead to necrosis.[18] Any remaining HRIG that cannot be administered into the local wound area should be injected intramuscularly at a site distant from vaccine administration. HRIG is prepared from human blood and screened for known viruses (e.g., human immunodeficiency virus, hepatitis). No cases of virus transmission from HRIG that is commercially available in the United States or Australia have been reported. HRIG should not be given to those with immunoglobulin A deficiencies and known antibodies of immunoglobulin A, because small amounts of immunoglobulin A may be present in HRIG and can cause a severe allergic reaction.

WORLD HEALTH ORGANIZATION POSTEXPOSURE PROPHYLAXIS GUIDELINES

In the United States, only regimens recommended by the Advisory Committee on Immunization Practices should be used. The World Health Organization has provided recommendations for rabies postexposure prophylaxis that also consider the cost and availability of vaccines and HRIG.[19,20] Per the World Health Organization, the indication for postexposure prophylaxis depends on the contact with the suspected rabid animal:

- Category I: touching or feeding animals, licks on intact skin (that is, no exposure)
- Category II: nibbling of uncovered skin, minor scratches or abrasions without bleeding
- Category III: single or multiple transdermal bites or scratches, contamination of mucous membrane with saliva from licks, licks on broken skin, exposure to bats

For category I exposures, no prophylaxis is required. For category II, immediate vaccination is recommended. For category III, immediate vaccination and administration of rabies immunoglobulin are recommended. Per the World Health Organization, factors that should be taken into consideration when deciding whether to initiate postexposure prophylaxis include the epidemiologic likelihood of the implicated

TABLE 157-7 Rabies Postexposure Prophylaxis Schedule—United States, 2010

Immunization Status	Treatment	Regimen*
Not previously immunized	Wound cleansing	Cleanse all wounds with soap and water; irrigate wounds with 9:1 diluted solution of povidone-iodine (if available).
	HRIG	Administer **20 IU/kg actual body weight.** If anatomically feasible, infiltrate the *full dose* around the wound(s) and give any remaining volume IM at an anatomic site distant from vaccine administration; do not give HRIG in the same syringe as vaccine. HRIG may partially suppress active production of rabies virus antibody, so **do not give more than the recommended dose.**
	Vaccine	HDCV or PCECV 1.0 mL (deltoid area†), one dose on days 0,‡ 3, 7, and 14.#
Previously immunized^f^	Wound cleansing	Cleanse all wounds with soap and water; irrigate wounds with 9:1 povidone-iodine solution.
	HRIG	HRIG should *not* be administered.
	Vaccine	HDCV or PCECV 1.0 mL (deltoid area†), one dose on days 0‡ and 3.

Abbreviations: HDCV = human diploid cell vaccine; HRIG = human rabies immunoglobulin; PCECV = purified chick embryo cell culture vaccine.

*These regimens are appropriate for all age groups, including children.

†The deltoid area is the only acceptable site of vaccination for adults and older children. For younger children, the outer aspect of the thigh (anterolateral aspect) may be used. Vaccine should never be administered in the gluteal area.

‡Day 0 is the day the first dose of vaccine is administered.

#Day 28 vaccine dose no longer recommended by the Advisory Committee on Immunization Practices, **unless the patient is immunocompromised** (see later section, Immunocompromised Persons). See http://www.cdc.gov/rabies/resources/acip_recommendations.html.

^f^Any persons with a history of preexposure prophylaxis with HDCV or PCECV; prior postexposure prophylaxis with HDCV or PCECV; or previous immunization with any other type of rabies vaccine and a documented history of antibody response to the prior immunization.

animal being rabid, the category of exposure (i.e., I, II, or III), and the clinical features of the animal, as well as its availability for observation and laboratory testing. In most situations in developing countries, the vaccination status of the implicated animal alone should not be considered when deciding whether to give or withhold prophylaxis.

For IM administration, the World Health Organization recommends the following postexposure regimens. The postexposure vaccination schedule is based on injecting 1 mL or 0.5 mL (volume depends on the type of vaccine) into the deltoid muscle (or anterolateral thigh in children <2 years of age) of patients with category II and III exposures. The recommended regimen consists of either a 5-dose or a 4-dose schedule:

- The five-dose schedule consists of one dose on each of days 0, 3, 7, 14, and 28.
- The four-dose schedule consists of two doses on day 0 (one dose in each of the two deltoid or thigh sites) followed by one dose on each of days 7 and 21.

An alternative for healthy, fully immunocompetent, exposed persons who receive wound care plus high-quality rabies immunoglobulin plus World Health Organization–prequalified rabies vaccines is a postexposure regimen consisting of four doses administered intramuscularly on days 0, 3, 7, and 14.

For intradermal administration, the World Health Organization recommends the following postexposure regimen: The two-site regimen prescribes injection of 0.1 mL at two sites (deltoid and thigh) on days 0, 3, 7, and 28. This regimen may be used for people with category II and III exposures in countries where the intradermal route has been endorsed by national health authorities.

POSTEXPOSURE PROPHYLAXIS IN SPECIAL POPULATIONS

Persons with Prior Rabies Immunization If exposed to rabies, persons previously vaccinated should receive two intramuscular doses (1 mL each) of vaccine, one immediately and one 3 days later.[14,17] "Previously vaccinated" refers to persons who have received one of the recommended preexposure or postexposure prophylaxis regimens of human diploid cell vaccine or purified chick embryo cell culture vaccine, or those who have received another vaccine and had a documented acceptable rabies antibody titer. HRIG is unnecessary and should not be given in these cases, because an anamnestic antibody response will follow the administration of a booster regardless of the prebooster antibody titer.

Immunocompromised Persons Immunization of immunocompromised persons presents special challenges. First, vaccines may represent a danger to the immunocompromised individual. Second, the immune response to vaccination may be insufficient. Higher doses or additional immunizations may be required, and even with these modifications, the immune response may be suboptimal. The severely immunocompromised are those who have congenital immunodeficiency, human immunodeficiency virus infection, leukemia or lymphoma, aplastic anemia, or generalized malignancy, or who are being treated with alkylating agents, antimetabolites, radiation, or large amounts of corticosteroids.[17]

Because rabies vaccine is formulated with inactivated virus, it does not represent a danger to immunocompromised persons and may be administered to such persons using the standard recommended doses and schedule (**Table 157-7**). However, a five-dose schedule should be used in immunocompromised persons.[17]

The recommendations for the use of HRIG are the same for immunocompromised and immunocompetent persons. However, corticosteroids, antimalarials, other immunosuppressive agents, and immunosuppressive illnesses can interfere with the development of active immunity and predispose the patient to developing rabies. **Immunosuppressive agents should not be administered during postexposure prophylaxis, unless they are essential for the treatment of other conditions.** When rabies postexposure prophylaxis is administered to persons receiving steroids or other immunosuppressive therapy, it is especially important that serum be tested for rabies antibody to ensure that an adequate response has developed.[12] To confirm the adequacy of the immune response, serum collected 1 to 24 weeks after the postexposure prophylaxis course should completely neutralize challenge virus at a 1:5 serum dilution, as measured by a rapid fluorescent focus inhibition test.[12] If no acceptable antibody response is detected, consult an infectious disease expert and appropriate public health officials.

Travelers Preexposure prophylaxis is recommended for certain international travelers based on the local incidence of rabies in the countries to be visited, the availability of appropriate antirabies biologicals, and the intended travel activity.[21,22] Such persons include veterinarians, animal handlers, field biologists, spelunkers, missionaries, and certain laboratory workers. **Chloroquine phosphate** (and possibly other structurally related antimalarials such as mefloquine, which is administered for malaria chemoprophylaxis) **may interfere with the antibody response to intradermal rabies vaccine administered for preexposure prophylaxis.** The IM route, not the intradermal route, should be used for people taking chloroquine concurrently (the intradermal route is not approved for use in the United States); ideally, the rabies preexposure vaccination series should be completed before beginning chloroquine.

Between 2001 and June 2010, six persons died in the United States from rabies after having been bitten by a dog (another died after being bitten by a fox) while visiting a foreign country. For this reason, all persons who have returned from abroad should be questioned regarding whether they received an animal bite or scratch in an area with endemic rabies. Persons bitten or scratched by an animal in an area with endemic rabies should receive appropriate postexposure prophylaxis if the injury has occurred within the known incubation period (which may rarely extend up to 5 or more years).

U.S. citizens and residents who are exposed to rabies while traveling in countries where rabies is endemic may sometimes receive postexposure prophylaxis with regimens or biologicals that are not used in the United States. If postexposure prophylaxis is begun outside the United States using a regimen or biological of nerve tissue origin not approved by the U.S. Food and Drug Administration, it may be necessary to provide additional treatment when the patient reaches the United States.[12] State and local health departments should be contacted for specific advice in such cases. The major modification used abroad, usually in an attempt to reduce cost, is the substitution of various schedules for intradermal injection or the use of vaccines not approved by the U.S. Food and Drug Administration.

Pregnant Women **Adverse pregnancy outcomes or fetal abnormalities have not been associated with rabies vaccination.** Because of the potential consequences of inadequately treated rabies exposure and because adverse events have not been associated with rabies postexposure prophylaxis during pregnancy, pregnancy is not considered a contraindication to rabies postexposure prophylaxis or HRIG.[12] If there is substantial risk of exposure to rabies, preexposure prophylaxis may also be indicated during pregnancy.

Children The dose of rabies vaccine for preexposure and postexposure prophylaxis is the same in infants and children as in adults (**Table 157-7**).[12] The dose of HRIG for postexposure prophylaxis is based on actual body weight. For small children with multiple bites, the calculated dose of HRIG may be insufficient to infiltrate all wounds. However, sterile saline can be used to dilute the volume twofold or threefold to permit thorough infiltration.[21]

CLINICAL RABIES

Rabies virus causes **acute encephalitis** in all warm-blooded hosts, including humans, and the outcome is almost always fatal. Although patients with rabies may manifest a variety of clinical symptoms and signs, the disease tends to follow a characteristic course (**Table 157-8**).

Most commonly, the incubation period after a bite ranges from 20 to 90 days.[2] However, incubation periods have been reported that are as short as 4 days and as long as 6 years. For patients who died from rabies in the United States between 1980 and 1996 and in whom a definite animal bite occurred, the median incubation period was 85 days (range, 53 to 150 days).[23] The incubation period is shorter when the site of the bite is on the head than when it is on an extremity.[2]

TABLE 157-8 Natural History of Clinical Rabies in Humans after Incubation Period

Clinical Stage	Defining Event	Usual Duration	Common Symptoms and Signs*
Prodrome	First symptom	2–10 d	Pain or paresthesia at site of bite Malaise, lethargy Headache Fever Nausea, vomiting, anorexia Anxiety, agitation, depression
Acute neurologic phase	First neurologic sign	2–7 d	Anxiety, agitation, depression Hyperventilation, hypoxia Aphasia, incoordination Paresis, paralysis Hydrophobia, pharyngeal spasms Confusion, delirium, hallucinations Marked hyperactivity
Coma	Onset of coma	0–14 d	Coma Hypotension, hypoventilation, apnea Pituitary dysfunction Cardiac arrhythmia, cardiac arrest
Death or recovery (extremely rare)	Death or initiation of recovery	Months (recovery)	Pneumothorax Intravascular thrombosis Secondary infections

*Not every symptom or sign may be present in each case.

CLINICAL FEATURES

During the prodrome, the symptoms and signs are nonspecific. Early in the course, some patients may report symptoms suggestive of rabies such as limb pain, limb weakness, and paresthesias at or near the presumed exposure site. The prodrome merges into the acute neurologic phase, which begins when the patient develops objective signs of CNS disease.

There are two clinical forms of rabies: an encephalitic form in 80% and a paralytic form in 20%.[11] In encephalitic rabies, there are often episodes of generalized arousal or hyperexcitability, disorientation, hallucinations, and bizarre behavior, often separated by lucid intervals. Autonomic dysfunction is common and includes hypersalivation, hyperthermia, tachycardia, hypertension, piloerection, cardiac arrhythmias, and priapism. Paralytic rabies generally begins with paresis in the bitten extremity with spread to quadriparesis and bilateral facial weakness. There is progression of paralytic rabies to coma and organ failure, typically with a longer clinical course than in encephalitic rabies.[11] About 50% of patients have classic hydrophobia, in which attempts to drink fluids result in severe spasms of the pharynx, larynx, and diaphragm.

Coma almost always occurs within 10 days of the onset of symptoms. Death occurs due to a variety of complications, including pituitary dysfunction, seizures, respiratory dysfunction with progressive hypoxia, cardiac dysfunction with dysrhythmias and arrest, autonomic dysfunction, renal failure, and secondary bacterial infections.

Only seven patients are known to have survived rabies. In all but one case, the patient had received either postexposure or preexposure prophylaxis with rabies vaccine (e.g., duck embryo, suckling mouse brain) before the onset of symptoms.

DIAGNOSIS AND TREATMENT

Rabies should be included in the differential diagnosis of any patient with unexplained acute, rapidly progressive encephalitis, especially in the presence of anatomic instability, dysphagia, hydrophobia, paresis, or parasthesias.[24-27] Diseases that may be confused with rabies include tetanus, poliomyelitis, Guillain-Barré syndrome, botulism, transverse myelitis, postvaccinal encephalomyelitis, intracranial mass lesions, cerebrovascular accidents, poisoning with atropine-like compounds, and infectious causes of viral encephalitis (e.g., herpes simplex, varicella zoster, arthropod-borne viral encephalitis such as eastern equine encephalitis). Emerging diseases that can be confused with rabies include West Nile virus (United States, Europe, Middle East, Africa), Toscana virus (Europe), Japanese encephalitis (Asia), enterovirus 71 (Asia), human herpes virus 6 (worldwide), chikungunya fever (Asia, Africa, Europe), Nipah virus (Asia), and Hendra virus (Asia).[28,29]

The diagnosis of rabies is frequently made postmortem. This occurs because of the rarity of the disease, the increasing number of persons without an obvious exposure, and clinical confusion with other disorders. Important clues to diagnosis include a history of an animal bite or bat exposure and the development of the pathognomonic signs of hydrophobia and aerophobia (precipitating grimacing and other signs by blowing air on the patient's face).

During the incubation period of rabies, no diagnostic test is available for animals or humans that will indicate infection. Once symptoms become evident, antigen and antibody testing of serum, cerebrospinal fluid, saliva, and tissue, such as cornea, brain biopsy, and skin from highly innervated locations (e.g., nuchal skin biopsy), can detect evidence of the disease.[4] Serum antibodies may be present as early as day 5 of clinical illness, but antibodies may be absent after 10 to 14 days or longer. CT of the brain is only useful to exclude other diseases. MRI of the brain may be normal or may show lesions in gray matter areas of the brain parenchyma, including the brainstem. Cerebrospinal fluid analysis often shows a mild mononuclear pleocytosis.

No specific therapy has been of demonstrated benefit in clinical rabies.[4] Treatment with rabies vaccine, rabies immunoglobulin, IV ribavirin, or interferon is not effective.[30] In animal models, use of corticosteroids shortens the incubation time and increases mortality, and for this reason **steroids are contraindicated**. Survival with normal neurologic function was reported for a 15-year-old girl in whom coma was induced and treatment with ketamine, midazolam, ribavirin, and amantadine was provided.[30] However, similar regimens have been used for more than 20 other patients without success.[30] Currently, treatment is directed at the clinical complications of the disease. Although rabies is not treatable, every attempt should be made to achieve rapid diagnosis, because it justifies public health measures to limit contacts with the patient and permits reconstruction of a history to identify others who may have been exposed to the same infective source.

REFERENCES

The complete reference list is available online at www.TintinalliEM.com.

CHAPTER 158 Malaria

Malcolm Molyneaux

INTRODUCTION

Malaria, a protozoan disease transmitted by the bite of the *Anopheles* mosquito, is one of mankind's most feared and serious afflictions. It is a leading cause of morbidity and mortality in many tropical areas of the world, especially in Africa. Approximately 55% of the world's population is exposed to the infection, which exerts its toll mainly on the young and the pregnant. Malaria is endemic or sporadic throughout most of the tropics and subtropics below an altitude of 1500 m, excluding the Mediterranean littoral, the United States, and Australia. Malaria is perhaps the most significant disease acquired through international travel to the tropics.

Five species of the genus *Plasmodium* infect humans: *Plasmodium vivax, Plasmodium ovale, Plasmodium malariae, Plasmodium falciparum,* and *Plasmodium knowlesi.* In 2012, there were an estimated 207 million cases of symptomatic malaria worldwide (80% of which occurred in Africa), with about 627,000 deaths, 90% of which occurred in Africa, and with nearly 77% of those occurring in young children.[1] The great majority of malaria deaths are due to *P. falciparum* infections, although both *P. vivax* and *P. knowlesi* can also cause fatal disease.

The incidence of malaria has decreased dramatically in some countries in recent years as a result of intensive control efforts (e.g., South Africa), but elsewhere there has been little change, and some areas have experienced increases or epidemics (e.g., Algeria, Venezuela). In the United States, more cases of imported malaria were identified in 2011 than in any year since 1971.[2] Obstacles to successful reduction of malaria worldwide include human factors (poverty, war, inadequate international cooperation), capacities of the mosquito vector (changing temperatures, insecticide resistance) and parasite characteristics (antimalarial drug resistance).

In an area of intense transmission, most malaria infections occur in children, who gradually acquire a considerable degree of immunity. In such areas, a high percentage of children may have asymptomatic parasitemia (**malaria infection**), and illness due to malaria (**malaria disease**) is commonly mild and only occasionally severe or life threatening. Nevertheless, the absolute burden of mortality is large because nearly all children are infected. Adults in such areas rarely develop severe or fatal disease.

By contrast, malaria due to *P. falciparum* is a medical emergency in a nonimmune host of any age, because the infection, if untreated, is likely to progress and to become life threatening. Once a *P. falciparum* infection has reached the stage of severe disease, there is a 5% to 30% risk of a fatal outcome, even if optimal treatment is then begun. The early clinical features of malaria are nonspecific, and malaria can mimic many other infections. A diagnosis of malaria must be considered in any person returning from the tropics with an unexplained febrile illness and must be considered in any resident in the tropics who develops a fever.

EPIDEMIOLOGY

Malaria transmission occurs in large areas of Central and South America, the Caribbean, sub-Saharan Africa, the Indian subcontinent, Southeast Asia, the Middle East, and Oceania. Certain species may predominate in a given geographic area.[3] For example, *P. vivax* is more common in the Indian subcontinent, whereas *P. falciparum* is the most prevalent form in Africa, Haiti, and New Guinea. *P. knowlesi* has been found in several countries in southeast Asia, including Malaysia, Myanmar (Burma), Thailand, the Philippines, and Singapore.[4]

The risk of contracting malaria varies considerably between regions. In 2011, the Centers for Disease Control and Prevention reported 1925 cases of malaria among persons in the United States.[2] Of 1655 imported cases where the region of acquisition was known, 1144 (69%) were acquired in Africa (63% of these in West Africa), 363 (22%) in Asia (68% of these in India), 104 (6.3%) in the Caribbean and Central America, 35 (2%) in South America, and 7 (<1%) in Oceania. *P. falciparum* accounted for 49% and *P. vivax* for 22% of all cases (although in many cases, the parasite species was not identified). Thus, almost half of all cases of malaria, including the majority of cases due to *P. falciparum,* were acquired from travels in West Africa, despite the fact that for every traveler to sub-Saharan Africa, at least 10 travelers visit potential malarious areas of Asia and South America each year. Complications developed in 14% of the reported cases of malaria identified in the United States in 2011, and five patients died (1.8% of the 275 severe cases).

P. knowlesi is a zoonosis. Macaques (old world monkeys) are the natural host. Members of the *Anopheles leucosphyrus* groups are equally attracted to humans and monkeys, which has given rise to human cases. The forest fringe habitat of this mosquito will hopefully limit the spread of this species of parasite.[5]

Resistance of *P. falciparum* to chloroquine has been widespread for many years.[6] Strains of *P. falciparum* have since become resistant to other chemotherapeutic agents, including pyrimethamine-sulfadoxine (no longer recommended as first-line treatment; can be used in pregnancy), quinine, mefloquine, and doxycycline.[7] Widespread mefloquine-resistant strains of *P. falciparum* have been seen in parts of Thailand, Myanmar (Burma), Cambodia, and China. Of greatest current concern is the observation in Cambodia and in parts of Thailand that parasites are slower to respond to artemisinin therapy than a few years ago.[8] There has not yet been evidence of impaired cure rates with artemisinin therapy, but worldwide vigilance is required to track the continuing efficacy of this important class of drugs. Resistance of *P. vivax* to chloroquine has also been identified in Southeast Asia.[9]

PATHOPHYSIOLOGY

The organism is transmitted primarily by the bite of an infected female *Anopheles* mosquito, which requires a blood meal every 3 to 4 days to nourish its eggs. This vector is most frequently found in tropical and subtropical regions below 1500 m (5000 ft) above sea level. Plasmodial sporozoites are injected into the host's bloodstream during the mosquito's blood meal and are carried through the bloodstream to the liver. Within hours, the hepatic parenchymal cells are invaded, and asexual reproduction of the parasite begins (pre-erythrocytic schizogony or exoerythrocytic stage). After thousands of daughter merozoites have been formed within a hepatocyte (amplification cycle), the cell ruptures, releasing daughter merozoites into the circulation, where they rapidly invade erythrocytes to begin the erythrocytic stage of the asexual cycle. In *P. vivax* and *P. ovale* infection, a portion of the intrahepatic forms are not released, but remain dormant as **hypnozoites**, which can reactivate after months or years to cause clinical relapses.

Once merozoites enter the erythrocytic stage, they do not reinvade the liver. A merozoite matures within the erythrocyte, feeding on hemoglobin and enlarging until it divides into about a score of daughter merozoites to form a schizont. Eventually, the infected erythrocyte lyses, merozoites are released, and these invade uninfected red blood cells, continuing and amplifying the infection.

A portion of the merozoites develop into sexual forms (gametocytes). Upon ingestion by another feeding *Anopheles* mosquito, male and female gametocytes undergo sexual reproduction within the vector's gut and migrate as infective sporozoites to her salivary glands. To maximize her blood meal, the mosquito injects her next victim with saliva containing an anticoagulant, which introduces the malarial infection. The rate at which parasites replicate and migrate in the mosquito is temperature dependent; at average environmental temperatures below about 15°C (59°F), the cycle does not complete before the death of the mosquito, and malaria transmission cannot occur.

The clinical signs of malaria first appear during the erythrocytic stage. The rupture of schizont-containing erythrocytes triggers an array of host cytokine responses, giving rise to fever and other features of the malarial illness. Because fever slows the rate of schizont formation, early-stage parasites tend to catch up with more mature stages, and therefore over time, schizont rupture may become synchronous, giving rise to the periodic fever characteristic of untreated malaria. Such periodicity rarely has time to develop when malaria is treated promptly with efficacious drugs.

Each species of *Plasmodium* has specific characteristics, including typical morphologic forms and selective red blood cell tropism (**Table 158-1**). Many of these characteristics are responsible for important pathophysiologic consequences.

Anemia can develop rapidly with *P. falciparum* infection because the percentage of erythrocytes parasitized can be overwhelming (erythrocytes of all ages are susceptible to invasion) and because the lifespan of uninfected erythrocytes is also reduced, while bone marrow erythropoiesis is slowed or halted. *P. falciparum* asexual parasites transport to the red cell surface proteins that can adhere to host endothelial receptors, resulting in the sequestration of mature parasites in the microvasculature of many tissues and organs. Sequestration may be enhanced by the impaired deformability of infected erythrocytes and consequent slowing of blood flow through microvessels. Sequestration benefits parasites by keeping them away from the spleen, but additional consequences for the host include metabolic deprivation and/or impaired perfusion of tissues, processes that are believed to contribute to many of the syndromes characteristic of

TABLE 158-1 Characteristics of Malaria-Causing *Plasmodium* Species

	P. falciparum	*P. vivax*	*P. ovale*	*P. malariae*	*P. knowlesi*
Clinical Characteristics					
Incubation period	8–25 d	8–27 d	9–17 d	15–30 d	Uncertain
Chloroquine resistance	Yes	Rare	No	No	No
Fatal attack	Yes	No	No	No	No
Relapse	No	Yes	Yes	No	No
Histologic Characteristics					
Asexual erythrocytic cycle	48 h	48 h	48 h	72 h	Uncertain
RBC preference	Reticulocytes (but can infect RBCs of all ages)	Reticulocytes	Reticulocytes	Older cells	All RBCs
Degree of parasitemia	High (multiple rings per RBC)	Low	Low	Low	Can be high
Ring forms and early trophozoites	Ring forms predominate; threadlike cytoplasm with double-chromatic dots	Amoeboid cytoplasm	Compact cytoplasm	Compact cytoplasm	Ring forms sometimes seen
Mature trophozoites	Rarely seen	Observed	Observed	Observed	Observed
Schizonts	Rarely seen	Observed	Observed	Observed	Observed
Gametocytes	Banana shaped	Round	Round	Round	Round
Circumference of infected red cell	Normal	Enlarged	Oval, with ragged (fimbriated) ends	Normal	Normal
Appearance of red cell cytoplasm	Normal	Stippled (fine Schuffner's dots)	Larger Schuffner's dots	Normal	Normal

Abbreviation: RBC = red blood cell.

severe falciparum malaria. Acidosis, for example, results from tissue hypoxia, to which sequestration, hypotension, and severe anemia may all contribute. Hypoglycemia occurs largely due to impaired hepatic gluconeogenesis, possibly enhanced by the consumption of glucose by actively metabolizing parasites and the diversion of glucose for the host's anaerobic glycolysis. Sequestration accounts for the paucity of observed mature parasites in the peripheral smear of patients infected with *P. falciparum*.

Although nearly all malaria transmission is mediated by mosquito vectors, plasmodia of any species may also be transmitted by transfusion of infected blood, by needlestick accident, or across the placenta from mother to fetus. In these cases, an exoerythrocytic phase is absent, and hypnozoites of *P. vivax* or *P. ovale* cannot develop.

Untreated, inadequately treated, or frequent malaria may lead to sequelae mediated by immunologic mechanisms, including massive splenomegaly with consequent hypersplenism, and glomerulonephritis leading to a nephrotic syndrome (attributed, without strong evidence, mainly to *P. malariae* infection). Thrombocytopenia (rarely sufficient to cause bleeding) is invariable in acute symptomatic malaria.

INCUBATION PERIOD

The incubation period between infection and symptoms varies with the species of parasite (Table 158-1). In the nonimmune, symptoms begin after an incubation period ranging from 7 days to several weeks or more. Incomplete suppression of disease by partially active chemoprophylaxis and partial immunity can prolong the incubation period to months or even years. For U.S. residents who developed malaria associated with travels abroad during 2011, disease became evident within 1 month after arrival home in 95% of *P. falciparum* cases, but in only 52% of *P. vivax* cases. The interval between arriving in the United States and becoming ill was between 3 and 12 months in 46% of *P. vivax* cases and 5% of *P. falciparum* cases. Six patients (0.6% overall) became ill more than 1 year after returning to the United States.[2]

CLINICAL FEATURES

UNCOMPLICATED MALARIA

The clinical hallmark of malaria is fever, with a prodrome of malaise, myalgia, headache, and chills.[10] In some patients, chest pain, cough, abdominal pain, or arthralgias may be prominent. Early symptoms are nonspecific and can easily be confused with a viral syndrome such as influenza or hepatitis or with bacterial sepsis. In a nonimmune individual, the illness usually progresses to include chills, followed by high-grade fever accompanied by nausea, orthostatic dizziness, and extreme weakness. After several hours, the fever abates and the patient develops diaphoresis and becomes exhausted. If the infection is untreated, the paroxysms of malaria—chills and fever followed by diaphoresis—may over time begin to occur at nearly regular intervals that correspond to the length of the asexual erythrocytic cycles (Table 158-1). The classic paroxysms of malaria are often lacking in malaria due to *P. falciparum* or in persons who received some form of chemoprophylaxis. The findings upon physical examination are also not specific for malaria. Most patients appear acutely ill with high fever, tachycardia, and tachypnea. Splenomegaly and abdominal tenderness are common. The liver may or may not be enlarged. Clinical signs that point to a diagnosis other than (or in addition to) malaria include lymphadenopathy and a maculopapular or petechial skin rash.

In children growing up in a malarious area, attributing an illness to malaria is particularly difficult because many children carry parasites without being unwell and because symptoms and signs of both mild and severe malaria are nonspecific.[11] In these circumstances, the higher the parasite density in the peripheral blood, the greater is the likelihood that malaria is the cause of the illness.

SEVERE (COMPLICATED) MALARIA

Malaria is described as severe or complicated when it includes one or more of the following syndromes in the context of a plasmodial infection, usually due to *P. falciparum*: coma with or without seizures ("cerebral malaria"), prostration, severe anemia, acidosis, hypoglycemia, acute renal failure, acute respiratory distress syndrome, pulmonary edema, jaundice, intravascular hemolysis, shock, and disseminated intravascular coagulation. The percentage of malaria cases imported to the United States that were classified as severe increased significantly from 18% of 1691 cases in 2010 to 22% of 1925 cases in 2011.[2]

Complications of malaria can develop rapidly in untreated *P. falciparum* infection or may supervene early in the course of treatment. Occasionally, one or more complications may constitute the presenting illness, when correct diagnosis may be both difficult and critically important. A patient with severe malaria is at risk of dying even with optimal case management. Case fatality rates range between 5% and 30% in patients receiving treatment for severe malaria according to the complications present and their intensity.

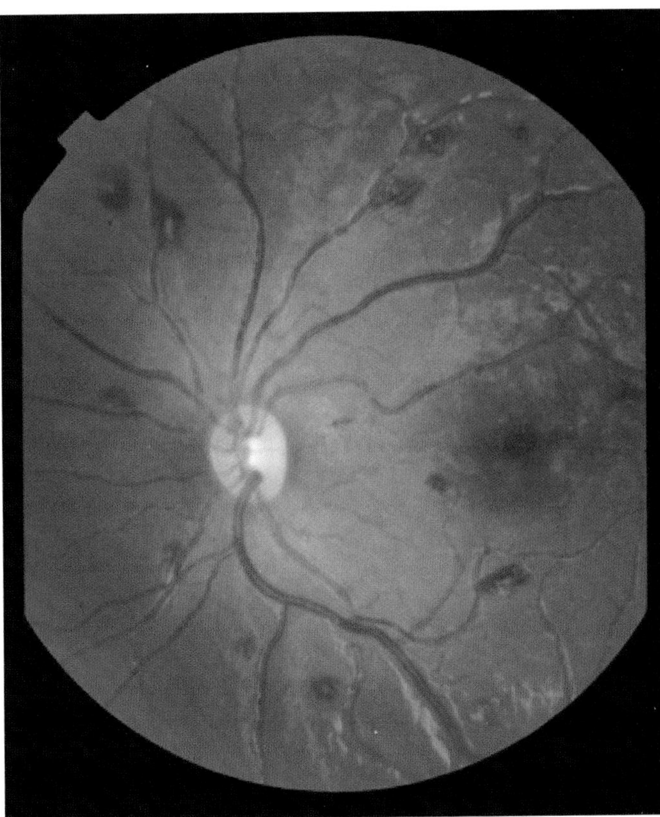

FIGURE 158-1. Retinal examination in a child with cerebral malaria. Note the patches of whitening around the fovea (dark area 2.5 disc diameters from the disc, right of field). Note also scattered white-centered hemorrhages. [Photo contributed by Ian McCormick, MD.]

When cerebral malaria is suspected, meningitis or encephalitis must be either excluded or treated, and the clinician must decide whether a lumbar puncture is safe. At lumbar puncture, the opening pressure is usually raised in children and normal in adults. The fluid is normal in appearance and on routine tests. In children in *P. falciparum*–endemic areas, asymptomatic parasitemia is common, so it is difficult to be sure that an illness is due to malaria. In a child with coma and parasitemia, the presence of a recently identified retinopathy (**Figure 158-1**) greatly strengthens confidence that malaria is the cause of the syndrome.[12] Among those who recover from cerebral malaria, up to 1 in 5 children and up to 1 in 20 adults may be left with, or may later develop, neurologic sequelae.

Infections caused by any species of *Plasmodium* can result in hemolysis, some degree of anemia, splenic enlargement, and, occasionally, splenic rupture.

The very young, the elderly, and pregnant women are at greatest risk of developing complications when infected with *P. falciparum*.[13] Additional risk factors for severe malaria include an immunocompromised state, asplenia, failure to take appropriate chemoprophylaxis, refusal of or delay in seeking medical care, and late or erroneous diagnosis.[14]

DIAGNOSIS

The diagnosis of malaria rests on a history of potential exposure in a malarious area, clinical symptoms, signs, and competent microscopic examination of well-prepared thick and thin blood films (**Figure 158-2**). Diagnosis based on clinical features alone has very low specificity and results in overtreatment.[1]

The three major questions to be answered by the blood smear are as follows: (1) Is there evidence of malaria? (2) If so, what is the density of parasitemia (correlates with prognosis)? (3) What species of malaria is responsible for the infection and, in particular, is *P. falciparum* present? Clues to the diagnosis of *P. falciparum* infection include the presence of small ring forms with double-chromatin dots within the erythrocyte,

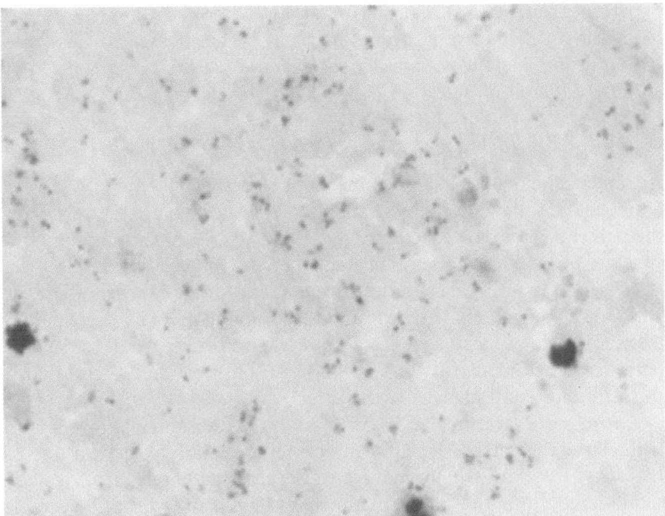

A

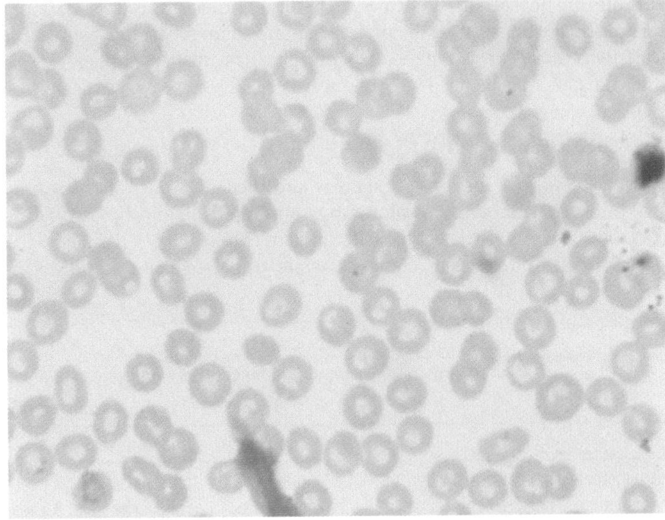

B

FIGURE 158-2. **A.** Thick and **B.** thin blood microscopy films from different children with malaria. The thick film shows numerous parasite nuclei, each with a faint blush of cytoplasm, seen either as a ring or as a smudge beside the nucleus. The thin film shows a single early ring stage of *P. falciparum* (center of field). The absence of dots in the erythrocyte cytoplasm and the normal size and shape of the erythrocyte distinguish this from *P. vivax* and *P. ovale*.

multiple infected rings in individual red blood cells, a paucity (usually absence) of mature trophozoites and schizonts on smear, and infected erythrocytes that are not enlarged and that have cytoplasm without basophilic stippling. In some (but not all) cases, gametocytes may be seen; in *P. falciparum* infection, these have a diagnostic crescent shape (banana shape). Parasite densities above 4% of erythrocytes are rare in malaria due to nonfalciparum species. Obtain smears daily to assess the efficacy of drug treatment.

P. knowlesi is usually misdiagnosed as the less aggressive *P. malariae*, because the two are identical under light microscopy and require polymerase chain reaction for differentiation. Any patient coming from Asia with a high parasite burden resembling *P. malariae* should be assumed to be harboring *P. knowlesi*.[4]

THICK BLOOD FILM

Place a small drop of blood (5 μL) on a microscope slide, spread it evenly to a diameter of ~1 cm, allow it to dry, and then stain, without initial fixation, with Fields or Giemsa stain. Record the result as the number of parasites seen per oil-immersion field (for an approximate indication of density) or per 200 white cell nuclei counted (a more accurate density of parasites can then be calculated once the WBC count is known). A thick blood film contains several layers of red cells (which are lysed by the staining procedure), allowing parasitemias down to ~40/μL to be detected by an expert microscopist.

THIN BLOOD FILM

A standard hematologic blood smear (fixed with methanol and stained with Giemsa) allows a single sheet of intact red cells to be scrutinized for the percentage of red cells parasitized, from which the number of parasites per microliter can be calculated when the red cell count is known. Because the red cells are not destroyed, a thin film allows both parasite and red cell morphology to be examined, enabling more confident identification of the species of plasmodium. A thin film may fail to detect a parasitemia with a density below ~1000/μL, but it is more useful than a thick film for counting very heavy infections.

A long and careful search for parasites is necessary before a film is declared "negative." In early infection, especially infection due to *P. falciparum*, in which mature-stage parasitized erythrocytes are sequestered from the bloodstream, parasitemia may be undetectable even in a competently read thick blood film. **In highly suspicious cases, failure to detect parasitemia is not an indication to withhold therapy.** If parasites are not seen in the stained thin smear, a thick smear must be done. If parasites are not seen on the first thick film, obtain repeat thick smears at least twice daily for as long as malaria remains a suspected diagnosis or until the patient is better. The first smear is positive in >90% of cases.[15]

ADDITIONAL DIAGNOSTIC TECHNIQUES

Newer techniques for rapid diagnosis and speciation include quantitative buffy coat fluorescent microscopy and rapid diagnostic tests (dipstick bedside tests) to detect parasite antigens (BinaxNOW®, ParaSight-F®) or to detect the parasite enzyme lactate dehydrogenase (OptiMal).[16] Sensitivity of rapid tests is excellent for *P. falciparum* malaria with high parasitemia levels, but poor for nonfalciparum malaria, and sensitively drops with lower parasitemia levels. Polymerase chain reaction–based techniques to detect parasite DNA are more sensitive than microscopy and are valuable for research studies but are rarely available for routine clinical purposes.

ADDITIONAL LABORATORY STUDIES

Nonspecific laboratory features of malaria include normochromic normocytic anemia with findings suggestive of hemolysis, a normal or mildly depressed total leukocyte count, thrombocytopenia, an elevated erythrocyte sedimentation rate, mild abnormalities in liver and renal functions, and a biologic false-positive Venereal Disease Research Laboratory test. In severe *P. falciparum* malaria, there may be hypoglycemia, severe anemia, hyperlactatemia, electrolyte disturbances, or evidence of acute renal failure or disseminated intravascular coagulation.

TREATMENT

Treatment decisions are based on the severity of the illness and the species of the infecting parasite determined by microscopic examination of thick and thin blood films.

UNCOMPLICATED (NONSEVERE) MALARIA DUE TO *P. FALCIPARUM*

Admit the patient to the hospital because severe disease can develop rapidly even after the start of specific therapy. Give analgesia if required (e.g., acetaminophen, 500 milligrams every 6 hours PO) and oral fluids. If the patient can take and retain drugs by mouth, begin a full course of oral antimalarial drugs without delay (**Table 158-2**). Artemisinin-containing combination therapies are considered the drugs of choice by the World

TABLE 158-2 Drug Options for Therapy of Uncomplicated *Plasmodium falciparum* Malaria

Treatment of choice is an artemisinin-containing combination therapy (ACT)		
Drug	**Adult Dose**	**Pediatric Dose**
Artemether-lumefantrine (CoArtem®; each tablet contains artemether 20 milligrams and lumefantrine 120 milligrams)	4 tablets twice daily for 3 d (the first 2 doses should be about 8 h apart)	5–15 kg: 1 tab initially, 1 tablet in 8 h, then 1 tablet every 12 h × 2 d 15–25 kg: 2 tablets initially, 2 tablets in 8 h, then 2 tablets every 12 h × 2 d 25–35 kg: 3 tablets initially, 3 tablets in 8 h, then 3 tablets every 12 h × 2 d >35 kg: follow adult dosing
Artesunate-amodiaquine (where available; not available in the United States; each adult tablet contains artesunate 100 milligrams and amodiaquine hydrochloride salt 270 milligrams)	2 tablets once daily for 3 d	5 to <9 kg: 1 tablet/day of artesunate (AS) 25 milligrams/amodiaquine (AQ) 67.5 milligrams 9 to <18 kg: 1 tablet/day of AS 50 milligrams/AQ 135 milligrams 18 to <36 kg: 1 tablet/day of AS 100 milligrams/AQ 270 milligrams ≥36 kg: 2 tablets/day of AS 100 milligrams/AQ 270 milligrams (adult dose)
Alternatives to ACT		
Drug	**Adult Dose**	**Pediatric Dose**
Atovaquone-proguanil (Malarone®; each adult tablet contains atovaquone 250 milligrams and proguanil 100 milligrams; each pediatric tablet contains atovaquone 62.5 milligrams and proguanil 25 milligrams)	4 tablets once daily for 3 d. Do not use for treatment if atovaquone-proguanil has been taken as chemoprophylaxis and the patient's current illness is a suspected treatment failure.	5–8 kg: 2 pediatric tablets × 3 d 9–10 kg: 3 pediatric tablets × 3 d 11–20 kg: 1 adult tablet × 3 d 21–30 kg: 2 adult tablets × 3 d 31–40 kg: 3 adult tablets × 3 d >41 kg: adult dose
Quinine sulfate (plus doxycycline or clindamycin)	650 milligrams PO every 8 h for 3–7 d	10 milligrams sulfate salt/kg, up to adult dose PO every 8 h for 3–7 d
Plus		
Doxycycline	100 milligrams PO every 12 h for 7 d	2.2 milligrams/kg (up to adult dose of 100 milligrams) PO every 12 h for 7 d
Or in children under age 8 y		
Clindamycin		7 milligrams/kg PO every 8 h for 7 d

Health Organization.[1,17] If a dose is vomited, the dose may be repeated; if it is vomited again, switch to parenteral therapy as for severe disease (see Table 158-3) until able to resume treatment by mouth. Maintain regular checks for the development of any complications (listed above under "Clinical Features"). Check blood daily for parasite density and for hemoglobin concentration. When stable, the patient may be discharged to complete the course of oral drugs at home; stress the importance of completing the course and of reporting back with any recurrence of symptoms.

The World Health Organization does not recommend chloroquine for the treatment of *P. falciparum* malaria due to changing resistance patterns and the superiority of artemisinin-containing combination therapies.[1,17] As of July of 2013, the Centers for Disease Control and Prevention recommend chloroquine for *P. falciparum* malaria imported from areas of low chloroquine resistance including Central America west of the Panama Canal, Haiti, the Dominican Republic, and parts of the Middle East.[18,19] Dose options are listed at the Centers for Disease Control and Prevention malaria Web site (http://www.cdc.gov/malaria/).

UNCOMPLICATED MALARIA DUE TO *P. VIVAX, P. MALARIAE, P. OVALE*, OR *P. KNOWLESI*

Admission to the hospital should not be necessary in most cases; however, if *P. knowlesi* is suspected, hospital admission is recommended. Dual infection with *P. falciparum* and any of the other species is possible. Make sure that the initial and subsequent slides are carefully scrutinized for evidence of *P. falciparum*, because severe disease may then develop even while on treatment. Give simple analgesia and fluids as required. Treat nonfalciparum malaria with chloroquine (each tablet contains 250 milligrams of salt = 150 milligrams of base); the adult dose is four tablets initially, then two tablets after 6 hours, then two tablets daily for 2 days. The pediatric dose is 16.7 milligrams (salt)/kg PO immediately, followed by 8.3 milligrams (salt)/kg PO at 6, 24, and 48 hours. Alternatively, an artemisinin combination therapy can be given (see Table 158-3 for dosage). *P. vivax* malaria acquired from an area with chloroquine resistance should be treated with artemisinin-containing combination therapy.[1]

Patients with *P. vivax* or *P. ovale* malaria require additional treatment to eradicate hypnozoites from the liver. This treatment can be given after full recovery from the initial illness; the most common agent used is primaquine phosphate. The adult dose is 30 milligrams of base per day for 14 days. First check the patient for glucose-6-phosphate dehydrogenase deficiency (glucose-6-phosphate dehydrogenase–deficient persons are at risk of hemolysis when treated with primaquine; an alternative management of relapsing malarias is chloroquine base 300 milligrams weekly for 6 months). Treatment with primaquine is not needed in patients with *P. falciparum* or *P. malariae* malaria because there are no dormant asexual forms in the liver. *P. vivax* or *P. ovale* infections that have been acquired by needlestick accident, blood transfusion, or transplacental infection do not need treatment with primaquine for the same reason.

SEVERE (COMPLICATED) MALARIA

Severe malaria is usually due to *P. falciparum*, but occasionally, it is due to *P. vivax* or *P. knowlesi*. The patients should be admitted to an appropriate level of intensive care. Both supportive and specific antimalarial therapies are urgent and critical to the patient's survival. Monitor the patient frequently; new complications may develop after the start of treatment.

Supportive Management Initial resuscitation may require oxygen for hypoxia, fluid replacement, IV glucose for hypoglycemia, blood transfusion for severe anemia or for disseminated intravascular coagulation, and occasionally intubation for severe respiratory distress or suspected raised intracranial pressure with altered mental status. Additional treatments for septic shock may be necessary (see chapter 151, "Sepsis"). Monitor to identify and treat seizures, hyperpyrexia, acute respiratory distress syndrome, or acute renal failure. Culture blood samples for bacterial infections, and give immediate parenteral antibiotics, because a bacterial co-infection cannot be ruled out by clinical assessment initially.

Specific Antimalarial Chemotherapy Initiate parenteral therapy with an efficacious antimalarial drug without delay. Options are listed in **Table 158-3**.

With any of the regimens in Table 158-3, continue the treatment by a parenteral route for at least 24 hours; thereafter, as soon as the patient is well enough to take drugs by mouth, switch to a complete course of the best available oral therapy (Table 158-2). If the patient remains unable to take oral therapy, the chosen parenteral therapy should be continued for a maximum of 7 days.

Do not delay treatment while awaiting laboratory confirmation, because the initial smear for *P. falciparum* may be negative, even on microscopy of a thick blood film, in a nonimmune individual. An unstable patient (abnormal vital signs, severe anemia, renal failure, pulmonary edema, acute respiratory distress syndrome, disseminated intravascular coagulation, acidosis, jaundice, hemoglobinuria, or seizures) with a clinical or travel history suggesting malaria should be started on artesunate (if available) or quinidine gluconate (Table 158-3) until a diagnosis of malaria can be ruled out.

In the United States, parenteral quinine should be reserved for individuals who develop, or who are considered to be at high risk of developing, cardiotoxicity while receiving IV quinidine.

To initiate a patient with severe malaria in the Centers for Disease Control and Prevention treatment protocol (United States only) using artesunate, contact the Centers for Disease Control and Prevention Malaria Hotline: 770-488-7788 (Monday–Friday, 9 a.m.–5 p.m., eastern time) or after hours, call 770-488-7100 and request to speak with a Centers for Disease Control and Prevention Malaria Branch clinician.[20]

IV artesunate is the drug of choice for severe malaria, according to the World Health Organization. Artesunate is rapidly effective and extremely

TABLE 158-3 Antimalarial Drug Options for Severe (Complicated) Malaria

Drug	Adult Dose	Pediatric Dose
Artesunate* (available from the CDC if quinidine fails to provide improvement; call 770-488-7788)	2.4 milligrams/kg IV at 0, 8, and 24 h, then daily. Artesunate can be given IM if necessary.	2.4 milligrams/kg IV at 0, 8, and 24 h, then daily. Artesunate can be given IM if necessary.
Quinidine gluconate (plus doxycycline or clindamycin)†	6.25 milligrams base (= 10 milligrams salt)/kg IV load over 2 h (maximum, 600 milligrams), follow with 0.0125 milligram base (= 0.02 milligram salt)/kg/min continuous infusion.	6.25 milligrams base (= 10 milligrams salt)/kg IV load over 2 h (maximum, 600 milligrams), follow with 0.0125 milligram base (= 0.02 milligram salt)/kg/min continuous infusion.
Plus		
Doxycycline	2.2 milligrams/kg IV (up to adult dose of 100 milligrams) every 12 h for 7 d.	2.2 milligrams/kg IV (up to adult dose of 100 milligrams) every 12 h for 7 d
Or in children under age 8 y		
Clindamycin		10 milligrams base/kg loading dose IV followed by 5 milligrams base/kg IV every 8 h for 7 d.

Abbreviation: CDC = Centers for Disease Control and Prevention.

*Artesunate is considered the drug of choice by World Health Organization guidelines.

†Quinine dihydrochloride is an alternative to quinidine gluconate (20 milligrams [salt]/kg infused IV over 2–4 hours, then 10 milligrams/kg every 8 hours, can be given IM if necessary, as 50 milligrams/mL solution).

potent against all erythrocyte stages. It does not cause cardiac toxicity or hypoglycemia. It is effective and is superior to IV quinine in both adults[21] and children.[22] Prompt treatment for severe malaria is critical, and artesunate's major limitation at present in the United States is its lack of timely availability.

RATES OF PARASITE CLEARANCE

With correct treatment, the parasite load in the peripheral blood should decrease rapidly during the first few days. This decrease is significantly faster with artemisinin drugs than with all other therapies, because artemisinin drugs kill early-stage as well as late-stage parasites. With artemisinin treatment, the parasite count usually decreases significantly within the first 12 hours, whereas with other drugs, this steep decrease may take 24 to 48 hours. In a patient treated with quinidine or quinine, the density of asexual parasites may be unchanged or even increased after 24 hours of therapy, but this is rarely the case in a person treated with an artemisinin therapy. Asexual forms of the parasite should not be detectable within 5 days of the start of any effective treatment course. Gametocytes, the sexual forms, which do not cause disease in the human host, may persist for several weeks after treatment and do not indicate treatment failure.

COMPLICATIONS OF TREATMENT

Complications of treatment are listed in **Table 158-4**.

Glucocorticoids are of no proven benefit for cerebral malaria and should not be used. Other unproven or harmful adjunctive therapies include heparin, iron chelators, pentoxifylline, and dichloroacetate.

Quinine and quinidine are potent inducers of insulin release and may cause severe hypoglycemia, especially during pregnancy. Sudden changes in orientation, sweating, tremor, tachycardia, or anxiety should prompt bedside glucose measurement and treatment accordingly. Cinchona alkaloids are myocardial depressants, so cardiac monitoring is needed during administration of quinidine or quinine. At least partial resistance to quinine has been reported in Southeast Asia, but it has not yet been identified in Africa.

DISPOSITION AND FOLLOW-UP

Many patients feel better after the first day or two of treatment for uncomplicated malaria. Emphasize the importance of completing the treatment, because partial therapy may fail to eliminate parasites and may be followed by recrudescence of infection. Advise the patient to report any recurrence of symptoms, because even completed treatment may fail or an unrecognized additional infection may emerge. An episode of malaria is an opportunity to advise an individual about how to prevent further infections. After severe malaria, review the patient at intervals for any sequelae. Survivors of acute kidney injury, acute respiratory distress syndrome, or severe anemia usually recover fully, but cerebral malaria may be followed by neurologic sequelae in a proportion of cases, especially in children.[23]

SPECIAL CONSIDERATIONS

PREGNANCY

Among nonimmune adults, those who are pregnant are at greater risk of developing severe disease than others. Pregnant women are at particular risk of anemia, hypoglycemia, and, especially in the third stage of labor, fluid overload. Artemisinin drugs are probably safe in pregnancy but are still subject to restriction in the first trimester. Quinidine and quinine can be used in pregnancy but carry a greater risk of causing hypoglycemia through stimulation of insulin secretion from hypertrophied pancreatic β-cells.

TABLE 158-4 Adverse Effects, Precautions, and Contraindications of Antimalarial Drugs

Drug	Minor Toxicity	Major Toxicity	Precautions/Contraindications
Chloroquine	Nausea/vomiting, diarrhea, pruritus, postural hypotension, rash, fever, headache, dizziness	Rare; hypotension and shock after parenteral therapy Retinopathy after prolonged use	Avoid in patients with severe psoriasis and some types of porphyria, caution with decreased liver function.
Quinine or quinidine	Cinchonism (nausea and vomiting, headache, tinnitus, dizziness, visual disturbance)	Hypotension, cardiac dysrhythmias, hypoglycemia, Coombs-positive hemolysis, abortions, neuromuscular paralysis (myasthenia)	Contraindicated in cardiac disease. Caution in pregnancy, myasthenia gravis.
Mefloquine	Nausea/vomiting, cramps, diarrhea, anorexia, dizziness, headaches, nightmares, and bradycardia	Rare unless underlying heart disease with bradycardia or the patient is on selected cardiotoxic medications (dysrhythmias, arrest); acute toxic confusional states may occur, as can seizures	Precaution during pregnancy and in children weighing <10 kg. Avoid if the patient is receiving quinidine. Avoid if the patient has heart conduction disturbance or if underlying seizure or major neuropsychiatric disorders.
Doxycycline	GI disturbances, phototoxicity, vaginal candidiasis	Rare; esophageal ulcerations if not taken with fluids	Contraindicated during pregnancy, in children <8 y of age. May depress prothrombin time in patients receiving anticoagulants.
Artemether-lumefantrine (Coartem®)	Headache, dizziness, anorexia, and asthenia	Rare; severe skin rash, QT prolongation	Avoidance with other drugs that may prolong QT interval. Drug interactions with cytochrome P-450 3A4 and cytochrome P-450 2D6.
Atovaquone-proguanil (Malarone®)	Nausea, vomiting, cramps, oral ulcers, headaches, dizziness	Rare serious allergic reactions and alopecia reported	Contraindicated in pregnancy and in children <5 kg (no safety data) and in patients with creatinine clearance <30.
Primaquine*	Nausea, vomiting, diarrhea, cramps, methemoglobinemia	Massive hemolysis in patients with G6PD deficiency Exacerbation of systemic lupus erythematosus or rheumatoid arthritis	Contraindicated in G6PD deficiency, pregnancy.

Abbreviation: G6PD = glucose-6-phosphate dehydrogenase.

*Terminal treatment for *Plasmodium vivax* and *Plasmodium ovale* infections only.

PREVENTION

In malaria-endemic areas, national efforts are aimed at identifying and correctly treating malaria cases while reducing transmission through widespread use of long-lasting insecticide-impregnated bednets and programs of indoor residual spraying with insecticides. Several countries have now achieved elimination of transmission within their borders, while many more are beginning to set elimination as a national target.

For nonimmune travelers, malaria is largely preventable through the use of personal protective measures and appropriate chemoprophylaxis. Travelers to malarious areas frequently do not use antimosquito measures or take antimalarial drugs.[24] Of the U.S. civilians who acquired malaria abroad during 2011, only 6% had followed a chemoprophylactic drug regimen recommended by the Centers for Disease Control and Prevention for the area to which they had traveled.[2] Persons who immigrated to the United States years ago from malarious areas often falsely assume that they are immune to disease.

Between dusk and dawn, travelers should remain in well-screened areas, use insecticide-impregnated mosquito nets, and wear long-sleeved, light-colored clothing. Nets impregnated with long-lasting insecticides are very effective, although resistance of mosquitoes to insecticides is an increasing concern. An insect repellent containing *N,N*-diethyl-*m*-toluamide (DEET) in concentrations no higher than 35% should be applied to exposed skin. DEET-based repellents are significantly more efficacious than non–DEET-based repellents.[25] Newer formulations of DEET exist with polymer encapsulation and sustained-release properties and provide long-acting protection at lower concentrations of DEET.

Appropriate chemoprophylaxis depends on the travel destination. If exposure to infected mosquitoes is likely, prophylaxis is warranted even if such exposure will be brief. Because recommendations change quite frequently and are area specific, anyone requiring advice for the prophylaxis appropriate for travel to a particular area should attend a travel clinic, or see current recommendations on the Centers for Disease Control and Prevention Web site (www.cdc.gov/malaria/travelers/drugs.html). Failure to take appropriate chemoprophylaxis is a significant risk factor for fatal infection.[26] Even with the rigorous use of antimosquito measures and chemoprophylaxis, malaria can be contracted or can recur.

Vaccines directed against various antigens and life-cycle stages of *P. falciparum* are being intensively investigated. Results of a multicountry phase III trial of the currently most developed vaccine candidate will be available by 2015 to allow a final decision about efficacy and deployment. This vaccine, which primarily aims to benefit infants and children in malarious areas, will at best have partial efficacy, so that it will complement but not replace other measures of prevention and control.[27]

PRACTICE GUIDELINES

Both the World Health Organization[17] and the Centers for Disease Control and Prevention[18,19] publish and update practice guidelines for the diagnosis and treatment of malaria.

REFERENCES

The complete reference list is available online at www.TintinalliEM.com.

Food and Waterborne Illnesses

Lane M. Smith
Simon A. Mahler

FOODBORNE ILLNESSES

INTRODUCTION AND EPIDEMIOLOGY

Foodborne illness occurs after consumption of a food contaminated with bacteria, viruses, parasites, chemicals, or biotoxins. As one example, in 2008, melamine-contaminated dairy products in China affected over 50,000 children. The World Health Organization estimates that more than two million children die every year from exposure to unsafe water or food.[1] Outbreaks from contaminated food are often widespread, and foodborne disease is a public health concern. International travel contributes to foodborne illnesses as travelers are exposed to new pathogens, and migrants may introduce diseases.[1]

The Centers for Disease Control and Prevention (CDC) estimates that foodborne diseases cause 1 in 6 Americans to get sick, leading to 128,000 hospitalizations and 3000 deaths in the United States each year.[2,3] Children have the highest frequency of foodborne illness. Viruses are the most common cause of foodborne disease, with the norovirus causing more than half of all cases and 26% of all admissions.[2] Other viral sources of infection include rotavirus, astrovirus, and enteric adenovirus.

Bacterial causes tend to be more severe, with nontyphoidal *Salmonella* triggering the most cases requiring admission or resulting in fatality.[3] Other common bacterial causes of foodborne illness include *Clostridium perfringens*, *Campylobacter* spp., *Toxoplasma gondii*, *Shigella*, *Staphylococcus aureus*, and Shiga toxin–producing *Escherichia coli*. Over the past decade, there has been little change in the overall incidence of foodborne pathogens aside from *Campylobacter*, which has been steadily increasing since 2001.[3] The most common foods associated with outbreaks reported in the United States are poultry, leafy vegetables, and fruits/nuts.[2,3]

PATHOPHYSIOLOGY

There are three basic mechanisms by which microbes cause illness. First, some pathogens such as *S. aureus*, *Bacillus cereus*, and *Clostridium botulinum* (botulism) produce toxins capable of causing illness. These preformed toxins are present in the food before ingestion and result in the rapid onset (1 to 6 hours) of symptoms. Preformed toxins such as staphylococcal enterotoxin exert their effect by stimulating the host immune system to release inflammatory cytokines within the intestine.[4] These cytokines are responsible for the accompanying nausea and vomiting.

The second method involves toxin production after ingestion, which interacts with intestinal epithelium as seen with *Vibrio*, *Shigella*, and Shiga toxin–producing *E. coli*. These cause diarrhea and lower GI symptoms (cramping and sometimes bloody diarrhea), with onset at approximately 24 hours after exposure. Some toxins produced by *Vibrio* and enterotoxigenic *E. coli* alter chloride and sodium transport across intestinal mucosal surfaces without destroying cells.[5] The resulting osmotic gradient produces a large fluid shift into the intestinal lumen, which overwhelms the absorptive capacity of the colon, causing watery diarrhea. Other toxins produced after ingestion by organisms such as *Shigella* and Shiga toxin–producing *E. coli* disrupt host cell protein production, which causes death of the intestinal epithelium, resulting in bloody diarrhea and extraintestinal symptoms.[6]

Finally, direct invasion of the intestinal epithelium is a common mechanism for the enteric viruses, *Salmonella*, enteroinvasive *E. coli*, and *Campylobacter*. These pathogens enter host cells and destroy intestinal epithelium.[7] This causes diarrhea due to transient malabsorption that is frequently bloody and accompanied by systemic symptoms such as fever. These viruses require ingestion of just a few viral particles to cause disease. The upper and lower GI symptoms from invasive organisms last from 24 hours to weeks (**Table 159-1**).

TABLE 159-1 Etiologic Agents for Foodborne Diseases and Usual Incubation Periods

1–6 Hours	6–24 Hours	24–48 Hours	2–6 Days	1–2+ Weeks
Astrovirus	*Bacillus cereus* diarrhea toxin	*Clostridium botulinum*	*Campylobacter*	*Brucella*
B. cereus preformed toxin	*Clostridium perfringens*	Enterotoxigenic *Escherichia coli*	*Shigella*	*Cryptosporidium*
Ciguatoxin	*Vibrio parahaemolyticus*	*Salmonella*	Enterohemorrhagic *E. coli*	*Entamoeba*
Heavy metals		*Trichinella*	*Vibrio cholerae*	*Giardia*
Monosodium glutamate			*Yersinia*	Hepatitis A
Norovirus				*Listeria*
Scromboid toxin				*Salmonella typhi*
Staphylococcus aureus toxin				
Tetrodotoxin				

The normal human digestive tract has physiologic defenses against foodborne diseases. The low gastric pH of 1 to 3 kills many ingested pathogens, while the normal intestinal flora competitively inhibits pathogens and secretes bactericidal fatty acids and other chemicals.[8,9] Normal intestinal motility prevents pathogens from having prolonged contact with mucosal surfaces and mixes organisms with mucous-containing protective glycoproteins. Immunologic tissues are also present in the GI tract to directly attack pathogens attempting transmural migration.[9]

Alteration of these protective mechanisms can increase susceptibility to foodborne disease. For example, proton pump inhibitors, histamine-2 (H_2) blockers, and antacids reduce gastric acid production. Recent antibiotic use, chemotherapy or radiation therapy, and recent surgery alter the intestinal flora. Decreased intestinal motility from narcotics, antiperistaltic drugs, and surgery may encourage pathogen growth and migration.[9]

CLINICAL FEATURES

Suspect a foodborne disease when two or more people in a household or close association (e.g., the same workplace or communal eating arrangement) simultaneously develop GI symptoms. The most common symptoms are nausea, vomiting, diarrhea, and abdominal cramping. Systemic symptoms of fever, dehydration, and malaise are also common in patients with severe foodborne infections.

Question patients about the types of food they have recently ingested, frequency of restaurant meals, consumption of public-vended or street-vended foods, ingestion of seafood, and consumption of raw foods. Additional questions include recent travel or camping, contact with food handlers, and diaper changing. Children who attend day care centers and residents of long-term care facilities are at increased risk for foodborne diseases. People working in the food industry are also frequent victims or sources; ask them about their personal hygiene and food-handling practices. Finally, seek a history of comorbidities or influencing therapies, including human immunodeficiency virus (HIV) infection or immunosuppressive drug use.

On exam, look for dehydration and a toxic appearance. Another priority is the identification of blood in the stool and the exclusion of alternative causes of symptoms such as appendicitis. The clinical features of specific foodborne infections are summarized in **Table 159-2**.

DIAGNOSIS

Most patients with foodborne diseases do not require diagnostic testing; illnesses are often self-limited. Routine testing for stool ova and parasites or cultures is not indicated.[10] However, electrolytes and a CBC are helpful in toxic patients or those with prolonged symptoms. Stool tests are obtained in the following clinical situations[10,11]:

- Watery diarrhea with signs of hypovolemia
- Bloody diarrhea
- Fever ≥38.5°C (101.3°F)
- Prolonged duration of illness >1 week
- Severe abdominal pain or tenderness
- Hospitalized patients or recent antibiotic use

TABLE 159-2 Clinical Features of Foodborne Infections

Clinical Presentation	Foodborne Pathogens
Gastroenteritis with vomiting as the primary symptom	Viral pathogens: *Norovirus, Rotavirus,* and *Astrovirus;* preformed toxins: *Staphylococcus aureus* and *Bacillus cereus*
Noninflammatory diarrhea (watery, nonbloody)	Can be any enteric pathogen, but classically: ETEC *Giardia* *Vibrio cholerae* Enteric viruses *Cryptosporidium* *Cyclospora*
Inflammatory diarrhea (grossly bloody, fever)	*Shigella* *Campylobacter* *Salmonella* EIEC Shiga toxin–producing *Escherichia coli* 0157:H7 and non-0157:H7 *Vibrio parahaemolyticus* *Yersinia* *Entamoeba*
Persistent diarrhea (>14 d)	Parasites: *Giardia* *Cyclospora* *Entamoeba* *Cryptosporidium*
Neurologic manifestations	Botulism (*Clostridium botulinum toxin*) Scombroid fish poisoning Ciguatera fish poisoning Tetrodotoxin Toxic mushroom ingestion Paralytic shellfish poisoning Guillain-Barré syndrome
Systemic illness	*Listeria monocytogenes* *Brucella* *Salmonella typhi* *Salmonella paratyphi* *Vibrio vulnificus* Hepatitis A, E

Abbreviations: EIEC = enteroinvasive *E. coli*; ETEC = enterotoxigenic *E. coli*.

- Elderly (≥70 years of age) or the immunocompromised
- Pregnant women or those with comorbidities such as inflammatory bowel disease

Routine stool cultures will identify *Salmonella*, *Campylobacter*, and *Shigella*. A single sample is usually sufficient, but be aware of local laboratory limitations. For example, most laboratories do not routinely culture enterotoxigenic *E. coli*, vibrios, and viruses. In 2009, the Centers for Disease Control and Prevention recommended that clinical laboratories culture all submitted stool specimens for Shiga toxin–producing *E. coli* and perform toxin assays for Shiga toxin.[12]

Testing for ova and parasites is indicated for the immunocompromised, patients with symptoms lasting longer than 2 weeks, community waterborne outbreaks, or men who have sex with men.[10,13] Because parasite excretion may not be continuous, three specimens separated by at least 24 hours may be needed to identify the causative pathogen.

Testing for fecal leukocytes has historically been performed to predict the presence of an invasive cause for acute diarrhea and increase stool culture yield. Unfortunately, several studies have shown that fecal leukocytes are neither sensitive nor specific for invasive disease, and they are a poor a predictor of response to antimicrobial therapy.[14,15] The neutrophil marker lactoferrin is a more sensitive, but less widely available, screening test for inflammatory cells in stool. If positive, fecal lactoferrin also increases the likelihood of positive stool cultures.[16,17] Direct antigen detection panels are available for specific viruses such as rotavirus, bacteria, and parasitic pathogens in many clinical laboratories.

TREATMENT

Most episodes of acute gastroenteritis require only adequate hydration and supportive care. The World Health Organization recommends initial therapy with a glucose-containing fluid (i.e., Pedialyte or equivalent) for oral rehydration.[18] Parenteral rehydration is recommended for patients with severe dehydration or continued vomiting and inability to tolerate oral fluids. Antiemetics may reduce vomiting, emergency department length of stay, and need for admission.[19,20] Antimotility medications, such as loperamide, may decrease illness duration for mild to moderate nonbloody diarrhea in adults without fever but are generally avoided in young children and patients with dysentery (fever and bloody diarrhea) due to concerns of prolonging the illness.[21]

Empiric antibiotics do not appear to dramatically alter the course of illness since most cases are viral or self-limited bacterial in origin. The 2001 Infectious Diseases Society of America guidelines recommend empiric treatment for patients with moderate to severe traveler's diarrhea, those with symptoms for more than 1 week, patients requiring hospitalization due to volume depletion, and immunocompromised hosts.[10] A common bacterial enteritis regimen is oral ciprofloxacin 500 milligrams twice daily or levofloxacin 500 milligrams once a day, each for 3 to 5 days. Azithromycin 500 milligrams once daily for 3 days is an alternative regimen.[10] Antibiotics and antimotility agents are contraindicated in patients with Shiga toxin–producing *E. coli* O157:H7 infection due to increased risk of hemolytic-uremic syndrome, especially in children and the elderly.[22] See **Tables 159-3, 159-4, 159-5, and 159-6** for more detailed treatment recommendations.

DISPOSITION AND FOLLOW-UP

Patients who appear toxic or have systemic symptoms, significant comorbidities, or severe dehydration with inability to tolerate oral fluids are admitted. Discharged patients should receive instructions on proper hygiene, notably frequent hand washing, to protect family members and contacts who are not ill. Patients discharged with pending stool culture or other studies should have a clear plan for follow-up.

SPECIAL POPULATIONS

Elderly patients, young children, and the immunocompromised are more likely to have severe illness, atypical presentations, and long-term sequelae. Patients with human immunodeficiency virus or other immunocompromised states can rapidly develop life-threatening symptoms. Thus, test more liberally and admit at a lower threshold. Pregnant patients have increased risk of complications, especially with *Listeria* infection, and may require further monitoring.[10]

SPECIAL CONSIDERATIONS

Enterohemorrhagic *E. coli* and Hemolytic-Uremic Syndrome Enterohemorrhagic *E. coli* that produces Shiga toxin is the most common cause of hemolytic-uremic syndrome in the United States.[22] The Shiga toxin–producing *E. coli* strain O157:H7 is most commonly associated with pediatric hemolytic-uremic syndrome, but other strains such as O104:H4 and O111 are associated with adult hemolytic-uremic syndrome–like illnesses. The Shiga toxin produced by these organisms halts protein synthesis in renal glomerular cells as the precipitating event in hemolytic-uremic syndrome. Toxin binding to the glomerular endothelium produces a thrombogenic environment leading to microangiopathic hemolysis through multiple cellular mechanisms.[23,24] Antibiotics may promote Shiga toxin release, which increases the incidence of hemolytic-uremic syndrome, and are avoided when this is suspected or identified. In addition, avoid antimotility agents. Treatment of hemolytic-uremic syndrome is supportive, with plasma infusion and exchange therapy showing some benefit. Approximately 50% of pediatric patients with hemolytic-uremic syndrome will require dialysis, and dehydration at the time of admission increases the frequency and duration of renal support.[25]

Scombroid and Ciguatera Poisoning **Scombroid fish poisoning** occurs after ingestion of fish of the family Scombridae (tuna, mackerel, and bonito). Other non-Scombridae fish such as mahi-mahi, bluefish, herring, and sardines are also implicated. The disease occurs when histidine is metabolized by bacteria into histamine and other bioactive amines. Improper temperature control allows high concentrations of these substances to accumulate in the fish. Symptoms usually begin 30 minutes to 24 hours after ingestion and include flushing, headache, abdominal cramping, vomiting, and diarrhea. Symptoms are usually self-limited for 12 to 48 hours. However, severe cardiac and respiratory symptoms may occur in the elderly or patients with comorbid conditions. Treatment is with antihistamines (H_1 and H_2 blockers) such as diphenhydramine and cimetidine. Laboratory testing is not needed in most cases.[26]

Ciguatera poisoning is caused by eating reef fish contaminated with the dinoflagellate *Gambierdiscus toxicus*, which produces ciguatoxin. The toxin is heat resistant and accumulates in large predatory fish such as grouper, snapper, amberjack, and barracuda. Ciguatoxin acts on sodium channels resulting in membrane depolarization. Nausea, vomiting, and diarrhea occur 1 to 24 hours after ingestion, followed by hypesthesias, paresthesias, numbness, malaise, generalized weakness, and sensitivity to temperature extremes. The latter is often described as a reversal of heat and cold sensation. Bradycardia and hypotension are also described.[27] The GI symptoms typically resolve over a few days, whereas the neurologic symptoms may persist in a waxing and waning pattern for 3 months to years.[28] Acute treatment is supportive. Mannitol has been used to treat severe cases, but the evidence is conflicting.[29,30]

Chronic Sequelae of Foodborne Illness About 2% to 3% of patients with foodborne diseases have chronic sequelae thought to be related to autoimmunity.[31,32] Protein virulence factors (superantigens) present in a number of foodborne pathogens can initiate extreme immune responses. *Salmonella, Shigella,* and *Campylobacter* have been associated with a seronegative reactive arthritis in about 2% of those infected.[33] *Campylobacter* infection is associated with Guillain-Barré syndrome with a reported rate as high as 30.4 per 100,000 cases.[32] Symptoms of Guillain-Barré syndrome typically occur 7 to 21 days after the GI symptoms resolve.[31,32] Other autoimmune disorders thought to be associated with superantigens from foodborne pathogens include multiple sclerosis, rheumatoid arthritis, psoriasis, and Graves' disease.[32] Infections with *Salmonella, Yersenia,* and *Campylobacter* may increase short- and long-term risk of death even after accounting for comorbid diseases.[33]

Prevention and Surveillance The Centers for Disease Control and Prevention tracks foodborne infections in the United States through **FoodNet**. The U.S. Food and Drug Administration and U.S. Department of Agriculture provide the Centers for Disease Control and Prevention

TABLE 159-3 Clinical Features, Diagnosis, and Management of Bacterial Foodborne Illness

Etiology	Signs and Symptoms	Duration of Illness	Associated Foods	Laboratory Testing	Treatment
Bacillus anthracis	Nausea, vomiting, bloody diarrhea, abdominal pain, malaise	Weeks	Poorly cooked meat	Blood	Ciprofloxacin or doxycycline IV + PCN, vancomycin, rifampin, or clindamycin
Bacillus cereus (preformed toxin)	Sudden onset of nausea, vomiting; can have diarrhea	24 h	—	Clinical diagnosis; assay must be ordered specifically	Supportive care
B. cereus (diarrheal toxin)	Watery diarrhea, cramping, nausea	1–2 d	Meats, gravies, stew, vanilla sauces	Not necessary	Supportive care
Brucella	Fever, chills, myalgias, arthralgias, weakness, bloody diarrhea	Weeks	Raw milk, unpasteurized goat's milk or cheese, contaminated meat	Serology, blood culture	Doxycycline 100 milligrams PO twice daily + streptomycin 1 gram IM for 14–21 d
Campylobacter	Diarrhea, cramping, nausea, vomiting, fever, often bloody diarrhea	2–10 d	Contact with raw poultry, undercooked poultry, unpasteurized milk, contaminated water	Routine stool culture; requires special media and temperature	Ciprofloxacin 750 milligrams PO twice daily or levofloxacin 500 milligrams PO daily or azithromycin 500 milligrams daily for 3–5 d
Clostridium botulinum (preformed toxin)	Vomiting, diarrhea, blurred vision, diplopia, dysphagia, descending muscle weakness, paralysis	Days to months	Canned foods, canned fish, foods kept warm in dishes, herbed oils, cheese sauce	Stool, serum, or food assay for toxin; stool culture	Supportive care (may require intubation), botulism antitoxin
C. botulinum—infants	Infants <12 mo, lethargy, weakness; poor feeding, head control, and suck	Variable	Honey, home canned vegetables, corn syrup	Stool, serum, or food for toxin; stool culture	Botulism immunoglobulin; antitoxin not recommended in infants
Clostridium perfringens	Watery diarrhea, nausea, cramping	1–2 d	Meat, poultry, dried or precooked foods, poor temperature control	Stools for enterotoxin, stool culture	Supportive care
Enterohemorrhagic *Escherichia coli* and Shiga toxin–producing *E. coli*, 0157:H7	Severe, often bloody diarrhea; abdominal pain; vomiting; little or no fever	5–10 d	Undercooked beef (hamburger), unpasteurized milk, juices, raw fruits and vegetables	Stool culture; may require special media; toxin assay	Supportive; avoid antibiotics due to risk of hemolytic-uremic syndrome
Enterotoxigenic *E. coli*	Watery diarrhea, cramping, vomiting	3–7 d	Water or food contaminated with human feces	Stool culture (specific testing)	Supportive; ciprofloxacin 500 milligrams PO twice per day or levofloxacin 500 milligrams PO once daily for 3 d
Listeria monocytogenes	Fever, myalgias, nausea, diarrhea; premature delivery if pregnant; meningitis	Variable	Fresh soft cheeses, poorly pasteurized dairy products, deli meats, hot dogs	Blood or CSF fluid culture; listeriolysin O antibody assay	Supportive care; ampicillin or penicillin G; TMP-SMX for PCN allergic
Salmonella	Diarrhea, vomiting, abdominal pain, fever, myalgia	4–7 d	Eggs, poultry, unpasteurized dairy products, raw fruits and vegetables, street-vended food	Routine stool culture	Supportive care; ciprofloxacin 500 milligrams PO twice daily or levofloxacin 500 milligrams once daily for 3–5 d; ceftriaxone IV for severe disease or immunocompromised; vaccine for *S. typhi*
Shigella	Abdominal cramping, fever, diarrhea with blood and mucus	4–7 d	Fecal contamination of any food or water, person to person, prepared food	Routine culture	Supportive care; ciprofloxacin 500 milligrams PO twice per day or levofloxacin 500 milligrams once per day for 3–5 d or azithromycin 500 milligrams PO daily for 3 d
Staphylococcus aureus (preformed toxin)	Sudden-onset severe nausea, vomiting, diarrhea, fever	1–2 d	Improperly refrigerated meats, potato or egg salad; left out pastries	Clinical diagnosis; assay for toxin; culture if indicated	Supportive care only
Vibrio cholerae	Profuse watery diarrhea and vomiting; life-threatening dehydration	3–7 d	Contaminated water, fish, shellfish, street-vended foods	Specifically ordered stool culture	Aggressive PO or IV fluid replacement, azithromycin 1 gram PO once or doxycycline 300 milligrams once or ciprofloxacin 1 gram PO once

(*Continued*)

TABLE 159-3 Clinical Features, Diagnosis, and Management of Bacterial Foodborne Illness (*Continued*)

Etiology	Signs and Symptoms	Duration of Illness	Associated Foods	Laboratory Testing	Treatment
Vibrio parahaemolyticus	Watery diarrhea, cramping, vomiting	2–5 d	Undercooked or raw fish or shellfish	Stool culture (special media required)	Supportive care; antibiotics in severe illness: ciprofloxacin 500 milligrams PO twice daily or TMP-SMX-DS PO twice daily or doxycycline 100 milligrams PO twice daily for 3 d
Vibrio vulnificus	Vomiting, abdominal pain, diarrhea, skin infections; can be fatal in liver disease or immunocompromised patients	2–8 d	Undercooked or raw fish or shellfish	Specifically ordered stool, blood, or wound cultures	See Table 159-8
Yersinia	Pseudoappendicitis, fever, abdominal pain, vomiting, diarrhea, rash	1–3 wk	Undercooked pork products, tofu, contaminated water	Stool, blood, or vomitus cultures (special media)	Supportive care; antibiotics usually not required; if septic: gentamicin 5 milligrams/kg IV daily + ceftriaxone 2 grams IV daily

Abbreviations: CSF = cerebrospinal fluid; DS = double strength; PCN = penicillin; TMP-SMX = trimethoprim-sulfamethoxazole.

TABLE 159-4 Clinical Features, Diagnosis, and Management of Viral Foodborne Illness

Etiology	Signs and Symptoms	Duration of Illness	Associated Foods	Laboratory Testing	Treatment
Hepatitis A	Diarrhea, jaundice, dark urine, flu-like illness, abdominal pain	2 wk to 3 mo	Shellfish, raw produce, contaminated water, infected contacts	Liver profile, bilirubin, positive immunoglobulin, and antihepatitis A antibodies	Supportive care; prevention with immunization
Norovirus, Rotavirus, and other enterovirus	Nausea, vomiting, abdominal cramping, diarrhea; sometimes fever, malaise, headache	12 h to 9 d	Fecally contaminated foods; foods touched by infected workers (salads, sandwiches, produce); shellfish	Clinical diagnosis; reverse transcriptase polymerase chain reaction and electron microscopy on stool for *Norovirus* are available but rarely used; stool immunoassay, serology, or enzyme-linked immunosorbent assay kits	Supportive care, good hygiene, adequate fluid replacement

TABLE 159-5 Clinical Features, Diagnosis, and Management of Parasitic Foodborne Illness

Etiology	Signs and Symptoms	Duration of Illness	Associated Foods	Laboratory Testing	Treatment
Cryptosporidium	Watery diarrhea, cramping, fever	Weeks to months—may be relapsing	Any contaminated uncooked food, water	Specific stool examination	Supportive care and HAART in HIV infected; consider nitazoxanide 500 milligrams PO twice daily for 3 d + azithromycin in patient with HIV and severe symptoms
Cyclospora	Watery diarrhea, weight loss, cramping, vomiting, fatigue	Weeks to months, relapsing	Various types of fresh produce	Specific stool examination	TMP-SMX-DS PO twice per day or ciprofloxacin 500 milligrams twice daily for 7–10 d; nitazoxanide 500 milligrams PO twice daily for 7 d In HIV patients: TMP-SMX-DS PO four times a day for 21 d
Entamoeba histolytica	Bloody diarrhea, frequent stools, lower abdominal pain	Weeks to months	Any contaminated uncooked food, water	Examination of stool for cysts and parasites; serology	Metronidazole 750 milligrams PO three times daily for 5–10 d or paromomycin 500 milligrams PO three times daily for 7 d or tinidazole 2 grams PO for 3 d or nitazoxanide 500 milligrams PO twice daily for 3 d
Giardia	Diarrhea, cramping, copious flatus	Months	Any contaminated uncooked food	Examination of stool for ova and parasites	Metronidazole 250 milligrams PO three times daily for 7–10 d or tinidazole 2 grams PO once or nitazoxanide 500 milligrams PO twice daily for 3 d or paromomycin 500 milligrams PO three times daily for 7 d or albendazole 400 milligrams PO once daily for 5 d

Abbreviations: HAART = highly active antiretroviral therapy; HIV = human immunodeficiency virus; TMP-SMX-DS = trimethoprim-sulfamethoxazole double-strength.

TABLE 159-6 Clinical Features, Diagnosis, and Management of Toxinogenic Foodborne Illness

Etiology	Signs and Symptoms	Duration	Foods	Laboratory Testing	Treatment
Ciguatera toxin	Abdominal pain, vomiting, diarrhea, paresthesias, reversal of hot and cold sensation, weakness, hypotension, bradycardia	Days to months	Large reef fish (barracuda most common)	Clinical diagnosis	Supportive care; high-dose atropine for bradycardia; IV mannitol for severe neurologic symptoms
Tetrodotoxin (puffer fish)	Paresthesias, headache, vomiting, diarrhea, abdominal pain, ascending paralysis, respiratory failure, death	Death in 4–6 h	Puffer fish	Detection of tetrodotoxin in fish	Emergent supportive care; anticholinesterases such as neostigmine and edrophonium
Scombroid (histamine)	Flushing, rash, burning sensation, dizziness, paresthesias	3–6 h	Pelagic fish—tuna, mackerel, swordfish, mahi-mahi	Clinical diagnosis, can assay for histamine in fish	Antihistamines, supportive care
Shellfish toxins	Diarrhea, vomiting, abdominal pain, fever, numbness, dizziness, myalgias, confusion, memory loss, coma	2 h to 3 d	Shellfish, mussels, clams	Detection of toxin in shellfish	Supportive care, self-limited

with data about the origin and distribution of food products, which allows investigators to determine the source of a foodborne outbreak.

The Food Safety Modernization Act was passed into law in 2011 to address the rise in foodborne diseases by preventing, rather than responding to, outbreaks of foodborne illness. The law gives the U.S. Food and Drug Administration broad regulatory authority to oversee how food is harvested and processed.[34]

WATERBORNE ILLNESSES

INTRODUCTION AND EPIDEMIOLOGY

Waterborne illnesses occur from ingestion or contact with contaminated water found in swimming pools, hot tubs, spas, and naturally occurring fresh and salt water during recreational use.[35] Numerous species of bacteria, viruses, and protozoans are introduced into the water by fecal contamination and are capable of causing waterborne infections. However, some species of bacteria are indigenous aquatic organisms such as *Pseudomonas aeruginosa, Vibrio, Aeromonas,* nontuberculous *Mycobacterium*, and *Legionella*. Schistosomiasis is common among children in Africa, Asia, and South America, because they are likely to play in infected water. There is concern about the relationship between pediatric urogenital or intestinal schistosomiasis (often acquired in childhood) and human immunodeficiency virus risk.[36]

There were 81 recreational waterborne disease outbreaks in the United States reported to the Centers for Disease Control and Prevention in 2009–2010, which resulted in at least 1326 cases of disease and 62 hospitalizations.[35] The vast majority of these outbreaks were from treated water sources such as swimming pools and water fountains. Approximately two thirds of the waterborne illnesses were gastroenteritis, and 25% were dermatologic diseases or chemical exposures. The most common pathogen associated with these outbreaks was *Cryptosporidium*, which accounted for half of all cases.[35] The most common noninfectious source of waterborne disease was exposure to pool chemicals.

BACTERIA AND WATERBORNE ILLNESS

Implementation of water disinfection and filtration treatments has significantly reduced waterborne outbreaks from enteric bacteria.[37] Waterborne infections from *Vibrio cholerae* and *Salmonella typhi* are now extremely rare in the developed world, but both remain a major cause of illness in developing nations.[37]

Several enteric bacteria are commonly implicated in waterborne disease outbreaks in the United States. *Campylobacter* is found in virtually all surface waters due to contamination from wild bird feces and is the most common bacteria associated with recreational waterborne disease outbreaks.[35,38] Several outbreaks of human campylobacteriosis have been reported from contaminated drinking water.[39] Shiga toxin–producing *E. coli* can also be transmitted from ingestion or contact with water contaminated by farm animal feces.[40] *Shigella* species, *Salmonella* species, and *Yersinia enterocolitica* are other enteric bacteria that can cause waterborne outbreaks.[36] Most enteric bacteria, including *E. coli* O157:H7 and *Campylobacter*, are susceptible to chlorination.

Although *V. cholerae* is an enteric organism acquired from water with fecal contamination, many *Vibrio* species are endemic in marine and estuarine waters. The cholera epidemic began in Haiti in October 2010 and continues, with over 600,000 cases and nearly 8000 deaths. Environmental reservoirs have been identified in Haiti, with concern that transmission could occur to the Dominican Republic and other parts of the Caribbean.[41] *Vibrio* species can cause diarrheal illnesses or skin infections. *Vibrio vulnificus* is associated with life- and limb-threatening necrotic wound infections. The organism is found predominantly along the Gulf Coast and is acquired by patients with open wounds that are exposed to seawater. The wound infections are associated with a high rate of sepsis and amputation. Cirrhosis and high iron levels are associated with worse outcome.[42]

Found in fresh and marine waters, *Aeromonas* species can cause gastroenteritis and wound infections.[43] The majority of wound infections are simple cellulitis, but necrotizing infections and septic arthritis occur.[44,45] In addition, immunocompromised patients may progress to develop peritonitis, cholangitis, and meningitis.[43]

P. aeruginosa is an opportunistic pathogen found in fresh water. Immunocompromised patients are at risk from waterborne disease due to *Pseudomonas*. In normal hosts, *Pseudomonas* can cause otitis externa, keratitis in contact lens wearers, and folliculitis.[46] Although *Pseudomonas* can contaminate drinking water, it does not appear to cause a diarrheal illness in normal hosts.[47]

Nontuberculous *Mycobacterium* are found in salt and fresh water and can cause illness.[48] *Mycobacterium marinum* is associated with granulomatous skin infections (**Figure 159-1**).[49] *Mycobacterium avium* complex is associated with GI, pulmonary, or disseminated disease in immunocompromised patients, particularly patients with human immunodeficiency virus.[36]

Legionella is a common inhabitant of fresh water, including water that meets the standards for drinking.[36] Infection occurs from inhalation of contaminated aerosols, resulting in one of two syndromes: Legionnaires' disease or Pontiac fever. Pontiac fever is a flulike illness contracted by breathing mist that comes from a water source (such as air conditioning cooling towers, whirlpool spas, and showers) contaminated with the bacteria. For further discussion of Legionnaires' disease, refer to the chapter 65, "Pneumonia and Pulmonary Infiltrates."

PROTOZOA AND WATERBORNE ILLNESS

Giardia lamblia is a common protozoal cause of waterborne disease in the United States that accounts for 20,000 cases of diarrheal disease annually.[36,50] It is frequently found in surface waters from mountain

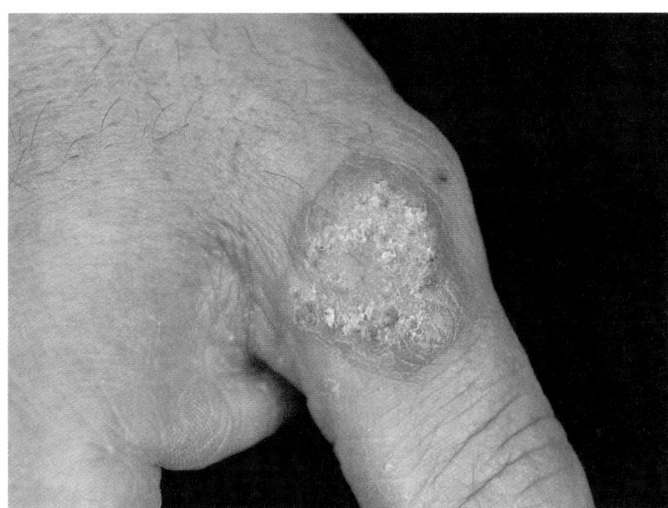

FIGURE 159-1. Skin infection from *Mycobacterium marinum*. A painful indurated plaque is noted on the dorsal surface of the proximal thumb. [Reproduced with permission from Wolff K, Johnson RA: *Color Atlas and Synopsis of Clinical Dermatology*, 5th ed. © 2005, McGraw-Hill, New York.]

streams to municipal reservoirs and is resistant to the levels of chlorination typically used in water treatment. Infected animals such as beavers may contribute to contamination of natural waters, which explains the term "beaver fever" used to describe giardiasis. Backpackers, campers, and travelers to disease-endemic areas are at high risk for waterborne giardiasis, as are children under 5 years of age.[50,51] Community outbreaks often start out as a waterborne disease, but subsequent transmission commonly occurs from person to person. *Giardia* is associated with acute and chronic forms of gastroenteritis, although many patients infected with *Giardia* remain asymptomatic.

Cryptosporidium is an intracellular protozoan parasite that is another common cause of waterborne illness in the United States.[52] The Centers for Disease Control and Prevention estimates that 748,000 cases of cryptosporidiosis occur each year and result in hospital admissions costing $45.8 million.[52] The inoculum required to cause infection is low, and large numbers of oocysts are excreted in the feces of infected hosts.[53] Standard doses of chlorine and zonation used in water treatment are not effective against *Cryptosporidium*, which explains its association with recreational water sources.[52] Water filtration reduces the number of oocysts, but occasionally enough remain to be infective. Infection with *Cryptosporidium* in a normal host results in a self-limited diarrheal illness, and many exposures are asymptomatic. Immunocompromised patients may experience chronic diarrhea or life-threatening complications.[51,53] *Cyclospora, Isospora,* and *Microspora* are other protozoan parasites that can cause severe disease in immunocompromised patients.[54,55]

Entamoeba histolytica is a protozoa that causes intestinal amebiasis. It is a significant waterborne pathogen in developing countries, but in the United States, it is most commonly seen in migrants, travelers to endemic areas, men who have sex with men, and institutionalized patients.[56,57] Symptoms range from asymptomatic infection to severe dysentery.[56] Fulminant colitis with bowel necrosis and perforation occurs in <1% of cases but has a mortality rate of >40%.[58] Seeding of the liver can occur, particularly in men with underlying liver disease, resulting in the formation of amoebic hepatic abscesses.[56,59]

ENTERIC VIRUSES AND WATERBORNE INFECTION

Enteric viruses are an important cause of waterborne disease. More than 100 enteric viruses pathogenic in humans have been reported, many of which can be transmitted via drinking water and recreational water.[60] Several enteric viruses, including the Norwalk virus and rotaviruses, are relatively chlorine resistant. Outbreaks have been associated with contamination of private wells and community water systems.[60]

Hepatitis A and E are associated with epidemic and sporadic infections from contaminated water. Infection from the hepatitis A virus typically results in an acute self-limited hepatitis that rarely develops into fulminant hepatic failure. The incidence of hepatitis A infections has decreased in the United States due to implementation of vaccination in high-risk adults and all children.[61] Hepatitis E is mostly confined to tropical and subtropical regions but is often complicated by cholestasis, and it causes significant morbidity and mortality in pregnant women.[62]

Noroviruses, including the Norwalk virus, are the leading cause of acute gastroenteritis across all age groups.[63] Outbreaks have been linked to contaminated drinking and recreational water, including on cruise ships.[64] Rotavirus and enteric adenoviruses are other important waterborne enteric viruses. Noroviruses, rotaviruses, and enteric adenoviruses typically cause a self-limited gastroenteritis, although dehydration from these infections can be severe in children.[36]

CLINICAL FEATURES

The majority of patients with waterborne disease present with nausea, vomiting, and diarrhea. Think of this cause in symptomatic patients with recent travel, outdoor activities such as camping or backpacking, recent recreational water use, or those using a private drinking water supply rather than municipal drinking water or bottled water. Patients with severe or chronic gastroenteritis symptoms may have immune deficiency such as human immunodeficiency virus or immunosuppressive drugs. In patients with bloody diarrhea, suspect invasive enteric bacteria as the cause.[11] Giardia and other protozoan parasites are suspected in patients with diarrhea lasting 2 or more weeks.[10]

Physical examination should focus on identifying signs of dehydration and any open skin wounds acquired in fresh or marine waters. Waterborne skin infections can range in severity from simple cellulitis to necrotizing fasciitis. Patients with *V. vulnificus* present after recent exposure to salt water and hemorrhagic bullae or signs of necrotizing infection (**Figure 159-2**).[43] Clinical features of waterborne pathogens are summarized in **Table 159-7**.

DIAGNOSIS

Diagnostic testing is usually not needed. Viral antigen tests for rotavirus may be helpful in children with severe or persistent symptoms to distinguish viral from bacterial pathogens. Testing of stool for ova and parasites is indicated in patients with recent travel to endemic countries, immunocompromised status, or diarrheal illness of 2 or more weeks; during community-wide waterborne outbreaks; or in men who have sex with men.[10,13] Because parasite excretion may not be continuous, three specimens separated by at least 24 hours may be needed to identify the causative pathogen.

The diagnosis of waterborne skin infections is based primarily on the patient's physical examination findings and history of water exposure. Identification of the causative agent can be attempted by Gram stain and

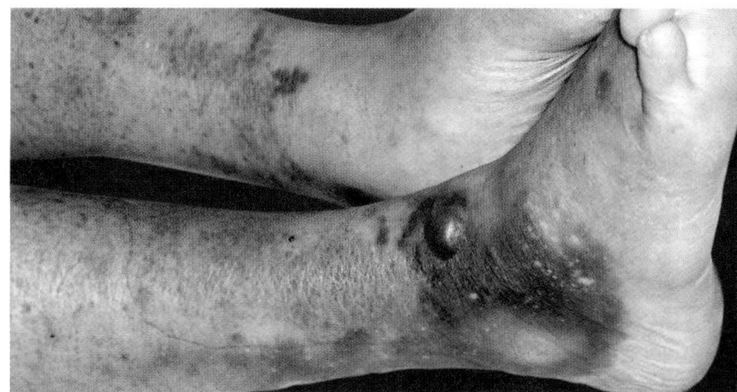

FIGURE 159-2. Skin infection from *Vibrio vulnificus. V. vulnificus* was cultured from the bulla aspirates from this patient with hemorrhagic and bullous skin lesions of the lower legs. [Reproduced with permission from Wolff K, Johnson R: *Fitzpatrick's Color Atlas and Synopsis of Clinical Dermatology*, 6th ed. © 2009 McGraw-Hill, New York.]

TABLE 159-7 Type of Transmission and Clinical Features Associated with Waterborne Pathogens

Pathogen	Drinking Water	Recreational Water	Clinical Features
Campylobacter	+	+	Gastroenteritis; can be associated with Guillain-Barré syndrome
Escherichia coli 0157: H7	+	+	Gastroenteritis; can be associated with hemolytic-uremic syndrome
Salmonella species	+	+	Gastroenteritis, typhoid fever
Shigella species	+	+	Gastroenteritis
Yersinia species	+	+	Gastroenteritis
Vibrio species	+	+	Gastroenteritis; skin infections
Aeromonas species	+	+	Gastroenteritis; skin infections
Pseudomonas	–	+	Skin infections, nosocomial infections
Nontuberculous *Mycobacterium*	+/–	+	Skin infections, disseminated disease in immunocompromised
Giardia	+	+	Acute and chronic gastroenteritis, asymptomatic carriage
Cryptosporidium	+	+	Acute and chronic gastroenteritis, severe among immunocompromised
Entamoeba	+	+	Acute and chronic gastroenteritis, rare fulminant colitis, liver abscess
Hepatitis A	+	+	Acute hepatitis; rare liver failure
Hepatitis E	+	+	Acute hepatitis; fulminant and severe in pregnancy
Enteric viruses	+	+	Gastroenteritis

+, potential source of infection; –, not potential source of infection

wound culture (acid-fast staining if *M. marinum* is suspected). Blood cultures are best reserved for systemically ill patients.

TREATMENT

In most cases of acute gastroenteritis from waterborne pathogens, treatment is limited to rehydration. Empiric antibiotic therapy is used for patients with moderate to severe disease, recent travel history, or symptoms lasting more than 1 week; those needing hospitalization; and immunocompromised hosts.[10] **Avoid antibiotics in cases of suspected *E. coli* O157:H7 due to an increased risk of development of hemolytic-uremic syndrome.** Appropriate antibiotics include 3 to 5 days of oral ciprofloxacin 500 milligrams twice daily, levofloxacin 500 milligrams once daily, or double-strength trimethoprim-sulfamethoxazole twice daily.[10] Azithromycin 500 milligrams orally once daily for 3 to 5 days is recommended for pregnant women, children, and patients with travel to areas with fluoroquinolone-resistant *Campylobacter* (Thailand).[10]

Antimotility agents can be given to patients or children >3 years old without signs of invasive bacterial infection (bloody stools or fever).[21,22] Probiotics, such as lactobacilli, may shorten the duration of diarrheal illnesses in adults and children.[65]

Infections from *Giardia* and *Entamoeba* are typically treated with metronidazole (Table 159-5). Paromomycin is an alternative to metronidazole in pregnant women.[66] Other alternatives for *Giardia* and *Entamoeba* treatment include tinidazole and nitazoxanide.[66] Albendazole is also effective for giardiasis, but not amebiasis. Infections from *Cryptosporidium* are generally self-limited and usually do not require specific treatment in immunocompetent patients. However, antimicrobial treatment with nitazoxanide or paromomycin is used in patients with prolonged infections, children, and the immunocompromised.[67] For immunocompromised patients with *Cryptosporidium*, nitazoxanide or paromomycin alone or in combination with azithromycin is used. Initiation of highly active antiretroviral therapy is the first priority for *Cryptosporidium* treatment in patients with human immunodeficiency virus.[68]

Treatment of waterborne skin infections includes empiric antibiotic administration (**Table 159-8**) and tetanus vaccination if needed. Consensus is that initial empiric antibiotic therapy should be broad spectrum, including clindamycin in combination with a fourth-generation cephalosporin, an extended-spectrum fluoroquinolone (i.e., moxifloxacin), or an antipseudomonal penicillin (i.e., piperacillin-tazobactam).[69,70] If *V. vulnificus* is suspected, treat with doxycycline and a fourth-generation cephalosporin.[42] Clarithromycin or doxycycline is indicated for most *M. marinum* infections, but severe cases require added rifampin or ethambutol.[49] Patients with evidence of necrotizing infections need immediate surgical consultation for operative debridement.[69]

DISPOSITION AND FOLLOW-UP

Most episodes of acute gastroenteritis secondary to waterborne pathogens are benign and self-limited. Patients with systemic symptoms, severe dehydration, significant comorbidities, or inability to tolerate oral fluids should be considered for admission. Patients with waterborne skin infections should be admitted for systemic illness, suspected necrotizing infections, or comorbidities such as immunocompromised states.

TABLE 159-8 Treatment of Waterborne Skin Infections

Pathogen	Clinical Features of Skin Infection	Treatment
Vibrio vulnificus	Cellulitis with hemorrhagic bullae, septicemia	Doxycycline 100 milligrams IV twice per day plus fourth-generation cephalosporin; necrotizing infections require emergent surgical debridement
Aeromonas species	Cellulitis, necrotizing wound infections	Mild infections: ciprofloxacin 500 milligrams PO twice per day; severe infections: ciprofloxacin 400 milligrams IV twice per day plus an IV antipseudomonal penicillin or fourth-generation cephalosporin; necrotizing infections require emergent surgical debridement
Pseudomonas aeruginosa	Hot-tub folliculitis, cellulitis in immunocompromised/diabetics	Hot-tub folliculitis is usually self-limited. Severe infection: ciprofloxacin 400 milligrams IV twice per day plus an IV antipseudomonal penicillin or fourth-generation cephalosporin
Mycobacterium marinum	Granulomatous skin infections	Clarithromycin 500 milligrams PO twice per day or doxycycline 100 milligrams PO twice per day for 3 mo; severe cases: combine with rifampin or ethambutol

PREVENTION AND SURVEILLANCE

The U.S. Safe Water Drinking Act of 1974 authorizes the Environmental Protection Agency to set national standards for U.S. public drinking water systems. The agency has set standards for 90 chemical, microbiologic, radiologic, and physical contaminants.[71] These include coliform counts, the presence of human enteric viruses, *Cryptosporidium*, and *Giardia*.

All public drinking water is required to be disinfected, which typically involves treatment with chlorine and ozone.[71] Enteric bacteria such as *E. coli* and *Campylobacter* are susceptible to these disinfection measures. However, pathogens such as protozoans and some enteric viruses are less susceptible to chlorine, and despite filtration, these pathogens may be present in sufficient quantities to cause disease.

Several recently developed vaccines are available to prevent waterborne infection from hepatitis A virus. An aggressive vaccination campaign in high-risk adults and all children has resulted in a decline in cases in the United States.[61]

REFERENCES

The complete reference list is available online at www.TintinalliEM.com.

CHAPTER 160 Zoonotic Infections

Bryan B. Kitch
John T. Meredith

INTRODUCTION

The World Health Organization defines zoonotic infections as those diseases and infections that are naturally transmitted from vertebrate animals to or from humans. Zoonotic infections are often encountered in emergency care. Ticks are one of the most important vectors of human infectious diseases in the world.

A zoonotic infection has presenting symptoms similar to many acute infections: fever, headache, myalgias, malaise, and weakness. Given this, a specific diagnosis is often difficult. Particular exposures or occupations that involve animal contact carry an increased risk of disease (**Table 160-1**). Recent travel, particularly in spring, summer, and early fall, or history of habitation in an underdeveloped country, are also risk factors. Zoonoses can occur at any time of the year, but in temperate climates, most zoonoses happen in the spring and summer.

Zoonoses that can present as an undifferentiated febrile illness are listed in **Table 160-2**.

TABLE 160-1 Risk Factors for Zoonotic Infection

Risk Category	Examples
Agricultural workers	Farmers, cattle ranchers, sheep ranchers, and migrant workers
Animal processing workers	Slaughterhouse workers, animal hide processors, and workers in manufacturing who deal with animal products
Outdoor enthusiasts	Forestry workers, lumbermen, surveyors, park rangers, hunters, spelunkers, and fishermen
Pet owners	Those living alongside a dog, cat, bird, rodent, rabbit, reptile, or fish
Professionals	Veterinarians, animal researchers, and animal handlers
Immunocompromised patients	Those with congenital immunodeficiencies, diabetes mellitus, alcoholism, renal failure, liver failure, cancer, splenectomy, or human immunodeficiency virus

TICKBORNE ZOONOTIC INFECTIONS

Ticks parasitize vertebrates in virtually every part of the world. Saliva of some tick species contains an anesthetic, as well as several inflammatory factors, and some species contain a toxin that paralyzes the host. Ticks feed for several days on the host, and their presence often goes unnoticed for a time, and many affected patients do not recall a history of a tick bite.[1] Tickborne diseases are often accompanied by a rash. Tickborne zoonoses have a geographic distribution (**Table 160-3**) and seasonal variation.

TICK REMOVAL, PROPHYLACTIC TREATMENT, AND PREVENTION OF TICK BITES

The most effective way to remove an embedded tick is manual extraction with tweezers or blunt angled forceps to grasp the tick as close to the skin surface as possible. Avoid puncturing or grasping the body of the tick, because this can lead to rupture of the tick and release of an infectious pathogen. Pull perpendicular to the skin with gentle traction, avoiding twisting or breaking the tick. Remove all portions of the tick because residual body parts can stimulate a granulomatous reaction and persistent infection. After complete removal of the tick, cleanse and disinfect the skin surface. Do not handle the extracted tick with bare hands. Do not use topical or injected lidocaine or pass sutures through the tick, and avoid the use of gasoline, kerosene, petroleum jelly, or fingernail polish, which all can increase infection or impair complete tick removal. Commercially available tick removal devices exist, with certain models having improved outcomes over the use of tweezers.[2] Save the removed tick in alcohol to aid in identification, especially if illness occurs.

Prophylactic treatment of a tick bite can be given only in select, not all, circumstances.[3] Recommended settings for prophylactic treatment include the ability to easily identify the tick as *Ixodes scapularis*, tick attachment for greater than 36 hours or with obvious tick engorgement, and a local tick bite in an area with *Borrelia burgdorferi* carrier rate of greater than 20%.[4] In these cases, use a *one-time dose* of doxycycline 200 milligrams for adults or 4 milligrams/kg in children for Lyme prophylaxis.

The best method to avoid tick bites is the application of topical DEET (N,N-diethyl-m-toluamide) to exposed skin and treatment of clothing with permethrin. Optimal DEET concentration is 15% to 33%, with less effectiveness if the DEET concentration is >35%. Apply to skin according to label directions.

ROCKY MOUNTAIN SPOTTED FEVER

The human disease-causing rickettsioses—the spotted fevers—include a number of different species identified in the Americas, Europe, Southwest Asia, Africa, Siberia, western Russia, and Australia. Disease names are based on species and geography: Mediterranean spotted fever, Israel spotted fever, Astrakhan fever, Siberian tick typhus, Queensland tick typhus, African tick bite fever, and so on.

Rocky Mountain spotted fever (RMSF) is one of the most severe of the tickborne illnesses in the United States, with peak occurrence occurring in June and July. The fatality rate for RMSF is currently less than 0.5%. Geographically, although reported widely and in both rural and urban settings any time of the year, more than 60% of reported cases originate from five states: North Carolina, Tennessee, Oklahoma, Missouri, and Arkansas.[5] The causative organism of RMSF is *Rickettsia rickettsii*, a pleomorphic, obligate intracellular organism, and the vectors in the United States are the very small *Dermacentor* (*D. variabilis* and *D. andersoni*, the American dog tick) and *Rhipicephalus sanguineus* ticks (the brown dog tick, found in the American southwest). Deer, rodents, horses, cattle, cats, and dogs are zoonotic hosts, with higher incidence in communities with free-roaming dog presence.[5] *Rickettsia parkeri* and

TABLE 160-2 Common Systemic Zoonotic Infections

Agent	Animal Reservoir	Physical Findings	Diagnostic Tests	Treatment
Aeromonas species	Fish, reptiles	Nonspecific fever, severe crepitant cellulitis with systemic toxicity, gastroenteritis	—	See chapter 159, "Food and Waterborne Illnesses"
Brucella canis	Dogs	Nonspecific fever	Serologic testing, blood culture	Doxycycline plus gentamicin or rifampin. TMP-SMX plus gentamicin in children
Capnocytophaga	Dogs and cats	Fever, septic shock, and meningitis from infected bite	Culture of bite wound	Amoxicillin-clavulanate or clindamycin. Pip-Tazo or a carbapenem plus clindamycin/vancomycin for shock
Chlamydophila psittaci	Birds	Fever, flulike illness, pneumonia, endocarditis, sepsis	Serologic testing and sputum culture	Doxycycline. Azithromycin and levofloxacin are alternatives
Coxiella burnetii	Cattle, sheep, goats. Occasionally cats	Fever, pneumonia, hepatitis, meningitis, endocarditis	Serologic testing, PCR	Doxycycline, with the possible alternative of a fluoroquinolone or macrolide
Ehrlichia species	Ticks	Nonspecific fever, sepsis, meningitis, hepatitis	Clinical diagnosis, serologic testing, peripheral blood smear, immunocytologic testing, PCR	Doxycycline recommended for all patients (even children and pregnancy). Rifampin is alternative.
Leptospira species	Birds, dogs, rodents	Fever, pneumonia, conjunctivitis, lymphadenopathy	Darkfield microscopic examination of body fluids, serologic testing	Penicillin G IV. Ceftriaxone IV alternative. Mild disease: oral doxycycline or amoxicillin or azithromycin
Francisella tularensis	Rabbits, cats, wild animals, biting insects	Fever, sepsis, meningitis, pneumonia, hepatitis, rash	Serologic testing (poses hazards to laboratory staff)	IV aminoglycosides. Alternative: Doxycycline or ciprofloxacin
Rickettsia rickettsii	Ticks	Fever, diarrhea, or typical presentation of Rocky Mountain spotted fever	Clinical diagnosis, rise in antibody titer between acute and convalescent serum, skin biopsy	Doxycycline or chloramphenicol
Salmonella enterica	Dogs, cats (rarely), reptiles (turtles)	Fever, abdominal pain, sepsis, cellulitis, meningitis, endocarditis, septic arthritis	Blood or stool culture	Fluoroquinolones or third-generation cephalosporins
Streptococcus iniae cellulitis	Fish, seafood	Fever, cellulitis	Wound culture, blood culture	β-Lactams except aztreonam. Alternatives: azithromycin, clindamycin, fluoroquinolones
Yersinia pestis	Dogs, cats, rodents	Bubonic: fever, headache, buboes, or pneumonic: cough, chills, dyspnea, shock	Blood culture, culture of suspected sites	Doxycycline, fluoroquinolone, gentamicin, streptomycin, or chloramphenicol

Abbreviations: PCR = polymerase chain reaction; Pip-Tazo = piperacillin-tazobactam; TMP-SMX = trimethoprim-sulfamethoxazole.

other members of the family are implicated in causing cases of possible RMSF and may be responsible for an increase in incidence as more cases are reported.

Clinical Features The diagnosis relies on epidemiologic features and the clinical exclusion of other diseases. Early signs and symptoms of RMSF are fever, headache, myalgia, and malaise. Additionally, other nonspecific findings include lymphadenopathy, abdominal pain, nausea, vomiting, diarrhea, and headache. Late in the disease course, confusion, meningismus, renal failure, respiratory failure, and myocarditis may occur. The classic clinical picture is the triad of fever, rash, and tick bite, but only about half of the patients can recall a tick bite.

The rash occurs on days 2 to 4 after the onset of fever but is absent in about 20% of patients. Most patients do not have a petechial rash when they seek initial medical care.[1] The rash occurs earlier in children than in adults and begins as small blanching erythematous to pink macules and becomes petechial later. This characteristic maculopapular rash begins on the hands, feet, wrists, and ankles, and then spreads centripetally up the trunk (see chapter 249, "Generalized Skin Disorders"). The *rash is not pathognomonic* and may occur in other illnesses. Additionally, the rash is easily overlooked early in infection and in those with dark skin. Another feature to recognize is the possibility of a nonexudative conjunctival injection with bilateral periorbital edema, resembling that found in toxic shock syndrome or Kawasaki's disease. Abdominal distention and organomegaly may exist on physical exam.[6]

Diagnosis and Treatment Immunoglobulin G– or immunoglobulin M–specific antibodies are not detectable in acute-phase serum. Laboratory abnormalities are usually nonspecific, but the **combination of normal white and red cell counts, thrombocytopenia, mild elevation of liver enzymes (aspartate aminotransferase and alanine aminotransferase), and hyponatremia suggests RMSF**, especially if the disease is advanced. Hypoalbuminemia may be present and is the cause of edema.[6] In addition to clinical patterns, diagnosis can be confirmed with a rise in antibody titer between acute and convalescent serum, skin biopsy with immunofluorescent testing, or culture, although none of these are useful for ED diagnosis.

Preferred treatment is doxycycline (**Table 160-4**). Given the relatively long half-life of doxycycline (18 to 21 hours), several days of a higher dose regimen may be required to achieve rapid therapeutic response in the critically ill patient. The risk of cosmetically perceptible tooth staining is small for a single course of treatment. **Doxycycline therapy is recommended by the American Academy of Pediatrics and by the Centers for Disease Control and Prevention as the treatment of choice for all rickettsial diseases, including RMSF, in children of all ages.**[1]

TICK PARALYSIS

Many tick species secrete neurotoxic substances from salivary glands of attached ticks. Tick paralysis occurs worldwide, in Australia, Africa, Europe, and North America, and is more common in children than adults. Prolonged tick attachment (5 to 7 days) can result in host paralysis. Symptoms are ascending weakness, beginning in the lower extremities, and moving upward to the trunk, upper extremities, and

TABLE 160-3 Tickborne Zoonotic Infections

Disease	Primary Vector	Animal Reservoir	Clinical Features	Geographic Distribution
Babesiosis	*Ixodes dammini, I. scapularis,* and *I. pacificus*	Cattle, horses, dogs, cats, rodents, deer	Fatigue, malaise, anorexia, nausea, headache, sweats, rigors, abdominal pain, emotional lability, depression, dark urine, hepatomegaly, fever, petechiae, ecchymosis, occasional rash, and occasionally, pulmonary edema	Northeast and north-central United States
Colorado tick fever	*Dermacentor andersoni* (wood tick)	Deer, marmots, porcupines	Fever, chills, headache, myalgias, nausea, vomiting, photophobia, abdominal pain, and occasional sore throat; also may have conjunctivitis, lymphadenopathy, hepatosplenomegaly, stiff neck, retro-orbital pain, weakness, and lethargy	Western and northwestern United States and southwestern Canada
Anaplasmosis	*I. scapularis, I. pacificus*	Dogs, deer, other mammals	Fevers, chills, malaise, headache, nausea, muscle aches, cough, sore throat, and pulmonary infiltrates (especially in children)	Japan, Malaysia, and the eastern, northeastern, and north-central United States
Ehrlichiosis	*Amblyomma americanum* (lone star tick)	Dogs, deer, other mammals	Fevers, chills, malaise, headache, nausea, muscle aches, cough, sore throat, and pulmonary infiltrates (especially in children)	Japan, Malaysia, Europe, and southeastern and south-central United States
Lyme disease (*Borrelia burgdorferi*)	*I. dammini*	Deer, sheep, deer mice	Erythema migrans, meningitis, encephalitis, neuropathy, and joint and heart symptoms	Atlantic central and north-central United States, Europe
Rocky Mountain spotted fever (*Rickettsia rickettsii*)	*D. andersoni* and *D. variabilis* (dog tick)	North American mammals	Petechiae, purpura, pulmonary infiltrates, jaundice, myocarditis, hepatosplenomegaly, meningitis, encephalitis, and lymphadenopathy	Most of the continental United States, although more prevalent in the southeast and south-central United States
Relapsing fever (*Borrelia* species)	*Ornithodoros* species	Human body lice, wild rodents, humans	Fever, chills, headache, myalgias, and arthralgias; pain, nausea, vomiting, and hypotension	Worldwide
Tularemia (*Francisella tularensis*)	*Dermacentor* spp. and *Amblyomma* spp.	Rabbits, deer, dogs	Pneumonia, regional lymphadenopathy and headache, cough, myalgias, arthralgias, nausea, vomiting, ulceration at inoculation site, and ocular findings	Northern hemisphere, North America, northern Asia, Europe

TABLE 160-4 Tickborne Zoonotic Infections and Specific Treatment

Tickborne Zoonotic Infection	Specific Treatment
Rocky Mountain spotted fever	Doxycycline 100 milligrams PO or IV twice a day for 7 d, or for 2 d after temperature normalizes. Some recommendations exist for an initial loading dose of 200 milligrams. For children weighing <45 kg, the dose is 2.2 milligrams/kg twice daily. Although doxycycline is contraindicated for use in pregnancy, it may be warranted in life-threatening situations. Chloramphenicol is an alternative; however, it has multiple toxic effects and contraindications, and may be difficult to obtain. Dosing is 50 milligrams/kg/d divided into 4 doses for 7 d.
Lyme disease	Primary stage or mild secondary: 14–21 d of doxycycline (100 milligrams PO twice a day), amoxicillin (500 milligrams PO 3 times a day in adults, 50 milligrams/kg/d divided 3 times a day in children), or cefuroxime (500 milligrams PO twice a day in adults, 30 milligrams/kg/d divided 3 times a day in children). Macrolides possible but less effective. Severe illness, CNS positive, or high-degree heart block: ceftriaxone 2 grams IV for 14–30 d. A single 200-milligram oral dose of doxycycline given within 72 h of a high-risk deer tick bite is effective in preventing Lyme disease.
Tickborne relapsing fever	Doxycycline (100 milligrams PO/IV twice a day for 7–10 d). Alternative: erythromycin (500 milligrams PO/IV 4 times a day for 7–10 d). Chloramphenicol is an alternate.
Colorado tick fever	Treatment is supportive.
Tularemia	Adults: streptomycin, 1 gram IM/IV twice a day, or gentamicin/tobramycin, 5 milligrams/kg IV divided every 8 h. Treat for 10 d. Children: streptomycin, 15 milligrams/kg IM twice daily (should not exceed 2 grams/d). Mild disease: ciprofloxacin 750 milligrams PO twice a day or doxycycline 100 milligrams PO twice a day. Treat for 21 d. Prophylaxis for lab exposures: doxycycline 100 milligrams PO twice a day or ciprofloxacin 500 milligrams PO twice a day. Treat for 14 d.
Babesiosis	Atovaquone (750 milligrams PO every 12 h) plus azithromycin (500 milligrams PO on day 1, then 250–1000 milligrams daily). Treat for 10 d. If relapse occurs, treat for the longer duration: 6 weeks or 2 weeks after negative blood smear. Severe disease in adults: clindamycin (1200 milligrams IV twice a day or 600 milligrams PO 3 times a day) + quinine (650 milligrams PO 3 times a day). Treat for 7–10 d.
Ehrlichiosis and anaplasmosis	Doxycycline, 100 milligrams PO twice a day for 7–14 d. For children weighing <45 kg, the dose is 2.2 milligrams/kg twice a day.

head over hours to days. Cerebrospinal fluid analysis is normal. Diagnosis is made upon finding a tick on the body. Tick removal leads to recovery in 24 hours.

LYME DISEASE

Lyme disease was probably first noted in Europe about 100 years ago, based on descriptions of the rash, erythema chronicum migrans. Lyme disease is the most common vectorborne zoonotic infection in the United States, with approximately 30,000 cases reported annually. Based on public health data and insurance information, the actual number of patients diagnosed with Lyme disease may be closer to 300,000 per year.[7] Lyme disease is reported in Europe, China, Japan, Australia, parts of Russia, and in all U.S. continental states, with 95% of the reported cases originating from just 13 states clustered in the northeast and upper midwest. Peak transmission occurs in May through August. The responsible organism is *B. burgdorferi*, a spirochete, and the vector is the *Ixodes* deer tick, also known as *black-legged tick*. The overall risk of Lyme disease after a deer tick bite is low, about 3% in endemic areas. However, the risk of infection is proportional to the length of time the tick feeds on the host, with minimal to no risk associated with tick attachment duration less than 36 hours.[4,8]

Clinical Features Lyme disease has three stages. The **first stage** is local and often characterized by **erythema migrans**: an erythematous plaque with central clearing. Erythema migrans develops in approximately 60% to 80% of cases.[1] It develops within 2 to 30 days at the site of the tick bite and is a result of a vasculitis. There may also be nonspecific symptoms of fever, chills, fatigue, myalgias, arthralgias, and lymphadenopathy. The rash may persist for up to 1 month and recur in the secondary stage of Lyme disease. Untreated erythema migrans resolves spontaneously in 3 to 4 weeks. This rash causes few symptoms and, depending on skin location, may go unnoticed by the patient.

The **second stage**, early disseminated disease, develops with the reproduction and spread of the *Borrelia* spirochete and occurs within a few days to months of the initial infection. This stage is characterized by fever, adenopathy, neuropathies, cardiac abnormalities, arthritic complaints, and skin lesions. Multiple annular/target-shaped skin findings occur in up to 50% of the patients infected and are the most characteristic component of the secondary stage of illness.

The most common neurologic symptom in the secondary stage of illness is the development of cranial neuritis, most often **unilateral or bilateral facial nerve palsy**. Facial palsy can also occur along with the initial rash of erythema migrans. Neuroborreliosis occurs in 15% of the untreated cases and can consist of periodic headache, neck stiffness, difficulty in mentation, cerebellar ataxia, myelitis, encephalitis, motor or sensory radiculoneuritis, mononeuritis multiplex, and facial palsy.[9] Asymmetric oligoarticular arthritis of the large joints, with a particular predilection for the knees, is another complication. Brief attacks of asymmetric oligoarticular arthritis are common in the untreated patient in the secondary stage of illness. Attacks are characteristically separated by months of remission. Cardiac abnormalities occur in up to 8% of patients and present as varying degrees of atrioventricular block, sometimes requiring the insertion of a temporary pacemaker for stabilization. Additionally, myopericarditis may also be a manifestation on initial presentation.

The **late disseminated stage** of illness occurs months to years after the initial infection and is characterized by chronic arthritis, myocarditis, subacute encephalopathy, axonal polyneuropathy, and leukoencephalopathy.[9] The advanced, chronic neurologic forms of Lyme disease can persist for over 10 years. Additionally, between 10% and 20% of patients treated with antibiotics can have persistent symptoms of disease, usually muscle and joint aches with fatigue. This entity is currently being studied but seems to be an autoimmune response persistent from the initial infection.

Diagnosis and Treatment Diagnosis is clinical early in disease when erythema migrans is present; testing is required to diagnose later stages of Lyme disease.[8] For the latter, use polymerase chain reaction testing, polyvalent fluorescence immunoassay, or Western immunoblot testing,[9] because *B. burgdorferi* is difficult to culture.

Treatment of Lyme disease is with doxycycline (preferred agent) or amoxicillin. Neurologic symptoms or persistent other manifestations require ceftriaxone therapy (Table 160-4). A previously marketed vaccine no longer exists, because it conferred no ongoing immunity.

EHRLICHIOSIS

Ehrlichiosis is a group of zoonotic diseases caused by the *Ehrlichia* genus, gram-negative pleomorphic coccobacilli that infect circulating leukocytes.[1] Infection due to *Ehrlichia chaffeensis* is also called *human monocytic ehrlichiosis*. The disease vector is the lone star tick, *Amblyomma americanum*. The major animal reservoir in North America is the white-tailed deer in the southeastern United States, with dogs and mice carrying several less common species of the pathogen.[10] Disease incidence has been on the rise, increasing from 0.8 to 3 cases/million in the United States in 2000 to 2007, partly attributed to increased recognition. It has also been described in Europe. The mortality rate in confirmed cases varies between 1% and 3% depending on causative agent.[10]

Symptoms usually develop within 1 to 2 weeks of a tick bite.[11] Clinical signs and symptoms are fever, headache, malaise, nausea, vomiting, diarrhea, abdominal pain, and arthralgias. Fever is present in the vast majority of cases (97%). Rash is present in 30% of adults and has no pathognomonic features, making it a nonspecific diagnostic clue.[12] With disease progression, a minority of patients go on to develop severe complications of renal failure, respiratory failure, and encephalitis. The acute phase of illness lasts less than 4 weeks, with the majority of patients recovering and proceeding on to a convalescent phase.

Laboratory studies can demonstrate leukocytopenia, thrombocytopenia, and elevation of hepatic enzymes. Diagnosis is made clinically but can be confirmed by laboratory testing once treatment has begun. Peripheral blood smear may show colonies of ehrlichiae in the white blood cells in 20% of infected patients. Polymerase chain reaction is specific but not sensitive and is best in the first week of illness. Antibody tests are expected to be negative in 85% of patients during initial infection. The gold standard test is immunofluorescence assay.[11]

Treatment is with doxycycline until 3 to 5 days after fever resolution or 10 to 14 days after resolution of CNS symptoms in severe disease. Rifampin is used in those with contraindications to doxycycline.[12]

ANAPLASMOSIS

Anaplasmosis is a tickborne disease caused by the bacteria *Anaplasma phagocytophilum*.[13] Older terms for the disease are *human granulocytic ehrlichiosis* and *human granulocytic anaplasmosis*. The vector is the black-legged tick, *I. scapularis*, as well as the western black-legged tick, *Ixodes pacificus*. The zoonotic reservoirs are deer, elk, and rodents, and the disease is prevalent in the upper midwestern and northeastern United States in the same areas where Lyme disease is present, with 90% of all reported anaplasmosis cases from only six states. Peak transmission occurs in the summer, specifically June and July. Incidence of reported cases has risen from 1.4 to 6.1 cases per million in the United States from 2000 to 2010. Case mortality rate has remained less than 1%.[14] Symptoms, developing within 1 to 2 weeks of the initial bite, are nonspecific and similar to those of ehrlichiosis or influenza—fever, chills, headache, and myalgias. Rash is rare in anaplasmosis and should clue the clinician to consider an alternative diagnosis.[14] Laboratory findings are nonspecific and should not alter the clinical decision to treat but may consist of leukocytopenia, thrombocytopenia, and elevation of hepatic enzymes. Confirmatory testing modalities are similar to those for ehrlichiosis. Treatment is with doxycycline, as noted in other tick infections (Table 160-4).

TICKBORNE RELAPSING FEVER

Relapsing fever is caused by several varieties of gram-negative *Borrelia* spirochetes. It was first described in West Africa and is now recognized worldwide. Within the United States, it is rarely found east of Texas.[15] *Ornithodoros* ticks (soft ticks that can survive for years between meals) are the vectors, and the principal zoonotic reservoirs are wild rodents, specifically tree squirrels and chipmunks.[16] The classic risk factor is sleeping in rustic mice-infested structures in the wilderness of the western United States. The initial presentation may be that of a rash or a 2- to 3-mm pruritic eschar at the site of a tick bite. An average incubation period of 7 days precedes the onset of fever, chills, cephalgia, myalgia, arthralgia, abdominal pain, and general malaise. Headache and myalgia occur in over 90% of cases.[16] Characteristically, the roughly 3-day-long febrile episodes are interspersed with 7-day-long afebrile periods, which may cycle one to four times before resolution.[16] Untreated, the disease is usually self-limited, with deaths occurring mostly at the extremes of age.

Leukocytosis and thrombocytopenia are the typical laboratory findings. Diagnosis is confirmed with the appearance of spirochetes on darkfield microscopy or Wright-Giemsa–stained peripheral blood smears, with a 70% sensitivity if obtained during a febrile period. Patients with relapsing fever may test false positive on Lyme disease assays due to protein cross-reactivity.[16]

The recommended treatment is with tetracycline or erythromycin. Use IV ceftriaxone for 10 to 14 days if any CNS involvement is seen.[16] Similar to Lyme disease, patients in an endemic area with a confirmed tick bite can receive postexposure doxycycline as effective prophylaxis.[17]

COLORADO TICK FEVER

Colorado tick fever is caused by an RNA virus of the genus *Coltivirus* in the family Reoviridae.[18] The principal vector is the wood tick, *D. andersoni*, and the zoonotic reservoirs are deer, marmots, and porcupines. The disease is endemic to the western mountainous regions of the United States and is limited to elevations between 4000 and 10,000 ft. Transmission to humans can occur with short periods of tick attachment. The incubation period is 3 to 5 days, and the onset of illness is characterized by fever, chills, headache, myalgias, and photophobia. There may be a macular or petechial rash in a minority of patients. The disease is self-limited, and complications are rare, although some patients may experience recurrent fever after 1 to 2 days of improvement. Diagnosis is most often based on history, clinical findings, and geography. Treatment is supportive.[18]

TULAREMIA

Tularemia is caused by a small gram-negative, nonmotile intracellular coccobacillus, *Francisella tularensis*. The disease is found in North America, northern Asia, and Europe. The zoonotic vectors are ticks of the *Dermacentor species* (wood tick, dog tick) and the *Amblyomma* species (lone star tick), as well as various flies. The principal zoonotic reservoirs are rabbits, hares, and deer.[18] Tularemia is contracted through tick/fly bites, by inhalation, or through open wounds while in contact with an infected zoonotic host. Incubation is often between 3 and 6 days but may range from 2 hours to 3 weeks. The clinical presentation depends on the method of inoculation, and the clinical forms are called *ulceroglandular, glandular, typhoidal, pneumonic, oculoglandular,* and *oropharyngeal*. The **ulceroglandular form** is the most common, occurring in 80% of cases,[18] and is characterized by a maculopapular skin lesion that ulcerates, followed by painful regional adenopathy and systemic symptoms. The **glandular form** consists of painful adenopathy without ulcerations. The **typhoidal form**, occurring in 20% to 30% of cases, consists of high fever, chills, cephalgia, and abdominal pain with an absence of skin and lymph involvement. Typhoidal tularemia is noted to have a slower tachycardia than would be expected given the fever magnitude. It is the form of the disease with highest morbidity, complications, and organ failure. The **oculoglandular form** and **pneumonic form** are the result of deposition into the eyes or inhalation of the *F. tularensis* bacterium. Pneumonic tularemia has up to a 50% mortality rate and is the most lethal form of disease.

Laboratory findings are nonspecific; confirmatory testing is difficult and poses health risks to laboratory staff. First-line treatment is with streptomycin; gentamicin, ciprofloxacin, imipenem, doxycycline, and chloramphenicol are alternative therapies. Prevention of exposure and early treatment are key measures to prevent adverse outcomes. Clinical suspicion should be high for this disease in endemic areas. Due to the ease of transmission and lethality, *F. tularensis* is a possible agent of biologic warfare/terrorism (Table 160-4).

BABESIOSIS

Babesiosis is a malaria-like disease transmitted by ticks, with the etiologic agents being protozoan parasites. *Babesia microti* is the most common causative organism in the United States, with sporadic cases caused by *Babesia duncani* on the Pacific coast.[19] The major zoonotic reservoirs are domesticated mammals, rodents, and deer. Ixodes ticks function as the principal vector globally. Babesiosis has been transmitted through blood transfusions and is the most common transmitted pathogen reported to the Food and Drug Association, with about 160 cases reported since 1979.[19] Clinically, the presentation occurs 1 to 4 weeks after exposure with generalized malaise, anorexia, fever, and chills that can progress to intermittent sweats, myalgia, headache, and hemolytic anemia. Splenectomy and immunosuppression are risk factors. Laboratory tests demonstrate hemolysis, liver dysfunction, anemia, thrombocytopenia, and renal failure. Co-infection with Lyme disease or anaplasmosis/ehrlichiosis is common; patients with severe disease or disease refractory to treatment should be considered for alternative etiologies of illness. Diagnosis is made by finding intraerythrocytic ring forms resembling malaria on a Giemsa- or Wright-stained peripheral blood smear, although false-negative results can occur when the level of parasitism is low. Treatment duration is typically for 7 to 10 days with atovaquone plus azithromycin or clindamycin, with quinine added for severely ill patients (Table 160-4).

ZOONOTIC ENCEPHALITIS AND MENINGITIS

Zoonotic encephalitis is most often an arboviral infection transmitted hematologically by an arthropod or insect vector from an animal host.[20] There are multiple distinct arboviruses that cause zoonotic encephalitis in the United States and Canada. Furthermore, encephalitis may be seen in the nonviral zoonotic infections of *Bartonella henselae, Brucella canis*, borreliosis, *Coxiella burnetii, Ehrlichia* species, listeriosis, leptospirosis, Lyme disease, RMSF, psittacosis, and toxoplasmosis.[20]

Often, the vector is a mosquito or tick, and the animal host is a small animal or bird. Rabies is an exception (see chapter 157, "Rabies"), as a virus that ascends peripheral nerve tracts after inoculation from an infected animal's bite.

The first clinical signs and symptoms are nonspecific: malaise, myalgia, and fever. These findings are followed by headache and a sudden decline in mental status. Head CT scan is usually normal. The cerebrospinal fluid is often abnormal, showing a slightly elevated opening pressure, normal to slightly elevated protein concentration, normal glucose levels, and predominance of lymphocytes. The electroencephalogram is abnormal, with diffuse bilateral slowing interrupted by occasional spike activity. Cerebrospinal fluid viral cultures are frequently sterile, and the infectious agent is rarely isolated from the cerebrospinal fluid. Enzyme-linked immunosorbent assay of serum can be used to detect most arboviral infections causing encephalitis.

Treatment is supportive and directed toward decreasing elevated intracranial pressure. Consider treatable causes of encephalitis, such as herpes simplex or varicella, in the differential diagnosis.

The West Nile virus is an arbovirus that can cause a flulike illness, West Nile fever or **West Nile virus encephalitis**. Infected mosquitoes transmit the virus to humans and other animals through bites. Approximately 20% of patients infected will develop symptomatic illness. Of those who do, less than 1% develop severe or potentially fatal infection.[21] West Nile is the most common arboviral infection in the United States. Although antibody responses can be measured to confirm disease, lab testing is usually not specific. Treatment for West Nile virus is supportive, with attention to the need for mechanical ventilation and management of elevated intracranial pressure or seizures (**Table 160-5**; see chapter 153, "Serious Viral Infections").

Zoonotic meningitis can be caused by brucellosis, listeriosis, plague, salmonellosis, tularemia, leptospirosis, Lyme disease, ehrlichiosis, Q fever, RMSF, or psittacosis. Cerebrospinal fluid is almost always abnormal, showing a slightly elevated opening pressure, normal to slightly elevated protein concentration, normal glucose levels, and predominance of lymphocytes. Treatment is directed toward the specific organism cultured from the cerebrospinal fluid. However, empiric antibiotic coverage should be administered immediately in

TABLE 160-5 Selected Zoonotic Infections and Specific Treatment

Selective Zoonotic Infections	Specific Treatment
West Nile virus encephalitis	Supportive care.
Brucellosis (*Brucella* species)	Mild disease: doxycycline, 100 milligrams PO twice a day for 6 weeks, + gentamicin, 5 milligrams/kg IV daily for 7 d. Alternative: doxycycline, 100 milligrams PO twice a day, + rifampin, 600–900 milligrams PO daily for 6 weeks. Joint involvement: doxycycline, 100 milligrams PO twice a day, + rifampin, 600–900 milligrams PO daily for 3 months, + gentamicin, 5 milligrams/kg IV once daily for first 7 d. Neurologic involvement: doxycycline, 100 milligrams IV/PO twice a day, + rifampin, 600–900 milligrams PO daily, + ceftriaxone, 2 grams IV twice a day. Treat until cerebrospinal fluid normalizes.
Psittacosis (*Chlamydophila psittaci*)	Doxycycline, 100 milligrams PO for 5–7 d. Alternative: azithromycin dose pack or levofloxacin, 750 milligrams PO for 5–7 d.
Q fever (*Coxiella burnetii*)	Doxycycline, 100 milligrams PO twice a day for 2–3 weeks. Alternative: consider 2–3 weeks of a fluoroquinolone or a macrolide.
Pasteurellosis (*Pasteurella multocida*)	Amoxicillin-clavulanate, 875/125 milligrams PO twice a day for 7–10 d. Alternative therapies based on culture data and presence of *Staphylococcus* co-infection. Often resistant to cephalexin, clindamycin, and macrolides.
Plague (*Yersinia pestis*)	Gentamicin, 5 milligrams/kg IV daily for 10 d. Alternative: streptomycin, 15 milligrams/kg IV/IM twice a day for 10 d. Postexposure prophylaxis: Doxycycline, 100 milligrams PO twice a day, or ciprofloxacin, 500 milligrams PO twice a day. Treat for 7 d.
Hantavirus	Treatment consists of supportive care with attention to adequate oxygenation.
Toxocariasis (*Toxocara canis*)	Moderate to severe disease: albendazole, 400 milligrams PO twice a day, with/without prednisone, 60 milligrams/d for allergic response. Treat for 5 days. Alternative: mebendazole, 100–200 milligrams PO twice a day for 21 d.
Dipylidiasis (dog tapeworm)	Praziquantel, 5–10 milligrams/kg PO, one-time dose. Alternative: niclosamide, 2 grams PO, one-time dose
Leptospirosis	Mild disease: doxycycline, 100 milligrams PO twice a day for 5–7 d. Alternative: azithromycin, 500 milligrams PO daily for 3 d. Severe disease: penicillin G, 1.5 million units IV every 6 h for 7 d, or ceftriaxone, 1–2 grams IV daily for 7 d. Alternative: doxycycline, 100 milligrams IV for 7 d.

any presumptive case of meningitis in an effort to reduce mortality and morbidity (see chapter 174, "Central Nervous System and Spinal Infections").

UPPER RESPIRATORY ZOONOTIC INFECTIONS

Recurrent pharyngitis in a household member can have a zoonotic source, sometimes the household pet. Case reports exist where domestic animals in cohabitation with humans were associated with group A streptococcal pharyngitis recurrence; however, current practice guidelines on infection can find no causal link.[22] **Prolonged exudative pharyngitis raises the suspicion of a zoonotic origin or atypical pharyngitis, particularly if the exudative pharyngitis includes systemic symptoms and leukocytosis, and is refractory to standard antistreptococcal therapy.** Dogs and domesticated farm animals can be the source of *Streptococcus* species, *Corynebacterium ulcerans, Yersinia* species, and viral vesicular stomatitis. All of these zoonoses can present as an exudative pharyngitis. Nondomesticated animals can be a source of exudative pharyngitis as a result of *Bordetella* species, *F. tularensis, Streptobacillus moniliformis,* and *Yersinia pestis.* Birds carry *Chlamydophila psittaci*, which can cause an atypical exudative pharyngitis in humans.

LOWER RESPIRATORY ZOONOTIC INFECTIONS

Zoonotic pneumonia presents as an atypical, community-acquired pneumonia with systemic symptoms. Most often, the presentation consists of productive or nonproductive cough, fever, chills, headache, myalgias, and a nonspecific rash. Symptoms can progress very rapidly. A detailed history is an important tool for the consideration of zoonotic pneumonia. Ask about animal exposure, occupation, and recent travel. Consider zoonotic pneumonia as a source of gram-negative community-acquired pneumonia and in any case of atypical pneumonia with systemic symptoms (**Table 160-6**).

ANTHRAX

Inhalation anthrax (*Bacillus anthracis*) is acquired most often from handling unsterilized, imported animal hides or imported raw wool; anthrax is generally fatal. Inhalation anthrax is a mediastinitis without alveolar involvement rather than pneumonia. Initial symptoms are similar to influenza with a slightly higher propensity for dyspnea. Illness can progress to respiratory failure in 2 to 3 days, with marked mediastinal and hilar edema. Anthrax vaccine is available primarily for populations at high risk of exposure to aerosolized *B. anthracis* spores such as military personnel and laboratory workers.[23] The protocol for **anthrax vaccination** consists of five intramuscular injections, three injections on day 0 and one each at weeks 2 and 4.[24] The vaccination is well tolerated by most patients.

A 60-day antibiotic course combined with a three-dose vaccination course used in postexposure prophylaxis could be effective in preventing anthrax postexposure, although this regimen is not presently approved by the Food and Drug Administration for this purpose.[24] Antibiotics typically used in inhalation anthrax are doxycycline or ciprofloxacin, plus an additional one or two agents for synergy, including penicillin G, vancomycin, rifampin, or other agents for which the strain is suspected to be sensitive. Cephalosporins are contraindicated due to resistance.[24]

TABLE 160-6 Zoonotic Pneumonias

Disease	Organism	Reservoirs	Treatment
Inhalation anthrax	*Bacillus anthracis*	Imported animal hides, raw wool, sick domestic animals	Adult initial treatment: ciprofloxacin, 400 milligrams IV every 12 h (alternative: doxycycline, 100 milligrams IV every 12 h or levofloxacin, 500 milligrams every 24 h), + clindamycin, 900 milligrams IV every 8 h, + rifampin, 300 milligrams IV every 12 h Plus one-time infusion raxibacumab, 40 milligrams/kg diluted over 2.25 h When clinically stable: ciprofloxacin, 500 milligrams PO twice a day, + clindamycin, 450 milligrams PO every 8 h, + rifampin, 300 milligrams PO twice a day Treat for 60 d
Brucellosis	*Brucella* species	Food animals and product handling, ingestion, inhalation	See Table 160-5
Psittacosis, ornithosis	*Chlamydophila psittaci*	Bird exposure—pet and pet shop, veterinarians, turkey farms	See Table 160-5
Q fever	*Coxiella burnetii*	Inhaled endospores from animal-contaminated soil; cat afterbirth, ticks	See Table 160-5
Tularemia	*Francisella tularensis*	Aerosol from dead birds, animals; bacteremic spread from bubo; ticks and biting flies	See Table 160-4
Leptospirosis	*Leptospira interrogans*	Domestic and wild animals, contaminated water, veterinarians, farmers	See Table 160-5
Pasteurellosis	*Pasteurella multocida*	Underlying respiratory disease; contact with cat, dog in home	See Table 160-5
Rocky Mountain spotted fever	*Rickettsia rickettsii*	Tick-associated, typical rash	See Table 160-4
Toxoplasmosis	*Toxoplasma gondii*	Contact with domestic food animals and pets, ingestion of cysts, pneumonia in immunocompromised persons	Severe disease: Pyrimethamine, 200 milligrams PO on d 1, followed by 50–75 milligrams PO every 24 h, + sulfadiazine, 1–1.5 grams PO every 6 h, + leucovorin, 5–20 milligrams 3 times weekly If ocular involvement, treat as above and add prednisone, 0.5 milligrams/kg PO twice a day Treat until 1–2 weeks after symptoms resolve, continue leucovorin for 1 week past that
Plague	*Yersinia pestis*	Contact with mammals and fleas; veterinarians; outdoor activities in endemic area; cats	See Table 160-5
Viral pneumonias			
Hantavirus pulmonary syndrome	Bunyaviridae	Rodent feces, urine, and saliva	Ventilator oxygenation or consideration of ribavirin
Influenza pneumonia	Influenza A	Aquatic fowl, pigs, horses, marine mammals	Supportive care; amantadine or rimantadine; oseltamivir if benefits outweigh risks

BRUCELLOSIS

Brucellosis (*Brucella* species) occurs most often from the consumption of unpasteurized dairy products. Another way of acquiring brucellosis is found in slaughterhouse workers exposed to aerosols containing *Brucella* bacteria.[25] In reference to the inhalation form of *Brucellosis*, this rare presentation is one of an upper respiratory infection with a cough, productive sputum, hoarseness of voice, dyspnea, and wheezing. There are no pathognomonic signs on chest x-ray, and a variety of findings may be present including pneumonia, adenopathy, effusion, granulomas, and effusion. With long-standing resolution, calcified granulomas may remain.[26] Doxycycline combined with rifampin is effective therapy; the recommended duration is 6 weeks to prevent recurrence[25] (Table 160-5).

PSITTACOSIS

Psittacosis (parrot fever, parrot disease, or ornithosis) is caused by *Chlamydophila psittaci*, an organism common to most birds and domesticated fowl. This disease is rare, with only a handful of cases reported annually in the United States, although underreporting is likely due to the often mild unrecognized form of disease.[27] Human acquisition is from the inhalation of dust from dried bird feces, feather dust, aerosolized avian respiratory secretions, or direct bird contact.[27] Psittacosis is characterized by an incubation period of 5 to 14 days followed by abrupt onset of fever, chills, cephalgia, myalgia, and generalized malaise. Pneumonia is atypical, with a nonproductive cough and lobar or interstitial infiltrates on chest radiograph. Extrapulmonary manifestations including endocarditis, hepatitis, cranial nerve palsies, and acute interstitial nephritis are possible. Diagnosis is made based on clinical suspicion for the disease and confirmation of isolation of *C. psittaci* from respiratory secretions or by IgM immunoassay. Doxycycline is the mainstay of treatment, with most patients responding rapidly to therapy. Tetracycline is also an option along with macrolides[27] (Table 160-5).

Q FEVER

Q fever (*Coxiella burnetii*) is a rickettsial infection acquired by aerosol inhalation primarily; however, arthropod vector transmission is possible.[28] The primary reservoirs are cattle, sheep, and goats, with bacterial shedding in urine, afterbirth products, and feces. The organism is highly resistant to environmental degradation. The disease is often self-limiting, with variable pulmonary manifestations and extrapulmonary findings. In addition to pulmonary infiltrates, severe headache, pericarditis, myocarditis, endocarditis, and a nonjaundiced hepatitis can occur. The majority of patients will have nonspecific infiltrates on chest x-ray.[28] Doxycycline is the treatment of choice for acute Q fever and is most effective in reducing duration of symptoms and risk of complications when initiated within the first 3 days of illness. Q fever may rarely progress to a chronic infective state with fatigue and extrapulmonary manifestations being predominant findings[28] (Table 160-5).

PASTEURELLOSIS

Pasteurellosis (*Pasteurella multocida*) is endemic to the normal oral flora of cats and most dogs. Classically, infection is associated with necrotizing cellulitis from bite wounds. Rarely bronchitis, bronchopneumonia, and suppurative pleural effusion occur as a result of pulmonary infection. Treatment is with amoxicillin-clavulanate, doxycycline, penicillin, or a third-generation cephalosporin (Table 160-5).

PULMONIC PLAGUE

Between 1000 and 2000 cases of plague are reported to the World Health Organization each year, with mortality rates reported as approximately 10%. Most human cases today are reported from sub-Saharan Africa. In the United States, plague (pulmonary form) (*Yersinia pestis*) is most often found in rock squirrels and ground rodents of the Southwest. Cats can be carriers of plague, whereas dogs are resistant to the disease. The principal vector is the rodent flea, with the majority of infected fleas globally found on black rats or brown sewer rats.[29] Humans and household pets can become infected when bitten by an infected flea or consuming other infected animals. Humans may also be infected by inhalation of animal secretions. Incubation period from a flea bite to disease ranges from 2 to 10 days. Often an eschar is found at the site of the flea bite, followed by the development of a bubo, an enlarged, suppurative, proximal lymph node. Sepsis and pneumonia from hematologic spread occur following the bubo appearance. The disease is rapidly fatal if not aggressively treated.

Start treatment at the time plague is suspected with parenteral streptomycin or gentamicin. Transition to oral therapy with doxycycline, ciprofloxacin, or chloramphenicol occurs when clinically improved. These agents can be used as initial therapy in those who cannot tolerate the preferred choice. Continue any therapy for at least 10 days or 2 days after resolution of fever[29] (Table 160-5).

HANTAVIRUS

Hantavirus, identified in 1977, is from the Sin Nombre virus, which belongs to the Bunyaviridae family of viruses. The deer mouse (*Peromyscus maniculatus*) is the primary vector in the southwestern United States.[30] Infected rodents excrete hantavirus in feces, urine, and saliva. Human infection occurs with the inhalation of dried, particulate feces, by contact with urine, or by a rodent bite. Clusters of hantavirus pulmonary syndrome have been reported in South America. In Asia, hantaviruses can cause hemorrhagic fever with renal syndrome—acute renal failure with concurrent thrombocytopenia, ocular abnormalities, and flulike symptoms. In the United States, the presentation of this zoonosis is that of hantavirus cardiopulmonary syndrome,[30] which consists of an initial flulike prodromal illness of 3 to 4 days in duration, rapidly followed by pulmonary edema, hypoxia, hypotension, tachycardia, and metabolic acidosis. Dizziness, nausea, vomiting, absence of cough, and thrombocytopenia are common and may help to differentiate hantavirus pulmonary syndrome from acute respiratory distress syndrome, bacterial pneumonia, and influenza pneumonia. Hantavirus pulmonary syndrome carries a very high mortality rate, which was previously estimated around 60% but has now improved to 30% with efforts toward prevention, recognition, and early aggressive care.[31] Diagnosis is with an immunofluorescent or immunoblot assay. Treatment is supportive.[32]

GI ZOONOTIC INFECTIONS

Many of the parasitic, bacterial, and viral organisms responsible for gastroenteritis share a zoonotic source in addition to a human source. These are discussed elsewhere.

HEPATITIS E

Hepatitis E virus is a nonenveloped virus with a single-strand RNA genome. Hepatitis E virus is global in distribution and is characterized by zoonotic as well as other means of transmission. When transmitted from animals, the origin is suspected to be boar, deer, and domestic pigs, cattle, sheep, goats, and ducks. Domesticated pigs are particularly susceptible to hepatitis E virus and provide a major source of exposure to humans, particularly in Japan. Further specifics of the disease can be found elsewhere in this text.

DERMATOLOGIC ZOONOTIC INFECTIONS

Dermatologic findings are common in zoonotic infections, because the skin is often the site of inoculation and may display focal findings. The common dermatologic infections of impetigo, ecthyma, and cellulitis can be transmitted zoonotically, as can human infestations with mites and lice. The dermatophytoses *Trichophyton verrucosum* and *Microsporum canis* account for the majority of zoonotic dermatophyte infections, with *M. canis* accounting for 15% of all human dermatophytoses. Chancriform lesions (ulcerations at the site of inoculation) can result from zoonotic infection of bacterial, mycobacterial, fungal, or viral etiology.

BACTERIAL ZOONOTIC SKIN INFECTIONS

The most well-described bacterial chancriform zoonotic lesions are *B. anthracis* (anthrax), *B. henselae* (cat-scratch disease), *Erysipelothrix rhusiopathiae* (erysipeloid), *F. tularensis* (tularemia), *Listeria monocytogenes* (listeriosis), *Mycobacterium marinum* (aquarium granuloma), and *Burkholderia mallei* (glanders).[33] The majority of these chancriform zoonotic infections occur in livestock workers, cattle ranchers, veterinarians, stable workers, horse trainers, slaughterhouse workers, poultry workers, and farmers. Significant zoonotic fungal infection is principally from *Blastomyces dermatitidis* (cutaneous blastomycosis) and *Sporothrix schenckii* (sporotrichosis). Dog and cat owners, along with veterinarians, are most at risk of contracting these two fungal zoonoses. All of the chancriform zoonotic infections most commonly appear at the site of inoculation, often the hands or forearms.

CUTANEOUS ANTHRAX

Cutaneous anthrax, also known as *woolsorter's disease*, accounts for 95% of all anthrax infections.[34] Cutaneous anthrax is most common in societies dependent on and in close contact with livestock and agriculture-based societies. Recently, localized outbreaks have been seen among injection drug users.[34] The hands and fingers are the most commonly infected areas of the body, but arms, lower legs, and feet can also be involved. Anthrax spores are deposited in a skin wound; in 1 to 5 days, a painless or pruritic macule develops at the inoculum site. The macule evolves into an ulcerative site with multiple serosanguineous vesicles. Vesicles contain the anthrax bacillus and are infectious. Gram stain or culture of the vesicular fluid is often diagnostic. The ulcer eventually progresses to a painless black eschar and falls off within 2 weeks. If purulence is present, suspect secondary bacterial superinfection. Untreated, mortality is between 5% and 20% with progression to shock possible. If the disease is thought to have been acquired naturally (i.e., bioterrorism not a concern), penicillin or amoxicillin for 3 to 7 days is the primary treatment.[35] Other patients are treated with oral ciprofloxacin for 60 days, with doxycycline as an alternative option.

VIRAL ZOONOTIC SKIN INFECTIONS

Zoonotic dermatoses of viral etiology include *Vaccinia* species (cowpox), *Paravaccinia* species (pseudocowpox), and bovine papular stomatitis. These cutaneous viral zoonoses often occur on the hands and forearms of patients who work closely with cattle, sheep, goats, or horses. Systemic zoonoses can be accompanied by dermatologic findings, usually a generalized maculopapular rash, which is common in bartonellosis, lymphocytic choriomeningitis, Colorado tick fever, leptospirosis, psittacosis, and

TABLE 160-7 Specific Zoonotic Dermatologic Findings

Zoonoses	Characteristic Rash
Aeromonas species	Crepitant cellulitis with systemic toxicity
Lyme disease	Erythema migrans at the focus of the tick bite
Rocky Mountain spotted fever	Maculopapular rash on soles and palms with centripetal spread, advanced characteristics of petechial hemorrhage and necrosis
Viral hemorrhagic fever	Petechial and purpuric rash

rickettsial infections. However, the maculopapular rash associated with most zoonotic infections is nonspecific and does not facilitate the diagnosis. Those zoonotic infections with specific dermatologic findings that can aid in diagnosis are infections from *Aeromonas* species, Lyme disease, RMSF, *Vibrio* species, and viral hemorrhagic fevers (**Table 160-7**).

ZOONOSES ACQUIRED FROM HOUSEHOLD PETS

Dogs and cats are the two most common household pets in North America and account for the majority of these zoonotic infections. Small rodents, pet birds, reptiles, and aquarium fish account for only a fraction of the zoonotic infections in the United States[36] (**Table 160-8**). Although pet owners often have close contact with their pets, pet-acquired zoonoses are rare and not often recognized.

HELMINTHS (WORMS)

Up to 50% of dogs are infected with at least one intestinal parasite, and 15% of adult dogs actively excrete *Toxocara canis*, the source of **toxocariasis** and visceral larva migrans.[36] Despite its prevalence in dogs, human toxocariasis is infrequently diagnosed, probably because infection is often subclinical. Typically, the only indication of infection is eosinophilia. Children may display fever, cough, nonspecific rash, and failure to thrive. Rarely, pulmonary infiltrates, hepatosplenomegaly, and seizures may occur. Diagnosis is by either biopsy of infected tissue or by enzyme-linked immunosorbent assay. Treatment in the symptomatic patient consists of albendazole or mebendazole (Table 160-5). Corticosteroids can be used to control the allergic component.

Other intestinal parasites that may be transmitted to humans from household pets include *Ancylostoma caninum* or *braziliense* (cutaneous larva migrans), *Echinococcus granulosus* (echinococcosis), and *Dipylidium caninum* (dipylidiasis or dog and cat tapeworm).[36]

Cutaneous larva migrans is often a self-limiting, pruritic, erythematous serpiginous rash caused by a migrating hookworm larva in the skin and is often acquired from fecally contaminated soil. Single-dose ivermectin is the preferred treatment in patients over 5 years of age. Multiple-dose albendazole is another option, as is topical thiabendazole. Although dogs and other carnivores are the definitive hosts for *E. granulosus*, echinococcosis is most common in areas of cattle and sheep ranching. This zoonosis involves multiple organ systems: liver, lung, muscle, bone, kidney, and brain. Typically, there is a unilocular cyst containing multiple larvae that enlarge over time. Definitive treatment is surgical; however, leakage of the cystic fluid can spread the infection and cause an anaphylactic reaction. Should the lesion not be anatomically favorable for unruptured excision, pharmacotherapy with benzimidazoles can be used, but recurrence is high.[37]

Dipylidiasis, caused by a tapeworm common to both dogs and cats, is found worldwide. Human infection is rare, requiring a human to swallow an infected flea. When infection does occur, it is often in children and presents with the nonspecific symptoms of diarrhea and pruritus ani. Occasionally, the cucumber-shaped proglottides are seen moving in the child's stool. Treatment is with praziquantel or niclosamide[36] (Table 160-5).

PROTOZOA

Cats are the host of the intracellular protozoan *Toxoplasma gondii*, which causes **toxoplasmosis**. Human toxoplasmosis can occur in three ways: by ingestion of uncooked or raw meat, especially pork or mutton containing the *Toxoplasma* cysts; by ingestion of the oocysts from cat and wild-animal feces; and transplacentally.[36] Transplacental transmission can result in congenital abnormalities of retinochoroiditis, hydrocephalus, hepatosplenomegaly, and thrombocytopenia in 10% of the children infected. The majority of children transplacentally infected with toxoplasmosis display no significant abnormalities. Nevertheless, pregnant women should limit their contact to only indoor cats and avoid contact with cat feces. The encysted trophozoite can become reactivated in a previously infected host if the host becomes immunocompromised. Treatment of acute chorioretinitis, of severely symptomatic patients, or in certain pregnancy conditions is with pyrimethamine (25 to 100 milligrams/d PO for 3 to 4 weeks) plus sulfadiazine (1.0 to 1.5 grams PO four times a day for 3 to 4 weeks) and folinic acid.[36,38]

SPECIAL POPULATION: IMMUNOCOMPROMISED PATIENTS

Immunocompromised patients include those with congenital immunodeficiencies, diabetes mellitus, chronic renal failure, or liver failure; splenectomized patients; chronic alcoholics; cancer patients; transplanted patients; and human immunodeficiency virus–positive

TABLE 160-8 Pet-Associated Zoonotic Infections

Dog	Cat	Bird	Rodent	Fish and Reptiles
Anthrax	Anthrax	Cryptococcosis	Leptospirosis	Erysipeloid
Brucellosis	Campylobacteriosis	Erysipeloid	Listeriosis	*Mycobacterium marinum*
Campylobacteriosis	Cryptosporidiosis	Listeriosis	Lymphocytic choriomeningitis	Salmonellosis
Cryptosporidiosis	Histoplasmosis	*Mycobacterium*	Murine typhus	*Streptococcus iniae* (fish)
Dirofilariasis	Pasteurellosis	Ornithosis (*Chlamydophila psittaci*)	Plague	Vibriosis
Echinococcosis	Plague	Salmonellosis	Rat-bite fever (*Streptobacillus moniliformis*)	
Histoplasmosis	Q fever	Tularemia	Salmonellosis	
Leptospirosis	Rabies	Viral encephalitis	Tularemia	
Pasteurellosis	Salmonellosis		Yersiniosis	
Rabies	Toxocariasis			
Rocky Mountain spotted fever	Tularemia			
Salmonellosis				
Toxocariasis				
Tularemia				
Yersiniosis				

TABLE 160-9 Zoonotic Infections in Immunocompromised Patients

Infection	Source	Clinical Findings	Antibiotic Treatment
Cat-scratch disease *Bartonella henselae*	Cats	Pyogenic granulomas, regional lymphadenopathy, and fever	Doxycycline or a macrolide
Bordetella *Bordetella bronchiseptica*	Dogs	Fever, pharyngitis, and cough	Azithromycin Alternatives: clarithromycin, TMP-SMX
Campylobacter *Campylobacter* species	Dogs, cats	Gastroenteritis and diarrhea	See chapter 159, "Food and Waterborne Illnesses."
Cryptococcus *Cryptococcus neoformans*	Bird droppings and cats	Flulike symptoms early, photophobia, headache, cranial nerve symptoms, and meningeal irritation later	Mild disease: fluconazole Severe: amphotericin B + flucytosine followed by fluconazole
Cryptosporidium	Dogs	Diarrhea	Immunocompetent host: nitazoxanide HIV positive: HAART only
Giardia *Giardia lamblia*	Dogs, cats	Gastroenteritis and diarrhea	See chapter 159.
Listeria *Listeria monocytogenes*	Livestock and dairy products	Sepsis and meningitis	Severe disease: ampicillin + gentamicin Gastroenteritis in at-risk population: amoxicillin or TMP-SMX
Mycobacterium			
M. avium	Pet birds	Pneumonia and gastroenteritis	Clarithromycin or azithromycin + ethambutol + rifampin
M. marinum	Fish	Cutaneous granulomas, skin ulcerations at distal extremities	Clarithromycin, minocycline, doxycycline, TMP-SMX, or rifampin + ethambutol
Rhodococcus *Rhodococcus equi*	Farm animals	Pneumonia and cavitating lung lesions	Two of the following agents: levofloxacin, rifampin, azithromycin, ciprofloxacin, imipenem, vancomycin
Salmonella *Salmonella* species	Dogs, cats, reptiles, and farm animals	Gastroenteritis, diarrhea, and sepsis	See chapter 159.
Toxoplasmosis *Toxoplasma gondii*	Cats	Pneumonia, brain abscesses, encephalitis, and ocular disease	Pyrimethamine + sulfadiazine + folinic acid

Abbreviations: HAART = highly active antiretroviral therapy; HIV = human immunodeficiency virus; TMP-SMX = trimethoprim-sulfamethoxazole.

patients. Of all of these patients, those undergoing chemotherapy and those with acquired immunodeficiency syndrome have the greatest risk of acquiring a zoonotic infection.[38] *Salmonella* and *Campylobacter* are the two most common infections acquired by immunocompromised patients from their pets, but the overall risk of transmission of *Salmonella* and *Campylobacter* from contact with pets is low. Additionally, *M. marinum* from aquatic pets and *Bartonella* from cats are also commonly acquired by immunocompromised patients. Other acquired zoonotic infections that immunocompromised patients are susceptible to include *T. gondii, Cryptosporidium, Giardia, Rhodococcus equi,* and *Bordetella bronchiseptica* (**Table 160-9**). With the exception of *Bartonella* (cat-scratch disease), most of these zoonotic infections are acquired by immunocompromised patients from sources other than exposure to animals.[38]

REFERENCES

The complete reference list is available online at www.TintinalliEM.com.

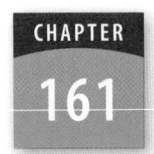

Global Travelers

Raghu Venugopal
Shawn D'Andrea

INTRODUCTION

Of returning travelers who become ill, many have neither serious nor exotic illnesses.[1] The most likely causes of acute symptoms are common problems such as upper respiratory infections, diarrheal illnesses, or reactions to stress, fatigue, or new medications. The ED physician often does not confirm the final diagnosis, but rather protects the health of the public from potentially communicable diseases, begins diagnostic and therapeutic interventions, and provides appropriate referral. Local or regional international health clinics are good resources for referral of patients who need more advanced evaluation, serologic testing, and long-term follow-up (see http://www.travelersvaccines.com/).

Key points for the initiation of ED care are the following:

1. Isolate and use personal protective precautions early when evaluating patients with suspected travel-related infections.
2. Most travelers do not have exotic diseases; think of common causes.
3. Malaria lurks in the febrile patient returning from travel, even in the presence of prophylaxis.

INITIAL EVALUATION OF THE RETURNING TRAVELER

RISK ASSESSMENT

Of travelers, 64% report one or more illnesses during travel, 26% are ill upon return, and 56% of those ill upon return develop symptoms after arrival in the United States.[2] Many disease incubation times are longer than the transit times.

Most travelers on vacation or business are abroad for <20 days, and <5% spend extended time overseas. Some travelers originate from disease-endemic nations, as tourists or newly arrived immigrants; these people are at risk of illness due to transit and exposure to areas with high rates of endemic infectious disease. Others at risk include nonvoluntary travelers, such as refugees and displaced persons, as well as landed immigrants returning from visiting their homeland. In all extended-duration travelers, consider endemic illnesses, even if they lived in the area previously. Travelers also have a risk of tropical illness due to increasing adventure-type travel to areas that were previously inaccessible (**Table 161-1**).

Diseases such as malaria are uncommon in the United States but are leading causes of mortality overseas. Other parasitic agents, such as helminths and rickettsia, also occur with increased frequency and severity in the tropics (see chapters 158 and 160, "Malaria" and "Zoonotic Infections"). Diagnosis of a tropical infection requires a unique set of tests, and therapy is organism specific.

Think of a potential bioterrorist agent as a cause of disease when factors suggest intentional release, such as divergence of the disease presentation from the typical epidemiology of the community and an atypical number of patients presenting with similar clinical syndromes. Examples of diseases that could be weaponized include anthrax, plague, viral hemorrhagic fevers, and tularemia (see chapters 9, "Bioterrorism" and 160).

INCUBATION PERIOD

The approximate incubation period (the time between exposure and signs and symptoms) can be helpful in assessing illness risk. For example, if fever begins >21 days after return or infected patient contact, yellow fever, viral hemorrhagic fevers (including Ebola, covered elsewhere), and other arboviruses (e.g., dengue fever) are unlikely, irrespective of the exposure history (**Table 161-2**). In comparison, schistosomiasis may cause symptoms 5 weeks after exposure. Many diseases have variable incubation depending on factors such as host immunity and the use of chemoprophylaxis and antipyretics.

HISTORY

Suspect imported disease in recent world travelers, and direct the history appropriately (Table 161-2 and **Table 161-3**). Note previous medical conditions because immunosuppression, age <5 years, advanced age, pregnancy, and diabetes often render the patient less tolerant of tropical infections.

Ask about the duration of travel (suggesting specific disease incubation periods) and destination or origin (suggesting possible cause), which can focus the differential diagnosis (**Table 161-4**). Other important considerations are the living conditions and locale of the traveler (rural areas have greater infectious risks of certain diseases), type of accommodation, and travel-related activities (suggesting possible exposure, **Table 161-5**).

Review any pretravel immunizations and preventive medications, high-risk behaviors, and prior medical conditions. Immunization history is relevant because proper vaccination against hepatitis A, hepatitis B, and yellow fever can effectively rule these out as causes of illness. Adherence to appropriate chemoprophylaxis reduces the risk of acquiring malaria—which is the most important tropical emergency—yet it cannot eliminate the possibility. Because of increasing malaria resistance, assume that the febrile returning traveler has malaria even if chemoprophylaxis was correctly taken.

A history of medications, herbs, and traditional medicines consumed is also useful information, because these may contain antipyretics that can alter disease presentation. If altered mental status exists, suspect cerebral malaria or meningitis and consider early empirical treatment for both until the diagnosis is confirmed.

TABLE 161-1 Risk of Infectious Exposure

High risk (1 in 10 travelers): diarrhea, upper respiratory illness, and noninfectious illnesses such as injuries and exacerbation of preexisting chronic diseases
Moderate risk (1 in 200 travelers): dengue fever, Chikungunya, enteroviral infection, gastroenteritis, giardiasis, hepatitis A, malaria, salmonellosis, sexually transmitted diseases, shigellosis
Low risk (1 in 1000 travelers): amebiasis, ascariasis, measles, mumps, enterobiasis, scabies, tuberculosis, typhoid, hepatitis B
Very low risk (1 in >1000 travelers): human immunodeficiency virus, anthrax, Chagas' disease, hemorrhagic fevers, pertussis, plague, typhus, hookworm

TABLE 161-2 Typical Incubation Periods for Selected Tropical Infections

Incubation Period	Infections Likely
<10 d (short incubation)	Traveler's diarrhea Dengue fever and arboviral infections Yellow fever Spotted fevers Anthrax Diphtheria Malaria Rabies Typhoid fever Meningococcal infections Plague Tularemia Typhus (louse- and flea-borne)
<21 d (intermediate incubation)	Leptospirosis Viral hemorrhagic fevers Malaria Enteric fevers (typhoid, paratyphoid) Typhus African trypanosomiasis
>21 d	Viral hepatitis (A, B, C, D, E) Malaria Acute HIV infection Amebic liver abscess Schistosomiasis (Katayama fever) Visceral leishmaniasis Filariasis
>Months	Tuberculosis Malaria Filariasis Viral hepatitis B, C HIV Visceral leishmaniasis Rabies Syphilis African and American (Chagas' disease) trypanosomiasis

Abbreviation: HIV = human immunodeficiency virus.

PHYSICAL EXAMINATION

When assessing vital signs, consider that antipyretics can mask fever. Evaluate the abdomen for hepatosplenomegaly or focal abdominal

TABLE 161-3 Travel-Specific Aspects of the Medical History

Pretravel information
Previous medical condition
Pediatric patient, diabetes, pregnancy, immunosuppression (especially human immunodeficiency virus [HIV]/acquired immunodeficiency syndrome or steroid use)
Pretravel consultation and preparation (self-treatment medications, vaccination history, prophylaxis, etc.)
Type and compliance with chemoprophylaxis, particularly malaria
History of routine childhood immunization (DPT, polio, MMR, HiB, etc.)
Nation of birth and citizenship
Travel information
Exact itinerary of departure and arrival (within the last 3–5 y may be relevant)
Season of travel (monsoon, dry season)
Destinations visited (including locations of transit or stopovers)
Urban or rural, altitude
Purpose of travel and activities in country
General purpose of visit or travel (e.g., "adventure travel" with high exposure to remote, natural elements)
Contacts and their health
Habitat and location of lodging (bednets, window screens, thatched roof, mud walls)
Crowded living or sleeping conditions
High-risk activities (e.g., medical care of displaced populations, spelunking in caves)
Opioid use or injection drug use
Sexual intercourse with high-risk sexual contacts (unprotected with anyone; with high-risk populations, e.g., commercial sex workers, in areas with high prevalence of HIV); dates and nature of sexual contact
Exposure to environment (swimming in fresh or salt water, hiking, trekking, digging, or soil contact, e.g., open-toed shoes or bare feet)
Consumption of high-risk foods (wild game or bush meat, raw or undercooked meats or fish, unpasteurized milk products, food from street vendors, natural sources of water, salads)
Exposure to dogs, birds, or rodents
Adverse incidents
Insect or animal bites
Saliva from animals to open wounds
Assault or trauma
Status and health of fellow travelers
Possible ill contacts
In-country medical consultations sought, remedies used, and procedures (injections, acupuncture, transfusions, dental procedures, body piercing, or tattooing)

Abbreviations: DPT = diphtheria, pertussis, and tetanus; HiB = *Haemophilus influenzae* type b; MMR = measles, mumps, and rubella.

discomfort. Examine for lymphadenopathy and inspect the skin for rashes, lesions, or pallor. Ophthalmologic examination for scleral icterus, conjunctival injection, or petechiae helps detect causes. Imported diseases should be suspected in the presence of high fever, signs of hemorrhage, diarrhea, shortness of breath, skin lesions, and neurologic disturbances. **Table 161-6** lists other signs of tropical illness.[3]

Usually one or more hallmark symptoms or signs are associated with specific infections, allowing categorization. These include fever, CNS complaints, abdominal pain, diarrhea, skin and eye complaints, and respiratory symptoms. It is important to identify diseases that may be rapidly fatal, easily treatable, and/or potentially contagious.

LABORATORY TESTING

Initial studies include a CBC with differential and platelet count, hepatic function tests, and urinalysis; thick and thin blood smears for malaria (and rapid antigen detection test); blood cultures, urine cultures, stool cultures, and stool analysis for WBCs, ova, and parasites; and a chest radiograph for fever and cough. The absolute eosinophil count is often

TABLE 161-4 Regional Tropical Illnesses

Africa: malaria, human immunodeficiency virus, TB, hookworm, tapeworm, roundworm, brucellosis, yellow fever (and other hemorrhagic fevers such as Lassa fever or Ebola), relapsing fever, schistosomiasis, tick typhus, filariasis, strongyloidiasis
Central and South America: malaria, relapsing fever, dengue fever, filariasis, TB, schistosomiasis, Chagas' disease, typhus
Mexico and the Caribbean: dengue fever, hookworm, malaria, cysticercosis, amebiasis
Australia, New Zealand: dengue fever, Q fever, Murray Valley encephalitis, Japanese encephalitis
Middle East: hookworm, malaria, anthrax, brucellosis
Europe: giardiasis, Lyme disease, tickborne encephalitis, babesiosis
China and East Asia: dengue fever, hookworm, malaria, strongyloidiasis, hemorrhagic fever, Japanese encephalitis

Abbreviation: TB = tuberculosis.

elevated to >500/mm^3 in parasitic diseases caused by worms. In a clinically well-appearing patient in whom malaria treatment is not begun but malaria is suspected, obtain blood for smear every 12 to 24 hours. Specific serologic tests are deployed selectively, such as erythrocyte sedimentation rate, purified protein derivative, syphilis test, human immunodeficiency virus test, and serology for arboviruses or rickettsiae.

Consult an infectious disease specialist early in the evaluation to optimize testing and follow-up. It is also wise to obtain an extra vial of serum in a red-top tube (for serology and immunology) during the initial evaluation. This specimen can be used later for comparison with convalescent-stage specimens.

DISEASES COMMONLY ASSOCIATED WITH FEVER

Although fever is nonspecific, it raises the suspicion for a serious infection (**Table 161-7**).[4,5] **Patients with fever after tropical travel have malaria until proven otherwise.** Other common serious infections are listed in **Table 161-8**.[6,7]

MALARIA

The classic clinical triad for all species of malaria is fever, splenomegaly, and thrombocytopenia.[8,9] Fever is typically irregular for the first week and later may demonstrate periodicity. Patients usually have continuous symptoms initially followed by episodic pyrexia every 2 to 3 days, depending on the infecting species. Periodicity is unusual with falciparum malaria. Serious malaria infections occur primarily in young children, pregnant women, the elderly, individuals never previously infected, and patients with comorbid medical problems. Because associated symptoms such as headache, cough, and GI problems mimic other conditions, malaria is a consideration in all febrile travelers.

Diagnosis is based on clinical presentation and confirmed with laboratory evidence of bloodborne protozoa. Patients with fever >38.5°C (101.4°F) of unclear origin and recent or past travel to an endemic area should be screened by blood smears and rapid antigen detection tests when available. Refer to chapter 158 for a detailed discussion of malaria diagnosis and treatment.

DENGUE FEVER

Dengue is the most serious febrile tropical disease after malaria. The World Health Organization reported a 30-fold increase in incidence of dengue in from the 1960s to the 2010s, with up to 50 million cases occurring annually worldwide.[10] Suspect dengue fever among travelers with fever developing within 2 weeks of travel. Dengue may be contracted more than once because each of the four strains offers no cross-protective immunity. Many cases are self-limiting, and the illness is not reportable in the United States.[11]

Dengue fever occurs in urban environments in most tropical nations and is transmitted by the peridomestic day-biting *Aedes aegypti* mosquito.

TABLE 161-5 Specific Exposures and Associated Tropical Infections

Contact/Exposure	Possible Infections
Untreated water, unpasteurized dairy products	Salmonellosis, shigellosis, hepatitis, amebiasis, brucellosis, listeriosis, TB
Raw or undercooked shellfish	Clonorchiasis, paragonimiasis, *Vibrio*, hepatitis A
Raw or undercooked animal flesh	Trichinosis (e.g., pig, horse, bear), *Salmonella*, enterohemorrhagic *Escherichia coli*
Raw vegetables, water plants (e.g., watercress)	Fascioliasis
Animal contact (and animal products)	Rabies, Q fever, tularemia, brucellosis, echinococcosis, anthrax, plague, Nipah virus, toxoplasmosis, herpes B encephalitis
Rodent contact	Hantavirus, viral hemorrhagic fevers, murine (endemic) typhus, Lassa fever, plague, leptospirosis
Arthropod vectors	
Mosquitoes	Malaria, dengue fever, Chikungunya, filariasis, yellow fever, and other arboviral infections
Ticks or mites	Rickettsioses, tularemia, scrub typhus, Crimean-Congo hemorrhagic fever, African tick bite fever
Reduviid (kissing) bugs	American trypanosomiasis (Chagas' disease)
Tsetse flies	African trypanosomiasis (African sleeping sickness)
Fleas	Typhus, plague
Sandflies	Leishmaniasis, sandfly fever
Freshwater exposure	Schistosomiasis, leptospirosis
Barefoot exposure	Strongyloidiasis, cutaneous larva migrans, hookworm
Sexual contacts	Human immunodeficiency virus, hepatitis B, syphilis, gonorrhea, chlamydia, herpes simplex
Infected persons contact	Viral hemorrhagic fever, enteric fever, meningococcal infection, TB

Abbreviation: TB = tuberculosis.

Urban dengue in the Americas, Africa, and the Indian subcontinent is usually classical dengue fever, whereas in Southeast Asia, it manifests as hemorrhagic fever and shock. Classic dengue fever presents after a typically short incubation period of 4 to 7 days with sudden high fever, headache, nausea, vomiting, myalgias, and rash usually lasting several days. Facial flushing, conjunctival injection (although uncommon), and retro-orbital pain can occur. After defervescence, a fine, pale, morbilliform rash develops on the trunk and spreads to the extremities and face. Small children may only present with a mild upper respiratory infection, and classic dengue may be confused with influenza, measles, or rubella. Although other causes of fever can present with a similar clinical picture, such as West Nile fever (transmitted by the *Culex* mosquito), West Nile fever causes lymphadenopathy, which is usually absent in dengue. **Dengue can also cause petechial hemorrhages indistinguishable from meningococcemia.**

Dengue hemorrhagic fever preferentially occurs among infants of immune mothers, children >1 year old, and those with second and subsequent infections. It begins as classical dengue with fever and myalgias. After 2 to 7 days, as pyrexia improves, lassitude, fatigue, and shock develop with an ensuing mortality that is >10%. Clinical features include pleural effusions and bleeding diathesis with epistaxis, purpura, petechia, and marked thrombocytopenia with elevated hematocrit because of vascular permeability. Dengue hemorrhagic fever may rapidly evolve into dengue septic shock, which is often fatal. Dengue septic shock is heralded by abdominal pain, severe emesis, mental status changes, and alternating severe pyrexia and hypothermia.

TABLE 161-6 Physical Findings in Selected Tropical Infections

Physical Finding	Likely Infection or Disease
Rash	Dengue fever, typhus, syphilis, gonorrhea, Ebola fever, brucellosis, Chikungunya, HIV seroconversion
Jaundice	Hepatitis, malaria, yellow fever, leptospirosis, relapsing fever
Lymphadenopathy	Rickettsial infections, brucellosis, HIV, Lassa fever, leishmaniasis, Epstein-Barr virus, cytomegalovirus, toxoplasmosis, trypanosomiasis
Hepatomegaly	Amebiasis, malaria, typhoid, hepatitis, leptospirosis
Splenomegaly	Malaria, relapsing fever, trypanosomiasis, typhoid, brucellosis, kala-azar, typhus, dengue fever, schistosomiasis
Eschar	Typhus, borreliosis, Crimean-Congo hemorrhagic fever, anthrax
Hemorrhage	Lassa, Marburg, or Ebola viruses; Crimean-Congo hemorrhagic fever; meningococcemia, epidemic louse-borne typhus

Abbreviation: HIV = human immunodeficiency virus.

Diagnosis of dengue is based on clinical findings; although serology is confirmatory, cross-reactivity often occurs with other flaviviruses. Enzyme-linked immunosorbent assay provides rapid confirmation of infection by day 6 of the illness. Laboratory abnormalities include leukopenia, thrombocytopenia, and hepatic dysfunction. In uncomplicated dengue fever, treatment is supportive and consists of fluids and analgesics. Only acetaminophen is recommended for managing pain and fever because **aspirin and other nonsteroidal anti-inflammatory drugs are contraindicated** due to anticoagulant properties.

TYPHOID FEVER

Enteric fever, or typhoid fever, is a serious infection diagnosed in roughly 400 travelers annually returning to the United States, with an additional 100 cases of paratyphoid. Typhoid and paratyphoid are caused by *Salmonella typhi* and *Salmonella paratyphi*, respectively.[12] **Once malaria is excluded, typhoid fever is commonly the cause of a febrile illness lasting >10 days.**[13] Imported cases occur in visiting friends and relatives and travelers from Mexico, Indonesia, Peru, and the Indian subcontinent. Vaccination before travel helps thwart acquisition, although protection wanes with time and revaccination is required.

The disease is transmitted in a dose-related fashion after food contamination by feces or urine from actively infected cases or healthy disease carriers. Incubation times and disease severity vary from 1 to 3 weeks. After ingestion, bacteria adhere to the small bowel mucosa, invade lymphoid tissues, and disseminate by lymphatics to the bone marrow, gallbladder, and spleen to reproduce in macrophages. Most pathology occurs in the gut as a consequence of inflammation, necrosis, and ulceration. Typhoid fever classically begins with fever and headache, and then progresses to high fever with chills, headache, cough, abdominal distention, myalgias, constipation, and prostration. The differential diagnosis includes malaria, typhus, viral hepatitis, amebic liver abscess, and other types of infective enteritis. In epidemics, patients can present with acute diarrhea and vomiting, headache, and meningeal signs. Most patients, however, present with constipation rather than diarrhea.

TABLE 161-7 Tropical Infectious Diseases Causing Fever among International Travelers

INCUBATION <2 WEEKS		
Disease	Distribution	Mode of Transmission
Undifferentiated fever		
Malaria	Most tropical and subtropical areas	Infected mosquito bite
Dengue	Tropics and subtropics, including urban areas	Infected mosquito bite
Chikungunya	Africa, Asia, and Caribbean	Infected mosquito bite
Spotted fever	Worldwide	Infected tick or mite bite
Scrub typhus	Asia, Australia	Infected mite bite
Leptospirosis	Widespread, mostly tropics	Percutaneous contact with animal urine or contaminated soil and water; ingestion
Typhoid fever	Developing countries, especially Indian subcontinent	Contaminated food/water ingestion
Acute HIV infection	Worldwide	Permucosal or percutaneous exposure to infective blood or fluids
African trypanosomiasis	East African form found in East and South Africa. West African form found in central and West Africa	Infective tsetse fly bite
Shigellosis	Widespread, most common in developing countries	Contaminated food/water ingestion
Salmonellosis	Widespread, most common in developing countries	Contaminated food/water ingestion
Campylobacteriosis	Widespread, most common in developing countries	Contaminated food/water ingestion
Fever with hemorrhage		
Meningococcemia	Widespread, highly prevalent in sub-Saharan meningitis belt in dry season from December to June	Via respiratory and oral secretions
Leptospirosis	Widespread, most common in tropical climate	Freshwater exposure
Crimean-Congo hemorrhagic fever	East and West Africa, Eurasia	Infected tick bite
Viral hemorrhagic fever	Worldwide	Contact with an infected patient, rodent, bat, tick, or mosquito
Other bacterial infection		
Fever with CNS involvement		
Meningococcemia	See listing above	See listing above
Rabies	Common in Africa, Asia, and Latin America	Infected animal saliva exposure
Malaria	See listing above	See listing above
Many viral and bacterial forms		
Arboviral encephalitis (Japanese encephalitis, tickborne encephalitis, dengue, West Nile, Murray Valley)	Worldwide	Infected mosquito or tick bite
Angiostrongyliasis	Widely scattered, most common in East Asia and Southeast Asia	Ingestion of contaminated food/water with snail or slug slime
Poliomyelitis	Primarily Africa and parts of Asia	Ingestion of feces-contaminated food/water
Fever with respiratory findings		
Influenza	Widespread; outbreaks on cruise ships	Direct or airborne droplet transmission
Severe acute respiratory syndrome	China, Hong Kong, other regions in East Asia	Direct or airborne droplet transmission
Legionellosis (legionnaires' disease)	Widespread; outbreaks in hotels and cruise ships	Inhalation or aspiration of infected droplets
Q fever	Worldwide	Inhalation of infective aerosol from animal source
INCUBATION 2–6 WEEKS		
Malaria	See listing above	See listing above
Typhoid fever	See listing above	See listing above
Hepatitis A and E	Widespread; most common in developing countries	Contaminated food/water ingestion
Acute schistosomiasis	Africa, Middle East, Southeast Asia, and Brazil	Penetration of skin by larval cercaria during freshwater exposure
Amebic liver disease	Widespread; developing countries	Ingestion of cysts usually in feces-contaminated food/water
Leptospirosis	See listing above	See listing above
African trypanosomiasis	See listing above	See listing above
Q fever	See listing above	See listing above
Acute HIV infection	Worldwide, increased risk in developing countries	Sexual exposure

(*continued*)

TABLE 161-7 Tropical Infectious Diseases Causing Fever among International Travelers (*Continued*)

Disease	Distribution	Mode of Transmission
INCUBATION >6 WEEKS		
Malaria	See listing above	See listing above
Tuberculosis	Worldwide	Inhalation
Hepatitis B	Widespread	Permucosal or percutaneous exposure to infective blood or fluids
Visceral leishmaniasis	Many parts of Africa, Asia, South America, and Mediterranean basin	Infective sand fly bite
Lymphatic filariasis	Widespread in tropical areas	Infected mosquito bite
Schistosomiasis	See listing above	See listing above
Amebic liver abscess	See listing above	See listing above
Rabies	Worldwide	Infected animal saliva exposure
African trypanosomiasis	See listing above	See listing above

Abbreviation: HIV = human immunodeficiency virus.

Bradycardia relative to fever is classic (but may be absent); after several days of fever, a pale red macular rash may appear on the trunk (**rose spots**) among fair-skinned individuals. As the disease progresses, splenomegaly develops. Patients may develop leukopenia and elevated liver enzymes, although most cases have nonspecific laboratory values. Complications include small bowel ulceration, anemia, disseminated intravascular coagulopathy, pneumonia, meningitis, myocarditis, cholecystitis, and renal failure. Sequelae include deafness, and neurologic involvement including psychosis, ataxia, and seizures can occur.[14]

Diagnosis is clinical and confirmed by culturing blood, urine, or stool (during the second week) or by rapid antigen testing. Although most cultures have a moderate yield, bone marrow culture is most sensitive, and organism identification is possible after antibiotic treatment.

Current treatment recommendations for typhoid fever include **fluoroquinolones** (ciprofloxacin), **cephalosporins** (cefixime and ceftriaxone), or **azithromycin**, with duration of treatment dependent on severity of illness. Currently, ampicillin, trimethoprim-sulfamethoxazole, and chloramphenicol are unreliable due to resistance. Nalidixic acid–resistant *S. typhi* strains are also associated with fluoroquinolone resistance; these organisms are found in both India and Southeast Asia. If typhoid meningitis is suspected, administer dexamethasone, 3 milligrams/kg IV loading dose over 30 minutes, followed by 1 milligram/kg IV every 6 hours for eight doses in addition to antibiotics. Supportive treatment includes IV rehydration and blood transfusion (if needed from GI losses). Untreated, mortality is 10% to 15%, mostly in young children.

RICKETTSIAL SPOTTED FEVERS

Rickettsial spotted fevers are transmitted by the bite, body fluid, or feces of ixodid arthropod ticks, and the ticks are widely globally distributed. Fleas and mites also transmit rickettsial infections. Among the eight major rickettsial infections, there is great variation in severity. Mortality without treatment approaches 25%, which is lowered to 5% with treatment (see chapter 160). Suspect scrub typhus (*Rickettsia orientalis*) after rural travel in the Asia-Pacific region and maritime Russia and African tick typhus (*Rickettsia conorii* var. *pijperi*) after travel to sub-Saharan Africa or the West Indies.

TABLE 161-8 Most Common Causes of Fever after Travel to Tropical Regions

Malaria
Respiratory tract infections (upper respiratory tract infections, pneumonia, legionnaires' disease, and influenza)
Diarrheal disease
Urinary tract infection
Dengue fever
Enteric fever (typhoid, paratyphoid fever)
Rickettsial infection
Infectious mononucleosis
Pharyngitis

Scrub Typhus and African Tick Typhus The mite bite, in the case of scrub typhus, or tick bite, with African tick typhus, may go unnoticed. After 3 to 14 days of incubation, patients develop fever, malaise, myalgias, severe headache, rash, nausea, and vomiting. The rash may be absent. Scrub typhus is characterized by a papule at the bite site. The papule later becomes necrotic and forms a crusted black "tache noire" eschar. As organisms disseminate, patients develop fever, malaise, headache, lymphadenopathy, and splenomegaly. African tick typhus presents like scrub typhus, but with much less severe symptoms and localized lymphadenopathy associated with an eschar. Diagnosis is clinical, and serologic tests are confirmatory. **Doxycycline**, 100 milligrams PO twice daily for 7 to 10 days, is the empirical treatment of choice, and chloramphenicol is an alternative. African tick typhus requires only 3 days of therapy and is often self-limited even without treatment. In severe cases of scrub typhus, death occurs from a multiorgan toxemia within 1 to 2 weeks of illness onset if untreated. Continue treatment for at least 5 days and for 48 hours after defervescence.

Typhus (Epidemic Louse-Borne Typhus) Typhus is a rickettsial louse-borne disease caused by *Rickettsia prowazekii*. Typhus is a different disease from the bacterial disease due to *S. typhi*, typhoid fever (see above). Epidemic louse-borne typhus is transmitted by the arthropod body louse. Typhus is widespread and found in Central Africa, Asia, and Central, North, and South America. It is also common in cold mountainous regions affected by famine, war, or mass population movement, where adequate clothing exists to harbor the louse or lice. Louse-borne disease occurs after louse body fluids and feces are rubbed into abrasions or after bites. Infection results in high fevers after an 8- to 12-day incubation period. Severe headache is common, and a maculopapular rash appears between days 4 and 7, generally sparing palms and soles. The rash may be hemorrhagic. Diagnosis starts on clinical grounds and is confirmed with serologic testing. Treatment is **doxycycline** (100 milligrams PO twice daily) or chloramphenicol (50 milligrams/kg/d PO in four divided doses) for 7 days and until 48 hours after defervescence. Untreated, mortality is as high as 60%.

LEPTOSPIROSIS (WEIL'S DISEASE)

Leptospirosis, or Weil's disease, follows mucous membrane or percutaneous exposure to freshwater contaminated by *Leptospira interrogans*. Infected animals excrete the spirochete in their urine. Infected patients typically have had contact with dogs; swam, rafted, or waded in contaminated surface water; or farmed or gardened in contaminated areas. Outbreaks commonly occur after flooding. Although the risk to most routine travelers is low, recent ecotourists and adventure travelers have become infected after intense water exposure.

The clinical course can be asymptomatic, but often symptoms illustrate a biphasic pattern. After an incubation of 2 to 20 days, high fever, severe headache, chills, myalgias, hepatitis (with or without jaundice), and nonspecific influenza-like symptoms develop. **Notable is conjunctival injection without purulent discharge.** Symptoms resolve in 4 to 7 days, followed several days later by the severe, icteric Weil's disease caused by circulating antibodies. The second phase lasts for up to 4 weeks and can include aseptic meningitis, renal failure, uveitis, rash, and, rarely, circulatory collapse. Isolation of leptospires from blood, urine, or cerebrospinal fluid is diagnostic, although sensitivity varies with duration of symptoms. Serology is most often used to confirm the diagnosis. Treatment reduces the severity and duration of symptoms and may prevent the second disease phase. Mild disease can be treated within the first 3 days of illness with PO **amoxicillin**, 500 milligrams four times daily, or **doxycycline**, 100 milligrams twice daily, whereas more severe cases require IV penicillin (1.5 million units every 6 hours), ceftriaxone (1 gram daily), or ampicillin (1 gram every 6 hours). Treatment duration is 7 to 14 days total. Consider empiric therapy with PO doxycycline or IV penicillin (or ampicillin) if leptospirosis is suspected.

RELAPSING FEVER

Relapsing fever is a bacterial infection caused by the spiral-shaped *Borrelia* species (*Borrelia recurrentis*) transmitted by lice or tick bites. It is rare among travelers, yet should be suspected in those who have contact with refugee and displaced populations. After being introduced by a louse or tick bite, *Borrelia* reproduce in body fluids and produce endotoxins affecting the liver, spleen, and capillaries. After incubation of 3 to 10 days, patients develop fever, chills, headache, myalgias, abdominal pain, and jaundice. In severe cases, mental status changes, meningoencephalitis, myocarditis, hepatic failure, and disseminated intravascular coagulopathy occur. After 5 to 7 days, fever may spontaneously abate, accompanied by hypotension, and, near day 14, fever may recur. The number of relapses varies, with 1 to 2 relapses in louse-borne fever, 3 to 6 relapses in tickborne fever, and up to 11 relapses in African varieties. Diagnosis is made by clinical suspicion and confirmed by identifying spirochetes blood peripheral smear, cerebrospinal fluid, or bone marrow. Spirochetes are best observed in blood when taken during the febrile period. Louse-borne and tickborne relapsing fever is treated with tetracycline, 500 milligrams PO every 6 hours for 10 days; doxycycline, 100 milligrams PO every 12 hours for 7 to 10 days; or erythromycin, 500 milligrams PO every 6 hours for 10 days. When CNS involvement is suspected, ceftriaxone, 2 grams IV, should be given every 24 hours.

DISEASES COMMONLY ASSOCIATED WITH FEVER AND HEMORRHAGE

Among the most feared tropical diseases are viral hemorrhagic fevers. However, viral hemorrhagic fevers are rare when compared with other febrile hemorrhagic infections such as malaria, dengue fever, meningococcemia, leptospirosis, plague, bacterial sepsis, and rickettsial fevers. ***Neisseria meningitidis*** **is the most common cause of acute hemorrhagic fever in temperate climates.** Among travelers, several treatable infections, including Lassa fever, meningococcemia, leptospirosis, and rickettsial infection, can cause fever associated with hemorrhage. Most people with viral hemorrhagic fevers, such as dengue, hantavirus (see chapter 160), Lassa, Ebola, Marburg, and Rift Valley, develop fever within 3 weeks after exposure. Establish a precise travel itinerary to estimate the incubation time. Viral hemorrhagic fever usually follows the bite of infected mosquitoes and ticks, close contact with rodent/bat excreta, or direct contact with infected, symptomatic individuals (the latter notably for Ebola).

In the event of a suspected viral hemorrhagic fever of tropical origin, institute control measures, including isolation in a negative-pressure room, the use of high-efficiency particulate-arresting respirators, and the use of gloves and gowns. **Immediately notify local public health officials for suspected contagious viral hemorrhagic fevers such as Marburg, Lassa, Ebola, or Crimean-Congo hemorrhagic fever.** If intentional bioterrorism is suspected, notify local law enforcement officials, the Federal Bureau of Investigation, and the Centers for Disease Control and Prevention (1-770-488-7100).

CRIMEAN-CONGO HEMORRHAGIC FEVER

This tickborne viral disease is common in Africa, eastern Europe, Asia, and the Middle East, especially in Turkey.[15] Agriculture workers are at greatest risk, but healthcare workers are the second most affected group. Mortality ranges from 3% to 30%.[15] The prehemorrhagic period is characterized by the sudden onset of fever, headache, myalgia, dizziness, and, possibly, mental confusion. The hemorrhagic period is short (2 to 3 days), develops rapidly, usually begins between the third to fifth day of disease, and may be accompanied by tender hepatomegaly. The most common bleeding sites are the nose, GI system (hematemesis, melena, and intra-abdominal), uterus (menometrorrhagia) and urinary tract (hematuria), and the respiratory tract (hemoptysis). Thrombocytopenia is common. Patients may have leukopenia and elevated liver enzymes, lactate dehydrogenase, and creatinine. Prothrombin time and activated PTT can be prolonged.

Diagnosis is clinical and confirmed with serology. Treatment is primarily supportive, including treatment of coagulopathy and respiratory support in severe cases.[15] Oral or IV forms of **ribavirin** are available and used in more severe cases; treat for 10 days (30 milligrams/kg as an initial loading dose, then 15 milligrams/kg every 6 hours for 4 days, and then 7.5 milligrams/kg every 8 hours for 6 days).[15]

YELLOW FEVER

Yellow fever, an acute zoonotic flavivirus, has a jungle monkey reservoir, and its equatorial belt lies in South/Central America and Africa. Recent outbreaks in Bolivia, Kenya, and Nigeria indicate that it could reappear in the southern United States, where the day-biting mosquito vector *A. aegypti* (also transmitting dengue) is endemic. Yellow fever vaccination is mandatory in endemic areas. Outbreaks are common near tourist areas and may occur among nonimmunized adventure travelers who travel to endemic areas.

Yellow fever ranges in severity from an undifferentiated self-limited flulike illness to a hemorrhagic fever that is fatal in 20% of cases. After an incubation of 3 to 6 days, patients develop fever, headache, myalgias, conjunctival injection, abdominal pain, prostration, facial flushing, and relative bradycardia. In most cases, patients recover, but in others, fever remission lasts a few hours to several days, followed by renewed high fever, vomiting, headache, back pain, shock, multiorgan failure, and bleeding diathesis. **The classic presentation is a triad of jaundice, black emesis, and albuminuria.** In severe cases, hypotension, shock, and metabolic acidosis develop, complicated by myocardial dysfunction and arrhythmias. Confusion, seizures, and coma are common in the late stages of the illness, and death can occur within 7 to 10 days after onset. The diagnosis is primarily clinical, although confirmation is possible through virus identification or rising antibody titers in recovering patients. Leukopenia and albuminuria are typical, direct bilirubin levels rise, and liver enzymes are elevated for several days during which time azotemia and oliguria ensue. Treatment is supportive, with fluid replacement and management of hematologic complications.

LASSA FEVER

Lassa fever, an arenavirus, was first detected in Lassa, Nigeria, and is spread by contact with bush rat excreta. Epidemics were noted with civil unrest and forced migration of populations. The likelihood of travelers becoming infected is low because it is primarily a disease of rural communities where bush rats thrive. Although Lassa fever is mostly found in rural West Africa, it has been exported to Europe and North America by infected patients. The disease is highly contagious through close contact with blood and body fluids.

After an incubation period of 3 to 16 days, the disease presents as a viral syndrome with insidious onset of fever, malaise, headache, sore throat, retrosternal chest pain, back pain, abdominal pain, and myalgias. Varied and nonspecific symptoms persist for 4 to 6 days, at which time the patient suddenly deteriorates and becomes gravely ill. Among those infected, 80% have few symptoms and 20% have severe multiorgan disease. The main features are high fever, severe prostration out of proportion to the fever, severe sore throat with dysphagia and yellow-white exudates, abdominal pain, diarrhea, and vomiting. Only one third of patients experience bleeding, which may include oozing from the gums, hematemesis, melena, hematochezia, hemoptysis, hematinuria, or brain hemorrhage. Diagnosis is made by enzyme-linked immunosorbent assay serology, culture, or immunohistochemistry. Strict patient isolation and use of personal protection by healthcare workers are necessary. Treatment is largely supportive, but patients with severe disease may benefit from early treatment with **ribavirin** IV or PO (see dose for Crimean-Congo hemorrhagic fever above in "Crimean-Congo Hemorrhagic Fever"). Survivors will defervesce within 10 days of disease onset and, except for sensorineural deafness, can make a complete recovery.

EBOLA

Periodic outbreaks of Ebola virus disease have been reported since 1976, when an outbreak occurred in the Democratic Republic of the Congo (Zaire). Since then, outbreaks have occurred in Gabon and Uganda, with the most recent large outbreak in multiple West African countries. Four Ebola species cause disease in humans. Symptoms begin 2 to 21 days after exposure with fever, myalgia, malaise, diarrhea, abdominal pain, and vomiting, and progress to hemorrhage, shock, and end-organ failure. Mortality is high, but those who recover have an antibody response that lasts about 10 years. Disease transmission is by direct contact with infected blood or body fluids, contaminated needles or syringes, or infected bats or primates. The virus is stable, with little mutation in current species compared to that in the epidemic of 1976. Diagnosis is by enzyme-linked immunosorbent assay serology, polymerase chain reaction, culture, or immunochemistry. Treatment is supportive, but vaccines are currently under development. Epidemic containment focuses on avoidance of exposure, and for healthcare workers, use of personal protective equipment. Hospital preparedness consists of the identification of potential exposed contacts by identifying travel and direct exposure history, determining disease signs and symptoms, and then isolating individuals with possible disease.

DISEASES COMMONLY ASSOCIATED WITH FEVER AND CENTRAL NERVOUS SYSTEM INVOLVEMENT

Fever with acute mental status changes, headache (**Table 161-9**), nuchal rigidity, and focal neurologic signs is associated with a number of serious infections. **CNS involvement with fever in travelers returning from malaria-endemic regions requires emergency presumptive treatment for both malaria and bacterial meningitis (see chapters 158 and 174, "Malaria" and "Central Nervous System and Spinal Infections").** The differential diagnosis for fever with CNS involvement includes malaria, bacterial meningitis, tuberculosis, typhoid fever, rickettsial infections, and rabies. Other causes are viral encephalitides, including Japanese and West Nile encephalitis, which often present similarly.

Patients with altered mental status suspected of tropical illness may demonstrate coma, decreased level of consciousness, meningeal signs, or seizures. Although seizures should arouse suspicion of cerebral malaria, suspect **cysticercosis** in those with long-term residence in Latin America and a first-time seizure. **Meningococcal meningitis** occurs with regularity in sub-Saharan Africa along the "meningitis belt" running from Ethiopia in the east to Senegal in the west, and pilgrims attending the Hajj in Saudi Arabia are also at risk of *Neisseria* meningitis. Aseptic meningitis may be caused by enteroviruses or, less commonly, typhoid fever, leptospirosis, or rickettsiae. Encephalitis may be caused by an arboviral infection, such as Japanese B encephalitis.

TABLE 161-9 Tropical Infectious Diseases Causing Severe Headache and Fever
Malaria
Rickettsial disease
Dengue fever
Typhoid fever
Human African trypanosomiasis

JAPANESE ENCEPHALITIS

Japanese encephalitis is a *Culex* mosquito-borne flavivirus infection that occurs in an epidemic or sporadic pattern over large areas of Asia and the western Pacific. It is rarely transmitted to U.S.-bound travelers because the vector breeds primarily in rural rice fields. Infected patients present with a sudden high fever, headache, nuchal rigidity, vomiting, and seizures (especially infants) after the incubation time of 5 to 15 days. A variety of pyramidal and extrapyramidal signs may develop soon after fever. If the outcome is fatal, it usually occurs in the first 10 days. Diagnosis is based on clinical suspicion, although virus can be isolated from cerebrospinal fluid, and antibody titers can rise. Treatment is supportive with IV fluid and electrolyte management, assisted respiration if necessary, anticonvulsants, and neuropsychiatric consultation during convalescence. Recovery may take months, and varying degrees of residual neurologic damage may persist indefinitely. Immunization is recommended for travelers to rural, endemic regions in Asia.

CYSTICERCOSIS

Cysticercosis is a systemic illness caused by dissemination of the larval form of the pork tapeworm, *Taenia solium*. The disease affects an estimated 50 million people worldwide. Endemic areas include Mexico, Latin America, sub-Saharan Africa, India, and East Asia. The incidence in the United States is increasing due to increased immigration from endemic areas and increased travel to endemic areas. Humans are definitive *T. solium* hosts and can carry the intestinal adult tapeworm. An intermediate host, usually a pig, ingests fecally shed egg-containing proglottids or *T. solium* eggs. Humans develop cysticercosis when they inadvertently ingest eggs from contaminated food or soil or eat undercooked pork.

Infestation can occur in almost any tissue. Involvement of the CNS, *neurocysticercosis*, is the most clinically important manifestation of the disease. Neurocysticercosis is a leading cause of new adult-onset seizures worldwide. Other symptoms of neurocysticercosis include obstructive hydrocephalus, meningoencephalitis, stroke-like focal deficits, headache, and visual or mental status changes. Noncontrast CT scan shows calcifications of inactive disease and can reveal mass effect or hydrocephalus. Antihelminthic agents are the mainstay of treatment (**praziquantel**, 50 milligrams/kg/d PO divided three times daily for 15 days). Use steroids in those with encephalitis, hydrocephalus, or vasculitis to avoid inflammation as cysts involute.

DISEASES COMMONLY ASSOCIATED WITH CHRONIC FEVER

Evaluate patients with chronic or relapsing fever lasting beyond 3 weeks after travel initially for non–travel-related infections, inflammatory diseases, and noninfectious disorders. Tropical illnesses that cause chronic fever include protozoal infections (such as trypanosomiasis, leishmaniasis, amebiasis, and malaria), typhoid or paratyphoid fever, and tuberculosis (**Table 161-10**).

HUMAN AFRICAN TRYPANOSOMIASIS (AFRICAN SLEEPING SICKNESS)

Sleeping sickness is caused by the two identical endemic protozoan subspecies, *Trypanosoma brucei gambiense* (responsible for most clinical cases) and *Trypanosoma brucei rhodesiense*, transmitted by the aggressive tsetse fly found in rural Africa. The tsetse fly is indigenous to vegetation near rivers, lakes, forests, and wooded savannah. After a bite, a localized inflammatory reaction occurs, followed in 2 to 3 days by a painless chancre that increases in size for 2 to 3 weeks and then gradually regresses. Trypomastigotes mature and divide in the blood and lymph after the development of the chancre and cause intermittent fever unresponsive to antimalarials. Malaise, rash, wasting, and eventual CNS involvement occur, causing behavioral and neurologic changes, encephalitis, coma, and death. Disease categorization depends on whether the

TABLE 161-10 Selected Causes of Chronic and Relapsing Fevers

Etiologic Organism	Organism Species
Bacterial	Bartonellosis Brucellosis Leptospirosis Q fever Relapsing fever Syphilis Tuberculosis Tularemia Typhoid fever
Fungal	Blastomycosis Coccidioidomycosis Cryptococcosis Histoplasmosis
Protozoan	Amebic liver disease Visceral leishmaniasis Malaria Human African and human American trypanosomiasis
Viral	Human immunodeficiency virus
Helminthic	Angiostrongyliasis Fascioliasis Schistosomiasis Toxocariasis Trichinosis

CNS has been invaded or not. Other complications include hemolysis, anemia, pancarditis, and meningoencephalitis.

Diagnosis is made by rapid evaluation of blood smears for the mobile parasite. Organisms can also be identified by aspiration of lymph nodes, chancres, or bone marrow or by CSF examination. The treatment of sleeping sickness varies according to the stage of illness. If the disease has not invaded the CNS, treat with pentamidine or suramin. If the CNS is invaded, treatment requires melarsoprol, eflornithine, or a combination of nifurtimox and eflornithine. Diagnosis and treatment need infectious disease consultation.

AMERICAN TRYPANOSOMIASIS (CHAGAS' DISEASE)

The protozoan *Trypanosoma cruzi* is found in up to 5% of emigrants from endemic parts of Latin America and is reported as far north as Texas. It is spread by the reduviid "kissing bug" or "assassin" bug. The bites typically happen nocturnally after the bug emerges from rural adobe walls or thatched roofs. Among travelers, it is rare; it causes an acute illness and, commonly, an asymptomatic infection with complications arising years later in the heart and GI tract. It is transmitted during a blood meal when the bug defecates trypanosome-infected feces around the meal site, causing a local inflammatory reaction and trypanosome inoculation after the host rubs the organism into the bite wound or into adjacent mucous membranes or conjunctiva. Infection can also be acquired by blood transfusion, by laboratory accidents, and congenitally.

Unilateral periorbital edema (Romaña sign) or painful cutaneous edema at the site of skin penetration (chagoma) is followed by a toxemic phase with parasitemia causing lymphadenopathy and hepatosplenomegaly. The acute phase generally lasts 2 to 4 weeks but may last up to 3 months. Next is a long, asymptomatic, latent phase when nerve ganglion cells are gradually destroyed, leading to depressed cardiac and GI function. Cardiac complications include myocarditis, dysrhythmias, cardiomyopathy, and sudden death. Chagas-induced heart disease is the leading form of congestive heart failure in much of Latin America. GI complications are megaesophagus or megacolon.

The acute phase diagnosis is made by examination of peripheral blood smears demonstrating motile parasites or by blood culture or muscle biopsy. In the chronic phase, serologic tests and tissue biopsy are useful. Treatment is available for acute, reactivated, or chronic cases. The two medications used are nifurtimox and benznidazole, which are available in the United States through the Centers for Disease Control and Prevention.

TABLE 161-11 Clinical Syndromes of Leishmaniasis

Visceral leishmaniasis (kala-azar or black fever): The most devastating and fatal form caused by *Leishmania donovani*. A progressive, chronic, and systemic disease with high mortality if untreated, but with a good prognosis if provided adequate care. Fatality is a result of secondary infections such as tuberculosis, pneumonia, and dysentery. It is typified by the pentad of fever, weight loss, hepatosplenomegaly, pancytopenia, and hypergammaglobulinemia.
Cutaneous leishmaniasis: Characterized by skin sores initially appearing as papules or nodules. These later ulcerate, especially on exposed skin surfaces, later leaving scars.
Mucocutaneous leishmaniasis (espundia): Chronic and relentless disease affecting the mucous membranes of the nose, mouth, and throat.
Diffuse cutaneous leishmaniasis: Typically chronic diffuse plaques or nodules, difficult to treat, and with few resulting deaths.

LEISHMANIASIS (VISCERAL)

Leishmania is an intracellular protozoan transmitted by *Lutzomyia* or *Phlebotomus* sandflies. The disease occurs sporadically in rural Africa, Asia, the Mediterranean basin, and Central/South America, and outbreaks occasionally occur, such as in Brazil, India, and the Sudan, which places resident expatriates and travelers at risk. The disease is a low risk to most travelers, although European travelers to nonendemic Mediterranean nations occasionally export cases. Suspect *Leishmania* in the military and their families living proximal to jungles, adventure travelers, field biologists, and emigrants from endemic zones.

The infecting species determines the pathology, ranging from a localized self-healing lesion to widespread, persistent, and potentially destructive disease. Four major clinical syndromes are recognized (**Table 161-11**).

The most important diagnostic information is patient origin and travel itinerary because endemic areas suggest the infection type. Definitive diagnosis requires reference laboratory expertise to isolate motile extracellular parasites aspirated from bone marrow, spleen, or lymph nodes, or on smears or sections taken from the ulcer edge by punch biopsy.

Treatment of visceral leishmaniasis by infectious disease consultants relies on factors such as the origin of the disease, type of disease, parasite species, and patient comorbidities. Treatment for visceral leishmaniasis is with agents such as **amphotericin B**, **pentavalent antimonials, or miltefosine**. Treatment of cutaneous leishmaniasis is either by local therapy, oral systemic therapy, or parenteral systemic therapy.

DISEASES COMMONLY ASSOCIATED WITH ABDOMINAL AND URINARY COMPLAINTS

Illnesses causing abdominal pain and diarrhea are common among world travelers because of infecting bacteria, viruses, soil-transmitted helminths, and other parasites. Most infections are caused by the consumption of undercooked or fecal-contaminated foods and are preventable by adequate hygiene, potable water, and careful food preparation.

SCHISTOSOMIASIS (BILHARZIA OR SNAIL FEVER)

Schistosomiasis, infection with a blood fluke found in Africa, the Middle East, South America, and Asia, infects >200 million people worldwide, with 20 million people suffering severe consequences. Suspect schistosomiasis in travelers with GI symptoms following exposure to freshwater in endemic zones. For most short-term travelers, the risk is low, although significant outbreaks now occur among adventure tourists, Peace Corps workers, and those who swim in infested streams and lakes. The larvae are released into freshwater by snails, which are intermediate hosts. Infection occurs by tiny, free-swimming cercariae that penetrate wet, unbroken skin or are ingested from slow-moving freshwater. Brief or even single exposures like washing or wading can cause infection in previously unexposed asymptomatic individuals. After inoculation, an immediate cercarial allergic and pruritic dermatitis occurs that can last days. In the following 4 to 8 weeks, fever occurs, accompanied by headache, cough, urticaria, diarrhea, hepatosplenomegaly, and hypereosinophilia (Katayama fever). Worms mature into adults in the venous blood and, for the next 30 to 40 years, deposit eggs into selective body tissues (*Schistosoma haematobium* in the bladder and *S. mansoni* and *S. japonicum* in the GI tract). Eggs are deposited throughout the brain, skin, liver, and GI tract. Eggs stimulate a vigorous immune response that results in clinical symptoms.

CNS symptoms include seizures, paralysis, and acute transverse myelitis. *S. haematobium* infection causes dysuria, frequency, and terminal hematuria, and can cause bladder scarring, calcification, and squamous cell carcinoma. *S. japonicum* and *S. mansoni* infections lead to hepatosplenomegaly, hepatic granulomas, and periportal fibrosis. *S. japonicum* and *S. mansoni* also can cause diarrhea, abdominal cramps, acute abdominal pain, and, late in the disease course, portal hypertension. *S. dermatitis*, a non–human-infecting schistosome, has cercariae that only penetrate the superficial skin, causing an irritation known as *swimmer's itch*.

Diagnosis is by detecting eosinophilia and is made primarily by microscopic identification of ova in mid-day urines or stool or in a biopsy specimen. Serologic antibody detection methods are highly accurate and are usually positive in light infections missed by egg detection. Offer treatment to symptomatic patients and seropositive travelers using **praziquantel**; some may require a second treatment. For swimmer's itch, no treatment is required.

CLONORCHIASIS (CHINESE OR ORIENTAL LIVER FLUKE)

Clonorchiasis, a trematoidal disease of the bile ducts, is caused by *Clonorchis sinensis* and follows ingestion of poorly cooked freshwater fish containing encysted larvae. Travelers are at low risk despite the tremendous prevalence among those living in endemic zones such as Southeast Asia. Once ingested, larvae mature into adults, migrate to bile ducts, survive for 30 or more years, and cause fibrosis. The extent of pathology is related to parasite burden, and among the millions infected, only few are symptomatic. Acute symptoms include anorexia and diarrhea and may progress in heavy infections to chronic bile duct obstruction, liver tenderness, and/or jaundice and, in advanced cases, biliary cirrhosis and cholangiocarcinoma. Diagnosis is made by detecting the characteristic embryonated eggs in stool or duodenal aspirate, and eosinophilia is common. Serologic tests using enzyme-linked immunosorbent assay have 70% sensitivity, and CT, abdominal ultrasonography, and upper endoscopy examinations are useful. Treatment is with praziquantel or albendazole.

DISEASES COMMONLY ASSOCIATED WITH ABDOMINAL PAIN AND DIARRHEA

Diarrhea and gastroenteritis are the most common travel ailments, affecting up to one half of travelers (**Table 161-12**). Traveler's diarrhea is especially common after travel to Africa, Asia, the Middle East, South and Central America, and Mexico. Diarrhea is typically accompanied by fever, flatulence, nausea, emesis, and abdominal pain, which is usually spasmodic and colicky. *Campylobacter jejuni* may cause severe and constant pain, and cholera may cause somatic muscle cramps. Nonbloody gastroenteritis and diarrhea are usually caused by bacteria or bacterial toxins, whereas dysentery usually results from toxigenic and invasive bacteria such as *Shigella*, *Salmonella*, *Campylobacter*, *Aeromonas*, *Escherichia coli*, or *Entamoeba histolytica* (**Table 161-13**). Traveler's diarrhea is not commonly due to viruses.

Acute abdominal pain among travelers should first be considered to be caused by nontravel causes with an expanded travel-based differential diagnosis. Give empiric therapy to those with pain and severe diarrhea using fluoroquinolones (ciprofloxacin or levofloxacin) before stool testing results are available, although regional resistance can occur and should be verified (see chapter 159, "Food and Waterborne Illnesses").

TABLE 161-12 Common Infectious Diseases Causing Diarrhea in Travelers

Cause	Organism	Comments
Acute (duration <2 wk)		
Viral	Norwalk-like virus Rotaviruses Enteroviruses	Often not diagnosed; may account for 5%–10% of acute traveler's diarrhea
Bacterial	*Escherichia coli* (enterotoxigenic or enteroaggregative) *Campylobacter jejuni* *Salmonella* *Shigella* *Vibrio* *Clostridium difficile*	Most common identified cause of acute traveler's diarrhea; 50%–70%
Parasitic	*Giardia lamblia* *Cryptosporidium parvum* *Entamoeba histolytica* *Cyclospora cayetanensis* *Isospora belli* *Balantidium coli* *Trichinella spiralis*	Accounts for <1%–5% of acute traveler's diarrhea
Chronic or persistent (duration >2–4 wk)		
Bacterial	See above	Rare cause of chronic diarrhea
Parasitic		
Microsporidial	*Enterocytozoon bieneusi* *Encephalitozoon intestinalis*	Almost exclusively in immunocompromised
Protozoal	*G. lamblia* *E. histolytica*	Most commonly identified cause Bloody diarrhea with fever; fecal WBCs are rare
Helminthic	*Trichuris trichiura* *Strongyloides stercoralis* *Fasciolopsis buski* *Schistosoma*	Rarely associated with chronic diarrhea; usually in persons with heavy parasite burdens

AMEBIASIS

Pathogenic species such as *E. histolytica* are found worldwide and disproportionately infect those living in low-income settings. Amebiasis is typically spread by asymptomatic carriers whose excrement contains the encysted organism. Short-term travelers are at low risk, but longer-term travelers, such as Peace Corps volunteers, are at higher risk. The disease is most severe among young children, the elderly, and pregnant women. Incubation times are typically 1 to 3 weeks for colitis and 2 weeks to

TABLE 161-13 Causes of Diarrhea with and without Fever or Blood

	With Fever	Without Fever
With blood	Bacillary dysentery *Campylobacter enterocolitis* *Salmonella enterocolitis* *Escherichia coli*	Amebiasis *Balantidium coli* *Schistosoma* *Trichuris*
Without blood	*Salmonella enteritis* Malaria (especially *Plasmodium falciparum*) Mild shigellosis *Campylobacter* infections Almost any infections in a child	*Staphylococcus aureus* *E. coli* (enterotoxigenic) *Clostridium perfringens* Viral infections of the gut Food toxins

several months for liver abscesses. Once cysts are ingested, amebic trophozoites invade the colon wall, lyse tissues, and cause necrotic abscesses.

Most infected people do not have symptoms. Symptoms range from alternating constipation and diarrhea over 1 to 3 weeks, to abdominal pain, bloody diarrhea, fever, dehydration, and weight loss. Extraintestinal metastases can infect the liver and, rarely, pericardium, lung, and brain. Colitis can lead to intestinal perforation and peritonitis. Complications such as liver abscesses may cause fever, right upper quadrant pain, or chronic, vague abdominal pain accompanied by weight loss. Hepatic abscesses can be fatal if the abscess ruptures.

Stool ova and parasite examination is diagnostic, and organisms are found either as motile trophozoites or cysts. It can be difficult to differentiate pathogenic organisms (*E. histolytica*) from benign organisms (*Entamoeba dispar*) without use of stool antigen detection tests. Serology for elevated antibody titers is almost uniformly sensitive for extraintestinal disease and 80% sensitive for invasive colon disease after 1 week of illness. Ultrasonography or CT scans may be useful to identify hepatic abscesses.

Treatment of asymptomatic cyst passers includes **iodoquinol**, 650 milligrams PO three times a day for 20 days; **paromomycin**, 500 milligrams PO three times a day for 7 days; or **diloxanide furoate**, 500 milligrams PO three times a day for 10 days. For **symptomatic disease**, choices include **metronidazole**, 500 to 750 milligrams PO three times a day for 5 to 10 days, or **tinidazole**, 1 gram PO twice a day for 3 days, followed by either iodoquinol or paromomycin in the doses and duration noted earlier. For **liver abscess**, treat with metronidazole, 750 milligrams PO or IV three times a day for 5 days, followed by iodoquinol or paromomycin as described above.

GIARDIASIS

Giardia lamblia is a flagellated protozoan infecting the small intestine and biliary tree. It is distributed worldwide and is food- or waterborne by fecal contamination with encysted parasites. It is common to rural areas with poor sanitation and impure surface water but has also occurred in day care settings in the United States. In Eastern Europe, it is a common cause of chronic traveler's diarrhea and can be contracted at camping sites and rural swimming areas. Long-term residents of tropical nations are at high risk, but short-term travelers are also at risk. Ingested parasites reside in the duodenum and may lead to malabsorption because of duodenal microvilli obstruction. Symptoms include abdominal cramping, flatulence, and foul-smelling, watery diarrhea without blood or mucus. Chronic infections cause weight loss and anemia, and a common complication is lactose intolerance. Diagnosis is by stool ova and parasites showing either motile trophozoites or cysts. *Giardia* antigen detection in stool has good sensitivity and specificity. Treatment is with **metronidazole** (250 milligrams PO three times daily for 5 to 7 days), **tinidazole** (2 grams PO for one dose), **quinacrine** (100 milligrams PO three times daily for 7 days), or **nitazoxanide** (500 milligrams twice daily for 3 days). In children, treat with tinidazole, 50 milligrams/kg up to 2 grams in a single dose, or metronidazole, 35 to 50 milligrams/kg/d PO up to 750 milligrams/dose, three times per day for 10 days. Treatment is not always successful regardless of drug used.

CHOLERA

Cholera is an acute diarrheal disease caused by the bacterium *Vibrio cholerae*. It is endemic and epidemic to many tropical nations. It is reported in Africa, Asia, Latin America, and most recently Haiti and Mexico. Epidemics occur after flooding or acute population displacement with disruption of the water-sanitation system. Transmission is by fecal contamination of water or food (including raw or poorly cooked seafood and shellfish). Significant bacterial ingestion is required to cause symptoms. The incubation time is 2 to 3 days, and symptoms result from sodium pump inhibition in the GI tract by the cholera toxin. Infection is usually mild but can be life-threatening, particularly among vulnerable populations, such as malnourished children, migrants, and those with chronic illness. Another group at risk are individuals with achlorhydria or those using medications decreasing gastric acidity. There is an asymptomatic carrier state.[16]

Severe disease is characterized by profuse, usually painless, watery diarrhea ("rice water stools"), severe dehydration, vomiting, leg cramps, and, occasionally, fever. Rapid fluid loss (up to 15 L/d) leads to extreme dehydration and shock. Without aggressive rehydration, death can occur within hours. With proper fluid resuscitation, almost no patients should die. Diagnosis is clinical, and when suspected, a rectal swab or stool specimen can be sent to a reference laboratory for culture confirmation. Rapid dipstick testing of stool is possible, but should be followed by confirmatory testing.

The cornerstone of treatment is aggressive fluid resuscitation with PO rehydration solution or IV fluids, coupled with correction of metabolic acidosis and hypokalemia. For those with severe illness, antibiotics can shorten the illness course, diminish vomiting, lessen volume resuscitation needs, and ensure that bacteria are eradicated from stool. **Doxycycline** is the antibiotic of choice, followed by azithromycin or erythromycin for children and pregnant women. Secondary transmission is rare, and close contacts should not be given antibiotics as prophylaxis.

PARASITIC HELMINTH (WORM) INFECTIONS

Major infestations are discussed here, and diagnosis and treatment are presented in **Table 161-14**.

In the patient in whom empirical therapy is chosen due to the appearance of a worm in fecal matter, treatment for nematodes can be considered. **By treating the adult patient empirically with albendazole, 400 milligrams twice daily for 3 days (with a single repeat dose in 2 weeks), a number of pathologies can be treated** (roundworm, pinworm, whipworm, and hookworm). Send stool samples for laboratory analysis to provide more focused treatment.

ASCARIASIS (ROUNDWORM)

The risk of infection with *Ascaris lumbricoides* to short-term travelers is low and suspected following ingestion of street vendor foods or vegetables fertilized by "night soil" (human feces) or animal feces. Eggs survive for years in moist soil, and transmission is typically fecal–oral or through poorly cooked food. Symptoms are usually minimal; a dry cough or pneumonia may occur as young worms are expectorated and migrate from the lungs to the esophagus and gut. A large worm burden can lead to malnutrition and weakness, and a mass of worms may lead to bowel obstruction. Wandering *Ascaris* also traverse internal organs, rarely leading to biliary obstruction, hepatic abscess, acute pancreatitis, acute appendicitis, or hypersensitivity pneumonitis. The diagnosis and treatment are described in Table 161-14.

ENTEROBIASIS (PINWORM, SEATWORM)

Enterobiasis vermicularis is a common tropical disease caused by a small intestinal parasite transmitted by the fecal–oral route and is often acquired from contaminated objects such as toys, utensils, and bedding. It is a common disease among U.S. children and is more likely to be peridomestic rather than after tropical travel. The disease is characterized by intense perianal itching. The diagnosis and treatment are found in Table 161-14.

TRICHURIS (WHIPWORM DISEASE)

Whipworm (*Trichuris trichiura*) is a nematode parasite of the large intestine distributed globally but most heavily in the tropics. Long-term travelers, former tropical residents, and visitors from the tropics are at high risk. It is obtained by ingesting contaminated soil or vegetables and is not transmissible from person to person. Light infestations are asymptomatic, and heavy infestations cause bloody diarrhea and rectal prolapse. Diagnosis and treatment are found in Table 161-14.

HOOKWORM

Hookworm is a common chronic nematodal infection caused by *Ancylostoma duodenale* and *Necator americanus*, which are globally distributed but most heavily in the tropics and subtropics. Because symptoms require large worm burdens, it is a low risk among short-term travelers. Hookworm causes chronic, severe anemia, especially in children. The cutaneous

TABLE 161-14 Common Parasitic Helminth (Worm) Infestations

Name	Source of Contamination	Human Symptoms	Diagnosis	Treatment
Ascaris lumbricoides (roundworm)	Fecal–oral contamination or poorly cooked food	Minimal symptoms; or pneumonia, malnutrition, biliary or bowel obstruction, hepatic abscess, appendicitis, etc.	Stool examination, serology.	Albendazole, 400 milligrams single dose *or* Mebendazole, 100 milligrams twice a day for 3 d or 500 milligrams single dose *or* Ivermectin, 150–200 micrograms/kg single dose
Enterobiasis (pinworm, seatworm)	Fecal–oral and from contaminated objects	Intense perianal itching	Visual inspection, cellophane tape swab of anus upon waking.	Albendazole, 400 milligrams single dose and repeat in 2 wk *or* Mebendazole, 100 milligrams single dose and repeat in 2 wk *or* Pyrantel pamoate, 11 milligrams/kg (up to 1 gram) single dose and repeat in 2 wk
Trichuris trichiura (whipworm)	Fecal–oral contamination	Asymptomatic; or bloody diarrhea, rectal prolapse	Stool examination.	Albendazole, 400 milligrams daily for 3 d *or* Mebendazole, 100 milligrams daily for 3 d or 500 milligrams single dose
Ancylostoma duodenale and *Necator americanus* (hookworm)	Contaminated soil, larvae penetrate the skin	Severe anemia; cutaneous larva migrans	Stool examination, may require serial exams.	Albendazole, 400 milligrams single dose *or* Albendazole, 400 milligrams twice a day for 3 d *or* Pyrantel pamoate, 11 milligrams/kg (maximum, 1 gram) daily for 3 d
Taenia solium (pork tapeworm), *T. saginata* (beef tapeworm), and *Diphyllobothrium latum* (fish tapeworm)	Raw or undercooked pork or beef or fish	Asymptomatic, abdominal pain, bowel obstruction; *Taenia* cysts in skin, eye, brain, heart (see "Cysticercosis" section, above)	Stool examination or serology. Serology may be negative if cysts are calcified.	Praziquantel, 5–10 milligrams/kg single dose
Strongyloides stercoralis (threadworm)	Contaminated soil, larvae penetrate skin	Cough, pneumonia, and wheezing; abdominal pain, bloody diarrhea	Stool examination or stool concentration methods; serology or sputum examination.	Ivermectin, 100 micrograms/kg/d for 2 d or Albendazole, 400 milligrams twice a day for 7 d

form is called *cutaneous larva migrans*. Transmission is by direct skin contact with soil contaminated by human feces, often in children with poor footwear exposed to raw sewage. Filariform larvae penetrate the skin. Microscopic examination of stool for eggs is the usual means of diagnosis. Diagnosis and treatment are found in Table 161-14.

CESTODES (TAPEWORMS)

Among the cestodes, taeniasis and cysticercosis are the most pathologic. Infections occur worldwide, but especially in the tropics, and risk is high among children, the mentally disabled, and immigrants or visitors from endemic nations. Risk to travelers is low but is increased with consumption of undercooked pork, fish, or beef.

Taenia solium* and *Taenia saginata* (Pork and Beef Tapeworm)** ***T. solium **(pork tapeworm)** is encountered in the United States in immigrants or visitors to or from Central America and the Middle East. *T. saginata* (beef tapeworm) is seen more often, especially in those who consume raw beef (e.g., steak tartare), particularly in Latin America, Eastern Europe, Africa, and Russia. Adult worms live in the small intestine. Infected patients can be asymptomatic or present with nausea and vomiting, headache, abdominal pain, pruritus, constipation, diarrhea, and intestinal obstruction. The larval stage of *T. solium* can cause clinical disease (cysticercosis), which can sometimes be fatal. *Taenia* cysts may be found in subcutaneous tissue, the eye, brain, and heart, and cause seizures and hydrocephalus. Radiographs of the soft tissues may reveal curvilinear calcifications indicative of cysts, and cysts can be seen in the meninges and brain parenchyma on CT scanning. Diagnosis and treatment are found in Table 161-14. For discussion of neurocysticercosis see the "Cysticercosis" section, above. *Dipylidium caninum* is discussed in the chapter 160.

Diphyllobothrium latum* (Fish Tapeworm)** ***Diphyllobothrium latum (fish tapeworm) is encountered in those consuming raw fish (e.g., sushi and sashimi) or gefilte fish. Diphyllobothrium can compete with the host for vitamin B_{12}, and patients can develop pernicious anemia. Most patients are asymptomatic, but some develop intestinal or biliary obstruction. Diagnosis and treatment are found in Table 161-14.

STRONGYLOIDES

Strongyloides stercoralis infects the small intestine. Distribution is worldwide, but infection is most common in humid tropics. Infection can develop in overseas military personnel, refugees, or immigrants. The risk is low in short-term travelers. Most infections cause minimal or no symptoms. However, fatalities may occur due to hyperinfection in elderly and immunocompromised patients and those with chronic disease. An upper GI series may reveal a deformed duodenal bulb, and *Strongyloides* may be confused with ulcer disease. Diagnosis and treatment are found in Table 161-14.

DISEASES COMMONLY ASSOCIATED WITH EYE OR SKIN COMPLAINTS

Skin complaints among travelers are common and nonspecific and have many causes. **Travel-related skin disease is generally caused by one of the following: (1) exacerbations of previous conditions (e.g., atopic dermatitis, psoriasis); (2) environmental conditions (e.g., photosensitivity,**

TABLE 161-15 Cutaneous Manifestations of Selected Infections

Appearance of Lesion	Possible Diagnosis
Maculopapular rash	Dengue fever
	Viral hemorrhagic fevers
	Leptospirosis
	Acute human immunodeficiency virus infection
Erythema chronicum migrans	Lyme disease
Rose spots	Typhoid fever
Pustules	Disseminated gonococcal infection
Petechiae, ecchymoses, hemorrhage	Meningococcemia
	Dengue fever
	Viral hemorrhagic fevers
	Yellow fever
	Rocky Mountain spotted fever
	Epidemic louse-borne typhus
	Leptospirosis
Eschar	Tick or scrub typhus
	Anthrax
Ulcer	Tularemia
	Cutaneous diphtheria
Urticaria	Helminthic infections

contact allergies); or (3) infective organisms causing infestations or infections.[16] The distribution and timing of the dermatosis may aid diagnosis of rashes associated with systemic illness (**Table 161-15**).[17] Among rashes reported by travelers, most are minor problems such as sunburn, phototoxic/sensitivity reactions, insect bites, and prickly heat, and are often self-limiting and necessitate symptomatic care. **The top 10 tropical travel dermatoses requiring specific therapy are cutaneous larva migrans, pyodermas due to staphylococcal or streptococcal ecthyma, arthropod-reactive dermatoses, myiasis, tungiasis, urticaria, febrile syndromes with rash, cutaneous leishmaniasis, scabies, and fungal infections.**[18] The risk of serious conditions tends to increase with the amount of time spent overseas, and thus short-term travelers rarely contract dermatoses such as filariasis, Buruli ulcer, yaws, and leprosy (Hansen's disease). To further aid diagnosis, travelers with dermatoses can fit into five syndromic and morphologic categories (**Table 161-16**).

Management includes arranging biopsy for patients with chronic ulcerative lesions. Beware of the rare patient presenting with anxiety of parasitosis regardless of travel history. The following are select dermatoses associated with tropical exposures.

ONCHOCERCIASIS (RIVER BLINDNESS)

River blindness is a chronic, nonfatal filarial disease leading to subcutaneous skin changes and blindness. It is caused by *Onchocerca volvulus*, a nematode transmitted by the female black fly, *Simulium* species, found near fast-moving rivers in parts of Central/South America and mostly equatorial Africa. Early treatment can prevent blindness and reduce systemic spread, because the incubation period from fly bite to microfilariae appearing in skin is often more than a year. Symptoms include intractable pruritus, altered skin pigmentation, skin nodules, lymphadenitis, and gradual visual impairment leading to blindness. Adult female worms reside in 2- to 3-cm painless nodules in skin and bones near joints, and release microfilariae that migrate through the skin, causing intense pruritus when they die, leading to chronic dermatitis, edema, and skin atrophy. Skin pigment changes result in "leopard skin," whereas loose pelvic skin is called "hanging groin." Blindness is a result of microfilariae migrating to the eye, invading it, and causing permanent damage when they die. Diagnosis is made by identification of microfilariae from a fresh skin biopsy, nodule biopsies, or in the urine. Slit-lamp examination may reveal microfilariae in the cornea, anterior chamber, or vitreous. Treatment is one dose of ivermectin, 150 micrograms/kg PO, which does not kill the adult worm, but when repeatedly dosed every 6 to 12 months, reduces morbidity by killing microfilariae, suppressing microfilariae release from adults, and preventing spread to eyes and skin. **Diethylcarbamazine citrate (DEC)** and **suramin** (which can kill adult worms and microfilariae) have serious side effects and are avoided. Surgical removal of nodules can reduce symptoms, reduce the worm burden, and, if removed from the frontal scalp, help prevent progression of visual impairment and blindness.

TABLE 161-16 Syndromic Categories of Travel-Related Dermatoses with Select Examples

Fever and rash (petechial or hemorrhagic): dengue fever, arboviruses, rickettsial infections (e.g., scrub typhus), Chikungunya, meningococcemia, leptospirosis, malaria, and erythema multiforme caused by drug reaction or common infection
Papular eruptions: insect bites, persistent lesions (chiggers), scabies, allergic drug reactions, cercarial dermatitis (swimmers), *Pseudomonas* folliculitis (hot-tubbing), onchocerciasis (long-term travel)
Persistent nodules: furunculosis, myiasis (movement within the lesion), chancroid, syphilis, systemic parasites/fungi
Migratory swellings or skin lesions: cutaneous larva migrans, strongyloidiasis (fast-moving and often on the buttocks), urticaria from various causes, and loa loa (rarely)
Ulcerative lesions: pyodermas, spider bites, chancroid and syphilis, cutaneous leishmaniasis

LOA LOA (EYE WORM)

Loiasis is caused by a filarial nematode confined to the rain forests of western and central Africa. It is a low risk to short-term travelers but should be suspected among immigrants, refugees, visiting nationals, and expatriates living several months or more in endemic zones. Among travelers, worm burden is usually low, and symptoms are related to hypersensitivity syndromes and not serious disease. The adult worms inhabit subcutaneous tissues, move about freely, and can live for up to 18 years after the patient's last possible exposure. They are spread from the bite of the *Chrysops* fly and take 1 year to mature. Infections are usually asymptomatic; however, at times, infections cause painful or itchy subcutaneous swellings near the face and extremities known as *Calabar swellings*. The most dramatic presentation is when a worm passes across the eye under the conjunctiva, thus coining the disease "eye worm."

Patients will complain of "something in their eye," intense irritation, pain, and swelling of the periorbital tissues. The worm usually moves out of the conjunctiva in 30 minutes, but it takes usually several days for symptoms to subside.

Diagnosis is made by clinical presentation and by evaluating daytime-drawn blood for distinctively sheathed microfilariae and high-grade eosinophilia. Treatment for microfilariae and adult worms is **diethylcarbamazine citrate,** 2 milligrams/kg PO three times daily for 3 weeks. In patients with very high microfilariae counts, diethylcarbamazine citrate may induce a sudden severe hypersensitivity and encephalitic syndrome, so treatment is begun with a very small dose. Alternatives are albendazole or blood filtration to remove large numbers of larvae. Surgical excision is not recommended because multiple worms may not be visible. Subconjunctival worms, however, can be removed from the eye with analgesia and fine tweezers.

CREEPING ERUPTION (CUTANEOUS LARVA MIGRANS)

This erythematous "creeping eruption" commonly occurs among tropical travelers and beach resort vacationers who walk barefoot or sit in beach sand contaminated by dog feces harboring the parasite *Ancylostoma braziliense*.[19] The lesions are typically slow moving, tracking, and serpiginous, and are a result of an inflammatory reaction from the worm, which is unable to complete its growth cycle in humans (it is only an effective parasite of dogs or cats). Pruritus causes sleeplessness and restlessness, and diagnosis is based on clinical presentation and eosinophilia. Treatment consists of **albendazole**, 400 milligrams daily for 3 to 7 days, or a single dose of ivermectin, 200 micrograms/kg once.

Liquid nitrogen freezing or surgical excision is not recommended because of scarring.

CUTANEOUS LEISHMANIASIS

Cutaneous leishmaniasis is the most important cause of chronic skin ulceration in the world and is spread by sandflies in tropical and subtropical regions of Latin America, Africa, the Middle East, and Asia. This should be suspected among travelers such as military personnel, biologists, ecotourists, and adventure travelers, and should be part of the differential diagnosis of cutaneous ulcers among travelers, foreign visitors, and immigrants from endemic areas. Although there are a variety of subtypes causing varying infections, the common presentation is of a small papule slowly enlarging and forming a painless shallow skin ulcer with a noticeable rolled edge like a volcano, with a raised edge and central crater, often with a scab. Diagnosis is made by tissue biopsy of the indurated ulcer margin or scraping of the base with material placed on a slide followed by Giemsa stain. Many forms are self-limiting; treat based on clinical presentation and in concert with infectious disease consultants or the Centers for Disease Control and Prevention Parasitic Diseases Branch.

BANCROFTIAN FILARIASIS (*WUCHERERIA BANCROFTI*)

Bancroftian filariasis, a filarial disease, is caused by nematodes residing in the subcutaneous tissues and lymphatics for up to 10 years. It is common to South America, Africa, and Asia and the risk to short-term travelers is low, although cases are imported by long-term travelers. It is transmitted by flies or mosquitoes permitting larvae to enter the puncture wound during their blood meal. Adult filariae then reside in lymphatics and produce microfilariae that migrate to the bloodstream at night. Because the incubation period is long, first symptoms usually develop after 6 months or later (up to 5 years). The most common symptom is recurrent bouts of "filarial fevers" lasting 2 to 3 weeks, associated with warmth and tenderness overlying a lymphatic vessel, followed by retrograde lymphangitis. The most frequently affected sites are extremities, breasts, and spermatic cord. As more attacks occur, lymphatics are chronically damaged, and the most important consequence is the disfiguring and ostracizing condition elephantiasis. Diagnosis depends on finding the sheathed microfilariae in a nocturnal peripheral blood smear. Serology is often useful in mild infections. Treatment is **diethylcarbamazine citrate**, 2 milligrams/kg three times daily for 3 weeks. This drug is well tolerated but can cause hypersensitivity reactions because of early antigen liberation, resulting in fever, headache, nausea, and urticaria. Symptoms can be reduced by starting with a small dose. Repeated treatment may be necessary.

DISEASES COMMONLY ASSOCIATED WITH PULMONARY COMPLAINTS

Returning travelers frequently develop respiratory complaints such as persistent cough, sinus congestion, and fever, and such nonspecific symptoms may be due to travel-related causes such as malaria, typhoid fever, typhus, and dengue. Common local respiratory pathogens, such as viral causes like influenza, and bacterial infections are the most common triggers. Risk factors for pulmonary disease include prolonged air travel with recirculation of dry cabin air and exposure to fellow travelers with infectious agents. Long-term travelers are at increased risk for tuberculosis that may manifest many years after travel. **In the ED, isolate the patient** because contagious infections such as tuberculosis, influenza, or coronaviruses, such as severe acute respiratory syndrome or Middle East respiratory syndrome, are possible. Also, have healthcare workers use personal protective devices.

Once public health threats are reasonably excluded, the evaluation is similar as for any nontravel patients. Additionally, ask about travel-related risk factors because a variety of pathogens such as viruses (viral hemorrhagic fevers), helminths (*Strongyloides*, *Schistosoma*, *Paragonimus*, *Ascaris*), and protozoa (*E. histolytica*, *Trypanosoma*, *Leishmania*) produce pulmonary symptoms or radiographic infiltrates.

MIDDLE EAST RESPIRATORY SYNDROME, SEVERE ACUTE RESPIRATORY SYNDROME, AND EMERGING INFECTIONS

Between September 2012 and February 2014, the World Health Organization reported a total of 182 cases of the Middle East respiratory syndrome coronavirus infection with 79 deaths[20]; cases now exist in the United States. Like the 2003 to 2004 outbreak of severe acute respiratory syndrome, Middle East respiratory syndrome is caused by a coronavirus. The Centers for Disease Control and Prevention defines clinical criteria for a suspected case of Middle East respiratory syndrome as follows:

- Fever (≥38°C, 100.4°F) and pneumonia or acute respiratory distress syndrome (based on clinical or radiological evidence);

  AND
- history of travel from countries in or near the Arabian Peninsula within 14 days before symptom onset;

  OR
- close contact with a symptomatic traveler who developed fever and acute respiratory illness (not necessarily pneumonia) within 14 days after traveling from countries in or near the Arabian Peninsula;

  OR
- is a member of a cluster of patients with severe acute respiratory illness (e.g., fever and pneumonia requiring hospitalization) of unknown etiology in which MERS-CoV [Middle East respiratory syndrome coronavirus] is being evaluated, in consultation with state and local health departments.[21]

Although not certain, Middle East respiratory syndrome is likely to be spread by "droplet infection," through exposure to respiratory droplets spread by a cough or sneeze from an infected person. Polymerase chain reaction can be used to detect Middle East respiratory syndrome coronavirus.

Preventative measures are aimed at reducing close contact with infected persons and nosocomial transmission. Hospitalized patients should be placed on airborne precautions, and healthcare providers should use gowns, gloves, eye protection, and respiratory protection with a minimum of an N95 mask.[22] Medical personnel treating patients suspected of infection with Middle East respiratory syndrome coronavirus should promptly notify local and state health departments of the case.

Treatment of Middle East respiratory syndrome is supportive care.

TUBERCULOSIS

Refugees and immigrants or expatriate workers (especially healthcare workers) returning from endemic areas are at higher risk of clinical tuberculosis (e.g., Eastern Europe, Africa, Asia). The risk of tuberculosis in travelers is approximately 3% per year of stay in endemic areas. High-risk sites for multidrug-resistant mycobacteria are Russia, Eastern Europe, Southeast Asia, China, southern Africa and South America. The initial ED management of suspected tuberculosis after respiratory isolation is discussed elsewhere (see chapter 67, "Tuberculosis").

PARAGONIMUS (LUNG FLUKE DISEASE)

Paragonimus westermani is a trematoidal infection primarily affecting the lungs. It is widely distributed, but is mostly found in the Far East and Southeast Asia (China is the major endemic site). It is uncommon in short-term travelers but should be considered among immigrants or long-term residents of Asia who are also at risk for tuberculosis and among travelers indulging in local exotic foods. Humans are infected by swallowing larvae contaminating raw or pickled crustaceans. Incubation lasts 6 to 12 weeks, as larvae migrate from the duodenum to the lungs, where they cause cough (sometimes with rusty sputum), pleuritic chest pain, and hemoptysis. Chest pain is often present, and fever with night sweats may occur during early infections, causing tuberculosis to be incorrectly diagnosed.

Chest radiographs demonstrate diffuse segmental infiltrates, nodules, ring cysts, or pleural effusions. Suspect paragonimiasis when no sputum smear acid-fast bacilli are found. If parasites do not reach the lung, diverse symptoms develop depending on fluke location. Symptoms include abdominal pain, diarrhea, migrating subcutaneous swelling, blindness, epididymis, testicular inflammation, and a variety of cerebral symptoms. Seizures can occur from intracranial encysted adults. Diagnosis is made by finding the characteristic eggs in sputum, urine, or stool, or by serologic tests. The treatment of choice is **praziquantel** or **bithionol**.

PARASITE-INDUCED BRONCHOSPASM

The most common helminths causing pulmonary symptoms are *Ascaris* and *Strongyloides*. A suggestive clinical history includes recent travel and ingestion of local food of uncertain quality. Suspicion should be raised by any new pulmonary symptoms such as cough or wheezing associated with patchy infiltrates on chest radiograph and hypereosinophilia. For diagnosis and treatment for each helminth, see previous respective sections.

REFERENCES

The complete reference list is available online at www.TintinalliEM.com.

CHAPTER 162 Occupational Exposures, Infection Control, and Standard Precautions

Charissa B. Pacella

INTRODUCTION

The U.S. Occupational Safety and Health Administration defines *occupational exposure* as a "reasonably anticipated skin, eye, mucous membrane, or parenteral contact with blood or other potentially infectious materials that may result from the performance of the employee's duties."[1] Blood is defined as "human blood, blood products, or blood components."[1] *Other potentially infectious materials* are defined as "human body fluids, such as saliva, semen, and vaginal secretions; cerebrospinal, synovial, pleural, pericardial, peritoneal, and amniotic fluids; any body fluids visibly contaminated with blood; unfixed human tissue or organs; HIV [human immunodeficiency virus] or HBV [hepatitis B virus] containing cell or tissue cultures, culture mediums, or other solutions; and all body fluids where it is difficult or impossible to differentiate between body fluids."[1] Healthcare workers should treat all bodily secretions, fluids, and tissues as potentially infectious.

The Hospital Infection Control Practices Advisory Committee of the Centers for Disease Control and Prevention lists select infections and conditions that may be encountered in the ED, along with recommended occupational exposure precautions.[2-4] The concept of *standard precautions* is built on the premise that healthcare workers cannot readily identify patients who are infected or at risk for infection. This is why using infection control practices and personal protective equipment during all patient care activities is key.

U.S. Occupational Safety and Health Administration federal regulations prescribe safeguards to protect workers and reduce risk of exposure to blood and body fluids.[5] Updated and detailed standards (known as the Bloodborne Pathogens Standard) are in Title 29 of the *Code of Federal Regulations* and amended by the Needlestick Safety and Prevention Act.[6,7] The standards require healthcare facilities (1) to develop a written exposure control plan, (2) to use engineering controls to reduce risk by removing the hazard or isolating the worker from exposure, (3) to use work practice controls to standardize and maximize the safety with which work tasks are performed, (4) to identify mechanisms for compliance with Title 29 standards, and (5) to communicate workplace hazards to those with potential for bloodborne disease exposures. The Centers for Disease Control and Prevention and U.S. Occupational Safety and Health Administration Web sites provide the most up to date information regarding current regulations and standards.

PORTALS FOR EXPOSURE

Portals for infectious disease entry are percutaneous, mucous membrane (oral, ocular, nasal, vaginal, or rectal), respiratory, and dermal. The risk of infection in an exposed healthcare provider depends on (1) the route (portal) of exposure, (2) the concentration (number of organisms) of the pathogen in the infectious material, (3) the infectious characteristics (virility) of the pathogen, (4) the volume (dose) of infectious material, and (5) the immunocompetence (susceptibility) of the exposed individual.

Percutaneous exposures pose the highest risk of transmission for bloodborne disease. Needle sticks and lacerations by sharp objects account for the majority of percutaneous injuries. Phlebotomy, initiation of IV access, manipulation of access devices, suturing, and medication injection all put workers at risk.

Mucous membrane exposures result from splatters, splashes, and sprays of blood and body fluids. Tasks associated with risk of mucous membrane exposure include wound management (hemorrhage control, exploration, irrigation, debridement), airway suctioning, nasogastric or orogastric tube placement, intubation, and specimen handling.

Respiratory exposures occur through inhalation of airborne or droplet particulate materials. Exposure risk grows when an individual is confined with an expectorating, coughing, or sneezing patient for prolonged periods or in a poorly ventilated environment.

Dermal exposure involves skin contact with patients (direct contact) or environmental surfaces or objects contaminated with infectious materials (indirect contact). The risk of infection increases if the contact involves a large surface area or nonintact skin (abraded, chapped, or excoriated). Drug-resistant organisms (e.g., methicillin-resistant *Staphylococcus aureus*, vancomycin-resistant enterococci) and parasites of the integument (e.g., scabies, lice) are transmitted by dermal exposure. Workplace activities associated with dermal exposure include patient examination, turning or moving patients, and changing linens or wound dressings. Healthcare workers are also at risk for hypersensitivity reactions to specific inert substances, notably latex, after prolonged or repeated dermal exposure.

INFECTION CONTROL

Infection control practices seek to prevent transmission of microbial agents and to provide a wide margin of safety for healthcare workers. **These practices include hand washing; use of personal protective equipment; cleaning, disinfecting, and sterilizing patient care equipment and environmental surfaces; decontamination and laundering of soiled uniforms, clothing, and patients' linens; disposal of needles, sharps, and infectious waste; and patient location.** Infection control measures that are simple, part of the routine work environment, and uniform across all situations have the greatest likelihood of compliance.

A complete infection control program includes administrative controls, equipment engineering, work practice controls, education of the workforce, and medical management.

Administrative controls organize, define, and direct infection control activities. The written infection control (exposure) plan defines all policies, procedures, and activities related to the education, prevention, and management of infectious diseases in the workforce. Initial and recurrent training in infectious disease hazards and risk activities must be provided to all healthcare workers.

Equipment engineering reduces employee exposure by removing hazards or isolating healthcare workers from exposure. Examples include self-sheathing needles, needleless drug administration devices, sharps containers, disposable airway equipment, syringe splash guards, and personal protective equipment. Medical safety devices reduce occupational exposures experienced by healthcare personnel and should be used whenever possible.

TABLE 162-1 Task-Specific Recommendations for Use of Personal Protective Equipment

Patient Care Activity	Disposable Gloves	Mask and Protective Eyewear	Impervious Gown
Measuring blood pressure	No*	No	No
Measuring pulse	No*	No	No
Measuring temperature	No*	No	No
Examination of bleeding patient	Yes	No†	No†
Wound management, dressing	Yes	No†	No†
Minor hemorrhage control	Yes	No†	No†
Profuse hemorrhage control	Yes	Yes	Yes
Cardiopulmonary resuscitation	Yes	No†	No†
Venipuncture	Yes	No	No
IV line placement	Yes	No	No
IM, SC, IV medication administration	Yes	No	No
Cricothyrotomy, needle decompression	Yes	Yes	No
Intubation, airway adjunct placement, suctioning	Yes	Yes	No†
Childbirth	Yes	Yes	Yes
Nasogastric or orogastric tube placement	Yes	Yes	No†
Specimen handling	Yes	No	No

*Use gloves if task performance includes possible contact with patient's blood, secretions, or body fluids.

†Use mask, protective eyewear, and impervious gown if possibility of splashing or spray exists.

Personal protective equipment is "specialized clothing or equipment which does not permit blood or potentially infectious substances to pass through or reach worker clothing, skin, eyes, mouth, or other mucous membranes under normal conditions of use."[1] Personal protective equipment includes examination gloves, facemasks, eye protection, face shields, and impervious gowns, leggings, and shoe covers. Personal protective equipment mitigates occupational exposures experienced by healthcare personnel; it limits but does not eliminate exposure risks. Recommendations for task-specific use of personal protective equipment are provided in **Table 162-1**.[8]

Work practice controls modify the performance of a task to minimize exposure to blood and blood-containing body fluids and infectious materials. Work practice controls include policies to guide disposal of needles and sharps containers (i.e., avoid shearing, bending, recapping, or breaking); disposal of contaminated linens, clothing, and infectious waste; disinfection of reusable equipment; and restriction of employee activities (eating, drinking, smoking, and application of cosmetics) in work areas where there is a reasonable likelihood of exposure to blood and body fluids.

Workforce education includes information about the agents of infectious disease, epidemiology, disease transmission, signs and symptoms, risky work activities, risk reduction strategies, and postexposure management. Education must occur at the time of initial employment, with recurrent training at specified intervals.

Medical management practices include preexposure preventive vaccinations, postexposure medical evaluation, testing, infectious disease counseling, disease prophylaxis, and referral. The U.S. Occupational Safety and Health Administration mandates preexposure vaccines at initial employee training and within 10 days of employment for all personnel at risk of exposure.[1] The Advisory Committee on Immunization Practices and the Hospital Infection Control Practices Advisory Committee make specific recommendations concerning the use of certain immunizing agents in healthcare personnel.[9]

TABLE 162-2 Outline for Management of Exposures to Blood or Body Fluids

Expedite medical evaluation.
Irrigate exposed areas with water; wash wounds with soap and water.
Obtain history regarding exposure circumstances, source patient, and vaccination history of exposed person (Table 162-3).
Obtain blood samples for laboratory studies (using consents when required) from exposed person; obtain urine pregnancy test for women of childbearing potential.
Order laboratory studies from source patient if known (using consents when required).
Determine need for tetanus immunization.
Determine need for hepatitis B PEP (Table 162-6).
Determine need for human immunodeficiency virus PEP (Table 162-7) and mechanism for dosing as rapidly as possible.
Counsel exposed person regarding risk of specific bloodborne pathogens and discuss risks/benefits of available treatment options.
Review dosing and side effects of recommended treatments (Table 162-8).
Arrange follow-up through employee health clinic within 72 h. Obtain expert consultation in appropriate cases (Table 162-9).

Abbreviation: PEP = postexposure prophylaxis.

EXPOSURE TO HEPATITIS B, HEPATITIS C, AND HUMAN IMMUNODEFICIENCY VIRUS

Once an infectious exposure has occurred, healthcare workers should have access to a plan for postexposure prophylaxis (PEP) medical management 24 hours a day. The plan should include immediate medical assessment, risk analysis, counseling, treatment and prophylaxis, and follow-up appropriate to the type and source of the exposure.[9-14]

An outline for a standardized initial approach is shown in **Table 162-2**.[11]

The medical record of care for the exposed patient (the occupational exposure report) should contain specific information relative to the exposure incident. Key elements include the circumstances of exposure, medical history of the source person, and medical history of the exposed person per Centers for Disease Control and Prevention recommendations (**Table 162-3**).[10]

INITIAL TREATMENT AND ASSESSMENT

Thoroughly wash exposed wounds and skin sites with soap and water, and irrigate mucous membranes with water. **Do not apply** caustics (bleach), antiseptics, or disinfectants directly to the wound.

TABLE 162-3 Recommendations for the Contents of the Occupational Exposure Report

Date and time of exposure.
Details of the procedure being performed, including where and how the exposure occurred; if related to a sharp device, the type and brand of device and how and when in the course of handling the device the exposure occurred.
Details of the exposure, including the type and amount of fluid or material and the severity of the exposure (e.g., for a percutaneous exposure, depth of injury and whether fluid was injected; for a skin or mucous membrane exposure, the estimated volume of material and the condition of the skin [e.g., chapped, abraded, intact]).
Details about the exposure source (e.g., whether the source material contained hepatitis B virus, hepatitis C virus, or HIV; if the source is HIV infected, the stage of disease and prognosis, history of antiretroviral therapy, viral load, and antiretroviral resistance information, if known).
Details about the exposed person (e.g., hepatitis B vaccination and vaccine-response status).
Details about counseling, postexposure management, and follow-up.

Abbreviation: HIV = human immunodeficiency virus.

TABLE 162-4 Factors to Consider in Assessing Healthcare Workers After Occupational Exposures

Type of exposure
Percutaneous injury
Mucous membrane exposure
Nonintact skin exposure
Bites resulting in blood exposure to either person involved
Type and amount of fluid/tissue
Blood
Fluids containing blood
Potentially infectious fluid or tissue (semen; vaginal secretions; and cerebrospinal, synovial, pleural, peritoneal, pericardial, and amniotic fluids)
Direct contact with concentrated virus
Infectious status of source
Presence of hepatitis B surface antigen
Presence of HCV antibody
Presence of HIV antibody
Susceptibility of exposed person
Hepatitis B vaccine and vaccine response status
HBV, HCV, and HIV immune status

Abbreviations: HBV = hepatitis B virus; HCV = hepatitis C virus; HIV = human immunodeficiency virus.

Evaluate the exposure event for the potential to transmit hepatitis B virus, hepatitis C virus, and human immunodeficiency virus (HIV) based on the type of body substance involved and the route and volume of the exposure (**Table 162-4**).[10] Blood, fluid containing visible blood, human tissue, or other potentially infectious material (including semen, vaginal secretions, and cerebrospinal, synovial, pleural, peritoneal, pericardial, and amniotic fluids) may transmit bloodborne viruses. Percutaneous injury or mucous membrane contact with these substances conveys risk for virus transmission. Dermal contact with these substances does not convey risk of virus transmission unless the skin is *not* intact (abraded, chapped, excoriated, open wound).

TESTING FOR EXPOSURE

Perform diagnostic testing to determine the hepatitis B virus, hepatitis C virus, and HIV infection status of an exposure source as soon as possible and with consent (**Table 162-5**).[10] If possible, obtain a rapid HIV-antibody on the exposure source; direct viral assays (HIV p24 antigen enzyme immunoassay, HIV RNA, hepatitis C virus RNA) are not recommended. Testing of needles or sharps instruments for contamination is also not recommended. If the exposure source is HIV positive, obtain additional information as available including CD4+ T-cell count, viral load, current and previous antiretroviral therapy, and history of antiretroviral resistance and prognosis to help identify optimal PEP regimen. If this information is not known at the time of exposure, do not delay the initiation of PEP, as changes in the regimen may be made on follow-up within 72 hours after exposure.[10]

TABLE 162-5 Evaluation of Occupational Exposure Sources

Known sources
Test known sources for hepatitis B surface antigen, anti–hepatitis C virus, and HIV antibody.
Direct virus assays for routine screening of source patients are *not* recommended.
Consider using a rapid HIV-antibody test.
If the source person is *not* infected with a bloodborne pathogen, baseline testing or further follow-up of the exposed person is *not* necessary.
For sources whose infection status remains unknown (e.g., the source person refuses testing), consider medical diagnoses, clinical symptoms, and history of risk behaviors.
Do not test discarded needles for bloodborne pathogens.
Unknown sources
For unknown sources, evaluate the likelihood of exposure to a source at high risk for infection.
Consider likelihood of bloodborne pathogen infection among patients in the exposure setting.

Abbreviation: HIV = human immunodeficiency virus.

HEPATITIS B VIRUS EXPOSURE AND PEP

Factors in the management of hepatitis B virus exposure include the hepatitis B surface antigen status of the source and the hepatitis B vaccination and vaccine response status of the exposed person. Following a percutaneous exposure, the estimated risks of hepatitis in unvaccinated healthcare workers are 22% to 31% (source patient positive for hepatitis B surface antigen and hepatitis B e antigen) and 1% to 6% (source patient positive for hepatitis B surface antigen and negative for hepatitis B e antigen). The estimated risk of transmission is lower following mucous membrane exposure, nonintact skin exposure, or an exposure involving nonbloody fluids or tissues.[10] Every unvaccinated healthcare worker exposed to blood or body fluids should receive the hepatitis B vaccine series. For the rest, recommendations for PEP following hepatitis B virus exposure vary according to the hepatitis B surface antigen status of the exposure source and the vaccination/vaccine-response status of the exposed person (**Table 162-6**).[10] If hepatitis B immunoglobulin is indicated, give it as soon as possible after the exposure (ideally within 24 hours); after 7 days, the effectiveness of hepatitis B immunoglobulin is unknown.

The **Hepatitis Hotline** provides guidance to clinicians with regard to the acute and chronic management of hepatitis (**1-888-443-7232, http://www.cdc.gov/hepatitis**).

HEPATITIS C VIRUS EXPOSURE

For occupational hepatitis C virus exposures, the Centers for Disease Control and Prevention recommends anti–hepatitis C virus testing of the source patient. Test the exposed person for anti–hepatitis C virus and alanine aminotransferase at baseline and follow-up (at 4 to 6 months), and testing for hepatitis C virus RNA may be performed at 4 to 6 weeks after exposure if needed to aid early diagnosis of hepatitis C virus. Confirm all positive anti–hepatitis C virus tests by enzyme immunoassay with supplemental testing (i.e., recombinant immunoblot assay). If the source patient is hepatitis C virus infected, the mean estimated risk of transmission is 1.8% after a percutaneous exposure (range 0% to 7%). Estimated risk of transmission is even lower following mucous membrane exposure, nonintact skin exposure, or an exposure involving nonbloody fluids or tissues.[10] Immunoglobulin and antivirals are not recommended for PEP after exposure to hepatitis C virus–positive blood.

Healthcare workers exposed to hepatitis B virus– or hepatitis C virus–infected blood do not need to take any precautions to prevent secondary transmission during the follow-up period; however, they should not donate blood, plasma, organs, tissue, or semen.

HIV EXPOSURE AND PEP

Healthcare workers potentially exposed to HIV should receive expedited evaluation and baseline testing for HIV. Factors in the management of HIV exposure include the type of exposure (percutaneous, mucous membrane, or dermal), the volume of the exposure (small or large), and the HIV status of the source. Risk of HIV transmission following percutaneous exposure increases with exposure to a larger quantity of blood as indicated by (1) a device visibly contaminated with blood, (2) a needle placed in the source patient's artery or vein, (3) a large-bore hollow needle, or (4) a deep injury.[16] If the source patient is HIV infected, the estimated risk of transmission is 0.3% after a percutaneous exposure and 0.09% after a mucous membrane exposure. Estimated risk of transmission following a nonintact skin exposure or an exposure involving nonbloody fluids or tissues is even lower.[14]

TABLE 162-6 Postexposure Prophylaxis for Percutaneous and Mucous Membrane Exposure to Hepatitis B Virus

Vaccination and Antibody Response Status of Exposed Workers	Treatment		
	Source Is HBsAg Positive	Source Is HBsAg Negative	Source Is Unknown or Not Available for Testing
Unvaccinated/nonimmune	HBIG* × 1 and initiate HB vaccine series	Initiate HB vaccine series	Initiate HB vaccine series
Previously vaccinated			
Previously vaccinated known responder†	No treatment	No treatment	No treatment
Previously vaccinated known nonresponder‡	HBIG × 1 and initiate revaccination or HBIG × 2#	No treatment	If known high-risk source, treat as if source were HBsAg positive
Previously vaccinated antibody response unknown	Test exposed person for anti-HBs[f] 1. If adequate,† no treatment is necessary 2. If inadequate,‡ administer HBIG × 1 and vaccine booster	No treatment	Test exposed person for anti-HBs[f] 1. If adequate,† no treatment is necessary 2. If inadequate,‡ administer vaccine booster and recheck titer in 1–2 mo

Note: Ideally, HBIG and first vaccination should be initiated within 24 hours of exposure. Persons who have previously been infected with hepatitis B virus are immune to reinfection and do not require postexposure prophylaxis.

Abbreviations: HB = hepatitis B; HBIG = hepatitis B immunoglobulin; HBsAg = hepatitis B surface antigen.

*Dose is 0.06 mL/kg IM.

†A responder is a person with adequate levels of serum antibody to HBsAg (i.e., anti-HBs ≥10 mIU/mL).

‡A nonresponder is a person with inadequate response to vaccination (i.e., serum anti-HBs <10 mIU/mL).

#The option of giving one dose of HBIG and reinitiating the vaccine series is preferred for nonresponders who have not completed a second three-dose vaccine series. For persons who previously completed a second vaccine series (≥6 doses) but failed to respond, two doses of HBIG are preferred one month apart.[15]

[f]Antibody to HBsAg.

If the source patient has a negative HIV antibody test, baseline testing and further follow-up of the exposed person are not normally necessary. If the source patient has a positive HIV antibody test, consider the source to be HIV positive *regardless of viral load* for the purpose of PEP and follow-up testing. Exposure to a source patient with an undetectable viral load does not eliminate the possibility of HIV transmission. If the source patient is suspected to have acute retroviral syndrome, consider the source to be HIV positive regardless of HIV test result.

PEP should be initiated as soon as possible; if later testing determines the source to be HIV negative, discontinue PEP. PEP is less effective if started more than 24 to 36 hours after exposure. The interval after which no benefit is gained is unknown, so start PEP even when the postexposure interval exceeds 36 hours.

The U.S. Public Health Service provides guidelines for PEP following occupational exposure to HIV.[14] Guidelines now recommend three (or more) tolerable antiretroviral drugs for all occupational exposures to HIV as shown in **Tables 162-7 and 162-8**. Anticipate side effects and consider preemptive prescribing of ameliorating medications to improve PEP regimen adherence.[14] Also, consult with a local expert or with the **National Clinicians' Post-Exposure Prophylaxis Hotline (PEPline at 1-888-448-7737)** for the more complex situations listed in **Table 162-9**. If a delay in obtaining expert input occurs, start postexposure therapy immediately, allowing later discontinuation based on new information or expert consultation. The optimal duration of PEP is unknown, but the Centers for Disease Control and Prevention recommends 4 weeks of treatment.[10]

Following an exposure to HIV, advise healthcare workers to be reevaluated within 72 hours to assess information about the source patient. Also, emphasize the importance of adherence to the PEP regimen for the duration of treatment. Similarly, recommend that all exposed healthcare personnel try to prevent secondary transmission, especially during the first 6 to 12 weeks after exposure, by doing the following: use condoms or exercise sexual abstinence; refrain from donating blood, plasma, organs, tissue, or semen; avoid pregnancy; and, if possible, avoid breastfeeding. Advise exposed workers to seek medical evaluation for any acute illness that occurs during the follow-up period, as this may signal the onset of acute retroviral syndrome. Follow-up testing includes HIV testing at baseline and at 6 weeks, 12 weeks, and 6 months after exposure, usually concluded 4 months after the exposure if a newer fourth-generation HIV p24 antigen-HIV antibody test is negative.

TABLE 162-7 Human Immunodeficiency Virus (HIV) Postexposure Prophylaxis (PEP) Regimens

Preferred HIV PEP Regimen	
Raltegravir (400 milligrams twice daily) ***plus*** Truvada® (tenofovir DF 300 milligrams + emtricitabine 200 milligrams once daily)	
Alternative Regimens	
May combine 1 drug or drug pair from the left column with 1 drug or drug pair from the right column. Prescribers unfamiliar with these agents/regimens should consult with a physician familiar with these agents and their toxicities.	
Raltegravir	Tenofovir DF + emtricitabine (Truvada®)
Darunavir + ritonavir	Tenofovir DF + lamivudine
Etravirine	Zidovudine + lamivudine (Combivir®)
Rilpivirine	Zidovudine + emtricitabine
Atazanavir + ritonavir	
Lopinavir/ritonavir (Kaletra®)	
The following alternative is a complete fixed-dose combination regimen	
Elvitegravir, cobicistat, tenofovir DF + emtricitabine (Stribild®)	
Other alternative antiretroviral regimens should be used for PEP only with expert consultation.	

TABLE 162-8 Drugs Commonly Used for Human Immunodeficiency Virus Postexposure Prophylaxis (PEP)

Drug (Trade Name; Abbreviation)	Dosage	Advantages/Disadvantages
Atazanavir (Reyataz®; ATV)	ATV 300 milligrams + RTV 100 milligrams once daily (preferred dosing for PEP) ATV 400 milligrams once daily without RTV	Well tolerated Jaundice (indirect hyperbilirubinemia), rash, nephrolithiasis, drug interactions, PR prolongation, absorption depends on low pH, must be given with food
Darunavir (Prezista®; DRV)	DRV 800 milligrams + RTV 100 milligrams once daily (preferred dosing for PEP) DRV 600 milligrams + RTV 100 milligrams twice daily	Well tolerated Rash (sulfonamide moiety), diarrhea, nausea, headache, hepatotoxicity, drug interactions, must be given with food and with RTV
Emtricitabine (Emtriva®; FTC)	200 milligrams daily Also component of fixed-dose combinations: Complera®, Stribild®, Truvada®	Well tolerated, minimal toxicity Skin discoloration, withdrawal may cause acute hepatitis exacerbation in the setting of chronic hepatitis B
Lamivudine (Epivir®; 3TC)	3TC: 300 milligrams twice daily (preferred dosing for PEP) Also component of fixed-dose combinations: generic combination lamivudine/zidovudine, Combivir®, Epzicom®, Trizivir®	Well tolerated, minimal toxicity Withdrawal may cause acute hepatitis exacerbation in the setting of chronic hepatitis B
Lopinavir/ritonavir (Kaletra®; LPV/RTV)	LPV/RTV: 400/100 milligrams = 2 tablets twice daily (preferred dosing for PEP) LPV/RTV: 800/200 milligrams = 4 tablets once daily (alternative dosing)	GI intolerance, nausea, vomiting, and diarrhea are common PR and QT prolongation reported Potential for serious or life-threatening drug interactions
Raltegravir (Isentress®; RAL)	400 milligrams twice	Well tolerated, minimal toxicity Insomnia, nausea, fatigue, headache, severe skin and hypersensitivity reactions
Rilpivirine (Endurant®; RPV)	25 milligrams once daily Also component of fixed-dose combination: Complera®	Well tolerated Depression, insomnia, rash, hypersensitivity, headache Potential for serious or life-threatening drug interactions Caution with H_2 blockers, antacids Coadministration with proton pump inhibitors is contraindicated May increase risk for torsade de pointes Must be given with food
Tenofovir DF (Viread®, TDF)	300 milligrams once daily Also component of fixed-dose combinations: Atripla®, Complera®, Stribild®, Truvada®	Well tolerated Asthenia, headache, diarrhea, nausea, vomiting Nephrotoxicity; should not be administered to individuals with acute or chronic kidney injury, or estimated glomerular filtration rate <60 Withdrawal may cause acute hepatitis exacerbation in the setting of chronic hepatitis B
Zidovudine (Retrovir®; ZDV, AZT)	300 milligrams twice daily Also component of fixed-dose combinations: generic lamivudine/zidovudine, Combivir®, Trizivir®	Side effects common and may impact adherence: nausea, vomiting, headache, insomnia, fatigue Anemia, neutropenia

TABLE 162-9 Situations for Which Expert Consultation for Human Immunodeficiency Virus (HIV) Postexposure Prophylaxis (PEP) Is Recommended

Delayed exposure report (>72 h after exposure)

Unknown source (e.g., needle in a sharps disposal container or laundry)

- Decide PEP case by case based on epidemiologic likelihood of HIV exposure.
- Do not test needles or instruments.

Known or suspected pregnancy or breastfeeding in the exposed person

- Provision of PEP should not be delayed awaiting expert consultation.

Toxicity of the initial PEP regimen

- Symptoms are often manageable without changing regimen by prescribing antimotility or antiemetic agents. Counseling and support are encouraged because anxiety may worsen side effects.

Serious medical illness in the exposed person

- Significant underlying illness (e.g., renal disease) or an exposed provider already taking multiple medications may increase the risk of toxicity and drug interactions.

Expert consultation can be made with local experts or by calling the National Clinicians' Post-Exposure Prophylaxis hotline at 1-888-448-7737.

OTHER COMMON OCCUPATIONAL EXPOSURES

Other infectious diseases require special precautions, preventative measures, and postexposure care in order to minimize the risk of occupational exposure. Common sources of other occupational exposures are listed in **Table 162-10**. Maintain high suspicion for disease in populations at risk, and institute isolation precautions promptly when disease is considered.

INFECTION PRECAUTIONS

The Centers for Disease Control and Prevention's Hospital Infection Control Practices Advisory Committee promulgates two tiers of precautions: standard and transmission based. Standard precautions assume a broad approach to healthcare personnel and patient protection by including agents transmitted by routes other than blood. Transmission-based precautions are designed for patients with documented or suspected transmissible pathogens for which additional protection beyond standard precautions is required. Transmission-based precautions are of three types: airborne, droplet, and contact. Transmission-based precautions are to be used in addition to, not in place of, standard precautions.[2-4]

TABLE 162-10 Other Common Occupational Exposures

Disease	Infective Material	Infection Control and PPE*	Vaccine Availability and Efficacy	Employee Vaccination and Testing	Post Exposure Management
Tuberculosis	Aerosolized bacilli and respiratory secretions	Airborne precautions	Yes (BCG) Limited efficacy Widely used outside U.S. Not recommended in U.S.	Vaccine not recommended in U.S. Routine testing (PPD) for those in high-risk areas every 6–12 months	Approximately 20% of exposed people become infected. CDC recommended prophylactic treatment after exposure, but research does not support that practice.[17]
Measles (rubeola)	Respiratory secretions and droplet nuclei	Airborne precautions	Yes Highly effective Monovalent or combination	Primary immunization recommended 2 doses >4 weeks apart	Previously unvaccinated individuals: Vaccine may prevent disease if given within 72 hours of exposure. IG conveys temporary immunity and may prevent or modify disease if given within 6 days of exposure.[18,19]
Mumps	Respiratory secretions	Droplet precautions	Yes Highly effective Monovalent or combination	Primary immunization recommended 2 doses >4 weeks apart	Previously unvaccinated individuals: Vaccine is unlikely to prevent disease but is not harmful and may protect in case of future exposure. IG is not effective and not recommended.[18]
Rubella	Respiratory secretions and contact	Droplet and contact precautions	Yes Highly effective Monovalent or combination	Primary immunization recommended 2 doses >4 weeks apart	Previously unvaccinated individuals: Vaccine is unlikely to prevent disease but is not harmful and may protect in case of future exposure. IG is not effective and not recommended.[18]
Varicella zoster (herpes zoster, chickenpox, shingles)	Respiratory secretions and aerosols from vesicular fluid	Airborne and contact precautions†	Yes Highly effective	Immunization (or evidence of immunity) recommended[20,21]	Previously unvaccinated individuals: Vaccine may prevent infection. VZIG conveys temporary immunity and may prevent or modify disease if given within 4 days. Employee should be on furlough from day 10–21 following exposure.[20]
Influenza	Respiratory secretions	Droplet precautions Recommend exclusion or reassignment of employees who are ill with fever and respiratory symptoms	Yes Efficacy varies annually	Annual immunization recommended[22,23]	Individuals not vaccinated within the past year: Vaccine will not prevent disease but is not harmful and may protect in case of future exposure. Consider oseltamivir or zanamivir for chemoprophylaxis in higher risk employees who experience a significant influenza exposure.[24]
Meningococcus	Respiratory secretions	Droplet precautions	Yes Not recommended without specific indication[25]	None recommended	Chemoprophylaxis should be reserved for individuals who performed mouth-to-mouth, intubated, or suctioned the patient without a mask in the setting of confirmed meningococcus.[26,27] Rifampin 10 milligrams/kg (max 600 milligrams/dose) every 12 hours for 2 days Ceftriaxone 250 milligrams in single dose Ciprofloxacin 500 milligrams in single dose
Severe acute respiratory syndrome[28]	Respiratory secretions and droplet nuclei	Airborne and contact precautions Eye shield	None available	None recommended	No disease-specific recommendations
Scabies (mites)	Direct and indirect contact	Contact precautions	None	None available	No disease-specific recommendations
Pediculosis (lice)	Direct and indirect contact	Contact precautions	None	None available	No disease-specific recommendations

Abbreviations: BCG = bacillus Calmette-Guérin; CDC = Centers for Disease Control and Prevention; IG = immunoglobulin; PPD = purified protein derivative; PPE = personal protective equipment; VZIG = varicella zoster immunoglobulin.

*Standard precaution should always be applied in addition to other recommended precautions.

†If all skin lesions can be covered completely, then contact precautions alone are acceptable.

STANDARD PRECAUTIONS

Standard precautions are exercised when caring for *all* patients and include hand washing/sanitization, gloves, mask and eye protection or face shield, gowns, handling of patient care equipment and linens, environmental controls, workplace controls, and patient location or placement depending on the indication.

Hand Washing Hand washing is required after touching blood, body fluids, secretions, excretions, and contaminated items *even if gloves are worn*. Wash hands immediately after gloves are removed, between patient contacts, and when otherwise indicated to avoid the transfer of organisms to other patients or environments. It may be necessary to wash hands between procedures on the same patient to prevent cross-contamination of different body sites. *Plain soap and water are recommended for routine use*. Washing with an antimicrobial agent or waterless antiseptic may be done for control of outbreaks or hyperendemic infections, but some pathogens, such as *Clostridium difficile*,[29] are not eradicated by alcohol-based antiseptics.

Gloves Use clean, nonsterile gloves when touching blood, body fluids, secretions, excretions, and contaminated items. Change gloves between tasks and procedures involving blood or other potentially infectious materials. Remove gloves and wash hands before touching noncontaminated items or environmental surfaces (e.g., phones, light switches, writing implements) or other patients.

Masks and Shields Facemasks, eye protection, and face shields that are fluid resistant are worn to protect mucous membranes of the eyes, nose, and mouth during patient care activities and procedures likely to generate splashes or sprays of blood, body fluids, secretions, excretions, and infectious materials. Replace masks that are soiled, moistened by the user's exhaled vapor, or contaminated by fluids as soon as possible. Protective function may be lost when the barrier device is completely saturated.

Gowns Clean, nonsterile gowns that are fluid resistant protect the worker's skin and clothing during patient care activities and procedures likely to generate splashes or sprays of blood, body fluids, secretions, and excretions. Replace soiled gowns as soon as possible because barrier protection is lost if the garment is saturated with contamination. Use sleeve protectors, booties, and leggings if exposure to a large volume of contamination or infectious material is anticipated.

Disposal Handle patient care equipment and linens soiled with blood, body fluids, secretions, and excretions specifically to avoid skin and mucous membrane exposure, contamination of clothing, and transfer of microorganisms to other patients and environments. Reusable items should be cleaned and reprocessed to eliminate infectivity. Promptly discard single-use items.

ENVIRONMENTAL AND WORK PRACTICE CONTROLS

Environmental controls include hospital procedures for the decontamination of objects in patient care areas. Clean and disinfect environmental surfaces, beds, bed rails, bedside equipment, and frequently touched surfaces between patient uses.

Workplace controls (work practice controls) include proper disposal of needles, scalpels, and other sharp instruments. Avoid recapping, excessive handling, and manipulation of sharp devices. Use self-sheathing devices and puncture-resistant containers, and replace sharps containers before they overflow. Patients who contaminate the environment or those who cannot assist in their own hygiene should be located in a private room if available.

AIRBORNE PRECAUTIONS

In addition to standard precautions, use airborne precautions for patients known or suspected of being infected with microorganisms transmitted by airborne droplet nuclei. Airborne precautions also apply to small-particle (<5 μm) residue of evaporated droplets containing microorganisms that remain suspended in the air and can be widely dispersed by air currents. Examples of infectious agents spread by this method are found in **Table 162-11**.[2]

TABLE 162-11 Airborne-Spread Infectious Diseases
Rubeola (measles)
Varicella (including disseminated zoster)
Tuberculosis

ISOLATION

Isolate ED patients requiring airborne precautions in an **airborne infection isolation room** with (1) monitored negative air pressure in relation to surrounding areas, (2) 6 to 12 air changes per hour, and (3) discharge of the room air to the outdoors or high-efficiency filtration of the air before it is circulated to other areas in the hospital. The patient must remain in the isolation room with the door closed. Limit the movement in and out of the room and transportation of the patient. When movement is unavoidable, the patient should wear respiratory protection to avoid contamination of other areas within the hospital. Healthcare workers entering the room must wear respiratory protection, such as a personalized, fitted mask with efficient filters (approved particulate respirator).

DROPLET PRECAUTIONS

In addition to standard precautions, use droplet precautions for patients known to have or suspected of having serious illnesses transmitted by large particle droplets (>5 μm). Droplets are generated during talking, sneezing, or coughing and during the performance of procedures. Examples of infectious agents spread by this method are listed in **Table 162-12**.[2,4]

ISOLATION AND FACE MASKS

Place the patient in a private room when possible. Prioritize patients with excessive cough and sputum production to available single-patient rooms. Special air handling and ventilation are not required, and the door may remain open. If a private room is not available, the patient may be placed in a room with other patients who have active infections with the same microorganism (i.e., cohorting). If cohorting is also not possible, place a mask on the patient and maintain a spatial separation of at least 3 ft (1 m) between the infected patient and other patients and visitors. Avoid placing patients with droplet precautions in the same room with patients at increased risk for adverse outcomes from infection. Limit the movement and transportation of patients with droplet precautions. When movement is required, place a face mask on the patient. Healthcare workers should wear face masks when working within 3 ft (1 m) of the patient. Healthcare workers should wear respiratory protection equivalent to a fitted N95 filtering respirator or higher level of protection during aerosol-generating procedures such as suctioning. Change protective attire and perform hand hygiene between contacts with all patients.

TABLE 162-12 Droplet-Spread Infectious Diseases
Invasive *Haemophilus influenzae* type B (including meningitis, pneumonia, epiglottitis, sepsis)
Invasive *Neisseria meningitidis* (including meningitis, pneumonia, sepsis)
Serious bacterial respiratory infections
Diphtheria (pharyngeal)
Mycoplasma pneumonia
Pertussis
Pneumonic plague
Streptococcal pharyngitis, pneumonia, scarlet fever
Serious viral infections
Adenovirus
Influenza (including H1N1)
Mumps
Parvovirus B19
Rubella

TABLE 162-13 Contact-Spread Infectious Diseases

Multidrug-resistant infections or colonization (GI, respiratory, skin, wound sites)
Enteric infections with low infective dose or prolonged environmental survival
Clostridium difficile
Enterohemorrhagic *Escherichia coli* 0157:H7
Shigella
Hepatitis A
Rotavirus
Respiratory syncytial virus
Parainfluenza virus
Enteroviral infections
Skin infections that are highly contagious or that may occur on dry skin:
Diphtheria (cutaneous)
Herpes simplex virus (neonatal or mucocutaneous)
Impetigo
Major, noncontained abscesses, cellulitis, decubiti
Pediculosis
Scabies
Staphylococcal furunculosis
Herpes zoster (disseminated or in an immunocompromised host)
Viral hemorrhagic conjunctivitis
Viral hemorrhagic infections (Ebola, Lassa, Marburg, Crimean-Congo hemorrhagic fever)

CONTACT PRECAUTIONS

In addition to standard precautions, use contact precautions when patients are known to have or suspected of having serious illnesses transmitted by direct patient contact or contact with items in the patient's environment. Examples of such infectious diseases are shown in **Table 162-13.**[2,4]

Change gloves whenever the examination and care of a patient result in contact with infectious materials and a high concentration of microorganisms (wound drainage or fecal material). When expecting contact with infectious materials (incontinence, dressing changes, attention to colostomy), wear a clean, nonsterile gown and gloves. Remove the gown and gloves before leaving the care area. Wash hands with an antimicrobial agent or waterless antiseptic after removal of gloves, and avoid contact with potentially contaminated environmental surfaces or items in the room after hand washing.

Limit transportation and movement of the patient. When movement is required, cover contaminated areas with large, bulky dressings. Bulky, adsorbent, leakproof dressings contain contaminated secretions and limit spread of disease.

Durable, multiuse medical equipment (e.g., blood pressure cuffs, stethoscopes, bedside commodes) should be dedicated to a single patient (or cohort of similarly infected patients). Personnel who use personal medical equipment (e.g., stethoscopes) should thoroughly clean these items between patient contacts to avoid contamination.

LATEX ALLERGY

Rubber latex is a manufactured polymer that exhibits excellent tensile strength, elasticity, and barrier capacity.[30] Rubber latex is in many medical products, including gloves (for surgery, examination, and housekeeping and cleaning), intravascular devices (balloon catheters, IV tubing, and ports), airway devices (nasopharyngeal airways, endotracheal tubes, and oxygen masks), tourniquets, blood pressure cuffs, ECG leads, tape, and dressings.

REACTIONS TO LATEX

Immune reactions to latex products may take three forms: irritant, contact dermatitis (type IV), and immunoglobulin E (type I).

Irritant reactions are nonimmune in nature and result in dry dermal erythema limited to the site of contact.

Contact dermatitis occurs as a result of dermal exposure to chemicals used in the manufacturing of latex products. Thirams and thiazoles are the most common chemicals to induce this type IV response. This reaction, which may extend beyond the site of contact, results in a dry dermal erythema, pruritus, weeping, and vesiculation. Such loss of skin integrity permits the access of latex proteins to the immune system and may result in an immunoglobulin E–mediated response.

An immunoglobulin E (type I) response is an immunologic reaction to protein allergens contained in latex. Clinical manifestations of such reactions include urticaria, asthma, rhinitis, angioedema, laryngeal edema, and anaphylaxis. Immunoglobulin E reactions may occur as a result of mucosal, dermal, contact, or inhalational exposure. Cornstarch powder, which serves as a lubricant to ease the donning of latex gloves, binds and aerosolizes protein allergens, leading to inhalation exposure.

At highest risk of developing immunoglobulin E–mediated latex allergy are those with high exposure to latex and who are atopic. Workers in industries that make rubber products (e.g., tire manufacturers and doll makers) and those who use rubber products (e.g., housekeepers, hairdressers, and healthcare workers) are at high risk of developing this allergy. Although anyone can develop latex allergy, those at higher risk have a history of multiple allergies, asthma, eczema, multiple food allergies, frequent surgical or dental procedures, spina bifida and related conditions of spinal dysraphism, urogenital anomalies, or sensitivity to ethylene oxide (a sterilizing agent).

LATEX-FREE PRODUCTS AND MINIMIZING LATEX ALLERGY

Many latex-free medical products exist on the market and may be substituted for currently used products. Prevention of disease in healthcare workers is critical and requires the use of synthetic or low-allergen powder-free gloves.[30,31] To protect themselves from latex exposure and allergy in the workplace, healthcare personnel may also use nonlatex gloves for workplace activities that do not involve contact with infectious materials, use synthetic or low-allergen powder-free gloves when handling infectious materials, avoid oil-based hand lotions or creams when wearing latex gloves (to prevent glove deterioration), wash hands with mild soap and dry thoroughly upon removal of latex gloves, frequently clean work areas and equipment contaminated with latex-containing dust, obtain education and training regarding latex allergy, and recognize the symptoms of latex allergy. Hypoallergenic latex gloves do not reduce the risk of latex allergy but do reduce reactions to chemical additives in latex.

RESOURCES FOR POSTEXPOSURE PROPHYLAXIS

The National Clinicians' Post-Exposure Prophylaxis Hotline offers 24-hour telephone consultation for physicians managing occupational exposures to bloodborne pathogens (888-448-7737, http://www.nccc.ucsf.edu). The Hepatitis Hotline provides guidance to clinicians with regard to the acute and chronic management of hepatitis (1-888-443-7232, http://www.cdc.gov/hepatitis).

Acknowledgments: The author thanks David M. Cline and Kathy J. Rinnert, the authors of this chapter in the previous edition of this book.

REFERENCES

The complete reference list is available online at www.TintinalliEM.com.

CHAPTER 163

Pharmacology of Antimicrobials

Ralph H. Raasch

ANTIBACTERIAL DRUGS

Effective antibacterial drugs can either inhibit the growth of (bacteriostatic) or kill (bactericidal) bacteria. Antibacterial effects result from the inhibition of cell wall synthesis, inhibition of intrabacterial protein synthesis, alteration in nucleic acid metabolism, or intrabacterial enzyme inhibition (**Table 163-1**). The drug mechanism of action does not necessarily correlate with bacteriostatic or bactericidal effects, because the latter are affected also by the concentration of antibiotic to which bacteria are exposed. Drugs of choice for most infections are not based on a bacteriostatic or bactericidal effect of an agent, but rather are chosen based on whether the drug reaches the site of infection in adequate quantities, the spectrum of the agent, its safety, and cost.

MECHANISMS OF ACTION

CELL WALL ACTIVE AGENTS

β-Lactam (penicillins, cephalosporins) and glycopeptide antibiotics (vancomycin, telavancin, teicoplanin) bind to receptors in the bacterial cell wall. The target receptors for penicillins and cephalosporins are called *penicillin-binding proteins*. Autolytic enzymes within the cell wall bind to penicillin-binding proteins; once activated, the enzymes damage the peptidoglycan component of the cell wall, creating weakening and eventual cell lysis. Glycopeptide antibiotics bind to a terminal dipeptide (alanine-alanine) in the cell wall peptidoglycan and prevent the necessary cross-linking for a competent cell wall structure. At usual doses, β-lactam and glycopeptide antibiotics are bactericidal. Resistance arises due to mutations in the penicillin-binding proteins, leading to reduced β-lactam binding (e.g., by oxacillin-resistant *Staphylococcus aureus* or penicillin-resistant *Streptococcus pneumoniae*) or changes to the terminal dipeptide (e.g., by vancomycin-resistant *Enterococcus faecium*) that reduce the level of binding. Daptomycin inserts a lipophilic part of the molecule into the cell wall of gram-positive bacteria, depolarizing the cell wall, which causes the leakage of intracellular content and a bactericidal effect.

The emergence of multidrug-resistant organisms (most commonly in species of *Pseudomonas, Acinetobacter,* and *Klebsiella*) has led to the renewed use of older, but more toxic drugs such as colistin and polymyxin B. These agents interact with the lipids within the cell wall, increasing cell wall permeability, which leads to a bactericidal effect because of the leakage of intracellular contents.

TABLE 163-1 Mechanisms of Action of Antibacterial Drugs

Cell wall active agents	*Nucleic acid inhibitors*
Penicillins	Fluoroquinolones
Vancomycin	Rifampin
Cephalosporins	Nitrofurantoin
Teicoplanin	***Enzyme inhibitors***
Telavancin	Fosfomycin
Daptomycin	Sulfonamides
Colistin	Trimethoprim
Polymyxin B	
Protein synthesis inhibitors	
Aminoglycosides	
Macrolides	
Linezolid	
Tetracyclines (including tigecycline)	
Clindamycin	
Quinupristin/dalfopristin	

PROTEIN SYNTHESIS INHIBITORS

Several classes of antibacterial drugs bind to ribosomes within bacteria, blocking necessary protein synthesis. Aminoglycosides and tetracyclines (including tigecycline) bind to the 30S ribosomal subunit, whereas macrolide antibiotics and clindamycin bind to the 50S subunit. Ribosomal binding inhibits transfer RNA function, decreasing the amount of protein synthesis. Ribosomal-binding drugs enter through the cell wall and bind in adequate concentrations to reversibly inhibit protein synthesis. Resistance mechanisms arise with reduced cell wall permeability, an active efflux pump that removes the antibiotic from the cell, or ribosomal-binding site mutations that decrease antibiotic affinity.

NUCLEIC ACID INHIBITORS

Fluoroquinolone antibiotics inhibit DNA gyrase, the enzyme responsible for DNA unwinding for transcription and recoiling during bacterial replication. Fluoroquinolones must reach the nucleus of the bacterial cell to provoke these effects; resistance can arise when cell wall permeability is reduced, active efflux occurs, or a DNA gyrase mutation has arisen that reduces fluoroquinolone binding. Rifampin is a broad-spectrum antimicrobial agent active against many gram-positive and gram-negative bacteria and mycobacteria. Rifampin (or rifampicin) inhibits RNA synthesis by binding to DNA-dependent RNA polymerase, thereby blocking the initiation of RNA chain formation. Nitrofurantoin is modified by bacterial metabolism to a compound that damages DNA. Susceptible bacteria rarely become resistant to nitrofurantoin.

ENZYME INHIBITORS

Sulfonamides and trimethoprim block sequential steps in the formation of folic acid. Sulfonamides inhibit dihydropteroate synthase, the enzyme that converts *p*-aminobenzoic acid to dihydrofolic acid; trimethoprim inhibits dihydrofolate reductase, the enzyme that converts dihydrofolic to tetrahydrofolic acid. Together, this paired action is an effective bactericidal process and not far removed from the intracellular actions of methotrexate. Fosfomycin inactivates enolpyruvate transferase, inhibiting cell wall synthesis; it is gaining resurgent popularity for single-dose treatment (3 grams orally) of uncomplicated urinary tract infections given the activity against the common pathogens involved. Resistance to these drugs arises by enzyme mutations that reduce the affinity of sulfonamide, trimethoprim, or fosfomycin to their respective enzyme targets.[1] These antibacterial drug mechanisms of action are summarized in **Figure 163-1**. **Table 163-2** summarizes the classification, names, and routes of the most common antibiotics within each antibiotic class.[1]

INDICATIONS IN THE ED AND DRUGS OF CHOICE

Drugs of choice for specific infections are based on clinical effectiveness and adverse events. Successful effectiveness is based on the knowledge of the likely bacterial pathogen responsible for a specific infection type and the usual antimicrobial spectrum of antibiotics. Alternate drugs of choice are selected in cases of resistance to an initial drug, a history of intolerance or allergy to the drug of choice, or because of a higher risk of adverse events. Taking into account those infections most likely to be present in ED patients and the most likely pathogens involved in these infections, **Table 163-3** summarizes drugs of choice for common infections.[2]

ANTIBIOTIC DOSAGE AND DOSAGE ADJUSTMENTS

Adequate drug dosage takes into account achievable serum and tissue levels plus the concentrations necessary (determined in the laboratory) to inhibit the growth of susceptible bacteria. Standard dosing guidelines usually result in successful treatment when a susceptible organism is present and barriers to drug penetration (i.e., abscess) are absent. If antibiotic penetration issues exist, such as in suspected meningitis,

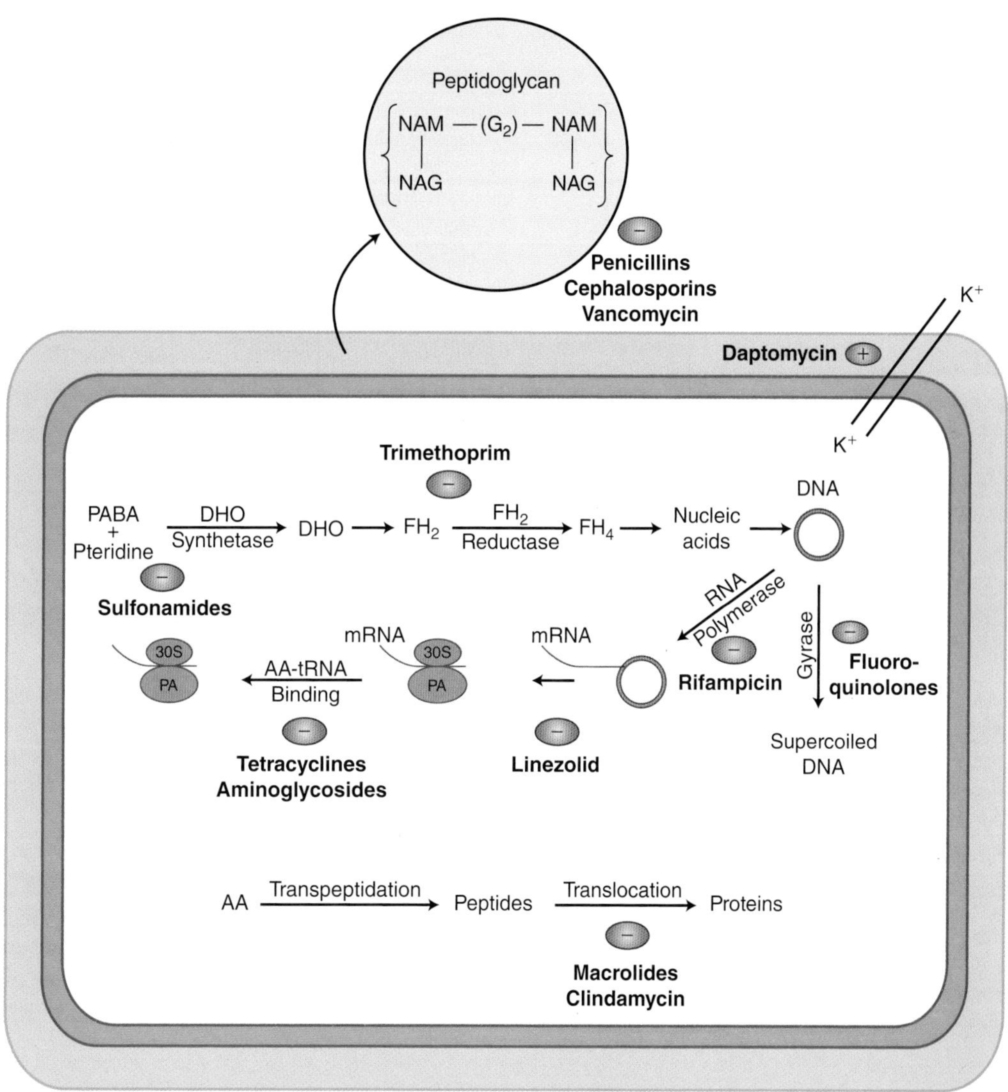

FIGURE 163-1. Mechanisms of action of antibacterial drugs. The peptidoglycan layer in the bacterial cell wall is a crystal lattice structure formed from linear chains of two alternating amino sugars, namely *N*-acetylglucosamine (GlcNAc or NAG) and *N*-acetylmuramic acid (MurNAc or NAM). Penicillins, cephalosporins, and vancomycin are cell wall active agents, preventing the necessary cross-linking within the peptidoglycan layer, rendering it incompetent. Other listed antibiotics exert their actions on cellular mechanisms within the bacteria as shown. AA = amino acids; DHO = dihydropteroate; FH_2 = dihydrofolate, FH_4 = tetrahydrofolate; (G_2) = glucose; K^+ = potassium; PA = peptide donor-acceptor site; PABA = *p*-aminobenzoic acid; + = enhance; − = inhibit.

endocarditis, or osteomyelitis, give the highest doses recommended to improve effect.

Dosage adjustments of many antibiotics are necessary for patients with renal disease to prevent adverse events from drug accumulation, most notably when using IV administration. Oral doses are typically lower, so toxic drug accumulation is less likely in those with renal dysfunction. Dosage modifications in liver disease are less clear because of limited ways to accurately assess decreases in drug elimination characteristics or rate. Fosfomycin in single-dose use for urinary tract infection requires no adjustment. Guidelines for dosing adjustment, primarily with IV therapy, are summarized in **Table 163-4**.[3]

ADVERSE EFFECTS AND CONTRAINDICATIONS OF ANTIBACTERIAL DRUGS

Allergic reactions and direct pharmacologic-based toxicity are the two general categories of adverse drug reactions to antibiotics.

Allergic reactions are not dose related, are unpredictable, and cannot be studied effectively in animal models. Allergic reactions vary from mild skin rashes to life-threatening events, such as toxic epidermal necrolysis or anaphylactic reactions. Drug fever, hepatitis, and interstitial nephritis are also examples of allergic drug reactions.

Direct dose-related toxicity is the result of the pharmacologic properties of the drug. These reactions are possible in any recipient if the dose or accumulated drug in the body is high. Dose-related adverse events typically are reversible once the antibiotic is discontinued. There is some predictability to these reactions, such as renal dysfunction caused by an aminoglycoside; these drugs are ideal candidates for appropriate dose adjustments of antibiotics (Table 163-4).

Certain adverse effects of antibiotics, such as pseudomembranous colitis, do not fall into either category; all antibiotics can cause this side effect. The common allergic and dose-related adverse effects of antibacterial drugs are summarized in **Table 163-5**.[3]

CONTRAINDICATIONS AND DRUG INTERACTIONS

DRUG ALLERGY

In general, previous allergy is a contraindication for use. This circumstance is most pertinent for patients with a penicillin or cephalosporin allergy; between 1% and 10% of patients report a penicillin allergy. Some agents exhibit cross-reactivity; those with penicillin or amoxicillin allergy have a higher risk of the same with oral first-generation cephalosporins, likely due to similarities in antibiotic side chain

TABLE 163-2 Classification of Antibacterial Drugs with Common Trade Names

Penicillins

Natural Penicillins	Aminopenicillins	Penicillinase-Resistant Penicillins	Antipseudomonal Penicillins	β-Lactam / β-Lactamase Inhibitor Combination	Monobactams and Carbapenems	Aminoglycosides	Fluoroquinolones
Penicillin G IV, PO	Ampicillin IV, PO	Oxacillin (Bactocill®) IV, PO	Piperacillin IV	Amoxicillin-clavulanic acid (Augmentin®) PO	Aztreonam (Azactam®) IV	Amikacin IV	Moxifloxacin (Avelox®) IV, PO
Penicillin V PO	Amoxicillin (Amoxcil®) PO	Dicloxacillin PO		Ticarcillin-clavulanic acid (Timentin®) IV	Ertapenem (Invanz®) IV	Gentamicin IV	Ciprofloxacin (Cipro®) IV, PO
		Nafcillin (Nallpen®) IV, PO		Ampicillin-sulbactam (Unasyn®) IV	Meropenem (Merrem®) IV	Neomycin (Neo-Fradin®) PO	Levofloxacin (Levaquin®) IV, PO
				Piperacillin-tazobactam (Zosyn®) IV	Imipenem (Primaxin®) IV	Streptomycin IM, IV	Gemifloxacin (Factive®) PO
					Doripenem (Doribax®) IV	Tobramycin IV	

Cephalosporins

First Generation	Second Generation	Third Generation	Fourth/Fifth Generation	Macrolides/Tetracyclines	Enzyme Inhibitors	Miscellaneous
Cefazolin (Ancef®) IV	Cefaclor PO Cefotetan IV	Ceftibuten (Cedax®) PO	Cefepime (Maxipime®) IV	Erythromycin (Erythrocin®) IV, PO	Trimethoprim-sulfamethoxazole (Bactrim®, Septra®) IV, PO	Clindamycin (Cleocin®) IV, PO
Cefadroxil PO	Cefuroxime axetil (Ceftin®) PO	Cefotaxime (Claforan®) IV	Ceftaroline (Teflaro®) IV	Azithromycin (Zithromax®) IV, PO	Trimethoprim PO	Metronidazole (Flagyl®) IV, PO
Cephalexin (Keflex®) PO	Cefprozil PO Cefoxitin (Mefoxin®) IV	Ceftazidime (Fortaz®, Ceptaz®, Tazicef®) IV		Clarithromycin (Biaxin®) PO	Fosfomycin (Monurol®) PO	Nitrofurantoin (Macrodantin®, Macrobid®) PO
	Cefuroxime (Zinacef®) IV	Ceftriaxone (Rocephin®) IV		Tetracycline PO		Quinupristin/dalfopristin (Synercid®) IV
		Cefpodoxime PO		Minocycline (Minocin®) PO		Vancomycin (Vancocin®) IV, PO
		Cefdinir PO		Doxycycline (Vibramycin®) IV, PO		Linezolid (Zyvox®) IV, PO
		Cefixime (Suprax®) PO		Tigecycline (Tygacil®) IV		Daptomycin (Cubicin®) IV

structure, with about a 10% cross-reactivity occurrence. However, true allergies, as documented by antibiotic skin tests, are less common than often stated, so obtaining a clear description is important before choosing alternate therapy. For example, a patient with a history of respiratory distress, wheezing, angioedema, or hives (an immediate-type hypersensitivity) during a previous course of β-lactam treatment may be at higher risk for a life-threatening reaction upon re-exposure to another β-lactam, particularly if the patient reacts to skin tests with the other β-lactam. Unfortunately, with the exception of penicillin, these antibiotic skin tests are not commercially available and not used in clinical practice. So in this case, it would be wise to avoid a penicillin or first-generation cephalosporin, although a carbapenem or third-generation cephalosporin would have little cross-reactivity. On the other hand, if the patient history is a mild maculopapular rash while taking amoxicillin or other penicillin (a delayed-type hypersensitivity reaction), treatment later with a cephalosporin would not likely provoke an allergic event. Similarly, a fainting spell with injection may not represent a drug allergy at all, although it clearly was an adverse event for that treatment interval. Note that sulfa moieties are contained in many other drugs, such as furosemide, thiazides, sulfonylureas (glyburide), and celecoxib. Despite package labeling that suggests cross-sensitivity in a patient who is allergic to sulfonamides is a risk, the frequency of any allergic reaction upon exposure to one of the nonantibiotic sulfas is not common. A patient allergic to sulfonamides is at a higher risk to develop another allergic reaction to another drug, including penicillins.[4] Several of the human immunodeficiency virus protease inhibitor agents also contain a sulfa moiety (amprenavir, fosamprenavir, tipranavir, darunavir), but the risk of cross-reactivity in a sulfonamide-allergic patient is not well known.[4]

DRUG INTERACTIONS

Drug interactions with antibacterial drugs derive from two mechanisms. The first mechanism is an inhibition of absorption of oral antibiotics. The best example of this interaction occurs when any of the tetracycline or fluoroquinolone antibiotics are given at the same time as divalent cations (Ca^{2+}, Mg^{2+}, Fe^{2+}). This reduces absorption, so these agents must not be given orally with calcium or iron preparations or with antacids.

Second, certain antibiotics can slow the metabolism of other drugs by inhibiting several of the hepatic cytochrome P450 enzymes in the liver. In particular, ciprofloxacin, clarithromycin, and trimethoprim-sulfamethoxazole are drugs that are able to provoke this enzyme inhibition. Summaries of these antibiotic contraindications and drug interactions are included in **Tables 163-6 and 163-7**.[3]

ANTIFUNGAL DRUGS

The mechanism of action of antifungal agents is primarily based on actions that decrease cell wall integrity. Amphotericin B and its lipid-based derivatives bind to cell wall ergosterol, increasing cell wall permeability that eventually results in cell lysis. Triazole antifungals (e.g., fluconazole, itraconazole) block ergosterol synthesis by inhibition of a fungal cytochrome P450–dependent enzyme. Echinocandin antifungals (caspofungin, micafungin, and anidulafungin) are other enzyme inhibitors; in this case, the inhibition is of β-glucan synthetase. β-Glucan, like ergosterol, is another necessary component of the cell wall of several fungal species. Flucytosine is an antimetabolite that disrupts DNA function after conversion intracellularly to 5-fluorouracil. These mechanisms of action of antifungal agents are illustrated in **Figure 163-2**.

TABLE 163-3 Antibiotics of Choice for Treatment of Common Adult Infections in the ED

Site/Type of Infection	Suspected Organisms	Drug of Choice	Alternative
Respiratory			
Pharyngitis	Group A streptococci	Penicillin V	Macrolide
Bronchitis,* otitis,* acute sinusitis*	*Streptococcus pneumoniae* *Haemophilus influenzae*	Amoxicillin, amox/clav, or cefuroxime	Macrolide or doxycycline
Epiglottitis	*H. influenzae*, Group A streptococci	Ceftriaxone	Cefuroxime
Community-acquired pneumonia			
Normal host	*S. pneumoniae*, viral, *Mycoplasma*	Azithromycin or doxycycline	Levofloxacin
Aspiration	Aerobes and anaerobes	Clindamycin	Pip/TZ, ceftriaxone plus metronidazole
Alcoholic	*S. pneumoniae*, *Klebsiella*	Ceftriaxone	Levofloxacin
Urinary tract infection	*Escherichia coli* and other enteric gram-negative rods	TMP/SMX†	Ciprofloxacin, cephalexin, nitrofurantoin, or fosfomycin (latter single dose 3 grams PO)
Sexually transmitted infections			
Urethritis	*Neisseria gonorrhea*, *Chlamydia*	Ceftriaxone, azithromycin	Cefixime, doxycycline
Genital ulcers	*Treponema pallidum*, herpes simplex virus	Penicillin G Acyclovir	Doxycycline Valacyclovir
Skin/soft tissue			
Cellulitis	Group A streptococci, *Staphylococcus aureus*	Cephalexin†	Dicloxacillin, clindamycin, TMP/SMX, or vancomycin
Necrotizing fasciitis	Polymicrobial	Imipenem or meropenem Plus vancomycin	—
Fresh/brackish water infections	Mixed flora, *Aeromonas*	TMP/SMX	Fluoroquinolone
Cat bite	*Pasteurella*, mixed flora	Amox/clav	Clindamycin and ciprofloxacin
Meningitis			
Normal host	*S. pneumoniae*, *Neisseria meningitidis*, *S. aureus*	Ceftriaxone and vancomycin	—
Immunocompromised or >50 y old	*Listeria*, *H. influenzae*	Add ampicillin	—
Acute abdomen (perforation)	Gram-negative rods, anaerobes, enterococci	Ampicillin/sulbactam or Pip/TZ	Cefoxitin or cefotetan or imipenem

Abbreviations: amox/clav = amoxicillin/clavulanate; Pip/TZ = piperacillin/tazobactam; TMP-SMX = trimethoprim-sulfamethoxazole.

**Note:* Many authorities question the need for antibiotics for uncomplicated presentations of these diseases; see appropriate chapters in this text to determine indications for treatment.

†Resistance to the listed antibiotic is a significant clinical issue; see chapter 152, "Soft Tissue Infections" for a discussion of alternatives for treatment in the event of known resistance in your community.

These agents for systemic fungal infections are summarized in **Table 163-8**. Multiple topical antifungal preparations are available, as summarized in **Table 163-9**, and are indicated for *Candida* or tinea infections.[1,3]

Of the various lipid-based amphotericin B preparations, liposomal amphotericin B (AmBisome®) is preferred because of a lower rate of infusion-related reactions and a lower frequency of renal dysfunction compared with the other lipid products. Because amphotericin B has the broadest antifungal spectrum of all these systemic agents, it is the preferred drug for empiric therapy until further diagnostics determine the pathogen involved. All amphotericin B infusions, whether conventional (infused over 4 hours) or lipid-based (infused over 2 hours), can be preceded by acetaminophen (650 milligrams PO) and diphenhydramine (Benadryl®, 25 to 50 milligrams PO or IV) given 30 minutes prior to attenuate development of fever and rash.

In addition to infusion-related reactions, amphotericin B also causes renal dysfunction. The lipid-based products reduce but do not eliminate the risk of renal toxicity. The kidney dysfunction created includes renal tubular acidosis and renal wasting of bicarbonate, potassium, and magnesium. When using this antifungal, monitor electrolyte levels and supplement as needed. Amphotericin B may elevate blood urea nitrogen and serum creatinine, although slightly less when using lipid-based products. If this occurs, reduce the daily dose or extend the infusion intervals to every other day if the creatinine level rises to >2.5 to 3.0 milligrams/dL.

Fluconazole, itraconazole, voriconazole, posaconazole, caspofungin, and micafungin do not provoke the renal dysfunction associated with amphotericin B. Occasionally, liver function test elevations and hepatitis result from triazole therapy, so patients on prolonged courses of these drugs should have liver function tests assessed monthly.

Triazoles (particularly itraconazole) can interact with other drugs metabolized by the cytochrome P450 system. In particular, warfarin, phenytoin, cyclosporine, and tacrolimus levels routinely increase in patients on itraconazole. Fluconazole is a less potent inhibitor of cytochrome P450, so interactions are less frequent. Flucytosine can cause reversible bone marrow suppression, with leukopenia and thrombocytopenia. Dose-modification issues are relevant for fluconazole and flucytosine. For creatinine clearance <50 mL/min, reduce fluconazole to 200 milligrams daily and flucytosine to 25 to 37.5 milligrams/kg every 12 hours; for creatinine clearance <10 mL/min, reduce flucytosine to 25 to 37.5 milligrams/kg every 24 hours.[3]

The pregnancy category for the amphotericin products is category B; for the triazoles, caspofungin, and flucytosine, the category is C.

ANTIVIRAL AGENTS

Advances in antiviral agents can treat infections caused by herpes simplex virus I and II, varicella-zoster virus, cytomegalovirus, influenza A and B, human immunodeficiency virus, and hepatitis B and C. **Table 163-10** summarizes the mechanism of action of the agents and spectrum of use for these drugs outside of human immunodeficiency virus and hepatitis.[1] Human immunodeficiency virus care is discussed elsewhere in the text, including postexposure prophylaxis. Uses for the non–human immunodeficiency virus antiviral agents for patients in the ED are summarized in **Table 163-11**. **Table 163-12** summarizes the drugs available and common side effects of drugs for hepatitis B and hepatitis C; dosing is usually outside ED care and not reviewed.[1,3,5,6]

TABLE 163-4 IV Dosage Guidelines for Selected Antibacterial Drugs in Adults

Drug	Major Route of Elimination	Maximum Daily IV Dose (grams)	Dose Adjustment for Creatinine Clearance (mL/min)		
			>50	10–50	<10
Ampicillin	Renal	12	1–2 grams every 4–8 h	1 gram every 6 h	1 gram every 12 h
Ampicillin/sulbactam	Renal	12	1.5–3 grams every 6 h	1.5–3 grams every 12 h	1.5–3 grams every 24 h
Aztreonam	Renal	8	1–2 grams every 6–8 h	1–2 grams every 12 h	1 gram every 12 h
Cefazolin	Renal	8	1–2 grams every 8 h	1 gram every 12 h	1 gram every 24 h
Cefotaxime	Renal	12	1–2 grams every 4–8 h	1–2 grams every 12 h	1 gram every 12 h
Ceftazidime	Renal	6	1–2 grams every 8 h	1–2 grams every 24 h	0.5 gram every 24 h
Ceftriaxone	Biliary	4	1–2 grams every 12–24 h	No adjustments	No adjustments
Cefepime	Renal	4	1–2 grams every 12 h	1–2 grams every 24 h	0.5–1 gram every 24 h
Ciprofloxacin	Renal	1.2	0.4 gram every 8–12 h	0.4 gram every 12 h	0.4 gram every 24 h
Levofloxacin	Renal	0.75	0.25–0.75 gram every 24 h	0.25–0.75 gram every 48 h	0.25–0.5 gram every 48 h
Clindamycin	Biliary	4.8	0.6–0.9 gram every 6–8 h In hepatic failure, limit dose to 0.6 gram every 8 h	No adjustments	No adjustments
Imipenem	Renal	2	0.5 gram every 6–8 h	0.5 gram every 12 h	0.5 gram every 24 h
Meropenem	Renal	3	0.5–1 gram every 8 h	0.5 gram every 12 h	0.5 gram every 24 h
Metronidazole	Biliary	2	0.5 gram every 6–8 h In hepatic failure, limit dose to 0.5 gram every 12 h	No adjustments	No adjustments
Nafcillin, oxacillin	Biliary	12	1–2 grams every 4–6 h	No adjustments	No adjustments
Penicillin G	Renal	24 MU	3–4 MU every 4 h	2 MU every 6 h	1 MU every 6 h
Piperacillin/tazobactam	Renal	18	3.375 grams every 6 h	2.25 grams every 6 h	2.25 grams every 8 h
Tobramycin, gentamicin	Renal	7 milligrams/kg per dose	Every 24 h	Every 36–48 h	Do not use
Vancomycin	Renal	15 milligrams/kg per dose	Every 12–24 h	Every 24–48 h	Use levels

Abbreviation: MU = million units.

TABLE 163-5 Antibacterial Adverse Effects

Antibiotic Class	Pregnancy Category*,†	Allergic Reactions	Dose-Related Effects
β-Lactams (penicillins, cephalosporins, monobactams, carbapenems)	B	Anaphylaxis, urticaria, rash, fever, serum sickness; hepatitis, nephritis, anemia, thrombocytopenia Cross-reactivity between penicillins and cephalosporins is <5%; little cross-reactivity between cephalosporin and aztreonam or imipenem	Diarrhea (amoxicillin/clavulanate), biliary sludging (ceftriaxone); phlebitis; seizures (imipenem, penicillin G); antiplatelet effects and hemolytic anemia; decreased vitamin K synthesis and disulfiram reaction (cefotetan); nausea, hypotension (rapid infusion of imipenem)
Aminoglycosides	C	Rare	Nephrotoxicity: incidence 10%–15%, usually reversible Ototoxicity: incidence 1%–5%, causes deafness and/or dizziness; toxicity is both dose- and duration-related
Macrolides	B/C	Cholestatic jaundice: associated with IV erythromycin	GI toxicity: nausea, vomiting, diarrhea, cramping—mostly with erythromycin
Clindamycin	B	Rash	Diarrhea—most common adverse effect; pseudomembranous colitis
Tetracyclines, including tigecycline	D	Rash (including photosensitivity), anaphylaxis, urticaria, fever, hepatitis	Nausea, vomiting, diarrhea; increase in blood urea nitrogen; deposits in and discolors teeth and bone (avoid in pediatrics); dizziness and vertigo (minocycline)
Vancomycin	C	Rash (rare)	Infusion-related reactions: phlebitis, "red-person syndrome" from rapid infusions—give 1 gram over 60 min; oto- and nephrotoxicity with high doses, or in combination with other oto or nephrotoxins
Fluoroquinolones	C	Rare	Nausea, vomiting, diarrhea; confusion, headache, seizures; tendonitis and tendon rupture; prolonged QT interval
Sulfonamides	X	Rash, Stevens-Johnson syndrome, exfoliative dermatitis (more common in acquired immunodeficiency syndrome); cholestatic hepatitis; bone marrow suppression	Nausea, vomiting, diarrhea; crystalluria (doses taken with insufficient fluids); hyperkalemia (with trimethoprim); kernicterus (in neonates)

*U.S. Food and Drug Administration Safety-in-Pregnancy Code: A: controlled human studies show no risk. B: no evidence of risk in humans; the chance of fetal harm is remote but remains a possibility. C: risk cannot be ruled out; well-controlled human studies are lacking, and animal studies have shown risk or are lacking; there is a chance of fetal harm if administered during pregnancy. D: positive evidence of risk; studies in humans have demonstrated fetal risk. X: contraindicated in pregnancy; the risk of fetal abnormalities outweighs the potential benefit of the drug.

†LactMed is an NLM database providing information on drugs and lactation http://toxnet.nlm.nih.gov/cgi-bin/sis/htmlgen?LACT

TABLE 163-6 Antibiotic Contraindications

Antibiotic Class	Contraindications
Aminoglycosides	Prior allergic or toxic reactions to aminoglycosides
Cephalosporins	Sensitivity to cephalosporins, imipenem (carbapenems), penicillins
Clindamycin	Sensitivity to clindamycin; meningitis (inadequate CNS penetration)
Fluoroquinolones	Sensitivity to fluoroquinolones; tendonitis or tendon rupture; use of QT interval–prolonging drugs (amiodarone, procainamide); myasthenia gravis
Macrolides	Sensitivity to macrolides; meningitis (inadequate CNS penetration)
Metronidazole	Sensitivity to metronidazole; first trimester of pregnancy
Penicillins	Sensitivity to penicillins, cephalosporins, imipenem (carbapenems)
Sulfonamides	Sensitivity to sulfonamides, pregnancy at term, lactation
Tetracyclines	Sensitivity to tetracyclines
Vancomycin	Sensitivity to vancomycin

Abbreviation: CNS = central nervous system.

Acyclovir, valacyclovir, famciclovir, and valganciclovir are oral drugs for the treatment of herpes simplex virus and cytomegalovirus infections. Of all, the absorption of acyclovir is less than others, requiring higher doses to achieve adequate blood and tissue levels to inhibit viral replication.

The development of new agents for hepatitis B and C infections has been similar to that of several of the antiretroviral drug classes. Effective drugs are analogues of nucleotides or nucleosides that result in nucleic

TABLE 163-7 Antibacterial Drug Interactions

Antibiotic Class	Drug Interactions
Aminoglycosides	Neuromuscular blockers—may prolong respiratory depression; loop diuretics—may increase auditory toxicity
Cephalosporins	Antacids—may reduce the oral absorption of cefaclor, cefdinir, and cefpodoxime Warfarin—cefotetan enhances the anticoagulant effect of warfarin
Fluoroquinolones	Antacids, iron salts, sucralfate—absorption of the fluoroquinolone is reduced by chelation Theophylline—metabolism is slowed by ciprofloxacin, may cause theophylline toxicity; warfarin elimination is slowed by fluoroquinolones—follow clotting times carefully
Macrolides	Clarithromycin can increase levels of warfarin, cyclosporine, lovastatin, theophylline—monitor additive effects carefully
Penicillins	Allopurinol—increased rash with ampicillin Aminoglycosides—when administered IV simultaneously, inactivation occurs Probenecid—reduced renal elimination of penicillin
Tetracyclines	Antacids, iron salts—bind to tetracycline and reduce oral absorption (occurs least with doxycycline) Oral contraceptives—failure
Trimethoprim-sulfamethoxazole	Warfarin—can prolong clotting times; phenytoin—increase in serum levels and possible toxicity
Vancomycin	Aminoglycosides—may increase risk of nephrotoxicity

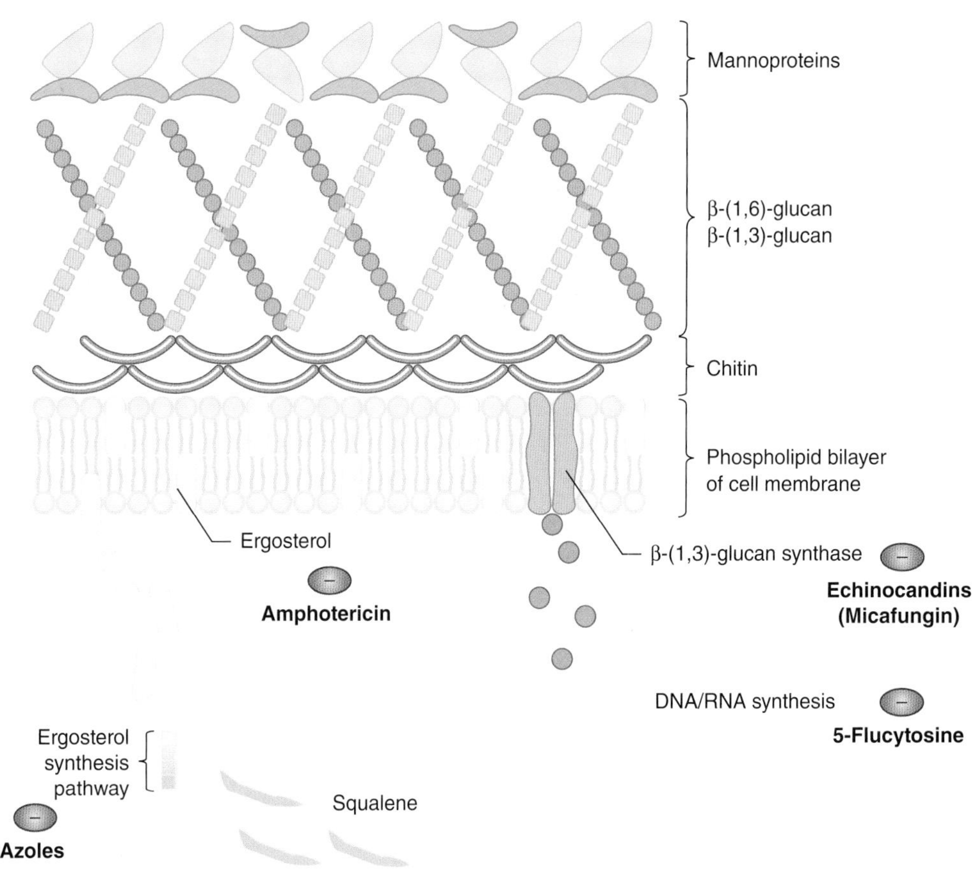

FIGURE 163-2. Mechanisms of action of antifungal agents.

TABLE 163-8 Antifungal Agents for Systemic Infections

Drug	Spectrum	Usual Doses
Amphotericin B, IV Conventional (Fungizone®) Lipid complex (Abelcet®) Liposomal (AmBisome®) Colloidal dispersion (Amphotec®)	*Aspergillus, Candida, Cryptococcus,* histoplasmosis, mucormycosis	0.5–1.0 milligram/kg/d 5.0 milligrams/kg/d 5.0 milligrams/kg/d 5.0 milligrams/kg/d
Triazoles		
Fluconazole (Diflucan®) IV, PO Itraconazole (Sporanox®) IV, PO Posaconazole (Noxafil®) PO Voriconazole (Vfend®) IV, PO	*Candida, Cryptococcus, Aspergillus* (not fluconazole), histoplasmosis, mucormycosis (posaconazole)	400–800 milligrams per day 200 milligrams twice daily 200 milligrams three times daily with food 6 milligrams/kg IV every 12 h for 2 doses, then 4 milligrams/kg IV every 12 h; 200 milligrams PO every 12 h
Echinocandins		
Anidulafungin (Eraxis®) IV Caspofungin (Cancidas®) IV Micafungin (Mycamine®) IV	*Aspergillus, Candida* (not *Cryptococcus*)	200 milligrams × 1, then 100 milligrams every day 70 milligrams × 1, then 50 milligrams every day 100 milligrams every day
Antimetabolite		
Flucytosine (Ancobon®), PO	*Candida, Cryptococcus* (should not be used as monotherapy)	25.0–37.5 milligrams/kg every 6 h

TABLE 163-9 Selected Topical Antifungal Agents

Class and Products	Dosage Forms	Comments
Allylamines/benzylamines		
Butenafine (Mentax®, Lotrimin® ultraTM) Naftifine (Naftin®) Terbinafine (Lamisil AT®)	1% cream, gel, solution, spray	Treatment for 1–4 wk for tinea
Imidazoles		
Clotrimazole (Lotrimin AF®, Mycelex 7®)	1% cream, lotion, 100- and 200-milligram vaginal suppositories	Topical (Candida, tinea) apply twice daily Vaginal suppository, 100 milligrams × 7 d or 500 milligrams at bedtime × 1
Miconazole (Micatin®, Monistat®)	2% cream, ointment, vaginal suppository	As above, except 200-milligram vaginal suppository × 3 d, or 500 milligrams once
Tioconazole (Vagistat-1®)	6.5% vaginal ointment	Application at bedtime × 1
Miscellaneous (for tinea only)		
Tolnaftate (Tinactin®, Ting®)	1% cream, solution, gel, powder, spray	Apply twice daily for 2–6 wk Less effective than imidazoles

TABLE 163-10 Antiviral Agents for Cytomegalovirus, Systemic Herpes, Varicella, and Influenza

HSV I and II, VZV	HSV I and II, VZV, Cytomegalovirus	Influenza A	Influenza A and B
Acyclovir (Zovirax®), valacyclovir (Valtrex®), famciclovir (Famvir®)	Valganciclovir (Valcyte®) Mechanism: nucleoside analogue (guanine); when phosphorylated, inhibits viral DNA polymerase	Amantadine (Symmetrel®), rimantadine (Flumadine®)	Oseltamivir (Tamiflu®), zanamivir (Relenza®)
Mechanism: purine nucleoside analogues; triphosphate form inhibits HSV DNA polymerase and viral DNA replication	Foscarnet (Foscavir®) Mechanism: inorganic pyrophosphate analogue that inhibits DNA polymerase Cidofovir (Vistide®) Mechanism: nucleotide analogue that inhibits viral DNA polymerase	Mechanism: inhibits uncoating of virus and uptake of nucleic acid by host cells	Mechanism: inhibitor of influenza virus neuraminidase with possible alteration in viral aggregation and release

Abbreviations: HSV = herpes simplex virus; VZV = varicella-zoster virus.

TABLE 163-11 Antiviral Therapy (Non–Human Immunodeficiency Virus) in the ED

Diagnosis	Drug	Dosage	Route
Herpes encephalitis	Acyclovir	10 milligrams/kg every 8 h × 10 d (adult) 500 milligrams/m² every 8 h (6 mo–12 y old)	IV
Mucocutaneous herpes (immunocompromised)	Acyclovir	5 milligrams/kg every 8 h × 7 d (adult) 250 milligrams/m² every 8 h (<12 y old)	IV
Varicella-zoster (immunocompromised)		Same as above for herpes encephalitis	IV
Herpes zoster (normal host)	Acyclovir, or famciclovir, or valacyclovir	800 milligrams five times/day × 7–10 d 500 milligrams three times daily × 7 d 1 gram three times daily × 7 d	PO PO PO
Varicella (chickenpox)	Acyclovir	20 milligrams/kg (≤800 milligrams) four times a day (adults and children >2 y old) × 5 d	PO
Influenza A	Amantadine	100 milligrams twice daily × 10 d (adults and children >9 y old) 4.4–8.8 milligrams/kg/d, but <150 milligrams/d (children 1–9 y old)	PO
	Rimantadine	100 milligrams twice daily × 7 d (adults and children >10 y old) 5 milligrams/kg/d, but <150 milligrams/d (children 1–10 y old)	PO
	Oseltamivir	75 milligrams twice daily (adults and children >12 y old) × 5 d Pediatrics (age 2 wk thru 12 y): based on weight Also active against influenza B	PO
	Zanamivir	10 milligrams (two inhalations) twice daily × 5 d (adults and children >6 y old) Also active against influenza B	Inhalation

TABLE 163-12 Antiviral Agents for Hepatitis B and Hepatitis C

Hepatitis B		Hepatitis C		
Interferons: interferon alfa-2b (Intron A®); peginterferon alfa-2a (Pegasys®)	Nucleotide or nucleoside analogues: Preferred agents: Entecavir (Baraclude®) 0.5–1 milligram PO daily Tenofovir (Viread®) 300 milligrams PO daily Alternate agents: Adefovir (Hepsera®) 10 milligrams PO daily Lamivudine (Epivir-HBV®) 100 milligrams PO daily Telbivudine (Tyzeka®) 600 milligrams PO daily	Interferons: Products for hepatitis B: Interferon alfa-2a (Roferon®) Peginterferon alfa-2b (Pegintron®) Interferon alfacon-1 (Infergen®)	Ribavirin (CoPegus®, Rebetol®) 800–1400 milligrams PO every day depending upon hepatitis C virus genotype and body weight	Enzyme inhibitors: Boceprevir (Victrelis®) 800 milligrams PO three times daily with food Simeprevir (Olysio®) 150 milligrams PO once daily with food Sofosbuvir (Sovaldi®) 400 milligrams PO once daily with or without food Sofosbuvir 400mg + ledipasvir 90mg (Harvoni®) one tablet PO once daily with or without food
Mechanism: immunostimulant; activates cytolytic T cells against infected hepatocytes Adverse effects: flu-like syndrome, nausea, diarrhea, fatigue, depression, myelosuppression	Mechanism: inhibitor of viral DNA polymerase Adverse effects: headache, fatigue, nausea, asthenia, abdominal pain and distention, insomnia, lactic acidosis, hepatomegaly, increased creatinine	Mechanism and adverse effects: See Hepatitis B	Mechanism: nucleoside analogue, inhibits hepatitis C virus polymerase Adverse effects: hemolytic anemia and pancytopenia, allergic reactions, dyspnea, pneumonitis, bacterial infections	Mechanism: boceprevir and simeprevir inhibit NS3/4A protease; sofosbuvir inhibits RNA polymerase Adverse effects: anemia, nausea, fatigue, headache, rash, pruritus ledipasvir inhibits NS5A protein

acid polymerase inhibition (for example, entecavir for hepatitis B or simeprevir for hepatitis C) or directly inhibit RNA polymerase (sofosbuvir for hepatitis C). These agents are used in combination (for example, sofosbuvir with ribavirin and peginterferon).

HYPERSENSITIVITY SYNDROME

Used in human immunodeficiency virus care, abacavir (Ziagen®, also contained in Trizivir® and Epzicom®) causes a hypersensitivity syndrome. This is more common in individuals who are positive for the major histocompatibility complex class I allele HLA-B*5701, and this allele is now screened before a patient is placed on abacavir.[5] The syndrome is characterized by rash and other systemic complaints. The reaction is reversible with discontinuation of abacavir. However, if the patient then takes abacavir again, life-threatening cardiovascular and respiratory insufficiency can develop.

Many other infrequent adverse reactions are possible but beyond the scope of one chapter. Multiple online sources can aid if needed.[3,5]

REFERENCES

The complete reference list is available online at www.TintinalliEM.com.

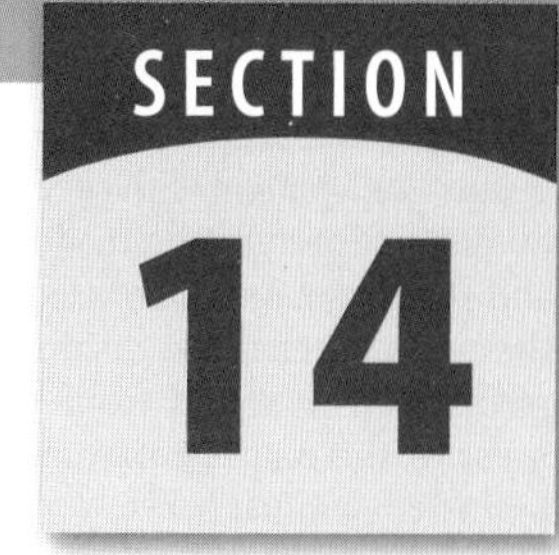

Neurology

CHAPTER 164 Neurologic Examination

J. Stephen Huff
Andrew D. Perron

INTRODUCTION

In most patients, the physical examination confirms thoughts formulated during history taking that are often the key to patient evaluation. Time of onset, symptom progression, associated complaints, and exacerbating factors are important historical points to guide appropriate examination and other testing. The neurologic examination does not exist in isolation from the general physical examination or imaging procedures, and it is unusual for the neurologic examination to delineate a problem not already suggested by the patient's history or general physical examination. Few findings of the neurologic examination are pathognomonic of clinical conditions or are sufficiently specific that examination alone secures the diagnosis. Further complicating the value of the neurologic examination is that the sensitivity and specificity of different examination techniques have not been rigorously investigated, and the degree of interobserver variability is not known. The uncooperative patient or patient with altered mental status presents additional challenges in performing a detailed examination.

The idea of performing a "complete" examination in the ED is impractical, because most frequently, a "complete" examination is neither required nor appropriate. An adequate examination is one that is sufficient for the task at hand. Examination of children follows the same framework as that for adults, but even more information is gathered indirectly by observation. For example, interacting with a child playing with a toy or other object allows the examiner to assess vision, extraocular motion, coordination, and strength as the child reaches for and grasps the toy.[1] Traditional neurologic formulation follows a three-tiered approach: (1) Is there a lesion of the nervous system? (2) Where is the lesion? (3) What is the lesion? The examination detailed in this chapter is arbitrarily divided into eight sections with basic and advanced levels described for each section.

ORGANIZATIONAL FRAMEWORK

Organization of the neurologic examination into a framework of subsections is a convenient technique. At the bedside, mentally review the framework as during the examination, and select more detailed tests as needed. Some of the tests grouped in a section assess several aspects of nervous system function, and listing of tests in a particular section is for organizational convenience. For example, visual field testing, although technically a test of higher cortical function, is listed with cranial nerve testing because the examining physician may find it easier to evaluate visual fields during that portion of the examination assessing cranial nerve function. One organizational scheme divides the examination into eight elements:

1. Mental status testing
2. Higher cerebral functions
3. Cranial nerves
4. Sensory examination
5. Motor system
6. Reflexes
7. Cerebellar testing
8. Gait and station

MENTAL STATUS TESTING

A mental status examination is part of every patient encounter. The observation may be brief and descriptive, such as, "The patient is awake, alert, and conversant," or it may be quite detailed. Mental status assesses the emotional and intellectual functioning of the patient. It is important to make some assessment of mental status, because the patient with an abnormal mental status cannot be relied on for an accurate medical history.

Major elements of mental status testing are assessment of appearance, mood, and insight; assessment for thought disorders or abnormal thought content such as hallucinations; and testing of the sensorium. *Sensorium* is a term for the appropriate awareness and perception of consciousness. Mental status testing is covered more fully in chapter 168, Altered Mental Status and Coma.

One key element in mental status testing is attention and memory assessment. Attention testing is performed with digit repetition. The average adult of normal intelligence should be able to repeat six or seven digits forward and four or five digits backward. Failure to do so may suggest confusion, delirium, or a problem with language perception. Often this represents a problem with attention rather than with memory. Memory is a complex process but is often simply broken into long-term and short-term activities. *Long-term memory* is recall of events of some months or years ago. *Short-term memory* is assessed by asking about events of the day or by three-object recall at 5 minutes. State three items in a neutral tone and ask the patient to repeat; reassess at 5 minutes to obtain a gross assessment of short-term memory function. Failure to repeat the items immediately after presentation is likely an indication of an attention problem rather than of a memory problem.

Evaluation by screening tools is described in chapter 168. Other screening tests for depression, substance abuse, and other problems are outside the scope of this chapter.

In general, patients with abnormal mental status, especially attention problems or disorientation, are more likely to have medical problems rather than functional or psychiatric causes. If a patient suffers from significant inattention, it is unlikely that the examiner will truly be able to determine whether the primary problem is one of cognition or attention.

HIGHER CEREBRAL FUNCTIONS

Higher cerebral functions test neurologic tasks that are thought to reside in the cerebral cortex. Language function defines the dominant hemisphere. The majority of the population is right-handed; for 90% of these patients, the left hemisphere is where language functions reside; hence, they are referred to as *left-hemisphere dominant*. Even in left-handed patients, most will be left-hemisphere dominant for language. Thus, a large cortical stroke affecting the cortex of the dominant hemisphere (the left hemisphere in most patients, whether they are left- or right-hand dominant) likely will affect language functions.

The nondominant hemisphere is concerned with spatial relationships. Often a nondominant hemispheric problem is suspected in the ED when the patient has consistent visual inattention to a care provider approaching from one side (usually the left since most patients are left-hemisphere dominant).

Higher cerebral function pragmatically involves the assessment of language. For a patient with speech that is difficult to understand, a fundamental distinction must be made between *dysarthria* and a *dysphasia* (aphasia and dysphasia are often used interchangeably in clinical practice). Dysarthria is a mechanical disorder of speech resulting from difficulty in the production of sound from weakness or incoordination of facial or oral muscles; this may result from a motor system problem (cortical, subcortical, brainstem, cranial nerve, or cerebellar), but it does not represent a disorder of higher cerebral function. Dysphasia is a problem of language resulting from cortical or subcortical damage; the portion of the brain concerned with comprehension, processing, or producing language is impaired.

There are many different types of aphasias, but a simplified scheme is sufficient for assessment. A description of aphasia into fluent, nonfluent, or mixed patterns is adequate for testing in the ED and for communicating with other physicians.

BASIC

Normal conversation monitoring for correct responses is the common screening examination for a language disorder. If suspicion of a language disorder exists, a series of assessments allows confirmation and categorization of the aphasia.

Test comprehension initially by the ability to follow simple commands. Asking the patient to identify common objects may also be part of the assessment. Use commonly available objects, such as a watch, a pen, or a glass, as a stimulus. Query the patient regarding the names of different parts of the objects. Ask the patient to demonstrate how an object is used. The inability to show how an object is used, assuming hearing and motor functions are intact, may represent an apraxia, defined as the inability to perform a willed act.

In a nonfluent aphasia (a rough synonym is motor or expressive aphasia), the speed of language and the ability to find the correct words may be impaired. A common type of nonfluent motor aphasia is known as *Broca's aphasia*. Speech may be halting and slow, with stops between words or word fragments.

In a fluent aphasia (a rough synonym is auditory or receptive aphasia), the quantity of word production is normal or even increased. Sentences may have normal grammatical structure with normal rhythm, and intonation may be clearly articulated. However, language is impaired, and the listener may be struck by peculiarities of conversation that lack appropriate content. Incorrect words may be substituted within sentences that may be sound-alike words or words with similar yet incorrect meanings. A global or mixed aphasia involves elements of fluent and nonfluent aphasias and is the most common type encountered in clinical practice.

Nondominant hemisphere problems may show problems of auditory or visual inattention or sensory inattention.

ADVANCED

Testing of mental status and cognitive function requires an appreciation of cultural context and language barriers. Further assessment of comprehension may involve showing the patient a picture (there are some standard stimuli, but almost any magazine photo may be used) and asking for the patient's interpretation of the picture while noting if the content is correctly described and if the sentence structure and word selection of the descriptions are correct.

Assessing the ability of the patient to repeat a phrase may be a key point in delineating some types of fluent aphasias. Typically, the ability to repeat short words is more impaired than the ability to repeat longer words. A classic test involves the patient repeating the phrase, "No ifs, ands, or buts." In one type of fluent aphasia, *Wernicke's aphasia*, comprehension is impaired, as is repetition.

Paraphasic errors may be further characterized in patients with fluent aphasia. A literal paraphasic error is one in which part of a word is replaced by an incorrect sound. The use of *spool* when *spoon* is meant is an example of a literal paraphasic error. At times, the errors may reach the point at which the substitutions are not understandable, and a neologism (a meaningless collection of syllables that takes the place of a word in conversation) is produced. Verbal paraphasic errors involve substitution of one correct word for another; for example, a patient may wish to use *spoon* in a sentence and substitute *fork* or even *bike*; the word is a correct word, but the meaning of the sentence is transformed erroneously.[2]

A patient aphasic in speaking will also be aphasic in written communication. Writing and drawing simple constructions may be revealing in some patients. A sequence of simple commands such as requesting the patient to draw a circle and then placing numbers like numbers on a clock may reveal constructional errors. A response consistent with dysfunction of the nondominant hemisphere might be numbering half the clock face and stopping or placing all the numbers around one half of the circle.

Impairment of sensory perception on the cortical level may involve the inability to distinguish objects by touch alone. Implied in this testing is that the primary sensory modalities (sharp, light touch, etc.) are intact. In cases of nondominant hemisphere lesions, the ability to identify objects placed in a hand, such as a coin, may be impaired.

SPECIAL CIRCUMSTANCES

Fluent aphasias may so severely impair communication that the patient is thought to be intoxicated or psychotic. Pay attention to the pattern of speaking—this may give the first indication of a language problem, and further constructional or language testing may demonstrate the presence of an aphasia.

CRANIAL NERVES

BASIC

A survey of the cranial nerves is an integral part of neurologic assessment. Much information may be gathered informally. Look for facial asymmetry (cranial nerve VII) at rest or with movement. Lingual movement (XII) and other facial movements may be inferred during conversation if articulation is good. However, a more formal approach often is used in examination. Most examiners start sequentially with cranial nerve II in testing; cranial nerve I (olfactory) testing has infrequent application in emergency medicine.

Cranial nerve II is the optic nerve active in the afferent function of light and visual perception. The optic nerve head is visible with direct ophthalmoscopy and may be inspected for abnormalities. Common tests for optic nerve function include visual acuity and stimulation for pupillary reactivity. The response to bright light stimulation involves direct and indirect (consensual) pupillary responses. This is a reflex arc, with the afferent limb being cranial nerve II and the efferent limb of the arc being cranial nerve III, which carries the pupilloconstrictors. A bright light directed into one eye should cause a brisk constriction of equal magnitude in both pupils. In the swinging flashlight test, observe the pupils as the light is slowly moved from one pupil to the other. A seemingly paradoxical dilation of one pupil as the light is moved onto that pupil may indicate optic nerve dysfunction of that eye; this is referred to as an *afferent pupillary defect* (see chapter 241, Eye Emergencies).

Cranial nerves III, IV, and VI are concerned with extraocular eye movements (see chapter 241). Tracing an object through a full-H pattern allows assessment of the different cranial nerves. Cranial nerve VI innervates the lateral rectus muscle, which abducts the globe, moving it laterally away from the midline; this lateral movement will be impaired or lost in the case of cranial nerve VI palsy. In fact, the unopposed adduction movement of medial rectus muscle innervated by cranial nerve III may result in the globe being medially deviated. Cranial nerve III innervates the extraocular muscles that adduct each eye and those that elevate and depress the globe. Impairment of cranial nerve III will reveal several abnormalities of extraocular movement, reflecting weakness in the innervated muscles. A complete paresis of cranial nerve III will show a dilated pupil in a globe deviated downward and outward. An isolated cranial nerve IV weakness may be hard to detect; cranial nerve IV supplies the superior oblique muscle that elevates and intorts the globe.

Cranial nerve III also carries the parasympathetic pupilloconstrictors to the eye; a lesion of cranial nerve III may impair those fibers, resulting in unopposed dilatation (by functioning sympathetic fibers reaching the eye by a circuitous path) and a pupil larger than in the unaffected eye.

Ptosis from levator muscle paralysis is another finding of cranial nerve III paresis.

Cranial nerve V has motor and sensory functions. It supplies the muscles of mastication and is assessed by appreciating the masseter bulk. The sensory component of cranial nerve V supplies the cornea; the corneal reflex is a reflex arc of cranial nerves V to VII. Cranial nerve VII supplies the muscles for facial movement as well as facial proprioception.

Cranial nerve VIII has auditory and vestibular afferent components. Cranial nerves IX and X are tested by observing pharyngeal musculature and gag reflexes. Cranial nerve XI is assessed by a shoulder shrug. Cranial nerve XII controls lingual movement and can be assessed by asking the patient to stick out the tongue and observing for any asymmetry of motion.

ADVANCED

In approximately 20% of the population, some degree of physiologic anisocoria is present on the order of 1 to 2 mm. Small differences in pupillary size in otherwise asymptomatic patients likely represent this normal variant. A peripheral lesion of cranial nerve VII will cause complete facial paralysis on the same side as the lesion. A cortical lesion (often stroke) results in weakness of the lower and midface on the opposite side of the injury, with preservation of motor function in the upper face ("central VIIth pattern"). This is due to the bilateral cortical upper motor neuron innervation of the forehead musculature present in most patients.

SPECIAL CIRCUMSTANCES

In the comatose patient, a **unilaterally dilated pupil** that is unreactive or reacts sluggishly to light may represent third nerve dysfunction or paresis from impingement of the oculomotor (III) nerve at the tentorium; this finding is consistent with the uncal herniation syndrome.

Vertigo often is a symptom from a vestibular system dysfunction but may result from a central nervous system disorder such as posterior circulation stroke. The horizontal head impulse test is a bedside maneuver to detect peripheral vestibular disease (see later discussion).[3] A normal (negative) finding of the horizontal head impulse test reliably identifies patients with a central cause of acute vertigo, but an abnormal test (positive) may occur with both peripheral and central causes of vertigo.[4] Two additional maneuvers are advocated in conjunction with the horizontal head impulse test to reliably exclude central causes of vertigo, examination for nystagmus and assessment for skew gaze.[5] Nystagmus that changes direction with gaze to either side is predictive of a central lesion, as is spontaneous vertical or multidirectional nystagmus.[6] Skew deviation refers to misalignment of the eyes. Though subtle at times, it may be unmasked by alternately covering each eye while the patient fixes gaze on the examiner.[7]

Assess the **horizontal head impulse test** by rapidly rotating the head to one side then the other; inability to maintain visual fixation during head rotation requires a rapid corrective jerking (saccade) back to the target; this is a positive horizontal head impulse test and suggests a peripheral vestibular lesion. Additional maneuvers help confirm the assessment. Observe the patient for nystagmus while looking ahead; if present while simply looking ahead, especially if vertical or direction-changing, a central cause of vertigo is likely. If **vertical skew gaze** is present or provoked by alternately covering each eye with the patient looking directly ahead, a central cause may be present. Again, a negative horizontal head impulse test (no corrective saccade observed) in the presence of acute vertigo suggests the possibility of a CNS lesion. The horizontal head impulse test has not been tested in the ED.

SENSORY EXAMINATION

BASIC

The sensory evaluation can be key in some patients with sensory complaints. The primary sensory modalities are light touch, pinprick, position, vibration, and temperature sense. Because of variability in neuroanatomy, at times, dissociation of these modalities occurs and allows localization of problems to anatomic areas within the CNS.

Practically establishing that touch or pinprick is perceived in all extremities is often the only sensory assessment needed in a screening examination. However, if touch or pinprick is not intact or if peripheral nerve or spinal cord injury is suspected, additional detailed examination is usually necessary.

Position testing is best used for the detection of peripheral neuropathy or posterior column spinal cord disease. Position and vibration sensations are conveyed in the posterior columns of the spinal cord, so that there is no need to test both position and vibration—just test one.

ADVANCED

Spinal cord dermatome levels are illustrated in **Figure 164-1**. If sensory alteration conforms to a level or selectively involves specific dermatomes, further localization to the peripheral nerve or nerve root may be possible.

If primary sensory modalities are intact, then testing of higher sensory functions may be pursued; these are covered in the section on Higher Cerebral Functions.

SPECIAL CIRCUMSTANCES

A few patterns of sensory loss are worthy of special mention. In cervical spinal cord injury or compression, an area of apparent sensory demarcation often appears to be just above the nipples. This transverse sensory level suggests a spinal cord lesion in the low cervical to high thoracic area. Most cervical dermatomes are represented in the upper extremity and not in the trunk (see Figure 164-1), and further testing is necessary to delineate the sensory level.

With suspected spinal cord injury, test the area of the perineum for sensation. The sacral dermatomes are distributed in an onion skin pattern around the perineum and are represented only in that region. The demonstration of a preserved island of sensation around the perineum may be the only sign of an incomplete spinal cord injury, which has a different prognosis than a complete spinal cord injury.

Some general comments may be made about patterns of sensory alterations. In general, a half-body sensory loss or alteration suggests cortical or subcortical lesions. A localized problem in one limb suggests a peripheral nerve or nerve root problem, although there are other possible locations of abnormalities in the CNS.[8]

MOTOR SYSTEM

There is more to evaluation of the motor system than simple assessment of strength. Muscle bulk and muscle tone are basic areas of assessment.

BASIC

Muscle tone may be characterized as normal, decreased, or increased. Assess tone by movement of muscle groups and appreciating any resistance to movement. Ask the patient to relax and not resist. Increased tone is greater than normal resistance to passive motion. **Cogwheeling** is transient increase or catching in resistance followed by release to the movement. Assess axial or truncal tone by standing behind the patient, grasping the shoulders, and gently moving the shoulders back and forth in a gentle rotation. A patient with normal tone will offer little resistance to repeated motions, and some spontaneous swing of the arms will be noted. A patient with increased axial tone (e.g., Parkinson's disease) may turn without the arm swing.

Simply having the patient hold the arms outstretched with palms upward and observing for any inward rotation or downward drift is a very sensitive sign for upper extremity weakness (**pronator drift**); this also may be assessed in unresponsive patients (**Figure 164-2**). If both arms are held outright at the same time, comparison is easy, with observation of the upper extremity of one side as opposed to the other. A similar maneuver may be performed in the lower extremities. Another sensitive test for a subtle hemiparesis is the forearm-rolling technique. With the forearms outstretched, ask the patient to make tight circles with each arm. The movements should be small and rapid. Asymmetry or slowness with one arm suggests a weak

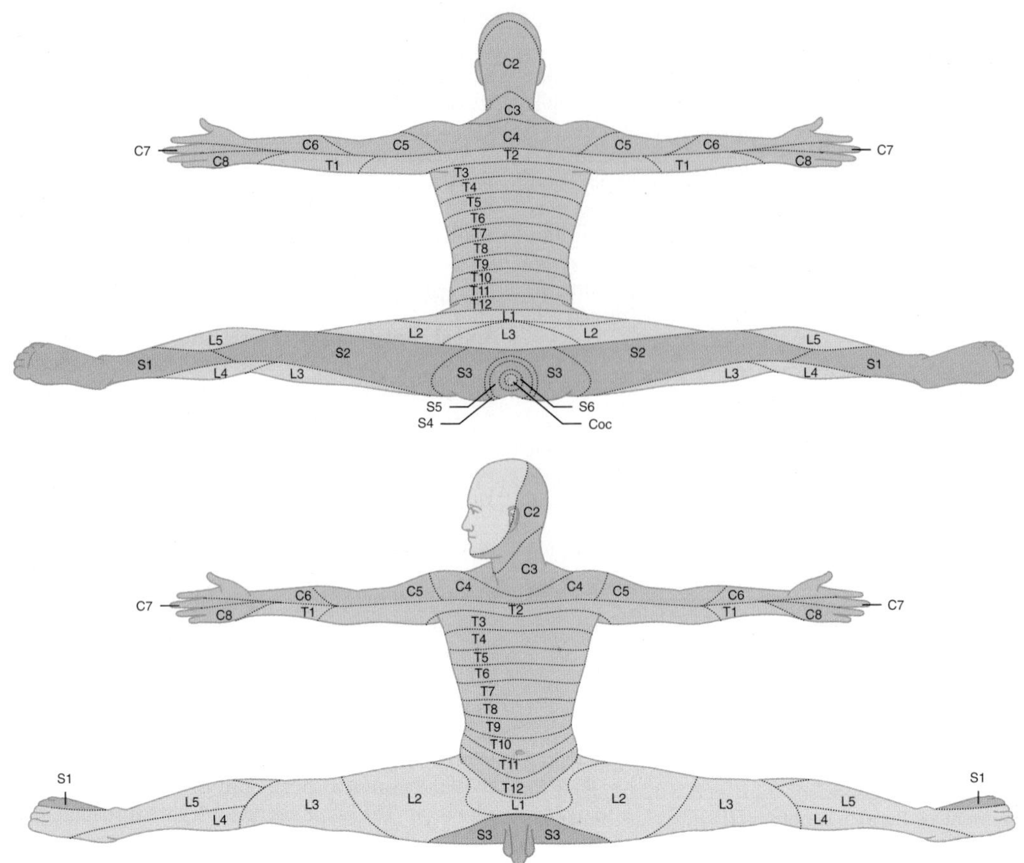

FIGURE 164-1. Sensory dermatomes.

limb.[9] Decreased speed of foot tapping also may suggest weakness and an upper motor neuron probem.[10]

Tremor can be difficult to characterize, and there are many types of tremor. Action tremors, those that are absent at rest but evident with action or sustained limb position, include those from caffeine, hyperthyroidism, and alcohol or sedative withdrawal. Essential familiar tremor is also an action tremor. Rest tremors characterize **Parkinson's disease**, with tremor present during rest, diminishing with willed movement, and then resuming with the new position.

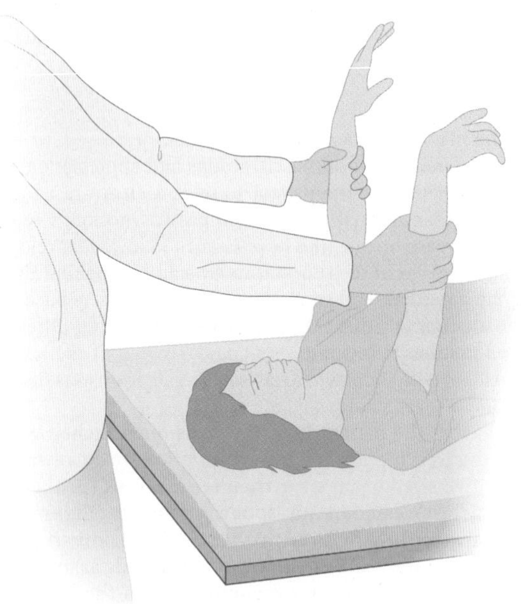

FIGURE 164-2. Testing for weakness in the comatose patient; diagram illustrates assessment of muscular tone in a patient with a right hemiplegia. A similar maneuver may be used in the conscious patient.

Assessment and recording of other motor strength are best done by description of the stimulus and response. For example, the fact that the patient is able to strongly resist elbow extension or elbow flexion against the examiner is an appropriate notation.

ADVANCED

Compare muscle mass or bulk of the affected area with muscle groups of the unaffected areas. If weakness or paralysis has been present for some time, muscle wasting or atrophy may be present. Brief, rapid twitches of small parts of a muscle may represent fasciculations, which may indicate a process involving the lower motor neurons.

A formal rating scale for muscle strength exists but is not straightforward to apply. A rating of 5 is assigned for normal strength, and a rating of 4 indicates weakness and the ability to contract the muscle against some resistance. Thus, a tremendous range of strength is covered within the range of the 4 rating; rating is often further roughly quantified by adding 4+ and 4− to that rating range. A rating of 0 represents complete paresis, and a rating of 1 indicates a minimal flicker of contraction. A rating of 2 is assigned for active movement of a muscle with gravity eliminated by limb repositioning (e.g., so that elbow flexion and contraction are demonstrated by a horizontal rather than by a vertical movement). A value of 3 is assigned to a muscle able to voluntarily demonstrate full motion against gravity only. It is better for the examiner to describe the strength of a muscle by noting the amount of resistance than by invoking what may be a little-used scale and erroneously applying a rating.

Listings of some muscle innervations, actions to test, and dermatomal representations are found in **Tables 164-1 and 164-2.**

TABLE 164-1 Muscle Innervation: Shoulder and Upper Extremity

Nerve	Action to Test	Muscle*
Long thoracic	Forward shoulder thrust	Serratus anterior
Dorsal scapular	Elevate scapula	Levator scapulae
Suprascapular	Arm external rotation	Infraspinatus; C5, C6
Axillary	Abduct arm (>90 degrees)	Deltoid; C5
Musculocutaneous	Flex and supinate arm	Biceps brachii
Ulnar	Ulnar flexion of hand	Flexor carpi ulnaris; C7, C8,† T1
	Flex DIP of fingers 4 and 5	Flexor digitorum profundus
	Thumb adduction	Adductor pollicis; C7, C8†
	Abduction of finger 5	Abductor digitorum minimi
	Opposition of finger 5	Opponens digitorum minimi
	Flexion of finger 5	Flexor digitorum minimi brevis
	Finger abduction and adduction	Interossei; C8, T1†
	Flex PIP and extend DIP of fingers 4 and 5	Lumbricals 3 and 4
Median	Forearm pronation	Pronator teres
	Radial hand flexion	Flexor carpi radialis; C7, C8, T1
	Hand flexion	Palmaris longus
	PIP flexion of fingers 2–5	Flexor digitorum superficialis
	Abduct thumb at the metacarpophalangeal	Abductor pollicis brevis
	Flex proximal phalanx thumb	Flexor pollicis brevis; C7, C8†
Anterior interosseous	Flex DIP fingers 2–5	Flexor digitorum profundus (radial)
	Flex thumb interphalangeal	Flexor pollicis longus
	Oppose thumb	Opponens pollicis; C8, T1†
	Flex PIP and extend DIP of fingers 2 and 3	Lumbricals 1 and 2
Posterior interosseous	Extension of digits 2–5	Extensor digitorum
	Ulnar hand extension	Extensor carpi ulnaris
	Thumb abduction	Abductor pollicis longus
	Thumb extension	Extensor pollicis longus and brevis
	Index finger extension	Extensor indicis proprius
Radial	Forearm extension	Triceps brachii; C6, C7,† C8
	Forearm flexion	Brachioradialis; C5, C6
	Radial hand extension	Extensor carpi radialis
	Forearm supination	Supinator

Abbreviations: DIP = distal interphalangeal joint; PIP = proximal interphalangeal joint.

*Dermatomal representations are listed after some muscles.

†Predominant dermatome.

TABLE 164-2 Muscle Innervation: Hip and Lower Extremity

Nerve	Action to Test	Muscle*
Femoral	Hip flexion	Iliopsoas; T12, L1,† L2, L3
	Leg extension	Quadriceps femoris; L2, L3,† L4
Obturator	Thigh adduction	Pectineus
		Adductor longus, brevis, magnus; L2, L3, L4
		Gracilis
Superior gluteal	Thigh abduction	Gluteus medius and minimus
	Thigh flexion	Tensor fascia lata
	Lateral thigh rotation	Piriformis
Inferior gluteal	Thigh abduction	Gluteus maximus
Sciatic (trunk)	Leg flexion	Biceps femoris; L5,† S1, S2
		Semitendinosus
		Semimembranosus
Deep peroneal	Foot dorsiflexion and supination	Tibialis anterior; L4, L5
	Toes 2–5 and foot extension	Extensor digitorum longus/brevis
	Great toe and foot dorsiflexion	Extensor hallucis longus
Superficial peroneal	Plantar flexion foot and eversion	Peroneus longus/brevis; L5, S1
Tibial	Plantar flexion and inversion	Posterior tibialis
	Flex distal phalanx toes 2–5	Flexor digitorum longus
	Flex distal phalanx great toe	Flexor hallucis longus
	Flex middle phalanx toes 2–5	Flexor digitorum brevis
	Flex proximal phalanx great toe	Gastrocnemius; L5, S1,† S2
	Knee flexion and ankle plantar flexion	Flexor hallucis brevis
	Ankle plantar flexion	Plantaris, soleus
Pudendal	Voluntary pelvic floor contraction	Perineal and sphincters; S3, S4

*Dermatomal representations are listed after some muscles.

†Predominant dermatome.

SPECIAL CIRCUMSTANCES

Although not classically described as part of the motor system examination, information regarding bladder tone and function is at times vital to the examiner. In patients with complaints of incontinence and low back pain, for example, discovery of a probable neurogenic bladder by demonstrating large US-assessed or postcatheterization **residual urine volume** might be a key to diagnosis of spinal cord compression. What is an abnormal postvoid residual bladder volume is difficult to say with certainty, and the literature is not clear on this point, but **in general, a volume of >100 mL, and certainly 200 mL, is cause for concern.**

REFLEXES

Muscle stretch reflexes are the least important part of the neurologic examination and offer little value when used in isolation. Correctly termed *muscle stretch reflexes*, the jerk or involuntary motor movement follows the stretching of intrafusal muscle spindle fibers by the strike of the reflex hammer and the involuntary muscle contraction that follows. Muscle stretch reflexes serve mainly to confirm evidence collected in other parts of the history or physical examination.

Depending on the force of the reflex hammer strike and local impact factors, an elicited reflex may seemingly change from moment to moment. Make sure the patient and the muscle tested are relaxed. Often several reflex strikes are performed. Record the best response.

BASIC

Muscle stretch reflexes are graded on a scale from 1 to 4 that is not rigorously defined, with 0 representing the absence of reflex, 2 or 3 being normal, and 4 representing hyperactive reflexes. Patterns of reflex abnormalities (e.g., upper vs. lower extremity, left vs. right) may suggest a location of a problem within the CNS or peripheral nervous system.

The **Babinski response** is the toe that moves upward in response to a mildly noxious stimulation applied to the lateral plantar or lateral aspect of the foot. The application of stimuli should not be hard or forceful. In

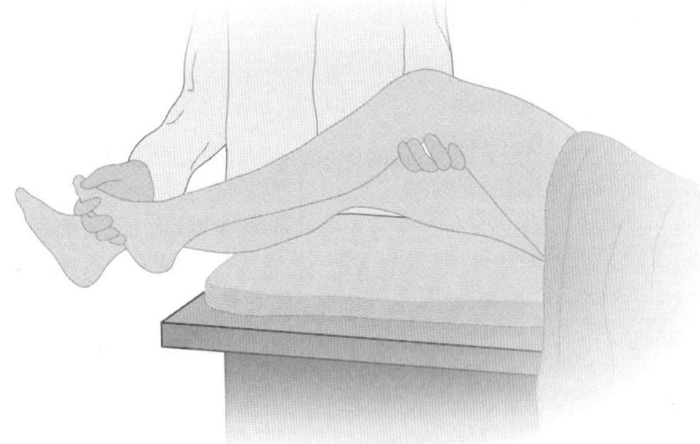

FIGURE 164-3. Method for eliciting ankle clonus.

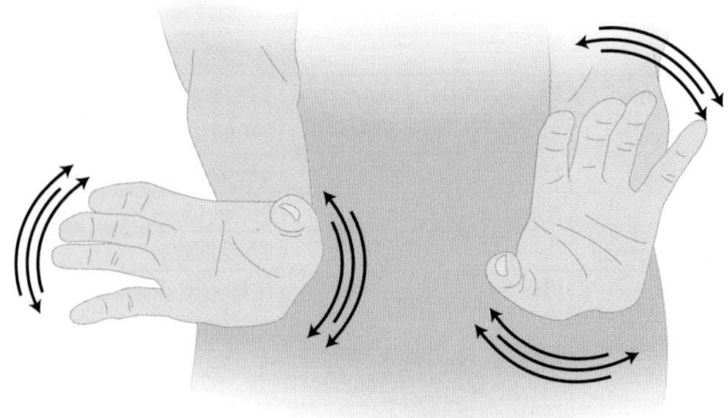

FIGURE 164-4. Pronation and supination test: cerebellar testing.

adults, the normal response of the toe is to move downward to plantar stimulation. The presence of a **Babinski's sign**—that is, the abnormal reflex with movement of the great toe upward and perhaps fanning of the other toes—is the classic indicator of an upper motor neuron lesion. The reliability and accuracy of a Babinski's sign have been called into question.[10] Asymmetry of rapid foot tapping, a little-used test, was found to be more accurate in one small study, with a slowing of foot tapping being the abnormal response.[10]

ADVANCED

Clonus is the rhythmic oscillation of a body part, typically the ankle, elicited by a brisk stretch (**Figure 164-3**). It is one sign of spasticity, in addition to a Babinski response (or slowing of foot tapping), increased muscle tone, and hyperactive muscle stretch reflexes. It may be seen in conditions of metabolic disturbance and primary neurologic dysfunction.

SPECIAL CIRCUMSTANCES

Disease processes involving upper motor neurons or their processes (cortical or spinal cord injuries) result in hyperactive reflexes, a Babinski response, and clonus. Processes injuring lower motor neurons, their axons, peripheral nerve roots, peripheral nerves, or the muscles themselves may result in hypoactive reflexes. However, in spinal cord injury or stroke, reflexes may take several hours or even days to become hyperactive, so the absence of these signs is not valuable in excluding acute spinal cord injury.

Spinal cord emergencies are high-risk clinical scenarios. Although the presence of a Babinski's sign and hyperreflexia are cardinal signs of upper motor neuron syndrome, the absence of these signs does not reliably exclude a diagnosis of spinal cord compression; pursue the diagnosis if historical or other physical examination findings suggest the possibility of this critical diagnosis.[11,12]

CEREBELLAR TESTING

The cerebellum is concerned with involuntary activities of the CNS and is a structure that helps with smoothing muscle movements and aiding with movement coordination. Very simply, the central cerebellar structures may be thought of as controlling coordination of posture and truncal movements (**axial coordination**). The lateral cerebellar structures are more coordinated with movements of the extremities (**appendicular coordination**).

BASIC

Rapidly alternating movements may be assessed by a variety of maneuvers. Hand-slapping tests, asking the patient to rapidly pronate and then supinate the forearm, and slapping the thigh with each movement is a commonly used test. The movements are normally small, and the hand slapping should be symmetric. Rapid pronation and supination of the hands is another test for dystaxia and dysmetria; the movements should be equal with both hands (**Figure 164-4**).

ADVANCED

Although usually included in cranial nerve testing, eye movements are useful in assessing cerebellar function, and abnormalities in their movements may suggest cerebellar dysfunction. Tracking an object slowly should show smooth, slow eye movements; breakup of the smooth movement may be evident and is analogous to the decompensation of movements that may occur in isolated cerebellar impairment. Similarly, if a patient is asked to look back and forth between two objects (finger-to-nose testing involves the patient looking back and forth quickly between the examiner's outstretched finger and nose), the eyes should quickly and conjugately look at the target without overshoot. These faster movements are, at least in part, reflective of intact cerebellar function. **Nystagmus** is rapid involuntary movements of the eyes that may be present with primary (straight-ahead) gaze or provoked by looking at extremes of gaze. Coarse nystagmus or other abnormalities of eye movements are at times present with cerebellar problems (see chapter 170, Vertigo, for a discussion of nystagmus).

GAIT AND STATION

It has been said that, if only one neurologic test could be performed, observation of the patient walking would be the most informative. The posture that the patient assumes when stationary defines the station of the patient. A variety of abnormal gaits and postures are discussed further in chapter 169, Ataxia and Gait Disturbances, as are different techniques of physical examination.

One feature common in many patients with cerebellar hemorrhage is the sudden inability to walk. Keep the possibility of cerebellar injury in mind when evaluating a patient with sudden onset of symptoms that include the inability to walk. Patients with cerebellar hemorrhage may also have severe nausea and vomiting and be massively diaphoretic. Their clinical condition is such that fine neurologic examination is simply not possible.

Acknowledgments: The authors would like to acknowledge the work of Dr. Greg Henry and Dr. Hugh S. Mickel, authors of chapters on this topic in previous editions of the study guide. Their chapters served as a check for completeness and provided some tabular information. J. Stephen Huff would like to acknowledge the influence of the late Dr. William DeMyer of Indiana University, whose instruction in the neurologic examination years ago stimulated an interest in this area.

REFERENCES

The complete reference list is available online at www.TintinalliEM.com.

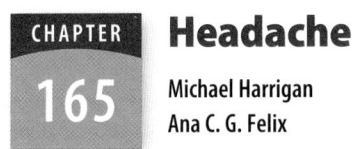

Headache

Michael Harrigan
Ana C. G. Felix

INTRODUCTION AND EPIDEMIOLOGY

Headache is the fifth most common symptom presenting to the ED in the United States, with a total of 2.1 million visits per year.[1] Overall, headaches affect people across all ethnic, geographic, and economic levels, with an estimated global prevalence of 47% in adults.[2]

In the ED, the approach to headache focuses on identifying patients at risk for rapid deterioration, morbidity, and mortality; rapidly identifying high-risk headache syndromes; and providing appropriate headache therapy.

PATHOPHYSIOLOGY

The brain parenchyma has no pain sensors.[3] Early theories postulating vasoconstriction and rebound vasodilatation as the cause of migraine have been refuted.[4] Numerous physiologic mechanisms play a role in the development of the various clinical headache syndromes. For example, occipital nerve irritation may lead to the development of occipital neuralgia.[5] Similarly, headaches associated with disturbances in intracranial pressure (both high and low) are related to compression of, or traction on, pressure-sensitive structures in the meninges.[6] The pathophysiologic mechanisms of other headache syndromes, such as migraine headaches, cluster headaches, and toxic and metabolic headaches, are less clear. Discussion of these mechanisms is beyond the scope of this chapter.

CLINICAL FEATURES

Most patients with headache have conditions that are painful but benign in etiology. Identifying those at high risk is the first step in management (**Table 165-1**). A high-risk cause for headache accounts for only 4% of all headaches but 10% to 14% of acute-onset ("thunderclap") headaches.[7,8] Although headaches are typically classified as **primary headaches** when there is no underlying cause (such as migraine or cluster headaches) and **secondary headaches** if associated with an underlying cause (such as tumor, meningitis, or subarachnoid hemorrhage), this distinction is not clinically useful in the ED setting.

TABLE 165-1 High-Risk Features for Headache: Clinical "Red Flags"

Onset	Sudden Trauma Exertion
Symptoms	Altered mental status Seizure Fever Neurologic symptoms Visual changes
Medications	Anticoagulants/antiplatelets Recent antibiotic use Immunosuppressants
Past history	No prior headache Change in headache quality, or progressive headache worsening over weeks/months
Associated conditions	Pregnancy or postpregnancy status Systemic lupus erythematosus Behçet's disease Vasculitis Sarcoidosis Cancer
Physical examination	Altered mental status Fever Neck stiffness Papilledema Focal neurologic signs

HISTORY

Features associated with high-risk headaches are as follows:

Patient Age Patients >50 years of age, with a new or worsening headache, represent a high-risk group. The incidence of migraine, cluster, and tension headaches decreases with age, raising the likelihood of ominous pathology for older patients.[9]

Onset of Symptoms The abrupt onset of severe headache, or **"thunderclap" headache**, requires immediate and thorough evaluation.[10] Thunderclap headache associated with intracerebral aneurysmal leak ("sentinel hemorrhage" or "herald bleed") may precede catastrophic aneurysmal rupture. Associated symptoms may include neck stiffness, nausea, vomiting, loss of consciousness, neurologic deficit, or altered mentation.[11] Onset of thunderclap headache during periods of exertion raises suspicion for subarachnoid hemorrhage or **arterial dissection** of the carotid or vertebrobasilar circulation. Headaches associated with the Valsalva maneuver may herald an intracranial abnormality.[12] Rarely, spontaneous intracranial hypotension and acute hydrocephalus associated with third ventricular colloid cyst may present with thunderclap headache.[13] Other causes for thunderclap headache are listed in **Table 165-2**.

Headache Quality A change in pattern, frequency, quality, or intensity of a preexisting headache syndrome needs the same evaluation as a new-onset headache syndrome.

Fever Fever raises concern for CNS infection, such as meningitis, encephalitis, or brain abscess. However, the absence of fever does not exclude a CNS infection, especially in patients at the extremes of age and with immunocompromised states.

Medication History Ask about over-the-counter medications, anticoagulants, antiplatelet agents, chronic steroids, immunomodulatory agents, or antibiotics (prescribed or not) to identify patients at high risk for infection (e.g., eculizumab and its elevated risk for meningococcal infection). Chronic use of analgesic and anti-inflammatory agents may result in **rebound or withdrawal headaches**. Medication overuse is defined as use >10 times a month and is notable for ergots, triptans, and opioids.[12] Anticoagulants and antiplatelet agents increase the risk for hemorrhage, both spontaneous and traumatic.[14] The recent use of antibiotics may present with a falsely reassuring clinical appearance due to partial treatment of a potentially dangerous CNS infection.

Prior Headache History A prior history suggestive of migraine, tension, or cluster-type headaches, and response to specific therapy, may obviate the need for extensive ED evaluation (**Tables 165-3 and 165-4**).

TABLE 165-2 Causes of Thunderclap Headache

Hemorrhage	Intracranial hemorrhage "Sentinel" aneurysmal hemorrhage Spontaneous intracerebral hemorrhage
Vascular	Carotid or vertebrobasilar dissection Reversible cerebral vasoconstriction syndrome (RCVS) Cerebral venous thrombosis Posterior reversible encephalopathy syndrome (PRES)
Other causes	Coital headache Valsalva-associated headache Spontaneous intracranial hypotension Acute hydrocephalus (e.g., colloid cyst obstructing third ventricle)[13] Pituitary apoplexy

TABLE 165-3 Clinical Features Suggestive of Migraine

Prior history of migraine	Moderate/severe intensity
Younger age	Unilateral
Multiple prior episodes	Throbbing
Aura and prodrome	Nausea/vomiting
Familiar triggers	Photophobia/phonophobia
Family history	Lasts hours
History of motion sickness	

Substance Use History Use of adrenergic agents such as cocaine, amphetamine, or derivative compounds such as methamphetamine increases risk of intracranial hemorrhage or the less common entity of reversible cerebral vasoconstriction syndrome.[15] Patients with a history of alcohol abuse are at increased risk of intracranial bleeding due to falls, interpersonal violence, and the potential for liver dysfunction associated with prolonged coagulation times and thrombocytopenia.

Family History Known aneurysm or sudden death in first-degree relatives raises the suspicion for intracranial aneurysm.[16] The incidence of aneurysm in patients with a family history is three to five times higher than in those without a family history. A personal or family history of autosomal dominant polycystic kidney disease also increases the risk for intracranial aneurysm. In patients with autosomal dominant polycystic kidney disease, aneurysmal rupture is more likely to occur at a younger age. The presence of migraine in a first-degree relative is associated with a two- to four-fold increased risk of developing migraine.[17]

PHYSICAL EXAMINATION

Vital Signs Headache is a common symptom associated with fever. For example, headache is seen in up to 60% of patients with upper respiratory tract infection symptoms.[7,18] However, the persistence of headache in the presence of a normalized temperature suggests consideration for further evaluation of a possible CNS infection. The presence of fever in association with neck stiffness and altered mental status represents the classic triad of meningitis. Ninety-five percent of patients with bacterial meningitis present with at least two of the four findings (classic triad plus headache).[19]

Severe hypertension can be associated with headache and the development of acute changes in mental status and neurologic function. Posterior reversible encephalopathy syndrome[20] and hypertensive urgency should be considered in such patients (see "Posterior Reversible Encephalopathy Syndrome" section).

Examination of the Head and Neck

Meningismus is an important clinical clue to the presence of infection or hemorrhage.[19] Examine the ears, nose, and throat to identify otitis media and sinusitis, both of which may cause headache and contribute to the extension of infection to the CNS. Palpate for scalp tenderness and tenderness over the temporal arteries to assess for possible temporal arteritis.

Examination of the Eye

Headache can occur with acute angle-closure glaucoma, scleritis, and endophthalmitis. Consider **acute angle-closure glaucoma** even when there is no focal ocular complaint, because the pain can be so severe the patient may fail to localize pain to the eye. Measure intraocular pressure to exclude glaucoma. Check visual acuity and visual fields and examine the pupils and eyelids, checking for signs of Horner's syndrome.

TABLE 165-4 Clinical Features Suggestive of Cluster Headache

At least 5 attacks that meet the following criteria:	Associated **ipsilateral symptoms** (at least one):
• Severe	• Lacrimation
• Unilateral	• Conjunctival injection
• Lasts 15–180 min (untreated)	• Nasal congestion or rhinorrhea
• Circadian/circannual pattern	• Ptosis and/or miosis
	• Edema of the eyelid and/or face
	• Sweating of the forehead and/or face

Funduscopic Examination

Papilledema can be seen in the presence of raised intracranial pressure. However, there is typically a delay in the onset of papilledema once intracranial pressure begins to elevate, and papilledema can persist once intracranial pressure returns to normal.[21] The ability to recognize papilledema by routine direct ophthalmoscopy alone (particularly with non-dilated pupils) is limited, but using a panoptic ophthalmoscope provides a more reliable view of the retina.[22] Bedside US of the optic nerve sheath can also assess for papilledema.[23,24] The presence of papilledema requires CT imaging before lumbar puncture.[25]

Neurologic Examination A baseline neurologic assessment includes the following: mental status assessment; cranial nerve examination, including pupillary examination (for asymmetry or ptosis, which may suggest third nerve compression by posterior communicating artery aneurysms); assessment for other cranial neuropathies (which may raise suspicion for carcinomatous meningitis); motor examination to detect extremity weakness (particularly subtle weakness with pronator drift); reflex examination for subtle asymmetry or a Babinski reflex; and gait and coordination testing (which may be impaired in cerebellar lesions).

DIAGNOSIS

There are many causes of headache, each of which is diagnosed and managed differently. See discussions of specific causes of headache below.

LABORATORY TESTING

Routine blood testing is of limited utility in the diagnosis of acute headache and should be guided by the patient's age, history, relevant comorbidities, and medication history.

The laboratory evaluation of patients with high-risk headaches may include basic metabolic profile, CBC, coagulation panel, erythrocyte sedimentation rate, and blood cultures for possible infection.

IMAGING

Selecting an appropriate imaging study depends on the history, physical examination findings, and differential diagnosis of headache,[26-28] as well as the resources available to the emergency provider. **Table 165-5** summarizes some of the American College of Radiology recommendations for

TABLE 165-5 Choice of Imaging Modality

Noncontrast Head CT	MRI of Brain With and Without Contrast
• Trauma	• New-onset headache *plus* focal neurologic deficit/papilledema
• Thunderclap headache	• Possible encephalitis
• New headache *plus* focal neurologic deficit or papilledema	• Possible vertebral/carotid dissection
• Chronic headache *plus* change in clinical features*	• Horner's syndrome
	• Valsalva or coital headache
	• Immunocompromised individual
	• Patient with cancer history/current cancer
	• Suspected temporal arteritis
	• Intracranial hypotension (low-pressure headache)
	• Headache with suspected intracranial complication of sinusitis/mastoiditis/oromaxillofacial origin
	• New-onset headache in pregnant woman (without contrast)
	• Headache of trigeminal autonomic origin
	• Chronic headache with *new* feature or focal deficit (CT can be first step)

appropriate imaging. When MRI is immediately unavailable and diagnostic uncertainty regarding the possibility of an underlying lesion prevails, further imaging may be necessary, the timing of which will depend on the clinical circumstances and likelihood of the patient being able to follow-up in a reliable fashion.[26]

If the patient presents with a typical history of headache that responds to typical measures and a normal neurologic examination, avoiding imaging may be prudent to reduce the risk for radiation exposure. For most patients in the ED with headache, a noncontrast head CT is the fastest and most appropriate initial imaging study, as well as the most sensitive for detecting acute intracranial hemorrhage.[28,29]

Contrast (iodinated contrast and gadolinium-based magnetic resonance contrast agents) is contraindicated for patients with renal insufficiency due to risk for renal toxicity and nephrogenic systemic fibrosis.[30] Gadolinium is also relatively contraindicated in pregnancy and breastfeeding women. **MRI** can be limited by claustrophobia. A discussion with the radiologist and/or radiology technical staff can clarify the safety of MRI in patients with devices or foreign bodies.

Magnetic resonance angiography is useful in detecting arterial disease (stenosis, congenital anomalies, dissection, CNS vasculitis) and should be considered in any case where there may be arterial pathology underlying the patient's symptoms. Discuss concerns for dissection with the radiologist to determine the most appropriate MRI method.

If MRI is unavailable or not clinically feasible, consultation with radiology regarding other appropriate imaging modalities is prudent.

LUMBAR PUNCTURE

After the clinical assessment, blood work, and imaging, the next step is to determine whether or not to perform a lumbar puncture (LP) and, if so, the timing of LP. LP can serve as both a diagnostic tool (as in meningitis, subarachnoid hemorrhage, intracranial hypotension, carcinomatous meningitis) and therapeutic tool (as in pseudotumor cerebri).

Ideally, perform the LP with the patient in the lateral decubitus position in order to allow for the accurate measurement of opening pressure. Seated LP does not allow for accurate assessment of opening pressure. Opening pressure provides critical information about the patient's intracranial pressure, should be performed routinely, and should be considered a routine procedure when performing LP.

The possibility of herniation in association with LP is a frequent concern of emergency providers. There is no randomized controlled trial assessing the question of when it is safe to perform an LP. The cumulative evidence suggests that in patients without a history of immunosuppression, who have a normal sensorium, and who have no focal neurologic deficits, it is safe to proceed with LP without imaging prior to LP.[31,32]

In the evaluation of patients with suspected acute bacterial meningitis, clinical signs of "impending" herniation are the best predictors of when to delay an LP because of the risk of precipitating herniation. Risk of an abnormal CT scan is elevated in patients with any of the following clinical features: a deteriorating or altered level of consciousness (particularly a Glasgow coma scale score of ≤11), brainstem signs (including pupillary changes, posturing, or irregular respirations), focal neurologic deficit, history of recent seizure, history of a preexisting neurologic disorder, or history of immunocompromised state. In patients with these clinical features, imaging prior to LP is appropriate, but antibiotic administration should not be delayed while imaging is obtained. In patients without such findings, it is usually safe to perform LP without performing a CT scan in cases of suspected bacterial meningitis.[33]

DISPOSITION AND FOLLOW-UP

Most patients with headache can be treated and released from the ED with an appropriate follow-up plan. Identification of potential barriers to follow-up is an important step in ensuring that proper follow-up will be available to all patients, particularly for patients with limited resources or other barriers to accessing medical care. For some patients, inpatient care or observation may be warranted until symptoms improve or until testing is completed. A follow-up plan is especially important for patients with high-risk conditions, such as temporal arteritis or idiopathic intracranial hypertension. Follow-up is similarly important for patients with chronic headaches, given the potential for substance abuse, overutilization of resources, and repeated unnecessary imaging with potentially harmful radiation.[27]

SPECIFIC CAUSES OF HEADACHE

MENINGITIS

Consider meningitis in patients with headache and the classic triad of fever, altered mentation, and neck stiffness.[19] The source of infection can be viral, bacterial, and less commonly, fungal or parasitic. Have a high index of suspicion for meningitis in those with immunosuppression (particularly acquired immunodeficiency syndrome, human immunodeficiency virus, cancer history, chemotherapy, chronic steroids), which may be associated with more insidious types of meningitis such as *Cryptococcus*. An LP is indicated for suspected meningitis. **If the LP is delayed (e.g., CT, coagulopathy, thrombocytopenia, agitation) and meningitis is strongly suspected, administer antibiotics without delay.**[25,34] For many patients who are awake, are alert with no evidence of papilledema or focal neurologic deficit, and have no history to suggest immunocompromised state or new-onset seizure, the head CT can be delayed until after the LP.[25]

SUBARACHNOID HEMORRHAGE

Subarachnoid hemorrhage resulting from rupture of an intracranial aneurysm carries only a 50% 30-day survival rate.[35,36] Approximately half of survivors have some degree of neurologic impairment. Early detection and appropriate management lead to improved clinical outcome. Only 1% of patients presenting to the ED with headache have subarachnoid hemorrhage. However, 10% to 14% of those complaining of the "worst headache of their life" have subarachnoid hemorrhage.[7,8] **Acute onset of a severe headache is subarachnoid hemorrhage until proven otherwise.**[10,11] Inquire about a family history as outlined above.[16] Obtain a noncontrast head CT as the first step in evaluation.[37] With third-generation CT equipment, CT scan done within 6 hours of headache onset is reported to have a sensitivity of 93% and specificity of 100%, with a negative predictive value of 99.4% and positive predictive value of 100%.[38] If head CT is negative for blood but suspicion for subarachnoid hemorrhage is strong, the next step is LP to detect blood or xanthochromia in the cerebrospinal fluid.[39] For further discussion, see chapter 166, "Spontaneous Subarachnoid and Intracerebral Hemorrhage." Consultation with a neurologist or neurosurgeon may be appropriate if the history is highly suggestive of subarachnoid hemorrhage, because both the CT and LP can be normal.[40-42] CT angiogram, magnetic resonance angiogram, MRI with fluid-attenuated inversion recovery/susceptibility-weighted images,[43,44] or four-vessel cerebral angiogram may be reasonable.[26]

SUBDURAL HEMATOMA AND INTRACEREBRAL HEMORRHAGE

Intracranial hemorrhage may occur with or without a history of trauma, in the context of new or progressive headache, with or without associated neurologic deficit. This is particularly important in the elderly, those with chronic alcohol and substance abuse, and patients using antiplatelet and anticoagulant agents. The antiplatelet agent clopidogrel increases the risk of acute intracranial bleeding immediately after trauma, so patients receiving antiplatelet agents and anticoagulants should be screened using head CT, regardless of symptoms. In a prospective trial of patients with blunt head trauma, 12% of those taking clopidogrel and 5.1% of those taking warfarin had acute intracranial hemorrhage noted on their initial CT scan. The risk of delayed intracranial hemorrhage was small in both groups (0 of 296 patients taking clopidogrel and 4 of 687 patients taking warfarin).[14]

Acute headache with associated vestibular symptoms (vertigo or ataxia) should be considered a cerebellar hemorrhage until proven otherwise. Cerebellar hemorrhages make up approximately 10% of all intracerebral hemorrhages and may require prompt surgical evacuation of the hematoma in order to prevent the rapid progression to severe disability or death.[45]

BRAIN TUMOR

Headache in the setting of brain tumor is caused, at least in part, by cerebrospinal fluid flow obstruction and intracranial hypertension.[46]

Clinical signs and symptoms suggesting brain tumor include abnormal neurologic examination, headache worsened by Valsalva maneuver, headache causing awakening from sleep, seizures, recent cancer diagnosis, or mental status change. Of course, the absence of these features does not exclude the possibility of a brain tumor. MRI with and without gadolinium is the study of choice for detecting brain tumors, but cost and limited access make it unfeasible in many settings. A noncontrast CT will identify large masses and edema associated with large masses, but may fail to identify smaller masses. Evaluate for potential barriers to access of medical care in clinical decision making, because additional imaging may be needed at follow-up.

CEREBRAL VENOUS THROMBOSIS

Cerebral venous thrombosis is a rare, but dangerous, cause of headache. Consider the diagnosis in patients presenting with new headache symptoms, especially in the presence of certain known risk factors. Cerebral venous thrombosis is more common in women, especially in the peripartum period, and in patients with a recent surgical history. It is associated with hypercoagulable states such as use of oral contraceptives, hematologic disorders, factor V Leiden homozygous mutation, protein S or protein C deficiency, and anti–thrombin III deficiency.[47] The presentation can vary widely, from a progressive headache developing over days to weeks to, in some instances, a "thunderclap" headache. Similarly, the patient's clinical appearance can be quite benign, especially early on in the course of the illness, or in more severe cases, patients may present with seizures, stroke symptoms, and even coma.[48,49]

In the presence of abnormal imaging (CT, MRI), focal neurologic deficit, or altered mental status, the diagnosis is made definitively with magnetic resonance venography. Given the rare nature of this diagnosis, it is likely that patients suffering from cerebral venous thrombosis may be undergoing evaluation for other causes of severe headache. An elevated LP opening pressure should raise suspicion of central venous thrombosis in the appropriate clinical setting and prompt further imaging with magnetic resonance venography or consultation with a neurologist.[50,51] LP can safely be performed in patients with central venous thrombosis.

POSTERIOR REVERSIBLE ENCEPHALOPATHY SYNDROME (PRES)

Patients with posterior reversible encephalopathy syndrome can present with severe headache, visual changes, seizures, and encephalopathy in the setting of marked blood pressure elevation (usually rapidly developing). It is most common in patients undergoing active treatment with immune-suppressing or -modulating medications or chemotherapeutic agents, as well as in patients with end-stage renal disease. Imaging with MRI typically shows evidence of symmetrical vasogenic edema in the occipital area of the brain, although other areas of the brain can be involved. Treatment involves blood pressure control and supportive care.[52]

REVERSIBLE CEREBRAL VASOCONSTRICTION SYNDROME

This condition is one of a short list of conditions that can mimic subarachnoid hemorrhage (Table 165-2). Characterized by the occurrence of one or more "thunderclap" headaches, the diagnosis should only be considered when the evaluation for subarachnoid hemorrhage has proven negative. The underlying pathophysiology of the syndrome is poorly understood, but it appears to coexist with a number of other cerebral angiopathies (including posterior reversible encephalopathy syndrome) that are characterized by diffuse cerebral vasospasm. The incidence is greater in women, and the peak age of onset is in the early 40s. Most patients will have more than one thunderclap headache over the course of a few weeks. Severe headache may be the only presenting feature, although some patients can present with seizure or focal neurologic deficit. The key diagnostic feature (multiple areas of cerebral vasoconstriction on cerebral angiography) is most commonly found on follow-up angiography between 2 and 3 weeks after symptom onset.[15]

TABLE 165-6 American College of Rheumatology Criteria for Diagnosis of Temporal Arteritis

Clinical Features	Comments
Age at disease onset ≥50 years	
New headache	Onset or type
Temporal artery abnormality	Tenderness to palpation of temporal arteries Decreased pulsation of temporal arteries
Erythrocyte sedimentation rate ≥50 mm/h	Westergren method
Abnormal artery biopsy (can be done after initiating steroids)	Vasculitis Predominance of mononuclear cell infiltration or granulomatous inflammation Multinucleated giant cells

In three published series, the rate of permanent neurologic disability was between 6% and 20%. Reversible cerebral vasoconstriction syndrome, although not widely known among nonneurologists, does not appear to be that rare. One prospective case series included 67 patients diagnosed at a single hospital over a 3-year period of data collection.[53,54]

Initial neuroimaging in these patients may show evidence of nonaneurysmal subarachnoid hemorrhage, ischemic stroke, or intracranial hemorrhage. However, head CT is most commonly normal in these patients. Ultimately, there will be magnetic resonance angiography evidence of cerebral vasoconstriction in all patients, but this may be delayed in appearance. As such, the clinical presentation of thunderclap headache without evidence of subarachnoid hemorrhage should be the main prompt to making this diagnosis or consulting with a neurologist.

TEMPORAL ARTERITIS

Temporal arteritis, also known as giant cell arteritis, is an inflammatory condition affecting the small and medium-sized intracranial and extracranial vessels. Primarily a disease of those >50 years old, its incidence increases with age. In addition to headache, associated symptoms may include fatigue, fever, proximal muscle weakness, jaw claudication, or transient ischemic attack symptoms, especially transient visual loss. Sedimentation rate may be elevated. Check intraocular pressure to exclude glaucoma. Diagnosis is made by the presence of three of the five criteria listed in **Table 165-6**, with a sensitivity of 93.5% and a specificity of 91.2%.[55] Begin treatment with prednisone, 60 milligrams PO daily, to minimize morbidity from visual impairment and stroke. Consult with an ophthalmologist to determine optic nerve function and a rheumatologist. It is important to ensure that there is rapid and appropriate follow-up for patients discharged from the ED, ideally with their primary care provider.

MIGRAINE

The most common non–life-threatening headache in the ED is **migraine** (Table 165-3). Migraine is defined as a headache of moderate to severe intensity that lasts hours (4 to 72 hours on average) and is usually unilateral, pulsatile in quality, typically associated with both photophobia and phonophobia, and generally made worse with physical activity. Migraine can be episodic or chronic and can occur with or without aura. The characteristics of migraine aura vary widely. Among the most common aura symptoms are lightheadedness and visual changes (scotoma and scintillations). Migraines usually start in childhood and peak around age 40 years, with gradual decline thereafter. Prevalence is about 5% for males and 15% to 17% for females.[9]

Chronic migraine is defined as 5 or more migraine headache days per month over the past 3 months. Migraine sufferers who present to the ED are more likely to be chronic headache sufferers.[56,57]

There are many effective treatment options for management of migraine headache, based on randomized controlled trials. Triptans are considered first-line abortive therapy for migraine. However, in the ED setting, most patients have failed abortive therapy and require rescue therapy.

TABLE 165-7 Treatment Options for Migraine Headache

Drug	Dosing	Contraindications	Precautions and Pregnancy Category	Notes
Ketorolac	30 milligrams IV or IM	History of peptic ulcer disease (especially in elderly)	Pregnancy Category B Avoid in third trimester	
Prochlorperazine	5–10 milligrams IV or PR		Pregnancy Category C Drowsiness Dystonic reactions	**Antiemetic** Concurrent: diphenhydramine
Metoclopramide	10 milligrams IV		Pregnancy Category B Drowsiness Dystonic reactions	**Antiemetic** Concurrent: diphenhydramine
Droperidol	2.5 milligrams IV slow, or 2.5 milligrams IM		Pregnancy Category C QT interval prolongation and/or torsade de pointes	Concurrent: diphenhydramine
Chlorpromazine	7.5 milligrams IV		Pregnancy not classified Hypotension Drowsiness Dystonic reactions	**Antiemetic** Pretreat with: normal saline bolus to minimize hypotension Concurrent: diphenhydramine
Magnesium sulfate	2 grams IV over 30 min		Pregnancy Category D but effective in pre-eclampsia and eclampsia	Nonvalidated
Methylprednisolone	125 milligrams IV or IM		Rescue therapy	Nonvalidated
Dexamethasone	6–10 milligrams IV		Rescue therapy	Adjunctive therapy to reduce recurrence
Sumatriptan	6 milligrams SC	Ischemic Heart Disease Uncontrolled hypertension Basilar or hemiplegic migraine	Pregnancy Category C	
Dihydroergotamine (DHE)	1 milligram IV over 3 min	Pregnancy Uncontrolled hypertension Ischemic Heart Disease Recent sumatriptan use (within 24 h)[61] Basilar or hemiplegic migraine	Pregnancy Category X Nausea Vomiting Diarrhea Abdominal pain	Pretreat with antiemetic
Valproate	500 milligrams IV	Pregnancy	Pregnancy Category X	Nonvalidated

ED Treatment of Migraine Initial treatment consists of IV hydration and repetitive IV treatment with nonsteroidal anti-inflammatory drugs and an antiemetic (**Table 165-7**). Many combinations are effective. **Combination with antihistamine (usually diphenhydramine 25 to 50 milligrams IV) is helpful,** because increased histamine levels correlate with migraine attacks, and diphenhydramine can also treat akathisias from antiemetics. Antihistamines alone are not helpful.[58]

Steroids can be useful to reduce the risk for headache recurrence after ED discharge.[59,60]

Opiates and barbiturate-containing compounds should not be used routinely for abortive migraine therapy unless other standard treatments fail. Not recommended for routine use are ergotamine and codeine- and tramadol-containing medications, as well as butorphanol and butalbital-containing medications.[62,63]

In **pregnancy**, there is scant data on treatment of migraine. In general, triptans are contraindicated; acetaminophen, opioids, or corticosteroids can be used. Metoclopramide (U.S. Food and Drug Administration Category B) may be used. Nonsteroidal anti-inflammatory drugs may be also used until the third trimester. Ergotamines and combination agents with caffeine and isometheptene are absolutely contraindicated in pregnant women.

Upon discharge from the ED, more than half of patients will have some residual headache, and there is an increased rate of recurrence of headache within the first 3 days after discharge.[59,60,64] Therefore, a prescription for abortive medications should form part of the discharge plan for patients being discharged from the ED with a diagnosis of migraine. Providers should be familiar with one or two fast-acting triptans (such as sumatriptan, sold as Imitrex™ in the United States, and rizatriptan, sold as Maxalt™ in the United States), as well as combinations of triptans, such as sumatriptan/naproxen (sold as Treximet™ in the United States), or combination drugs, such as Midrin™ (acetaminophen, 325 milligrams/dichloralphenazone, 100 milligrams/isometheptene, 65 milligrams).

OCCIPITAL NEURALGIA

Occipital neuralgia is characterized by paroxysms of lancinating pain at the back of the head, in the distribution of the greater and/or lesser occipital nerve. Patients describe the pain as stabbing or electric shock–like in quality, with hypersensitivity in the distribution of the affected nerve. Most cases are attributed to chronic neck tension or unknown causes. However, the condition can be associated with osteoarthritis or degenerative disease of the upper cervical spine. Occipital nerve block typically results in marked improvement of symptoms, and the results can persist for weeks after the injection. The procedure is both diagnostic and therapeutic. The procedure can be performed with ease in any setting and requires minimal expertise.

IDIOPATHIC INTRACRANIAL HYPERTENSION (PSEUDOTUMOR CEREBRI SYNDROME)

Idiopathic intracranial hypertension, also known as pseudotumor cerebri, is most common in obese women. The incidence is 19.3 per 100,000 obese women between the ages of 20 and 44 years and has increased along with the obesity epidemic. The most prominent symptoms include headache (84%), transient visual obscurations (68%), back pain (53%), and pulsatile tinnitus (52%). Only 32% of patients report visual loss. Untreated, idiopathic intracranial hypertension can lead to permanent visual impairment if not recognized and treated appropriately.[65]

The diagnostic criteria include papilledema with an otherwise normal neurologic examination and elevated opening pressure on LP (>25 cm H_2O in adults and >28 cm H_2O in children), in the setting of normal cerebrospinal fluid composition and normal imaging (having excluded other causes of raised intracranial pressure). Treatment is focused on preservation of vision. A variant of pseudotumor has been identified that does not present with papilledema but may present with the other clinical features of pseudotumor cerebri, along with abducens nerve palsy (unilateral or bilateral). In the absence of either papilledema or abducens nerve palsy, the diagnosis of pseudotumor without papilledema can be made if at least three of the following neuroimaging findings are present: empty sella, flattening of the posterior aspect of the globe, distention of the perioptic subarachnoid space with or without a tortuous optic nerve, and transverse venous sinus stenosis.[66]

LP is necessary to make the diagnosis of idiopathic intracranial hypertension, and concomitant removal of a volume of cerebrospinal fluid can provide temporary relief of symptoms. However, subjective improvement of symptoms after LP is not reliable in establishing the diagnosis.[66] Perform the LP with the patient in the lateral decubitus position, without sedation (which may cause mild hypercapnia and, subsequently, an elevated cerebrospinal fluid pressure measurement). The knees should be extended for measurement of cerebrospinal fluid pressure, and the base of the manometer should be level with the right atrium. Elevated cerebrospinal fluid pressures can occur in the setting of the Valsalva maneuver, such as breath holding and crying, and if the pressure is measured in the sitting position. Cerebrospinal fluid can be removed in multiple aliquots, measuring cerebrospinal fluid pressure after each removal, until a target pressure of 15 to 20 cm H_2O is achieved. Determine the opening pressure. **In general, removal of 1 mL of cerebrospinal fluid will lower the cerebrospinal fluid pressure by about 1 cm H_2O.**[67] To avoid lowering the pressure excessively, first remove 1 mL for every 1 cm H_2O reduction desired, and then remeasure cerebrospinal fluid pressure. Excess cerebrospinal fluid removal can result in intracranial hypotension and a "low-pressure headache," which may require epidural blood patch for relief.

Oral acetazolamide can be effective in lowering intracranial pressure and decreasing the symptoms of idiopathic intracranial hypertension. Treatment is typically started at 250 to 500 milligrams twice a day.[68] The dose can be increased to as much as 4 grams/d, but dose escalation is associated with significant side effects (paresthesias, fatigue, decreased libido, metallic taste) and should be done under the supervision of a neurologist or ophthalmologist for ongoing monitoring of papilledema and visual field testing to minimize the risk of visual loss.[69] Long-term interventional management may include cerebrospinal fluid shunting and optic nerve sheath fenestration for failing vision. For obese patients, weight loss is recommended.[69]

INTRACRANIAL HYPOTENSION

The headache of intracranial hypotension (low-pressure headache) is most commonly associated with recent dural penetration, either during LP, epidural anesthesia, or any operative procedure that involves opening the dura. Using a noncutting needle reduces the risk of post-LP headache.[70] Rarely, intracranial hypotension can occur spontaneously or in association with head or spine trauma.[71-73] Clinical features include headache that increases in severity with upright posture but improves or resolves in the supine position. Associated symptoms, such as alterations in hearing or vision, nausea, vomiting, diplopia, and visual changes, may occur. MRI, with and without contrast, confirms the diagnosis by showing diffuse enhancement of the meninges. The LP, if performed, should have an opening pressure <6 cm H_2O. Most patients experience spontaneous resolution of their symptoms. Evidence to support treatments, including IV fluid resuscitation and IV caffeine, is limited. The most effective therapy for low-pressure headache is an epidural blood patch, typically performed by anesthesiologists.[71,74]

CARCINOMATOUS MENINGITIS

About 5% to 10% of patients with cancer develop leptomeningeal metastases. In addition to headache, cranial nerve abnormalities (typically more than one) and other neurologic findings may be present. Risk factors for carcinomatous meningitis include aggressive lymphoma subtypes and uncontrolled systemic disease. In suspected patients, the appropriate testing would include MRI with and without contrast (to evaluate for meningeal enhancement). Obtain MRI before LP because MRI evidence of meningeal enhancement is common after LP and may confound the diagnosis. LP may reveal an elevated opening pressure (>20 cm H_2O). Cerebrospinal fluid analysis should include cytology (solid tumors) or flow cytometry (hematologic tumors). Malignant cells degrade quickly, so timely review of cerebrospinal fluid is important.[75]

CLUSTER HEADACHE

Cluster headaches (Table 165-4) occur in about 0.4% of the general population and can mimic dental pain. More common in men, cluster headaches typically start in adulthood and tend to occur in "clusters," with a circadian and circannual pattern, recurring daily for more than a week and remitting for at least 4 weeks. Episodes are typically unilateral and excruciating, but brief and self-limited. Up to 10% of patients will experience a more chronic form, with fewer episodes of remission. Associated **ipsilateral symptoms are common** (Table 165-4), and a distinguishing feature of this headache is the need for the patient to "pace," in contrast to the patient with migraine, who prefers to lie still in a quiet and dark room. Treatment consists of 100% oxygen administered at 12 L/min for 15 minutes through a nonrebreathing facemask.[76,77] Sumatriptan, 6 milligrams SC, can also be used.

HYPERTENSIVE HEADACHE

There is no compelling evidence linking mild to moderate **hypertension** with headache. Several studies using ambulatory blood pressure monitoring have found no association between mild to moderate high blood pressure (systolic blood pressure <180 mm Hg and/or diastolic blood pressure <120 mm Hg) and patient self-reported headache.[78] Uncontrolled hypertension can be associated with headache, especially in conditions where there is a rapid and marked rise in blood pressure, such as pheochromocytoma, posterior reversible encephalopathy syndrome,[20] hypertensive crisis, pre-eclampsia, and eclampsia.[78]

METABOLIC CAUSES OF HEADACHE

Metabolic headaches are hallmarked by deterioration in the setting of a disorder of homeostasis and typically improve after resolution of the disorder of homeostasis (**Table 165-8**).[78]

COITAL HEADACHE

Coital headache, also known as orgasmic headache, is a thunderclap headache that occurs at orgasm. Coital headache is considered benign with no specific treatment needed. Recovery is complete. However, the diagnosis is one of exclusion, to ensure that other causes of thunderclap headache are not missed, including subarachnoid hemorrhage and reversible cerebral vasoconstriction syndrome.[79] The clinical diagnosis of coital headache is one of exclusion and cannot be made without imaging. If MRI is unavailable or not clinically feasible, consultation with radiology regarding other appropriate imaging modalities is prudent.[26]

VALSALVA-ASSOCIATED HEADACHE

Valsalva maneuver may trigger thunderclap headache, a diagnosis made when the headache is only associated with cough, straining, or a Valsalva maneuver, with normal neuroimaging. Symptomatic cough headache is the diagnosis made when an underlying pathology (usually a type I Chiari malformation) is likely to be the cause of the headache.[80]

PITUITARY APOPLEXY

Pituitary tumor apoplexy is a rare clinical diagnosis, that is usually due to spontaneous hemorrhage or infarction of a preexisting pituitary adenoma.[81] The earliest symptom is sudden, severe headache.

TABLE 165-8 Metabolic Causes of Headache

History	Examples	Treatment
Hypoxia/hypercapnia	High altitude	Acetaminophen/ibuprofen Acetazolamide 125–250 milligrams twice a day Steroids (dexamethasone) Prophylaxis: acetylsalicylic acid, 320 milligrams at 4-h intervals, starting 1 h prior to ascent; repeat 3 times
	Air travel	Nonsteroidal anti-inflammatory drugs (NSAIDs), pseudoephedrine, and nasal decongestants
	Pulmonary disease Congestive heart failure Sleep apnea	
Dialysis		NSAIDs/analgesics during dialysis
Autonomic dysreflexia (typical in quadriplegia)		Seated position Remove/loosen clothing Scrutinize for bladder distension/bowel impaction
Other	Hypothyroidism Fasting Cardiac cephalgia (associated with myocardial ischemia)	

The headache location tends to be retro-orbital, bifrontal, or suboccipital. Between 63% and 100% of patients will experience headache.[81] Associated symptoms may include ophthalmoplegia, reduced visual acuity, visual field defects, altered consciousness, meningismus, and nausea and vomiting. CT (noncontrast) and MRI may show a sellar mass and hemorrhage. In the first 1 to 2 hours, the hyperacute hemorrhage may be easier to see on CT than MRI. Pituitary adenomas and cerebral aneurysms have a co-occurrence rate of 7.4%.[81] Pituitary tumor apoplexy requires immediate treatment with corticosteroids and urgent neurosurgical consultation. The treatment usually requires consultations from endocrinology, ophthalmology, and neurology with intensive care monitoring.

THIRD VENTRICLE COLLOID CYSTS

Colloid cysts of the third ventricle are a rare cause of acute neurologic deterioration and sudden death. The colloid cyst is usually congenital, slow growing, and benign, accounting for about 0.2% to 2% of all intracranial tumors, but it is the most common tumor of the third ventricle.[82] The usual clinical presentation is a history of severe paroxysmal and episodic attacks of (typically frontal) headache associated with nausea and vomiting. The presumptive cause is the intermittent obstruction of cerebrospinal fluid flow through the foramina of Monro with associated rapid increase in intracranial pressure.[83]

SINUSITIS

Classic features of purulent nasal discharge, nasal or facial congestion, hyposomia, or anosmia with or without fever, along with headache, ear pain or fullness, halitosis, and dental pain, allow for clinical diagnosis of **sinusitis**,[84] and treatment with antibiotics is warranted.

REFERENCES

The complete reference list is available online at www.TintinalliEM.com.

CHAPTER 166 Spontaneous Subarachnoid and Intracerebral Hemorrhage

Jeffrey L. Hackman
Anna M. Nelson
O. John Ma

INTRODUCTION

Although nontraumatic subarachnoid and intracerebral hemorrhages account for a relatively small portion of ED visits, a missed diagnosis can produce devastating results. Early recognition and aggressive management may improve outcomes.

Subarachnoid hemorrhage is the leakage of blood into the subarachnoid space, most often due to a ruptured intracranial aneurysm. The classic presentation is a sudden, severe headache.

Intracerebral hemorrhage, or hemorrhagic stroke, typically presents as an acute neurologic deficit, often accompanied by headache. The features and treatment of subarachnoid and intracerebral hemorrhage are discussed in this chapter. Management of intracerebral hemorrhage is very different from the management of ischemic stroke. Ischemic stroke is discussed in chapter 167, Stroke Syndromes.

SUBARACHNOID HEMORRHAGE

EPIDEMIOLOGY

About 75% of subarachnoid hemorrhages are caused by a ruptured aneurysm. In about 20%, a cause is not identified.[1] The remaining causes are related to a variety of miscellaneous conditions, including arteriovenous malformations, sympathomimetic drugs, and other less common causes. About 20% of patients with one aneurysm will have an additional aneurysm, which makes identification of the initial aneurysm important.

Two percent of family members of patients with subarachnoid hemorrhage will develop the same disease. This risk rises with increasing number of family members involved or with a family history of adult polycystic kidney disease.[1] Hypertension and smoking increase the risk. Additional risk factors are listed in **Table 166-1**.

PATHOPHYSIOLOGY

Cerebral aneurysms are focal arterial pouches typically located in areas of bifurcation of the circle of Willis. While the precise pathophysiology is not known, many factors have been associated with aneurysmal development and rupture. Such factors include familial/genetic predisposition, cellular aberrations in vascular wall repair or remodeling, and aberrations in local blood flow.[2] While it is not possible to predict rupture risk of a particular aneurysm, larger aneurysms (>5–10 mm) are more likely to rupture than smaller aneurysms.[2,3]

TABLE 166-1 Risk Factors for Subarachnoid Hemorrhage

Hypertension
Smoking
Excessive alcohol consumption
Polycystic kidney disease
Family history of subarachnoid hemorrhage
Coarctation of the aorta
Marfan's syndrome
Ehlers-Danlos syndrome type IV
α_1-Antitrypsin deficiency

CLINICAL FEATURES

Patients with subarachnoid hemorrhage classically present to the ED with a severe headache of acute onset (termed a "thunderclap" headache) that reaches maximal intensity within minutes. Typically, the headache persists for several days, but may resolve in a shorter period.[1] Subarachnoid hemorrhage is diagnosed in 11% to 25% of patients who present to the ED with a thunderclap headache.[4,5] **Even if a patient is not experiencing the "worst ever" headache, a headache that is different in intensity or quality from past headaches raises concern for subarachnoid hemorrhage.** Headaches associated with loss of consciousness, seizure, diplopia or other neurologic signs, or nuchal rigidity also require clinical investigation.[6] Less frequently, patients may present with nausea and vomiting, altered mental status, photophobia, or symptoms suggestive of ischemic stroke. Approximately 20% of patients develop their symptoms while engaged in activities that cause increased blood pressure, such as exercise, sexual intercourse, or defecation. Isolated, uncomplicated true syncope without head trauma, headache, seizure, neurologic deficits, nuchal rigidity, or other symptoms of subarachnoid hemorrhage does not require evaluation for subarachnoid hemorrhage. In the absence of blunt trauma, subhyaloid retinal hemorrhage is pathognomonic of subarachnoid hemorrhage but is not commonly seen.

DIAGNOSIS

Patients with subarachnoid hemorrhage who are misdiagnosed at their initial ED visit have worse outcomes than those who are diagnosed early.[7,8] Misdiagnosis is associated with normal mental status (present in about half of patients with subarachnoid hemorrhage) and smaller size of hemorrhage.[8] Complications of missed diagnosis include repeat hemorrhage and obstructive hydrocephalus. Symptomatic improvement following analgesics does not exclude life-threatening causes of headache.[9] **Table 166-2** lists the differential diagnosis of subarachnoid hemorrhage.

Imaging The initial diagnostic modality of choice when subarachnoid hemorrhage is suspected is a noncontrast CT of the head (**Figures 166-1** and **166-2**). **The sensitivity of CT in diagnosing subarachnoid hemorrhage is highest shortly after symptoms begin and is estimated to be 98% within 6 to 12 hours of the onset of symptoms.** Sensitivity decreases to about 91% to 93% at 24 hours and continues to decline rapidly thereafter, reaching 50% at 1 week.[6,9] Newer-generation CT scanners provide increased sensitivity for detecting subarachnoid hemorrhage, especially in the setting of (1) patients presenting within 6 hours of symptom onset, and (2) greater availability of a timely interpretation by a neuroradiologist.[10-12] For suspected subarachnoid hemorrhage, a negative head CT is typically followed by LP (see later discussion).

CT/CT angiography (CTA) and MRI/MRA are options after a negative head CT, when these studies are clinically appropriate and available.[13] In a small study, two of 116 patients had an aneurysm discovered by CTA after normal findings on both CT and LP.[14] The probability of excluding a subarachnoid hemorrhage following CT/CTA is about 99.4%.[15]

TABLE 166-2 Differential Diagnosis of Subarachnoid Hemorrhage
Vascular (other intracranial hemorrhage, ischemic stroke or transient ischemic attack, arterial dissection, venous thrombosis)
Drug toxicity
Infection (meningitis, encephalitis)
Intracranial tumor
Intracranial hypotension
Metabolic derangements
Primary headache syndromes (benign thunderclap headache, migraine, cluster headache)
Hypertensive disorders

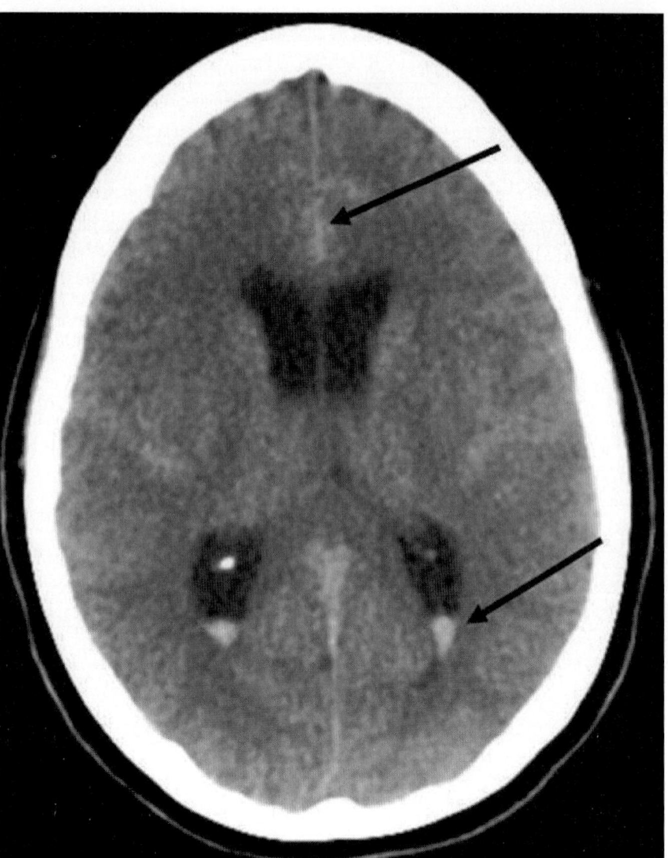

FIGURE 166-1. Diffuse subarachnoid hemorrhage with associated ventricular hemorrhage. *Top arrow* indicates blood in interhemispheric fissure. *Bottom arrow* indicates blood in lateral ventricle. [Image used with permission of James Anderson, MD, Department of Radiology, Oregon Health & Science University.]

Important consequences of this diagnostic pathway include the detection of incidental aneurysms, as opposed to clinically significant bleeds, with the background incidence of aneurysms in the population (2% to 6%) exceeding that of the morbidity and mortality associated with subarachnoid hemorrhages.[16] The major disadvantage of CT/CTA is ionizing radiation. The usefulness of MRI, particularly fluid-attenuated inversion recovery MRI sequences, is limited.[17] A negative MRI result would still need to be followed by an LP.[18] The major disadvantages of MRI/MRA at this time are availability, time to perform the examination, and cost.

Lumbar Puncture Most authorities recommend CSF analysis when a patient with suspected subarachnoid hemorrhage has a normal result on head CT.[19,20] Another advantage of LP is the ability to identify other causes of headache such as meningitis or idiopathic intracranial hypertension. The disadvantages of LP include post-LP headache and inability to perform the procedure in the patient with coagulopathy or thrombocytopenia.

The two CSF tests of greatest interest are the presence of xanthochromia and RBC count. **Xanthochromia** is a yellow appearance of the CSF due to the enzymatic breakdown of blood releasing bilirubin. Any exposure of the CSF to light prior to interpretation can increase the rate of bilirubin degradation, which decreases any xanthochromia present.[1] Similarly, a delay in processing the CSF specimen may result in the development of xanthochromia following a traumatic LP. CSF is evaluated for xanthochromia with visual inspection, the standard technique in most U.S. laboratories, or by spectrophotometry, which may have superior sensitivity but approximately 75% specificity, resulting in additional unnecessary diagnostics for false positives.[21] The utility of the

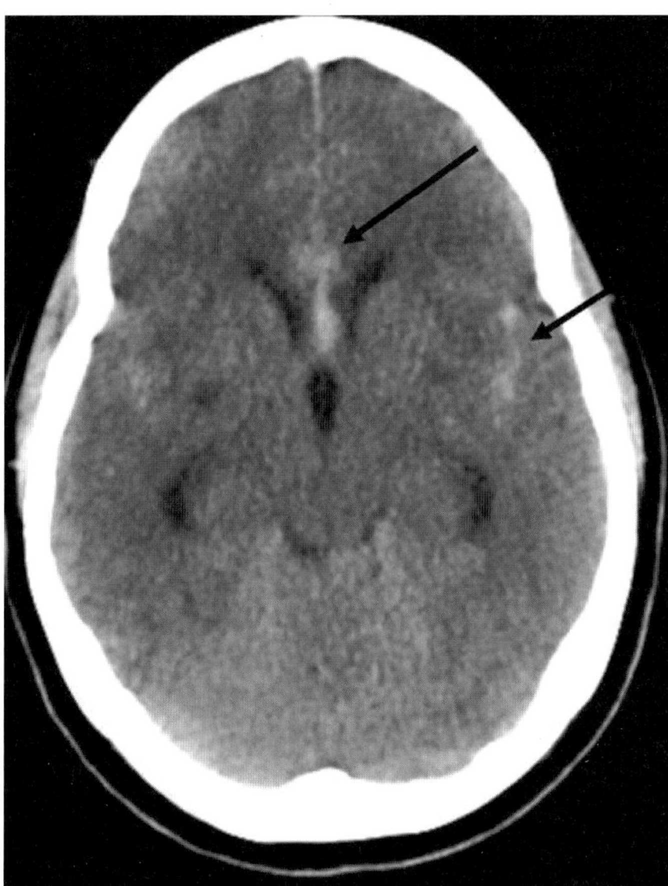

FIGURE 166-2. Scattered subarachnoid hemorrhages (*arrows*). [Image used with permission of James Anderson, MD, Department of Radiology, Oregon Health & Science University.]

test is further limited in that it takes approximately 12 hours for xanthochromia to develop in CSF.[22]

The RBC count in the third or fourth tube of CSF is commonly used to identify subarachnoid hemorrhage. Several issues can make interpreting CSF results challenging. The number of RBCs that constitutes a "positive" LP result has never been clearly defined, nor has the number of RBCs that may be attributed to a "traumatic" LP. One study showed that approximately 10% or 15% of LPs are traumatic, using cutoffs of 400 and 1000 RBCs, respectively.[23] A comparison of cell counts between consecutive tubes or between tubes 1 and 4 is sometimes used to differentiate subarachnoid hemorrhage from a traumatic LP. A small study, however, demonstrated that a 25% reduction in RBCs between tubes 1 and 4 may occur even in cases of confirmed subarachnoid hemorrhage.[24] Another small study found that RBCs <100 in the final tube effectively ruled out subarachnoid hemorrhage, whereas an RBC count of >10,000 in the final tube was associated with an increase in the odds of subarachnoid hemorrhage by a factor of 6.[25]

In general, **normal findings on head CT, the absence of xanthochromia, and zero or few RBCs ($<5 \times 10^6$ RBCs/L) in the CSF help reliably exclude subarachnoid hemorrhage.**[26] A normal head CT result with a positive finding of xanthochromia or elevated RBC count should be considered diagnostic of subarachnoid hemorrhage. **Unfortunately, the literature remains unclear on the precise threshold number of RBCs needed in the CSF to be considered diagnostic of subarachnoid hemorrhage.**

Subarachnoid Hemorrhage Grading Scales Many different subarachnoid hemorrhage grading scales exist. Those most widely used include the Hunt and Hess scale and the World Federation of Neurosurgical Societies scale (**Table 166-3**). A higher grade on either scale indicates a higher likelihood of poor outcome.

TREATMENT

Medical management of the subarachnoid hemorrhage patient in the ED should occur in a monitored critical care area and should target the prevention of complications. Check the Glasgow Coma Scale and pupillary responses regularly because a decrease of 1 Glasgow Coma Scale point can indicate the onset of complications.[1] Intracerebral and extracerebral complications of subarachnoid hemorrhage include rebleeding, vasospasm, cerebral infarction, cerebral edema, hydrocephalus, intracranial hypertension, fluid status and electrolyte abnormalities, respiratory failure, myocardial dysfunction, thromboembolism, and sepsis.[27]

The risk of rebleeding is greatest in the first 24 hours and can be reduced by adequate blood pressure control; however, the ideal target blood pressure and antihypertensive agent remain unclear. If known, maintain the patient's prehemorrhage blood pressure; otherwise, a mean arterial pressure of <140 mm Hg is a reasonable target while avoiding hypotension.[28] Because blood pressure may fluctuate through the course of the disease, a titratable IV antihypertensive is preferred. **Labetalol** and **nicardipine** are most often used, with neither showing clear superiority. **Avoid nitroprusside and nitroglycerin** because they increase cerebral blood volume and intracranial pressure.[29,30] Pain medications and antiemetics also play an important role in maintaining the alert patient's comfort and blood pressure. There is debate regarding the use of antifibrinolytics to prevent rebleeding after subarachnoid hemorrhage, with evidence supporting short- but not long-term use, although generally, these are not used because there is a risk of increased cerebral ischemia.[31]

Vasospasm is most common 2 days to 3 weeks after subarachnoid hemorrhage. A modest protective benefit is seen with administration of nimodipine, 60 milligrams PO every 4 hours, and this therapy should be initiated within 96 hours of symptom onset unless contraindicated due to allergy, nonfunctioning GI tract, or hepatic disease. Clinical trials of other novel treatments, including statins, magnesium, and endothelin receptor antagonist, have not demonstrated significant reductions in mortality.[32-36]

Delayed cerebral ischemia is associated with hypothermia, hyperthermia, and hyperglycemia. Prevent these conditions with the appropriate use of warming or cooling blankets, antipyretics, or insulin when indicated.

TABLE 166-3 Grading Scales for Subarachnoid Hemorrhage

Grade	Hunt-Hess Scale	World Federation of Neurosurgical Societies Scale
1	Mild headache, normal mental status, no cranial nerve or motor findings	GCS of 15, no motor deficits
2	Severe headache, normal mental status, may have cranial nerve deficit	GCS of 13 or 14, no motor deficits
3	Somnolent, confused, may have cranial nerve or mild motor deficit	GCS of 13 or 14, with motor deficits
4	Stupor, moderate to severe motor deficit, may have intermittent reflex posturing	GCS of 7–12, with or without motor deficits
5	Coma, reflex posturing or flaccid	GCS of 3–6, with or without motor deficits

Abbreviation: GCS = Glasgow Coma Scale score.

(*Source:* Reproduced with permission from Hemphill JC: Neurologic critical care, in Fauci AS, Braunwald E, Kasper DL, et al (eds): *Harrison's Principles of Internal Medicine, 17th ed.* © McGraw-Hill Inc., New York, 2008.)

Approximately 5% to 20% of patients with subarachnoid hemorrhage have at least one seizure. Consideration of seizure prophylaxis is currently supported by several clinical guidelines; however, this topic remains controversial and should be determined in conjunction with the intensivist or neurosurgeon who will manage the patient.[37]

DISPOSITION AND FOLLOW-UP

Admit all patients diagnosed with subarachnoid hemorrhage to an intensive care unit in consultation with a neurosurgeon. In the absence of another indication for admission, patients who have normal findings on head CT and CSF analysis within 2 weeks of occurrence of initial symptoms may be safely discharged from the ED.[1,38] Consider consultation with a neurosurgeon for patients who present >2 weeks after the sudden onset of a severe headache causing suspicion for subarachnoid hemorrhage if the initial workup yields normal findings.[1]

INTRACEREBRAL HEMORRHAGE

EPIDEMIOLOGY

Spontaneous intracerebral hemorrhage causes 8% to 11% of all acute strokes and is twice as common as subarachnoid hemorrhage. Like subarachnoid hemorrhage, intracerebral hemorrhage carries a high morbidity and mortality. Seven-day mortality is approximately 30%, 1-year mortality about 55%, and 10-year mortality approximately 80%.[39] Among those who survive, only one in five will be functionally independent at 1 year. There has been no recent change in mortality after intracerebral hemorrhage. This may be because the increased use of anticoagulation for atrial fibrillation to prevent ischemic stroke contributes to poorer outcomes in those patients taking anticoagulants who develop intracerebral hemorrhage.[39] Intracerebral hemorrhage occurs more than two times more frequently in blacks than in whites, which may be related to the higher prevalence of hypertension in blacks.[40] Anticoagulation with warfarin is a significant risk factor for intracerebral hemorrhage, with an annual intracerebral hemorrhage incidence of 0.3% to 0.6% in those taking the drug, and plays a role in 6% to 16% of all cases of intracerebral hemorrhage. Among patients taking warfarin, the risk of intracerebral hemorrhage nearly doubles for each 0.5 increase in international normalized ratio above 4.5. Intracerebral hemorrhage occurs in approximately 3% to 9% of patients treated with tissue plasminogen activator for acute ischemic stroke.[28] Current information suggests that major bleeding events occur at a similar rate with warfarin and direct thrombin inhibitors.[41]

PATHOPHYSIOLOGY

Risk factors for intracerebral hemorrhage include long-standing hypertension, arteriovenous malformations, arterial aneurysm, anticoagulant therapy, use of sympathomimetic drugs (particularly cocaine and phenylpropanolamine), intracranial tumors, and amyloid angiopathy in the elderly. Current smoking and increased frequency of smoking also raise the risk of intracerebral hemorrhage, but the etiology of this increased risk has not been as well defined as in ischemic stroke.[42]

CLINICAL FEATURES

Intracerebral hemorrhage may be clinically indistinguishable from cerebral infarction, subarachnoid hemorrhage, and ischemic stroke. In intracerebral hemorrhage, headache, nausea, and vomiting often precede the neurologic deficit, and in contrast to subarachnoid hemorrhage, the headache onset is usually more insidious. **In hypertensive intracerebral hemorrhage, bleeding is usually localized to the putamen, thalamus, pons, or cerebellum (in decreasing order of frequency)**, and clinical examination findings may be relatable to those areas. **Cerebellar hemorrhage** is commonly associated with dizziness, vomiting, marked truncal ataxia, gaze palsies, and depressed level of consciousness. Patients with cerebellar hemorrhage are more likely to have rapidly progressive symptoms and may require more aggressive intervention than patients with other forms of intracerebral hemorrhage.

DIAGNOSIS AND IMAGING

The differential diagnosis of intracerebral hemorrhage is similar to that of subarachnoid hemorrhage. The history, rapidity of progression of symptoms, and other clinical features may suggest that intracerebral hemorrhage is more likely than subarachnoid hemorrhage or ischemic stroke, but these features are not adequate alone to make a clinical diagnosis. CT and MRI each have areas of superiority in evaluating a patient for intracerebral hemorrhage. **CT is optimal for demonstrating hemorrhage extension into the ventricles, whereas MRI is superior for demonstrating underlying structural lesions.** Either modality is considered acceptable as the initial study for diagnosing intracerebral hemorrhage.[28] Widespread availability of CT makes a noncontrast CT the initial study of choice in most EDs (**Figure 166-3**). The addition of contrast may allow identification of masses or aneurysms.

Cerebral angiography may be useful in selected patients in stable condition who do not require urgent surgery, particularly those in whom no obvious cause of bleeding is identified and those younger than 45 years of age without hypertension.[43]

Additional tests should be performed to exclude coexisting pathology or facilitate surgery, if necessary, including a complete blood count, electrolyte levels, creatinine level, glucose level, electrocardiogram, chest radiograph,

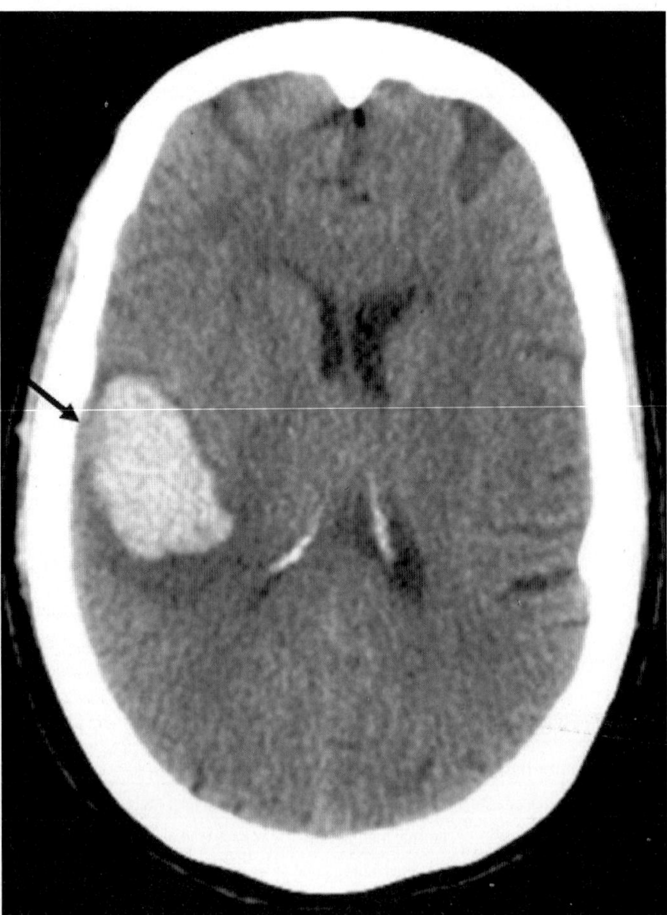

FIGURE 166-3. Large right-sided parietal intraparenchymal hemorrhage (*arrow*). [Image used with permission of James Anderson, MD, Department of Radiology, Oregon Health & Science University.]

TABLE 166-4 Suggested Guidelines for Treating Elevated Blood Pressure in Spontaneous Intracranial Hemorrhage

Clinical Circumstances	Management
SBP >200 mm Hg or MAP >150 mm Hg	Consider aggressive reduction of blood pressure with continuous IV infusion.
SBP >180 mm Hg or MAP >130 mm Hg and evidence or suspicion of elevated ICP	Consider monitoring ICP and reducing blood pressure using intermittent or continuous IV medications to keep cerebral perfusion pressure >60–80 mm Hg.
SBP >180 mm Hg or MAP >130 mm Hg and no evidence or suspicion of elevated ICP	Consider a modest reduction of blood pressure (e.g., MAP of 110 mm Hg or target blood pressure of 160/90 mm Hg) using intermittent or continuous IV medications.

Abbreviations: ICP = intracranial pressure; MAP = mean arterial pressure; SBP = systolic blood pressure.

coagulation studies, and blood type and screen. A urine pregnancy test and screen for drugs of abuse should be performed as appropriate.

TREATMENT

Treatment of patients with intracerebral hemorrhage should occur in a monitored critical-care area with appropriate urgency. Patients with cerebellar hemorrhage are at particularly high risk of rapid deterioration and may require rapid intervention.[44] Maintain close attention to the patient's airway, monitoring of neurologic status, management of hyperthermia with antipyretics, administration of antiepileptic medications if seizures occur, aggressive management of hyperglycemia (>160 milligrams/dL), blood pressure management, and reversal of coagulopathy (if present). Management of elevated intracranial pressure should include raising the head of the bed 30 degrees and providing appropriate analgesia and sedation. If more aggressive reduction of intracranial pressure is required—such as administration of osmotic diuretics or intubation with neuromuscular blockade and mild hyperventilation—invasive intracranial pressure monitoring is generally indicated. Current guidelines for blood pressure management are listed in **Table 166-4**.[28] **The INTERACT2 study demonstrated no reduction in the rate of death or severe disability among patients assigned to rapid (within 1 hr) reduction of blood pressure to <140 mm Hg; however the study showed better functional outcomes in those with rapid BP reduction.**[45]

Reverse Coagulopathy Given the complexity and variety of antiplatelet and anticoagulation agents in current use, institutional protocols should be available with clear algorithms listing the indications for, and dosing of, reversal agents (**Table 166-5**). If the coagulopathy is related to heparin use, administer protamine at approximately 1 milligram per 100 units of heparin, adjusted based on the time since the heparin was last given. For patients taking warfarin, provide reversal no matter what the value of the international normalized ratio. For further discussion, see chapter 239, Thrombotics and Antithrombotics. Several options exist for reversing warfarin-induced coagulopathy: vitamin K, fresh frozen plasma, recombinant factor VIIa, and prothrombin complex concentrates. Preferred route of administration of vitamin K is the PO route, since IV and SC routes can cause anaphylaxis. Vitamin K takes many hours to be effective. Fresh frozen plasma has a faster onset but contains variable amounts of clotting factors, and the dose of 15 mL/kg requires a large volume infusion that most patients cannot tolerate. **Fresh frozen plasma can be available for rapid administration as universal donor (AB+) without the need for type and cross-match.**

Recombinant factor VIIa does not improve survival or functional outcome after intracerebral hemorrhage.[46] **Prothrombin complex concentrates** are effective and rapidly reverse oral anticoagulants; however, morbidity and mortality remain high even when the coagulopathy is reversed.[47]

TABLE 166-5 Reversal of anticoagulation for Intracerebral Hemorrhage

Anticoagulant	Reversal Agent	Comment
Warfarin	Vitamin K 2.5–5 milligrams PO	Full effect in 24 h; IV can cause anaphylaxis; allergic reactions also reported with IM and SC dosing
	Fresh frozen plasma 2 units IV	Full dose 15 mL/kg limited by volume
	Prothrombin complex concentrate (PCC) 50 IU/kg IV	Dose-related risk of thromboembolism; available as 3- (II, IX, X) and 4- (II, VII, IX, X) factor PCC; use what is available in your institution
Aspirin and adenosine diphosphate receptor agonists	Obtain consultation if available when considering platelet infusion	CAUTION: platelet reversal may cause coronary or arterial thrombosis; use only if benefits outweigh risk
Unfractionated heparin (UFH)	1 milligram protamine/100 units of UFH; maximum dose, 50 milligrams; calculate last 3 h of heparin dose to determine protamine dose because heparin has short half-life	Infusion rate ≤5 milligrams/min; risk of hypersensitivity in patients with fish allergy or prior protamine exposure: premedicate with hydrocortisone 500 milligrams IV and diphenhydramine 50 milligrams IV
Low-molecular-weight heparin (LMWH)	If last dose within 8 h, give 1 milligram protamine/1 milligram LMWH; maximum dose, 50 milligrams If last dose 8–12 h ago, give 0.5 milligram protamine/1 milligram LMWH If last dose ≥12 h ago, do not give protamine	See above protamine cautions. Infusion rate ≤5 milligrams/min; higher infusion rates can cause hypotension or bradycardia
Direct thrombin inhibitor or factor Xa inhibitors	No effective reversal agent	Consult hematology While activated charcoal 1 gram/kg can bind apixaban, rivaroxaban, or dabigatran if these drugs were taken in last 2 h, risk of CNS deterioration and pulmonary aspiration typically prohibit use in CNS bleed

Manage intracerebral hemorrhage related to fibrinolytic therapy with standard intracerebral hemorrhage treatment along with platelet and cryoprecipitate infusions, although little evidence exists to guide therapy in these cases.[28]

DISPOSITION AND FOLLOW-UP

Admit all patients to an intensive care unit in consultation with a neurosurgeon.

REFERENCES

The complete reference list is available online at www.TintinalliEM.com.

CHAPTER 167 Stroke Syndromes

Steven Go
Daniel J. Worman

INTRODUCTION AND EPIDEMIOLOGY

In the United States, 795,000 people experience strokes annually (one stroke every 40 seconds).[1] Of these events, 77% are primary strokes, whereas 23% represent recurrent strokes.[1] In addition to the human costs, the financial implications of stroke are enormous—strokes accounted for an estimated $36.5 billion of total expenditures in the United States in 2010. Despite these grim statistics, from 2000 to 2010, the annual stroke death rate fell 35.8%.[2] With the growing use of stroke units, thrombolysis, and other new therapies, there is increased hope for patients with acute stroke who present to the ED.

PATHOPHYSIOLOGY

Stroke is generally defined as any disease process that interrupts blood flow to the brain. Injury is related to the loss of oxygen and glucose substrates necessary for high-energy phosphate production and the presence of mediators of secondary cellular injury. Subsequent factors, such as edema and mass effect, may exacerbate the initial insult.

ANATOMY

An understanding of the diagnosis and treatment of stroke begins with a working knowledge of the relevant vascular supply and neuroanatomy of the brain.

The arterial supply to the brain is illustrated in **Figures 167-1 and 167-2**.

The vascular supply is divided into anterior and posterior circulations. Clinical findings in stroke are determined by the location of the lesion(s) (**Table 167-1**), but the degree of collateral circulation may cause variations in the specific clinical symptoms and their severity.

STROKE TYPE

Stroke results from two major mechanisms: ischemia and hemorrhage. Ischemic strokes account for 87% of all strokes and are categorized by cause: thrombotic, embolic, or hypoperfusion related. Hemorrhagic strokes are subdivided into intracerebral (accounting for 10% of all strokes) and nontraumatic subarachnoid hemorrhage (accounting for 3% of all strokes)[1] (**Table 167-2**). The final common pathway for all of these mechanisms is altered neuronal perfusion. Neurons are exquisitely sensitive to changes in cerebral blood flow and die within minutes of complete cessation of perfusion—hence, the current treatment emphasis on rapid reperfusion strategies.

PREHOSPITAL CARE

The early detection of stroke must begin with the general public. In general, stroke knowledge among laypersons remains suboptimal and has led to several educational initiatives to raise stroke awareness.[3]

Three of the more commonly used prehospital tools are the Cincinnati Prehospital Stroke Scale,[4] the Los Angeles Prehospital Stroke Screen,[5] and the Melbourne Ambulance Stroke Screen (**Table 167-3**).[6]

Time is a critical component in the care of stroke patients. EMS personnel should quickly ascertain the time of onset of the patient's symptoms, giving particular attention to bystander accounts to clarify details, because stroke patients may be poor historians. Family members and/or witnesses to the event should be urged to come to the ED as soon as possible to provide further medical information to the treating physician. Time at the scene should be limited: EMS personnel should rapidly stabilize the patient's condition and transport the patient to a facility capable of optimally managing acute stroke, being sure to notify the receiving facility of the patient's condition and estimated time of arrival. In some cases, it may be necessary to bypass closer, but less capable, facilities in order to increase the chances of the patient receiving the best possible care.[7]

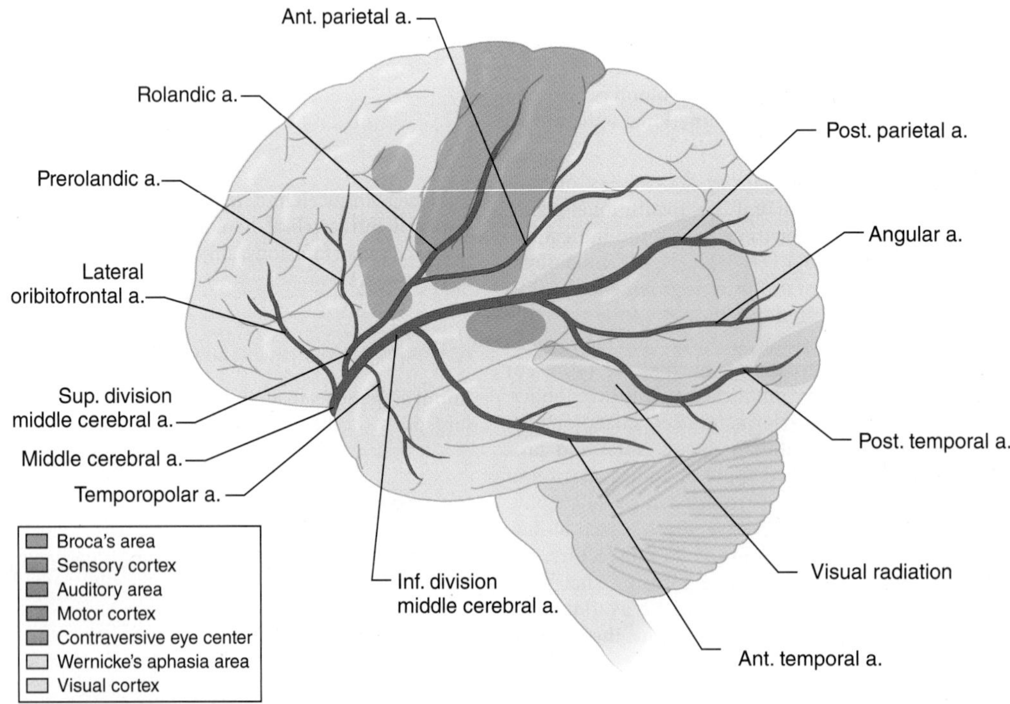

FIGURE 167-1. Cerebral hemisphere, lateral aspect. Note the branches and distribution of the middle cerebral artery and the principal regions of cerebral localization. The middle cerebral artery bifurcates into a superior and inferior division. a. = artery; ant. = anterior; inf. = inferior; post. = posterior; sup. = superior. [Modified with permission from Fauci AS, Braunwald E, Kasper DL, et al: *Harrison's Principles of Internal Medicine, 17th ed.* New York, McGraw-Hill Professional, 2008.]

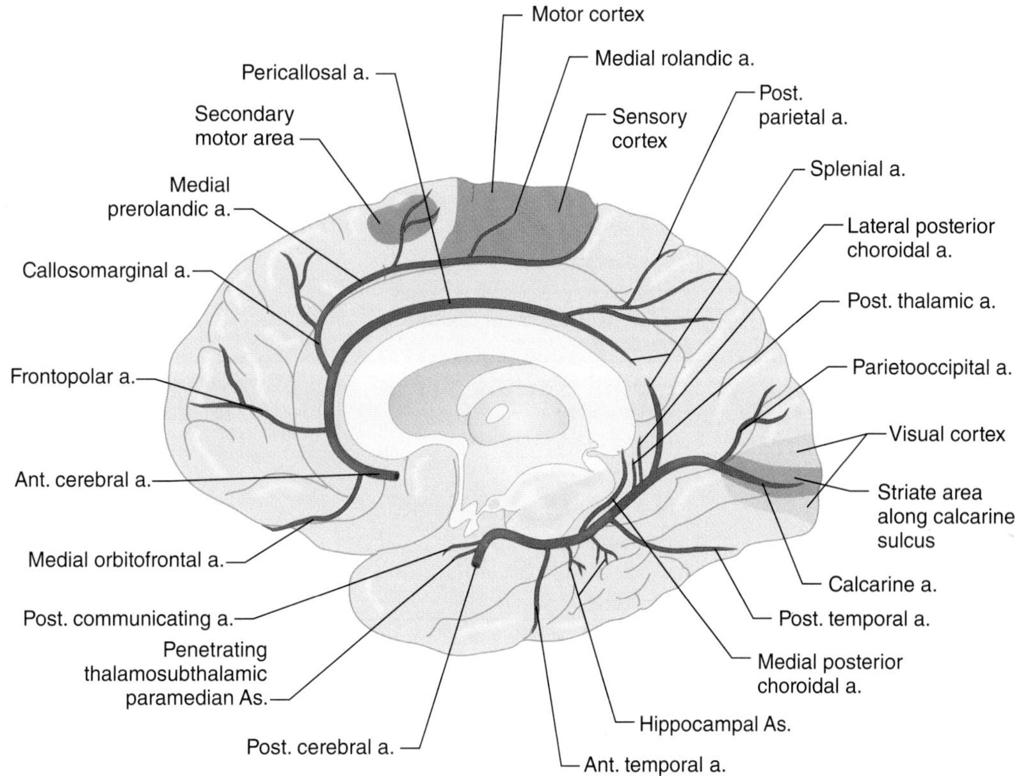

FIGURE 167-2. Cerebral hemisphere, medial aspect. Note the branches and distribution of the anterior cerebral artery, posterior cerebral artery, and the principal regions of cerebral localization. a. = artery; ant. = anterior; post. = posterior. [Reproduced with permission from Fauci AS, Braunwald E, Kasper DL, et al: *Harrison's Principles of Internal Medicine,* 17th ed. New York, McGraw-Hill Professional, 2008.]

CLINICAL FEATURES

The diagnosis of stroke in the ED rests on the bedrock of a focused, accurate history and physical examination.[8] The clinical presentation of stroke can range from the obvious (facial droop, arm drift, abnormal speech[8]) to the subtle (generalized weakness, lightheadedness, vague sensory changes, altered mental status). Women account for slightly more than half of new or recurrent strokes in the United States,[9] and modest gender differences exist in terms of presenting signs and symptoms.[10,11] In general, women tend to report diffuse, nontraditional symptoms and are less likely to report traditional symptoms when compared to men, but evidence of these distinctions is limited (**Table 167-4**).[10-12]

TABLE 167-1 Anterior and Posterior Circulation of the Brain

Circulation	Major Arteries	Major Regions of Brain Supplied
Anterior (internal carotid system)	Ophthalmic	Optic nerve and retina
	Anterior cerebral	Frontal pole
		Anteromedial cerebral cortex
		Anterior corpus callosum
	Middle cerebral	Frontoparietal lobe
		Anterotemporal lobe
Posterior (vertebral system)	Vertebral	Brainstem
	Posteroinferior cerebellar	Cerebellum
	Basilar	Thalamus
	Posterior cerebral	Auditory/vestibular structures
	Medial temporal lobe	Visual occipital cortex

HISTORY

The timing of symptom onset, the presence of associated symptoms, and the medical history may point toward a particular mechanism of stroke. For example, sudden onset of symptoms suggests an embolic or hemorrhagic stroke, whereas a stuttering or waxing and waning deficit suggests a thrombotic or hypoperfusion-related stroke. A history of Valsalva maneuver immediately preceding a thunderclap headache or sudden onset of symptoms suggests a ruptured cerebral aneurysm, whereas a recent history of neck trauma or manipulation suggests cervical artery dissection. Risk factors for vessel thrombus include hypertension, diabetes mellitus, and coronary atherosclerotic disease. In contrast, atrial fibrillation, valvular replacement, or recent myocardial infarction suggests embolism. Transient neurologic deficits occurring in the same vascular distribution suggest underlying vascular disease consistent with a thrombotic stroke, whereas transient deficits involving different vascular distributions suggest embolism. Although adjunctive history can be helpful in determining the type of stroke, exhaustive or unduly prolonged attempts to elicit nonessential history should not delay therapy.

Accurately determine the time of symptom onset. Time of onset is frequently misreported as the time a patient was *discovered* with symptoms or the time of awakening (if symptoms were noted upon awakening). For the purposes of thrombolysis, if a patient awakens with the symptoms of stroke, **the time of onset is the last known time when the patient's condition was at baseline.**[7]

Exclude as many **stroke mimics** as possible (**Table 167-5**).[7,8,13] After stroke mimics are excluded, if acute stroke is still the most likely diagnosis and if the symptom onset is within the recommended time limits for thrombolytic therapy, elicit information pertaining to inclusion and exclusion criteria for thrombolytic therapy (see Table 167-11[7,14] and Table 167-12[7,15] for the criteria for administration of recombinant tissue plasminogen activator [rtPA] in acute ischemic stroke).

TABLE 167-2 Stroke Classification

Stroke Type	Mechanism	Major Causes	Clinical Notes
Ischemic			
Thrombotic	Narrowing of a damaged vascular lumen by an in situ process—usually clot formation	Atherosclerosis Vasculitis Arterial dissection Polycythemia Hypercoagulable state Infection (human immunodeficiency virus infection, syphilis, trichinosis, tuberculosis, aspergillosis)	Symptoms often have gradual onset and may wax and wane. Common cause of transient ischemic attack.
Embolic	Obstruction of a normal vascular lumen by intravascular material from a remote source	Valvular vegetations Mural thrombi Paradoxical emboli Cardiac tumors (myxomas) Arterial-arterial emboli from proximal source Fat emboli Particulate emboli (IV drug use) Septic emboli	Typically sudden in onset. Account for 20% of ischemic strokes.
Hypoperfusion	Low–blood flow state leading to hypoperfusion of the brain	Cardiac failure resulting in systemic hypotension	Diffuse injury pattern in watershed regions. Symptoms may wax and wane with hemodynamic factors.
Hemorrhagic			
Intracerebral	Intraparenchymal hemorrhage from previously weakened arterioles	Hypertension Amyloidosis Iatrogenic anticoagulation Vascular malformations Cocaine use	Intracranial pressure rise causes local neuronal damage. Secondary vasoconstriction mediated by blood breakdown products or neuronal mechanisms (diaschisis) can cause remote perfusion changes. Risks include advanced age, history of stroke, and tobacco or alcohol use. More common in those of Asian or African descent.
Nontraumatic subarachnoid	Hemorrhage into subarachnoid space	Berry aneurysm rupture Vascular malformation rupture	May be preceded by a sentinel headache ("warning leak").

PHYSICAL EXAMINATION

Airway, breathing, and circulation are the top priorities. Next, the goals of examination are to confirm the diagnosis of stroke, exclude stroke mimics, and identify comorbidities. Fever should prompt an investigation for potential infection. CNS infections (meningitis, encephalitis) may mimic a stroke, or an infection such as aspiration pneumonia or a urinary tract infection may be a complication of the stroke. Look for meningismus, signs of emboli (Janeway lesions and Osler nodes), and bleeding diatheses (ecchymoses or petechiae). A funduscopic examination may identify signs of papilledema (suggesting a mass lesion, cerebral vein thrombosis, or hypertensive crisis) or preretinal hemorrhage (consistent with subarachnoid hemorrhage).

TABLE 167-3 Prehospital Stroke Scales

Cincinnati Prehospital Stroke Scale (If *any* of the three items is abnormal, sensitivity = 66%, specificity = 87% for acute stroke.)	1. Facial droop (abnormal: one side of face does not move as well as other side) 2. Arm drift (abnormal: one arm does not move or one arm drifts down compared with the other) 3. Speech (abnormal: slurred, inappropriate words or mute)
Los Angeles Prehospital Stroke Screen (If answers to *all* items 1–6 are "Yes" or "Unknown," sensitivity = 91% [95% confidence interval (CI) 76%–98%], specificity = 97% [95% CI 93%–99%] for acute stroke.)	1. Age >45 y 2. No history of seizure disorder 3. New onset of neurologic symptoms in last 24 h 4. Patient ambulatory at baseline (prior to event) 5. Blood glucose level of 60–400 milligrams/dL 6. Obvious asymmetry in *any* of the following examinations: facial smile/grimace, grip, arm strength
Melbourne Ambulance Stroke Screen (If answers to *all* items 1-4 are "Yes" PLUS at least one of 5-8 is present, sensitivity = 90% [95% CI: 81%-96%), specificity = 74% [95% CI: 53%-88%] for acute stroke.)	1. Age > 45 y 2. No history of seizure/epilepsy 3. Not wheelchair-bound/bedridden at baseline 4. Blood Glucose 50-400 mg/dL 5. Unilateral facial droop 6. Unilateral hand grip weakness 7. Unilateral arm drift 8. Abnormal speech

TABLE 167-4 Selected Stroke Symptoms

Traditional symptoms	Sudden numbness or weakness of face, arm, or leg—especially unilateral*
	Sudden altered mental status†
	Sudden aphasia
	Sudden memory deficit or spatial orientation or perception difficulties
	Sudden visual deficit or diplopia*
	Sudden dizziness, gait disturbance, or ataxia*
	Sudden severe headache with no known cause
Nontraditional symptoms	Loss of consciousness or syncope
	Generalized weakness†
	Shortness of breath
	Sudden pain in the face, chest, arms, or legs
	Seizure
	Falls or accidents
	Sudden hiccups
	Sudden nausea
	Sudden fatigue
	Sudden palpitations
	Altered mental status

*More common in men.

†More common in women.

Look for findings suggestive of possible cardiac or vascular disease, such as rales, an S_3 gallop, or carotid bruit.

The National Institutes of Health Stroke Scale (NIHSS) is the standard tool for documenting the severity of a stroke. The **NIHSS** is an 11-category (15-item) neurologic evaluation (score range of 0 to 42) that is quick to use (5 to 10 minutes), yields reproducible results, has a high interrater reliability, and provides a score that correlates with infarct volume[16] (**Table 167-6**).[17,18] An Adobe Acrobat (pdf) file of the NIHSS, as well as detailed instructions for its use, are readily available for download from the National Institute of Neurological Disorders and Stroke (NINDS) Web site (http://www.ninds.nih.gov/doctors/nih_stroke_scale.pdf). In addition, NIHSS calculators are available on the Internet[19] and for use with mobile devices.[20,21] A modified NIHSS, which omits the redundant and least reliable items, produces clinical results similar to those for the full NIHSS[18] and is easier to use (score range of 0 to 31). An important caveat is that the NIHSS is weighted toward the detection of anterior circulation strokes as opposed to posterior circulation strokes.[22] This is because common symptoms of posterior strokes (cranial nerve deficits and ataxia) receive fewer points, and ataxia is often scored as absent by raters if weakness is present. For example, one study[23] found that the NIHSS score associated with a favorable outcome was ≤5 for posterior circulation strokes and ≤8 for anterior circulation strokes. In addition, the NIHSS has a bias toward detection of dominant hemisphere strokes.[24]

ISCHEMIC STROKE SYNDROMES

ANTERIOR CEREBRAL ARTERY INFARCTION

Occlusion of the anterior cerebral artery is uncommon (0.5% to 3% of all strokes[25]), but when unilateral occlusion occurs, it can cause contralateral sensory and motor symptoms in the lower extremity, with sparing of the hands and face. In addition, a left-sided lesion is typically associated with akinetic mutism and transcortical motor aphasia (repetition ability retained), whereas right-sided infarction can result in confusion and motor hemineglect. Bilateral occlusion can cause a combination of the above symptoms, but was particularly associated with mutism, incontinence, and poor outcome in one small series.[26]

TABLE 167-5 Stroke Mimics

Disorder	Distinguishing Clinical Features
Seizures/postictal paralysis (Todd's paralysis)	Transient paralysis following a seizure, which typically disappears quickly; can be confused with transient ischemic attack. Seizures can be secondary to a cerebrovascular accident.
Syncope	No persistent or associated neurologic symptoms.
Meningitis/encephalitis	Fever, immunocompromised state may be present, meningismus, detectable on lumbar puncture.
Complicated migraine	History of similar episodes, preceding aura, headache.
Brain neoplasm or abscess	Focal neurologic findings, signs of infection, detectable by imaging.
Epidural/subdural hematoma	History of trauma, alcoholism, anticoagulant use, bleeding disorder; detectable by imaging.
Subarachnoid hemorrhage	Sudden onset of severe headache.*
Hypoglycemia	Can be detected by bedside glucose measurement, history of diabetes mellitus.
Hyponatremia	History of diuretic use, neoplasm, excessive free water intake.
Hypertensive encephalopathy	Gradual onset; global cerebral dysfunction, headache, delirium, hypertension, cerebral edema.
Hyperosmotic coma	Extremely high glucose levels, history of diabetes mellitus.
Wernicke's encephalopathy	History of alcoholism or malnutrition; triad of ataxia, ophthalmoplegia, and confusion.
Labyrinthitis	Predominantly vestibular symptoms; patient should have no other focal findings; can be confused with cerebellar stroke.
Drug toxicity (lithium, phenytoin, carbamazepine)	Can be detected by particular toxidromes and elevated blood levels. Phenytoin and carbamazepine toxicity may present with ataxia, vertigo, nausea, and abnormal reflexes.
Bell's palsy	Neurologic deficit confined to isolated *peripheral* seventh nerve palsy; often associated with younger age.
Ménière's disease	History of recurrent episodes dominated by vertigo symptoms, tinnitus, deafness.
Demyelinating disease (multiple sclerosis)	Gradual onset. Patient may have a history of multiple episodes of neurologic findings in multifocal anatomic distributions.
Conversion disorder	No cranial nerve findings, nonanatomic distribution of findings (e.g., midline sensory loss), inconsistent history or examination findings.

*Although subarachnoid hemorrhage is a type of stroke, it has special considerations in terms of diagnosis and management. See chapter 166, "Spontaneous Subarachnoid and Intracerebral Hemorrhage."

MIDDLE CEREBRAL ARTERY INFARCTION

The middle cerebral artery is the vessel most commonly involved in stroke, and clinical findings can be quite variable, depending on exactly where the lesion is located and which brain hemisphere is dominant. (In right-handed patients and in up to 80% of left-handed patients, the left hemisphere is dominant.) A middle cerebral artery stroke typically presents with hemiparesis, facial plegia, and sensory loss contralateral to the affected cortex. These deficits variably affect the face and upper extremity more than the lower extremity. If the dominant hemisphere is involved, aphasia (receptive, expressive, or both) is often present. If the nondominant hemisphere is involved, inattention, neglect, extinction on double-simultaneous stimulation, dysarthria without aphasia, and constructional apraxia (difficulty in drawing complex two-dimensional or three-dimensional figures) may occur. A homonymous hemianopsia and gaze preference toward the side of the infarct may also be seen, regardless of the side of the infarction.

POSTERIOR CEREBRAL ARTERY INFARCTION (DISTAL POSTERIOR CIRCULATION)

The classic symptoms and signs of posterior circulation strokes include ataxia, nystagmus, altered mental status, and vertigo, but presentation

TABLE 167-6 National Institutes of Health Stroke Scale (NIHSS)

Instructions	Scale Definition
1a. Level of consciousness (LOC)* The investigator must choose a response if a full evaluation is prevented by such obstacles as an endotracheal tube, language barrier, or orotracheal trauma/bandages. A 3 is scored only if the patient makes no movement (other than reflexive posturing) in response to noxious stimulation.	0 = Alert; keenly responsive. 1 = Not alert, but arousable by minor stimulation to obey, answer, or respond. 2 = Not alert; requires repeated stimulation to attend, or is obtunded and requires strong or painful stimulation to make movements (not stereotyped). 3 = Responds only with reflex motor or autonomic effects or is totally unresponsive, flaccid, and areflexic.
1b. LOC questions The patient is asked the month and his or her age. The answer must be correct—there is no partial credit for being close. Aphasic and stuporous patients who do not comprehend the questions are given a score of 2. Patients unable to speak because of endotracheal intubation, orotracheal trauma, severe dysarthria from any cause, language barrier, or any other problem not secondary to aphasia are given a score of 1. It is important that only the initial answer be graded and that the examiner not "help" the patient with verbal or nonverbal cues.	0 = Answers both questions correctly. 1 = Answers one question correctly. 2 = Answers neither question correctly.
1c. LOC commands The patient is asked to open and close the eyes and then to grip and release the nonparetic hand. Substitute another one-step command if the hands cannot be used. Credit is given if an unequivocal attempt is made but not completed due to weakness. If the patient does not respond to command, the task should be demonstrated to him or her (pantomime) and the result scored (i.e., follows no, one, or two commands). Patients with trauma, amputation, or other physical impediments should be given suitable one-step commands. Only the first attempt is scored.	0 = Performs both tasks correctly. 1 = Performs one task correctly. 2 = Performs neither task correctly.
2. Best gaze Only horizontal eye movements are tested. Voluntary or reflexive (oculocephalic) eye movements are scored, but caloric testing is not done. If the patient has a conjugate deviation of the eyes that can be overcome by voluntary or reflexive activity, the score is 1. If a patient has an isolated peripheral nerve paresis (cranial nerve III, IV, or VI), the score is 1. Gaze is testable in all aphasic patients. Patients with ocular trauma, bandages, preexisting blindness, or other disorder of visual acuity or fields should be tested with reflexive movements, and a choice made by the investigator. Establishing eye contact and then moving about the patient from side to side will occasionally clarify the presence of a partial gaze palsy.	0 = Normal. 1 = Partial gaze palsy; gaze is abnormal in one or both eyes, but forced deviation or total gaze paresis is not present. 2 = Forced deviation, or total gaze paresis not overcome by the oculocephalic maneuver.
3. Visual Visual fields (upper and lower quadrants) are tested by confrontation, using finger counting or visual threat, as appropriate. Patients may be encouraged, but if they look at the side of the moving fingers appropriately, this can be scored as normal. If there is unilateral blindness or enucleation, visual fields in the remaining eye are scored. Score 1 only if a clear-cut asymmetry, including quadrantanopia, is found. If the patient is blind from any cause, score 3. Double simultaneous stimulation is performed at this point. If there is extinction, patient receives a score of 1, and the results are used to respond to item 11.	0 = No vision loss. 1 = Partial hemianopia. 2 = Complete hemianopia. 3 = Bilateral hemianopia (blind including cortical blindness).
4. Facial palsy* Ask—or use pantomime to encourage—the patient to show teeth or raise eyebrows and close eyes. Score symmetry of grimace in response to noxious stimuli in the poorly responsive or noncomprehending patient. If facial trauma/bandages, orotracheal tube, tape, or other physical barriers obscure the face, these should be removed to the extent possible.	0 = Normal symmetric movements. 1 = Minor paralysis (flattened nasolabial fold, asymmetry on smiling). 2 = Partial paralysis (total or near-total paralysis of lower face). 3 = Complete paralysis of one or both sides (absence of facial movement in the upper and lower face).
5. Motor arm The limb is placed in the appropriate position: extend the arms (palms down) 90 degrees (if sitting) or 45 degrees (if supine). Drift is scored if the arm falls before 10 s. The aphasic patient is encouraged using urgency in the voice and pantomime, but not noxious stimulation. Each limb is tested in turn, beginning with the nonparetic arm. Only in the case of amputation or joint fusion at the shoulder, the examiner should record the score as untestable (UN) and clearly write the explanation for this choice. 5a. Left arm 5b. Right arm	0 = No drift; limb holds 90 (or 45) degrees for full 10 s. 1 = Drift; limb holds 90 (or 45) degrees, but drifts down before full 10 s; does not hit bed or other support. 2 = Some effort against gravity; limb cannot get to or maintain (if cued) 90 (or 45) degrees, drifts down to bed, but has some effort against gravity. 3 = No effort against gravity; limb falls. 4 = No movement.
6. Motor leg The limb is placed in the appropriate position: hold the leg at 30 degrees (the patient is always tested supine). Drift is scored if the leg falls before 5 s. The aphasic patient is encouraged using urgency in the voice and pantomime, but not noxious stimulation. Each limb is tested in turn, beginning with the nonparetic leg. Only in the case of amputation or joint fusion at the hip, the examiner should record the score as untestable (UN) and clearly write the explanation for this choice. 6a. Left leg 6b. Right leg	0 = No drift; leg holds 30-degree position for full 5 s. 1 = Drift; leg falls by the end of the 5-s period but does not hit bed. 2 = Some effort against gravity; leg falls to bed by 5 s, but has some effort against gravity. 3 = No effort against gravity; leg falls to bed immediately. 4 = No movement.

(*Continued*)

TABLE 167-6 National Institutes of Health Stroke Scale (NIHSS) (*Continued*)

Instructions	Scale Definition
7. Limb ataxia* This item is aimed at finding evidence of a unilateral cerebellar lesion. Test with the patient's eyes open. In case of visual defect, ensure that testing is done in the intact visual field. The finger-nose-finger and heel-shin tests are performed on both sides, and ataxia is scored only if present out of proportion to weakness. Ataxia is absent in the patient who cannot understand or is paralyzed. Only in the case of amputation or joint fusion, the examiner should record the score as untestable (UN) and clearly write the explanation for this choice. In case of blindness, test by having the patient touch the nose from an extended arm position.	0 = Absent. 1 = Present in one limb. 2 = Present in two limbs.
8. Sensory† Sensation or grimace to pinprick when tested, or withdrawal from a noxious stimulus in the obtunded or aphasic patient. Only sensory loss attributed to stroke is scored as abnormal, and the examiner should test as many body areas (arms [not hands], legs, trunk, face) as needed to check accurately for hemisensory loss. A score of 2, "severe or total sensory loss," should be given only when a severe or total loss of sensation can be clearly demonstrated. Stuporous and aphasic patients will therefore probably score 1 or 0. The patient with brainstem stroke who has bilateral loss of sensation is scored 2. If the patient does not respond and is quadriplegic, score 2. Patients in a coma (item 1a score = 3) are automatically given a 2 on this item.	0 = Normal; no sensory loss. 1 = Mild-to-moderate sensory loss; patient feels pinprick is less sharp or is dull on affected side, or there is loss of superficial pain with pinprick, but patient is aware of being touched. 2 = Severe to total sensory loss; patient is not aware of being touched on face, arm, and leg.*
9. Best language A great deal of information about comprehension is obtained during the preceding sections of the examination. For this scale item, the patient is asked to describe what is happening in the test picture, to name the items on the test naming sheet, and to read from the test list of sentences. Comprehension is judged from responses here as well as responses to all of the commands in the preceding general neurologic examination. If vision loss interferes with the tests, ask the patient to identify objects placed in the hand, repeat, and produce speech. The intubated patient should be asked to write. The patient in a coma (item 1a score = 3) automatically scores 3 on this item. The examiner must choose a score for the patient with stupor or limited cooperation, but a score of 3 should be used only if the patient is mute and follows no one-step commands.	0 = No aphasia; normal. 1 = Mild-to-moderate aphasia; some obvious loss of fluency or facility of comprehension, without significant limitation on ideas expressed or form of expression. However, reduction of speech and/or comprehension makes conversation about provided materials difficult or impossible. For example, in conversation about provided materials, examiner can identify picture or naming card content from patient's response. 2 = Severe aphasia; all communication is through fragmentary expression; great need for inference, questioning, and guessing by listener. Range of information that can be exchanged is limited; listener carries burden of communication. Examiner cannot identify materials provided from patient's response. 3 = Mute, global aphasia; no usable speech or auditory comprehension.
10. Dysarthria* If the patient is thought to be normal, an adequate sample of speech must be obtained by asking the patient to read or repeat words from the test list. If the patient has severe aphasia, the clarity of articulation of spontaneous speech can be rated. Only if the patient is intubated or has other physical barriers to producing speech, the examiner should record the score as untestable (UN) and clearly write an explanation for this choice. Do not tell the patient why he or she is being tested.	0 = Normal. 1 = Mild-to-moderate dysarthria; patient slurs at least some words and, at worst, can be understood with some difficulty. 2 = Severe dysarthria; patient's speech is so slurred as to be unintelligible in the absence of or out of proportion to any dysphasia, or is mute/anarthric.
11. Extinction and inattention Sufficient information to identify neglect may be obtained during the prior testing. If the patient has a severe vision loss preventing visual double simultaneous stimulation and the responses to cutaneous stimuli are normal, the score is 0. If the patient has aphasia but does appear to attend to both sides, the score is 0. The presence of visual spatial neglect or anosognosia may also be taken as evidence of abnormality. Because the abnormality is scored only if present, the item is never scored as untestable.	0 = No abnormality. 1 = Visual, tactile, auditory, spatial, or personal inattention or extinction to bilateral simultaneous stimulation in one of the sensory modalities. 2 = Profound hemi-inattention or extinction in more than one modality; patient does not recognize own hand or orients to only one side of space.

*Shaded cells indicate items not included in the modified NIHSS.[18]

†Scale for item 8 is compressed to two elements (0 = normal; 1 = abnormal) for modified NIHSS.[18]

Source: National Institute of Neurological Disorders and Stroke (NINDS) Web site (http://www.ninds.nih.gov/doctors/nih_stroke_scale.pdf). Accessed January 18, 2014.

can sometimes be rather subtle.[27] Crossed neurologic deficits (e.g., ipsilateral cranial nerve deficits with contralateral motor weakness) may indicate a brainstem lesion. According to an analysis of a large stroke registry,[28] symptoms of posterior cerebral artery involvement include unilateral limb weakness, dizziness, blurry vision, headache, and dysarthria. Common presenting signs include visual field loss, unilateral limb weakness, gait ataxia, unilateral limb ataxia, cranial nerve VII signs, lethargy, and sensory deficits.[28] Visual field loss, classically described as contralateral homonymous hemianopsia and unilateral cortical blindness, is thought to be specific for distal posterior circulation stroke because the visual centers of the brain are supplied by the posterior cerebral artery. Light-touch and pinprick sensation deficits, loss of ability to read (alexia) without agraphia, inability to name colors, recent memory loss, unilateral third nerve palsy, and hemiballismus have also been reported. Motor dysfunction, although common, is typically minimal, which can keep some patients from realizing they have had a stroke.

BASILAR ARTERY OCCLUSION (MIDDLE POSTERIOR CIRCULATION)

Occlusion of the basilar artery most commonly presents with symptoms of unilateral limb weakness, dizziness, dysarthria, diplopia, and headache.[28] The most common presenting signs are unilateral limb weakness, cranial nerve VII signs, dysarthria, Babinski sign, and oculomotor signs.[28] Dysphagia, nausea or vomiting, dizziness, and Horner's syndrome are positively correlated with basilar artery occlusion.[28] Basilar artery occlusion can also rarely cause **locked-in syndrome**, which occurs with bilateral pyramidal tract lesions in the ventral pons and is characterized by complete muscle paralysis except for upward gaze and blinking. Basilar artery occlusions have a high risk of death and poor outcomes.[29]

VERTEBROBASILAR INFARCTION (PROXIMAL POSTERIOR CIRCULATION)

Patients with vertebrobasilar infarction most commonly present with symptoms of dizziness, nausea or vomiting, headache, dysphagia, unilateral limb weakness, and unilateral cranial nerve V symptoms.[28] Common presenting signs include unilateral limb ataxia, nystagmus, gait ataxia, cranial nerve V signs, limb sensory deficit, and Horner's syndrome.[28] For further discussion of vertigo, see chapter 170, "Vertigo."

CEREBELLAR INFARCTION

Patients with cerebellar infarction can present with very nonspecific symptoms and frequently present with dizziness (with or without vertigo), nausea and vomiting, gait instability, headache, limb ataxia, dysarthria, nystagmus, and cranial nerve abnormalities.[30] Mental status may vary from alert to comatose. Because CT is inadequately sensitive for posterior fossa lesions, **obtain a diffusion-weighted MRI (DWI-MRI) when this diagnosis is suspected**. A CT angiogram or magnetic resonance angiogram is useful to characterize any vascular lesion once the diagnosis is made. The clinical presentation and course of cerebellar infarction can be frustratingly difficult to predict, but the clinician must remain vigilant to the possibility of rapid deterioration secondary to increased brainstem pressure caused by cerebellar edema. Therefore, extremely close serial examinations (especially looking for gaze palsy and altered mental status) and prompt neurologic and neurosurgical bedside consultations are needed. **Obtain early neurosurgical consultation for patients with cerebellar infarction.** Cerebellar edema can lead to rapid deterioration with herniation, and consultation is required to determine the need for emergency posterior fossa decompression in these patients. Acute **obstructing hydrocephalus** requires treatment of elevated intracranial pressure and emergent surgical decompression.[30]

LACUNAR INFARCTION

Lacunar infarcts are pure motor or sensory deficits caused by infarction of small penetrating arteries and are commonly associated with chronic hypertension and increasing age. The presentation is variable based on the location and size of the lesions. The prognosis is generally considered more favorable than for other stroke syndromes.

CAROTID AND VERTEBRAL ARTERY DISSECTION

Carotid or vertebral artery dissection is an uncommon but important cause of stroke (10% to 25% of cases), especially in young and middle-aged patients.[31] A history of neck trauma in the days to weeks prior to presentation is a prominent risk factor. The trauma is usually minor[32] (e.g., manipulative therapy of the neck[33] or sport-related trauma[34]). Other risk factors include connective tissue disease,[35] history of migraine,[36] large vessel arteriopathies,[37] and hypertension.[38]

The typical first symptom of patients with carotid or vertebral artery dissection is unilateral **headache** (68%), neck pain (39%), or face pain (10%),[39-41] which can precede other symptoms by hours to days (median, 4 days).[42] New-onset headache or neck pain of unclear etiology is such an important symptom that imaging of the neck vessels is recommended by some as part of initial evaluation.[41] **Symptoms may be transient or persistent.** The median time between an initial presentation of neck pain and the development of other neurologic symptoms is 14 days, but if headache is the first symptom, other neurologic symptoms follow within a median time of 15 hours.[42]

Carotid Artery Dissection The headache is most commonly in the frontotemporal region and, due to its variable quality and severity, may mimic subarachnoid hemorrhage (i.e., "thunderclap" headache), temporal arteritis, or preexisting migraine. A partial Horner's syndrome (miosis and ptosis) has traditionally been linked to carotid artery dissection, but in reality, it occurs in only about 25% of patients and is a sign accompanying other disorders besides stroke.[43] Associated cranial nerve palsies have been reported in 12% of carotid artery dissections.[44] Carotid dissection can progress to cause cerebral ischemia or, rarely, retinal infarction.

Vertebral Artery Dissection Vertebral artery dissection commonly presents with neck pain (66%) and headache (65%), both of which can be unilateral or bilateral.[40] The headache is typically occipital, but can rarely present with pain on an entire side of the head or in the frontal region.[39] Other symptoms and signs may include unilateral facial paresthesia, dizziness, vertigo, nausea/emesis, diplopia and other visual disturbances, ataxia, limb weakness, numbness, dysarthria, and hearing loss. Cervical radiculopathy (typically a peripheral motor deficit at the C5 level) is a rare presentation (1%) and can also involve multiple levels and sensory findings.[45] Untreated vertebral artery dissection may result in infarction in regions of the brain supplied by the posterior circulation.

MRI/magnetic resonance angiography and CT/CT angiography are the diagnostic modalities of choice for suspected carotid, vertebral, or basilar artery dissection.[46] Choice of study is usually determined by consultation with the neurologist and radiologist.[47] Color duplex US may not detect important vascular lesions.[48,49]

Treatment of Carotid and Vertebral Artery Dissection In the absence of contraindications, carotid and vertebral artery dissection has been traditionally treated with IV heparin followed by warfarin (to maintain an INR of 2.0 to 3.0). This treatment has persisted despite the absence to date of published, high-quality randomized controlled trials comparing anticoagulation with other potentially more effective treatment modalities.[50] In 2012, the nonrandomized arm (88 patients) of the Cervical Artery Dissection in Stroke Study was published along with a meta-analysis of previous trials.[51] These preliminary results showed no difference between anticoagulation and antiplatelet therapy in terms of prevention of stroke after cervical artery dissection. Nonrandomized data regarding endovascular approaches to cervical artery dissection have been published, but no randomized controlled trial has been published yet. Therefore, pending the availability of new randomized controlled trial data, administer either anticoagulant or antiplatelet therapy in the ED in conjunction with appropriate specialist consultation.

HEMORRHAGIC STROKE SYNDROMES

INTRACEREBRAL HEMORRHAGE

Intracerebral hemorrhage may be clinically indistinguishable from ischemic infarction, but the two conditions are distinct clinical entities in terms of management, with higher levels of morbidity and mortality for hemorrhage than for ischemic infarction.[52,53] Therefore, perform imaging to differentiate between the two. Headache, nausea, and vomiting often precede the neurologic deficit, and the patient's condition may quickly deteriorate (see chapter 166, "Spontaneous Subarachnoid and Intracerebral Hemorrhage").

CEREBELLAR HEMORRHAGE

Cerebellar hemorrhage may be clinically indistinguishable from cerebellar infarction. The same clinical presentation and management considerations detailed earlier in this chapter apply (see "Cerebellar Infarction").

SUBARACHNOID HEMORRHAGE

Subarachnoid hemorrhage is typically characterized by a severe occipital or nuchal headache. Patient history includes the recent sudden onset of a maximal-intensity headache in many cases. Careful history taking may reveal activities associated with a Valsalva maneuver, such as defecation, sexual activity, weight lifting, or coughing, at stroke onset. For further information, see chapter 166.

STROKE DIAGNOSIS

Mimics (Table 167-5)[7,8,13] can often be distinguished from stroke by careful history taking and physical examination, bedside tests, observation, and appropriate imaging. However, it can be difficult to distinguish conditions with focal transient symptoms (e.g., seizure) from transient ischemic attack (TIA).

INITIAL DIAGNOSTIC EVALUATION

The classic mantra, "**time is brain**,"[54] explains the current American Heart Association/American Stroke Association (AHA/ASA) stroke guidelines Class IB recommendation to enact "an organized protocol for the emergency evaluation of patients with suspected stroke" in which "the goal is to evaluate and to decide treatment within 60 minutes of the patient's arrival in an ED."[7] Creation of a multidisciplinary "stroke team" is encouraged, and the culture of the institution should be aligned to encourage rapid diagnosis and treatment of stroke. Train triage personnel to suspect stroke and to quickly activate a stroke critical pathway that includes specific standing orders and procedures. Implement the critical pathway immediately upon that patient's arrival, beginning in the triage area. Notify the emergency physician, the ED charge nurse, and the CT and laboratory technicians immediately when acute stroke is suspected. Do not delay the workup because ED beds are overcrowded or the emergency physician is currently otherwise engaged, and move the patient to a monitored bed as soon as feasible.

Concurrent with focused history taking and physical examination, perform a prioritized group of interventions and diagnostic studies rapidly in the ED when acute stroke is suspected (**Table 167-7**).

Nonessential testing should NOT delay performing brain imaging **within 25 minutes of the patient's arrival (Table 167-8)**.[7]

IMAGING

Brain Imaging Obtain emergency non-contrast-enhanced CT for suspected acute stroke. **Most acute ischemic strokes are not visualized by a noncontrast brain CT in the early hours of a stroke.**[8] Therefore, the utility of the first brain CT is primarily to exclude intracranial bleeding, abscess, tumor, and other stroke mimics, as well as to detect current contraindications to thrombolytics (e.g., evidence of more than one-third middle cerebral artery territory involvement).

The CT scan should be reviewed by the most expert interpreter available within 45 minutes of patient arrival, especially if thrombolytic therapy is being considered.[7] The identification of subtle hemorrhage, infarctions involving more than one third of the middle cerebral artery territory, and early cerebral infarction requires expertise. Telemedicine consultation is an excellent option, because reports indicate

TABLE 167-8 AHA/ASA Time Recommendations for Acute Ischemic Stroke

Intervention	Time Goal (from ED arrival)
Begin ED physician evaluation	10 min
Activation of stroke team	15 min
Begin head CT	25 min
Complete head CT interpretation	45 min
Begin rtPA administration	1 h
Admission to stroke unit	3 h

Abbreviations: AHA/ASA = American Heart Association/American Stroke Association; rtPA = recombinant tissue plasminogen activator.

TABLE 167-7 Core ED Interventions for Suspected Acute Stroke

Intervention/Evaluation	Rationale/Discussion
All patients	
Assessment of *a*irway, *b*reathing, *c*irculation	Immediate life threats must be addressed before other interventions are undertaken. Actively manage airway if necessary.
Establishment of IV access	IV access is necessary for possible thrombolytic therapy.
Oxygen administration (if hypoxia is present)	Routine oxygen supplementation is not indicated in mild to moderate stroke,[55] and should only be given to keep oxygen saturation >94%.[7]
Cardiac monitoring	Dysrhythmias, especially atrial fibrillation, are not infrequent in acute stroke and may predict 3-month mortality.[56,57] Prophylactic administration of antiarrhythmic agents is not indicated.
Bedside glucose determination	To rapidly rule out hypoglycemia mimicking stroke. Treat hypoglycemia (<60 milligrams/dL) with IV dextrose. **This is the only laboratory test result required prior to thrombolytic therapy**[7] *unless* the patient is taking/possibly taking oral anticoagulation therapy or heparin, or if there is a suspicion of thrombocytopenia or other bleeding diatheses (Table 167-11).
Pulse oximetry	To detect hypoxia.
ECG	Acute coronary syndrome, dysrhythmias (atrial fibrillation, in particular), ECG changes, and elevated troponin T levels are frequently associated with acute stroke.[58] ECG abnormalities may also predict 3-mo mortality.[56] A large study (n = 9180) of consecutive stroke patients revealed that 2.3% suffered a subsequent myocardial infarction with 64.9% morbidity/mortality compared with 35.8% in the entire cohort.[59]
Noncontrast brain CT or MRI	To exclude intracerebral hemorrhage, frank hypodensity (especially more than one third of the middle cerebral artery territory) (CT) or hyperdensity of ischemia (MRI),[7] abscess, and tumor. (See discussion in "Imaging" section of this chapter.)
CBC including platelet count	To detect polycythemia, thrombocytosis, or thrombocytopenia.
Coagulation studies	To detect preexisting coagulopathy in hemorrhagic stroke or when thrombolytics are being considered (Table 167-11).
Electrolyte levels	To detect electrolyte-imbalance stroke mimics (particularly Na^+ and Ca^{2+}).
Cardiac enzyme levels	See "ECG" earlier in this table.
Nothing by mouth (NPO) order	To protect against aspiration.
Strict bedrest in the ED	To protect against falls and seizures (in the period immediately after stroke). In patients who can maintain oxygenation, supine position has been recommended to possibly improve cerebral blood flow[7,60]; however, this remains controversial.[61] Head of bed elevation to 15 to 30 degrees may be used in patients at risk for hypoxia, airway compromise, aspiration, or suspected increased intracranial pressure.[7]
Selected patients	
Urinalysis and/or chest radiograph (if infection suspected)	To detect infectious stroke mimics or stroke-associated infections. Routine chest radiography is not recommended.[7]
Pregnancy test (if female of childbearing age)	Pregnancy influences diagnosis and management considerations.
Toxicology screen and/or blood alcohol level (if ingestion suspected)	To detect stroke mimics as well as potential causes of stroke such as ingestion of a sympathomimetic (e.g., cocaine, methamphetamine, phencyclidine).
Lumbar puncture (if infection or subarachnoid hemorrhage suspected)	To detect stroke mimics. Thrombolytics should not be given before or after a lumbar puncture because of increased risk of post–lumbar puncture epidural hematoma.

excellent interobserver agreement in CT readings between telemedicine stroke neurologists and neuroradiologists.[62]

Diffusion-weighted MRI is superior to non–contrast-enhanced CT or other types of MRI (T1/T2 weighted, fluid-attenuated inversion recovery) in the detection of acute infarction.[63,64] However, at this time, the ED role of MRI for acute stroke is limited because of MRI's uncertain accuracy in detecting acute hemorrhage,[65] lack of rapid availability,[66] patient-specific contraindications (lack of cooperation, claustrophobia, metallic implants or pacemakers, and diminished access to the patient), relative inexperience in some practitioners in interpreting MRI scans in acute stroke, and cost-effectiveness. In addition, thrombolytic inclusion/exclusion criteria were originally developed using CT findings,[67] although the use of MRI-based rtPA selection criteria continues to be explored.[68,69] Postthrombolysis diffusion-weighted MRI may be useful in differentiating stroke from other diagnoses such as TIA and stroke mimics (including coronary artery disease) in patients who have received rtPA.[70]

Despite these caveats, the current AHA/ASA acute ischemic stroke guidelines recommend either non–contrast-enhanced CT or MRI as the initial imaging in the acute stroke patient.[7] However, **in the vast majority of EDs, a non–contrast-enhanced CT is the most readily available imaging study and is the *only* imaging study necessary prior to administration of rtPA.**[71]

Vascular Imaging The current AHA/ASA acute ischemic stroke guidelines state that vascular imaging is "strongly recommended" only in patients eligible for endovascular therapies, but these studies should not delay rtPA administration.[7] With the advent of endovascular therapies (intra-arterial thrombolysis and clot retrieval/disruption), identifying the presence of intracranial large-vessel stenosis or occlusion is important for therapeutic decisions. CT angiography, digital subtraction angiography, or magnetic resonance angiography can detect intracranial arterial stenosis.[72] Some centers perform CT angiography after non–contrast-enhanced CT to identify lesions amenable to endovascular treatment.[71]

Perfusion Studies In acute ischemic stroke, the area of irreversible brain infarct (core) is surrounded by ischemic tissue that may potentially be salvageable, regardless of the time of onset of symptoms. The size of this penumbra region cannot be ascertained clinically, so perfusion CT and MRI can be used to measure the size of the penumbra and to guide further therapy for patients who fall outside the time ranges for thrombolysis or where the time of symptom onset is unclear.[73] To date, the impact of perfusion studies on therapy is mixed.[74,75]

GENERAL TREATMENT OF ACUTE ISCHEMIC STROKE

STANDARD TREATMENT

Initial ED stabilization and interventions are listed in Table 167-7. Many of these interventions are consensus based. Not all patients will be eligible for systemic rtPA, so it is important to follow general treatment principles whether or not rtPA is given.

DEHYDRATION

Dehydration can contribute to poor stroke outcomes secondary to increased blood viscosity, hypotension, renal impairment, and venous thromboembolism.[76] Correct dehydration with IV isotonic crystalloid.[7] Routine volume expansion and hemodilution do not appear to improve outcomes in stroke patients[77] and should probably not be done except perhaps in patients with hyperviscous states. For euvolemic patients, provide maintenance fluids.

HYPOXIA

The 2013 AHA/ASA consensus guidelines recommend oxygen administration to patients in stable condition only as necessary to maintain oxygen saturation >94% and to maintain normoxia.[7] Routine normobaric oxygen administration does not appear to improve short- or long-term outcomes in mild to moderate stroke,[55,78] and oxygen administration has been associated with increased stroke mortality.[79] Hyperbaric oxygenation is not currently recommended.[7]

HYPERPYREXIA

Fever is associated with increased morbidity and mortality in stroke, possibly due to increased metabolic demand and free radical production.[80] Identify the source of fever and treat with acetaminophen.[7]

HYPERTENSION

Based on consensus opinion, the current AHA/ASA acute stroke guidelines[7] dichotomize recommendations for hypertensive therapy based on the potential for acute reperfusion intervention. **For patients who are not candidates for thrombolytics or reperfusion measures, the guidelines call for *permissive hypertension*, with no active attempts made to lower blood pressure unless the systolic blood pressure is >220 mm Hg or the diastolic blood pressure is >120 mm Hg or if the patient has another medical condition that would benefit from lowering blood pressure. If the decision has been made to initiate blood pressure control, a suggested target is a 15% reduction in systolic blood pressure for the first 24 hours.**[7]

Conversely, blood pressure control is essential prior to, during, and after thrombolytic therapy. A systolic blood pressure >185 mm Hg or a diastolic blood pressure >110 mm Hg is a contraindication to the use of rtPA[15,67] because elevated blood pressure is associated with hemorrhagic transformation of ischemic stroke.[81] **Therefore, if a patient is a candidate for rtPA, actively attempt to lower blood pressure to meet these entry parameters.** An approach to management of arterial hypertension is detailed in **Table 167-9**[7] and **Table 167-10.**[7] If the target arterial blood pressures for rtPA administration cannot be reached with these measures, **then the patient is no longer a candidate for rtPA therapy**.

HYPERGLYCEMIA

The current AHA/ASA guidelines recommend the maintenance of blood glucose from 140 milligrams/dL (7.77 mmol/L) to 180 milligrams/dL (9.99 mmol/L).[7] Avoid, and treat, hypoglycemia (<60 milligrams/dL [3.33 mmol/L]).

Hyperglycemia is common in acute stroke,[82] and glycemic control has been recommended based on data that associate less favorable outcomes with hyperglycemia.[83] However, glycemic control must avoid hypoglycemia, which in itself can result in brain dysfunction.[84]

TABLE 167-9 Management of Hypertension before Administration of Recombinant Tissue Plasminogen Activator (rtPA)

If the patient is a candidate for rtPA therapy, the target arterial blood pressures are:
systolic blood pressure ≤185 mm Hg and diastolic blood pressure ≤110 mm Hg

Drug	Comments
Labetalol, 10–20 milligrams IV over 1–2 min, may repeat ×1	Use with caution in patients with severe asthma, severe chronic obstructive pulmonary disease, congestive heart failure, diabetes mellitus, myasthenia gravis, concurrent calcium channel blocker use, hepatic insufficiency. May cause dizziness and nausea. Pregnancy category C (D in second and third trimesters).
or	
Nicardipine infusion, 5 milligrams/h, titrate up by 2.5 milligrams/h at 5- to 15-min intervals; maximum dose: 15 milligrams/h; when desired blood pressure attained, reduce to 3 milligrams/h	Use with caution in patients with myocardial ischemia, concurrent use of fentanyl (hypotension), congestive heart failure, hypertrophic cardiomyopathy, portal hypertension, renal insufficiency, hepatic insufficiency (may need to adjust starting dose). Contraindicated in patients with severe aortic stenosis. Can cause headache, flushing, dizziness, nausea, reflex tachycardia. Pregnancy category C.

If the target arterial blood pressures for rtPA administration cannot be reached with these initial measures, then ***the patient is no longer a candidate for rtPA therapy***.

TABLE 167-10 Management of Hypertension during and after Administration of Recombinant Tissue Plasminogen Activator (rtPA)

Blood Pressure Monitoring Frequencies	
Time after Start of rtPA Infusion	**Frequency of Blood Pressure Monitoring**
0–2 h	Every 15 min
3–8 h	Every 30 min
9–24 h	Every 60 min
Drug Treatment of Hypertension during and after Administration of rtPA	
If systolic blood pressure is >180–230 mm Hg or diastolic blood pressure is >105–120 mm Hg	Labetalol, 10 milligrams IV followed by infusion at 2–8 milligrams/min. *or* Nicardipine infusion, 5 milligrams/h, titrate up by 2.5 milligrams/h at 5- to 15-min intervals; maximum dose 15 milligrams/h.
If blood pressure is not controlled by above measures or if diastolic blood pressure >140 mm Hg	Consider sodium nitroprusside infusion (0.5–10 microgram/kg/min). Continuous arterial monitoring advised; use with caution in patients with hepatic or renal insufficiency. Increases intracranial pressure. Pregnancy category C.

ASPIRIN

The current AHA/ASA guidelines recommend the oral administration of aspirin (initial dose is 325 milligrams) within 24 to 48 hours after stroke onset.[7] However, no antiplatelet agent (including aspirin) should be given within 24 hours of rtPA therapy. In addition, some experts recommend that oral aspirin therapy be deferred until swallowing studies can be done to avoid potential aspiration.[7] When the results of the International Stroke Trial[85] and the Chinese Acute Stroke Trial[86] are combined (40,000 patients), these studies demonstrate significant reduction in mortality and morbidity rates (at 4 weeks and 6 months) when aspirin is administered to acute ischemic stroke patients within 48 hours.[87] The benefit seems due mainly to reduction of recurrent stroke. The number needed to treat is 100, but aspirin is cost-effective and adds no risk to the outcome of ischemic stroke.[87]

THROMBOLYSIS BACKGROUND

NINDS STUDY

The National Institutes of Health/NINDS study[67] was a randomized double-blind trial comparing IV rtPA with placebo. The drug was administered within 3 hours of symptom onset, with approximately one half of patients treated within 90 minutes. Outcomes were measured using four different neurologic outcome scales (including the NIHSS) and a global statistic. Although there was no difference in the treatment and control groups at 24 hours, at 3 months, the odds ratio (OR) for a favorable outcome in patients treated with rtPA was 1.7 (95% confidence interval [CI] 1.2 to 2.61; $P = .008$), an 11% to 13% absolute risk reduction benefit (number needed to treat = 8 to 9, for tPA <3 hours). Put another way, 31% to 50% of the patients receiving rtPA (depending on the scale used) had a favorable outcome at 3 months compared with 20% to 38% of patients given placebo. Benefit was found regardless of ischemic stroke subtype and was sustained 1 year after therapy. Symptomatic intracerebral hemorrhage attributable to rtPA occurred in 6.4% of patients in the rtPA group (45% mortality), whereas symptomatic intracerebral hemorrhage occurred in 0.6% of those in the placebo group (50% mortality). Despite this increased rate of intracerebral hemorrhage, the mortality rate at 3 months was not significantly different for the treatment and placebo groups (17% vs. 21%, respectively; $P = .30$), and the percentage of patients left severely disabled was lower among those receiving rtPA.[67] The NINDS trial represented the first randomized placebo-controlled trial that showed benefit of IV rtPA in acute stroke. Prior trials using different thrombolytic agents, different dosing of rtPA, or different treatment windows failed to show benefit or showed harm. **Based largely on the NINDS data, in 1996 the U.S. Food and Drug Administration approved the use of IV rtPA in acute ischemic stroke within 3 hours of stroke onset.** As of this writing, although the European Medicines Agency has approved rtPA use from 3 to 4.5 hours after symptom onset, the Food and Drug Administration has denied approval for this application.[107] Confidentiality regulations have prevented the release of the rationale for these decisions.[7]

Concerns have been raised about the NINDS trial results.[108] The NINDS trial, although well designed, was relatively small and studied 624 patients total, 312 of whom received rtPA. As a result of chance, there existed an imbalance in baseline stroke severity between the two groups that apparently favored the rtPA group. Therefore, the NINDS investigators commissioned an independent reanalysis of the data[109] in 2004 that took this imbalance into account. This reanalysis found that, despite the imbalance, the originally described benefit of rtPA held. The authors concluded that "these findings support the use of tPA to treat patients with acute ischemic stroke within 3 hours of onset."[109] However, they did concede the need to collect further data to determine which particular stroke subgroups would benefit from or be harmed by rtPA. In 2009, a graphic reanalysis of the NINDS trial data set was published,[110] which showed very small differences in the treatment and placebo group outcomes, with a slight favoring of rtPA treatment. Therefore, the authors concluded that the reported NINDS results could have resulted from confounding alone. However, the methodology of this reanalysis was challenged in a subsequent graphic reanalysis of the NINDS data that supported the original results,[111] although these critiques have also been challenged in turn.[112]

SUBSEQUENT THROMBOLYTIC TRIALS

The European Cooperative Acute Stroke Study III (ECASS III) demonstrated efficacy with an expansion of the rtPA treatment window to 4.5 hours.[15] The OR favored patients treated with rtPA (OR = 1.34; 95% CI 1.02 to 1.76), and the post hoc analysis, which adjusted for confounding variables, yielded similar statistical results (OR = 1.42; 95% CI 1.02 to 1.98). Although the incidence of intracerebral hemorrhage was higher in the rtPA group than the placebo group (27% vs. 17%) and the incidence of symptomatic hemorrhage was also higher in the rtPA group (2.4% vs. 0.2%; 7.9% vs. 3.5% when the NINDS definition of symptomatic hemorrhage was used), mortality was similar in both groups (7.7% in the rtPA group and 8.4% in the control group). The number needed to treat for benefit was 14. Based on these data, AHA/ASA issued a 2009 scientific advisory[113] that recommended rtPA should be administered to eligible patients who present between 3 and 4.5 hours of an acute stroke, as long as they meet the ECASS III criteria. However, rtPA administration >3 hours after symptom onset is still considered "off label" in the United States because the Food and Drug Administration has declined approval[107] (see Table 167-12).

In 2012, the third International Stroke Trial (IST-3)[114] was published, making it the largest (3035 patients) rtPA in ischemic stroke randomized controlled trial to date. Patients in the treatment group were given the standard dose of rtPA up to 6 hours after stroke onset, with 72% of them receiving rtPA after 3 hours. The exclusion criteria were loosened, including eliminating any upper age limit and the broadening of the acceptable blood pressure range prior to rtPA (systolic 90 to 220 mm Hg; diastolic 40 to 130 mm Hg).[115] The trial showed no difference at 6 months in the primary outcome measure, Oxford Handicap Score (0 to 2; alive and independent): 37% versus 34% (OR = 1.13; 95% CI 0.95 to 1.35; $P = .181$) in the treatment versus control groups, respectively. However, a secondary ordinal analysis showed a favorable shift in Oxford Handicap Score scores (indicating less disability) in the treatment group at 6 months. Although symptomatic intracranial hemorrhage occurred in 7% of rtPA patients versus 1% of controls ($P < .0001$) and 11% of deaths occurred within 7 days in rtPA patients versus 7% in controls ($P < .001$), mortality at 6 months was the same (27%) in both treatment and control groups. The favorable shift in Oxford Handicap Score in rtPA patients appeared to last at least 18 months and was associated with higher overall self-reported health, with no increased mortality.[116] Interestingly, a subgroup analysis in IST-3 revealed that patients receiving thrombolytics between 3 and 4.5 hours after symptom onset actually had a nonstatistical trend toward a *worse* functional outcome compared with controls than those receiving rtPA less than 3 hours and from 4.5 to 6 hours after symptom onset.[114]

Finally, in a 2012 systematic review and meta-analysis that included **12 randomized controlled trials of rtPA** in ischemic stroke (7012 patients), the authors concluded that rtPA-treated stroke patients were more likely to have favorable outcomes than controls and that early treatment was better than late treatment, with possible benefit up to 6 hours after symptom onset.[117]

THROMBOLYSIS: INDICATIONS, EXCLUSIONS, DOSAGE, AND COMPLICATIONS

The decision to administer rtPA must be made rapidly and accurately. There must be careful identification of the time of symptom onset, defined as the **last moment the patient was known to be at baseline**. Taking the patient and family chronologically through the events immediately prior to the stroke is particularly helpful in unclear cases. **Thrombolytic use in stroke is not recommended when the time of onset cannot be reliably determined.** As of this writing, strokes recognized upon awakening (up to 29.6% of strokes[118]) should be clocked from the time at which the patient was last known to be without symptoms. Preliminary studies of thrombolysis in these so-called "wake-up" strokes have been published[119-121] that suggest some of these patients might benefit from rtPA, but these results await confirmation by randomized controlled trials.

The patient must be evaluated carefully for indications and exclusions for rtPA therapy (**Table 167-11** and **Table 167-12**), and the findings must be documented meticulously, preferably on preprinted assessment forms. The decision to administer rtPA is made by assessing multiple factors, including the numerical NIHSS score. A score between 4 and 22 is commonly used as one of the criteria for rtPA administration. However, some patients may have a lower NIHSS score, yet have a potentially disabling condition (e.g., aphasia, hemianopia, gait disturbance). Some studies have also shown poor outcomes for untreated minor strokes.[122-124] Thus, interpret an NIHSS score in the total context of the individual patient when making treatment decisions.

In the previous AHA/ASA stroke guidelines,[14,113] the exclusion criteria hewed very closely to those published by the NINDS and ECASS III trials. However, in the current recommendations,[7] several of the previous exclusion criteria have been reclassified as **"relative exclusion criteria"** on the basis of "recent experience." The guidelines urge that the risks versus anticipated benefits of proposed rtPA therapy should be carefully considered if any of the relative contraindications are present prior to administration of the drug. When faced with such patients, obtain emergency consultation with a physician with acute stroke expertise, whether on site or via telemedicine,[125,126] because local treatment varies and patient care decisions should be individualized.

A bedside blood glucose is required prior to rtPA; however, do not withhold rtPA because other laboratory results are still pending unless there is reason to suspect a pathologic or iatrogenic coagulopathy. Administer rtPA to eligible patients even if endovascular therapies are being considered.[7]

The total dose of rtPA is 0.9 milligram/kg IV, with a maximum dose of 90 milligrams; administer 10% of the dose as a bolus over 1 minute, with the remaining amount infused over 60 minutes. Perform blood pressure and neurologic checks every 15 minutes for 2 hours after starting the infusion. Table 167-10 outlines the emergent management of hypertension during and after administration of thrombolytics. **Do not give anticoagulants or antiplatelet agents in the initial 24 hours following treatment**,[7] because only rtPA trials without early aspirin have shown benefit. Admit patients to a specialized stroke unit (if available) or an intensive care unit familiar with the use of thrombolytic drugs and neurologic monitoring. If post-rtPA bleeding is suspected, halt further rtPA administration and perform an emergent CT. Order a CBC with platelet count, coagulation studies, fibrinogen level, and typing and cross-match for packed red blood cells, cryoprecipitate or fresh frozen plasma, and platelets. Emergent neurology, neurosurgery, and hematology consultations, as needed, are appropriate. Be prepared to treat the possible rtPA side effect of angioedema.

OTHER TREATMENT MODALITIES

Therapeutic hypothermia, induced hypertension, endovascular therapies, carotid endarterectomy/stenting, and emergency hemicraniectomy for massive infarcts are modalities that are being studied, but as of this writing, benefits are unproven.

Mild **therapeutic hypothermia** is associated with improved neurologic outcomes in comatose patients who survive cardiopulmonary arrest.[88] Consequently, there is much interest in the potential benefit of induced hypothermia in acute stroke, but evidence-based data about effectiveness are not available at this time.[89]

Animal data[90] and preliminary trials have suggested that implementing **drug-induced hypertension** in an effort to increase blood flow to the ischemic penumbra may benefit outcomes from acute ischemic stroke.[91,92] However, there are insufficient data to recommend this modality at this time.[7]

There is intense interest in **endovascular therapies**, primarily intra-arterial thrombolysis and mechanical clot disruption/extraction. Potential advantages of endovascular therapies include an expanded treatment window, a treatment for patients with non–time-based contraindications to IV rtPA, an ability to specifically evaluate the occluded vascular territory, use of lower total doses of thrombolytic drugs, and the possibility of mechanical clot disruption. However, indications, timing, and exclusions have yet to be established. Endovascular treatments are still considered investigational,[93] but they may be considered in patients ineligible for rtPA.

The Interventional Management of Stroke III (IMS III) trial[94] was designed to compare IV rtPA followed by endovascular treatment (including mechanical clot extraction devices) versus IV rtPA alone, but this study was terminated in 2012 after 656 subjects were enrolled due to lack of power to find statistical significance.[95] The Systemic Thrombolysis for Acute Ischemic Stroke (SYNTHESIS Expansion) trial[96] showed no difference between endovascular therapy versus IV rtPA. The Mechanical Retrieval and Recanalization of Stroke Clots Using Embolectomy (MR RESCUE) trial[74] showed no benefit to endovascular therapy in patients chosen by presence of ischemic penumbra.

In TIA patients with medically treated high-grade internal carotid artery lesions, **carotid endarterectomy** should be performed promptly, because surgical benefit is greatest within 2 weeks of the TIA.[97] The Carotid Revascularization Endarterectomy versus Stenting Trial (CREST)[98] and the International Carotid Stenting Study (ICSS)[99] suggest that **carotid stenting** is a viable alternative to endarterectomy, especially in patients <70 years old[98] or in patients with higher surgical risks.[99] The evidence-based role of carotid endarterectomy/stenting in acute stroke, on the other hand, is still not currently defined.[7,100]

Patients with a massive middle cerebral artery infarct are not candidates for thrombolytic therapy and have an 80% mortality rate. A pooled analysis of data from three European trials (Decompressive Surgery for the Treatment of Malignant Infarction of the Middle Cerebral Artery [DECIMAL], Decompressive Surgery for the Treatment of Malignant Infarction of the Middle Cerebral Artery [DESTINY], and Hemicraniectomy After Middle Cerebral Artery Infarction With Life-Threatening Edema Trial [HAMLET]) showed that decompressive hemicraniectomy was associated with better outcomes than medical therapy.[101] However, the Hemicraniectomy and Durotomy upon Deterioration Infarction-Related Swelling (HeADDFIRST) pilot trial[102] revealed less mortality at 180 days (40%) in patients with medical treatment than previously reported (50% to 70%).[103] In addition, there was no statistical difference between the medically managed patients in this trial and the patients who underwent hemicraniectomy plus medical treatment (36%).[102] These results may suggest a possible benefit to standardized medical management in these patients. At this time, the decision to perform surgery must be made on an individual basis; therefore, evidence-based indications for decompressive surgery in acute stroke have not yet been established.

There are currently insufficient data to recommend the use of dipyridamole, ticlopidine, or clopidogrel (either alone or in combination with aspirin) in early acute stroke. Antiplatelet therapy is contraindicated in acute hemorrhagic stroke.

TABLE 167-11 American Heart Association (AHA)/American Stroke Association (ASA) 2013 Inclusion/Exclusion Criteria for IV Recombinant Tissue Plasminogen Activator (rtPA) in Acute Ischemic Stroke

Inclusion Criteria	
Measurable diagnosis of acute ischemic stroke	Use of NIHSS score recommended. Major strokes (NIHSS score >22) are more likely to have poor outcomes.
Onset of symptoms <3 h prior to rtPA administration	Must be *well established* and is defined as the time of the witnessed onset of symptoms or the time the patient was last known at baseline.
Age ≥18 y	No clear upper age limit.
Exclusion Criteria	
Significant head trauma or prior stroke in previous 3 mo Symptoms suggest subarachnoid hemorrhage Arterial puncture at noncompressible site ≤7 d ago History of previous intracranial hemorrhage Intracranial neoplasm, arteriovenous malformation, or aneurysm* Seizure with postictal residual neurologic impairments thought to be due to the seizure Recent intracranial or intraspinal surgery* Pretreatment systolic blood pressure >185 mm Hg *or* diastolic blood pressure >110 mm Hg despite therapy (see Table 167-9) Active internal bleeding*	
Platelet count <100,000/mm³	If patient has no history of thrombocytopenia, rtPA may be given before this lab result is available; however, rtPA should be stopped if the platelet count is <100,000/mm³.
Use of heparin within preceding 48 h *and* a prolonged activated partial thromboplastin time (aPTT) greater than upper limit of normal	
International normalized ratio (INR) >1.7 or partial thromboplastin time (PTT) >15 s	Oral anticoagulant use in and of itself is not a contraindication to rtPA. If patient is not taking oral anticoagulant or heparin, rtPA may be given before this lab result is available; however, rtPA should be stopped if these lab tests come back elevated above normal limits.
Current use of direct thrombin inhibitors or direct factor Xa inhibitors with elevated sensitive laboratory tests (such as aPTT, INR, platelet count, and ecarin clotting time [ECT]; thrombin time [TT]; or appropriate factor Xa activity assays)*	
Blood glucose level <50 milligrams/dL (2.7 mmol/L)	
Non–contrast-enhanced CT (NECT) demonstrates multilobar infarction (hypodensity >1/3 cerebral hemisphere)	Do not give rtPA if CT shows acute intracranial hemorrhage or neoplasm.
Relative Exclusion Criteria	
Only minor or rapidly improving stroke symptoms (clearing spontaneously)	Some patients may have a lower NIHSS score but have a potentially disabling condition (e.g., aphasia, hemianopia). Some studies have shown poor outcomes for untreated minor strokes.[122-124]
Pregnancy	No randomized controlled trials have been published regarding safety or efficacy of rtPA for ischemic stroke in pregnancy. Case series have reported mixed results.[127-129]
Seizure at onset with postictal residual neurologic impairments	rtPA can be given if the residual impairments are thought to be secondary to the stroke as opposed to the seizure.[7,130]
Major surgery or serious trauma within preceding 14 d†	
Previous GI or urinary tract hemorrhage within preceding 21 d†	
Previous myocardial infarction within preceding 3 mo†	Rationale for this criterion was a statement indicating that myocardial rupture can result if rtPA is given within a few days of acute myocardial infarction.[14]
Former Exclusion Criteria from 2007 AHA/ASA Guidelines[14]	
Evidence of acute trauma (fracture)	
Failure of the patient or responsible party to understand the risks and benefits of, and alternatives to, the proposed treatment after a full discussion	

*New exclusion criteria for 2013 AHA/ASA guidelines.

†Changed from absolute contraindication from 2007 AHA/ASA guidelines.

Abbreviation: NIHSS = National Institutes of Health Stroke Scale.

DISPOSITION

Admit all acute stroke patients to monitored care units familiar with the care of stroke patients, preferably to specialized stroke units at designated stroke centers. The use of stroke units has been associated with decreased complications and length of stay, improved daily function, decreased rate of discharge to long-term care facilities, and increased likelihood of being able to live at home in the long term—with the benefit being independent of thrombolytic use.[104-106] If a patient with acute stroke presents to a facility that lacks these resources, consider transferring the patient to a higher level of care after the patient's condition has stabilized and IV rtPA has been given, as indicated—the "drip and ship" model. Emergent, early consultation with an experienced stroke physician at the accepting institution is desirable in these circumstances.

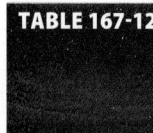

TABLE 167-12 American Heart Association (AHA)/American Stroke Association (ASA) 2013 Additional Inclusion/Exclusion Criteria for IV Recombinant Tissue Plasminogen Activator (rtPA) in Acute Ischemic Stroke for Patients Presenting within 3 to 4.5 Hours after Onset

Additional Inclusion Criteria
Measurable diagnosis of acute ischemic stroke
Onset of stroke symptoms 3–4.5 h before initiation of rtPA administration
Additional Exclusion Criteria
Age >80 y
Severe stroke as assessed clinically (e.g., NIHSS score >25) or by appropriate imaging techniques (i.e., involving >1/3 of middle cerebral artery territory)
Taking an oral anticoagulant regardless of international normalized ratio
History of previous ischemic stroke and diabetes mellitus
Exclusion Criterion from ECASS III Not Included in Current AHA/ASA Guidelines
Blood glucose >400 milligrams/dL

Abbreviation: ECASS III = European Cooperative Acute Stroke Study III; NIHSS = National Institutes of Health Stroke Scale.

TABLE 167-13 ABCD² Score to Predict Very Early Stroke Risk after Transient Ischemic Attack

Criteria	Points
*A*ge ≥60 y	0 = Absent
*A*ge ≥60 y	1 = Present
*B*lood pressure ≥140/90 mm Hg	0 = Absent
*B*lood pressure ≥140/90 mm Hg	1 = Present
*C*linical features	0 = Absent
*C*linical features	1 = Speech impairment without unilateral weakness
*C*linical features	2 = Unilateral weakness (with or without speech impairment)
*D*uration	0 = Absent
*D*uration	1 = 10–59 min
*D*uration	2 = ≥60 min
*D*iabetes	0 = Absent
*D*iabetes	1 = Present
	Total Score: 0–7

ANTIPLATELET THERAPY

STROKE

The current AHA/ASA guidelines recommend the oral administration of aspirin (initial dose is 325 milligrams) within 24 to 48 hours after stroke onset.[7] However, no antiplatelet agent (including aspirin) should be given within 24 hours of rtPA therapy. In addition, some experts recommend that oral aspirin therapy be deferred until swallowing studies can be done to avoid potential aspiration.[7] When the results of the International Stroke Trial[85] and the Chinese Acute Stroke Trial[86] are combined (40,000 patients), these studies demonstrate significant reduction in mortality and morbidity rates (at 4 weeks and 6 months) when aspirin is administered to acute ischemic stroke patients within 48 hours.[87] The benefit seems mainly due to reduction of recurrent stroke. The number needed to treat is 100, but aspirin is cost-effective and adds no risk to the outcome of ischemic stroke.[87]

There are currently insufficient data to recommend the use of dipyridamole, ticlopidine, or clopidogrel (either alone or in combination with aspirin) in early acute stroke. Antiplatelet therapy is contraindicated in acute hemorrhagic stroke.

TRANSIENT ISCHEMIC ATTACK (TIA)

TIA is defined as follows: "a transient episode of neurological dysfunction caused by focal brain, spinal cord, or retinal ischemia, without acute infarction."[131] This tissue-based definition recognizes that although TIA symptoms typically last less than 1 to 2 hours, duration of symptoms is an unreliable discriminator between TIA and infarction. A TIA should be viewed as analogous to unstable angina—that is, an ominous harbinger of a potential future vascular event. In fact, the adjusted OR for stroke <1 month after TIA is 30.4 (95% CI 10.4 to 89.4)[132] and the overall 90-day stroke risk after TIA is about 9.2% to 9.5%.[133-135] Some data suggest that 50% of these subsequent events occur within 2 days after presentation to the ED.[133] Published risk factors associated with increased risk for subsequent stroke include hypertension, diabetes mellitus, symptom duration of ≥10 minutes, weakness, and speech impairment.[133] A study of admitted patients found increased risk with male sex, age ≥65 years, hyperlipidemia, and dysarthria.[136]

TIA DIAGNOSIS

View TIAs as ominous signs of cerebral vascular disease indicating a high risk of stroke in the near future.[131] In 2007, the ABCD² scoring system was intended to replace two previous scoring scales (California score and ABCD score) (**Table 167-13**).[137]

Johnston et al[137] initially reported a 2-day risk of subsequent stroke as: 1% (ABCD² score 0 to 3), 4.1% (score 4 to 5), and 8.1% (score 6 to 7). The 7-day risk of stroke was 1.2% (ABCD² score 0 to 3), 5.9% (score 4 to 5), and 11.7% (score 6 to 7).

Based on these data, it was hoped that the ABCD² score could be used to risk-stratify low-risk patients for outpatient workup of TIA. However, subsequently published studies have produced conflicting conclusions as to the ABCD² score's predictive value for subsequent stroke after TIA.[138,139] A meta-analysis (>16,000 patients)[140] found inadequate positive and negative likelihood ratios (1 to 2 and 0.5 to 1, respectively) to be of practical use when deciding stroke risk in a given patient. Overall, the ABCD² score identified high-risk patients poorly and had only modest success in predicting low-risk patients, and the study author's cautioned against solely relying on the ABCD² score to risk-stratify patients.[140] In an attempt to improve accuracy of ABCD², the presence of two or more TIA events at 7 days (ABCD³) and diffusion-weighted MRI (ABCD³-I) have been added to the scoring system. Although one study demonstrated the superiority of these new scales to predict stroke,[141] the addition of these two data points limits the usefulness of these scales in the ED during initial presentation.

In summary, although the ABCD² score has been recommended for use by major guidelines,[131] definitive evidence-based admissions thresholds have yet to be determined. Therefore, some experts recommend that most TIA patients be hospitalized to monitor and educate them, begin antiplatelet therapy (unless contraindicated), rapidly treat subsequent stroke, assess stroke risk factors, implement preventative measures, and perform endarterectomy in appropriate patients.[131] Others recommend beginning the workup in the ED, starting antiplatelet therapy in appropriate patients, educating the patient and family regarding risk modification, and giving explicit return precautions.[142] The specific approach to a patient must be individualized and may depend not only on medical factors, but also available healthcare resources and the patient's social situation.

TIA TREATMENT

Antiplatelet Agents After TIA, the use of aspirin to prevent vascular events is historically well accepted. Current practice includes dipyridamole plus aspirin (reasonable as a first choice), clopidogrel, and aspirin alone. The selection of a particular antiplatelet regimen is a multifactorial decision based on comorbid conditions, bleeding risk, prior drug use, and cost.

A very large meta-analysis (>88,000 patients)[143] concluded that aspirin plus dipyridamole was superior to aspirin alone for prevention of vascular events after stroke or TIA. Aspirin plus dipyridamole was associated with more hemorrhagic events than dipyridamole (relative risk = 1.83; 95% CI 1.17 to 2.81), but was associated with fewer hemorrhagic events than aspirin and clopidogrel (relative risk = 0.38; 95% CI 0.25 to 0.56). However, a trial of 5170 patients found that the combination of clopidogrel and aspirin was superior to aspirin alone for reducing the risk of stroke in the first 90 days without increasing the risk of hemorrhage.[144] A trial (the Platelet-Oriented Inhibition in New TIA and Minor Ischemic Stroke [POINT] trial) is currently in progress to investigate this comparison as well.[145]

Anticoagulation Adjusted-dose oral anticoagulation with warfarin has been the historical therapy of choice for stroke prevention in patients with nonvalvular atrial fibrillation and TIA; however, an assessment of warfarin anticoagulation for stroke prevention in the United States demonstrated a dismal rate of optimal anticoagulation control.[146] This has led to multiple randomized controlled trials of novel anticoagulants, which have been shown to have equivalent efficacy but with less risk of intracranial hemorrhage compared to warfarin.[147] The risk of recurrent stroke in the presence of atrial fibrillation without anticoagulation is low, probably <5% over the next 48 hours; moreover, the risk of hemorrhagic transformation of an acute stroke is also greatest in the first 48 hours. Consequently, **in the setting of acute atrial fibrillation, anticoagulation therapy typically should not be started in the ED but should be initiated in the inpatient setting.**

Multiple studies have demonstrated that, although unfractionated heparin may help prevent recurrent stoke, its potential benefits are outweighed by the increased risk of intracranial hemorrhage. Multiple studies of low-molecular-weight heparin and heparinoids have found similarly disappointing results. A Cochrane systematic review of 24 randomized trials (23,748 patients) found no net benefit of anticoagulants in acute stroke.[148] In addition, a meta-analysis of seven trials focused specifically on anticoagulant use in acute cardiothrombotic stroke and found no overall benefit.[149] **Therefore, the use of unfractionated heparin, low-molecular-weight heparin, or heparinoids for emergent treatment of a specific stroke subtype or TIA cannot be recommended based on available evidence, even in the presence of atrial fibrillation.**[150]

SPECIAL POPULATIONS

STROKE OR TIA WITH CONCURRENT ACUTE MYOCARDIAL INFARCTION

The co-occurrence of acute myocardial infarction and acute stroke has implications for acute treatment in the ED. There is little published information on co-occurrence of the two conditions, and treatment must be extrapolated. Troponin T elevation in acute stroke is likely to be related to acute myocardial infarction if renal failure and symptomatic heart failure are excluded and is associated with worse clinical outcomes.[151] However, the newer highly sensitive troponin assays do not appear to add additional prognostic information if a fourth-generation troponin assay is normal.[152] Although anticoagulation with heparin is not recommended for the treatment of acute stroke, heparin does reduce extension or reinfarction in the setting of acute myocardial infarction (relative risk = 0.40; number needed to treat = 33).[153] However, the risk of mortality, the need for revascularization procedures, major or minor bleeding, and recurrent angina appear to be similar with and without heparin. Weigh the risks when requested to initiate heparin therapy by the cardiologist and when advised by the neurologist that heparin may induce hemorrhagic transformation. Consider the patient's baseline cardiac and neurologic status. The balance often swings to the preservation of cardiac status.

SICKLE CELL DISEASE

Stroke afflicts both adults and children with sickle cell disease, with an overall prevalence of 3.8%,[154] compared to the overall prevalence of 2.8% (age ≥20 years) in the general population in the United States.[1] Sickle cell disease is the most common cause of ischemic stroke in children. Patients homozygous for hemoglobin S have the highest incidence of stroke (0.61 in 100 patient-years), but all genotypes are at increased risk.[154] The highest incidence of hemorrhagic stroke in these patients occurs from ages 20 to 29.[154]

Cerebral aneurysms and arterial abnormalities also occur with increased frequency in patients with sickle cell disease, and careful evaluation for subarachnoid hemorrhage is mandated for patients presenting with headache and neurologic findings. Initial management is similar to that for stroke patients without sickle cell disease, but care should also be taken to treat the underlying sickle cell disease with oxygen administration, hydration, and pain control, if necessary. Although evidence is limited, expert consensus recommends exchange transfusion in sickle cell patients with acute ischemic stroke, with the goal of reducing hemoglobin S levels to <30%.[155,156] The same therapy has been recommended in hemorrhagic stroke in order to reduce vasospasm and secondary ischemic infarction.[155] Sickle cell disease is not currently considered a contraindication to rtPA therapy in eligible adults. In any event, emergent consultation with a hematologist and a stroke neurologist is in order, and admission to a stroke unit setting is indicated.

YOUNG ADULTS

Exercise particular care when evaluating young adults (age 15 to 50 years) with acute stroke. In this group, **cervical arterial dissection** accounts for 20% of all ischemic strokes and may often be preceded by only minor trauma. The young adult with a cardioembolic event may have mitral valve prolapse, rheumatic heart disease, or paradoxical embolism as the originating cause. Migrainous stroke (infarction associated with typical migraine attack, among those with established recurrent migraines) is also a possibility in this age group. Some members of this population are at risk for ischemic stroke from substance abuse. Heroin, cocaine, amphetamines, and other sympathomimetic drugs are often implicated. Human immunodeficiency virus is also a risk factor for stroke in young adults.[157]

PREGNANT WOMEN

Women are at increased risk of ischemic and hemorrhagic stroke during pregnancy and the postpartum period (up to 6 weeks after birth). Potential contributors to this increased risk include the presence of preeclampsia or eclampsia, hypertension, diabetes,[158] sickle cell disease, and drug abuse, as well as the venous stasis, edema, and hypercoagulable state that naturally occur.[9] Following birth, decreases in blood volume, alterations in hormonal status, and the potential for amniotic fluid embolism also contribute.[159] The number of antenatal strokes is approximately 34 per 100,000 deliveries,[160] with an adjusted relative risk in one series of 2.4 compared with nonpregnant females.[161] Interestingly, the overall risk for all types of stroke is far greater during 6 weeks postpartum than during pregnancy itself, with adjusted relative risks versus nonpregnant females of 8.7 and 28.3 for ischemic and hemorrhagic stroke, respectively.[161] Presentation of acute stroke is similar to that in nonpregnant patients, although pregnant patients are particularly susceptible to cerebral venous thrombosis, especially during delivery or the postpartum period, and may present primarily with a headache. MRI is generally considered the safest brain imaging study,[162] but the benefits of an emergent non–contrast-enhanced CT clearly outweigh the risks to the fetus in this setting if MRI is not immediately available. A head CT exposes the fetus to <1 rad. For further discussion, see chapter 99, "Comorbid Disorders in Pregnancy." rtPA does not cross the placenta, and there are reports of successful IV rtPA use for stroke in pregnant patients.[128,163-165] ED treatment of stroke in pregnant women should ideally involve early consultation with obstetricians, stroke neurologists, and neonatologists, as appropriate.

REFERENCES

The complete reference list is available online at www.TintinalliEM.com.

CHAPTER 168

Altered Mental Status and Coma

J. Stephen Huff

INTRODUCTION

Disorders of consciousness may be divided into processes that affect either *arousal* or *content of consciousness*, or a combination of both. Arousal behaviors include wakefulness and basic alerting. Anatomically, neurons responsible for these arousal functions reside in the reticular activating system, a collection of neurons scattered through the midbrain, pons, and medulla. The neuronal structures responsible for the content of consciousness reside in the cerebral cortex. Content of consciousness includes self-awareness, language, reasoning, spatial relationship integration, emotions, and the myriad complex integration processes that make us human. One simplistic model holds that dementia is failure of the content portions of consciousness with relatively preserved alerting functions. Delirium is arousal system dysfunction with the content of consciousness affected as well. Coma is failure of both arousal and content functions. Psychiatric disorders and altered mental states may share features such as hallucinations or delusion. Some distinctions between the different states are summarized in **Table 168-1**.

Mental status is the clinical state of emotional and intellectual functioning of the individual. The mental status evaluation may be divided into six areas (**Table 168-2**). Testing the mental status is done both formally and informally in patient evaluation by emergency physicians.[1] Assessment of higher mental or cognitive functions requires specific tests. Screening tests are described in the Diagnosis subsections under Delirium, Dementia, and Coma.

DELIRIUM

INTRODUCTION

Delirium, acute confusional state, acute cognitive impairment, acute encephalopathy, altered mental status, and other synonyms all refer to a transient disorder with impairment of attention and cognition. The patient has difficulty focusing, shifting, or sustaining attention. Confusion may fluctuate (**Table 168-1**).

The incidence of delirium in ED populations is not clear. It is estimated that 10% to 25% of elderly hospitalized patients have delirium at the time of admission.[2,3] The literature suggests that up to one quarter of all ED patients aged 70 years or older have impaired mental status or delirium and contends that routine evaluation is not satisfactory to identify many of these patients.[4,5]

TABLE 168-1 Features of Delirium, Dementia, and Psychiatric Disorder

Characteristic	Delirium	Dementia	Psychiatric Disorder
Onset	Over days	Insidious	Sudden
Course over 24 h	Fluctuating	Stable	Stable
Consciousness	Reduced or hyperalert	Alert	Alert
Attention	Disordered	Normal	May be disordered
Cognition	Disordered	Impaired	May be impaired
Orientation	Impaired	Often impaired	May be impaired
Hallucinations	Visual and/or auditory	Often absent	Usually auditory
Delusions	Transient, poorly organized	Usually absent	Sustained
Movements	Asterixis, tremor may be present	Often absent	Absent

TABLE 168-2 Six Elements of Mental Status Evaluation

Appearance, behavior, and attitude
Is dress appropriate?
Is motor behavior at rest appropriate?
Is the speech pattern normal?
Disorders of thought
Are the thoughts logical and realistic?
Are false beliefs or delusions present?
Are suicidal or homicidal thoughts present?
Disorders of perception
Are hallucinations present?
Mood and affect
What is the prevailing mood?
Is the emotional content appropriate for the setting?
Insight and judgment
Does the patient understand the circumstances surrounding the visit?
Sensorium and intelligence
Is the level of consciousness normal?
Is cognition or intellectual functioning impaired?

PATHOPHYSIOLOGY

Pathologic mechanisms producing delirium are complex and are thought to involve widespread neuronal or neurotransmitter dysfunction. There are four general causes[6]:

1. Primary intracranial disease
2. Systemic diseases secondarily affecting the CNS
3. Exogenous toxins
4. Drug withdrawal

CLINICAL FEATURES

Delirium or acute confusional state generally develops over days. Attention, perception, thinking, and memory are all altered. Alertness is reduced as manifested by difficulty maintaining attention and focusing concentration. The patient may appear quite awake, but attention is impaired. Activity levels may be either increased or decreased. The patient may fluctuate rapidly between hypoactive and hyperactive states. **Symptoms may be intermittent, and it is not unusual for different caregivers to witness completely different behaviors within a brief time span.** The sleep-wake cycles are often disrupted, with increased somnolence during the day and agitation at night, or "sundowning." Tremor, asterixis, tachycardia, sweating, hypertension, and emotional outbursts may be present. Hallucinations tend to be visual, although auditory hallucinations can also occur.[2,3,7]

DIAGNOSIS

Both historical and physical examination findings indicating delirium are necessary to confirm the diagnosis. Obtaining a history from caregivers, spouse, or other family members is the primary method for diagnosing delirium.[2,3,7] **The acute onset of attention deficits and cognitive abnormalities fluctuating in severity throughout the day and worsening at night is virtually diagnostic of delirium.** Examine medication history, including over-the-counter medications taken and prescribed medications, in detail. Check for drug interactions. Assess for an underlying process, such as pneumonia or urinary tract infection. Ancillary testing should include serum electrolyte levels, hepatic and renal studies, urinalysis, CBC, and a chest radiograph. Order a head CT if a mass lesion such as subdural hematoma is suspected; follow this by performing a lumbar puncture if meningitis or subarachnoid hemorrhage is considered.

One key tool for detecting delirium is the mental status examination and other cognitive screening instruments.[8-12] These tests are valuable in directing the physician to study aspects of attention and memory that might not otherwise be formally tested. Parts of the Mini-Mental State Examination are sometimes used in the ED.[8-10] The complete test takes 7 to 10 minutes to administer, but copyright restrictions limit reproduction and use.[11] Age, education, chronic cognitive impairment, and verbal abilities all may affect scores. The Mini-Mental State Examination does not detect mild impairment. The median positive and negative likelihood ratios for the test are 6.3 and 0.19, respectively.[11] Several other shorter evaluation tools have been proposed.[9-12] The **Quick Confusion Scale** has been tested in ED patients, yields scores that correlate well with those on the Mini-Mental State Examination ($r = 0.61$ in one study[10] and 0.783 in another[9]), and takes <3 minutes to administer. The patient does not need to read, write, or draw to complete the test[10] (**Table 168-3**).

Depression may resemble hypoactive delirium, with withdrawal, slowed speech, and poor results on cognitive testing present in both conditions. However, rapid fluctuation of symptoms is common in delirium but generally absent in depression. In addition, clouding of consciousness is absent in patients with depression. **Patients with depression are oriented and able to perform commands.**

TABLE 168-3 The Quick Confusion Scale

Item	Score (Number Correct)	¥ (Weight)	=	(Total)
What year is it now?	0 or 1 (Score 1 if correct, 0 if incorrect)	×2	=	_____
What month is it?	0 or 1	×2	=	_____
(Present memory phrase): Repeat this phrase after me and remember it: "John Brown, 42 Market Street, New York."				
About what time is it? (Answer correct if within 1 h.)	0 or 1	×2	=	_____
Count backward from 20 to 1.	0, 1, or 2	×1	=	_____
Say the months in reverse.	0, 1, or 2	×1	=	_____
Repeat the memory phrase (each underlined portion correct is worth 1 point).	0, 1, 2, 3, 4, or 5	×1	=	_____
Final score is the sum of the totals.			=	_____

Notes:

15 is the top score; a score <15 may indicate the need for additional assessment.	
Scores highest number in category indicates correct response; lower scoring indicates increased number of errors.	
Item 1. What year is it now?	Score 1 if answered correctly, 0 if incorrect.
Item 2. What month is it?	Score 1 if answered correctly, 0 if incorrect.
Item 3. About what time is it?	Answer considered correct if within 1 h; score 1 if correct, 0 if incorrect.
Item 4. Count backward from 20 to 1.	Score 2 if correctly performed; score 1 if one error, score 0 if two or more errors.
Item 5. Say the months in reverse.	Score 2 if correctly performed; score 1 if one error, score 0 if two or more errors.
Item 6. Repeat memory phrase: "John Brown, 42 Market Street, New York."	Each underlined portion correctly recalled is worth 1 point in scoring; score 5 if correctly performed; each error drops score by 1.
Final score is the sum of the weighted totals; items 1, 2, and 3 are multiplied by 2 and summed with the other item scores to yield the final score.	

TABLE 168-4 Important Medical Causes of Delirium

Infectious	Pneumonia Urinary tract infection Meningitis or encephalitis Sepsis
Metabolic/toxic	Hypoglycemia Alcohol ingestion Electrolyte abnormalities Hepatic encephalopathy Thyroid disorders Alcohol or drug withdrawal
Neurologic	Stroke or transient ischemic attack Seizure or postictal state Subarachnoid hemorrhage Intracranial hemorrhage CNS mass lesion Subdural hematoma
Cardiopulmonary	Congestive heart failure Myocardial infarction Pulmonary embolism Hypoxia or carbon dioxide narcosis
Drug related	Anticholinergic drugs Alcohol or drug withdrawal Sedatives-hypnotics Narcotic analgesics Selective serotonin or serotonin-norepinephrine reuptake inhibitors Polypharmacy

An unusual cause of confusional state, but one that is suspected to be underrecognized, is **nonconvulsive status epilepticus**, or **complex partial status epilepticus**. This twilight state may persist for hours or even months. Suspicion and electroencephalography are required for recognition.[10] (See chapter 171, Seizures, for further discussion of nonconvulsive status epilepticus.)

TREATMENT

Direct treatment at the underlying cause. Common medical causes of delirium are listed in **Table 168-4**. Multiple causes may be present in a given patient.

Environmental manipulations such as adequate lighting, psychosocial support, and mobilization may be helpful in enhancing the patient's ability to interpret the surroundings correctly.[2,6,7] Sedation may be needed. Haloperidol is a frequent initial choice at a dose of 5 to 10 milligrams PO, IM, or IV with reduced dosing of 1 to 2 milligrams in the elderly. Repeat at 20- to 30-minute intervals as needed. Benzodiazepines such as lorazepam, 0.5 to 2.0 milligrams PO, IM, or IV, may be used in combination with haloperidol in doses of 1 to 2 milligrams, with the dose varying widely depending on the age and size of the patient and the degree of agitation. Chapter 287, Acute Agitation, provides further discussion on management of agitation.

DISPOSITION AND FOLLOW-UP

Admit the patient into the hospital for further treatment and additional diagnostic testing unless a readily reversible cause for the acute mental status change is discovered and treatment initiated. This decision is individualized with consideration of patient characteristics, the resources in the home or healthcare facility, and the patient's safety.

DEMENTIA

INTRODUCTION

Dementia implies a loss of mental capacity. Psychosocial level and cognitive abilities deteriorate, and behavioral problems develop. The largest categories of dementia are idiopathic dementia (Alzheimer's disease) and vascular dementia, which are essentially diagnoses of exclusion. However, other, more treatable disorders may cause or simulate dementia.

The typical course of dementia is slow with insidious symptom onset. The abrupt onset of symptoms or rapidly progressive symptoms should prompt a search for other diagnoses. Presentation to the ED is usually precipitated by some sentinel event. Hallucinations, delusions, repetitive behaviors, and depression are all common.

PATHOPHYSIOLOGY

Most cases of dementia in the United States are due to Alzheimer's disease, a neurodegenerative disorder of unknown etiology. The pathophysiology is complex, with a reduction in neurons in the cerebral cortex, increased amyloid deposition, and the production of neurofibrillary tangles and plaques. Other neurodegenerative diseases have their own unique pathologies. Vascular dementia accounts for the next largest number of dementia cases. The pathology is that of cerebrovascular disease with multiple infarctions. A listing of different types of dementia is provided in **Table 168-5**.

TABLE 168-5 Classification of Dementia by Cause

Degenerative
Alzheimer's disease
Huntington's disease
Parkinson's disease
Vascular
Multiple infarcts
Hypoperfusion (cardiac arrest, profound hypotension, others)
Subdural hematoma
Subarachnoid hemorrhage
Infectious
Meningitis (sequelae of bacterial, fungal, or tubercular)
Neurosyphilis
Viral encephalitis (herpes, human immunodeficiency virus), Creutzfeldt-Jakob disease
Inflammatory
Systemic lupus erythematosus
Demyelinating disease, others
Neoplastic
Primary tumors and metastatic disease
Carcinomatous meningitis
Paraneoplastic syndromes
Traumatic
Traumatic brain injury
Subdural hematoma
Toxic
Alcohol
Medications (anticholinergics, polypharmacy)
Metabolic
Vitamin B_{12} or folate deficiency
Thyroid disease
Uremia, others
Psychiatric
Depression (pseudodementia)
Hydrocephalic
Normal-pressure hydrocephalus (communicating hydrocephalus)
Noncommunicating hydrocephalus

CLINICAL FEATURES

Impairment of memory, particularly recent memory, is gradual and progressive. Remote memories are often preserved. Impairment of memory and orientation with preservation of motor and speech abilities is said to be characteristic of the onset of dementia associated with Alzheimer's disease. Degenerative dementias are divided into early, middle, and late stages. Early in the disease, complaints of memory loss, naming problems, or forgetting of items is common. The middle stage shows progression of these problems plus loss of reading, decreased performance in social situations, and loss of direction. The late stage of the illness may include extreme disorientation, inability to perform self-care tasks, and personality change. Clinical features may include affective symptoms such as depression and anxiety, behavioral disorders, and speech difficulties.

Patients with vascular or multi-infarct dementia often show similar symptoms, but may have findings on physical examination of exaggerated or asymmetric deep tendon reflexes, gait abnormalities, or weakness of an extremity.

DIAGNOSIS

General physical examination does not determine the diagnosis of dementia but may be helpful in identifying associated causes.[13] The presence of focal neurologic signs may suggest vascular dementia or a mass lesion. Increased motor tone and other extrapyramidal signs such as rigidity or a movement disorder may suggest Parkinson's disease. Perform mental status testing as outlined earlier.

Laboratory assessment typically includes a CBC, comprehensive metabolic profile, urinalysis, thyroid function tests, serum vitamin B_{12} level, and serologic testing for syphilis (in patients at risk).[14,15] Other helpful laboratory tests may include erythrocyte sedimentation rate, serum folate level, human immunodeficiency virus testing, and chest radiography. Consider CT or MRI imaging in every patient at some point in the diagnostic evaluation. Perform lumbar puncture if the diagnosis is not readily apparent.

Diagnosis of probable vascular dementia requires signs of cerebrovascular disease. The relationship between stroke and cognitive decline must be temporally related, with dementia within 3 months of the stroke or abrupt deterioration in memory and other cognitive abilities. A fluctuating, stepped course suggests vascular dementia.[16]

The possibility of a concurrent medical condition suddenly causing cognitive functioning to deteriorate should be strongly considered and often is the thrust of investigation in the ED. Urinary tract infection, congestive heart failure, and hypothyroidism are just a few of the conditions that may cause a mildly demented but functioning individual to show rapid decline. The symptoms overlap with those of delirium as discussed earlier in the Clinical Features section under Delirium, and the two conditions may overlap.[3,7] Consider depression imitators, the so-called treatable causes of dementia (included in **Table 168-5**), in the differential diagnosis.

Depression may coexist with dementia, and also consider depression-imitating dementia (pseudodementia). Arrange appropriate inpatient or outpatient follow-up for further behavioral health evaluation. If depression is severe, consider hospital admission.

TREATMENT

All types of dementia are treatable, at least to some degree, by environmental or psychosocial interventions. Antipsychotic drugs are used to manage psychotic and nonpsychotic behaviors, but adverse drug effects complicate treatment. Reserve antipsychotic drugs for patients with persistent psychotic features or those with extreme disruptive or dangerous behaviors.[3,17] Coordinate treatment with caregivers who are in a position to monitor the patient's behavior patterns over time.

Treatment of vascular dementia is limited to treatment of risk factors, including hypertension.

Normal-pressure hydrocephalus is suggested by the presence of excessively large ventricles on head CT and can prompt consideration of a trial of lumbar puncture with cerebrospinal fluid drainage or ventricular shunting. **Consider normal-pressure hydrocephalus if urinary incontinence and gait disturbance develop early in the disease process.**

DISPOSITION AND FOLLOW-UP

A new diagnosis of dementia may be entertained in the ED, but the depth of the required diagnostic evaluation usually exceeds the time available during the ED visit. A decision to admit or to arrange an outpatient diagnosis is the usual disposition after the major differential diagnostic possibilities have been eliminated. Direct attention toward the presence of delirium or a treatable cause of dementia. Consider hospital admission if comorbid medical problems, a rapidly progressive or atypical clinical course, or an unsafe or uncertain home situation exists.

COMA

INTRODUCTION

Coma is a state of reduced alertness and responsiveness from which the patient cannot be aroused.[18,19] The Glasgow Coma Scale (**Table 168-6**; see also chapter 257, Head Trauma) is a widely used clinical scoring system for alterations in consciousness. Advantages are the simplicity of the scoring system and assessment of separate verbal, motor, and eye-opening functions. Disadvantages include lack of acknowledgment of hemiparesis or other focal motor signs and lack of testing of higher cognitive functions. Interrater variability has been noted in assessments using the **Glasgow Coma Scale.**[20] Another coma scale, the FOUR (*F*ull *O*utline of *U*n*R*esponsiveness) score, has been used in intensive care units and has the advantages of assessing simple brainstem functions and respiratory patterns, as well as eye and motor responses.[21] Causes of coma likely to be encountered in the ED are noted in **Table 168-7**.

PATHOPHYSIOLOGY

The pathophysiology of coma is complex. Coma can result from deficiency of substrates needed for neuronal function (as with hypoglycemia or hypoxia). With systemic causes, the brain is globally affected, and signs that localize dysfunction to a specific area of the brainstem or cortex are usually lacking. With primary CNS causes, coma may result from a brainstem disorder such as hemorrhage or from bilateral cortical dysfunction. Signs localizing to specific areas of CNS dysfunction such

TABLE 168-7 Differential Diagnosis of Coma

Coma from causes affecting the brain diffusely
Encephalopathies
- Hypoxic encephalopathy
- Metabolic encephalopathy
- Hypertensive encephalopathy

Hypoglycemia
Hyperosmolar state (e.g., hyperglycemia)
Electrolyte abnormalities (e.g., hypernatremia or hyponatremia, hypercalcemia)
Organ system failure
- Hepatic encephalopathy
- Uremia/renal failure

Endocrine (e.g., Addison's disease, hypothyroidism, etc.)
Hypoxia
Carbon dioxide narcosis
Toxins
Drug reactions (e.g., neuroleptic malignant syndrome)
Environmental causes—hypothermia, hyperthermia
Deficiency state—Wernicke's encephalopathy
Sepsis

Coma from primary CNS disease or trauma
Direct CNS trauma
- Diffuse axonal injury
- Subdural hematoma
- Epidural hematoma

Vascular disease
- Intraparenchymal hemorrhage (hemispheric, basal ganglia, brainstem, cerebellar)

Subarachnoid hemorrhage
Infarction
- Hemispheric, brainstem

CNS infections
Neoplasms
Seizures
- Nonconvulsive status epilepticus
- Postictal state

TABLE 168-6 Glasgow Coma Scale

Component	Score	Adult	Child <5 y	Child >5 y
Motor	6	Follows commands	Normal spontaneous movements	Follows commands
	5	Localizes pain	Localizes to supraocular pain (>9 mo)	
	4	Withdraws to pain	Withdraws from nail bed pressure	
	3	Flexion	Flexion to supraocular pain	
	2	Extension	Extension to supraocular pain	
	1	None	None	
Verbal	5	Oriented	Age-appropriate speech/vocalizations	Oriented
	4	Confused speech	Less than usual ability; irritable cry	Confused
	3	Inappropriate words	Cries to pain	Inappropriate words
	2	Incomprehensible	Moans to pain	Incomprehensible
	1	None	No response to pain	
Eye opening	4	Spontaneous	Spontaneous	
	3	To command	To voice	
	2	To pain	To pain	
	1	None	None	

as hemiparesis or cranial nerve abnormalities may be present. Unilateral hemispheric disease, such as stroke, should not alone result in coma. The function of the brainstem and/or both hemispheres must be impaired for unresponsiveness to occur.

The herniation syndromes are models for alterations of consciousness, but their mechanisms are unknown. In **uncal herniation syndrome**, the medial temporal lobe shifts to compress the upper brainstem, which results in progressive drowsiness followed by unresponsiveness.[19,22] The ipsilateral pupil is sluggish, eventually becoming dilated and nonreactive as the third cranial nerve is compressed by the medial temporal lobe. Hemiparesis may develop ipsilateral to the mass from compression of the descending motor tracts in the opposite cerebral peduncle. **Central herniation syndrome** is characterized by progressive loss of consciousness, loss of brainstem reflexes, decorticate posturing, and irregular respiration.[19] Because midline shift without herniation, as demonstrated by neuroimaging, seems to correlate with a decreased level of consciousness, vascular compression due to local cerebral edema or local increased intracranial pressure (ICP) may be an underlying mechanism for these syndromes.

A diffuse increase in ICP can cause diffuse CNS dysfunction. Cerebral blood flow is constant at mean arterial pressures (MAPs) of 50 to 100 mm Hg due to the process of cerebral autoregulation. At MAPs outside this range, cerebral blood flow may be reduced, and diffuse ischemia may develop. **Cerebral perfusion pressure is equal to the MAP minus the ICP (cerebral perfusion pressure = MAP − ICP).** In extreme uncontrolled elevation of the ICP, cerebral perfusion pressure is diminished as the ICP approaches the MAP, which causes brain ischemia.

Particularly in unresponsive patients with a history of seizures, the possibility of ongoing nonconvulsive seizures must be considered. Subtle status epilepticus or ictal coma may represent transformed generalized convulsive status epilepticus. Electrical seizures may continue in the absence of clinical seizures.[23]

CLINICAL FEATURES

The clinical features of coma vary with both the depth of coma and the cause. For example, a patient in a coma with a hemispheric hemorrhage and midline shift may have decreased muscle tone on the side of the hemiparesis. The eyes may conjugately deviate toward the side of the hemorrhage. **With expansion of the hemorrhage and surrounding edema, increase in ICP, or brainstem compression, unresponsiveness may progress to a complete loss of motor tone and loss of the ocular findings as well.**

A variety of abnormal breathing patterns may be seen in the comatose patient.[19] They offer little information in the acute setting. Pupillary findings, the results of other cranial nerve evaluation, hemiparesis, and response to stimulation are all part of the clinical picture that need assessment. These findings can assign the cause of the coma into a probable general category—diffuse CNS dysfunction (toxic-metabolic coma) or focal CNS dysfunction (structural coma). A further division of structural coma into hemispheric (supratentorial) or posterior fossa (infratentorial) coma is often possible at the bedside.

Toxic-Metabolic Coma Many different toxic and metabolic conditions cause coma. The diffuse CNS dysfunction is reflected by the lack of focal physical examination findings that point to a specific region of brain dysfunction. For example, in toxic-metabolic coma, if the patient demonstrates either spontaneous movements or reflex posturing, the movements are symmetric without evidence of hemiparesis. Muscle stretch reflexes, if present, are symmetric. Pupillary response is generally preserved in toxic-metabolic coma. Typically the pupils are small but reactive. If extraocular movements are present, they are symmetric. If extraocular movements are absent, however, this sign is of no value in differentiating toxic-metabolic from structural coma. A notable exception is severe sedative poisoning as from barbiturates; the pupils may be large, extraocular movements absent, muscles flaccid, and the patient apneic, which simulates the appearance of brain death.

Coma from Supratentorial Lesions Coma caused by lesions of the hemispheres, or supratentorial masses, may present with progressive hemiparesis or asymmetric muscle tone and reflexes. The hemiparesis may be suspected with asymmetric responses to stimuli or asymmetric extensor or flexor postures. Uncal herniation syndrome, as described earlier in Pathophysiology, is an example of a supratentorial syndrome. Frequently, however, large acute supratentorial lesions are seen without the features consistent with temporal lobe herniation. Coma without lateralizing signs may result from decreased cerebral perfusion secondary to increased ICP. Reflex changes in blood pressure and heart rate may be observed with increased ICP or brainstem compression. Hypertension and bradycardia in a comatose patient may represent the Cushing reflex from increased ICP.

Coma from Infratentorial Lesions Posterior fossa or infratentorial lesions comprise another structural coma syndrome. **An expanding lesion, such as cerebellar hemorrhage or infarction, may cause abrupt coma, abnormal extensor posturing, loss of pupillary reflexes, and loss of extraocular movements.** The anatomy of the posterior fossa leaves little room for accommodating an expanding mass. Early brainstem compression with loss of brainstem reflexes may develop rapidly. Another infratentorial cause of coma is pontine hemorrhage, which may present with the unique signs of pinpoint-sized pupils.

Pseudocoma Pseudocoma or psychogenic coma is occasionally encountered and may present a perplexing clinical problem. Adequate history taking and observation of responses to stimulation reveal findings that differ from those in the syndromes described in the previous sections. Pupillary responses, extraocular movements, muscle tone, and reflexes are shown to be intact on careful examination. Tests of particular value include responses to manual eye opening (there should be little or no resistance in the truly unresponsive patient) and extraocular movements. Specifically, if avoidance of gaze is consistently seen with the patient always looking away from the examiner, or if nystagmus is demonstrated with caloric vestibular testing, this is strong evidence for nonphysiologic or feigned unresponsiveness.

DIAGNOSIS

In the approach to the comatose patient, perform stabilization, diagnosis, and treatment actions simultaneously. Examination, laboratory procedures, and neuroimaging allow differentiation between structural and metabolic causes of coma in almost all patients in the ED. History and physical examination findings allow that initial assignment in many patients, but liberal use of CT scanning is encouraged because exceptions to the tentative clinical diagnosis are frequent.

Address airway, breathing, and circulation immediately. Consider reversible causes of coma, such as hypoglycemia or opiate overdose. Access all available historical sources (EMS personnel, caregivers, family, witnesses, medical records, etc.) to aid in diagnosis.

The tempo of onset of the coma is of great diagnostic value. Abrupt coma suggests abrupt CNS failure with possible causes such as catastrophic stroke or seizures. A slowly progressive onset of coma may suggest a progressive CNS lesion such as tumor or subdural hematoma. Metabolic causes, such as hyperglycemia, may also develop over several days.

Address general examination and measurement of vital signs (including oxygen saturation and temperature) following stabilization and resuscitation. General examination may reveal signs of trauma or suggest other diagnostic possibilities for the unresponsiveness. For example, a toxidrome may be present that suggests diagnosis and treatment, such as the opiate syndrome with hypoventilation and small pupils.

Neurologic testing deviates from the standard examination. Fine tests of weakness, such as testing for pronator drift of the outstretched upper extremities, are not possible in the unresponsive patient. However, asymmetric findings on examination of cranial nerves through pupillary examination, assessment of corneal reflexes, and testing of oculovestibular reflexes may suggest focal CNS lesions. Abnormal extensor or flexor postures are nonspecific for localization or cause of coma but suggest profound CNS dysfunction. Asymmetric muscle tone or reflexes raise the suspicion of a focal lesion. **The goal of the physician is to rapidly determine if the CNS dysfunction is from diffuse impairment of the brain or if signs point to a focal (and perhaps surgically treatable) region of CNS dysfunction.**

CT is the neuroimaging procedure of choice. Acute hemorrhage is readily identified, as is midline shift and mass lesions. Consider lumbar puncture if CT scan findings are unremarkable and subarachnoid hemorrhage or CNS infection is suspected. Suspect basilar artery thrombosis in a comatose patient with "normal" results on head CT, in which the only finding may be a hyperdense basilar artery.[24] MRI or cerebral angiography is needed to make the diagnosis of basilar artery thrombosis.

SPECIAL CONSIDERATIONS IN COMA

If trauma is suspected, maintain stabilization of the cervical spine during assessment. If protection of the airway is in doubt or the coma state is likely prolonged, then protect the airway by intubating the patient. Rapid-sequence intubation techniques are discussed at length in chapter 29, Intubation and Mechanical Ventilation. **ingestions, infections, and child abuse in the appropriate clinical setting.**

Patients who have had generalized seizures and remain unresponsive may be in a continuing state of electrical seizures without corresponding motor movements. This is called **nonconvulsive status epilepticus** or **subtle status epilepticus** and can be described as electromechanical dissociation of the brain and body. **If the motor activity of the seizure stops and the patient does not awaken within 30 minutes, then consider nonconvulsive status epilepticus.** Obtain neurologic consultation and electroencephalography.[23]

TREATMENT

Treatment of coma involves identification of the cause of the brain failure and initiation of specific therapy directed at the underlying cause. Attend to airway, ventilation, and circulation. Evaluate and treat for readily reversible causes of coma, such as hypoglycemia and opioid toxicity.

Antidotes Rapid point-of-care glucose determination can identify the need for dextrose. Although thiamine should be administered before glucose infusion in patients with a suspected history of alcohol abuse or malnutrition, thiamine is not necessary for all patients. Routine use of flumazenil in coma of unknown cause is not recommended.[25] Naloxone, the opiate antagonist, is useful in coma because typical signs of opiate overdose may be absent.

Increased Intracranial Pressure If history, physical examination, or neuroimaging findings suggest increased ICP, specific steps can reduce or ameliorate any further rise in ICP. Any noxious stimulus, including "bucking" the ventilator, can increase ICP, so use paralytic and sedative agents. A general recommendation is to keep the head elevated about 30 degrees and at midline to aid in venous drainage. **Mannitol** (0.5 to 1.0 gram/kg IV) can decrease intravascular volume and brain water and may transiently reduce ICP. In cases of brain edema associated with tumor, dexamethasone, 10 milligrams IV, reduces edema over several hours. Hyperventilation with reduction of partial pressure of arterial carbon dioxide can reduce cerebral blood volume and transiently lower ICP. Current recommendations are to avoid excessive hyperventilation (partial pressure of arterial carbon dioxide ≤35 mm Hg) during the first 24 hours after brain injury. Brief hyperventilation may be necessary for refractory intracranial hypertension. Data to recommend specific therapy are lacking, and preferences among individuals and institutions vary greatly, so communicate early with consultants and admitting physicians.

DISPOSITION AND FOLLOW-UP

Patients with readily reversible causes of coma, such as insulin-induced hypoglycemia, may be discharged if home care and follow-up care are adequate and a clear cause for the episode is suspected. Admit patients with persistent altered consciousness. Most institutions depend on emergency physicians to stabilize the patient's condition and correctly assign a tentative diagnosis so that the patient may be admitted to the proper specialty service. If the appropriate service is not available, then consider transfer to another hospital after patient stabilization.

REFERENCES

The complete reference list is available online at www.TintinalliEM.com.

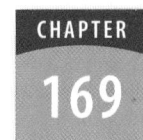

Ataxia and Gait Disturbances

J. Stephen Huff

INTRODUCTION

Ataxia and gait disturbances may be symptoms of many disease processes and generally are not themselves diagnoses. **Ataxia** is uncoordinated movement. A **gait disorder** is an abnormal pattern or style of walking. The presenting problem may be articulated by the patient or family as weakness, dizziness, stroke, falling, or another nonspecific chief complaint. Such symptoms must always be viewed in the context of the patient's overall clinical picture. This chapter reviews the more common causes of acute ataxia and gait disorders (**Table 169-1**).

PATHOPHYSIOLOGY

Clinicians erroneously tend to think that ataxia and gait disorders result primarily from cerebellar lesions. However, such disorders result from many systemic or focal conditions that affect different elements of the central and peripheral nervous systems. Cerebellar lesions may indeed cause ataxia, but isolated lesions of the cerebellum are not the most common cause of these complaints. Ataxias are classified as either motor (cerebellar) or sensory.

TABLE 169-1 Common Etiologies of Acute Ataxia and Gait Disturbances
Systemic conditions
Intoxications with diminished alertness
Ethanol
Sedative-hypnotics
Intoxications with relatively preserved alertness (diminished alertness at higher levels)
Phenytoin
Carbamazepine
Valproic acid
Heavy metals—lead, organic mercurials
Other metabolic disorders
Hyponatremia
Inborn errors of metabolism
Wernicke's disease
Disorders predominantly of the nervous system
Conditions affecting predominantly one region of the CNS
Cerebellum
Hemorrhage
Infarction
Degenerative changes
Abscess
Cortex
Frontal tumor, hemorrhage, or trauma
Hydrocephalus
Subcortical
Thalamic infarction or hemorrhage
Parkinson's disease
Normal pressure hydrocephalus
Spinal cord
Cervical spondylosis and other causes of spinal cord compression
Posterior column disorders
Conditions affecting predominantly the peripheral nervous system
Peripheral neuropathy
Vestibulopathy

MOTOR ATAXIAS

Motor ataxias (also referred to as **cerebellar ataxias**) are usually caused by disorders of the cerebellum. The sensory receptors and afferent pathways are intact, but integration of the proprioceptive information is faulty. Involvement of the lateral cerebellum (one of the cerebellar hemispheres) may lead to a motor ataxia of the ipsilateral limb. Lesions affecting primarily the midline portion of the cerebellum often cause problems with axial muscle coordination, which is reflected in difficulty maintaining a steady upright standing or sitting posture.

There are many reports of lesions in what would seem to be unlikely locations producing motor ataxia. Supratentorial infarctions, particularly small, deep infarctions, and lacunae of the posterior limb of the internal capsule have been reported to cause isolated hemiataxia. It is postulated that interruption of either ascending or descending cerebellar to cortical pathways are the cause of this motor-type ataxia.[1] Small infarctions or hemorrhages in thalamic nuclei may produce a clinical picture of motor- or cerebellar-like ataxia with hemisensory loss. These effects are seen contralateral to the lesion.[2] Lesions affecting the frontal lobe, such as tumor or cystic masses, may cause a motor ataxia of the contralateral extremities through poorly understood mechanisms.[3] Nontraumatic spinal cord compression may present with gait ataxia or abnormality.[4]

SENSORY ATAXIAS

Sensory ataxias are due to failure of transmission of proprioception or position sense information to the CNS. Failure may arise from disorders affecting the peripheral nerves, spinal cord, or cerebellar input tracts. Coordinated motor performance is faulty, even though motor systems and the cerebellum are intact. Sensory ataxias may be somewhat compensated by visual sensory information. Loss of visual information leads to the observation that sensory ataxias often worsen in poor lighting conditions and may be brought out during examination.

GAIT DISORDERS

No organized classification scheme exists for gait disorders, and different authors categorize abnormal gaits in descriptive terms. A **cerebellar or motor ataxic gait** is widely based with unsteady and irregular steps, and compensation to barriers in the environment may be lacking. The **gait of sensory ataxia** resulting from loss of proprioception is notable for abrupt movement of the legs and slapping impact of the feet with each step. A variety of other terms are used to describe abnormal gaits.

An **apraxic gait** is one in which the patient seemingly has lost the ability to initiate the process of walking, an "ignition failure." This may occur with right or nondominant hemispheric lesions. Frontal lobe dysfunction may result in a similar gait and may be seen in normal pressure hydrocephalus.[5]

The term **festinating gait** is used to describe narrowly based miniature shuffling steps and is common in Parkinson's disease. An abnormal gait with outward swinging or circumabduction of the leg suggests a mild **hemiparesis** reflecting the asymmetric weakness of the proximal lower extremity muscles. Bilateral weakness of the trunk and pelvic girdle muscles may result in a **waddling gait** from failure to maintain the normal position of the pelvis relative to the lower extremities.

A functional gait disorder is one in which the patient is unable to walk normally, although all motor pathways, sensory pathways, and cerebellar functions may be demonstrated to be functioning normally. The underlying problem is often a conversion disorder. Functional gaits may be bizarre, at times resembling a person balancing on a tightrope and seemingly threatening to fall but not falling. A dramatic functional gait with flailing movements without falling actually demonstrates that strength, balance, and coordination are intact.

A unifying concept defines gait disorders according to the level of processing of neurologic information (**Table 169-2**).[6,7] The classification scheme is not ideal but does allow a thoughtful approach to patient diagnosis.

TABLE 169-2 Classification of Gait Disorders

Low-level gait disorders
Musculoskeletal problems
Arthritic gait or other joint or skeletal problems
Muscle weakness
Peripheral sensory problems
Sensory ataxic gait
Vestibular problems
Middle-level gait disorders
Hemiplegia
Paraplegia
Motor or cerebellar ataxia
Parkinson's disease
Dystonia, chorea, other movement disorders
High-level gait disorders
Senile gait (cautious gait)
Frontal ataxic gait
Apraxic gait (gait ignition failure)
Frontal disequilibrium

Low-level gait disturbance refers to disorders of proprioception or dysfunction of the musculoskeletal system. **Middle-level gait disturbance** causes distortion of appropriate interaction of postural and motor processes or synergies. This might include stroke with paralysis, cerebellar dysfunction, or diseases of the basal ganglia such as Parkinson's disease. **High-level gait disturbances** seemingly involve structures or processes that choose the appropriate responses for the support surface, body position in space, and intention of the patient. Cautious gait, apraxic gait, and the frontal gait disorder conceptually fall into this group with pathology that correlates with lesions in the frontal cortex or thalamus. This latter group is the least understood and the source of clinical confusion.

CLINICAL FEATURES

HISTORY

Collect historical information about the entire symptom constellation, and ask about headache, nausea, fever, weakness, or numbness. A history of fever, review of medication history, or family history of ataxia may lead to the diagnosis in individual cases. The nature of onset of symptoms and the time course of the process guide the pace of investigations. For example, abrupt onset of gait difficulty in a patient with severe headache, drowsiness, nausea, and vomiting should suggest an acute process within the CNS, possibly a hemorrhage into the cerebellum. The possible consequences of that diagnosis are severe and may require immediate attention. At the other extreme, a patient without significant medical history who is brought to the ED with a stumbling gait after an episode of binge drinking requires examination but may need nothing other than observation unless history or physical examination suggest trauma or some alternative cause for the symptoms.

PHYSICAL EXAMINATION

The following discussion of the neurologic examination assumes that the gait disorder is the dominating abnormality. Physical examination including testing of cranial nerves, mental status, sensation, and the motor system is necessary and may yield findings that lead to an unanticipated diagnosis.

General physical examination of a patient with ataxia or gait disturbance should include determination of orthostatic vital signs. Orthostatic hypotension may be present in hypovolemia, diabetic neuropathy, and other neurologic syndromes. Especially in the elderly, fluid replacement for simple hypovolemia may correct many symptoms of unsteadiness.

Gait testing is one of the most important parts of the directed neurologic examination. Observe the patient sitting upright in the stretcher, and then have the patient rise, stand, walk, and turn around. The patient should be asked to walk at a normal speed, then walk on the heels, and then the toes. Tandem gait is toe-to-toe walking and also tests many elements of the nervous system. **Do not assume a normal examination without observing ambulation.**

Cerebellar functions are tested by asking the patient to perform smooth voluntary movements and rapidly alternating movements. Dyssynergia (breakdown of movements into parts), dysmetria (inaccurate fine movements), or dysdiadochokinesia (clumsy rapid movements) may indicate a lateral cerebellar lesion. The rapid thigh-slapping test particularly examines rapidly alternating movements. This is correctly performed by asking the patient to pat the thigh with the palm then the back of the same hand in alternating fashion, making a sound with each rapid slap. The maneuver is performed with each hand in turn. The finger-to-nose test may be helpful in distinguishing between cerebellar and posterior column (proprioceptive) lesions. Performing this test with the eyes closed tests proprioception in the upper extremity. A test for cerebellar function that emphasizes the lower extremities is the heel-to-shin test. In cerebellar disease, the heel may initially overshoot the other shin or knee, and the action is done with a series of jerky movements. In posterior column disease, there may be difficulty locating the knee, and the movement down the shin typically weaves from side to side or falls off. Another test commonly used for cerebellar function is the Stewart-Holmes rebound sign (with sudden release of the flexed forearm, the individual fails to check the movement). Another example of rebound phenomena is when a tapped outstretched arm oscillates back and forth for several cycles.

The Romberg test is primarily a test of sensation, and if positive may distinguish sensory from motor ataxia. While standing with arms outstretched and eyes open, observe the patient for signs of unsteadiness. The feet should be narrowly spaced, and the posture should be easily maintained. The inability to maintain a steady standing posture (or, in extreme cases, a seated position) confirms that an ataxia is present but does not yet give any information about the type of ataxia. Then ask the patient to close the eyes, to eliminate visually orienting information. If the ataxia worsens with the loss of visual input, then the Romberg sign is present or positive, suggesting sensory ataxia with a problem of proprioceptive input (posterior column, vestibular dysfunction), or a peripheral neuropathy. Further neurologic examination is indicated to confirm the suspicion of sensory ataxia. In patients who show little or no change in unsteadiness with eye closure (Romberg test–negative), a motor ataxia is suggested, with possible localization of that problem to the cerebellum. Note that many normal individuals will have some small increase in unsteadiness with eye closure.

Historically, tabes dorsalis (neurosyphilis) was a common cause of sensory ataxia. In tabes dorsalis, the posterior columns and posterior spinal roots degenerate, primarily in the lumbosacral region. The loss of proprioceptive information from the lower extremities renders the patient dependent on visual cues for correct gait. The classic description is that of a patient who walks slowly with wide gait while staring at the ground. In darkness or with interruption of vision, the patient is unable to walk. The gait in this condition is peculiar, with the foot first raised and then slapped to the ground with each step. These abnormalities reflect the loss of proprioceptive information from the posterior roots and posterior columns. Consider vitamin B_{12} deficiency in patients with evidence of posterior column disease. If the deficiency is left untreated, an initial unsteady gait may progress to weakness, spasticity, and ataxia. The finding of a megaloblastic anemia may be a clue, but the neuropathy may precede the anemia.

Sensory examination in a patient with unsteady gait or movements should include position or vibration testing (posterior columns), as well as testing sensation to pinprick. Testing of the deep tendon reflexes will serve largely to discover asymmetry or spasticity that might suggest an alternative diagnosis. Acute cerebellar injury may result in muscle hypotonia for a few days or weeks.[8]

Nystagmus is seen in many different disorders due to lesions in a variety of different locations of the CNS, but the presence of nystagmus does suggest that the pathologic process is intracranial (CNS or vestibular) and not in the spinal cord or peripheral nervous system (see chapter 170, Vertigo).

DIAGNOSIS

Assuming a primary complaint of ataxia, the first task is to determine whether the ataxia is sensory or motor and whether the primary process is systemic or within the nervous system. If the ataxia is thought to result from problems within the nervous system, the next question is one of localization to the peripheral nervous system versus the CNS and perhaps to a more specific anatomic location. Finally, the tempo of the illness, comorbid diseases, and other clinical findings guide investigations and may allow a disease-specific diagnosis.

A patient with acute gait failure over hours to days needs thorough evaluation in the ED, often requiring CT scan and MRI, or lumbar puncture if cerebrospinal fluid infection is suspected. Acute ataxia or gait disturbance may also be evaluated by consultation if available, and possible admission, in contrast to a patient with gradual loss of abilities over weeks or months where outpatient referral and evaluation may be more appropriate.

SPECIAL POPULATIONS

THE GERIATRIC PATIENT

The gait changes with advancing age. A typical constellation includes gait slowing, shortening of the stride, and widening of the base. This results in the appearance of a guarded gait—that is, the gait of someone about to slip and fall. Many patients are aware of the loss of speed and adaptive balance and acknowledge the need to be careful. The nature of the senile gait is not fully understood but may represent a mild degree of neuronal loss, failing proprioception, slowing of corrective responses, or weakness of the lower extremities. Senile gait disorder is thought to exist in up to one fourth of the elderly population. Some authorities divide this disorder into components of gait ataxia with mild truncal instability and widened gait, and gait slowing with diminished spontaneous arm swing and bradykinesia.[9] However, elements of the senile gait are also found in neurodegenerative diseases, so consider the possible presence of a neurodegenerative disorder such as Parkinson's disease or normal pressure hydrocephalus in elderly patients with gait impairment.[9] Patients unable to walk or care for themselves, or with increasing falls at home need admission for supportive care.

THE ALCOHOLIC PATIENT

A history of alcoholism or malabsorption problem in the patient with ataxia or gait disorder raises the possibility of a potentially remedial nutritional problem. If acute motor ataxia is present with confusion or eye movement abnormalities, consider **Wernicke's disease** and administer IV thiamine.[10] The entity of alcoholic cerebellar degeneration (sometimes referred to as rostral vermis syndrome, because a portion of the cerebellar vermis is preferentially affected) may represent the same nutritional deficiency and not the direct toxic effects of alcohol.

CHILDREN

In evaluating children with acute ataxia or gait disorder, examination must exclude weakness and musculoskeletal disorders. The child may be awake, alert, and playful but is visibly unsteady or wobbly sitting on a stretcher. The differential diagnosis is extensive (**Table 169-3**). Acute or deteriorating presentation generally mandates an aggressive search for the underlying cause and will likely need inpatient management.[11]

Intoxications are a cause of ataxia in children, and the ingestion may be surreptitious. History should include queries about any medications in the household. Acute ataxia may follow immunizations, viral illnesses, or varicella and also has been rarely reported in the preeruptive phase of varicella.[12] Most children are in the 2- to 4-year-old range. Acute cerebellar ataxia of childhood is thought to be a postinfectious demyelinating disorder. The onset of gait ataxia is abrupt, and only occasionally is fever present at the time ataxia begins.

TABLE 169-3 Causes of Acute Ataxia in Children, Roughly in Order of Frequency

Cause	Example
Drug intoxication	Ethanol Isopropyl alcohol Phenytoin Carbamazepine Sedatives Lead, mercury
Idiopathic	Acute cerebellar ataxia of childhood
Infection and inflammation	Varicella Coxsackievirus A and B Mycoplasma Echovirus Postinfectious inflammation Postimmunization
Neoplasm	Neuroblastoma Other CNS tumors
Paraneoplastic	Opsoclonus-myoclonus syndrome
Trauma	Subdural or epidural posterior fossa hematoma
Congenital or hereditary	Pyruvate decarboxylase deficiency Friedreich's ataxia Hartnup disease
Hydrocephalus Cerebellar abscess Labyrinthitis/vestibular neuronitis Transverse myelitis Meningoencephalitis	

The latency from the prodromal illness to the onset of ataxia is from 2 days to 2 weeks. Other neurologic findings encountered included truncal ataxia, dysmetria, and, uncommonly, cranial nerve abnormalities. Patients with ataxia following varicella appear to have uniform excellent recovery compared with patients with acute cerebellar ataxia from other causes who may have some residual problems.[13] Little workup is needed if the ataxia occurs in the convalescent phase of varicella, and antiviral medications are not indicated. Otherwise, neuroimaging, lumbar puncture, and consultation are advisable. One study showed that although roughly half of the patients had cerebrospinal fluid inflammatory changes with pleocytosis or elevated immunoglobulin G index, MRI identified inflammatory changes in the cerebellum in only a minority of cases.[12] Another small report noted MRI abnormalities not only in the cerebellum, but also in other areas of the CNS. This "syndrome" may in fact consist of several subgroups, some of which involve transient demyelination.[14]

Posterior fossa mass lesions and other CNS masses may present with ataxia, although usually some abnormality of cranial nerves or strength will be discovered with careful examination. Attention is needed to exclude abnormalities on physical examination that might suggest problems not localized to the cerebellum. Abnormal ocular movements should increase the suspicion of a mass lesion. Acute ataxia associated with rapid chaotic eye movements (opsoclonus) and myoclonic extremity jerks of the head and extremities are the striking syndrome of opsoclonus-myoclonus. This may be a postviral syndrome but is often a paraneoplastic syndrome associated with a neuroblastoma located in the abdomen or chest.[10]

Unusual metabolic disorders such as pyruvate decarboxylase complex deficiency may present with ataxia. Family history may or may not suggest a metabolic disorder. Typically, the onset is gradual, but abrupt decompensations may occur. Other systemic or CNS abnormalities will be present.

REFERENCES

The complete reference list is available online at www.TintinalliEM.com.

Vertigo

Brian Goldman

INTRODUCTION AND EPIDEMIOLOGY

Dizziness is a common complaint in patients >40 years old, leading to roughly 10 million visits to ambulatory care settings and 25% of ED visits.[1] Dizziness can lead to falls in elderly patients. The symptoms may persist and be incapacitating. Patients may use various terms for the complaint: dizziness may mean vertigo, syncope, presyncope, weakness, giddiness, anxiety, or a disturbance in mentation.

Vertigo is the perception of movement (rotational or otherwise) where no movement exists. **Syncope** is a transient loss of consciousness accompanied by loss of postural tone with spontaneous recovery. **Near-syncope** is light-headedness with concern for an impending loss of consciousness. **Psychiatric dizziness** is defined as a sensation of dizziness not related to vestibular dysfunction that occurs exclusively in combination with other symptoms as part of a recognized psychiatric symptom cluster.[2] **Disequilibrium** refers to a feeling of unsteadiness, imbalance, or a sensation of "floating" while walking.

Acute vestibular syndrome is a symptom complex consisting of vertigo, nausea and vomiting, intolerance to head motion, spontaneous nystagmus, unsteady gait, and postural instability caused by injury to peripheral or central vestibular structures. To be called acute vestibular syndrome, the associated vertigo must persist for at least 24 hours, thus excluding causes of transient vertigo such as benign paroxysmal positional vertigo (BPPV). Acute vestibular syndrome may be peripheral or central in origin. Clinical findings that distinguish central from peripheral causes include focal neurologic deficits such as hemiparesis, hemisensory loss, or gaze palsy. **The most common peripheral cause of acute vestibular syndrome is vestibular neuronitis. The most common central cause is ischemic stroke of the posterior fossa (brainstem or cerebellar), followed by demyelination. There is growing evidence that a significant number of patients with central acute vestibular syndrome are misdiagnosed in the ED.** A systematic review estimated that roughly 25% of patients presenting with acute vestibular syndrome have had a stroke.[3]

The time-honored paradigm of evaluating dizziness is based largely on the patient's subjective description. More recently, objective bedside physical examination has emerged as a more reliable way of arriving at the correct diagnosis.[4]

PATHOPHYSIOLOGY

The CNS coordinates and integrates sensory input from the visual, vestibular, and proprioceptive systems. Vertigo arises from a mismatch of information from two or more of the involved senses, caused by dysfunction in the sensory organ or its corresponding pathway.

Visual inputs provide spatial orientation. Proprioceptors help relate body movements and indicate the position of the head relative to that of the body. The vestibular system (via the otoliths) establishes the body's orientation with respect to gravity. The cupulae's sensors track rotary motion. The three semicircular canals sense orientation to movement and head tilts and are filled with a fluid called *endolymph*. The endolymphatic sac produces glycoproteins that create an osmotic

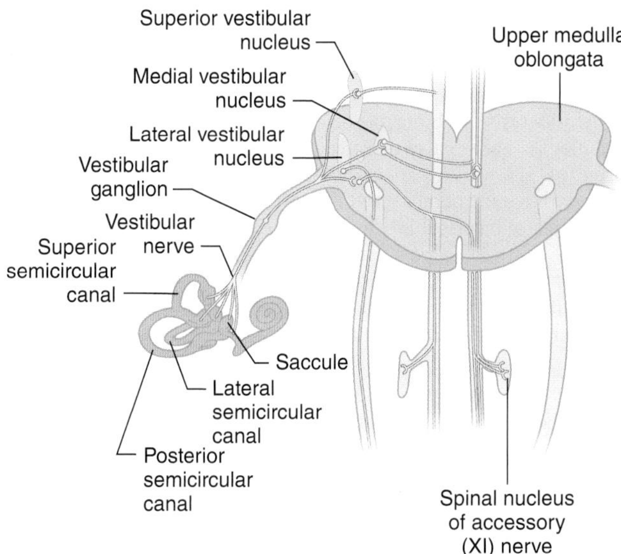

FIGURE 170-1. Vestibular innervation.

sink necessary to maintain flow. The movement of fluid in the semicircular canals causes specialized hair cells inside the canals to move, causing afferent vestibular impulses to fire. Sensory input from the vestibular apparatus travels to the nucleus of the eighth cranial nerve (**Figure 170-1**).

The medial longitudinal fasciculus, the red nuclei, the cerebellum, the parietal lobes, and the superior temporal gyrus of the cerebral cortex integrate the various sensory inputs. Connections between these structures and the oculomotor nuclei that drive the vestibulo-ocular reflex complete the system. The vestibulo-ocular reflex prevents visual blurring from head movements and body sway.

Balanced input from the vestibular apparatus on both sides is the norm. Unilateral lesions of the vestibular apparatus as well as excessive unilateral firing due to abnormal motion of the endolymph produce imbalanced activity and vertigo. Rapid head movements accentuate the imbalance. Symmetric bilateral damage does not usually produce vertigo but may lead to truncal or gait instability.

The most striking clinical sign associated with vertigo is **nystagmus**, a rhythmic movement of the eyes that has both a fast and a slow component, with direction named by its fast component. The slow component is due to the vestibulo-ocular reflex and is generated by excitation of the semicircular canal, producing eye movement away from that canal. The fast component of nystagmus is caused by the cortex, which exerts a quick corrective movement in the opposite direction. Vestibular disorders produce nystagmus that is provoked when the affected side is in the dependent position, and the characteristic pattern is vertical and rotational or horizontal. **Vertical nystagmus by itself usually indicates a brainstem abnormality.** However, an atypical pattern of nystagmus in the absence of other signs of CNS disease does not necessarily indicate central pathology.[5]

The prevalence of dizziness increases with age and is due to decreases in visual acuity, proprioception, and vestibular input, plus an increase in free-floating otoconia within the semicircular canals that cause BPPV. Older patients are also more likely to take medications that cause dizziness.

PHYSIOLOGIC VERTIGO

Physiologic vertigo results from a mismatch of visual, proprioceptive, and vestibular input. This may be the pathogenesis of motion sickness as well as the transient visual vertigo associated with watching a film that captures the visual sensation of motion, by attending complex visual environments, such as shopping malls, and by viewing complex floor or wallpaper patterns.

CLINICAL FEATURES

The conditions that cause acute undifferentiated vertigo are summarized in **Table 170-1**. Vertigo is usually categorized as "peripheral" or "central," and making the distinction between the two is the most important part of the evaluation. **Peripheral vertigo is caused by disorders affecting the vestibular apparatus and the eighth cranial nerve, whereas central vertigo is caused by disorders affecting central structures, such as the brainstem and the cerebellum.** Peripheral vertigo tends to cause distressing symptoms, but is seldom life threatening; the reverse tends to be true for central vertigo. Disorders causing central vertigo often require urgent diagnostic imaging or consultation with a neurologist or neurosurgeon.

Some of the features that distinguish peripheral causes from central causes (mainly cerebrovascular disease) are found in **Table 170-2. Note that many of the so-called distinguishing features of peripheral acute vestibular syndrome may also be found in some patients with cerebrovascular disease.**[6]

HISTORY

An approach to vertigo is shown in **Figure 170-2**. Try to obtain an unprompted description of the patient's "dizziness" and avoid leading questions that bias the patient's responses. However, the initial description may not be a reliable predictor of underlying pathology.[7]

Patients with acute vestibular syndrome have continuous vertigo or dizziness for more than 24 hours. Thus, the list excludes causes of brief transient episodes such as BPPV, Ménière's syndrome, and transient ischemic attack. If the patient has experienced true vertigo, determine whether the vertigo is of peripheral or central origin, and determine the temporal pattern and precipitating causes (**Table 170-3**). Peripheral vertigo is more likely than central vertigo to be intense and to be associated with nausea, vomiting, diaphoresis, tinnitus, hearing loss, and photophobia.

Headache is generally not a feature of peripheral causes of acute vestibular syndrome but is associated with central causes. Dizziness and

TABLE 170-1 Causes of Acute Undifferentiated Vertigo

Vestibular/otologic	Benign paroxysmal positional vertigo
	Traumatic: following head injury
	Infection: labyrinthitis, vestibular neuronitis, Ramsay Hunt syndrome
Systemic conditions with vestibular/otologic effects	Ménière's syndrome
	Neoplastic
	Vascular
	Otosclerosis
	Paget's disease
	Toxic or drug-induced: aminoglycosides
Neurologic	Vertebrobasilar insufficiency or vertebral artery dissection
	Lateral Wallenberg's syndrome
	Anterior inferior cerebellar artery syndrome
	Neoplastic: cerebellopontine angle tumors
	Cerebellar disorders: hemorrhage, degeneration
	Basal ganglion diseases
	Multiple sclerosis
	Infections: neurosyphilis, tuberculosis
	Epilepsy
	Migraine headaches
	Cerebrovascular disease
General	Hematologic: anemia, polycythemia, hyperviscosity syndrome
	Toxic: alcohol
	Chronic renal failure
	Metabolic: thyroid disease, hypoglycemia

TABLE 170-2 Differentiating Peripheral from Central Causes of Acute Undifferentiated Vertigo

	Peripheral	Central
Onset	Sudden or insidious	Sudden
Severity of vertigo	Intense spinning	Ill defined, less intense
Prodromal dizziness	Occurs in up to 25%; often single episode	Occurs in up to 25%; recurrent episodes suggest transient ischemic attacks
Intolerant of head movements/Dix-Hallpike maneuver	Yes	Sometimes
Associated nausea/diaphoresis	Frequent	Variable
Auditory symptoms	Points to peripheral causes	May be present
Proportionality of symptoms	Usually proportional	Often disproportionate
Headache or neck pain	Unusual	More likely
Nystagmus	Rotatory-vertical, horizontal	Vertical
CNS symptoms/signs	Absent	Usually present
Head impulse test	Abnormal	Usually normal
HINTS examination (combined horizontal head impulse test, nystagmus, and test of skew)	Normal on all three bedside tests	Abnormal on at least one of three bedside tests

headache suggest migraine but also occur with vertebral artery dissection or aneurysm.[8]

Head trauma and medications can precipitate episodes of dizziness or interfere with central adaptation. Recent head or neck trauma is a risk factor for **dissection of the vertebral artery**. In patients with acute vertigo, a recent history of trauma should spark concern for dissection even if pain is absent.

Evaluate the following groups for central vertigo: older patients, those with hypertension or cardiovascular disease, those with other risk factors for stroke, or those taking warfarin. Patients with acute vestibular syndrome and more than one vascular risk factor appear to be at increased risk of stroke. Although age is a known risk factor for stroke, patients age 50 and older with symptoms of acute vertigo and no neurologic signs are more likely to have vestibular neuronitis than stroke.[9] However, age per se does not rule out stroke as the cause of central acute vestibular syndrome. In a study of patients with cerebellar infarctions who were misdiagnosed on initial ED presentation, half of the patients misdiagnosed were younger then 50 years of age who presented with headache and vertigo. All of the patients misdiagnosed had either an incomplete or a poorly documented neurologic examination. Almost all of the patients had a CT scan of the brain that was initially interpreted as normal. The overall mortality was 40%; among survivors, 50% had disabling neurologic sequelae. This study underscores the need for a careful neurologic assessment in all such patients.[10]

PHYSICAL EXAMINATION

Perform complete ear, neurologic, and vestibular examinations in patients presenting with vertigo or dizziness. Examine the external auditory canal and tympanic membrane for evidence of otitis media, cholesteatoma, and other pathology. Test for hearing, and also perform Webber and Rinne testing. Hearing loss usually points to peripheral causes such as vestibular neuronitis and Ménière's syndrome. However, auditory symptoms and signs may also be due to ischemia of the inner ear associated with cerebrovascular disease.

When assessing patients with acute vestibular syndrome, keep the possibility of cerebrovascular disease in mind. The presence of focal neurologic deficits indicates a central etiology. However, focal deficits are not uniformly present in central vertigo. A systematic review found focal neurologic deficits in 80% of patients with acute vestibular syndrome caused by stroke.[3] In the **HINTS** study, neurologic (e.g., facial palsy, hemiparesis, limb ataxia) or oculomotor (e.g., internuclear ophthalmoplegia, gaze palsy, vertical nystagmus) abnormalities were reported in 51% of 76 patients with a central cause and none of 25 patients with a peripheral cause.[8] The presence of gait unsteadiness and severe truncal ataxia (inability to sit unaided with arms crossed) suggests vertigo due to stroke. A positive Romberg test is rarely found in patients with peripheral vertigo. The absence of focal neurologic deficits in some patients with central acute vestibular syndrome has led to growing interest in other methods of bedside testing.

HINTS Testing HINTS testing is an important advance in the rapid assessment of ED patients with acute vestibular syndrome. **HINTS** is an acronym that stands for horizontal head impulse test, nystagmus, and test of skew—three bedside tests that when taken together reliably help distinguish central (usually stroke) from peripheral acute vestibular syndrome.

The horizontal head impulse test is also known as the **Halmagyi head thrust** and, by itself, is the most helpful bedside test for distinguishing central from peripheral vertigo. The Halmagyi head thrust assesses the vestibulo-ocular reflex. Ask the patient to fixate on a visual target, while the examiner rotates the patient's head rapidly first from the center position to 40 degrees left and back again to the center position. Repeat the test on the right side. Carefully watch the patient's eyes for the response to the maneuver. The intact vestibulo-ocular reflex compensates for the rotational head thrust by rapidly and smoothly moving the eyes in the direction **opposite** to the head thrust. This is the normal physiologic response to a passive head thrust; an intact vestibulo-ocular reflex maintains fixation of the eyes with respect to the patient's environment. Thus, the patient will be able to maintain his or her gaze on the visual target throughout the head thrust.

If the vestibulo-ocular reflex is impaired, then the patient will not be able to maintain his or her gaze on the visual target, and the patient will exhibit a rapid simultaneous movement of both eyes (known as a **saccade**) in order to reacquire fixation upon the visual target. This is an abnormal response to the horizontal head impulse test.[11]

Thus, in a patient with no symptoms or signs of acute vestibular syndrome, a normal horizontal head impulse test (i.e., no corrective saccade) means that the vestibulo-ocular reflex is normal. **In a patient with acute vestibular syndrome, an abnormal response horizontal head impulse test (i.e., a corrective saccade) usually indicates a peripheral vestibular lesion, while no corrective saccade is highly suspicious for a stroke.**[12] In the HINTS study, the head impulse test had both a sensitivity and specificity comparable to that of MRI.[8]

The second part of HINTS testing that helps predict central acute vestibular syndrome is direction-changing horizontal nystagmus on lateral gaze. An abnormal response, which consists of right-beating nystagmus on right gaze and left-beating nystagmus on left gaze with or without nystagmus when the patient looks straight ahead, is believed to represent failure of gaze-maintaining structures located in the brainstem and the cerebellum. Direction-changing nystagmus has low sensitivity but high specificity for correctly identifying central causes of acute vestibular syndrome. The third part of HINTS testing is known as skew deviation or skew and refers to vertical ocular misalignment during the alternate cover test. Skew deviation only occurs in the presence of right-left imbalance in sensory inputs from the vestibular system to the oculomotor syndrome. As with direction-changing nystagmus, skew deviation is not sensitive but is highly specific for central acute vestibular syndrome.

All three bedside tests (horizontal head impulse test, nystagmus, and skew) have been combined into the HINTS battery of tests that define a clinical prediction rule for stroke. Just one finding specific for central acute vestibular syndrome on any of the three tests that make up the HINTS battery is considered 100% sensitive and 96% specific for stroke.[8] A cross-sectional study of patients with acute vestibular syndrome at high risk for stroke found that HINTS testing substantially outperformed ABCD2 risk scoring for stroke diagnosis in the ED and also outperformed MRI obtained within the first 2 days of symptom onset.[13] A current review concluded that with appropriate training in the

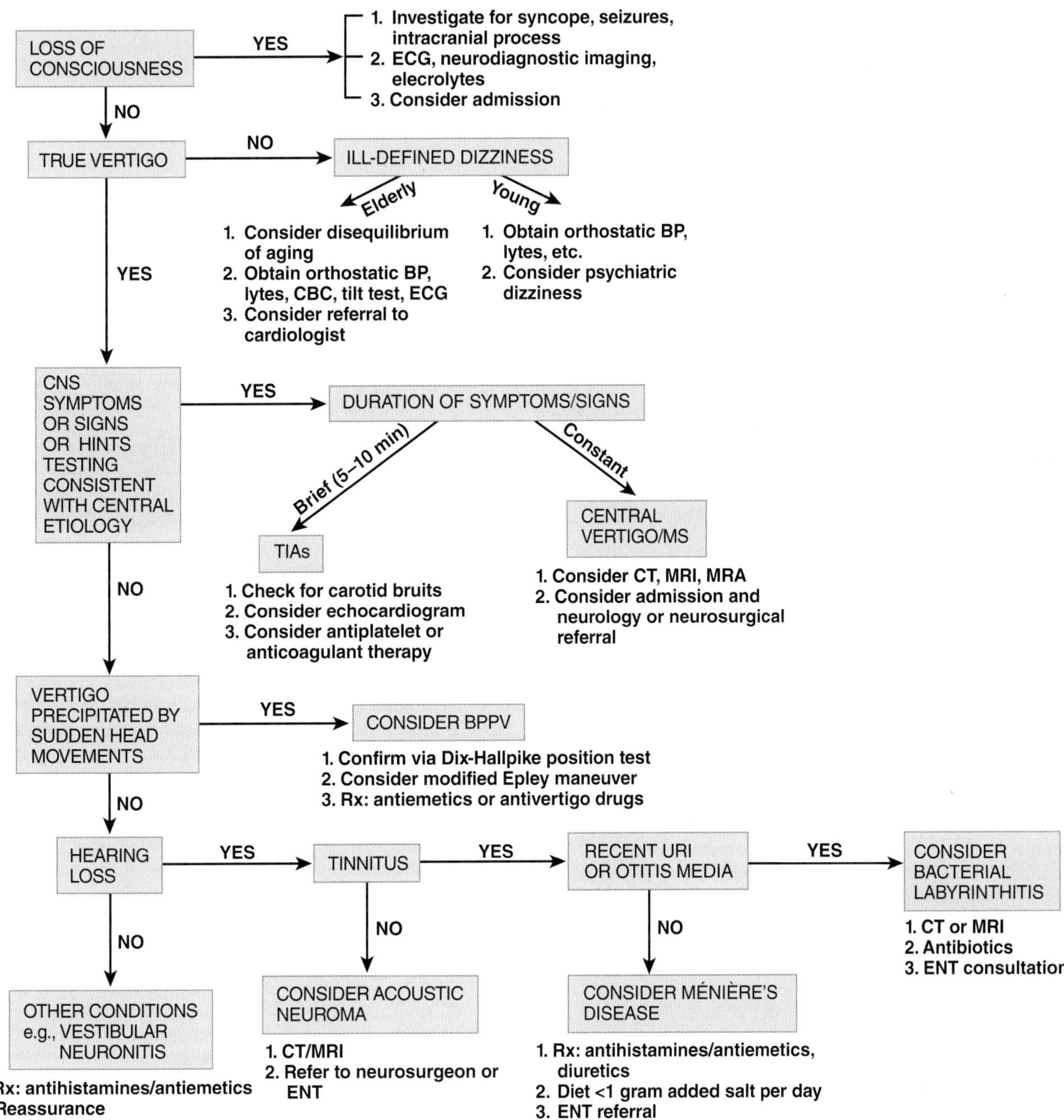

FIGURE 170-2. Guideline approach to vertigo. BP = blood pressure; BPPV = benign paroxysmal positional vertigo; CBC = complete blood count; CNS = central nervous system; ENT = ear, nose, and throat; MRA = magnetic resonance angiography; MS = multiple sclerosis; Rx = treatment; TIAs = transient ischemic attacks; URI = upper respiratory infection.

technique, it is reasonable to use HINTS testing as a tool to distinguish central from peripheral vertigo.[14]

Dix-Hallpike Maneuver **The diagnosis of BPPV involving the posterior canal is aided by the Dix-Hallpike position test.** Do not perform this test on patients with carotid bruits, a history of prior cerebrovascular disease, or risk factors or concern for vertebrobasilar insufficiency, because the Dix-Hallpike maneuver carries a theoretical risk of precipitating a stroke. In addition, use caution in patients with spinal injury or cervical spondylosis. The test may provoke vertigo. Pretreatment with 50 milligrams of dimenhydrinate IM or IV may make the test more tolerable but will not obliterate nystagmus. Have patients keep their eyes open at all times and stare at the examiner's nose or forehead. Start with the patient seated upright on the examining table. To test the right posterior semicircular canal, rotate the head 30 to 45 degrees to the right. Keeping the head in this position, rapidly bring the patient supine until the head is 20 degrees below the level of the examining table. Rotatory nystagmus following a latency of no more than 30 seconds is considered a positive test; the nystagmus exhibits rapid eye torsions toward the affected ear and lasts for 10 to 40 seconds. Return the patient to the upright sitting position, and repeat the test on the left side. **The side exhibiting the positive test is the side of the lesion.**[15]

TABLE 170-3 Temporal Patterns of Vertigo

Pattern	Conditions
Seconds	Benign paroxysmal positional vertigo, postural hypotension
Minutes	Transient ischemic attacks
Hours	Ménière's syndrome
More than 24 hours	Acute vestibular syndrome: peripheral or central

TABLE 170-4 Imaging and Ancillary Testing for Vertigo and Dizziness

Condition	Suggested Tests
Bacterial labyrinthitis	CBC, blood cultures, CT scan, or MRI for possible abscess; lumbar puncture if meningitis suspected
Vertigo associated with closed head injury	CT scan or MRI
Near-syncope	ECG, Holter monitor, CBC, glucose, electrolytes, renal function, table tilt testing
Cardiac dysrhythmias	ECG, Holter monitor
Suspected valvular heart disease	ECG, echocardiography
Nonspecific dizziness; disequilibrium of aging	CBC, electrolytes, glucose, renal function tests
Thyrotoxicosis	Thyroid-stimulating hormone, triiodothyronine, thyroxine
Cerebellar hemorrhage, infarction, or tumor	CT or MRI
Vertebral artery dissection	Cerebral angiogram to include neck vessels or MRA
Vertebrobasilar insufficiency	ECG, cardiac monitoring, echocardiogram, carotid Doppler, MRI, MRA

Abbreviation: MRA = magnetic resonance angiography.

DIAGNOSIS

IMAGING AND ANCILLARY TESTS

Patients with signs or symptoms concerning for central vertigo require emergent imaging and laboratory investigations (**Table 170-4**). CT alone is not adequate because it does not visualize the brainstem well.[16] MRI is more sensitive than CT.[17] For patients who may have vertebrobasilar insufficiency, MRI with magnetic resonance angiography of the head, neck vessels, and circle of Willis; duplex US of the carotid arteries; and neurologic consultation are indicated. Detailed cochleovestibular testing can be done by a specialist.

TREATMENT

SYMPTOMATIC TREATMENT FOR PERIPHERAL VERTIGO

Short-term treatment with antiemetic and vestibular suppressant pharmacotherapy is a mainstay for patients with peripheral vertigo (**Table 170-5**).[18] Withdraw such treatments as soon as possible to facilitate central vestibular compensation.[19]

DRUG THERAPY

Pharmacotherapy is used to treat specific conditions, reduce symptoms, or enhance vestibular compensation. Drugs with anticholinergic effects can be quite effective for vertigo. The agent of choice is transdermal scopolamine. H_1 antihistamines are commonly prescribed drugs for their anticholinergic effects. H_2 antihistamines are not effective. Calcium channel blockers (Table 170-5) possess antihistaminic and antidopaminergic activity and are indicated for the symptomatic relief of vertigo in patients not responding to scopolamine or antihistamines and are also indicated for vestibular migraine. Neuroleptics such as promethazine and metoclopramide reduce nausea and vomiting by blocking brainstem dopaminergic receptors. They too are indicated as second-line treatment. **Do not use prochlorperazine and chlorpromazine in vertigo caused by orthostatic hypotension.** Ondansetron, a serotonin 5-HT_3 receptor antagonist, has been used to treat intractable vertigo in brainstem disorders as well as vertigo due to multiple sclerosis.

Small doses of benzodiazepines such as diazepam and clonazepam may be used sparingly to relieve severe anxiety accompanying vertigo. However, these agents bind to γ-aminobutyric acid receptors in the CNS and thus may impair vestibular compensation. Benzodiazepines are given for central ocular motor disorders that cause nystagmus.

Methylprednisolone is indicated for vestibular neuronitis. However, the antiviral drug valacyclovir has not been proven to be efficacious in clinical trials. Anticonvulsant drugs are indicated for prophylaxis of vestibular migraine; gabapentin is indicated for dizziness associated with multiple sclerosis.

Antihistamines can cause sedation and anticholinergic adverse effects. Antidopaminergic neuroleptic agents can induce or exacerbate orthostatic hypotension. These drugs also cause somnolence and acute dystonia and can exacerbate anticholinergic adverse effects. Avoid using medications with overlapping anticholinergic and antidopaminergic effects in combination. Do not treat patients with nonvertiginous dizziness and disequilibrium of aging with antivertigo medications.

DISORDERS CAUSING PERIPHERAL VERTIGO

Peripheral vertigo produces an intense sensation of spinning or hurtling toward the ground or surrounding walls of abrupt onset. It is worsened by rapid movement and by changes in head position and is frequently associated with nausea, vomiting, diaphoresis, bradycardia, and hypotension.

BENIGN PAROXYSMAL POSITIONAL VERTIGO

BPPV is a mechanical disorder of the inner ear causing transient vertigo (with autonomic symptoms) and associated nystagmus that is precipitated by certain head movements. The lifetime prevalence of BPPV is 2.4% with a 1-year incidence of 0.6%, with women and patients over the age of 50 more likely to be affected. The mean duration of an episode is 2 weeks; 86% of patients affected seek medical attention.[20]

BPPV is believed to be caused by inappropriate activation of a semicircular canal, typically the posterior semicircular canal and typically unilateral, by the presence of free-floating particles or otoconia. The otoconia become displaced from the utricular macula by aging, head trauma, or labyrinthine disease. The particles tend to clump in the long arm of the posterior semicircular canal of the endolymph system. Once the clump reaches sufficient mass, changes in head position cause gravitation of the particles, which creates a plunger effect on the endolymph, causing the cupula to be displaced. This results in inadvertent neural firing, causing both vertigo and nystagmus.

The onset of BPPV is sudden and is precipitated by rolling over in bed, lying supine, leaning forward, looking up at the sky or ceiling, or turning the head. Because the symptoms fatigue, they tend to be worse in the morning. Patients may eliminate the offending activities. There is no associated hearing loss or tinnitus and no physical findings on examination of the external auditory canal.

Several findings support a diagnosis of BPPV (**Table 170-6**). There is a latency period of 1 to 5 seconds between assuming the offending head position and onset of vertigo and nystagmus. Both the vertigo and nystagmus crescendo to a peak of intensity and then subside within 5 to 40 seconds. Unlike vestibular neuronitis, the head thrust test in BPPV is normal and there is no spontaneous nystagmus. The Romberg test is negative, and the gait is normal. Posterior canal **BPPV can be diagnosed using the Dix-Hallpike test** (see "Physical Examination" section).[15] Symptoms disappear with repeated testing. The supine roll test (Pagnini-McClure test[21]) for horizontal canal BPPV is done as follows: place the patient supine, turn the head to the right and observe for nystagmus, and then turn the head back to neutral position. Repeat by turning the head to the left. The side with the most prominent nystagmus is the side of the affected canal.

BPPV involving the anterior semicircular canal is rare, and the Dix-Hallpike maneuver may elicit downbeating nystagmus with the affected ear up. However, any downbeating nystagmus should raise strong suspicion for a cerebellar or brainstem lesion (**Table 170-7**).[21] Patients with isolated BPPV often undergo many tests with little or no diagnostic yield.[22]

TABLE 170-5 Pharmacotherapy of Vertigo and Dizziness

Category	Drug	Dosage	Indications	Advantages	Disadvantages
Anticholinergics	Scopolamine	0.5 milligram transdermal patch (behind ear) three to four times a day	Vertigo, nausea	Useful if patient is vomiting	Sometimes difficult to obtain
Antihistamines	Dimenhydrinate	50–100 milligrams IM, IV, or PO every 4 h	Vertigo, nausea	Inexpensive	Drowsiness/anticholinergic effect
	Diphenhydramine	25–50 milligrams IM, IV, or PO every 4 h	Vertigo, nausea	Inexpensive	Drowsiness/anticholinergic effect
	Meclizine	25 milligrams PO two to four times a day	Vertigo, nausea		Drowsiness/anticholinergic effect
Antiemetics	Hydroxyzine	25–50 milligrams PO four times a day	Vertigo, nausea	Inexpensive	Drowsiness/anticholinergic effect
	Metoclopramide	10–20 milligrams IV, PO three times a day	Vertigo, nausea	Effective, versatile	Occasional extrapyramidal effect
	Ondansetron	4 milligrams IV two to three times a day; 8 milligrams PO twice a day			
	Promethazine	25 milligrams IM, PO, or PR three to four times a day	Vertigo, nausea	Useful if vomiting	Occasional extrapyramidal effect
Benzodiazepines	Diazepam	2–5 milligrams PO two to four times a day	Central vertigo, anxiety related to peripheral vertigo	Inexpensive	Dependency, may impair vestibular compensation
	Clonazepam	0.5 milligram PO two times a day	Central vertigo, anxiety related to peripheral vertigo	Inexpensive	Dependency, may impair vestibular compensation
Calcium antagonists	Cinnarizine	25 milligrams PO two to three times a day	Peripheral vertigo, vestibular migraine	Nonsedating	Lesser clinical experience
	Nimodipine	30 milligrams PO two times a day	Peripheral vertigo, vestibular migraine	Nonsedating	Lesser clinical experience
	Flunarizine	20 milligrams PO two times a day	Ménière's syndrome	Well tolerated	Not available in the United States
Vasodilators	Betahistine	48 milligrams PO three times a day for up to 6–12 mo	Ménière's syndrome	Well tolerated	Little evidence of efficacy for other causes of peripheral vertigo
Corticosteroids	Methylprednisolone	100 milligrams/d tapered by 20 milligrams/d every fourth day	Vestibular neuronitis	Well tolerated	Efficacy largely unproven; adverse effects associated with corticosteroids
Antivirals	Valacyclovir	1000 milligrams three times a day for 7 d	Vestibular neuronitis	Well tolerated	Efficacy largely unproven
Anticonvulsants	Carbamazepine	200–600 milligrams/d	Vestibular paroxysmia	Inexpensive	Monitor CBC and liver function tests
	Topiramate	50–100 milligrams/d	Vestibular migraine prophylaxis	Well tolerated	Not well evaluated; does not abort acute vertigo
	Valproic acid	300–900 milligrams/d	Vestibular migraine prophylaxis	Well tolerated	Not well evaluated; does not abort acute vertigo
	Gabapentin	300 milligrams four times per day	MS associated dizziness	Reduces acquired pendular nystagmus of multiple sclerosis	Known adverse effect profile
β-Blockers	Metoprolol	100 milligrams/d	Vestibular migraine prophylaxis	Long experience	Known adverse effect profile

Perform the particle-repositioning maneuver (or Epley maneuver) for patients with posterior canal BPPV in the ED.[23] **This maneuver uses gravity to induce the particles to move along the semicircular canals until they end up inside the utricle where unlikely to cause vertigo.** It is indicated in patients with suspected BPPV plus a positive Dix-Hallpike test (**Figure 170-3**). Do not perform these maneuvers in patients with neck or cervical spine abnormalities, or if carotid or vertebral dissection is suspected.

TABLE 170-6 Supportive Findings in Benign Paroxysmal Positional Vertigo

Latency period of <30 s between the provocative head position and onset of nystagmus.
The intensity of nystagmus increases to a peak before slowly resolving.
Duration of vertigo and nystagmus ranges from 5–40 s.
If nystagmus is produced in one direction by placing the head down, then the nystagmus reverses direction when the head is returned to the sitting position.
Repeated head positioning causes both the vertigo and accompanying nystagmus to fatigue and subside.
Abnormal horizontal head impulse test indicating abnormal vestibule-ocular reflex function.
HINTS testing not indicative of stroke.

Abbreviation: HINTS = horizontal head impulse test, nystagmus, and test of skew.

TABLE 170-7 Benign Paroxysmal Positional Vertigo (BPPV)

Canal Affected by BPPV	Frequency (%)	Diagnostic Maneuver	Nystagmus (direction named by fast component)
Posterior	85	Dix-Hallpike, affected ear down	Upbeat, affected ear down
Horizontal	10–17	Supine roll test (Pagnini-McClure test)	Horizontal, changes direction when head is turned to right or left while supine
Anterior	1	Dix-Hallpike, affected ear up	Downbeating, great concern for brainstem or cerebellar lesions

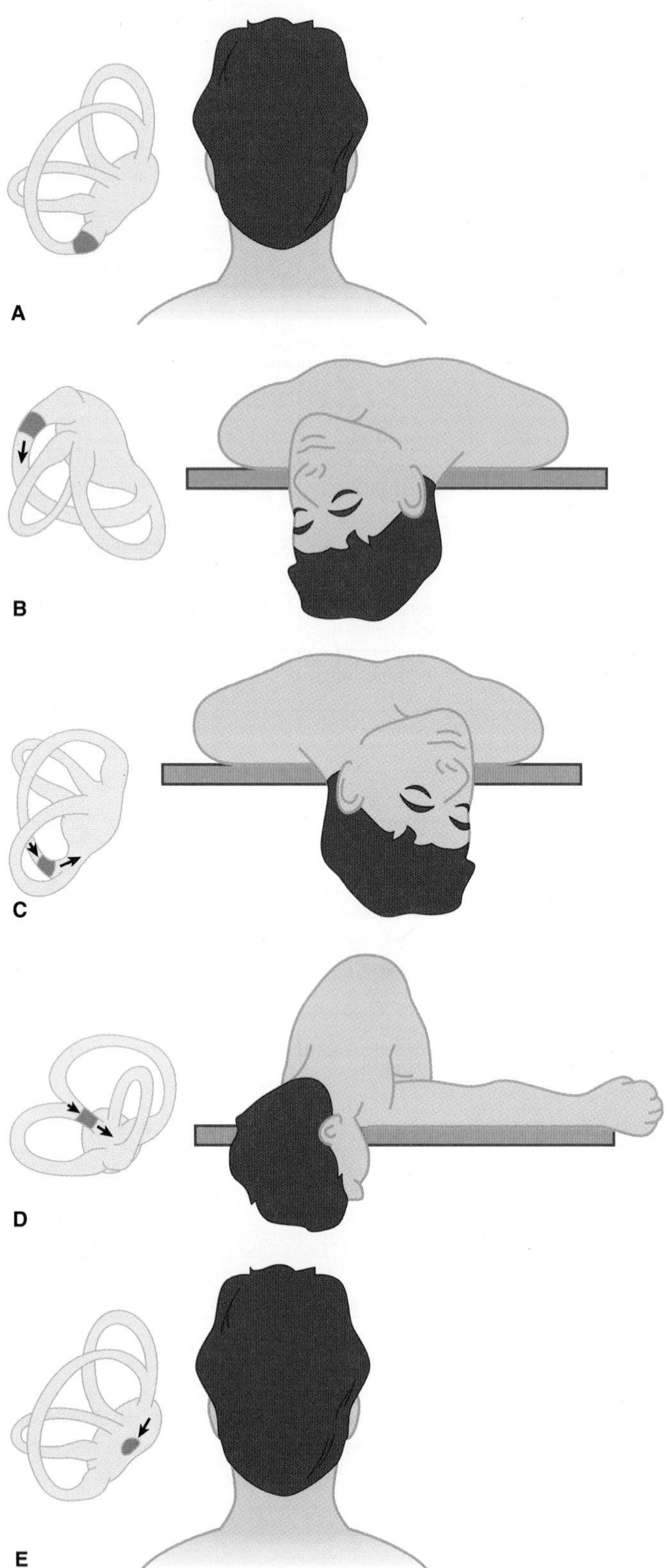

FIGURE 170-3. A through C. Dix-Hallpike position test; D, E. Epley Maneuver. Turn onto unaffected side. Hold position for 60 secs.

The affected ear is determined by the side of the positive Dix-Hallpike position test. Antihistamines or antiemetics administered before the maneuver may improve patient comfort. Seat the patient in the Dix-Hallpike position test, and turn the head 45 degrees toward the affected ear. Gently bring the patient to the recumbent position with the head hanging roughly 20 degrees below the examining table. Gently rotate the head 45 degrees to the midline. Then rotate the head a further 45 degrees to the unaffected side. The patient rolls onto the shoulder of the unaffected side, at the same time rotating the head a further 45 degrees. Return the patient to the sitting position and return the head to the midline. Wait 5 minutes after each portion of the maneuver to permit the particles to traverse their intended course. Observe for nystagmus in the same direction as during Dix-Hallpike testing. Nystagmus in the opposite direction suggests the particles have moved back toward the cupula; this portends an unsuccessful maneuver. Repeat the maneuver until both the vertigo and the accompanying nystagmus have disappeared. A home treatment device has been found to enable patients with an established diagnosis of BPPV to perform the maneuver themselves safely and effectively.[24]

While the Epley maneuver is safe and effective for posterior canal BPPV, relapses are common. Adverse effects include light-headedness and exacerbation of vertigo.

Most episodes of BPPV resolve spontaneously after a few days. Refer patients with persistent symptoms to an otolaryngologist.

MÉNIÈRE'S SYNDROME

Ménière's syndrome is a disorder associated with an increased endolymph within the cochlea and labyrinth. It tends to occur in older men and women with equal prevalence. The disease is usually unilateral but may become bilateral over time. The precise pathogenesis is unknown, but evidence suggests that patients have difficulty regulating the volume, flow, and composition of endolymph. The onset is usually sudden, with associated nausea, vomiting, and diaphoresis, with attacks lasting from 20 minutes to 12 hours. The frequency of attacks varies from several times per week to several times per month. Other associated symptoms include tinnitus, diminished hearing, and fullness in one ear. Between attacks, the patient is usually well, although decreased hearing may persist.

Ménière's syndrome is managed symptomatically with antihistamines and betahistine; combination therapy with triamterene and hydrochlorothiazide is also recommended in confirmed cases. Ménière's syndrome is the only condition for which betahistine has proven efficacy. A high-dose regimen of at least 48 milligrams three times daily has been shown to provide long-term prophylaxis.[25] Calcium channel blockers may also be used (Table 170-5). None of these drug treatments improves hearing. Intratympanic gentamicin administration may provide significant immediate and long-term relief.[26] Refer patients for treatment to an otolaryngologist. Attacks of vertigo are generally controllable, but tinnitus and hearing loss tend to be unresponsive to therapy.[27]

PERILYMPH FISTULA

A perilymph fistula is an opening in the round or oval window that permits pneumatic changes in the middle ear to be transmitted to the vestibular apparatus. Trauma, infection, or a sudden change in the pressure inside the ventricular system may cause the tear. The diagnosis is suggested by the sudden onset of vertigo associated with flying, scuba diving, severe straining, heavy lifting, coughing, or sneezing. Associated symptoms may include hearing loss. **The diagnosis is confirmed by nystagmus elicited by pneumatic otoscopy (Hennebert sign).**

Perilymph fistula is managed with symptomatic treatment and bed rest and referral to an ear, nose, and throat specialist for surgical repair (emergent referral for patients with acute associated hearing loss).

VESTIBULAR NEURONITIS

Vestibular neuronitis, a disorder of suspected viral etiology, is the second most common cause of peripheral vertigo. Unlike BPPV and Ménière's syndrome, vestibular neuronitis typically lasts several days and does not recur. The onset is sudden, often with a current or recent viral illness. Intense vertigo may require bedrest for several days. Unilateral loss of hearing and tinnitus may occur. Positive findings on physical examination include positive head thrust and horizontal or mild torsional nystagmus. The Romberg test is negative; however, the gait tends to be slow, cautious, and widely based. The condition remits spontaneously with no recurrence. Treatment is symptomatic. Both methylprednisolone and valacyclovir have been recommended, but there is insufficient evidence that these agents enhance recovery.[28]

VESTIBULAR GANGLIONITIS

Vestibular ganglionitis is believed to be caused by a neurotrophic virus such as varicella zoster reactivated years following initial infection. Herpes zoster oticus, also known as the Ramsay Hunt syndrome, is a neuropathic disorder thought to be associated with vestibular ganglionitis. It is characterized by deafness, vertigo, and facial nerve palsy. **The diagnosis is confirmed by the presence of grouped vesicles on an erythematous base inside the external auditory canal.** Treat this disorder with antiviral therapy started within 72 hours of the appearance of vesicles along with symptomatic treatments.

LABYRINTHITIS

Labyrinthitis, an infection of the labyrinth, causes peripheral vertigo associated with hearing loss. Viral labyrinthitis (associated with measles and mumps) has a course that is similar to vestibular neuronitis. Serous labyrinthitis occasionally causes vertigo.

Bacterial labyrinthitis may be a sequela of otitis media, in which bacteria and toxins diffuse across the membrane of the round window. Possible antecedents for bacterial labyrinthitis include otitis media with fistula, meningitis, mastoiditis, cholesteatoma, and dermoid tumor. **The hallmarks of this disease include sudden onset of vertigo with associated hearing loss and middle ear findings.**

Patients with bacterial labyrinthitis are at risk for meningitis and require antibiotics and referral to an ear, nose, and throat specialist for admission and possible surgical drainage.

OTOTOXICITY

Various drugs have been found to be ototoxic (**Table 170-8**).[29] Aminoglycoside antibiotics produce hearing loss and peripheral vestibular dysfunction by accumulating inside the endolymph, causing the death of cochlear and vestibular hair cells. However, because both inner ears are affected, vertigo is uncommon. Clinical manifestations include ataxia and oscillopsia (defined as the inability to maintain visual fixation while moving). The damage is usually irreversible but is dose- and duration-dependent. Loop diuretics (furosemide and ethacrynic acid) also cause irreversible vestibular toxicity and ototoxicity. *N*-Acetylcysteine administered orally may help prevent aminoglycoside-induced ototoxicity in hemodialysis patients.[30] Cytotoxic agents such as vinblastine and cisplatin cause vestibular damage; however, newer platinums, such as carboplatin, are less likely to do so. The antiarrhythmic drug quinidine and antimalarial drugs derived from quinine, such as chloroquine and mefloquine, also can cause vestibular symptoms that may be irreversible.

Reversible causes of vestibular damage and ototoxicity include nonsteroidal anti-inflammatory drugs, salicylates, minocycline, erythromycin, and some fluoroquinolones. Isolated cases of unsteady gait have been observed with antiviral drugs such as abacavir as well as antiparasitic agents. Solvents and other chemicals such as propylene glycol, toluene, mercury, and hydrocarbons can cause both peripheral and central vestibular symptoms.

TABLE 170-8 Ototoxic and Vestibulotoxic Agents

Agent	Dose Dependent	Reversible
Aminoglycosides	Yes	Usually not; possible improvement with *N*-acetylcysteine
Erythromycin	No	Yes
Minocycline	No	Yes
Fluoroquinolones	No	Yes
Nonsteroidal anti-inflammatory drugs; salicylates	Yes	Yes
Loop diuretics	No	Can be irreversible
Cytostatic drugs	Yes	No
Antimalarials	No	Yes
Anticonvulsants	Yes	Yes

Drugs that sometimes induce a central vestibular syndrome include tricyclic antidepressants, neuroleptics, opiates, and alcohol. Anticonvulsants cause dizziness and ataxia, especially in older patients. Lamotrigine may cause less dizziness.[31] Phenytoin, toluene, and cancer chemotherapy agents can cause irreversible cerebellar toxicity. Phencyclidine is a recreational drug that causes central vestibular symptoms, including nystagmus and ataxia.

In general, most patients adapt to chronic vertigo by relying on intact proprioception and vision. However, **benzodiazepines and neuroleptics that are often used as antivertigo therapy may exacerbate symptoms by delaying or inhibiting such compensation.** Thus, avoid using this therapy on a long-term basis. Refer patients with suspected ototoxicity to an otolaryngologist.

EIGHTH NERVE LESIONS AND CEREBELLOPONTINE ANGLE TUMORS

Lesions of the eighth cranial nerve such as meningiomas and acoustic schwannomas may produce mild vertigo. The onset is usually gradual and remains constant until central compensation takes place. Hearing loss usually precedes the vertigo. Tumors of the cerebellopontine angle such as acoustic neuromas, meningiomas, and dermoids may also cause vertigo. **These usually present with deafness and ataxia, as well as ipsilateral facial weakness, loss of the corneal reflex, and cerebellar signs.** All such patients require urgent diagnostic imaging as well as referral to a neurosurgeon.

POSTTRAUMATIC VERTIGO

Acute posttraumatic vertigo and unsteady gait are caused by a direct injury to the labyrinthine membranes. The onset of vertigo is immediate and is accompanied by nausea and vomiting. There may be a concomitant fracture of the temporal bone. Vertigo associated with a closed head injury warrants CT or MRI to exclude an intracranial hemorrhage. Vertigo due to direct labyrinthine trauma tends to resolve within several weeks. Closed head trauma also can displace otoconia from the utricular maculae, precipitating an attack of BPPV. Postconcussive syndrome can be associated with unsteadiness of gait and a vague sense of dizziness. These patients may be treated symptomatically, with referral to a specialist if symptoms fail to resolve.

VERTIGO AFTER COCHLEAR IMPLANTATION

Vertigo is a well-known complication of cochlear implantation. The etiology is likely multifactorial and includes the dislodging of otoconia and the introduction of bone dust into the labyrinth.[32]

DISORDERS CAUSING CENTRAL VERTIGO

Central vertigo is caused by disorders affecting the cerebellum and the brainstem. These include cerebrovascular disease, hemorrhage, migraine, demyelination, and neoplasms. Central vertigo is unlikely to be associated with tinnitus and hearing impairment. Nystagmus is more likely to be vertical than horizontal or rotatory and may be present in the absence of vertigo.

CEREBELLAR HEMORRHAGE AND INFARCTION

Cerebellar hemorrhage typically causes acute vertigo and ataxia along with headache, nausea, and vomiting. Instead of intense vertigo, patients tend to complain of a sense of side-to-side or front-to-back motion. Patients may have truncal ataxia and may not be able to sit without support. Romberg testing and tandem gait will be abnormal. Occasionally, there may be a sixth cranial nerve palsy or conjugate eye deviation away from the side with the hemorrhage. Cerebellar infarction has a similar clinical presentation. Such patients require emergent MRI, and those with cerebellar hemorrhage require emergent neurosurgical consultation.

WALLENBERG'S SYNDROME

A lateral medullary infarction (Wallenberg's syndrome) of the brainstem can cause vertigo as part of its clinical presentation. **Classic ipsilateral findings include facial numbness, loss of corneal reflex, Horner's syndrome, and paralysis or paresis of the soft palate, pharynx, and larynx (causing dysphagia and dysphonia).** Contralateral findings include loss of pain and temperature sensation in the trunk and limbs. Occasionally, lesions of the sixth, seventh, and eighth cranial nerves can occur, causing vertigo, nausea, vomiting, and nystagmus. These patients require emergent MRI and neurologic consultation.

VERTEBROBASILAR INSUFFICIENCY

Transient ischemic attack of the brainstem due to vertebrobasilar insufficiency can produce vertigo that may closely mimic peripheral vestibular disorders. Focal neurologic signs may be absent in more than half of patients.[3] Patients have typical risk factors for cerebrovascular disease. As with transient ischemic attacks in general, the vertigo may be of sudden onset and typically lasts from minutes to hours and should resolve completely within 24 hours. Vertebrobasilar insufficiency–induced vertigo may be accompanied by diplopia, dysphagia, dysarthria, bilateral long-tract signs, and bilateral loss of vision. Unlike other causes of central vertigo, vertebrobasilar insufficiency may be provoked by position. Turning the head partially occludes the ipsilateral vertebral artery. **If the contralateral artery is stenotic, head turning could cause transient ischemia to the brainstem, resulting in vertebrobasilar insufficiency.** Order a brain MRI and consult a neurologist in patients suspected of having vertebrobasilar insufficiency.

VERTEBRAL ARTERY DISSECTION

Vertebral artery dissection can lead to a stroke involving the posterior circulation. **The most common symptoms of vertebral artery dissection are dizziness, headache, and neck pain.** However, one in four patients with dissection present without headache.[3] Unlike vestibular migraine, the onset of headache is often sudden and severe. Recent head or neck trauma is a known risk factor. A history of trauma (e.g., motor vehicle crash, diving injury, or even coughing or sneezing) along with headache and dizziness should spark concern for underlying dissection. It is a rare but recognized complication of chiropractic neck manipulation.[33] The age of presentation is usually less than 50 years. Patients with suspected dissection require emergent diagnostic imaging and referral.

MULTIPLE SCLEROSIS

Demyelinating disease can present with vertigo that lasts several hours to several weeks and is usually nonrecurrent. The vertigo is mild, with nystagmus the most prominent finding on physical examination. Such patients require confirmatory testing with MRI as well as vestibular evoked myogenic potentials plus urgent referral to a neurologist.

NEOPLASMS

Neoplasms of the fourth ventricle can cause brainstem signs and symptoms, including vertigo. Such tumors include ependymomas in younger patients and metastases in older patients. These patients require diagnostic imaging while in the ED and should be referred to a neurosurgeon.

VESTIBULAR MIGRAINE

There is an epidemiologic link between vertigo and migraine. A disproportionate number of patients presenting to a dizziness clinic have a history of migraine, and the prevalence of vertigo is increased in patients with migraine. Vertigo can be a symptom of an aura, an analog or equivalent of the headache phase itself, or an associated symptom with the migraine prodrome. Basilar migraine is a migraine variant in which the aura has clinical manifestations similar to those of vertebrobasilar insufficiency. Vestibular migraine is the most common cause of recurrent spontaneous vertigo and should be considered in almost any patient with dizziness and headache.

The diagnostic criteria for migraine-related vertigo include a history of vertigo not attributable to other known conditions and a present or past history of migraine or a strong family history. In a first episode, cerebrovascular disease may have to be excluded.

Acute episodes are treated with acetaminophen and antiemetics. Frequent attacks may be managed with prophylactic agents such as metoprolol, topiramate, or valproic acid. **Avoid using ergotamine preparations or sumatriptan in patients with basilar migraine.**

Patients with Ménière's syndrome also have an increased prevalence of migraine. Therefore, patients who fail to respond to therapy specific for Ménière's syndrome may benefit from therapy for vertigo associated with migraine headaches.

SPECIAL CONSIDERATIONS

DISEQUILIBRIUM OF AGING

Disequilibrium of aging (sometimes referred to as "psychomotor disadaptation syndrome") manifests as ill-defined dizziness and gait unsteadiness. It is associated with age-related loss of hearing, balance, proprioceptive input, and vision, resulting in an alteration of postural reactions, reactional hypertonia, gait modifications, and fear of falling.[34] Other factors include a decline in central integration and processing, as well as a decrease in motor responses. Symptoms may be precipitated or exacerbated by diminished ambient light (with worsening of symptoms at night), unfamiliar surroundings, and the use of benzodiazepines and drugs with anticholinergic effects such as tricyclic antidepressants and neuroleptic agents. Refer these patients to an internist or gerontologist.

CONVULSIVE DISORDERS

Nonconvulsive status epilepticus, which is characterized by altered mental status without loss of consciousness or tonic-clonic phenomena yet associated with electroencephalographic evidence of seizure activity, may also produce nonvertiginous dizziness. Symptoms may last for hours to days. Refer patients with suspected convulsive disorders to a neurologist.

HYPERVENTILATION SYNDROME

Patients with primary hyperventilation may experience nonvertiginous dizziness or near-syncope during an episode. Diagnostic clues include paresthesias and carpopedal spasm.

PSYCHIATRIC DIZZINESS

Psychiatric dizziness presents as part of a recognized psychiatric disorder or symptom complex that is not related to known vestibular disorders. Dizziness, which can be chronic, is often reported by patients with primary and secondary anxiety disorders, especially panic disorder.[35] The diagnosis is made by exclusion of other more serious causes of dizziness.

DISPOSITION AND FOLLOW-UP

Discharge patients with peripheral vertigo from the ED once symptoms are controlled. Patients can be referred for vestibular rehabilitation therapy, an exercise-based program that promotes CNS compensation for peripheral vertigo. **Vestibular exercises are indicated for patients with BPPV, chronic vertigo, and psychiatric dizziness.** A Cochrane systematic review concluded that vestibular rehabilitation is safe and effective for unilateral peripheral vestibular vertigo.[33]

Refer all patients with a first episode of peripheral vertigo to their primary care physician or an otolaryngologist for further testing. Refer patients with BPPV who have had a particle-repositioning maneuver to an otolaryngologist for follow-up.

All patients with central vertigo require neuroimaging and other diagnostic testing to establish the diagnosis; life-threatening central causes of vertigo (e.g., stroke, cerebellar hemorrhage) require emergent diagnostic imaging and neurologic or neurosurgical consultation while in the ED. Outpatient psychiatric consultation may be considered for patients with psychiatric dizziness.

REFERENCES

The complete reference list is available online at www.TintinalliEM.com.

Seizures

Joshua G. Kornegay

INTRODUCTION AND PATHOPHYSIOLOGY

A seizure is an episode of abnormal neurologic function caused by inappropriate electrical discharge of brain neurons. Neuronal electrical discharge, in its most simple form, can be thought of as the homeostasis of glutaminergic (excitatory) and γ-aminobutyric acid (inhibitory) activity. The seizure is the clinical attack experienced by the patient in the setting of inappropriate excitatory activity. Some patients with "epileptic" electroencephalographic (EEG) discharges may not experience any overt clinical symptoms. Some seizure-like episodes may be due to causes other than abnormal brain electrical activity, but such attacks are not true seizures.

Epilepsy is a clinical condition in which an individual is subject to recurrent seizures. It implies a fixed, more excitatory condition of the brain with a lower seizure threshold. The term *epileptic* does not refer to an individual with recurrent seizures caused by reversible conditions such as alcohol withdrawal, toxins, hypoglycemia, or other metabolic derangements.

Primary, or *idiopathic*, seizures are those in which no evident cause can be identified. *Secondary*, or *symptomatic*, seizures are a consequence of an identifiable neurologic condition, such as a mass lesion, previous head injury, or stroke. Electrical stimulation of the brain, convulsant potentiating drugs, profound metabolic disturbances, or a sharp blow to the head all may cause *reactive seizures* in otherwise normal individuals. Reactive seizures are generally self-limited, and a reactive seizure is not considered to be a seizure disorder or epilepsy.

There are further definitions of seizures based on clinical factors: a **provoked seizure** has an acute precipitating event within 7 days of the insult; an **unprovoked seizure** has no acute precipitating factor or may result from a very remote incident; **status epilepticus** is seizure activity for ≥5 minutes or two or more seizures without regaining consciousness between seizures[1]; and **refractory status epilepticus** is persistent seizure activity despite the IV administration of adequate amounts of two antiepileptic agents.

SEIZURE CLASSIFICATION

The International League Against Epilepsy recommends dividing seizures into two major groups: *generalized seizures* and *partial seizures* (**Table 171-1**). When there are inadequate data to categorize the seizure, the seizure is considered *unclassified.*

GENERALIZED SEIZURES

Generalized seizures are thought to be caused by a nearly simultaneous activation of the entire cerebral cortex, perhaps caused by an electrical discharge originating deep in the brain and spreading outward. The attacks begin with abrupt loss of consciousness. Loss of consciousness may be the only clinical manifestation of the seizure (as in absence attacks), or there may be a variety of motor manifestations (e.g., tonic posturing, clonic jerking of the body and extremities).

TABLE 171-1 Classification of Seizures
Generalized seizures (consciousness always lost)
Tonic-clonic seizures (grand mal)
Absence seizures (petit mal)
Others (myoclonic, tonic, clonic, or atonic seizures)
Partial (focal) seizures
Simple partial (no alteration of consciousness)
Complex partial (consciousness impaired)
Partial seizures with secondary generalization (Jacksonian march)
Unclassified (inadequate information)

Generalized tonic-clonic seizures (grand mal) are the most familiar and dramatic of the generalized seizures. **In a typical attack, the patient suddenly becomes rigid (tonic phase), trunk and extremities are extended, and the patient falls to the ground.** As the tonic phase subsides, there is increasing coarse trembling that evolves into a symmetric, rhythmic (clonic) jerking of the trunk and extremities. Patients are often apneic during this period and may be cyanotic. They often urinate and may vomit. As the attack ends, the patient is left flaccid and unconscious, often with deep, rapid breathing. Typical attacks last from 60 to 90 seconds; bystanders generally overestimate the duration of the seizure. Consciousness returns gradually, and postictal confusion, myalgias, and fatigue may persist for several hours or more.

Absence seizures (petit mal) are very brief, generally lasting only a few seconds. **Patients suddenly develop altered consciousness but no change in postural tone. They appear confused, detached, or withdrawn, and current activity ceases.** They may stare or have twitching of the eyelids. They may not respond to voice or to other stimulation and may exhibit involuntary movements or lose continence. The attack ceases abruptly, and the patients typically resume previous activity without postictal symptoms. Patients and witnesses may be unaware that anything has happened. Classic absence seizures occur in school-age children and are often attributed by parents or teachers to daydreaming or inattention. The attacks can occur as frequently as 100 or more times daily and may result in poor school performance. They usually resolve as the child matures. Similar attacks in adults are more likely to be minor complex partial seizures and should not be termed absence. The distinction is important because the causes and treatment of the two seizures are different.

PARTIAL (FOCAL) SEIZURES

Partial seizures are due to electrical discharges beginning in a localized region of the cerebral cortex. The discharge may remain localized or may spread to involve nearby cortical regions or the entire cortex. Focal seizures are more likely to be secondary to a localized structural lesion of the brain.

In simple partial focal seizures, the seizure remains localized, and consciousness and mentation are not affected. It is possible to deduce the likely location of the initial cortical discharge from the clinical features at the onset of the attack. For example, unilateral tonic or clonic movements limited to one extremity suggest a focus in the motor cortex, whereas visual symptoms suggest an occipital focus. Bizarre olfactory or gustatory hallucinations suggest a focus in the medial temporal lobe. Such sensory phenomena, known as *auras,* are often the initial symptoms of attacks that then become more widespread, termed *secondary generalization.*

Complex partial seizures are focal seizures in which consciousness or mentation is affected. They are often caused by a focal discharge originating in the temporal lobe and are sometimes referred to as *temporal lobe seizures*. Complex partial seizures are commonly misdiagnosed as psychiatric problems because symptoms can be so bizarre. **Symptoms may include automatisms, visceral symptoms, hallucinations, memory disturbances, distorted perception, and affective disorders.** Common automatisms include lip smacking, fiddling with clothing or buttons, or repeating short phrases. Visceral symptoms often consist of a sensation of "butterflies" rising up from the epigastrium. Hallucinations may be olfactory, gustatory, visual, or auditory. There may be complex distortions of visual perception, time, and memory. Affective symptoms may include intense sensations of fear, paranoia, depression, elation, or ecstasy. Because such seizures result in alterations of thinking and behavior, they were previously referred to as *psychomotor seizures,* but to avoid any confusion with psychiatric illness, the term *complex partial seizure* is preferred.

As noted, a focal seizure may spread to involve both hemispheres, mimicking a typical generalized seizure. For the purpose of classification, diagnosis, and treatment, such attacks are still regarded as focal seizures. In some patients, the discharge may spread so rapidly that no focal symptoms are evident, and the correct diagnosis may depend entirely on demonstration of the focal discharge on an EEG recording.

CLINICAL FEATURES

HISTORY

When a patient presents after the event, the first step is to determine whether the episode was truly a seizure. Obtain a careful history of the details of the attack from the patient and any bystanders who witnessed the attack. Inquire about the physical description of the attack, because witnesses may mislabel the activity and mistake nonseizure activity as a seizure.

Important avenues of inquiry include the presence of a preceding aura, abrupt or gradual onset, progression of motor activity, loss of bowel or bladder control, presence of oral injury, and whether the activity was localized or generalized and symmetric or unilateral. Ask about the duration of the episode and determine the presence of postictal confusion or lethargy.

Next, determine the clinical context of the episode. If the patient is a known epileptic, clarify the baseline seizure pattern. If the attack is consistent with the previous seizure pattern, identify precipitating factors of the current seizure. **Common precipitating factors include missed doses of antiepileptic medications; recent alterations in medication, including dosage change or conversion from brand name; sleep deprivation; increased strenuous activity; infection; electrolyte disturbances; and alcohol or substance use or withdrawal.**

If there is no previous history of seizures, a more detailed inquiry is needed. Symptoms such as unexplained injuries, nocturnal tongue biting, or enuresis suggest previous unwitnessed or unrecognized seizures. Ask about a history of recent or remote head injury. Ask about any previous similar episodes that may be suspect as seizures. Persistent, severe, or sudden headache suggests intracranial pathology. Pregnancy or recent delivery raises the possibility of eclampsia. A history of metabolic or electrolyte abnormalities, hypoxia, systemic illness (especially cancer), coagulopathy or anticoagulation, exposure to industrial or environmental toxins, drug ingestion or withdrawal, and alcohol use may point to predisposing factors (**Table 171-2**).

TABLE 171-2 Common Causes of Provoked (Secondary) Seizures
Trauma (recent or remote)
Intracranial hemorrhage (subdural, epidural, subarachnoid, intraparenchymal)
Structural CNS abnormalities
Vascular lesion (aneurysm, arteriovenous malformation)
Mass lesions (primary or metastatic neoplasms)
Degenerative neurologic diseases
Congenital brain abnormalities
Infection (meningitis, encephalitis, abscess)
Metabolic disturbances
Hypo- or hyperglycemia
Hypo- or hypernatremia
Hyperosmolar states
Uremia
Hepatic failure
Hypocalcemia, hypomagnesemia (rare)
Toxins and drugs (many)
Cocaine, lidocaine, antidepressants, theophylline, isoniazid
Mushroom toxicity (*Gyromitra* spp.)
Hydrazine (rocket fuels)
Alcohol or drug withdrawal
Eclampsia of pregnancy (may occur up to 8 weeks postpartum)
Hypertensive encephalopathy
Anoxic-ischemic injury (cardiac arrest, severe hypoxemia)

PHYSICAL EXAMINATION

Immediately obtain a complete set of vital signs and a point-of-care glucose determination. In the post-seizure setting, focus the initial exam on checking for injuries, especially to the head or spine, as a result of the seizure itself. A posterior shoulder dislocation is an injury that is easy to overlook. Lacerations of the tongue and mouth, dental fracture, and pulmonary aspiration are also frequent sequelae.

Perform a directed, complete neurologic examination and subsequent serial examinations. Follow the patient's level of consciousness and mentation closely to avoid missing nonconvulsant status epilepticus (see below). **A transient focal deficit (usually unilateral) following a simple or complex focal seizure is referred to as *Todd's paralysis* and should resolve within 48 hours.**

DIAGNOSIS

Clinical features that help to distinguish seizures from other, nonseizure attacks include:

- Abrupt onset and termination. Some focal seizures are preceded by auras that can last 20 to 30 seconds, but most attacks begin abruptly. Attacks reported to develop over several minutes or longer should be regarded with suspicion. Most seizures last only 1 or 2 minutes, unless the patient is in status epilepticus.
- Lack of recall. Except for simple partial seizures, patients usually cannot recall the details of an attack.
- Purposeless movements or behavior during the attack.
- Most seizures, except for simple absence attacks or simple partial seizures, are followed by a period of postictal confusion and lethargy.

DIFFERENTIAL DIAGNOSIS

Many episodic disturbances of neurologic function may be mistaken for seizures (seizure mimics). A complete review of these conditions is too lengthy for inclusion here, but several important entities are mentioned (**Table 171-3**).

Syncope usually presents with prodromal symptoms, such as lightheadedness, diaphoresis, nausea, and "tunnel vision." However, cardiac syncope may occur suddenly without any prodromal warning. Syncope may be associated with injury, incontinence, or even brief tonic-clonic activity. Recovery is usually rapid, with no postictal-like symptoms. For further discussion see chapter 52, "Syncope."

Pseudoseizures can be extremely difficult to distinguish from true seizures and may occur in a patient who also has a documented seizure disorder. Pseudoseizures are psychogenic in origin and are often associated with a conversion disorder, panic disorder, psychosis, impulse control disorder, Munchausen syndrome, or malingering. Suspect the

TABLE 171-3 Paroxysmal Disorders: Differential Diagnosis
Seizures
Syncope
Pseudoseizures or psychogenic seizures
Hyperventilation syndrome
Migraine headache
Movement disorders

diagnosis of pseudoseizures when seizures occur in response to emotional upset or only occur with witnesses present. These attacks are often bizarre and highly variable. Patients often are able to protect themselves from noxious stimuli during the attack. Characteristic movements include side-to-side head thrashing, rhythmic pelvic thrusting, and clonic extremity motions that are alternating rather than symmetric. Incontinence and injury are uncommon, and there is usually no postictal confusion. Patients will often stop the seizure-like activity on command. Accurate diagnosis of pseudoseizures may require prolonged EEG or video monitoring to demonstrate normal EEG activity during an attack. The lack of a lactic acidosis or elevated prolactin level drawn within 10 to 15 minutes of the cessation of seizure-like activity makes true seizures much less likely.

Hyperventilation syndrome can be misdiagnosed as a seizure disorder. A careful history will reveal the gradual onset of the attacks with shortness of breath, anxiety, and perioral numbness. Such attacks may progress to involuntary spasm (especially carpopedal) of the extremities and even loss of consciousness, although postictal symptoms are rare. Asking the patient to hyperventilate often reproduces the episodes.

Movement disorders, such as dystonia, chorea, myoclonic jerks, tremors, or tics, may occur in a variety of neurologic conditions. Consciousness is always preserved during these movements, and the patient can often temporarily suppress the movements.

Migraine headaches may be preceded by an aura similar to that seen in some partial seizures. The most common migraine aura is the scintillating scotoma. Migraine headaches may also be accompanied by focal neurologic symptoms, such as homonymous hemianopsia or hemiparesis. However, active movement disorders are inconsistent with migraine.

LABORATORY TESTING

Individualize the use of laboratory studies. **In a patient with a well-documented seizure disorder who has had a single unprovoked seizure, the only tests that may be needed are a glucose level and pertinent anticonvulsant medication levels.**

In the case of an adult with a first seizure or unclear seizure history, more extensive studies are usually needed and depend on the clinical context. Obtain serum glucose, basic metabolic panel, lactate, calcium, magnesium, a pregnancy test, and toxicology studies. Consider assays for anticonvulsant drug levels. A seizure may result in a lactate-driven, wide anion gap metabolic acidosis.[2] Most lactate abnormalities will clear within 30 minutes. The prolactin level may also be elevated for a brief period (15 to 60 minutes) immediately after a seizure.[3] These tests can prove helpful in distinguishing true seizures from a pseudoseizure.

Interpret the results of anticonvulsant levels with caution. If the patient history is limited, a positive serum assay for anticonvulsant drugs suggests (but does not prove) the presence of a chronic seizure disorder. The usual therapeutic and toxic levels indicated in laboratory reports are helpful only as rough guides. **The therapeutic level of a drug is the level that provides adequate seizure control without unacceptable side effects.** A marked change in previously stable drug levels may indicate noncompliance, a change in medication, malabsorption of a drug, or ingestion of a potentiating or competing drug. A very low serum anticonvulsant drug level suggests noncompliance with medication and is the most common cause of a breakthrough seizure.

IMAGING

Obtain a CT scan of the head in the ED for patients with a first-ever seizure or a change in established seizure patterns to evaluate for a structural lesion. A noncontrast CT is an appropriate screening tool.[4,5] Obtain a CT scan if there is any concern for an acute intracranial process based on history, comorbidities, or findings on physical examination. **Concern for an acute intracranial process is an important indication for obtaining CT imaging, even if there is a coexistent metabolic process.**

Because many important processes, such as tumors or vascular anomalies, may not be evident on noncontrast studies, a follow-up contrast-enhanced CT or MRI is often needed. Almost one-quarter of adults with new-onset seizure will have visualized pathology on follow-up MRI, with rates increasing to as high as 53% in those with onset of a focal seizure.[6] The timing of further imaging studies can be discussed with the consulting neurologist.

Obtain other radiographic studies as indicated by the clinical presentation to avoid missing injuries acquired as a result of the seizure. Obtain radiographs of the cervical spine if there is suspicion of head or neck trauma. Chest radiographs may reveal primary or metastatic tumors or aspiration. Shoulder radiographs may help rule out posterior dislocations. Special examinations, such as cerebral angiography, are rarely part of the ED evaluation.

LUMBAR PUNCTURE

Lumbar puncture in the setting of an acute seizure is indicated if the patient is febrile or immunocompromised or if subarachnoid hemorrhage is suspected and the noncontrast head CT is normal. For further discussion, see chapters 166, "Spontaneous Subarachnoid and Intracerebral Hemorrhage" and 174, "Central Nervous System and Spinal Infections."

ELECTROENCEPHALOGRAPHY

Although EEG is very helpful, it is often not readily available in most EDs. Emergent EEG can be considered in the evaluation of a patient with persistent, unexplained altered mental status to evaluate for nonconvulsive status epilepticus, subtle status epilepticus, paroxysmal attack when a seizure is suspected, or ongoing status epilepticus after chemical paralysis for intubation. Patients in whom an emergent EEG is warranted typically require neurologic consultation and admission to a critical care setting.

TREATMENT OF UNCOMPLICATED SEIZURES

PATIENTS WITH ACTIVE SEIZURES

Typically, little is required during the course of an active seizure other than supportive and patient protective measures. If possible, turn the patient to the side to reduce the risk of aspiration. It is usually not necessary or even possible to ventilate a patient effectively during a seizure, but once the attack subsides, clear the airway. Suction and airway adjuncts should be readily available. **It is not necessary or recommended to give IV anticonvulsant medications during the course of an uncomplicated seizure.** Most seizures will self-resolve within 5 minutes. Any unnecessary sedation at this point will complicate the evaluation and result in a prolonged decrease in level of consciousness.[7] Seizures that fail to abate after 5 minutes are considered status epilepticus and require more aggressive medical interventions (see "Status Epilepticus" section, below).

PATIENTS WITH A HISTORY OF SEIZURES

Proper management of a patient with a well-documented seizure disorder who presents after one or more seizures depends on the particular circumstances of the case. Identify and correct potential precipitants that may lower the seizure threshold. Many seizures occur because of failure to take anticonvulsant medication as prescribed. Some anticonvulsants have very short serum half-lives, and missing even a single dose may result in a sharp drop in serum levels. If anticonvulsant levels are very low, supplemental doses are appropriate, and the regular regimen can be restarted or adjusted. A loading dose is also frequently provided. Without a loading dose, the patient may not achieve anticonvulsant effects for days to weeks and is at risk for subsequent seizures. Because there are no data comparing parenteral versus oral replacement, this issue is left to the discretion of the medical provider[8] and should be based on knowledge of pharmacology. For example, the oral loading dose of phenytoin is 20 milligrams/kg given in three divided doses every 2 to 4 hours, a time frame not acceptable for a typical ED stay, so the IV route is needed to achieve the proper loading dose.

In the known or suspected noncompliant patient, obtain a serum anticonvulsant level before administering a supplemental or loading dose to avoid drug toxicity. **If anticonvulsant levels are adequate and the patient has had a single attack, specific treatment may not be needed if the seizure pattern and frequency fall within the expected range for the patient.** If anticonvulsant levels are not locally available (e.g., levetiracetam or lacosamide), and there is a missed dose or noncompliance, give the usual dose in the ED before discharge.

Even well-controlled patients may have occasional breakthrough seizures. Attempt to identify any precipitants or conditions that have lowered the seizure threshold. If none is found, a change or adjustment of medication may be needed and should be made in consultation with the patient's primary care physician or neurologist. If the maintenance dose is increased, ensure follow-up within 1 to 3 days. There are no specific guidelines for the duration of ED observation in the situation of an individual with a prior history of seizures. Some clinicians discharge patients with seizures resulting from nontherapeutic anticonvulsant levels after administration of a loading dose of an anticonvulsant if vital signs are normal and the mental status has returned to baseline. Ideally, discharge patients with a reliable family member or friend and with medical follow-up arranged, as above.

PATIENTS WITH A FIRST UNPROVOKED SEIZURE

Guidelines do not recommend hospital admission or initiation of anticonvulsant therapy in the patient with a first unprovoked seizure, as long as the patient has returned to neurologic baseline.[1,8] The most important predictors of seizure recurrence are the underlying cause of the seizure and the results of the EEG. The decision to begin outpatient treatment with antiepileptics depends on the risk of recurrent seizures weighed against the risk–benefit ratio of anticonvulsant therapy. In general, patients with a first unprovoked seizure who have a normal neurologic examination, no acute or chronic medical comorbidities, normal diagnostic testing including noncontrast head CT, and normal mental status can safely be discharged from the ED. Initiation of antiepileptic medication may be deferred to the outpatient setting where further studies, including an EEG and MRI, can be performed.[1,4,8] Consider consultation and/or admission for patients who do not meet the above criteria.

Patients with provoked (secondary) seizures due to an identifiable underlying condition (Table 171-2) often require admission and should generally be treated to minimize seizure recurrence.

The ideal initial antiepileptic regimen is a single-drug therapy that controls seizures with minimum toxicity. If treatment is initiated, drug selection is based on the type of seizure and should be done in consultation with a neurologist. Antiepileptic agents, such as valproate, lamotrigine, topiramate, levetiracetam, and oxcarbazepine, are options for adults with new-onset seizures.[5,9] Consider developing common protocols between emergency medicine and neurology when treatment of new-onset seizures is initiated from the ED.

Instruct discharged patients to take precautions to minimize the risks for injury from further seizures. Swimming, working with hazardous tools or machines, and working at heights should be prohibited. Driving is prohibited until cleared by the neurologist or primary care physician. Driving privileges should conform to state law, and it may be up to the emergency physician to document seizure activity with the Department of Motor Vehicles.

SPECIAL POPULATIONS

HUMAN IMMUNODEFICIENCY VIRUS

Mass lesions, encephalopathy, herpes zoster, toxoplasmosis, *Cryptococcus*, neurosyphilis, and meningitis are all seen more frequently in this population and can all provoke seizure activity.[10,11]

Perform an extensive investigation for the cause of the seizure. If no space-occupying lesion is identified on noncontrast head CT scan and there is no evidence of increased intracranial pressure, perform a lumbar puncture to exclude CNS infection. If no explanation for seizures is found, then obtain a contrast-enhanced head CT or MRI.

NEUROCYSTICERCOSIS

Neurocysticercosis is caused by a CNS infection with the larval stage of the tapeworm *Taenia solium* and is the most common cause of provoked (secondary) seizures in the developing world.[12] The most common form of disease is parasitic invasion of brain parenchyma and cyst formation. Over 1 to 2 years, the cyst degenerates and becomes fibrotic, leaving a focal area of scar and calcification. Seizures are the most common clinical manifestation of neurocysticercosis and most frequently occur as the parasite is degenerating. In 80% to 90% of cases, the lesions resolve within 3 to 6 months, leaving the patient free of seizures. Up to 20% of patients will continue to have seizures and require ongoing therapy with antiepileptic medications.[12]

In most cases, neuroimaging in neurocysticercosis is nondiagnostic. CT or MRI may demonstrate a 1- to 2-cm cystic lesion with thin walls and a 1- to 3-mm mural nodule (the parasite), a localized area of ring-like enhancement with surrounding edema, a calcified lesion, or hydrocephalus. Definitive diagnosis relies on a combination of the patient's clinical picture, exposure history, serologic testing, and neuroimaging.

Seizures in neurocysticercosis are typically controlled by antiepileptic monotherapy. Definitive treatment of neurocysticercosis is controversial and highly variable, depending on the number, location, and viability of the parasites within the CNS.[13,14] Antiparasitics (praziquantel and albendazole) and steroids are best initiated in consultation with an infectious disease specialist or neurologist.

PREGNANCY

The management of seizures (or control of epilepsy) during pregnancy requires a multidisciplinary approach. Most seizures in pregnancy are not first-time seizures, and initial evaluation is generally as discussed earlier, with the addition of an obstetric evaluation to determine gestational age and fetal well-being.

When a woman beyond 20 weeks of gestation develops seizures in the setting of hypertension, edema, and proteinuria, the condition is defined as *eclampsia*. Magnesium sulfate has long been used to treat eclampsia with good results. In eclamptic women, magnesium sulfate infusion compared to diazepam and phenytoin resulted in a >50% reduction in recurrence of seizures and a lower incidence of pneumonia, intensive care unit admission, and assisted ventilation.[15-17] Detailed discussion of seizures in pregnancy is discussed in chapter 100, "Maternal Emergencies after 20 Weeks of Pregnancy and in the Postpartum Period."

ALCOHOL ABUSE

Seizures and alcohol use are associated through missed doses of medication, sleep deprivation as an epileptogenic trigger, increased propensity for head injury, toxic co-ingestions, electrolyte abnormalities, and withdrawal seizures. Benzodiazepines in doses sufficient to manage withdrawal symptoms will usually afford adequate protection from acute seizures. These doses are often very large and need to be given in an escalating fashion.[18] Evaluate and treat the alcohol-abusing patient with a first seizure as any other patient with a first-time seizure. Detailed discussion of alcohol withdrawal seizures is provided in chapter 292, "Substance Use Disorders."

STATUS EPILEPTICUS

Status epilepticus can occur in patients with a history of seizures or can be a first epileptic event. The most common causes of status epilepticus include subtherapeutic antiepileptic levels; preexisting neurologic conditions, such as prior CNS infection, trauma, hemorrhage, or stroke; acute stroke; anoxia or hypoxia; metabolic abnormalities; and alcohol or drug intoxication or withdrawal.[19]

Status epilepticus is a single seizure ≥5 minutes in length or two or more seizures without recovery of consciousness between seizures.[1,20,21] After 5 minutes, seizures are less likely to spontaneously terminate, less likely to be controlled with antiepileptic drugs, and more likely to cause neuronal damage. **Status epilepticus is a neurologic**

emergency, and treatment should be initiated in all patients with continuous seizure activity lasting more than 5 minutes.

As seizures surpass the 5-minute mark, dramatic changes occur at the cellular level. Decreased expression and internalization of γ-aminobutyric acid receptors, coupled with increased expression of both glutamine and *N*-methyl-D-aspartate receptors, lead to a greatly diminished seizure threshold.[22,23] The blood–brain barrier is also compromised, leading to CNS penetration of potassium and albumin, both of which are hyperexcitatory CNS chemicals.[24] After 20 minutes, hypotension, hypoxia, metabolic acidosis, hyperthermia, and hypoglycemia are present. Additionally, cardiac dysrhythmias, rhabdomyolysis, and pulmonary edema can develop.[25] After 2 hours of seizure activity, neurotoxic amino acids and calcium are released into cells, leading to permanent neuronal necrosis and apoptosis.[22] The hyperexcitatory milieu makes standard antiseizure therapies much less effective in seizure termination.

In **nonconvulsive status epilepticus**, the patient is comatose or has fluctuating abnormal mental status or confusion, but no overt seizure activity is present. The diagnosis is challenging and is typically made by EEG. Findings suggestive of nonconvulsive status epilepticus include a prolonged postictal period after a generalized seizure; subtle motor signs such as twitching, blinking, and eye deviation; fluctuating alterations in mental status; or unexplained stupor and confusion in the elderly.[25]

Epilepsia partialis continua is focal tonic-clonic seizure activity with normal alertness that most commonly affects the distal leg or arm.

TREATMENT OF STATUS EPILEPTICUS

The goal of treatment is seizure control as soon as possible and within 30 minutes of presentation (**Figure 171-1**). Examination; identification of potential causes; checking the airway, breathing, and circulation; and treatment all begin simultaneously. Direct a focused history and physical examination toward possible causes and subsequent injuries.

Establish large-bore IV access and determine a bedside glucose. Administer normal saline, avoiding IV fluids containing glucose because phenytoin is not compatible with glucose-containing solutions. Place the patient on oxygen, a cardiac monitor, a pulse oximeter, and end-tidal capnography.

In established status epilepticus, consider endotracheal intubation for airway protection, oxygenation, and ventilation. If a paralytic agent is used for intubation, use a short-acting agent so as not to mask ongoing seizure activity. Arrange for continuous EEG monitoring as soon as possible after paralytic agents have been used.

Initial laboratory evaluation includes blood glucose, a metabolic panel including calcium and magnesium, lactate, and if appropriate, a pregnancy test, a toxicology screen, and anticonvulsant levels.

Administer glucose IV if hypoglycemia is suspected or confirmed. Monitor temperature continuously, and treat hyperthermia with passive cooling. Place a urinary catheter to monitor urine output, and insert a nasogastric tube to help prevent aspiration.

If toxic ingestion is suspected as the cause of seizures, proceed with GI decontamination (as appropriate). Do not attempt lumbar puncture during status epilepticus. **If bacterial meningitis or encephalitis is suspected, start empiric antibiotic or antiviral therapy.** Status epilepticus can induce a brief peripheral leukocytosis as well as a mild cerebrospinal fluid pleocytosis. Radiographic studies, such as a CT scan, will usually need to be delayed until seizures are controlled.

ANTICONVULSANT DRUGS IN STATUS EPILEPTICUS

The drugs most often used in the therapy of status epilepticus are the benzodiazepines (lorazepam or, if not available, diazepam) and phenytoin or fosphenytoin (Figure 171-1). Benzodiazepines are used in patients with continuous or very frequent seizures to temporarily control the seizures until more specific agents can be given. IV lorazepam (2 to 4 milligrams) and IV diazepam (5 to 10 milligrams) have equal efficacy in controlling status epilepticus.[8] Compared to diazepam, lorazepam has a slightly slower onset (3 vs 2 minutes) but a significantly longer duration of action (12 to 24 hours vs 15 to 60 minutes) and is associated with fewer seizure

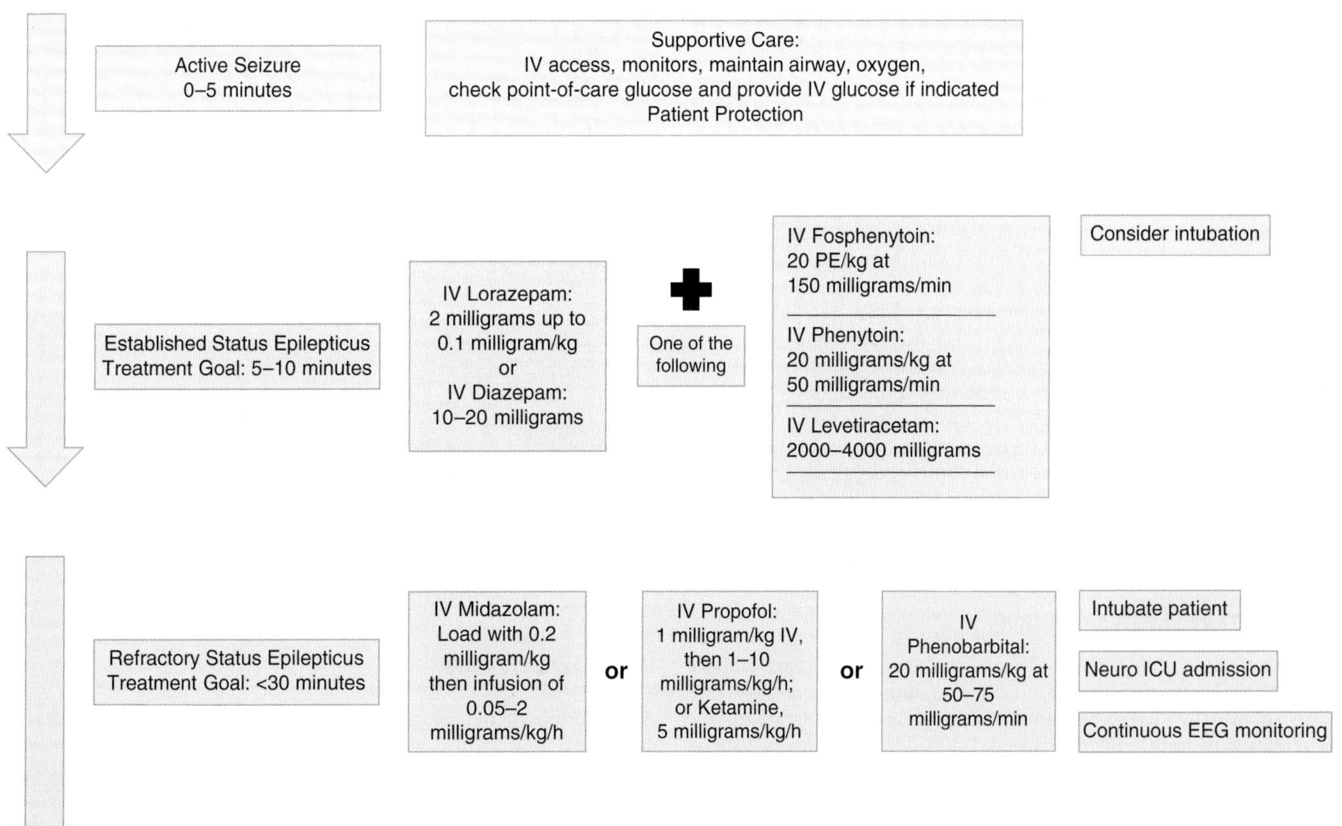

FIGURE 171-1. Guidelines for management of active seizures and status epilepticus. ICU = intensive care unit; PE = phenytoin equivalents.

recurrences. In one prehospital study, IM midazolam demonstrated decreased seizure time and fewer intensive care unit admissions when compared to lorazepam if no IV access was available[26]; however, **IV lorazepam is still considered the initial agent of choice.** Lorazepam is also more effective than phenytoin or phenobarbital as the initial drug.[27] Respiratory depression and hypotension may occur, especially in young children and in patients taking alcohol, barbiturates, narcotics, or other sedatives. In patients with difficult IV access and emergent need for seizure control, there may be a role for rectal diazepam gel or buccal midazolam. Although there have been no trials in adults, rectal diazepam has been used by EMS providers in children with good success for years, and recent trials of buccal midazolam (0.5 milligram/kg, up to 10 milligrams) show more efficacy than rectal diazepam in the pediatric population.[28,29]

In established status epilepticus, follow benzodiazepines with a longer-acting antiepileptic agent: fosphenytoin or phenytoin, levetiracetam, valproate, or lacosamide. One of these antiepileptic agents should be started within 20 minutes of diagnosis.[1]

Fosphenytoin is a water-soluble prodrug of phenytoin that is converted to phenytoin in the plasma. Fosphenytoin has similar time of onset, effectiveness, and cardiac effects as phenytoin. It has much fewer infusion-site reactions due to the lack of propylene glycol and ethanol as the diluents. Fosphenytoin may be infused quickly, and for that reason, it is preferred over phenytoin. Fosphenytoin dosing is expressed as phenytoin equivalents (PE) to prevent confusion. The loading dose is 20 PE/kg, which can be infused at 150 PE/minute over 10 to 15 minutes.[9] Fosphenytoin can also be given IM, which may be useful if the patient does not have IV access.

The loading dose for **phenytoin** is 20 milligrams/kg IV. Doses in excess of the usual 1000 milligrams are often required. Due to myocardial depression from its propylene glycol diluent, phenytoin is typically infused no faster than a rate of 25 milligrams per minute (taking about 1 hour to administer). The rate may be increased to 50 milligrams per minute during status epilepticus as long as hypotension does not develop. Place patients on a cardiac monitor, with blood pressure assessments every 5 to 15 minutes during the infusion and every 15 minutes for 1 hour after infusion.[30] Phenytoin should not be mixed with any glucose-containing IV fluid and should not be given IM due to erratic absorption. The drug is contraindicated in patients with second- or third-degree atrioventricular block. Other adverse effects include infusion site reactions, hypotension, and cardiac dysrhythmias. If side effects develop, stop the infusion and restart at a lower rate after side effects have resolved.

Valproic acid is effective but has serious side effects compared to the agents listed above. The U.S. Food and Drug Administration has issued a black box warning for hepatic failure and pancreatitis, and valproic acid should not be administered along with phenytoin. The dose is 20 milligrams/kg IV.[1,9,22,31,32]

Levetiracetam is very effective, is quick to administer, and has few interactions and side effects. The precise mechanism of action is unknown, but it may inhibit voltage-dependent calcium channels and facilitate γ-aminobutyric acid inhibitory transmission. The dose is 20 milligrams/kg IV. Although it is not yet approved by the Food and Drug Administration for status epilepticus, it is rapidly gaining favor as a first-line drug for established status epilepticus.[1,9,33-35]

Lacosamide is a potential alternative for status epilepticus with limited availability and limited data on its use. The dose is 200 milligrams IV given over 15 minutes.[1,36]

REFRACTORY STATUS EPILEPTICUS

Refractory status epilepticus is defined as persistent seizure activity despite the IV administration of adequate amounts of two antiepileptic agents and usually exceeds 60 minutes.[1] One study found that up to 31% of patients with status epilepticus went on to develop refractory status epilepticus.[37]

Various approaches to refractory status epilepticus have been suggested (Figure 171-1).[1,7,9,22,32-43] Overall, there are few controlled trials that strongly support a single agent or combination of agents. Current recommendations include propofol, midazolam, and barbiturates such as phenobarbital or pentobarbital given as infusions.[1] All of these agents can lead to hypotension, sometimes requiring concomitant vasopressor use, and require intubation. Ideally, treatment is in consultation with a neurologist and in an intensive care setting, because advanced respiratory support, cardiovascular support, and EEG monitoring are all needed.

Propofol is a widely used, lipophilic, general anesthetic that has come into favor for refractory status epilepticus. It can be started as an infusion at typical rates of 2 to 10 milligrams/kg/h and titrated up to effect seizure cessation. Propofol has the added benefit of a short half-life, allowing for quicker neurologic recovery after seizure control is achieved. At higher doses (>40 milligrams/kg/h), patients are at increased risk for hemodynamic instability, including hypotension, as well as propofol infusion syndrome.[1,7,9,22,39]

Midazolam is an easily titrated, infusible benzodiazepine that can also be used in the ongoing treatment of refractory status epilepticus. Midazolam can be started at 0.05 to 0.4 milligram/kg/h and is titrated up to seizure cessation.[1,9,40] Midazolam can accumulate in peripheral soft tissues, particularly with renal insufficiency, leading to a prolonged recovery period.

Barbiturates, such as **phenobarbital** (up to 20 milligrams/kg IV) or **pentobarbital**, may be considered as third-line drugs in patients whose seizures are not controlled despite full loading doses of benzodiazepines and other agents. However, **patients in refractory status may not respond to barbiturates.** One study found no added seizure control with phenobarbital.[32] A subsequent meta-analysis showed improved seizure control with pentobarbital compared to propofol or midazolam but no differences in mortality.[38] Respiratory depression and hypotension are more common when using barbiturates, especially at higher doses or when diazepam or lorazepam is also given.[1,9,22] Additionally, midazolam and propofol have the advantage over barbiturates of having a shorter half-life and rapid clearance, allowing for earlier extubation and clinical assessment.[1] For these reasons, current recommendations are to use propofol and midazolam infusions as first- and second-line agents, respectively, in refractory status epilepticus with barbiturates as third-line agents.[1,9,22,39,40]

Finally, **ketamine** may also be considered as a third-line agent in refractory status epilepticus. Ketamine is an *N*-methyl-D-aspartate receptor antagonist and helps block the hyperexcitatory pathway, which is thought to be a greater culprit in refractory status epilepticus. Ketamine can be administered as a bolus dose of 0.5 to 4.5 milligrams/kg or as an infusion up to 5 milligrams/kg/h. Multiple case reports and one retrospective study have demonstrated its safe use and likely benefit in terminating refractory status epilepticus.[22,41-43]

REFERENCES

The complete reference list is available online at www.TintinalliEM.com.

Acute Peripheral Neurologic Disorders

Phillip Andrus
J. Michael Guthrie

INTRODUCTION

Acute peripheral neurologic lesions are a diverse group of disorders. By definition, they involve injury or disease in sensory and motor fibers outside of the central nervous system (CNS) extending to the neuromuscular junction. The peripheral nervous system (PNS) serves sensory, motor, and autonomic functions. Thus, the patient with a peripheral nerve lesion may have deficits in any combination of these functions. **Exclude central processes, such as stroke or spinal cord injury, before considering an acute peripheral lesion.**

DISTINGUISHING CENTRAL AND PERIPHERAL LESIONS

Use CNS and PNS neuroanatomy principles to distinguish lesions. Peripheral nerves contain varying amounts of motor, sensory, and autonomic fibers and follow well-described paths that make them prone to typical injuries. Thus, peripheral nerve lesions are more likely to be confined to one limb and to present with the involvement of multiple sensory modalities and motor symptoms. A typical example would be a nerve compression syndrome presenting with weakness, numbness, and tingling that developed after the arm was held in an unusual position for a prolonged period. However, weakness and numbness can be seen in both peripheral and central disorders. Hyporeflexia sometimes occurs with acute central lesions, but hyperreflexia and spasticity invariably develop with time. PNS disorders, like CNS diseases, can affect bulbar structures, resulting in diplopia, dysarthria, or dysphagia. Despite the overlap, CNS disorders have other features not seen in peripheral disease. For example, aphasia, apraxia, and vision loss are hallmarks of cortical disease. Most CNS lesions will result in upper motor neuron signs: hyperreflexia, hypertonia (spasticity), and extensor plantar (Babinski) reflexes. Perhaps the most important distinguishing component is the examination of deep tendon reflexes. Dorsiflexion of the great toe with fanning of remaining toes and flexion of the leg is a pathologic Babinski's sign, indicating a central disruption of the pyramidal tract. Although there can be many similarities between patients with CNS and PNS lesions, the distinctions are clear (**Table 172-1**). Lateralization of weakness, hyperreflexia, positive Babinski's sign, or any other CNS finding requires further investigation for a central rather than peripheral disorder.

LOCALIZING PERIPHERAL NERVE LESIONS

Patients with peripheral nerve disorders frequently require diagnostic evaluation unavailable during the initial ED encounter. A careful history and physical examination will exclude critical diagnoses and point toward the appropriate management.

TABLE 172-1 Differentiating Central Nervous System from Peripheral Nervous System Disorders

	Central	Peripheral
History	Cognitive changes Sudden weakness Nausea, vomiting Headache	Weakness confined to one limb Weakness with associated pain Posture- or movement-dependent pain Weakness after prolonged period in one position
Physical Examination		
Reflexes	Brisk reflexes (hyperreflexia) Babinski's sign Hoffman's sign	Hypoactive reflexes Areflexia
Motor	Asymmetric weakness of ipsilateral upper and lower extremity Facial droop Slurred speech	Symmetric proximal weakness
Sensory	Asymmetric sensory loss in ipsilateral upper and lower extremity	Reproduction of symptoms with movement (compressive neuropathy) All sensory modalities involved
Coordination	Discoordination without weakness	Loss of proprioception

HISTORY

The elements required to localize the process will usually include the following: symmetry; proximal versus distal symptoms; sensory, motor, or autonomic involvement; and mono- versus polyneuropathy. Sensory symptoms may include numbness, tingling, dysesthesias, pain, or ataxia. Motor symptoms manifest as weakness. Autonomic disability may present as orthostasis, bowel or bladder dysfunction, gastroparesis, or sexual dysfunction. Associated findings will frequently narrow the differential diagnosis or suggest a specific diagnosis. For example, in the setting of a recent viral infection or vaccination, consider Guillain-Barré syndrome. Is there a history of diabetes or subacute trauma? Does the patient with thrush or wasting and undiagnosed immunodeficiency have a human immunodeficiency virus (HIV)-associated neuropathy? Patients with an attached tick may have tick paralysis.

PHYSICAL EXAMINATION

Perform a comprehensive neurologic examination on patients with peripheral nerve disorders, paying particular attention to the specific area and distribution involved. Evaluate for hypotonia, muscle wasting, fasciculations, and hyporeflexia. Is there focal weakness? What is the perception of light touch, vibration, and position sense? If there are sensory deficits, what spinal nerve levels do they involve?

DIAGNOSIS

Many patients with peripheral nerve disorders will require electromyography and nerve conduction velocity studies. Electromyography is used to differentiate primary muscular or neuromuscular junction problems from peripheral nerve disorders. Nerve conduction velocity studies, which measure the speed of conduction by observing the response to nerve stimulation by distally placed electrodes, can differentiate between axonal loss and demyelination. Combined with the history and physical examination, these tests allow the consultant to better localize the lesion and make a firm diagnosis. Lumbar puncture and cerebrospinal fluid (CSF) analysis are frequently required to confirm the diagnosis in acute or subacute inflammatory and infectious processes. In certain cases, nerve biopsy may be required. In cases where biopsy is considered, MRI can direct the biopsy site to the area of greatest utility.

TREATMENT

Management of PNS disorders depends on the specific diagnosis. However, a few general principles apply. Initiate supportive care for severe, life-threatening neuromuscular diseases in the ED. Monitor patients with the potential for respiratory failure, aspiration, and cardiac dysrhythmias. **For patients at risk for diaphragmatic failure, measure baseline forced vital capacity or negative inspiratory pressure in the ED to assess whether there is an immediate need for respiratory support or admission to an intensive care unit.** Admit patients with acute peripheral neurologic conditions if there is potential respiratory or autonomic compromise, or with severe or rapidly progressing weakness. If a peripheral disorder is suspected and the patient does not require admission, arrange for neurologic follow-up within 7 to 10 days.

ACUTE PERIPHERAL NEUROPATHIES

GUILLAIN-BARRÉ SYNDROME

Guillain-Barré syndrome is an acute polyneuropathy characterized by immune-mediated peripheral nerve myelin sheath or axon destruction. The prevailing theory is that antibodies directed against myelin sheath and axons of peripheral nerves are formed in response to a preceding viral or bacterial illness. Symptoms are at their worst in 2 to 4 weeks, and recovery can vary from weeks to a year.

Clinical Features Classically, Guillain-Barré syndrome is preceded by a viral illness, followed by **ascending symmetric weakness or paralysis and areflexia or hyporeflexia**. Paralysis may ascend to the diaphragm, compromising respiratory function and requiring mechanical ventilation in one third of patients. Autonomic dysfunction may be present as well.

TABLE 172-2 Diagnostic Criteria for Classic Guillain-Barré Syndrome

Required
Progressive weakness of more than one limb
Areflexia
Suggestive
Progression over days to weeks
Recovery beginning 2–4 weeks after cessation of progression
Relative symmetry of symptoms
Mild sensory signs and symptoms
Cranial nerve involvement (Bell's palsy, dysphagia, dysarthria, ophthalmoplegia)
Autonomic dysfunction (tachycardia, bradycardia, dysrhythmias, wide variations in blood pressure, postural hypotension, urinary retention, constipation, facial flushing, anhydrosis, hypersalivation)
Absence of fever at onset
Cytoalbuminologic dissociation of cerebrospinal fluid (high protein and low white cell count)
Typical findings on electromyogram and nerve conduction studies

TABLE 172-3 Managing Respiratory Failure in Guillain-Barré Syndrome

Indications for intubation
Vital capacity <15 mL/kg
Declining one breath count
Pao_2 <70 mm Hg on room air
Bulbar dysfunction (difficulty with breathing, swallowing, or speech)
Aspiration
Indications for admission to intensive care unit
Patients with 4 or more of the following findings: inability to stand, inability to lift the head, inability to lift the elbows, insufficient cough, time from symptom onset to hospital admission <7 days or elevated liver enzymes
Autonomic dysfunction
Bulbar dysfunction
Initial vital capacity <20 mL/kg
Initial negative inspiratory force less than −30 cm of water
Decrease of >30% of vital capacity or negative inspiratory force
Inability to ambulate
Treatment with plasmapheresis

Abbreviation: Pao_2 = partial pressure of arterial oxygen.

There are several variants of Guillain-Barré syndrome. The **Miller-Fisher syndrome** variant is associated with ***Clostridium jejuni* infection**. It is preceded by diarrhea and is characterized by ophthalmoplegia, ataxia, and decreased or absent reflexes. Weakness is less severe and the disease course is milder than Guillain-Barré syndrome. Antibody testing for *C. jejuni* can confirm the diagnosis. Acute motor axonal neuropathy is a pure motor variant, also associated with *C. jejuni* infection, and is seen in Japan and China. Another variant is acute motor and sensory axonal neuropathy, with loss of both motor and sensory function. This variant begins abruptly, progresses rapidly, and has a prolonged course and poor prognosis.

Diagnosis The diagnosis is mostly historical, but lumbar puncture and electrodiagnostic information can improve confidence in the diagnosis. **Table 172-2** lists the specific diagnostic criteria.

CSF analysis shows high protein levels (>45 milligrams/dL) and WBC counts typically <10 cells/mm^3, with predominantly mononuclear cells. When there are >100 cells/mm^3, other considerations include HIV, Lyme disease, syphilis, sarcoidosis, tuberculous or bacterial meningitis, leukemic infiltration, or CNS vasculitis. Electrodiagnostic testing demonstrates demyelination. Nerve biopsy reveals a mononuclear inflammatory infiltrate. If MRI is performed to rule out alternative diagnoses, it will show enhancement of affected nerves.

Treatment The first step in management is assessment of respiratory function. Airway protection in advance of respiratory compromise decreases the incidence of aspiration and other complications. A well-established monitoring parameter is vital capacity, with normal values ranging from 60 to 70 mL/kg. A simple bedside assessment of respiratory status is obtained by trending values reached when the patient counts from 1 to 25 with a single breath. **Avoid depolarizing neuromuscular blockers like succinylcholine for intubation in Guillain-Barré syndrome due to the risk of a hyperkalemic response.**

Both IV immunoglobulin and plasmapheresis shorten the time to recovery. Neither has been shown to be superior to the other, nor are they more efficacious when used together. There are adverse effects seen with both modalities of treatment. IV immunoglobulin has been associated with thromboembolism and aseptic meningitis; plasmapheresis is associated with hemodynamic instability, but a lower rate of relapse. In general, IV immunoglobulin is more widely available and less cumbersome to administer. Corticosteroids are of no benefit and may be harmful.[1]

Disposition Admit patients with acute Guillain-Barré syndrome to a unit where cardiac, respiratory, and neurologic functions can be monitored. Even if a patient does not initially meet the criteria for intubation, intensive care unit admission may still be indicated in order to avoid sudden, unmonitored respiratory failure (**Table 172-3**).[2]

BELL'S PALSY AND UNILATERAL FACIAL PARALYSIS

Bell's palsy or idiopathic facial nerve palsy is the most common cause of unilateral facial paralysis. There are 23 to 25 cases per 100,000 annually, affecting men and women equally. Cranial nerve VII, the facial nerve, supplies motor innervation to the muscles of expression of the face and scalp, the stapedius muscle, and taste to the anterior two thirds of the tongue. The cause of Bell's palsy is not clear. Herpes simplex virus DNA and antigens have been discovered around the facial nerve of affected patients. However, antiviral medications are ineffective, casting doubt on the once predominant theory that herpes simplex virus is responsible for the disease.

Clinical Features **Idiopathic Bell's palsy may be preceded by pain around or behind the ear.** Onset of facial paralysis is acute, with maximal symptoms in 2 to 3 days. Facial numbness or hyperesthesia can accompany paralysis. Subtle dysfunction of cranial nerves V, VIII, IX, and X may be associated; for example, patients may also complain of decreased taste or hyperacusis due to paralysis of the stapedius muscle. On exam, patients will have facial droop, effacement of wrinkles and forehead burrows, and inability to completely close the eye. Recurrent idiopathic Bell's palsy occurs in a small number of patients.

Diagnosis Diagnosis of idiopathic Bell's palsy is based on the history and physical exam and is a diagnosis of exclusion of other conditions that can cause facial palsy. **The most important alternative diagnoses to exclude are ear infections and stroke.** Always perform an ear examination to identify otitis media and malignant otitis, and palpate the mastoids for tenderness, because infections of the ear and mastoids can affect the mastoid, tympanic, labyrinthine, or meatal segments of the cranial nerve VII (**Figure 172-1**).

When a central process causes facial paralysis, the forehead will be spared, as the forehead is supplied by cranial nerve VII arising near the pontomedullary junction, with crossed innervation. Peripheral facial nerve palsies will manifest as weakness throughout the facial nerve distribution, including the forehead. **Middle cerebral artery ischemia or stroke** consists of hemiparesis, facial plegia sparing the forehead, and sensory loss all contralateral to the affected cortex. **Rarely, a brainstem stroke may mimic Bell's palsy if the stroke affects the area where the facial nerve wraps around the abducens (cranial nerve VI) nucleus.** Brainstem stroke findings include peripheral facial nerve palsy and ipsilateral gaze palsy due to ischemia of the abducens nucleus. So, **test extraocular muscle function for all patients suspected of having Bell's palsy. Any patient with facial paralysis sparing the forehead or inability to abduct an eye should undergo neuroimaging to assess for stroke.** No imaging or laboratory testing is needed in patients with high suspicion of Bell's palsy unless further studies are required to exclude alternative diagnoses.

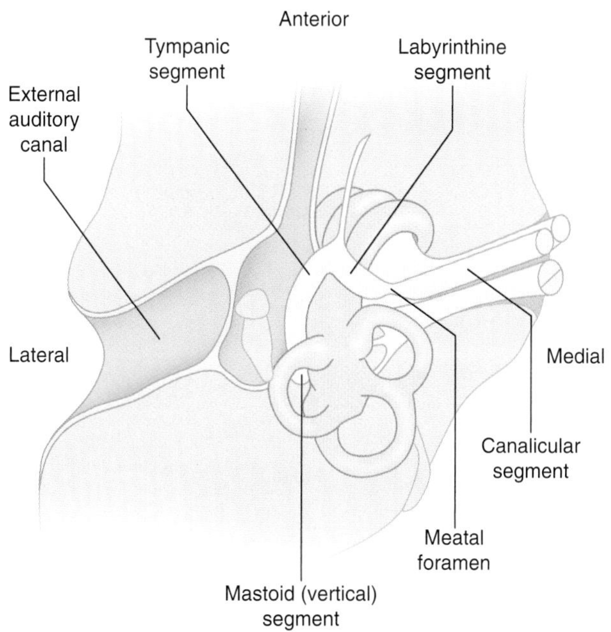

FIGURE 172-1. Relationships of cranial nerve VII to the inner and middle ear. [Adapted with permission from Lalwani AK (ed): *Current Diagnosis & Treatment in Otolaryngology-Head & Neck Surgery*, 3rd ed. McGraw-Hill, Inc., 2012. Sect XVI Facial Nerve Chapter 70. Figure 70-3, Part A.]

A number of viral infections and other disorders have been associated with Bell's palsy (e.g., mumps, Epstein-Barr virus, rubella, Lyme disease; see later discussion) but are suspected by associated signs and symptoms.

Treatment and Disposition Treatment with corticosteroids increases the frequency of complete recovery.[3] The dose of prednisone is 1 milligram/kg per day PO for 7 days. There is no benefit from antiviral medications, either alone or in addition to steroid therapy.[4] There is insufficient evidence to support acute surgical decompression. The greatest risk to patients with facial paralysis is corneal abrasions and keratitis due to eyelid weakness and incomplete eye closure. Patch the affected eye if there is incomplete closure, and provide instructions for ophthalmology follow-up to determine when the patch can be removed. Make sure there is no lid movement under the eye patch. Provide patients with ocular lubricants, including a tear replacement for daytime and a more viscous topical lubricant for sleep.

Most patients begin to recover within 3 weeks, but about 15% will have permanent paralysis. Ensure follow-up within 7 days with a primary care physician or ear, nose, and throat specialist.

RAMSEY HUNT SYNDROME (HERPES ZOSTER OTICUS)

Ramsey Hunt syndrome is a herpes zoster infection of the geniculate ganglion. Signs and symptoms include unilateral facial nerve palsy, severe pain, and a vesicular eruption on the face. Ramsey Hunt syndrome may be indistinguishable from Bell's palsy if paralysis precedes the vesicular eruption. Cranial nerve VIII may also be involved with associated vertigo, nausea, and hearing loss. As opposed to classic Bell's palsy, when active herpes zoster is suspected, treatment is with both steroids (prednisone 1 milligram/kg per day PO for 7 days) and antivirals (famciclovir 500 mg PO three times a day for 7 days or valacyclovir 1 gram PO three times a day for 7 days).[5]

ACUTE NEUROPATHIES OF LYME DISEASE

Lyme disease may cause a broad range of nervous system disease, both peripheral and central, acute and chronic. Consider Lyme disease as the causative agent in patients who have facial palsy with erythema migrans, tick bite, or arthritis. Some patients will have bilateral facial palsy. Multifocal Lyme polyradiculopathy may occur in the acute phase of Lyme infection. Signs and symptoms include burning and painful neuropathy, plexopathy, and other mononeuropathies.

Diagnosis is based on history of tick bite and a physical examination that uncovers an attached tick or erythema chronicum migrans rash (see Figure 251-18). If CSF is obtained, it will show the mononuclear pleocytosis typical of Lyme infection. Treatment is with doxycycline 100 milligrams twice daily for 14 to 21 days. Facial nerve palsies in Lyme disease represent the secondary stage of illness and require 1 month of treatment with doxycycline (100 milligrams PO twice a day) or amoxicillin, cefuroxime, ceftriaxone, or azithromycin.

FOCAL MONONEUROPATHIES

Focal mononeuropathies are most likely due to focal nerve compression, although systemic processes may also lead to mononeuropathy. Diabetes is the most common systemic cause of noncompressive focal neuropathy. Focal mononeuropathy can occur at any point of compression along the course of a peripheral nerve, but most commonly occurs along the ulnar, median, radial, lateral femoral cutaneous, and peroneal nerves.

MEDIAN MONONEUROPATHY (CARPAL TUNNEL SYNDROME)

The most common form of any focal mononeuropathy is median mononeuropathy, or carpal tunnel syndrome. Carpal tunnel syndrome results from compression of the median nerve at the wrist where it traverses the carpal tunnel. The boundaries of the carpal tunnel are the carpal bones and the flexor retinaculum. The most common etiology is injury due to repetitive use, but other causes include diabetes mellitus, pregnancy, amyloidosis, obesity, renal failure, rheumatoid arthritis, hypothyroidism, trauma, and edema.

Clinical Features The classic signs of carpal tunnel syndrome are pain, paresthesias, and numbness in the distribution of the median nerve—the palmar aspect of the thumb, index, middle, and radial aspect of the fourth finger. Patients may report symptoms in the entire hand, but careful examination will reveal preserved sensation in the fifth and ulnar fourth digits. Symptoms are worsened by extension and flexion of the wrist and are worse at night. Weakness and wasting of the muscles of the thenar eminence may be noted on exam.

Diagnosis Provocative testing, such as Tinel's sign and Phalen's maneuvers, can confirm the diagnosis of carpal tunnel syndrome (**Figure 172-2**). **Tinel's sign** detects irritated nerves by percussing over the nerve and eliciting tingling. Tapping on the palmar aspect of the wrist will result in an electric shock sensation shooting into the hand when there is compression of the median nerve. **Phalen's maneuver** is positive for carpal tunnel syndrome when holding the wrists in flexion for 60 seconds evokes or worsens symptoms. Electrodiagnostic testing demonstrates slowing of nerve conduction across the carpal tunnel. Testing is typically performed on an outpatient basis to confirm the diagnosis or to aid in the decision for operative repair.

Treatment and Disposition The initial treatment of carpal tunnel syndrome is conservative. Encourage evaluation of workplace ergonomics. Provide a wrist splint, with the wrist in neutral position (**Figure 172-3**). Nonsteroidal anti-inflammatory drugs are often given. Refer to a hand surgeon if splinting is not effective, for steroid injection and consideration for surgical repair.

ULNAR MONONEUROPATHY (CUBITAL TUNNEL SYNDROME AND GUYON'S CANAL SYNDROME)

The ulnar nerve extends from the medial cord of the brachial plexus and courses through the cubital tunnel behind the medial epicondyle at the elbow before entering the forearm. At the wrist, it passes through Guyon's canal, bounded by the hamate and pisiform bones and the ligament connecting them. It supplies cutaneous innervation to the medial palm via the superficial terminal branch and to the fifth and medial fourth

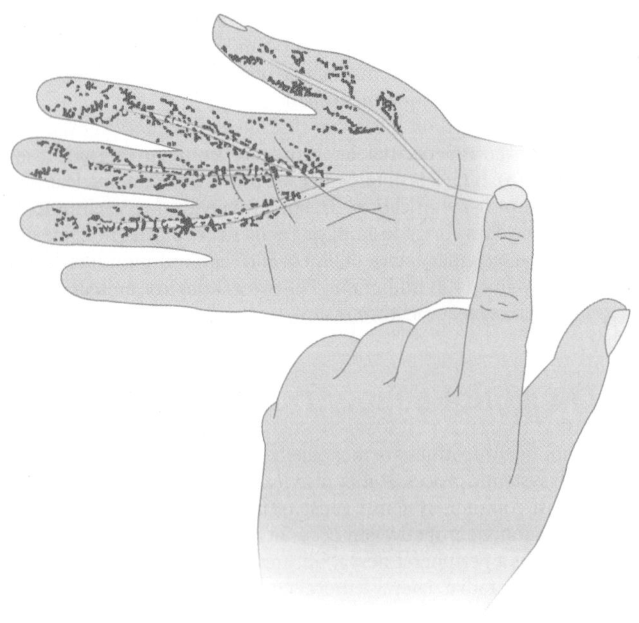

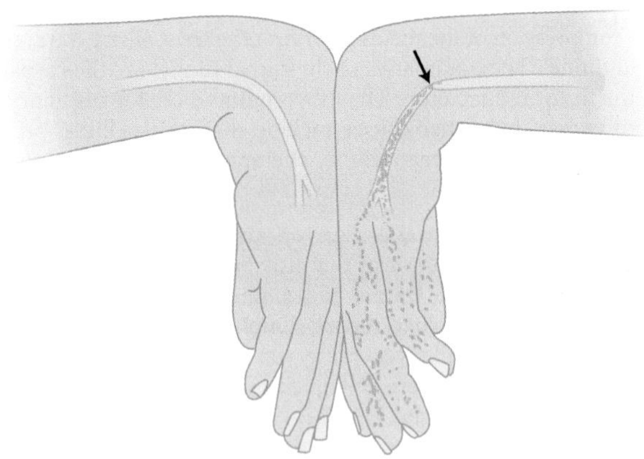

FIGURE 172-2. **A.** Tinel's sign for median nerve compression. The Tinel test is performed by tapping the volar surface of the wrist over the median nerve. **B.** Phalen's maneuver. Phalen's maneuver is performed by compressing the opposing dorsal surfaces of the hands with the wrists flexed together as shown. This causes tingling over the median nerve distribution. [Reproduced with permission from Simon RR, Sherman SC, Koenigsknecht SJ: Wrist. In: *Emergency Orthopedics: The Extremities, 5th ed.* © 2007, McGraw-Hill Inc., New York.)

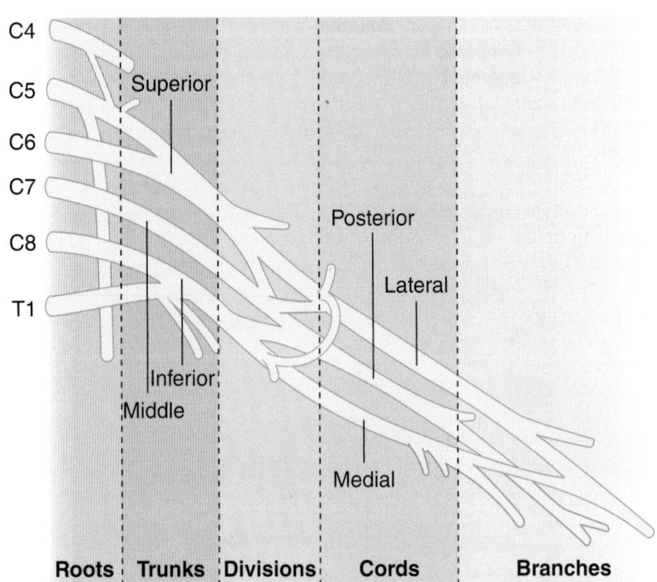

FIGURE 172-3. The anatomy of the brachial plexus. [Reproduced with permission from Reichman EF, Tolson DR: Regional nerve blocks, in Reichman EF, Simon RR (eds): *Emergency Medicine Procedures*. New York, McGraw-Hill, 2004.]

fingers via the deep terminal branch and innervates the palmaris brevis muscle. The ulnar nerve is most vulnerable to repetitive stress, inflammation, and trauma in the cubital tunnel and at Guyon's canal.

Cubital tunnel syndrome is the most common ulnar mononeuropathy and the second most common compressive mononeuropathy. It results from pressure on the ulnar nerve at the medial epicondyle.

Guyon's canal syndrome is caused by entrapment of the ulnar nerve in Guyon's canal of the wrist. It is also called **"handlebar palsy,"** because it occurs in cyclists from prolonged compression of the wrist against the handlebars.

Clinical Features The classic symptoms of ulnar mononeuropathy include tingling in the fifth and lateral fourth fingers. With time, numbness and weakness of the intrinsic muscles of the hand develop. In severe cases, paralysis and wasting of the intrinsic muscles of the hand may occur.

Diagnosis Provocative testing is useful. Ulnar compression is possible if tapping on the cubital tunnel at the elbow provokes symptoms. A positive elbow flexion sign is seen when symptoms recur within 3 minutes of the elbow being held in flexion with the wrist in extension. **Froment's sign** is an inability of the thumb to oppose or put pressure against the index finger. To perform this test, ask the patient to hold a piece of paper between thumb and index finger. If you can pull the paper away or the thumb flexes at the interphalangeal joint to compensate for weakness of the adductor pollicis brevis, the test is positive. In the patient with suspected **cubital tunnel syndrome**, consider C8 entrapment and thoracic outlet syndrome. C8 entrapment can be differentiated by the presence of neck pain and worsening symptoms with neck flexion. Thoracic outlet syndrome worsens with shoulder abduction. Electrodiagnostic testing serves to precisely localize the lesion. In Guyon's canal syndrome, or handlebar palsy, compression of the ulnar nerve is more likely to spare sensory fibers that branch off before the canal. It presents as intrinsic weakness without sensory symptoms. Diagnosis of Guyon's canal syndrome is difficult, and MRI can sometimes aid in diagnosis.

Treatment and Disposition In most cases of ulnar nerve mononeuropathy, the goal of treatment in the ED is to initiate conservative treatment and to ensure proper diagnosis and appropriate follow-up, usually with an orthopedist. Pain is not a common component of this syndrome, but anti-inflammatory medication may alleviate symptoms. Reduce repetitive use at work and home, and eliminate habits that cause pressure on the elbow or wrist.

DEEP PERONEAL NERVE ENTRAPMENT

The deep peroneal nerve may become entrapped at three locations along its course: the fibular head, anterior to the ankle joint as it passes beneath the extensor retinaculum (anterior tarsal tunnel syndrome), and distal to this point. Compression of the deep peroneal nerve may result from proximal fibular fracture or habitual crossing of the legs. Patients develop foot drop or numbness of the web between the great and second toes. Conservative treatment is recommended initially—provide a splint or brace to maintain the foot at a right angle with the leg. Prompt follow-up with a neurologist is important because nerve conduction studies should be performed to differentiate this syndrome from lumbar root or motor neuron disease.

MERALGIA PARESTHETICA

Meralgia paresthetica is entrapment of the lateral femoral cutaneous nerve in the inguinal canal. Entrapment causes numbness and pain of the anterolateral thigh. The cause can be pelvic (pregnancy, enlarging mass, aneurysm), extrapelvic (trauma, tight garment or belt, obesity), or systemic (diabetes). On examination, the patient may complain of hyperesthesia in the area of pain, and Tinel's sign may be evident when percussing over the anterior superior iliac spine. The **pelvic compression test** also supports this diagnosis: turn the patient on his or her side, compress the pelvis, and if the patient's symptoms are relieved after 30 seconds of lateral compression of the pelvis, the diagnosis is confirmed.

Conservative management with nonsteroidal anti-inflammatory drugs, weight loss, relief from tight garments, and physiotherapy is usually successful. Local injection of lidocaine and corticosteroid near the insertion of the inguinal ligament into the anterior superior iliac spine provides relief. Surgical decompression or nerve resection may be required for relief of symptoms.

PLEXOPATHIES

The cervical, brachial, and lumbosacral plexuses are formed by the convergence of nerve roots, which then branch into peripheral nerves. In the case of the brachial plexus, the process of mixing and dividing is repeated in the stages of trunks and cords before peripheral nerves take off. Plexopathies share many of the same causes, the most common being trauma, surgery, neoplasm, and radiation therapy. Despite this similarity, plexopathies differ significantly in diagnosis and management.

BRACHIAL PLEXOPATHY

The brachial plexus, formed by the C5-T1 nerve roots, is the most common site of plexopathy. The brachial plexus is made complex by the nerve roots merging into upper middle and lower trunks, which split and merge into lateral posterior and medial cords that split again and form five peripheral nerves (see Figure 172-3). Injury at each of these anatomic locations will result in differing symptoms. Brachial plexopathies generally manifest as weakness first, but pain and paresthesias may also develop. On examination, the patient has weakness in various distributions of the brachial plexus. The upper trunk is the more common site of involvement, affecting strength of proximal arm and shoulder musculature. Infraclavicular plexopathy due to trauma is frequently associated with injury to the axillary vessels. Causes of brachial plexopathy include trauma (penetrating trauma, humeral neck fracture, severe traction injury, or dislocation), shoulder reduction, neoplasm (Pancoast tumor), radiation, or surgery. A **"burner"** is burning pain involving one upper extremity, sometimes with numbness, paresthesias, or weakness, occurring after trauma to the neck and shoulder. It can occur in football players and other athletes during sports. A burner can be a brachial plexopathy, caused by traction to the shoulder or an injury to the cervical nerve roots caused by neck flexion-hyperextension. Brachial plexopathies can also result from cervical rib compression, midshaft clavicular fracture, or penetrating trauma. Assessment consists of careful neurologic examination, spine imaging, and consultation with neurology, neurosurgery, or orthopedics, depending on the specific injury identified.

LUMBOSACRAL PLEXOPATHY

The L1-S4 nerve roots form the lumbosacral plexus. Causes of lumbosacral plexopathy are less likely traumatic and more likely to include radiation, diabetic amyotrophy, aortic aneurysm, retroperitoneal hemorrhage, or compression from arteriovenous malformations. The differential diagnosis also includes the **cauda equina and conus medullaris syndromes**. Lesions affecting the lumbar portion of the plexus result in weakness of hip adduction and flexion and knee extension, decreased sensation at the top and inner thigh, and decreased patellar reflexes. Lesions affecting the sacral portion of the plexus result in inability to abduct the thigh at the hip joint, weakness of hip extension and knee flexion, and decreased sensation of the back of the thigh and below the knee. Plain radiographs of the lumbar spine are useful to screen for spine compression from degenerative or neoplastic disease. Perform MRI when cord injury or compression is considered. See chapter 279, Neck and Back Pain, for detailed discussion of epidural compression syndromes, cauda equina syndrome, and conus medullaris syndrome. CT of the abdomen will exclude aortic aneurysm, psoas muscle masses, and retroperitoneal hemorrhage, which also present with asymmetric lower extremity weakness. Management of plexopathies is usually directed at the underlying cause.

CERVICAL PLEXOPATHY

The cervical plexus, formed by the C1-C4 nerve roots, is the least common plexopathy. Apart from trauma or neoplasm, the condition is occasionally seen postoperatively due to positioning during surgery. Patients may have few symptoms. Neoplastic lesions may cause a deep boring and constant pain. Due to anatomic parameters, electrodiagnostic assessment is difficult and unreliable. Order a CT or MRI scan if a neoplastic process is considered. The management of cervical plexopathy is usually nonoperative.

NEUROMUSCULAR JUNCTION DISORDERS

BOTULISM

Botulism is a toxin-mediated neuromuscular junction disorder that causes acute weakness leading to respiratory failure. In 2010, the Centers for Disease Control and Prevention reported 112 cases of botulism. Of these, 76% were infantile botulism, 15% were wound botulism, and 8% were food borne.[6] Botulism affects infants between the ages of 1 week and 11 months and has been implicated as a cause of sudden infant death syndrome. The causative organism, *Clostridium botulinum*, is an anaerobic spore-forming bacterium found in soil and honey. In suitable environments, these spores germinate and release toxin that irreversibly binds the presynaptic membrane of peripheral and cranial nerves, inhibiting the release of acetylcholine at the peripheral nerve synapse. Three of the eight known toxins, types A, B, and E, produced by *C. botulinum* cause human disease. The most commonly implicated is toxin A, which is also used cosmetically in injection form. Most cases of botulism are isolated events associated with improperly preserved canned foods. In adults, botulism results from ingestion of preformed toxin. Infantile botulism occurs due to ingestion of spores that germinate in the higher pH of the infant GI tract. Botulism can result from wound infections, mostly occurring in injection drug users. In 2010, every reported case of wound botulism but one was due to injection drug use.[7] Toxin type E is associated with preserved or fermented fish and marine mammals, and the latter are the most important sources of botulism in Alaska, Japan, Russia, and Scandinavia. *C. botulinum* is classified as a category A bioweapon by the Centers for Disease Control and Prevention, among the most lethal.[7]

Clinical Features Onset of symptoms occurs 6 to 48 hours after the poisoning with toxin. Patients experience nausea, vomiting, abdominal cramps, and diarrhea or constipation, which may easily be misdiagnosed as an acute gastroenteritis. **Classically, botulism produces a descending, symmetric paralysis.** Since the disorder is at the neuromuscular junction, there is no sensory deficit and no pain. The muscles first affected are the cranial nerves and bulbar muscles. The patient presents with diplopia, dysarthria, and dysphagia and may report blurred vision. Deep tendon reflexes are normal or diminished. Toxin-mediated decrease in cholinergic output causes anticholinergic symptoms, such as constipation, urinary retention, dry skin and eyes, and hyperthermia. **Pupils are often dilated and nonreactive to light.** Pupillary findings provide an important point of differentiation from myasthenia gravis, which does not affect the pupil. Infantile botulism presents as constipation, poor feeding, lethargy, and weak cry; consequently, this diagnosis must be in the differential of the "floppy" infant.

Diagnosis The diagnosis of botulism is made based on clinical findings and exclusion of other processes. The toxin can be identified in both serum and stool, but the assay is not commonly available. If the suspected food source is available, it should be tested for toxin.

Treatment and Disposition Initial treatment is supportive. Secure the airway if there is respiratory compromise. In several retrospective cohort studies, botulinum equine antitoxin was associated with decreased number of days on the ventilator and in the hospital, and it is most effective when used early.[7] The Centers for Disease Control and Prevention recommend giving one 10-mL vial of trivalent equine antitoxin as soon as the diagnosis is made. Human botulism immunoglobulin has been shown to decrease mechanical ventilation requirements and length of intensive care unit and hospital stays.[9]

Patients diagnosed with botulism require admission to the intensive care unit and intubation for respiratory failure. Report suspected cases to the local health department so that further exposures can be prevented.

TICK PARALYSIS

Tick paralysis, or tick toxicosis, is an uncommon disease caused by a poorly defined neurotoxin secreted in the saliva of several tick species. It is most common in spring and summer and in the Pacific Northwest, western, and southeastern states. Most cases are in children.

Clinical Features Initially, 4 to 7 days after tick attachment, patients experience nonspecific influenza-like symptoms including malaise and weakness. These symptoms progress to ataxia and then an **ascending weakness and paralysis** without sensory involvement. Infants and children may be listless or irritable. When the bulbar nerves and diaphragm become involved, respiratory failure ensues.

Diagnosis Tick paralysis is diagnosed based on typical symptoms and when the culprit tick is located. **Perform a complete body search for ticks before initiating treatment for other possible diagnoses.** The most common tick attachment site is the scalp. If no tick is found, the differential diagnosis of acute ataxia and ascending flaccid paralysis without sensory involvement includes Guillain-Barré syndrome, botulism, spinal cord tumor, and poliomyelitis.

Misdiagnosis of tick paralysis can lead to failure to find and remove the tick and unnecessary therapies such as central venous access, plasma exchange, and IV immunoglobulin. Tick paralysis and Guillain-Barré syndrome are indistinguishable even with nerve conduction studies.[10]

Treatment and Disposition Treatment involves complete removal of the attached tick. Remove ticks by taking hold of the very head of the tick with tweezers and applying gentle steady traction.

Admit patients with respiratory distress to the intensive care unit, and admit all patients to the hospital to ensure symptoms do not progress. Local wound care and supportive care (including intubation and mechanical ventilation if necessary) result in excellent recovery within hours to days.[10]

INFLAMMATORY MYOPATHIES

Although not acute peripheral neurologic lesions, polymyositis and dermatomyositis present with similar symptoms to many peripheral neuropathies. These diseases are rare inflammatory myopathies causing symmetric weakness that progresses over weeks to months.

Clinical Features Patients develop weakness of the proximal limbs, trunk, and neck. Some experience dysphagia, myalgias, and rarely dyspnea when the respiratory muscles become involved. Sensation and reflexes are normal, and the ocular muscles are usually spared. Occasionally cardiac muscle may be involved with cardiomyopathy, heart failure, and conduction disturbances. The findings of dermatomyositis are similar with the addition of a diffuse violaceous rash often on the face and trunk.

Diagnosis Diagnosis is mainly clinical, but certain laboratory findings are characteristic such as elevated erythrocyte sedimentation rate, elevated creatinine kinase, and leukocytosis. The differential diagnosis includes Lambert-Eaton syndrome, endocrinopathies, toxic myopathies, and infectious myopathies.

Treatment and Disposition To prevent irreversible muscle damage, both polymyositis and dermatomyositis require treatment with systemic corticosteroids or other immunosuppressants.

Admit patients with rhabdomyolysis, respiratory distress, or profound weakness. Otherwise, patients may be discharged with neurology or rheumatology follow-up within 7 days.

SUBACUTE AND ACUTE ON CHRONIC PERIPHERAL NERVE LESIONS

Neuropathies can also be associated with an underlying medical disorder, such as HIV and diabetes.

HUMAN IMMUNODEFICIENCY VIRUS–ASSOCIATED PERIPHERAL NEUROLOGIC DISEASE

HIV infection, its complications, and its pharmacologic treatments are associated with a number of peripheral neurologic disorders. The most common of these, HIV neuropathy and antiretroviral drug–induced neuropathy, are chronic processes that do not cause sudden disability or symptoms. HIV-infected patients have a high rate of mononeuritis multiplex and an inflammatory myopathy resembling polymyositis. In late-stage acquired immunodeficiency syndrome, almost all patients manifest neuropathy. Patients in the early stages of HIV infection have greater susceptibility to Guillain-Barré syndrome. The presentation is similar to that of the non–HIV-infected patient. Treatment is the same as in non-HIV Guillain-Barré syndrome, with an emphasis on identifying patients who are likely to need intubation and mechanical ventilation early in the ED stay followed by close monitoring of respiratory function.

CYTOMEGALOVIRUS RADICULITIS

In the latter stages of acquired immunodeficiency syndrome, cytomegalovirus may acutely infect the lumbosacral nerve roots, causing a polyradiculopathy or cauda equina syndrome. Evidence of systemic cytomegalovirus infection, including retinitis, is almost always present. As opposed to the more common chronic neuropathy of HIV, patients with cytomegalovirus radiculitis become acutely weak, with primarily lower extremity involvement, and may have variable degrees of bowel and bladder dysfunction. The examination shows primarily lower extremity weakness and hyporeflexia, with decreased sensation in the lower extremities and groin. Rectal tone may be impaired. Lumbar puncture reveals a pleocytosis with predominantly polymorphonuclear cells and modestly increased protein. Viral DNA is detected by polymerase chain reaction in most patients and is highly specific. MRI of the lumbosacral spine demonstrates swelling and clumping of the cauda equina. Imaging is recommended to exclude mass lesions of the lower spine or nerve roots. Early identification is important, as antiviral treatment is effective. The treatment of cytomegalovirus radiculitis is IV ganciclovir, started at 5 milligrams/kg every 12 hours for 3 to 6 weeks. Treatment can be initiated before definitive diagnosis.

DIABETIC PERIPHERAL NEUROPATHY

Diabetes mellitus remains the most common cause of noncompressive focal neuropathy. A variety of mechanisms contribute to the pathophysiology of diabetic neuropathy. Chronic hyperglycemia and glycemic variability lead to oxidative stress and neuroinflammatory processes that result in a variety of neuropathic syndromes.

Diabetic peripheral neuropathy is the term used for any neuropathy in a type 1 or type 2 diabetic patient. The most common manifestation of diabetic peripheral neuropathy is a distal symmetric polyneuropathy, but it may also lead to focal neuropathies and mononeuropathy multiplex. Diabetic peripheral neuropathy is an example of a distal axonopathy resulting in length-dependent, centripetal "dying back" of the affected nerves. This phenomenon produces the typical stocking and glove distribution of diabetic neuropathy.

Hyperglycemic neuropathy is seen in newly diagnosed diabetics and normally improves with glycemic control. Insulin neuritis is a reversible condition characterized by acute limb pain and paresthesias associated with rapid glycemic control with insulin. Painful diabetic neuropathy is usually intermittent and worse at night. It can be experienced variably as pins and needles, throbbing, burning, achy, or cramping. Duration is less than 6 months. After 6 months, the same process is termed chronic painful diabetic neuropathy. Diabetic neuropathic cachexia is a rare syndrome causing weight loss and painful dysesthesias of the limbs and trunk.

Diabetic amyotrophy is a lumbosacral plexopathy seen in patients with a long-standing history of diabetes and presents with back pain followed by weakness. Patients report the acute onset of ipsilateral back pain, followed within days by progressive leg weakness. Sensory findings are absent. The examination reveals decreased leg power in a variety of patterns reflecting impairment of plexus function with relatively

TABLE 172-4 Medications Used in the Treatment of Painful Diabetic Neuropathy

Class	Starting Dose	Notes
Anticonvulsants	Pregabalin, 50 milligrams three times daily	May cause somnolence, dizziness, weight gain
	Gabapentin, 300 milligrams at bedtime	Similar adverse effects to pregabalin
Antidepressants	Duloxetine, 30 milligrams daily	Consider with concomitant depression
	Desipramine, 10–25 milligrams before bedtime	Tricyclic antidepressant with fewest side effects
Topical therapy	Capsaicin, 0.075% up to four times daily	Apply using gloved hand Cut in half to save cost
	Lidocaine, 5% two to four patches daily	
Opioids	Oxycodone CR®, 10 milligrams twice daily	May cause constipation, somnolence
	Tramadol, 50 milligrams twice daily	Avoid in patients with seizure or on selective serotonin reuptake inhibitor

symmetric sensation. There may be muscle wasting in affected limbs in long-standing disease. Deep tendon reflexes may be diminished on the affected side. Bowel and bladder functions are not affected.

There is a clear relationship between glycemic control and neuropathy. The Diabetes Control and Complications Trial demonstrated a 60% reduction in risk of developing neuropathy with tight glycemic control, which persisted for 8 years.[11] Emphasize strict foot care to the diabetic who has already developed neuropathy. Neuropathy-associated anesthesia may result in inadvertent trauma and subsequent development of ulcers, cellulitis, fasciitis, osteomyelitis, and eventual amputation. Symptomatic management is an ED patient's most immediate concern. Nonsteroidal anti-inflammatory drugs are ineffective in treating neuropathic pain and are relatively contraindicated in the diabetic patient due to their renal and cardiac effects. Narcotics carry addictive potential. Tricyclic antidepressants, anticonvulsants, and topical capsaicin all have proven beneficial (**Table 172-4**). Best evidence supports the use of duloxetine, venlafaxine, amitriptyline pregabalin, gabapentin valproate, tramadol, or oxycodone.[12]

Acknowledgment: The authors gratefully acknowledge the contributions of Andy Jagoda, MD, who authored this chapter in the 7th edition.

REFERENCES

The complete reference list is available online at www.TintinalliEM.com.

Chronic Neurologic Disorders

Daniel A. Handel
Sarah Andrus Gaines

AMYOTROPHIC LATERAL SCLEROSIS

Amyotrophic lateral sclerosis (ALS), often called *Lou Gehrig's disease*, causes rapidly progressive muscle atrophy and weakness resulting from the degeneration of both upper and lower motor neurons. ALS leads to varying degrees of spasticity, hyperreflexia, and muscle paralysis, eventually resulting in pulmonary complications and the need for mechanical ventilatory support. Because there is no cure, clinicians attempt to slow disease progression and preserve function as much as possible. Medical management is directed at preventing pulmonary infections and forestalling terminal respiratory failure.

PATHOPHYSIOLOGY

Since 2009, 13 genes and loci have been identified that are associated with the disease.[1] Inclusions in the TAR DNA-binding protein-43 have been found in both ALS and frontotemporal dementia.[2] Environmental exposures are suspected to increase the risk of ALS, but no specific ones have been identified to date.[3]

Gross CNS pathology includes frontal cortical atrophy, degeneration of both the corticospinal and spinocerebellar tracts, a reduction in large cervical and lumbar motor neurons, and cranial nerve nuclei degeneration. Both motor and sensory peripheral nerves undergo axonal degeneration and segmental demyelination, including motor end plate and axon terminal involvement.

CLINICAL FEATURES

Upper motor neuron demyelination and dysfunction cause limb spasticity, hyperreflexia (including Babinski sign and a brisk jaw-jerk reflex), and emotional lability. Limb weakness, a lower motor neuron dysfunction, is the first symptom in 65% of patients.[4] Other associated lower motor neuron dysfunctions include atrophy, cramps, fasciculations, dysarthria, dysphagia, and difficulty in mastication. At the time of initial presentation, asymmetric extremity cramping, fatigue, weakness, muscle fasciculations, and atrophy can be seen, especially in the upper extremities.[5] Facial weakness, dysarthria, tongue weakness, atrophy, and fasciculations can be seen with bulbar lower motor neuron dysfunction. Despite these profound motor findings, sensory and cognitive function is usually spared. Regardless of the initial symptoms, widespread motor and respiratory dysfunction progresses within weeks to months. Significant extremity atrophy occurs, as well as fasciculations, hyperreflexia, foot drop, and claw deformity of the hand. Patients also may develop monotonous speech caused by tongue atrophy, despite the relative sparing of facial and eye movements. Some patients eventually diagnosed as having ALS present initially with cervical or back pain consistent with an acute compressive radiculopathy. Despite successful operative intervention, significant muscle wasting consistent with motor neuron dysfunction develops shortly after the procedure.[6] **Progressive respiratory muscle weakness initially causes exertional dyspnea and eventual dyspnea at rest.** Overt dementia and parkinsonism may occur in up to 15% of patients, especially those with ALS. Other cognitive problems, such as apathy, poor attention and motivation, and altered social skills, may be noted.

DIAGNOSIS

The clinical diagnosis of ALS is suggested when there are signs of both upper and lower motor neuron dysfunction, including weakness, muscle atrophy, fasciculations, and hyporeflexia without other CNS dysfunction.[7] Given the complexity of diagnosing ALS, the median time to diagnosis is 14 months.[1] ALS-like symptoms can be seen with other systemic illnesses, such as diabetes, dysproteinemia, thyroid and parathyroid dysfunction, vitamin B_{12} deficiency, heavy metal toxicity, and vasculitis, as well as CNS and spinal cord tumors. The diagnosis requires the exclusion of other inflammatory neuropathies, such as myasthenia gravis. Refer patients with signs suggesting ALS to a neurologist for definitive diagnosis. The Amyotrophic Lateral Sclerosis Functional Rating Scale (revised) is reliable for diagnosis of ALS.[8] Electromyography, nerve conduction velocity studies, spinal fluid analysis, and neuromuscular biopsies are useful diagnostic studies. MRI excludes other disease processes but does not confirm the diagnosis of ALS.[9]

TREATMENT

Therapy is designed to enhance muscle function, especially those that support breathing, swallowing, and speech, in order to avoid malnutrition, recurrent aspiration, or choking. Riluzole, which modulates the excitotoxin glutamate, may prolong survival.[10-13] It is most useful in patients with a clear diagnosis of ALS whose symptoms have been present for <5 years, with a forced vital capacity >60% of predicted, who do not have a tracheostomy. Guidelines on care and treatment of ALS patients are available.[12,13]

Optimizing pulmonary function, including the eventual use of long-term assisted ventilation, is an important part of enhancing the quality of life as diaphragm weakness progresses.[12] Many ALS patients will find some benefit from regular progressive resistance exercise, which may provide an anti-inflammatory effect, a neuroendocrine effect, or beneficial effects on CNS plasticity and myofiber remodeling.[14]

DISPOSITION

Typically, patients with ALS will not present to the ED undiagnosed unless there is extremely rapid disease progression or a long period without medical care. **Emergency management usually is required for acute respiratory failure, aspiration pneumonia, choking episodes, or trauma related to extremity weakness. Blood gas determination does not reliably predict impending respiratory failure**, because mild hypoxia and hypercarbia may exist throughout the disease course. **A forced vital capacity <25 mL/kg, or a 50% decrease from predicted normal, increases the risk of aspiration pneumonia and respiratory failure.** Provide treatment to improve pulmonary function (e.g., nebulized medications, steroids, antibiotics, assisted ventilation, and intubation). Because the need for long-term ventilatory assistance rarely reverses, establish or confirm the patient's preference regarding intubation through patient and family conversation, a living will, or power of attorney for health care. Hospital admission is indicated with impending respiratory failure, pneumonia, the inability to control secretions, or a worsening overall status that requires social service intervention for long-term placement.

MYASTHENIA GRAVIS

Myasthenia gravis is an autoimmune disease characterized by muscle weakness and fatigue, which is seen especially with repetitive use of voluntary muscles. Acetylcholine receptor antibodies impair receptor function at the neuromuscular junction, causing muscle weakness, most often in proximal muscles. This weakness is generally relieved by rest and requires long-term immunotherapy. The diagnosis of cholinergic and myasthenic crises and the aggressive management of respiratory complications associated with a myasthenic crisis are the most important issues for the ED management of myasthenia gravis patients. Occasionally a first diagnosis of myasthenia gravis can be suspected in the ED if increasing muscle weakness is noted during the ED stay or is reported by the patient to occur over the day.

PATHOPHYSIOLOGY

In the normal neuromuscular junction, acetylcholine release by the nerve fiber causes a localized end plate potential that leads to muscle fiber contraction. In myasthenia gravis, there is a marked decrease in the number and function of the muscle fiber acetylcholine receptors, despite normal nerve anatomy and function. Failure to respond to acetylcholine stimulation causes decreased muscle fiber potential amplitudes, leading to decreased muscle strength. Acetylcholine receptor autoantibodies are seen in approximately 80% of patients.[15] These antibodies react with the acetylcholine receptor. Disease severity can be correlated with acetylcholine receptor autoantibody levels. The autoantibodies cause accelerated acetylcholine receptor degradation, dysfunction, and blockade.

Either dysfunction of the **thymus gland** or an immune response to exogenous infectious antigens causes the pathologic autoimmune response. The thymus is abnormal in most patients with myasthenia gravis, most often as thymic hyperplasia or a thymoma. Thymectomy resolves or improves the symptoms in most patients, especially those with a thymoma. It is likely that the acetylcholine receptor autoantibodies arise after exposure to similar antigens, such as those caused by herpes simplex virus or bacterial infection, causing a pathologic attack on the acetylcholine receptor proteins.

CLINICAL FEATURES

The symptoms of myasthenia gravis can mimic the symptoms seen in many other chronic neurologic disorders, and some call it "the great imitator." **Most myasthenia gravis patients have general weakness, especially of the proximal extremity muscle groups, neck extensors, and facial or bulbar muscles.** Although ptosis and diplopia are the most common presenting symptoms, limb weakness and oropharyngeal symptoms, such as dysphagia, dysarthria, dysphonia, and dyspnea, can also be seen initially or occur over time. Ocular signs can include Cogan lid twitch (in which the eyes are lowered for 10 to 20 seconds, then droop or twitch when the patient attempts to raise them); ptosis; cranial nerve III, IV, or VI weakness; gaze palsies; internuclear or complete ophthalmoplegia; and end-gaze nystagmus.[16] Symptoms can fluctuate throughout the day, usually worsening as the day progresses or with prolonged muscle group use, such as with prolonged reading or prolonged chewing during a meal. Despite the presence of profound muscle weakness, there usually is no deficit in sensory, reflex, or cerebellar functioning. **Myasthenia gravis in elderly patients can be misdiagnosed as ischemic stroke, especially when new-onset facial weakness is seen.**[17]

Although weakness is typically focal and mild to moderate in severity, rarely, undiagnosed patients with myasthenia gravis may present with extreme weakness in the muscles of respiration, resulting in respiratory failure. **This life-threatening situation, termed *myasthenic crisis*, can be seen before diagnosis or as a result of inadequate drug therapy or drug tolerance.**

DIAGNOSIS

Consider the diagnosis of myasthenia gravis in any patient who complains specifically of ocular disturbances or proximal limb muscle weakness not associated with systemic causes of generalized fatigue. Involvement of the facial muscles or muscles of mastication and swallowing may suggest myasthenia gravis, as well as the observations that the symptoms fluctuate, often worsening as the day progresses, and are alleviated by rest.[18] The differential diagnosis includes congenital myasthenia gravis, Lambert-Eaton syndrome (seen with small-cell lung tumors), drug-induced myasthenia (e.g., penicillamine, procainamide, quinines, aminoglycosides), botulism, thyroid disorders, and other causes of ocular disorders, such as intracranial mass lesions.

The diagnosis is established through the administration of edrophonium chloride (an acetylcholinesterase inhibitor); electromyography, which demonstrates a postsynaptic neuromuscular junctional dysfunction with repetitive nerve stimulation; and serologic testing for acetylcholine receptor antibodies. **In the presence of abnormal neuromuscular transmission, edrophonium or neostigmine is expected to improve muscle strength in objectively weak limb, ocular, and pharyngeal muscles.** Because these drugs can actually cause profound weakness in the presence of other disorders that impair neuromuscular transmission, be prepared to provide ventilatory support or perform endotracheal intubation as a complication of pharmacologic testing. Electromyographic testing with repetitive nerve stimulation demonstrates a rapid reduction in the size of the muscle action potential, a finding that correlates with the clinical observation of enhanced weakness with prolonged or repetitive muscle use.

TREATMENT

Treatment includes administration of the acetylcholinesterase inhibitors pyridostigmine or neostigmine, thymectomy, chronic immune suppression with corticosteroids or azathioprine, and acute immune modulation using plasma exchange or IV immunoglobulin when indicated.[19-21] A favorable response to thymectomy can occur in patients with a thymoma, a limited response to acetylcholinesterase inhibitor therapy, and a short time interval between diagnosis and operative intervention.[22,23] Most patients show improvement with oral corticosteroids in the short term, although high-dose steroids sometimes result first in more weakness before improvement. Azathioprine or mycophenolate[24] can supplement chronic oral steroid therapy and lowers the steroid dose.[24,25] Severe symptoms, such as those that would require hospital admission, might require the use of IV immunoglobulin[26,27] or a combination of high-dose steroids and plasma exchange.

TABLE 173-1 Drugs to Avoid in Myasthenia Gravis

Steroids	Adrenocorticotropic hormone,* methylprednisolone,* prednisone*
Anticonvulsants	Phenytoin, ethosuximide, trimethadione, paraldehyde, magnesium sulfate, barbiturates, lithium
Antimalarials	Chloroquine,* quinine*
IV fluids	Sodium lactate solution
Antibiotics	Aminoglycosides, fluoroquinolones,* neomycin,* streptomycin,* kanamycin,* gentamicin, tobramycin, dihydrostreptomycin,* amikacin, polymyxin A, polymyxin B, sulfonamides, viomycin, colistimethate,* lincomycin, clindamycin, tetracycline, oxytetracycline, rolitetracycline, macrolides, metronidazole
Psychotropics	Chlorpromazine,* lithium carbonate,* amitriptyline, droperidol, haloperidol, imipramine
Antirheumatics	D-Penicillamine, colchicine, chloroquine
Cardiovascular	Quinidine,* procainamide,* β-blockers (propranolol, oxprenolol, practolol, pindolol, sotalol), lidocaine, trimethaphan; magnesium; calcium channel blockers (verapamil)
Local anesthetics	Lidocaine,* procaine,*
Analgesics	Narcotics (morphine, hydromorphone, codeine, Pantopon, meperidine)
Endocrine	Thyroid replacement*
Eye drops	Timolol,* echothiophate
Others	Amantadine, diphenhydramine, emetine, diuretics, muscle relaxants, central nervous system depressants, respiratory depressants, sedatives, procaine,* phenothiazines
Neuromuscular blocking agents	Tubocurarine, pancuronium, rocuronium, gallamine, dimethyl tubocurarine, succinylcholine, decamethonium

Note: See also discussion on eMedicine from WebMD by William D. Goldenberg, MD, available at: http://emedicine.medscape.com/article/793136-overview#a1.

*Case reports implicate drugs in exacerbations of myasthenia gravis

Muscle weakness usually does not return to normal even with the use of immunomodulators. Variability in the amount of muscle weakness occurs in response to asthma exacerbations, infections, menstruation, pregnancy, emotional stress, hot weather, and other disorders that alter the response to medication, such as pulmonary, renal, and GI disease.

Many drugs used in the ED affect neuromuscular function—especially common antibiotics (**Table 173-1**). Make sure that myasthenia gravis patients being treated for other conditions receive their usual dose of cholinergic inhibitors, such as pyridostigmine, while waiting in the ED. The suggested pyridostigmine dose is 60 to 90 milligrams PO every 4 hours. **If a dose is missed, the next dose is usually doubled. If the patient cannot take oral medications or is intubated, administer one-thirtieth of the PO dose (2 to 3 milligrams) of pyridostigmine by slow IV infusion. The usual IV dose for neostigmine is 0.5 milligram.** Consult a neurologist to determine the optimal IV dose, rate of infusion, and timing of repeat pyridostigmine or neostigmine dosing.

TABLE 173-2 Edrophonium Testing in Myasthenia Gravis

	Myasthenic Crisis	Cholinergic Crisis
Pathology	Undermedication, decrease in acetylcholine receptor causes decreased stimulation by ACh	Overmedication, excess anticholinesterase drugs, overstimulation by ACh
Finding after edrophonium administration	Visible improvement in muscle contractibility, fusion of diplopia, or resolution of ptosis	Worsening of symptoms, muscle weakness, and possible respiratory paralysis
Implication of edrophonium test finding	Patient positive for myasthenia gravis, undermedication of anticholinesterase drugs	Overmedication has occurred, possibly due to insufficient effect from anticholinesterase drugs
Clinical treatment required based on test results	Increase in anticholinesterase drugs, such as pyridostigmine and neostigmine	Treat with atropine; if respiratory paralysis occurs, assist with ventilation

Abbreviation: ACh = acetylcholine.

The most significant ED complication of myasthenia gravis is respiratory failure, which is usually precipitated by infection, surgery, or the rapid tapering of immunosuppressive drugs. Although intubation should be considered in patients with a low forced vital capacity or in the presence of abnormal blood gas analysis, this decision is made primarily on clinical grounds. Because of the increased sensitivity of myasthenia gravis patients to neuromuscular junction inhibitors and an unpredictable reaction to succinylcholine in particular,[28] **avoid the administration of depolarizing or nondepolarizing paralytic agents** in preparation for intubation. Patients with myasthenia are extremely sensitive to these agents, and the paralytic effects can be expected to persist at least two to three times longer than in normal patients. Consider using short-acting agents such as etomidate, fentanyl, or propofol in smaller doses.[29] Intubation using deep inhalational anesthetics, including halothane, isoflurane, or sevoflurane, is also a possible strategy. If paralytic agents are absolutely necessary, consider using one-half the dose of these agents, although there are no clinical studies supporting this recommendation.

Up to 15% to 20% of myasthenia gravis patients will undergo a myasthenic crisis requiring acute emergency intervention.[30] Myasthenic crisis, which occurs either because of disease exacerbation or inadequate drug therapy, must be distinguished from cholinergic crisis, which is caused by excessive cholinergic effects of the drugs used to treat the disease. This differentiation can be made in the ED by the use of edrophonium chloride testing (**Table 173-2 and Figure 173-1**).

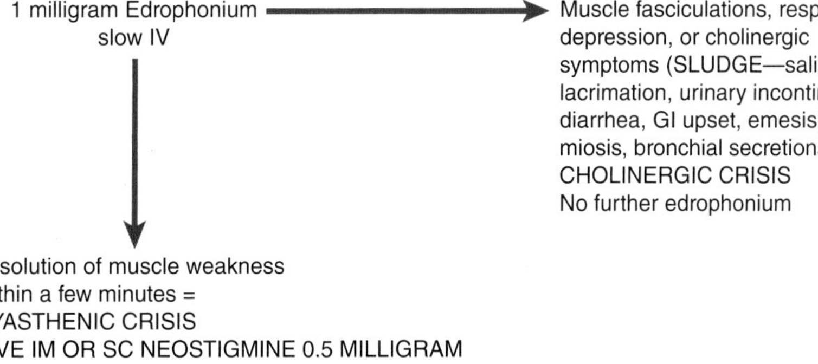

FIGURE 173-1. Edrophonium test for myasthenic versus cholinergic crisis.

Edrophonium is used for this purpose because of its rapid onset (30 seconds) and the short duration of effects (5 to 10 minutes). **A positive result, one that suggests that the symptoms are caused by a myasthenia exacerbation, is characterized by the resolution of muscle weakness within a few minutes.** To ensure that the patient does not react adversely to the edrophonium test (as a result of excessive baseline cholinergic effects), administer only 1 milligram by slow IV push initially. The development of muscle fasciculations, respiratory depression, or cholinergic symptoms within a few minutes of this test dose of edrophonium suggests that the baseline muscle weakness is related to a cholinergic crisis, rather than a myasthenic crisis, and further edrophonium administration is contraindicated. If there is no evidence of adverse cholinergic effects, up to 10 milligrams of edrophonium can then be given in order to demonstrate benefit in the face of a presumed myasthenic crisis. In other words, if the symptoms improve with the 1-milligram edrophonium test dose, then the testing is considered positive for myasthenic crisis, and additional edrophonium therapy can be provided to reverse the effects of myasthenia gravis itself. Neostigmine can then be given IM or SC in 0.5- to 2.0-milligram doses, with clinical effectiveness by 30 minutes and lasting for up to 4 hours. Alternatively, 15-milligram neostigmine tablets can be given PO, each having a clinical effect comparable with that of a 0.5-milligram parenteral neostigmine injection.

In children, the total edrophonium IV dose is 0.15 milligram/kg, not to exceed 10 milligrams. To test adverse cholinergic effects with a test dose in children, give an initial IV edrophonium dose one tenth that of the total dose. For children weighing <75 lb (34 kg), a test dose of 1 milligram is appropriate, and a total dose of 5 milligrams can be used in 1-milligram increments. In infants, or when IV access is not available in children <75 lb (34 kg), the IM edrophonium test dose is 0.5 to 2.0 milligrams.

If giving edrophonium to patients with cardiac disease, place the patient on a cardiac monitor and pulse oximetry, have the crash cart with atropine available, and have intubation equipment prepared. Edrophonium may cause bradycardia, atrioventricular block, atrial fibrillation, and cardiac arrest. Although atropine will counteract the muscarinic effects (miosis, lacrimation, salivation, bradycardia) of edrophonium, it will not reverse the nicotinic effects (skeletal muscle paralysis) of a cholinergic crisis. Acute respiratory failure can result from either acute myasthenic crisis or acute cholinergic crisis. Patients with cholinergic crisis who worsen with edrophonium test dose administration may require immediate intubation and management of excessive secretions and acute bronchospasm.

DISPOSITION

When determining final disposition, consider other complications of muscle weakness in patients with myasthenia gravis, such as impaired swallowing, aspiration pneumonia, dehydration, and decubitus ulcers.

PRACTICE GUIDELINES

The American Academy of Neurology provides a guideline on medical treatment of the ocular symptoms involved in myasthenia gravis, as well as a summary of thymectomy indications.[31] Additionally, the European Federation of Neurological Societies has formulated a versatile therapeutic plan for treatment.[32] Cyclosporin and cyclophosphamide significantly improve myasthenia gravis, whereas azathioprine, mycophenolate, and tacrolimus have not been found to provide significant benefit.[33] Corticosteroids are stated to be useful short-term.[34]

MULTIPLE SCLEROSIS

Multiple sclerosis (MS) is a neurologic disorder that causes variable motor, sensory, visual, and cerebellar dysfunction as a result of multifocal areas of CNS myelin destruction. Paresthesias, gait difficulty, extremity weakness, poor coordination, and vision disturbances occur most often with a relapsing and remitting clinical course. Despite the lack of a definitive cure, immunosuppression and immunomodulation provide adequate symptomatic relief in the majority of patients, such that most have only mild to moderate lifetime morbidity and a reduction in overall life expectancy of only 5 to 10 years.[35]

Three clinical courses are noted in patients with MS. Up to 90% have a relapsing and remitting course, with relapses lasting weeks to months. The remaining patients have either a relapsing and progressive course or a chronically progressive clinical course, the latter of which is more common with advanced age.

PATHOPHYSIOLOGY

The cause of MS is unknown. It is best described as an inflammatory disorder resulting in scattered neuron demyelination. The most frequently postulated theory is a genetic predisposition triggered by a virus (such as herpes or human T-cell leukemia virus type I), heavy metals, or other environmental toxins that induce an immune-mediated neuronal inflammation and demyelinization.[36] There is no risk of MS from vaccinations.[37] MS causes a dysfunction in oligodendrocytes such that the axonal myelin sheaths are damaged, slowing nerve impulse conduction. Scattered cerebral and spinal plaques cause gliosis primarily in the white matter, with relative axon sparing.

Plaques occur in multiple areas, including the cerebrum, brainstem, spinal cord, and cranial nerves. Lesions in the corticospinal tracts, posterior columns, and spinothalamic tracts will cause upper motor neuron, proprioception/vibration, and pain/temperature dysfunction, respectively. Cranial nerve lesions result in optic neuritis, as well as facial motor and sensory deficits.

CLINICAL FEATURES

MS is suggested when a young person presents multiple times with neurologic symptoms that suggest different areas of pathology, often with resolution of the earlier symptoms. For most patients, lower extremity symptoms are more severe than upper extremity symptoms. For example, a young person might complain of an inability to walk on a street without tripping over a curb or a sense of clumsiness with physical activity. **The physical examination may reveal decreased strength, increased tone, hyperreflexia, clonus, a positive Babinski reflex, a decrease in both vibration sense and joint proprioception, and a reduction in pain and temperature sensation.** Although sensory and motor deficits are present initially in only one third of patients, all patients will experience these findings at some point during the disease course. Patients describe these deficits as a heaviness, weakness, stiffness, or extremity numbness. **Lhermitte sign** is commonly experienced during the course of MS and is described as an electric shock sensation, a vibration, or a pain radiating down the back and often into the arms or legs resulting from the flexion of the neck. Rarely, patients with established MS may present with acute transverse myelitis, with complete or near-complete loss of motor function. Cerebellar lesions may cause a kinetic tremor, dysmetria, or truncal ataxia. Vertigo may develop as a result of brainstem lesions.

Optic neuritis, which usually causes acute or subacute central vision loss, may be the initial sign of MS in up to 30% of patients. Vision loss, which occurs over several days and is usually unilateral, often is preceded by retrobulbar pain or extraocular muscle pain that may be reproduced with periorbital palpation. Optic neuritis may cause an afferent pupillary defect, or **Marcus Gunn pupil**. This is found when a light directed into the affected eye causes pupil dilation instead of constriction (see chapter 241, "Eye Emergencies"). The optic disc may be pale. Although ocular pain most often resolves over several days, it may take months for the vision disturbances to resolve. Most patients at some time experience blurred vision, compromised color vision, and/or eye pain due to optic neuritis. Nystagmus, diplopia, and internuclear ophthalmoplegia are often seen. Internuclear ophthalmoplegia usually causes abnormal eye adduction bilaterally and horizontal nystagmus. When bilateral internuclear ophthalmoplegia is seen acutely in an otherwise healthy young person, it is highly suggestive of MS.

Dysautonomias can cause vesicourethral dysfunction, resulting in urinary retention, urgency, frequency, detrusor–external sphincter dyssynergia, and stress or overflow incontinence. GI dysfunction can cause constipation and fecal incontinence. Sexual dysfunction, especially in males, may be a presenting symptom and correlates with other types of urologic dysfunction. Cognitive and emotional changes, including dementia, decreased motivation, depression, and bipolar mood disorders, occur in many patients. Cerebral MS, which affects only 5% of MS patients, can cause a severe, disabling decrease in intellect as well as seizures. Overall, the incidence of generalized seizures is the same in patients with MS as in the general population. Simple partial seizures are twice as common in patients with MS than in the general population. Treatment can cause seizures, and the treatment of seizures can worsen symptoms of MS.[38]

MS symptoms often worsen with increases in body temperature, as occurs with exercise, fever, or even hot baths. Visual acuity may worsen with increases in body temperature. Most initial attacks or exacerbations of MS will progress over several days, peak at about 1 week, and resolve over several weeks to months. Complete recovery from an acute exacerbation occurs more commonly early in the course of the disease than it does in later years.

DIAGNOSIS

The diagnosis of MS is suggested when a patient has either two or more prolonged or worsening episodes of neurologic dysfunction that suggest distinct white matter pathology or spinal cord dysfunction in two or more distinct locations.[39] Optic, cerebrospinal fluid, and neuroimaging findings, as well as typical features such as dysautonomias, all suggest the diagnosis. Symptoms that mimic MS are seen with systemic lupus erythematosus, Lyme disease, neurosyphilis, human immunodeficiency virus disease, and Guillain-Barré syndrome, which is associated with peripheral nervous system demyelination. MS progression is often monitored with the Expanded Disability Status Scale and the Multiple Sclerosis Functional Composite scores.[40]

Nearly all patients will demonstrate some nervous system pathology on MRI neuroimaging. T2-weighted scans demonstrate multiple discrete lesions in the supratentorial white matter, homogeneous borders surrounding the ventricles, or infratentorial or spinal cord lesions.[41] Although CT is not as sensitive as MRI, it may show cerebral atrophy, ventricular enlargement, and low-density focal lesions in the cerebrum, brainstem, or optic nerves. Cerebrospinal fluid protein and gamma-globulin concentrations can be elevated. A slight increase in cerebrospinal fluid WBCs (up to 25/mm^3) can also be seen, most of which are T lymphocytes.

TREATMENT

Consult a neurologist for diagnosis or treatment. Treatment modalities include mitoxantrone, glucocorticoids, natalizumab, interferon-β, and glatiramer.[42] Mitoxantrone has been associated with bone marrow and cardiac toxicity.[43] High-dose methylprednisolone therapy shortens the duration of exacerbations.[44,45] There is a 1:1000 incidence of progressive multifocal leukoencephalopathy with natalizumab treatment.[46] IV immunoglobulin is suggested for postpartum exacerbations and for patients with relapsing-remitting disease in whom other therapies such as interferon-β and glatiramer are not tolerated.[47]

DISPOSITION

Prioritize management at identifying the complications of acute exacerbations, such as respiratory distress, optic neuritis, pulmonary infections, severe constipation, and worsening muscle weakness. Use rapid sequence induction and the Sellick maneuver for endotracheal intubation because of an increased aspiration risk as a consequence of decreased gastric motility. Also, because many patients with MS have labile autonomic nervous system function, be prepared to treat hypotension in the setting of rapid sequence induction, emergency intubation, mechanical ventilation, and surgical anesthesia. Treat seizures with standard anticonvulsant medications and management protocols. Reduce fever to minimize the weakness associated with elevated temperature. **Test for urinary tract infections and pyelonephritis, especially in patients with residual urine volumes >100 mL.** Obtain a postvoid residual urine volume and a urine culture, and initiate antibiotic therapy whenever there is clinical evidence of a urinary tract infection or significant bacteriuria. When feasible, discharged patients should manage elevated residual urine volumes with intermittent sterile catheterization as opposed to chronic placement of a urinary drainage catheter. **Hospitalize for a disease exacerbation or for IV antibiotic or steroid therapy.** Admission is also indicated when depression or suicidal ideation require inpatient management.

PRACTICE GUIDELINES

The American Academy of Neurology has published guidelines describing the use of MRI in MS diagnosis, treatment with natalizumab and mitoxantrone, and the utility of the measurement of interferon-β antibody levels. These guidelines conclude the following: The use of natalizumab reduces clinical features such as relapse rate and disease severity but is associated with adverse effects.[48] Mitoxantrone has modest beneficial clinical effects that must be balanced against adverse effects.[49] The presence of MRI-identifiable lesions at the time of symptom onset is associated with later definitive MS diagnosis.[50] The European Federation of Neurological Societies also provides similar guidelines that address neuroimaging, MS treatment options, and the use of interferon-β antibody levels.[51-54] The Cochrane Collaboration has published reviews outlining the use of amantadine, azathioprine, corticosteroids, cyclophosphamide, mitoxantrone, and dietary interventions, as well as the treatment of ataxia. These reviews conclude the following:

1. The use of amantadine to reduce fatigue in MS patients is not substantiated.[55]
2. Azathioprine is a useful alternative to interferon-β in patients who frequently relapse and require steroid therapy.[56]
3. There is no clear benefit to the use of oral or IV steroids in the treatment of optic neuritis in MS patients, although quicker recovery of vision may occur with IV therapy.[57]
4. Cyclophosphamide does not prevent the progression of MS symptoms, and its use is associated with significant adverse effects.[58]
5. Mitoxantrone modestly reduces MS patient disease progression and relapse frequency and should be considered for patients with worsening disability caused by MS.[59]
6. Dietary regimens and vitamin supplementation have yet to demonstrate clinical benefit for MS patients.[60]
7. There are insufficient data to support any specific therapies for the treatment of ataxia and/or tremors that occur in MS patients.[61]

LAMBERT-EATON MYASTHENIC SYNDROME

Lambert-Eaton myasthenic syndrome is an autoimmune disorder that causes fluctuating weakness and fatigue, especially of the proximal limb muscles. Patients with Lambert-Eaton myasthenic syndrome may show some improvement in strength with sustained or repeated exercise. For example, when the patient is asked to grasp the examiner's hand, the squeeze becomes more forceful over several seconds—this is termed the **Lambert sign**. Lambert-Eaton myasthenic syndrome is sometimes associated with an antibody attack of P/Q-type voltage-gated calcium channels of axon nerve terminals.[62,63] These channels are integral to the release of acetylcholine during the action potential, and thus any calcium ion flow impairment results in muscle weakness. Lambert-Eaton myasthenic syndrome diagnosed in the absence of these anti-P/Q–type voltage-gated calcium channel antibodies is termed *seronegative*. It is hypothesized that seronegative Lambert-Eaton myasthenic syndrome is also incited by autoantibodies.[64] Patients often complain of myalgias, muscle stiffness (especially in the hip and shoulders), paresthesias, metallic tastes, and autonomic symptoms (e.g., dry mouth and impotence) caused by muscarinic cholinergic insufficiency. Although eye movements are unaffected, pupillary reflexes can be abnormal. Motor reflexes may be diminished. The sensory examination can be normal, but because the disease is associated with malignancy, paraneoplastic or chemotherapy-induced neuropathy can lead to a superimposed sensory deficit.

Lambert-Eaton myasthenic syndrome is predominantly a disease associated with older men with a history of cigarette smoking and lung cancer. The syndrome can precede detection of malignancy by several years. Approximately half of patients have concurrent small-cell lung cancer. Diagnosis is confirmed by electromyography. Small-cell lung cancer in Lambert-Eaton myasthenic syndrome patients correlates strongly with more rapid disease progression.[65] Electromyography is abnormal as a result of diseased calcium channels at the cholinergic nerve terminals. Reduced compound muscle action potentials that increase by >100% following maximal voluntary action on electrophysiologic testing helps to confirm the diagnosis.[66]

TREATMENT

Treatment is mostly supportive. Progression to respiratory or bulbar failure is rare. Neuromuscular transmission can also be enhanced with 3,4-diaminopyridine, which is considered first-line treatment.[67,68] Immunosuppression with corticosteroids, IV immunoglobulin, guanidine, aminopyridines, and azathioprine also can be used to reduce symptom severity.[69,70] Hospital admission is indicated when infectious complications occur or when severe disability requires inpatient immunotherapy.

PRACTICE GUIDELINES

Guidelines suggest that treatment with either 3,4-diaminopyridine or IV immunoglobulin could provide some benefit by improving muscle strength and compound muscle action potential amplitudes.[71-73]

PARKINSON'S DISEASE

Parkinson's disease is an extrapyramidal movement disorder characterized by a resting tremor, cogwheel rigidity, bradykinesias or akinesias, and impaired postural reflexes. The disease is associated with a reduced number of functional dopaminergic receptors in the substantia nigra. Drug therapy is designed to enhance central dopaminergic activity, thus decreasing the relative excess in central cholinergic activity. Even though multiple drug and surgical therapies can be used to minimize symptoms, the disease still progresses without symptom remission in most patients.

PATHOPHYSIOLOGY

Parkinson's disease is characterized by the presence of cellular cytoplasmic inclusions, termed *Lewy bodies,* and extracellular pigment granules that stimulate macrophage activity. In the pigmented areas of the midbrain, especially the substantia nigra, there is depigmentation, dopaminergic neuron loss, and gliosis. These cellular changes result in the loss of functional dopaminergic receptors, causing a decrease in the overall level of striatal dopamine.

CLINICAL FEATURES

The clinical diagnosis of Parkinson's disease is based on the presence of one or more of four hallmark neurologic signs identified in the mnemonic ***TRAP*: resting *tremor*, cogwheel *rigidity*, bradykinesia or *akinesia*, and impairment in *posture* and equilibrium**. Besides these signs, there also may be facial and postural changes, voice and speech abnormalities, depression, and muscle fatigue. Before diagnosis, most patients will have symptoms for months to years, including a general feeling of slowness or stiffness and/or difficulties with handwriting and other skills that require manual dexterity. The first stage of the disease is the premotor phase that includes reduced olfaction and constipation. This is followed by the motor phase, which responds to L-dopa in the honeymoon phase of the disease. When patients start to see motor complications, they experience fluctuations and dyskinesia. In late-stage disease, patients experience motor disabilities, freezing of their gait, falls, incontinence, orthostatic hypotension, and dementia.[74]

Patients typically will complain initially of a unilateral resting tremor of the upper extremity. The tremor is a repetitive low-amplitude movement usually involving the fingers and thumb, but also of the legs or face, that occurs five or more times per minute, described as **"pill rolling."** Tremors can dissipate when intentional movement is performed, which differentiates it from the kinetic tremor of other neurologic disorders. For example, on physical examination, the resting tremor of Parkinson's disease will become less prominent as the patient performs the finger-to-nose test, and tremor resumes once this purposeful movement is ended and the limb is supported and at rest. Cogwheel rigidity is elicited by causing passive movement of the limb through a full range of motion. As the limb is moved, its muscles develop an increased tone, and a ratchet-like movement is noted. Bradykinesia, the general sense of slowness of voluntary movement, is often felt to be the most debilitating symptom. The most severely affected patients can develop akinesia, the inability to perform the movements necessary for daily living, such as turning over in bed, rising from a seated position, or walking. When the disorder impairs postural reflexes, patients may have an impaired ability to turn or change direction while walking or may lose their balance and fall. Patients are also commonly affected by impulse control disorders.[75]

DIAGNOSIS

The clinical diagnosis of Parkinson's disease is straightforward, if all of the TRAP symptoms are present. The symptoms of Parkinson's disease also can be seen in postencephalitis patients and those with other infections such as neurosyphilis, subacute spongiform encephalopathy, and acquired immunodeficiency syndrome. Parkinsonism can occur as a result of street drugs, toxins, neuroleptic drugs, hydrocephalus, head trauma, and more rare and complex neurologic disorders.

In **drug-induced Parkinson's disease**, akinesia is the most common sign, with resting tremor less commonly observed. Other characteristics of drug-induced parkinsonism include a history of drug ingestion known to interfere with central dopamine activity, short interval between symptom onset and maximal disability, bilateral presentation of motor dysfunction, and the presence of other drug-related motor abnormalities.

There is no definitive laboratory or neuroimaging study that is pathognomonic for diagnosis. CT and MRI most often only show CNS atrophy.

TREATMENT

Currently available therapies do not change the underlying pathology but can reduce symptoms. Therapies include anticholinergics, such as trihexyphenidyl and benztropine; drugs that increase central dopamine levels, such as amantadine, levodopa, and carbidopa; and dopamine receptor agonists, such as bromocriptine and pergolide. Ergot agonists are no longer recommended, as newer agents have replaced them.[76] When symptoms cause severe motor dysfunction, the monoamine oxidase inhibitor selegiline and the catechol methyltransferase inhibitors entacapone and tolcapone may be effective.

Levodopa, which is converted into dopamine by decarboxylases that are present peripherally, can cause symptoms such as anorexia, nausea, and vomiting due to increases in peripheral dopamine levels. When levodopa is combined with carbidopa, a peripheral decarboxylase inhibitor, smaller doses of levodopa are required for effectiveness, reducing side effects. Over time, the effectiveness of levodopa will diminish, requiring the additional use of dopamine receptor agonist therapy. Individuals who are fully mobile, in the "on" state, can suddenly convert to the "off" state and become akinetic, especially in the morning shortly after rising and before taking the initial daily dose. This "on-off" phenomenon is treated by the use of controlled-release preparations of the combined carbidopa-levodopa therapy. Human aromatic L-amino acid decarboxylase allows for more effective levodopa conversion to dopamine without the adverse effects of high doses of levodopa.[77] Other dopamine agonists that have been found to be effective as monotherapy included piribedil, pramipexole, ropinirole, rotigotine, and cabergoline.[78]

When drug effectiveness diminishes over time or when significant motor or psychiatric complications occur, a "drug holiday" lasting approximately 1 week is often attempted. Despite the fact that withdrawal of dopaminergic therapy can worsen symptoms, functioning actually can improve once therapy is resumed, with improvement lasting weeks to months. Deep brain stimulation can treat advanced disease with motor disabilities and can improve quality of life.[79]

The treatment for drug-induced parkinsonism is termination of the causative agents. Patients who are refractory to optimal drug therapy for all types of Parkinson's disease may benefit from pallidotomy, a stereotactic neurosurgical procedure that enhances medical therapy effectiveness and reduces dyskinesia severity.[80,81] Thalamic stimulation or thalamotomy is useful for patients with severe tremor.

SPECIAL CONSIDERATIONS

Although most patients with Parkinson's disease present to the ED already diagnosed, some might present undiagnosed with motor or sensory symptoms that may not be attributed immediately to the disorder. Patients may experience motor symptoms such as freezing episodes, dysphagia, or abnormalities of whole-body movement. Sensory complaints may include akathisias, paresthesias, muscles aches, or extremity pain. Although severe pain is usually related to the loss of medication efficacy, it can be a prominent symptom of undiagnosed Parkinson's disease. Complications related to motor, gait, and truncal disabilities include deep venous thrombosis, pulmonary embolism, aspiration pneumonia, compressive neuropathies, and trauma from frequent falls. Autonomic disturbances, such as orthostatic hypotension, intestinal motility disorders, and bladder dysfunction, can occur, as well as facial seborrhea. Behavior abnormalities caused by frontal lobe dysfunction and dementia also are seen.

Dyspnea, respiratory distress, and pneumonia are more likely during the "off" periods, when drug efficacy is reduced. The most common cause of death in severe Parkinson's disease is respiratory failure.

Dopaminergic therapy toxicities can include cardiac dysrhythmias, orthostatic hypotension, dyskinesias, and dystonias. Psychiatric and sleep disturbances, including nightmares, auditory and visual hallucinations, paranoia, and psychosis, are related to the treatment dose and duration and can be improved by a reduction in dosage or a drug holiday. Depression and panic attacks are common and can occur in patients independent of dopaminergic therapy. Psychotropics (such as haloperidol) that can cause tardive dyskinesia must be used carefully, if at all, in patients with Parkinson's disease.

Adjustment of chronic therapies should be done in consultation with the patient's primary care physician or neurologist, who can often help to determine which symptoms reflect dopaminergic excess and whether prior drug holidays have improved the patient's symptoms.

POLIOMYELITIS AND POSTPOLIO SYNDROME

Poliomyelitis is a neurotropic enterovirus that causes paralysis through motor neuron destruction, muscle denervation, and atrophy. Indigenously acquired wild poliovirus was eradicated from the United States in 1979 and from the Western Hemisphere in 1991. However, the disease is still endemic in India, Pakistan, Afghanistan, and Nigeria.[82] Postpolio syndrome, also called *postpoliomyelitis progressive muscular atrophy*, is an important sequela of acute poliomyelitis. This disorder is characterized by the recurrence of motor symptoms, following a latent period of several decades, after the resolution of the motor symptoms caused by the initial infection.

Mass immunization with the inactivated poliovirus vaccine or attenuated oral poliovirus vaccine has dramatically reduced the incidence of polio, but polio outbreaks still occur in populations that are not consistently or adequately immunized. Immunocompromised patients are at greater risk for contracting polio after exposure to children who were vaccinated with the attenuated oral poliovirus vaccine. With the use of attenuated oral poliovirus vaccine, some immunized children will develop polio, as will some young adults who are exposed to children who have been vaccinated with the attenuated oral poliovirus vaccine; immunocompromised patients are at greater risk for this. In developing countries, recent intramuscular injections, tonsillectomy, and strenuous exercise all are associated with increased polio infection severity.

Postpolio syndrome is expected to affect up to 100,000 of the 250,000 U.S. adults with a history of polio. Because most cases of polio occurred before mass immunization, patients diagnosed now with postpolio syndrome most likely will be >50 years old. Disease onset is 20 to 35 years after the initial infection. Although postpolio syndrome most often occurs after a stable, disease-free period of 20 to 30 years, current retrospective reviews claim 35 years.[83] There are risk factors that predict an earlier onset of postpolio syndrome. These include advanced age at the time of initial polio infection, greater residual motor disability, residual bulbar or respiratory signs, and the occurrence of recent injuries that require limb immobilization. Postpolio syndrome is a diagnosis of exclusion.[84]

PATHOPHYSIOLOGY

In developed countries, the viral transmission of polio is oral to oral, whereas in developing countries, where the sanitation is poor, the transmission is fecal to oral. Acutely, the polio enterovirus enters the body through the GI tract and reproduces in the GI lymphoid tissue, termed *gut-associated lymphoid tissue*. Oral secretion of the virus takes place for several days, whereas stool excretion can last for several weeks.

At a critical concentration, the virus spreads to the large motor nuclei of the spinal cord, the brainstem, and the reticular formation. The vestibular and brainstem motor nuclei, hypothalamus, thalamus, cerebellum, and precentral motor cerebral cortex also can be infected by the poliovirus. There is loss of infected neurons. Neuron loss then causes a cycle of muscle denervation and reinnervation, resulting in loss of muscle function.

The cause of the postpolio syndrome is unknown. The motor neuron degeneration is thought to be a result of dysfunction in the individual nerve axons in surviving motor neurons.

CLINICAL FEATURES

Acute Poliomyelitis Polio infection is asymptomatic in >90% of cases. The majority of **symptomatic polio infections** involve only a minor viral illness that causes no paralysis, termed *abortive polio*. After an incubation period of a few days, symptoms may include fever, malaise, headache, sore throat, and GI symptoms. Some of the patients who experience the minor viral illness, especially young children, may develop aseptic meningitis as the infection resolves. Only 1% to 2% of all poliovirus infections result in the major illness associated with neurologic involvement. Often there is resolution of the minor viral illness symptoms before development of neurologic symptoms, so that it is difficult to identify the preceding minor viral illness. Muscle pain, stiffness, and weakness during the early viral syndrome may be premonitory of later paralysis.

When the major illness occurs, most commonly the spinal cord anterior horn cells are affected, causing asymmetric proximal limb weakness, especially in the lower extremities. **Flaccid and weak muscles, absent tendon reflexes, and fasciculations characterize spinal polio.** Although polio patients note pain, paresthesias, and transient sensory abnormalities, sensory deficits are usually not found on clinical examination. Maximal paralysis usually occurs within 5 days, and muscle wasting then occurs over several weeks. Autonomic dysfunction, including sweating disturbances, urine retention, delayed gastric emptying, and constipation, is commonly found. Most spinal polio patients will demonstrate improved motor function, with resolution of the paralysis occurring within the first year after the acute infection.

Up to 20% of polio patients with paralysis will develop bulbar polio, which can cause speech, swallowing, facial muscle, and extraocular muscle dysfunction. Acute polio infection also can cause encephalitis and can disturb the reticular formation, resulting in cardiac dysrhythmias, blood pressure alterations, hypoxia, and hypercarbia. Patients who survive the acute episode of encephalitis normally recover without residual effects.

Consider **acute paralytic poliomyelitis** whenever an at-risk patient develops an acute febrile illness, aseptic meningitis, and asymmetric flaccid paralysis associated with the loss of deep tendon reflexes and normal sensation. As with other causes of aseptic meningitis, the cerebrospinal fluid reveals pleocytosis during the first week after paralysis onset. The cerebrospinal fluid white cell count can elevate into the hundreds, with a predominance of neutrophils early in the disease course. Although the poliovirus can be cultured from the cerebrospinal fluid early in the disease course, throat and rectal swabs provide a greater yield. When a particular viral serotype is identified, serial serum antibody titers can be used to verify the cultures.

The most important cause of paralysis on the differential diagnosis that must be considered and excluded is Guillain-Barré syndrome, which, unlike the acute polio infection, causes more symmetric muscle weakness. Acute paralysis can result from peripheral neuropathies caused by infectious mononucleosis, Lyme disease, or porphyria. Paralysis also can result from inflammatory myopathies, electrolyte abnormalities, toxins, or other viruses, such as coxsackieviruses, mumps, echoviruses, and nonpolio enteroviruses. Paralysis also can result from acute spinal cord compression, vascular lesions, and transverse myelitis, all of which should produce a sensory level and sphincter disturbances. In children, it is necessary to exclude spinal muscular atrophy, which can be undiagnosed until it is manifested by dramatic limb weakness caused by an acute febrile illness.

Postpolio Syndrome Patients with **postpolio syndrome** complain of muscle fatigue, joint pain, worsening of skeletal deformities, or weakness in muscles that were spared during the initial viral infection.[85] When muscle weakness is observed, atrophy, pain, and fasciculations may be noted both in previously unaffected muscle groups and in those previously involved. Patients may also develop new bulbar, respiratory, or sleep difficulties. For example, laryngeal muscle weakness can cause progressive dyspnea, dysphagia, and/or hoarseness. Some patients complain of abnormal movements in sleep that disturb normal sleep, requiring therapy with benzodiazepines or dopaminergic drugs.[86] These symptoms occur independently of any concurrent neurologic, orthopedic, psychiatric, or systemic medical illness.

To diagnose postpolio syndrome, the patient should have a history of acute paralytic poliomyelitis with stable recovery of motor function associated with residual muscle atrophy, weakness, and areflexia with normal sensation in at least one limb. Additionally, there should be new muscle symptoms or weakness not attributable to an acute injury, neuropathy, radiculopathy, or systemic, neurologic, or psychiatric illness.

Treatment of the new muscle weakness seen with postpolio patients is primarily symptomatic, with the use of analgesic and anti-inflammatory medications. Most patients with postpolio syndrome benefit from muscle training[87] and daily exercise.[88] An additional therapeutic option is lamotrigine (Lamictal). When used in conjunction with an exercise routine, lamotrigine may improve the quality of life in postpolio patients.[89]

Acknowledgments: The authors would like to thank Edward P. Sloan for his work on previous editions of this chapter.

REFERENCES

The complete reference list is available online at www.TintinalliEM.com.

CHAPTER 174 Central Nervous System and Spinal Infections

Mary E. Tanski
O. John Ma

BACTERIAL MENINGITIS

INTRODUCTION AND EPIDEMIOLOGY

Bacterial meningitis is a life-threatening emergency that affects 1.38 out of 100,000 people, with a case fatality rate of 14.3%.[1] Although the incidence of bacterial meningitis has declined significantly since the initiation of vaccination programs, the disease is still prevalent and associated with significant morbidity and mortality.[2-4] In the United States, the most common causes of bacterial meningitis are *Streptococcus pneumoniae* (58.0%), group B *Streptococcus* (18.1%), *Neisseria meningitidis* (13.9%), *Haemophilus influenzae* (6.7%), and *Listeria monocytogenes* (3.4%).[1] *Escherichia coli* in the neonatal population and *Mycobacterium tuberculosis* in immunocompromised hosts are also important considerations.[5]

PATHOPHYSIOLOGY

Organisms enter the cerebrospinal fluid either through hematogenous or direct contiguous spread. In hematogenous spread, bacteria colonize the upper airway and invade the bloodstream, gradually making their way to the subarachnoid space. The subcapsular components of *S. pneumoniae*, *H. influenzae* type b, and *N. meningitides* induce an inflammatory cascade, and leukocyte toxins cause cellular swelling and inflammation of the brain and meninges.[6] Blood–brain barrier permeability increases, allowing protein and water to enter and leading to vasogenic edema. Cerebrospinal fluid drainage is inhibited by reduced absorption of the arachnoid granules with resultant obstruction and hydrocephalus, and cerebrospinal fluid is forced into the periventricular parenchyma causing interstitial edema. Disruption of cell membrane homeostasis causes cytotoxic edema. As the brain and meninges rest in a fixed-volume skull, this leads to an elevation in intracranial pressure. Vasculitis decreases cerebral blood flow and can cause ischemia and thrombosis. Additionally, neurons are directly injured by free radicals from granulocytes and endothelial cells.[7]

In direct contiguous spread, organisms gain entry into the cerebrospinal fluid from adjacent infections such as sinusitis, brain abscess, or otitis media. Organisms can also enter directly with penetrating traumatic injury, through congenital defects, or during neurosurgical procedures. In these cases, the organisms and their pathophysiologic effects vary.

Important risk factors for bacterial meningitis are listed in **Table 174-1**.

CLINICAL FEATURES

The presentation of fever, headache, stiff neck, and altered mental status is commonly seen in patients with bacterial meningitis. Although most patients have at least two of four of these symptoms, their absence does not exclude meningitis. Headache is the most common symptom and is seen in more than 85% of patients. Fever is the second most common symptom.[7] Seizures and focal neurologic deficits are seen in 25% to 30% of patients.

History Assess historical data in order to elicit risk factors suggestive of certain pathogens. *N. meningitidis* is associated with close living

TABLE 174-1 Important Risk Factors for Bacterial Meningitis
Acute or chronic otitis media
Sinusitis
Immunosuppression/splenectomy
Alcoholism
Pneumonia
Diabetes mellitus
Cerebrospinal fluid leak
Pneumonia
Endocarditis
Neurosurgical procedure/head injury
Indwelling neurosurgical device/cochlear implant
Advanced age
Malignancies
Liver disease
Unvaccinated to *Haemophilus influenzae* type b, *Neisseria meningitidis*, or *Streptococcus pneumoniae*

quarters, such as in military barracks and college dormitories. Unvaccinated patients are at risk for *H. influenzae*. Consider *L. monocytogenes* in older adults and alcoholics.[8] Penetrating head trauma makes *S. pneumoniae* more likely. *Staphylococcus aureus*, coagulase-negative staphylococci, and streptococci are the most commonly implicated organisms after craniotomy, whereas coagulase-negative staphylococci are commonly seen after ventriculoperitoneal shunt and spinal surgery.[4] Immunocompromised patients, such as those with human immunodeficiency virus, on chronic steroids, or with a history of splenectomy, are susceptible to meningitis with encapsulated organisms.

Physical Examination Evaluate for focal neurologic dysfunction such as hemiparesis, facial asymmetry, visual field deficits, or disordered eye movements. Increased intracranial pressure can cause papilledema, decreased venous pulsations, or cranial nerve palsy especially involving cranial nerves 3, 4, 6, and 7. Assess for meningeal irritation with Brudzinski sign (flexion of hips and knees in response to passive neck flexion) and Kernig sign (contraction of the hamstrings in response to knee extension while the hip is flexed). Examine the skin for cutaneous stigmata such as petechiae, splinter hemorrhages, and pustules, and consider aspirating to send for culture.[9] Percuss the sinuses and examine the ears for signs of primary infection.

DIAGNOSIS

Lumbar Puncture The diagnosis of meningitis is based on cerebrospinal fluid results obtained by lumbar puncture (LP). Withhold LP if there is coagulopathy, as evidenced by thrombocytopenia or anticoagulant or antithrombotic use, until coagulopathy is corrected. As a general rule, a platelet count ≤20,000/μL (and some prefer ≤50,000/μL) or INR ≥1.5 is a contraindication to performing an LP on an emergent basis.[10] The risk of bleeding complications such as epidural hematoma resulting from LP in the presence of aspirin, antiplatelet agents, and nonsteroidal anti-inflammatory drugs is not known, and risks and benefits of LP must be considered in such circumstances.[11,12] Send cerebrospinal fluid for studies including Gram stain and culture, cell count with differential, glucose, and protein.[7] Typical cerebrospinal fluid findings for bacterial, viral, fungal, and neoplastic meningitides are listed in **Table 174-2**,[13-16] but there is considerable overlap in findings.

Laboratory Testing Bacterial meningitis is associated with an elevated opening pressure >170 mm H_2O, and WBCs are elevated greater than 1000/mm³ with a neutrophilic predominance. Gram stain is positive in 60% to 80% of patients before antibiotics are initiated, with a significant decline once antibiotics have been started. Cerebrospinal fluid protein is often elevated above 200 milligrams/dL, and glucose is often decreased below 40 milligrams/dL or the glucose serum–to–cerebrospinal fluid ratio is <0.4.[13-15] Although it is not specific for bacterial meningitis, cerebrospinal fluid lactate is a promising indicator to assist with differentiation between aseptic and bacterial meningitis.[16]

Sterilization of the cerebrospinal fluid is possible within 2 hours of initiating parenteral antibiotics in meningococcal and 6 hours in pneumococcal meningitis, highlighting the importance of timely LP.[17] Without antibiotics, Gram stain is positive in 60% to 80% of cases, but in patients treated with antibiotics, the Gram stain is positive in 7% to 41%.[15] Cerebrospinal fluid culture is positive in 80% to 90% of cases if cerebrospinal fluid analysis is preformed before antibiotics are initiated, although results are not available during the course of the ED stay. **However, when bacterial meningitis is considered, never withhold empiric antibiotic therapy in order to collect the cerebrospinal fluid sample.**[18]

Rapid latex agglutination tests can be used to detect bacterial antigens and improve bacterial identification. These tests are available for *S. pneumoniae, group* B streptococci, *H. influenzae, E. coli*, and *N. meningitides*, but are associated with false-positive and false-negative results and limited sensitivity and specificity. Polymerase chain reaction testing is highly sensitive for organisms such as *S. pneumoniae, N. meningitides*, group B streptococci, *H. influenzae, L. monocytogenes*, and *M. tuberculosis* but does not provide information on antimicrobial susceptibility.[7] Serum procalcitonin, C-reactive protein, and cerebrospinal fluid lactate concentrations have been studied as adjuncts to diagnosis of bacterial meningitis with negative cerebrospinal fluid examinations, but are not a substitute for decision making in the treatment of an individual patient.[19] If suspicion is great despite negative initial cerebrospinal fluid results, admit for empiric antibiotic treatment and consider repeat LP.[13]

CT Scan before Lumbar Puncture Perform the LP as soon as possible to secure the diagnosis of meningitis. Concern about the complication of cerebral herniation from LP has led to controversy regarding whether patients require a CT scan of the brain prior to the procedure.[15]

Risk factors for brain herniation are listed in **Table 174-3**. Order a head CT prior to LP in patients exhibiting any of these high-risk criteria. Although a CT scan can help identify contraindications for an LP, a normal CT scan does imply that there is no risk of herniation with LP if a patient exhibits clinical predictors of impending herniation such as deteriorating mental status, posturing, irregular respirations and pupillary changes, or seizures.[20]

TREATMENT

After addressing airway, breathing, and circulation status, immediately initiate empiric antibiotic therapy if bacterial meningitis is clinically suspected. **Never delay administration of empiric antibiotic therapy for neuroimaging or to perform LP, because antibiotic treatment takes precedence over definitive diagnosis.**[6] Obtain blood cultures to assist in identification of the organism and to help guide inpatient therapy if it will not delay time to antibiotics. Base antibiotic selection on the clinical scenario including age, immunization status, living conditions, and past medical history.

Empiric Treatment for Presumptive Bacterial Meningitis The empiric antibiotic regimen for adults between 18 and 49 years of age is a third-generation cephalosporin, such as ceftriaxone, 2 grams IV, plus vancomycin, 15 milligrams/kg IV, to cover the common pathogens *S. pneumoniae* and *N. meningitides*. For adults over the age of 50 years who

TABLE 174-2 Cerebrospinal Fluid (CSF) Diagnostic Evaluation

	Opening Pressure (<170 mm H_2O)*	Color (clear)	Gram Stain (negative)	Cell Count (<5 WBC, 0 PMN)	Glucose (>40 mg/dL)	Protein (<50 mg/dL)	Cytology (negative)
Bacterial	Elevated	Cloudy, turbid	Positive (60%–80% before antibiotic, 7%–41% after antibiotic)	>1000–2000/mm³ WBC, neutrophilic predominance, >80% PMN	<40 mg/dL, CSF/blood glucose ratio <0.3–0.4	>200 mg/dL	Negative
Viral	Normal	Clear or bloody	Negative	<300/mm³ WBC, lymphocytic predominance, <20% PMN	Normal	<200 mg/dL	Negative
Fungal	Normal to elevated	Clear or cloudy	Negative	<500/mm³	Normal to slightly low	>200 mg/dL	Negative
Neoplastic	Normal	Clear or cloudy	Negative	<300/mm³	Normal to slightly low	>200 mg/dL	Positive

*Normal values and findings are in parentheses.

Abbreviation: PMN, polymorphonuclear lymphocyte.

TABLE 174-3 Criteria for Obtaining Head CT before Lumbar Puncture[6,15,20]

Criteria
Altered mental status or deteriorating level of consciousness
Focal neurologic deficit
New-onset seizure
Papilledema
Immunocompromised state
Malignancy
History of focal CNS disease (stroke, focal infection, tumor)
Concern for mass CNS lesion
Age >60 y

are immunocompromised, add ampicillin, 2 grams IV, to cover *L. monocytogenes*.[6] If patients have a severe allergy to penicillin, options include replacing ceftriaxone with chloramphenicol and substituting ampicillin with trimethoprim-sulfamethoxazole. Consider adding acyclovir if herpes simplex virus (HSV) encephalitis is suspected.[13] Use a fourth-generation cephalosporin, such as cefepime, plus vancomycin for patients who have recently undergone neurosurgery.[14] Initiate antibiotics as soon as possible in order to increase survival and reduce morbidity.[3,7]

The second priority is administration of steroids to patients with presumptive pneumococcal meningitis. Administration of dexamethasone before or with the first dose of antibiotics has been shown to reduce cerebrospinal fluid inflammation, reduce the risk of morbidity and mortality in adults, and reduce hearing loss and other neurologic sequelae in children, especially with *S. pneumoniae* infection.[8,21] The recommended dosage of dexamethasone is 10 milligrams IV for adults.[21]

Current guidelines provide no recommendation for the most common ED situation, in which the first dose of empiric antibiotics is given before LP is performed or before results of LP are received. Common sense suggests that dexamethasone could be administered just before, or concurrently with, empiric antibiotics to patients with strong suspicion for bacterial meningitis or to patients in whom grossly purulent cerebrospinal fluid is obtained at the time of LP. Infectious Disease Society of America guidelines state that dexamethasone should not be given to adults who have already received antibiotics.

SPECIAL SITUATIONS

Bacterial Meningitis Resulting from Sinusitis or Otitis The prevalent use of antibiotics has decreased the frequency of suppurative intracranial complications from sinusitis and otitis, but bacterial meningitis resulting from these diseases still occurs. The virulence of the affecting organism and host factors, such as immunocompromised state, influence spread to the CNS. In the ear, bacteria can spread through endolymphatic channels, bony erosions, or osteothrombophlebitis of small vessels. Thrombophlebitis of veins is a common mechanism by which bacteria disseminate from the sinuses; this may result in cavernous sinus thrombosis or empyema.[22] CT imaging is very sensitive for sinusitis and permits earlier diagnosis with demonstration of air-fluid levels in the involved sinuses. CT is nonspecific, however, and should be interpreted with the clinical background in mind (**Figure 174-1**). Infections are often polymicrobial. Initiate empiric antibiotic therapy with fluoroquinolones, such as levofloxacin or moxifloxacin, or with a third-generation cephalosporin, such as ceftriaxone, plus metronidazole.[23] Invasive infections and those with intracranial spread require emergency consultation for surgical drainage.

Additional Adjunctive Treatment for Bacterial Meningitis Monitor patients with meningitis closely for complications or signs of clinical deterioration, especially evaluating their respiratory and neurologic status.[8] Treat hyperpyrexia and manage seizures with anticonvulsants. Avoid hypotonic fluids, and monitor serum sodium level serially to detect syndrome of inappropriate antidiuretic hormone or cerebral salt wasting.[7,21] Closely evaluate for signs of increased intracranial pressure and vasculopathy that may lead to brain ischemia. If signs of elevated intracranial pressure are detected, elevate the bed to 30 degrees, use 25% mannitol or hypertonic 3% saline for diuresis, and consider a trial of mild hyperventilation.[7] Measurement of intracranial and systemic arterial pressure may be useful in severe cases to monitor cerebral perfusion pressure. Consider admission to the intensive care unit to ensure proper level of care.[8]

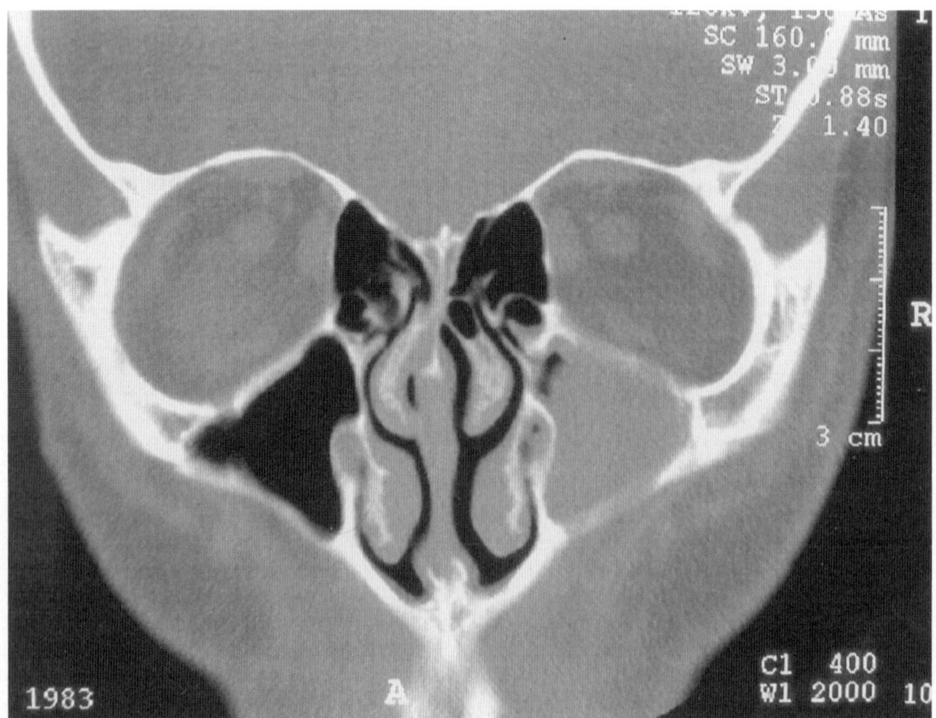

FIGURE 174-1. Acute sinusitis with opacification of the maxillary sinus. [Reproduced with permission from Brunicardi FC, Andersen D, Billiar T, et al: *Schwartz's Principles of Surgery*, 8th ed. New York, McGraw-Hill.]

Chemoprophylaxis for Those Exposed to Bacterial Meningitis Bacterial meningitis is spread by droplets, and risk for developing bacterial meningitis after exposure is estimated to be 500 to 800 times higher than the general population.[14] Chemoprophylaxis has been shown to decrease transmission of *N. meningitidis* by 89% in close contacts. Chemoprophylaxis is recommended for individuals who have been exposed to patients diagnosed with *N. meningitidis* and *H. influenzae*.[9] It is not recommended for patients diagnosed with pneumococcal meningitis.[14] Close contacts include housemates, individuals exposed to secretions (shared utensils or toothbrushes, kissing, mouth-to-mouth resuscitation), and individuals who intubated the patient without a facemask. To be most effective, initiate chemoprophylaxis within 24 hours of contact. Risk of infection after a period of 2 weeks from exposure is considered rare, and prophylaxis is not recommended after this time period. Treatment options for high-risk contacts include rifampin 10 milligrams/kg to a maximum of 600 milligrams per dose every 12 hours for four doses, ciprofloxacin 500 milligrams orally once, or ceftriaxone 250 milligrams IM once.[9] Instruct all patients who receive chemoprophylaxis to seek medical attention immediately if they develop any symptoms of illness or meningitis.

DISPOSITION AND FOLLOW-UP

Admit all patients diagnosed with bacterial meningitis and those highly suspected of having meningitis to the hospital on droplet isolation.

VIRAL MENINGITIS

INTRODUCTION

Viral meningitis typically presents with subacute headache and fever and findings of meningeal irritation, such as nuchal rigidity. Several viruses can cause viral meningitis, including nonpolio enteroviruses, HSV, varicella-zoster virus, cytomegalovirus, adenovirus, and human immunodeficiency virus. Specific diagnosis depends on isolation of the virus or positive results on immunoassay of the cerebrospinal fluid. Nonpolio enteroviruses (echovirus, coxsackievirus, and enterovirus) typically are seen in summer through fall and account for more than 90% of all cases of viral meningitis.[4]

LABORATORY TESTING

Viral meningitis is associated with normal opening pressures and a negative Gram stain. WBCs are <300/mm^3 with a lymphocytic predominance, and usually less than 20% polymorphonuclear lymphocytes.[20] Protein is often slightly elevated, but not typically above 200 milligrams/dL, and cerebrospinal fluid glucose is normal. The percentage of polymorphonuclear cells may be higher in early viral meningitis, and in some cases, glucose levels may be decreased.[13] Consider partially treated bacterial meningitis if a patient with symptoms consistent with meningitis had previously been treated with antibiotics and the LP suggests aseptic meningitis. Viral culture is insensitive, so if a viral etiology is suspected, send for molecular testing by polymerase chain reaction from the cerebrospinal fluid.[4] Polymerase chain reaction testing is available for HSV, enterovirus, and other viral organisms.

DISPOSITION AND FOLLOW-UP

There can be overlap of cerebrospinal fluid findings with early bacterial meningitis and partially treated bacterial meningitis, making specific diagnosis for some cases of viral meningitis difficult in the ED. Although supportive care is the mainstay of treatment for viral meningitis, it is appropriate to admit the toxic-appearing patient to the hospital for empiric antibiotic therapy until culture results return in situations of diagnostic uncertainty. HSV-2 meningitis can cause necrotizing encephalitis and neurologic deficits.[4] Admit patients with diagnosed or suspected HSV-2 meningitis after beginning treatment with acyclovir 10 milligrams/kg IV every 8 hours.[8]

FUNGAL CNS INFECTIONS

Over the past 30 years, the incidence of fungal CNS infections has been increasing, likely due to acquired immunodeficiency syndrome as well as an increase in patients on immunosuppressants due to stem cell and organ transplants.[24] The most common cause of fungal meningitis is *Cryptococcus neoformans*, followed by *Coccidioides immitis*, which can be seen in immunocompetent hosts as well as the immunocompromised.[4,24] *Aspergillus* and *Candida* are most often discovered in immunocompromised hosts. Mucormycoses can be seen especially in diabetics from direct extension of sinus infection.

LABORATORY TESTING

The cerebrospinal fluid analysis of fungal meningitis shows lymphocytic predominance, an elevated opening pressure, low glucose, and slightly increased protein.[5,25] Significant elevations in opening pressure are often seen in cryptococcal meningitis. Gram stain is negative, and WBC is usually <500/mm^3. Consider fungal testing especially for immunocompromised patients where fungal etiologies are suspected, including India ink staining and serum cryptococcal antigen testing, cytology, and histopathology.[5] Send cerebrospinal fluid for *Borrelia* antibodies in patients with suspected Lyme disease and for acid-fast stain and culture for suspected mycobacteria in tuberculous meningitis.

Patients often have a prolonged symptom course. Use fungal stain and culture for diagnosis if a fungal etiology is suspected, and look for elevated opening pressure during LP. Consider CT or MRI to search for intracranial complications such as granulomas or abscesses.

TREATMENT

Treatment for fungal infections is dependent on diagnosis through LP. Amphotericin is the agent of choice in cryptococcal meningitis. Use fluconazole or itraconazole for *C. immitis*. Treat *Candida* meningitis with amphotericin B and flucytosine.[5]

VIRAL ENCEPHALITIS

Viral CNS infections can also cause viral encephalitis, which is an infection and inflammation of the brain parenchyma.[4] Viral encephalitis is clinically distinguished from viral meningitis with presence of neurologic findings such as altered level of consciousness, focal weakness, or seizures, although the two often coexist.

The causes of viral encephalitis vary year to year and across geographical locations, with an incidence of 3.5 to 7.5 per 100,000 people.[26] Immune status, exposure to insects or animals, and travel history play a key role in determining the etiology. An underlying cause, however, is found in only about a third of cases.[25] HSV accounts for 40% to 50% of cases where a cause is determined. HSV-1 is responsible for most cases of HSV encephalitis; HSV-2 frequently causes aseptic meningitis but is not usually associated with development of encephalitis.[26] Other viral pathologic agents in North America include Epstein-Barr virus, cytomegalovirus, and rabies. Common arboviral encephalitides include La Crosse encephalitis, St. Louis equine encephalitis, Western equine encephalitis, and West Nile virus.

PATHOPHYSIOLOGY

Immunocompromised patients such as those with organ or stem cell transplants are susceptible to new or reactivated infections with HSV and varicella-zoster virus. Impaired immune status also plays a role in cytomegalovirus encephalitis. The arboviruses are transmitted by mosquitoes and ticks. Rabies is transferred by the bite of an infected animal and leads to severe encephalitis and a very high mortality rate.[4] Common to all is preliminary viral invasion of the host at a site where replication takes place that is outside the CNS. Most viruses then reach the nervous system hematogenously during viremia. However, at least three important viruses—rabies, HSV, and herpes zoster virus—reach the spinal cord and eventually the brain by traveling backward within axons from a distal site, where they gain access to nerve endings. Once in the brain, disruption of neural cell functions by the virus and by the effects of the host's inflammatory responses ensue. Gray matter is predominantly affected, resulting in cognitive and psychiatric signs, lethargy, and seizures.

CLINICAL FEATURES

Consider encephalitis in patients exhibiting behavioral changes, new psychiatric symptoms, cognitive deficits, or seizures.[25] Although the triad of headache, fever, and altered mental status may be seen, it is not invariably present. Assess for signs of clinical syndromes outside the CNS. Rash or skin vesicles suggest herpes zoster, and skin vesicle culture may be useful for diagnosis. Lymphadenopathy or splenomegaly points to Epstein-Barr virus, which can be picked up on serologic testing. New onset of psychiatric symptoms and behavioral changes may be attributable to HSV. MRI, electroencephalogram, and polymerase chain reaction of the CSR could assist in making the diagnosis.

Physical Examination Examine for signs of meningeal irritation and increased intracranial pressure and for neurologic findings that reflect the areas of involvement. Carefully assess mental status and cognition. Encephalitis may show regional tropism. HSV involves limbic structures of the temporal and frontal lobes with prominent psychiatric features, memory disturbance, and aphasia. Some arboviruses predominantly affect the basal ganglia, causing choreoathetosis and parkinsonian movements. Involvement of the brainstem nuclei that control swallowing leads to the hydrophobic choking response characteristic of rabies encephalitis.[27]

DIAGNOSIS

Neuroimaging studies such as MRI or CT, electroencephalography, and LP are important in ruling out mass occupying lesions and making the diagnosis of encephalitis. MRI is more sensitive than CT. Obtain an MRI to help exclude lesions such as brain abscesses, and examine for findings suggestive of HSV encephalitis, such as involvement of the gray matter in the medial temporal and inferior frontal lobes (**Figure 174-2**). Electroencephalogram findings are generally nonspecific but can be useful in cases such as HSV encephalitis where an almost pathognomonic picture of periodic, asymmetric sharp waves is seen in the setting of acute febrile encephalopathy.[25] LP is the most useful diagnostic procedure in the ED once imaging studies exclude the increased intracranial pressure and the risk of uncal herniation.

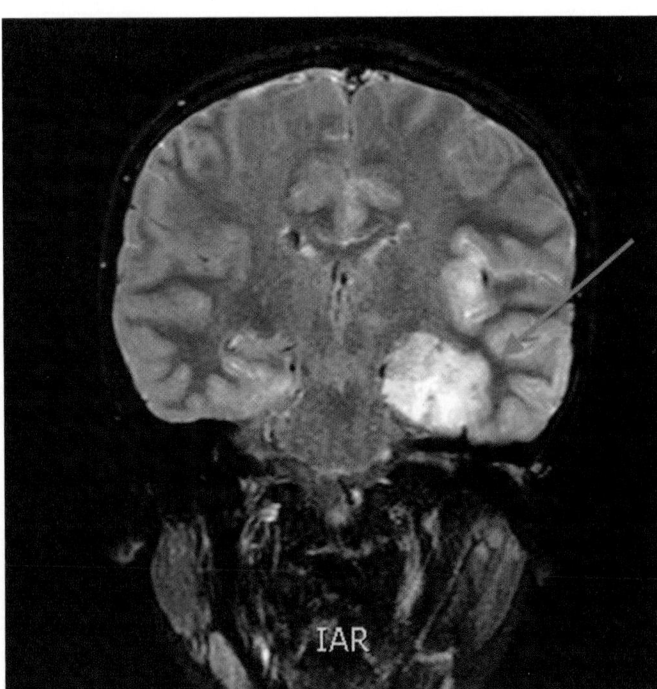

FIGURE 174-2. Fluid-attenuated inversion recovery hyperintensity in the left temporal lobe and left insula (arrow) suggests the diagnosis of herpes encephalitis. [Photo contributed by Elizabeth Yutan, Department of Radiology, Oregon Health & Science University.]

Consider bacterial meningitis in the differential diagnosis when fever and meningeal symptoms predominate. A late-summer encephalopathy suggests the possibility of arbovirus encephalitis, and an animal bite for which no antirabies treatment was administered has relevance for rabies. Suspect subarachnoid hemorrhage with acute onset of severe headache as the presenting sign. Lyme disease, tuberculosis, and fungal and neoplastic meningitis are in the differential diagnosis in less fulminant cases. If focal neurologic signs are present, consider brain abscess, empyema, or cavernous sinus thrombosis as possible causes.

TREATMENT

The antiviral of choice for HSV encephalitis is high-dose acyclovir at 10 milligrams/kg IV.[8,26] Initiate treatment as soon as possible because the prognosis of HSV encephalitis is correlated with neurologic condition at the time antivirals are initiated. Treat varicella-zoster virus with acyclovir, 10 to 15 milligrams/kg IV. Patients with herpes zoster virus encephalitis may also benefit from acyclovir therapy. Treat patients with cytomegalovirus encephalitis with ganciclovir, 5 milligrams/kg IV.[27] There are no known treatments for arbovirus encephalitis; consider initiating treatment with acyclovir empirically until a cerebrospinal fluid diagnosis is made.[8] Rabies encephalitis is rare but neurologically devastating, and once symptomatic, it is usually fatal.

DISPOSITION AND FOLLOW-UP

Prognosis of viral encephalitides depends on the causative virus and host factors. Older adults and those who are immunocompromised are more likely to have an adverse outcome. Admit patients with encephalitis to the hospital. Patients may require intensive care unit care if they have signs of altered mental status or coma.

BRAIN ABSCESS

INTRODUCTION

A brain abscess begins as a focal area of cerebritis, which develops into a central pus-filled cavity ringed by a layer of granulation tissue and an outer fibrous capsule in a period of about 14 days.[28] It is surrounded by edematous brain tissue infiltrated with inflammatory cells. A brain abscess is a pathologic response typical of a relatively competent immune system against a bacterial invader. Focal brain infections from other organisms, such as granulomas due to tuberculosis, necrotic lesions of toxoplasmosis in immunocompromised patients, or cystic lesions of cysticercosis, are not abscesses in the pathologic sense.

PATHOPHYSIOLOGY

Organisms reach the brain hematogenously, from direct contiguous infection, or by direct seeding by neurosurgery or penetrating trauma. Hematogenous spread accounts for 15% to 30% of cases, direct spread from infection accounts for 25% to 50%, and trauma or surgery for 8% to 20%. The route is unknown in 15% to 20% of cases.[28,29] Direct spread usually results in an isolated brain abscess, whereas hematogenous seeding results in multiple abscesses.

Investigate for the source of the brain abscess in order to determine the likely bacterial etiology and to treat the source itself. Otogenic brain abscesses are often caused by gram-negative rods and are located adjacent to the temporal lobe or cerebellum. Sinogenic or odontogenic abscesses are often caused by anaerobic and microaerophilic streptococci and are commonly located in the frontal lobes. Abscesses formed from hematogenous spread are usually polymicrobial, with anaerobic and microaerophilic streptococci commonly represented. Direct implantation or traumatic injuries yield staphylococci, with Gram-negative rods also seen in cases related to neurologic surgery.[25]

CLINICAL FEATURES

History Presenting features of brain abscess are nonspecific, and patients are generally appear nontoxic. Headache is the most common feature, with fever as a close second. Although most patients present with one or more findings of headache, fever, altered mental status, focal neurologic symptoms, seizures, or balance changes, the classic triad of headache, fever, and focal neurologic deficit is present in <25% of all patients.[28,29] The nonspecific presentation contributes to both severity and outcome of brain abscesses because diagnosis and treatment are often delayed.[30] Symptoms reflect the infectious and neurologic (focal and mass-effect producing) aspects of the disease and are often present for 1 to 8 weeks.[28] The presentation may be dominated by the origin of the infection (e.g., ear or sinus pain). Seizure occurs in 25% to 34% of patients.[31]

Physical Examination Examine for focal neurologic signs that demonstrate the site of the lesion; for example, a frontal lobe lesion presenting with hemiparesis, a temporal lobe lesion presenting with homonymous superior quadrant visual field deficits or aphasia, or a cerebellar lesion presenting with limb incoordination or nystagmus. Focal signs are present in approximately 60% of patients. Assess for potential sites of origin, which may raise suspicion of brain abscess when the presentation is otherwise nonspecific (e.g., otitis media, sinus tenderness, evidence of pulmonary suppuration, or right-to-left shunting) in a patient with subacute headache and lethargy.

DIAGNOSIS

Neuroimaging is essential to the diagnosis of brain abscess and is one instance where a contrast-enhanced head CT scan is preferred over a noncontrast study in the ED. A noncontrast CT scan may only show a hypodense low-attenuation abnormality with mass effect, but later in the course, CT may show a peripheral ring.[28] A head CT with IV contrast shows one or several thin, smooth rings of enhancement surrounding a low-density central area and surrounded by edema (**Figure 174-3**). MRI usually demonstrates a ring whether or not gadolinium enhancement is used. Both CT and MRI are highly sensitive; CT is often more readily available in the ED. Avoid LP if clinical suspicion is high or focal neurologic deficits are present to prevent potential herniation in the case of increased intracranial pressure. If possible, obtain cultures of blood and other sites of infection to guide future management.

The differential diagnosis is broad because of the nonspecific symptoms of brain abscess. A sudden onset with focal features may suggest cerebrovascular disease. Prominent fever, stiff neck, and altered mental status may suggest meningitis or encephalitis. A protracted course with features of increased intracranial pressure may suggest neoplasm. Brain neoplasm, subacute brain hemorrhage, and other focal brain infections, such as toxoplasmosis, may mimic the imaging findings of brain abscess.

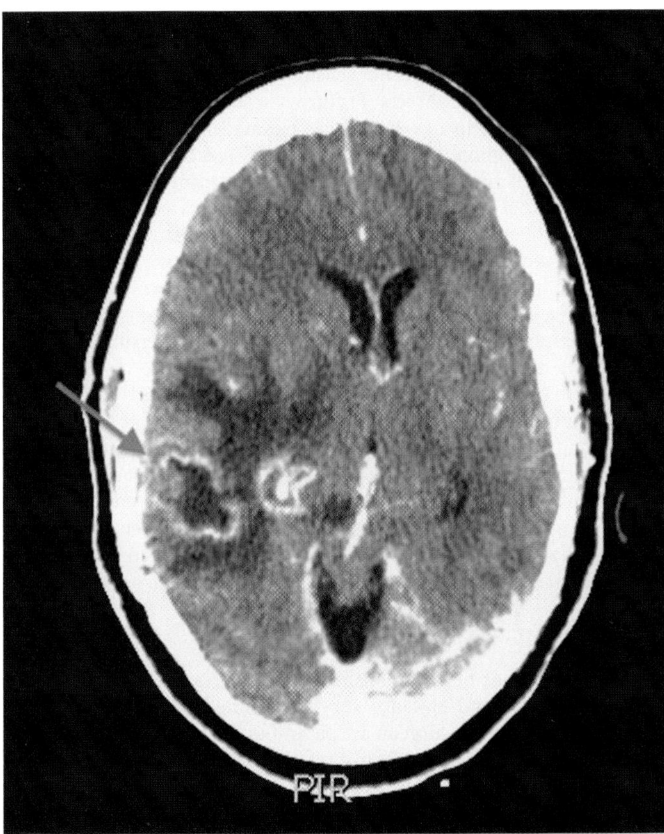

FIGURE 174-3. Ring-enhancing brain abscess with surrounding edema (arrow). [Photo contributed by David Peterson, Department of Radiology, Oregon Health & Science University.]

TREATMENT

Early combination empiric antibiotic therapy is important (**Table 174-4**). A multidisciplinary approach with neurosurgery and infectious disease consultations will help guide treatment selection. Aminoglycosides, macrolides, and first-generation cephalosporins are not effective treatment for brain abscess. Treatment with steroids is controversial.

DISPOSITION AND FOLLOW-UP

Neurosurgery involvement is paramount in the treatment and management decisions. Patients with small abscesses <2.5 cm, with good clinical condition with a Glasgow coma score >12, and who have an etiology that is known may be treated with IV antibiotics alone.[32] Aspiration may be done by the neurosurgical team to elucidate the causative organism. Total excision is less necessary with improved imaging, although it is preformed in the setting of increased intracranial pressure or after failed medical management or aspiration.[5]

EPIDURAL ABSCESS

INTRODUCTION AND EPIDEMIOLOGY

Spinal epidural abscess is a collection of pyogenic material that accumulates in the epidural space between the dura and vertebral periosteum and often leads to devastating neurologic outcomes.[33,34] Spinal epidural abscess is a rare diagnosis and accounts for 0.2 to 1.2 cases per 10,000 hospital admissions. The incidence has doubled in the past two decades, largely attributed to factors such as an increasing proportion of immunocompromised patients, more prevalent IV drug use, a larger number of spinal procedures being preformed, and improved imaging modalities for detection.[35,36] Despite improvement in diagnosis and treatment, mortality remains high at 2% to 20%.[33] *S. aureus* is the most commonly involved bacteria and is responsible for 70% of cases with a higher proportion of methicillin-resistant *S. aureus* seen in patients with implantable devices.[33,36] Other pathogens include *Staphylococcus epidermidis*, streptococcal species, and gram-negative bacilli, which is especially prevalent in IV drug users. Mycobacteria and fungi causing spinal epidural abscess are rare.

PATHOPHYSIOLOGY

Spinal epidural abscess arises from hematogenous spread through blood circulation 25% to 50% of the time, with soft tissue, urine, and respiratory infections contributing in the majority of cases. In general, hematogenously spread epidural abscesses are more likely to be found in the posterior epidural space. Ten to 30% of spinal epidural abscesses are caused by direct extension from infected adjacent tissue, such as psoas abscess, vertebral diskitis, or vertebral osteomyelitis. Direct extension often infects the anterior portion of the spinal column.[33,37] Fifteen to 22% of spinal epidural abscesses are caused iatrogenically from neurosurgical procedures, including percutaneous diagnostic and therapeutic techniques. Trauma contributes to a small proportion of spinal epidural abscesses, with the remainder of cases without an identifiable source.[35,36]

Most spinal epidural abscesses affect the thoracic and lumbar spine, where the epidural space is wider with a larger venous plexus.

TABLE 174-4 Guidelines for Empiric Treatment of Brain Abscess Based on Presumed Source

Presumed Source	Primary Empiric Therapy	Alternative Therapy
Otogenic	Cefotaxime 2 grams IV every 4–6 h or ceftriaxone 2 grams IV every 12 h PLUS metronidazole 500 milligrams IV every 8 h	Piperacillin/tazobactam 4.5 grams IV every 6 h
Odontogenic	Penicillin G 4 million units IV every 4 h	Ceftriaxone 2 grams IV every 12 h PLUS metronidazole 500 milligrams IV every 6 h
Sinogenic	Cefotaxime 2 grams IV every 6 h or ceftriaxone 2 grams IV every 12 h PLUS metronidazole 500 milligrams IV every 8 h	No recommendation
Penetrating trauma	Cefotaxime 2 grams IV every 6 h or ceftriaxone 2 grams IV every 12 h PLUS metronidazole 500 milligrams IV every 8 h ± rifampin 10 milligrams/kg every 24 h	No recommendation
After neurosurgical procedure	Vancomycin loading dose 25–30 milligrams/kg IV loading dose or linezolid 600 milligrams IV every 12 h PLUS ceftazidime 2 grams IV every 8 h ± rifampin 10 milligrams/kg every 24 h	Can substitute linezolid 600 milligrams IV every 12 h instead of vancomycin. Can substitute meropenem 2 grams IV every 8 h OR piperacillin/tazobactam 4.5 grams IV every 6 h OR cefepime 2 grams IV every 8 h for ceftazidime.
Unknown source	Cefotaxime 2 grams IV every 6 h PLUS metronidazole 500 milligrams IV every 6 h	No recommendation

Note: See also http://www.hopkins-abxguide.org; accessed June 18, 2014.

The cervical spine is affected only 5% to 20% of the time, although morbidity and neurologic devastation are much greater in these cases.[38]

Mechanisms for spinal cord neurologic sequelae are uncertain and are thought to be from a combination of direct compression from the abscess itself, ischemia due to compression of spinal veins and arteries, and septic thrombophlebitis.[33]

CLINICAL FEATURES

Back pain is the most common presenting complaint and is seen in 70% to 90% of cases. Fever is another common symptom, followed by the presence of a neurologic deficit. However, the classic triad of back pain, fever, and neurologic symptoms is seen in a minority of patients (8% to 37%) on initial presentation.[33,36] Typically, patients with spinal epidural abscess progress through four stages in a period ranging from hours to days. Stage 1 consists of back pain, fever, and localized spinal tenderness. Stage 2 is composed of spinal irritation, including radicular pain, hyperreflexia, and nuchal rigidity. Stage 3 involves the bowel and bladder, with symptoms of fecal or urinary incontinence, as well as focal neurologic deficits such as motor weakness. Finally, in stage 4, paralysis ensues.[33,36]

HISTORY

Screen any patient presenting with back pain, fever, or neurologic complaint for spinal epidural abscess. Patients may have a history of chronic back pain or may offer a mechanism of mild trauma as an explanation for their symptoms, which can distract from a diagnosis of spinal epidural abscess. Similarly, neck pain or stiffness is often thought to be meningitis or encephalitis, causing cervical spinal epidural abscess to be overlooked.

Carefully search for back pain red flags in the patient's history, including immunocompromised states, such as human immunodeficiency virus or diabetes, and immunosuppressant medications, such as steroids or chemotherapy. Elicit a history of recent systemic illness or infection. Inquire about any current or former IV drug use, which can make patients higher risk for spinal epidural abscess development from *Pseudomonas* species. Solicit information about prior spinal surgeries or procedures, including LPs, epidurals, spinal injections, or anesthesia. Ask about any changes in bowel or bladder habits, specifically episodes of bladder fullness or urinary or fecal incontinence.[36,39]

PHYSICAL EXAMINATION

Perform a thorough physical examination starting with a general assessment of sources of infection, including observation of the skin and palpation of soft tissues for signs of infection. Palpate the spine searching for tenderness to palpation, especially in the midline, which may suggest spinal epidural abscess. Complete a full neurologic examination, including sensory dermatome testing and motor evaluation including ambulation. Check reflexes for hyper- or areflexia. Evaluate for symptoms of cauda equine syndrome. Perform a rectal examination looking for decreased rectal tone, which has a sensitivity of 60% to 80%, and an evaluation of perianal sensation for saddle anesthesia, which has a sensitivity of 75%.[40]

DIAGNOSIS

Diagnosis is delayed in many patients with spinal epidural abscess due to nonspecific presenting symptoms and the rarity of diagnosis. Send blood for laboratory studies including blood culture, CBC, erythrocyte sedimentation rate, and C-reactive protein. Leukocytosis is seen in only 60% to 75% of patients and is not sensitive or specific enough for a diagnosis of spinal epidural abscess. Erythrocyte sedimentation rate is much more sensitive and, in one study, was elevated in 110 of 117 patients diagnosed with spinal epidural abscess.[41] C-reactive protein has the advantage of rising faster than erythrocyte sedimentation rate and returns to normal sooner as well, but some labs have a delay in resulting C-reactive protein. Do not withhold further diagnostics and treatment pending C-reactive protein.[36] Blood cultures are positive in 40% of cases and may be helpful for inpatient teams. Do not perform LP if there is suspicion for spinal abscess. Cerebrospinal fluid culture is positive less than a quarter of the time, and LP poses the risk of traversing an abscess and causing meningitis or a subdural infection.[36]

MRI with gadolinium is the gold standard imaging study for the diagnosis of spinal epidural abscess and has a sensitivity and specificity greater than 90%.[37] If MRI is not available, consider emergent transfer to an appropriate referral center. In patients with contraindications to MRI, CT with myelography can be useful to localize epidural compression but is limited in its ability to distinguish abscess from other compressive lesions.[36] Plain radiographs are not sensitive or specific for diagnosis of spinal epidural abscess.[37]

TREATMENT

Once diagnosis has been established, prompt treatment is essential to reduce morbidity and enhance survival. Immediate consultation and evaluation with a spine surgeon are paramount, and if a spine surgeon is not available, emergent transfer to a referral center is appropriate.[36] Neurologic outcome is correlated with degree of neurologic deficit prior to treatment, so time is of the essence.

There are no conclusive data regarding surgery versus conservative antibiotic therapy, and practices vary considerably from immediate operative therapy to conservative IV antibiotic therapy.[37] Patients with neurologic deficits usually require evacuation of the abscess with decompressive laminectomy, debridement, and long-term IV antibiotics, and some studies have shown improved outcomes with emergent surgery.[35] Patients who are neurologically intact or who have had neurologic deficits for >72 hours may be candidates for conservative treatment or CT-guided aspiration depending on the spinal surgeon's practice, with the understanding that if they develop neurologic deficits or decompensate immediate surgical therapy is likely required.[35]

Start empiric antibiotic therapy if there will be an unavoidable delay for surgery or if the patient exhibits neurologic dysfunction or signs of sepsis. Appropriate empiric antibiotics can include a combination of vancomycin, 25 to 30 milligrams/kg loading dose and then 15 milligrams/kg every 12 hours, to cover methicillin-resistant *S. aureus* along with ceftazidime, 2 grams IV every 8 hours, or cefepime, 2 grams IV every 12 hours.[33,42] Consider adding gentamicin, 5 milligrams/kg IV every 24 hours, if the spinal epidural abscess occurred after a neurosurgical procedure.[42] Once cultures return, an infectious disease consult may be helpful to determine long-term antibiotic choice and duration.

DISPOSITION AND FOLLOW-UP

Admit patients diagnosed with spinal epidural abscess directly to the operating room for spinal surgery. If the patient will receive conservative therapy, then admit to the intensive care unit for close monitoring, neurologic checks, and further management in conjunction with the spinal surgery team.

Lumbar Puncture Checklist

1. Assess patient for risk factors or clinical signs of increased intracranial pressure, as in Table 174-3. If signs or risk factors are present, order noncontrast head CT prior to lumbar puncture (LP) to assess for risk of herniation.
2. Assess clinically and/or evaluate laboratory results to ensure no signs of coagulopathy or thrombocytopenia.
3. Obtain informed consent from patient or medical decision maker, and document discussion of risks and benefits.
4. Gather supplies including LP tray with two spinal needles, four cerebrospinal fluid (CSF) tubes, manometer with three-way valve, local anesthetic, syringe with 18-guage needle to draw up anesthetic and 25-guage needle to inject anesthetic, 0.5% chlorhexidine/70% alcohol, sterile gloves, mask, cap, and drape.
5. Position patient properly (if right-handed, position in left lateral decubitus position, and if left-handed, place in right lateral decubitus position). Maintain the patient's head in a neutral position and flex the patient's knees to their chest.
6. Assess the patient's anatomy in the midline, searching for a palpable area between the vertebrae L4/5 or L5/S1 for spinal needle insertion.
7. Ensure sterile technique: apply mask and cap, carefully wash hands, and don sterile gloves.
8. Prepare LP tray and open CSF tubes so they are ready for fluid collection. Prepare manometer by connecting the two tubes and loosening the manometer tap.
9. Carefully cleanse the patient's skin over desired lumbar puncture area in a circular fashion three times.
10. Anesthetize the space starting with a small intradermal bleb of lidocaine, and advance to slightly deeper areas drawing back on the syringe before injecting the anesthetic.
11. Insert spinal needle into the anesthetized space with the stylet in place. Slowly advance, maintaining a horizontal plane, with a trajectory slightly cephalad until mild resistance is felt at the ligamentum flavum with a subsequent "give" while entering the subarachnoid space.
12. Remove the stylet and wait for CSF to drip from the needle. If it does not drip, replace the stylet and advance an additional 2 mm, and check again for CSF. If resistance is felt, bone is likely being hit. In this case, withdraw the needle to the subcutaneous tissue and palpate landmarks to ensure you are midline, change the angle slightly cephalad, and attempt again.

Lumbar Puncture Checklist (*Continued*)

13. Once CSF is visualized, attach the manometer to the spinal needle for a measurement of opening pressure.
14. Once opening pressure is measured, remove the manometer and collect the CSF, approximately 1 mL in each tube in the order of tubes 1 to 4. Note the color and consistency of the CSF as it drips into the collection tube.
15. Once CSF is collected, replace the stylet into the spinal needle and remove the spinal needle.
16. Apply a sterile dressing to the procedure site.

REFERENCES

Boon JM, Abrahams PH, Meiring JH, Welch T: Lumbar puncture: anatomical review of a clinical skill. *Clin Anat* 17: 544, 2004. [PMID: 15376294]

Doherty CM, Forbes RB: Diagnostic lumbar puncture. *Ulster Med J* 83: 93, 2014. [PMID: 25075138]

Roos K: Lumbar puncture. *Semin Neurol* 23: 105, 2003. [PMID: 12870112]

REFERENCES

The complete reference list is available online at www.TintinalliEM.com.

CHAPTER 175 Central Nervous System Procedures and Devices

Jay G. Ladde

LUMBAR PUNCTURE

Lumbar puncture is considered the gold standard diagnostic procedure to assist clinicians with the evaluation of subarachnoid hemorrhage, meningitis, and other neurologic conditions. Anxiolytics, such as benzodiazepines, may be administered to improve patient comfort, relaxation, and cooperation. Contraindications to lumbar puncture are listed in **Table 175-1**.

If an anxiolytic is used, give a short-acting agent to avoid clouding subsequent clinical assessment. Antiseptic technique should be strictly observed. Scrub the site with povidone-iodine and allow to dry thoroughly to avoid introduction of the chemical and the subsequent production of chemical arachnoiditis.

In adults, a transverse line drawn between the iliac crests crosses the spine at the L4 spinous process. The L4-L5 interspace is the most commonly used interspace for lumbar puncture, although one can also select the L3-L4 interspace. Palpate the L4-L5 interspace while the patient is curled as tightly as possible in a fetal position. Alternatively, the patient may be seated on the edge of a bed or cart leaning over a tray stand. This latter technique is particularly useful when landmarks are uncertain due to body habitus.

Use a $3^{1}/_{2}$-inch atraumatic 22-gauge needle in adults. Use of a needle larger than 20-gauge may double the incidence of post–lumbar puncture headache compared with a smaller needle. The use of an atraumatic or pencil-point needle (such as a Whitacre or Sprotte needle) is associated with fewer post–lumbar puncture headaches than a conventional cutting needle[1,2] (**Figure 175-1**). Also, a smaller needle size using the stylet is associated with reduced frequency of post–lumbar puncture headaches.[1]

TECHNIQUE

Assemble all equipment. Then properly position the patient and identify the patient's L4-L5 interspace. Now put on your sterile gown, mask, and gloves. Next, apply povidone-iodine to the area and let dry. Apply sterile

TABLE 175-1 Contraindications to Lumbar Puncture

Contraindications
Skin infection near the site of lumbar puncture
CNS lesion causing increased intracranial pressure, or spinal mass
Platelet count <20,000 mm³ is an absolute contraindication; platelet counts >50,000 mm³ are safe for lumbar puncture*
International normalized ratio ≥1.5*
Administration of unfiltrated heparin or low-molecular-weight heparin in past 24 h*
Hemophilia, von Willebrand's disease, other coagulopathies*
Trauma to lumbar vertebrae

*Correct clotting factor and/or platelet levels before lumbar puncture.

drapes. Anesthetize the skin with 1% lidocaine by raising a skin bleb, then directing the needle toward the umbilicus, and injecting the anesthetic in a fan-shaped area around the proposed lumbar puncture site. Make sure to pull back on the plunger to check for blood return before injecting to avoid intravascular injection. Recheck the patient's position, making sure the patient is perpendicular to the horizontal and not slanted. Check the needle and make sure that it is the correct size and that the stylet is easily removed and reinserted. Identify that the needle bevel (Quincke needle) or notch (Whitacre needle) is facing the ceiling. Put together the manometer, making sure you know how the stopcocks work. Assuming you are right-handed, identify the interspinous space with your left hand and position the needle at the L4-L5 interspace, parallel to the horizontal, and direct it firmly and slowly toward the patient's umbilicus. As the needle advances, you may feel a slight "pop," indicating that you have pierced the ligamentum flavum and dura mater. Remove the stylet, note draining cerebrospinal fluid (CSF), and attach the manometer to measure the opening pressure. After collecting at least 1 mL in each of four tubes, disconnect the manometer and replace the stylet before withdrawing the spinal needle (**Figure 175-2**). Do not aspirate because slight negative pressure may facilitate herniation.[1]

If unable to penetrate the subarachnoid space, it is best to withdraw the needle completely, out of the skin, and direct the needle again. In some patients (for example, those who are extremely obese or who have degenerative disease of the spine), it is particularly difficult to successfully perform a lumbar puncture. The use of US guidance or even consultation of a radiologist to perform under fluoroscopy may be necessary.

US imaging of the interspinous processes is superior to palpation with regard to fewer failed attempts.[3] A 5- to 10-MHz linear probe is applied in the sagittal plane to identify the dorsal spinous processes, and the midline is then marked with a sterile marking pen. Lumbar puncture is then performed as outlined above.

For results to be meaningful, measure the opening pressure with the patient lying extended on his or her side. Pressures measured with the patient still curled in extreme flexion or sitting may be artificially elevated. Normal pressure is <170 mm H_2O. Careful repositioning (straightening the curled patient or helping the seated patient to a lying position on his or her side) can be safely performed with the needle in place. Obtain accurate pressure readings only when the patient is in a calm state if possible. Shouting, crying, or coughing can elevate the pressure falsely.[1]

Obtain four tubes, each containing at least 1 mL of CSF. Obtain red and white blood cell counts with differential for tubes 1 and 4. Tube 4 may also be used for culture and Gram staining. Tube 2 is sent for determination of protein and glucose levels. Save tube 3 for other studies that may be required. **Table 175-2** lists normal CSF findings. See chapters 166, "Spontaneous Subarachnoid and Intracerebral Hemorrhage" and 174, "Central Nervous System and Spinal Infections" for further discussion of CSF interpretation.

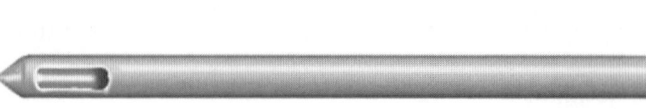

TABLE 175-2 Normal Cerebrospinal Fluid Values

Parameter	Value
Opening pressure	50–170 mm H_2O
Appearance	Clear (can be clear with up to 400 cells/mm³)
Xanthochromia	None
Red blood cells	≤5/mm³
WBCs	≤5/mm³ (no polymorphonuclear leukocytes)
Glucose level	>40 milligrams/dL or 60%–70% of serum glucose level
Protein level	<50 milligrams/dL
Gram stain and culture results	Negative

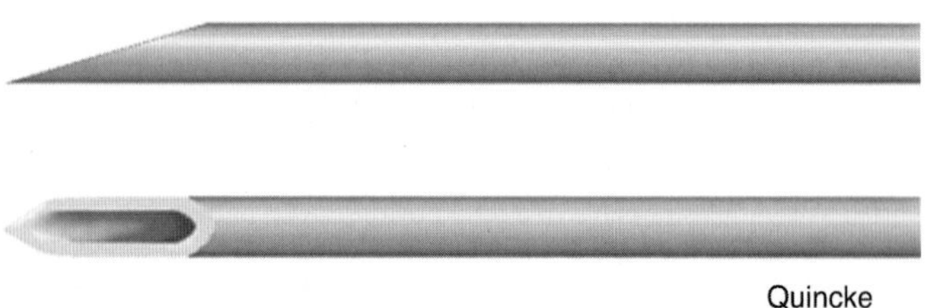

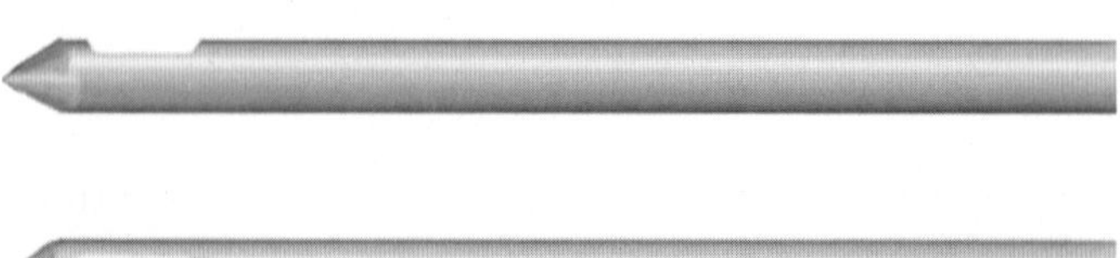

FIGURE 175-1. Two types of needle for lumbar puncture. The Quincke is a bevel-type needle, and the Whitacre is a pencil-point needle.

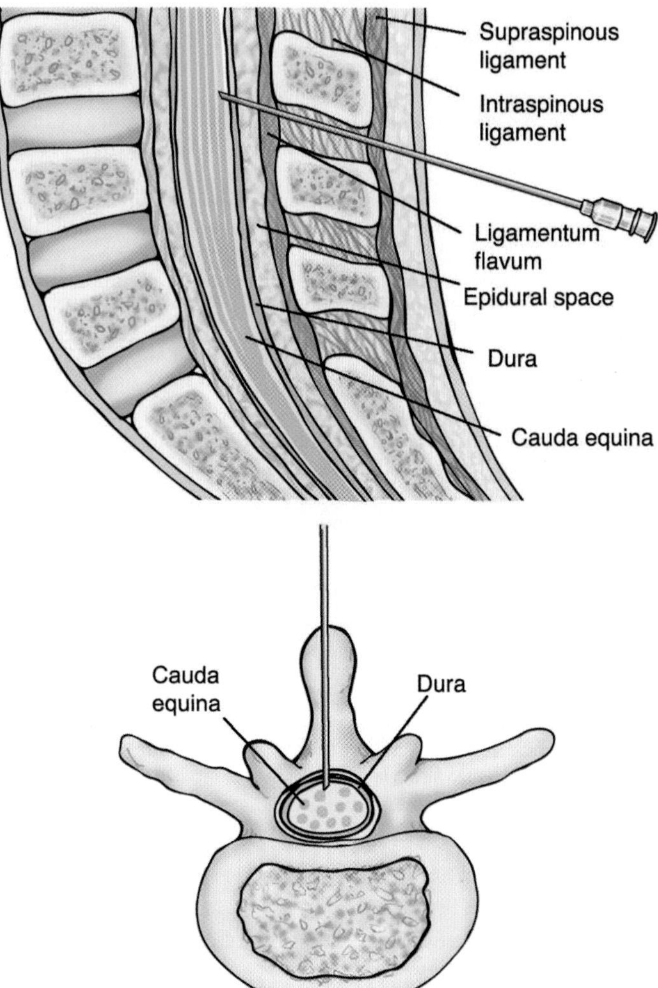

FIGURE 175-2. Anatomy of the lumbar spinal interspaces for lumbar puncture.

COMPLICATIONS OF LUMBAR PUNCTURE

Local discomfort is to be expected; radicular pain indicates that the needle is too lateral, which necessitates repositioning. Spinal hematoma is a particularly ominous complication. The development of severe or persistent back pain after the procedure, radicular pain, new neurologic symptoms, or sphincter disturbance indicates that a spinal hematoma may be present. Most present within the first 6 hours.[1] Management includes MRI of the spine and neurosurgical consultation.

Post–lumbar puncture headache is the most common complication of lumbar puncture. The cause is thought to be continuous CSF leakage from the dural puncture site. Traction on bridging vessels, dura, and nerves causes headache. Post–lumbar puncture headache usually begins 24 to 48 hours after the procedure and is located in the frontal or occipital area. It is pressure-like and throbbing, with variable intensity. It is intensified when the patient is sitting or standing upright and with Valsalva maneuvers such as coughing. The headache improves or resolves when the patient is supine. It can be associated with nausea, vomiting, and even vertigo and tinnitus. Risk factors for post–lumbar puncture headache include use of a large needle size (>22 gauge), use of a cutting (Quincke) needle, multiple attempts, and failure to replace the stylet when withdrawing the needle.[1,2] Post–lumbar puncture headache does not seem to be related to the opening pressure, the volume of CSF removed, or bed rest after the procedure. Postprocedural bed rest does not prevent this complication.[4] Diagnosis is clinical. Most headaches resolve with rest in the supine position, maintenance of hydration, and administration of antiemetics and analgesics.[1] IV caffeine (500 milligrams IV of caffeine sodium benzoate) is commonly administered, but whether or not it improves headache is controversial.[5] Persistent headache (>24 hours) can be treated with an epidural blood patch. In this procedure, usually performed by an anesthesiologist, a needle is introduced into the epidural space, and 20 to 30 mL of the patient's blood is injected into the epidural space.

CEREBROSPINAL FLUID SHUNTS

Mechanical shunting is the primary treatment for hydrocephalus. Placement of a CSF shunt is the most common pediatric neurosurgical procedure performed in the United States. It is also the neurosurgical procedure with the highest incidence of postoperative complications.[6] Many types of CSF shunt systems exist (**Figures 175-3, 175-4, and 175-5**). Most systems consist of three components, beginning with a silastic tube passed into the ventricle via a burr hole. This tubing is tunneled subcutaneously to a valve chamber. The valve chamber, the second component, establishes a pressure gradient that ensures drainage of fluid away from the ventricle. The valve chamber, or in some cases a separate reservoir, allows access to the shunt system for patency testing, pressure measurement, CSF sampling, medication injection (e.g., chemotherapy, antibiotics), or contrast administration. Distal tubing, which is the third component, connects the valve chamber to a drainage point. The most common drainage site is the peritoneal cavity. Other drainage sites include the right atrium, gallbladder, pleural cavity, and ureter.

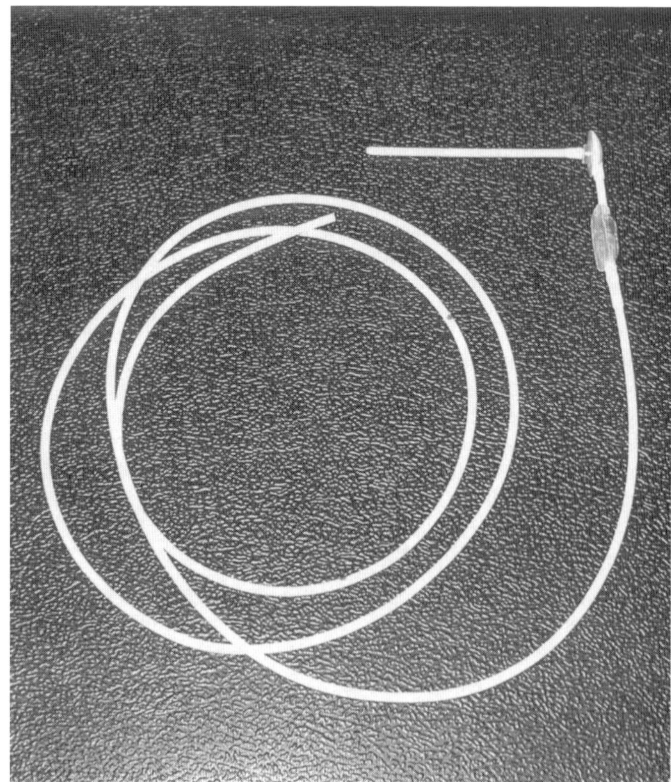

FIGURE 175-4. Typical ventriculoperitoneal shunt.

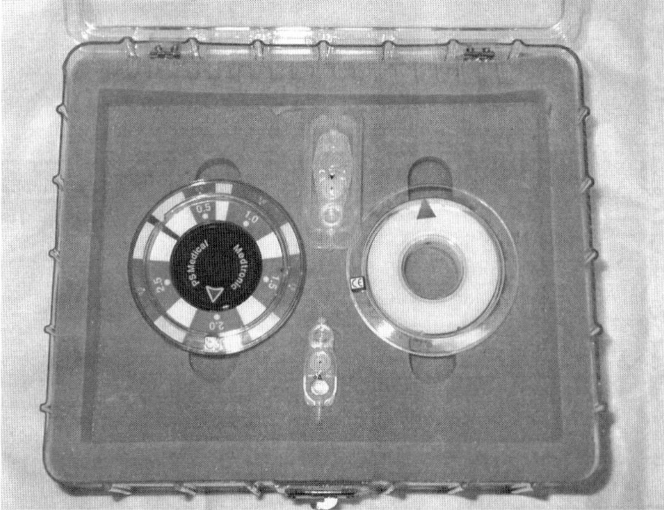

FIGURE 175-3. Example of a shunt kit. Circular objects on the left are a locator and a pressure/performance indicator. Circular object on the right is an adjustment tool. All three are needed to adjust the settings. Two sizes of valves are shown in the middle.

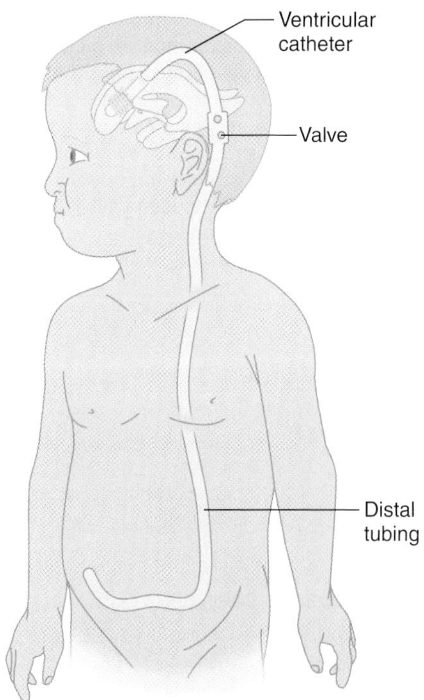

FIGURE 175-5. Ventriculoperitoneal shunt system.

Programmable shunt valves allow for easier control of flow rates, which is particularly useful in previously difficult cases that required frequent adjustments. The valve can be adjusted and tested using a locator and indicator tool to determine the pressure programmed into the valve. An adjustment tool can then be used to increase or decrease the valve's pressure or performance as needed. Typical nonadjustable pressure-type valves are available with low, medium, and high settings. These valves open at a pressure gradient of 2 to 4, 4 to 6, and 8 to 10 cm H_2O for the low, medium, and high settings, respectively. The adjustable valves typically have five preset pressure settings that can be selected or adjusted as clinically warranted. The patient (or family) should have been given a card that documents initial settings and any subsequent adjustments. Pressure setting can also be confirmed by radiography using the radiopaque dials on the valve.

Exposure to strong magnetic fields and some MRI units can change the valve pressure setting, so all patients should have the setting verified after any exposure to strong magnetic fields. Controversy still exists as to whether programmable valves offer an advantage over traditional valves in reducing the number of revisions and extending shunt life.[7-9]

CSF SHUNT MALFUNCTION

Shunt malfunctions are the most common complications encountered with CSF shunts. Shunt malfunction can be due to obstruction, mechanical failure, overdrainage, loculation of ventricles, or abdominal complications.

Obstruction **Obstruction is the most common type of shunt malfunction.** The most frequent location of obstruction is the proximal tubing, followed by the distal tubing, and then the valve chamber. Proximal obstructions usually occur within the first years after shunt insertion. **Table 175-3** lists the common causes of CSF shunt obstruction.

Distal obstruction is the most frequently encountered obstruction in shunts in place for >2 years.[6] Shunt obstruction usually manifests with signs and symptoms of increased intracranial pressure. Infants generally present with vomiting, irritability, and a bulging fontanelle.[10] Older children and adults may present with cephalgia, nausea, vomiting, lethargy, ataxia, and cranial nerve palsies.[10]

Mechanical Failure Mechanical failure of shunts can be secondary to fracture, disconnection, migration, or misplacement. Typically, fractures appear in distal tubing many years after shunt placement; this is due to both degradation of tubing and stress from the growth of the patient.[6] The most common location for a fracture is along the clavicle or lower ribs.[6] Patients present with mild symptoms of increased intracranial pressure. Local symptoms of pain, mild erythema, and edema over the affected area are not uncommon. In fact, it not unusual for a fracture to be found incidentally because the shunt tract often serves as a conduit between the fractured segments.[6] Disconnection often occurs shortly after insertion and manifests as increased intracranial pressure and fluid at the skin site around the disconnection. Migration occurs when a properly placed catheter migrates to a position in which drainage is compromised partially or completely. Misplacement entails the placement of the catheter into brain parenchyma, the choroid plexus, or the temporal horns; it usually manifests postoperatively with evidence of failure.

TABLE 175-3 Causes of CSF Shunt Obstruction

Proximal obstruction
Tissue debris
Choroid plexus
Clot
Infection
Catheter tip migration
Localized immune response to the tubing
Distal obstruction
Kinking or disconnection of the tube
Pseudocyst formation
Infection

Overdrainage Overdrainage and the slit ventricle syndrome are seen in approximately 5% of patients with shunts. Because of overdrainage, the tissues actually occlude the orifices of the proximal shunt apparatus. As intracranial pressure increases, the same occluding tissue is disengaged, which allows drainage to resume. This phenomenon is cyclical and is responsible for the episodic or waxing and waning aspect of the presenting complaint. Patients present with episodes of elevated intracranial pressure caused by a transient obstruction of the ventricular catheter from a collapsed ventricle. Decreased cerebral compliance may prevent the ventricles from fully expanding as intracranial pressure and volume increase, which further contributes to ventricular collapse. The rate of this complication is lower for currently used shunt systems with antisiphon devices and programmable shunt valves.[8,11]

Loculation Separate, noncommunicating CSF accumulations may develop within a ventricle so that the shunt device is not able to drain the entire ventricular system, leaving behind enlarging pockets of fluid that may have compressive sequelae. Trapped fourth ventricle syndrome occurs when the fourth ventricle becomes loculated, presumably from closure of the sylvian aqueduct.[6] Patients present with typical symptoms of increased intracranial pressure as well as symptoms of brainstem compression, including poor feeding, disconjugate gaze, and difficulty swallowing.

Abdominal Complications Several abdominal processes can secondarily result in shunt malfunction. The most commonly encountered complication is malfunction due to pseudocyst formation. Pseudocysts are localized abdominal fluid collections that form around the peritoneal catheter. Infection is the major cause, with an infection rate of 40%.[12] They often are asymptomatic until they enlarge substantially enough to cause abdominal pain.

CLINICAL PRESENTATION

Symptoms of CSF shunt malfunction usually develop over several days, although rapid deterioration within 24 hours has been reported. **Clinical features include mental status changes, headache, nausea, vomiting, abdominal pain, lethargy, decreased intellectual performance, ataxia, coma, and autonomic instability.** Often, the presenting complaint is vague. No single sign or symptom is accurate in predicting shunt malfunction, although a decrease in level of consciousness may have the highest correlation with shunt malfunction.[6] As intracranial pressure increases, paralysis of upward gaze, dilated pupils, and papilledema may develop. Paralysis of upward gaze (or sundowning) is caused by impingement on the brainstem by the third ventricle as it engorges. Symptoms of slit ventricle syndrome are exacerbated or precipitated when the patient stands or exercises due to excessive CSF drainage and are relieved when the patient lies down or is in the Trendelenburg position.

SHUNT EVALUATION

Identification of shunt type is important, although frequently difficult. Many different types exist, and appropriate assessment depends on the apparatus implanted. For example, many flow control valves have a high set resistance so that flow is quite slow but steady. Conversely, such a flow pattern might indicate obstruction in a low-resistance shunt.[13] Evaluate shunt function by manual testing and radiologic studies. Palpation of the shunt allows the physician to locate the valve chamber. Shunt patency is evaluated somewhat differently for each type of device depending on features such as the presence of valves or dome- or cylinder-shaped reservoirs. Generally, testing follows intuitive expectations but still may prove perplexing to inexperienced clinicians. For a simple device, once the chamber is located, it is gently compressed and observed for refill. **Difficulty compressing the chamber indicates distal flow obstruction, whereas slow refill, defined as refill requiring >3 seconds after compression, generally indicates a proximal obstruction.** Compression is inaccurate for identifying shunt obstruction because up to 40% of obstructed shunts show normal refill during manual palpation.[4] Furthermore, positive predictive value has been found to be as low as 12% for shunt pumping.[13] In any case, further evaluation is required.

A shunt series of plain radiographs includes anteroposterior and lateral radiographs of the skull and an anteroposterior view of the chest and

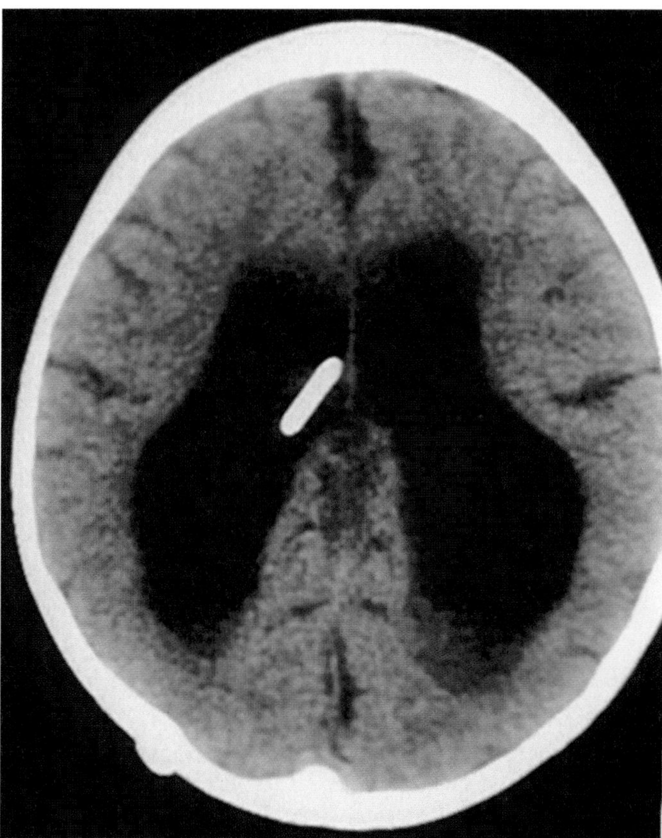

FIGURE 175-6. CT may reveal a persistent hydrocephalus despite the presence of a shunt, which suggests a malfunction. Comparison CTs are helpful when available.

abdomen (for ventriculoperitoneal shunts). Although plain radiography will identify kinking, migration, or disconnection of the shunt system, CT is required to evaluate ventricular size (**Figures 175-6 and 175-7**). **Compare with previous CT scans because many patients with shunts have an abnormal baseline ventricular size.** In one series using either CT or both CT and plain radiography, 24% of patients with documented shunt malfunction showed no radiologic evidence of the malfunction.[14] In another series, radiographs were shown to have a sensitivity of 20% and a negative predictive value of 22%; CT had a sensitivity of 83% and a negative predictive value of 95%.[15] Therefore, in patients with suggestive clinical features, unremarkable findings on CT and/or radiographic shunt series cannot be relied on to exclude shunt obstruction. Thus, **obtain neurosurgical consultation whenever shunt malfunction is suspected.**

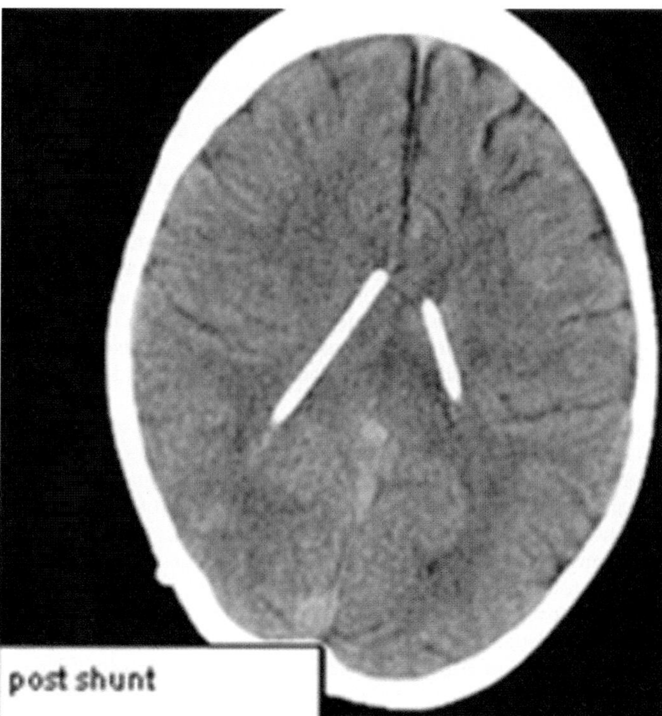

FIGURE 175-7. Slit ventricle syndrome often presents with waxing and waning symptoms. The CT is often helpful in distinguishing it from other causes of malfunction.

Perform a shunt tap to make the diagnosis of shunt malfunction, exclude infection, or alleviate life-threatening increased intracranial pressure. Unless a CNS emergency exists, the shunt tap should be performed by a neurosurgeon to avoid damage to the valve apparatus. Emergency physicians should be prepared to perform a shunt tap if a neurosurgeon is unavailable or if a shunt tap is needed to control life-threatening increased intracranial pressure.

To perform a shunt tap, locate and sterilely prepare the site over the valve system or reservoir of the shaved scalp. A 23-gauge needle or butterfly attached to a manometer is inserted into the reservoir. If no fluid returns or flow ceases, a proximal obstruction is likely. Measure the opening pressure while the reservoir outflow is occluded. An opening pressure of ≥20 cm H_2O indicates a distal obstruction, whereas low pressures indicate a proximal obstruction. The normal basal intracranial pressure is 12 ± 2 cm H_2O.

Flash MRI has assumed a growing role in serial examination for shunt function to obviate some of the radiation exposure associated with CT. In certain institutions, single-shot T2-weighted MRI has become the initial imaging modality of choice. With the advent and widespread use of programmable shunts, the concern over shunt failure after MRI exists. The MRI magnetic field can change the valve-pressure setting in programmable valves. Newer programmable valves do not reprogram even at a 3-T magnetic field.[6] In general, the settings of a programmable valve should be checked by the neurosurgeon after a patient undergoes MRI.

TREATMENT OF SHUNT MALFUNCTION

Surgical intervention is generally required in cases of shunt obstruction. As a temporizing measure, intracranial pressure can be lowered by standard methods of hyperventilation and osmotic diuresis (mannitol). **If these measures fail and surgical intervention is not immediately available, intracranial pressure can be lowered by removing CSF via the reservoir if the malfunction is distal.** To prevent choroid plexus bleeding, CSF should be removed slowly, and the process should be discontinued when intracranial pressure reaches 10 to 20 cm H_2O. Stable patients in whom obstruction is suspected require admission and neurosurgical consultation. Observe patients for any neurologic changes, abdominal complaints, or fever.

SHUNT INFECTION

Infection rates range between 0.6% and 21% per procedure.[16-19] The highest infection rates are found in the very young and old and in patients who have had multiple shunt revisions. There is a 26% recurrence rate of shunt infection.[20] Patients who develop shunt infections demonstrate impairment in intellectual development compared with those who do not develop infection. Half of all shunt infections present within the first 2 weeks of placement, 70% present within 2 months, and 80% present within 6 months of placement. Up to 10% of shunt infections present >1 year after surgery.

CSF shunt infections can be categorized into internal and external infections. External infections involve the subcutaneous tract around the shunt, which is usually tender, and there is often an associated fluid collection within the skin. An internal infection involves the shunt and the CSF contained within that shunt. Patients with CSF shunts have a higher risk of developing meningitis from typical pathogens (e.g., *Streptococcus pneumoniae*, and *Neisseria meningitidis*) than the general population. This increased risk may be due to disruption of the blood–brain barrier by foreign material. Shunt infections are reduced with the use of antibiotic-impregnated catheters.[21,22]

The mortality is low if shunt infection is diagnosed and treated in a timely fashion. However, if ventriculitis develops, mortality ranges from 30% to 40%, which underscores the need for prompt diagnosis and aggressive management.[23]

BACTERIOLOGY

CSF shunt infections are typically caused by low-virulence organisms. In adults, the most commonly cultured agent is *Staphylococcus epidermidis*, which accounts for nearly half of all shunt infections, followed by *Staphylococcus aureus* and *Propionibacterium acnes*.[18,20] Gram-negative, anaerobic, and mixed infections account for approximately 5% to 10% of shunt infections. Gram-negative infections are associated with the highest mortality. *Candida* accounts for a small number of infections and should be considered in premature newborns, immunosuppressed patients, and patients on long-term, broad-spectrum antibiotics. It is associated with a 5.8% mortality rate.[20]

CLINICAL FEATURES

The clinical presentation varies with the virulence of the organism and the severity of the infection. Typically, patients present with symptoms of obstruction and meningeal symptoms, including mental status changes, headache, nausea, vomiting, neck stiffness, and irritability. Fever and abdominal pain may also be present. These signs are not universally noted. In fact, the finding of fever is highly variable, and meningismus may be present in only one third of patients with shunt infection.[18] Abdominal pain may be the predominant symptom in patients with ventriculoperitoneal shunts. Swelling, erythema, and tenderness along the site of the shunt tubing are highly suggestive of external shunt infection.[13]

Shunt nephritis involves a chronic complication of vascular shunts. Typically, patients develop a chronic bacteremia from coagulase-negative *Staphylococcus* leading to an immune response. The patient presents with a nephritic syndrome with fever episodes and increased urinary sediment. Treatment of the underlying infection leads to complete resolution of the renal disorder.[18]

DIAGNOSIS

A shunt tap is required to exclude CSF shunt infection (Figure 175-7). **A traditional lumbar puncture often misses CSF shunt infection** and has no meaningful role in the evaluation when shunt infection is suspected.

Analysis of fluid from infected CSF shunts usually reveals an elevated leukocyte count, elevated protein level, and normal glucose level. Almost one fifth of patients evaluated for shunt malfunction have positive CSF culture results despite normal results on CSF analysis. Other (non-CSF) laboratory values are rarely helpful in diagnosing CSF shunt infection. CT and plain radiographs of the shunt (shunt series) are required to exclude mechanical shunt malfunction, which often coexists with shunt infection.[24] Abdominal US or CT is indicated if an abdominal fluid collection, pseudocyst, or abscess is suspected. In patients with ventriculoatrial shunts, blood cultures are helpful in identifying the offending organism. In most other cases, hematogenous dissemination of infection is rare, thus rendering blood cultures of limited value.[24]

TREATMENT

Patients with CSF shunt infection or suspected shunt infection require emergent neurosurgical consultation and admission. Until the infecting agent is identified, therapy with broad-spectrum antibiotics effective against typical pathogens (e.g., ceftriaxone and vancomycin) is recommended. Rifampin has been given along with vancomycin for treatment of recurrent gram-positive infections because it easily penetrates the CSF. Early removal of the colonized device is important.

HALO DEVICES

The halo vest provides one of the most rigid types of cervical immobilization available. The halo vest consists of a lightweight radiolucent ring attached to a lightweight adjustable vest. Current vests allow adjustment of the cervical spine in multiple planes. Titanium pins that do not interfere with MRI are stronger, lighter, and more expensive than older stainless steel pins. Pins are usually tightened to 8 lb of pressure (**Figure 175-8**).[25]

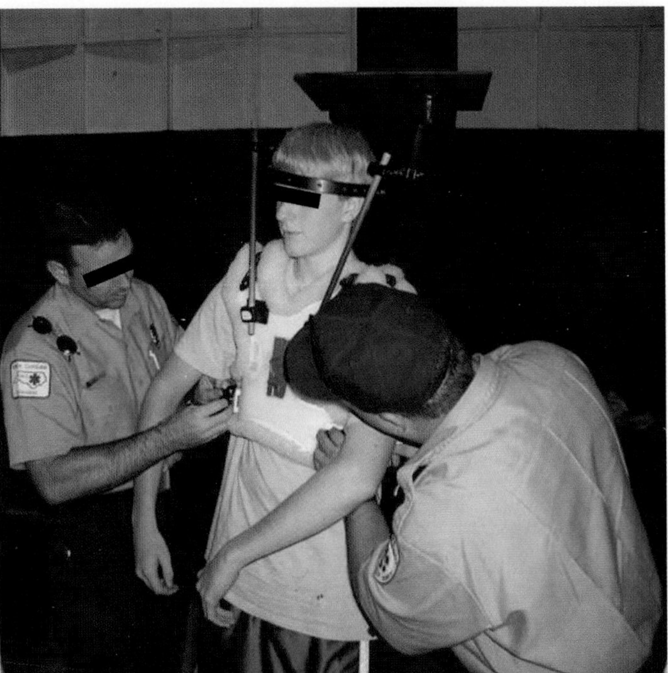

FIGURE 175-8. Demonstration of halo device application by emergency medical technicians at a high school assembly. [Reproduced with permission from North Carolina SAFETeens, Inc.]

Halo devices are indicated for stabilization of an unstable cervical spine, including stabilization of fractures, dislocations, and subluxations, and alignment of severe kyphotic and scoliotic spines. A halo is not applied if there is a sensory deficit that extends beneath the halo vest because this leads to a higher risk of skin breakdown and infection. Pin sites are chosen to avoid nerves, vessels, and muscle while placing the pins in the thickest area of the calvaria possible. Four pins are generally used. The anterior pins are placed in the frontal or temporal regions. Posterior pins are placed in sites approximately opposite to the anterior pin sites.

COMPLICATIONS

Pin loosening is the most common complication encountered in the ED.[26] Obtain neurosurgical consultation and exclude infection of the pin site. **If pin loosening has caused movement of the halo device, assume that the cervical spine is unstable, immobilize the cervical spine using an alternative technique, and obtain radiographs to assess for proper alignment.** Tangential plain radiography, CT, or MRI can be used to exclude penetration of a pin through the inner table of the skull. Pin-site infection is the second most frequently encountered complication. It occurs in approximately 10% to 20% of patients with halo devices.[26] Nearly 50% of infections occur in the first 4 weeks after halo placement, and 60% involve the anterior pins. Careful examination is required to differentiate a localized pin-site infection from less common, more serious infections (<1% of cases), such as cellulitis, osteomyelitis, and abscess formation.[26] Consider these more serious infections if there is persistent pain, continued drainage despite antibiotic therapy, clear drainage, or a history of a fall. Patients with cellulitis often present with fever and systemic signs and symptoms of infection. Patients with osteomyelitis usually have a prolonged infection, pin-site loosening, and radiologic abnormalities. Patients who develop an abscess usually have neurologic changes and evidence of intertable penetration (CSF leak, trauma).

Local pin-site infections are commonly managed with local wound care. The skin around the pin site must be pulled away to allow thorough cleaning of the skin beneath the pin and the skin–pin interface with soap and water four times a day. Obtain culture specimens from the wound site and administer antibiotics effective against skin pathogens (e.g.,

Staphylococcus and *Streptococcus* species). If local infection does not respond to treatment or if cellulitis, osteomyelitis, or abscess is suspected, obtain neurosurgical consultation for admission, IV antibiotics, and possible surgical intervention.

Pin-site discomfort occurs in up to 20% of patients.[26] It is most commonly a result of local inflammation. However, consider infection (localized or systemic) in each case. Sensory and motor deficits or paresthesias indicate nerve damage or pressure, whereas painful mastication indicates temporalis muscle inflammation, which often indicates too lateral a placement of pins. If infection is excluded, a short course of analgesics is recommended. Neurosurgical consultation is required if pain continues or a serious complication is suspected.

Ring migration or loss of immobilization occurs in 10% to 13% of patients. Suspect loss of immobilization in patients complaining of neck pain and change in fit or position of the ring or vest. Immediately immobilize the cervical spine using an alternative technique (e.g., hard collar plus backboard) and obtain radiographs to assess for changes in alignment. Obtain neurosurgical consultation for reapplication of the halo device.

Skin breakdown and pressure sores occur in 11% to 30% of patients. If either is present, inspect the vest for adequate padding and strap position. Urgent referral to a neurosurgeon for refitting may be required.

Dysphagia occurs in 1% to 2% of patients with halo devices.[26,27] Immobilization that holds the head in exaggerated extension is the usual cause of the dysphagia. Halo adjustment will remedy this problem. Alternatively, dysphagia can occur following anterior displacement of a bone graft. This diagnosis can be made by plain radiography or a swallowing study, and emergency surgical intervention is required.

Dural punctures occur in 1% to 2% of patients and are a result of halo system trauma.[26,27] This is rarely attributable to postapplication trauma because newer pin tighteners are designed to fail when torque exceeds 8 lb. Symptoms include headache, malaise, or visual changes. Physical examination may reveal a CSF leak or evidence of skull fracture. All patients with dural punctures require admission and neurosurgical consultation. Treatment includes elevation of the head, IV antibiotics, and pin removal.

In rare cases, CPR is required in patients with halo devices. To perform chest compressions, remove the anterior portion of the vest. Instructions for removing the halo vest are printed on the front of most vests. Intubation is performed with the halo in place. Emergent or semiemergent intubation was required 13% of the time in one series.[27] If orotracheal intubation is unsuccessful, other airway management options include nasotracheal intubation, laryngeal mask airway, and cricothyrotomy.

SPECIAL POPULATIONS

Use of halo devices carries a special risk in the elderly patient. A mortality rate of 21% is reported in patients >79 years of age.[28] Rates of serious complications, such as respiratory depression (8% of cases) and dysphagia (11% of cases), are much higher in elderly patients.[28]

OTHER CENTRAL NERVOUS SYSTEM DEVICES

INTRATHECAL BACLOFEN INFUSION DEVICES

Generalized dystonia occurs in 15% to 25% of patients with cerebral palsy. Baclofen, a γ-aminobutyric acid agonist that acts at the level of the spinal cord by impeding the release of excitatory neurotransmitters, decreases spasticity. Oral baclofen offers patients only mild relief because of its inability to cross the blood–brain barrier and its poor lipid solubility. Intrathecal administration (**Figure 175-9**) is more effective, requires lower dosages, and leads to higher CSF levels. Intrathecal baclofen reduces spasticity and improves gait, sitting ability, and upper extremity function in most patients.[29] Intrathecal baclofen pumps are also used to treat spasticity related to spinal cord injury, multiple sclerosis, brain injury, cerebrovascular accidents, and perinatal infection sequelae.[29,30] Complications observed in patients receiving continuous intrathecal baclofen can be divided into medication-related, mechanical, and infection-related complications and are listed in **Table 175-4**.

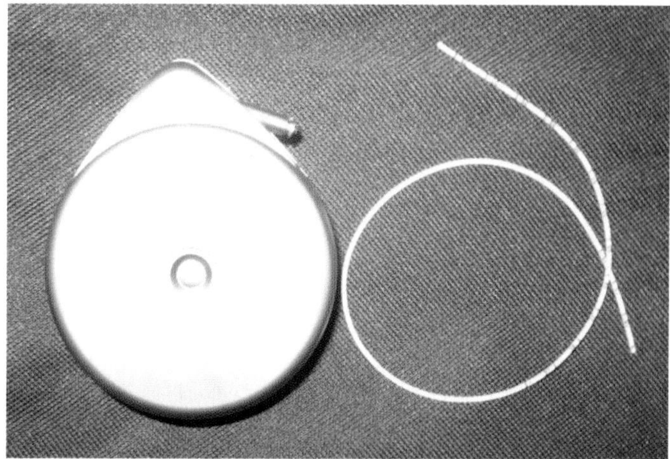

FIGURE 175-9. Typical baclofen pump.

When a complication occurs disrupting the administration of baclofen, withdrawal symptoms can be severe and life-threatening, including extreme hypertonicity and spasms that may lead to rhabdomyolysis. The apparent accelerated spasticity should signal to the provider that a potential complication has arisen. Oral baclofen, dantrolene, and oral or parenteral benzodiazepines may be used to alleviate these symptoms. Complications occur in approximately 20% to 30% of all cases. Infectious complications occur more frequently in children, revised pumps, and those placed subcutaneously.[31,32] Infection rate is 10%, with most infections presenting during the first month after placement.[29] Most infections are caused by *Staphylococcus* species, with a recent increase in methicillin-resistant *S. aureus*.[33] Serious infections and meningitis may arise even without local symptoms.[33] The majority of infections require neurosurgical consultation and IV antibiotics. Direct concerns about baclofen pumps to the neurosurgeon.

IMPLANTABLE CENTRAL NERVOUS SYSTEM STIMULATORS

The pathogenesis of Parkinson's disease is thought to involve unregulated activity of the subthalamic nucleus and globus pallidus interna. High-frequency stimulation with implantable CNS devices is being used for suppression of parkinsonian and essential tremors. Neurostimulation is typically used if drug therapy has failed to control tremors. Neurostimulation is as efficient at controlling tremors as classic thalamotomy but is less invasive. Deep brain stimulation studies have shown a 40% to 75% improvement in motor scores as well as improvement of rigidity, bradykinesia, and postural instability.[34] Reported complication rates range from 7% to 65%, with

TABLE 175-4 Complications of Intrathecal Baclofen Infusion

Medication related
Hypotension
Bradycardia
Apnea
Oversedation
Respiratory depression
Mechanical
Pump pocket effusions
Pump failure
Catheter extrusion
Catheter dislodgement
Infection
Local infection
Meningitis
Cerebrospinal fluid fistula formation

a decline in the number of reported complications as physician experience increases.[34] Infection rates approach 3% to 10%.[34] Patients may present to the ED with varied complaints, including problems related to the subcutaneous pulse generator, temporary or permanent paresthesias, dysarthria, disequilibrium, or failure of the neurostimulator to suppress tremors. Neurosurgical consultation is needed because these complaints may represent lead displacement or migration requiring surgical correction or replacement. If the diagnosis remains uncertain, observation with the stimulator in the off position may be required to help differentiate mechanical failure from an acute neurologic deficit.[34]

SPINAL CORD STIMULATION

Spinal cord stimulation is an established modality for treating chronic back pain, multiple sclerosis pain, complex regional pain syndromes, phantom pain, diabetic neuropathy, postherpetic neuralgia, angina pectoris, intractable pain associated with some malignancies, and the pain syndromes associated with vascular disease. Multicontact electrodes are placed in the epidural space, and the distal end of the electrode is connected to an internalized pulse generator. The therapeutic response is thought to be a result of stimulation of one of several dorsal tracts as well as activating the release of inhibitory neurotransmitters.[35,36] Complications include dural puncture, spinal cord compression, CSF leak, hemorrhage, infection, abscess, epidural fibrosis, migration, interruption of wires, corrosion of contacts, and battery failure. The most frequent complication is device failure, accounting for 17% to 25% of complications.[37] The rate of infection is reported between 2.5% and 5%.[36] Patients with these devices should not undergo MRI.

PERIPHERAL NERVE STIMULATION

Peripheral nerve stimulators are used to treat neuropathic pain disorders in patients with chronic intractable pain such as with occipital neuralgia. The device is similar to other stimulators except that the electrodes are placed in the subcutaneous tissue overlying the peripheral nerves. Case reports of interference of stimulators causing pauses in cardiac pacemakers exist and thus must be considered in patients with both a pacemaker and stimulator and a new conduction abnormality.[38]

Acknowledgment: The author gratefully acknowledges the contributions of Dr. Joseph Pagane, the co-author of this chapter in previous editions.

REFERENCES

The complete reference list is available online at www.TintinalliEM.com.

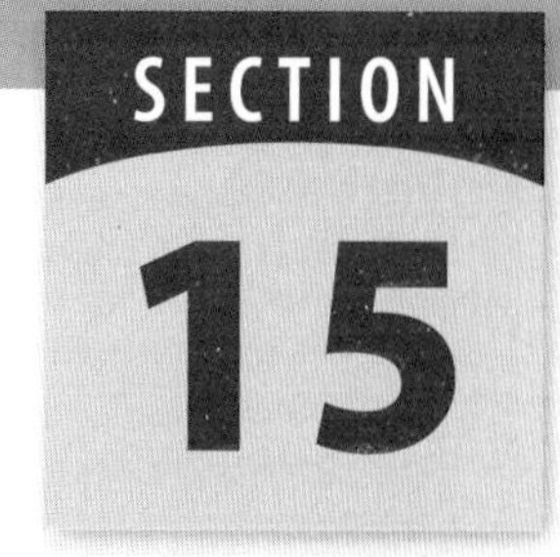

Toxicology

CHAPTER 176 General Management of Poisoned Patients

Shaun Greene

INTRODUCTION

Poisoning is a worldwide problem that consumes substantial health care resources and causes many premature deaths. The burden of serious poisoning is carried by the developing world[1,2]; however, poisoning-related morbidity and mortality is also a significant public health concern in the developed world.[3-9]

Unintentional poisoning deaths in the United States are increasing, especially as a result of prescription analgesics. This increase has been ascribed to increasing prescription rates and aging of the baby-boom population.[10-12] U.S. poison control centers documented 2.38 million human exposures in 2010, with 1146 associated deaths.[13] Prevention is the key to reducing unintentional poisoning deaths. Pharmacists can that ensure medications are labeled correctly, anticipate potential drug interactions, and educate patients to use medications safely. To prevent pediatric deaths from poisoning, parents have the responsibility to ensure that poisons are placed in childproof, labeled containers stored in adult-only accessible nonfood storage areas. Teachers and healthcare providers can provide age-appropriate education to children about the dangers of poisons. After an exposure, poison control centers staffed by highly trained individuals can provide customized advice to healthcare providers and the public. Poison control centers also participate in prevention, education, and toxico-surveillance activities.

Exposures occur most commonly by ingestion; other routes include inhalation, insufflation, cutaneous and mucous membrane exposure, and injection. Some exposures have minimal risk. The criteria used to determine whether the exposure is nontoxic are: (1) an unintentional exposure to a clearly identified single substance, (2) where an estimate of dose is known, and (3) a recognized information source (e.g., a poison control center) confirms the substance as nontoxic in the reported dose. Asymptomatic patients with nontoxic exposures may be discharged after a short period of observation, providing they have access to further consultation and a safe discharge destination.

Serious clinical effects occur in <5% of acutely poisoned patients presenting to developed-world hospitals, and in-hospital mortality rates are <1%.[9,13]

RESUSCITATION

Resuscitation is the first priority in any poisoned patient. After resuscitation, a structured risk assessment is used to identify patients who may benefit from an antidote, decontamination, or enhanced elimination techniques. Most patients only require provision of good supportive care during a period of observation in an appropriate environment.

Treatment of cardiac arrest in poisoned patients follows Advanced Cardiac Life Support guidelines with the addition of interventions potentially beneficial in toxin-induced cardiac arrest (**Table 176-1**).[14] Prolonged resuscitation is generally indicated, as patients are often young with minimal preexisting organ dysfunction. Utilization of extracorporeal cardiac and respiratory assist devices until organ toxicity resolves may be life-saving.

Stabilization of airway, breathing, and circulation represents initial priorities. Compromised airway patency or reduced respiratory drive may lead to inadequate ventilation; provision of a mechanical airway and assisted ventilation is vital in these circumstances. IV crystalloid bolus (10 to 20 mL/kg) is first-line treatment of hypotension. Since most patients without toxin-induced fluid loss are generally not fluid depleted, avoid administration of excess fluid. Persisting hypotension despite an adequate volume infusion may respond to a specific antidote. Otherwise, cautious administration of an inotropic agent is indicated. Inotrope choice is guided by knowledge of the toxin's toxicodynamic properties and assessment of circulatory status (e.g., cardiac pump failure versus vasodilatory shock).

ANTIDOTES

Stabilization of airway, breathing, and circulation allows further assessment of blood glucose concentration, temperature, and conscious state. Although the proper use of antidotes (**Table 176-2**) is important, only a few are indicated before cardiopulmonary stabilization (e.g., naloxone for opiate toxicity, cyanide antidotes for cyanide toxicity, and atropine for organophosphate poisoning).

HYPOGLYCEMIA

Treat hypoglycemia with IV dextrose (glucose). Patients at risk of Wernicke's encephalopathy also require thiamine, but do not require that it be administered before the dextrose.[15] Altered mental status when hypoglycemia cannot be excluded is an indication for IV dextrose. Supplemental oxygen, thiamine, glucose, and naloxone are often administered empirically as a cocktail in cases of altered mental status. Although relatively safe and affordable in the developed world, this approach may not be cost-effective in developing countries. The decision to administer an antidote should be made after a rapid collateral history is obtained and targeted examination completed. Altered mental status not responding to an antidote or not consistent with exposure history requires further investigation. Metabolic, infective, and surgical (e.g., intracranial injury) causes of altered mental status should be considered.

CARDIAC ARRHYTHMIAS

In general, antiarrhythmic drugs are not first-line treatment for toxin-induced arrhythmias, as most antiarrhythmic drugs have proarrhythmic and negative inotropic properties. Most toxin-induced arrhythmias respond to correction of hypoxia, metabolic/acid–base abnormalities, and administration of an antidote (e.g., digoxin Fab). Sodium bicarbonate is administered for sodium-channel blocker toxicity with cardiovascular complications, such as wide QRS complex tachyarrhythmias. Ventricular tachyarrhythmias may respond to overdrive pacing.

SEIZURES

Drug-induced seizures are treated with titrated doses of IV benzodiazepines, with the exception that isoniazid-induced seizures require pyridoxine. Metabolic disorders, such as hypoglycemia and hyponatremia, can also produce seizures and should be rapidly excluded. Barbiturates are second-line agents for benzodiazepine-resistant seizures (once isoniazid-induced seizures are excluded). **There is no role for phenytoin in the treatment of toxin-induced seizures; it has neither theoretical nor proven efficacy, and may worsen toxicity.**[16]

TABLE 176-1 Potential Interventions in Toxin-Induced Cardiac Arrest[15]

Toxin or Toxin/Drug Class	Intervention
Toxins with a specific antidote (examples)	Antidote
Digoxin	Digoxin Fab
Organophosphates	Atropine
Envenomation	Antivenom
Sodium channel blocker or wide-complex tachycardia	Sodium bicarbonate
Calcium channel blocker or β-blocker	High-dose insulin
Local anesthetic agents Lipophilic cardiotoxins	IV lipid emulsion
Other Therapies to Consider	
Cardiac pacing Intra-aortic balloon pump Extracorporeal membrane oxygenation	

AGITATION

Agitation is treated with titrated doses of benzodiazepines. Large doses may be required and are appropriate in monitored settings where advanced airway interventions are available if required. Although antipsychotic agents are often used as second-line agents for toxin-induced agitation, they have theoretical disadvantages, including anticholinergic and extrapyramidal effects.[17] Droperidol has been associated (rarely) with QT interval prolongation and cardiac arrhythmias.

HYPERTHERMIA AND HYPOTHERMIA

Patients with core temperatures of >39°C (>102.2°F) require aggressive active cooling measures to prevent complications such as rhabdomyolysis, organ failure, and disseminated intravascular coagulation. Sedation, neuromuscular paralysis, and intubation are required if active measures are ineffective. Several toxidromes associated with hyperthermia are treated with specific pharmaceutical agents: sympathomimetic (benzodiazepines), serotonin (cyproheptadine[18]), and neuromuscular malignant syndrome (bromocriptine[19]).

TABLE 176-2 Common Antidotes Used in Resuscitation of the Acutely Poisoned Patient

Antidote	Pediatric Dose	Adult Dose	Indication
Calcium chloride 10% 27.2 milligrams/mL elemental Ca	0.2–0.25 mL/kg IV	10 mL IV	Calcium channel antagonists
Calcium gluconate 10% 9 milligrams/mL elemental Ca	0.6–0.8 mL/kg IV	10–30 mL IV	Hypermagnesemia Hypocalcemia
Cyanide antidote kit			
Amyl nitrite	Not typically used	1 ampule O_2 chamber of ventilation bag 30 s on/30 s off	Cyanide Hydrogen sulfide (use only sodium nitrite)
Sodium nitrite (3% solution)	0.33 mL/kg IV	10 mL IV	Cyanide
Sodium thiosulfate (25% solution)	1.65 mL/kg IV	50 mL IV	Cyanide
Dextrose (glucose)	0.5 gram/kg IV	1 gram/kg IV	Insulin Oral hypoglycemics
Digoxin Fab Acute toxicity	1–2 vials IV	5–10 vials	Digoxin and other cardioactive steroids
Flumazenil	0.01 milligram/kg IV	0.2 milligram IV	Benzodiazepines
Glucagon	50–150 micrograms/kg IV	3–10 milligrams IV	Calcium channel blockers β-Blockers
Hydroxocobalamin	70 milligrams/kg IV (maximum 5 grams). Can be repeated up to 3 times. Administer with sodium thiosulfate.		Cyanide Nitroprusside
IV lipid emulsion 20%	1.5 mL/kg IV bolus over 1 min (may be repeated two times at 5-min intervals), followed by 0.25 mL/kg per minute	100-mL IV bolus over 1 min, followed by 400 mL IV over 20 min	Local anesthetic toxicity Rescue therapy for lipophilic cardiotoxins
Methylene blue	1–2 milligrams/kg IV Neonates: 0.3–1.0 milligram/kg IV	1–2 milligrams/kg IV	Oxidizing toxins (e.g., nitrites, benzocaine, sulfonamides)
Naloxone	As much as required Start: 0.01 milligram IV	As much as required Start: 0.1–0.4 milligram IV	Opioids Clonidine
Pyridoxine	Gram for gram if amount isoniazid ingested is known		Isoniazid
	70 milligrams/kg IV (maximum 5 grams)	5 grams IV	*Gyromitra esculenta* Hydrazine
Sodium bicarbonate	1–2 mEq/kg IV bolus followed by 2 mEq/kg per h IV infusion		Sodium channel blockers Urinary alkalinization
Thiamine	5–10 milligrams IV	100 milligrams IV	Wernicke's syndrome Wet beriberi

Drug-induced coma with subsequent immobility and environmental exposure or inherent drug toxicity (opioids, phenothiazines, ethanol) may produce hypothermia. A core temperature <32°C (<90°F) is an indication for active rewarming.

NALOXONE

Naloxone is a nontoxic, diagnostic, and therapeutic antidote. It is a competitive opioid antagonist administered IV, IM, or intranasally[20] to reverse opioid-induced deleterious hypoventilation. Naloxone can be used as a diagnostic agent when history and/or examination findings (respiratory rate of <12 breaths/min is a predictor of response to naloxone) suggest possible opioid exposure. Naloxone is titrated to clinical effect using bolus doses, typically 0.1 to 0.4 milligrams. Large initial bolus doses may precipitate vomiting and aspiration, acute opioid withdrawal, or an uncooperative, agitated patient. Miosis is an unreliable indicator of naloxone's adequate clinical effect, as some opioids do not affect pupil size. Doses are titrated to achieve desirable ventilation and conscious state (adequate respiratory rate, normal arterial oxygen saturations on room air, and verbal or motor response to voice). Although naloxone may reverse the effects of opioids for 20 to 60 minutes, the effect of many opioids will outlast this time frame with possible return of respiratory depression. Patients should be observed for 2 to 3 hours after administration of IV naloxone.

INTRAVENOUS LIPID EMULSION

Animal studies demonstrate the potential for IV lipid emulsion to act as an antidote for lipophilic toxins. Provision of an intravascular "lipid sink" is postulated as the predominant mechanism, as sequestration of lipophilic toxins prevents target receptor interaction. Human case reports indicate that IV lipid emulsion may provide benefit in cases of potentially life-threatening toxicity from a local anesthetic agent, haloperidol, tricyclic antidepressant, lipophilic β-blocker, or calcium channel blocker.[21] **Currently, IV lipid emulsion can be considered in life-threatening cardiotoxicity caused by lipophilic cardiotoxins that is resistant to conventional therapies.**

RISK ASSESSMENT

Following initial resuscitation and stabilization, a risk assessment is performed to predict course of clinical toxicity, interventions required, and patient disposition. Risk assessment is formulated using history, examination, and ancillary test results. Acute poisoning is a dynamic process; therefore, risk assessment may change with time and requires ongoing review.

HISTORY

Patients may not provide a clear history due to psychiatric illness, clinical effects of exposure, and fear of arrest or repercussions from family or friends. Information including identity of substances, doses, and route of exposure is crucial in formulating a risk assessment. Obtain collateral information from family, friends, previous medical records, and usual healthcare provider. Prehospital emergency services can provide information regarding empty medication containers or the scene environment (smells, particular materials or substances present). If possible, obtain knowledge of hobbies, occupation, presence of a suicide note, and recent changes in patient behavior.

EXAMINATION

A systematic physical examination can yield important clues to the nature and potential severity of an exposure (**Table 176-3**). Examine the skin folds, body cavities if appropriate, and clothing for retained tablets or substances.

TOXIDROMES

Substances belonging to a particular pharmaceutical/chemical class often produce a cluster of symptoms and signs, or "toxidrome" (**Table 176-4**), enabling the identification of potential toxins when a clear history is unavailable.

TABLE 176-3 Examination of the Poisoned Patient

Organ System	Examination	Example of Finding (Possible Significance)
General appearance	General demeanor and dress Signs of injury Odors Mental state Nutritional state Temperature	Unkempt (psychiatric illness) Scalp hematoma (intracranial injury) Malnourished (IV drug use, HIV infection) Smell of bitter almonds (cyanide toxicity)
Central nervous	Conscious state Pupil size and reactivity Eye movements Cerebellar function/gait	Miosis (opioids, organophosphates, phenothiazines, clonidine intoxication) Nystagmus/ataxia (anticonvulsant and ethanol toxicity)
Cardiovascular	Heart rate/blood pressure Cardiac auscultation	Murmur (endocarditis/IV drug abuse)
Respiratory	Oxygen saturation Respiratory rate Chest auscultation	Fever/crepitations/hypoxia (aspiration pneumonia) Bronchorrhea/crepitations/ hypoxia (organophosphate toxicity)
Gastrointestinal	Oropharynx Abdomen Bladder	Urinary retention (anticholinergic toxicity) Oral cavity burns (corrosive ingestion) Hypersalivation (cholinergic toxidrome)
Peripheral nervous	Reflexes Tone Fasciculations Tremor Clonus	Tremor/fasciculations (lithium toxicity) "Lead pipe" rigidity (neuromuscular malignant syndrome) Clonus/hyperreflexia (serotonin toxicity)
Dermal/peripheral	Bruising Cyanosis Flushing Dry/moist skin Injection sites Bullae	Bruising (coagulopathy, trauma, coma) Flushing /warm, dry skin (anticholinergic toxicity) Warm, moist skin (sympathomimetic toxicity) Bullae (prolonged coma, barbiturates)

DIAGNOSTIC TESTING

A serum acetaminophen concentration is a routine screening test in poisoned patients. Early acetaminophen poisoning is often asymptomatic and does not have a readily identifiable toxidrome at the time when antidotal treatment is most efficacious. Acetaminophen screening is especially important in patients presenting with altered mental status or a self-harm ingestion, for whom an accurate history may not be available.

An electrocardiogram is a useful test to detect cardiac conduction abnormalities and identify patients at increased risk of toxin-induced adverse cardiovascular events.[22]

Measurement of drug or toxin concentrations in body fluids is not required in most poisonings, but in some exposures, measurement of serum drug concentrations does influence management (**Table 176-5**).

Toxicologic screening tests of the urine and/or blood can be done in a central laboratory or performed with point-of-care drug screening

TABLE 176-4 Common Toxidromes

Toxidrome	Examples of Agents	Examination Findings (most common in bold)
Anticholinergic	Atropine, *Datura* spp., antihistamines, antipsychotics	**Altered mental status, mydriasis, dry flushed skin, urinary retention, decreased bowel sounds, hyperthermia, dry mucous membranes** Seizures, arrhythmias, rhabdomyolysis
Cholinergic	Organophosphate and carbamate insecticides Chemical warfare agents (Sarin, VX)	**Salivation, lacrimation, diaphoresis, vomiting, urination, defecation, bronchorrhea, muscle fasciculations, weakness** Miosis/mydriasis, bradycardia, seizures
Ethanolic	Ethanol	**Central nervous system depression, ataxia, dysarthria, odor of ethanol**
Extrapyramidal	Risperidone, haloperidol, phenothiazines	**Dystonia, torticollis, muscle rigidity** Choreoathetosis, hyperreflexia, seizures
Hallucinogenic	Phencyclidine Psilocybin, mescaline Lysergic acid diethylamide	**Hallucinations, dysphoria, anxiety** Nausea, sympathomimetic signs
Hypoglycemic	Sulfonylureas Insulin	**Altered mental status, diaphoresis, tachycardia, hypertension** Dysarthria, behavioral change, seizures
Neuromuscular malignant	Antipsychotics	**Severe muscle rigidity, hyperpyrexia, altered mental status** Autonomic instability, diaphoresis, mutism, incontinence
Opioid	Codeine Heroin Morphine	**Miosis, respiratory depression, central nervous system depression** Hypothermia, bradycardia
Salicylate	Aspirin Oil of Wintergreen (methyl salicylate)	**Altered mental status, respiratory alkalosis, metabolic acidosis, tinnitus, tachypnea, tachycardia, diaphoresis, nausea, vomiting** Hyperpyrexia (low grade)
Sedative/hypnotic	Benzodiazepines Barbiturates	**Central nervous system depression, ataxia, dysarthria** Bradycardia, respiratory depression
Serotonin	SSRIs MAOIs Tricyclic antidepressants Amphetamines Fentanyl St. John's wort	**Altered mental status, hyperreflexia and hypertonia (>lower limbs), clonus, tachycardia, diaphoresis** Hypertension, flushing, tremor
Sympathomimetic	Amphetamines Cocaine Cathinones	**Agitation, tachycardia, hypertension, hyperpyrexia, diaphoresis** Seizures, acute coronary syndrome

Abbreviations: MAOI = monoamine oxidase inhibitor; SSRI = selective serotonin reuptake inhibitor.

assays.[23] However, the results seldom directly influence patient management, and toxicology screening has limitations (**Table 176-6**).

Toxicologic screening may be appropriate for medicolegal reasons, especially in pediatric cases when inappropriate drug administration or nonaccidental injury is suspected. A positive urine drug screen for an illicit substance is an indication to involve local child protection services.

TABLE 176-5 Drug Concentrations That May Assist Patient Assessment or Management

Acetaminophen	Methanol
Carbamazepine	Methotrexate
Carbon monoxide	Paraquat
Digoxin	Phenobarbital
Ethanol	Phenytoin
Ethylene glycol	Salicylate
Iron	Theophylline
Lithium	Valproic acid
Methemoglobin	

TABLE 176-6 Limitations of Toxicologic Drug Screening Assays

Nonspecific	Most tests use enzyme-immunoassays that only detect *typical* drugs within a class: opioids, amphetamines, benzodiazepines, cannabinoids, cocaine, barbiturates. Amphetamine screens do not detect methylenedioxy-methamphetamine. Opioid screens do not detect meperidine. Benzodiazepine screens do not detect flunitrazepam.
Time frame	Drugs may be detected days to weeks after exposure. A positive test may not account for current clinical findings.
Cross-reactivity	Carbamazepine, cyproheptadine, and chlorpromazine test positive for tricyclic antidepressants. Selegiline, methylphenidate, and pseudoephedrine test positive for amphetamines.
Noninclusive	A negative drug screen does not exclude a rare exposure.
Sampling error	Assay may be negative if dilute urine is tested.

DECONTAMINATION

Decontamination is required for toxic exposures affecting large dermal areas. Healthcare providers wearing personal protective equipment (if indicated) or observing universal precautions (gown, gloves, eye protection) should assist with undressing and washing the patient using copious amounts of water. Contaminated clothing is collected, bagged, and properly disposed. Decontamination ideally occurs in a separate area adjacent to the ED, minimizing cross-contamination.

OCULAR DECONTAMINATION

Eye exposures may require local anesthetic (e.g., 0.5% tetracaine) instillation and lid retractors to facilitate copious irrigation with crystalloid solution. Alkalis produce greater injury than acids due to deep tissue penetration via liquefaction so that prolonged irrigation (1 to 2 hours) may be required. Ten minutes after irrigation (allowing equilibration of crystalloid and conjunctival sac pHs), conjunctival sac pH is tested. Irrigation continues until pH is <7.4. Ophthalmologic consultation is indicated for all ocular alkali injuries.

GASTROINTESTINAL DECONTAMINATION

Gastric decontamination is not a routine part of poisoned-patient management; there is minimal evidence demonstrating positive benefit, and there are associated complications (**Table 176-7**). Gastric decontamination may be considered in individual patients after a three-question risk-benefit analysis: (1) Is this exposure likely to cause significant toxicity? (2) Is gastrointestinal decontamination likely to change clinical outcome? (3) Is it possible that gastrointestinal decontamination will cause more harm than good?[24]

Emesis Traditionally, ipecac syrup was administered to induce vomiting, theoretically emptying the stomach of poisons. No published evidence supports the induction of emesis, and adverse outcomes associated with emesis are documented.[25] The American Association of Poison Control Centers guideline[25] comments that ipecac may be used in rare circumstances in remote locations, but this recommendation has been questioned.[26] There is no role for the induction of emesis in the ED.[27]

Orogastric Lavage Once a widely practiced intervention, attempted removal of ingested toxin from the stomach by aspiration of fluid placed via an orogastric tube is now rarely indicated. No published evidence demonstrates that orogastric lavage changes outcome, and the procedure has numerous complications.[28] Gastric lavage may be considered in cases of ingestion of a life-threatening amount of poison within the previous hour where institution of supportive care and antidotal therapy would not ensure full recovery. When orogastric lavage is performed in a resuscitation area:

- Ensure a protected airway if consciousness level is reduced.
- Use a 36 to 40F-gauge orogastric tube (22 to 24F in children).
- Position the patient on the left side with the head down 20 degrees.
- Pass lubricated tube down the esophagus a distance equal to that between chin and xiphoid process.
- Confirm tube position by insufflation of air.
- Gently lavage with 200 mL (10 mL/kg in children) of warm tap water.
- Continue until returned fluid is clear.
- Consider administration of activated charcoal via orogastric tube before removal.

Single-Dose Activated Charcoal Super-heating carbonaceous material produces activated charcoal, a highly porous substance, which is suspended in solution and given PO as a slurry. Toxins within the gastrointestinal lumen are adsorbed onto the activated charcoal and carried through the gastrointestinal tract, limiting absorption.[29] Activated charcoal does not effectively adsorb metals, corrosives, and alcohols. The decision to give activated charcoal requires individual patient risk assessment and is not considered routine management.

Activated charcoal may be effective when given >60 minutes after ingestion of substances known to slow gastrointestinal motility (e.g., anticholinergics)[30] or after massive ingestion of a substance associated with bezoar formation (e.g., salicylates). Activated charcoal mixed with ice cream improves palatability for children. Activated charcoal can be administered to intubated patients using an orogastric or nasogastric tube. There are insufficient published data supporting the routine use of a cathartic agent added to activated charcoal.[31]

TABLE 176-7 Indications, Contraindications, and Complications of Gastrointestinal Decontamination Procedures

Orogastric Lavage	
Indications	Rarely indicated Consider for recent (<1 hour) ingestion of life-threatening amount of a toxin for which there is no effective treatment once absorbed
Contraindications	Corrosive/hydrocarbon ingestion Supportive care/antidote likely to lead to recovery Unprotected airway Unstable, requiring further resuscitation (hypotension, seizures)
Complications	Aspiration pneumonia/hypoxia Water intoxication Hypothermia Laryngospasm Mechanical injury to gastrointestinal tract Time consuming, resulting in delay instituting other definitive care
Activated Charcoal	**Adults 50 grams orally, children 1 gram/kg orally**
Indications	Ingestion within the previous hour of a toxic substance known to be adsorbed by activated charcoal, where the benefits of administration are judged to outweigh the risks
Contraindications	Nontoxic ingestion Toxin not adsorbed by activated charcoal Recovery will occur without administration of activate charcoal Unprotected airway Corrosive ingestion Possibility of upper gastrointestinal perforation
Complications	Vomiting Aspiration of the activated charcoal Impaired absorption of orally administered antidotes
Whole-Bowel Irrigation	**Polyethylene glycol 2 L/h in adults, children 25 mL/kg per hour (maximum 2 L/h)**
Indications (potential)	Iron ingestion >60 milligrams/kg with opacities on abdominal radiograph Life-threatening ingestion of diltiazem or verapamil Body packers or stuffers Slow-release potassium ingestion Lead ingestion (including paint flakes containing lead) Symptomatic arsenic trioxide ingestion Life-threatening ingestions of lithium
Contraindications	Unprotected airway Gastrointestinal perforation, obstruction or ileus, hemorrhage Intractable vomiting Cardiovascular instability
Complications	Nausea, vomiting Pulmonary aspiration Time consuming; possible delay instituting other definitive care

Whole-Bowel Irrigation Polyethylene glycol is an osmotically balanced electrolyte solution. Administration in large quantities mechanically forces substances through the gastrointestinal tract, limiting toxin absorption.[32] Polyethylene glycol can be administered orally to cooperative, awake patients, but consider formal airway control if consciousness is likely to deteriorate. Minimize risk of pulmonary aspiration during whole-bowel irrigation by patient positioning (head up 30 degrees), ensuring bowel sounds are present during fluid administration, 1:1 nursing with suctioning of the oral cavity during infusion, and utilization of cuffed endotracheal tubes.

Evidence supporting whole-bowel irrigation is limited to volunteer studies and case reports[32] from which potential indications have been developed (**Table 176-7**). Nonsurgical treatment of asymptomatic body drug packers using whole-bowel irrigation is increasingly common, although no randomized clinical trials exist.[33] An antiemetic such as the prokinetic agent metoclopramide may be required to control polyethylene glycol–induced gastric distension and vomiting. The endpoint of whole-bowel irrigation treatment is clear rectal effluent and imaging demonstrating absence of foreign bodies.

ENHANCED ELIMINATION

MULTIDOSE ACTIVATED CHARCOAL

Multidose activated charcoal increases elimination of toxins with enteroenteric, enterohepatic, or enterogastric recirculation. Lipophilic drugs with low volume of distribution, protein binding, and molecular weight may pass down a concentration gradient between intravascular space and activated charcoal in the gut lumen. Multidose activated charcoal may also adsorb residual intraluminal toxins; this is more likely for substances slowing gastric motility or forming bezoars (**Table 176-8**). Although animal studies, volunteer studies, case reports, and case series demonstrate increased elimination rates (in some cases comparable to those of hemodialysis or charcoal hemoperfusion) of carbamazepine, dapsone, phenobarbital, quinine, and theophylline, there is limited evidence that multidose activated charcoal changes clinical outcome.[34]

Multidose activated charcoal may be administered by an orogastric or nasogastric tube to intubated patients. Regular aspiration of stomach contents helps avoid gastric distension. Multidose activated charcoal should not be given when bowel sounds are absent. Continued requirement for further multidose activated charcoal should be reviewed regularly during therapy.

URINARY ALKALINIZATION

Alkaline urine favors ionization of acidotic drugs within renal tubules, preventing resorption of the ionized drug back across the renal tubular epithelium and enhancing elimination through the urine.[35] Urinary alkalinization is most effective for weak acids primarily eliminated by the renal tract that are also readily filtered at the glomerulus and have small volumes of distribution (**Table 176-8**). Hypokalemia will reduce the effectiveness of urinary alkalinization. The primary indication for urinary alkalinization is moderate to severe salicylate toxicity when criteria for hemodialysis have not been met. Urinary alkalinization for adult patients can be instituted as follows:

- Correct any existing hypokalemia.
- Administer a 1 to 2 mEq/kg IV sodium bicarbonate bolus.
- Infuse 100 mEq of sodium bicarbonate mixed with 1 L of D5W at 250 mL/h.
- 20 mEq of potassium chloride may be added to the solution to maintain normokalemia.
- Monitor serum potassium and bicarbonate every 2 to 4 hours to detect hypokalemia or excessive serum alkalinization.
- Check urine pH regularly (every 15 to 30 minutes), aiming for a pH of 7.5 to 8.5.
- A further IV bolus of 1 mEq/kg of sodium bicarbonate may be necessary if sufficient alkalinization of the urine is not achieved.

Although urinary acidification can enhance the elimination of weak bases including amphetamines and phencyclidine, associated risks (e.g., rhabdomyolysis) outweigh potential benefit. Forced diuresis has no indication for any poisoning, with the exception of chlorophenoxy herbicides (see chapter 201, Pesticides).

TABLE 176-8 Indications, Contraindications, and Complications of Enhanced Elimination Procedures

Multidose Activated Charcoal	Initial dose: 50 grams (1 gram/kg children), repeat dose 25 grams (0.5 gram/kg children) every 2 hours
Indications	Carbamazepine coma (reduces duration of coma)
	Phenobarbital coma (reduces duration of coma)
	Dapsone toxicity with significant methemoglobinemia
	Quinine overdose
	Theophylline overdose if hemodialysis/hemoperfusion unavailable
Contraindications	Unprotected airway
	Bowel obstruction
	Caution in ingestions resulting in reduced gastrointestinal motility
Complications	Vomiting
	Pulmonary aspiration
	Constipation
	Charcoal bezoar, bowel obstruction/perforation
Urinary Alkalinization	
Indications	Moderate to severe salicylate toxicity not meeting criteria for hemodialysis
	Phenobarbital (multidose activated charcoal superior)
	Chlorophenoxy herbicides (2-4-dichlorophenoxyacetic acid and mecoprop): requires high urine flow rate 600 mL/h to be effective
	Chlorpropamide: supportive care/IV dextrose normally sufficient
Contraindications	Preexisting fluid overload
	Renal impairment
	Uncorrected hypokalemia
Complications	Hypokalemia
	Volume overload
	Alkalemia
	Hypocalcemia (usually mild)

EXTRACORPOREAL REMOVAL

Extracorporeal removal techniques, including hemodialysis, hemoperfusion, and continuous renal replacement therapies, have limited indications in poisoned patients (**Table 176-9**). These procedures require a critical care setting, are expensive and invasive, are not always available, and have complications. Extracorporeal removal techniques were utilized in less than 0.1% of cases reported to U.S. poison control centers in 2010.[13]

A toxin must possess a number of properties to be effectively removed by an extracorporeal technique in a clinically meaningful timeframe: low volume of distribution (<1.0 L/kg), low molecular weight (<500 Da), relatively low protein binding, and low endogenous clearance.[36] In general, extracorporeal removal must improve endogenous clearance rate by >30% to be clinically beneficial. Hemoperfusion uses a charcoal (or other adsorbent) filter, which comes into direct contact with blood, partially overcoming molecular weight and protein-binding limitations.

Continuous renal replacement therapies (including venovenous hemofiltration and venovenous hemodiafiltration) are widely available and easily instituted in most hospitals. However, there is sparse evidence demonstrating any benefit in poisoning, primarily due to slow clearance rates.[36] A patient who requires extracorporeal removal should undergo hemodialysis or hemoperfusion, if available. Continuous renal replacement therapy can be used if hemodialysis or hemoperfusion is unavailable or will not be

TABLE 176-9 Indications, Contraindications, and Complications of Extracorporeal Removal Techniques

Hemodialysis	**Movement of solute down a concentration gradient across a semipermeable membrane**	
Toxin requirements	Low volume of distribution, low protein binding, low endogenous clearance, low molecular weight	
Indications	**Life-threatening poisoning by:** Lithium Metformin lactic acidosis Phenobarbital Salicylates Valproic acid	Methanol/ethylene glycol Metformin-induced lactic acidosis Potassium salts Theophylline
Contraindications	Hemodynamic instability Infants (generally)	Poor vascular access Significant coagulopathy
Hemoperfusion	**Movement of toxin from blood, plasma, or plasma proteins onto a bed of activated charcoal (or other adsorbent)**	
Toxin requirements	Low volume of distribution, low endogenous clearance, bound by activated charcoal	
Indications	**Life-threatening poisoning caused by:** Theophylline (high-flux hemodialysis is an alternative) Carbamazepine (multidose activated charcoal or high-efficiency hemodialysis also effective) Paraquat (theoretical benefit only if instituted early after exposure)	
Contraindications	Hemodynamic instability Infants (generally) Poor vascular access	Significant coagulopathy Toxin not bound to activated charcoal
Continuous Renal Replacement Therapies	**Movement of toxin and solute across a semipermeable membrane in response to hydrostatic gradient. Can be combined with dialysis.**	
Indications (potential)	Life-threatening ingestions of toxins when hemodialysis or hemoperfusion is indicated, but is unavailable, or hemodynamic instability precludes their utilization	
Contraindications	Hemodynamic instability or hemoperfusion is available Poor vascular access Significant coagulopathy	
Complications of Extracorporeal Removal Techniques		
Fluid/metabolic disruption	Limited by hypotension (not continuous renal replacement therapy)	
Removal of antidotes	Infection/bleeding at catheter site	
Limited availability	Intracranial hemorrhage secondary to anticoagulation	

tolerated (e.g., due to hypotension).[36] Extracorporeal removal techniques including high-flux hemodialysis are constantly evolving, so discussion with an intensivist or nephrologist may be beneficial when this approach is considered.

DISPOSITION

Planning for patient disposition from the ED should be part of initial risk assessment. Admission is indicated if the patient has persistent and/or severe toxic effects or will require a prolonged course of treatment. In most cases, a 6-hour observation period is sufficient to exclude the development of serious toxicity. Onset of clinical toxicity can be delayed after a number of exposures, including (but not limited to) modified-release preparations of calcium channel antagonists, selective norepinephrine reuptake inhibitors (tramadol, venlafaxine), and newer antipsychotics (amisulpride); hence a period of extended observation is indicated. In the developed world, toxicity will resolve within 24 hours in most poisoned patients requiring noncritical care inpatient management, and so these patients can be efficiently and safely managed in a toxicology or short-stay ward, if available. Patients who have deliberately self-poisoned require appropriate mental health assessment before disposition.

REFERENCES

The complete reference list is available online at www.TintinalliEM.com.

Cyclic Antidepressants

Frank LoVecchio

INTRODUCTION

Cyclic antidepressants were the first-generation of drugs developed to treat depression. Their use for treating depression has declined greatly as safer agents have been developed. Cyclic antidepressants are now occasionally used to treat obsessive-compulsive disorder, attention-deficit disorder, panic and phobia disorders, anxiety disorders, and a variety of other conditions.

In 2013, cyclic antidepressants were the most commonly identified antidepressants associated with overdose-related deaths.[1,2] Roughly half of all cyclic antidepressant exposures involve other drugs as well, and most co-ingestants increase the incidence and severity of cyclic antidepressant overdose toxicity.

Eight cyclic antidepressants are currently available in the United States (**Table 177-1**), with more agents available in other countries. Therapy is initially started at the lowest therapeutic level and slowly increased until the desired therapeutic response is achieved. This approach allows patients to become acclimated to adverse effects such as sedation and dry mucous membranes. Two related antidepressants, amoxapine and maprotiline, have structural differences from traditional cyclic antidepressants but have similar toxicity in overdose. Cyclobenzaprine is a muscle relaxant that is almost structurally identical

TABLE 177-1 Cyclic Antidepressants and Related Drugs

Generic Name	Typical Adult Outpatient Daily Dose (milligrams)	Recommended Maximal Adult Outpatient Daily Dose (milligrams)	Active Metabolites
Amitriptyline	75–150	300	Nortriptyline
Amoxapine*	50–300	400	7-Hydroxyamoxapine (minor) 8-Hydroxyamoxapine (major)
Clomipramine	25–50	250	Desmethylclomipramine
Cyclobenzaprine*	15–30	30	None
Desipramine	75–200	300	None
Doxepin	75–300	300	Desmethyldoxepin
Imipramine	75–200	300	Desipramine
Maprotiline*	75–150	225	Desmethylmaprotiline
Nortriptyline	75–150	150	None
Protriptyline	15–60	60	None
Trimipramine	75–200	300	Desmethyltrimipramine

*See text for clarification.

TABLE 177-3 Pharmacologic Profile of Cyclic Antidepressants

Pharmacologic Activity	Clinical Presentation
Antagonism of postsynaptic histamine receptors	Sedation
Antagonism of postsynaptic muscarinic receptors	Sedation, coma, agitation, confusion, hallucinations, ataxia, seizures, mydriasis, dry mucous membranes, dry skin, flushed skin, tachycardia, mild hypertension, hyperthermia, ileus, urinary retention, tremor
Antagonism of postsynaptic α-adrenergic receptors	Sedation, miosis, orthostatic hypotension, reflex tachycardia
Inhibition of norepinephrine reuptake	Agitation, mydriasis, diaphoresis, tachycardia, early hypertension
Inhibition of serotonin reuptake	Sedation, mydriasis, myoclonus, hyperreflexia (see later discussion of inhibition of amine reuptake and chapter 178, "Atypical and Serotonergic Antidepressants")
Inhibition of voltage-gated sodium channels	Impaired conduction, wide QRS complex, other conduction abnormalities; impaired cardiac contractility; wide-complex tachycardia, Brugada pattern, ventricular ectopy Hypotension
Inhibition of voltage-gated rectifier potassium channels	Prolongation of QT interval, ventricular ectopy, torsades de pointes

to amitriptyline but lacks antidepressant activity, and serious toxicity from overdose is rare.[3]

Cyclic antidepressant–related drug toxicity can occur at therapeutic dosages from one or more of seven possible mechanisms (**Table 177-2**).

PHARMACOLOGY

The cyclic antidepressants are named after their chemical structure, which consists of a three-ring central structure plus a side chain, thus the common term *tricyclic antidepressants*. Maprotiline is a tetracyclic (also termed a *heterocyclic*), with a four-ring central structure plus a side chain. Cyclic antidepressants are subdivided into two categories: tertiary and secondary amines. Tertiary amines have two methyl groups at the end of the side chain. The five tertiary amines—amitriptyline, clomipramine, doxepin, imipramine, and trimipramine—are generally more potent in blocking reuptake of serotonin compared with norepinephrine. Tertiary tricyclics also cause more anticholinergic side effects (e.g., constipation or blurred vision) and are also highly sedating because of their central effects on histamine receptors.

Secondary amines—desipramine, nortriptyline, and protriptyline—have one methyl group at the end of the side chain and are more potent in blocking reuptake of norepinephrine. Desipramine is the active (demethylated) metabolite of imipramine, and nortriptyline is the active (demethylated) metabolite of amitriptyline. The tetracyclic maprotiline has a side chain identical to that of the secondary amines; thus it is more potent in blocking reuptake of norepinephrine.

TABLE 177-2 Mechanisms for Cyclic Antidepressant Drug Toxicity at Therapeutic Dosages

Administration of high therapeutic dosages to naive individuals
Drug interactions with medications sharing similar pharmacologic actions
Elevated levels of cyclic antidepressants due to genetically slow hepatic metabolism
Drug interactions with other medications that inhibit hepatic metabolism (cytochrome P-450 system)
Additional toxicity from other active ingredients (e.g., antipsychotics) contained in some combination cyclic antidepressant formulations
Preexisting cardiovascular or CNS disease that predisposes patients to toxicity
Development of serotonin syndrome, usually in combination with serotoninergic medications

Amoxapine has a three-ring central structure and a side chain that differs from the other tricyclics. It is a potent norepinephrine reuptake inhibitor and also blocks postsynaptic dopamine receptors. Thus, it is the only antidepressant that has antipsychotic effects and can produce seizures with minimal warning and normal QRS complex.

Cyclic antidepressants are nonselective agents with multiple pharmacologic effects (**Table 177-3**) with considerable variation in potency at therapeutic dosages.[4] However, these differences become less important at the higher plasma levels typically seen in overdose. Inhibition of amine reuptake (norepinephrine, serotonin) and antagonism of postsynaptic serotonin receptors are believed to produce the therapeutic effects of these agents. The remaining pharmacologic actions are seemingly without therapeutic benefit in treating major depression but significantly contribute to cyclic antidepressant–related adverse effects and overdose toxicity.

ANTIHISTAMINIC EFFECTS

Cyclic antidepressants are potent inhibitors of peripheral and central postsynaptic histamine receptors.[4] Antagonism of central histamine receptors produces sedation and contributes significantly to the depressed level of consciousness and coma frequently seen in cyclic antidepressant overdose.

ANTIMUSCARINIC EFFECTS

Cyclic antidepressants are competitive inhibitors of acetylcholine at central and peripheral muscarinic receptors but not at nicotinic receptors.[4] Thus, they are antimuscarinic agents and not truly anticholinergic drugs. Central antimuscarinic symptoms vary from agitation to delirium, confusion, amnesia, hallucinations, slurred speech, ataxia, sedation, and coma. Peripheral antimuscarinic symptoms include dilated pupils, blurred vision, tachycardia, hyperthermia, hypertension, decreased oral and bronchial secretions, dry skin, ileus, urinary retention, increased muscle tone, and tremor. Antimuscarinic symptoms are especially common when cyclic antidepressants are combined with other medications that also have antimuscarinic activity, such as antihistamines, antipsychotics, antiparkinsonian drugs, antispasmodics, and some muscle relaxants. Antimuscarinic symptoms and signs are common findings in cyclic antidepressant overdose, making them an important clinical marker for toxicity, but these effects are not directly responsible for cyclic antidepressant–related deaths, and they do not require specific therapy other than supportive care.[5]

INHIBITION OF α-ADRENERGIC RECEPTORS

Inhibition of postsynaptic central and peripheral α-adrenergic receptors is a characteristic action of most cyclic antidepressants.[4] Cyclic antidepressants have a much greater affinity for α_1-adrenergic than for α_2-adrenergic receptors. Inhibition of α_1-receptors produces sedation, orthostatic hypotension, and pupillary constriction. This action frequently offsets pupillary dilatation induced by antimuscarinic activity. Thus patients with cyclic antidepressant toxicity can present with mid-sized or small pupils despite having other antimuscarinic signs. Orthostatic hypotension is often associated with reflex tachycardia. The antihypertensive effect of clonidine can be negated by cyclic antidepressants because of their ability to block the binding of clonidine to α_2-receptors.

INHIBITION OF AMINE REUPTAKE

Inhibition of amine reuptake is believed to be the most important mechanism for treating depression.[6] Cyclic antidepressants are potent inhibitors of norepinephrine and serotonin reuptake but produce little inhibition of dopamine reuptake, except for amoxapine, which does inhibit dopamine reuptake. Inhibition of neurotransmitter reuptake leads to increased synaptic levels and subsequent augmentation of the neurotransmitter response. Inhibition of norepinephrine reuptake is thought to produce the early sympathomimetic effects occasionally seen in some cyclic antidepressant overdoses and may contribute to the development of cardiac dysrhythmias. Myoclonus and hyperreflexia are attributed to increased serotonin activity. Serotonin syndrome results from increased serotonin brainstem activity that can be produced by cyclic antidepressants that are particularly potent serotonin uptake inhibitors, such as clomipramine and amitriptyline (see chapter 178). In general, cyclic antidepressants produce serotonin syndrome only when used in combination with other serotonergic agents.

SODIUM CHANNEL BLOCKADE

Cyclic antidepressant–induced cardiotoxicity is the most important factor contributing to patient mortality.[7] Cardiac conduction abnormalities occur during cyclic antidepressant poisoning because inhibition of the fast sodium channels in the His-Purkinje system and myocardium decreases conduction velocity, increases the duration of repolarization, and prolongs absolute refractory periods. Severe sodium channel blockade culminates in depressed myocardial contractility, hypotension, various types of heart blocks, cardiac ectopy, bradycardia, widening of the QRS complex, and/or the Brugada pattern. Mechanisms that contribute to hypotension during overdose include decreased contractility from reduced calcium release during depolarization within the ventricular myocytes and peripheral vasodilatation from blockade of α_1-adrenergic receptors. Rapid influx of sodium is necessary for the release of intracellular calcium stores and subsequent myocardial contractility. Some of the negative chronotropic effects of sodium channel blockade can be attenuated by the sinus tachycardia secondary to antimuscarinic activity.

Cyclic antidepressant cardiotoxicity produces ECG changes, such as prolongation of the PR interval and QRS duration, frontal plane right axis deviation, and the Brugada pattern (incomplete right bundle-branch block with ST-segment elevation in leads V_1 to V_3).[7,8] The right axis deviation is most pronounced in the terminal 40 milliseconds of limb leads, demonstrated by a terminal R wave in ECG lead aVR and an S wave in ECG lead I. The Brugada pattern is seen in approximately 10% to 15% of all patients with significant cyclic antidepressant overdose admitted to an intensive care unit but is rarely seen in other types of overdose.[8,9] **Therefore, the Brugada pattern strongly suggests a cyclic antidepressant overdose.**

Slow electrical conduction can produce various types of heart blocks. Local changes in electrical conduction can predispose to ventricular dysrhythmias by establishing reentry loops. Bradycardia, when accompanied by QRS complex widening, indicates profound sodium channel blockade.

POTASSIUM CHANNEL ANTAGONISM

Cyclic antidepressants block myocardial potassium channels and inhibit the efflux of potassium during repolarization.[7] This effect is seen on the ECG as QT interval prolongation, which is more pronounced at slower heart rates.[10,11] Torsades de pointes is rarely seen in cyclic antidepressant overdoses in the presence of sinus tachycardia, which is partially protective against severe QT interval prolongation and after-potential generation.

PHARMACOKINETICS

All cyclic antidepressants share similar pharmacokinetic properties.[4] They are highly lipophilic, readily cross the blood–brain barrier, and achieve peak plasma levels between 2 and 6 hours after ingestion at therapeutic doses. In overdose, GI absorption can be prolonged because of the antimuscarinic effect on gut motility. Bioavailability is only 30% to 70% because of extensive first-pass hepatic metabolism. Cyclic antidepressants are highly protein bound to α_1-acid glycoproteins, with a large apparent volume of distribution, ranging from 10 to 50 L/kg. Tissue cyclic antidepressant levels are commonly 10 to 100 times greater than plasma levels, and only 1% to 2% of the total body burden of cyclic antidepressants is found in the blood. These pharmacokinetic properties explain why it is unproductive to attempt removal of cyclic antidepressants by hemodialysis, hemoperfusion, peritoneal dialysis, or forced diuresis.

Cyclic antidepressants are eliminated almost entirely by hepatic oxidation, which consists of *N*-demethylation of the amine side-chain groups and hydroxylation of ring structures. The removal of a methyl group from the tertiary amine side chain usually produces an active metabolite designated by the desmethyl prefix (Table 177-1). Clinical toxicity from cyclic antidepressants usually lasts longer than explained by the activity of the parent drug because of the production of active metabolites. These active metabolites often have different pharmacologic activities compared with the parent compounds. Secondary amines such as desipramine, nortriptyline, and protriptyline are not believed to have active metabolites. Amoxapine and maprotiline both have active metabolites. Some cyclic antidepressants undergo enterohepatic circulation prior to their eventual oxidation, conjugation, and renal elimination, but this does not significantly contribute to their toxicity.

The average elimination half-life of cyclic antidepressants is approximately 24 hours (range, 6 to 36 hours) at therapeutic dosages, but this can increase to 72 hours after overdose. Inhibition of cyclic antidepressant metabolism by other drugs that use the same hepatic enzymes can prolong the half-life of cyclic antidepressants.

Cyclic antidepressants undergo significant postmortem drug redistribution.[12] Plasma levels can increase significantly after death as tissue binding sites release cyclic antidepressants back to the blood. This is a time-dependent process, and therefore, the diagnostic accuracy of postmortem cyclic antidepressant levels is inversely proportional to the time after death at which the measurement sample was obtained, among other factors.

TOXICITY

Therapeutic dosages of cyclic antidepressants are variable, generally ranging from 1 to 5 milligrams/kg per day (Table 177-1). Ingestions of <1 milligram/kg are generally nontoxic.[13] Life-threatening symptoms usually occur with ingestions of >10 milligrams/kg in adults, and fatalities are commonly associated with ingestions of >1 gram. Children are particularly susceptible to antimuscarinic effects and show clinical toxicity at lower dosages.[5] The majority of adult intentional ingestions and pediatric accidental exposures of >2.5 milligrams/kg are expected to result in some clinical toxicity based on the low therapeutic index of cyclic antidepressants.[13] In addition, patients at higher risk for cyclic antidepressant toxicity include patients who have co-ingested cardiotoxic or sedative-hypnotic medications, geriatric patients, and patients with underlying heart or neurologic disease.

Desipramine is the most potent sodium channel blocker among the cyclic antidepressants and is able to precipitate severe cardiotoxicity (e.g., wide QRS complex, hypotension) without producing significant antimuscarinic symptoms. It is associated with a higher case-fatality rate than the other cyclic antidepressants.[14] Amoxapine and maprotiline have historically been associated with greater toxicity than other cyclic antidepressants, especially in regard to causing seizures.[14]

Quantitative measurement of plasma levels of cyclic antidepressants is helpful in monitoring long-term drug therapy, but results are rarely available during the time of patient evaluation. Patients with a combined plasma level of parent cyclic antidepressant and metabolite of >1000 nanograms/mL (>3500 nmol/L) are at greater risk for developing seizures and cardiotoxicity. However, the severity of clinical toxicity does not always correlate with the degree of plasma cyclic antidepressant elevation.[7] Serious toxicity rarely develops at therapeutic levels, typically 75 to 300 nanograms/mL (300 to 1000 nmol/L) for most agents.

CLINICAL FEATURES

The clinical presentation of cyclic antidepressant toxicity varies from mild antimuscarinic symptoms to severe cardiotoxicity secondary to sodium channel blockade. Antimuscarinic symptoms commonly serve as markers for cyclic antidepressant toxicity (e.g., dry mouth and axillae, sinus tachycardia), but they alone are rarely responsible for fatalities. Moreover, antimuscarinic symptoms are not uniformly present in cyclic antidepressant toxicity. Altered mental status is the most common symptom reported after cyclic antidepressant exposure.[5,15-17] A Glasgow coma scale score of <8 in the ED is a strong predictor of serious complications such as seizures and cardiac dysrhythmias.[6,7] Sinus tachycardia is the most frequent dysrhythmia noted in cyclic antidepressant toxicity, occurring in up to 70% of symptomatic patients.[7,15-17]

Mild to moderate cyclic antidepressant toxicity presents as drowsiness, confusion, slurred speech, ataxia, dry mucous membranes and axillae, sinus tachycardia, urinary retention, myoclonus, and hyperreflexia. Antimuscarinic syndrome is classically associated with decreased bowel sounds and ileus, but bowel function is fairly resistant to inhibition, so the presence of active bowel sounds does not exclude antimuscarinic syndrome. Mild hypertension is occasionally present and rarely requires treatment. Overflow urinary incontinence may be mistaken for normal micturition in diaper-dependent children or older adults.

Most cyclic antidepressant overdose fatalities occur within the initial hours after ingestion, often before the patient reaches the hospital. **If serious toxicity is going to occur, it almost always is seen within 6 hours of ingestion and consists of the following features: coma, cardiac conduction delays, supraventricular tachycardia, hypotension, respiratory depression, ventricular tachycardia, and seizures.**[14] Secondary complications from serious toxicity include aspiration pneumonia, pulmonary edema, anoxic encephalopathy, hyperthermia, and rhabdomyolysis. Seizures are more commonly reported in maprotiline and trimipramine overdoses.[18] Seizures are usually generalized, of brief duration, and occur with other signs of serious toxicity.[6] **The exception to this rule is amoxapine overdoses; this agent can cause status epilepticus without warning or QRS complex widening.** Cyclobenzaprine overdoses are usually characterized by prolonged CNS sedation and antimuscarinic toxicity with minimal cardiotoxicity compared to amitriptyline.[3]

DIAGNOSIS

Cyclic antidepressant toxicity is diagnosed using a combination of four criteria: history of exposure, clinical symptomatology, characteristic ECG findings, and positive cyclic antidepressant urine drug screen results. Other toxic exposures may produce similar symptoms, signs, and ECG changes; the essential point is that the initial treatment for toxicity due to any of these medications is identical and should not be delayed until definitive drug test results become available. At least half of all cyclic antidepressant exposures involve coingestion of other substances, which can significantly increase or alter toxic manifestations.

False-positive results on qualitative cyclic antidepressant urine drug screens occur for carbamazepine, cetirizine, cyclobenzaprine, cyproheptadine, diphenhydramine, hydroxyzine, quetiapine, and phenothiazines (e.g., thioridazine).[19] The false-positive cyclic antidepressant screen result is generally dose dependent and is more common following a supratherapeutic dose of these medications. Most of these medications are structurally similar to cyclic antidepressants, producing the same ECG abnormalities and clinical toxicity in overdose as cyclic antidepressants. Conversely, false-negative results on cyclic antidepressant drug tests are extremely unusual with clinical toxicity.

ECG abnormalities are common with cyclic antidepressant toxicity and are useful in identifying patients at increased risk for seizures and ventricular dysrhythmias.[20] The classic ECG with cyclic antidepressant toxicity shows sinus tachycardia, right axis deviation of the terminal 40 milliseconds, and prolongation of the PR, QRS, and QT intervals (**Figure 177-1**). Right axis deviation is demonstrated as a positive terminal R wave in lead aVR and a negative S wave in lead I (Figure 177-1). **This classic ECG pattern is seen frequently in moderate to severe cyclic antidepressant toxicity, but its absence does not eliminate the possibility of toxicity, and life-threatening complications can occur in the absence of significant ECG abnormalities, especially following amoxapine ingestion.** Moderate prolongation of the QT interval is noted frequently, even at therapeutic cyclic antidepressant dosages. Nonspecific ST-segment and T-wave abnormalities are observed commonly in cyclic antidepressant overdose. Less common ECG abnormalities include right bundle-branch block and high-degree atrioventricular blocks. The Brugada pattern is seen in roughly 10% to 15% of patients with cyclic antidepressant poisoning who require intensive care unit admission.

The risk of seizures increases if the QRS complex is >100 milliseconds, and ventricular dysrhythmias are more common if the QRS duration is >160 milliseconds.[7,20] Widening of the QRS complex from baseline and positive deflection of the terminal QRS complex in lead aVR are usually seen together but can occur independently of each other. The development of right axis deviation of the terminal 40 milliseconds and/or QRS complex widening appear to be less predictive of cyclic antidepressant–induced cardiotoxicity in young children because pediatric ECGs tend to have a wider range of acceptable variant features, and this complicates the identification of cyclic antidepressant toxicity on the ECG.

ECG abnormalities develop within 6 hours of ingestion and typically resolve over 36 to 48 hours.[7] These ECG abnormalities in isolation are not 100% specific for cyclic antidepressant toxicity, so because prior ECGs may not be available for comparison, any observed ECG abnormalities should be assumed attributable to cyclic antidepressant exposure and managed accordingly.

TREATMENT

Evaluate patients for alterations of consciousness, hemodynamic instability, and respiratory impairment. Establish an IV line, initiate continuous cardiac rhythm monitoring, and obtain serial ECGs. Suggested laboratory studies include serum electrolytes, creatinine, and glucose. To identify co-ingestants, obtain serum acetaminophen and salicylate levels. Blood gas measurement is required for symptomatic patients. In patients with antimuscarinic symptoms, urinary catheterization may be required to prevent urinary retention, and a nasogastric tube may be needed if ileus is present. **Patients who are initially asymptomatic may deteriorate rapidly and therefore should be monitored closely for 6 hours.** Treatment recommendations (**Table 177-4**) are based primarily on cohort or case-control studies resulting in only moderate strength of evidence for those measures discussed below.[21]

GI DECONTAMINATION

Do not use ipecac syrup or gastric lavage.[13,22-24] **Give a single 1 gram/kg dose of activated charcoal PO** if patients are awake, have a patent airway, and arrive within 1 hour of ingestion.[13,25] Activated charcoal effectively binds cyclic antidepressants and decreases absorption. Neither multidose activated charcoal nor whole-bowel irrigation is warranted.[22,26] Asymptomatic patients with reliable histories of minimal cyclic antidepressant ingestion can be treated with activated charcoal alone and observed for toxicity.

SODIUM BICARBONATE

Sodium bicarbonate is used to treat cardiac conduction abnormalities, ventricular dysrhythmias, or hypotension refractory to IV fluid.[21] **Administer sodium bicarbonate as an initial IV bolus of 1 to 2 mEq/kg,** and repeat until patient improvement is noted or until blood pH is between 7.50 and 7.55 (**Figure 177-2**). Additional

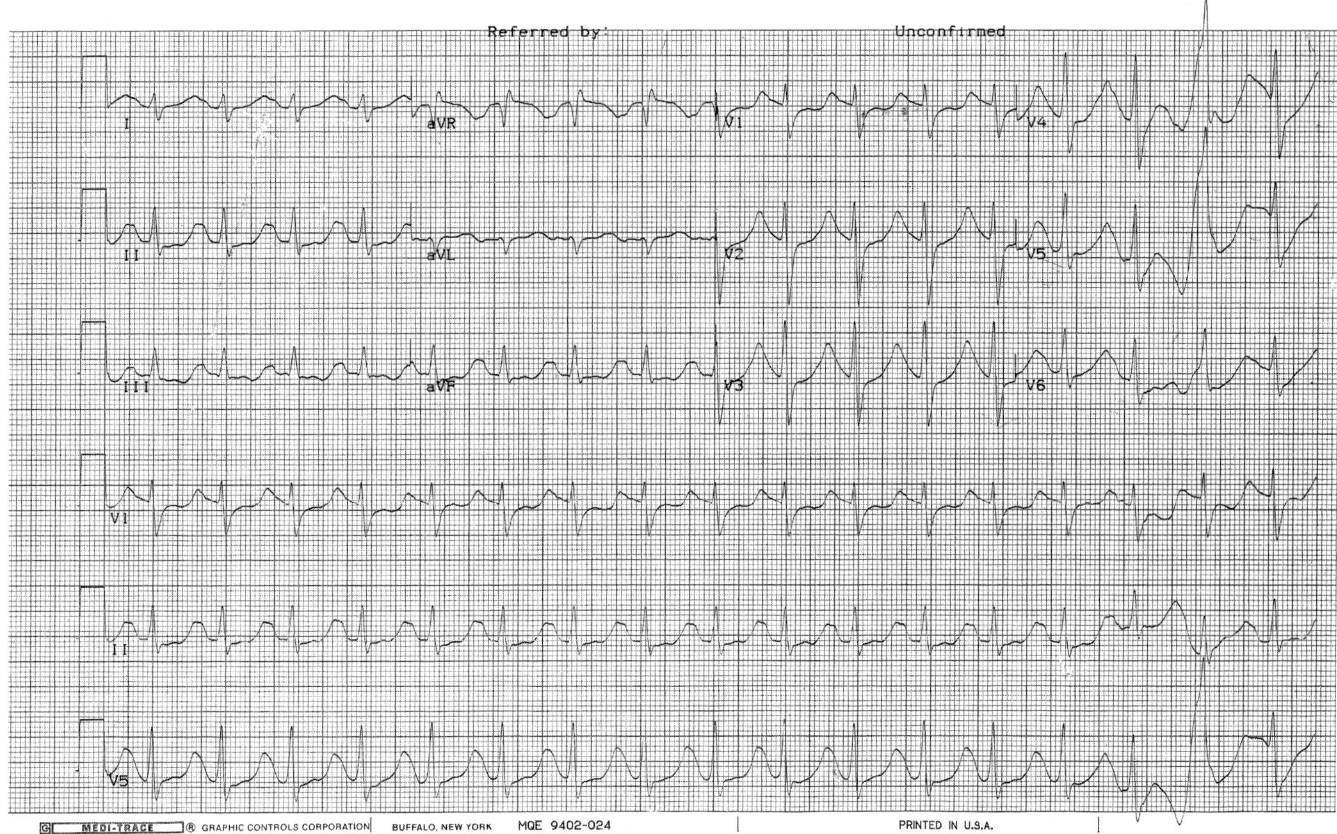

FIGURE 177-1. Twelve-lead ECG showing classic cyclic antidepressant ECG abnormalities: sinus tachycardia; prolonged PR, QRS, and QT intervals; and right axis deviation of the terminal 40 milliseconds of the QRS complex.

alkalization beyond this point can be deleterious to oxygen extraction and serum electrolytes.

As an alternative of repeat boluses, continuous infusions of sodium bicarbonate can be administered as 150 mEq added to 1 L of 5% dextrose in water (or 100 mEq added to 5% dextrose in 0.45% saline, creating a slightly hypertonic solution with the sodium bicarbonate added) and infused IV at a rate of 2 to 3 mL/kg per hour. Adjustments in the IV rate are made based on blood pH measurements and clinical response to therapy. Monitor serum electrolytes during the sodium bicarbonate infusion. Hypernatremia is not of particular concern using this dose of sodium bicarbonate.[16] Serum potassium will decrease during sodium bicarbonate therapy, and IV potassium supplementation may be required.[16]

ALTERED LEVEL OF CONSCIOUSNESS

Antagonism of postsynaptic muscarinic, histaminic, and α-adrenergic receptors contributes to the development of depressed mentation in cyclic antidepressant overdose. Coma from cyclic antidepressant toxicity

TABLE 177-4 Treatment of Cyclic Antidepressant Overdose

Treatment	Dose	Indication	Comments
GI decontamination	Activated charcoal 1 gram/kg PO	Within 1 h of ingestion as long as airway is stable and patient is awake	Do not give multidose charcoal; do not do whole-bowel irrigation
Initial treatment of hypotension or dysrhythmias	Sodium bicarbonate, 1–2 mEq/kg IV bolus; repeat bolus or add 150 mEq in 1 L 5% dextrose in water at 2–3 mL/kg per hour	For dysrhythmias, conduction abnormalities (QRS >100 ms), or hypotension refractory to IV fluid	Keep blood pH 7.50–7.55
Hypokalemia	Replace potassium as needed	Serum potassium <3.5 mEq/L	Bicarbonate will decrease potassium
Seizures or agitation	Benzodiazepines for seizures or agitation	Phenobarbital 10–15 milligrams/kg for seizures refractory to benzodiazepines; watch for hypotension; secure airway with intubation	Do not give physostigmine, flumazenil, or phenytoin
Hypotension	Treat hypotension with normal saline, up to 30 mL/kg	Use norepinephrine or epinephrine if refractory to IV normal saline	Case reports of glucagon, 1 milligram IV bolus
Torsades de pointes and refractory dysrhythmias	Magnesium sulfate 2 grams IV; 3% saline 1–3 mL/kg IV over 10 min; overdrive pacing	Consider lipid emulsion for refractory dysrhythmias, but no convincing evidence of effectiveness	**Do not give** class I antiarrhythmics (i.e., procainamide, lidocaine, phenytoin, flecainide), β-blockers, calcium channel blockers, or class III antiarrhythmics (i.e., amiodarone, sotalol, ibutilide)

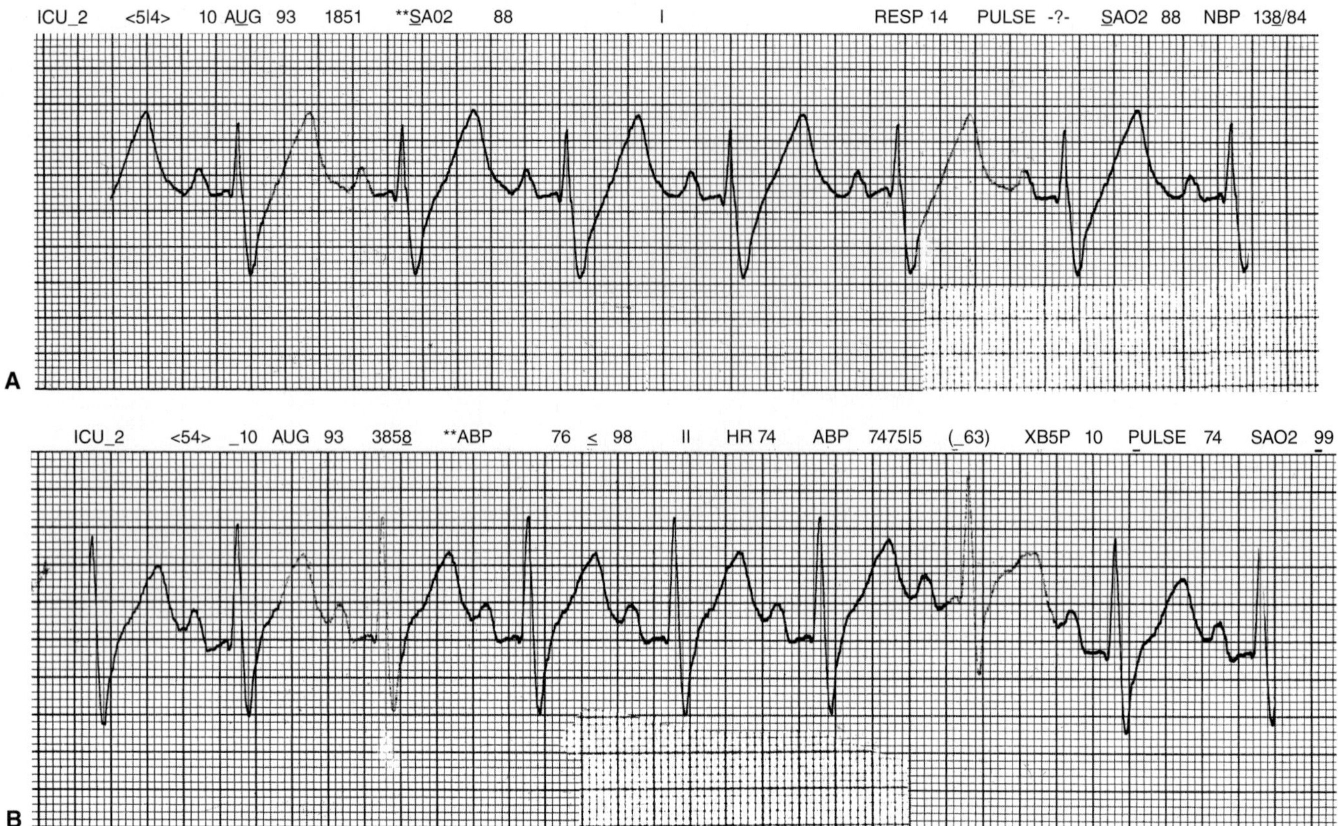

FIGURE 177-2. ECG before and after bicarbonate treatment. **A.** Cardiac rhythm strip of a patient with a wide QRS complex recorded 3 hours after ingestion of amitriptyline. **B.** Narrowing of the QRS complex in the same patient after administration of an IV bolus of sodium bicarbonate.

typically is rapid in onset and is a predictive factor for cardiotoxicity and/or seizures.[6] Pulmonary aspiration is common among comatose cyclic antidepressant overdose patients. Agitation is observed commonly prior to the onset of coma, as well as during awakening. Agitation is best controlled with reassurance, decreased environmental stimulation, and benzodiazepines. **Do not give flumazenil or physostigmine for mixed cyclic antidepressant–benzodiazepine or cyclic antidepressant–anticholinergic overdoses, respectively.**

SEIZURES

Most seizures occur within the first 3 hours following ingestion and are typically generalized and of brief duration.[6] Multiple seizures are reported in approximately 10% to 30% of cases of cyclic antidepressant overdose. Focal seizures and status epilepticus are atypical and should prompt further neurologic evaluation. Seizures are especially common with maprotiline and amoxapine ingestions and require aggressive management, because status epilepticus is frequently associated with these two particular antidepressants.[14] **Benzodiazepines (e.g., diazepam, lorazepam) are the anticonvulsants of choice to stop seizure activity.** Barbiturates (e.g., phenobarbital) are indicated to treat seizures resistant to benzodiazepines. The initial IV dose of phenobarbital is 10 to 15 milligrams/kg, but this can be increased in patients with continued seizure activity and adequate blood pressure. Other therapy for refractory seizures includes continuous-infusion midazolam or propofol. Hypotension is a major side effect of IV phenobarbital administration.

Endotracheal intubation and respiratory support are typically required when benzodiazepines are combined with barbiturates or propofol. **Phenytoin, sodium bicarbonate, and physostigmine do not stop cyclic antidepressant–induced seizures.** Neuromuscular blockers will stop the physical manifestations of seizures and their secondary effects, which include metabolic acidosis, hyperthermia, rhabdomyolysis, and renal failure, but they do not stop brain seizure activity. Therefore, following the induction of muscle paralysis, continue anticonvulsant therapy and consider electroencephalographic monitoring.

HYPOTENSION

Hypotension should be treated initially with isotonic crystalloid fluids in IV boluses in increments of 10 mL/kg to a maximum of 30 mL/kg.[21] With impaired cardiac contractility, pulmonary edema can develop if excessive fluids are administered. Hypotension that does not improve with appropriate fluid challenges should be treated with sodium bicarbonate (regardless of QRS complex duration). Vasopressors should be used when hypotension is unresponsive to fluids and sodium bicarbonate therapy. **Norepinephrine and epinephrine are the most effective vasopressors because they directly compete with the cyclic antidepressants at the α-adrenergic receptors.** Start the IV infusion at 1 microgram/min and titrate according to blood pressure. Vasopressin can be tried if there is no response to norepinephrine or epinephrine.[27] Dopamine is less effective than norepinephrine in reversing cyclic antidepressant–induced hypotension because it has primarily indirect α-adrenergic agonist activity and, at lower dosages, promotes vasodilation through its β-adrenergic and dopaminergic actions.

Placement of a pulmonary artery catheter for monitoring in patients whose hypotension is refractory to fluid, sodium bicarbonate, and vasopressor therapy may precipitate life-threatening conduction abnormalities and ventricular dysrhythmias as the catheter passes through the right ventricle. Mechanical support of the circulation with cardiopulmonary bypass, overdrive pacing, or aortic balloon pump assistance may be warranted in patients with refractory hypotension, although no studies document the effectiveness of these measures. There are isolated case reports suggesting that glucagon administered as 1 milligram IV boluses might be effective in patients with refractory cyclic antidepressant–induced hypotension.[28]

CARDIAC CONDUCTION ABNORMALITIES AND DYSRHYTHMIAS

Cyclic antidepressants frequently alter cardiac rate, conduction, and contractility. These negative cardiac effects are increased with acidosis, which occurs in patients with respiratory depression or seizures. Asymptomatic patients with sinus tachycardia, isolated PR interval prolongation, or first-degree atrioventricular block do not require specific pharmacologic therapy. Conduction blocks greater than first-degree atrioventricular block are worrisome because they can progress rapidly to complete heart block secondary to impaired infranodal conduction.

The controversial issue is whether asymptomatic or mildly toxic patients with isolated QRS complex prolongation should be treated with sodium bicarbonate therapy.[21] There are no controlled human trials demonstrating benefits in otherwise asymptomatic patients with QRS complex prolongation. Nonetheless, many physicians use sodium bicarbonate therapy in asymptomatic or minimally toxic patients with cyclic antidepressant overdose if the QRS duration is >100 milliseconds. Hyperventilation represents a reasonable alternative to sodium bicarbonate therapy in the setting of renal failure, pulmonary edema, or cerebral edema, although hyperventilation is less effective in reversing toxicity.[29]

Ventricular dysrhythmias should be treated with sodium bicarbonate. Consider 3% hypertonic saline, 1 to 3 mL/kg IV over 10 minutes, to decrease ventricular ectopy or dysrhythmia in a patient with cardiotoxicity refractory to sodium bicarbonate therapy.[30]

Torsades de pointes should be treated initially with 2 grams of IV magnesium sulfate. Identify and treat electrolyte disorders that are associated with torsades de pointes. Overdrive pacing may be considered for refractory tachydysrhythmias. Older case reports indicate that IV isoproterenol may be of some benefit when overdrive pacing is not available. **The following medications are contraindicated in the treatment of cyclic antidepressant–induced dysrhythmias: all class I antiarrhythmic agents, β-blockers, calcium channel blockers, and all class III antiarrhythmic agents. Lidocaine, a sodium channel blocker, has unclear benefits in cyclic antidepressant–induced dysrhythmias, and there are no convincing data to support its effectiveness.**

LIPID EMULSION

Cyclic antidepressants are highly lipid soluble, and it has been postulated that intravenous lipid emulsion creates a "lipid sink" that sequesters the drug and prevents toxicity.[31] Case descriptions report both benefit[32-36] and complications.[31,37] Currently, there is no consensus or convincing evidence for the use of lipid emulsion in cyclic antidepressant toxicity.[21,38,39] In patients with cardiotoxicity refractory to other measures, it seems reasonable to infuse a 20% lipid emulsion in an amount based on that recommended for local anesthetic systemic toxicity: 100 mL IV bolus (1.5 mL/kg) over 2 to 3 minutes, followed by an infusion of 18 mL (0.25 mL/kg) per minute to a total dose of 10 mL/kg.[40]

DISPOSITION AND FOLLOW-UP

Patients who remain asymptomatic after 6 hours of observation do not require hospital admission for toxicologic reasons.[13] All symptomatic patients require hospital admission to a monitored bed. Patients demonstrating signs of moderate to severe toxicity should be admitted to an intensive care unit. Hospitalized patients can be cleared medically after 24 hours if they are asymptomatic, with a normal or baseline ECG, normal mental status, and resolution of all antimuscarinic symptoms. Patients with an intentional overdose require mental health evaluation.

REFERENCES

The complete reference list is available online at www.TintinalliEM.com.

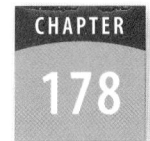

Atypical and Serotonergic Antidepressants

Frank LoVecchio
Erik Mattison

INTRODUCTION

Atypical and serotonergic antidepressants are commonly referred to as *newer* or *second-generation antidepressants*, to distinguish them from the first-generation monoamine oxidase inhibitors and cyclic antidepressants. As a group, these antidepressants are the most popular form of psychopharmacologic therapy for the treatment of major depression, obsessive-compulsive disorder, panic disorders, and eating disorders.[1] These antidepressants produce less severe toxicity in overdose and are associated with fewer fatalities than either cyclic antidepressants or monoamine oxidase inhibitors.[2,3] This favorable overdose profile is tempered by the U.S. Food and Drug Administration black box warning regarding the use of some agents by patients <24 years old due to increased suicidal ideation and behavior.

PHARMACOLOGY

This group of antidepressants is a heterogeneous collection of drugs that differ significantly in chemical structure, mechanism of action, pharmacokinetic characteristics, and adverse effect profile.[1] Nonetheless, they also share many important similarities.

Most possess serotonergic activity and, especially in combination with other serotonergic agents, have the potential to produce serotonin syndrome. Thus, they all carry specific warnings about this syndrome, particularly against their combination with monoamine oxidase inhibitors and other high-potency agents.

Most of these antidepressants do not significantly inhibit cardiac sodium, calcium, or potassium ion channels, with a lower risk for cardiac toxicity, which in large part explains their greater safety in overdose compared with cyclic antidepressants. These agents do not inhibit monoamine oxidase activity and are not associated with tyramine-like reactions. Unlike monoamine oxidase inhibitor toxicity, indirect sympathomimetics can be used for hypotension induced by these atypical antidepressants.

These agents have negligible affinity for acetylcholine, dopamine, γ-aminobutyric acid, glutamate, and β-adrenergic receptors. Although their exact mechanism of action remains poorly understood, it is traditionally attributed to inhibition of neurotransmitter reuptake or interruption of negative feedback loops.

These antidepressants are metabolized primarily by hepatic enzyme systems (cytochrome P-450 pathways). If two drugs are given that interact with a common metabolic pathway, drug levels can increase or decrease depending on the interaction. In addition, hepatic dysfunction can lead to elevated drug levels and subsequent drug toxicity. These antidepressants are not detected by routine hospital serum and urine drug screens. Specialty laboratories can measure parent drug and metabolite plasma levels, but this information is useful only for the confirmation of suspected drug overdose. Specific levels are not immediately available, nor do they affect patient management. Postmortem drug redistribution is likely to occur with these agents, which affects forensic investigation.

ATYPICAL ANTIDEPRESSANTS

The atypical antidepressants have unique chemical structures different from each other and from the other antidepressant classes (**Table 178-1**). They possess some unique clinical features at therapeutic doses and with overdoses.

TABLE 178-1 Atypical Antidepressants

Agent	Recommended Maximum Daily Adult Dose (milligrams)	Elimination Half-Life (h)	Major Active Metabolite
Bupropion	450	10–21	Hydroxybupropion
Mirtazapine	45	20–40	Desmethylmirtazapine
Trazodone	400	3–6 (first phase) 5–9 (second phase)	*Meta*-chlorophenylpiperazine

TABLE 178-2 Treatment of Bupropion Overdose

IV access, cardiac rhythm monitor, and ECG
Anticipate seizures; be prepared to treat with benzodiazepines
Single-dose activated charcoal if ingestion within 1 h, especially if extended-release formulation
Sodium bicarbonate for QRS complex prolongation >110 ms
Magnesium sulfate for QTc interval prolongation >500 ms
Consider IV lipid emulsion therapy for refractory cardiovascular instability

BUPROPION

Bupropion has a monocyclic phenylaminoketone chemical structure that resembles the phenylethylamines (e.g., amphetamine), but does not produce stimulant effects or drug-addictive behavior at therapeutic dosages. The therapeutic mechanism of action of bupropion is primarily inhibition of neuronal reuptake of norepinephrine and dopamine with very minimal serotonergic activity.[4]

Bupropion is absorbed rapidly after oral administration, with peak plasma levels within 2 hours for regular-release tablets and within 3 hours for sustained-release preparations. Bupropion undergoes extensive first-pass hepatic metabolism, is highly protein bound, has an extremely large volume of distribution, and readily crosses the blood–brain barrier. The active metabolite, hydroxybupropion, although less potent than bupropion, preferentially inhibits norepinephrine reuptake and may contribute to seizure development.

Bupropion antidepressant therapy is well tolerated. It does not produce mental status depression, orthostatic hypotension, or cardiovascular changes, or impair sexual function at therapeutic dosages. The most commonly reported adverse effects at therapeutic dosages are mild and include dry mouth, dizziness, agitation, nausea, headache, constipation, tremor, anxiety, confusion, blurred vision, and increased motor activity.[5] Seizures with therapeutic dosages are rare, but the incidence increases drastically at dosages of >450 milligrams/d. Bupropion infrequently produces catatonia, hallucinations, psychosis, and paranoia, which are likely related to its dopaminergic activity. Abrupt discontinuation of bupropion has not been associated with withdrawal symptoms, but as a dopamine agonist, it may pose a slight theoretical risk of precipitating neuroleptic malignant syndrome after discontinuation.

Clinical Features Bupropion differs from other atypical antidepressants in that it has a narrow therapeutic index. Toxicity can occur at dosages equal to or just slightly greater than the maximum therapeutic dose of 450 milligrams/d. **Conversely, significant toxicity is not expected in pure bupropion overdose with adult ingestions of <450 milligrams.** The most commonly reported symptoms in pure bupropion overdose include agitation, dizziness, tremor, nausea and vomiting, drowsiness, and tachycardia.[6,7] Mild hyperthermia is reported occasionally. Sinus tachycardia is the most common ECG abnormality seen following overdose, but QRS widening and QT interval prolongation have been reported.[8] Hypotension is unexpected in pure bupropion overdoses but has been reported in mixed-drug overdoses. Hypertension may occur but is usually of only mild to moderate severity. Coma and cardiac arrest have been reported in severe bupropion overdoses.

Seizures are more common with bupropion toxicity than with other atypical antidepressants[7,9] and usually are accompanied by other signs such as sinus tachycardia or altered mental status.[6,7,10] Unfortunately, **seizures can develop suddenly in otherwise asymptomatic patients**. Seizures usually occur within the first 1 to 4 hours after ingestion of immediate-release bupropion, but their appearance may be delayed for up to 8 hours.[6] Ingestions of extended-release preparations may predispose patients to seizures up to 24 hours after exposure.[10]

Treatment Establish a peripheral IV line, initiate cardiac rhythm monitoring, and obtain an ECG (**Table 178-2**). GI decontamination with activated charcoal is recommended provided it can be done within 1 hour of ingestion.[7] There is no evidence to support multidose activated charcoal or whole-bowel irrigation, even in overdoses of sustained-release products. Ipecac syrup is contraindicated due to the risk of seizures. Early onset of generalized seizures should be anticipated in all cases of bupropion ingestion and treated with benzodiazepines followed by phenobarbital, if necessary.

Hospital admission is recommended for all patients with seizures, persistent sinus tachycardia, or lethargy. Asymptomatic patients who have ingested only regular-release bupropion should be observed for 8 hours before discharge. **Adult patients ingesting >450 milligrams of extended-release bupropion require monitoring for at least 24 hours.**[10]

MIRTAZAPINE

Mirtazapine is a tetracyclic compound structurally unrelated to other currently available antidepressants. In contrast to other atypical antidepressants, mirtazapine does not inhibit neuronal amine uptake.[1] Instead, it blocks central presynaptic α_2-adrenergic receptors and postsynaptic 5-HT_2 and 5-HT_3 receptors. This has the therapeutic effect of increasing central norepinephrine and serotonin neurotransmission. Mirtazapine has a high affinity for blocking histamine-1 receptors and a moderate affinity for blocking muscarinic receptors. These effects commonly produce somnolence, especially in overdose.

Mirtazapine has a pharmacokinetic profile similar to other atypical antidepressants. It is absorbed rapidly with peak plasma levels within 2 hours after ingestion. Bioavailability is approximately 50% due to significant first-pass hepatic metabolism. The elimination half-life for mirtazapine is shorter in males than females, attributed to decreased cytochrome P-450 metabolism in females. Mirtazapine is highly protein bound (85%) and has a large volume of distribution (5 L/kg). Agranulocytosis is a rare but potentially serious complication of chronic mirtazapine use.

Clinical Features Mirtazapine produces limited toxicity in overdose; the most common features are sedation, confusion, sinus tachycardia, and mild hypertension.[11-13] The risk of coma and respiratory depression is greatest at larger doses or when mirtazapine is combined with other sedative drugs.[13] Cardiac abnormalities such as sinus tachycardia or QT interval prolongation are rarely of clinical significance.[11-13]

Treatment Isolated mirtazapine overdose is managed with supportive care alone in the majority of ingestions.[11-13] Administer single-dose activated charcoal if the ingestion has occurred within the past hour. Ipecac syrup is contraindicated, and multidose activated charcoal or whole-bowel lavage is unnecessary. Symptomatic patients should be admitted to a monitored bed, but significant cardiac toxicity is very unlikely. Asymptomatic patients can be discharged after 6 hours of observation.

TRAZODONE

Trazodone is a triazolopyridine derivative that is structurally unrelated to other antidepressants. The antidepressant action is believed to be due to a combination of serotonin reuptake inhibition and antagonism of postsynaptic serotonin type 2 (5-HT_2) receptors.[1] Trazodone is a moderately potent nonselective α-adrenergic receptor blocker with at least five times greater affinity for α_1-adrenergic than α_2-adrenergic receptors. Consequently, trazodone is frequently associated with orthostatic hypotension, which is maximal within the first 6 hours after ingestion, so the harmful consequences can be minimized by taking the medication at bedtime. Sedation, which is a common side effect of trazodone therapy, is believed to be secondary to inhibition of central α-adrenergic and histamine receptors.

Trazodone is absorbed rapidly and completely, with peak plasma levels occurring between 1 and 2 hours following oral administration. It is highly protein bound (89% to 95%) and has a moderate volume of distribution (1.2 L/kg). Trazodone primarily undergoes hepatic oxidation by the cytochrome P-450 isoenzyme system producing one active metabolite, *meta*-chlorophenylpiperazine, which has a complex pharmacologic profile, including inhibition of serotonin uptake, stimulation and inhibition of multiple postsynaptic serotonin receptors, and interactions with other neurotransmitter systems.

The adverse effect profile for trazodone during therapeutic use is very favorable except that **trazodone is one of the most common causes of drug-induced priapism,** with an estimated incidence ranging from 1 to 10 per 10,000 patients. Trazodone should be discontinued immediately in any patient with a history of increased frequency of, increased duration of, or inappropriate penile or clitoral engorgement. Rare case reports describe reversible elevation of liver enzyme levels, jaundice, and abnormal liver histologic findings in association with trazodone therapy. Trazodone has been reported occasionally to be arrhythmogenic during therapeutic use, especially in patients with underlying cardiac risk factors such as conduction abnormalities or ischemic heart disease.

Clinical Features The most common symptom of acute trazodone poisoning is CNS depression. Other neurologic symptoms include ataxia and dizziness, and rarely, coma and seizures. Coma and seizures are more common when another epileptogenic drug is co-ingested. Pupils are usually of normal size and remain reactive. Trazodone-induced neurologic symptoms show marked improvement within 6 to 12 hours after ingestion and almost always resolve by 24 hours. Orthostatic hypotension is the most frequently reported cardiovascular abnormality noted in trazodone overdose and usually responds to fluid administration. The most common ECG abnormality is moderate prolongation of the QT interval.[14] Polymorphic ventricular tachycardia (torsades de pointes) has been reported in rare cases.[15] Commonly reported GI complaints include nausea, vomiting, and nonspecific abdominal pain. Respiratory depression is unlikely with pure trazodone overdoses.

Treatment Establish IV access, initiate cardiac rhythm monitoring, and obtain an ECG (**Table 178-3**). GI decontamination with single-dose activated charcoal can be used in appropriate patients who present within 1 hour. Patients who ingest >2 grams of trazodone or co-ingest other substances are at increased risk for serious toxicity with coma, seizures, respiratory arrest, cardiac dysrhythmias, and cardiac arrest.

Hypotension is treated initially with isotonic IV fluid administration. For persistent hypotension, use a direct-acting vasopressor (e.g., norepinephrine). Drugs with β-adrenergic receptor activity (e.g., dopamine) theoretically can worsen the hypotension in the presence of trazodone-induced α-adrenergic receptor antagonism. Treat QT interval prolongation and/or torsades de pointes dysrhythmia with IV magnesium sulfate, followed by cardiac pacing as needed.[15]

Patients who have remained asymptomatic for at least 4 to 6 hours can be discharged safely from the ED, provided that necessary psychiatric evaluation has been completed or arranged. Patients with neurologic and/or cardiac symptoms require hospital admission to a monitored bed.

TABLE 178-3 Treatment of Trazodone Overdose

Treatment of Trazodone Overdose
IV access, cardiac rhythm monitor, and ECG
Single-dose activated charcoal if ingestion within 1 h
Treat seizures with IV benzodiazepines
IV fluids for hypotension
Direct-acting vasopressor (norepinephrine) for persistent hypotension and circulatory shock
Magnesium sulfate for QTc interval prolongation and/or torsades de pointes

SELECTIVE SEROTONIN REUPTAKE INHIBITORS

Selective serotonin reuptake inhibitors (SSRIs) are a structurally heterogeneous group of drugs that share selective affinity for inhibiting presynaptic serotonin reuptake without significantly affecting norepinephrine or dopamine reuptake (**Table 178-4**).[1] As with most antidepressants, acute alterations in biogenic amine levels do not correlate with immediate clinical response to drug therapy. It is currently believed that secondary receptor and cellular compensatory mechanisms play an important role in their mechanism of action. SSRIs are essentially devoid of direct presynaptic or postsynaptic receptor interactions. Thus they are associated with fewer unwanted pharmacologic actions, in contrast with cyclic antidepressants.

SSRIs are the most common form of pharmacotherapy for depression in the United States.[1] This class of antidepressants is the most frequently reported to be involved in drug overdoses, but fatalities are uncommon due to the high therapeutic index of these drugs.[2,3]

The SSRIs have similar pharmacokinetic profiles, including rapid and complete oral absorption, peak plasma levels occurring 4 to 8 hours after ingestion (except citalopram and escitalopram, which achieve peak plasma levels at 2 to 4 hours), significant first-pass hepatic metabolism, a high degree of protein binding (except citalopram and escitalopram), and a large volume of distribution. Fluoxetine is unique in that the active metabolite, norfluoxetine, is as potent as the parent compound. The half-life of norfluoxetine is 7 to 14 days, so the clinical effects of fluoxetine may last for up to 5 weeks after the last dose due to norfluoxetine.

The SSRIs are metabolized almost entirely by the hepatic cytochrome P-450 isoenzyme system, and these agents can inhibit the metabolism of other drugs dependent on that system. **The most serious drug-related adverse effect of SSRI psychopharmacotherapy is serotonin syndrome** (see "Serotonin Syndrome" below).

Adverse effects with therapeutic doses include hyponatremia, which is believed to be secondary to inappropriate secretion of antidiuretic hormone.[1] Sexual dysfunction (e.g., anorgasmia) is a relatively common adverse effect and is reversible with drug discontinuation. Priapism has been reported but is extremely rare. A withdrawal syndrome consisting of nonspecific neurologic, psychiatric, and GI symptoms has been described in conjunction with abrupt discontinuation. It is less likely to occur with fluoxetine due to its long-acting metabolite. Paroxetine is more likely to be associated with weight gain and sexual dysfunction.

Other neurologic adverse effects associated with SSRIs include headache, sedation, insomnia, dizziness, weakness or fatigue, tremor, and

TABLE 178-4 Selective Serotonin Reuptake Inhibitors

Agent	Recommended Maximum Daily Adult Dose (milligrams)	Elimination Half-Life (h)	Active Metabolite
Citalopram	40	35	Monodesmethylcitalopram Didesmethylocitalopram
Escitalopram	20	27–32	Desmethylcitalopram
Fluoxetine	80	96–144	Norfluoxetine
Fluvoxamine	300	16	None
Paroxetine	50	21	None
Sertraline	200	26	Desmethylsertraline

nervousness.[1] Seizures are uncommon but have been reported with all of these agents, with citalopram associated with the highest incidence of seizures among the SSRIs.[1] Serotonin has varying effects on the dopaminergic system. In many cases, extrapyramidal symptoms such as dystonic reactions, akathisia, dyskinesia, hypokinesia, and parkinsonian symptoms have been reported in association with SSRI therapy.[16] Consequently, SSRIs should be used cautiously with antipsychotic agents because they can potentiate antidopaminergic activity. Patients taking SSRIs commonly report GI complaints, such as nausea, diarrhea, constipation, vomiting, and anorexia. Other adverse effects less commonly reported include dry mouth, increased sweating, and blurred vision.

CLINICAL FEATURES

The greatest amount of human SSRI overdose experience has been with fluoxetine.[17] Information from case series involving the other SSRIs is consistent with the information accumulated on fluoxetine.[18,19] Fortunately, all of the SSRIs are characterized by a high therapeutic index, and fatalities are uncommon with pure overdoses.[2,3] Most adult and pediatric patients remain asymptomatic following SSRI overdose. The most common clinical features in symptomatic patients from overdose include nausea, vomiting, sedation, tremor, and sinus tachycardia. Less frequently observed are mydriasis, seizures, diarrhea, agitation, hallucinations, hypertension, and hypotension.

Sinus bradycardia is observed more frequently in fluvoxamine overdoses than in overdoses of other SSRIs. **Prolongation of the QRS complex and QT interval occurs in association with significant citalopram and escitalopram ingestions.[20-24]** Other SSRIs have been reported rarely to produce similar ECG abnormalities. In most cases, the ECG abnormalities gradually resolve over 24 hours. Tachycardia, mild hypotension, and lethargy are seen more commonly when SSRIs are combined with ethanol. Mixed-drug ingestions can produce a wide variety of additional symptoms depending on the toxicity of the co-ingestant. **About 10% of instances of serotonin syndrome occur as a consequence of acute overdose.**

TREATMENT

In patients who intentionally overdose, establish a peripheral IV line, initiate cardiac rhythm monitoring, and obtain an ECG (**Table 178-5**). Pure SSRI overdoses are associated with limited toxicity except for the infrequent development of life-threatening complications such as generalized seizures and serotonin syndrome. Based on the high therapeutic index and unlikelihood of serious toxicity, treatment with single-dose activated charcoal is logical for patients presenting within 1 hour of ingestion. Gastric lavage, ipecac syrup, multidose activated charcoal, and whole-bowel irrigation are not recommended.

Benzodiazepines are recommended as initial anticonvulsant therapy, followed by phenobarbital if seizures persist. Aside from citalopram and, potentially, escitalopram, the SSRIs generally have very little effect on the QRS or QT intervals. Activated charcoal decreases QTc prolongation after citalopram overdose.[20] Delayed-onset serotonin syndrome and extrapyramidal reactions are possibilities, especially with sustained-release compounds.

Patients should be observed for 6 hours, during which time supportive care is generally adequate. Hospital admission with continuous cardiac rhythm monitoring is recommended for all patients who remain tachycardic, have altered mental status, ingested citalopram or escitalopram, demonstrate cardiac conduction abnormalities, or have features of the serotonin syndrome.

TABLE 178-5 Treatment of Selective Serotonin Reuptake Inhibitor Overdose

IV access, cardiac rhythm monitor, and ECG
Single-dose activated charcoal if ingestion within 1 h
Treat seizures with IV benzodiazepines
Sodium bicarbonate for prolonged QRS complex
Magnesium sulfate for QTc interval prolongation and/or torsades de pointes

SEROTONIN/NOREPINEPHRINE REUPTAKE INHIBITORS

The serotonin/norepinephrine reuptake inhibitors (SNRIs) available in the United States are venlafaxine (a bi-cyclic compound that is structurally different from other antidepressants), desvenlafaxine (an analog of the known active metabolite of venlafaxine), duloxetine, and a new agent levomilnacipran (**Table 178-6**).[1]

In contrast to the SSRIs, these agents are primarily nonselective inhibitors of serotonin and norepinephrine reuptake with a very small amount of dopamine reuptake inhibition.[1] These drugs have no significant direct effect on presynaptic or postsynaptic neurotransmitter receptors. The SNRIs differ in their degree of protein binding and apparent volume of distribution, from venlafaxine with 27% protein binding and 6 to 7 L/kg volume of distribution, to duloxetine with 95% protein binding and a 1640 L/kg volume of distribution. Venlafaxine is absorbed the fastest after ingestion, achieving peak levels at 2 hours, whereas duloxetine reaches peak blood levels 6 to 10 hours after ingestion.

The adverse effect profile during therapeutic use for these medications is similar to that for SSRIs.[25] Venlafaxine is a notable exception, able to produce mild to moderate hypertension when dosages exceed 225 milligrams/d, probably secondary to inhibition of norepinephrine reuptake. Duloxetine appears to have more GI side effects, such as nausea, dizziness, and vomiting, but causes less hypertension than venlafaxine.[26]

CLINICAL FEATURES

All SNRIs cause sympathetic nervous system stimulation via inhibition of norepinephrine reuptake, which predisposes patients to tachycardia, hypertension, diaphoresis, tremor, and mydriasis. Most of these effects are of moderate severity and can usually be managed with supportive care alone.[27] Patients may display alterations in level of consciousness, with mild to moderate sedation being fairly common and progressing to coma on rare occasions. Generalized seizures are more common after overdose with venlafaxine than after most SSRI exposures.[9] Seizures are particularly worrisome because they tend to occur early after ingestion. Subclinical rhabdomyolysis has been observed in about 25% of patients without seizures and 60% of patients with seizures following a venlafaxine overdose.[28] Large overdoses of venlafaxine can produce severe global impairment of left ventricular systolic contraction with a markedly reduced ejection fracture.[29]

ECG abnormalities are common following intentional SNRI overdoses. Sinus tachycardia is the most common ECG abnormality observed, but QRS widening and QT interval prolongation have also been reported.[8] Mortality is low in isolated overdose.[30]

TREATMENT

Establish a peripheral IV line, initiate cardiac rhythm monitoring, and obtain an ECG (**Table 178-7**). Single-dose activated charcoal is logical therapy for most SNRI overdoses.[31] Gastric lavage and ipecac syrup are contraindicated due to the potential for seizures and aspiration. Consider whole-bowel irrigation with a large venlafaxine ingestion.[31] Benzodiazepines are the anticonvulsants of choice. Hypertension and sinus tachycardia rarely require specific pharmacologic therapy, and β-blockers have the theoretical disadvantage of allowing unopposed α-adrenergic receptor stimulation. Treat hypotension with fluids and direct-acting α-agonists.

TABLE 178-6 Serotonin/Norepinephrine Reuptake Inhibitors

Agent	Recommended Maximum Daily Adult Dose (milligrams)	Elimination Half-Life (h)	Major Active Metabolites
Desvenlafaxine	100	11	None
Duloxetine	120	12	None
Levomilnacipran	120	12	None
Venlafaxine	375	5	Desmethylverlafaxine

TABLE 178-7 Treatment of Serotonin/Norepinephrine Reuptake Inhibitor Overdose

IV access, cardiac rhythm monitor, and ECG
Single-dose activated charcoal if ingestion within 1 h
Consider whole-bowel irrigation with large (>4000 milligrams) venlafaxine overdoses
Treat seizures with IV benzodiazepines
IV fluids for rhabdomyolysis
Sodium bicarbonate for prolonged QRS complex
Magnesium sulfate for QTc interval prolongation
IV fluids and direct-acting vasopressors for hypotension

Asymptomatic patients should be observed for 6 hours. Symptomatic patients should be admitted to a monitored bed. Patients ingesting extended-release preparations require additional observation for at least 24 hours due to the possibility of delayed onset of toxicity.

SEROTONIN SYNDROME

Serotonin syndrome is a potentially life-threatening adverse drug reaction to serotonergic medications. It can be produced by any drug or, more commonly, by a combination of drugs that increase central serotonin neurotransmission (**Table 178-8**).[32-36] Antidepressants are the drug class most commonly associated with serotonin syndrome. This important fact can be easily overlooked if the patient does not have a history of depression and is taking the medication for treatment of a different disorder. Serotonin syndrome is characterized by a combination of alterations in cognition and behavior, autonomic nervous system function, and neuromuscular activity.[32-36] The degree of abnormality in any one area is highly variable. The stimulation of specific postsynaptic serotonin receptors is required for full expression of this syndrome, primarily the 5-HT_{1A} and 5-HT_{2A} receptors, but other receptor subtypes may contribute. Drugs that block postsynaptic serotonin receptors are incapable of inducing this syndrome and are often used as a form of treatment.

TABLE 178-8 Serotonergic Drugs

Antidepressants
Monoamine oxidase inhibitors: phenelzine, tranylcypromine, isocarboxazid, pargyline, rasagiline, and selegiline
Selective serotonin reuptake inhibitors: fluoxetine, sertraline, paroxetine, fluvoxamine, citalopram, and escitalopram
Serotonin/norepinephrine reuptake inhibitors: venlafaxine, desvenlafaxine, levomilnacipran, and duloxetine
Cyclic antidepressants: amitriptyline, clomipramine, desipramine, doxepin, imipramine, nortriptyline, protriptyline, and trimipramine
Miscellaneous: trazodone (moderate potency), bupropion (low potency)

Other Agents	
Amantadine (low potency)	L-Tryptophan and 5-hydroxytryptophan (high potency)
Amphetamines (moderate potency)	Lysergic acid diethylamide (moderate potency)
Bromocriptine (low potency)	Meperidine (high potency)
Buspirone (moderate potency)	Mescaline (moderate potency)
Carbamazepine (low potency)	Metoclopramide (low potency)
Cocaine (moderate potency)	Pentazocine (low potency)
Codeine (low potency)	Pergolide (low potency)
Dextromethorphan (high potency)	Reserpine (low potency)
Fentanyl (moderate potency)	St. John's wort (moderate potency)
Levodopa (moderate potency)	Sumatriptan and related triptans (high potency)
Linezolid (high potency)	Tramadol (high potency)
Lithium (high potency)	

TABLE 178-9 Clinical Features of Serotonin Syndrome

	Major	Minor
Cognitive	Altered level of consciousness Agitation	Insomnia Restlessness Anxiety
Autonomic	Hyperthermia Diaphoresis	Tachycardia Hypertension or hypotension Tachypnea Mydriasis
Neuromuscular	Muscle rigidity Hyperreflexia Myoclonus Tremor	Akathisia Incoordination

CLINICAL FEATURES

The triad of cognitive, autonomic, and neuromuscular effects is a classic feature of the serotonin syndrome (**Table 178-9**). The vast majority of serotonin syndrome cases occur in patients taking serotonergic drugs at therapeutic dosages, but approximately 10% of cases develop after an overdose of serotonergic medication. Serotonin syndrome usually occurs within 2 to 24 hours after the dosage of a serotonin agonist (e.g., a monoamine oxidase inhibitor or an SSRI) has been increased or after a second serotonergic agent (e.g., dextromethorphan) has been added.

The importance of serotonin syndrome in emergency practice is twofold. First, the diagnosis of serotonin syndrome is very challenging because of its nonspecific symptomatology.[37] Mild cases of serotonin syndrome frequently are misinterpreted as other psychiatric and medical disorders, and severe cases are often misdiagnosed as neuroleptic malignant syndrome.[38,39] Without proper recognition of patients at risk for serotonin syndrome, emergency physicians may inadvertently precipitate serotonin syndrome by administering serotonergic agents (e.g., meperidine, tramadol, dextromethorphan). To prevent iatrogenic precipitation of the serotonin syndrome, the emergency provider can use drug databases and other resources to evaluate for potential drug interactions.

The severity of serotonin syndrome varies (**Table 178-10**). The most commonly reported signs and symptoms associated with serotonin syndrome are altered mental status, hyperthermia, and increased muscle tone.[32-36] **Myoclonus is a common finding in serotonin syndrome and is an important distinguishing feature, because myoclonus is rarely seen in other conditions that mimic serotonin syndrome** (see chapters 179, "Monoamine Oxidase Inhibitors," and 180, "Antipsychotics").[38,39]

Muscle rigidity, when present, is especially prominent in the lower extremities, which serves as another valuable clinical marker for serotonin syndrome. Patients with ataxia should be examined carefully for lower extremity hypertonia. Unilateral muscle rigidity and focal neurologic findings are not expected. Seizures are always generalized and usually short-lived. Hyperthermia is usually of moderate severity, but temperatures >41°C (106°F) have been reported and are a marker of a poor prognosis. Hypertension is twice as common as hypotension and is associated with a more favorable prognosis.

There are no confirmatory laboratory tests for serotonin syndrome. Therefore, the diagnosis of serotonin syndrome is based entirely on

TABLE 178-10 Severity Pattern of Serotonin Syndrome

Category	Clinical Features
Mild	Mild agitation, mild fever (<40°C), tremor, myoclonus, hyperreflexia, diaphoresis, mydriasis, elevated blood pressure and heart rate
Moderate	Marked agitation, hyperthermia (>40°C), myoclonus, hyperreflexia, ocular clonus, increased bowel sounds
Severe	Hyperthermia (>41.1°C), delirium, marked muscle rigidity, marked swings in blood pressure and heart rate

TABLE 178-11 Treatment of Serotonin Syndrome

Stop all serotonergic therapy
Initiate cardiopulmonary monitoring, establish peripheral IV access, and obtain ECG
IV fluid rehydration
External cooling measures for hyperthermia
Benzodiazepines for agitation
Use short-acting IV antihypertensives (nitroprusside or esmolol) for severe hypertension
Use direct-acting IV vasopressors (norepinephrine, epinephrine, or phenylephrine) for hypotension resistant to IV fluid resuscitation
Consider cyproheptadine for moderate to severe clinical features refractory to supportive care

clinical assessment and exclusion of other psychiatric and medical conditions. Published diagnostic criteria for serotonin syndrome emphasize exposure to a known serotonergic drug and the presence of muscle clonus alone or at least one or two of the other common features.[32-36]

TREATMENT

The cornerstone of treating serotonin syndrome is discontinuing all serotonergic drugs and providing appropriate supportive care (Table 178-11).[32-36] All patients with serotonin syndrome should be admitted to the hospital until their symptoms have completely resolved. Severely ill patients require admission to an intensive care unit. Approximately 25% of patients require endotracheal intubation and ventilatory support. Most patients show dramatic improvement within 24 hours of symptom onset. Mortality varies according to the severity of the syndrome and aggressiveness of care.[33-36] The most common cause of death is severe hyperthermia.

Benzodiazepines are nonspecific serotonin antagonists and can be used to decrease patient discomfort and promote muscle relaxation. Patients with severe serotonin syndrome should be sedated, undergo neuromuscular blockade with a nondepolarizing agent, have an endotracheal tube placed, be started on mechanical ventilation, and be admitted to the intensive care unit.

Cyproheptadine appears to be the most effective antiserotonergic agent in humans.[33-36] Unfortunately, it is available only in an oral tablet or syrup formulation, so it is usually given via a nasogastric tube in severely symptomatic patients. The initial dose is 8 to 12 milligrams, with repeat doses of 2 milligrams every 2 hours until clinical improvement is seen. Cyproheptadine therapy should be discontinued if no response is observed after administration of 32 milligrams during the first 24 hours. Patients who respond to cyproheptadine are usually given 4 to 8 milligrams every 6 hours for 48 hours to prevent relapse.

Chlorpromazine is an antagonist of 5-HT_{2A} receptors and has been successfully used to treat serotonin syndrome.[33,35] The advantage of chlorpromazine is that it is available in a parenteral form, but a potential disadvantage is that it can cause hypotension. It also blocks dopamine receptors, which can promote muscle rigidity, lower seizure threshold, and exacerbate neuroleptic malignant syndrome. The use of dopamine agonists (e.g., bromocriptine) has no accepted role in treating patients with serotonin syndrome.[34] Dantrolene is a nonspecific muscle relaxant that is used occasionally in the management of serotonin syndrome, but clinical benefit is unproven.[34]

Patients with muscle rigidity, seizures, or hyperthermia should be monitored closely for rhabdomyolysis and/or metabolic acidosis. Clinical features of the serotonin syndrome usually resolve within 24 hours after the inciting drug is stopped, an exception being fluoxetine, due to its long half-life and that of the active metabolite. Once a patient recovers from serotonin syndrome, avoid future exposure to serotonergic drugs (Table 178-4), although the risk of recurrence is unknown.

REFERENCES

The complete reference list is available online at www.TintinalliEM.com.

CHAPTER 179 Monoamine Oxidase Inhibitors

Frank LoVecchio

INTRODUCTION

Monoamine oxidase inhibitors (MAOIs) were the first class of antidepressants, but current use of these agents is primarily limited to treating atypical and refractory cases of depression (**Table 179-1**).[1] Newer antidepressants have a more favorable side effect profile, less overdose toxicity, and no dietary restrictions. The declining popularity of oral MAOIs for the treatment of depression is partially offset by increasing use of agents in this class for the treatment of Parkinson's disease.[2] In addition, a transdermal method of selegiline administration is approved for use in major depression and appears to avoid some of the worrisome aspects associated with traditional oral therapy.[3-5]

Safety and effectiveness of MAOIs in children have not been established, and the four agents used for treatment of depression have the identical U.S. Food and Drug Administration–mandated black box warning stating that patients <24 years old may have increased suicidal thinking and behavior while taking any type of antidepressant medication.

MAOIs are associated with tyramine reactions, serotonin syndrome, and medication incompatibilities that are unique to this class of antidepressants. Overdoses of MAOIs are considered life-threatening emergencies, and **even one pill could potentially kill a toddler**. The onset of clinical toxicity is often delayed to between 6 and 24 hours after ingestion, which can lead to misdiagnosis and mismanagement.

MAOI antidepressants with improved safety and tolerability, such as moclobemide, are available in Canada, Australia, and Europe, but not the United States. **St. John's wort (*Hypericum perforatum*)** contains many active ingredients, some of which have the ability to inhibit monoamine oxidase and block serotonin reuptake.[6] St. John's wort is considered generally safe when taken at recommended dosages, but even modest monoamine oxidase inhibition may become clinically significant in overdose, may contribute to serotonin syndrome, or may participate in a drug–drug interaction.

Some medications have monoamine oxidase inhibition as an unrelated pharmacologic action, such as linezolid, procarbazine, furazolidone, and methylene blue.[7,8] Patients taking these medications have the potential to develop serotonin syndrome when they are combined with other serotonergic agents.

PHARMACOLOGY

Monoamine oxidase is an intracellular enzyme bound to the outer mitochondrial membrane.[9,10] It has been identified in most human cells except erythrocytes, which do not contain mitochondria. Monoamine oxidase removes amine groups from both endogenous and exogenous biogenic amines. This oxidative deamination process is the primary mechanism by which endogenous biogenic amines, such as norepinephrine, dopamine, and serotonin, become inactivated. A second important function of monoamine oxidase is to decrease the systemic availability of absorbed dietary biogenic amines (e.g., tyramine) via hepatic and intestinal metabolism. Thus, inhibition of monoamine oxidase leads to the accumulation of neurotransmitters in presynaptic nerve terminals (both centrally and peripherally) and increased systemic availability of dietary amines. Monoamine oxidase has a negligible role in metabolizing circulating catecholamines, either secreted endogenously (e.g., by the adrenal gland) or administered parenterally (e.g., epinephrine). Circulating catecholamines are metabolized by the enzyme catechol-O-methyltransferase that is located extraneuronally and is not affected by MAOIs.

Monoamine oxidase exists as two different isoenzymes, designated *monoamine oxidase isoenzyme A* (MAO-A) and *monoamine oxidase isoenzyme B* (MAO-B). Each isoenzyme has its own relative preference for different neurotransmitters, dietary amines, and inhibitory drugs.[9]

TABLE 179-1 U.S. Food and Drug Administration Approved Monoamine Oxidase Inhibitors

Agent	Indication	Formulation	Average Daily Therapeutic Dose	Maximum Daily Therapeutic Dose	Selectivity
Isocarboxazid	Major depression	10-milligram tablet	10–40 milligrams	60 milligrams	Nonselective
Phenelzine	Major depression	15-milligram tablet	45–75 milligrams	90 milligrams	Nonselective
Tranylcypromine	Major depression	10-milligram tablet	20–40 milligrams	60 milligrams	Nonselective
Selegiline	Major depression	6 milligrams, 9 milligrams, and 12 milligrams per 24-h patch	6 milligrams per 24-h patch	12 milligrams per 24-h patch	Nonselective (as a skin-patch formulation)
Rasagiline	Parkinson's disease	0.5- and 1.0-milligram tablets	0.5–1.0 milligram	1 milligram	MAO-B
Selegiline	Parkinson's disease	5-milligram tablet	10 milligrams	10 milligrams	MAO-B (as an oral formulation)
		1.25-milligram oral disintegrating tablet	1.25 milligrams	2.5 milligrams	MAO-B (as an oral formulation)
Moclobemide*	Major depression, social anxiety	150- and 300-milligram tablets	300 milligrams	600 milligrams	MAO-A

Abbreviations: MAO-A = monoamine oxidase isoenzyme A; MAO-B = monoamine oxidase isoenzyme B.

*Not available in the United States.

During normal physiology, MAO-A is primarily responsible for the breakdown of serotonin and norepinephrine, whereas MAO-B preferentially metabolizes phenylethylamine; MAO-A and MAO-B have equal ability to metabolize dopamine or tyramine. These preferences are entirely dose dependent and can be overcome at higher substrate concentrations or inhibitor doses (e.g., selegiline).

Overall, the human brain contains more MAO-B, and this predominance increases with advancing age. Dopaminergic neurons lack MAO-B activity and have limited MAO-A activity,[2] but significant MAO-B activity is present in surrounding astrocytes and glial cells. Thus dopamine inactivation depends on astrocyte and glial cell metabolism. Serotonergic neurons exclusively contain MAO-B, which allows more serotonin to be recycled while metabolizing more other nonserotonin neurotransmitters. Intestinal monoamine oxidase activity is mostly due to MAO-A, whereas approximately equal proportions of both isoenzymes are found in the liver, affording the body protection against ingested exogenous amines that can cause toxicity (e.g., tyramine reaction).

Blockade of MAO-A in the GI tract is responsible for a severe hypertensive crisis that can occur after patients on MAOIs ingest foods containing the sympathomimetic tyramine. Tyramine is usually metabolized in the GI tract, but the blockade of MAO-A allows it to flow into the general circulation. Although the accepted "MAOI diet" has been liberalized in recent years,[11] there are still several dietary restrictions to which patients on these medications must adhere.

MAOIs share structural similarities with endogenous amines that allow them to act as potential substrates for the enzyme. The antidepressant activity of phenelzine, tranylcypromine, isocarboxazid, and transdermal selegiline has been primarily attributed to their ability to increase norepinephrine and serotonin neurotransmission by increasing presynaptic concentrations of both amines. Their antidepressant effect correlates with >80% MAO-A inhibition. Additional mechanisms by which they exert their therapeutic effects are probably related to delayed postsynaptic receptor modifications (e.g., downregulation), indirect release of neurotransmitters, and inhibition of neurotransmitter reuptake.

The therapeutic benefit of selective MAO-B inhibitors in Parkinson's disease is related to increased striatal dopamine neurotransmission and protection against neuronal damage from oxidative stress.[2] MAO-B inhibition of >80% correlates with the observed therapeutic effect of selegiline and rasagiline in Parkinson's disease. At therapeutic doses, there is limited inhibition of MAO-A with modest effects on norepinephrine and serotonin metabolism.[2] However, at large doses (e.g., selegiline >20 milligrams/d) increasing MAO-A inhibition increases presynaptic norepinephrine and serotonin concentrations and thus has the potential to produce drug-related toxicity similar to that of the nonselective agents (phenelzine, tranylcypromine, and isocarboxazid).

Traditional MAOIs, such as isocarboxazid, phenelzine, tranylcypromine, rasagiline, and selegiline, form irreversible covalent bonds with the enzyme, rendering it permanently inactive. Once an irreversible inhibitor drug has been discontinued, it takes approximately 2 weeks before new enzyme synthesis restores activity to 50% of normal and up to 40 days to regain 100% activity.[10] Reversible inhibitors, on the other hand, competitively inhibit enzyme activity. After the reversible inhibitor drug is stopped, monoamine oxidase function recovers over a period of hours as the drug–enzyme complex spontaneously dissociates. Moclobemide and toloxatone are reversible MAOIs available in most of the world, but not in the United States.

PHARMACOKINETICS

MAOI tablets are absorbed rapidly and completely from the GI tract but have relatively low bioavailability because of a large first-pass effect of hepatic metabolism.[10] The skin patch form of selegiline allows for more parent drug to bypass first-pass liver metabolism; this results in elevated blood levels that have nonselective monoamine oxidase activity, and hence, it works as an antidepressant.[4] The oral form of selegiline has lower blood levels secondary to first-pass effects, retains its MAO-B selectivity, and does not have antidepressant qualities. Metabolism by hepatic cytochrome P-450 predisposes MAOIs to potential interactions with other drugs requiring similar hepatic enzyme pathways. Peak drug levels usually occur within 1 to 3 hours of ingestion. These drugs are highly protein bound and have relatively large volumes of distribution. Elimination half-life is relatively short, and an important feature of clinical toxicity is that it is usually delayed until well after most of the drug has already been metabolized. **Hence, blood levels do not correlate with clinical toxicity.**

Selegiline has many active metabolites, including desmethylselegiline, amphetamine, and methamphetamine.[5,12] Tranylcypromine does not produce amphetamine metabolites at normal therapeutic doses, but amphetamine has been noted in the serum following tranylcypromine overdose. Phenelzine metabolism results in multiple active metabolites such as β-phenylethylamine, which is metabolized by MAO-B. Rasagiline does not have any active metabolites.[2] Transdermal selegiline offers the advantage of continuous absorption over a 24-hour period without any peak effects. However, its absorption can be drastically increased by external heat application (e.g., sauna, heating pad).[4,5] The pharmacokinetic profile of most MAOIs indicates that attempts at extracorporeal removal (e.g., hemodialysis) or administration of repeat doses of activated charcoal would be unsuccessful in significantly reducing plasma drug levels.

DRUG INTERACTIONS

Long-term MAOI therapy predisposes to many potentially significant drug–drug interactions; some have been well established, whereas others are based on single case reports or solely on theoretical considerations.[11] Controlled human studies are impossible due to the life-threatening nature of these reactions, and animal studies often have limited applicability to human toxicity. **Therefore, emergency physicians should never administer medications to patients taking MAOIs unless absolutely necessary.** Compatibility should always be confirmed before a new drug is administered, and the lowest effective dose should be used.

Drug–drug interactions involving MAOIs can be grouped into two categories: pharmacodynamic or pharmacokinetic. The most common pharmacodynamic reaction involves indirect-acting sympathomimetics. They have the potential to produce a hyperadrenergic condition similar to the tyramine reaction and can be found in over-the-counter preparations, drugs of abuse, and some prescription products. Pharmacokinetic interactions have been noted between certain drugs and MAOIs because these drugs are metabolized through the cytochrome oxidase enzyme system and thus can inhibit the metabolism of each other. A notable example of this type of drug interaction is the ability of ciprofloxacin and cimetidine to inhibit the metabolism of rasagiline, which can double its serum concentration.[2] Tranylcypromine and phenelzine have been shown to increase insulin release and predispose to hypoglycemia, especially in patients taking oral sulfonylurea agents.

SEROTONIN SYNDROME

Serotonin syndrome (see chapter 178, "Atypical and Serotonergic Antidepressants") is a rare, potentially life-threatening, often iatrogenic reaction. It occurs most commonly when MAOIs are combined with other serotonergic agents. **The important principle for emergency physicians is not to use meperidine, dextromethorphan, tramadol, linezolid, propoxyphene, a selective serotonin reuptake inhibitor, or a selective serotonin-norepinephrine reuptake inhibitor in a patient on MAOI therapy.** Patients should be warned about concomitant use of illicit drugs in general but especially, cocaine, MDMA (3,4-methylenedioxy-methamphetamine popularly known as ecstasy), and methamphetamine. Even after a patient discontinues therapy, 2 weeks are required before 50% of monoamine oxidase enzyme activity returns. **Consequently, there should be at least a 2-week abstinence period between the time an MAOI is discontinued and when any contraindicated drug is started; this recommendation is particularly important to prevent the development of serotonin syndrome.**

Awareness of which medications are generally considered safe for patients taking MAOIs is useful (**Table 179-2**). Aspirin, acetaminophen, ibuprofen, morphine, and most antibiotics have been used in combination with MAOIs without complications. Morphine should be given in decreased dosages due to impairment of morphine metabolism and enhancement of opiate effects. Direct-acting sympathomimetic agents (e.g., norepinephrine) can be given with caution, but use the lowest possible effective dosage. Direct-acting sympathomimetics do not rely on the release of neurotransmitters for their activity, and circulating sympathomimetics do not require monoamine oxidase for deactivation.

TABLE 179-2 Medications Considered Safe in Combination with Monoamine Oxidase Inhibitors*

Direct-Acting Sympathomimetics	Miscellaneous Drugs
Albuterol aerosol	Acetaminophen
Dobutamine	Antibiotics (except linezolid and furazolidone)
Epinephrine	Barbiturates
Isoproterenol	Benzodiazepines
Methoxamine	Calcium channel blockers
Norepinephrine	Corticosteroids
Terbutaline	Lidocaine
Vasopressin	Morphine
	Nitroglycerin
	Nitroprusside
	Nonsteroidal anti-inflammatory drugs
	Phentolamine
	Procainamide

*Always use the lowest effective dosage.

CLINICAL FEATURES

MAOIs have a low ratio of toxic to therapeutic dose. This characteristic predisposes patients to significant drug toxicity with ingestions just slightly larger than normal therapeutic doses. For isocarboxazid, phenelzine, or tranylcypromine, acute ingestions of 1 to 2 milligrams/kg may produce mild to moderate toxicity, ingestions more than 2 to 3 milligrams/kg can be life-threatening, and the lethal dose is estimated to be between 4 and 6 milligrams/kg.[13] Selegiline overdose experience is extremely limited, but because selectivity is lost after a 30-milligram ingestion, it should be assumed to produce toxicity similar to that of the traditional nonselective MAOIs.[12] Rasagiline is a far more selective MAO-B inhibitor than selegiline. It was given to healthy volunteers at doses 20 times the normal therapeutic dose without any significant toxicity. However, there are no published cases of rasagiline overdose, so prudence dictates that it should be subject to the same precautions as other agents in this class. Toxicity from moclobemide overdose alone is usually mild, even with large ingestions. But when combined with a serotonergic agent, serotonin syndrome is common and can be severe.[14]

An important clinical aspect of MAOI overdose is that the appearance of toxic symptoms is characteristically delayed to between 6 and 12 hours after ingestion, and the delay can be as long as 24 hours. The delayed onset of toxicity is attributed to the gradual accumulation of norepinephrine and serotonin in the brain and peripheral sympathetic neurons. Symptoms of MAOI overdose are most consistent with a hyperadrenergic state secondary to excessive stimulation of α-adrenergic and β-adrenergic receptors, but symptoms related to excessive serotonin receptor activity are also seen. Patients receiving long-term therapy may show earlier signs of toxicity due to preexisting enzyme inhibition. In severe cases, the hyperadrenergic state can be followed rapidly by hypotension and CNS depression resembling a sympatholytic condition. Toxicity usually persists for 1 to 4 days after ingestion.

Published descriptions of MAOI toxicity indicate tremendous variation in presentation: **there is no "typical" presentation of MAOI toxicity and no orderly progression of symptoms.**[12,13,15,16] The initial symptoms of overdose are reported to include headache, agitation, irritability, nausea, palpitations, and tremor. The earliest signs of toxicity include sinus tachycardia, hyperreflexia, hyperactivity, fasciculations, mydriasis, hyperventilation, nystagmus, and generalized flushing. In cases of moderate toxicity, opisthotonus, muscle rigidity, diaphoresis, chest pain, hypertension, diarrhea, hallucinations, combativeness, confusion, marked hyperthermia, and trismus may become evident. A peculiar ocular finding described as "ping-pong gaze" has been observed in some cases of MAOI toxicity and refers to bilateral wandering horizontal eye movements.[17] The cause for this gaze disorder is unknown, and it resolves gradually as the patient improves. Because the signs and symptoms of acute MAOI toxicity are often nonspecific and thus can easily be misattributed to other conditions, even in its most severe form, toxicity can resemble numerous other conditions, which can lead to misdiagnosis (**Table 179-3**).

Severe toxicity is accompanied by coma, seizures, bradycardia, hypotension, hypoxia, and worsening hyperthermia. Hypotension is an ominous finding and commonly remains resistant to therapy. Fetal death, cerebral edema, pulmonary edema, and intracranial hemorrhage have been reported in association with MAOI overdoses. The most common ECG abnormality seen with toxicity is sinus tachycardia, but T-wave abnormalities are occasionally seen. Moclobemide overdose may produce QT interval prolongation but without associated dysrhythmias.[18] Death is usually secondary to multiorgan failure.

DIAGNOSIS

MAOI overdose is a clinical diagnosis based solely on history. Plasma drug levels do not correlate with clinical toxicity, nor are such tests routinely available in most hospital laboratories. Routine urine drug

TABLE 179-3 Differential Diagnosis of Monoamine Oxidase Inhibitor Overdose

Intoxications	Medical conditions	Adverse drug reactions
Amphetamines	Heat stroke	Dystonic reactions
Antimuscarinics	Hypoglycemia	Malignant hyperthermia
Cathinone	Hyperthyroidism	Serotonin syndrome
Cocaine	Pheochromocytoma	Tyramine reaction
Methylphenidate		Spontaneous hypertensive crisis
MDMA (3,4-methylene-dioxymethamphetamine)	**Withdrawal states**	Neuroleptic malignant syndrome
	Ethanol (delirium tremens)	Malignant catatonia
Phencyclidine	Sedative-hypnotics	**Infectious diseases**
Phenylpropanolamine	Clonidine	Encephalitis
Strychnine	β-Blockers	Meningitis
Theophylline		Rabies
Tricyclic antidepressants (early)		Sepsis
		Tetanus

screens do not detect drugs of this class. Selegiline is likely to produce amphetamine metabolites, which can be detected on most urine drug screens. Tranylcypromine has the potential to produce amphetamine metabolites in overdose, but these are rarely detected. Laboratory tests can assist in the differential diagnosis and identify possible complications, including hypoxia, rhabdomyolysis, renal failure, hyperkalemia, metabolic acidosis, hemolysis, and disseminated intravascular coagulation. Leukocytosis and thrombocytopenia are seen commonly with toxicity.

The differential diagnosis includes drugs and medical conditions capable of producing a hyperadrenergic state, altered mental status, and/or muscle rigidity (Table 179-3). In addition, toxicity can be associated with a sympatholytic presentation. As noted, MAOI toxicity is difficult to diagnose without a history of exposure to the drug.

An elevated blood pressure in a patient receiving long-term MAOI therapy presents a dilemma. At therapeutic doses, hypertension can result from tyramine reactions, spontaneous hypertensive crisis, or serotonin syndrome.[9] Tyramine reactions are likely to occur in close relation to ingestion of food or drugs containing indirect sympathomimetics. Spontaneous hypertensive crisis is a rare condition, usually occurring in relation to recent drug dosing.[9] Serotonin syndrome most commonly occurs shortly after exposure to other serotonergic agents and usually is associated with significant cognitive-behavioral and neuromuscular abnormalities.

TREATMENT

GENERAL CARE

There are no known antidotes for MAOI toxicity. ED management therefore is directed toward supportive care and early treatment of complications. Place at least one preferably large-bore peripheral IV line and a cardiac monitor. Obtain laboratory studies, especially to identify hyperkalemia, metabolic acidosis, and rhabdomyolysis. Onset of toxicity is usually gradual and delayed, sometimes up to 24 hours after ingestion. However, the abrupt development of seizures, coma, respiratory insufficiency, hyperadrenergic storm, and cardiovascular collapse is possible. For any given dose of inhibitor, toxicity is predicted to be greater for patients with significant underlying medical problems, children, the elderly, and patients co-ingesting other drugs.

There is no accepted need or best method for GI decontamination in an MAOI overdose.[19] Ipecac syrup is contraindicated.[20] Gastric lavage is generally not recommended.[19,21] MAOIs are absorbed rapidly, so delayed gastric lavage or whole-bowel irrigation is unlikely to be of clinical benefit.[22] **If presentation is within 1 hour, consider activated charcoal administered as a single dose**, but multidose administration is not expected to be useful.[23] Hemodialysis, hemoperfusion, and peritoneal dialysis have no established role in the treatment of MAOI poisoning. Urinary acidification is not recommended because it is ineffective in enhancing MAOI elimination and predisposes to acute renal failure secondary to myoglobin precipitation within renal tubules.

HYPERTENSION

Treat hypertension only with short-acting IV antihypertensive agents because of the potential for development of precipitous hypotension. In many cases, an intra-arterial catheter is required for accurate blood pressure monitoring. The recommended antihypertensive agents are phentolamine and nitroprusside. Phentolamine is a nonspecific α-adrenergic receptor blocker usually administered in 2.5- to 5.0-milligram IV boluses every 10 to 15 minutes until the elevated blood pressure is controlled. It also can be given as a continuous infusion (0.2 to 0.5 milligram/min) for maintenance therapy. Phentolamine use is commonly associated with reflex tachycardia.

Nitroprusside is as effective as phentolamine. It is given as a continuous IV infusion starting at a rate of 1 microgram/kg per minute and is then titrated according to blood pressure response. Prolonged administration of high doses of nitroprusside can predispose to cyanide toxicity, but this potential complication is not relevant to initial treatment. Nitroglycerin is indicated for the relief of anginal chest pain and in patients with signs of myocardial ischemia. β-Blockers pose a theoretical risk of increasing blood pressure through unopposed vasoconstriction and are relatively contraindicated.

HYPOTENSION

Hypotension indicates a poor prognosis after MAOI overdose. Give IV normal saline fluid boluses initially. **When vasopressors are required, a direct-acting agent such as norepinephrine is preferred, and all indirect-acting agents such as dopamine should be avoided.** Patients receiving long-term MAOI therapy usually demonstrate an increased sensitivity to vasopressors, so use low initial dosages.

DYSRHYTHMIAS

Sinus tachycardia rarely calls for specific drug therapy unless it is producing cardiac ischemia. Lidocaine and procainamide are the most effective antiarrhythmics for treating the ventricular dysrhythmias seen with toxicity. Bradycardia may degrade quickly into asystole in the later stages of toxicity and requires pacemaker placement. Pharmacologic treatment of bradycardia includes atropine, isoproterenol, and dobutamine.

SEIZURES

Benzodiazepines such as lorazepam and diazepam are the anticonvulsants of choice in treating MAOI-induced seizures. Barbiturates such as phenobarbital are as effective as benzodiazepines but may cause hypotension, especially at higher dosages. Phenytoin is generally ineffective in stopping drug-induced seizures. General anesthesia and muscle paralysis may be necessary in cases of status epilepticus to prevent the metabolic acidosis, hyperthermia, and rhabdomyolysis that commonly accompany persistent seizure activity. Muscle paralysis is best accomplished using nondepolarizing neuromuscular blocking agents, because the action of succinylcholine may be enhanced by these MAOIs. **Vecuronium is preferred to pancuronium** because of the latter's propensity to produce elevations in heart rate and blood pressure. Electroencephalographic monitoring is required when muscle paralysis is used to control the peripheral manifestations of seizure activity.

HYPERTHERMIA

Antipyretics are not effective in lowering drug-induced fever. Benzodiazepines such as lorazepam or diazepam are useful first-line agents to reduce muscle hyperactivity and thus decrease secondary heat production. Increasing evaporative and conductive heat loss is essential for the successful treatment of drug-induced hyperthermia. This is best accomplished by using cool mist sprays and evaporative fans or cooling blankets.

Hyperthermia is often resistant to treatment as long as there is persistent muscle rigidity. Muscle paralysis (using nondepolarizing agents) should be considered when diffuse rigidity is refractory to benzodiazepine therapy. Anecdotally, dantrolene is an effective relaxant in resistant cases of muscle rigidity, given at a dose of 0.5 to 2.5 milligrams/kg IV every 6 hours, but should only be used when other measures have failed to relieve muscle rigidity.

DISPOSITION AND FOLLOW-UP

All patients with intentional MAOI overdoses or accidental ingestions of isocarboxazid, phenelzine, or tranylcypromine >1 milligram/kg require admission to an intensive care unit or equivalent. Patients with accidental exposures of <1 milligram/kg still require hospital admission but, because they are less likely to develop life-threatening complications, can be admitted to a bed with less frequent monitoring. Consultation with a medical toxicologist and regional poison control center is strongly recommended. Asymptomatic patients should be monitored for at least 24 hours before discharge. Dietary and medication restrictions should be followed meticulously during the hospitalization. All patients should be instructed to avoid contraindicated foods and medications for a minimum of 2 weeks after MAOI drug exposure. Patients who require transfer to hospitals with intensive care units should be transferred as soon as possible to avoid the problems anticipated with delayed onset of toxicity. All patients being transferred should be accompanied by medical personnel capable of performing advanced life support and airway management. **Even a single MAOI tablet may produce life-threatening drug interactions under the right circumstances.**

TYRAMINE REACTION

Tyramine is an exogenous dietary amine that is normally metabolized by intestinal and hepatic monoamine oxidase.[11,24,25] Tyramine can be found in small amounts in many foods but is present at much higher levels in aged, cured, smoked, pickled, or fermented dietary products. The body normally has multiple levels of protection to prevent tyramine and other similar exogenous amines from entering the systemic circulation, but this protection is lost once the normal activity of MAO-A is inhibited by >80%. Therefore, all nonselective inhibitors predispose to tyramine reactions; however, tranylcypromine is associated more frequently with tyramine reactions than either phenelzine or isocarboxazid. Selective MAO-B inhibitors and reversible inhibitors are associated with a much lower incidence of tyramine reactions because they leave intestinal and hepatic MAO-A unaffected to metabolize tyramine. Selegiline (MAO-B selective) is unlikely to produce a tyramine reaction if taken in oral form at therapeutic doses, but at elevated doses, its selectivity is lost and it functions the same as the nonselective inhibitors. Dietary restrictions are unnecessary with rasagiline because of its greater selectivity for MAO-B at therapeutic dosages.[2]

Tyramine is structurally similar to amphetamine and is classified as an indirect sympathomimetic. Like most indirect sympathomimetics, tyramine enters the presynaptic neuron through amine uptake pumps. Once inside the neuron, indirect sympathomimetics are capable of releasing presynaptic stores of norepinephrine and, to a lesser degree, serotonin and dopamine. Tyramine also can displace epinephrine from the adrenal gland. A similar effect occurs with ingestion of foods that contain large amounts of dopamine, such as broad (fava) beans. It has been reported that <30% of patients taking MAOIs adhere to the recommended tyramine-restricted diet. In addition, approximately 4% to 8% of adherent patients experience a tyramine reaction during their course of therapy. Many of the previously restricted food sources are no longer considered dangerous, and newer guidelines call for avoiding only a few high-risk food groups such as meats or fish that are not fresh, sauerkraut, aged meats and cheeses, alcohol (tap or unpasteurized beers), pickled fish (herring), concentrated yeast extracts, banana peels, soy sauce, tofu, and broad beans.[11,24,25]

The tyramine reaction is typically of rapid onset, occurring within 15 to 90 minutes of ingestion of the dietary amine. The severity of this reaction is highly variable and is partially related to the total amount of tyramine ingested. **The hallmark symptom of the tyramine reaction is a severe occipital or temporal headache.** Other associated symptoms include hypertension, diaphoresis, mydriasis, neck stiffness, pallor, neuromuscular excitation, palpitations, and chest pain. Most symptoms resolve gradually over 6 hours without specific therapy, but fatalities have been reported in rare cases, usually due to intracranial hemorrhage or myocardial infarction. An ECG should be obtained for all patients with tyramine-associated chest pain. Focal neurologic findings or a persistent, severe headache warrants investigation with a CT scan of the head.

In cases of severe hypertension, the recommended drug is phentolamine, given as 2.5- to 5.0-milligram IV doses every 5 to 15 minutes until the blood pressure is controlled. The half-life of phentolamine is approximately 20 minutes, and its duration of action is <1 hour. Nitroprusside is another rapidly acting direct vasodilator that is administered as a continuous IV infusion (1 to 4 micrograms/kg per minute). In cases of moderate hypertension, nifedipine and prazosin have been reported to be effective. Recommendations for the treatment of accelerated chronic hypertension discourage the use of nifedipine due to concerns of excessive blood pressure reduction, but these concerns may not apply to the acute hypertension seen in tyramine reactions. β-Adrenergic blockers are contraindicated because of unopposed α-receptor stimulation. Hospital admission should be strongly considered for patients whose symptoms do not resolve completely within 6 hours of onset. Patients who are asymptomatic after 4 hours of observation can safely be discharged home.

REFERENCES

The complete reference list is available online at www.TintinalliEM.com.

CHAPTER 180 Antipsychotics

Michael Levine
Frank LoVecchio

ANTIPSYCHOTICS

INTRODUCTION

Developed starting in the 1950s, the typical antipsychotics are effective against the positive signs of psychosis (e.g., delusions, hallucinations, disorganized thought), but they provided no treatment for the negative signs (e.g., avolition, alogia, social withdrawal). In addition, numerous adverse side effects associated with these agents lead to poor patient compliance. The second-generation drugs, or atypical antipsychotics, have been available starting in the 1990s. These drugs are characterized by minimal extrapyramidal side effects when taken at effective dosages and have activity against the negative signs of schizophrenia (**Table 180-1**). Third-generation agents are being developed to minimize the adverse side effects seen with the first- and second-generation agents.

Antipsychotics were originally referred to as *major tranquilizers*, because of their ability to calm patients, but because they are not simply sedatives, this term is inappropriate. These drugs were also termed *neuroleptics*, which refers to their ability to slow movement. With the advent of the atypical antipsychotics, it became clear that antipsychotic properties do not necessarily parallel neuroleptic properties. For this reason, the preferred term is *antipsychotics*. Although *antipsychotic* is a useful term, these drugs are sometimes administered to treat other conditions, such as agitation, nausea and emesis, various headache conditions; to suppress hiccups; and to control various involuntary motor disorders, such as Tourette's syndrome, Huntington's chorea, and basal ganglia disorders.

TABLE 180-1 Common Antipsychotics

First-Generation or Typical Antipsychotics	
Phenothiazines	
Aliphatic compounds	Chlorpromazine Levomepromazine Methotrimeprazine Promazine Promethazine Triflupromazine
Piperazines	Flupentixol Fluphenazine Perphenazine Prochlorperazine Trifluoperazine
Piperidines	Mesoridazine Thioridazine
Nonphenothiazines	
Butyrophenones	Droperidol Haloperidol
Diphenylbutylpiperidine	Pimozide
Dihydroindolone	Molindone
Thioxanthenes	Chlorprothixene Flupenthixol Thiothixene Zuclopenthixol
Second-Generation or Atypical Antipsychotics	
Benzadines	Amisulpride Remoxipride Sulpiride
Benzepines	Clozapine Loxapine Olanzapine Quetiapine
Indoles	Iloperidone Risperidone Sertindole Ziprasidone
Third-Generation Antipsychotic	
Quinolinone	Aripiprazole

PATHOPHYSIOLOGY

Currently more than 50 different antipsychotics are available worldwide. Classification by structure is difficult; a more useful method is classification according to their relative receptor-binding profiles (**Table 180-2**).[1] **In overdose, the clinical toxicity is primarily an exaggerated effect of the pharmacologic activity.**

Virtually all antipsychotics bind to (and inhibit) presynaptic and postsynaptic dopamine-2 (D_2) receptors in the CNS. When antipsychotic treatment is initiated, blockade of the D_2 receptor results in increased production and release of dopamine from the presynaptic cell. However, with continued use, depolarization inactivation occurs, and decreased production and release develop, along with continued postsynaptic receptor blockade.

The blockade of dopamine receptors in different regions of the brain produces varying effects. Blockade of D_2 receptors in the mesocortical and mesolimbic system is associated with antipsychotic efficacy, whereas D_2 receptor blockade in the area postrema (chemotactic trigger zone) is responsible for antiemetic activity. Aripiprazole is different for other antipsychotics; it is a partial D_2-agonist, with specific effects dependent on the concentration of dopamine. At low levels of dopamine, aripiprazole will stimulate the D_2 receptors, and at high levels of dopamine, aripiprazole will inhibit the D_2 receptors.

Blockade of the D_2 receptors in other regions of the brain produces many of the adverse effects associated with antipsychotics. Antagonism of the D_2 receptors in the tuberoinfundibular region is associated with hyperprolactinemia, which can cause galactorrhea, gynecomastia, and sexual dysfunction.[1] Blockade of the D_2 receptors in the nigrostriatal region is associated with the development of extrapyramidal symptoms. Agents with greater D_2 receptor affinity (e.g., haloperidol or fluphenazine) have a greater likelihood of inducing extrapyramidal symptoms, whereas agents with less receptor affinity (e.g., clozapine) are less likely to cause extrapyramidal symptoms. Blockade of the D_2 receptors in the anterior hypothalamus (preoptic area) can produce alterations in body temperature.

In addition to blocking dopamine receptors, many antipsychotics have activities at the α-adrenergic, muscarinic, histaminergic, and serotoninergic receptors. Antagonism of the α_1-adrenergic receptors leads to orthostatic hypotension and reflex tachycardia. Antagonism of the muscarinic receptors can produce anticholinergic symptoms, including hyperthermia, tachycardia, mydriasis, dry mucosal membranes, and urinary retention. Blockade of the histaminergic receptors primarily results in sedation.

Among the first-generation antipsychotics, potency is inversely related to the likelihood of sedation but directly correlated with extrapyramidal effects. Therefore, high-potency agents such as haloperidol, fluphenazine, and thiothixene are less sedating but more likely to cause extrapyramidal symptoms than are lower potency agents such as chlorpromazine and thioridazine.

Antagonism of the serotonin receptors is associated with a reduced likelihood of inducing extrapyramidal symptoms.[2] Because serotonin receptor antagonism inhibits dopamine release in the nigrostriate and prefrontal cortex, blockade of the serotonin subtype 2A (5-HT_{2A}) receptors is associated with increased efficacy in treatment of negative symptoms, while providing reduced risk of extrapyramidal symptoms. Agents that are partial 5-HT_{1A} receptor agonists, such as ziprasidone and aripiprazole, have similar effects.

PHARMACOKINETICS

Most of the antipsychotics have similar pharmacokinetic profiles. After oral administration, absorption occurs rapidly, the drugs undergo significant first-pass metabolism, and peak plasma concentrations typically occur within 1 to 6 hours. Following IM injection, peak plasma concentrations typically occur within 60 minutes for immediate-release products, but can be delayed up to 1 day with depot preparations. Nearly all antipsychotics have high protein binding and a large volume of distribution. Metabolism is primarily through the cytochrome P-450 enzyme system, with isoenzymes 2D6, 1A2, and 3A4 accounting for the majority of drug metabolism. Because of the near-complete hepatic metabolism of these drugs, renal impairment rarely requires dosage adjustments (notable exceptions include sulpiride and remoxipride).

CLINICAL FEATURES

Isolated overdose of antipsychotics is rarely fatal, and most patients develop only mild to moderate symptoms.[3-6] Toxicity is largely a function of the dose ingested, habituation, comorbid conditions, and age. Following overdose, CNS depression is frequent but is less severe in patients receiving long-term therapy, because tolerance to the sedative effects develops after days to weeks of regular use. CNS effects range from lethargy, ataxia, dysarthria, and confusion to coma with respiratory depression in cases of severe overdose.[5,6] The ingestion of a single pill of some of the atypical or typical antipsychotics can cause significant CNS and respiratory depression in young children.[7] Respiratory depression is more common in multidrug overdoses.

Paradoxical agitation and delirium may occur in mixed overdoses, especially those involving agents with antimuscarinic properties.

TABLE 180-2 Relative Receptor Affinity of Selected Antipsychotics

		Receptor				
Agent	Brand Name in the United States	D_2	H_1	M_1	α_1-Adrenergic	5-HT_{2A}
Aripiprazole	Abilify®	3+	2+	0	2+	3+
Asenapine	Saphris®	3+	3+	0	3+	3+
Chlorpromazine	Thorazine®	2+	2+	1+	3+	3+
Clozapine	Clozaril®	1+	3+	3+	3+	3+
Fluphenazine	Prolixin®	3+	0	0	0	0
Haloperidol	Haldol®	2+	0	0	1+	1+
Iloperidone	Fanapt®	3+	2+	0	0	3+
Loxapine	Loxitane®	1+	3+	2+	3+	3+
Lurasidone	Latuda®	3+	0	0	2+	3+
Mesoridazine	Serentil®	2+	3+	1+	3+	?
Olanzapine	Zyprexa®	2+	2+	3+	2+	3+
Prochlorperazine	Compazine®	2+	1+	0	1+	0
Paliperidone	Invega®	3+	3+	0	2+	3+
Quetiapine	Seroquel®	1+	3+	3+	3+	1+
Risperidone	Resperdal®	3+	3+	0	2+	3+
Sertindole	Serdolect®	3+	0	0	1+	3+
Thioridazine	Mellaril®	2+	2+	3+	3+	2+
Ziprasidone	Geodon®	3+	0	0	3+	0

Notes: 0 = no affinity; 1+ = slight affinity; 2+ = moderate affinity; 3+ = high affinity; ? = unknown.

Abbreviations: D_2 = dopamine-2; H_1 = histamine-1; 5-HT_{2A} = serotonin subtype 2A; M_1 = muscarinic-1.

Seizures occur in approximately 1% of individuals after overdose, with the incidence higher for loxapine and clozapine. Gastric pharmacobezoars have been reported with quetiapine extended-release overdose.[8]

Many of the antipsychotics have antimuscarinic properties (Table 180-2). Thus, patients can manifest signs or symptoms that are consistent with **antimuscarinic toxicity**, including tachycardia, dry mucous membranes, dry skin, mydriasis, decreased bowel sounds, urinary retention, agitation, delirium, and hyperthermia. Due to the α-adrenergic antagonism of many of these agents, mydriasis expected with pure anticholinergic agents is less likely to be present.

The most common cardiovascular manifestations of antipsychotic overdose are **sinus tachycardia and orthostatic hypotension**. **ECG changes** include prolongation of the PR, QRS, and QT intervals, depressed ST segments, T-wave abnormalities (widening, flattening),[9] and increased U-wave amplitude. Ventricular dysrhythmias are rare,[7] with the exception of amisulpride (not available in the United States) overdoses.[10]

DIAGNOSIS

Routine laboratory analysis should include a CBC, basic chemistry tests, and a pregnancy test for women of childbearing age. Obtain an ECG to assess the conduction intervals. Obtain a CBC for a patient with a fever while taking clozapine or chlorpromazine, even if in therapeutic amounts.

TREATMENT

Treatment for patients with antipsychotic poisoning is largely supportive.[3-6] For patients who are known to have ingested or are suspected of having ingested a significant amount, establish IV access and monitor cardiac rhythm. Patients with respiratory depression should receive ventilatory support. Patients with depressed consciousness should receive oxygen supplementation, continuous pulse oximetry, assessment of blood glucose, and consideration for administration of naloxone and thiamine. Seizures should be treated with a benzodiazepine such as lorazepam.

Treat hypotension with aggressive fluid resuscitation. Adults without previously known or suspected cardiac disease should receive at least 1 to 2 L of isotonic crystalloid. Children should receive 20 to 40 mL/kg. If hypotension persists, direct-acting α-adrenergic agonists, such as **phenylephrine or norepinephrine**, are the preferred vasopressors for treatment. Dopamine, an indirect-acting vasopressor, is not recommended as a first-line agent for treatment of hypotension following an antipsychotic overdose.

Patients with a QT_c interval of >500 milliseconds are at increased risk for **torsade de pointes**.[11,12] Assuming there are no contraindications to magnesium supplementation, and regardless of the serum magnesium level, adults with a QT_c interval of >500 milliseconds should receive **magnesium sulfate**, 2 grams IV over 10 minutes.[5] Patients with torsade de pointes should receive 2 grams of magnesium sulfate as a bolus, followed by an infusion of 2 to 4 milligrams/min, regardless of the magnesium concentration. Overdrive pacing can also be useful, especially in cases that prove refractory to magnesium.[13]

Patients with an intraventricular conduction delay (e.g., prolonged QRS complex) and ventricular arrhythmias should be treated with **sodium bicarbonate**, 1 to 2 mEq/kg IV bolus, followed by intermittent boluses or a continuous infusion. Lidocaine is an acceptable alternative or second-line agent for ventricular dysrhythmias. Do not use types Ia (e.g., quinidine, procainamide), Ic (e.g., propafenone), III (e.g., amiodarone), and IV antiarrhythmics in patients with cardiac conduction disturbances or ventricular arrhythmias, because their use can potentiate such cardiotoxicity. Consider **intravenous lipid emulsion** for severe quetiapine overdoses with cardiovascular instability refractory to conventional therapy.[14-16]

DISPOSITION AND FOLLOW-UP

Following ingestion, observe the patient for at least 6 hours. Because of the potential for orthostatic hypotension, obtain orthostatic pulse and blood pressures prior to disposition. The patient can be judged free of toxicity if there are no mental status changes, pulse and blood pressure abnormalities, orthostatic hypotension, and QT_c interval prolongation after 6 hours of observation from the time of ingestion.[17] Patients with evidence of toxicity (e.g., sinus tachycardia or QT interval prolongation) should be admitted to a monitored bed for observation. Patients who develop severe symptoms (e.g., seizure, respiratory depression, hypotension, acidosis) during the observation period in the ED should be admitted to an intensive care unit.

ADVERSE EFFECTS OF THERAPEUTIC DOSING

CARDIOVASCULAR

Both atypical and typical antipsychotics can affect myocardial conduction and repolarization. At therapeutic dosages, this is usually evidenced by prolongation of the QT interval. Of the typical agents, thioridazine, pimozide, and IV haloperidol cause the greatest degree of QT prolongation.[11,18] The prescribing information for haloperidol contains a warning that QT interval prolongation and torsade de pointes can occur, especially when administered IV or in doses higher than typically used. The warning advises caution when treating patients who have other QT interval–prolonging conditions or are taking drugs known to prolong the QT interval. This warning also emphasizes that haloperidol is not approved for IV administration and that electrocardiographic monitoring is recommended if IV haloperidol is given. Among the atypical antipsychotics, ziprasidone, sertindole, and amisulpride are associated with the greatest degree of QT prolongation in therapeutic dosing.[11,18]

EXTRAPYRAMIDAL SYMPTOMS

Extrapyramidal symptoms result from D_2 receptor blockade in the basal ganglia (nigrostriatal region). Although high-potency typical agents cause the highest rate of extrapyramidal symptoms, all antipsychotic agents are capable of producing these symptoms.[19] Blockade of the 5-HT_{2C} receptors may contribute to the induction of extrapyramidal symptoms as well by inhibiting dopamine release in the nigrostriatal and mesolimbic pathways. Many of the atypical antipsychotic agents bind to the 5-HT_{2C} receptors.

Extrapyramidal symptoms can be classified into three major patterns: (1) early-onset reversible syndromes, (2) delayed-onset reversible syndromes, and (3) potentially irreversible syndromes. The early-onset reversible syndromes typically start within hours to days and include **acute dystonia** and **akathisia**. The delayed-onset reversible syndromes occur days to weeks after the antipsychotic is started and include **parkinsonism** and neuroleptic malignant syndrome. The potentially irreversible syndromes typically begin months to years after therapy is started and include **focal perioral tremor** and **tardive dyskinesia**.

Acute dystonia is a hyperkinetic movement disorder characterized by intermittent, uncoordinated, involuntary contractions of the muscles of the face, tongue, neck, trunk, or extremities. Clinical manifestations include tongue protrusions, facial grimacing, trismus, oculogyric crisis, blepharospasm, opisthotonus, tortipelvis, and abnormal postures and gait. Although distressing to patients, these effects are not life threatening.

Akathisia is a subjective sensation of motor restlessness. It typically occurs within minutes to days of initiating or increasing the dose of an antipsychotic.[20,21] Occasionally, akathisia can be misinterpreted as increasing agitation related to an underlying psychiatric condition and can thereby prompt additional medication administration. Although akathisia is more likely to occur with the use of high-potency D_2 receptor antagonists, it can occur with large doses, rapid escalation of doses, or parenteral administration of all antipsychotics.[22]

The treatment of **akathisia** or **acute dystonia** includes the administration of diphenhydramine, 25 to 50 milligrams, or benztropine, 1 to 2 milligrams, either orally or parenterally, with parenteral administration preferred in severe cases. Benzodiazepines may serve as adjunctive therapy or can be used primarily if there is a concern about the administration of anticholinergic agents. Because of the prolonged effects of the dystonia-inducing agent, oral therapy with either diphenhydramine or benztropine should be continued for approximately 2 days after parenteral treatment.

Parkinsonism typically occurs weeks to months after initiation of therapy. It is characterized by cogwheel-type muscle rigidity, pill-rolling tremor, mask facies, shuffling gait, bradykinesia or akinesia, and cognitive impairment. It occurs in up to 13% of patients receiving long-term antipsychotic therapy. Treatment of drug-induced parkinsonism may involve lowering the dosage of a typical antipsychotic, changing to an atypical agent, adding an anticholinergic agent such as diphenhydramine or benztropine, or adding an agent that enhances dopaminergic activity (e.g., amantadine).

Perioral lip tremor, termed the *rabbit syndrome*, is an uncommon late-onset extrapyramidal adverse effect of antipsychotics. **Tardive dyskinesia** is a late-onset extrapyramidal syndrome that can range from reversible to partially reversible to irreversible. Clinical observation suggests that if patients take these drugs long enough, the majority develop the disorder. Tardive dyskinesia is characterized by painless, stereotyped, repetitive movements of the orofacial structures. There can be occasional tongue protrusion, lip smacking, facial grimacing, and choreoathetosis of the trunk and limbs. Although tardive dyskinesia can occur with any antipsychotic agent, it is more common with the typical agents. In young patients, the observed annual occurrence rate of tardive dyskinesia is about 3% to 5% with the typical antipsychotics. In elderly patients, tardive dyskinesia can develop in up to 25% during the first year of haloperidol therapy. The occurrence rate for tardive dyskinesia with the atypical agents is about one tenth that with the first-generation antipsychotics.

Because the symptoms of tardive dyskinesia may be irreversible, the best treatment is the use of steps to minimize its occurrence.[19] Early detection and prompt withdrawal of the antipsychotic increase the likelihood of complete recovery. Unlike with drug-induced parkinsonism, anticholinergic agents exacerbate tardive dyskinesia and should not be used.

OTHER ADVERSE EFFECTS

Therapeutic use of atypical antipsychotics is linked with the development of type 2 diabetes mellitus and diabetic ketoacidosis.[19,23-26] There is some suggestion that the risk is greatest with olanzapine.[27] Atypical antipsychotics are associated with weight gain and intra-abdominal obesity, abnormal glucose regulation, and insulin resistance.[28] Nonalcoholic steatohepatitis has been reported with the therapeutic use of risperidone and olanzapine, and pancreatitis has been associated with the use of clozapine. Hyperprolactinemia is more common with the typical antipsychotics, but can occur with the atypical antipsychotics as well, manifesting as menstrual disturbances and galactorrhea in females and gynecomastia in males.[29] Amisulpride, paliperidone, and risperidone are the most likely of the atypical antipsychotics to induce hyperprolactinemia.

Phenothiazines are associated with leukopenia in up to 0.8% and agranulocytosis in 0.05% of patients.[30] Several atypical antipsychotics have also been associated with agranulocytosis, with the highest incidence in patients taking clozapine, in whom leukopenia occurs in 3% and agranulocytosis in 0.8%. Due to these adverse effects, clozapine can only be prescribed within a strictly monitored program.

Seizures have been associated with several antipsychotics, primarily chlorpromazine, loxapine, and clozapine.[31-33] The risk of seizure appears to be dose dependent.

NEUROLEPTIC MALIGNANT SYNDROME

Neuroleptic malignant syndrome is a rare but potentially fatal idiosyncratic complication of antipsychotic drug therapy.[34,35] Neuroleptic malignant syndrome is not the result of overdose. It most often occurs shortly after the start of therapy or after a dosage adjustment, and the antipsychotic serum concentration is usually within the therapeutic range. Neuroleptic malignant syndrome is associated with all the typical antipsychotics and most of the commonly available atypical antipsychotics, including aripiprazole, clozapine, olanzapine, risperidone, and ziprasidone.[36,37] The incidence is about 1 to 2 cases per 10,000 patients treated.[35]

Neuroleptic malignant syndrome typically develops over a period of 1 to 3 days and is characterized by the tetrad of fever, muscular rigidity, autonomic dysfunction, and altered mental status (including lethargy, agitation, mutism, or coma). The rigidity is typically described as lead-pipe and cogwheel rigidity, similar to that observed with parkinsonism.

Major diagnostic criteria for neuroleptic malignant syndrome are fever and muscle rigidity (**Table 180-3**). An international consensus panel includes two criteria that embody important concepts about this syndrome: (1) recent dopamine antagonist exposure or dopamine agonist withdrawal, and (2) negative evaluation for other causes.[38] Common

TABLE 180-3 Diagnostic Criteria for Neuroleptic Malignant Syndrome

	Caroff and Mann*	Levenson†	American Psychiatric Association‡
Major criteria	Fever >38°C (100.4°F)	Fever	Fever
	Muscle rigidity	Muscle rigidity	Muscle rigidity
		Elevated CK level	
Minor criteria	Change in mental status	Tachycardia	Diaphoresis
	Tachycardia	Abnormal blood pressure	Dysphagia
	Hypertension or hypotension	Tachypnea	Tremor
	Tachypnea or hypoxia	Leukocytosis	Incontinence
	Diaphoresis or sialorrhea	Diaphoresis	Altered mental status
	Tremor	Altered mental status	Mutism
	Incontinence		Tachycardia
	Increased CK level or myoglobinuria		Labile blood pressure
	Leukocytosis		Leukocytosis
	Metabolic acidosis		Elevated CK level
Diagnostic requirement	Both major and at least 5 minor criteria must be present, and treatment with an antipsychotic must have been within 7 d of symptom onset (or 2–4 wk with a depot agent).	All 3 major criteria or 2 major and 4 minor criteria must be present.	Both major and at least 2 minor criteria must be present.

Abbreviation: CK = creatine kinase.

*Caroff SN, Mann SC: Neuroleptic malignant syndrome. *Med Clin North Am* 77: 185, 1993.

†Levenson JL: Neuroleptic malignant syndrome. *Am J Psychiatry* 142: 1137, 1985.

‡American Psychiatric Association: *Diagnostic and Statistical Manual of Mental Disorders*, 4th ed, text revision. Washington, DC: American Psychiatric Association, 2000:795.

laboratory abnormalities include elevated creatine kinase level, leukocytosis, elevated levels of hepatic transaminases, hypernatremia or hyponatremia, metabolic acidosis, myoglobinuria, elevated BUN and creatinine levels, and decreased serum iron level.[39]

Treatment is primarily supportive.[34,35,40,41] Withdraw any antipsychotics and potentiating drugs, such as anticholinergics, antihistamines, or lithium. Consider and evaluate for other medical conditions that can present in a similar manner, including CNS infection, other drug-induced hyperthermic syndromes, serotonin syndrome, anticholinergic poisoning, and sympathomimetic toxicity.[40,41] Reduce the patient's temperature with external cooling measures; pharmacologic antipyretics such as acetaminophen are not beneficial in lowering the temperature associated with this syndrome. Sedation is very important to decrease agitation and sympathetic activity; a benzodiazepine, such as lorazepam, is recommended.[34,40,41]

Airway and breathing difficulties should be anticipated, and patients with excessive secretions, dysphagia, decreased airway reflexes, acidosis, or hypoxia should be intubated. In addition, strongly consider intubating patients with fever and rigidity, because muscular paralysis reduces the muscle contraction and thereby reduces the fever. **When patients with neuroleptic malignant syndrome are intubated, nondepolarizing agents (e.g., rocuronium) are preferred over depolarizing agents (e.g., succinylcholine).**

Complications from profound muscle rigidity are responsible for most deaths in neuroleptic malignant syndrome. Prompt reduction in muscle rigidity can be expected to minimize the occurrence of complications such as rhabdomyolysis, renal failure, respiratory failure, disseminated intravascular coagulation, and cardiovascular collapse. The role of specific pharmacotherapy is unclear. For each therapy reported effective, none has clearly been shown to be superior to supportive care alone.[34,40,41]

Pharmacologic therapies described in case reports and series include amantadine, bromocriptine, and dantrolene. **Dantrolene** (1.0 to 2.5 milligrams/kg IV load, followed by 1 milligram/kg IV every 6 hours) should primarily be used for more severe cases of neuroleptic malignant syndrome in which the rigidity is pronounced. Dantrolene should not be used concurrently with calcium, because this increases the risk of cardiovascular collapse.[6] **Bromocriptine**, a centrally acting dopamine agonist, can reduce fever and muscle rigidity in neuroleptic malignant syndrome and possibly shorten the duration.[42] This drug is only available in an oral preparation and may require administration by a nasogastric tube. Adverse sides effects of hypotension, vomiting, and worsening of psychosis are limiting factors to the routine use of bromocriptine.[41]

Acknowledgment: The authors would like to thank Dr. Richard A. Harrigan and Dr. William J. Brady, who authored this chapter in previous editions.

REFERENCES

The complete reference list is available online at www.TintinalliEM.com.

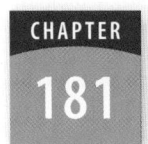

Lithium

Sandra M. Schneider
Daniel J. Cobaugh
Benjamin D. Kessler

INTRODUCTION

Lithium is one of the most effective medications for the continuous treatment of bipolar disorder. It is particularly useful for the treatment of acute manic episodes and reduces rates of suicide associated with affective disorders.[1-3] Off-label uses for lithium include augmentation of the action of other antidepressant drugs and treatment of aggression, posttraumatic stress disorder, and pediatric conduct disorders. Lithium for the treatment of Alzheimer's disease is under investigation.[4] Lithium toxicity most often results from accidental or intentional overdose, increased dose, or reduction in renal clearance of lithium.

PHARMACOLOGY

The specific pharmacologic effect responsible for the therapeutic benefit in bipolar disorder and mania is unknown.[5] Lithium competes with other similar cations, including sodium, potassium, magnesium, and calcium, and displaces them from intracellular and extracellular sites. Interference with sodium ions at the sodium channel and the sodium-potassium pump on the cell membrane is responsible for lithium's adverse effect on myocardial electrical activity. Lithium inhibits arginine vasopressin, an effect that is responsible for polyuria and nephrogenic diabetes insipidus seen during lithium therapy. Some toxic effects of lithium may be due to inhibition of 3-glycogen synthase kinase, which is present in high quantities in the brain.[5] Other pharmacologic effects include inhibition of inositol monophosphatase and reduction of the concentration of inositol in the cytoplasm, inhibition of adenylate cyclase and reduction of intracellular cyclic adenosine monophosphate and possibly cyclic guanosine monophosphate, and interference with the release and reuptake of norepinephrine at the nerve terminal site. Lithium may enhance serotonin release, particularly from the hippocampus, and has been implicated in serotonin syndrome when combined with other medications that alter serotonin metabolism.

Lithium is excreted by the kidneys, so medications that reduce glomerular function have the potential to contribute to lithium toxicity, particularly thiazide diuretics.[6] **Neuromuscular blocking agents such as succinylcholine, vecuronium, and pancuronium may result in a prolonged neuromuscular blockade when given to patients receiving long-term lithium therapy.**

PHARMACOKINETICS

After oral ingestion of therapeutic doses, lithium is rapidly and almost completely absorbed, although delayed absorption may occur with sustained-release products and after ingestion of a large number of tablets.[7] Lithium is not bound to plasma proteins and has an initial volume of distribution of 0.6 L/kg, which is similar to that of body water, but over time this can increase to 0.9 L/kg as the ion distributes throughout the body. Ingestion of a single tablet of lithium carbonate 300 milligrams containing 8.12 mEq of lithium ion will acutely raise serum lithium levels by about 0.2 mEq/L (0.2 mmol/L) in a 70-kg adult.

Lithium distribution into and out of the brain is slower, resulting in neurologic effects that do not correlate with serum levels. The lithium concentrations in the brain and in the serum may differ by twofold to threefold.[8] Continuation of toxic effects, even after hemodialysis, can be due to the drug's slow movement out of the CNS. Therefore, **serum levels do not predict CNS levels and only roughly correlate with clinical symptoms**.

The elimination half-life after a single dose of lithium is about 18 to 24 hours in young adults and almost twice that in the elderly.[7] After continued therapy of longer than a year, the lithium elimination half-life increases, up to almost 60 hours in all ages. Lithium is not metabolized and is excreted unchanged, primarily in the urine. Like other cations of similar size, lithium is reabsorbed in the proximal tubule.

Renal insufficiency is a critical factor in the development of lithium toxicity. Changes in fluid and electrolyte status can impact lithium clearance; sodium and water loss due to heat or exercise may lead to lithium retention. The elderly are particularly prone to toxicity because of their decreased volume of distribution and reduced renal clearance. Elderly patients are at risk for lithium toxicity when concomitantly treated with either loop diuretics or angiotensin-converting enzyme inhibitors.[9]

CLINICAL FEATURES

ADVERSE EFFECTS OF CHRONIC LITHIUM THERAPY

Adverse effects during therapeutic lithium use are common, occurring in up to 90% of treated patients. **The most frequent adverse effects include fine postural hand tremor, fatigue, polyuria due to loss of urinary concentration ability, hypothyroidism, and hyperparathyroidism with hypercalcemia.**[10-12] Worsening of a baseline tremor and development of ataxia or dysarthria are important signals of developing toxicity and may signal a need to decrease the dose of lithium. Long-term lithium treatment can lead to electroencephalographic changes, including diffuse slowing, an increase in theta and delta waves, and a decrease in alpha activity.

Lithium is a common cause of drug-induced nephrogenic diabetes insipidus, which is prevalent in up to 40% of patients receiving long-term lithium treatment and occurs through decreased expression of aquaporin-2 in the distal tubule of the nephron.[13,14] This leads to decreased urinary concentrating ability, which is usually compensated in patients by increased thirst. The defect in the distal nephron can also result in an inability to acidify the urine, causing an incomplete distal renal tubular acidosis without acidemia. Long-term lithium treatment can lead to a progressive nephropathy, with a mild reduction in glomerular filtration[12,15] and about a 1% absolute risk of requiring renal replacement therapy.[15,16] Maintaining serum lithium levels below 0.8 mEq/L (0.8 mmol/L) may reduce long-term renal damage.[17]

GI side effects, including nausea, vomiting, and diarrhea, are common at initiation of treatment, are generally transient, and can be decreased by giving the lithium dose with food or dividing the dose over the day. Development of these symptoms during the course of treatment, on the other hand, may signal toxicity or may cause volume depletion and induce toxicity.

ECG abnormalities commonly reported with lithium use include QT interval prolongation, T-wave flattening or inversion, and significant bradycardia.[18]

Hypothyroidism is the most prevalent endocrine dysfunction, occurring at a rate almost six times that in the general populace.[12,19] Hyperparathyroidism and hypercalcemia are frequently reported and can be associated with stimulation of hyperplasia or adenomas.[20]

TOXIC EFFECTS

Lithium toxicity can be divided into three main categories: acute toxicity in naïve patients, acute-on-chronic toxicity in those who take lithium long term and take an acute intentional overdose, and chronic toxicity developing in patients receiving long-term lithium therapy who experience a change in lithium dosage or decreased renal clearance.[21-24] Decreases in glomerular filtration or intravascular volume depletion are a precipitating cause in nearly all cases of chronic toxicity. Other factors may also contribute to the development of lithium toxicity (**Table 181-1**).[25]

Recognizing lithium toxicity may be challenging, particularly in patients with chronic toxicity.[26,27] There is only an approximate correlation between serum levels and clinical symptoms.[24] Common symptoms are increased tremor, muscle fasciculations, clonus, choreoathetosis, ataxia, muscle weakness, dysarthria, agitation, and lethargy (**Table 181-2**).[25,27,28] It may be difficult to distinguish between lithium toxicity and organic delirium.[29] Although most patients present with a slowing of cognitive function, cases of lithium toxicity presenting with mania or auditory, visual, and tactile hallucinations have been reported. As toxicity worsens, confusion, lethargy, stupor, seizures, and finally coma develop.

TABLE 181-1 Factors Precipitating the Development of Lithium Toxicity

Decreased glomerular filtration: renal injury or failure, heart failure, sepsis
Volume depletion: diuretic use, vomiting, diarrhea, diaphoresis, decreased oral intake
Drug–drug interaction, including polypharmacy

TABLE 181-2 Lithium Toxicity

Toxicity	Clinical Features	Typical Lithium Level (mEq/L or mmol/L)*
Mild	Nausea, vomiting, fatigue, lethargy, fine tremor	1.5–2.5
Moderate	Confusion, agitation, dysarthria, ataxia, hypertonia, hyperreflexia, nystagmus, muscular weakness	2.5–3.5
Severe	Coma, seizures, myoclonus, hyperthermia, cardiovascular collapse	>3.5

*Lithium levels have only an approximate correlation with severity.

Lithium toxicity commonly produces distal renal tubule dysfunction, with decreased response to arginine vasopressin, so that patients may develop significant polyuria compensated by polydipsia. Alteration of this balance can lead to electrolyte disturbances such as hypernatremia, volume depletion, and renal insufficiency.

GI symptoms such as nausea, vomiting, diarrhea, bloating, or generalized abdominal pain are common in both acute and chronic toxicity. Cardiac abnormalities are more common in acute toxicity and can cause hypotension, bradycardia, and ventricular dysrhythmias, presenting as syncope.[30,31] Chronic lithium toxicity may be associated with rare cases of ventricular tachycardia.[32] ECG changes with a prolonged QT interval, transient ST-segment depression, or T-wave inversion are seen in some patients. Less common toxic effects include hyperthermia, hypothermia, peripheral neuropathy, and severe leukopenia. Rare cases of adult respiratory distress syndrome have been associated with acute lithium toxicity.[33]

Up to 10% of patients with severe lithium toxicity die, generally of respiratory failure or cardiovascular collapse. Most patients recover, with toxic effects resolving as the body burden of lithium decreases. Permanent cerebellar and basal ganglia damage may develop. A syndrome of irreversible lithium-effectuated neurotoxicity has been described after lithium toxicity and involves various degrees of neurologic dysfunction after cessation of lithium use for at least 2 months. These patients have truncal ataxia, ataxic gait, scanning speech, and diffuse incoordination.[28] Short-term memory loss, dementia, and a tremor of the hands and head accompany the cerebellar signs.

DIAGNOSIS

Acute lithium overdoses present with more GI toxicity and less neurologic toxicity because of the slower accumulation into the brain after ingestion and distribution in body water. With time, as CNS lithium levels rise, neurologic findings increase after GI symptoms abate. Patients with acute overdose may have markedly elevated serum concentrations that do not correlate well with either symptom severity or prognosis.

Patients with chronic toxicity display earlier and more prominent neurologic effects in association with lower serum concentrations. Serum lithium levels in such patients correlate better with degree of toxicity, but the clinical condition of the patient is the most important factor.[34] Lithium toxicity has even been reported at therapeutic levels.

Acute-on-chronic ingestions occur in patients who are undergoing treatment with lithium and ingest an additional amount. These patients can have both GI and neurologic symptoms and signs.

Monitor lithium serum concentrations and obtain serial serum measurements during observation and treatment. Collect blood samples for measurement of serum lithium concentration in the appropriate tube to avoid falsely increased levels; collection in tubes containing lithium-heparin may cause false elevation in lithium level.[18] Therapeutic lithium levels are considered to be 0.6 to 1.2 mEq/L (0.6 to 1.2 mmol/L). The toxic range varies according to the clinical circumstance, with most patients manifesting toxic effects at levels >2 mEq/L (>2 mmol/L).

A 12-lead ECG may be helpful in identifying a level >1.2 mEq/L (>1.2 mmol/L); QT_c interval >440 milliseconds and diffuse T-wave inversions have positive likelihood ratios of 7 and 4, respectively.[35]

Lithium-induced hypothyroidism can be severe, precipitating myxedema crisis, so check thyroid-stimulating hormone and thyroid hormone levels in patients with altered level of consciousness.[36]

TREATMENT

Initial stabilization of the patient's condition includes protection of the airway and provision of ventilatory and hemodynamic support. Establish IV access, initiate cardiac rhythm monitoring, obtain an ECG, and order renal function tests, fluid and electrolyte levels, calcium levels, magnesium levels, CBC, thyroid-stimulating hormone and thyroid hormone levels if altered level of consciousness, pregnancy test where applicable, and serum levels of lithium and other possible co-ingestions. Subsequent treatment depends on clinical severity (**Table 181-3**).

TABLE 181-3 Management of Lithium Toxicity

IV saline infusion	Used in essentially all patients with toxicity Reestablishes euvolemia and normal lithium renal elimination
Whole-bowel irrigation	Used in awake patients who ingest sustained-release lithium preparations
Sodium polystyrene sulfonate	Consider in awake patients with mild to moderate toxicity
Hemodialysis	Used for patients with severe toxicity Also used for patients with renal failure, patients who cannot tolerate IV saline infusion, and patients with high elevated serum lithium levels (>4.0 mEq/L in any type of overdose and >2.5 mEq/L in chronic toxicity)
IV benzodiazepines	Used for seizures seen in severe toxicity

Treat seizures with IV benzodiazepines, such as lorazepam. Obtain toxicology and neurology consultation for refractory seizures. Phenytoin is ineffective in controlling drug-induced seizures.

Gastric lavage has no role in most cases of lithium overdose because the sustained-release preparations are often too large and the immediate-release preparations are too rapidly absorbed.[37] Ipecac syrup is no longer recommended.[38] Whole-bowel irrigation with polyethylene glycol solution at 2 L/h is effective in removing lithium from the body after an acute ingestion of sustained-release preparations, as long as there is no alteration of mental status.[39,40] **GI decontamination is useless in patients with chronic toxicity.**

IV administration of normal saline is critical, because nearly all patients with significant toxicity have some sodium and volume deficit.[41] Typical adult dosing is an IV bolus of normal saline, 20 mL/kg, followed by continuous infusion at 1.5 to 2 times the maintenance rate. Volume repletion reestablishes normal renal elimination kinetics of lithium. Diuretic-induced diuresis does not enhance lithium elimination, and in fact, loop and thiazide diuretics promote water loss, which is followed by lithium retention.

Sodium polystyrene sulfonate (Kayexalate®), an exchange resin, binds lithium, relieves a modest amount of the body burden of lithium, and shortens elimination half-life.[42,43] Doses used in observational studies, mostly in patients with chronic toxicity, are 30 grams dissolved in 120 mL of water, orally, every 4 to 6 hours. This approach is not widely used because oral drugs are to be avoided in patients with impaired mental status due to the risk of aspiration, the potential for hypokalemia and constipation, and the effectiveness of other therapies.

Anecdotal treatment with sodium bicarbonate and acetazolamide (both for urinary alkalinization) and aminophylline has no proven benefit.

Lithium can be removed by hemodialysis, but there is much debate over the threshold for initiating this treatment.[44] Hemodialysis is indicated in patients with symptoms of severe toxicity, those who cannot tolerate treatment with IV fluids, or those whose renal function is impaired and who lack the ability to eliminate lithium. Extracorporeal treatment is recommended for severe toxicity (coma, seizures, life-threatening dysrhythmias) or a serum lithium level > 4.0 mEq/L (> 4 mmol/L) in the presence of renal insufficiency. Consult with a medical toxicologist or nephrologist for patients who have little decrease or increase in serum lithium level after 6 hours of IV saline administration or for patients who have ingested sustained-release preparations.

The goal of hemodialysis is to reduce the body burden of lithium. Because of the intracellular concentration of lithium, redistribution after hemodialysis is expected and an increase in serum levels after hemodialysis is common. Therefore, monitor serum lithium levels for up to 8 hours after hemodialysis. If symptoms of toxicity recur or worsen or if the levels rise significantly, consider repeat hemodialysis. Peritoneal dialysis has been used for treatment of lithium toxicity in the past, but the clearance rates are approximately the same as through normal renal clearance (**Table 181-4**).

TABLE 181-4 Reported Lithium Clearance in Normal Adults with Acute Toxicity

Therapy	Elimination Half-Life (h)	Clearance (mL/min)
No treatment	18–42*	10–40*
IV saline	13–20	–
Sodium polystyrene sulfonate	12–20	–
Peritoneal dialysis	12–16	10–15
Hemodialysis	4–6	70–170

*Longer elimination half-lives and reduced clearance rates are seen in older adults and in patients with acute-on-chronic toxicity.

DISPOSITION

Admission decisions are made by considering such issues as the presence and persistence of factors predisposing the patient to toxicity, the acuity of the toxicity, and the circumstances that led to the toxicity.[45] Asymptomatic patients with acute ingestions should be monitored for 4 to 6 hours, with serial serum lithium levels measured. Admit patients with serum lithium levels of >1.5 mEq/L (>1.5 mmol/L) after an acute ingestion. **Any patient with an *acute* ingestion of a sustained-release preparation should be admitted regardless of serum lithium level.**

Patients with mild toxicity who have no additional risk factors may be managed with IV saline treatment for 6 to 12 hours, often in an observation unit. Once repeated serum lithium levels decrease to <1.5 mEq (<1.5 mmol/L), such patients can be discharged after psychiatric evaluation, if needed. Patients with moderate toxicity require admission, and patients with severe toxicity require intensive care.

Patients taking lithium may seek care in the ED for conditions not related to mental health or lithium toxicity. Take care to avoid prescribing any drugs that negatively impact glomerular filtration and renal function. Thiazide diuretics, nonsteroidal anti-inflammatory drugs, angiotensin-converting enzyme inhibitors, and angiotensin receptor blockers are some common agents that have the potential for lithium interaction promoting toxicity.[6,46]

REFERENCES

The complete reference list is available online at www.TintinalliEM.com.

CHAPTER 182 Barbiturates

Chip Gresham
Frank LoVecchio

INTRODUCTION

Barbiturate toxicity has historically been associated with the highest risk of morbidity and mortality among all sedative-hypnotics. Barbiturates are still the most common class of antiepileptic drugs used in developing countries, but their use is declining due to the introduction of safer, less toxic sedative-hypnotics, such as benzodiazepines, and second-generation anticonvulsants.[1] Status epilepticus,[2] severe ethanol and sedative withdrawal syndromes,[3-5] and toxicologic seizures[6] are typically managed with benzodiazepines, but barbiturates have a useful role as a second-line agent. They are still used in combination drugs (i.e., butalbital) and alone (i.e., secobarbital) for the treatment of tension and migraine headaches,[7,8] although the efficacy of either is controversial.[9] Barbiturates are used in the pharmacologic management of refractory intracranial hypertension from focal and diffuse brain injury, but evidence of improved outcomes has been modest.[10]

PHARMACOLOGY

Barbiturates are generally classified according to their duration of action, which is primarily dependent on lipid solubility and tissue distribution rather than the elimination half-life (**Table 182-1**).

Barbiturates readily distribute throughout the body to most tissues, crossing the blood–brain barrier and placenta, and are excreted in breast milk. Fetal blood barbiturate concentrations closely reflect maternal plasma levels, creating the potential for fetal withdrawal syndrome.[11] Most barbiturates are metabolized in the liver to inactive metabolites primarily through routes involving the cytochrome P450 system. The elimination half-life of barbiturates can be greatly shortened in infants and children and very prolonged in the elderly and in patients with liver or renal disease. Chronic barbiturate use induces activity of the cytochrome P450 enzymes and may accelerate the metabolism of other therapeutic drugs, such as oral contraceptives, anticoagulants, and corticosteroids, when taken concurrently.

Barbiturates' main action is the depression of activity in the CNS and musculoskeletal system. In the CNS, this is accomplished by enhancing the action of the primary inhibitory neurotransmitter γ-aminobutyric acid at its receptor.[12] When γ-aminobutyric acid binds to its chloride channel receptor, it causes it to open, resulting in depolarization, which temporarily stabilizes the resting membrane potential and inhibits the firing of new action potentials. Barbiturates bind to the α subunit of the γ-aminobutyric acid receptor, causing an increase in the duration of time that the cell membrane chloride channel is open, resulting in prolonged depolarization and prolonged inactivity.

Benzodiazepines bind to a different site on the α subunit of the γ-aminobutyric acid receptor and increase the frequency with which the chloride channel opens. Increased duration, as opposed to increased frequency, is one of the reasons cited for increased morbidity and mortality with barbiturate overdoses compared to benzodiazepines.

Barbiturates inhibit both the activity of the excitatory neurotransmitter, glutamate, at the glutamate receptor and calcium-mediated excitatory neurotransmitter release at the presynaptic terminal. Blockade of the calcium channel may contribute to the cardiac contractility impairment seen with barbiturate overdoses. Barbiturates also have effects on voltage-dependent sodium and potassium channels, but in concentrations typically far above the therapeutic range.[13] These effects may contribute to the toxicity or paradoxical actions seen with some barbiturate drugs in overdoses.

CLINICAL FEATURES

Mild to moderate barbiturate intoxication closely resembles alcohol intoxication and toxicity of other sedative-hypnotics; drowsiness, disinhibition, ataxia, slurred speech, and mental confusion are common features that escalate with increasing dose. The progressive neurologic depression seen with *severe* barbiturate intoxication predictably manifests as a range from stupor to coma to complete neurologic unresponsiveness, including the absence of a corneal reflex and deep tendon reflexes.

The most common vital sign abnormalities seen in overdose are respiratory depression, hypothermia, and hypotension, with respiratory depression usually occurring first. Abnormal temperature control and respiratory depression are centrally mediated phenomena, whereas hypotension is primarily a result of decreased vascular tone. Pulse rate, pupil size, light reactivity, and nystagmus are variable. GI tract motility is slowed, resulting in delayed gastric emptying and ileus. Skin bullae, sometimes referred to as "barb blisters" or "coma blisters," are uncommon and may indicate nothing more than the effects of local skin pressure, although hypoxia has been implicated as well.[14] Coma blisters are not specific to sedative-induced coma; they have been reported after surgery,[15] from other causes of coma,[16] and even without coma.[17]

Early deaths in barbiturate overdose result from respiratory arrest and cardiovascular collapse. Common complications include hypoglycemia (perhaps due to starvation), pulmonary edema, aspiration pneumonia, and acute lung injury. Current mortality rates range between 1% and 3%; death usually results from multiple organ system failure. Lethal doses are estimates (Table 182-1), but severe poisoning can be assumed if more

TABLE 182-1 Selected Properties of Commonly Used Barbiturates

	Long Acting*		Intermediate Acting*		Short Acting*		Ultrashort Acting*	
Agent	Barbital†	Phenobarbital†	Amobarbital	Butalbital	Pentobarbital	Secobarbital	Thiopental	Methohexital
pK_a	7.4	7.24	7.75	7.6	7.96	7.90	7.6	7.9
Major route of detoxification	Renal (33%)	Renal (30%)	Hepatic	Hepatic	Hepatic	Hepatic	Hepatic	Hepatic
Plasma protein binding (%)	5	20	ND	45	35	44	80	73
Volume of distribution (L/kg)	0.7	0.7	1.05	0.8	1.0	1.5	1.4–6.7	1.1
Hypnotic dose PO (milligrams)	300–500	100–200	50–200	100–200	50–100	100–200	50–100 IV	50–120 IV
Duration of action (h)	>6	>6	3–6	3–4	<3	<3	5–10 min	5–7 min
Plasma half-life (h)	48	24–96	14–42	35–88	21–42	20–28	6–26	1–2
Fatal dose, approximate (grams)‡	2–6	5	3–6	2–5	3–6	3–6	ND	ND
Reported lethal serum levels (milligrams/L)	>100	>80	13–96	13–26	10–169	5–52	10–400	98

Abbreviation: ND = no data.

*This classification scheme is a convention only; it preceded the discovery that the elimination half-lives do not conform to the apparent duration of action.

†Only drugs responsive to alkaline diuresis.

‡In nontolerant individuals.

than 10 times the hypnotic dose has been ingested in a single exposure in an intolerant patient.[18] As with other sedative-hypnotics, the toxic properties of barbiturates may be enhanced in the presence of benzodiazepines or alcohol. Conversely, the depressive effects may be protective in a mixed-stimulant overdose.[19]

DIAGNOSIS

Laboratory evaluation in barbiturate overdose should include determination of glucose levels, blood chemistries, CBC, arterial blood gas (if indicated), toxicology screen, chest radiograph, and an electrocardiogram. Urine drug screens most commonly use the immunoassay methodology, and a false-positive result on the barbiturate screen has been reported with ibuprofen and naproxen.[20] If important, confirm a positive urine screen using a more accurate method, such as gas chromatography–mass spectrometry.

Barbiturate serum levels are useful in establishing the diagnosis of a comatose patient; however, acute treatment decisions should be clinically based. Serum barbiturate levels reported in lethal overdoses vary widely, and measurements are not reliable in predicting clinical course after an overdose because they do not reflect brain barbiturate concentrations and may underestimate the clinical condition of a patient in the setting of polydrug exposure.[21] Barbiturate levels are also invalid in chronic barbiturate abusers who have developed physiologic tolerance and in patients with renal or hepatic disease who have decreased clearance.[18]

TREATMENT

In a barbiturate overdose, the initial priorities are airway management and supportive care. Once pulmonary and cardiovascular function has been stabilized, options for increasing drug clearance are considered.

AIRWAY ASSESSMENT AND INITIAL STABILIZATION

Assess the patient's mental status and airway stability. Intubation with mechanical ventilation in severe sedative-hypnotic overdose is often required. Barbiturate toxicity results in decreased cardiac output and vascular tone, often resulting in profound hypotension. Volume expansion with intravenous crystalloids is the mainstay for circulatory support in the absence of cardiac failure. If fluid resuscitation fails to correct hypotension, administer vasopressors such as dopamine or norepinephrine. Hypothermia between 30°C (86°F) and 36°C (96.8°F) is common and should be monitored via continuous core temperature and treated with rewarming measures.

ACTIVATED CHARCOAL

A single dose of activated charcoal should be given to cooperative, clinically stable patients who present within 1 hour of acute oral overdose.[22] Multidose activated charcoal is beneficial in reducing serum phenobarbital concentrations; however, no significant difference in clinical outcome has ever been demonstrated. Current consensus guidelines are to consider multidose activated charcoal if a patient has ingested a life-threatening amount of phenobarbital.[23] A typical adult regimen for multidose activated charcoal is an initial dose of 50 to 100 grams PO followed by 12.5 to 25 grams PO every 4 hours. Concurrent administration of cathartic agents remains unproven and is discouraged (see chapter 176, General Management of Poisoned Patients). Careful attention to and monitoring of the patient's airway is important to decrease the risk of aspiration or bowel obstruction.

FORCED DIURESIS

Forced diuresis is not recommended because of the risks of sodium and fluid overload and lack of proven efficacy.

URINARY ALKALIZATION

Urinary alkalization (see chapter 176) does enhance the clearance of phenobarbital and primidone (which is metabolized to phenobarbital). The treatment is less effective than multidose activated charcoal in reducing serum levels, does not improve clinical outcomes, and **is not effective for shorter-acting barbiturates.**[24] In barbiturate poisoning, urinary alkalization is not a first-line treatment and has only a minor, if any, role.[25,26]

EXTRACORPOREAL ELIMINATION

Hemodialysis, hemoperfusion, and hemodiafiltration can enhance elimination of phenobarbital but are reserved for patients who are deteriorating despite aggressive supportive care.[26-28] **These modalities are not useful for poisoning from barbiturates other than phenobarbital.** Exchange transfusion has also been reported to be useful in neonatal phenobarbital toxicity.[29]

DISPOSITION AND FOLLOW-UP

Mild to moderate barbiturate intoxication responds well to general supportive care, including a single dose of activated charcoal, if appropriate. Improvement in neurologic status and vital signs over 6 to 8 hours signals eventual patient discharge or transfer. When indicated, obtain mental health assessment. For a long-acting agent such as phenobarbital, serial serum levels should be obtained during the initial 6 hours after an overdose before concluding the patient can be safely discharged or transferred. Evidence of toxicity after 6 hours will require hospital admission, and patients with severe toxicity should go to the intensive care unit. Consult with a medical toxicologist or local poison center to assist in the care of barbiturate-poisoned patients.

SPECIAL CONSIDERATIONS

BARBITURATE WITHDRAWAL SYNDROME

Barbiturates are notorious for their rapid development of tolerance, high liability for physical dependence and abuse, and multiple drug interactions. Abrupt discontinuation of barbiturates in a chronically dependent user will produce minor withdrawal symptoms within 24 hours and major life-threatening symptoms within 2 to 8 days. The severity of the withdrawal reflects the degree of physical dependence and drug half-life. Cessation of short-acting barbiturates results in more severe abstinence symptoms than stopping long-acting barbiturates. Such effects are consistent with the clinical observation that the brain has more time to adapt to gradually declining drug concentrations.

Clinical manifestations of barbiturate withdrawal mimic those described for alcohol withdrawal. *Minor symptoms* include anxiety, restlessness, depression, insomnia, anorexia, nausea, vomiting, muscle twitching, abdominal cramping, and sweating. *Major symptoms* include psychosis, hallucinations, delirium, generalized seizures, hyperthermia, and cardiovascular collapse.

Priorities in the treatment of major withdrawal symptoms are cardiovascular stabilization and seizure control. Seizures may be treated with benzodiazepines but are more effectively treated with barbiturates. Due to the associated mortality, gradual in-hospital detoxification is needed.

NEONATAL WITHDRAWAL

Infants born to mothers physically dependent on barbiturates are at risk for dependence and subsequently withdrawal. Withdrawal may manifest within the first to third days of life.[11] Signs and symptoms include high-pitched crying, vomiting, diarrhea, tremors, and, possibly, seizures. Withdrawal is treated with gradually decreasing doses of phenobarbital.[11]

REFERENCES

The complete reference list is available online at www.TintinalliEM.com.

Benzodiazepines

Dan Quan

INTRODUCTION

Benzodiazepines, to varying degrees, have in common six major pharmacologic effects: sedative, hypnotic, anxiolytic, amnestic, anticonvulsant, and muscle relaxant.[1] Benzodiazepines are commonly used for the short-term treatment of anxiety, insomnia, seizures, and alcohol and sedative-hypnotic withdrawal.[2-5] The long-term benefits of benzodiazepines for psychiatric disorders are controversial.[6,7] Midazolam, a benzodiazepine with a short duration of action, is also used for procedural sedation and general anesthesia (**Table 183-1**).

Isolated benzodiazepine overdose has low mortality, and death is rare.[8] However, increased rates of morbidity do result from mixed overdose, especially in combination with opioids. **Isolated overdose with high-potency short-acting agents, such as alprazolam, temazepam, and triazolam, is associated with higher incidences of intensive care unit admissions, coma, and mechanical ventilation with toxicity compared to other benzodiazepines, such as diazepam.**[9] In the ED, parenteral administration of benzodiazepines may result in significant complications, particularly respiratory depression and hypotension, especially when combined with opioids or other sedatives.

PHARMACOLOGY

Benzodiazepines stimulate the α subunit of the postsynaptic γ-aminobutyric acid ($GABA_A$) receptor in the CNS. Stimulation of this receptor affects the ligand-gated chloride channel on the cell membrane, altering the transmembrane resting potential to below stimulation threshold and rendering the postsynaptic neuron less excitable. Stimulation of this $GABA_A$ receptor leads to inhibitory effects throughout the neuraxis, producing the typical clinical effects of sedation, anxiolysis, anticonvulsant activity, and striated muscle relaxation.

In general, benzodiazepines are well absorbed from the GI tract. The onset of action after oral ingestion is limited more by the rate of absorption from the GI tract than by the relatively rapid passage from the bloodstream into the brain. With the exception of lorazepam and midazolam, IM injection of benzodiazepines results in unpredictable absorption. IV administration of midazolam and lorazepam has an onset of action in 1 to 5 minutes. Diazepam may be administered rectally, and midazolam may be administered intranasally or intrabuccally, with variable rates of absorption by those routes.

Benzodiazepines are relatively lipid-soluble, with some variation among the agents. Increased lipid solubility is associated with more rapid diffusion across the blood–brain barrier. After single doses, the more highly lipophilic benzodiazepines have a shorter onset of action but also a shorter duration of activity. This short duration of activity occurs because of rapid egress of the drug from the brain and bloodstream into inactive tissue storage sites. For this reason, the serum half-life is not a good indicator of the duration of action in an acute ingestion.

Benzodiazepine derivatives undergo hepatic metabolism through different pathways depending on the agent. Hepatic biotransformation occurs through either oxidation or conjugation; both pathways may be used by some derivatives. Oxidation often produces active metabolites that prolong the pharmacologic effects of the parent compounds. Oxidation is more susceptible to impairment by such factors as disease states (chronic liver disease), demographic characteristics (advanced age), and concurrent treatment with drugs that affect metabolism (estrogen, isoniazid, ethanol, ketoconazole, cimetidine, and phenytoin). Conjugation is a rapid process that generally produces inactive metabolites. Examples of agents that undergo conjugation primarily include lorazepam, oxazepam, and temazepam. These agents may be safer in these susceptible groups such as those patients with hepatic dysfunction.

There is conflicting evidence on how benzodiazepines affect fetal development.[10-12] In general, the cohort studies did not find an increase in congenital malformations, but the case-control studies did show a small increase, especially for cleft lip and palate. This difference is ascribed to the higher sensitivity of case-control studies in identifying an association with specific conditions. The effect on fetal outcome of large doses of benzodiazepines taken for suicide attempts by pregnant women is not clear. Retrospective reviews of overdose with four different benzodiazepines, albeit with relatively small numbers, did not find an increased incidence of congenital abnormalities in the offspring.[13-16]

Chronic use of benzodiazepines during pregnancy can result in **withdrawal syndrome** in the infant after birth such as "floppy baby syndrome" (sedation, hypotonia, apnea, cyanosis, hypothermia) and neonatal withdrawal (restlessness, hypertonia, tremors).[17] Nearly all benzodiazepines enter breast milk, and therefore, caution should be exercised in patients taking benzodiazepines.[10,11]

Administration of benzodiazepines in patients with comorbid conditions such as hepatic dysfunction or the elderly may cause significant effects. Those with hepatic dysfunction may have impaired metabolism, causing increased clinical effects. Elderly patients taking benzodiazepines are at increased risk for falls, cognitive impairment, delirium, fractures, and motor vehicle accidents.[12,18]

TABLE 183-1 Benzodiazepines

Generic Name	Time to Peak Effect (hours)[†]	Elimination Half-Life (hours)[‡]	Duration of Action (hours)	Active Metabolite Half-Life (hours)	Oral Dose Equivalents in Milligrams to Diazepam 10 Milligrams
Short Acting					
Alprazolam*	1–2	6–12	4–7	No	0.5
Midazolam*	IV 1–2 min IM 10-15 min PO 0.5–1	3–6	IV 2 IM 4–6 PO 4–6	Yes	5
Oxazepam*	0.3–0.5	5–10	3–6	No	20
Tetrazepam	1–3	15	6–8	No	50–100
Triazolam*	0.25–0.5	2–5	6–7	No	0.25–0.50
Intermediate Acting					
Bromazepam	1–3	10–20	<12	Yes	5–6
Cinolazepam	0.5–2	9	9	No	40
Estazolam*	1	10–24	<12	No	1–2
Flunitrazepam	0.25–0.3	18–24	4–6	Yes (36–200)	1
Loprazolam	0.5–4	6–12	<12	No	1–2
Lorazepam*	IV 5–20 min IM 20–30 min PO 0.5–1	9–16	6–8	No	1
Lormetazepam	0.5–2	10–12	<12	No	1–2
Nimetazepam	0.25–0.5	14–30	<12	No	5
Nitrazepam	0.5–5	16–48	<12	No	10
Premazepam	2	10–13	<12	No	3.75
Temazepam*	1.5	9–12	5–20	No	20
Long Acting					
Chlordiazepoxide*	2	5–30	5–30	Yes (36–200)	25
Clonazepam*	0.3–0.5	20–80	<12	No	0.5
Clorazepate*	1–2	48	8–24	Yes (36–200)	15
Cloxazolam	2–5	65	18–50	No	1–2
Diazepam*	IV 1–5 min PO 15–45 min PR 5–45 min	20–50	IV 0.25–1 PO 12–24 —	Yes (36–200)	10
Flurazepam*	0.5–1	2	12	Yes (50–100)	15–30
Flutoprazepam	0.5–2	60–90	24	Yes	2–3
Halazepam	1–3	—	12–24	Yes (30–100)	20–40
Ketazolam	2.5–3	30–100	12–24	Yes (36–200)	15–30
Medazepam	—	36–150	10–12	Yes (36–200)	10
Nordazepam	2	40–50	12–14	Yes (50–120)	10
Phenazepam	1.5–4	60	12	Yes	1
Pinazepam	1–2	20–25	12–24	Yes (40–100)	20
Prazepam	2–6	40–80	12–24	Yes (36–200)	10–20
Quazepam*	0.5–2	27–41	12–24	Yes (28–80)	20

*Available in the United States.

[†]After oral ingestion, unless otherwise specified.

[‡]Parent compound.

Drug–drug interactions with benzodiazepines occur mainly with drugs that affect the **cytochrome P450 pathway**, specifically CYP3A4 and CYP2C19. For example, drugs such as ketoconazole or cimetidine are CYP3A4 inhibitors and may increase benzodiazepine blood levels, increasing their duration of action and/or clinical effect. Benzodiazepines themselves have not been implicated in affecting cytochrome P450 enzymes and, therefore, are unlikely to interfere with metabolism of other agents.

CLINICAL FEATURES

The clinical presentation of benzodiazepine intoxication is nonspecific and may be highly variable because of the frequent co-ingestion of other agents. Except for additive effects, drug interactions of benzodiazepines with other sedative-hypnotics are unusual.

The predominant manifestations of benzodiazepines are neurologic and are characterized by somnolence, dizziness, slurred speech, confusion, ataxia, incoordination, and general impairment of intellectual function. Prolonged coma is atypical and should prompt suspicion of intoxication with other agents or a non–toxin-related medical condition. In the elderly, infants and children, protein-deficient persons, and those with hepatic disease, the neurologic effects of benzodiazepines may be prolonged or enhanced.

Paradoxical reactions, including excitement, anxiety, aggression, hostile behavior, rage, and delirium, have been reported but are quite uncommon. Paradoxical reactions may occur more with hyperactive children and in psychiatric patients. Benzodiazepines may have a disinhibiting effect, which, in the presence of various extrinsic factors, can lead to such actions as aggressive or hostile behavior. Other effects that have been reported and that have unclear etiologies include headache, nausea, vomiting, chest pain, joint pain, diarrhea, and incontinence.

Benzodiazepines may cause short-term anterograde amnesia; this effect may be desired, especially in procedural sedation.[12] Agents most often associated with anterograde amnesia are lorazepam, midazolam, and triazolam, although this may occur with the other benzodiazepines.

Uncommonly, respiratory depression and hypotension may occur, generally with either parenteral administration or in the presence of co-ingestants. IV administration is more likely to cause serious cardiorespiratory effects with rapid administration of large doses. In addition, the elderly and those with underlying cardiorespiratory disease are more susceptible to adverse effects of IV administration.

Propylene glycol as a diluent in parenteral preparations of diazepam and lorazepam may cause severe metabolic acidosis (lactic acidosis), nephrotoxicity, and hyperosmolar states when infused at doses >1 milligram/kg per day for an extended period of time.[19,20] During such treatment, an osmolar gap >10 is predictive of elevated propylene glycol concentrations.[20] Treatment of propylene toxicity is generally supportive but may require hemodialysis.[21]

Extrapyramidal reactions have been associated with the use of midazolam. Various allergic, hepatotoxic, and hematologic reactions also have been reported, but they are infrequent. In general, benzodiazepines have no long-term organ-system toxicity other than that which can be ascribed to indirect effects from neurologic or cardiorespiratory depression.

DIAGNOSIS

Toxicologic testing in benzodiazepine ingestion is of limited value. Serum benzodiazepine levels do not correlate well with the clinical state, so serum level measurement is not routinely indicated. Qualitative testing with urine drug screens is typically designed to identify major metabolites of most benzodiazepines, such as oxazepam, temazepam, or nordiazepam, and not the parent compound.[22] Depending on the antibody specificity used in the immunoassay, a false-negative test can occur and is commonly seen with midazolam and flunitrazepam. A urine benzodiazepine screen can usually detect a short-acting agent (e.g., lorazepam) up to 3 days and a long-acting agent (e.g., diazepam) up to 30 days after ingestion. Thus, detection of a benzodiazepine agent taken in the recent past may not correctly identify the toxicologic cause of the patient's current condition. False-positive benzodiazepine urine drug screens have been reported with oxaprozin and sertraline, although improved immunoassay techniques have reduced this potential interference.[23,24]

TREATMENT

GENERAL MEASURES

Benzodiazepines often are ingested with other agents, and the history is frequently inaccurate. Therefore, in patients with depressed or altered mental status, other metabolic and toxicologic possibilities should be considered (see chapter 176, General Management of Poisoned Patients). Do not induce emesis in benzodiazepine overdose because mental status depression may develop and increase the risk for pulmonary aspiration. Activated charcoal binds benzodiazepines effectively and may be considered. Gastric lavage, elimination enhancement by forced diuresis, hemodialysis, or hemoperfusion is not effective. Monitor neurologic and respiratory status and provide mechanical ventilation if necessary. Aspiration pneumonitis may be caused by severe respiratory and neurologic depression.

TABLE 183-2 Contraindications to Flumazenil

Overdose of unknown agents
Suspected or known physical dependence on benzodiazepines
Suspected cyclic antidepressant overdose
Co-ingestion of seizure-inducing agents
Known seizure disorder
Suspected increased intracranial pressure

BENZODIAZEPINE ANTAGONIST

Flumazenil is a unique selective antagonist of the central effects of benzodiazepines, although there have been inconclusive claims that it may be effective in reversing the neurologic toxicity from other drugs.[25] Potential clinical applications include the reversal of coma in benzodiazepine overdose and reversal of iatrogenic benzodiazepine-induced sedation during procedural sedation.[22,26] Its use in benzodiazepine toxicity may obviate the need for tracheal intubation and respiratory support.[27]

However, some toxicologists advocate that flumazenil has limited utility in the ED, noting it is useful mainly in reversing the effects of short-acting benzodiazepines administered for diagnostic and therapeutic procedures.[28] Even in such cases, management is usually accomplished safely and easily by allowing the effects of the benzodiazepine to subside without antidotal administration. Although the plasma elimination half-life of flumazenil is approximately 1 hour, its duration of action is variable and depends on the dose of flumazenil and the benzodiazepine administered. **Recurrent benzodiazepine toxicity may result once the effects of flumazenil have worn off.** This is less likely for a benzodiazepine with a short duration of action, such as midazolam. The dose **of flumazenil is 0.2 milligram IV**, which can be repeated every minute, titrated according to response or to a total dose of 3 milligrams.

Several considerations should limit the empiric administration of flumazenil to a poisoned patient (**Table 183-2**). There is a higher incidence of side effects, albeit generally minor, when flumazenil is administered to an unconscious patient presenting to the ED.[27] Of greater importance, generalized seizures have occurred in patients given flumazenil after co-ingestions of benzodiazepines and seizure-inducing agents, particularly cyclic antidepressants.[29] Seizure activity after flumazenil administration also has occurred in patients physically dependent on benzodiazepines and in patients receiving benzodiazepines for control of a seizure disorder. The putative explanation for this convulsive activity is either the reversal of the cerebroprotective and anticonvulsive effects of benzodiazepines or the precipitation of a benzodiazepine withdrawal syndrome.

Flumazenil-precipitated seizures in patients who are chronically taking benzodiazepines should be treated aggressively with another $GABA_A$ receptor agonist because the benzodiazepine site on the receptor is antagonized. **Anticonvulsants such as phenobarbital or propofol are recommended for flumazenil-induced seizures.** Careful monitoring of the patient's respiratory and mental status is necessary during treatment and may require securing the airway.

Another reason to avoid empiric administration of flumazenil in overdose patients is that the history is often unreliable or unavailable. The apparent overdose may be caused instead by an intracranial mass lesion. **Flumazenil is contraindicated in patients with a suspected elevation of intracranial pressure, such as in severe head injury, due to its adverse effect on cerebral hemodynamics.**

DISPOSITION AND FOLLOW-UP

Indications for observation or hospital admission include significant alterations in mental status, respiratory depression, and hypotension. If mental status depression persists or is profound, other agents or conditions must be considered. Although many clinicians use the 6-hour principle for observation of stable patients after ingestion, there is insufficient literature to recommend a specific duration for appropriate ED observation to conclude the patient is safe for discharge or transfer after a benzodiazepine overdose.

BENZODIAZEPINE ABUSE AND WITHDRAWAL

Physiologic addiction to benzodiazepines may occur, particularly with prolonged use and high doses.[30] Benzodiazepines are usually abused by individuals who abuse other psychoactive drugs and use the benzodiazepine to augment the effects of the primary agent or to counter its adverse effects. In addition, those with alcohol addiction may abuse benzodiazepines.

Benzodiazepine withdrawal may occur on abrupt discontinuation and is more likely in patients with prolonged use and high doses. Because of the long biologic half-life of several derivatives, withdrawal manifestations may not occur for several days to more than 1 week after discontinuing the benzodiazepine. Unfortunately, it is often difficult to distinguish between withdrawal and underlying symptoms for which the drugs were prescribed initially.

Reported withdrawal manifestations include anxiety, irritability, insomnia, nausea, vomiting, tremor, sweating, and anorexia. Serious manifestations, including confusion, disorientation, psychosis, and seizures, also have been reported. For patients with an acute organic brain syndrome, a history of possible benzodiazepine withdrawal always should be pursued. Withdrawal reactions may be avoided by gradually tapering the medication, although there is no consensus benzodiazepine tapering method, including the length of time to taper.[31,32] It appears that slow tapering over weeks to months may be preferred. Treatment of acute withdrawal reactions may be accomplished by drug substitution or by reintroduction of a benzodiazepine with subsequent tapering.[33] Benzodiazepine equivalent dosing should be considered if treatment with benzodiazepine substitution is performed. Withdrawal from high-potency benzodiazepines, such as alprazolam, may require higher doses of traditional benzodiazepines (e.g., IV diazepam) to achieve the appropriate clinical response.

REFERENCES

The complete reference list is available online at www.TintinalliEM.com.

Nonbenzodiazepine Sedatives

Michael Levine
Dan Quan

INTRODUCTION

The term *sedative-hypnotic* refers to any drug designed to produce sedation and sleepiness. These drugs can be divided into the benzodiazepines (see chapter 183, Benzodiazepines) and nonbenzodiazepines (**Table 184-1**).

One is most likely to encounter toxicity from these sedative drugs as part of accidental or nonaccidental overdose, as well as after an assault or trauma. Many nonbenzodiazepines were developed and are marketed for the treatment of insomnia.[1] The sedative effect of other agents, including antihistamines (e.g., diphenhydramine, doxylamine), antidepressants (e.g., amitriptyline, trazodone, and mirtazapine), and antipsychotics (e.g., quetiapine), are also used to promote sleep.

Three sedative agents used in the past have been removed from the legal U.S. and Canadian markets: ethchlorvynol, glutethimide, and methaqualone. However, comments on the Internet suggest these drugs might be available to North American customers from locations in Eastern Europe, Africa, Asia, and South America.[2]

TABLE 184-1 Sedative-Hypnotics

Name	Time to Peak Plasma Levels	Oral Bioavailability	Elimination Half-Life
Buspirone	40–90 min	<5%	2–3 h
Carisoprodol	1.5 h	Unknown	2 h
Chloral hydrate	30 min	Unknown	4 min for chloral hydrate and 6–10 h for trichloroethanol
γ-Hydroxybutyrate	30–60 min	25%	0.3–1 h
Melatonin	30–60 min	15%	40–50 min
Meprobamate	3.6 h	Unknown	10 h
Ramelteon	45 min	2%	1–2.6 h
Tasimelteon	0.5–3 h	Unknown	1.3 h
Zaleplon	0.7–1.4 h	30%	0.9–1.2 h
Zolpidem	1–2 h	65%–70%	1.4–4.5 h
Zopiclone	1.5–2 h	75%–80%	5–6 h
Eszopiclone	1–1.5 h	75%–80%	6–7 h

BUSPIRONE

Buspirone is approved by the U.S. Food and Drug Administration for treatment of anxiety disorders.[3] Other off-label uses include treatment of depression and nicotine dependence. Buspirone is a partial agonist at the serotonin-1A receptor and an antagonist of the dopamine-2 receptor. The resultant effect on serotonin and dopamine neurotransmitter levels is complex, depending on the concentration of the drug and specific brain location, but overall effects are primarily suppression of CNS serotoninergic activity and enhancement of dopaminergic and, possibly, noradrenergic activity.

The typical starting dose for buspirone is 5 milligrams PO three times daily, and the maximum recommended total daily dose is 60 milligrams. Following ingestion, absorption is rapid and nearly complete, with significant first-pass metabolism in the liver, primarily via oxidation, resulting in a low bioavailability. Metabolism of buspirone, by cytochrome P3A4, produces several metabolites, including one active metabolite. Primary elimination is renal, with additional substantial fecal elimination.

Common adverse effects with buspirone use include sedation, GI discomfort, vomiting, and dizziness. In therapeutic dosing, buspirone does not appear to cause psychomotor depression and has not been associated with any potential for abuse or withdrawal.[4]

The effects observed with a buspirone overdose would likely be an exaggeration of adverse effects observed during therapeutic dosing. In general, the drug is well tolerated in overdose, and the treatment is largely supportive.[5] Animal toxicity studies indicate the potential for buspirone to provoke seizures, and one human case report noted the occurrence of a generalized tonic-clonic convulsion approximately 36 hours after a buspirone overdose (**Table 184-2**).[6] **Because of its serotoninergic properties, buspirone has been associated with serotonin syndrome.**[7]

CARISOPRODOL AND MEPROBAMATE

Carisoprodol and its primary active metabolite meprobamate have been used since the 1950s. Carisoprodol is marketed as a centrally acting muscle relaxant, whereas meprobamate is marketed as an anxiolytic drug.

The exact mechanism of action of carisoprodol is not known; animal data demonstrate its ability to block interneuronal activity within the spinal cord and descending reticular formation. Other evidence suggests that the primary mechanism of action is simply related to sedation.[8] Carisoprodol may also have direct γ-aminobutyric acid activity, independent of its metabolite meprobamate.[9]

The recommended dose of carisoprodol is 200 to 350 milligrams PO up to four times daily. Following ingestion, carisoprodol is rapidly

TABLE 184-2 Selected Aspects of Nonbenzodiazepine Overdose

Agent	Features Commonly Seen with Overdose	Unique Toxicologic Effects
Buspirone	Sedation	Generalized seizures (rare) Serotonin syndrome (possible)
Carisoprodol	Sedation, coma, cardiovascular collapse, pulmonary edema	Myoclonic jerks
Meprobamate	Sedation, coma, cardiopulmonary depression	Gastric bezoar with prolonged coma
Chloral hydrate	Coma	Cardiac instability, ventricular dysrhythmias, sensitivity to catecholamines, GI distress, hemorrhagic gastritis
γ-Hydroxybutyrate	Amnesia, sedation, seizure, coma, cardiac and respiratory depression	Steep dose–response curve Sudden awakening
Melatonin	Sedation, disorientation	None observed
Ramelteon	Sedation	None observed
Tasimelteon	Unknown	Limited experience, headache (possible)
Zolpidem	Sedation, coma possible	Limited experience, vomiting
Zaleplon	Sedation, incoordination	Limited experience, headache (possible)
Zopiclone and eszopiclone	Sedation	Limited experience, methemoglobinemia and hemolytic anemia (large overdoses)

absorbed, with an onset of action within 30 minutes and a duration of action between 2 and 6 hours. Several formulations are marketed, sometimes combined with aspirin, caffeine, or codeine. Following metabolism in the liver, the carisoprodol metabolites are renally excreted.

The recommended dose of meprobamate is 400 milligrams PO three or four times daily, with a maximum total daily dose of 2400 milligrams. Following ingestion, meprobamate is rapidly absorbed, with a duration of action of 6 to 10 hours. Following metabolism in the liver, the metabolites and 10% to 20% of the unchanged drug are eliminated by the kidneys.

With a carisoprodol overdose, sedation, coma, cardiovascular collapse, and pulmonary edema have been reported. **Myoclonic jerks are commonly observed and appear somewhat unique to carisoprodol; occasional jerking movements of the extremities in a sedated or comatose patient suggest carisoprodol toxicity.** Serotoninergic features of carisoprodol intoxication have been noted, but the mechanism by which these symptoms and signs are produced is not understood.[10] Treatment of carisoprodol overdose and toxicity is supportive.

With meprobamate overdose, sedation, coma, and cardiopulmonary depression are seen, but the myoclonic jerks described above are not. **Ingestion of a large number of meprobamate tablets has been reported to form a gastric bezoar, and prolonged coma has been attributed to such retained drug within the stomach.** If this occurs, endoscopic removal of the mass or multidose activated charcoal would appear useful.

Carisoprodol and meprobamate have significant potential for abuse and dependence.[11] A withdrawal syndrome has been described in which patients can develop tremor, anxiety, insomnia, and anorexia, usually within 12 to 48 hours of abstinence. Visual and auditory hallucinations and seizures have been described during withdrawal, although these later effects are observed less consistently.

CHLORAL HYDRATE

Chloral hydrate was first marketed as a sedative in 1869, making it the oldest sedative hypnotic agent still available. It remained quite popular until the early 1900s, when barbiturates largely supplanted its use. Chloral hydrate is primarily used for procedural sedation in young children because of its relatively wide therapeutic index, the lack of significant respiratory depression, and the ability for oral administration,[12] although it is not without risk.[13]

The hypnotic dose in adults is 500 to 1000 milligrams PO. For children the hypnotic dose is 50 milligrams/kg PO and the sedation dose is 80 to 100 milligrams/kg PO.[12] Following ingestion, chloral hydrate is quickly absorbed and rapidly reduced to trichloroethanol, an active metabolite, via alcohol dehydrogenase. Trichloroethanol is further oxidized to trichloroacetic acid, which is an inactive compound. Renal excretion of chloral hydrate is minimal.

Co-ingested chloral hydrate and ethanol have a synergistic effect. The metabolism of ethanol results in increased amounts of the reduced form of nicotinamide adenine dinucleotide, which, in turn, promotes the conversion of chloral hydrate to trichloroethanol. In addition, because of competition by chloral hydrate for alcohol dehydrogenase, there is decreased metabolism of ethanol. These interactions result in more elevated levels of both trichloroethanol and ethanol than would be seen if either was ingested alone. The resultant profound sedation yields the terms "**knock-out drops**" or "**Mickey Finn**" for this combination.

At therapeutic doses, chloral hydrate results in mental status depression, but airway and respiratory reflexes are not impaired. Paradoxical hyperactivity occurs in 1% to 2% and vomiting is seen in 3% to 10% of children given doses of 50 to 100 milligrams/kg PO.

With an overdose, chloral hydrate can produce coma. **An important feature of chloral hydrate overdose is cardiovascular instability, manifested by decreased cardiac contractility, myocardial electrical instability, and increased sensitivity to catecholamines.**[14] Commonly encountered cardiac dysrhythmias include premature ventricular contractions, ventricular fibrillation, torsade de pointes, and asystole. GI irritation, including nausea, vomiting, and hemorrhagic gastritis, has been observed. A diagnostic clue is the common presence of a pear-like odor.

Treatment of chloral hydrate overdose and toxicity is largely supportive. With coma, endotracheal intubation may be necessary. **IV β-adrenergic blockers should be used to treat ventricular dysrhythmias seen with chloral hydrate overdose.**[15] Torsade de pointes should be managed with IV magnesium sulfate or ventricular overdrive pacing.

Chronic consumption of chloral hydrate can result in dependency and addiction. A withdrawal state, similar to ethanol, has been described.

γ-HYDROXYBUTYRATE

γ-Hydroxybutyrate (GHB) is an endogenous molecule as well as a drug. GHB was originally used as an IV anesthetic, primarily in several European countries. In recent years, it has been marketed as a drug for body builders to improve body mass and reduce fat, as well as for use as a hypnotic, antidepressant, anxiolytic, and cholesterol-lowering drug.[16] GHB has been found in drug-facilitated sexual assaults.[17] Sodium oxybate (the sodium salt of GHB) is currently approved only for use within a highly regulated setting for the treatment of narcolepsy.[18] In some European countries, GHB or sodium oxybate is used as a treatment for alcohol dependence and withdrawal.[19] GHB can be formulated as a clear liquid or in solid form as a capsule, tablet, or white powder. GHB has many vernacular names, including **"liquid ecstasy," "Georgia Home Boy," "G,"** and **"Grievous Bodily Harm."**

Sodium oxybate is categorized a Schedule III drug by the U.S. Food and Drug Administration when used to treat narcolepsy, but GHB used for any purpose is considered a Schedule I drug. To circumvent laws, GHB precursors, namely γ-butyrolactone and 1,4-butanediol, have been introduced into the drug scene.[20] Following ingestion, lactonase enzymes in the blood convert γ-butyrolactone into GHB. Depending on the level of lactonase enzyme activity, this conversion can be rapid and produce a faster onset of symptoms compared with GHB. The conversion of 1,4-butanediol to GHB is a two-step process: conversion via alcohol dehydrogenase to γ-hydroxybutyraldehyde with subsequent conversion via aldehyde dehydrogenase to GHB.

GHB undergoes metabolism via GHB dehydrogenase to succinic acid semialdehyde, which, in turn, can either get converted to succinic acid, to enter the Krebs cycle, yielding carbon dioxide and water, or be converted to γ-aminobutyric acid, a primary inhibitory neurotransmitter. A small percentage of GHB will be excreted unchanged in the urine.

Following ingestion, GHB is rapidly absorbed from the GI tract, with peak plasma concentration occurring within an hour.[20] GHB has a relatively low oral bioavailability due to significant first-pass metabolism. After absorption, GHB follows a two-compartment model, in which the initial serum levels decline due to redistribution. There is a subsequent slower decline in the serum concentrations following metabolic degradation. Because of its short half-life, GHB is difficult to detect in the urine >6 hours after ingestion and is virtually nondetectable >12 hours after ingestion.[21] GHB has minimal protein binding and readily crosses the blood–brain barrier and placenta.

The body produces some endogenous GHB, both as a precursor and a breakdown product of γ-aminobutyric acid. At physiologic concentrations, GHB binds to a unique receptor, which is distinct from γ-aminobutyric acid receptors. When the concentration of GHB in the brain exceeds the physiologic micromolar concentration, GHB can bind to (and activate) the γ-aminobutyric acid subunit B receptors.

GHB has a steep dose–response curve with a narrow therapeutic ratio; doses of 10 milligrams/kg result in short-term amnesia, doses of 20 to 30 milligrams/kg result in sedation and drowsiness, and doses exceeding 50 milligrams/kg result in seizure, coma, respiratory depression, and cardiac depression.[22] Bradycardia, hypothermia, and either miosis or mydriasis can occur.[20] During recovery, the patients often wake up surprisingly quickly as opposed to the more prolonged awakening phase seen after an overdose with other sedatives. Despite co-ingestants being commonly encountered, most patients fully regain consciousness within 6 hours. The co-ingestion of ethanol can worsen hypoxia and possibly result in a longer elimination half-life of GHB.[23]

Treatment is largely supportive.[20] Intubation is generally unnecessary, even in patients with severely depressed consciousness (Glasgow Coma Scale score ≤8) because patients are usually able to protect their airway and maintain ventilation.[24] Once the patient is awake and alert, assuming no co-ingestants or secondary complications such as aspiration, the patient can be medically discharged or transferred. **Physostigmine or neostigmine is not recommended for reversal of known or suspected GHB intoxication.**[25] Fomepizole (a competitive antagonist of alcohol dehydrogenase) has little benefit in 1,4-butanediol overdoses because preventing metabolism of the ingested drug into GHB is of little benefit due to the short expected duration of symptoms.

Chronic GHB use is associated with a withdrawal syndrome characterized by two often distinct phases.[20,26] The first phase is typified by insomnia, confusion, GI distress, anxiety, and tremor. This first stage can be observed as soon as 2 hours after the last dose in patients who habitually use GHB. The second stage, which can occur in 2 to 3 days after the last dose, is characterized by tachycardia, hypertension, diaphoresis, tremor, confusion, hallucinations, and paranoia. The withdrawal state can last anywhere from 3 days to 2 weeks. The short latency period between the last dose and the onset of symptoms is helpful in distinguishing ethanol withdrawal from GHB withdrawal.

Toxicologic detection of GHB can be difficult because of its short half-life, the complexity of assay methodology, and the presence of the endogenous compound. If needed, toxicologic confirmation should be performed with blood or urine collected as soon as the individual arrives in the ED.[21]

MELATONIN

Melatonin is an endogenous hormone that is normally secreted by the pineal gland and is believed to be involved with the circadian sleep–wake cycle.[27] Melatonin is available without prescription in tablets or capsules at doses ranging from a physiologic dose of 0.3 milligram up to a pharmacologic dose of 10 milligrams.

Two primary melatonin receptor subtypes are found in the human CNS.[27] The MT_1 receptor is located primarily in the hypothalamic suprachiasmatic nucleus and is involved in the effect melatonin has on circadian rhythm. The MT_2 receptor is found primarily in the retina, presumably involved in the interaction between incoming light, melatonin, and the circadian cycle. The MT_2 receptor is also found in the hypophysial pars tuberalis and is possibly responsible for the effects of melatonin on reproduction.

Following ingestion, peak plasma melatonin concentrations occur within 40 to 50 minutes. Melatonin has a short plasma half-life and a short duration of action in therapeutic doses. Melatonin is metabolized by initial conversion to O-desmethylmelatonin and 6-hydroxymelatonin. Both are subsequently conjugated as either a glucuronide or a sulfate and then excreted by the kidneys.

At therapeutic dosing, side effects from melatonin include fatigue, headache, dizziness, and irritability.[28] Data on melatonin overdoses are limited, but overdose would be expected to result in an exaggeration of therapeutic effects, primarily sedation and disorientation without any significant life-threatening effects.[29]

RAMELTEON

Ramelteon is a highly selective agonist at the melatonin MT_1 and MT_2 receptors, marketed for the treatment of insomnia.[30] Ramelteon has no significant activity at the γ-aminobutyric acid, dopamine, serotonin, norepinephrine, or opiate receptor sites. An active metabolite does have weak activity at the serotonin-2B receptor, but is thought to be clinically insignificant.

Ramelteon is rapidly absorbed following oral administration, but oral bioavailability is <2% due to extensive first-pass metabolism. Hepatic metabolism of ramelteon yields four metabolites, one of which is active. Metabolism is primarily through cytochrome P1A2 enzyme, with minor contributions via P2C and P3A4. The coadministration of P1A2 inhibitors such as fluoroquinolones and verapamil has been shown to increase ramelteon concentrations. Protein binding is extensive, the volume of distribution is large, and excretion is primarily renal.

In overdose, sedation would be expected and treatment is supportive.[31] Ramelteon has not been associated with any potential for abuse and has minimal risk for producing withdrawal symptoms or rebound insomnia.[30]

TASIMELTEON

Tasimelteon is an agonist at melatonin MT_1 and MT_2 receptors used for treatment of non–24-hour sleep–wake disorder, a syndrome characterized by insomnia or excessive sleepiness from abnormal synchronization between the 24-hour light–dark cycle and the endogenous circadian rhythms of sleep and wakefulness.[32] The majority of patients with this syndrome are totally blind. Ramelteon and tasimelteon may have benefit in sleep disorders associated with comorbid psychiatric, neurologic, and cardiovascular conditions.[33]

The recommended dose of tasimelteon is 20 milligrams taken on an empty stomach before bedtime, at the same time every night. After ingestion, peak concentrations occur within 0.5 to 3 hours. There is a large volume of distribution, high protein binding, and extensive metabolism with an elimination half-life of 1.3 hours.

There is no reported experience with tasimelteon overdose. Adverse effects reported during clinical trial suggest headache may occur. There has been no observed findings suggestive of abuse potential, physical dependence, or withdrawal during clinical trials.

ZOLPIDEM, ZALEPLON, AND ZOPICLONE

Zolpidem, zaleplon, and zopiclone are three nonbenzodiazepine sedative-hypnotics used to treat insomnia.[1,28] All three promote sleep by enhancing CNS γ-aminobutyric acid activity but differ in their pharmacodynamic and pharmacokinetic profiles.

All three drugs bind to the benzodiazepine binding site on the postsynaptic γ-aminobutyric acid subtype A1 receptor, although they have different binding affinities to the α-1 and α-2 subunits.[34] Zaleplon has a very short half-life (about 1 hour), as opposed to the somewhat longer half-lives of zolpidem and zopiclone (Table 184-1).

All three drugs were initially promoted as an improvement upon benzodiazepines for the treatment of insomnia. They were to be safer, produce less psychomotor impairment with therapeutic doses, and be not addictive and not associated with a withdrawal state. With experience, all three drugs have been found to impair psychomotor function,[35,36] create tolerance and dependence, and be associated with withdrawal states characterized by insomnia, anxiety, agitation, and delirium.[34] **Zaleplon, presumably because of its shorter elimination half-life, appears to produce less tolerance and withdrawal symptoms than zolpidem or zopiclone.**[37]

Zolpidem undergoes hepatic metabolism into three inactive metabolites, so dosage restrictions are recommended for those with hepatic impairment and those with chronic renal insufficiency. Common adverse effects include somnolence and nausea. Because of occasional psychomotor impairment, individuals should not drive or engage in hazardous activity the day following use of zolpidem. There are numerous reports of sleep walking or vivid dreams after its consumption. Following overdose, sedation (including coma) and vomiting can occur. Fatalities usually occur with co-ingestants, rather than with zolpidem by itself.[38]

Zaleplon absorption occurs rapidly (Table 184-1) but can be delayed if zaleplon is co-ingested with a high-fat meal. Following absorption, zaleplon undergoes extensive first-pass metabolism in the form of oxidation via aldehyde oxidase to form inactive metabolites. Elimination is primarily renal, with some fecal elimination as well. In therapeutic doses, zaleplon is not associated with any dependence or withdrawal state when taken for up to 5 weeks.[39] At doses up to 10 milligrams, no psychomotor or memory impairment is observed, but a dose of 20 milligrams is associated with some impairment. Reports of overdose with zaleplon are limited, but one could expect sedation, incoordination, and, possibly, headache to occur.

Zopiclone is not currently available in the United States, but **eszopiclone**, the *S*-configuration and active isomer of zopiclone, is marketed. Zopiclone is rapidly absorbed and hepatically metabolized into active (*N*-oxide metabolite) and inactive (*N*-dimethyl metabolite) compounds. Nearly half of the parent drug is excreted in the lungs following decarboxylation. Reports of zopiclone or eszopiclone overdose indicate sedation to be the primary observed effect.[40] Prolonged coma was reported in an elderly patient who ingested a large amount of eszopiclone.[41] Rare cases of methemoglobinemia and mild hemolytic anemia have been reported after large zopiclone overdoses.[42]

HISTORICAL SEDATIVES

Ethchlorvynol was marketed during the 1950s as an alternative to barbiturates. In 1999, the remaining U.S. manufacturer stopped production and sales of the drug, but availability elsewhere in the world is suggested by mention on Internet sites. Following ingestion, ethchlorvynol is rapidly absorbed from the GI tract with a biphasic distribution process, characterized by an initial phase of adipose tissue deposition followed by a redistribution out of adipose stores and back into the plasma. Ethchlorvynol has a plasma half-life of 10 to 25 hours, undergoes hepatic metabolism, and is renally excreted. At therapeutic dosing, sedation and nystagmus can occur. Overdose can be characterized by prolonged deep coma, hypothermia, hypotension, bradycardia, and cardiovascular collapse. Similar to other severe coma states, bullous lesions have been seen with ethchlorvynol overdose. Abusers have been reported to inject the drug, sometimes producing acute pulmonary edema. Ethchlorvynol overdose may produce a vinyl-like odor that can be a useful diagnostic clue. Treatment is largely supportive, but charcoal hemoperfusion has been used in massive overdoses. Ethchlorvynol is associated with both tolerance and physical dependence, and a withdrawal state has been described.

Glutethimide was withdrawn from the market in 1999 when the remaining U.S. manufacturer stopped production and sales. Availability overseas is suggested by listings on the Internet for sales of this drug. A unique aspect of this drug was that the combination of oral glutethimide with codeine produced a euphoria considered similar to that induced by heroin. A characteristic of glutethimide overdose is the ability to produce a deep coma with periods of cyclic responsiveness. The cause of these cycles has been ascribed to an active metabolite, but evidence is not convincing. Following ingestion, absorption is variable and plasma half-life is 10 to 12 hours. Glutethimide possesses antimuscarinic properties, so toxic patients may have tachycardia, hypertension, mydriasis, urinary retention, and intestinal ileus. Treatment is primarily supportive. Chronic glutethimide abuse is associated with the development of psychosis and seizures.

Methaqualone was withdrawn from the U.S. market in 1984 when the remaining manufacturer stopped production. Continued use and abuse of methaqualone in South Africa is a significant problem, with the drug often mixed with cannabis and smoked. As with the other two sedatives of historical interest, availability in other countries is suggested by Internet sites. A unique feature of a methaqualone overdose is muscular hyperactivity, with hyperreflexia and clonus and a lower rate of respiratory depression and hypotension compared with other sedatives. In severe overdoses, prolonged supportive treatment is often required. Chronic methaqualone abuse can produce both tolerance and habituation, and abstinence can provoke seizures.

Acknowledgment: The authors would like to thank Dr. Raquel M. Schears for her work on the previous edition of this chapter.

REFERENCES

The complete reference list is available online at www.TintinalliEM.com.

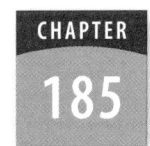

Alcohols

Jennifer P. Cohen
Dan Quan

INTRODUCTION

All alcohols cause clinical inebriation, with the strength of the inebriating effects directly proportional to the alcohol's molecular weight; hence, at the same concentration, isopropanol is more intoxicating than ethanol (**Figure 185-1**).

Primary toxicity can be due to the parent compound (ethanol and isopropanol) or to toxic metabolites (ethylene glycol and methanol). **Ethanol** and **isopropanol** are the most common alcohols ingested; their principal effects are GI irritation and intoxication; and they do not in themselves produce metabolic acidosis. **Methanol** and **ethylene glycol** are toxic alcohols because they cause serious physiologic morbidity.

ETHANOL

INTRODUCTION

Ethanol (CH_3CH_2OH, molecular weight 46.07) is a colorless, volatile liquid that is the most frequently used and abused drug in the world. Morbidity from acute ethanol intoxication is usually related to secondary injuries rather than direct toxic effects. Toxicity most commonly occurs from ingestion, but ethanol may also be absorbed via inhalation or percutaneous exposure.

Ethanol is readily available in many different forms. A standard alcoholic beverage, such as 12 oz (355 mL) of beer (2% to 6% ethanol by volume), 5 oz (148 mL) of wine (10% to 20% ethanol by volume), or 1.5 oz (44 mL) of 80-proof spirits (40% ethanol by volume), contains about 15 grams of ethanol. Ethanol may be found in high concentrations in many other common household products such as mouthwash (may contain up to 75% ethanol by volume), colognes and perfumes (up to 40% to 60%), and as a diluent or solvent for medications (concentration varies widely between 0.4% and 65%). Such products are often flavored or brightly colored and may be attractive to children.

PATHOPHYSIOLOGY

Ethanol is rapidly absorbed after oral administration, and blood levels peak about 30 to 60 minutes after ingestion. The presence of food in the stomach prolongs absorption and delays the peak blood level. High

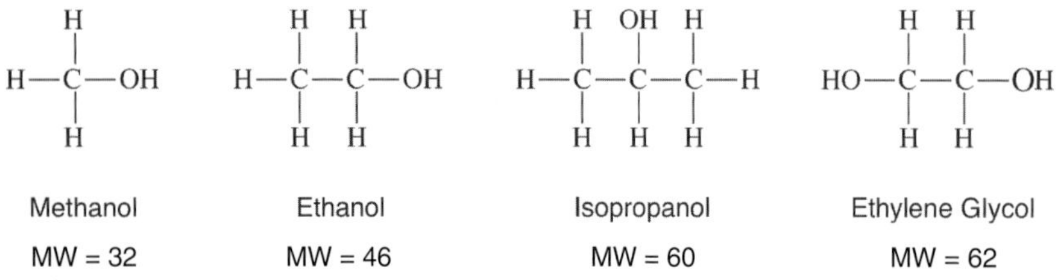

Methanol	Ethanol	Isopropanol	Ethylene Glycol
MW = 32	MW = 46	MW = 60	MW = 62

FIGURE 185-1. Chemical structures of the common alcohols.

concentrations of ethanol in the stomach may cause pylorospasm delaying gastric emptying. Some ethanol is broken down in the stomach by gastric alcohol dehydrogenase, which lowers the amount available for absorption. This enzyme is present at higher levels in men than in women, which may account for the fact that women usually develop a higher blood ethanol level than men after consuming the same dose per kilogram of body weight. The volume of distribution of ethanol is also gender dependent due to difference in body fat percentages: 0.6 L/kg in men and 0.7 L/kg in women.

Ethanol is a CNS depressant[1] that enhances the inhibitory neurotransmitter γ-aminobutyric acid receptors and blockade of excitatory *N*-methyl-D-aspartic acid receptors. Modulation of these systems leads to the development of tolerance, dependence, and a withdrawal syndrome when ethanol intake ceases in dependent individuals.

Because of the phenomenon of tolerance, blood ethanol levels correlate poorly with degree of intoxication. Although death from respiratory depression may occur in nonhabituated individuals at concentrations of 400 to 500 milligrams/dL (87 to 109 mmol/L), some alcoholic individuals can appear minimally intoxicated at blood concentrations as high as 400 milligrams/dL (87 mmol/L).[2] Although Canada, Mexico, and the United States have adopted 80 milligrams/dL (17 mmol/L) as the legal definition of intoxication for the purposes of driving a motor vehicle, impairment may occur with levels as low as 50 milligrams/dL (11 mmol/L), especially in nonhabituated individuals.[3]

Ethanol is predominantly eliminated by hepatic metabolism, with about 10% excreted in the urine, exhaled breath, and sweat. **Alcohol dehydrogenase** (**Figure 185-2A**) is the major enzyme involved in the metabolism of ethanol, producing acetaldehyde. At low ethanol concentrations, this process follows first-order kinetics,[4] but as concentrations rise, alcohol dehydrogenase becomes saturated and metabolism switches to zero-order kinetics—a fixed amount is metabolized per unit of time. Also, as ethanol concentrations rise, the hepatic microsomal oxidizing system (specifically, cytochrome P-450 2E1 [CYP2E1]) plays a more important role in metabolism.

Both alcohol dehydrogenase and CYP2E1 are inducible and thus are more active in chronic ethanol users. Therefore, rates of ethanol elimination from the blood vary from about 20 milligrams/dL per h (4 mmol/L per h) in nonhabituated individuals[5] to up to 30 milligrams/dL per h (6 mmol/L per h) in individuals with chronic alcoholism.

CLINICAL FEATURES

The hallmark of ethanol toxicity is clinical inebriation.[6] Behavioral disinhibition may initially appear as euphoria or agitation and combativeness. As intoxication becomes more severe, slurred speech, nystagmus, ataxia, and decreased motor coordination develop. Severe intoxication may cause respiratory depression and coma. Nausea and vomiting often occur in conjunction with neurologic depression.

Ethanol causes peripheral vasodilation and flushed, warm skin. Vasodilation causes heat loss to the environment promoting hypothermia. Vasodilation may also lead to orthostatic hypotension and reflex tachycardia. Ethanol-induced hypotension is usually mild and transient, so significant or persistent hypotension warrants investigation for alternative causes.

Ethanol ingestion may cause hypoglycemia, usually in children and malnourished individuals due to low glycogen stores and reduced gluconeogenesis. The metabolism of ethanol by alcohol dehydrogenase requires the presence of the oxidized form of nicotinamide adenine dinucleotide (NAD^+), which is then converted into its reduced form (NADH). The metabolism of a significant amount of ethanol increases the NADH/NAD^+ ratio, which then promotes the conversion of pyruvate to lactate, diverting pyruvate away from the gluconeogenesis pathway (**Figure 185-2B**).

When a chronic alcoholic suddenly stops consuming calories in the form of either ethanol or food, the body uses alternative fuel sources and begins to break down adipose tissue. This metabolism of fatty acids results in ketoacidosis (see chapter 226, Alcoholic Ketoacidosis).

DIAGNOSIS

Ethanol-intoxicated patients often have other disease processes, such as infections and traumatic injuries, so perform a detailed physical examination, looking especially for evidence of trauma, and obtain as much history as possible. Uncomplicated ethanol intoxication improves over a few hours. **If depressed mental status fails to improve or deteriorates, consider other causes of altered mental status and evaluate aggressively.**[7,8]

The clinical assessment guides the selection of laboratory tests. For altered levels of consciousness, obtain a point-of-care glucose level. Ethanol levels are not necessarily required in cases of mild or moderate intoxication when no other abnormality is suspected, but measure serum alcohol levels in patients with altered mental status of unclear cause. Clinical judgment of ethanol intoxication is unreliable, and self-reported drinking is also unreliable, particularly around levels of 100 milligrams/dL (22 mmol/L)[9,10] or in alcohol-tolerant patients.[11] In isolated ethanol intoxication, the presence of horizontal gaze nystagmus has a sensitivity of 70% to 80% for a blood ethanol level of 80 milligrams/dL (17 mmol/L) and a sensitivity of 80% to 90% for blood ethanol levels >100 milligrams/dL (22 mmol/L).[12-14]

Ask about concomitant drug use, especially cocaine. The attraction of abusing these drugs together may relate to the formation of the cocaine metabolite cocaethylene that, although less potent than the parent compound, has a half-life that is three to five times longer.[15] The risk of sudden death among users of both drugs simultaneously is higher than that among cocaine users alone.

Ethanol ingestion is the most common cause of an osmolar gap on serum electrolyte analysis (see chapter 17, Fluids and Electrolytes) and

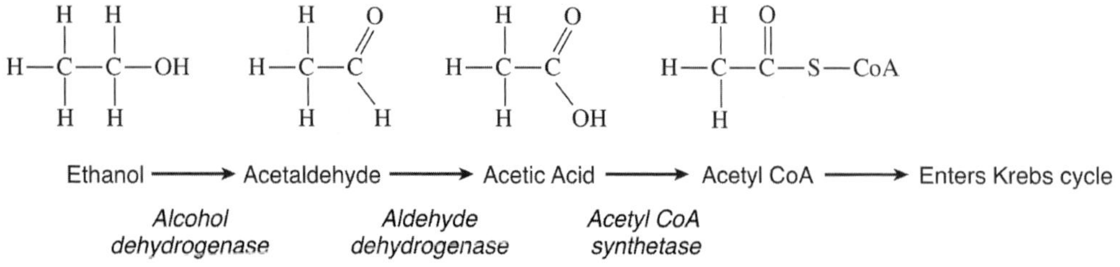

Ethanol → Acetaldehyde → Acetic Acid → Acetyl CoA → Enters Krebs cycle

Alcohol dehydrogenase (Ethanol → Acetaldehyde); *Aldehyde dehydrogenase* (Acetaldehyde → Acetic Acid); *Acetyl CoA synthetase* (Acetic Acid → Acetyl CoA)

FIGURE 185-2A. Metabolism of ethanol. CoA = coenzyme A.

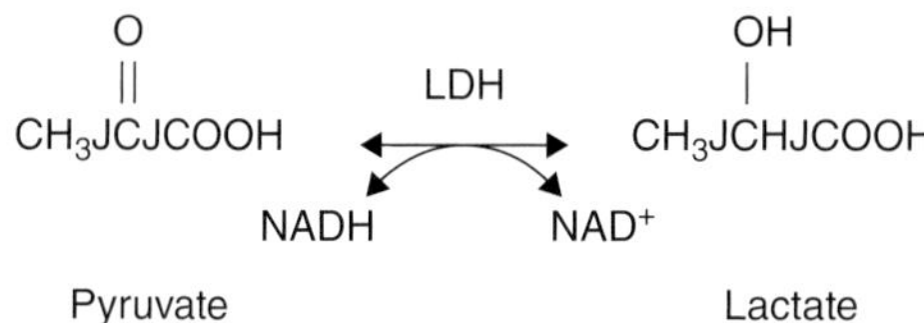

FIGURE 185-2B. Conversion of pyruvate to lactate. LDH = lactate dehydrogenase; NAD^+ = oxidized form of nicotinamide adenine dinucleotide; NADH = reduced form of nicotinamide adenine dinucleotide.

may be associated with a mild metabolic acidosis,[16] but a significant anion gap metabolic acidosis suggests the presence of lactic acidosis, ketoacidosis, or methanol or ethylene glycol toxicity.

TREATMENT

Management is observation until sobriety.[6] Activated charcoal is not useful since ethanol is rapidly absorbed; consider activated charcoal only if toxic adsorbable substances have been coingested.

Treat hypoglycemia with IV glucose 0.5 to 1 grams/kg. Although acute **Wernicke's encephalopathy** can be precipitated by prolonged sustained administration of IV carbohydrate, there is no evidence that a single dose of IV glucose can cause this syndrome.[17,18] The prevalence of vitamin deficiencies in acutely intoxicated ED patients is low and does not justify the routine use of IV vitamin-containing fluids.[19] However, long-term drinkers are sometimes treated with IV fluids containing magnesium, folate, thiamine, and multivitamins, termed a ***banana bag*** because of the yellow color imparted by the multivitamin mixture. Wernicke's encephalopathy is characterized by abnormal mental status, ataxia, and nystagmus, and requires daily treatment with thiamine, 100 milligrams, until normal diet is resumed. **Fluid administration does not hasten alcohol elimination**, so establishment of IV access for fluid administration alone is unnecessary in uncomplicated mild to moderate intoxication.[20,21]

Metadoxine, which is not currently available in the United States but is available in Latin America, Mexico, Asia, Africa, and Eastern Europe, enhances the metabolism of ethanol and accelerates recovery.[6,22] Metadoxine is an ion pair between pyrrolidone carboxylate and pyridoxine. A dose of 900 milligrams IV is reported to double the rate at which ethanol blood levels decrease with time compared with the patient's own metabolism.[23,24]

DISPOSITION AND FOLLOW-UP

Patients with acute ethanol intoxication as the only clinical problem require ED observation until sober. Prior to discharge, reassess for an underlying mental health disorder, such as suicidal or homicidal ideation, that requires further care or hospital admission. Clinical judgment, rather than a serum ethanol level, determines the appropriateness of discharge. Discharge the patient in the care of a responsible companion. Patients treated for alcohol intoxication should not be responsible for their own transportation home.

ISOPROPANOL

INTRODUCTION

Isopropanol (CH_3CHOCH_3, molecular weight 60.10), also known as ***isopropyl alcohol*** and ***2-propanol***, is a colorless, volatile liquid with a bitter, burning taste and an aromatic odor. It is found in many common, inexpensive household products, such as **rubbing alcohol** (usually 70% isopropanol). Isopropanol is widely used in industry as a solvent and disinfectant and is a component of a variety of skin and hair products, jewelry cleaners, detergents, paint thinners, and deicers.

Poisoning usually results from ingestion[25] but may also occur after inhalation or dermal exposure in poorly ventilated areas or during alcohol sponge bathing. **Isopropanol is approximately twice as potent as ethanol in causing CNS depression, and its duration of action is two to four times that of ethanol.** As a result, it is often used as a substitute intoxicant by alcoholics as well as in suicide attempts.

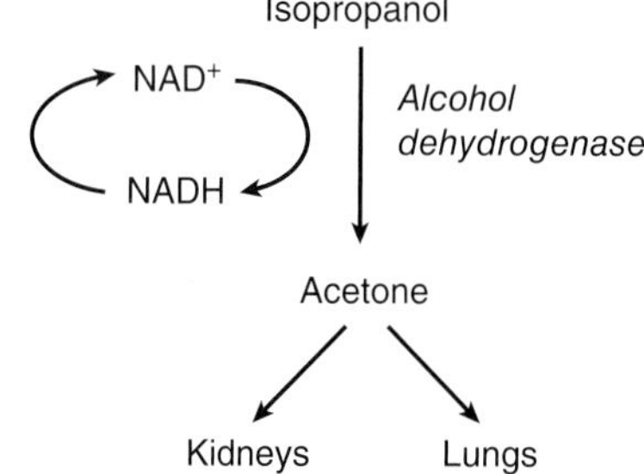

FIGURE 185-3. Metabolism of isopropanol. NAD^+ = oxidized form of nicotinamide adenine dinucleotide; NADH = reduced form of nicotinamide adenine dinucleotide.

PATHOPHYSIOLOGY

Isopropanol is rapidly absorbed from the GI tract. Its peak blood levels occur 30 to 120 minutes after ingestion, and its volume of distribution is similar to that of ethanol. The major pathway for the metabolism of isopropanol is in the liver by alcohol dehydrogenase (50% to 80%), with the remainder excreted unchanged in the urine. Isopropanol is metabolized to a ketone, not an acid (**Figure 185-3**).

Ketosis and an osmolar gap without acidosis are the hallmarks of isopropanol toxicity.[25,26] The principal metabolite, acetone, does not cause eye, kidney, cardiac, or metabolic toxicity, although high levels of acetone may contribute to CNS depression. Acetone is excreted primarily by the kidneys, with some excretion through the lungs. It takes about 30 to 60 minutes after isopropanol ingestion for acetone to appear in the serum and about 3 hours for it to be detectable in the urine.[27]

Isopropanol metabolism most closely follows concentration-dependent (first-order) kinetics. The elimination half-life of isopropanol in the absence of ethanol is 6 to 7 hours, whereas the elimination half-life of acetone is 17 to 27 hours.[28] The long half-life of acetone may contribute to the prolonged mental status depression often associated with isopropanol poisoning. The toxic dose of 70% isopropanol is approximately 1 mL/kg, although as little as 0.5 mL/kg may cause symptoms. The minimum lethal dose for an adult has been reported as approximately 2 to 4 mL/kg, but survival has been reported following ingestions of up to 1 L. **Children are especially susceptible to toxic effects and may develop symptoms after as little as three swallows of 70% isopropanol.**[29]

CLINICAL FEATURES

The primary clinical toxicities of isopropanol are CNS depression caused by both the parent compound and acetone, and gastric irritation from isopropanol itself.[25,26] Onset of symptoms occurs within 30 to 60 minutes after ingestion, with peak effects in a few hours and duration of symptoms for many hours longer, possibly due to the contribution of acetone. As with the metabolism of any alcohol by alcohol dehydrogenase, the increased NADH/NAD^+ ratio may produce hypoglycemia.

Gastric irritation appears early and is a striking feature of isopropanol ingestions. GI symptoms range from nausea, vomiting, abdominal pain, and acute pancreatitis to hemorrhagic gastritis and upper GI bleeding. Severe poisoning is marked by early onset of coma, respiratory depression, and hypotension; rhabdomyolysis and renal failure have also been reported.

Massive ingestion may cause hypotension secondary to peripheral vasodilation. In infants and small children, if isopropanol is used to clean the skin, chemical burns can result and systemic symptoms can occur from dermal absorption.

DIAGNOSIS

Obtain point-of-care glucose testing and other testing as directed by the history and physical examination. Assess for upper and lower GI bleeding. Suspect isopropanol poisoning if the fruity odor of acetone or the smell of rubbing alcohol is present on the breath. Other signs are elevated osmolar gap, ketonuria, and ketonemia without acidosis. An increased anion gap or metabolic acidosis is not due to isopropanol intoxication, so if either is present, investigate for another cause.

A spurious increase in serum creatinine level as a result of acetone's interference with the colorimetric creatinine assay is sometimes seen.[30,31]

Serum isopropanol and acetone levels may be assessed, although isopropanol levels may not be readily available from hospital laboratories. Isopropanol levels of 50 milligrams/dL (8 mmol/L) are often associated with intoxication in individuals who are not habituated to ethanol, but alcoholic patients may be considerably more resistant to the CNS effects of isopropanol.

TREATMENT

Treatment is supportive. Do not administer activated charcoal or perform gastric lavage unless indicated by coingestion of an additional toxic substance. **Do not administer fomepizole or ethanol**, because the metabolite (acetone) is no more toxic than isopropanol itself, and preventing isopropanol metabolism may prolong CNS toxicity.

Monitor for respiratory depression, and intubate and ventilate as needed. Hypotension usually responds to IV fluids. Obtain blood for type and cross-match if needed to treat GI bleeding.

Consider hemodialysis if hypotension is refractory to conventional therapy or when the isopropanol level is >400 milligrams/dL (>66 mmol/L).[25] However, there is no consensus regarding the need for hemodialysis even in life-threatening situations.[31] Hemodialysis eliminates both isopropanol and acetone.

DISPOSITION AND FOLLOW-UP

Patients with lethargy or prolonged CNS depression should be admitted to the hospital. Those who remain asymptomatic for 4 to 6 hours after ingestion may be discharged with referral for substance abuse counseling or mental health evaluation as indicated.

METHANOL AND ETHYLENE GLYCOL

INTRODUCTION

Methanol and **ethylene glycol** are similar in that the parent compounds possess minor toxicity (both causing inebriation and some direct gastric irritation) but the major toxicity occurs when the liver metabolizes these compounds to substances that cause metabolic acidosis and end-organ damage.[25,32-34] Treatment is primarily directed toward halting the formation of these toxic metabolites. **Table 185-1** provides a summary comparison of methanol and ethylene glycol metabolism, clinical features, and treatment.

Methanol Methanol, the simplest alcohol (CH_3OH, molecular weight 32.05), is a colorless, volatile liquid with a distinctive "alcohol" odor. Methanol is used in the synthesis of other chemicals and may be found in automotive windshield cleaning solution, solid fuel for stoves and chafing dishes, model airplane fuel, carburetor cleaner, gas line antifreeze, photocopying fluid, and solvents. Trivial amounts are found in fruits and vegetables, aspartame-containing products, and fermented spirits.

Most cases of methanol poisoning occur by ingestion, and most contemporary exposures in the United States occur from unintentional ingestion of windshield washer fluid and other automotive cleaning products.[35,36] Worldwide, there are outbreaks of poisoning from contaminated alcoholic beverages.[37,38] Persons who wish to consume ethanol but have no access to it for financial or other reasons may consume methanol as an alternative, either intentionally or unintentionally (due to improper or confusing labeling containing the word *alcohol*). Methanol may be systemically absorbed after inhalation or dermal exposure, but this rarely causes significant clinical toxicity. **Hence, extensive evaluation or observation is not required after minor skin or inhalational exposures.**

Ethylene Glycol Ethylene glycol [$CH_2CH_2(OH)_2$, molecular weight 62.07] is a colorless, odorless, sweet-tasting liquid. It was considered

TABLE 185-1 Features of Methanol and Ethylene Glycol Toxicity and Treatment

	Methanol	Ethylene Glycol
Sources	Windshield cleaners; gas line antifreeze, solvents, solid fuel for stoves, adulterated alcoholic beverages, moonshine	Glycerin substitute, hydraulic fluid, antifreeze, adulterated alcoholic beverages, adulterated toothpaste (diethylene glycol)
Absorption	30–60 min	1–4 h
Metabolism (untreated)	Decreases 8.5 milligrams/dL per h (2.7 mmol/L per h)	Elimination half-life ≈ 3–8 h
Minimum lethal dose	1 gram/kg or about 100 mL in an adult	1.1 to 1.7 grams/kg or about 100 mL in an adult
Metabolism	Methanol → formaldehyde → formic acid	Ethylene glycol → glycoaldehyde → glycolic acid → glyoxylic acid → oxalic acid
Toxic effects	Formic acid blocks oxidative phosphorylation; metabolic acidosis from formic and lactic acids	Metabolic acidosis and tissue toxicity from glycolic acid and calcium oxalate tissue damage
Clinical features	Inebriation from parent compound, then 12–14 h later: metabolic acidosis; blurred or snow field vision; nausea, vomiting, abdominal pain	Inebriation from parent compound, then 4–12 h: CNS effects, hypocalcemia, metabolic acidosis; 12–24 h: multisystem organ failure; 24–72 h: renal failure
Diagnosis	Methanol level >20 milligrams/dL (>6 mmol/L) Early: unexplained osmolal gap >10 mOsm/kg H_2O Later: elevated anion gap metabolic acidosis	Ethylene glycol level >20 milligrams/dL (>3.2 mmol/L) Early: unexplained osmolal gap >10 mOsm/kg H_2O Later: elevated anion gap metabolic acidosis and calcium oxalate crystals in urine
Treatment	Fomepizole 15 milligrams/kg IV over 30 min and then 10 milligrams/kg IV over 30 min every 12 h OR Ethanol 10 mL/kg of 10% IV ethanol @ 100 milligrams/kg per h to keep ethanol level >150 milligrams/dL Folic acid 1 milligram/kg IV every 4–6 h (up to 50 milligrams per dose), continue until toxicity resolved IV sodium bicarbonate to maintain serum pH >7.30 See text for indications for hemodialysis	Fomepizole 15 milligrams/kg IV over 30 min and then 10 milligrams/kg IV over 30 min every 12 h OR Ethanol 10 mL/kg of 10% IV ethanol @ 100 milligrams/kg per h to keep ethanol level >150 milligrams/dL Pyridoxine 50–100 milligrams IV every 6 h for 24–48 h Thiamine 100 milligrams IV every 6 h for 24–48 h Magnesium sulfate 2 grams IV (once) IV sodium bicarbonate to maintain serum pH >7.20 See text for indications for hemodialysis

nontoxic in the early 1900s until the first case of toxicity was reported in 1930.[39] Ethylene glycol has many contemporary uses as a glycerin substitute, preservative, component of hydraulic brake fluid, foam stabilizer, component for chemical synthesis, and most commonly an automotive coolant (antifreeze).

Virtually all ethylene glycol toxicity results from ingestion, because the chemical has a low vapor pressure and does not penetrate skin well.[40] Its sweet taste renders ethylene glycol an attractive ingestant for children and pets. Other common exposure scenarios include ingestion as an ethanol substitute when ethanol is unavailable, and intentional suicidal ingestions.[36]

PATHOPHYSIOLOGY

Methanol After ingestion, methanol is rapidly absorbed, with peak blood levels achieved within 30 to 60 minutes, although there has been a case report of delayed peak at 8 hours after a large ingestion.[41] Methanol is rapidly distributed among body water with a volume of distribution of 0.6 to 0.77 L/kg. Without treatment, the minimum lethal dose in humans is thought to be approximately 1 gram/kg or 1.25 mL/kg. With treatment, survival has been reported after much larger ingestions. **The dose required to cause permanent visual impairment in an adult is estimated to be about a mouthful (24 grams or 30 mL).**

Methanol is metabolized in the liver by alcohol dehydrogenase to formaldehyde, and then by aldehyde dehydrogenase to formic acid (**Figure 185-4**). First-order kinetics is present at very low methanol concentrations, with an elimination half-life of 1.8 to 3.0 hours.[42] At higher methanol concentrations, metabolism switches to zero-order kinetics, and blood methanol level decreases at a fixed rate, roughly 8.5 milligrams/dL per h (2.7 mmol/L per h).[43] Very small amounts of the unchanged parent compound may also be exhaled in vapor form.

Formic acid is the metabolite responsible for the toxicity and metabolic acidosis that occurs with methanol poisoning. Acidosis correlates well with formic acid levels both in its magnitude and in the timing of its development. Formic acid's main mechanism of toxicity is its binding to cytochrome oxidase and blockade of oxidative phosphorylation. This leads to anaerobic metabolism and development of lactic acidosis.[20] In addition, metabolism of methanol increases the NADH/NAD$^+$ ratio, which favors the conversion of pyruvate to lactate and thereby worsens lactic acidosis. Early in the course of methanol poisoning, more of the acidosis is due to formic acid itself, whereas later on, as cellular aerobic respiration is blocked and more lactate builds up, the contribution of lactate becomes more significant.[44]

Formic acid's inhibition of cytochrome oxidase increases with decreasing pH, so acidemia worsens the blockade of aerobic metabolism. Falling pH also favors the undissociated form of formic acid (as opposed to formate ion), which moves more readily across tissue barriers. Therefore, at lower pH, more formic acid can enter the brain and ocular tissues, worsening CNS depression as well as retinal and optic nerve injury. Lower pH may also prolong formic acid elimination by increasing tubular reabsorption.[45]

Ethylene Glycol Ethylene glycol is rapidly absorbed from the GI tract, and blood levels generally peak 1 to 4 hours after ingestion. Ethylene glycol distributes rapidly with a volume of distribution of 0.5 to 0.8 L/kg. Based on animal studies and a limited number of case reports, the minimum lethal dose in humans is estimated to be 1.0 to 1.5 mL/kg or 1.1 to 1.7 grams/kg (approximately 100 mL in an adult).[39]

Like methanol, ethylene glycol itself has minor toxicity (it is a stronger inebriant than both methanol and ethanol and causes gastric irritation), and it is the hepatic oxidation of ethylene glycol that creates the toxic metabolites responsible for metabolic acidosis and end-organ damage. The liver metabolizes about 80% of an ingested dose, whereas the other 20% is excreted unchanged in the urine. When metabolism is unblocked, ethylene glycol has first-order metabolic kinetics with an elimination half-life of roughly 3 to 8 hours.

Like the other alcohols, ethylene glycol is metabolized sequentially by alcohol dehydrogenase to glycoaldehyde, followed by metabolism with aldehyde dehydrogenase to glycolic acid (**Figure 185-5**). The subsequent conversion of glycolic acid to glyoxylic acid is the rate-limiting step for the elimination of ethylene glycol. Glycolic acid is the toxic metabolite, and its buildup is responsible for most of the metabolic acidosis. Once glycolic acid is converted to glyoxylic acid, it can be metabolized by one of several pathways. The major pathway is the conversion of glyoxylic acid to oxalic acid. Oxalic acid can complex with calcium, which leads to hypocalcemia and precipitation of calcium oxalate crystals in tissues and urine.[46] **End-organ damage from ethylene glycol poisoning is thought to be due to direct cytotoxicity of glycolic acid (although the exact mechanism of this is unclear) and tissue damage from precipitation of calcium oxalate crystals.**[46,47]

CLINICAL FEATURES

Methanol **Methanol poisoning is characterized by CNS depression, metabolic acidosis, and visual changes.**[25] However, multiple other organ systems are also affected.[25] Coma, seizure, and severe metabolic acidosis on presentation predict a poor outcome in methanol poisoning.[48,49] Severity of poisoning correlates more with the level of acidosis than with the methanol level.

Because methanol itself is not toxic, but requires metabolism to formic acid before tissue damage occurs, clinical signs and symptoms may be significantly delayed after exposure, often by 12 to 24 hours. Because ethanol competes for alcohol dehydrogenase, formation of the toxic

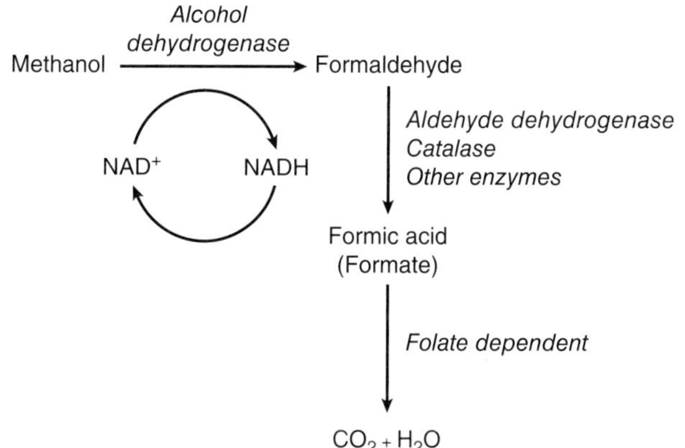

FIGURE 185-4. Metabolism of methanol. NAD$^+$ = oxidized form of nicotinamide adenine dinucleotide; NADH = reduced form of nicotinamide adenine dinucleotide.

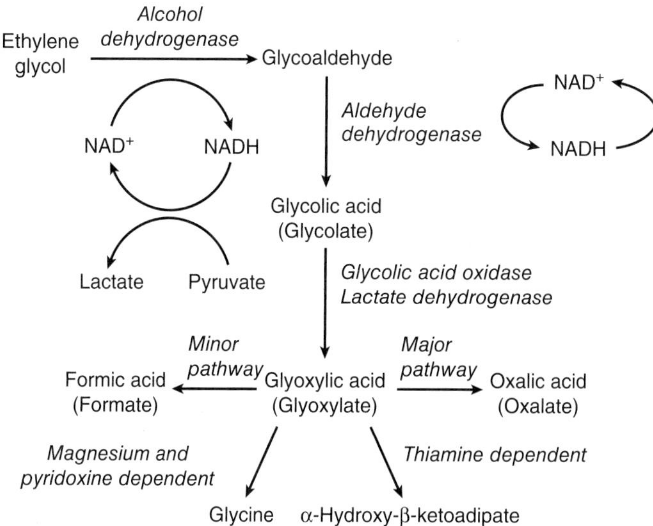

FIGURE 185-5. Metabolism of ethylene glycol. NAD$^+$ = oxidized form of nicotinamide adenine dinucleotide; NADH = reduced form of nicotinamide adenine dinucleotide.

metabolites from methanol will be delayed if ethanol has also been ingested.

Methanol is only a mild inebriant, and patients with tolerance to ethanol also demonstrate tolerance to methanol's intoxicating effects. Neurologic symptoms seen with methanol toxicity include headache, vertigo, dizziness, and seizures. Retinal and optic nerve tissue seem to be especially sensitive to the toxic effects of formic acid. **Ocular toxicity may present as photophobia or blurred or "snow field" vision**, with clinical findings including papilledema, nystagmus (rare), and nonreactive mydriasis once permanent damage has occurred.[50]

Head CT may demonstrate bilateral putamen necrosis, subcortical white matter damage, and other patterns of brain injury from methanol poisoning.[51,52] Intracranial hemorrhages may occur in rare cases, so obtain a noncontrast head CT first when considering heparin for hemodialysis or for other reasons.[53] **Delayed parkinsonism and polyneuropathies can occur.**[54]

Cardiovascular toxicity includes tachycardia and hypotension, which may progress to shock. Initially, patients often demonstrate tachypnea and shortness of breath while attempting to compensate for the metabolic acidosis, but over time, this may progress to respiratory failure.

Methanol is irritating to the GI tract and may cause abdominal pain, anorexia, nausea, vomiting, pancreatitis or gastritis. Transaminitis is usually mild and transient.[44] Rhabdomyolysis, renal failure, coma, and shock can occur in severe cases.[55]

Ethylene Glycol **Ethylene glycol poisoning is characterized by CNS depression, metabolic acidosis, and renal failure.**[25,56] However, multiple other organ systems may be affected.[25,56] Clinical poisoning has historically been divided into three stages, although timing may vary and stages may overlap.

The first or "neurologic" stage typically begins 30 minutes to 12 hours after ingestion due to the intoxicating effects of the ethylene glycol parent compound, and may range from mild depression to seizure and coma. Patients with tolerance to the depressant effects of ethanol may also exhibit relative tolerance to the inebriating effects of ethylene glycol. Patients are often described as appearing intoxicated (with ataxia, confusion, and slurred speech) but without an ethanol odor on the breath. Ethylene glycol is directly irritating to the GI tract, so abdominal pain, nausea, and vomiting may be present.

The generation of toxic metabolites generally takes 4 to 12 hours, or more if ethanol was coingested. CNS tissue effects of glycolic acid and calcium oxalate crystals include cerebral edema, basal ganglia hemorrhagic infarction, and meningoencephalitis.[57] Hypocalcemia, which occurs when calcium combines with oxalate, may contribute to seizures. Metabolic acidosis appears as toxic metabolites are generated.

The second or "cardiopulmonary" stage begins 12 to 24 hours after ingestion and is characterized by tachycardia and possibly hypertension. Tachypnea compensates for metabolic acidosis. Glycolate and oxalate crystal deposition in tissues leads to multiorgan system failure, including heart failure, acute lung injury, and myositis. Hypocalcemia, if present during any stage, may cause prolongation of the QT interval, myocardial depression, and arrhythmias. Most deaths occur during this stage.

The third or "renal" stage is often delayed 24 to 72 hours after ingestion and is characterized by renal failure due to calcium oxalate crystal deposition in the proximal tubules, the most common major complication of serious ethylene glycol poisoning. Short-term hemodialysis is often required, and it may take weeks to months for the kidneys to recover. Delayed neuropathies may occur 5 to 20 days after ethylene glycol poisoning.[54,58,59]

DIAGNOSIS OF METHANOL OR ETHYLENE GLYCOL POISONING

Laboratory tests for a patient with suspected methanol or ethylene glycol poisoning should include blood ethanol levels, arterial blood gas analysis, chemistry panel, calculation of anion and osmolar gaps, serum osmolarity, and creatine kinase level. Serum ketone, β-hydroxybutyrate (if available), and lactate levels are helpful if a metabolic acidosis or an osmolar gap is present. Falsely elevated lactate results have been seen with some point-of-care analyzers in patients with severe ethylene glycol poisoning.[60,61] Check point-of-care glucose level. Measure serum acetaminophen and salicylate levels in patients with an intentional overdose. **Consider methanol or ethylene glycol poisoning in a patient with an unexplained acidosis** (see chapter 15, Acid-Base Disorders).

Acidosis will not be present immediately after exposure. The parent compounds must be converted to toxic metabolites before the acidosis develops; this may be delayed by hours to over a day, especially if ethanol is coingested.

Methanol and Ethylene Glycol Levels **The best laboratory test for diagnosing methanol or ethylene glycol poisoning is measurement of the specific serum level of the alcohol.**[34]

Asymptomatic individuals following methanol ingestion usually have levels of <20 milligrams/dL (<6 mmol/L), and CNS symptoms may appear as levels rise above that. Ocular problems are associated with methanol levels of >50 milligrams/dL (>16 mmol/L), and the risk of fatality rises with levels >150 to 200 milligrams/dL (>47 to 62 mmol/L). However, toxicity associated with a given level depends greatly on how long after ingestion the level was measured. A level of 50 milligrams/dL (16 mmol/L) obtained 3 hours after ingestion implies a much smaller ingestion and less toxicity than if the same value was obtained 12 hours after ingestion.[62]

Asymptomatic individuals following ethylene glycol ingestion usually have peak levels <20 milligrams/dL (<3.2 mmol/L). As with methanol, toxicity associated with a given level depends greatly on how long after ingestion the level was measured. More useful are factors indicating metabolic dysfunction such as acidosis.

Osmolar Gap In many hospital and clinical laboratories, methanol and ethylene glycol levels are not available in a timely manner to assist with initial medical decision making. In such circumstances, the **osmolar gap** may be used as a surrogate marker for toxic alcohol levels (**Table 185-2**).[63] This calculation determines the difference between the measured serum osmoles and the calculated osmoles. Methanol and ethylene glycol, but not their metabolites, are osmotically active and will contribute to the measured serum osmolarity.

For accurate calculation of the osmolar gap, obtain blood samples for a basic serum chemistry panel (including blood urea nitrogen, glucose, and sodium levels), measurement of ethanol level, and measurement of serum osmolarity simultaneously. **Using a previously obtained specimen to measure serum osmolarity ("add-on" tests) is not acceptable, because any toxic alcohols present may have volatilized since the sample was obtained.** In addition, the freezing point depression method must be used to measure serum osmolarity, rather than the vapor pressure method, which can miss volatile substances such as toxic alcohols. There is considerable variation in baseline osmolar gap in healthy subjects depending on the formula used for calculation,[64] so the range of "normal" values is −14 to +10 mOsm/kg H_2O, and ranges may differ among clinical laboratories. In general, an osmolar gap of more than 10 to 15 mOsm/kg H_2O raises concern for toxicity. An osmolar gap of >50 mOsm/kg H_2O is highly suggestive of either methanol or ethylene glycol poisoning and is associated with increased mortality.[65]

The osmolar gap is highest when the parent toxic alcohol level is at its peak (roughly 30 to 60 minutes after ingestion), before significant metabolism has occurred (**Figure 185-6**). As the time since ingestion increases and the parent compound is metabolized, the osmolar gap will

TABLE 185-2 Substances That Contribute to the Osmolar Gap

Substance	Molecular Weight	mOsm/kg H_2O with a Serum Concentration of 100 milligrams/dL	Conversion Factor
Ethanol	46	22	4.6
Isopropanol	60	17	6.0
Methanol	32	31	3.2
Ethylene glycol	62	16	6.2

Notes: Calculated serum osmolarity = 2 × sodium + (blood urea nitrogen/2.8) + (glucose/18) + (ethanol/4.6) + (isopropanol/6.0) + (methanol/3.2) + (ethylene glycol/6.2)

Osmolar gap = measured serum osmolarity − calculated serum osmolarity

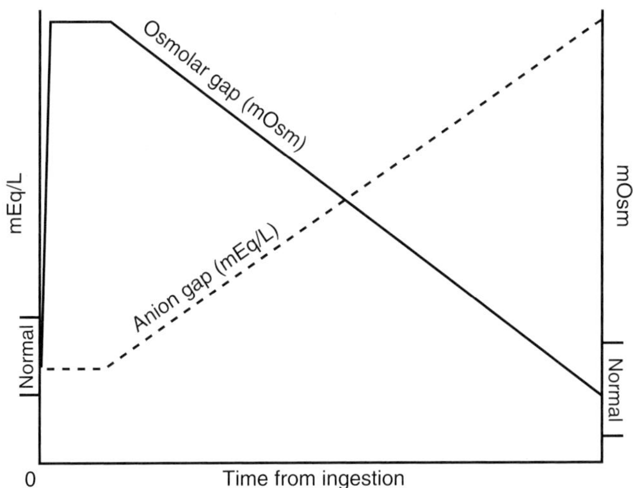

FIGURE 185-6. Relative changes in anion and osmolar gaps over time from ingestion of a toxic alcohol.

decrease. Hence, later-presenting patients may not have significant osmolar gaps. As metabolism occurs, acid metabolites build up and an anion gap metabolic acidosis develops as the osmolar gap narrows. There may be a time period in the middle range when the patient has both an osmolar gap and an anion gap.[66]

Although the osmolar gap may be helpful in conjunction with the rest of the clinical picture, it has many shortcomings and cannot be relied on to definitively diagnose or exclude a toxic alcohol poisoning.[63,67,68] Other conditions such as ketoacidosis, shock, and sepsis may cause an elevated osmolar gap.[69] Also, forgetting to account for ethanol is a common error when calculating the osmolar gap.

As noted, the range of normal variation in osmolar gap is wide and dependent on the formula used for calculation, so a toxic concentration of methanol or ethylene glycol may be present with an osmolar gap in the normal range.[67-69] For example, 1 milligram/dL (0.3 mmol/L) of methanol will raise serum osmolarity by 0.34 mOsm/kg H_2O.[20] Therefore, a methanol concentration of 50 milligrams/dL (15 mmol/L)—generally accepted to be toxic—will raise serum osmolarity 17 mOsm/kg H_2O. If a given patient's baseline was low to begin with, this methanol concentration would not create an abnormal osmolar gap.

Anion Gap The positively charged cations in the serum are electrically balanced by the negatively charged anions. In the clinical laboratory, not all cations and anions are routinely measured, and the level of measured cations is usually greater than that of measured anions; the difference is termed **unmeasured anions**. The predominant serum cation measured is sodium, which is almost completely balanced by the measured charged chloride and bicarbonate anions; the difference is termed the **anion gap**, consisting mostly of serum proteins, phosphate, sulfate, organic acids, and conjugate bases of ketoacids (see chapter 15, Acid-Base Disorders).

$$\text{Anion gap} = Na^+ - (Cl^- + HCO_3^-)$$

The normal anion gap varies according to the methodology used, and the physician should use the values established by the clinical laboratory. **In most clinical settings, an anion gap >15 mEq/L should be considered abnormal.** As noted, it takes time for the acidotic metabolites to become present, as much as 12 to 16 hours following methanol ingestion, so a normal anion gap does not exclude the diagnosis.

Urinary Fluorescence Urinary fluorescence under an ultraviolet or Wood's lamp has been anecdotally taught to be a helpful sign of ethylene glycol poisoning because most antifreeze products contain sodium fluorescein as an additive to aid in the detection of radiator leaks. Not all ethylene glycol products contain fluorescein; the fluorescence may be short-lived (lasting about 4 hours after ingestion); and the ability of the physician to detect fluorescence is affected by many technical factors.[70] Thus, the absence of urinary fluorescence cannot exclude an ethylene glycol ingestion. In addition, false-positive results occur, because many types of glass or plastic containers fluoresce on their own, and numerous foods, medications, toxins, and endogenous substances may cause urinary fluorescence.[71,72]

Calcium Oxalate Crystals for Ethylene Glycol Approximately half of patients poisoned with ethylene glycol demonstrate either monohydrate or dihydrate calcium oxalate crystals on urinalysis.[73] These are often misread as hippurate crystals. If present, they start to appear 4 to 6 hours after ingestion and may persist for days, especially in patients with renal failure. The monohydrate form is more common, and the dihydrate form is more specific for ethylene glycol poisoning.

TREATMENT

Because toxic alcohols are absorbed so rapidly, gastric decontamination is unlikely to be of benefit, and there is no evidence to support its routine use.[39,44,74] Activated charcoal may be used if there is a coingestant known to adsorb to charcoal.

The basic principles of treatment for both methanol and ethylene glycol poisoning are performing initial resuscitation, providing cardiopulmonary support, correcting acidosis, preventing formation of toxic metabolites, and enhancing the clearance of the parent compound and toxic metabolites.

Correct Acidosis Correcting acidosis may improve the outcome in patients poisoned with methanol because acidosis worsens the toxicity of formate; rapid improvement in visual and other systemic symptoms has been reported with correction of acidosis. In addition, alkalinization may help increase formic acid clearance by decreasing reabsorption in the proximal renal tubules.[45] However, the benefits of alkalinization may be equivocal if the patient is treated with metabolic blockade and hemodialysis. When used in methanol poisoning, give IV sodium bicarbonate infusions to maintain a serum pH of >7.30.[44] There is no evidence that alkalinization is specifically beneficial in ethylene glycol poisoning, but it seems reasonable to use sodium bicarbonate IV if there is a severe metabolic acidosis with pH <7.20.

Metabolic Blockade Because laboratory confirmation may take time and because prompt treatment is important to prevent the formation of toxic metabolites, the decision to block metabolism often must be made before the diagnosis is secure (**Table 185-3**).[75] Start treatment while sorting out the clinical picture to protect the patient from serious toxicity, such as blindness or renal failure. Treatment with either ethanol or fomepizole greatly slows the elimination of methanol and ethylene glycol. Because hepatic oxidation is inhibited, elimination is determined by first-order renal excretion, and the elimination half-life averages 52 hours (range 22 to 87 hours) for methanol (compared to an elimination

TABLE 185-3 Indications for Metabolic Blockade with Fomepizole or Ethanol

1. Elevated plasma levels: methanol >20 milligrams/dL (>6 mmol/L) or ethylene glycol >20 milligrams/dL (>3 mmol/L)
2. If methanol or ethylene glycol level not available:
   A. Documented or suspected significant methanol or ethylene glycol ingestion with ethanol level lower than approximately 100 milligrams/dL (22 mmol/L)*
   B. Coma or altered mental status in patient with unclear history and:
      (1) Unexplained serum osmolar gap of >10 mOsm/L
      or
      (2) Unexplained metabolic acidosis *and* ethanol level of <100 milligrams/dL (<22 mmol/L)*

*If serum ethanol level is >100 milligrams/dL (>22 mmol/L), patient will be protected from the formation of toxic metabolites by coingestion of ethanol, and specific metabolic blockade treatment can be delayed until toxic alcohol level is available. If the ethanol level is likely to fall to <100 milligrams/dL before the toxic alcohol results are back, then initiate metabolic blockade.

half-life without metabolic blockade of 1.8 to 3 hours) and 13 to 20 hours for ethylene glycol (compared to an elimination half-life without metabolic blockade of 3 to 8 hours).[39,45,76,77]

Metabolic Blockade with Fomepizole The initial step in the metabolism of methanol (see **Figure 185-4**) or ethylene glycol (see **Figure 185-5**) is performed by alcohol dehydrogenase. This enzyme is competitively inhibited by either ethanol or **fomepizole** (4-methyl-1H-pyrazole).[76] Both ethanol and fomepizole have a much higher affinity for alcohol dehydrogenase than does methanol or ethylene glycol. Although ethanol was traditionally administered for metabolic blockade in methanol and ethylene glycol poisonings, fomepizole has supplanted ethanol for this purpose in many institutions. The primary advantage of fomepizole is the lack of side effects such as CNS depression, GI irritation, and hypoglycemia caused by ethanol therapy.[78-80] Fomepizole is less susceptible to dosing errors than ethanol.[81] The primary limiting factor to fomepizole use is the increased cost of the drug relative to ethanol, which may reduce availability in resource-poor locations.

Fomepizole is dosed with an initial loading dose of 15 milligrams/kg IV administered over 30 minutes, followed by additional doses of 10 milligrams/kg IV (also infused over 30 minutes) every 12 hours. Fomepizole is continued until the toxic alcohol level is <20 milligrams/dL (methanol <6 mmol/L or ethylene glycol <3 mmol/L) and the metabolic acidosis has resolved. Fomepizole is believed to induce its own metabolism, so it is recommended that the dose be increased to 15 milligrams/kg every 12 hours if treatment lasts >48 hours.[44,82] More frequent dosing (every 4 hours) is required during hemodialysis because fomepizole is removed during this procedure. Fomepizole does not require frequent monitoring of serum levels or dosage adjustments necessary with ethanol treatment.

Adverse effects from fomepizole are rare; mild and transient nausea, headache, dizziness, and injection site irritation are most commonly reported.[76] The safety of fomepizole in pregnancy is unknown, so the risks and benefits to fetus and mother of fomepizole therapy should be weighed against those of the alternative treatments. Reports show good efficacy of fomepizole therapy in children.[83]

Metabolic Blockade with Ethanol If fomepizole is not available or its use is contraindicated (i.e., the patient has a known allergy), ethanol may be used to inhibit toxic alcohol metabolism. Ethanol may be administered PO or IV.[84] Although ethanol may prevent toxic alcohol metabolism at blood levels as low as 30 milligrams/dL (7 mmol/L), the general recommendation is to maintain a target ethanol level of 100 to 150 milligrams/dL (22 to 33 mmol/L).[44] Extremely elevated toxic alcohol levels may reduce the effectiveness of alcohol dehydrogenase inhibition by ethanol, and ethanol levels of >150 milligrams/dL (>33 mmol/L) may be required to effectively block production of the toxic metabolites. Achieving the desired ethanol level may be difficult because individual response to ethanol administration varies considerably depending on baseline ethanol consumption.

The loading dose of IV ethanol is 800 milligrams/kg (10 mL/kg of 10% IV solution). Maintenance dosing varies depending on the patient's baseline ethanol use but generally averages 100 milligrams/kg per h (1.2 mL/kg per h of 10% IV solution) with ranges between 70 and 150 milligrams/kg per h (0.8 to 2 mL/kg per h of 10% IV solution). The oral loading dose (PO or via nasogastric tube) using 80-proof liquor is 1.5 to 2 mL/kg followed by maintenance dosing of 0.2 to 0.5 mL/kg per h. **Do not use oral ethanol preparations IV.** Serum ethanol concentrations should be monitored every 1 to 2 hours. All maintenance doses need to be doubled for patients undergoing hemodialysis.

With severe adult poisoning and when fomepizole therapy may be delayed or transport time to the hospital may be long, administration of three or four 1-oz (30-mL) "shots" of 80-proof liquor should raise blood ethanol concentrations sufficiently to block toxic alcohol metabolism in a 70-kg adult.[20] Maintenance dosages are approximately one to two shots per hour.

Ethanol treatment is continued until the toxic alcohol level is <20 milligrams/dL (methanol <6 mmol/L or ethylene glycol <3 mmol/L) and the metabolic acidosis has resolved. The disadvantage of using ethanol is the induction of a state of inebriation, so patients require close monitoring for neurologic and respiratory depression. Individual metabolic variations make dosing complicated, and frequent serum level monitoring and dosage adjustments are required. Children and malnourished individuals are particularly at risk for the development of hypoglycemia, although with careful monitoring, this complication is rare.[79] Administration of the 10% IV ethanol solution requires central venous access, because it is hyperosmolar and irritating to peripheral veins. Use of less concentrated solutions, such as 5% IV ethanol solutions, may require administration of large fluid volumes.

TABLE 185-4 Indications for Hemodialysis after Methanol or Ethylene Glycol Ingestion

Refractory metabolic acidosis: pH <7.25 with anion gap >30 mEq/L and/or base deficit less than −15
Visual abnormalities*
Renal insufficiency
Deteriorating vital signs despite aggressive supportive care
Electrolyte abnormalities refractory to conventional therapy
Serum methanol or ethylene glycol level of >50 milligrams/dL†

*Applies only to methanol; visual abnormalities may not resolve immediately, so their persistence in the absence of other indications once hemodialysis is started is *not* an indication for continued hemodialysis.

†Although previously considered an indication for hemodialysis, there are reports of patients with levels of ≥50 milligrams/dL (methanol ≥15 mmol/L or ethylene glycol ≥7.5 mmol/L) being successfully treated with fomepizole with or without bicarbonate and no hemodialysis.

Hemodialysis Hemodialysis can rapidly clear the toxic alcohols and metabolites, as well as correct acid-base disorders, thereby shortening the duration of metabolic blockade treatment.[39,44,85-87] Conversely, with fomepizole, patients can receive prolonged treatment with few side effects and without the need for hemodialysis and attendant risks.[88]

Hemodialysis may be required emergently for patients with severe acidosis, visual changes, hemodynamic instability, or renal failure (**Table 185-4**).[39,44,89,90] A serum level of ≥50 milligrams/dL (methanol ≥15 mmol/L or ethylene glycol ≥7.5 mmol/L) is considered an indication for hemodialysis, but this criterion has been questioned because many patients with high methanol or ethylene glycol levels have been effectively treated without hemodialysis.[56,88,91,92] Consider the entire clinical picture, rather than making a decision based only on a serum level. Some rebound in toxic alcohol levels may occur after hemodialysis is stopped, so it is recommended that metabolic blockade therapy be continued for several hours after cessation of dialysis, with blood level rechecked to ensure that the toxic alcohol level remains low.[39,44]

Vitamin Therapy Adjunctive treatment with B vitamins (including folate) is recommended to help clear the toxic metabolites of methanol and ethylene glycol more quickly, although no solid evidence exists to indicate that this treatment is necessary or even helpful.[93]

In methanol poisoning, high doses of folate or folinic acid may facilitate breakdown of formic acid into carbon dioxide and water (see **Figure 185-4**). Experimental animals with very large folate stores do not develop acidosis and toxicity from methanol poisoning unless they are artificially depleted of folate. Theoretically, increasing folate stores should hasten the detoxification of formate and prevent it from accumulating and causing end-organ damage. Folinic acid, the activated form of folic acid, is preferred, but folic acid may be used if the former is not available. Recommended dosing is 1 milligram/kg (up to 50 milligrams) IV every 4 to 6 hours.[44]

In ethylene glycol poisoning, adjunctive therapy with pyridoxine, thiamine, and magnesium may be used to facilitate metabolism of glyoxylate to nontoxic glycine and α-hydroxy-β-ketoadipoic acid (see **Figure 185-5**). Magnesium can be given as a one-time dose of magnesium sulfate 2 grams IV. The two B vitamins are given in large doses: thiamine, 100 milligrams IV, and pyridoxine, 50 to 100 milligrams IV, both every 6 hours for 2 days.[94]

Visual impairment can be a permanent complication of methanol poisoning.[95,96] Although treatment with fomepizole or ethanol and bicarbonate can prevent ocular toxicity, there is no other proven therapy to prevent or restore established visual damage.[95]

DISPOSITION AND FOLLOW-UP

Because of the complex management decisions required with methanol or ethylene glycol poisoning, consultation with a medical toxicologist or a regional poison control center is strongly recommended. Symptoms of methanol or ethylene glycol intoxication may be delayed, particularly if ethanol has been coingested. A patient with suspected ethylene glycol ingestion should be observed and monitored for 6 hours. If no ethanol is present, the patient remains completely asymptomatic, there is no osmolar gap, and no metabolic acidosis develops, the patient can be discharged. Methanol toxicity may be delayed longer, so a patient with suspected methanol ingestion should be observed for 12 hours using the same criteria. A patient with significant signs and symptoms should be admitted to an intensive care setting. Patients seen at facilities unable to provide hemodialysis or intensive care should be transferred as soon as possible, if in sufficiently stable condition, to institutions capable of providing such care. Suicidal patients should receive a psychiatric evaluation when their condition improves and prior to discharge.

REFERENCES

The complete reference list is available online at www.TintinalliEM.com.

CHAPTER 186 Opioids

Guillermo Burillo-Putze
Oscar Miro

INTRODUCTION

Opioids refers broadly to all compounds related to opium that possess analgesic and sedative properties. **Opiate** describes the opioid alkaloids found naturally in the opium poppy plant, *Papaver somniferum*. The term **narcotic** refers to a broader group of agents, predominantly used by law enforcement to designate a variety of controlled substances with abuse or addictive potential; use of this term in medical practice is discouraged.

Opioid abuse is a significant public health issue in the United States with a dramatic increase in prescription opioid use and abuse in the past 10 years.[1,2] Opioids most frequently involved in reported toxic drug exposures were, in order of number of cases recorded, tramadol, oxycodone, methadone, morphine, buprenorphine, and hydrocodone.[3] Deaths were primarily associated with exposure to methadone, oxycodone, and morphine. The majority of prescription opioid overdose deaths were associated with diversion, doctor shopping, and nonmedical use.

PHARMACOLOGY

Opioids modulate nociception in the terminals of afferent nerves in the CNS, peripheral nervous system, and GI tract. Opioids are agonists at the three primary opioid receptors: μ (mu), κ (kappa), and δ (delta). Opioid receptors are similar to other G protein–coupled receptors; they are transmembrane proteins that undergo conformational change when activated by external molecules, and this change then alters some aspect of intracellular function. Opioid receptors vary widely in morphology and distribution. Also, the specificity and affinity of an opioid for a particular receptor are variable. For example, tramadol possesses 1/6000 the affinity of morphine at the μ-receptor site.

Stimulation of the μ-receptors results in analgesia, sedation, miosis, respiratory depression, cough suppression, euphoria, and decreased GI motility. Stimulation of κ-receptors results in weaker analgesia, sedation, miosis, decreased intestinal motility, dysphoria, and hallucinations. Stimulation of the δ-receptors results in some analgesia and antidepressant effect. **All currently available opioid agonists possess μ-receptor activity and result in some degree of respiratory depression.**

There is interplay between opioid receptors and other transmembrane receptors found in the nervous system. One example is that opioid binding to μ-receptors in the nucleus accumbens results in the localized release of dopamine (the "dopamine pleasure pathway"). A second example is that the analgesic effect of morphine is enhanced in the presence of *N*-methyl-D-aspartate receptor blockers such as amantadine. A third example is the induction of mast cell histamine release by morphine and meperidine.

Opioids can be categorized as naturally occurring compounds (termed *opiates*), chemical modifications of natural compounds (semisynthetic), and completely artificial compounds (synthetic) (**Table 186-1**). Some opioids are agonists at all opioid receptors (e.g., morphine and hydromorphone), whereas others are partial agonists–antagonists (e.g., pentazocine, butorphanol, and nalbuphine) at the opioid receptors.

PHARMACOKINETICS

Opioids are readily absorbed, achieving peak blood levels 30 to 60 minutes after ingestion of standard oral formulations. Sustained-release forms take longer after ingestion to achieve peak blood levels; for example, morphine sulfate controlled-release tablets take about 90 minutes to reach peak blood levels compared with 30 minutes for standard morphine tablets. After GI absorption, most opioids undergo first-pass hepatic metabolism, so bioavailability can vary from as low as 10% to as high as 80% after PO administration. Thus, at equal doses, most opioids are more potent given parenterally than PO. The opioids with good oral bioavailability are codeine, oxycodone, methadone, hydromorphone, and tapentadol.

The metabolism of codeine, meperidine, methadone, morphine, oxycodone, and propoxyphene is mostly hepatic and subject to drug interactions and genetic variations. For example, antiretroviral medications can enhance the metabolism of methadone, which results in lower plasma methadone concentrations. As another example, codeine is metabolized to morphine via cytochrome P-450 isoenzyme 2D6, an enzyme with genotypic and phenotypic variability. Patients with rapid cytochrome P-450 enzyme 2D6 metabolism produce more morphine after a fixed dose of codeine.[4] These interactions and genetic variations may influence the therapeutic effect of opioids (see chapter 35, "Acute Pain Management").

In drug misuse, unconventional routes of administration (insufflating or injecting ground opioid tablets, heating fentanyl patches or applying more than one patch to the skin) may alter the drug's pharmacokinetics and often increase the rate of opioid absorption. Similarly, in cases of opioid overdose resulting in high plasma levels, the pharmacokinetics are altered due to enzymatic saturation. This may increase the severity of poisoning, delay the onset, and prolong the duration of action, as compared with the expected therapeutic actions.[5]

CLINICAL FEATURES

The full opioid intoxication toxidrome includes respiratory and mental status depression, analgesia, miosis, orthostatic hypotension, nausea and vomiting (especially in opioid-naïve patients), histamine release resulting in localized urticaria (Figure 186-1) and bronchospasm, ileus secondary to decreased GI motility, and urinary retention secondary to increased vesical sphincter tone.[6] The depression in mental status can be profound. The respiratory depression is characterized by slow and shallow respirations that can produce hypercarbia, hypoxia, and cyanosis. Miosis is not universally present from intoxication with every opioid; normal or even enlarged pupils have been documented secondary to diphenoxylate, meperidine, morphine, pentazocine, and propoxyphene toxicity. Mydriasis may also signal severe cerebral hypoxia or result from co-ingestants. Other possible findings include pulmonary edema, hypothermia, rhabdomyolysis, compartment syndrome, myoglobinuric renal failure, and seizures associated with overdoses of tramadol, propoxyphene, and meperidine.

Opioid-induced acute lung injury, previously known as *noncardiogenic pulmonary edema*, is an uncommon complication associated with heroin overdose.[6,7] Acute lung injury can occur immediately or be delayed up to 24 hours after heroin overdose and presents with tachypnea, rales, decreased oxygen saturation, and bilateral pulmonary infiltrates with a normal cardiac silhouette on chest radiograph. The incidence of acute

TABLE 186-1 Classification and Characteristics of Major Pharmaceutical Opioids

	Oral Dose Equianalgesic to Morphine 10 milligrams SC (milligrams)	Parenteral Dose Equianalgesic to Morphine 10 milligrams SC (milligrams)	Duration of Analgesic Action* (h)	Elimination Half-Life* (h)
Opiate				
Codeine	200	120	4–6	2.5–4
Morphine	30	10	3–4	2–4
Semisynthetic				
Buprenorphine	4 SL	0.3	6–24	20–44
Hydrocodone	30	Not available	4–6	8
Hydromorphone	7.5	1.5	2–4	2–3
Oxycodone	20	Not available	3–6	3–4
Oxymorphone	6	1.5	4–6	7–11
Synthetic				
Diphenoxylate	2.5	Not available	Not applicable	2 h for diphenoxylate and 12–14 h for difenoxin†
Fentanyl	0.125	0.100	1	3–4
Levorphanol	1	2	1–3	10–11
Meperidine	300	100	1–3	3–4
Methadone	20	10	4–8	12–18
Pentazocine	150	50 SC	3–4	2–4
Propoxyphene	130	Not available	4–6	6–12
Tapentadol	75	Not available	4–6	4–5
Tramadol	100	100	4–6	5–7

*Initial doses in therapeutic amounts.

†Active metabolite.

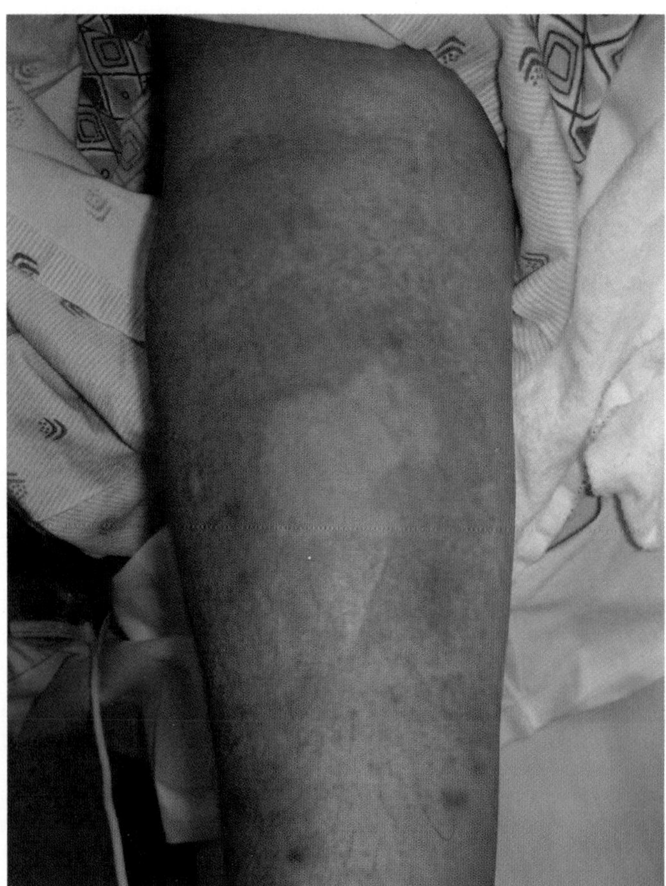

FIGURE 186-1. Urticaria on a forearm from local histamine release due to IV morphine. [Photo used with permission of J. S. Stapczynski, MD.]

lung injury is 10% in patients with severe heroin overdose requiring naloxone.[8] The pathophysiology of heroin-induced acute lung injury is poorly understood, but some degree of direct capillary injury is suspected. Treatment includes oxygen supplementation and ventilatory support, either noninvasive or invasive modalities, and positive end-expiratory pressure. Additional naloxone, diuretics, and digoxin are not indicated.

The combination of meperidine, tramadol, or dextromethorphan with monoamine oxidase inhibitors, selective serotonin reuptake inhibitors, or linezolid can result in **serotonin syndrome** (see chapter 178, Atypical and Serotonergic Antidepressants).[9] Serotonin syndrome is characterized by disorientation, hyperthermia, autonomic instability, hyperreflexia, and muscle rigidity, especially in the lower extremities. Although uncommon, deaths have been reported. Naloxone is not effective in treating opioid-induced serotonin syndrome.[9,10]

DIAGNOSIS

The combination of coma, miosis, and respiratory depression strongly suggests opioid intoxication, and in many clinical scenarios, evidence of opioid use is present. The combination of a respiratory rate of <12 breaths/min, miosis, and circumstantial evidence of opioid use (drug paraphernalia, needle marks, presence of a tourniquet, bystander corroboration) was highly sensitive for opioid overdose.[11]

Listen for auscultatory findings suggestive of pulmonary edema. Undress the patient completely and look for hidden opioids or drug-use paraphernalia, check for fentanyl patches on all parts of the body, including mucous cavities, and palpate muscle groups to detect signs of compartment syndrome.

The differential diagnosis of opioid intoxication includes toxicologic exposure to agents that produce similar findings, such as clonidine, organophosphates and carbamates, phenothiazines and atypical antipsychotic medications, sedative-hypnotic medications, and carbon monoxide. Clonidine overdoses are characterized by coma, bradycardia, hypotension, miosis, and periods of apnea that respond to tactile or auditory stimulation. Organophosphate and carbamate overdoses cause the cholinergic toxidrome: miosis, muscle fasciculations, profuse vomiting and diarrhea, and sweating. Phenothiazines, olanzapine, and risperidone cause neurologic depression and miosis from decreased adrenergic tone.[12] γ-Hydroxybutyrate intoxication is associated with profound CNS depression, bradypnea, and, occasionally, miosis. Sedative-hypnotic agents and carbon monoxide cause profound neurologic depression but are not usually associated with miosis. Hypoglycemia, hypoxia, CNS infections, postictal states, and pontine and intracranial hemorrhages should also be considered in the differential diagnosis.

OPIOID SCREENS

A qualitative urine opioid screen may aid in the diagnosis, but available tests have limitations. The assay in most commercially available urine opioid screens recognizes morphine.[13] Therefore, morphine and those opioids that are metabolized to morphine, such as codeine and heroin, are readily detected. However, the semisynthetic opioids hydrocodone and oxycodone are usually not detected by urine opioid screens, and essentially all synthetic opioids also are not routinely detected. A specific urine assay is required to detect oxycodone or methadone.

Urine opioid screens can have false-positive results.[13] Depending on the threshold level, ingestion of poppy seeds contained in baked goods can lead to a false-positive test result. Rifampin, rifampicin, quinine, diphenhydramine, and fluoroquinolones have been reported to cause false-positive urine opioid screen results, presumably by interfering with the immunoassay technique. An opioid analogue, dextromethorphan, can produce a positive result on the urine opioid screen. Prescription drugs reported to cause a false-positive result with the methadone urine drug screen include chlorpromazine, clomipramine, diphenhydramine, doxylamine, ibuprofen, quetiapine, thioridazine, and verapamil.

A urine opioid screen can be positive up to 2 to 3 days after a single use of codeine, morphine, or heroin. The methadone-specific screen can be positive up to 3 days after ingestion. Thus, detection of an opioid agent taken in the recent past may not correctly identify the toxicologic cause of the patient's current condition. Plasma acetaminophen concentration should be obtained in all suicidal ingestions and all cases of combination opioid-acetaminophen overdoses.

TREATMENT

Airway protection and ventilatory maintenance are the most important treatment steps for opioid intoxications, because respiratory depression is the major morbidity and the cause of essentially all the mortality.[6] Use bag-valve mask ventilatory support as needed to initially maintain adequate oxygenation and ventilation. After adequate ventilation is ensured, administer naloxone (**Table 186-2**). In fully awake patients or after the airway is protected with an endotracheal tube in unresponsive patients, administer single-dose activated charcoal, 1 gram/kg PO, if an opioid ingestion occurred within the hour. Endotracheal intubation is a therapeutic option in some cases of opioid overdose with severe respiratory depression unresponsive or poorly responsive to naloxone or in cases in which acute lung injury is suspected.[6] Intubation offers the advantages of protection of the airway, easy access for suctioning, provision of an alternate route of administration for some medications, and total airway control. Rapid-sequence intubation, omitting anesthetic-sedative agents, is the preferred technique.

Under special circumstances, delayed and multiple doses of activated charcoal may be useful, as in diphenoxylate hydrochloride–atropine sulfate overdoses and in cases of large ingestions of sustained-release preparations.[14]

TABLE 186-2 Opioid Antagonists

Drug	Route	Initial Dose*	Onset of Action	Duration of Action†
Naloxone	IV	0.1–0.4 milligrams if breathing spontaneously	1–2 min	20–90 min
		2 milligrams if apneic		
	IM or SC	2 milligrams	5–6 min	
	Intranasal	2 milligrams (1 milligram in each nostril)	6–8 min	
	Nebulized	2 milligrams in 3 mL normal saline	5 min	
Nalmefene	IV	0.1–0.5 milligrams if breathing spontaneously	2–5 min	Up to 4 h
		2 milligrams if apneic	2–5 min	8 h
	IM or SC	1 milligram	5–15 min	4–6 h
Naltrexone	PO	50 milligrams	30–60 min	24 h
		100 milligrams	30–60 min	48 h
		150 milligrams	30–60 min	72 h

*See text regarding subsequent dosing.

†Duration dependent on amount of opioid agonist present.

NALOXONE

Naloxone, a derivative of oxymorphone, is a pure competitive antagonist at all opioid receptors, with particular affinity for μ-receptors. Naloxone therefore fully reverses all the effects of opioids, including respiratory depression, CNS depression, miosis, and analgesia. Naloxone also antagonizes opioid-induced seizures, except those induced by meperidine, propoxyphene, or tramadol. The elimination half-life of naloxone is 60 to 90 minutes, but the duration of action is as short as 20 minutes if a large amount of opioid agonist is present.

Naloxone has poor oral bioavailability but is well absorbed when given by injection (IV, SC, or IM), inhaled, or deposited on mucosa (intratracheally or intranasally, but not sublingual). Inhaled naloxone by nebulization is reasonably effective in reversing depressed mental status and respirations in opioid toxicity, with about 10% requiring additional rescue parenteral naloxone.[15-17] Intranasally administered naloxone provides a pharmacokinetic profile similar to that of IM or SC naloxone and is used by EMS personnel and in bystander naloxone administration programs.[18-20]

Naloxone effectiveness is dependent on the dose administered and the amount of opioid that needs to be reversed. A small starting dose of naloxone, 0.1 milligram IV, is recommended in opioid-dependent patients who present with mental status depression but with minimal respiratory depression, because larger doses can induce opioid withdrawal symptoms in opioid-dependent patients. An initial dose of naloxone, 0.4 milligram IV, is recommended in non–opioid-dependent patients who present with mental status depression but with minimal respiratory depression. Subsequent doses of naloxone of 0.1 to 0.4 milligram IV are administered until the desired effect is reached. Incremental dosing of naloxone mitigates the precipitation of acute opioid withdrawal.[21]

An initial dose of naloxone, 2 milligrams IV, should be administered to patients presenting with apnea or near-apnea and cyanosis, regardless of drug use history. Repeated doses of 2 milligrams IV every 3 minutes are recommended until a maximum of 10 milligrams IV is reached or respiratory depression is reversed. Exposures to synthetic opioids, such as propoxyphene, fentanyl, pentazocine, or dextromethorphan, and to sustained-release preparations may require these larger-than-ordinary doses. Toxicity from leaking opioid-containing packets in the intestinal tract (i.e., in "body packers") can be extremely severe, and such patients require large and sustained naloxone doses until the drug-containing packets are expelled or removed.

The duration of action of naloxone is often shorter than that of the offending opioid, so naloxone infusions are occasionally required to support respiration over several hours as the opioid is metabolized. This is especially true for certain long-acting opioids, such as buprenorphine, methadone, and propoxyphene; for exposures to sustained-release preparations; and for ingestions of dermal patches. A continuous infusion should be considered only if the patient responded to the initial naloxone bolus and subsequently required repeat administration. **To calculate the naloxone continuous infusion dose, determine the "wake-up dose" and administer two thirds of that dose per hour by IV infusion.** Adjustments may be required if the patient develops respiratory depression (by repeating a bolus and increasing infusion rates) or withdrawal symptoms (by decreasing infusion rates). It is recommended that patients on naloxone infusions be admitted to a monitored unit.

Naloxone has a remarkable safety profile. Although adverse effects are seen in about one third of patients who receive it for a suspected opioid overdose, serious complications are rare.[22] The most common adverse effects associated with naloxone are anxiety, nausea, vomiting, diarrhea, abdominal cramps, piloerection, yawning, and rhinorrhea, related to the precipitation of the opioid withdrawal syndrome. Careful dosing of naloxone can prevent the precipitation of opioid withdrawal symptoms.[21,23]

Naltrexone, an oral opioid antagonist, is primarily used to maintain opioid abstinence after detoxification. Naltrexone may be useful in preventing delayed respiratory depression in opioid-naïve methadone-intoxicated patients in resource-limited locations.[24] The elimination half-life for the two major active metabolites of naltrexone is 10 to 13 hours, but the duration of action is dose-dependent and longer.

Nalmefene, both an oral and parenteral opioid antagonist, has not been available in the United States since August 2008. The elimination half-life is about 11 hours. In the suspected opioid-dependent adult with mental status and respiratory depression, the initial nalmefene dose is 0.1 milligram IV. If no withdrawal occurs, a dose of 0.5 milligram is given, followed by 1 milligram in 2 to 5 minutes if mental status or respirations are still depressed.

DISPOSITION AND FOLLOW-UP

The optimal observation period after an opioid intoxication is determined by the history and clinical picture. Naloxone-responsive injection drug users with presumed heroin intoxication can be safely discharged 1 to 2 hours after administration of naloxone if they have independent mobility, oxygen saturation on room air >92%, respiratory rate >10 breaths/min, pulse rate >50 beats/min, normal temperature, and a Glasgow coma scale score of 15.[25]

In cases of exposure to opioids other than heroin, an observation period of 4 to 6 hours in the ED is recommended after the last naloxone administration. In long-acting opioid overdose, observation should be extended for a minimum of 8 hours.[4] Moderate to severely symptomatic patients usually require hospital admission to monitored settings and may require continued administration of naloxone. A behavioral health evaluation is needed in cases with suicidal intent.

SPECIAL CONSIDERATIONS

BUPRENORPHINE

Buprenorphine is a partial agonist at μ-receptors, with decreased intrinsic activity that causes its clinical effects to plateau at higher dosages.[26] Buprenorphine has high affinity for and slow dissociation from the μ-receptor, which results in a long duration of action. Furthermore, other opioid agonists (such as heroin) or antagonists (such as naloxone) cannot easily displace buprenorphine from the μ-receptor. Buprenorphine has poor oral bioavailability because of extensive first-pass metabolism and is therefore administered SL or parenterally. The most frequently prescribed SL buprenorphine formulation is in combination with naloxone in a 4:1 ratio. Because naloxone has poor bioavailability from PO or SL administration, it was introduced into the preparation to discourage and limit parenteral abuse of the buprenorphine portion while not interfering with therapeutic use in the form of the SL tablet.

Buprenorphine can be associated with three distinct clinical scenarios. First, the opioid-naïve patient who overdoses on buprenorphine will experience mental status depression, nausea, vomiting, miosis, and respiratory depression (usually with a plateau). In this situation, naloxone may not be fully effective in reversing mental status and respiratory depression.[27] **Because of the long duration of action of buprenorphine, readministration of naloxone and naloxone infusions is frequent, and admission to the hospital is necessary in symptomatic patients.** The second possible scenario is buprenorphine exposure in the opioid-dependent patient still under the influence of the opioid agonist. In this case, buprenorphine will precipitate opioid withdrawal symptoms, because the partial agonist buprenorphine behaves like an antagonist in the presence of an agonist. Buprenorphine-induced withdrawal is best managed with symptom-driven therapy, including antiemetics, nonopioid analgesics, antidiarrheals, and nonbenzodiazepine sedatives for insomnia. The third possible clinical scenario is buprenorphine exposure in the opioid-dependent patient undergoing withdrawal, in whom buprenorphine will act as a partial agonist and alleviate the symptoms of opioid withdrawal. This forms the basis for buprenorphine detoxification and maintenance therapy. Thus, **buprenorphine is unique in that it can both induce and treat opioid withdrawal, depending on the timing of its administration.**

METHADONE

Methadone is synthetic opioid used as replacement therapy in opioid-dependence and for chronic pain. The initial analgesic duration is 4 to 8 hours with an elimination half-life of 12 to 18 hours. With repetitive dosing, analgesic action duration and elimination half-life increase to about 22 to 36 hours and up to 59 hours, respectively. The long duration of activity enables once-a-day dosing during chronic therapy. Methadone has a higher risk for overdose-related deaths than other opioids, often with co-ingestants.[28,29]

Methadone has several drug–drug interactions that can precipitate toxicity or withdrawal in patients on chronic therapy.[30] Interactions between methadone and human immunodeficiency virus medications are common and complex, creating potential for both increased toxicity and withdrawal. The relevant interactions for emergency physicians include ciprofloxacin, fluconazole, ketoconazole, and omeprazole, which can increase toxicity. Drug–methadone interactions that have potential to precipitate withdrawal include macrolide (especially clarithromycin), phenobarbital, phenytoin, spironolactone, and verapamil.

Methadone prolongs the QT interval prolongation in acute overdose or during long-term methadone treatment, providing the substrate for cardiac dysrhythmias, such as torsade de pointes.[31] In patients with acute methadone overdose resulting in QT interval prolongation, serum electrolyte imbalances should be corrected and the patient should be admitted to a monitored bed until the condition resolves. Patients on long-term methadone therapy who develop a QT_c interval of >450 milliseconds but <500 milliseconds do not require a dosage adjustment, but electrolyte imbalances should be corrected if present, and patients should be followed on an outpatient basis with frequent ECGs. In patients on long-term methadone therapy who develop a QT_c interval of >500 milliseconds, any electrolyte imbalances should be corrected, methadone dosage reduction or discontinuation should be considered, and other contributing factors should be eliminated.[32]

Acute methadone overdoses present similar to other opioid intoxications, but the duration can be much longer.[33] Naloxone infusions are often required with close neurologic and respiratory monitoring, or oral naltrexone can be used in resource-limited circumstances.[24]

PROPOXYPHENE

Propoxyphene and its metabolite, norpropoxyphene, are cardiotoxic and neurotoxic.[34] Propoxyphene overdoses produce sodium channel blockade, causing QRS interval prolongation, atrioventricular conduction block with bradycardia, prolonged QT interval, and ventricular bigeminy. Seizures have been reported in about 10% of overdoses. Propoxyphene is usually combined with acetaminophen or salicylates, so levels of those drugs should be checked in an overdose.

As in other overdoses that involve sodium channel blockade, propoxyphene-induced QRS interval prolongation should be treated with sodium bicarbonate, 1 mEq/kg IV.[35] Seizures should be treated with benzodiazepine or phenobarbital. Naloxone will not reliably reverse the cardiotoxicity or terminate propoxyphene-induced seizures.[36]

TRAMADOL

Tramadol overdoses are associated with lethargy, nausea, tachycardia, and seizures.[37,38] At doses exceeding 500 milligrams, coma, hypertension, respiratory depression, and apnea are seen.[10,39] Features consistent with serotonin syndrome have been seen in isolated tramadol overdoses.[40] Tramadol-induced seizures are common, and naloxone is ineffective in preventing them. Fortunately, tramadol-induced seizures are usually single and anticonvulsants are not necessary.[41,42] Dependence during chronic therapy and withdrawal symptoms upon discontinuation have been reported with tramadol.[43]

MIXED AGONISTS-ANTAGONISTS

The mixed agonists-antagonists include pentazocine, butorphanol, and nalbuphine. These agents have variable but mostly antagonist activity at the μ-receptor. They may cause significant respiratory depression in overdose, and naloxone will reverse this respiratory depression. Mixed agonists-antagonists usually precipitate withdrawal when taken by an opioid-dependent individual, which reduces their potential for abuse. Pentazocine overdose can cause seizures.[44]

DIPHENOXYLATE HYDROCHLORIDE–ATROPINE SULFATE

Diphenoxylate hydrochloride–atropine sulfate is a frequently prescribed antidiarrheal agent. The medication is formulated as a combination tablet or liquid, containing diphenoxylate, 2.5 milligrams, and atropine, 0.025 milligram, in each tablet or 5 mL of liquid. In an overdose, initially the anticholinergic toxidrome dominates the clinical picture (see chapter 202, "Anticholinergics"). The second phase of intoxication is characterized by the opioid toxidrome. Children <6 years of age can be symptomatic after ingestion of a single tablet. In pediatric patients, absorption can be delayed up to 6 to 12 hours in some cases because of the effect of atropine on GI motility. Current recommendations are that all children <6 years of age be admitted to the hospital and be closely observed for 24 hours after ingestion of a combination tablet of diphenoxylate and atropine. Older children and adults should be observed in the ED for 6 hours. Administration of activated charcoal is recommended unless contraindicated.

MIXED DRUGS AND CONTAMINANTS

Illicitly obtained heroin is often mixed with other compounds, such as cocaine, scopolamine, clenbuterol, and fentanyl, which may contribute to heroin overdose toxicity. Adulterants found in illicit heroin may include strychnine, quinine, lactose, and talc. Scopolamine is an antimuscarinic agent that produces the anticholinergic toxidrome. Clenbuterol is a long-acting β-adrenergic agonist similar to albuterol and is used in veterinary medicine. Heroin-fentanyl mixtures (colloquially called **China-white**) resulted in hundreds of deaths among injection drug users in metropolitan areas of the United States during 2007.[45] A potent neurotoxin, 1-methyl-4-phenyl-1,2,3,-tetrahydropyridine, has been used as a meperidine adulterant, producing parkinsonism in users.[46]

Starting in Russia in 2010, episodes of deaths and gangrene were reported associated with intravenous desomorphine or **"Crokodile,"** a synthetic alternative to heroin crudely made from codeine tablets with a high concentration of tissue-toxic impurities. The colloquial name is derived from the appearance of the skin after it is injected.[47]

KRATOM

Kratom (*Mitragyna speciosa*) has mitragynine as its principal alkaloid, with stimulating effects at low doses (cocaine-like effect) and sedative effects (opioid-like effect) at high doses.[48] Regular kratom use can lead to dependence, craving, and withdrawal symptoms.[49,50] Kratom can produce serious toxicity or even death, often associated with interaction with other drugs, such as nasal decongestants, over-the-counter drugs, and benzodiazepines.[51] Krypton, a combination containing kratom, desmethyltramadol, and caffeine has been associated with fatalities.[52]

TABLE 186-3 Opioid Withdrawal

Onset: Within Hours	Onset: 12 h	Onset: 24–36 h
Peak effects: 36–72 h	Peak effects: 72 h	Peak effects: 72 h
Anxiety	Irritability	Insomnia
Yawning	Tremor	Muscle spasms
Drug craving	Piloerection	Abdominal pain
Lacrimation	Mydriasis	Nausea, vomiting, diarrhea
Rhinorrhea		
Diaphoresis		
Myalgias		

Kratom is available in smoke shops and on the Internet.[53] Kratom preparations are used as self-management of chronic pain, as replacement therapy for opioid analgesics, and for opioid and alcohol withdrawal symptoms.[54]

OPIOID WITHDRAWAL

Downregulation of endogenous endorphins, dynorphins, and opioid receptors occurs with long-term use of opioids. Abrupt cessation of opioid use does not allow time for upregulation of receptors and results in increased neuronal firing and the opioid withdrawal syndrome.

Opioid withdrawal usually starts with feelings of anxiety, yawning, lacrimation, diaphoresis, rhinorrhea, and diffuse myalgias (**Table 186-3**),[55] progressing to piloerection, mydriasis, nausea, profuse vomiting, diarrhea, and abdominal cramping. Opioid withdrawal reactions are very uncomfortable but are not life-threatening and rarely fatal. Vomiting and aspiration of gastric contents can cause pneumonitis and dehydration. Onset of withdrawal is usually within 6 to 12 hours of last heroin use and within 30 hours of last methadone exposure. It can be precipitated by the administration of antagonists such as naloxone or naltrexone or the administration of partial agonists such as buprenorphine. Opioid withdrawal symptoms usually peak on the third day of abstinence and resolve by the fifth or sixth day. Subjective and objective opiate withdrawal scales can be used to monitor the severity of symptoms and signs and guide therapy.[56]

Symptoms of opioid withdrawal can be rendered more tolerable by the administration of the central α_2-agonist clonidine, antiemetics, and antidiarrheal agents.[57] Clonidine may be used at a dose of 5 micrograms/kg PO if the blood pressure is >90 mm Hg systolic. Multidrug regimens are sometimes used in ambulatory detoxification programs to control withdrawal symptoms.[58,59]

The management of opioid-dependent individuals hospitalized for medical or surgical reasons remains controversial. Detoxification from opioids during the course of an acute medical illness is usually unsuccessful, and alleviation of withdrawal symptoms with opioid replacement is generally the goal. Daily administration of a verified dose of methadone PO (or half the verified dose IM if the patient cannot take oral medications) is recommended to inhibit withdrawal symptoms and reduce craving. This applies only to individuals who are enrolled in a methadone treatment program and in whom the dose can be verified. A habitual user who is not receiving methadone maintenance therapy can be given methadone 20 milligrams PO or 10 milligrams IM. These doses should inhibit withdrawal symptoms but not induce euphoria. Buprenorphine, 0.3 to 1.2 milligrams IV or IM every 6 hours, can safely be administered to a medically ill opioid-dependent patient experiencing withdrawal who will be admitted to the hospital.[60] **No methadone or buprenorphine should be administered to an opioid-dependent patient until withdrawal symptoms appear.**

REFERENCES

The complete reference list is available online at www.TintinalliEM.com.

CHAPTER 187

Cocaine and Amphetamines

Jane M. Prosser
Jeanmarie Perrone

INTRODUCTION

Historical records of indigenous cultures in South America describe early stimulant use by chewing leaves of the *Erythroxylum coca* plant, a practice that continues today. Cocaine was first used therapeutically in 1884 for ophthalmologic procedures. Amphetamines were first synthesized in 1887, and in 1932 they were first marketed medicinally in an inhaler form as a bronchodilator. Use of methamphetamine to enhance physical and intellectual performance began in the 1930s. These drugs have limited therapeutic roles but are widely used as drugs of abuse. Clinical effects and toxicity are due to sympathetic nervous system stimulation.

PHARMACOLOGY

COCAINE

Cocaine is the naturally occurring alkaloid found in *E. coca*, a plant indigenous to South America. The water-soluble hydrochloride salt is absorbed across all mucosal surfaces, including oral, nasal, GI, and vaginal epithelium; thus, cocaine can be topically applied, swallowed, or injected IV. The hydrochloride (salt) form is most often insufflated (snorted) or injected IV. The freebase form of cocaine can be prepared in several ways. A common method uses an alkali, such as sodium bicarbonate, to produce "crack cocaine," a freebase form that is stable to pyrolysis that, when smoked, produces the popping sound that characterizes its name. The onset and duration of action vary with the route of administration (**Table 187-1**).

When cocaine is insufflated nasally, the delayed and prolonged effect is a result of vasoconstrictive properties that limit mucosal absorption as well as the swallowing of a portion of the insufflated cocaine, which is then absorbed from the stomach. GI absorption is also delayed by vasoconstriction, producing delayed peak effect.

Cocaine is primarily metabolized to ecgonine methyl ester by plasma cholinesterase. Relative deficiency of this enzyme may predispose affected patients to life-threatening toxicity.[1] Benzoylecgonine is the other major metabolite excreted in the urine and is the target compound detected in routine urine toxicology screens. Cocaethylene is a long-acting metabolite formed when cocaine is used in combination with ethanol. Cocaethylene has vasoconstrictive properties similar to those of cocaine.

Cocaine is both a CNS stimulant and a local anesthetic.[2,3] Central effects are mediated by enhancement of excitatory amino acids and blockade of presynaptic reuptake of norepinephrine, dopamine, and serotonin. The excess of neurotransmitters at postsynaptic receptor sites leads to sympathetic activation, producing the characteristic physical findings of mydriasis, tachycardia, hypertension, and diaphoresis, and predisposing to dysrhythmias, seizures, and hyperthermia. Cocaine use produces a euphoria associated with enhanced alertness and a general sense of well-being. It is thought that the psychological addiction, drug craving, and withdrawal effects are mediated by interference with dopamine and serotonin balance in the CNS. Subsequent dopamine depletion at the nerve terminals may account for the dysphoria and depression associated with long-term abuse.

Like other local anesthetics, cocaine inhibits conduction of nerve impulses by blocking fast sodium channels in the cell membrane. Cocaine also has quinidine-like effects on conduction, causing QRS-complex widening and QT-interval prolongation. Thus, in large doses, cocaine may exert a direct toxic effect on the myocardium, resulting in negative inotropy and wide-complex dysrhythmia.

TABLE 187-1 Pharmacokinetics of Cocaine

Route of Exposure	Onset of Action	Peak Action	Duration of Action
IV	<1 min	3–5 min	30–60 min
Nasal insufflation (snorting)	1–5 min	20–30 min	60–120 min
Inhalation (smoking)	<1 min	3–5 min	30–60 min
GI	30–60 min	60–90 min	Unknown

Source: Reproduced with permission from Hoffman RS, Howland MA, Lewin NA, Nelson LS, Goldfrank LR: *Goldfrank's Toxiciologic Emergencies,* 10th ed, © 2015 by McGraw-Hill, Inc., New York.

TABLE 187-2 Pharmacokinetics of Methamphetamine

Route of Exposure	Onset of Action	Peak Action	Duration of Action
IV	15–30 s	30 min	10–12 h
Nasal insufflation (snorting)	3–5 min	1–2 h	10–12 h
Inhalation (smoking)	10–30 s	5–10 min	8–12 h
GI	15–20 min	2–3 h	10–12 h

AMPHETAMINES

Amphetamines comprise a broad class of structurally similar derivatives of phenylethylamine.[4] The derivative methamphetamine, also known as "ice," is abused by ingestion, IV injection, inhalation, or nasal insufflation. Absorption and peak effects vary with the route (**Table 187-2**). Modification of the basic amphetamine structure produces substances with additional psychoactive properties.[4] Over 50 such "designer" amphetamines have been created (**Table 187-3**), primarily for hallucinogenic effects (see chapter 188, "Hallucinogens"). Methamphetamine and the designer amphetamines may have effects that persist for up to 12 hours or longer.

Synthetic (or substituted) cathinones, often termed "**bath salts**," are designer drugs derived from naturally occurring amphetamine analogs found in the *Catha edulis* plant. Cathinones stimulate the release and block the reuptake of norepinephrine, dopamine, and serotonin at synapses in the brain, producing stimulant effects similar to cocaine and amphetamines.[5-7] Commonly abused substituted cathinones include mephedrone, methylenedioxypyrovalerone, and methylone, although the composition in bath salts sold for use by abusers varies widely. Stimulant medications for attention-deficit disorder, such as methylphenidate and dextroamphetamine, are available in both immediate- and extended-release formulations. Abusers may crush the extended-release tablet to separate the active agent from the extended-release matrix to achieve a rapid onset of action after insufflation or injection.[8]

Amphetamines enhance the release and block the reuptake of catecholamines at the presynaptic terminal and may also directly stimulate catecholamine presynaptic and postsynaptic receptors.[9] Some amphetamine metabolites inhibit monoamine oxidase, increasing cytoplasmic concentrations of norepinephrine. Certain amphetamine derivatives can also induce release of serotonin and affect central serotonin receptors.

TABLE 187-3 Commonly Abused Designer Amphetamines

Abbreviation	Chemical Name
MDMA	3,4-methylenedioxymethamphetamine
MDA	3,4-methylenedioxyamphetamine
MDEA	3,4-methylenedioxyethamphetamine
PMA	Paramethoxyamphetamine
DOB	4-bromo-2,5-dimethoxyamphetamine
2CB	4-bromo-2,5-dimethoxyphenylethylamine
STP or DOM	4-methyl-2,5-dimethoxyamphetamine

These serotonergic effects account for the hallucinogenic properties of some amphetamine derivatives such as MDMA (3,4-methylenedioxymethamphetamine) and mescaline (3,4,5-trimethoxyphenethylamine). Downregulation of dopamine receptor activity with long-term use may contribute to the withdrawal phenomenon. Mortality from amphetamine toxicity is a result of hyperthermia, dysrhythmias, seizures, hypertension (intracranial hemorrhage or infarction), and encephalopathy.

Stimulants such as methylphenidate, ephedrine, pseudoephedrine, and phenylpropanolamine produce toxic syndromes similar to those caused by cocaine and amphetamines.[10-15] Ephedrine is derived from ephedra or ma huang (*Ephedra sinica*) and is an indirect-acting sympathomimetic that was advertised as a "natural" stimulant in health food supplements and promoted for dieting, energy, and maintenance of alertness. Cardiovascular and neurologic toxicity associated with psychosis, severe hypertension, and several deaths prompted the U.S. Food and Drug Administration in 2004 to ban the sale of ephedra in dietary supplements.

CLINICAL FEATURES

The clinical features of cocaine and amphetamine toxicity are the result of their sympathomimetic, vasoconstrictive, psychoactive, and local anesthetic properties affecting a variety of organ systems.[2-4,9]

CARDIOVASCULAR

Cocaine induces dysrhythmias, myocarditis, cardiomyopathy, and acute coronary syndromes.[16] Other vascular complications include aortic rupture and aortic and coronary artery dissection. Even at relatively low doses, cocaine induces vasoconstriction in coronary arteries, contributing to cocaine-induced chest pain.[17] Coronary vasoconstriction is exacerbated by β-adrenergic blockade and antagonized by phentolamine, which suggests mediation through stimulation of α-adrenergic receptors.[18] This effect is further potentiated by cigarette smoking. In addition to promoting vasospasm, cocaine potentiates acute coronary syndrome by increasing atherogenesis through increased platelet aggregation, thrombogenesis, and accelerated atherosclerosis.

The patient most at risk for cocaine-associated acute coronary syndrome is a male between 20 and 40 years old, who is a cigarette smoker and who regularly uses cocaine.[19,20] All routes of cocaine administration are associated with chest pain, acute coronary syndrome, ST-elevation myocardial infarction, and non–ST-elevation myocardial infarction. Atypical chest pain is common.

Acute coronary syndromes and aortic dissection are also reported in association with ephedrine, phenylpropanolamine, and amphetamine use.[21] Mitral and aortic valve abnormalities associated with use of the amphetamine combination phentermine-fenfluramine prompted a voluntary recall of these drugs. Cardiopulmonary toxicity from other amphetamine diet aids has also been reported.

Dysrhythmias induced by cocaine can result from sympathomimetic stimulation, blockade of the sodium channel during depolarization, inhibition of the potassium channel during repolarization, and effects on calcium channel current.[16,22] Sympathomimetic-induced dysrhythmias are tachycardias, such as sinus tachycardia, reentrant supraventricular tachycardia, and atrial fibrillation and flutter. Sodium channel blockade produces a rightward shift of the terminal portion of the QRS complex as seen on the frontal plane ECG leads, a pattern similar to that of cyclic antidepressants.[23] Progressive toxicity may induce a complete right bundle-branch block or a prolonged QRS >120 ms that, when combined with sinus tachycardia, produces a wide-complex tachycardia. Cocaine can induce the ECG appearance of the **Brugada** pattern, although it is not clear whether this is strictly a toxic effect or if the sodium channel–blocking effect of cocaine unmasked an underlying genetic predisposition to the Brugada syndrome.[24]

Potassium channel blockade impairs repolarization, prolonging the QT interval on the ECG.[23] The effects of cocaine on calcium channel current are dose dependent and complex, but at concentrations associated with clinical toxicity, prolongation of both depolarization and repolarization is seen, as well as enhanced dispersion in repolarization.[22] Delayed repolarization and enhanced dispersion promote early afterpotentials that can trigger reentrant dysrhythmias, such as ventricular tachycardia and a variant, torsades de pointes.

Takotsubo syndrome, transient apical ballooning of the left ventricle, has been associated with cocaine use. The physiology is not clearly understood but has been attributed to the effects of a sympathomimetic surge on the myocardium after cocaine use.[25]

CNS

Neurologic syndromes associated with cocaine abuse include seizures, intracranial infarctions, and hemorrhages. Hyperadrenergic tone induces severe transient hypertension, hemorrhage, or focal vasospasm, and, sometimes, exacerbation of underlying abnormalities of cerebral blood vessels. Cerebral vasoconstriction following cocaine administration has been observed using magnetic resonance angiography.[26]

Other CNS manifestations reported after cocaine use include spinal cord infarctions, cerebral vasculitis, and intracranial abscesses. Choreoathetosis and repetitive movements (termed "crack dancing") are associated with cocaine and amphetamine intoxication and appear related to dopamine dysregulation. Acute dystonic reactions following cocaine use and withdrawal are also observed. Unilateral blindness has been reported secondary to central retinal artery occlusion, and bilateral blindness can be caused by diffuse vasospasm. A syndrome of corneal abrasions and ulcerations secondary to smoke and irritation is known as "crack eye." Keratitis caused by methamphetamine use has been described as well.

"Cocaine washout" is a syndrome that may occur in patients after a prolonged crack binge and results from depletion of neurotransmitters. Patients have a depressed level of consciousness but can be aroused to normal with stimulation. Resolution of lethargy can take up to 24 hours.

Amphetamine, phenylpropanolamine, and ephedrine use are associated with intracranial hemorrhage, infarction, encephalopathy, and seizures.[4,9] Amphetamines can also cause a CNS vasculitis resulting in focal neurologic deficits. A profound paranoid psychosis can be seen with long-term amphetamine abuse and withdrawal.

PULMONARY

Respiratory effects of cocaine use are more common in patients who smoke crack cocaine. Pulmonary hemorrhage, barotrauma, pneumonitis, asthma, and pulmonary edema have been observed.[27] Pneumomediastinum, pneumothorax, and pneumopericardium result from barotrauma secondary to performance of the Valsalva maneuver after inhalation or nasal insufflation in an attempt to enhance drug effect. Pneumonitis, asthma, and bronchiolitis may be an immunologic phenomenon or may result from numerous adulterants in illicit preparations.

Inhalation of crack cocaine is associated with new-onset bronchospasm, likely the result of local airway irritation.[28,29] Acute lung injury associated with cocaine use is multifactorial and may be catecholamine-mediated because a similar syndrome has been described in patients with adrenergic excess from pheochromocytoma and intracranial hemorrhage. Upper airway irritation and a "thermal" uvulitis can occur in patients smoking crack cocaine.

GI

Cocaine-induced mesenteric vasospasm may produce intestinal ischemia, bowel necrosis, ischemic colitis, and splenic infarctions. In addition, GI ulceration, bleeding, and perforation occur in association with cocaine use. Advanced tooth decay (termed "meth mouth") is common in habitual methamphetamine users. The reasons are presumably multifactorial and are related to poor oral hygiene, persistent dry mouth, consumption of high-carbohydrate carbonated beverages, jaw clenching, and tooth grinding. The belief that contamination with acidic or corrosive substances from the manufacturing process is responsible for this condition is not supported by analysis of illicitly produced methamphetamine.

ENDOCRINE

MDMA users may develop hyponatremia due to drug-induced secretion of vasopressin in the setting of overhydration with water. There is limited evidence suggesting that synthetic cathinones may cause similar effects, and they have been associated with several deaths.

RENAL

Cocaine or amphetamine use may cause traumatic and nontraumatic rhabdomyolysis.[30,31] In cocaine-induced rhabdomyolysis, up to one-third of patients develop acute kidney failure.[31] Risk factors for rhabdomyolysis include altered mental status, seizures, dysrhythmias, and hemodynamic instability. Stimulants may further exacerbate renal injury by producing hyperthermia, vasoconstriction, hypotension, and hypovolemia. Renal infarction has been described following IV cocaine use.

PREGNANCY

Cocaine is a potent vasoconstrictor that affects uteroplacental blood flow. Cocaine abuse during pregnancy is associated with an increased incidence of spontaneous abortions, abruptio placentae, fetal prematurity, and intrauterine growth retardation.[32,33] Both spontaneous abortions and abruptio placentae appear to occur from placental vasoconstriction and increased uterine contractility, with concomitant maternal hypertension. A breastfed infant can become intoxicated secondary to maternal cocaine use. Methamphetamine abuse during pregnancy has detrimental effects on fetal growth.

DIAGNOSIS

Cocaine or amphetamine intoxication can usually be suspected based on the symptoms and signs of the sympathomimetic toxidrome: agitation, mydriasis, diaphoresis, tachycardia, tachypnea, hypertension, and possibly hyperthermia. Mental status can range from normal to severely agitated and paranoid. Lethargy or coma suggests a postictal state or intracranial hemorrhage. Symptoms such as chest pain, palpitations, dyspnea, headache, or focal neurologic complaints suggest end-organ toxicity. Without a history of cocaine or other stimulant use, it may be difficult to distinguish this presentation from other conditions with catecholamine excess, such as withdrawal from alcohol or sedative-hypnotic drugs (**Table 187-4**). Lactic acidosis may be present following seizures or as a result of vasoconstriction and hypoperfusion. As with all intoxicated patients, consider occult trauma and hypoglycemia.

TABLE 187-4 Differential Diagnosis of Cocaine or Amphetamine Toxicity

Toxicologic	Phencyclidine toxicity
	Hallucinogen toxicity
	Anticholinergic toxicity
	Sedative-hypnotic withdrawal
	Serotonin syndrome
	Neuroleptic malignant syndrome
Intracranial	Ischemic stroke
	Intracranial hemorrhage
	Traumatic brain injury
	Encephalitis or meningitis
	Cerebral vasculitis
	Neoplasm
Endocrine	Hypoglycemia
	Pheochromocytoma
	Hyponatremia
	Thyrotoxicosis
Psychiatric	Acute psychosis
Other	Heat stroke
	Hypoxia

Concomitant use of alcohol and other drugs frequently alters the clinical presentation. For example, a patient using both opioids and stimulants may present with a decreased level of consciousness and few if any other diagnostic features of catecholamine excess. When the opioid effects are reversed with naloxone, the stimulant effects are unmasked, often with impressive findings.

LABORATORY EVALUATION

Laboratory studies and imaging are directed by clinical findings. Obtain a chemistry panel and creatine kinase level in a patient with agitation or elevated temperature to evaluate for possible metabolic acidosis, renal failure, or rhabdomyolysis. Hyponatremia, often with altered mental status, occasionally occurs after the use of hallucinogenic amphetamines such as MDMA or mescaline. For chest pain, obtain an ECG and serum levels of cardiac biomarkers. If the patient is hyperthermic (>104°F or 40°C), coagulation and liver function studies should be performed. Altered mental status typically requires CT of the head.

Urine drug screens to confirm cocaine or amphetamine use are readily available, but interpretation requires knowledge of pharmacology and the testing method.[34] Most of the rapid urine screening tests for cocaine are highly specific for cocaine metabolites (such as benzoylecgonine) and exhibit little cross-reactivity to the parent compound or other metabolites. Commonly available urine drug screens for the cocaine metabolite benzoylecgonine are sensitive at very low levels, and cocaine use within the past 24 to 72 hours is typically detected, depending on dose. Cocaine can be detected in habitual users by more sensitive techniques (radioimmunoassay, gas chromatography) for up to 2 weeks after last use of the drug.

Most urine amphetamine screens detect amphetamine, dextroamphetamine, methamphetamine, and, with decreasing sensitivity, 3,4-methylenedioxyethamphetamine, MDMA, and 3,4-methylenedioxyamphetamine. Synthetic cathinones may be detected, but results are too variable to be clinically useful due to variation in both laboratory analyzers as well as "bath salt" preparations. Commercial urine drug screens for amphetamine are sensitive to 1000 nanograms/mL, and amphetamine use within the past 48 hours is usually detected. However, interfering substances and other phenylethylamine compounds cross-react with amphetamine immunoassays, which limits their specificity. For example, excessive use of certain nasal inhalers that contain cross-reacting stimulant-class drugs may lead to positive results on immunoassays. Patients who take the nonprescription decongestants pseudoephedrine or phenylephrine or use prescription stimulants for attention-deficit disorder or narcolepsy can have a positive urine amphetamine result. Many drugs, such as bupropion, chlorpromazine, promethazine, thioridazine, trazodone, desipramine, and doxepin, have metabolites that react with the amphetamine immunoassay. Other drugs, such as labetalol, isometheptene, ranitidine, ritodrine, and trimethobenzamide, possess enough structural similarity to the basic amphetamine form to react with the immunoassay as well.

TREATMENT

Follow the standard protocol for poisoned patients (see chapter 176, "General Management of Poisoned Patients"). Establish IV access, and provide oxygen administration for hypoxia. The cornerstone of therapy is monitoring of vital signs, treatment of medical complications, supportive care, and adequate sedation to prevent self-harm and allow for testing and imaging (**Table 187-5**).[35] Treat hyperthermia with cool-mist spray and fans or cooling blankets (see chapter 210, "Heat Emergencies").[36] Aggressive IV hydration is the primary treatment for rhabdomyolysis (see chapter 89, "Rhabdomyolysis"). Seizures are initially treated with benzodiazepines, and status epilepticus requires aggressive treatment (see chapter 171, "Seizures"). Obtain head CT to identify intracranial pathology as the cause of seizures.

SEDATION

Benzodiazepines are the cornerstone of therapy for sedation. Lorazepam, 2 milligrams IV, or diazepam, 5 milligrams IV, can be administered and titrated with repeated doses to decrease the excess autonomic

TABLE 187-5 Management of Sympathomimetic Toxicity

Vital sign monitoring
Supportive care and prevent self-harm
Benzodiazepines for sedation
Aggressive cooling for hyperthermia
IV fluid for rhabdomyolysis
Anticonvulsants for seizures
Evaluate chest pain and treat ACS
Phentolamine for uncontrolled hypertension
Targeted therapy for dysrhythmias
IV lipid emulsion for refractory dysrhythmias

Abbreviation: ACS = acute coronary syndrome.

and neural stimulation. Antipsychotics such as haloperidol, droperidol, and chlorpromazine are not first-line therapy because they may lower the seizure threshold, contribute to hyperthermia, and increase QT prolongation and the risk of ventricular dysrhythmias. However, if benzodiazepines are ineffective, antipsychotics are often necessary to control agitation and destructive and dangerous behavior.

CHEST PAIN

Chest pain characteristics in cocaine users are no different than in patients with atherosclerotic heart disease. Question chest pain patients about the use of cocaine.[37] Cocaine users with suspected acute coronary syndrome are managed with aspirin and nitroglycerin (see chapter 49, "Acute Coronary Syndromes").[37,38] Additional therapy is guided by the ECG. **Oral or intravenous calcium channel blockers (diltiazem, 20 milligrams IV) are recommended in patients with ST-segment elevation or depression.**[37]

Use of β-adrenergic antagonists ("β-blockers") in the management of cocaine-associated myocardial ischemia or infarction is controversial.[37-39] Case reports suggested that β-blockers may create the potential for unopposed stimulation of α-adrenergic receptors that worsens coronary and peripheral vasoconstriction, hypertension, and possibly ischemia.[37,38] Conversely, large observational studies of patients with cocaine-related chest pain did not find an increased incidence of adverse effects in patients who received a β-blocker in the ED.[40-42] Labetalol (a mixed α-adrenergic and β-adrenergic antagonist) has been suggested for use by some in cocaine-associated chest pain because it does not appear to induce coronary artery vasoconstriction, even though β-adrenergic blocking activity predominates over α-adrenergic blocking activity. **The 2014 AHA/ACC Guidelines recommend that β-blockers not be administered to patients with signs of acute intoxication unless they are also receiving coronary artery vasodilator therapy (e.g., IV nitroglycerin).**[38]

Emergent coronary angiography is recommended if ST segments remain elevated despite nitroglycerin and calcium channel blocker therapy.[37] Fibrinolytic therapy may be used for cocaine-induced ST segment elevation myocardial infarction, if no other contraindications exist and coronary angiography is not available.[37]

DYSRHYTHMIAS

Target antidysrhythmic therapy according to the probable pathogenesis of the dysrhythmia.[43] Sinus tachycardia is generally responsive to sedation, cooling, and intravenous fluid rehydration, and specific β-blocker therapy is rarely necessary. Use a calcium channel blocker to treat reentrant supraventricular tachycardia as well as to control the ventricular rate in atrial fibrillation or flutter.

A wide-complex tachycardia with clinical evidence of cocaine toxicity can be assumed to be due to sodium channel blockage and treated with sodium bicarbonate, a 1 to 2 mEq/L IV bolus followed by either intermittent boluses or an infusion.[43,44] The frequency of boluses or the rate of infusion is guided by clinical response and serum pH; do not alkalinize the serum above a pH of 7.55 with sodium bicarbonate. Lidocaine in standard doses can be used in refractory cases of wide-complex tachycardia; theory and animal models suggest harmful interaction, but clinical experience has documented safety.[43]

Magnesium, lidocaine, and overdrive pacing have all been reported to be successful in cocaine-induced torsades de pointes. It seems reasonable, although unproven, to administer magnesium in patients with a prolonged corrected QT interval to prevent torsades from occurring.

In cases of severe cocaine toxicity, with persistent cardiovascular instability and/or refractory wide-complex tachycardias, intravenous lipid emulsion therapy has been reported to rapidly terminate the dysrhythmia and stabilize the cardiovascular system,[45,46] although failure has been reported also.[47] No recommendations on dose can be made from such limited clinical experience, so it seems reasonable to use the standard IV 20% lipid protocol developed for local anesthetic systemic toxicity: 100 mL (1.5 mL/kg) IV bolus over 2 to 3 minutes followed by an infusion of 18 mL (0.25 mL/kg) per minute until clinical improvement is seen or a total dose of 10 mL/kg has been given.

HYPERTENSION

Treat severe hypertension not responding to sedation with a sodium nitroprusside infusion (initial dose, 0.3 microgram/kg per minute) or phentolamine (initial dose, 2.5 to 5.0 milligrams IV). Blood pressure may be lowered aggressively if the patient does not have chronic hypertension. Treatment for refractory hypertension is similar to that for hypertensive emergencies except that β-adrenergic blockers are not used (see chapter 57, "Systemic Hypertension").

BODY STUFFERS AND BODY PACKERS

Cocaine and other drugs can be internally concealed.[48] Patients who swallow cocaine following police pursuit to conceal the evidence are termed "body stuffers." The swallowed packets are often poorly wrapped and can leak or perforate.[49] "Body packers" swallow a large number of well-sealed packets in order to smuggle drugs across international borders. Both methods can result in severe toxicity and death.[35,49]

Management of an asymptomatic cocaine body packer brought in by police or customs officials is a treatment dilemma.[48] CT is the best imaging modality to identify the packets.[50] If the patient shows no signs of toxicity, give single-dose activated charcoal and institute whole-bowel irrigation with polyethylene glycol electrolyte solution to gently hasten packet elimination.[35,51] Continue whole-bowel irrigation until passage of the last packet, and then obtain a confirmatory CT to ensure that all containers have passed. For symptomatic patients, provide sedation and symptomatic care, and obtain immediate surgical consultation for operative removal of the packets. Do not consult for endoscopy or colonoscopy because endoscopic manipulation may rupture the packets.[48,49]

DRUG INTERACTIONS

Because cocaine is metabolized by plasma cholinesterase, co-administration of drugs such as succinylcholine and mivacurium that are also metabolized by plasma cholinesterase may lead to unpredictable rates of metabolism, leading to foreshortened or prolonged effects.

Both lidocaine and cocaine are local anesthetics and act as sodium channel antagonists. It is thought that the neurotoxic effects of both occur by similar mechanisms. Despite theoretical risk in treating cocaine-induced dysrhythmias with lidocaine, it has been used safely in patients with cocaine-associated myocardial infarction.

Monoamine oxidase inhibitors block the degradation of intracellular catecholamines, increasing adrenergic neurotransmitters in the presynaptic terminals. Amphetamines are indirect-acting sympathomimetic amines that induce the release of stored catecholamines and are also weak inhibitors of monoamine oxidase. Thus, patients taking monoamine oxidase inhibitors who subsequently use amphetamines or phenylpropanolamine (and to a lesser extent cocaine) may precipitate an acute syndrome of excessive catecholamine release that results in severe hypertension, tachycardia, hyperthermia, agitation, tremors, and possible severe neurotoxicity.

WITHDRAWAL

Cocaine withdrawal is characterized by irritability, paranoid ideation, and depression.[52] Although symptoms during cocaine withdrawal are generally milder than those during amphetamine withdrawal, psychological addiction may be particularly strong. Methamphetamine withdrawal is characterized by drowsiness, lethargy, hunger, tremor, and chills. There is considerable potential for long-term depression and suicide. Symptoms of withdrawal are strongest during the first 48 hours, but milder symptoms can last up to 2 weeks. Although pharmacologic adjuncts, such as antidepressants, adrenergic antagonists, or dopaminergic agents, are sometimes used during cocaine or amphetamine withdrawal, there are no data confirming efficacy.[52,53]

DISPOSITION AND FOLLOW-UP

Disposition depends on initial patient presentation, response to therapy, the nature of the stimulant involved, and expected duration of effect. Patients demonstrating resolution of toxicity and clear sensorium in the absence of focal complaints or end-organ damage should be advised of the medical risks of drug abuse and referred to appropriate detoxification, counseling, and social support services.

Patients who present with adrenergic excess following recent cocaine use and who respond to initial sedation may be expected to improve completely during a period of observation in the ED because of the relatively limited duration of cocaine effects. In contrast, amphetamines have a longer duration of effect and produce prolonged toxicity, which necessitates observation or hospitalization.

REFERENCES

The complete reference list is available online at www.TintinalliEM.com.

CHAPTER 188 Hallucinogens

Katherine M. Prybys
Karen N. Hansen

INTRODUCTION AND EPIDEMIOLOGY

The term *hallucinogen* is misleading. Hallucinogenic compounds rarely produce true hallucinations—but rather, users experience profound distortions in body image, sensory perception, and time perception, in addition to rapid, intense alterations in mood, increased intensity of any emotions, and heightened suggestibility. *Hallucinogen* is sometimes used interchangeably with the term *psychedelic*.

Hallucinogens are widely perceived as safe by the public. However, these substances can cause dangerous physiologic effects resulting in serious health consequences.[1-3] The identity, purity, and amount of hallucinogenic compound is usually uncertain, and individual response can be unpredictable.

Hallucinogens in current use consist of both natural and synthetic compounds.[4] The proliferation of "designer drugs"—chemical analogs or derivatives of illicit drugs marketed to circumvent existing drug laws—is a growing problem. Manufacturers of designer drugs try to circumvent U.S. federal drug laws by stamping their product with advisories such as "not intended for human consumption" or by identifying the products as plant food, bath salts, or potpourri. Prosecution through the Federal Analog Act, a section of the Controlled Substance Abuse Act, can occur only if the drug is "intended for human consumption." Because of this limitation in federal law, some states have moved to ban the sale of such drugs.

Conditions that mimic hallucinogen intoxication include alcohol or benzodiazepine withdrawal, anticholinergic poisoning, thyrotoxicosis, central nervous system infections, structural brain lesions, acute psychosis, hypoglycemia, and hypoxia.[5] Some prescription and nonprescription medications can cause hallucinations. The identity of street drugs is often misrepresented, and substitutions or adulteration of product is common.[6,7]

Drug-induced psychosis may be difficult to distinguish from primary psychotic disorders.[8,9] A patient with substance-induced psychosis is more likely to have a diagnosis of dependence on any drug, report visual hallucinations, and have a history of parental drug abuse.[9]

GENERAL APPROACH TO TREATMENT

Start by assessing the patient's general medical condition and stabilizing the vital signs. Identify and correct hypoxia and hypoglycemia. Obtain a core temperature to recognize hyperthermia. Obtain serum chemistries and if the patient is agitated, obtain creatine phosphokinase to identify rhabdomyolysis. Obtain an electrocardiogram to identify QT interval prolongation.

Gastric decontamination is not needed in most cases because most hallucinogens are rapidly absorbed and because most patients with adverse effects do not present until several hours after the drug was taken. However, consider administration of oral activated charcoal for ingestions occurring within the previous hour or longer when gastric emptying is delayed, such as with anticholinergic poisonings (e.g., nutmeg ingestion).

Reassurance and a calm, supportive environment can often sufficiently soothe the agitated patient. Pharmacologic sedation and possibly physical restraints may be necessary in order to ensure the safety of the patient and the ED staff and to facilitate evaluation and treatment. **Benzodiazepines** are the preferred agents for the treatment of hallucinogenic-induced agitation and delirium because they possess no significant drug interactions, have no dystonic or anticholinergic adverse effects, do not prolong the QT interval or promote arrhythmias, and are reversible by flumazenil if over sedation occurs. Start with diazepam 5 to 10 milligrams PO or IV, or lorazepam 1 to 2 milligrams PO, IM, or IV. Give repeated doses as needed, and monitor blood pressure and respiration. Tachycardia and hypertension often respond to sedation with benzodiazepines alone. Severe hypertension can be treated with IV nitroprusside. Correct electrolyte abnormalities and treat dehydration and hypovolemia with normal saline infusion. Treat symptomatic arrhythmias using standard antiarrhythmic protocols. Active cooling measures should be initiated for patients with significant hyperthermia. Treatment of severe agitation, hyperthermia, or seizures may require neuromuscular paralysis and endotracheal intubation. Seizures are treated with benzodiazepines or propofol. Patients with rhabdomyolysis require aggressive IV hydration to maintain urine output.

DISPOSITION AND FOLLOW-UP

Compared with other abused psychoactive agents, hallucinogens have some of the largest acute safety ratios when lethal doses are measured against the doses customarily used to produce the desired hallucinogenic effects.[10] Most patients seen in the ED due to adverse reactions from hallucinogen use can be discharged into the custody of family or friends if they are lucid and in medically stable condition after a period of observation. Patients with persistent psychotic symptoms or comorbid psychiatric illnesses require psychiatric evaluation.

COMMON HALLUCINOGENS

Common hallucinogens are listed in **Table 188-1**.

LYSERGIC ACID DIETHYLAMIDE

Lysergic acid diethylamide is a potent psychoactive drug. As little as 25 micrograms produces psychedelic effects. The hallucinogenic effects are believed to be mediated through agonism at the serotonin type 2 ($5\text{-}HT_2$) receptor.[11,12]

Lysergic acid diethylamide is a colorless, tasteless, odorless, water-soluble substance that is sold in various forms, but most commonly as small squares of dried blotter paper printed with colorful graphics and

TABLE 188-1 Common Hallucinogens

Drug	Typical Hallucinogenic Dose	Duration of Action	Clinical Features	Complications	Specific Treatment
Lysergic acid diethylamide	20–80 micrograms	8–12 h	Mydriasis Tachycardia Anxiety Muscle tension	Coma Hyperthermia Coagulopathy Persistent psychosis Hallucinogen persisting perception disorder	Reassurance Benzodiazepines
Psilocybin	5–100 mushrooms 4–6 milligrams of psilocybin	4–6 h	Mydriasis Tachycardia Muscle tension Nausea and vomiting	Seizures (rare) Hyperthermia (rare)	Reassurance Hydration Benzodiazepines
Mescaline	3–12 "buttons" 200–500 milligrams of mescaline	6–12 h	Mydriasis Abdominal pain Nausea/vomiting Dizziness Nystagmus Ataxia	Rare	Supportive Benzodiazepines
Methylenedioxymethamphetamine ("Ecstasy")	50–200 milligrams	4–6 h	Mydriasis Bruxism Jaw tension Ataxia Dry mouth Nausea	Hyponatremia Hypertension Seizures Hyperthermia Arrhythmias Rhabdomyolysis	Benzodiazepines Hydration Active cooling Dantrolene Specific serotonin antagonists
Synthetic cathinone derivatives ("bath salts")	50–300 milligrams of mephedrone	2–4 h	Agitation Tachycardia Hypertension Diaphoresis Mydriasis	Paranoia Panic reactions Hyperthermia Seizures Hyponatremia Rhabdomyolysis	Benzodiazepines Hydration Active cooling
Phencyclidine ("angel dust")	1–9 milligrams	4–6 h	Small or midsized pupils Nystagmus Muscle rigidity Hypersalivation Agitation Catatonia	Coma Seizures Hyperthermia Rhabdomyolysis Hypertension Hypoglycemia	Benzodiazepines Hydration Active cooling
Marijuana (cannabis)	5–15 milligrams of tetrahydrocannabinol	2–4 h	Tachycardia Conjunctival injection	Acute psychosis (rare) Panic reactions (rare)	Supportive Benzodiazepines
Synthetic cannabinoids ("K2," "Spice")	2–5 milligrams of JWH-018	3–4 h	Tachycardia Conjunctival injection	Acute psychosis Panic reactions Seizures (rare) Arrhythmias (rare)	Supportive Benzodiazepines
Bromo-benzodifuranyl-isopropylamine (Bromo-DragonFLY)	200–800 micrograms	10–14 h	Agitation Hallucinations	Seizures Vasoconstrictor with necrosis and gangrene	Supportive Benzodiazepines

cartoons that have been perforated and soaked in liquid lysergic acid diethylamide solution. Each square typically delivers a dose of 20 to 80 micrograms. Other forms include "microdots" (tiny tablets), "windowpane" (gelatin sheets), impregnated sugar cubes or candy, and small bottles of "breath drops" (the drug in solution).

The psychedelic effects begin within 30 minutes of ingestion, peak within 4 hours, and last between 8 to 12 hours.[13,14] Sympathomimetic stimulation with mydriasis and elevations of pulse, blood pressure, and temperature usually precede the psychedelic effects.[13,14] Marked facial flushing, mild gastric distress, piloerection, increased muscle tension, and hyperreflexia may occur. In massive overdoses, coagulopathy, hyperthermia, seizure, coma, and respiratory arrest have been reported.[15]

The psychedelic effects of lysergic acid diethylamide depend on the user's prevailing mood, expectations, and surrounding environment. Effects may be perceived as pleasurable or horrifying. Profound distortions in perception of sensory stimuli, time, emotions, and memories occur and may cause users to experience paranoia, depression, extreme panic, or an acute psychotic reaction known as a *dysphoric reaction* or "bad trip." Dangerous and impulsive behavior is possible, resulting in serious physical trauma or suicide. Prolonged and sometimes permanent psychosis, known as "flashbacks" or "hallucinogen persisting perception disorder," can result.[16]

The typical user is usually conscious, alert, and able to provide history of the drug ingestion.[13] Diagnosis is based on history of use, the presence of sympathomimetic signs, and reported psychedelic effects. Lysergic acid diethylamide can be detected in the urine for several days after ingestion using specific radioimmunoassay and enzyme immunoassay techniques. Reassurance and observation in a quiet, safe environment are generally the only interventions required to manage a dysphoric reaction. Oral or parenteral benzodiazepines are indicated for patients with extreme agitation or signs of excessive sympathomimetic stimulation. Patients with paranoid or psychotic symptoms lasting longer than 8 to 12 hours may require hospital admission. Medical complications due to massive overdose are rare, and recovery is usually rapid and requires only supportive care.[13-15]

PSILOCYBIN

Psilocybin is a naturally occurring hallucinogenic compound found in at least six genera of mushrooms, but most notably the *Psilocybe* genus. Psilocybin is an indolalkylamine that is metabolized to the pharmacologically active compound psilocin. Both psilocybin and psilocin are believed to act as serotonin type 2 receptor agonists similar to lysergic acid diethylamide.

Psilocybin-containing mushrooms grow naturally in the southern United States and Europe but can also be grown from kits sold over the Internet.[17] Most species of psilocybin-containing mushrooms turn bluish when bruised, but this is not a definitive method of identification or determination of potency. Psilocybin-containing mushrooms may be dried or cooked without losing potency. Hallucinogenic mushrooms sold on the street are often nonpsychoactive mushrooms that have been adulterated with lysergic acid diethylamide or phencyclidine.[6] Because of the variation in mushroom size and concentration of psychoactive compounds, there is little correlation between the number of mushrooms ingested and the hallucinogenic effects. A user may ingest as few as five or as many as 100 mushrooms for a single "dose."

Hallucinogenic effects begin within 30 minutes of ingestion and last 4 to 6 hours.[18,19] The hallucinogenic effects are similar to, although less powerful than, those produced by lysergic acid diethylamide. Other common effects include mydriasis, tachycardia, nausea, and vomiting. Serious medical complications are extremely rare but include seizures, hyperthermia, rhabdomyolysis, and renal failure.[20] Mistaken identity and ingestion of highly toxic mushrooms is possible and can lead to serious outcomes.[21]

Management is supportive. There is no routinely available screening test for psilocybin or psilocin in the urine. If the patient's symptoms are not consistent with psilocybin ingestion, consider the possibility that a toxic mushroom (see Chapter 219, Mushroom Poisoning) or other psychoactive substances were ingested.[21]

MESCALINE AND PEYOTE

Mescaline is found in many cacti, most notably the Mexican Peyote cactus (*Lophophora williamsii*) and the Peruvian San Pedro cactus (*Trichocereus pachanoi*). Peyote is used in Native American religious ceremonies, and its legal use is restricted to the Native American Church. Mescaline is a phenylethylamine, structurally related to amphetamines, making it chemically distinct from lysergic acid diethylamide.[22] Mescaline is believed to act as a serotonin type 2 receptor agonist, but is much less potent than lysergic acid diethylamide.

Peyote is most commonly sold as raw cactus or "buttons," 2- to 3-cm discs sliced off of the top of the cactus. Each button contains approximately 45 milligrams of mescaline. A typical hallucinogenic dose is 200 to 500 milligrams. Pills or capsules sold on the street as "mescaline" are unlikely to be genuine and may instead contain lysergic acid diethylamide or phencyclidine.[6]

Peyote is bitter tasting and causes uncomfortable physical side effects within an hour of ingestion—including nausea, vomiting, abdominal discomfort, diaphoresis, dizziness, nystagmus, ataxia, and headache—that generally resolve after about 2 hours. Adrenergic stimulation causes mydriasis and mild elevations in pulse, blood pressure, and temperature. Hallucinogenic effects begin several hours after ingestion and persist for 6 to 12 hours. Significant morbidity or mortality caused by the physiologic effects of mescaline has not been observed, but death can result from aberrant behavior while under the influence of the drug.[23] Mescaline-intoxicated patients are managed supportively. Routine urine drug screens do not detect mescaline.

HALLUCINOGENIC AMPHETAMINES

More than 50 "designer" amphetamines have been created for their hallucinogenic properties. Best known is **methylenedioxymethamphetamine**, a synthetic phenylethylamine derivative structurally related to both amphetamines and mescaline and commonly known by the street name "**Ecstasy.**" Other designer amphetamines include methylenedioxyamphetamine and methylenedioxyethamphetamine ("**Eve**"). Methylenedioxymethamphetamine is known for both its psychedelic properties and unique effects on mood and intimacy, which has led to its reputation as a "love drug" popular in dance clubs.[24] Methylenedioxymethamphetamine has complex effects, interacting with dopamine, norepinephrine, acetylcholine, and β_2-adrenergic and serotonin type 2A receptors, and affecting the release of several hormones, including prolactin, oxytocin, adrenocorticotrophic hormone, dehydroepiandrosterone, and antidiuretic hormone.[25]

Methylenedioxymethamphetamine is usually ingested as tablets in doses of 50 to 200 milligrams. The drug is colorless and tasteless—properties lending to its use as a date-rape drug.[26] Symptoms occur within 30 minutes of ingestion and last about 4 to 6 hours. These include feelings of euphoria, inner peace, enhanced sociability, verbosity, and heightened sexual interest. The drug rarely causes actual hallucinations but can produce sensory effects such as alterations in the intensity of colors or sensation of textures. Other common effects include mydriasis, tachycardia, and elevated blood pressure, as well as nausea, jaw tension, bruxism, dry mouth, muscle aches, and ataxia. Current urinary amphetamine immunoassays incorporate a specific monoclonal antibody for methylenedioxymethamphetamine and should routinely detect this drug.

Methylenedioxymethamphetamine and related amphetamines can produce serious complications and death.[27-30] As with other amphetamines, large-quantity overdoses can cause severe hypertension, intracranial hemorrhage, and ischemia in the heart or brain.[27] Fatal arrhythmias and sudden cardiac death have been reported, both with and without underlying cardiac disease.[27,28] The most frequently cited causes of death are hyperthermia and hyponatremia.[31-34] A syndrome of methylenedioxymethamphetamine toxicity manifested by hyperthermia, seizures, disseminated intravascular coagulation, rhabdomyolysis, and hepatotoxicity has been described.[35] This pattern shares many features of the serotonin syndrome, and **combining methylenedioxymethamphetamine with selective serotonin reuptake inhibitors (see Chapter 178, Atypical and Serotonergic Antidepressants) or monoamine oxidase inhibitors (see Chapter 179, Monoamine Oxidase Inhibitors) can precipitate serotonin syndrome.**[36]

Hyponatremia is predominantly due to excessive water consumption and inappropriate antidiuretic hormone secretion.[31,32] Excessive water drinking from thirst can occur if the drug is taken at hot and crowded club venues, with vigorous dancing and profuse sweating.[31,33] Persistent neurotoxic effects are possible from chronic methylenedioxymethamphetamine use. Neuropsychiatric studies of habitual users demonstrate long-lasting cognitive impairment and mood dysfunction, including memory impairment, diminished learning ability, and depression.[37]

Gastrointestinal decontamination with activated charcoal may be useful if the drug was ingested within 60 minutes of ED arrival.[38] Hypertension and tachycardia often respond to benzodiazepines. Severe hypertension is treated with IV phentolamine or nitroprusside. Rapid IV titration with high doses of benzodiazepines or propofol may be required to control symptoms in patients with refractory agitation or seizures. Arrhythmias are managed with standard therapy.

Check serum electrolyte concentrations and anticipate and treat abnormalities, especially hyponatremia (see Chapter 17, Fluids and Electrolytes). Hyperthermia is managed with cooling measures and fluid resuscitation.[32,33] Patients with temperatures exceeding 40°C (104°F) have increased morbidity and mortality, so rapid cooling is important.[39] Although there is no evidence from controlled studies, expert opinion and case reports support the use of dantrolene when methylenedioxymethamphetamine-induced hyperthermia is refractory to sedation and active cooling.[38,40-42] Specific serotonin antagonists, such as methysergide or cyproheptadine, have been suggested for patients with features of the serotonin syndrome following methylenedioxymethamphetamine use.[43]

SYNTHETIC CATHINONE DERIVATIVES

In the fall of 2010, U.S. Poison Control Centers began receiving calls regarding synthetic cathinone derivatives, and use has increased dramatically since then.[44,45] Cathinone is a naturally occurring alkaloid extracted from the leaves of the *Catha edulis* plant (khat) native to areas of Africa and the Middle East. Cathinone and synthetic derivatives, including mephedrone, methylenedioxypyrovalerone, and methylone, are chemically similar to amphetamines. These drugs likely stimulate the release and inhibit the uptake of biogenic amines such as norepinephrine, dopamine, and serotonin.

Synthetic cathinone derivatives are abused by individuals seeking a "legal" high with stimulatory effects similar to those of cocaine or methylenedioxymethamphetamine. These drugs are often labeled as "**bath salts**" or "**plant food**," with fanciful names such as "**Vanilla Sky**" or "**Ivory Wave**." They are often labeled as "not for human consumption" in an attempt to avoid federal regulations.

Synthetic cathinones can be nasally insufflated ("snorted"), ingested, or injected. Duration of effects depends on method of use—1 to 2 hours with nasal insufflation and up to 4 hours if ingested.[46] Approximately 20% of users report adverse effects including sweating, palpitations, nausea, headache, and dizziness.[46] Agitation is common, and paranoia, panic attacks, and aggression—including violent behavior—have been reported. Sympathomimetic toxicity, with dilated pupils, tachycardia, and hypertension, is common. Hyperthermia, seizures, hyponatremia, rhabdomyolysis, and deaths have been reported.[46-50] Synthetic cathinones are not detected on routine urine toxicology screens.

Treatment is primarily supportive, including cardiovascular monitoring; benzodiazepines as needed for agitation, sympathomimetic effects, or seizures; and cooling for hyperthermia. Admission to a monitored or intensive care unit setting is appropriate for patients with persistent symptoms.

In September 2011 the U.S. Drug Enforcement Administration issued an emergency order to place three synthetic cathinones (mephedrone, methylenedioxypyrovalerone, and methylone) temporarily into Schedule 1 under the Controlled Substances Act, making the manufacture, sale, or possession of these agents illegal.[51]

PHENCYCLIDINE

Phencyclidine is a synthetic piperidine derivative, structurally related to ketamine. Phencyclidine does not fit easily into a single classification, combining features of hallucinogens, depressants, and stimulants.[52] Unlike classic hallucinogens, phencyclidine causes a clouding of the sensorium rather than heightened sensory awareness. The primary pharmacologic action is blockade of *N*-methyl-D-aspartate receptor channels. At high concentrations, phencyclidine also interacts with other receptors and channels, including the opioid, acetylcholine receptor and voltage-gated electrolyte channels, and exhibits sympathomimetic effects by blocking reuptake of norepinephrine and dopamine.

Phencyclidine is easily and inexpensively synthesized. Powdered ("**angel dust**") or liquid ("**dippers**") drug is often combined with tobacco, marijuana, or other leafy materials and smoked. Phencyclidine can also be ingested orally, snorted, or intravenously injected.[53] Phencyclidine may be unknowingly ingested, because it is often sold as another drug or used to adulterate another illicit drug product.[17] The onset of action depends on the mode of administration. With smoking the onset is about 5 minutes and effects generally last 4 to 6 hours. With large doses, effects can persist for days due to its lipid solubility and accumulation in fat stores.[54,55]

Patients may experience CNS stimulation or depression, with clinical presentations ranging from physically violent to catatonic or comatose states.[53,56] A combination of cholinergic, anticholinergic, and sympathomimetic effects causes a confusing clinical toxidrome. Phencyclidine is often coadministered with other drugs such as crack cocaine ("**beam me up**"), marijuana ("**crystal supergrass**"), or ethanol, which also complicates the clinical picture.[54] The most common findings in phencyclidine-intoxicated patients are nystagmus and hypertension (generally mild), each occurring in almost 60% of cases.[54] Feelings of detachment (dissociation) from the environment and self may give the user feelings of strength, power, and invulnerability. Violent actions, agitation, bizarre and unpredictable behavior, and hallucinations or delusions are frequent. Diaphoresis, tachycardia, muscle rigidity, dystonic reactions, ataxia, and a decreased response to painful stimuli can occur. About 10% of patients are described as comatose.[55] Pupil size is variable, but widely dilated pupils are uncommon.[54]

Medical complications from phencyclidine toxicity are frequent.[52,56,57] Seizures occur in about 3% of patients, and rhabdomyolysis, occasionally producing acute renal failure, is reported in up to 70%.[55] Hypoglycemia, hypertension causing intracerebral hemorrhage, hyperthermia causing hepatic necrosis, and multiorgan failure can occur.[54,55,57,58] Violent behavior can result in self-injury.

Evaluate patients with suspected phencyclidine toxicity for occult injury, hypoglycemia, and rhabdomyolysis.[52,53,56] Phencyclidine can be detected by commercially available urine drug screens up to 8 days after single use and up to several weeks after long-term use.[59] Cough and cold medications (dextromethorphan, diphenhydramine, and doxylamine), analgesics (ibuprofen, meperidine, and tramadol), and psychotropics (imipramine, mesoridazine, thioridazine, and venlafaxine) cross-react with the drug screen and produce false-positive results.

Sedation and physical restraints are frequently required to control violent and aggressive behavior. Parenteral benzodiazepines are preferable to physical restraints because fighting against restraints may contribute to rhabdomyolysis.

Treatment is generally supportive. Treat seizures with benzodiazepines. Status epilepticus or seizures refractory to benzodiazepines may require intubation and treatment with propofol or barbiturates. Treat hyperthermia with active cooling measures. Hypertension usually responds to sedation, but severe hypertension can be treated with nitroprusside. Rhabdomyolysis is treated with aggressive hydration and close monitoring of urine output.

Patients exhibiting only minor clinical features of phencyclidine intoxication and no medical complications can be discharged when behavior normalizes.[52,53,55,56]

MARIJUANA OR CANNABIS

Marijuana or cannabis consists of the dried leaves and flowers of the hemp plant *Cannabis sativa*. **Hashish** is prepared from the dried resin from the flower tops of this plant. The psychoactive ingredient in marijuana is tetrahydrocannabinol.[60]

Marijuana is most often smoked[61] but can also be ingested. Symptoms persist for 2 to 4 hours after smoking, or longer if ingested. Clinical effects include drowsiness, euphoria, heightened sensory awareness, paranoia, and distortions of time and space. Hallucinations do not usually occur at usual doses. Common physiologic effects of marijuana are mild tachycardia, injected conjunctiva, bronchodilation, orthostatic hypotension, and impaired motor coordination.[62] Medical complications, such as panic reactions, brief toxic psychoses, pneumomediastinum, and pneumothorax, are rare. Acute cardiac events associated with marijuana use have been reported,[63,64] possibly the result of aging in the population of marijuana users and the increasing availability of medical marijuana.

Marijuana is used for treatment of medical conditions such as glaucoma and chemotherapy-related nausea and to promote weight gain in patients with HIV infection and AIDS.

Chronic cannabis use is associated with psychiatric, respiratory, cardiovascular, and bone effects.[65] Cyclic vomiting syndrome can be due to marijuana use.[66-68] Symptoms are often misdiagnosed as gastroparesis or opiate withdrawal, and cannabis cessation results in symptomatic recovery.

Acute psychiatric symptoms due to marijuana use can generally be managed with reassurance alone, but benzodiazepines can be used for severe symptoms. Standard urine drug screens are unreliable indicators of acute marijuana intoxication. High lipid solubility results in extensive deposition within body fat and slow excretion in the urine. After a single use, tetrahydrocannabinol is detected by commercially available urine screens for up to 3 days. With long-term use, cannabinoids can be detected up to 30 days or longer after abstinence.[69] Ibuprofen, naproxen, pantoprazole, and efavirenz, a non-nucleoside reverse transcriptase inhibitor used to treat HIV infection, can produce false-positive results on the urine cannabinoid screen.

SYNTHETIC CANNABINOIDS

Synthetically produced cannabinoid-receptor agonists have been created for hallucinogenic use and are generally combined with herbal blends and labeled as "**Spice**" or "**K2**."[47] These products contain a variety of compounds that are active at the cannabinoid receptors but are not structurally related to tetrahydrocannabinol. One of the first synthetic cannabinoids (1-pentyl-1H-indol-3-yl)-1-naphthalenyl-methanone, goes by the term JWH-018 for the initials of J.W. Huffman, who developed this compound to investigate drug-receptor interactions.[70]

Products containing synthetic cannabinoids are sold in shops and on the Internet labeled as "incense" and "not for human consumption." The appeal of such products is driven by the desire for a legal "high" that is not detectable by current urine drug assays.

The product is usually rolled in paper and smoked in a manner similar to marijuana. Effects begin within minutes and may last for several hours, generally disappearing within 4 hours.[47] Most users will not seek or require medical attention, but some have experienced adverse reactions, with anxiety and tachycardia being the most common.[72] Other reported adverse effects include hypertension, diaphoresis, tremulousness, and agitation.[72,73] Synthetic cannabinoids can precipitate psychosis in patients with prior mental illness.[74] Symptoms are usually self-limited and short-lived, and treatment is supportive.

In March 2011 the U.S. Drug Enforcement Administration placed five synthetic cannabinoid compounds (JWH-018, JWH-073, JWH-200, CP-47,497, and cannabicyclohexanol) into Schedule 1, criminalizing their sale or use.[75] These will likely be replaced in the illegal hallucinogen marketplace by other related molecules in this class.

DESIGNER ALKALOIDS

Bromo-benzodifuranyl-isopropylamine, or **Bromo-DragonFLY**, is a phenethylamine hallucinogen.[76] Bromo-DragonFLY stimulates serotonin receptors in the brain, similar to lysergic acid diethylamide. Bromo-DragonFLY was developed as a research chemical to study the relationship between molecular structure and psychedelic activity. The name comes from its chemical structure, two furanyl rings with double bonds and a side amphetamine arm, which gives it the appearance of a dragonfly. In 2005, Bromo-DragonFLY became available in human experimental markets and was soon diverted to hallucinogenic use.

Bromo-DragonFLY is sold as white to pink powder that can be snorted, smoked, or injected. Bromo-DragonFLY may also be sold on blotter paper, similar to lysergic acid diethylamide, which has led to confusion in users mistakenly consuming Bromo-Dragon-FLY instead. The hallucinogenic dose of Bromo-DragonFLY ranges from 200 to 800 micrograms, with the onset of action within 20 to 90 minutes and a duration of hallucinogenic effects up to 10 to 14 hours. Toxicity includes agitation, hallucinations, and tonic-clonic seizures that may be delayed in onset.[77] Bromo-DragonFLY acts as a long-acting vasoconstrictor that can cause necrosis and gangrene several weeks after use. Bromo-DragonFLY has been associated with fatalities in several countries.[78] Two similar compounds, 2C-B-FLY and 3C-B-FLY, are also abused as hallucinogens.

Benzylpiperazine and trifluoromethylphenylpiperazine are synthetic phenylpiperazine analogues used as substitutes for amphetamine-derived designer drugs.[47,79] These two compounds are usually combined and sold as "**Legal X**" in attempt to mimic the effects of methylenedioxymethamphetamine. These drugs are legally available in many countries. Clinical effects include sympathomimetic effects such as palpitations, agitation, anxiety, confusion, dizziness, headache, tremor, mydriasis, insomnia, urinary retention, vomiting, and seizures.[47,80] Deaths have been associated, but in most cases, recovery occurs with supportive care and benzodiazepines.[81]

LESS COMMONLY ABUSED HALLUCINOGENS

Other drugs with hallucinogenic properties (**Table 188-2**) are enjoying increasing popularity because of information disseminated on the Internet that promotes the use of these "natural" psychoactive agents.[47,82]

SALVIA

Salvia divinorum ("**salvia**," "**Sally**," "**magic mint**") is a perennial herb in the mint family.[83] Salvia is sold as seeds, plant cuttings, whole plants,

TABLE 188-2 Less Commonly Abused Hallucinogens

	Typical Route of Use	Onset of Action	Duration of Action	Additional Features of Acute Toxicity
Salvia divinorum: salvinorin A	Smoking of dried leaves Chewed leaves held in SL or buccal location	20–60 s (smoking) 10–20 min (SL or buccal)	20–30 min (smoking) 30–90 min (SL or buccal)	Headache
Toad venom or eggs: bufotoxins	Ingestion of toad venom extract or food made with toad eggs	30–60 min (nausea and vomiting)	1–3 d (untreated)	Abdominal pain, vomiting Sympathomimetic effects Features similar to cardiac glycoside toxicity
Ipomoea species (morning glory): lysergic acid amide	Ingestion of seeds	1–2 h	6–10 h	None
Nutmeg: myristicin	Ingestion of seeds or ground spice	3–6 h	6–24 h	Some features resemble anticholinergic toxicity
Datura species (Jimson weed and angel's trumpet): scopolamine, atropine, and hyoscyamine	Ingestion of seeds Smoking dried plant parts	1–3 h (ingestion) 5 min (smoking)	24–48 h	Anticholinergic effects
Ketamine	Snorting dried powder or smoking of powder admixed with marijuana or tobacco	5–15 min (nasal insufflation) 1–3 min (smoking)	45–60 min (nasal insufflation) 30–45 min (smoking)	Sympathomimetic effects
Dextromethorphan	Ingestion of liquid Nasal insufflation of powder	20–60 min (ingestion)	4–6 h (ingestion)	Nausea, vomiting, and diarrhea

fresh and dried leaves, and liquid extracts purported to contain the active ingredient salvinorin A. Although salvia and salvinorin A are not currently regulated under the U.S. Controlled Substance Act, a number of states have placed controls on the plant and extract. When chewed, the leaf mass and juice are retained within the mouth, and absorption of the active ingredient is rapid, causing clinical effects within 5 to 10 minutes. Dried leaves, as well as extract-enhanced leaves, can be smoked. Smoking pure salvinorin A at a dose of 200 to 500 micrograms results in effects that begin within 30 seconds and last up to 30 minutes. Desired effects include perceptions of bright lights, vivid colors and shapes, body movements, and object distortions.[47,84,85] Adverse effects may include dysphoria, incoordination, dizziness, and slurred speech.[86] Treatment is supportive.

BUFOTOXINS

Bufotoxins (bufotenine and 5-methoxy-dimethyltryptamine) are hallucinogenic tryptamines found in the venom, skin, and eggs of many toads (e.g., *Bufo alvarius*, *Bufo marinus*).[87] Toad venom has also been used as an aphrodisiac ("**love stone**" or "**rock hard**") and in some traditional Chinese medicines (*chan su* and *kyushin*). Venom can be obtained by "milking" the toad's parotid glands and drying the liquid venom to form an extract. 5-Methoxy-dimethyltryptamine is a powerful psychedelic whereas bufotenine has weaker effects. In addition to psychoactive substances, the venom contains cardioactive steroids (bufagins or bufadienolides), catecholamines (epinephrine and norepinephrine) and noncardiac sterols (e.g., cholesterol). Bufagins are **cardioactive steroids** that can cause cardiac toxicity similar to digoxin.[88] Toxicity from toad venom varies considerably depending on the toad species and its geographic location.

Symptoms of toad venom poisoning occur almost immediately. Effects may be restricted to local gastrointestinal irritation, with copious salivation, nausea, vomiting, and abdominal discomfort persisting for hours. Systemic toxicity may develop due to sympathomimetic effects. Cardiac toxicity is similar to acute digoxin poisoning, with hyperkalemia, bradycardia, atrioventricular conduction block, ventricular tachycardia, ventricular fibrillation, and cardiac arrest.[89,90]

Serum digoxin immunoassay often yields a positive result. Bradyarrhythmias are initially treated with atropine and may require pacemaker placement. Antiarrhythmic drugs should be used for ventricular arrhythmias. Digoxin-specific Fab antibody treatment has been effective in animal models and human cases.[91,92]

MORNING GLORY SEEDS AND *IPOMOEA* SPECIES

Morning glory seeds (*Ipomoea violacea*, *Ipomoea tricolor*, and others) contain lysergic acid amide (ergine), a compound closely related to lysergic acid diethylamide. The seeds can be ingested for their hallucinogenic effects; typically several hundred seeds are ingested as one "dose." Physical and psychologic manifestations closely resemble the effects of lysergic acid diethylamide, and patients are managed similarly.

MYRISTICIN

Nutmeg is the dried seed from the tropical *Myristica fragrans* tree. Accidental or intentional ingestion of large amounts of nutmeg can cause delirium with hallucinations.[93] The hallucinogenic properties of nutmeg may be due to the component myristicin, but the mechanism is not well understood. Ingestion of one to three nutmegs or 5 to 15 grams of the ground spice produces psychologic effects that begin 3 to 6 hours later and lasts for 6 to 24 hours. Symptoms include tachycardia, flushing, dry mouth, nausea, and abdominal pain. Signs and symptoms may resemble anticholinergic poisoning, but pupils are usually small or midsized. Management is supportive care.

DATURA SPECIES

Jimson weed (*Datura stramonium*) and **angel's trumpet** (*Datura candida*) are plants that originated in the United States and Mexico but have spread worldwide throughout other areas with warm and temperate climates. All *Datura* species contain the anticholinergic alkaloids atropine, scopolamine, and hyoscyamine. Seeds or other parts of the plant can be ingested or smoked and produce delirium, hallucinations, and seizures along with other classic anticholinergic effects, such as mydriasis, tachycardia, dry mouth and skin, blurred vision, urinary retention, and hyperthermia (see chapter 202, Anticholinergics).[94,95] Gastric emptying is often delayed, and the small, plentiful seeds can become trapped among the gastrointestinal folds after ingestion; thus **gastric decontamination can be an important therapy.** Whole-bowel irrigation is also recommended for patients who have ingested a large number of seeds. Medications with anticholinergic properties, such as phenothiazines, should be avoided. Physostigmine, a reversible acetylcholine esterase antagonist, is effective treatment for severe anticholinergic poisoning.[95]

KETAMINE AND DEXTROMETHORPHAN

Ketamine and dextromethorphan are chemically related to phencyclidine. Ketamine and phencyclidine are described as dissociative drugs because they distort perceptions of sight and sound and produce feelings of detachment from the environment and self.[53,96] Ketamine, known by the street names "**vitamin K**" and "**special K**," can be abused by SC or IM injection, nasal insufflation of the dried powder, or smoking of the dried power admixed with marijuana or tobacco.[97] Ketamine abusers may come to the ED because of anxiety, palpitations, and chest pain.[98]

Dextromethorphan, available in over-the-counter cough-suppressant products, has become popular among adolescents.[99,100] A large quantity must be ingested for the user to experience hallucinogenic effects. Abuse among youths has prompted many states to enact restrictions regarding the age of the buyer and the maximum amount purchasable, and most retailers and pharmacists keep cough medicines containing dextromethorphan behind the counter. **Cold and cough products often contain other ingredients, such as antihistamines and acetaminophen, so investigate for toxic amounts of a co-ingestant in any patient who has ingested hallucinogenic doses of dextromethorphan.** Medical care is primarily supportive.

REFERENCES

The complete reference list is available online at www.TintinalliEM.com.

CHAPTER 189 Salicylates

Rachel Levitan
Frank Lovecchio

INTRODUCTION

The widespread availability of aspirin or acetylsalicylic acid in prescription and over-the-counter preparations can lead to both accidental and intentional toxicity. Morbidity and mortality increase significantly when the condition is not rapidly identified, if there is a delay to starting treatment, or if poisoned patients are not treated aggressively.

In additional to aspirin oral preparations, numerous forms of salicylate are available as karyolitic agents, liniments, flavoring agents, and combination products. These products may contain salicylate, methyl salicylate, or acetylsalicylic acid, but regardless of the product, all formulations are rapidly converted to salicylate once ingested.[1] Five mL of oil of wintergreen contains 7 g of aspirin and can be deadly to a toddler. Liniments and products used in hot vaporizers have high concentrations of methyl salicylate, and an ingestion of 5 to 10 mL can be lethal for an infant or a toddler.[2] Even though salicylate is poorly absorbed after ingestion of bismuth subsalicylate (Peptobismol®), significant exposures can occur from massive ingestions, such as in patients with human immunodeficiency virus/acquired immunodeficiency syndrome taking this medication for chronic diarrhea.[3]

PATHOPHYSIOLOGY

After ingestion of therapeutic doses in standard tablet formulation, absorption is variable and dependent on dosage form, presence of food, and gastric pH, with peak salicylate levels usually occurring in 1 to 2 hours. In overdose, peak serum salicylate concentrations may not be reached for hours. Enteric-coated aspirin exhibits erratic absorption in therapeutic doses, and peak levels may be delayed for hours after an overdose.[4] Salicylate itself impairs gastric emptying, which may account for delayed absorption in some cases[5] and create the potential for gastric bezoar formation, which can provide an additional source of ongoing absorption.[6] Ingestion of methyl salicylate or other liquid formulations may have much more rapid absorption and achieve peak levels more rapidly.

After absorption, aspirin is hydrolyzed to salicylic acid (salicylate) and is distributed throughout body tissues with 50% to 80% being bound to serum proteins. As salicylate concentrations increase and saturate protein-binding sites, free (unbound) concentrations of salicylate increase. In solution, salicylate exists in equilibrium between the ionized and nonionized state; only the unbound, nonionized salicylate can readily cross cell membranes. At physiologic pH (7.40), almost all salicylate is ionized, but acidemia will increase the nonionized fraction, enabling more salicylate to cross cell membranes and, importantly, substantially increasing brain salicylate concentration.[7] Patients with identical total salicylate serum concentrations may vary greatly in their degree of toxicity depending on their tissue burden, plasma protein concentrations, pH, and other factors.

Salicylate undergoes hepatic metabolism; however, this process rapidly becomes saturated even within the therapeutic ranges of drug use and changes to zero order kinetics; a set amount of salicylate is eliminated per unit of time.[8] Increased fraction of unbound salicylate also enhances renal clearance, making the kidney the major route of elimination during toxicity. Nonionized salicylate can be resorbed by renal tubules. Serum alkalinization can be used to keep salicylate in the plasma compartment and out of tissues, and urinary alkalinization can be used to enhance renal elimination. If the urine pH is above 7.5, more salicylate molecules in the urine will be ionized compared with the renal tubular cell pH of 7.4, and reabsorption across the urinary tubule will be reduced. This pH difference will also enhance secretion of nonionized salicylate down the concentration gradient.

Salicylate toxicity affects many physiologic systems (**Table 189-1**).

Salicylate directly stimulates the medullary respiratory center to produce tachypnea, hyperpnea, and respiratory alkalosis.[9] As toxicity worsens, inhibition of metabolism produces an acidosis that overwhelms the alkalosis. **Classically the acid-base disturbance associated with salicylate poisoning is mixed: early respiratory alkalosis, followed by an elevated anion gap metabolic acidosis, and possibly late respiratory acidosis.** Co-ingestion or administration of CNS depressants may blunt this initial respiratory stimulation. Salicylate stimulates skeletal muscle metabolism, which causes an increase in oxygen consumption and carbon dioxide production. Neurologic toxicity may impair ventilation so that it is unable to keep pace with increased carbon dioxide production, leading to respiratory acidosis—usually a late and ominous finding. Decreased ventilation can also be related to co-ingestions or iatrogenic medication.

TABLE 189-1 Pathophysiology of Salicylate Toxicity

Pathophysiology of Salicylate Toxicity
Local gastric irritation
Stimulation of the chemoreceptor zone
Stimulation of medullary respiratory center
Stimulation of skeletal muscle metabolism
Uncoupling of oxidative phosphorylation
Enhancement of lipolysis
Inhibition of Krebs cycle
Increased vascular permeability
Mobilization of glycogen stores
Inhibition of gluconeogenesis
Reversible ototoxicity

Salicylate affects both central and peripheral glucose homeostasis. Although salicylate causes mobilization of glycogen stores, resulting in hyperglycemia, it is also a potent inhibitor of gluconeogenesis. Therefore, normoglycemia is the most common finding, hyperglycemia can occur, and hypoglycemia is a rare possibility during toxicity.[10] Animal studies demonstrate that toxic doses of salicylate produce a profound decrease in brain glucose concentration despite normal serum glucose concentrations.[7,11] This suggests that a patient may be relatively neuroglucopenic even if the blood glucose is normal.

Salicylate can cause corrosive injury of the GI tract with abdominal pain, nausea, and vomiting and occasional hematemesis. This can all lead to volume loss, metabolic alkalosis, and hypokalemia. Gastric perforation has been reported after significant aspirin ingestion.[12] Salicylate-induced acute lung injury (noncardiogenic pulmonary edema) has been observed in humans. Antiplatelet activity is a well-known, often desired effect of aspirin (but not other salicylate products), but hemorrhage is a rare complication of acute, single, massive overdose. Large doses of all salicylates may cause significant hypoprothrombinemia resulting from inhibition of vitamin K–dependent functions.[13]

Salicylate ototoxicity is common, and tinnitus often occurs with levels >20 milligrams/dL (1.4 millimol/L). Although classically described as tinnitus or "ringing in the ears," in practice most patients will describe decreased sounds or that their hearing is "muffled." The exact mechanism causing this is unknown, and hearing effects are not permanent. Cardiac arrhythmias are a rare complication of salicylate poisoning.[14]

CLINICAL FEATURES

Clinical manifestations of salicylate toxicity depend on the dose ingested, duration of exposure, age, and comorbidities of the patient.[7,15] In children and the elderly, end-organ toxicity can be seen with smaller doses and lower serum levels following an acute overdose. Chronic toxicity can produce insidious and severe neurologic changes that do not correlate well with dose or serum salicylate level. Patients with even a mild toxicity can become critically and severely ill if acidemia or dehydration develops.

INTOXICATION IN CHILDREN

In general, when the duration of salicylate intoxication is between 12 to 24 hours, metabolic acidosis and acidemia (pH <7.35) occur primarily in children <4 years old, and nearly all children <1 year old have acidosis. Young children can have a respiratory alkalosis, but this is often transient and missed because of their smaller ventilatory reserves.[16] In older children (>4 years old), the acid-base disturbance is usually a mixed disturbance with respiratory alkalosis, increased anion gap metabolic acidosis, and alkalemia (pH >7.45).

Chronic or "therapeutic" (repeated dose) pediatric salicylate poisonings are more serious and are associated with a higher mortality than acute salicylism.[7,15,17] Often, several days may elapse between the initial salicylate administration and the onset of symptoms. There is frequently a coincidental illness that prompted salicylate administration, and children usually appear more ill than those with acute intoxication. The presenting features are usually fever, hyperventilation, and altered mental status with volume depletion, acidosis, and severe hypokalemia.[15] Young children are prone to hyperpyrexia, which indicates a worse prognosis.[17] Renal failure may be a significant complication, but pulmonary edema is unusual in the pediatric population.[15,17] Chronic salicylism is often mistaken for an infectious process, and the resultant delay in diagnosis may account for the more severe clinical picture.

The diagnosis may be delayed if a history of salicylate ingestion is not available. The differential diagnosis includes diabetic ketoacidosis, sepsis, iron intoxication, and toxic alcohol poisoning.

INTOXICATION IN ADULTS

Acute salicylate intoxication in adults is often due to intentional ingestion. The typical clinical presentation includes nausea, vomiting, tinnitus, hearing loss, sweating, and hyperventilation. Patients with tinnitus or hearing loss following an acute ingestion usually have an elevated serum salicylate value.[18]

Most adult patients with acute salicylate overdose have a mixed acid-base disturbance of alkalemia with respiratory alkalosis and metabolic acidosis. As toxicity progresses, acidosis worsens. CNS dysfunction manifests as agitation, lethargy, confusion, seizure, or coma. CNS dysfunction leading to cerebral edema is an ominous development and a sign of severe toxicity, requiring rapid and aggressive treatment.[7,19] Despite treatment and decreasing serum salicylate levels, patients may worsen and die from progressive neurologic impairment, possibly because of increasing CNS salicylate levels.

Salicylate-induced vomiting can produce a metabolic alkalosis. Other rare complications of salicylate toxicity include rhabdomyolysis, gastric perforation, and GI hemorrhage. Poor prognostic factors for acute salicylate toxicity include coma, fever, respiratory acidosis, seizure, and cardiac dysrhythmias.

Chronic salicylate intoxication (from repeated excessive dosing) in adults often presents with neurologic abnormalities such as lethargy, altered mental status, irritability, and hallucinations, particularly in the elderly.[20] Toxicity can develop even with small increases in doses due to saturable kinetics. Clinical features of chronic intoxication include hyperventilation, tremor, papilledema, agitation, paranoia, bizarre behavior, memory deficits, confusion, and stupor. Nausea and vomiting are less common than in acute salicylate toxicity, whereas increased liver function tests and increased prothrombin time are more common. Neurologic abnormalities in chronic salicylate poisoning may be nonspecific and may often mislead physicians. Chronic salicylism should be considered in a patient with unexplained neurologic or behavioral dysfunction, especially in the presence of a mixed acid-base disturbance, tachypnea, dyspnea, or unexplained pulmonary edema.[21] Compared with acute toxicity, adults with chronic salicylate toxicity have a higher tissue burden of salicylate leading to more significant toxicity at a lower serum concentration.

The distinction between acute and chronic salicylate toxicity may not always be clear. A patient may present many hours after an acute severe salicylate overdose, when altered mental status, acidosis, elevated prothrombin time, and a "therapeutic" serum salicylate concentration appear more consistent with a chronically poisoned patient. Significant toxicity may be evident despite declining or "therapeutic" serum salicylate concentrations. In these situations, the patient's clinical status is most important when assessing the severity of toxicity (**Table 189-2**).

Chronic salicylism may develop in patients taking carbonic anhydrase inhibitors for treatment of glaucoma. The normal anion gap (hyperchloremic) metabolic acidosis produced by carbonic anhydrase inhibitors increases the volume of distribution for salicylate and facilitates its entry into the CNS, causing toxicity at a "therapeutic" serum salicylate concentration.

The differential diagnosis of a triple-mixed acid-base disturbance of increased anion gap acidosis, metabolic alkalosis, and respiratory alkalosis seen in salicylate toxicity is limited. However, in clinical practice or at early stages of toxicity, this classic acid-base disturbance may be difficult to appreciate. The differential is very broad and includes but is not limited to sepsis, diabetic ketoacidosis, renal and hepatic failure, alcoholic ketoacidosis, poisoning by methanol and ethylene glycol, iron, theophylline, and caffeine.

TABLE 189-2 Severity Grading of Salicylate Toxicity in Adults

	Mild	Moderate	Severe
Acute ingestion (dose)	<150 milligrams/kg	150–300 milligrams/kg	>300 milligrams/kg
End-organ toxicity	Tinnitus Hearing loss Dizziness Nausea/vomiting	Tachypnea Hyperpyrexia Diaphoresis Ataxia Anxiety	Abnormal mental status Seizures Acute lung injury Renal failure Cardiac arrhythmias Shock

DIAGNOSIS

Diagnosis of salicylate toxicity is made by correlating a careful history, physical examination, and thoughtful ancillary testing. Supportive laboratory findings include an anion-gap metabolic acidosis and elevated serum salicylate levels. **The Done nomogram is misleading and can grossly underestimate toxicity; it *should not be used.***

TOXICOLOGIC TESTING

A pitfall in treating salicylate toxicity is reliance on a single serum level. Salicylate toxicity can evolve rapidly. In patients with moderate or severe poisoning, it is prudent to obtain serial serum salicylate concentrations approximately every 1 to 2 hours, until the concentrations are declining and the patient's clinical status stabilizes.[22,23] Enteric-coated or modified-release preparations are formulated to remain intact in the acidic gastric environment but to dissolve in the alkaline intestinal fluids. Drug release is therefore primarily a function of gastric emptying, and peak levels may not be reached until up to 60 hours after ingestion in an overdose.[4]

Commercially available tests can qualitatively detect salicylate in the urine, but these tests have limitations, and a qualitative level does not help determine whether the patient is therapeutic or intoxicated with salicylate and cannot help guide treatment. Similarly, the ferric chloride test is very sensitive to small quantities of salicylic acid, but a positive test result does not indicate salicylate poisoning or toxicity. Serum salicylate levels should always be obtained in patients with salicylate or suspected salicylate toxicity.

Commercially available tests for serum salicylate concentration are very accurate; the only reported significant interference has been with diflunisal (a nonsteroidal anti-inflammatory drug), which produces false-positive results for significantly high serum salicylate concentrations.[24] Another pitfall is that units for measuring salicylate are not universal. Traditionally stated in milligrams/dL, measurement units can vary by laboratory and institution, with the potential for patients to be mistakenly diagnosed as "salicylate toxic" if the physician mistakenly assumes the unit of measurement used.

ADDITIONAL ANCILLARY TESTING

Essential laboratory tests include electrolytes, glucose, BUN, and creatinine. Arterial blood gases, chest and abdominal radiograph, ECG, CBC, serum calcium level, and urinalysis with urine pH determination should be obtained as clinically indicated. As in any ingestion, consider testing for acetaminophen as well, especially considering the number of combination products available in the market. Some enteric-coated medications are radiopaque and may be visible on an abdominal radiograph.[25]

A normal anion gap does not exclude salicylate toxicity in patients with an unknown ingestion. Mixed ingestions that include aspirin and the timing of exposure can alter "classic" metabolic disturbances. A negative anion gap metabolic acidosis may be noted in salicylate toxicity due to aberrant reading of salicylate ions as chloride ions by analyzer electrodes.[26]

TREATMENT

GENERAL MEASURES

Treatment priorities are (1) immediate resuscitation with stabilization of airway, breathing, and circulation; (2) correction of volume depletion and metabolic derangements; (3) GI decontamination; and (4) reduction in body salicylate burden.[22,23] Salicylate absorption is reduced by the administration of activated charcoal both for regular and modified-release formulations. A single dose of activated charcoal, 1 to 2 grams/kg, should be administered to appropriate patients who have ingested potentially toxic amounts of salicylate.[22,27,28] There are no convincing data to support the use of repeated or multiple doses of activated charcoal in salicylate overdose.[29]

Patients with severe salicylate intoxication are usually significantly volume depleted, have serious acid-base disturbances, and require aggressive IV volume and electrolyte replacement. Careful assessment of a patient's volume and electrolyte status is important, particularly in the elderly or in patients with a history of cardiac disease. Volume replacement is initially undertaken with normal saline or lactated Ringer's with administration of an initial bolus of 20 mL/kg. The average adult who presents several hours after ingestion is dehydrated by at least 4 to 6 L.

ALKALINIZATION

Systemic and urinary alkalinization are beneficial for salicylate toxicity, although the precise mechanism is debated.[23,30] As initial fluid resuscitation is undertaken, patients should undergo treatment with sodium bicarbonate with a goal of a serum pH of ~7.5. Hypokalemia is common, and potassium should be added to the infusion after adequate urine output has been established. Serum potassium should be maintained in the 4.0 to 4.5 mEq/L range.

Urinary salicylate clearance is directly proportional to urine flow rate, but, more importantly, it is logarithmically proportional to urine pH.[30] Urine alkalinization is more effective in enhancing salicylate elimination than forced diuresis and avoids the potential complication of fluid overload that may result from the large intravenous volume given to increase urine flow, especially in those with marginal cardiac reserve or cardiac performance. Urinary alkalinization should be considered as first-line treatment for patients with moderately severe salicylate poisoning.[22,31]

Hydration and alkalinization should be initiated simultaneously in patients with severe salicylate intoxication. A common approach is to volume restore patients with normal saline or lactated Ringer's to a target urine output of 1 to 2 mL/kg per hour. Concurrently, in a second IV line, an IV bolus of sodium bicarbonate (1 to 2 mEq/kg) is given followed by a continuous infusion (three ampules of either 44 or 50 mEq/ampule of sodium bicarbonate added to 1 L of 5% dextrose in water). Unless there is a contraindication, potassium should be added to the bicarbonate fluid as well. The infusion is run at two to three times maintenance and adjusted to maintain the urine pH >7.5 (**Figure 189-1**).

In moderate and severe overdoses, the patient's cardiopulmonary and neurologic status should be assessed frequently. Serum salicylate, urine pH, and electrolyte concentrations should be checked every 1 to 2 hours.[22,23] Once the serum salicylate concentration peaks and begins to decrease on serial measurement, repeat measurement can be obtained every 4 to 6 hours.

OTHER MEASURES

Patients with salicylate-induced acute lung injury (noncardiogenic pulmonary edema) should be managed as are patients with acute lung injury from other causes. Pulmonary edema begins to improve concomitantly with the lowering of serum salicylate concentrations. This suggests that aggressive efforts toward rapid elimination by hemodialysis may be beneficial in this subset of patients.[32] In addition, early hemodialysis enables removal of salicylate without the volume challenge that accompanies sodium bicarbonate administration, and it avoids the possibility of aggravating lung injury.

When a patient with severe salicylate toxicity requires endotracheal intubation, mechanical ventilation, and sedation, it is important to maintain hyperventilation; ventilator settings should not be based on standard age- and weight-based nomograms. Before intubation and mechanical ventilation, most patients with severe salicylate toxicity have a respiratory alkalosis. Controlling the ventilatory rate and volume to "normal" ranges produces a decrease in serum pH and causes a rapid shift of salicylate into the CNS. It is important to maintain respiratory alkalosis during

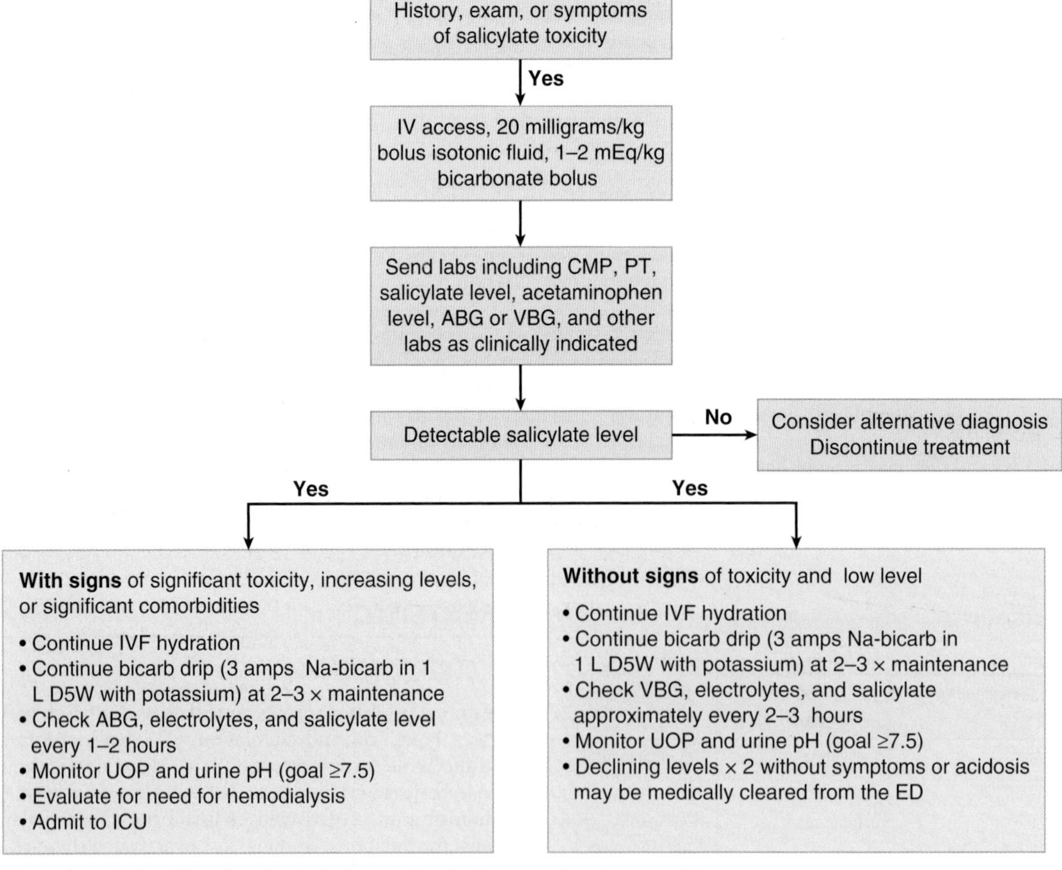

FIGURE 189-1. Management of salicylate poisoning. ABG = arterial blood gas; bicarb = bicarbonate; CMP = comprehensive metabolic panel; D5W = 5% dextrose in water; ICU = intensive care unit; IVF = intravenous fluids; PT = prothrombin time; UOP = urinary output; VBG = venous blood gas.

mechanical ventilation. Use the minimal amount of safe sedation that allows a patient to continue over-breathing the ventilator. Consider one to two ampules (88 to 100 mEq) of bicarbonate bolus immediately prior to intubation as a basic buffer for the transient decrease in ventilation that occurs during rapid-sequence induction intubation.

Hemorrhagic complications are rarely seen following single massive salicylate overdoses, but chronic administration of large doses may cause significant hypoprothrombinemia. However, even in this circumstance, hemorrhage is rarely seen in clinical practice or in animal experiments. When bleeding does occur, it rarely appears to be a contributing factor in mortality from salicylate toxicity. Patients with clinically significant bleeding should be treated with fresh frozen plasma. Observations in animals and humans indicate that administering large doses of vitamin K after the development of hypoprothrombinemia has little or no effect on the prothrombin time when serum salicylate concentration is high.

HEMODIALYSIS

Hemodialysis is considered the extracorporeal technique of choice for the treatment of serious salicylate toxicity because hemodialysis can correct acid-base and electrolyte abnormalities while rapidly reducing the body salicylate burden.[33,34] Anticipating the possible need for hemodialysis, thoughtful planning and prompt consultation with the nephrology service are strongly advised because of intrinsic delays to its immediate implementation. **Indications for hemodialysis include clinical deterioration or failure of improvement despite intensive supportive care, lack of success in establishing an alkalinization of serum and urine, renal insufficiency or renal failure, severe acid-base disturbance, altered mental status, and patients with acute lung injury. Consider hemodialysis for salicylism requiring respiratory and ventilatory support.**[34]

Serum salicylate concentration should not be the sole determinant in the decision to initiate hemodialysis; however, patients with acute toxicity and serum salicylate concentrations >100 milligrams/dL (>7.2 millimol/L), chronic patients with concentrations >60 milligrams/dL, (>4.3 millimol/L) and symptomatic patients with lower serum salicylate concentrations should be considered candidates for hemodialysis. Consider the early use of hemodialysis in patients who are elderly, have chronically ingested aspirin, have altered mental status, have acidemia, or have comorbidities (e.g., coronary artery disease or chronic obstructive pulmonary disease).

Emergency hemodialysis places a significant demand on the cardiovascular system, and hypotensive patients or those with underlying cardiac disease may not be able to tolerate the hemodynamic intensity of 4-hour hemodialysis treatments. Less demanding but a longer therapy, such as hemofiltration, hemodiafiltration, or sustained low-efficiency dialysis, may be used until hemodialysis can be tolerated. Once initiated, extracorporeal elimination techniques should be continued until the serum salicylate level is <20 milligrams/dL (<1.4 millimol/L).

DISPOSITION AND FOLLOW-UP

A patient may be discharged from the ED once it can be determined that the patient had an inconsequential salicylate overdose; and this requires demonstration of serial declining salicylate levels. Patients who have overdosed on enteric-coated or modified-release preparations of aspirin should be treated regardless of initial serum salicylate concentrations and be observed for approximately 24 hours, with serial serum salicylate concentrations until a declining level is confirmed. Salsalate overdoses may warrant an even longer period of observation.[35] Although the determination of serial salicylate concentrations offers valuable information regarding the effectiveness of the treatment implemented, it is not a substitute for clinical evaluation of a patient, and management decisions should not be solely based on a particular serum salicylate concentration. Early consultation with a clinical toxicologist or the regional poison control center is recommended.

REFERENCES

The complete reference list is available online at www.TintinalliEM.com.

Acetaminophen

Oliver L. Hung
Lewis S. Nelson

INTRODUCTION AND EPIDEMIOLOGY

Acetaminophen (*N*-acetyl-*p*-aminophenol or paracetamol) is the most popular over-the-counter analgesic and is one of the most common toxic exposures reported to poison centers. Acetaminophen is available as a sole agent or combined with a variety of other medications prepared in many different forms, such as tablets, capsules, gels, and liquids. Poisonings often occur because of the erroneous belief that this medication is benign or because the victim was unaware that acetaminophen was an ingredient in the ingested preparation.[1] The U.S. Acute Liver Failure Study Group found that acetaminophen poisoning was the cause of acute liver failure in 18% of cases initially judged to be of unknown cause.[2] Acetaminophen–opioid combination products have been implicated in chronic overuse, likely due to an increasing opioid requirement leading to concomitantly increasing acetaminophen exposure. In response to these safety concerns, the U.S. Food and Drug Administration recently limited the prescription acetaminophen–opioid combination preparation strength to 325 milligrams per dosage unit and now requires a boxed warning to notify consumers of the potential risk for serious liver toxicity.[3]

During 2010, the American Association of Poison Control Centers received reports of 66,473 exposures to acetaminophen–opioid combinations and 73,307 exposures to acetaminophen alone.[4] There were 65 deaths attributed to isolated ingestions of acetaminophen combinations and 60 deaths attributed to isolated acetaminophen ingestions.[4] Combining ED, hospital, and poisoning databases, an estimated 450 deaths occur each year in the United States due to acetaminophen overdose, and approximately 100 of them are unintentional, primarily due to supratherapeutic dosing of child preparations.[5]

PHARMACOLOGY AND DOSING

ORAL ACETAMINOPHEN

The recommended maximum total daily dose is 3900 milligrams in adults using 325-milligram acetaminophen (regular strength) and 3000 milligrams when using the 500-milligram acetaminophen (extra strength) preparation. Adults should not use acetaminophen for more than 10 consecutive days unless directed by their physician. **For children, the recommended acetaminophen dose is 10 to 15 milligrams/kg every 4 to 6 hours as needed, with a maximum daily dose of 75 milligrams/kg or five doses in a 24-hour period.** In 2011, the infant acetaminophen formulation (80 milligrams/0.8 mL concentration) was discontinued to minimize the risk for medication error. All pediatric, both infant and child, acetaminophen liquid preparations are now standardized to a concentration of 160 milligrams/5 mL.

Patients with insufficient glutathione stores (e.g., alcoholics and acquired immunodeficiency syndrome patients) and patients with induced cytochrome P-450 enzymatic activity (e.g., alcoholics and those taking concurrent anticonvulsant or antituberculous medications) may be at greater risk for developing acetaminophen-induced hepatotoxicity following overdose (as opposed to therapeutic dosing described earlier). Although the evidence supporting this risk is not definitive, it may be prudent to reduce acetaminophen dosage for this population. In contrast, children, because of their greater ability to metabolize acetaminophen through hepatic sulfation, may be at decreased risk for developing hepatotoxicity following a moderate overdose.[6,7]

After ingestion of therapeutic doses, acetaminophen is rapidly absorbed from the GI tract, and peak serum concentrations are usually achieved within 30 minutes to 2 hours. In an overdose, peak serum concentrations are usually achieved within 2 hours, but delayed absorption of acetaminophen occurs following overdoses of preparations in which acetaminophen is combined with propoxyphene or diphenhydramine, as well as those with altered-release kinetics such as extended-release preparations.[8-11] In therapeutic amounts, acetaminophen has nearly 100% bioavailability, is approximately 20% bound to serum proteins, has a volume of distribution of around 0.85 L/kg, and has an elimination half-life of approximately 2.5 hours. The therapeutic concentration for the antipyretic effect of acetaminophen is between 10 and 20 micrograms/mL (66 to 132 micromoles/L), but therapeutic concentrations for analgesia are not established.

Oral acetaminophen appears to be nontoxic when administered following therapeutic dosing guidelines. Both retrospective and prospective studies have yielded inconsistent results concerning the risk of acute liver injury with repeated use of therapeutic acetaminophen doses.[12] The prospective studies, which are better controlled than the retrospective ones, find a slight increase in liver injury but no evidence of increased hepatic failure or death when using therapeutic acetaminophen doses for sustained periods.[13] For **alcoholic patients**, no evidence of liver injury was seen when treated with the recommended maximal daily dose of acetaminophen for 3 consecutive days.[14,15]

IV ACETAMINOPHEN

An **IV acetaminophen** formulation was approved by the U.S. Food and Drug Administration in 2010 for adults and children 2 years of age or older. The recommended dosing of IV acetaminophen for adults or children weighing more than 50 kg is 650 milligrams every 4 hours or 1000 milligrams every 6 hours, with a maximum total daily dose of 4 grams. For adults or children weighing less than 50 kg, the recommended dosing is 12.5 milligrams/kg every 4 hours or 15 milligrams/kg every 6 hours (maximum individual dose of 750 milligrams), with a maximum total daily dose of 75 milligrams/kg or 3750 milligrams. Peak concentrations following IV administration occur at the end of the 15-minute infusion period.[16] Compared to a similar dose of oral acetaminophen, IV acetaminophen achieves a 70% greater maximum concentration but provides a similar total drug exposure.[16]

ACETAMINOPHEN METABOLISM

In therapeutic amounts, acetaminophen is primarily metabolized by the liver through sulfation (20% to 46%) and glucuronidation (40% to 67%), with <5% undergoing direct renal elimination. Normally, a small percentage is also oxidized by the cytochrome P-450 system to a reactive metabolite, *N*-acetyl-*p*-benzoquinoneimine (**NAPQI**). This is quickly detoxified by hepatic glutathione to a nontoxic acetaminophen-mercapturate compound that is renally eliminated (**Figure 190-1**). After acetaminophen overdose, hepatic metabolism through glucuronidation and sulfation may be saturated, and a larger proportion of acetaminophen is therefore metabolized by cytochrome P-450 to NAPQI, depleting intracellular glutathione. When hepatic stores of glutathione decrease to <30% of normal, NAPQI binds to other hepatic macromolecules, and hepatic necrosis ensues. Although the clinical manifestations of acetaminophen toxicity are classically delayed, hepatic injury actually occurs early, within 12 hours of exposure.

Within the hepatic lobule, cytochrome P-450 is concentrated within hepatocytes surrounding the terminal hepatic vein and is least concentrated within hepatocytes surrounding the portal triad. As a result, acetaminophen-induced hepatic injury develops in the characteristic pattern of centrilobular necrosis. Hepatic injury can be identified by microscopic evidence as well as immunofluorescent staining of NAPQI-hepatic protein adducts within hepatocytes. Observed hepatocyte damage typically progresses with cell lysis on the second day after an acute toxic exposure, releasing hepatic enzymes, such as transaminases, and NAPQI-hepatic protein adducts into the circulation where they are detectable in the serum. This corresponds generally to the development of overt clinical toxicity.

CLINICAL FEATURES OF ACETAMINOPHEN TOXICITY

The initial clinical findings of acetaminophen toxicity are nonspecific and delayed in onset.

FOUR STAGES OF ACETAMINOPHEN TOXICITY

The clinical presentation of human acetaminophen poisoning can be roughly divided into four stages (**Table 190-1**). During the first 24 hours after exposure (stage 1), patients often have minimal and nonspecific symptoms of toxicity, such as anorexia, nausea, vomiting, and malaise. **Hypokalemia and metabolic acidosis** may be seen during the first 24 hours and correlate with a high 4-hour acetaminophen concentration.[17-20] By days 2 to 3 (stage 2), symptoms seen in stage 1 often improve, but clinical signs of hepatotoxicity may occur, including right upper quadrant abdominal pain and tenderness, with elevated serum transaminases. Even without treatment, most patients with mild to moderate hepatotoxicity recover without sequelae. However, by days 3 to 4 (stage 3), some patients will progress to fulminant hepatic failure.[21,22] Characteristic stage 3 findings include metabolic acidosis, coagulopathy, renal failure, encephalopathy, and recurrent GI symptoms. Patients who survive the complications of fulminant hepatic failure begin to recover over the next 2 weeks (stage 4), with complete resolution of hepatic dysfunction in survivors after 1 to 3 months.

Acetaminophen may also cause acute, extrahepatic toxic effects, presumably because of the presence of cytochrome P-450 or similar enzymes (e.g., prostaglandin H synthase) in other organs. Ingestion of massive doses of acetaminophen (e.g., 4-hour acetaminophen concentrations >800 micrograms/mL or >5300 micromoles/L) is associated with the altered sensorium and a metabolic acidosis with an elevated lactate that can occur in the absence of either liver failure or hypotension.[23] Renal insufficiency occurs in 1% to 2% of patients following acetaminophen overdose, usually after hepatic failure is evident.[24-26] In rare cases, isolated renal injury, cardiac toxicity, and pancreatitis may occur.[27,28]

DIAGNOSIS

Acute acetaminophen poisoning is diagnosed by the serum acetaminophen concentration and estimating the time since ingestion.

A toxic exposure to acetaminophen is suggested when a patient ≥6 years old ingests (1) >10 grams or 200 milligrams/kg as a single ingestion, (2) >10 grams or 200 milligrams/kg over a 24-hour period, or (3) >6 grams or 150 milligrams/kg per 24-hour period for at least 2 consecutive days. For children <6 years old, ingestion of 200 milligrams/kg or more of acetaminophen as a single ingestion or over an 8-hour period, or of 150 milligrams/kg per 24-hour period for the preceding 48 hours is considered a toxic exposure. These values are empiric and not validated in human trials, but they are widely used as recommendations for emergency evaluation. Even though a patient's history of the amount ingested may be unreliable, a patient report of >10 to 12 grams ingested was associated with a 4-hour acetaminophen concentration above 150 micrograms/mL (1000 micromoles/L) in 40% to 70% of toxic exposures.[29,30]

Due to the widespread availability of acetaminophen-containing products, the delayed clinical manifestations after overdose, and the serious complications of acute toxicity without antidotal therapy, **measurement of a serum acetaminophen concentration is recommended for all patients presenting to the ED with an intentional overdose.**[31,32] Potentially toxic acetaminophen levels have been seen in ED overdose patients who denied ingesting acetaminophen.[33,34] Empirical testing of all patients with intentional overdoses may be cost-effective, as the estimated cost of treating a single patient for complications of acetaminophen-induced hepatotoxicity is judged to outweigh the cost of routine laboratory testing all intentional overdose patients. A qualitative acetaminophen urine screen can also be used to identify potential acetaminophen overdose patients.[35]

THE RUMACK-MATTHEW NOMOGRAM

The implication of a measured acetaminophen concentration is determined by plotting the value on the Rumack-Matthew nomogram (**Figure 190-2**).[36] This nomogram was derived from a retrospective analysis of oral acetaminophen overdose patients and their clinical outcomes. The original nomogram line separating possible toxicity from unlikely toxicity was based on a 4-hour acetaminophen concentration of

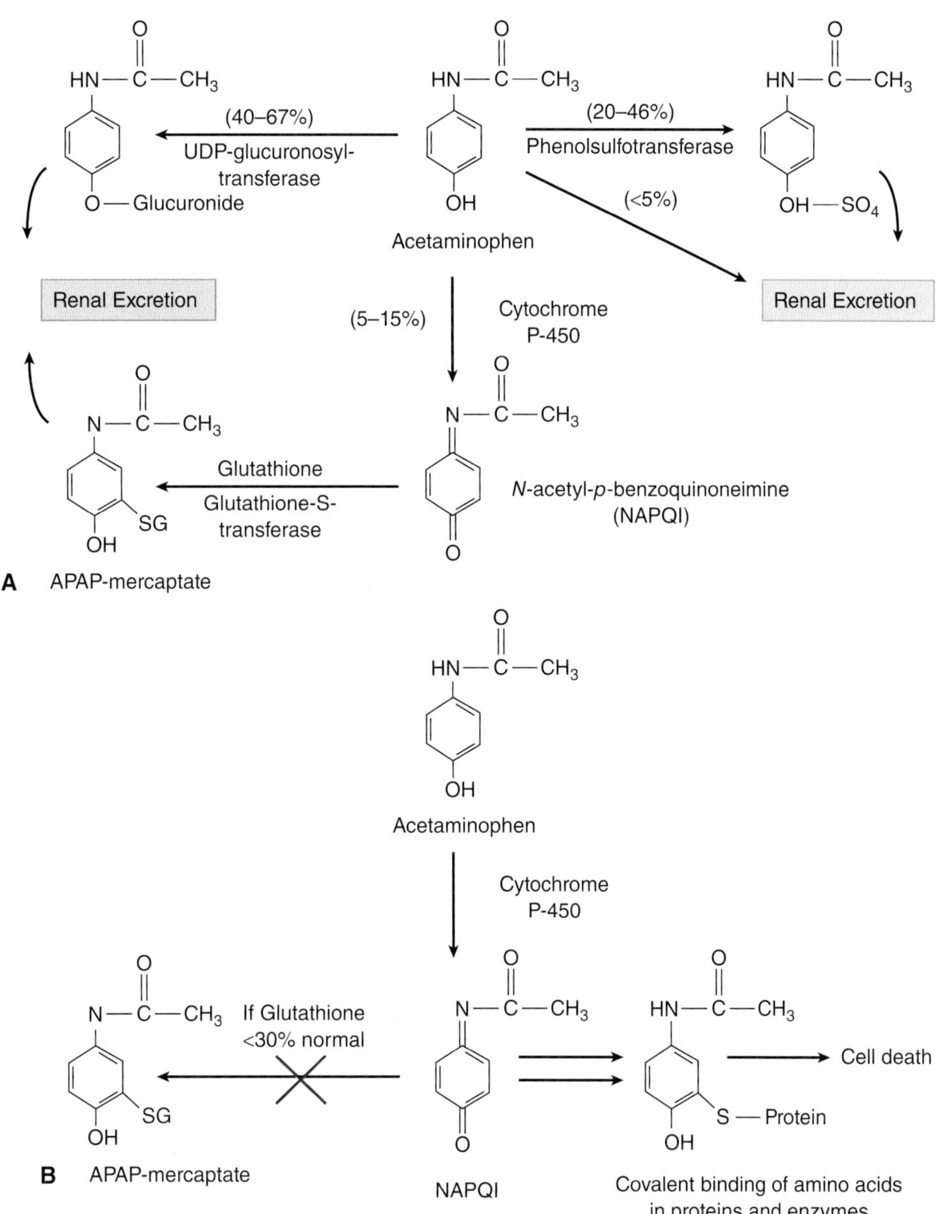

FIGURE 190-1. Acetaminophen metabolism. **A.** After ingestion of therapeutic amounts, predominant metabolism is via glucuronidation and sulfation. The small amount of *N*-acetyl-*p*-benzoquinoneimine (NAPQI) generated is conjugated with glutathione to a nontoxic compound. **B.** After ingestion of large amounts, glucuronidation and sulfation are saturated, and an increased amount of NAPQI is generated. Detoxification of NAPQI to a nontoxic compound soon depletes glutathione stores, leaving excess NAPQI to bind to intracellular proteins, causing cell death. APAP = *N*-acetyl-*p*-aminophenol (acetaminophen).

TABLE 190-1 Clinical Stages of Acute Acetaminophen Toxicity

	Stage 1	Stage 2	Stage 3	Stage 4
Timing	First 24 h	Days 2–3	Days 3–4	After day 5
Clinical manifestations	Anorexia Nausea Vomiting Malaise	Improvement in anorexia, nausea, and vomiting Abdominal pain Hepatic tenderness	Recurrence of anorexia, nausea, and vomiting Encephalopathy Anuria Jaundice	Clinical improvement and recovery (7–8 d) *or* Deterioration to multi-organ failure and death
Laboratory abnormalities	Hypokalemia	Elevated serum transaminases Elevated bilirubin and prolonged prothrombin time if severe	Hepatic failure Metabolic acidosis Coagulopathy Renal failure Pancreatitis	Improvement and resolution *or* Continued deterioration

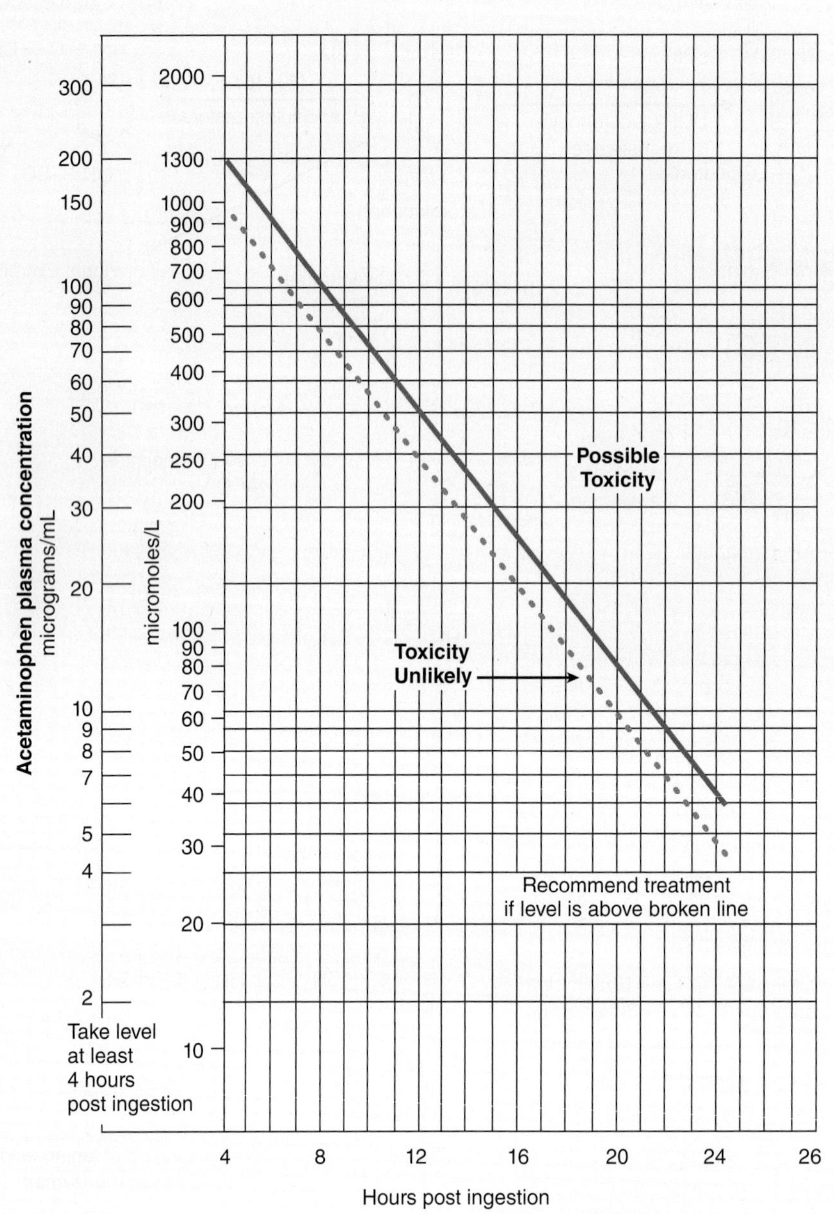

FIGURE 190-2. Rumack-Matthew nomogram.

200 micrograms/mL (1300 micromoles/L), but was subsequently modified by moving the line to a 4-hour acetaminophen concentration of 150 micrograms/mL (1000 micromoles/L) to increase the safety margin for treatment decisions. **The nomogram only directly applies to an acetaminophen concentration obtained after a single oral exposure and during the window between 4 hours and 24 hours postingestion.** Outcome prediction using this nomogram cannot be applied to acetaminophen concentrations obtained outside this 20-hour window or with chronic or recurrent exposures. Obtaining multiple acetaminophen concentrations following acute overdose is rarely indicated in the absence of hepatotoxicity.[37,38] An initial concentration below the nomogram line may rarely "cross the line" in patients who ingest acetaminophen preparations known to have prolonged absorption kinetics.[11] However, the clinical significance of "crossing the line" in this fashion is unknown. Similarly, because the nomogram was constructed and verified by using only a single serum concentration, the clinical implications of a concentration above the line that falls below it on repeat analysis are unknown.

Based on data obtained before the widespread use of antidotal therapy, patients with serum acetaminophen concentrations above the original line (4-hour postingestion concentration >200 micrograms/mL or >1300 micromoles/L) were observed to have a 60% risk of developing hepatotoxicity (defined as alanine aminotransferase >1000 IU/mL), a 1% risk of renal failure, and a 5% risk of mortality.[39] In addition, patients with extremely high serum acetaminophen concentrations (above a parallel line coinciding with a 4-hour postingestion concentration of 300 micrograms/mL or 2000 micromoles/L) were observed to have a 90% risk of developing hepatotoxicity. The prediction of a safe outcome below the nomogram line corresponding to a 4-hour postingestion concentration of 150 micrograms/mL (1000 micromoles/L) was confirmed in patients who did not receive antidotal therapy; the incidence of hepatotoxicity in patients with acetaminophen concentrations below this nomogram line was 1%, and all patients recovered without complications.[38]

A method to determine potential toxicity from IV acetaminophen overdose has not been established. Fortunately, the European experience with IV acetaminophen suggests that these overdoses appear to be rare in-hospital occurrences that are likely to occur following an error in calculating the acetaminophen dose in pediatric patients.[40-42] However, the available clinical data for evaluating IV acetaminophen overdose remain limited to several published case reports.[42] Because the Rumack-Matthew nomogram was solely derived from oral acetaminophen overdose patients, strictly applying the nomogram to determine toxicity following IV acetaminophen overdose may not be appropriate at this time.

TREATMENT

GI DECONTAMINATION

Treatment of acetaminophen poisoning consists primarily of the timely use of the antidote acetylcysteine and supportive care.[1,36,37] For most cases of acetaminophen poisoning, adequate GI decontamination consists of the early administration of activated charcoal orally or through a nasogastric tube.[1,43,44] Inducing emesis by administering ipecac syrup is undesirable because it delays the administration of the oral antidote. In addition, more aggressive forms of decontamination, such as gastric lavage or whole-bowel irrigation, are unnecessary because of the rapid GI absorption of acetaminophen and the great success of treating acetaminophen poisoning with acetylcysteine.

ACETYLCYSTEINE

The mainstay for the prevention or treatment of acetaminophen toxicity is the administration of acetylcysteine.[1,45-47] The current "standard" acetylcysteine protocols were developed from primarily observational trials, and it is not clear if they represent the most effective regimens.[48]

Although its mechanisms of action are not fully understood, acetylcysteine is thought to have two important beneficial effects.[47,48] In early acetaminophen poisoning (<8 hours after ingestion), acetylcysteine averts toxicity by preventing the binding of NAPQI to hepatic macromolecules. Acetylcysteine may do this by acting as a glutathione precursor or substitute, or a sulfate precursor, or it may directly reduce NAPQI back to acetaminophen. In established acetaminophen toxicity or >24 hours after acetaminophen ingestion, acetylcysteine diminishes hepatic necrosis by acting as an antioxidant, decreasing neutrophil infiltration, improving microcirculatory blood flow, or increasing tissue oxygen delivery and extraction.

If acetylcysteine is given within 8 hours of an acute acetaminophen ingestion, it is nearly 100% effective in preventing the development of hepatotoxicity.[39] The longer the initiation of acetylcysteine therapy is delayed beyond 8 hours after ingestion, the greater the risk of developing hepatotoxicity.[49] **Even up to 24 hours following acetaminophen ingestion, however, acetylcysteine treatment is associated with a lower risk of hepatotoxicity than historical controls.**[39]

Clinical experience suggests that patients with poor glutathione reserves, such as alcoholics and the chronically ill, have similar excellent clinical outcomes when the standard treatment guidelines are applied to their care. As such, there is no need to alter the use of the acetaminophen treatment nomogram or modify the dosing of acetylcysteine for these patients.

The weight of evidence suggests that **acetylcysteine therapy is both safe and efficacious during pregnancy** and that the approach to treating a pregnant patient following an acetaminophen overdose should remain the same. Although an ovine model demonstrated that acetylcysteine is unable to cross the placenta, there are data in humans establishing that it does.[50] Acetylcysteine treatment has never been associated with fetal malformations in humans, but fetal demise and malformations have been described following delayed acetylcysteine treatment after acetaminophen overdose in first-trimester pregnant women.[51]

IV Acetylcysteine IV acetylcysteine has been used to supplant oral administration due to its greater ease of administration, greater patient acceptance, equivalent efficacy, and shorter duration of treatment for many cases of acetaminophen poisoning.[52-55] The major limitation of IV acetylcysteine is the occurrence of drug-related anaphylactoid reactions (occurring during the first 2 hours of administration), which in mild cases is treated with diphenhydramine and in severe cases is treated by temporarily slowing/stopping the acetylcysteine infusion.[56] The risk of anaphylactoid reaction from IV acetylcysteine ranges from 4% to 17%.[57-60] Asthmatics appear to have a greater risk of anaphylactoid reactions during IV acetylcysteine therapy, whereas overdose patients with high acetaminophen concentrations appear to have a lower risk of developing anaphylactoid reactions.[59-62] Approximately 13% of patients treated with IV acetylcysteine develop nausea and vomiting.[63] Rare complications, including status epilepticus, hemolytic uremic syndrome, cerebral edema, and death, have been reported following massive overdose of IV acetylcysteine.[64-67]

The standard regimen for IV acetylcysteine utilizes a 20-hour protocol with a loading dose of 150 milligrams/kg over 15 minutes to 1 hour, followed by a first maintenance dose of 50 milligrams/kg infused over 4 hours, and then followed by a second maintenance dose of 100 milligrams/kg infused over 16 hours (**Table 190-2**). Administering the initial dose over an hour appears to minimize the incidence of drug-related adverse effects, particularly anaphylactoid responses, although this belief has not been substantiated when prospectively studied.[58] Because the three-phase dosing regimen for IV acetylcysteine may result in dosing errors and produce side effects due to the initial high infusion rate, alternative dosing regimens are being explored.[68-70]

TABLE 190-2 Acetylcysteine Dosing Regimens

	Oral	IV Adult	IV Pediatric (<40 kg)
Preparation	Available as 10% and 20% solutions. Dilute to 5% solution for oral administration.	Available as 20% solution.	Available as 20% solution. Dilute to 2% solution by mixing 50 mL in 450 mL 5% dextrose in water.
Loading dose	140 milligrams/kg.	150 milligrams/kg in 200 mL 5% dextrose in water infused over 15–60 min.	150 milligrams/kg (7.5 mL/kg) infused over 15–60 min.
Maintenance dose	70 milligrams/kg every 4 h for 17 doses.	50 milligrams/kg in 500 mL 5% dextrose in water infused over 4 h (12.5 milligrams/kg per hour). *followed by* 100 milligrams/kg in 1000 mL 5% dextrose in water infused over 16 h (6.25 milligrams/kg per hour).	50 milligrams/kg (2.5 mL/kg) infused over 4 h (12.5 milligrams/kg per hour). *followed by* 100 milligrams/kg (5 mL/kg) infused over 16 h (6.25 milligrams/kg per hour).
Duration of therapy	72 h.	20 h.	20 h.
Comments	Dilute with powdered drink mix, juice, or soda. Serve chilled. Drink through a straw to reduce disagreeable smell.	Monitor for drug-related adverse effects and anaphylactoid reactions.	Monitor for drug-related adverse effects and anaphylactoid reactions. 500 mL of the 2% solution prepared as described above is enough to treat a 33-kg child for the full 20-h course.

IV acetylcysteine is commercially available as a 20% solution and requires dilution to a 2% solution for infusion into a peripheral vein. Both 5% dextrose in water and half-normal saline can be used as diluents.[71] **Given the volume and hypotonicity of fluid required, children and small adults should be carefully monitored to avoid fluid overload and hyponatremia during treatment.**[52]

Despite the lack of randomized direct comparisons, IV acetylcysteine is as effective and safe as oral therapy for patients with early acetaminophen poisoning, as compared with retrospective cohorts and historical controls.[54,72-75] IV acetylcysteine is the route of choice for patients with acetaminophen-induced fulminant hepatic failure, because oral acetylcysteine has not been adequately studied in this setting.[76] There is the potential for delayed hepatic toxicity after the completion of acetylcysteine therapy, especially the 20-hour IV protocol.[77]

Oral Acetylcysteine The standard 72-hour oral acetylcysteine regimen used in the United States consists of a loading dose of 140 milligrams/kg followed by maintenance doses of 70 milligrams/kg every 4 hours for 17 additional doses (**Table 190-2**). It may still be appropriate in certain patients, such as those at high risk for anaphylactoid responses to the IV formulation and asthmatics. The taste is disagreeable, and some patients with persistent nausea and vomiting may require concomitant antiemetics such as ondansetron.

EXTRACORPOREAL ELIMINATION

Case reports describe the use of extracorporeal detoxification in patients presenting late after a serious acetaminophen overdose to both remove the drug and treat the hepatic encephalopathy.[78,79] The role of such therapy in the overall management of serious acetaminophen toxicity remains to be defined.

TREATMENT GUIDELINES BASED ON TIME TO ED PRESENTATION

Treatment guidelines for oral acetaminophen poisoning are based on the time to presentation to the ED after ingestion: <4 hours, between 4 hours and 24 hours, and unknown time or >24 hours before presentation (Figure 190-3).[37] In toxic overdoses, the risk of hepatotoxicity increases with the lag time between ingestion and initiation of acetylcysteine therapy.[49] The optimal outcome with acetylcysteine therapy is seen if it is administered within 8 hours after ingestion, so the optimal "decision-time window" for treatment is between the 4-hour acetaminophen concentration measurement and 8-hour goal to initiate acetylcysteine.[39] No further acetaminophen serum measurements are necessary once the need for acetylcysteine therapy has been determined until the completion of the course of therapy.

Presentation Within 4 Hours of Ingestion For patients who present to the ED within 4 hours and are likely have a significant acetaminophen overdose, treatment begins with GI decontamination (usually activated charcoal) while awaiting the 4-hour postingestion acetaminophen concentration. If the clinical laboratory can report an acetaminophen concentration within 8 hours postingestion, wait for the serum acetaminophen concentration and plot the result on the nomogram to determine whether acetylcysteine therapy is necessary. If the acetaminophen concentration will not be available by 8 hours postingestion, empirically initiate acetylcysteine therapy without waiting for the result. Subsequently, when the acetaminophen concentration

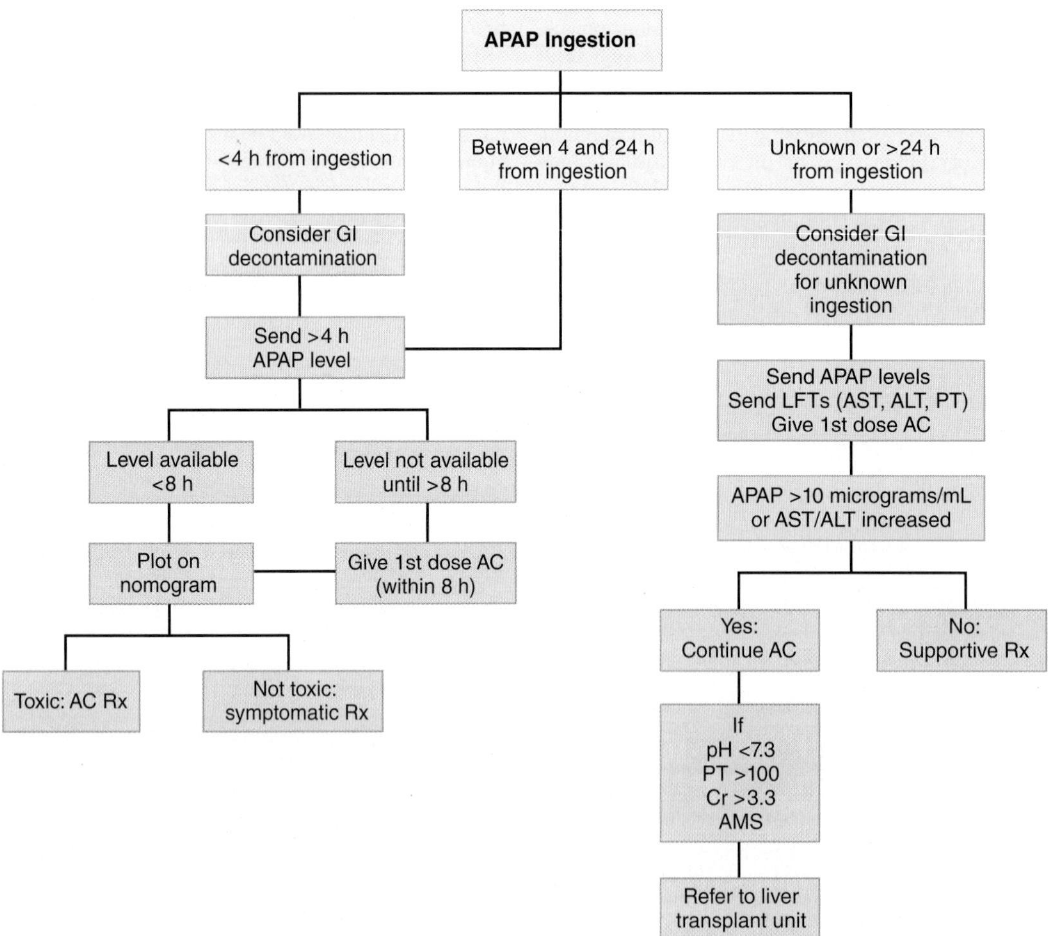

FIGURE 190-3. Treatment guidelines for acetaminophen (APAP) ingestion. All times noted are postingestion. AC = acetylcysteine; ALT = alanine aminotransferase; AMS = altered mental status; AST = aspartate aminotransferase; Cr = creatinine; LFTs = liver function tests; PT = prothrombin time; Rx = treatment.

is determined, the need for acetylcysteine therapy can be determined with the use of the nomogram.

Presentation >4 and <24 Hours After Ingestion For patients who present >4 hours but <24 hours following acetaminophen ingestion, determine the serum acetaminophen concentration as soon as possible. GI decontamination may be performed, particularly for suspected coingestants, but it may have limited effectiveness because of the delay in presentation. If the laboratory can determine the acetaminophen concentration within 8 hours postingestion, await the acetaminophen concentration and plot the result on the nomogram to determine if acetylcysteine therapy is necessary. Otherwise, empirically administer acetylcysteine.

Presentation >24 Hours After Ingestion or Time of Ingestion Unknown For patients in whom the time of acetaminophen ingestion remains unknown or is >24 hours or for those with suggestive clinical findings of acetaminophen poisoning, a serum acetaminophen concentration and serum transaminase, bilirubin, and prothrombin time tests should be determined. Initiate acetylcysteine therapy as soon as possible while awaiting laboratory results. In this scenario, a detectable acetaminophen concentration (>10 micrograms/mL or >66 micromoles/L) suggests that the patient may be at risk for developing hepatotoxicity. Similarly, elevated serum transaminases suggest the possibility of ongoing hepatic toxicity. Therefore, continued acetylcysteine therapy is indicated if the acetaminophen concentration is measurable or if the serum transaminases are elevated. If serum acetaminophen concentration is <10 micrograms/mL (<66 micromoles/L) and the serum transaminases are not elevated, then acetylcysteine can be discontinued.

DISPOSITION AND FOLLOW-UP

Many experts recommend **rechecking serum acetaminophen and transaminase levels** at the completion of acetylcysteine therapy with continuation of acetylcysteine infusion at the rate of 6.25 milligrams/kg per hour until the serum acetaminophen concentration is not detectable or is less than 10 micrograms/mL (66 micromoles/L) and transaminase concentrations are normal or rapidly decreasing.[48,55]

All patients requiring acetylcysteine therapy should be admitted to the hospital until the completion of the therapy. In general, admission to a hospital floor bed is adequate unless the coingestant is of concern, hepatotoxicity is severe, or the patient is suicidal and 24-hour direct observation cannot be arranged. Patients who are not at risk for developing acetaminophen-induced hepatotoxicity (e.g., acetaminophen concentration below the nomogram or unmeasurable acetaminophen concentration with normal hepatic transaminase concentrations) should be observed in the ED for 4 to 6 hours to exclude potentially toxic coingestants before disposition. Psychiatric evaluation should be considered for patients with intentional acetaminophen overdoses. Cases of acetaminophen ingestion or toxicity should be reported to the regional poison control center for both data collection purposes and assistance with management.

SPECIAL CONSIDERATIONS

FULMINANT HEPATIC FAILURE

Unfortunately, a small percentage of patients who overdose with acetaminophen will develop fulminant hepatic failure. Acetaminophen poisoning is the number one cause of acute liver failure, accounting for 39% to 46% of cases in the United States.[80,81] The mortality rate for patients with acetaminophen-induced fulminant hepatic failure without acetylcysteine therapy is estimated to be between 5% and 80%. Most fatalities occur on days 3 to 5 after overdose and are attributed to hepatic complications such as cerebral edema, hemorrhage, shock, acute lung injury, sepsis, and multi-organ failure. Patients who eventually survive fulminant hepatic failure generally begin to show evidence of recovery by days 5 to 7. Survivors will eventually develop complete hepatic regeneration without any persistence of hepatic impairment.

Acetylcysteine treatment decreases the incidence of cerebral edema, reduces vasopressor requirements, and improves survival in acetaminophen-induced fulminant hepatic failure.[76,82] Acetylcysteine also appears to be beneficial in the treatment of other forms of hepatic failure, including viral hepatitis and alcoholic cirrhosis.[83]

Prognostic indicators associated with the highest risk of mortality from acetaminophen-induced fulminant hepatic failure include metabolic acidosis (arterial pH <7.30) despite fluid and hemodynamic resuscitation, or a combination of coagulopathy (prothrombin time >100 seconds), renal insufficiency (serum creatinine >3.3 milligrams/dL or >292 micromoles/L), and grade III or IV hepatic encephalopathy.[84] Other predictors of a poor prognosis include an Acute Physiology and Chronic Health Evaluation II score >15, elevated serum lactate (>26 milligrams/dL or >3.0 mmol/L) after fluid resuscitation, and elevated serum phosphate (>3.71 milligrams/dL or >1.2 mmol/L) on the second day after ingestion.[85-87] Multifactor scoring systems have also been developed to predict hepatotoxicity in single and staggered overdoses.[88-90]

Treatment for acetaminophen-induced fulminant hepatic failure includes acetylcysteine therapy, correction of coagulopathy and acidosis, monitoring for and aggressive treatment of cerebral edema, and early patient referral to a liver specialty/transplant center. Unlike the treatment of early acetaminophen toxicity, IV acetylcysteine therapy should be continued past the 20-hour standard regimen until the patient recovers, receives a liver transplant, or dies.

MULTIPLE-DOSE AND EXTENDED-RELEASE ACETAMINOPHEN INGESTIONS

Patients with staggered acetaminophen ingestions and liver injury often have delayed presentation to the hospital and a higher rate of adverse outcomes.[91] **Multiple closely spaced acetaminophen ingestions and extended-release acetaminophen ingestions represent two unique aspects of acetaminophen poisoning for which the Rumack-Matthew nomogram cannot be readily applied because a single time of ingestion does not exist.** A conservative approach is to assume that a single ingestion occurred at the earliest possible time stated by the patient, with the acetaminophen concentration plotted on the Rumack-Matthew nomogram based on this artificial time and treatment decisions made accordingly. For example, if the patient ingests five doses of 50 milligrams/kg of acetaminophen over a 4-hour period beginning 8 hours ago, a single acetaminophen ingestion is assumed to have occurred 8 hours ago, and the serum concentration accordingly is plotted on the nomogram.

Extended-release acetaminophen formulations consist of a bilayered tablet containing a 325-milligram immediate-release outer layer and a 325-milligram slow, continuous-release, highly compressed inner layer. Because there are little clinical data concerning overdose with these preparations, treatment guidelines remain conservative, and the manufacturer recommends obtaining a second acetaminophen concentration 4 to 6 hours after the first concentration in those situations in which the first measured concentration (4 to 8 hours postingestion) is elevated but below the nomogram line.[92,93] A full course of acetylcysteine therapy should be instituted (or continued if already started) if the second acetaminophen concentration is above the nomogram line. If the initial concentration is above the nomogram line, standard therapy should be administered, and there is no need to obtain a second concentration.

IV ACETAMINOPHEN OVERDOSE

Accepted guidelines for treatment of IV acetaminophen overdose do not currently exist in the United States. The local poison center should be contacted for guidance following any suspected IV acetaminophen overdose.

REFERENCES

The complete reference list is available online at www.TintinalliEM.com.

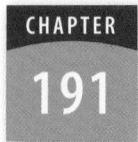

Nonsteroidal Anti-Inflammatory Drugs

Joseph G. Rella
Wallace A. Carter

INTRODUCTION

Nonsteroidal anti-inflammatory drugs (NSAIDs) are among the most widely used class of drugs in the United States, and all share inhibition of the cyclooxygenase enzyme as a mechanism of action. NSAIDs are effective antipyretics, analgesics, and anti-inflammatory agents. Because of their large therapeutic window, acute ingestion with overdoses rarely produces serious complications.[1,2] The morbidity from NSAIDs in acute overdose is far overshadowed by complications of NSAIDs at therapeutic doses, which include GI bleeding, drug-induced renal failure, and atherosclerotic heart disease.[3-6] Due to their increased risk for cardiovascular disease, rofecoxib and valdecoxib were withdrawn from the U.S. market in 2004 and 2005, respectively.

PHARMACOLOGY

OVERVIEW

NSAIDs are structurally varied compounds with common therapeutic effects (**Table 191-1**). NSAIDs reversibly inhibit the enzyme cyclooxygenase, which is responsible for the production of prostaglandins from arachidonic acid (**Figure 191-1**). The anti-inflammatory effect of NSAIDs is through the inhibition of prostaglandin production, and they may also inhibit neutrophil migration via unclear mechanisms. NSAIDs are antipyretics through inhibition of prostaglandin E_2 in the hypothalamus. NSAIDs attenuate prostaglandin-mediated hyperalgesia and local pain fiber stimulus.

CYCLOOXYGENASE

Two isoforms of cyclooxygenase (abbreviated COX-1 and COX-2) vary in presence and distribution.[7] COX-1 is present with steady level of activity and is found primarily in blood vessels, kidneys, and stomach. In contrast, COX-2 is not normally found to a significant degree in human tissue with the possible exception of the brain and kidneys, unless its production is induced by local inflammation.

Cyclooxygenase inhibitors can be categorized as nonselective, partially selective, or selective regarding their inhibition of COX enzyme isoforms (Table 191-1). Most NSAIDs nonselectively inhibit both COX-1 and COX-2. COX-1 inhibition is responsible for most of the unwanted GI side effects of NSAIDs. Drugs, such as etodolac and meloxicam, were created to inhibit preferentially COX-2, theoretically reducing the unwanted GI effects. Unfortunately, the COX-2–selective compounds do not appear to be more effective mediators of inflammation or analgesia and are still associated with GI side effects in addition to usually being more expensive.[8,9]

PHARMACOKINETICS

All NSAIDs are rapidly absorbed from the GI tract, and most achieve peak serum levels within approximately 2 hours. They are highly protein bound in the plasma, have low volumes of distribution (approximately 0.2 L/kg), and cross the blood–brain barrier. NSAIDs undergo metabolism mainly in the liver via glucuronic acid conjugation or via liver enzymes before elimination in the urine or feces. Plasma half-lives of NSAIDs range from 2 hours for ibuprofen to greater than 50 hours for the long-acting agents piroxicam and phenylbutazone (Table 191-1). Creation of active metabolites may prolong the therapeutic effect beyond that of the parent compound.

Ingestion of large amounts of some drugs, such as ibuprofen and naproxen, exhibits slower absorption, taking 3 to 4 hours to achieve peak plasma levels. As greater amounts of NSAIDS are absorbed in large overdoses, greater fractions of free drug become available for toxicity in a nonlinear manner because protein binding is limited.

TABLE 191-1 Nonsteroidal Agents Available in the United States

Class and Agent	Half-Life with Therapeutic Doses of Standard Oral Tablets or Capsules[*] (h)
Nonselective NSAIDs	
Salicylates	
Aspirin	6 (salicylic acid)
Diflunisal	8–12
Salsalate	16
Acetic acids	
Diclofenac	2
Indomethacin	4–5
Ketorolac	5
Meclofenamate	1–2 (15[†])
Mefenamic acid	2
Nabumetone	<1 (22–26[†])
Sulindac	8 (16[†])
Tolmetin	5
Propionic acids	
Fenoprofen	3
Flurbiprofen	6–8
Ibuprofen	2
Ketoprofen	2–4
Naproxen	12–17
Oxaprozin	16–45 (38–57[‡])
Pyrazolones	
Phenylbutazone	72
Oxicams	
Piroxicam	50
Partially selective COX-2 inhibitors	
Etodolac	6–8
Meloxicam	20–24
Selective COX-2 inhibitors	
Celecoxib	11
Rofecoxib	17
Valdecoxib	8–11

Abbreviation: COX-2 = cyclooxygenase 2.
[*]Not sustained-release or enteric-coated preparations.
[†]Half-life of active metabolite.
[‡]Half-life of protein-bound drug.

Topical NSAIDS Topical NSAIDS are well absorbed through the skin and reach therapeutic levels in synovial fluid. They provide good pain relief for osteoarthritis, with very low blood levels and no toxic effects described to date.[10,11]

SIGNIFICANT DRUG–DRUG INTERACTIONS

Aspirin Daily aspirin therapy reduces the incidence of recurrent myocardial infarction and stroke via impairment of platelet aggregation. Ibuprofen administered three times per day competitively inhibits this aspirin effect on platelets via its interaction with the thromboxane pathway, undermining its cardioprotective effect. This observation may extend to other NSAIDs but not to diclofenac or the COX-2 inhibitors.[12]

Antihypertensive Agents NSAIDs can decrease the effectiveness of some antihypertensives including angiotensin-converting enzyme

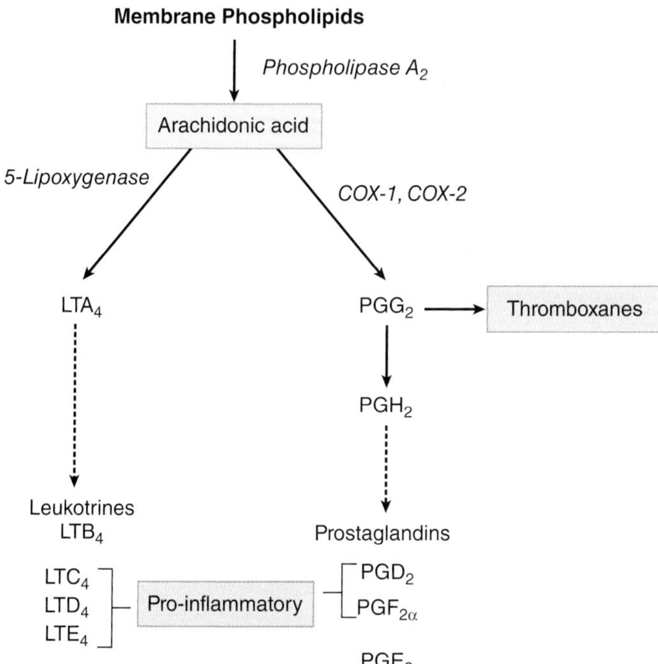

FIGURE 191-1. The arachidonic acid cascade is the primary pathway for the formation of arachidonic acid within cells from which inflammatory mediators—prostaglandins, leukotrienes, and thromboxanes—are generated. NSAIDs target this cellular mechanism to produce their anti-inflammatory effect. COX = cyclooxygenase; LT = leukotriene; PG = prostaglandin.

inhibitors, diuretics, and α- and β-adrenergic antagonists. Inhibition of prostaglandin synthesis is believed to be a central mechanism for these effects. Lower prostaglandin levels result in alterations in the renin-angiotensin system causing decreased renal sodium clearance, water retention, and changes in vascular tone.[13]

Warfarin Warfarin and NSAIDs have several important interactions that may increase the risk of bleeding.[14] Some NSAIDs may displace warfarin from plasma proteins, but the effect is small and does not lead to increased anticoagulation. The selective COX-2 inhibitors at therapeutic doses also elevate prothrombin times, likely through decreased elimination of warfarin. Other nonselective NSAIDs have not been reported to change warfarin protein binding or elimination, but their use is not recommended in warfarin users because they inhibit platelet aggregation and can significantly increase the risk of bleeding.

Decreased Renal Clearance of Drugs NSAIDs may also decrease renal clearance via inhibition of renal prostaglandin synthesis, decreasing their vasodilatory effect, causing a decrease in renal blood flow and glomerular filtration rate, and ultimately decreasing the rate of elimination of certain drugs. Therefore, NSAID use can lead to increased concentrations of consequential drugs such as lithium, methotrexate, and metformin. NSAIDs are a potential risk factor in the development of metformin-associated lactic acidosis, a rare complication of metformin therapy with a high mortality.[15]

CLINICAL FEATURES

TOXICITY AT THERAPEUTIC DOSES

NSAIDs are generally safe drugs but have a number of well-reported side effects at therapeutic doses (**Table 191-2**). It is generally believed that indomethacin and other long-acting agents, such as piroxicam, are responsible for a greater proportion of side effects, whereas the propionic acid agents, such as ibuprofen, are responsible for fewer side effects.

Central Nervous System CNS adverse effects at therapeutic doses include headache, cognitive difficulties, behavioral change, and aseptic meningitis.[16,17] Acute psychosis has been reported with indomethacin and sulindac use, which is hypothesized to result from the structural similarity of these NSAIDs to serotonin.

TABLE 191-2 NSAID Toxicity at Therapeutic Doses

Organ System	Clinical Toxicity
CNS	Behavioral changes, cognitive difficulties, headache, psychosis, aseptic meningitis
Cardiovascular	Increased risk of myocardial infarction and risk of sudden death following myocardial infarction
Pulmonary	Bronchospasm, hypersensitivity pneumonitis, pulmonary edema
GI	Dyspepsia,* nausea,* heartburn,* gastritis, gastric and duodenal erosions, mucosal bleeding,* gastric and duodenal perforation
Hepatic	Spectrum of hepatic injury ranging from asymptomatic elevation of serum transaminases to fulminant hepatic failure
Renal	Sodium and water retention,* hyperkalemia, azotemia,* acute tubular necrosis, interstitial nephritis, renal failure
Hematologic	Increased risk of bleeding, bone marrow suppression, aplastic anemia, agranulocytosis, red cell aplasia, hemolytic anemia, thrombocytopenia
Dermatologic	Maculopapular rashes, photosensitivity reactions, Stevens-Johnson syndrome, toxic epidermal necrolysis
Bone	Delayed wound and fracture healing
Reproductive	Slowed uterine contractions, premature closure of ductus arteriosus, fetal intracranial hemorrhage, necrotizing enterocolitis, oligohydramnios

*Common side effects.

Patients with NSAID-induced aseptic meningitis may experience symptoms of headache, fever, and neck stiffness occurring within hours of a therapeutic dose.[16-18] Cerebrospinal fluid analysis of these patients finds elevated WBC counts and protein levels with normal or decreased glucose levels. Symptoms resolve after NSAID use is stopped and in some cases recur with repeat NSAID challenges.[18,19] This phenomenon is most often seen in patients who have underlying autoimmune diseases, such as systemic lupus erythematosus, and is thought to be a hypersensitivity reaction. Exclusion of an infectious cause is necessary before the diagnosis of NSAID-induced aseptic meningitis can be assigned. Agents associated with aseptic meningitis include celecoxib, diclofenac, ibuprofen, ketoprofen, naproxen, rofecoxib, sulfasalazine, sulindac, and tolmetin.

Cardiovascular Increased cardiovascular events, including myocardial infarction, have been reported with long-term use of both nonselective NSAIDs and selective COX-2 agents.[20] The observed risk increase is variable among the different agents, but risk is dose and duration dependent, as well as more profound in patients with established coronary artery disease.[20,21] Selective COX-2 inhibitors are associated with a doubling of the relative risk of myocardial infarction and heart failure.[22] For nonselective NSAIDs, no increase in major vascular events has been observed with naproxen, whereas ibuprofen and diclofenac regimens were associated with a relative risk for major vascular events as much as 1.5 that of placebo.[22] A stepped-care approach to NSAID use for managing musculoskeletal symptoms in those with known cardiovascular disease or risk factors is recommended.[22,23] Begin therapy with medications not associated with increased cardiovascular effects, such as acetaminophen, and progress carefully to nonselective NSAIDs, or for patients over 75 years of age, use a topical rather than oral NSAID.[24-26]

Pulmonary NSAIDs have been associated with adverse pulmonary reactions, including bronchospasm in asthmatics, hypersensitivity pneumonitis, and pulmonary edema. Patients with NSAID-related hypersensitivity pneumonitis may complain of fever, cough, and shortness of breath. Chest radiographs may show pulmonary infiltrates, and blood work may show leukocytosis and eosinophilia. Cessation of NSAID use resolves the symptoms, whereas rechallenging causes recurrence. NSAIDs implicated in hypersensitivity pneumonitis include diclofenac, diflunisal, naproxen, piroxicam, and sulindac. The mechanism of NSAID-mediated pneumonitis is also thought to be an immune-mediated hypersensitivity reaction.

NSAID-induced bronchospasm is a well-described phenomenon in patients with reactive airways disease. The spectrum of this reaction ranges from rhinitis to severe bronchospasm with laryngeal edema.[27] Patients with underlying reactive airways disease and nasal polyps are at greater risk for these complications. The mechanism of this hypersensitivity reaction to NSAIDs in asthmatics does not appear to be immunoglobulin E–mediated but rather may result from excessive production of leukotrienes.

Gastrointestinal The greatest morbidity caused by therapeutic use of NSAIDs is GI.[9,28] These effects derive from inhibition of cytoprotective gastric prostaglandins resulting in injuries ranging from dyspepsia, heartburn, and nausea, to life-threatening bleeding.[5] During long-term therapy (>3 months), endoscopic ulcers are observed in 10% to 30% of patients, but only 1% to 2% experience serious ulcer complications, such a bleeding or perforation. Patients at higher risk for GI bleeding include those with a history of ulcers, those taking high doses of NSAIDs or corticosteroids, and the elderly.[29-31] Reduced incidence of GI side effects has been observed with celecoxib, but not other COX-2–selective agents, such as rofecoxib.

Hepatic Clinically apparent liver injury caused by NSAIDs is most likely idiosyncratic and rare, occurring in 1 to 10 cases per 100,000 prescriptions.[32,33] More commonly, asymptomatic elevations of serum transaminases are seen in up to 18% of users taking NSAIDs over a long period. Diclofenac and sulindac are the two NSAIDs most commonly linked to hepatotoxicity. Stopping the drug should lead to complete recovery while also avoiding other NSAIDs that may cause recurrence.

Renal NSAIDs exert many toxic effects on the kidney.[5,6] COX inhibition decreases prostaglandin synthesis, leading to vasoconstriction of the renal vascular supply with resultant reversible prerenal azotemia. Continued use may lead to acute tubular necrosis. Interstitial nephritis may result from NSAID-associated activation of inflammatory cells. Glomerular injury may be caused by caused by proinflammatory leukotrienes stimulated by NSAIDs resulting in alteration of glomerular permeability. Chronic renal injury in the form of patchy necrosis, as well as medullary ischemia, is associated with chronic, large cumulative doses of NSAIDs, resulting from chronic inhibition of vasodilatory prostaglandins. Additionally, chronic interstitial fibrosis, hyperkalemia, and hyponatremia may be caused by NSAID use.[34]

Hematologic Nonselective NSAIDs inhibit platelet formation of thromboxane A_2, a potent stimulator of platelet aggregation, resulting in qualitative platelet deficiencies. The new COX-2 inhibitors have far fewer antiplatelet effects than traditional NSAIDs, which may explain why an increase in cardiac and neurovascular events in patients taking the COX-2 inhibitor rofecoxib was observed versus the nonselective COX-1 inhibitor naproxen. Most NSAIDs decrease platelet aggregation only when significant concentrations of the drug are present, and therefore, increased bleeding tendencies from NSAIDs are not widely reported.

Bone marrow suppression and aplastic anemia are rare hematologic complications of almost all NSAIDs with indomethacin, diclofenac, and phenylbutazone responsible for most reported cases. NSAID use has also resulted in agranulocytosis, hemolytic anemia, red cell aplasia, and thrombocytopenia.

Dermatologic NSAIDs account for approximately 10% to 27% of all cutaneous drug reactions.[35] The agents most frequently involved in dermatologic complications include benoxaprofen, phenylbutazone, and piroxicam. Drug reactions to NSAIDs range from benign maculopapular rashes to Stevens-Johnson syndrome and toxic epidermal necrolysis. NSAIDs are among the most commonly implicated drugs in cases of toxic epidermal necrolysis, accounting for up to one third of drug-related cases. NSAIDs of all types (oral and topical) can cause photosensitivity reactions including increased sensitivity to sun exposure (phototoxic) and true photoallergic reactions (see chapter 249, "Generalized Skin Disorders"). Ketoprofen and piroxicam are the most frequently involved in photoallergic reactions. Isoxicam was removed from the U.S. market after fatal skin reactions.

Bone Controversy surrounds the use of NSAIDs for control of pain resulting from a fractured bone. Although NSAIDs are well known to treat musculoskeletal pain effectively, bone healing is a complex cascade of events that involves prostaglandins' influence on the balance between bone formation and resorption.[36] With conflicting results regarding wound healing, some orthopedists recommend delayed administration of NSAIDs for 3 to 4 weeks following a fracture, using judicious doses, and possibly avoiding NSAIDs altogether in cases of spinal fusion.[37]

Reproductive Prostaglandins are found in high concentration in the uterus at term and have a stimulatory effect on normal labor. NSAIDs will impair uterine motility through inhibition of prostaglandin synthesis. Although NSAIDs are not believed to be teratogenic in humans, they cross the placenta in late pregnancy. One of the most significant effects of fetal exposure to NSAIDs is premature constriction of the ductus arteriosus that may result in fetal pulmonary hypertension. Other reported effects of in utero exposure to NSAIDs include fetal intracranial hemorrhage, necrotizing enterocolitis, oligohydramnios, and renal dysfunction. NSAID-induced inhibition of platelet aggregation may place the fetus and the mother at increased risk for peripartum hemorrhage. **The safest recommendation is to avoid NSAID use during pregnancy, especially during the third trimester.**

TOXICITY WITH ACUTE OVERDOSE

Although the vast majority of patients with acute overdoses suffer little morbidity, some fatalities occur with massive NSAID ingestions that often include the clinical features of altered mental status, metabolic acidosis, and shock.[38-41] Historically, phenylbutazone was most commonly associated with severe toxicity following an overdose, and although it was withdrawn from the U.S. market in the 1970s, it is still available from veterinary sources and in other countries. By a wide margin, ibuprofen is the most common agent currently reported in NSAID overdoses. Patients who develop symptoms following an ibuprofen overdose usually ingest more than 100 milligrams/kg, and initial symptoms predominantly include abdominal pain, nausea, and vomiting, all beginning within 4 hours of ingestion (**Table 191-3**). Most patients who manifest severe toxicity, including apnea, coma, and metabolic acidosis, ingest more than 400 milligrams/kg. There is limited published experience concerning acute overdose of COX-2 inhibitors, but they are assumed to have similar profiles as the nonselective NSAIDs.

Central Nervous System CNS manifestations of acute NSAID overdose are usually minimal, although patients with significant overdose may have headache, diplopia, nystagmus, and altered mental status including coma.[17] Mefenamic acid has been identified as a drug with high potential for seizures in overdose.[42] Muscle twitching and seizures that are responsive to benzodiazepines have been reported.

Cardiovascular Acute NSAID overdose can result in hypotension and bradydysrhythmia. NSAIDs are not known to be a primary cause of dysrhythmias, but fluid and electrolyte abnormalities provoked by NSAID toxicity may induce cardiac rhythm abnormalities. Cardiovascular dysfunction from acute NSAID overdose is responsive to conventional critical care management.

Metabolic Electrolyte and acid-base abnormalities may occur in acute NSAID overdoses. Alterations in serum electrolytes may develop

TABLE 191-3 NSAID Toxicity after an Acute Overdose

Initial symptoms within 4 h after ingestion	Abdominal pain, nausea, vomiting
CNS	Headache, nystagmus, diplopia, altered mental status, coma, muscle twitching, and seizures (mefenamic acid)
Cardiovascular	Hypotension, shock, bradydysrhythmia
Metabolic	Hyperkalemia, hypocalcemia, hypomagnesemia
GI and hepatic	Continued abdominal pain, nausea, vomiting, hepatic injury, pancreatitis (rare)
Renal	Acute kidney injury

secondary to decreased prostaglandin synthesis or from NSAID-induced renal failure. Sodium and water retention may lead to volume overload in patients with preexisting cirrhosis, heart failure, or renal failure. Hyperkalemia, hypocalcemia, and hypomagnesemia have been reported in NSAID overdoses complicated by acute renal failure.

Increased anion gap metabolic acidosis has been observed with large overdoses of ibuprofen and naproxen, which may be due to these NSAIDs and their metabolites being weak acids. Concurrent lactic acid production in the setting of NSAID-induced seizures and shock may exacerbate the acidosis in some cases.

GI and Hepatic Patients presenting after acute NSAID overdose may have abdominal pain, nausea, and vomiting, but life-threatening GI hemorrhage is not a typical finding after acute overdoses. Overdose may also result in hepatic injury, as measured by cholestasis and elevated transaminase levels. Rare cases of pancreatitis have been reported after overdoses of ibuprofen, naproxen, and indomethacin.[43-45]

Renal NSAID overdose rarely causes acute kidney injury but may place a stressed renal system at risk for failure. The clinical presentation may include hematuria and oliguria. Most patients with acute renal failure due to an NSAID overdose have eventual recovery of renal function, but some may need long-term dialysis.

TREATMENT

Most patients who present following an NSAID overdose will be asymptomatic. Follow the general principles for managing the poisoned patient (see chapter 176, "General Management of Poisoned Patients"), including screening for possible co-ingestants, consultation with a toxicologist, and consideration of GI decontamination. Attempt to ascertain whether the amount of drug ingested was less than 100 milligrams/kg (unlikely to result in toxicity) or more than 400 milligrams/kg (significant risk for toxicity).

Asymptomatic NSAID ingestions usually require minimal laboratory evaluation and supportive care (**Figure 191-2**). GI decontamination is best accomplished with activated charcoal and may be considered depending on the perceived risk of severe ingestion and clinical condition. Gastric lavage is not useful in the majority of cases but may be considered for a patient who has ingested a massive quantity within the past hour, especially mefenamic acid or phenylbutazone. Fluid and electrolyte replacement is given as necessary. Consider screening for potentially dangerous co-ingestants by measuring the serum acetaminophen and salicylate levels and obtaining a 12-lead ECG.

Patients who are symptomatic with altered mental status, seizures, shock, respiratory distress, or cardiac dysrhythmias require aggressive resuscitation and stabilization (Figure 191-2). Establish an airway as needed, institute mechanical ventilation when necessary, treat hypotension with fluid boluses and/or vasopressors, and manage seizures initially with IV benzodiazepines. Consider gastric lavage for recent ingestions involving mefenamic acid or phenylbutazone. Whole-bowel irrigation is recommended for severe overdose with enteric-coated formulations. Multidose activated charcoal has no proven benefit in symptomatic NSAID overdoses. Hemodialysis, hemofiltration, or charcoal hemoperfusion are not effective in enhancing elimination because NSAIDs are highly protein bound. Likewise, manipulation of serum and urine pH through IV alkalinization is not beneficial in enhancing renal elimination.

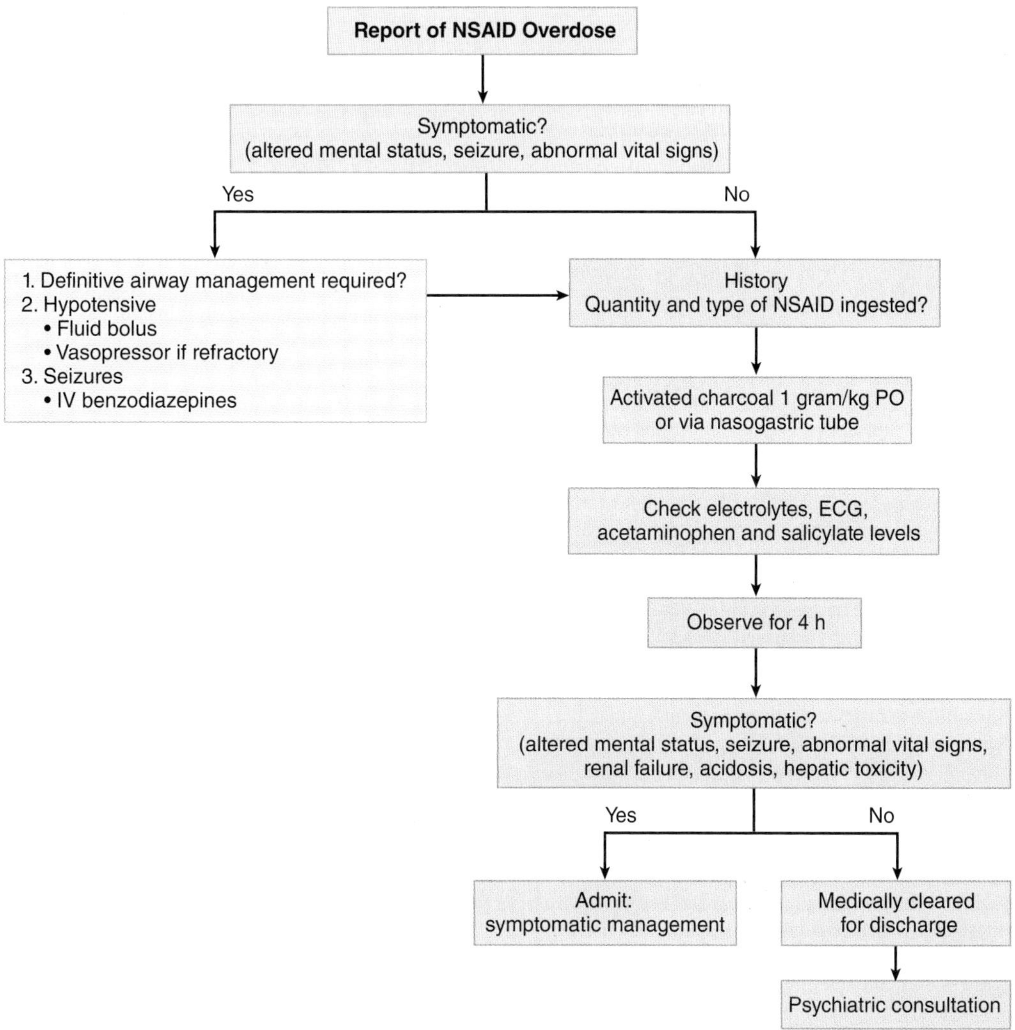

FIGURE 191-2. Approach to treatment of acute nonsteroidal anti-inflammatory drug (NSAID) overdose.

Patients with symptomatic NSAID overdoses should have a serum chemistry panel, hepatic profile, CBC, coagulation profile, and serum salicylate and acetaminophen levels measured. Serum NSAID levels do not correlate with observed toxicity or outcomes, so serum levels for specific NSAIDs are not indicated.

DISPOSITION AND FOLLOW-UP

Most patients with asymptomatic NSAID ingestions can be safely discharged after a 4-hour period of observation. Patients with a symptomatic overdose (altered mental status, abnormal vital signs, electrolyte abnormalities, or acute renal failure) should be admitted for observation and supportive care. All overdoses should be reported to the regional poison control center both for management assistance and for statistical tracking. The majority of NSAID overdoses will not cause significant sequelae. Even patients with major symptoms have a good prognosis if they overcome the initial insult.

REFERENCES

The complete reference list is available online at www.TintinalliEM.com.

CHAPTER 192

Methylxanthines and Nicotine

Chip Gresham
Daniel E. Brooks

INTRODUCTION

Methylxanthines include **caffeine**, **theophylline**, **theobromine**, and **nicotine**. These agents are plant-derived alkaloids with ubiquitous use in beverages (caffeine in coffee and soda), foods (theobromine in chocolate), tobacco products (nicotine), and medications (theophylline and caffeine). Newer methylxanthine derivatives include pentoxifylline (improves peripheral blood flow) and doxofylline (a bronchodilator).[1,2] All methylxanthines have shared pharmacologic properties and very similar pharmacodynamic effects.

METHYLXANTHINES

EPIDEMIOLOGY

Caffeine (1,3,7-trimethylxanthine), a methylxanthine and structural analog of adenosine, is the most commonly used psychoactive drug in the world and the only one that can be legally purchased by children. It is found in varying amounts in beverages and "energy-enhanced" foods, such as candy bars, potato chips, and oatmeal (**Table 192-1**).[3] Nearly 6 billion caffeinated "energy drinks" were purchased in the United States in 2012.[4] Many "energy drinks" contain guarana, a plant whose seeds contain high concentrations of caffeine and other methylxanthines. Drinks with guarana may not list caffeine as an ingredient.[5] Other uses for caffeine include apnea of prematurity, analgesic adjuncts, appetite suppression for weight loss, sleep prevention, and diuresis.

Theophylline (1,3-dimethylxanthine) and its water-soluble salt, **aminophylline**, were used extensively in the past for the treatment of asthma and chronic obstructive pulmonary disease. However, theophylline's use has declined due to its narrow therapeutic window and the development of safer agents. Theophylline is still used in patients with debilitating bronchospastic disease, particularly outside the United States, and has been studied for the treatment of other diseases, including acute mountain sickness and contrast-induced nephropathy.[6,7]

Theobromine (3,7-dimethylxanthine) is found in the seeds of *Theobroma cacao*, from which chocolate and cocoa are derived; and *Commelia thea*, from which teas are steeped; and is an ingredient in numerous "energy drinks" in addition to caffeine. There are very few cases of human toxicity, but theobromine has been associated with atrial fibrillation.[8]

TABLE 192-1 Caffeine Content of Various Products

Source	Caffeine Content (milligrams)
Coffee (8 oz or 240 mL, brewed)	60–120
Tea (8 oz or 240 mL, brewed)	20–90
Colas, caffeinated (8 oz or 240 mL)	20–40
Dark chocolate (1 oz or 30 mL)	5–35
"Higher caffeine energy drinks" (8–24 oz)	70–505
Acetaminophen-aspirin-caffeine tablet	65
Nonprescription antidrowsiness tablet	200

PHARMACOLOGY

Caffeine is most commonly consumed orally; however, it can be administered rectally or parenterally. Theophylline is usually taken orally, although its absorption may be affected by food. It is available as an elixir or as extended-release and controlled-release tablets. Controlled-release tablets can result in erratic or rapid absorption. Theophylline can also be administered IV as aminophylline.

All methylxanthines are rapidly absorbed with early peak levels; they cross the blood–brain barrier and placenta and are excreted in breast milk (**Table 192-2**). Half-lives are only accurate at therapeutic concentrations and vary based on several factors, including drug level, age extremes, smoking, organ system dysfunction (e.g., cirrhosis), infection, and cytochrome P-450 inhibition (**Table 192-3**).

Methylxanthines exhibit Michaelis-Menten kinetics; that is, metabolism changes from first-order to zero-order kinetics at increased concentrations such that a fixed amount, not percentage, of drug is eliminated per unit of time, making accurate half-life calculations impossible following an overdose. This also explains why patients who chronically use theophylline may develop a large increase in serum theophylline concentration with only a small increase in dose. Methylxanthines are metabolized in the liver by the cytochrome P-450 1A2 pathway. Theophylline undergoes significant enterohepatic recirculation, so toxic serum levels can be maintained longer than anticipated.

TABLE 192-2 Pharmacokinetics of Methylxanthines

Parameter	Caffeine	Theophylline
Therapeutic serum concentration	5–20 micrograms/mL (25–100 micromoles/L)	8–20 micrograms/mL (44–110 micromoles/L)
Bioavailability (oral)	~100%	~100%
Oral peak absorption (h) (delayed in overdose)	0.5–1.0	1–2 (up to 8 h with sustained release preparations)
Volume of distribution (L/kg)	~0.6	~0.5
Protein binding	~35%	~60%
Major active metabolites	Paraxanthine Theobromine Theophylline	Caffeine (only if <6 mo old)
Clearance	Hepatic	<1 y old: 50% hepatic and 50% renal >1 y old: 90% hepatic and 10% renal
Half-life (accurate only at therapeutic concentrations)	Neonates: >50 h <1 y old: 20 h >1 y old: 5 h	Neonates: 20–30 h Children and adults: 5 h > 60 y old: 10 h

TABLE 192-3 Factors Affecting Theophylline Clearance

	Increases Theophylline Clearance	Decreases Theophylline Clearance
Medications	Barbiturates Benzodiazepines (suspected) Carbamazepine Phenytoin St. John's wort	Cimetidine Ethanol (coingested) Erythromycin (all macrolides suspected) Oral contraceptives Propranolol (metoprolol suspected) Fluoroquinolones (most) Verapamil
Medical conditions		Cirrhosis Heart failure Pneumonia (other infections suspected)
Other	Hyperthyroid Tobacco Marijuana (cannabis)	Pregnancy Obesity Fever (suspected)

CLINICAL FEATURES OF TOXICITY

Theophylline has the most potential for significant toxicity, followed by caffeine and then theobromine. The underlying pathophysiology involves adenosine antagonism, increased endogenous adrenergic stimulation, and, at toxic levels, phosphodiesterase inhibition (**Table 192-4**).

The main organ systems involved in methylxanthine toxicity are GI, neurologic, cardiovascular, and metabolic (**Table 192-5**).

GI Toxic Effects **Nausea and vomiting** are reported in >70% of acute overdoses.[9] Theophylline can also induce esophageal reflux by decreasing lower esophageal sphincter pressure.

Neurologic Toxic Effects **Methylxanthine-induced seizures** can be severe and refractory to treatment. First-time seizures in the setting of heavy caffeinated "energy drink" consumption have been reported.[4,10] In theophylline toxicity, incidence of seizures is approximately 50% when serum levels are >40 micrograms/mL (>200 micromoles/L) during chronic therapy and >120 micrograms/mL (>600 micromoles/L) after an acute ingestion.[9] Seizures at a lower serum concentration, even as low as 20 micrograms/mL (100 micromoles/L), are more likely in chronic toxicity due to relatively higher tissue levels. In chronic toxicity, seizures can occur without prior neurologic symptoms of tremor or agitation.

Cardiovascular Toxic Effects Methylxanthines induce the release of endogenous catecholamines, stimulating β-adrenergic receptors, resulting in increased inotropy and chronotropy, vasodilation, hypotension, and reflex tachycardia. Sinus tachycardia is the most common cardiac manifestation of both caffeine and theophylline use and toxicity. Atrial fibrillation and supraventricular tachycardia are described with excessive caffeine intake.[11,12] Theophylline toxicity may result in atrial arrhythmias such as multifocal tachycardia and fibrillation/flutter. Ventricular ectopy are more common with chronic toxicity and in patients with advanced age or underlying cardiac dysfunction.[13] Ventricular fibrillation and tachycardia are rare.

TABLE 192-5 Clinical Manifestations of Methylxanthine Toxicity

Organ System	Manifestation
GI	Nausea Vomiting Gastritis
Neurologic	Headache Tremor Agitation Seizure
Cardiovascular	Hypotension Tachycardia Atrial arrhythmias Ventricular ectopy
Metabolic	Hypokalemia Metabolic acidosis Hyperglycemia Hyperthermia Rhabdomyolysis

Metabolic Toxic Effects Methylxanthine toxicity is associated with hypokalemia, hyperglycemia, and metabolic acidosis. Hypokalemia is most common in acute overdose, due to increased catecholamines. Rhabdomyolysis has been reported in caffeine and theophylline overdoses, presumably due to the hypermetabolic state, agitation, and seizures.

Chronic use of methylxanthines, particularly caffeine, can lead to tolerance, dependence, or withdrawal. Caffeine withdrawal syndrome has a varied course depending on use. Withdrawal symptoms typically start at 6 to 24 hours after the last dose, peak at about 36 hours, and can last for several days. Headache and fatigue are the most common symptoms and are seen after either chronic use or short-term, high-dose exposures. **Caffeine withdrawal headaches** can be debilitating and should be included in the differential diagnosis of ED patients with headache.

DIAGNOSIS OF TOXICITY

Caffeine Toxicity There is no clearly defined toxic dose or level of caffeine. Following a single ingestion of 120 milligrams of caffeine, an average peak serum concentration of 3 micrograms/mL (15 micromoles/L) results at 1 hour. Caffeine doses around 120 milligrams enhance arousal and performance of both cognitive and psychomotor skills.[14]

Ingestions of 100 to 150 milligrams/kg or serum levels >100 micrograms/mL (>500 micromoles/L) are likely to cause life-threatening toxicity, and an acute ingestion of >200 milligrams/kg can be lethal.[5,15] Serum caffeine concentrations are not readily available in most clinical

TABLE 192-4 Methylxanthine Mechanisms of Action and Toxicity

	Adenosine Antagonism	Increased Catecholamines	Inhibition of Phosphodiesterase
Mechanism	Inhibition of adenosine-1 and adenosine-2 > adenosine-3 receptors	Increased circulating catecholamines (epinephrine and norepinephrine)	Phosphodiesterase inhibition (at toxic levels)
Effect	Decreased adenosine activity Increased excitatory neurotransmitters activity	Stimulation of β_1 and β_2 receptors	Increased concentration of cyclic adenosine monophosphate and catecholamine effects
Therapeutic effect	Bronchodilation	Bronchodilation	No role at therapeutic doses
Clinical toxicity	Vasoconstriction Arrhythmias Seizures	Tachycardia Vasodilation Hypotension	Enhanced β-adrenergic effects

TABLE 192-6 Methylxanthine Toxicity Classifications

	Acute Toxicity	Acute on Chronic Toxicity	Chronic Toxicity
Clinical scenario	Acute exposure: one-time ingestion of a bottle of theophylline or caffeine tablets	Acute exposure in a person chronically using that methylxanthine: an acute ingestion of a bottle of theophylline in a patient taking theophylline	An ongoing exposure to a stable amount with bioaccumulation; typically due to decreased clearance: a newly prescribed medication inhibits theophylline metabolism, leading to slowly increasing tissue concentrations
Risk of clinical effects	Variable, depends on amount	High, depends on amount ingested and comorbidities	High, depends on tissue level of drug, age, and comorbidities
Timing of peak serum concentration	Often delayed for many hours	Usually delayed	Often immediately available
Correlation of peak serum concentration with clinical effects	Moderate correlation	Moderate correlation	Weak correlation

settings and offer little in terms of clinical decision making, so management of caffeine toxicity is guided by clinical findings.

Theophylline Toxicity Although there is an established therapeutic serum concentration for theophylline, clinical effects are determined by the amount of free drug in tissue, not the serum. **The best predictor of major theophylline toxicity after an acute overdose—seizures, hypotension, or cardiac arrhythmias—is the peak serum concentration. In chronic toxicity, although serum levels are elevated, the level itself does not necessarily predict major toxicity.** An elevated theophylline level is more likely to be associated with major toxicity in those >65 years old (odds ratio, 7.8; 95% confidence interval, 2.9–21.1) than in those 30 to 65 years old (odds ratio, 3.2; 95% confidence interval, 1.03–10.1).[16] In an acute ingestion, monitor serial theophylline levels to establish a trend in absorption, document the peak concentration, and assist in the medical clearance of patients as peak levels may be delayed many hours following a massive, acute overdose (**Table 192-6**). Conversely, management decisions should be based on symptoms and the patient's clinical condition, not on drug levels alone.

TREATMENT

As with the majority of poisoned patients, there are three main components to caring for a patient with methylxanthine toxicity: resuscitation (stabilizing cardiovascular and pulmonary function), GI decontamination to interrupt continued absorption (when appropriate), and minimizing end-organ effects. Supportive care and an appropriate observation period are required to prevent secondary sequelae. Monitor patients in a high-acuity setting. Treatments specific to methylxanthines, particularly theophylline, include use of activated charcoal, treatment of arrhythmias and seizures, and enhanced elimination.

Initial ancillary studies should include ECG, serum electrolytes, creatinine, urea, glucose, and total creatinine kinase. Other laboratory tests may be required based on patient presentation, available medications, and comorbidities. After an intentional ingestion, consider comorbid poisonings, such as with acetaminophen or salicylate. Consult with a medical toxicologist or a regional poison control center to discuss optimal, case-specific treatment.

GI Decontamination Consider GI decontamination when dealing with a potentially life-threatening **theophylline** poisoning provided there are no contraindications, such as an unprotected airway, intractable nausea or vomiting, ileus, bowel obstruction, or need for emergent endoscopy (**Table 192-7**).[17] In **caffeine** ingestion, there is little benefit to GI decontamination because of the rapid absorption and associated nausea.

Ondansetron is the preferred antiemetic to control any associated nausea or vomiting. Do not use phenothiazines (i.e., promethazine) because these agents lower the seizure threshold. Ranitidine can be used to decrease gastric acid hypersecretion. **Do not give cimetidine as it can prolong methylxanthine half-life.**

Multidose activated charcoal can enhance theophylline elimination by interrupting enterohepatic recirculation.[18] Consult with a toxicologist or poison center regarding the use of whole-bowel irrigation for the ingestion of sustained-release preparations.[19] Endoscopic removal of a slow-release, theophylline-containing bezoar may be necessary. Ipecac syrup, cathartics, and gastric lavage after theophylline ingestion have no proven benefit, have potential adverse effects, and are not recommended.[20,21]

Seizures Due to adenosine antagonism, seizures may be difficult to control, particularly with theophylline toxicity. Benzodiazepines, such as lorazepam 2 to 4 milligrams IV or diazepam 5 to 10 milligrams IV in adults, are first-line agents. Repeated, larger doses may be necessary. Barbiturates, such as phenobarbital 10 to 20 milligrams/kg IV in adults, should be used if escalating doses of benzodiazepines are ineffective. At high doses, benzodiazepines and barbiturates can compromise the airway or lead to respiratory depression, so maintain a low threshold for endotracheal intubation. Phenytoin is not useful or recommended.[22]

Patients who fail to respond to anticonvulsant therapy should be sedated, intubated, and paralyzed with a neuromuscular blocking agent; general anesthesia may be required. Paralyzed patients should have an electroencephalogram to monitor for continued seizure activity. Due to the severity of theophylline-induced seizures, some toxicologists recommend prophylactic use of a γ-aminobutyric acid agonist (e.g., lorazepam) to raise seizure threshold in patients presenting with markedly elevated theophylline levels, but this approach has not been validated in human studies.

Cardiovascular Support Manage hypotension initially with IV fluids. The most commonly reported methylxanthine-induced tachyarrhythmias are atrial fibrillation and supraventricular tachycardia, presumably due to excessive β-adrenergic stimulation. Ventricular arrhythmias are uncommon.[23] Cardioselective β-blockers (esmolol or metoprolol) are an option for serious supraventricular dysrhythmias if routine interventions (vagal maneuvers, adenosine) are ineffective. Nonspecific β-blockers, such as propranolol, can lead to bronchospasm, so cardioselective β-blockers, such as esmolol or metoprolol, are preferred.

Enhanced Elimination The use of enhanced elimination techniques can prevent or help treat significant toxicity following methylxanthine poisonings. Multidose activated charcoal is recommended for toxic or potentially toxic theophylline ingestions.[18]

TABLE 192-7 GI Decontamination for Methylxanthine Toxicity

GI Decontamination Technique	Indication*	Dosing
Activated charcoal (single dose)	Acute ingestion	<12 y old: 0.5–1.0 gram/kg PO >12 y old: 25–100 grams PO
Multidose activated charcoal (requires close observation)	Acute ingestion	Normal activated charcoal loading dose, followed by: 0.25–0.5 gram/kg PO every 2–4 h for 12 h (frequency and duration may vary)
Whole-bowel irrigation using iso-osmolar polyethylene glycol electrolyte solution	Acute ingestion of sustained-release preparations	9 mo–6 y: 25 mL/kg per hour 6–12 y old: 1000 mL/h >12 y old: 1500–2000 mL/h Duration: 4–6 h or until clear rectal effluent

*Consider contraindications; for details see http://www.clintox.org/positionstatements.cfm.

Hemodialysis is safe and is as efficacious as hemoperfusion for the treatment of theophylline toxicity.[24] Hemodialysis is also effective for massive caffeine ingestions and pentoxifylline toxicity.[25,26]

Hemodialysis is readily available in many centers and provides fluid and electrolyte correction. The criteria for using hemodialysis in methylxanthine toxicity vary, but most experts suggest that a methylxanthine-induced life-threatening event, such as seizures or intractable arrhythmias, is an indication. **In addition, we suggest that dialysis should be considered when (1) after an acute ingestion, a symptomatic patient has a serum theophylline level >90 micrograms/mL (>500 micromoles/L), or (2) a chronic toxicity patient has a serum theophylline level >40 micrograms/mL (>220 micromoles/L) with significant symptoms or comorbidities.** Published experience suggests that most patients who receive hemodialysis **after** a methylxanthine-induced life-threatening event, such as a seizure or arrhythmia, will continue to have them, whereas as few as 5% of patients who received hemodialysis **before** manifesting severe toxicity will go on to develop a life-threatening event.[27]

Supportive Care Treat vomiting with antiemetics, and correct volume depletion with isotonic fluids. Hypokalemia may not require treatment unless there are clinical findings such as ECG changes, cardiac ectopy, or muscle weakness, because potassium is shifted intracellularly and total body potassium is only mildly depleted. Provide continuous cardiac monitoring until toxicity has resolved. Assess for hyperthermia, rhabdomyolysis, and compartment syndrome, and provide specific treatment. Patients who are sedated and paralyzed should undergo continuous electroencephalographic monitoring to evaluate for occult sustained or recurrent seizures.

DISPOSITION AND FOLLOW-UP

Following an intentional or accidental methylxanthine ingestion, patients are judged nontoxic when they are asymptomatic, have a normal physical examination and vital signs, and, if available, have normal or decreasing serum concentrations. Patients who remain asymptomatic for at least 6 hours after an acute ingestion of immediate-release tablets can be considered nontoxic. Patients with an ingestion of sustained-release medication should be monitored for 12 hours or longer. Patients with intentional ingestions should receive a behavioral health or psychiatric evaluation to assist with appropriate disposition and follow-up.

NICOTINE

EPIDEMIOLOGY

Nicotine is the primary alkaloid in tobacco, a product produced from the dried leaves of plants in the genus *Nicotiana*. Tobacco is consumed as smoked (i.e., cigarettes) or smokeless (i.e., chewing tobacco) products.[28] A typical cigarette contains approximately 20 milligrams of nicotine but only about 1 milligram is absorbed during smoking. Nicotine gums usually contain 2 or 4 milligrams per piece; formulation and mastication assist in higher absorption compared to smoking a cigarette. There is no consensus on the estimated lethal dose of nicotine, but experts do agree that while nicotine is potentially toxic, accidental ingestion of tobacco products, even in children, rarely results in serious outcomes.[29] Other nicotine sources include smoking cessation products (gums, patches, nasal inhalers), pesticides, traditional remedies, and plants, including dermal exposures during tobacco harvest causing "green-tobacco sickness."[30]

PHARMACOLOGY

Nicotine is rapidly absorbed in the lungs, as well as across mucous membranes, the intestinal tract, and intact skin. Smoking tobacco leads to a peak serum nicotine concentration of approximately 40 nanograms/mL (250 micromoles/L), depending on depth of inhalation. Nicotine crosses the blood–brain barrier and affects the CNS within seconds of smoking. Absorption across mucous (oral) membranes is slower than absorption from smoking and is further delayed by acid in the stomach. Therapeutic use of a 4-milligram piece of nicotine gum leads to a peak nicotine concentration of about 10 nanograms/mL (60 micromoles/L) at approximately 45 minutes.[31] The half-life of nicotine is variable, averaging approximately 2 hours in adults. Metabolism is by the liver, mainly by cytochrome P-450 2A6, with 85% being converted to **cotinine**.

TABLE 192-8 Clinical Effects of Nicotine Toxicity

	Signs and Symptoms of Nicotine Toxicity*	
Organ System	**Immediate (<1 h)**	**Delayed (>1 h)**
GI	Hypersalivation Nausea Vomiting	Diarrhea
Cardiovascular	Tachycardia Hypertension	Arrhythmias Bradycardia Hypotension
Neurologic	Tremor Headache Ataxia	Hypotonia Seizure Coma
Respiratory	Bronchorrhea	Hypoventilation Apnea

*Onset of toxicity is varied and can be delayed for hours following dermal exposure.

Once absorbed, nicotine binds to nicotinic acetylcholine receptors throughout the body, including the central nervous, autonomic, and neuromuscular systems. Early in toxicity, nicotine acts as an agonist, activating these ion channels, leading to increased neuronal firing with release of neurotransmitters, including acetylcholine, dopamine, glutamate, norepinephrine, and serotonin. At higher concentrations and/or as toxicity persists, the acetylcholine receptors are inhibited by persistent membrane depolarization, ultimately leading to receptor inactivation.

CLINICAL FEATURES OF TOXICITY

In overdose, nicotine mainly affects the GI, cardiovascular, neurologic, and respiratory systems (**Table 192-8**). Nausea and vomiting are the most common effects and can limit absorbed amounts following ingestion. Early effects are due to acetylcholine receptor activation and include tremor, dizziness, tachycardia, and bronchorrhea. Delayed effects, manifesting after larger exposures, occur due to receptor inactivation and include bradycardia, arrhythmias, hypoventilation, and coma. Seizures are possible and are due to centrally mediated actions.

Nicotine poisoning in children usually results from the ingestion of tobacco or nicotine-containing products. **A child who ingests one or more intact cigarettes, or three or more cigarette butts, has a 90% chance of becoming symptomatic, usually within 30 minutes.**[32] More severe poisonings, such as ingestion of nicotine-containing pesticides or abuse of dermal patches, can result in seizures, respiratory failure, hypotension, arrhythmias, and death. Because nicotine freely crosses the placenta and is found in small concentrations in breast milk, neonatal withdrawal is possible.[33]

Green-tobacco sickness is characterized by nausea, vomiting, weakness, dizziness, and headaches, due to the dermal absorption of nicotine during tobacco harvesting.[30] Onset of symptoms may be delayed for several hours. Patients with significant comorbidities, particularly underlying cardiovascular or seizure disorders, are theoretically at higher risk for morbidity.

Chronic nicotine use has been associated with insulin resistance in diabetics, increased cardiovascular risks, arrhythmias, and the potential for withdrawal.[34] Nicotine withdrawal manifests with irritability, depression, drowsiness, trouble sleeping, increased appetite, and headaches, with symptoms peaking at 2 to 3 days after last use. Withdrawal can occur in smokers as well as smokeless tobacco and nicotine gum users.

DIAGNOSIS OF TOXICITY

The diagnosis of acute nicotine toxicity is based on reliable history and physical examination, with laboratory analysis being of little value. Qualitative toxicologic screening assays can detect nicotine and cotinine in the urine but may only reflect exposure.

TABLE 192-9 Treatment of Nicotine Toxicity

Clinical Condition	Intervention	Considerations
Nausea, vomiting, gastritis	Antiemetics Proton pump inhibitors	Ondansetron, 4 milligrams IV Pantoprazole, 40 milligrams IV
Tremor, seizures	Benzodiazepines	Lorazepam, 1–2 milligrams IV Diazepam, 5–10 milligrams IV
Hypotension	Fluid resuscitation	Monitor and replace serum electrolytes
Hypoventilation	Intubation and mechanical ventilation	—
Withdrawal	Nicotine replacement therapy	Requires outpatient follow-up

TREATMENT OF TOXICITY

The treatment of nicotine toxicity is symptomatic. Fortunately, because nicotine has a very short half-life, symptoms typically resolve rapidly. Cardiovascular and ventilatory support may be required in severe toxicity (**Table 192-9**). Benzodiazepines may be used for seizures, and endotracheal intubation and mechanical ventilation may be required if significant neuromuscular weakness or respiratory depression develops. Ipecac syrup or activated charcoal is not recommended. Decontamination with soap and water may be beneficial following dermal exposures. There is no role for enhanced elimination or urine acidification.

Nicotine withdrawal can be distressing but is not life threatening. Treatment options include the use of nicotine replacement therapy and antidepressants.

DISPOSITION AND FOLLOW-UP

Monitor patients with known or suspected nicotine toxicity; the length of observation depends on the type of product ingested. Patients who remain asymptomatic with normal vital signs after 3 hours from an acute ingestion of nicotine-containing product (except intact transdermal patches) can be discharged from medical care. **Those who ingest intact transdermal patches should be observed longer, at least 6 hours.** Patients with intentional ingestions should receive a behavioral health or psychiatric evaluation to assist with appropriate disposition and follow-up.

REFERENCES

The complete reference list is available online at www.TintinalliEM.com.

Digitalis Glycosides

Michael Levine
Aaron B. Skolnik

INTRODUCTION

The medicinal benefits of cardiac glycosides have been recognized for centuries, and even with other alternative medications, digitalis preparations, such as digoxin, are still used for the treatment of atrial fibrillation and symptomatic congestive heart failure.[1] In addition to availability as pharmaceuticals, cardiac glycosides are also found in plants such as foxglove, oleander, red squill, and lily of the valley. Similar cardioactive steroids are also found in the skin of toads in the Bufonidae family and in some herbal medications. Despite declining use of digoxin, the prevalence of patients diagnosed with digoxin toxicity has remained constant, and the use of digoxin-specific antibody fragments has increased.[2] Digitoxin, a cardiac glycoside similar in structure to digoxin but with a longer half-life, is no longer commercially available in the United States, but is available in Canada and elsewhere in the world.

PATHOPHYSIOLOGY

Digoxin is a cardiac glycoside available for oral or intravenous use. Following oral absorption, digoxin reaches a maximal serum concentration 1 to 3 hours after ingestion. It is approximately 25% protein bound and has a large volume of distribution (6 to 7 L/kg). The drug is primarily eliminated through the kidneys.

Digoxin, like other cardiac glycosides, inhibits sodium-potassium ATPase.[3] This inhibition results in increased intracellular sodium and increased extracellular potassium. As a result of the increased intracellular sodium, the sodium-calcium antiporter is not able to effectively remove calcium from the myocyte. Consequently, there is an increase in intracellular calcium, which augments inotropy. The increased intracellular calcium can contribute to delayed after-depolarizations, which may lead to premature ventricular contractions and dysrhythmias. In addition, there is a decreased refractory period of the myocardium, which increases automaticity and hence is associated with an increased risk of dysrhythmias. Furthermore, cardiac glycosides shorten atrial and ventricular repolarization, thereby decreasing the refractory period and thus increasing automaticity.

Cardiac glycosides also increase vagal tone via action at the carotid body, thereby reducing conduction through the sinoatrial and atrioventricular nodes. In toxic concentrations, cardiac glycosides can increase sympathetic tone. Digoxin can reduce plasma renin concentrations in patients with advanced heart failure, thereby resulting in peripheral vasodilation.[4] In contrast, in those without heart failure, digoxin can cause vasoconstriction. This difference is likely due to increased sensitivity of the carotid baroreceptors in patients with advanced, chronic heart failure.[5]

CLINICAL FEATURES

Digoxin has a narrow therapeutic index, and toxicity results from an exaggeration of its pharmacologic activity. The timing and clinical presentation of acute versus chronic digoxin toxicity differ significantly (**Table 193-1**).[6] In addition to cardiac manifestations such as syncope and dysrhythmia, digoxin toxicity may present with GI distress, dizziness,

TABLE 193-1 Clinical Presentation of Digitalis Glycoside Toxicity

	Acute Toxicity	Chronic Toxicity
Clinical history	Intentional or accidental ingestion	Typically elderly cardiac patients taking diuretics; may have renal insufficiency
GI effects	Nausea and vomiting, abdominal pain, anorexia	Nausea, vomiting, diarrhea, abdominal pain
CNS effects	Headache, dizziness, confusion, coma	Fatigue, weakness, confusion, delirium, and coma are often prominent features
Cardiac effects	Bradydysrhythmias or supraventricular tachydysrhythmias with atrioventricular block	Almost any ventricular or supraventricular dysrhythmia can occur; ventricular dysrhythmias are common
Electrolyte abnormalities	Hyperkalemia	Normal, decreased, or increased serum potassium, hypomagnesemia
Digoxin level	Marked elevation (if obtained within 6 h)	Minimally elevated or within "therapeutic" range

headache, weakness, malaise, delirium, or confusion. Thus, an elderly patient taking digoxin who presents with mental status changes should be evaluated for toxicity.

ACUTE TOXICITY

Patients with acute digoxin toxicity tend to have more abrupt onset of symptoms than those with chronic toxicity. In acute cardiac glycoside poisoning, there may be an asymptomatic period of several hours before the onset of symptoms. GI symptoms, such as nausea, vomiting, anorexia, and vague abdominal pain, are often the earliest manifestations of acute toxicity. Increased central vagal tone typically produces cardiac manifestations such as bradydysrhythmias or atrioventricular block. Neurologic manifestations such as weakness or confusion can occur independently of the blood pressure. The classic description of digoxin toxicity includes viewing yellow-green halos around objects, termed *xanthopsia*. However, patients more frequently describe nonspecific changes in their color vision.[7]

Hyperkalemia is an important finding in acute toxicity and may develop due to inhibition of sodium-potassium ATPase. Digoxin levels obtained with the first 6 hours following an acute ingestion may be falsely elevated as the level represents a predistribution level rather than reflecting the amount ingested. **Overall, the severity of acute toxicity correlates most closely with the degree of hyperkalemia and correlates poorly with the early serum digoxin levels.**[8]

CHRONIC TOXICITY

Chronic toxicity occurs most typically in the elderly and is often the result of drug–drug interactions or declining renal function. Some of the more common drug interactions that predispose to chronic digoxin toxicity include calcium channel antagonists, amiodarone, β-receptor antagonists, diuretics, indomethacin, clarithromycin, quinidine, procainamide, and erythromycin. In particular, interaction between digoxin and clarithromycin contributes to increased hospitalizations for digoxin toxicity in elderly patients.[9] A common scenario involves a patient starting to take a diuretic, which results in mild dehydration and hypokalemia; dehydration reduces the clearance of digoxin, and hypokalemia increases susceptibility to digoxin, resulting in chronic toxicity.

Decreases in renal function and lean body mass associated with aging may alter the pharmacokinetics of digoxin, leading to toxicity at normally therapeutic doses.[10] This population may also possess a higher risk due to coexisting diseases and polypharmacy.[10,11]

The patient with chronic digoxin toxicity often has vague and nonspecific signs and symptoms compared to the patient with acute digoxin toxicity. GI symptoms may occur but may be less pronounced. **Neurologic manifestations, such as weakness, fatigue, confusion, or delirium, are more prominent features in chronic toxicity.**[6,12]

DIAGNOSIS

The diagnosis of digoxin toxicity is a composite picture, using history, physical examination, and laboratory studies; no single element excludes or confirms the diagnosis. In patients with heart failure and normal renal function, daily digoxin doses are usually between 125 and 250 micrograms. Digoxin toxicity can occur with a single ingestion of 1 to 2 milligrams in an adult, and fatalities have been reported following an acute ingestion of 10 milligrams in an adult and 4 milligrams in a child.

Differential diagnosis includes other toxins that may induce bradydysrhythmias such as calcium channel antagonists, β-receptor antagonists, class IA antidysrhythmics (procainamide and quinidine), class IC antidysrhythmics (flecainide and encainide), clonidine and other imidazolines, and organophosphate or carbamate insecticide poisoning. Glycoside-containing and other cardiotoxic plants should also be considered (e.g., foxglove, squill, lily of the valley, oleander, rhododendron, monkshood, tobacco, false hellebore, and yew berry). Sick sinus syndrome, with its combination of supraventricular dysrhythmias and cardiac conduction blocks, can also mimic digoxin toxicity. Hyperkalemia from any cause may produce bradycardia and abnormal cardiac conduction and should be considered in the differential diagnosis.

ELECTROCARDIOGRAM

Almost any cardiac dysrhythmia may be observed in digoxin toxicity, with the exception of rapidly conducted atrial dysrhythmias.[13,14] **The most common dysrhythmia in digoxin toxicity is premature ventricular contractions.** Ventricular dysrhythmias occur more frequently in chronic than in acute poisonings. Although rare and not pathognomonic for digoxin toxicity, bidirectional ventricular tachycardia should be investigated for possible toxicity because only a few xenobiotics are known to produce this unique dysrhythmia, digoxin included.

Four specific electrocardiographic findings are seen with therapeutic levels of digoxin and are not indicators of toxicity, although they may also be seen in poisoned patients. These findings include T-wave changes such as flattening or inversion, QT-interval shortening, a "scooped" appearance of the ST segment with ST-segment depression, and an increase in U-wave amplitude (**Figure 193-1**).[14]

LABORATORY

In acute poisonings, the serum potassium and digoxin levels can provide useful diagnostic information.[15] As noted, acute poisoning of the sodium-potassium ATPase pump may result in markedly elevated serum potassium levels, and the serum potassium level is a better indicator of end-organ toxicity and a better prognostic indicator than the serum digoxin level in this circumstance.[8]

With chronic toxicity, in contrast to acute poisoning, the serum potassium and digoxin levels are less diagnostic. In these patients, the serum potassium is usually normal or low due to concomitant diuretic therapy, but may be elevated due to renal insufficiency. Thus, in the setting of chronic toxicity, measured serum potassium is more reflective of underlying comorbidities than the degree of inhibition of sodium-potassium ATPase by digoxin. Also, the serum digoxin level does not correlate with the clinical manifestations and *may be within therapeutic ranges* despite significant cardiac toxicity.

Serum digoxin levels should be interpreted in the overall clinical context and not relied upon as the sole indicator of the presence or absence of toxicity. Generally accepted therapeutic digoxin levels are 0.5 to 2.0 nanograms/mL (1.0 to 2.6 nmol/L), with corresponding toxic levels above 2.5 nanograms/mL (above 3.2 nmol/L). Due to a relatively slow distribution phase, high digoxin levels sampled from the serum following a recent acute ingestion are not always an accurate indicator of concentration at receptor sites. Serum levels are most reliable when obtained 6 hours after ingestion, when distribution is complete.[15] However, given the preceding limitations, it is still common that the higher the serum level, the greater is the likelihood of toxicity.[16] **Importantly, the serum digoxin level should not be the sole factor in establishing the diagnosis of digoxin toxicity, so do not wait for a digoxin level before implementing therapy in an unstable patient.**

Digoxin-like immunoreactive substances are substances that can be found in certain individuals that cross-react with the digoxin assay, artificially elevating the serum digoxin level, even in the absence of cardiac glycosides. Digoxin-like immunoreactive substances may be found in neonates, third-trimester pregnant women, patients with subarachnoid hemorrhage, and patients with renal or hepatic dysfunction. In addition, naturally occurring cardiac glycosides and cardioactive steroids from plants and animals may cross-react with digoxin assays. The degree of cross-reactivity is variable, and no reproducible correlation has been established between serum levels of these substances and toxicity.[17]

TREATMENT

Management of a digoxin-poisoned patient includes general supportive care, treatment of specific complications of toxicity, prevention of further drug absorption, enhancement of drug elimination, antidote administration when indicated, and safe disposition (**Table 193-2**).[6] Although patients with intentional or accidental ingestions may present with no symptoms, life-threatening complications of toxicity should be anticipated. Management of the asymptomatic patient should focus on preventing drug absorption and closely monitoring for the development of toxicity. Continuous cardiac monitoring, IV access, and frequent

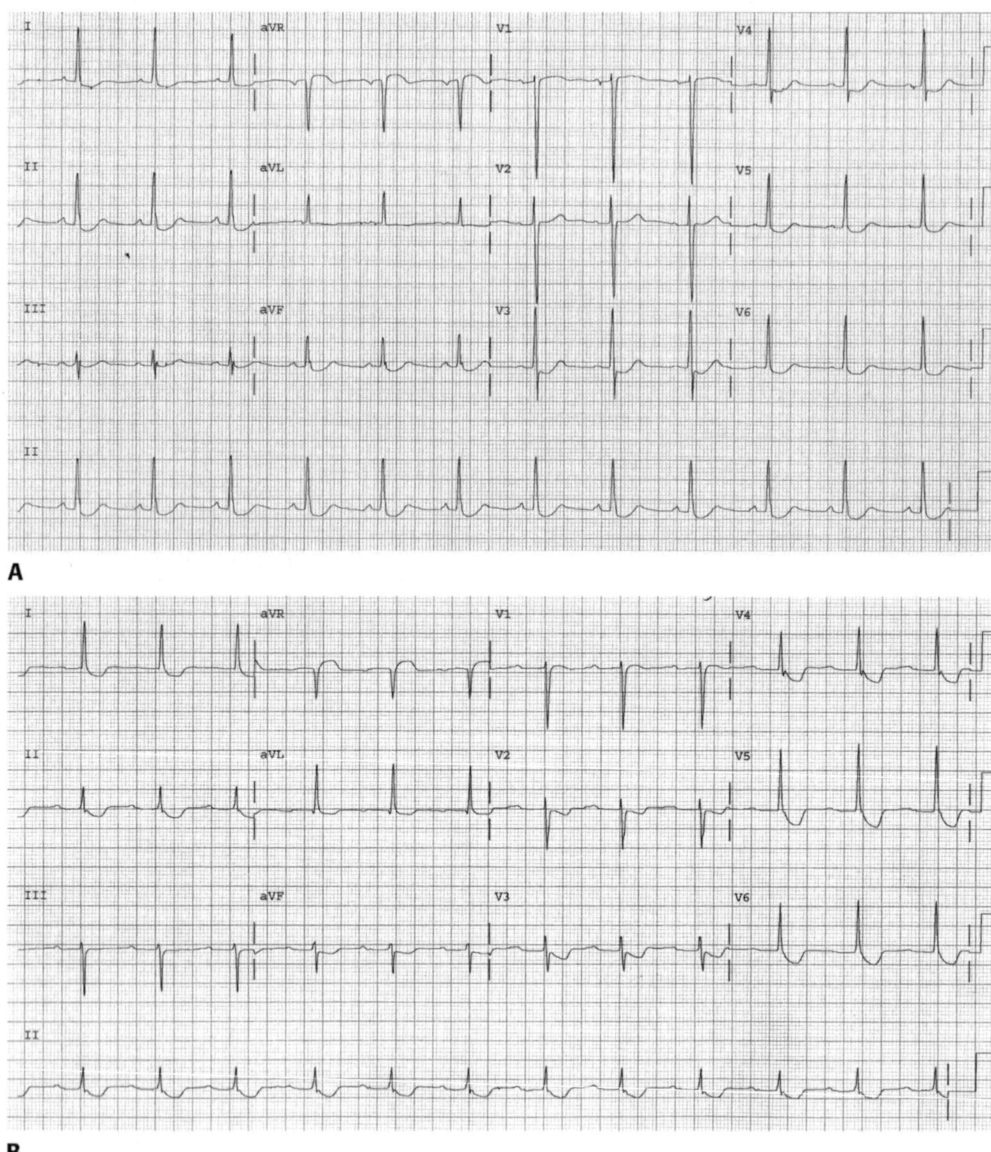

FIGURE 193-1. ECG demonstrating findings seen with digoxin use. **A.** ECG shows scooping of ST segments and small U waves with a serum digoxin level of 0.9 nanogram/mL (1.15 nmol/L). **B.** ECG shows scooping of ST segments, flattening of T waves, and first-degree atrioventricular block with a serum digoxin level of 1.2 nanograms/mL (1.54 nmol/L).

reevaluations should be provided for any patient with a potentially toxic ingestion of digoxin.

For the patient with life-threatening dysrhythmias, identify and rapidly correct conditions such as hypoxia, hypoglycemia, hypovolemia, and electrolyte abnormalities. IV magnesium may counteract ventricular irritability seen with cardiac-glycoside toxicity.[18] Use atropine and/or transvenous cardiac pacing as a temporizing treatment for bradydysrhythmias while preparing or obtaining digoxin-specific antibody fragments.[19]

Digoxin-specific antibody fragments (digoxin-Fab) are the treatment of choice in acute poisoning with hyperkalemia (potassium >6.0 mEq/L) and in acute or chronic toxicity with any life-threatening dysrhythmia.[20-22] Hyperkalemia is not typically the cause of the death; it is a predictor of severe poisoning and increased mortality. Treatment of digoxin-induced hyperkalemia with insulin, dextrose, sodium bicarbonate, or exchange resins does not reduce mortality.[8]

Administration of calcium salts in cardiac glycoside–induced hyperkalemia is controversial. Older literature indicated an increased incidence of ventricular dysrhythmias and a higher mortality when calcium was administered to digoxin-toxic patients. However, data from an animal model and retrospective review of a limited number of human patients with digoxin toxicity who received IV calcium found no increase in ventricular dysrhythmias or mortality.[23-25] **In summary, hyperkalemia in acute digoxin poisoning indicates severe toxicity and digoxin-Fab should be given to reduce mortality.**

In chronic toxicity, hypokalemia and hypomagnesemia should be corrected, because both predispose to digoxin toxicity.

GI DECONTAMINATION AND ENHANCED ELIMINATION

Administrating activated charcoal may have utility in early acute ingestion of digoxin.[22] Activated charcoal may be of benefit following the acute ingestion of yellow oleander, although results of large, randomized trials have been mixed.[26] Gastric lavage is not recommended; asystole has been reported in a digoxin-toxic patient, presumably from vagal stimulation during lavage, and no clinical benefit has been demonstrated. Cathartics, forced diuresis, hemodialysis, and hemoperfusion have no role in enhancing elimination of digitalis glycosides. In patients with chronic renal failure who develop digoxin toxicity, there are limited data for the use of binding resins such as cholestyramine to help enhance elimination.[27,28]

DIGOXIN-SPECIFIC ANTIBODY FRAGMENTS (DIGOXIN-FAB)

Digoxin-Fab are derived from ovine antibodies to digoxin. Following IV infusion, the antibody fragments bind digoxin in the plasma and

TABLE 193-2 Overview: Treatment of Digitalis Glycoside Poisoning

Asymptomatic patients
Obtain accurate history
Secure IV access
Initiate continuous cardiac monitoring
GI decontamination: activated charcoal, 1 gram/kg PO, can be considered in an awake, alert, cooperative patient who presents within 1 h of ingestion
Frequent reevaluation
Symptomatic patients
Obtain accurate history
Secure IV access
Initiate continuous cardiac monitoring
GI decontamination: activated charcoal, 1 gram/kg PO, in an awake, alert, cooperative patient who presents within 1 h of ingestion
Bradydysrhythmias
Atropine: 0.5–1.0 milligram IV as a temporizing measure for bradydysrhythmias while awaiting digoxin-specific Fab antibodies
Transcutaneous pacing while awaiting digoxin-specific Fab antibodies for symptomatic bradycardia that does not respond to atropine
Digoxin-specific antibody fragments: IV infusion (see discussion below for dose)
Cardiac arrest
CPR with current advanced cardiac life support protocols
Digoxin-specific antibody fragments: IV bolus (5–10 vials if amount ingested is unknown)

distribute widely throughout the body, removing digoxin from tissues. In severely poisoned patients after digoxin-Fab administration, 90% will show reversal or significant improvement in life-threatening dysrhythmia; in most cases, clinical improvement occurs within 1 hour. Patients in cardiac arrest had a 50% survival when receiving digoxin-Fab during the resuscitation, which is significantly better than historical survival with treatment with conventional therapies.[20] Because of cross-reactivity with other cardiac glycosides, digoxin-Fab are also beneficial in treating digitoxin, foxglove, and oleander poisonings, although large doses have sometimes been required.[17,26] Indications for digoxin-Fab are life-threatening dysrhythmias (including hemodynamically significant bradydysrhythmias unresponsive to standard therapy) and hyperkalemia in excess of 6 mEq/L associated with acute poisoning.

Digoxin-Fab administration is associated with few adverse effects.[20,21] Cardiogenic shock has been reported in patients dependent on digoxin for inotropic support.[29] In addition, ventricular response to atrial fibrillation may be increased. Hypokalemia may develop rapidly as digoxin toxicity is reversed. Mild, acute hypersensitivity reactions, including rash, flushing, and facial swelling, have been reported. No incidences of serum sickness or anaphylaxis have been observed, even in patients with repeated administration.[29] Skin testing has not proven to be useful in predicting allergic responses and may delay urgently needed treatment.[30] Failures to digoxin-Fab therapy have been attributed to inadequate dosing, moribund state before administration, and incorrect diagnosis of digoxin toxicity.[29]

A full neutralizing dose of digoxin-Fab is based on an estimation of the total-body load of digoxin, which can be calculated from either the dose ingested or a steady-state serum digoxin level (**Table 193-3**). In an acute poisoning, each vial of digoxin-Fab reverses approximately 0.5 milligram of ingested digoxin. In hemodynamically stable patients, half the calculated full neutralizing dose is infused, and the other half is given if an adequate clinical response is not seen in 1 to 2 hours.[31] Observational studies report that a total of 200 to 480 milligrams of digoxin-Fab (5 to 12 vials) were required to effectively treat severely digoxin-toxic patients.[20] When the ingested dose is unknown and serum level is unavailable, 10 vials are recommended as initial treatment in life-threatening situations. Digoxin-Fab are administered IV through a 0.22-mm filter over 30 minutes, except in cardiac arrest, when the dose is given as an IV bolus.

TABLE 193-3 Calculation of Digoxin-Specific Antibody Fragment Full Neutralizing Dose

Based on suspected amount ingested	Digoxin body load (milligrams) = 0.8 × suspected ingested amount (milligrams)*
	Digoxin body load (milligrams) = serum digoxin concentration (nanograms/mL) × 5.6 L/kg × weight (kg)/1000
	One vial (about 40 milligrams) of digoxin-Fab neutralizes 0.5 milligram of digoxin ingested
Based on total serum digoxin concentration	Number of vials = serum concentration (nanograms/mL) × patient weight (kg)/100

*0.95 should be used instead of 0.8 if the preparation is an elixir or gel tablet; 1 should be used if the cardiac glycoside is digitoxin.

Calculations of a full neutralizing dose may overestimate the amount of digoxin-Fab necessary, and smaller doses may adequately eliminate digoxin from the central compartment.[32] An alternative approach in acute poisoning with a hemodynamically stable patient is to give an 80-milligram (two vials) bolus of digoxin-Fab, evaluate the effect, and repeat the dose every 30 to 60 minutes as necessary until dysrhythmias have resolved and potassium has normalized. Such a protocol may reverse toxicity with less than half of a calculated full neutralizing dose.

In chronic toxicity, an acceptable approach in the hemodynamically stable patient is to give a 40-milligram (one vial) bolus of digoxin-Fab and repeat after 1 hour if the patient is still symptomatic. One to three vials (40 to 120 milligrams) of digoxin-Fab are often adequate in reversing chronic toxicity.[32]

Total serum digoxin levels obtained following digoxin-Fab administration have little correlation with clinical toxicity. Because most laboratory assays do not distinguish between antibody-bound and unbound digoxin, total serum levels obtained following digoxin-Fab administration may increase 10- to 20-fold.[20] However, because the Fab-digoxin complex is not pharmacologically active, this increased level does not correlate with clinical toxicity. The Fab-digoxin complex is eliminated by renal excretion.[33]

In the presence of renal failure, the Fab-digoxin complex may persist in the circulation for prolonged periods.[34] Recurrent toxicity can occur up to 10 days after digoxin-Fab administration in patients with renal failure as the complex degrades. Due to the large molecular weight of the Fab-digoxin complex (45,000 to 50,000 Da), hemodialysis does not enhance its elimination, although plasma exchange may be of benefit.[33,35,36] New liver support devices incorporating albumin-based dialysis and plasma filtration would be expected to be able to clear the Fab-digoxin complex on the basis of molecular weight alone; some devices have been reported to clear substances up to 100 kDa.[37] However, there is no experience using this technique with digoxin-poisoned patients.

DISPOSITION AND FOLLOW-UP

Extended observation with serial digoxin and potassium levels is recommended for anyone with a confirmed acute ingestion. Asymptomatic patients should be observed until the serum digoxin level is decreasing on serial measurements and the potassium level has remained normal. Patients with signs of toxicity or a history of a large (>6 milligrams in an adult) ingested dose should be admitted to a monitored unit. Consultation with a medical toxicologist or the regional poison control center is recommended. Patients receiving digoxin-Fab require intensive care unit observation for 6 to 12 hours.[31] Patients in renal failure who receive digoxin-Fab may be at risk of delayed toxicity, as the Fab-digoxin complex can dissociate several days later. Finally, patients with suspected suicidality should undergo behavioral health or psychiatric evaluation before discharge.

REFERENCES

The complete reference list is available online at www.TintinalliEM.com.

CHAPTER 194

Beta-Blockers

Jennifer L. Englund
William P. Kerns II

INTRODUCTION

β-Adrenergic receptor antagonists (β-blockers) are medications used in the treatment of various cardiovascular, neurologic, endocrine, ophthalmologic, and psychiatric disorders. Among all the exposures to cardiovascular agents, β-blocker exposures were the leading cause of poison center calls and ranked among the top three in this class as a cause of severe toxicity and mortality.[1]

PHARMACOLOGY

The β-adrenergic receptors are membrane glycoproteins present as three subtypes in various tissues (**Table 194-1**). These receptors play a critical role in cardiovascular physiology by modulating cardiac activity and vascular tone.

During times of stress (i.e., catecholamine release), β-adrenergic receptor stimulation increases myocardial and vascular smooth muscle cell activity through a sequence of intracellular events (**Figure 194-1**).[2,3]

The β-receptor is coupled to a stimulatory G_s protein. This G_s protein stimulates adenylate cyclase, which in turn catalyzes the formation of cyclic adenosine monophosphate, the so-called *intracellular second messenger*. Increased cyclic adenosine monophosphate ultimately phosphorylates the L-type calcium channel, which leads to channel opening and calcium entry into the cell. Extracellular calcium is then coupled to the ryanodine receptor to carry the calcium current to the sarcoplasmic reticulum, which then releases its stored calcium. This process is termed *calcium-induced calcium release*. Stored calcium becomes available to participate in mechanical contraction via the actin and myosin complex. Like the cardiac myocyte, the vascular smooth muscle uses L-type calcium channels to regulate intracellular calcium and subsequently coordinate vascular tone. To prevent overdrive of the cell, phosphodiesterase breaks down cyclic adenosine monophosphate to adenosine 5′-monophosphate, thus removing the stimulus for calcium channel opening, and the contractile process ceases.

The β-blockers modulate the activity of myocyte and vascular smooth muscle contraction by decreasing calcium entry into the cell.[2,3]

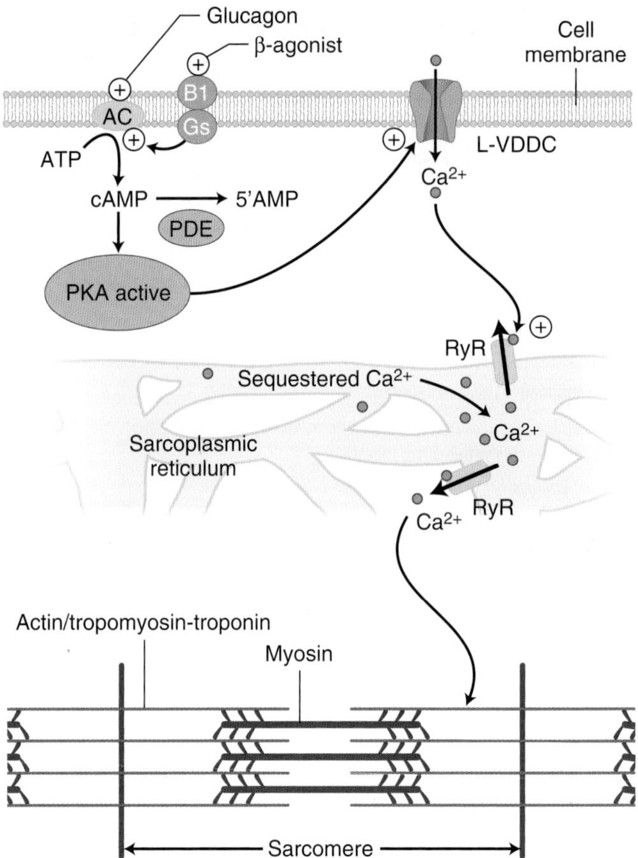

FIGURE 194-1. Cardiac myocyte $β_1$-receptor and calcium signaling. Following myocyte depolarization, extracellular calcium (Ca^{2+}) enters the cell via the L-type or voltage-gated calcium channel (L-VDCC) and binds to the ryanodine receptor (RyR) in the sarcoplasmic reticulum, causing an efflux of sequestered Ca^{2+} out of the sarcoplasmic reticulum into the cytosol. Free Ca^{2+} binds to troponin that allows the myosin and actin interaction, resulting in contraction of the cardiac myocyte. Binding of a β-agonist to the $β_1$-adrenergic receptor (B1) on the cell surface activates the Gs protein. The Gs protein then activates adenylate cyclase (AC), which converts adenosine triphosphate (ATP) to cyclic adenosine monophosphate (cAMP). The increased cAMP activates protein kinase A (PKA). Activated PKA serves as further stimulus for the L-VDCC opening. Glucagon independently activates adenylate cyclase. cAMP is metabolized by phosphodiesterase (PDE) into inactive adenosine 5′-monophosphate (5′AMP).

TABLE 194-1 Location and Activity of β-Adrenergic Receptors

β-Receptor Type	Location	Agonism	Antagonism
$β_1$	Myocardium	Increases inotropy	Decreases inotropy
		Increases chronotropy	Decreases chronotropy
	Kidney	Stimulates renin release	Inhibits renin release
	Eye	Stimulates aqueous humor production	Inhibits aqueous humor production
$β_2$	Bronchial smooth muscle	Causes bronchodilation	Causes bronchospasm
	Visceral smooth muscle	Relaxes uterus	—
		Causes ileus	
	Skeletal muscle	Increases force of contraction	—
		Stimulates glycogenolysis	
	Liver	Stimulates glycogenolysis and gluconeogenesis	Inhibits glycogenolysis and gluconeogenesis
	Vascular	Vasodilation	Minimal vasoconstriction
$β_3$	Adipose tissue	Stimulates lipolysis	Inhibits lipolysis
	Skeletal muscle	Stimulates thermogenesis	Inhibits thermogenesis

Therapeutically, β-blockade lessens the work performed by the diseased or injured myocardium and lowers elevated blood pressure. On the other hand, excessive β-blockade may lead to profound pump failure, with bradycardia, decreased contractility, and hypotension.[2]

The pharmacologic properties of various β-blockers influence their spectrum of action, adverse drug reactions, and toxicity (**Table 194-2**).[4,5] These properties include receptor selectivity, sodium channel blockade (also known as *membrane-stabilizing activity*), lipid solubility, protein binding, and partial agonist activity (also known as *intrinsic sympathomimetic activity*). For example, highly lipid-soluble agents, such as propranolol, readily cross the blood–brain barrier and achieve high concentrations in brain tissue.[2,3] This may contribute to the more severe CNS manifestations of mental status depression, seizures, and coma seen after an overdose of such agents.[2,3] Several β-blockers inhibit myocardial sodium channels, similar to quinidine and cyclic antidepressants, rendering these drugs potentially more cardiodepressant following overdose.[3] However, in massive overdoses, all β-blockers can be severely cardiodepressive.[6]

Although $β_1$ cardioselective medications have less risk of unwanted $β_2$ effects, such as bronchospasm, selectivity is often lost following large overdoses.[3] Several β-blockers like pindolol have partial agonist activity, causing weak stimulation of the β-receptor, with a lessor

TABLE 194-2 β-Blocker Pharmacologic Profiles

Agent	β_1 Selectivity	Lipophilicity	Partial Agonism	Protein Binding (%)	Sodium Channel Blockade	Half-Life (h)
Acebutolol	+	Moderate	+	25	+	3–4
Atenolol	+	Weak	0	6–16	0	6–9
Betaxolol	+	High	0	55	±	14–22
Bisoprolol	++	Moderate	0	30–40	0	9–12
Carvedilol	0	Moderate	0	>95	±	7–10
Esmolol	+	Weak	0	55	±	9 min
Labetalol	+	Weak	0	50	±	3–4
Metoprolol	++	Moderate	0	12	±	3–4
Nadolol	0	Weak	0	30	0	12–24
Nebivolol	+++	Moderate	0	98	0	8–27
Oxprenolol	0	Moderate	++	80	+	1–2
Pindolol	0	High	++	40–60	±	3–4
Penbutolol	0	High	+	80–98	0	5–20
Propranolol	0	High	0	>90	++	3–4
Sotalol	0	Weak	0	Minimal	0	12
Timolol	0	High	±	10–60	0	4–5

Abbreviations: + = some activity; ++ = strong activity; ± = possible activity; 0 = no activity.

tendency for bradycardia during therapeutic use.[4] Some β-blockers, such as labetalol and carvedilol, are also antagonists at α_1-adrenergic receptors, which can result in exaggerated hypotension during therapeutic use. Sotalol is unique among β-blockers in its ability to block potassium channels important for repolarization, as do other class III antiarrhythmic drugs.[2-4]

In addition to having cardiopulmonary effects, β-blockers also alter metabolism in the liver, skeletal muscle, and adipose tissue. Under normal conditions, the heart uses free fatty acids as its primary energy source, but during times of stress, it switches to using carbohydrates to maintain metabolism. Inhibition of glycogenolysis and gluconeogenesis reduces the availability of carbohydrates for use by metabolically active cells. Although hypoglycemia can occur as a consequence of β-blocker toxicity, it is actually uncommon.[2] In the presence of adequate glucose stores, euglycemia and hyperglycemia are more common than hypoglycemia.

Clinically relevant pharmacokinetic characteristics include drug formulation (regular or extended release), rate of drug absorption, protein binding, lipid solubility, elimination mostly by hepatic metabolism, and volume of distribution. These properties determine onset of symptoms, duration of symptoms, target organ toxicity, and potential treatment modalities.

CLINICAL FEATURES

Toxicity due to β-blockers can produce a spectrum of clinical symptoms (**Table 194-3**).[2,3,7] The timing of symptom appearance depends upon the formulation. Absorption of regular-release β-blockers occurs rapidly, often with peak effects within 1 to 4 hours. However, delays of up to 6 hours following acute ingestion have occurred.[8] Experience is limited regarding onset of symptoms with poisoning following an ingestion of sustained-release β-blocker formulations, but based on other sustained-release cardiac drugs, it is assumed that symptoms may be delayed >6 hours after ingestion.[2,3] Co-ingestants that alter gut function, such as opioids and anticholinergics, may affect absorption of β-blockers and subsequent onset of symptoms.[2]

The primary organ system affected by β-blocker toxicity is the cardiovascular system, and the hallmark of severe toxicity is bradycardia and shock.[2,3,7,9] Bradycardia due to sinus node suppression or conduction abnormalities occurs in virtually all significant β-blocker intoxications, although ingestion of β-blockers with partial agonist activity may initially present with hypertension and tachycardia.[9] The β-blockers with sodium channel antagonism can worsen conduction abnormalities, causing a wide-complex bradycardia (especially when the QRS interval is >100 milliseconds).[9]

The cardiotoxic profile of sotalol is different from that of other β-blockers due to its ability to block potassium channels and prolong the QT interval.[3] Thus, sotalol is more often associated with ventricular dysrhythmias, including premature ventricular contractions, bigeminy, ventricular tachycardia, ventricular fibrillation, and torsades de pointes.[3]

β-Blockers also affect the CNS and pulmonary system. Neurologic manifestations include depressed mental status, coma, and seizures.[2] These symptoms most likely occur as a result of a combination of hypoxia due to poor perfusion, sodium channel antagonism, and direct neuronal toxicity.[2] More lipophilic β-blockers, such as propranolol, cause greater neurologic toxicity than the less lipophilic agents.[9] Seizures are generally brief, and status epilepticus is rare.[2] Nonselective β-blockers may antagonize the β_2-receptor in bronchial smooth muscle causing bronchospasm. Similarly, in large ingestions of cardioselective β-blockers, the β_1 selectivity may be lost.

TABLE 194-3 Common Findings with β-Blocker Toxicity

- Cardiovascular
  - Hypotension
  - Bradycardia
  - Conduction delays and blocks (first-degree atrioventricular block)
  - Ventricular dysrhythmias (sotalol)
  - Asystole
  - Decreased contractility
- CNS
  - Depressed mental status
  - Coma
  - Psychosis
  - Seizures
  - Respiratory arrest
- Pulmonary
  - Bronchospasm
- Electrolytes
  - Hypoglycemia
  - Hyperkalemia

TABLE 194-4 Toxicologic Causes of Bradycardia and Hypotension

Cause	Differentiating Features
Calcium channel blockers	Elevated lactate level and hyperglycemia
Naturally occurring cardiac glycosides (oleander, foxglove, lily of the valley, rhododendron, and toad-derived bufotoxin)	Ventricular ectopy May cross-react with digoxin immunoassay
Class IC antiarrhythmic drugs (propafenone)	Wide-complex bradycardia
Clonidine	Opioid-like manifestations: coma, miosis, decreased respirations
Cyanide	Profound metabolic acidosis and elevated lactate level
Digoxin (acute)	Hyperkalemia Elevated level on digoxin immunoassay
Organophosphates	Muscarinic toxidrome

DIAGNOSIS

The diagnosis of β-blocker toxicity is primarily made on clinical grounds, including patient history, physical examination findings, and results of basic diagnostic testing. Patients commonly present with a history of intentional overdose or therapeutic misadventure. The diagnosis may be more challenging in the case of polypharmacy "heart or blood pressure medication" overdose or with suspected chronic drug toxicity in the patient on multiple cardiovascular drugs. Exposure to other drugs and toxins can present with bradycardia and hypotension, but useful features can help differentiate toxicity from these agents from that due to β-blockers (**Table 194-4**).

Laboratory testing is recommended to assess renal function, glucose level, oxygenation, and acid-base status. Although specific β-blocker drug levels might be of value for later confirmation of an ingestion, these levels are not helpful initially because they do not correlate with the degree of toxicity and are generally not available in a timely fashion to affect acute management.[2,3,7] False-positive amphetamine results can be seen on urine drug screens from labetalol, because one of its metabolites is structurally similar to amphetamine and methamphetamine.[10] Cardiac function is evaluated with a 12-lead ECG, rhythm monitor, and bedside cardiac US.[11] A drug-induced Brugada pattern may be observed in an overdose of propranolol, a β-blocker that also affects cardiac sodium channels.[12]

TREATMENT

GENERAL MANAGEMENT

Evaluate patients with suspected β-blocker overdose in a critical-care area of the ED with appropriate monitoring because these patients may experience abrupt cardiovascular collapse or neurologic depression. If orotracheal intubation is needed, the drugs used to sedate and paralyze may worsen hypotension in the face of an already depressed myocardium.[2,3,7]

GI DECONTAMINATION

Although there is little evidence to support routine GI decontamination following overdose of most substances, ingestion of a significant quantity of β-blockers with the risk of severe toxicity is a circumstance in which decontamination should be considered.[13] Activated charcoal may be of benefit if it can be given within 1 hour after ingestion and the patient is able to maintain the airway.[14,15] There may be an additional window of opportunity for activated charcoal therapy following ingestion of sustained-release β-blockers. Ipecac syrup and cathartic agents are not recommended.[16] Gastric lavage is not recommended.[13] Whole-bowel irrigation may be beneficial after a large ingestion of an extended-release product.[17]

PHARMACOLOGIC TREATMENT

Specific pharmacologic therapies are directed at restoring perfusion to critical organ systems by improving myocardial contractility, increasing heart rate, or both.[2,3,7] This is done through fluid resuscitation and administration of glucagon, adrenergic agonists, high-dose insulin, calcium, and phosphodiesterase inhibitors (**Figure 194-2**). Individual pharmacologic therapies have variable effectiveness and are often used simultaneously.[7] Aggressive measures such as hemodialysis, hemoperfusion, cardiac pacing, placement of intra-aortic balloon pumps, and extracorporeal circulatory support have also been used when patients are refractory to pharmacologic therapy.[18]

GLUCAGON

Glucagon is a first-line agent in the treatment of acute β-blocker–induced bradycardia and hypotension.[2,19] Glucagon, produced in the pancreatic α-cells from proglucagon, independently activates myocardial adenylate cyclase, bypassing the impaired β-receptor (Figure 194-1). Effects from an IV bolus of glucagon are seen within 1 to 2 minutes, reach a peak in 5 to 7 minutes, and have a duration of action of 10 to 15 minutes.[2,3] Due to the short duration of effect, a continuous infusion is often necessary after bolus administration. The bolus dose of glucagon is 3 to 10 milligrams (30 to 150 micrograms/kg in children), and if a response is not seen within 15 minutes, a repeat bolus can be given. If a beneficial effect is seen from the glucagon bolus, a continuous infusion of 1 to 5 milligrams/h (20 to 70 micrograms/kg per hour in children) can be used to maintain this effect. Glucagon infusion should be titrated to rate to achieve adequate hemodynamic response. There is no identified maximum therapeutic dose or duration of treatment.[19]

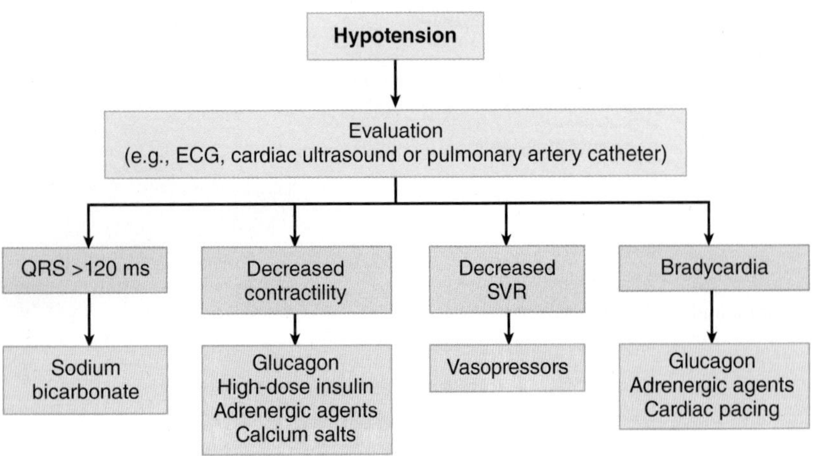

FIGURE 194-2. Management strategies in β-blocker toxicity. Cardiac function is evaluated using ECG, cardiac US, and/or central hemodynamic monitoring. For wide QRS interval, consider sodium bicarbonate therapy. For impaired myocardial contractility, consider glucagon, high-dose insulin, adrenergic agents, and calcium therapy. For decreased systemic vascular resistance, consider vasopressors, such as norepinephrine, epinephrine, dopamine, and phenylephrine. For bradycardia, consider glucagon, adrenergic agents, and cardiac pacing. (See text for details.) SVR = systemic vascular resistance.

The amount of glucagon required to treat a significant β-blocker overdose may exceed the total amount available at any given hospital.[19] The positive inotropic and chronotropic effects of glucagon may not be maintained for a prolonged period due to possible tachyphylaxis. Nausea and vomiting are commonly reported side effects of high-dose glucagon therapy and may be related to esophageal sphincter relaxation. Intubation prior to glucagon administration may be warranted in any patient with altered mental status to limit the risk of aspiration.[2,3,7]

Prior to 1998, glucagon was derived from porcine and bovine pancreas and contained other pancreatic compounds such as insulin and phenol as a preservative.[2] The contribution of this insulin content to the original glucagon's overall efficacy is unclear (see discussion below in "High-Dose Insulin Therapy"). Since 1998, glucagon has been produced via recombinant technology and is devoid of insulin or phenol.

ADRENERGIC RECEPTOR AGONISTS

The β-adrenergic receptor agonists—such as norepinephrine, dopamine, epinephrine, and isoproterenol—are used routinely to treat β-blocker toxicity.[2,19] However, results have been variable even when dosages far exceed those recommended in standard guidelines for cardiac resuscitation.[3] The most effective adrenergic receptor agonists may be norepinephrine and epinephrine due to their chronotropic and vasopressor effects. Phenylephrine may also be beneficial as a vasopressor. Although isoproterenol may increase heart rate, it does so at the expense of vasodilation. Dobutamine has a similar downside: potential improvement in inotropy but worsening of hypotension due to vasodilation.

HIGH-DOSE INSULIN THERAPY

High-dose insulin therapy, sometimes called hyperinsulinemia-euglycemia therapy, is an important treatment modality for β-blocker toxicity.[17,20-22] Insulin acts as an inotrope by facilitating myocardial utilization of glucose, the desired energy substrate during stress, in contrast to glucagon, epinephrine, and calcium, which promote free fatty acid utilization.[20-23] In animal models, high-dose insulin therapy improved survival in severe β-blocker overdose compared with glucagon, epinephrine, or vasopressin administration.[24,25] The most consistent cardiodynamic effect in these models was an increase in contractility.

High-dose insulin therapy dosing used for treatment of β-blocker toxicity is much higher than that used for traditional glucose control in diabetes (**Table 194-5**). The initial dose is regular insulin 1 unit/kg IV bolus and is followed by a continuous infusion of 0.5 to 1 unit/kg per hour that is titrated to the desired hemodynamic response of a heart rate at least 50 beats/min and systolic blood pressure of at least 100 mm Hg (13.3 kPa).[20-22] The maximum dose has not yet been established, although an animal model of propranolol overdose[26] found that cardiac output increased in a dose-response manner when the insulin dose was raised from 1 to 10 units/kg per hour, and human case reports have used doses this high.[22]

TABLE 194-5 Protocol for High-Dose Insulin Therapy in Severe β-Blocker Overdose

Check serum glucose, and if <200 milligrams/dL (<11 mmol/L), administer 50 mL of 50% dextrose (0.5 gram/mL) in water IV (children 1 mL/kg of 25% dextrose).
Administer regular insulin 1 unit/kg IV bolus.
Begin regular insulin infusion at 0.5–1.0 unit/kg per hour along with dextrose 10% (0.1 gram/mL) in water at 200 mL/h (adult) or 5 mL/kg per hour (pediatric).
Titrate infusion rate up to 10 units/kg per hour according the hemodynamic goal of HR >50 beats/min and SBP >100 mm Hg (>13.3 kPa).
Monitor serum glucose every 15–20 min.
Titrate dextrose infusion rate to maintain serum glucose level between 100 and 200 milligrams/dL (5.3 and 10.7 mmol/L).
Once dextrose infusion rates have been stable for 60 min, glucose monitoring may be decreased to hourly.
Monitor serum potassium level and start IV potassium infusion if serum potassium level is <2.8 mEq/L (<2.8 mmol/L).
Maintain serum potassium between 2.8 and 3.2 mEq/L (2.8 and 3.2 mmol/L).

Abbreviations: HR = heart rate; SBP = systolic blood pressure.

The onset of action with high-dose insulin therapy is reported to be 15 to 45 minutes, but a delayed response of several hours has been noted.[20] High-dose insulin therapy is continued until resolution of toxicity; the duration of high-dose insulin therapy infusion described in case reports ranges from 9 to 49 hours.[22] The insulin infusion can be gradually weaned or abruptly halted. Reinstitute the insulin infusion if the heart rate or blood pressure falls after cessation of high-dose insulin therapy.

Potential adverse effects from high-dose insulin therapy are hypoglycemia and lowered serum potassium. Dextrose infusion is used to prevent hypoglycemia and often required during the duration of therapy.[22] Serum potassium is monitored and supplemental replacement is given if the level is below 2.8 mEq/L (2.8 mmol/L).[20,22] An increase in the dextrose infusion rate required to maintain serum glucose between 100 and 200 milligrams/dL (5.3 and 10.7 mmol/L), along with signs of clinical improvement, may be an indication that metabolic status is normalizing; that is, that the stress response is diminishing, the heart is reverting back to basal energy substrates, and extra insulin is no longer needed.

INTRAVENOUS LIPID EMULSION THERAPY

Intravenous lipid emulsion therapy, also known as fat emulsion therapy or lipid rescue, is effective in treating toxicity from local anesthetics, calcium channel blockers, typical and atypical antipsychotics, cyclic and other antidepressants, and some β-blockers.[27-29] The exact mechanism is not fully understood, but the likely explanation is that lipid emulsion acts as a pharmacologic sink, by sequestering lipophilic drugs into a separate lipid compartment, and the amount of free drug available to target tissues is reduced ("lipid sink" model).[30] Other potential mechanisms may include supplying the myocardium with free fatty acids and phospholipids, increasing myocardial contractility by increasing myocyte calcium concentration, and elevating blood pressure by central sympathetic activation.

Animal models suggest that intravenous lipid emulsion may be most effective in the lipophilic β-blockers (Table 194-2), such as propranolol and carvedilol, and may be less effective in more hydrophilic agents, such as metoprolol and atenolol.[31]

The dosing regimen for intravenous lipid emulsion is based on treatment of local anesthetic systemic toxicity. The standard 20% lipid emulsion is given as a 1.5 mL/kg bolus over 1 minute, followed by a infusion at 0.25 mL/kg per minute.[30] If the blood pressure remains low, an additional 1.5 mL/kg bolus may be repeated followed by an increase in the infusion rate to 0.5 mL/kg per minute. The recommended upper limit is about 10 mL/kg over the initial 30 minutes. If the patient's hemodynamic stability is dependent on continued lipid infusion, the treatment may be continued beyond this level. Duration of therapy has not been fully established. If cardiac arrest occurs, a bolus dose can be given during the resuscitation.

Adverse effects reported with the use of lipid emulsion for the treatment of overdose and toxicity include lipemia causing interference with laboratory analysis, hypertriglyceridemia, pancreatitis, and possibly acute lung injury, acute renal failure, deep vein thrombosis, and cardiac arrest.[32-34] Lipid emulsion may clog the hemofiltration filter precluding renal replacement therapy during the infusion and until the lipid has been cleared from the blood.[35] Given the current understanding and limited clinical experience using intravenous lipid emulsion as an antidote, this treatment should be reserved for refractory shock.

ATROPINE

Atropine, a muscarinic blocker, is unlikely to be effective in the management of β-blocker–induced bradycardia and hypotension, although its use is unlikely to cause harm.[3,4,7] Its use may be beneficial for co-ingestants.

CALCIUM

Canine studies and limited case reports suggest that calcium therapy may reverse depression of the myocardium via positive inotropic action, although with few chronotropic effects.[2,3] Calcium administration is not routinely recommended in β-blocker overdose, but may be considered in patients with refractory shock unresponsive to other therapies. Calcium for IV administration is available in two forms, gluconate and chloride, both in a 10% solution. A 10-mL dose of 10% calcium chloride solution contains three times more elemental calcium, 13.6 mEq (6.8 mmol), than 10 mL of 10% calcium gluconate solution, 4.5 mEq (2.23 mmol). Thus, one 10-mL ampule of 10% calcium chloride equals three 10-mL ampules of 10% calcium gluconate.

Potential adverse effects of calcium therapy include hypercalcemia, conduction blocks, worsening bradycardia, and inefficient cardiac energetics during shock (see "High-Dose Insulin Therapy"). Most patients tolerate transient increases in total calcium level without difficulty, and conduction blocks are rare. Severe soft tissue injury associated with inadvertent IV infiltration of the chloride formulation is the most concerning adverse event. Thus, calcium chloride is ideally given via a central line. Calcium gluconate is only rarely associated with tissue injury and is the preferred form for peripheral administration.

The optimum dose of calcium in β-blocker toxicity is unknown. Animal studies and limited human studies suggest that large amounts of calcium are needed to treat drug-induced cardiac toxicity, but these data come from experience derived from treating calcium channel blocker toxicity.[2,3] The recommended dose of 10% calcium gluconate is 0.6 mL/kg given over 5 to 10 minutes, followed by a continuous infusion of 0.6 to 1.5 mL/kg per h.[2,3] The equivalent dosage of 10% calcium chloride is 0.2 mL/kg given via central line over 5 to 10 minutes, followed by a continuous infusion of 0.2 to 0.5 mL/kg per h. Ionized calcium levels should be checked every 30 minutes initially and then every 2 hours to achieve an ionized calcium level of twice the normal value.[2]

PHOSPHODIESTERASE INHIBITORS

Phosphodiesterase inhibitors such as milrinone have been used to treat β-blocker toxicity. These agents inhibit the breakdown of cyclic adenosine monophosphate, thereby sustaining intracellular calcium levels (Figure 194-1).[2,3] In animal models, phosphodiesterase inhibitors produce positive inotropic effects without increasing myocardial oxygen demand but have no appreciable effect on heart rate. Compared with glucagon, phosphodiesterase inhibitors do not provide any additional benefit and therefore have no advantage over glucagon. However, if glucagon is not available or pharmacy stores have been exhausted, a phosphodiesterase inhibitor is a reasonable alternative. In the setting of a β-blocker overdose, milrinone is administrated as a continuous IV infusion, starting with a 50 micrograms/kg IV bolus, followed by an IV infusion of 0.375 to 0.75 micrograms/kg per minute for milrinone.[36]

SODIUM BICARBONATE

Sodium bicarbonate is used to treat severe acidosis and wide QRS-interval dysrhythmias secondary to sodium channel blockade. β-Blockers with sodium channel–blocking ability (Table 194-2) can interfere with ventricular depolarization, predisposing to cardiac dysrhythmias. When the QRS interval is longer than 120 to 140 milliseconds, it is reasonable to administer sodium bicarbonate.[2] The suggested dose is a rapid bolus of 2 to 3 mEq/kg over 1 to 2 min.[2,3,6] Thus, a 70-kg adult receives a bolus of 140 to 210 mEq of sodium bicarbonate, or three to four ampules (50 mL each) of 8.4% sodium bicarbonate. Repeat boluses or an infusion may be required to maintain the QRS interval at <120 milliseconds.

CARDIAC PACING

Internal or external pacing may be considered to treat bradycardia in the setting of β-blocker toxicity.[2,3] Electrical capture and restoration of blood pressure is not always successful, potentially due to the lack of intracellular calcium needed for contraction.[2,3] Cardiac pacing may be most beneficial in treating torsades de pointes associated with sotalol toxicity.

EXTRACORPOREAL ELIMINATION (HEMODIALYSIS)

The high degree of protein binding and lipid solubility of β-blockers, as well as their large volume of distribution, renders extracorporeal drug removal useless for most drugs in this class. Acebutolol, atenolol, nadolol, and sotalol may be amenable to removal through hemodialysis owing to their lower protein binding, water solubility, and lower volume of distribution.[37]

EXTRACORPOREAL CIRCULATION

Occasionally, extreme means of resuscitation, including extracorporeal circulation (extracorporeal membrane oxygenation) and intra-aortic balloon pumps, have been successful when pharmacologic measures have failed to reverse cardiogenic shock.[38,39]

TREATMENT OF SOTALOL TOXICITY

Treatment of sotalol toxicity may require pharmacologic measures different from those required for other β-blockers due to its potassium channel effects. In addition to the therapies discussed above, magnesium supplementation, lidocaine, and cardiac overdrive pacing may be of specific benefit.

SUMMARY

No one particular treatment is consistently effective in cases of β-blocker toxicity, and multiple simultaneous treatment measures may be required to resuscitate the critically ill patient. Tailor therapy based on the ECG, bedside cardiac US, and/or central hemodynamic monitoring. The goal of resuscitation is to improve hemodynamics and organ perfusion. Specific end points of therapy may include a cardiac ejection fraction of 50% or greater, a reduction of the QRS interval to <120 milliseconds, a heart rate of >50 to 60 beats/min, a systolic blood pressure of >90 to 100 mm Hg (12.0 to 13.3 kPa) in an adult, a urine output of 1 to 2 mL/kg per hour, and improved mentation.

DISPOSITION AND FOLLOW-UP

Patients who develop altered mental status, bradycardia, conduction delays, or hypotension should be managed in an intensive care unit. A patient who ingests a sustained-released β-blocker product warrants admission and monitoring for the development of delayed toxicity.[2,3,9] Patients ingesting an overdose of regular-release β-blocker tablets who remain asymptomatic and have normal vital signs for 6 hours after ingestion can be deemed medically safe for discharge or admission to a psychiatric facility.[9]

REFERENCES

The complete reference list is available online at www.TintinalliEM.com.

Calcium Channel Blockers

Alicia B. Minns
Christian Tomaszewski

INTRODUCTION

Calcium channel blockers (CCBs) are commonly used for the treatment of hypertension and angina pectoris and for ventricular rate control in supraventricular dysrhythmias. Less common uses include prophylactic treatment of migraine headaches, treatment of arterial vasospasm due to Raynaud's disease, esophageal spasm, and pulmonary hypertension.[1] For the last 50 years, CCBs have accounted for more poisoning deaths than any other cardiovascular drug and are the second most common cause of prescription drug poisoning death.

PHARMACOLOGY

Intracellular calcium is the primary stimulus for smooth and cardiac muscle contraction and for impulse formation in sinoatrial pacemaker cells. At therapeutic concentrations, CCBs bind to the subunit of the L-type calcium channel, causing the channel to favor the closed state and thereby decreasing calcium entry during the plateau phase (phase 2) of the transmembrane action potential. At very high concentrations, some CCBs (notably verapamil) may occupy the channel canal and completely block calcium entry. The result is profound smooth muscle relaxation, weakened cardiac contraction, blunted cardiac automaticity, and intracardiac conduction delay.[1] Clinically, these effects produce hypotension and bradycardia. Animal data suggest that verapamil overdose also impairs myocardial carbohydrate intake, which contributes to the negative cardiac inotropy.[2]

The three main pharmacologic classes of CCBs are phenylalkylamines (verapamil and gallopamil), benzothiazepines (diltiazem), and dihydropyridines (nifedipine, amlodipine, and most newer agents—aranidipine, azelnidipine, barnidipine, benidipine, cilnidipine, clevidipine, efonidipine, felodipine, lacidipine, lercanidipine, manidipine, nicardipine, nilvadipine, nimodipine, nisoldipine, nitrendipine, and pranidipine).

All of these drugs relax vascular smooth muscle, reduce pacemaker activity, and decrease cardiac contractility; however, these effects occur at different dose ranges for each drug. In addition, all three classes increase coronary blood flow in a dose-dependent fashion.[3] Each group binds a different region of the calcium channel and has different affinities for calcium channels in various tissues. Verapamil is the most potent negative inotrope of all CCBs, causing at least equal depression of heart contraction and vascular smooth muscle dilatation at any concentration.[4] This combined cardiovascular effect may be one reason that verapamil overdose causes more deaths than all other CCBs combined.

Dihydropyridines bind more selectively to vascular smooth muscle calcium channels than to cardiac calcium channels and therefore relax smooth muscle at concentrations that produce almost no negative inotropy. The differences in the effects of these agents is the reason for preferential use of specific agents in particular clinical situations.[5] For example, verapamil and diltiazem are used to manage hypertension, to achieve rate control in atrial flutter and atrial fibrillation, and to abolish supraventricular reentrant tachycardias. Dihydropyridines are typically used to treat diseases with increased peripheral vascular tone such as hypertension, Prinzmetal's angina, and vasospasm after subarachnoid hemorrhage.[1]

The original three CCBs—verapamil, nifedipine, and diltiazem—all have relatively short serum half-lives (**Table 195-1**). Consequently, extended-release formulations have been developed for all of these agents. Because extended-release formulations prolong drug absorption, onset of symptoms may be delayed and toxicity may be prolonged following overdose.[6,7] Several of the newer dihydropyridines have prolonged duration of action, and therefore are generally not formulated as extended-release products. Because newer formulations are released frequently, it is helpful to contact a regional poison control center for help in determining if a given product ingested in an overdose is formulated as an extended-release preparation.

TABLE 195-1 Oral Calcium Channel Blockers

	Metabolism	Half-Life (standard preparation, not extended-release)	Maximum Recommended Adult Daily Dose (milligrams)
Verapamil*	Liver extensively	2–5 h	480
Diltiazem*	Liver extensively	3–5 h	480 for regular-release and 540 for extended-release
Nifedipine*	Liver	2 h	180 for regular-release and 90 for extended-release
Amlodipine	Liver extensively	30–50 h	10
Felodipine*	Liver extensively	9 h	10
Isradipine	Liver	8 h	10
Nicardipine*	Liver extensively	8–14 h	120
Nimodipine	Liver extensively	Early: 1–2 h Terminal: 8–9 h	360
Nisoldipine*	Liver extensively	7–12 h	34

*Also available in extended-release preparations.

CLINICAL FEATURES

The most prominent and life-threatening effects are an extension of the therapeutic effects on the cardiovascular system, particularly myocardial depression and peripheral vasodilation. Hypotension is the most common physiologic abnormality after overdose.[8,9] Patients with moderate verapamil or diltiazem poisoning often have sinus bradycardia, varying degrees of atrioventricular block, and hypotension. Atrioventricular block occurs more often with verapamil than with diltiazem or nifedipine.[10] Mild or moderate dihydropyridine overdoses usually cause peripheral vasodilatation with resultant hypotension and reflex tachycardia.[10] In severe overdose, any of these agents may cause complete heart block, depressed myocardial contractility, and vasodilatation that ultimately results in cardiovascular collapse.

Pulmonary and CNS effects are generally secondary to decreased myocardial function and impaired organ perfusion. Cardiogenic pulmonary edema is sometimes observed in severe overdoses, especially if large volumes of crystalloid are infused during resuscitation. Acute lung injury (noncardiogenic pulmonary edema) has also been reported.[11,12] Seizures, delirium, and coma have been described and are presumed to be secondary to cerebral hypoperfusion. Alteration in consciousness in the absence of hypotension should not be attributed to CCB toxicity; prompting an evaluation for other causes. GI symptoms, such as nausea and vomiting, are uncommon.[13]

DIAGNOSIS

POTENTIAL TOXICITY

Estimations have been made of the lowest doses and mean doses ingested that produce toxicity (**Table 195-2**).[7] A history of ingestion that is near these doses should be considered potentially toxic, and doses in excess of the lowest toxic dose reported should be expected to produce toxicity.[7] Adults receiving long-term therapy with CCBs can develop hypotension, bradycardia, or cardiac conduction abnormalities if they ingest twice their regular daily dose.[14] It is hypothesized that patients receiving long-term CCB therapy have comorbidities and may be taking additional medications, such as other antihypertensives, that render these patients sensitive to the adverse effects of an additional amount of their CCB. Children may be sensitive to CCB toxicity, and deaths have been reported after ingestion of a single tablet: nifedipine, 10 milligrams, in a 14-month-old child[15] and verapamil, 25 milligrams, in a 7-day-old infant.[16] **Therefore, all pediatric CCB ingestions should be referred for medical attention and observation.**

Extended-release preparations are increasingly used for patient convenience and enhancing patient adherence to the drug regimen. These preparations complicate the management of overdosed patients by delaying the onset of toxicity. Therefore, it is important to determine the exact formulation of the ingested agent to guide management decisions. If the history cannot identify the exact formulation, the clinician should assume it is extended-release and modify treatment in a conservative way. In a review of CCB overdose cases, 52% of patients ingested extended-release preparations, and of these, 8% had no evidence of toxicity on initial evaluation but developed delayed toxicity 6 hours or later

TABLE 195-2 Single-Ingestion Toxicity from Calcium Channel Blockers

Agent	Lowest Toxic Dose (adult)	Mean Toxic Dose (adult)	Mean Toxic Dose (pediatric)
Verapamil	720 milligrams	2708 milligrams	16 milligrams/kg
Diltiazem	420 milligrams	2167 milligrams	5.7 milligrams/kg
Nifedipine	50 milligrams	245 milligrams	8.0 milligrams/kg

TABLE 195-3 Differential Diagnosis of Bradycardia, Atrioventricular Block, and Hypotension

Hypothermia
Acute coronary syndrome
Hyperkalemia
Cardiac glycoside toxicity
β-Blocker toxicity
Antiarrhythmic drugs class IA and IC toxicity
Central α-adrenergic agonist (clonidine or tetrahydrozoline) toxicity

TABLE 195-4 General Treatment for Calcium Channel Blocker Toxicity*

Treatment	Comments
Monitoring	Initiate cardiopulmonary monitoring and obtain ECG
Point-of-care glucose	If altered mental status, and also in anticipation of insulin therapy
Naloxone	If signs of opioid toxicity
Single-dose activated charcoal	If ingestion within 1 h and no vomiting or altered mental status; for children even if one tablet ingested
Multidose activated charcoal	For extended-release preparations
IV crystalloid for hypotension	Overaggressive treatment can cause pulmonary edema
Endotracheal intubation	Early intubation if altered mental status or hemodynamic instability

*See Figure 195-1 for treatment of severe toxicity.

after ingestion.[10] In addition to the exact formulation ingested, other important aspects in the history are the time of ingestion and the possibility of co-ingestants that may contribute to toxicity.

ECG findings include sinus bradycardia, varying degrees of atrioventricular block, and slowing of intraventricular conduction. Reflex tachycardia is commonly seen with low to moderate toxic ingestions of dihydropyridines, whereas junctional rhythms and ventricular escape rhythms are frequently noted in severe overdoses with verapamil or diltiazem.

Laboratory testing is done to assess the overall metabolic state of the patient; none is crucial in the acute management of CCB toxicity. Hyperglycemia is often noted after CCB ingestion, which differentiates it from β-blocker ingestion, which is typically euglycemic or sometimes hypoglycemic.[17] CCBs inhibit calcium-mediated insulin secretion from the beta islet cells in the pancreas, impeding the use of carbohydrates, and also increase insulin resistance by unclear mechanisms.[18]

Systemic hypoperfusion may cause a lactate acidosis with an elevated anion gap and low serum bicarbonate level. Hypokalemia may be observed in severe overdoses. Serum calcium levels are usually normal. Ionized serum calcium levels may be followed during treatment with intravenous calcium preparations, but the optimum serum calcium level for patients with severe CCB poisoning is unknown. CCB serum concentrations are not routinely available and are not used in management. Screen blood and urine for other potential toxins after suicidal overdose.

DIFFERENTIAL DIAGNOSIS

A few conditions and other drug toxicities can produce bradycardia, atrioventricular block, and hypotension (**Table 195-3**). Hypothermia should be detected during vital sign assessment. Myocardial infarction may be evident on the initial or subsequent ECG. Suspect hyperkalemia in patients with renal failure.

It may be difficult to distinguish CCB toxicity from cardiac glycoside toxicity; patients may be taking these drugs for the same indications and at the same time (see chapter 193, "Digitalis Glycosides"). In general, patients with chronic digoxin poisoning have greater ventricular excitation, including rate and ectopy, than patients with CCB toxicity. In acute overdose, digoxin toxicity may be distinguished by hyperkalemia. However, because the main manifestation of acute cardiac glycoside poisoning is heart block and bradycardia, bedside differentiation may be difficult.

Toxicity from β-adrenergic antagonists may be clinically indistinguishable from CCB toxicity (see chapter 194, "Beta-Blockers"). In general, β-blocker toxicity is not as severe, and patients tend to have low to normal glucose and normal to elevated serum potassium levels. However, these findings are not consistent enough to have diagnostic value. Fortunately, the treatment for these two poisonings is similar, with calcium, adrenergic agonists, glucagon, insulin, and pacing considered useful therapy for both.[19]

TREATMENT

Institute cardiopulmonary monitoring and obtain an ECG (**Table 195-4**). Evaluate patients with altered mental status for hypoglycemia and opioid toxicity. Decreased level of consciousness following CCB ingestion is a result of cerebral hypoperfusion or co-ingestion. Administer oral activated charcoal if within 1 hour of ingestion or in cases of extended-release preparations, as long as there are no contraindications such as altered mental status or vomiting. Provide early airway management in patients with mental status change or hemodynamic instability. Endotracheal intubation may minimize the risk of aspiration associated with GI decontamination. Vomiting is not only associated with decontamination, but glucagon administration also often precipitates vomiting. Finally, early airway management allows the physician to concentrate on treating the often-precipitous cardiovascular collapse without having to perform a "crash airway" procedure.

Following airway management, provide cardiovascular stabilization. The goal of treating bradycardia is to increase end-organ perfusion rather than restoring a specific heart rate; some patients with heart rates in the 30 to 40 beats/min range can maintain adequate blood pressure and perfusion, and therefore require only monitoring rather than a specific intervention. Conversely, patients may respond to cardiac pacing with an increase in heart rate to 90 to 100 beats/min without improvement in blood pressure or perfusion and require additional therapy to improve inotropy.

Therapies to increase heart rate include medications and cardiac pacing. Atropine alone is rarely effective for CCB-induced bradycardia, but administration is commonly recommended.[10] Calcium salts may improve both heart rate and blood pressure, but the response is variable. Transcutaneous and transvenous pacing may be attempted and are often successful in restoring an acceptable rate but may have little to no effect in correcting hypotension. However, pacing is indicated for hypotensive patients with severe bradycardia (heart rate <30 beats/min).

Administer IV crystalloid for hypotension, but overaggressive fluid administration may produce or worsen pulmonary edema. Persistent hypotension after treatment of bradycardia, administration of calcium salts, and infusion of crystalloid should be treated with adrenergic vasopressors. Recommendations for additional therapies are based on animal data and human case reports or series, with the caution that case reports often document the use of multiple therapies simultaneously.[19-21]

GI DECONTAMINATION

CCBs bind well to charcoal, and activated charcoal should be given to adults following any potentially significant ingestion if within an hour of ingestion.[22] Give activated charcoal after accidental ingestion of verapamil in children, because life-threatening toxicity has been reported following ingestion of a single tablet. Multiple-dose activated charcoal may be considered in the setting of ingestion of an extended-release preparation.

Ipecac syrup to induce emesis is not recommended.[22] Routine gastric lavage has no proven benefit in CCB ingestions. However, because large CCB overdoses are often life-threatening and may not respond to therapy, some toxicologists recommend gastric lavage for a patient who presents within 60 minutes of ingesting an amount significantly in excess of toxicity (Table 195-2) or for any patient who requires intubation after CCB ingestion. However, evidence for improvement in outcomes after gastric lavage is lacking.

Whole-bowel irrigation is frequently advocated for ingestion of extended-release CCBs.[23] Case reports note that a large amount of medication may be recovered. Given the potential for severe toxicity, consider whole-bowel irrigation for patients with large ingestions of extended-release products, although complications from whole-bowel irrigation may contribute to hemodynamic instability.[24]

CALCIUM SALTS

Exogenous calcium increases the extracellular calcium concentration and increases the transcellular gradient, driving calcium intracellularly through unblocked calcium channels. Administration of calcium salts has improved blood pressure in animal models and in human case reports of CCB toxicity.[23,25-28] However, the effect of calcium salts on the heart rate of patients with CCB toxicity is variable.

Calcium chloride is preferred to calcium gluconate because it provides triple the amount of calcium on a weight-to-weight basis. However, calcium chloride is best administered through a central venous line, because peripheral extravasation can result in severe soft tissue necrosis. Calcium chloride is usually given as a 1-gram (10 mL of 10% solution) IV bolus over 5 minutes in adults (pediatric dose is 15 milligrams/kg or 0.15 mL/kg of the 10% solution). Calcium gluconate can be given at three times this amount. **The effects of calcium administration may be transient, and repeat dosing up to every 10 to 20 minutes is commonly required. Alternatively, a continuous infusion of calcium chloride 2 to 6 grams/h may also be used in adults (pediatric dose is 10 to 40 milligrams/kg per hour).** Serum calcium levels should be measured every 1 to 2 hours, and a calcium concentration goal of approximately 1.5 to 2 times normal should be achieved. However, for patients who do not respond to other therapies, it is reasonable to continue calcium administration even when serum calcium levels are considerably elevated.

An acceptable level for hypercalcemia has not been defined. Published case reports of CCB poisoning describe survival following administration of 30 grams of calcium chloride over 12 hours resulting in a serum calcium level of 23 milligrams/dL (5.94 mmol/L)[23] and death from iatrogenic hypercalcemia with a serum calcium level of 32.3 milligrams/dL (8.07 mmol/L).[29] A safe but effective dose of calcium salts to use in the treatment of CCB toxicity is unclear. If repeat dosing or continuous infusions are used, hypercalcemia and/or hypophosphatemia can occur. Although monitoring of serum calcium and phosphorus concentrations during repeated or prolonged calcium therapy is recommended, it is unclear if such electrolyte abnormalities have clinical consequence or should be treated.

ADRENERGIC AGENTS

Patients who do not respond to calcium administration or who require repeated doses are usually given adrenergic agonists (Figure 195-1).[19-21] Although animal data suggest that other therapies may lead to better metabolic function and better survival in severe poisonings, adrenergic agonists have several advantages. Physicians and nurses are familiar with these agents, therapy can be initiated quickly, and most patients respond favorably. This prevents a period of nontreatment while the supplies for more esoteric therapies are gathered. Given the availability of adrenergic agonists and the familiarity of clinicians with their use, adrenergic agonists are the first line of treatment for persistent hypotension following CCB ingestion.

No single adrenergic vasopressor is consistently effective. A response may occur with dopamine, epinephrine, norepinephrine, vasopressin, dobutamine, and isoproterenol.[30-32] Patients with decreased contractility and peripheral vasodilatation, especially in the face of relative bradycardia, may benefit from an agent with both α- and β-agonist effects, such as epinephrine or norepinephrine (Figure 195-1). Phosphodiesterase inhibitors such as amrinone, milrinone, and enoximone have also been reported to improve blood pressure in animal studies and human case reports.[33-36]

When standard doses are inadequate, it is reasonable to use high doses or multiple agents titrated to achieve a systolic blood pressure >90 mm Hg (>12 kPa), although there is the risk of ischemic complications.[32]

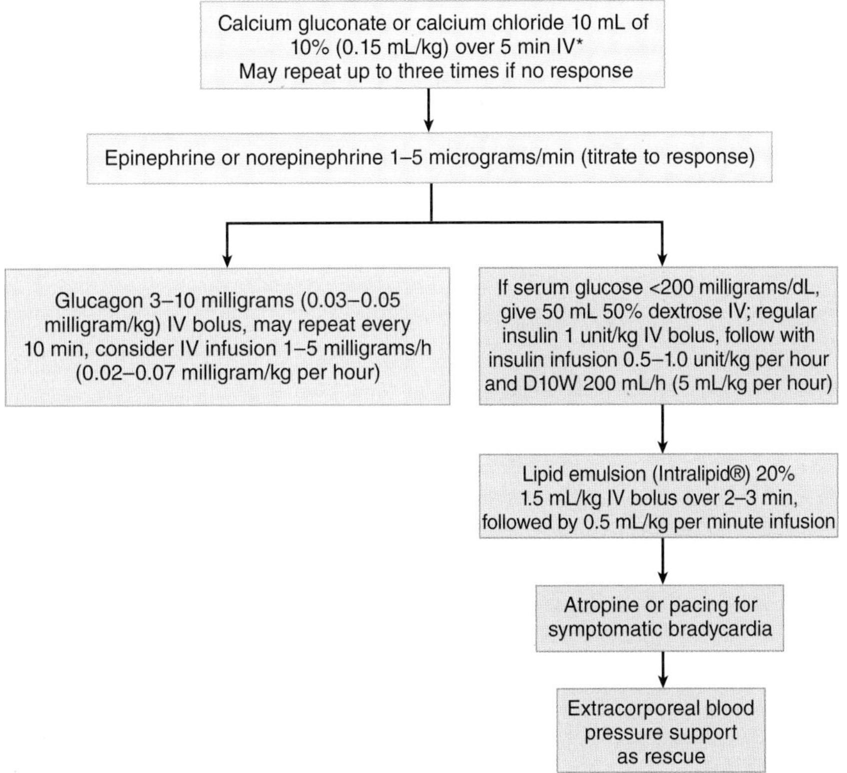

FIGURE 195-1. Treatment algorithm for severe calcium channel blocker toxicity, for stepwise or simultaneous therapy. *Calcium chloride provides three times as much elemental calcium as calcium gluconate; monitor for ventricular arrhythmias in concomitant digoxin toxicity. D10W = 10% dextrose in water.

Alternatively, another approach, such as high-dose insulin, glucagon, or lipid-emulsion, can be considered.

HIGH-DOSE INSULIN THERAPY

High-dose insulin therapy, also known as hyperinsulinemia-euglycemia therapy, is a promising treatment for the myocardial suppression associated with CCB poisoning.[37-46] Potential mechanisms of action include positive inotropic effects of insulin, increased calcium entry, and improved myocardial use of carbohydrates as an energy source.[18] Insulin increases intracellular transport of glucose into cardiac and skeletal muscle and has inotropic properties.[39] There are no clinical trials comparing high-dose insulin therapy directly to other treatments, but multiple human case reports show that high-dose insulin therapy improves perfusion in CCB poisoning unresponsive to other therapies, with a therapeutic response noted with 15 to 30 minutes.[39-45] The main adverse effect is potential hypoglycemia, which is easily detected with point-of-care glucose testing and treated with dextrose. When to institute therapy is unclear; some toxicologists recommend high-dose insulin therapy if the patient is refractory to standard doses of vasopressors, and others advocate it as first-line therapy. **Given benefit seen in animal models and clinical reports, high-dose insulin therapy should be considered if the patient does not respond to vasopressor therapy** (Figure 195-1).

Doses of insulin used for high-dose insulin therapy are greater than that for diabetic treatment (**Table 195-5**).[46] An initial insulin bolus is followed by a continuous infusion along with a dextrose infusion to prevent hypoglycemia (Table 195-5). The hemodynamic response to high-dose insulin therapy is usually seen in 15 to 45 minutes, so the infusion rate may be increased if no clinical improvement is seen within that time. Monitor the serum glucose concentrations and adjust the dextrose infusion to maintain an acceptable glucose range. Monitor serum potassium and replace as needed. Maintain the high-dose insulin therapy infusion until toxicity has resolved; durations of 9 to 49 hours may be necessary. The insulin infusion may either be weaned gradually or stopped abruptly and reinstituted if toxicity recurs. Dextrose supplementation may be required for up to 24 hours after the infusion is discontinued due to persistent elevated insulin concentrations.

GLUCAGON

Glucagon, a hormone synthesized by the pancreas, is the therapy of choice for β-adrenergic blocker poisoning because of its ability to bypass the β-adrenergic receptor and stimulate cardiac activity (see chapter 194). In CCB poisoning, the inhibition is downstream from glucagon's binding site, and therefore, glucagon theoretically offers no advantage over other agents. Nevertheless, glucagon administration improves blood pressure in animal models, and several case reports have also noted improvement in hemodynamics after glucagon therapy.[47-50] However, failure to respond has also been reported.[40]

The recommended glucagon dose is an IV bolus of 3 to 10 milligrams in adults and 0.03 to 0.05 milligram/kg in children (Figure 195-1). A response is usually seen within 15 minutes. If there is no response, the bolus dose may be repeated. If there is hemodynamic improvement, a maintenance infusion should be initiated at 1 to 5 milligrams/kg per hour in adults and 0.02 to 0.07 milligram/kg per hour in children.

The main adverse effects of glucagon are vomiting and hyperglycemia. Therefore, endotracheal intubation should be strongly considered prior to initiation of glucagon therapy in a patient with altered mental status. Also, an antiemetic such as ondansetron may be empirically administered. Because of the large amounts of glucagon required, hospital supplies of the drug are often rapidly depleted, and it may be necessary to contact other institutions for additional drug.

TABLE 195-5 Protocol for High-Dose Insulin Therapy in Severe Calcium Channel Blocker Overdose

Check serum glucose, and if <200 milligrams/dL (<11 mmol/L), administer 50 mL of 50% dextrose (0.5 gram/mL) in water IV (children, 1 mL/kg of 25% dextrose).
Administer regular insulin 1 unit/kg IV bolus.
Begin regular insulin infusion at 0.5–1.0 unit/kg per hour along with dextrose 10% (0.1 gram/mL) in water at 200 mL/h (adult) or 5 mL/kg per hour (pediatric).
Titrate insulin infusion rate up to 10 units/kg per hour according the hemodynamic goal of HR >50 beats/min and SBP >100 mm Hg (>13.3 kPa).
Monitor serum glucose every 15–20 min.
Titrate dextrose infusion rate to maintain serum glucose level between 100 and 200 milligrams/dL (5.3 and 10.7 mmol/L).
Once dextrose infusion rates have been stable for 60 min, glucose monitoring may be decreased to hourly.
Monitor serum potassium level and start IV potassium infusion if serum potassium level is <2.8 mEq/L (<2.8 mmol/L).
Maintain serum potassium between 2.8 and 3.2 mEq/L (2.8 and 3.2 mmol/L).

Abbreviations: HR = heart rate; SBP = systolic blood pressure.

INTRAVENOUS LIPID EMULSION THERAPY

Lipid emulsion therapy was first described in the management of local anesthetic toxicity. Lipid emulsions appear to create a pharmacologic sink for fat-soluble drugs.[51] Therapy may also provide fatty acid substrate for cardiac energy supply and improve myocyte function by increasing intracellular calcium levels. Lipid emulsion therapy prolongs survival in an animal model of verapamil poisoning,[52] and several case reports also describe benefit in CCB ingestions unresponsive to standard therapy.[53,54] There are many different commercial lipid emulsion preparations, with the major components typically being soybean oil, egg yolk phospholipids, and glycerin. Consult with the poison control center or pharmacist when considering lipid emulsion therapy.

The recommended dose is a 20% lipid emulsion given as a 1.5 mL/kg bolus over 2 to 3 minutes, followed by an 0.25 mL/kg per minute infusion. If the blood pressure remains low, an additional 1.5 mL/kg bolus may be repeated followed by an increase in the infusion rate to 0.5 mL/kg per minute. The recommended upper limit for lipid emulsion infusion is about 10 mL/kg over the initial 30 minutes. If the patient's hemodynamic stability is dependent on continued lipid infusion, the treatment may be continued.[55] Case reports suggest that if sudden cardiac arrest occurs in the setting of overdose, a bolus can be given in the hope of restoring spontaneous circulation. In addition to interference with laboratory parameters, there are rare adverse effects such as hypertriglyceridemia, hypoxemia (with high doses), and hyponatremia.[21]

EXTRACORPOREAL CIRCULATORY SUPPORT

Patients who do not respond to the aforementioned therapies may benefit from circulatory support measures, such as the placement of intra-aortic balloon pumps, the use of left ventricular assist devices, and even extracorporeal circulatory support, which may provide adequate blood pressure to allow clearance of the drug and resolution of symptoms.[21,56,57] Hemodialysis or hemoperfusion is not beneficial in the treatment of CCB overdoses.[58]

DISPOSITION AND FOLLOW-UP

In general, patients usually manifest toxicity within 6 hours of ingestion of non–extended-release products. Therefore, those who are asymptomatic and who have normal vital signs after a 6-hour observation period can be discharged after appropriate psychiatric evaluation.[22] Toxicity may be delayed for up to 12 hours after ingestion of extended-release products.[6,7] **As a rule, patients who ingest potentially toxic amounts of extended-release products should be monitored for 12 to 24 hours.** Contact the regional poison control center for assistance with management.

REFERENCES

The complete reference list is available online at www.TintinalliEM.com.

CHAPTER 196

Antihypertensives

Frank Lovecchio
Dan Quan

INTRODUCTION

An estimated 30% of adults in the United States have hypertension; thus, antihypertensives are medications commonly found in patient homes.[1] Several classes of drugs used to treat hypertension are discussed in this chapter: diuretics, sympatholytic agents, angiotensin-converting enzyme inhibitors (ACEIs), angiotensin II receptor blockers (ARBs), and vasodilators (**Table 196-1**). Calcium channel blockers and β-blockers, also used in the treatment of hypertension, are discussed elsewhere (see chapters 195, "Calcium Channel Blockers," and 194, "Beta-Blockers").

For most of these agents, life-threatening toxicity is not expected in acute overdose.[2] In nearly all cases, good supportive care is adequate. The initial approach to the patient with potential overdose of an antihypertensive drug is fairly uniform. Secure the airway as necessary, establish IV access, provide continuous cardiac monitoring, and obtain an ECG. A bolus of crystalloid solution is first-line treatment for hypotension. If a vasopressor is required, a direct-acting drug such as norepinephrine is preferred. If pulmonary aspiration is not a concern, activated charcoal can be given within the first hour. Although there is usually no specific therapy for initial management of these drugs in overdose, the different classes of antihypertensives are distinct in their potential for causing metabolic derangements and adverse effects.

DIURETICS

Acetazolamide, a carbonic anhydrase inhibitor diuretic, is not used for management of hypertension. Acetazolamide may be indicated for management of high-altitude disease or glaucoma (in oral or topical preparations). Carbonic anhydrase plays a role in the renal proximal tubule sodium-hydrogen exchange. In the proximal tubule, [Na^+] is reabsorbed from the tubule in exchange for [H^+]. Carbonic anhydrase in the proximal tubule brush border catalyzes the conversion of H_2CO_3 (formed from [H^+] and [HCO_3^-] present within the tubular lumen) to H_2O and CO_2. The CO_2 is then reabsorbed. Inhibition of carbonic anhydrase reduces the amount of [H^+] available for exchange, so that more [Na^+] and [HCO_3^-] stays within the tubular lumen and is eliminated. Because sodium can be reabsorbed distally, the most clinically significant effect of carbonic anhydrase inhibition is loss of urinary bicarbonate with the development of a non–anion gap metabolic acidosis. Overdose experience is limited, and treatment is supportive.

Diuretics initially control hypertension by increasing elimination of salts, but their mechanism of action in long-term blood pressure control is not clear. All diuretics cause increased sodium elimination, which results in the potential for hyponatremia, hypokalemia, hypomagnesaemia, and hypovolemia.

Thiazides, like hydrochlorothiazide, inhibit sodium chloride reabsorption in the renal distal convoluted tubule. Decreased sodium reabsorption leads to increased excretion of potassium and the possibility of hypokalemia. Calcium regulation is also affected by thiazide diuretics via two separate mechanisms: (1) inhibition of vitamin D synthesis and thus decreased calcium absorption from the GI tract, and (2) increased renal absorption of calcium. The net result, however, is calcium retention and potentially hypercalcemia.[3] Glucose intolerance is noted at higher doses.

Loop diuretics, such as furosemide and bumetanide, are used more frequently for control of edema and pulmonary congestion than for management of high blood pressure. Loop diuretics inhibit the activity of the sodium-potassium-chloride symporter (a type of cotransporter that facilitates transport across a plasma membrane) in the renal loop of Henle, where 25% of the filtered sodium load is typically reabsorbed. A secondary effect of the inhibition of this symporter is decreased calcium and magnesium reabsorption, which results in hypocalcemia, hypokalemia, and hypomagnesemia.

Triamterene, amiloride, spironolactone, and eplerenone are referred to as potassium-sparing diuretics for their ability to cause a sodium chloride diuresis without increased potassium secretion. Triamterene and amiloride inhibit sodium channels in the distal renal tubule and collecting duct, which play a role in both reabsorbing sodium and secreting potassium. These drugs may be used in conjunction with other stronger diuretics for management of hypertension. Triamterene has been associated with rare cases of crystalline nephropathy.[4]

Spironolactone and eplerenone are antagonists of mineralocorticoids, such as aldosterone. Mineralocorticoid antagonists increase elimination of sodium and retention of hydrogen and potassium. Spironolactone is typically used to treat heart failure and hepatic cirrhosis. In the acute overdose setting, hyperkalemia and hypotension are the most serious clinical manifestations of these drugs.

Clinical manifestations of excessive diuresis include tachycardia, hypotension (orthostatic or supine), electrolyte abnormalities, and generalized weakness. The ECG may show changes caused by these electrolyte abnormalities (see chapter 17, "Fluids and Electrolytes"). A widened QRS interval or peaked T waves may suggest hyperkalemia, such as from a potassium-sparing diuretic. A prolonged QT interval may indicate hypokalemia, hypomagnesemia, or hypocalcemia, which may be caused by a loop diuretic.

The first priority of therapy is restoration of plasma volume. Administer an isotonic crystalloid solution bolus, such as 0.9% saline. If life-threatening hyperkalemia is encountered, provide standard management and fluid resuscitation.

In addition to causing direct toxicity, diuretics may potentiate toxicity from other medications. Mechanisms include decreased renal clearance of drugs or creation of a metabolic state that changes a particular drug's effect. **Diuretics and ACEIs can increase the risk of lithium toxicity** by reducing lithium elimination (see chapter 181, "Lithium").[5] Because hypokalemia exacerbates digoxin toxicity, non–potassium-sparing diuretics may exacerbate arrhythmias seen in chronic digoxin poisoning or other antiarrhythmics (see chapter 193, "Digitalis Glycosides").

SYMPATHOLYTIC AGENTS

Catecholamines produced by the sympathetic nervous system play a key role in maintaining blood pressure. Drugs with action at α-adrenergic receptors are used to diminish peripheral sympathetic tone in order to decrease blood pressure. There are two subtypes of α-adrenergic receptors. Stimulation of the α_1-adrenergic receptors causes vasoconstriction of arterioles and veins, increasing peripheral vascular resistance and elevating blood pressure. Stimulation of the α_2-adrenergic receptors produces different effects in the peripheral and central nervous systems. In the peripheral nervous system, stimulation of the α_2-receptors produces vasoconstriction and increases blood pressure. In the CNS, stimulation of the α_2-receptors at presynaptic sympathetic terminals inhibits the release of catecholamines, thereby decreasing sympathetic tone, promoting peripheral vasodilation, and decreasing blood pressure.

Doxazosin, prazosin, and terazosin antagonize α_1-adrenergic receptors, reducing peripheral vascular resistance. Although the aforementioned drugs are used for the treatment of hypertension, other members of this class, such as **tamsulosin**, are used exclusively for management of benign prostatic hyperplasia and as an adjunct in nephrolithiasis management. Because an increase in peripheral vascular resistance is required to maintain blood pressure when changing from a supine to an upright position, it is not surprising that the most typical adverse effect observed with α_1-adrenergic antagonists is orthostatic hypotension, particularly within 30 to 90 minutes after ingestion, and is most prominent after taking the first dose.[6]

Although orthostatic hypotensive episodes may be associated with lightheadedness and adverse events such as falls resulting in hip fracture, patients rarely come to the ED with prolonged hemodynamic instability. Patients who do present with hypotension associated with α_1-adrenergic antagonist use should be placed supine and receive a crystalloid bolus. Based on the mechanism of action of these drugs, phenylephrine, an α_1-adrenergic agonist, is an ideal agent if blood pressure does not improve with IV fluids.

TABLE 196-1 Summary of Antihypertensive Drugs

Class	Drug	Mechanism of Action	Clinical Presentation with Toxicity	Comments
Diuretics	Acetazolamide	Inhibition of proximal tubule sodium-hydrogen exchange	Hypovolemia Non–anion gap metabolic acidosis	
	Chlorothiazide Chlorthalidone Hydrochlorothiazide Indapamide Metolazone	Inhibition of distal tubule sodium chloride absorption	Hypovolemia Hypokalemia Hypercalcemia	Metabolic complications, such as hypokalemia, glucose intolerance, and hyperuricemia seen with increased therapeutic thiazide doses.
	Bumetanide Furosemide	Inhibition of sodium-potassium-chloride symporter in renal loop of Henle	Hypovolemia Hypocalcemia Hypokalemia Hypomagnesemia	
	Amiloride Triamterene	Inhibition of sodium absorption and potassium elimination in renal distal collecting duct	Hypovolemia Hyperkalemia	
	Eplerenone Spironolactone	Mineralocorticoid antagonist	Hypovolemia Hyperkalemia	
Sympatholytics	Doxazosin Prazosin Tamsulosin Terazosin	α_1-Adrenergic receptor antagonist	Hypotension	Phenylephrine may be used for refractory hypotension.
	Clonidine Guanabenz Guanfacine	α_2-Adrenergic receptor agonist Imidazoline receptor agonist μ-Receptor opioid agonist	Hypotension Bradycardia Neurologic depression	Dopamine considered agent of choice for hypotension. Phenylephrine may be used for refractory hypotension.
	Oxymetazoline Tetrahydrozoline	Imidazoline receptor agonist	Hypotension, Bradycardia, and Neurologic depression	
	Guanadrel Methyldopa Reserpine	Decreased norepinephrine release	Hypotension Bradycardia Hemolytic anemia (idiosyncratic reaction to methyldopa)	
ACE inhibitors	Benazepril Captopril Enalapril Fosinopril Moexipril Perindopril Quinapril Trandolapril	Inhibition of ACE Inhibition of bradykininase	Hypotension Hyperkalemia Angioedema (idiosyncratic) Cough (idiosyncratic)	Epinephrine, corticosteroids, and antihistamines have no proven benefit in ACEI-induced angioedema. Icatibant 30 milligrams SC or C1 esterase inhibitor [human] 1000 U IV are effective in ACEI-induced angioedema.
Angiotensin receptor blockers	Candesartan Eprosartan Irbesartan Losartan Telmisartan Valsartan	Angiotensin II receptor antagonist	Hypotension Hyperkalemia Angioedema (less common than with ACE inhibitors)	Epinephrine, corticosteroids, or antihistamines have no proven benefit in ARB-induced angioedema.
Vasodilators	Hydralazine	Arteriolar vasodilation	Hypotension Lupus-like syndrome (idiosyncratic reaction to hydralazine)	
	Minoxidil	Arteriolar vasodilation	Tachycardia Increased myocardial oxygen demand	
	Sodium nitroprusside	Arteriolar and venous vasodilation (via nitric oxide release)	Hypotension Tachycardia Thiocyanate toxicity (after prolonged infusion) Cyanide toxicity (very rare)	Thiosulfate should be administered if cyanide toxicity is considered. Many pharmacies mix sodium nitroprusside and thiosulfate to avert cyanide toxicity.

Abbreviation: ACE = angiotensin-converting enzyme.

CLONIDINE

Clonidine is the most commonly used α_2-adrenergic agonist. Clonidine is available in an oral formulation and as a transdermal patch. This class of drugs, which also includes guanabenz and guanfacine, stimulates α_2-adrenergic receptors in the CNS, inhibiting release of catecholamines in the periphery, which results in decreased heart rate, contractility, and peripheral vascular resistance. Clonidine shares the imidazoline functional group with the nasal spray decongestant oxymetazoline and topical eye vasoconstrictor medication tetrahydrozoline. **Inappropriately ingesting oxymetazoline or tetrahydrozoline can result in toxicity similar to clonidine poisoning.**[7,8] In addition to hemodynamic effects, clonidine also possesses opioid agonist properties at the μ-receptor.[9] For this reason, clonidine is used in some opioid-dependent patients to ameliorate symptoms of withdrawal.

Clonidine poisoning typically results from either intentional overdose or exploratory pediatric poisoning.[10,11] **Even a single tablet may cause significant symptoms in a child.**[12,13] Toxicity can develop from ingesting clonidine patches.[14,15] Compounded ointments used for chronic pain may contain clonidine that when applied to small children or to adults in excessive quantity may produce toxicity.[16,17]

Shortly after an ingested overdose of clonidine, the peripheral α_2-adrenergic stimulation may cause hypertension.[11,18] By the time of presentation, however, the clinical manifestations of central α_2-adrenergic stimulation and imidazoline toxicity are present with bradycardia and hypotension.[10] Clonidine may produce miotic pupils in a manner similar to opioids.[19] Hypothermia may occur as a result of opioid or adrenergically mediated pathways. Somnolence is typical and may progress to apnea in severe cases.[7,10,20] Although clonidine is intended to be dosed twice daily, symptoms may last days with an overdose.

Focus on ventilatory and hemodynamic support in clonidine toxicity. Clonidine-induced respiratory and neurologic depression has variable response to naloxone, and its use is unlikely to be helpful.[21-25] Bradycardia may be treated with atropine. When encountered, hypertension should be treated only if it is severe and prolonged. Because hypertension may unpredictably give way to hypotension, a drug that can be immediately discontinued, such as nitroprusside, should be used. Hypotension associated with clonidine typically responds well to crystalloid fluid resuscitation. Theoretically, a direct α_1-adrenergic agonist such as phenylephrine may be appropriate in cases of refractory hypotension, but dopamine is a better choice.

METHYLDOPA

Methyldopa is also a centrally acting antihypertensive, although it has a unique mechanism. Methyldopa is a dopamine analog that, in the CNS, is converted in two steps to α-methylnorepinephrine, which in turn substitutes for norepinephrine in adrenergic neuron secretory vesicles. In the CNS, α-methylnorepinephrine stimulates presynaptic α_2-adrenergic receptors, reducing peripheral sympathetic tone. In therapeutic dosing, the peak effect of methyldopa is delayed for 6 to 8 hours, because time is required for methyldopa to pass into the brain and be converted to its active form. Methyldopa use is also associated with hemolytic anemia, of autoimmune etiology, which occurs during long-term therapeutic use.[26,27] If symptomatic hypotension is encountered in association with methyldopa, IV crystalloid solution should be administered. In cases of refractory, severe hypotension, a direct-acting vasopressor such as norepinephrine should be administered.

GUANADREL AND RESERPINE

Guanadrel and reserpine are antihypertensives that interfere with the release of catecholamines from synaptic terminals. Guanadrel, which has no intrinsic sympathetic activity, substitutes for norepinephrine in presynaptic storage vesicles. Reserpine inhibits formation of biogenic amine storage vesicles in central and peripheral neurons. In each case, there is a decreased capacity to release catecholamines in response to a sympathetic stimulus. Sympathetic tone is diminished, and peripheral vascular resistance decreases. There is little experience with these drugs in overdose. However, because the common mechanism of both drugs is a decrease in circulating catecholamines, it would seem reasonable to administer boluses of crystalloid as first-line therapy and to use a direct-acting vasopressor, such as norepinephrine or phenylephrine, to treat refractory hypotension.

ANGIOTENSIN-CONVERTING ENZYME INHIBITORS AND ANGIOTENSIN RECEPTOR BLOCKERS

Angiotensin II raises blood pressure by several mechanisms, including triggering aldosterone release, increasing response to catecholamines, and acting as a direct vasoconstrictor. Angiotensin II is created in a two-step process. In the first step, renin, released by the kidneys, cleaves angiotensinogen, forming angiotensin I. The second step uses angiotensin-converting enzyme, which separates the carboxy terminus off angiotensin I, forming angiotensin II. Inhibition of this conversion at either step results in decreased blood pressure.

ACEIs are thought to slow the progression of diabetic glomerulopathy and have been shown to improve mortality and left ventricular function when administered after myocardial infarction. Members of this large class of drugs can be identified by their shared "-pril" suffix: benazepril, captopril, enalapril, fosinopril, moexipril, perindopril, quinapril, and trandolapril. Inhibition of angiotensin-converting enzyme results in decreased production of angiotensin II, which causes vasodilation. Despite their widespread use, these medications have not been associated with significant morbidity in overdose. ACEIs can cause hyperkalemia in therapeutic dosing. If hypotension is encountered, initial therapy focuses on basic management, including administration of boluses of crystalloid and vasopressors for refractory cases.

Captopril, and possibly other ACEIs, are thought to inhibit the metabolism of the enkephalins, a group of endogenous opioids. Naloxone, a μ-opioid antagonist, may reverse captopril-associated hypotension[28] but is not universally effective.[29]

ARBs produce vasodilatation and increase renal salt elimination. Members of this class end with the suffix "-artan" and include losartan, candesartan, irbesartan, valsartan, telmisartan, and eprosartan. When they are taken therapeutically, the peak antihypotensive effect of agents in this class is not observed for 4 weeks. Typically these drugs are not associated with significant morbidity in overdose. There are no reported cases of ARBs causing life-threatening hypotension. Like ACEIs, ARBs can cause hyperkalemia, which results from decreased aldosterone production. This effect is typically seen in patients with renal insufficiency.[23]

Persistent dry cough occurs in 5% to 20% of patients treated with ACEIs.[30] Cough typically develops within a few weeks after ACEI therapy is started and is more common in women, and the rate of occurrence or severity does not correlate with dose. Cough will usually resolve in 1 to 4 weeks after the drug is stopped, although resolution may take up to 3 months for some patients. The only effective treatment is discontinuing the ACEI, substituting a different antihypertensive. ARBs are not associated with an increased incidence of chronic cough and may be used in patients with ACEI-induced cough.[31]

Angioedema is the most consequential adverse effect associated with ACEIs and ARBs (see chapter 14, "Anaphylaxis, Allergies, and Angioedema").[32,33] Angioedema is an idiopathic reaction that occurs in 0.1% to 0.7% of patients prescribed these drugs.[33,34] Because these agents are widely used, this small percentage represents a large number of events. Patients present with swelling of the lips, larynx, pharynx, tongue, or vocal cords, which can range in severity from mild to airway compromise. Symptoms develop over several hours and may not resolve for 24 hours or longer. **The absence of urticaria differentiates angioedema from allergic anaphylaxis**. The mechanism is thought to be related to inhibition of ACE-mediated degradation of bradykinin, a peptide associated with vasodilatation and tissue edema, and accumulation of substance P and other prostaglandins. ARBs do not inhibit bradykinin, so the exact pathophysiology of angioedema associated with drugs from this class is not clear. **The mean time from first use to development of angioedema has been reported as about 2 years,**[35] **but angioedema can occur at any time during therapy,** with 12% of patients developing this reaction in the first week of ACEI use.

Management of ACEI-induced angioedema begins with evaluation of the airway. If the patient has difficulty breathing, stridor, or severe oropharyngeal edema, secure the airway, usually by intubation. Edema of the oral cavity or oropharynx (especially the tongue) is the best predictor of the need for airway intervention.[36] Fiberoptic-guided laryngoscopy is recommended because it requires minimal sedation and provides direct visualization in an edematous airway. **Regardless of the method employed, a skilled operator should secure the airway early because angioedema can progress rapidly and anatomic landmarks may become obscured.**

Allergic reaction drugs, such as epinephrine, antihistamines, and corticosteroids, are often given but not likely beneficial because ACEI-induced angioedema is not mediated by immunoglobulin E.[33] Icatibant, a bradykinin-2 antagonist, is effective in reducing swelling; the dose is 30 milligrams SC.[37] C1 esterase inhibitor [human] 1000 U IV is also effective.[38] Plasma or fresh frozen plasma contains angiotensin-converting enzyme, so the administration of plasma is thought to degrade high levels of bradykinin with subsequent resolution of angioedema. Two units of fresh frozen plasma in adults are reported to resolve ACEI-induced angioedema in 2 to 4 hours.[39,40] Ecallantide is a recombinant protein that inhibits kallikrein and is approved for use in hereditary angioedema. However, ACEI-induced angioedema is caused by the persistence of bradykinin due to lack of metabolism rather than overproduction, so it is not likely that ecallantide would be effective.

Patients with milder symptoms should be observed and managed medically. There is no consensus regarding the disposition of patients with ACEI-associated angioedema who do not require ED airway intervention. Patients with milder swelling only around the lips or face should be observed for 12 to 24 hours and discharged when swelling is regressing. Patients should be instructed that angioedema can recur if they continue to take the same agent or switch to another agent of the same class.[41,42] **After an episode of angioedema, the safest and recommended course of action is to discontinue all ACEIs and ARBs.**

VASODILATORS

HYDRALAZINE AND MINOXIDIL

Hydralazine is an antihypertensive agent most commonly used during pregnancy. Hydralazine relaxes arteriolar smooth muscle but does not affect venous smooth muscle or epicardial coronary arteries. Hydralazine is metabolized to an inactive compound by hepatic acetylation. Roughly half of Americans are fast acetylators and therefore require a higher dose to achieve a given clinical effect. The peak effect of the drug is seen 30 to 120 minutes after ingestion, although effects may last as long as 12 hours. The most common adverse effects of hydralazine overdose result from vasodilatation, but serious events are rare. Hydralazine overdose with mild hypotension may develop ST-segment depressions on ECG.[43] This myocardial ischemia is thought to result from a steal syndrome in which peripheral vasodilatation is accompanied by reflex tachycardia without an increase in epicardial blood flow, so that myocardial demand increases while coronary perfusion does not. Because of this reflex tachycardia, hydralazine should not be used for treatment of acute coronary syndrome or cocaine-associated chest pain.

Patients on continuous treatment with hydralazine are at risk for development of a lupus-like syndrome. The mechanism is thought to be formation of autoantibodies, but it is not known how hydralazine contributes to this process. Risk factors include high dose, female gender, slow-acetylator phenotype, and white ethnic background. Symptoms of this syndrome include arthralgia, arthritis, fever, and pericardial effusion. Management includes administration of anti-inflammatories and discontinuation of the drug.

Minoxidil is a potent antihypertensive generally used only for resistant cases of hypertension. Minoxidil is better known for its topical formulation as a treatment for male pattern baldness. Minoxidil is metabolized to minoxidil sulfate, which in turn relaxes smooth muscle by opening potassium channels and causing hyperpolarization. Like hydralazine, minoxidil has little effect on venous smooth muscle. Peripheral vasodilatation results in reflex tachycardia and increased cardiac output. Reduced renal perfusion causes fluid retention. For this reason, minoxidil is usually prescribed with a β-blocker and diuretic. Overdose of minoxidil is associated with hypotension, common reflex tachycardia, and occasional myocardial ischemia in a manner similar to hydralazine.[44-46]

Hypotension from either hydralazine or minoxidil is treated with IV crystalloid fluids. Vasopressors should be avoided if possible, because severely poisoned patients may have coronary ischemia. If blood pressure is refractory to fluid resuscitation, an α_1-adrenergic agonist, such as phenylephrine or midodrine,[46] is preferable to a β-adrenergic agonist, such as dopamine, to minimize tachycardia and prevent increased myocardial oxygen demand.

SODIUM NITROPRUSSIDE

Sodium nitroprusside is administered IV for hypertensive emergencies.[47,48] Nitroprusside derives its activity from the release of nitric oxide, an endogenous mediator of vasodilation, which stimulates smooth muscle guanylyl cyclase to produce cyclic guanosine monophosphate. The onset of action is roughly 30 seconds, and the offset is 3 minutes. Nitroprusside dilates both arteriolar and venous smooth muscle. In the ED, hypotension is the adverse effect most likely to be observed. If hypotension occurs, the infusion should be stopped immediately. If signs of cerebral hypoperfusion are present, place the patient supine or possibly in the Trendelenburg position. Because of the very brief duration of action of the drug, little else is generally necessary after discontinuing the drug.

When nitric oxide is released from nitroprusside, cyanide is produced as well. As long as the nitroprusside infusion rate is not above 2 to 5 micrograms/kg per minute, the cyanide is usually of little consequence, because it is immediately metabolized by rhodanese to thiocyanate, a much less toxic metabolite. At higher infusion rates over several days, the ability of rhodanese to detoxify cyanide may become overwhelmed.[49] Administration of sodium thiosulfate, which serves as a substrate for rhodanese, can be protective for patients requiring a high rate of nitroprusside administration. Cyanide toxicity may manifests as confusion, lactic acidosis, and progression to cardiovascular collapse. If the clinician is concerned about cyanide toxicity, the infusion should be discontinued, and sodium thiosulfate should be administered.

Over time, the thiocyanate generated by detoxification of cyanide can itself cause toxicity. Thiocyanate toxicity, although much more common than cyanide toxicity during nitroprusside treatment, is unlikely to occur in the ED. Thiocyanate, which is eliminated by the kidney with a half-life of 3 to 7 days, usually does not accumulate until infusion has continued for several days. The most important predictors of toxicity are rate of production (nitroprusside infusion rate) and rate of elimination (renal function). Thiocyanate toxicity may manifest as nausea, fatigue, and CNS depression.

FENOLDOPAM

Fenoldopam is a selective dopamine-1 agonist used for hypertensive emergencies, although its clinical utilization in the United States has remained low.[50,51] Fenoldopam is administered parenterally and acts as a vasodilator and diuretic.[47,48] Fenoldopam has a half-life of approximately 5 minutes, and after infusion is instituted, steady-state serum levels are reached in about 30 to 60 minutes. If hypotension is encountered after fenoldopam administration, the infusion should be stopped immediately and a fluid bolus administered.

REFERENCES

The complete reference list is available online at www.TintinalliEM.com.

CHAPTER 197 Anticonvulsants

Frank LoVecchio

INTRODUCTION

Anticonvulsants, or antiepileptics, are used to treat acute seizures and prevent convulsions in patients with epilepsy. The first generation of antiepileptics was developed between 1939 and 1980 (**Table 197-1**). Since 1993, 15 additional agents have been introduced into clinical use, termed the "second and third generation" of antiepileptic drugs. In general, these new anticonvulsants have fewer serious adverse side effects and fewer drug interactions than the first-generation agents. The first-generation drugs have an established therapeutic range for serum levels that can guide therapy during long-term management and that correlate with acute toxicity from an overdose. Consistent therapeutic levels have not been established for the second- and third-generation anticonvulsants, and serum levels are not a useful guide to therapy.

This chapter reviews the pharmacology, clinical features, and treatment for commonly used anticonvulsants. Disposition recommendations depend on the resolution of clinical toxicity, but patients with intentional overdose need mental health evaluation in the ED before discharge.

PHENYTOIN AND FOSPHENYTOIN

Phenytoin is a primary anticonvulsant for partial and generalized tonic-clonic seizures. It is useful in the treatment of non–drug-induced status epilepticus in conjunction with rapidly acting anticonvulsants.[1] Phenytoin has been used to prevent seizures due to head trauma (in the immediate post-traumatic period) and in the management of some chronic pain syndromes. Serious complications are extremely rare after intentional phenytoin overdose if supportive care is provided. Most phenytoin-related deaths have been caused by rapid IV administration or hypersensitivity reactions.

Phenytoin is available in oral and injectable forms. Phenytoin has poor solubility in water, so the vehicle for the parenteral formulation is 40% propylene glycol and 10% ethanol, adjusted to a pH of 12 with sodium hydroxide. The acute cardiovascular toxicity seen with IV phenytoin infusion has frequently been ascribed to the propylene glycol diluent. Other limitations with parenteral phenytoin are the irritating nature of the vehicle and a tendency to precipitate in IV solutions. **Fosphenytoin** (a disodium phosphate ester of phenytoin) is a prodrug that is converted to phenytoin by phosphatases in the body with a conversion half-life of 10 to 15 minutes. **The advantage with parenteral fosphenytoin is that it is soluble in aqueous solutions, is buffered to a pH of 8.8, is nonirritating to the tissues, and can be given by IM injection.**[2]

TABLE 197-1 Anticonvulsant Drugs

First Generation	Second and Third Generation
Carbamazepine	Eslicarbazepine acetate
Ethosuximide	Ezogabine or retigabine
Phenobarbital	Felbamate
Phenytoin and fosphenytoin	Gabapentin
Primidone	Lacosamide
Valproate	Lamotrigine
	Levetiracetam
	Oxcarbazepine
	Pregabalin
	Rufinamide
	Stiripentol
	Topiramate
	Tiagabine
	Vigabatrin
	Zonisamide

PATHOPHYSIOLOGY

Mechanism of Action Phenytoin exerts its anticonvulsant effect by blocking voltage-sensitive and frequency-dependent sodium channels in the neurons, suppressing repetitive neuronal activity, and preventing the spread of a seizure focus.[3] At higher concentrations, phenytoin delays activation of outward potassium currents in nerves and prolongs the neuronal refractory period. It also may exert an anticonvulsant effect by influencing calcium channels and γ-aminobutyric acid receptors or by inhibiting adenosine reuptake.

Pharmacokinetics Phenytoin is a weak acid with a pK_a of 8.3. In the acid milieu of the stomach and even at physiologic pH, more of the drug is nonionized, and its aqueous solubility is limited. Absorption after oral ingestion is slow, variable, and often incomplete, especially after an overdose. Different phenytoin preparations can possess major differences in bioavailability. **Consequently, it may be necessary to obtain serial measurements of serum level in suspected overdose to determine peak levels.** Peak levels typically occur between 3 and 12 hours after a *single therapeutic* oral dose.

After absorption, phenytoin is distributed throughout the body, with a volume of distribution of 0.6 to 0.8 L/kg. Brain tissue concentrations equal those in plasma within about 10 minutes of IV infusion and are correlated with therapeutic effects, whereas cerebrospinal fluid and myocardium equilibrate within 30 to 60 minutes.

Protein Binding Phenytoin is extensively (about 90%) bound to plasma proteins, especially albumin. The free, unbound form is the biologically active moiety responsible for the drug's clinical effect and toxicity. The unbound fraction of the drug is greater in neonates, the elderly, pregnant women, renal failure, hypoalbuminemia (cirrhosis, nephrosis, malnutrition, burns, trauma, or cystic fibrosis), and hyperbilirubinemia. Drugs that displace phenytoin from binding sites (salicylate, valproate, phenylbutazone, tolbutamide, and sulfisoxazole) also result in an increased unbound fraction.

Patients with decreased protein binding have higher levels of free phenytoin and experience a greater biologic effect despite lower levels of total phenytoin. Free phenytoin concentrations are more useful in predicting toxicity. **Corrected serum phenytoin levels** (the concentration that would be present if a patient's serum albumin level were normal) can be calculated as follows: corrected phenytoin concentration = (measured phenytoin concentration × 4.4)/(albumin concentration), with phenytoin concentration measured in micrograms/mL and the albumin concentration measured in grams/dL.

Metabolism After absorption and distribution, only 4% to 5% of phenytoin is excreted unchanged in the urine. The remainder is metabolized by hepatic microsomal enzymes, primarily hydroxylated through a series of inactive compounds. The metabolism of phenytoin is capacity limited (dose dependent). At plasma concentrations of <10 micrograms/mL, elimination is **first-order kinetics** (a fixed *percentage* of drug metabolized per unit of time). At higher concentrations, including those in the therapeutic range of 10 to 20 micrograms/mL, the metabolic pathways may become saturated, and the elimination may change to **zero-order kinetics** (a fixed *amount* metabolized per unit of time). With zero-order kinetics, small increases in maintenance doses may saturate the enzyme systems, markedly prolonging the half-life of phenytoin, and result in a disproportionate increase in the plasma level. **Thus incremental dose increases should be limited to 30 to 50 milligrams at a time, and levels should be carefully monitored when it is necessary to raise phenytoin doses above 300 milligrams (or above 5 milligrams/kg) per day.**

Concomitant use of drugs that inhibit or enhance hepatic microsomal activity may result in an increase or decrease of phenytoin level, respectively. Phenytoin also affects the metabolism of various other agents (**Table 197-2**).

TABLE 197-2 Phenytoin Drug Interactions (Partial List)

Phenytoin increases serum levels of	Phenytoin levels are increased by
Acetaminophen	Amiodarone
Acetazolamide	Chloramphenicol
Amiodarone	Cimetidine
Oral contraceptives	Disulfiram
Primidone	Fluconazole
Zidovudine	Isoniazid
Phenytoin increases toxicity of	Oral anticoagulants
Carbamazepine	Phenylbutazone*
Oral anticoagulants	Salicylate (high dose)*
Phenytoin decreases serum levels of	Trimethoprim
Cyclosporine	**Phenytoin levels are decreased by**
Disopyramide	Antineoplastic drugs
Doxycycline	Calcium
Ethanol (chronic use)	Ethanol
Furosemide	Diazepam
Glucocorticoids	Diazoxide
Levodopa	Folic acid
Methadone	Phenobarbital
Mexiletine	Rifampin
Quinidine	Sucralfate
Theophylline	Sulfonamides*
Valproate	Theophylline
	Tolbutamide*
	Valproate*

*These drugs displace phenytoin from its protein-binding sites, thus increasing the free phenytoin fraction, although the total phenytoin level may decrease.

Propylene Glycol and Ethanol Diluents Propylene glycol is a potent myocardial depressant and vasodilator and also enhances vagal tone. This chemical can cause coma, seizures, circulatory collapse, ventricular dysrhythmias, atrioventricular node depression, and hypotension in experimental animals.[4] Other toxic effects from propylene glycol include hyperosmolality, hemolysis, and lactic acidosis.[5] The ethanol diluent fraction of parenteral phenytoin may precipitate a reaction in patients taking disulfiram.

CLINICAL FEATURES

Central Nervous System Toxicity As toxic phenytoin levels are reached, inhibitory cortical and excitatory cerebellar and vestibular effects begin to occur. The initial sign of toxicity is usually nystagmus, which is seen first on forced lateral gaze and later becomes spontaneous (**Table 197-3**).[6] Vertical, bidirectional, or alternating nystagmus may occur with severe intoxication. A decreased level of consciousness is common, with initial sedation, lethargy, ataxic gait, and dysarthria.[6] This may progress to confusion, coma, and even apnea in a large overdose. Nystagmus may disappear as the level of consciousness decreases, and complete ophthalmoplegia and loss of corneal reflexes may occur. Therefore, absence of nystagmus does not exclude severe phenytoin toxicity. Nystagmus returns as serum drug levels decrease and coma lightens.

Paradoxically, very high levels of phenytoin may be associated with seizures, although this is a rare occurrence, and such phenytoin-induced seizures are usually brief and generalized and almost always are preceded by other signs of toxicity, especially in acute overdose.[7]

Cerebellar stimulation and alterations in dopaminergic and serotonergic activities may cause acute dystonias and movement disorders, such as opisthotonos and choreoathetosis. Hyperactive deep tendon reflexes, clonus, and extensor toe responses also may be elicited. Chronic neurologic toxicity includes peripheral neuropathy and cerebellar degeneration with ataxia.

TABLE 197-3 Clinical Features of Phenytoin Toxicity

Central nervous system	Dizziness, tremor (intention), visual disturbance, horizontal and vertical nystagmus, diplopia, miosis or mydriasis, ophthalmoplegia, abnormal gait (bradykinesia, truncal ataxia), choreoathetoid movements, irritability, agitation, confusion, hallucinations, fatigue, coma, encephalopathy, dysarthria, meningeal irritation with pleocytosis, seizures (rare)
Peripheral nervous system	Peripheral neuropathy, urinary incontinence
Hypersensitivity (anticonvulsant hypersensitivity syndrome)	Eosinophilia, rash, pseudolymphoma (diffuse lymphadenopathy), systemic lupus erythematosus, pancytopenia, hepatitis, pneumonitis
Gastrointestinal	Nausea, vomiting, hepatotoxicity
Dermatologic	Hirsutism, acne, rashes (including Stevens-Johnson syndrome)
Other organs	Fetal hydantoin syndrome, gingival hyperplasia, coarsening of facial features, hemorrhagic disease of the newborn, hyperglycemia, hypocalcemia
Parenteral toxicity	May cause hypotension, bradycardia, conduction disturbances, myocardial depression, ventricular fibrillation, asystole, and tissue necrosis from infiltration

Cardiovascular Toxicity Cardiovascular complications have been almost entirely limited to cases of IV administration, in large part due to the constituents of the parenteral vehicle, or in rare cases of chronic oral toxicity.[8] Cardiac toxicity after oral phenytoin overdose in an otherwise healthy patient has not been reported and, if observed, is due to other causes (e.g., hypoxia and other drugs).[8]

Reported cardiovascular complications include hypotension with decreased peripheral vascular resistance, bradycardia, conduction delays progressing to complete AV nodal block, ventricular tachycardia, primary ventricular fibrillation, and asystole. ECG changes include increased PR interval, widened QRS interval, and altered ST segments and T waves. Cardiovascular toxicity is more common in the elderly, those with underlying cardiac disease, and the critically ill. Guidelines for parenteral phenytoin administration stress a slow rate of infusion and constant monitoring (**Table 197-4**).

TABLE 197-4 Guidelines for Phenytoin or Fosphenytoin Loading

IV	Loading dose is 18 milligrams/kg as phenytoin or fosphenytoin PE.*
	Mix total dose in 150–200 mL of normal saline.
	Keep phenytoin concentration <6 milligrams/mL or fosphenytoin PE concentration <25 milligrams/mL.
	Administer phenytoin through Millipore filter using an infusion pump.
	Rate of administration should not exceed 25–50 milligrams/min of phenytoin or 150 milligrams/min of fosphenytoin PE.
	Use a slower rate of infusion in patients with cardiovascular disease.
	Monitor the blood pressure and cardiac rhythm continually during the infusion.
	In the event of complications, immediately stop the infusion and administer isotonic crystalloid and other treatment as indicated.
IM	Administer 15 milligrams/kg fosphenytoin PE preparation in one or multiple IM sites.
PO†	Loading dose is 20 milligrams/kg.
	Phenytoin tablets or suspension may be used.
	Patient must be conscious with an intact gag reflex and not actively seizing or vomiting.
	Administer the total amount in one dose.

Abbreviation: PE = phenytoin equivalents.

*For simplicity, the pharmaceutical concentration and dose of fosphenytoin is expressed in PE, with 150 milligrams fosphenytoin = 100 milligrams PE.

†Unlike with IV loading, not all patients will reach a therapeutic level with oral loading.

Even though fosphenytoin does not contain the propylene glycol diluent, cardiovascular toxicity can occur with IV administration. Hypotension is seen in about 8%, and rare cases of bradycardia, AV nodal block, and asystole have been observed.[2,10,11]

Vascular and Soft Tissue Toxicity IM injection of *phenytoin* may result in localized crystallization of the drug with hematoma, sterile abscess, and myonecrosis at the injection site. IV extravasation may produce skin and soft tissue necrosis, compartment syndrome, and limb gangrene. Delayed bluish discoloration of the affected extremity ("purple glove syndrome") followed by erythema, edema, vesicles, bullae, and local tissue ischemia has been described.[12]

Hypersensitivity Reactions Hypersensitivity reactions usually occur within 1 to 6 weeks of beginning phenytoin therapy and can present as a febrile illness with skin changes (erythema multiforme, toxic epidermal necrolysis or Stevens-Johnson syndrome) and internal organ involvement (hepatitis, rhabdomyolysis, acute interstitial pneumonitis, renal failure, lymphadenopathy, leukopenia and/or disseminated intravascular coagulation). **Patients with a history of previous hypersensitivity reactions should not receive phenytoin, and because of similar reactions to phenobarbital, lamotrigine, felbamate, and carbamazepine, these anticonvulsants should also be avoided.**

Miscellaneous Effects Gingival hyperplasia is relatively common and is associated with poor dental hygiene (gingivitis and dental plaques). Because of the risk of fetal hydantoin syndrome, oral phenytoin therapy should never be initiated in a pregnant patient without consultation with and close follow-up by a neurologist and obstetrician.

DIAGNOSIS

The therapeutic phenytoin serum level is 10 to 20 micrograms/mL (40 to 80 micromoles/L), which generally corresponds to a free phenytoin level of 1 to 2 micrograms/mL.[13] Although 50% of patients achieve reduction in seizure frequency below these levels, some patients require levels as high as 20 micrograms/mL for adequate control. The ratio of toxic dose to therapeutic dose for phenytoin is rather low, and there is wide individual variability in the levels required to cause adverse effects. In general, toxicity is correlated with increasing plasma levels (**Table 197-5**).

TREATMENT

The initial treatment of severe oral phenytoin overdose is similar to that for ingestion of other drugs. Correct acidosis (respiratory or metabolic) to decrease the active free phenytoin fraction. Multidose activated charcoal may decrease drug half-life but does not decrease time to recovery and does not change outcome in overdose patients.[14] Seizures may be treated with IV benzodiazepines or phenobarbital, with the caution that seizures are uncommon in phenytoin overdose. **For patients with severe and persistent toxicity, hemodialysis and hemoperfusion can produce substantial improvement in neurologic toxicity.**[15-17]

Cardiac monitoring after isolated oral ingestion is unnecessary. Atropine and temporary cardiac pacing may be used for symptomatic bradyarrhythmias associated with IV phenytoin. Hypotension that occurs during IV administration of phenytoin or fosphenytoin usually responds to discontinuation of the infusion and administration of isotonic crystalloid.

TABLE 197-5 Correlation of Plasma Phenytoin Level and Toxic Effects

Total Plasma Level (micrograms/mL)	Toxic Effects
<10	Usually none
10–20	Occasional mild nystagmus
20–30	Nystagmus
30–40	Ataxia, slurred speech, nausea and vomiting
40–50	Lethargy, confusion
>50	Coma, seizures

DISPOSITION AND FOLLOW-UP

Phenytoin has a long and erratic absorption phase after oral overdose, so the decision to discharge or medically clear a patient for psychiatric evaluation cannot be based on one serum level. After acute ingestions, serum level should be measured every few hours. Patients with serious complications after an oral ingestion (seizures, coma, altered mental status, or significant ataxia) should be admitted for further evaluation and treatment. Those with mild symptoms should be observed in the ED and discharged once their levels of phenytoin are declining and they are clinically well. Mental health or psychiatric evaluation should be obtained, as indicated, in cases of intentional overdose.

Patients with symptomatic chronic intoxication should be admitted for observation unless signs are minimal, adequate care can be obtained at home, drug levels are decreasing, and 6 to 8 hours have elapsed since the patient's last therapeutic dose. Phenytoin therapy should be stopped in all cases, and if toxicity continues to resolve, serum level may be reassessed in 2 to 3 days to guide resumption of therapy. Surgical consultation should be obtained for patients with significant extravasation of IV phenytoin or with other signs of local vascular or tissue toxicity after infusion.

CARBAMAZEPINE

Carbamazepine is a primary anticonvulsant used in the treatment of partial and tonic-clonic seizures. Other uses include trigeminal neuralgia, chronic pain disorders, manic disorder, and bipolar disorder.

PATHOPHYSIOLOGY

Carbamazepine inhibits sodium channels and interferes with muscarinic acetylcholine receptors, nicotinic acetylcholine receptors, *N*-methyl-D-aspartate receptors, and central nervous system adenosine receptors.[3] Carbamazepine may relieve neuropathic pain through blockade of synaptic transmission in the trigeminal nucleus. Carbamazepine also possesses anticholinergic, antiarrhythmic, antidepressant, sedative, and neuromuscular-blocking properties. It has central antidiuretic effects, which may lead to the syndrome of inappropriate antidiuretic hormone secretion. Carbamazepine is a potent cytochrome P-450 enzyme inducer and enhances its own metabolism over time.

Carbamazepine is an iminostilbene derivative that is chemically and structurally similar to imipramine. Gastrointestinal absorption is slow, and peak serum concentrations usually occur within 8 hours but may be as late as 12 hours after ingestion. A therapeutic carbamazepine concentration is 4 to 12 micrograms/mL.[18]

Carbamazepine has a protein binding of about 80% and a volume of distribution of 0.8 to 1.2 L/kg. It is metabolized by liver cytochrome P-450 isoenzymes to an active metabolite (10,11-epoxide). The epoxide concentration comprises 15% of the parent compound in adults and slightly higher in children. The epoxide metabolite is responsible for much of the neurotoxicity seen in overdose. Autoinduction of the enzymes that metabolize carbamazepine occurs with about 1 month of continuous use. Because of this, the drug's half-life shortens over time: the half-life after an isolated carbamazepine dose is about 35 hours, much longer than the 10 to 20 hour half-life at steady state after 3 to 5 weeks of continuous therapy.[17]

CLINICAL FEATURES

After an overdose, the delayed and erratic absorption due to anticholinergic properties (which delay gastrointestinal motility) and low water solubility can cause delayed clinical deterioration or a crescendo-decrescendo clinical course.[19] Manifestations of acute toxicity include mental status depression, ataxia, nystagmus, ileus, hypertonicity with increased deep tendon reflexes, dystonic reactions, and an anticholinergic toxidrome.[19-21] Paradoxical seizures can occur in patients with high carbamazepine concentrations and an underlying seizure disorder. There are sporadic reports of left ventricular dysfunction with heart failure and transient heart block (without hemodynamic compromise). **Cardiac arrhythmias are rarely seen, but carbamazepine is one of the few drugs that can potentially cause both a wide QRS interval and seizures.** Laboratory abnormalities seen with acute overdose include hyponatremia, hyperglycemia, and transient elevation of serum liver enzyme levels.

Adverse effects occur in 25% of patients receiving long-term carbamazepine therapy. Mild transient leukopenia may occur during the first month of treatment. This is unrelated to the more serious side effect of aplastic anemia, which has a reported incidence of 1 to 5 per million patient-years, approximately 11 times higher than in the normal population. Mild liver enzyme elevation occurs in up to 10% of patients on long-term therapy. Stevens-Johnson syndrome and toxic epidermal necrolysis are reported with about the same frequency as aplastic anemia.

DIAGNOSIS

Serum carbamazepine concentrations are not linearly correlated with poisoning severity. However, serum concentrations of >40 micrograms/mL are associated with an increased risk of serious complications such as seizures, respiratory failure, coma, and cardiac conduction defects.[22] Serum concentrations higher than 60 to 80 micrograms/mL may be fatal. The seriousness of toxicity should be judged by the clinical status of the patient, not by the serum concentration.[20-22]

Because the chemical structure of carbamazepine is related to imipramine, **carbamazepine can cause a false-positive tricyclic antidepressant result on a urine drug screen.**[23] Both carbamazepine and epoxide metabolite are measured by the standard enzyme-multiplied immunoassay to determine serum levels.

TREATMENT

Activated charcoal may be considered if the patient is not obtunded and presents within 1 hour of ingestion, because delayed absorption is possible.[14] Multidose activated charcoal may decrease drug half-life but does not decrease time to recovery or change outcome in overdose patients.[24] **In patients with severe toxicity and multiorgan dysfunction, hemodialysis, hemoperfusion, or hemodiafiltration is effective.**[25-31] Although cardiac conduction delays are rare, if conduction delay is noted on the electrocardiogram, sodium bicarbonate treatment seems reasonable.

DISPOSITION AND FOLLOW-UP

Patients can be medically cleared from the ED if at least two carbamazepine measurements obtained a few hours apart show decreasing levels (preferably below 15 micrograms/mL) and the patient is awake, ambulatory, and free of cardiac conduction abnormalities.

VALPROATE

Valproate (or valproic acid) is used to treat tonic-clonic seizures, absence seizures, partial complex seizures, and post-traumatic epilepsy. Valproate is also used in migraine headache prophylaxis, to control manic episodes in bipolar disorder, and to treat neuropathic pain.

PATHOPHYSIOLOGY

Valproate affects neurotransmitters and the function of electrically excitable cells.[3] Valproate increases γ-aminobutyric acid concentrations, reduces release of γ-hydroxybutyrate, and blocks *N*-methyl-D-aspartate receptors.[32] Valproate prolongs recovery of inactivated sodium channels, enhances potassium conductance, and reduces T-type calcium current firing.

With standard preparations at therapeutic doses, peak serum concentrations occur within 4 hours after ingestion. If the enteric-coated or controlled-release formulation has been ingested, peak serum concentration may be delayed for 12 to 17 hours.[33]

Valproate is metabolized by the liver by glucuronic acid conjugation and mitochondrial beta oxidation. Valproate enters mitochondria by using L-carnitine as a cofactor. Protein binding is extensive and influenced by serum concentration, with 90% of the drug protein bound at concentrations of 40 micrograms/mL. Valproate is an eight-carbon fatty acid and has a small volume of distribution of 0.13 to 0.23 L/kg. The half-life of valproate is 8 to 21 hours but may be two or three times longer after overdose.[33-36]

CLINICAL FEATURES

After an overdose with acute toxicity, the most frequent sign is CNS depression, ranging from drowsiness to coma.[35] Other findings include respiratory depression, hypotension, hypoglycemia, hypocalcemia, hypernatremia, hypophosphatemia, and anion gap metabolic acidosis that may persist for days. Toxicity to the liver produces elevated serum levels of aminotransferases, ammonia, and lactate. Pancreatitis may occur, and thrombocytopenia may be clinically significant and severe.[35]

Valproate increases renal ammonia production and blocks hepatic ammonia metabolism. Hyperammonemia in the absence of liver failure has been reported following valproate overdose and during long-term therapy.[37,38] Cerebral edema has been seen in acute overdose.[34,35] During long-term therapeutic use, increased serum liver enzyme levels occur in >50% of patients with therapeutic valproate serum concentrations. Liver enzyme levels typically normalize with dosage reduction or discontinuation of the drug. Hepatic failure, histologically evident as microvesicular steatosis, occurs in about 1 in 20,000 patients receiving long-term therapy.[39-41] Valproate-induced hepatotoxicity may be either intrinsic and benign (reversible, reproducible, and dose dependent) or idiosyncratic and fatal (unpredictable, not dose dependent, with a long latent period). Children <3 years of age who are receiving multiple antiepileptic agents and have additional medical problems are at highest risk for fatal hepatotoxicity, with an incidence of about 1 in 500. Serum levels of transaminases and ammonia should be checked in children on valproate therapy who demonstrate somnolence or lethargy.

DIAGNOSIS

Therapeutic valproate concentrations are 50 to 100 micrograms/mL. Although serum concentration does not correlate well with either seizure control or toxicity, adverse side effects increase as concentrations rise above 150 micrograms/mL, and coma may occur with levels above 800 micrograms/mL. When serum valproate concentrations are measured, the enzyme-multiplied immunoassay technique yields higher values than gas-liquid chromatography, so a consistent analytic methodology should be used when monitoring treatment. Serum ammonia and glucose concentrations should be measured with suspected valproate toxicity. **Valproate is eliminated partly as ketone bodies and may cause a positive test result for ketones in the urine or blood.**

TREATMENT

Single-dose activated charcoal alone is sufficient for the vast majority of patients with a valproate overdose. Consider multidose activated charcoal and/or whole-bowel irrigation after ingestion of enteric-coated, delayed-release preparations to prevent the ongoing absorption that may occur from delayed capsule or tablet dissolution.[14,42] Because of delayed peak serum levels after an overdose, serial concentrations should be measured.

Administration of high-dose naloxone has been reported to reverse valproate-induced neurologic depression, possibly by reversal of valproate-induced release of endogenous opioids or reversal of valproate-induced blockade of γ-aminobutyric acid uptake.[43,44] Because the serious toxic effects of valproate involve more than just these two mechanisms, naloxone is unlikely to be helpful in the management of a comatose patient after valproate overdose.

Overdose patients have been given **L-carnitine** in an attempt to increase valproate metabolism by beta oxidation, and this therapy appears to hasten the resolution of coma, prevent hepatic dysfunction, and reverse mitochondrial metabolic abnormalities in patients with acute valproate intoxication.[45-47] Administration of L-carnitine 100 milligrams/kg IV initially followed by infusions of 50 milligrams/kg every 8 hours is recommended in cases of valproate toxicity with lethargy, coma, hyperammonemia, and hepatic dysfunction.[46] For patients receiving long-term valproate therapy, oral carnitine administration reverses carnitine deficiency, decreases elevated ammonia levels, and reduces lethargy.

Hemoperfusion and hemodiafiltration have been used to treat severe valproate overdose.[48-52] Although valproate should not be amenable to dialysis due to significant protein binding, unbound (free) drug is markedly increased in overdose, and removal of valproate from this pool appears beneficial. During hemoperfusion and hemodiafiltration treatment, elimination half-life ranges from 1.7 to 3 hours compared with 4.8 to 21 hours in patients before and after extracorporeal therapy. Clinical comparison of extracorporeal detoxification with supportive care reports a benefit to extracorporeal removal.[53]

DISPOSITION AND FOLLOW-UP

Assess valproate levels every few hours until a decline in the level is noted and the patient is asymptomatic.

SECOND- AND THIRD-GENERATION ANTICONVULSANTS

As a group, the second- and third-generation anticonvulsants are less toxic in acute overdose than the first-generation agents, and most of the serious complications reported occur in cases of mixed ingestion.[54] Some specific acute toxic effects are notable (**Table 197-6**).

ESLICARBAZEPINE ACETATE

Eslicarbazepine acetate is a prodrug drug for eslicarbazepine, an anticonvulsant that stabilizes sodium-dependent channels in their inactivated state.[55,56] Eslicarbazepine acetate has a half-life of 10 to 20 hours and possesses modest and possible clinically relevant drug interactions with phenytoin, carbamazepine, and oral contraceptives.[55-57] Symptoms of vertigo, ataxia, and hemiparesis have been observed after accidental overdose. Eslicarbazepine acetate is available in Europe but not in the United States as of March 2012.

EZOGABINE

Ezogabine (generic name in the United States) or **retigabine** (generic name in Europe) activates voltage-gated potassium channels in the brain, a unique mechanism among the anticonvulsants.[55,56,58] Ezogabine has a half-life of 6 to 10 hours and possesses drug interactions with phenytoin, carbamazepine, and lamotrigine.[55-57] Side effects seen with ezogabine therapy include dizziness, fatigue, confusion, tremor, and ataxia.[58] Increased rate of urinary retention and slight increase in QT interval have been reported. There is limited experience with overdose, but agitation, irritability, and aggressive behavior have been noted.

FELBAMATE

Felbamate was the first of the second-generation antiepileptics.[54] However, shortly after its introduction in 1993 it received a "black box warning" because of the association with aplastic anemia (with an incidence 100 times higher than in the general population) and hepatic failure. Hence it is only recommended when other treatment regimens have failed. The proposed mechanism of action of felbamate is inhibition at γ-aminobutyric acid receptors and excitation at *N*-methyl-d-aspartic acid receptors. Felbamate has a half-life of 20 to 23 hours and possesses drug intersections with the first-generation anticonvulsants and oral contraceptives. In overdose, the symptoms are usually mild, but in large ingestions, felbamate can crystallize in the kidney, producing crystalluria, hematuria, and possibly acute renal failure.[59-61] Treatment is supportive.

GABAPENTIN

Gabapentin, as its name suggests, increases γ-aminobutyric acid levels in the brain. It also has indirect effects on calcium channels located on the postsynaptic terminal. Gabapentin has a half-life of 5 to 9 hours and possesses drug interactions with cimetidine and antacids. With an overdose, gabapentin produces little toxicity, usually drowsiness, ataxia, nausea, and vomiting that resolve in about 10 hours.[62] Depressed level of consciousness has been described in a patient with end-stage renal disease who ingested multiple doses of gabapentin over 2 days without intervening hemodialysis; hemodialysis was associated with rapid recovery.[63] The only reported suicide from gabapentin overdose is controversial.[64]

LACOSAMIDE

Lacosamide affects voltage-gated sodium channels in the central nervous system.[65] Lacosamide has a half-life of 12 to 16 hours and has no significant drug interactions.[56,57] During therapeutic use, adverse reactions are usually mild to moderate and typically include dizziness, headache, nausea, and diplopia.[65] There is limited clinical experience with lacosamide overdose, but serious toxicity after an isolated overdose would not be expected to occur.

LAMOTRIGINE

Lamotrigine inhibits sodium channels in CNS neurons and likely has the same effect in the heart.[55] Lamotrigine has a half-life of 15 to 35 hours and interacts with the first-generation antiepileptics.[57] Autoimmune

TABLE 197-6 Unique Aspects of Overdose With Second- and Third-Generation Anticonvulsants

Drug (Generation)	Effects
Eslicarbazepine acetate (3rd)*	Vertigo, ataxia, hemiparesis
Ezogabine or retigabine (3rd)	Agitation, irritability, aggressive behavior
Felbamate (2nd)	Crystalluria, hematuria, aplastic anemia, liver failure
Gabapentin (2nd)	Drowsiness, ataxia, nausea, vomiting
Lacosamide (3rd)	Limited experience; serious toxicity unlikely
Lamotrigine (2nd)	Drowsiness, vomiting, ataxia, and dizziness; serious neurologic and cardiovascular toxicity with co-ingestants; "Stevens-Johnson syndrome"
Levetiracetam (2nd)	Lethargy, coma, respiratory depression
Oxcarbazepine (2nd)	Little toxicity from isolated oxcarbazepine overdose
Pregabalin (2nd)	Drowsiness and depressed level of consciousness
Rufinamide (2nd)	Limited experience; serious toxicity unlikely
Stiripentol (2nd)*	No information
Tiagabine (2nd)	Rapid onset of lethargy, coma, seizures, and status epilepticus; myoclonus, muscular rigidity, and delirium
Topiramate (2nd)	Somnolence, vertigo, agitation, and mydriasis; seizures and status epilepticus; metabolic acidosis
Vigabatrin (2nd)	Drowsiness, unconsciousness, coma
Zonisamide (2nd)	Little toxicity from isolated zonisamide overdose

*Not available in the United States as of March 2012.

reactions, such as Stevens-Johnson syndrome, have occurred during therapeutic use. With an overdose, the clinical course is usually benign, and the most common effects are drowsiness, vomiting, ataxia, and dizziness.[66,67] Serious neurologic and cardiovascular toxicity is rare, but has been reported after lamotrigine overdose, sometimes with coingestants.[68-72] Neurologic toxicity includes oculogyric crisis, provoking of seizures,[70,74-77] status epilepticus, and coma. Cardiac toxicity includes QRS complex widening,[78] AV nodal block,[79] and cardiovascular collapse.[72,77] Acute pancreatitis has been reported in association with a lamotrigine overdose.[80] Treatments used in lamotrigine overdose include **activated charcoal** to reduce absorption,[81] **sodium bicarbonate for QRS complex widening, magnesium sulfate for QT interval prolongation, and IV lipid emulsion** to remove active drug from binding sites and sequester it in a lipid sink.[82,83]

LEVETIRACETAM

The mechanism of action of **levetiracetam** is not known. Levetiracetam has a half-life of 6 to 8 hours and possesses drug interaction only with phenytoin. During therapeutic use, the major side effect is somnolence, usually seen during the initial 4 weeks of therapy.[84] There are few reports of levetiracetam overdose, and the most common symptom is lethargy that can progress to coma and respiratory depression.[85-88] Recovery is usually rapid with supportive care alone.

OXCARBAZEPINE

Oxcarbazepine inhibits voltage-sensitive sodium channels in the nervous system.[89] Oxcarbazepine has a half-life of 8 to 15 hours and interacts with phenytoin, lamotrigine, and oral contraceptives.[56,57] During therapeutic use, hyponatremia and drug rash can be seen. There appears to be little toxicity from isolated oxcarbazepine overdose; most of the serious neurologic depression has been seen with mixed ingestions.[90-93]

PREGABALIN

Pregabalin has a mechanism of action similar to that of gabapentin, increasing γ-aminobutyric acid levels in the brain in addition to having indirect effects on calcium channels located on the postsynaptic terminal. Pregabalin has a half-life of 5 to 7 hours and possesses drug interactions with ethanol, lorazepam, and oxycodone.[56,57] During long-term therapeutic use, the most commonly reported side effects are somnolence and dizziness; serious adverse effects are rare. There is little reported experience with pregabalin overdose; depressed level of consciousness appears to be the major symptom.[94,95] Similar to the experience with gabapentin, toxicity from pregabalin has been reported in patients with end-stage renal failure but resolves with dialysis.[96]

RUFINAMIDE

Rufinamide inhibits the activity of sodium channels, prolonging their inactive state.[97] Rufinamide has a half-life of 6 to 10 hours and has drug interactions with other anticonvulsants—phenytoin, carbamazepine, valproate, phenobarbital, and lamotrigine—as well as with oral contraceptives.[56,57] During long-term therapy, commonly reported adverse reactions include headache, dizziness, fatigue, and somnolence. There is limited clinical experience with rufinamide overdose, but given the lack of symptoms seen with doses of more than six times the recommended amount, toxicity would not be expected after an isolated overdose.

STIRIPENTOL

Stiripentol inhibits the reuptake of γ-aminobutyric acid into the presynpatic neuron, thereby increasing γ-aminobutyric acid concentrations in the synaptic cleft and promoting γ-aminobutyric acid activity. Stiripentol has a half-life of 5 to 13 hours and possesses modest drug interactions with valproate and clobazam.[56,57] Side effects during therapeutic use include drowsiness, ataxia, tremor, anorexia, nausea, and vomiting. Transient aplastic anemia and leukopenia have occurred. There is no information on clinical overdose with this medication. Stiripentol is available in Europe and Canada, but not in the United States as of March 2012.

TIAGABINE

Tiagabine inhibits the reuptake of γ-aminobutyric acid into the presynpatic neuron, thereby increasing γ-aminobutyric acid concentrations in the synaptic cleft and promoting γ-aminobutyric acid activity. Tiagabine has a half-life of 5 to 8 hours and interacts with most of the first-generation antiepileptics, including phenytoin, valproate, carbamazepine, phenobarbital, and primidone.[56,57] In overdose, tiagabine can cause the rapid onset of neurologic toxicity, including lethargy, coma, and seizures.[98-101] Tiagabine overdose can provoke status epilepticus, even in patients without an underlying seizure disorder.[102-105] Other signs seen in tiagabine overdose include myoclonus, muscular rigidity, and delirium.[98] Recovery usually occurs in about 24 hours.

TOPIRAMATE

Topiramate inhibits γ-aminobutyric acid receptors in addition to affecting sodium channels in the brain. Topiramate has a half-life of 20 to 30 hours and possesses drug interactions with other anticonvulsants—phenytoin, valproate, carbamazepine, phenobarbital, and primidone—as well as with oral contraceptives.[56,57] Adverse effects observed during therapeutic use include promotion of renal stone formation and glaucoma. In overdose, topiramate can produce somnolence, vertigo, agitation, and mydriasis.[106-108] Seizures and status epilepticus have been reported.[109,110] **A unique aspect of topiramate overdose is the production of a non-anion gap metabolic acidosis.**[111-113] The cause is inhibition of renal carbonic anhydrase, and because of the long half-life of topiramate, metabolic acidosis can last up to 7 days. However, this effect is completely reversible, and no permanent sequelae have been seen.

VIGABATRIN

Vigabatrin is a structural analog of γ-aminobutyric acid that increases brain concentrations of this neurotransmitter. Vigabatrin has a half-life of 5 to 7 hours and has a modest drug interaction with phenytoin.[56,57,114] During chronic therapy, vigabatrin may worsen mood and exacerbate psychosis. Sedation, headache, and weight gain are common side effects. After acute overdose, drowsiness, unconsciousness, and coma are described in the majority of cases.[115]

ZONISAMIDE

Zonisamide inhibits voltage-sensitive sodium channels in CNS neurons.[116] Zonisamide has a long half-life, 50 to 70 hours, and possesses drug interactions with most of the first-generation antiepileptics, including phenytoin, valproate, carbamazepine, phenobarbital, and primidone.[56,57] Serious adverse effects during therapeutic use include the promotion of renal stone formation and a drug-induced rash. Isolated zonisamide overdose is associated with lethargy.[117,118] A death ascribed to zonisamide overdose was actually a mixed ingestion that included mirtazapine, diphenhydramine, and caffeine.[119]

REFERENCES

The complete reference list is available online at www.TintinalliEM.com.

Iron

Stephanie H. Hernandez
Lewis S. Nelson

INTRODUCTION

Iron supplements are widely available, particularly in homes with small children and young women. The attractiveness of the bright color and sugar coating of the tablets and their initial distribution in non–child-resistant vials made children susceptible to ingestion. The 1997 Federal requirement that all iron-containing pharmaceuticals containing more than 30 milligrams of elemental iron be distributed only in blister packs reduced the reported incidence of iron ingestion and deaths in young children.[1,2] This requirement was removed in 2003, but blister packs remain in common use along with child-resistant bottles, and serious iron poisonings in young children have remained low.[2] Women of childbearing age are at risk for intentional iron overdose due to the availability of iron and increased stress during pregnancy and the postnatal period.[3] Children with inadvertent overdoses[4,5] and adults with intentional overdose[6] are at risk of serious toxicity or death.

PHARMACOLOGY

Total-body iron store averages about 4 grams in adults; the range is between 2 and 6 grams, with less iron in women than in men. About two thirds of the body's iron is incorporated into hemoglobin, and the remainder is found in other iron-containing proteins such as myoglobin, cytochromes, and other enzymes and cofactors, or is stored as ferritin. The recommended daily intake of iron is about 8 milligrams for boys, adult men, and nonmenstruating women; 18 milligrams for menstruating women; and 27 milligrams for pregnant females.[7] Because excess iron is toxic, the body uses several mechanisms to maintain iron homeostasis: serum protein binding, intracellular storage, and, most importantly, regulation of GI tract absorption.[8]

The oral bioavailability of iron depends on the formulation ingested. Inorganic iron has <10% bioavailability, with ferrous iron (Fe^{2+}) better absorbed than ferric iron (Fe^{3+}). Common ionic formulations include ferrous chloride, ferrous fumarate, ferrous gluconate, ferrous lactate, and ferrous sulfate (**Table 198-1**). Nonionic formulations include carbonyl iron and iron polysaccharide (iron dextran). Most dietary iron is in the ferric form and chelated to the heme moiety. Following ingestion, the ferric ion is separated from heme and reduced to ferrous iron by a brush border ferrireductase. Chelated iron, such as that found in meat, is more readily absorbed than the iron in ionic preparations. Commercially available formulations of iron chelated with amino acids (e.g., glycinate) mimic the benefits of dietary meat for iron absorption (Table 198-1).

Ferrous iron is transported into enterocytes by a membrane proton-coupled metal transporter.[7] Within the enterocyte, ferrous iron is oxidized to ferric iron. Transferrin, a serum protein, serves as a carrier and moves ferric iron from the enterocytes into the circulation and transports iron through the body. The serum total iron-binding capacity assay primarily measures the amount of serum transferrin and is generally two to three times the normal serum iron concentration (50 to 170 micrograms/dL or 9 to 30 micromol/L). Iron is stored within the body in the form of ferritin, a large intracellular storage protein that can reversibly bind as many as 4500 molecules of iron. Ferritin can also be incorporated by phagolysosomes to form hemosiderin granules. In adults, about 0.5 to 1 gram of elemental iron is stored as ferritin and hemosiderin, primarily in the bone marrow, spleen, and liver. In iron deficiency, iron is mobilized from ferritin and transported via transferrin to the hematopoietic cells in the spleen and bone marrow, where it is incorporated into appropriate molecules.[8] Under normal conditions, unbound iron, or free iron, does not exist within the body, and essentially all circulating plasma iron is normally bound to transferrin.

There is no physiologic mechanism for removal of iron once it has entered the body.[7] Regulation of GI iron uptake and limitation of absorption by sloughing of mucosal cell containing surplus iron are the principal mechanisms for maintaining physiologic iron concentrations.[7]

TABLE 198-1 Iron Formulations and Elemental Iron Composition

	Iron Formulation	Elemental Iron Composition
Ionic	Ferrous fumarate (PO)	33%
	Ferrous chloride (PO)	28%
	Ferrous sulfate (PO)	20%
	Ferrous lactate (PO)	19%
	Ferrous gluconate (PO)	12%
	Ferrous gluconate (IV)	1.25%
Nonionic	Carbonyl iron (PO)	98%
	Iron polysaccharide (PO)	46%
	Ferric hydroxide dextran (IV)	10% or 20%
	Iron sucrose (IV)	2%
Chelated	Ferrous bisglycinate (PO)	20%
	Iron glycinate (PO)	27%

Example: A 325-milligram ferrous sulfate tablet is 20% elemental iron and contains 65 milligrams of elemental iron per tablet. Iron sucrose is a 2% elemental iron solution and contains 20 milligrams of elemental iron per 1 mL.

PATHOPHYSIOLOGY

Iron is a potent catalyst for the production of oxidants such as free radicals.[9] Through this mechanism, iron is a direct GI tract irritant and causes vomiting, diarrhea, abdominal pain, mucosal ulceration, and bleeding soon after a significant ingestion. As the mucosal surface is injured, the regulatory enterocyte barrier is compromised, and free iron passes unimpeded into the blood, becoming systemically available.

Free iron disrupts critical cellular processes and induces acidosis and widespread organ toxicity. It enters the mitochondria, where it inhibits oxidative phosphorylation by disrupting the electron transport chain, which results in metabolic acidosis with an elevated lactate. Production of toxic hydroxyl radicals, induction of membrane lipid peroxidation, liberation of hydrogen ions from reduction of ferrous iron, and hypotension all contribute to the metabolic acidosis seen with acute iron toxicity. Hepatotoxicity occurs as the portal blood supply delivers a large amount of iron to the liver. In addition, coagulopathy unrelated to hepatotoxicity may occur through inhibition of thrombin formation and the effect of thrombin on fibrinogen. Myocardial and vascular dysfunction result from vasodilation, negative ionotropic effect, and direct myocardial iron deposition.

TOXICITY

The amount of ingested elemental iron correlates with the potential for toxicity (**Table 198-2**). Toxic effects are reported after oral doses as low as 10 or 20 milligrams/kg of elemental iron. **In general, moderate toxicity occurs at doses of 20 to 60 milligrams/kg of elemental iron, and**

TABLE 198-2 Predicted Toxicity of Iron Ingestion

Predicted Clinical Effects	Elemental Iron Dose*	Serum Iron Concentration†
Nontoxic or mild GI symptoms	<20 milligrams/kg	<300 micrograms/dL (<54 micromol/L)
Expected significant GI symptoms and potential for systemic toxicity	20–60 milligrams/kg	300–500 micrograms/dL (54–90 micromol/L)
Moderate to severe systemic toxicity	>60 milligrams/kg	>500 micrograms/dL (>90 micromol/L)
Severe systemic toxicity and increased morbidity		>1000 micrograms/dL (>180 micromol/L)

*Elemental iron dose by history.
†Serum iron concentration obtained within 4–6 h of ingestion.

severe toxicity can be expected following ingestion of >60 milligrams/kg of elemental iron.[6] The most commonly prescribed formulation, a ferrous sulfate 325-milligram tablet, contains 65 milligrams of elemental iron, and approximately 20 to 35 tablets would be expected to produce moderate toxicity after an acute ingestion in an adult. Pediatric multivitamins typically contain 10 to 18 milligrams of elemental iron per tablet, and this reduced amount is associated with a near absence of fatalities after ingestion of iron-containing pediatric multivitamins in children compared with adult iron supplements.[10] Ferric chloride poisoning can occur with occupational inhalation, accidental ingestion through mislabeling, and suicidal ingestion.[11] Ingestion of commercially available chemical hand warmers, containing 95 to 120 grams of reduced elemental iron (not an iron salt), may cause corrosive injury of the esophagus and stomach[12] and result in significant iron absorption with potential toxicity.[13]

Exceptions to the correlation of ingested dose and toxicity include chelated iron and carbonyl iron. Despite their increased iron content, chelated sources of supplemental iron are less toxic than nonchelated iron in overdose, because the ligand sterically limits the iron from participating in redox reactions.[14] Similarly, carbonyl iron is a nonionic iron molecule that does not participate in redox reactions, and the limited experience with overdose of carbonyl iron suggests a lower incidence of toxicity compared with ingestion of an equivalent amount of ionic iron.[15]

CLINICAL FEATURES

Five stages of clinical toxicity are traditionally described, although in more practical terms, acute iron toxicity can be considered to manifest in two clinical stages: local GI tract toxicity and systemic toxicity.

Stage 1 of iron poisoning is characterized by abdominal pain, vomiting, and diarrhea.[16] Iron is directly irritating and corrosive to the GI tract and typically induces vomiting within the first few hours following ingestion. Vomiting is the clinical sign most consistently associated with acute iron toxicity. Patients with symptoms of gastric irritation may either recover over several hours or progress to systemic toxicity. **The absence of GI symptoms within 6 hours of ingestion essentially excludes a significant iron ingestion.**

Stage 2, or the "latent" stage, does not always occur. If present, this stage is a 6- to 24-hour interval following ingestion during which GI symptoms may resolve and falsely reassure the patient and physician. However, this is not a truly quiescent phase. Patients with significant toxicity have ongoing clinical illness and progressive systemic deterioration because of volume loss and worsening metabolic acidosis, despite the absence of GI symptoms. Alternatively, the resolution of GI findings may signal the end of mild poisoning, and in such a circumstance, the results of the patient's laboratory studies should be normal.

Stage 3 is characterized by systemic toxicity from iron-induced disruption of cellular metabolism with resultant shock and lactic acidosis. Iron-induced coagulopathy may worsen bleeding and hypovolemia. The coagulopathy may be biphasic, with prolonged prothrombin time and partial thromboplastin time within the first 24 hours. This initial coagulopathy appears to be reversible with chelation therapy, because it is free iron that initially interferes with the activity of factors in the coagulation cascade. Subsequent coagulopathy is from iron-induced hepatic injury that reduced coagulation factor production. During stage 3, renal failure, cardiomyopathy, and failure of other critical organ systems may also occur.

Stage 4, the hepatic stage, develops 2 to 5 days following ingestion.[6,17] It results from iron uptake by the reticuloendothelial system with local lipid peroxidation; it manifests as elevation of aminotransferase levels and may progress to hepatic failure.

Stage 5 refers to delayed sequelae, including gastric outlet obstruction secondary to the corrosive effects of iron on the pyloric mucosa. Delayed sequelae are rare and occur 4 to 6 weeks after ingestion.[16]

DIAGNOSIS

LABORATORY TESTING

Laboratory tests should include CBC, determination of serum electrolyte levels, renal and liver function studies, coagulation function tests, serum glucose, and serum iron levels, with the understanding that these results are to assess the overall condition of the patient, because **iron toxicity is largely a clinical diagnosis.**

Arterial blood gas analysis and serum lactate determination are usually unnecessary in mild cases, because determination of serum electrolyte levels (anion gap evaluation) usually yields all the important information. However, in patients with moderate to severe toxicity or in those with respiratory compromise, arterial blood gas results yield useful information regarding the patient's acid-base status. With moderate to severe ingestions, the blood bank should perform blood typing and screening in anticipation of potential need.

Interpret serum iron levels to assess toxicity and direct management with caution. **In general, serum iron levels measured within 4 to 6 hours after an acute ingestion correlate with the severity of toxicity** (Table 198-2), **but low serum iron levels do not necessarily mean absence of toxicity.** Serum iron levels may be low because of variable times to peak level following ingestions of different iron preparations, and treatment with deferoxamine can artificially lower serum iron levels. **Serum total iron-binding capacity has little value in the assessment of iron-poisoned patients.** It becomes falsely elevated in the presence of elevated serum iron levels or deferoxamine, and significant organ damage occurs despite exceeding the serum iron level.

IMAGING

Standard ferrous sulfate tablets and reduced iron are radiopaque and frequently visible on routine radiographs,[12,13] and this may help guide GI decontamination when present. However, many iron preparations are not routinely detected, including pediatric chewable and liquid preparations, and absence of radiopaque material on radiographs does not exclude iron ingestion.[2]

TREATMENT

Iron poisoning is a clinical diagnosis. Signs and symptoms consistent with iron poisoning should guide treatment, rather than serum iron concentrations alone (**Figure 198-1**). Patients who are asymptomatic on ED arrival, have not ingested a potentially toxic amount, and have normal findings on physical examination can be observed and do not require specific medical treatment. Patients who vomit once or twice from the gastric irritant effects of iron but who are otherwise asymptomatic can also be observed and may require no specific treatment.

Patients with clinical toxicity should first be stabilized with attention to airway, breathing, and circulation, after which GI decontamination and chelation therapy with deferoxamine may proceed.[2,18] Antiemetics such as metoclopramide or ondansetron should be used for repetitive vomiting. Patients with persistent vomiting and abnormal vital sign values or other signs of poor perfusion or shock should undergo aggressive fluid resuscitation and treatment with deferoxamine. Coagulopathy should be treated with parenteral vitamin K_1 and/or fresh frozen plasma, as indicated. Significant blood loss may require transfusion.

GI DECONTAMINATION

Do not use ipecac syrup because it may obscure the initial signs of clinical toxicity and is not proven to be more effective at gastric emptying than is iron-induced vomiting.[19] **Do not give activated charcoal, cathartics, oral sodium bicarbonate, or phosphosoda.** Activated charcoal does not adsorb significant amounts of iron in an overdose to prevent toxicity, and its use may complicate endoscopy if that becomes necessary.[19] Cathartics should not be given. Orogastric lavage may not be effective if the ingested tablets are large or if several hours have elapsed since ingestion, but it may be useful in rare cases if performed shortly after large ingestion, prior to significant vomiting, or if a modified-release formulation was ingested.[2,20] There are no data to support the efficacy of oral sodium bicarbonate or phosphosoda in forming insoluble iron salts and preventing absorption.[2,19]

Radiopaque tablets visible on radiography indicate potential for progressive toxicity and can guide decontamination measures

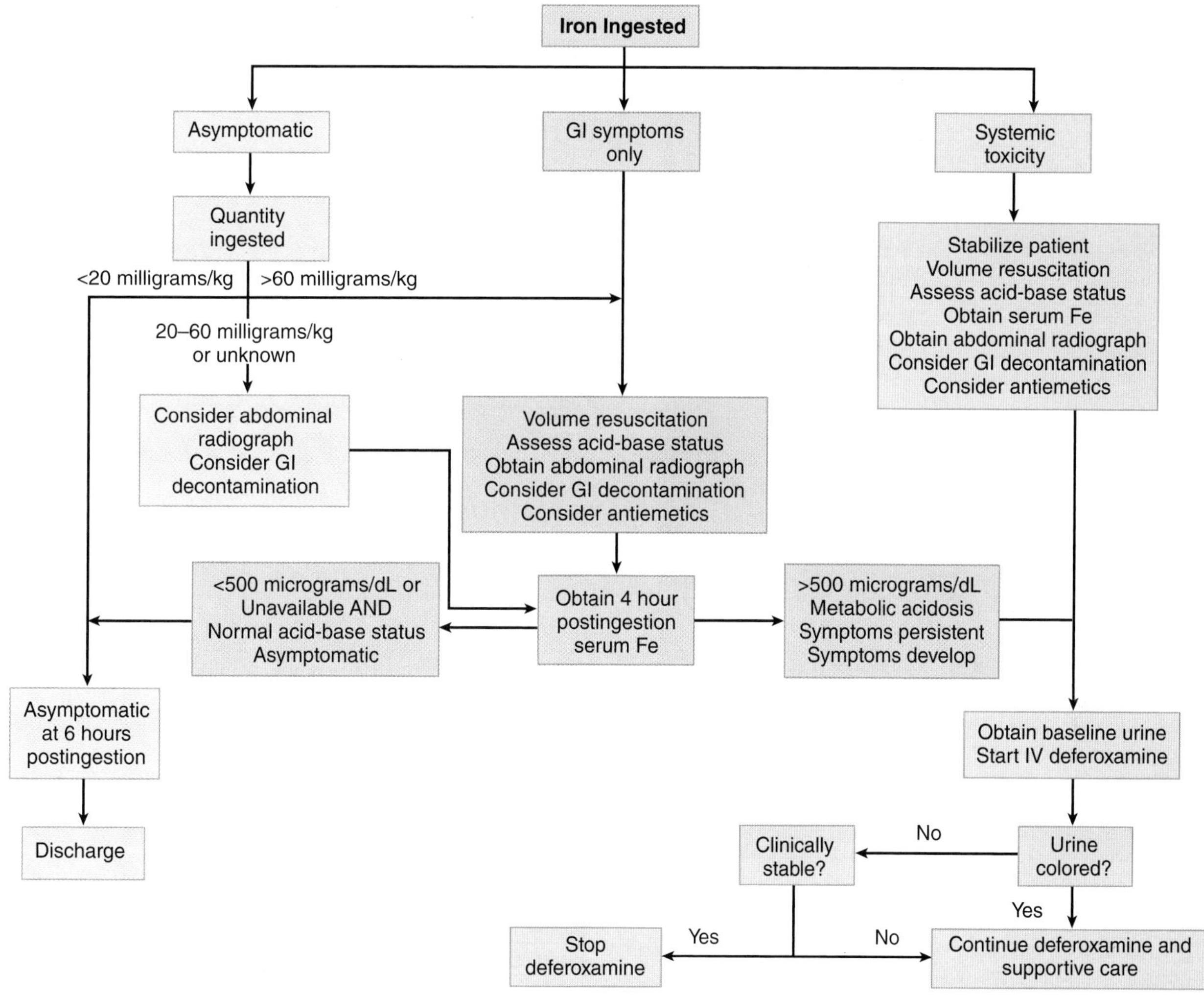

FIGURE 198-1. Algorithm for clinical management of iron ingestion.

(**Figure 198-2**). Whole-bowel irrigation with a polyethylene glycol solution is effective in children with large iron ingestions.[2,21] Administration of 250 to 500 mL/h in children or 2 L/h in adults by nasogastric tube may clear the GI tract of iron pills before absorption can occur.[21] Endoscopy can remove large iron loads or an iron-containing gastric bezoar.[22,23] Laparoscopic gastrotomy may be a rare option for removal of an iron-containing gastric bezoar in profoundly ill patients when other measures are unsuccessful or impractical.[24]

DEFEROXAMINE

Deferoxamine is chelating agent derived from *Streptomyces pilosus* used to treat iron toxicity. Deferoxamine binds free iron, iron from plasma, and iron from inside cells and mitochondria, but not iron bound to organic molecules. Upon binding, it forms the complex ferrioxamine, which is renally excreted. Deferoxamine can be safely administered to children and pregnant women.[3] Although deferoxamine binds a small amount of iron (9 milligrams of elemental iron for each 100 milligrams of deferoxamine) and thus chelates only a small fraction of the total amount of iron ingested, removing this small but critical amount of iron often proves clinically effective in restoring cellular function. Deferoxamine may work by other mechanisms in addition to binding excess iron, and complete binding of ingested iron is not the goal of therapy.

Administration of deferoxamine is indicated in the iron-poisoned patient with systemic toxicity, persistent emesis, metabolic acidosis, progressive symptoms, or a serum iron level predictive of moderate to severe toxicity (Figure 198-1).[2,18] The manufacturer recommends IM administration for all patients not in shock,[25] but most toxicologists advise IV administration rather than IM administration because of the unreliability of IM absorption and enhanced iron excretion following IV administration.[2,18]

The initial deferoxamine adult dose is 1000 milligrams (children 50 milligrams/kg) IV. Begin the infusion slowly, starting at 5 milligrams/kg per hour to avoid producing a rate-related drop in blood pressure. Aggressive volume resuscitation may be required in the volume-depleted, hypotensive, iron-toxic patient who is in need of deferoxamine. **Hypotension is not a contraindication to IV deferoxamine administration.**

The infusion rate of deferoxamine IV can be increased up to 15 milligrams/kg per hour as tolerated. The recommended amount of deferoxamine for an acute iron overdose is a total of 360 milligrams/kg or 6 grams in an adult during the first 24 hours, typically ordered as 500-milligram infusions over 4 to 8 hours after the initial 1000-milligram dose.[18,25] Amounts larger than this are associated with complications, including mucormycosis, renal insufficiency or failure,[26] pulmonary toxicity,[27] and sepsis from *Yersinia enterocolitica*, which may be related to duration of therapy.

As ferrioxamine is excreted, the urine color changes to what is classically called "vin rosé" but is more typically a brown or rusty hue.[28] Theoretically, the disappearance of the "vin rosé" color means that the patient no longer has significant toxicity because there is no more free iron available to be complexed with deferoxamine and excreted. False-negative results, color-change latency, and difficulty in visualizing a color change can limit the utility of this test.[18]

There is uncertainty regarding the duration of deferoxamine therapy.[2,18,25] Recommended endpoints include clinical recovery and normal iron levels, measurement of normal iron-to-creatinine ratios, and clinical recovery with normal iron level in conjunction with normal urine color. **Clinical**

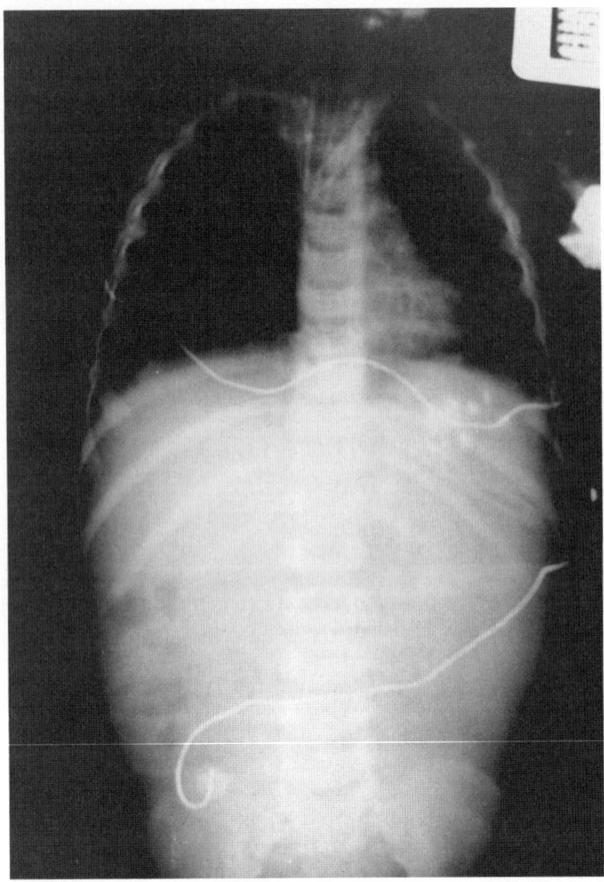

FIGURE 198-2. A 17-month-old boy came to the hospital with lethargy and hematemesis following a large ingestion of iron supplement pills. [Reproduced with permission from Nelson LS, Lewin NA, Howland MA, Hoffman RS, Goldfrank LR, Flomenbaum NE: *Goldfrank's Toxicologic Emergencies*, 9th ed. © 2011 by McGraw-Hill, Inc., New York.]

recovery of the patient is probably the most important factor guiding the decision to terminate therapy because measured iron levels are artificially depressed by the presence of deferoxamine and urine color change can be unreliable. Continue deferoxamine therapy in patients who continue to exhibit severe iron toxicity after 24 hours of treatment, using a decreased rate to avoid the associated risks mentioned earlier.

OTHER THERAPIES

Oral iron chelators—**deferiprone** and **deferasirox**—reduce iron absorption when administered simultaneously or within 1 hour of iron ingestion.[29] However, there is no evidence of benefit in human overdoses, and oral chelation therapy would theoretically be of use only when taken promptly after the iron ingestion; thus their use is limited by the time to presentation for treatment and the significant vomiting expected with clinical iron toxicity. **Oral iron chelating agents should NOT replace intravenous deferoxamine when chelation is indicated in clinical iron toxicity.**

Although hemodialysis and hemofiltration do not remove iron, such treatment may be necessary to remove the deferoxamine–iron complex in patients with renal failure who are unable to excrete the complex in their urine.[18,30,31] Severe iron poisoning can be treated with exchange transfusion in addition to deferoxamine therapy.[32]

DISPOSITION AND FOLLOW-UP

Patients who have not ingested a potentially toxic amount of iron, who remain asymptomatic (other than vomiting once or twice from the gastric irritant effects of iron), and who have normal findings on physical examination for a period of 6 hours can be safely discharged or transferred for appropriate mental health evaluation. Patients who receive deferoxamine therapy should be admitted to the intensive care unit. The regional poison control center should be contacted for both data collection purposes and assistance with management.

REFERENCES

The complete reference list is available online at www.TintinalliEM.com.

CHAPTER 199

Hydrocarbons and Volatile Substances

C. William Heise
Frank LoVecchio

INTRODUCTION

Hydrocarbons are a diverse group of organic compounds consisting primarily of carbon and hydrogen atoms. The two basic forms of hydrocarbons are aliphatic (straight- or branched-chain carbon arrangement) or aromatic (carbon arranged in a ring). Hydrocarbons are in many household and occupational products (**Table 199-1**). While all hydrocarbons can be toxic, aromatic and halogenated hydrocarbons are

TABLE 199-1 Common Products That Contain Hydrocarbons

Hydrocarbon (state at room temperature)	Commercial Use
Aliphatic – linear structure, toxicity varies depending on volatility	
Gasoline (petrol) – liquid	Motor fuel
Kerosene (paraffin) – liquid	Stove and lamp fuel
Mineral seal oil – liquid	Furniture polish
Petroleum ether – liquid	Industrial solvent
Diesel fuel – liquid	Motor fuel
n-Hexane – liquid	Plastic cement, rubber cement
Methane, butane, propane, and ethane – gas	Fuel
Mineral spirits (white spirits) – liquid	Solvent, paint thinner
Turpentine – liquid	Solvent, paint thinner
Mineral oil (liquid paraffin) – liquid	Lubricant, laxative
Paraffin wax – solid	Industrial uses, candles
Petroleum jelly (petrolatum or soft paraffin) – solid	Skin lotion
Aromatic – ring structure, high toxicity	
Benzene – liquid	Chemical intermediate, gasoline (small amount, 0.8% on average)
Toluene – liquid	Airplane glue, plastic cement, acrylic paint
Xylene – liquid	Solvent, cleaning agent, degreaser
Halogenated – high toxicity	
Carbon tetrachloride – liquid	Solvent, refrigerant, aerosol propellant
Chloroform – liquid	Solvent, chemical intermediate
Methylene chloride – liquid	Paint stripper, varnish remover, aerosol paint, degreaser
Trichloroethylene – liquid	Spot remover, degreaser, typewriter correction fluid
Trichloroethane – liquid	Spot remover, degreaser, typewriter correction fluid
Tetrachloroethylene (perchloroethylene) – liquid	Dry cleaning agent, degreaser

TABLE 199-2 Commonly Abused Volatile Substances

Product	Volatile Agent
Acrylic spray paint	Toluene
Adhesives, glue	Toluene, trichloroethylene
Aerosol propellants	Propellants and butane
Cigarette lighter refills	Butane
Degreasing agents	Trichloroethylene
Dry cleaning agents	Tetrachloroethylene
Fire extinguishers	Bromochlorodifluoromethane
Inhalational anesthetics	Nitrous oxide, halothane
Lighter fluid	Naphtha
Motor fuel	Gasoline (petrol)
Nitrites ("poppers")	Isobutyl nitrite, amyl nitrite
Paint stripper	Methylene chloride
Plastic modeling cement	Methyl ethyl ketone, toluene
Spot removers	Trichloroethylene, trichloroethane
Typewriter correction fluid	Trichloroethane, trichloroethylene

associated with the most severe systemic toxicity. Volatile agents are associated with the highest aspiration risk. Identification of the specific hydrocarbon or class can help anticipate specific potential toxicity and guide management.

Chain length and branching determine the phase of the hydrocarbon at room temperature. Short-chain aliphatic compounds (up to 4 carbons), such as methane, ethane, propane, and butane, are gases; intermediate-chain aliphatic compounds (5 to 19 carbons), such as solvents, lamp oil, lighter fluid, and gasoline, are liquid; and long-chain aliphatic compounds (>19 carbons), such as waxes, are solids. Liquid hydrocarbons account for most exposures seen in the ED.[1]

Most hydrocarbon exposures occur as liquid ingestions or inhalations and usually have a benign clinical course.[1,2] Serious toxicity and deaths associated with hydrocarbon exposure are usually due to ingestions rather than inhalation. Symptoms and signs of pulmonary injury develop in up to 50% of the children who ingest hydrocarbons,[3,4] and hydrocarbon aspiration can produce acute respiratory distress syndrome.[5] Suicidal injection of gasoline or kerosene with severe multi-organ toxicity has been reported.[6,7]

Volatile substances, usually hydrocarbon solvents contained in household or commercial products, can be inhaled for their euphoric effects (**Table 199-2**).[8] Abusers are typically teenagers and younger adults, especially those in lower socioeconomic groups.[9] Inhalation occurs by three different methods: (1) in "huffing," the individual soaks a rag with the inhalant and then places it over the mouth and nose; (2) in "bagging," the individual puts the hydrocarbon in a bag (usually a plastic bag) and repeatedly inhales deeply from the bag; and (3) in "sniffing," the hydrocarbon is directly inhaled via the nostrils.[10] In addition to causing deaths, abuse of volatile agents is associated with crimes such as homicide, sexual assault, and child abuse.[11] The most commonly abused volatile hydrocarbons are paints, solvents, and gasoline.

PATHOPHYSIOLOGY

The toxic potential of hydrocarbons depends on their physical characteristics (viscosity, surface tension, and volatility), chemical characteristics (aliphatic, aromatic, or halogenated), presence of toxic additives (pesticides or heavy metals), routes of exposure, concentration, and dose. The physical characteristics contribute the most to aspiration risk.

Viscosity refers to the general "thickness" of a liquid; fluids with a lower viscosity flow more easily than ones with high viscosity. Viscosity is measured in Saybolt universal seconds (SUS); fluids such as gasoline, kerosene, mineral seal oil, and turpentine have low viscosity (<60 SUS), whereas diesel fuel, grease, mineral oil, paraffin wax, and petroleum jelly have high viscosity (>100 SUS).[12] Surface tension refers to the property where liquid molecules tend to cohere to each other. Liquids with high surface tension in contact with a solid surface tend to ball up, creating the smallest surface area rather than spreading out. Volatility refers to the ability of the liquid or solid to vaporize and is inversely related to the boiling point; highly volatile liquids have a low boiling point. **Ingestion of liquids with low viscosity and surface tension and high volatility increases the risk for aspiration because these substance can flow easily, spreading out widely on the oral mucosa, and vaporize at body temperature. Inhalation of aromatic hydrocarbons or halogenated hydrocarbons can result in systemic absorption and the potential for significant toxicity.**

CLINICAL FEATURES

Ingestion or aspiration of hydrocarbons mainly impairs the pulmonary system, but depending on the specific compound, the central nervous, peripheral nervous, GI, cardiovascular, renal, hepatic, dermal, and/or hematologic systems may be affected (**Table 199-3**).[13]

PULMONARY TOXICITY

Hydrocarbon aspiration causes chemical pneumonitis by direct toxicity to the pulmonary parenchyma and alteration of surfactant function. Destruction of alveolar and capillary membranes results in increased vascular permeability and edema. The clinical manifestations of pulmonary aspiration are usually apparent soon after exposure from irritation of the oral mucosa and tracheobronchial tree. Symptoms include coughing, choking, gasping, dyspnea, and burning of the mouth. Patients with these symptoms should be assumed to have aspirated.

Signs include tachypnea, grunting respirations, wheezing, or retractions depending on the severity of aspiration. An odor of the hydrocarbon may be noted on the patient's breath. Hyperthermia of ≥39°C (≥102.2°F) is likely and may occur initially or 6 to 8 hours after exposure. The fever is usually an inflammatory response due to pneumonitis. Necrotizing pneumonitis and hemorrhagic pulmonary edema may develop within minutes to hours in patients with severe aspiration. In most fatalities, these complications occur rapidly. With less severe damage, symptoms usually subside within 2 to 5 days, except in the case of pneumatoceles and lipoid pneumonias, the symptoms of which may persist for weeks to months.

Although in most patients with clinically significant aspiration chest radiographic results eventually are abnormal, the time course of radiographic changes varies, and correlation with physical examination findings may be poor. Changes may be seen as early as 30 minutes after aspiration, but **the initial radiograph in a symptomatic patient may be deceptively clear. Conversely, an asymptomatic patient can still have abnormal chest radiographic findings later during the clinical course.**

TABLE 199-3 Clinical Manifestations of Hydrocarbon Exposure

System	Clinical Manifestations
Pulmonary	Tachypnea, grunting respirations, wheezing, retractions
Cardiac	Ventricular dysrhythmias (may occur after exposure to halogenated hydrocarbons and aromatic hydrocarbons)
Central nervous	Slurred speech, ataxia, lethargy, coma
Peripheral nervous	Numbness and paresthesias in the extremities
GI and hepatic	Nausea, vomiting, abdominal pain, loss of appetite (mostly with halogenated hydrocarbons)
Renal and metabolic	Muscle weakness or paralysis secondary to hypokalemia in patients who abuse toluene
Hematologic	Lethargy (anemia), shortness of breath (anemia), neurologic depression/syncope (carbon monoxide from methylene chloride), cyanosis (methemoglobinemia from amine-containing hydrocarbons)
Dermal	Local erythema, papules, vesicles, generalized scarlatiniform eruption, exfoliative dermatitis, "huffer's rash," cellulitis

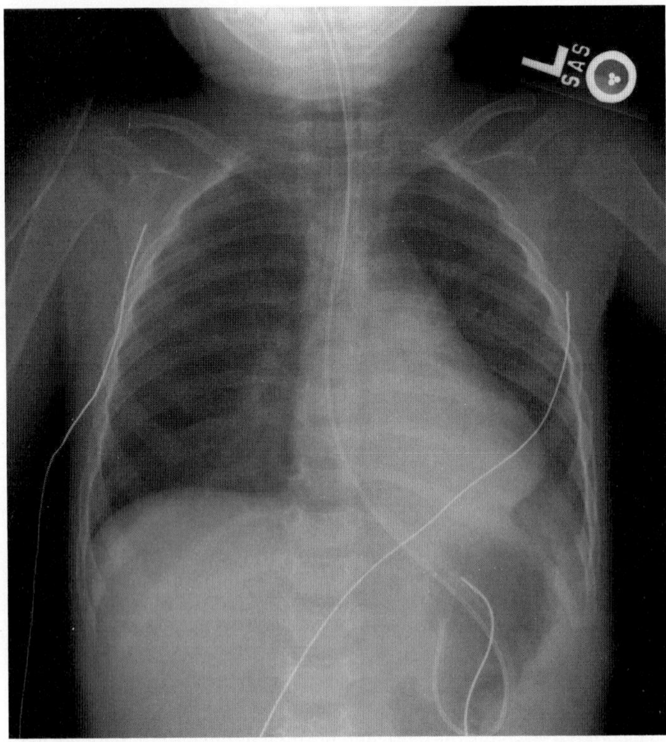
A

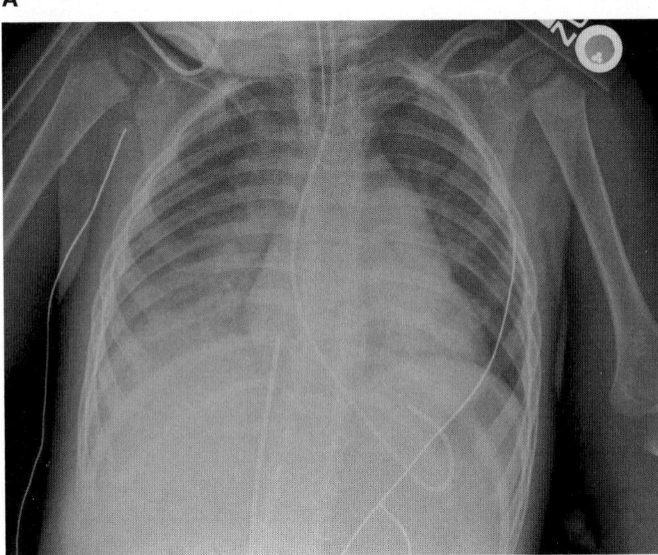
B

FIGURE 199-1. Two chest radiographs of a child who aspirated lamp oil and developed aspiration pneumonitis. **A.** Day 1: intubated, left lower lobe infiltrates. **B.** Day 3: intubated, worsening perihilar and bibasilar patchy infiltrates and new right small pleural effusion.

Radiographic changes usually appear by 2 to 6 hours and are almost always present by 24 hours, if they are to occur (**Figure 199-1**). The most common radiologic finding is bilateral infiltrates at the bases with multilobar involvement more common than single-lobe involvement and right-sided involvement more common than left-sided involvement.[14-16] Hydrocarbon-induced aspiration pneumonitis can lead to lung necrosis and the creation of a pneumatocele.[17]

CARDIAC TOXICITY

Life-threatening dysrhythmias, such as ventricular tachycardia and ventricular fibrillation, may occur with systemic absorption. Dysrhythmias occur most commonly after exposure to halogenated hydrocarbons and aromatic hydrocarbons. Exposure to short-chain aliphatic hydrocarbons occasionally causes dysrhythmias (ventricular fibrillation).[10] The most worrisome acute complication found in solvent abusers is "**sudden sniffing death syndrome**" and occurs within minutes of exposure.[8] The mechanism of toxicity is believed to be catecholamine sensitization of the heart by hydrocarbons (especially halogenated hydrocarbons), resulting in ventricular dysrhythmias.[8,10,18] Other mechanisms for sudden death include simple asphyxia, respiratory depression, and vagal inhibition. Ventricular akinesia and polymorphic ventricular dysrhythmias have also been described after overdose of chloral hydrate (a halogenated aliphatic hydrocarbon).[18]

CNS TOXICITY

CNS effects, primarily depression of consciousness, result from: (1) a direct toxic response to the systemic absorption of the hydrocarbon, (2) an indirect result of severe hypoxia secondary to aspiration, (3) simple asphyxiation due to the displacement of oxygen by the volatile hydrocarbon, and/or (4) volatile substance abuse with a plastic bag that prevents adequate oxygenation. Systemic effects occur through GI absorption, the inhalation of highly volatile petroleum distillates, or direct dermal penetration.

Signs of neurologic toxicity include slurred speech, ataxia, lethargy, and coma.[13] Although hydrocarbons are central neurologic depressants, they often have an initial excitatory effect manifested as hallucinations, tremor, agitation, and convulsions. Individuals who abuse volatile solvents or workers who experience long-term hydrocarbon exposure may present to the ED complaining of recurrent headaches, ataxia, emotional lability, cognitive impairment, or psychomotor impairment.

PERIPHERAL NERVOUS SYSTEM TOXICITY

Exposure to *n*-hexane, methyl *n*-butyl ketone, and other six-carbon aliphatic hydrocarbons is associated with the development of a characteristic peripheral polyneuropathy caused by demyelinization and retrograde axonal degeneration.[19] Onset of symptoms may be delayed for weeks, and toxicity is attributed to a metabolite, 2,5-hexanedione, produced by the cytochrome P-450–mediated biotransformation of the parent compounds. This neurotoxic metabolite is thought to inhibit glutaraldehyde-3-phosphate dehydrogenase, which supplies energy for axonal transport.

Clinically, the patient may complain of chronic numbness and paresthesias in the extremities. The key component in making the diagnosis is a history of exposure to solvents, usually through occupations and hobbies. The compound *n*-hexane is found in solvents used in the printing, shoemaking, textile, and furniture industries, as well as in gasoline, quick-drying glues, and rubber cement.[20]

GI AND HEPATIC TOXICITIES

Most hydrocarbons are GI irritants. Vomiting, which occurs in many patients with aliphatic hydrocarbon ingestions, increases the risk of pulmonary aspiration. Gastric perforation has been reported after accidental ingestion of chlorofluorocarbons.[21]

Hepatic damage resulting from ingestion of halogenated hydrocarbons is well described.[22,23] **Chlorinated hydrocarbons, such as carbon tetrachloride, methylene chloride, trichloroethylene, and tetrachloroethylene, are especially hepatotoxic.** For example, carbon tetrachloride causes centrilobular liver necrosis similar to acetaminophen toxicity. Free radical metabolites of these agents that cause lipid peroxidation are apparently responsible for hepatocellular destruction. The time course of hepatic dysfunction with acute exposures appears similar to that of acetaminophen hepatotoxicity—within 24 to 48 hours after ingestion.

Clinically, patients may come to the ED complaining of nausea, vomiting, abdominal pain, or loss of appetite. Depending on the severity, the physical examination may reveal a patient with jaundice, lethargy, and/or abdominal tenderness, especially in the right upper quadrant. Results of serum transaminase tests and other hepatic synthetic function tests may be abnormal within 24 hours after ingestion.

RENAL AND METABOLIC TOXICITIES

Solvent abuse and occupational exposure to hydrocarbons may result in renal dysfunction. **Chlorinated hydrocarbons, such as chloroform,**

carbon tetrachloride, and trichloroethylene, are also nephrotoxic. Toluene, an aromatic hydrocarbon that is commonly abused, may cause renal tubular acidosis in patients who inhale toluene-containing substances.[8,24] The mechanism of toluene-induced renal tubular acidosis is not clear. The typical metabolic profile of renal tubular acidosis is a normal anion gap hyperchloremic acidosis with hypokalemia and a urine pH of >5.5. The metabolites of toluene (hippuric acid and benzoic acid) can be the cause of an elevated anion gap metabolic acidosis.[25]

Clinically, habitual toluene abusers may complain of muscle weakness caused by hypokalemia.[26] The serum potassium level may be so low (<2 mEq/L) that severe weakness develops, occasionally resulting in muscle paralysis. Significant rhabdomyolysis may also result.[27] **Toluene abuse should be considered in individuals (especially young patients) who come to the ED with symptoms similar to hypokalemic periodic paralysis.**[24,26]

HEMATOLOGIC TOXICITY

Hydrocarbon-induced hemolysis rarely occurs after the acute ingestion of gasoline, kerosene, and tetrachloroethylene, and after inhalation of mineral spirits. Exposure to benzene (an aromatic hydrocarbon) is associated with an increased incidence of hematologic disorders, including aplastic anemia, acute myelogenous leukemia, and multiple myeloma.[28] Naphthalene exposure is associated with hemolytic anemia. Delayed methemoglobinemia is associated with occupational exposure to hydrocarbons containing amine functional groups such as aniline (see chapter 207, "Dyshemoglobinemias").[29] Delayed carboxyhemoglobinemia is associated with **methylene chloride** exposure due to its metabolism to carbon monoxide, which takes a few hours.[30] This is unlike ordinary carbon monoxide exposure from exogenous sources in which the maximum carboxyhemoglobin level occurs at the time of the exposure. **Clinically, patients may come to the ED with malaise, headache, dyspnea, or cyanosis depending on the exposure and the severity of the toxicity.**

DERMAL TOXICITY

Dermal toxicity from exposure to hydrocarbons is most often associated with the short-chain aliphatic, aromatic, and halogenated hydrocarbons. These agents act as primary irritants and as sensitizers. Occasionally, highly permeable hydrocarbons can penetrate the skin, resulting in systemic toxicity. Skin findings can range from local erythema, papules, and vesicles to a generalized scarlatiniform eruption and an exfoliative dermatitis (Table 199-3). A "huffer's rash" may be noted over the face of patients who habitually abuse the volatile hydrocarbons.[8] Frostbite of the face may develop during the inhalational abuse of fluorinated agents. A defatting dermatitis, similar to chronic eczematoid dermatitis, may occur.

Cellulitis and sterile abscesses have been associated with the injection of hydrocarbons, and even a small amount of injected hydrocarbon can cause significant injury.[31] Hydrocarbon-induced soft tissue necrosis has recently been seen in patients using "**krokodil**," desomorphine synthesized from codeine with the use of hydrocarbon solvents.[32] Dermal exposure to heated high-viscosity, long-chain aliphatics, such as tar, asphalt, or bitumen, presents a particularly challenging problem because of their association with thermal burns, hyperthermia, and difficulty with decontamination.[33] Tar burns are discussed in the chapter 217, "Chemical Burns."

DIAGNOSIS

Diagnosis of hydrocarbon toxicity incorporates the findings of the history, physical examination, bedside cardiac and pulmonary monitoring, laboratory tests, and chest radiography. Determine the specific hydrocarbon-containing product, because identification can help anticipate specific potential toxicity and guide management. Pulse oximetry is useful to evaluate oxygenation status, and arterial blood gas analysis can be used to assess ventilation and acid-base status. Cardiac rhythm monitoring and an ECG are indicated in symptomatic patients and patients who ingest halogenated hydrocarbons. A chest radiograph is indicated in a symptomatic patient after hydrocarbon aspiration.

There are no specific quantitative hydrocarbon tests in standard use when evaluating suspected hydrocarbon intoxication. A basic metabolic panel is indicated in patients with a history of toluene abuse or in whom electrolyte abnormalities and renal insufficiency are suspected. Obtain hepatic function studies, serum ammonia, and prothrombin time in patients who ingest or inhale halogenated hydrocarbons. A CBC is indicated if anemia, bleeding disorder, hemolysis, or leukemia is considered. Measure carboxyhemoglobin level in patients with exposure to methylene chloride; repeat measurements may be necessary. Determination of methemoglobin level is indicated in patients with exposure to hydrocarbons containing amine functional groups. Abdominal radiographs may show evidence of ingestion of chlorinated hydrocarbons such as carbon tetrachloride or chloroform because of the radiopaque nature of polyhalogenated substances.[22]

An outpatient nerve conduction study and electromyography can be considered in patients who present with chronic numbness and paresthesias in the extremities and who have a history of *n*-hexane exposure.

TREATMENT

Securing the airway and maintaining ventilation are the critical maneuvers in patients who present with respiratory depression and/or significant neurologic depression (**Table 199-4**). Swelling of the lips and tongue due to irritant effect or freeze injuries can complicate airway management. Administer oxygen to correct hypoxia. Inhaled β_2-agonists may also be useful, especially in the setting of bronchospasm, but their role in the treatment of hydrocarbon pneumonitis has not been studied. Positive end-expiratory pressure or continuous positive-pressure airway ventilation may sometimes be required to maintain oxygenation, but may increase the potential for further injury from barotrauma, such as the development of pneumatoceles or pneumothorax. In cases of severe pulmonary aspiration resulting in refractory hypoxemia, treatment

TABLE 199-4 Management of Hydrocarbon Exposures

Airway and breathing	Secure airway. Antidotes: Administer oxygen for carboxyhemoglobinemia and methylene blue for methemoglobinemia. Provide supplemental oxygen. Administer inhaled β_2-agonists. Ventilatory support: Provide positive end-expiratory pressure or continuous positive airway pressure as needed to achieve adequate oxygenation.
Cardiac	Circulation: Administer IV crystalloid fluid for initial volume resuscitation of hypotensive patients. Do not use catecholamines in cases of halogenated hydrocarbon exposure. Consider propranolol, esmolol, or lidocaine for ventricular dysrhythmias induced by halogenated hydrocarbon exposure. Consult the poison control center, toxicologist, and other appropriate specialists as needed.
Decontamination	Dermal: Remove hydrocarbon-soaked clothes, decontaminate skin with soap and water, and decontaminate eyes with saline irrigation. GI: Not indicated. See discussion below.
Other	Laboratory tests: Order CBC, basic metabolic panel, liver function tests (serum transaminase, bilirubin, albumin levels), prothrombin time, partial thromboplastin time, carboxyhemoglobin level, methemoglobin level, and/or radiologic studies as indicated (see text). Correct electrolyte abnormalities. Do not give steroids Administer blood products as needed.

with high-frequency jet ventilation or extracorporeal membrane oxygenation has proved successful according to case reports.[34,35] Surfactant therapy has been used to treat acute lung injury from hydrocarbon aspiration.[36-38]

Treat hypotension with aggressive fluid resuscitation. **Avoid administration of catecholamines such as dopamine, norepinephrine, and epinephrine. Catecholamines may cause dysrhythmias, especially after exposure to halogenated hydrocarbons and aromatic hydrocarbons.** Hydrocarbon-induced dysrhythmias are generally seen shortly after the exposure, especially with inhalational use. Continuous cardiac monitoring should be initiated, and an ECG should be obtained. For hydrocarbon-induced ventricular dysrhythmias, class IA (procainamide) or class III (amiodarone, bretylium, and sotalol) antiarrhythmics should be avoided because of the risk of QT-interval prolongation.[18] Propranolol, esmolol, and lidocaine have been reported to treat these ventricular dysrhythmias successfully.[10,18,39]

There is no benefit to gastric lavage because risks of aspiration far outweigh any theoretical benefits.[40] Activated charcoal does not adsorb hydrocarbons well and poses a risk for vomiting and aspiration, so charcoal is not recommended either. In the rare case where the hydrocarbon was combined with a highly toxic substance, such as a pesticide, or is highly toxic itself, such as an aromatic or halogenated chemical, and ingestion has occurred in the last hour or less, consult with the poison center first, as even in that situation, benefit from gastric lavage is unproven.

There is no clear evidence that corticosteroids are helpful in hydrocarbon-induced pneumonitis.[13] One meta-analysis advocating low-dose steroids for acute lung injury and respiratory distress[41] has been criticized because the patients were not generally treated with current lung-protective ventilation strategies.[42] Antibiotics are not indicated unless there is clinical suspicion of superimposed bacterial pneumonitis.

In dermal exposures, decontamination is preferably done at the scene or before entering the ED to avoid spreading fumes to patient treatment areas. The patient needs to be fully undressed to prevent ongoing contamination from hydrocarbon-soaked clothes. Make sure staff wear protective gloves and aprons to prevent secondary exposure, especially to organophosphate-containing mixtures. Dermal decontamination with soap and cold water, and eye decontamination with saline irrigation should be performed.

DISPOSITION AND FOLLOW-UP

Consult a medical toxicologist or regional poison control center for all symptomatic or asymptomatic exposures to aromatic hydrocarbons or hydrocarbons with toxic additives. In cases of inhalation or aspiration of **nonhalogenated aliphatic hydrocarbons**, asymptomatic patients may be discharged home after about 6 to 8 hours of observation with instructions to return if delayed symptoms develop.

Further observation or hospitalization is required for patients who are symptomatic after hydrocarbon exposure. For pediatric hydrocarbon ingestions, the presence of wheezing, altered consciousness, or tachypnea within 2 hours predicts the need for further treatment.[43] Hospitalization is also recommended for those who ingest hydrocarbons capable of producing delayed complications (e.g., halogenated hydrocarbons causing hepatic toxicity) or hydrocarbons with toxic additives (organophosphates and organic metal compounds). Patients with suicidal intent or with complications of solvent abuse need behavioral health evaluation.

REFERENCES

The complete reference list is available online at www.TintinalliEM.com.

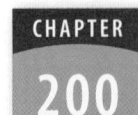

Caustic Ingestions

Nicole C. Bouchard
Wallace A. Carter

INTRODUCTION AND EPIDEMIOLOGY

Caustics are substances that cause both functional and histologic damage on contact with body surfaces. Many household and industrial chemicals have caustic potential. Caustics are broadly classified as alkalis (pH >7) or acids (pH <7). In developed nations, increased education and product regulation (especially of acids) have decreased morbidity and mortality from caustic exposures in both adults and children. However, in underdeveloped parts of the world, exposure to caustics remains a significant problem.[1-4] The challenges to exposure prevention and patient care include relative lack of childproof containers, easy and unregulated access to highly corrosive substances, cultural-specific propensities to ingest caustics in suicide attempts, sheer high volume of cases, delays to care in rural settings, malnutrition, financial resources of hospitals and families to provide the services needed, and poor follow-up.[4] Alkaline ingestions predominate in the developed world,[5] whereas acid ingestions are more common in developing countries.[6]

Caustic exposures tend to fall into three distinct groups: (1) intentional teen or adult ingestions with suicidal ideation[7]; (2) unintentional ingestions (the majority of which are by curious children in the toddler age group)[8]; and (3) other incidental, often occupational or industrial contact exposures. The majority of reported exposures are unintentional or accidental, but although less frequent, intentional ingestions account for the majority of serious injuries.[1] The geographic variation in caustic ingestion circumstances, such as involved substances, intention, age of the patient, and extent of evaluation, make it difficult to create encompassing recommendations or a consensus approach.[4,9,10]

Many chemicals used in industry have caustic potential (**Table 200-1**). Household caustics are often less concentrated forms of industrial strength cleansers.

TABLE 200-1 Common Caustic Compounds

Alkali	Found in
Sodium hydroxide	Industrial chemicals, drain openers, oven cleaners
Potassium hydroxide	Drain openers, batteries
Calcium hydroxide	Cement, hair relaxers, and perm products
Ammonium hydroxide	Hair relaxers and perm products, dermal peeling/exfoliation, toilet bowl cleaners, glass cleaners, fertilizers
Lithium hydroxide	Photographic developer, batteries
Sodium tripolyphosphate	Detergents
Sodium hypochlorite	Bleach
Acids	
Sulfuric acid	Automobile batteries, drain openers, explosives, fertilizer
Acetic acid	Printing and photography, disinfectants, hair perm neutralizer
Hydrochloric acid	Cleaning agents, metal cleaning, chemical production, swimming pool products
Hydrofluoric acids	Rust remover, petroleum industry, glass and microchip etching, jewelry cleaners
Formic acid	Model glue, leather and textile manufacturing, tissue preservation
Chromic acid	Metal plating, photography
Nitric acid	Fertilizer, engraving, electroplating
Phosphoric acid	Rust proofing, metal cleaners, disinfectants

PATHOPHYSIOLOGY

The degree to which a caustic substance produces tissue injury is determined by a number of factors: pH, concentration, duration of contact, volume present, and titratable acid or alkaline reserve. Acids tend to cause significant injuries at a pH <3 and alkalis at a pH >11. The physical properties of the product formulation (i.e., liquid, gel, granular, or solid) can influence the nature of the contact with the tissue. Following ingestion, solid or granular caustics often injure the oropharynx and proximal esophagus, whereas liquid alkali ingestions are characterized by more extensive esophageal and gastric injuries. *Titratable acid or alkaline reserve* refers to the amount of acid or base required to neutralize the agent; the greater this value, the greater is the potential for tissue injury.

Esophageal mucosal burns from caustic ingestions are classified by a visual endoscopic grading system: **grade 1 burns** involve tissue edema and hyperemia; **grade 2 burns** include ulcerations, blisters, and whitish exudates, which are subdivided into grade 2A (noncircumferential) and 2B (deeper or circumferential) lesions; and **grade 3 burns** are defined by deep ulcerations and necrotic lesions. Following the initial mucosal injury, tissue remodeling occurs over roughly 2 months. In mild cases, normal esophageal function is restored, but in severe cases, dense scar tissue forms, resulting in stricture formation. Esophageal strictures are a source of significant morbidity and may require long-term treatments with dilations, stenting, or surgery. Early phases of remodeling, particularly days 2 to 14, are associated with increased tissue friability and higher risk of perforation, both spontaneous and iatrogenic.

ALKALI INJURIES

Following caustic alkali exposures, the hydroxide ion easily penetrates tissues, causing immediate cellular destruction via protein denaturation and lipid saponification. This is followed by thrombosis of local microvasculature that leads to further tissue necrosis. Alkali injuries induce a deep tissue injury called **liquefaction necrosis**. Severe intentional alkali ingestion may cause deep penetration into surrounding tissues with resultant multisystem organ injuries, including esophageal injury, gastric perforation, and necrosis of abdominal and mediastinal structures. Severe injuries to the pancreas, gallbladder, small intestine, and mediastinum after intentional ingestion have been reported. Solid alkali ingestions, such as some lye preparations, have a greater potential for oropharyngeal and proximal esophageal tract injury and less for distal injury.

The most common household alkali is **bleach**, a 3% to 6% sodium hypochlorite solution with a pH of approximately 11. Household liquid bleach is minimally corrosive to the esophagus and rarely causes significant injury beyond grade 1 esophageal burns. Esophageal stricture was not observed as a complication of household bleach ingestion in a series involving almost 400 patients.[11] However, ingestion of industrial strength bleach containing much higher concentrations of sodium hypochlorite may result in gastric and esophageal necrosis. Bleach ingestion may cause emesis secondary to gastric irritation and/or pneumonitis after aspiration. Pulmonary irritation related to chlorine gas production in the stomach or when mixed with other substances may also occur.[12,13] A common reaction is the production of the highly irritating **chloramine gas** when bleach and ammonia household cleaners are combined.[14]

ACIDS

Injuries by strong acids produce **coagulation necrosis**. Dissociated hydrogen ions and their associated anions penetrate tissues, leading to cell death and eschar formation. This process is believed to limit continued hydrogen ion penetration and protect against deeper injury. When ingested acids settle in the stomach, gastric necrosis, perforation, and hemorrhage may result. Although it was previously thought that acids were esophagus-sparing with most tissue injury concentrated in the stomach, endoscopy following an acid ingestion finds a similar incidence of gastric and esophageal injury.[15-17] Despite relatively less tissue destruction, strong acid ingestion results in high-grade gastric injuries (secondary to pylorospasm and pooling) and a higher mortality rate compared with strong alkali ingestions. Acid ingestion is sometimes complicated by systemic absorption of acid with associated metabolic acidosis, hemolysis, and renal failure.[18]

Hydrofluoric acid is a unique ingestion discussed in chapter 217, Chemical Burns (see Hydrofluoric Acid).

CLINICAL FEATURES

The cardinal features of caustic ingestion are a chemical burn to the oral mucosa,[19] sometimes associated with chemical burns to the skin or eyes from splashes or dribbling (see chapters 217, Chemical Burns and 241, Eye Emergencies). Pharyngeal burns from ingestion produce pain, odynophagia, drooling, and vocal hoarseness. Dyspnea may be caused by edema of the upper airway, aspiration of the caustic substance into the tracheobronchial tree, or inhalation of fumes, particularly acids. Esophageal burns produce dysphagia, odynophagia, and chest pain. Ocular burns are painful, reduce visual acuity, and produce visible damage to the anterior structures of the eye.

HISTORY

The key priority is rapid airway assessment and stabilization. Following that, obtain a directed history to determine the type and amount of caustic ingested and the presence of coingestants. Determine if the ingestion was intentional or unintentional.

PHYSICAL EXAMINATION

Look for signs of respiratory distress or circulatory shock. With ingestions, look for signs of pharyngeal injury (mucosal burns, drooling), respiratory injury (dysphonia, coughing, stridor, wheezing), and gastric injury (vomiting, epigastric tenderness) (**Figure 200-1**).[5,19-24] Streaks of caustic burns on the face or chest are called "dribble burns" (**Figure 200-2**).

DIAGNOSIS

Conflicting data exist on the reliability of presenting signs and symptoms to predict upper GI injuries.[25-29] **Intentional ingestions are associated with higher grades of GI tract injury, with or without clinically obvious signs.**[30] The incidence of serious GI injury after pediatric unintentional ingestions has been the focus of many studies.[5,25-27,29,31,32] Although serious esophageal injury can occur in the absence of oral burns, essentially all children with serious esophageal injuries (grade 2 or 3) after accidental caustic ingestion have some initial sign or symptom, such as stridor, drooling, or vomiting.[26,27,29] Pain alone is an inconsistent predictor of severity of injury, and pain may be absent initially and early in the clinical course.

Assess for hemodynamic instability. Causes of shock include GI bleeding, complications of GI perforation, volume depletion, and toxicity from coingestants. Examine for peritoneal signs due to hollow viscous perforation. Consider mediastinitis in patients complaining of chest discomfort, and palpate the chest wall and neck for signs of subcutaneous emphysema. Inspect the eyes for ocular burns and the skin for splash and dribble burns.

LABORATORY TESTING

For children who accidentally ingest common household alkalis (e.g., bleach) or acids (e.g., toilet bowl cleaner), the need for ancillary testing is only necessary in patients with signs or symptoms of significant injury: drooling, respiratory distress, or vomiting. For an intentional ingestion, or one from a strong acid or alkali, laboratory evaluation should include a venous or arterial blood gas, electrolyte panel, hepatic profile, complete blood count, coagulation profile, lactate, and blood type and screen. Caustic ingestions can cause an **anion gap acidosis** based on lactate production due to direct tissue injury or shock. Strong acid ingestions may be associated with both severe anion gap (e.g., sulfuric acid) and nongap acidoses (e.g., hydrochloric acid). Obtain acetaminophen and salicylate levels to screen for potential coingestants in suicidal patients. An ECG is indicated following a hydrofluoric acid exposure to check for QT-interval prolongation from hypocalcemia.

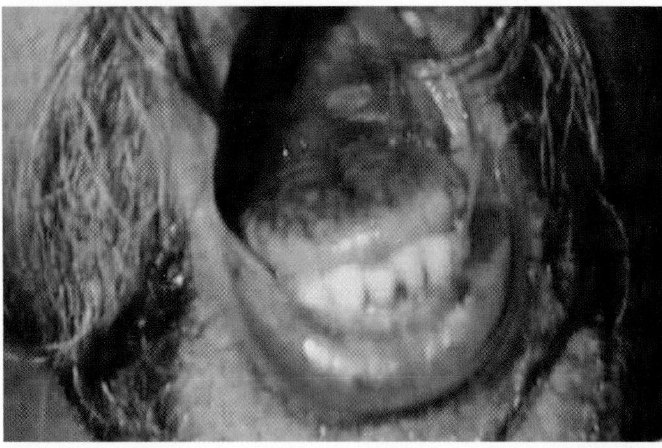

A

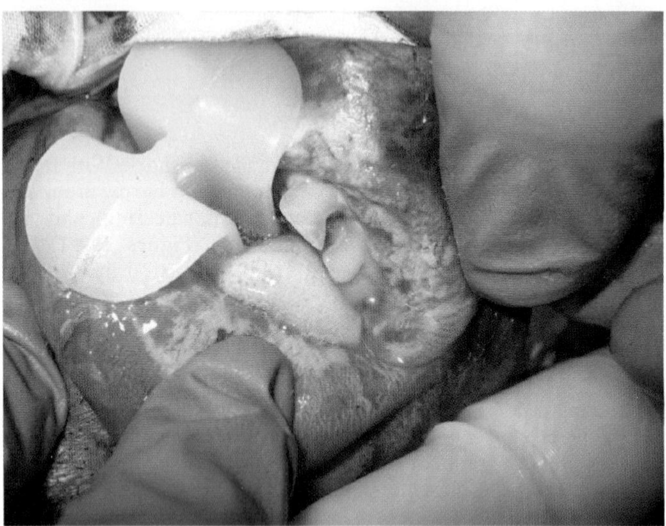

B

FIGURE 200-1. Acid ingestion. **A.** Moderate intraoral burns on buccal mucosa and tongue. **B.** Lingual burns.

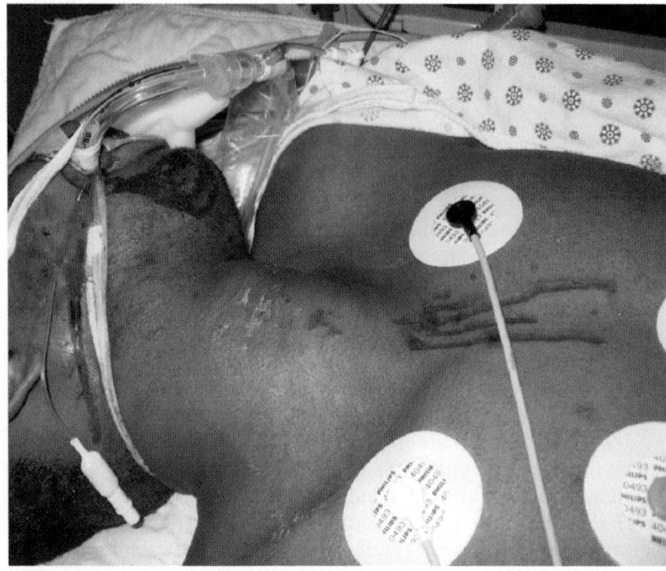

FIGURE 200-2. Acid ingestion. Dermal dribble burns on upper chest.

IMAGING

Obtain a chest radiograph in patients with chest pain, dyspnea, or vomiting to check for peritoneal and mediastinal air. Thoracoabdominal CT scanning is useful to assess for esophageal injury after ingestion of strong caustics or if intra-abdominal perforated viscus is suspected. Endoscopy is the gold standard for identifying the severity of esophageal injury. IV and oral contrast-enhanced CT scanning is an alternative when endoscopy is not readily available or during the postingestion time period when the risk of esophageal perforation by endoscopy is increased (see Endoscopy section).[33] Because oral contrast can interfere with subsequent endoscopic visualization, it is best to discuss the need for oral contrast administration with the endoscopist prior to the CT study. Ultrasound can be used to evaluate and follow-up corrosive gastric injury if there is perforation or severe edema preventing endoscopy.[34]

ENDOSCOPY

Endoscopy is the gold standard for evaluating the location and severity of injury to the esophagus, stomach, and duodenum after caustic ingestion. The controversy has been who needs endoscopy and when should it be done.[28,29,32,35,36] **Patients with intentional caustic ingestions should undergo early endoscopy because ingestions with suicidal intent carry the highest risk of clinically important injury.** In unintentional ingestions, particularly by children, the decision to perform endoscopy is not clear cut.[28,29,32,35,36] Most children with serious caustic esophageal injury will be symptomatic,[32] and although there is a correlation between clinical findings and corrosive severity, lack of symptoms is judged by some authors not to be an adequate predictor of no injury.[8,31,37] **Early endoscopy is recommended after unintentional caustic ingestions in adults and children with signs or symptoms of serious injury such as stridor or significant oropharyngeal burns and/or vomiting, drooling, or food refusal, with or without oropharyngeal burns.**[26,28,29,32,35,36,38]

The general purpose of endoscopy is diagnosis.[39-46] Early endoscopy permits grading of injuries, helps guide treatment, and predicts future morbidity (**Table 200-2**). Early endoscopy is safe and may decrease the time that patients will be without nutritional support. This is particularly important in children with low glycogen stores and in high-grade injuries, where caloric requirements will be high.

Tissue friability after a caustic burn increases significantly at 24 to 48 hours after injury and is maximal between days 5 and 14. **Most experts agree that endoscopy should be performed early after ingestion, ideally <12 hours and not >24 hours after ingestion to avoid iatrogenic perforation.**[36,47] Traditionally, endoscopists have terminated their examination at the first sign of severe esophageal injury (grade 2B or 3). Experienced operators using smaller, flexible endoscopes with minimal insufflation of air can decrease the incidence of perforation, permitting more distal visualization documenting all injuries to the esophagus, stomach, and duodenum.

TREATMENT

AIRWAY

The first priority is airway maintenance. Patients with respiratory distress may have significant oral, pharyngeal, and/or laryngotracheal injuries that require emergent airway management. If emergency airway management precedes patient decontamination, prevent exposure to the ED staff. Caustic airway injuries are difficult airways. Ideally, patients with potential airway injuries should have fiberoptic evaluation of the airway before intubation to determine the extent of the damage, but this may not always be possible. **Blind nasotracheal intubation is contraindicated** due to the potential for exacerbating airway injuries. **Oral intubation with direct visualization is the first choice for definitive airway management.** For potential airway compromise, establish a secure endotracheal airway early rather than risk greater difficulty later when secondary effects of injury, such as edema, complicate the situation.

TABLE 200-2 Correlation of Esophageal Injury Grade with Morbidity and Interventions

Endoscopic Injury Grade	Grade 1 Esophageal Injury	Grade 2A Esophageal Injury	Grade 2B and 3 Esophageal Injuries
Future morbidity	No risk of strictures or carcinoma	Strictures tend not to occur	At risk for hemorrhage and perforation (early), strictures (delayed), and carcinoma (late)
Nutritional support	Diet as tolerated	If unable to tolerate PO, provide nutritional support via nasogastric, orogastric, or percutaneous feeding tube *or* Total parenteral nutrition	Initiate early percutaneous feeding tube *or* Total parenteral nutrition
General interventions	Supportive care	Admission recommended, supportive care	Intensive care unit admission recommended; may require additional imaging or surgical exploration for gastric injuries

Cricothyrotomy may be needed if oropharyngeal edema, tissue friability, and bleeding make intubation difficult or impossible.

Avoid laryngeal mask airways, combination tubes with pharyngeal and tracheal balloons, retrograde intubation, and bougies because these devices/techniques can increase tissue damage or cause perforation.

DECONTAMINATION, NEUTRALIZATION, AND DILUTION

The ED staff should take precautions to prevent ongoing injury to the patient and staff from continued caustic exposure. ED staff involved should wear protective gowns, gloves, and masks with face shields. Standard decontamination, with removal of soiled or soaked clothing and copious irrigation with towels and soap (as needed), is adequate in most cases. Vomiting may re-expose patient and staff to the caustic agent.

Gastric decontamination with activated charcoal is contraindicated if a caustic is the only ingestion. Charcoal does not adhere well to most caustics and will impede visualization when endoscopy is performed. However, activated charcoal may be considered when coingestants pose a risk for severe systemic toxicity.[48] **Ipecac syrup is contraindicated**, because vomiting will result in repeat exposure of the airway and GI mucosa to the caustic agent and could precipitate perforation.[49]

In general, do not insert nasogastric tubes until after endoscopic evaluation. With high-grade esophageal burns, feeding tubes may be inserted under endoscopic guidance if clinically indicated.

Dilution and neutralization therapy are not recommended in the prehospital setting or ED because there is no proven human benefit and potential risk of gastric distension, vomiting, and perforation.[50-53]

FLUID RESUSCITATION

Establish large-bore IV access and resuscitate with crystalloids. Coingestants, bleeding, and third spacing, as well as metabolic disarray from acid-base derangements, can lead to shock. Central venous access may be required for monitoring of resuscitation.

SYSTEMIC STEROIDS AND PROPHYLACTIC ANTIBIOTICS

There is currently no evidence of consistent benefit from systemic steroids, so steroids are not recommended as part of ED treatment.[54-60]

The ability of steroids to inhibit the inflammatory response led to the hypothesis that steroids may decrease stricture formation after caustic ingestion, and animal models have suggested benefit. However, individual human trials and pooled meta-analysis have not shown benefit for injury,[54-60] and steroids may increase the risk of infection, perforation, and hemorrhage.[56]

One criticism of pooled meta-analysis data is that the individual studies did not clearly distinguish between grade 1 and 2A lesions, which do not typically lead to strictures, and grade 2B and 3 injuries, which might theoretically benefit from steroids.[59]

There is no current evidence to support the ED administration of prophylactic antibiotics after caustic ingestions in humans. However, in protocols in which steroids are used or in grade 2B or 3 injury, addition of penicillin or another antibiotic that covers oral flora has been part of treatment regimen.[56,61] Because steroids have largely fallen out of favor, the need for antibiotics in the ED is rare.

SURGERY AND ESOPHAGEAL STENTING AND DILATION

Major ingestions of caustic agents may result in perforation of the GI tract or extensive tissue necrosis requiring emergency surgery.[62-67] Laparotomy is generally preferred over laparoscopic evaluation for posterior gastric visualization. The indications for emergency laparotomy include esophageal perforation, peritoneal signs, or free intraperitoneal air. Large-volume ingestions (>150 mL), signs of shock, respiratory distress, persistent lactic acidosis, ascites, and pleural fluid may be other indications for surgical exploration.[62]

For grade 2B and 3 injuries without obvious perforation, recommendations include a period of esophageal rest,[68] early gastrostomy for enteral feeding,[38,69] and dilation therapy (in the first 3 weeks) with or without stenting.[70-73] Once strictures form, they may be difficult to treat and require stenting and/or multiple balloon dilatations or bouginage.[9] Controversy exists about the most appropriate treatment for esophageal stricture (i.e., long-term repetitive dilation therapy versus surgery).[9,72-74]

TREATMENT OF SYSTEMIC TOXICITY

Morbidity or death from alkali injuries usually results from the complications of direct tissue necrosis, but acid ingestions may result in additional systemic toxicity from absorption of the acid.[18] Acid-base disorders (increased anion gap or normal anion gap acidosis depending on acid ingested), hemolysis, coagulopathy, and renal failure may result. In cases of systemic toxicity, traditional critical-care principles should be applied to optimize the patient's hemodynamics. Acute lung injury (noncardiogenic pulmonary edema) may follow caustic ingestions as a complication of local or systemic effects.

NUTRITIONAL SUPPORT

Nutritional support is often necessary following a severe caustic injury to the esophagus or stomach. Support can be achieved by percutaneous (usually jejunostomy) feeding, nasoenteral feeding, or total parenteral nutrition.[61,75]

EXPERIMENTAL THERAPIES

Animal experiments have found that drugs affecting collagen deposition, including interferon-α-2b, octreotide, β-aminopropionitrile, colchicine, *N*-acetylcysteine, and D-penicillamine,[9,76] can prevent esophageal strictures after caustic alkali ingestion. Pentoxifylline, a local inflammatory and microcirculation mediator, has experimental benefit. Mitomycin C, a fibroblast proliferation inhibitor, has been used topically on strictures with some success.[9] Oral agents to coat and protect the GI tract from insult, including sucralfate, bismuth subsalicylate, and sodium polyacrylate, are beneficial in animal experiments. None of these agents have been evaluated in controlled human clinical trials, and no specific recommendation can be made regarding their use. H_2

blockers and proton pump inhibitors are often used in the treatment protocol,[61] but no evidence supports or refutes their use.

DISEASE COMPLICATIONS

Short-term prognosis is worse with grade 3 GI injury, systemic complications, and age >65 years.[47,77] Most long-term sequelae from caustic exposure are related to injuries to the GI tract. Acid ingestions may scar the pylorus and result in gastric outlet obstruction. Caustic alkali ingestions may result in esophageal strictures, which may result in dysphagia, odynophagia, and malnutrition. Persistent drooling, reluctance to eat, severe oropharyngeal burns, and persistent fever correlate with the development of esophageal stricture after accidental caustic ingestion in children.[78]

Patients with grade 3 caustic injuries to the esophagus have about a 1000-times increased risk for squamous cell cancer of the esophagus that can occur decades after the initial ingestion and resulting esophageal injury.[79] Because cancer can develop if a portion of the esophagus remains after reconstructive surgery for esophageal stricture, total removal of the esophagus is recommended.[80]

DISPOSITION AND FOLLOW-UP

Admit all patients with symptomatic caustic ingestions. Patients with grade 1 injuries can be discharged from hospital after endoscopy, provided they can tolerate oral fluids and food. Grade 2A injuries warrant hospitalization to ensure that symptoms and injury do not progress. Grade 2B and 3 injuries are significant, require enteral or parenteral nutrition, and have an early risk for bleeding or perforation; admit to an intensive care unit.[61] Organ perforation or extensive necrosis is an indication for surgery. Contact the regional poison control center for data collection purposes and assistance with management.

SPECIAL CONSIDERATIONS

LAUNDRY DETERGENT POD INGESTIONS

Laundry detergent pods, also known as capsules, liquitabs, or sachets, have been available in Europe for over a decade and were introduced to the U.S. market in 2010.[81,82] Each pod contains concentrated detergent within a dissolvable plastic membrane. An individual pod may have internal chambers that contain a stain remover and brightener separate from the detergent. Exposure to the concentrated preparation in these pods is more likely to produce symptoms than exposure to traditional laundry detergent products.[83]

Dermal or ocular exposure to the contents can produce irritation of the skin, conjunctiva, or cornea. **Ingestion by young children can produce serious toxicity with profuse vomiting, respiratory distress, and neurologic depression.**[84] The etiology of these systemic symptoms is unknown. Caustic injury to the pharynx and esophagus can produce difficulty swallowing with drooling and aspiration during recovery.[85] Treatment is supportive with airway protection and mechanical ventilation. In severe cases, ventilation may be required for days.

Acknowledgment: The authors wish to thank Dr. G. Richard Bruno for his contributions to this chapter in previous editions.

REFERENCES

The complete reference list is available online at www.TintinalliEM.com.

CHAPTER 201 Pesticides

Guillermo Burillo-Putze
Santiago Nogue Xarau

Pesticides include insecticides, herbicides, and rodenticides.[1] Pesticide toxicity results from intentional, accidental, and occupational exposures. More than 300,000 pesticide-poisoning deaths occur each year worldwide, with insecticides accounting for the majority of deaths.[2] **Pesticides are marketed as multiple formulations, often under shared brand names; therefore, complex clinical syndromes can result from exposure to both active and other ingredients.** Ingredients in proprietary formulations, such as petroleum distillates, are inert to pests during typical exposures, but can be toxic to humans, especially with excessive amounts. Pesticides have class-specific toxicities, with many having both local and systemic effects. Management often includes consultation with a hazardous materials and toxins database or with a poison control center. Supportive care is of utmost importance in pesticide poisonings, but for some compounds, antidotes are essential.

The World Health Organization classifies pesticides according to toxicity based on the median lethal dose for oral and dermal exposure in rats. This classification has been criticized because human case-fatality rates display large variation for compounds within the same chemical and/or World Health Organization toxicity classification.[3] **Toxicity classification should not be used to predict severity after human exposure.**

INSECTICIDES

Chemical insecticides are toxic to the nervous system, with acute and chronic manifestations, as well as delayed sequelae after acute exposure. Six major classes of insecticides are in common use (**Table 201-1**). Other compounds used to control insects include repellants.

ORGANOPHOSPHATES

Commonly used organophosphates include diazinon, acephate, malathion, parathion, and chlorpyrifos and many others in different countries. Organophosphate and carbamate compounds are the insecticides most commonly associated with systemic illness.[4,5] Potency among organophosphates varies; highly potent compounds, such as parathion, are used primarily in agriculture, whereas those of intermediate potency, including coumaphos and trichlorfon, are used in animal care. Diazinon and chlorpyrifos were phased out from household use in the United States in 2000 due to neurotoxicity, particularly on the developing brains of children, but they continue to be used in many other parts of the world.[6] The organophosphate structure can be modified into chemical agents of mass destruction (see chapter 8, Chemical Disasters).

Organophosphate poisoning results primarily from accidental exposure in the home, recently sprayed or fogged areas using pesticide applicators, agriculture, industry, and the transport of these products.[4] Inadvertent exposure can occur from flea-dip products in pet groomers and children and from contaminated food. In addition, these chemicals are involved in intentional poisonings from homicides and suicides.[7] Systemic absorption of organophosphates occurs by inhalation and after mucous membrane, transdermal, transconjunctival, and GI exposure.

Pathophysiology Organophosphate and carbamate compounds inhibit the enzyme cholinesterase.[1] Acetylcholinesterase (true or red

TABLE 201-1 Insecticides and Repellants

Insecticides	Repellants
Organophosphates	Amitraz
Carbamates	*N,N*-diethyl-3-methylbenzamide (DEET)
Organochlorines	
Pyrethrins/pyrethroids	
Neonicotinoids	
Nereistoxin analogs	

blood cell acetylcholinesterase) is found primarily in erythrocyte membranes, nervous tissue, and skeletal muscle. Plasma cholinesterase (pseudocholinesterase or butyrylcholinesterase) is found in the serum, liver, pancreas, heart, and brain. Inhibition of cholinesterase leads to acetylcholine accumulation at nerve synapses and neuromuscular junctions, resulting in overstimulation of acetylcholine receptors. This initial overstimulation is followed by paralysis of cholinergic synaptic transmission in the CNS, in autonomic ganglia, at parasympathetic and some sympathetic nerve endings (e.g., sweat glands), and in somatic nerves. Excess acetylcholine results in a ***cholinergic crisis*** that manifests as a central and peripheral clinical toxidrome.

Organophosphate compounds bind irreversibly to acetylcholinesterase, thus inactivating the enzyme through the process of phosphorylation. *Aging* is a term describing the permanent, irreversible binding of the organophosphorus compound to the cholinesterase. The time to aging is highly variable among different agents and can range from minutes to a day or more. **Once aging occurs, the enzymatic activity of cholinesterase is permanently destroyed,** and new enzyme must be resynthesized over a period of weeks before clinical symptoms resolve and normal enzymatic function returns. **Antidotes must be given before aging occurs to be effective.**

Clinical Features Clinical presentations depend on the specific agent involved, the quantity absorbed, and the route of exposure.[7,8] Organophosphate insecticide poisoning can have substantial variability in clinical course, response to treatment, and outcome.[7] Four clinical syndromes are described following organophosphate exposure: **acute poisoning, intermediate syndrome, chronic toxicity, and organophosphate-induced delayed neuropathy.**[9]

In **acute organophosphate poisoning**, most poisoned patients are symptomatic within the first 8 hours and nearly all within the first 24 hours. Organophosphate agents such as malathion are associated with local irritation of the skin and respiratory tract with resulting dermatitis and wheezing, respectively, without evidence of systemic absorption.

Acute organophosphate poisoning results in CNS, muscarinic, nicotinic, and somatic motor manifestations (**Table 201-2**). In mild to moderate poisoning, symptoms occur in various combinations. Time to symptom onset varies according to exposure route; it is most rapid with inhalation and least rapid with transdermal absorption; however, dermatitis or skin excoriation may hasten this. Symptoms can occur within minutes after massive ingestion that is uniformly fatal.

CNS symptoms of cholinergic excess include anxiety, restlessness, emotional lability, tremor, headache, dizziness, mental confusion, delirium, hallucinations, and seizures. Coma with depression of respiratory and circulatory centers may result. Inhibition of acetylcholinesterase in the parasympathetic system produces muscarinic effects (**Table 201-3**).

Acetylcholine is the presynaptic neurotransmitter at nicotinic receptors in the sympathetic ganglia and adrenal medulla. Inhibition of acetylcholinesterase at these locations results in sympathetic stimulation, producing pallor, mydriasis, tachycardia, and hypertension. In most patients, parasympathetic stimulation usually predominates, but mixed autonomic effects are common.

TABLE 201-3 Mnemonics for the Muscarinic Effects of Cholinesterase Inhibition

S	Salivation
L	Lacrimation
U	Urinary incontinence
D	Defecation
G	GI pain
E	Emesis
D	Defecation
U	Urination
M	Muscle weakness, miosis
B	Bradycardia, bronchorrhea, bronchospasm
E	Emesis
L	Lacrimation
S	Salivation
"Killer B's"	Bradycardia, bronchorrhea, bronchospasm

Nicotinic stimulation at neuromuscular junctions results in muscle fasciculations, cramps, and muscle weakness. This syndrome may progress to paralysis and areflexia, making it difficult to detect seizure activity. Respiratory muscle paralysis can lead to ventilatory failure.

Abdominal pain is common with rare cases of pancreatitis and peritonitis.[10] The clinical course may be complicated by broncho-aspiration of gastric contents contributing to respiratory distress. Many of these insecticide preparations contain hydrocarbons that act as solvents, and in cases of aspiration, they cause lipoid pneumonia, with severe respiratory failure.

More lipid-soluble organophosphates may not produce immediate symptoms of toxicity, but instead produce delayed sequelae. Low-grade chronic organophosphate exposures occur among farm workers, pesticide manufacturing plant workers, exterminators, and patients taking cholinergic ophthalmologic preparations.[11] Symptoms and signs are often less dramatic and nonspecific, occurring without the cholinergic syndrome.

An **intermediate syndrome** may occur 1 to 5 days after an organophosphate exposure, reported in up to 40% of patients following ingestion.[12] Clinical features include paralysis of neck flexor muscles, muscles innervated by the cranial nerves, proximal limb muscles, and respiratory muscles; respiratory support may be needed. Symptoms or signs of cholinergic excess are absent in this syndrome. Electromyography may assist in making the diagnosis.[13] Aggressive, early antidote therapy and supportive measures may prevent or ameliorate the severity of this syndrome. Symptoms usually resolve within 7 days. Nerve gas poisoning has not been reported to cause the intermediate syndrome.

Chronic toxicity is seen primarily in agricultural workers with daily exposure, manifesting as symmetrical sensorimotor axonopathy.[14] This mixed sensorimotor syndrome may begin with leg cramps and progress

TABLE 201-2 Acute Organophosphate Poisoning Severity Grading*

Severity	Butyrylcholinesterase Activity (% normal) Measured from Plasma	Acetylcholinesterase Activity (% normal) Measured from Red Blood Cells	Clinical Features	Typical Initial Atropine Amount to Control Symptoms
Mild	40–50	50–90	Lightheadedness, nausea, headache, dyspnea Lacrimation, rhinorrhea, salivation, diaphoresis	<2 milligrams IV/IM
Moderate	10–40	10–50	Restless, confusion, vomiting, diarrhea, drowsiness Autonomic instability: bradycardia or tachycardia, hypotension or hypertension, miosis or mydriasis Muscle fasciculations Bronchorrhea and bronchospasm	2–10 milligrams IV/IM
Severe	<10	<10	Coma, seizures, flaccid paralysis, urinary or fecal incontinence, respiratory arrest	>10 milligrams IV/IM

*The correlation between cholinesterase activity, clinical symptoms, and atropine dose is inconsistent, and treatment should be guided predominately by clinical symptoms.

to weakness and paralysis, mimicking features of the Guillain-Barré syndrome.

Organophosphate-induced delayed neuropathy is characterized by cognitive dysfunction, impaired memory, mood changes, autonomic dysfunction, peripheral neuropathy, and extrapyramidal signs.[11] Chronic fatigue syndrome and multiple chemical sensitivity have been reported in some patients, predominantly female, after exposure to very low doses of organophosphate insecticides.[15] Children are at greater risk of toxicity when exposed due to smaller body size and lower baseline levels of cholinesterase activity.

Chemical warfare nerve agents, such as soman, sarin, tabun, and VX, are organophosphate compounds that inactivate acetylcholinesterases. They are rapid acting and extremely potent; death can occur within minutes of inhalation or dermal exposure, as occurred in the subway terrorist attack in Tokyo 1985. Soman ages within minutes, giving little time to administer antidotes.

Diagnosis **Diagnosis and treatment are based on history and the presence of a suggestive toxidrome; laboratory cholinesterase assays and reference laboratory testing for specific compounds take time and have limitations, and waiting for results delays administration of potentially life-saving therapy.** Diagnosis is often difficult due to a constellation of clinical findings that can be variable in both acute and chronic poisonings. Point-of-care testing tools are in development.[16]

Noting a characteristic hydrocarbon or garlic-like odor may assist in diagnosis. The cholinergic toxidrome may vary depending on the predominance of muscarinic, nicotinic, and CNS manifestations and the severity of the intoxication. Organophosphate insecticide poisoning should be considered in the differential diagnosis of a patient with altered mental status and pinpoint pupils. **Miosis and muscle fasciculations are considered reliable signs of organophosphate toxicity.**

Cholinesterase activity is used to assess potential toxicity, with red cell acetylcholinesterase enzymatic activity a more accurate indicator of synaptic cholinesterase inhibition, but plasma butyrylcholinesterase is easier to assay and more available (**Table 201-2**). The degree of cholinesterase inhibition necessary to produce symptomatic illness is variable, so although cholinesterase levels should correlate with toxicity, there is large individual variability in baseline measurements, and standardization of normal ranges among laboratories is poor, so deviation from a symptomatic patient's baseline may be significant when values are reported within the normal range for the testing laboratory.

When the cholinesterase function falls gradually, as in chronic exposure, clinical symptoms may be subtle. Plasma butyrylcholinesterase levels may be depressed in genetic variants, chronic disease states, liver dysfunction, cirrhosis, malnutrition and low serum albumin states, neoplasm, infection, and pregnancy. Red blood cell acetylcholinesterase is affected by factors that influence the circulating life of erythrocytes such as hemoglobinopathies. Unless pralidoxime is given before aging occurs, plasma butyrylcholinesterase takes up to 4 to 6 weeks and red blood cell acetylcholinesterase takes as long as 90 to 120 days to return to baseline after exposure.

Routine laboratory test abnormalities are nondiagnostic but may include evidence of pancreatitis, hypo- or hyperglycemia, leukocytosis, and abnormal liver function. In severe cases, a chest radiograph may show pulmonary edema. The ECG may be abnormal and correlate with the degree of toxicity and outcome. Common abnormalities include ventricular dysrhythmias, torsade de pointes, and idioventricular rhythms. Atrioventricular blocks and prolongation of the QT interval are common. A prolonged QT_c interval correlates with severity and mortality in severe organophosphate poisoning.[17] Electromyography may identify and quantify acetylcholinesterase inhibition at neuromuscular junctions.

Treatment Treatment consists of airway control, intensive respiratory support, general supportive measures, decontamination, prevention of absorption, and the administration of antidotes (**Table 201-4**).[9,18,19] **Therapy should not be withheld pending determination of cholinesterase levels.**

In cases of acute cutaneous exposure, protective clothing must be worn to prevent secondary poisoning of healthcare workers.[20]

TABLE 201-4 Treatment for Organophosphate Poisoning

Decontamination	Protective clothing must be worn to prevent secondary poisoning of healthcare workers. Handle and dispose of all clothes as hazardous waste. Wash patient with soap and water. Handle and dispose of water runoff as hazardous waste.
Monitoring	Cardiac monitor, pulse oximeter, 100% oxygen.
Gastric lavage	No proven benefit (see text).
Activated charcoal	No proven benefit (see text).
Urinary alkalinization	No proven benefit (see text).
Atropine	1–3 milligrams IV in an adult or 0.01–0.04 milligram/kg IV (but never <0.1 milligram per dose) in children. Repeat every 5 min until tracheobronchial secretions attenuate. Followed by continuous infusion to maintain the anticholinergic state. Dose varies from 0.4 to 4 milligrams/h IV infusion in adults.
Pralidoxime	No proven benefit (see text). 1–2 grams for adults or 20–40 milligrams/kg IV (up to 1 gram) in children, mixed with normal saline and infused over 5–10 min. Followed by continuous infusion: 500 milligrams/h in adults or 5–10 milligrams/kg per hour in children.
Seizures	Benzodiazepines IV.

Neoprene or nitrile gloves should be used instead of latex. Patients with suspected exposure must be removed from the contaminated environment. All clothes and accessories must be removed completely, placed in plastic bags, and disposed of as hazardous materials.[21] The patient is immediately decontaminated externally with copious amounts of a mild detergent such as dishwashing liquid and water. Decontamination includes the scalp, hair, fingernails, skin, conjunctivae, and skin folds. Body fluids should be treated as contaminated. Abrasion or irritation of the skin should be avoided. Contaminated runoff water should be contained and disposed of as hazardous material. Instruments used can be decontaminated using chlorine bleach.

Patients with acute exposures should be placed on oxygen, a cardiac monitor, and pulse oximeter. A 100% nonrebreather mask will optimize oxygenation in the patient with excessive airway secretions and bronchospasm; however, atropine administration should not be delayed or withheld if oxygen is not immediately available.[22] Gentle suction will assist in clearing airway secretions from hypersalivation, bronchorrhea, or emesis. Coma, seizures, respiratory failure, excessive respiratory secretions, or severe bronchospasm necessitate endotracheal intubation. An IV line should be established with baseline blood sampling and determination of cholinesterase levels. **A nondepolarizing agent should be used when neuromuscular blockade is needed. Succinylcholine is metabolized by plasma butyrylcholinesterase, and therefore, prolonged paralysis may result.** Hypotension is initially treated with fluid boluses of isotonic crystalloid.

Gastric lavage is widely used in Asia following organophosphate ingestion despite the lack of evidence for improved outcome.[19,23] Given the sometimes rapid onset of symptoms after ingestion, it is unlikely that gastric lavage will be of benefit except in patients who present within 2 hours after a large ingestion. Activated charcoal is sometimes recommended because organophosphates do bind in vitro, although there is no evidence that single or multiple doses of activated charcoal improve patient outcome.[19] Urinary alkalinization is often used in Brazil and Iran for organophosphate poisoning, but there is no controlled evidence that shows benefit.[19] Hemodialysis, hemofiltration, and hemoperfusion are of no proven value.[19]

Atropine is the antidote for significant organophosphate poisonings (Table 201-4).[9,18,19] Atropine, a competitive antagonist of acetylcholine at central and peripheral muscarinic receptors, will reverse the effects secondary to excessive cholinergic stimulation. **The dose is repeated every 5 minutes until copious tracheobronchial secretions attenuate; large**

amounts may be necessary, in the order of hundreds of milligrams in massive ingestions. Pupillary dilatation is not a therapeutic end point. **Tachycardia is not a contraindication to the use of atropine in organophosphorus poisoning because tachycardia can occur secondary to bronchospasm or bronchorrhea with hypoxia, which can be reversed with atropine.**

The initial atropine should be IV when possible, but 2 to 6 milligrams IM should be considered when IV access is not possible. Normally, this initial dose of atropine should produce antimuscarinic symptoms; therefore, absence of anticholinergic symptoms after an initial dose is indicative of organophosphate poisoning. Once an effective amount of atropine has been given, an infusion should be started to maintain an anticholinergic state; the dose required varies according to severity,[24] and prolonged therapy may be necessary. **Importantly, atropine does not reverse muscle weakness.**

Glycopyrrolate, an alternate anticholinergic agent, may be used, but dosing is not well defined, and there is no proven benefit compared to atropine.[19] Nebulized atropine or ipratropium may be used to improve pulmonary symptoms. Glycopyrrolate and ipratropium do not cross the blood–brain barrier and are ineffective in treating central neurologic symptoms.

Compounds called *oximes* are used to displace organophosphates from the active site of acetylcholinesterase, thus reactivating the enzyme.[9,18,19] Pralidoxime is the oxime in common use, ameliorating muscarinic, nicotinic, and CNS symptoms. Importantly, pralidoxime reverses muscle paralysis if given early, before aging occurs. If possible, blood samples for acetylcholinesterase levels are obtained before administration of pralidoxime, but it is **important that pralidoxime be administered as soon as possible before permanent and irreversible aging occurs.** Although pralidoxime is more effective in acute than in chronic intoxications, it is recommended for use even after >24 to 48 hours after exposure.

Response to pralidoxime therapy with a decrease in muscle weakness and fasciculations and relief of muscarinic effects with atropine usually occurs within 10 to 40 minutes of administration. Pralidoxime can also be given by the IM route. A continuous infusion is preferable to repeated bolus dosing if paralysis does not resolve after the initial dose or if paralysis returns. The pralidoxime dose recommended by the World Health Organization is a 30-milligram/kg IV bolus followed by an IV infusion of 8 milligrams/kg per hour.

Pralidoxime should be continued for 24 to 48 hours while monitoring acetylcholinesterase levels. Despite theoretical and experimental benefit and worldwide clinical use, current evidence is inadequate to show that oximes, such as pralidoxime, reduce mortality or complication rate in acute organophosphate poisoning.[19,25,26] **Pralidoxime is not recommended for asymptomatic patients or for patients with known carbamate exposures presenting with minimal symptoms.**

Seizures are treated with airway protection, oxygen, atropine, and benzodiazepines.[19] **Atropine may prevent or abort seizures due to cholinergic overstimulation that occur within the first few minutes.** Pulmonary edema and bronchospasm are treated with oxygen, intubation, positive-pressure ventilation, atropine, and pralidoxime. Succinylcholine, ester anesthetics, and β-adrenergic blockers may potentiate poisoning and should be avoided.

Disposition and Follow-Up Minimal exposures may require only decontamination and 6 to 8 hours of observation in the ED to detect delayed effects. Reexposure should be avoided because sequential exposures can have cumulative toxicity, so patients returning to work should be limited from further exposure. All clothing, including shoes and belts, should be discarded properly as hazardous materials and not returned to the patient; recrudescence of poisoning has occurred from contaminated clothes and leather, even after washing or cleaning.[21]

Admission to the intensive care unit is necessary for significant poisonings. Most patients respond to pralidoxime therapy with an increase in acetylcholinesterase levels within 48 hours. If there is no posthypoxic brain damage, and if the patient is treated early, symptomatic recovery occurs in 10 days. If toxins are fat soluble, the patient may be symptomatic for prolonged periods of time and dependent on continuous pralidoxime infusion. During this period, which may last weeks while awaiting resynthesis of new enzyme, supportive care and respiratory support may be needed. The end point of therapy is determined by the absence of signs and symptoms on withholding pralidoxime therapy.

Following an acute exposure, the patient may have neurologic sequelae, such a paresthesias or limb weakness, along with nonspecific symptoms lasting days to months.[27] Death from organophosphate poisoning usually occurs in 24 hours in untreated patients, usually from respiratory failure secondary to paralysis of respiratory muscles,[28] neurologic depression, or bronchorrhea.

CARBAMATES

The carbamate insecticides (aldicarb, carbofuran, carbaryl, ethienocarb, fenobucarb, oxamyl, methomyl, pirimicarb, propoxur, and trimethacarb) are cholinesterase inhibitors that are structurally related to the organophosphate compounds.[1] These agents are primarily used as insecticides, but illegally imported rodenticides may contain aldicarb.[29]

Pathophysiology Carbamates can be toxic after dermal, inhalation, and GI exposure. Carbamates transiently and reversibly bind to and inhibit the cholinesterase enzyme. Regeneration of enzyme activity by dissociation of the carbamyl-cholinesterase bond occurs within minutes to a few hours involving rapid, spontaneous hydrolysis of the carbamate-cholinesterase bond. Therefore, aging does not occur, and as a major difference from organophosphate poisoning, new enzyme does not need to be synthesized before normal function is restored after carbamate poisoning.

Clinical Features **In adults, symptoms of acute carbamate poisoning are similar to the cholinergic syndrome observed with organophosphate agents but are of shorter duration.** Because carbamates do not effectively penetrate the CNS in adults, less central toxicity is seen, and seizures do not occur. However, in children, presentation of acute carbamate poisoning differs, with a predominance of CNS depression and nicotinic effects. Carbamates can also produce the intermediate syndrome.[12]

Diagnosis Diagnosis is based on clinical history and findings. Measurement of acetylcholinesterase activity is generally not helpful because enzymatic activity may return spontaneously to normal 4 to 8 hours after a carbamate exposure.

Treatment Initial treatment of carbamate poisoning is the same as for organophosphorus compounds. Atropine is the antidote of choice and is administered for muscarinic symptoms. Atropine is usually all that is necessary while waiting for the carbamylated acetylcholinesterase complex to dissociate spontaneously and recover function, usually within 24 hours. Therapy usually is not needed for more than 6 to 12 hours.

The use of pralidoxime in carbamate poisoning is controversial. The carbamate-binding half-life to cholinesterase is approximately 30 minutes, and irreversible binding does not occur; therefore, there is little need for pralidoxime. Human case reports and some but not all animal studies suggest that pralidoxime may potentiate the toxicity of carbamates, such as carbaryl.[30] Therefore, pralidoxime should be avoided in known single-agent carbaryl poisonings. However, pralidoxime should be considered in mixed poisonings with an organophosphorus compound and a carbamate or if the type of insecticide is unknown.

Disposition and Follow-Up Because carbamate poisonings have transient cholinesterase inhibition and rapid enzyme reactivation, the clinical course tends to be more benign than seen with organophosphates, and most patients recover completely within 24 hours. However, patients with depressed levels of consciousness have a significant mortality,[31] and methomyl poisoning is associated with a high risk of cardiac arrest at presentation and subsequent death after resuscitation.[32]

In mild poisonings, observation suffices, and the patient may be discharged with follow-up. Moderate poisonings necessitate 24 hours of observation that includes evaluation for possible concomitant exposure to or toxicity from inactive ingredients or vehicles such as hydrocarbons.

ORGANOCHLORINES

Dichlorodiphenyltrichloroethane (DDT) is the prototype insecticide of these chlorinated hydrocarbons. Chlordane, heptachlor, dieldrin, and aldrin are compounds used for termite and roach control. Most have been restricted or banned in the United States, Europe, and many other countries because of their persistence in the environment, long half-life in the human body, and toxicity. Worldwide, these insecticides continue to be used. Hexachlorocyclohexane (lindane) is a general garden organochlorine insecticide that is also used in some countries to treat scabies and head lice infestations. This compound is well absorbed by ingestion and inhalation. Dermal absorption occurs, particularly if the skin is abraded or repeated applications are used. Children and the elderly can develop neurotoxicity and seizures with therapeutic use of lindane.

Pathophysiology Organochlorines are central neurologic stimulants that can be toxic after dermal, inhalation, and GI exposures. The physical state of the agent, whether a liquid or a solid, and the type of vehicle affect transdermal absorption. Organochlorines antagonize γ-aminobutyric acid–mediated inhibition of the central neurons, leading to hyperexcitability with repetitive neuronal discharges following the action potential. Organochlorines are highly lipid soluble and accumulate in human tissues. Most are capable of inducing the hepatic microsomal enzyme system. Therefore, the therapeutic efficacy of other chemicals and drugs that are inactivated by this system is reduced in the presence of organochlorines.

Clinical Features **Neurologic symptoms predominate in acute organochlorine intoxication.**[33] Mild poisoning presents with dizziness; ataxia; fatigue; malaise; headache; neurologic stimulation with hyperexcitability, irritability, and delirium; apprehension; tremulousness; myoclonus; and facial paresthesias. Fever is common. More severe exposures may result in seizures, coma, renal injury, and death.[34] Seizures may occur early, without prodromal syndromes, and are usually short lived, although some patients may have status epilepticus. Organochlorines are used dissolved in hydrocarbon solvents that, by themselves, can cause sedation, coma, and pneumonitis from aspiration. Sensitization of the myocardium to endogenous catecholamines with cardiac dysrhythmia can occur from both organochlorines and the solvents. Chronic neurotoxic effects from low-level exposure to the organochlorine compound chlordane include deficits in tests of balance, reaction time, and verbal recall.

A related agent, the halogenated pyrrole chlorfenapyr, has two unusual features. First, it is a prodrug that is converted into the active form after absorption by the insect. Second, it manifests biphasic neurotoxicity.[35] Initial symptoms are nonspecific and include headaches, body aches, drowsiness, and weakness; these symptoms last for a few days, followed by a latent period of apparent recovery. Around the seventh day after ingestion, neurologic symptoms recur with rapidly progressing paralysis and stupor leading to coma with a fatal outcome. No treatment is effective once the delayed symptoms start. The requirement for metabolism to an active toxin and the latent period suggest it may be possible to develop an agent to inhibit this metabolic conversion and reduce the risk of progression to the delayed fatal neurologic course.

Diagnosis History is important, and valuable information can be obtained from the package label regarding the product and vehicle involved. Laboratory evaluation generally is not helpful, but organochlorines can be detected in the serum and urine by specialty laboratories.

Treatment Treatment includes administration of oxygen, with intubation indicated to treat hypoxia secondary to seizures, aspiration, and respiratory failure. Benzodiazepines are indicated for seizure control. Dysrhythmia control may be indicated, but epinephrine should be avoided because both organochlorines and organic solvents can sensitize the myocardium to endogenous catecholamines. Hyperthermia is managed by external cooling techniques. Removal of clothing and skin decontamination with mild detergent and water are important. Avoid using oils on the skin because they promote absorption. Activated charcoal and possibly gastric lavage in large, recent ingestions are potentially useful. The exchange resin cholestyramine is potentially useful for symptomatic patients exposed to chlordecone.

Disposition and Follow-Up Exposed patients should be observed for 6 hours and admitted to the hospital if signs of toxicity develop or if ingestion involved a hydrocarbon.

PYRETHRINS AND PYRETHROIDS

Pyrethroid use and poisonings have increased since the phase-out of organophosphate insecticides for use in human dwellings. Pyrethrins are naturally occurring active extracts derived from the chrysanthemum plant. Pyrethroids are synthetic analogues of the pyrethrins with greater potency and environmental persistence, but are considered safer than organochlorine and organophosphate insecticides.[36] Pyrethroids are used commonly as aerosols in automated insect sprays in public areas; therefore, inhalation is the most common source of exposure. These agents are available as dusts and liquids in a hydrocarbon base. Pyrethrins are common ingredients in over-the-counter household insecticides, pediculicides, and scabicides. They are rapidly metabolized and therefore are of low toxicity in humans.

Pathophysiology Toxicity results from dermal absorption, inhalation, or ingestion. Pyrethroids block the sodium channel at the neuronal cell membrane, causing repetitive neuronal discharge.[1,37] Additional effects include inhibition on γ-aminobutyric acid receptors, increased nicotinic cholinergic transmission, norepinephrine release, and interference with sodium–calcium exchange across cell membranes. Pyrethrin antigens are cross-antigenic with ragweed pollen, so allergic reactions are common after exposure

Clinical Features These compounds can cause dermal, pulmonary, GI, and neurologic illness. **Allergic hypersensitivity reactions are the most common effects of pyrethrins, producing dermatitis, bronchospasm, rhinitis, hypersensitivity pneumonitis, or anaphylaxis.**[36,38] Skin contact may lead to paresthesias and burning within 30 minutes of exposure that usually dissipates within 24 hours. These compounds are well absorbed but are rapidly metabolized in the liver, usually resulting in minimal systemic toxicity.

Systemic toxicity can occur from occupational poisonings and following large intentional ingestions. Features of systemic toxicity include fatigue and lethargy, nausea and vomiting, paresthesias, hyperexcitability, tremors, muscle fasciculations, pulmonary edema, respiratory failure, and seizures.[39,40]

Diagnosis Diagnosis is dependent on a history of exposure. Differential diagnosis includes allergic reactions and ingestions with neurologic stimulants. Laboratory tests have no diagnostic value.

Treatment Treatment includes removal from exposure; dermal, ocular, and GI decontamination; treatment of allergic manifestations; and supportive care.

Disposition and Follow-Up Disposition is usually related to the severity of asthmatic and allergic manifestations. The clinical course is usually benign, and hospitalization is not necessary for most accidental exposures.

NEONICOTINOIDS

Neonicotinoids are structurally similar to nicotine, acting as agonists at the postsynaptic acetylcholine receptor. Neonicotinoids have high affinity for the receptors within the insect CNS, producing paralysis and death. Commercially available agents from this family include imidacloprid, thiamethoxam, clothianidin, acetamiprid, thiacloprid, dinotefuran, and nitenpyram.

Data regarding human toxicity are limited to case reports. Toxicity from imidacloprid poisoning is relatively mild to moderate in most cases, with symptoms of nausea, emesis, diarrhea, and headache.[41] However, uncommon cases of respiratory failure, encephalopathy, hypotension, rhabdomyolysis, and renal failure have occurred.[42-44] Toxicity from acetamiprid poisoning has been associated with severe nausea and vomiting, muscle weakness, hypothermia, convulsions, and hypothermia.[45] Treatment is supportive.

NEREISTOXIN ANALOGS

Analogs of nereistoxin are considered low-toxicity insecticides. Agents in common use include nensultap, cartap, thiocyclam and thiosultap. These insecticides induce neurotoxicity by promoting extracellular calcium influx and stimulating the release of intracellular calcium from the sarcoplasmic reticulum.

Case reports of toxicity from occupational skin exposure report nausea, vomiting, muscles tremors, dyspnea, and mydriasis. Intentional ingestions are associated with depressed level of consciousness, muscle fasciculations and spasms, seizures, hypotension, and hypoxia.[46-48]

Animal studies suggest that sulfhydryl-containing compounds, such as l-cysteine, acetylcysteine, d-penicillamine, and dimercaprol, are effective antidotes, but human data are lacking, and suggested doses are conjectures. Recovery from severe toxicity associated with coma is possible, although death from multiple organ failure may occur.

AMITRAZ

Amitraz is a topical insecticide and acaricide, as well as an insect repellant. Amitraz is used as a spray on agricultural crops and as a wash-solution to treat ectoparasites found on farm animals, dogs, and cats. Amitraz possesses agonist activity at the postsynaptic α_2-adrenergic receptor, and interacts with the neuromodulator octopamine, inhibits monoamine oxidase, and impairs prostaglandin synthesis.

The clinical manifestations following human overdose include mental status depression, bradycardia, respiratory depression, miosis, hypotension, and hypothermia.[49,50] Mechanical ventilation may be required, and with supportive therapy, recovery is expected.

N,N-DIETHYL-3-METHYLBENZAMIDE (DEET)

DEET is used extensively as an over-the-counter insect repellant that comes in a variety of product formulations ranging in concentrations from 5% to 100%. When used as directed, they are generally safe. Toxicity can occur with ingestion or prolonged exposure on covered or damaged skin. DEET is absorbed through the skin and is a neurotoxin that causes seizures after large ingestions and extensive dermal exposures of high-concentration products. Small children are most susceptible to systemic toxicity from skin absorption. Skin absorption occurs within 2 hours of topical application, but peak concentrations may be delayed several hours.

Systemic toxicity is rare but manifests as restlessness, insomnia, altered behavior, confusion, neurologic depression, slurred speech, ataxia, tremors, muscle cramps, hypertonia, and seizures occurring with or without prodrome. DEET-induced hypotension and bradycardia have been reported with heavy dermal or oral exposure. Treatment includes benzodiazepines for seizures, skin decontamination with mild detergent and water, and activated charcoal for recent ingestions. Most patients recover with supportive care.

HERBICIDES

Herbicides are used to kill weeds. Mechanisms of plant toxicity includes inhibition of photosynthesis, respiration, protein synthesis, or growth stimulation mimicking plant hormones called *auxins*. Some classes pose a health hazard to humans (**Table 201-5**). Herbicidal formulations contain multiple ingredients such as organic solvents, surfactants, and preservatives that may have their own toxic effects; these may not be always disclosed on the product label.

TABLE 201-5 Selected Herbicide Classes that Pose Potential Harm to Humans

Chlorophenoxy compounds
Bipyridyls: paraquat and diquat
Urea-substituted
Organophosphates
Glyphosate

CHLOROPHENOXY HERBICIDES

Chlorophenoxy herbicides are synthetic plant hormones. The most commonly used compounds are 2,4-dichlorophenoxyacetic acid (2,4-D) and 4-chloro-2-methylphenoxy-acetic acid. 2,4,5-Trichlorophenoxy acetic acid (2,4,5-T) has been banned in the United States because of its contamination with 2,3,7,8,-tetrachlorodibenzo-*p*-dioxin. The aerially applied defoliant Agent Orange used during the Vietnam War was a mixture of 2,4-D and 2,4,5-T. These compounds are effective against broadleaf plants and are used as weed killers on lawns and grain crops.

Pathophysiology The metabolic pathway or mechanism related to human toxicity is unknown. Toxicity can result from dermal contact, inhalation, or ingestion. Systemic absorption can produce neurologic, cardiac, and skeletal muscle toxicity.

Clinical Features Local exposure leads to eye and mucous membrane irritation that may last for days. After ingestion, nausea, vomiting, and diarrhea occur. Pulmonary toxicity may produce dyspnea, tachypnea, and signs of pulmonary edema. Cardiovascular findings include hypotension, tachycardia, and dysrhythmias. Mental status changes and seizures may occur. Muscle toxicity manifests as muscle tenderness, fasciculations, myotonia, and rhabdomyolysis. The patient may become hyperthermic. Peripheral neuropathy has been described in the recovery phase after acute exposure and with chronic exposure.

Diagnosis Diagnosis is based on a history of exposure. Ancillary tests generally are nonspecific but may demonstrate a metabolic acidosis, rhabdomyolysis, or evidence of hepatorenal dysfunction. Toxin levels are not immediately available. Differential diagnosis includes other causes of acute myopathy.

Treatment Treatment is supportive, including decontamination measures and respiratory support for myopathic-related respiratory failure.[51,52] Urinary alkalinization will increase the elimination of these compounds and is recommended for severely poisoned patients.[53] Hemodialysis can also be used to enhance chlorophenoxy herbicide clearance. Patients should be monitored for rhabdomyolysis and treated as necessary.

Disposition and Follow-Up Severe toxicity and serious complications are not common following chlorophenoxy herbicides. Because toxic effects usually appear within 4 to 6 hours, patients with mild symptoms can be observed and discharged after that time. Significant toxicity warrants admission.

BIPYRIDYL HERBICIDES

The bipyridyl compounds, **paraquat and diquat**, are nonselective contact herbicides. Both are used widely and are responsible for significant morbidity if ingested.[54] Paraquat is a fast-acting, nonselective herbicide. It is used for killing grass and weeds; is manufactured as a liquid, granules, or an aerosol; and is commonly combined with diquat and other herbicides. Most products contain a blue dye, a stenchant, and an emetic. Ingestion is responsible for the majority of paraquat deaths,[54] although deaths have been reported after transdermal exposure. Inhalation exposure to sprays can be very irritating to conjunctiva and the airway but are unlikely to cause systemic toxicity.

Pathophysiology Paraquat is a severe local irritant and devastating systemic toxin.[55] There is minimal transdermal absorption of paraquat in the absence of preexisting skin lesions. Ingested paraquat is absorbed rapidly, particularly if the stomach is empty. Plasma concentration peaks within minutes to 2 hours after ingestion. Paraquat is then distributed to most organs, with the highest concentrations found in the kidneys and lungs. A lethal oral dose of the 20% concentrate solution is about 10 to 20 mL in an adult and 4 to 5 mL in a child.

Paraquat actively accumulates in the alveolar cells of the lungs, where it is transformed into a reactive oxygen species, the superoxide radical.[55] This anion is responsible for lipid peroxidation that leads to degradation of cell membranes, cell dysfunction, and necrosis. Lung injury has two phases. An initial destructive phase is characterized by loss of type I and type II alveolar cells, infiltration by inflammatory cells, and hemorrhage. These changes may be reversible. The later, proliferative phase is characterized by fibrosis in the interstitium and alveolar spaces. Paraquat and oxygen enhance each other's toxicity by sustaining the redox cycle. Myocardial injury and necrosis of the adrenal glands may occur.

TABLE 201-6 Paraquat Toxicity from Ingestion

Category	Clinical Features	Approximate Amount Ingested
Mild	Asymptomatic or nausea, vomiting, and diarrhea. Renal and hepatic injury minimal or absent. Decreased pulmonary diffusion capacity may be present. Complete recovery expected.	<20 milligrams/kg or <7.5 mL of 20% concentrated solution in average adult
Severe	Initially nausea, vomiting, diarrhea, abdominal pain, mouth and throat ulceration. Positive colorimetric test for paraquat in the urine. 1–4 d: renal failure, hepatic impairment, hypotension. 1–2 wk: cough, hemoptysis, pleural effusion, pulmonary fibrosis. Survival possible, but majority of cases die within 2–3 wk from pulmonary failure.	Between 20 and 40 milligrams/kg or between 7.5 and 15 mL of 20% concentrated solution in average adult
Fulminant	Initially nausea, vomiting, diarrhea, and abdominal pain. Rapid development of renal and hepatic failure, GI ulceration, pancreatitis, toxic myocarditis, refractory hypotension, coma, convulsions. Death from cardiogenic shock and multiorgan failure within 1–4 d.	>40–50 milligrams/kg or >15–20 mL of 20% concentrated solution in average adult

Diquat has a similar structure and mechanism as paraquat. Formulations containing diquat do not contain the dye, stenching agent, or emetic usually added to paraquat. The lethal dose for diquat is similar to that of paraquat, but there is less occurrence of pulmonary injury and fibrosis because of diquat's lower affinity for pulmonary tissue. Diquat is caustic to the skin and GI tract, and exposure can result in renal and liver necrosis.

Clinical Features Clinical features depend on the route of exposure and amount. Paraquat's severe caustic effects produce local skin irritation and ulceration of epithelial surfaces. Severe corrosive corneal injury may result from eye exposure. Upper respiratory tract exposure may result in mucosal injury and epistaxis. Inhalation may lead to cough, dyspnea, chest pain, pulmonary edema, epistaxis, and hemoptysis. Respiratory symptoms may persist for several weeks after inhalation exposure.

Ingestion causes GI irritation and mucosal damage with ulcerations (**Table 201-6**). A burning sensation of the lips or mouth may occur within a few minutes to hours followed by ulceration 1 to 2 days later. Nausea, vomiting, diarrhea, buccopharyngeal pain, esophageal pain, and abdominal pain may develop. Hypovolemia occurs from GI fluid losses and decreased oral intake.

Multisystem effects include GI tract corrosion, acute renal failure, cardiac failure, hepatic failure, and extensive pulmonary injury. The effects can be evident within a few hours following large ingestions, but, more typically, manifestations of renal failure and hepatocellular necrosis develop between the second and fifth days, with progressive pulmonary fibrosis leading to refractory hypoxemia 5 days to several weeks later. Metabolic (lactic) acidosis is common as a result of pulmonary effects (hypoxemia) and multisystem failure.

Diagnosis Early diagnosis and therapy are important. Obtain details of the exposure, including accidental or intentional, route of exposure, concentration of the product, time of occurrence, and estimated amount. The differential diagnosis includes exposure to other corrosive agents and herbicides. Qualitative and quantitative analyses for paraquat in urine and blood can assist in the diagnosis, and nomograms are used for predicting survival based on plasma paraquat concentration and time of ingestion.[55] A commercially available semi-qualitative colorimetric test (Paraquat Test Kit®; Syngenta CTL, Surrey, United Kingdom) can be done on urine or plasma to detect paraquat within a few hours after ingestion; such detection indicates potentially severe course. Serial pulmonary function tests, chest radiographs, and arterial blood gas determinations, including alveolar-arterial gradient, and arterial lactate may be used to monitor toxicity.[56]

Laboratory abnormalities generally reflect multiorgan necrosis. Chest radiographs may show pneumomediastinum or pneumothorax due to corrosive rupture of the esophagus. Radiographic abnormalities of diffuse consolidation indicating parenchymal injury on the chest radiograph may not parallel the severity of clinical symptoms. Upper GI endoscopy should be performed to identify the extent and severity of mucosal lesions.

Treatment The goal of early and vigorous decontamination is to prevent absorption and pulmonary toxicity. Any exposure to paraquat is a medical emergency, with hospitalization indicated even if the patient is asymptomatic. Early treatment is mainly supportive but is an important determinant of survival. Do not administer supplemental oxygen unless the patient is severely hypoxic, because added oxygen stimulates superoxide radical formation and promotes oxidative stress.

Remove clothing and decontaminate skin with mild detergent and water. Take care to avoid skin abrasions that may increase absorption. If there is conjunctival irritation, irrigate with copious amounts of water or saline. Fluid and electrolytic losses can occur from GI tract damage, vomiting, and cathartics. Maintain intravascular volume and urine output to prevent prerenal kidney injury. Pain associated with oropharyngeal lesions should be treated with opioids. Emesis is common, and there is no proven benefit to gastric lavage.[55] In patients with pharyngeal or esophageal burns, prophylactic placement of a nasogastric tube for subsequent enteral nutrition is recommended.[55]

Immediate GI decontamination with absorbents that bind paraquat is indicated in patients with a protected airway. A single dose of activated charcoal (1 to 2 grams/kg), diatomaceous fuller's earth (1 to 2 grams/kg in 15% aqueous suspension), or bentonite (1 to 2 grams/kg in a 7% aqueous slurry) should be used.[55] **Charcoal hemoperfusion can remove paraquat and has been recommended to be started as soon as possible and continued for 6 to 8 hours, but there is no evidence to show that prognosis is improved.**[55] Repeated pulse doses of glucocorticoids and cyclophosphamide may improve survival in severe cases.[57-59]

Supportive care includes airway protection, maintaining intravascular volume, pain relief, treatment of renal failure and complications, and treatment of infection. Maintaining renal function will assist in avoiding toxic accumulation in other tissues.

Treatment for diquat poisoning is similar to that for paraquat, and despite the lower toxicity for diquat, mortality approaches 50% following intentional diquat ingestion.

Disposition and Follow-Up Outcome is determined by the amount ingested; therefore, intentional ingestions tend to have a worse prognosis.[60] Prognosis is worse ingesting a highly concentrated liquid formulation on an empty stomach. Conversely, ingestion of dilute solid formulations rarely cause death.

UREA-SUBSTITUTED HERBICIDES

Urea-substituted herbicides such as chlorimuron, diuron, fluometuron, and isoproturon are inhibitors of photosynthesis and have low systemic toxicity. In humans, methemoglobinuria may occur with ingestion.[61] Treatment includes decontamination, supportive care, and treatment for methemoglobinemia with methylene blue, as appropriate (see chapter 207, "Dyshemoglobinemias").

ORGANOPHOSPHATE HERBICIDES

In addition to their use as insecticides, some organophosphate compounds are effective herbicides. Butiphos is used commonly as a cotton defoliant before mechanical harvesting. Treatment is identical to that for organophosphate insecticides.

GLYPHOSATE

Glyphosate is the active ingredient in many widely used preparations available for consumer use on lawns and gardens. A problem with lawn and garden chemicals is that some products sold using a common or group brand name may contain different active ingredients; a common brand name may contain either glyphosate or the more toxic herbicide diquat.

Glyphosate can produce severe toxicity with massive ingestions of the diluted product or ingestions of concentrated solutions.[62] Preparations

TABLE 201-7 Nonanticoagulant Rodenticides

Rodenticide	Toxicity	Mechanism	Clinical Effects	Treatment
Arsenic	Severe	Binds sulfhydryl groups on proteins	Dysphagia, muscle cramps, nausea and vomiting, bloody diarrhea, cardiovascular collapse, altered mental status, seizures, and late peripheral neuropathies	Gastric lavage, activated charcoal, catharsis, chelation therapy using succimer, dimercaprol, or penicillamine
Barium carbonate and other soluble forms such as barium chlorides, hydroxides, and sulfides	Severe	Depolarizing neuromuscular blockade	Onset occurs within 1–8 h with nausea, vomiting, diarrhea, abdominal pain, dysrhythmias, respiratory failure, muscular weakness, paresthesias, and paralysis	Gastric lavage with sodium or magnesium sulfate added to lavage solution to convert carbonate to less toxic sulfate; potassium replacement
Elemental or yellow phosphorus	Severe, early cardiac and neurologic toxicity is a poor prognostic sign	Caustic; uncouples oxidative phosphorylation	Skin irritation, cutaneous burns, oral burns, abdominal pain, hematemesis, possible "smoking" luminescent vomitus and stool, garlicky odor, direct toxic effects on the myocardium, kidney, and peripheral vessels, cardiovascular collapse; late neurologic depression with multisystem toxicity and hepatorenal syndrome	Gastric lavage with dilute potassium permanganate solution may convert phosphorus to less toxic phosphates; activated charcoal; avoid emesis
N-3-Pyridylmethyl-*N′*-*p*-nitrophenylurea (PNU or Vacor)	Severe	Destroys pancreatic β cells within hours of ingestion by interfering with nicotinamide metabolism	Within 24 h of ingestion, GI symptoms, perforation, autonomic nervous system dysfunction, insulin-deficient hyperglycemia or diabetic ketoacidosis, dysrhythmias, neuropathies	Nicotinamide (niacinamide) IV or IM is an antidote; lavage for recent ingestions; activated charcoal and insulin for treatment of hyperglycemia and ketoacidosis
Sodium fluoroacetate (SFA)[67]	Severe	Blocks Krebs cycle	Nausea, vomiting, apprehension, lactic acidosis, seizures, coma, respiratory depression, cardiac dysrhythmias, and pulmonary edema; electrocardiographic abnormalities include ST-segment and T-wave changes, tachycardia, premature ventricular contractions, ventricular tachycardia, and ventricular fibrillation; hyperkalemia and hypocalcemia are common	Activated charcoal, seizure and dysrhythmia control, and supportive care; experimental regimens include glycerol monoacetate, calcium gluconate, sodium succinate, and ethanol loading; consultation with a toxicologist is recommended
Strychnine	Severe	Competitive antagonism of the inhibitory neurotransmitter glycine at the postsynaptic brainstem and spinal cord motor neuron	Restlessness, muscle twitching, painful extensor spasms, opisthotonos, trismus, inability to swallow, and facial grimacing; medullary paralysis and death can follow	Airway control, quiet environment (minimize sensory stimulation), and activated charcoal; avoid lavage (may precipitate seizures); benzodiazepines, barbiturates, analgesia; neuromuscular blockage if necessary
Tetramine[68-70]	Severe	Blocks γ-aminobutyric acid receptors in the CNS	Rapidly acting; initial features include headache, nausea, dizziness, fatigue, anorexia, numbness, and listlessness; severe symptoms include loss of consciousness, seizures, and coma; death usually caused by respiratory failure	The median lethal dose for tetramine is ~0.1 milligram/kg; 6–12 milligrams sufficient to kill an adult; no antidote; supportive care; benzodiazepines or barbiturates for seizures
Thallium sulfate[71]	Severe	Combines with mitochondrial sulfhydryl groups, interfering with oxidative phosphorylation	Early GI symptoms: nausea, vomiting, and abdominal pain; after 2–5 d, painful paresthesias, myalgias, muscle weakness, headache, lethargy, tremors, ataxia, delirium, seizures, and coma; death from respiratory failure and dysrhythmias; alopecia after approximately 2 wk; chronic neurologic sequelae	Supportive care; multiple doses of activated charcoal or Prussian blue (potassium ferric hexaniacinate) to interrupt enterohepatic circulation and increase elimination in stool; hemodialysis
Zinc or aluminium phosphide[72-76]	Severe	Combines with water and stomach acid to produce phosphine gas; cellular toxicity and necrosis to the GI tract, kidney, and liver if ingested and to the lungs if inhaled	Immediate nausea, vomiting, epigastric pain, phosphorous or fishy breath, black vomitus, and GI irritation or ulceration; myocardial toxicity, shock, and acute lung injury; agitation, coma, seizures, hepatorenal injury, metabolic acidosis, hypocalcemia, tetany	Gastric lavage with potassium permanganate or combination coconut oil and sodium bicarbonate; magnesium sulfate IV[77]; treat acidosis and hypocalcemia; consider acetylcysteine[78]; supportive care
α-Naphthyl-thiourea (ANTU)	Moderate	Increases alveolar capillary permeability, causing pulmonary edema	Dyspnea, cyanosis, cough, pleuritic chest pain, noncardiogenic pulmonary edema, and pleural effusion	Supportive care; activated charcoal
Cholecalciferol (vitamin D_3)	Moderate	Mobilization of calcium from bones	Hypercalcemia, osteomalacia, and systemic metastatic calcifications	Treat hypercalcemia with IV normal saline, furosemide, steroids, calcitonin, and biphosphates as needed
Bromethalin	Low	Uncouples oxidative phosphorylation in CNS mitochondria, interrupting nerve conduction	Muscle tremors, myoclonic jerks, contractions of flexor muscles, ataxia, and focal motor seizures; personality changes, confusion, and coma	Decontamination; benzodiazepines for seizures
Norbormide or dicarboximide	Low	Irreversible smooth muscle vasoconstriction	Tissue hypoxia and ischemia	Supportive care; decontamination
Red squill	Low (limited toxicity in humans due to early onset of emesis with gastric emptying)	Blocks sodium-potassium adenosine triphosphatase (similar to digoxin poisoning)	Nausea, protracted vomiting, diarrhea, abdominal pain; massive ingestion causes hyperkalemia, atrioventricular block, ventricular irritability with dysrhythmias, and death	Treat as digoxin toxicity (atropine, external pacing, digoxin-specific antibody fragments, activated charcoal)

may contain the toxic surfactant polyoxyethyleneamine, which is a corrosive, and the combination is more toxic than glyphosate alone. Inhalational exposures cause respiratory irritation. Dermal absorption is poor, so symptomatic poisonings are generally from ingestion.

Clinical effects include mucous membrane irritation and erosions with nausea, vomiting, abdominal pain, and diarrhea.[63] Widespread organ failure with refractory cardiovascular collapse and dysrhythmias has been reported. Respiratory distress requiring intubation, metabolic acidosis, tachycardia, renal failure, and hyperkalemia portend a fatal outcome.

Treatment includes activated charcoal following a recent ingestion and supportive care, with attention to support of oxygenation and ventilation, ameliorating complications due to the corrosive effects on the GI tract, treating hyperkalemia, and supporting the circulation. Intravenous lipid emulsion is reported as useful in preventing hypotension[64] and treating refractory hypotension.[65] Hemodialysis may be supportive when severe acidosis and acute kidney injury are present.[66]

Patients with small, asymptomatic ingestions can be discharged after 6 hours of observation. Significant GI symptoms, altered level of consciousness, hypoxemia, metabolic acidosis, and cardiovascular abnormalities indicate admission to an intensive care unit.

RODENTICIDES

A number of agents with distinct toxicities are used as rodenticides. Rodenticides are commonly classified based on whether they are anticoagulants or nonanticoagulants. Although intentional ingestions are often associated with significant morbidity and mortality, most unintentional exposures occur in young children and result in minimal or no toxicity.

NONANTICOAGULANTS

A number of nonanticoagulant rodenticides have been used throughout history. Many have been discontinued, although poisonings still occur from old product stored in garages, barns, and homes (**Table 201-7**).

ANTICOAGULANTS

Warfarin-type anticoagulants were the first generation of anticoagulant rodenticides and distributed commonly disguised as yellow corn meal or rolled oats.[79] **Most one-time warfarin rodenticide ingestions are insignificant accidental poisonings and do not cause any bleeding problems. Significant coagulopathy requires large amounts in a single exposure or a repetitive exposure over several days.** Following a single large ingestion, onset of the anticoagulant effect takes place within 12 to 48 hours. Warfarin's biologic half-life is approximately 42 hours.

Therapy is not necessary for ingestion of a single mouthful of a warfarin rodenticide. For potentially toxic recent ingestion, consider activated charcoal. Obtain a baseline prothrombin time and INR determination and repeat it in 12 to 24 hours. Vitamin K_1 (phytonadione) administration is indicated if the INR is >2.0. The suggested total PO daily dose is 1 to 5 milligrams in children and 20 milligrams in adults, administered in two to four divided doses.

Second-generation superwarfarins and the indandione derivatives were introduced when rodent resistance to warfarin began to appear.[79] They are currently responsible for approximately 80% of human rodenticide exposures reported in the United States. Their mechanisms are the same as that of warfarin, but they are more potent, have more prolonged anticoagulant activity, and therefore have the potential to be highly toxic. Poisonings involving the indandione derivatives pindone, diphacinone, chlorophacinone, and valone have toxic and clinical characteristics similar to those of the superwarfarins.

The **superwarfarins** include the 4-hydroxy-coumarins brodifacoum, diphenacoum, coumafuryl, and bromadoline. These are readily available over the counter as grain-based bait. After intentional ingestions, adults often develop a coagulopathy within 24 to 48 hours. **Because the biologic half-life of brodifacoum is approximately 120 days, a single ingestion may result in marked anticoagulation effects for weeks to months.**[80] Intentional repeated ingestions can cause severe bleeding.

The diagnosis may not be readily apparent. Some patients may not report an intentional ingestion. Small children and depressed patients with an unexplained coagulopathy and/or bleeding should raise suspicion of superwarfarin poisoning. Although the prothrombin time and INR are usually monitored, large doses of warfarin can also cause prolongation of the activated partial thromboplastin time. **Superwarfarins are not detected by warfarin assays, but specific serum assays are available in reference laboratories.**

Unintentional superwarfarin ingestions in the pediatric patient are unlikely to result in significant toxicity.[81] Obtain a baseline INR and repeat 24 and 48 hours after ingestion. For acute intentional ingestions, gastric lavage is indicated for early presentations, and activated charcoal should be administered. Obtain a baseline INR and repeat in 12 and 24 hours. If the INR is elevated but there is no active hemorrhage, oral vitamin K_1 is recommended. Because of the extended half-life of the anticoagulant, prolonged therapy with high doses of vitamin K_1 may be required to maintain hemostasis.[82,83] Initial daily doses of 1 to 5 milligrams in children and 20 milligrams in adults are recommended with titration to maintain a normal INR. Doses up to 100 milligrams per day for 10 months have been reported. Upon discontinuation of vitamin K_1 therapy, serial INR determinations are required to ensure that further therapy is not needed.

Patients with acute hemorrhage may require repletion of volume losses with normal saline or blood transfusions. Fresh frozen plasma should be used if bleeding is severe or unresponsive to vitamin therapy. Vitamin K_1, 10 milligrams, should be administered by slow IV infusion to minimize the risk of a hypotensive reaction. Forms of vitamin K other than vitamin K_1 are ineffective because the conversion of these other forms to the active form is blocked by superwarfarins. Administration of prothrombin complex concentrates or recombinant activated factor VII can be considered for patients with ongoing hemorrhage despite fresh frozen plasma and vitamin K_1 therapy.

For asymptomatic patients who have accidentally ingested a superwarfarin, follow-up in 24 and 48 hours for coagulation studies should be arranged. Prevention measures should be emphasized.

CONSULTATION

Consultation with a poison control center or medical toxicologist is recommended to assist in patient management and to collect data for surveillance reports. When consulting, precise communication of the specific product name from the container label is essential to identify both active and inert ingredients. As noted, confusion can arise because similar brand names are used for more than one agent.

REFERENCES

The complete reference list is available online at www.TintinalliEM.com.

Anticholinergics

Dan Quan
Frank Lovecchio

INTRODUCTION

Approximately 620 compounds have anticholinergic properties, including prescription drugs, over-the-counter medications, and plants (**Table 202-1**). Many of these substances possess anticholinergic activity as either a direct therapeutic effect or an adverse effect, in addition to their primary or predominant pharmacologic effect. Atropine (D,L-hyoscyamine), hyoscyamine, and scopolamine (L-hyoscine) are natural alkaloids that represent prototypical anticholinergic compounds.

Antihistamine (particularly diphenhydramine) overdose is the most common overdose that produces anticholinergic toxicity.[1] Toxicity in

TABLE 202-1 Major Groups of Substances with Anticholinergic Activity

Class and Subclass	Prototypical Agent(s)
Cyclic antidepressants	Amitriptyline hydrochloride, imipramine hydrochloride, doxepin hydrochloride
Antihistamines	
Ethanolamines	Diphenhydramine, dimenhydrinate
Ethylenediamines	Tripelennamine
Alkylamines	Chlorpheniramine
Piperazines	Loratadine, meclizine, cetirizine
Phenothiazines	Prochlorperazine, promethazine
Antiparkinson drugs	
Tropanes	Benztropine mesylate
Piperidines	Trihexyphenidyl
Antipsychotics	
Phenothiazines	Chlorpromazine, thioridazine, perphenazine
Nonphenothiazines	Clozapine, olanzapine, molindone, loxapine, quetiapine
Antispasmodics	
Cyclohexane carboxylic acids	Dicyclomine
Quaternary ammonium	Methantheline bromide
Belladonna alkaloids	
Tropanes	Atropine, homatropine, scopolamine hydrobromide
Pyrrolidines	Glycopyrrolate
Mydriatics	
Phenylacetates	Cyclopentolate hydrochloride
Pyridines	Tropicamide
Skeletal muscle relaxants	
Tricyclics	Cyclobenzaprine hydrochloride
Ethylamines	Orphenadrine citrate
Plants	
Datura species	*Datura stramonium* (Jimson weed), *Datura candida* (angel's trumpet)
Mandragora species	*Mandragora officinarum* (mandrake)
Brugmansia species	*Brugmansia suaveolens* (angel's tear, maikoa, or white angel's trumpet), *Brugmansia versicolor* (angel's tear or angel's trumpet)
Mushrooms	
Amanita species	*Amanita muscaria*, *Amanita pantherina*

children may result from accidental ingestion of an anticholinergic medication, administration of hyoscyamine-containing agents to treat colic, the topical use of diphenhydramine-containing salves, and therapeutic application of a transdermal hyoscine patch.[2-5] In the elderly, therapeutic doses of one or multiple medications with anticholinergic properties may produce anticholinergic symptoms or ileus without all the signs of the anticholinergic toxidrome.[6,7] Ophthalmologic instillation of anticholinergic mydriatic agents can cause toxicity, especially in the elderly or young children; thus patients are instructed to lie down and apply 5 minutes of gentle pressure on the nasolacrimal duct when instilling these agents.[8]

Atropine is the antidote for a cholinergic syndrome produced from a nerve agent or an organophosphate insecticide.[9] Use of high-dose atropine by someone without cholinesterase poisoning may result in anticholinergic toxicity within 1 hour. This occurred in Israel during the first Gulf War in 1991 when frightened civilians dosed themselves with atropine fearing an incoming Scud missile chemical weapon attack.

Plant poisonings may result in an anticholinergic toxidrome. In Taiwan, the anticholinergic toxidrome is most commonly associated with plant exposures.[10] Belladonna alkaloid-containing plants have potent anticholinergic effects producing toxicity 1 to 4 hours after ingestion or sooner if smoked. Alkaloid plants are abused for their hallucinogenic effects.[11,12] Group anticholinergic plant poisonings are common in adolescents seeking these psychoactive hallucinogenic effects.[13,14] Inadvertent poisoning from the ingestion of belladonna-contaminated herbal teas and Chinese traditional medicines has been reported.[15,16] Ingestion of seeds and berries, sometimes due to mistaken identity, can produce anticholinergic toxicity.[17,18] Anticholinergics have been substituted for other abused psychoactive drugs and then sold to unwitting customers.[19] Adulteration of commonly abused drugs, such as heroin or cocaine, with scopolamine or atropine has been observed.[20-22]

PHARMACOLOGY

Anticholinergic drug absorption can occur after ingestion, smoking, or ocular use. With oral ingestion, the onset of anticholinergic toxicity usually occurs within 1 to 2 hours. Because muscarinic blockade slows gastric emptying and decreases GI motility, absorption and peak clinical effects are often delayed. An example is diphenoxylate-atropine (e.g., Lomotil®), an antidiarrheal agent that may present with toxicity up to 12 hours after ingestion.

Cholinergic receptors exist as two major subtypes: muscarinic receptors and nicotinic receptors. Muscarinic receptors are found predominantly on autonomic effector cells that are innervated by postganglionic parasympathetic nerves, on some ganglia, and in the brain, particularly the hippocampus, cortex, and thalamus. Nicotinic receptors are found at peripheral autonomic ganglia, neuromuscular junctions, and also the brain. Acetylcholine is the neurotransmitter that modulates both receptor types. Five genes encode for muscarinic receptors through G protein receptor activation; four seem to be physiologically active (**Table 202-2**).

The structure of nicotinic receptors is complex, composed of several subunits that are encoded by multiple genes. The subunits are combined into four main families of nicotinic receptors: the muscle type, found at the neuromuscular junction; the ganglion type, found in autonomic ganglia; and two brain types, found in the CNS.

Anticholinergic drugs and plant toxins competitively inhibit or antagonize the binding of the neurotransmitter acetylcholine to muscarinic acetylcholine receptors. The term *anticholinergic* is technically a misnomer; a more accurate term is *antimuscarinic* agents, because anticholinergic agents do not antagonize the effects at nicotinic acetylcholine receptors, such as at the neuromuscular junction. Clinical manifestations from these drugs are modulated through disturbances in the CNS (central effects) and the parasympathetic nervous system (peripheral effects) (**Table 202-3**).

The signs and symptoms of anticholinergic toxicity are a result of both central and peripheral cholinergic blockade. The *central anticholinergic*

TABLE 202-2 Muscarinic Receptors

Receptor	Target Organ	Receptor Action When Stimulated
M_1	Autonomic ganglia Brain Salivary glands Stomach	Decreases activity in autonomic ganglia Increases salivary and gastric acid secretion
M_2	Heart	Decreases sinus node rate and slows conduction through the atrioventricular node Decreases the force of atrial contraction and possibly ventricular contraction
M_3	Smooth muscle Endocrine/exocrine glands Iris	Bronchospasm Mild vasodilation Increases saliva and gastric acid production Constricts the pupil
M_4	CNS	Multiple actions
M_5	Has not been elucidated	

TABLE 202-3 Muscarinic and Antimuscarinic Effects

Organ	Stimulation or Muscarinic Effect	Antagonism or Antimuscarinic Effect
Brain	Complex interactions Possible improvement in memory	Complex interactions Impairs memory Produces agitation, delirium, and hallucinations Fever
Eye	↓ pupil size (miosis) ↓ intraocular pressure ↑ tear production	↑ pupil size (mydriasis) ↑ intraocular pressure Loss of accommodation (blurred vision)
Mouth	↑ saliva production	↓ saliva production Dry mucous membranes
Lungs	Bronchospasm ↑ bronchial secretions	Bronchodilation
Heart	↓ heart rate Slows atrioventricular conduction	↑ heart rate Enhances atrioventricular conduction
Peripheral vasculature	Vasodilation (modest)	Vasoconstriction (very modest)
GI	↑ motility ↑ gastric acid production Produces emesis	↓ motility ↓ gastric acid production
Urinary	Stimulates bladder contraction and expulsion of urine	↓ bladder activity Promotes urinary retention
Skin	↑ sweat production	↓ sweat production (dry skin) Cutaneous vasodilation (flushed appearance)

syndrome refers to the clinical state when the central effects of muscarinic receptor antagonism predominate, with fever, agitation, delirium, and coma. The *peripheral anticholinergic syndrome* refers to the syndrome seen with peripheral muscarinic antagonism, such as tachycardia, flushed dry skin, dry mouth, ileus, and urinary retention.

The full range of clinical manifestations associated with anticholinergic overdose may only be partly explained by muscarinic receptor blockade. Many of these anticholinergic agents possess activity at other cell membrane receptors, and toxicity after overdose can be a mixture of multiple pharmacologic mechanisms. For example, the clinical findings associated with cyclic antidepressant overdose are only partly characterized by the anticholinergic effects that vary considerably among different cyclic antidepressants. The most life-threatening complications of cyclic antidepressant overdose are a result of the sodium-channel blocking effects on the heart, producing wide-complex tachydysrhythmias, not the anticholinergic effects.

Intravenous injection of antihistamines, particularly those affecting the H_1 histamine receptor antagonists (diphenhydramine), seems to cause euphoria in some patients. This effect may be attributed to the drug increasing dopamine levels in the nucleus accumbens area of the brain that stimulates the reward and motivation system.[23]

CLINICAL FEATURES

The classic features of the anticholinergic toxidrome can be stated as:

- Dry as a bone
- Red as a beet
- Hot as a hare
- Blind as a bat
- Mad as a hatter
- Stuffed as a pipe

Dry skin (especially dry axillae) and dry mucous membranes (e.g., dry mouth) are the typical peripheral clinical manifestations, the result of impaired sweat gland and salivary gland secretions, respectively. The skin may be warm and flushed (red) from cutaneous vasodilatation. Other typical peripheral features of muscarinic blockade include hypoactive or absent bowel sounds secondary to decreased peristalsis and GI motility. A palpable bladder or enlargement on bedside US secondary to urinary retention may be seen.

Sinus tachycardia is usually present. More malignant dysrhythmias are less common. Ingestions of large amounts of diphenhydramine have been associated with wide-complex tachydysrhythmias from a sodium-channel blocking effect and not from an anticholinergic effect.[24,25] Diphenhydramine overdose has been reported to cause QT-interval prolongation.[26,27] Dilated pupils are often a delayed clinical finding (12 to 24 hours) that may not be observed despite the presence of other anticholinergic signs.

The **delirium** of the central anticholinergic syndrome is characterized by restlessness, irritability, disorientation, confusion, agitation, auditory and visual hallucinations, and incoherent speech. The anticholinergic toxic patient has great difficulty interacting appropriately with environmental stimuli. Lilliputian ("little people") hallucinations have been described in this setting. Repetitive picking at the bed clothes or imaginary objects is also characteristic. A characteristic feature of anticholinergic delirium is dysarthria, manifested by a staccato speech pattern and difficult-to-comprehend speech. This may be exacerbated by severe dysphasia from decreased mucous secretion. High-pitched cries may sometimes be heard. Patients may also exhibit jerking movements of the extremities and seizures.

Although this delirium is usually accompanied by the peripheral manifestations discussed above, clinical presentations vary, and tachycardia without delirium or delirium without tachycardia may occur. "Agitated depression" can occur from both central excitation and depression. Depression is usually associated with higher doses, and features include lethargy, somnolence, and coma. Overdose with olanzapine, an atypical antipsychotic with significant anticholinergic properties, produces unpredictable fluctuations in mental status, from somnolence to agitation lasting hours.[28]

Agitation-induced hyperthermia is a worrisome complication of anticholinergic toxicity, and its development may be significantly potentiated by decreased sweating and the inability to dissipate heat. A markedly elevated body temperature may lead to multisystem organ dysfunction and rhabdomyolysis, resulting in liver, kidney, and brain injury and coagulopathy. Fatalities associated with anticholinergic overdose are characterized by severe agitation, status epilepticus, hyperthermia, wide-complex tachydysrhythmias (usually from sodium channel–blocker effect), and cardiovascular collapse.[29]

The risk of toxicity for most anticholinergic agents is dose related. For example, severity of diphenhydramine overdose correlates with the amount ingested, with moderate symptoms occurring after ingestion of 300 milligrams[30] and 7.5 milligrams/kg in children,[31] and severe symptoms seen only after ingestions of 1000 milligrams or more in adults.[30]

DIAGNOSIS

DRUG SCREENING

In patients with altered mental status, obtain routine laboratory evaluation, including measurement of electrolytes, glucose, creatine kinase, and pulse oximetry. In most cases of isolated anticholinergic toxicity, these tests should be normal. Limited urine drugs-of-abuse screening generally does not detect anticholinergic agents, although some rapid screens may produce positive results for cyclic antidepressants due to the structural similarities of some anticholinergic compounds, particularly diphenhydramine and hydroxyzine. Comprehensive urine drug screens, usually performed by thin layer chromatography or mass spectrometry, may detect most antihistamines and phenothiazines, although such testing does not usually detect plant alkaloids, scopolamine, or atropine. A positive drug screen for an anticholinergic agent only indicates exposure, such as a therapeutic dose, and does not necessarily imply an overdose or supratherapeutic ingestion.

DIFFERENTIAL DIAGNOSIS

The differential diagnosis of anticholinergic toxicity includes life-threatening presentations such as viral encephalitis, Reye's syndrome, head trauma, alcohol and sedative-hypnotic withdrawal, postictal state, other intoxications, neuroleptic malignant syndrome, and an acute psychotic disorder. The difference between anticholinergic toxicity and sympathomimetic toxicity (e.g., cocaine toxicity or delirium tremens) can be subtle, because patients with either may develop tachycardia, mydriasis, and delirium. The presence of red dry skin and the absence of bowel sounds suggest anticholinergic poisoning.[32] At times, patients presenting with acute psychotic disorders may have an abnormal mental status, suggesting anticholinergic toxicity, but true delirium and attention deficits are much more characteristic of the latter condition. Other CNS disorders, such as viral encephalitis, may also affect cholinergic outflow and produce similar anticholinergic clinical signs not related to a toxic exposure.[33]

TREATMENT

Treatment of anticholinergic toxicity primarily includes observation, monitoring, and good supportive care (**Table 202-4**). Temperature monitoring and treatment of hyperthermia are essential. GI decontamination with activated charcoal may be warranted to decrease absorption if the ingestion occurred within 1 hour. Although the benefit of activated charcoal is equivocal after 1 hour from ingestion, the decreased gut motility associated with anticholinergic ingestions may warrant charcoal administration beyond this 1-hour window.[34-36] Multidose activated charcoal is not recommended in patients with impaired GI motility, such as with anticholinergic toxicity.[37] Ipecac syrup is contraindicated in an anticholinergic overdose, and its use in any overdose patient should be abandoned.[31,38]

The major therapeutic challenge in the treatment of moderate to severe anticholinergic poisoning involves obtaining adequate control of the agitated individual. Inadequate sedation may lead to worsening hyperthermia, rhabdomyolysis, and traumatic injuries. Although physical restraints may be required to gain initial control, **pharmacologic sedation is strongly recommended**, because prolonged use of physical restraints in the struggling and agitated patient may lead to further complications.

Pharmacologic sedation should begin with IV administration of a benzodiazepine, such as lorazepam or diazepam. Benzodiazepines are not a specific antidote, and some patients may be refractory to large doses. Phenothiazines should be avoided because of their own anticholinergic effects. In severe cases of agitation when adequate sedation cannot be achieved without impairing respiration, mechanical ventilation and deep sedation may be necessary.

Intravenous sodium bicarbonate should be used to treat wide-complex tachydysrhythmias.[24,25] Class IA antiarrhythmic agents should be avoided because of their own sodium-channel blockade properties.

Physostigmine is a reversible acetylcholinesterase inhibitor (mechanistically related to the carbamate insecticides) that crosses the blood–brain barrier because of its lipophilic tertiary ammonium properties. Acetylcholinesterase inhibition results in acetylcholine accumulation that reverses both central and peripheral anticholinergic effects. Using physostigmine to reverse anticholinergic toxicity is controversial.[39,40]

The major adverse effects of physostigmine—profound bradycardia and seizures—were historically touted as common, but evidence for this belief is lacking.[41] Importantly, **the risk of these adverse effects appears greater in patients without anticholinergic toxicity, so accurate diagnosis of anticholinergic toxicity is important before administering physostigmine.**[40,41]

Evidence for benefits of physostigmine in anticholinergic toxicity is mixed. Retrospective analysis of 52 patients[42] and case reports[43-45] found that physostigmine was significantly better in controlling agitation and reversing delirium compared with benzodiazepines and was associated with fewer complications and a shorter recovery time. There was no difference in adverse effects between the two groups. Conversely, a different case series did not find that physostigmine use reduced complications or shortened length of stay in 17 patients with severe agitation and delirium after Jimson weed ingestion.[46] However, no adverse effects or complications were observed from physostigmine use.

Physostigmine can be used in cases of severe agitation and delirium from pure anticholinergic toxicity, especially in cases necessitating physical restraints and resistant to benzodiazepines. The adult dose of physostigmine is 0.5 to 2 milligrams (pediatric dose is 0.02 milligram/kg with a maximum dose of 2 milligrams) by slow IV administration over 5 minutes. When effective, a significant decrease in agitation may be apparent within 15 to 20 minutes. Provide continuous cardiac monitoring before and during administration of physostigmine to assess for potential bradycardia. Monitor the patient for signs of cholinergic excess, such as diarrhea, urination, miosis, bradycardia, bronchospasm, bronchorrhea, emesis, lacrimation, and salivation. **In cases of uncertain anticholinergic poisoning, a diagnostic challenge with physostigmine is *not* recommended because of the small but increased risk of adverse effects in patients *without* anticholinergic toxicity.**[40,41]

Physostigmine may be repeated in the same dose if required. Patients who remain asymptomatic for more than 6 hours after the first dose of physostigmine will not require repeat physostigmine dosing.[47] Contraindications to physostigmine use include asthma, nonpharmacologically mediated intestinal or bladder obstruction, cardiac conduction disturbances, and suspected concomitant sodium-channel antagonist poisoning.

DISPOSITION AND FOLLOW-UP

Patients with mild symptoms of anticholinergic toxicity that resolve after 6 hours of ED observation may be considered for disposition. Because the duration of action of physostigmine is generally shorter than the duration of action of many anticholinergic agents, the reversal effect may dissipate, resulting in recurrent toxicity. Most symptomatic patients, including those patients who have received physostigmine, require hospital observation for at least 24 hours.

REFERENCES

The complete reference list is available online at www.TintinalliEM.com.

TABLE 202-4 Treatment of Anticholinergic Toxicity

Action	Agent	Comments
GI decontamination	Activated charcoal	May be more effective due to the decreased GI motility.
Sedation	Benzodiazepines	Decreases the risk of hyperthermia, rhabdomyolysis, and traumatic injuries.
Wide-complex tachyarrhythmias	Sodium bicarbonate	Arrhythmia due to sodium-channel blockade; avoid class IA antiarrhythmics (procainamide).
Cholinesterase inhibition	Physostigmine	Use for cases of severe agitation or delirium; avoid when cardiac conduction abnormalities are present (see "Treatment" section).

CHAPTER 203 Metals and Metalloids

Heather Long
Lewis S. Nelson

INTRODUCTION

Acute metal and metalloid toxicity is uncommon but can cause significant morbidity and mortality if unrecognized and inappropriately treated. **Metals** are chemical elements that possess three general properties: (1) they are a good conductor of heat and electricity, (2) they are able to form cations, and (3) they can combine with nonmetals through ionic bonds. The term *heavy metal* has a historical tradition in clinical medicine, but has been criticized by chemists as lacking in a precise definition or scientific merit. An alternative term, *toxic metal*, which also lacks firm definition, is sometimes used instead. In clinical toxicology, the following metals, noted in ascending atomic weight, are usually considered under the concept of "heavy" or "toxic" metal poisoning: beryllium, vanadium, cadmium, barium, osmium, mercury, thallium, and lead, with lead and mercury being the metals most clinically significant concerning human poisoning.

Metalloids are chemical elements with properties intermediate to those of metals and nonmetals. Although there is no precise definition, metalloids tend to have these two general properties: (1) they are semiconductors of electricity, and (2) they form amphoteric oxides. In order of ascending atomic weight, the following elements are generally considered metalloids: boron, silicon, germanium, arsenic, antimony, tellurium, and polonium; arsenic is the most clinically significant metalloid.

Exposure to either metals or nonmetals can be from (1) the pure element, (2) an organic compound containing the toxic element (defined as those compounds that contain carbon), or (3) an inorganic compound containing the element (defined as those that do not contain carbon). Depending on the metal or metalloid, potential toxicity is affected by which chemical form is responsible for the exposure.

Because of their effects on numerous enzymatic systems in the body, the metals and metalloids often present with protean manifestations primarily affecting five systems: neurologic, cardiovascular, GI, hematologic, and renal. Effects on the endocrine and reproductive systems are less clinically apparent. **It is important to recognize an initial "index case" of metal poisoning to prevent others from being poisoned when the metal source is environmental or industrial (Table 203-1).**

TABLE 203-1 Sources of Metal and Metalloid Poisoning

Element	Source
Lead	
Elemental, inorganic	Soldering; battery burning/reclamation; bronzing; brass-making; glassmaking; ingesting ceramic lead glaze; stripping old paint; "deleading" homes; "moonshine" whiskey; liquids in improperly glazed pottery; contaminated herbal medications and cosmetics; indoor shooting ranges; ingestion of paint chips, lead-laden floor dust, lead foreign bodies; lead bullets in abdomen or joint spaces
	Workers at risk: jewelers, painters, lead burners and smelters, including stained glass designers, pipe cutters, pigment makers, printers, welders, pottery makers, radiator repair personnel, battery reclamation workers, construction workers
Organic	Leaded gasoline (tetraethyl lead)
Arsenic	
Inorganic (arsenite [trivalent] or arsenate [pentavalent])	Insecticides, rodenticides, herbicides, mining, smelting/refining, Ayurvedic and homeopathic medicines, well water contaminated by leaching mineral ores and/or industrial waste
Organic	Seafood, parasitical medicines (veterinary)
Gas (arsine)	Mining smelting/refining, semiconductor industry; made by mixing acids with arsenic-containing insecticides
Mercury	
Elemental	Battery and thermometer manufacture; sphygmomanometer repair; dentistry; jewelry and lamp manufacture; photography; mercury mining; manufacture of scientific instruments
Inorganic (mercury salts)	Cosmetic products, especially skin-lightening products; taxidermy; fur processing; tannery work; chemical laboratories; manufacture of explosives, fireworks, disinfectants, button batteries, inks, and vinyl chloride
Organic (methyl mercury, ethyl mercury, and phenyl mercury)	Contaminated seafood; embalming; manufacture of drugs, fungicides, bactericides; handling of insecticides; pesticides, coated seeds; use of chlor-alkali process; working with wood preservatives

LEAD

EPIDEMIOLOGY

Lead is the most common cause of chronic metal poisoning and remains a major environmental contaminant, especially in developing countries. Exposure to lead can occur from inhalation or ingestion, and both inorganic and organic forms of lead produce clinical toxicity. Nonpaint sources include foreign medications, herbal and dietary supplements, Ayurvedic medications, traditional remedies, metallic charms, and cosmetics, especially products from Asia and Africa.[1] Although no safe blood lead level has been identified, the Centers for Disease Control and Prevention reference value for an elevated level is ≥5 micrograms/dL (0.24 micromol/L).[2]

The United States has banned lead in household paints, gasoline, plumbing systems, food, and drink cans; created lead abatement programs; and enforced standards for industrial use of lead.[2,3] Elevated blood levels in children age 1 to 5 years old are associated with residence in urban dwellings, residence in dwellings built before 1974 (especially those built before 1946), poverty, non-Hispanic black race or ethnicity, and higher population density.[4] Chronic lead exposure and toxicity in children is a significant public health problem because of the effect on intellectual development.[5] Worldwide, 16% of all children are estimated to have lead levels >10 micrograms/dL (0.48 micromol/L). Common sources in low-income countries are substandard or marginal living conditions near landfills and industries such as smelters, mines, and refineries, and leaded gasoline. Child labor in highly polluted conditions is another source of exposure.[4] In developing countries, informal recycling of used lead-acid batteries and processing of gold ore rich in lead have caused mass lead poisonings.[6,7]

PHARMACOLOGY

Absorption of inorganic lead is usually via the respiratory and GI tracts; skin absorption is negligible. Dietary deficiencies in calcium, iron, copper, and zinc may contribute to increased GI absorption in children. There is usually minimal absorption of lead from bullets or shot lodged in bone or muscle, but increased absorption and toxicity have been reported when bullets or shot are in constant contact with body fluids, such as synovial fluid or cerebrospinal fluid. Absorption of organic lead can occur after inhalation, ingestion, and dermal exposure. Exposure to organic lead can occur from sniffing gasoline (see chapter 199, "Hydrocarbons and Volatile Substances"), which may contain tetraethyl lead ("leaded gasoline"). After absorption, tetraethyl lead is metabolized to inorganic lead and triethyl lead; the latter is responsible for the neurotoxicity from leaded gasoline.

Greater than 90% of the total body lead is stored in bone, where it easily exchanges with the blood. Lead can be transferred across the placenta, a process exacerbated by increased bone turnover during pregnancy. Excretion of lead occurs slowly; the biologic half-life of lead in bone has been estimated to be 30 years.

PATHOPHYSIOLOGY

Lead toxicity primarily affects the nervous, cardiovascular, hematopoietic, and renal systems. In the CNS, the toxic effects of lead include (1) injuries to astrocytes, with secondary damage to the microvasculature and resultant disruption of the blood–brain barrier, cerebral edema, and increased intracranial pressure; (2) decreases in cyclic adenosine monophosphate and protein phosphorylation, which contribute to memory and learning deficits; and (3) alteration with calcium homeostasis, which leads to spontaneous and uncontrolled neurotransmitter release.[8] In the peripheral nervous system, lead causes primary segmental demyelination, followed by secondary axonal degeneration, mostly of the motor nerves.[9]

In the cardiovascular system, small but statistically significant increases in the prevalence of hypertension and atherosclerotic vascular disease are found in individuals with elevated blood lead levels.

In the hematopoietic system, lead interferes with porphyrin metabolism, which may contribute to lead-induced anemia. Coexisting iron deficiency may act synergistically with lead toxicity to produce a more profound anemia and, in children, may be more important than lead as the cause of a microcytic anemia. Hemolytic anemia also occurs as a result of inhibition of red blood cell pyrimidine 5′-nucleotidase, an enzyme responsible for clearing cellular RNA degradation products.

In the kidney, lead affects the proximal tubule, producing Fanconi's syndrome with aminoaciduria, glycosuria, phosphaturia, and renal tubular acidosis.[10] Chronic interstitial nephritis and increased uric acid levels are due to increased tubular reabsorption of urate. Chronic lead toxicity has been linked to gout and chronic renal failure.

Lead adversely affects osteoblast and osteoclast function in bone. With chronic lead exposure, increased calcium deposition at growth plates may be seen as "**lead lines**" on radiographs of long bones. Lead-induced adverse effects on the reproductive system include increased fetal wastage, premature rupture of membranes, depressed sperm counts, abnormal or nonmotile sperm, and sterility.

CLINICAL FEATURES

Signs and symptoms of lead toxicity vary according to the type of exposure (acute vs chronic) and, to a lesser extent, according to the age of the individual and type of lead (inorganic vs organic) involved (**Table 203-2**). Young children are more susceptible than adults to the effects of lead. Encephalopathy, a major cause of morbidity and mortality, may begin dramatically with seizures and coma or develop indolently over weeks to months with decreased alertness and memory progressing to mania and delirium.[11] Encephalopathy due to lead poisoning typically occurs in toddlers age 15 to 30 months old with blood lead levels >100 micrograms/dL (4.8 micromol/L) but has been reported with blood lead levels of 70 micrograms/dL (3.4 micromol/L) or lower.

GI and hematologic manifestations occur more frequently with acute than with chronic poisoning, and the colicky abdominal pains may be associated with concurrent hemolysis. Patients may complain of a metallic taste and, with long-term exposure, have bluish-gray gingival lead lines. Lead toxicity also causes constitutional symptoms, including arthralgias, generalized weakness, and weight loss. Delayed cognitive development can occur in infants and children whose blood lead levels are 10 micrograms/dL (0.48 micromol/L) or higher.[12] Conversely, adult and pediatric patients may be asymptomatic in the face of significantly elevated blood lead levels.

With organic lead poisoning, neurologic abnormalities predominate. Symptoms range from behavioral changes, with irritability, insomnia, restlessness, and nausea and vomiting, to tremor, chorea, convulsions, and mania.

DIAGNOSIS

Exposure history, whether occupational or environmental, related to recent travel or immigration, a hobby, or a retained lead bullet, is the most important clue in making the diagnosis. The clinician should focus on symptoms, developmental and dietary histories (in children), pica, and any house or day care remodeling. Occupational, travel, medication, dietary supplement, cosmetic, and hobby histories should be elicited for adults being evaluated and for children who may be exposed to lead secondarily from these adult activities. Toxicity due to retained lead bullets may manifest several decades after being shot. Hyperthyroidism, pregnancy, fever, reinjury, or immobilization of the affected extremity can promote lead release from these retained objects after years of dormancy. **The combination of abdominal or neurologic dysfunction with a hemolysis should raise suspicion for lead toxicity. Consider the diagnosis in all children presenting with encephalopathy.**

The definitive diagnosis rests on finding an elevated blood lead level, with or without symptoms. The blood lead level is the best single test for evaluating lead toxicity, and levels at or >5 micrograms/dL (0.24 micromol/L) are considered elevated in children. Screening may be performed on fingerstick capillary blood, but because of the potential for environmental lead contamination, elevated levels always should be confirmed on a venous blood sample.[13] The edetate calcium disodium provocation test and testing for erythrocyte protoporphyrin (e.g., free erythrocyte protoporphyrin, zinc protoporphyrin) are no longer recommended.

Although it is important to order a blood lead level for confirmatory diagnosis and assistance in monitoring therapy, the laboratory turnaround time for results may be days. **Diagnostic studies in the ED should therefore focus on evaluation for anemia and examination of radiographs for evidence of lead exposure.**

The anemia from lead toxicity can be normocytic or microcytic, possibly with evidence of hemolysis, such as an elevated reticulocyte count and increased serum-free hemoglobin. Basophilic stippling in red blood cells from impaired clearing of cellular RNA degradation products is sometimes seen in lead-poisoned patients. This finding is nonspecific for lead toxicity; it is also found in arsenic toxicity, sideroblastic anemia, and the thalassemias. **Anemia and basophilic stippling occur variably, and their absence does not exclude lead toxicity.**

Following acute or subacute ingestion of lead, abdominal radiographs may show radiopaque material in the GI tract. In children, radiographs of long bones, especially of the knee, may reveal horizontal, metaphyseal "lead lines," which represent failure of bone remodeling rather than deposition of lead.

The differential diagnosis of lead toxicity includes causes of encephalopathy, such as Wernicke's encephalopathy; withdrawal from ethanol and other sedative-hypnotic drugs; meningitis; encephalitis; human immunodeficiency virus infection; intracerebral hemorrhage; hypoglycemia; severe fluid and electrolyte imbalances; hypoxia; arsenic, thallium, and mercury toxicity; and poisoning with cyclic antidepressants, anticholinergic drugs, ethylene glycol, or carbon monoxide. The abdominal pains of lead toxicity can mimic sickle cell crisis, the hepatic porphyrias, and even appendicitis. Chronic lead toxicity can mimic major depression, hypothyroidism, polyneuritis, gout, iron deficiency anemia, and learning disability.

TABLE 203-2 Clinical Features of Lead Poisoning

System	Clinical Manifestations
CNS	Acute toxicity: encephalopathy, seizures, altered mental status, papilledema, optic neuritis, ataxia
	Chronic toxicity: headache, irritability, depression, fatigue, mood and behavioral changes, memory deficit, sleep disturbance
Peripheral nervous system	Paresthesias, motor weakness (classic is wrist drop), depressed or absent deep tendon reflexes, sensory function intact
GI	Abdominal pain (mostly with acute poisoning), constipation, diarrhea, toxic hepatitis
Renal	Acute toxicity: Fanconi's syndrome (renal tubular acidosis with aminoaciduria, glucosuria, and phosphaturia)
	Chronic toxicity: interstitial nephritis, renal insufficiency, hypertension, gout
Hematologic	Hypoproliferative and/or hemolytic anemia; basophilic stippling (rare and nonspecific)
Reproductive	Decreased libido, impotence, sterility, abortions, premature births, decreased or abnormal sperm production

TREATMENT

Patients with appropriate signs and symptoms and an elevated blood lead level are classified as lead toxic and should be treated.

Lead-induced encephalopathy is rare but causes serious morbidity and mortality. In severely toxic patients, standard life support measures should be instituted. Seizures are treated with benzodiazepines and general anesthesia, if necessary. Lumbar puncture may precipitate cerebral herniation and should be performed carefully, if at all, with the removal of only a small amount of cerebrospinal fluid. If lead encephalopathy is suspected, initiate chelation therapy promptly (i.e., in the ED) without waiting for the results of a blood lead level (**Table 203-3**). If abdominal films demonstrate radiopaque flecks consistent with lead, whole-bowel irrigation with a polyethylene glycol electrolyte solution should be instituted. Larger lead bodies, such as fishing sinkers and jewelry, may require endoscopic or surgical removal.

Chelation therapy for lead toxicity uses dimercaprol (previously known as *British anti-Lewisite*), edetate calcium disodium (sometimes

TABLE 203-3 Guidelines for Chelation Therapy in Lead-Poisoned Patients*

Severity (blood lead level [micrograms/dL])	Dose
Encephalopathy	Dimercaprol, 75 milligrams/m² (or 4 milligrams/kg) IM every 4 h for 5 d *and* Edetate calcium disodium, 1500 milligrams/m² per day via continuous infusion or in 2–4 divided doses IV for 5 d; start 4 h after dimercaprol
Symptomatic and/or Adults: blood lead >100 Children: blood lead >69	Dimercaprol *and* Edetate calcium disodium (as described above) *or* Edetate calcium disodium (alone) *or* Succimer (as described below)
Asymptomatic Adults: blood lead 70–100 Children: blood lead 45–69	Succimer, 350 milligrams/m² (or 10 milligrams/kg) PO every 8 h for 5 d, then every 12 h for 14 d
Asymptomatic Adults: blood lead <70 Children: blood lead <45	Routine chelation not indicated; remove patient from source of exposure

*General guidelines. Consult with medical toxicologist or regional poison center for specifics and dosing.

abbreviated *CaNa₂-EDTA*), and succimer (also known as *dimercaptosuccinic acid*) (Table 203-3). Another chelating agent, penicillamine, has not received approval for use in the treatment of lead toxicity by the U.S. Food and Drug Administration, but there is published experience demonstrating benefit, and penicillamine is used in Europe for lead poisoning. **The chelation dosing schedules are guided by the blood lead levels, the presence or absence of symptoms, and the age of the patient.** Adverse side effects from chelation therapy are common, and consultation with a medical toxicologist is recommended to assist in management.

Dimercaprol crosses the blood–brain barrier and is indicated when neurotoxicity or high blood lead levels are present. Dimercaprol is administered IM and is typically used with edetate calcium disodium to prevent lead from being transported into the brain. **The diluent for dimercaprol includes peanut oil, and therefore, dimercaprol should be used with great caution in patients with peanut allergy.** Side effects of dimercaprol include hypertension; fever, pain, and sterile abscess at injection site; nausea; vomiting; diarrhea; abdominal pain; headache; lacrimation; rhinorrhea; and hemolysis in glucose-6-phosphate dehydrogenase–deficient patients. Side effects with dimercaprol are dose dependent and occur in up to 65% of treated patients using recommended doses.

Edetate calcium disodium can be used as a single agent in the treatment of lead toxicity, although there is some concern that mobilization of lead from bone by this agent may lead to increased transport of lead into the brain. Edetate calcium disodium does not cross the blood–brain barrier, and therefore, dimercaprol, which does cross, should be given before and during the entire course of edetate calcium disodium when there are CNS symptoms. **An important precaution is to not confuse this product for treatment of lead toxicity with edetate disodium, used to treat hypercalcemia.** This confusion can lead to serious toxicity and even death, if the wrong drug is used. Side effects from edetate calcium disodium include renal toxicity (especially if dehydrated), dermatitis, headache, fever, chills, and myalgias.

Succimer, an oral analog of dimercaprol, effectively chelates lead. Although succimer does not cross the blood–brain barrier, its use as a sole agent is not associated with exacerbation of lead-induced encephalopathy.[14] Some toxicologists consider succimer the preferred chelator for lead poisoning in all but the most severe cases. Its advantages include oral administration without increasing lead absorption from the GI tract, no serious adverse effects, and minimal chelation of essential metals. Repeat treatment may be necessary after a 2-week drug-free period. Side effects from succimer include nausea, vomiting, diarrhea, abdominal pain, rash, pruritus, sore throat, rhinorrhea, drowsiness, paresthesias, transient elevations in serum transaminases and alkaline phosphatase, thrombocytosis, and eosinophilia.

Chelation was not associated with any increased risk of birth defects in the few published cases, and pregnant women with elevated blood lead levels should be chelated following the same guidelines (Table 203-3).[15] Neonatal blood lead levels may be elevated despite maternal chelation, and similarly, neonates should also be chelated following birth.

DISPOSITION AND FOLLOW-UP

Removal of the source of lead is the most important action for all individuals with lead poisoning, and patients should not be returned to their former environments until appropriate lead decontamination and abatement measures have been addressed. Family members and coworkers should be evaluated for occult lead toxicity. Hospital admission is recommended for (1) children with symptoms or with a blood lead level >70 micrograms/dL (>3.4 micromol/L), (2) adults with central neurologic symptoms, and (3) patients with suspected lead toxicity when returning to the environment is considered dangerous.

Approximately 85% of patients who suffer lead-toxic encephalopathy develop permanent central neurologic damage, including seizures, mental retardation in children, and cognitive deficits in adults. Abdominal colic usually subsides within days after beginning chelation therapy, and other acute manifestations clear within 1 to 16 weeks with therapy. Lead-induced nephropathy may be partly reversible with chelation therapy.

ARSENIC

EPIDEMIOLOGY

Arsenic is a nearly tasteless, odorless metalloid that causes significant acute and chronic toxicity worldwide.[16] Arsenicals are found in a variety of compounds and industries (Table 203-1) and continue to be used as a means for homicide and suicide.

Arsenic exists in elemental, inorganic salts, organic salts, and gaseous forms. Elemental and organic forms have little to no toxicity, whereas inorganic compounds, including arsenite (trivalent or As^{3+}) and arsenate (pentavalent or As^{5+}), are highly toxic. Arsine is a colorless, nonirritating toxic gas encountered in the semiconductor industry, ore smelting, and refining processes and is produced when arsenic-containing insecticides are mixed with acids.

PHARMACOLOGY

Arsenic is well absorbed by GI, respiratory, and parenteral routes and may be absorbed through nonintact skin. Due to its water solubility, pentavalent arsenic (arsenate) is more readily absorbed through mucous membranes, such as the GI tract, than is trivalent arsenic (arsenite), which penetrates the skin more readily due to its increased lipid solubility. After absorption, arsenic localizes in erythrocytes and leukocytes or binds to serum proteins. Within 24 hours, redistribution into the liver, kidney, spleen, lung, GI tract, muscle, and nervous tissues occurs, with subsequent integration into hair, nails, and bone. Elimination from the blood is rapid, and excretion is predominantly renal. Toxicity of the various forms is partly determined by excretory rates, with the more toxic arsenite being excreted at a slower rate than arsenate or the organic arsenical compounds. Arsenic crosses the placenta and is teratogenic in animals and humans.

PATHOPHYSIOLOGY

Ingested or absorbed arsenic reversibly binds with sulfhydryl groups found in many tissues and enzyme systems. Acute exposure produces dilatation and increased permeability of small blood vessels, resulting in GI mucosal and submucosal inflammation and necrosis, cerebral edema and hemorrhage, myocardial tissue destruction, and fatty degeneration of the liver and kidneys. Subacute or chronic exposure can cause a primary peripheral axonal neuropathy with secondary demyelination. Inhaled arsine attaches to sulfhydryl groups of hemoglobin, producing an acute hemolytic anemia with resulting jaundice, abdominal pain, and hemoglobinuria-induced acute renal failure.[17]

CLINICAL FEATURES

The signs and symptoms of toxicity vary with the form, amount, and concentration ingested and the rates of absorption and excretion of the various arsenical compounds (**Table 203-4**).

With acute toxicity, clinical effects usually develop within minutes to hours of ingestion. Severe gastroenteritis with nausea, vomiting, and cholera-like diarrhea is the hallmark of acute poisoning and may last several days to weeks, frequently necessitating hospitalization. Patients may complain of a metallic taste. Hypotension and tachycardia secondary to volume depletion, capillary leak, and myocardial dysfunction occur in moderate to severe cases. The ECG may demonstrate nonspecific ST-segment and T-wave changes with a prolonged QT interval, although these findings are more common in chronic intoxication. Ventricular tachycardia with a *torsade de pointes* morphology has been reported.[18] Secondary myocardial ischemia may occur, leading to an erroneous diagnosis of primary myocardial infarction. Acute encephalopathy, acute respiratory distress syndrome, acute kidney injury, and rhabdomyolysis may ensue.

Survivors of acute poisonings and patients who are poisoned slowly may develop subacute toxicity, typically presenting with complaints of weakness, muscle aches, abdominal pain, memory loss, personality changes, periorbital and extremity edema, or skin rash, often with a history of gastroenteritis occurring 1 to 6 weeks earlier.[19] Central neurologic symptoms include headache, confusion, delirium, and personality changes. Chronic encephalopathy with delirium, hallucinations, disorientation, agitation, and confabulation resembling Korsakoff's syndrome may occur. Peripheral neuropathy develops in a stocking-glove distribution and is initially sensory, with motor symptoms developing later. Patients with severe poisoning can develop an ascending paralysis mimicking Guillain-Barré syndrome. Dermatologic manifestations vary and include morbilliform rash, alopecia, and desquamation. Mees lines (1- to 2-mm–wide transverse white lines in the nails) due to disrupted keratinization of the nail matrix may be seen 4 to 6 weeks after an acute ingestion.

Chronic toxicity from arsenic occurs with ongoing low-level occupational or environmental exposure and has been linked to the development of hypertension, peripheral vascular disease, diabetes mellitus, epidermoid cancer, respiratory tract cancer, hepatic angiosarcoma, and, possibly, leukemia. Dermatologic manifestations are prominent and include hyperpigmentation, hyperkeratosis of the palms and soles, Bowen's disease, and squamous and basal cell carcinomas. Perforation of the nasal septum has been found in workers exposed occupationally to arsenic.

TABLE 203-4 Clinical Features of Arsenic Toxicity

Onset of Symptoms	Clinical Features
Acute toxicity (10 min to several hours)	GI: nausea, vomiting, cholera-like diarrhea
	Cardiovascular: hypotension; tachycardia; dysrhythmias, including torsade de pointes; secondary myocardial ischemia
	Pulmonary: acute respiratory distress syndrome
	Renal: acute renal failure
	Central neurologic: encephalopathy
Subacute toxicity (1–3 wk after acute exposure or with chronic exposure)	Central neurologic: headache, confusion, delirium, personality changes
	Peripheral neurologic: sensory and motor neuropathy
	Cardiovascular: QT-interval prolongation
	Pulmonary: cough, alveolar infiltrates
	Dermatologic: rash, alopecia, Mees lines
Chronic toxicity (ongoing low-level occupational or environmental exposure)	Dermatologic: hyperpigmentation, keratoses, Bowen's disease, squamous and basal cell carcinoma
	Cardiovascular: hypertension, peripheral arterial disease
	Endocrine: diabetes mellitus
	Oncologic: lung and skin cancer

DIAGNOSIS

The diagnosis is easily missed without a history of known exposure to arsenic. Physicians rarely encounter arsenic toxicity, and unfortunately, criminal poisonings often go undetected. The diagnosis of **acute arsenic poisoning should be considered in a patient with hypotension that was preceded by severe gastroenteritis**. The diagnosis of chronic arsenic toxicity should be considered in a patient with a peripheral neuropathy, typical skin manifestations, or recurrent bouts of unexplained gastroenteritis.

An abdominal radiograph may demonstrate intestinal radiopaque metallic flecks in cases of arsenic ingestions. The ECG often reveals a prolonged QT interval, especially in subacute poisoning. The CBC may reveal a normocytic, normochromic, or megaloblastic anemia, and/or a thrombocytopenia. The WBC count may be elevated in acute toxicity and decreased in chronic toxicity. A relative eosinophilia and red cell basophilic stippling may be observed. Elevated reticulocyte counts are found in cases with a component of hemolytic anemia.

Definitive diagnosis of acute poisoning depends on finding elevated arsenic levels in a 24-hour urine collection. All urinary measurements of metals should be collected in metal-free containers after a 5-day seafood-free diet. Normal urinary arsenic level is below 50 micrograms/L (0.67 micromol/L), and total urinary arsenic excretion in an unexposed patient typically does not exceed 100 micrograms/d (1.3 micromol/d). If the baseline urinary level is within normal limits and arsenic intoxication is still suspected, hair and nail clippings should be harvested for laboratory analysis. Due to the rapid distribution of arsenic in tissues, blood arsenic levels are unreliable.

Include arsenic toxicity in the differential diagnosis for septic shock, encephalopathy, peripheral neuropathy (including Guillain-Barré syndrome), Addison's disease, hypo- and hyperthyroidism, patients with the previously mentioned dermatologic manifestations, Korsakoff's syndrome, persistent gastroenteritis and/or cholera-like diarrhea, porphyria, other metal toxicities such as thallium and mercury, and unexplained, prolonged malaise and weakness.

TREATMENT

Acute arsenic toxicity is a life-threatening illness requiring aggressive management. The first task is to stabilize circulatory function, because hypotension and dysrhythmias are the chief causes of death. Hypotension, usually due to volume depletion, should be managed initially with crystalloid volume replacement, and vasopressor therapy with dopamine or norepinephrine may be required. Overhydration should be avoided because pulmonary and cerebral edema can occur. Ventricular tachycardia and fibrillation may be treated with lidocaine, amiodarone, and electrical defibrillation as necessary. Magnesium sulfate, isoproterenol, and overdrive pacing therapies should be considered for torsade de pointes. Drugs that prolong the QT interval, including classes IA (procainamide, quinidine, and disopyramide), IC, and III antidysrhythmics, should be avoided. Potassium, calcium, and magnesium levels should be monitored and corrected as necessary to prevent further prolongation of the QT interval and exacerbation of torsade de pointes dysrhythmias.

Gastric lavage with a large-bore orogastric tube should be performed in cases of acute ingestion, and activated charcoal, although it poorly adsorbs arsenic, may be effective if co-ingestants were taken. Whole-bowel irrigation should be considered if abdominal radiographs reveal intestinal radiopaque materials consistent with arsenic. Seizures can be treated with benzodiazepines and general anesthesia as necessary.

Initial management of chronic toxicity should be directed toward prevention of further arsenic absorption and GI decontamination, if appropriate. In cases of suspected homicidal intent, patients should be

TABLE 203-5 Guidelines for Chelation Therapy in Arsenic-Poisoned Patients

Chelator	Dose
Dimercaprol	3–5 milligrams/kg IM every 4 h for 2 d, followed by 3–5 milligrams/kg IM every 6–12 h until able to switch to succimer
Succimer	10 milligrams/kg PO every 8 h for 5 d, followed by 10 milligrams/kg PO every 12 h

advised to avoid food and drinks prepared by others, and visitor contact with hospitalized patients should be monitored carefully.

Chelation therapy for arsenic toxicity uses dimercaprol or succimer (**Table 203-5**). Treat patients with acute arsenical poisoning or severe, life-threatening toxicity with dimercaprol until the clinical condition stabilizes and succimer, the less toxic oral chelating agent, can be substituted.[20] **Do not delay chelation in severely ill patients until laboratory confirmation because chelation is most effective when given within minutes to hours of exposure.** Conversely, hold chelation therapy in clinically stable patients with suspected chronic arsenic toxicity pending diagnosis. Chelation with the oral agent succimer may lower the tissue content of arsenic and speed urinary excretion but does not appear to decrease morbidity or mortality in chronic arsenic poisoning.[20] Early consultation with a regional poison control center or medical toxicologist for assistance with treatment and chelation is recommended.

Patients with acute arsine poisoning are managed with blood transfusions, exchange transfusion to remove the nondialyzable arsine, and hemodialysis for the acute kidney injury.[17] Chelation therapy has no role in the management of arsine toxicity.

DISPOSITION AND FOLLOW-UP

Hospitalization is recommended for (1) patients with acute or life-threatening known or suspected arsenic poisoning, (2) chronically poisoned patients requiring dimercaprol therapy, and (3) patients in whom suicidal or homicidal intent is suspected. In patients with acute arsenic toxicity, prognosis may be influenced favorably by the rapid institution of dimercaprol therapy. Recovery from arsenical neuropathy appears to be related more to the initial severity of symptoms than to institution of chelation therapy, although in patients who do recover, dimercaprol appears to significantly shorten the duration of illness. Often, neurologic recovery occurs slowly over months to years. Normalization of hematologic values can occur in the absence of any specific therapy. Dermatologic manifestations of chronic toxicity are unresponsive to chelation.[20]

MERCURY

EPIDEMIOLOGY

Mercury occurs in inorganic and organic forms. Inorganic mercury compounds are subdivided into elemental mercury (quicksilver), mercurous (Hg^{+}) salts (e.g., mercurous chloride or calomel), and mercuric (Hg^{2+}) salts (e.g., cinnabar or mercuric sulfide). Organic mercurials exist as short- and long-chained alkyl and aryl compounds. The short-chained alkyls, such as methyl mercury and ethyl mercury, are more toxic to humans, with dimethyl mercury being lethal in small amounts. All forms of mercury are toxic but differ in the means of exposure, routes of absorption, constellations of clinical findings, and responses to therapy (Table 203-1).[21,22]

PHARMACOLOGY

Elemental mercury is absorbed primarily by vapor inhalation. Vacuuming elemental mercury, as from a broken thermometer or fluorescent light bulb, causes volatilization due to both the heat and the airflow through the canister. Absorption by the GI tract is usually negligible so that **swallowing mercury contained in a glass thermometer (elemental mercury) does not produce adverse effects unless the mucosa is damaged.** Elemental mercury can be absorbed dermally. IM injections of mercury can induce abscess and granuloma formation. Slow absorption and delayed systemic toxicity after IM injections of elemental mercury have been reported.[23] IV injections have produced mercury pulmonary and systemic emboli.[24] Elemental mercury crosses the blood–brain barrier, where it is ionized and trapped in the CNS.

Inorganic mercury salts are absorbed primarily through the GI tract, but they may also be absorbed across intact skin.[25] Mercuric salts deposit in the ionized form primarily in the kidney, followed by the liver and spleen. Mercury salts do not enter the CNS in consequential amounts nor do they cross the placenta.

Organic mercury compounds are also primarily absorbed by the GI tract. The highly lipid-soluble short-chained alkyls easily cross membranes, accumulating in red blood cells, the CNS, liver, kidney, and fetus. Longer-chained alkyl and the aryl compounds are biotransformed into inorganic mercuric ions in the body. Therefore, toxicity with these compounds more closely resembles inorganic mercury toxicity.

Inorganic and the aryl organic mercurials are eliminated in the urine and feces. The short-chained alkyl compounds are excreted primarily in the bile, where they undergo significant enterohepatic circulation.

PATHOPHYSIOLOGY

Mercury binds with sulfhydryl groups, affecting a diverse number of enzyme and protein systems. Methyl mercury also inhibits choline acetyl transferase, which catalyzes the final step in the production of acetylcholine and may produce symptoms of acetylcholine deficiency.[26] Mercuric salts produce proximal renal tubular necrosis.[21]

CLINICAL FEATURES

The clinical effects of mercury poisoning depend on the form and, in some cases, the route of administration.[21,22] In general, the neurologic, GI, and renal systems are predominantly affected.

Elemental Mercury Acute symptoms following inhalation of elemental mercury vapor include shortness of breath, fever/chills, cough, nausea, vomiting, diarrhea, metallic taste, headaches, weakness, and blurry vision. In severe cases, patients may develop acute lung injury and severe respiratory distress. Following metabolism of ingested or injected elemental mercury to inorganic salts, patients may also develop signs of inorganic mercury toxicity, including tremor and renal failure.

Inorganic Mercury Mercury salts are caustic, and an acute ingestion produces a severe hemorrhagic gastroenteritis with abdominal pain often associated with a characteristic graying of the oral mucosa and metallic taste. Shock and cardiovascular collapse may rapidly ensue. Acute kidney injury results from both direct toxicity of the mercury ions and from decreased renal perfusion due to shock.

GI symptoms of chronic inorganic mercury toxicity include metallic taste, burning sensation in the mouth, loose teeth, mucosal lesions and fissures, excessive salivation, and nausea. Hallmarks of chronic neurologic toxicity include tremor, neurasthenia, and erethism.[21,22] *Neurasthenia* is characterized by fatigue, depression, headaches, and difficulty concentrating. *Erethism* refers to behavioral changes characterized by shyness, emotional lability, irritability, insomnia, and delirium. Chronic renal toxicity ranges from reversible proteinuria to the nephrotic syndrome. Acrodynia, also known as *pink disease*, is an immune-mediated reaction characterized by a generalized rash; edema and erythema of the palms, soles, and face; excessive sweating; fever; irritability; splenomegaly; and generalized hypotonia with particular weakness of the pelvic and pectoral muscles.

Organic Mercury The short-chained alkyl compounds, methyl, dimethyl, and ethyl mercury, have the most devastating effects on the CNS. After a latent period of weeks to months, orofacial paresthesias are a common initial symptom, followed by headache, tremor, and fatigue. In severe cases, patients may develop ataxia, muscle rigidity and spasticity, blindness, hearing deficits, and dementia.[21,22] Although less prominent than the neurotoxicity, mild GI, renal, and pulmonary abnormalities may develop with organic mercury poisoning.

DIAGNOSIS

An occupational exposure history, in either the index patient or a household member, along with typical physical findings, especially tremor or a constellation of signs and symptoms suggesting erethism or acrodynia,

TABLE 203-6 Guidelines for Chelation Therapy in Mercury-Poisoned Patients

	Elemental and Inorganic Mercury	Organic Mercury
Severe acute poisoning	Dimercaprol, 5 milligrams/kg IM every 4 h for 2 d, followed by 2.5 milligrams/kg IM every 6 h for 2 d, followed by 2.5 milligrams/kg IM every 12–24 h until clinical improvement occurs or until able to switch to succimer therapy	Succimer, 10 milligrams/kg PO every 8 h for 5 d, then every 12 h for 14 d
Mild acute poisoning and chronic poisoning	Succimer, 10 milligrams/kg PO every 8 h for 5 d, then every 12 h for 14 d	No proven benefit for chelation therapy

suggests mercury toxicity. Ingestion of mercuric chloride can produce a rapidly fatal course and should be considered in a patient presenting with a corrosive gastroenteritis.[27] Often, however, the diagnosis of mercury toxicity is subtle, arrived at only after many other diagnoses have been investigated.

For poisoning from all forms of mercury, except short-chained alkyls, a 24-hour urinary measurement of mercury should be performed after a 5-day seafood-free diet. A seafood meal (contaminated with mercury) can temporarily elevate the mercury level to the toxic range until the mercury is eliminated. Most unexposed individuals will have 24-hour urine mercury levels <10 to 15 micrograms/L (<0.05 to 0.075 micromol/L). A level >20 micrograms/L (>0.1 micromol/L) may indicate meaningful exposure.

Short-chained alkyl mercury compounds are excreted predominantly by the bile, rendering urinary measurements invalid to assess toxicity from these agents. Laboratory diagnosis after this exposure rests on finding elevated whole-blood mercury levels, because these compounds concentrate in erythrocytes. Whole-blood mercury levels are normally <5 micrograms/L (<0.025 micromol/L).

Although elevated blood or urine values are necessary to confirm the diagnosis, they correlate poorly with toxicity and are unable to distinguish the asymptomatic exposure from mercury poisoning. Furthermore, because of significant redistribution within the body, blood or urine levels do not represent total-body burden. They are most useful in confirming exposure and in following the effects of chelation therapy (see "Treatment," below).

MRI findings in methyl mercury toxicity from ingestion of contaminated seafood include marked atrophy of the visual cortex, cerebellar vermis and hemispheres, and postcentral cortex.[28]

Behavioral changes or tremor similar to those caused by mercury can be seen with hypothyroidism, apathetic hyperthyroidism, metabolic encephalopathy, senile dementia, adverse effects of therapeutic drugs (such as lithium, theophylline, or phenytoin), Parkinson's disease, delayed neuropsychiatric sequelae of carbon monoxide poisoning, lacunar infarction, cerebellar degenerative disease or tumor, and ethanol or

TABLE 203-7 Miscellaneous Metal Poisoning: Unique Manifestations and Treatments of Patients Poisoned by Less Common Metals

Metal	Poisoning Source	Acute Clinical Manifestations	Chronic Clinical Manifestations	Specific Treatment
Bismuth	Antidiarrheals (bismuth subsalicylate), impregnated surgical packing paste	Abdominal pain, acute renal failure	Myoclonic encephalopathy	Dimercaprol (limited evidence)
Cadmium	Contaminated soil in cadmium-rich areas; alloys used in welding, soldering, jewelry, and batteries	Ingestion: hemorrhagic gastroenteritis Inhalation: pneumonitis, acute respiratory distress syndrome	Proteinuria, osteomalacia (itai-itai or ouch-ouch disease), lung cancer (questionable)	Ingestion: succimer (limited evidence; not generally indicated) Pneumonitis: chelation not indicated
Chromium	Corrosion inhibitors (e.g., heating systems), pigment production, leather tanning, metal finishing, dietary supplements, prosthetic joints	Skin irritation and ulceration, contact dermatitis; GI irritation, renal and pulmonary failure	Mucous membrane irritation, perforation of nasal septum, chronic cough, contact dermatitis, skin ulcers ("chrome holes"), lung cancer	Acetylcysteine (animal studies suggest efficacy as chelator)
Cobalt	"Hard metal dust" (tungsten–cobalt mixture), flexible magnets, drying agents, prosthetic joints	Contact dermatitis, asthma	Hard metal lung disease (spectrum ranging from alveolitis to fibrosis), cardiomyopathy, thyroid hyperplasia	Acetylcysteine (animal studies suggest efficacy as chelator)
Copper	Leaching from copper pipes and containers; fungicide (copper sulfate); welding (copper oxide)	Ingestion: resembles iron poisoning; blue vomitus (copper salts), hepatotoxicity, hemolysis, methemoglobinemia Inhalation: metal fume fever (self-limited fever, chills, cough, dyspnea)	Hepatotoxicity (childhood cirrhosis or idiopathic copper toxicosis)	Dimercaprol for hepatic or hematologic toxicity Succimer in mild poisoning
Silver	Colloidal (metallic) silver used for medicinal purposes as oral solutions, aerosols, and douches; cauterizing and antiseptic agent (silver nitrate); jewelry, wire	Mucosal irritation (silver oxide and nitrate)	Argyria (permanent skin discoloration due to silver deposition and melanocyte stimulation)	Selenium (possible role)
Thallium	Rodenticides (use prohibited in the United States); contaminated herbal products; medical radioisotope (miniscule dose); most poisonings related to homicide	Early: nausea, vomiting, abdominal pain, tachycardia Intermediate (>24 h): painful ascending neuropathy, cardiac dysrhythmias, altered mental status Delayed (2 wk): alopecia	Sensorimotor neuropathy, psychosis, dermatitis, hepatotoxicity	Multidose activated charcoal Prussian blue, 125 milligrams/kg PO every 12 h (usually dissolved in 50 mL of 15% mannitol)
Zinc	Smelting, electroplating, military smoke bombs, zinc lozenges, welding/galvanizing (zinc oxide)	Ingestion: nausea, vomiting, abdominal pain (resembles iron poisoning) Inhalation: mucosal irritation, metal fume fever (zinc oxide)	Copper deficiency, sideroblastic anemia, neutropenia	Edetate calcium disodium Supportive care for metal fume fever

sedative-hypnotic drug withdrawal. Corrosive gastroenteritis can be caused by iron, arsenic, phosphorus, acids, or alkali ingestion. Cerebral palsy, intrauterine hypoxia, and teratogenic effects of therapeutic and illicit drugs and environmental contaminants should be considered when evaluating an infant thought to be affected in utero by short-chained alkyl mercury compounds.

TREATMENT

General therapeutic measures include removal from exposure and supportive therapy, including supplemental oxygen and IV hydration. Hemodialysis does not enhance mercury clearance but may be indicated for treatment of acute kidney injury.

For **elemental mercury**, the severe respiratory failure following inhalation of volatilized elemental mercury or aspiration of elemental mercury may require endotracheal intubation and positive-pressure ventilation.

For ingestion of **inorganic mercury salts**, treat with aggressive IV hydration and GI decontamination, including gastric lavage if the patient has not had significant emesis, and consider activated charcoal. Given the profuse diarrhea that may ensue, a cathartic is not indicated.

For **organic mercury** toxicity, institute gastric decontamination in the setting of acute ingestion. Neostigmine may improve motor function in methyl mercury–poisoned patients by improving acetylcholine levels at the neuromuscular junction.[26]

Chelation is indicated if it can be given within a few hours after ingestion of mercury salts.[20] Chelation therapy for chronic exposures, especially to organic mercury, is much less effective. A history of significant mercury exposure, signs and symptoms consistent with mercury poisoning, and elevated blood or urine mercury levels may assist in the decision making and help determine duration of treatment for chronic mercury toxicity. Dimercaprol and succimer are the preferred chelators for mercury poisoning (**Table 203-6**).

The chelation regimen is adjusted according to clinical response and development of adverse reactions. Adverse reactions with dimercaprol increase with dose and include nausea, vomiting, headache, paresthesias, and diaphoresis. Fever is frequently seen in children during dimercaprol therapy. The dimercaprol-mercury complex is dialyzable, and hemodialysis may be helpful in patients receiving dimercaprol who have diminished renal function. Plasma exchange transfusion also was beneficial in a case of mercuric chloride ingestion.[27] **Dimercaprol is contraindicated in methyl mercury poisoning due to the potential for exacerbation of central neurologic symptoms.** Succimer is generally well tolerated. Consultation with a poison control center or medical toxicologist is recommended for further assistance with chelation treatment.

DISPOSITION AND FOLLOW-UP

Hospital admission is recommended for (1) patients known or suspected to have ingested mercury salts, (2) patients known or suspected to have inhaled elemental mercury vapor with pulmonary injury, and (3) patients requiring dimercaprol therapy.

Outcome depends on the form of mercury and the severity of toxicity. Mild cases of elemental and mercury salt poisoning and very mild cases of organic mercury toxicity may have complete recovery. Death can occur in severe cases of mercuric chloride poisoning and with dimethyl mercury exposure. Most patients with symptomatic organic mercury poisoning are left with residual neurologic deficits. Environmental decontamination and removal of the patient, family members, and coworkers from a site of ongoing contamination play a critical role in preventing injury to others.

OTHER METALS AND METAL SALTS

Other metals and their salts may cause toxicity (**Table 203-7**). Metal salts typically cause early GI irritation (nausea, vomiting, diarrhea, cramping, and hemorrhage) with subsequent neurologic, renal, hematologic, and cutaneous abnormalities. Symptoms are often vague, and without an explicit history of metal salt exposure, patients are usually misdiagnosed.[29] Treatment universally involves removal of the patient from the source, topical decontamination, administration of activated charcoal (if exposure involves ingestion), and supportive care, including aggressive fluid and electrolyte repletion and hemodialysis, if required. Indications for chelation and its efficacy in treating metal toxicity vary with the specific metal (Table 203-7).[30] Consult with a medical toxicologist or a regional poison control center for specific indications and drug doses.

REFERENCES

The complete reference list is available online at www.TintinalliEM.com.

Industrial Toxins

Chip Gresham
Frank LoVecchio

INTRODUCTION AND EPIDEMIOLOGY

A **hazardous chemical** is defined by the U.S. Occupational Safety and Health Administration as any chemical that has been scientifically shown to be a health hazard (causes acute or chronic health effects) or a physical hazard (combustible liquid, explosive, flammable, etc.). This federal agency estimates that there are 575,000 chemicals in the workplace, with 53,000 being potentially hazardous.[1] Considering that unplanned exposures and contamination can occur at any time during manufacturing, transport, storage, usage, or disposal of these chemicals, inevitably, emergency physicians can expect to occasionally be responsible for the management and care of a hazardous materials patient (see chapter 5, Disaster Preparedness).[2]

When managing a patient exposed to an industrial chemical, it is helpful to refer to the Material Safety Data Sheet and adhere to the recommendations regarding decontamination. Although the Material Safety Data Sheet will also include "first aid" recommendations (**Table 204-1**), the provider should also consult with a medical toxicologist or a regional poison control center to discuss case-specific hazards, optimal treatments, and dispositions. Contacting the regional poison control center facilitates data collection and analysis of toxicologic exposures. While many exposures produce immediate effects, some agents may result in delayed onset of symptoms that require at least 24 hours of observation (**Table 204-2**).

This chapter discusses common industrial toxins that produce primarily respiratory toxicity (**Table 204-3**) and those that cause metabolic toxicity. Toxic chemicals discussed elsewhere include nerve agents and

TABLE 204-1 Agents Absorbed through Intact Skin That May Result in Systemic Toxicity*

Acrylamide	Methyl bromide
Acrylonitrile, acetonitrile, propionitrile	Methylene chloride (slow)
Aniline	Nerve agents
Chlordane	Nitrates
Dinitrophenol	Nitrobenzene
Hydrocarbons: benzene, gasoline, toluene, xylene (all slowly absorbed)	Pesticides
Hydrogen cyanide, cyanide salts	Phenol
Hydrogen fluoride (hydrofluoric acid)	T2 toxin (biologic)
Metals (organic mercury, thallium)	

*Many toxins may be absorbed through abraded skin.

TABLE 204-2 Toxins with Delayed Onset of Symptoms or Requiring Prolonged Monitoring

Agent	Potential Delayed Toxicity
Acrylonitrile, acetonitrile, propionitrile	Cyanide toxicity
Aniline	Methemoglobinemia
Arsine	Hemolysis
Benzene	Bone marrow suppression and leukemia
Cadmium	Pulmonary toxicity
Chlorine	Pulmonary edema
Ethylene oxide	Pulmonary edema and neurotoxicity
Halogenated solvents	Hepatorenal toxicity
Hydrofluoric acid	Pulmonary edema, dermal burns, electrolyte changes (hypocalcemia)
Hydrogen sulfide	Pulmonary edema
Metals	Hepatorenal, neurotoxicity
Methanol	Neurologic, acid-base disturbance
Methyl bromide	Pulmonary edema
Methylene chloride	Carbon monoxide toxicity, dysrhythmias
Organophosphates (highly lipid soluble), or dermal exposure to nerve agents	Cholinergic toxicity
Nitrogen oxides	Pulmonary edema, methemoglobinemia
Paraquat	Pulmonary edema/fibrosis
Phosgene	Pulmonary edema
Phosphine	Pulmonary edema
Zinc phosphide	Pulmonary edema

vesicants (see chapter 8, Chemical Disasters); hydrocarbons (see chapter 199, Hydrocarbons and Volatile Substances); acids and alkalis (see chapter 200, Caustic Ingestions); organophosphates and carbamates (see chapter 201, Pesticides); metals (see chapter 203, Metals and Metalloids); oxidants (see chapter 207, Dyshemoglobinemias); and carbon monoxide (see chapter 222, Carbon Monoxide).

Several factors render children sensitive to chemical exposures.[3-5] Children have increased exposure to respiratory toxins because their minute volumes are higher, resulting in greater inhalational exposure. The smaller airway diameters and lesser ability to clear secretions render children more susceptible to inhaled toxins. Dermal absorption after exposure is also increased, because their skin is thinner and more permeable and they have a larger body surface-to-mass ratio. Children also are at risk for profound dehydration, resulting from vomiting and diarrhea secondary to toxic exposures. Many emergency protocols and antidote kits were developed for healthy adults, so dosing and care for pediatric exposures is usually scaled down from that used in adults.

A pregnant woman should be treated as any other adult patient because the best care for the fetus is proper care of the mother.[6] Consult an obstetrician if there is a significant exposure or evidence of systemic toxicity.

RESPIRATORY TOXINS

Determinants of airborne agent toxicity primarily include factors such as concentration of the inhaled toxin, duration of exposure, and whether the exposure occurred in an enclosed space. Other influential factors include vapor density, allergic or nonallergic bronchospastic response, exertional state or metabolic rate of the victim, and unique host susceptibility such as underlying reactive airway disease, history of smoking, or extreme age. Aspiration of gastric contents may cause further pulmonary insult.

General management of the patient with toxic inhalation injury begins with removal from the source, supplemental oxygen for hypoxemia, and inhaled bronchodilators for bronchospasm. The physical examination should include inspection of the upper airway for evidence of singed nasal hair, soot in the oropharynx, facial or oropharyngeal burns, stridor, hoarseness, dysphagia, cough, carbonaceous sputum, tachypnea, retractions, accessory muscle use, wheezing, or cyanosis. Because of the potential for sudden deterioration in patients with upper airway injury, there should be a low threshold for endotracheal intubation. Irrigate the eyes and skin as appropriate.

Copious airway secretions, hypoxia, bronchospasm, and pulmonary edema should be anticipated. Prophylactic antibiotics and steroids are not *routinely* indicated following toxic gas inhalation. Steroids can be given if the patient has underlying reactive airway disease or toxin-induced bronchospasm, and prophylactic steroids and antibiotics can be considered after **nitrogen dioxide** exposure.[7]

TABLE 204-3 Toxic Industrial Exposures That Cause Respiratory Symptoms

Agent	Irritant	Signs/Symptoms/Findings	Treatment
Phosgene	Mild/none	I—Eye and upper airway irritation; possibly none D—Dyspnea, noncardiogenic pulmonary edema	Supplemental oxygen only if hypoxemic (Sa_{O2} <92%) Respiratory supportive care Consider nebulized β-agonists Mandatory rest Ocular care
Chlorine	Yes	I—Eye and upper airway irritation, nausea and vomiting (low-level exposure) D—Pulmonary edema (high-level exposure)	Humidified oxygen Respiratory supportive care Consider nebulized β-agonists Consider nebulized sodium bicarbonate Ocular care
Nitrogen dioxide	Yes	I—Dyspnea with transient improvement D—Worsening dyspnea due to pulmonary edema 24–72 h after exposure; methemoglobinemia	Humidified oxygen Respiratory supportive care Consider early corticosteroid treatment
Ammonia	Yes	I—Coughing, hoarseness, bronchospasm, eye and upper airway irritation	Humidified oxygen Consider nebulized β-agonists Consider nebulized anticholinergics Respiratory supportive care Ocular care

Abbreviations: D = delayed; I = immediate; Sa_{O2} = arterial oxygen saturation.

Pertinent laboratory studies include arterial blood gas analysis with carboxyhemoglobin, methemoglobin, and lactate levels; whole-blood cyanide levels if persistent acidosis occurs (although this will not change immediate management); electrocardiogram monitoring; and chest radiography. The role for diagnostic or therapeutic bronchoscopy in inhaled toxin exposure is controversial.

Many highly toxic gases produced in large quantities in the industrial sector are potential agents for malicious use. Toxic gases of particular concern are those used in the battlefield or stockpiled—phosgene, chlorine, or ammonia. Additional toxicity can result from products of combustion such as hydrocarbons (see chapter 199, Hydrocarbons and Volatile Substances) or carbon monoxide (see chapter 222, Carbon Monoxide).

PHOSGENE

Phosgene was first used as a chemical agent of warfare in World War I, where it was responsible for 80% of all chemical gas fatalities. While stockpiled for potential use in World War II, it was never used in combat. Phosgene is no longer stockpiled by the U.S. military; however, it has widespread use in manufacturing and industry as a chemical precursor in the production of plastics, pharmaceuticals, dyes, polyurethane, and pesticides.[8,9] The heating of chlorinated fluorocarbons (Freon®) will also form phosgene gas and has caused poisonings in the refrigerator/air conditioner manufacturing and repairing industry.[10]

Phosgene release and contamination can be insidious. The gas is relatively water insoluble and therefore has poor warning properties. Only mild initial eye, nose, throat, and upper airway irritation are expected, and these may be entirely absent.[8] Classically, when released, it forms a white cloud with a characteristic odor of newly mown hay. The major injury is an acid burn to lower airways as phosgene reaches the alveoli and hydrolyzes to carbon dioxide and hydrochloric acid.[11] Acylation of alveolar capillary membranes results in diffuse capillary leak and noncardiogenic pulmonary edema, which may be delayed for up to 24 hours.[11,12] Symptoms are typically dyspnea and chest tightness. If the exposure is massive, immediate dyspnea and mucous membrane and eye irritation may occur. The onset of dyspnea or pulmonary edema within 4 hours of exposure suggests a very poor prognosis.[11]

Recovery usually occurs with respiratory supportive care and management of acute lung injury (noncardiogenic pulmonary edema).[13] Do not provide supplemental oxygen until symptoms and signs of hypoxia develop or arterial oxygen saturation falls, and then administer at the lowest fraction of inspired oxygen to maintain arterial oxygen saturation above 94%.[14] There is no benefit from IV and inhaled steroids or nebulized acetylcysteine.[15] Nebulized β-agonists may reduce lung inflammation if given within 1 hour of exposure.[13,16] Exertion increases pulmonary edema from phosgene, so rest is mandatory.[12] If patients require intubation and mechanical ventilation for respiratory failure, a protective ventilation strategy with low tidal volume, low plateau pressures, and high positive end expiratory pressure should be used.[17,18] Observe and monitor even asymptomatic patients for 24 hours after acute exposure.

CHLORINE

Chlorine is widely available in the industrial sector, in the setting of laboratories, paper manufacturing, swimming pool chemical distribution, and municipal water treatment.[19-22] Chlorine gas also has potential for use by terrorists.[23] When dispersed, this dense green-yellow gas has an acrid, pungent odor and, unlike phosgene, has excellent warning properties. Chlorine gas has intermediate water solubility, which is consistent with the observation that moderately exposed World War I soldiers exhibited both central airway damage and pulmonary edema.[24]

Early inflammatory injury results from the formation of hydrochloric and hypochlorous acids and oxidants upon contact with moist membranes.[25] Immediate ocular and upper airway irritation along with nausea and vomiting are common following mild exposures.[19,26] More significant exposure results in coughing, hoarseness, and pulmonary edema, usually within 6 hours, with some exposures leading to acute respiratory distress syndrome.[20,27] Severe exposures may produce pulmonary infiltrates or edema visible on radiographs or CT scan.[28]

Care is primarily supportive, with the use of humidified oxygen and bronchodilators as needed. Prophylactic antibiotics are not recommended. Nebulized sodium bicarbonate as a neutralizing therapy may improve pulmonary function during the initial 4 hours of treatment, but the long-term benefits are unproven.[21,29,30] Uncontrolled studies of both parenteral and inhaled steroids show improvement in airway resistance and arterial oxygenation but no improvement in the outcome with severe lung injury.[7] Chlorine causes dermal injury at high concentration, and skin decontamination may be required. In patients with ocular symptoms, the cornea should be evaluated for a chemical burn. A moderately symptomatic patient should be observed for 24 hours, monitoring for delayed onset of respiratory complications.

NITROGEN DIOXIDE

Nitrogen dioxide and other **nitrogen oxides** are encountered in the form of silo gas (**"silo filler disease"**), as products of combustion, in industrial processes, or as components of military blast weapons, smokes, and obscurants.[31,32] These oxides have limited water solubility that results in primarily lower airway toxicity.[33] An exposure to a high concentration may only produce very mild initial discomfort. Slow conversion of nitrogen dioxide to nitric acid in the alveoli results in delayed alveolar injury and pulmonary edema.[31,34-36] A triphasic illness typically is seen with initial dyspnea and flulike symptoms, transient improvement, and then worsening dyspnea, which heralds the onset of pulmonary edema 12 hours after exposure.[32,34,36-38] **Methemoglobinemia** has been reported from nitrogen oxide exposure. Case reports describe benefit with early corticosteroid treatment for acute lung injury following nitrogen dioxide exposure,[38] although overall evidence is inconclusive.[7]

AMMONIA

Ammonia is widely available; it is found in household and industrial chemicals and fertilizers and is used in the synthesis of plastics and explosives.[39] Ammonia is a highly water-soluble, colorless, alkaline, corrosive gas with a characteristic pungent odor that rapidly reacts with wet surfaces to form ammonium hydroxide. Ammonia has good warning properties due to its odor and immediate symptoms of mucous membrane, eye, and throat irritation. Lower airway involvement resulting in bronchospasm, pulmonary edema, residual reactive airway disease, and even permanent lung injury have been described following massive exposures, especially in those who are entrapped in enclosed spaces.[40]

Treatment is supportive with humidified oxygen, bronchodilators, and anticholinergics.[41] Concentrated ammonia, such as 8.4% ammonia hydroxide, is hazardous to the eyes, and symptomatic patients should undergo ocular irrigation followed by evaluation for corneal burns.

CYANIDE

Cyanide has an infamous history. It was the agent used by Nazi Germany (Zyklon B) in the gas chambers during the Holocaust, by Jim Jones in the mass cult suicide at the People's Temple in Guyana (commonly called "Jonestown"), for murder in over-the-counter drug-tampering incidents, and at the World Trade Center bombing in 1993.[42,43] Cyanide can be generated through natural and industrial processes (**Table 204-4**).

PATHOPHYSIOLOGY

Cyanide inhibits many metabolic processes, with its most toxic effect from binding with very high affinity to the ferric ion cytochrome a_3 portion of cytochrome oxidase within the mitochondria, resulting in an abrupt cessation of electron transport and oxidative phosphorylation, thus inhibiting cellular respiration.[43] This results in significantly impaired ATP production, even in the presence of sufficient oxygen, and profound disruption of aerobic metabolism. Thus following an acute exposure, organs and tissues with high oxygen consumption are the first and most severely affected.

TABLE 204-4 Sources of Cyanide

Sources of Cyanide
Burning of: wool, nylon, silk, acrylic, polyurethane, melamine, polyacrylonitrile, polyamide plastics
Industries: fabrication of plastics, electroplating, mining, photography, precious metal reclamation, solvents, hair removal from hides
Fumigants and fertilizers
Vermin extermination: cyanide spread into burrows and dens
Chemistry laboratories
Medicinal: Laetrile,* sodium nitroprusside
Plants: seeds from *Prunus* species (apricots, cherries, plums, peaches), cassava, bamboo shoots
Illicit phencyclidine manufacturing
Cigarette smoke
Vehicle exhausts

*No longer available in the United States, but widely available via the Internet and sold outside the United States.

TABLE 204-5 Signs and Symptoms of Acute Cyanide Toxicity

System / Sign	Severity
Cardiovascular	
Tachycardia	Mild
Hypertension	↓
Bradycardia	↓
Hypotension	↓
Cardiovascular collapse	↓
Asystole	Severe
CNS	
Headache	Mild
Drowsiness	↓
Seizures	↓
Coma	Severe
Pulmonary	
Dyspnea	Mild
Tachypnea	↓
Apnea	Severe

Adverse physiologic effects due to chronic subacute cyanide exposure are poorly defined. Studies of workers chronically exposed to cyanide demonstrated a higher incidence of thyroid disease and vitamin B_{12} deficiency.

Cassava, a tropical root that is the food staple in many countries, contains the cyanogenic glycosides *linamarin* and *lotaustralin* that liberate cyanide when metabolized in the body.[44] Chronic exposure to **dietary cyanide** is linked to tropical ataxic neuropathy and is endemic in countries where cassava consumption is high.[45,46] The combination of chronic tobacco use and a diet poor in cyanide-scavenging carotenes is associated with the development of optic neuropathy.[47] Techniques to reduce cyanoglucoside content in the raw tuber and different processing methods to reduce levels in prepared food have promise to reduce toxicity.[48]

Natural products, such as cyanogenic foods, or manmade sources, such as cigarettes, result in low cyanide concentrations in humans. Smokers' whole-blood levels of cyanide are roughly 2.5-fold higher than nonsmokers' levels.[49] The primary mechanism for detoxification of cyanide is its metabolism in the liver by rhodanese to thiocyanate, a nontoxic compound that is renally excreted. Toxicity occurs when this mechanism is rapidly overwhelmed.

CLINICAL FEATURES

Clinical presentation of the cyanide-poisoned patient depends on the cyanide-containing compound, the route of exposure, the concentration to which the patient is exposed, and the time since exposure. The onset of symptoms following inhalational exposure to hydrogen cyanide gas is immediate.[50] Exposure to concentrations <50 parts per million causes restlessness, anxiety, palpitations, dyspnea, and headache.[51] Higher concentrations of hydrogen cyanide gas cause severe dyspnea, loss of consciousness, seizures, and cardiac dysrhythmias. Coma, cardiovascular collapse, and death may occur immediately on exposure to very high levels. The median lethal dose for humans from hydrogen cyanide gas is estimated to be 200 parts per million for a 30-minute exposure and 600 to 700 parts per million for a 5-minute exposure.[51] The onset of symptoms following ingestion of a cyanide salt typically occurs within minutes. The median lethal dose of potassium or sodium cyanide in an untreated adult is estimated at 140 to 250 milligrams, but death has been reported with ingestion of as little as 50 milligrams, and survival has been reported in much larger ingestions when antidotes are used.[51]

The typical seriously poisoned patient has an altered level of consciousness and is hyperventilating, hypotensive, and bradycardic (**Table 204-5**).[42,52] Cutaneous manifestations vary, but, importantly, the patient is not initially cyanotic, as cyanide does not significantly alter the oxygen-carrying capacity of hemoglobin. However, cyanosis does follow if there is significant respiratory compromise or arrest. A smell of **bitter almonds** supports the diagnosis of cyanide poisoning, but reliability varies because only approximately 60% to 80% of the population can detect the odor. **Cherry-red skin color** has been described as a result of the increased venous hemoglobin oxygen saturation, but this is uncommon.

Severe unexplained metabolic acidosis is a consistent clinical feature (Table 204-6). In victims of smoke inhalation, toxic cyanide levels correlate with plasma lactate levels >90 milligrams/dL (>10 mmol/L), independent of the carbon monoxide level.[53] The decision to institute antidotal treatment of cyanide poisoning must be made long before confirmatory laboratory studies can be obtained. Although cyanide levels are not closely correlated with toxicity, they can be used to retrospectively confirm a clinical diagnosis or for forensic purposes. A variety of methods are available to measure cyanide in the environment and in biologic fluids,[54] but whole-blood cyanide level is the most commonly available test.[51]

Symptoms of poisoning are delayed following the ingestion of compounds that require metabolic activation to release free cyanide, such as **acetonitrile**, a solvent sold commercially as a cosmetic nail remover,[55] and **amygdalin** from apricot pits.[56] The slow release of cyanide by the spontaneous degradation of **sodium nitroprusside**, which is increased by exposure to sunlight, also results in delayed toxicity, particularly during prolonged or high-dose infusions.[57]

TABLE 204-6 Anticipated Laboratory Findings in Cyanide Poisoning

Test	Result	Cause
Serum electrolytes	Elevated anion gap	Lactic acidosis from anaerobic metabolism
Arterial blood gases	Metabolic acidosis Normal Pa_{O_2}	Oxygenation initially normal
Lactate	>90 milligrams/dL (>10 mmol/L)	Correlates with toxic cyanide level
Measured oxygen saturation by co-oximetry	Normal	Hemoglobin retains normal oxygen-carrying capacity
Measured arterial-mixed venous oxygen difference	Decreased	Decreased tissue oxygen consumption
Whole-blood cyanide level	Toxic >0.5 microgram/mL (>12 micromoles/L) Fatal >2.5 micrograms/mL (>60 micromoles/L)	Note: plasma cyanide levels are roughly one tenth of the whole-blood cyanide levels.
Fire victims	Elevated carboxyhemoglobin level	Carbon monoxide generated by incomplete combustion Synergistic toxicity with cyanide

Abbreviation: Pa_{O_2} = partial pressure of arterial oxygen.

TREATMENT

There are multiple antidotes for cyanide toxicity with variation in regional availability.[52,58-60] The two antidotes most commonly used in the United States are the **cyanide antidote kit** (containing nitrites and thiosulfate) and **hydroxocobalamin**. Aggressive supportive care with 100% oxygen, crystalloids, and vasopressors for hypotension is important.[61] Treat profound acidemia with sodium bicarbonate, because it enhances the effect of the nitrites and thiosulfate.[62]

The cyanide antidote kit has been well established for cyanide poisoning in the United States and is based on experimental and chemical principles developed by Chen and colleagues in 1933.[63,64] The antidotes contained in the cyanide treatment kit include ampules of amyl nitrite for inhalation, 10-mL vials of 3% sodium nitrite (300 milligrams), and 50-mL vials of 25% sodium thiosulfate (12.5 grams) (**Table 204-7**).

The decision to administer the cyanide antidote kit is straightforward when faced with a comatose, bradycardic patient with a clear history of cyanide exposure. More difficult management decisions arise in patients with smoke inhalation who have or may have carbon monoxide exposure as well as suspected cyanide exposure, and patients who are critically ill and acidotic without any known history of cyanide exposure. Consultation with a toxicologist or the regional poison control center is advised.

Nitrites The rationale for using nitrites is based on their ability to form methemoglobin, which binds cyanide more avidly than the ferric iron of cytochrome oxidase. This process removes cyanide from the cytochrome and enables the mitochondria to reactivate electron transport and oxidative metabolism.[65] Although this is believed to be the main mechanism of action of nitrites in cyanide poisoning, the vasodilatory effects may contribute to its effects.[66,67] **Inhaled amyl nitrite is a temporizing measure when an IV line is not available, but amyl nitrite is not needed when sodium nitrite can be given IV.** Inhalation of the amyl nitrite ampule generates approximately 5% methemoglobin, while sodium nitrite IV generates approximately 8% to 20%.[68] Nitrites do have significant side effects, including hypotension and the development of excessive methemoglobinemia.[58,62,69] **However, hypotension is not a contraindication to nitrite therapy in severe cyanide poisoning.**

In children, the sodium nitrite dose is adjusted according to the hemoglobin level to keep the methemoglobin level less than 30% (**Table 204-8**).[51,69] Aggressive sodium nitrite treatment has resulted in the death of a child from methemoglobinemia after a nonlethal ingestion of cyanide.[51,69] If hemoglobin values are not available, the empiric dose of sodium nitrite for a child less than 25 kg is based on the 10-gram hemoglobin concentration.[69]

Theoretically, nitrites are relatively contraindicated in victims of smoke inhalation who have or are thought to have concomitant carbon monoxide poisoning because the induction of methemoglobinemia will further decrease oxygen delivery. In cases such as these where increased methemoglobinemia would be potentially harmful, consider withholding the nitrites and giving only the sodium thiosulfate or using hydroxocobalamin.[70]

TABLE 204-7 Treatment of Cyanide Poisoning in Adults

100% oxygen	
IV crystalloids and vasopressors for hypotension	
Sodium bicarbonate for acidemia	
AND	
Cyanide antidote kit	Amyl nitrite inhaler; crack vial and inhale over 30 s.*
	Sodium nitrite 3% solution: 10 mL (300 milligrams) IV given over no less than 5 min.†
	Sodium thiosulfate 25% solution: 50 mL (12.5 grams) IV.
	Repeat sodium thiosulfate once at half dose (25 mL) if symptoms persist.
OR	
Hydroxocobalamin	5 grams IV over 15 min.
	If needed, may repeat 5 grams for a total of 10 grams.

*Not necessary if IV is in place.

†Avoid nitrites in the presence of severe hypotension if diagnosis is unclear; consider sodium thiosulfate or hydroxocobalamin.

TABLE 204-8 Treatment of Cyanide Poisoning in Children

100% oxygen	
IV crystalloids and vasopressors for hypotension	
Sodium bicarbonate for acidemia	
AND	
Cyanide antidote kit	Amyl nitrite inhaler; crack vial and hold in front of nose for 15–30 s.*†
	Sodium nitrite 3% solution: adjusted according to hemoglobin level, given IV over no less than 5 min†‡ (monitor methemoglobin level <30%).
Hemoglobin (grams/100 mL)	**Sodium Nitrite 3% Solution (mL/kg)**
7	0.19
8	0.22
9	0.25
10	0.27
11	0.30
12	0.33
13	0.36
14	0.39
Sodium thiosulfate 25% solution: 1.65 mL/kg IV.	
Repeat sodium thiosulfate once at half dose (0.825 mL/kg) if symptoms persist.	

*Not necessary if IV is in place.

†Consider withholding nitrites if suspected concomitant carbon monoxide poisoning.

‡Avoid nitrites in the presence of severe hypotension if diagnosis is unclear.

Sodium Thiosulfate After the administration of sodium nitrite, infuse sodium thiosulfate. Sodium thiosulfate enhances the activity of the enzyme rhodanese, a mammalian enzyme that likely evolved in response to the ubiquitous presence of cyanide in nature. Rhodanese catalyzes the transfer of sulfate from sodium thiosulfate to cyanide to form thiocyanate, a less toxic form that is excreted by the kidneys.[58,62,63] Animal studies using lethal doses of cyanide demonstrate that the therapeutic effects of sodium nitrite and sodium thiosulfate are synergistic.[62-64]

Sodium thiosulfate has very limited toxicity in comparison with nitrites and is a safer empirical therapy when the diagnosis is not clear. It may also be useful as a sole therapy for victims of inhalation injury where there is concern that the induction of methemoglobinemia in the setting of carbon monoxide exposure may further reduce oxygen carrying capacity.[71] However, sodium thiosulfate alone was not effective in an animal model of cyanide-induced shock, suggesting that such isolated therapy is not useful for serious human toxicity.[72]

Hydroxocobalamin Because of the side effects of nitrites, an effort has been made to develop equally efficacious but less toxic therapies.[58-60] **Hydroxocobalamin (vitamin B_{12a})**, was approved in 2006 by the U.S. Food and Drug Administration. Hydroxocobalamin is a metalloprotein with a cobalt center that binds cyanide, removing it from cytochrome oxidase and forming cyanocobalamin, which is then eliminated via the kidneys. Because of its low toxicity and its efficacy, **it is thought to be ideal in cases where the diagnosis of cyanide poisoning is uncertain or in cases where the induction of methemoglobinemia (i.e., concomitant exposure to carbon monoxide) may be detrimental.**[73-75]

The dose of hydroxocobalamin in an adult patient is 5 grams IV over 15 minutes. A second dose of 5 grams IV may be repeated once (for a total of 10 grams) if the patient's condition warrants.[76] Side effects associated with hydroxocobalamin include transient hypertension, a reddish discoloration of the skin and mucous membranes, and rare anaphylactic reactions. Due to the discoloration of body fluids caused by hydroxocobalamin,[77] interference with chemistry and co-oximetry tests[78,79] and with hemodialysis machines has been reported.[80]

The combination of hydroxocobalamin followed by sodium thiosulfate led to a faster return to baseline of the mean arterial pressure in animal models when compared to sodium nitrate and sodium thiosulfate; however, there was no difference in mortality.[81] A follow-up study in the same animal model found that reversing cyanide-induced shock resided with the hydroxocobalamin alone.[72]

Other Antidotes **Dimethylaminophenol** is a rapid methemoglobin inducer developed in Germany for the treatment of cyanide poisoning.[58-60,62] Clinical efficacy is similar to sodium nitrite. The adult dose is 250 milligrams (5 mL of 5% solution) IV over 1 minute, used in combination with sodium thiosulfate.

Dicobalt edetate is a cobalt compound with a high affinity for cyanide. Although highly effective as a cyanide antidote, the toxicity of dicobalt edetate is greater when cyanide is not present, limiting its use to cases where the presence of cyanide is unequivocal.[42,43,58-60,62] The adult dose for dicobalt edetate is 300 milligrams IV over approximately 1 minute. If there is inadequate clinical response after 5 minutes, a second dose of 300 milligrams IV may be given.

Cobinamide, a precursor to cobalamine, is highly effective in a mouse model of cyanide poisoning.[82] A potential advantage is that cobinamide sulfite can be administered as an IM injection and could be useful in the prehospital setting.

Hyperbaric Oxygen The data on hyperbaric oxygen for cyanide poisoning are conflicting.[83-85] Although there are reports in the literature that support its use, studied patients had received multiple therapies, so improvement cannot be contributed solely to hyperbaric oxygen. In addition, animal studies of cyanide poisoning show no benefit of hyperbaric oxygen over 100% oxygen.[62] The timing, lack of science, and impracticality make hyperbaric oxygen therapy an unproven endeavor in acute cyanide toxicity.

Gastric Decontamination Patients with a history of ingestion may benefit from activated charcoal, which should be considered only in patients who are alert, have a patent airway, and present within 1 hour of ingestion.

DISPOSITION AND FOLLOW-UP

All patients who receive cyanide antidotal therapy should be admitted for observation. Patients who have ingested a substance that may result in delayed toxicity (up to 6 hours) should also be admitted. Full recovery is anticipated in many cases of severe poisoning in which treatment is initiated rapidly and cardiac arrest has not yet occurred. Recovery despite cardiac arrest also has been reported, but anoxic encephalopathy may ensue. Successful organ transplant has been reported after death secondary to cyanide poisoning.[86]

HYDROGEN SULFIDE

Hydrogen sulfide is a colorless, flammable gas that may be encountered in industries such as oil and gas or as a natural product of organic decomposition, such as sewer or manure gas.[87,88] Hydrogen sulfide can be made by mixing common household products, and in Japan, this method was associated with a rash of attempted suicides in 2008.[89] Regardless of its source, it is among the most common causes of fatal gas inhalation exposures. Fatal exposures usually occur in enclosed spaces that may claim additional victims as would-be rescuers are poisoned upon entering. Large industrial or natural releases of hydrogen sulfide may produce fatalities in unconfined spaces.[90]

The mechanism of toxicity is similar to that of cyanide, with disruption of oxidative phosphorylation through inhibition of cytochrome oxidase a_3, except this impairment reverses rapidly when hydrogen sulfide exposure ceases.[91] Cellular asphyxia and impaired ATP production promote anaerobic metabolism with lactate accumulation and metabolic acidosis.

Hydrogen sulfide is one of the few chemical asphyxiants that also possesses irritative properties, such that respiratory and ocular irritation are common following exposure.[88,92] The characteristic odor of "rotten eggs" may not be noticed due to olfactory fatigue from persistent low-level exposures or from olfactory paralysis seen at high hydrogen sulfide levels. In high concentrations, rapid loss of consciousness, seizures, and death occur after only a few breaths.[93] Delayed pulmonary edema and corneal injury should be anticipated with massive exposures.

Treatment begins with removal from the source, administration of high-flow oxygen, and decontamination of the skin and eyes, as appropriate.[94] For patients still conscious, symptoms resolve with this treatment alone. For patients with altered sensorium or impaired cardiovascular function after hydrogen sulfide exposure, administration of **sodium nitrite** 300 milligrams IV can produce rapid improvement.[88,94] The concept is that low-level methemoglobin formation may enhance conversion of sulfide to the less toxic sulfmethemoglobin. An animal model of lethal hydrogen sulfide toxicity found benefit with hydroxocobalamin, but human treatment experience is needed before this agent can be recommended.[95,96] Hyperbaric oxygen therapy for hydrogen sulfide toxicity has been described in multiple published case reports, but there is no evidence that it is superior to standard oxygen therapy.[84,97]

REFERENCES

The complete reference list is available online at www.TintinalliEM.com.

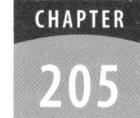

CHAPTER 205 Vitamins and Herbals

Rick Tovar

INTRODUCTION

Vitamins and herbal preparations, particularly those sold in health food stores, are considered by many to be innocuous but may have potential toxicity when taken in excessive amounts over a period of time. Also, herbal preparations may contain toxic contaminants that can cause acute poisoning.

Hypervitaminosis from the fat-soluble vitamins A, D, and E can produce chronic toxicity (after weeks to months of excessive ingestion) or subacute toxicity (after days to a few weeks). Of the water-soluble vitamins, niacin, pyridoxine, and ascorbate are associated with toxicity (**Table 205-1**).

VITAMIN A

Dietary vitamin A is usually found in two forms: retinyl palmitate (an ester) from animal sources or carotenoids found in plants. After ingestion, the ester form is hydrolyzed in the gastrointestinal tract to retinol. Retinol is then absorbed into intestinal mucosal cells, where it then combines with a fatty acid to again become a retinyl ester. Carotenoids are dark-colored compounds found in plants. Plants containing the carotenoids have β-carotene, which is the vegetable compound most efficiently converted to retinol. The liver contains approximately 95% of body vitamin A stores.

Vitamin A forms part of the visual pigments of the retina (rhodopsin and iodopsin), is important for the formation of mucus-secreting cells in the columnar epithelium, maintains bone growth, and maintains cellular membrane stability. The recommended dietary allowance ranges from 4000 international units (IU) for women to 5000 IU for men.

Hypervitaminosis A generally occurs in either the supplement or dietary forms.[1] The chronic form of vitamin A toxicity is usually due to excessive supplement use, although there have been case reports of acute toxicity due to ingestion of mammal organs (e.g., fish liver).[2] When the total dose is similar, water-miscible preparations are more toxic than oily preparations because of better absorption.[3] There is variability among patients in the amounts necessary to develop hypervitaminosis; hemodialysis patients can develop hypercalcemia with lower doses of vitamin A supplementation due to decreased renal clearance of retinol.[4] Thus the minimum dose that may cause toxicity in humans is not established.

TABLE 205-1 Symptoms of Hypervitaminosis

Vitamin	Symptoms
Vitamin A	Subacute toxicity: red peeling rash, headache, vomiting Chronic toxicity: blurred vision, appetite loss, abnormal skin pigmentation, hair loss, dry skin, pruritus, long-bone pain, bone fractures, rare cases of pseudotumor cerebri, hypercalcemia, and hepatic failure
Vitamin D	Subacute toxicity: hypercalcemia, anorexia, nausea, abdominal pain, lethargy, weight loss, polyuria, constipation, confusion, and coma
Vitamin E	Chronic toxicity: coagulopathy in patients on warfarin, nausea, fatigue, headache, weakness, and blurred vision
Vitamin K	Acute toxicity: anaphylactoid reactions if given in parenteral form (rare)
Vitamin B_1 (thiamine)	No toxicity observed with ingestion of large doses
Vitamin B_2 (riboflavin)	No toxicity observed with ingestion of large doses
Vitamin B_3 (niacin)	Acute toxicity: niacin flush, dose >100 milligrams, redness, burning, and itching of the face, neck, and chest; rarely hypotension Chronic toxicity: doses >2000 milligrams/d, abnormalities of liver function, impaired glucose tolerance, hyperuricemia, skin dryness and discoloration
Vitamin B_6 (pyridoxine)	Subacute and chronic toxicity: doses >1–3 grams/d orally or more over several weeks, peripheral neuropathy with unstable gait, numbness of the feet, similar symptoms in the hands and arms, marked loss of position and vibration senses
Vitamin B_{12}	No toxicity observed with ingestion of large doses. With large IV doses: erythema of skin, mucous membranes, serum, and urine. Rare anaphylactoid reactions. Possible interference with serum colorimetric lab studies.
Folate	No toxicity observed with ingestion of large doses. Masking of macrocytic anemia from vitamin B_{12} deficiency with large doses of folate.
Vitamin C (ascorbate)	Chronic toxicity: nephrolithiasis (controversial), intrarenal deposition of oxalate crystals with renal failure; large doses can produce diarrhea and abdominal cramps.

Symptoms of hypervitaminosis A include blurred vision, appetite loss, abnormal skin pigmentation, loss of hair, dry skin, pruritus, long-bone pain, and an increased incidence of bone fractures. **Massive doses can additionally cause pseudotumor cerebri, hypercalcemia, and hepatic failure.**[5]

The treatment of hypervitaminosis A includes discontinuation of the vitamin and supportive care. Acute ingestions may be treated with oral activated charcoal.

β-Carotene, a precursor of vitamin A, may be rarely associated with toxicity but does not generally cause hypervitaminosis A. In diabetic patients and patients with hypothyroidism, however, large doses of β-carotene can cause a yellowish discoloration of the skin, which fades once β-carotene is stopped. This phenomenon is occasionally seen in infants and toddlers who consume large amounts of carrots and other pigmented vegetables.

VITAMIN D

Dietary vitamin D is ingested as a provitamin, either ergocalciferol (vitamin D_2) or cholecalciferol (vitamin D_3). Both forms are essentially bioequivalent. These provitamins are then converted to calcitriol (1, 25-dihydroxycholecalciferol), the physiologically active form of vitamin D. The major function of calcitriol is to elevate plasma calcium and phosphorus levels, enabling normal bone mineralization.

The recommended dietary allowance for vitamin D is approximately 400 IU, and therapeutic doses sometimes exceed 5000 IU. Infants may develop hypercalcemia from doses as low as 2000 IU, but adults require much higher doses before toxicity develops.[6,7] **The main toxicity from hypervitaminosis D is hypercalcemia,** and clinical findings include anorexia, nausea, abdominal pain, lethargy, weight loss, polyuria, constipation, confusion, and coma. Symptoms from massive doses of 1000 to 3000 IU/kg per day can develop in 2 to 8 days.

Treatment of hypervitaminosis D includes discontinuation of vitamin D, reduction of the calcium intake, and reduction of serum calcium levels. Pamidronate disodium, a bisphosphonate, inhibits osteoclastic bone resorption and can be used to treat the hypercalcemia.[10,11]

VITAMIN E

Vitamin E activity is not limited to one compound; eight different fat-soluble, naturally occurring alcohols (called tocopherols and tocotrienols) have vitamin E activity, but α-tocopherol is the most active form. Because it is rapidly oxidized, α-tocopherol protects other molecules from being oxidized and thus is termed an *antioxidant*.[10] Foods high in vitamin E include wheat germ, corn, soybean, sunflower seed, cod liver, and others.

Vitamin E is absorbed and distributed through the body similarly to other fat-soluble vitamins: from the intestines and then through lymphatic chylomicrons. The recommended dietary allowance is about 15 milligrams (or 22.4 IU) of α-tocopherol in adults with an increase to 19 milligrams per day during lactation.

Vitamin E is thought to be nontoxic at daily doses of up to 600 IU. The most significant clinical effect of vitamin E at doses higher than 1000 IU per day taken on a long-term basis is the ability to antagonize the effects of vitamin K.[11] Specifically, vitamin E acts as a competitive inhibitor of vitamin K–dependent γ-carboxylation. This effect is only clinically significant in those patients taking warfarin.[12] Additionally, through the production of thromboxane, high levels of vitamin E inhibit platelet aggregation. **Patients being treated with warfarin should be cautioned about ingesting large amounts of vitamin E.** Patients not undergoing treatment with warfarin may rarely have bleeding from large amounts of vitamin E. Other effects in adults who take large doses for a long period of time include nausea, fatigue, headache, weakness, and blurred vision.[13] These symptoms resolve weeks after discontinuation of the vitamin.

VITAMIN K

Vitamin K activity is found in several compounds of varied origin: phylloquinone or vitamin K_1, which is naturally produced by plant sources; menaquinone or vitamin K_2, which is produced by bacterial sources; and menadione or vitamin K_3, a synthetic chemical that is a vitamin precursor of vitamin K_2. Because large doses of menadione are toxic, the use of menadione supplements is banned in the United States for human use but can still be found in animal feed. The gastrointestinal absorption of vitamin K requires the presence of bile and pancreatic juice. Between 10% and 80% of ingested vitamin K is absorbed. It is thought that most of the vitamin K stores in the body are derived from plant sources (K_1). Furthermore, if one has an adequate dietary intake of vitamin K_1, eradication of the gut bacteria will not lead to a deficiency of vitamin K.[14] The recommended dietary allowance of vitamin K is small, about 1 microgram/kg per day. Because most adults consume a diet that contains 300 to 500 micrograms, vitamin K deficiency states are uncommon. In contrast to the other fat-soluble vitamins, vitamin K is not stored in the body to any significant extent.

Vitamin K is required for the production of several factors involved in the coagulation cascade: factor II (prothrombin), factor VII (proconvertin), factor IX (Christmas factor), and factor X (Stuart-Prower factor), and proteins C, S, and Z. Warfarin compounds inhibit vitamin K activity, thereby producing a coagulopathy.

The main concern about vitamin K toxicity is the adverse reactions seen with the IV form. The only recommended form of vitamin K for both oral and parenteral use is K_1. Because vitamin K is fat soluble, it must be given parenterally in a lipid-soluble form. Toxicity from IV vitamin K_1 injection is due to the aqueous colloidal suspension formulation[15] producing rare anaphylactoid reactions and reported deaths.[16]

The absorption of IM vitamin K_1 is erratic and therefore not recommended. PO vitamin K is equal in efficacy to the SC route. Therefore, SC injection of vitamin K is recommended only when the patient is hemodynamically stable and unable to take the oral form. The IV form is usually reserved for serious or life-threatening bleeding due to warfarin.[17]

Toxicity from oral vitamin K is rare, although doses exceeding 500 micrograms per day are associated with skin rashes. Treatment from excessive vitamin K includes stopping the drug and monitoring prothrombin times for patients on warfarin.

VITAMIN B_1 (THIAMINE)

Vitamin B_1, or thiamine, is converted by the body to thiamine pyrophosphate, which acts as a cofactor for several metabolic reactions, including transketolations. Food sources of thiamine include fruits, grain, meats, fish, and milk, among others. The recommended dietary allowance for thiamine is 1.5 milligrams.[18]

Intestinal absorption of thiamine is greatest in the jejunum. Thiamine is not stored in the body to any significant extent. Because of renal excretion (water solubility), there is no toxicity to the ingestion of large doses of thiamine over prolonged periods.

The two main clinical concerns with thiamine include the precipitation of Wernicke's encephalopathy and anaphylactoid reactions. Older literature observed the "precipitation" of Wernicke's encephalopathy in patients with thiamine deficiency with prolonged (not acute) treatment with hypertonic IV glucose.[19] However, there was no observed precipitation of Wernicke's encephalopathy from a single or repeated bolus of IV glucose, even in patients with an altered mental status.[20] Furthermore, thiamine uptake into nerve cells is slower than that of glucose uptake, making pretreatment with thiamine low in efficacy in the prevention of a Wernicke's encephalopathy.[21] **In summary, IV glucose is unlikely to precipitate Wernicke's encephalopathy in patients with altered mental status.**

The issue of IV thiamine toxicity is based on older literature that noted anaphylactoid reactions, likely due to the diluent and contaminants.[22] The current pure aqueous forms of thiamine for IV use very rarely result in anaphylactoid adverse reactions.[23] Therefore, IV use of thiamine is both safe and clinically efficacious. Conversely, PO and IM thiamine is absorbed unpredictably in the emergency setting.

VITAMIN B_2 (RIBOFLAVIN)

Riboflavin is excreted through the urine, and toxicity has not been reported regardless of the amount ingested.[24]

VITAMIN B_3 (NIACIN)

There are two active forms of niacin—nicotinic acid and nicotinamide—which, in conjunction with thiamine and riboflavin, have antipellagra activity. Niacin, thiamine, and riboflavin all function as coenzymes in energy metabolism. Niacin becomes part of the coenzymes nicotinamide-adenine dinucleotide and nicotinamide-adenine dinucleotide phosphate; both are required in all major metabolic pathways in which there is oxidative breakdown of amino acids, fatty acids, and other compounds, including the oxidation of ethanol.

Niacin is found primarily in poultry, meat, and fish, with lesser amounts in plants. Niacin deficiency causes changes first in cells of the skin, followed by impairment of nervous system and GI function. Deficiency states create symptoms such as anorexia, anxiety, depression, irritability, and weakness.

Nicotinic acid in the range of 100 to 200 times the recommended dietary allowance of 20 milligrams lowers serum cholesterol and β-lipoprotein, but nicotinamide does not. Large niacin doses can also deplete cardiac muscle glycogen and can cause liver toxicity. Some patients experience a frightening "niacin flush" when taking a dose of >100 milligrams. **The niacin flush, caused by prostaglandin D_2 and E_2 release with subsequent vasodilation, is characterized by face, neck, and chest burning, itching, and erythema.**[25] **Rarely, hypotension may occur.**[26] An adult-strength aspirin may decrease the prostaglandin surge caused by niacin.[27]

Higher niacin doses may additionally cause nausea, abdominal cramping, diarrhea, and headache. Even higher doses >2000 milligrams per day over a prolonged period can produce abnormalities of liver function, impaired glucose tolerance, hyperuricemia, and skin changes such as dryness and discoloration. These subacute and chronic symptoms resolve within days to weeks after stopping treatment.

VITAMIN B_6 (PYRIDOXINE)

Vitamin B_6 is a necessary cofactor for many enzymatic processes. The active form of pyridoxine is pyridoxal-5-phosphate. Dietary deficiency of pyridoxine is classically characterized by cheilosis, glossitis, seborrheic dermatitis, and stomatitis. Severe dietary deficiency can lead to altered mental status and seizures.[27] Dietary deficiency in infants can result in seizures (as a consequence of a reduced synthesis of γ-aminobutyric acid), anemia (caused by impaired synthesis of heme), xanthurenic aciduria (because of reduced formation of hydroxyanthranilic acid), cystathioninuria (because of decreased cleavage of cystathionine to cysteine and homoserine), and homocystinuria (because of impaired formation of cystathionine). Deficiency states can be induced through ingestion of antagonists to vitamin B_6 such as isoniazid, hydrazines (rocket fuels and the toxic mushroom *Gyromitra esculenta*), cycloserine, and penicillamine.

Vitamin B_6 in high doses >1 gram/d over more than several weeks will cause nerve damage.[28-30] Initial symptoms are an unstable gait and numbness of the feet. This is followed by similar symptoms in the hands and arms. There may be a marked loss of position and vibration senses. After withdrawal of the vitamin, recovery occurs within several months, although some patients may have residual neurologic impairment. **There is no evidence that a single 5-gram IV dose of pyridoxine (the usual dose given for hydrazine exposure) will cause any type of nerve damage.**[31]

Vitamin B_6 also can cause intestinal inactivation of levodopa in patients receiving that medication for Parkinson's disease. Patients should be instructed not to take this vitamin at the same time as the medication.

VITAMIN B_{12} (CYANOCOBALAMIN)

Vitamin B_{12} deficiency can result in hematologic, neurologic, and psychiatric effects.[32] The common hematologic disorders include megaloblastic anemia and pancytopenia. The neurologic disorders commonly observed include paresthesias, peripheral neuropathies, and dorsal spinal cord column demyelination. Psychiatric symptoms include depression, dementia, and psychosis.

Partially because of the size and complexity of the vitamin B_{12} molecules, deficiencies of this water-soluble vitamin result more from absorption problems than from dietary insufficiencies.[32] Absorption depends on the production of intrinsic factor by the parietal cells of the stomach. Vitamin B_{12}–intrinsic factor complexes are initially formed in the stomach. The complexes pass to the ileum, where the intrinsic factor attaches to the intestinal epithelium, facilitating the absorption of the vitamin B_{12}. Vitamin B_{12} is stored in the liver in such quantities that it takes several years for pernicious anemia to develop in an individual who is a strict vegetarian and ingests little B_{12} or in someone unable to produce intrinsic factor.[32]

Until recently, it was believed that vitamin B_{12} had a wide therapeutic index for harm. **With the advent of the use of vitamin B_{12} as an antidote for cyanide poisoning, there have been a few case reports of direct vitamin B_{12} toxicity given in the recommended dose of 5 grams IV to adults, producing erythema of the skin, mucous membranes, urine, and serum.**[33] Rare cases of anaphylactoid reactions have also been reported. Hydroxocobalamin can also interfere with colorimetric lab tests, including those that test for carbon monoxide.[34]

BIOTIN

Biotin is required by all organisms but can be synthesized only by bacteria, yeasts, molds, algae, and some plant species. Those taking chronic antibiotics and those on extremely low-calorie diets are at risk of developing a biotin deficiency. For such individuals, 100 to 300 micrograms of biotin per day is recommended. There is no known toxicity to biotin overdosage.[35]

FOLATE

Folate or folic acid is essential for the production of DNA, RNA, and proteins. Folate is found in fresh leafy green vegetables, yeasts, and liver. Recommended daily allowance for folate in nonpregnant adults is 0.4 milligram. After ingestion, folate is actively absorbed in the small and large intestine. Both deficiencies of vitamin B_{12} and folate can result in megaloblastic (macrocytic) anemia. Large doses of folic acid given to an individual with an undiagnosed vitamin B_{12} deficiency could correct megaloblastic anemia but leave the individual at risk of developing irreversible neurologic damage. Such cases of neurologic progression in vitamin B_{12} deficiency have been mostly seen at folate doses of 5 milligrams and above.[36]

VITAMIN C (ASCORBATE)

The major form of vitamin C, ascorbate or ascorbic acid, is a strong reducing agent that participates in hydroxylation reactions such as those necessary for the formation of collagen. **Scurvy** is due to vitamin C deficiency and results in collagen, protein, and lipid metabolism abnormalities. Additionally, the presence of vitamin C in the intestines increases the absorption rate of iron, so those with a vitamin C deficiency will also be iron depleted.

Vitamin C, which is found primarily in fruits and vegetables, is absorbed through the jejunum and ileum. Large doses of vitamin C can lower the frequency of gout attacks.[37] It is controversial whether high-dose vitamin C is responsible for an increased risk of oxylate renal kidney stones.[38] Intrarenal deposition of oxalate crystals has been reported to cause renal failure in patients with chronic high-dose ascorbate ingestion.[39] Large doses of vitamin C may produce diarrhea and abdominal cramps, which subside with discontinuation. **Megadoses of vitamin C may result in false-negative guaiac testing of feces and may give falsely elevated glucose levels on dipstick testing.**

HERBAL AGENTS

Herbal preparations have long been used by traditional cultures, and their use appears to be increasing in developed countries.[40] In developed countries, herbal preparations have been looked upon as a natural and inexpensive alternative to common Western pharmaceuticals. Unfortunately, many studies funded by the National Center for Complementary and Alternative Medicine have not supported the use of herbal medications for treatment of depression (St. John's wort),[41] dementia (Ginkgo biloba),[42] prostatic hypertrophy (saw palmetto),[43] osteoarthritis (glucosamine and chondroitin),[44] and the common cold (Echinacea).[45] In addition, no herbal is completely free of adverse side effects or the potential for herb–drug interactions.[46] This can be a problem because many patients are reluctant to divulge that they are taking herbal preparations to medical providers.[47]

Although the U.S. Food and Drug Administration (FDA) has some regulatory oversight of herbal preparations, regulation is not as strict as that for drugs. Instead, herbs are classified as dietary supplements by the Dietary Supplemental Health and Education Act of 1994.[48] Unlike drugs, where the manufacturer must prove safety before marketing, the FDA needs to show that a dietary supplement is unsafe before it may take steps to restrict its sale or remove it from the market. Herbal agents can be classified as generally safe, potentially toxic, and toxic (**Table 205-2**).[49-52] Many herbal agents have specific liver, eye, and cardiovascular toxicities.[53-58]

TABLE 205-2 Some Generally Safe Herbal Agents

Agent	General Use	Rare Adverse Effect
Chamomile	Antispasmodic	Anaphylaxis if patient allergic to ragweed
Chondroitin	To treat arthritis	May cause GI upset
Echinacea	To treat or prevent upper respiratory or urinary tract infections	Anaphylaxis if patient allergic to daisies May deplete vitamin stores
Feverfew	To prevent migraines	Suddenly discontinuing may precipitate migraine If chewed, may cause mouth sores If applied to skin, may cause dermatitis
Garlic	To treat hypertension, colic, and hyperlipidemia	Hypotension, rash, nausea, vomiting, diarrhea; death has been reported in massive doses in children
Ginkgo	To treat dementia, vertigo, and Raynaud's disease	May inhibit platelet aggregation and interact with warfarin May cause GI upset
Ginseng	To treat impotence, fatigue, ulcers, and stress	May interact with warfarin Lowers blood glucose May cause insomnia, nervousness
Glucosamine	To treat arthritis	Allergic reaction
Kava	Used for sedation and to relieve sore throat pain	Hepatotoxicity
St. John's wort	To treat depression	Phototoxicity May interact with serotonin reuptake inhibitors; avoid tyramine-containing foods
Valerian	Used for sedation	Interacts with other sedating drugs May have paradoxical stimulant effect

TABLE 205-3 Some Potentially Toxic Herbal Agents

Agent	General Use	Adverse Effect
Black cohosh	To delay or treat menopause	Nausea, vomiting, dizziness, weakness
Chaparral (creosote bush)	Antioxidant effects, analgesia	Potentially hepatotoxic and nephrotoxic
Comfrey	Bone and teeth building, variety of other uses	Potentially hepatotoxic
Ephedra	Weight loss	Hypertension; contraindicated for patients with hypertension, diabetes, or glaucoma
Hawthorn	Congestive heart failure	Additive toxicity with prescribed cardioactive steroids
Juniper	Diuretic	Hallucinogenic; may also cause renal toxicity, nausea, and vomiting
Lobelia	As an expectorant or for treatment of asthma	Anticholinergic syndrome
Nutmeg	Dyspepsia, muscle aches, and arthritis	Hallucinations, GI upset, agitation, coma, miosis, and hypertension
Pennyroyal	Rubefacient, delaying menses, abortifacient	Hepatotoxicity
Pyrrolizidine alkaloids	Pulmonary ailments	Hepatic veno-occlusive disease
Sabah	Weight loss	Pulmonary toxicity
Wormwood	Dyspepsia	Absinthism: restlessness, vertigo, tremor, paresthesias, delirium
Yohimbe	Aphrodisiac	Hallucinations, weakness, hypertension, and paralysis

TABLE 205-4 Some Likely Herb–Drug Interactions

Herb	Herb Used for	Drug	Effect of Interaction
Cayenne (Capsicum)	Arthritis, neuralgia, analgesic	Angiotensin-converting enzyme inhibitors	Increased cough
		Theophylline sustained-release	Increased absorption
Dan shen (salvia)	Reduction of lactation	Warfarin	Decreased warfarin metabolism
Ephedra	Energizer, weight loss, asthma, sinus congestion	Monoamine oxidase inhibitors	Increased toxicity
		Sympathomimetics	Additive effect
Ginkgo	Dementia, peripheral arterial disease, tinnitus	Aspirin Warfarin	Increased risk of bleeding
Grapefruit juice	For vitamin C activity	Amiodarone Benzodiazepines Calcium channel blockers Carbamazepine Clomipramine Cyclosporine Dextromethorphan Ethinyl estradiol 3-hydroxy-3-methyl-glutaryl-CoA reductase inhibitors ("statins") Phosphodiesterase type 5 inhibitors (erectile dysfunction drugs) Quinidine Sertraline	Increased drug availability of any one of these drugs because of inhibition of intestinal CYP3A4
Kava	Sedative/anxiolytic	Caffeine Fluvoxamine Theophylline	Increased levels from inhibition of CYP1A2
Licorice in chronic, high doses	Respiratory disorders, hepatitis, inflammatory diseases, infections	Antihypertensives	Decreased effect (can cause pseudohyperaldosteronism by inhibiting 11-β-dehydrogenase)
		Diuretics	Increased potassium loss, myopathy
		Prednisolone	Increased drug levels
St. John's wort	Depression	Cyclosporine	Decreased serum levels; transplant rejection
		Digoxin	Decreased serum level
		Indinavir	Decreased serum level
Yohimbine	Erectile dysfunction, sexual potency	Clonidine	Decreased effect
		Cyclic antidepressants	Enhanced autonomic and central effects of yohimbe

Abbreviation: CYP = cytochrome P-450.

Although herbal preparations can cause direct toxicity from the herb itself, it is much more common that the patient becomes ill from the contamination, misuse, overuse, or misidentification of the herbal preparation.[59] Herbal preparations can cause either direct toxicity (**Table 205-3**) or indirect toxicity from herb–drug interactions (**Table 205-4**).[52] Reported contaminants in herbal preparations include lead, selenium, and cyanide.[62-66]

Much of the available literature on herb–drug interactions is anecdotal and nonreproducible, but there are some herb–drug interactions that, because of numerous clinical reports, animal studies, and/or controlled clinical studies, can be deemed to be "likely" (**Table 205-4**).[61] Although not usually of clinical relevance, certain herbals may also interfere with assays for therapeutic drugs.[67-69]

REFERENCES

The complete reference list is available online at www.TintinalliEM.com.

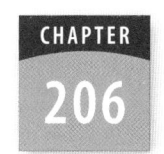

Antimicrobials

Joseph G. Rella
Wallace A. Carter

INTRODUCTION

Adverse effects associated with antimicrobials occur primarily in three circumstances: side effects with therapeutic dosing, acute toxicity resulting from excessive dosing, and subacute to chronic effects from sustained therapeutic use. Side effects can be immunologic (allergic) or nonimmunologic (pharmacologic or idiosyncratic) in nature. Antibiotics cause more reported allergic reactions than other drugs, possibly due to their high frequency of use that is often in a repeated and interrupted fashion. Sometimes a diluent or other chemical constituent in the formulation of a drug causes the adverse effect.

Most patients who sustain an acute antimicrobial overdose remain asymptomatic, and observation is generally all that is required. Measurement of drug levels is not helpful for management but may be

TABLE 206-1 Select Antimicrobial Toxicities and Their Specific Treatments

Drug	Acute Toxicity	Special Therapy for Symptomatic Overdose
Antibacterials		
Penicillin	Seizures (50 million units or more IV)	Benzodiazepines
Amoxicillin	Crystalluria, hematuria, acute renal failure	IV fluid
Cephalosporins	Encephalopathy, seizures	Benzodiazepines
Chloramphenicol	Cardiovascular collapse	Hemodialysis
Fluoroquinolones	Seizures	Benzodiazepines
Macrolides	Prolonged QT interval, torsades de pointes arrhythmia	Magnesium sulfate
Sulfonamides	Methemoglobinemia	Methylene blue
Vancomycin	"Red man syndrome" (anaphylactoid response)	Slow or stop infusion, antihistamines
Antimalarials		
Chloroquine	Seizures, QRS-complex and QT-interval prolongation, hypotension, hypokalemia	Epinephrine, diazepam
Quinine (quinidine)	Sodium-potassium channel blockade, α-adrenergic antagonism, hypoglycemia, ototoxicity, ophthalmic toxicity	Multidose activated charcoal, sodium bicarbonate, dextrose, octreotide
Primaquine	Methemoglobinemia, hemolysis	Methylene blue
Antituberculous medications		
Isoniazid	Inhibition of γ-aminobutyric acid synthesis and functional deficiency pyridoxine, seizures	Benzodiazepines, high-dose pyridoxine

confirmatory. Levels are available for several antibiotics such as chloroquine, isoniazid, and quinine. Ancillary testing should be based on the substance ingested and the clinical condition of the patient, such as methemoglobin concentrations for patients with dapsone or chloroquine toxicity.[1] Some antimicrobials are associated with specific, significant toxicities following an acute ingestion and may require particular therapy (**Table 206-1**).

Consider GI decontamination for patients suspected of ingesting a toxic amount of a potentially dangerous antimicrobial agent. Single-dose activated charcoal without sorbitol given orally or via nasogastric tube is most beneficial within 1 hour of the ingestion.[2,3] Multidose activated charcoal is indicated in symptomatic patients who have ingested dapsone or quinine.[4] Hemodialysis or hemoperfusion is effective at reducing concentrations of dapsone,[5,6] chloramphenicol, cefepime,[7,8] and possibly pentamidine.[9]

ANTIBACTERIALS

PENICILLINS, CEPHALOSPORINS, AND OTHER β-LACTAM AGENTS

Acute overdoses of penicillins and cephalosporins mainly produce nausea, vomiting, and diarrhea but are rarely life threatening. Large doses of penicillins or cephalosporins may produce seizures through γ-aminobutyric acid inhibition, and seizures are managed by administration of benzodiazepines or barbiturates. Seizures resulting from intrathecal doses of penicillins or cephalosporins may require cerebral spinal fluid exchange for treatment. Imipenem may cause seizures in overdose or at therapeutic doses, and these are treated in the same manner. Agitation, encephalopathy, absence seizures, and nonconvulsive status epilepticus have been reported with cefazolin, ceftazidime, cefuroxime, and cefepime.[8,10,11] Patients most at risk for adverse neurologic effects from β-lactams are those with renal failure, those with underlying CNS abnormalities, and those receiving high-dose therapy.[11,12] Amoxicillin overdose may produce crystal-induced interstitial nephritis, hematuria, and renal failure; treatment is supportive with IV fluids.[13-16]

Amoxicillin-clavulanate can cause rare cases of cholestatic hepatitis (1 to 6 weeks following initiation) and pancreatitis.[17] Treat with supportive care and withdrawal of the drug. Penicillins are associated with bone marrow suppression, hemolysis, interstitial nephritis, and vasculitis.[18] Cephalosporins, particularly cefaclor, are associated with serum sickness and can cause acute hemolytic crisis. Cephalosporins with the *N*-methylthiotetrazole side chain, such as cefazolin and cefotetan, can produce a disulfiram-like reaction as the side chain is released.

Two particular acute adverse reactions to procaine penicillin G are the Jarisch-Herxheimer reaction and Hoigne's syndrome. The Jarisch-Herxheimer reaction can begin within a few hours following antibiotic treatment of Lyme disease or early syphilis. This reaction is characterized by headache, fever, myalgias, and rash; is usually limited to 24 hours; and results from antigen released from lysed bacteria.[19] Hoigne's syndrome begins within minutes after an intramuscular or intravascular injection of procaine penicillin G. This syndrome is characterized by extreme apprehension, fear, hallucinations, illusions, hypertension and tachycardia, and seizures. The cause of this reaction is unclear, but the effects occur in the absence of other signs of anaphylaxis. Amoxicillin and ceftriaxone has been reported to produce a similar reaction.

CLINDAMYCIN

The lincosamide class includes clindamycin and lincomycin, and its main acute toxicities are nausea, vomiting, and diarrhea. Although all antibiotics have been associated with depletion of normal gut flora that allows for proliferation of *Clostridium difficile*, clindamycin is among those antibiotics that carry a higher risk for this infection, along with potential complications of pseudomembranous colitis and toxic megacolon.[20] Clindamycin is also associated with two forms of liver injury: (1) transient elevations of serum aminotransferases and (2) acute idiosyncratic liver injury characterized by jaundice, alanine transaminase levels 2 to 12 times over baseline, fever, and rash. This latter form of injury usually shows minimal cell injury on liver biopsy and is not associated with liver failure.[21]

FLUOROQUINOLONES

Acute overdose of fluoroquinolones rarely produces life-threatening effects. Seizures are a rare consequence of fluoroquinolone use, possibly due to γ-aminobutyric acid inhibition or through sequestration of magnesium, which may also result in prolongation of the QT interval and cause torsades de pointes. Fluoroquinolones are associated with acute renal failure, possibly through a hypersensitivity reaction where risk factors include concomitant use of renin-angiotensin–blocking agents.[22] Crystal-induced nephropathy has been reported with therapeutic doses of ciprofloxacin.[23] Caution is advised when using in children due to potential problems with developing cartilage and bone. In adults, tendon rupture has been attributed to fluoroquinolone use for up to 120 days following start of treatment. Discontinue the antibiotic in those who complain of painful or swollen tendons. Fluoroquinolones are also associated with dysglycemia, rash, serum sickness, and tinnitus.[11]

LINEZOLID

The first member of a new class of antibiotic, synthetic oxazolidinones, linezolid inhibits monoamine oxidase and can lead to serotonin syndrome when used concurrently with other serotonergic medications such as selective serotonin reuptake inhibitors.[24]

Chronic therapy longer than 28 days is associated with peripheral neuropathy and optic neuropathy with loss of central vision and loss of color and visual acuity. Lactic acidosis can occur, especially in patients with numerous comorbidities including sepsis and cirrhosis. Linezolid is also associated with anemia, thrombocytopenia and pancytopenia, and cholestatic hepatitis.[25]

MACROLIDES AND KETOLIDES

Although the most common adverse reaction to macrolide use is GI distress, QT-interval prolongation with potential for torsades de pointes is the most important.[26,27] The mechanism for this effect is blockade of the delayed rectifier potassium currents and has resulted from use of erythromycin, clarithromycin, telithromycin, and, to a lesser extent, azithromycin. Erythromycin and clarithromycin, but not azithromycin, also inhibit the cytochrome P-450 3A4 enzyme, which can result in severe drug interactions. Additionally, macrolides are associated with high-frequency sensorineural hearing loss, cholestatic hepatitis, and rarely pancreatitis.[28]

TRIMETHOPRIM-SULFAMETHOXAZOLE

These two antimicrobials work together for their antibiotic effect and are associated with many commonly reported adverse effects. Among them are allergic reactions, hematologic disorders, hypoglycemia, methemoglobinemia, rhabdomyolysis, and psychosis. Trimethoprim-sulfamethoxazole is also associated with idiosyncratic acute liver injury with a clinical pattern suggestive of a drug allergy or hypersensitivity mechanism and is particularly common among HIV-infected patients.[29]

VANCOMYCIN

Red man syndrome is an anaphylactoid response related to rate of intravenous vancomycin infusion that can include angioedema, chest pain, dyspnea, flushing, pruritus, and urticaria. Rarely, this syndrome can also cause seizures and cardiovascular collapse. Most symptoms resolve within 15 minutes when the infusion is stopped. Continuing the infusion at a slower rate or with increased dilution can help decrease recurrence. Pretreatment with diphenhydramine is also helpful.[30]

ANTIFUNGALS

TRIAZOLES

Antifungal agents such as fluconazole, clotrimazole, and miconazole are not expected to produce severe toxicity in acute overdose settings. Uncommon adverse reactions such as hepatotoxicity can occur, rarely leading to liver failure and death. Liver injury is hepatocellular and can be accompanied by eosinophilia, fever, and rash. Recovery begins with stopping the drug and may take as long as 3 to 4 months. These antifungals are also associated with neutropenia and thrombocytopenia, and they inhibit cytochrome P-450 3A4, potentiating toxicity from other pharmaceuticals.

AMPHOTERICIN B

Amphotericin B is used for progressive, life-threatening fungal infections and is rarely encountered in the ED. Acute overdoses are associated with fever, headache, nausea, vomiting, rigors, hypotension and tachycardia, anemias, dysrhythmias, electrolyte wasting, nephrotoxicity, neuropathy, and cardiac arrest.[31]

ANTIMALARIALS

CHLOROQUINE AND HYDROXYCHLOROQUINE

Chloroquine toxicity usually begins within 3 hours of ingestion with nausea, vomiting, and diarrhea.[32] Cardiovascular collapse may be precipitous, with QRS-complex prolongation and atrioventricular nodal blockade. Hypotension may be more severe than that seen with quinine overdose and is accompanied by respiratory depression and hypokalemia. Neurologic toxicity may include headache, obtundation, and seizures.

Aggressive supportive care is needed. A decreased mortality rate has been demonstrated in chloroquine overdose treated with early intubation, gastric lavage, deep sedation with benzodiazepines, and vasoactive pressor support with epinephrine to maintain a systolic blood pressure of 100 mm Hg (13.3 kPa).[33-35]

MEFLOQUINE

Mefloquine is used for prophylaxis or treatment of drug-resistant malaria and is associated with a variety of complications. In addition to GI distress, mefloquine is a rare cause for cardiac depression and severe CNS events, including seizures, hallucinations, and psychosis. Milder CNS effects, such as headache, insomnia, and vivid dreams, occur in up to 25% of patients. Mefloquine is not recommended as first-line therapy and is contraindicated in patients with seizures or psychiatric disorders.[36]

PRIMAQUINE

Primaquine is associated with GI distress and may cause hemolytic anemia and methemoglobinemia, especially in a glucose-6-phosphate dehydrogenase–deficient population. Granulocytosis, granulocytopenia, hypertension, dysrhythmia, and neurologic depression are rare complications associated with overdose.[37,38]

QUININE

The cardiac toxicity of quinine includes both sodium and potassium channel antagonism, which may result in widened QRS-complex intervals, torsades de pointes, hypotension, syncope, and sudden death.[39] Quinine also has significant ocular toxicity in acute overdose and blindness may result from serum levels >10 to 15 micrograms/mL (31 to 46 micromol/L).[40,41] Ototoxicity from quinine can produce symptoms that range from tinnitus to deafness.[42] Hypoglycemia may also result from hyperinsulinemia.

Sodium bicarbonate to maintain a serum pH of 7.55 is the mainstay of treatment for quinine-induced cardiac toxicity while avoiding class IA, IC, and III antidysrhythmic agents. **Quinine overdose is one of the few drugs for which multiple-dose activated charcoal is truly indicated.**[4]

ATOVAQUONE-PROGUANIL

Atovaquone-proguanil (Malarone) is most often associated with GI distress and headache. It is quite well tolerated and is considered safe during pregnancy and breastfeeding.

ANTIPARASITICS

Most antiparasitics, such as albendazole, mebendazole, and thiabendazole, have minimal toxicity following an acute overdose, usually only producing abdominal pain, nausea, and vomiting. Levamisole, an antihelminthic that was discontinued in the United States in 1999 due to agranulocytosis, has been a common adulterant in illicit cocaine. Complications found among cocaine users stemming from the levamisole contaminant include leukocytoclastic vasculitis, cutaneous necrotizing vasculitis, and thrombotic vasculopathy without vasculitis.[43]

ANTITUBERCULOUS MEDICATIONS

ISONIAZID

First-line medications used to treat both latent and active tuberculosis include isoniazid, rifampin, ethambutol, and pyrazinamide. Of these, isoniazid is associated with high morbidity and mortality in overdose.[44,45] At therapeutic doses, adverse effects from isoniazid include neuropathy and hepatic injury.

The clinical symptoms of acute isoniazid overdose typically begin with nausea, mental status changes, and ataxia, which may be seen as early as 30 minutes after ingestion. These symptoms may progress to **the three classic features of acute isoniazid overdose: seizures, metabolic acidosis, and protracted coma.**[46,47] Seizures typically follow acute isoniazid ingestions of greater than 20 to 30 milligrams/kg. Isoniazid-induced seizures are generalized tonic-clonic in nature and are often refractory to standard anticonvulsive therapy with benzodiazepines and barbiturates. The mechanism for isoniazid-induced seizures is a functional deficiency of pyridoxine (vitamin B_6) and inhibition of the synthesis of γ-aminobutyric acid, the primary CNS inhibitory neurotransmitter. Seizures with therapeutic doses of isoniazid have been reported in patients,[48] presumably due to very low vitamin B_6 levels.[49] Although the metabolic acidosis that accompanies isoniazid-induced seizures is likely due to motor activity, the lactic acidemia may not resolve as rapidly as with other more typical epileptic seizures.

Consider isoniazid overdose in patients with refractory seizures.[44] Isoniazid-induced seizures are treated with a combination of benzodiazepines and pyridoxine. The dose of **pyridoxine** is a gram-for-gram equivalent to the amount of isoniazid ingested.[50] For patients who ingest an unknown quantity of isoniazid, the recommended dose of pyridoxine is 5 grams IV in adults and 70 milligrams/kg (maximum 5 grams) in pediatric patients. Pyridoxine may be administered at a rate of approximately 1 gram IV every 2 to 3 minutes until the seizures stop or the maximum dose has been given. After the seizures have ceased, the remainder of the pyridoxine dose should be given over the following 4 to 6 hours to limit recurrent seizures.

Adequate single-dose therapy of pyridoxine should be effective to stop most seizures, but patients who do not receive adequate pyridoxine dosing may have repeat seizures. Pyridoxine may also assist in reversing isoniazid-induced comas. Hospitals where tuberculosis is endemic should ensure that an adequate supply of intravenous pyridoxine is maintained to treat overdoses.[51] If only pyridoxine tablets are available, they may be crushed and administered by nasogastric tube.

Phenytoin has no role in treating seizures originating from isoniazid overdose, and there is little role for sodium bicarbonate treatment of the metabolic acidosis resulting from isoniazid toxicity. Because most isoniazid-induced toxicity occurs within 2 hours of ingestion, patients who remain asymptomatic for 6 hours after ED presentation are safe for medical clearance.

OTHER ANTITUBERCULOSIS AGENTS

Other antituberculous medications are associated with a variety of adverse reactions of a milder nature. **Ethambutol** toxicity is also primarily GI in nature, but additionally may cause unilateral or bilateral ocular toxicity including blurred vision, disruption of color perception, and loss of peripheral vision. **Rifampin** infrequently causes severe toxicity and is most often associated with GI symptoms. Acute toxicity has been associated with flushing, angioedema, and neurologic effects including numbness, extremity pain, ataxia, and weakness. Rifampin has been presumptively implicated in producing acute kidney injury with proteinuria.[52] **Pyrazinamide** is not associated with any toxic effects following an acute overdose.

REFERENCES

The complete reference list is available online at www.TintinalliEM.com.

CHAPTER 207 Dyshemoglobinemias

Brenna M. Farmer
Lewis S. Nelson

INTRODUCTION

Dyshemoglobinemias are disorders in which the hemoglobin molecule is functionally altered and prevented from carrying oxygen. The most clinically relevant dyshemoglobinemias are carboxyhemoglobin, methemoglobin, and sulfhemoglobin.[1] Carboxyhemoglobin is created during carbon monoxide exposure and, because of its unique importance and prevalence, is usually considered an environmental emergency (see chapter 222, "Carbon Monoxide").

METHEMOGLOBINEMIA

PATHOPHYSIOLOGY

The iron moiety within deoxyhemoglobin normally exists in the ferrous (bivalent or Fe^{2+}) state. Ferrous iron avidly interacts with compounds seeking electrons, such as oxygen or other oxidizing agent, and in the process is oxidized to the ferric (trivalent or Fe^{3+}) state. Hemoglobin in the ferric form is unable to bind oxygen for transport and is termed *methemoglobin*. Under normal circumstances, <1% to 2% of circulating hemoglobin exists as methemoglobin; higher concentrations define the condition of *methemoglobinemia*.

Methemoglobin accumulation is enzymatically prevented by the rapid reduction of the ferric iron back to the ferrous form. Cytochrome b_5 reductase is primarily responsible for this reduction, in which reduced nicotinamide adenine dinucleotide donates its electrons to cytochrome b_5, which subsequently reduces methemoglobin to hemoglobin (**Figure 207-1**). This pathway is responsible for reducing nearly 95% of methemoglobin produced under typical circumstances. Methemoglobinemia occurs when this enzymatic reduction is overwhelmed by an exogenous oxidant stress, such as a drug or chemical agent (**Table 207-1**).

Methemoglobin can also be reduced by a second enzymatic pathway using the reduced form of nicotinamide adenine dinucleotide phosphate (or NADPH) and NADPH-methemoglobin reductase.[2] This pathway is normally of minimal importance and is responsible for less than 5% of total reduction under typical circumstances. However, this enzyme and pathway are crucial for the antidotal effect of methylene blue (Figure 207-1).

The limited role for NADPH partially explains why patients with glucose-6-phosphate dehydrogenase deficiency with a resultant deficiency in NADPH are **not** at increased risk of developing methemoglobinemia, although they are at risk of developing hemolysis following exposure to an oxidant stress. To a very limited extent, nonenzymatic reduction systems, such as vitamin C and glutathione, may participate in the reduction of methemoglobin to hemoglobin.

The primary clinical effect of methemoglobin is to reduce the oxygen content of the blood. Because hemoglobin-bound oxygen accounts for the vast majority of an individual's oxygen-carrying capacity, as the methemoglobin concentration rises, oxygen-carrying capacity to the tissues falls. Patients with methemoglobinemia are often more symptomatic than patients who suffer from a simple anemia that produces an equivalent reduction in oxygen-carrying capacity. This is caused by a leftward shift in the oxyhemoglobin dissociation curve, the consequence of which is a reduced release of oxygen from the erythrocyte to the tissue at a given partial pressure of oxygen (**Figure 207-2**).[2]

The oxyhemoglobin dissociation curve of blood with a 50% reduction in erythrocytes (i.e., anemia) follows a curve similar to that of nonanemic blood; although the oxygen content is lower, unbinding of half of the oxygen (50% oxygen saturation) occurs at the same Po_2. With 50% methemoglobin, the leftward shift of the oxyhemoglobin dissociation curve means that hemoglobin is less willing to give up its oxygen, so that tissue hypoxia is more severe than in those with a 50% anemia.

Acquired Methemoglobinemia Drugs in conventional doses rarely produce clinically significant methemoglobinemia, although subclinical methemoglobinemia may go unrecognized (Table 207-1). Benzocaine is the local anesthetic most commonly associated with methemoglobinemia.[3-5] Methemoglobin induction with sodium nitrite is a therapeutic goal in the management of patients suffering from cyanide poisoning (see chapter 204, "Industrial Toxins"). Certain compounds, particularly dapsone,[6] require metabolism to the "active" oxidant, and there may be substantial delay until toxicity is evident. Occupational methemoglobinemia usually involves exposure to aromatic compounds, primarily amino- and nitro-substituted benzenes.[7] Routes of absorption are typically dermal or inhalational due to the high lipophilicity and volatility of these compounds, respectively.

Neonates and infants are more susceptible to methemoglobin accumulation because of undeveloped methemoglobin reduction mechanisms. This accounts for the relatively common development of methemoglobinemia in infants given certain nitrogenous vegetables (e.g., spinach) or well water that contains high nitrate levels (generally from fertilizer use). Bacteria within the GI flora convert nitrate to the nitrite form, which is a more potent oxidant. Another common cause of acquired infantile methemoglobinemia is gastroenteritis, which presumably is caused by an increased oxidant burden originating in the GI tract.[8]

Hereditary Methemoglobinemia Hereditary methemoglobinemia results from either an enzymatic deficiency (i.e., cytochrome b_5 reductase)

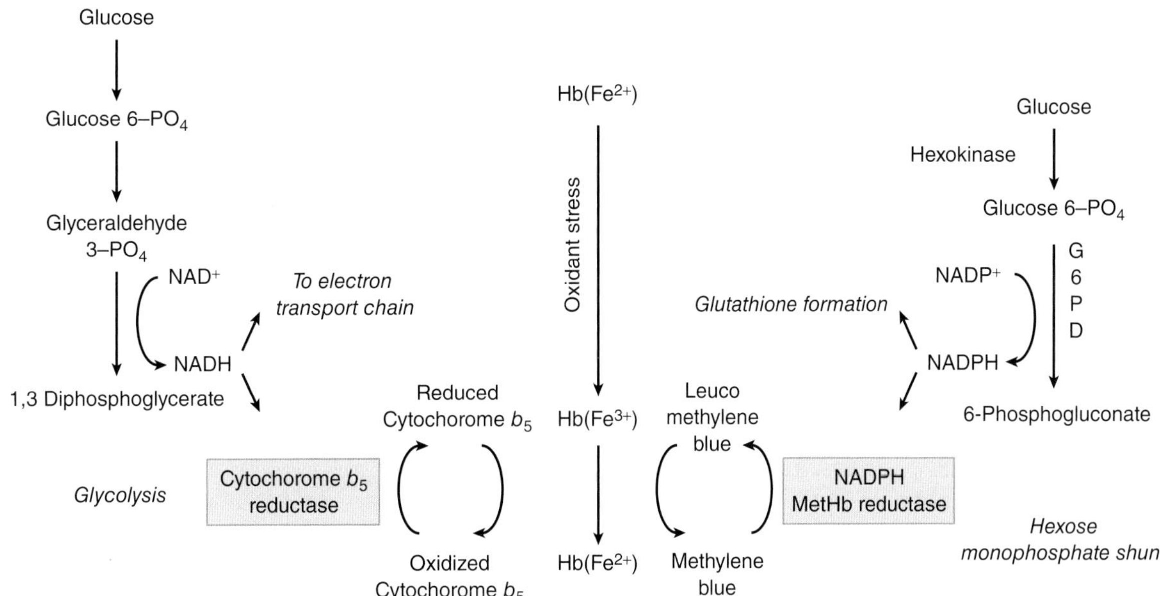

FIGURE 207-1. Methemoglobin formation and mechanism of action of methylene blue. G6PD = glucose-6-phosphate dehydrogenase; $Hb(Fe^{2+})$ = hemoglobin; $Hb(Fe^{3+})$ = methemoglobin; NAD^+ = oxidized nicotinamide adenine dinucleotide; NADH = reduced form of nicotinamide adenine dinucleotide; $NADP^+$ = nicotinamide adenine dinucleotide phosphate; NADPH = reduced form of nicotinamide adenine dinucleotide phosphate; PO_4 = phosphate.

or from the presence of an amino acid substitution within the hemoglobin molecule itself, termed *hemoglobin M*.[1] Patients with cytochrome b_5 reductase deficiency develop methemoglobin levels of 20% to 40%. Cyanosis in these individuals begins at birth, but they remain asymptomatic and develop normally.

Hemoglobin M, an abnormal form of hemoglobin, has altered tertiary structure so that the heme iron exists in an environment favoring the ferric form. This disorder only occurs in the heterozygous form, because the homozygous form is incompatible with life. As with cytochrome b_5 reductase deficiency, patients develop profound cyanosis but tolerate the elevated methemoglobin concentrations well due to compensatory mechanisms.

TABLE 207-1 Drugs Causing Methemoglobinemia

Oxidant	Comments
Analgesics	
Phenazopyridine	Commonly reported
Phenacetin	Rarely used
Antimicrobials	
Antimalarials	Common
Dapsone	Hydroxylamine metabolite formation is inhibited by cimetidine
Local anesthetics	
Benzocaine	Most commonly reported of the local anesthetics
Lidocaine	Rare
Prilocaine	Common in topical anesthetics
Dibucaine	Rare
Nitrates/nitrites	
Amyl nitrite	Cyanide antidote kit and used to enhance sexual encounters
Isobutyl nitrite	Used to enhance sexual encounters
Sodium nitrite	Cyanide antidote kit
Ammonium nitrate	Cold packs
Silver nitrate	Excessive topical use
Well water	Problem in infants, due to nitrate fertilizer runoff
Nitroglycerin	Rare
Sulfonamides	
Sulfamethoxazole	Uncommon

CLINICAL FEATURES

Healthy patients who have normal hemoglobin concentrations do not usually develop clinical effects until the methemoglobin level rises above 20% of the total hemoglobin.[9] At methemoglobin levels between 20% and 30%, anxiety, headache, weakness, and light-headedness develop, and patients may exhibit tachypnea and sinus tachycardia. Methemoglobin levels of 50% to 60% impair oxygen delivery to vital tissues, resulting in myocardial ischemia, dysrhythmias, depressed mental status (including coma), seizures, and lactate-associated metabolic acidosis. Levels above 70% are largely incompatible with life.

Cyanosis associated with methemoglobin is often described as a gray discoloration of skin, with a detection threshold for methemoglobin of 1.5 grams/dL, corresponding to methemoglobin levels between 10% and 15% in a nonanemic individual (**Figure 207-3**). Methemoglobin levels above 20% will discolor the blood a chocolate brown.[10]

Anemic patients may not exhibit cyanosis until the methemoglobin level rises well above 10% because cyanosis detection is dependent on the level of methemoglobin, not the percentage. Anemic patients may likewise suffer significant symptoms at lower methemoglobin concentrations because the relative percentage of hemoglobin in the oxidized form is greater. Patients with preexisting cardiopulmonary diseases that impair oxygen delivery will also manifest symptoms with less significant elevations in their methemoglobin levels. Conversely, compensatory mechanisms that shift the oxyhemoglobin dissociation curve to the right, such as acidosis or elevated 2,3-diphosphoglycerate, may result in somewhat better toleration of methemoglobin.

DIAGNOSIS

Consider methemoglobinemia in patients with cyanosis, particularly if cyanosis does not improve with supplemental oxygen (**Figure 207-4**).[4-6,9] A useful clue is that patients with methemoglobin-associated cyanosis generally are less symptomatic than equivalently appearing patients with hypoxemia-induced cyanosis. This is due to the more deeply pigmented color of methemoglobin compared with deoxyhemoglobin; it takes about 5 grams/dL of deoxyhemoglobin to cause cyanosis, which

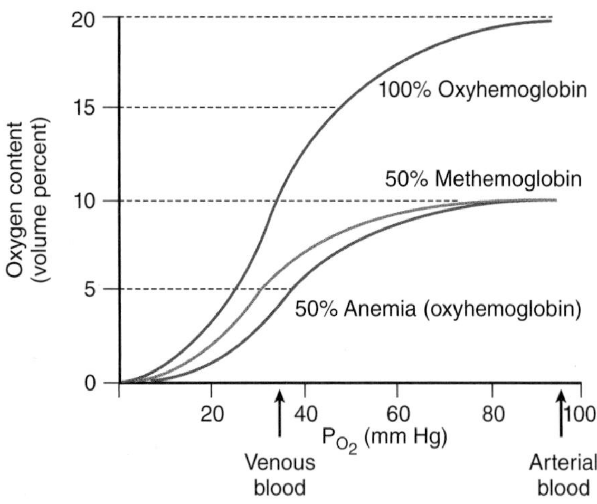

FIGURE 207-2. Oxyhemoglobin dissociation curve.

equates to an oxygen-carrying capacity of approximately 67% of normal, compared with the cyanosis visible with a methemoglobin concentration of 1.5 grams/dL, which equates to an oxygen-carrying capacity of 90% of normal. Blood containing methemoglobin has a characteristic "chocolate brown" color when phlebotomized. Detection of this discoloration is improved when compared directly with normal blood.[10]

Pulse oximetry results are not accurate in patients with methemoglobinemia.[11] The standard pulse oximeter uses two wavelengths of light, 660 nm and 940 nm, to calculate the percentage of oxyhemoglobin. Methemoglobin is also detected by these wavelengths, and light absorption by methemoglobin confounds the calculation for the oxyhemoglobin percentage. **In patients with methemoglobinemia, the pulse oximeter will report a falsely elevated value for arterial oxygen saturation percentage.** The specific values vary by oximeter,[3,11] but typically trend to approximately 85%.[11]

Pulse co-oximeters are commercially available that use additional wavelengths of light to measure the total hemoglobin concentration and percentages of carboxyhemoglobin and methemoglobin.[11] When first released, accuracy for methemoglobinemia levels was progressively unreliable with increasing hypoxemia,[12] but the new probes[13] appear to have corrected the problem.[11]

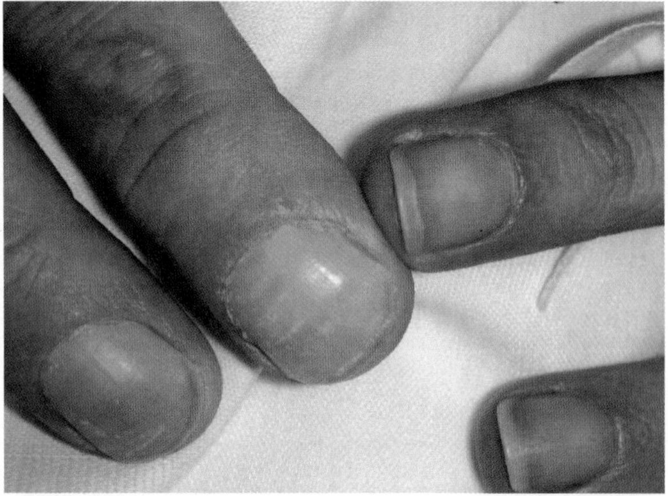

FIGURE 207-3. Methemoglobinemia due to dapsone. Gray-blue discoloration of the patient's fingernails compared with that of the physician. With the patient on supplemental oxygen, the pulse oximeter reported an oxygen saturation of 93%. Arterial blood gas measurement reported a Pa_{O_2} of 307 mm Hg, a calculated oxygen saturation of 99.8%, and a measured methemoglobin of 12%. [Photo Contributed by J. S. Stapczynski, MD.]

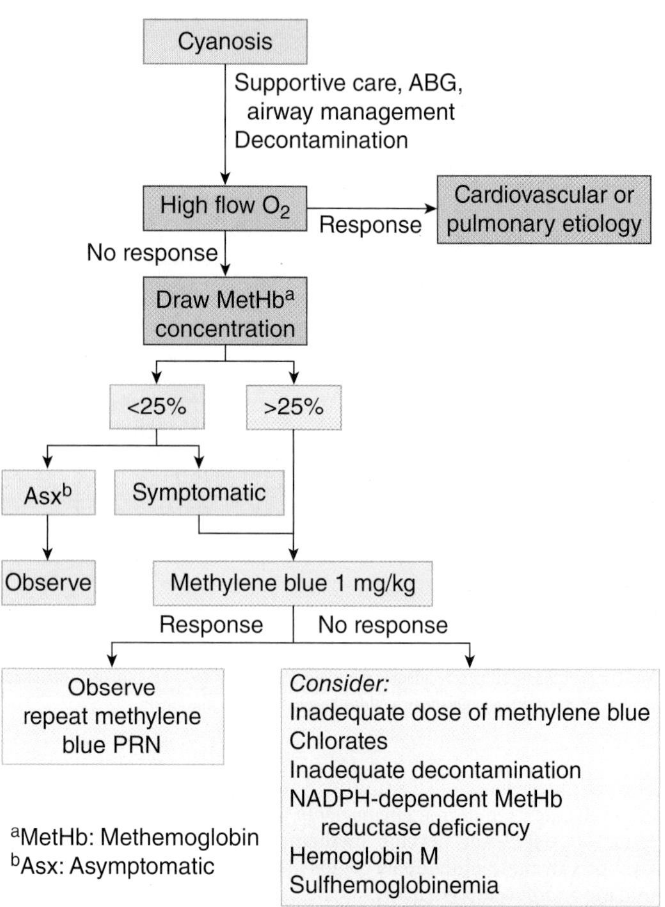

FIGURE 207-4. Toxicologic approach to the cyanotic patient. ABG = arterial blood gas; NADPH = reduced form of nicotinamide adenine dinucleotide phosphate. [Reproduced with permission from Nelson LS, Lewin NA, Howland MA, Hoffman RS, Goldfrank LR, Flomenbaum NE (eds): *Goldfrank's Toxicologic Emergencies*, 9th ed. McGraw-Hill, Inc., 2011; Figure 127-7, p. 1704.]

Definitive identification of dyshemoglobinemias requires co-oximetry, a spectrophotometric method capable of differentiating among oxyhemoglobin, deoxyhemoglobin, carboxyhemoglobin, and methemoglobin species.[9] This widely available test can be performed on a venous or arterial specimen.

Arterial blood gas results may be initially deceptive because the partial pressure of oxygen, a measure of dissolved, not bound, oxygen, is normal. Thus, calculation of oxygen saturation from measured partial pressure by the blood gas analyzer will produce a falsely elevated result.

TREATMENT

Patients with methemoglobinemia require supportive measures to ensure oxygen delivery and the administration of appropriate antidotal therapy, if indicated (**Table 207-2**). Gastric decontamination is of limited value, because there often is a substantial time interval between exposure to the toxic agent and the development of methemoglobin. If a source of continuing GI exposure is suspected, decontamination is indicated, and in most stable patients, a single dose of activated charcoal is likely sufficient. Dermal decontamination should be used as indicated. **Antidotal therapy with methylene blue is reserved for symptomatic patients or for those asymptomatic patients with methemoglobin levels >25%.**

Methylene blue indirectly accelerates the enzymatic reduction of methemoglobin by NADPH-methemoglobin reductase. NADPH-methemoglobin reductase reduces methylene blue to leucomethylene blue, which is then capable of directly reducing the oxidized iron (Fe^{3+}) back to the ferrous state (Fe^{2+}) (Figure 207-1). The initial methylene blue dose is 1 milligram/kg (0.1 mL/kg of the 1% solution or approximately

TABLE 207-2 Management of Methemoglobinemia

Management of Methemoglobinemia
Assess airway, breathing, and circulation; exclude other causes of cyanosis
Insert an IV line
Administer oxygen
Attach the patient to a cardiac and pulse oximeter or co-oximeter
Obtain an ECG
Decontaminate the patient as needed
Administer methylene blue: if symptomatic or methemoglobin >25%
Consider: cimetidine for patients taking dapsone

7 mL in an adult) IV over 5 minutes. The infusion should be slow because rapidly administered doses of methylene blue are painful. Clinical improvement should be seen within 20 minutes, and as the methemoglobin level falls, the most severe signs and symptoms will resolve first. Resolution of the cyanosis occurs later only after the methemoglobin concentration falls below 1.5 grams/dL. Repeat dosing of methylene blue is acceptable, if cyanosis has not cleared in 1 hour. Serotonin toxicity (syndrome) is a rare risk when methylene blue is administered to patients on serotonergic drugs such as antidepressants.[14]

Treatment failures may result if the patient has glucose-6-phosphate dehydrogenase deficiency, because this enzyme is critical for the production of NADPH by the hexose monophosphate shunt (Figure 207-1). Hemolysis may impede a response to methylene blue, which requires an intact erythrocyte to be effective. Oxidant drugs with long serum half-lives, such as dapsone with a half-life of approximately 50 hours, produce prolonged oxidant stress to the red blood cell. Therefore, dapsone-exposed patients may require repetitive dosing of methylene blue. Because the hydroxylamine metabolite of dapsone is responsible for the production of methemoglobin, inhibition of its formation by cytochrome P450 with cimetidine,[6] in standard doses, is generally recommended.

In rare instances, patients may be deficient in NADPH-methemoglobin reductase, the required enzyme for methylene blue activation. Lastly, treatment failure may occur in patients with sulfhemoglobinemia, which is clinically indistinguishable from methemoglobinemia, but which is not responsive to methylene blue. Patients who do not respond to methylene blue should be treated supportively. If clinically unstable, the use of packed red cell transfusions or exchange transfusions may be indicated.

SULFHEMOGLOBINEMIA

PATHOPHYSIOLOGY

Sulfhemoglobinemia is a rare condition that occurs when a sulfur atom irreversibly binds to the porphyrin ring of the heme moiety and induces the permanent oxidation of iron to the ferric (Fe^{3+}) state.[1] Many of the agents responsible for sulfhemoglobinemia are identical to those associated with methemoglobin. Because many of these drugs or chemicals do not contain sulfur, the origin of sulfur is speculative; hypotheses include alteration of intestinal flora with production and absorption of hydrogen sulfide and/or glutathione.[15] Historically, sulfhemoglobinemia was most often associated with acetanilide, phenacetin, sulfonamide, and a proprietary mixture that contained sodium bromide. Because these drugs are rarely used and the sodium bromide component in the proprietary mixture was removed in 1975, contemporary cases of drug-induced sulfhemoglobinemia are now most often reported with phenazopyridine, dapsone, metoclopramide, and sumatriptan.[16,17] Sulfhemoglobinemia has been associated with industrial chemicals, such as trinitrotoluene, hydroxylamine sulfate, dimethyl sulfoxide, and hydrogen sulfide.[18]

CLINICAL FEATURES

Patients with sulfhemoglobinemia can have a clinical presentation similar to those with methemoglobinemia. However, the disease process itself is substantially less concerning because, although the reduction in the patient's oxygen-carrying capacity is quantitatively similar, the sulfhemoglobin oxygen dissociation curve is shifted rightward, not leftward as in methemoglobinemia, favoring the release of hemoglobin-bound oxygen to the tissue with sulfhemoglobinemia. Because of the milder symptoms, speculation is that cases of sulfhemoglobinemia are often missed.[19]

DIAGNOSIS

The pigmentation of the blood by sulfhemoglobin is substantially more intense than other colored hemoglobin species; only 0.5 gram/dL of sulfhemoglobin is needed to produce a cyanosis equivalent to that produced by 1.5 grams/dL of methemoglobin or 5 grams/dL of deoxyhemoglobin. The color of blood drawn from a patient with sulfhemoglobinemia has been described as dark greenish-black. **In sulfhemoglobinemia, standard pulse oximetry tends to report a falsely low value for arterial oxygen saturation percentage.**[20] The diagnosis of sulfhemoglobinemia may be difficult to confirm. Standard co-oximetry may not differentiate sulfhemoglobin from methemoglobin because of similar spectral absorbance, and specialized settings are required to reliably measure sulfhemoglobin concentration.[21]

TREATMENT

Sulfhemoglobin persists for the life of the red cell and the level is not reduced by treatment with methylene blue. Most patients require only supportive care, although exchange transfusion or packed red cell transfusion is occasionally recommended for patients with severe toxicity.

REFERENCES

The complete reference list is available online at www.TintinalliEM.com.

Environmental Injuries

CHAPTER 208 Cold Injuries

Michael T. Paddock

INTRODUCTION

The occurrence of cold-related injuries depends on the degree of cold exposure, as well as environmental and individual factors. Frostbite is the prototypical freezing injury and is seen when ambient temperatures are well below freezing. Nonfreezing cold injuries occur as a result of exposure to wet conditions when temperatures are above freezing. The most common nonfreezing cold injuries are trench foot and chilblains. Although frostbite may result in permanent tissue damage, nonfreezing cold injuries are characterized by usually mild but uncomfortable inflammatory lesions of the skin. This chapter describes the occurrence, risk factors, treatment, and prevention of the nonfreezing cold injuries—trench foot and immersion foot, chilblains or pernio, panniculitis, and cold urticaria—and the freezing injury—frostbite.

NONFREEZING COLD INJURIES

TRENCH FOOT

Trench foot and its more severe variant, immersion foot, are rare conditions in civilians but can be a significant problem in military operations. The pathophysiology of trench foot is multifactorial but involves direct injury to soft tissue sustained from prolonged cooling, accelerated by wet conditions. The peripheral nerves seem to be the most sensitive to this form of injury.

Early symptoms progress from tingling to numbness of the affected tissues. On initial examination, the foot is pale, mottled, anesthetic, pulseless, and immobile, with no immediate change after rewarming. A hyperemic phase begins within hours after rewarming and is associated with severe burning pain and reappearance of proximal sensation. As perfusion returns to the foot over 2 to 3 days, edema and possibly bullae form, and hyperemia may worsen. Anesthesia frequently persists for weeks and may be permanent. In more severe cases, tissue sloughing and gangrene may develop. Hyperhidrosis and cold sensitivity are common late features and may persist for months to years. Severe cases may be associated with prolonged convalescence and permanent disability.[1]

Treatment is supportive, but vasodilator drugs may be tried. Oral prostaglandins can increase skin temperatures, which suggests improved circulation.[2] Feet should be kept clean, warm, dryly bandaged, elevated, and closely monitored for early signs of infection. Prophylaxis for trench foot includes keeping warm, ensuring good boot fit, changing out of wet socks several times a day, never sleeping in wet socks and boots, and, once early symptoms are identified, maximizing efforts to warm, dry, and elevate the feet.

CHILBLAINS OR PERNIO

Chilblains, or pernio, are characterized by mild but uncomfortable inflammatory lesions of the skin caused by long-term intermittent exposure to damp, nonfreezing ambient temperatures. Symptoms are precipitated by acute exposure to cold.[3] The most common areas affected are the feet (toes), hands, ears, and lower legs. Chilblains are primarily a disease of women and children, and although rare in the United States, the disease is common in the United Kingdom and other countries with a cold or temperate, damp climate.[3] In addition, young females with Raynaud's phenomenon and other immunologic abnormalities such as lupus erythematosus, as well as those in households with inadequate heating and lack of warm clothing, are at greatest risk. Some studies suggest that a low body mass index may be associated with increased risk.[3,4]

Early symptoms progress from tingling to numbness of the affected tissues. The cutaneous manifestations, which appear up to 12 to 24 hours after acute exposure, include localized edema, erythema, cyanosis, plaques, nodules, and, in rare cases, ulcerations, vesicles, and bullae. Patients may complain of pruritus and burning paresthesias. Rewarming may result in the formation of tender blue nodules, which may persist for several days.

Management is supportive. The affected skin should be rewarmed, gently bandaged, and elevated. Some European studies support the use of nifedipine, 20 milligrams PO three times daily; pentoxifylline, 400 milligrams PO three times daily; or an analog of prostaglandin E_1, limaprost, 20 micrograms PO three times daily, as both prophylactic and therapeutic treatment for local cold injury.[2,5] Topical corticosteroids (0.1% triamcinolone cream) are also effective.[6]

PANNICULITIS

Panniculitis is characterized by mild degrees of necrosis of the subcutaneous fat tissue that develops during prolonged exposure to temperatures just above freezing. It is observed in children (e.g., "popsicle panniculitis" of the cheeks) and on the thighs and buttocks of young women involved in equestrian activities.[7] During resolution of the mild inflammation, adipose fibrosis may result in cosmetic defects, such as unevenness of the skin. There is no effective treatment for the injury.

COLD URTICARIA

Cold urticaria is a distinctive example of hypersensitivity to cold air or water, which in rare cases may lead to fatal anaphylaxis.[8] Most cases are idiopathic,[9] but they can also be associated with increased affinity of immunoglobulin E to mast cells and viral infections.[9] The diagnosis can be confirmed with the cold water test during follow-up. Young adults and children and those with atopy or other forms of inducible urticaria are most commonly affected.[8,10]

Cold urticaria is treated similarly to urticarial lesions from other causes. Antihistamines (H1) are recommended for acute cases, although higher than usual dosing may be required.[11] Other potential therapies include leukotriene receptor antagonists (zafirlukast, montelukast)[12,13] and topical capsaicin. For persistent cold urticaria, ketotifen or doxantrazole may be tried, but oral preparations of these mast cell stabilizers are not available in the United States. Prescribe epinephrine autoinjectors for patients with a history of cold-induced anaphylaxis.

FREEZING INJURIES

EPIDEMIOLOGY

Groups at high risk for frostbite include military personnel, winter sports enthusiasts, outdoor workers, the elderly, the homeless, people who abuse drugs or alcohol, and those with psychiatric disorders. Individual attributes, such as anthropometry, physiology, behavior, and general health, affect an individual's likelihood of developing cold-related injuries[14,15] (**Table 208-1**).

TABLE 208-1 Factors Influencing the Likelihood of Frostbite

Factors
Environmental
Temperature
Wind
Wetness
Contact with cold objects or liquids (e.g., metals, petroleum, oil, lubricants)
Duration of cold exposure
Geographical area
Hypoxia
Altitude
Physical/Anthropometric Characteristics
Age
Gender
Race
Behavioral
Cold acclimatization
Alcohol use
Fatigue
Dehydration
Smoking
Use of protective ointments
Inappropriate or wet clothing
Constrictive clothing (e.g., tight boots)
Prolonged stationary posture
Health-Related/Physiologic
Raynaud's phenomenon
Vibration-induced white finger
Cold-induced vasodilation reactivity
Other peripheral vascular diseases
Diabetes
Peripheral neuropathies
Certain medications (e.g., vasoconstrictive drugs)
Previous cold injury
Psychiatric disorders or altered mental status

The areas most commonly affected by frostbite are the head (31% to 39.1% of cases), hands (20% to 27.9%), and feet (15% to 24.9%).[16-18] Studies vary regarding which of these sites is most commonly affected, with military personnel reporting higher incidences of foot and hand involvement than civilians.[18] Although most cases of frostbite are mild (frostnip), 12% of cases are more severe (**Table 208-2**).

RISK FACTORS FOR FROSTBITE

Age and Gender Both age and gender influence the incidence of frostbite. Among Finnish teens, twice as many teenage boys as girls report having had frostbite of at least blister grade during the previous year (4.1% of boys and 2.4% of girls).[19] Young men entering the military service report a cumulative lifetime incidence of 44%.[16] Although frostbite injuries occur more frequently in men as they age, the same is not true of women.[19] In general, the occurrence of frostbite is higher in men than in women,[19,20] which is possibly related to different occupational and leisure time activity patterns. The smaller size of women and their larger surface area–to–mass ratio increase the cooling rate, which makes women more susceptible to cooling and cold injuries.[15,21]

TABLE 208-2 Body Parts Affected by Frostbite (Lifetime Cumulative Incidence)

Degree of Frostbite	Number of Frostbite Episodes			
	All	Head	Hands	Feet
All frostbite cases	2555 (44%)	1668 (31%)	1154 (20%)	810 (15%)
First degree	2333 (41%)	1462 (28%)	1064 (19%)	738 (14%)
Higher than first degree, deep	671 (12%)	459 (9%)	213 (4%)	174 (3%)

Notes: Study population = 5839. Some persons had multiple locations and degrees of frostbite.

Temperature and Windchill The incidence of frostbite among civilians is governed by latitude of residence, the annual number of days on which the ambient temperature is below −15°C (5°F), and the length of daily cold exposure.[19] In the United States, the majority of occupational outdoor cold injuries occur during the few coldest days of winter. Wind strongly increases the injury rate. Rates of injury begin to increase when temperatures fall below −12°C (10.4°F) and wind speeds exceed 4.5 m/s (10 mph).[22] Wind markedly increases the cooling rate by increasing convective heat loss and reducing the insulation value of clothing, thus increasing the risk of frostbite. In addition, the colder temperatures at high altitudes, combined with high wind speeds, increase the risk of frostbite. Frostbite risk is clearly increased above 5182 m (17,000 ft).[23,24]

The National Weather Service windchill temperature index provides the relative risk for frostbite and predicted time for freezing risk at given air temperatures and wind speeds. The risk of frostbite is <5% when the ambient temperature is above −15°C (5°F), but increased surveillance is warranted when the windchill temperature falls below −27°C (−16.6°F).[15]

Frostbite most often occurs at environmental temperatures below −20°C (−4°F). Exposure times for injury vary from hours to several days depending on magnitude of exposure, degree of protective clothing, and physical activity level.

Skin temperature is <0°C (<32°F) when frostbite occurs. Of note, the risk of finger frostbite increases linearly from 5% to 95% when temperature at the skin surface decreases from −4.8°C to −7.8°C (23.4°F to 18.0°F).[25] In addition to ambient temperature and wind, merely touching cold materials (e.g., metal) is a risk factor for frostbite. Contact cooling is dependent on the surface temperature, type of material, duration of contact, and several individual factors. Frostbite can develop within 2 to 3 seconds when metal surfaces that are at or below −15°C (5°F) are touched.[26] Touching surfaces at ambient temperatures of <0°C (<32°F) with bare hands is not recommended. Other factors that increase heat loss and cooling rate and raise the risk of frostbite are wetting of the skin and contact with supercooled liquids (petroleum, oil).

Behavioral and Physiologic Risk Factors for Cold Injuries Multiple behavioral factors influence the risk of cold-related injuries. Alcohol consumption and smoking increase the occurrence of frostbite.[19,23] Inappropriate clothing (e.g., lack of gloves, headgear, or scarf, or wet clothes), constrictive clothing, and prolonged stationary posture increase the incidence of both freezing and nonfreezing injuries. Interestingly, the use of protective ointments is associated with an increased risk of frostbite on the head and face.[17]

Among military personnel, lower level of education or training and lower military rank, as well as situational misjudgments, accidental situations, fatigue, and insufficient nutrition, are all associated with a higher incidence of frostbite.[17] U.S. military studies suggest that black soldiers and those from warmer climatic regions are more susceptible to frostbite.[18]

Certain disease states, such as peripheral vascular disease, atherosclerosis, arteritis, Raynaud's disease, vibration-induced white finger, hypovolemia, diabetes, vascular injury secondary to trauma or infection, and previous cold-related injuries, may predispose to cold-related injury.[16,17,23] In addition, medications that affect the circulation, such as vasoconstrictors, may increase the risk of frostbite[14,19] (Table 208-1).

PATHOPHYSIOLOGY

It is generally agreed that freezing alone is usually not sufficient to cause tissue death, and often the consequences of thawing contribute markedly to the degree of injury. The depth of tissue freezing depends on the temperature, the duration of exposure, and the velocity of freezing.

TABLE 208-3 Classification of Frostbite Injuries

First degree	Numbness, central pallor with surrounding erythema and edema, desquamation, dysesthesia
Second degree	Blisters of the skin with surrounding edema and erythema
Third degree	Tissue loss involving the entire thickness of the skin; hemorrhagic blisters
Fourth degree	Tissue loss involving the entire thickness of the part, including deep structures, resulting in the loss of the part

Endothelial damage, beginning at the point of thaw, is the likely critical event in frostbite. Immediately after freezing and thawing, an arachidonic acid cascade forms and promotes vasoconstriction, platelet aggregation, leukocyte sludging, and erythrostasis, which results in venule and arterial thrombosis and subsequent ischemia, necrosis, and dry gangrene.[27] The necrosis of tissue following frostbite either is due to cellular injury or is secondary to a vascular lesion.[28]

Frostbite injury can be divided into three zones. The *zone of coagulation* is the most severe and is usually distal, and the damage is irreversible. The *zone of hyperemia* is the most superficial, is typically proximal, has the least cellular damage, and generally recovers without treatment in <10 days. The *zone of stasis* is the middle ground and is characterized by severe, but possibly reversible, cell damage. It is this middle zone for which treatment may have benefit if the circulation in the frozen area can be restored.

Tissue susceptibility to frostbite varies. The least to most sensitive tissues are, in order, cartilage, ligament, blood vessel, cutis, epidermis, bone, muscle, nerve, and bone marrow.

CLINICAL FEATURES AND DIAGNOSIS

Frostbite injuries are frequently classified by the depth of injury and amount of tissue damage based on appearance after rewarming (**Table 208-3**). Visual determination of tissue viability is difficult during the first few weeks after the injury, and viable tissue can often be identified only after gangrenous tissue has demarcated and sloughed.

First-degree injury (frostnip) is characterized by partial skin freezing, erythema, mild edema, lack of blisters, and occasional skin desquamation several days later. The patient may complain of stinging and burning, followed by throbbing. Prognosis is excellent. **Second-degree injury** is characterized by full-thickness skin freezing, formation of substantial edema over 3 to 4 hours, erythema, and formation of clear blisters filled with fluid rich in thromboxane and prostaglandins (**Figure 208-1**). The blisters form within 6 to 24 hours, extend to the end of the digit, and usually desquamate and form hard black eschars over several days. The patient complains of numbness, followed later by aching and throbbing. Prognosis is good. **Third-degree injury** is characterized by damage that extends into the subdermal plexus. Hemorrhagic blisters form and are associated with skin necrosis and a blue-gray discoloration of the skin (**Figure 208-2**). The patient may complain that the involved extremity feels like a "block of wood," which is followed later by burning, throbbing, and shooting pains. Prognosis is often poor. **Fourth-degree injury** is characterized by extension into subcutaneous tissues, muscle, bone, and tendon. There is little edema. The skin is mottled, with nonblanching cyanosis, and eventually forms a deep, dry, black, mummified eschar. Vesicles often present late, if at all, and may be small, bloody blebs that do not extend to the digit tips. The patient may complain of a deep, aching joint pain. Prognosis is extremely poor (**Figures 208-3** and **208-4**).

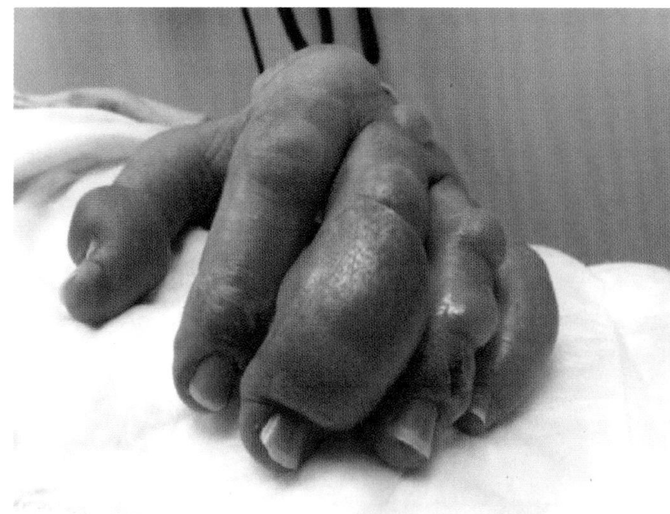

FIGURE 208-2. Second- and third-degree frostbite in the hand with blisters. [Photo contributed by Edward Lew, MD.]

DIAGNOSIS

Frostbite may occur anywhere on the skin but is generally limited to the distal part of the extremities, face, nose, and ears. The injured area looks

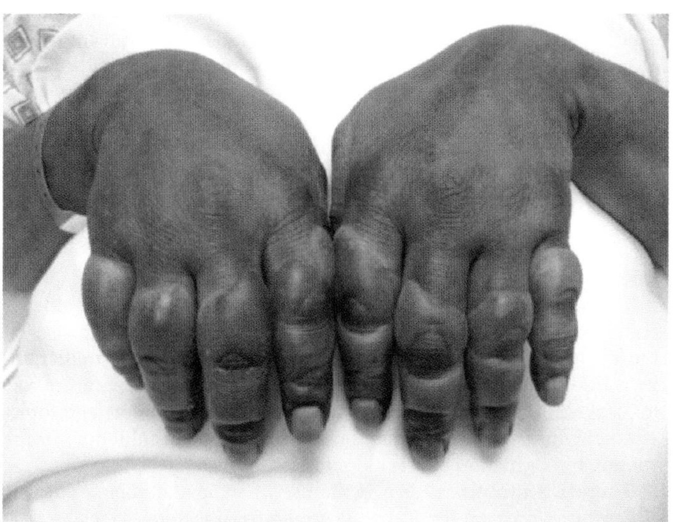

FIGURE 208-1. Second-degree frostbite in the hand with blisters. [Photo contributed by Scott Sherman, MD.]

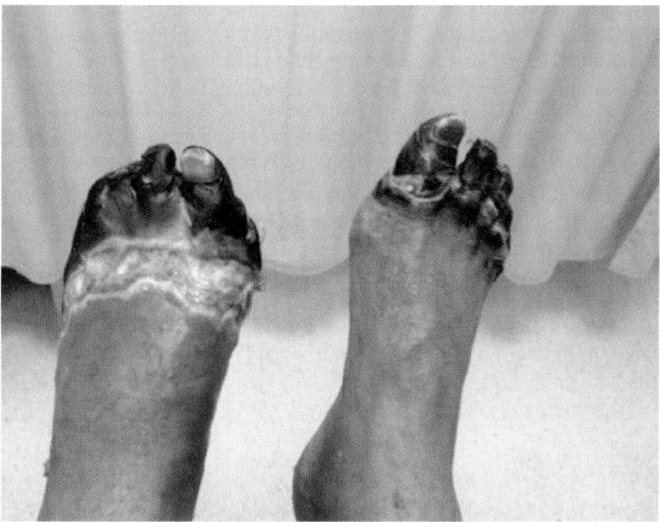

FIGURE 208-3. Third- and fourth-degree frostbite of bilateral feet. [Photo contributed by Edward Lew, MD.]

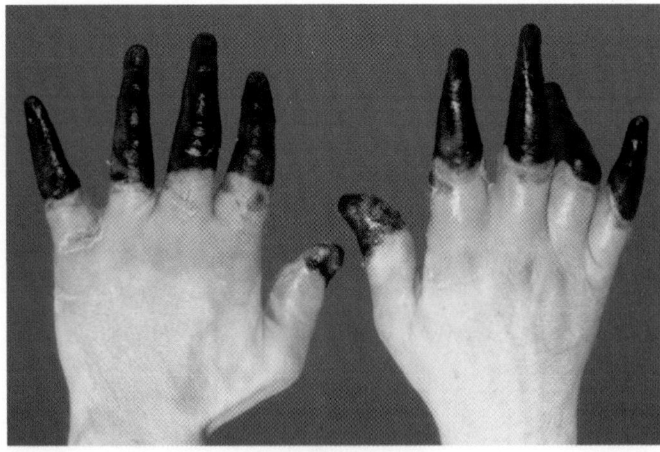

A

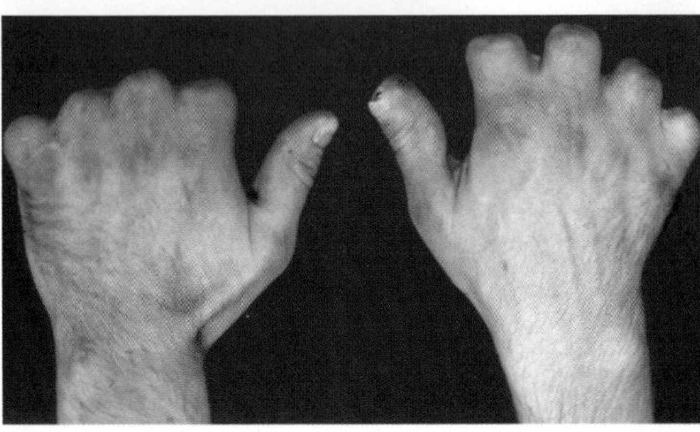

B

FIGURE 208-4. **A.** Fourth-degree frostbite 1 month after injury. Note the clear demarcation line in the fingers. **B.** The same hands 2 months later after surgical treatment.

pale and waxy and feels hard and cold. Patients frequently complain of stinging and numbness.

Because it is initially difficult to estimate the depth of the cold injury, early injuries are best classified simply as either superficial or deep. Prognostic considerations of ultimate tissue loss should take into account duration of exposure, environmental conditions (temperature, wind, and precipitation), type of clothing worn, level of physical activity, possible contact with metal or moisture, and associated use of recreational drugs, alcohol, or tobacco in addition to physical findings. Patients with frostbite may have concomitant cold-related problems such as hypothermia and dehydration, and patients with hypothermia may also have frostbite.

Although some chemical liquids and burn injuries may cause blister formation, a history of cold exposure differentiates chemically induced blisters from cold-induced injuries.

The diagnosis of frostbite is clinical. **No specific laboratory tests are indicated when treating patients with frostbite**, and specific laboratory evaluation should be guided by the clinical situation including associated trauma or medical illness. Early imaging is rarely helpful, either for diagnostic or prognostic purposes, although the use of technetium-99 scintigraphy may have prognostic value outside of the ED setting.[29]

TREATMENT

Prehospital Care Initial field management of frostbite includes prevention of further cold injury, hypothermia, and dehydration. Remove wet and constrictive clothing, cover with dry clothing, and protect against wind. In mild cases, and if the patient is conscious, warm drinks can be administered. Do not heat the frozen area, because dry heat may cause further injury. Do not attempt rewarming until the risk of refreezing is eliminated.[30,31] Refreezing will cause even more severe damage and is an important concern. Provide analgesia, because the rewarming process is very painful. Immobilize and elevate frozen extremities, and handle gently. Do not ambulate on edematous and blistered feet. Home remedies such as rubbing the affected area or rubbing snow on frostbitten tissue increase tissue damage.[30,31] Locally applied creams should not be used in the field.

ED Management Rapid rewarming is the first definitive step of frostbite therapy and should be initiated as soon as possible.[30,31] Place the injured extremity in gently circulating water heated to a temperature of 37°C to 39°C (98.6°F to 102.2°F), for approximately 20 to 30 minutes, until the distal extremity is pliable and erythematous.[30,31] Frostbitten faces can be thawed using moistened compresses soaked in warm water. Some patients may tolerate immersion of the ears in a bowl or pool of warmed water. **Anticipate severe pain during rewarming and treat with parenteral opiates.**

Local care is directed toward tissue preservation and infection prevention. Management of clear blisters and the use of prophylactic antibiotics are somewhat controversial. The blister fluid is rich in destructive thromboxane and prostaglandins. Although removal theoretically limits damage from these chemicals and enables access to the underlying tissue for topical therapy, not all experts agree that removal is indicated. Hemorrhagic blisters should not be debrided, because this often results in tissue desiccation and worse outcome. However, there is some controversy as to whether aspiration is helpful. Both blister types should be treated with **topical aloe vera cream** every 6 hours, which helps to combat the arachidonic acid cascade.[30,31] Affected digits should be separated with cotton and wrapped with sterile, dry gauze. Other affected areas should be dressed in bulky, loose-fitting dry gauze dressings to allow room for the expected subsequent edema. Elevation of the involved extremities helps decrease edema and pain.

Tetanus immunization status should be assessed and appropriate vaccination administered if needed, because frostbite is a tetanus-prone wound (see chapter 156, "Tetanus").

Because microvascular thrombosis plays a role in tissue injury, thrombolysis has been advocated by some for use in cases at risk for proximal or multiple digit amputations[32,33] and, when given after rapid rewarming, appears to reduce digit amputations.[30,34-36] The evidence in support of IV or intra-arterial tissue plasminogen activator is limited to retrospective studies, and bleeding risks must be weighed against potential benefit.

The role of prophylactic antibiotics is unclear. The edema that is present on the first several days after injury does appear to predispose to infection. *Staphylococcus aureus*, *Staphylococcus epidermidis*, and β-hemolytic streptococci account for nearly half of infections, but anaerobes, *Pseudomonas*, and *Enterococcus* are important pathogens as well. Therapy with penicillin G, 500,000 units IV every 6 hours for 48 to 72 hours, is recommended in several successful protocols and seems to be beneficial. However, infection prophylaxis using topical bacitracin may be as good as or better than IV penicillin. The use of silver sulfadiazine cream also has been advocated by some, but it has not been shown to be consistently beneficial. One disadvantage of using topical antibiotics is that they complicate the concurrent use of aloe vera cream.

Several agents besides aloe vera cream have been recommended to battle the arachidonic acid cascade and thereby limit tissue damage. The most commonly advocated oral medication is ibuprofen, 12 milligrams/kg/d PO in divided doses. Animal studies suggest possible future roles for oral methimazole (a thromboxane synthetase inhibitor) and topical 1% methylprednisolone acetate (a phospholipase A2 inhibitor) in preventing the formation of arachidonic acid.

Another controversial area is the use of sympathetic blockade with either intra-arterial reserpine or surgical sympathectomy to relieve vasospasm and edema. There is no role for early sympathectomy. Prolonged sympathetic blockade using a long-acting anesthetic drug (bupivacaine) may improve blood flow to the hand, relieve pain, and speed recovery.

TABLE 208-4 Treatment of Frostbite

Core Treatment
1. Immersion in or application of water at 37°C to 39°C (98.6°F to 102.2°F) until affected area is pliable and erythematous; do not begin rewarming until risk of refreezing is eliminated
2. Parenteral narcotics for pain management
3. Topical aloe vera cream every 6 h
3. No blister or soft tissue debridement acutely
4. Meticulous local care
5. Tetanus immunization
6. Ibuprofen, 12 milligrams/kg/d PO, in divided doses
Optional Treatment
1. Topical bacitracin ointment for infection prophylaxis
2. Penicillin G, 500,000 units IV every 6 h, for prophylaxis for susceptible organisms
3. Topical silver sulfadiazine cream for prophylaxis (do not use on face)

Continuous epidural anesthesia may relieve peripheral vasospasm and perhaps prevent retrograde arterial and venous thrombosis.

Heparin and hyperbaric oxygen therapy appear to be of little value, although case reports of improvement in isolated cases have been published.[37,38] IV low-molecular-weight dextran has theoretical benefits, but dose and effectiveness have not been validated.[39]

Early surgical intervention is not indicated in the management of frostbite. Premature surgery has been an important contributor to unnecessary tissue loss and poor results in the past. This is due primarily to the inability to assess the depth of frostbite at early stages and the fact that the blackened, mummified carapace protects the underlying regenerating tissue. Limited early escharotomy may be indicated if the eschar is preventing adequate range of motion or circulation. Fasciotomy is rarely, if ever, indicated.

Table 208-4 presents the core treatment of frostbite.

SEQUELAE

Up to 65% of persons with frostbite injuries experience sequelae from their injuries.[1] Sequelae may be seen in patients with mild injuries but are generally more intense with more severe frostbite. The most typical sequelae are hypersensitivity to cold, pain, and ongoing numbness. Neuropathies have also been described. The clinical and functional limitations associated with late sequelae are dependent on the type and severity of the frostbite injury and the related anatomic deformities and amputations.

DISPOSITION AND FOLLOW-UP

Because it is difficult to determine the extent of frostbite on initial examination, it is best to be conservative when contemplating admission. Consider social and medical issues. The homeless or elderly, especially when unable to care for themselves adequately, should never be discharged into subfreezing temperatures. If the frostbite is extensive and the hospital and staff are not equipped to treat injury of that degree of severity, consider transfer to a tertiary hospital after initial rewarming and treatment.

Patients with only superficial local frostbite may be discharged home if social circumstances allow. Patients with deeper frostbite injuries should be hospitalized. At discharge from the ED, patients must be provided with sufficient guidelines for self-care and clear instructions for close short-term and long-term follow-up, preferably with local burn center or plastic surgery providers. They must also be instructed to contact their doctor at an early stage if problems or concerns arise. Patients who are discharged from the ED should be treated with topical aloe vera cream and oral ibuprofen and encouraged not to smoke or drink alcohol. **Table 208-5** lists prevention strategies.

TABLE 208-5 Cold Injury Prevention Strategy

Risk Assessment
Assessment of environmental conditions
Assessment of expected duration of exposure and physical activity level
Risk Management
Raising of awareness
Identification of susceptible population groups, education to recognize personal warning signals of adverse cooling, provision of training and information, distribution of learning and guidance materials
Organizational Preventive Measures
Advance planning; appropriate scheduling of activities; assessment of physical activity level; provision of facilities for warming; establishment of mandatory clothing changes, breaks, etc.
Technical Preventive Measures
Attention to shelters, tools, external heating, work areas, slippery surfaces, lighting, etc.
Protective Clothing
Whole-body protection, hand and footwear, head protection, face and respiratory protection, use of personal protective equipment together with cold protective clothing
Health Care
Individual recommendations based on special needs

REFERENCES

The complete reference list is available online at www.TintinalliEM.com.

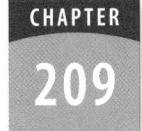

Hypothermia

Doug Brown

INTRODUCTION AND EPIDEMIOLOGY

Accidental hypothermia is an involuntary drop in core temperature below 35°C (<95°F) and can often be associated with significant morbidity and mortality.[1] **Therapeutic hypothermia**, also called targeted temperature management, is a purposeful drop in core temperature usually performed with the hope of ameliorating tissue damage associated with an ischemic event.[2,3]

Accidental hypothermia can be subclassified as primary, due to simple environmental exposure, or secondary, due to impaired thermoregulation (**Table 209-1**). Primary accidental hypothermia is commonly seen in cold climates, whereas secondary accidental hypothermia can be seen worldwide. The true incidence of accidental hypothermia and its related morbidity and mortality remain unknown.[4]

HYPOTHERMIA CLASSIFICATION

Historically, hypothermia has been classified as mild, moderate, severe, and profound, based on core temperature, shivering, level of consciousness, and vital signs.[5-7] Unfortunately, there is considerable variation in clinical features at any given temperature, and a reliable core temperature is sometimes unavailable during initial assessment. Shivering is particularly unreliable because it may be present or absent across a wide temperature range. The modified staging system (mild, moderate, severe, hypothermia stage IV)[5-7] described in **Table 209-2** is a hybrid of the Swiss[7] and classical systems[5] that is based primarily on level of consciousness, the presence or absence of vital signs, and core temperature (when available).

TABLE 209-1 Causes of Secondary Hypothermia

Predominantly Increased Heat Loss
Burns
Iatrogenic (i.e., blood transfusions and other cold infusions, cooling blankets, inadequate insulation)
Recent birth
Predominantly Impaired Thermogenesis
Impaired shivering (i.e., advanced or very young age, malnutrition, physical exhaustion, neuromuscular disease)
Multifactorial
Medications and toxins (i.e., alcohol, anesthetic agents, narcotics, sedatives, vasodilators)
Metabolic and endocrine disorders (i.e., alcoholic or diabetic ketoacidosis, hypoadrenalism, hypoglycemia, hypopituitarism, hypothyroid, lactic acidosis, Wernicke's encephalopathy)
Neurologic (i.e., space-occupying lesion, stroke, spinal cord injury)
Sepsis (small subset of sepsis cases, more common in the elderly or cachectic patient)
Shock
Trauma

PATHOPHYSIOLOGY

Body temperature is tightly regulated by a combination of behavioral, neuroendocrinologic, and cardiovascular responses to cold stress. Core temperature will fall when the amount of heat lost to the environment exceeds the amount of heat produced.

HEAT LOSS

Heat is lost from a warm body by conduction, convection, evaporation, and radiation. Conduction occurs when a warm body makes direct contact with a cold object. Conductive heat loss can be minimized by avoiding contact with cold or poorly insulated objects (e.g., metal backboards or stretchers). Convective cooling occurs when a fluid (usually air or water) comes in contact with a warm body. The amount of heat lost via convection can be considerable and is proportional to the amount of fluid that flows around the body, the specific heat capacity of the fluid, and the temperature difference between the fluid and the body. Practically, the emergency physician needs to understand that exposure to cool air or water will result in heat loss, that water can absorb a large amount of heat in a short period of time, and that windy conditions or flowing water can significantly increase the rate of cooling. Evaporative heat loss occurs due to the energy required for water to phase change from a liquid to a gas. The amount of heat lost to evaporation is proportional to the temperature difference between the body and the air and the wind speed over the body and is inversely proportional to the humidity. Therefore, a warm moist body exposed to cold, dry, windy air will lose a significant amount of heat. A vapor barrier (e.g., a plastic bag or sheet), placed around the patient, effectively prevents evaporative cooling but is often not practical when repeated access to the patient's skin is required. Radiant cooling occurs because all warm bodies "radiate" heat, in the form of electromagnetic waves. Increasing the temperature of the room can minimize radiant heat loss, and some losses can be recovered using special reflective fabrics (likely low yield in most clinical situations). In summary, it is important to minimize heat loss in the hypothermic patient, and a basic understanding of the physics of heat transfer can be helpful. Practically, heat loss can be minimized by heating the room, removing wet clothes, drying the patient (or wrapping the patient in a vapor barrier), providing insulation, and protecting the patient from wind.

HEAT CONSERVATION AND PRODUCTION

The most important responses to cold include behavior (e.g., putting on warm clothing, seeking a warm environment), peripheral vasoconstriction, increased metabolic rate, and muscular thermogenesis (voluntary or shivering). Shivering is a remarkably efficient method of heat production, and care is required to preserve this important

TABLE 209-2 Staging and Treatment of Accidental Hypothermia

Stage	Clinical Symptoms	Typical Core Temperature	Treatment
Mild (HT I)	Conscious, shivering	35–32°C	Warm environment and clothing, warm sweet drinks, and active movement (if possible) HT I patients with significant trauma or comorbidities or those suspected of secondary hypothermia should receive HT II treatment
Moderate (HT II)	Impaired consciousness* (may or may not be shivering)	<32–28°C	Active external and minimally invasive rewarming techniques (warm environment; chemical, electrical, or forced air heating packs or blankets; warm parenteral fluids) Cardiac and core temperature monitoring Minimal and cautious movements to avoid arrhythmias Full-body insulation, horizontal position, and immobilization
Severe (HT III)	Unconscious*, vital signs present	<28°C	HT II management plus: Airway management as required Preference to treat in an ECMO/CPB center, if available, due to the high risk of cardiac arrest Consider ECMO/CPB in cases with cardiac instability that is refractory to medical management Consider ECMO/CPB for comorbid patients who are unlikely to tolerate the low cardiac output associated with HT III
HT IV	Vital signs absent	Cardiac arrest is possible below 32°C; the risk increases substantially below 28°C and continues to increase with ongoing cooling	CPR and up to three doses of epinephrine and defibrillation (further dosing guided by clinical response) Airway management Transport to ECMO/CPB† Prevent further heat loss (insulation, warm environment, do not apply heat to head) Active external and minimally invasive rewarming (see HT II) during transport is recommended but controversial; do not apply heat to head

Abbreviations: CPB = cardiopulmonary bypass; ECMO = extracorporeal membrane oxygenation; HT = hypothermia.

*Consciousness may be impaired by comorbid illness (e.g., trauma, CNS pathology, toxic ingestion) independent of core temperature.

†Transfering an HT IV patient to an ECMO/CPB center may reduce mortality by 40% to 90% (number needed to treat, ~2); if ECMO/CPB is not available within a few hours of transport,[6,8] consider on-site rewarming with hot packs or forced air blankets, warm IV fluid, ± warm thoracic lavage, ± warm bladder lavage, and ± warm peritoneal lavage; do not apply heat to the head.

source of heat. Unfortunately, shivering can be suppressed by medications (e.g., analgesics, sedatives), by the application of warming devices (e.g., hot packs, forced air blankets, warm humidified air), if energy stores are exhausted, or if the core temperature drops below a critical level (~31°C).[5] The suppression of shivering by various warming methods is one of the reasons why the rewarming literature is so controversial.

CONTINUED CORE COOLING

Core temperature may continue to drop after a patient is removed from the cold environment,[9,10] a process often referred to as afterdrop. The amount of continued core cooling will depend on the stage of hypothermia, the degree of thermoregulatory dysfunction, the ongoing cold stress (often significant in the prehospital care environment), and the physics of heat transfer (heat from the relatively warmer core will be transferred to the cooler periphery by direct conduction or by convection from blood flow). The relative importance of the various mechanisms and the impact of various rewarming techniques are the source of much debate, due in part to the desire to avoid iatrogenic core cooling. Historically, there was concern that rewarming or active movement could cause convection of cold blood from the periphery to the core with a potential increase in morbidity. Careful experimental studies have demonstrated an ~1°C drop in core temperature during minimally invasive rewarming when shivering is inhibited with narcotics[11] or during exercise,[12] but case series have not demonstrated any clinically significant afterdrop or morbidity when minimally invasive rewarming is used.[6,13] In general, healthy uninjured patients who are able to shiver and have adequate fuel reserves (or can drink warm sweet drinks) will be able to self-rewarm once removed from further cold stress. In contrast, patients who have lost the ability to shiver are at significant risk of further temperature decline unless active rewarming is used.[6,14,15] The use of aggressive immersion rewarming techniques such as hot baths or showers should likely be avoided due to the potential risks of vasodilatory hypotension or convective cooling.[16]

SECONDARY HYPOTHERMIA

Cases of secondary hypothermia can be conveniently organized into those caused predominantly by increased heat loss, those caused predominantly by impaired thermoregulation, and those caused by multiple factors (Table 209-1). This classification is somewhat arbitrary, but in general, the multifactorial cases have a higher risk of missed diagnosis and are less likely to fully resolve with rewarming and supportive care. Iatrogenic causes of hypothermia deserve special attention, particularly in trauma patients, where the loss of just a few degrees of core temperature can create a profound coagulopathy and more than double patient mortality.[17] Massive transfusion and large-volume crystalloid resuscitation are common iatrogenic causes of hypothermia unless proper fluid warmers are used. Inadequate insulation, repeated or prolonged exposure to the cool air of the resuscitation or operating room, and inadequate core temperature monitoring all contribute to iatrogenic heat loss, which may increase morbidity and mortality.

COLD PHYSIOLOGY

The body attempts to preserve normothermia through mechanisms such as increased metabolic rate, peripheral vasoconstriction, increased preshivering muscle tone, or shivering. As the core temperature drops below ~35°C, progressive impairment occurs affecting all of the body's organ systems. CNS impairment can progress from poor judgment, amnesia, and dysarthria, to ataxia and apathy, unconsciousness, areflexia, and eventually electroencephalographic arrest.[5] Paradoxical undressing is a potentially deadly behavior that occurs in up to 30% of fatal hypothermia cases.[18] Below ~29°C, the pupils may become dilated and fixed, and below ~23°C, corneal reflexes may be absent; neither are reliable for neurologic prognosis in hypothermia.[5]

Cardiorespiratory Responses Cardiovascular responses to cold include profound peripheral vasoconstriction and an initial increase in heart rate and blood pressure, usually followed by progressive bradycardia, hypotension, and myocardial irritability. Below ~32°C, the risk of cardiac arrest increases as malignant cardiac arrhythmias become more common, particularly below 28°C.[19] The term *rescue collapse* is used to describe cardiac arrest that can commonly occur during extrication, transport, or treatment of a deeply hypothermic patient. The cause of rescue collapse is multifactorial but ultimately related to the profound irritability of the cold myocardium. Atrial fibrillation and flutter are expected arrhythmias and not necessarily markers of cardiac instability.[6] ECG changes in hypothermia are variable but classically include bradycardia with prolonged PR, then QRS widening, and then prolonged QT_c. ECGs are often complicated by muscle tremors or shivering, and hypothermia can cause almost any heart block or atrial or ventricular arrhythmias. The classic **Osborn J waves (Figure 209-1)** usually occur below 32°C, can be misdiagnosed as ST elevation myocardial infarction, and can also be caused by intracranial pathology or sepsis.[5] Occasionally patients may be in a low-flow state, with a very difficult to detect pulse that may provide some oxygen delivery. Asystole is the common final arrhythmia, but in accidental hypothermia, it does not exclude the possibility of a successful resuscitation.[6]

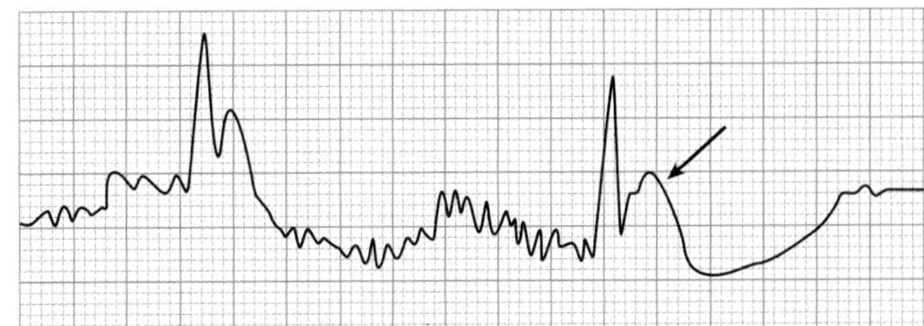

FIGURE 209-1. ECG strip from a patient with a temperature of 25°C (77°F) showing atrial fibrillation with a slow ventricular response, muscle tremor artifact, and Osborn (J) wave (*arrow*).

Respiratory changes include initial tachypnea, followed by a progressive decrease in minute ventilation and eventual respiratory arrest. Pulmonary edema is an inconsistent complication of hypothermia but is common after resuscitation from stage IV hypothermia.

Metabolic Responses The renal response to hypothermia is termed *cold diuresis* and is a response to vasoconstriction-induced hypervolemia. It results in significant fluid losses, which may be further increased in patients with a history of cold water immersion or alcohol intoxication.[5] Rhabdomyolysis is a potential complication of hypothermia[20]; however, the clinician should always exclude a missed compartment syndrome or extensive frostbite when an elevated creatine kinase is detected. Hypothermia can also cause muscle rigidity, termed *pseudo-rigor mortis*; hence, rigor mortis cannot be used as a reliable marker of death in the cold patient. Hypothermia has a somewhat dramatic impact on coagulation and blood viscosity, and these effects are often under-recognized by clinicians because blood samples are heated to 37°C prior to analysis. Coagulopathy is a concern below 34°C, particularly in trauma patients in whom hypothermia can compromise the chance for a surgical cure and exponentially increase mortality,[17] partly due to poor activity of clotting factors and platelet dysfunction.[21] Hypothermic patients can also be hypercoagulable from a combination of increased viscosity, hemoconcentration, and an inflammatory cascade similar to disseminated intravascular coagulation; these factors can put hypothermic patients at an increased risk for venous thromboembolic disease as well as coronary and cerebral artery occlusion.[5]

Cellular oxygen consumption decreases as core temperature drops and, in an otherwise healthy patient who has adequate oxygen delivery prior to cooling, may provide protection against ischemia. It is estimated that cerebral oxygen requirements are approximately 50% at 28°C, 19% at 18°C, and 11% at 8°C.[5,22] This neuroprotective effect of hypothermia is exploited in certain cardiac surgeries. The most dramatic technique is deep hypothermic circulatory arrest, where patients are cooled to ~18°C and cardiac arrest is induced and maintained for up to ~30 minutes.[23] The combination of the potential to survive prolonged periods of ischemia, with the uncertainty of knowing if a patient has been in a low-flow state (difficult to detect cardiac activity that provides some oxygen delivery) versus cardiac arrest, increases the complexity of termination of resuscitation decisions for hypothermic patients unless the history clearly indicates death prior to cooling.

CLINICAL FEATURES

Patients with hypothermia will feel cold to touch; they will have a core temperature less than 35°C and may have a history of cold exposure or a history of a condition associated with secondary hypothermia (Table 209-1). Hypothermia can be staged clinically using level of consciousness and vital signs (Table 209-2). Measure the core temperature as soon as possible. If the core temperature deviates significantly from the clinical features of the stage, then consider alternative diagnoses. For example, if a patient has a core temperature of 33°C but is unconscious, hypothermia is unlikely the main cause of coma.

CORE TEMPERATURE MEASUREMENT

Make sure that the device being used to measure core temperature is capable of extreme measurements and is properly calibrated (thermistor devices are usually preferred). Temperature measurement at different body sites will yield different readings depending on local perfusion and environmental conditions. In the intubated patient, the lower third of the esophagus (~24 cm below the larynx in an adult) is the preferred site for core temperature measurement, because it closely mirrors the cardiac temperature.[5] In the absence of an esophageal probe, a rectal probe inserted to a depth of 15 cm or a bladder probe is adequate, but realize that these temperatures often lag behind true core temperature during rewarming and that bladder or peritoneal lavage may falsely elevate the reading. Oral and infrared tympanic temperature measurements do not correlate well with core temperature and should not be used. When an accurate core temperature measurement is not available, management decisions should be made based on clinical staging (Table 209-2). Ongoing core temperature monitoring should be implemented as soon as possible for all moderate through severe hypothermia patients (stages II to IV).

DIAGNOSIS

Hypothermia causes dysfunction of every organ system, so the potential list of differential diagnoses is broad. A practical approach is to focus the differential diagnosis using a combination of history, physical exam, and expected degree of dysfunction for the clinical stage and measured core temperature. For the patient with absent vital signs, if the history indicates normothermic cardiac arrest prior to cooling, then hypothermia can be excluded as the cause of cardiac arrest, regardless of the patient's core temperature (**Figure 209-2**). Similarly, in the patient with absent vital signs, asystole, and an accurate core temperature above 32°C, accidental hypothermia is *not* the cause of cardiac arrest. Classic diagnostic dilemmas in relation to accidental hypothermia often revolve around impaired cognitive function, level of consciousness, or declaration of death. Intoxication, head injury, and CNS infection are three examples of conditions that impair neurologic function directly but can also cause secondary hypothermia and cold-related neurologic dysfunction. Vigilance is required with any decreased level of consciousness, particularly if the degree of neurologic impairment does not match the stage of hypothermia. Areflexia or paralysis should not be attributed to hypothermia until spinal injury has been ruled out.

Carefully consider secondary causes of accidental hypothermia, particularly if the measured core temperature is lower than expected based on the cold exposure history or the patient is slow or fails to rewarm with appropriate therapy. Tachycardia or tachypnea can be a marker of secondary pathology in moderate and severe hypothermia (stages II and III), because bradycardia with or without bradypnea is the normal response to hypothermia below a core temperature of ~32°C. Intoxication and sepsis are two common causes of secondary hypothermia, and depending on the patient presentation, routine screening and, in some cases, empiric therapy may be reasonable. Classic causes such as adrenal failure and myxedema coma are comparatively rare, and empiric testing or therapy is likely unwarranted in the absence of good historical or laboratory evidence. Hyperglycemia that persists after rewarming may indicate secondary pathology such as diabetic ketoacidosis or pancreatitis. The appropriate breadth of workup will vary considerably depending on the particular patient and the degree of clinical uncertainty.

Declaration of Death Declaration of death in the presence of hypothermia is particularly challenging due to the ability of hypothermia to mimic death (can cause fixed and dilated pupils, stiffness resembling rigor mortis, absent reflexes, or respiratory arrest) or cause death that may be reversible. **Figure 209-3** provides a triage tool for stage IV (absent vital signs) patients, to assist with clinical decision making. In general, patients with obvious signs of irreversible death or who are frozen solid, have a history of normothermic arrest with subsequent cooling, or have a potassium level >12 mmol/L are extremely unlikely to benefit from resuscitative efforts, and death can be declared without rewarming.[6] An exception to the above statement is the child with simultaneous normothermic cardiac arrest and very rapid accidental cooling (e.g., a child pinned underwater in an icy creek); in such a case, prolonged resuscitation and expert consultation may be appropriate (see "Special Considerations/Special Populations, Children").[24]

LABORATORY TESTING AND IMAGING

Laboratory testing and imaging studies should be targeted based on history, physical examination, and the differential diagnosis. It seems reasonable that every hospitalized hypothermia patient undergo point-of-care glucose testing, but additional routine tests are not necessarily required. An ECG should be obtained for moderate and severe hypothermia (stages II and III) patients, and a chest x-ray is likely reasonable depending on the suspicion for conditions such as aspiration or pulmonary edema. For cases where secondary hypothermia is suspected, measuring CBC, serum electrolytes, creatinine, glucose, lactate, lipase, thyroid-stimulating hormone, random cortisol level, osmolality, and levels of potential intoxicants (e.g., ethanol, aspirin, acetaminophen) and calculation of the anion and osmolar gap may be reasonable depending on clinical suspicion. Patients with suspected sepsis may benefit from blood culture. For patients with suspected compartment syndrome, frostbite, or prolonged immobility, measure serum creatinine kinase. Severe hypothermia (stages III and IV) patients should be considered critically ill, and therefore, expanded laboratory testing including CBC, electrolytes, pH, lactate, blood gas levels, and creatine kinase may be considered. For patients in cardiac arrest (stage IV), a serum potassium level ≥12 mmol/L is strongly associated with nonsurvival.[6]

HYPOTHERMIA EFFECTS ON LABORATORY VALUES

Laboratory results from hypothermic patients can be difficult to interpret due to the fact that high, low, or "normal" values may be appropriate in different patients. In an otherwise healthy patient with primary hypothermia, most laboratory values will normalize with rewarming; therefore, treat the patient, not the numbers. For complex cases or those that do not respond to usual therapy, it may be helpful to have a sense of the "expected" abnormalities associated with hypothermia. Hematocrit classically increases ~2%/°C, secondary to decreased circulating plasma volume.[5] WBC counts may be normal or decreased due to sequestration or secondary causes such as sepsis. Electrolyte abnormalities are inconsistent, and cold blood may be prone to sampling hemolysis; hence rewarming and ongoing monitoring are often the best strategy. Glucose levels are somewhat unpredictable with an early rise being common secondary to catecholamine-induced gluconeogenesis and hypothermia-induced insulin resistance. This increase is classically followed by a drop with the onset of resource depletion and metabolic failure.[5] Acid-base disturbances in hypothermia are complex; some hypothermic patients will be acidotic, whereas others may be alkylotic, and both conditions may be an appropriate physiologic response to cooling[5] or may be a marker of secondary pathology. Blood gas analyzers rewarm samples to 37°C, and in rewarmed samples, the partial pressure of gases increases and the pH is lower, compared with the cold in vivo sample (correction usually not required, see stage III treatment for details). It is also important to note that the coagulopathy of

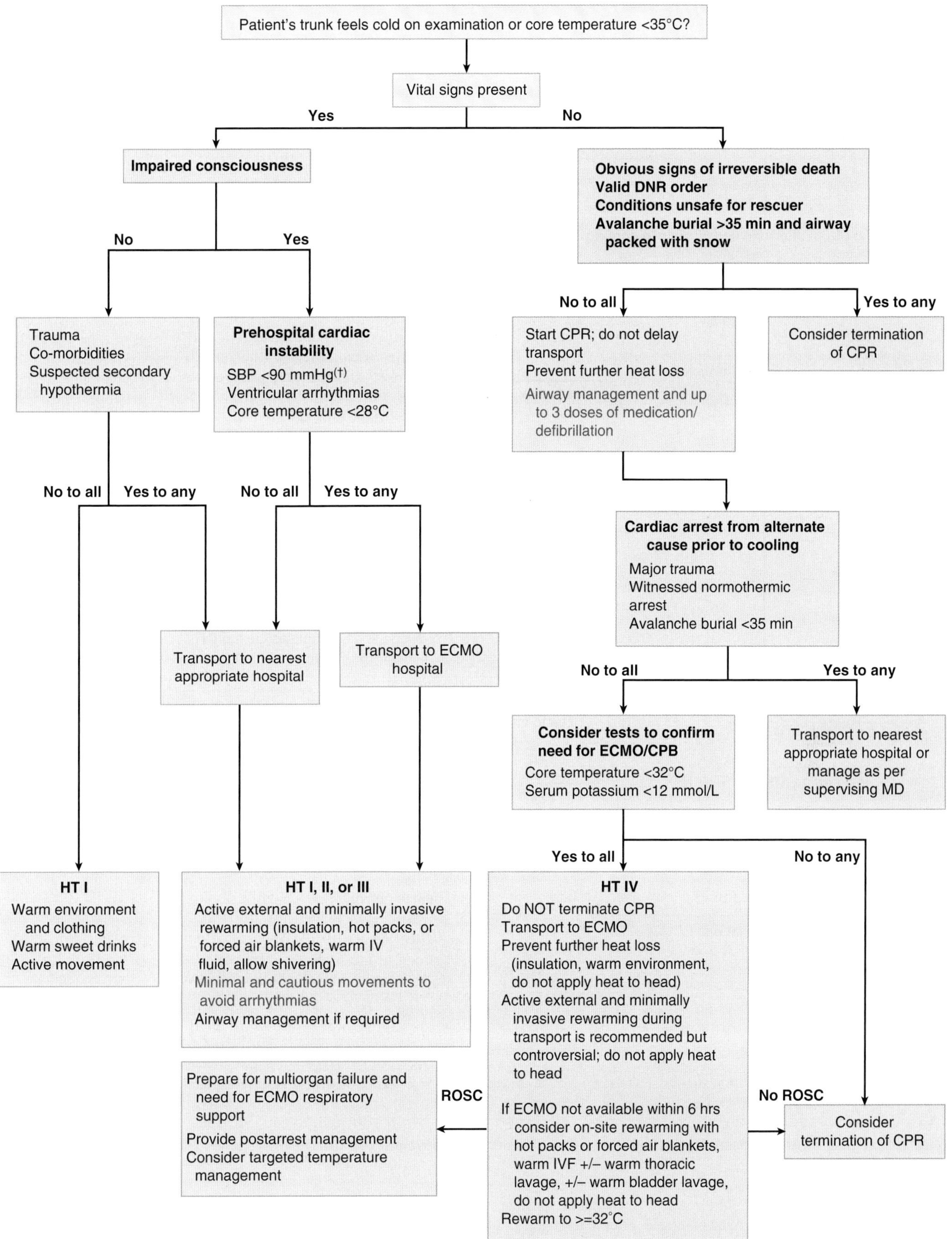

FIGURE 209-2. Transport and management of accidental hypothermia.[6] CPB = cardiopulmonary bypass; DNR = do not resuscitate; ECMO = extracorporeal membrane oxygenation; HT = hypothermia; ROSC = return of spontaneous circulation; SBP = systolic blood pressure. [© Doug Brown, MD, FRCPC.]

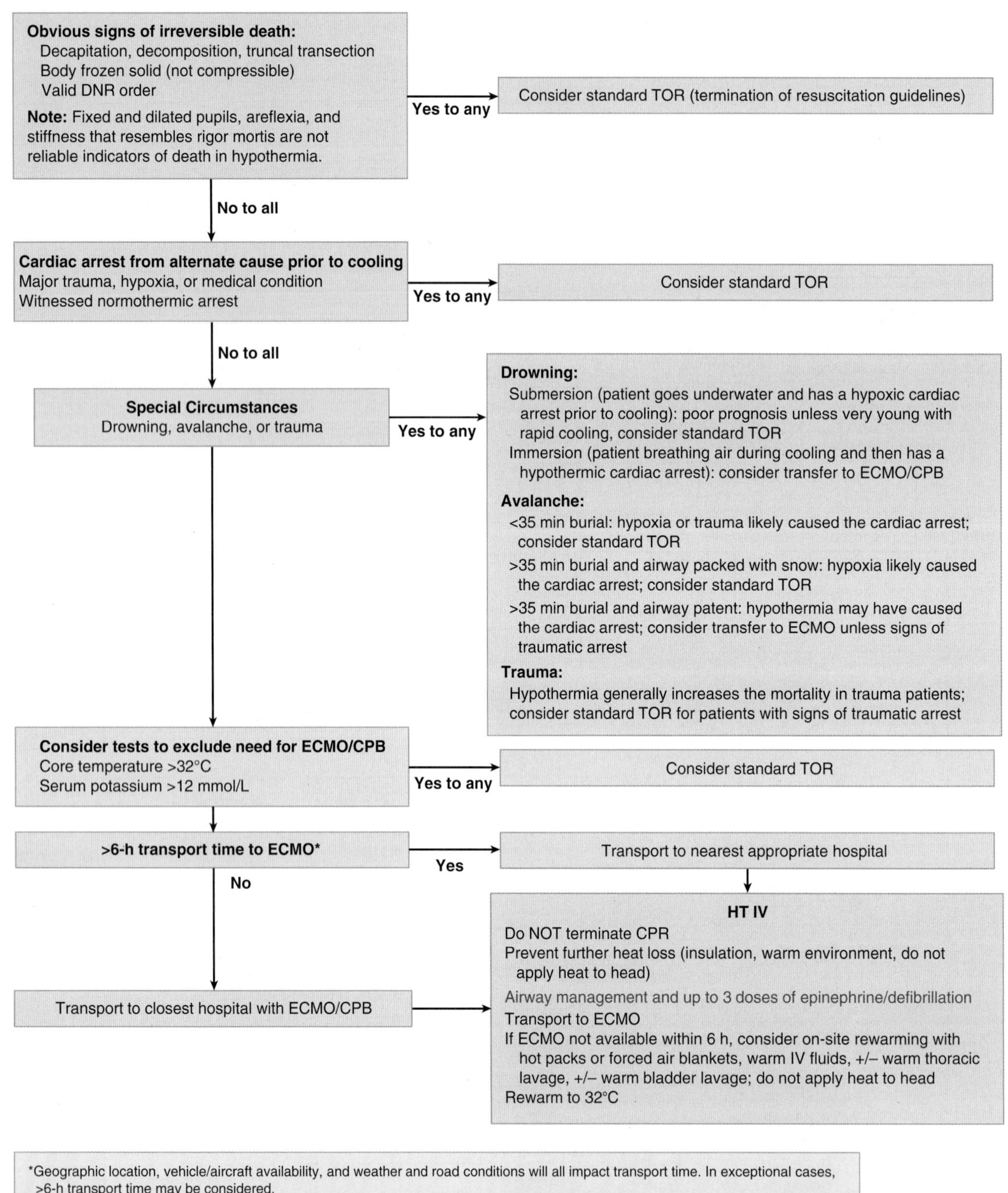

FIGURE 209-3. Triage tool for hypothermia (HT) patients with absent vital signs. CPB = cardiopulmonary bypass; DNR = do not resuscitate; ECMO = extracorporeal membrane oxygenation. [© Doug Brown, MD, FRCPC.]

hypothermia (see earlier section, "Cold Physiology") will not be apparent on laboratory results due to the warming of samples prior to testing.

TREATMENT

Treatment of accidental hypothermia varies depending on the clinical stage, but the general principles include basic or advanced life support, prevention of further heat loss, transport to an appropriate facility if indicated, rewarming (Table 209-2 and Figure 209-2), and in secondary hypothermia, treatment of the underlying cause.

MILD HYPOTHERMIA (STAGE I)

Otherwise healthy stage I patients (conscious, shivering, core temperature ≥32°C) can often be rewarmed locally using a warm environment, provision of dry clothes, warm sweet drinks, and active movement. Stage I patients with traumatic injuries or significant medical comorbidities or in whom secondary hypothermia is suspected should be transported to the nearest appropriate hospital and managed as per stage II guidelines.

MODERATE HYPOTHERMIA (STAGE II)

Stage II patients (impaired consciousness, may or may not be shivering, core temperature ~28 to 32°C) require careful handling, prevention of further heat loss, active external and minimally invasive rewarming (warm environment; forced air, electrical, or chemical warming blankets; warm parenteral fluids), cardiac monitoring, and core temperature monitoring (**Figure 209-4**). Careful handling to decrease the risk of cardiac arrhythmia becomes important for stage II and III patients, due to the increasing irritability of the cold myocardium. For all stages of hypothermia, warmed crystalloids (38 to 42°C) should be titrated based on clinical volume status. It should be noted that significant volume might be required during rewarming and that warmed IV fluids do not provide significant heat but do prevent iatrogenic cooling. Atrial fibrillation, atrial flutter, and bradycardia are common in accidental

Hospital Resuscitation Checklist:

☐ Cardiac monitor & careful handling
☐ Core temperature monitoring (esophageal, rectal or bladder)
☐ If cardiac arrest, ventricular dysrhythmia, core temp < 28°C or unstable:
- do not stop resuscitation, seek expert consultation
- potential for good outcome despite prolonged resuscitation, ideally transfer to ECMO center if indicated

☐ Minimally invasive rewarming:
  ☐ Hypothermia burrito (see below, preference for forced air warming blankets)
  ☐ +/– Bladder lavage
    (3-way Foley, 40°C saline, 2–4 L/hr by gravity)
    [confirm volume in = volume out, will invalidate bladder and rectal temperature measurements]
☐ IV Fluid Resuscitation: (crystaloid, 38–42°C)
  ☐ Titrate fluids to clinical volume status (avoid over-resuscitation)
  ☐ 10–20 mL/kg (~1 L) to start (may be reasonable)
  ☐ Additional 10–20 mL/kg per ~3°C core temp increase (may be required)
☐ Hypothermia is NOT a contraindication to airway management
☐ Avoid hyperoxia (titrate FiO_2 to 92–98%)
☐ If central venous access is required, keep the tip of the catheter (and guidewire) far from the heart (femoral, shallow internal jugular or shallow subclavian)
☐ Avoid vasopressors during early resuscitation (relative hypotension may be physiologic depending on core temperature, consider expert consultation)

Minimally Invasive Rewarming: (hypothermia burrito)

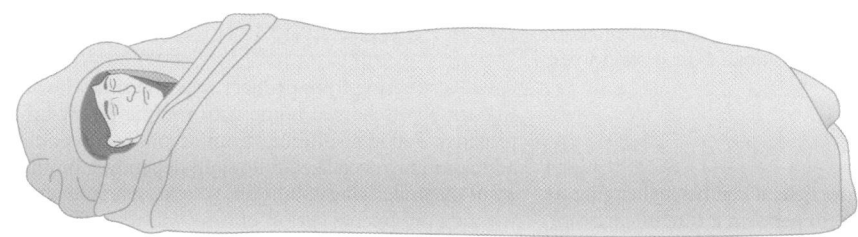

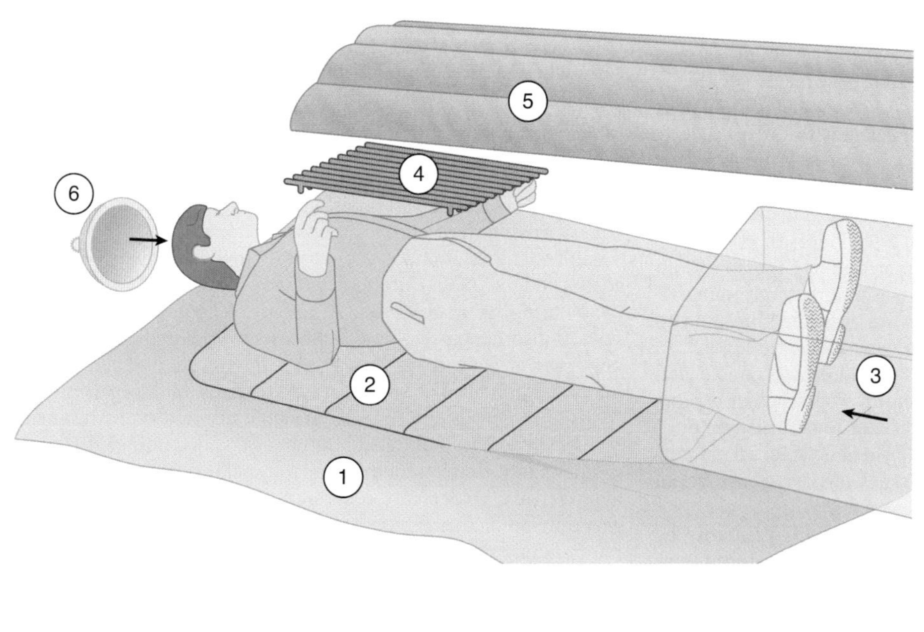
1 Outer wind & waterproof wrap +/– reflective tarp (prehospital only)
2 Insulation or heating pad*
3 Replace wet clothes if practical, otherwise wrap patient in plastic
4 Forced air, chemical or electrical heating device(s)*
5 Insulating blanket
6 Insulate the head**
* To avoid burns, keep heating device temperatures < ~40°C.
** If in cardiac arrest, do not apply heat to the head (allow warm oxygenated blood to rewarm the brain centrally).

FIGURE 209-4. Practical tips for rewarming patients with moderate and severe hypothermia. ECMO = extracorporeal membrane oxygenation. [© Doug Brown, MD, FRCPC.]

hypothermia, do not usually require specific therapy, and typically resolve with rewarming. Vasopressors are usually not indicated in early resuscitation because hypothermia already provides maximal vasoconstriction and the addition of vasopressors may increase the risk of arrhythmia. Vasopressors may be indicated later in resuscitation, if rewarming-induced vasodilation cannot be managed with fluids and is contributing to significant hypotension. Special care is required when assessing the risk-to-benefit ratio of sedatives and analgesics. Many medications will inhibit shivering, decrease sympathetic tone, and/or cause vasodilatation, all of which can contribute to a further drop in core body temperature.[12,25] Depending on the stage of hypothermia, the degree of thermoregulatory dysfunction, the cold stress, and the physics of heat transfer, continued core cooling is possible despite appropriate treatment, particularly in the prehospital care setting. Such a failure to rewarm should trigger the clinician to reconsider secondary causes of hypothermia and ensure that ongoing heat losses have been ameliorated (uninsulated backboard, wet clothing, cool or windy environment) and that rewarming techniques are actually delivering significant heat.

SEVERE HYPOTHERMIA (STAGE III)

Stage III (unconscious, vital signs present, core temperature <~28°C) patients require the same treatment as stage II patients and will often require intubation for airway protection (Table 209-2). The role of invasive vascular rewarming methods that do not support circulation (dialysis, venovenous extracorporeal membrane oxygenation, and commercial temperature management systems) remains uncertain due to unproven benefits and the potential for procedure- and device-related morbidity.[26] The use of body cavity lavage rewarming has mostly been replaced by minimally invasive rewarming methods for stable patients and by arterial-venous extracorporeal membrane oxygenation (ECMO) or cardiopulmonary bypass (CPB), where available, for unstable patients or those in cardiac arrest.[6] For stable patients who are slow to rewarm, it is reasonable to use warm saline (38 to 42°C) bladder lavage because the potential for morbidity is very low, particularly when compared with peritoneal, thoracic, gastric, or rectal lavage. The use of warm humidified gases for ventilation is recommended; however, it does not contribute significantly to rewarming.[27,28] Other invasive interventions, such as advanced airway management and central line placement, should be performed if required, despite the slight risk of triggering a malignant arrhythmia (avoid guidewire or catheter tip contact with the heart).[6]

Stage III patients are at high risk for cardiac arrest, so patients with a core temperature <28°C, hypotension out of proportion to the degree of hypothermia, or ventricular arrhythmias should be transferred to an ECMO/CPB center if one is available within a few hours of transport[6,8] unless comorbidities, such as major trauma, necessitate transfer to an alternate center. For stage III patients with vital signs, the minimum sufficient circulation is unknown, and there is no accepted threshold to transition a potentially unstable patient with vital signs onto ECMO. In studies involving mostly healthy young people, patients with stable vital signs do well with minimally invasive rewarming,[29] but in older comorbid populations (who may have poor tolerance for low cardiac output), there is emerging evidence that ECMO may be beneficial for all patients with a core temperature <28°C (see "Special Considerations/Special Populations, ECMO/CPB" below).[30]

Treat acid-base disturbances in hypothermic patients primarily by rewarming and reassessment. For the intubated patient, respiratory parameters should target an uncorrected P_{CO_2} of 40 mm Hg (this is known as an alpha-stat strategy, where correction factors are *not* applied to account for the temperature difference between patient temperature and blood gas analysis temperature).[5,31,32] Do not give bicarbonate to correct pH, unless there is a clear alternate indication, as in certain toxic ingestions.

STAGE IV

Because hypothermia induces a low-flow state, it can be challenging to detect a pulse in a hypothermic patient, so perform a careful check for signs of life. If any breathing, movement, or pulse is detected, watchful waiting and supportive care are recommended; otherwise, start CPR. High-quality CPR, prevention of further heat loss, and transfer to an ECMO/CPB center when possible are the most important priorities for stage IV patients. When transfer to ECMO/CPB is definitely not available and the patient is in cardiac arrest, thoracic lavage with normal saline (38 to 42°C) using a single or dual chest tube method may be the second best rewarming strategy when combined with ongoing CPR.[33]

Controversy exists regarding the use of epinephrine and defibrillation in hypothermic cardiac arrest. The European Resuscitation Council 2010 guidelines recommend up to three defibrillation attempts, to withhold epinephrine until the core temperature exceeds 30°C, and to double the dose frequency until the temperature is above 35°C.[27] In contrast, the American Heart Association 2010 guidelines state that it may be reasonable to use vasopressors during cardiac arrest.[28] Given the conflicting animal and human data that each recommendation is based on, a reasonable approach is to use standard advanced cardiac life support protocols for up to three cycles and, in the absence of clinical response, defer further defibrillation or epinephrine until core temperature increases significantly or the patient's clinical status changes.

One of the major challenges with stage IV hypothermia is to select the patient with cardiac arrest caused by hypothermia for prolonged resuscitation while avoiding futile resuscitation for patients with normothermic cardiac arrest and subsequent cooling. Measuring a serum potassium >12 mmol/L or a core temperature >32°C can help to avoid futile resuscitation, but in their absence, the clinician is dependent on the history and physical to select the patients who may benefit from prolonged resuscitation (Figure 209-3).

Stage IV patients with return of spontaneous circulation should be rewarmed to ≥32°C and get standard postarrest management[28] with consideration given to targeted temperature management[3] or therapeutic hypothermia[2] based on institutional preference. Patients rewarmed to ≥32°C without return of spontaneous circulation who are in asystole can be considered for termination of resuscitation in the absence of other causes of reversible cardiac arrest.

DISEASE COMPLICATIONS

Early complications are those that develop during the rewarming process, whereas late complications occur after rewarming. Most early complications have been described in the previous "Cold Physiology" section and can be minimized by handling patients carefully and using minimally invasive or extracorporeal rewarming techniques. Early ECMO/CPB-related complications are mostly related to cannulation and include bleeding, vessel perforation, dissection, and distal limb ischemia.[30] Possible late complications are numerous and can affect most organ systems. Common respiratory complications include pulmonary edema and infection. Common cardiac complications include prolonged hypotension or arrhythmias. A variety of neurologic injuries, such as seizure disorders, peripheral neuropathy, impaired cognitive function, or persistent vegetative state, are possible in cases of severe or prolonged ischemia. Similar to other critically ill patients, multiorgan failure is possible, including, but not limited to, acute respiratory distress syndrome, renal failure, liver failure, rhabdomyolysis, disseminated intravascular coagulopathy, bowel ischemia, and adrenal insufficiency.[1] With stage IV hypothermia, colder core temperatures and longer durations of CPR generally predict increased complications. Cardiac stunning and respiratory failure requiring ECMO support are two important potential late complications of stage IV hypothermia due to the resource intensity required for management.[25]

DISPOSITION AND FOLLOW-UP

Patients suffering from primary hypothermia who are rewarmed in the ED can be discharged home with routine follow-up by a primary care provider. Patients suffering from secondary hypothermia may require admission or specialized follow-up depending on the nature and severity of the underlying condition. Patients who are unable to be rewarmed within a reasonable period of time will require admission with cardiac and core temperature monitoring (stage III and IV patients require a critical care setting).

SPECIAL CONSIDERATIONS/SPECIAL POPULATIONS

CHILDREN

Pediatric stage IV hypothermia patients require special consideration, and in general, expert consultation is warranted prior to termination of resuscitation. They have a larger surface area–to–body mass ratio, which means they have the potential to cool more rapidly than adults. Additionally, children may have an increased ability to tolerate and recover from hypoxic brain injury. Therefore, prolonged resuscitation may be indicated, even in cases of normothermic hypoxic cardiac arrest, if there is simultaneous very rapid cooling. The classic outlier in the literature is the case of a 2.5-year-old girl who went immediately under the water of a 5°C creek and suffered a normothermic hypoxic cardiac arrest but was rapidly cooled (pinned against a rock under fast-flowing cold water); 66 minutes later, she was removed from the water in cardiac arrest, received 3 hours of CPR, had a core temperature of 19°C, was successfully resuscitated using ECMO/CPB, and had a good neurologic outcome.[24]

ECMO/CPB

The use of ECMO/CPB for the management of stage IV hypothermia can dramatically improve survival for patients, with a number needed to treat of ~2 (absolute risk reduction of death 50% to 90%).[6,8] Well-selected patients treated in an ECMO/CPB center have an ~50% to 100% survival rate, compared with a rate of ~10% to 30% if treated in a center without extracorporeal rewarming.[6,35] Hypothermic patients have tolerated prolonged periods of CPR (≥5 hours) with a good neurologic outcome.[8,36,37] The combination of improved outcomes with extracorporeal rewarming and the prolonged patient tolerance for CPR argue for the early identification of stage III and IV patients and priority transfer to an ECMO/CPB center. Unfortunately, many physicians are not aware of this benefit, and many healthcare systems are not prepared to transfer patients in cardiac arrest. The creation of critical care pathways that outline triage, initial management, transport destinations, and care goals within a given healthcare systems have the potential to improve outcomes, in a similar manner to cardiovascular care pathways.[38] A recent *New England Journal of Medicine* current concepts article[6] provides a preliminary framework, but considerable local and regional work is still required to create a functional system. The Bernese Algorithm,[39] although somewhat dated, is one of the only published hypothermia care pathways. The provincial health authority in British Columbia, Canada, is currently creating a clinical practice guideline and care pathway, which will likely be published and available for download at the authors' Web site in the future.

DROWNING, AVALANCHE, AND TRAUMA

Drowning, avalanche burial, and trauma are three situations that warrant special consideration in the context of hypothermia. Patients removed from cold water should be extracted in a horizontal position in an effort to decrease the risk of orthostatic and hydrostatic changes triggering rescue collapse. The majority of drowning is **submersion**, where the patient immediately goes under the water, suffers a hypoxic cardiac arrest, and then develops hypothermia. With the exception of children, who may undergo simultaneous hypoxic cardiac arrest and rapid cooling,[24] most submersion patients are unlikely to benefit from prolonged resuscitation (normothermic hypoxic cardiac arrest with brain death prior to cooling). The less common **immersion** patient may benefit from prolonged resuscitation; this patient is initially immersed in cold water but able to breathe air, cooling ensues, and the patient eventually suffers a presumed hypothermic cardiac arrest and may or may not become secondarily submerged. An amazing immersion case series took place on a single day in Denmark in 2011. Seven adolescent school children wearing personal floatation devices were found in cardiac arrest, in 2°C water, after a dragon boat accident. All seven were successfully resuscitated using ECMO after prolonged CPR and the neurologic outcome was good in six out of the seven cases.[35] See chapter 215, "Drowning," for detailed discussion of drowning.

With **avalanche** burial, most episodes of cardiac arrest are caused by asphyxia or trauma.[40] Avalanche burial results in much slower cooling than cold water exposure, and it will take from 35 minutes to several hours for the patient's core temperature to drop below 32°C (assuming initial normothermia). Therefore, if the patient is recovered in cardiac after less than 35 minutes of burial, hypothermia is not the cause of cardiac arrest. For patients recovered after 35 minutes of burial, in the absence of obvious traumatic death, an airway packed with snow, or an accurate core temperature >32°C, accidental hypothermia may be the cause of cardiac arrest and prolonged resuscitation may be indicated. Cardiac arrest secondary to blunt trauma has a dismal prognosis (<1% survival),[41] and a core temperature <35°C further increases the odds of death by at least 2.4.[17] Therefore, it is reasonable to apply normothermic termination of resuscitation guidelines to patients suspected of blunt traumatic arrest, even in the presence of hypothermia.

AUSTERE ENVIRONMENTS

In the rare circumstances of stage IV hypothermia in an austere environment, when ongoing CPR during transport is not possible, it may be reasonable to transport without CPR (particularly if the patient has pulseless electrical activity) until such a time as CPR can be maintained or a definitive care center is reached. The decision to not perform CPR in an austere environment may be risky given that prehospital CPR is performed in the vast majority of stage IV hypothermia literature; however, there are two published cases that have shown good outcomes despite CPR interruptions[36,42] and one case where CPR was not performed at all during transport.[43] Interestingly there has been considerable historical and ongoing expert opinion controversy about whether or not to perform CPR for stage IV patients with pulseless electrical activity, even in the nonaustere setting.[44,45] Presumably those who advocate against CPR fear an undetectable perfusing rhythm that could be terminated by starting CPR. Given that a rescuer has carefully checked for a pulse or signs of life for 60 seconds, that starting CPR will generate a palpable pulse and provide ~40% of cerebral blood flow,[46] that CPR has been shown to be safe in normothermic nonarrested patients,[47] that in the absence of adequate cerebral blood flow a deeply hypothermic patient is likely to suffer irreversible hypoxic injury after 30 to 60 minutes,[22] and that CPR is performed in the vast majority of stage IV hypothermia literature, it is this author's opinion that the benefits of CPR far outweigh the risks for the patient with absent vital signs, regardless of the ECG findings.

Acknowledgment: I thank my hypothermia mentors: Jeff Boyd, Hermann Brugger, Peter Paal, and Ken Zafren.

REFERENCES

The complete reference list is available online at www.TintinalliEM.com.

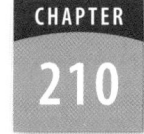

Heat Emergencies

Frank LoVecchio

INTRODUCTION AND EPIDEMIOLOGY

Heat emergencies represent a continuum of disorders from heat cramps to heat stress that, when severe, culminate in heat stroke. In most circumstances, heat emergencies can be avoided through common sense, public education, and prevention.

The incidence of heat-related emergencies varies with the weather, although this is not an absolute requirement.[1] During heat waves and severe droughts, fatality rates spike.[1] Heat stroke is likely seen less among persons who live in warmer climates than travelers to these areas because of physiologic acclimatization and cultural adaptation of the former to heat.

From 1999 to 2003, an average of 688 heat-related deaths per year from exposure to extreme heat were reported in the United States.[1] The heat wave during the summer of 2003 is estimated to have caused 14,800 deaths in France.[2] In the Russian heat wave in July/August 2010, there were an estimated 15,000 deaths, with additional morbidity from associated forest fires and smoke injury.[3]

PATHOPHYSIOLOGY

MECHANISMS OF HEAT TRANSFER

Body temperature is regulated through the delicate balance of heat production, accumulation, and dissipation. Heat is generated by cellular metabolism and the mechanical work of skeletal muscle. Heat accumulates from radiation from the sun and direct contact with hot objects and is absorbed when the ambient temperature rises above body temperature. As core temperature rises, the autonomic nervous system is stimulated to promote sweating and cutaneous vasodilatation.

The body has several mechanisms for dissipating heat to the environment, including radiation (the transfer of heat by electromagnetic waves from a warmer object to a colder object), conduction (heat exchange between two surfaces in direct contact), convection (heat transfer by air or liquid moving across the surface of an object), and evaporation (heat loss by vaporization of water, or sweat).

Radiation and evaporation dissipate most body heat at lower ambient temperatures (<35°C [<95°F]). Conduction of heat into a layer of ambient air surrounding the skin ends rapidly as soon as that layer acquires similar temperature as the skin surface. This results in creation of an "insulator zone" of warmed air through which little heat may be lost. Removing the warmed air next to the skin and replacing it with cooler air may increase conductive heat loss by convection. When conduction is coupled with convection, rates of heat energy transfer from the body increase. Conduction of heat into water is many times more efficient than conduction into air of the same temperature.

The effect of wind on heat loss depends on wind velocity. Wind moves heat away from the skin by convection, but above 32.2°C (90°F) and 35% humidity, convection does not remove heat well.[4] This is why the use of fans alone is not effective in preventing heat stroke during periods of high environmental temperature and humidity.

When the external temperature rises to >35°C (>95°F), the body can no longer radiate heat to the environment and becomes dependent on evaporation for heat transfer. As humidity increases, the potential for evaporative heat loss decreases. Sweat that drips from the skin does not provide any cooling benefit and only exacerbates dehydration. As a result, the combination of high temperature and high humidity essentially blocks the two main physiologic mechanisms that the body uses to dissipate heat.

RESPONSE TO HEAT STRESS

The body maintains a core temperature between 36°C and 38°C (96.8°F and 100.4°F). Native thermal regulation mechanisms begin to fail at core temperatures of <35°C (<95°F) and >40°C (>104°F).[5] It is possible to maintain core temperatures of 40°C to 42°C (104.0°F to 107.6°F) for short periods without adverse effect.[5]

The physiologic response to heat stress consists of four primary mechanisms: dilatation of blood vessels, particularly in the skin; increased sweat production; decreased heat production; and behavioral heat control. As the core temperature of the body rises, the sympathetic outflow of the posterior hypothalamus is inhibited, which leaves unopposed the sympathetic outflow from the anterior hypothalamus. Sympathetic flow from the anterior hypothalamus results in decreased vascular tone throughout the body, particularly in the cutaneous circulation.

During exercise in conditions of hyperthermia, the heart rate increases to compensate for the decrease in stroke volume from the cutaneous vascular dilation and to maintain cardiac output.[6] Patients with underlying cardiovascular disease or pharmacologic or physiologic impairment of these mechanisms may not be able to elevate cardiac output. Heat stress may also result in arrhythmias, myocardial ischemia, and exacerbation of congestive heart failure.

Elevated cholinergic stimulation to the skin results in increased sweat production. Sharp increases in the rate of sweat production normally occur with core temperature elevations above 37°C (98.6°F). As a general rule, for every pound of weight lost by sweating, 500 mL of fluid should be consumed. Endurance athletes can perspire at a rate of up to 1.5 L/h.[7] Cutaneous vascular dilation and sweating increase as the body temperature rises until a homeostatic stall of heat production and input with heat dissipation is reached and the body's temperature stops rising.[8] Interestingly, sweating activation in older individuals begins at 1.5°C (34.7°F) higher than that in younger individuals.[9]

MEDICATIONS

Medications often interfere with heat-removal mechanisms. Notable drugs are anticholinergic agents, diuretics, phenothiazine, β-blockers, calcium channel blockers, and sympathomimetic agents.[10] Anticholinergic agents impair sweating and the cardiovascular response to heat. Diuretics lead to volume depletion and decreased cardiac output. Phenothiazines have anticholinergic properties and deplete central stores of dopamine, which interfere with the hypothalamic thermoregulatory center. Medications such as β-blockers and calcium channel blockers decrease the cardiovascular response to heat and reduce peripheral blood flow and the ability to sweat. Sympathomimetics cause cutaneous vasoconstriction and inhibit sweating. Alcohol inhibits secretion of antidiuretic hormone, which leads to dehydration, and blunts the psychological heat-avoidance response. Heroin, cocaine, and amphetamines disrupt the function of endogenous endorphins and adrenocorticotropic hormones that are involved in heat adaptation mechanisms. Amphetamines and cocaine increase muscle activity and lead to heat production. Lysergic acid diethylamide and phencyclidine act on the CNS to induce a hypermetabolic state.[10]

ACCLIMATION

Acclimation is the adaptation of the body to environmental changes. It involves a number of physiologic and biochemical adjustments that allow an individual to withstand heat stresses that would otherwise result in substantial morbidity and mortality.

Acclimation lowers the thermal set point in the hypothalamus, which triggers the onset of sweating at lower core temperatures in the acclimated human. In addition, the maximal rate of sweat production is dramatically increased to 1.5 to 3.0 L/h and can be sustained for longer periods.[7] Aldosterone secretion is boosted, and sodium conservation results from more efficient reabsorption from the sweat. Plasma volume expands, heart rate decreases for any given heat load, and exercise tolerance improves. Dilation of cutaneous blood vessels occurs at a lower core temperature to promote earlier cooling.

In most individuals, acclimation can be achieved over 7 days to several weeks.[11-13] Moderate exercise in a hot, dry environment for 60 to 100 minutes each day is probably the optimal approach to achieve acclimation. To maintain heat and exercise-induced adaptive responses, heat exposure needs to continue intermittently at least on 4-day intervals. Simple exposure to a hot environment for 1 to 4 hours a day also may result in acclimation within 2 weeks. Once removed from the hot environment, the body will de-acclimate to the original physiologic parameters within 1 to 2 weeks.[12]

MODELS OF HEAT INJURY

The pathology of heat stroke is not completely understood, and although heat stroke is triggered by hyperthermia, there is evidence that secondary endotoxemia triggers a systemic inflammatory response, coagulopathy, and multiorgan failure.[14,15]

Heat exhaustion and heat stroke occur when the body's thermoregulatory responses are impaired or overwhelmed and are no longer capable of maintaining homeostasis. Excessive heat is directly toxic to cells, causes an acute-phase reaction with release of inflammatory cytokines, and damages vascular endothelium. Nearly all cells respond to sudden heating by producing heat stress proteins, whose mechanism of action is still not completely understood.[14,15]

Escalating cellular temperature results in denaturation of proteins, interruption of cellular processes, and cell death. Temperatures of

>41.6°C (>106.9°F) can produce cellular injury in hours. As temperature rises, cellular damage occurs more quickly and extensively. Temperatures >49°C (>120.2°F) typically result in immediate cell death and tissue necrosis.[15] The enhanced vascular permeability due to damaged vascular endothelium results in activation of the coagulation cascade and disseminated intravascular coagulation.

Classic heat injury occurs during periods of high environmental heat stress. Physical exertion is not required if the heat gain occurs at environmental temperatures and humidity levels that overwhelm the native heat loss mechanisms. The increase in core temperature seen in this setting is often slow, occurring over a period of hours to days. Because of this slow rise in heat burden, volume and electrolyte abnormalities are common. High-risk populations include the elderly, the young, and those with psychological, physiologic, and pharmacologic impairments of heat loss mechanisms (e.g., diabetes; Raynaud's disease; drugs such as anticholinergics, diuretics, antipsychotics, cocaine). Epidemiologic studies of classic heat injury typically identify the elderly, living alone or without social support and without air-conditioning.[16]

Exertional heat injury usually affects individuals who are participating in athletic events or performing jobs under conditions of high heat stress. Risk factors include dehydration, concurrent illness, obesity, wearing too much clothing, and poor cardiovascular fitness. In this setting, heat production and heat gain from the environment exceed the capacity of heat removal processes. Physical exercise is the most common single source of internal heat production. Without an efficient cooling mechanism, progressive dehydration and hyperpyrexia continue to the level of cardiovascular and metabolic failure.

Confinement hyperpyrexia is a special category of nonexertional hyperpyrexia and can occur in several circumstances, such as when children are left inside cars, when stowaways are abandoned inside closed vehicles or railroad cars, and when workers are occupationally exposed to heat inside enclosed spaces. Between July 2000 and June 2001 in the United States, 1960 nonfatal heat injuries and 78 fatalities were reported in children who were left intentionally in motor vehicles during hot days.[17] Nonventilated vehicle compartments in a hot environment may reach temperatures of 54°C to 60°C (129.2°F to 140.0°F) in <10 minutes.[17] Infants have less capacity than adults to deal with heat stress and, if left in motor vehicles for only a matter of minutes, may accumulate a critical heat burden. During 2000, nearly 500 individuals died attempting to cross the Mexico-U.S. border through the desert, locked in closed vehicle compartments and then abandoned by smugglers, with >50% of these deaths due to heat stroke. A particularly dangerous region is southern Arizona, which accounts for 22% of all southwest border deaths of illegal immigrants. In the August 2003 heat wave in France, a risk factor for heat stroke mortality was heat exposure at home or in a non–air-conditioned healthcare facility.[18]

CLINICAL FEATURES AND TREATMENT

Heat emergencies comprise a range of disorders from minor (heat edema, prickly heat, heat cramps, and heat exhaustion) to major (heat stroke).

MINOR HEAT ILLNESSES

Heat Edema **Heat edema** is a self-limited process manifested by mild swelling of the feet, ankles, and hands that appears within the first few days of exposure to a hot environment. Heat edema is due to the cutaneous vasodilatation and orthostatic pooling of interstitial fluid in gravity-dependent extremities. An increase in the secretion of aldosterone and antidiuretic hormone in response to the heat stress contributes to the mild edema. In general, heat edema is found in elderly nonacclimatized individuals who are physically active after a period of sitting while traveling in a vehicle or airplane. Occasionally, heat edema occurs after prolonged standing. It is commonly seen in healthy travelers just arriving from a colder climate. The edema is mild and does not impair or interfere with normal activities. Very rarely, pitting edema of the ankles may develop but does not progress to the pretibial region.

History and physical examination are usually sufficient to exclude systemic causes of edema, and no further testing or treatment except removal from heat source is needed. In the elderly, new pedal edema from heat should be differentiated from early congestive heart failure or deep venous thrombosis. Heat edema usually resolves spontaneously in a few days. No special treatment is necessary, but elevation of the legs and the use of support hose facilitate removal of the interstitial fluid. Diuretics are not effective and can predispose to volume depletion, electrolyte abnormalities, or more serious heat emergencies.[8]

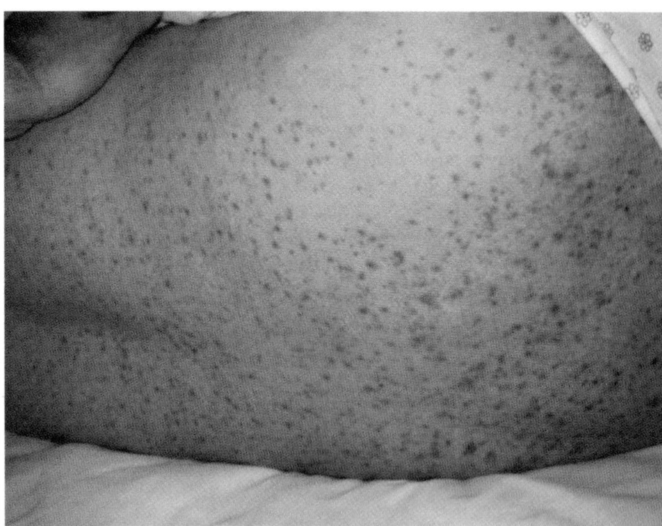

FIGURE 210-1. Miliaria rubra (prickly heat). [Image used with permission of Peter Lio, MD.]

Prickly Heat **Prickly heat** is a pruritic, maculopapular, and erythematous rash over normally clothed areas of the body. Also known as *lichen tropicus*, *miliaria rubra*, or *heat rash*, it is an acute inflammation of the sweat ducts caused by blockage of the sweat pores by macerated stratum corneum (**Figure 210-1**). The sweat ducts become dilated under pressure and ultimately rupture, producing superficial vesicles in the malpighian layer of the skin on a red base. Itching is the predominant clinical feature during this phase and can be treated successfully with antihistamines. Wearing clean, light, and loose-fitting clothing and avoiding sweat-generating situations can prevent prickly heat. Calamine lotion or topical steroids can be of benefit. Chlorhexidine in a light cream or salicylic acid cleaning may provide some relief.[19]

With prolonged or repeated heat exposure, a keratin plug fills the sweat duct, causing obstruction in the stratum malpighian layer. When the duct ruptures a second time, the resultant vesicle will be driven deeper into the dermis. This vesicle simulates the white papules of piloerection and is not pruritic. This is known as the *profunda* stage of prickly heat (miliaria profunda) and can readily advance into a chronic dermatitis. Infection with *Staphylococcus aureus* or methicillin-resistant *S. aureus* is a common complication. The skin can be desquamated by applying 1% salicylic acid to the affected area three times a day.

Heat Cramps **Heat cramps** are painful, involuntary, spasmodic contractions of skeletal muscles, usually those of the calves, although they may involve the thighs and shoulders. These cramps usually occur in individuals who are sweating profusely and replace fluid losses with water or other hypotonic solutions. Heat cramps may occasionally occur during exercise or, more commonly, during a rest period after several hours of vigorous physical activity. Nonacclimated or unconditioned individuals who are just starting manual labor in a hot environment are at risk for heat cramps. Although heat cramps are self-limited and do not cause significant morbidity, the pain associated with them can precipitate an ED visit. In general, heat cramps are short in duration, are limited to a definitive group of muscles, and almost never involve enough muscle mass to cause rhabdomyolysis.

The pathogenesis of heat cramps is believed to involve a relative deficiency of sodium, potassium, or magnesium and fluid at muscle level. The production of large amounts of sweat, which has a high sodium content, coupled with inadequate sodium replacement results in cellular hyponatremia. This in turn produces muscle cramps with calcium-dependent muscle relaxation. Patients with severe heat cramps may have hyponatremia and hypochloremia.[20] Rhabdomyolysis is rare and occurs secondary to diffuse and protracted muscle spasm.[15]

Treatment consists of fluid and salt replacement (PO or IV) and rest in a cool environment. For mild cases, or if an overwhelming number of patients require treatment, a 0.1% to 0.2% saline solution can be given PO. Two 650 milligram salt tablets dissolved in a quart of water provide a 0.1% saline solution.[13,20] Many electrolyte solution drinks (sports drinks) are commercially available and are much more palatable. Patients with more severe symptoms require IV rehydration with normal saline. Heat cramps can be prevented by maintaining adequate dietary salt intake or by drinking commercial electrolyte beverages. Salt tablets by themselves should not be used, because the tablets are a gastric irritant and cause nausea and vomiting.

Heat Stress Heat stress occurs in two different ways, through water depletion and through sodium depletion, but often is characterized by a combination of both. Water depletion tends to occur in the elderly and in persons working in hot environments with inadequate water replacement. Salt depletion heat exhaustion tends to occur in unacclimatized individuals who replace fluid losses with large amounts of hypotonic solutions.

Heat stress presents with symptoms that include headache, nausea, vomiting, malaise, dizziness, and muscle cramps as well as signs of dehydration, such as tachycardia and orthostatic hypotension or near-syncope. Heat cramps and/or rhabdomyolysis are present on rare occasions. Because of the ill-defined and nonspecific symptoms, heat stress is often a diagnosis of exclusion.

On physical examination, the temperature may be normal or elevated, usually not above 40°C (104°F). Patients with heat exhaustion do not manifest signs of CNS impairment.

Laboratory studies almost universally demonstrate hemoconcentration, although the specific electrolyte abnormalities seen depend on the ratio of fluid and electrolyte losses to intake. Patients who have had no fluid intake of any kind exhibit hypernatremia, whereas those who partly rehydrate with salt-containing fluids develop isotonic hypovolemia with normal sodium and chloride levels. Serum potassium and magnesium levels are variable.

Heat stress is treated with volume and electrolyte replacement and rest. Removal from the heat-stressed environment is essential. Patients with mild heat stress may be treated with oral electrolyte solutions. Rapid infusion of moderate amounts of IV fluids (1 to 2 L of normal saline) may be necessary in patients who demonstrate significant tissue hypoperfusion. Ideally, the choice of IV solution should be guided by laboratory determinations, but isotonic salt solutions may be used until specific electrolyte abnormalities are identified. In general, hospitalization is not required. Patients with congestive heart failure or severe electrolyte disturbances may require admission, because of the time needed to correct their fluid and/or electrolyte deficits.

Heat stress can progress to heat stroke even after the patient is removed from the hot environment. Therefore, patients with heat stress who do not respond to approximately 30 minutes of fluid replacement and removal from the hot environment should be cooled until the core temperature drops to 39°C (102°F).

HEAT STROKE

Heat stroke is an acute life-threatening emergency with high mortality and is fatal if left untreated (**Table 210-1**).

TABLE 210-1 Signs and Symptoms of Heat Emergencies

Heat Cramps	Heat Stress	Heat Stroke
Muscle cramps	Symptoms seen in heat cramps plus:	Symptoms seen in heat stress plus:
Normal to mildly elevated temperature	Normal to elevated temperature (<40°C [<104°F])	Elevated temperature (>40°C [>104°F])
Sweating	Nausea, vomiting, headache, malaise, dizziness	Neurologic abnormalities: inappropriate behavior, confusion, delirium, ataxia, coma, seizures
	Orthostatic hypotension	
		Anhidrosis or sweating

TABLE 210-2 Differential Diagnosis of Heat Stroke

Infection	*Neurologic*
Sepsis syndrome	Hypothalamic bleeding or infarct
Meningitis	Cerebrovascular accident
Encephalitis	Status epilepticus
Malaria	*Toxicologic*
Typhoid	Anticholinergic toxidrome
Tetanus	Sympathomimetic overdose
Endocrine	Salicylate overdose
Thyroid storm	Serotonin syndrome
Pheochromocytoma	Malignant hyperthermia
Diabetic ketoacidosis	Neuroleptic malignant syndrome
	Withdrawal syndromes—alcohol and benzodiazepine withdrawal

The cardinal features of heat stroke are hyperthermia (>40°C [>104°F]) and altered mental status. Although patients presenting with classic (nonexertional) heat stroke may exhibit anhidrosis, the absence of sweat is not considered a diagnostic criterion because sweat is present in over half of patients with heat stroke.[15]

The CNS is particularly vulnerable in heat stroke. The cerebellum is highly sensitive to heat, and ataxia can be an early neurologic finding. Virtually any neurologic abnormality may be present in heat stroke, including irritability, confusion, bizarre behavior, combativeness, hallucinations, plantar responses, decorticate and decerebrate posturing, hemiplegia, status epilepticus, and coma. Seizures are quite common, especially during cooling. Neurologic injury is a function of the maximum temperature reached and the duration of exposure.[15]

The distinction between exertional and classic (nonexertional) heat stroke is not clinically important, because immediate cooling and support of organ system function is the therapeutic goal for both. A delay in cooling increases the mortality rate.

DIAGNOSIS

There are no diagnostic tests for heat stroke, and the differential diagnosis is extensive. Therefore, the diagnosis of heat stroke is determined by history and clinical presentation, and exclusion of other processes (**Table 210-2**).

LABORATORY EVALUATION

Diagnostic studies are directed toward detecting end-organ damage and excluding other diseases. Helpful studies include a CBC, comprehensive metabolic panel with arterial blood gas analysis, coagulation profile, creatine phosphokinase level, myoglobin level, urinalysis, ECG, and chest radiograph. Lumbar puncture and CT of the head may be indicated to rule out other causes of altered mental status. The partial pressure of arterial carbon dioxide is often <20 mm Hg due to hyperventilation. Patients with exertional heat stroke often have lactic acidosis, and hypoglycemia may occur.

TREATMENT

The goals of therapy are immediate cooling and aggressive support of organ system function.

PREHOSPITAL CARE

Remove the patient from the hot environment immediately, and perform standard resuscitation measures. Check point-of-care glucose if there is altered mental status. Start cooling by removing clothing and implementing one of the following methods: spray the patient with water and provide airflow over the patient (ideal method but not always practical during transportation); place wet towels or sheets over the patient's body; or place ice on the patient. Administer a bolus of normal saline (1 to 2 L) if hypotension is present.[15] Online medical direction is helpful when transport times are long and when EMS personnel in the given region rarely encounter heat stroke.

ED MANAGEMENT

Initial Resuscitation Continue standard resuscitation measures. Administer IV fluids at a rate that ensures adequate urine output. In elderly patients or patients with cardiovascular disease, consider invasive monitoring. Check glucose levels. Monitor core temperature with an electronic rectal thermometer, temperature probe–equipped urinary drainage catheter, or esophageal thermometer.

Cooling Techniques Currently, only physical methods of cooling are recommended, and there is no evidence to support one particular approach over another. In clinical practice, the primary physical cooling procedure is one that allows easy patient access, is readily available, is tolerated well by the patient, and is effective (**Table 210-3**). With all cooling methods, the goal is to reduce the core temperature to approximately 39°C (102.2°F) and to avoid overshoot hypothermia. If the initial cooling method used does not lower temperature quickly, try another method.[15,21]

Evaporative Cooling **Cooling by evaporation** is practical and comfortable for the patient compared with other methods. Remove patient clothing and spray cool water (~15°C [59°F]) on most of the patient's body surface. Directing a fan over the patient facilitates evaporation. If the skin temperature is reduced below 30°C (86°F), shivering will result in more heat production, and peripheral vasoconstriction will impair evaporation. To prevent hypothermic overshoot, some recommend using either tepid water warmed to 40°C (104°F) or exposing the patient to hot air (45°C [113°F]) with the fan.[21] This method is the foundation of several cooling units such as the **Makkah cooling unit**, which is widely used in the Middle East to treat pilgrims traveling to Mecca who succumb to heat stroke. The Makkah cooling unit is composed of a large hammock with built-in sprinklers that spray cool water (15°C [59°F]) over the patient's body and powerful fans that blow warm air (45°C [113°F]) over the patient. The main problems with the Makkah cooling method are cost, portability, and the fact that evaporation rates are reduced in very humid environments.

The two main difficulties associated with evaporative cooling are shivering and the inability of cardiac electrodes to adhere to the skin. Shivering is treated primarily with short-acting benzodiazepines and secondarily with phenothiazines. Phenothiazines may lower the seizure threshold and cause hypotension, and their anticholinergic properties impair sweating.

Immersion Cooling **Immersion cooling** is performed by placing the undressed patient into a tub of ice water deep enough to cover the trunk and extremities, while keeping the patient's head out of the water. Problems associated with immersion cooling include shivering, displacement of monitoring leads, and inability to perform defibrillation or resuscitative procedures. Also, a tub or receptacle large enough to accommodate the patient may not be readily available. The efficiency of immersion cooling has been documented primarily in young, healthy patients without comorbid diseases. The efficacy and safety of immersion in patients with classic (nonexertional) heat stroke and patients with significant comorbid diseases (e.g., coronary artery disease) have not been established.

Massage with ice water is an alternative for patients who cannot tolerate immersion, although its effectiveness as a single modality for cooling remains unclear.[21]

Invasive Cooling Measures When evaporation or immersion methods are not sufficient, invasive cooling may be considered. The most rapid method of cooling a heat stroke victim is cardiopulmonary bypass, although lack of availability and logistical problems are major disadvantages. Cold water gastric lavage, cold water urinary bladder lavage, and cold water rectal lavage are other adjunctive measures that can be performed in the ED but require patient cooperation, are labor intensive, have the potential for inducing water intoxication, and are of questionable efficacy. Cold water peritoneal lavage is yet another option, but its effectiveness has not been validated.

Other Cooling Measures **Cooling blankets** work slowly and should not be a sole treatment for heat stroke. IV infusion of cold fluids alone is not considered effective treatment. Applying ice packs to the neck, axillae, and groin does not lower temperature quickly enough to be used alone. There are no studies on the effectiveness of antipyretics. Dantrolene is not indicated for treatment of heat stroke.[21]

TABLE 210-3 Summary of Cooling Techniques

Cooling Method	Advantages	Disadvantages	Recommendations
Evaporative cooling	Provides effective cooling	Can cause shivering	Strongly recommended
	Readily available	Less effective in humid environments	
	Practical	Makes it difficult to maintain electrode positions	
	Well tolerated		
Immersion cooling	Provides effective cooling	Can cause shivering	Recommended
		Poorly tolerated	
		Not compatible with resuscitation settings	
Ice packs on neck, axillae, and groin	Practical	Cooling times longer than other modalities	Can be used as adjunct cooling method
	Can be added to other cooling methods	Poorly tolerated	
Cardiopulmonary bypass	Provides fast and effective cooling	Invasive	Recommended in severe or resistant cases when available
		Not readily available	
		Setup is labor intensive	
Cooling blankets	Easy to apply	Have limited cooling efficacy	Not recommended when other methods available
		Impede use of other cooling methods	
Cold water gastric, urinary bladder, rectal, or peritoneal lavage	—	Invasive	Effectiveness and safety not established
		Labor intensive	
		May lead to water intoxication	
		Human experience is limited	

COMPLICATIONS

Heat stroke causes both early and late complications (**Table 210-4**). Hypotension is a common initial finding. Usually the blood pressure will rise in response to fluid bolus and body cooling. The combination of low cardiac output and elevated central venous pressure warrants the use of vasoactive catecholamines such as dopamine or dobutamine if a 20 cc/kg fluid bolus does not result in improvement. Once the central venous pressure reaches 12 to 14 mm Hg and cooling is initiated, dopamine or dobutamine may be used to maintain a normal blood pressure. Inotropes that cause severe vasoconstriction by α-adrenergic stimulation, such as norepinephrine, may impede cooling by redirecting blood flow away from the skin.

Fluid and electrolyte abnormalities vary depending on the type of onset and duration of the disorder, any underlying disease (especially cardiovascular disease), and any prior use of medications, such as diuretics. Hypokalemia due to total-body depletion of potassium may be noted, and hyperkalemia may result from acute renal failure and rhabdomyolysis. Hypernatremia is seen in severely dehydrated patients, whereas hyponatremia occurs in patients who hydrate with oral hypotonic solutions.

Hematologic disorders may be apparent clinically and on laboratory evaluation. Findings of abnormal hemostasis include purpura, petechiae, and conjunctival, GI, renal, or pulmonary hemorrhage. Coagulation studies may show thrombocytopenia, hypoprothrombinemia, and hypofibrinogenemia. Thermal injury to the vascular endothelium can cause increased platelet aggregation, changes in capillary permeability, thermal deactivation of plasma proteins resulting in a decreased level of clotting factors, disseminated intravascular coagulation, and fibrinolysis.[15,22]

Thermal injury to the liver is a common finding in heat stroke, although jaundice does not always develop. Delayed elevation of hepatic enzyme levels, peaking 24 to 72 hours after the thermal insult, is attributed to centrilobular necrosis. Glucose homeostasis is affected. Hepatic damage is almost always reversible, with a full recovery.

Renal failure results from direct thermal injury to the kidney, rhabdomyolysis, or volume depletion. Clinically, this is manifested by oliguria, microscopic hematuria, proteinuria, myoglobinuria, and granular or red cell casts in the urine. Early volume expansion decreases the detrimental renal effects of heat stroke.

Adult respiratory distress syndrome requires ongoing respiratory support until cooling has been accomplished. Cardiac muscle injury may also occur. The presence of hypotension, low cardiac output, and a falling cardiac index is associated with a poor prognosis.

Seizures may occur during cooling and can be controlled with benzodiazepines.

Mortality correlates with the degree of temperature elevation, time to initiation of cooling measures, and the number of organ systems affected. In one prospective cohort study, the risk of death increased substantially in patients who presented with anuria (hazard ratio, 5.24; 95% confidence interval, 2.29-12.03), coma (hazard ratio, 2.95; 95% confidence interval, 1.26-6.91), or cardiovascular failure (hazard ratio, 2.43; 95% confidence interval, 1.14-5.17).[23]

TABLE 210-4 Complications of Heat Stroke

	Early	Late
Vital signs	Hypotension	—
	Hypothermic overshoot	
	Hyperthermic rebound	
Muscular	Rhabdomyolysis	—
Neurologic	Delirium/coma	Cerebral edema
	Seizure	Encephalopathy
		Persistent neurologic deficit
Cardiac	Heart failure	Myocardial injury
Pulmonary	Pulmonary edema	Acute respiratory distress syndrome
Renal	Oliguria	Renal failure, rhabdomyolysis
GI	—	Intestinal ischemia or infarction
		Pancreatic injury
		Hepatic dysfunction
Metabolic	Hypokalemia	Hyperkalemia
	Hypernatremia	Hypocalcemia
	Hyponatremia	Hyperuricemia
Hematologic	—	Thrombocytopenia
		Disseminated intravascular coagulation

DISPOSITION AND FOLLOW-UP

Patients with minor heat emergency syndromes (heat edema, heat cramps, or heat stress) require only ED treatment along with clear discharge instructions and outpatient follow-up. However, patients with underlying diseases, such as congestive heart failure or renal failure, and patients with severe electrolyte imbalance may require hospital admission. No decision rules exist to guide disposition decisions.

Patients with heat stroke require admission to a unit providing care at a level appropriate to the patient's condition. Patients who are intubated, are in hemodynamically labile condition, require invasive hemodynamic monitoring, or need continued cooling should be admitted to the intensive care unit. If the receiving health care facility is unable to provide the services needed for quality care, then transfer the patient to a higher-level facility.

SPECIAL POPULATIONS

Populations at higher risk of developing heat emergencies include the elderly, young children, athletes, persons with limited mobility, alcoholic individuals, and people taking antipsychotics, major tranquilizers, anticholinergics, antiparkinsonian agents, cardiovascular medications (β-blockers, calcium channel blockers, and vasodilators), or over-the-counter sleeping aids or stimulants.[10] Other risk factors for exertional heat emergencies include obesity, dehydration, and vigorous exertion in the heat without proper training and acclimatization.

In addition, individuals with a history of heat stroke are at greater risk for another episode. Patients with congenital absence of sweat glands, progressive systemic scleroderma, hyperthyroidism, and pheochromocytoma are also at increased risk for heat stroke.

Elderly persons who lack mobility, have preexisting medical illness, take medications that may affect thermoregulation or ambulation, live in housing that is without thermal insulation, or sleep on the top floor are particularly susceptible to heat stress.[18]

Young children lack adequate thermoregulatory and sweating capabilities, do not instinctively replace their fluid losses or limit exercise in extreme heat, and may be unable to remove themselves from risky environments such as a closed car in the sun. Teenagers and preadolescents are at risk because they may use poor judgment when exercising in high heat and humidity and may push themselves to the limit. Early season high school heat stroke deaths are most likely to occur during the first 4 days of practice; children require 10 to 14 days to achieve an appropriate acclimatization response.

Athletes should be prescreened about risk factors for heat illness (sickle cell disease, prior heat illness, dehydration) and be acclimated to heat gradually over 1 to 2 weeks. Although there are no standardized guidelines for return to play after heat stroke, depending on the severity of the episode, a rest period of at least 1 week, followed by medical clearance and then gradual progression of activity, is suggested.[13]

PREVENTION

Behavioral control of temperature regulation is important. As individuals begin to feel hot and uncomfortable when exposed to heat stress, they may take actions to find a cool environment. Public education regarding heat-related illness should capitalize on this response mechanism.

Populations with no home air-conditioning have a higher risk for a serious heat illness than populations with air-conditioning. Taking "heat breaks" in an air-conditioned location for periods as short as 2 hours a day decreases the likelihood of heat stroke among those with no home air-conditioning.

Acclimation protocols to decrease the frequency of heat-related illness have been developed for personnel (e.g., military, firefighters, laborers, and disaster relief workers) who are preparing to deploy to hot environments.

Avoidance of strenuous exercise during periods of high environmental heat stress, as judged by the heat index chart, coupled with acclimation, hydration, breaks from the heat, and education, will prevent exertional heat injury.

Serious heat-related illnesses are preventable. General recommendations for the individual include (1) decreasing or rescheduling strenuous activity for cooler parts of the day; (2) wearing light and loose-fitting clothing; (3) increasing carbohydrate intake and decreasing protein intake to decrease endogenous heat production; (4) drinking plenty of fluids, even when not thirsty; (5) avoiding alcoholic beverages; (6) using salt tablets as well as fluids; (7) avoiding direct sunlight; and (8) taking advantage of the shade. Community health officials and governmental leaders should recognize the need to educate the public, coordinate and plan the implementation of these measures in advance, and avoid resorting to crisis management.

Acknowledgment: The authors acknowledge James S. Walker and David E. Hogan for their contributions to this chapter.

REFERENCES

The complete reference list is available online at www.TintinalliEM.com.

CHAPTER 211 Bites and Stings

Aaron Schneir
Richard F. Clark

INTRODUCTION AND EPIDEMIOLOGY

The phylum Arthropoda is the largest division of the animal kingdom. The phylum includes insects (bees, wasps, hornets, flies, mosquitoes, bedbugs, fire ants, caterpillars, fleas), arachnids (spiders, scorpions, chiggers, ticks), and crustaceans (shrimp, lobsters, crabs). Venomous bites and stings from arthropods are a significant worldwide problem.[1] In the United States, the American Association of Poison Control Centers reported almost 50,000 cases of exposures to arthropods in 2012.[2] Some of these were listed as resulting in major or severe reactions, including severe pain, neurotoxicity, or other signs and symptoms. Fatalities among these exposures are rarely reported to poison centers and usually result from allergic reactions to Hymenoptera stings. Toxic reactions to multiple stings by members of the order Hymenoptera and severe systemic allergic reactions to one or more stings or bites of other insects, such as deerflies, blackflies, horseflies, and kissing bugs, can all present as emergency, life-threatening situations.[3] Other arthropod bites and envenomations merit review either because they cause specific organ system toxicity or because they can result in transmission of infectious disease. This chapter discusses the most common and serious arthropod bites and envenomations. Tick bites are discussed in the "Tickborne Zoonotic Infections" section of chapter 160, "Zoonotic Infections: Tickborne Zoonotic Infections."

HYMENOPTERA (WASPS, BEES, AND ANTS)

More fatalities result from stings by these insects than by stings or bites by any other arthropod. There are three major subgroups or superfamilies of medical importance: (1) Apidae, which includes the honeybee and bumblebee; (2) Vespidae, which includes yellow jackets, hornets, and wasps; and (3) Formicidae, or ants.

BEES AND WASPS (APIDAE AND VESPIDAE)

Apids, such as honeybees and bumblebees, are usually docile, stinging only when provoked. A female honeybee is capable of stinging only once (male bees have no stinger), because its stinger has multiple barbs that cause the sting apparatus to detach from the bee's body, which leads to evisceration and eventual death.

Africanized honeybees, or so-called killer bees, are now found in most of the southern and warmer regions of the United States extending from coast to coast. These bees are hybrids of African bees that escaped from laboratories in Brazil during the 1950s and have successfully spread northward along the coasts and temperate regions of the continent. Their venom is no more toxic than that of their American counterpart, but Africanized hybrid honeybees are more aggressive, and a hive can respond to a perceived threat with >10 times the number of bees that respond from a hive of typical North American bees. An attack from Africanized bees can lead to massive stinging, resulting in multisystem damage and death from severe venom toxicity.[4,5]

Most of the allergic reactions reported each year due to Hymenoptera occur from vespid (wasp, hornet, and yellow jacket) stings. These arthropods nest in the ground, in trees, or in walls; have volatile tempers; and may be disturbed by work taking place around the nest. As with bees, only the females have adapted a stinger from the ovipositor on the posterior aspect of the abdomen. Although vespids also possess barbed stingers, they have the ability to withdraw their stingers from the victim, which permits multiple stings.

Venom Hymenoptera venom contains several components.[6] Although histamine is one of those components, other substances are now recognized as more important. Melittin, a known membrane-active polypeptide that can cause degranulation of basophils and mast cells, constitutes >50% of the dry weight of bee venom. Protein enzymes such as phospholipase and hyaluronidase may account for most systemic reactions.[7,8] Because all Hymenoptera share many of these components, cross-sensitization may occur in individuals allergic to one species. Yellow jacket venom is perhaps the most potent sensitizer.

Clinical Features The most common response to Hymenoptera venom is a local reaction: pain, slight erythema, edema or urticaria, and pruritus at the sting site. A severe local reaction may involve one or more neighboring joints. A local reaction occurring in the mouth or throat can produce airway obstruction. Stings around the eye or on the lid may result in the development of an anterior capsule cataract, atrophy of the iris, lens abscess, perforation of the globe, glaucoma, or refractive changes. When local reactions become increasingly severe, the likelihood of future systemic reactions appears to increase, and if skin test results are positive, immunotherapy may be warranted.

Anaphylaxis Symptoms range on a continuum. Criteria for anaphylaxis are presented in **Table 211-1**, and detailed discussion of anaphylaxis is provided in chapter 14, "Anaphylaxis, Allergies, and Angioedema." Most reactions develop within the first 15 minutes, and nearly all occur within 6 hours. Initial mild symptoms may progress swiftly to shock. There is no correlation between systemic reaction and the number of stings. Symptoms include nausea, vomiting, and diarrhea; light-headedness and syncope; involuntary muscle spasms; edema without urticaria; and, rarely, seizures. Respiratory distress and cardiac arrest can result. Urticaria and bronchospasm do not need to be present. In general, the shorter the interval between the sting and the onset of symptoms, the more severe is the reaction. Fatalities that occur within the first hour after the sting usually result from airway obstruction or hypotension.

Renal and hepatic failure and disseminated intravascular coagulation can result from massive bee stings. Creatine phosphokinase concentrations can reach 100,000 IU/L or more in cases in which rhabdomyolysis occurs from direct venom toxicity.[5] Toxic reactions are believed to occur due to a direct multisystem effect of the venom. Symptoms usually subside within 48 hours but may last for several days in severe cases, and some effects, such as rhabdomyolysis, can be delayed. We recommend **hospital admission or observation for victims with**

TABLE 211-1 Clinical Criteria for Anaphylaxis

1. Acute onset of an illness (minutes to several hours) with involvement of the skin and/or mucosal tissue (e.g., hives/urticaria, pruritus, flushing, swollen lips, tongue, or uvula) associated with at least one of the following: Respiratory compromise (e.g., dyspnea, wheeze, stridor) *or* Reduced blood pressure *or* Associated symptoms of organ dysfunction (e.g., hypotonia, syncope, incontinence)
2. Two or more of the following that occur rapidly after exposure to a likely allergen for that patient (minutes to several hours): Involvement of the skin and/or mucosal tissue Respiratory compromise Reduced blood pressure or associated symptoms Persistent GI symptoms (e.g., cramps, vomiting)
3. Anaphylaxis should be suspected when patients are exposed to a known allergen and develop hypotension

>100 stings, for those with substantial comorbidities, and for those at extremes of age.

Delayed Reaction A delayed reaction, appearing 5 to 14 days after a sting, consists of serum sickness–like signs and symptoms of fever, malaise, headache, urticaria, lymphadenopathy, and polyarthritis.[9] Frequently, the patient has forgotten about the encounter and is puzzled by the sudden appearance of symptoms. This reaction is believed to be immune complex mediated.

Unusual Reactions Infrequently, a reaction to Hymenoptera venom produces neurologic, cardiovascular, and urologic symptoms, with signs of encephalopathy, neuritis, vasculitis, and nephrosis. Guillain-Barré syndrome has been reported as a possible consequence of a Hymenoptera sting. Identification of the offending insect can be difficult, except for the honeybee, which predictably leaves its stinger with venom sac attached in the lesion. In general, definitive insect identification is unnecessary, because signs and symptoms of envenomation are similar for all species of Hymenoptera. If edema persists at the sting site, then consider secondary cellulitis. Severe local reactions on the foot or ankle can be misdiagnosed as gout if the insect sting is not visible.

General Treatment If the bee stinger is present in the wound, remove it. Although conventional teaching suggested scraping the stinger out to avoid squeezing remaining venom from the retained venom gland into the tissues, involuntary muscle contraction of the gland continues after evisceration, and the venom contents are quickly exhausted. Immediate removal is the important principle, and the method of removal is irrelevant. Wash the sting site thoroughly with soap and water to minimize infection. For local reactions, intermittent application of ice packs at the site diminishes swelling and delays the absorption of venom while limiting edema. Oral antihistamines and analgesics may limit discomfort and pruritus. Nonsteroidal anti-inflammatory drugs can be effective in relieving pain. Standard doses of opioid analgesics also can be administered. If edema is significant, elevation and rest of the affected limb should limit swelling unless secondary infection develops, in which case antibiotics are necessary. In local tissue reactions, there is often significant inflammatory erythema and swelling, which make it difficult to distinguish from infection. As a general rule, infection is uncommon. We recommend **hospital admission or observation for victims with >100 stings, for those with substantial comorbidities, and for those at extremes of age.**

Anaphylaxis Treatment Although the initial signs and symptoms of a systemic reaction may be mild, the victim's condition can deteriorate rapidly in a matter of minutes. Administer IM epinephrine, 0.3 to 0.5 milligram (0.3 to 0.5 mL of 1:1000 concentration) in adults and 0.01 milligram/kg in children (up to 0.3 milligram). Massage the injection site to hasten absorption. **To avoid mishaps in dosing, many EDs now stock adult and pediatric EpiPens, which provide a standard adult or pediatric dose (EpiPen, 0.3 milligram epinephrine; EpiPen-Jr, 0.15 milligram epinephrine for children <30 kg).** Provide aggressive fluid resuscitation with crystalloids. Antihistamines, histamine-2 receptor antagonists, and steroids are also commonly given. See chapter 14 for detailed discussion. Antivenoms have been studied for the treatment of mass bee attacks but are not yet commercially available.[10]

Long-Term Management and Preventive Care Results of skin tests and radioallergosorbent tests are not fully reliable for determining which patients are at risk for systemic reaction during future encounters with Hymenoptera (**Table 211-2**) but should be coupled with information from the clinical history.[8,11] Patients with negative test results may have been sensitized by the skin tests themselves. Every patient who has had a systemic reaction should be provided with an insect sting kit containing premeasured epinephrine and should be carefully instructed in its use. The physician should stress that the patient must inject the epinephrine at the first sign of a systemic reaction. Physicians should also advise their patients who are allergic to insects to wear identification (e.g., medical alert tags) describing their severe allergy. They should also be advised to follow up with an allergist.

ANTS

There are five known species of fire ants (*Solenopsis*) in the United States: the native species *Solenopsis aurea*, *Solenopsis geminata*, and *Solenopsis xyloni*, and at least two imported species, *Solenopsis invicta* and *Solenopsis*

TABLE 211-2 Long-Term Management for Patients with Reactions to Hymenoptera Stings

Type of Reaction	Risk of Systemic Reaction on Subsequent Stings	Perform Skin Testing?	Results of Skin Testing	Recommended Treatment
Never stung	Minimal	No		None
Local reaction				
Minor local reaction: immediate pain, swelling, and itching at sting site, resolves in 1 d	Minimal	No		None
Extensive local reaction: swelling develops 24–48 h after sting and resolves in 3–7 d	<10%	No		Epinephrine syringe
Systemic reaction				
Adult (urticaria, angioedema, anaphylaxis)	High	Yes	+	Venom immunotherapy plus epinephrine syringe
			–	Epinephrine syringe
Child (urticaria and mild angioedema)	Low	Yes	+	Venom immunotherapy or epinephrine syringe
			–	Epinephrine syringe
Child (anaphylaxis)	Moderate	Yes	+	Venom immunotherapy plus epinephrine syringe
			–	Epinephrine syringe

TABLE 211-3 Medically Important Spider Bites and Treatment

Spider	Bite Features	Complications	Treatment
Loxosceles: brown recluse spider, corner spider (worldwide distribution)	Painless bite, usually firm erythematous lesion that heals with little or no scar over days to weeks	Occasional hemorrhagic blister at 24 h; dermatonecrosis; systemic effects rare, mostly in in children, at 24–72 h	No validated treatments
Widow spider: black widow, redback, button spider (worldwide distribution);	Pinprick bite; pain can spread to entire extremity; target lesion 1–2 cm	Acetylcholine and norepinephrine release; muscle cramps extending to trunk, back, and abdomen; hypertension, tachycardia	*Latrodectus* antivenom, species specific; derived from horse serum; Fab antivenom available in Mexico
Armed spider: banana spider (Central and South America)	Intense pain at bite site	Severe pain, sympathetic and parasympathetic effects; priapism; vertigo, visual disturbances	Antivenom available in Brazil
Funnel-web spider (Australia)	Severe pain, with wheal and erythema at site; very rapid envenomation	Parasympathetic effects, muscle fasciculation; pulmonary edema; cerebral edema; death can occur within minutes	Compressive elastic bandage; funnel-web spider antivenom
Tarantula (worldwide)	Painful bite with local erythema and edema	Barbed hairs can penetrate cornea and conjunctivae; contact dermatitis from hairs	Ophthalmology consult for red eye and pain

richteri. These two imported species entered the United States through Mobile, Alabama, in the 1930s, have now become well established throughout the Gulf Coast states, and are spreading throughout the southwest.[12] Fire ants inhabit loose dirt and breed 9 to 10 months of the year. One mature nest can produce 200,000 ants during a 3-year period, which accounts for rapid spread. The venom of the fire ant is almost entirely an insoluble alkaloid. There is possible cross-reactivity between the venoms of fire ants and those of other Hymenoptera, and individual stings may produce systemic toxicity in sensitized individuals.

Fire ants are characterized by their tendency to swarm when provoked, and they may attack in great numbers. Fire ants in a swarm most often position themselves on their victim and sting simultaneously in response to an alarm pheromone released by one or several individuals. Immobilized or elderly patients can become rapidly covered by swarms, with multiple severe stings or death.[13] Each sting usually results in a papule that becomes a sterile pustule in 6 to 24 hours. Localized necrosis, scarring, and secondary infection can result. Rarely, a systemic reaction manifested by urticaria and angioedema can occur. Fatalities and other severe reactions have been reported to occur rapidly following single stings from ants, but most occur in patients with a history of prior venom allergy and prior cardiopulmonary disease, and injectable epinephrine was not given.[14,15] Rhabdomyolysis and renal failure have also been reported after massive fire ant stings.[16]

Estimated hypersensitivity to fire ant venom occurs in 16% of the general population, with some crossover with those sensitized to the stings of other Hymenoptera. Treatment of fire ant stings consists of local wound care.[13] In systemic reactions, treat for anaphylaxis. Desensitization may be necessary in patients exhibiting potentially life-threatening reactions to these arthropods. The wearing of socks or cotton tights seems to provide more protection from fire ant stings than the use of insect repellants.[17]

SPIDERS (ARANEAE)

Although nearly 40,000 species of spiders have been described worldwide, medically significant envenomations have been described in only a few dozen (**Table 211-3**). Spiders are carnivores, and venom probably evolved for paralyzing prey. The vast majority of spiders pose little harm to humans because their venom-injecting fangs are too small to penetrate human skin, the amount of venom injected is too little to produce toxicity, or the venom itself has little effect on mammalian cells. Even if a reaction is elicited, it is often local, and systemic toxicity is confined to a few specific species (Table 211-3 and **Figure 211-1**).

SPIDERS CAUSING NECROTIC ARACHNIDISM (*LOXOSCELES*)

Loxosceles are brown spiders that have a worldwide distribution. Native species exist in the United States (Figure 211-1), and of these, *Loxosceles reclusa* (the brown recluse spider) occupies the largest geographic area and accounts for the majority of significant envenomations. In South America, particularly Brazil, *Loxosceles laeta* and *Loxosceles intermedia* account for most significant envenomations. Envenomation outside of endemic areas is unusual.[18] *Loxosceles* spiders are nocturnal; are shy; are found both indoors and outdoors in dark, dry areas such as basements, closets, and woodpiles; and may bite when threatened. A pigmented, violin-shaped pattern on the cephalothorax of the brown recluse is often present (**Figure 211-2**). However, this characteristic is considered

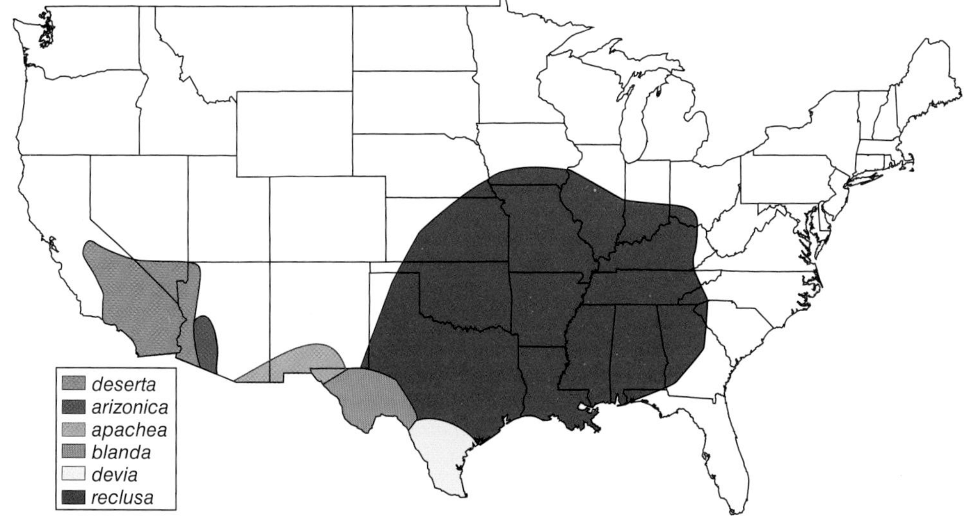

FIGURE 211-1. Range of recluse (genus *Loxosceles*) spiders in the United States.

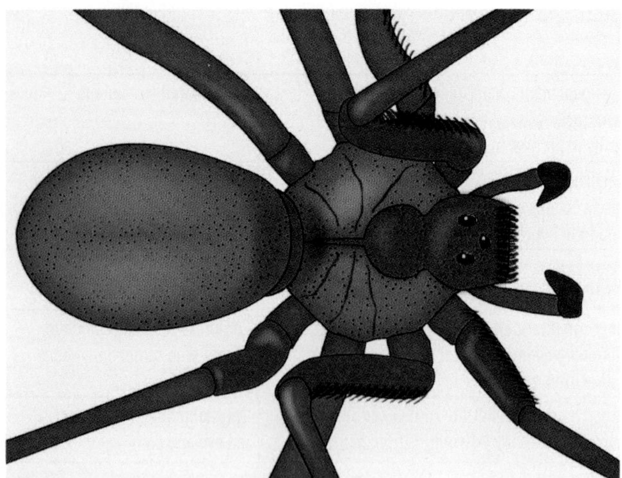

FIGURE 211-2. Close-up look at the characteristic fiddle-shaped back marking on the brown recluse spider (*Loxosceles reclusa*).

unreliable and often misinterpreted. *Loxosceles* species are most accurately identified by their eye pattern, which consists of six paired eyes (one anterior pair and two lateral pairs).[18] Most other U.S. spiders have eight eyes arranged in two rows of four. The venom of the brown recluse contains multiple enzymes, including hyaluronidase and sphingomyelinase D, which is the major enzyme responsible for necrosis. Significant necrotic wounds are rare but possible through neutrophil activation, platelet aggregation, and thrombosis. Although both local and systemic complications of *Loxosceles* envenomation have been well described, the perceived threat of the brown recluse far exceeds its actual danger. For more information about recluse spiders see http://spiders.ucr.edu.

Clinical Features Bites by *Loxosceles* spiders are described as initially painless, which often prohibits possible identification of the spider. The most common manifestation of a bite is a mild erythematous lesion that may become firm and heal with little or no scar within several days or weeks. Occasionally, a more severe local reaction occurs, beginning with mild to severe pain several hours after the bite, accompanied by localized erythema, pruritus, and swelling. A hemorrhagic blister then forms, surrounded by vasoconstriction-induced blanched skin (**Figure 211-3**). By day 3 or 4, the hemorrhagic area may become ecchymotic, which leads to the "red, white, and blue" (erythema, blanching, and ecchymosis) sign. The ecchymotic area may become necrotic, with eschar formation by the end of the first week. The necrotic, slowly healing ulcers may not reach maximum size for many weeks after envenomation and can occasionally result in a significant cosmetic defect requiring skin grafting.

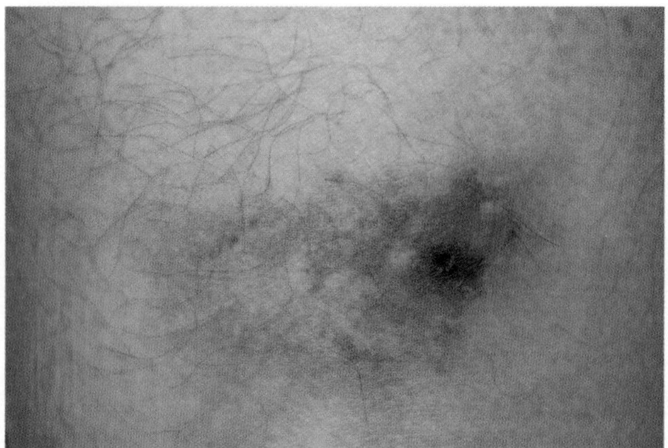

FIGURE 211-3. Early brown recluse spider bite (approximately 8 hours old) with a violaceous center surrounded by a faint spreading erythema. [Photograph by Lawrence B. Stack, MD. Reproduced with permission from Knoop KJ, Stack LB, Storrow AB, Thurman RJ: *The Atlas of Emergency Medicine*, 3rd ed, © 2009 by McGraw-Hill, Inc., New York.]

Although significant systemic effects are not uncommon after bites of *L. laeta*, the predominant South American species, they rarely occur after bites of the brown recluse, the predominant U.S. species. Systemic effects, the hallmark of which is hemolysis, are seen more often in children and typically occur 24 to 72 hours after the bite. Other effects include nausea, vomiting, fever, chills, arthralgias, thrombocytopenia, rhabdomyolysis, hemoglobinuria, and renal failure. Disseminated intravascular coagulation and death are extremely rare.

Correct diagnosis of a brown recluse envenomation without definitive spider identification is difficult. Although the presence of a consistent clinical picture in an endemic area is suggestive, it is likely that a myriad of infectious and noninfectious conditions are misdiagnosed as brown recluse bites.[18] In patients who are suspected of having been bitten and who exhibit signs and symptoms of envenomation, obtain a CBC, BUN and creatinine, and coagulation profile. Assays to detect envenomation have been used in research, but a commercial test is not currently available.

Treatment Treatment of a possible necrotic spider bite should include the usual supportive measures, including pain medication. Antibiotics are indicated if signs of infection exist. However, secondary infections are uncommon. Arrange follow-up for serial wound evaluation. If ulceration develops, surgical debridement is delayed until clear margins are established, often 2 to 3 weeks after the bite.

Patients with systemic symptoms following a bite warrant hospitalization. Various treatments have been advocated for brown recluse spider bites, including antihistamines, antivenom, colchicine, dapsone, hyperbaric oxygen, surgical excision, steroids, and topical nitroglycerin. None of these therapies have clear benefit, and most wounds from the brown recluse are self-limiting and heal without any medical intervention. Administration of the leukocyte inhibitor dapsone continues to be advocated by some despite lack of supporting research and known adverse effects, including hemolysis and methemoglobinemia. Early antivenom administration after envenomation is efficacious in animal models.[19] However, the delayed time in which patients typically present after envenomation, the current inability to definitively identify an envenomation, and the inability to prognosticate the development of dermatonecrosis, which in itself is rare, greatly limits its potential use.

An equine-derived antivenom is commonly used in Brazil; however, its efficacy is unclear. In the United States, there is no commercially available *Loxosceles* antivenom.

HOBO SPIDER (*ERATIGENA AGRESTIS;* FORMERLY *TEGENARIA AGRESTIS*)

A native of Europe and central Asia, the hobo or northwestern brown spider is now found in the Pacific Northwest of the United States and southern British Columbia. It is not aggressive.[20] Hobo spiders are brown with gray markings and have a 7- to 14-mm body length and a 27- to 45-mm leg span. They live in moist, dark areas such as woodpiles and basements.

Little documentation supports the occurrence of necrosis from hobo spider bites.[18] In its native European habitat, it is not considered poisonous to humans, and venom analysis comparing European to U.S. species has confirmed no unique differences. Confirmed bites have demonstrated localized erythema, itching, pain, and swelling.[20]

There is no diagnostic test for hobo spider envenomation, and there is no proven treatment.

WIDOW SPIDERS (*LATRODECTUS*)

Latrodectus or "widow" spiders have a worldwide distribution. In the United States, the black widow is the most well known, although of the five *Latrodectus* species found commonly in the United States, only three (*Latrodectus mactans*, *Latrodectus variolus*, and *Latrodectus hesperus*) are actually black. Other varieties may be predominantly brown (*Latrodectus geometricus*) or red (*Latrodectus bishopi*). An orange-red hourglass-shaped marking characterizes many of the *Latrodectus* species

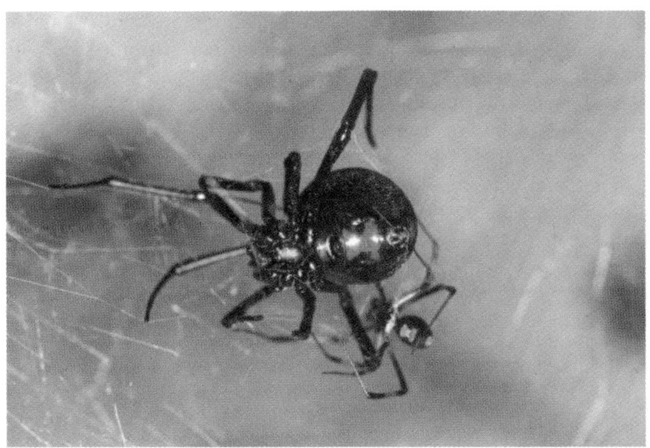

FIGURE 211-4. Black widow spider (*Latrodectus mactans*) with offspring. Note characteristic hourglass marking on abdomen. [Photograph by Lawrence B. Stack, MD. Reproduced with permission from Knoop KJ, Stack LB, Storrow AB, Thurman RJ: *The Atlas of Emergency Medicine*, 3rd ed, © 2009 by McGraw-Hill, Inc., New York.]

(**Figure 211-4**). Female spiders are relatively large, with a body size ranging up to 1.5 cm in length and leg spans of 4 to 5 cm. The male spider is approximately one-third the size of the female and lighter in color, and his bite cannot penetrate human skin. Black widow spiders are found most often in woodpiles, basements, garages, and sheds. *Latrodectus* will aggressively defend her web, particularly when guarding her eggs. Most black widow bites occur between April and October and are usually seen on the hands and forearms.

The black widow spider injures its victim and its prey with highly potent venom. The most active component of the venom is α-latrotoxin, which acts through both calcium-dependent and calcium-independent pathways leading to receptor stimulation, pore formation, and ultimately massive release of neurotransmitters (predominantly acetylcholine and norepinephrine).[21] Acetylcholine release accounts for neuromuscular manifestations, and norepinephrine release accounts for the cardiovascular manifestations.

Clinical Features Most *Latrodectus* bites are felt immediately as a pinprick sensation at the bite site, followed by increasing local pain that may spread quickly to include the entire bitten extremity. Erythema appears approximately 20 to 60 minutes after the bite. In many bites, a small, <5-mm erythematous macule develops that may evolve into a larger target lesion with a blanched center and surrounding erythema (**Figure 211-5**). The clinical syndrome is called *latrodectism*. Victims frequently complain of muscle cramp–like spasms in large muscle groups, although physical examination of the "cramping" extremity rarely reveals rigidity. The pain often increases progressively, becomes generalized, and can involve the trunk, back, and abdomen. Localized diaphoresis near the site of envenomation can be seen. Severe abdominal wall musculature pain and cramping are well described. Hypertension and tachycardia are common, and systemic symptoms include headache, nausea, vomiting, diaphoresis, photophobia, and dyspnea. Rarely reported complications include atrial fibrillation, myocarditis, priapism, and death. The pain with envenomation can be severe and intermittent and, if untreated, often lasts for a day. Occasionally, symptoms may persist for several days.

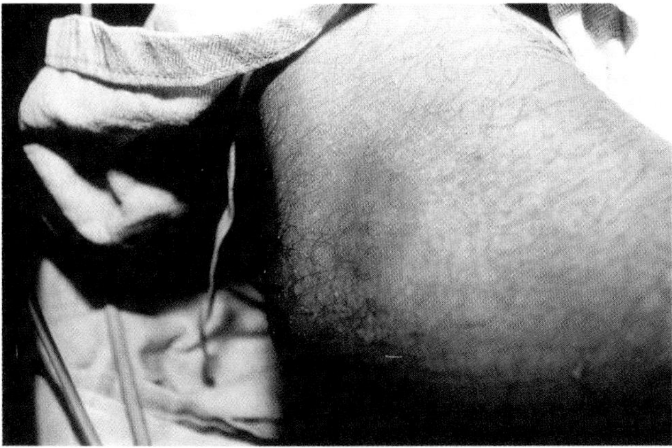

FIGURE 211-5. Black widow spider bite on the knee. [Photograph by Gerald O'Malley, DO. Reproduced with permission from Knoop KJ, Stack LB, Storrow AB, Thurman RJ: *The Atlas of Emergency Medicine*, 3rd ed, © 2009 by McGraw-Hill, Inc., New York.]

Because an immediate pinprick sensation is usually reported with *Latrodectus* bites, it is common for the offending spider to be identified. In the absence of a witnessed bite, a clinical diagnosis can be made based on characteristic symptoms and signs. There is no confirmatory laboratory test.

Treatment Cleansing of the bite site is reasonable. Pain and muscle spasms can generally be controlled with liberal doses of opioids and benzodiazepines.[22] Although IV calcium has been advocated to relieve symptoms, a retrospective review of patients with *Latrodectus* envenomation indicated that this treatment is ineffective.[22] For severe envenomations, admission may be required for continued analgesia. The most effective therapies for severe envenomation are parenteral opioids and *Latrodectus* antivenom.

Administration of ***Latrodectus* antivenom** often causes rapid resolution of symptoms and can significantly shorten the course of illness. Even in severely symptomatic cases of *Latrodectus* envenomation, patients can often be discharged from the ED after a short observation period when antivenom is administered. Successful treatment of latrodectism with antivenom has been described even with administration 90 hours after envenomation.[23] Antivenin *Latrodectus mactans* is not contraindicated in pregnancy.[24]

Latrodectus antivenom is produced in at least three countries with specificity for indigenous species: Redback (*Latrodectus hasselti*) Spider Antivenom (CSL Ltd., Melbourne, Australia), Button Spider Antivenom (South African Vaccine Producers Institute, Edenvale, South Africa), and Antivenin *Latrodectus mactans* (Merck & Co., Inc., Whitehouse Station, NJ). It is likely that the antivenom to one species would be clinically effective in treating the bites of the others. Indications, amount, and route of administration vary according to product. Antivenin *Latrodectus mactans* and Button Spider Antivenom are administered IV, and Redback Spider Antivenom is typically administered by IM injection. An Australian-based study using Redback Spider Antivenom found minimal clinical difference between IV and IM routes.[25]

Latrodectus antivenom is derived from horse serum, and hypersensitivity reactions are possible. Redback antivenom is the most frequently used antivenom in Australia, and adverse reactions are rare. Until recently one death from anaphylaxis had been reported after administration of Antivenin *Latrodectus mactans* in the United States. Analysis attributed this to the antivenom being administered undiluted via IV push to an asthmatic patient with known allergies to multiple medications. Slow administration of diluted Antivenin *Latrodectus mactans* has generally been considered safe.[26] However, two additional cases of anaphylaxis to Antivenin *Latrodectus mactans* have been described despite dilution and slow administration.[27,28] In one of these cases, the anaphylaxis resulted in cardiac arrest, and despite successful resuscitation, the patient later died.[27] Such cases should be kept in mind, particularly because *latrodectism* itself is rarely life-threatening. A F(ab)2 antivenom [Antivenin Latrodectus Equine Immune F(ab)2 (Analatro)], expected to be less immunogenic and safer than whole-antibody products, is currently commercially available in Mexico. At the time of writing, it is not approved in the United States.[29]

ARMED SPIDERS (*PHONEUTRIA*)

The armed spiders are found throughout South America and Costa Rica. The majority of clinically important bites have been described in Brazil. The spiders are solitary, nocturnal, do not construct a web, and possess potent neurotoxic venom. They have been reported to hide in banana bunches during shipping and can bite workers handling these bananas at their destination. When threatened, they assume a characteristic aggressive position by raising their four front legs, displaying their fangs, bristling their leg spines, and moving position to continually face their threat. The best-known armed spider, *Phoneutria nigriventer* (banana spider), is large, with a body size up to 3.5 cm and leg length up to 6 cm. *P. nigriventer* venom contains a mixture of potent neurotoxins that produce CNS, spinal cord, and autonomic effects.

Most *P. nigriventer* bites produce no significant symptoms. Significant envenomation produces local symptoms (severe pain) followed by sympathetic stimulation (tachycardia, hypertension), parasympathetic hyperactivity (nausea, vomiting, diaphoresis, salivation), spinal cord impairment (priapism), and CNS effects (vertigo, visual changes). Children and the elderly are at highest risk for serious envenomation. Pulmonary edema, shock, and death are rare.[30] Most healthy adults recover in 1 to 2 days.

In most cases, supportive care is adequate. Local anesthetic infiltration at the bite site can control pain. A polyvalent antivenom (Instituto Butantan, São Paulo, Brazil) is available for cases of severe envenomation from *P. nigriventer*.

FUNNEL-WEB SPIDERS (*ATRAX/HADRONYCHE*)

Funnel-web spiders are arguably the most deadly spiders in the world. Fortunately, they exist in a localized geographical location in eastern Australia, and no fatalities have been reported since the introduction of antivenom in 1981.[31] The spiders are so named because they construct a cylindrical web that extends into a recess, such as a burrow in the ground or a hole in a tree.

Funnel-web spiders have a shiny black body and long fangs, and females can grow up to 4 cm in body length. Females stay close to their webs, but the smaller and more aggressive males tend to wander, especially during the summer following a rain. *Atrax* venom contains a potent mixture of neurotoxins with neuromotor and autonomic effects.

Clinical Features *Atrax* bites may result in local reaction with immediate pain, followed by wheal formation and surrounding erythema. Later, localized sweating and piloerection may be observed. The vast majority of *Atrax* bites do not result in significant envenomation or systemic toxicity. The onset of severe envenomation is rapid and unlikely to begin after 2 hours.[31] Symptoms and signs of systemic toxicity include perioral paresthesias, parasympathetic hyperactivity (nausea, vomiting, diaphoresis, salivation, lacrimation, bronchorrhea), neuromuscular stimulation (muscle fasciculation, tremors, spasms, weakness), and CNS toxicity (altered level of consciousness). Death after *Atrax robustus* envenomation has been reported as a result of cardiac arrest, hypotension, or pulmonary failure occurring between 15 minutes and 3 days after a bite.

Treatment To reduce venom absorption and systemic toxicity from a bite on an extremity, apply a compressive elastic bandage to the entire length of the limb, and splint the extremity to prevent movement.[32] Immobilize the victim and transport promptly to the hospital.

The specific treatment for systemic toxicity is Funnel-Web Spider Antivenom (CSL Ltd., Melbourne, Australia). If the patient has signs of systemic toxicity upon arrival or develops them after the compressive elastic bandage is carefully removed, antivenom should be administered until symptoms improve. Supportive therapy for hypotension (IV fluid), bronchorrhea (atropine), tremors and agitation (benzodiazepines), and hypertension and tachycardia (β-blockers) may be necessary, but antivenom is the only therapy known to consistently improve survival.

TARANTULAS (THERAPHOSIDAE)

Tarantulas are large, hairy spiders belonging to the family Theraphosidae that are popular as pets. The hairs found on the abdomen of most species of tarantulas in North and South America resemble a velvety covering and are used defensively. When threatened, tarantulas may flick these hairs a short distance with their two back legs. Although North American tarantula hairs rarely penetrate human skin, the hairs can imbed deeply into the conjunctiva and cornea and can cause inflammation in all levels of the eye, from conjunctiva to retina. **Patients who manifest a red eye and pain after handling a tarantula should be examined to determine if offending barbed hairs are present in the cornea or conjunctiva.** Although hairs are sometimes easily seen on slit-lamp examination, they may at times be very difficult to detect. Therapy includes surgical removal of the hairs and topical application of steroids to control inflammation. Ophthalmia nodosa is a granulomatous, nodular reaction that can occur in cases of ocular exposure to tarantula hairs.[33] Patients may also develop a diffuse contact dermatitis from indirect exposure to hair while cleaning a tarantula cage. Bites from tarantulas are typically painful, with local erythema and edema, and some patients describe local joint stiffness following bites on nearby areas. Systemic symptoms other than fever are unusual.

OTHER SPIDERS

Yellow sac spiders (*Cheiracanthium*) are medium-sized, typically yellow spiders that have a worldwide distribution. A few species are commonly found in homes. The most common symptoms of a bite are local sharp pain. Minor erythema, swelling, and pruritus may occur at the bite site. Dermatonecrotic lesions are rare.[34]

Wolf spiders (*Lycosa*) are small- to medium-sized (3- to 5-mm body length) ground-dwelling spiders with a worldwide distribution. The venom produces local pain and occasionally induration and erythema, but no systemic symptoms and no skin necrosis.

Jumping spiders (family Salticidae) are typically small (<15 mm), brightly colored, and very active spiders with a worldwide distribution. A bite may produce pain, swelling, pruritus, and erythema with resolution in 2 days.

Daddy long-legs spiders (family Pholcidae) are common cellar and outbuilding dwellers along the Pacific coast and in southwestern deserts. There are no case reports of human envenomation.

SCORPIONS (SCORPIONIDAE)

Scorpions have a worldwide distribution, and highly toxic species are found in Africa, India, Mexico, North Africa, South America, the Middle East, and the Caribbean island of Trinidad. The toxins of the *Centruroides* and *Parabuthus* scorpions exhibit primarily neuromuscular effects, but toxins of the *Androctonus*, *Buthus*, and *Mesobuthus* scorpions exhibit cardiovascular effects.[35] Several species of scorpions are found in the warmer parts of the southern United States, but most species cause little more than localized pain. In the United States, only *Centruroides sculpturatus* (bark scorpion), found throughout Arizona, New Mexico, and parts of Texas and California, possesses venom potent enough to cause systemic toxicity.

CLINICAL FEATURES

Most stings cause localized pain at the bite site, and systemic toxicity occurs in <10% of stings. Scorpion venom contains many toxins, but the toxins with the most serious medical effects can open neuronal sodium channels and cause prolonged and excessive depolarization. Somatic and autonomic (parasympathetic and sympathetic) systems are affected (**Table 211-4**).[35] **Infants and young children are at highest risk for severe systemic symptoms**, which can be life threatening. Motor hyperactivity is nearly universal when symptoms are systemic and may present as restlessness or uncontrollable jerking of the extremities that appears to be seizure-like activity. Peripheral nervous system toxicity includes abnormal oculomotor function, loss of pharyngeal muscle control, uncoordinated neuromuscular activity with respiratory compromise, and tongue fasciculations. Hypersalivation is common and, combined with cranial nerve dysfunction, can threaten airway integrity. Cardiovascular toxicity from systemic envenomation includes tachycardia, hypertension, pulmonary edema, and cardiogenic shock.

DIAGNOSIS

Diagnosis is clinical. Laboratory studies are needed in severe envenomation to identify organ system involvement.

TREATMENT

Treatment is described in Table 211-4. Administer opioids for pain control and short-acting benzodiazepines for sedation as needed. In Latin

TABLE 211-4 Scorpion Bite Effects and Treatment

Clinical Effect	Pathophysiology	Treatment	Comments
Local effects only	Pain at bite site	Acetaminophen, nonsteroidal anti-inflammatory drug, local lidocaine without epinephrine at sting site	
Dermatonecrosis over hours or days	Local necrosis, in 20% systemic features, myoglobinuria; similar to *Loxosceles* spider envenomation		*Habromys lepturus* of Iran
Tachycardia, hypertension, mydriasis	Excess catecholamines	Antivenom*; prazosin	
Agitation and anxiety	Neuromuscular agitation	Benzodiazepines	
Pulmonary edema	Catecholamine-induced cardiac injury, myocardial depression; cardiogenic shock	Antivenom*; nitroglycerin or prazosin†; dobutamine† for cardiogenic shock	*Androctonus, Buthus, Mesobuthus,* and *Tityus* scorpions
Hypotension, bradycardia, salivation, sweating, abdominal pain, diarrhea, pancreatitis	Cholinergic effects	Atropine	*Tityus* species
Oculomotor abnormalities, uncoordinated neuromuscular activity, muscle spasms	Neuromuscular excitation	Antivenom*; benzodiazepines	*Centruroides* scorpions, also *Parabuthus* and *Tityus*
Multiorgan failure			Supportive care

*Role of antivenom not clear once systemic toxicity established, as antivenom binds toxin but does not reverse established injury.

†Role of vasodilators not clear; concern if using vasodilators with dobutamine.

America and India, the vasodilator prazosin is used to counteract the adrenergic surge that can lead to hypertension and resultant pulmonary edema. Envenomations in North Africa, on the other hand, are thought to develop pulmonary edema from systolic dysfunction, and the use of dobutamine may be helpful.[36] Scorpion antivenom directed against different species has been produced for research or clinical use in many other countries. Recommendations for use and dosing of these products vary widely. Like all animal-derived antivenom, both immediate and delayed allergic reactions, including serum sickness, are possible. A randomized, double-blind study from Arizona in children suffering from significant neurotoxic effects of *Centruroides* stings demonstrated that an intravenous scorpion-specific antibody resolved the clinical syndrome within 4 hours and significantly reduced the need for concomitant sedation.[37] The antivenom Anascorp® is a F(ab) equine preparation that is approved by the Food and Drug Administration in the United States but currently is quite expensive and should be restricted to patients with severe systemic symptoms.

CHIGGERS (TROMBICULIDAE)

Chigger infestations result from mite larvae feeding on host skin cells. Mites are found in almost every habitat and are 0.3 to 1.0 mm in length, and the larvae attach themselves to host skin with mandibular structures. They tend to attach in areas where an obstacle like tight-fitting clothing is met, such as at the tops of socks, the leg bands of underwear, the waistband, or the edges of a bra. Once attached, the larvae release digestive enzymes to liquefy epidermal cells. The combination of digestive enzymes secreted by the mite and subsequent host immune response produces the "chigger bite."

CLINICAL FEATURES

Although diseases such as rickettsialpox and scruff typhus have been spread by mite vectors, the major clinical manifestation of chigger infestation is most often intense pruritus. The attached chigger may be seen initially as a bright red fleck on the skin, and it, along with the larvae, may be easily scratched off. Lesions are intensely pruritic and often appear as grouped papules or papulovesicles. The localized allergic response may last for weeks, and significant excoriation may occur at the site from intense scratching.

The diagnosis of chigger infestation may be difficult, because many other arthropods cause similar clinical manifestations. The history of outdoor exposure combined with the presence of signs and symptoms localized to areas of snug-fitting clothing may be helpful.

TREATMENT

Treatment is primarily symptomatic to control the itching and consists of oral antihistamines and topical steroids. Oral steroids may be helpful in severe cases. Chiggers themselves may be killed with permethrin and other topical scabicides. If secondary infection occurs, antibiotics are indicated.

MOSQUITOS, FLIES, FLEAS, AND LICE (DIPTERA)

MOSQUITOES

Mosquitoes penetrate skin with the piercing motion of a bayonetlike proboscis. The actual puncturing of the skin surface causes minimal trauma and frequently is not felt by the host. A local anesthetic is injected into the wound that causes local tissue damage and local hypersensitivity. Bites can lead to both immediate and delayed reactions. An immediate skin reaction includes redness, a wheal, and itching. A delayed reaction can occur and usually consists of edema and pruritus. The immediate reaction tends to be of short duration, whereas a delayed reaction may persist for hours, days, and even weeks. Severe local reactions with skin necrosis are possible. Patients can acquire allergy to mosquito saliva constituents and develop symptoms consisting of an escalating reaction to seasonal exposures with increasingly pronounced edematous and pruritic lesions, sometimes accompanied by fever, malaise, generalized edema, severe nausea and vomiting, and necrosis with resulting scarring. Treatment is symptomatic with antihistamines and nonsteroidal anti-inflammatory drugs.

The greatest danger from mosquitoes is the transmission of disease. Even with extensive pest control programs, arbovirus infections and malaria are epidemic in many parts of the world. Chikungunya virus, dengue, Japanese B encephalitis, yellow fever, and various types of equine encephalitis are among the many viruses transmitted by mosquitoes. In addition, West Nile virus has recently spread west across North America. Malaria is also encountered frequently in patients in the United States after travel and in immigrant populations from areas where malaria is endemic. Insect repellents offer some protection from mosquito bites.

FLIES

Bloodsucking flies range in size from the tiny sand fly, approximately 1 to 3 mm in length, to horseflies, which can be >2 cm. All flies stab and pierce the skin, causing some degree of pain and pruritus. Several species, such as deerflies, blackflies, horseflies, and sand flies, can produce allergic reactions, although these are rarely as severe as those produced by Hymenoptera venom. There is also the possibility of myiasis (infestation of tissue with fly larvae, i.e., botfly) from fly bites, but this condition is rare in the United States.

The diagnosis of fly bite depends chiefly on the patient's history and a knowledge of the arthropods that frequent the area of encounter. Treatment for most local reactions to Diptera bites is symptomatic, and treatment of systemic reactions is the same as for reactions to Hymenoptera venom. Application of cold compresses may alleviate localized edema. Secondary infection of Diptera bites can occur, and antibiotics may be necessary in some cases. Oral antihistamines may be helpful in relieving pruritus from fly bites, but topical steroids can be used when local reactions are severe, and oral steroids are indicated when systemic hypersensitivity symptoms are present.

FLEAS (SIPHONAPTERA)

Bites of fleas, lice, and scabies mites produce lesions so similar that diagnosis is often difficult. Flea bites are frequently found in zigzag lines, especially on the legs and in the waist area. The lesions most often have a hemorrhagic-appearing center surrounded by erythematous and urticarial patches. Flea bites are usually quite pruritic, and red spots can persist at bite sites for some time.

The main concern in the treatment of these bites is the possibility of secondary infection. Children may develop impetigo as a complication. The lesions should be washed thoroughly with soap and water. Children with flea bites should have their fingernails cut short to prevent scratching. To relieve discomfort and itching, local application of calamine, cool soaks, and oral or topical antihistamines may be helpful. For severe discomfort, application of a topical steroid cream or spray may be necessary. If secondary infection develops, topical or oral antibiotics may be needed.

KISSING BUGS AND BED BUGS (HEMIPTERA)

The order Hemiptera includes two blood-sucking families of arthropods with medical importance. These are Reduviidae (reduviids, or "kissing" bugs) and Cimicidae ("bed bugs" and their relatives). Various species of kissing bugs are found predominantly in the southern United States and Central and South America. The common name "kissing bugs" derives from their habit of feeding at night on any exposed surface of a sleeping victim, commonly the face. Bed bugs are also nocturnal feeders, and their distribution is worldwide. Recently, there has been a worldwide major resurgence in bed bug infestations, particularly in developed countries. This has been attributed to immigration, international travel, and insecticide resistance.[38] Both bugs are attracted to warm bodies and hide near beds. Bed bugs are found in nearby cracks and crevices. Kissing bugs of Central and South America are vectors of Chagas' disease (trypanosomiasis). Although transmission of many diseases to humans has been attributed to bed bugs, there is little evidence to support it. The transmission of hepatitis B does appear at least theoretically possible.[38]

Clinical Features Bites from both bugs are typically painless. Erythematous papules, bullae, and wheals may develop. A linear bite pattern on the skin is well described with bed bugs, and telltale brown or black patterns of excrement may be found on bed linen. A thorough search of bedding and nearby cracks and crevices will often reveal the bugs. Bed bugs are notoriously difficult to eradicate. One study demonstrated the potential for ivermectin (oral antiparasitic drug) administration to help eradicate those bed bugs that are feeding on the patient.[39]

Treatment Treatment of both types of bite is symptomatic. Cool compresses, topical steroids, and antihistamines can be used to relieve associated pruritus. Some individuals become highly sensitive to kissing bugs and react with systemic allergic symptoms following a bite. They should be treated as previously outlined for Hymenoptera envenomation.

CATERPILLARS AND MOTHS (LEPIDOPTERA)

Lepidopterism refers to the adverse effects resulting from contact with butterflies, moths, or their caterpillars. Caterpillars, the larval stage of moths and butterflies, are responsible for the vast majority of symptomatic exposures. For protection, they may have either hairs or spines that can be attached to venom glands. The spines and hairs may cause mechanical irritation, whereas the venom can produce additional symptoms. Although isolated exposures are most common, particularly in children who may be attracted to the colored or "furry" appearance of caterpillars, there are multiple species that under the right conditions can cause "epidemics" of cutaneous or systemic exposures. A couple of moth species, most notably the *Hylesia* genus in Venezuela (responsible for the "Caripito itch"), can cause local irritant or allergic reactions.

CLINICAL FEATURES

Most reactions to Lepidoptera are mild and self-limited. The vast majority of caterpillars are harmless to humans. Pruritus from localized "caterpillar dermatitis" and occasional diffuse urticaria are the predominant symptoms of exposures to the hairs and venom. The puss caterpillar (*Megalopyge opercularis*) is found in the southeastern United States and accounts for most of the serious envenomations in that country. After initial contact, intense local burning pain, rather than pruritus, is typical. A gridlike pattern of hemorrhagic papules may be seen within 2 to 3 hours of these exposures and may last for several days. Regional lymphadenopathy is common, and the affected limb can swell considerably. Other potential symptoms include headaches, fever, hypotension, and convulsions. No deaths have been reported. Ingestions of the hickory tussock caterpillar (*Lophocampa caryae*), found in the eastern United States, have been reported, with symptoms ranging from drooling to diffuse urticaria. Spines have been visualized in the oropharynx and even the esophagus in some of these patients, requiring endoscopy to aid in removal.[40] Two species of *Lonomia* caterpillars, found primarily in Brazil and Venezuela, are capable of causing potentially fatal coagulation defects.

TREATMENT

Treatment is symptomatic and supportive. Spines can be removed using adhesive tape. Antipruritic or topical anesthetic preparations, topical steroids, and oral antihistamines are typically used. For symptomatic ocular and oral exposures, removal of hairs may be necessary, and endoscopy has been described. Anaphylaxis is rare but would be treated in the typical manner. An antivenom specifically for *Lonomia obliqua* is available in Brazil to reverse coagulopathy.[41]

BLISTER BEETLES (COLEOPTERA)

Although the order Coleoptera includes a large number and variety of beetles, clinically significant envenomation occurs only from those that contain a vesicant (blister beetles). Blister beetles are found worldwide, including the United States. The most well-known blister beetle is the "Spanish fly" (*Cantharis vesicatoria*), found in Spain.

CLINICAL FEATURES

Blister beetles contain a highly potent vesicant (either cantharidin or pederin) that can be exuded or released if the beetle is brushed against, pressed, or crushed on the skin. **For this reason, a blister beetle should be removed from the skin by blowing or flicking.** Cantharidin-containing preparations are used medicinally in wart removal. Application of these substances in low concentration is without adverse effect.[42] However, higher concentrations or contact with the beetle's venom may cause local inflammation, leading to bullae formation. Severe conjunctivitis may also occur if cantharidin or pederin contacts the eyes from contaminated hands. The majority of described cases of blister beetle dermatosis are from seasonal outbreaks due to pederin-containing beetles.[43] At least one outbreak has been described in the United States. Topical exposure to blister beetles can cause a vesiculobullous eruption typical of a vesicant. Pederin-containing dermal exposures result in a more delayed (up to 36 to 72 hours) but more painful and symptomatic eruption than those from cantharidin-containing beetles. Due to the delay in onset of symptoms and signs, misdiagnosis is common. High concentrations of cantharidin preparations may result in dermal absorption and systemic toxicity. Systemic toxicity is well described following the ingestion, either of the whole beetle or of cantharidin-containing preparations. Severe vomiting, hematemesis, abdominal pain, and diarrhea may occur, followed by dysuria, hematuria, oliguria, and renal failure. Although the exact mechanism by which cantharidin produces systemic toxicity is unknown, the vesicant action likely explains most of the findings. Direct cardiac toxicity with large ingestions of cantharidin is possible, and deaths have been reported. Fortunately, most preparations sold as "Spanish fly" for their purported aphrodisiac properties have very low concentrations of cantharidin. The local vascular congestion and urethral inflammation that occur following ingestion may be interpreted by some as enhanced sexuality.

TREATMENT

Treatment is supportive. The skin should be irrigated thoroughly after topical exposure to remove any persistent vesicant, followed by local wound care. Patients who are symptomatic after ingestion should be admitted and treated supportively.

REFERENCES

The complete reference list is available online at www.TintinalliEM.com.

CHAPTER 212 Reptile Bites

Richard C. Dart
Julian White

INTRODUCTION AND EPIDEMIOLOGY

An estimated 1.5 to 3 million bites and possibly greater than 100,000 deaths occur each year in the world from venomous snakes.[1] The American Association of Poison Control Centers reports an average of 6000 bites each year, approximately 2000 of them by venomous snakes. Because of underreporting, the true number of snakebites is possibly as high as 45,000 per year in the United States, with 7000 to 8000 by venomous snakes.[2] The major venomous snakes of the world can be divided into three groups: Viperidae (vipers and pit vipers), Elapidae (includes Hydrophiinae, or sea snakes; see chapter 213, titled "Marine Trauma and Envenomation"), and the diverse group of non–front-fanged colubrid snakes (former family Colubridae, now split into several families).

In the United States, most snakebites occur in the warm summer months, when snakes and victims are most active. In the past, it was estimated that mortality from venomous snakebite approached 25%. Because of the availability of antivenom and advances in emergency and critical care, mortality rates today are <0.5%; approximately five deaths occur per year.[3]

Except for bites by imported species, North American venomous snakebites involve the pit vipers (Crotalinae subfamily of Viperidae) or coral snakes (Elapidae family). The crotaline snakes are represented by the rattlesnakes (*Crotalus* species), pygmy rattlesnakes, and massasauga (*Sistrurus* species), as well as the copperheads and water moccasins (*Agkistrodon* species). Venomous snakebites from imported exotic species are infrequent but may occur in zoo personnel as well as in amateur herpetologists. A regional poison control center can provide information on snake identification, expected toxicity, and location of antivenom.

CROTALINAE (PIT VIPER) BITES

The crotaline snakes are called pit vipers because of bilateral depressions or pits located midway between and below the level of the eye and the nostril (**Figure 212-1**). The pit is a heat receptor that guides strikes at warm-blooded prey or predators. Crotaline snakes are also distinguished by the presence of two fangs that fold against the roof of the mouth, in contrast to the coral snakes, which have shorter, fixed, erect fangs. Within the pit viper group, the rattle distinguishes the rattlesnake from other crotaline snakes. The mistaken belief that rattlesnakes always rattle before striking has persisted for centuries. In truth, many strikes occur without a warning rattle.

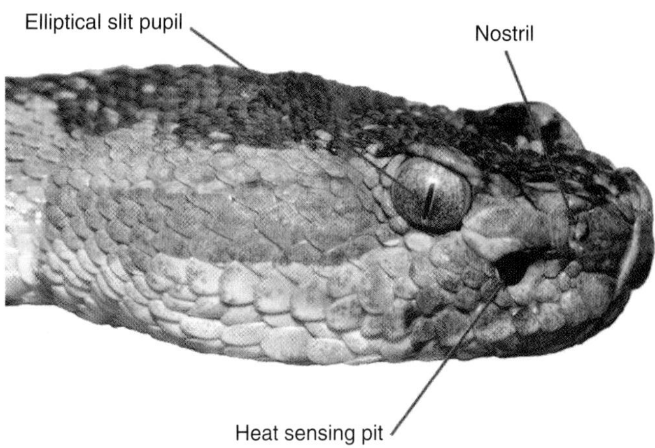

FIGURE 212-1. Pit viper.

PATHOPHYSIOLOGY

Crotaline venom is a complex enzyme mixture that causes local tissue injury, systemic vascular damage, hemolysis, fibrinolysis, and neuromuscular dysfunction, resulting in a combination of local and systemic effects. Crotaline venom quickly alters blood vessel permeability; this leads to loss of plasma and blood into the surrounding tissue, which causes hypovolemia. Crotaline venom activates and consumes fibrinogen and platelets, causing a coagulopathy. In some species, specific venom fractions block neuromuscular transmission, which leads to cranial nerve weakness (e.g., ptosis), respiratory failure, and altered sensorium.

CLINICAL FEATURES

Up to 25% of crotaline snakebites are dry bites: venom effects do not develop. The manifestations of crotaline envenomation involve a complex interaction of the venom and the victim. The species and size of the snake, the age and size of the victim, the time elapsed since the bite, and characteristics of the bite or bites (location, depth, and number; the amount of venom injected) all affect the clinical evolution. The severity of envenomation following a crotaline bite is therefore variable. An initially minimal bite may evolve into a more serious bite and require large amounts of antivenom.

The cardinal manifestations of crotaline envenomation are the presence of one or more fang marks, localized pain, and progressive edema extending from the bite site.[2] Other early symptoms and signs are nausea and vomiting, weakness, oral numbness or tingling of the tongue and mouth, dizziness, and muscle fasciculation. Systemic effects include tachypnea, tachycardia, hypotension, and altered level of consciousness. In general, local swelling at the bite site becomes apparent within 15 to 30 minutes, but in some cases, swelling may not start for several hours. In severe cases, edema can involve an entire limb within an hour. In less severe cases, edema may progress over 1 to 2 days. Edema near an airway or in a muscle compartment may threaten life or limb without causing systemic effects. Rapid onset of angioedema may occur.

Progressive ecchymosis may also develop because of leakage of blood into subcutaneous tissue. Ecchymoses may appear within minutes or hours, and hemorrhagic blebs may be seen within several hours. Hemoconcentration often develops as a result of fluid extravasation into subcutaneous tissue, followed by a decrease in hemoglobin level over several days as intravascular volume is restored.

DIAGNOSIS

The diagnosis of snakebite is based on the presence of fang marks and a history consistent with exposure to a snake (e.g., walking through a field). **Snake envenomation involves the presence of a snakebite plus evidence of tissue injury. Clinically, the injury may be manifest in three ways: local injury (swelling, pain, ecchymosis), hematologic abnormality (thrombocytopenia, elevated prothrombin time, hypofibrinogenemia), or systemic effects (e.g., oral swelling or paresthesias, metallic or rubbery taste in the mouth, hypotension, tachycardia).** Abnormalities in any one of these areas indicate that venom effect is developing. The absence of any of these manifestations for a period of 8 to 12 hours following the bite indicates a dry bite.

TREATMENT

FIRST AID

First aid measures should never substitute for definitive medical care or delay the administration of antivenom (**Table 212-1**). Take all patients bitten by a pit viper to a healthcare facility. **Avoid dangerous first aid treatments such as suction and incision.** Do not use Snake Bite Kit and similar products because they contain cups that produce little suction and seal poorly on digits. The blade in the kit, or any method of incision, can injure digital nerves, arteries, and tendons. The Sawyer Extractor (Sawyer Products, Inc., Safety Harbor, FL) suction pump is said to remove venom without incision, but safety and efficacy of the product are questioned.[4] Electric shock treatment of the bite site is dangerous and ineffective and can cause electrical injuries. Ice water immersion worsens the venom injury.

Do not use tourniquets because they obstruct arterial flow and cause ischemia. Constriction bands may be useful, especially when immediate medical care is not available. A constriction band is an elastic bandage or Penrose drain, thick rope, or piece of clothing wrapped circumferentially above the bite, applied with enough tension to restrict superficial venous and lymphatic flow while maintaining distal pulses and capillary filling. **Apply the band snugly but loose enough to avoid arterial compromise.** A constriction band can delay venom absorption without causing increased swelling.[5]

PREHOSPITAL MANAGEMENT

In the prehospital phase, immobilize the limb, establish IV access in another limb, administer oxygen, and transport the victim to a medical facility. Do not remove tourniquets or constricting bands until antivenom is available.

Institute advanced life support measures as indicated. If the patient is hypotensive, rapidly administer IV isotonic fluids. Continue to immobilize the limb in a neutral position during transport to reduce further venom absorption. Consult with a physician or poison control center familiar with the management of snake envenomation for most cases.

ED MANAGEMENT

Antivenom is the mainstay of therapy for venomous snakebites[2,6] (Table 212-2). Antivenom is composed of heterologous antibodies derived from the serum of animals immunized with the appropriate snake venoms. The antibodies bind and neutralize the venom molecules.

TABLE 212-1 Recommended First Aid Measures for Snakebite

Retreat well beyond striking range. Many victims are bitten again while trying to capture the snake.
Remain calm. Movement will increase venom absorption.
Immobilize the extremity in a neutral position below the level of the heart.
Ensure prompt transport to a medical facility whether or not there are signs of envenomation.
Constriction bands (see text) can be applied if there is no nearby medical facility.

TABLE 212-2 Clinical Features and Treatment of Reptile Envenomation

Reptile	Clinical Findings	Antivenom
Crotaline snake (pit viper)	Fang marks Local tissue injury Fibrinolysis Thrombocytopenia Systemic effects	Crotalidae Polyvalent Immune Fab
Coral snake	Neurologic dysfunction	Antivenom (*Micrurus fulvius*)
Elapid snake	Coagulopathy for some species Systemic effects, primarily neurologic dysfunction Cardiac arrhythmias and dysfunction Local injury for some species	Each species has monovalent or polyvalent antivenoms
Gila monster	Local pain and swelling Infections from retained teeth Systemic effects	No antivenom available

Crotalidae Polyvalent Immune Fab (Ovine) (FabAV) is used in the United States; equine-derived products (Antivenom [Crotalidae] Polyvalent; see below) are no longer available. FabAV is produced by immunizing herds of sheep with one of four crotaline snake venoms: eastern diamondback (*Crotalus adamanteus*), western diamondback (*Crotalus atrox*), Mojave (*Crotalus scutulatus*), or cottonmouth (*Agkistrodon piscivorus*). The immune serum is harvested from each group and then digested with papain to produce antibody fragments (Fab and Fc). The more immunogenic Fc portion of the antibody is eliminated during purification. The four individual monospecific Fab preparations are combined to form the final antivenom product.

Treat all patients with bites who develop progressive signs and symptoms with antivenom promptly. **Progression is defined as worsening of local injury (e.g., pain, ecchymosis, or swelling), abnormal results on laboratory tests (e.g., worsening platelet count, prolonged coagulation times, or decreased fibrinogen level), or systemic manifestations (e.g., unstable vital signs or abnormal mental status) (Table 212-3).**

Administer FabAV IV as a large "initial control" dose followed by three smaller maintenance doses (**Figure 212-2**). **Initial control is cessation of progression of three clinical evaluation parameters: local effects, systemic effects, and hematologic abnormalities.** The initial dose is four to six vials, which may be repeated to establish initial control of the envenomation. After initial control has been established, two-vial maintenance doses are recommended (Figure 212-2). After reconstitution, dilute each

TABLE 212-3 Laboratory Evaluation in Crotaline or Elapid Snakebite

CBC*
INR or prothrombin time*
PTT*
Fibrinogen level*
Fibrin degradation product levels
Serum electrolyte levels
Glucose level
BUN level
Platelet count
Creatine kinase level
ECG†
Arterial blood gas analysis‡

*Should be performed as soon as possible and repeated within 12 h.

†Suggested for patients >50 y of age and patients with a history of heart disease.

‡Should be performed if any signs or symptoms of respiratory compromise are evident.

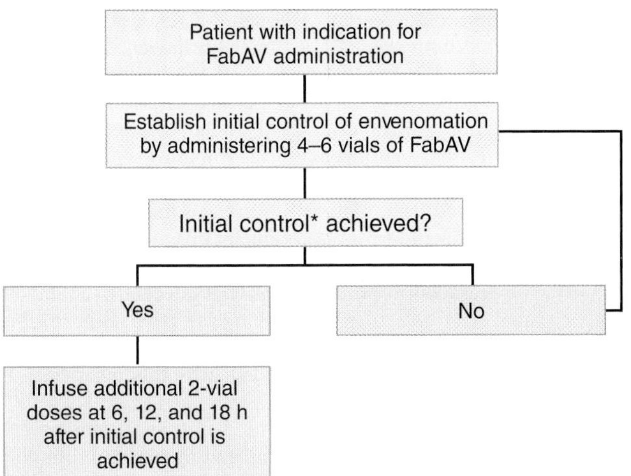

FIGURE 212-2. Administration of Crotalidae Polyvalent Immune Fab (Ovine) (FabAV). *Initial control is cessation of progression of all components of envenomation: local effects, systemic effects, and coagulopathy.

dose of FabAV in 250 mL of crystalloid and infuse over 1 hour. **The total volume, but not the number of vials, may be reduced in small children.**[7] **If IV access is unavailable, consider intraosseous administration.**

Do not inject antivenom directly into a digit, or IM, because venom-induced hypovolemia may retard absorption of antivenom. Hospital pharmacies in those regions of the United States where venomous snakes are prevalent should maintain adequate stocks of antivenom. Unfortunately, many hospitals stock insufficient amounts of antivenom, even in endemic areas.[8]

The package insert is useful as a guide for antivenom preparation. Give antivenom in a critical care facility such as an ED or intensive care unit, under direct physician supervision, and with resuscitative drugs and equipment immediately available (including epinephrine). The incidence of acute reactions to FabAV is <10%.[9] If an acute allergic reaction occurs, stop the infusion immediately and administer antihistamines (both histamine-1 and histamine-2 receptor blockers). Epinephrine should be readily available and administered for anaphylaxis.

Continue to observe for progression of edema and systemic signs of envenomation during and after antivenom infusion. Measure limb circumference at several sites above and below the bite, and outline the advancing border of edema with a pen every 30 minutes. These measures serve as an index of the progression as well as a guide for antivenom administration. Repeat laboratory determinations every 4 hours or after each course of antivenom therapy, whichever is more frequent. Additional doses of FabAV may be warranted if the patient's condition worsens. FabAV has been formally tested only in the treatment of rattlesnake bites. Initial case reports support its efficacy in treatment of copperhead snakebites.[10]

The value of aggressive supportive care cannot be overemphasized. Administer isotonic fluid resuscitation followed by vasopressor agents for hypotension. **Antivenom is the best treatment for hematologic abnormalities, but if active bleeding occurs, blood component replacement may be necessary.** Compartment syndrome is another complication of snakebite: increased compartment pressure may occur when venom is injected or spreads into a compartment. This is often manifested by severe pain, localized to a compartment and usually resistant to opiate analgesia. **Table 212-4** presents the suggested treatment of compartment syndrome.[11] The use of fasciotomy is controversial, and there is no firm evidence supporting its use.

Clean the bite wound and determine the need for tetanus immunization. Obtain wound specimens for culture and administer antibiotics if signs of infection are present. Although antibiotic prophylaxis is recommended by some authors, the data available do not support its use.[12] Steroids are not effective and could be harmful. Steroids should be reserved for the treatment of allergic reactions or serum sickness.

Serum sickness develops in about 5% of patients after FabAV treatment. The symptoms are fever, rash, and arthralgias. Start oral prednisone, 1 milligram/kg/d, and taper over 1 to 2 weeks.

TABLE 212-4 Management of Compartment Syndrome Caused by Crotalinae Snake Envenomation*†

Determine intracompartmental pressure.
If pressure is not elevated, continue standard management.
If signs of compartment syndrome are present and compartment pressure is >30 mm Hg:
Elevate limb.
Administer mannitol, 1–2 grams/kg IV over 30 min.
Simultaneously administer *additional* FabAV, 4–6 vials IV over 60 min.
If elevated compartment pressure persists another 60 min, consider fasciotomy.

Abbreviation: FabAV = Crotalidae Polyvalent Immune Fab (Ovine).

*Elevated compartment pressure is caused by the action of the venom on the tissues, and thus management of compartment syndrome due to snakebite is unique; therefore, the most effective treatment is to neutralize the venom, which may reduce the compartment pressure.

†The mannitol and antivenom deliver a high osmotic load, and fluids and electrolyte levels need careful monitoring. The administration of mannitol and antivenom must be completed promptly so that, if ever needed, fasciotomy may be performed as early as possible.

DISPOSITION AND FOLLOW-UP

It cannot be overemphasized that one can easily be deceived by a bite that initially appears innocuous. Unremarkable physical examination and laboratory test results at presentation do not reliably exclude significant envenomation. **Observe patients for at least 6 to 8 hours in the ED before determining disposition.**

Discharge patients with dry bites who have been observed for 6 to 8 hours with instructions to return if pain, swelling, or bleeding develop. Admit patients with severe or life-threatening bites and patients receiving antivenom to an intensive care unit; the general ward is appropriate for patients with mild or moderate envenomations who have completed or do not require further antivenom therapy.

Patients are ready for discharge from the hospital when swelling begins to resolve, coagulopathy has been reversed, and the patient is ambulatory. Physical therapy for the bitten part (particularly the hand) is recommended after swelling has lessened and coagulopathy has resolved. Outpatient follow-up is necessary to monitor for infection and serum sickness, and as with all antivenoms, the patient should be advised of the symptoms of serum sickness prior to discharge and advised to report if such symptoms develop.

ELAPID SNAKEBITE

U.S. CORAL SNAKEBITES

U.S. coral snakes include the eastern coral snake (*Micrurus fulvius fulvius*), the Texas coral snake (*Micrurus fulvius tenere*), and the Arizona (Sonoran) coral snake (*Micruroides euryxanthus*). The eastern coral snake is found primarily in the southeastern United States. The Texas and Arizona coral snakes are found primarily in the states that bear their names. Coral snakes account for 20 to 25 bites a year.

All coral snakes are brightly colored with black, red, and yellow rings. The red and yellow rings touch in coral snakes, but they are separated by black rings in nonvenomous snakes, which led to the well-known rhyme, **"Red on yellow, kill a fellow; red on black, venom lack." This rule is not always true outside of the United States.**

Coral snake venom is primarily composed of neurotoxic components that do not cause marked local injury (Table 212-2). Admit potential victims of coral snakebite to the hospital for observation, because venom effects may develop hours after a bite and are not easily reversed. Administer three to five vials of Antivenin (*Micrurus fulvius*) to patients who have definitely been bitten, because it may not be possible to prevent further effects or reverse effects once they develop.[13] Additional doses of coral snake antivenom are reserved for cases in which symptoms or signs of coral snake envenomation appear. Because respiratory failure may result from clinical effects of the neurotoxin, baseline and serial measurement of pulmonary function parameters (such as inspiratory pressure and vital capacity), in addition to intensive care observation, may be useful. Prolonged ventilatory support may be required in severe cases. Observe the patient closely for signs of respiratory muscle weakness and hypoventilation. Bites by the Sonoran coral snake are mild, and antivenom is not usually needed.

ELAPID BITES WORLDWIDE

Elapids are found throughout the world in warm climates. Elapids occur in Australia, New Guinea, Asia, Africa, and the Americas. All sea snakes are elapids (subfamily Hydrophiinae). Medically significant groups include some venomous snakes of Australia (tiger snakes [*Notechis*], brown snakes [*Pseudonaja*], taipans [*Oxyuranus*], death adders [*Acanthophis*], "black" snakes [*Pseudechis*], copperheads [*Austrelaps*], rough scaled snake [*Tropidechis carinatus*], broad headed snakes [*Hoplocephalus*]), cobras (*Naja*), mambas (*Dendroaspis*), kraits (*Bungarus*), coral snakes (*Micrurus*), and a variety of less common genera/species.[14]

Elapid bites produce systemic effects, particularly neurologic effects: tremor, salivation, dysarthria, diplopia, bulbar paralysis with ptosis, fixed and constricted pupils, dysphagia, dyspnea, and seizure.[14] Some groups like the cobra species also produce pain and local injury and necrosis, which may be more clinically prominent than systemic effects.[14] The immediate cause of death is usually paralysis of respiratory muscles. Signs and symptoms may be delayed up to 12 or more hours.

PATHOPHYSIOLOGY

The Elapidae possess nonretractile small- to medium-sized paired fangs that have grooved, often enclosed venom channels rather than hollow venom ducts.[14] It is thought that the Elapidae exert voluntary control over the injection of venom, hence the frequent occurrence of a dry bite.

The venom of the Australian elapids contains several important components.[14,15] Neurotoxins (tiger snake, taipan, and death adder) act at the neuromuscular junction and cause descending symmetric flaccid paralysis. Signs usually develop within 2 to 12 hours after the bite and may include ptosis, partial ophthalmoplegia (diplopia), dysarthria, loss of facial expression, and loss of airway control, as well as respiratory paralysis in severe cases. The procoagulant toxins (brown snake, tiger snake, taipan) act as prothrombin converters, leading to a venom-induced consumptive coagulopathy with fibrinogen depletion and variable thrombocytopenia. Intracranial hemorrhage is a recognized complication.

The brown snake can cause rapid collapse and death.[15,16] Renal impairment or failure may also result from snakebite. The mechanisms are poorly understood and may include hypotension, myoglobinuria, coagulopathy, and direct renal toxicity.[14,15] Myolysins (tiger snake, taipan, mulga snake) are structurally related to the neurotoxins but instead produce rhabdomyolysis, which may result in muscle pain, weakness, myoglobinuria, renal failure, and hyperkalemia.[14,15] Rarely, a venom-induced thrombotic microangiopathy may complicate brown and tiger envenomation.[16-18] Local tissue destruction is uncommon with the bite of any Australian species, although mild to moderate ecchymosis and swelling may occur.[15]

CLINICAL FEATURES

The severity of elapid envenomation cannot be estimated by the clinical appearance of the bite site or initial symptoms.[14-17] Even with severe envenomation patients may initially feel well and manifest few clinical features. Initial symptoms include nausea, vomiting, headache, abdominal pain, diplopia, dysphonia, progressive muscle weakness, discolored urine, and seizures.[15] Young children may not provide a history of snakebite, so a high index of suspicion for elapid snakebite is needed if a child develops symptoms of toxicity in a region populated with elapids.[15]

DIAGNOSIS

The diagnosis requires correlation of history, clinical features of envenomation, and laboratory investigations. Laboratory tests often determine if the patient requires antivenom treatment.[14-17] Key tests include prothrombin time, INR, activated PTT, D-dimer, fibrinogen, fibrin degradation products, hemoglobin, platelet count, electrolytes, renal function test, and creatine kinase and should be performed prior to removal of first aid, 1 hour after removal of first aid, and at 6 hours and 12 hours after bite (earlier if abnormalities or clinical symptoms/signs develop).[15,19] Look for evidence of procoagulant coagulopathy (prolonged prothrombin time and activated PTT, high INR, raised D-dimer/fibrin degradation products, low fibrinogen), anticoagulant coagulopathy (abnormal prothrombin time, activated PTT, and INR, but normal fibrinogen, D-dimer/fibrin degradation products), platelet effects, rhabdomyolysis (grossly elevated creatine kinase, myoglobinuria), renal damage (abnormal renal function tests, reduced urine output), hyponatremia, and hemolytic-uremic syndrome–like syndrome (thrombocytopenia, anemia, intravascular hemolysis).[15] A Snake Venom Detection Kit (bioCSL, Parkville, Victoria, Australia) is available to identify snake venom identified at the bite site or in the urine, correlated to venom immunotype (which corresponds to "monovalent" antivenom type), for use exclusively with Australian and New Guinea snakes.[15] Positive Snake Venom Detection Kit identification of venom at the bite site or in the urine assists in selecting a "monovalent" antivenom, but does not represent an indication for antivenom therapy without other evidence of systemic venom effects.[15] World Health Organization guidelines on treating snakebite in Asia and Africa are a useful resource on diagnosis and treatment for these regions and are available online.[20,21]

TREATMENT

FIRST AID

In Australia and New Guinea, pressure bandaging and immobilization of the involved limb is used. The principle is to contain the venom locally and prevent venom transport by lymphatic vessels. Wrap an elastic bandage firmly over the bite site and then extend it to cover the entire limb (bandage pressure similar to that used for sprains: firm, but not tourniquet tight).[15] Splint the limb to prevent movement, an essential part of the method. Examination of lymphatic flow rates with simulated venom has demonstrated that, even if the upper or lower limb is appropriately bandaged and immobilized, walking will hasten systemic envenoming.[22] **Use of tourniquets is contraindicated.** In the rare circumstance that a bite is inflicted on the trunk, apply firm pressure to the affected area without restricting breathing.

Outside of Australia and New Guinea, the choice of first aid is more nuanced. If the bite is from an elapid that may cause local tissue damage or is from an unidentified snake, then pressure bandaging and immobilization may increase local tissue injury.[14] Omit the pressure bandage but splint the bitten part.

ED MANAGEMENT

Any history suggestive of snakebite should prompt appropriate first aid and transport to a medical facility with appropriate medical expertise, laboratory facilities, and antivenom supplies. Maintain pressure bandage immobilization (or immobilization only) until envenomation is excluded or until the patient can receive antivenom.[15] If the patient's condition deteriorates immediately after removal of first aid measures, reapply and give antivenom. Once antivenom is infusing, remove the pressure bandage so that antivenom can reach the envenomed area. There is no evidence that venom is inactivated by being trapped at the bite site.[15]

Antivenom should be given only in cases in which there is clear clinical or laboratory evidence of systemic envenomation. Clinical indications for immediate antivenom therapy include evidence of neurotoxic effects (ptosis, cranial nerve involvement, progressive muscle weakness, or diaphragmatic involvement), coagulopathy, rhabdomyolysis, renal failure, cardiac collapse, significant local tissue injury, or vomiting unresponsive to antiemetics.[14,15] In the absence of clinical or laboratory evidence of systemic envenomation, remove the first aid measures and observe the patient for at least

12 hours, longer for some species.[15,19] Repeat laboratory tests 1 hour after removing the first aid measures and at intervals thereafter dictated by the patient's condition.

For Australian elapid snakebites, there is only one producer (CSL Ltd, Melbourne, Australia), producing five "monovalent" antivenoms corresponding to the five venom immunotypes, a polyvalent antivenom that covers all of the five venom immunotypes, plus a sea snake antivenom that is effective for all sea snake species globally.[14,15] The initial dose of antivenom is controversial, but simply following the product instructions is prudent. Similarly, the initial dose of antivenom for non-Australian snakes should be based on manufacturer recommendations. For patients presenting with severe envenomation, higher initial doses may be warranted. Always administer antivenom IV. **If IV access is unavailable, consider intraosseous administration.** IM administration is strongly discouraged due to slow absorption and potential complications of anticoagulation. Dilute antivenom about 1:10 in normal saline (lower dilution in small children or cardiac-compromised adults), then commence the infusion slowly, looking for evidence of adverse reaction (rash, wheeze, hypotension, angioedema); gradually increase the rate to give the entire dose over 20 to 30 minutes (longer if high volume antivenom).[14,15] Give the same dose to children as adults. Skin testing before antivenom administration is not recommended,[14,15] and equipment for treatment of anaphylaxis should be at the bedside. Hypersensitivity is an uncommon complication of antivenom therapy in Australia.[23-25] Elsewhere, antivenoms may have high rates of adverse reactions. A 5-day course of prednisolone may be prescribed to reduce the incidence of serum sickness, but clear evidence of efficacy is lacking.[15]

Antivenom cannot reverse some venom effects, such as established presynaptic neurotoxic paralysis, renal failure, and rhabdomyolysis. It is therefore important to give antivenom as soon as indicated. If this is not possible, support respiration and renal function as clinically required. Advanced flaccid paralysis usually requires protection of airway and respiratory support for periods of days to months.

When indicated, give monovalent or polyvalent antivenom immediately in sufficient doses to improve coagulation values. Pregnancy is not a contraindication to antivenom therapy.

GILA MONSTER BITES

Gila monsters are slow-moving lizards that inhabit the desert in the southwestern United States. They possess venom as potent as rattlesnake venom but lack the apparatus to inject it effectively. Instead of fangs, they have short, grooved teeth down which their venom flows. Therefore, envenomation requires a prolonged bite. Gila monsters bite tenaciously and may be difficult to remove from the bitten extremity, so fractures and deep injury are possible.

There are few if any documented deaths from Gila monster bite. Most bites result in local pain and swelling only, which worsens over several hours and then subsides over several more hours. Dislodged teeth often contaminate the wound. Occasionally, a more severe syndrome of systemic toxicity develops, including weakness, light-headedness, paresthesia, and diaphoresis. Severe hypertension may occur, which also resolves over several hours.

First aid involves removal of the reptile from the bite site without sustaining another bite. This may require force. It helps to place the animal on a solid surface, because it often loosens its grip when it is no longer suspended in midair. Once the animal is removed, standard local wound care is sufficient, with care taken to remove any teeth in the wound. Radiographs should be considered if bony injury is possible. Update tetanus immunization status and give antibiotics if infection develops.

REFERENCES

The complete reference list is available online at www.TintinalliEM.com.

Marine Trauma and Envenomation

John J. Devlin
Kevin Knoop

MARINE TRAUMA

Human contact with the marine environment is becoming more frequent as recreational and commercial use of the world's oceans increases. In addition to the hazards of drowning and cold exposure, the marine environment provides the habitat for dangerous marine fauna. Many marine animals have evolved sharp teeth and spines or venom glands for defense and predation. Encounters with marine life may result in traumatic injury or envenomation, requiring emergency medical management. Providing care for these conditions may be further complicated by the marine environment's geographic isolation from locations with definitive health care.

EPIDEMIOLOGY

Epidemiologic information typically is organized by geographic region. The most common reported U.S exposures are to jellyfish (31%), stingrays (16%), venomous fish (including lionfish, catfish, and others) (28%), and gastropods (6%).[1] However, data likely favor the reporting of more severe injuries and the exclusion of common minor injuries. Human impact may be altering the geographic distribution of marine fauna as climate change affects migration patterns and artificial waterways connect previously separated bodies of water and their ecosystems.[2,3]

The International Shark Attack File recorded 2074 unprovoked shark attacks between 1960 and 2013, with the United States reporting the most attacks of any country and Florida reporting the most attacks of any state.[4] Despite the public perception, the risk of shark attack is extremely small compared with almost any other injury. There are probably between 70 and 100 shark attacks worldwide each year, with between 5 and 15 deaths.[4,5] Although the incidence of shark attacks has steadily risen since 1900, the mortality has fallen from 40% in the 30 years following World War II to current rates of approximately 10% to 20%.[6] Death is usually a result of a lack of prehospital resuscitation, hemorrhagic shock, or drowning.

Other marine creatures have been reported to attack humans, typically in defense of territory rather than for feeding. The great barracuda (*Sphyraena barracuda*) is the only barracuda species implicated in human attacks.[6] Moray eels, found in tropical to temperate waters, can inflict severe puncture wounds or lacerations, commonly to the hands of inquisitive divers. Other marine vertebrates known to cause traumatic injuries to humans include giant groupers, sea lions, seals, crocodiles, alligators, and piranhas. Some fish with sharp spines and fins (needlefish, wahoo, and triggerfish) can inadvertently injure humans. Wounds resulting from interactions with such creatures are a combination of crush injury, abrasion, puncture, and/or laceration.

BACTERIOLOGY OF MARINE SOFT TISSUE INFECTIONS

Marine soft tissue infections are often polymicrobial, halophilic gram-negative infections that may be resistant to first- and second-generation penicillins and cephalosporins.[7] Infecting bacteria are numerous and can vary with the environment, type of injury, and marine organism. Bacteria include staphylococci, streptococci, *Aeromonas hydrophilia*, *Escherichia coli*, *Pseudomonas* species, *Erysipelothrix* species, *Chromobacterium*, *Edwardsiella*, *Shewanella*, *Mycobacterium* species, *Mycoplasma* species, and *Vibrio* species.[8-10] Culture results can refine antibiotic treatment. Marine-associated infections are frequently diagnosed late because the history of marine exposure or injury is poorly recalled, and patients are often initially given inappropriate antibiotics, which potentially increases the morbidity of an already virulent infection. Patients with underlying conditions such as liver disease, immunosuppression, and diabetes are more susceptible to halophilic *Vibrio* infections.[11] *Vibrio* skin infections can progress rapidly from initial contact and local painful inflammation, through subepidermal bullae containing hemorrhagic fluid and vasculitis, to necrosis and small-vessel thrombosis, bacteremia, and septicemia.[8,11]

MAJOR MARINE TRAUMA

Encounters with sharks, skates, stingrays, barracuda, Moray eels, and giant grouper can result in major trauma. Of these animal-related injuries, shark bites are the best characterized.[12,13] Shark attacks can result in neurovascular injury and significant tissue loss. Sharks typically attack the appendages (be they seals or humans), which tend to dangle lower than the head and torso while the victim is swimming on the surface. In 70% of surface swimmers, only the lower limb is involved. The upper limb can be subsequently injured when the victim tries to fend off the attacker. Sharks are unable to chew their prey and so sequentially strip it.[5] In more serious attacks, substantial tissue loss and extremity amputation are common.

Stingrays possess spined tails that reflexively whip upward when stepped on or startled. These encounters typically result in foot and ankle injuries. However, serious thoracoabdominal injuries have been reported, such as the sensationalized 2006 death of naturalist Steve Irwin. Morbidity and mortality result from penetrating trauma to internal organs.[14-16] Rarely, spine tips are retained in stingray wounds.

Victims of marine animal–associated trauma should be removed sufficiently from the water to allow immediate resuscitation. As in military settings, place a tourniquet on limbs with evidence of uncontrolled arterial hemorrhage, because the survival benefit after tourniquet placement outweighs the low risk of neurologic injury from compression.[17] At the hospital, manage injuries according to institutional trauma protocols.[12]

However, there are two caveats for marine injuries. First, teeth and spines may be retained in bone and soft tissue and be a source of infection. Obtain plain radiographs of all injured regions to identify fractures, periosteal stripping, and retained foreign bodies. If radiographs are unremarkable but there is still a high clinical suspicion for a retained foreign body, US may be helpful. US may be particularly helpful in identifying radiolucent fragments of sea urchin spines and stingray barbs.[18,19] Second, the mouths and integument of marine fauna can be heavily colonized with marine bacteria. Wounds should be swabbed and specimens sent for culture. Many marine microorganisms require special selective media for culture and sensitivity testing, so alert the microbiology laboratory that a marine-acquired organism might be present. Infections from marine microorganisms can be more serious than usual soft tissue infections. Irrigate open wounds and debride devitalized tissue. **Do not suture lacerations or puncture wounds sustained in marine environments. Provide early antibiotic treatment** for wounds from major trauma, in those at risk for infection, in the immunocompromised or those with hepatic disease, and for established infection (**Tables 213-1 and 213-2**).[8,9,11,20,21] Provide postexposure tetanus prophylaxis.[22] Obtain early surgical consultation for thorough debridement for suspected *Vibrio vulnificus* infections or any necrotizing infection. Regardless of the antibiotic choice, close clinical follow-up is essential to identify treatment failures early.

MINOR MARINE TRAUMA

Most marine injuries and stings do not cause serious injury. Treatment depends on the agent and the seriousness of injury (Table 213-2). Coral cuts are probably the most common injuries sustained underwater and usually involve the hands, forearms, elbows, and knees (**Figure 213-1**). The initial reaction to a coral cut is stinging pain, erythema, and pruritus. Within minutes, the break in the skin may be surrounded by an erythematous wheal, which fades over 1 to 2 hours. With or without treatment, the local reaction of red, raised welts and local pruritus may progress to cellulitis with ulceration and tissue sloughing. The wounds heal slowly over 3 to 6 weeks.

TABLE 213-1 Recommendations for Antibiotic Treatment of Marine-Associated Wounds

No Antibiotic Indicated	Prophylactic/Outpatient Antibiotics	Hospital Admission for IV Antibiotics
Healthy patient	Late wound care	Predisposing medical conditions
Prompt wound care	Large lacerations or injuries	Long delays before definitive wound care
No foreign body	Early or local inflammation	Deep wounds, significant trauma
No bone or joint involvement		Wounds with retained foreign bodies
Small or superficial injuries		Progressive inflamatory change Penetration of periosteum, joint space, or body cavity Major injuries associated with envenomation Systemic illness

Promptly and vigorously irrigate cuts to remove all foreign matter. Fragments that remain can become embedded and increase the risk of infection or foreign-body granuloma. Clean superficial wounds daily. Give antibiotics if infection develops (Tables 213-1 and 213-2).

MARINE ENVENOMATIONS

Venomous marine animals produce venom in specialized glands. The venom can then be applied to or injected parenterally into other organisms using a specialized venom apparatus. Venom is not a pure substance but a mixture of mainly protein and peptide toxins. The effect of a specific toxin depends on its site of action; it may be neurotoxic, hemotoxic, dermatotoxic, cytotoxic, or myotoxic. Unlike thermostable ingestible seafood poisons, marine venoms are typically high-molecular-weight, heat-labile proteins.[23]

STINGRAYS AND VENOMOUS FISH

STINGRAYS

All stingrays' tails house venomous spines.[15] Inflicted lacerations allow the injection of venom. Stingray injuries cause immediate intense local pain that may radiate and last for many hours. There is often significant bleeding depending on the site of injury, and the wound may be erythematous or dusky. Systemic effects are uncommon but have been reported and relate more to the systemic response to severe pain. Submerging the affected extremity in **hot water between 110°F (43.3°C) and 114°F (45.6°C)** can denature the venom protein and provide pain

TABLE 213-2 Antibiotics for Marine-Associated Wound Infections*

For All: Staphylococci and Streptococci Coverage	Seawater Associated: *Vibrio* Species Coverage	Freshwater Associated: *Aeromonas* Species Coverage
First-generation cephalosporin	Fluoroquinolone	Fluoroquinolone
or	*or*	*or*
Methicillin-resistant *Staphylococcus aureus* coverage depending on prevalence	Third-generation cephalosporin	Trimethoprim-sulfamethoxazole
		or
		Carbapenems

*The choice of antibiotic is not clear-cut, and there are no robust evidence-based treatment guidelines. Antibiotic sensitivities vary, and there is considerable discrepancy between the in vitro antibiotic susceptibility data and clinical outcomes. Antibiotic choices should reflect the frequent polymicrobial nature of marine infections.

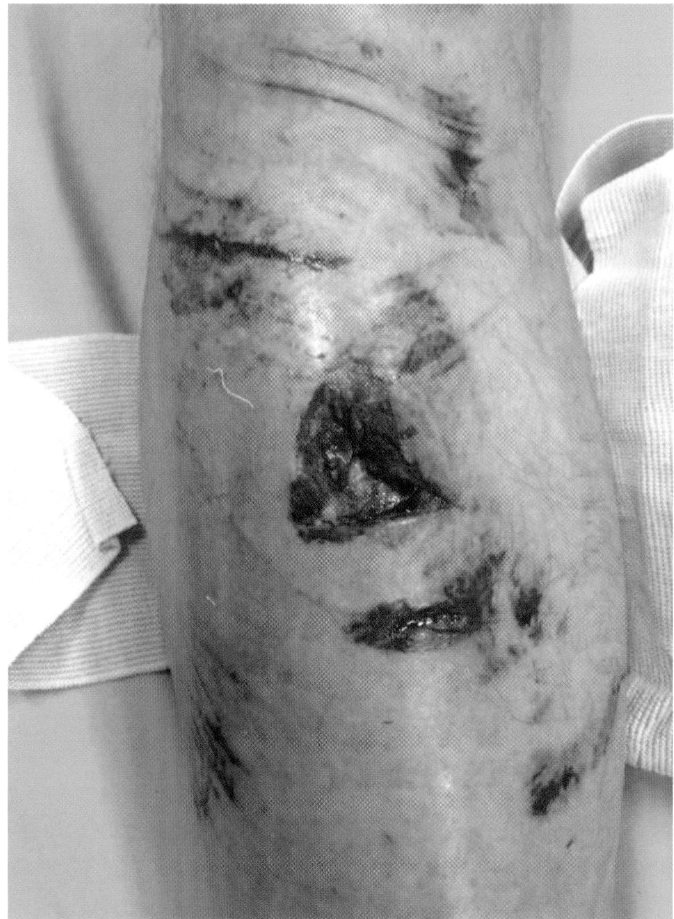

FIGURE 213-1. These injuries occurred when the swimmer was thrown up against coral by wave action. Coral wounds should be evaluated for retained foreign body. [Photo contributed by Kaitlin Pala, MD.]

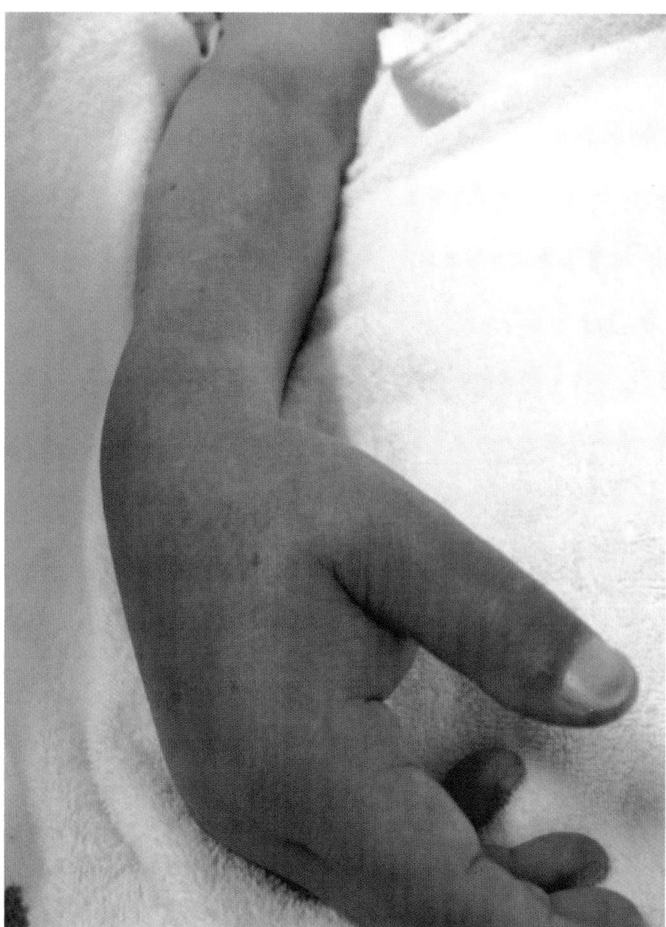

FIGURE 213-2. Significant edema and erythema of the right hand after stonefish sting to the thumb. [Photo contributed by Anthony Morocco, MD.]

relief within 10 to 30 minutes.[24,25] Topical lidocaine can be applied for additional pain relief.

VENOMOUS FISH STINGS

Venomous fish are found in tropical and, less commonly, temperate oceans and private aquariums. The important venomous fish include stonefish, weeverfish, scorpionfish, and lionfish. The effects of the stings range from severe with stonefish to minimal with some types of catfish and other fish with nonvenomous spines.[16,26]

Stonefish (*Synanceia* species) and scorpionfish (Scorpaenidae) occur throughout tropical and warmer temperate oceans from the central Pacific, west through the Indo-Pacific, to the East African coastline. They are a diverse group of fish, with differing habitats, swimming patterns, and ability to camouflage.[16,26] The venom apparatus varies among species but most have 5 to 15 dorsal spines. Stonefish are stationary bottom dwellers usually frequenting shallow water.

Clinical effects are characterized by immediate severe and increasing local pain, which may radiate proximally. Untreated, the pain typically peaks at 30 to 90 minutes and persists for 4 to 6 hours, but this varies considerably for different fish. The wound site usually has significant local edema and erythema (**Figure 213-2**). Nonspecific systemic effects such as sweating, nausea, vomiting, and even syncope may occur. Extensive tissue necrosis is not seen unless a secondary infection develops.

Weeverfish (or weaverfish) are all saltwater fish and are the most venomous fish in the temperate zone. They are found in the Mediterranean and European coastal areas and are bottom dwellers that sting when stepped on. Their five to seven envenoming dorsal spines can penetrate leather boots, producing pain severity similar to stonefish injuries. Wounds may eventually necrose.

TREATMENT OF VENOMOUS FISH AND STINGRAY INJURIES

Irrigate the wound immediately, and remove any visible pieces of the spine or integumentary sheath. Control bleeding and immerse in hot water immersion as soon as possible (**Table 213-3**). During the hot water soak, the wound can be explored and foreign material removed. Provide oral or parenteral analgesics as needed. The wound can also be infiltrated with lidocaine **without epinephrine,** or a regional nerve block can be applied to help control pain.

Once pain is controlled, cleanse the wound using an aseptic technique, reexplore and remove foreign material, and debride necrotic tissue. Obtain soft tissue imaging when possible, to visualize retained foreign material.

The conclusions of the few study series involving venomous fish stings and the experience of aquarium workers are that most injuries are minor and do not require antibiotics.[26] Although some authors routinely recommend antibiotic prophylaxis, the majority do not unless the wound is large or there is considerable foreign material. This situation is more likely with stingray wounds, which have the greatest potential to cause necrosis and infection. Prevention of infection by careful cleaning of the wound and debridement, if required, is more important. An **antivenom exists for stonefish envenomation** (CSL Ltd., Melbourne, Australia) and should be used in cases of severe systemic reactions to stonefish and possibly other venomous fish.[27,28] Although it is registered for IM and IV administration, IV is more likely to be effective, based on experience with other antivenoms. The antivenom is prepared from horse serum, so be prepared to treat anaphylaxis.

SEA SNAKES

There are numerous species of sea snakes that are closely related to terrestrial elapids, all of which are venomous. They occur in the tropical and warm temperate Pacific and Indian Oceans. None are found in the

TABLE 213-3 Early Treatment of Marine Envenomations

Organism	Detoxification	Further Treatment
Penetrating Envenomations		
Catfish, lionfish, scorpionfish, stingray	Hot water immersion*, topical lidocaine	Usual wound care†; irrigate with seawater or normal saline (NS) Observe for development of systemic symptoms **Carefully assess for deep penetration from stingray spines**
Stonefish, weeverfish	Hot water immersion*, topical lidocaine	Usual wound care†; irrigate with seawater or NS **Stonefish antivenom** for severe systemic reaction (CSL Ltd., Melbourne, Australia); be prepared to treat anaphylaxis
Sea snake	—	Pressure immobilization **Polyvalent sea snake antivenom** (CSL Ltd., Melbourne, Australia) for systemic reaction; be prepared to treat anaphylaxis Supportive care; observe for 8 h for myotoxicity and neurotoxicity; may need intensive care unit (ICU) care
Blue-ringed octopus	—	Pressure immobilization; flaccid paralysis and respiratory failure can develop in minutes. Provide respiratory support and ICU care
Cone snail	—	Pressure immobilization; observe for paralysis and respiratory failure; supportive care
Sea urchin and starfish	Hot water immersion*, topical lidocaine	Explore wound and remove any spines, tufts, or pincers
Fireworms	Topical 5% acetic acid (vinegar)	Consider topical corticosteroids Remove bristles
Nonpenetrating Envenomations		
Fire coral, hydroids	Irrigate with seawater or saline	Topical corticosteroids for itching
Portuguese man-of-war, bluebottle jellyfish	Hot water immersion*, seawater irrigation, topical lidocaine Remove tentacles and nematocysts	Topical corticosteroids for itching Observe for development of systemic symptoms Supportive care
Box jellyfish (Indo-Pacific *Chironex* species and Australian *Carukia* species)	Hot water immersion* Irrigate with saline or seawater Topical 5% acetic acid (vinegar)‡ Remove tentacles and nematocysts Topical lidocaine	Topical corticosteroids for itching Observe for development of systemic symptoms Supportive care
Irukandji syndrome (Australian, *Carukia* species)	Irrigate with saline or seawater Hot water immersion* Remove tentacles and nematocysts	Administer ***Chironex*** **antivenom**; be prepared for anaphylaxis Magnesium for cardiac arrest Parenteral opioids for pain

*Hot water immersion = 111°F (43.3°C) to 114°F (45.6°C) water until pain is relieved.

†Usual wound care = Irrigate, explore, debride, consider antibiotics and analgesics, update tetanus immunization, elevate extremity.

‡Controversial; depends on species.

Atlantic Ocean, the Caribbean, or North American coastal waters, except Hawaii. Probably the most important species medically is the beaked sea snake (*Enhydrina schistosa*), which has caused fatalities in Southeast Asia.

Sea snakes can be distinguished from land snakes by their flat tails and valve-like nostril flaps and from eels by the presence of scales and the absence of gills and fins. The venom apparatus consists of two to four short, hollow maxillary fangs, and a pair of associated venom glands. About 20% of bites cause significant envenomation, and up to 40% of these are potentially fatal without treatment. The venom of sea snakes contains neurotoxins and myotoxins; one tends to dominate the clinical features. However, there are no toxins that affect coagulation.

Bites are typically painless and may go unnoticed. Symptoms typically become apparent 30 minutes to 4 hours after the bite. The first complaint is usually related to myotoxicity, with severe myalgia and nonspecific muscle weakness. Other symptoms include nausea, vomiting, and malaise. The muscle pain may become so severe that movement is limited, which is typified by trismus that develops in the jaw. Immobility secondary to pain should be distinguished from weakness or paralysis caused by neurotoxicity. Rhabdomyolysis and secondary renal failure develop in more severe cases, which may be complicated by hyperkalemia. In some sea snake envenomations, neurotoxicity has been reported without myotoxicity, with ascending flaccid or spastic paralysis accompanied by ophthalmoplegia, ptosis, facial paralysis, and pupillary changes. Death is most commonly a result of respiratory failure.

Diagnosis of a sea snake bite is based on the combination of snake identification and the presence of a puncture bite wound that was initially painless and occurred in or near the water. Suspect envenomation if severe myalgia develops. The presence of myoglobinuria and an elevated creatine kinase level is also typical, indicating rhabdomyolysis. Neurotoxic symptoms are rapid in onset and usually appear within 2 to 3 hours. If no symptoms develop by 6 to 8 hours, envenomation is unlikely to have occurred.

First aid treatment is pressure immobilization of the affected limb.[29] Elastic bandages are preferred.[30] Administer **polyvalent sea snake antivenom (CSL Ltd., Melbourne, Australia)** for systemic envenomation.[28] The antivenom is made from horse serum, so be prepared to treat anaphylaxis. Intensive supportive care and monitoring of renal, metabolic, and respiratory functions are critical.

OCTOPUS INJURIES

Injuries from the octopus or squid are unusual. All octopuses have venom, but the only dangerous octopus is the blue-ringed octopus. The venom tetrodotoxin, introduced by a bite, causes respiratory arrest within minutes. Treatment is supportive. Pressure immobilization at the bite area is the recommended first-aid treatment.

The bite of the Australian blue-ringed octopus (*Hapalochlaena* species) has caused at least two deaths. The saliva of the octopus contains tetrodotoxin and produces effects clinically identical to those of tetrodotoxin poisoning seen most commonly with puffer fish ingestion.[31,32] Octopus bites typically occur on the upper extremity, almost always when the animal is picked up (**Figure 213-3**). The bite causes small, painless puncture marks and many go unnoticed. In most cases, no symptoms develop or only mild local numbness and paresthesia occur. In more severe envenomations, vomiting and progressive flaccid paralysis with eventual respiratory failure may begin within 10 minutes of envenomation.[33] Wrap the limb with a lymphatic occlusive bandage to provide pressure immobilization until definitive care is reached. Treatment is supportive, with mechanical ventilation as required, and full recovery usual occurs over 1 to 5 days. No antivenom or antidote is available.

CONE SNAIL INJURIES

Cone snails have intricate shell patterns, making them attractive to handle. Cone snails are predators that feed by injecting a potent mixture of neurotoxins using detachable, dart-like radicular teeth. Stings by cone snails are very rare. Most stings occur after prolonged contact with the shell or when breaking the shell. With significant envenomation, local pain is followed immediately by local numbness, which quickly spreads from the extremity to the trunk and then to the head and neck region. Partial paralysis develops within 30 minutes, progressing to complete voluntary muscle paralysis and respiratory failure. Mortality following *Conus geographus* envenomation may be as high as 65%.[34] Less severe envenomations cause muscle pain, partial paralysis, or ataxia, or in mild cases only local effects. Treatment is pressure immobilization with a lymphatic-occlusive bandage until definitive care is reached.

SEA URCHINS AND STARFISH

Sea urchins are found in all oceans, and most sea urchins have solid nontoxic spines. Injury from the spines causes localized pain, which is exacerbated by pressure, even if there are no retained spines in the wound[35] (**Figure 213-4**). If a spine enters a joint, it may cause severe synovitis. Wounds from black sea urchin spines may leave a black discoloration of the skin. Contact with the venomous spines causes immediate, intense burning pain, with erythema, swelling, and often bleeding of the skin surrounding the puncture sites. The acute pain usually subsides over hours. Secondary infection and granuloma formation from remaining spine fragments are well-described delayed effects. Systemic features have been reported rarely, often when multiple spines are involved, but may be due to severe pain.

Some starfish have surface spines, tufts, or pincers. The crown-of-thorns starfish (*Acanthaster planci*) can be found on most reefs in the Indo-Pacific region and has caused outbreaks of envenomation in Japan and Australia.[1] Crown-of-thorn starfish are covered with sharp, rigid spines that can passively deliver a variety of substances when they penetrate skin. This includes venom produced in special glandular tissue, mucus, bacteria, and dermal tissue. Injury by the spines causes severe burning pain, often greater than expected for the mechanical injury, and lasts 1 to 2 hours. Other local effects include bleeding, erythema, and mild edema. In more severe cases, particularly with multiple punctures, the wound may become dusky or discolored. Pruritus and persisting edema can occur, perhaps as a result of allergy. Systemic effects are uncommon but may include paresthesias, nausea, vomiting, lymphadenopathy, and muscular paralysis.[1,6]

Treatment is immediate immersion in hot water to tolerance (45°C [113°F]) for 30 to 90 minutes or until pain is relieved. Topical or locally injected lidocaine can provide additional pain relief. Give analgesics. Remove retained spines or tufts as well as possible, without causing more tissue injury. Soft tissue radiographs, US, or MRI may be helpful in locating retained spines. US may be particularly helpful in identifying radiolucent fragments of sea urchin spines.[19] Arrange follow-up, because further surgical removal of spines may be required if there are ongoing symptoms. Spines in joints require immediate orthopedic consultation.

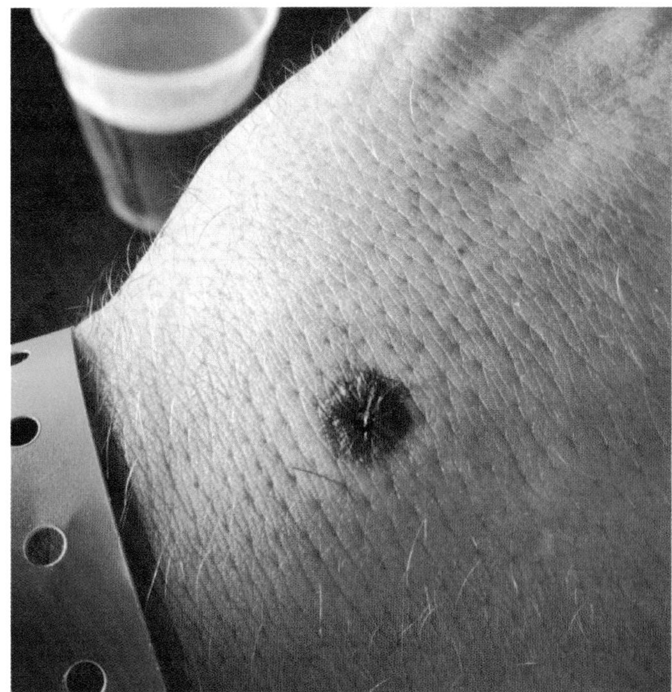

A

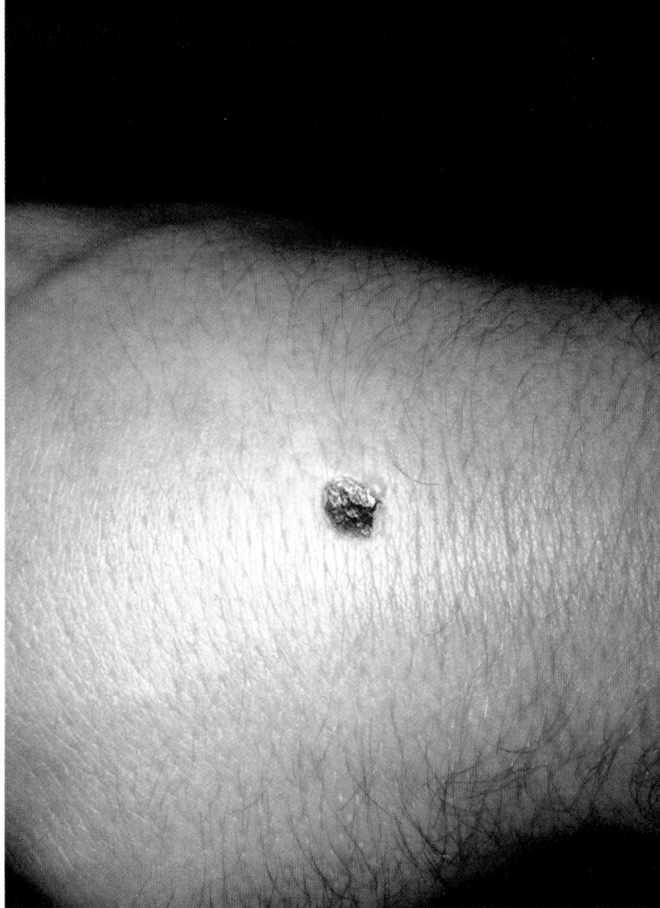

B

FIGURE 213-3. This acute octopus bite (**A**) was initially treated with ciprofloxacin, but persisted with a scab (**B**) and regional adenopathy for several months. After treatment with doxycycline, adenopathy resolved, but a chronic nonhealing ulcer remained despite multiple specialty consultants. [Photo contributed by Steven Whelpley, MD.]

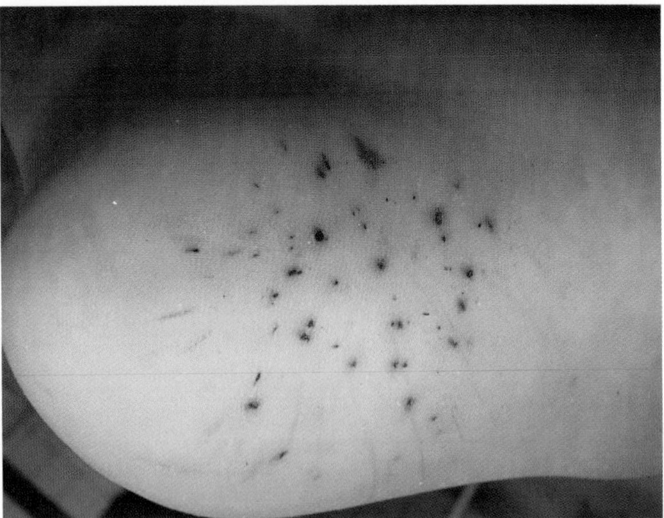

FIGURE 213-4. Sea urchin sting in the foot showing the entry sites. [Used with permission of Vidal Haddad Jr., MD, PhD.]

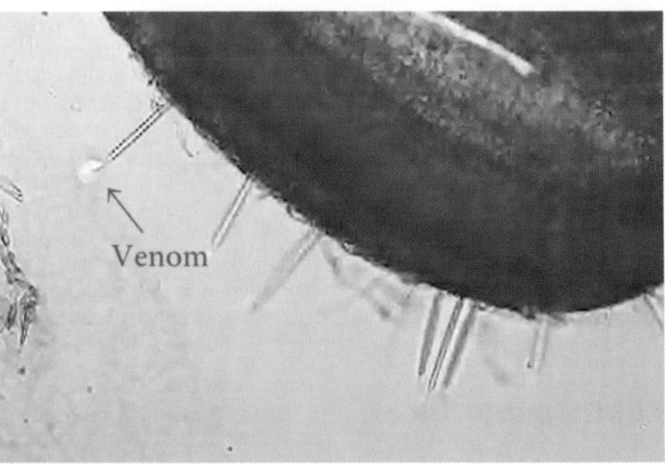

FIGURE 213-5. Nematocyst. Photomicrograph of anemone tentacle showing discharged nematocysts. Note venom ejected upon discharge. [Used with permission of Destin Sandlin, Smarter Every Day, full video may be viewed at: https://www.youtube.com/watch?v=7WJCnC5ebf4.]

FIREWORMS OR BRISTLEWORMS

Fireworms, or bristleworms, are segmented worms covered with cactus-like bristles that can penetrate the skin. These bristles easily detach in the skin and can be difficult to remove. Envenomation causes intense inflammation with a burning sensation and erythema. Untreated, the pain generally resolves within a few hours, but erythema may last for 2 to 3 days. Bristles should be removed with forceps or adhesive tape. Vinegar (5%) may be applied topically. The inflammatory response may require a course of corticosteroids.

HYDROIDS AND FIRE CORAL

Hydroids are colonies of tiny jellies attached to a feather-like or seaweed-like base. They are abundant on seaweed, reefs, pilings, floating docks, or lines. Coastal storms can break off feather hydroid branches and cause infestation of a local swimming area. Fire corals look like corals, are often mistaken for seaweed, and are small brush-like growths on rocks and coral itself. Contact with nematocysts or stinging threads results in an immediate sting after even a superficial brush contact, followed by itching pain, associated with the development of painful wheals and urticaria after 30 minutes. The welts may last for up to a week but leave no permanent mark. With more extensive exposure, blistering and a hemorrhagic and zosteriform reaction can occur. Lesions crust over after a few days. Vinegar can inhibit nematocyst discharge. Pain relief can be provided with analgesics. Treat itching with topical steroids.

JELLYFISH

There are many types of jellyfish, but the most important groups affecting humans are the Portuguese man-of-war or bluebottle jellyfish, the box jellyfish, and those jellyfish causing Irukandji syndrome.

Jellyfish are characterized by their unique stinging nematocysts[34] (**Figure 213-5**), which number in the thousands and are found mainly on the tentacles, but also in lesser numbers on the body or bell. The nematocyst contains a minute dose of venom, in some cases highly potent, and a harpoon-like mechanism. A physical or chemical stimulus triggers the rapid release of a hollow, sharply pointed, threadlike tube from the nematocyst, which penetrates the skin and delivers venom subcutaneously. There are a number of genera causing local and systemic reactions, off the coasts of Russia, Japan, Brazil , Uruguay, and Argentina—all with similar toxic effects.

The clinical features of jellyfish envenomation vary in severity. The severity depends on the venom dose, the marine species, and the victim (age and size). Mild envenomation results in bothersome acute skin reactions, with immediate stinging pain and erythema or wheal formation at the site. Lesions usually resolve spontaneously over days to a couple of weeks, with occasional postinflammatory hyperpigmentation.

Treatment of jellyfish stings is not well studied, and results are often conflicting. A treatment helpful for one species may worsen effects from another species. Irrigation with seawater to remove nematocysts and hot water immersion and application of topical lidocaine appear to be the most universally beneficial treatments. Other applications, such as sodium bicarbonate or vinegar, may worsen stinging from some species.

PORTUGUESE MAN-OF-WAR AND BLUEBOTTLE JELLYFISH

This group of jellyfish (*Physalia* species) has a large gas-filled float, which suspends multiple tentacles. The nematocysts are found on the tentacles but not on the float. *Physalia* species are the most widely distributed jellyfish and are responsible for thousands of human envenomations in Florida, parts of Asia and Africa, Australia, and Western Europe.[1,2,36] All species occur in swarms in shallow water and usually cause stings in the surf or are washed up on the shore. Nematocysts from fractured tentacles may remain active for months.

The Portuguese man-of-war is a multitentacled jellyfish common in the Atlantic, with tentacles that can be as long as 30 m. The bluebottle jellyfish is smaller and single-tentacled and found commonly in Australia and Hawaii.

Stings from *Physalia* species cause immediate, intense pain that often fades over an hour but may persist for many hours, particularly with larger specimens. The sting causes a characteristic linear erythematous eruption, classically referred to as a "string of pearls" pattern.[35] Respiratory distress and death have been reported following *Physalia* envenomation, and delayed effects have been reported in rare instances.[36,37]

Treatment is to first wash the area with seawater and then immerse in hot water, as the venom is heat labile. In general, vinegar is not recommended for *Physalia* stings. Remove tentacles and nematocysts by scraping the skin with a sharp object (e.g., razor or credit card) or by applying adhesive tape.[38] If adhesive tape is used, the adherent nematocysts can later be identified.

There is no specific antidote for *Physalia* envenomation, and care is supportive.

BOX JELLYFISH AND IRUKANDJI SYNDROME

The box jellyfish is the most dangerous jellyfish and includes two important members: the Indo-Pacific box jellyfish (*Chironex fleckeri*) and the

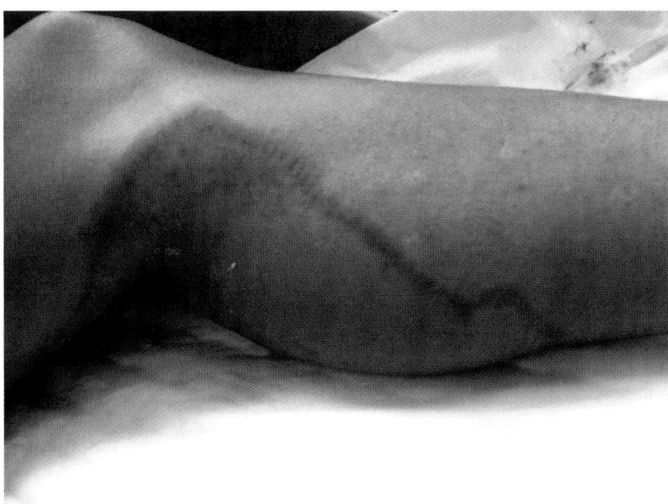

FIGURE 213-6. Box jellyfish sting. This 24-year-old woman was snorkeling off of Koh Tao, Thailand, when she was stung by a box jellyfish 15 minutes prior to this photograph being taken. She presented with severe extremity pain and chest tightness. [Photo contributed by Sittidet Toonpirom, MD, and Rittirak Othong, MD.]

Australian jellyfish (*Carukia barnesi)* that causes **Irukandji syndrome**.[39,40] Box jellyfish are also found in the Philippines, Japan, and the U.S. Atlantic coast. The Hawaiian box jellyfish (*Carybdea alata*) causes numerous stings to beachgoers in Hawaii, although no deaths have been confirmed from this organism.[41]

The Indo-Pacific box jellyfish (*Chironex*) has been described as the world's most venomous animal.[42] It has caused over 80 deaths in the past century.[43] The exact mechanism of toxicity and toxins involved in death—which occurs rapidly, often within 20 minutes—remains unclear, but a primary cardiotoxic role is likely.[42] Severe reactions or death can occur following skin contact with tentacles, especially in children.[39,44] However, the vast majority of stings are mild to moderate, consisting of skin welts and immediate, sometimes severe pain.[39] The toxic skin reaction may be quite intense, with rapid formation of wheals, vesicles, and a darkened reddish brown or purple whip-like flare pattern with stripes 8 to 10 mm wide. With more severe stings, blistering occurs, and superficial necrosis develops after 12 to 18 hours. Severe box jellyfish stings cause a pathognomonic crosshatched pattern, classically referred to as a "frosted ladder" pattern (**Figure 213-6**). Following the acute toxic reaction, a delayed hypersensitivity reaction occurs in approximately 60% of cases, with papular urticaria at the sting sites.[39,45]

The Australian jellyfish (*C. barnesi)* causes the **Irukandji syndrome**.[40] The sting initially causes mild local effects with localized pain and erythema. Approximately 20 to 30 minutes later, severe generalized pain in the abdomen, back, chest, head, and limbs develops. The pain is usually associated with systemic signs of catecholamine excess, including tachycardia, hypertension, sweating, piloerection, and agitation. In severe cases, cardiogenic shock with pulmonary edema and serum troponin elevation occur.[40,44]

Treatment **Treatment** consists of deactivation of attached nematocysts, tentacle removal, reversal of venom effects if possible, and symptomatic and pain relief. All victims with systemic signs or symptoms should be observed for ongoing envenomation or delayed reactions (Table 213-3).

Irrigate with seawater or normal saline to deactivate undischarged nematocysts. After deactivation, visible tentacles can be removed. Do not irrigate with freshwater because the hypotonic solution is thought to stimulate nematocyst discharge. Best methods for removal are scraping the skin with a sharp object (e.g., razor or credit card) or application of adhesive tape.[38] If adhesive tape is used, the adherent nematocysts can later be identified. Treat with hot water immersion (111°F [43.3°C] to 114°F [45.6°C]) and apply topical lidocaine.[46]

Effective topical decontaminants appear to be species specific.[46,47] Because the species is often unknown, the geographic location of the envenomation guides decontamination. In Indo-Pacific waters, **particularly those surrounding Australia,** nematocyst deactivation therapy with 5% acetic acid (vinegar) is recommended,[43,48] and 5% acetic acid is the first-line management recommendation by the Australian Resuscitation Council.[43,49]

Treatment for severe *Chironex* envenomation (Irukandji syndrome) consists of standard resuscitative measures and administration of sheep-derived antivenom specific for *C. fleckeri* (CSL Ltd., Melbourne, Australia).[39] Be prepared to treat anaphylaxis. Fatalities despite antivenom administration may be related to the rapidity of onset of cardiovascular collapse after *Chironex* envenomation.[27] Therefore, antivenom should be administered IV as early as possible. The initial dose may be repeated if there is no clinical response, and some clinicians recommend three or more doses in severe envenomations associated with cardiovascular collapse.[44] Magnesium improves outcome in animal studies and should be considered in refractory cases of severe *Chironex* envenomation with cardiac arrest.[40,45]

Severe generalized pain in Irukandji syndrome requires titrated IV opioid analgesia, often with large and repeat doses. Magnesium bolus and infusion have been used for treatment of the pain and hypertension associated with Irukandji syndrome.[45,50] However, adverse effects due to hypermagnesemia have been reported, and the treatment has not been as effective as originally suggested.[50] All patients should have an ECG and troponin testing on admission, and echocardiography is useful in patients with myocardial involvement. Pulmonary edema should be managed with oxygen supplementation, positive-pressure ventilation, and inotropes

In waters surrounding the United States, application of 5% acetic acid solutions to tentacles from *Chrysaora* species appear to increase nematocyst discharge.[51,52] For *Chrysaora* or *Cyanea*, a slurry of baking soda (sodium bicarbonate) is thought to be effective. Traditionally, acetic acid solutions were thought to deactivate North American *Physalia* species nematocysts.[52] However, one review of North American and Hawaiian jellyfish envenomation management has questioned the use of acetic acid, concluding that "vinegar may not be an ideal agent because it causes pain exacerbation," but may be considered in *Physalia* species envenomations, whereas "hot water and lidocaine appear more universally beneficial in improving pain symptoms and are preferentially recommended."[46] The venoms are heat labile, and heat reduces toxicity in most jellyfish envenomations.[36,41,47]

MARINE DERMATITIS

SPONGES

Thousands of sponge species exist, but few are medically important. A number of sponges produce toxic secretions (crinotoxin—slimes or surface liquids), including fire sponges (*Tedania* species) and *Neofibularia* species in Australia, which cause skin irritation and dermatitis referred to as *stinging sponge dermatitis*.[53] Minor effects from sponges are likely due to simple mechanical irritation by the spicules. There is often no initial sensation following contact, but after a few minutes to hours, an itching or burning sensation develops. The stinging or itching sensation usually increases in intensity over 2 to 3 days and may become almost unbearable. The effects are usually confined to the area of contact or just adjacent to it. There may be associated local joint stiffness, and an acute inflammatory reaction with erythema and edema develops when symptoms are severe. Untreated mild reactions subside over 3 to 7 days. Papules, vesicles, and bullae may develop in some cases, followed by desquamation of the area days to weeks later, which is most commonly reported with fire sponges.[53] Treatment is irrigation, analgesia, and topical corticosteroids for itching or inflammation.[53]

SEABATHER'S ERUPTION

Seabather's eruption is a vesicular or morbilliform pruritic allergic dermatitis resulting from contact with larvae of the sea anemone or jellyfish in Atlantic ocean areas. Dermatitis typically occurs within 24 hours after saltwater exposure, and involves skin surfaces covered by bathing suits, swim caps, or fins. Divers may be affected on the neck when floating in water churned by boat propellers that have ground floating jellyfish into fragments. Dermatitis persists for 2 to 14 days and resolves spontaneously. If contact is suspected, shower after removing the bathing or diving suit.

SEA CUCUMBERS

Direct contact with sea cucumbers may induce a contact dermatitis, which is usually mild. Immerse the extremity in hot water. The greatest risk is to the corneas and conjunctivae, which may become intensely inflamed. For ocular exposure, irrigate copiously with normal saline or fresh water.

Acknowledgement: The authors gratefully acknowledge Paul S. Auerbach, Geoffrey K. Isbister, and David G. Caldicott for contributions to this chapter from previous editions.

REFERENCES

The complete reference list is available online at www.TintinalliEM.com.

CHAPTER 214 Diving Disorders

Brian Snyder
Tom Neuman

INTRODUCTION

Millions of recreational, commercial, and scientific dives are logged annually, and the vast majority of dives are completed without incident. However, there are physiologic effects and injuries relatively unique to the underwater environment. Generally, these effects and injuries are secondary to pressure changes on the submerged human body and the breathing of compressed gas.[1] This chapter outlines the most common diving injuries: barotrauma of descent (otic, sinus, and pulmonary), barotrauma of ascent (pulmonary overinflation syndromes and arterial gas embolism), decompression sickness, immersion pulmonary edema, oxygen toxicity, and nitrogen narcosis.

THE GAS LAWS

Understanding diving injuries requires familiarity with the three relevant gas laws most pertinent to diving: Boyle's law, Dalton's law, and Henry's law.

Boyle's law states that given a constant temperature, the pressure and volume of an ideal gas are inversely related. That is, if pressure is doubled, the volume of gas is halved. This law is stated as: $P_1V_1 = P_2V_2$.

Pressure can be measured in a variety of units. The International System of Units defines pressure using the pascal (Pa). Other commonly used units of pressure include millimeters of mercury (mm Hg), torr, pounds per square inch (psi), bar, or atmosphere (atm): 1 atm = 760 mm Hg = 760 torr = 14.7 psi = 1.013 bar = 101,325 Pa = 101.325 kPa. Additionally, pressure in diving settings is often described using feet of seawater (fsw) or meters of seawater (see below). In this chapter, we use atm, mm Hg, and fsw for pressure units.

Because of the high density of water, a relatively small change in depth causes a great change in pressure. The weight of seawater produces a change of 1 atm for each 33 ft of depth. For freshwater, pressure increases 1 atm for each 34 ft of depth. Therefore, the pressure exerted on a diver at a depth of 33 ft in seawater = 1 atm for the seawater + 1 atm for the atmosphere above the water = 2 atmospheres absolute (ATA). A diver at 165 ft of seawater would experience 6 ATA of pressure (1 atm for each 33 ft of seawater = 5 atm + 1 atm for atmospheric pressure at sea level).

Thus, **Boyle's law** dictates as a diver descends in the water column, the volume of air-containing structures will decrease. For example, if the lungs contain volume *V* at the surface, a diver who descends to 33 ft of seawater holding his or her breath would have a lung volume of $^1/_2V$. If the diver then breathes compressed air at this depth (from scuba equipment or from a surface-supplied source of gas), lung volume would return to *V*. If the diver then ascends to the surface without exhaling, lung volume would be 2*V* at the surface. This pressure–volume relationship governed by Boyle's law is important in the etiology of injuries due to barotrauma and produces the volume changes of bubbles in the tissues and circulation that are associated with recompression (hyperbaric) therapy.

Dalton's law states that the total pressure exerted by a mixture of gases is the sum of the partial pressures of each gas. Therefore, the partial pressure of a given component of a gas mixture will increase as the ambient pressure increases, although the proportion of gas in the mixture remains constant. The partial pressure of nitrogen in air at sea level is approximately 600 mm Hg or 0.79 ATA (the fraction of nitrogen in air, 0.79 × 760 mm Hg or 1 ATA). At a depth of 99 fsw, the partial pressure of nitrogen in air would be 4 × 600 = 2400 mm Hg (or 3.16 ATA).

Henry's law, which states that at equilibrium the quantity of a gas in solution in a liquid is proportional to the partial pressure of the gas, along with Dalton's law, explains the uptake of inert gas into tissues when breathing compressed air at depth. It is the uptake of inert gas that is intrinsic to the development of decompression sickness.

BAROTRAUMA OF DESCENT

The clinical conditions resulting from barotrauma of descent are barotitis (ear squeeze), external ear squeeze, sinus barotrauma, inner ear barotrauma, and face, tooth, or dry-suit squeeze (**Table 214-1**).

PATHOPHYSIOLOGY

During descent, the volume of gas in all air-containing body cavities decreases. The air space in the middle ear makes the tympanic membrane the tissue most commonly affected by this phenomenon, if active measures such as "clearing the ears" with a Valsalva or other maneuvers are not successful.[2] As the volume of gas decreases, the tympanic membrane is bent inward, causing a feeling of fullness or pain in the ear. Forcing air through the Eustachian tube with a Valsalva maneuver will equalize the pressure between the middle ear and external ear canal by filling the middle ear with additional gas. Generally, divers who experience pain in an ear during descent will attempt to clear the ear and, if unsuccessful, will ascend to decrease the pressure differential and attempt equalizing again. If the diver is unsuccessful in equalizing and continues the descent, prolonged pain and injury to the tympanic membrane may result, known as barotitis or "ear squeeze."

BAROTITIS (EAR SQUEEZE)

Barotitis can range from symptoms of pain or fullness without otoscopic changes, to hemorrhage within the tympanic membrane or hemorrhage into the middle ear with hemotympanum. Ultimately, the tympanic membrane may rupture, resulting in relief of the pain but also possibly causing an influx of water into the middle ear. This, in turn, might cause calorically induced vertigo and potential panic, drowning, or other injury.

Barotitis is treated conservatively with analgesics and decongestants. If tympanic membrane rupture occurs, antibiotics can be prescribed, especially if the diving occurred in contaminated water. Divers with perforated tympanic membranes should refrain from diving until the perforation heals. Most such perforations heal without difficulty, but referral to an otolaryngologist is appropriate for individuals with larger perforations or when healing does not occur. Divers with barotitis without perforation

TABLE 214-1 Summary of Barotrauma of Descent and Ascent

Barotrauma	Clinical Features	Treatment
Barotrauma of descent		
Otic barotrauma ("ear squeeze")	Pain, fullness, vertigo, conductive hearing loss from inability to equalize middle ear pressure	Decongestants, consider antibiotics
Sinus barotrauma ("sinus squeeze")	Pain over affected sinus, possible bleeding from nares	Decongestants, consider antibiotics
Inner ear barotrauma	Sudden onset of sensorineural hearing loss, tinnitus, severe vertigo after forced Valsalva	Head of bed up, no nose blowing, antivertigo medications, and urgent otolaryngology consultation as some surgeons advocate early exploration
Barotrauma of ascent		
Pulmonary overinflation syndromes (pulmonary barotrauma)	Dyspnea, chest pain, subcutaneous air, extra-alveolar air on radiograph; usually occurring secondary to rapid or uncontrolled ascent	Pneumomediastinum requires only symptomatic care and does not require recompression Pneumothorax requires drainage and does not require recompression (if recompression is instituted for treatment of arterial gas embolism, then the pneumothorax must be drained before recompression)
Arterial gas embolism	Neurologic symptoms occurring immediately after uncontrolled or rapid ascent or neurologic symptoms in the setting of pulmonary barotrauma	Airway, breathing, circulation, high-flow oxygen, IV hydration, immediate recompression (hyperbaric oxygen), consider adjunctive lidocaine Any neurologic symptom in the setting of documented pulmonary barotrauma must be treated as an arterial gas embolism

should refrain from diving until the diver is again able to equalize the pressure in the affected middle ear.

EXTERNAL EAR SQUEEZE

If the external canal is occluded by cerumen or an ear plug, the inability to equalize pressure between the external canal and the tympanic membrane causes the bending of the tympanic membrane outward, producing an injury called "external ear squeeze" that produces pain and tympanic membrane hemorrhage.

SINUS BAROTRAUMA

If the ostia to the sinuses are occluded, air cannot enter the sinuses during descent to equalize the increasing pressure. This causes pain and mucosal edema and can lead to submucosal hemorrhage and stripping of the sinus mucosa from bone, hemorrhage (often causing bleeding from the nose into the mask), and, rarely, paresthesias in the infraorbital nerve distribution. A similar traumatic neuropathy can occur to the facial nerve with middle ear barotrauma. Sinus barotrauma is treated with conservative measures, including decongestants and, possibly, antibiotics.

INNER EAR BAROTRAUMA

The inner ear is also susceptible to barotrauma, occasionally causing significant, long-term damage. If a diver attempts a forceful Valsalva maneuver to equalize the middle ear against an occluded Eustachian tube, the pressure differential between the cerebrospinal fluid, transmitted through the vestibular and cochlear structures and the middle ear air space, can cause rupture of the oval or round window, fistulization of the window, tearing of the vestibular membrane, or a combination of such injuries. Additionally, if the diver is able to open the Eustachian tube in this situation, a rapid increase in middle ear pressure may occur. This pressure wave is transmitted to the inner ear and can also cause a similar injury. Divers with inner ear barotrauma will generally present with unilateral roaring tinnitus, sensorineural hearing loss, and profound vertigo. A "fistula test" may be positive—that is, insufflation of the tympanic membrane on the affected side causes the eyes to deviate to the contralateral side. Because this injury usually occurs on descent and divers will provide a history of difficulty clearing the ears, this condition can usually be easily differentiated from other causes of vertigo, such as inner ear decompression sickness, cerebral arterial gas embolism, or alternobaric vertigo (discussed below).

Immediate complications of inner ear barotrauma are potential panic or disorientation, leading to possible drowning or a rapid ascent that predisposes the diver to pulmonary barotrauma. Divers with barotraumatic injuries to the inner ear require urgent otolaryngologic evaluation. Treatment is controversial, with some authors advocating immediate exploration and others suggesting a trial of bed rest (head upright), medications to control vertigo, and mechanical measures to reduce cerebrospinal fluid pressure spikes (e.g., stool softeners, no nose blowing). These authors reserve exploration for patients whose symptoms do not respond to conservative therapy or patients with severe hearing defects or significant abnormalities on an oculo-nystagmogram. Divers with potential inner ear barotrauma who will be treated with hyperbaric oxygen for decompression sickness or cerebral arterial gas embolism require emergent tympanostomy, because hyperbaric treatment will recreate the same pressure differentials that caused the injury, potentially causing more perilymph leakage and, possibly, worsening the injury.[2]

FACE SQUEEZE, TOOTH SQUEEZE, AND DRY-SUIT SQUEEZE

Other air-containing structures can be compressed during descent, producing "squeeze" symptoms. A face squeeze occurs when air is not added to the facemask during descent, causing the face and eyes to be forced into the collapsing mask. This can produce facial bruising, conjunctival injection or hemorrhage, changes in vision, and, rarely, retrobulbar hemorrhage. The latter could be a true ophthalmologic emergency. A tooth squeeze occurs when air spaces inside a tooth—due to decay, a filling, or an abscess—become compressed during descent. A dry-suit squeeze occurs when suit folds are compressed into the underlying skin, producing local trauma manifested by painful red streaks.

BAROTRAUMA OF ASCENT

The clinical conditions of barotrauma of ascent are alternobaric vertigo, pulmonary barotrauma, arterial gas embolism, and decompression sickness (Table 214-1).

ALTERNOBARIC VERTIGO

During ascent, the physics of gas in air-containing organs is, of course, opposite that of descent—that is, air will expand as the pressure decreases. Air will flow through the ostia of the sinuses, and the expanding air in the middle ear will open the Eustachian tube (much like during takeoff in an airplane). Should air be trapped temporarily in one middle ear cavity, the pressure differential may cause unequal vestibular impulses to the brain, resulting in vertigo (alternobaric vertigo). This is usually transient and generally requires no specific treatment.

PULMONARY BAROTRAUMA

Air also expands within the lungs with ascent. If a diver breathing compressed air ascends with a closed glottis (holds breath, coughs, vomits), most frequently seen in a rapid, panicked, out-of-air ascent, the expanding air may cause parenchymal lung injury. This can occur even in shallow water (e.g., a swimming pool). Pulmonary barotrauma, also called *pulmonary overinflation* or *burst lung syndrome*, can lead to pneumomediastinum. This generally only requires symptomatic treatment and may be subtle on the chest radiograph.[3] Mediastinal air can track superiorly into the neck, resulting in subcutaneous air on physical examination or air on a cervical spine radiograph. Pulmonary overinflation injury can cause pneumothorax, requiring aspiration or air or tube thoracostomy. If air enters the pulmonary venous circulation, embolization of the gas through the arterial system occurs. The most sensitive end-organ to such embolization is the brain, and *cerebral arterial gas embolism* is the term applied to this condition, although the air emboli distribute to other tissues and organs.[4] **Any neurologic symptom or sign referable to the circulation to the CNS in the setting of barotrauma associated with ascent should be considered to be secondary to cerebral arterial gas embolism.** The symptoms, signs, and treatment are discussed below in the section "Arterial Gas Embolism."

Pulmonary barotrauma (**Figure 214-1**) can occur without a rapid ascent or closed glottis in divers with congenital cysts, obstructive pulmonary disease, or other processes that cause air trapping.

OTHER BAROTRAUMAS OF ASCENT

An air pocket underneath a tooth may equilibrate with ambient pressure while diving, only to expand during ascent. This produces severe pain and may dislodge a filling or fracture a tooth. Swallowed air during diving may expand during ascent, rarely producing gastric distention and abdominal cramps.

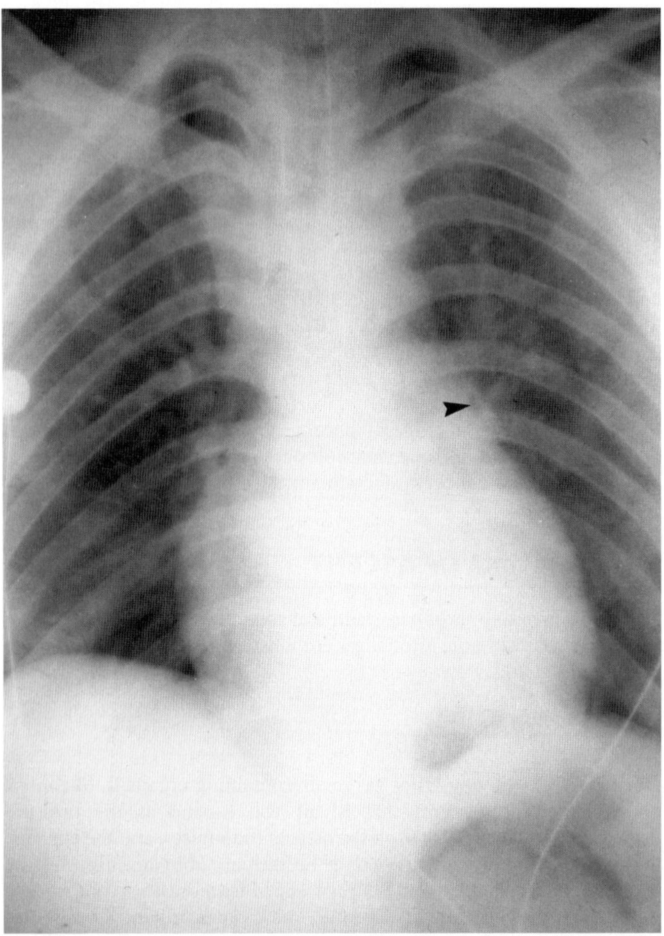

FIGURE 214-1. Pulmonary barotrauma. Note the air in the mediastinum in this radiography (*arrow*). There is also air in the soft tissues of the neck.

DECOMPRESSION SICKNESS

The pathophysiology of decompression sickness is related to the obstructive and inflammatory effects of inert gas bubbles in tissues and the vascular system.[4] Decompression sickness may occur in divers breathing compressed air, caisson workers, high-altitude pilots, or astronauts. Bubbles may form when a body with additional inert gas in solution experiences a decrease in ambient pressure that causes liberation of the gas. Uptake of inert gas occurs at different rates in different tissues.

The U.S. Navy publishes dive tables to provide the limits to a dive (measured by bottom depth and time) that can be undertaken without a decompression stop ("no decompression" or "no stop" dives). Other Navy tables provide a variety of decompression schedules for longer dives. A multitude of dive computers, often using proprietary mathematical models, provide divers with relatively safe diving limits. Decompression sickness is unlikely to occur if the limits of the dive tables or dive computer are followed, but compliance with dive table limits or a dive computer does not completely eliminate risk.

Bubbles are necessary but not sufficient by themselves to cause decompression sickness; bubbling occurs after many dive profiles that do not lead to decompression sickness. Obviously, there must be a threshold at which the bubble load causes symptoms. The exact mechanism of bubble formation is not known, although preexisting gas micronuclei in the circulation likely form a nidus for gas accumulation. This is inferred, because the energy required to form bubbles de novo is much higher than the energy state caused by the saturation of inert gas in tissue.[5] Bubbles may form directly in tissues or the circulation (usually the low-pressure venous circulation). Classically, it is thought that bubbles directly obstruct blood flow, leading to direct ischemia. Also, the air–blood and air–endothelial interfaces initiate a variety of inflammatory and thrombotic processes; activate the endothelium, leading to neutrophil adhesion and activation; and change the permeability of the endothelium, resulting in third spacing of fluid. In addition, decompression stress induces the production of microparticles, which are lipid bilayer–enclosed membranous vesicles extruded from vascular endothelial and other cells. Injection of these microparticles in animal models creates a clinical condition consistent with decompression sickness.[6]

There are no current definitive diagnostic criteria for decompression sickness. The San Diego Diving and Hyperbaric Organizations criteria use a point system to identify dive injuries resulting in decompression sickness with a high degree of specificity.[7] This is helpful to create databases of divers with decompression sickness to study outcomes and allow study of adjunctive therapies. Unfortunately, this system has relatively low sensitivity. Studies of therapies for decompression sickness often lack an acceptable case definition of decompression sickness.

CLINICAL FEATURES

The most commonly used classification divides decompression sickness into two (or sometimes three) main groups (**Table 214-2**). We focus on type I and II for clarity. **Type I** is also called "pain-only" decompression sickness and involves the joints, extremities, and skin ("cutis marmorata"). Lymphatic obstruction can occur in type I, causing lymphedema, which usually takes days to resolve despite recompression therapy. **Type II** involves the CNS (mainly the spinal cord in compressed air divers and the brain in high-altitude decompressions), vestibular symptoms ("staggers"), and cardiopulmonary symptoms ("chokes"). To further complicate the nomenclature and classification of decompression sickness, it can also occur when an arterial gas embolism (see below) causes inert gas to come out of solution after a dive profile that would otherwise not be expected to cause decompression sickness (called type III).[8] Some advocate the use of the alternate term *decompression illness*, instead of differentiating between decompression sickness and cerebral arterial gas embolism, to encompass all pathologic syndromes following a reduction in ambient pressure.[1]

Generally, the symptoms of decompression sickness occur minutes to several hours after surfacing, but in rare cases, symptoms can occur

TABLE 214-2 Classification of Decompression Sickness (DCS)

Classification	Clinical Features	Comments
Type I: "pain-only" DCS	Deep pain in joints and extremities, unrelieved but not worsened with movement	Usually single joint, most commonly knees and shoulders
	Skin changes—mottling, pruritus, and color changes	Lymphatic obstruction can occur and takes days to resolve despite recompression therapy
Type II: "serious" DCS	Pulmonary ("chokes")—cough, hemoptysis, dyspnea, and substernal chest pain	
	Cardiovascular collapse can occur	
	Neurologic—sensation of truncal constriction® ascending paralysis, usually rapid in onset	Has a tendency to affect the lower cervical and thoracic regions may see scattered lesions
		Autonomic dysfunction seen
	Vestibular ("staggers")—vertigo, hearing loss, tinnitus, and disequilibrium	Usually occurs after deep, long dives
Type III: combination of DCS and arterial gas embolism	Symptoms of DCS II noted above plus a variety of stroke syndromes, symptoms, and signs	Symptoms occur on ascent or immediately upon surfacing Symptoms of arterial gas embolism may spontaneously resolve

days after diving. Symptoms occurring between dives may improve during a subsequent dive (as recompression has occurred) but get worse upon resurfacing (as the inert gas load has increased and ambient pressure has decreased). Flying with the resultant decrease in ambient pressure may precipitate or worsen symptoms. For this reason, divers are generally advised to refrain from flying for at least 12 to 24 hours after the last dive depending on the nature of the diving exposure.[9]

Pain Divers with type I decompression sickness typically describe a deep pain, unrelieved but not worsened with movement. This pain can be attributed to or confused with pain caused by injury, potentially making accurate diagnosis difficult. Pain is thought to be due to distention from bubbles in ligaments or fascia, intramedullary bubbles at the ends of long bones, or the activation of stretch receptors caused by bubbles in tendons. The mechanism of simple distention of tissues is supported by the rapid improvement of symptoms with recompression. Common pain locations are knees and shoulders, and most often, only a single joint is involved. Decompression sickness in commercial and military divers, caisson workers, and aviators tends to manifest most often as joint pain. Sport divers, who usually perform multiple dives, often over a period of days, are more prone to spinal cord effects.

Poorly localized and difficult-to-describe back or abdominal pain may herald the more serious signs of spinal cord involvement.

Pulmonary Symptoms Pulmonary symptoms, generally seen usually only after more prolonged exposures, are caused by large numbers of pulmonary artery bubbles and include symptoms of cough, hemoptysis, dyspnea, and substernal chest pain. Cardiovascular collapse can occur.

Neurologic Symptoms The classic description of divers with neurologic decompression sickness (type II) can begin with a sensation of truncal constriction or girdle-like pain. Often a wooly feeling begins in the feet, developing into an ascending paralysis, producing symptoms of transverse myelitis. This form is usually rapid in onset and has a tendency to affect the lower cervical and thoracic regions. However, in type II decompression sickness, neurologic deficits do not necessarily cause distinct spinal cord syndromes (i.e., an anterior or posterior spinal artery syndrome), nor will a definitive level necessarily be found, as lesions may be scattered throughout the spinal cord.[10] Autonomic involvement, with resulting incontinence and sexual dysfunction, is not uncommon. The pathophysiology of spinal cord decompression sickness seems to be initial bubbling in the low-pressure venous plexus system that first impedes and then obstructs venous outflow from the cord. Decreasing venous blood flow prevents dissolved nitrogen in spinal cord tissues from egressing, and in situ bubbles within the spinal cord develop (called *autochthonous bubbles*).

Vestibular Symptoms Vestibular decompression sickness usually occurs after deep, long dives, although it has been reported in sport divers. Signs are vertigo, hearing loss, tinnitus, and disequilibrium. The vestibular syndrome can be differentiated from inner ear barotrauma mainly by the history, because patients with inner ear barotrauma develop symptoms in the water and, generally, immediately after a forced Valsalva maneuver to equalize the middle ear pressure.[11]

Other, nonspecific symptoms such as headache, nausea, dizziness, or unusual fatigue are also reported. It may be difficult to differentiate fatigue from decompression sickness from the expected fatigue from the exertion of diving.

Patent Foramen Ovale The association between decompression sickness and patent foramen ovale is unclear. There appears to be an increased prevalence in patients with inner ear and cutaneous decompression sickness. It is reasonable to screen divers with recurrent, unexplained decompression sickness for a patent foramen ovale. Closure of a large defect will reduce arterialization of venous gas emboli, although it has yet to be shown if such closure will reduce the incidence of subsequent decompression sickness.[12]

ARTERIAL GAS EMBOLISM

Arterial gas embolism occurs when air enters the left side of the vascular system. In the setting of diving, this most often results from pulmonary barotrauma. Arterial gas embolism can also occur as a complication of certain medical procedures, such as central vascular catheterization and cardiac bypass. Air inadvertently introduced into the venous circulation can cross from the right side of the circulation from intracardiac or pulmonary arteriovenous shunts. Air bubbles may also arterialize through these same shunts, sometimes making the source of arterial bubbles difficult to determine.[13] Whatever the source, when air embolizes systemically, distribution depends mainly on blood flow and not gravity.

Clinical Features The most dramatic effect of arterial gas embolism is on the brain, resulting in a variety of stroke syndromes, symptoms, and signs, depending on the part of the brain affected. Rarely, diving-related arterial gas embolism from pulmonary barotrauma causes immediate apnea and cardiac arrest. The mechanism of cardiovascular collapse appears to be air in the entirety of the large arteries and veins of the central vascular bed.[14] The effects of arterial gas embolism secondary to pulmonary barotrauma usually occur on ascent or immediately upon surfacing. If the victim does not die immediately, the symptoms of cerebral arterial gas embolism often include loss of consciousness, seizure, blindness, disorientation, or hemiplegia. Symptoms may spontaneously improve as the gas enters the venous cerebral circulation after a spike in blood pressure. Sometimes, by the time the patient reaches the clinician, the only signs that remain are subtle defects. In particular, parietal lobe signs and symptoms are easily overlooked. A cascade of inflammatory processes also occurs in air embolism, just as in decompression sickness.[4]

Laboratory Testing The hematocrit may elevate from hemoconcentration and third spacing of fluids. The creatine phosphokinase (and other enzymes such as lactate dehydrogenase, alanine aminotransferase, and aspartate aminotransferase) will become elevated secondary to the systemic distribution of bubbles. The degree of elevation of creatine phosphokinase corresponds to the embolism severity. Cardiac troponins may also be elevated and most likely do not represent occlusive coronary artery disease.[4]

Treatment of Decompression Sickness and Arterial Gas Embolism **The treatment includes administering 100% oxygen, increasing tissue perfusion with IV fluids, and rapid recompression.** Some advocate placing patients with air embolism in the Trendelenburg position or in the left lateral decubitus position to "trap" air in the left ventricle. By the time the victim is brought onto the dive boat or the ambulance arrives, the air has usually been distributed, and the Trendelenburg position merely increases intracranial pressure, decreases cerebral perfusion, and interferes with other first aid measures. Nonetheless, some divers with arterial gas embolism have collapsed when placed in a sitting or standing position. **As a result, a supine position—not Trendelenburg position—is recommended for patients with arterial gas embolism.** Vomiting patients should be placed in the lateral decubitus position to prevent aspiration.

Recompression therapy with hyperbaric oxygen treats by several mechanisms. See the chapter 21, titled "Hyperbaric Oxygen Therapy" for detailed discussion. The administered pressure decreases the size of bubbles, and the high partial pressure of oxygen in solution increases inert gas washout from bubbles and tissue. Mass action dictates a gas will travel down pressure gradients; therefore, nitrogen will move from bubbles with a high partial pressure of nitrogen into plasma, where it will travel to the lungs and be exhaled. Conversely, oxygen from plasma with a high partial pressure of oxygen will enter bubbles, but ultimately will diffuse into cells and be metabolized, further reducing bubble size. Hyperbaric oxygen also decreases tissue edema, increases oxygen delivery to ischemic tissues, and reduces neutrophil adhesion to the endothelium and neutrophil activation.[15]

Recompression using the U.S. Navy Treatment Table 6 is a commonly used method of management for decompression sickness, employing a maximal treatment pressure of 2.8 ATA (60 fsw). Table 6 is also used for air embolism, although some advocate an initial pressurization to 6 ATA (165 fsw) to maximize bubble compression, then continuation at 2.8 ATA (U.S. Navy Table 6A). Different treatment tables are used in other parts of the world, and there is some experience using lower treatment pressures for decompression sickness in monoplace chambers with reportedly comparable results.[16] Some patients may benefit from repeated treatments if symptoms do not fully resolve. Recompression should occur as soon as possible, and it should not be withheld in cases with delayed presentation.[4] Additionally, for divers who have missed needed decompression stops because of an emergency ascent or nonadherence to appropriate diving tables, it may be appropriate for them to undergo recompression therapy *even if asymptomatic*. U.S. Navy Table 5 recompression would usually be adequate in such a circumstance.

The administration of IV lidocaine as a therapeutic adjunct for cerebral arterial gas embolism has been advocated, because it appears to decrease neuropsychiatric deficits when given during anesthesia for cardiac procedures requiring bypass,[17-19] since bypass operations commonly cause the entry of air into the arterial system. Dosing of lidocaine in this setting is not standardized, although typical cardiac dosing is commonly used.[20]

The **Divers Alert Network** (telephone: 1-919-684-9111; Web site: http://www.diversalertnetwork.org) has staff available 24 hours a day to provide assistance to divers and to help clinicians treat patients with decompression sickness or arterial gas embolism. The Divers Alert Network can provide information and the location of the nearest recompression facility around the world.

SPECIAL CONSIDERATIONS

ASTHMA

There is some debate over the safety of diving for individuals with asthma. Although the relative risk of pulmonary barotrauma may be higher in asthmatics (possibly as much as twice that of the general diving population), the absolute risk is still low because of the rarity of pulmonary barotrauma in diving (approximately 1 in 125,000 dives).[21] A physician who specializes in diving medicine should examine divers or potential divers with asthma, and an exercise pulmonary function test should be performed. Asthmatics can be cleared for diving if, using their usual medications, they have a normal exercise pulmonary function test and if they understand the potential increased risk of pulmonary barotrauma.[22] A diver who develops a lung injury that cannot be explained by the circumstances of the dive (i.e., the diver did not have a rapid, breath-holding ascent) should be evaluated for congenital or acquired structural lung disease and should probably no longer dive.

IMMERSION PULMONARY EDEMA

Pulmonary edema can occur while diving. Because the first reported cases occurred in cold water, this condition was first described as "cold water" or "cold-induced" pulmonary edema. However, many cases have subsequently been reported in warm water, up to 27°C (80.6°F).[23] Typical symptoms of pulmonary edema (dyspnea, chest discomfort, coughing up pink frothy secretions) occur at depth and usually improve over time or with standard treatments for pulmonary edema. The cause is unknown despite human studies.[24] This syndrome generally occurs in divers with no structural or ischemic heart disease, but diagnostic evaluation for heart conditions is indicated for those with risk factors for underlying heart disease. Immersion pulmonary edema is not caused by decompression and is not treated with recompression therapy. Interestingly, some divers will experience repeated episodes, whereas others may never experience another episode.

NITROGEN NARCOSIS

Inert gas narcosis occurs when air is breathed at a depth of 100 fsw or greater. Symptoms include loss of fine motor skills and high-order mental processes as well as behavior similar to that seen in alcohol intoxication. Symptoms increase as depth is increased beyond 100 fsw. Divers have codified this increase in symptoms as the "martini rule" (with many variations). A common description is that each 33 ft of depth (1 ATA) in excess of 100 fsw is the equivalent to drinking one martini. Nitrogen narcosis can cause divers to engage in dangerous or foolish activities during deep dives. At depths greater than 300 fsw, unconsciousness may occur from the anesthetic effect of nitrogen. At depths greater than 200 fsw, helium is often used in place of nitrogen in gas mixtures to prevent nitrogen narcosis.

OXYGEN TOXICITY

Oxygen toxicity usually affects the lungs or brain, depending on the partial pressure of oxygen delivered and duration of exposure. Pulmonary oxygen toxicity generally occurs at lower partial pressures of oxygen but with longer exposures, whereas cerebral oxygen toxicity occurs at high partial pressures with generally short exposures. Pulmonary oxygen toxicity can occur at partial pressures of oxygen at or below 1 ATA, for example, in patients requiring prolonged mechanical ventilation with high fractions of inspired oxygen. Pulmonary oxygen toxicity is unusual in diving.

Cerebral oxygen toxicity most often occurs with partial pressures of oxygen >1.4 ATA in the water. Some divers may breathe "nitrox" or *oxygen-enriched air* with fractions of oxygen of 32% to 36%. Therefore, cerebral oxygen toxicity can occur at lesser depths and actually is the factor that limits diving depth with nitrox. Additionally, there are rebreather systems (*closed-circuit systems*), with the diver breathing within a continuous circuit of gas that has a very high fraction of oxygen (>95%), with carbon dioxide being scrubbed out. With these systems, cerebral oxygen toxicity can occur at depths as little as 25 ft.

Signs and symptoms of cerebral oxygen toxicity include twitching, nausea, paresthesias, dizziness, and seizures. If a seizure develops in the water as the initial manifestation of cerebral oxygen toxicity, drowning may result. High partial pressures of oxygen are used clinically in hyperbaric chambers (2.4 ATA, 2.8 ATA, and sometimes 3.0 ATA), but cerebral oxygen toxicity in this setting is rare, reported in <1 per 1000 patients. This is because patients in hyperbaric chambers are dry, warm, and at rest, while divers are wet, often cold, and exerting themselves—and all of these latter factors exacerbate cerebral oxygen toxicity. Cerebral oxygen toxicity is affected by partial pressure of arterial carbon dioxide and cerebral blood flow and may be caused by an increase in nitric oxide production, although this is still an area of active investigation.[25]

Besides nitrogen narcosis and oxygen toxicity, other gas-related conditions important in diving medicine are toxicity from carbon monoxide and the adverse effects of elevated partial pressures of carbon dioxide. Additional issues, especially with very deep dives, include heat loss from breathing helium and the high-pressure nervous syndrome, characterized by tremor and loss of fine motor function caused by the direct effects of pressure.

OTHER CONDITIONS

Injuries and medical conditions occurring during and immediately after compressed air diving are often misattributed as decompression sickness or cerebral arterial gas embolism. Be aware that any medical condition can occur under the water. Acute myocardial infarction, pulmonary embolism, stroke, seizure, encephalitis, and even appendicitis have been erroneously attributed to diving. True diving accidents or cardiac sudden death can be misattributed to drowning—a common final pathway of submersion.[26]

REFERENCES

The complete reference list is available online at www.TintinalliEM.com.

CHAPTER 215 Drowning

Stephen John Cico
Linda Quan

INTRODUCTION AND EPIDEMIOLOGY

Drowning is submersion in a liquid medium resulting in respiratory difficulty or arrest.[1] As with other causes of accidental death, drowning injury typically involves otherwise healthy, young individuals, but can involve individuals of any age or background.

Worldwide, drowning accounts for >500,000 deaths annually and is the leading cause of injury death among children <15 years of age. In the United States, there are >500,000 drowning events each year and 1100 deaths, which makes drowning the second leading cause of unintentional death of individuals from birth to age 19 years old.[2,3] However, the rate of drowning deaths has decreased over the past 40 years. In 1970, there were nearly 8000 deaths due to drowning in the United States,[4] and education with public awareness has been the major contributor to the decreased incidence. The vast majority of victims survive submersion events, with effects ranging from minimal or transient injury to profound neurologic insult.

Drowning incidence peaks in three age groups: The highest is in children <5 years old, the second peak is in those aged 15 to 24 years, and the third peak is in the elderly. Toddlers drown primarily after falling into swimming pools or open water, but they also drown in bathtubs and buckets in the home. Physicians also need to evaluate for intentional drowning (child abuse) or factitious disorder by proxy (formerly Munchausen's by proxy). In teenagers and adults, suicide, homicide, and domestic violence can be causes of drowning. The elderly also have an increased risk of bathtub drowning, often related to comorbid medical conditions or medications. Even in coastal areas, most drownings take place in warm, freshwater bodies of water (especially swimming pools).

TABLE 215-1 Disorders and Injuries Associated with Drowning

Disorders Associated with Drowning
Alcohol or other intoxicants
Syncope (e.g., due to hyperventilation prior to underwater diving)
Seizures
Cardiac conditions (e.g., dysrhythmias including prolonged QT syndromes, Brugada's syndrome, ischemic heart disease)
Dementia
Intentional (suicide, homicide, child abuse or neglect in young children)
Injuries Associated with Drowning
Spinal cord injuries due to diving into shallow water, significant falls from heights, or boating/personal watercraft mishaps
Hypothermia
Aspiration
Respiratory failure, insufficiency, or distress

Additional injuries or disorders that either precipitate or are associated with drowning events are shown in **Table 215-1**.

PATHOPHYSIOLOGY

After submersion, the degree of hypoxic insult to the central nervous system determines the ultimate outcome. It was previously thought that parasympathetic activation of the **diving reflex** (i.e., bradycardia, apnea, peripheral vasoconstriction, and central shunting of blood flow) provided transient protection during submersion. The diving reflex is strongest in infants <6 months of age, but the effects decrease with age.[5] In adults, vertical immersion (head out) and vertical submersion (head under) activate both the sympathetic and parasympathetic systems, which blunts any effect of the diving reflex.[6] Furthermore, physiologic stress associated with submersion also activates the sympathetic nervous system. Thus, the diving reflex is not protective. Cerebral protection in cold water submersions most likely results from rapid central nervous system cooling before significant hypoxic damage occurs.

Physiologic scoring systems[7,8] to predict drowning outcome have been devised but are not clinically helpful. The vast majority of patients who arrive at the hospital with stable cardiovascular signs and awake, alert neurologic function survive with minimal disability, whereas those who arrive with unstable cardiovascular function and coma do poorly because of the hypoxic-ischemic insult. Predictors are not accurate for the 15% to 20% of drowning victims whose condition on arrival is between these two extremes.[9]

End organs can also be affected by hypoxemia and metabolic acidosis. Aspiration of substances such as contaminated foreign material, particulate matter, bacteria, vomitus, or chemical irritants can affect eventual pulmonary recovery. **Electrolyte abnormalities are seldom significant and are usually transient unless there is significant hypoxia, central nervous system depression, renal injury from hemoglobinuria, or myoglobinuria.**[8,9] Hematologic values are usually normal unless there has been massive hemolysis. Disseminated intravascular coagulation can be a complicating factor in drowning outcome but usually occurs following severe hypoxic insult.

TREATMENT

PREHOSPITAL CARE

Rapid resuscitation of a drowning victim (quickly restoring ventilation and oxygenation) optimizes outcome. After safe removal of the victim from the water, CPR should be initiated as quickly as possible. Trauma as a cause of drowning is uncommon, and most injured drowning patients have a history of trauma or signs of injury on examination.[10] Cervical spine injury is rare (0.5%) in drowning unless there is a history of diving, falling from a significant height, or motorized vehicle crash.[11] Use cervical spine precautions if the history warrants it.

Administer high-flow oxygen by facemask if the patient is breathing or by positive-pressure bag-valve mask ventilation if the patient is not breathing. For patients who do not recover spontaneous respiratory effort, endotracheal intubation and positive-pressure ventilation are necessary.

All patients with drowning amnesia for the event, loss of or depressed consciousness, or an observed period of apnea, as well as those who require a period of artificial ventilation, should be transported to an ED for evaluation, even if they are asymptomatic at the scene. The patient should be warmed and monitored, and IV access should be established (**Figure 215-1**).

ED MANAGEMENT

Upon the patient's arrival at the ED, **assess and secure the airway, provide oxygen, determine core temperature, and assist ventilation as necessary**. If the patient is hypothermic, administer warmed isotonic IV fluids and apply warming adjuncts (e.g., blankets, overhead warmers, warming devices). Address any associated injuries. **Because cervical injury is rare without a history of diving or associated trauma, routine cervical immobilization and CT of the brain are not necessary.**[11]

Patients who present to the ED with a Glasgow Coma Scale score of >13 and an oxygen saturation of ≥95% are at low risk for complications (Figure 215-1) and should be observed for 4 to 6 hours. If the pulmonary examination does not reveal rales, rhonchi, wheezing, or retractions and arterial oxygen saturation on room air remains ≥95%, the patient can be safely discharged home. Laboratory studies and radiographs are unnecessary and are not predictive of discharge.[12] The patient should be told to return if fever, mental status changes, or pulmonary symptoms occur. If, after 4 to 6 hours, the patient develops an oxygen requirement, the findings on pulmonary examination are abnormal (rales, rhonchi, wheeze, retractions, etc.), or the patient's condition deteriorates, reassessment and admission or transfer to a monitored bed are needed.

Patients who present to the ED with a Glasgow Coma Scale score of <13 should be maintained on supplemental oxygen and ventilatory support as needed. If high-flow oxygen (fraction of inspired oxygen of 40% to 60%) cannot maintain an adequate partial pressure of arterial oxygen (>60 mm Hg in adults, >80 mm Hg in children), then intubate the patient and provide positive-pressure ventilation. Chest radiography and laboratory studies should be done to evaluate for pulmonary aspiration and other complications (Figure 215-1). Although aspiration is common, prophylactic antibiotics have not been shown to improve outcome and may be associated with resistant infections.[13] Continuous cardiac monitoring, pulse oximetry, temperature monitoring, and frequent reassessments should be performed for all patients. Hypothermia is a concern in patients who have been submerged in cold water (see chapter 209, Hypothermia).

If the patient is normothermic upon arrival in the ED and in cardiopulmonary arrest or asystole, serious thought should be given to discontinuing resuscitation efforts because recovery without profound neurologic complications is rare.[14,15]

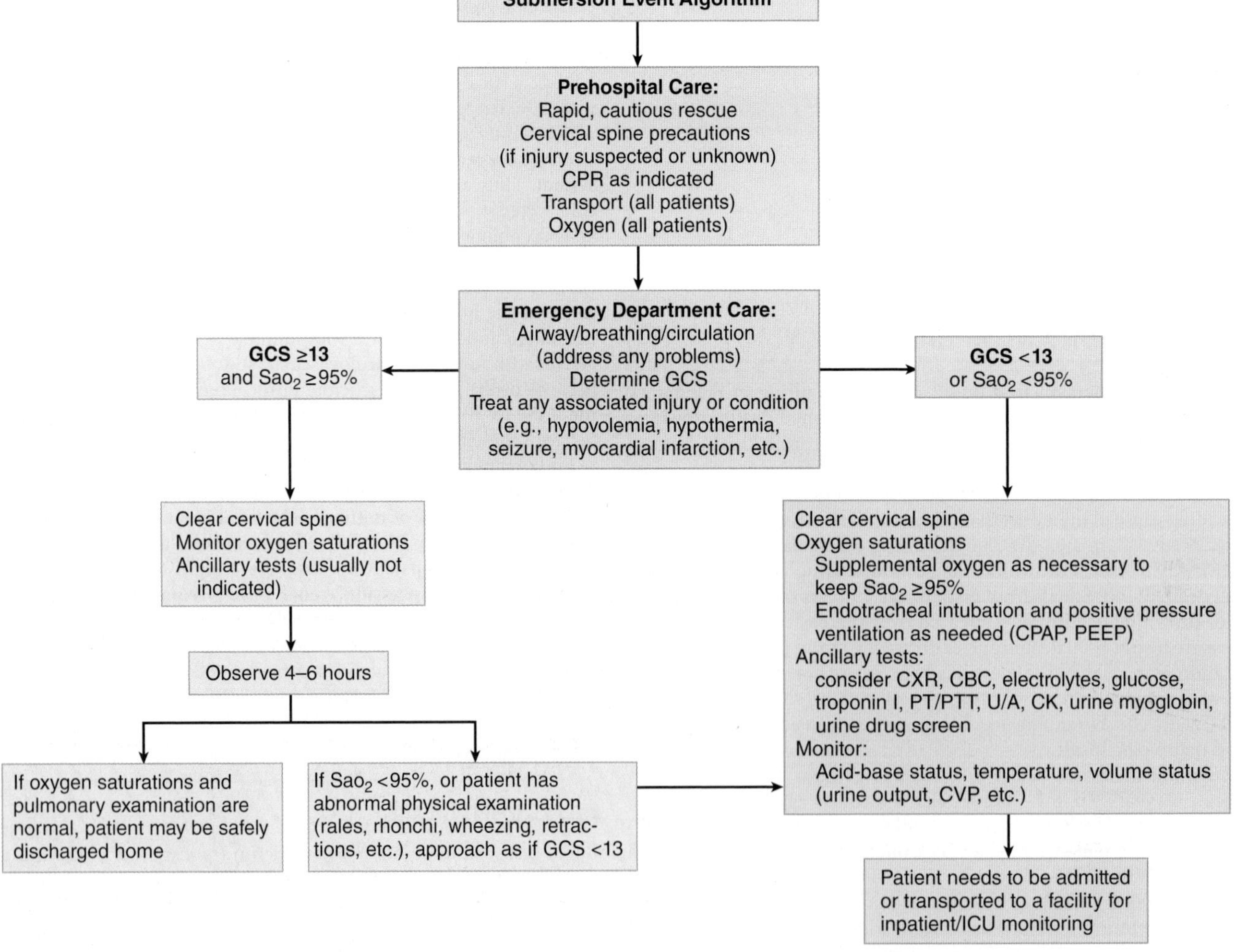

FIGURE 215-1. Drowning event algorithm. CBC = complete blood count; CK = creatine kinase; CPAP = continuous positive airway pressure; CVP = central venous pressure; CXR = chest radiograph; GCS = Glasgow Coma Scale score; ICU = intensive care unit; PEEP = positive end-expiratory pressure; PT = prothrombin time; PTT = partial thromboplastin time; Sao_2 = oxygen saturation (via pulse oximetry); U/A = urinalysis.

CONTINUED MANAGEMENT

Hospital management of drowning victims is largely supportive.[16] All drowning victims who require ED resuscitation should be admitted to an intensive care unit for continuous cardiopulmonary and frequent neurologic monitoring. Most victims of significant submersion injury benefit from mechanical ventilation. Supernormal levels of positive end-expiratory pressure may be used to recruit fluid-filled lung units and aid oxygenation. Most patients demonstrate rapid improvement in oxygenation in the first 24 hours. Patients presenting with a significant aspiration pattern or cardiovascular collapse are predisposed to develop acute respiratory distress syndrome. Although prophylactic antibiotics lack supporting evidence, delayed pulmonary infection, particularly among patients requiring mechanical ventilation, is a risk, and unusual organisms, including *Aeromonas* species, should be considered if treatment is initiated. Care should be taken to avoid lung overdistention and ventilator-associated barotrauma.

For patients who have been resuscitated from cardiac arrest, the hemodynamic response to exogenously administered epinephrine is frequently short-lived, and most require a continuous infusion of dopamine or epinephrine in the ED or intensive care unit. Invasive (pulmonary artery catheter) or noninvasive (echocardiogram) measurement of ventricular function is often instructive. Hemodynamic recovery, when it occurs, can be expected within 48 hours. Patients demonstrating no hemodynamic recovery after 48 hours may slowly improve over the first week but are more likely to have long-term neurologic damage.[17]

Results of "brain resuscitation" after significant warm water drowning have been disappointing.[9,16] The degree of cerebral edema is largely determined by the duration of the anoxic or ischemic insult at the time of submersion. Efforts to control cerebral edema, including the use of mannitol, loop diuretics, hypertonic saline, fluid restriction, and mechanical hyperventilation, have not shown benefit.[16] Controlled hypothermia, barbiturate "coma," and intracranial pressure monitoring do not improve outcome in pediatric drowning victims.[9] Although rare, complete or near-complete neurologic recovery after asystole has been reported in both children and adults after icy water submersion episodes.

PROGNOSIS, DISPOSITION, AND FOLLOW-UP

Family members should be counseled about likely outcome. Based on initial presentation, resuscitation, laboratory data, and serial examinations, experienced practitioners should be able to provide accurate predictions of outcomes in most cases.[17] There are no standardized terms for describing drowning incidents.[1] This chapter uses the terms *asymptomatic* and *symptomatic drowning.*

ASYMPTOMATIC DROWNING

Drowning victims who are asymptomatic or mildly symptomatic can be observed for 4 to 6 hours. If the findings of pulmonary examination and oxygen saturation on room air remain normal, patients can be discharged home. If deterioration is going to occur, it will do so within the 4- to 6-hour observation period.[12,18,19] No data are available regarding long-term outcomes, but it is unlikely that there are any measurable adverse effects. Patients and/or parents should be advised to seek medical care for any respiratory complaints or fever.

SYMPTOMATIC DROWNING

Because submersion duration is frequently unknown or only estimated, the extent of required resuscitation is often the most objective measure of the degree of anoxic or ischemic insult (Table 215-2). Details of initial presentation and resuscitation are frequently strong prognostic indicators.

For patients who require hospital admission, if the submersion victim does not require cardiopulmonary resuscitation at the scene or in the ED, complete recovery within 48 hours is expected. A small fraction of patients with significant aspiration may develop severe, even life-threatening acute respiratory distress syndrome.

Victims requiring bystander CPR at the scene have a guarded prognosis. Of scene-resuscitated pediatric victims, about 20% later die in the hospital, and about 5% are left with severe hypoxic-ischemic encephalopathy.[15,20] Those victims who demonstrate continuous neurologic and cardiovascular improvement after hospital admission generally make a good recovery. Frequently, neurologic and cardiovascular examinations are normal within 24 hours of the drowning event. Victims who later die in the hospital usually demonstrate deteriorating cardiovascular and neurologic status.

TABLE 215-2 Factors Associated with Poor Resuscitation Prognosis in Near-Drowning

Need for bystander CPR at scene
CPR in the ED
Asystole at scene or in ED after warming

Victims undergoing CPR in the ED have a poor prognosis. Prolonged (>30 minutes) CPR in drowning victims indicates significant anoxic or ischemic insult to the heart, brain, and other vital organs. Complete neurologic recovery is rare, with only anecdotal reports of neurologic recovery after ED CPR of pediatric drowning victims. Asystole, whether noted at the scene or in the ED, is a near-universal sign of poor prognosis in both adult and pediatric drowning injury.[16,21]

For the emergency physician, the answers to the questions of whom and how vigorously to resuscitate remain challenging.[16,20] **Complete or near-complete neurologic recovery after asystole has been reported in both children and adults after drowning in icy water, although such occurrences are rare** and documented mostly in case reports or small series. A large series of 1377 open-water drowning victims found *no* intact survivors among the group submerged for more than 15 minutes, whether in warm or cold water, and there were no survivors of submersion greater than 60 minutes.[22] There was also no difference in survival for children compared with adults in several studies, which contradicts the common belief that pediatric patients do better than adults.[7,21] For asystolic victims of drowning with short submersion durations (i.e., a few minutes) and short transport times who receive CPR en route, a vigorous resuscitation attempt is reasonable.[23] CPR should be abandoned if no response is noted. Conversely, because of the poor prognosis for intact neurologic survival, ED resuscitation attempts can reasonably be withheld from asystolic victims of drowning with longer submersion and transport times.[15,20]

PREVENTION

Submersion episodes in children <1 year of age are best prevented by parental vigilance during bathing. Child abuse or neglect, particularly bathtub drownings in young children, and those with atypical presentations, should be considered.[24] Bath seats may give parents a false sense of reassurance. Parents should never leave infants in bath seats unattended.[25] Bathtub drownings are rare outside of the toddler age range, so abuse or seizures should be suspected.[26] Among preschool children, adult supervision in conjunction with properly installed and maintained four-sided pool fences that completely isolate the pool could prevent 50% to 90% of drownings.[27,28]

Teen and young adult drownings may be reduced by avoiding alcohol and illicit drug use, which has been implicated in 40% of all adult drownings and 75% of boating-related adult drownings.[29] The use of personal flotation devices decreases boating-related drowning deaths.[30] Practical experience suggests that the ability to swim protects against teen and adult drowning, but evidence only supports the efficacy of swimming lessons for decreasing drowning death in young children.[31] Efforts to decrease risk-taking behavior in the high-risk adolescent and young adult age groups need to be developed.

Swimmers with seizure disorders must be constantly monitored by an experienced professional or competent bystander while they are in the water.

In the elderly, drowning locations closely parallel those of infant and toddler drowning. Adequate pool fencing and bathtub handrails are important preventive measures for the elderly population and patients with premorbid conditions.

Acknowledgment: The authors gratefully acknowledge that portions of this chapter are based on previous work by Bruce E. Haynes, Alan L. Causey, and Mark A. Nichter (dec.)

REFERENCES

The complete reference list is available online at www.TintinalliEM.com.

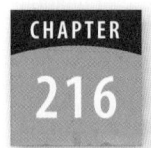

Thermal Burns

E. Paul DeKoning

EPIDEMIOLOGY

An estimated 450,000 individuals in the United States receive medical treatment each year for burn injuries. Although 40,000 patients require hospitalization and more than 60% of those are treated at one of 127 specialized burn centers,[1] the vast majority of burn patients are treated in the acute setting by emergency physicians and discharged with outpatient follow-up.[2,3]

Nearly 70% of burn victims are male,[1] and risk is highest between the ages of 18 and 35. Seventy-seven percent of all injuries are accounted for by fire or scalding; 43% of scald injuries occur in children less than 5 years of age.[4] Although overall survival exceeds 96%, fire, burn, and smoke inhalation still account for approximately 3400 deaths each year in the United States.[1] Elderly patients understandably have a disproportionately higher death rate.[4-6] The risk of death from a major burn increases with larger burn size, older age, the presence of inhalation injury, and female sex.[6]

The Centers for Disease Control and Prevention lists the following groups as being at increased risk of fire-related injuries and death: children ≤4 years of age, adults ≥65 years of age, African Americans and Native Americans, persons living in rural areas, persons living in manufactured homes or substandard housing, and persons living in poverty.[7]

Care of the acute burn–injured patient has improved significantly over the last several decades.[8,9] The rate of hospital admissions has decreased owing to improvements in both the acute care provided in the ED and outpatient care at specialized burn centers. Only approximately 4% of those treated in specialized burn treatment centers die from their injuries or associated complications.[4,10]

PATHOPHYSIOLOGY

Skin consists of two layers: the epidermis and the dermis (**Figure 216-1**). Skin thickness varies both by age and anatomic location: it is relatively thinner at extremes of age, whereas it is thicker on the palms, soles, and upper back. Thus, the depth and severity of thermal injury varies by both the age of the victim and the anatomic location exposed.

Skin functions as a semipermeable barrier to evaporative water loss, protects against environmental assault, and aids in the control of body temperature, sensation, and excretion. Partial-thickness thermal injury disrupts these barrier functions and contributes to free water deficits. This effect may be significant with moderate to large burns.

Thermal injury results in a spectrum of local and systemic homeostatic disorders that contribute to burn shock (**Table 216-1**). These include disruption of normal cell membrane function, hormonal alterations, acid-base disturbance, hemodynamic changes, and hematologic derangement.

The fluid and electrolyte abnormalities seen in burn shock are largely the result of alterations of cell membrane potential causing intracellular influx of water and sodium, and extracellular migration of potassium, secondary to dysfunction of the sodium pump. In patients with burns greater than 60% of total body surface area, depression of cardiac output results in a lack of response to aggressive volume resuscitation. Although

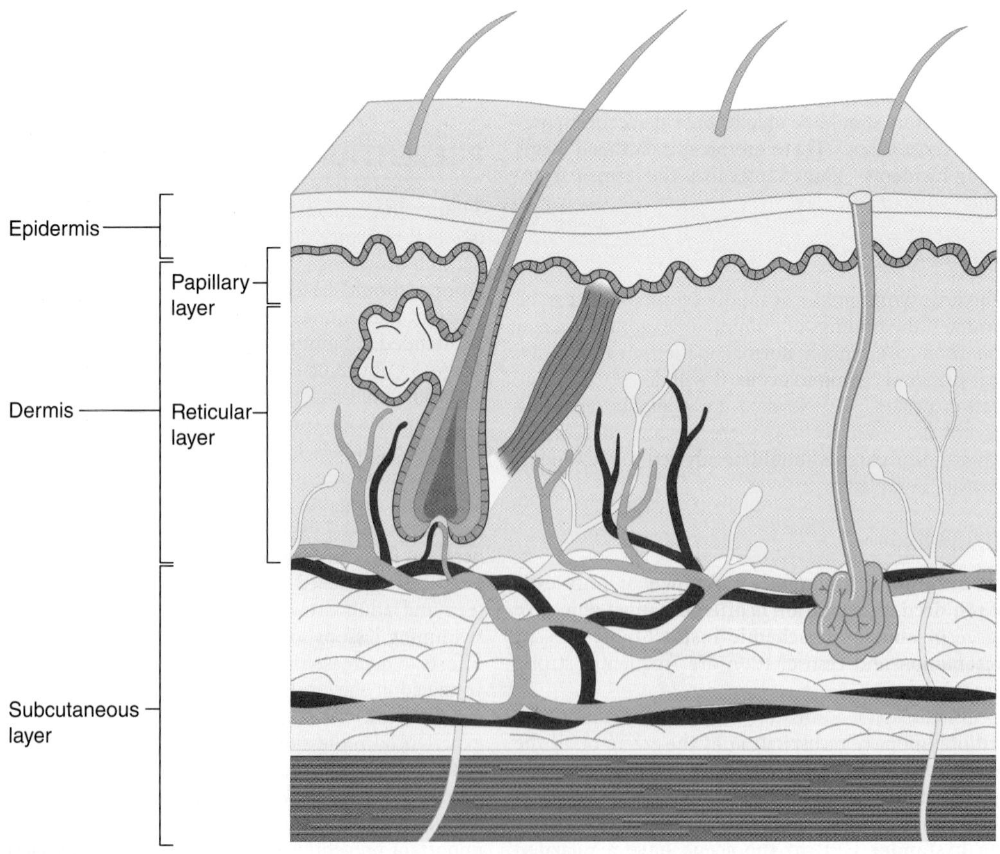

FIGURE 216-1. Layers of the skin.

TABLE 216-1 Physiologic Effects of Thermal Injury

Disruption of sodium pump
Intracellular influx of sodium and water
Extracellular efflux of potassium
Depression of myocardial contractility (>60% of body surface area burned)
Increased systemic vascular resistance
Metabolic acidosis
Increase in hematocrit and increased blood viscosity
Secondary anemia from erythrocyte extravasation and destruction
Local tissue injury
Release of histamines, kinins, serotonins, arachidonic acids, and free oxygen radicals

disputed by others, Baxter and Shires[11] have explained this phenomenon on the basis of circulating myocardial depressants. Systemic vascular resistance is increased. A significant metabolic acidosis may be present even in the early stages of a large burn injury. Massive thermal injury results in an increase in hematocrit with increased blood viscosity during the early phase, followed by anemia from erythrocyte extravasation and destruction. Surprisingly, however, transfusion is seldom required for patients with isolated burn injury, and aggressive transfusion has been associated with increased morbidity and mortality.[12-14]

Thermal injury is progressive. Local effects of thermal injury include the liberation of vasoactive substances, disruption of cellular function, and formation of edema. The subsequent systemic response alters the neurohormonal axis and further extends the injury. Implicated in these events are histamine, kinin, serotonin, arachidonic acid metabolites, and free oxygen radicals. These substances exert their primary effects at the local level and cause progression of the burn wound. **Although many factors may influence prognosis, the severity of the burn, the presence of inhalation injury, associated injuries, the patient's age, comorbid conditions, and acute organ system failure are most important.**[5,6] Cell damage occurs at temperatures of >45°C (113°F) owing to denaturation of cellular protein. The size and depth of the resulting burn are functions of the burning agent, its temperature, and the duration of exposure. Burn wounds are described as having three zones: the zone of coagulation, in which tissue is irreversibly destroyed with thrombosis of blood vessels; the zone of stasis, in which there is *stagnation* of the microcirculation; and the zone of hyperemia, in which there is *increased* blood flow. The zone of stasis can become progressively more hypoxemic and ischemic if resuscitation is not adequate. In the zone of hyperemia, there is minimal damage to the cells and spontaneous recovery is likely.

CLINICAL FEATURES

BURN SIZE

The size of a burn injury is quantified as the percentage of body surface area involved.[9] The **Rule of Nines** is a simple and commonly used method to calculate burn size (**Figure 216-2**), It divides the body into segments that are approximately 9% or multiples of 9%, with the perineum forming the remaining 1%. Because of the proportionately larger heads and smaller legs of infants and children, this method must be modified in pediatric burn injury.

A second method assumes that **the area of the back of the *patient's* hand is approximately 1% of their total body surface area. The number of "hands" that equal the area of the burn can approximate the percentage of body surface area burned.** A third and more precise method uses the **Lund-Browder burn diagram** (**Figure 216-3**). This allows an accurate age-adjusted determination of burn size for a given depth, allowing for the anatomical differences of children.[15]

Experienced burn care nurses and physicians can reliably estimate burn size regardless of the method used. Although it is common for inexperienced individuals to estimate burn size incorrectly when patients are first assessed in the ED, it remains a vital determinant of both fluid resuscitation and the need for ultimate transfer.

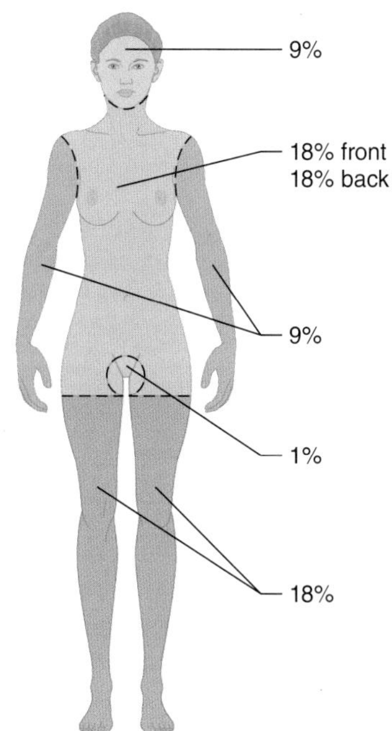

FIGURE 216-2. Rule of Nines diagram for estimation of adult burn size.

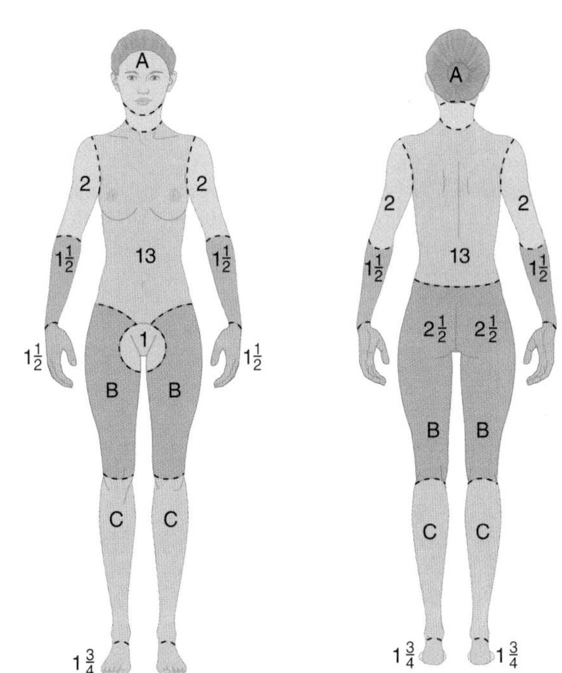

Relative percentages of areas affected by growth (age in years)

	0	1	5	10	15	Adult
A: half of head	$9\frac{1}{2}$	$8\frac{1}{2}$	$6\frac{1}{2}$	$5\frac{1}{2}$	$4\frac{1}{2}$	$3\frac{1}{2}$
B: half of thigh	$2\frac{3}{4}$	$3\frac{1}{4}$	4	$4\frac{1}{4}$	$4\frac{1}{2}$	$4\frac{3}{4}$
C: half of leg	$2\frac{1}{2}$	$2\frac{1}{2}$	$2\frac{3}{4}$	3	$3\frac{1}{4}$	$3\frac{1}{2}$

Second-degree ________________ and

Third-degree ________________ =

Total percent burned ______

FIGURE 216-3. Lund-Browder diagram for estimation of burn size.

TABLE 216-2 Burn Depth Features Classified by Degree of Burn

Burn Depth	Histology/Anatomy	Example	Healing
Superficial (first degree)	Epidermis	Sunburn	7 d
	No blisters, painful		
Superficial partial-thickness (superficial second degree)	Epidermis and superficial dermis	Hot water scald	14–21 d, no scar
	Blisters, very painful		
Deep partial-thickness (deep second degree)	Epidermis and deep dermis, sweat glands, and hair follicles	Hot liquid, steam, grease, flame	3–8 wk, permanent scar
	Blisters, very painful		
Full-thickness (third degree)	Entire epidermis and dermis charred, pale, leathery; no pain	Flame	Months, severe scarring, skin grafts necessary
Fourth degree	Entire epidermis and dermis, as well as bone, fat, and/or muscle	Flame	Months, multiple surgeries usually required

BURN DEPTH

The depth of a burn has historically been described in degrees: first, second, third, and fourth (**Table 216-2**). However, a classification of burn depth according to the need for surgical intervention has become the accepted approach in burn treatment centers: superficial partial-thickness, deep partial-thickness, and full-thickness burns[8] (**Table 216-3**). Determination of burn depth requires clinician judgment using commonly observed wound features. There is no objective method of measuring burn depth, and burn wound biopsy is not routine practice.

A superficial burn involves only the epidermal layer of skin. Sunburn is frequently given as an example, even though it is caused by ultraviolet light instead of thermal injury.[16] **The burned skin is red, painful, and tender without blister formation.** Superficial burns usually heal in about 7 days without scarring and require only symptomatic treatment (**Figure 216-4**).

Partial-thickness burns extend into the dermis and are subdivided into superficial partial-thickness (**Figure 216-5**) and deep partial-thickness burns (**Figure 216-6**).

In superficial partial-thickness burns, the epidermis and the superficial dermis (papillary layer) are injured while the deeper layers of the dermis, hair follicles, and sweat and sebaceous glands are spared. Superficial partial-thickness burns are often caused by hot water scalding. **The skin is blistered, and the exposed dermis is red and moist.** These wounds are exceedingly painful to touch. The dermis is well-perfused with intact capillary refill. Healing typically occurs in 14 to 21 days, scarring is usually minimal, and there is full return of function.

Deep partial-thickness burns extend into the deep dermis (reticular layer) (Figure 216-6). Hair follicles and sweat and sebaceous glands are damaged, but their deeper portions usually survive. Hot liquids (e.g., oil or grease), steam, or flame usually cause this type of injury. **The skin may be blistered, and the exposed dermis is pale white to yellow in color. The burned area does not blanch; it has absent capillary refill and absent pain sensation.** Deep partial-thickness burns may be difficult to distinguish from full-thickness burns. Healing takes 3 weeks to 2 months; scarring is common and related to the depth of the dermal injury. Surgical debridement and skin grafting may be necessary to obtain maximum function.

Full-thickness burns involve the entire thickness of the skin (**Figure 216-7**). All epidermal and dermal structures are destroyed. These injuries are typically caused by flame, hot oil, steam, or contact with hot objects. **The skin is charred, pale, painless, and leathery.**

TABLE 216-3 Burn Depth Features: American Burn Association Burn Classification

Burn Classification	Burn Characteristics	Disposition
Major burn	Partial-thickness >25% BSA, age 10–50 y	Burn center treatment
	Partial-thickness >20% BSA, age <10 y or >50 y	
	Full-thickness >10% BSA in anyone	
	Burns involving hands, face, feet, or perineum	
	Burns crossing major joints	
	Circumferential burns of an extremity	
	Burns complicated by inhalation injury	
	Electrical burns	
	Burns complicated by fracture or other trauma	
	Burns in high-risk patients	
Moderate burn	Partial-thickness 15%–25% BSA, age 10–50 y	Hospitalization
	Partial-thickness 10%–20% BSA, age <10 y or >50 y	
	Full-thickness burns ≤10% BSA in anyone	
	No major burn characteristics present	
Minor burn	Partial-thickness <15% BSA, age 10–50 y	Outpatient treatment
	Partial-thickness <10% BSA, age <10 y or >50 y	
	Full-thickness <2% in anyone	
	No major burn characteristics present	

Abbreviation: BSA = body surface area.

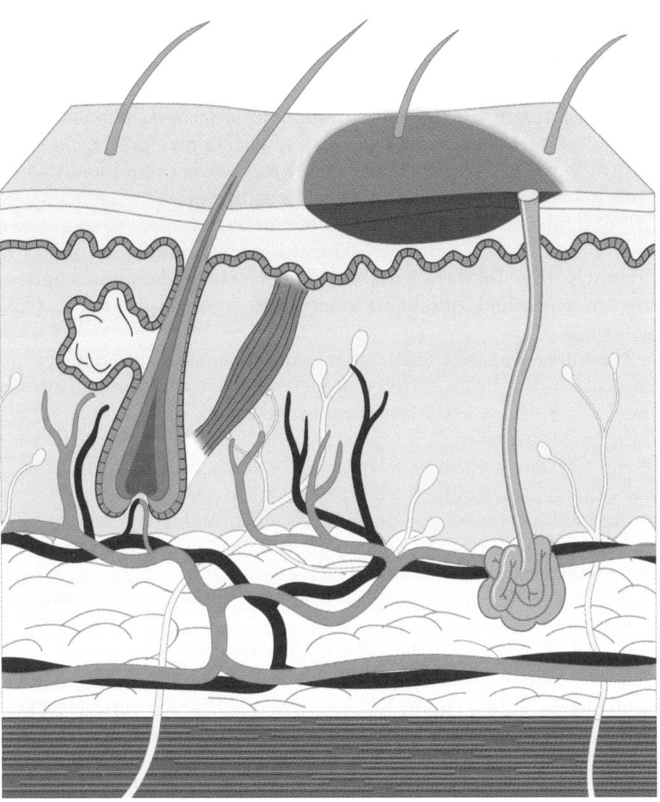

FIGURE 216-4. Superficial burn.

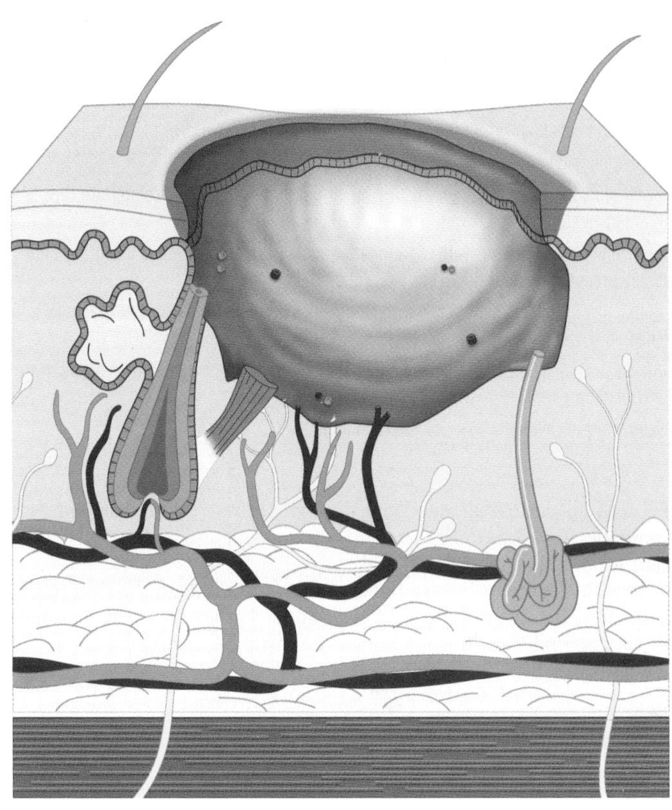

FIGURE 216-6. Deep partial-thickness burn.

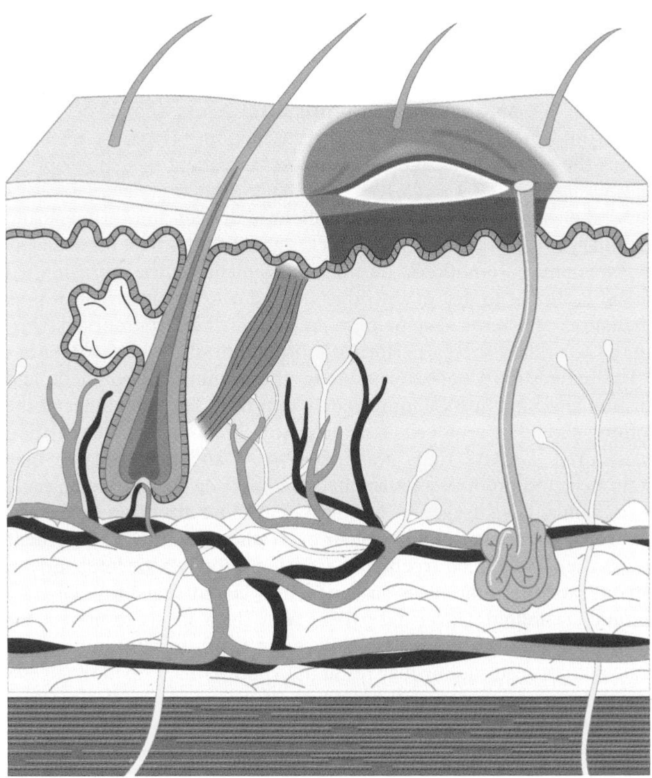

FIGURE 216-5. Superficial partial-thickness burn.

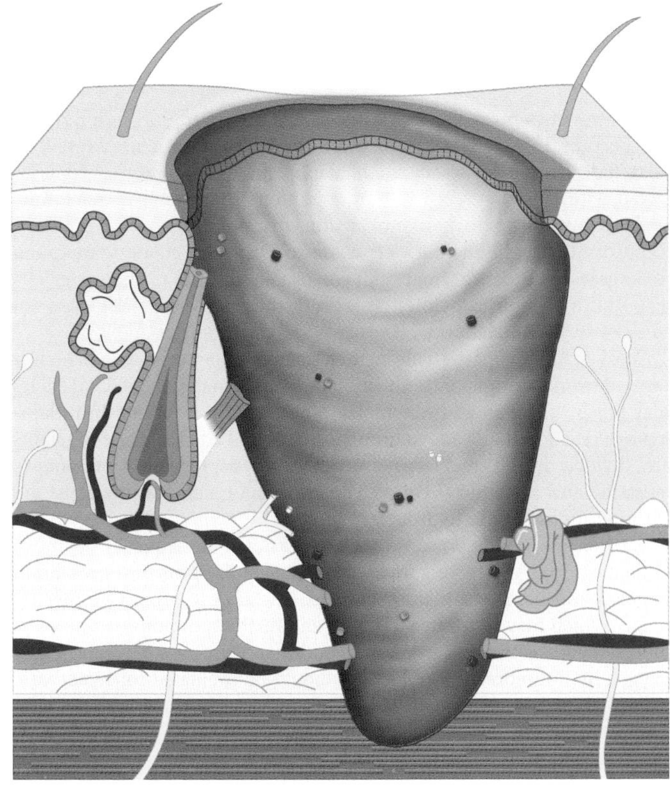

FIGURE 216-7. Full-thickness burn.

TABLE 216-4 American Burn Association Burn Unit Referral Criteria

Full-thickness/third-degree burns in any age group
Electrical burns, including lightning injury
Chemical burns
Inhalation injury
Burn injury in patients with preexisting medical disorders that could complicate management, prolong recovery, or affect mortality
Burn injury in any patients with concomitant trauma (such as fractures) in whom the burn injury poses the greatest risk of morbidity or mortality
Burn injury in children in hospitals without qualified personnel or equipment to care for children
Burn injury in patients who will require special social, emotional, or long-term rehabilitative intervention
Burn injury in children <10 y and adults >50 y of age

Because all dermal elements are destroyed, these injuries do not heal spontaneously. Surgical repair and skin grafting are necessary; significant scarring is the norm.

Fourth-degree burns are those that extend through the skin to the subcutaneous fat, muscle, and even bone. These are devastating, life-threatening injuries. Amputation or extensive reconstruction is sometimes required.

BURN CENTER TRANSFER

The American Burn Association provides guidelines for referral to a burn center, in addition to indications based on burn depth (**Table 216-4**).[9,17] Children <10 years of age and adults >50 years are considered high-risk patients. Patients with significant comorbidities, such as heart disease, diabetes, or chronic pulmonary disease, are also likely to require prolonged care and should be considered for transfer to a burn unit. Burn severity, underlying medical and social conditions, and the capabilities of the institution initially receiving the patient must all be considered in the decision to transfer the patient to a burn unit. As always, use clinical judgment. While some institutions may transfer all burn patients to a burn center, others may choose to care for patients with minor and some moderate burns locally.

INHALATION INJURY

As treatment of burn shock and sepsis has improved, inhalation injury has become the main cause of mortality in burn patients. Most fire-related deaths are due to smoke inhalation.[5,6,10] Inhalation injury is associated with closed-space fires and conditions that decrease mentation, such as overdose, alcohol intoxication, drug abuse, and head injury. Exposure to smoke includes exposure to heat, particulate matter, and toxic gases.[18] Direct thermal injury is usually limited to the upper airway; thermal injuries below the level of the vocal cords can occur in cases of steam inhalation.

Smoke contains particulate matter, usually <0.5 μm in size, which is formed from incomplete combustion of organic material. Small particles may reach the terminal bronchioles, where they can initiate an inflammatory reaction that leads to bronchospasm and edema. Toxic inhalants are divided into three large groups: tissue asphyxiants, pulmonary irritants, and systemic toxins.[18] The two major tissue asphyxiants are carbon monoxide and hydrogen cyanide.

Carbon monoxide poisoning is a well-known consequence of smoke inhalation injury. Severe carbon monoxide poisoning produces brain hypoxia and coma. Comatose patients lose airway protective mechanisms, which may result in aspiration and further pulmonary injury. All patients with suspected carbon monoxide exposure should receive 100% oxygen by nonrebreather mask and should be evaluated for hyperbaric oxygen therapy (see chapter 222, "Carbon Monoxide"). Hydrogen **cyanide** is formed by the combustion of nitrogen-containing polymers such as wool, silk, polyurethane, and vinyl. Cyanide binds to and uncouples mitochondrial oxidative phosphorylation, which leads to profound tissue hypoxia. Specific treatment for cyanide toxicity may be required (see chapter 204, "Industrial Toxins").

Inhalation injury damages endothelial cells, produces mucosal edema of the small airways, and decreases alveolar surfactant activity, resulting in bronchospasm, airflow obstruction, and atelectasis. Bronchospasm may occur early. Although lower airway edema may not be clinically evident for up to 24 hours, upper airway edema can occur rapidly. Over time, tracheal and bronchial epithelial sloughing occurs. Approximately half of intubated burn patients admitted to burn centers develop acute respiratory distress syndrome.[19] **Therefore, when inhalation injury is present, careful fluid resuscitation guided by hemodynamic monitoring can help avoid pulmonary edema and acute respiratory distress syndrome.**

The initial diagnosis of smoke inhalation is made from a history of exposure to fire in an enclosed space and physical signs that include facial burns, singed nasal hair, soot in the mouth or nose, hoarseness, carbonaceous sputum, and expiratory wheezing. No single method for diagnosing the extent of inhalation injury exists. Measurement of arterial carboxyhemoglobin is used to document prolonged exposure to products of incomplete combustion. The chest radiograph may be normal initially. Bronchoscopy and radionuclide scanning may also be helpful in evaluating the full extent of injury.

Treat suspected inhalation injury *prior to* definitive diagnosis. Provide humidified oxygen (100%) by facemask. Obtain arterial blood gas concentrations, ***including carboxyhemoglobin levels***. Control of the upper airway is achieved by prompt endotracheal intubation. Indications for intubation include (1) full-thickness burns of the face or perioral region, (2) circumferential neck burns, (3) acute respiratory distress, (4) progressive hoarseness or air hunger, (5) respiratory depression or altered mental status, and (6) supraglottic edema and inflammation on bronchoscopy. Additionally, consider the patient's anticipated clinical course.

BURN TREATMENT

The management of patients with *moderate to major* burns can be divided into three phases: (1) prehospital care, (2) ED resuscitation and stabilization, and (3) admission or transfer to a specialized burn center.

PREHOSPITAL CARE

The basis of prehospital care of the burn-injured patient consists of the following: (1) stop the burning process; (2) assess and, if necessary, secure the airway; (3) initiate fluid resuscitation; (4) relieve pain; (5) protect the burn wound; and (6) transport the patient to an appropriate facility.

On-site assessment of a burned patient is divided into primary and secondary surveys. In the primary survey, identify and treat immediately life-threatening conditions. Initial management of the burn-injured patient is similar to that of any other trauma patient: airway, breathing, circulation, and cervical spine immobilization where appropriate. During the secondary survey, perform a thorough head-to-toe evaluation.

The patient must be extricated from the burning environment, and burning clothing must be immediately removed. The remainder of the clothing should be removed after the airway, breathing, and circulation are secured. Remove rings, watches, jewelry, and belts because they retain heat and produce a tourniquet-like effect on the extremity, causing ischemia. Give oxygen by facemask. **Pay close attention to the airway: rapid deterioration may occur even when the initial assessment judges the airway to be acceptable.** Consider prophylactic intubation in patients with perioral burns sustained in a closed-space fire. Give IV isotonic crystalloid. Cover the patient with clean sheets to protect the wound. While early cooling can reduce the depth of burn and reduce pain, uncontrolled cooling may result in hypothermia. Provide analgesia according to protocol or with direction of the online medical control physician. Transport the patient to the nearest ED capable of caring for a burn-injured patient or, if none is available, to the nearest ED for stabilization and subsequent transfer.

ED MANAGEMENT

INITIAL ASSESSMENT

Obtain a directed history from the patient and EMS personnel to determine the burning agent(s), involvement of chemicals, the duration of exposure, and if the injury was sustained in an open or enclosed space. Assess for loss of consciousness, risk of blast injury from explosion, contact with electricity, or other trauma. Assess the adequacy of, or need for, cervical immobilization. Obtain the general history, including past medical and surgical illnesses, chronic disease, allergies, medications, and tetanus immunization status.

Quickly assess the patient's respiration and circulation and initiate stabilization (**Table 216-5**). Examine the patient for signs of inhalation injury, as evidenced by respiratory distress, facial burns, carbonaceous sputum, singed nasal hair, and soot in the mouth. **If there is any evidence of airway compromise with swelling of the neck, burns inside the mouth, or wheezing, perform early endotracheal intubation.**

Assess the adequacy of circulation by noting the blood pressure, pulse rate, capillary refill time, mental status, and urinary output. Insert IV lines in unburned areas, but when this is not possible, a burned area can be used and resuscitation started according to a burn fluid resuscitation formula.

During the secondary examination, perform a head-to-toe assessment, including examination of the eye for corneal burns. Estimate and record the size and depth of the burn injury. In patients with partial-thickness burns of >20% of body surface area, nasogastric tube insertion is routinely required due to frequent development of ileus. Insert a urinary catheter to measure urinary output and to prevent urinary retention in patients with perineal burns.

Routine laboratory tests, including a CBC and measurement of electrolyte, BUN, creatinine, and glucose levels, should be performed. In patients with moderate/severe burns or suspected inhalation injury, obtain an arterial blood gas analysis, carboxyhemoglobin level, serum creatine kinase, urinalysis for myoglobin, chest radiograph, and ECG. Fiberoptic bronchoscopy is indicated in suspected inhalation injury and in intubated patients for both diagnostic and therapeutic purposes. Additional radiographs should be taken as indicated for other suspected trauma.

Treat suspected inhalation injury with humidified 100% oxygen, intubation and ventilation, bronchodilators, and aggressive pulmonary toilet; hyperbaric oxygen may be necessary for severe carbon monoxide poisoning.

Burn injury in the pregnant woman is associated with significant morbidity to mother and child. The outcome of the pregnancy is determined by the extent of injury to the mother. Spontaneous termination of pregnancy is common in large–body surface area burns. Resuscitation requirements may exceed those estimated using common guidelines. Fetal monitoring and early consultation with the obstetrician and burn specialist are recommended.

FLUID RESUSCITATION

The burn shock resuscitation formulas in use today are derived from laboratory studies of burn shock and resuscitation, and the utility of such formulas has been called into question.[20] Although the importance of early fluid resuscitation is supported by clinical experience,[20,21] no consensus exists on the appropriate assessment of resuscitation and its effect on outcome.[20] Additionally, over-resuscitation is not without consequence. In general, resuscitation should be guided by monitoring cardiorespiratory status and urine output rather than strict adherence to a formula. **The following formulas are a guide for fluid resuscitation of the burn-injured patient. Monitor and adjust according to individual patient response.**

The Baxter or Parkland formula is likely the most widely used thermal injury resuscitation regimen in North America.[8,9] This formula calls for 4 mL of lactated Ringer's solution multiplied by the percentage of body surface area burned (partial- and full-thickness burns only) multiplied by patient body weight in kilograms. Half of the total is administered in the first 8 hours after injury and the remainder during the following 16 hours (**Table 216-6**). Volumes may be large, and hemodynamic monitoring techniques should be used to protect against inadvertent volume overload.

Patients with thermal injury and concomitant multisystem trauma and those with inhalation injuries generally require fluid resuscitation in excess of calculated needs. Burn patients with preexisting cardiac or pulmonary disease require much greater attention to fluid management. Monitor fluid resuscitation closely by frequent assessment of vital signs, cerebral and skin perfusion, pulmonary status, and urinary output, as well as hemodynamic monitoring. Urine output should be 0.5 to 1.0 mL/kg/h.

Because the ED is primarily responsible for initial fluid resuscitation, discussion with burn specialists may be helpful in avoiding early under- or over-resuscitation. Patients with major burns can quickly receive excessive IV fluid during the prehospital and ED phases, particularly if two large-bore peripheral catheters are in place with fluid infusing at a wide-open rate. Document total fluid infused and titrate infusion to the patient's response. Clear documentation of fluid resuscitation should accompany all patients transferred to burn centers.

There are several methods of calculating fluid resuscitation for infants and children. The Parkland formula can be modified to maintain a urinary output of 1 mL/kg/h. Alternatively, a pediatric maintenance rate for 24 hours can be calculated, and an additional 2 to 4 mL/kg multiplied by

TABLE 216-6 Parkland Formula for Fluid Resuscitation

Adults
LR 4 mL × weight (kg) × % BSA burned* over initial 24 h
Half over the first 8 h from the time of burn
Other half over the subsequent 16 h
Example: 70-kg adult with 40% second- and third-degree burns:
4 mL × 70 kg × 40 = 11,200 mL over 24 h
Children
LR 3 mL × weight (kg) × % BSA burned* over initial 24 h plus maintenance
Half over the first 8 h from the time of burn
Other half over the subsequent 16 h

Abbreviations: BSA = body surface area; LR = lactated Ringer's solution.

*Partial- and full-thickness burns only.

TABLE 216-5 ED Care of Patients with Major Burns

Airway	Breathing	Circulation	Adjuncts
Reevaluation of airway	Continuous pulse oximetry with supplemental O_2	Establishment of two large-bore peripheral IV lines in unburned skin	Placement of Foley catheter
Early intubation for any sign of breathing difficulty, airway burn, swelling, or suspected inhalation injury			Insertion of nasogastric tube
	Determination of carboxyhemoglobin level	IV administration of lactated Ringer's solution using Parkland or other burn resuscitation formula	Administration of tetanus booster
	Bronchoscopy if inhalation injury is a concern	Cardiac monitoring	Assessment for other trauma using Advanced Trauma Life Support guidelines
	Mechanical ventilation as needed		Pain control

percentage of body surface area burned is then added to the total. The entire amount is infused over the first 24 hours. In children weighing <25 kg, a goal urine output of 1.0 mL/kg/h is necessary. Add 5% dextrose to maintenance fluids for children weighing <20 kg due to smaller glycogen stores.[8]

Two additions or modifications to isotonic crystalloid resuscitation have been studied: adjuvant colloid and hypertonic saline. However, neither improves patient outcome. Adjuvant colloid given along with isotonic crystalloid resuscitation is not beneficial and is associated with decreased glomerular filtration rate.[22] Discussion of the use of adjuvant colloid continues, but it is used very little in North America and the United Kingdom,[23] although Israeli investigators have reported favorable results with the addition of colloid to their burn formulas.[24] Use of hypertonic saline has been associated with an increased rate of renal failure and death.[25] In an effort to decrease burn edema, protein loss, and abdominal compartment syndrome, investigators have also studied the efficacy of *permissive hypovolemia* in reducing burn edema and the multiple organ dysfunction that follows.[26] This practice necessitates invasive monitoring and is of interest, but it is not standard of care and should not be used in ED resuscitation at this time.

Electrical injuries, incineration burns, and associated crush injuries may produce rhabdomyolysis and myoglobinuria, leading to renal failure. Acute renal failure occurs in approximately 15% of patients admitted to burn centers and is associated with severe burns (mean body surface area involvement of 48%).[27] Therapy to limit renal damage from myoglobinuria should be initiated as outlined in chapter 89, "Rhabdomyolysis."

WOUND CARE

After evaluation and resuscitation of the patient, attend to burn wounds.[2] Initially, wounds are best covered with a clean, dry sheet. Later, small burns can be covered with a moist saline-soaked dressing while the patient is awaiting admission or transfer. The soothing effect of cooling on burns is most likely due to local vasoconstriction. Cooling stabilizes mast cells and reduces histamine release, kinin formation, and thromboxane B_2 production. For large burns, sterile drapes are preferred, because application of saline-soaked dressings to a large area can cause hypothermia.

Consult the admitting service or burn center early. Avoid the use of antiseptic dressings in the ED, because the admitting service will need to assess the wound. Wound care for transferred patients should be discussed with the accepting burn center. Do not delay transfer for wound debridement. For transferred patients, the referring facility should follow the accepting regional burn center's treatment protocol if available.

Escharotomy Patients with circumferential deep burns of the limbs may develop compromise of the distal circulation, particularly after initiation of resuscitation. The distal vascular status of such patients must be monitored closely, including pulses, capillary refill, pulse oximetry, and skin temperature. Doppler flow testing may likewise be useful. If vascular compromise is evident, escharotomy is indicated. The eschar is incised with a scalpel to the level of the fat on the mid-lateral portion of the limb, using care to avoid incising the fascia (i.e., fasciotomy). Elevated compartment pressures can be clinically evident. The incision may be extended to the hand and fingers (**Figure 216-8**). Escharotomy may provoke substantial soft tissue bleeding. Consider consultation by phone with a burn surgeon.

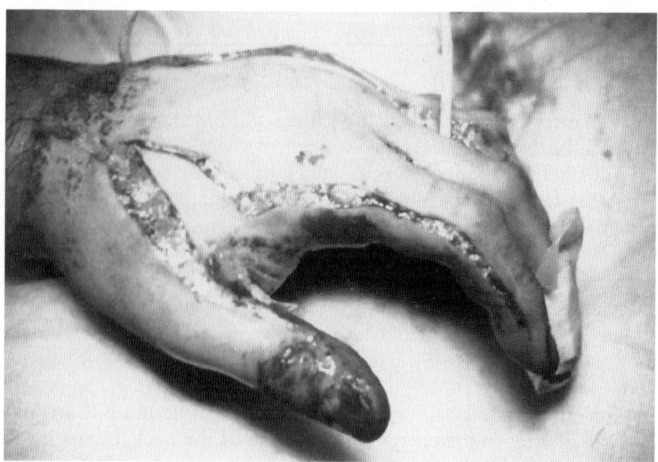

FIGURE 216-8. Escharotomy of the hand.

If there are circumferential burns of the chest and neck, eschar may restrict ventilation. An escharotomy of the chest wall should be performed to allow adequate ventilation. Incisions are made at the anterior axillary line from the level of the second rib to the level of the twelfth rib. These two incisions should be joined transversely so the chest wall can expand (**Figure 216-9**).

PAIN CONTROL

Burn injuries are exceedingly painful, and superficial partial-thickness burns are the most painful. Burn injury not only makes an otherwise already injured area and surrounding tissue more painful, but also causes hyperalgesia, chiefly mediated by A fibers. Local cooling may be soothing but does not provide pain control and can cause hypothermia;[28] additional pain management should be provided.

During the acute phase, the preferred route for most medication is IV. Opioids (e.g., morphine, fentanyl, hydromorphone) are the mainstay of treatment, and relatively large dosages may be required. Anxiolytic agents may also be given. Ensure adequate analgesia for patients being discharged, including a regimen for both background and breakthrough pain associated with dressing changes. Achieving adequate pain control is required for patients being considered for discharge.

CARE OF MINOR BURNS

Minor burns typically qualify for ambulatory care. Minor burns should be isolated, should not cross joints or be circumferential, and should not meet criteria for burn center care. Consider the patient's social situation and medical comorbidities when electing ambulatory care. Treatment of minor burns is listed in **Table 216-7**. Even in patients with burn injury <10% body surface area, patients at the extremes of age and/or patients with significant comorbidities, challenging social situations, or inadequate pain control should be treated as inpatients and possibly transferred to a burn center. Additionally, the patient's reliability should be considered as an important factor in deciding whether outpatient treatment is appropriate. Care of minor burns in discharged patients requires appropriate wound care instructions, adequate pain control, and coordination between the ED and the physician who will see the patient in follow-up.[2]

Because burns are painful, appropriate analgesia is required. After appropriate analgesia, clean the burn wound with mild soap and water or dilute antiseptic solution. Debride ruptured blisters. Also debride

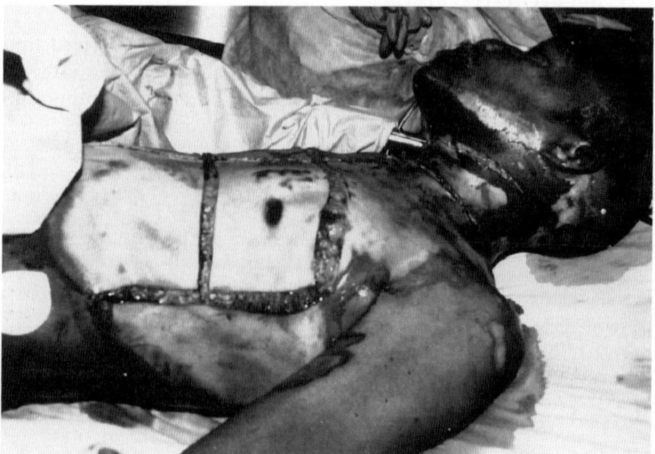

FIGURE 216-9. Escharotomy of the chest wall.

TABLE 216-7 ED Care of Minor Burns
Provide appropriate analgesics before burn care and for outpatient use
Cleanse burn with mild soap and water or dilute antiseptic solution
Debride wound as needed
Apply topical antimicrobial:
1% silver sulfadiazine cream (not on the face or in patients with a sulfa allergy)
Bacitracin ointment
Triple-antibiotic ointment (neomycin, polymyxin B, bacitracin zinc)
Consider use of synthetic occlusive dressings
Provide detailed burn care instructions with follow-up in 24–48 h

large intact blisters or those over very mobile joints. Small blisters on nonmobile areas should be left intact. Tetanus immunization status should be assessed, and tetanus toxoid and/or immunoglobulin should be administered as needed.

Topical antimicrobials play an important role in reducing bacterial colonization and enhancing the rate of healing in burns.[8,9] A wide variety of topical agents are commonly used for minor burns. The most common is 1% silver sulfadiazine due to its easy application and minimal toxicity. It should not be used in patients with sulfa allergy or glucose-6-phosphate dehydrogenase deficiency, in pregnant patients near term, or in premature or young infants less than 2 months of age. Excretion into breast milk is not known; thus, silver sulfadiazine should be used with caution in nursing mothers. Do not use it on the face because it can stain the skin gray. When dressings are changed, remove silvadene to avoid gray discoloration, cleanse the skin, and apply new silvadene.

There are less costly and equally effective alternatives to silver sulfadiazine.[29,30] Alternative topical agents include bacitracin and triple-antibiotic (neomycin, polymyxin B, and bacitracin zinc) ointments. Although 8.5% mafenide acetate cream and 0.2% nitrofurazone ointment are available for topical application, these are not good choices for treatment of large burns in an outpatient setting. Mafenide penetrates the eschar well and is useful in treating patients with invasive infections, but it is a carbonic anhydrase inhibitor and can cause metabolic acidosis. Nitrofurazone is supplied in a polyethylene glycol vehicle that can be toxic if absorbed in patients with compromised renal function. Mafenide and nitrofurazone have little utility in the ED management of the acutely burn-injured patient. **Dressings should ideally be changed twice daily, gently removing residual ointment, for as long as the wounds continue to weep, then daily until healing is complete.**

Synthetic occlusive dressing is an alternative method of managing partial-thickness burns in outpatients. Wounds are cleansed and debrided prior to application of these dressings (e.g., Biobrane, Dow Hickam Pharmaceuticals, Sugar Land, TX; Tegaderm, 3M Health Care, St. Paul, MN; DuoDERM, Bristol-Myers Squibb, New York, NY). This strategy is most appropriate for clean burns on flat surfaces. The goal is for the dressing to adhere to the wound and act as artificial skin. Adherence is important because most bacteria causing infection wound infections produce fibrinolytic agents. Wounds should be reevaluated at 24 to 48 hours for adherence. The dressing is left in place until spontaneous separation of the dressing occurs. Wounds treated with synthetic occlusive dressings are well tolerated by patients, require few dressing changes, and heal with good appearance.[31]

Reassess burn wounds at 24 hours for depth and extent of burn. Explain the follow-up visit schedule and prescribe analgesics. Discharge instructions should include home burn care, pain control, and the symptoms and signs of infection. Burned extremities should be elevated for 24 to 48 hours to prevent edema. Advise patients to return to the ED with signs or symptoms of infection or if pain is inadequately controlled. Patients with deep partial-thickness, full-thickness, and mixed-thickness burns not requiring admission should be referred to a plastic surgeon or burn care specialist in 2 to 4 days for reevaluation and consideration for skin grafting.

REFERENCES

The complete reference list is available online at www.TintinalliEM.com.

CHAPTER 217 Chemical Burns

Anthony F. Pizon
Michael J. Lynch

INTRODUCTION AND EPIDEMIOLOGY

More than 25,000 products are capable of producing chemical burns. Exposures occur both occupationally and in homes. As many as 10% of all burn center admissions are the result of chemical burns. Although a smaller percentage of total burns, the mortality is high and may account for as many as 30% of all burn deaths.[1] Careful individual attention is required for chemical burn treatment due to the nature of concomitant tissue injury and chemical exposure.

PATHOPHYSIOLOGY

The skin is a barrier and transition zone between the internal and external environments. Although the outer stratum corneum layer of the skin functions as an excellent barrier against many chemicals, some penetrate it readily. Chemicals can produce burns, dermatitis, allergic reaction, thermal injury, and/or systemic toxicity.

Most chemicals produce tissue damage by their chemical reaction rather than by thermal injury. Certainly, some chemicals produce significant heat by means of an exothermic reaction. However, most skin damage is the result of the chemical's unique characteristics. Unlike thermal burns, chemical burn injuries require tailored evaluations and treatments based on the specific agent involved. Multiple factors influence tissue damage and percutaneous absorption of chemicals (**Tables 217-1 and 217-2**).

Most chemical burns are caused by acids or alkalis. At similar volumes and manner of contact, alkalis usually produce far more tissue damage than acids. **Acids tend to cause coagulation necrosis with protein precipitation and form a tough leathery eschar.** The eschar typically limits deeper penetration of the agent. **Alkalis produce liquefaction necrosis and saponification of lipids.** The result is a poor barrier to chemical penetration and deeper, ongoing burns. Other chemical injuries occur by various pathophysiologic mechanisms. Some chemical agents cause injury by more than one mechanism (**Table 217-3**).

Death early after severe chemical burns is usually related to hypotension, acute renal failure, and shock as a result of fluid loss. However, systemic toxicity and subsequent morbidity and mortality may also occur if chemicals are absorbed. Acidosis, hypotension, hyperkalemia, dysrhythmia, and shock can occur with systemic absorption of acids (**Table 217-4**).

GENERAL APPROACH TO CHEMICAL BURNS

The initial goal of treatment is to remove the patient from the exposure and prevent any further chemical exposure. If not performed prior to arrival, remove all exposed clothing immediately. With few exceptions, aggressive irrigation with water is the cornerstone of initial treatment for chemical burns. Chemical agents will continue to damage tissue until they are removed or inactivated. Dry chemical particles such as lime should be brushed away before irrigation. Sodium metal and related compounds should be initially covered with mineral oil or excised, because water can cause a severe exothermic reaction. Dilution of phenol (carbolic acid) with water may enhance penetration. **For the most**

TABLE 217-1 Factors Influencing Tissue Damage
Concentration of agent
Quantity of agent
Duration of contact
Mechanism of action
Extent of penetration

TABLE 217-2 Factors Influencing Percutaneous Absorption of Chemicals

Body site
Areas of thin skin (i.e., genitalia, face, and skinfolds are particularly vulnerable)
Amount of surface area
Integrity of skin
Increased vulnerability: traumatized skin, elderly skin, dehydration, inflammation
Nature of the chemical
Lipid solubility, pH, concentration
Duration of contact
Poor irrigation, chemical-soaked garments, occlusive dressings

part, however, use of water or saline to irrigate a chemical burn should not be delayed while searching for other treatment agents and should ideally begin immediately at the scene of the accident. Almost universally, earlier irrigation means a better prognosis.

Hospital personnel should maintain universal precautions while decontamination is ongoing. At the very minimum, mask, face shield, chemical-resistant gown, gloves, and water-impervious boots should be worn at all times. The exact personal protective equipment worn will ultimately depend on the specific agent involved.

The amount of elapsed time to initiate dilution or removal of chemical agents is directly related to the eventual depth and degree of injury. Wounds irrigated 3 minutes after contact with some chemicals have a twofold greater chance of becoming full-thickness burns than wounds irrigated within 1 minute of chemical contact. The time required for irrigation varies. Severe alkali burns may require several hours of irrigation. Use pH indicator paper to determine continued presence of alkali or acid in burn wounds and possible need for further irrigation. Irrigation should continue until pH is neutral or near neutral.

Although thermal energy is produced in an exothermic reaction when using water irrigation, copious amounts of water will decrease the rate and intensity of the chemical reaction and dissipate the heat.[2] Continue irrigation at a gentle flow to avoid continued skin contact with chemicals. After irrigation and debridement of remaining particles and devitalized tissue, apply topical antimicrobial agents to affected areas, and provide tetanus immunization as needed. Other than measures specific for a particular chemical burn, treatment following initial therapy is similar to that of thermal burns (**Table 217-5**). Aggressive fluid replacement is needed if extensive chemical burns are sustained. Analgesics may be needed, and in the case of allergic responses to chemicals, epinephrine, antihistamines, and steroids may be required.

ACID BURNS

Do not limit the examination of a patient with a significant chemical acid burn to the skin because acids may cause respiratory and mucous membrane irritation as well. Furthermore, skin absorption of some compounds may occur and result in systemic signs and symptoms.

With the exception of hydrofluoric acid, strong acids produce coagulation necrosis from the denaturation of proteins in the superficial tissue. Injury severity is related to the physical characteristics of the acid. Most substances with a pH <2 are strong corrosives. Other important tissue-damaging properties of acids include concentration, molarity, and complexing affinity for hydroxyl ions. The higher each of these factors is, the greater is the tissue damage. **Contact time with the skin is the most important chemical burn feature that healthcare professionals may alter.** For example, instantaneous skin decontamination of 18M sulfuric acid will cause no burn, but a 1-minute exposure can cause full-thickness skin damage.

TABLE 217-3 Classification of Chemicals

Classification of Chemical Damage	Mechanism of Injury
Acids	Protein denaturation as proton donors
Alkalis	Protein denaturation as proton acceptors
Organic solvents	Disruption of cellular membranes
Inorganic solvents	Scavenge ions and salt production within tissues

TABLE 217-4 Systemic Effects Associated with Chemical Burns

Chemical	Systemic Toxicity
Hydrofluoric acid	Hypocalcemia, hypomagnesemia, hyperkalemia, cardiac arrhythmias, sudden death
Tannic acid, chromic acid, formic acid, picric acid, phosphorus	Hepatic necrosis, nephrotoxicity
Cresol	Methemoglobinemia, massive hemolysis, multiple organ failure
Gasoline	Severe pulmonary, cardiovascular, neurologic, renal, and hepatic complications
Phenol (carbolic acid)	Cardiovascular and central nervous system toxicity
Sodium nitrate, potassium nitrate	Severe methemoglobinemia with refractory cyanosis
Dichromate solution	Liver failure, acute renal failure, death despite hemodialysis

ACETIC ACID

The dilute (<40%) acetic acid solution found in hair-wave neutralizer solutions is perhaps the most common cause of chemical burns to the scalp in women. Prolonged contact, especially with an already damaged scalp, can cause a partial-thickness burn that heals slowly and is prone to infection. Initial treatment is copious water irrigation. Oral antibiotics should be prescribed if the scalp burn has created open skin lesions.

CARBOLIC ACID (PHENOL)

Phenol (carbolic acid), a corrosive organic acid used widely in industry and medicine, denatures proteins and causes chemical burns characterized by a relatively painless white or brown coagulum. Paradoxically, dilute phenol penetrates tissue more readily than the concentrated form. Systemic absorption may result in life-threatening cardiac dysrhythmias or seizures. The unpleasant, acrid odor of phenol, detectable in air at 0.047 parts per million, and its low volatility help prevent airborne exposure. Although commercially available in concentrations up to 90%, even dilute solutions of 1% to 2% phenol may cause a burn if contact is prolonged or extensive. Chemically related phenolic compounds that induce skin damage include cresol, creosote, and cresylic acid.

Coagulation necrosis of the involved area is common. Necrotic tissue may delay absorption temporarily, but phenol may become entrapped under the eschar. Remove contaminated clothing and begin water irrigation immediately. Water lavage alone may not be totally effective, because the necrotic coagulum inhibits water penetration to the deeper layers.

Decontamination is more effective by the use of an undiluted polyethylene glycol solution of molecular weight 200 to 400 or by a gentle wash with isopropyl alcohol. Adequate supplies of either irrigation solution should remain stored for such use. Either irrigation solution reduces the extent of cutaneous corrosion and also decreases systemic toxicity. **An isopropyl alcohol rinse is equivalent to polyethylene glycol in removing phenol.**[3] The advantage of isopropyl alcohol is its ready availability. If neither polyethylene glycol nor isopropyl alcohol is available in adequate supplies, large volumes of water should be used.

CHROMIC ACID

Chromium hexavalent compounds (Cr^{6+}) are powerful oxidizers. The chromate ion in chromic acid produces a chronic penetrating ulcerating lesion of the skin. Associated signs and symptoms of chromic acid

TABLE 217-5 Treatment of Select Chemical Burns

Chemical	Treatment	Comments
Acids		
All acid burns require prompt decontamination and copious irrigation with water		
Acetic acid	Copious irrigation	Consider systemic antibiotics for extensive scalp burns
Phenol (carbolic acid)	Copious irrigation	Isopropyl alcohol may also be used
	Sponge with undiluted polyethylene glycol 200–400	
Chromic acid	Copious irrigation	Observe for systemic toxicity
Formic acid	Copious irrigation	Dialysis may be needed for severe toxicity
Hydrofluoric acid	Copious irrigation	Consider intradermal injection of 10% calcium gluconate or intra-arterial calcium gluconate for severe cases
	10% calcium gluconate intradermal	Monitor serum calcium and magnesium in severe exposure
	Topical calcium gluconate gel	25 mL of 10% calcium gluconate in 75 mL of sterile water-soluble lubricant (K-Y jelly or US jelly)
Nitric acid	Copious irrigation	Consult with burn specialist
Oxalic acid	Copious irrigation	Evaluate serum electrolytes and renal function
	IV calcium may be required	Cardiac monitoring for serious dermal exposure
Alkalis		
All alkali burns require prompt decontamination and copious, prolonged irrigation with water		
Portland cement	Prolonged copious irrigation	May need to remove cement particles with a brush, such as a preoperative scrubbing brush
Elemental Metals		
Water is generally contraindicated in extinguishing burning metal fragments embedded in the skin		
Elemental metals (sodium, lithium, potassium, magnesium, aluminum, and calcium)	Cover metal fragments with sand, foam from a class D fire extinguisher, or mineral oil	
	Excise metal fragments that cannot be wiped away	
Hydrocarbons		
Gasoline	Decontamination	
Tar	Cool before removal	Baby oil can be used
	Remove using antibiotic ointment containing polyoxylene sorbitan (polysorbate)	
Vesicants		
Mustards	Decontaminate	If limited water supply, adsorbent powders (flour, talcum powder, fuller's earth) can be applied to the mustard and then wiped away with a moist towel
	Copious irrigation	
Reducing Agents		
Alkyl mercury compounds	Copious irrigation	Blister fluid is high in metallic mercury content
	Debride, drain, and copiously irrigate blisters	
Lacrimators		
Tear gas	Copious irrigation	May cause respiratory symptoms if inhaled
Pepper spray	Copious irrigation	May cause respiratory symptoms if inhaled
Miscellaneous		
White phosphorus	Remove clothing	Systemic toxicity is a significant concern
	Copious irrigation, keep exposed skin areas wet or submerged until all particles have been removed due to risk of ignition when exposed to air	
	Debride visible particles	
Airbag	Prolonged copious irrigation	

exposure are conjunctivitis, lacrimation, and ulceration of the nasal septum. Systemic chromium toxicity can cause liver or renal failure, GI bleeding, coagulopathy, and CNS disturbances. Significant symptoms may occur after only 1% to 2% body surface area burns. **A 10% body surface area cutaneous burn caused by chromic acid can be fatal due to systemic toxicity.** Any acute skin exposure to chromic acid should be treated with copious water irrigation and observation for systemic effects. Aggressive excision is the best method for prevention of systemic effects because depth of the burn is difficult to determine and absorption of chromium may continue after irrigation.[4]

FORMIC ACID

Formic acid in 60% solution is used by acrylate glue makers, cellulose formate workers, and tanning workers. Formic acid produces coagulation necrosis of the skin. Systemic effects, including decreased respiration, anion gap metabolic acidosis, and hemolysis have been reported.[5] Treatment includes immediate decontamination and irrigation with water. Systemic toxicity may require intravenous sodium bicarbonate for the metabolic acidosis or exchange transfusions for severe hemolysis.

HYDROCHLORIC AND SULFURIC ACIDS

The dermal toxicity of hydrochloric acid and sulfuric acid is so well recognized that early decontamination and water irrigation usually prevent severe burns to the skin. These acids can burn the skin dark brown or black. Toilet bowl cleaners may contain 80% solutions of sulfuric acid, and some drain cleaners may be 95% to 99% sulfuric acid solutions. Munitions, chemical, and fertilizer manufacturers commonly use 95% to 98% sulfuric acid solutions in their industrial processes. Automobile battery fluid is 25% sulfuric acid. Most household bleaches are only 3% to 6% hypochlorite solutions, which, although acidic, cause little damage unless they are in contact with skin for a prolonged time. Treatment is the same as for formic acid burns.

HYDROFLUORIC ACID

Hydrofluoric acid is used in the production of high-octane fuel, etching and frosting glass, semiconductors, microelectronics/microinstruments, germicides, dyes, plastics, tanning, and fireproofing material and is used in cleaning stone and brick buildings. It is also a very effective rust remover.

Unlike other acids, hydrofluoric acid penetrates deeply and will cause progressive tissue loss. It produces burns in two ways. First, hydrogen ions cause direct cellular damage as other acids do through protein denaturation. Second, free fluoride ions scavenge intracellular cations, such as calcium and magnesium, disrupt cellular membranes, and inhibit the sodium/potassium/ATPase. This leads to systemic hypocalcemia, hypomagnesemia, and hyperkalemia. Locally, free fluoride ions cause spontaneous depolarization of nerve tissue and severe pain. Pain will persist until all free fluoride ions have been neutralized.

The dermal effects may not be immediately noted and appear to be more related to the concentration of hydrofluoric acid than to the duration of exposure. Solutions >50% produce immediate pain and tissue destruction. Solutions <20% may not produce signs and symptoms until 12 to 24 hours after exposure. The skin often develops a blue-gray appearance with surrounding erythema.

The treatment of hydrofluoric acid burns consists of two phases. The first, immediate phase is copious water irrigation of the affected skin for 15 to 30 minutes. This may be the only treatment that is needed if the hydrofluoric acid solution is <20% concentration, the duration of exposure was very brief, and decontamination is begun immediately. Severe, persistent pain denotes a more serious injury requiring the second phase of treatment.

The second phase of treatment is aimed at replacing calcium and magnesium and detoxifying the enzyme-poisoning fluoride ion. Two ions—calcium (Ca^{2+}) and magnesium (Mg^{2+})[6]—bind the fluoride ion and curtail its toxic effects. However, the overwhelming clinical experience to date has been with calcium gluconate, so it is the agent of choice. Calcium gluconate can be administered as a topical preparation, subcutaneous/intradermal injection, or intra-arterial infusion. A calcium gluconate gel made with a water-soluble lubricant is generously applied to the affected skin. **The topical preparation is made by mixing 3.5 grams of calcium gluconate powder in 5 oz of water-soluble lubricant, or 25 mL of 10% calcium gluconate in 75 mL of water-soluble lubricant.** Calcium chloride or calcium carbonate can be substituted if no calcium gluconate is available. The main limitation of topical therapy is the impermeability of the skin to calcium, and therefore, topical therapy is limited to use in mild, superficial burns. Most importantly, topical therapy should not delay intradermal or intra-arterial injections for severe burns.

Treatment with intradermal injection of a 10% calcium gluconate solution through a 27-gauge needle into the hydrofluoric acid–burned skin is a very effective treatment. **A typical dose of 0.5 mL of 10% calcium gluconate per square centimeter of burned skin is recommended.** Pain relief is nearly immediate, and, indeed, the elimination of pain may be used as a guide for further therapy. Recurrence of pain indicates the need for further therapy. Unfortunately, injection therapy has several disadvantages: (1) only limited amounts of calcium are delivered to the tissue; (2) hyperosmolarity and inherent toxicity of free calcium ions cause more pain initially, and more tissue damage is possible if calcium is not bound to fluoride; (3) vascular compromise can result if too much fluid is injected, especially into digits; and (4) rapid penetration of hydrofluoric acid beneath the nail requires nail removal to administer the calcium gluconate into the nail bed adequately. **Acute hydrofluoric acid contamination of the hands, feet, digits, or nails requires consultation with a medical toxicologist and plastic surgeon.**

Intra-arterial infusion of calcium gluconate may be used to prevent tissue necrosis and stop the pain associated with hydrofluoric acid burns.[7] This should be performed as soon as possible after the initial burn, preferably within 6 hours of insult. Place an intra-arterial catheter in the appropriate vascular supply (the brachial artery if the entire hand is affected) and connect to a three-way stopcock to which is attached an arterial pressure-monitoring device and the infusion syringe of calcium gluconate. A 50-mL syringe may be filled with 10 mL of a 10% calcium gluconate solution and 40 mL of 5% dextrose in water and infused over 4 hours. The arterial pressure-monitoring device ensures that the catheter has not dislodged from the lumen of the cannulated artery. Repeat infusion may be needed if pain recurs within 4 hours. Intra-arterial infusion avoids the disadvantages of local infiltration therapy, but it has its own disadvantages: it is an invasive vascular procedure that (1) may result in arterial spasm or thrombosis, (2) requires more time and hospital resources, and (3) requires experience in the technique.

Inhalation of hydrofluoric acid can cause immediate or delayed pulmonary injury. All cases of suspected inhalation injury should be admitted for observation even if asymptomatic. Nebulized calcium gluconate may be attempted in these cases, but no controlled studies exist for its use. **The solution is made by adding 1.5 mL of 10% calcium gluconate solution into 4.5 mL of sterile water or saline and is administered by nebulizer.**

Ocular exposure to hydrofluoric acid requires water irrigation for at least 30 minutes and requires emergent ophthalmologic consultation. An animal study suggests that calcium-containing irrigation fluids for eye exposures may be harmful.[8] Therefore, standard eye irrigation practices should be used. The possibility of severe injury and eye necrosis should not be taken lightly. In severe ocular exposures, systemic absorption is possible as well.

Systemic toxicity from dermal hydrofluoric acid exposure can result in ventricular fibrillation as a result of systemic acidosis, hyperkalemia, hypomagnesemia, and hypocalcemia. **In major hydrofluoric acid burns, immediately administer IV calcium and magnesium, using standard slow IV rates, before laboratory results are available.** Once patients develop hypocalcemia or hypomagnesemia, it is very difficult to restore these electrolyte deficiencies. Cardiac monitoring, IV access, and electrolyte monitoring should be performed in all cases of significant hydrofluoric acid dermal burns (**Table 217-6**).

METHACRYLIC ACID

Methacrylic acid, found in many artificial nail cosmetic products, can produce severe dermal burns, usually in preschoolers. Emergency treatment is copious water irrigation.

TABLE 217-6 Options for Treatment of Hydrofluoric Acid Skin Burns

1. Copious irrigation for 15–30 min immediately.
2. Application of calcium gluconate gel, 25 mL of 10% calcium gluconate in 75 mL of water-soluble lubricant.
3. Further treatment options as dictated by patient response:
    a. Dermal injection of 10% calcium gluconate at the rate of 0.5 mL/cm^2 of skin surface using a small-gauge needle.
    b. Arterial infusion over 4 h (40 mL of 5% dextrose in water with 10 mL of 10% calcium gluconate).
    c. Consider supplemental magnesium and calcium IV.

NITRIC ACID

Nitric acid is used in industry for casting iron and steel, electroplating, engraving, and fertilizer manufacturing. Upon contact with skin, nitric acid can produce tissue damage by oxidation and may turn the skin yellowish as it is burned. Emergency treatment consists of copious water irrigation and standard burn care (see chapter 216, "Thermal Burns").

OXALIC ACID

Oxalic acid is used for leather tanning and blueprint paper. Oxalic acid binds calcium and prevents muscle contraction. The wounds should be irrigated with water, and IV calcium may be required. Serum electrolytes and renal function should be evaluated, and cardiac monitoring should be instituted after serious dermal exposure.

ALKALI BURNS

Alkalis penetrate skin deeper and longer than acids and present a greater danger of toxicity from systemic absorption. Wounds may initially look superficial only to become full-thickness burns in 2 to 3 days. Alkalis combine with protein and lipids in tissue to form soluble protein complexes and soaps that permit passage of hydroxyl ions deep into tissue. Soft, gelatinous, friable, brownish eschars are often produced (**Figure 217-1**). Strong alkalis have a pH >12.

LYES

Strong, corrosive alkalis ("lyes") include ammonium, barium, calcium, lithium, potassium (caustic potash), and sodium (caustic soda) hydroxides. Lyes are widely used in industry and are found in home products such as drain and toilet cleaners, detergents, and paint removers. The urine sugar reagent tablet Clinitest® (Bayer) contains anhydrous sodium hydroxide.[9] Ammonium hydroxide is used in the production of synthetic fibers and extensively in agriculture. Exposure to these chemicals can result in severe toxicity including mucous membrane, ocular, dermal, GI, and inhalational/pulmonary injury. As a mode of assault, lyes have a lower mortality rate than gunshot wounds or stabbings, but victims often suffer long-term pain, scarring, and blindness. Suicidal ingestion of lye may result in rapid death from upper airway occlusion. Late morbidity related to esophageal and gastric necrosis may be minimized by early surgical intervention with esophagogastrectomy. The mainstay of treatment is immediate, voluminous, and persistent irrigation.[10] **Lyes are extremely corrosive and penetrating. Burns require copious irrigation for long periods of time.**

LIME

Lime (calcium oxide) is found in agricultural products and cements. There is considerable variability of lime content in different grades of cement, with fine to textured masonry cement having more lime than concrete. Lime is converted by water to the alkali calcium hydroxide. Upon skin contact, lime draws water out of the skin. **All dry lime particles should be brushed away before irrigation. Even a small amount of water may generate an exothermic reaction resulting in calcium hydroxide formation and tissue injury.** Brisk irrigation with a large volume of water (taking care to avoid splashing in eyes) should be used and will permit dissipation of heat.

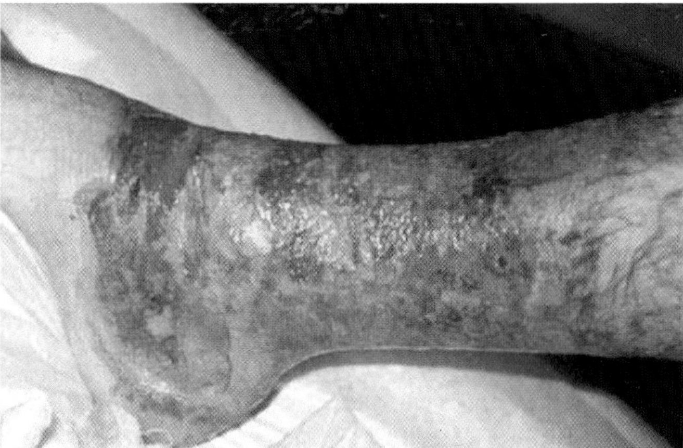

FIGURE 217-1. Deep alkali burn. [Reproduced with permission from http://www.burnsurgery.org/Modules/initial_mgmt/sec_6.htm.]

PORTLAND CEMENT

Portland cement, which accounts for a major proportion of the cement used in the United States, is a mixture of sand, lime, and other metal oxides. In the presence of water, calcium hydroxide, sodium hydroxide, and potassium hydroxide may all be formed. Workers who kneel in wet cement or get cement in their boots may discover burns hours after initial contact. In addition, skin may become irritated from gritty material, and a contact dermatitis may develop in individuals sensitive to the chromate contained in the material. Treatment of cement burns may require cleaning the wound with a brush, such as a preoperative scrubbing brush, to remove cement particles imbedded in the dermis. Careful attention to appropriate donning of personal protective equipment should be emphasized to patients suffering dermatitis or burns from contact with cement.

METALS

Foundry workers are sometimes burned by molten metal, which may spill or splash on body parts and run down into the boots. Elemental metals, sodium, lithium, potassium, magnesium, aluminum, phosphorus, and calcium may all cause burns. When exposed to air, some elemental metals spontaneously ignite. **Water is generally contraindicated in extinguishing burning metal fragments embedded in the skin because the resultant explosive exothermic reaction can lead to significant tissue injury. Burning metal may be extinguished with a class D fire extinguisher, smothered with sand, or covered with mineral oil.** Wound debridement should include excision of metal fragments that cannot be wiped away. Metal fragments should be placed in mineral oil to prevent further ignition.

HYDROCARBONS

GASOLINE

Hydrocarbons cause a fat-dissolving corrosive injury to the skin referred to as defatting dermatitis. Gasoline, a complex mixture of alkanes, cycloalkanes, and aromatic hydrocarbons, is the most common hydrocarbon burn treated in the ED.

A hydrocarbon chemical burn typically resembles a thermal scald or a partial-thickness burn, although full-thickness burns can result from prolonged contact with gasoline.[11] During extremely cold weather, topical gasoline exposure may lead to frostbite when rapid gasoline evaporation causes heat loss from the skin. Systemic effects of hydrocarbon absorption include neurologic, pulmonary, cardiovascular, GI, and hepatic injuries. For further discussion, see chapter 199, "Hydrocarbons and Volatile Substances."

The primary treatment is decontamination by removing saturated clothing and irrigating exposed skin with soap and water. Otherwise, management is as for a thermal burn.

HOT TAR

Hot tar is derived from long-chain petroleum and coal hydrocarbons. Roofing tars and asphalt are heated to temperatures up to 500°F (260°C), and the burns sustained are usually more thermal than chemical. Although the surface area size of the burn is usually small, solidified material stuck to skin and hair is difficult to remove. **If hot, the tar should be cooled to prevent continued thermal injury.** Manual mechanical debridement can be painful and destructive to skin structures. Polyoxylene sorbitan (polysorbate), contained in many antibiotic ointments, is an emulsifying agent that can be used to remove tar. Industrial removal agents such as De-Solv-It®, a citrus and petroleum distillate, are also effective in tar removal. Baby oil is also effective for tar removal.

VESICANTS (DIMETHYL SULFOXIDE, CANTHARIDES, AND SULFUR MUSTARD)

Dimethyl sulfoxide, cantharides, and mustard gas are vesicant or drying agents. Skin burns with edema and blister formation occur due to production of ischemia and anoxic necrosis at the site of contact. Dimethyl sulfoxide is a water-soluble organic solvent used in industry. It is available without prescription and is used topically for sprains, bruises, minor burns, and joint pain. Due to its chemical composition and solubility, dimethyl sulfoxide can penetrate barrier surfaces such as nitrile gloves. Cantharides ("Spanish Fly") is occasionally used for its supposed aphrodisiac effects. Sulfur mustard is a vesicant historically used in chemical warfare. An alkylating agent, exposure results in inhibition of cellular enzymatic activity, leading to necrosis. For further discussion, see chapter 8, "Chemical Disasters."

Skin damage following vesicant exposure can be severe and result in deep skin penetration, edema, blisters, ulcers, and serious morbidity. Immediate, copious irrigation with water or saline may mitigate the extent of tissue injury. Skin can also be decontaminated by using adsorbent powders such as flour, talcum powder, and fuller's earth if the supply of water is limited. These powders adsorb the mustard from the skin and should be wiped away with a moist towel. Almost any material can be used to brush the vesicant away from skin. The military uses M258A1 kits for skin decontamination. These kits contain three sets of towelettes, one of each containing phenol, sodium hydroxide, and sodium benzene sulphonochloramine (chloramine). Chloramine produces "free" chlorine, which inactivates sulfur mustard. Povidone iodine shows great promise in the prevention and early treatment of skin damage caused by sulfur mustard. Human data are currently lacking, but in animal models, both prevention of burns and immediate (<10 minutes) treatment of exposure yielded impressive skin protection.[12]

POTASSIUM PERMANGANATE

Potassium permanganate is an oxidizing agent that is mildly irritating in dilute solution, but in concentrated solution, it can produce dermal burns with a thick, brownish purple eschar of coagulated protein. Burns should be copiously irrigated with water.

ALKYL MERCURY COMPOUNDS

Alkyl mercury compounds, which are reducing agents used in disinfectants, fungicides, and wood preservatives, can produce dermatitis or burn lesions. Lesions typically are erythematous with blister formation. The blister fluid is high in metallic mercury content. The burning process continues as long as the agent remains in contact with skin. Partial-thickness burns deepen if the blister fluid is allowed to remain, so the blisters should be debrided, drained, and copiously irrigated. Repeated or prolonged exposure to topical mercury compounds may lead to systemic mercury toxicity.

LACRIMATORS OR TEAR GAS

Lacrimators, or tear gas, such as 2-chloroacetophenone, o-chlorobenzylidene malonitrile, and oleoresin capsicum (pepper spray), cause skin and mucosal irritation within 20 to 60 seconds of exposure and can lead to development of contact dermatitis. Although the skin injury is usually limited, inhalation and eye injuries may be severe. Treatment of skin exposure is rapid removal from the offending agent followed by saline irrigation. Ocular irritation is treated with copious water irrigation, followed by slit-lamp examination for corneal damage. Arrange ophthalmology follow-up in 24 hours. High concentrations of lacrimators cause structural damage of the cornea. Inhalation injuries are treated with respiratory support including oxygen and bronchodilators. There is no role for steroid therapy.[13]

WHITE PHOSPHORUS

White phosphorus is used as an incendiary in munitions and fireworks and as a component of insecticides, rodenticides, and fertilizers. It ignites spontaneously when exposed to air and is rapidly oxidized to phosphorus pentoxide. Burns caused by both its solid and liquid forms are seen in both the military and civilian populations. In munitions, white phosphorus is solid, but some of it may liquefy with detonation. Death has been reported in burns covering <10% body surface area.

Flaming droplets of inorganic phosphorus may embed beneath the skin. The heat of the reaction causes tissue destruction. Particles continue to oxidize slowly until debrided, neutralized, or completely oxidized. As long as phosphorous is exposed to air, it will continue to burn. Remove contaminated clothing and visible particles, and copiously irrigate burns with normal saline or water. Skin exposed to white phosphorus must remain wet or immersed in water until completely debrided to prevent further injury. **Wood's lamp** examination aids identification of remaining phosphorus as it fluoresces. **Copper sulfate solution should not be used despite its ability to detoxify phosphorous because it causes hemolysis and increases mortality.**

White phosphorus burns are characterized by slow healing and ongoing burning, necessitating early and aggressive treatment. Systemically absorbed phosphorous is a serious concern. Hypocalcemia, hyperkalemia, and hepatic and renal injury all have been reported. Even patients with small burns should be considered for admission or transfer to a burn center for aggressive hydration, monitoring, and further treatment.[14] Treatment providers should take care to wear protective equipment and avoid direct contact with the patient's clothing, feces, and emesis.

AIRBAG BURNS

Approximately 8% of individuals suffering injuries related to airbag deployment are burned. Airbags deploy by ignition of solid propellant—sodium azide and cupric oxide—that creates an exothermic reaction leading to rapid inflation of the airbag. Many other gases are created during activation, including corrosives such as sodium hydroxide, nitric oxide, ammonia, and multiple hydrocarbons. An airbag is deflated within 2 seconds of inflation through exhaust side ports on the bag. Burns associated with airbags include friction, thermal, and chemical burns.[15] Sodium hydroxide produced during airbag activation can cause chemical keratitis. Full-thickness skin burns have been reported. Perform slit-lamp examination for eye irritation to detect keratitis. Treatment of airbag chemical burns is similar to any alkali burn: immediate and copious water irrigation.

OCULAR BURNS

Chemical burns to the eyes are ocular emergencies requiring immediate treatment.[16]

If the nature of the chemical is not known, use pH paper to determine the presence of acid or alkali. Acid quickly precipitates the superficial tissue proteins of the eye, producing the typical "ground glass" appearance of the cornea. **Damage sustained secondary to acid burns is, in most cases, immediate and limited to the area of contact.** The posterior segment of the eye rarely suffers injury, but prolonged exposure, highly concentrated solution, or exposure to hydrofluoric acid may lead to deeper penetration and permanent injury.

Alkali burns are generally more severe, frequently with unsightly and disastrous results. Higher pH, more concentrated solution, and longer duration of exposure are associated with greater injury. **In a short period of time, strong alkalis can penetrate the cornea, anterior chamber, and retina, with destruction of all sensory elements, thus causing complete blindness** (see Figure 241-50 in chapter titled "Eye Emergencies").

The penetration of alkali can continue for hours to days, resulting in globe perforation. The vessels of the conjunctiva and sclera as well as collecting veins of the anterior chamber may be destroyed, leading to secondary glaucoma. Second- and third-degree burns of surrounding tissue can complicate the burn.

Treatment of eye burns should not be delayed. Immediate treatment is copious and continuous water irrigation at the scene, in transport, and at the hospital. Eye-irrigation kits may be used. Although specific solutions may be beneficial in irrigation of the injury, delay in irrigation cannot be justified. Sterile water or saline is recommended. **In general, 1 to 2 L of normal saline for each eye for 30-minute continuous irrigation is the minimum treatment. Neutralizing substances should not be used.**

Acid burns may not require as much volume or treatment time as alkali burns. For treatment of severe alkali burns, 24 hours or more of continuous irrigation may be necessary. Checking the pH in the conjunctival sac to see whether it has returned to 7.4 is helpful in determining need for further irrigation. However, extended 2- to 3-hour irrigation, despite apparent conjunctival pH correction, is recommended in the setting of strong alkaline or hydrofluoric acid burns with obvious examination abnormality to correct anterior chamber pH as well as conjunctival pH. **During irrigation, the eyelid may have to be held open manually or with retractors due to severe orbicularis spasm (see chapter 241).** The eyelids should be everted. **Sweep the fornices with a wet cotton applicator to remove any particulate matter, especially if the pH is not responding well to irrigation.**

Pain control with topical anesthetics during evaluation and treatment is necessary. Systemic opioids may be necessary for severe pain or associated injuries. **Emergency ophthalmology consultation is needed for corneal burns.** For additional discussion, see chapter 241.

IATROGENIC CHEMICAL BURNS

Iatrogenic chemical burns have been caused by the use of potassium permanganate at an inappropriately high concentration to treat dermatologic problems. Dimethyl sulfoxide used as a transcutaneous vehicle for minor sprains has caused burns. Patients in the operating room may develop burns from skin preparation solutions. Thimerosal, which has a high mercury content, is the most common agent implicated. Mechanical abrasion of the skin from scrubbing and from pooling of the skin preparation agent under the torso or tourniquet predisposes patients to burns. Blister formation, skin sloughing, and eschar development have been reported in neonates when isopropyl alcohol pledgets were substituted for conducting paste beneath limb electrocardiograph electrodes. Silver nitrate used to cauterize umbilical granulomas in infants reportedly has caused periumbilical burns.

REFERENCES

The complete reference list is available online at www.TintinalliEM.com.

Electrical and Lightning Injuries

Caitlin Bailey

INTRODUCTION

Electrical injuries are divided into high-voltage injuries (≥1000 V), low-voltage injuries (<1000 V), and electric arc flash burns, which by definition do not result in passage of current through the tissues. Lightning injury is an extreme and unique form of electrical injury. This chapter also discusses injuries caused by electronic control devices, such as the **Taser®**. Burns from electrical accidents can result from heating due to electric current flow through tissues, explosions, and burning of flammable liquids, clothes, and other objects. Burns are discussed in the chapter 216, "Thermal Burns."

EPIDEMIOLOGY

Approximately 6500 electrical injuries occur per year in the United States, accounting for 4% of total burns. Of these, the majority are work related (61%), mostly industrial injuries. The overall complication rate is 10.6%, with the fewest complications among children age 1 to 5 years (2%).[1] The most common high-voltage injuries in the United States are also work related and include arc burns in electricians and high-voltage injuries in power line workers.[2] The Electrical Safety Foundation International estimates that contact with electric current caused nearly 1800 workplace fatalities between 2003 and 2010.[3] High-voltage power line injuries are particularly disabling because they often lead to deep-muscle necrosis and the need for fasciotomy and amputation.[2]

BASICS OF CURRENT FLOW

Electric current is the movement of electrical charges. **Table 218-1** lists a few key terms related to electricity.

Current flow is measured in amperes. Current flow is driven by an electrical potential difference, which is measured in volts. Intervening material between two or more contact points resists electric current flow; this resistance is measured in ohms. Ohm's law describes the relationship between current (I), voltage (V), and resistance (R) and states that the *current* through a conductor between two points is directly proportional to the potential difference or voltage drop across the two points and inversely proportional to the resistance between them. For example, a person who grasps a grounded pipe in one hand and a metal cable connected to a 120-V source in the other hand will experience a current flow through the body, the magnitude of which varies inversely with the resistance of the circuit. If the total resistance from the power source, through the person, and to ground is estimated to be 1000 Ω, the current would be I = (120 V)/(1000 Ω) = 0.120 A = 120 mA.

Conductors are materials that allow electric current to flow easily. Insulators are materials that do not allow electric current flow. Most biologic materials conduct electricity to some extent. Tissues with high fluid and electrolyte content conduct electricity better than tissues with less fluid and electrolyte content. Bone is the biologic tissue with the greatest resistance to electric current, whereas nerves and vascular structures have low resistance. Dry skin has high resistance, but sweaty or wet skin has much less resistance.

Many of the physiologic effects of electric shock are related to the amount, duration, and type of current (alternating current [AC] or direct current [DC]) and the path of current flow (**Table 218-2**). DC current flows in a constant direction, whereas AC current alternates direction in a cyclical fashion. **Standard household electricity is AC. Electricity in batteries and lightning is DC. Low-frequency (50- to 60-Hz) AC can be more dangerous than similar levels of DC because the alternating current fluctuations can result in ventricular fibrillation.** The identification of electric shock as due to AC or DC is also important

TABLE 218-1 Electrical Terms and Units of Measure

Term	Unit of Measure
Electric current Movement of electrical charges	Amperes
Current flow Driven by voltage or electrical potential difference	Volts
Resistance Hindrance to flow of current	Ohms
Ohm's law (current = voltage/resistance) The current is proportional to voltage. The current is inversely proportional to resistance.	—

TABLE 218-2 Effects of Current

Effect	Current Path	Minimum Current: 60 Hz AC (mA)*
Tingling sensation, minimal perception	Through intact skin	0.5–2.0
Pain threshold	Through intact skin	1–4
Inability to let go: tetanic contractions of hand and forearm tighten grasp, decreasing skin resistance	From hand through forearm muscles into trunk	6–22
Respiratory arrest: can be fatal if prolonged	Through chest	18–30
Ventricular fibrillation	Through chest	70–4000
Ventricular standstill (asystole): similar to defibrillation; if current stops, sinus rhythm may resume	Through chest	>2000

*Ranges are approximate and depend on various factors.

to reconstruct the mechanism of injury. AC current can produce muscular tetany, during which the victim cannot let go of the electrical source. Both AC and DC current can hurl the victim away from the current source, which results in severe blunt force injury.

For current to flow through an individual, a complete circuit must be created from one terminal of a voltage source to a contact area on the body, through the subject, and then from another contact on the person to the other terminal of the voltage source (or to a ground that is connected to the voltage source). Current flows through a person from one contact area to another along multiple, somewhat parallel paths. For example, electrical power source contacts just on the left hand and left leg would result in current flow through those limbs and the trunk, including the heart, muscles of respiration, and other tissues in the trunk. Current would not flow through the other limbs or head, because they are not in an electrically conductive path between the two power source contacts. The pattern of current flow through the body, if known, can be used to raise or lower suspicion of injury to certain body parts; for instance, hand-to-hand flow involves crossing the thorax and heart, raising the suspicion for cardiac involvement.

An exception to the requirement that a circuit be present occurs with electrostatic discharge. Electrostatic discharge is the transfer of excess charge to or from a person or object to another object and results when objects at different potentials come into direct contact with each other. An example is static electricity, which can cause pain and reflex movements.

MECHANISMS OF ELECTRICAL INJURY

HIGH- AND LOW-VOLTAGE INJURIES

The risk for serious and fatal electrical injury increases with voltage, especially >600 V (Table 218-2). High voltage is usually defined as >1000 V. Power lines in U.S. residential areas typically carry 7620 V AC. This is stepped down by transformers to 240 V AC before entering most residential and nonindustrial buildings. **In the United States, home outlets are 120 V, and in Europe and Australia, they are 240 V.** Urban subway electrical third rails may be 600 V or more AC or DC. High-voltage injuries are more often associated with severe musculoskeletal, visceral, and nervous system injury than are low-voltage injuries.

Electricity-induced injuries can occur via several mechanisms: (1) direct tissue damage from the electrical energy, (2) tissue damage from thermal energy, and (3) mechanical injury from trauma induced by a fall or muscle contraction.

ELECTRICAL BURNS

Electrical burns are severe when high voltages are involved, because only a fraction of a second of current flow is necessary for severe damage to occur.[4] Burns are less common with low-voltage injuries, because low-voltage contact produces little heat energy in the skin and other tissues.[5]

ELECTRIC ARC INJURIES

Electricity arcing from one conductor to another may radiate enough heat to burn and even kill persons 10 or more feet from the arc. There can also be a blast force that throws the person. Arcs that do contact a person directly will have heating due to current flow through the body, in addition to the flash burn and mechanical blast forces. Serious burns often result.[6] The voltages that create an electric arc are usually in the thousands of volts. Temperatures as high as 20,000°C (35,000°F) are created. Serious, and sometimes fatal, burns may result from heat radiated by the arc and clothing ignited by the arc.

TETANIC CONTRACTIONS

Electric current can induce sustained muscular contraction, or tetany. The overall effect varies according to type (AC or DC), frequency, voltage, and extent of contact.[4,7] For example, AC current flowing through the forearm can cause flexor tetany of the fingers and forearm that overpowers actions of the extensor muscles. Forceful muscle contractions can cause fractures and joint dislocations, especially around the shoulders.[8] If the hand and fingers are properly positioned, the hand will grasp the conductor tightly, leading to prolonged, low-resistance contact with the power source because the person cannot let go. This allows current to flow for many seconds or minutes.

The increased duration of contact and the decreased contact resistance caused by a tight sustained grasp greatly increase the heat-related damage to deep tissues. Heating due to electric current builds over time. Because heating is directly proportional to the duration of current flow and proportional to the square of the current amplitude (until burning and other tissue changes occur), a person who is unable to let go of a conductor for 30 seconds receives about 90 times as much tissue heating as a person who recoils from the voltage source in one third of a second. To make injury still more severe, a tight grasp on a conductor decreases contact resistance, which leads to an increase in current flow. Thus, heat-related injury to deep tissues is often more than a hundred times worse when there is a history of the patient's being unable to let go of the conductor.

Current flow through the trunk and legs may cause brief, but strong, opisthotonic (arching) posturing and leg movements. The person appears to be thrust from the voltage source due to these muscle contractions and may sustain mechanical trauma in addition to electrical injury. If a person does manage to hold on to a high-voltage source, severe tissue damage occurs.

CLINICAL FEATURES OF ELECTRICAL INJURY

Electric current can induce immediate cardiac dysrhythmias, respiratory arrest, and seizures. Current that traverses the chest vertically (hand to foot or head to toe) or horizontally (hand to hand) can produce arrhythmias and respiratory arrest.

CARDIAC DYSRHYTHMIAS

Fatalities due to asystole or ventricular fibrillation usually occur prior to arrival in the ED.[5] **Asymptomatic patients with normal ECGs on arrival to the hospital do not develop later dysrhythmias after low-voltage (<1000 V) injuries.**[9-13] However, nerve and deep-muscle injuries are relatively common following contact with voltages >400 V. Therefore, carefully examine for peripheral nervous system and CNS function and burns, and check for elevated serum creatine phosphokinase.

CNS, SPINAL CORD, AND PERIPHERAL NERVOUS SYSTEM INJURY

Neurologic impairment is common in electrical injuries, occurring in approximately 50% of patients with high-voltage injuries.[2] Nerve tissue has the lowest resistance in the body, encouraging electrical passage through these tissues and causing associated damage. Given the multi-system dysfunction present in many electrical injury patients, document a neurologic exam, if possible, before intubation and sedation.

Brain Injury Electrocution can result in a broad range of CNS dysfunction. Transient loss of consciousness is common and may be followed by seizures. Victims may be confused and agitated or deeply comatose and require airway protection. Patients may also demonstrate focal neurologic deficits such as quadriplegia, hemiplegia, aphasia, or visual disturbances. Obtain head and cervical spine CT to rule out traumatic etiologies for these deficits; MRI may be necessary for purely electrical damage. Electrical injury can cause blindness[14] due to occipital lobe injury as well as direct injury to the optic nerve.[15,16] Neurologic deficits may be transient, but survivors may have persistent difficulties with attention, working memory, and learning.[17]

Spinal Cord Injury Spinal cord injury can occur in up to 8% of high-voltage electrical injuries.[18] Spinal cord injuries can be the result of compressive vertebral fractures, sometimes at multiple levels.[19] However, damage can also occur due to purely electrical damage without fractures, through direct cellular damage as well as vascular injury.[20] With electrical trauma, initial spinal cord MRI results do not necessarily correlate with prognosis. MRI findings may be normal in electrical trauma patients with permanent spinal cord injury,[21-23] although newer MRI imaging protocols may detect abnormalities silent on standard MRI.[24] With mechanical trauma, emergency MRI after spinal cord injury provides accurate prognostic information regarding neurologic function.

Neurologic deterioration can occur days to months after the initial injury[25-27] and generally has incomplete resolution. There is a motor predominance in deficit in most of these cases. Delayed onset of spinal cord dysfunction may be due to progressive vascular injury (especially to the spinal artery branch supplying the anterior horn cells) or delayed cell membrane damage via the cumulative effect of free radicals (electroporation), leading to progressive demyelination.[21,28] The clinical features may take the form of transverse myelitis, amyotrophic lateral sclerosis, or a Guillain-Barré–like illness.[29]

Peripheral Nerve Injury Peripheral nerve injuries often involve the hands after the individual touches a power source. Paresthesias may be immediate and transient or delayed in onset, appearing up to 2 years after injury.[2,30] Extensive peripheral nerve damage may occur with minimal thermal injury. Electrical contact with the palm produces median or ulnar neuropathy more often than radial nerve injury.[31] Brachial plexus lesions have also been reported. Persistent symptoms related to peripheral nerve damage can occur despite normal results on nerve conduction studies.[32]

CUTANEOUS BURNS

Cutaneous burns are often seen at the electrical contact areas (often referred to as *entry* and *exit wounds* in the case of DC current, or *contact wounds* in the case of AC current). Many seriously injured patients have burns on either the arm or skull, paired with burns on the feet. Burns are typically painless, gray to yellow, depressed areas. Most patients with burns from electrical injury need admission and care by a burn specialist. See chapter 216 for detailed discussion of management of cutaneous burns.

ORTHOPEDIC INJURY

Fractures may be caused by tetanic muscle contractions or associated falls. Fractures may be missed on initial assessment due to altered mental status and the overall severity of systemic illness. A comprehensive tertiary survey should be performed when clinically feasible to detect orthopedic injuries. Although fractures are more likely to result from high-voltage injury, fractures of the wrist, forearm, humerus, femoral necks, shoulders, and scapulae have been reported from exposure to household voltages (120 to 220 V AC) without associated trauma.[7,33,34] Posterior shoulder dislocations are commonly seen with electrical injury.

VASCULAR AND MUSCLE INJURY

Vascular and muscle injuries occur most commonly in the setting of high-voltage injury, such as power line contact. Electric current passing along peripheral arteries may cause early spasm and persistent deficits in endothelial and smooth muscle function,[35] as well as subsequent thrombosis, stenosis, or aneurysm formation. Because of concomitant vascular and muscular destruction, **patients with high-voltage shocks are at significant risk for development of compartment syndrome, even if the contact (or arcing) lasted <1 second.** Compartment syndrome has also been noted in patients with injuries from 120 V AC or higher who sustain contact for longer than a few seconds. Patients typically exhibit ongoing muscle pain with movement.[6]

Contact with >1000 V, prehospital cardiac arrest, crush injury, and full-thickness skin burns are associated with significant tissue damage requiring surgical intervention. Fasciotomy and amputation are frequent sequelae of high-voltage injuries, occurring in 29% and 41% of patients in one study.[36] High-voltage electrical injury is associated with rapid loss of body fluids into the areas of tissue damage, requiring aggressive resuscitation.

COAGULATION DISORDERS

Thermal injury or tissue necrosis from electric current can cause a variety of coagulation disorders. Low-grade disseminated intravascular coagulation may be a result of hypoxia, vascular stasis, rhabdomyolysis, and release of procoagulants from damaged tissue. Transient coagulopathies have also been reported with high-voltage injury, including acquired, transient factor X deficiency.[37] Electrical injury may unmask underlying vascular injury and has been reported in association with ischemic stroke at low voltage.[38]

BLAST INJURY

Electric arcs in the industrial environment or near a power line can produce a strong blast pressure, similar to those seen in other types of explosions.[39] Cognitive complaints following blast injury may resemble those that result from moderate mechanical head trauma. Mechanisms of brain injury include mechanical trauma related to the blast and arterial air emboli associated with blast-related alveolar disruption (see chapter 7, "Bomb, Blast, and Crush Injuries").

INHALATION INJURY

Chemical toxins such as ozone can be produced by coronas and arcs. Acute effects of ozone exposure include mucous membrane irritation, temporarily reduced pulmonary function, and pulmonary hemorrhage and edema. Fires and explosions associated with electric incidents may lead to inhalation of carbon monoxide and other toxic substances.

OCULAR INJURY

Electrical shock can cause a wide range of ocular trauma, most commonly to the cornea (epithelial erosion/defect, keratitis, scarring), as well as uveitis, retinal detachment, macular edema, optic nerve damage, and intraocular bleeding and thrombosis.[15,40,41] Obtain a full ophthalmologic evaluation for any electric shock patient with an ocular complaint to document related injury. Cataract formation has been described weeks to years after electrical injury to head, neck, or upper chest.[7] Cataracts have also occurred after electric arc or flash burns.

AUDITORY INJURY

The auditory system may be damaged by current or by hemorrhage in the tympanic membrane, middle ear, cochlea, cochlear duct, and vestibular apparatus. Delayed complications include mastoiditis, sinus thrombosis, meningitis, and brain abscess. Hearing loss may be immediate or develop later as a result of complications. Hearing should be briefly checked in the ED, with follow-up formal testing arranged for any patient who appears to have a deficit.

GI INJURY

Pain due to bowel perforation and intra-abdominal hemorrhage may be attributed to more obvious coexisting injuries.[42] There are reports in the literature of lethal intra-abdominal injuries from electric current that were found only at autopsy. Ileus may develop in association with spinal cord injury.

SCENE AND PREHOSPITAL CARE

Table 218-3 outlines prehospital care of the patient with electrical injury.

RESCUER SAFETY

Stay away from downed power lines. The scene of a high-voltage electric incident contains many hazards for rescue personnel. Power lines are almost never insulated, although a line may appear to be insulated because of atmospheric contaminants deposited on the line over time. Electrocution is possible when walking on ground near a downed power line because of voltage gradients in the ground. **Stay at least 10 m (32 ft) from downed power lines. Even this distance is not without risk.**

Reapplication of voltage to downed lines sometimes occurs as circuit breakers automatically reset, which makes the lines physically jump many feet with great force. This danger may be mitigated by placing a heavy object over the line, but this maneuver itself is fraught with risk.

Support structures may be electrically alive. Metal cables that support telephone and power poles are normally grounded, but may be energized if they are broken or disconnected from a ground attachment and contact is made with a nearby power line.

Victims still in contact with a source of voltage may transmit an electric current to would-be rescuers. It is best first to turn off the source of electricity if it can be done quickly. If this cannot be done quickly, precautions must be taken to prevent electrical injury to the rescuer. With voltages above about 600 V, dry wood and other materials may conduct significant amounts of electric current and therefore cannot be used to remove the person from a voltage source. A rescuer standing on the ground touching any part of a vehicle that is in contact with a power line is likely to be killed or seriously injured. Electric shock is not prevented in this situation by the rescuer's wearing rubber gloves and boots, unless these are designed for the voltage present and have been recently tested for insulation integrity. Persons inside a vehicle in contact with a power line are likely to be killed as they step out of the vehicle and may also receive a shock if they touch objects at different potentials inside the vehicle.

SCENE RESUSCITATION AND STABILIZATION

Rescue breathing for line workers in respiratory arrest on utility power poles should be initiated by rescuers while the injured individual is still on the pole as long as the injured worker and rescuers are no longer in contact with the energized line. As soon as the patient is lowered to the ground, chest compressions can be done if there is cardiac and respiratory arrest.

Low-voltage AC can produce ventricular fibrillation by direct stimulation of the heart, or it can occur after several minutes of respiratory arrest resulting from paralysis of respiratory muscles (Table 218-2). **High-voltage AC and DC are more likely to produce transient ventricular asystole.** Asystole sometimes reverts spontaneously to normal sinus rhythm with pulses, but prolonged apnea may continue. **Apnea with pulses** sometimes occurs in linemen working above the ground near high-voltage lines. Supporting respirations above ground may be all that is needed to stabilize the patient. Maintain vigorous resuscitation efforts for cardiac arrest from electric shock, because there may be insignificant tissue damage despite the potentially lethal dysrhythmia.[43]

Maintain spinal immobilization during resuscitation to the extent possible, because spinal fractures can be caused by tetanic muscle contractions, falls, and other secondary trauma.

TABLE 218-3 Scene and Prehospital Care

Stay at least 10 m (32 ft) from downed power lines, jumping power lines, and support structures.
Turn off the source of electricity prior to rescue, if possible.
If electrical source cannot be quickly turned off, take precautions to prevent electrical injury to the rescuer.
Wear gloves and shoes rated for the power line voltage.
Initiate rescue breathing and resuscitation efforts while injured person is still on pole, if no contact with source of electricity is assured.
Maintain spinal immobilization of injured person, if possible.

ED DIAGNOSIS AND TREATMENT

Provide the usual evaluation (airway, breathing, circulation) and resuscitation for major trauma victims. Maintain spinal immobilization during resuscitation until adequate imaging and examination can be done.

Treat cardiac arrhythmias according to accepted advanced life support guidelines. Institute ED cardiac monitoring for patients with high-voltage injuries as well as all symptomatic patients.[9,10] Cardiac complications are more common in patients with high-voltage injuries and in those with loss of consciousness and include ventricular and atrial dysrhythmias, bradydysrhythmias, and QT-interval prolongation.[44-46] **Admission for cardiac monitoring is not needed for asymptomatic patients with normal ECG on presentation after a low-voltage electrical injury.**

Assess for tissue damage and identify associated complications. A careful vascular and neurologic examination of involved extremities is important. Normal findings on initial assessment do not exclude serious injury or the possibility of delayed spinal cord injury following high-voltage contact.

Focus next on systematic assessment and treatment, especially for injuries specific to or common in electrical injury, as outlined in **Table 218-4**. Laboratory and radiographic evaluation of high-voltage injuries should follow standard trauma guidelines (see chapters in Section 21, "Trauma," and Section 22, "Injuries to Bones and Joints").

TABLE 218-4 Assessment and Treatment of Complications Associated with Electrical Injuries

Organ or System	Assessment/Treatment/Comments
Circulatory	Start with Parkland fluid resuscitation formula.*
Renal	Initiate fluid resuscitation.
Myoglobinuria	Initiate fluid resuscitation†
Central and peripheral nervous	Order head CT if mental status is abnormal; assess for spinal cord and peripheral nerve injury.
Skin	Assess and treat cutaneous burns.*
Musculoskeletal	Perform careful assessment of spine, pelvis, long bones, and joints. Assess for compartment syndrome and need for fasciotomy.
Vascular	Spasm may occur leading to delayed thrombosis, aneurysm formation, or muscle damage.
Coagulation	Treat coagulation disorders by eliminating the precipitating factor through early surgical debridement. If bleeding is present, replace coagulation factors.‡
Lungs	Assess for inhalation injury, carbon monoxide, or alveolar injury from blast.
Eyes	Document complete eye examination. Delayed cataracts may develop.
Ears	Assess for blast injury. Document hearing. Middle and inner ear disorders and hearing loss may occur.
GI	Intra-abdominal injury may occur from current or blast.
Lips and oral cavity	Watch for delayed bleeding.

*Refer to chapter 216, "Thermal Burns."
†Refer to chapter 89, "Rhabdomyolysis."
‡Refer to chapter 254, "Trauma in Adults."

TABLE 218-5 GI Injury in Electrocution

When to Suspect GI Injury
Electrical burns of the abdominal wall
History of a fall, nearby explosion, or other mechanical trauma
Evaluation
US and CT
Surgical consult as indicated
Treatment
Ileus: nasogastric tube insertion
Stress (Curling) ulcer prophylaxis: histamine-2 blockers, antacids, proton pump inhibitors
Monitoring for development of ileus, bowel perforation, hemorrhage, and other delayed complications
Surgical management as appropriate

In the case of **low-voltage injuries**, laboratory testing and imaging are usually not required unless the patient is symptomatic or has abnormal physical examination findings. Symptoms such as chest pain, palpations, loss of consciousness, altered mental status, confusion, weakness, dyspnea, abdominal pain, burn with subcutaneous damage, vascular compromise, or abnormal results on ECG require further testing.

FLUID RESUSCITATION

Fluid resuscitation guided by the Parkland formula (4 mL/kg multiplied by the percentage of body surface area burned, administered over 24 hours) is a reasonable starting point in fluid management. Extensive deep tissue damage resulting from high-voltage injury may be present even when the cutaneous burn seems limited. Therefore, fluid requirements are often greater than predicted by the Parkland formula and physical examination.

MYOGLOBINURIA

Patients with suggestive symptoms or high-voltage injury should be monitored for the onset of compartment syndrome, rhabdomyolysis, and renal failure. If myoglobinuria is suspected, institute aggressive IV fluid resuscitation to maintain a urinary output of between 1 and 2 mL/kg/h, with attention to correction and prevention of electrolyte abnormalities. Evidence of effectiveness of sodium bicarbonate is not well documented. Initial IV rate in the adult is up to 1.5 L/h (more if there is hypotension or obvious blood loss). Maintain a high urine output until serum creatine kinase level is less than five times normal or urine myoglobin measurements return to normal. **Monitor serum, not urine, pH.** Urine pH measurements are influenced by hemochromogens in the urine and, therefore, may not be useful.

Prognostic factors associated with the need for a fasciotomy within 24 hours of injury are (1) myoglobinuria, (2) burns over 20% of total body surface area, or (3) a full-thickness burn over 12% body surface area.[36] Presence of any one of these three factors is predictive of development of the need for fasciotomy.

GI INJURY

GI injuries should be suspected in all patients with a history of electrical burns to the abdominal wall or mechanical trauma associated with the electrical injury. **Table 218-5** summarizes an approach to GI injury.

DISPOSITION AND FOLLOW-UP

LOW-VOLTAGE INJURIES <600 V

Although there is no universally accepted protocol for management and disposition of patients with low-voltage injuries, **in general, asymptomatic patients who sustain an electric shock of ≤240 V AC can be discharged home if they have a normal ECG on presentation and normal examination findings.**[9,10] Patients who feel unwell or have any new ECG abnormality should be monitored for 6 hours and reassessed.[9,10]

HIGH-VOLTAGE INJURIES

All patients having contact with ≥600 V AC should be admitted for observation, even if there is no apparent injury. Routine cardiac monitoring is not required unless the patient is symptomatic or the initial ECG findings are abnormal. Low-voltage injury patients with symptoms beyond superficial skin injury or abnormal lab/ECG results may have systemic injury and require admission as well. Patients with extensive cutaneous burns should be transferred to a specialized burn center after initial trauma stabilization. This is especially true in children.[47]

SPECIAL POPULATIONS

PREGNANT WOMEN

In addition to the measures recommended above, in pregnant women beyond 20 to 24 weeks of gestation, monitor fetal heart rate and uterine activity for at least 4 hours because of the possibility of mechanical trauma related to the electric shock and electrical discharge to the fetus.[48-50]

CHILDREN

Children are more likely to sustain household current electrical injury than high-voltage injury. Overall outcome appears to be better, including a lower incidence of amputation and fasciotomy than in adults, although skin grafts may be required (25% in one 10-year study of pediatric burn center referrals).[47]

Oral and Lip Burns Serious oral injury can occur in a child who places the end of a power cord in the mouth. The electric field and current flow created between the two wires near the end of the cord can produce high temperatures and significant tissue damage. Most injuries are unilateral, involving the lateral commissure, tongue, and/or alveolar ridge[4,51,52] (**Figure 218-1**). Systemic complications of oral burns are uncommon. **Vascular injury to the labial artery is not immediately apparent** because of vascular spasm, thrombosis, and overlying eschar. Severe bleeding from the labial artery occurs in up to 10% of cases when the eschar separates, usually after 5 days. For this reason, children with this injury are sometimes

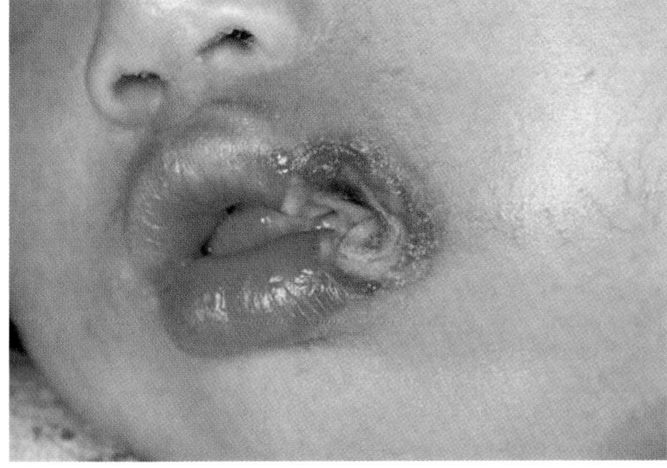

FIGURE 218-1. Oral burn in a child from power cord. A 2-year-old boy sustained a third-degree burn to the commissure of the mouth after biting down on an electrical cord. This photograph was taken 3 days after initial treatment. [Reproduced with permission from Shah BR, Lucchesi M: *Atlas of Pediatric Emergency Medicine*. © 2006 by McGraw-Hill, Inc., New York.]

admitted to the hospital. However, some authors believe that outpatient management is adequate in the right circumstances.[53] If the parents are reliable, can monitor the child, and can be shown how to control bleeding, outpatient management may be considered. Parents should be educated that bleeding may occur up to 2 weeks after injury. Prior to discharge, however, specialty consultation should be obtained and follow up secured, because of the risk of deforming scar formation during the healing process, in which new cells tend to migrate medially, reducing the span of mouth opening. Splinting and other measures are often needed to prevent the development of this deformity and dysfunction. Home care includes saline or hydrogen peroxide rinses and gentle swabbing to debride necrotic tissue and promote formation of healthy granulation tissue. Topical application of petrolatum-based antibiotics may have a soothing effect.

Hand Wounds Children who sustain hand wounds from electrical outlet injuries with no other injury and no evidence of cardiac or neurologic involvement can be discharged after local wound care is provided and careful follow up ensured. A child with a home situation of equivocal safety or reliability should be admitted.

LIGHTNING INJURIES

Lightning causes approximately 500 injuries each year in the United States, with an average of 51 deaths per year over the last 20 years (1984 to 2013).[54] Lightning fatalities constitute fewer than 3% of weather-related deaths, which are more commonly due to extreme heat or cold.[55] Lightning fatalities are most common in fishermen, but also occur in other outdoor recreational activities such as golf and camping.[54] Lightning injury reporting is inexact and biased toward the more severe and fatal events. Approximately 70% to 90% of persons struck by lightning survive, but as many as three quarters of these survivors have permanent sequelae.[56,57]

Lightning most often occurs during thunderstorms in association with large cumulonimbus clouds. However, approximately 10% of lightning occurs without rain and when the sky is blue.[58] In addition, lightning can occur during dust storms, sandstorms, tornados, hurricanes, snowstorms, and nuclear explosions, and in the clouds over volcanic eruptions. Lightning injuries can also occur while riding in airplanes. Lightning injury associated with indoor telephone use during lightning storms has been reported. A study in Australia identified up to 80 such injuries yearly without any reported fatalities.[59]

Even though lightning is electrical energy, lightning injuries differ substantially from high-voltage electrical injuries seen in association with human-generated sources. There are differences in injury patterns, injury severity, and emergency treatment[48,60,61] (**Table 218-6**).

PATHOPHYSIOLOGY

Lightning often travels over the surface of the body in a phenomenon called *flashover* and is therefore less likely to cause internal cardiac injury or muscle necrosis than is human-generated electrical energy. Wet skin may actually decrease the risk of internal injury, helping the current travel along the outside of the body. Flashover explains how victims may survive a lightning strike with little or no injury. Lightning causes internal injury through blunt mechanical force, current flow through the body, and other mechanisms. The large current flow in lightning creates a pulsed magnetic field that can induce current flow in a nearby person[62] and can produce destructive effects.

Lightning emits brief but intense thermal radiation that produces rapid heating and expansion of the surrounding air. Tympanic membrane perforation and internal organ contusion may occur. Vaporization of sweat from the skin can occur with tearing of clothing, giving the appearance of an assault.[63] Lightning may inflict thermal injury as moisture on the victim's skin is transformed into steam, as electric current flows through deeper tissues, and through resistance heating of metal objects on the body or in clothing pockets. Lightning may melt metallic objects on the victim. Lightning can be conducted along metal fences, bleachers, plumbing pipes, and other structures. Intense photic stimulation may damage the retina or produce cataracts.

STUNNING (KERAUNOPARALYSIS)

Neurologic and muscular "stunning," referred to as *keraunoparalysis*, can follow lightning strike and may initially produce a variety of neurologic signs and symptoms.[64] Keraunoparalysis is associated with successful resuscitation after cardiorespiratory arrest. In cases of keraunoparalysis that resolve within an hour, there can be lower limb weakness that is greater than upper limb weakness. Other extremity-related signs and symptoms include sensory abnormalities, pallor, coolness, and diminished and absent pulses. Excessive autonomic nervous system stimulation may be responsible for these transient symptoms.[65] In some cases, keraunoparalysis persists for a longer time. In such cases, there is typically amnesia and "neurotic" behavior that slowly clears over a week. More persistent and sometimes permanent sequelae can include muscular weakness and pain, photophobia, and disturbances of neurologic control.[62]

TYPES OF LIGHTNING STRIKES

Lightning strikes in a number of different ways, some of which injure multiple victims. A *direct strike* occurs when the victim is struck directly by the lightning discharge. A *side flash* occurs when a nearby object is

TABLE 218-6 Comparison of Lightning and Electrical Injuries

Factor	Lightning	High-Voltage AC	Low-Voltage AC
Current duration	10 μs to 3 ms	Generally brief (1–2 s), but may be prolonged	0.3 s or many minutes
Typical voltage and current range	10 million to 2 billion V, 10 to 200,000 A	600–200,000 V, <1000 A	<600 V, usually <20–30 A
Current characteristics	Unidirectional (DC)	Alternating (AC)	Alternating (AC)
Current pathway	Skin flashover; deeper pathways can result in burns	Horizontal (hand to hand), vertical (hand to foot)	Horizontal (hand to hand), vertical (hand to foot)
Tissue damage	Superficial and minor if no deep-tissue pathway	Deep-tissue destruction	Sometimes deep-tissue destruction
Initial rhythm in cardiac arrest	Asystole	Asystole more than ventricular fibrillation	Ventricular fibrillation
Renal involvement	Myoglobinuria is uncommon, and renal failure is rare	Myoglobinuria and renal failure are relatively common	Myoglobinuria and renal failure occur occasionally
Fasciotomy and amputation	Rarely necessary	Relatively common	Sometimes necessary
Blunt injury	Caused by explosive shock wave that can throw the person and cause eardrum rupture	Caused by falls, being thrown from current source, tetanic contractions	Caused by tetanic contraction, falls, being thrown from current source
Immediate cause of death	Prolonged apnea, blunt injury, deep-tissue burns	Prolonged apnea, ventricular fibrillation, blunt injury, deep-tissue burns	Ventricular fibrillation, prolonged apnea, blunt injury

Abbreviations: AC = alternating current; DC = direct current.

struck and current then traverses through the air to strike the victim. A side flash may injure multiple victims at once, as when a group huddles close to a structure that is struck. A *contact strike* occurs when lightning strikes an object the victim is holding and current is transferred from the object through the person to the ground. Lightning injury from indoor telephone use during a lightning storm is an example of contact strike. A *ground current* occurs when lightning hits the ground and current is transferred through the ground to nearby victims. The amount of electrical voltage and current decrease as the distance between the victim and strike point increases. This ground current can create a *stride potential* or step voltage between the victim's separated feet. The foot closer to the strike point will experience a higher electrical potential than the foot further away. Therefore, electric current can enter one foot, travel up that leg, through the torso, and down the other leg and exit the other foot. This can resuit in isolated neurovascular injury to the legs. Recently, a fifth mechanism, in which a weak *upward streamer* does not become connected to the completed lightning channel, was implicated in a fatal lightning injury.[66]

Immediate cardiac arrest from lightning strike results from depolarization of the myocardium and sustained asystole. Immediate respiratory arrest after lightning strike may be a result of depolarization and paralysis of the medullary respiratory center. **Both cardiac and respiratory arrest may be present without evidence of external injury.** Although cardiac automaticity may spontaneously return, concomitant respiratory arrest may persist and lead to a secondary hypoxic cardiac arrest. The duration of apnea, rather than the duration of cardiac arrest, appears to be the critical prognostic factor. Prolonged respiratory support with frequent monitoring of pulses can be effective in this situation.

CARE AT THE SCENE

Lightning can produce multiple victims because of multiple lightning strikes, stride potentials, and side flashes.[60] **In contrast to patients with cardiac arrest caused by mechanical trauma, persons with lightning injury who appear to be dead (in respiratory arrest, with or without cardiac arrest) should be treated first.** Such victims may have little physical damage, and they have a reasonable chance of successful resuscitation. Use of automated external defibrillators and other defibrillators along with CPR can be lifesaving. **Prolonged CPR is sometimes successful.**

During a storm, power lines may fall to the ground as a result of high winds, lightning-related damage to power lines and their support structures, and vehicular damage to power line support structures. Therefore, a person thought to have been hit by lightning may actually have been shocked by the stride potential related to a nearby power line lying on the ground. If a downed power line is found, safety precautions are important. Physical findings suggestive of lightning injury may be subtle or nonexistent. Therefore, information about the scene of the accident may be just as informative as examination of the patient.

ED DIAGNOSIS AND TREATMENT

The usual advanced cardiac and trauma treatment principles apply, including assessment and stabilization of the airway, breathing, and circulation. Lightning victims in cardiac arrest have a better prognosis than those in cardiac arrest from coronary artery disease, so aggressive resuscitative efforts are indicated.[43] Hypotension is not an expected finding following lightning injury and warrants an investigation for hemorrhagic blood loss. A careful secondary examination should be done to detect occult injuries.[67] Cutaneous burns may help identify the current path and suggest potential organ injury. Initial ancillary studies include CBC, serum electrolyte levels, creatinine level, BUN level, glucose level, creatine kinase level, urinalysis, and ECG. Imaging studies (plain radiography, US, or CT) should be performed as dictated by suspected injuries. Other ancillary studies may be indicated depending on clinical circumstances.

CARDIAC EFFECTS

In the victim with spontaneous circulation, hypertension and tachycardia are common findings, presumably because of sympathetic nervous system activation. Specific treatment is usually not necessary, because blood pressure and pulse rate will spontaneously decrease. Cardiac effects reported after lightning injury include global depression of myocardial contractility, coronary artery spasm, pericardial effusion, and atrial and ventricular arrhythmias. The ECG may show acute injury with ST-segment elevation and QT-interval prolongation. T-wave inversions may be seen, especially in the presence of neurologic injury. Myocardial infarction after lightning injury is unusual. CPR, automated external defibrillators, and other resuscitative measures should be used promptly.[43] Prolonged resuscitative efforts are sometimes successful.

NEUROLOGIC INJURY

Many lightning-strike victims are rendered unconscious or have temporary lower extremity paralysis. Seizures may result from the passage of electric current through the brain or may be the result of mechanical brain injury or hypoxia. The most lethal neurologic injuries involve heat-induced coagulation of the cerebral cortex, development of epidural or subdural hematoma, and intracerebral hemorrhage.

Autonomic dysfunction caused by lightning may produce pupillary dilation or anisocoria not related to brain injury, and these signs have no prognostic significance in comatose lightning-strike victims. Most neurologic injury related to lightning strike can be classified as immediate and transient or delayed and permanent, although some effects may be immediate and permanent. Transient effects that typically resolve in 24 hours include loss of consciousness, confusion, amnesia, and extremity paralysis. Delayed and often progressive disorders include seizures, muscular atrophy and amyotrophic lateral sclerosis, parkinsonian syndromes, progressive cerebellar ataxia, myelopathy with paraplegia or quadriplegia, and chronic pain syndromes.[28] Lightning can cause intracranial injury directly when passing through the head, as well as by secondary trauma. Therefore, CT scan is indicated in cases of coma, altered mental status, or persistent headache or confusion.

VASCULAR EFFECTS

Vasomotor spasm in an extremity is sometimes seen as a local response to lightning exposure. Possible mechanisms include sympathetic nervous stimulation, local arterial spasm, and ischemia of peripheral nerves. Skin color changes, from white to blue to red, may occur in extremities after lightning strike. Such changes are presumably from cycles of vasoconstriction and vasodilatation, with pallor and cyanosis followed by hyperemia. Severe vasoconstriction is thought to be responsible for loss of pulses, mottling of skin, coolness of extremities, loss of sensation, and paralysis due to ischemia of peripheral nerves. As vasoconstriction resolves spontaneously, these signs and symptoms often resolve. Because skeletal muscle injury is rare in lightning strike, compartment syndromes are less likely. If doubt exists, the presence of compartment syndrome and the need for fasciotomy may be confirmed by measurement of intracompartmental pressures and close clinical monitoring.

OCULAR INJURY

Ophthalmic injuries are common in lightning-strike victims, and lightning-induced cataracts are the most frequently observed ocular sequelae.[68] Cataracts caused by lightning are usually bilateral. Cataract formation without evidence of current flow through the head or eyes, such as after brief exposure to an electric arc, has been described. Perhaps this is a result of damage of the lens by radiant energy. Cataracts may form weeks to years after the lightning injury. Lightning can affect any part of the eye, producing hyphema, vitreous hemorrhage, corneal abrasion, uveitis, retinal detachment or hemorrhage, macular holes, and optic nerve damage. A patient with discomfort or visual changes deserves a careful examination with follow-up.

AUDITORY INJURY

Blast effect producing tympanic membrane rupture is relatively common. Victims sustaining lightning strike via a conventional corded telephone are at higher risk for otologic injury, including persistent tinnitus,

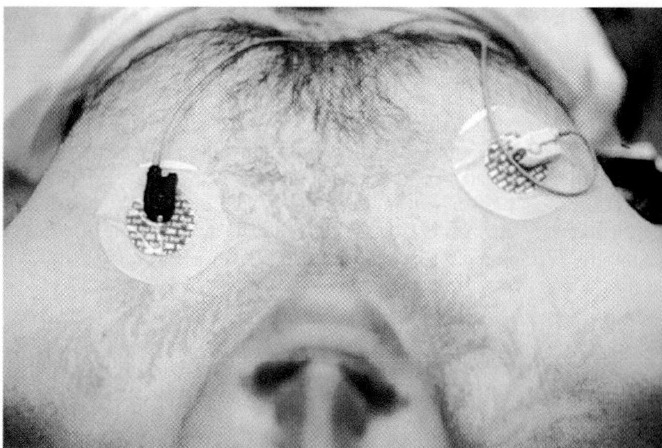

FIGURE 218-2. Lichtenberg figures with lacy ferning pattern seen on the upper chest. [Reproduced with permission from Knoop KJ, Stack LB, Storrow AB: *The Atlas of Emergency Medicine, 2nd ed.* © 2002 by McGraw-Hill, Inc., New York.]

sensorineural deafness, ataxia, vertigo, and nystagmus.[59] In patients who are sleeping with an ear or eye on the ground near a lightning strike, temporary deafness or blindness can result.

MUSCULOSKELETAL INJURY

A variety of skeletal fractures can be seen from the blunt force injury associated with lightning strike. Intense myotonic contractions can produce shoulder dislocations. Rhabdomyolysis after lightning strike is unusual. Spinal fractures can be caused by tetanic muscle contractions, as well as by falls and other secondary trauma. Therefore, maintain spinal immobilization during retrieval and resuscitation, to the extent possible under the circumstances, until spinal stability can be assessed. Because spinal fractures often occur at multiple levels in the same patient, image the entire vertebral column when a fracture is found at one level.

CUTANEOUS INJURY

There are six main dermatologic manifestations of lightning injury. **Lichtenberg figures** are considered pathognomonic for lightning strike and consist of a superficial feathering or ferning pattern (**Figure 218-2**). These figures are the result of electron showering over the skin and are not true thermal burns; they disappear within 24 hours. *Flash burns* are similar to those found in arc welders, appearing as mild erythema, and may involve the cornea. *Punctate burns* (**Figure 218-3**) look similar to cigarette burns in that they are usually <1 cm and are full-thickness burns. *Contact burns* occur when metal close to the skin is heated from the lightning current. *Superficial erythema* and *blistering burns* have been described. *Linear burns*, <5 cm wide, occur in areas of skin folds such as the axilla or groin. Contact wounds characteristic of electrical injury from human-produced sources are not commonly seen in lightning injuries. Cutaneous wounds are treated with customary wound or burn care, including tetanus prophylaxis, irrigation, debridement, and dressing.

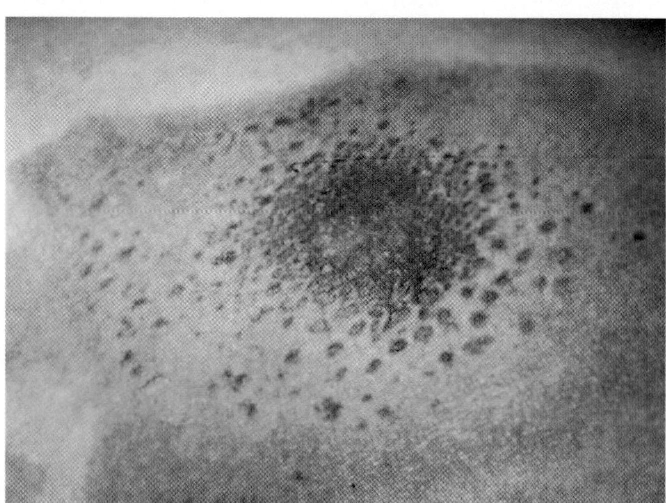

FIGURE 218-3. Punctate lightning burns. [Reproduced with permission from Knoop KJ, Stack LB, Storrow AB: *The Atlas of Emergency Medicine, 2nd ed.* © 2002 by McGraw-Hill, Inc., New York.]

PREVENTION

Safety recommendations include anticipating possible lightning storms (using resources such as the National Oceanic and Atmospheric Administration Weather Radio) and seeking safe shelter **indoors** when lightning is first seen or thunder is heard. Safer shelters include large structures with plumbing or electrical wiring, and fully enclosed metal vehicles. Dangerous locations to avoid include trees and other tall structures, open fields, open vehicles, and other open structures. During lightning storms, it is important to avoid being in or near water and to avoid contact with metal or wire fences and other conductive objects.[58]

DISPOSITION AND FOLLOW-UP

Patients should be carefully assessed for injuries. ECG and other monitoring is indicated as for any electric shock. Admission should be considered for most patients with persistent muscle pain, as well as those with persistent neurologic, cardiac rhythm, or vascular abnormalities. Follow-up is recommended to assess delayed effects of lightning, even for patients with no apparent injury.

SPECIAL POPULATIONS

In some cases, fetal injury and death have been noted to follow lightning strike with little or no maternal injury. One review reported that among 11 pregnant women who survived being struck by lightning, there were five cases of fetal death in utero, abortion, stillbirth, or neonatal death.[49] Abruptio placentae has also been reported. Monitoring of maternal uterine activity and fetal heart rate is recommended for at least 4 hours after a lightning strike to a pregnant woman. Such monitoring will alert the physician to the development of abruptio placentae, which can occur following any physical trauma.

INJURY DUE TO ELECTRONIC CONTROL DEVICES

Electronic control devices (also known as conductive energy devices), such as the cattle prod, stun gun, and the Taser®, can lead to injuries. Approximately 11% of "legal intervention injuries" (i.e., injuries sustained while being taking into custody) are related to electronic control devices, and the incidence is increasing. The vast majority of patients injured by electronic control devices are treated and released, but 6% are hospitalized.[69] TASER International, Inc. (Scottsdale, AZ), produces a series of devices that deliver high-voltage, low-amperage electrical pulses, typically at 10 to 20 cycles per second (subtetanic rate). The pulses are designed to induce involuntary muscle contraction, neuromuscular incapacitation, and/or pain. The likelihood of electrical injury is minimal;[70-73] however, reports have been published attributing cardiac arrest to these devices.[74,75] In addition, falls or other forceful movements resulting from electric current can lead to injury, as can use in flammable and other hazardous environments. Some devices shoot wires with fishhook-like barbs on the ends that penetrate and hook into the skin; penetrating injuries can result from this mechanism.

CLINICAL FEATURES

Most electronic control device injuries are limited to superficial punctures, minor lacerations, and cutaneous burns. Reported significant injuries have included skull penetration,[76] eye perforation,[77,78] retinal detachment,[79] testicular torsion,[80] miscarriage,[81] and pneumothorax,[80] as well as blunt trauma from falls and burns. Burns may occur when electronic control devices are used in flammable environments or used to incapacitate someone on a hot surface.

Clinical evaluation should address the underlying agitation underlying the use of the electronic control device. Patients may be agitated due to stimulant intoxication or other causes of medical delirium (including alcohol withdrawal or thyroid storm) and should be fully evaluated for both the underlying cause and the metabolic consequences of delirium, including hyperthermia, electrolyte abnormalities, rhabdomyolysis, and acidosis.[82]

TREATMENT AND DISPOSITION

Cardiac monitoring and other testing is not needed just because an electronic control device has been used. An initial ECG should be obtained if the patient is symptomatic. A series of human studies have suggested that electronic control devices do not cause or worsen hyperthermia, hyperkalemia, hypoxia, acidosis, and a variety of other problems often seen with in-custody deathsm,[83-86] but many underlying medical conditions may be at play in the patient who has required electronic control device discharge for restraint. The physician should try to determine why the electronic control device was used and obtain a history of the patient's behavior. Careful evaluation and monitoring are needed in the ill-appearing patient with the differential considerations of agitated delirium.

Patients who have calmed down, have no history of loss of consciousness or significant cardiac disease, and appear well can usually be discharged with no ECG or other testing beyond vital signs and a physical examination.

Patients with a history of severe agitation may be discharged if they have calmed down, maintained stable vital signs for 2 hours, and have a normal 12-lead ECG, electrolytes, arterial blood gas, and creatine phosphokinase. Those with abnormal labs, a history of loss of consciousness or significant underlying cardiac disease, and abnormalities on ECG should be admitted for further observation.

REFERENCES

The complete reference list is available online at www.TintinalliEM.com.

CHAPTER 219 Mushroom Poisoning

Anne F. Brayer
Lynette Froula

INTRODUCTION AND EPIDEMIOLOGY

Mushrooms are a common toxic exposure, with >6600 poisonous mushroom exposures and six deaths reported to poison control centers in 2012 and more than half occurring in children <6 years of age.[1]

Fortunately, the majority of reported mushroom exposures have a benign outcome.[2,3] To prevent mushroom poisoning, avoid eating wild mushrooms. There are no easily recognizable differences between nonpoisonous and poisonous mushrooms. Mushroom toxins are not heat labile and so are not destroyed or deactivated by cooking, canning, freezing, drying, or other means of food preparation.

Depending on the type of mushroom, adverse effects from ingestion range from mild GI symptoms to major cytotoxic effects resulting in organ failure and death. Toxicity varies based on the amount ingested, the age of the mushroom, the season, the geographic location, and the way in which the mushroom was prepared prior to ingestion. One person may show significant effects, whereas others may be asymptomatic after ingesting the same mushroom (**Table 219-1**).

Mushroom toxicity is divided into early toxicity (within 2 hours after ingestion) and delayed toxicity (6 hours to 20 days later).

Mushroom poisoning occurs in four main groups of individuals: young children who ingest poisonous mushrooms inadvertently, wild mushroom foragers, individuals attempting suicide or homicide, and individuals looking for a hallucinatory "high." Identification of the mushroom ingested may be difficult and time consuming. Very often, foragers mix different species of mushrooms together, so it is not always clear that the species being identified is the same one that was ingested. Therefore, direct treatment by a patient's symptoms rather than by attempts at mushroom identification. Treatment for mushroom poisoning is based on case reports and small series.[3]

Nearly all fatalities in the United States and Europe occur from ingestion of mushrooms of the *Amanita* species (*Amanita phalloides*, *Amanita virosa*, and *Amanita bisporigera*).[4] If *Amanita* ingestion is suspected, identification of the species may be helpful but is difficult because there are many *Amanita* mushrooms that are nontoxic. *Amanita* species generally have warts on the cap (remnants of the membrane covering the emerging mushroom), which give it a spotted appearance. The gills are "free," ending before the stem begins. The stem characteristically has a membrane ring around it and widens as it enters the soil. In most cases, the stem of the mushroom is contained in a cup or volva, which may be underground (**Figures 219-1, 219-2, and 219-3**).

EARLY-ONSET GI SYMPTOMS

PATHOPHYSIOLOGY

Most wild mushroom ingestions cause mild GI irritation, and mushrooms that cause GI irritation can be of many types. In North America and in almost every country, *Chlorophyllum molybdites* is particularly common and is sometimes mistaken for an *Amanita*.[3] Many little brown mushrooms found commonly in lawns, and often accidentally ingested by children, are in this category. *Omphalotus*, *Boletus*, *Entoloma*, *Gomphus*, *Hebeloma*, *Lactarius*, and *Verpa* genera are other examples for this group (**Figure 219-4**). The actual toxin varies with the species of mushroom, but most toxins are poorly described.

CLINICAL FEATURES

The majority of mushroom-induced intoxications are mild and do not prompt a visit to the ED. *C. molybdites*, however, is an exception that may cause severe symptoms.[5] Typically, patients present with acute onset of vomiting and diarrhea <2 hours after ingesting the mushroom. There may be intestinal cramping, chills, headaches, and myalgias. Diarrhea is usually watery, but occasionally bloody with fecal leukocytes. Most commonly, symptoms are mild and self-limited. Symptoms usually resolve within 24 hours but may last up to several days. Vomiting and diarrhea can cause dehydration and electrolyte imbalance. The presentation may be confused with acute gastroenteritis or acute food poisoning if the patient does not offer the history of mushroom ingestion.

TREATMENT

Treat symptomatic toxic mushroom ingestion with activated charcoal 0.5 to 1.0 gram/kg, PO or by nasogastric tube. There is no role for prophylactic decontamination therapy of asymptomatic patients.[6] Other treatment is largely supportive and includes IV fluid and electrolyte replacement when necessary. Antiemetics can be given, but do not give antidiarrheal agents, because they may prolong exposure to the toxin.[2] In most cases, symptoms are self-limited, resolving within 12 to 24 hours. Some cases of *Amanita smithiana* ingestion present with early GI symptoms (between 30 minutes and 12 hours) and can progress to renal failure within 3 to 5 days.[7]

Once vomiting has subsided and the patient is tolerating oral fluids, discharge from the ED is safe. Rarely, symptoms may persist and hospitalization may be needed for fluid and electrolyte replacement. Recommend outpatient follow-up within 5 days, and provide return precautions (urinary changes, lumbar or flank pain).[7]

TABLE 219-1 Mushrooms: Symptoms, Toxicity, and Treatment

Symptoms	Mushrooms	Toxicity	Treatment
GI symptoms			
Onset <2 h	*Chlorophyllum molybdites* *Omphalotus illudens* *Cantharellus cibarius* *Amanita caesarea*	Nausea, vomiting, diarrhea (occasionally bloody)	IV hydration Antiemetics
Onset 6–24 h	*Gyromitra esculenta* *Amanita phalloides, Amanita bisporigera*	Initial: nausea, vomiting, diarrhea Day 2: rise in AST, ALT levels Day 3: hepatic failure	IV hydration, glucose; monitor AST, ALT, bilirubin, BUN, and creatinine levels, prothrombin time, partial thromboplastin time For *Amanita:* activated charcoal Consider penicillin G, 300,000–1,000,000 units/kg/d Silymarin, 20–40 milligrams/kg/d Consider cimetidine, 4–10 grams/d Consider hyperbaric oxygen therapy
Muscarinic syndrome Onset <30 min	*Inocybe* *Clitocybe*	SLUDGE syndrome (**s**alivation, **l**acrimation, **u**rination, **d**efecation, **G**I hypermotility, and **e**mesis)	Supportive; atropine, 0.01 milligram/kg, repeated as needed for severe secretions
CNS excitement Onset <30 min	*Amanita muscaria* *Amanita pantherina*	Intoxication, dizziness, ataxia, visual disturbances, seizures, tachycardia, hypertension, warm dry skin, dry mouth, mydriasis (anticholinergic effects)	Supportive; sedation with diazepam, 0.1 milligram/kg IV for children; diazepam, 2–5 milligrams IV, or phenobarbital, 30 milligrams IV for adults
Hallucinations Onset <30 min	*Psilocybe* *Gymnopilus*	Visual hallucinations, ataxia	Supportive; sedation with diazepam, 0.1 milligram/kg or 5 milligrams IV for adults, or phenobarbital, 0.5 milligram/kg or 30–60 milligrams IV for adults
Disulfiram reaction 2–72 h after mushroom, and <30 min after alcohol	*Coprinus*	Headache, flushing, tachycardia, hyperventilation, shortness of breath, palpitations	Supportive; IV hydration β-Blockers for supraventricular tachycardia Norepinephrine for refractory hypotension
Dermatitis 1–2 d after ingestion	Shiitake	Whip-like, linear, erythematous wheals, blanching erythematous patches, scattered petechiae, pruritus	Oral antihistamines, 0.1% triamcinolone ointment twice daily; spontaneously resolves within 1–3 wk

Abbreviations: ALT = alanine aminotransferase; AST = aspartate aminotransferase.

EARLY-ONSET NEUROLOGIC SYMPTOMS

PATHOPHYSIOLOGY

Several classes of mushrooms can cause neurologic symptoms. These include the hallucinogenic mushrooms ("magic mushrooms") that contain the chemical psilocybin, which is rapidly dephosphorylated by alkaline phosphatase to the more psychoactive chemical psilocin.[8] Psilocin acts on serotonergic neurons in the CNS, causing effects similar to those of lysergic acid diethylamide. Mushrooms of the *Psilocybe* genus, which are the most commonly ingested in this class, are small brown or gold mushrooms that commonly grow on dung in warmer climates throughout the Pacific Northwest and southeastern United States as well as warm regions of Central America, South America, Asia, and Australia.[9] They characteristically turn a greenish blue when bruised or cut. They may also be cultivated at home from purchased spores. Nontoxic mushrooms may also be laced with phencyclidine or lysergic acid diethylamide and sold as hallucinogenic mushrooms.

Mushrooms containing the isoxazole derivatives ibotenic acid and muscimol also possess neurologic effects, which are thought to be mediated by

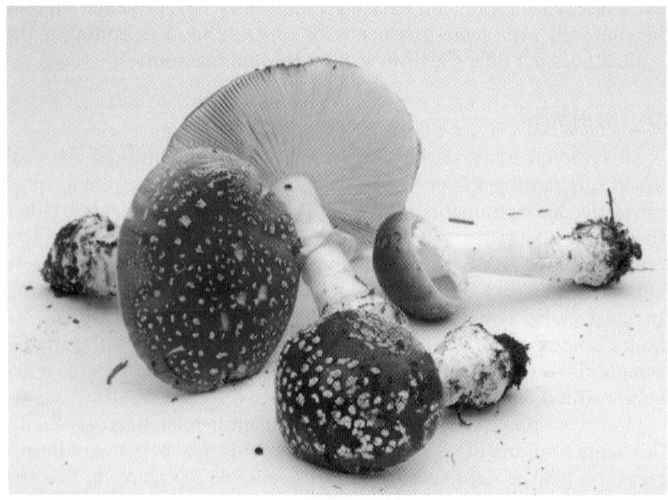

FIGURE 219-1. *Amanita muscaria.* [Photo used with permission of Jilber Barutciyan.]

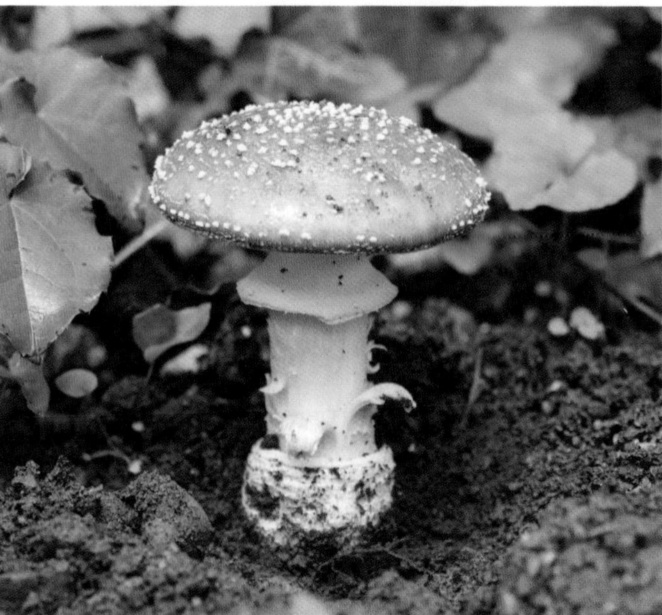

FIGURE 219-2. *Amanita pantherina.* [Photo used with permission of Jilber Barutciyan.]

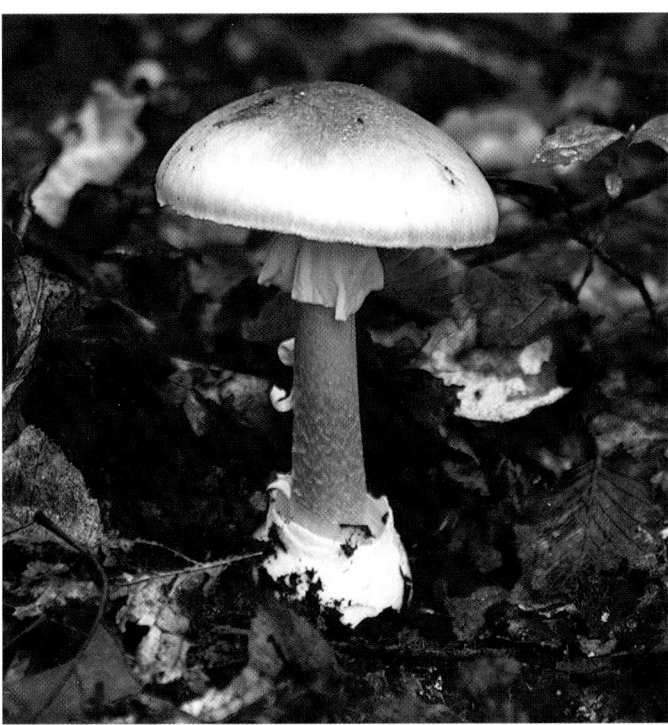

FIGURE 219-3. *Amanita phalloides.* [Photo used with permission of Jilber Barutciyan.]

γ-aminobutyric acid and anticholinergic activity. *Amanita muscaria* is the principle representative of this group of mushrooms and is easily identified (Figure 219-1). It has an orange or red cap with white warts (remnants of the universal veil present in young specimens), as well as a ring (annulus) and cup (volva) on the stem. *Amanita pantherina*, another member of the group, is 5 to 14 cm in length and diameter, with a white to brown cap, and has the ring and cup on the stem (Figure 219-2). Both specimens grow under trees in woodlands throughout North America.

CLINICAL FEATURES

Symptoms typically develop within 2 hours of ingestion of hallucinogenic mushrooms. Euphoria, a heightened imagination, a loss of the sense of time, and visual distortions or hallucinations are common. Tachycardia and hypertension may be noted because of the presence of phenylethylamine in psilocybin-containing mushrooms.[10] Fever and seizures have been reported in rare cases. Symptoms generally last 4 to 6 hours but can persist up to 12 hours.[11] There are infrequent reports of flashbacks for up to 4 months after ingestion, particularly in association with other substances that alter cognition such as alcohol or marijuana.[9]

Patients ingesting isoxazole-containing mushrooms usually present with symptoms within 30 minutes of ingestion. Signs of muscarinic poisoning are the first apparent (nausea, vomiting, diarrhea, vasodilation, diaphoresis, salivation). These are replaced by an atropine-like symptom complex about 30 minutes after ingestion (mydriasis, xerostomia, elevated temperature, increased blood pressure), along with drowsiness, amentia, dizziness, photosensitivity, euphoria, motor hyperactivity, ataxia, muscle jerking, hallucinations, and delirium with difficulty with perception of size, time, and place. Seizures have been reported in children. Symptoms are typically self-limited, resolving within 4 to 6 hours after ingestion. Headache and fatigue are reported to occur the day following ingestion, with headache lasting up to a few weeks.[9]

TREATMENT

Treatment for ingestion of hallucinogenic mushrooms is largely supportive. Place the patient in a darkened, quiet room, devoid of visual stimuli, and provide reassurance. If sedation is required, benzodiazepines such as diazepam or lorazepam are preferred. Do not give anticholinergic agents because they may aggravate delirium.

Treat symptomatic ingestion of isoxazole-containing mushrooms with activated charcoal. Do not give syrup of ipecac because of the potential for CNS depression and seizures, which place the patient at risk for aspiration. In patients with severe vomiting and diarrhea, replace fluids and electrolytes. Appropriately restrain patients who are agitated, and provide sedation as necessary with benzodiazepines (diazepam or lorazepam). Treat seizures with benzodiazepines.

Consider treatment with physostigmine only for patients with severe anticholinergic symptoms. Physostigmine can produce bradycardia, hypotension, and seizures, so administration should be reserved for severely symptomatic patients. The dose is 1 to 2 milligrams IV in adults and 0.5 milligram IV in children, administered slowly. Monitor continuous cardiorespiratory effects and blood pressure during administration. Base the decision to discharge from the ED on duration of symptoms and need for ongoing pharmacologic sedation or intubation.

EARLY-ONSET MUSCARINIC SYMPTOMS

Muscarine was the first mushroom toxin to be identified.[12] Mushrooms of the *Inocybe* and *Clitocybe* genera are common causes of muscarinic poisoning (**Figure 219-5**). The *Inocybe* mushrooms are small brown

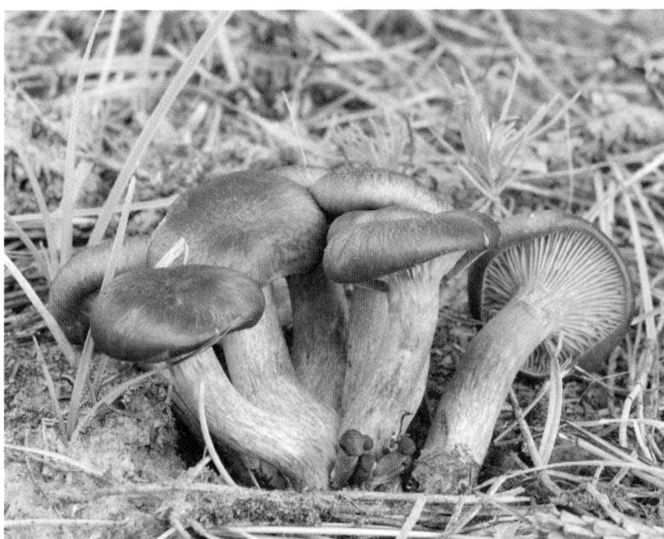

FIGURE 219-4. *Omphalotus olearius.* [Photo used with permission of Jilber Barutciyan.]

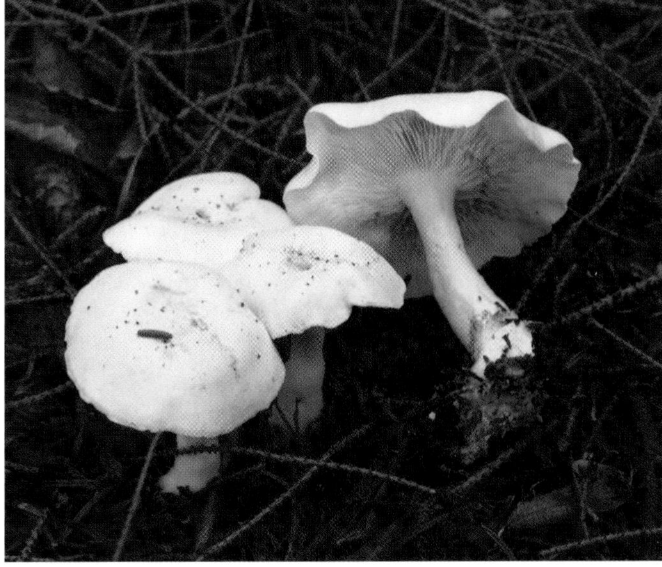

FIGURE 219-5. *Clitocybe candicans.* [Photo used with permission of Jilber Barutciyan.]

mushrooms with conical caps, typically found under hardwoods and conifers. The *Clitocybe* mushrooms are usually found individually on lawns and in parks and are white to gray, with a cup-shaped cap. *A. muscaria*, despite its name, contains far less muscarine than these other groups and only rarely causes cholinergic poisoning symptoms. Isoxazole-containing mushrooms can cause transient muscarinic symptoms early after ingestion.

PATHOPHYSIOLOGY

Muscarine is a parasympathomimetic compound that is heat stable and acetylcholine like. It is not degraded by cholinesterase and, therefore, has a long duration of action.[13] Acetylcholine receptors on the heart, apocrine glands, and smooth muscle are activated by muscarine.[12] Mushrooms containing muscarine cause neurologic symptoms and muscarinic or cholinergic effects.

CLINICAL FEATURES

The symptoms of muscarinic intoxication are characterized by the **SLUDGE syndrome** (salivation, lacrimation, urination, defecation, GI hypermotility, and emesis). In addition to the SLUDGE syndrome, patients with muscarine ingestions can develop diaphoresis, muscle fasciculations, miosis, bradycardia, and bronchorrhea. Symptoms typically present within 30 minutes of ingestion and spontaneously resolve in 4 to 12 hours.

TREATMENT

In most cases, muscarinic symptoms are mild and self-limited. Supportive care is sufficient. Because emesis is a common presenting symptom, activated charcoal administration is often difficult. Patients with severe vomiting may require IV fluid and electrolyte replacement.

Atropine is an antidote for muscarinic symptoms and can be administered to patients with severe symptoms. It can be effective in treating bradycardia and hypotension unresponsive to IV fluid administration. Atropine is helpful in the treatment of diaphoresis, increased oral secretions, and bronchorrhea. It may also help reduce GI cramping, emesis, and diarrhea. The dose is 0.5 to 1.0 milligram IV for adults and 0.01 milligram/kg IV for children (minimum dose, 0.1 milligram; maximum does, 1 milligram). The dose can be repeated as necessary to control bronchorrhea, bradycardia, or hypotension. Large doses may be necessary to treat severe toxicity. Patients should be carefully monitored during administration. Oxygen and inhaled β agonists (albuterol) are recommended for the treatment of patients with increased pulmonary secretions and bronchospasm.

Because symptoms of muscarinic poisoning frequently resolve within 12 hours of ingestion, many patients can be safely discharged from the ED after observation when symptoms have subsided.

DELAYED-ONSET GI SYMPTOMS

Mushrooms of two different genera, *Gyromitra* and *Amanita*, cause significant toxicity, which characteristically presents several hours after ingestion. *Gyromitra esculenta* (the false morel) is an uncommon cause of poisoning in North America, but is more common in Scandinavia and Europe.[4] *G. esculenta* has a brown convoluted top resembling a brain and is often mistaken for the tasty morel mushroom. *A. phalloides* and *A. bisporigera* are common in the Northern Hemisphere and are particularly common from north central Europe through the Middle East. Mushrooms of these species are found throughout the West Coast, Midwest, and parts of the Northeast of the United States. Immigrants may mistake these mushrooms for edible varieties common in eastern Asia. Mushrooms of the *Amanita* genus are responsible for 95% of deaths associated with mushrooms. Toxic ingestions in North America occur most commonly in the autumn.

PATHOPHYSIOLOGY

Gyromitrin (*N*-methyl-*N*-formylhydrazone) is a volatile heat-labile toxin and primarily responsible for symptoms. Gyromitrin concentration decreases significantly after boiling and desiccation.[14] Gyromitrin is hydrolyzed in the stomach to form *N*-methyl-*N*-formylhydrazine and *N*-methylhydrazine. *N*-Methylhydrazine is chemically identical to rocket fuel, and workers exposed to this compound develop CNS toxicity. *N*-Methylhydrazine binds to pyridoxine and interferes with enzymes that require pyridoxine as a cofactor. γ-Aminobutyric acid is lowered in the CNS, which may be a cause of associated seizures. *N*-Methyl-*N*-formylhydrazine is converted into a free radical in the liver and causes local hepatic necrosis by blocking the activity of the cytochrome P-450 system, glutathione, and other hepatic enzyme systems.[14] These two chemicals explain the CNS and hepatic dysfunction characteristic of gyromitrin toxicity. The cause of the initial GI symptoms is not known.

A. phalloides contains several phallotoxins and amatoxins. Phallotoxin is a bi-cyclic peptide that alters the enterocyte cellular membrane, thereby causing early GI symptoms. Its effect is limited to the GI tract, because it is not absorbed by the intestine.[15] Amatoxins are bi-cyclic octapeptides that are rapidly absorbed through the intestinal mucosa. They are carried to the liver and undergo enterohepatic circulation, which results in prolonged toxin exposure after ingestion. Nine amatoxins have been identified, but α-amanitin (amanitin) appears the most physiologically active.[2] Kinetic studies in humans show that α-amanitin is cleared from the plasma within 48 hours.[16] Concentrations in the plasma are quite small. Amatoxins are not protein bound, but are actively transported into hepatocytes, where they bind to RNA polymerase II and inhibit the formation of messenger RNA. Free radical formation may also be involved in toxicity.[17] α-Amanitin has the greatest effect on cells that undergo rapid protein synthesis and turnover, including cells of the GI tract mucosa, hepatocytes, and renal tubular epithelium.[18] In adults, the dose that causes 50% mortality is 0.1 milligram/kg of body weight, which is commonly contained in a single mushroom.[15]

Pathologic changes are noted in both gyromitrin and amatoxin toxicity. Patients who ingest gyromitrin-containing mushrooms show diffuse hepatocellular damage and interstitial nephritis. Patients who ingest amatoxin-containing mushrooms show fatty degeneration of the liver, with intranuclear collection of lipids and extensive hepatic necrosis. Electron microscopy shows vacuolization of the mitochondria and clumping of the chromatin in the nucleoli. There are extensive lipid peroxidation changes in both the nucleus and the cytoplasm.

CLINICAL FEATURES

The distinctive characteristics of gyromitrin-containing mushroom toxicity are intense GI signs and symptoms (nausea, vomiting, and watery diarrhea) that develop 6 to 24 hours after ingestion, typically between 6 and 8 hours.

Hypovolemia is common during this phase of toxicity. In severe cases, hepatic failure is evident on day 3 and may result in death as early as day 7. Serum transaminase levels may be significantly elevated. **Hypoglycemia** occurs during the GI phase and again in the acute hepatic failure phase.

Initial GI symptoms can be accompanied by dizziness, headache, seizures, incoordination, and muscle cramps. The initial GI symptoms resolve within 2 to 5 days.[5] In a mild ingestion, the neurologic symptoms persist for several days and resolve without sequelae.

Patients who ingest amatoxin-containing mushrooms also have delayed onset of GI symptoms (6 to 24 hours). The gastroenteritis is intense, often requiring fluid and electrolyte replacement. There are four stages in amatoxin poisoning. The first (latent) stage is characterized by the absence of any signs or symptoms and lasts up to 24 hours after ingestion. During the 12 to 24 hours of the second stage, GI symptoms such as intense cramping abdominal pain, nausea, vomiting, and diarrhea dominate the clinical picture. Both stools and vomitus may become bloody. Although right upper quadrant tenderness and hepatomegaly may be noted, results of liver function tests are usually normal. Patients who present during this stage are frequently misdiagnosed with gastroenteritis. The third, or convalescent, phase lasts 12 to 24 hours. During this stage, the patient feels and looks better, but levels of liver enzymes, such as aspartate aminotransferase, alanine aminotransferase, and bilirubin, begin to rise, heralding the onset of liver damage. Renal function may also deteriorate. In the fourth and final stage, which begins 2 to 4 days after ingestion, transaminase levels rise dramatically, and liver and renal function deteriorate. Hyperbilirubinemia, coagulopathy, hypoglycemia, acidosis, hepatic encephalopathy, and hepatorenal syndrome are noted.[2]

In both *Gyromitra* and *Amanita* toxicity, prothrombin time may be elevated and unresponsive to administration of vitamin K or fresh frozen plasma. Amylase and lipase elevation suggests pancreatic damage, although symptomatic pancreatitis is rare. Abnormal laboratory findings in amatoxin poisoning include a decrease in neutrophils, lymphocytes, and platelets, and abnormal thyroid function results. Hypophosphatemia (primarily noted in children), hypocalcemia, and elevated insulin levels occur. None of these laboratory abnormalities correlates with clinical disease, and their cause is unknown.

The mortality from *Gyromitra* ingestion is estimated at 15% to 35% and is generally attributed to hepatic failure, renal failure, or fluid and electrolyte disorders.[5] More recently, mortality has been reduced to 10% to 15%, because of improved care for hepatic failure and liver transplantation. Patients who survive severe hepatic failure from amatoxin may develop signs of chronic active hepatitis with persistent elevation in liver transaminase levels, development of anti–smooth muscle antibodies, and presence of cryoglobulins. No prolonged effects from gyromitrin toxicity have been reported.

DIAGNOSIS

The diagnosis of gyromitrin toxicity is generally assumed from the clinical features and the identification of the mushroom ingested, either by the patient or from samples. Identification of *Amanita* species generally requires a trained mycologist. The **Meixner colorimetric test** is used to look for the presence of amatoxin. A drop of fresh mushroom pulp, methanol extract from dried mushrooms, or gastric material is placed on a high-lignin paper (e.g., newspaper) and allowed to dry. A drop of 10-N or 12-N hydrochloric acid is then applied to catalyze the reaction of the amatoxin with the lignin in the paper. The area will turn blue within 1 to 2 minutes if amatoxins are present, but the appearance of color may be delayed up to 30 minutes if the amatoxin concentration is low.[2] Although the test is sensitive, it is not very specific, and other nontoxic mushrooms may give a positive test result. Tests using thin-layer chromatography, high-performance liquid chromatography, and radioimmunoassay have been developed to detect amatoxin. Unfortunately, these assays are not generally available to clinicians and are used most often in research settings.[2] Amatoxin can be detected in plasma, urine, GI tract contents, and feces. However, its presence merely confirms amatoxin poisoning. Levels do not appear to correlate with clinical severity, and amatoxin is not detected in many patients, presumably because of rapid clearance.

TREATMENT

Administer activated charcoal to patient presenting with severe vomiting and diarrhea within a few hours of mushroom ingestion. Repeated doses of charcoal for at least the first 24 hours may be effective, particularly in the presence of amatoxin (because it undergoes enterohepatic circulation).[15] Fluid and electrolyte replacement is mandatory. Glucose level should be monitored and glucose replaced as needed. **Hypoglycemia is one of the most common causes of death in early mushroom toxicity.**

All patients who have ingested amatoxin- or gyromitrin-containing mushrooms should be closely monitored for 48 hours for the development of hepatic and renal failure. Electrolyte levels, liver enzyme levels, and prothrombin time should be monitored several times a day. Patients should be treated with a low-protein diet and should receive standard supportive therapy for hepatic failure. Fresh frozen plasma and vitamin K can be used for the treatment of prolonged prothrombin time, but in many cases, coagulopathy does not respond to treatment.

Patients who develop hepatic failure should be monitored closely, and in severe cases, preparations should be made for liver transplantation. Although no firm criteria exist, progressive coagulopathy, encephalopathy, and renal failure despite maximal medical therapy are frequently listed indications for emergency liver transplantation.[19] Many patients have met these criteria and survived without transplantation, and many patients have died without meeting these criteria. Liver transplantation, however, does provide the only option for patients in fulminant hepatic failure and has been quite successful. Auxiliary liver transplantation has also been used. In this case, a portion of the damaged liver is removed and a temporary transplant provided, which allows time for the native liver to regenerate.[20]

Gyromitrin-Specific Treatment Treat the neurologic symptoms associated with gyromitrin with high-dose pyridoxine. **Pyridoxine** provides the cofactor required for the regeneration of γ-aminobutyric acid. High doses of pyridoxine, 25 milligrams/kg IV over 30 minutes up to a maximum of 25 grams/d, are recommended, but doses of pyridoxine in excess of 40 grams are associated with severe peripheral neuropathy.[21,22] Pyridoxine does not affect the development or course of hepatic failure, and there is no specific therapy for gyromitrin-induced hepatic failure.

Amatoxin-Specific Treatment Although multiple modalities have been tried in the past with mixed results, **activated charcoal**, *silybinum marianum,* and ***N*-acetylcysteine** are emerging as the best-supported treatment modalities.[15,23] Early in the clinical course, repeated dosing of activated charcoal is thought beneficial by reducing the absorption of amatoxin as it undergoes enterohepatic circulation. *Silybinum marianum,* a milk thistle isolate, is also thought to prevent toxicity by interfering with transmembrane transport during enterohepatic circulation and inhibiting the binding of α-amanitin to hepatocytes.[15,23] There is some evidence that *silybinum* has additional hepatoprotective effects that result from stimulating protein synthesis and inhibiting tumor necrosis factor-α release in damaged liver cells.[23] It is given as a loading dose of 5 milligrams/kg over 1 hour followed by 20 milligrams/kg/d for 6 days. This treatment is not currently approved by the U.S. Food and Drug Administration; it is available in Europe, and phase II/III clinical trials are in progress in the United States.[15] *N*-Acetylcysteine is also beneficial as a means of reducing reactive metabolites by providing sulfhydryl groups for this purpose. It is given intravenously in three sequential doses of 150 milligrams/kg over 1 hour, 50 milligrams/kg over 4 hours, and 100 milligrams/kg over 16 hours.

Despite these therapies, amatoxin toxicity may lead to fulminant liver failure. In cases of amatoxin-induced liver failure, the amatoxin itself is rapidly absorbed and excreted, which limits the utility of hemoperfusion and/or hemodialysis. The Molecular Adsorbent Recirculation System™ can support liver function while hepatocytes recover or until transplantation becomes feasible.[24] Although randomized controlled trials are not available, numerous case reports have shown improved liver functioning coinciding with this device.[24] Orthotopic liver transplantation (the entire organ is replaced with a graft) and auxiliary partial orthotopic liver transplantation (a portion of the native liver is removed and replaced with a graft until recovery occurs) are both surgical options.[15]

High-dose penicillin G and ceftazidime have both demonstrated a capacity for decreasing the uptake of amanitin by hepatocytes.[18,25] However, these therapies appear to be less effective than using *silybinum* alone.[23] Thioctic acid is a free radical scavenger and has been used for many years but has not yet gained support in the literature.

Patients suspected of ingesting amatoxin- or gyromitrin-containing mushrooms should be admitted and monitored for 48 hours, with monitoring of hepatic and renal function.

DELAYED-ONSET RENAL FAILURE

Delayed-onset renal failure is seen after ingestion of *Cortinarius* (*Cortinarius orellanus, Cortinarius speciosissimus,* and *Cortinarius gentilis*) and *A. smithiana* mushrooms.[26] *Cortinarius* species are found primarily in Europe. This mushroom is often mistaken for a pine mushroom and grows commonly in the Pacific Northwest. *A. smithiana* mushrooms are common in forest areas of western North America.[7]

PATHOPHYSIOLOGY

Orellanine and ortinarin A and B are the nephrotoxic compounds in species of *Cortinarius* (*C. orellanus, C. speciosissimus,* and *C. gentilis*). These toxins are heat stable, and their mechanisms of action are not well known. Orellanine and its derivatives are believed to inhibit protein synthesis in the kidneys. Histopathologic examination indicates interstitial nephritis with edema and leukocyte infiltration, tubular necrosis, basal membrane rupture, and fibrosis without glomerular injury in patients poisoned with orellanine-containing mushooms.[18,22,27]

Allenic norleucine (aminohexadienoic acid) and chlorocrotylglycine are the nephrotoxins found in *A. smithiana*.[26] Allenic norleucine has been shown to induce renal tubular epithelial necrosis and tends to exert its effect earlier than orelline in cultured cell lines.[7]

CLINICAL FEATURES

Patients who ingest mushrooms containing nephrotoxins often present initially with GI symptoms, including nausea, vomiting, and nonbloody diarrhea. Symptoms begin several hours to days after ingestion and may persist for 3 days. Occasionally, paresthesias, abnormal taste, and cognitive dysfunction are reported. Symptoms of renal failure, including lumbar and flank pain, oliguria, or more rarely polyuria, begin between 3 and 20 days after ingestion. Patients who ingest *A. smithiana* tend to develop GI symptoms earlier, with a range of symptom onset between 30 minutes and 12 hours (median, 5 to 6 hours). Orellanine ingestion tends to present with GI symptoms later, with a range of 12 hours to 14 days after ingestion. Similarly, renal failure is noted to develop earlier in allenic norleucine cases (within 3 to 5 days) and occurs within 4 to 15 days of orellanine ingestion.[7] Orellanine poisoning can be confirmed by thin-layer chromatography of renal biopsy specimens or by plasma assays for orellanine or orelline, but these tests are not commonly available in clinical practice.[5] Many patients who ingest these mushrooms never develop renal dysfunction, which suggests variability in host sensitivity to their toxic effects. Consider allenic norleucine or orellanine toxicity from wild mushroom ingestion in a patient with unexplained acute renal failure.

TREATMENT

There is no specific treatment for patients who develop renal failure from ingestion of *Cortinarius* or *A. smithiana* mushrooms. Monitor urine output and electrolyte, calcium, magnesium, BUN, and creatinine levels. Hemodialysis is indicated for refractory hyperkalemia, refractory acidosis, uremic symptoms, or severe renal dysfunction. Supportive hemodialysis may be required, but many patients experience a spontaneous return of normal renal function. Because spontaneous improvement is reported, renal transplantation should be withheld for several months to monitor patient response. Renal transplantation has been used in several patients with good success.[28]

Monitor patients suspected of ingesting orellanine- or ortinarin-containing mushrooms for at least 72 hours for electrolyte abnormalities and renal failure.

DELAYED-ONSET DISULFIRAM REACTION

Perhaps most interesting, although clinically least important, is a mushroom toxin contained in the *Coprinus* genus. This mushroom, which is very common in North America, is known as "inky cap" or "shaggy mane." It is a tall, white, thin mushroom with a shaggy cap. As the mushroom ages, the cap liquefies and blackens, and black liquid drips from the necrosing cap. The mushroom contains coprine, which is chemically related to disulfiram.

PATHOPHYSIOLOGY

Coprine causes inhibition of alcohol dehydrogenase within 2 hours of ingestion, and activity may last up to 72 hours. If alcohol is consumed during this sensitive period, patients develop a typical disulfiram reaction. Mushrooms ingested at the same time as alcohol produce no toxicity.

CLINICAL FEATURES

Because of the delay between mushroom consumption and alcohol consumption, few patients link their symptoms to the ingestion of a mushroom. Symptoms include headache, paresthesias of distal extremities, metallic taste, flushing, palpitations, chest pain, nausea, vomiting, and diaphoresis and generally occur within minutes to several hours after alcohol consumption. Symptoms generally last for 2 to 4 hours but may last up to 2 days.[5] Most symptoms are mild. Diagnosis is made based on presence of the symptom complex and its association with alcohol consumption.

Because alcohol is readily absorbed from the GI tract, GI decontamination has no role and charcoal administration is not beneficial. Patients occasionally become hypotensive and respond to administration of IV fluids or, in refractory cases, norepinephrine. Excessive sympathetic activity can be inhibited by β-blockers.[5]

Most cases are self-limited, and patients can be discharged once they can tolerate oral fluids. Prior to discharge, educate patients about the link between alcohol consumption and mushroom ingestion.

SHIITAKE DERMATITIS

Shiitake dermatitis is a well-known entity in Japan, China, and Korea, and cases have been reported in Europe and the United States.[29,30] Shiitake dermatitis is a characteristic flagellate erythema appearing as whip-like, linear wheals that appear within 1 or 2 days of ingesting raw or cooked shiitake mushrooms. The rash tends to be pruritic and can also involve branching patches of erythema and scattered petechiae. The pathophysiology is not fully understood but is thought to be toxin-induced, involving the thermolabile polysaccharide lentinan that is found in the shiitake mushroom. Skin biopsy results are nonspecific.[29,30] Allergy testing in affected individuals is negative.[30]

Treat symptoms with 0.1% triamcinolone ointment twice daily and oral antihistamines. Regardless of treatment, the rash resolves spontaneously without hyperpigmentation in 1 to 4 weeks.[29,30]

The rash is self-limited, and no sequelae have been reported.

SPECIAL POPULATIONS

Toxic mushroom exposure during pregnancy has been reported.[28] In one series, a slightly lower birth weight was noted in infants born to mothers with toxic mushroom exposure than in infants of mothers with no such exposure. Most infants appeared to be healthy and developmentally normal, in keeping with the findings that amatoxins do not cross the placental barrier.[31,32]

REFERENCES

The complete reference list is available online at www.TintinalliEM.com.

Poisonous Plants

Betty C. Chen
Lewis S. Nelson

INTRODUCTION

Common poisonous and injurious plants number in the hundreds and have a wide variety of toxicities. This chapter focuses on the most important plant-related exposures clinically relevant to emergency medicine (**Tables 220-1 and 220-2**).[1,2] Individual plants are discussed in terms of their pathophysiology, clinical features (toxidromes), and treatment.[3] Highly poisonous plants (Table 220-1) are highlighted in depth below, and brief reviews are provided for other common poisonous plants. Table 220-2 organizes common poisonous plants according to toxin structure.

TABLE 220-1 Some Highly Poisonous Plants

Some Highly Poisonous Plants
Poison hemlock (*Conium maculatum*)
Yew (*Taxus spp.*)
Foxglove (*Digitalis purpurea*)
Oleander (*Nerium oleander*)
Castor bean (*Ricinus communis*)
Rosary pea (*Abrus precatorius*)
Water hemlock (*Cicuta maculata*)
Buckthorn (*Karwinskia humboldtiana*)

EPIDEMIOLOGY

In 2012, the American Association of Poison Control Centers received 49,374 reports of plant exposures. Of these cases, 31,920 involved children less than 5 years of age. There were an additional 2918 nonexposure calls that provided information about plants to callers.[2] The vast majority of exposures (96%) are unintentional ingestions. Cutaneous and ophthalmic exposures are common but generally go unreported. Although inhalational exposures are possible, they are rarely reported.

Unfortunately, obtaining an accurate plant exposure history can be difficult. Most exposures occur in children and are usually unwitnessed. Uncertainty typically surrounds these cases, particularly whether ingestion truly occurred. The timing and amount of exposure is also difficult to quantify in many of these situations. Furthermore, even when a plant is available, identification errors are common and may require a botanist's expertise. In fact, data from the National Poison Data System demonstrate that medical providers and poison centers are unable to identify plants more than 22% of the time.[2]

CLINICAL FEATURES

Classification of plants and their toxicities is complex. The most straightforward approach for emergency physicians is to classify toxic plants by the mechanism of action of the toxin and then to further subclassify based on the specific toxin. This will help predict the toxicologic effects. The reverse process can be used if the patient presents with clinical findings (Table 220-2). Unfortunately, attributing one toxicologic syndrome

TABLE 220-2 Classification of Poisonous Plants

Classification	Mechanism of Toxicity	Example Plant Species
Alkaloids	Solanine and chaconine	Green potato leaves, American nightshade, black nightshade (Solanaceae)
	Anticholinergics	Deadly nightshade (*Atropa belladonna*) Angel's trumpet or jimsonweed (*Datura* spp.) Henbane (*Hycoscyamus niger*) Mandrake (*Mandragora officinarum*)
	Cholinergics	Calabar bean (*Physostigma venenosum*) Pilocarpus (*Pilocarpus* spp.)
	Nicotinic and nicotine-like	Tobacco (*Nicotiana* spp.) Poison hemlock (*Conium maculatum*) Golden chain (*Laburnum anagyroides*) Blue cohosh (*Caulophyllum thalictroides*) Lupin (*Lupinus* spp.)
	Psychotropics	Peyote (*Lophophora williamsii*) Nutmeg and mace (*Myristica fragrans*) Morning glory (*Agyreia* spp. and *Ipomoea* spp.) Hawaiian baby woodrose seeds (*Argyreia nervosa*)
	Hepatotoxic pyrrolizidines	Comfrey (*Symphytum officinale*) Sassafras (*Sassafras albidum*) Ragwort (*Heliotropium* spp.)
	Sodium channel modulators	Monkshood (*Aconitum* spp.) Larkspur (*Delphinium* spp.) False or green hellebore (*Veratrum* spp.) Yew (*Taxus* spp.)
	Antimitotic alkaloids and resins	Autumn crocus (*Colchicum autumnale*) Mayapple (*Podophyllum peltatum*) Wild mandrake (*Podophyllum emodi*) Glory lily (*Gloriosa superba*) Madagascar periwinkle (*Catharanthus roseus*)
Glycosides	Cardioactive steroids or cardiac glycosides	Foxglove (*Digitalis purpurea*) Lily of the valley (*Convallaria majalis*) Oleander (*Nerium oleander*) Christmas rose (*Helleborus niger*) Milkweed (*Asclepias* spp.) Squill (*Urginea maritime and Urginea indica*) Yellow oleander (*Thevetia peruviana*)
	Cyanogenic glycosides	Almond, apricot, and cherry pits (*Prunus* spp.) Tapioca plant, cassava (*Manihot esculenta*) Elderberry (*Sambucus canadensis*) Hydrangea (*Hydrangea macrophylla*)
	Saponins	Holly (*Ilex* spp.)
	Salicylates	Poplar species (*Populus* spp.) Willow species (*Salix* spp.)
Proteins, peptides, and lectins	Toxalbumins	Castor bean (*Ricinus communis*) Rosary pea (*Abrus precatorius*) Pokeweed (*Phytolacca americana*) Black locust (*Robinia pseudoacacia*) American mistletoe (*Phoradendron flavescens*) European mistletoe (*Viscum album*) Black vomit nut (*Jatropha curcas*)
	Hypoglycin	Ackee fruit (*Blighia sapida*)
Carboxylic acids	Calcium oxalate crystals	Dumbcane (*Dieffenbachia* spp.) Philodendron (*Philodendron* spp.) Caladium (*Caladium* spp.) Jack in the pulpit (*Arisaema triphyllum*) Elephant's ear (*Colocasia* spp.) Rhubarb (*Rheum raponticum*)
Alcohols	Convulsants	Water hemlock (*Cicuta maculate*)
Phenols and phenylpropanoids	Coumarins and derivatives	Sweet clover (*Melilotus* spp.) Tonka beans (*Dipteryx* spp.) Sweet-scented bedstraw (*Galium triflorum*) Red clover (*Trifolium pretense*)
	Capsaicin	Cayenne pepper (*Capsicum* spp.)
	Demyelination	Buckthorn or coyotillo (*Karwinskia humboldtiana*)
Terpenoids and resins	Grayanotoxin (sodium channel blockers)	Azalea and rhododendron (*Rhododoendron* spp.), mountain laurel (*Kalmia latifolia*)
	Kava lactones	Kava kava (*Piper methysticum*)
	Thujone	Wormwood (*Artemisia absinthium*)
	Anisatin	Star anise (*Illicum* spp.)
	Tetrahydrocannabinol	Marijuana (*Cannabis sativa*)

per plant oversimplifies the complexity of plant chemistry, because plants often contain multiple toxic compounds, each of which produces its own toxicologic effects.

Moderate systemic effects as a consequence of plant-related exposures occur in about 1% of patients. Severe life-threatening effects or disabling injuries are extremely uncommon and occur in only about 0.04% of patients. Death occurs in <0.001% of patients.

Dermatitis and GI irritation are the most commonly reported effects of plant toxicity. GI complaints occur commonly following ingestion, and additional toxic symptoms may accompany or follow. Although dermatitis is another commonly reported finding of plant toxicity, systemic toxicity rarely follows (see Table 220-3).

TREATMENT

Most plant-related exposures can be managed with supportive care. In patients able to tolerate oral administration and believed to have potentially concerning exposures, administer activated charcoal to prevent absorption of toxin from the GI tract. Because of the uncertainty surrounding plant exposures, observe asymptomatic or minimally symptomatic patients for 4 to 6 hours in the ED. Discharge asymptomatic patients and those with resolved minor toxicity after observation, with strict return precautions if symptoms develop. Admit those with more than minimal findings because toxicity may continue to evolve. This approach is generally applied to all patients with plant exposure because the scientific literature lacks adequate data to provide less conservative recommendations. There are few antidotes available to treat poisonings by plant toxins; none are unique to plant exposures but rather are generalized from use in other poisonings.

Report all exposures to the regional poison control center to obtain assistance with plant identification, to obtain assistance with patient management, and to enable collection of accurate data on toxic plant exposures. Unfortunately, data reported by the National Poison Data System does not require confirmation of exposure, and the incidence of adverse effects is diluted by inconsequential or unconfirmed ingestions.

NICOTINIC AND NICOTINE-LIKE TOXINS (POISON HEMLOCK)

In *Phaedo*, Plato details the death of Socrates: after drinking a potion consisting of the extracts of poison hemlock (*Conium maculatum*), he slowly develops paralysis and dies. All parts of poison hemlock contain coniine and similar alkaloids that are structurally and functionally analogous to nicotine. Overstimulation of nicotine receptors can rapidly progress from seemingly mild symptoms to death from respiratory failure. Symptoms may occur within hours. Mild effects include nervousness and tremor due to sympathomimetic stimulation. As toxicity progresses, patients exhibit more pronounced sympathomimetic features, parasympathetic findings, and paralysis from nicotinic receptor stimulation at the neuromuscular junction. Typically, ingestion of poison hemlock is due to misidentification because of its similarity in appearance to wild carrot or Queen Anne's lace (*Daucus carota*), parsley (*Petroselinum crispum*), parsnip (*Pastinaca sativa*) roots, or anise (*Pimpinella anisum*). Although most ingestions are unintentional, there are case reports of toxicity from intentional use by patients for a presumed opioid-like effect or for intentional self-harm.[4-6] Treatment consists of GI decontamination with activated charcoal and supportive care, which may include respiratory support and administration of IV fluids, antidysrhythmics, and anticonvulsants.

SODIUM CHANNEL TOXINS (YEW, RHODODENDRON, LAUREL, MONKSHOOD, LARKSPUR)

A number of plants across different classifications cause sodium channel effects that result in cardiac, respiratory, GI, and CNS effects. Yew (*Taxus* spp.) contains taxine alkaloids in all parts of the shrub except the aril, which is the berry's red fleshy portion. The hard seed inside of the berry contains taxine alkaloids that block sodium and calcium channels.[7,8] Few symptoms are to be expected if ingestions are small or if berries are consumed without crushing the central seed. However, large ingestions can lead to more serious effects.

Grayanotoxins are terpenoids, which inhibit the opening of sodium channels, and are found in the leaves, flowers, and nectar of several plants such as azaleas and rhododendron (*Rhododendron* spp.). They are also found in in the mountain laurel (*Kalmia latifolia*). Ingestion of the leaves, flower, or honey from the nectar of the flower can result in toxicity.[9]

Aconite, found in monkshood (*Aconitum* spp.) and larkspur (*Delphinium* spp.), is an alkaloid that activates cardiac, and less so neuronal, sodium channels. Monkshood is sometimes used in traditional Chinese medicine as an inotrope. False or green hellebore (*Veratrum* spp.) is often confused for leeks by foragers, and these plants contain veratridine and other assorted veratrum alkaloids, which function similarly to aconite.

Regardless of the particular alkaloid or terpenoid and its specific mechanism of cardiac toxicity, findings after ingestion include salivation, lacrimation, bradycardia or tachycardia, cardiac dysrhythmias, hypotension, hyperkalemia, paresthesias, muscle weakness, respiratory failure, seizures, and potentially death.[8-10]

Early after ingestion, activated charcoal may decrease absorption from the GI tract. No antidote is available, and symptomatic patients should receive supportive care such as IV fluids or vasopressors if hypotensive. Atropine is effective for bradycardia, but antiarrhythmics, such as amiodarone, carry variable efficacy, as reported in the literature. Cardioversion for wide complex dysrhythmias can be attempted in unstable patients with the understanding that instability may persist and dysrhythmias may recur given the underlying channelopathy. Case reports describe successful use of extracorporeal membrane oxygenation in treating critically ill patients with refractory cardiac toxicity from yew posioning.[8,11,12]

CARDIOACTIVE STEROIDS (FOXGLOVE, OLEANDER)

Cardioactive steroids are found in many plants, including foxglove (*Digitalis* spp.), oleander (*Nerium* spp.), dogbane (*Apocynum cannabinum*), lily of the valley (*Convallaria majalis*), and milkweed (*Asclepias* spp.). Cardioactive steroids, sometimes called cardiac glycosides, inhibit the sodium/potassium–adenosine triphosphatase pump. Acute toxicity closely resembles that from digoxin and includes early GI symptoms followed by cardiac dysrhythmias. Serum digoxin concentrations may be used to qualitatively confirm cardioactive steroid exposure due to cross-reaction with the laboratory assay, but the absolute value holds little clinical quantitative value. Early after ingestion, oral activated charcoal may decrease systemic exposure by preventing absorption.[13] Assess serum potassium concentration and obtain an ECG to aid in prognosis and therapy. Administer digoxin immune Fab fragments to patients with a serum potassium >5 mEq/L after an acute overdose or any cardiac dysrhythmia.[14] Antidote dosing should be empiric (unlike with digoxin), and the digoxin concentration should not be used to calculate dosing, because the assay is not an accurate reflection of toxin burden. Avoid transvenous pacing and calcium administration for the increased theoretical risks of inducing a dysrhythmia. Traditional treatments for hyperkalemia such as insulin, calcium, sodium bicarbonate, or hemodialysis are usually unnecessary if digoxin immune Fab is administered.

TOXALBUMINS (CASTOR BEAN, RICIN)

Ricin and abrin are examples of toxalbumins that can be extracted from the castor bean (*Ricinus communis*) and rosary pea (*Abrus precatorius*), respectively. Ricin, in particular, is a potential biologic weapon and has been implicated in a number of attempted assassinations.

These toxalbumins are proteins, peptides, or lectins, which exert their toxicity by entering cells and inhibiting protein synthesis. The clinical syndrome associated with the toxalbumins depends on quantity as well as route of exposure. Although one castor bean contains enough ricin to kill, its toxicity is typically limited following ingestion. Even if the castor bean is chewed to break the protective hard shell that sequesters the toxin, the enteral absorption of ricin is poor and tends to limit toxicity to diarrhea and abdominal pain. Although delayed systemic toxicity is possible following large ingestions, these symptoms tend to occur more in parenteral exposures. Systemic organ dysfunction includes cardiac, neurologic, hepatic, and renal sequelae. Inhalational exposures are rapidly progressive and can result in life-threatening respiratory failure, circulatory collapse, and death within 36 hours.[15]

Treat toxalbumin ingestion by administration of activated charcoal followed by a lengthy observation period. All routes of exposure can be fatal, but hydration and aggressive supportive care significantly reduce mortality. More information about ricin can be found at the Centers for Disease Control and Prevention Web site (http://www.bt.cdc.gov/agent/ricin/).

Toxalbumins are found in a number of other plants such as American mistletoe (*Phoradendron flavescens*) and European mistletoe (*Viscum album*). The leaves and stems contain phoratoxin and viscumin, both of which are less potent than ricin. The berries also contain low levels of toxins that may result in gastroenteritis following large doses. These berries are abundant in homes during the holiday season and are attractive to children. Fortunately, significant morbidity after berry ingestion is rare, although single incidents of seizure, gait instability, hepatotoxicity, and death have been reported.[16] Provide GI decontamination with activated charcoal accompanied by fluid and electrolyte monitoring for minimally symptomatic patients.

CONVULSANTS (WATER HEMLOCK)

Cicutoxin is a diol found in the water hemlock (*Cicuta maculata*), western water hemlock (*Cicuta douglasii*), and hemlock water dropwort (*Oenanthe crocata*). These plants are often mistaken for wild parsnip, turnip, or parsley, causing toxicity through dermal or enteric absorption. All parts of the plant are poisonous, with the highest concentration of cicutoxin in the tuber. Cicutoxin's mechanism of action is not fully understood. However, it may impair γ-aminobutyric acid receptor or potassium channel function. Toxicity can manifest as early as 15 minutes following exposure. Mild symptoms include GI discomfort, followed by bradycardia, hypotension, respiratory distress, seizures, and death. Seizures may be severe and refractory to conventional anticonvulsant therapy. The mortality rate may be as high as 30%.[17] Treatment consists of GI decontamination with activated charcoal and supportive care. Treat seizures with γ-aminobutyric acid agonists such as benzodiazepines or barbiturates.

DEMYELINATING ANTHRACENONES (BUCKTHORN)

Buckthorn or coyotillo (*Karwinskia humboldtiana*), which is found in the southwestern United States, Mexico, Central America, and the Caribbean, contains demyelinating anthracenones that lead to progressive muscle weakness that resembles Guillain-Barré syndrome. Weakness occurs weeks after ingestion, rendering GI decontamination futile in symptomatic patients. In severe cases, respiratory paralysis can lead to death without respiratory support. There is no antidote, and treatment is largely supportive until recovery.[9]

BELLADONNA ALKALOIDS (NIGHTSHADE, JIMSONWEED, HENBANE)

Deadly nightshade (*Atropa belladonna*), jimsonweed (*Datura* spp.), and henbane (*Hyoscyamus niger*) all contain atropine-like alkaloids such as hyoscyamine and scopolamine. Ingestion or smoking results in antimuscarinic effects such as tachycardia, hyperthermia, mydriasis, decreased bowel sounds, urinary retention, altered mental status, and dry, flushed skin. Severe poisoning can include seizures, coma, and death. Onset of effects depends on route of exposure, but findings should be evident within 4 hours. Exposures most commonly are intentional, such as through experimentation with the plant's hallucinogenic properties.[18]

Treatment is largely supportive. Benzodiazepines are useful in calming patients, but avoid antipsychotics such as haloperidol to prevent further antimuscarinic activity. Physostigmine inhibits cholinesterase, resulting in increased synaptic concentrations of acetylcholine that can overcome the muscarinic antagonism from the atropine-like alkaloids. Physostigmine is generally indicated only for patients with moderate to severe symptoms. Improvement in symptoms may be transient, and patients can require repeat dosing if symptoms recrudesce. Patients who receive physostigmine improve faster and require shorter hospitalizations than patients receiving sedative-hypnotics.

ANTIMITOTIC ALKALOIDS (AUTUMN CROCUS, GLORY LILY, MAYAPPLE)

Colchicine is contained in all parts of the autumn crocus (*Colchicum autumnale*) and glory lily (*Gloriosa superba*). Colchicine halts cellular mitosis by inhibiting microtubule formation. Gastroenteritis, which may be delayed (2 to 24 hours), is followed by multisystem organ failure. Common effects include coagulopathy, bone marrow suppression with granulocytopenia and thrombocytopenia, cardiac dysrhythmias, cardiogenic shock, acute respiratory distress syndrome, hepatic failure, delirium, seizures, coma, and death. If patients survive, alopecia and neuropathy may develop. Mild toxicity is expected if GI symptoms begin >9 hours after ingestion.[19,20]

Podophyllin is an extract of the roots of the mayapple plant (*Podophyllum peltatum*). This extract contains a mixture of toxins including podophyllotoxin, which inhibits topoisomerase II and microtubule formation. Toxicity is characterized by obtundation, coagulopathy, hematologic suppression, renal failure, GI irritation, hepatotoxicity, and death.[9]

Early after ingestion, pursue aggressive GI decontamination because there is no antidote and toxicity can be fatal due to multisystem organ involvement. Due to its delayed onset, observe exposed patients for a prolonged period. In addition to GI decontamination with activated charcoal, treatment usually requires aggressive fluid resuscitation and aggressive supportive care. Colchicine-specific Fab fragments have been used in colchicine-poisoned patients with some success experimentally but are not commercially available.

CALCIUM OXALATE (ELEPHANT'S EAR)

Many common household ornamental plants contain crystalline calcium oxalate. Examples include dumbcane (*Dieffenbachia* spp.), elephant's ear (*Colocasia* spp.), and philodendron (*Philodendron* spp.). The calcium oxalate crystals are needle-shaped and are packaged in raphides that also contain proteolytic enzymes and other chemicals. The contents are extruded when the plant is injured, causing both direct trauma from the crystals and inflammation due to the chemicals' effects.

Ingestion of calcium oxalate–containing plants results in immediate oropharyngeal pain and swelling. This pain usually limits the amount of plant ingested. In serious cases, the swelling can involve upper airway structures and cause respiratory compromise due to obstruction.[21] Ocular exposures to the calcium oxalate–containing plants result in ocular pain, corneal injury, and conjunctivitis. Pain and swelling can last up to 8 days.

Patients with oropharyngeal swelling and pain following ingestion tend to improve with supportive care. Anti-inflammatories may decrease swelling and provide analgesia. Topical treatments such as ice, ice water, and ice cream are soothing and can be given in patients with stable, patent airways. Patients at risk of airway obstruction must be closely monitored and should be quickly intubated if progressing. Consider steroid administration; however, there are no trials demonstrating outcome improvement with steroid use.

CYANOGENIC PLANTS (*PRUNUS* SPECIES)

Several thousand plants, including many common vegetables and fruits, contain cyanogenic compounds, such as amygdalin. Fortunately, the toxins are either sequestered in nonconsumed portions of the foods (seeds) or exist in quantities that are not clinically significant. Amygdalin is found in the leaves, bark, and seeds of those fruits of the *Prunus* species, including pears, apples, plums, peaches, and apricots. Although the aril (fruit portion) of these plants is nontoxic, ingestion of the other portions of the plants and their seeds can result in the liberation of hydrogen cyanide from amygdalin in the GI tract. Linamarin and lotaustralin are present in cassava (*Manihot esculenta*) and are similarly hydrolyzed to liberate hydrogen cyanide.[9,22] If prepared correctly, the cyanogenic glycosides can be hydrolyzed prior to ingestion, thereby liberating the cyanide prior to consumption.[23,24] Initial effects may be slightly delayed and include GI irritation, followed by signs of tissue hypoxia. Rapid progression of toxicity can occur, and treatment for cyanide poisoning should be initiated immediately.

CAPSAICIN (PEPPERS)

Capsicum peppers contain capsaicin, a phenylpropanoid toxin that causes irritation, burning, and pain upon contact with skin and mucous membranes. This toxin enhances the release of substance P from small unmyelinated nerve fibers, which stimulate nociceptors that cause the sensation of burning or heat. Contact typically occurs as a result of self-inoculation while preparing peppers or exposure to spraying of pepper extracts in self-defense. Decontaminate affected areas by irrigation with copious amounts of water and gentle hand soap. Ocular exposures may require aggressive decontamination and ophthalmologic evaluation. Analgesics may be necessary.

MISCELLANEOUS GI TOXINS

Solanine and chaconine are glycoalkaloids that are present in many common plants and vegetables of the *Solanum* species. Unripe eggplant, green potatoes, and their sprouts contain a small amount of these heat-labile glycoalkaloids. Ingestion may cause GI effects such as vomiting, diarrhea, and abdominal pain, which can be delayed as long as 24 hours. CNS symptoms such as hallucinations, delirium, and obtundation are reported.[25] There is no definitive antidote for solanine or chaconine poisoning, and supportive care is usually sufficient.

Pokeweed (*Phytolacca americana*) contains phytolaccatoxin and similar phytotoxins in the leaves and roots. The mature berries are less toxic. Exposures can occur when foragers mistake the roots for other nontoxics such as parsnips or horseradish. Pokeweed is often prepared in poke salad or pokeroot tea. Toxicity is avoided if prepared by parboiling young greens. Incorrect preparation results in GI upset from direct mucosal irritation. Nausea, vomiting, hemorrhagic gastritis, abdominal pain, and profuse diarrhea may last for 48 hours.[26] Severe intoxications may rarely result in coma and death. Treatment is supportive. A nonconsequential lymphocytosis develops approximately 3 days after ingestion and typically resolves within 2 weeks.

Ackee fruit grows on the *Blighia sapida* tree, and it is a common ingredient in West African and Jamaican cuisine. Unripe ackee fruit contains the heat-stable toxins hypoglycin A and B. Hypoglycin A inhibits free fatty acids from entering the mitochondria, impairs substrate formation for gluconeogenesis, and prevents conversion of glutamate to γ-aminobutyric acid. The resulting clinical syndrome, which is characterized by severe vomiting and hypoglycemia, is Jamaican vomiting sickness. Severe cases develop acidemia, seizures, and encephalopathy.[9,27] Administer IV dextrose or a carbohydrate-heavy meal to hypoglycemic patients. Treat seizures liberally with benzodiazepines. However, seizures may be refractory to benzodiazepines if γ-aminobutyric acid concentrations are critically low. Rarely, chronic toxicity from hypoglycin A can lead to cholestatic hepatitis or fulminant liver failure.[9,28] Admit symptomatic patients for close monitoring and treatment.

Holly (*Ilex* spp.) exposures are in the top 10 plants reported to poison control centers.[2] Although the leaves are nontoxic, the attractive berries contain a mixture of toxins. The most consequential of this mixture are saponins, glycosides that cause abdominal pain, vomiting, and diarrhea. If fewer than six berries are ingested, minimal toxicity should follow.[29] Large ingestions with severe GI upset may result in electrolyte abnormalities. For symptomatic patients, treatment is supportive.

PLANT-INDUCED DERMATITIS

Dermal exposure to a number of plants can result in an undesired dermatitis. These exposures are some of the most commonly reported plant-related concerns reported to poison control centers in the United States.[2] Classification by mechanism of action can guide therapy (**Table 220-3**), but often, exposure to a single plant can result in injury due to multiple mechanisms.

MECHANICAL INJURY

Specialized plant structures can injure the dermis and serve as a nidus for entry of toxins. Needle-shaped crystals, such as calcium oxalate crystal bundles, are found in a number of common plants, including dumbcane (*Dieffenbachia* spp.) and philodendron (*Philodendron* spp.). Needles of pineapples (*Bromeliaceae* spp.) and the hairs of stinging nettles (*Urtica dioica*) directly pierce the dermis, and chemical irritants in these structures cause further dermal injury (see below).

IRRITANT DERMATITIS

Phorbol esters found in the sap of plants of the Euphorbiaceae (spurge) can cause dermal irritation following contact. Symptoms such as erythema and bullae may develop shortly after direct contact. The phorbol esters can penetrate the dermis upon contact. Ocular injuries and GI injury can also occur upon exposure or ingestion. Occasionally, aerosolized irritants can cause dermatitis or respiratory distress. Exposures to poinsettia (*Euphorbia pulcherrima*) are typically well tolerated.[30] Pineapples (*Bromeliaceae* spp.), stinging nettles (*U. dioica*), and dumbcane (*Dieffenbachia* spp.) all introduce irritants such as proteolytic

TABLE 220-3 Plant-Induced Dermatitis

Dermatitis Classification	Mechanism of Injury	Specific Plants
Mechanical injury		
	Calcium oxalate	Dumbcane (*Dieffenbachia maculate*)
		Philodendron (*Philodendron* spp.)
	Raphides and trichomes	Stinging nettles (*Urtica dioica*)
		Velvet bean or cowhage (*Mucuna pruriens*)
		Pineapple (*Bromeliaceae* spp.)
Irritant dermatitis	Phorbol esters	Cow's horn (*Euphorbia grandicornis*)
		Poinsettia (*Euphorbia pulcherrima*)
		Manchineel tree (*Hippomane mancinella*)
	Other chemical irritants	Stinging nettles (*U. dioica*)
		Velvet bean or cowhage (*M. pruriens*)
		Pineapple (*Bromeliaceae* spp.)
Contact dermatitis		
	Urushiol oleoresins	Ginkgo (*Ginkgoaceae*)
		Poison ivy, oak, and sumac (*Toxicodendron* spp.)
		Mango (*Mangifera indica*)
		Pistachio (*Pistacia vera*)
		Cashew (*Anacardium occidentale*)
	Miscellaneous antigens	Peruvian lily (*Alstroemeria* spp.)
		Narcissus and daffodils (*Narcissus* spp.)
		Tulips (*Tulipa* spp.)
		Primroses (*Primula* spp.)
Phytophotodermatitis		
	Furocoumarins	Cow parsnip (*Heracleum lanatum*)
		Wild parsnip (*Pastinaca sativa*)
		Lime (*Citrus aurantiifolia*)

enzymes and other proinflammatory chemicals such as histamine, acetylcholine, and 5-hydroxytryptamine.[10]

ALLERGIC CONTACT DERMATITIS

Many plants can cause allergic contact dermatitis after repeat exposure. Sensitization occurs after a resin binds to skin proteins and forms an antigen. Reexposure then stimulates a T-cell–mediated immune response.

Poison ivy, poison oak, and poison sumac (*Toxicodendron* spp.) are ubiquitous sources of the antigenic resin urushiol. Ginkgo (*Ginkgoaceae*), mango (*Mangifera indica*), pistachio (*Pistacia vera*), and cashew (*Anacardium occidentale*) are common foods with urushiol. In sensitized individuals, reexposure can result in urticaria and pruritus. Over 12 to 48 hours, symptoms may progress to varying degrees of vesiculobullous formation. Treatment usually consists of drying agents and local topical steroids, but systemic steroids may be necessary in severe cases. Some exposures can result in type I hypersensitivity or anaphylaxis.

Tulips (*Tulipa* spp.) and daffodils (*Narcissus* spp.) contain the glycoside tuliposide A. After hydrolysis, an allergen causes tulip fingers or daffodil itch with chronic reexposure, a painful and pruritic condition.

PHYTOPHOTODERMATITIS

Phytophotodermatitis occurs when furocoumarins are activated by sunlight and produce symptoms that resemble sunburn in the acute phase; erythema and bullae are common. When these symptoms heal, hyperpigmentation persists for months. The mechanism is unknown. Exposure can be directly through the dermis, or furocoumarins can be deposited in the skin following ingestion and subsequent systemic circulation. Many plants, including common foods, can cause phytophotodermatitis, including numerous citrus fruits, celery, carrots, and herbs.[9]

REFERENCES

The complete reference list is available online at www.TintinalliEM.com.

CHAPTER 221 High-Altitude Disorders

Peter H. Hackett
Christopher B. Davis

INTRODUCTION AND EPIDEMIOLOGY

Millions of people annually visit mountainous areas of the western United States at altitudes of >2440 m (>8000 ft). In addition, tens of thousands travel to high-altitude regions in other parts of the world. Adventure travel to mountainous regions is booming.[1] Physicians working or traveling in or near these locations are likely to encounter high-altitude illness or preexisting conditions that are exacerbated by altitude. Although the focus of this chapter is hypoxia-related problems, patients in the mountain environment may require care for associated illnesses such as hypothermia (see chapter 209, "Hypothermia"), frostbite (see chapter 208, "Cold Injuries"), trauma, ultraviolet keratitis, dehydration, and lightning injury (see chapter 218, "Electrical and Lightning Injuries").

High altitude (>2440 m [>8000 ft]) is a hypoxic environment. Because the concentration of oxygen in the troposphere remains constant at 21%, the partial pressure of oxygen (P_{O2}) decreases as a function of the barometric pressure. In Denver at 1610 m (5280 ft), air pressure is 17% less than at sea level. The air of Aspen, Colorado, 2440 m (8000 ft), has 26% less oxygen than sea level. At 5490 m (18,000 ft), there is half the available oxygen, whereas on top of Mount Everest, there is only one third. Oxygen supplementation prevents symptoms of altitude illness during hypobaric exposure, and therefore, hypoxia, not hypobaria per se, is responsible for illness.

Altitude may be divided into stages according to physiologic effects. *Intermediate altitude*, 1520 to 2440 m (5000 to 8000 ft), produces decreased exercise performance and increased alveolar ventilation without major impairment in arterial oxygen transport. Acute mountain sickness (AMS) occurs at and above 2130 to 2440 m (7000 to 8000 ft) and sometimes at lower altitudes in particularly susceptible individuals. Patients who have limitations in ventilatory response such as some neuromuscular diseases or those with preexisting hypoxemia may become more symptomatic in this range of altitude. *High altitude,* 2440 to 4270 m (8000 to 14,000 ft), is associated with decreased arterial oxygen saturation (Sa_{O2}); marked hypoxemia may occur during exercise and sleep. Most cases of altitude-related medical problems occur in this elevation range, because of the availability of overnight tourist facilities located at these heights. *Very high altitude,* 4270 to 5490 m (14,000 to 18,000 ft), is uncommon in the United States but is encountered by visitors to the mountainous regions of South America and the Himalayas. Abrupt ascent can be dangerous, and a period of acclimatization is required to prevent illness. *Extreme altitude,* >5490 m (>18,000 ft), is experienced only by mountain climbers and is accompanied by severe hypoxemia and hypocapnia. At this height, progressive physiologic deterioration eventually outstrips acclimatization, and sustained human habitation is impossible. **Because hypoxemia is maximal during sleep, the sleeping altitude is the critical altitude to consider.**

PHYSIOLOGY AND PATHOPHYSIOLOGY OF ALTITUDE ACCLIMATIZATION

Acutely hypoxic individuals become dizzy, faint, and rapidly unconscious if hypoxic stress is sufficient (Sa_{O2} <65%). Captain Hawthorne Gray, in an attempt to set the record for highest hot air balloon flight in 1927, lost consciousness and died when his balloon rose to >12,200 m (>40,000 ft). However, individuals given days to weeks to acclimatize can tolerate surprising degrees of hypoxemia and function quite well. Although the fundamental process of this acclimatization takes place in the metabolic machinery of cells and mitochondria, acute "stress" responses are critical while allowing cells time to adjust.

VENTILATION

The primary initial adaptation is defense of alveolar P_{O2} through increased ventilation. The hypoxic ventilatory response is modulated by the carotid body, which senses a decrease in arterial oxygenation and signals the central respiratory center in the medulla to increase ventilation. The vigor of this inborn response relates to successful acclimatization and increased performance. Respiratory depressants or stimulants may affect hypoxic ventilatory drive, as does chronic hypoxia, which eventually blunts the response. A low hypoxic drive may allow extreme hypoxemia to develop during sleep. Initial hyperventilation is attenuated quickly by respiratory alkalosis, which acts as a brake on the respiratory center. As renal excretion of bicarbonate compensates for the respiratory alkalosis, pH returns toward normal, and ventilation continues to increase. The process of maximizing ventilation, termed *ventilatory acclimatization*, culminates after 4 to 7 days at a given altitude. With continuing ascent to higher altitudes, the central chemoreceptors reset to progressively lower values of partial pressure of carbon dioxide, and the completeness of acclimatization can be gauged by the partial pressure of arterial carbon dioxide. Acetazolamide, which forces a bicarbonate diuresis, greatly facilitates this process. An appreciation of the normal values for blood gases and acid-base status with acclimatization at various altitudes is necessary to distinguish abnormalities (**Table 221-1**).

BLOOD

Within 2 hours of ascent to altitude, serum erythropoietin level increases and results in increased red cell mass over days to weeks. This adaptation has no importance during initial acclimatization when acute altitude illness develops; however, excessive red cell mass may develop over a period of weeks to months leading to chronic mountain polycythemia. Shifts in

TABLE 221-1 Blood Gas Concentrations at Various Altitudes

Altitude	Pa_{O2} (mm Hg)	Sa_{O2} (%)	PaC_{O2} (mm Hg)
Sea level	90–95	96	40
5000 ft (1520 m)	75–81	95	35.6
7500 ft (2290 m)	69–74	92–93	31–33
15,000 ft (4570 m)	48–53	86	25
20,000 ft (7000 m)	37–45	76	20
25,000 ft (7620 m)	32–39	68	13
29,000 ft (8840 m)	26–33	58	9.5–13.8

Abbreviations: Pa_{O2} = partial pressure of arterial oxygen; PaC_{O2} = partial pressure of arterial carbon dioxide; Sa_{O2} = arterial oxygen saturation.

the oxyhemoglobin dissociation curve are thought to be minimal at altitude because of balancing physiologic effects. Hypoxia causes an increase in the level of 2,3-diphosphoglyceric acid and shifts the curve to the right. Respiratory alkalosis shifts the curve to the left. Naturally occurring left-shifted hemoglobin is advantageous at high altitude; a given partial pressure of oxygen will yield higher oxygen saturation and facilitate loading of oxygen onto hemoglobin in the pulmonary capillary.

FLUID BALANCE

Peripheral venous constriction on ascent to altitude causes an increase in central blood volume that triggers baroreceptors to suppress secretion of antidiuretic hormone and aldosterone and induces a diuresis. Combined with the bicarbonate diuresis from the respiratory alkalosis, the result is decreased plasma volume and a hyperosmolality (serum osmolality of 290 to 300 mOsmol/L) that results from a reset of the osmolar center of the brain. The hemoconcentration also increases oxygen-carrying capacity of the blood. Clinically, diuresis and hemoconcentration are considered a healthy response, whereas antidiuresis is associated with AMS and may contribute to edema formation.

CARDIOVASCULAR SYSTEM

Stroke volume decreases initially, and increased heart rate maintains cardiac output. Maximum exercising heart rate declines at altitude proportional to the decrease in maximum oxygen consumption (Vo_2max). Cardiac muscle in healthy persons can withstand extreme levels of hypoxemia (partial pressure of arterial oxygen [Pa_{O2}] of <30 mm Hg) without evidence of ST-segment changes or ischemic events. Blood pressure typically increases mildly on ascent secondary to increased sympathetic tone, but labile blood pressure is also possible.

The pulmonary circulation constricts with exposure to hypoxia. Although pulmonary vasoconstriction is advantageous during conditions of regional alveolar hypoxia, such as pneumonia, it poses a disadvantage during the global hypoxia of altitude exposure, increasing to a variable degree pulmonary vascular resistance and pulmonary artery pressure. A hyperreactive response increases susceptibility to high-altitude pulmonary edema.

Cerebral blood flow transiently increases on ascent to altitude (despite the hypocapnic alkalosis), which increases oxygen delivery to the brain. This response, however, is limited by the increase in cerebral blood volume, which may increase intracranial pressure and aggravate symptoms of altitude illness.

EXERCISE CAPACITY

Exercise capacity, as measured by Vo_2max, drops dramatically on ascent to altitude, approximately 10% for each 1000-m (3280-ft) altitude gain above 1500 m (4920 ft). During acclimatization, submaximal endurance increases appreciably after 10 days, but Vo_2max does not. The mechanism of this decrement might be lack of adequate oxygen supply to the muscle cells due to the low driving pressure for diffusion of oxygen from the capillary. Another theory suggests that the CNS limits muscle activity to preserve its own oxygenation.

LIMITATIONS TO ACCLIMATIZATION

There are limits to acclimatization. Even those who are by nature good acclimatizers cannot tolerate the hypoxia of extreme altitude for long. Miners in South America report that they cannot live at altitudes >5800 m (>19,000 ft) because of weight loss, increasing lethargy, poor-quality sleep, weakness, and headache. High-altitude mountaineers cannot survive for more than a few days at >8000 m (>26,200 ft) without supplemental oxygen because of rapid deterioration of physiologic functioning. Considerable weight loss due to loss of fat and lean body mass is unavoidable. Other factors limiting the ability to adapt to extreme altitude include right ventricular strain from excessive pulmonary hypertension, intestinal malabsorption, impaired renal function, polycythemia leading to microcirculatory sludging, and prolonged cerebral hypoxia. Even at more modest altitudes, some individuals acclimatize poorly due to genetic and epigenetic factors. One phenotype is blunted carotid body function that leads to inadequate ventilation at high altitude.

SLEEP AT HIGH ALTITUDE

Sleep stages III and IV are reduced at altitude, whereas sleep stage I is increased. More time is spent awake, with a significant increase in arousals, but with only slightly less rapid eye movement time. Frequent nighttime awakenings are a common source of bitter complaints from skiers and others, but they are innocuous and improve with time at altitude. The typical periodic breathing (Cheyne-Stokes respiration) in those sleeping at >2700 m (>8860 ft) consists of 6- to 12-second apneic pauses interspersed with cycles of vigorous ventilation. Intervals of apnea of >20 seconds have been observed at extreme altitudes. Interestingly, the frequent awakenings are not necessarily related to sleep periodic breathing, and they are not related to AMS either. Quality of sleep and arterial oxygenation during sleep improve with acclimatization and with acetazolamide.

HIGH-ALTITUDE SYNDROMES

High-altitude syndromes are those attributed directly to the hypoxia: acute hypoxia, AMS, pulmonary edema, cerebral edema, retinopathy, peripheral edema, sleeping problems, and a group of neurologic syndromes. Other syndromes occurring at high altitude, which are not necessarily related to hypoxia, include thromboembolic events (which may be attributable to dehydration, prolonged incapacitation, polycythemia, and cold), high-altitude pharyngitis and bronchitis, and ultraviolet keratitis. **Although the different hypoxic clinical syndromes overlap, all share a fundamental mechanism, all are seen in the same setting of rapid ascent in unacclimatized persons, and all respond to the same essential therapy: descent and oxygen.**

ACUTE HYPOXIA

The syndrome of acute hypoxia occurs in the setting of sudden and severe hypoxic insult, such as accidental decompression of a pressurized aircraft cabin or failure of the oxygen system used by a pilot or high-altitude mountaineer. Sudden overexertion precipitating arterial desaturation, acute onset of pulmonary edema, carbon monoxide poisoning, and sleep apnea may result in relatively acute hypoxia as well. Unacclimatized persons become unconscious at an Sa_{O2} of 50% to 60%, a Pa_{O2} of less than approximately 30 mm Hg, or a jugular venous P_{O2} of <15 mm Hg. Acute hypoxia reverses with immediate administration of oxygen, rapid descent, and correction of the underlying cause. Symptoms of acute hypoxia reflect the sensitivity of the CNS to this insult: dizziness, light-headedness, and dimmed vision progressing to loss of consciousness. Hyperventilation increases the time of useful consciousness during acute alveolar hypoxia.

ACUTE MOUNTAIN SICKNESS

AMS is a syndrome characterized by headache along with some combination of GI disturbance, dizziness, fatigue, or sleep disturbance

TABLE 221-2 Lake Louise Acute Mountain Sickness (AMS) Self-Questionnaire*

1. Headache	Score
No headache—0	
Mild headache—1	
Moderate headache—2	
Severe headache, incapacitating—3	
2. GI symptoms	Score
No symptoms—0	
Poor appetite or nausea—1	
Moderate nausea or vomiting—2	
Severe nausea and vomiting, incapacitating—3	
3. Fatigue/weakness	Score
Not tired or weak at all—0	
Mild fatigue or weakness—1	
Moderate fatigue or weakness—2	
Severe fatigue or weakness, incapacitating—3	
4. Dizzy/light-headedness	Score
No dizziness/light-headedness—0	
Mild dizziness/light-headedness—1	
Moderate dizziness/light-headedness—2	
Severely light-headed, fainting/passing out—3	
5. Difficulty sleeping	Score
Slept well—0	
Did not sleep as well as usual—1	
Woke many times, poor night's sleep—2	
Could not sleep at all—3	
Total symptom score	

*Diagnosis of AMS requires headache plus 1 or more of the above symptoms.

Mild AMS: score of 2–4

Moderate AMS: score of 5–9

Severe AMS: score of 10–15

Source: Reproduced with permission from Roach RC, Bartsch P, Hackett PH, Oelz O; the Lake Louise AMS Scoring Consensus Committee: The Lake Louise Acute Mountain Sickness Scoring System, in Sutton J, Houston C, Coates G (eds): *Hypoxia and Mountain Medicine: Proceedings of the 8th International Hypoxia Symposium*. Burlington, VT: Pergamon Press, 1992, p. 272.

(Table 221-2). It occurs in the setting of more gradual and less severe hypoxic insult than in acute hypoxia syndrome. Its incidence varies by location, ease of access to the high-altitude environment, rate of ascent, and sleeping altitude. One study found a 25% incidence of AMS in physicians attending a continuing-education meeting held at 2100 m (6900 ft) in Colorado. Other studies at resorts at altitudes between 2220 and 2700 m (7280 and 8860 ft) claim an incidence between 17% and 40%, and a sleeping altitude of 2740 m (9000 ft) seems to be a threshold for an increase in attack rate.[2] Approximately 40% of trekkers in Nepal on the path to Mount Everest experience AMS, and climbers on Mount Rainier have a very high incidence of 70% because of the rapidity of ascent.

In addition to rate of ascent and sleeping altitude, inherent factors determine individual susceptibility to AMS. Blunted carotid body response and low vital capacity are examples. Age has little influence on incidence, with children being as susceptible as adults, although those >50 years of age tend to have less AMS. Women are just as likely to develop mountain sickness but appear to have less pulmonary edema. Obesity has recently been linked to the development of AMS, possibly due to greater nocturnal oxygen desaturation.[3] Susceptibility to AMS generally is reproducible in an individual on repeated exposures. Persons living at intermediate altitudes of 1000 to 2000 m (3300 to 6600 ft) already are partially acclimatized and do much better than lowlanders on ascent to higher altitudes. There is no relationship between susceptibility to AMS and physical fitness.

PATHOPHYSIOLOGY

AMS is due to hypobaric hypoxia, but the exact sequence of events leading to illness is unclear. Cerebral vasodilation appears to be the initiating event. Vasodilation occurs in the brain in all persons ascending to high altitude, thus increasing cerebral blood flow and blood volume. Whether this is solely sufficient to cause the symptoms of mild AMS is unclear. However, in persons who progress to high-altitude cerebral edema, vasogenic edema is evident as increased T2 signal on MRI.[4] The leaky blood–brain barrier in high-altitude cerebral edema is due either to loss of autoregulation leading to overperfusion, or to increased permeability caused by mediators such as vascular endothelial growth factor or bradykinin. A combination of these two processes is also possible. The fact that dexamethasone so effectively treats AMS also supports the notion of vasogenic edema. An alternative notion is that the trigeminal-vascular system is triggered by hypoxic vasodilation or by noxious agents such as nitric oxide or free oxygen radicals.

CLINICAL FEATURES

The diagnosis of AMS is based on an appropriate setting paired with characteristic symptoms. The setting is rapid ascent of an unacclimatized person to 2000 m (6560 ft) or higher. On arrival the person typically feels light-headed and slightly breathless, especially with exercise. Symptoms develop between 1 and 6 hours later, but sometimes are delayed for 1 or 2 days (especially after a night's sleep). Symptoms of mild AMS are remarkably similar to those of an alcohol hangover. Headaches are usually bifrontal and worsen with exertion, bending over, or performing a Valsalva maneuver. GI symptoms include anorexia, nausea, and sometimes vomiting, especially in children. The chief constitutional symptoms are lassitude and weakness. The person with AMS can be irritable and often wants to be left alone. Sleepiness and a deep inner chill also are common. The Lake Louise AMS self-report questionnaire can be helpful in following the severity of the illness (Table 221-2).

As the illness progresses, headache becomes more severe while vomiting and oliguria develop. Lassitude may progress so that the victim requires assistance in eating and dressing. The onset of ataxia and altered level of consciousness heralds high-altitude cerebral edema. Coma may ensue within 12 hours if treatment is delayed. The diagnosis of AMS can be difficult in preverbal children and should be a diagnosis of exclusion.[5]

Physical findings in mild AMS are nonspecific. Heart rate and blood pressure are variable and usually in the normal range, although postural hypotension may be present. **Presenting percent Sa_{O_2} is typically normal or slightly low for a given altitude, and percent Sa_{O_2} overall correlates poorly with the diagnosis of AMS.** Localized rales are detectable in up to 20% of persons with AMS. Fundoscopy reveals venous tortuosity and dilatation, and retinal hemorrhages are common at altitudes >5000 m (>16,400 ft) and in those with pulmonary and cerebral edema. Facial and peripheral edema sometimes accompanies AMS.

The differential diagnosis in this setting includes hypothermia, carbon monoxide poisoning, pulmonary or CNS infection, dehydration, migraine, and exhaustion. Carbon monoxide poisoning may have a presentation very similar to that of AMS and is not uncommon in mountain towns in the winter. Reduced oxyhemoglobin levels complicate hypoxia from high altitude, and the effects are additive. Hypoxia may trigger a migraine headache in patients with a personal or family history of migraine.[6] Headache from AMS often dissipates within 10 to 15 minutes with supplemental oxygen administration, unlike headaches from other causes. Providers may find this to be a useful diagnostic maneuver.

The average duration of AMS at a Colorado resort (3000 m or 9840 ft) was 15 hours, with a range of up to 94 hours. Half of those affected with AMS chose to self-medicate.[2] At higher sleeping altitudes the illness may last much longer, up to weeks if untreated, and is more likely to progress to pulmonary or cerebral edema. Eight percent of those with AMS at 4270 m (14,000 ft) in Nepal developed cerebral or pulmonary edema or both.[7]

TREATMENT

The goals of treatment (**Table 221-3**) are to prevent progression, treat symptoms, and improve acclimatization. Early diagnosis is essential. Initial

TABLE 221-3 Suggested Treatment Options for High-Altitude Illness

Mild AMS	No further ascent
	Descent to lower altitude or acclimatization at same altitude
	Acetazolamide, 125–250 milligrams PO twice a day, to speed acclimatization
	Symptomatic treatment as necessary with analgesics and antiemetics
Moderate/severe AMS	Immediate descent for worsening symptoms
	Low-flow oxygen if available
	Acetazolamide, 250 milligrams PO twice a day, and/or dexamethasone, 4 milligrams PO every 6 h
	Hyperbaric therapy
High-altitude cerebral edema	Immediate descent or evacuation
	Oxygen 2–4 L/min or titrated to Sa_{O_2} >90%
	Dexamethasone, 8 milligrams PO, IM, or IV, then 4 milligrams every 6 h
	Hyperbaric therapy if patient cannot descend
High-altitude pulmonary edema	Immediate descent or evacuation
	Oxygen 4 L/min or titrated to Sa_{O_2} >90%
	Nifedipine, 30 milligrams PO extended release every 12 h if no oxygen or descent*
	Hyperbaric therapy if patient cannot descend
	Measures to minimize patient exertion and keep patient warm
	Dexamethasone if cerebral signs present, 4 milligrams PO every 6 h
Periodic breathing/ insomnia	Acetazolamide, 62.5–125.0 milligrams PO at bedtime as needed

Abbreviations: AMS = acute mountain sickness; Sa_{O_2} = arterial oxygen saturation.

*Drug therapy is unnecessary if oxygen is available.

clinical presentation does not predict eventual severity, and all persons with AMS must be observed carefully for progression. **The three principles of treatment are (1) do not proceed to a higher sleeping altitude in the presence of symptoms, (2) descend if symptoms do not abate or become worse despite treatment, and (3) descend and treat immediately in the presence of a change in consciousness, ataxia, or pulmonary edema.** Descent is the definitive treatment for all forms of altitude illness. However, descent is not always an option, nor is it always necessary.

Descent and Oxygen Mild AMS is self-limited and generally improves with an extra 12 to 36 hours of acclimatization if ascent is halted. Remarkably, a drop in altitude of only 300 to 1000 m (980 to 3280 ft) usually is effective. Evacuation to a hospital or to sea level is unnecessary except in the most severe cases. To simulate descent, portable hyperbaric bags are being used in various locations to treat high-altitude illness. The patient is inserted into the fabric chamber, and a pressure of 0.9 kg/2.5 cm^2 (2 lb/in.^{2}) is achieved by means of a manual or automated pump, equivalent to a drop in altitude of 1500 m (4920 ft). A valve system creates sufficient ventilation to avoid carbon dioxide accumulation or oxygen depletion.

Oxygen effectively relieves symptoms, but it is generally unavailable in the field or reserved for those with moderate to severe AMS in order to conserve supplies. Oxygen supplementation quickly relieves headache and dizziness. Nocturnal administration of low-flow oxygen (0.5 to 1 L/min) is particularly helpful and efficient. The combination of oxygen and descent provides optimal therapy, especially in more severe illness.

Medical Therapy Pharmacologic treatment offers an alternative to descent or oxygen administration in patients with mild to moderate AMS. Acetazolamide acts by inhibiting the enzyme carbonic anhydrase. In the kidney, acetazolamide reduces reabsorption of bicarbonate, causing a bicarbonate diuresis and metabolic acidosis that stimulates ventilation. As a result, Pa_{O_2} is higher. Acetazolamide thus reverses the deleterious effects of hypobaric hypoxia. The drug also maintains cerebral blood flow despite greater hypocapnia.

The treatment regimen for AMS varies: 125 milligrams PO twice daily is effective for some individuals, whereas others may require 250 mg PO twice daily. Side effects are more common with higher doses and include peripheral paresthesias and sometimes nausea or drowsiness. Although acetazolamide contains a sulfhydryl moiety, cross-reactivity in those with sulfa antibiotic allergy is uncommon. Nevertheless, individuals with a history of anaphylaxis to sulfa antibiotics should avoid acetazolamide. Treatment should be continued until symptoms of AMS resolve. It can always be restarted if symptoms return. Because the drug inhibits carbonic anhydrase on the tongue, carbonated beverages such as soda or beer may have an altered flavor.

Symptomatic treatment of AMS is often sufficient. Aspirin, 650 milligrams, acetaminophen, 650 to 1000 milligrams (with or without codeine), or ibuprofen, 600 to 800 milligrams, is effective for headache. Aspirin is effective for prophylaxis of headache in persons who are not exercising.[8] Ondansetron orally disintegrating tablets, 4 to 8 milligrams every 4 to 6 hours, effectively treat nausea and vomiting associated with AMS and should be the first-line antiemetic in this setting.

Dexamethasone, 4 milligrams PO, IM, or IV every 6 hours, is quite effective for mountain sickness, but is best reserved for cases of moderate to severe AMS because of potential side effects. Also dexamethasone does not aid acclimatization and may result in some rebound symptoms when discontinued. A short taper period may prevent rebound. The administration of acetazolamide to speed acclimatization and a brief course of dexamethasone to treat illness is a useful combination. Another useful treatment regimen but one that is not yet validated is a one-time dose of dexamethasone followed by a course of acetazolamide.

Frequent nighttime awakening is a common nuisance at high altitude. Before bedtime, acetazolamide, 62.5 to 125 milligrams, improves sleep oxygenation and reduces apneic periods, thereby improving sleep quality. The newer nonbenzodiazepine sleep agents can also be used. These include zolpidem, 5 to 10 milligrams, zolpidem controlled-release, 6.25 to 12.5 milligrams, or eszopiclone, 1 to 2 milligrams. These drugs are safe at altitude and do not depress ventilation. Diphenhydramine, 25 to 50 milligrams before bedtime, is a safe over-the-counter alternative (**Table 221-4**).

PREVENTION

Graded ascent with adequate time for acclimatization is the best prevention. A recommendation for those visiting moderate-altitude resorts in the western United States is to spend a night at an intermediate altitude of 1500 to 2000 m (4920 to 6560 ft) (Denver or Salt Lake City) before sleeping at altitudes >2500 m (>8200 ft). Mountaineers and trekkers should avoid abrupt ascent to sleeping altitudes over 3000 m (9840 ft) and then allow 2 nights for each 1000-m (3230-ft) gain in camp altitude starting at 3000 m (9840 ft). Other preventative measures include avoiding overexertion, alcohol, and respiratory depressants. Prophylactic acetazolamide benefits those with a history of AMS or those with forced rapid ascent to sleeping altitude above 2500 m. Because the drug prevents AMS by enhancing ventilatory acclimatization, fear of masking serious illness is unwarranted. The drug should be started 24 hours before the ascent and should be continued for the first 2 days at altitude. It can be restarted if illness develops. Acetazolamide reduces the symptoms of AMS by approximately 75% in persons ascending rapidly to sleeping altitudes of >2500 m (>8200 ft). An alternative for those with anaphylaxis to sulfa is dexamethasone, 4 milligrams PO every 12 hours, starting the day of ascent and continuing for the first 2 days at altitude. Conflicting evidence exists on the use of ginkgo biloba for AMS prevention. A few studies indicate that 100 milligrams twice a day started 3 to 5 days before ascent is effective in preventing AMS, but other studies have shown no benefit.[9] Lack of standardization of gingko preparations likely explains conflicting results, and the active ingredient is still unknown. Despite the variable results, ginkgo is a safe option for those who desire a natural alternative.

Preacclimatization Although graded ascent is the most effective means of preventing altitude illness, this strategy is not always feasible. Numerous preacclimatization strategies have been proposed using intermittent exposure either to hypobaric hypoxia by use of hypobaric chambers or normobaric hypoxia through commercially available low-oxygen

TABLE 221-4 Medications for High-Altitude Illnesses

Agent	Indication	Dosage	Adverse Effects	Comments
Acetazolamide	Prevention of AMS	125–250 milligrams PO twice a day beginning 24 h before ascent and continuing during ascent and for at least 48 h after arrival at highest altitude	Common: paresthesias, polyuria, altered taste of carbonated beverages Less common: drowsiness, nausea	Can be taken episodically for symptoms (speeds acclimatization); no rebound effect; pregnancy category C, avoid in breastfeeding
	Treatment of AMS	250 milligrams PO every 8–12 h		
	Pediatric AMS	5 milligrams/kg/d PO in divided doses every 8–12 h		
	Periodic breathing	125 milligrams PO 4 h before bedtime		
Dexamethasone	Treatment of AMS	4 milligrams every 6 h PO, IM, or IV	Mood changes, hyperglycemia, dyspepsia	Rapidly improves AMS symptoms; can be life-saving in HACE, may improve HACE enough to facilitate descent; no value in HAPE; pregnancy category C but preferably avoided in pregnancy or breastfeeding
	HACE	8 milligrams initially, then 4 milligrams every 6 h PO, IM, or IV		
	Pediatric HACE	0.15 milligram/kg every 6 h PO, IM, or IV, not to exceed 16 milligrams/d		
Tadalafil	Prevention of HAPE	10 milligrams PO twice a day starting 1 d prior to ascent and continuing for 2–4 d at maximum sleeping altitude	Headache, hypotension (less than with nifedipine), priapism (rare), visual/hearing change or loss (extremely rare)	More effectively blunts hypoxic pulmonary vasoconstriction than sildenafil; better tolerated than nifedipine; pregnancy category B
Nifedipine	Prevention of HAPE	20–30 milligrams extended-release PO every 12 h	Reflex tachycardia, hypotension (uncommon)	
	Treatment of HAPE	30 milligrams extended-release formulation PO every 12 h		No value in AMS or HACE; not necessary if supplemental oxygen available; pregnancy category C

Abbreviations: AMS = acute mountain sickness; HACE = high-altitude cerebral edema; HAPE = high-altitude pulmonary edema.

tents or breathing masks. The overall goal is to reduce the incidence of altitude illness and to improve exercise performance on ascent to altitude. These strategies vary considerably in their use of hypoxic "dose" (simulated altitude), duration of exposure, and overall number of exposures over a period of days. Although many of these strategies induce physiologic responses suggestive of acclimatization, only a few are able to demonstrate a significant decrease in AMS incidence.[10-12] Short-term exposure to hypoxia of less than 6 hours per day has not been shown to be efficacious in preventing mountain sickness. The most efficient and effective preacclimatization strategy has yet to be determined.

HIGH-ALTITUDE CEREBRAL EDEMA

High-altitude cerebral edema is defined as progressive neurologic deterioration in someone with AMS or high-altitude pulmonary edema. It is characterized by altered mental status, ataxia, stupor, and progression to coma if untreated. Headache, nausea, and vomiting are not always present. Because of raised intracranial pressure, focal neurologic signs, such as third and sixth cranial nerve palsies, may result. High-altitude cerebral edema at intermediate altitudes is all but nonexistent with the rare case likely precipitated by severe hypoxia associated with high-altitude pulmonary edema and/or a preexisting space-occupying cerebral lesion.

High-altitude cerebral edema is usually associated with pulmonary edema. Pathologically, necropsies have described severe, diffuse cerebral edema with multiple small hemorrhages and sometimes thrombosis.

Treatment of high-altitude cerebral edema is oxygen supplementation, descent, and steroid therapy (Tables 221-3 and 221-4). Descent is the highest priority. Acetazolamide may be used as an adjunct, but immediate reversal of the illness is the goal. Improving acclimatization comes later. In acutely ill patients who cannot descend, a combination of steroids, supplemental oxygen, and a hyperbaric bag is optimal therapy but rarely available. Persons remaining ataxic or confused after descent should be admitted to hospital. The possibility of encephalitis or meningitis, stroke, or subarachnoid hemorrhage should be considered in patients whose condition does not improve with treatment. Comatose patients require an advanced airway. Typically the partial pressure of arterial carbon dioxide is already low and the pH high, and hyperventilation could produce cerebral ischemia. Evidence is lacking for the use of hypertonic saline, loop diuretics, or mannitol in high-altitude cerebral edema. Coma may persist for days, even for weeks, after evacuation to lower altitude, yet the patient may still recover. Persistent coma is unusual, however, and mandates exclusion of other possible causes. MRI findings of high-altitude cerebral edema include reversible white matter edema evidenced by increased T2 signal, especially in the splenium of the corpus callosum (**Figure 221-1**).[4] In contrast, hemosiderin depositions in the corpus

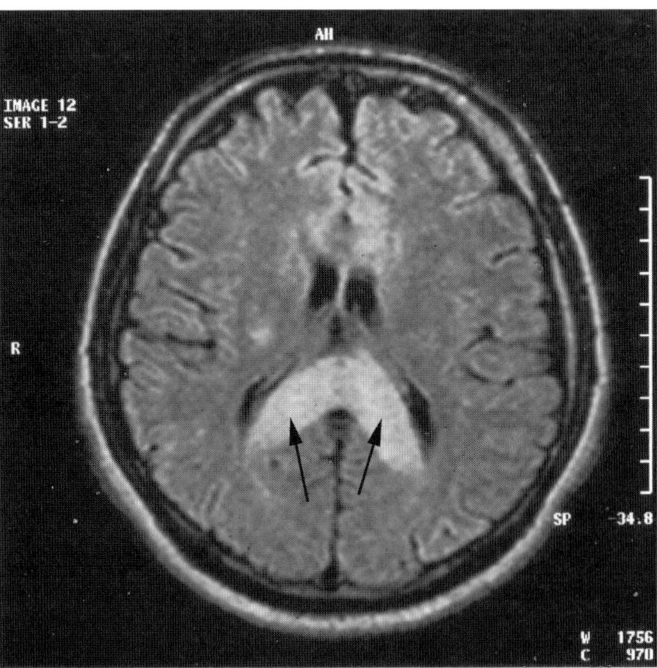

FIGURE 221-1. MRI of a 34-year-old male high-altitude mountaineer with high-altitude cerebral edema. The *arrows* indicate the markedly increased T2 signaling in the splenium of the corpus callosum indicating edema.

callosum may be detected by MRI for years after a case of high-altitude cerebral edema; this may be useful in the setting of diagnostic uncertainty.[13]

HIGH-ALTITUDE PULMONARY EDEMA

High-altitude pulmonary edema is the most lethal of the altitude illnesses. The cause of death is usually lack of early recognition, misdiagnosis, or inability to descend to a lower altitude. The condition is easily reversible with descent and oxygen administration.

The incidence of high-altitude pulmonary edema varies from less than 1 in 10,000 skiers in Colorado to 2% to 3% of climbers on Mount McKinley; an incidence of 15% was reported in some regiments of the Indian army that were airlifted to high altitude during the Indian-Chinese war. Women appear less susceptible than men. Risk factors include heavy exertion, rapid ascent, cold, excessive salt ingestion, use of a respiratory depressant, a previous history indicating inherent individual susceptibility, and pulmonary hypertension. Genetic factors include diminished lung epithelial sodium channel activity, excessive hypoxic pulmonary hypertension, and immunogenetic factors.[14,15] Pulmonary hypertension from any cause greatly predisposes to high-altitude pulmonary edema. As a result, high-altitude pulmonary edema has been reported in patients with intracardiac shunts (atrial septal defect, patent ductus arteriosus, patent foramen ovale), congenital absent pulmonary artery, drug-induced pulmonary hypertension (phentermine), and chronic venous thrombotic disease.[16,17] Preexisting respiratory infection may predispose children to high-altitude pulmonary edema.[18]

PATHOPHYSIOLOGY

High-altitude pulmonary edema is a noncardiogenic, hydrostatic edema; left ventricular function is normal. Left ventricular end-diastolic pressure, wedge pressures, and left atrial pressures are low to normal, cardiac output is low, and pulmonary vascular resistance and pulmonary artery pressure are markedly elevated. The culprit in high-altitude pulmonary edema is high microvascular pressure. Pulmonary hypertension is an essential component, but not all persons with pulmonary hypertension develop high-altitude pulmonary edema. Other factors that play a role include pulmonary venous constriction and uneven arterial vasoconstriction, which leads to overperfusion of some areas of the lung vasculature. Inflammation is not present early in the course of high-altitude pulmonary edema, as measured by the chemical composition of bronchoalveolar lavage fluid, but appears to be a secondary finding later in the illness.[19] Predisposed individuals have a low hypoxic ventilatory response and an abnormal pulmonary circulation response to hypoxia, and tend to experience high-altitude pulmonary edema on repeated exposures to high altitude.

CLINICAL FEATURES

The differential diagnosis of shortness of breath at altitude is broad. This includes pneumonia, pulmonary embolism, myocardial infarction, congestive heart failure, mucous plugging, and bronchitis. Early in the course of high-altitude pulmonary edema, the individual develops a dry cough, decreased exercise performance, dyspnea on exertion, and increased recovery time from exercise. Localized rales, usually in the right mid-lung field, are common. Resting percent Sa_{O2} is often 10 to 20 points lower than normal for a given altitude and will drop further with exertion. Late in the course of the illness, tachycardia, tachypnea, dyspnea at rest, marked weakness, productive cough, cyanosis, and more generalized rales develop. As hypoxemia worsens, altered mental status and eventually coma develop.

Early diagnosis is critical, and decreased exercise performance and dry cough are enough to raise the suspicion of early high-altitude pulmonary edema. Progression of dyspnea with exertion to dyspnea at rest is a hallmark of high-altitude pulmonary edema. The typical victim is strong and fit and may or may not have symptoms of AMS before the onset of high-altitude pulmonary edema. The condition typically worsens at night and is most commonly noticed on or after the second night at a new altitude. Rales are not audible in 15% of persons with high-altitude pulmonary edema at rest but can be elicited immediately after a short bout of exercise. Low-grade fever is common, and tachycardia and tachypnea generally correlate with the severity of illness. On cardiac auscultation, a prominent P_2 and right ventricular heave may be appreciated. ECG may reveal right-axis deviation and a right ventricular strain pattern consistent with acute pulmonary hypertension. Chest radiographic findings progress from interstitial to localized alveolar to generalized alveolar infiltrates as the illness progresses from mild to severe (**Figure 221-2**). The absence of infiltrates should alert the clinician to the possibility of an alternate diagnosis.

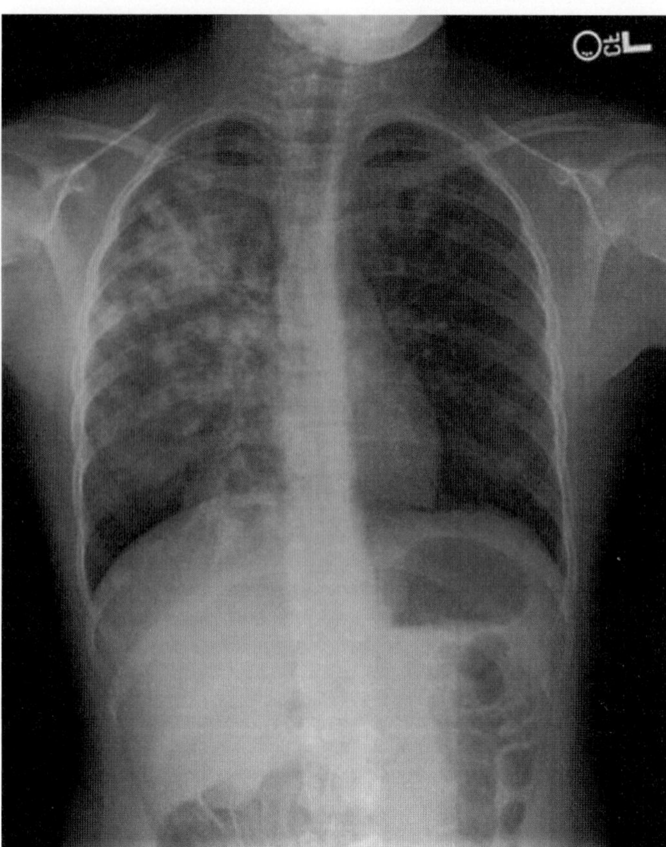

FIGURE 221-2. Chest radiograph of an 11-year-old girl with reentry high-altitude pulmonary edema at 2670 m (8750 ft).

TREATMENT AND PREVENTION

The key to successful treatment of high-altitude pulmonary edema (Tables 221-3 and 221-4) is early recognition, because the condition in its early stage is easily reversible. The optimal therapy depends on the environmental setting, evacuation options, availability of oxygen or hyperbaric units, and ease of descent. **Immediate descent is the treatment of choice, but this is not always possible.** During descent, exertion by the patient must be minimized. Reports of patients dying during descent probably are related to overexertion that offsets the benefit of lower altitude. Oxygen supplementation produces excellent results and can completely resolve the pulmonary edema without descent to a lower altitude, but it may require 36 to 72 hours to do so. In settings such as Colorado ski resorts, for example, keeping the patient at altitude but on oxygen is a practical option. The required quantities of oxygen are rarely available to trekking, mountaineering, and back country skiing groups, however. Oxygen immediately lowers pulmonary artery pressure and improves arterial oxygenation. Its use is lifesaving when descent is not an option; in such cases, rescue groups should make delivery of oxygen to the victim the highest priority.

As in the treatment of AMS and high-altitude cerebral edema, the portable hyperbaric bag is a useful adjunct to therapy when immediate descent is not possible.

Bed rest may be adequate for very mild cases, and bed rest with supplemental oxygen may suffice for moderate illness, as long as the safety of the patient can be ensured by the presence of a medical facility, adequate oxygen, or immediate descent capability should the patient's condition deteriorate.[20] Because cold stress elevates pulmonary artery pressure, the patient should be kept warm. The use of an expiratory positive airway pressure mask increases Sa_{O2} by 10% to 20% in high-altitude pulmonary edema patients by enhancing alveolar recruitment. The mask is lightweight, is well tolerated, and may be a useful adjunct to descent. Continuous positive airway pressure or bilevel positive airway pressure ventilation would likely work as well.

Because oxygen supplementation and descent are so effective, experience with drugs has been limited. Several studies have demonstrated that nifedipine, either as a 10-milligram capsule or 30-milligram extended-release formulation, reduces pulmonary artery pressure by 30% to 50% but increases Sa_{O2} only slightly.[21] Nifedipine, 20 milligrams (slow-release preparation) every 8 hours while ascending, provides effective prophylaxis in those who have previously experienced high-altitude pulmonary edema.[22] Nitric oxide lowers pulmonary artery pressure and redistributes blood away from edematous areas but is rarely available.[23]

The phosphodiesterase-5 inhibitors sildenafil and tadalafil blunt hypoxic pulmonary vasoconstriction.[24] Tadalafil, 10 milligrams PO twice a day 24 hours prior to ascent, effectively prevents high-altitude pulmonary edema in susceptible individuals.[25] These agents may also prove to be useful for treatment of high-altitude pulmonary edema when oxygen is unavailable.

Inhaled salmeterol twice a day reduces the incidence of high-altitude pulmonary edema by 50% in persons with previous repeat episodes of high-altitude pulmonary edema.[26] The mechanism is presumed to be upregulation of the epithelial sodium channel and increased clearance of alveolar fluid, a known effect of β-agonists. Although these agents have not yet been studied for the treatment of high-altitude pulmonary edema, given their likely benefit and safety and ease of use, treatment of high-altitude pulmonary edema with β-agonists is reasonable. **None of these agents is as effective as oxygen administration or descent, which still remain the treatments of choice.**

Hospitalization is warranted for severe illness that does not respond immediately to descent, especially if cerebral edema is present. Intubation, oxygen supplementation with a high fraction of inspired oxygen (FIO_2), and positive end-expiratory pressure ventilation are rarely required. Antibiotics are indicated for coexisting infection when present. Measurement of brain natriuretic peptide level or echocardiography may be needed to exclude a cardiac component of edema in persons with potential heart failure. Patients with high-altitude pulmonary edema who do not make the usual rapid improvement or who develop the condition at <2500 m (<8200 ft) should be evaluated for pulmonary emboli or other anatomic abnormalities, such as congenital absence of a pulmonary artery or intracardiac shunt. Echocardiography with bubble contrast material can assess for the presence or absence of shunting from a patent foramen ovale or other cardiac abnormality.

Adequate discharge criteria are progressive clinical and radiographic improvement and a Pa_{O2} of 60 mm Hg or an Sa_{O2} of >90%. Residual effects such as fibrosis or abnormal pulmonary function tests have not been reported. An episode of high-altitude pulmonary edema is not a contraindication to subsequent ascent, but patients should be counseled regarding the advisability of staged ascent; prophylaxis with acetazolamide along with tadalafil, sildenafil, or nifedipine; and the importance of recognizing early signs and symptoms.

PERIPHERAL EDEMA

Swelling of the face and distal extremities is common at high altitude. Peripheral edema was reported in 18% of trekkers at 4200 m (13,800 ft) in Nepal and was twice as common in women.[7] It often was associated with AMS but not in all cases. The presence of peripheral edema should raise suspicion of altitude illness and prompt a thorough examination for pulmonary and cerebral edema. The problem can be treated with diuretics but will resolve spontaneously with descent. The mechanism is presumably similar to that of fluid retention altitude illness but with edema formation peripherally rather than in the brain and lung.

HIGH-ALTITUDE RETINOPATHY

Retinal abnormalities described at high altitude include retinal edema, tortuosity and dilatation of retinal veins, disc hyperemia, retinal hemorrhage, and, rarely, cotton-wool exudates. Retinal hemorrhages are asymptomatic, except for rarely occurring macular hemorrhages, and are not considered an indication for descent unless vision changes are present. They resolve spontaneously in 10 to 14 days. Hemorrhages are common at sleeping altitudes of >5000 m (>16,400 ft) and occur at lower altitudes in persons with altitude illness.

HIGH-ALTITUDE BRONCHITIS

Many unacclimatized persons exercising at altitudes of >2500 m (>8200 ft) develop a dry, hacking cough. Breathing high volumes of dry, cold air may induce respiratory heat loss, secretions, and bronchospasm. As in cough-variant asthma, fast-acting β-agonists, such as albuterol, delivered by metered-dose inhaler may provide relief from these coughing spasms. Prophylactic use of long-acting β-agonists and inhaled steroids may be useful for prevention of debilitating cough for those staying at altitude for long periods. Those staying at ski resorts or indoors at altitude may find humidifiers helpful. Wearing a silk balaclava or a scarf of similar material across the nose and mouth that is sufficiently porous to allow large-volume ventilation but that traps some moisture and heat may help ameliorate this bothersome high-altitude condition.

CHRONIC MOUNTAIN POLYCYTHEMIA/CHRONIC MOUNTAIN SICKNESS

Monge's disease, also called *chronic mountain sickness*, has been recognized in all high-altitude locations of the world. Both long-term high-altitude residents and lowlanders who relocate to high altitude may develop this condition after variable lengths of residence. Males have a much higher incidence, and incidence increases with age. The disease is characterized by excessive polycythemia for a given altitude, which causes symptoms such as headache, muddled thinking, difficulty sleeping, impaired peripheral circulation, drowsiness, and chest congestion. The diagnosis is based on presence of the characteristic symptoms and a hemoglobin value greater than expected for the altitude, generally over 20 to 22 grams/dL. Any problem causing hypoxemia at sea level causes greater hypoxemia at altitude, and the cause of chronic mountain polycythemia can be traced to problems such as chronic obstructive pulmonary disease and sleep apnea in 50% of patients. "Pure" chronic mountain polycythemia is attributed to idiopathic hypoventilation based on diminished ventilatory drive.

Therapy includes phlebotomy, relocation to a lower altitude, or home oxygen use. Respiratory stimulants such as acetazolamide (250 milligrams PO twice a day) and medroxyprogesterone acetate (20 to 60 milligrams PO per day) also have been used successfully. The response to respiratory stimulants supports the role of hypoventilation in this disorder.

ULTRAVIOLET KERATITIS (SNOW BLINDNESS)

Ultraviolet A and ultraviolet B light penetrate the atmosphere to a greater degree at high altitude because there is less cloud cover, less water vapor, and less particulate matter in the air. Radiation increases roughly 5% for every 300 m (980 ft) gained and is exacerbated by reflection back from snow. The cornea absorbs ultraviolet radiation of <300 nm (ultraviolet B), and high levels can cause corneal burns in 1 hour. Symptoms may not become apparent for 6 to 12 hours. Severe pain, a foreign-body or gritty sensation, photophobia, tearing, marked conjunctival erythema, chemosis, and eyelid swelling comprise the main symptoms of photokeratitis. Ultraviolet keratitis generally is self-limited and heals within 24 hours, but the condition is sufficiently painful to warrant administration of systemic analgesics. Application of cold compresses also may provide some relief. Prevention cannot be overemphasized, because this condition can be disabling, especially in hazardous terrain. Sunglasses should transmit <10% of ultraviolet B light. Side shields are necessary if one is traveling on snow, and polarizing lenses help by absorbing glare. Makeshift protection can be fashioned by cutting narrow horizontal slits in cardboard, foam, or any available material ("Eskimo sunglasses").

SPECIAL POPULATIONS

INDIVIDUALS WITH ILLNESSES AGGRAVATED BY HIGH ALTITUDE

Chronic Lung Disease Patients with chronic obstructive pulmonary disease ascending to altitude often report increased dyspnea and reduced exercise performance. Patients with hypoxemia, pulmonary hypertension, disordered control of ventilation, and sleep-disordered breathing at sea level may require supplemental oxygen at altitude because of greater alveolar hypoxia. Patients who are oxygen dependent at sea level will need to increase their F_{IO_2}. The required F_{IO_2} can be calculated by multiplying low-altitude F_{IO_2} by the ratio of low-altitude barometric pressure to high-altitude barometric pressure. This will ensure the delivery of the same P_{O2} as at low altitude. Although no data exist to suggest that persons with chronic obstructive pulmonary disease are more likely to develop AMS or high-altitude pulmonary edema, these patients may simply avoid travel to high altitude. In fact, persons with mild to moderate chronic obstructive pulmonary disease already are partially acclimatized and may do well at modest altitude. High altitude per se does not exacerbate asthma, and persons with chronic bronchospasm often report easier breathing at high altitude due to lower air density and/or cleaner air. Patients with allergic asthma do better at high altitude because of reduced allergens.

Arteriosclerotic Heart Disease A healthy heart and cardiovascular system can tolerate even extreme hypoxia remarkably well. Examinations of numerous ECGs, echocardiograms, heart catheterization findings, and exercise test results demonstrate no cardiac ischemia or cardiac dysfunction in healthy persons at high altitude, even when Pa_{O2} is <30 mm Hg. Those with arteriosclerotic disease may not have the same adaptive capabilities and intuitively seem more likely to experience acute cardiac events. Epidemiologic data, however, do not support this supposition. Long-term residence at high altitude reduces morbidity and mortality from arteriosclerotic heart disease,[27] and visitors apparently do not have increased risk of acute myocardial infarction. Ischemia may be provoked with less exercise during the first few days at 2500 m (8200 ft) among persons with coronary artery disease; however, after 5 days of acclimatization, patients perform at their sea-level exercise capacity without increased or early-onset angina.[28] A cohort of individuals who underwent revascularization for acute coronary syndrome 6 months previously were able to perform symptom-limited exercise testing after rapid ascent to 3,454 m without ECG evidence of myocardial ischemia or significant arrhythmia.[29]

Congestive heart failure may worsen in tourists arriving at the moderate altitude of ski resorts; this is related to fluid retention rather than depressed ventricular function from hypoxia. Therefore, patients with congestive heart failure should maintain or increase their diuretic dosage during travel to high altitude, and clinicians may consider administering low-flow oxygen during sleep to patients with congestive heart failure, at least for the first few nights after arrival at altitude. Individuals who have undergone coronary artery bypass grafting have trekked to altitudes of >5000 m (>16,400 ft) without problems.

Ascent to altitude produces a mild increase in blood pressure in normotensive and hypertensive persons secondary to increased sympathetic tone. However, the magnitude of blood pressure response varies significantly and is quite unpredictable. Patients should continue hypertensive medications at altitude, and blood pressure monitoring might be prudent. Occasionally, hypertensive medication dosages may need to be temporarily adjusted. No data suggest that hypertensive patients have a higher risk for any of the altitude illnesses, and in general, hypertension is not a contraindication to altitude exposure.

Neurologic Syndromes of High Altitude Until recently, most neurologic events at high altitude were attributed to high-altitude cerebral edema or AMS. Clearly, this has been a diagnostic oversimplification. Other syndromes now recognized as related to high altitude include altitude syncope, cerebrovascular spasm (migraine equivalent), cerebral arterial or venous thrombosis (infarct), transient ischemic attack, and cerebral hemorrhage. These syndromes are characterized by more focal neurologic findings than in cerebral edema, although differentiation in the field may be difficult. Other symptoms may be due to exacerbation or unmasking of underlying disease. Cortical blindness and various focal neurologic signs, such as transient hemiparesis or hemiplegia, also occur. **Focal neurologic signs should be thoroughly evaluated and not attributed to altitude illness.**

Other symptoms may be due to exacerbation or unmasking of underlying disease, such as previously asymptomatic brain tumors and epilepsy. Presumably, space-occupying lesions become symptomatic because of increased brain volume at altitude. Hyperventilation (hypocapnic alkalosis), which is commonly used to induce seizure activity on electroencephalography, may explain unmasking of seizure disorder at altitude, whereas changes in cerebral blood flow may exacerbate preexisting vascular lesions such as aneurysm or arteriovenous malformation, leading to spontaneous intracerebral hemorrhage.

In the field, it is reasonable to treat neurologic events as if cerebral edema were present, with rapid descent to lower altitude, oxygen supplementation, administration of steroids, and evacuation to hospital if symptoms persist. It is prudent to avoid use of agents that may contribute to hypotension and decrease cerebral perfusion.

Sickle Cell Disease Even the modest cabin altitude of pressurized aircraft (1500 to 2000 m [5000 to 6600 ft]) may cause persons with hemoglobin SC and sickle cell–thalassemia disease to experience vaso-occlusive crisis. Exposure to high altitude thus requires oxygen supplementation for such individuals. Although sickle cell trait is not considered a risk factor for increased altitude-related problems, splenic infarction syndrome during heavy exercise at altitude has been reported in individuals with the trait. Left upper quadrant pain should alert the physician at high altitude to consider splenic infarction syndrome.

Pregnant Women Pregnant women who live at high altitude have an increased prevalence of hypertension, delivery of low-birth-weight infants, and neonatal hyperbilirubinemia in their offspring. However, an increased incidence of pregnancy complications in lowlanders who visit high altitude has not been reported. The normal Pa_{O2} of the fetus is 29 to 33 mm Hg, and the mild maternal hypoxia induced by traveling to resort-type altitudes does not generate significantly more hypoxic stress. Few data exist regarding exercise in pregnant women at altitudes of >2500 m (>8200 ft), so a conservative approach should be used.[30] Pregnant women should avoid altitudes at which Sa_{O2} falls to <85%, such as a sleeping altitude of 3000 m (10,000 ft) or higher.[30] Perhaps of more concern than mild hypoxia is the fact that high-altitude locations are often remote from medical facilities. Patients need to be aware that without access to sophisticated medical care, complications may be associated with more serious consequences. Patients with high-risk pregnancies should be managed at low altitude.

REFERENCES

The complete reference list is available online at www.TintinalliEM.com.

CHAPTER 222

Carbon Monoxide

Gerald Maloney

INTRODUCTION

Carbon monoxide is one of the most common toxic exposures that emergency physicians will encounter. It is the most common cause of fatal poisoning, via either intentional (suicidal) or accidental exposure in the United States, and may be the most common worldwide cause of fatal poisoning.[1] Despite much clinical experience and several randomized trials, there is a great deal of controversy about the ideal approach for management.

EPIDEMIOLOGY

Exact statistics for carbon monoxide poisoning are difficult to determine, mainly due to incomplete reporting. Data from the American Association of Poison Control Centers Toxic Exposure Surveillance System in 2012[2] reported 13,038 exposures, with 54 deaths. However, this information is limited, as many exposures and some deaths are not reported to the local poison control center. It is also unclear how often patients with mild carbon monoxide poisoning are misdiagnosed and thus are not included in the database. Data from the Centers for Disease Control and Prevention paint a much broader picture of exposures than the Toxic Exposure Surveillance System database. The most recent large epidemiologic report from the Centers for Disease Control and Prevention on the subject, which reviewed data on non–fire-related carbon monoxide exposures, revealed 5149 deaths, for an average of 430 deaths per year.[3] Interestingly, the incidence of carbon monoxide exposure has not decreased despite more widespread use of carbon monoxide detectors.[3]

In the past, vehicular emissions were the major source of carbon monoxide poisoning in adults. Currently, nonvehicular sources have become more common as use of catalytic converters has reduced carbon monoxide in vehicular exhaust emissions[4] (**Table 222-1**)

Peak incidence occurs in the fall and winter months, generally due to increased use of space heaters, wood-burning stoves, charcoal burning for heat, or portable generators without adequate ventilation.[3] Additional sources of carbon monoxide exposure include air conditioners, portable generators in camping tents, exhaust on motorboats, and Zamboni machines used in ice rinks.[5-7] Exposures have been reported in persons riding in the back of pickup trucks, as well as in vehicles with an exhaust pipe occluded by snow.

It is believed that carbon monoxide poisoning is probably the most pressing danger from smoke inhalation and is a major contributor to fire-related deaths. Although carbon monoxide poisoning most commonly affects adults in the third to fifth decades, it may be seen across age groups, and it is not uncommon for entire families to be affected.

Another source for carbon monoxide poisoning is methylene chloride, which is found in varnishes and paint strippers, and in Christmas ornaments as a bubbling fluid. Routes of exposure are inhalation or ingestion, and the methylene chloride is metabolized in the liver to carbon monoxide. As a result of ongoing production, persistent elevation of carboxyhemoglobin occurs despite oxygen therapy.[8] Time to peak carbon monoxide levels may be 8 hours or longer.

TABLE 222-1 Sources of Carbon Monoxide

Automotive exhaust
Motorboat exhaust
Propane-fueled heaters
Wood- or coal-burning stoves or heaters
Structure fires
Gasoline-powered generators or motors
Natural gas–powered heaters/furnaces/generators
Methylene chloride
Forklifts

PATHOPHYSIOLOGY

Carbon monoxide is typically described as a colorless, odorless gas. It is normally present in air at 10 ppm or less, perhaps higher in urban areas. There are multiple industries in which there may be occupational exposure to carbon monoxide. The Occupational Safety and Health Administration set a permissible exposure level of carbon monoxide of 50 ppm averaged over an 8-hour shift (https://www.osha.gov/pls/oshaweb/owadisp.show_document?p_table=STANDARDS&p_id=10366). Toxicity generally begins at levels of 100 ppm.

Carbon monoxide is also an endogenous substance, with production occurring in the body during the normal breakdown of heme. Normal physiologic carbon monoxide levels from this process are ~1% in healthy nonsmokers. This physiologic production can be increased in hemolysis or sepsis. Baseline levels in smokers of up to 10% have been reported.

The most easily quantified physiologic effect seen after carbon monoxide exposure is its binding to hemoglobin. The binding affinity of normal adult hemoglobin for carbon monoxide is approximately 200 times that of oxygen. Binding is higher for fetal hemoglobin, which may account for potentially more severe fetal toxicity.[9] Approximately 85% of carbon monoxide is bound to hemoglobin; the remaining carbon monoxide is dissolved in plasma or bound intracellularly, often to myoglobin. Carbon monoxide binds to hemoglobin to form carboxyhemoglobin. There are mathematical models for predicting the half-life of carboxyhemoglobin; these have been evaluated in both volunteer human models and actual carbon monoxide–poisoned patients. Quoted half-lives of carboxyhemoglobin on room air at normal atmospheric pressure range from 249 to 320 minutes.[7] On 100% oxygen at atmospheric pressure, this is reduced to an average of 74 to 80 minutes.[10] The exception to this is carboxyhemoglobin generated by methylene chloride exposure, which can have a half-life of up to 13 hours due to ongoing metabolic production.[8]

Carboxyhemoglobin does not participate in oxygen delivery to the cells, and as carboxyhemoglobin levels increase, relative anemia and hypoxia occur. Further, carbon monoxide shifts the oxyhemoglobin dissociation curve to the left, impairing oxygen release to the tissues. However, these features alone do not fully explain the physiologic effects of carbon monoxide or its delayed neurologic sequelae. Patients with corresponding levels of hypoxia, or anemia, who are not carbon monoxide poisoned, do not have similar short- and long-term effects seen with carbon monoxide poisoning. This indicates that there is a separate toxicity to carbon monoxide irrespective of the level of carboxyhemoglobin. Carboxyhemoglobin appears to be more a marker for the degree of poisoning than the primary cause of injury itself. The best experimental evidence of this involved dogs that were given carbon monoxide by inhalation to produce carboxyhemoglobin levels of 80%.[11] Exchange transfusion of this blood into healthy dogs produced no symptoms, suggesting that something other than simply the carboxyhemoglobin level is at play in explaining the full range of toxic effects.

As carboxyhemoglobin level rises, there is an increase in body burden of carbon monoxide. Ten to 15% of the carbon monoxide is dissolved unbound into plasma, a large proportion of which ultimately moves into the intracellular compartment. Like hemoglobin, myoglobin has a greater affinity for carbon monoxide than it does for oxygen, and myoglobin will bind to carbon monoxide with approximately 60 times the affinity of oxygen. Carbon monoxide inhibits intracellular cytochrome oxidase, interfering with cellular respiration and adenosine triphosphate generation. This results in a relative uncoupling of oxidative phosphorylation and the generation of elevated lactate levels, resulting in a lactic acidosis. Carbon monoxide also causes endothelial dysfunction and vasodilatation through the release of guanylate cyclase and nitric oxide. Carbon monoxide–induced nitric oxide release may in fact be one of the key factors in the cytotoxic effects of carbon monoxide poisoning. The release of guanylate cyclase and nitric oxide can contribute to hypotension. The combination of relative hypoxia and hypotension can cause ischemia-reperfusion injury in cardiac myocytes, as well as neuronal tissue. The damaged endothelium attracts neutrophils and triggers an inflammatory cascade, resulting in lipid peroxidation and ultimately neuronal cell death. This complex intracellular process explains many of the clinical effects of carbon monoxide.[7] Rhabdomyolysis, acute myocardial infarction, and neuronal cell death are a result of this cellular toxicity. Cells in the basal ganglia are particularly sensitive to this neurotoxic effect, demonstrated by the globus pallidus lesions sometimes seen on cranial CT imaging.

CLINICAL FEATURES

The clinical presentation of carbon monoxide poisoning is protean, which likely leads to misdiagnosis in many cases (**Table 222-2**). An unconscious patient pulled from a house fire or from a running car in a closed garage does not present a diagnostic dilemma; the patient with "flu-like" symptoms or the elderly person presenting with syncope and ischemic changes on their ECG may be more difficult to diagnose. Given the lack of any predictable clinical toxidrome for carbon monoxide poisoning, a strong clinical suspicion remains the best initial method of detection.

History may be strongly suggestive, such as use of a propane heater in an apartment associated with a headache at home but relieved with exit from the home. Symptoms such as a new-onset seizure, syncope, myocardial infarction, or cardiac arrest may not be helpful. Sometimes, concurrent symptoms in other members of the household, or even pets, can be a clue. However, even within a household, different persons may manifest different symptoms, depending on age, comorbid disease, and proximity to the source of carbon monoxide. Occupational history may help, particularly in cases due to less common causes such as methylene chloride exposure. Exposure to any gas- or propane-powered motors, especially if working inside enclosed facilities, or fumes from methylene chloride, which is used as a varnish or paint stripper, may serve as a clue in patients with nonspecific symptoms. **Carbon monoxide poisoning should be in the differential diagnosis for comatose patients, patients with mental status changes, and those with an unexplained elevated anion gap metabolic acidosis or lactic acidosis.**

Physical exam findings are diverse. The classically touted finding of cherry red oral mucosa is rarely seen in living patients. Vital signs may demonstrate mild fever, tachycardia, tachypnea, hypertension, or hypotension. Severe poisoning may present with respiratory or cardiac arrest. Neurologic findings, which are generally thought of as being one of the hallmark signs for this poisoning, are also variable, ranging from mild headache and confusion to irritability, seizures, focal neurologic deficits, and coma. Retinal hemorrhages have been reported with severe poisoning. Skin findings include bullous lesions, generally seen in patients with prolonged immobility from pressure necrosis, although a direct toxic effect of carbon monoxide on epidermal tissue is also possible. Carbon monoxide poisoning may be obscured by other findings, such as trauma or severe burns. A comatose patient removed from a fire scene should be assumed to have carbon monoxide poisoning until proven otherwise, even in the absence of cutaneous or airway burns.

Although most discussions of carbon monoxide poisoning focus on acute exposure, chronic carbon monoxide poisoning, generally from occupational sources, must also be considered. Symptoms are usually more insidious, such as trouble concentrating, personality changes, or memory loss, and can be difficult to diagnose. Patients with chronic carbon monoxide poisoning are at risk of carbon monoxide–related neurotoxicity and may have long-term neuropsychiatric issues.

TABLE 222-2 Signs and Symptoms of Acute Carbon Monoxide Poisoning

Headache	Visual disturbances
Vomiting	Confusion
Ataxia	Dyspnea/tachypnea
Seizure	ECG changes/dysrhythmias
Syncope	Retinal hemorrhage
Chest pain	Bullous skin lesions
Focal neurologic deficit	

DIAGNOSIS

The diagnosis is best made by measuring carboxyhemoglobin levels. Although carboxyhemoglobin in and of itself may not be the most significant factor in carbon monoxide–mediated injury, obtaining free plasma carbon monoxide is rarely feasible. Thus, carboxyhemoglobin serves as a marker of severity of exposure and can help to stratify patients at risk for delayed sequelae. **Co-oximetry, which measures total hemoglobin as well as oxyhemoglobin, methemoglobin, and carboxyhemoglobin saturation, is the only accurate measurement tool.** Routine arterial blood gas analyzers without co-oximetry calculate, rather than measure, saturation, and will not differentiate the contribution of dyshemoglobinemias to total saturation. As a result, the oxygen saturation may appear artificially high. There is excellent correlation between arterial and venous carboxyhemoglobin levels, and thus, a venous blood gas with co-oximetry is sufficient in most cases.[12]

Interpreting carboxyhemoglobin levels can be challenging and needs to take into consideration time and duration of exposure, time from exposure to presentation, treatment (such as high-flow oxygen) rendered en route, and clinical symptoms. Although a markedly elevated level, such as 50%, is a clear indicator of severe intoxication, a level of 10% in a patient who experienced serious symptoms a few hours earlier presents a dilemma in terms of diagnosis and appropriate disposition. Symptomatology and carboxyhemoglobin levels do not always correlate well: levels as high as 47% have been reported in minimally symptomatic patients, whereas levels as low as 10% have been reported in comatose patients in whom the diagnosis of carbon monoxide poisoning was ultimately confirmed.[13]

Standard pulse oximetry is unreliable in the diagnosis of carbon monoxide poisoning. The wavelengths for carboxyhemoglobin fall into the same range of those for oxyhemoglobin, and standard pulse oximetry does not differentiate the two. As a result, the oxyhemoglobin saturation by pulse oximetry reading will appear artificially high[14] (**Figure 222-1**). The **pulse oximetry gap** is a measure of this discordance. When the pulse oximetry values are compared to the oxygen saturation on an arterial blood gas, the oxygen saturation on the pulse oximeter will be higher than the saturation on the arterial blood gas.

Data on currently available pulse co-oximeters are mixed. Until a large, randomized, and well-designed study looking at the accuracy of these devices in an ED setting can be performed, it is not recommended to rely solely on pulse co-oximeters to exclude carbon monoxide poisoning.[15-17]

Other laboratory and diagnostic testing can be also be informative. Elevated lactate from the interference in the electron transport chain, an unexplained elevated anion gap metabolic acidosis, elevated creatine phosphokinase, or elevated troponin may trigger an investigation for

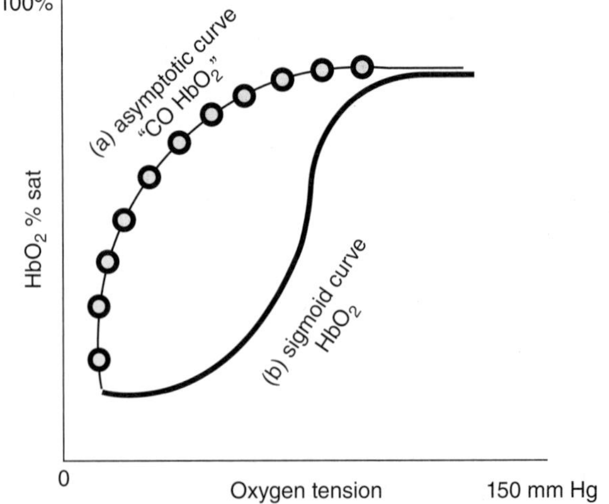

FIGURE 222-1. Carboxyhemoglobin "shift to the left" reshaping of the oxyhemoglobin (HbO_2) dissociation curve. (**A**) Carbon monoxide (CO)–affected HbO_2 dissociation curve (asymptotic) and (**B**) normal HbO_2 dissociation curve (sigmoid).

carbon monoxide poisoning. Concomitant cyanide poisoning may be seen in patients rescued from structure fires. Neuron-specific enolase or S100B,[18] CNS proteins that are released in greater quantities into the plasma when neuronal injury has occurred, and cerebrospinal fluid myelin basic protein are markers for carbon monoxide neurotoxicity. However, these tests may be more useful in determining prognosis than diagnosis and are rarely available for use in ED clinical decision making.

Electrocardiographic findings may range from entirely normal to acute injury patterns, such as ST elevation myocardial infarction. There does not appear to be any classic carbon Monoxide ECG pattern. Few patients with acute myocardial infarction due to carbon monoxide poisoning have occlusive lesions identified at cardiac catheterization.[19]

Radiographic imaging is generally of limited utility and is usually more helpful in establishing an alternative diagnosis. There is, however, one radiographic finding that has been specifically associated with carbon monoxide poisoning, and that is lesions in the globus pallidus. Lesions are generally bilateral and symmetric and are usually noted in severely poisoned patients.[7]

TREATMENT

Initial resuscitation of the carbon monoxide–poisoned patient does not differ from initial resuscitation of any other critically ill patient. **If carbon monoxide poisoning is strongly suspected based on history, immediately provide supplemental oxygen in the highest concentrations available.**

Conditions for the application of hyperbaric oxygen treatment have not been clearly identified. Despite years of experience using hyperbaric oxygen and several clinical trials, identifying individuals who can benefit from HBO is challenging. The most recent comprehensive review on the subject is a Cochrane review from 2011.[20] Six clinical trials were reviewed. Two of the six demonstrated a benefit in terms of decreased neurologic sequelae; the remaining four trials failed to demonstrate a benefit. All studies had various methodologic flaws. The only trials to include sham dives (diving but at room air instead of high-concentration oxygen) were the two positive trials (Weaver and Scheinkestel). These two positive trials were stopped early due to reported clear benefit; however, they did not test multiple hypotheses and had significant heterogeneity in their treatment protocols. The four negative trials were smaller, methodologically heterogeneous, and suffered from problems with long-term follow-up. Given the lack of conclusive evidence-based data, the best guidance comes from consensus recommendations from multiple professional groups (**Table 222-3**). Recommendations consider multiple factors such as carboxyhemoglobin level, comorbid conditions (including pregnancy), stability of the patient, and location of the nearest center with emergency hyperbaric capabilities.

The rationale behind hyperbaric oxygen therapy stems from early studies demonstrating its effectiveness in decreasing carboxyhemoglobin levels. Initial studies on both volunteers and poisoned patients in the 1940s demonstrated that use of hyperbaric oxygen at 2.5 atmospheres of pressure lowered the effective half-life of carboxyhemoglobin to an average of 24 minutes due to a competitive displacement of carbon monoxide from its binding sites by the increased concentration of oxygen.[10] The clinical logic that led to recommendations for routine use centered on the premise that rapid reduction in carboxyhemoglobin levels meant that carbon monoxide was being cleared from the system and that toxicity could be reversed. Neurotoxicity is the endpoint most commonly studied; however, not all studies use the same assessment tools or follow-up periods. Scheinkestel et al[21] were unable to demonstrate any conclusive prevention of delayed neurologic sequelae with use of hyperbaric oxygen, whereas Weaver et al[22] saw a significant reduction in neurologic sequelae (cerebellar dysfunction and cognitive sequelae).

The consensus recommendations for consideration of hyperbaric oxygen therapy are listed in Table 222-3. The decision to initiate hyperbaric oxygen needs to occur in conjunction with a specialist in hyperbaric medicine. The Undersea and Hyperbaric Medicine Society maintains a list of chambers at the following Web site: www.hyperbariclink.com. For complete discussion of hyperbaric oxygen, see the chapter 21, "Hyperbaric Oxygen Therapy."

TABLE 222-3 Commonly Used Indications for Referral for Hyperbaric Oxygen Treatment

Pregnancy with carboxyhemoglobin level >15%
Carboxyhemoglobin >25%
Syncope
Evidence of acute myocardial ischemia
Confusion/altered mental status
Seizure
Coma
Focal neurologic deficit

DISPOSITION

Three distinct categories of carbon monoxide–poisoned patients exist: (1) those with minimal intoxication, with mild or no symptoms throughout their clinical course; (2) those with symptoms attributable to carbon monoxide poisoning but without any high-risk features that suggest a need for hyperbaric oxygen referral; and (3) those with signs of serious toxicity for whom consultation with a specialist in hyperbaric medicine should be considered.

Those with minimal intoxication, who are asymptomatic initially or after a period of brief observation, may be sent home if the exposure is not a suicide attempt and discharge is to a safe environment. If there is a suspected source of carbon monoxide poisoning, contact other potentially exposed persons for ED evaluation, and notify the fire department to measure ambient levels of carbon monoxide at the source site. Once the safety of the discharge destination is established, the patient may be discharged.

Those with more serious symptoms, such as headache or vomiting, or those with an elevated carboxyhemoglobin level but no high-risk features (Table 222-3) should be treated with supplemental oxygen, have pertinent labs checked, and be observed for several hours. After 4 hours of observation, patients may be discharged home if symptoms have resolved, assessment is otherwise benign, and discharge is to a safe environment.

Patients who require referral for possible hyperbaric oxygen therapy need consultation with a hyperbaric specialist and stabilization as best as possible prior to transfer. Critically ill or unstable patients should continue to receive high-concentration normobaric oxygen and should be reassessed prior to transfer.

SPECIAL POPULATIONS

Children may be more susceptible to the effects of carbon monoxide due to a higher percentage of fetal hemoglobin as well as higher metabolic rates.[7] The indications for referral of pediatric patients for HBO therapy are similar to those for adults. HBO has been used in children with a good safety profile.

Pregnant women should be referred to a hyperbaric center at carbon monoxide levels of 15% to 20% because fetal morbidity has been demonstrated at lower levels than usual due to the high affinity of carbon monoxide for fetal hemoglobin.[7]

The elderly, particularly those with serious comorbid disease, are also at higher risk from carbon monoxide poisoning. In patients with known coronary artery disease, even low levels of carboxyhemoglobin (4% to 6%) can cause ECG changes and myocardial ischemia.[7] Some of the elderly may also be at risk due to use of alternate heating sources, particularly during the winter.

PREVENTION

Preventive measures center on education. Educate the public about the dangers of using wood- or coal-burning appliances to heat their homes during the winter and about using adequate ventilation, and review warning signs and symptoms of carbon monoxide exposure. A relatively inexpensive preventative measure is the use of carbon monoxide detectors in the home; some municipalities have even given these away through the fire department. Local fire departments are generally willing to screen for elevated carbon monoxide levels in homes. Many educational resources are available on the Internet (http://www.cdc.gov/co/guidelines.htm; http://www.carbonmonoxidekills.com; http://www.usfa.dhs.gov/citizens/all_citizens/co/index.shtm).

REFERENCES

The complete reference list is available online at www.TintinalliEM.com.

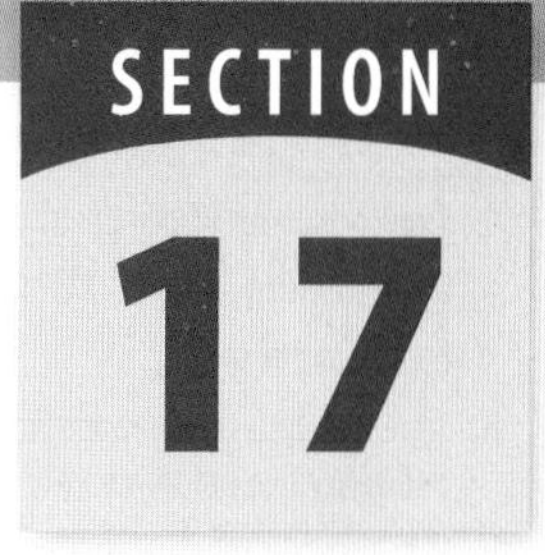

Endocrine Disorders

CHAPTER 223

Type 1 Diabetes Mellitus

Nikhil Goyal
Adam B. Schlichting

INTRODUCTION AND EPIDEMIOLOGY

During 2002–2005, 15,600 people under 20 years of age were newly diagnosed with type 1 diabetes annually in the United States.[1] Classification of diabetes (American Diabetes Association) is shown in **Table 223-1**.[2,3]

PATHOPHYSIOLOGY

Type 1 diabetes is characterized by almost no circulating insulin and the failure of β-cells to respond to insulinogenic stimuli. This accounts for only 5% to 10% of all cases of diabetes and is mostly diagnosed in children and young adults, with peaks before school age and at puberty. Immune-mediated destruction of β-cells causes 90% of these cases, and the remainder have no known cause. Spontaneous ketoacidosis almost always develops in untreated cases, and insulin is required for survival. It is often not possible to clearly classify patients as type 1 or type 2 in the ED.[3]

Chapter 224, Type 2 Diabetes Mellitus, discusses type 2 diabetes mellitus in detail. Hyperglycemia is present in all types of diabetes mellitus and is the main factor responsible for complications. Therefore, maintaining euglycemic control is the cornerstone of management.

DIAGNOSIS

The American Diabetes Association criteria for diagnosis are listed in **Table 223-2**.[2,3] Any one of these can be used to make the diagnosis. Patients with a fasting plasma glucose of 100 milligrams/dL to 125 milligrams/dL (5.6-7.0 mmol/L), a hemoglobin A1C of 5.7% to 6.4%, or a 2-hour plasma glucose of 140 to 199 milligrams/dL (7.8-11.0 mmol/L) as part of an oral glucose tolerance test are classified as having *prediabetes*.[2]

Glycated hemoglobin represents the average blood glucose level over the period of red blood cell half-life. The glycated hemoglobin assay may not be accurate for diagnosis of diabetes in patients with increased red blood cell turnover such as thalassemia, anemia, chronic kidney or liver disease, pregnancy, or in patients who have had heavy bleeding or received a transfusion within the preceding 3 months.[2]

In the ED, it is common to encounter isolated elevations of blood glucose with no established relationship to a meal ("casual plasma glucose," as defined by the American Diabetes Association). Ask about symptoms of hyperglycemia and refer to a primary care physician.

TREATMENT

Type 1 diabetes is characterized by an absolute insulin deficiency, so some form of insulin is required for survival. In addition to insulin, patients with type 1 diabetes may also be treated with prandial injections of pramlintide, a synthetic form of the β-cell–produced hormone amylin, which aids in suppressing glucagon secretion.[4] Patients with type 1 diabetes may also benefit from β-cell transplantation, pancreas transplantation, or combined kidney/pancreas transplantation. Other noninsulin agents are useful in type 2 diabetes and are discussed separately in chapter 224.

INSULIN

Currently, all insulin sold in the United States is of human type and manufactured using recombinant DNA technology (bovine or porcine insulin can still be obtained via special permission from the U.S. Food and Drug Administration). Modern insulin is highly pure and stable, and vials in use can be kept up to 30 days at room temperature. All types of insulin are standardized to a concentration of 100 units/mL ("U100"). When extremely high doses of insulin are required, a concentration of 500 units/mL ("U500") of regular insulin can also be used in consultation with an endocrinologist.

Although unmodified "regular" insulin was the first type of insulin used, many new insulin analogues have now become available (**Table 223-3**, **Figure 223-1**).[5,6] There can be considerable variability in the onset and duration of action depending on the dose (e.g., regular insulin has a longer duration of action with larger doses), site of injection, degree of exercise, and presence of circulating anti-insulin antibodies. Use of insulin analogues and highly pure insulin preparations has reduced the emergence of anti-insulin antibodies.

A physiologic regime of insulin generally starts with half of the daily requirement given as basal insulin (once-daily long-acting, or twice-daily intermediate-acting insulin) and a prandial dose of rapid-acting insulin administered 5 to 30 minutes before a meal.[5] Prandial dosing is most often based on the amount of carbohydrate that is about to be consumed, for example, 1 unit of insulin for each 15 grams of carbohydrate; this is known as "carb counting." Alternatively, some patients may be on a simplified, fixed amount of insulin for each meal.

Methods of Insulin Administration Insulin can be given as intermittent dosing, IV infusion, or continuous subcutaneous infusion using an insulin pump.

Intermittent insulin doses are given with a syringe or pen. The syringe method is the least expensive, but requires care and precision to give the correct dose. Pens provide more accurate dosing.

SC injection is the most common method of insulin administration. Absorption varies due to regional circulatory differences, and frequent use of a single site may lead to fibrosis or lipodystrophy. Therefore, patients are asked to limit injections to one region of the body, but rotate sites within that region.

IV administration of regular insulin leads to almost instantaneous effect on plasma glucose and is the recommended method of administration in hyperglycemic crises—diabetic ketoacidosis and hyperglycemic hyperosmolar nonketotic state.

INSULIN PUMPS (CONTINUOUS SC INSULIN INFUSION)

The use of an insulin pump (**Figure 223-2**) (continuous SC insulin infusion) is common, with estimates as high as 40% of U.S. patients with type 1 diabetes using insulin pumps.[7] An insulin pump is a small device (about the size of a pager) that delivers fixed doses of rapid-acting insulin at a basal rate (generally, 0.5 to 1.5 units/h) by a flexible tube attached to a subcutaneous catheter. **Table 223-4** lists manufacturers of insulin pumps available in the United States. The pump is usually attached to the patient's clothing. However, one manufacturer produces an insulin pump that does not use tubing, but is directly attached to the patient with adhesive.[8] The reservoir needs to be refilled every few days, and the catheter is changed by the patient every 3 days or so.

The basal rate of insulin can be varied throughout the day, for example, increased to counteract an early morning cortisol surge or decreased before exercising. The continuous basal insulin delivery

TABLE 223-1 Etiologic Classification of Diabetes Mellitus

I. Type 1 diabetes (β-cell destruction, usually leading to absolute insulin deficiency)
   a. Immune mediated
   b. Idiopathic
II. Type 2 diabetes (may range from predominantly insulin resistance with relative insulin deficiency to a predominantly secretory defect with insulin resistance)
III. Other specific types, such as
   a. Genetic defects of β-cell function
   b. Genetic defects in insulin action
   c. Diseases of the exocrine pancreas (pancreatitis, trauma, cystic fibrosis, etc.)
   d. Endocrinopathies (Cushing's syndrome, pheochromocytoma, hyperthyroidism, somatostatinoma, glucagonoma, etc.)
   e. Drug- or chemical-induced (interferon-α, β-adrenergic agonists, diazoxide, phenytoin [Dilantin®], glucocorticoids, nicotinic acid, pentamidine, thiazides, thyroid hormone, pyrinuron [Vacor®], etc.)
   f. Infections (congenital rubella, cytomegalovirus, etc.)
   g. Uncommon forms of immune-mediated diabetes
   h. Other genetic syndromes sometimes associated with diabetes (Down's syndrome, Klinefelter's syndrome, Turner's syndrome, etc.)
IV. Gestational diabetes mellitus

eliminates the need for long-acting insulin injection such that the pump delivers all insulin required by the patient in the form of rapid-acting insulin. Rarely, patients requiring exceptionally high doses of insulin using an insulin pump, patients who wish to be disconnected from their pump for extended periods of time, or patients at higher risk of hyperglycemia or diabetic ketoacidosis (e.g., young children) may also inject a once- or twice-daily long-acting insulin.[9,10] **The pump can be manually activated to deliver a bolus for hyperglycemia and for prandial dosing.** Insulin pumps are most appropriate for motivated patients who are mechanically adept, well educated about diabetes and carbohydrate counting, and able to monitor their capillary glucose four to six times a day.

Several models of insulin pumps are also capable of continuous glucose monitoring. These devices measure interstitial glucose concentrations and transmit glucose values to the pump or other display device. Interstitial glucose values are adjuncts to capillary glucose monitoring and still require manipulation of the insulin pump to administer insulin. Interstitial glucose is a proxy for serum glucose and is better for monitoring trends than absolute glucose level. **Capillary or serum glucose levels should be monitored in the ED, and interstitial glucose values should not be relied upon for diagnostic purposes.**

Insulin Pump Complications Insulin pump delivery can fail for a variety of reasons (disconnection, empty reservoir, kinked catheter, priming errors), although modern pumps have built-in alarms to detect these conditions.[11] **Because pumps use only rapid-acting insulin, onset of ketoacidosis can be very rapid after pump failure—an hour or less. If the pump is defective or needs to be removed for a procedure such as MRI, give the patient either a dose of rapid-acting insulin or long-acting insulin, especially if the insulin pump is to be interrupted for over an hour.**

Patients being switched from multiple daily injections of insulin to insulin pumps are typically handled as outpatients and will require special attention if presenting to the ED in this transition period. Specific considerations for patients on insulin pumps presenting with hyperglycemia or hypoglycemia are discussed later in this chapter.

Other important complications of insulin pump therapy include cellulitis at the infusion site or lipodystrophy. ED patients with nondiabetes complaints who are incidentally found to have hyperglycemia or hypoglycemia should be allowed to treat themselves (they should have been previously instructed by their endocrinologist) either by administering an insulin bolus through the insulin pump or by consuming carbohydrates.

PRAMLINTIDE

In addition to prandial insulin, patients with type 1 diabetes who are unable to achieve optimal glucose control using insulin or insulin analogues may also be treated with prandial injections of pramlintide, a synthetic form of the hormone amylin, which is produced by β-cells. Amylin promotes satiety, slows gastric emptying, aids in suppressing glucagon secretion,[4] and reduces hemoglobin A1C levels.[12] In initial studies of pramlintide, there was a significant increase in the occurrence of severe hypoglycemia, especially during the first 4 weeks of therapy and when insulin doses were not reduced.[13] **If insulin doses are reduced by about 25% with initiation of pramlintide, the risk of hypoglycemia could be eliminated.**[12,14]

TRANSPLANTS

There are three methods of pancreas transplantation: simultaneous pancreas and kidney, pancreas after kidney, and pancreas transplant alone.[15] In 2010, 350 pancreas transplants and 828 combined kidney/pancreas transplants were performed in the United States.[16] Long-term immunosuppression with medications such as sirolimus and tacrolimus is required.

Another promising modality is islet cell transplantation. One of the most successful protocols is the Edmonton protocol, which has led to insulin independence in type 1 diabetics.[17] Insulin independence is short lived, however; by 2 years post-transplantation, 76% of patients again required the use of exogenous insulin.[17]

TABLE 223-2 American Diabetes Association Criteria for the Diagnosis of Diabetes

A1C ≥6.5%*	The test should be performed in a laboratory using a method that is NGSP certified and standardized to the DCCT assay.
Or Fasting plasma glucose ≥126 milligrams/dL (7.0 mmol/L)*	Fasting is defined as no caloric intake for at least 8 h.
Or Casual plasma glucose ≥200 milligrams/dL (11.1 mmol/L) **and** symptoms of hyperglycemia	Classic symptoms of hyperglycemia include polyuria, polydipsia, and unexplained weight loss.
Or 2-h plasma glucose ≥200 milligrams/dL (11.1 mmol/L) during an oral glucose tolerance test (OGTT)*	OGTT must be performed as described by the World Health Organization.

Abbreviations: A1C = glycated hemoglobin; DCCT = Diabetes Control and Complications Trial; NGSP = National Glycohemoglobin Standardization Project.

*Should be confirmed by repeat testing unless unequivocal hyperglycemia is present.

GLYCEMIC COMPLICATIONS IN INSULIN-DEPENDENT PATIENTS

The major hyperglycemic emergencies, hyperosmolar hyperglycemic state and diabetic ketoacidosis, are discussed in chapters 227, "Hyperosmolar Hyperglycemic State" and 225, "Diabetic Ketoacidosis," respectively. Here we discuss the common ED presentation of an "abnormal lab value" (i.e., a patient with no acute symptoms of hyperglycemia who was found to have elevated plasma glucose on laboratory or point-of-care testing).

HYPERGLYCEMIA IN PREVIOUSLY DIAGNOSED TYPE 1 DIABETICS

For patients with type 1 diabetes with hyperglycemia noted on multiple ED visits, refer to the primary physician for insulin dose adjustment. In the interim, ask patients to keep a daily record of every meal, every dose of insulin administered (along with type of insulin), and blood glucose

TABLE 223-3 Commonly Used Insulin Preparations, Their Pharmacokinetics and Unique Features*

Category of Insulin or Analogue	Name	Pharmacokinetics Onset (hour)	Peak (hour)	End (hour)	Unique Properties
Rapid acting	Insulin lispro (Humalog®)	0.1–0.25	1.0–1.5	4	Fixed duration of action, regardless of dose Useful in patients allergic to insulin and other analogues[13-15]
	Insulin aspart (NovoLog®)	0.1–0.25	1–2	4–6	More stable than other rapid-acting insulins
	Insulin glulisine (Apidra®)	0.1–0.25	1.0–1.5	3–4	Antiapoptotic; may counteract β-cell destruction[16]
Short acting	Regular insulin (Humulin R®, Novolin R®)	0.25–1.0	2–4	6–8	—
Intermediate acting	NPH (Humulin N®, Novolin N®)	2–4	6–7	10–20	Inexpensive
	Insulin detemir (Levemir®)	1–3	9–?	6–24	Action is relatively constant with gentle peak
Long acting	Insulin glargine (Lantus®)	1.5	No peak	24+	Cannot be mixed with other insulins in same syringe
Mixtures	70/30 Humulin®/Novolin® (70% NPH, 30% regular)	0.5–1.0	3–12	10–20	—
	50/50 Humulin®/Novolin® (50% NPH, 50% regular)	0.5–1.0	2–12	10–20	—
	75/25 Humalog® (75% NPL, 25% lispro)	0.2–0.5	1–4	10–20	—
	50/50 Humalog® (50% NPL, 50% lispro)	0.2–0.5	1–4	10–20	—
	70/30 NovoLog Neutral® (70% protamine aspart, 30% aspart)	0.2–0.5	1–4	10–20	—

Note: All brand names are copyrighted by their respective owners.

Abbreviations: NPH = neutral protamine Hagedorn; NPL = neutral protamine lispro.

*Ultralente and Lente insulins are no longer available in the United States.

levels four times a day (after rising in the morning, before lunch, before dinner, and at bedtime).

If an insulin dose adjustment is made in the ED, the basic regime should be a once- or twice-daily dose of long- or intermediate-acting insulin, combined with prandial doses of rapid-acting insulin. The magnitude of increase in the basal insulin dose should be tailored to the degree of hyperglycemia in the patient. **The total daily dose of insulin is estimated at 0.2 to 0.4 units/kg/day,** with half given as basal insulin such as insulin glargine and half to be given in divided doses preprandially.

A conservative supplemental prandial dose of rapid-acting insulin can be calculated as follows: 1 unit per 50 milligrams/dL above target

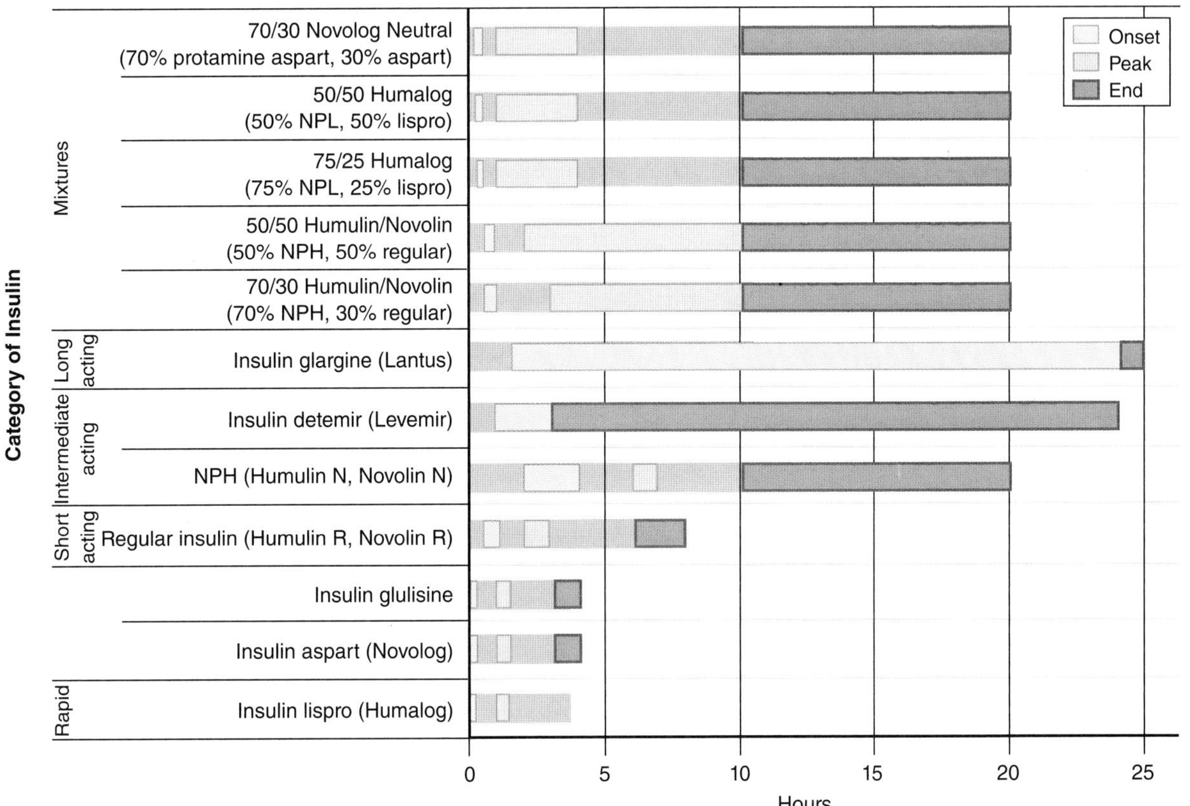

FIGURE 223-1. Insulins: onset, peak, and duration of action. NPH = neutral protamine Hagedorn; NPL = neutral protamine lispro.

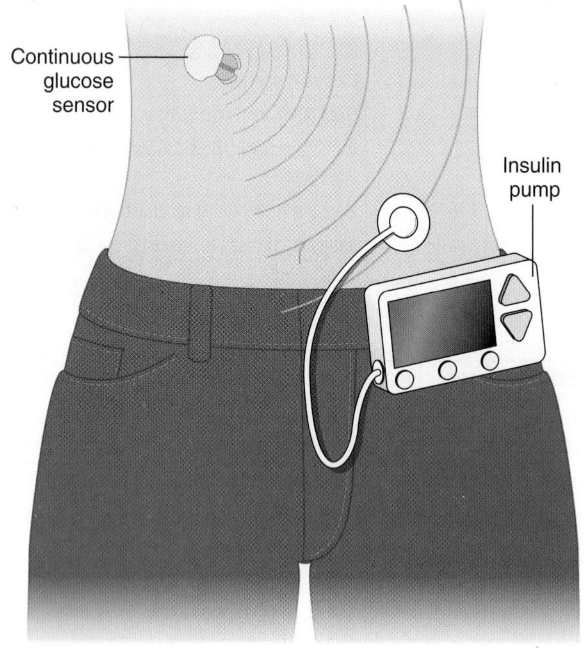

FIGURE 223-2. Schematic illustration of insulin pump.

glucose level for type 1 diabetics, and 1 unit per 30 milligrams/dL above target glucose level for type 2 diabetics.[18]

If the patient is using neutral protamine Hagedorn insulin, then inspect the neutral protamine Hagedorn vial; if frosting is noted on the sides of the bottle, this may indicate denaturation, which renders the insulin ineffective and can lead to diabetic ketoacidosis. Give a new prescription and discard the old vial.

Patients Using Insulin Pumps At this time, there are no published guidelines for the ED management of patients with insulin pumps who present to the ED with diabetic emergencies. **We recommend that patients using insulin pumps who present to the ED with either hyperglycemia or hypoglycemia should be treated the same as patients who are on multiple daily doses of insulin, and the insulin pump should not be disabled.**

Hyperglycemia in Patients Using Insulin Pumps For treatment of hyperglycemia, have the patient give a bolus of rapid-acting SC insulin using the pump (see insulin dosing as previously described).

Once the patient has been stabilized, ask about dietary indiscretions and search for infections. Ask specific questions about the insulin pump: when was the insulin reservoir filled; when was the infusion set last changed; is the insertion site of the infusion set periodically changed? Examine the device thoroughly to ensure the pump is on, the reservoir is not empty, no alarms are indicated, the tubing is not kinked, and the infusion site is well attached to the skin. The patient or caregiver may provide useful information on operation of the pump, pump diagnostics, and how to disconnect it if necessary. All pumps have a toll-free telephone number for 24-hour technical support from the manufacturer (**Table 223-4**). If there is suspicion for pump malfunction, consult endocrinology for consideration of replacement of the insulin pump with long-acting basal insulin.

TABLE 223-4 Manufacturers of Insulin Pumps Available in the United States With Their 24-Hour Phone Numbers

Manufacturer	Website	Telephone Number
Animas	http://www.animas.com	(877) 937-7867
Insulet OmniPod	http://www.myomnipod.com	(800) 591-3455
Medtronic MiniMed	http://www.medtronicdiabetes.net	(800) 646-4633
Nipro Diabetes Systems Amigo	http://amigoinsulinpump.com	(888) 651-7867
Roche Accu-Chek	http://www.accu-chekinsulinpumps.com	(800) 280-7801
Sooil DANA	http://www.sooil.com	(866) 747-6645 ext. 102

Diabetic Ketoacidosis in Patients Using Insulin Pumps In the case of diabetic ketoacidosis in a patient on an insulin pump, assume a problem with the pump, disconnect the pump, and start an IV insulin infusion and follow protocols for diabetic ketoacidosis treatment. Once the diabetic ketoacidosis has resolved, give a dose of long-acting insulin 1 hour before stopping the insulin drip unless the insulin pump is to be re-initiated—in that case, re-start pump therapy 1 hour before stopping the IV insulin drip. In order to re-initiate pump therapy, make sure that the pump is working appropriately by running diagnostics on the device, that the insulin reservoir is filled with fresh insulin, and that a new SC insulin infusion catheter has been placed. See chapter 225, for further discussion of transition of insulin dosing in diabetic ketoacidosis.

Check serum glucose levels every 30 to 60 minutes.

HYPOGLYCEMIA IN INSULIN-DEPENDENT PATIENTS

Hypoglycemia (plasma glucose <70 mg/dL) is a complication of intensive insulin therapy and is the major adverse effect of tight glycemic control. Apart from insulin administration, diabetics are prone to hypoglycemia because the surge of glucagon is absent in type 1 diabetes, and epinephrine secretion can be blunted as a result of neuropathy, age, or autonomic dysfunction due to frequent hypoglycemic episodes in the past.

Older insulin regimens used once- or twice-daily injections of neutral protamine Hagedorn or Lente insulin as the basal insulin and regular insulin as the prandial dose. Often premixed combinations (70/30, 75/25, 50/50) were used. These schedules mandated fixed meal times and activity schedules, so it was not unusual to develop hypoglycemia with missed meals and unusual stress. Use of modern physiologic regimes of insulin administration has significantly reduced the incidence of hypoglycemia. However, many patients remain on premixed dosing due to familiarity, or financial or insurance coverage limitations.

Determine the cause of hypoglycemia. Common causes include inadequate intake of food, inaccurate administration of insulin, infection, renal failure, acute coronary syndrome, unusual physical or mental stress, and so forth. Identify the timing and administration of insulin in relation to meals. There is a great variation in the pattern of hypoglycemic signs and symptoms from patient to patient; however, individual patients tend to experience the same pattern from episode to episode. Common neuroglycopenic symptoms include drowsiness, confusion, dizziness, tiredness, inability to concentrate, and difficulty speaking. Adrenergic symptoms such as tremor, sweating, anxiety, nausea, palpitations, feelings of warmth, and shivering are also seen, as are other symptoms such as hunger, weakness, and blurred vision.[19]

***Hypoglycemic unawareness* or *hypoglycemia-associated autonomic failure* occurs when diabetic patients have deficient counterregulatory hormone excretion, resulting in a lack of symptoms of hypoglycemia.**[3] This results in frequent episodes of hypoglycemia and profound hypoglycemic episodes. β-Blocker medication may also contribute to this condition, as the drug masks typical sympathetic symptoms of hypoglycemia.

Treatment of Hypoglycemia Glucose is the preferred treatment, although any glucose-containing carbohydrate may be used. The initial dose is 15 to 20 grams (PO, PR, or IV) that can be repeated if hypoglycemia persists after 15 minutes. In comatose patients, the IV or PR route is obviously necessary.

Pure fructose does not cross the blood–brain barrier, and protein has a negligible contribution to serum glucose—both are ineffective in treating hypoglycemia. Rectal syrup or honey is also an effective treatment. Once hypoglycemia has resolved, have the patient eat a meal or carbohydrate snack. **Table 223-5** lists the glucose content of commonly used oral agents.

Glucagon emergency kits are available for caregivers or family members of patients with type 1 diabetes for emergency situations. One milligram IM glucagon stimulates glycogenolysis and is usually effective in 10 to 15 minutes. Once the patient is alert enough to swallow,

TABLE 223-5 Glucose Content of Agents Available at Home

Agent	Dose/Route	Glucose Content
Fruit juice	1 cup PO	Variable depending on type of juice and manufacturer
		6 oz Mott's® apple juice: 21 grams sugar
Honey	1 tbsp PO/PR	17 grams sugar
Cake icing	2 tbsp PO	24 grams sugar
Sugar-containing soda	12 oz (one can) PO	(non-diet) Pepsi® = 41 grams sugars
		(non-diet) Sprite® = 38 grams sugars
		(non-diet) Coke® Classic = 40.5 grams sugars
Glucose tablets (commercially available)	Four tablets PO	16 grams carbohydrates

give oral glucose immediately. **Glucagon is not effective in glycogen-depleted patients**, and glucagon may induce nausea and vomiting, which can make it difficult to consume oral glucose subsequently.

Patients with a significant overdose of a long-acting agent should be admitted for monitoring of glucose levels. Most patients can be discharged if caregivers and family members can monitor symptoms and capillary glucose levels.

Hypoglycemia in Patients Using Insulin Pumps Treat hypoglycemia just as in other patients. **Do not discontinue the pump, as diabetic ketoacidosis can rapidly develop.** Please see section *General Considerations* for patients using insulin pumps, under *Hyperglycemia* (earlier).

If a patient on an insulin pump is to be made NPO, the insulin pump should *not* be removed and glucose levels should be checked every 30 to 60 minutes. If the patient has hypoglycemic episodes while NPO, the pump basal rate can be reduced, but this is best done in consultation with the endocrinologist.

SPECIAL CONSIDERATIONS

UNDIAGNOSED DIABETIC

A long asymptomatic period is common for type 2 diabetes, but type 1 diabetes typically has a short symptomatic period before the disease becomes overt. If the patient is newly identified with severe and symptomatic hyperglycemia (>250 to 300 milligrams/dL or 13.8-16.7 mmol/L), insulin should be administered in the ED. Insulin can be given even if it is not known at the time whether the patient has type 1 or type 2 diabetes. Patients with severe or symptomatic hyperglycemia should be given insulin and admitted or placed in an observation unit for further glucose control and education.

A low dose of regular or rapid-acting insulin (1 unit SC for every 30 milligrams/dL above glucose of 250 to 300 milligrams/dL) may be given to reduce hyperglycemia and a long-acting insulin (e.g., 0.1 to 0.2 units/kg of insulin glargine) should be given in the ED to prevent diabetic ketoacidosis.

For patients without severe and symptomatic hyperglycemia, regular or rapid acting insulin can be given to reduce the glucose to 250 milligrams/dL or so. Normoglycemia does not necessarily need to be achieved in the ED. Then the patient may be discharged with a prescription for metformin[3,20] and referral to their physician or clinic within 24 hours for further care. For further discussion of type 2 diabetes care and noninsulin antidiabetic agents such as metformin, see chapter 224.

GLUCOCORTICOID-INDUCED DIABETES

The American Diabetes Association defines glucocorticoid-induced hyperglycemia as an "other specific type" of diabetes. Patients receiving glucocorticoids are at risk of developing hyperglycemic crises, including hyperosmolar hyperglycemic nonketotic syndrome and diabetic ketoacidosis.

Patients with type 1 diabetes who are started on glucocorticoids before discharge from the ED will likely develop hyperglycemia. They should be informed about warning signs of hyperglycemia and advised to seek close follow-up with their primary physician, with frequent monitoring of blood glucose at home and additional prandial doses of insulin. Routine increase in basal insulin dosage is not indicated.

Although previously undiagnosed diabetics may develop hyperglycemia while on glucocorticoid therapy, the hyperglycemia will often resolve spontaneously once the glucocorticoid course is completed. If hyperglycemia is persistent or symptomatic, medication may be required after failure of dietary modification and exercise.

FALSELY ELEVATED CAPILLARY GLUCOSE

Peritoneal dialysis solutions using icodextrin interfere with many point-of-care capillary glucose measurement systems. These often result in falsely elevated readings, and there have been many reports of severe hypoglycemia due to insulin administration in response to such readings. **Obtain a central laboratory plasma glucose measurement for all peritoneal dialysis patients.**

"DEAD IN BED" SYNDROME

First described in 1991, the phenomenon of "dead in bed" syndrome can occur in typically young adults with uncomplicated type 1 diabetes who go to sleep in normal health and unexpectedly die, only to be found later in an undisturbed bed, without evidence of terminal struggle or seizure.[21,22] On autopsy, patients are found to be hypoglycemic but typically have no other pathologic findings. Several theories regarding the etiology of this phenomenon have been proposed, most of which implicate a terminal arrhythmia as a result of a hypoglycemia-induced prolonged QT_c,[23] possibly worsened by undiagnosed autonomic neuropathy.[21] The occurrence of dead in bed syndrome should reinforce to the emergency physician the lethal effects of hypoglycemia and the importance of avoiding hypoglycemia and hypoglycemic unawareness. By seeking consultation from endocrinology for young patients with type 1 diabetes presenting with hypoglycemia or instructing the patient to decrease their insulin dose until they follow up with their endocrinologist, it may be possible to decrease the risk of dead in bed syndrome.

REFERENCES

The complete reference list is available online at www.TintinalliEM.com.

Type 2 Diabetes Mellitus

Mohammad Jalili
Mahtab Niroomand

INTRODUCTION AND EPIDEMIOLOGY

Type 2 diabetes mellitus (T2DM) is a complex, chronic metabolic disorder characterized by hyperglycemia and associated with a relative deficiency of insulin production, along with a reduced response of the target tissues to insulin. It is a major public health issue and an important contributor to morbidity and mortality all over the world.[1] The top three countries with the highest number of diabetic patients are, in decreasing order, India, China, and the United States.[2] Epidemiology is summarized in **Table 224-1**.

T2DM is more common among women than men, and its prevalence increases by age. The prevalence of T2DM among youth is rising dramatically. Investigators attribute this rise to patterns of obesity and lack of physical activity. Native Americans, blacks, and Americans of Mexican or Japanese ethnicity are more commonly affected by T2DM than non-Hispanic whites (**Figure 224-1**).

TABLE 224-1 Epidemiology of Type 2 Diabetes Mellitus (T2DM)

T2DM Epidemiology Fact Sheet
Prevalence of T2DM can vary depending on geography, age, sex, and race/ethnicity.
In up to 30% of the affected people, the disease is undiagnosed.
Prevalence of T2DM is rising globally, with a greater increase in the developing countries.
There is an alarming trend toward increasing prevalence of T2DM among youth.
T2DM patients show a greater risk of mortality than nondiabetic subjects.
Diabetes is the leading cause of blindness, end-stage renal disease, and nontraumatic lower limb amputations.

Diabetes reduces the life expectancy of its victims by approximately 10 years. Mortality and morbidity increase because of increased risk of cardiovascular disease, heart disease and stroke, visual impairment, renal disease, and amputations. The utilization of health care, including emergency care, is higher in patients with diabetes compared with that of nondiabetic subjects. The relative risk is estimated to be 1.23 (95% confidence interval [CI], 1.08–1.39) before the diagnosis and 2.41 (95% CI, 2.18–2.66) after diagnosis is made.[3]

PATHOPHYSIOLOGY

T2DM is a complex heterogeneous metabolic disorder, characterized by chronic elevation of plasma glucose levels. The pathogenesis is complex and involves interaction of both genetic (usually polygenic) and environmental (often lifestyle-related) factors. The most important pathophysiologic features of T2DM are *decreased insulin sensitivity* (insulin resistance) and *impaired insulin secretion* (**Figure 224-2**).

It is generally believed that, in T2DM, fasting hyperglycemia is caused by increased production of glucose by liver, which is not suppressed because of hepatic resistance to insulin action. Normally, after meals, glucose uptake in peripheral tissues increases and glucose production by gluconeogenesis and glycogenolysis decreases. Insulin acts both directly and indirectly to inhibit gluconeogenesis and glycogenolysis. In T2DM, owing to hepatic resistance to insulin, the liver is programmed to both overproduce and underuse glucose.

However, postprandial hyperglycemia results from several mechanisms: abnormal insulin secretion by pancreatic β cells in response to a meal, impaired regulation of hepatic glucose production, and reduced glucose uptake by peripheral tissues, particularly the skeletal muscle, that are insulin sensitive.[4]

Insulin resistance is the diminished tissue response to insulin at one or more sites in the complex pathways of hormone action and requires higher than normal plasma insulin levels to maintain normoglycemia. The major sites of insulin resistance in T2DM are the liver, skeletal muscle, and adipose tissue.

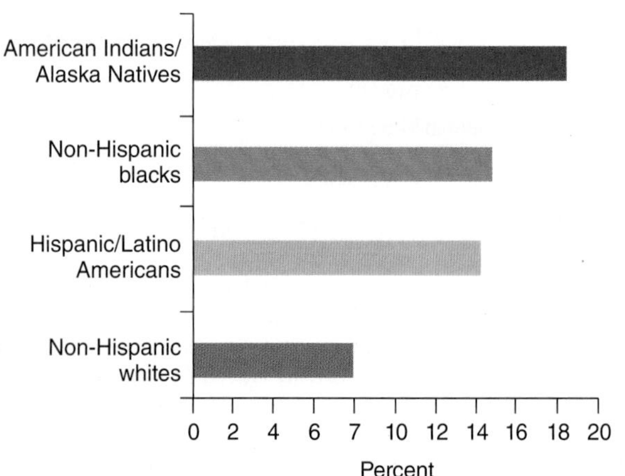

FIGURE 224-1. Estimated age-adjusted total prevalence of diabetes in people age 20 years or older, by race/ethnicity—United States, 2005. [Reproduced from the Centers for Disease Control and Prevention: National diabetes fact sheet: general information and national estimates on diabetes in the United States, 2005. Atlanta, GA: U.S. Department of Health and Human Services, Centers for Disease Control and Prevention, 2005.]

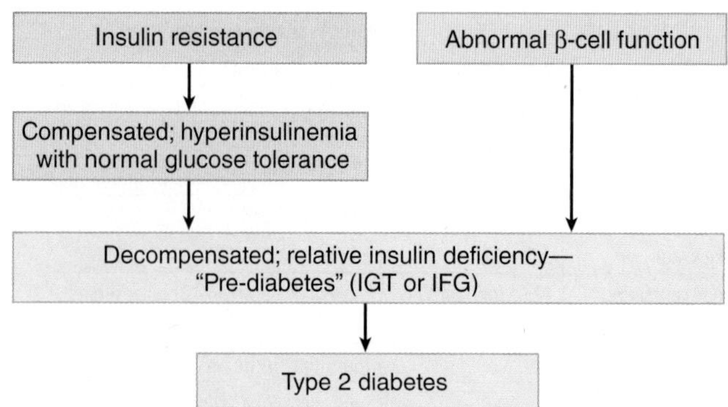

FIGURE 224-2. Pathophysiology of type 2 diabetes mellitus. IFG = impaired fasting glucose; IGT = impaired glucose tolerance.

Insulin secretion is usually impaired and generally insufficient to compensate for insulin resistance.[2] The mechanism behind impaired insulin release in T2DM is complicated and includes glucotoxic and lipotoxic effects, as well as deposition of amyloid within islet cells. *Glucotoxic effect* refers to increased exocytosis of insulin due to increased cytosolic calcium concentration, which occurs when β-cell metabolism of glucose generates adenosine triphosphate that closes adenosine triphosphate–sensitive K^+ channels and leads to depolarization of the membrane and hence opening of voltage-dependent Ca^{2+} channels. Exposure to increased levels of free fatty acid, as frequently found in diabetic patients, may also impair β-cell function, leading to impairment of insulin secretion (lipotoxic effect).[5]

The **incretin hormones** *glucagon-like peptide-1* (GLP-1) and *glucose-dependent inslinotropic polypeptide*, secreted by intestinal L cells following glucose intake, stimulate pancreatic β cells and are responsible for 50% to 70% of total insulin secretion. In people with T2DM, the incretin system is functionally impaired,[6,7] leading to hyperglycemia.

Chronic hyperglycemia is the cornerstone of **microvascular complications**. The causative role of chronic hyperglycemia in the development of **macrovascular complications** is less well defined, and other factors such as dyslipidemia and hypertension that often accompany T2DM may also play an important part in these complications.[8]

The increased prevalence of **infection** is primarily attributed to phagocyte dysfunction, including impaired adherence, chemotaxis, phagocytosis, bacterial killing, and respiratory burst.[9] Other abnormalities include nonenzymatic glycation of immunoglobulins and reduced T-lymphocyte populations.

CLINICAL FEATURES

The classic symptoms, which are usually mild and nonspecific, include fatigue, weakness, polyuria, polydipsia, polyphagia, and blurred vision. Most patients with T2DM are overweight, beyond their 30s, and suffer from other comorbid conditions such as hypertension, cardiovascular disease, dyslipidemia, and polycystic ovary syndrome. Clues in the patient's past medical history that are suggestive of diabetes mellitus include frequent superficial infections and slow healing of skin lesions after minor trauma.

Acute complications include diabetic ketoacidosis, hyperosmolar hypertonic nonketotic state, and hypoglycemia. Diabetic ketoacidosis and hyperosmolar hypertonic nonketotic state are covered elsewhere in this book (see chapters 225 and 227), and hypoglycemia, which in most cases is actually a complication of the treatment of diabetes, is discussed separately at the end of this chapter in the "Hypoglycemia" section.

Chronic complications are categorized as microvascular, macrovascular, and nonvascular complications (**Table 224-2**). One of the chronic complications of diabetes may be the reason for the patient presentation to the ED or may be found during review of systems and physical examination. A brief

TABLE 224-2 Chronic Complications of Type 2 Diabetes Mellitus

Vascular Complications
Microvascular complications
- Retinopathy
- Neuropathy
- Nephropathy

Macrovascular complications
- Coronary artery disease
- Cerebrovascular disease
- Peripheral vascular disease ("diabetic foot")

Nonvascular Complications
- Infections
- Dermatologic changes
- Urinary tract involvement
- Sexual dysfunction
- GI involvement (gastroparesis, diarrhea)
- Cataract/glaucoma
- Other: Obstructive sleep apnea, depression, fractures, hearing impairment, cognitive impairment, nonalcoholic fatty liver disease and hepatocellular carcinoma, periodontal disease

review of the manifestations of the involvement of various organ systems by diabetes will be presented here.

CARDIOVASCULAR COMPLICATIONS

Diabetes-related atherosclerosis (macrovascular complication) affects all major vascular territories, notably the coronary, cerebral, and peripheral arteries. In individuals with diabetes, the risk of coronary artery disease is two- to fourfold of nondiabetics, and the prognosis is worse than in nondiabetics. Diabetes blunts the cardiovascular benefit of female gender. **"Silent ischemia" (the absence of chest pain despite myocardial ischemia) is common in diabetic patients. It is also common for myocardial infarction to present with atypical or less impressive symptoms such as weakness, fatigue, and confusion.** Patients may suffer from pain in unusual locations or with lower than expected severity. This may explain the increased incidence of medically unrecognized acute myocardial infarction in diabetics compared with nondiabetics (40% vs 25%). The risk of heart failure is increased two to five times in individuals with diabetes (age- and risk factor–adjusted hazard ratio of 1.82 in men and 3.73 in women, according to the Framingham Heart Study). *Diabetic cardiomyopathy* refers to changes in myocardium, distinct from ischemic myocardial injury, which render it more susceptible to ischemia and less able to recover after an ischemic insult.

The incidence of peripheral arterial disease is increased in diabetic patients by a factor of two to four. Diabetes also affects the distribution of atherosclerosis in the lower limb, affecting tibial and peroneal arteries, as well as femoral and popliteal arteries. Claudication, critical limb ischemia and tissue loss, and, finally, amputation are the manifestations of this disorder.

RENAL COMPLICATIONS

Diabetic nephropathy is a major cause of morbidity and mortality. It affects 5% to 40% of patients with T2DM and is present in approximately 7% of the cases at the time of diagnosis. Although this complication is more common in type 1 diabetes, due to the fact that the overwhelming majority of diabetics are type 2, >80% of diabetic patients in renal replacement programs have this form of the disease. Clinically, diabetic nephropathy is characterized as a triad of hypertension, proteinuria (mainly albuminuria), and ultimately renal impairment. Other renal conditions associated with diabetes include urinary tract infections and papillary necrosis. Patients with **renal papillary necrosis** may be asymptomatic and not notice the sloughed papillary tissue excreted in their urine, or they may present with flank pain, hematuria, fever, and chills, symptoms similar to acute pyelonephritis. Urinalysis reveals necrotic fragments of renal papilla, along with red blood cells, white blood cells, and bacteria.

NEUROLOGIC COMPLICATIONS

Diabetics have a threefold increase in the risk of stroke, and diabetes increases the risk of recurrent stroke and stroke-related dementia. Diabetic neuropathy is a set of heterogeneous clinical syndromes, affecting various regions of the nervous system, singly or combined. Clinical manifestations of diabetic neuropathy can be nonspecific and mimic those seen in many other diseases. **Diabetic neuropathy** is a diagnosis of exclusion and should be labeled as such only after other forms of neuropathy, such as chronic inflammatory demyelinating polyneuropathy, B_{12} deficiency, hypothyroidism, and uremia, have been excluded. In most patients, this disorder is silent and goes undetected for long times, and less than half of patients with T2DM will develop symptomatic polyneuropathy in the 10 years after diagnosis. Neurologic disturbances in diabetes have been classified as subclinical neuropathy, diffuse clinical neuropathy, and focal neuropathy. Most common forms of diffuse neuropathies include chronic sensorimotor distal symmetric polyneuropathy and the autonomic neuropathies. Focal neuropathies consist of mononeuropathies and entrapment syndromes.

The most frequent symptoms of neuropathy are burning pain, electrical or stabbing sensations, paresthesia, hyperesthesia, and deep aching pain. Up to half of the patients are asymptomatic, and presence of neuropathy is discovered only on physical examination or when the patient presents with a painless foot ulcer. Physical examination usually reveals that perception of vibration, pressure, pain, and temperature is lost, more commonly in the feet and lower limbs with a symmetric stocking and glove pattern. The most significant morbidity associated with this type of neuropathy is foot ulceration.

Diabetic mononeuropathies usually have a sudden onset and are associated with pain. They may affect a large peripheral nerve such as ulnar, median, peroneal, or medial plantar nerves (as a result of entrapment) or an isolated cranial nerve, especially the third, fourth, or sixth cranial nerve (due to microvascular infarct). It may be difficult in the ED to differentiate the signs and symptoms of diabetic mononeuropathy from a transient ischemic attack or cerebrovascular accident, and imaging and other modalities are needed for diagnosis. The incidence of carpal tunnel syndrome is increased in diabetics.

Autonomic neuropathy may cause dysfunction of every part of the body and represents various clinical entities such as resting tachycardia, exercise intolerance, orthostatic hypotension, diarrhea, constipation, gastroparesis diabeticorum, erectile dysfunction, and neurogenic bladder. **Gastroparesis** is clinically manifested as nausea, vomiting, bloating, and easy satiety. Autonomic diarrhea is defined as at least 3 weeks of increased stool frequency and/or liquidity.

Proximal motor neuropathy with resultant weakness of the proximal muscles of the lower limbs and spontaneous or percussion-provoked muscle fasciculation may also be seen in diabetic patients. This disorder is believed to occur secondary to a variety of other diseases. These diseases are in turn more common in patients with diabetes mellitus than in the general population, and so proximal motor neuropathy may not be a primary component of diabetic neuropathy. Proximal motor neuropathy primarily affects the elderly and may begin, gradually or abruptly, with pain in the thighs and hips or buttocks.

INFECTIOUS COMPLICATIONS

Many common infections (such as pneumonia, soft tissue infections, and urinary tract infections) occur with greater frequency and severity in patients with diabetes. Infectious agents in these cases are usually similar to those seen in the nondiabetic population, but some organisms are more commonly encountered in these patients (*Staphylococcus aureus* and *Mycobacterium tuberculosis* in pneumonia, and *Candida* species in urinary tract infections). Still, there are several rare infections that almost exclusively occur in diabetics. This includes malignant otitis externa, emphysematous cholecystitis and pyelonephritis, and rhinocerebral mucormycosis. **Rhinocerebral mucormycosis** is an invasive fungal infection of the nasal and paranasal sinuses, sometimes involving the palate and adjacent tissues. The onset is sudden and rapidly progressive. Patients present with periorbital or perinasal pain, blood-tinged nasal discharge, unilateral headache, increased tearing, swelling of eyelids and conjunctiva, and decreased vision. Physical signs can include black eschar on the nasal mucosa or hard palate due to ischemia, proptosis, and, if the infection progresses, cranial nerve involvement or seizures. Patients with **malignant otitis externa** usually present with unilateral otalgia, decreased hearing, purulent ear discharge, and, sometimes, fever. Examination reveals a tender, inflamed external auditory canal with a mass of granular-appearing tissue. The infection can progress and involve the mastoid, temporal bone, or base of the skull, leading to osteomyelitis, meningitis, venous sinus thrombosis, or subdural emphysema. MRI or CT can define the extent of anatomic involvement. This infection is frequently due to *Pseudomonas aeruginosa*, but staphylococci, fungi, and other gram-negative organisms also have been isolated. **Emphysematous cholecystitis** may manifest as fever and abdominal pain. Abdominal radiographs may reveal gas within the gallbladder and biliary tree. Unexplained fever in diabetic patients, with or without abdominal pain, should be evaluated with US to search for cholecystitis. The causative agents are most frequently a *Clostridium* species in addition to streptococci, *Escherichia coli*, and *Pseudomonas*. **Emphysematous pyelonephritis** is a rare, life-threatening infection with gas production in renal parenchyma and around the kidney. Signs and symptoms include fever, clinical toxicity, flank pain, and, sometimes, a palpable mass.

FOOT AND LOWER EXTREMITY COMPLICATIONS

Diabetic foot ulceration results from interaction of many factors, including peripheral neuropathy, excessive plantar pressure, repetitive trauma, peripheral vascular disease, and wound-healing disturbances.[10,11] Ulcers act as a portal of entry for bacteria, resulting in cellulites and abscess formation. Aerobic gram-positive cocci (especially *S. aureus*) are the predominant pathogens in diabetic foot infections. Gram-negative rods may be encountered in patients with chronic wounds or those who have recently received antibiotic therapy. Those with foot ischemia or gangrene may be infected with obligate anaerobic microorganisms.[12]

Foot complaints in a diabetic require a thorough foot examination. Ulcer characteristics, including dimensions, depth, appearance (erythema, swelling, and purulence), and location, should be described. Hair and nail growth, calluses, corns, foot deformities, sensation, and vascular status (palpation of pedal and popliteal pulses) should be assessed. It is sometimes difficult to distinguish between lower extremity ulcers resulting from vascular insufficiency and those due to diabetes. **Venous ulcers** are typically present above the malleoli with irregular borders. **Arterial ulcers** are often found on the toes or the shins, with pale, "punched-out" borders. These ulcers are typically painful in the absence of coexisting neuropathy. **Diabetic ulcers**, on the other hand, usually occur at areas of increased pressure (e.g., sole of the foot) or friction (due to footwear).[13] **Any ulceration found should be unroofed and probed using a blunt-ended rigid sterile probe to determine the depth.** The ability to probe to bone through the ulcer suggests the strong possibility of osteomyelitis and deep-space soft tissue infection. Purulence or inflammation suggests infection, and both aerobic and anaerobic cultures should be taken from purulent drainage or material curetted from the base of the wound. Such specimens are preferable to wound swab specimens, which are often contaminated with colonizing bacteria and often do not identify the infected organism(s).

The diagnosis of **osteomyelitis** in patients with diabetic foot ulcer remains a challenge. When the wound can be probed to the underlying bone, presence of osteomyelitis is almost certain. Radiographs, although not very sensitive, should be obtained in patients with deep or long-standing ulcers to exclude osteomyelitis, subcutaneous gas, foreign bodies, and Charcot joints. MRI can identify osteomyelitis if radiographs are negative but clinical suspicion is high. **Table 224-3** shows the diagnostic utility of physical examination, laboratory, and basic radiographic testing in the diagnosis of osteomyelitis in patients with diabetic foot ulcer.

TABLE 224-3 Diagnostic Accuracy of Physical Examination, Laboratory, and Imaging Investigations for Lower-Extremity Osteomyelitis in Patients with Diabetic Foot Ulcers*

Finding	Positive LR (95% CI)	Negative LR (95% CI)
Ulcer area >2 cm^2	7.2 (1.1–49)	0.48 (0.31–0.76)
Positive "probe-to-bone" test	6.4 (3.6–11)	0.39 (0.20–0.76)
Erythrocyte sedimentation rate (with a cutoff of 70 mm/h)	11 (1.6–79)	0.34 (0.06–1.90)†
Plain radiograph	2.3 (1.6–3.3)	0.63 (0.51–0.78)
MRI	3.8 (2.5–5.8)	0.14 (0.08–0.26)

Abbreviations: CI = confidence interval; LR = likelihood ratio.

*Bone biopsy is considered the gold standard.

†95% CI crosses 1.0.

OPHTHALMOLOGIC COMPLICATIONS

Ocular complications of diabetes are summarized in **Figure 224-3**.

Retinopathy is divided into proliferative and nonproliferative forms. In the nonproliferative stage, changes in retinal vessels (vasodilation, microaneurysm formation, and leakage) occur and lead to accumulation of lipid in the outer plexiform layer (hard exudates) and hemorrhage in different layers of the retina (flame-shaped hemorrhage in the nerve fiber layer; dot-and-blot hemorrhage in deeper layers of the retina). Microinfarctions of the retina result in cotton-wool spots (soft exudates). In severe forms of the nonproliferative stage, venous tortuosity and beading occur. The proliferative stage is characterized by formation of new abnormal blood vessels (neovascularization) across the retinal surface and optic disc. These fragile new blood vessels may bleed into the vitreous, causing a vitreous hemorrhage. **Ocular hemorrhage in diabetic retinopathy after thrombolytic therapy is extremely uncommon,[14] and retinopathy should not be considered a contraindication. The indications and potential complications of thrombolytic therapy should be discussed with the patient before its administration.** Neovascularization can also affect the iris (rubeosis iridis), leading to severe glaucoma. Traction retinal detachment may result from contraction of the fibrous tissue that accompanies neovascularization.

Other ocular manifestations of diabetes include recurrent styes, blepharoconjunctivitis, and xanthelasma, fatty deposits in the subcutaneous tissue of the lids. Impaired corneal sensitivity can predispose to bacterial corneal ulcers, neurotropic ulcers, and difficulties with contact lenses. Cataracts and open- and narrow-angle glaucoma are more common in diabetics.

DERMATOLOGIC COMPLICATIONS

Skin manifestations of diabetes generally appear in patients with known diabetes, but they may also be the first presenting sign of diabetes or even precede the diagnosis by many years.[15] Protracted wound healing and skin ulcerations are the most common skin manifestations. Dermatologic complications of diabetes can be grouped as noninfectious (such as acanthosis nigricans, necrobiosis lipoidica, diabetic dermopathy, scleredema, and granuloma annulare), infectious (e.g., erythrasma, necrotizing fasciitis, and mucormycosis), and resulting from treatment of diabetes (e.g., lipoatrophy, lipohypertrophy, and various skin reactions as adverse effects of oral antidiabetics).

Common infections include cellulitis, furuncles and carbuncles, and candidiasis. Serious infections usually develop due to the combination of poorly controlled serum glucose, vascular insufficiency, and tissue hypoxia. Serious and rapidly progressive infections in diabetics include **necrotizing fasciitis** and **Fournier's gangrene**. See chapter 152, "Soft Tissue Infections" for further discussion. **Table 224-4** summarizes the cutaneous manifestations of diabetes.

PRINCIPLES OF EVALUATION

Look for diabetes in the presence of symptoms suggestive of hyperglycemia, detailed above, in the undiagnosed diabetic. It is reasonable to check the glucose level in patients with certain presentations such as

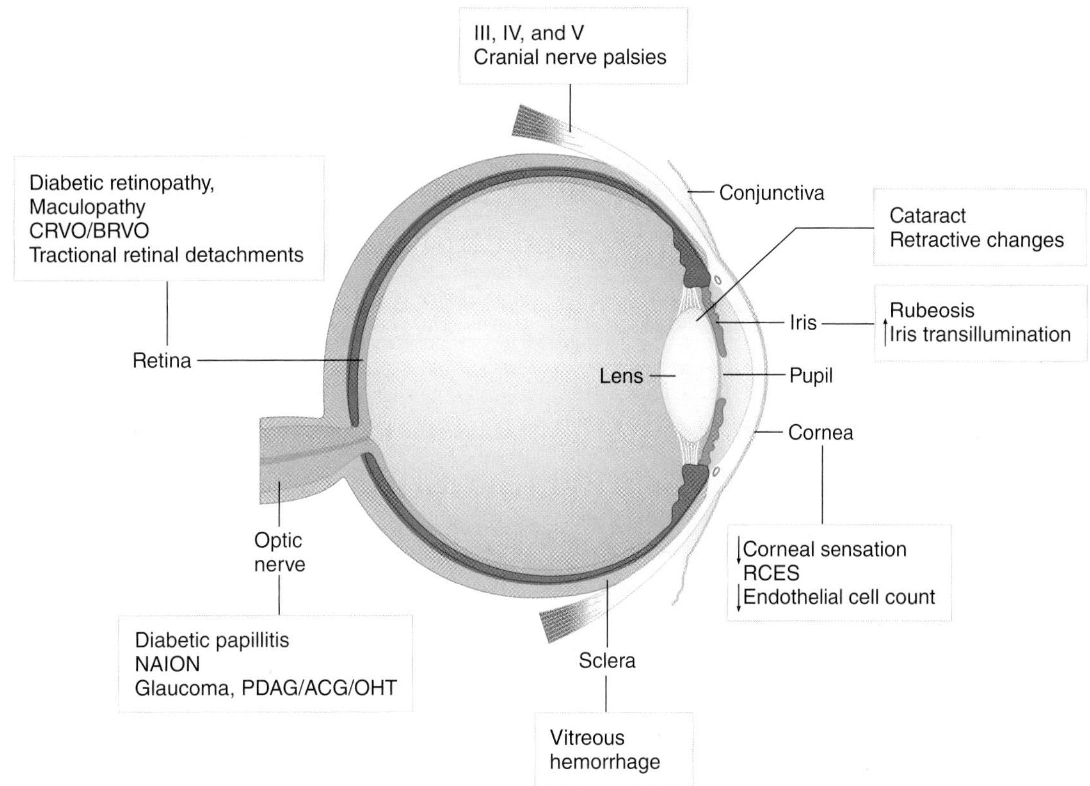

FIGURE 224-3. Common eye abnormalities in diabetes. ACG = angle-closure glaucoma; BRVO = branch retinal vein occlusion; CRVO = central retinal vein occlusion; NAION = nonarteritic ischemic optic neuropathy; OHT = ocular hypertension; POAG = primary open-angle glaucoma; RCES = recurrent corneal erosion syndrome.

unexplained cellulitis, foot ulcers, frequent candidal infections, and unexplained neuropathy.

When evaluating a patient with established diabetes mellitus in the ED, in addition to complaint-directed history and physical examination, special attention can be given to diabetes-related aspects. Assessment can include questions about prior diabetes care, presence or absence of diabetes complications and diabetes-related comorbidities, and assessment of the patient's knowledge about the disease. Elements of the history and physical examination relative to T2DM are presented in **Tables 224-5 and 224-6**.

TABLE 224-4 Cutaneous Manifestations of Diabetes Mellitus

Noninfectious	
Acanthosis nigricans	Hypertrophic, hyperpigmented, velvety plaques in body folds such as the neck, axillae, and groin.
Diabetic dermopathy ("shin spots")	Four to five dull red macules or papules, 5–12 mm in diameter, predominantly on the lower extremities, with a hyperpigmented scar.
Necrobiosis lipoidica	Oval violaceous patch with a red border and a yellow-brown central area, which then atrophies; prominent telangiectasias; may ulcerate.
Scleredema adultorum of Buschke	Asymmetric nonpitting induration of the skin, predominantly on the posterolateral aspects of the neck, shoulders, and upper back.
Granuloma annulare	A ring of small, firm, flesh-colored or red papules, most frequently found on the lateral or dorsal surfaces of the hands and feet.
Yellow skin (carotenodermia)	Skin of patients with diabetes may appear yellowish, secondary to deposition of carotenoids in the elastic tissue of the skin.
Diabetic bullae	Unilateral or bilateral tense, serous blisters of varying sizes from 0.5–3.0 cm, on the planter surfaces and margins of the feet.
Acrochordons (skin tags)	Soft tissue fibromas with a predilection for eyelids, neck, and axilla.
Infectious	
Necrotizing fasciitis	Typically of mixed bacterial origin, most common organisms: *Streptococcus pyogenes, Staphylococcus aureus,* anaerobic streptococci, and *Bacteroides.*
Malignant external otitis	Tenderness of the pinna and periauricular area, swollen external auditory canal, purulent discharge; *Pseudomonas aeruginosa.*
Erythrasma	Pruritic red-brown patch in the axilla or groin; *Corynebacterium minutissimum.*
Rhinocerebral mucormycosis	Fever, facial cellulitis, periorbital edema, proptosis, and blindness, facial numbness, black eschar in nasal mucosa or palate; mortality up to 50%.
Complications of diabetes treatment	
Lipoatrophy	Loss of subcutaneous fat at the insulin injection site.
Lipodystrophy	Localized hypertrophy of subcutaneous fat.
Skin reaction to oral hypoglycemic agents	Pruritus, erythema multiforme, erythema nodosum, urticaria, morbilliform rash, lichenoid eruptions, and photosensitivity.

TABLE 224-5 Elements of the Medical History in Patients with Type 2 Diabetes Mellitus

Key Elements of Medical History	
Past medical history	Cardiovascular disease, hypertension, dyslipidemia, foot lesion, ophthalmologic diseases, nephropathy, neuropathy, cerebrovascular disease
Prior diabetes care	Type of treatment and recent changes in the regimen; prior glycated hemoglobin A levels; blood sugar self-monitoring results; frequency, severity, and cause of hyper- or hypoglycemic episodes; diet and exercise history
Drug history	Oral hypoglycemic agents, insulin, diuretics, β-adrenergic agonists, β-adrenergic blockers
Social history	Smoking, substance abuse
Review of systems	Skin: dryness, pruritus, color changes, ulcers Weight loss GI: constipation, diarrhea, nausea, gastric fullness GU: urinary retention/incontinence, changes in amount of urine, and sexual dysfunction (impotence) Visual changes Numbness, dizziness, and weakness Chest pain

DIAGNOSIS

Diagnosis of diabetes can be done in three ways: by a fasting plasma glucose; a random glucose; or 2 hours after an oral glucose tolerance test (OGTT). An oral glucose tolerance test is reserved for patients in whom diabetes is strongly suspected despite a normal or impaired fasting glucose.[16] A hemoglobin A_{1c} (HbA_{1c}) level ≥6.5 can also diagnose diabetes, and HbA_{1c} is used to monitor the effectiveness of treatment.

Current criteria for the diagnosis of diabetes are summarized in **Table 224-7**. Impaired fasting glucose and impaired glucose tolerance are usually referred to as *prediabetes* and denote hyperglycemia not sufficient to meet diagnostic criteria for diabetes but significant for being risk factors for future diabetes and for cardiovascular disease.[17]

TREATMENT

Treatment of T2DM can be discussed under three topics: the day-to-day prevention of hyperglycemia (long-term management of hyperglycemia); prevention and management of chronic complications; and acute therapy of severe hyperglycemia and life-threatening metabolic decompensation (i.e., hyperosmolar hypertonic nonketotic state and diabetic ketoacidosis). Diabetic ketoacidosis and hyperosmolar hypertonic nonketotic state are discussed elsewhere in this book (see chapters 225 and 227, respectively).

The American Diabetes Association recommends that the goal of treatment in nonpregnant adults should be an HbA_{1c} value <7%. Other guidelines, such as that of the American College of Endocrinology, have recommended lower levels.[17] With respect to fasting, premeal, and postprandial targets, the American Diabetes Association suggestions are summarized in **Table 224-8**.[18]

TABLE 224-6 Elements of the Physical Examination in Patients with Type 2 Diabetes Mellitus

Key Elements of Physical Examination	
General	Height, weight, and body mass index
Vital signs	Blood pressure (including orthostatic measurement)
Head, eye, ear, nose, and throat examination	Funduscopy (to look for hemorrhage or proliferative retinopathy); visual acuity; intraocular pressure; thyroid palpation
Skin	Intertriginous areas (to look for acanthosis nigricans), insulin injection sites, lancet puncture sites, nonhealing wounds, cellulitis, tinea
Cardiovascular	Auscultation of the carotid arteries and abdomen for bruits; assessment of peripheral pulses (especially dorsalis pedis and posterior tibial pulses)
Foot examination	Signs of skin breakdown on the feet, signs of infection, determination of proprioception and vibration, monofilament sensation, presence/absence of patellar and Achilles reflexes

TABLE 224-7 Diagnostic Criteria for Diabetes

Test	Impaired Fasting Glucose (milligrams/dL)	Impaired Glucose Tolerance (milligrams/dL)	Diabetes* (milligrams/dL)
Fasting plasma glucose†	100–125 (5.5–6.9 mmol/L)	—	≥126 (≥6.9 mmol/L)
2-h OGTT	—	140–199 (7.8–11 mmol/L)	≥200 (≥11 mmol/L)
Random‡ plasma glucose concentration	—	—	≥200 (≥11 mmol/L) plus symptoms of diabetes#
$HgbA_{1c}$	5.7–6.4%		≥6.5%

Abbreviations: $HgbA_{1c}$ = hemoglobin A_{1c}; OGTT = oral glucose tolerance test (75-gram glucose load).

*In the absence of unequivocal symptoms of hyperglycemia, these criteria should be confirmed on a subsequent day.

†Fasting is defined as no caloric intake for at least 8 hours.

‡Random is defined as any time of the day without regard to time since last meal.

#The classic symptoms of hyperglycemia include polyuria, polydipsia, and unexplained weight loss.

NEWLY DIAGNOSED DIABETIC IN THE ED

The consensus statement on management of T2DM by the American Diabetes Association and the European Association for the Study of Diabetes recommends metformin in combination with lifestyle changes, as well as timely augmentation of therapy with additional agents (including other oral antidiabetic agents and insulin) to achieve recommended levels of glycemic control. This should be done in conjunction with the control of the symptoms of acute hyperglycemia and treatment of the underlying or exacerbating conditions. **Metformin can be safely initiated at a dose of 500 milligrams per day for patients whose T2DM has been newly diagnosed in the ED, provided that the serum creatinine level is ≤1.4 milligrams/dL.** The dose can be increased as needed in 500-milligram increments each week to a maximum of 2 grams per day. If admission is not warranted and exacerbating factors have been sought and effectively addressed, however, the initiation of pharmacotherapy can also be left to the primary care physician at 24- to 48-hour follow-up.

ACUTE THERAPY OF SEVERE HYPERGLYCEMIA

Acute hyperglycemia is defined as a blood glucose level of >300 milligrams/dL (>16.7 mmol/L). In this situation, the patient may have excessive urine output, weight loss, fatigue, blurred vision, or prominent neuropathic symptoms. Older patients may develop volume depletion, with acute mental status changes, hypovolemic shock, and acute renal insufficiency. Common precipitants include drug interaction with glucose-altering

TABLE 224-8 Glycemic Goals

Parameter	American Diabetes Association Recommended Target
Premeal plasma glucose	70–130 milligrams/dL (3.8–7.2 mmol/L)
Postprandial plasma glucose	<180 milligrams/dL (<10 mmol/L)
Hemoglobin A_{1c}	<7.0%

medications (most commonly, corticosteroids, sympathomimetics, diuretics, anticonvulsants, salicylates, and β-adrenergic receptor agonists), infections, acute illnesses such as acute coronary syndrome or CNS ischemia, or changes in or noncompliance with the prescribed drug regimen. Volume repletion, IV regular insulin, correction of electrolyte imbalance, and specific therapies directed toward any identified underlying cause of hyperglycemia are the components of treatment.

Regular human insulin is administered IV because absorption of SC insulin in a volume-depleted patient can be erratic. SC administration of insulin in non–volume-depleted patients is acceptable. Insulin lispro is an excellent alternative to regular human insulin. However, insulin lispro does not currently have U.S. Food and Drug Administration approval for IV administration, although many clinicians do use it. Typically, an initial bolus dose of 0.1 to 0.15 unit/kg IV or SC of regular human insulin or insulin lispro is given, which may be repeated in 1 to 2 hours if glucose levels have not fallen at least 50 milligrams/dL (2.8 mmol/L).

Patients should have a rapid therapeutic response to insulin, and, with improved glycemic control, many patients may become more responsive to oral therapies and may be able to switch to oral agents alone after using insulin initially. When initial therapy with insulin can be discontinued because of recovery from an acute illness or marked improvement of metabolic control, a standard oral therapy approach may be instituted.

MANAGEMENT OF HYPERGLYCEMIA IN ED OBSERVATION OR ED BOARDING

With many admitted patients boarding in the ED for longer periods, EPs frequently encounter patients with random blood glucose of 140 mg/dL (7.8 mmol/L) or higher on routine lab tests. The patient may or may not be a known diabetic. Stress and decompensation of diabetes may contribute to the pathophysiology of this problem, or it may be iatrogenic, resulting from either inadvertent cessation of antihyperglycemic medications or administration of hyperglycemia-inducing drugs such as glucocorticoids or vasopressors. Whatever the mechanism, emergency physicians may be called upon to control the patient's blood glucose. There is some evidence that in patients who are later admitted, paying careful attention to high blood glucose levels in the ED leads to better glycemic control in the hospital.

In critically ill patients, insulin infusion is usually required. The goal is to maintain blood glucose in the range of 140 to 180 mg/dL (7.8 to 10 mmol/L). More stringent control (with blood glucose <110 mg/dL [<6 mmol/L]) may actually increase mortality and is not recommended.

In patients who are not in a critical condition, subcutaneous insulin with a premeal glucose target of less than 140 mg/dL (7.8 mmol/L) and random blood glucose of less than 180 mg/dL (10 mmol/L) is recommended. In most patients with T2DM admitted for an acute illness, oral hypoglycemic agents should be discontinued and insulin substituted. However, writing orders for sliding scale insulin for admitted patients can lead to undesirable levels of hypoglycemia and hyperglycemia. Sliding scale insulin should not be used for more than 12 to 24 hours, and scheduled subcutaneous insulin therapy, consisting of basal (long- or intermediate-acting) insulin, in combination with bolus/prandial (rapid- or short-acting) insulin, should be substituted. A total dose of 0.2 to 0.5 U/kg/d is usually required based on the age and renal function of the patient. Half of this dose is administered as basal once or twice a day, and the remaining is given in three equally divided doses before each meal (only if the patient is eating). If the desired target blood glucose is not achieved, correction insulin should also be added to the scheduled insulin regimen.[19]

DISPOSITION AND FOLLOW-UP

Guidelines for admission considerations are listed in **Table 224-9**. Diabetic patients may need admission for conditions that in nondiabetics are usually treated on an outpatient basis.

Patients who present with new-onset T2DM without evidence of metabolic decompensation, acute hypoglycemia, or hyperglycemia and do not meet the aforementioned criteria for admission should see their primary care provider within 24 to 48 hours as a general rule to arrange for education, dietary evaluation, and initiation or refinement of appropriate therapy for glycemic control. Metformin can be safely initiated at a dose of 500 milligrams/d for patients whose T2DM has been newly diagnosed in the ED, provided that the serum creatinine level is ≤1.4 milligrams/dL. General discharge instructions for all diabetic patients, new or established, are detailed in **Table 224-10**.

TABLE 224-9 Disposition/Guidelines for Hospital Admission

Inpatient care for type 2 diabetes mellitus is generally appropriate for the following clinical situations:
Life-threatening metabolic decompensation such as diabetic ketoacidosis or hyperglycemic hyperosmolar nonketotic state
Severe chronic complications of diabetes, acute comorbidities, or inadequate social situation
Hyperglycemia (>400 milligrams/dL [>22 mmol/L]) associated with severe volume depletion or refractory to appropriate interventions
Hypoglycemia with neuroglycopenia (altered level of consciousness, altered behavior, coma, seizure) that does not rapidly resolve with correction of hypoglycemia
Hypoglycemia resulting from long-acting oral hypoglycemic agents
Fever without an obvious source in patients with poorly controlled diabetes

ANTIDIABETIC PHARMACOTHERAPY

There are five classes of antidiabetic agents: insulin and four classes of oral antidiabetic agents. Oral agent classification is based on mechanism of action: agents that cause insulin sensitization primarily in the liver, agents that cause insulin sensitization primarily in peripheral tissues, agents that promote secretion of insulin, and agents that slow the absorption of carbohydrates (**Tables 224-11 and 224-12**). Combined formulations are available that mix drugs from different classes of antihyperglycemic agents (metformin plus a thiazolidinedione or a secretagogue).

METFORMIN

Metformin is the only biguanide available in the United States (phenformin and buformin, other drugs of this class, are still available in some countries). Its precise mechanism of action is unknown. It has been suggested that metformin activates adenosine monophosphate–activated protein kinase and hence reduces hepatic insulin resistance. The resulting effect is decreased gluconeogenesis and glucose production in the liver. Some effect on improving insulin sensitivity in peripheral tissues has inconsistently been suggested. Metformin is usually started at a dose

TABLE 224-10 Discharge Instructions and Follow-Up Care

Follow a healthy diet.
Self-monitor blood glucose regularly.
Take insulin or oral hypoglycemic agents as directed.
Reduce weight where appropriate.
Cease smoking where appropriate.
Exercise regularly in the absence of contraindications, such as foot ulcers.
Practice good general foot care (check regularly for minor trauma and hot spots, keep nails trimmed properly, and wear well-fitted shoes). Wear a Medic-Alert bracelet or necklace.
Be able to recognize symptoms of high blood sugar, such as frequent urination, thirst, dizziness, headache, nausea or vomiting, abdominal pain, lethargy, or blurry vision.
Be able to recognize symptoms of low blood sugar, including fatigue, headache, drowsiness, agitation, pale or moist, visual changes, or loss of consciousness.
Know how to help yourself or others with low blood sugar by self-administering or giving an awake person (who can swallow without gagging or choking) candy, fruit juice, or sugar or by calling an emergency phone number (e.g., 911) if the affected person is not able to respond.

TABLE 224-11 Oral Antidiabetic Agents' Classification According to Their Mechanism of Action

Mechanism of Action	Class	Examples
Insulin sensitizers with primary action in the liver	Biguanides	Metformin
Insulin sensitizers with primary action in peripheral tissues	Thiazolidinediones (glitazones)	Pioglitazone, rosiglitazone
Insulin secretagogues	Sulfonylureas	Glyburide, chlorpropamide, glipizide
	Glinides	Repaglinide, nateglinide
Carbohydrate absorption slowing agents	α-Glucosidase inhibitors	Acarbose, miglitol

of 500 milligrams once daily (with a meal) and can be titrated upward slowly to a maximum dose of 2 grams/d. Due to its short duration of action, metformin is generally taken at least twice daily. The most common adverse effects are GI: nausea, diarrhea, crampy abdominal pain, metallic taste, and dysgeusia. **Another rare side effect of metformin is lactic acidosis, which almost exclusively occurs in patients with renal insufficiency. Metformin is eliminated by the kidney in unchanged form and so is contraindicated in patients with an estimated glomerular filtration rate of <40 mL/min.** In those with a glomerular filtration rate between 40 and 60 mL/min, half the recommended dose should be given. Because metformin does not increase insulin levels, it is not associated with a significant risk of hypoglycemia. Other contraindications include congestive heart failure requiring drug therapy, hepatic insufficiency, any form of acidosis, severe hypoxemia, and alcohol abuse. **Take care when administering metformin simultaneously with nephrotoxic agents such as contrast dye. Withhold metformin for 48 hours *after* IV contrast administration.**

GLITAZONES

Glitazones (thiazolidinediones) work through binding and modulation of the activity of peroxisome proliferator-activated receptors. This nuclear receptor influences the differentiation of fibroblasts into adipocytes and lowers free fatty acid levels. Thus, thiazolidinediones improve insulin sensitivity and reduce free fatty acid levels. Pioglitazone and rosiglitazone have replaced the first drug of this class, troglitazone, because they are believed to be safer. thiazolidinediones are well tolerated, and their only significant adverse effects are weight gain and fluid retention. Liver function should be assessed before beginning thiazolidinedione therapy. This class of drugs is contraindicated in the presence of active hepatocellular disease and in patients with unexplained serum alanine aminotransferase levels >2.5 times the upper limit of normal. Thiazolidinediones can affect bone turnover in animals, and an observational study has recently shown bone loss in older female diabetics who are treated with thiazolidinediones.[20] Thiazolidinediones may lead to macular edema, as well as increased risk of bone fracture and bladder cancer.[21]

SULFONYLUREAS

Sulfonylureas are the oldest class of oral antidiabetic agents.[3] They bind to the sulfonylurea receptor, a subunit of the adenosine triphosphate–sensitive potassium channel on plasma membrane of pancreatic β cells, causing a series of reactions, thereby leading to insulin secretion (exocytosis of insulin granules). Drugs in this class can be divided into first- and second- generation agents. First-generation sulfonylureas include chlorpropamide, tolbutamide, tolazamide, and acetohexamide. The second generation of this class includes drugs with higher potency and fewer adverse effects and drug–drug interactions (namely, glipizide, glyburide, gliclazide, and glimepiride). **Hypoglycemia** is the major adverse effect of sulfonylureas (highest risk seen with glyburide), and other side effects like allergic reactions, GI intolerance, hyponatremia, or alcohol flushing are very rare and drug dependent.[3]

REPAGLINIDE

Repaglinide is an insulin secretagogue, structurally distinct from the sulfonylureas. It binds to pancreatic β cells and stimulates insulin release. Repaglinide is absorbed more rapidly and so produces faster and briefer stimulus to insulin secretion. However, it has a prolonged effect on fasting glucose. The maximum dose of this drug is 2 milligrams taken with each meal. Repaglinide has an almost completely biliary elimination, and therefore, it can be used safely in patients with renal insufficiency.

NATEGLINIDE

Nateglinide, a phenylalanine derivative, has an even shorter duration of action than repaglinide. It has a specific effect on postprandial glucose and almost no effect on fasting glucose. This drug is used as 120-milligram tablets taken with each meal.

ACARBOSE AND MIGLITOL

Acarbose and miglitol inhibit the final step of carbohydrate digestion at the brush border of intestinal epithelium through competitive inhibition of α-glucosidases. This action delays the absorption of carbohydrates and consequently decreases the postprandial glucose peak and insulin response to the meal. They have only a modest effect on blood glucose reduction and commonly cause flatulence. Their advantage is lowering postprandial glucose without increasing weight or hypoglycemic risk.

TABLE 224-12 Some Properties of Classes of Antihyperglycemic Agents

Parameter	Secretagogues	Metformin	a-Glucosidase Inhibitors	Thiazolidinediones	Insulin
Mechanism of action	Potentiate insulin secretion	Suppresses liver glucose production	Delay intestinal carbohydrate absorption	Improve insulin sensitivity (fat, liver, and muscle)	Suppresses glucose production; enhance glucose uptake
Hemoglobin A_{1c} reduction (%)	1.5–2.0	1.5–2.0	0.5–1.0	0.75–2.0	Limited by hypoglycemia only
Adverse effects	Hypoglycemia, weight gain	Nausea, diarrhea, lactic acidosis	Flatulence, diarrhea	Edema, congestive heart failure, weight gain, anemia	Hypoglycemia, weight gain
Nonglycemic effects	None	Reduces CV risk markers; limits weight gain	Reduce CV risk markers	Reduce CV risk markers	Reduces CV risk markers
Evidence for benefit					
Microvascular	Strong	Strong	None	None	Strong
Macrovascular	None	Moderate	Weak	Weak	Moderate

Abbreviation: CV = cardiovascular.

INSULIN

Decreased secretion of insulin due to declining β-cell function eventually makes oral antidiabetic agents ineffective in achieving glycemic control and leads to the need for insulin therapy. Insulin can be used to supplement endogenous production of insulin both in the basal and postprandial state. Traditionally, insulin has been used for the treatment of T2DM when nutritional therapy and oral agents have failed to control blood glucose levels. There is, however, an increasing trend toward the initiation of insulin at an earlier stage of the disease. Besides when therapy with oral agents fails to achieve the glycemic target, insulin may be used in the treatment of T2DM in several other situations: during the perioperative period in a diabetic patient, for treatment of acute hyperglycemic crises, and even as the initial therapy in severe hyperglycemia. There are several formulations of insulin available, with different pharmacokinetics. See chapter 223, "Type 1 Diabetes Mellitus" for detailed discussion of insulins.

INCRETIN ANALOGUES

In humans, *glucagon-like peptide*, GLP-1, mediates the process by which oral glucose has a greater stimulatory effect on insulin secretion than parenteral glucose (the so-called *incretin effect*). GLP-1, among other antihyperglycemic actions, enhances endogenous insulin secretion in response to oral caloric intake. GLP-1 analogues (also referred to as *incretin analogues* or *incretin mimetics*) are used in the treatment of diabetes. An important feature of incretin-related therapies is that this class of drugs increases insulin secretion only in the presence of hyperglycemia. **Exenatide** (Byetta™) is a synthetic peptide with 53% amino acid similarity to GLP-1 and is indicated for therapy of T2DM patients who do not achieve adequate glycemic control on metformin, sulfonylurea, thiazolidinedione, or a combination of the two. Exenatide may be used with metformin or in combination with both metformin and a sulfonylurea.[22,23] It has also been used in combination with insulin to enhance glycemic control. Exenatide exerts its HbA_{1c}-lowering and weight reduction effects through several mechanisms: It suppresses glucagon secretion, slows gastric emptying, reduces food intake, and promotes β-cell proliferation. Exenatide is administered at a dose of 5 to 10 micrograms twice daily as SC injection in the abdomen, thigh, or arm. Dose adjustment is necessary in patients with end-stage renal failure (creatinine clearance of <30 mL/min). It is contraindicated in the presence of medullary thyroid cancer.

Liraglutide (Victoza®) is a GLP-1 receptor agonist that is injected at a dose of 0.6 to 1.2 milligrams once a day, so some prefer it over exenatide. It is contraindicated in the presence of medullary thyroid cancer or in those with multiple endocrine neoplasia. Pancreatitis is a reported adverse effect.

Dipeptidyl peptidase IV inhibitors are a distinct yet similar class of medications. These agents prolong the action of native GLP-1 by inhibiting its metabolism by dipeptidyl peptidase IV. They are administered orally. Saxagliptin, sitagliptin, and vildagliptin are available preparations. A safety alert was issued for saxagliptin in February 2014 due to possible association with heart failure.

AMYLIN ANALOGUES

Amylin is a neuroendocrine peptide that is normally cosecreted with insulin from the pancreatic β cells. It has a complementary action for insulin in regulating plasma glucose. In T2DM, secretion of amylin diminishes and is delayed in advanced stages of the disease. Pramlintide is the synthetic analogue of amylin with several metabolic effects: It (1) suppresses endogenous secretion of glucagon, especially in the postprandial state, thereby decreasing postprandial hepatic glucose production; (2) reduces the rate of gastric emptying; (3) decreases appetite and induces satiety; and (4) reduces postprandial glucose levels.[24] **Pramlintide** is used as a 120-microgram SC injection at mealtime in patients with type 1 diabetes as well as patients with T2DM who are treated with insulin, but who are very vigilant with insulin dosage and blood glucose monitoring. It carries a Food and Drug Administration black box warning; if given with insulin therapy, it can induce severe hypoglycemia, especially within 3 hours of insulin administration.

PREVENTION AND MANAGEMENT OF CHRONIC COMPLICATIONS

Emergency physicians can reinforce patient education and provide access to additional resources as necessary (**Table 224-13**). Interventions that may be initiated or augmented in the ED for chronic complications are briefly discussed below.

CARDIOVASCULAR COMPLICATIONS

Angiotensin II receptor blockers and angiotensin-converting enzyme inhibitors are the preferred antihypertensive agents in patients with T2DM. Although β-blockers may potentially mask hypoglycemic symptoms, they are safe in most patients with diabetes. Central adrenergic antagonists and α-adrenergic blockers may worsen orthostatic hypertension in those with autonomic neuropathy. For treatment of hypertension in diabetic patients, nondihydropyridine calcium channel blockers (i.e., verapamil and diltiazem) are preferred over the dihydropyridine group (i.e., amlodipine and nifedipine).

When acute coronary syndrome occurs in the setting of diabetes, the management is very much the same as in nondiabetic patients. Although proliferative retinopathy is considered a relative contraindication to thrombolytic therapy by some, the risk of intraocular bleeding is thought to be very low.[14]

RENAL COMPLICATIONS

Angiotensin-converting enzyme inhibitors are effective in preventing and slowing the progression of diabetic nephropathy, regardless of their effect on blood pressure. In addition, they can reduce major cardiovascular disease outcomes in patients with diabetes.

NEUROLOGIC COMPLICATIONS

A number of pharmacologic agents are effective for the symptomatic treatment of painful polyneuropathies: cyclics (e.g., amitriptyline, nortriptyline, and imipramine), anticonvulsants (gabapentin, carbamazepine, pregabalin), topical capsaicin (a substance P inhibitor), and duloxetine. Among these drugs, pregabalin and duloxetine have Food and Drug Administration indication for treatment of painful diabetic neuropathy (**Table 224-14**).

Several interventions can improve the quality of life but do not affect the underlying pathology or natural history of the disease process. Dietary modifications and prokinetic agents (e.g., metoclopramide, erythromycin), which decrease gastric emptying time, may improve symptoms of gastroparesis. Treatments for erectile dysfunction include phosphodiesterase type 5 inhibitors, such as sildenafil, and intracorporal or intraurethral prostaglandins[5] (**Table 224-15**).

VACCINATION

For patients with diabetes, vaccinations are recommended, according to the Centers for Disease Control and Prevention Advisory Committee on Immunization Practices (http://www.cdc.gov/vaccines/recs), against influenza annually in the fall and at least once with the pneumococcal polyvalent vaccine. Repeat pneumococcal vaccination is indicated for patients 65 years of age or older provided that their initial vaccination was administered >5 years ago and also in the setting of nephrotic syndrome, chronic renal disease, and other immunocompromised states, such as after transplantation.[17]

LOWER EXTREMITY AND FOOT COMPLICATIONS

From a clinical standpoint, foot ulcers can be classified as non–limb-threatening, limb-threatening, or life-threatening infections. Non–limb-threatening infection is defined as one that is small (<2 cm of surrounding cellulitis or inflammation), does not involve deep structures or bone, and is the result of recent injury to a well-perfused limb. The patient has no signs of systemic toxicity or leukocytosis. Limb-threatening infections are characterized by the presence of >2 cm of

TABLE 224-13 American Diabetes Association Recommendations for Prevention and Management of Diabetes Complications

Risk Factor/Complication	Screening	Treatment
Blood pressure control	Blood pressure should be measured at every routine diabetes visit.*	If 120 ≤ SBP ≤ 139 and DBP ≤80, start lifestyle therapy. If SBP ≥140 or DBP ≥80 (confirmed on 2 separate days), begin pharmacologic (ACEI or ARB) plus lifestyle therapy.
Lipid management	Fasting lipid profile should be measured at least annually.	Lifestyle modifications recommended for all patients. For diabetics: With overt CVD† Age >40 y old and one or more other CVD risk factors† With low-density lipoprotein >100 milligrams/dL Start statin therapy.
Smoking	—	Smoking cessation recommended for all patients.
CVD	—	Treat risk factors (as above). Antiplatelet therapy in diabetic patients with: History of CVD 40 y of age or more Additional risk factors‡
Nephropathy	Annual assessment of urine albumin excretion and serum creatinine	Optimize glucose and blood pressure control. ACEI or ARB in case of microalbuminuria Reduction of protein intake in case of chronic kidney disease
Retinopathy	At diagnosis and annual comprehensive eye examination	Optimize glucose and blood pressure control. Prompt referral of patients with any level of macular edema, severe nonproliferative diabetic retinopathy, or any proliferative diabetic retinopathy; laser photocoagulation therapy in selected patients
Neuropathy	At diagnosis and annual screening for distal symmetric polyneuropathy; at diagnosis screening for diabetic autonomic neuropathy	Improved glycemic control Symptomatic treatment

Abbreviations: ACEI = angiotensin-converting enzyme inhibitor; ARB = angiotensin II receptor blocker; CVD = cardiovascular disease; DBP = diastolic blood pressure; SBP = systolic blood pressure.

*High readings (≥130/80 mm Hg) should be confirmed on a separate day.

†Regardless of baseline lipid levels.

‡Including family history of CVD, hypertension, smoking, dyslipidemia, and albuminuria.

surrounding cellulitis or inflammation, with associated ascending lymphangitis, deep full-thickness ulceration or abscess, a large area of necrotic tissue, involvement of deep structures or bone, gangrene adjacent to the ulcer, or critical lower extremity ischemia (i.e., absence of palpable pulses). Life-threatening infection has clinical signs of sepsis, including fever, leukocytosis, hypotension, tachycardia, tachypnea, altered mental status, and metabolic abnormalities ranging from hypoglycemia to diabetic ketoacidosis and hyperosmolar hypertonic nonketotic state (**Table 224-16**).

Management of foot ulcers requires a multidisciplinary approach. Principles of management include debridement of necrotic tissues, avoidance of pressure points, management of infection (**Table 224-17**) and/or ischemia, management of medical comorbidities, proper wound handling, and surgery.

Treatment of noninfected chronic wounds mostly relies on avoidance of weight bearing and nonadherent padded dressings. Prophylactic antibiotics are not recommended, as this is costly and may result in adverse drug effects and the emergence of resistant organisms. Clinical signs of

TABLE 224-14 Drugs Used in the Treatment of Symptomatic Diabetic Autonomic Neuropathy

Class	Examples	Typical Dosages*
Tricyclic drugs	Amitriptyline	10–75 milligrams at bedtime
	Nortriptyline	25–75 milligrams at bedtime
	Imipramine	25–75 milligrams at bedtime
Anticonvulsants	Gabapentin	300–1200 milligrams twice a day
	Carbamazepine	200–400 milligrams twice a day
	Pregabalin†	100 milligrams twice a day
5-Hydroxytryptamine and norepinephrine uptake inhibitor	Duloxetine†	60–120 milligrams daily
Substance P inhibitor	Capsaicin cream	0.025–0.075% applied twice a day or four times a day

*Dose response may vary; initial doses need to be low and titrated up.

†Has U.S. Food and Drug Administration indication for treatment of painful diabetic neuropathy.

TABLE 224-15 Symptomatic Treatment of Selected Autonomic Neuropathies in Diabetic Patients

Manifestation of Autonomic Neuropathy	Treatment
Gastroparesis	Frequent small meals, prokinetic agents (e.g., erythromycin, metoclopramide)
Diarrhea	Soluble fiber, anticholinergic agents, cholestyramine
Constipation	Dietary fiber supplementation, bulking agents, stool softener
Neurogenic bladder	Bethanechol, intermittent catheterization
Erectile dysfunction	Psychological counseling, phosphodiesterase inhibitors (e.g., sildenafil)
Postural hypotension	Increasing salt intake (in the absence of hypertension), elastic stockings, or fludrocortisone
Anhydrosis	Scopolamine, emollients, skin lubricants

TABLE 224-16 Clinical Practice Pathways for Diabetic Foot Ulcer and Infection

Extent of Infection	Characteristics	Diagnostic Procedures	Treatment
Non–limb-threatening infection	<2 cm cellulitis	Cultures from base of ulcer (with tissue specimen if possible)	Outpatient management with follow-up in 24–72 h
	Superficial ulcer	Diagnostic imaging (radiography, MRI, nuclear scans as indicated)	Debridement of all necrotic tissue and callus
	Mild infection	Serologic testing	Wound care/dressing
	No systemic toxicity	CBC with differential	Empiric antibiotic coverage, modified by culture findings
	No ischemic changes	ESR	Appropriate off-loading of weight bearing
	No bone or joint involvement	Comprehensive metabolic panel	Wound care continued with packs, dressings, and debridement as needed
	Does not probe to bone		Hospital admission if infection progresses or systemic signs or symptoms develop
			Refer to podiatrist for follow-up care, special shoes, and prostheses as needed
Life- or limb-threatening infection	>2 cm cellulitis	Deep culture from base of ulcer/wound with tissue specimen if possible	Hospital admission
	Deep ulcer		Surgical debridement with resection of all necrotic bone and soft tissue
	Odor or purulent drainage from wound	Diagnostic imaging (radiography, MRI, nuclear scan, bone scan, leukocyte scan, arteriography)	Exploration and drainage of deep abscess
	Fever	Serologic testing	Empiric antibiotic coverage, modified by culture findings
	Ischemic changes	CBC with differential	Surgical resection of osteomyelitis
	Lymphangitis, edema	ESR	Wound care continued with packs, dressings, debridement as needed
	Sepsis or septic shock	Comprehensive metabolic panel	
		Blood cultures	Foot-sparing reconstructive procedures
			Refer to podiatrist for follow-up care, special shoes, and prostheses as needed

Abbreviation: ESR = erythrocyte sedimentation rate.

infection include prominent discharge, local erythema, and cellulites. The patient should be referred to a specialist in diabetes-related foot care within a few days to consider the need for debridement, total contact casting, further evaluation of any bony deformity or neuropathy, and evaluation for peripheral vascular disease.

Non–limb-threatening infections can usually be managed in the outpatient setting with appropriate minor debridement and administration of oral antibiotic therapy (Table 224-17). Application of well-padded dressing and avoidance of pressure to the affected area are necessary for adequate wound healing.

Treatment of limb-threatening infections requires hospitalization, IV antibiotics (Table 224-17), and surgical debridement. Empiric antibiotic therapy should be directed against the predominant pathogens, *Staphylococcus* and *Streptococcus* species. Include coverage for aerobic gram-negative and anaerobic bacteria when gangrenous, ischemic, or malodorous wounds are present. The use of topical antibiotics is generally not recommended. In the absence of palpable pedal pulses, vascular ultrasonography is needed. Further studies can include the ankle-brachial index, toe pressures, or measurement of transcutaneous oxygen tension. Immediate surgical consultation is indicated for incision and debridement, possible revascularization, or amputation.

HYPOGLYCEMIA

PATHOPHYSIOLOGY

Although there is no fixed laboratory definition of hypoglycemia, **it is clinically defined as follows: (1) symptoms consistent with the diagnosis; (2) symptoms associated with a low glucose level, usually <50 milligrams/dL (<2.7 mmol/L); and (3) symptoms resolve with glucose administration**.

Although the human brain depends on glucose as its primary source of energy, it is unable to synthesize or store glucose, accounting for the common manifestation of hypoglycemia as altered mental status. Physiologic response to low blood glucose includes suppression of insulin secretion and release of the counterregulatory hormones (e.g., glucagon and epinephrine). These responses are modified with increasing age. Renal clearance of insulin decreases with age, and this may enhance the risk of hypoglycemia in the elderly. On the other hand, in subjects with T2DM, counterregulatory hormones are secreted at higher blood glucose levels (compared with nondiabetics and those with type 1 diabetes mellitus), resulting in some protection against hypoglycemia in patients with T2DM. Improved glycemic control through insulin therapy lowers the blood glucose level threshold for the counterregulatory response and offsets this protective effect of diabetes.

CLINICAL FEATURES

Hypoglycemia is usually a complication of treatment. It occurs most frequently with insulin and sulfonylureas. **Hypoglycemia is not a common side effect of treatment with glitazones, glinides, or α-glucosidase inhibitors.**[25] Among sulfonylureas, the risk of hypoglycemia depends on the pharmacokinetic properties of each agent. Chlorpropamide, glyburide (glibenclamide), and long-acting glipizide are long-acting sulfonylureas and are associated with more episodes of hypoglycemia. Hypoglycemia is rarely, if ever, encountered in patients using only metformin. Risk factors for severe hypoglycemia in patients with T2DM include age, past history of vascular disease, renal failure, decreased food ingestion, alcohol consumption, and drug interactions.

The clinical manifestations of hypoglycemia are divided into two broad categories: *neuroglycopenic* and *autonomic*. Neuroglycopenic manifestations include alterations in consciousness, lethargy, confusion, combativeness, agitation, seizures, focal neurologic deficits, and unresponsiveness. **Autonomic** findings consist of anxiety, nervousness, irritability, nausea, vomiting, palpitations, and tremor. Cholinergic nervous system stimulation also may occur and result in manifestations such as sweating, changes in pupil size, bradycardia, and salivation. **Table 224-18** lists various medical conditions that may be mistaken for hypoglycemia. The rapidity of onset of the hypoglycemic event determines, in part, the presentation. A gradual onset of hypoglycemia results from a relatively slow decrease in the serum glucose and the development of the neuroglycopenic signs and symptoms.

TABLE 224-17 Antimicrobial Therapy in Infected Diabetes-Related Lower Extremity Ulcers

Non–limb-threatening*
Cephalexin, 500 milligrams PO every 6 h, 10-d course
Or
Clindamycin, 300–450 milligrams PO every 6–8 h, 10-d course
Or
Dicloxacillin, 500 milligrams PO every 6 h, 10-d course
Or
Amoxicillin-clavulanate, 875/125 milligrams PO every 12 h, 10-d course
Or
Clarithromycin 500 milligrams PO every 12 h *(in severe penicillin allergy)*
Limb-threatening*
Oral regimen†:
(Ciprofloxacin *or* levofloxacin *or* moxifloxacin) *plus* clindamycin
Or
Trimethoprim-sulfamethoxazole *plus* amoxicillin-clavulanate
IV regimens:
Ampicillin-sulbactam, 3 grams every 6 h
Or
Piperacillin-tazobactam 4.5 grams every 6–8 h
Or
Clindamycin, 900 milligrams every 6 h *plus* (ciprofloxacin, 400 milligrams every 8–12 h *or* ceftriaxone, 1 gram every 12 h)
Life-threatening*
IV regimens:
Imipenem-cilastatin, 500 milligrams every 6 h
Or
Meropenem 1 gram every 8 h
Or
Vancomycin, 15–20 milligram/kg every 12 h, *plus* metronidazole, 500 milligrams every 8 h, *plus* (aztreonam, 2 grams every 6–8 h *or* ciprofloxacin 400 milligrams every 8–12 h) *(if MRSA coverage is warranted)*

Abbreviation: MRSA = methicillin-resistant *Staphylococcus aureus*.

Note: Adjust all dosages for renal/hepatic function and monitor blood levels where appropriate.

*See the section "Lower Extremity and Foot Complications" for definitions.

†This approach is acceptable under special circumstances with close follow-up.

Conversely, a sudden drop in the blood sugar level will produce anxiety, diaphoresis, tremor, and the other hyperepinephrinemic findings. In most cases of hypoglycemia, however, CNS dysfunction predominates, with some degree of alteration in the level of awareness accompanied by diaphoresis and tachycardia.

TABLE 224-18 Differential Diagnosis of Hypoglycemia

Stroke
Transient ischemic attack
Seizure disorder
Traumatic head injury
Brain tumor
Narcolepsy
Multiple sclerosis
Psychosis
Sympathomimetic drug ingestion
Hysteria
Altered sleep patterns and nightmares
Depression

DIAGNOSIS

Diagnosis of hypoglycemia is very straightforward. **Hypoglycemia should always be considered early (including the prehospital setting) as a potential cause of altered mental status.** Failure to determine the blood glucose level early in the evaluation can result in a delayed or missed diagnosis with associated morbidity because of CNS injury or unnecessary invasive procedures and therapies. The diagnosis can easily be confirmed using bedside glucose testing. The accuracy of bedside reflectance tests is acceptable although less reliable at extremely low and high glucose levels. Glucose values of whole blood are approximately 15% less than that of serum or plasma. This discrepancy is a result of the relatively low glucose concentration in red blood cells. Whenever possible, a serum sample should be sent to the laboratory for confirmation of the bedside test result immediately before IV dextrose therapy. **In diabetic patients who develop hypoglycemia while taking the usual dose of sulfonylurea, an underlying cause should be suspected.** Drug interactions, decreased metabolism of the drug, and decreased drug excretion are common precipitating causes.[26]

TREATMENT

Regardless of the cause, management of hypoglycemia in the ED includes prompt diagnosis and PO or IV administration of rapidly metabolized carbohydrates (i.e., glucose or dextrose). In patients with altered mental status, 50% dextrose in water is administered IV as a bolus dose of 50 mL, which provides 25 grams of glucose. This dose may be repeated if hypoglycemia persists. When the patient regains consciousness, carbohydrates should be continued to prevent recurrence of hypoglycemia. This can be accomplished through PO administration of long-acting carbohydrates or continuous IV infusion of dextrose (10% dextrose in water at a rate to maintain the serum glucose >100 milligrams/dL [5.55 mmol/L]). Blood glucose should be determined every 30 minutes for the first 2 hours, looking for rebound hypoglycemia. If hyperglycemia is maintained by slow administration of dextrose, the infusion may be reduced and eventually withdrawn.

Failure to respond to parenteral glucose administration should prompt consideration of other causes of hypoglycemia, such as sepsis, toxin, insulinoma, hepatic failure, or adrenal insufficiency. Hypoglycemia resulting from sulfonylureas is much more challenging than insulin-induced hypoglycemia. Hemodialysis and charcoal hemoperfusion, although mentioned in case reports, are not routinely recommended for sulfonylurea overdose.

Octreotide is a somatostatin analog and is able to suppress insulin secretion. It can be used successfully for the treatment of sulfonylurea-induced hypoglycemia. It is superior to glucose and diazoxide in preventing recurrent hypoglycemia. The ideal dosage and interval of octreotide are not well defined. Recommendations vary from a single 50- to 100-microgram SC injection after a single hypoglycemic episode, to serial SC injections (50 to 100 micrograms every 6 to 8 hours) or constant IV infusion (125 micrograms/h) after a second hypoglycemic episode. Some suggest that the addition of octreotide, 50 micrograms SC, to standard therapy may result in a decrease in frequency of hypoglycemic episodes and an increase in mean plasma glucose.[27] **Octreotide is only recommended after initial glucose therapy has been initiated for sulfonylurea-induced hypoglycemia and can be considered when the response to dextrose is inadequate. It is primarily used to reduce the risk of recurrent hypoglycemia.**

Glucagon is a Food and Drug Administration–approved alternative that may be used SC or IM in the absence of IV access. SC injection of this polypeptide hormone can cause an approximate 100 milligrams/dL (5.55 mmol/L) increase in serum glucose of hypoglycemic patients. Response to glucagon therapy is generally slower when compared with IV dextrose, requiring 7 to 10 minutes for normalization of mental status. Additionally, the response to glucagon administration may be short lived. **In adults, glucagon is administered at the dose of 1 milligram as an SC or IM injection.** Intranasal glucagon has also been used safely in some studies for the treatment of hypoglycemia. Glucagon should be used cautiously in patients with sulfonylurea-induced hypoglycemia.

Diazoxide has also been used in the treatment of refractory sulfonylurea-induced hypoglycemia. It acts by directly inhibiting insulin secretion from pancreatic β cells. Diazoxide may cause hypotension and so should be administered as a slow IV infusion (300 milligrams over 30 minutes every 4 hours).

DISPOSITION AND FOLLOW-UP

Patients who experience hypoglycemia due to sulfonylureas, non–short-acting insulins, or meglitinides should be admitted for serial glucose monitoring and treatment.

REFERENCES

The complete reference list is available online at www.TintinalliEM.com.

Diabetic Ketoacidosis

Andrew L. Nyce
Cary L. Lubkin
Michael E. Chansky

INTRODUCTION AND EPIDEMIOLOGY

Diabetic ketoacidosis (DKA) is an acute, life-threatening complication of diabetes mellitus. DKA occurs predominantly in patients with type 1 (insulin-dependent) diabetes mellitus, but 10% to 30% of cases occur in newly diagnosed type 2 (non–insulin-dependent) diabetes mellitus, especially in African Americans and Hispanics.[1,2] Between 1993 and 2003, the yearly rate of U.S. ED visits for DKA was 64 per 10,000 with a trend toward an increased rate of visits among the African American population compared with the Caucasian population.[3] Europe has a comparable incidence. A better understanding of the pathophysiology of DKA and an aggressive, uniform approach to its diagnosis and management have reduced mortality to <5% of reported episodes in experienced centers.[4] However, mortality is higher in the elderly due to underlying renal disease or coexisting infection and in the presence of coma or hypotension.

PATHOPHYSIOLOGY

Figure 225-1 illustrates the complex relationships between insulin and counterregulatory hormones. DKA is a response to cellular starvation brought on by relative insulin deficiency and counterregulatory or catabolic hormone excess (**Figure 225-1**). Insulin is the only anabolic hormone produced by the endocrine pancreas and is responsible for the metabolism and storage of carbohydrates, fat, and protein. Counterregulatory hormones include glucagon, catecholamines, cortisol, and growth hormone. Complete or relative absence of insulin and the excess counterregulatory hormones result in hyperglycemia (due to excess production and underutilization of glucose), osmotic diuresis, prerenal azotemia, worsening hyperglycemia, ketone formation, and a wide-anion-gap metabolic acidosis.[4]

INSULIN

Ingested glucose is the primary stimulant of insulin release from the β cells of the pancreas. Insulin's main action occurs at the three principal tissues of energy storage and metabolism—the liver, adipose tissue, and skeletal muscle. Insulin acts on the liver to facilitate the uptake of glucose and its conversion to glycogen while inhibiting glycogen breakdown (glycogenolysis) and suppressing gluconeogenesis. The net effect of these actions is to promote the storage of glucose in the form of glycogen. Insulin increases lipogenesis in the liver and adipose cells by producing triglycerides from free fatty acids and glycerol while inhibiting

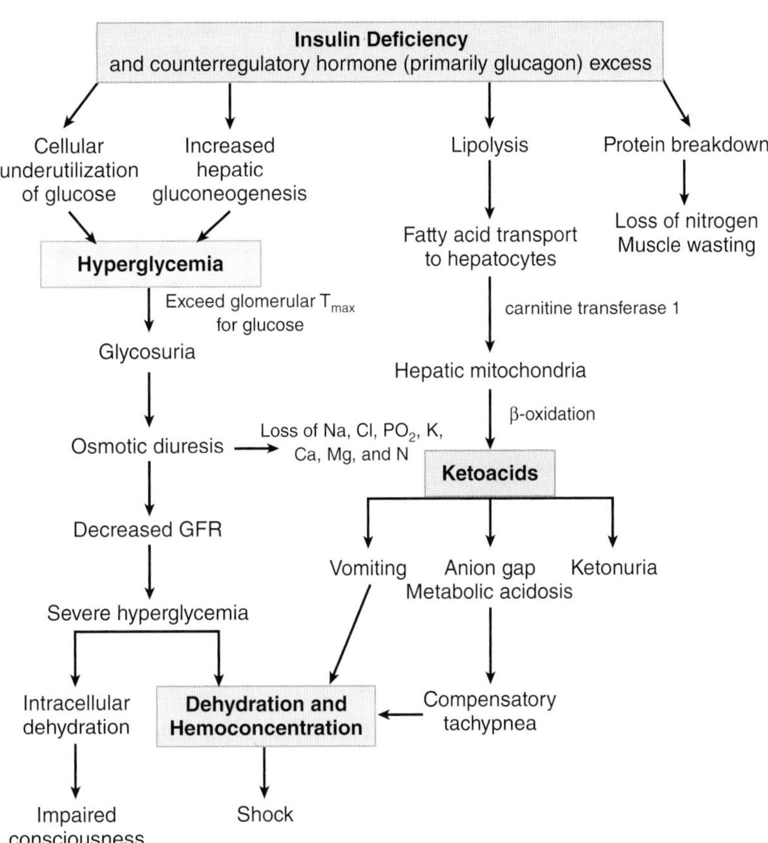

FIGURE 225-1. Insulin deficiency. Pathogenesis of diabetic ketoacidosis secondary to relative insulin deficiency and counterregulatory hormone excess. GFR = glomerular filtration rate.

the breakdown of triglycerides. Insulin stimulates the uptake of amino acids into muscle cells with subsequent incorporation into muscle protein while preventing the release of amino acids from muscle and hepatic protein sources.

Deficiency in insulin secretion due to loss of islet cell mass is the predominant defect in type 1 diabetes mellitus. In the initial stages of diabetes mellitus, the secretory failure of β cells impairs fuel storage and may be evident only during a glucose tolerance test. As levels of insulin decrease, fuel stores are mobilized during fasting, resulting in hyperglycemia. When pancreatic β-cell reserve is present, hyperglycemia may trigger an increase in insulin and a return to normal glucose concentration. With further disease progression, hyperglycemia can no longer trigger an increase in insulin activity. Despite the presence of elevated intravascular glucose, in the absence of insulin, cells are unable to use glucose as a fuel source. The body responds by breaking down protein and adipose stores to try to produce a usable intracellular fuel. Loss of the normal physiologic effects of insulin leads to secretion of catabolic (counterregulatory) hormones and resulting hyperglycemia and ketonemia.

KETOACIDOSIS

The response to cellular starvation seen with insulin insufficiency is increased levels of glucagon, catecholamines, cortisone, and growth hormone. Glucagon is the primary counterregulatory hormone. The catabolic effects of these hormones include increased gluconeogenesis and glycogenolysis, breakdown of fats into free fatty acids and glycerol, and proteolysis with increased levels of amino acids. Increased levels of glucogenic precursors, such as glycerol and amino acids, facilitate gluconeogenesis, worsening hyperglycemia.

Free fatty acids released in the periphery are bound to albumin and transported to the liver, where they undergo conversion to ketone bodies. The primary ketone bodies **β-hydroxybutyrate** (βHB) and **acetoacetic acid** (AcAc) account for the metabolic acidosis seen in DKA. The two are in equilibrium: **AcAc + NADH ⇌ βHB + NAD**. AcAc is metabolized to **acetone**, another major ketone body. Depletion of hepatic glycogen stores favors ketogenesis. Low or absent insulin levels decrease the ability of the brain and cardiac and skeletal muscle to use ketones as an energy source, increasing ketonemia. The persistently elevated serum glucose level eventually causes an osmotic diuresis. The resulting volume depletion worsens hyperglycemia and ketonemia.

The renin-angiotensin-aldosterone system, activated by volume depletion, exacerbates renal potassium losses already occurring from osmotic diuresis. In the kidney, chloride is retained in exchange for the ketoanions being excreted. The loss of ketoanions represents a potential loss of bicarbonate. In the face of marked ketonuria, a superimposed hyperchloremic acidosis is also present. As adipose tissue is broken down, prostaglandins I_2 and E_2 are produced. Both account for paradoxical vasodilation that occurs despite profound levels of volume depletion.

CAUSES OF DKA

Factors known to precipitate DKA are listed in **Table 225-1**.[4] Additional risk factors include poor economic background, lack of insurance or minority status, drug abuse, depression, and the presence of an eating disorder. In many patients, no clear precipitating cause is found.[4]

TABLE 225-1 Important Causes of Diabetic Ketoacidosis

Omission or reduced daily insulin injections
Dislodgement/occlusion of insulin pump catheter
Infection
Pregnancy
Hyperthyroidism, pheochromocytoma, Cushing's syndrome
Substance abuse (cocaine)
Medications: steroids, thiazides, antipsychotics, sympathomimetics
Heat-related illness
Cerebrovascular accident
GI hemorrhage
Myocardial infarction
Pulmonary embolism
Pancreatitis
Major trauma
Surgery

CLINICAL FEATURES

The clinical manifestations of DKA are related directly to hyperglycemia, volume depletion, and acidosis. The metabolic alterations of DKA tend to evolve within 24 hours.[4] Osmotic diuresis gradually leads to volume loss in addition to renal losses of sodium, chloride, potassium, phosphorous, calcium, and magnesium. Initially, patients may compensate by increasing fluid intake, and polyuria and polydipsia are usually the only symptoms until ketonemia and acidosis develop. As acidosis progresses, ventilation is stimulated physiologically by acidemia to diminish the P_{CO_2} and to counter metabolic acidosis. Acidosis combined with the effects of prostaglandins I_2 and E_2 leads to peripheral vasodilation despite profound levels of volume depletion. Prostaglandin release is also felt to play a role in unexplained nausea, vomiting, and abdominal pain that are seen frequently at presentation, especially in children. Vomiting, which may be a maladaptive physiologic response to diminish the acid load, unfortunately exacerbates potassium losses. As volume depletion progresses, poor absorption of SC insulin renders its administration ineffective. Impaired mental status may develop and is most likely multifactorial, related to metabolic acidosis, hyperosmolarity, low extracellular fluid volume, and poor hemodynamics. **Alteration of consciousness has been reported to correlate better with elevated serum osmolality (>320 mOsm/L or >320 mmol/kg) than with severity of metabolic acidosis.**[5]

Tachycardia, orthostasis or hypotension, poor skin turgor, and dry mucous membranes result from volume depletion. **Kussmaul respirations**, increased rate and depth of breathing, may be observed. Acetone produces the characteristic fruity odor on the breath found in some patients. The absence of fever does not exclude infection. Hypothermia is present occasionally because of peripheral vasodilation.

Abdominal pain and tenderness associated with DKA generally correlates with the level of acidosis. Pain can be due to gastric dilatation, ileus, or pancreatitis, but any other acute abdominal disorder can also develop. Due to the frequency of abdominal pain and the presence of an elevated serum amylase or lipase level in both DKA and pancreatitis, distinguishing these two conditions may be difficult. An elevated serum lipase level is more specific to pancreatitis, but it may also be elevated in DKA.

DIAGNOSIS

A blood glucose level >250 milligrams/dL (13.8 mmol/L), an anion gap >10 mEq/L (>10 mmol/L), a bicarbonate level <15 mEq/L (<15 mmol/L), and pH <7.3 with moderate ketonuria or ketonemia constitute the diagnosis of DKA.[4,6] Patients may sometime present with **"euglycemic ketoacidosis"** (glucose <300 milligrams/dL or <16.6 mmol/L), such as those who present just after receiving insulin, type 1 diabetics who are young and vomiting, patients with impaired gluconeogenesis (alcohol abuse or liver failure), patients with low caloric intake/starvation, patients with depression, or pregnant patients. Euglycemic DKA has recently been described as an adverse effect of sodium-glucose cotransporter 2 (SGLT-2) inhibitors (canaglifozin and others). Check blood ketones, venous pH, bicarbonate levels and anion gap) to avoid missing euglycemic DKA, because the degree of hyperglycemia may not be significant (**Table 225-2**).[7]

DIFFERENTIAL DIAGNOSIS

The differential diagnosis of DKA (**Table 225-3**) includes any cause of a high anion gap metabolic acidosis. Patients with hyperosmolar, nonketotic coma tend to be older, have a more prolonged course, and have prominent mental status changes. Serum glucose levels generally are much higher (>600 milligrams/dL or >33.3 mOsm/L), and there is little

TABLE 225-2 Risk Factors for Diabetic Ketoacidosis Patients with Initial Glucose < 300 milligrams/dL (16.6 mmol/L) (Euglycemic Ketoacidosis)
Patients presenting shortly after receiving insulin
Type 1 diabetics who are young and vomiting
Patients with impaired gluconeogenesis (alcohol abuse or liver failure)
Low caloric intake/starvation
Depression
Pregnancy

to no anion gap metabolic acidosis.[4] The ketosis in alcoholic ketoacidosis and starvation ketosis tend to be milder, and the serum glucose level is usually low or normal. βHB predominates in alcoholic ketoacidosis, so the urinary ketone test may be negative or trace positive.

If an ingestion cannot be excluded, serum osmolarity or drug-level testing is required. Renal failure, anion gap acidosis, and liver function abnormalities may be due to acetaminophen toxicity. Depending on the hemodynamic status, lactic acidosis (poor perfusion) may occur simultaneously with DKA; in these cases, determination of the serum lactate level is indicated. **Patients on metformin with new-onset renal insufficiency are at risk for developing type B (aerobic) lactic acidosis.**

LABORATORY TESTING

Obtain a rapid bedside glucose determination, a urine test strip, and an electrocardiogram to check for hyperkalemia, and obtain a CBC, serum electrolytes, BUN and creatinine, urinalysis, venous blood gas, and phosphate/magnesium/calcium levels. Calculate the anion gap. Blood cultures and other laboratory tests should be done as clinically indicated. Arterial blood gas determinations are optional but may be required for the diagnosis and monitoring of critically ill patients.

Ketone Bodies In DKA, elevated serum levels of βHB and AcAc cause acidosis and ketonuria (ketonemia). The **nitroprusside** reagent normally used to detect urine and serum ketones **only detects AcAc**; acetone is only weakly reactive and βHB not at all. Gas chromatography can be used to detect serum acetone but is expensive and time-consuming.

NADH accumulation in mitochondria, as may occur with lactic acidosis or alcohol metabolism, favors the βHB side of equilibrium noted earlier (**AcAc + NADH ⇌ βHB + NAD**). Paradoxically, as the patient is being treated and clinically improves, ketone levels will increase as the body converts the more acidic βHB to AcAc. Therefore, the blood ketone test (Acetest®) that uses the nitroprusside reaction is not a reliable measure for diagnosis or monitoring of DKA. Although not widely available, a new point-of-care capillary blood ketone test for βHB levels may be more sensitive and specific than traditional testing for urine ketones.[6,8] As point-of-care capillary blood ketone testing for βHB becomes more widespread, this test may offer an alternative approach for the diagnosis and monitoring of DKA management compared to traditional measurements of serum HCO_3, anion gap, and pH.[9]

Acid-Base Abnormalities DKA leads to a wide-anion-gap metabolic acidosis. Hyperchloremic acidosis also occurs on the basis of ketoanion exchange for chloride in the urine and is especially common in patients who maintain good hydration status and glomerular filtration rate despite ketoacidosis. Metabolic alkalosis may occur secondary to vomiting, osmotic diuresis, and concomitant diuretic use. Rarely, some patients with DKA may present with normal-appearing [HCO_3^-] or even an elevated [HCO_3^-], if coexisting metabolic alkalosis is severe enough to mask the acidosis. In such situations, an elevated anion gap may be the only clue to the presence of an underlying metabolic acidosis otherwise masked by the concomitant volume contraction–related metabolic alkalosis.

Venous pH has essentially replaced arterial blood gases in the assessment of the acid-base status of the DKA patient. A strong correlation exists between venous and arterial pH in patients with DKA, and the arterial blood gas value does not impact therapy.[10] **Venous pH is about 0.03 lower than arterial pH.** Venous pH obtained during routine phlebotomy should be used to avoid arterial puncture, which is painful and may cause arterial vascular complications.

A low P_{CO_2} determination usually reflects respiratory compensation for metabolic acidosis. If it is lower than explained by the degree of acidosis, a primary respiratory alkalosis exists, which may be an early indication of pulmonary disease (e.g., pneumonia, pulmonary embolus) or sepsis as a possible trigger of DKA. Chapter 15, Acid-Base Disorders, details how compensatory changes in P_{CO_2} can be distinguished from a primary respiratory alkalosis.

Potassium Total-body potassium is depleted by renal losses. **However, the measured serum potassium level is normal or elevated in most patients[4] because of two important factors**: extracellular shift of potassium secondary to acidemia and increased intravascular osmolarity caused by hyperglycemia. Although the actual incidence of initial hypokalemia in DKA is not known, a few studies report an occurrence of 4% to 6%.[5,11,12] **The decrease in serum potassium during therapy is reported to be about 1.5 mEq/L (1.5 mmol/L) and parallels the drop in glucose and the dose of insulin.**[5,11]

Electrocardiogram changes of hyperkalemia or hypokalemia may be seen. The electrocardiogram also should be evaluated for ischemia because myocardial infarction may precipitate DKA.

Sodium and Other Electrolytes Osmotic diuresis leads to excessive renal losses of sodium chloride in the urine. However, the presence of hyperglycemia tends to artificially lower the serum sodium levels. **Standard teaching is that 1.6 mEq (1.6 mmol) should be added to the reported sodium value for every 100 milligrams (5.55 mmol) of glucose >100 milligrams/dL (>5.5 mmol/L). However, the correction factor is probably 2.4, especially for blood glucose levels >400 milligrams/dL (>22.2 mOsm/L).**[13] Osmotic diuresis also causes urinary losses and total-body depletion of phosphorous, calcium, and magnesium. Hemoconcentration frequently leads to initially elevated levels of these electrolytes in serum. As therapy progresses, lower serum levels of each will be evident.

Other Laboratory Values Serum creatinine frequently may be elevated factitiously if the laboratory assay for creatinine is interfered with by the nitroprusside assay. Some elevation in creatinine is expected due to prerenal azotemia. Liver function studies may be elevated because of fatty infiltration of the liver, which gradually corrects as the acidosis is treated. Leukocytosis is often present because of hemoconcentration and stress. However, a WBC count >25,000 mm^3 and/or an absolute band count of 10,000 mm^3 or more is suggestive of infection. Elevation of C-reactive protein may reflect the proinflammatory state found in DKA; elevated levels of cytokines may also be present.

TABLE 225-3 Differential Diagnosis for Diabetic Ketoacidosis
Alcoholic ketoacidosis
Starvation ketoacidosis
Renal failure
Lactic acidosis
Ingestions
Salicylates
Ethylene glycol
Methanol

TREATMENT

The diagnosis of DKA should be suspected at triage, and aggressive fluid therapy should be initiated before receiving the laboratory results[4] (**Figure 225-2**). Place patients on a cardiac monitor and begin at least one large-bore (16- to 18-gauge) IV infusion of normal saline. A second IV line with 0.45% normal saline at minimal rate to keep the IV line open can be considered. The goals of therapy are (1) volume repletion, (2) reversal of the metabolic consequences of insulin insufficiency, (3) correction of electrolyte and acid-base imbalances, (4) recognition and

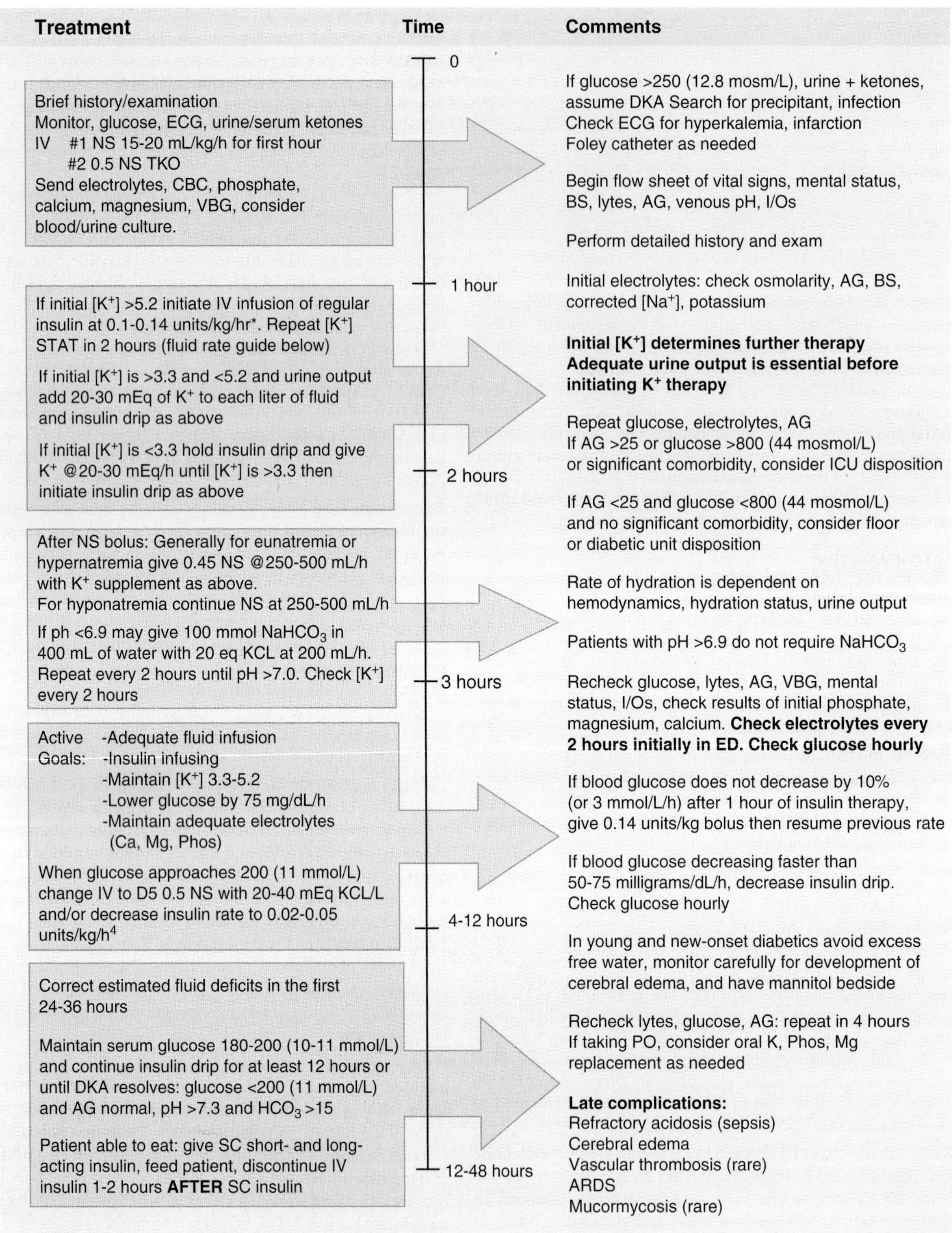

Treatment
Time
Comments
0
Brief history/examination
Monitor, glucose, ECG, urine/serum ketones
IV #1 NS 15-20 mL/kg/h for first hour
#2 0.5 NS TKO
Send electrolytes, CBC, phosphate, calcium, magnesium, VBG, consider blood/urine culture.
If glucose >250 (12.8 mosm/L), urine + ketones, assume DKA Search for precipitant, infection
Check ECG for hyperkalemia, infarction
Foley catheter as needed
Begin flow sheet of vital signs, mental status, BS, lytes, AG, venous pH, I/Os
Perform detailed history and exam
1 hour
If initial [K+] >5.2 initiate IV infusion of regular insulin at 0.1-0.14 units/kg/hr*. Repeat [K+] STAT in 2 hours (fluid rate guide below)
If initial [K+] is >3.3 and <5.2 and urine output add 20-30 mEq of K+ to each liter of fluid and insulin drip as above
If initial [K+] is <3.3 hold insulin drip and give K+ @20-30 mEq/h until [K+] is >3.3 then initiate insulin drip as above
Initial electrolytes: check osmolarity, AG, BS, corrected [Na+], potassium
Initial [K+] determines further therapy
Adequate urine output is essential before initiating K+ therapy
Repeat glucose, electrolytes, AG
If AG >25 or glucose >800 (44 mosmol/L) or significant comorbidity, consider ICU disposition
2 hours
If AG <25 and glucose <800 (44 mosmol/L) and no significant comorbidity, consider floor or diabetic unit disposition
After NS bolus: Generally for eunatremia or hypernatremia give 0.45 NS @250-500 mL/h with K+ supplement as above.
For hyponatremia continue NS at 250-500 mL/h
If ph <6.9 may give 100 mmol NaHCO3 in 400 mL of water with 20 eq KCL at 200 mL/h. Repeat every 2 hours until pH >7.0. Check [K+] every 2 hours
Rate of hydration is dependent on hemodynamics, hydration status, urine output
Patients with pH >6.9 do not require NaHCO3
3 hours
Recheck glucose, lytes, AG, VBG, mental status, I/Os, check results of initial phosphate, magnesium, calcium. Check electrolytes every 2 hours initially in ED. Check glucose hourly
Active Goals: -Adequate fluid infusion
-Insulin infusing
-Maintain [K+] 3.3-5.2
-Lower glucose by 75 mg/dL/h
-Maintain adequate electrolytes (Ca, Mg, Phos)
When glucose approaches 200 (11 mmol/L) change IV to D5 0.5 NS with 20-40 mEq KCL/L and/or decrease insulin rate to 0.02-0.05 units/kg/h4
If blood glucose does not decrease by 10% (or 3 mmol/L/h) after 1 hour of insulin therapy, give 0.14 units/kg bolus then resume previous rate
If blood glucose decreasing faster than 50-75 milligrams/dL/h, decrease insulin drip. Check glucose hourly
4-12 hours
In young and new-onset diabetics avoid excess free water, monitor carefully for development of cerebral edema, and have mannitol bedside
Correct estimated fluid deficits in the first 24-36 hours
Maintain serum glucose 180-200 (10-11 mmol/L) and continue insulin drip for at least 12 hours or until DKA resolves: glucose <200 (11 mmol/L) and AG normal, pH >7.3 and HCO3 >15
Patient able to eat: give SC short- and long-acting insulin, feed patient, discontinue IV insulin 1-2 hours AFTER SC insulin
Recheck lytes, glucose, AG: repeat in 4 hours
If taking PO, consider oral K, Phos, Mg replacement as needed
Late complications:
Refractory acidosis (sepsis)
Cerebral edema
Vascular thrombosis (rare)
ARDS
Mucormycosis (rare)
12-48 hours

FIGURE 225-2. Timeline for the typical adult patient with suspected diabetic ketoacidosis (DKA). *IV insulin infusion <1.0 units/kg/hr may require a bolus dose of regular insulin (0.1 unit/kg)[4]. AG = anion gap; ARDS = acute respiratory distress syndrome; BS = blood sugar; ECG = electrocardiogram; ICU = intensive care unit; I/Os = inputs/outputs; NS = normal saline; TKO = to keep vein open; VBG = venous blood gas.

treatment of precipitating causes; and (5) avoidance of complications. **The order of therapeutic priorities is volume first and foremost, correction of potassium deficits, and then insulin administration.** Metabolic disturbances should be corrected at the approximate rate of occurrence or over 24 to 36 hours.

Meeting the goals of safely replacing deficits and supplying missing insulin requires monitoring every 2 hours of electrolytes (glucose, potassium, and anion gap), vital signs, level of consciousness, and volume input/output until recovery is well established. **The goal of treatment is glucose <200 milligrams/dL (<11.1 mmol/L), bicarbonate ≥18 mEq/L (≥18 mmol/L), and venous pH >7.3.**

VOLUME REPLETION

Fluid helps restore intravascular volume and normal tonicity, perfuse vital organs, improve glomerular filtration rate, and lower serum glucose and ketone levels.[4] Rehydration improves the response to low-dose insulin therapy.[4] The average adult patient has a water deficit of 100 mL/kg (5 to 10 L) and a sodium deficit of 7 to 10 mEq/kg (7 to 10 mmol/L/kg).[4] Normal saline is the most frequently recommended fluid for initial volume repletion even though the extracellular fluid of the patient is initially hypertonic.[14] Normal saline does not provide "free water" to correct intracellular fluid loss, but it does prevent an excessively rapid fall in extracellular osmolarity and the potential devastating transfer of excessive water into the CNS. After initial resuscitation with normal saline, change fluids to 0.45% normal saline once the corrected serum sodium is normal or elevated.[6,7]

Based on clinical suspicion alone and before initial electrolyte results, **administer the initial fluid bolus of isotonic saline at a rate of 15 to 20 mL/kg/h during the first hour** unless there are mitigating circumstances.[6] The rate of hydration should depend on hemodynamic stability, hydration status, urine output, and serum electrolytes. After the initial bolus, administer normal saline at 250 to 500 cc/h in hyponatremic patients, or give 0.45% normal saline at 250 to 500 cc/h for eunatremic and hypernatremic patients.[7] **In general, the first 2 L are administered rapidly over 0 to 2 hours, the next 2 L over 2 to 6 hours, and then an additional 2 L over 6 to 12 hours.** This replaces approximately 50% of the total water deficit over the first 12 hours, with the remaining 50% water deficit to be replaced over the subsequent 12 hours. When the blood glucose level is 250 milligrams/dL (13.8 mmol/L), change to 5% dextrose in 0.45% normal saline. Patients without extreme volume depletion can be managed safely with a more modest fluid replacement regimen such as 250 to 500 mL/h for 4 hours. Consider central venous pressure or pulmonary artery wedge pressure monitoring in the elderly or in those with heart or renal disease. Excess fluid may contribute to the development of adult respiratory distress syndrome and cerebral edema.

POTASSIUM REPLACEMENT

Patients in DKA usually present with profound total-body potassium deficits in the range of 3 to 5 mEq/kg (3 to 5 mmol/kg).[4] This deficit is created by insulin deficiency, metabolic acidosis, osmotic diuresis, and frequent vomiting. Only 2% of total-body potassium is intravascular. The initial serum concentration is usually normal or high because of the intracellular exchange of potassium for hydrogen ions during acidosis, the total-body fluid deficit, and diminished renal function. **Initial hypokalemia indicates severe total-body potassium deficits, and large amounts of replacement potassium are usually necessary in the first 24 to 36 hours.**

Correction of the acidosis predicts the change in serum potassium concentration. **For each 0.1 decrease in pH, serum potassium concentration rises approximately 0.5 mEq/L (0.5 mmol/L)**, and the same relationship holds as the pH increases. This can be used as a guide for estimating the serum potassium concentration when pH balance is restored.

Hypokalemia During initial therapy for DKA, the serum potassium concentration may fall rapidly, primarily due to the action of insulin promoting reentry of potassium into cells and, to a lesser degree, the dilution of extracellular fluid, correction of acidosis, and increased urinary loss of potassium. If these changes occur too rapidly, precipitous hypokalemia may result in fatal cardiac arrhythmias, respiratory paralysis, paralytic ileus, and rhabdomyolysis. **The rapid development of severe hypokalemia is potentially the most life-threatening electrolyte derangement during the treatment of DKA.**[4]

As a general guideline, an initial serum potassium level >3.3 mEq/L (>3.3 mmol/L) but <5.2 mEq/L (<5.2 mmol/L) (before fluid resuscitation and insulin, coupled with urine output) calls for 20 to 30 mEq/L (20 to 30 mmol/L) for at least 4 hours to keep K^+ between 4 and 5 mEq/L (4 and 5 mmol/L).[6] Because the most rapid changes occur during the first few hours of therapy, measure the plasma potassium level initially every 2 hours. If oliguria or renal insufficiency is present, withhold or decrease potassium replacement.

Initial hypokalemia (<3.3 mEq/L or <3.3 mmol/L) is uncommon but necessitates a more aggressive replacement before insulin therapy.[4] In this setting, give potassium IV at 20 to 30 mEq/h (20 to 30 mmol/h) and hold insulin until $[K^+]$ is ≥3.5 mEq/L (≥3.5 mmol/L).[6,7] There is no advantage to using potassium phosphate (K_2PO_4) compared to potassium chloride because K_2PO_4 may result in hypocalcemia and metastatic precipitation of calcium phosphate in tissues. Oral potassium replacement is safe and effective and is the preferred route of replacement as soon as the patient can tolerate oral fluids. In DKA, initial potassium replacement is usually by an intravenous line. Each institution may have specific guidelines for potassium replacement, but a general approach is a rate no faster than 10 mEq/h (10 mmol/h) via peripheral IV or 20 mEq/h (20 mmol/h) via central line access. Continuous electrocardiogram monitoring is generally recommended while replacing potassium in the severely hypokalemic patient. During the first 24 hours, 100 to 200 mEq or mmol of KCl is usually required.

Hyperkalemia **Obtain an electrocardiogram immediately and check for signs of hyperkalemia once DKA is suspected.**

Giving potassium to a patient in a hyperkalemic potentiating state (i.e., acidemia, insulin deficiency, volume contraction, renal insufficiency) may dangerously increase the extracellular potassium level and precipitate fatal dysrhythmias. The initial measurement of serum electrolytes, electrocardiogram review for signs of hyperkalemia, and the presence of urine output determine initial potassium therapy. An initial serum potassium level >5.2 mEq/L usually reflects a more profound acidemia and volume depletion, or renal insufficiency. Fluid and insulin therapy alone usually will lower the serum potassium level rapidly. Albuterol nebulization can provide an additional quick potassium-lowering effect. See chapter 17, Fluids and Electrolytes, for further treatment of hyperkalemia.

INSULIN

Low-dose regular insulin administration by an infusion pump is simple and safe, ensures a steady blood concentration of insulin, allows flexibility in adjusting the insulin dose, and promotes a gradual fall in serum glucose and ketone body levels.[4] The half-life of IV insulin is 4 to 5 minutes, with an effective biologic half-life at the tissue level of approximately 20 to 30 minutes.

IV Insulin After the initial fluid bolus, or simultaneously in a second IV line, **administer insulin at a rate of 0.1 to 0.14 unit/kg/h with no insulin bolus once hypokalemia ([K+] <3.3 mEq/L [<3.3 mmol/L]) is excluded.** An alternative insulin regimen is 0.1 unit/kg bolus IM, if it is difficult to establish another IV line,[9] followed by a drip rate at 0.1 unit/kg/h.[7] An IV loading dose of insulin is not recommended in children and new-onset young adult diabetics and is optional in adults.[9,15] Plasma glucose concentration typically decreases by 50 to 75 milligrams/dL/h (2.8 to 4.2 mmol/L/h), but if the blood glucose fails to drop by 10% 1 hour after initial therapy, or 3 mmol/L/h, (assuming adequate hydration), give a 0.14 unit/kg bolus and resume insulin drip rate.[6,7] **Another option is to increase the insulin infusion rate by 1 unit/h.**[9] The incidence of nonresponse to low-dose continuous IV insulin administration is 1% to 2%, with infection being the primary reason for failure to respond.

Resolution of hyperglycemia usually occurs earlier than resolution of the anion gap, so **once the serum glucose is 200 milligrams/dL (11 mmol/L), add dextrose to the IV fluids and reduce the insulin drip rate to 0.02 to 0.05 unit/kg/h.** Maintain the serum glucose between 150 and 200 milligrams/dL (8.3 and 11 mmol/L) until the resolution of DKA.[7] Occasionally a 10% dextrose solution may be needed to maintain glucose levels.[9] **Continue the insulin infusion until the resolution of DKA—glucose <200 milligrams/dL (<11 mmol/L) and two of the following: a serum bicarbonate level >15 mEq/L, a venous pH >7.3, and/or a normal calculated anion gap.**[7] Monitor laboratory values every 1 to 2 hours to ensure that insulin is being administered in the desired amount.

Transition from IV Insulin After DKA Correction **A transition from the IV insulin infusion to SC insulin is necessary to avoid relapse to hyperglycemia or DKA when the insulin infusion is stopped.** Relapse can occur quickly, within an hour after IV insulin is stopped, due to the short duration of action of IV insulin. The method of insulin transition varies, and there is no set protocol. Once the patient eats, the glucose infusion can be stopped. In patients who can eat, the transition should include a short-acting and long-acting insulin given when DKA has resolved. It is best to collaborate with the inpatient team or endocrinologist to develop a protocol for the transition to SC insulin. One method consists of giving 10 units of SC regular insulin 30 to 60 minutes before the insulin infusion is stopped and 80% of the usual long-acting insulin dose 1 to 2 hours before discontinuing the IV insulin infusion. Another method is to give 50% of the usual long-acting insulin dose 2 hours before the IV insulin infusion is stopped (see Figure 223-1, for onset and duration of action of long-acting insulins). If the patient is a newly diagnosed diabetic, one can estimate a starting dose of long-acting insulin at 0.1 to 0.2 unit/kg. Additional glucose coverage can be provided with short-acting insulin as needed. Continue glucose checks every hour for 2 hours. Further intervals for glucose checks and the need for additional SC regular insulin dosing depend on the patient's response and institutional protocols.

SC Insulin In uncomplicated mild to moderate DKA, the use of rapid-acting SC insulin may be another treatment option, although the standard treatment remains continuous IV insulin.[4,7,16] The dose of SC rapid-acting insulin is an initial injection of 0.2 unit/kg followed by 0.1 unit/kg every hour, or an initial dose of 0.3 unit/kg followed by 0.2 unit/kg every 2 hours until blood glucose is <250 milligrams/dL (<13.8 mmol/L). Then, the insulin dose is decreased by half and administered every 1 or 2 hours until resolution of DKA.[4,7] This can avoid intensive care admissions and lower hospital costs, but still requires close nursing monitoring that is difficult to accomplish in the ED or in a regular hospital bed.

HYPOPHOSPHATEMIA

Serum phosphate levels often are normal or increased on presentation of DKA and do not reflect the total-body phosphate deficits secondary to enhanced urinary losses.[11] Phosphate (similar to glucose and potassium) reenters the intracellular space during insulin therapy, resulting in low phosphate concentrations. Hypophosphatemia is usually most severe 24 to 48 hours after the start of insulin therapy. Acute phosphate deficiency (<1.0 milligram/dL) can result in hypoxia, skeletal muscle weakness, rhabdomyolysis, hemolysis, respiratory failure, and cardiac dysfunction.

There is no established role for initiating IV K_2PO_4 for DKA in the ED.[4,7,11] In general, do not give IV phosphate unless the serum phosphate concentration is <1.0 milligram/dL (0.323 millimol/L). Significant hypophosphatemia tends to develop many hours into therapy, after the patient is already admitted. Undesirable side effects from IV phosphate administration include hyperphosphatemia, hypocalcemia, hypomagnesemia, metastatic soft tissue calcifications, hypernatremia, and volume loss from osmotic diuresis. If *absolutely* necessary (a phosphate level <1.0 milligram/dL early in therapy), IV phosphate replacement should be administered as IV K_2PO_4, 2.5 to 5 milligrams/kg (0.08 to 0.16 millimol/kg).[17] Monitor serum calcium level if giving supplemental phosphate.

HYPOMAGNESEMIA

Osmotic diuresis may cause hypomagnesemia and deplete magnesium stores from bone. Hypomagnesemia may inhibit parathyroid hormone secretion, causing hypocalcemia and hyperphosphatemia. If the serum magnesium concentration is <2.0 mEq/L (<1.0 mmol/L) or symptoms are suggestive of hypomagnesemia, give magnesium sulfate 2 grams IV over 1 hour. Obtain serum magnesium and calcium levels on presentation and 24 hours into therapy. Monitor levels every 2 hours if there is initial hypomagnesemia or hypocalcemia or if symptoms suggestive of hypomagnesemia or hypocalcemia occur.

BICARBONATE

Acidotic patients routinely recover from DKA without alkali therapy, as fluid and insulin therapy inhibit lipolysis and resolve ketoacidosis without added bicarbonate.[4] **Give bicarbonate if the initial pH is ≤6.9, but do not give bicarbonate if the pH is ≥7.0.**[7,16,18,19]

Severe metabolic acidosis is associated with numerous cardiovascular (impaired contractility, vasodilation, and hypotension) and neurologic (cerebral vasodilation and coma) complications. Theoretical advantages of bicarbonate include improved myocardial contractility, elevated ventricular fibrillation threshold, improved catecholamine tissue response, and decreased work of breathing. The disadvantages of bicarbonate include worsening hypokalemia, paradoxical CNS acidosis, worsening intracellular acidosis, impaired (shift to left) oxyhemoglobin dissociation, hypertonicity and sodium overload, delayed recovery from ketosis, elevation of lactate levels, and possible precipitation of cerebral edema. During DKA treatment, hydrogen ion production ceases when ketogenesis stops; excessive hydrogen ions are eliminated through the urine and respiratory tract. Ketone body metabolism results in the endogenous production of alkali.

The decision to use bicarbonate in DKA patients should be based on the clinical condition and pH of the patient. Potential benefits of bicarbonate in the elderly with cardiovascular instability must be balanced against the potential disadvantages.[4] There may be selected patients who benefit from cautious alkali therapy, including those with decreased cardiac contractility and peripheral vasodilatation, and patients with life-threatening hyperkalemia and coma. Patients with severe acidosis may be at higher risk for clinical deterioration, so **adults with a pH <6.9 can be given 100 mEq (100 mmol) of sodium bicarbonate in 400 mL of water with 20 mEq (20 mmol) KCl at 200 mL/h for 2 hours until the venous pH >7.0.** If the pH remains <7.0 despite the infusion, repeat the infusion until pH >7.0.[6,7] Remember to check [K^+] every 2 hours. Severe acidosis (pH <7.0) and worsening pH despite aggressive therapy for DKA should prompt investigation for other causes of metabolic acidosis (see chapter 15).

DISEASE COMPLICATIONS

COMPLICATIONS RELATED TO ACUTE DISEASE

In general, the greater the initial serum osmolality, BUN, and blood glucose concentrations, and the lower the serum bicarbonate level (<10 mEq/L), the greater the mortality.

Infection and myocardial infarction are the main contributors to mortality. Additional factors that increase morbidity include old age, severe hypotension, coma, and underlying renal and cardiovascular disease. Severe volume depletion leaves the elderly at risk for deep venous thrombosis.

COMPLICATIONS RELATED TO THERAPY

Major complications related to therapy of DKA are listed in **Table 225-4.** These include hypoglycemia, hypokalemia, hypophosphatemia, acute respiratory distress syndrome, and cerebral edema. A gradual return to normal metabolic balance will diminish the likelihood of such outcomes.

Acute respiratory distress syndrome is a rare complication of therapy but can develop, particularly in the elderly and those with impaired myocardial contractility. Overly aggressive fluid therapy decreases plasma oncotic pressure and raises left atrial end-diastolic pressure, favoring a shift of fluid across the pulmonary capillary membrane.

In very young children, new-onset diabetics, and adolescents with DKA, **cerebral edema** remains the most common and feared cause of mortality[20-24] (see chapter 145, Diabetes in Children). Young age and new-onset diabetes (particularly in young adolescents) are the only identified potential risk factors. There are no evidence-based recommendations for adults.[4] Cerebral edema is often seen when the patient appears to be improving clinically and biochemically, and carries a high mortality.[22-24] One hypothesis is that the osmotic diuresis promotes loss of water and sodium from both intra- and extracellular spaces. Hyperglycemia leads to a hyperosmolar extracellular state. Brain cells enzymatically produce osmotically active particles that protect cells from further loss of water and shrinkage. During therapy with IV fluid and insulin, water moves into brain cells faster than osmotically active particles can dissipate, promoting cellular swelling.

There are no specific presentation or treatment variables that predict or contribute to the development of cerebral edema.[21,22] Gradual replacement of water and sodium deficits and slow correction of hyperglycemia may lessen the risk.

TABLE 225-4 Potential Pitfalls During Treatment of DKA

Pitfall	Guideline (See Text for Details)
Delay in diagnosis	Blood glucose may be 250–300 milligrams/dL (13.8–16.6 mmol/L); urine ketones may initially be negative
Unrecognized precipitating illness	Check electrocardiogram for infarction; examine patient for site of infection
Inadequate fluids	Majority of adult patients tolerate 15–20 cc/kg/h normal saline for first hour (1–2 L normal saline), additional fluids by clinical condition/serum Na^+
Unrecognized low K^+	Check K^+ prior to insulin; K^+ supplement before insulin for $[K^+]$ <3.3
Overemphasis on insulin	Follow insulin guidelines
Hypoglycemia	Goal for glucose decrease 50–75 milligrams/dL/h (2.8–4.2 mmol/L); add dextrose when glucose <250 milligrams/dL (<13.8 mmol/L)
Unrecognized electrolyte derangements	During first 6 hours of treatment, check glucose hourly and electrolytes every 2 hours
Overzealous use of bicarbonate and phosphate	$NaHCO_3$ not indicated for pH >6.9; no routine indication for phosphate supplementation
Recurrent DKA	Avoid stopping insulin drip until anion gap resolves. Give subcutaneous insulin, feed patient, stop insulin drip 1–2 h before stopping insulin drip.
Cerebral edema **NOT** recognized early	See **Table 225-5**. Very young and new-onset patients at risk; perform frequent neurologic checks for mental status change

Premonitory symptoms are severe headache, incontinence, change in arousal or behavior, pupillary changes, blood pressure changes, seizures, bradycardia, or disturbed temperature regulation. Any change in neurologic function early in therapy is an indication for IV mannitol (1 to 2 grams/kg).[24] Mannitol should be given before respiratory failure or obtaining confirmatory CT scans because serious morbidity and mortality may be prevented. Hypertonic saline (3%), 5 to 10 mL/kg over 30 minutes, may be an alternative to mannitol.[20,22] Intubation and fluid restriction are generally necessary. There are no data supporting glucocorticoid use in DKA-related cerebral edema.

LATER COMPLICATIONS

Metabolic acidosis refractory to routine therapy may be secondary to unrecognized infection (lactic acidosis), rarely insulin antibodies, or improper preparation or administration of the insulin drip. Shock that is unresponsive to aggressive fluid therapy suggests gram-negative bacteremia or silent myocardial infarction. Hyperchloremic non–anion gap metabolic acidosis can develop during therapy due to rapid volume expansion in the face of reduced bicarbonate. In addition, bicarbonate equivalents are excreted in the urine as ketones and are replaced with chloride provided by the normal saline. This emphasizes the importance of monitoring the anion gap during therapy. The non–anion gap metabolic acidosis resolves during recovery as bicarbonate is regenerated and excess chloride is excreted in the urine.

Late vascular thrombosis may occur in any muscular artery, although the cerebral vessels appear to be most susceptible. Volume depletion, low cardiac output, increased blood viscosity, and underlying atherosclerosis may predispose the elderly to this complication. Thrombosis may occur several hours or days after institution of therapy and after resolution of ketoacidosis. Despite this increased risk, no studies support prophylactic anticoagulant use, although some experts suggest the use of heparin may be beneficial in DKA if there is no associated bleeding disorder.[7,14]

Mortality in DKA results mainly from sepsis or pulmonary and cardiovascular complications in the elderly and fatal cerebral edema in children and young adults (**Table 225-6**).

TABLE 225-5 Best Practice to Prevent Cerebral Edema

Slow reduction of osmolality during treatment
Avoid large volumes of hypotonic fluid
Drop blood glucose slowly during treatment
Do not allow plasma Na^+ to fall during treatment
Avoid unnecessary bicarbonate during treatment
Avoid hypoxia, hypo-K^+, PO_4, Mg

DISPOSITION AND FOLLOW-UP

The great majority of patients require hospitalization in a monitored setting where there is nursing experience with IV insulin infusions. In many institutions, patients are cared for initially in an intensive or intermediate care unit. A select group of patients with an anion gap of <25, a glucose level of <600 milligrams/dL (<33.3 mmol/L), and no comorbidity at the time of disposition decision may be managed safely on an inpatient unit with nursing expertise using insulin infusions and managing diabetic patients. Some institutions may have protocols for the use of SC rapid-acting insulin on a medical floor. Patients presenting early in the course of their illness who can tolerate oral liquids may be managed safely in the ED or observation unit and discharged after 6 to 12 hours of therapy.

SPECIAL POPULATIONS

RECURRENT DKA PATIENTS

Patients who present to the ED with recurrent episodes of DKA should have barriers to care access addressed while in the ED or during their hospital stay. In urban settings, insulin noncompliance is a major trigger for recurrent DKA. Cocaine is an independent risk factor for DKA, and patients who use illicit drugs may benefit from drug rehabilitation.[6,7] Using social workers to assist patients with drug access and affordability, drug rehabilitation when indicated, and education provided by the diabetic care team can promote improved glycemic control.[26]

PATIENTS WITH INSULIN PUMPS

See chapter 223, for a detailed discussion of insulin pumps. **Patients with insulin pumps who are suspected to have DKA should have their pumps disconnected and turned off and should be treated just like any other patient. Reinstitution of pump therapy should start in the same time frame as switching over to SC insulin in the non–pump user.**

TABLE 225-6 Complications of Diabetic Ketoacidosis

Related to Acute Disease	Related to Therapy	Later Complications
Loss of airway	Hypokalemia	Recurrent anion gap metabolic acidosis
Sepsis	Hypophosphatemia	Non–anion gap metabolic acidosis
Myocardial infarction	Acute respiratory distress syndrome	Vascular thrombosis
Hypovolemic shock	Cerebral edema	Mucormycosis
	Hypoglycemia	

DKA IN PREGNANCY

DKA in pregnancy is a leading cause of fetal loss, with a fetal mortality rate of approximately 30%.[25,26] Several physiologic changes make diabetic pregnant women prone to DKA. Maternal fasting serum glucose levels are normally lower, which leads to relative insulin deficiency and an increase in baseline free fatty acid levels in the blood. DKA is triggered at lower sugar levels in pregnancy.[24] Pregnant women normally have increased levels of counterregulatory hormones. In addition, the chronic respiratory alkalosis seen in pregnancy leads to decreased bicarbonate levels due to a compensatory renal response, resulting in a decrease in buffering capacity. Pregnancy is associated with vomiting and urinary tract infections, which can precipitate DKA. Maternal hyperglycemia causes fetal hyperglycemia and osmotic diuresis. Maternal acidosis causes fetal acidosis, decreases uterine blood flow and fetal oxygenation, and shifts the oxygen-hemoglobin dissociation curve to the right. Maternal hypokalemia also can lead to fetal dysrhythmias and death. **Correction of maternal hyperglycemia, acidosis, and electrolyte balance are the first priorities.**

REFERENCES

The complete reference list is available online at www.TintinalliEM.com.

Alcoholic Ketoacidosis

William A. Woods
Debra G. Perina

INTRODUCTION

Alcoholic ketoacidosis is a wide anion gap metabolic acidosis, most often associated with acute cessation of alcohol consumption after chronic alcohol abuse, and is typically associated with nausea, vomiting, and vague GI complaints.[1] Metabolism of alcohol combined with little or no glycogen reserves results in elevated ketoacid levels. Although alcoholic ketoacidosis is usually seen in chronic alcoholics, it has been described in first-time binge drinkers. Repeated episodes can occur.[2] Although with proper treatment this illness is self-limited, death has been reported from presumed excessive ketonemia.[2-4]

PATHOPHYSIOLOGY

Ethanol metabolism requires nicotinamide adenine dinucleotide (NAD) and the enzymes alcohol dehydrogenase and aldehyde dehydrogenase to convert ethanol to acetyl coenzyme A. Acetyl coenzyme A may be metabolized directly, resulting in ketoacid production; used as substrate for the Krebs cycle; or used for free fatty acid synthesis (**Figure 226-1**).

Alcoholic ketoacidosis occurs when NAD is depleted by ethanol metabolism, resulting in inhibition of the aerobic metabolism in the Krebs cycle, depletion of glycogen stores, ketone formation, and lipolysis stimulation. Ethanol metabolism results in NAD depletion manifesting as a higher ratio of the reduced form of nicotinamide adenine dinucleotide (NADH) to NAD. When glycogen stores are depleted in a patient stressed by concurrent illness or volume depletion, insulin secretion is also suppressed. Under these same conditions, glucagon, catecholamine, and growth hormone secretion are all stimulated. This hormonal milieu inhibits aerobic metabolism in favor of anaerobic metabolism and stimulates lipolysis. Acetyl coenzyme A is metabolized to the ketoacids, β-hydroxybutyrate (βHB) and acetoacetate.

NAD is used in the conversion of βHB to acetoacetate (AcAc + NADH $\rightleftharpoons$ βHB + NAD). Due to the depletion of NAD, βHB is the predominant ketone product formed. Normally, the ratio of acetoacetate to βHB is 1:1; however, in alcoholic ketoacidosis, the ratio can be 1:7 or higher.[5] Once the NADH:NAD returns to normal, lactate levels decrease and acetoacetate increases.[1] The ratio of βHB to acetoacetate is also much higher in alcoholic ketoacidosis than in diabetic ketoacidosis.[1] The high NADH:NAD ratio also results in increased lactate production, so lactate levels are higher than normal in alcoholic ketoacidosis but not as high as in shock or sepsis. Acetoacetate is metabolized to acetone so that acetone and its metabolites are elevated and may cause an osmolal gap.

Ketone production can be further stimulated in malnourished, vomiting patients or in those who are hypophosphatemic.[6] Both conditions are seen commonly in alcoholic patients with alcoholic ketoacidosis.

CLINICAL FEATURES

The typical history is an episode of heavy drinking followed by vomiting and an acute decrease in alcohol consumption. The most common symptoms are nausea, vomiting, and nonspecific abdominal pain.[2] Associated gastritis or pancreatitis may occur. Mental status changes are typically secondary to other causes, such as toxic ingestion, hypoglycemia, alcohol-withdrawal seizures, postictal state, or unrecognized head injury.

DIAGNOSIS

Diagnosis is made in the appropriate clinical setting and is based on laboratory evaluation. Laboratory evaluation should include CBC; electrolyte panel with calcium, phosphate, and magnesium; ethanol, methanol, and isopropyl alcohol levels; hepatic enzymes; lipase; and serum ketones. Determination of serum lactic acid level and serum osmolality also may be helpful. Diagnosis is made by the criteria listed in **Table 226-1**, with metabolic acidosis, positive serum ketones, elevated anion gap, and a low or mildly elevated serum glucose level. Patients frequently have hypophosphatemia, hyponatremia, and/or hypokalemia. Most patients also will have elevated bilirubin and liver enzyme levels due to liver disease from a long history of chronic ethanol use. BUN levels frequently are elevated due to relative volume depletion. The nitroprusside reagent used to measure urine and serum ketones measures acetoacetate. Acetone is

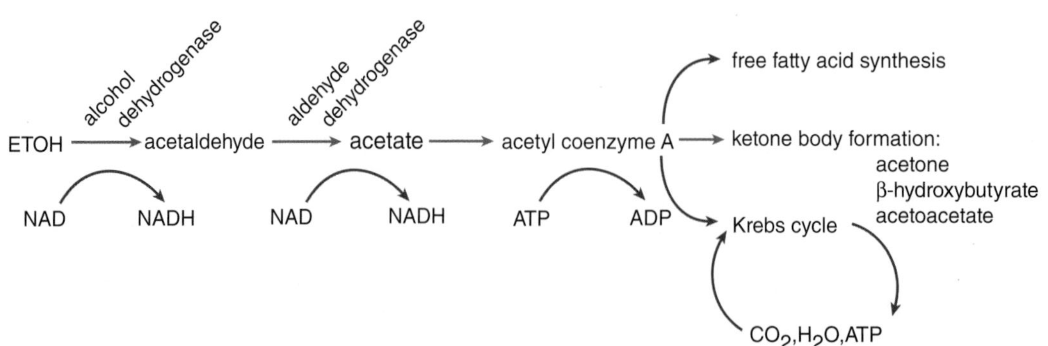

FIGURE 226-1. Ethanol metabolism. ADP = adenosine diphosphate; ATP = adenosine triphosphate; ETOH = ethanol; NAD = nicotinamide adenine dinucleotide; NADH = the reduced form of nicotinamide adenine dinucleotide.

TABLE 226-1 Diagnostic Criteria for Alcoholic Ketoacidosis*

Low, normal, or slightly elevated serum glucose
Binge drinking ending in nausea, vomiting, and decreased intake
Wide anion gap metabolic acidosis
Positive serum ketones*
Wide anion gap metabolic acidosis without alternate explanation

*The absence of ketones in the serum based on the nitroprusside test does not exclude the diagnosis.

weakly reactive, and βHB is not detected at all. So, the initial ketone levels may be low or negative in alcoholic ketoacidosis. With recovery, acetoacetate increases and assays become positive.[1] A small to moderate anion gap is invariable in alcoholic ketoacidosis. **Without routine evaluation of the anion gap in every patient at risk for alcoholic ketoacidosis, the diagnosis can be easily missed.** The anion gap is usually 16 to 33, with a mean of 21,[2] and is due to ketonemia, primarily from βHB. The osmolal gap may be slightly elevated because acetone and its metabolites cause an osmolal gap (<20 mmol/kg).[1] Consider co-ingestions or other causes of anion gap acidosis if the anion gap fails to close with ongoing treatment. Mild lactic acidosis may be present due to a shift to pyruvate metabolism toward lactate[1].

DIFFERENTIAL DIAGNOSIS

Table 226-2 and chapter 15, Acid-Base Disorders, list the most important causes of metabolic acidosis that should be excluded to diagnose alcoholic ketoacidosis.

Alcoholic ketoacidosis should be differentiated from other alcohol ingestions. Methanol and ethylene glycol ingestions do not produce ketosis, and acidosis tends to be severe. Isopropyl alcohol ingestion results in production of ketones. The presence of a large osmolal gap suggests acute isopropyl, ethanol, methanol, or ethylene glycol ingestion. If the blood alcohol level is known, then its contribution to any osmolal gap can be calculated. **Each 100 milligrams/dL (21.7 mmol/L) of ethanol raises the osmolal gap by 22.** Details of osmolal gap are discussed in chapter 17, Fluids and Electrolytes.

The presence of a mixed acid-base disturbance suggests a comorbid disorder. Common concurrent illnesses are dehydration and electrolyte disturbances from vomiting and reduced intake, pancreatitis, gastritis or upper GI bleeding, seizures, alcohol withdrawal, pneumonia, sepsis, and hepatitis.

Starvation ketosis occurs in patients with diminished carbohydrate intake, resulting in lipolysis and ketonuria. Ketone bodies appear after about 3 days of fasting but can appear earlier in the presence of stress and dehydration. Metabolic acidosis and ketonemia are rare in starvation ketosis, but ketonuria is common.[7]

TABLE 226-2 Differential Diagnosis for Alcoholic Ketoacidosis

Alternative diagnosis	Alternative or concomitant diagnosis
Lactic acidosis	Methanol ingestion
Uremia	Ethylene glycol ingestion
Secondary lactic acidosis	Isopropanol ingestion
Sepsis	Pancreatitis
Hypotension	Gastritis
Salicylic acid ingestion	Upper GI bleeding
Toxic alcohol ingestion	Seizures
Diabetic ketoacidosis	Ethanol withdrawal
Starvation ketosis	Pneumonia
	Sepsis
	Hepatitis

(Reproduced with permission from Soffer A, Hamburger S: Alcoholic ketoacidosis: a review of 30 cases. *J Am Med Women's Assoc* 37: 106, 1982.)

TABLE 226-3 Treatment of Alcoholic Ketoacidosis

Administer 5% dextrose in normal saline for rehydration. Then change to 5% dextrose in half normal saline as maintenance until oral intake resumes.
Replace potassium and magnesium.
Optional: 50–100 mg thiamine and 1 mg folate IV concurrent with, or after, glucose administration (see text below).
Avoid bicarbonate therapy unless pH <7.1 and unresponsive to fluid and glucose administration.
Consider other causes of anion gap acidosis if the anion gap is <20 mEq/L or fails to close with ongoing treatment.

TREATMENT

Therapy consists of both glucose administration and volume repletion (**Table 226-3**). Fluids alone do not correct the ketoacidosis as fast as fluids and glucose administered together. Glucose stimulates insulin production, which stops lipolysis and halts further ketone formation. Glucose also increases oxidation of NADH to NAD, thereby further stopping ketone production. The fluid of choice is 5% dextrose in normal saline. Once fluid and electrolyte losses are replaced, change fluids to 5% dextrose in half normal saline until oral intake is assured.[1] Patients with alcoholic ketoacidosis are not hyperosmolar. Unlike treatment of diabetic ketoacidosis, cerebral edema is of little concern with large volumes of fluid administration. Even with vigorous fluid resuscitation, in our review of the literature, cerebral edema has not been reported among those being treated for alcoholic ketoacidosis.

Insulin is of no proven benefit and can even be dangerous, as patients often have depleted glycogen stores and normal or low glucose levels. **Sodium bicarbonate is not indicated unless patients are severely acidemic, with a pH <7.0.** Severe acidemia is unlikely to be explained by alcoholic ketoacidosis alone. Mildly elevated osmolal gaps can exist, but it is important to consider co-ingestions, or other causes of anion gap acidosis, if the gap fails to close with ongoing fluid and carbohydrate treatment. Hypophosphatemia is common in alcoholics and can retard the resolution of acidosis because phosphorus is necessary for mitochondrial utilization of glucose for oxidation of NADH. However, phosphate replacement generally is unwarranted in alcoholic ketoacidosis unless levels are very low (<1.0 milligram/dL or <0.323 mmol/L).[6] Serum ketone levels correlated with clinical status may be used to help guide therapy because an increasingly positive reaction signifies improvement.

The prevalence of key vitamin deficiencies in alcohol-dependent patients is unknown but is probably low.[8] Some feel that the practice of routine administration of **IV thiamine** or **multivitamins** in the ED is necessary to prevent the theoretical precipitation of Wernicke's disease,[9] whereas others feel that vitamin supplementation in the ED should be reserved for those with confirmed deficiencies or who are truly at high risk for such deficiencies.[10] If vitamins are given, they can be provided concurrently with, or after, the administration of glucose.[11] Oral vitamin supplementation has also been described, with IM thiamine added to the oral regimen.[8] Administration of magnesium sulfate should be guided by laboratory results. Acidosis should clear within 12 to 24 hours.

DISPOSITION AND FOLLOW-UP

Patients with an uncomplicated ED course may be safely discharged home if there is resolution of acidosis and the patient is able to tolerate oral fluids. Patients should receive counseling on alcohol dependence, be encouraged to use multivitamins, and be offered treatment in an alcohol detoxification program. Patients with a complicated course, underlying illnesses, or persistent acidosis should be admitted for further evaluation and treatment (**Table 226-3**).

REFERENCES

The complete reference list is available online at www.TintinalliEM.com.

CHAPTER 227

Hyperosmolar Hyperglycemic State

Charles S. Graffeo

INTRODUCTION AND EPIDEMIOLOGY

The **hyperosmolar hyperglycemic state (HHS)** is characterized by progressive hyperglycemia and hyperosmolarity typically found in a debilitated patient with poorly controlled or undiagnosed type 2 diabetes mellitus, limited access to water, and commonly, a precipitating illness. A number of terms, including ***hyperosmolar hyperglycemic nonketotic state/coma/syndrome*** and ***nonketotic hyperglycemic coma***, are used to describe HHS. The syndrome does not necessarily include ketosis or coma, and we will use the terminology adopted by the American Diabetes Association.[1] Most cases of HHS occur in the elderly with comorbid organ or metabolic diseases, and about 70% of patients have been previously diagnosed as diabetics. However, the incidence in children is increasing, with the common risk factors being obesity and African American race.[2]

PATHOPHYSIOLOGY

The basic pathophysiology of diabetes is discussed in chapter 223, Type 1 Diabetes Mellitus, and chapter 224, Type 2 Diabetes Mellitus. The development of HHS is attributed to three main factors: (1) insulin resistance and/or deficiency; (2) an inflammatory state with marked elevation in proinflammatory cytokines (C-reactive protein, interleukins, tumor necrosis factors) and counterregulatory hormones (growth hormone, cortisol) that cause increased hepatic gluconeogenesis and glycogenolysis; and (3) osmotic diuresis followed by impaired renal excretion of glucose.[3]

In a patient with type 2 diabetes, physiologic stresses combined with inadequate water intake in an environment of insulin resistance or deficiency lead to HHS. As serum glucose concentration increases, an osmotic gradient develops, attracting water from the intracellular space into the intravascular compartment, causing cellular dehydration. The initial increase in intravascular volume is accompanied by a temporary increase in the glomerular filtration rate. As serum glucose concentration increases, the capacity of the kidneys to reabsorb glucose is exceeded, and glucosuria and osmotic diuresis occur. During osmotic diuresis, significant urinary loss of sodium and potassium, as well as more modest losses of calcium, phosphate, and magnesium may occur. As volume depletion progresses, renal perfusion decreases, and the glomerular filtration rate is reduced. Renal tubular excretion of glucose is impaired, which further worsens hyperglycemia. A sustained osmotic diuresis may result in total body water losses that often exceed 20% to 25% of total body weight, or approximately 8 to 12 L in a 70-kg patient.

The relative lack of severe ketoacidosis in HHS is poorly understood and has been attributed to three possible mechanisms: (1) higher levels of endogenous insulin than are seen in diabetic ketoacidosis, which inhibits lipolysis; (2) lower levels of counterregulatory "stress" hormones; and (3) inhibition of lipolysis by the hyperosmolar state itself. Evidence of significant ketoacidosis in a patient thought to have type 2 diabetes should bring into question the possibility of variants of type 1 diabetes, such as latent autoimmune diabetes in adults.[4] Additionally, a greater proportion of ketosis-prone type 2 diabetes has been described in black, Hispanic, and other populations.[5,6] This growing body of evidence identifying ketosis-prone type 2 diabetes has prompted a call by some for the reclassification of diabetes mellitus.[7]

CLINICAL FEATURES

HISTORY AND COMORBIDITIES

The typical patient with HHS is usually elderly with comorbid medical conditions who is often referred by a caretaker for fever, other abnormalities in vital signs, and/or mental status changes that have evolved over days or weeks. Complaints are often nonspecific and may include weakness, anorexia, fatigue, dyspnea, or chest or abdominal pain. Many patients have previously undiagnosed or poorly controlled type 2 diabetes precipitated by pneumonia or urinary tract infection. Underlying cardiovascular, respiratory, renal, or neurologic disease is common. Psychiatric patients taking antipsychotics or lithium may present a particular risk, and HHS should be considered as part of the medical screening process for ED psychiatric patients.[8]

HHS is associated with a host of conditions (**Table 227-1**) and drugs (**Table 227-2**) that may predispose to hyperglycemia and volume depletion.

TABLE 227-1 Conditions That May Precipitate Hyperosmolar Hyperglycemic State
Diabetes
Infection, especially pneumonia or urinary tract infection
Myocardial infarction
Renal insufficiency
Cerebrovascular events
Mesenteric ischemia
GI hemorrhage
Pulmonary embolism
Pancreatitis
Severe burns
Parenteral or enteral alimentation
Peritoneal or hemodialysis
Heat-related illness
Rhabdomyolysis

PHYSICAL EXAMINATION

The physical manifestations associated with HHS are nonspecific. Generally, clinical signs of volume depletion such as poor skin turgor, dry mucous membranes, sunken eyes, and hypotension will correlate with the degree of hyperglycemia and hyperosmolality.

Normothermia or hypothermia is common due to vasodilation, and hypothermia is a poor prognostic sign. HHS may develop in those who have sustained a physiologic stress, such as a cerebrovascular accident, severe burns, a myocardial infarction, infection, or other acute illness. Up to 15% of patients may present with seizures, which are typically focal, although generalized seizures may occur. The degree of lethargy and coma has a linear relationship to serum osmolality. Patients with coma tend to be older and have higher osmolality, more severe hyperglycemia, acidosis, and greater volume contraction.[9]

DIAGNOSIS AND DIFFERENTIAL DIAGNOSIS

HHS is "defined" by severe hyperglycemia with serum glucose usually >600 milligrams/dL (>33.3 mmol/L), an elevated calculated plasma osmolality of >315 mOsm/kg (>315 mmol/kg), serum bicarbonate

TABLE 227-2 Some Drugs That May Predispose Individuals to the Development of HHS
Diuretics
Lithium
β-Blockers
Mannitol
Chlorpromazine
Cimetidine
Glucocorticoids
Second-generation antipsychotics (ziprasidone, quetiapine, etc.)
Phenytoin
Calcium channel blockers

TABLE 227-3 Diagnostic Criteria for Diabetic Ketoacidosis (DKA) and Hyperosmolar Hyperglycemic State (HHS)

	DKA	HHS
Plasma glucose	>250 milligrams/dL (>13.8 mmol/L)	>600 milligrams/dL (>33.3 mmol/L)
Serum bicarbonate	≤18 mEq/L (<18 mmol/L)	>15 mEq/L (>15 mmol/L)
Urine acetoacetate*	+	– or small
Serum ketones†	+	– or small
Serum osmolality‡	Variable	>320 mOsm/kg (>320 mmol/kg)
Anion gap#	>12 mEq/L (>12 mmol/L)	<12 mEq/L (<12 mmol/L)
Arterial/venous pH	<7.30	>7.30

*Nitroprusside method.

†Gas chromatography method or nitroprusside method.

‡Osmolality calculation: 2(measured [Na^+] + glucose (milligrams/dL or mmol/L)/18.

#Anion gap calculation: [Na^+] – [Cl^-] + [HCO_3^-].

>15 mEq/L (>15 mmol/L), an arterial pH >7.3, and serum ketones that are negative to mildly positive in a 1:2 dilution (by nitroprusside method). These values, however, are fairly arbitrary. Metabolic acidosis or ketonemia associated with HHS is likely to be due to tissue hypoperfusion (lactic acidosis), starvation ketosis, and azotemia in various combinations, although there is growing evidence for ketosis-prone type 2 diabetic subgroups. **It is important to recognize the potential for a variety of mixed acid-base patterns in patients with HHS.**

A comparison of the laboratory features of diabetic ketoacidosis and HHS is shown in **Table 227-3**.

LABORATORY TESTING AND IMAGING

Tailor laboratory tests to the patient and the clinical findings. A comprehensive metabolic profile, calculated and measured serum osmolality, urine osmolality, lactic acid, serum ketones, magnesium, CBC with differential, and blood and urine cultures should all be considered. In addition, cardiac markers, total creatine phosphokinase, arterial or venous blood gas, thyroid function studies, procalcitonin, and coagulation profiles might be needed. Chest radiographs and electrocardiograms are generally recommended. Diagnostic studies, such as CT, lumbar puncture, and toxicologic studies, should be patient specific.

In general, electrolyte abnormalities vary. Initially, contraction alkalosis due to a profound water deficit may occur. An anion gap metabolic acidosis is often attributable to sepsis, poor tissue perfusion, starvation ketosis, or renal impairment.

Sodium Serum sodium level varies and is not a reliable indicator of the degree of volume contraction. Hyperglycemia has a dilutional effect on measured serum sodium: **Serum Na^+ decreases by approximately 1.6 mEq/L (1.6 mmol/L) for every 100 milligrams/dL (5.6 mmol/L) increase in serum glucose >100 milligrams/dL (5.6 mmol/L) (Formula 222-1).**

Formula for glucose in mg/dL

$$\text{Corrected}\,[Na^+] = \text{Measured}\,[Na^+] + \frac{1.6 \times (\text{glucose in mg/dL} - 100)}{100}$$

Formula for glucose in mmol/L

$$\text{Corrected}\,[Na^+] = \text{Measured}\,[Na^+] + \frac{1.6 \times (\text{glucose in mmol/L} - 5.6)}{5.6}$$

FORMULA 227-1. Formula for correction of sodium in presence of severe hyperglycemia.

For glucose levels >400 milligrams/dL (22.2 mmol/L), a correction factor of 2.4 may be more accurate.

Osmolality Serum osmolality correlates positively with severity of disease as well as mental status changes and coma. A calculated effective serum osmolality excludes osmotically inactive urea, which is usually included in laboratory measures of osmolality (**Formula 227-2**).

$$2[Na^+] + \frac{\text{glucose}}{18}$$

FORMULA 227-2. Formula for calculation of serum osmolality in presence of severe hyperglycemia.

The normal serum osmolality range is approximately 275 to 295 mOsm/kg. Values >300 mOsm/kg are usually indicative of significant hyperosmolality, and those >320 mOsm are commonly associated with alterations in cognitive function.

Potassium On average, potassium losses range from 4 to 6 mEq/kg, although deficits can be as high as 10 mEq/kg body weight. Despite these total body deficits, initial serum laboratory measurements may be normal or even high in the presence of acidemia. Initial values may be reported as normal with volume contraction and with metabolic acidosis when intravascular [H^+] ions are exchanged for intracellular [K^+] ions. As intravascular volume is replaced and acidemia is reversed, [K^+] deficiency becomes more apparent.

Other Laboratory Testing Hypomagnesemia is common, and serum magnesium levels should be monitored and replaced as appropriate.[10] Consequences of hypophosphatemia, such as CNS abnormalities, cardiac dysfunction, and rhabdomyolysis, are uncommon and usually associated with serum phosphate levels below 1.0 milligram/dL. Routine replacement of phosphate, unless severe, is usually unnecessary, and replacement may lower ionized calcium levels.[11] Prerenal azotemia is common, with plasma blood urea nitrogen:creatinine ratios often exceeding 30:1. Leukocytosis is variable but is usually due to infection or hemoconcentration.

TREATMENT

Improvement of tissue perfusion is the key to effective recovery in HHS. **Treatment includes correction of hypovolemia, identifying and treating precipitating causes, correcting electrolyte abnormalities, gradual correction of hyperglycemia and hyperosmolarity, and frequent monitoring.** The therapeutic plan must be carefully considered and adjusted for concurrent medical illnesses such as left ventricular dysfunction and renal insufficiency. Data flow sheets that document chronological clinical and laboratory parameters are important adjuncts to successful patient management.

Due to the potential for complications associated with patient comorbidities, rapid therapy should be reserved for potentially life-threatening electrolyte abnormalities only. A protocol for treating severely ill patients likely requiring intensive care unit–level care is shown in **Figure 227-1.**

FLUID RESUSCITATION

Fluid resuscitation replenishes intravascular volume, improves tissue perfusion, and decreases serum glucose about 35 to 70 milligrams/dL/h. **Begin normal saline infusion before insulin therapy is started.**

The average fluid deficit in HHS is in the range of 20% to 25% of total body water, or 8 to 12 L. In the elderly, approximately 50% of body weight is due to total body water. By using the patient's usual current weight in kilograms, normal total body water and water deficit can be calculated. **One half of the fluid deficits should be replaced over the initial 12 hours and the balance over the next 24 hours when possible.** The actual rate of fluid administration should be individualized for each patient, based on the presence of renal and cardiac impairment. **Begin fluid resuscitation with 0.9% normal saline at a rate of 15 to 20 mL/kg/h during the first hour, followed by rates from 4 to 14 mL/kg/h.** Limit the rate of volume repletion during the first 4 hours to <50 mL/kg of normal saline. Patients

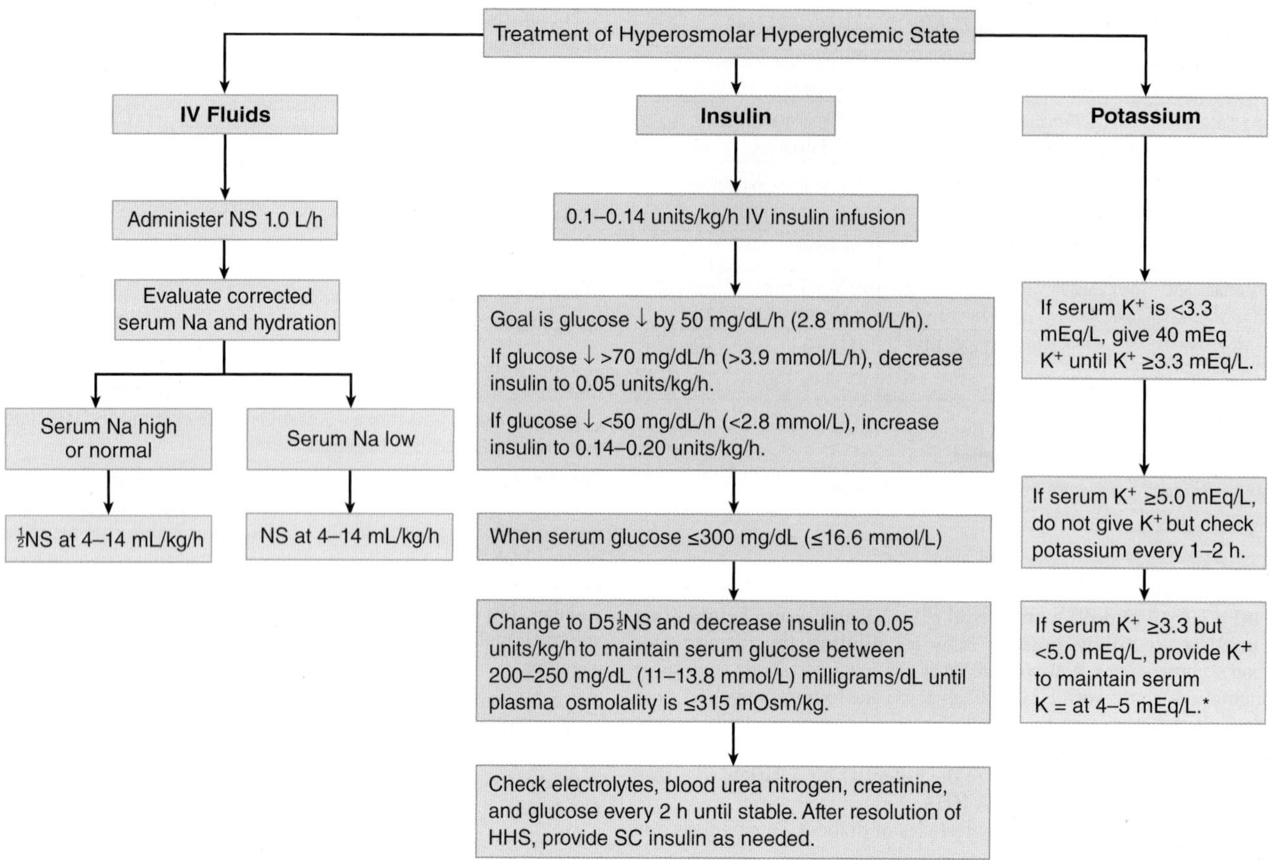

FIGURE 227-1. Protocol for the management of severely ill adult patients with hyperosmolar hyperglycemic state (HHS). *Concentrations of K^+ ≥20 mEq/L should be administered via central line. D5½NS = 5% dextrose in half normal saline; HHS = hyperosmolar hyperglycemic state; NS = normal saline.

with cardiac disease may require a more conservative rate of volume repletion. Once hypotension, tachycardia, and urinary output improve, 0.45% NaCl can be used to replace the remaining free water deficit. Urinary bladder catheterization and intravascular arterial and central venous access should be considered for monitoring progress in the critically ill.

ELECTROLYTES

Hypokalemia is a risk for dysrhythmia and should be anticipated, and potassium should be replaced during volume repletion and insulin administration. If the initial serum potassium measurement is <3.3 mEq/L, begin potassium supplementation and withhold insulin therapy until potassium is replenished.

In general, replace potassium at a rate of 10 to 20 mEq/h. For life-threatening hypokalemia, infusion rates of up to 40 mEq/h may be needed. If properly diluted, infusions of potassium through peripheral IV lines are well tolerated; however, the central venous line route is preferred when available and decreases the risk of extravasation. Monitor serum potassium levels every hour until a steady state has been achieved.

Sodium deficits are replenished fairly rapidly, considering the amount of normal saline given during IV fluid replacement. Replace **magnesium deficits** with 1 to 2 grams of magnesium given over 1 hour. Phosphate should only be replaced if the phosphate level is <1.0 milligram/dL (<1.0 mmol/L). The dose of IV potassium phosphate is 2.5 to 5 milligrams/kg (0.08 to 0.16 mmol/kg) over 6 hours. **Sodium bicarbonate** is recommended only if serum pH is <7.0.[1] Adverse effects of bicarbonate include hypokalemia, hypocalcemia, and abrupt changes in CNS pH levels.

INSULIN

Begin insulin after fluid resuscitation has begun. Intravascular volume may be further depleted as insulin causes a shift of osmotically active glucose into the intracellular space, bringing free water with it.

The absorption of insulin by the IM or SC route is unreliable in patients with HHS, and a continuous infusion of regular insulin is recommended. Although initiation of insulin therapy with a bolus of 0.1 unit/kg followed by a continuous infusion of 0.1 unit/kg/h is included as a treatment option in the current American Diabetes Association recommendations, there is no proven benefit over a simple continuous infusion beginning at >0.1 unit/kg/h.[1] The addition of bolus dosing of insulin is included as a recommendation when initial glucose levels have not dropped by 10% in the first hour of treatment. With adequate hydration and insulin therapy, the goal of therapy is to maintain a steady rate of decline in the glucose concentration of 50 to 75 milligrams/dL/h (2.8–4.1 mmol/L/h). With adequate hydration, the insulin infusion may be doubled every hour until a steady glucose decline as described above is achieved. If glucose falls too rapidly, decrease the infusion rate by half, to 0.05 or 0.07 unit/kg/h. Once serum glucose decreases to <300 milligrams/dL (<16.6 mmol/L), change the IV solution to 5% dextrose in half normal saline, and reduce the insulin infusion to 0.02 to 0.05 unit/kg/h until serum osmolality is <315 mOsm/kg and glucose is maintained between 200 and 300 milligrams/dL (11.1–16.6 mmol/L). Once the patient is mentally alert and able to eat, considerations for SC insulin dosing can be made.

DISEASE COMPLICATIONS

Despite cerebral edema representing >50% of fatalities in children with diabetic ketoacidosis, **cerebral edema is an uncommon complication in adults with HHS.** There are little data on the incidence of or clinical indicators that may predispose to cerebral edema in adults. The current recommendation is to limit the rate of volume repletion during the first 4 hours to <50 mL/kg of normal saline. Monitor the patient's mental status during treatment, and obtain a stat head CT if mental deterioration develops during treatment. While there are no evidence-based treatments for cerebral edema, mannitol as an osmotic agent remains the most practical option.

More common complications, such as hypoglycemia, hypokalemia, and pulmonary edema, are generally associated with overzealous resuscitation and inadequate monitoring.

DISPOSITION AND FOLLOW-UP

When considering the patient population predisposed to developing HHS (debilitated patients with multiple comorbidities), intensive care unit monitoring for the initial 24 hours of care is usually the most appropriate ED disposition. Patients without significant comorbid conditions and who demonstrate a good response to initial therapy as evidenced by documented improvement in vital signs, urine output, electrolyte balance, and mentation may be considered for step-down admission.

REFERENCES

The complete reference list is available online at www.TintinalliEM.com.

CHAPTER 228

Hypothyroidism

Alzamani Mohammad Idrose

INTRODUCTION AND EPIDEMIOLOGY

Hypothyroidism is a clinical syndrome caused by insufficient thyroid hormone production, which slows cell metabolism. Hypothyroidism is common in areas where iodine deficiency is common, particularly inland areas where there is no access to marine foods. In iodine-sufficient areas, chronic autoimmune destruction of thyroid gland (e.g., Hashimoto's thyroiditis) and iatrogenic causes from treatment of Graves' disease are the leading causes of hypothyroidism (after thyroidectomy or radioactive iodine ablation). The prevalence of hypothyroidism increases with age, and the disorder is nearly 10 times more common in females than in males.[1] Subclinical hypothyroidism is more prevalent than overt hypothyroidism in all age groups and can be seen in 4% to 15% of women, especially the elderly.[2,3]

Hypothyroidism occurs in 1% to 32% of patients taking amiodarone.[1]

PATHOPHYSIOLOGY

Primary hypothyroidism is caused by the intrinsic dysfunction of the thyroid gland, and this is the most common type. **Secondary hypothyroidism** is caused by a deficiency of thyroid-stimulating hormone from the pituitary gland or deficiency of thyrotropin-releasing hormone from the hypothalamus. **Table 228-1** lists common causes of hypothyroidism. **Euthyroid sick syndrome or low thyroxine syndrome**, also called nonthyroidal illness, is the term used for patients with low triiodothyronine and thyroxine levels and a normal or low thyroid-stimulating hormone level, but who are clinically euthyroid. This condition is found in critically ill patients or those with severe systemic illness.

Triiodothyronine is the major form of thyroid hormone. The ratio of triiodothyronine to thyroxine released in the blood is about 10:1. Peripherally, triiodothyronine is converted to the active **thyroxine**, which is three to four times more potent than triiodothyronine. The half-life of triiodothyronine is 7 days, and the half-life of thyroxine is about 1 day.

TABLE 228-1 Common Causes of Hypothyroidism

Primary Hypothyroidism (disorders of thyroid gland)	Secondary Hypothyroidism (disorders at hypothalamic-pituitary axis)
Autoimmune etiologies (Hashimoto's)	Panhypopituitarism
Thyroiditis (subacute, silent, postpartum)*	Pituitary adenoma
Iodine deficiency	Infiltrative causes (e.g., hemochromatosis, sarcoidosis)
After ablation (surgical, radioiodine)	
After external radiation	Tumors impinging on the hypothalamus
Infiltrative disease (lymphoma, sarcoid, amyloidosis, tuberculosis)	History of brain irradiation Infection (e.g., tuberculosis of the brain)
Other Causes	
Congenital	
Drugs affecting thyroid gland function	
Amiodarone	
Lithium	
Potassium perchlorate	
Iodine (in patients with preexisting autoimmune disease)	
α-Interferon	
Interleukin-2	
Idiopathic	

*Self-limiting etiologies, often preceded by hyperthyroid phase before getting into hypothyroid phase.

CLINICAL FEATURES OF HYPOTHYROIDISM

Symptoms can manifest in all organ systems and range in severity based on the degree of hormone deficiency (**Table 228-2**).

The common clinical features of hypothyroidism are listed in **Table 228-2**. Additional cardiopulmonary findings include angina, bradycardia, distant heart sounds from pericardial effusion, low voltage on the electrocardiogram, pleural effusions, cardiomyopathy, or hypoventilation.

Figures 228-1 and **228-2** show some characteristic findings of myxedema.

Table 228-3 describes the differences between primary and secondary hypothyroidism.

TABLE 228-2 Symptoms and Signs of Hypothyroidism

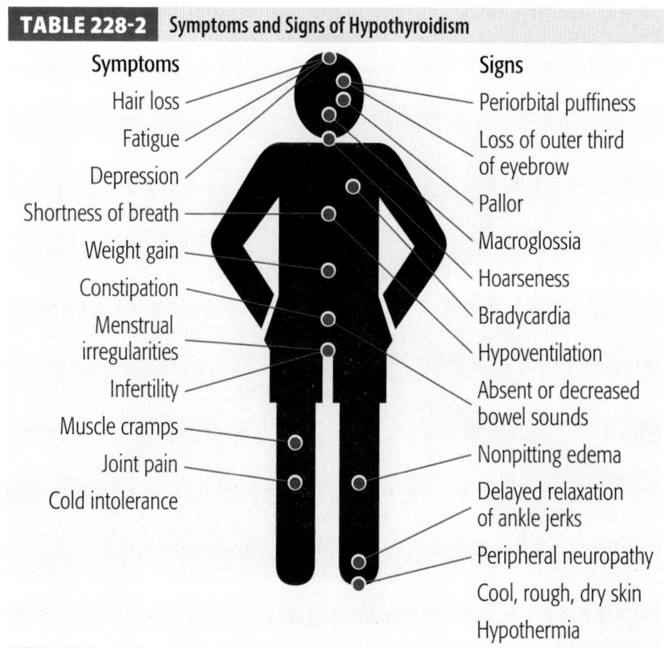

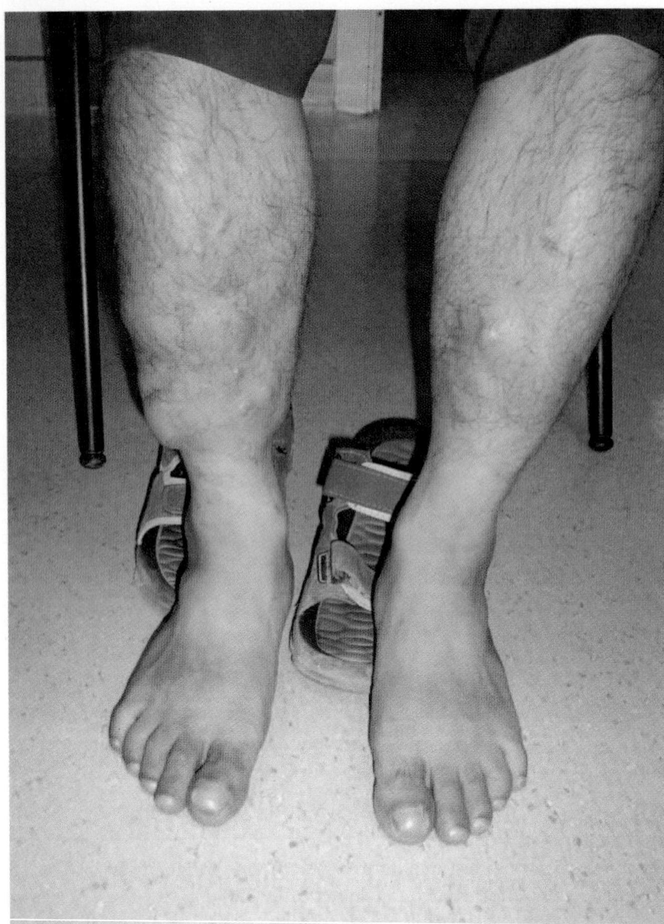

FIGURE 228-1. Myxedema (non-pitting edema) in a patient with hypothyroidism. [Image used with permission of Dr. Zanariah Hussein.]

CLINICAL FEATURES OF MYXEDEMA CRISIS

Myxedema crisis is a state of metabolic and multiorgan decompensation characterized by uncorrected hypothyroidism, mental status changes or coma, and hypothermia (usually <35.5°C [95.9°F]).[1] In hypothyroid patients, myxedema coma can be precipitated by a number of conditions, including infection, anesthetic agents, cold exposure, trauma, myocardial infarction or congestive heart failure, cerebrovascular accident, GI hemorrhage, metabolic conditions, hypoxia, hypercapnia, hyponatremia, hypoglycemia, surgery, burns, medications (e.g., β-blockers, sedatives, narcotics, phenothiazine, amiodarone), or thyroid medication noncompliance.

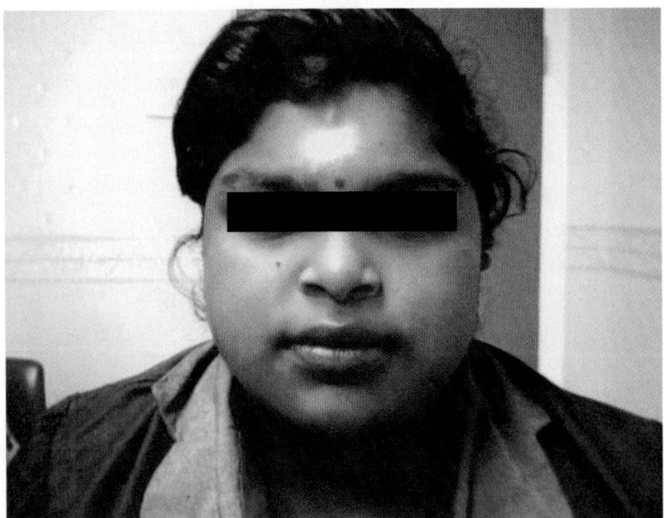

FIGURE 228-2. Hypothyroidism patient with facial swelling. [Image used with permission of Dr. Zanariah Hussein.]

TABLE 228-3 Differentiation of Primary and Secondary Hypothyroidism

Point of Difference	Primary Hypothyroidism	Secondary Hypothyroidism
Previous thyroid operation	Yes	None
Obese	More obese	Less obese
Hypothermia	More common	Less common
Voice	Coarse	Less coarse
Pubic hair	Present	Absent
Skin	Dry and coarse	Fine and soft
Heart size	Increased	Normal
Menses and lactation	Normal	No lactation, amenorrhea
Sella turcica size	Normal	May be increased
Serum TSH	Increased	Decreased
Plasma cortisol	Normal	Decreased
Response to TSH	None	Good
Response to levothyroxine without steroids	Good	Poor response

Abbreviation: TSH = thyroid-stimulating hormone.

The characteristic hypothyroid habitus is evident, as well as bradycardia, hypotension, hypothermia, hypoventilation, and altered mental status or coma. Blood pressure is quite variable, but of patients in full myxedema coma, half initially exhibit clinical shock with systolic pressure <100 mm Hg.[4,5] The capillaries are "leaky," and this may contribute to hypotension. Infection may be present even though fever, tachycardia, sweating, and leukocytosis may not be evident, because bradycardia and hypothermia mask these signs. Respiratory insufficiency and altered mental status can result from carbon dioxide narcosis. Pleural effusions are frequently demonstrable. Other potential respiratory problems include upper airway obstruction from glottic edema, vocal cord edema, and macroglossia. Metabolism of tranquilizers, sedatives, and anesthetics is reduced in hypothyroidism, and the exaggerated effects of such medications can also contribute to altered mental status. **Hypothermia is so common in myxedema that a normal temperature should suggest an underlying infection.** Hypothyroid habitus, absence of shivering, and pseudomyotonic reflexes (prolonged relaxation phase of deep tendon reflex—at least twice as long as the contraction phase) may help distinguish myxedematous from accidental hypothermia.

DIAGNOSIS

The diagnosis of hypothyroidism is based on laboratory testing. The diagnosis of myxedema crisis is clinical. The differential diagnoses include sepsis, depression, adrenal crisis, congestive heart failure, hypoglycemia, cerebrovascular accidents, hypothermia, drug overdose, and meningitis.

LABORATORY EVALUATION AND IMAGING

The baseline levels of thyroid-stimulating hormone, thyroxine, triiodothyronine, and cortisol levels should be drawn before initiating treatment. This facilitates eventual diagnosis as well as response to treatment.

High thyroid-stimulating hormone, with low total or free thyroxine and triiodothyronine, confirms primary hypothyroidism (thyroid gland etiology). Low thyroid-stimulating hormone with low total or free thyroxine and triiodothyronine points toward secondary hypothyroidism (hypothalamic–pituitary etiology). The assay of free thyroxine and triiodothyronine is preferable, as the result is more accurate and is not affected by protein binding.

Thyroid hormone levels may also be altered as a result of interactions with drugs such as amiodarone, lithium, ethionamide, α-interferon, and interleukin-2. Nevertheless, thyroid function usually normalizes after discontinuation of these drugs. Ideally, thyroid function tests should be obtained before initiating therapy with these agents and periodically thereafter.

Hypothyroidism may be associated with pernicious anemia, and thus macrocytic anemia may be evident. However, if menorrhagia after hypothyroidism is severe, anemia may be microcytic from iron deficiency. **Hyponatremia** due to increased antidiuretic hormone and impaired free water clearance is common. **Hypoglycemia** is common because of decreased gluconeogenesis, decreased insulin clearance, and concomitant adrenal insufficiency or growth hormone deficiency. Arterial blood gases typically show hypoxemia, hypercapnia, metabolic acidosis from tissue hypoxia, and respiratory acidosis from hypoventilation due to muscle weakness.

Further laboratory assessment depends on the differential diagnosis, comorbidities, and search for precipitating factors. Electrocardiogram is necessary to identify myocardial infarction or bradyarrhythmias or heart block. Chest radiograph is needed to identify pneumonia, pleural effusion, or cardiomegaly.

TREATMENT OF SYMPTOMATIC HYPOTHYROIDISM

If a patient has symptoms of hypothyroidism or has been noncompliant with thyroid medication, and hypothyroidism can be confirmed by thyroid function tests done in the ED, oral levothyroxine may be started. Full replacement dose for patients without cardiac disease is 1.6 micrograms/kg.[6] The average starting dose for healthy adults younger than 50 is 50 micrograms of oral levothyroxine once a day. For those older than 50 years or with cardiac disease, the initial dose is lower, 12.5 to 25 micrograms once a day. For all adults, the dose is adjusted by 12.5- to 25-microgram increments at 4- to 6-week intervals. Instruct the patient to follow up with the primary care physician for monitoring and further dose adjustments in a month.

TREATMENT OF MYXEDEMA CRISIS

Management of myxedema crisis is shown in **Table 228-4**. **The treatment includes supportive care, thyroid hormone replacement (supplementing with thyroxine, triiodothyronine, or combination of both), and identification and treatment of precipitating factors.**

THYROID HORMONE REPLACEMENT FOR MYXEDEMA CRISIS

Administer thyroid hormone upon clinical suspicion of myxedema crisis, as confirmatory laboratory thyroid hormone levels will not be available initially. Thyroxine is the usual replacement. Triiodothyronine alone can be given if it is available, but should be avoided in the elderly or those with cardiac disease. Triiodothyronine and thyroxine together can be given if the patient has persistent hemodynamic instability or poor respiratory effort. Because myxedema crisis is such a rare condition, there are no clear recommendations for the use of thyroxine alone, combined thyroxine and triiodothyronine, or triiodothyronine alone.

Thyroid hormone replacement should initially be given IV because severe or even mild hypothyroidism results in decreased intestinal motility and GI absorption. Once the patient has received IV replacement, intestinal motility should recover, and oral medication can be given.

Thyroxin (Levothyroxine) The dose is 4 micrograms/kg IV, with the usual dose from 200 micrograms to a maximum of 500 micrograms IV. The onset of action for IV thyroxine is between 6 and 8 hours. The advantages of thyroxine are a smooth, slow, and steady onset of action and its widespread availability. Disadvantages include the fact that extrathyroidal conversion of thyroxine to triiodothyronine may be reduced in myxedema coma. The onset of action of thyroxine is longer than that of triiodothyronine.

Triiodothyronine (Liothyronine) For triiodothyronine (liothyronine), start at 20 micrograms IV followed by 10 micrograms IV every 8 hours until oral medication can be given. The advantage of triiodothyronine over thyroxine is the fact that deiodinase conversion of thyroxine to the active hormone triiodothyronine is reduced in myxedema crisis. IV triiodothyronine also has a rapid onset of action, between 2 and 4 hours. In a primate study, triiodothyronine crossed the blood–brain barrier more readily than thyroxine.[7] However, the disadvantages of triiodothyronine are a more potent effect, fluctuating serum levels, and the fact that triiodothyronine is more likely to cause cardiac arrhythmias or myocardial infarction than thyroxine. Avoid replacement with triiodothyronine in patients with cardiac disease. If triiodothyronine is given, provide continuous cardiac monitoring and obtain interval electrocardiograms to identify myocardial ischemia.

TABLE 228-4 ED Treatment for Myxedema Crisis

Supportive care

Airway, breathing, and circulation support: ensure airway control, oxygen, IV access, and cardiac monitor

IV therapy: dextrose for hypoglycemia; water restriction for hyponatremia

Vasopressors: if indicated (ineffective without thyroid hormone replacement)

Hypothermia: treated with passive rewarming

Steroids: hydrocortisone (due to increased metabolic stress; 100–200 milligrams IV)

Thyroid replacement therapy (see discussion of Thyroid Hormone Replacement in text)

IV thyroxine (levothyroxine) at 4 micrograms/kg (typically between 200 and 500 micrograms as initial dose), followed in 24 h by 100 micrograms IV, then 50 micrograms IV until oral medication is tolerated. **Thyroxine is readily available. Thyroxine is preferred in the elderly and those with cardiac disease. Starting dose in the elderly is 100 micrograms IV.**

OR

IV triiodothyronine (liothyronine) at a dose of 20 micrograms IV followed by 10 micrograms IV every 8 h until the patient is conscious. **Start with no more than 10 micrograms IV for the elderly or those with coronary artery disease.**

Triiodothyronine is less preferred in patients with cardiac disease, as its potency could precipitate cardiac arrhythmias or infarction.

Note: *Either thyroxine or triiodothyronine alone can be used, but in patients with persistent hemodynamic instability or poor respiratory effort, both can be given simultaneously. When used together, the dose of thyroxine is 200 micrograms IV and triiodothyronine is 20 micrograms IV.*

↓

Identify and treat precipitating and comorbid factors

- Infections
- Sedatives
- Cold exposure
- Trauma
- Myocardial infarction or congestive heart failure
- Cerebrovascular accident
- Gastrointestinal hemorrhage
- Hypoxia
- Hypercapnia
- Hyponatremia
- Hypoglycemia

DISPOSITION AND FOLLOW-UP

Myxedema crisis carries a high mortality rate, ranging from 30% to 60% depending on comorbid diseases. Factors such as advanced age, bradycardia, and persistent hypotension suggest a poor prognosis. All patients with myxedema coma require intensive care unit admission. Milder hypothyroidism patients may only be discharged with a clear plan of management and followed up by either an endocrinologist or primary care physician.

SPECIAL POPULATIONS

PREGNANT WOMEN

Overt hypothyroidism is seen in about 1% to 2% of pregnant women.[8] Subclinical hypothyroidism is seen in another 2.5%.[9]

Most cases of hypothyroidism during pregnancy have the same cause as in hypothyroidism in general. Pregnancy increases the requirement of thyroid hormone because of the increased rate of metabolism in the mother and the transplacental transport of thyroid hormone, which is essential for the development and maturation of the different organs of the fetus. For women who are being treated for hypothyroidism, the dose of thyroxine should be increased approximately by 30% as soon as the pregnancy is confirmed.[10]

Thyroid function test results during pregnancy may be difficult to interpret. This is because pregnant patients may have a higher production of thyroid hormone from stimulation of the gland by human chorionic gonadotropin, which has a similar structure to that of thyroid-stimulating hormone. On top of that, increased estrogen during pregnancy results in higher levels of thyroid-binding globulin, which transports thyroid hormone in the blood. Therefore, a normal thyroid hormone level in a pregnant woman may not mean the patient is euthyroid, especially if the patient has symptoms of hypothyroidism. Thyroid hormone replacement may still be required in this case.

Hypothyroidism is diagnosed in pregnancy if patients have symptoms and, in general, have high levels of thyroid-stimulating hormone and low free thyroxine. Subclinical hypothyroidism in pregnancy can be identified if the test results show high levels of thyroid-stimulating hormone and normal free thyroxine. Subclinical hypothyroidism should be treated to ensure healthy pregnancy.

Synthetic thyroxine, which is identical to the thyroxine made by the thyroid gland, is used for pregnant women. It is safe for the fetus. Pregnant women with existing hypothyroidism require an increased dose of thyroxine during pregnancy, and the thyroid function is usually checked every 8 weeks.

ELDERLY PATIENTS

Age, the presence of cardiac comorbidities, and a high dose of thyroxine are associated with a poor outcome in myxedema crisis.[10] Standard doses of thyroxine, and especially of triiodothyronine, can precipitate cardiac arrhythmias. Start with no more than half the recommended dose of thyroxine or triiodothyronine for elderly patients.

PATIENTS WITH CARDIAC DISEASE

Thyroxine has fewer cardiac effects than triiodothyronine. Thyroxine is the preferred choice for thyroid hormone replacement in patients with heart disease.

THE ASYMPTOMATIC PATIENT WITH A PALPABLE NODULE IDENTIFIED IN THE ED

Solitary thyroid nodules are a common physical finding in the general population. Although most are benign colloid nodules that will disappear over time, a small percentage of solitary nodules are thyroid carcinomas. Biopsy results identify 70% of nodules to be benign, 5% to be malignant, and the remainder to be cytologically indeterminate.[11] Therefore, referral for fine-needle aspiration biopsy is indicated for all patients with palpable nodules.

LEVOTHYROXINE OVERDOSE

Synthetic levothyroxine is the most widely used agent for thyroid replacement. Deaths from overdose have not been reported. When taken in overdose, symptoms do not occur until 24 hours later as a result of metabolic conversion of thyroxine to triiodothyronine. Treatment is not standardized. For acute ingestion, activated charcoal can be given. Cholestyramine can decrease fecal elimination, and propranolol can control tachycardia and anxiety. Contact your local poison control center for specific treatment recommendations.

Acknowledgment: The author gratefully acknowledges the contributions of Horace K. Liang, the author of this chapter in the previous edition.

REFERENCES

The complete reference list is available online at www.TintinalliEM.com.

Hyperthyroidism

Alzamani Mohammad Idrose

INTRODUCTION AND EPIDEMIOLOGY

Thyroid hormone affects all organ systems and is responsible for increasing metabolic rate, heart rate, and ventricle contractility, as well as muscle and central nervous system excitability. Two major types of thyroid hormones are thyroxine and triiodothyronine. Thyroxine is the major form of thyroid hormone. The ratio of thyroxine to triiodothyronine released in the blood is 20:1. Peripherally, thyroxine is converted to the active triiodothyronine, which is three to four times more potent than thyroxine.

Hyperthyroidism refers to excess circulating hormone resulting only from thyroid gland hyperfunction, whereas thyrotoxicosis refers to excess circulating thyroid hormone originating from any cause (including thyroid hormone overdose).

Thyroid storm is the extreme manifestation of thyrotoxicosis. This is an acute, severe, life-threatening hypermetabolic state of thyrotoxicosis caused either by excessive release of thyroid hormones causing adrenergic hyperactivity or altered peripheral response to thyroid hormone following the presence of one or more precipitants.

The mortality of thyroid storm without treatment is between 80% and 100%, and with treatment, it is between 15% and 50%.

Primary hyperthyroidism is caused by the excess production of thyroid hormones from the thyroid glands. Secondary hyperthyroidism is caused by the excess production of thyroid-releasing hormones or thyroid-stimulating hormones in the hypothalamus and pituitary, respectively (**Tables 229-1** and **229-2**).

In the case of thyroid storm, the most common underlying cause of hyperthyroidism is Graves' disease (85% of all hyperthyroidism cases in the United States). It is caused by the thyrotropin receptor antibodies that stimulate excess and uncontrolled thyroidal synthesis and secretion of thyroid hormones. It occurs most frequently in young women (10 times more common in women compared with men) at any age group.[1]

PATHOPHYSIOLOGY

The pathophysiologic mechanisms underlying the shift from uncomplicated thyrotoxicosis to thyroid storm are not entirely clear. However, they involve adrenergic hyperactivity either by increased release of thyroid hormones (with or without increased synthesis) or increased receptor sensitivity. Many of the signs and symptoms are related to adrenergic hyperactivity. Patients with thyroid storm reportedly have relatively higher levels of free thyroid hormones as opposed to those with uncomplicated thyrotoxicosis. The total thyroid hormone level may or may not be increased in these patients.

When there is excess of thyroid hormones, circulating thyroxin and triiodothyronine are taken into the cytoplasm of cells. Thyroxin is converted to its active form, triiodothyronine. Within the cytoplasm, the triiodothyronine then exerts its effect by passing into the nucleus and binding to thyroid hormone receptors or thyroid hormone–responsive elements to induce gene activation and transcription.[2] The receptors receiving the hormone will stimulate changes specific to the tissue.

TABLE 229-1 Causes of Hyperthyroidism: Primary and Secondary Hyperthyroidism

Primary Hyperthyroidism	
Graves' disease (toxic diffuse goiter) (**Figure 229-1**)	Most common of all hyperthyroidism (85% of all cases) Associated with diffuse goiter, ophthalmopathy, and local dermopathy
Toxic multinodular goiter	Second most common cause of hyperthyroidism
Toxic nodular (adenoma) goiter (**Figure 229-2**)	An enlarged thyroid gland that contains a small rounded mass or masses called nodules with overproduction of thyroid hormone
Thyroiditis	Inflammation of the thyroid gland
Hashimoto's thyroiditis	Initially gland is overactive (hyperthyroidism state), but this is usually followed by a state of hypothyroidism
Subacute painful thyroiditis (de Quervain's thyroiditis)	
Subacute painless thyroiditis	
Radiation thyroiditis	
Secondary Hyperthyroidism	
Thyrotropin-secreting pituitary adenoma	Thyroid gland stimulated to produce hormones

In the pituitary gland, thyroid hormones exert negative regulation on the transcription of the genes for the subunit and the common subunit of thyroid-stimulating hormone, resulting in thyroid-stimulating hormone suppression.

During thyroid storm, precipitants such as infection, stress, myocardial infarction, or trauma will multiply the effect of thyroid hormones by freeing thyroid hormones from their binding sites or increasing receptor sensitivity.

THYROID STORM PRECIPITATION

The precipitants of thyroid storm are as shown in **Table 229-3.** In some patients undergoing radioactive iodine therapy for hyperthyroidism, thyroid storm may ironically occur following treatment due to withdrawal of antithyroid drugs, release of thyroid hormones from damaged thyroid follicles, or the effect of radioactive iodine itself.

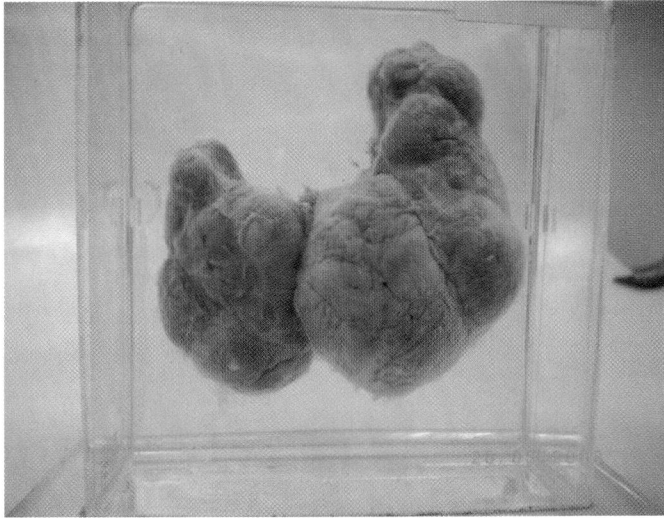

FIGURE 229-1. Pathology specimen of Graves' disease: most common cause of hyperthyroidism. Diffuse swelling is evident. [Image used with permission of the University of Malaya Pathology Museum.]

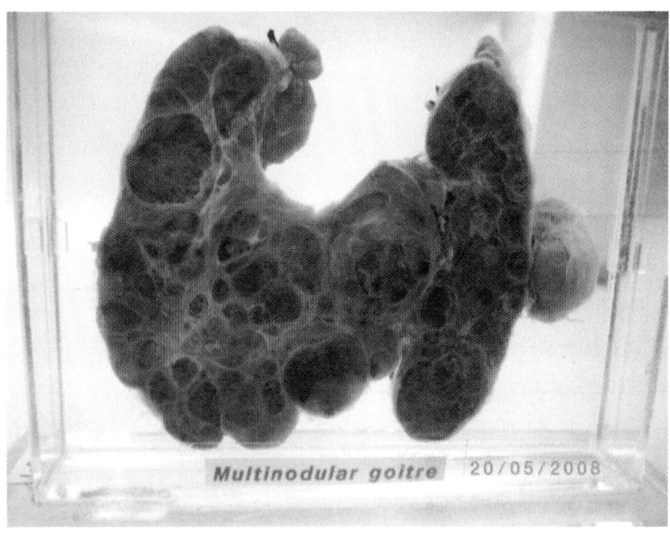

FIGURE 229-2. Pathology specimen of multinodular goiter: second most common cause of hyperthyroidism. Multinodular appearance can be seen. [Image used with permission of the University of Malaya Pathology Museum.]

CLINICAL FEATURES

HISTORY AND COMORBIDITIES

The patient may only complain of constitutional symptoms such as generalized weakness and fatigue. Heat intolerance, diaphoresis, fever, voracious appetite but poor weight gain, anxiety, emotional lability, palpitations, diarrhea, and hair loss are common historical features. If there is a history of hyperthyroidism, ask about treatment and compliance with medication.

PHYSICAL EXAMINATION

In general, patients often appear toxic and agitated. The signs and symptoms of hyperthyroidism patients are as shown in **Table 229-4**.

TABLE 229-2 Other Causes of Hyperthyroidism

Nonthyroidal Disease	
Ectopic thyroid tissue (struma ovarii)/teratoma	A rare form of mature teratoma that contains mostly thyroid tissue
Metastatic thyroid cancer	Stimulates production of thyroid hormones
Human chorionic gonadotropin	Secreting hydatidiform mole
Drug Induced	
Iodine	Iodine-induced thyrotoxicosis (called *Jod-Basedow disease*) After treatment of endemic goiter patients with iodine or stimulation of thyroid hormones from use of iodine-containing agents such as radiographic contrast agents
Amiodarone	Contains iodine; may cause either thyrotoxicosis or hypothyroidism
α-Interferon Interleukin-2	During treatment for other diseases, such as viral hepatitis and human immunodeficiency virus infection
Thyrotoxicosis factitia	Munchausen-like; thyroid hormone is taken by patient to fake illness
Ingestion of meat containing beef thyroid tissue	Cow thyroid tissue contains thyroid hormones
Excessive thyroid hormone ingestion	

TABLE 229-3 Precipitants of Thyroid Storm

Systemic insult	**Cardiovascular insult**
Infection	Myocardial infarction
Trauma	Cerebrovascular accidents
General surgery	Pulmonary embolism
Endocrinal insult	**Obstetrics related**
Diabetic ketoacidosis	Parturition
Hyperosmolar coma	Eclampsia
Drug or hormone related	**Radioactive iodine therapy**
Withdrawal of anti-thyroid medication	
Iodine administration	
Thyroid gland palpation	
Ingestion of thyroid hormone	
Unknown cause in up to 25% of cases	

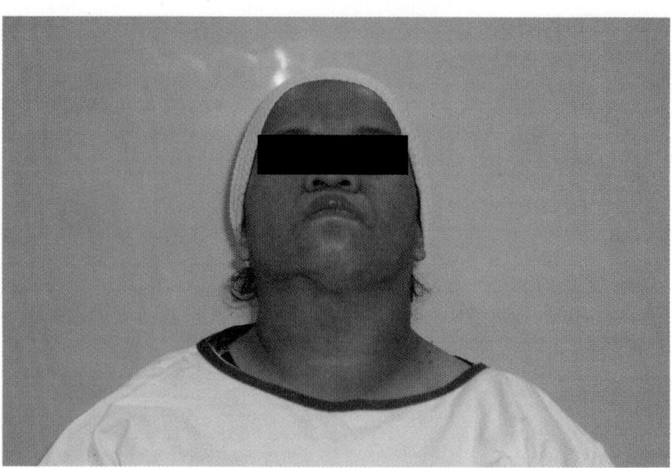

FIGURE 229-3. Goiter with hyperthyroidism symptoms: patient has large solitary toxic adenoma on the left lobe.

TABLE 229-4 Symptoms and Signs of Thyrotoxicosis

Affected System	Symptoms	Signs
Constitutional	Lethargy Weakness Heat intolerance	Diaphoresis Fever Weight loss
Neuropsychiatric	Emotional lability Anxiety Confusion Coma Psychosis	Fine tremor Muscle wasting Hyperreflexia Periodic paralysis
Ophthalmologic	Diplopia Eye irritation	Lid lag Dry eyes Exophthalmos Ophthalmoplegia Conjunctival infection
Endocrine: thyroid gland (**Figure 229-3**)	Neck fullness Tenderness	Thyroid enlargement Bruit
Cardiorespiratory	Dyspnea Palpitations Chest pain	Widened pulse pressure Systolic hypertension Sinus tachycardia Atrial fibrillation or flutter High output heart failure
Gastrointestinal	Diarrhea Yellowish sclera	Hyperactive bowel sound Jaundice
Reproductive	Oligomenorrhea Decreased libido	Gynecomastia Telangiectasia
Gynecologic	Menorrhagia Irregularity	Sparse pubic hair
Hematologic	Pale skin	Anemia Leukocytosis
Dermatologic	Hair loss	Pretibial myxedema* Warm, moist skin Palmar erythema Onycholysis

*Pretibial myxedema may be present in 5% of patients with Graves' disease.

As for thyroid storm, the additional signs and symptoms apart from those evident in thyrotoxicosis are as shown in **Table 229-5**.

Fever is often present in thyroid storm and may be quite high. It may herald the onset of thyrotoxic crisis in previously uncomplicated disease. Palpitations, tachycardia, and dyspnea are common. A pleuropericardial rub may be heard. The direct inotropic and chronotropic effects of thyroid hormone on the heart cause increased blood volume, increased contractility, and increased cardiac output. Enhanced contractility produces elevations in systolic blood pressure and pulse pressure, leading to a dicrotic or water-hammer pulse. Atrial fibrillation occurs in 10% to 35% of thyrotoxicosis cases.[3,4]

The severity of exophthalmos does not necessarily parallel the magnitude of thyroid dysfunction but reflects the responsible autoimmune process. Not all hyperthyroidism patients present with goiter. A goiter is not present with exogenous administration of thyroid hormone and apathetic thyrotoxicosis. Likewise, the presence of a goiter does not necessarily confirm the diagnosis of thyrotoxicosis. Thyroid gland tenderness can be found in inflammatory conditions such as subacute thyroiditis.[5]

DIAGNOSING THYROID STORM

Thyroid storm is a clinical diagnosis for patients with preexisting hyperthyroidism. In determining whether or not a patient has thyroid storm, the main systems to concentrate on are the **thermoregulatory system**

TABLE 229-5 Presenting Signs and Symptoms of Thyroid Storm

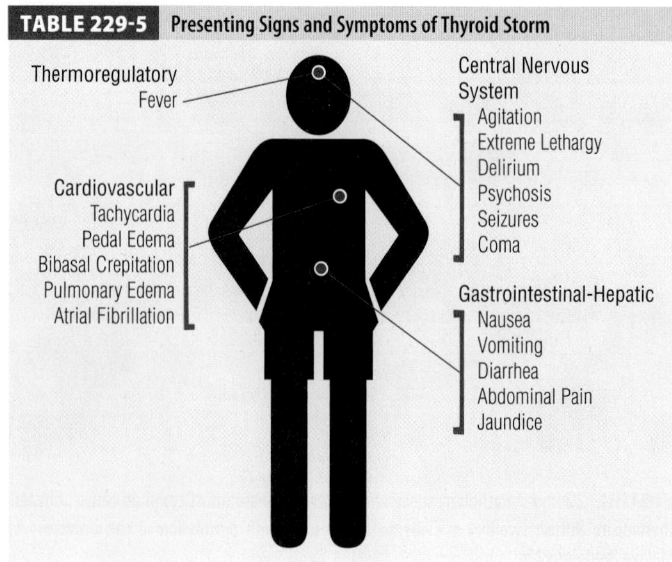

(rise in temperature), **CV system** (ranging from tachycardia to atrial fibrillation and congestive cardiac failure), **CNS** (ranging from being agitated to seizure), and the **GI-hepatic system** (ranging from nausea to vomiting and jaundice) (**Table 229-5**). **Table 229-6** provides a scoring system for thyroid storm as compared with severe thyrotoxicosis. A score ≥45 is highly suggestive of thyroid storm. The system is sensitive in picking up thyroid storm but is not very specific.

DIFFERENTIAL DIAGNOSIS

The differential diagnosis of thyroid storm is shown in **Table 229-7**.

LABORATORY TESTING

Serum Thyroid-Stimulating Hormone Level In **primary hyperthyroidism**, the thyroid-stimulating hormone level is low as a result of the negative feedback mechanism toward a high thyroid hormone level. Nevertheless, a low thyroid-stimulating hormone level by itself is not diagnostic, as serum thyroid-stimulating hormone may be reduced as a result of chronic liver or renal disease or the effect of certain drugs such as glucocorticoids, which reduce thyroid-stimulating hormone secretion.

In **secondary hyperthyroidism**, thyroid-stimulating hormone is increased because of increased production in the pituitary.

Free Thyroid Hormone Levels: Free Thyroxine and Free Triiodothyronine A low thyroid-stimulating hormone with an elevated free thyroxine confirms primary hyperthyroidism. A high thyroid-stimulating hormone with high free thyroxine denotes secondary causes of hyperthyroidism. On the other hand, a low thyroid-stimulating hormone with a normal free thyroxine but elevated free triiodothyronine is also diagnostic of triiodothyronine thyrotoxicosis. Triiodothyronine thyrotoxicosis occurs in <5% of patients who have thyrotoxicosis in North America.[5] Total thyroid hormone levels are not necessarily acutely elevated when the transition from uncomplicated thyrotoxicosis to thyroid storm occurs.

Triiodothyronine Resin Uptake Triiodothyronine resin uptake estimates free thyroxine levels by measuring unoccupied thyroxine-binding globulin sites and is also used to account for changes in binding protein concentration. A higher triiodothyronine resin uptake value means less thyroxine-binding globulin is available, implying the presence of hyperthyroidism.

Total Thyroid Hormone Level of Thyroxine and Triiodothyronine Total serum thyroxine and triiodothyronine (bound and unbound) are increased in thyrotoxicosis. Eighty percent of circulating triiodothyronine is derived from mono-deiodination of thyroxine in peripheral tissues, whereas 20% emanates from direct thyroidal secretion. Both thyroxine and triiodothyronine are then bound to proteins in the form of thyroxine-binding globulin, transthyretin, and albumin. Only a small fraction of the hormones are free and unbound. Laboratory measurement of total triiodothyronine and total thyroxine measures mainly protein-bound hormone concentrations. In thyroid storm, total thyroid hormone level may or may not be increased. Results also may be affected by conditions that affect protein binding. With the improved assays for free thyroxine and free triiodothyronine, there is now little indication to measure total triiodothyronine and total thyroxine.

Thyroid Antibody Titers Thyroid-stimulating antibodies are detected in Graves' disease. Thyroid antibody titers (to thyroid peroxidase or thyroglobulin) will help determine diagnosis.

Ancillary Tests Obtain a CBC, electrolytes, glucose, and renal and liver function tests to identify comorbidities, but start treatment upon suspicion of the diagnosis. In thyroid storm, CBC typically shows leukocytosis with shift to the left. Hyperglycemia tends to occur because of a catecholamine-induced inhibition of insulin release and increased glycogenolysis and rapid intestinal absorption of glucose. Mild hypercalcemia and elevated alkaline phosphatase can occur because of hemoconcentration and enhanced thyroid hormone–stimulated bone resorption.[6]

Thyrotoxicosis also induces liver enzyme metabolism, causing raised liver enzymes. A high serum cortisol value is an expected finding in thyrotoxic individuals. This should be the normal reaction of an adrenal

TABLE 229-7 Differential Diagnosis for Thyroid Storm

Infection and sepsis
Sympathomimetic ingestion (e.g., cocaine, amphetamine, ketamine drug use)
Heat exhaustion
Heat stroke
Delirium tremens
Malignant hyperthermia
Malignant neuroleptic syndrome
Hypothalamic stroke
Pheochromocytoma
Medication withdrawal (e.g., cocaine, opioids)
Psychosis
Organophosphate poisoning

TABLE 229-6 Burch and Wartofsky's Diagnostic Parameters and Scoring Points for Thyroid Storm

Diagnostic Parameters	Scoring Points
1. Thermoregulatory dysfunction	
Temperature °C (°F)	
37.2–37.7 (99–99.9)	5
37.7–38.3 (100–100.9)	10
38.3–38.8 (101–101.9)	15
38.9–39.4 (102–102.9)	20
39.4–39.9 (103–103.9)	25
≥40 (≥104.0)	30
2. CNS effects	
Absent	0
Mild (agitation)	10
Moderate (delirium, psychosis, extreme lethargy)	20
Severe (seizures, coma)	30
3. GI-hepatic dysfunction	
Absent	0
Moderate (diarrhea, nausea/vomiting, abdominal pain)	10
Severe (unexplained jaundice)	20
4. CV dysfunction	
Tachycardia (beats/min)	
90–109	5
110–119	10
120–129	15
≥140	25
5. Congestive heart failure	
Absent	0
Mild (pedal edema)	5
Moderate (bibasilar rales)	10
Severe (pulmonary edema)	15
6. Atrial fibrillation	
Absent	0
Present	10

Scoring system:
Score of ≥45: Highly suggestive of thyroid storm.
Score of 25–44: Suggestive of impending storm.
Score of <25: Unlikely to represent thyroid storm.
(Reproduced with permission from Burch HB, Wartofsky L. Life-threatening thyrotoxicosis. Thyroid storm. *Endocrinol Metab Clin North Am* 22: 263, 1993.)

gland to a body under stress. The finding of an abnormally low cortisol level in a patient with Graves' disease should raise suspicion of coincidental adrenal insufficiency.

Imaging Chest radiograph can be done to rule out infection as a precipitant for thyroid storm. A thyroid sonogram with Doppler flow can be done to assess thyroid gland size, vascularity, and the presence of nodules. Typically, a thyroid gland secreting excessive hormones would be enlarged. On the other hand, in the setting of subacute, postpartum thyroiditis, silent thyroiditis, or exogenous causes of hyperthyroidism, the thyroid gland is not expected to be enlarged. Nuclear medicine imaging with iodine-131 would reveal a greatly increased uptake of radioiodine as early as 1 or 2 hours after administration of the agent. CT of the brain may be necessary to exclude neurologic conditions if diagnosis is uncertain, as CNS abnormalities causing altered mental status may precipitate thyroid storm.

Electrocardiogram in Thyrotoxicosis Electrocardiogram findings in thyrotoxicosis most commonly include sinus tachycardia and atrial fibrillation. Sinus tachycardia occurs in approximately 40% of cases.[4] Atrial fibrillation occurs in 10% to 35% of thyrotoxicosis patients—more commonly in patients >60 years old with underlying structural heart disease.[4] Premature ventricular contractions and heart blocks may be present. Atrial premature contractions and atrial flutter may also occur.

TREATMENT

The order of therapy in treating thyroid storm is very important with regard to the use of thionamide and iodine therapy. **Inhibition of thyroid gland synthesis of new thyroid hormone with a thionamide should be initiated before iodine therapy to prevent the stimulation of new thyroid hormone synthesis that can occur if iodine is given too soon.**

Treatment aims are as follows:

1. Supportive care
2. Inhibition of new hormone synthesis
3. Inhibition of thyroid hormone release
4. Peripheral β-adrenergic receptor blockade
5. Preventing peripheral conversion of thyroxine to triiodothyronine

The treatment recommendations are shown in **Table 229-8**, with specific comments in the following sections.

TREATMENT AIM 1: SUPPORTIVE CARE

Fluid losses could result from the combination of fever, diaphoresis, vomiting, and diarrhea. Check blood glucose and if blood sugar is relatively low, IV fluids with dextrose (isotonic saline with 5% or 10% dextrose) may be given to replenish glycogen stores.

Cholestyramine Cholestyramine is used to inhibit thyroid hormone reabsorption. Thyroid hormone is metabolized mainly in the liver, where it is conjugated to glucuronides and sulfates. These conjugation products are then excreted in the bile. Free hormones are released in the intestine and finally reabsorbed, completing the enterohepatic circulation of thyroid hormone. In states of thyrotoxicosis, there is increased enterohepatic circulation of thyroid hormone. Cholestyramine is an anion exchange resin that decreases reabsorption of thyroid hormone from the enterohepatic circulation. Cholestyramine in combination with methimazole or propylthiouracil, causes a more rapid decline in thyroid hormone levels than standard therapy with thionamides alone.[1]

TREATMENT AIM 2: INHIBITION OF NEW THYROID HORMONE SYNTHESIS

Thionamides Thionamides used for the treatment of thyrotoxicosis are either methimazole or propylthiouracil. Thionamide therapy decreases the synthesis of new hormone production but also has immunosuppressive effects.[7] Thionamides inhibit synthesis of thyroid hormones by preventing organification and trapping of iodide to iodine and by inhibiting coupling of iodotyrosines.

Methimazole has a longer half-life than propylthiouracil, permitting less frequent dosing. It presents in free form in the serum, whereas 80% to 90% of propylthiouracil is bound to albumin.[7]

The dose for methimazole is 40 to 100 milligrams given PO as loading dose followed by 20 milligrams every 4 hours. The total daily dose that should be given is 120 milligrams/d. If given PR, 40 milligrams should be crushed in aqueous solution. Although there are no commercially available parenteral formulations of the thionamides, there are case reports of methimazole being administered IV in circumstances in which the PO and PR routes of administration could not be used.[8] Methimazole was shown to have similar pharmacokinetics for both PO and IV use in normal subjects and in subjects with hyperthyroidism. In some centers, only carbimazole (which is the prodrug of methimazole) is available. If methimazole is not available, carbimazole can be used with the same potency.[9] The initial dose is 40 to 60 milligrams, followed by a maintenance dose of between 5 and 20 milligrams daily.

As for propylthiouracil, the dose for thyroid storm is 600 to 1000 milligrams given PO as a loading dose followed by 200 to 250 milligrams every 4 hours. The total daily dose that should be given is between 1200 and 1500 milligrams/d. The drug can be given by nasogastric tube or PR. Outside the thyroid gland, only propylthiouracil, not methimazole, can inhibit conversion of thyroxine to triiodothyronine.

Warning on Use of Propylthiouracil The U.S. Food and Drug Administration (FDA) in 2009 notified healthcare professionals of the risk of serious liver injury, including liver failure and death, with the use of propylthiouracil in adults and children. There is an increased risk of hepatotoxicity with propylthiouracil when compared with methimazole.10 Since 2010, the FDA has added a boxed warning to the prescribing information of propylthiouracil to include information about reports of severe liver injury and acute liver failure, some of which have been fatal. The FDA recommends that propylthiouracil be reserved for patients who cannot tolerate methimazole.

Propylthiouracil is preferred only in the case of pregnant patients during the first trimester, as methimazole use during this period had been associated with teratogenicity.[11] Nevertheless, methimazole is again suggested for use during the second and third trimesters of pregnancy. If propylthiouracil is used, signs and symptoms of liver injury should be closely monitored, especially in the first 6 months of therapy initiation. Its use must be discontinued immediately in cases of suspected liver injury. Propylthiouracil should not be used in children unless the patient is allergic to or intolerant of methimazole and no other treatment options are available.

TREATMENT AIM 3: INHIBITION OF HORMONE RELEASE

Iodine Lugol solution, potassium iodide, ipodate (Oragrafin®), or lithium carbonate can be given to stop thyroid hormone release. **Thionamide therapy must be instituted first and these drugs only given at least 1 hour later.** Iodine therapy blocks the release of prestored hormone and decreases iodide transport and oxidation in follicular cells. Lugol solution can be given 30 to 40 drops/d divided three to four times a day. One may start with 8 to 10 drops initially. Lugol solution provides 8 milligrams of iodide per drop.

Iodinated radiographic contrast dyes that contain ipodate (Oragrafin®) 0.5 to 3 grams/d orally or IV iopanoic acid (Telepaque®) 1 gram every 8 hours for the first 24 hours followed by 500 milligrams twice a day have also been used to inhibit hormone release, and they also have the added property to effectively prevent conversion of thyroxine to triiodothyronine.

Nevertheless, iodine-containing solution should not be given to patients with iodine overload or iodine-induced hyperthyroidism or those with amiodarone-induced thyrotoxicosis. Lithium or potassium perchlorate may be used instead.

TREATMENT AIM 4: PREVENTING PERIPHERAL CONVERSION OF THYROXINE TO TRIIODOTHYRONINE

The peripheral conversion of thyroxine to triiodothyronine, which is responsible for 85% of triiodothyronine present in the circulation, is blocked by propylthiouracil, propranolol, and glucocorticoid. Nevertheless, for propylthiouracil and propranolol, this effect is not quantitatively significant. Therefore, glucocorticoids such as hydrocortisone or dexamethasone are essential in treatment. Glucocorticoid use in thyroid storm also improves survival rates.[2,12] In patients who have severe thyrotoxicosis, especially in conjunction with hypotension, treatment with glucocorticoids is a standard practice because of the possibility of relative adrenal insufficiency.

TABLE 229-8 Treatment for Thyroid Storm

1. **Supportive care**

   General: oxygen, cardiac monitoring

   Fever: external cooling; acetaminophen 325–650 milligrams PO/PR every 4–6 h (aspirin is contraindicated because it may increase free thyroid hormone)

   Dehydration: IV fluids, IV isotonic saline with 5% dextrose may be used to replace glycogen depletion if blood sugar is low

   Nutrition: glucose, multivitamins, thiamine, including folate can be considered (deficient secondary to hypermetabolism)

   Cardiac decompensation (atrial fibrillation, congestive heart failure): rate control and inotropic agent, diuretics, sympatholytics as required

2. **Inhibition of new thyroid hormone synthesis with thionamides**

   Methimazole 40 milligrams given PO as loading dose and followed by 25 milligrams every 4 h. Total daily dose should be given: 120 milligrams/d. If given PR, 40 milligrams should be crushed in aqueous solution.

   (Avoid methimazole for pregnant women in first trimester as it can cause teratogenic effect. It can only be used in second and third trimester of pregnancy.)

   or

   PTU, a loading dose of 600–1000 milligrams given PO and followed by 200–250 milligrams every 4 h. Total daily dose should be given: 1200–1500 milligrams/d. Drug can be given via nasogastric tube or PR. (PTU also blocks peripheral conversion of thyroxin to triiodothyronine.)

   (PTU is used for pregnant women in first trimester. PTU also has a boxed warning issued by the U.S. Food and Drug Administration in 2010 regarding its rare but severe side effect toward liver function. Methimazole is preferred as first-line treatment unless contraindicated.)

3. **Inhibition of thyroid hormone release (at least 1 h after step 2)**

   Lugol solution 8–10 drops PO every 6–8 h

   or

   Potassium iodide (SSKI) five drops PO every 6 h

   or

   IV iopanoic acid (Telepaque®), 1 gram every 8 h for first 24 h, then 500 milligrams twice a day

   or

   Ipodate (Oragrafin®), 0.5–3 grams/d PO (especially useful with thyroiditis or thyroid hormone overdose)

   or

   Lithium carbonate (if allergic to iodine or agranulocytosis occurs with thionamides), 300 milligrams PO every 6 h (1200 milligrams/d) and subsequently to maintain serum lithium at 1 mEq/L

4. **β-Adrenergic receptor blockade**

   Propranolol IV in slow 1- to 2-milligram boluses, which may be repeated every 10 to 15 min until the desired effect is achieved. For less toxic patient, PO dose of 20 to 120 milligrams per dose or 160 to 320 milligrams/d in divided doses (contraindicated in bronchospastic disease and congestive heart failure)

   or

   Esmolol 500 micrograms/kg IV bolus, then 50–200 micrograms/kg/min maintenance

   or

   Reserpine 2.5–5.0 milligrams IM every 4–6 h, preceded by 1-milligram test dose while monitoring blood pressure (use if β-blocker contraindicated but avoid in congestive heart failure or hypotension and cardiac shock)

   or

   Guanethidine 30–40 milligrams PO every 6 h (use if β-blocker contraindicated but avoid in congestive heart failure, hypotension, and cardiac shock)

5. **Preventing peripheral conversion of thyroxine to triiodothyronine**

   Hydrocortisone 100 milligrams IV initially, then 100 milligrams three times/d until stable (also for adrenal replacement due to hypermetabolism)

   or

   Dexamethasone 2 milligrams IV every 6 h

6. **Treat precipitating event**

   All triggers of thyroid storm should be searched and treated accordingly (infection, myocardial infarct, diabetic ketoacidosis, etc.).

7. **Definitive therapy**

   Radioactive iodine ablation therapy or surgery may be necessary.

Note: Replacement therapy: dialysis and plasmapheresis are last resorts for patients who do not respond to treatments 1–5.

Abbreviation: PTU = propylthiouracil.

TREATMENT AIM 5: β-ADRENERGIC RECEPTOR BLOCKADE

Propranolol can be given IV in slow 1- to 2-milligram boluses, which may be repeated every 10 to 15 minutes until the desired effect is achieved. Orally, propranolol therapy usually begins at 20 to 120 milligrams per dose or 160 to 320 milligrams/d in divided doses.

The contraindications to peripheral blockade are the same as those for other medical conditions. Exercise caution in patients with congestive cardiac failure and thyrotoxic cardiomyopathy. Complicated patients with both a tachydysrhythmia and congestive heart failure can be managed first with rate control and an inotropic agent.

ALTERNATIVE TREATMENTS

Several alternative therapeutic agents are considered when the first-line therapies of thionamides, iodide, β-blockers, and glucocorticoids fail or cannot be used owing to toxicity or contraindicated conditions.

Alternative Drugs for Inhibition of New Hormone Synthesis or Release • *Potassium Perchlorate* Potassium perchlorate blocks thyroid uptake of iodine and thus interferes with the production of new hormones The perchlorate anion, ClO4–, is a competitive inhibitor of iodide transport. The recommended dose is 0.5 gram of potassium perchlorate per day.13 It is used in amiodarone-induced thyrotoxicosis for which iodine replacement is contraindicated. However, it has side effects of aplastic anemia and nephrotic syndrome.

Lithium In situations in which there is a contraindication to giving iodine (e.g., hypersensitivity to iodine), an alternative such as lithium can be used. In severe thyroid storm conditions, lithium can also be used in combination with propylthiouracil or methimazole. Lithium inhibits thyroid hormone release from thyroid gland. Lithium also has effects on the thyroid gland that decrease thyroid hormone synthesis, thereby increasing intrathyroidal iodine content and inhibiting coupling of iodotyrosine residues that form thyroxine and triiodothyronine. In thyroid storm, the dosing for lithium is 300 milligrams every 8 hours. To avoid lithium toxicity, lithium level should be monitored regularly every day to maintain a concentration of approximately 0.6 to 1.0 mEq/L (0.6-1.0 mmol/L). Very frequent monitoring of serum lithium levels is mandatory, especially because the serum lithium concentrations may change as the patient is rendered more euthyroid.

Alternative Drugs for Peripheral Blockade of β-Receptor: Reserpine and Guanethidine Reserpine or guanethidine can be used, usually in severe asthmatic patients needing treatment for thyroid storm, as they do not block β-receptors. These agents would be indicated only in rare situations in which β-adrenergic receptor antagonists are contraindicated and when there is no hypotension or evidence of central nervous system–associated mental status changes.[2] Side effects of both medications include hypotension and diarrhea.

Reserpine is an alkaloid agent that depletes catecholamine stores in sympathetic nerve terminals and the central nervous system. It can have central nervous system depressant effects. In severe asthmatics, IM reserpine, 2.5 milligrams every 4 hours, may be considered in lieu of peripheral blockade.[13] Guanethidine inhibits the release of catecholamines. Dosing for guanethidine in thyroid storm is 30 to 40 milligrams PO every 6 hours.

Thyroid Hormone Removal In patients who have contraindications to propylthiouracil and methimazole, such as a prior severe reaction, direct removal of thyroid hormone has been described. Plasmapheresis, charcoal hemoperfusion, resin hemoperfusion, and plasma exchange have been found to be effective in rapidly reducing thyroid hormone levels in thyroid storm.[13,14]

IDENTIFY PRECIPITATING FACTORS

Search for infection in febrile thyrotoxic patients. Obtain an electrocardiogram to identify myocardial infarction, ischemia, or arrhythmia.

In cases of thyroid storm precipitated by diabetic ketoacidosis, myocardial infarction, pulmonary embolism, or other acute processes, appropriate management of the specific underlying problem should proceed along with the treatment of the thyrotoxicosis.[2]

DEFINITIVE THERAPY

Definitive therapy with radioactive iodine ablation may not be able to be done for several weeks or months after treatment with iodine for thyroid storm. Close follow-up and monitoring should continue, with plans for definitive therapy to prevent a future recurrence of life-threatening thyrotoxicosis.[2]

GUIDE FOR PREPARATION OF THYROTOXIC PATIENTS FOR EMERGENCY SURGERY

In the event that a patient has thyrotoxicosis background and requires emergent surgery, the recommendation of drug supplementation is as shown in **Table 229-9**. The supplementation is important, as surgery in a patient with hyperthyroidism may precipitate thyroid storm.

ADVERSE SIDE EFFECTS FROM ANTITHYROID DRUGS

Common adverse side effects of the antithyroid drugs are shown in **Table 229-10**.

TABLE 229-9 Rapid Preparation of Thyrotoxic Patients for Emergent Surgery

Drug Class	Recommended Drug	Dosage	Mechanism of Action	Continue Postoperatively?
β-Adrenergic blockade	Propranolol	40–80 milligrams PO 3 to 4 times a day	β-Adrenergic blockade; decreased thyroxine-to-triiodothyronine conversion (high dose)	Yes
	or			
	Esmolol	50–100 micrograms/kg/min	β-Adrenergic blockade	Change to PO propranolol
Thionamide	Propylthiouracil	200 milligrams PO every 4 h	Inhibition of new thyroid hormone synthesis; decreased thyroxine-to-triiodothyronine conversion	Stop immediately after near-total thyroidectomy; continue after nonthyroidal surgery
	or			
	Methimazole	20 milligrams PO every 4 h	Inhibition of new thyroid hormone synthesis	Stop immediately after near-total thyroidectomy; continue after nonthyroidal surgery
Oral cholecystographic agent	Iopanoic acid	500 milligrams PO twice a day	Decreased release of thyroid hormone; decreased thyroxine-to-triiodothyronine conversion	Stop immediately after surgery
Corticosteroid	Hydrocortisone	100 milligrams PO or IV every 8 h	Vasomotor stability; decreased thyroxine-to-triiodothyronine conversion	Taper over first 72 h
	or			
	Dexamethasone	2 milligrams PO or IV every 6 h	Vasomotor stability; decreased thyroxine-to-triiodothyronine conversion	Taper over first 72 h
	or			
	Betamethasone	0.5 milligram PO every 6 h, IM or IV	Vasomotor stability; decreased thyroxine-to-triiodothyronine conversion	Taper over first 72 h

(Reproduced with permission from Langley RW, Burch HB: Perioperative management of the thyrotoxic patient. *Endocrinol Metab Clin of North Am* 32: 519, 2003. Copyright Elsevier.)

TABLE 229-10 Common Adverse Side Effects from Antithyroid Drugs

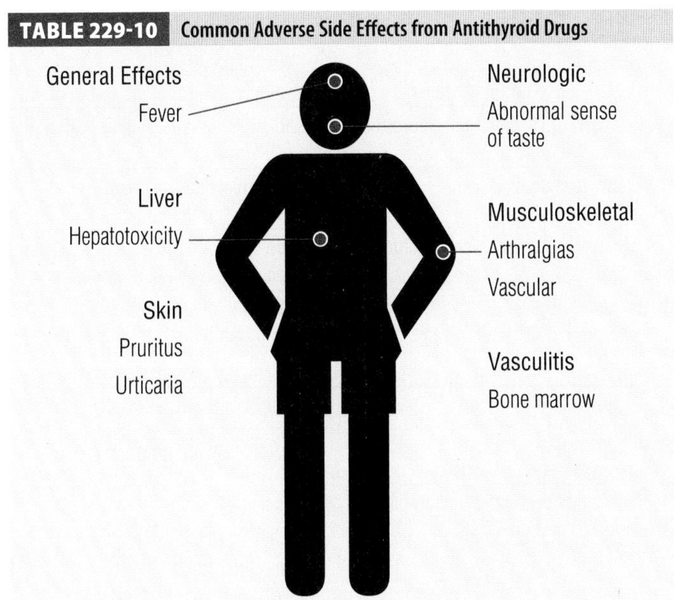

After surgery, the precipitating event should be determined, and definitive therapy of thyrotoxicosis should be planned.

DISPOSITION AND FOLLOW-UP

Thyroid storm patients typically require admission to the intensive care unit. Patients with thyroid storm often have concomitant diseases precipitating the attack and require close monitoring. Complete recovery may take 1 week until circulating levels of thyroid hormones are depleted. Stable hyperthyroid patients with minimal symptoms can only be discharged for follow-up either by an endocrinologist or primary care physician, if the patient is already on medication with a clear plan of follow-up.

SPECIAL POPULATIONS

ELDERLY PATIENTS

Older patients may present with "apathetic" thyrotoxicosis (i.e., with some atypical symptoms, including weight loss, palpitations, weakness, dizziness, syncope, memory loss, and physical findings of sinus tachycardia or atrial fibrillation).[5] Signs and symptoms of this condition are few and subtle, and the initial appearance of disease may be single-organ failure (e.g., congestive heart failure), producing diagnostic confusion by pointing to diagnoses other than thyrotoxicosis.

DRUG INTERACTIONS IN THYROTOXIC PATIENTS

Many drugs interfere with protein binding, including heparin, furosemide, phenytoin, carbamazepine, diazepam, salicylates, opiates, estrogens, and nonsteroidal anti-inflammatory drugs. Because of this interference with total thyroid hormone levels, free hormone concentrations are preferable in the diagnosis of thyrotoxicosis.[6]

THYROTOXIC PATIENTS AND AMIODARONE

Amiodarone is an essential anti-arrhythmic drug used in the ED. Amiodarone is also a precipitant of thyroid storm. It is 37% organic iodine by weight, and as such, can have many effects on thyroid function. Normal maintenance doses result in iodine loads of 10 to 20 times the normal dietary requirement of iodine. Chronic use of amiodarone causes either a hypothyroid or a thyrotoxic state in 20% to 30% of patients.[15]

THYROTOXIC PATIENTS WITH ATRIAL FIBRILLATION

The issue of anticoagulation in atrial fibrillation in the setting of thyrotoxicosis is controversial. Studies assessing the incidence of embolic events in thyrotoxic patients who have atrial fibrillation have yielded conflicting information regarding the incidence of embolism. Thyrotoxic patients who have atrial fibrillation may not be at greater risk for embolic events, compared with age-matched patients who have atrial fibrillation due to other causes.[16] Therefore, standard therapy with warfarin or aspirin would be indicated. Thyrotoxic patients may require a lower maintenance dose of warfarin than euthyroid patients because of increased clearance of vitamin K–dependent clotting factors.[17]

REFERENCES

The complete reference list is available online at www.TintinalliEM.com.

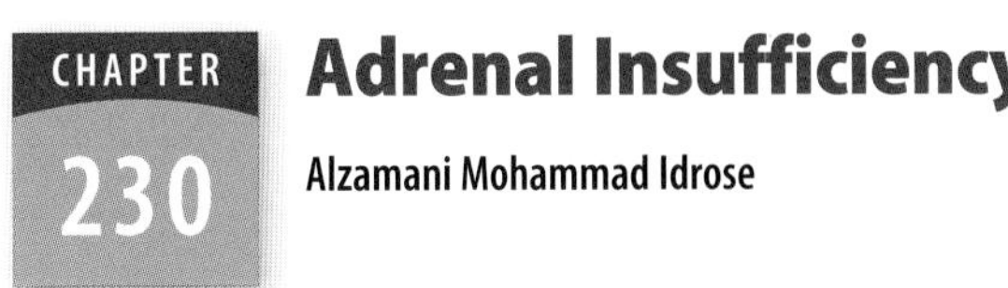

CHAPTER 230 Adrenal Insufficiency

Alzamani Mohammad Idrose

INTRODUCTION

The adrenal gland synthesizes steroid hormones in the cortex and catecholamines in the medulla. **Adrenal insufficiency** is deficiency of adrenal gland hormone production in the cortex. **Primary adrenal insufficiency,** or Addison's disease, is due to intrinsic adrenal gland dysfunction and results in decreased cortisol, aldosterone, and sex hormone production. The condition is rare, with prevalence ranging from 39 to 144 cases per million population.[1]

Secondary adrenal insufficiency is due to hypothalamic-pituitary dysfunction with failure to secrete corticotropin-releasing hormone and/or adrenocorticotropic hormone. This disorder results in cortisol deficiency only.

Adrenal crisis is a life-threatening exacerbation of adrenal insufficiency when an increased demand fails to increase hormone production.

ADRENAL GLAND PHYSIOLOGY

The adrenal gland is made up of the cortex and medulla producing steroid hormones and catecholamines, respectively. The adrenal cortex produces three categories of steroids: the glucocorticoids (**cortisol**), mineralocorticoids (**aldosterone**), and gonadocorticoids (**sex hormones**). Glucocorticoids are produced in the zona fasciculata, and mineralocorticoids and gonadocorticoids are produced in the zona glomerulosa and zona reticularis of the adrenal cortex. The adrenal medulla produces adrenaline, noradrenaline, and a small amount of dopamine in response to stimulation by sympathetic preganglionic neurons.

Cortisol is secreted in response to direct stimulation by adrenocorticotropic hormone. Adrenocorticotropic hormone secretion is stimulated by corticotropin-releasing factor released from the hypothalamus. Secretion occurs in a diurnal rhythm, with higher levels secreted in the morning and lower levels in the evening. In normal circumstances, the daily cortisol equivalent is about 20 milligrams/d of hydrocortisone. Plasma cortisol suppresses the release of adrenocorticotropic hormone through negative feedback inhibition. Cortisol facilitates the stress response by affecting the heart, vascular bed, water excretion, electrolyte balance, potentiation of catecholamine action, and control of water distribution. It affects fat, protein, and carbohydrate metabolism by stimulating glycogenolysis and neoglycogenesis. It is involved in immunologic and inflammatory responses and affects calcium metabolism. It promotes growth and development but, in excess, interferes with the GI tract mucosa maintenance, leading to peptic ulcer.

Aldosterone secretion is controlled primarily by the renin-angiotensin system and serum potassium concentration. The renin-angiotensin system controls aldosterone levels in response to changes in

TABLE 230-1 Causes of Primary Adrenal Insufficiency

Primary Adrenal Insufficiency	Examples
Autoimmune	Isolated adrenal insufficiency or associated with polyglandular insufficiencies (polyglandular autoimmune syndrome type I or II)
Adrenal hemorrhage or thrombosis	Necrosis caused by meningococcal sepsis Coagulation disorders Overwhelming sepsis (Waterhouse-Friderichsen syndrome)
Drugs	*Adrenal enzyme inhibitors (affect those with limited pituitary or adrenal reserve)* Etomidate Aminoglutethimide (can be used by body builders) Mitotane (orphan drug used to treat adrenocortical carcinoma) Ketoconazole
Infections	Tuberculosis Fungal, bacterial sepsis Acquired immunodeficiency syndrome involving adrenal glands
Infiltrative disorders	Sarcoidosis Hemochromatosis Amyloidosis Lymphoma Metastatic cancer
Surgery	Bilateral adrenalectomy Bariatric surgery
Hereditary	Adrenal hypoplasia Congenital adrenal hyperplasia Adrenoleukodystrophy Familial glucocorticoid deficiency

volume, posture, and sodium intake. Serum potassium (hyperkalemia) influences the adrenal cortex directly to increase aldosterone secretion. Aldosterone maintains sodium and potassium plasma concentrations. It regulates extracellular volume and controls sodium and water balance.

Gonadocorticoids include androgen hormones and estrogen. Androgens produced include testosterone, dehydroepiandrosterone, and dehydroepiandrosterone sulfate, which are present in both men and women. In women, androgens are produced in the adrenal glands as well as the ovaries and promote the development of sex characteristics such as axillary and pubic hair and libido. In men, most androgens (testosterone) are produced in the testes. Androgens made by the adrenal glands are less important for normal sexual function.

PRIMARY ADRENAL INSUFFICIENCY

Causes of primary adrenal insufficiency (Addison's disease) are shown in **Table 230-1**. Approximately 90% of the gland must be destroyed for clinical adrenal insufficiency to develop.[2] In the United States, autoimmune disorders are responsible for most cases of primary adrenal insufficiency.[1,3] Autoimmune disorders may occur as an isolated process or as a component of polyglandular autoimmune syndrome types I and II. **Polyglandular autoimmune syndrome type I** is associated with candidiasis, hypoparathyroidism, and adrenal failure. **Polyglandular autoimmune syndrome type II** consists of Addison's disease plus either an autoimmune thyroid disease or type 1 diabetes mellitus associated with hypogonadism, pernicious anemia, celiac disease, or primary biliary cirrhosis.

In terms of infection, worldwide, tuberculosis is the most common cause of primary adrenal insufficiency. Human immunodeficiency virus may cause adrenal insufficiency through opportunistic infections (principally cytomegalovirus) or use of medications, such as ketoconazole.

TABLE 230-2 Causes of Secondary Adrenal Insufficiency

Secondary Adrenal Insufficiency (hypothalamic-pituitary dysfunction)	Examples
Sudden cessation of prolonged glucocorticoid therapy	Chronic use of steroid inhibits CRH and ACTH production
Pituitary necrosis or bleeding	Postpartum pituitary necrosis (Sheehan's syndrome)
Exogenous glucocorticoid administration	Causes decreased production of CRH at hypothalamus and ACTH at pituitary
Brain tumors	Pituitary tumor Hypothalamic tumor Local invasion (craniopharyngioma)
Pituitary irradiation Pituitary surgery Head trauma involving the pituitary gland	Disrupts corticotropin-releasing hormone and ACTH production capacity in hypothalamic-pituitary axis
Infiltrative disorders of the pituitary or hypothalamus	Sarcoidosis Hemosiderosis Hemochromatosis Histiocytosis X Metastatic cancer Lymphoma
CNS infections involving hypothalamus or pituitary	Tuberculosis Meningitis Fungus Human immunodeficiency virus

Abbreviations: ACTH = adrenocorticotropic hormone; CRH = corticotropin-releasing hormone.

Secondary adrenal insufficiency can develop through inhibition of the hypothalamus-pituitary-adrenal axis.[4-7]

Infiltrative diseases such as amyloidosis, hemosiderosis, and bilateral metastasis from cancer may also cause primary adrenal insufficiency. Thrombosis and/or hemorrhage of the adrenals may occur as a complication of anticoagulation therapy, sepsis, disseminated intravascular coagulation, meningococcemia (Waterhouse-Friderichsen syndrome), or antiphospholipid syndrome.[8-10]

SECONDARY ADRENAL INSUFFICIENCY

Causes of secondary adrenal insufficiency are shown in **Table 230-2**. Secondary adrenal failure is usually characterized by depressed adrenocorticotropic hormone secretion, which reduces cortisol production, but aldosterone levels remain normal because of preserved stimulation by both the renin-angiotensin axis and potassium. Adrenal sex hormone production is also preserved. Intracranial disorders such as brain tumor, pituitary disease, postpartum pituitary necrosis, or major head trauma may affect the hypothalamic-pituitary function, resulting in secondary adrenal insufficiency.[11]

The most common cause of secondary adrenal insufficiency is long-term therapy with pharmacologic doses of glucocorticoids. Severity of adrenal suppression is variable and depends on the dose and potency of the glucocorticoid and the time of day the drug was taken (suppression is greater when taken in the evening). Recovery of the hypothalamus-pituitary-adrenal axis may take a few months to 1 year after steroid cessation. Although hypothalamus-pituitary-adrenal axis suppression is related to duration of treatment, steroid dose, and total cumulative dose, there is no strict correlation with any of these factors.[12] Some critically ill patients demonstrate reduced cortisol clearance and suppression of adrenocorticotropic hormone release.[13]

ADRENAL CRISIS

Adrenal crisis is shock refractory to volume resuscitation and pressors. It can result from acute destruction of the hypothalamic-pituitary axis or the adrenal glands or from acute stressors in the setting of underlying primary or secondary adrenal insufficiency. Reported stressors include

TABLE 230-3 Difference between Primary and Secondary Adrenal Insufficiency

Presentation	Primary	Secondary
Volume depletion and hypotension	Marked	Not as severe unless crisis is present
Serum potassium	Hyperkalemia	Hypokalemia
Serum sodium	Hyponatremia (due to salt wasting)	Hypernatremia (aldosterone functioning) or hyponatremia (due to water retention)
Cushingoid appearance	Absent	May be present (if due to long-term glucocorticoid use)
Symptoms of other pituitary hormone deficiencies (e.g., hypothyroidism and amenorrhea)	Absent	May be present (depends on the hypothalamic-pituitary site of lesion)
Skin pigmentation	Present (due to high ACTH level)	Absent

Abbreviation: ACTH = adrenocorticotropic hormone.

acute infection, especially gastrointestinal infection; surgery; extreme physical activity; acute severe injury or burns; and cessation of chronic glucocorticoid replacement.[14]

CLINICAL FEATURES

Primary and secondary adrenal insufficiency have dissimilar clinical presentations. These are depicted in **Table 230-3**. **Primary adrenal insufficiency** presents with symptoms of diminished cortisol, aldosterone, and gonadocorticoids, and increased adrenocorticotropic hormone, which causes skin hyperpigmentation. On the other hand, **secondary adrenal insufficiency** presents with symptoms of diminished cortisol only and possibly with related symptoms of intracranial lesions (e.g., headache, visual changes, galactorrhea).

Cortisol deficiency symptoms include weight loss, lethargy, weakness, mental status changes, and GI symptoms (anorexia, nausea, vomiting, abdominal pain, and diarrhea). **Aldosterone deficiency symptoms** include dehydration, syncope, salt craving, and hypotension (usually with orthostatic changes). **Gonadocorticoid deficiency symptoms** are observed more in women, who present with decreased axillary and pubic hair and decreased libido.

ADRENAL CRISIS

Acute adrenal crisis is characterized by severe hypotension refractory to vasopressors. Other symptoms include severe abdominal pain, nausea, and vomiting, mimicking an acute abdomen. CNS symptoms of confusion, disorientation, and lethargy may be present. There may be associated sepsis, even without fever. Consider adrenal crisis in situations of unexplained hypotension, especially in patients with a history of glucocorticoid therapy; those with acquired immunodeficiency syndrome, tuberculosis, autoimmune disease, or severe head trauma; those with a history of chronic fatigue and hyperpigmentation; and those with disorders known to cause acute adrenal crisis (as seen in Tables 230-1 and 230-2).

LABORATORY STUDIES AND IMAGING

Obtain a bedside glucose determination to identify hypoglycemia. Obtain CBC, full chemistries, hepatic function studies, ECG, and urinalysis. Additional studies are determined by the presumptive underlying source such as sepsis, hemorrhage, or CNS abnormality.

Primary adrenal insufficiency is typically characterized by hyponatremia and hyperkalemia due to aldosterone deficiency. **Secondary adrenal insufficiency** is characterized by either hypernatremia from functioning aldosterone causing sodium reabsorption in kidney or hyponatremia following water retention, and hypokalemia. In both primary and secondary adrenal insufficiency, cortisol deficiency is a common sequela, and hypotension or hypoglycemia may present. Mild metabolic acidosis is evident due to tissue hypoxia from hypovolemia and hypotension. ECG changes are generally related to potassium imbalances (e.g., prolonged QT, peaked T waves, and heart block in hyperkalemia in primary adrenal insufficiency, or inverted T waves and presence of U wave in hypokalemia in secondary adrenal insufficiency). An abdominal CT scan can identify adrenal gland hemorrhage or infarction.

Serum cortisol or adrenocorticotropic hormone levels are not usually readily available at ED presentation. If available, a serum cortisol >18 micrograms/dL generally rules out adrenal insufficiency.[15] The adrenocorticotropic hormone stimulation test measures serum cortisol after stimulation by synthetic adrenocorticotropic hormone (cosyntropin). Serum cortisol rises significantly in secondary, but not in primary, insufficiency. Serum corticotropin (adrenocorticotropic hormone) level[14] measurement also helps differentiate between primary and secondary adrenal insufficiency. A high adrenocorticotropic hormone level is seen in primary adrenal insufficiency, but adrenocorticotropic hormone is low in secondary adrenal insufficiency.

TREATMENT

ADRENAL INSUFFICIENCY

For **primary insufficiency**, treatment requires daily dosing of glucocorticoid and mineralocorticoid, usually for life. Androgen replacement may be recommended for women. The goal of treatment is to stabilize hormone levels and relieve symptoms. Mineralocorticoids are replaced with an oral, synthetic mineralocorticoid drug such as fludrocortisone (Florinef®). The dose is tailored to manage blood pressure and fluid balance. For **secondary insufficiency**, only glucocorticoid replacement is required.

ADRENAL CRISIS

The recommended treatment is outlined in **Table 230-4**. Begin therapy immediately in any suspected case of adrenal crisis, because prognosis is related to the rapidity of treatment onset. Give IV fluids early to treat hypotension. If hypoglycemia is present, give dextrose-containing solutions.

TABLE 230-4 Treatment Guide for Adrenal Crisis

Administer IV Fluids for Hypotension

Use dextrose-containing saline if hypoglycemic.

↓

Give Steroids

Hydrocortisone (100-milligram bolus) is the drug of choice for cases of adrenal crisis or insufficiency, especially for underlying primary insufficiency (provides both glucocorticoid and mineralocorticoid effects).

or

Dexamethasone, 4-milligram bolus (preferred if rapid adrenocorticotropic hormone stimulation test is contemplated).

↓

Consider Vasopressors

Administer only after steroid therapy in patients unresponsive to aggressive fluid resuscitation (choice of norepinephrine, dopamine, or phenylephrine [Neo-Synephrine®]).

↓

Consider Steroid Supplementation

Patients may require lifelong glucocorticoids ± mineralocorticoid ± androgen supplementation.

↓

Determine Underlying Cause

Investigate as appropriate—sepsis, adrenal hemorrhage, CNS abnormality.

↓

Optimize Maintenance Dosage of Steroids

During periods of stress, increase maintenance doss of chronic steroids to three times the daily dose, to satisfy increased physiologic need for cortisol.[16]

Hydrocortisone is the steroid drug of choice for cases of adrenal crisis or insufficiency because it provides both glucocorticoid and mineralocorticoid effects. IV hydrocortisone (100-milligram minimum bolus) can be administered. Alternatively, IV dexamethasone (4-milligram bolus) may be given rapidly if adrenocorticotropic hormone stimulation test is contemplated as part of diagnostic strategy. Give vasopressors only after steroid therapy in patients unresponsive to fluid resuscitation.

Determine the underlying cause. For **primary adrenal insufficiency**, abdominal CT scan may be performed to evaluate the adrenal glands. Consider retroviral screening if HIV is under consideration. Consider chest radiography to assess for bronchopneumonia or tuberculosis. For **secondary adrenal insufficiency**, a head CT or MRI, as well as blood tests of pituitary hormones, may be required.

For patients receiving chronic steroids, increase the maintenance dose during periods of stress (e.g., illness, surgery, trauma, GI upset) to satisfy the increased physiologic need for cortisol. Dosage recommendations vary and are based on expert opinion. **A typical stress dose is three times the daily maintenance dose of glucocorticoid.** Mineralocorticoid dosage generally stays the same. Endocrinology consultation can be helpful for further recommendations.

DISPOSITION AND FOLLOW-UP

Admit patients with adrenal crisis to an intensive care unit for careful clinical monitoring, IV steroid administration, and confirmation of diagnosis and identification of etiology. Discharge can only be considered for mild cases of adrenal insufficiency with identified etiologies and after a clear plan of management is established, often with endocrinology consultation.

SPECIAL POPULATIONS

PATIENTS ON CHRONIC CORTICOSTEROIDS

Hypothalamus-pituitary-adrenal axis function is inhibited with chronic use of steroids. Always consider adrenal insufficiency in patients with chronic steroid use presenting with any acute illness. Hypothalamus-pituitary-adrenal axis function should recover within about 1 month after the last dose of steroid intake, but may be longer in some cases. Patients who receive steroids by topical, intranasal, inhalational, or PR routes are not at risk for hypothalamus-pituitary-adrenal axis suppression.

PATIENTS WITH CHRONIC ADRENAL INSUFFICIENCY WITH ACUTE ILLNESS OR INJURY

Patients with chronic adrenal insufficiency who present to the ED with a minor illness or injury require special attention to steroid dosing.[15] In normal circumstances, about 20 milligrams/d of hydrocortisone is equivalent to the daily production of cortisol. For a minor illness or injury, triple the daily glucocorticoid dose for 24 to 48 hours until symptoms improve.[16] Increasing the mineralocorticoid dose, if the patient is receiving one, is usually not necessary. Arrange follow-up care in 24 hours with the primary care physician or endocrinologist. Patients should return to the ED if nausea, vomiting, fever, weakness, or any other untoward symptoms develop, or if they cannot retain their medications.

PREGNANCY WITH ADRENAL INSUFFICIENCY

Most women with primary adrenal insufficiency are able to undergo healthy pregnancy, labor, and delivery. They need to take medications on schedule with close monitoring of mother and fetus. Some may require adjustment of glucocorticoid doses, especially during the third trimester and during labor. Women with hyperemesis gravidarum may need to switch from oral medication to parenteral medication until symptoms subside.

REFERENCES

The complete reference list is available online at www.TintinalliEM.com.

SECTION 18

Hematologic and Oncologic Disorders

CHAPTER 231 Anemia

John C. Ray
Robin R. Hemphill

INTRODUCTION

Anemia is a common medical problem worldwide, affecting approximately one quarter of the world's population, especially children, pregnant and premenopausal women, the elderly, and the chronically ill.[1-7] Anemia is not so much a disease as a sign or symptom. There are three broad causes of anemia: (1) blood loss, (2) decreased red blood cell production, and (3) increased red blood cell destruction.

PATHOPHYSIOLOGY

Anemia is a reduced concentration of red blood cells (RBCs) from the normal ranges based on age, gender, and race.[8] In healthy persons, normal erythropoiesis ensures that the concentration of RBCs present is adequate to meet the body's demand for oxygen and that the destruction of RBCs balances the production. The average life of the circulating erythrocyte is approximately 110 to 120 days. Any process or condition that results in the loss of RBCs, that impairs RBC production, or that increases RBC destruction will result in anemia if the body cannot produce enough new cells to replace those lost (**Table 231-1**). It is not uncommon for more than one mechanism to produce anemia in the same individual.

Quantification of the erythrocyte concentration is reflected in (1) RBC count per microliter, (2) hemoglobin concentration, and (3) hematocrit (percentage of RBC mass to blood volume). Normal RBC values for adults vary between genders, with small variations for ethnicity and age (**Table 231-2**).

The body responds to anemia in several ways in order to blunt the effect of a reduction in the oxygen-carrying capacity. The mechanisms vary, depending on the rapidity of onset, the degree of anemia, and the underlying condition of the patient. In acute forms of anemia that result from intravascular volume loss, the peripheral vasculature compensates by vasoconstriction, while the central vasculature vasodilates to help preserve blood flow to vital organs.[9] As the condition worsens, systemic small-vessel vasodilation will occur, allowing increased blood flow to tissues. These mechanisms result in decreased systemic vascular resistance, increased cardiac output, and often tachycardia. Along with these changes, the RBCs themselves enhance their ability to release oxygen to the tissues. If the anemia is chronic in nature, there is commonly an increase in plasma volume that maintains total blood volume at a constant level.

TABLE 231-1 Classification of Anemia

Mechanism	Example
Loss of red blood cells by hemorrhage	Acute GI bleeding
Increased destruction	Sickle cell disease Drug-induced autoimmune hemolytic anemia
Impaired production	Nutritional deficiency anemia (iron, folate) Aplastic or myelodysplastic anemia
Dilutional	Rapid IV crystalloid infusion

TABLE 231-2 Normal Red Blood Cell Values for Adults

	Male	Female
Red blood cell count (million/mm^3)	4.5–6.0	4.0–5.5
Hemoglobin (grams/dL)	14–17	12–15
Hematocrit (%)	42–52	36–48
Mean corpuscular volume (fL)	78–100	78–102
Mean corpuscular hemoglobin (picograms/cell)	25–35	25–35
Mean corpuscular hemoglobin concentration (grams/dL)	32–36	32–36
Red cell distribution width (%)	11.5–14.5	11.5–14.5
Reticulocytes (%)	0.5–2.5	0.5–2.5

Note: Normal values may vary depending on the equipment used, patient's age, and the altitude of the equipment location.

Finally, anemia will result in the stimulation of erythropoietin as a result of tissue hypoxia and breakdown products from RBC destruction. New immature erythrocytes, known as reticulocytes, will appear in the blood within 3 to 7 days.

CLINICAL FEATURES

The severity of signs and symptoms related to anemia depends on several factors: the rate of development of anemia (acute vs chronic), the extent of anemia that is present, the age and general physical condition of the patient, and other existing comorbidities. Children and young adults, for example, may tolerate a significant decline in RBC volume with minimally altered vital signs until they become acutely hypotensive, whereas elderly patients frequently have other comorbidities that make physiologic compensation challenging.[3,4] Patients with chronic and slowly developing anemia may have no complaints even with hemoglobin levels as low as 5 to 6 grams/dL. Typically, most otherwise healthy adults will be symptomatic when hemoglobin levels decrease to about 7 grams/dL.

Patients with chronic anemia may note weakness, fatigue, dizziness, lethargy, dyspnea with minimal exertion, palpitations, and orthostatic symptoms. Specific historical features can be helpful in the identification and diagnosis of anemia; a history of recent trauma, hematochezia, melena, hemoptysis, hematemesis, hematuria, or menorrhagia suggests possible anemia. More subtle historical features include relevant comorbidities such as peptic ulcer disease, chronic liver disease, and chronic renal disease. Specific inquiries about the use of antiplatelet agents, anticoagulants, and nonsteroidal anti-inflammatory agents should be made.

Physical exam findings that may be present in patients with clinically significant anemia include tachycardia; skin, nail bed, and mucosal pallor; systolic ejection murmur; bounding pulse; and widened pulse pressure (**Figure 231-1**). Signs of easy bleeding or bruising suggest a coagulation disorder. Evidence of jaundice and hepatosplenomegaly suggests hemolysis. Unusual skin ulcerations, peripheral neuropathy, or neurologic signs such as ataxia or altered mental status may be evidence of nutritional deficiencies. Additional manifestations may depend on comorbid illnesses. For example, a patient with preexisting angina may find that episodes of chest pain are markedly worsened when anemia is present.

Patients who develop an acute, severe anemia may have all the signs and symptoms noted above and, in addition, may have hypotension, resting and exertional dyspnea, palpitations, diaphoresis, anxiety, or severe weakness that may progress to lethargy and altered mental status.

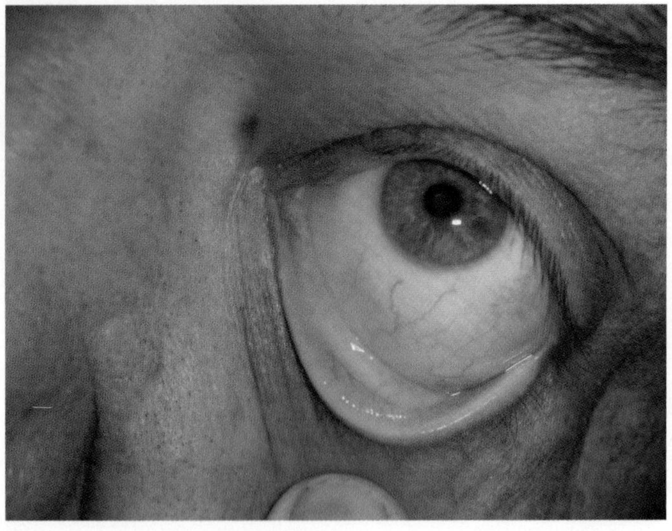

A

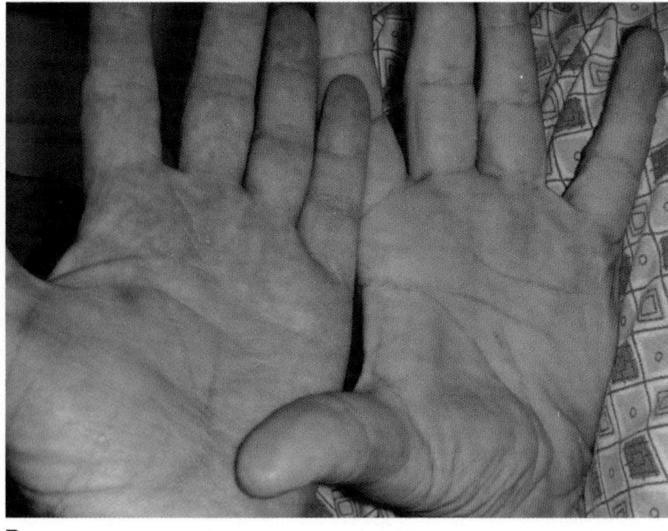

B

FIGURE 231-1. Pale conjunctiva (**A**) and palms (**B**) in patient with anemia. In **B**, the physician's hand is on the left for comparison with the patient's hand on the right. [Image used with permission of J. Stephan Stapczynski, MD.]

They may also complain of thirst and will usually have decreased urine output. Loss of >40% of blood volume from trauma or spontaneous hemorrhage can lead to severe symptoms that are due more to intravascular volume depletion than to anemia.[10] In healthy patients, myocardial oxygen delivery usually is not limited until hemoglobin concentration is 50% or less of normal.

DIAGNOSIS

The diagnosis is established by a finding of decreased RBC count, hemoglobin, and hematocrit on the routine CBC. It is rarely essential that a specific cause of anemia be established in the ED. However, appropriate assessment initiated in the ED can help expedite a diagnosis and should therefore be started before the transfusion of packed RBCs.[6,8]

The initial evaluation of a patient newly diagnosed with anemia includes several steps. First, look for a source of bleeding, including the most common internal sites—GI or uterine bleeding. If there is no physical or historical evidence of GI or uterine bleeding, then review RBC indices provided with the CBC, reticulocyte count, and peripheral blood smear (**Table 231-3**). The mean corpuscular volume is the most useful guide to the possible etiology of an anemia and is used to classify the anemic process as microcytic, normocytic, or macrocytic. Other useful diagnostic tests include the red cell distribution width and reticulocyte count. The serum ferritin is the most useful test for the diagnosis of iron deficiency anemia.[11] Following this initial classification, additional tests can lead to a specific diagnosis (**Figures 231-2, 231-3,** and **231-4**).[5,7,8,12-15]

TABLE 231-3 Laboratory Tests in the Evaluation of Anemia

Test	Interpretation	Clinical Correlation
MCV	Measure of the average RBC size.	Decreased MCV (microcytosis) is seen in chronic iron deficiency, thalassemia, anemia of chronic disease, and lead poisoning.
		Increased MCV (macrocytosis) can be due to vitamin B_{12} or folate deficiency, alcohol abuse, liver disease, reticulocytosis, and some medications (see "Diagnosis" section).
MCH	Measure of the amount of hemoglobin in average RBC.	—
RDW	Measures the size variability of the RBC population.	In early deficiency anemia (iron, vitamin B_{12}, or folate), may be increased before the MCV becomes abnormal.
MCHC	Measure of hemoglobin concentration in average RBC.	Low MCHC can be seen in iron deficiency anemia, defects in porphyrin synthesis, and hemolytic anemia.
Ferritin	Ferritin is a protein in the body that binds to iron. Serum levels serve as an indication of the amount of iron stored in the body.	Low serum ferritin is associated with iron deficiency anemia and helps differentiate this anemia from other causes.
Reticulocyte count	These RBCs of intermediate maturity are a marker of production by the bone marrow.	Decreased reticulocyte count reflects impaired RBC production.
		Increased counts are a marker of accelerated RBC production.
Peripheral blood smear	Allows visualization of the RBC morphology.	May guide to new diagnosis of diseases such as sickle cell disease.
	Allows evaluation for abnormal cell shapes.	Aids in the diagnosis of entities such as hemolytic anemia.
	Allows examination of the WBCs and platelets.	May guide the diagnosis of other diseases that cause anemia.
Direct and indirect Coombs test	Direct Coombs test is used to detect antibodies on RBCs.	Direct Coombs test is positive in autoimmune hemolytic anemia, transfusion reactions, and some drug-induced hemolytic anemia.
	Indirect Coombs test is used to detect antibodies in the sera.	Indirect Coombs test is routinely used in compatibility testing before transfusion.

Abbreviations: MCH = mean corpuscular hemoglobin; MCHC = mean corpuscular hemoglobin concentration; MCV = mean corpuscular volume; RBC = red blood cell; RDW = red cell distribution width.

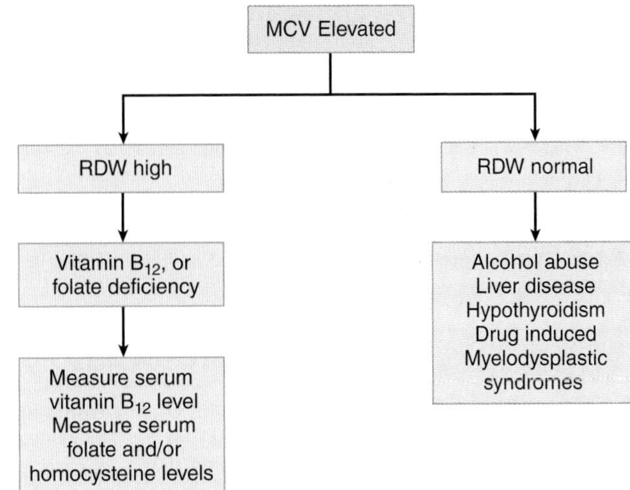

FIGURE 231-2. Evaluation of macrocytic anemia. MCV = mean corpuscular volume; RDW = red cell distribution width.

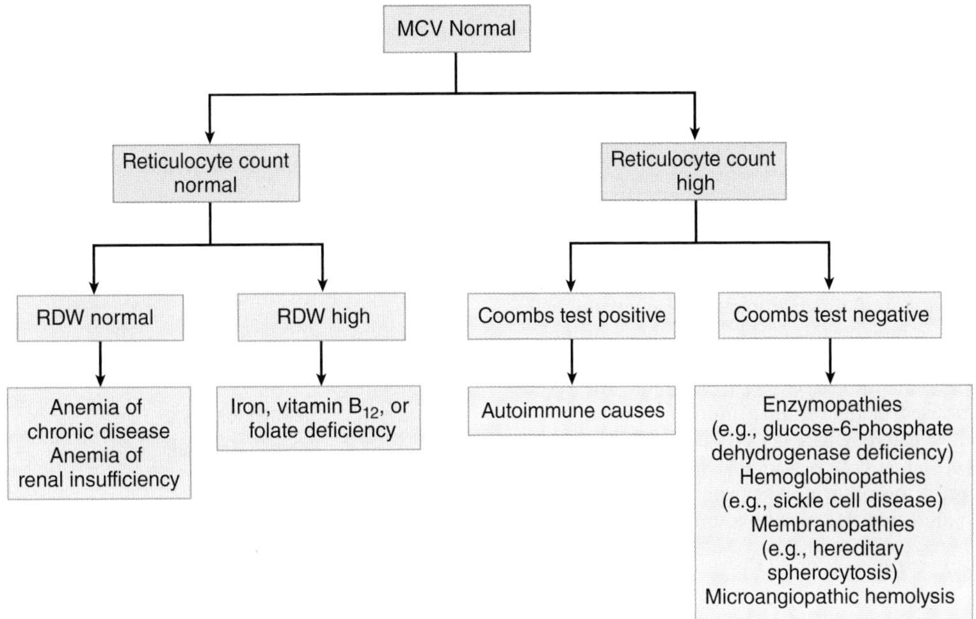

FIGURE 231-3. Evaluation of normocytic anemia. MCV = mean corpuscular volume; RDW = red cell distribution width.

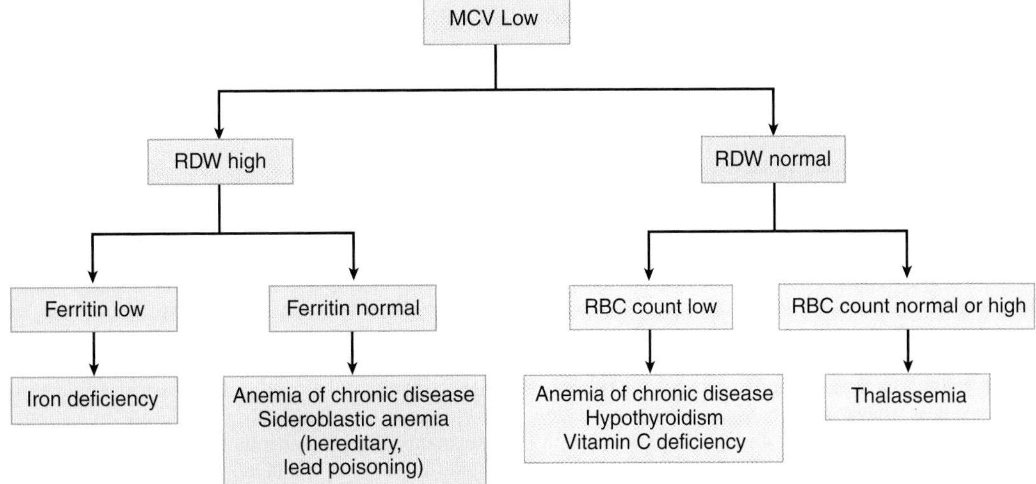

FIGURE 231-4. Evaluation of microcytic anemia. MCV = mean corpuscular volume; RBC = red blood cell; RDW = red cell distribution width.

TABLE 231-4 Treatment for Specific Anemias

Anemia Type	Treatment (Adult Doses)
Iron deficiency anemia	Elemental iron, 200–300 milligrams PO daily (e.g., ferrous sulfate, 325 milligrams PO, 3–4 tablets taken on an empty stomach over the course of day); reticulocyte count should increase within 4–7 d and peak at 10 d; sustained treatment after correction of anemia is usually necessary to replenish iron stores.
Cyanocobalamin (vitamin B_{12}) deficiency anemia	Cyanocobalamin, 1000 micrograms IM per week for 8 wk and every month thereafter; reticulocyte count should increase within 4 d and peak at 7 d. Oral replacement with 2000 micrograms daily is also effective (see "Treatment" section).
Folate deficiency anemia	Folate, 1 milligram PO daily (doses up to 5 milligrams may be needed for patients with malabsorption); reticulocyte count should increase within 4 d with normalization of hemoglobin level in 1–2 mo.
Sideroblastic anemia	Evaluate for reversible causes, including alcohol or other drug toxicity, or toxin exposure. Discontinue any offending agents. Treatment is mainly supportive, consisting primarily of blood transfusions to maintain the hemoglobin level. A trial of pyridoxine at pharmacologic doses (500 milligrams PO daily) may be helpful, with response most commonly seen in cases resulting from ethanol abuse or the use of pyridoxine antagonists. Some patients with hereditary, X-linked sideroblastic anemia also respond to pyridoxine. Improvement with pyridoxine is rare for sideroblastic anemia of other causes.
Aplastic anemia	Supportive care, including transfusion if appropriate. Referral for further workup.
Anemia of chronic disease	Supportive care, including transfusion if appropriate. Referral for further workup and evaluation for underlying disease.

Macrocytosis can result from multiple causes; most common are alcohol abuse, liver disease, vitamin B_{12} and/or folate deficiency, and hypothyroidism.[14,15] A variety of medications can affect folate absorption or metabolism and produce macrocytosis. Drugs include phenytoin, valproate, trimethoprim, sulfamethoxazole, and metformin. The reverse transcriptase inhibitors used to treat human immunodeficiency virus infection can also produce macrocytosis, but they do so without causing anemia. Reticulocytes are larger than mature RBCs, so automated blood cell counters can report a mean corpuscular volume value above the normal range when an increased reticulocyte count is present.

TREATMENT

The treatment of anemia depends on the etiology, symptoms, and clinical status of the patient. In the ED, anemia that requires the most urgent attention results from acute blood loss.[10] All patients who have ongoing blood loss and anemia should have their blood typed and cross-matched, so that information is available for transfusion, if needed (see chapter 238, "Transfusion Therapy"). The decision to transfuse RBCs must be individualized for each patient, taking into account clinical symptoms, age of the patient, presence of comorbid disease, and the likelihood of further blood loss.[16-20] In general, patients who are symptomatic and hemodynamically unstable and show evidence of tissue hypoxia and/or limited cardiopulmonary reserve should have RBCs transfused. In most settings, patients with anemia resulting from acute blood loss benefit when transfused at hemoglobin levels of 6 to 8 grams/dL. Liberal transfusion strategy (defined as a hemoglobin threshold of 9.5 to 10 grams/dL) is not associated with clinical benefit, so a hemoglobin value threshold of 6 to 8 grams/dL for RBC transfusion is recommended in most circumstances.[21]

ED patients with chronic anemia or a newly diagnosed anemia of uncertain etiology not caused by acute blood loss may not require immediate transfusion unless they are hemodynamically unstable, hypoxic, or have acidosis or ongoing cardiac ischemia. In a patient with newly diagnosed anemia of uncertain etiology, obtain laboratory studies for hematologic evaluation before transfusion. Consultation with a hematologist may be beneficial to guide this evaluation. The subsequent evaluation of some patients with chronic anemias or anemias of uncertain etiology can be made more difficult by transfusion, so transfusion should not be undertaken unless specifically indicated.

Treatment for nutritional deficiency anemias usually produces a reticulocyte response in 4 to 7 days (**Table 231-4**). Standard therapy for iron or folate deficiency uses oral replacement. Vitamin B_{12} replacement has traditionally been intramuscular because of concern that malabsorption of the vitamin, a common predisposing condition for vitamin B_{12} deficiency, would limit the effectiveness of oral replacement.[22] However, oral doses of 2000 micrograms of vitamin B_{12} per day are as effective as the intramuscular route in achieving the desired clinical response.[23,24]

DISPOSITION AND FOLLOW-UP

Patients with anemia from ongoing blood loss should be admitted to the hospital for further evaluation and treatment. Patients with isolated anemia that is chronic or newly diagnosed and not related to blood loss do not necessarily require hospital admission if they are asymptomatic and hemodynamically stable, they have minimal comorbid disease, and close follow-up can be arranged. Patients newly diagnosed with anemia who also have abnormalities in the WBC or platelet count should have hematologic consultation and should probably be admitted.

REFERENCES

The complete reference list is available online at www.TintinalliEM.com.

Tests of Hemostasis

Stephen John Cico
Robin R. Hemphill

THE BLEEDING PATIENT

Most bleeding seen in the ED is a result of trauma—local wounds, lacerations, or other structural lesions—and the majority of traumatic bleeding occurs in patients with normal hemostatic mechanisms.[1] In these patients, specific assessment of hemostasis is unnecessary. However, some ED patients have abnormal bleeding due to impaired hemostasis. Identifying these patients requires attention to the history and physical findings.[2-4] Generally speaking, when patients have spontaneous bleeding from multiple sites, bleeding from untraumatized sites, delayed bleeding several hours after trauma, and bleeding into deep tissues or joints, the possibility of a bleeding disorder should be considered.

Important historical data that aid in identifying a congenital bleeding disorder include the presence of unusual or abnormal bleeding in the patient and other family members and any occurrence of excessive bleeding after dental extractions, surgical procedures, or trauma.[5] Many patients with abnormal bleeding have an acquired disorder, such as liver disease, renal disease, or drug use (particularly ethanol, aspirin, nonsteroidal anti-inflammatory drugs, antiplatelet drugs, oral anticoagulants, antibiotics, and other salicylate-containing products).[2-4] Many supplements and herbal preparations, including garlic, ginseng, ginkgo biloba, ginger, and vitamin E, can also increase bleeding tendencies.

The site of bleeding may provide an indication of the hemostatic abnormality. Mucocutaneous bleeding, including petechiae, ecchymoses, epistaxis, GI or GU bleeding, or heavy menstrual bleeding, is characteristic of qualitative or quantitative platelet disorders. Purpura is often associated with thrombocytopenia and commonly indicates a systemic illness. Bleeding into joints and potential spaces, such as between fascial planes and into the retroperitoneum, and delayed bleeding are most commonly associated with coagulation factor deficiencies. Patients who demonstrate both mucocutaneous bleeding and bleeding in deep spaces may have disorders such as disseminated intravascular coagulation, in which both platelet abnormalities and coagulation factor abnormalities are present (see chapters 233, "Acquired Bleeding Disorders," 234, "Clotting Disorders," and 235, "Hemophilias and von Willebrand's Disease").

Common laboratory tests for hemostasis have their limitations.[6,7] They are generally useful and reliable for identifying disorders of coagulation factor function and quantitative platelet availability. However, tests of qualitative platelet function show a significant biologic variation, so that standardization has been difficult to achieve.[8,9] In addition, liver disease and renal failure—two conditions that increase the potential for abnormal hemorrhage—may not give rise to consistent and measurable abnormal results on routine tests of hemostasis.[10-12]

THE PATIENT WITH A THROMBUS

Presentation of a patient to the ED with a disorder due to an intravascular thrombosis, such as a deep venous thrombosis or pulmonary embolus, suggests the potential for an underlying hypercoagulable state (see chapter 234). Premature coronary artery disease and acute coronary syndrome in individuals as young as teenagers have also been linked to hypercoagulable conditions. However, many, if not most, occurrences of intravascular thrombosis are not due to exaggerated hemostasis, but rather are due to local conditions, with blood vessel wall injuries, local inflammation, or vascular stasis provoking the thromboembolic event.[13,14]

The susceptibility to hypercoagulation may be acquired or genetically transmitted. Common acquired hypercoagulable disorders include essential thrombocythemia, polycythemia vera, paroxysmal nocturnal hemoglobinuria, antiphospholipid syndrome, and cancer (often occult at the time of acute thrombosis). Inherited hypercoagulable disorders include factor V Leiden, prothrombin mutations, hyperhomocysteinemia, and deficiencies of protein C, protein S, and antithrombin. Patients with inherited hypercoagulable conditions tend to have venous thrombosis, whereas those with acquired disorders can have both arterial and venous clots.

Proteins C and S are vitamin K–dependent antihemostatic factors made in the liver, associated with disorders leading to deficiencies of these proteins inherited in an autosomal manner. Protein C is activated by thrombin and functions with protein S to stop fibrin formation and to stimulate the process of fibrinolysis. Antithrombin is also an antihemostatic protein that blocks activated coagulation factors. Elevated homocysteine level is also a known risk factor for thromboembolism.

Laboratory tests for a hypercoagulable diathesis show wide biologic variation, and standardization among laboratories has been difficult to achieve. The clinical utility of testing patients for suspected hypercoagulable conditions is dependent on the specific disorder.[13-15]

NORMAL COAGULATION

The normal hemostatic system consists of a complex process that limits blood loss through the formation of a platelet plug (primary hemostasis) and the production of cross-linked fibrin (secondary hemostasis), which strengthens the platelet plug. These reactions are counterregulated by the fibrinolytic system, which limits the size of the fibrin clot that is formed and thereby prevents excessive clot formation. Congenital and acquired abnormalities occur in all these systems. The affected patient may have excessive hemorrhage, excessive thrombus formation, or both.

PRIMARY HEMOSTASIS

Primary hemostasis is the platelet interaction with the vascular subendothelium that results in the formation of a platelet plug at the site of injury. Required components for this to occur are normal vascular subendothelium (collagen), functional platelets, normal von Willebrand factor (connects the platelet to the endothelium via glycoprotein Ib), and normal fibrinogen (connects the platelets to each other via glycoprotein IIb and IIIa) (**Figure 232-1**). Primary hemostasis begins within 20 seconds of injury, is short-lived, and requires secondary hemostasis for clot stabilization.

SECONDARY HEMOSTASIS

Secondary hemostasis consists of the tightly regulated reactions of the plasma coagulation proteins. The final product is cross-linked fibrin, which is insoluble and strengthens the platelet plug formed in primary hemostasis (**Figure 232-2**).

Secondary hemostasis is also known as the *coagulation cascade*. The inactivated coagulation proteins (factors) are identified by Roman numerals, and after activation, the activated factor is designated by *a*. There are two independent activation pathways. The contact system is known as the *contact activation pathway* or *intrinsic pathway*, and the tissue factor system is known as the *tissue factor pathway* or *extrinsic pathway*. The pathways merge at the point of activation of factor X. Medications such as rivaroxaban (Xarelto®) and apixaban (Eliquis®) inhibit the activity of factor Xa. The combination of factor Xa, factor Va, phospholipid, and calcium ("thrombinase complex") more efficiently catalyzes the conversion of prothrombin to thrombin than free factor Xa. In turn, thrombin catalyzes the conversion of fibrinogen to fibrin monomer. Medications such as bivalirudin (Angiomax®) or dabigatran (Pradaxa®) are direct thrombin inhibitors. The *common pathway* describes the steps from factor X activation to cross-linked fibrin formation.

THE FIBRINOLYTIC SYSTEM

The fibrinolytic system regulates the hemostatic mechanism by limiting the size of the fibrin clots that are formed (**Figure 232-3**). Tissue plasminogen activator (tPA), released from endothelial cells, is the principal physiologic trigger for the fibrinolytic process, converting plasminogen, synthesized in the liver and adsorbed in the fibrin clot, to plasmin. Plasmin degrades fibrinogen and fibrin monomer into low-molecular-weight fragments known as fibrin degradation products and degrades cross-linked fibrin into D-dimers.

Other physiologic inhibitors of hemostasis with clinical relevance include antithrombin and the protein C–protein S system. Antithrombin is a protein that forms complexes with all the serine protease coagulation factors (factors XIIa, XIa, Xa, IXa, and thrombin), thereby inhibiting their function. Heparin potentiates this interaction, and this is the basis for its use as an anticoagulant. Proteins C and S are vitamin K–dependent factors that are produced in the liver. Activated protein C binds to the cell-surface-bound protein S, and this complex is capable of inactivating the two plasma cofactors factors Va and VIIIa and inhibiting their participation in the coagulation cascade. A single amino acid substitution in factor V, a condition named factor V Leiden, prevents activated protein C from binding and inhibiting the activity of factor Va. Thus, patients with this inherited condition have prolonged thrombogenic factor Va activity. Factor V Leiden, deficiency or defects in antithrombin, protein C, and protein S produce a potentially hypercoagulable condition and predispose the patient to venous thromboses.

DIAGNOSIS

Before embarking on a sequence of hemostatic testing, evaluate the patient in three areas: (1) Is the bleeding abnormal? (2) Is there a current medical condition associated with increased hemorrhage? (3) Is there a structural cause that explains the bleeding?[13-17]

The basic laboratory tests obtained for a patient with a suspected abnormal bleeding disorder are a CBC and platelet count, prothrombin time, and activated partial thromboplastin time (**Table 232-1**). The

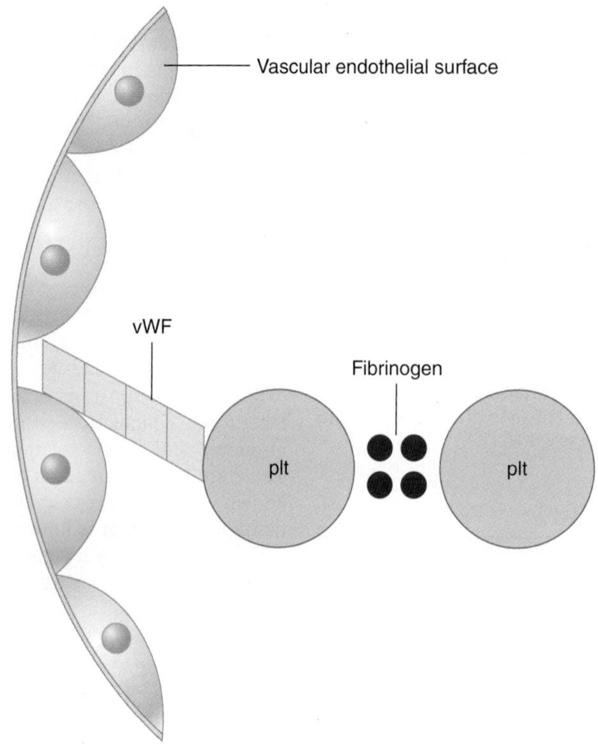

FIGURE 232-1. Primary hemostasis. plt = platelet; vWF = von Willebrand factor.

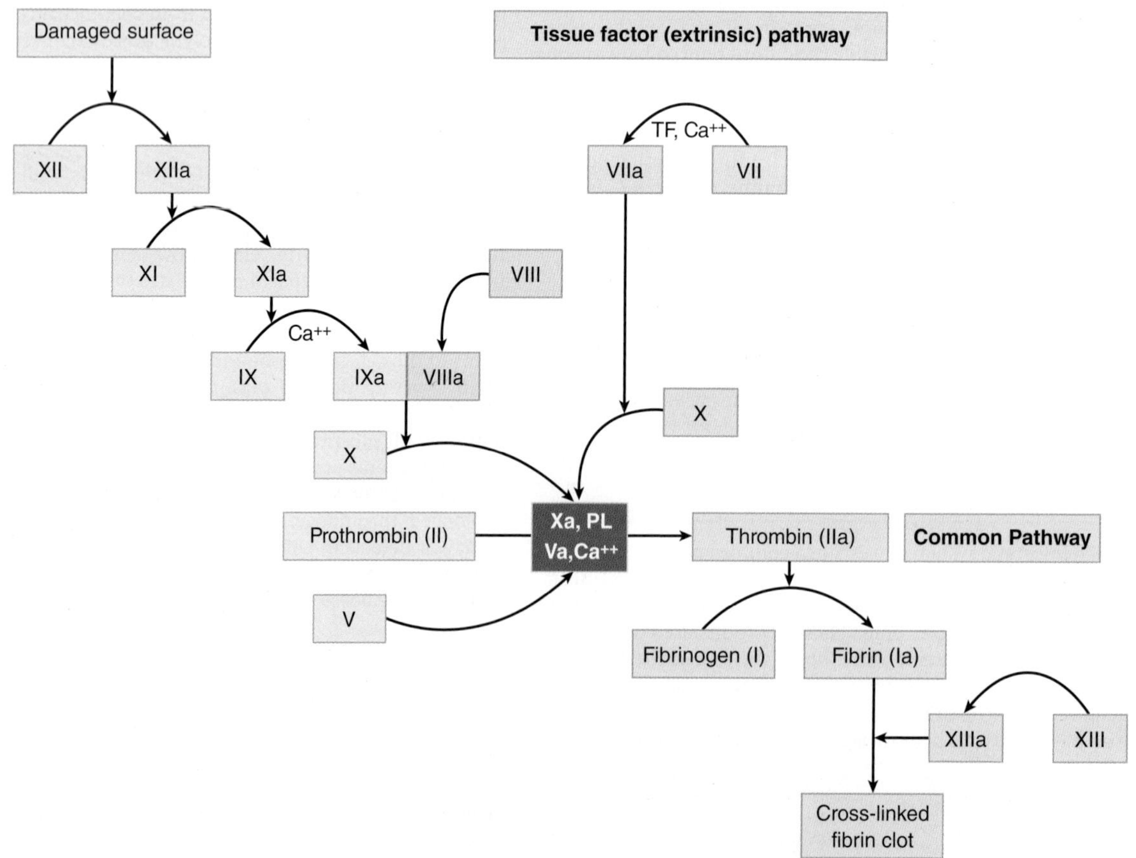

FIGURE 232-2. Secondary hemostasis. Ca^{2+} = calcium; fibrinogen is factor I; PL = phospholipid surface (often platelets); prothrombin is factor II.

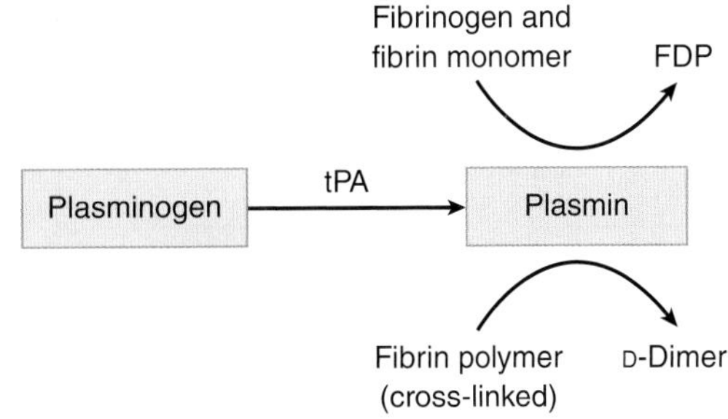

FIGURE 232-3. The fibrinolytic system. FDP = fibrin degradation product; tPA = tissue plasminogen activator.

TABLE 232-1 Initial Tests of Hemostasis

Screening Tests	Reference Value	Component Measured	Clinical Correlations
Primary Hemostasis			
Platelet count	150–400/mm^3 (150–400 × 10^9/L)	Number of platelets per mm^3	*Decreased platelet count (thrombocytopenia)*: bleeding usually not a problem until platelet count is <50,000/mm^3 (50 × 10^9/L); high risk of spontaneous bleeding, including CNS bleeding, seen with count of <10,000/mm^3 (10 × 10^9/L); usually due to decreased production or increased destruction of platelets
			Elevated platelet count (thrombocytosis): commonly a reaction to inflammation or malignancy, and occurs in polycythemia vera; can be associated with hemorrhage or thrombosis
Bleeding time (BT)	Variable	Interaction between platelets and the subendothelium	*Prolonged BT* caused by:
	Typically 2.5–10.0 min using a BT template		Thrombocytopenia (platelet count <50,000/mm^3 or 50 × 10^9/L)
			Abnormal platelet function (von Willebrand's disease, antiplatelet drugs, uremia, liver disease)
Secondary Hemostasis			
Prothrombin time (PT) and international normalized ratio (INR)	PT: 11–13 s; depends on reagent	Extrinsic system and common pathway—factors VII, X, V, prothrombin, and fibrinogen	*Prolonged PT* most commonly caused by:
	INR: 1.0	INR = 1.7 corresponds to approximately 30% activity of coagulation factors as a whole	Warfarin (inhibits production of vitamin K–dependent factors II, VII, IX, and X)
			Liver disease with decreased factor synthesis
			Antibiotics that inhibit vitamin K–dependent factors (moxalactam, cefamandole, cefotaxime, cefoperazone)
Activated partial thromboplastin time (aPTT)	22–34 s	Intrinsic system and common pathway—factors XII, XI, IX, VIII, X, V, prothrombin, and fibrinogen	*Prolonged aPTT* most commonly caused by:
	Depends on type of thromboplastin reagent used		Heparin therapy
	"Activated" with kaolin		Factor deficiencies (factor levels have to be <30% of normal to cause prolongation)
Fibrinogen level	Slightly variable according to specific test	Protein made in liver; converted to fibrin as part of normal coagulation cascade	Low levels seen in disseminated intravascular coagulation
	Typically 200–400 milligrams/dL (2–4 g/L)		Elevated in inflammatory processes (acute-phase reactant)
Thrombin clotting time (TCT)	10–12 s	Conversion of fibrinogen to fibrin monomer	*Prolonged TCT* caused by:
			Low fibrinogen level
			Abnormal fibrinogen molecule (liver disease)
			Presence of heparin, fibrin degradation products, or a paraprotein (multiple myeloma); these interfere with the conversion
			Occasionally seen in hyperfibrinogenemia
"Mix" testing	Variable	Performed when results on one or more of the above screening tests is prolonged; the patient's plasma ("abnormal") is mixed with "normal" plasma and the screening test is repeated	*If the mixing corrects* the screening test result: one or more factor deficiencies are present
			If the mixing does not correct the screening test result: a circulating inhibitor is present

TABLE 232-2 Additional Hemostatic Tests

Test	Reference Value	Component Measured	Clinical Correlations/Comments
Fibrin degradation product (FDP) and D-dimer levels	FDP: variable depending on specific test, typically <2.5–10 micrograms/mL (2.5–10 milligrams/L)	FDP test: measures breakdown products from fibrinogen and fibrin monomer	Levels are elevated in diffuse intravascular coagulation, venous thrombosis, pulmonary embolus, and liver disease, and during pregnancy
	D-Dimer: variable depending on specific test, typically <250–500 nanograms/mL (250–500 micrograms/L)	D-Dimer test: measures breakdown products of cross-linked fibrin	
Factor level assays	60%–130% of reference value (0.60–1.30 units/mL)	Measures the percent activity of a specified factor compared to normal	To identify specific deficiencies and direct therapeutic management
Protein C level	Variable	Level of protein C in the blood	Vitamin K dependent
	Typically 60%–150% of reference value		Increases with age
			Values higher in males than females
			Deficiency associated with thromboembolism in people <50 y of age
Protein S level	Variable	Level of protein S in the blood	Vitamin K dependent
	Typically 60%–150% of reference value		Increases with age
			Values higher in males than females
			Deficiency associated with thromboembolism in people <50 y of age
Factor V Leiden (FVL)	Variable	Screening test looks for activated protein C resistance, and confirmatory test analyzes DNA sequence of factor V gene	FVL not inactivated by activated protein C
		Screening assay uses activated partial thromboplastin time with and without added activated protein C	Heterozygotes have 7× and homozygotes have a 20× increased lifetime risk of venous thrombosis
			Mutation associated with thromboembolism in people <50 y of age
Antithrombin level	Variable depending on specific test	Measures level of antithrombin in the blood	Not vitamin K dependent; patients with deficiency require higher dosages of heparin for anticoagulation therapy
	Typically 20–45 milligrams/dL (200–450 milligrams/L)		Deficiency associated with thromboembolism in people <50 y of age
Antiphospholipid antibodies	IgG <23 GPL units/mL and IgM <11 MPL units/mL	Tests for antibodies that bind to phospholipids	*Lupus anticoagulant*: elevated in systemic lupus erythematosus (SLE) and other autoimmune diseases
		Lupus anticoagulant	*Anticardiolipin antibody*: elevated in SLE, other autoimmune diseases, syphilis, and Behçet's syndrome
		Anticardiolipin antibody	Increased risk of spontaneous abortions, fetal loss, and fetal growth retardation
Anti–factor Xa activity	During therapeutic anticoagulant use: 0.7–1.1 units/mL	Inhibition of factor Xa activity	Used to monitor low-molecular-weight heparin therapy, and newer anticoagulants such as apixaban and rivaroxaban
	During prophylactic anticoagulant use: 0.2–0.3 units/mL		May be elevated in renal dysfunction
Platelet function assay	88–183 s	Tests for platelet adhesion and aggregation	Affected by uremia, anemia, thrombocytopenia, antiplatelet medications, and von Willebrand's disease
	Variable		Initial test done with epinephrine. A prolonged test is repeated using ADP, and if normal <122 s, indicates probable aspirin effect
Peripheral blood smear	Qualitative and quantitative based on visualization	Estimates quantity and appearance of platelets, WBCs, and red blood cells	Allows identification of clumped platelets, abnormal cells interfering with coagulation (leukemia)
			Operator dependent
Dilute Russell viper venom time	23–27 s	Venom directly activates factor X and converts prothrombin to thrombin when phospholipid and factor V are present	Prolonged in the presence of antiphospholipid antibodies
Inhibitor screens	Variable	Verifies the presence or absence of antibodies directed against one or more of the coagulation factors	*Specific inhibitors*: directed against one coagulation factor, most commonly against factor VIII
			Nonspecific inhibitors: directed against more than one coagulation factor; example is lupus-type anticoagulant
Des-γ-carboxyprothrombin or PIVKA II (protein induced by vitamin K absence or antagonism) test	Variable	Measures inactive under-carboxylated form of prothrombin	Increased in vitamin K–deficient states, such as hemorrhagic disease of the newborn
			Increased in overdoses of warfarin or cholestatic liver diseases that can respond to vitamin K therapy

Abbreviations: ADP = adenosine diphosphate; GPL = 1 microgram of affinity-purified immunoglobulin G anticardiolipin antibody from an original index serum; IgM, immunoglobulin M; MPL = 1 microgram of affinity-purified immunoglobulin M anticardiolipin antibody from an original index serum.

results of these tests, coupled with clinical evaluation, should enable formulation of a differential diagnosis.[18] Additional studies are ordered as indicated (**Table 232-2**). Obtain hematologic consultation if the differential diagnosis or the laboratory approach is unclear. In patients with postoperative bleeding, the basic laboratory tests for coagulation are of little help in assessment or management.[19]

REFERENCES

The complete reference list is available online at www.TintinalliEM.com.

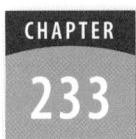

Acquired Bleeding Disorders

Robert W. Shaffer
Sally A. Santen

INTRODUCTION

Normal regulation of bleeding is a complex process involving platelets and the coagulation system (see chapter 232, "Tests of Hemostasis"). Platelet defects typically manifest with petechiae and mucosal bleeding, whereas coagulation defects usually present as spontaneous or excessive hemorrhage. Management of significant acquired bleeding disorders should be discussed with a hematologist because there are often subtleties in diagnosis and treatment.

ACQUIRED PLATELET DEFECTS

Circulating platelets provide the initial defense against bleeding. Acquired platelet disorders may be quantitative (decreased number of circulating platelets) or qualitative (poorly functioning platelets). Both significant thrombocytopenia and qualitative platelet dysfunction are commonly manifested by the presence of nonpalpable petechiae, often most pronounced in the lower extremities and in areas where blood flow is restricted. Other typical findings may include purpura, mucosal bleeding (gingival, epistaxis), menorrhagia, hemoptysis, hematuria, and hematochezia, whereas deep tissue bleeding and hemarthrosis are less common.

Securing circulatory stability is the primary treatment priority in the bleeding patient. Once this is done, the history, physical examination, and directed laboratory testing are used to define the clinical syndrome. Recent illness, symptoms, and medications are potentially relevant in the patient who appears to have a platelet disorder. Physical examination should assess for additional bleeding sites and the type of bleeding. Assess for lymphadenopathy, splenomegaly, pallor, or jaundice that suggests diagnoses such as leukemia, lymphoma, systemic lupus erythematosus, infectious mononucleosis, or hemolytic anemia.

THROMBOCYTOPENIA

Quantitative defects that result in thrombocytopenia are caused by decreased production, increased destruction, splenic sequestration, platelet loss, or a combination (**Table 233-1**).[1] The etiologies of thrombocytopenia are diverse, and the pathologic mechanism is not always initially clear. Viral infections may impair thrombopoiesis due to direct infection of the megakaryocyte, toxic effects of viral proteins or cytokines, hemophagocytosis, or production of antibodies that bind to platelets and enhance immune destruction.[2] A drug history is important, because many medications have been implicated in causing thrombocytopenia or impairing platelet function (**Table 233-2**).[3,4]

A CBC will establish the presence and degree of thrombocytopenia and determine whether other hematologic cell lines are affected. A peripheral smear should be examined to assess platelet morphology and evaluate other cell lines. Rarely, in vitro platelet agglutination occurs, which leads to spuriously low platelet counts reported by automated cell counters (pseudothrombocytopenia) when collected in ethylenediaminetetraacetic acid–coated blood tubes; this can be detected by the presence of platelet clumping on a peripheral smear. In this case, a correct platelet count may be obtained by using citrated or heparin-anticoagulated blood tubes.

Testing for human immunodeficiency virus and hepatitis C virus is recommended in cases of isolated thrombocytopenia, as low platelets may be the only readily apparent manifestation in early infections.[5] If the etiology of low platelets remains unclear, further laboratory testing to evaluate for disorders such as hemolysis and disseminated intravascular coagulation (DIC) may be needed. Although usually not necessary in instances of isolated thrombocytopenia, bone marrow biopsy may be obtained when malignancy or other bone marrow pathologies are of concern.

When circulating platelet levels decrease to below 10,000 to 20,000/mm^3 (10 to 20 × 10^9/L), the risk of spontaneous bleeding becomes con-

TABLE 233-1 Pathophysiology of Acquired Thrombocytopenia

Mechanism	Associated Clinical Conditions
Decreased platelet production	Marrow infiltration (tumor or infection)
	Viral infections (rubella, HIV, hepatitis C, others)
	Drugs (Table 233-2)
	Radiation
	Vitamin B_{12} and/or folate deficiency
Increased platelet destruction	Immune thrombocytopenia
	Thrombotic thrombocytopenic purpura
	Hemolytic-uremic syndrome
	Disseminated intravascular coagulation
	Viral infections (HIV, mumps, varicella, Epstein-Barr virus)
	Drugs (Table 233-2)
Platelet loss	Excessive hemorrhage
	Hemodialysis, extracorporeal circulation
Splenic sequestration	Sickle cell disease, cirrhosis

Abbreviation: HIV = human immunodeficiency virus.

TABLE 233-2 Drugs That Produce Thrombocytopenia or Impair Platelet Function

Produce Thrombocytopenia	Impair Function
Heparin 4+	Aspirin
Gold salts 4+	Nonsteroidal anti-inflammatory drugs
Sulfa-containing antibiotics 4+	Glycoprotein IIb–IIIa agents: ticlopidine and clopidogrel
Quinine and quinidine 4+	
Ethanol (chronic use) 4+	Penicillins and cephalosporins
Aspirin 3+	Calcium channel blockers
Indomethacin 3+	β-Adrenergic blockers: propranolol
Rifampin 2+	Nitroglycerin
Abciximab and eptifibatide 2+	Antihistamines
Thiazides and furosemide 2+	Phenothiazines
Acyclovir 2+	Cyclic antidepressants
Procainamide 2+	
Digoxin 2+	
Cimetidine and ranitidine 2+	
Phenytoin and valproate 1+	
Penicillins/cephalosporins 1+	

Note: 4+ to 1+ indicates relative incidence, from more frequent to less frequent, based on case reports.

cerning, particularly for intracranial hemorrhage. Additional risk factors for bleeding include age, comorbid illness (i.e, renal disease, liver disease, connective tissue disease, peptic ulcer disease, hypertension), fall risk, and lifestyle activity. With the exception of a few specific disease processes, platelet transfusion in the nonbleeding patient should be considered when counts fall below 10,000/mm³ (10 ×10⁹/L), or higher if other comorbid illnesses are present.[6] The cause of the platelet deficiency may also influence the risk of bleeding. At a given platelet level, patients with immune thrombocytopenia (ITP) typically bleed less than patients with aplastic anemia, as the younger platelets present in ITP are more effective in hemostasis.[7]

Immune Causes of Thrombocytopenia ITP is an acquired immune-mediated disorder in which circulating platelets typically fall to very low levels.[3,8] ITP results from antiplatelet antibodies that attack platelet surface glycoproteins such as glycoprotein IIb/IIIa, leading to peripheral platelet destruction. There is evidence that the same antibodies lead to impaired platelet production by megakaryocytes.[9] Despite very low platelet counts, the circulating platelets are not functionally impaired.

Immune thrombocytopenia may be classified as primary (formerly known as *idiopathic thrombocytopenic purpura*) or secondary when associated with other medical conditions (autoimmune disorders, infections) or drug exposures.[8] This distinction is of clinical importance, as management of the underlying disorder or discontinuation of the drug in cases of secondary ITP may lead to normalization of the platelet count.

Primary ITP may occur at any age, with equal prevalence between genders, with the exception of those age 30 to 60 years, in which women predominate. Primary ITP is classified by duration of illness: newly diagnosed (diagnosis to 3 months), persistent (3 months to 12 months), and chronic (>12 months).[8] The majority of adults with primary ITP progress to chronic illness.

The most common presenting sign of ITP is a petechial rash (**Figure 233-1A**). Mild epistaxis, gingival bleeding (**Figure 233-1B**), and menorrhagia in women of childbearing age may also be seen. Except for petechiae and bruising, the patient should have a normal physical examination.

The CBC should demonstrate normal cell lines except for the platelets. A mild anemia may be seen if bleeding is present. The peripheral smear should show large, well-granulated platelets, although they will be few in number. Bone marrow biopsy is not indicated unless clinical features are atypical. If the evaluation supports the diagnosis of primary ITP, then additional testing in the ED is not required.

Treatment for ITP is initiated based on the risk of bleeding (**Table 233-3**). Major bleeding complications in patients with platelets >50,000 /mm³ (>50 × 10⁹/L) are uncommon. As most fatal bleeding complications occur when platelet counts fall below 30,000/mm³ (30 × 10⁹/L), experts and guidelines recommend this level as the threshold for initiating treatment of ITP in adults.[5,6,9-11] Bleeding risk correlates with lower platelet counts and patient age greater than 60, a prior history of bleeding, certain chronic illnesses, and use of medications that alter hemostasis all heighten this risk. Therefore, certain patients may benefit from medical treatment despite a platelet count exceeding 30,000/mm³ (30 × 10⁹/L). For all patients with primary ITP, bleeding risk should be minimized, including avoiding use of antiplatelet medications when possible, maintenance of good blood pressure control, optimized treatment of exacerbating comorbid conditions (i.e., liver disease, renal disease), and addressing fall risks.

About two thirds of children with primary ITP will have spontaneous resolution within 6 months of diagnosis.[11] An antecedent viral infection is commonly reported. Additionally, the measles-mumps-rubella vaccination has been associated with the development of acute ITP, although this is rare and occurs in less than 1 per 25,000 doses given.[12] The risk of severe bleeding complications appears to be rare in children, regardless of their absolute platelet count.[5,8,13] Children without signs of active bleeding and good psychosocial support typically do not require hospitalization or medical treatment. Good anticipatory guidance should be provided to the family, and the child should abstain from contact sports or activities that might place them at risk for head injury.

First-line treatment for primary ITP generally includes corticosteroids, typically prednisone 1 milligram/kg per day for 4 weeks (shorter courses may be considered for children).[5,9-11,13] Initial response may not be seen for 4 to 14 days, and peak effect can be expected between 7 and 28 days. IV immunoglobulin may also be considered, either alone or in combination with corticosteroids, at a dose 1 g/kg/per day for 3 days. Initial response to IV immunoglobulin is more rapid than corticosteroids, occurring between 1 and 3 days, with peak effect seen between 2 and 7 days. Side effects of IV immunoglobulin may include aseptic meningitis, transient neutropenia, acute kidney injury, and transfusion reactions/hypotension.

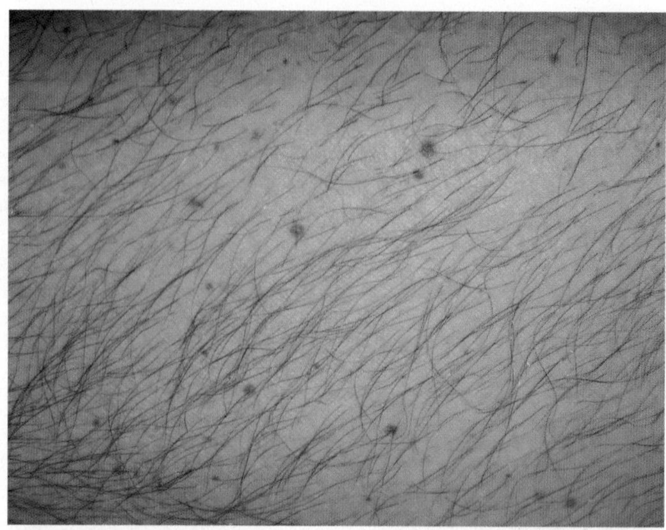

A

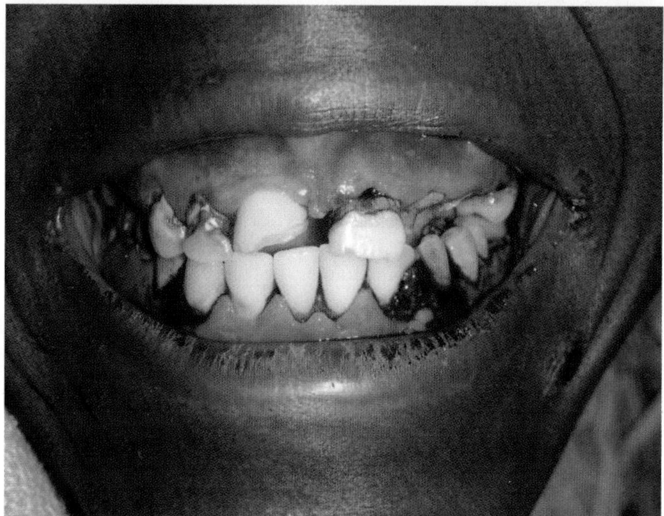

B

FIGURE 233-1. Two patients with idiopathic thrombocytopenic purpura. **A.** Petechiae with platelet count of 3000/mm³ (3 × 10⁹/L). **B.** Gingival bleeding with platelet count of 5000/mm³ (5 × 10⁹/L). [Image used with permission of J. Stephan Stapczynski, MD.]

TABLE 233-3 Treatment of Immune Thrombocytopenia

Platelet transfusion	<10,000–20,000/mm³ (<10–20 × 10⁹/L) prophylactically to prevent bleeding <50,000/mm³ (<50 × 10⁹/L) if actively bleeding <20,000–50,000/mm³ (<20–50 × 10⁹/L) if patient requires diagnostic puncture <50,000–100,000/mm³ (<50–100 × 10⁹/L) if patient requires invasive procedure
Corticosteroids	Prednisone, 1 milligram/kg PO per day for 21 days then tapered, or dexamethasone, 20 milligrams/m² IV per day for 4 d
IV immunoglobulin	1 gram/kg IV per day for 3 d
Splenectomy	Considered for refractory cases

Anti-Rho(D) immunoglobulin at 50 to 75 micrograms/kg for a single dose may also be considered as a first-line treatment strategy in patients who are Rh(D) positive and have not undergone splenectomy.[14] Initial response rate and peak effect are similar to that seen with IV immunoglobulin. Mild hemolysis can be expected, and rare serious or even fatal cases of intravascular hemolysis, DIC, and renal failure have been reported with anti-Rho(D) use, prompting the U.S. Food and Drug Administration to administer a warning pertaining to its use in 2010. Second-line treatment modalities include splenectomy and use of newer agents, such as the monoclonal antibody rituximab, which blunts the autoimmune destruction of platelets, and thrombopoietin receptor agonists, which stimulate platelet production (i.e., romiplostin, eltrombopag).

In the event of life-threatening hemorrhage where hemostasis must be achieved rapidly, IV corticosteroids (such as dexamethasone) and IV immunoglobulin should be administered concomitantly.[13] Platelet transfusions should be initiated, and doses two to three times the typical dose might be required due to persistent autoimmune destruction.[6] Platelet transfusions may need to be repeated frequently until bleeding subsides or targeted treatment modalities take effect. Emergent splenectomy may be considered if all other treatment options are exhausted.

Drug-Induced Immune Thrombocytopenia Over 200 drugs have been implicated in causing immune-mediated suppression of platelet production or increased platelet destruction (Table 233-2).[3,4] The clinical presentation is similar to ITP, and the thrombocytopenia may severe. Drug-induced thrombocytopenia typically occurs 5 to 14 days following initiation of a drug, but may occur sooner if there has been recent prior exposure. A careful history should not only include prescribed medications, but also herbal remedies and food and beverage use (i.e., quinine in tonic water, alcohol use, tahini). Chronic alcohol use is a common cause of thrombocytopenia. Platelet counts typically normalize with cessation of the causative agent. Heparin-induced thrombocytopenia causes a significant drop in platelets, but patients are paradoxically hypercoagulable due to platelet activation (see chapter 239, "Thrombotics and Antithrombotics").

Nonimmune Causes of Thrombocytopenia Thrombocytopenia may occur from various non–immune-mediated causes (Table 233-1). In thrombotic thrombocytopenic purpura and hemolytic-uremic syndrome, thrombotic microangiopathy occurs when vessel injury results in deposition of platelet-fibrin thrombi (see chapters 143 "Oncologic and Hematologic Emergencies in Children" and 237, "Acquired Hemolytic Anemia"). DIC is also a well-described cause of platelet destruction. In patients with marked hemorrhage, large-volume fluid resuscitation may lead to a dilutional thrombocytopenia. Additionally, certain bacterial, rickettsial, and viral infections can cause direct toxic destruction of platelets. Thrombocytopenia specific to pregnancy may be a result of the hemolysis–elevated liver enzymes–low platelets (HELLP) syndrome, pre-eclampsia, or gestational thrombocytopenia (see chapter 100, "Maternal Emergencies after 20 Weeks of Pregnancy and in the Postpartum Period"). Finally, an enlarged spleen can sequester a significant portion of the platelet pool.

Thrombocytopenia is present in up to 70% of patients with chronic liver disease.[15] The etiology appears multifactorial. Patients often have underlying medical conditions related to their liver disease such as alcohol use, viral hepatitis, or nutritional deficiencies that impair platelet production. Thrombopoietin, which is produced by hepatocytes, may be decreased. Portal hypertension may lead to splenic sequestration. Endotoxemia from infection may promote platelet aggregation. Some patients also demonstrate platelet autoantibodies. The degree of quantitative thrombocytopenia may be mitigated by an increased level of circulating von Willebrand factor that is typically seen, which promotes platelet adhesion. For this reason, routine platelet transfusion is not recommended in the absence of clinically significant bleeding. However, a platelet count of >50,000/mm³ (>50 × 10⁹/L) should be achieved prior to invasive procedures (i.e., lumbar puncture, surgery, liver biopsy).[16]

FUNCTIONAL PLATELET DISORDERS

Several disease processes can cause acquired qualitative or functional abnormalities of platelets (**Table 233-4**).[17] In the myeloproliferative diseases, platelets are often dysfunctional, even if the platelet count is normal or elevated. Patients can have prolonged bleeding times and clinically significant bleeding. To control acute bleeding, transfusion should be considered to raise the level of normal platelets to 50,000/mm³ (50 × 10⁹/L). In macroglobulinemia and related disorders, the elevated level of viscous proteins interferes with platelet function. Patients with clinically significant bleeding may require plasmapheresis to reduce the protein level and correct hemostatic function.

TABLE 233-4 Clinical Conditions Associated with Qualitative Platelet Abnormalities

Uremia
Liver disease
Disseminated intravascular coagulation
Antiplatelet antibodies (immune thrombocytopenia, systemic lupus erythematosus)
Cardiopulmonary bypass
Myeloproliferative disorders (thrombocytosis, polycythemia vera, chronic myeloid leukemia, acute lymphocytic or myelogenous leukemia)
Dysproteinemias (multiple myeloma, Waldenström's macroglobulinemia)
von Willebrand's disease (congenital or acquired)

Many drugs can influence platelet function (Table 233-2 and **Table 233-5**). Of these, the most commonly used are aspirin, which produces an irreversible impairment in platelet aggregation, and the nonsteroidal anti-inflammatory drugs, clopidogrel and ticlopidine, which produce temporary impairment in platelet adhesion and aggregation (see chapter 239).

Thrombocytosis, a platelet count exceeding 500,000/mm³ (500 × 10⁹/L), can be seen in many disorders including inflammatory reactions, malignancy, polycythemia, and postsplenectomy. Platelet function can be normal or abnormal depending on the underlying condition. Therefore, thrombocytosis can be associated with bleeding (mucosal, ecchymotic, GI) or thromboembolic (deep venous thrombosis, portal or mesenteric thrombosis, splenic vein thrombosis) manifestations. However, these events are unusual, even with platelet counts in excess of 1,000,000/mm³ (1000 × 10⁹/L).

ACQUIRED COAGULATION DISORDERS

Acquired coagulation disorders can result from underlying medical disease and autoimmune factor inhibitors.

LIVER DISEASE

Acute and chronic liver disease is commonly associated with laboratory tests of impaired coagulation. Hepatocytes synthesize all of the coagulation factors and related regulatory proteins, with the exception of factor VIII and von Willebrand factor. Diseases affecting the hepatic parenchyma may result in a decreased synthesis of these factors, including the vitamin K–dependent carboxylation of factors II (prothrombin), VII, IX, and X. Because vitamin K is a fat-soluble vitamin, malabsorption can occur with processes that interfere with the absorption of fat-soluble vitamins, including impaired bile acid metabolism (i.e., primary biliary cirrhosis), intrahepatic or extrahepatic cholestasis, and treatment with

TABLE 233-5 Duration of Antiplatelet Activity

Drug	Onset	Duration of Effect
Aspirin	1 h	Up to 7 d
Most nonsteroidal anti-inflammatory drugs	1 h	1 d
Piroxicam	1 h	2 d
Ticlopidine or clopidogrel	1–2 d	4–7 d

bile acid binders. Thus, prolonged prothrombin time is common in patients with decompensated hepatic function. Despite marked prolongations of prothrombin time and activated partial thromboplastin time (PTT) seen in advanced liver disease and cirrhosis, these tests poorly predict onset and severity of bleeding, including bleeding from esophageal varices or invasive procedures or surgery.[16,18-20] Although there may be marked reduction in procoagulant proteins in liver disease, there is typically a parallel decrease in the endogenous anticoagulant proteins such as protein C and antithrombin. Therefore, primary hemostasis may be relatively maintained. In fact, patients with liver disease may be susceptible to both increased bleeding and thrombosis. Patients with liver disease and cirrhosis are twice as likely to develop unprovoked deep venous thrombosis and have a relatively high incidence of portal venous thrombosis.[21]

In the actively bleeding patient with liver disease, attention to volume and circulatory status is paramount. Transfusion of packed red blood cells should be used to maintain an adequate hemoglobin and hemodynamic stability. Fresh frozen plasma transfusions or platelets should be transfused if significant hemorrhage (e.g., from esophageal varices) is associated with a coagulopathy or thrombocytopenia with a platelet count below 60,000/mm^3 (60 × 10^9/L).[16] Plasma transfusions should be used cautiously because they may incite thrombosis and expand intravascular volume, exacerbating portal hypertension and increasing the severity of variceal bleeding. There is no evidence that recombinant activated factor VII or four-factor prothrombin complex concentrate (Kcentra®) provides benefit.[22] The benefit of vitamin K in these patients has also been called into question, and its routine use is not substantiated.[22,23]

Primary prevention of bleeding in patients with liver disease should focus on medical optimization of their risk factors, rather than treatment of abnormal tests of coagulation or thrombocytopenia.[16,18] These include management and prevention of portal hypertension, treatment of esophageal varices, management of primary causes for liver disease (i.e., alcohol use, hepatitis C), optimization of renal function, and management and prevention of sepsis/infection.

RENAL DISEASE

Patients with renal disease frequently manifest disorders of hemostasis. Early renal impairment has been associated with a tendency for thrombosis relating to increased production of procoagulant factors as well as decreased formation of tissue plasminogen activator.[24] In advanced renal disease, bleeding complications are of particular concern due to qualitative platelet dysfunction from decreased ability to adhere to damaged endothelium and aggregate. Patients with chronic kidney disease are at increased risk for minor bleeding (mucosal and cutaneous) and major bleeding (intracerebral and GI hemorrhage). Serum prothrombin time, activated PTT, and platelet counts are often normal, although bleeding time will usually be prolonged. Abnormalities in platelet function can be due to direct effects of uremic toxins and impaired drug elimination. Anemia itself has been associated with platelet dysfunction. Thrombocytopenia can occur from dialysis, and the heparin used may also potentiate bleeding.

Desmopressin is the most common agent used to correct bleeding in patients with uremic platelet dysfunction, producing an increase in serum von Willebrand factor and enhancing the platelet's ability to aggregate.[25] The dose is 0.3 milligram/kg SC or IV, with a rapid onset and duration of action lasting at least 4 hours. Side effects are generally mild and include headache, flushing, minor hypotension, tachycardia, nausea, abdominal cramps, and local site reaction. Other strategies that improve platelet function include the use of cryoprecipitate, conjugated estrogens, erythropoietin to improve anemia, and hemodialysis to remove toxins.[24] Platelet transfusions alone are generally ineffective because the infused platelets quickly acquire the platelet defect. Cryoprecipitate and platelet transfusions should be reserved for life-threatening bleeding and should be used in combination with packed red blood cells, desmopressin, and conjugated estrogens.

DISSEMINATED INTRAVASCULAR COAGULATION

DIC is an acquired syndrome characterized by inappropriate and widespread activation of the coagulation system resulting in intravascular thrombin generation, small vessel thrombosis, and consumption of clotting factors and platelets.[26] Concomitant activation of the fibrinolytic system also occurs, resulting in the breakdown of fibrin clots and subsequent bleeding. DIC is associated with a wide variety of precipitating disorders (**Table 233-6**).

TABLE 233-6 Common Conditions Associated with Disseminated Intravascular Coagulation (DIC)

Clinical Setting	Comments
Infection Bacterial Viral Fungal	Probably the most common cause of DIC; 10%–20% of patients with gram-negative sepsis have DIC; endotoxins stimulate monocytes and endothelial cells to express tissue factor; Rocky Mountain spotted fever causes direct endothelial damage; DIC more likely to develop in asplenic patients or cirrhosis; septic patients are more likely to have thrombosis than bleeding.
Carcinoma Adenocarcinoma Lymphoma	Malignant cells may cause endothelial damage and allow the expression of tissue factor as well as other procoagulant materials; most adenocarcinomas tend to have thrombosis (Trousseau's syndrome), whereas prostate cancer tends to have more bleeding; DIC is often chronic and compensated.
Acute leukemia	DIC most common with promyelocytic leukemia; blast cells release procoagulant enzymes; there is excessive release at time of cell lysis (chemotherapy); more likely to have bleeding than thrombosis.
Trauma	DIC especially with brain injury, crush injury, burns, hypothermia, hyperthermia, rhabdomyolysis, fat embolism, hypoxia. Massive bleeding can occur.
Organ injury Liver disease Pancreatitis	May have chronic compensated DIC; acute DIC may occur in the setting of acute hepatic failure; tissue factor is released from the injured hepatocytes. Pancreatitis can activate the coagulation cascade.
Pregnancy	Placental abruption, amniotic fluid embolus, septic abortion, intrauterine fetal death (can be chronic DIC); can have DIC in hemolysis–elevated liver enzymes–low platelets (HELLP) syndrome.
Vascular disease	Large aortic aneurysms (chronic DIC can become acute at time of surgery), giant hemangiomas, vasculitis, multiple telangiectasias.
Envenomation	DIC can develop with bites of rattlesnakes and other vipers; the venom damages the endothelial cells; bleeding is not as serious as expected from laboratory values.
Acute lung injury (ALI) or adult respiratory distress syndrome	Microthrombi are deposited in the small pulmonary vessels; the pulmonary capillary endothelium is damaged; 20% of patients with ALI develop DIC, and 20% of patients with DIC develop ALI.
Transfusion reactions, such as acute hemolytic reaction	DIC with severe bleeding, shock, and acute renal failure.

Pathogenesis Although the diseases triggering DIC are diverse, the common pathway of these illnesses is that they lead to an inappropriate loss of localization or compensated control in the intravascular activation of coagulation (**Figure 233-2**). Immune, inflammatory, and coagulant pathways are involved. Damaged endothelial cell walls trigger activation of the intrinsic clotting cascade, leading to thrombin generation and subsequent intravascular fibrin clot deposition. Increased thrombin generation leads to consumption of anticoagulant regulatory proteins (i.e., protein C, protein S, and antithrombin), further potentiating thrombosis and ischemic tissue damage. Production of thrombin and fibrin indirectly activates tissue plasminogen activator and the counterregulatory fibrinolytic system. When hyperfibrinolysis occurs, the hemostatic clots dissolve and bleeding ensues.

Clinical Features Clinical features of DIC vary with the underlying precipitating illness.[27] Hypercoagulation may predominate in certain conditions such as sepsis, where signs of ischemic end-organ failure are common, and physical findings in these patients may include cutaneous gangrene or thrombotic purpura. In other instances such as DIC associated

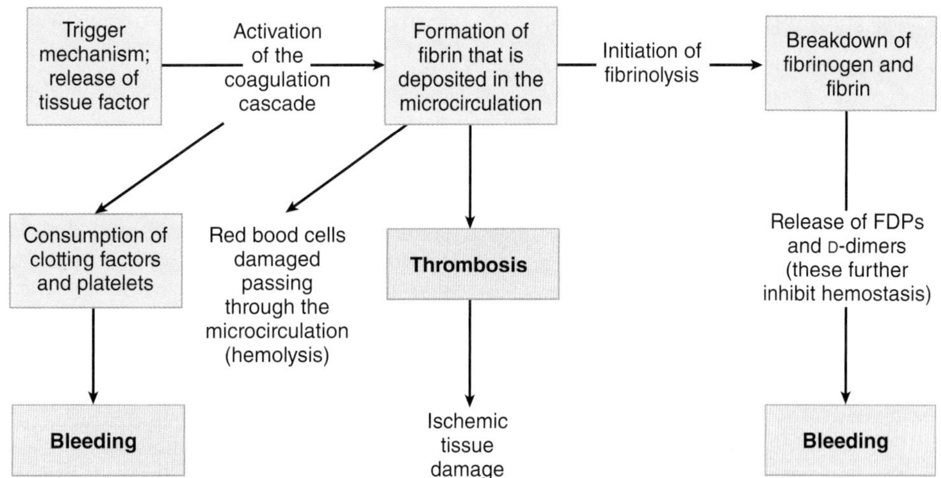

FIGURE 233-2. Pathophysiology of disseminated intravascular coagulation. Refer to "Pathogenesis" section under "Disseminated Intravascular Coagulation" for details. FDPs = fibrin/fibrinogen degradation products.

with leukemia, hyperfibrinolysis may predominate and clinical features may include petechiae, ecchymoses, oozing from catheter or venipuncture sites, or hematuria. Certain DIC-related disorders such as trauma and obstetric complications tend to have both strong hypercoagulation and hyperfibrinolysis elements and lead to major bleeding complications (i.e., wounds, intracranial, GI). Yet other conditions may be associated with mild and compensated DIC in which outward signs of thrombosis and bleeding are subclinical.

Laboratory Findings The typical laboratory results in acute DIC (**Table 233-7**) include thrombocytopenia, prolonged prothrombin time, low fibrinogen level, and elevation of fibrin-related markers (i.e., D-dimer, fibrin degradation products, soluble fibrin). The most commonly observed abnormality is thrombocytopenia; a progressive drop in the platelet count is sensitive, although not specific, for DIC. Depletion of coagulation factors is reflected by a prolonged prothrombin time. Fibrinogen is an acute-phase reactant and may be normal or elevated in early DIC. Scoring systems have been developed and validated to aid in the diagnosis (**Table 233-8**).[28,29]

Differential Diagnosis Primary fibrinolysis is a rare syndrome whereby plasmin and fibrinolysis occur without the production of thrombin. Severe liver disease will also manifest with coagulation abnormalities and low platelets. These two entities can be differentiated from DIC based on clinical history and laboratory tests. The hematologic abnormalities in liver disease should be relatively stable in contrast to the worsening abnormalities associated with acute DIC. Additionally, the D-dimer assay will usually be normal or minimally elevated in both primary fibrinolysis and liver disease, but is often significantly elevated in DIC.

Treatment Paramount to the management of DIC is the elimination of the underlying disorder whenever possible. Treatment strategies in DIC include blood product support and strategies to modulate thrombin formation (**Table 233-9**).[26,27,29] Generally speaking, blood products should only be administered when there is evidence of bleeding.

TABLE 233-7 Laboratory Abnormalities Characteristic of Disseminated Intravascular Coagulation (DIC)[28]

Studies	Result
Most Useful	
Platelet count	Usually low, or dropping
Prothrombin time	Prolonged
Fibrinogen level	Usually low (fibrinogen is an acute-phase reactant, so may actually start out elevated), fibrinogen level <100 milligrams/dL (<1 gram/L) correlates with severe DIC
Fibrin degradation products and D-dimer*	Elevated
Helpful	
Activated partial thromboplastin time	Usually prolonged
Thrombin clotting time	Prolonged (not sensitive)
Fragmented red blood cells	Should be present (not specific)
Specific factor assays	Extrinsic pathway factors are most affected (VII, X, V, and II)
Factor II, V, VII,† X	Low
Factor VIII (acute-phase reactant)	Low, normal, high
Factor IX	Low (decreases later than other factors)

*Levels may be chronically elevated in patients with liver or renal disease.

†Factor VII is usually low early because it has the shortest half-life.

TABLE 233-8 International Society on Thrombosis and Haemostasis Scoring System for DIC When Associated Condition Known to Cause Disseminated Intravascular Coagulation (DIC) Is Present[29]

Test	Points
Platelet count	
>100,000/mm³ (>100 × 10⁹/L)	0
50,000–100,000/mm³ (50–100 × 10⁹/L)	1
<50,000/mm³ (<50 × 10⁹/L)	2
Fibrin-related marker (D-dimer, fibrin degradation products)	
Normal	0
Mildly elevated	2
Markedly elevated	3
Prothrombin time prolongation	
<3 s	0
3–6 s	1
>6 s	2
Fibrinogen level	
>100 milligrams/dL (>1 gram/L)	0
<100 milligrams/dL (<1 gram/L)	1

Note. A score of ≥5 is compatible with overt DIC. A score <5 is suggestive (not affirmative) for nonovert DIC.

TABLE 233-9 Treatment of Disseminated Intravascular Coagulation (DIC)

Treat underlying precipitating disorder: volume resuscitation, antibiotics, external cooling
Platelet transfusions for thrombocytopenia <50,000/mm³ (<50 × 10⁹/L) and active bleeding
Fresh frozen plasma for prolonged PT or aPTT (>1.5) or low fibrinogen (<100 milligrams/dL [1 gram/L])
Fibrinogen concentrate for persistent low fibrinogen <100 milligrams/dL (<1 gram/L)
Vitamin K for prolonged PT
Consider LMWH when thrombotic events dominate clinical picture
Consider tranexamic acid for trauma-related DIC

Abbreviations: aPTT = activated partial thromboplastin time; LMWH = low molecular weight heparin; PT = prothrombin time.

Platelet transfusions are recommended in actively bleeding patients who have platelet counts below 50,000/mm³ (50 × 10⁹/L) and may be considered in those considered to be at high risk for bleeding (such as DIC resulting from chemotherapy) when platelet counts fall below 10,000 to 20,000/mm³ (10 to 20 × 10⁹/L). Plasma should be administered in bleeding patients when prothrombin time/activated PTT exceeds 1.5 times normal or when fibrinogen levels fall below 150 milligrams/dL (1.5 grams/L). The initial recommended dose is 15 mL/kg, although there is some evidence that 30 mL/kg may be superior when volume overload is not of concern. Fibrinogen concentrate should be considered when hypofibrinogenemia persists despite use of plasma. Patients with a prolonged prothrombin time should receive parenteral vitamin K.

There is no proven benefit in DIC with other coagulation factor products, such as three- or four-factor prothrombin complex concentrate or recombinant factor VIIa. Although there is no evidence demonstrating improved outcomes, low-molecular-weight heparin may be considered in patients with DIC where thrombotic complications predominate the clinical picture or in patients with evidence of early compensated DIC.[29] Patients with DIC are at very high risk for developing venous thromboembolism, and routine prophylaxis with low-molecular-weight heparin, in the absence of major bleeding, is recommended. Antifibrinolytic medications (i.e., tranexamic acid) should generally be avoided in patients with DIC. One notable exception is in trauma-related DIC, where their use reduces mortality.[30]

CIRCULATING INHIBITORS OF COAGULATION

Acquired inhibitors of blood coagulation, also known as *circulating anticoagulants*, are antibodies directed against one or more of the coagulation factors. Although inhibitors may develop spontaneously in previously healthy patients with normal hemostasis, most inhibitors develop in patients with hereditary bleeding disorders who receive transfusion of plasma products. Inhibitors have been described for most of the coagulation factors; the two most common inhibitors are factor VIII inhibitors and antiphospholipid antibodies. Factor VIII inhibitors are "specific" inhibitors, directed only against factor VIII, as opposed to antiphospholipid antibodies, including lupus anticoagulant and anticardiolipin antibodies, which are "nonspecific" inhibitors directed against several of the coagulation factors. Lupus anticoagulant and anticardiolipin antibodies often result in thrombosis (see chapter 234, "Clotting Disorders").

Factor VIII Inhibitors Factor VIII inhibitors most commonly develop in patients with hemophilia A (see chapter 235, "Hemophilias and von Willebrand's Disease"), but can also develop spontaneously in patients with previously normal hemostasis, a condition termed *acquired hemophilia*.[31,32] The incidence of spontaneously arising inhibitors is rare—estimated at 1.4 cases per 1 million persons per year. Although uncommon, it is important to recognize this clinical entity because the mortality rate approaches 22%. The majority of acquired hemophilia cases, approximately 85%, occur in the elderly. In about half of cases, inhibitors develop in association with preexisting disorders, such as autoimmune disorders (systemic lupus erythematosus, rheumatoid arthritis, ulcerative colitis) and lymphoproliferative disorders (multiple myeloma, Waldenström's macroglobulinemia, benign monoclonal gammopathy of uncertain significance), and in patients with allergic drug reactions (penicillins, sulfonamides, phenytoin).

Patients without a prior bleeding history who develop factor VIII inhibitors can present with massive spontaneous ecchymoses, hematomas, and hematuria. Laboratory studies classically show a normal prothrombin time, normal thrombin clotting time, and a greatly prolonged activated PTT that does not correct with mixing. A factor VIII–specific assay will show very low or absent factor VIII activity. Other factor-specific assays should be normal or only slightly decreased. Quantitative measurement of the inhibitor by the Bethesda inhibitor assay is important for the emergency management of bleeding episodes. Long-term management of acquired factor VIII inhibitors is with steroids, IV immunoglobulin, cytotoxic agents, or rituximab to suppress antibody production. A hematologist should direct the management of an acute, clinically significant bleeding episode.

There is no proven therapy to control bleeding episodes in patients with acquired factor VIII inhibitors.[33] Treatment options include administration of factor VIII, three- or four-factor prothrombin complex, recombinant factor VIIa, desmopressin acetate, and plasmapheresis. Additionally, the use of aspirin, nonsteroidal anti-inflammatory drugs, and intramuscular injections should be avoided and conservative therapies should be considered, including compression and immobilization of the bleeding site.[31,32]

REFERENCES

The complete reference list is available online at www.TintinalliEM.com.

CHAPTER 234 Clotting Disorders

Jessie G. Nelson
Robin R. Hemphill

INTRODUCTION

Most patients who develop an arterial or venous thrombosis do so because of local factors (e.g., a focal atherosclerotic lesion producing a thrombus in an coronary artery) or major systemic events (e.g., trauma, surgery, or prolonged immobilization). However, several inherited genetic mutations predispose patients to venous thromboembolism with some studies finding up to 50% of patients with venous thromboembolism having a thrombophilia (**Table 234-1**).[1] Importantly, risk for clotting from genetic, acquired, and environmental factors is additive or even multiplicative; a patient with mild deficiency may develop a deep venous thrombosis when started on estrogen.[2]

PATHOPHYSIOLOGY

Several physiologic systems ensure that blood clots do not extend beyond the necessary area. The two most clinically important pathways involve antithrombin and protein C (see Figures 232-1 and 232-2 and **Table 234-2**). Antithrombin is a plasma-based protein that inhibits several activated coagulation factors, primarily thrombin, factor Xa, and factor IXa. Both unfractionated heparin and low-molecular-weight heparin possess anticoagulant activity by increasing the rate by which antithrombin inhibits these factors: approximately 2000- to 4000-fold for thrombin, about 500- to 1000-fold for factor Xa, and about a million-fold for factor IXa. Protein C is a vitamin K–dependent plasma protein that binds to the endothelial cell surface and is activated by thrombin. Activated protein C cleaves both factor Va and factor VIIIa, inhibiting both the common pathway and the intrinsic pathway. Protein S, another vitamin K–dependent plasma protein, is a cofactor that increases the inhibitory action of activated protein C by about 20-fold.

TABLE 234-1 Hypercoagulable States

Inherited	Acquired
Activated protein C resistance due to factor V Leiden mutation	Pregnancy Oral contraceptives/hormone replacement therapy
Prothrombin gene mutation 20210A	Malignancy
Protein C deficiency	Heparin-induced thrombocytopenia
Protein S deficiency	Antiphospholipid syndrome
Antithrombin deficiency	Warfarin-induced skin necrosis
Hyperhomocysteinemia, severe	Hyperviscosity syndromes
	Human immunodeficiency virus (HIV)

CLINICAL FEATURES

Thrombophilic disorders are rarely diagnosed in the ED. Instead, the emergency physician's primary responsibilities are to (1) recognize higher risk of thrombosis in patients with a known thrombophilia, and (2) obtain pertinent information to suspect an undiagnosed hypercoagulable state (**Table 234-3**).[3]

DIAGNOSIS

Laboratory testing specific for hypercoagulable conditions is not helpful in an ED setting.[4,5] Some factor levels cannot be reliably measured in the setting of acute thrombosis or while the patient is taking a vitamin K antagonist such as warfarin. The focus is to suspect the thrombophilia, refer for evaluation, and appropriately manage acute thrombosis. The ED diagnostic approach to individual episodes of suspected thrombosis in a thrombophilic patient is site specific (e.g., cerebral circulation, coronary circulation, or peripheral venous system). **Using a normal serum D-dimer level to exclude venous thromboembolism in patients with known hypercoagulable disorders has not been validated.**

TABLE 234-2 Functions of Coagulation Proteins in Protein C and Antithrombin Systems

Factor	Function	Pertinent Disorders
Prothrombin (factor II)	Precursor to thrombin, which converts fibrinogen to fibrin.	Prothrombin mutations, 20210A and others
Factor V, activated	Complexes with Factor Xa, calcium, and phospholipid to convert prothrombin to thrombin.	Activated protein C resistance due to factor V Leiden mutation
Protein C, activated	Cleaves activated factors Va and VIIIa.	Congenital protein C deficiency Activated protein C resistance due to factor V Leiden mutation Neonatal purpura fulminans Warfarin-induced skin necrosis
Protein S	Cofactor for activated protein C. Cofactor for tissue factor pathway inhibitor (which inhibits extrinsic pathway of coagulation). Counteracts factor Xa's protection of factor Va from degradation.	Congenital protein S deficiency Neonatal purpura fulminans Warfarin-induced skin necrosis
Antithrombin	Inhibits thrombin, factor Xa, and factor IXa. Binds heparins, leading to increased antithrombin activity.	Antithrombin deficiency
Phospholipids	Present on cell membranes of endothelial cells that line blood vessels. The activity of several proteins in the coagulation cascade is enhanced when bound to phospholipids.	Antiphospholipid syndrome

TABLE 234-3 Features Suggestive of Thrombophilia

Early thrombosis (age 45 y and younger)
Recurrent thrombotic events or fetal loss
Family history of thrombosis or recurrent fetal loss
Thrombosis in unusual location (mesenteric, cerebral, axillary, or portal veins)

TREATMENT AND DISPOSITION

Initial management and disposition of individual episodes of confirmed thrombosis in a patient with thrombophilia is similar to that of a patient without known thrombophilia. Duration of treatment does differ (**Table 234-4**).

Patients not currently on anticoagulation should consider prophylactic anticoagulants for high-risk situations such as surgery, pregnancy and the postpartum period, and prolonged travel. Estrogen-based oral contraceptive pills and hormone replacement therapy should be avoided in patients with known thrombophilia because of the thrombotic risk.

SPECIFIC CONDITIONS ASSOCIATED WITH THROMBOPHILIA

INHERITED CLOTTING DISORDERS

ACTIVATED PROTEIN C RESISTANCE (FACTOR V LEIDEN)

Activated protein C resistance caused by the factor V Leiden mutation is the most prevalent inherited hypercoagulable disorder; approximately 5% of the U.S. population of European descent is heterozygous for this mutation.[6] In this disorder, the gene for factor V has a single point mutation that makes factor Va resistant to inhibition by activated protein C (factor V Leiden). This leads to overabundant conversion of prothrombin to thrombin. Factor V Leiden is inherited in an autosomal dominant pattern, with most patients being heterozygous for the mutation. Heterozygotes for factor V Leiden have a sevenfold increased risk of deep venous thrombosis compared with noncarriers, with homozygotes having a 20-fold increase in risk. Factor V Leiden is more highly associated with deep vein thrombosis than pulmonary embolism[6] and has been observed in up to 21% of patients with first-time deep venous thrombosis.[7] Activated protein C resistance also produces pregnancy complications such as

TABLE 234-4 Management of Inherited and Acquired Thrombophilias

Situation	Management
First episode of thrombosis	Unfractionated heparin or low-molecular-weight heparin for 5 d and/or until therapeutic anticoagulation achieved with an oral anticoagulant. Continue anticoagulation for 6 mo to 2 y; some advocate lifelong treatment.
Second episode of thrombosis	Lifelong anticoagulation.
Pregnancy	Begin unfractionated heparin or low-molecular-weight heparin at diagnosis of pregnancy. May use warfarin in postpartum period.
Active malignancy	Use low-molecular weight heparin for treatment of venous thromboembolic events
Oral contraception	Avoid.
Hormone replacement therapy	Avoid.

severe pre-eclampsia, placental abruption, fetal growth restriction, and stillbirth.

PROTHROMBIN GENE MUTATION

The most common mutation of the prothrombin gene (20210A) leads to increased prothrombin biosynthesis with about a 30% increase in circulating prothrombin levels, creating a hypercoagulable state. Prothrombin mutations are inherited in an autosomal dominant manner with mutations in the prothrombin gene present in about 2% of Caucasians.[2] Heterozygotes account for up to 10% of patients with initial episodes of deep venous thrombosis.[7] Patients with prothrombin gene mutation present with increased risk of venous thromboembolism and pregnancy complications, similar to activated protein C resistance from factor V Leiden.

ANTITHROMBIN DEFICIENCY

Several mutations to the antithrombin gene exist, many leading to antithrombin deficiency. Two percent of patients with a history of thrombosis have an antithrombin deficiency,[8] and it is more prevalent in Asian populations. Antithrombin deficiency is classified into two main groups. In type 1, the measured level of antithrombin is diminished, whereas patients with type 2 have a normal amount of antithrombin, but the function is greatly diminished due to conformational changes in the protein. Antithrombin deficiency is inherited in an autosomal dominant fashion. Heterozygous patients have a fivefold increased risk of thrombotic events, typically pregnancy complications and venous thromboembolism. Homozygous antithrombin deficiency is incompatible with life.

PROTEIN C AND S DEFICIENCIES

Protein C and protein S deficiencies, like antithrombin deficiency, are transmitted in an autosomal dominant fashion, but with more varied clinical presentations. Prevalence can only be estimated, because not all patients with heterozygous defects develop inappropriate thrombosis. Heterozygous protein C deficiency is thought to be present in 1:250 to 1:500 people, and heterozygous protein S deficiency is estimated to occur in about 1:500 individuals.[9] Homozygous protein C or S deficiency is rare and presents as neonatal purpura fulminans. Patients with heterozygous protein C or S deficiency are at higher risk for venous thromboembolism, and like antithrombin deficiency, these disorders can be associated with either decreased total amount of protein C or S or decreased functional activity. In general, lower protein function is associated with higher risk and frequency of thrombotic events. Protein C and S deficiency, like antithrombin deficiency, is more prevalent in the Japanese and Chinese populations with up to 65% percent of adults with venous thromboembolism having a deficiency of protein C, protein S, or antithrombin.[9]

Patients with heterozygous protein C or S deficiency are at higher risk for warfarin-induced skin necrosis because warfarin inhibits protein C and S synthesis. Warfarin-induced skin necrosis is rare and is prevented by both avoiding loading doses of warfarin and continuing heparin products until the INR is therapeutic. Therefore, any patient who develops warfarin-induced skin necrosis should be evaluated for protein C or S deficiency.

HYPERHOMOCYSTEINEMIA

Three enzymes are involved in the metabolism of homocysteine: methylenetetrahydrofolate reductase, cystathionine β-synthase, and methionine synthase. Inherited functional deficiency in the first two enzymes is associated with an increased risk of both arterial and venous thrombosis, as well as atherosclerosis.[2] The presence of elevated homocysteine in the blood is a marker of the functional enzyme deficiency. Heterozygotes for a variant mutation in either methylenetetrahydrofolate reductase or cystathionine β-synthase are found in approximately 15% of individuals with European, Middle Eastern, and Asian ancestry, compared with approximately 1% to 2% of African Americans.

Patients with profound hyperhomocysteinemia, generally because of homozygous inheritance of a dysfunctional enzyme, have the condition termed *congenital homocystinuria*, and have significant skeletal and ocular problems as well as mental retardation, developmental delay, and thrombotic events. Heterozygotes for a dysfunctional enzyme do not have the skeletal, ocular, or mental complications, but have a two- to fourfold increased risk for venous thrombosis. As with other hypercoagulable disorders, the presence of hyperhomocysteinemia can combine with other thrombotic conditions to greatly increase the risk of venous thrombosis; factor V Leiden mutation combined with hyperhomocysteinemia produces about a 20-fold increase in the risk for venous thrombosis.[2,10]

ACQUIRED CLOTTING DISORDERS

PREGNANCY AND ESTROGEN USE

The coagulation changes in pregnancy (**Table 234-5**) represent an adaptive measure to prevent excessive hemorrhage with delivery.[11] Many of these changes are anatomic in nature, whereas some are related to the relatively high estrogen state. These changes promoting thrombosis are similar but less profound in women taking oral contraceptive and hormone replacement therapy.

The exact mechanism of how exogenous estrogen therapy leads to a hypercoagulable state is complex and not completely understood, but higher doses of estrogen clearly confer a higher risk for clotting. The current low doses for estrogens in oral contraceptives are associated with a smaller but still clinically significantly increased risk of thrombosis. Estrogen use has been associated with modest increases in several procoagulant proteins (factors VII, VIII, X, prothrombin, and fibrinogen) as well as decreases in anticoagulant proteins (antithrombin, protein S, protein C). Use of oral contraceptives or hormone replacement therapy in a patient with known heterozygosity for factor V Leiden puts the patient at an even higher risk for thrombosis, approximately a 15-fold increase.

MALIGNANCY

Malignancy is associated with increased risk for thrombus formation, but the exact mechanisms are not completely understood.[12,13] For patients with the new diagnosis of cancer, the risk of venous thromboembolism is highest in the first 3 months after diagnosis, with an odds ratio of about 50. Some types of cancers are more likely to promote thrombosis than others, with pancreatic, brain, acute myelogenous leukemia, gastric, esophageal, gynecologic, kidney, and lung cancers having the highest association with thrombosis. Cancer also increases the incidence of arterial thrombotic events, such as myocardial infarction and ischemic stroke.[12] Other manifestations of hypercoagulability in cancer patients include chronic disseminated intravascular coagulation, nonbacterial thrombotic endocarditis, migratory superficial thrombophlebitis, and thrombotic microangiopathy. Chemotherapy itself can also affect coagulation in many ways, such as downregulation of proteins C and S, induction of tissue factor production by endothelial cells, and direct cell damage.

Use low-molecular-weight heparin for the initial treatment of venous thromboembolism in patients with active cancer.[13] Long-term anticoagulation following the diagnosis of venous thromboembolism in these patients should be with a low-molecular-weight heparin for 6 months as opposed to warfarin.[13] Prophylactic anticoagulation for primary prevention

TABLE 234-5 Factors Contributing to Hypercoagulable State in Pregnancy

Anatomic	Hematologic
Venous occlusion from gravid uterus.	Increased thrombin generation from placental secretion of tissue factor
Trauma to pelvic veins during delivery.	
Tissue injury during surgical delivery.	Increased production of procoagulant proteins
Left iliac vein crosses over left iliac artery, leading to relative compression (left leg deep venous thrombosis is three times more likely than right in pregnant patients).	Decreased free and total protein C
	Increased platelet activation and platelet turnover

of venous thromboembolism in ambulatory medical oncology patients is not recommended.[13]

HEPARIN-INDUCED THROMBOCYTOPENIA

Heparin-induced thrombocytopenia is a consumptive coagulopathy in which components of the clotting cascade are inappropriately activated, forming arterial and venous thrombus.[14] Platelet factor 4 is a cell-signaling molecule that plays a central role in this syndrome. Platelet factor 4 neutralizes heparin and heparin-like endogenous compounds, and the heparin–platelet factor 4 combination inhibits local antithrombin activity, thereby promoting coagulation. Heparin-induced thrombocytopenia develops when patients develop antibodies against the heparin–platelet factor 4 complex. A complex of heparin, platelet factor 4, and the antibody binds to platelets, activating them. The platelets then form small microparticles that initiate clot formation. The measured platelet count falls because platelets are bound in both small and large clots. Also, the heparin–platelet factor 4 antibody complex can stimulate endothelial cells and monocytes to release tissue factor, which further triggers the coagulation cascade.

The typical presentation of heparin-induced thrombocytopenia has the platelet count falling to 50,000 to 60,000/mm^3 (50 to 60 × 10^9/L) within 5 to 15 days after starting heparin treatment. Despite the low platelet counts, the patient is hypercoagulable for days to weeks, even after heparin is stopped. Rarely, patients can develop a rapid-onset presentation within hours of initiation of heparin.

With more outpatients being treated with heparin products for venous thromboembolism or other thrombophilias, patients with heparin-induced thrombocytopenia may present to the ED with this syndrome.[14] The diagnosis of heparin-induced thrombocytopenia hinges on laboratory findings and cannot be definitely diagnosed on clinical grounds alone.[15] Thrombocytopenia is almost universally present (with the exception being patients with preexisting thrombocytosis). Suspect the syndrome when platelets have dropped approximately 50% from a recent value in a patient currently or recently taking a heparin product. All heparin products, both unfractionated and low-molecular-weight, must be stopped. These patients need anticoagulation because the risk for thrombosis is highest in the first week after diagnosis.[14] Vitamin K antagonists, such as warfarin, should be avoided in acute heparin-induced thrombocytopenia because these can increase the risk of microvascular thrombosis acutely due to transient relative protein C deficiency. Hematology consultation should be sought.

WARFARIN-INDUCED SKIN NECROSIS

Warfarin inhibits the production of vitamin K–dependent coagulation factors, with the serum levels of the individual factors decreasing according to their half-life. Upon initiation of warfarin, protein C is decreased before most of the procoagulant proteins. This decrease in protein C leads to a transient relative protein C deficiency, which can lead to clinically significant hypercoagulability.

Warfarin-induced skin necrosis presents with painful, red lesions usually located over the extremities, breasts, trunk, or penis.[16] Lesions typically start with an initial central erythematous macule, extending over hours to a localized edema, developing central purpuric zones and then necrosis. Prevention of this complication is one of the reasons loading doses of warfarin are avoided. Thrombin inhibitors, such as low-molecular-weight heparin, should be administered and continued until therapeutic anticoagulation is achieved with warfarin.[16] Rarely, warfarin-induced skin necrosis occurs despite appropriate initiation of heparin treatment. When it does, approximately one-third of patients will prove to have an inherited protein C deficiency.

ANTIPHOSPHOLIPID SYNDROME

Antiphospholipid syndrome (APS) is an autoimmune disorder that is a cause of acquired thrombophilia.[17] Many of the specific antibodies discovered have targets that are not phospholipids, but rather proteins that interact with phospholipids, such as prothrombin, protein C, and protein S. The most common specific antibodies associated with APS are β_2-glycoprotein I and lupus anticoagulant. Lupus anticoagulant was initially discovered in patients with systemic lupus erythematosus and prolongation of the activated thromboplastin time; hence, the name *lupus anticoagulant*. However, in vivo, the lupus anticoagulant acts as a procoagulant and is associated with thrombosis.[17]

Prevalence of APS is about 40 to 50 cases per 100,000 persons. Up to 5% of normal, healthy young people have antiphospholipid antibodies; this number increases with age and comorbid conditions, but only a minority of these patients develops APS. Antiphospholipid antibodies are positive in approximately 13% of patients with stroke, 11% with myocardial infarction, and 9.5% with deep venous thrombosis.[18] As with most autoimmune disorders, APS is more common in women and is diagnosed from a combination of laboratory findings and clinical findings (**Table 234-6**).

TABLE 234-6 Clinical Manifestations of Antiphospholipid Syndrome

System	Examples
Venous	Deep venous thrombosis: extremities, cerebral, portal, hepatic, renal, retinal
Arterial	Premature atherosclerosis Acute coronary syndrome Ischemic stroke Vascular stenosis or occlusion: extremities, aorta, renal, retinal
Obstetric	Fetal loss: often after 10-wk gestation Preterm labor Low birth weight Pre-eclampsia
Neurologic	Stroke Migraine Sneddon's syndrome—clinical triad of stroke, hypertension, and livedo reticularis Cognitive dysfunction Subcortical dementia Chorea Dysphagia Guillain-Barré syndrome Seizures Optic neuritis
Skin	Livedo reticularis
Cardiac	Valvular abnormalities (Libman-Sacks endocarditis) Syndrome X (angina-like chest pain, cardiac stress test positive for ischemia, normal coronary angiography)
Skeletal	Osteonecrosis
Renal	Thrombotic microangiopathy Renal artery or vein thrombosis Renal artery stenosis with hypertension
Pulmonary	Pulmonary embolus Pulmonary hypertension (from recurrent emboli)
GI	Budd-Chiari syndrome (hepatic vein thrombosis) Mesenteric ischemia Hepatic infarction Acalculous cholecystitis with gallbladder necrosis
Hematologic (other than thrombosis)	Bleeding diathesis (rare) Acquired hypoprothrombinemia Thrombocytopenia Hemolytic anemia
Catastrophic antiphospholipid syndrome	Fulminant multisystem organ failure

Most patients with APS have no other predisposing conditions (primary APS). However, many patients with APS also have other conditions thought to be associated with their APS (secondary APS). Typical conditions include other rheumatologic or autoimmune disorders such as systemic lupus, infections, and drug exposures (e.g., phenytoin, hydralazine, cocaine).

Although most patients with APS present with isolated, recurrent thrombotic events, about 1% have a rapidly progressive form known as *catastrophic antiphospholipid syndrome,* representing acceleration in the pathophysiologic processes of APS with widespread small-vessel occlusions in multiple organs.[19] It is unknown why some APS patients develop such a severe course. Common triggers include infection, trauma, anticoagulation problems, and cancer. However, 40% of the time, no obvious trigger can be found. Mortality of catastrophic APS is approximately 50% despite treatment.

Obviously, APS patients with recurrent thrombotic events need lifelong anticoagulation. Pregnant women with APS need anticoagulation with subcutaneous unfractionated or low-molecular-weight heparin or low-dose aspirin therapy. Because many normal healthy patients have antiphospholipid antibodies, prophylaxis without a personal history of thrombosis is not recommended. In the rare event of catastrophic APS, a multipronged approach involving anticoagulation, steroids, plasmapheresis, and/or IV γ-globulin is typically used.

HYPERCOAGULABILITY ASSOCIATED WITH OTHER DISORDERS

Many other conditions are associated with increased risk of clotting. Patients with **nephrotic syndrome** have an increased risk of hypercoagulability for complex reasons. In several cases, this is simply a matter of increased urinary excretion of anticoagulant proteins. The nephrotic syndrome can also lead to increased endothelial injury and platelet aggregation. Patients with several different forms of **vasculitis**, such as Behçet's syndrome, antineutrophil cytoplasmic antibody–associated vasculitis, and granulomatosis with polyangiitis have a slightly increased risk of thrombosis. **Hyperviscosity syndromes,** such as essential thrombocythemia, polycythemia vera, Waldenström's macroglobulinemia, multiple myeloma, and sickle cell disease, also place patients at increased risk for thrombosis. Most risk factors for cardiovascular disease, such as smoking and diabetes, are also risk factors for venous thromboembolism to varying degrees.[20] **Diabetes** alone slightly increases the risk for thrombosis in younger patients without other obvious risks for thrombosis.[21] Patients with **human immunodeficiency virus** have a 2- to 10-fold increased risk for venous thromboembolism compared to the general population.[22]

REFERENCES

The complete reference list is available online at www.TintinalliEM.com.

CHAPTER 235 Hemophilias and von Willebrand's Disease

Robin R. Hemphill

INTRODUCTION

Hemophilias are bleeding disorders due to deficiency in one of the factors present in the clotting cascade.[1,2] The most common factor abnormalities are of factor VIII (**hemophilia A**) or factor IX (**hemophilia B**). **von Willebrand's disease** is a related defect of the von Willebrand factor.[3]

These hereditary bleeding disorders typically appear early in life, and adult patients will usually be able to relate a history of a bleeding problem. However, patients with mild forms of inherited disease may be unaware of a bleeding disorder until stressed by significant trauma or development of another hemostatic problem.

Systemic bleeding disorders should be suspected in patients with severe bleeding related to trivial trauma or minor surgery, or spontaneous bleeding, particularly when the bleeding occurs in joints or muscle. Unusual bleeding or bruising at multiple areas should also raise concern about a coagulopathy. Medications can be responsible for unmasking a mild bleeding diathesis.

The pattern of bleeding can suggest a likely cause. Patients with easy bruising, gingival bleeding, epistaxis, hematuria, GI bleeding, or heavy menses are more likely to have a deficiency or dysfunction of the platelets. Conversely, patients with spontaneous deep bruises, hemarthrosis, retroperitoneal bleeding, or intracranial bleeding are more likely to have a coagulation factor deficiency. In factor-deficient patients, bleeding associated with trauma may be delayed, due to inadequate fibrin clot formation that inadequately stabilizes the initial platelet thrombus. Patients with von Willebrand's disease may present with features of both platelet and clotting factor problems.

HEMOPHILIA

EPIDEMIOLOGY

The genes that encode factors VIII and IX are located on the long arm of the X chromosome. A genetic mutation in the factor VIII gene produces hemophilia A, occurring in about 1 in 5000 male births in the United States. A mutation in the factor IX gene causes hemophilia B, affecting approximately 1 in 25,000 male births in the United States. Together, these two forms of hemophilia make up about 99% of patients with inherited coagulation factor deficiencies. Hemophilia A and B are clinically indistinguishable from each other, and specific factor testing is required to identify the type.

Because hemophilia A and B are X-linked disorders, hemophilia is overwhelmingly a disease of men, with women typically being asymptomatic carriers. Only rarely do women have severe disease. While these disorders are genetic and usually inherited, a family history of bleeding may be absent because approximately one third of new cases of hemophilia arise from a spontaneous gene mutation.

PATHOPHYSIOLOGY

Bleeding manifestations in patients with all forms of hemophilia are directly attributable to the decreased plasma activity levels of either factor VIII or IX (**Table 235-1**). Those with factor activity levels of 0.3 to 0.4 IU/mL (30% to 40% of normal) may never be aware that they have hemophilia, or they might manifest unusual bleeding only after major surgery or severe trauma. Unless there is another underlying disease, patients with hemophilia do not have problems with minor cuts and abrasions, as hemostasis from these injuries is achieved by platelet activation and the formation of the primary hemostatic plug (see chapter 232, "Tests of Hemostasis").

Bleeding is the major complication of hemophilia, but as a result of frequent exposure to blood products, many hemophiliacs in the past were infected with viral hepatitis or human immunodeficiency virus, and had, in addition, complications related to these chronic infections; currently available factor replacement products have essentially eliminated the risk of seroconversion.

CLINICAL FEATURES

Depending on the severity of the disease, both hemophilia A and B are characterized by easy bruising and spontaneous recurrent bleeding into the joints and muscles.[1,2] Although the joints and muscles are the most common areas into which bleeding occurs, hemorrhage may also occur in other areas (**Table 235-2**). Trauma or a surgical procedure can result in prolonged and difficult-to-control bleeding.

Although adults often know that they have hemophilia, young children may not have been diagnosed before they present to the ED with a bleeding episode. Family history may reveal a bleeding disorder on the mother's side. Hemophilia should be suspected in an infant or child who presents with excessive bruising or with bleeding into the joints, muscles, or CNS that is spontaneous or out of proportion to the history of trauma. Because factor level determines the severity of disease, those

TABLE 235-1 Hemophilia Severity

Disease Severity	Percentage of Factor VIII or IX Activity (% of Normal)	Clinical Features
Severe	<0.01 IU/mL (<1%)	Severe spontaneous bleeding, difficult to control if trauma
Moderate	0.01–0.05 IU/mL (1%–5%)	Usually bleeding from trauma; may bleed spontaneously
Mild	0.06–0.40 IU/mL (6%–40%)	Bleeding after trauma

with mild hemophilia may come to medical attention only when they have a significant surgical procedure or trauma or have started a medication with antihemostatic effects.

Congenital hemophilia in neonates can be manifest as excess bleeding after circumcision or as intracranial hemorrhage, usually associated with traumatic delivery.[4,5] In infants and mobile children, nonpatterned bruising can suggest hemophilia. An irritable infant with hemophilia can be difficult to evaluate; if no other source is found, there should be a presumption of occult bleeding.

DIAGNOSIS

Hemophilia is diagnosed starting with the clinical suspicion of a bleeding disorder. Screening tests, such as the **prothrombin time**, which measures the extrinsic coagulation cascade, will be normal, whereas the **activated partial thromboplastin time**, which measures the intrinsic coagulation cascade, is usually abnormal. However, patients with mild hemophilia and factor levels above 0.3 to 0.4 IU/mL (30% to 40% of normal) may have an activated thromboplastin time within the test reference range. **Bleeding time in both forms of hemophilia will be normal and therefore not helpful**. The diagnosis is confirmed by quantitative measurement of factor VIII or IX levels below 0.50 IU/mL (<50% normal). If mild hemophilia A is suspected, a variant of von Willebrand's disease characterized by abnormal binding of factor VIII and von Willebrand factor should be excluded by special binding tests or genetic analysis.

For patients with established hemophilia, hemostatic testing (e.g., prothrombin time, activated partial thromboplastin time) is unlikely to yield new information and is not routinely indicated. Female carriers of a hemophilic gene can be suspected by family history and confirmed by DNA mutation analysis performed at specialized centers. Prenatal diagnosis is possible using chorionic villus sampling performed between 9 and 14 weeks of gestation or amniocentesis done at 15 to 17 weeks to detect the genetic mutation.

TABLE 235-2 Hemophilia Bleeding Manifestations

Site	Comments
Hemarthroses	Most common site, more frequent in hinged joints (elbows, knees, ankles) than in multiaxial joints.
Soft tissue	Bleeding into soft tissues or muscle; bleeding can dissect along fascial planes; most dangerous in the neck (airway compromise), limbs (compartment syndromes), eye (retro-orbital hematoma), spine (epidural hematoma), and retroperitoneum (circulatory shock).
Mucocutaneous bleeding	Delayed bleeding after dental extractions; spontaneous bleeding from the nose, pharynx, GI tract, or lungs is uncommon.
CNS	Intracranial bleeding is the most common cause of hemorrhagic death in hemophiliacs of all age groups; subdural hematomas occur spontaneously or with minimal trauma.
Hematuria	Common, usually not serious, and a specific bleeding site is rarely found.
Hemophilic pseudotumor	Unresolved or undertreated hematomas erode into adjacent bones resembling bone cysts or malignancy; may compress adjacent nerves and vessels.

HEMOPHILIA TREATMENT

General Principles Treatment of patients with hemophilia relies on either the early replacement of missing factors or, for those who have mild factor VIII deficiency, stimulating the body to secrete clotting factor from intracellular stores. **Begin replacement before or at the same time as other resuscitative and diagnostic maneuvers for intracranial, intrathoracic, intra-abdominal, retroperitoneal, ocular, or airway bleeding, as sustained bleeding raises the risk for morbidity and death (Table 235-2).** Bleeding into the neck, tongue, or retropharynx can compromise the airway. Suspected intracranial hemorrhage, either spontaneous with an acute severe headache or following blunt head injury, should receive immediate factor replacement therapy followed by noncontrast head CT. Complaints of back, thigh, groin, or abdominal pain may be symptoms of retroperitoneal bleeding. Hemorrhage into the iliopsoas muscle is a common form of retroperitoneal bleeding seen in hemophiliacs, and patients may describe hip pain and have difficulty straightening their leg, preferring to keep it in a flexed, externally rotated position. An **iliopsoas muscle bleed** can compress and damage the femoral nerve, cause anemia of blood loss, or produce circulatory shock.

The initial manifestations of bleeding can be subtle. Simple injuries, such as ankle and wrist sprains, may at first appear benign, and several hours may pass before hemarthrosis is apparent. **So, while there may not be physical signs of bleeding into a joint, patients reliably report when bleeding is occurring.** Prompt treatment of hemarthroses can prevent or reduce the long-term sequelae of hemophilic arthropathy. If a large hemarthrosis is already present, consultation with an orthopedist for appropriate splinting and rehabilitation may improve the outcome once the bleeding has been controlled.[6]

Compartment syndromes can result from bleeds within the fascial compartments of the extremities. Compartment pressures can be safely measured **after** the patient has received factor replacement.

Many patients and their families administer factor concentrate therapy at home. Patients are taught to self-treat or seek care at the first symptom before little outward evidence develops. Take patient concerns seriously. Many patients will have an established management plan for acute bleeding episodes in the medical record. Regional hemophilia foundations, associations, and centers often maintain a database that can be contacted for patient-specific information.

Bleeding episodes are terribly painful, so provide adequate pain control whether or not there is a history of opiate abuse.

When treating patients with hemophilia for other reasons, some general principles apply. Do not place central venous access or arterial lines without factor replacement. Similar rules apply to arterial blood gases, lumbar puncture, and other invasive procedures. Do not give IM injections unless factor replacement is given and maintained for several days. As a general rule, do not give compounds that contain aspirin or nonsteroidal anti-inflammatory drugs for pain relief. If a hemophiliac patient requires interhospital transfer, initiate factor replacement **before** transfer, and do not delay factor replacement with attempts to obtain imaging. Most hemophilia centers prefer to be consulted **anytime** a patient with hemophilia presents to the ED, especially if there is an uncertainty about the need for factor replacement.

Hemophilia Factor Replacement Therapy For patients with hemophilia, there are two sources for factor replacement therapy: recombinant technology from hamster cell lines and purification from human plasma (**Table 235-3**).[1,2,7,8] The highest level of purity and the lowest risk for human viral contamination are found with the recombinant factor concentrates: no transmission of human immunodeficiency virus, hepatitis B virus, or hepatitis C virus has been reported with the current products available in the United States. However, recombinant products may have a higher risk for the development of inhibitor antibodies than plasma-derived products.[9-11] It remains possible for even the highly treated and purified plasma-derived products to potentially transmit viruses such as hepatitis A and the highly heat-resistant parvovirus B19.[1,2,7,8] Opinions vary as to the preferred product,[12,13] and

TABLE 235-3 Hemophilia Replacement Factor Products

Hemophilia Type	Available Products* (Manufacturer/Distributor)
Hemophilia A	*Recombinant Factor VIII Concentrates*
	Advate® (Baxter)
	Helixate FS® (Bayer/CSL Behring)
	Kogenate FS® (Bayer)
	Recombinate® (Baxter)
	Xyntha® (Pfizer)
	Human Plasma-Derived Factor VIII Concentrates
	Hemofil M® (Baxter)
	Monoclate-P® (CSL Behring)
	Human Plasma-Derived Factor VIII Concentrates That Contain von Willebrand Factor
	Alphanate® (Grifols)
	Humate-P® (CSL Behring GmbH)
	Koate-DVI® (Grifols/Kedrion Biopharma)
Hemophilia B	*Recombinant Factor IX Concentrate*
	BeneFIX® (Pfizer)
	Human Plasma-Derived Factor IX Concentrates
	AlphaNine SD® (Grifols)
	Mononine® (CSL Behring)

*Commercial trade names provided for ease of specific identification.

current World Federation of Hemophilia guidelines do not express a preference.[2] In the United States, the National Hemophilia Foundation position is that recombinant factor concentrates are the preferred treatment for hemophilia despite a cost higher than plasma-derived products.[14] **Where possible, the treating physician should use the product that the patient uses at home.**

The dosing regimen used in the hemophilic patient is empiric based on the clotting factor volume of distribution, the half-life of the factor, and the hemostatic level of factor required to control the bleeding (**Table 235-4**).[15,16] Clotting factor is dosed in units of activity; 1 IU of factor represents the amount present in 1 mL of normal plasma. In hemophilia A, 1 IU of factor VIII per kilogram of body weight raises the plasma level by approximately 0.02 IU/mL (2%). The half-life of factor VIII is approximately 8 to 12 hours. For hemophilia B, 1 IU of factor IX per kilogram of body weight will raise the plasma level by approximately 0.01 IU/mL (1%). The half-life of factor IX is approximately 16 to 24 hours.

Factor concentrates are supplied as lyophilized powder in single-use glass vials containing a range of amounts, from 250 to 4000 IU per vial. Calculation of the amount of factor is done using the patient's weight, baseline factor level, the desired factor level, and, to avoid wasting factor, rounding up doses to the next vial. For patients with moderate and severe hemophilia and baseline factor levels below 0.05 IU/mL (5%), the presence of such low levels can be discounted when calculating initial dosing guided by these formulae:

Factor VIII dose = Desired factor VIII level × weight (kg) × 0.5
Factor IX dose = Desired factor IX level × weight (kg)

For major bleeding, high levels of factor replacement are required and continued until bleeding stops (**Table 235-4**). Repeat doses are usually given as intermittent bolus therapy every 8 to 24 hours, or 6 to 12 hours in patients under 6 years of age.

For less severe bleeding in soft tissue, muscle, or joints, a lesser amount of factor replacement is necessary; usually three doses over 1 to 2 days are sufficient to control bleeding. In addition to factor replacement, extremity and joint bleeding may benefit from splinting followed by physical therapy.[6] Cryotherapy has no proven benefit in hemarthroses.[17]

There may be rare instances in which a patient presents with what appears to be a previously undiagnosed bleeding disorder. In these cases, treatment with **fresh frozen plasma** is appropriate to control bleeding until definitive studies can be done. Fresh frozen plasma contains all of the plasma clotting factors, with an average concentration of 1 IU/mL. However, one bag (about 200 mL) of fresh frozen plasma will only raise the factor levels by 3% to 5% in an average adult, so volume overload can complicate extensive factor replacement using this product.

Special Considerations • *Oral and Mucosal Bleeding* Oral bleeding from hemophilia is more common in children than in adults. For an oral bleed, the area should be identified, cleaned of inadequate clot, and solution of **topical bovine thrombin** sprayed on to the site or applied in conjunction with a saturated absorbable gelatin sponge. Repeat doses should be limited because repetitive application of topical bovine thrombin can induce antibodies to factor V, resulting in a syndrome of severe bleeding and thrombosis, which can rarely be fatal. Factor replacement may be required, dosed according to the severity of bleeding. Antifibrinolytic agents, such as **aminocaproic acid** and **tranexamic acid**, are useful adjunctive therapies with a low rate of adverse effects.[2] For very superficial mucosal injuries, it may be possible to manage the bleeding with antifibrinolytic therapy alone. The dose of aminocaproic acid is 75 to 100 milligrams/kg every 6 hours for children, and 6 grams every 6 hours for adults, given PO or IV. The dose of tranexamic acid is 10 milligrams/kg IV three times per day for 1 to 7 days. Tranexamic acid should be used with caution if hematuria is present because ureteral obstruction due to clot formation has been reported.[7]

Mild Hemophilia A Patients with **mild hemophilia A** (factor levels of 5% of normal or greater) who have mild bleeding may not always require factor replacement.[1,2,18] Rather, they may be treated with desmopressin, which

TABLE 235-4 Initial Factor Replacement Guidelines in Moderate and Severe Hemophilia

Severity and Site	Desired Factor Level to Control Bleeding	Hemophilia A Initial Dose (IU/kg)	Hemophilia B Initial Dose (IU/kg)	Comments
Minor: skin (deep laceration)	—	—	—	Abrasions and superficial lacerations usually do not require factor replacement. Treat with pressure and topical thrombin.
Minor: early hemarthrosis, mild muscle bleeding, mild oral bleeding	0.2–0.4 IU/mL (20%–40%)	10–20	20–30	Repeat dose every 12–24 h for 1–3 d until bleeding episode is resolved. Typical duration of replacement is 1–3 d.
Moderate: definite hemarthrosis, moderate muscle bleeding, moderate oral bleeding	0.3–0.6 IU/mL (30%–60%)	15–30	25–50	Orthopedic consult may be required for splinting, physical therapy, and follow-up. Typical duration of replacement is 3–5 d.
Major: retropharyngeal, GI, intra-abdominal, intrathoracic, retroperitoneal	0.6–1.0 IU/mL (60%–100%)	30–50	30–50	Repeat dose every 8–24 h until resolution of bleeding episode. May require replacement for up to 10 d.
CNS	1.0 IU/mL (100%)	50	50–100	Treat before CT. Early neurosurgical consultation.

TABLE 235-5 Desmopressin Treatment of Mild Hemophilia A and von Willebrand Disease

Patient	IV Preparation	Nasal Preparation
<2 y	Not recommended	Not recommended
<50 kg weight	0.3 micrograms/kg IV over 30 min	Single spray 150 micrograms in one nostril
>50 kg weight	0.3 micrograms/kg IV over 30 min; maximum dose, 20 micrograms	One spray 150 micrograms in each nostril (total dose, 300 micrograms)

stimulates the release of von Willebrand factor from endothelial storage sites promoting an increase of factor VIII in the plasma (**Table 235-5**).[19,20] A concentrated intranasal preparation is available and can be used at home.[21] IV or intranasal desmopressin will increase the factor VIII level by two to four times. Desmopressin treatment can be repeated in 24 hours, but with repetitive use, the patient's stores of factor VIII will become depleted, and subsequently, the effect will be less. Desmopressin is an antidiuretic agent, and fluid restriction may be needed during use.[19]

Hematuria **Hematuria** is common in hemophilia but is typically not severe.[22] Rest and hydration are important to ameliorate the degree of bleeding. Factor replacement is indicated for gross hematuria. There is evidence that hemophiliacs are at increased risk for nephrolithiasis, suggesting that renal imaging is indicated for patients with symptoms of renal colic or new-onset hematuria.[23]

Factor Inhibitors **Factor inhibitors**, antibodies against replacement factors, tend to occur most commonly in severe hemophiliacs.[2] Inhibitors not only interfere with the effectiveness of factor replacement therapy, but also can cause anaphylaxis during factor administration in patients with hemophilia B.[24] The use of factor replacement in hemophilic patients with inhibitors is guided by the concentration of inhibitor (measured in Bethesda inhibitor assay units) and the type of response the patient has to factor concentrates. ED physicians should query hemophiliacs about whether they have known inhibitors.

The overriding principle in treating patients with inhibitors is close consultation with a hematologist. In patients with an inhibitor titer <5 Bethesda inhibitor assay units and who are not vigorous antibody responders, some hematologists may recommend giving an increased dose of factor in an attempt to overwhelm the existing antibody. Alternative therapies include human plasma-derived activated prothrombin complex concentrates and recombinant activated factor VII (**Table 235-6**).[25-27] Activated prothrombin complex concentrate contains factors II, IX, and X, mostly nonactivated, and factor VII, primarily in the activated form. Activated factor VII, either from human plasma or recombinant, when complexed with tissue factor, activates factor X. Factor Xa, in concert with factor Va, calcium, and phospholipid, promotes the conversion of prothrombin to thrombin, which ultimately leads to the formation of a hemostatic plug composed of cross-linked fibrin. Even without tissue factor, activated factor VII can bind to the surface of activated platelets stimulating the conversion of factor X to factor Xa.

TABLE 235-6 Replacement Therapy for Hemophilia A and B in Patients With Inhibitors

Type of Product*	Initial Dose	Dosing Interval	Comments
Human plasma-derived activated prothrombin complex concentrate FEIBA NF® (Baxter)	50–100 units/kg	6–12 h	Total daily doses should not normally exceed 200 units/kg
Recombinant activated factor VII NovoSeven RT® (Novo Nordisk)	90 micrograms/kg	2 h	Repeat until hemostasis achieved or therapy judged ineffective

*Commercial trade names provided for ease of specific identification.

Acquired Hemophilia **Acquired hemophilia** occurs when autoantibodies are created against factor VIII, resulting in inactivation of this factor and a hemorrhagic tendency.[28,29] This rare disorder is associated other conditions in about 40% of reported cases, such as autoimmune diseases, cancer, drugs (e.g., penicillin, sulfonamides, ciprofloxacin, phenytoin, clopidogrel), or the postpartum period. Acquired hemophilia occurs equally in both genders with a median age of 60 to 70 years. The bleeding pattern in acquired hemophilia is usually widespread cutaneous purpura and internal bleeding, with hemarthroses being less common, a difference from congenital hemophilia.

The autoantibodies are typically polyclonal IgG4 antibodies that form complexes with factor VIII in a manner that enables some residual factor VIII activity, causing a poor correlation between measured factor activity and bleeding severity. The laboratory findings include a prolonged activated partial thromboplastin time and a low factor VII level.[30] The autoantibody of acquired hemophilia has different kinetics of interaction with factor VII, enabling a differentiation between the inhibitor antibody sometimes seen in congenital hemophilia and antiphospholipid antibodies by mixing studies (see chapter 232).

Treatment of acute bleeding is with activated prothrombin complex concentrates or recombinant activated factor VII (**Table 235-6**).[30,31] Suppression of antibody formation is initiated with prednisone plus either cyclophosphamide or azathioprine. Most patients respond and maintain remission after the immunosuppressives are tapered and discontinued; relapse occurs in about 20%.[32]

Postpartum Acquired Hemophilia **Postpartum acquired hemophilia** is a rare condition with severe hemorrhagic potential.[33] The risk is highest with the first pregnancy, and presentation is typically 2 months after delivery with persistent vaginal bleeding being the most common presenting symptom. Treatment for hemorrhage is with activated prothrombin complex concentrates or recombinant activated factor VII (**Table 235-6**). Production of the autoantibodies will spontaneously cease over many months, achieving complete remission. Immunosuppressants will reduce time to remission. Recurrence with subsequent pregnancies is uncommon.

DISPOSITION AND FOLLOW-UP

Many hemophilic patients are able to judge the severity of bleeding, self-administer replacement therapy, and monitor the response at home.[1,2] Such patients may likely be discharged after initial treatment in the ED for typical joint, soft tissue, or nasal hemorrhage. Relative indications for hospital admission include treatment requiring multiple factor replacement doses or necessity for parenteral pain management. Patients with bleeding in the CNS, neck, pharynx, retropharynx, or retroperitoneum, or those with a potential compartment syndrome should be admitted. Given the complexity of treatment, consultation or transfer to a hemophilia treatment center is recommended.

VON WILLEBRAND'S DISEASE

EPIDEMIOLOGY

von Willebrand's disease is the most common inherited bleeding disorder, present in 1% of the population.[27] However, most patients have a mild defect, and clinically significant bleeding occurs in only about 1% of those with the disease. Congenital von Willebrand's disease is heterogeneously inherited and variably expressed, and although there are multiple variants, it can be classified into three major groups (**Table 235-7**).[34,35] An acquired form of von Willebrand's disease occurs when autoantibodies develop against von Willebrand factor, resulting in rapid clearance of the antibody–von Willebrand factor complex from the circulation.

PATHOPHYSIOLOGY

von Willebrand factor is a glycoprotein that, unlike most other coagulation factors, is synthesized, stored, and then secreted by the vascular endothelial cells. von Willebrand factor serves two key roles in normal

TABLE 235-7 von Willebrand Disease Classification and Treatment

Type	Frequency	Defect	Treatment
1	70%–80% of cases	Normal vWF is present, but in decreased quantity (approximately 20%–50% normal levels)	Desmopressin and, if no response, consider the measures below
2	10%–15% of cases	The vWF is abnormal and dysfunctional	vWF-containing concentrate or cryoprecipitate if vWF-containing product is not available
3	<10% of cases	Almost no vWF is present	vWF-containing concentrate or cryoprecipitate if vWF-containing concentrate is not available

Abbreviation: vWF = von Willebrand factor.

hemostasis: as a cofactor for platelet adhesion and as the carrier protein for factor VIII.[3,36] Circulating von Willebrand factor does not bind directly to platelets, but, when exposed to the subendothelial matrix, von Willebrand factor undergoes a structural change, allowing it to bind to platelet glycoprotein Ib. This interaction between von Willebrand factor and platelet glycoprotein Ib leads to platelet activation and adhesion to other platelets, as well as to the damaged endothelium. As a carrier protein, von Willebrand factor protects factor VIII from proteolytic degradation within the plasma. A defect in von Willebrand factor that diminishes factor VIII binding can produce a clinical presentation similar to mild hemophilia A.

CLINICAL FEATURES

Skin and mucosal bleeding is common in people with von Willebrand's disease, particularly in children and adolescents.[35] Examples of bleeding include recurrent epistaxis, gingival bleeding, unusual bruising, GI bleeding, and menorrhagia in young women. Hemarthrosis is not typical unless severe disease is present. In mild cases of von Willebrand's disease, the patient may be unaware of the disease until after a surgical procedure or injury when unexpected bleeding occurs.

DIAGNOSIS

Tests used to diagnose von Willebrand's disease include bleeding time, activated partial thromboplastin time, factor VIII coagulant activity, von Willebrand factor antigen level, and von Willebrand factor activity.[37,38] The common abnormalities seen in von Willebrand's disease include prolonged bleeding time, low or normal von Willebrand factor antigen, and low von Willebrand factor activity. The prothrombin time should be normal, and about half of patients have a mildly prolonged activated partial thromboplastin time. Diagnostic testing can be complicated, and misdiagnosis can occur from errors in specimen handling, storage, processing, and laboratory testing proficiency. Also, variability in von Willebrand factor levels can sometimes make von Willebrand's disease difficult to differentiate from mild hemophilia A.

TREATMENT

Desmopressin: Nontransfusional Therapy **Desmopressin** has become the primary therapy for many patients with type 1 von Willebrand's disease.[20,21,39,40] For other types of von Willebrand's disease, desmopressin may still work in conjunction with plasma products that contain von Willebrand factor, but hematologists tend to recommend either one or the other. Desmopressin induces the release of von Willebrand factor from storage sites within the endothelium. In responsive individuals, it causes a transient two- to four-fold increase in von Willebrand factor. Desmopressin also has an effect on the endothelium that promotes hemostasis. IV and concentrated nasal spray preparations of desmopressin are available (**Table 235-5**).[21] Desmopressin may be repeated in 24 hours, but the response to subsequent doses diminishes as vWF stores become depleted. Fluid restriction for 24 hours after desmopressin administration is important to prevent hyponatremia.[39] Medications with known antiplatelet effects should be avoided, including aspirin, nonsteroidal anti-inflammatory drugs, antiplatelet agents, heparin, and some antibiotics.

Transfusional Therapies Plasma derivatives that contain von Willebrand factor are used for those type I patients who do not (or no longer) respond to desmopressin or have type II or III von Willebrand's disease.[14,40,41] Because of the risk of viral contamination, factor VIII concentrates that contain multimeric von Willebrand factor and have undergone viral inactivation processes are preferred at a dose of 30 to 50 IU/kg (**Table 235-3**). Cryoprecipitate also contains von Willebrand factor, but because it does not undergo viral inactivation, cryoprecipitate should only be used in life-threatening emergencies when appropriate factor VIII concentrates are not available.[14] Platelet transfusions may benefit patients with certain types of von Willebrand's disease (type III) who do not respond to von Willebrand factor–containing plasma products.[42]

Additional Therapy Patients with von Willebrand's disease with significant epistaxis should be treated with desmopressin or transfusion therapy as needed to control bleeding. If unsuccessful, intranasal topical therapy or cauterization may be necessary (see chapter 244, "Nose and Sinuses") in some cases. Menorrhagia is a common complaint in young women with von Willebrand's disease. Oral contraceptives can help raise von Willebrand factor levels and limit the degree of menstrual bleeding. For dental injury or planned procedures in the oral cavity, an antifibrinolytic agent can be used. **Aminocaproic acid** can be taken orally and **tranexamic acid** can be made into a mouthwash, to be used for 5 to 10 days after the injury or surgical procedure.

DISPOSITION AND FOLLOW-UP

In most patients with von Willebrand's disease, the acute bleeding episodes can be controlled with local measures and desmopressin; such patients can usually be discharged. The unusual von Willebrand's disease patient with almost no von Willebrand factor activity is typically handled like a patient with hemophilia. Relative indications for hospital admission include treatment requiring multiple factor replacement doses or necessity for parenteral pain management. Patients with bleeding in the CNS, neck, pharynx, retropharynx, or retroperitoneum or those with a potential compartment syndrome should be admitted.

REFERENCES

The complete reference list is available online at www.TintinalliEM.com.

Sickle Cell Disease and Hereditary Hemolytic Anemias

Jean Williams-Johnson
Eric Williams

INTRODUCTION

Hereditary anemias result from defects in hemoglobin production, abnormalities in red blood cell (RBC) metabolism, or changes within RBC membrane structure. Increased hemolysis occurs because the RBCs produced are either abnormal or sustain damage after release from the bone marrow, and are removed from the circulation, primarily by the spleen. Depending on the compensatory rate of production, the concentration of circulating erythrocytes may decrease, resulting in anemia.

Inherited hemoglobin disorders are comprised of two main groups: disorders with abnormal hemoglobin structure (e.g., sickle cell disease) and disorders of abnormal hemoglobin production (e.g., the thalassemias). These disorders are widely prevalent; an estimated 7% of the world's population are carriers of an abnormal hemoglobin gene.[1] These genetic abnormalities result in hemoglobin that tends to gel or crystallize, possesses abnormal oxygen-binding properties, or is readily oxidized to methemoglobin, rendering the RBC susceptible to hemolysis.

SICKLE CELL DISEASE

Sickle cell disease (SCD) is a worldwide public health problem.[2] An estimated 250 million people (approximately 4.5% of the world population) are carriers of the sickle cell gene,[3] with 60 million new carriers of sickle cell and 1.2 million new individuals with SCD diagnosed every year.[4] SCD affects predominantly people of African Equatorial descent, although it is also found in persons of Mediterranean, Indian, and Middle Eastern origin.[5,6] SCD affects approximately 70,000 people in the United States, and about 2 million Americans are sickle cell gene carriers.[7]

The overall life expectancy of patients in the United States with SCD is now >50 years,[8] an improvement attributed to early diagnosis (antenatal and neonatal screening), parental education about complications, close monitoring in clinics and follow-up, immunizations, prophylactic penicillin to prevent pneumococcal septicemia, and increased use of drugs such as hydroxyurea.[9]

PATHOPHYSIOLOGY

The normal adult RBC contains three forms of hemoglobin: HbA, HbA_2, and fetal hemoglobin (HbF) (**Table 236-1**). Normal hemoglobin consists of a tetramer of four polypeptide chains, which are pairs of dissimilar chains (two α-globin chains and two non–α-globin chains). HbA accounts for approximately 96% to 98% of adult hemoglobin and consists of two α- and two β-globin chains. HbA_2 accounts for approximately 2.0% to 3.5% of adult hemoglobin and is composed of two α- and two δ-globin chains. HbF is composed of two α- and two γ-globin chains. HbF production peaks in utero and starts declining just before birth, reaching a baseline of <1% at approximately 48 weeks of age. Because of the 120-day life span of the normal RBC, HbF is the predominant form in the circulation for approximately the first 4 months of life. The α-globin chains are coded by four genes, two each on chromosomes 16, whereas the β-, γ-, and δ-globin chains are coded by two genes, one each on chromosomes 11.

SCD is caused by the presence of an abnormal β-globin chain.[10] The specific mutation is an adenine-to-thymine substitution in the codon that results in the hydrophobic amino acid, valine, replacing the hydrophilic amino acid glutamic acid in the sixth amino acid position of the β-globin chain. As a result, under deoxygenated conditions, valine becomes buried in a hydrophobic pocket on an adjacent chain. The globin chains then join together, and HbS polymerizes, deforming the RBC and producing the characteristic sickled appearance (**Figure 236-1**).

The distorted sickle cell results in premature RBC destruction (life span of about 20 days) and also increases the viscosity of blood, leading to obstruction within the microvasculature (Figure 236-1). The overall effect is chronic, ongoing hemolysis and episodic periods of vascular occlusion, resulting in tissue ischemia affecting many organ systems. Although the sickle cell gene results from a single base substitution, there is tremendous variability in the phenotypic expression of this mutation.[6,11,12]

SCD is seen in patients who are homozygous for the sickle gene or who are double heterozygous with another hemoglobin variant (e.g., HbSC). **Sickle cell anemia** refers to homozygosity of the mutation, also termed *HbSS* or *SS disease.*

People with **sickle cell trait** (HbAS, heterozygous with one gene for the sickle mutation) have a normal life span and usually are asymptomatic, although complications occur, grouped as definite, probable, or possible.[13] Definite associations include renal medullary carcinoma, hematuria and renal papillary necrosis, hyposthenuria, splenic infarcts, and exercise-related deaths. Probable associations include venous thromboembolic events, pregnancy-related complications, and complicated

TABLE 236-1 Composition of Normal Human Hemoglobin and Hemoglobin Variants

Syndrome	Types of Hemoglobin (Hb) Present	Percentage within the Red Blood Cell	Hemoglobin Tetramer Composition (globin chains)
Normal adults	HbA	96–98	Two α-chains and two β-chains
	HbA_2	3.0–3.5	Two α-chains and two δ-chains
	HbF	0.5–0.8	Two α-chains and two γ-chains
Sickle cell trait (heterozygous)	HbA	60–65	Two α-chains and two β-chains
	HbAS	35–40	Two α-chains, one normal β-chain, and one sickle β-chain
	HbF	0.5–0.8	Two α-chains and two γ-chains
Sickle cell disease (homozygous)	HbS	80–90	Two α-chains and two sickle β-chains
	HbA_2	2–4	Two α-chains and two γ-chains
	HbF	2–20	Two α-chains and two γ-chains

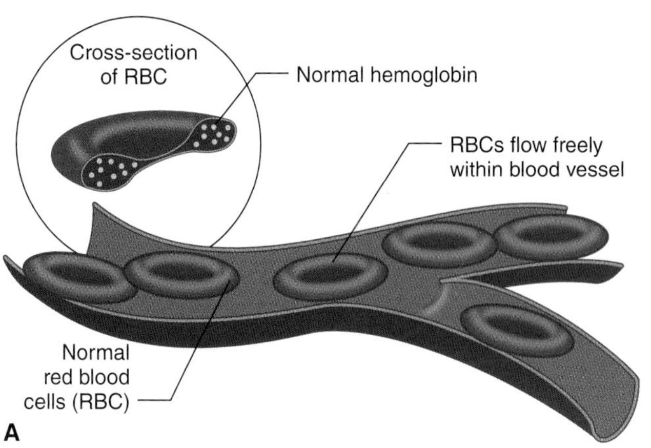

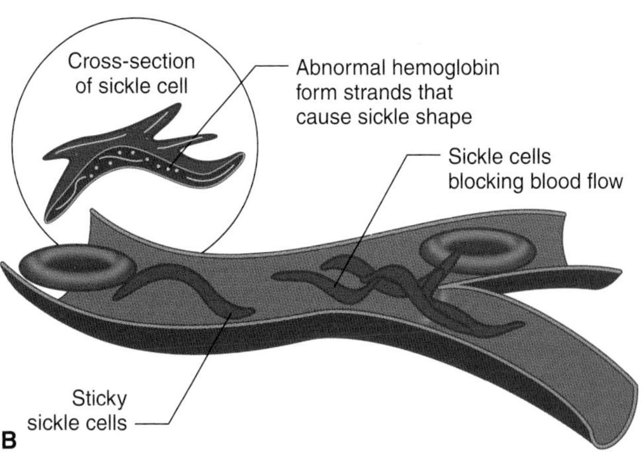

FIGURE 236-1. Intravascular blood flow of normal and sickle red blood cells (RBCs). **A.** Normal RBCs flowing freely in a blood vessel. **B.** Abnormal, sickled RBCs clumping and blocking blood flow in a blood vessel. (Other cells also may play a role in this clumping process.)

hyphema. Possible associations include retinopathy, acute chest syndrome, and asymptomatic bacteruria.[13] Many of the associations are seen only under conditions of severe tissue hypoxia, acidosis, dehydration, or hypothermia.

Polymerization of deoxygenated HbS, deforming the red cell into a sickled shape that causes microvascular sludging and obstruction (vaso-occlusion), is the major pathophysiologic process in SCD.[10] Vascular obstruction worsens hypoxia and causes acidosis in the microcirculation that contributes to further sickling. The sickling process is initially reversible when the HbS is reoxygenated, but with repeated episodes of sickling, the red cell membrane is permanently damaged, and the cell remains irreversibly sickled. Anywhere from 5% to 50% of the circulating erythrocytes in a patient with SCD can be irreversibly sickled cells. The sickling process is inhibited by the presence of HbF and other hemoglobin variants.[14] Structural and antigenic changes on the RBC membrane cause an abnormal tendency for the erythrocyte to catalyze plasma coagulation factors and adhere to vascular endothelium in SCD.

CLINICAL FEATURES

Because newborn screening occurs in the United States and in most developed countries, the majority of patients who present to the ED will already know that they have the sickle cell trait or disease. Although SCD can produce a wide spectrum of manifestations, vaso-occlusive crisis accounts for the majority of ED presentations as the sickled RBCs restrict the blood flow to various organs, thus causing ischemic pain and organ damage.[10,15,16] Patients may also present to the ED with life-threatening complications such as stroke, aplastic crisis, acute chest syndrome, and sepsis[17,18] (**Table 236-2**).

TABLE 236-2 Complications of Sickle Cell Anemia

Neurologic	Ischemic or hemorrhagic stroke Cerebral aneurysm Chronic pain syndrome Neuropathic pain syndrome
Eye	Retinopathy
Pulmonary	Acute chest syndrome Pulmonary hypertension
Cardiac	Cardiomegaly
Abdominal, GI	Mesenteric ischemia Hepatic infarction Cholelithiasis Intrahepatic cholestasis Splenic sequestration
Renal, GU	Hematuria Renal infarction Papillary necrosis Renal failure Priapism
Musculoskeletal	Acute vaso-occlusive pain crisis; bone, joint, and muscle pain Osteomyelitis Avascular necrosis of femoral head
Dermatologic	Leg ulcers
Infection	Osteomyelitis Pneumonia Urinary tract infection
Hematologic	Chronic hemolysis Acute hemolytic crisis Aplastic crisis Hypercoagulability: pulmonary embolism and venous thrombosis

Vaso-Occlusive Pain Crisis Acute vaso-occlusive pain crisis is a common problem in patients with SCD.[10,16] The initiating event may not be identifiable, but stressors such as infection, cold, dehydration, and altitude have been implicated. As a result of intravascular sickling and small-vessel occlusion, infarction of bone, viscera, and soft tissue occurs. This is manifested as diffuse bone, muscle, and joint pain and, in some cases, symptoms related to a specific affected organ. **Initial management of these patients includes aggressive pain management, appropriate hydration, and an assessment for a treatable cause of the current crisis as well as a search for additional complications (Table 236-3).**[1,18-20]

The CBC and reticulocyte count assess the degree of anemia and whether the marrow is still producing red cells. If the reticulocyte count is not available, the presence of polychromasia in the peripheral blood smear can be used to provide evidence of continued RBC production. It is common for SCD patients to have a low-grade temperature as well as a modestly elevated leukocyte count during a painful crisis, potentially confounding detection of an infection. A leukocyte count >20,000/mm^3 (> 20 × 10^9/L) with an increased number of bands is not typical for sickle crisis alone; this combination suggests a potential infection. Mild elevations in serum bilirubin and lactate dehydrogenase levels are common due to chronic hemolysis.

Supplemental oxygen has no proven benefit, unless the patient is systemically hypoxemic.[18,20] SCD patients during a painful crisis may be hypovolemic due to their disease (deficient renal concentrating ability) or crisis (anorexia, vomiting, or fever), so PO or IV rehydration may be necessary. No hydration regimen has proven capable of shortening the duration or severity of a painful sickle cell attack.[21] After rehydration, maintenance PO or IV (5% dextrose in 0.5 normal saline) should be provided.

Treatment of acute, moderate to severe pain usually requires opioids,[1,10,16,18-20] usually parenteral, but sustained-release oral morphine may be as effective as parenteral morphine.[22] Potent opioids, such as morphine or hydromorphone, are recommended, but meperidine, with the potential for neurotoxicity (seizures) from accumulation of the metabolite normeperidine, is not.[20] Some patients, because of prior opioid treatment, may be very tolerant, and large doses may be required to achieve adequate analgesia. Regular doses of analgesics for a few hours to several days typically are required. Patient-controlled analgesia has been used in selected patients. Nonsteroidal anti-inflammatory drugs can be used for their probable additive effect in pain management of sickle cell crisis.[18] Low-dose ketamine by continuous IV infusion is a potential adjuvant analgesic in acute pain crisis.[23]

Tinzaparin, a low-molecular-weight heparin that has antithrombotic, anti-inflammatory, and endovascular effects may be considered in protracted vaso-occlusive crises[1,24]; the recommended dose is 175 IU/kg SC daily for 2 to 7 days.

A recommended practice is to develop an individualized assessment and treatment protocol for specific patients who frequently present to the ED with painful crises.[20]

RBC transfusion to reduce the concentration of HbS-containing erythrocytes does not shorten the duration or reduce the risk of complications of routine acute vaso-occlusive painful crisis.[25] Furthermore, transfusion involves significant expense, the risk of bloodborne disease transmission, and the potential for iron overload and exposes the patient to the minor RBC antigens, with the potential to induce antibodies that prevent or complicate future transfusions (see chapter 238, "Transfusion Therapy").[26,27] Transfusion for sickle cell crisis or complications is reserved for specific indications such as aplastic crisis, pregnancy, stroke, respiratory failure, and general surgery.[10,28,29] Transfusion protocols in SCD are categorized as aggressive (decreasing HbS to <30%) and conservative (increasing hemoglobin to >10 grams/dL or 100 g/L); for most indications, there is no clinical difference between aggressive or conservative protocols.[29]

Hydroxyurea (hydroxycarbamide) successfully reduces the frequency and severity of painful crises in SCD.[8,30-33] Hydroxyurea blocks the synthesis of DNA and impairs cell division. It also increases the production of HbF to levels that are protective and preventive of RBC sickling. Hydroxyurea is indicated for young adults who have three or more

TABLE 236-3 Guidelines for the Assessment and Management of Acute Vaso-Occlusive Crisis

History	Duration and location of pain History of fever Presence of focal swelling or redness Precipitation factors for acute episode Medications taken for pain relief
Physical examination	Assess degree of pain Inspect sites of pain, looking for swelling, warmth, redness General: respiratory distress, pallor, hydration, jaundice, rash Vital signs: especially temperature, pulse oximetry Respiratory: lung sounds Heart: cardiomegaly and systolic murmur common with chronic anemia Abdomen: tenderness, organomegaly
Ancillary tests	Obtain if moderate to severe pain, focal pathology is present, or pain is atypical for acute episode CBC, leukocyte differential, reticulocyte count, urinalysis Chest radiograph, if signs of lower respiratory tract pathology Blood cultures and additional blood tests: as indicated by clinical condition
General management	Bed rest, provide warmth and a calm, relaxing atmosphere Distractions where appropriate: television, music, etc. Oral fluids: typically about 3 L/d IV fluids to correct dehydration or if reluctant to drink or vomiting is present Oxygen: not routinely required unless hypoxemia is present Encourage deep breathing, incentive spirometry
Pain management	Use analgesics appropriate to degree of pain Acetaminophen for mild pain Nonsteroidal anti-inflammatory drug for mild to moderate pain (avoid if renal insufficiency is present) Opioids for moderate to severe pain; typical initial doses include: Morphine, 0.3 milligram/kg PO or 0.1–0.15 milligram/kg IV Hydromorphone, 0.06–0.08 milligram/kg PO or 0.015–0.020 milligram/kg IV Reassess response in 15–30 min; may repeat with one fourth to one half of the initial dose
Consider adjuvant therapy	Medication to prevent constipation Antiemetic Anxiolytic Tinzaparin
Disposition and follow-up	Consider admission to the hospital if: Acute chest syndrome is suspected Sepsis, osteomyelitis, or other serious infection is suspected WBC count is >30,000/mm^3 Hemoglobin level is <5 grams/dL Platelet count is <100,000/mm^3 Pain is not under control after 2 to 3 rounds of analgesics in the ED
	Consider discharge if: Pain is under control and patient can take oral fluids and medications Appropriate oral analgesics are available Patient is able to comply with home care instructions Patient has resources for follow-up

hospitalizations for vaso-occlusive crisis in the preceding 12 months.[8,31] Daily prophylactic penicillin V reduces the incidence of infections and reduces mortality from sepsis in children but with little benefit in adults.[34]

Bone Pain Bone pain is common during a sickle cell crisis and is usually located in the back and the extremities.[35] The pain will be diffuse, without focal signs of inflammation; therefore redness, warmth, or swelling suggests infection such as cellulitis or osteomyelitis. Localized hip pain with difficulty ambulating suggests aseptic necrosis of the femoral head; approximately 30% of SCD patients develop femoral head damage by age 30 years old. Joint effusions are occasionally seen in painful sickle cell crisis, and arthrocentesis is often necessary to differentiate this complication from infection. Plain radiographs may show evidence of aseptic necrosis or osteomyelitis, whereas bone infarcts usually are not visible on radiographs. A radionuclide bone scan or MRI may be necessary to differentiate infection from infarction.

Acute Chest Syndrome **Acute chest syndrome** is defined as a new infiltrate on chest radiograph in association with one other new sign or symptom: fever >38.5°C (101.3°F), cough, wheezing, tachypnea, or chest pains.[36-38] In adults, acute chest syndrome occurs most commonly 1 to 3 days after hospitalization for an acute pain crisis. Acute chest syndrome is the leading cause of death in patients with SCD in the United States.[39] Although this phenomenon occurs most often as a single episode, some patients may experience multiple attacks, resulting in chronic lung disease.[40] Also, symptoms may vary with repeated episodes.

Acute chest syndrome has multiple potential etiologies; most commonly, the syndrome is precipitated by pulmonary infections, fat emboli, and rib infarction.[37,38,40] Acute chest syndrome may also result from iatrogenic causes, such as aggressive hydration for sickle cell painful crisis producing pulmonary edema and opioid use depressing inspiratory effort and promoting atelectasis.

Infectious pathogens were identified in patients admitted to the hospital with acute chest syndrome in a national study.[36] The two most common organisms identified were the atypical pneumonia pathogens *Chlamydia pneumoniae* and *Mycoplasma pneumoniae*.[36] Other organisms associated with acute chest syndrome include *Staphylococcus aureus*, *Haemophilus influenzae*, *Klebsiella pneumoniae*, adenoviruses, influenza viruses, parainfluenza viruses, respiratory syncytial viruses, cytomegalovirus, and parvovirus B19.[36] Traditionally, *Streptococcus pneumoniae* was considered the most frequent cause of pulmonary infection in SCD patients, but this pathogen is now rare in cases of acute chest syndrome, presumably due to the use of pneumococcal immunization and prophylactic penicillin therapy.

Abundant evidence for fat embolism as a possible cause for acute chest syndrome includes bony slivers and marrow fat found in the pulmonary vasculature at autopsy, fat droplets within endothelial cells identified in lung biopsy specimens collected via bronchoscopy in living patients, and elevated serum levels of free fatty acids and circulating secretory phospholipase A_2, a potent inflammatory mediator originating from the bone marrow.[41] It is postulated that reduced blood flow to the bone marrow during a vaso-occlusive crisis results in ischemia and necrosis, so that pieces of necrotic marrow embolize and become lodged in the pulmonary vasculature, playing a role in the pathophysiology of acute chest syndrome.

The combination of both ischemia and hypoxia in the pulmonary circulation promotes the production of free radicals, which further results in the upregulation of endothelial adhesion molecules such as vascular cell adhesion molecule-1. This activation causes binding of sickled RBC and leukocytes to the endothelium, which further increases the cycle of vaso-occlusion. The acute chest syndrome is the final result of several pathogenic processes exerting their effects individually and collectively in a vicious cycle, creating regional hypoxia, acidosis, and lung injury (**Figure 236-2**).

Respiratory symptoms are usually present, including cough, shortness of breath, chest pain, and fever, although the clinical presentation may vary.[37,38] Chest radiographs are important to identify the presence of a new patchy infiltrate; any lobe can be affected. The radiographic changes often lag behind the clinical features, so the radiograph may be initially normal, and the clinical severity of disease and the extent of hypoxia may not correlate with radiographs.

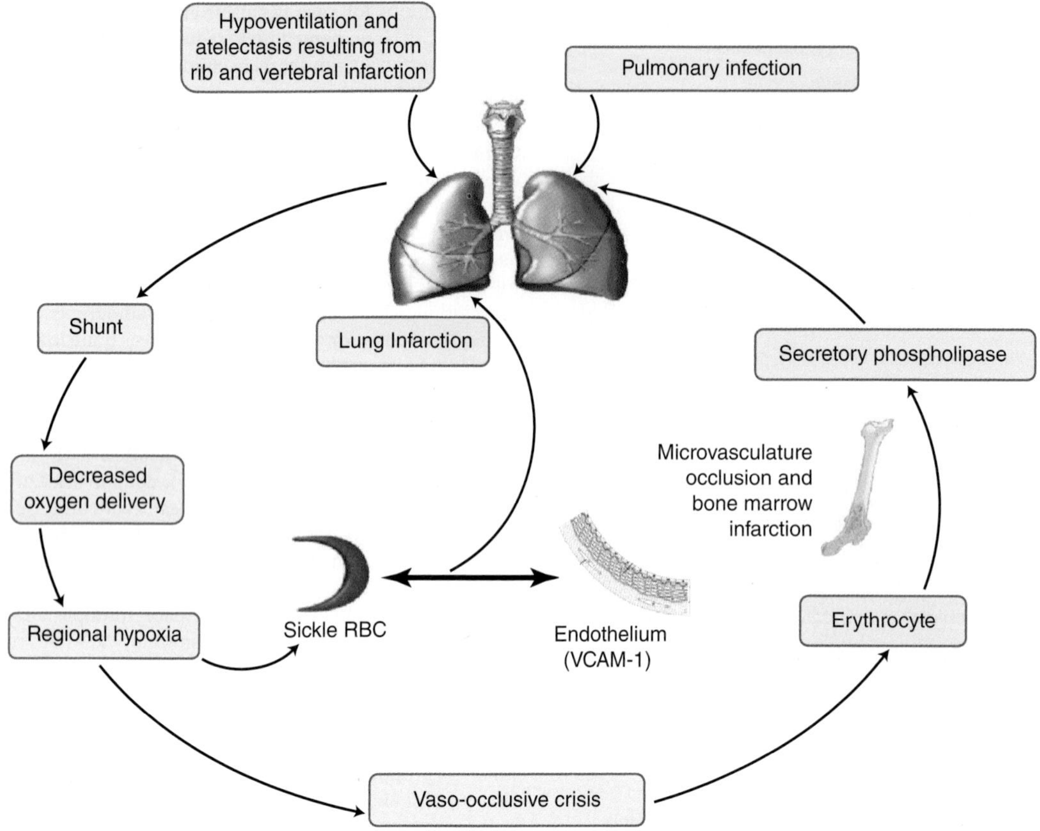

FIGURE 236-2. Pathogenesis of acute chest syndrome. NO = nitric oxide; RBC = red blood cell; VCAM-1 = vascular cell adhesion Molecule-1.

Acute chest syndrome is treated with supportive care (oxygen, analgesics, hydration), antibiotics, and exchange transfusion (**Table 236-4**).[37,38,40] Oxygen should be administered, especially if hypoxemia is demonstrated. Pain control initially requires high doses of parenteral opioids but requires careful monitoring to prevent both oversedation and hypoventilation. Dehydration results in increased plasma osmolarity and intracellular dehydration of RBCs, resulting in the further propagation of the sickling phenomenon. Supportive IV fluid therapy (up to 1.5 times maintenance) in the form of hypotonic solution facilitates free water passage into the relatively hypertonic red cells so that the resultant osmotic swelling decreases the mean corpuscular hemoglobin concentration and reduces the tendency for sickling.

Antibiotics are recommended irrespective of cultures, and many experts believe that patients with acute chest syndrome should receive a full course of empirical broad-spectrum antibiotics to treat pathogens commonly associated with community-acquired pneumonia,[37,38] but no specific regimen has proven superior.[42] Bronchospasm may accompany acute chest syndrome and can persist after recovery, indicating that bronchial hyperactivity can be a marker of lung injury in some patients. Inhaled β_2-adrenergenic agents can be used if wheezing occurs.[43]

Transfusion therapy is believed to be lifesaving in acute chest syndrome, but there are no firm evidence-based recommendations for its use,[44] and currently accepted indications for exchange transfusion in acute chest syndrome are based on empirical observations.[37,38,40] Exchange transfusion appears more advantageous, particularly in patients with relatively high hemoglobin (>9.0 grams/dL or 90 grams/L). Exchange transfusion decreases the concentration of sickled hemoglobin while maintaining an unchanged whole-blood viscosity and resulting in little iron gain. Exchange transfusion is usually reserved for severe crises signaled by deterioration of the patient's partial pressure of arterial oxygen (Pa_{O_2}) to <60 mm Hg (<8 kPa) with the goal to decrease the HbS level to <30%.

Hydroxyurea reduces the occurrence of acute chest syndrome primarily by stimulating an increase in HbF, with other therapeutic effects such as inhibiting sickle polymerization, increasing the deformability of RBC, and reducing the adhesion of sickle cells to vascular endothelium.[30-32,37,38]

Inhaled nitric oxide is beneficial in acute chest syndrome,[37,40] apparently due to its vasodilatory effects that improve the coordination between ventilation and perfusion in the damaged lung regions with minimal systemic absorption. In addition, nitric oxide reduces adhesion of RBCs and leukocytes to endothelial cells by decreasing the activity of vascular cell adhesion molecule-1.

Abdominal Crisis Generalized and constant abdominal pain is a common complaint during an acute sickle cell crisis, and it may be difficult to distinguish from focal abdominal problem, such as cholecystitis or appendicitis. **With a vaso-occlusive crisis, there should be accompanying musculoskeletal pain, the patient can frequently identify that the pain is similar to prior episodes, and there should not be physical evidence of peritonitis.** Repeated abdominal examinations should be done to assess for progression of tenderness and development of peritoneal signs.

Hepatic infarction may produce jaundice and abdominal pain, which can be difficult to distinguish from hepatitis or cholecystitis. Biliary disease is common because pigment-related cholelithiasis is seen in 30% to 70% of SCD patients. Severe right upper quadrant pain and marked elevations of bilirubin may be due to intrahepatic cholestasis, which rarely may progress to hepatic failure.

GU System Vaso-occlusive events involving the kidneys are often asymptomatic and likely account for the frequent finding of microscopic hematuria seen in SCD patients.[45] Infarction in the renal medulla may cause flank pain, renal colic–type pain, and costovertebral angle tenderness, mimicking pyelonephritis.[46] Papillary necrosis may result in either gross or microscopic hematuria, but RBC casts are uncommon. Renal imaging studies generally are necessary for correct diagnosis. Both renal medulla infarction and papillary necrosis are treated with IV fluids to maintain urine flow and close monitoring of hemoglobin levels to ensure that anemia does not worsen. Urinary tract infections are common in SCD patients, and routine urinalysis is recommended when these patients present to the ED.

TABLE 236-4 Assessment and Treatment of Acute Chest Syndrome

History	Major presenting symptoms: dyspnea, fever, cough
	Accompanying chest, rib, bone, or joint pain
	Assess degree or severity of pain
	Recent or previous sepsis, infection, pneumonia, or hospitalization
	Prior history of acute chest syndrome, especially if required intubation and ventilatory support
	Potentially infectious contacts
	Current medications
	Immunization history: especially pneumococcal and *Haemophilus influenzae* type b
	Baseline hemoglobin level and arterial oxygenation saturation
Physical examination	General: respiratory distress, pallor, hydration, jaundice, rash
	Vital signs: especially temperature, pulse oximetry
	Respiratory: chest wall, lung sounds
	Heart: cardiomegaly and systolic murmur common with chronic anemia
	Abdomen: tenderness, organomegaly
Ancillary tests	CBC, leukocyte differential, reticulocyte count, serum electrolytes, renal function, urinalysis
	Cross-match sample: if RBC transfusion is contemplated
	Arterial blood gas: if moderate to severe respiratory distress and/or hypoxemia on pulse oximetry
	Chest radiography
	Blood cultures
	Additional blood tests: as indicated by clinical condition
Treatment	Oxygen: adjust according to pulse oximetry
	Oral hydration: preferable
	IV hydration: use hypotonic fluids, use a rate and dose at approximately 1.5 times maintenance (aggressive IV fluids can worsen acute chest syndrome)
	Analgesics: if needed, generally potent parenteral opioids are used, monitor for signs of respiratory suppression
	Antibiotics: empiric antibiotics recommended to cover community-acquired pneumonia pathogens
	Transfusion: use if severe acute anemia is present
Exchange transfusion	Consider when
	Severe acute chest syndrome on admission and past history of requiring ventilatory support: useful to prevent intubation
	Deterioration despite above management: useful to prevent intensive care unit admission
	Patient already intubated and on ventilatory support: useful to shorten duration of ventilatory need
	Suspected or confirmed fat or bone marrow embolism

Priapism occurs in up to 30% of males with SCD. Patients with stuttering priapism (recurrent episodes that last <3 hours often with a pattern of increasing frequency and severity) are treated with oral adrenergic agents or hormonal analogues.[47] Patients with a major episode (sustained erection lasting >4 hours) are treated with fluid hydration, pain control, corporal aspiration, and intracorporal installation of a dilute α-adrenergic agonist solution (see chapter 93, "Male Genital Problems"). Transfusions, either simple or exchange, have no proven benefit for sickle cell–associated priapism.[47]

ADDITIONAL SYSTEMIC MANIFESTATIONS OF SICKLE CELL DISEASE

Splenic Infarction The spleen is particularly susceptible to the vaso-occlusive effects of sickled cells, and over time, microinfarctions result in a spleen that is essentially nonfunctional by age 5.[48] This renders these patients at risk for serious infections and sepsis from encapsulated organisms. Therefore, immunizations, prophylactic penicillin therapy, and parental education are critical to minimize the risk of infection and prompt early evaluation of fever in these patients. As SCD patients grow into teenage years, their risk of overwhelming sepsis decreases, but they remain predisposed to infection.

Splenic Sequestration Splenic sequestration is an important cause of significant morbidity and occasional mortality in SCD, with its occurrence being more common in children than in adults.[49] This syndrome manifests by the sudden enlargement of the spleen with an acute fall in the hemoglobin level due to sequestration of the blood volume within the spleen. Left upper quadrant pain may or may not be present. Symptoms include tachycardia, hypotension, pallor, and lethargy, and the spleen is usually enlarged and firm. Platelets also may be sequestered, resulting in moderate thrombocytopenia. The reticulocyte count should remain elevated.

Therapy includes volume resuscitation, which may mobilize some of the RBCs trapped within the spleen. Simple RBC transfusion or exchange transfusion may be necessary. An investigation for a precipitating infection should be done. Rarely, splenectomy is necessary. Unfortunately, recurrence of this syndrome is common.

Hemolytic Anemia Patients with SCD have a chronic hemolytic state due to the shape of the red cells. The baseline hemoglobin level is often between 6 and 9 grams/dL (60 to 90 grams/L), and the reticulocyte count is between 5% and 15%. With infections, the hemolytic process may worsen, and hemoglobin may drop from the previous baseline. Typically, erythrocyte production will increase in response to the increased RBC destruction, but it may not be enough to compensate for the increased hemolysis. Acutely, the patient may notice symptoms of worsening fatigue, shortness of breath, dyspnea on exertion, and scleral icterus. These symptoms may be worsened if other comorbid diseases are present. It is uncommon for the hemolysis to be so severe as to require transfusion.

Aplastic Crisis Aplastic crisis results when the production of RBCs declines significantly, producing a rapid decrease in the hemoglobin level with reticulocytopenia.[15] The most common cause of aplastic crisis appears to be infection, specifically from human parvovirus B19. Folate deficiency and bone marrow necrosis also may play a role. Aplastic crisis is more common in children than in adults. Patients generally will present with increasing fatigue and pallor and no evidence of increased hemolysis. The hemoglobin level will be unusually low, and few or no reticulocytes will be present; reticulocyte count is typically <0.5%. The leukocyte and platelet levels are usually normal. This syndrome is usually self-limiting, and the marrow will begin producing RBCs spontaneously within 1 week. Transfusion may be required in the interim.

Neurologic Disorders Ischemic and hemorrhagic stroke, as well as subarachnoid hemorrhage, are more common in patients with SCD.[50] The risk of stroke in children with SCD is >200 times greater than those without SCD,[51] and approximately 10% of patients with SCD experience a stroke before age 20 years old. The cause of stroke in most patients is cerebral infarction due to occlusion or narrowing of large cerebral vessels.[52] Silent cerebral infarcts visible on MRI have been observed in over a third of SCD patients by age 14, associated with decreased intellectual ability, poor academic achievement, and risk of progression to overt stroke.[53] Hemorrhagic strokes and subarachnoid hemorrhage most commonly occur in the third decade of life.[51] Cerebral aneurysms are also more common in SCD patients, perhaps due to local vessel occlusion or ischemia.

Acute stroke in a SCD patient is treated with emergent simple or partial exchange transfusion. Unfortunately, children who suffer a stroke are at 70% to 90% risk for recurrence, so chronic transfusion therapy is indicated to prevent recurrent stoke after the initial event.[53]

Chronic pain syndromes in SCD patients are associated with avascular necrosis and leg ulcers.[54] Neuropathic pain has been reported in SCD patients; the most commonly reported location is the mental nerve, with numbness of the chin and mandibular bone pain.[54]

Infections Patients with SCD are functionally asplenic after early childhood, rendering them susceptible to infections from encapsulated organisms, such as *H. influenzae* and *S. pneumoniae*.[48,55] Other common infections associated with SCD include pneumonia caused by these organisms as well as *M. pneumoniae*, meningitis, and osteomyelitis due to *Salmonella typhimurium*, *S. aureus*, and *Escherichia coli*. Although low-grade fever is not uncommon during an acute crisis, unexplained fevers of >38°C (100.4°F) require evaluation for bacterial infection and consideration for early treatment with broad-spectrum antibiotics. In addition to *H. influenzae* immunization, patients with SCD should be encouraged to receive yearly influenza vaccinations and remain up to date with pneumococcal immunization, and children should be maintained on prophylactic daily oral penicillin.[34]

Cardiac Complications Cardiomegaly is common and correlates with the degree of chronic anemia. Additionally, cardiac dysfunction may occur from microinfarcts and hemosiderin deposition from hemolysis and blood transfusion.[56] Cardiac contractility is enhanced to maintain adequate systemic oxygen delivery, producing a widely radiating systolic ejection murmur. SCD patients have laboratory evidence of coagulation overactivation, and there appears to be increased risk for pulmonary embolism and venous thrombosis.[57,58] Baseline D-dimer levels are increased in the steady-state in SCD patients, and levels are much higher during pain crisis.[59]

Dermatologic Chronic, poorly healing leg ulcers around the malleoli are common in older sickle cell patients.[60] Minor injury, impaired microcirculation due to repeated sickling episodes and microinfarcts, and infections all contribute to the development and persistence of these ulcers. No systemic or topical therapy has proven superior to achieve complete healing.[61]

VARIANTS OF SICKLE CELL DISEASE

SICKLE CELL–HEMOGLOBIN C DISEASE

HbC results from a single point mutation in the β-globin chain gene; lysine is substituted for glutamic acid at the sixth position. The prevalence of the HbC gene is approximately 1 per 5000 in African Americans but is as high as 16% in parts of West Africa.[62] Deoxygenated HbC has the tendency to precipitate inside the RBC, forming crystals that decrease cell deformability and increase blood viscosity. Patients with HbC trait (heterozygous for the HbC gene, or *HbAC*) are asymptomatic, and those with HbC disease (homozygous for the HbC gene, or *HbCC*) typically have a mild hemolytic anemia, abundant target cells,[63] and sporadic episodes of musculoskeletal pain, splenomegaly, dental infarctions, and angioid retinopathy.[64]

The heterozygous sickle cell variant, sickle cell–hemoglobin C (*HbSC*), results when the gene for HbS is inherited from one parent and the gene for HbC is inherited from the other parent. These individuals have almost equal amounts of HbS and HbC but no HbA. Because HbC does not polymerize as readily as HbS, HbSC disease generally has less severe clinical consequences than sickle cell anemia (HbSS).[65] These patients have a milder chronic hemolytic anemia and, as a consequence, milder reticulocytosis. The peripheral smear shows abundant target cells and a few sickle cells.

The complications of HbSC disease are similar to sickle cell anemia, although usually less severe. As opposed to sickle cell anemia, adult patients with HbSC disease often have splenomegaly. HbSC disease patients are susceptible to a proliferative retinitis that is visible on funduscopy as angioid streaks (jagged, reddish brown, subretinal lines that taper outward from the optic nerve), representing breaks in the brittle Bruch membrane.[64] Cracks in the membrane lead to impairment of the choriocapillaries that may produce loss of photoreceptor cells and lead to impaired vision.

SICKLE CELL–HEMOGLOBIN O-ARAB DISEASE

Hemoglobin O-Arab is a hemoglobin variant resulting from substitution of lysine for glutamic acid at position 121 of the β-globin chain. Hemoglobin O-Arab is widespread in the Middle East, is present in the Balkans, and occasionally occurs in African Americans.[6] Patients heterozygous for hemoglobin O-Arab (*HbAO-Arab*) have no clinical problems. Patients homozygous for hemoglobin O-Arab (*HbOO-Arab*) or heterozygous for sickle cell–hemoglobin O-Arab (*HbSO-Arab*) are clinically similar to patients with sickle cell anemia, having severe hemolytic anemia and recurrent vaso-occlusive crises, and children have the potential to develop sickle cell dactylitis and splenic sequestration crises.

THALASSEMIA

The thalassemias are a diverse group of hereditary disorders caused by defective synthesis of globin chains, resulting in an inability to produce normal adult hemoglobin.[66-68] The hallmark of these disorders is a microcytic, hypochromic, hemolytic anemia. These disorders are most common in those of Mediterranean, Middle Eastern, African, and Southeast Asian descent. Globalization as a result of migration has led to changing demographics, and persons who have thalassemia syndromes and heterozygote carriers now reside in all parts of the world. Similar to other hemoglobin disorders, namely SCD and glucose-6-phosphokinase deficiency, the high prevalence of thalassemia phenotypes is thought to be protective against malaria.[69]

The thalassemia syndromes are categorized depending on the globin chain affected or the abnormal hemoglobin produced. Thus, β-globin gene mutations give rise to **β-thalassemia** and α-globin mutations cause **α-thalassemia**.[68]

The β-thalassemias have diminished production of the β-globin chain, which allows unmatched α-globin chains to accumulate as α-tetramers in the immature RBC. These tetramers are very insoluble, and their precipitation damages the developing erythroid precursor cells, resulting in early death. The cells that are produced have decreased hemoglobin, which accounts for the hypochromia and target cell formation seen in thalassemias. Over 200 different mutations with variable impact on β-globin production have been identified associated with β-thalassemia.

Patients with α-thalassemia develop an excess of β-globin chains that accumulate as β-tetramers called *hemoglobin H*. Hemoglobin H is more soluble and stable so that in severe α-thalassemia, ineffective erythropoiesis is less of a problem, and increased destruction of the cells due to the structural abnormality is more prominent.

Both forms of thalassemia are characterized by varying degrees of anemia depending on the amount of ineffective erythropoiesis and premature destruction of the circulating RBCs. The hypoxia associated with severe anemia triggers compensatory mechanisms in an attempt to increase RBC production. This causes enlargement of the reticuloendothelial organs and expansion of the bone marrow cavity, leading to osteopenia.

β-Thalassemia has three clinical syndromes representing mutations in one or both β-globin genes: β-thalassemia major (Cooley's anemia), β-thalassemia intermedia, and β-thalassemia minor.[66,67,70-72] Because there are four α-globin genes, two each inherited from the individual parents, the genetics and clinical consequences of the α-thalassemias are determined by five genotypic possibilities.[73] A normal individual has four functioning α-globin genes, the silent α-thalassemia carrier has three normal functioning α-globin genes and one dysfunctional gene, the patient with α-thalassemia trait has two normal functioning α-globin genes and two dysfunctional genes, and the patient with hemoglobin H disease has one normal functioning α-globin gene and three dysfunctional genes. Individuals with a defect in all four α-globin genes, called *Hb Bart's*, have a disorder that is incompatible with life, producing stillborn or severely distressed infants. Outside of this most severe form, individuals with either α- or β-thalassemia can be minimally to severely affected due to the specific genotype and whether the mutation produces complete or partial reduction in globin chain production.[66,67]

α-THALASSEMIA CARRIER AND TRAIT

Patients who are α-thalassemia carriers and with α-thalassemia trait have no clinical symptoms or physical findings, and patients with α-thalassemia trait are detected by the finding of microcytic RBCs and a borderline to slightly low hemoglobin level.[67]

HEMOGLOBIN H DISEASE

Hemoglobin H disease is a disorder with one functional α-globin chain gene.[73] Hemoglobin H disease usually presents in the neonatal period

TABLE 236-5 Drugs That Produce Oxidative Stress on Red Blood Cells at Therapeutic Doses

	Definite Association	Possible Association
Sulfonamides	Sulfacetamide Sulfamethoxazole Sulfanilamide	Sulfasalazine Sulfadimidine Glibenclamide
Antimalarials	Primaquine Pamaquine	Chloroquine
Urinary agents	Nitrofurantoin Nalidixic acid Phenazopyridine	
Miscellaneous antibiotics	Dapsone	Ciprofloxacin Chloramphenicol
Mothballs	Naphthalene	
Miscellaneous drugs	Methylthionium chloride (methylene blue)	Vitamin K analogues Ascorbic acid

with a severe hypochromic anemia. Later in life, the clinical picture includes a hypochromic, microcytic anemia with jaundice and hepatosplenomegaly. These patients may not require regular transfusions, but under conditions of increased oxidative stress, which may cause precipitation of the unstable hemoglobin H resulting in hemolysis, a transfusion may be necessary. Most affected individuals will know their diagnosis, and the emergency physician needs only to provide supportive care and blood transfusion when necessary. Medications that may precipitate hemolysis should be avoided in this population (**Table 236-5**).

β-THALASSEMIA MINOR (β-THALASSEMIA TRAIT)

Patients with β-thalassemia minor are heterozygous for the β-globin mutation and have only mild microcytic anemia.[66,67] Splenomegaly may be present but is not common. On blood smear, these patients may have microcytosis and hypochromia as well as basophilic stippling. An elevated HbA_2 level, typically 4% to 6%, confirms the diagnosis. These patients generally will not have clinical manifestations and may only come to attention during an evaluation for a mild anemia.

β-THALASSEMIA INTERMEDIA

β-Thalassemia is the result of genetic combination of β-gene mutations producing microcytic moderate anemia (blood hemoglobin usually >7 g/dL), splenomegaly, and intense bone marrow hyperplasia. HbF levels are elevated.[70,71] Clinical symptoms tend to be milder and delayed compared to thalassemia major. Transfusion requirements are variable and complications from iron overload are less extreme.

β-THALASSEMIA MAJOR (COOLEY'S ANEMIA)

In β-thalassemia major, both β-globin genes are defective, and production of β-globin chains is severely impaired. Newborn infants with β-thalassemia major are usually well because HbF is predominant during the first few months of life. Symptoms emerge during the second 6 months of life when β-globin production would be expected. The RBCs of these children show a low mean corpuscular volume with microcytic and hypochromic cells. Variation in size and shape of the RBCs will be notable (increased RBC distribution width), as will be the presence of nucleated cells. HbF levels remain elevated, often >90% in untransfused individuals. This diagnosis should be considered in any child with a severe microcytic anemia and the appropriate ethnic background.

Affected children develop hepatosplenomegaly, jaundice, and expansion of the erythroid marrow causing bone changes and osteoporosis, and possess increased susceptibility to infection.[72] The anemia is severe and requires regular, lifelong blood transfusions, with resultant challenges of alloimmunization.[27] Transfusions and enhanced iron absorption eventually cause iron overload that is the etiology of most of the morbidity and mortality associated with the thalassemia. Untreated iron overload results in hemochromatosis with cardiac, hepatic, and endocrine dysfunction.[66,67,72,74] Treatment is chelation, with parenteral (desferrioxamine)[75] or oral (deferiprone and deferasirox)[76,77] agents.

For those with a known diagnosis who present to the ED with significant symptoms related to anemia or hemolysis, consider transfusion along with a search for precipitating events.

SICKLE CELL–β-THALASSEMIA DISEASE

Sickle cell–β-thalassemia disease, a heterozygous sickle cell variant, occurs when the gene for sickle hemoglobin is inherited from one parent and a gene for β-thalassemia is inherited from the other parent. The frequency of sickle cell–β-thalassemia disease is about 1 per 1600 African American births. The severity of the disease depends on the functionality of inherited β-thalassemia gene. Between 80% and 90% of affected individuals have a β-thalassemia gene that results in the production of some normal β-chains; thus, some normal HbA is made. Such patients have a mild hemolytic anemia with near-normal hemoglobin levels, few crises, and minimal organ damage. Those 10% to 20% of patients who inherit a β-thalassemia gene that inhibits all β-globin production have severe hemolytic anemia and vaso-occlusive symptoms comparable with patients with SCD.

GLUCOSE-6-PHOSPHATE DEHYDROGENASE DEFICIENCY

Glucose-6-phosphate dehydrogenase (G6PD) deficiency is the most common enzymopathy of RBCs in humans; worldwide it affects >400 million people.[78] Although the deficiency affects all ethnicities, it has been found mainly among persons of African, Asian, or Mediterranean ancestry, a distribution suggestive of an ability to protect against malaria.[79] The disease has many forms, with >400 variants.[78]

G6PD deficiency is an X-linked inherited disorder that primarily affects males. Females must have two defective genes to be severely affected, but because expression of this gene is variable, women with one abnormal gene may still show some symptoms. Most adults are usually asymptomatic, but some may have intermittent hemolytic anemia, and a few have chronic hemolysis.

G6PD is an enzyme that catalyzes the oxidation of glucose 6-phophogluconate while concomitantly being responsible for the production of nicotinamide adenine dinucleotide phosphate, a required cofactor for maintaining glutathione in its reduced state. Glutathione in the reduced state acts as a scavenger for harmful oxidative cell metabolites and, with the help of the enzyme glutathione peroxidase, converts harmful peroxide to water. G6PD-deficient RBCs are therefore susceptible to oxidative stress; oxidization of the sulfhydryl groups causes hemoglobin to precipitate within the cell. The precipitated hemoglobin is recognized by the presence of **Heinz bodies** on the peripheral blood smear (**Figure 236-3**). The affected RBCs are removed from the circulation by the spleen. Oxidant damage also occurs at the RBC membrane, producing both extravascular and intravascular hemolysis.

CLINICAL FEATURES

The clinical expression of G6PD variants encompasses a spectrum of hemolytic syndromes. The likelihood of developing hemolysis and disease severity are determined by the degree of the enzyme deficiency (**Table 236-6**).

A serious complication of G6PD deficiency is neonatal jaundice occurring during the first week of life. The elevated bilirubin induces neurotoxicity that can result in permanent neurologic sequelae (kernicterus). Phototherapy can be used to lower the serum bilirubin concentration.

Class III variants are the most prevalent G6PD mutations, with acute hemolytic events that are usually self-limited and well tolerated, so the variant condition may remain undetectable.[78]

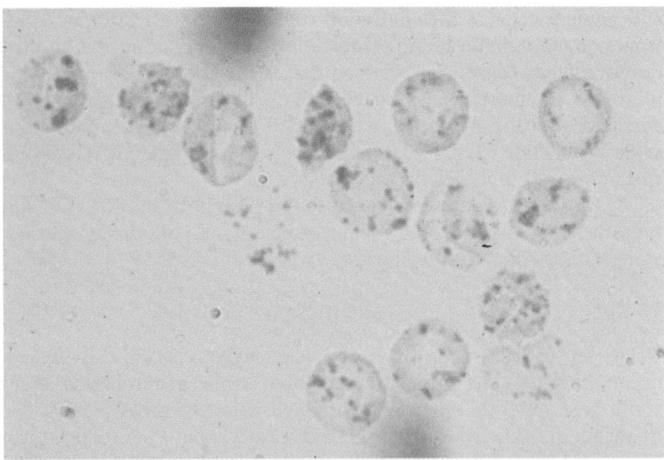

FIGURE 236-3. Heinz bodies. Blood mixed with hypotonic solution of crystal violet. Precipitates of denatured hemoglobin within the cells. [Reproduced with permission from Lichtman M, Beutler E, Kaushansky K, et al: *Williams Hematology*, 7th ed. Copyright © 2006, McGraw-Hill Inc., New York.]

Aside from favism and drug-induced hemolytic anemia, infection is the most common cause of hemolysis in G6PD-deficient individuals. There is also an increased incidence of pigmented gallstones and splenomegaly in patients with G6PD deficiency.

DIAGNOSIS

G6PD deficiency should be established by the demonstration of decreased enzyme activity through quantitative assay rather than the amount of enzyme protein present. In societies with a high prevalence of G6PD deficiency, neonatal screening programs for this disorder are appropriate.

Helpful ancillary tests to evaluate patients with acute symptoms include a CBC and reticulocyte count (to evaluate level of anemia and bone marrow function), serum bilirubin levels, serum aminotransferases (to exclude other causes of jaundice), and lactate dehydrogenase (elevated in hemolysis and a marker of hemolytic severity).

TREATMENT

Treatment of the patient with G6PD deficiency is determined by the patient's overall clinical condition. If the illness is severe, then blood transfusion with packed RBCs may be warranted.

In patients with known G6PD deficiency, infections should be treated aggressively and oxidant drugs avoided. **There is solid evidence to implicate seven currently used medications as causing acute hemolysis in patients with G6PD deficiency: dapsone, phenazopyridine, nitrofurantoin, primaquine, rasburicase, methylthioninium chloride (methylene blue), and tolonium chloride (toluidine blue).**[80] There is no evidence that other oxidant drugs (Table 236-5) in therapeutic doses are associated with increased hemolysis in G6PD-deficient patients.[80] Human immunodeficiency virus–positive patients should be screened for G6PD deficiency before dapsone is used for prophylaxis of *Pneumocystis jiroveci* pneumonia.

TABLE 236-6 World Health Organization Classification of Glucose-6-Phosphate Dehydrogenase (G6PD) Variants

Class I variants: severe enzyme deficiency (<1% of normal activity) and have chronic hemolytic anemia.
Class II variants, such as G6PD Mediterranean: severe enzyme deficiency (1%–10% normal activity), associated with acute intermittent hemolytic episodes.
Class III variants, such as G6PD A−: moderate enzyme deficiency (10%–60% of normal activity) with intermittent hemolysis usually associated with stressors such as infection or drugs.
Class IV variants: no enzyme deficiency (60%–150% normal activity), no hemolysis or other clinical significance.
Class V variants: increased enzyme activity (>150% normal activity), no clinical significance.

HEREDITARY SPHEROCYTOSIS

Hereditary spherocytosis is the result of an erythrocyte membrane defect and is the most prevalent hereditary hemolytic anemia among people of northern European descent.[81] The disease typically is inherited in an autosomal dominant pattern, although a less common autosomal recessive variant exists, and up to 20% of hereditary spherocytosis patients are the result of an apparent spontaneous mutation. The abnormal shape of the RBC results from molecular abnormalities in the cytoskeleton of the cell membrane, most commonly from mutations in the genes for the proteins spectrin and ankyrin.[82,83] These abnormalities result in RBCs with a microspherocytic shape that is not pliable enough to pass through the spleen. This results in an increased rate of destruction and a compensatory increase in RBC production.

CLINICAL FEATURES

The clinical spectrum of hereditary spherocytosis is divided into those with (1) mild disease, occurring in about 20% with an autosomal dominant inheritance; (2) moderate disease, occurring in about 75% with primarily autosomal dominant inheritance; and (3) severe, occurring in approximately 5% with an autosomal recessive inheritance.[84,85] The main complications include aplastic or megaloblastic crises, hemolytic crisis, cholecystitis or cholelithiasis, and neonatal hemolysis with jaundice.[84,85]

Neonatal jaundice during the first week of life occurs in 30% to 50% of those with hereditary spherocytosis. After the neonatal period, the symptoms and signs depend on the severity of ongoing hemolysis. Patients with mild disease usually have a normal hemoglobin level and little or no splenomegaly but are susceptible to hemolytic or aplastic episodes triggered by infection. Patients with moderate disease have mild to moderate anemia, modest splenomegaly, periodic episodes of hemolysis with jaundice, and an increased incidence of pigmented gallstones. The rare patient with severe hereditary spherocytosis has significant hemolytic anemia requiring episodic blood transfusions, chronic jaundice, and an enlarged spleen.

DIAGNOSIS

The peripheral blood smear shows spherocytes with a normal to low mean corpuscular volume and increased mean corpuscular hemoglobin concentration (>36%). The diagnosis of hereditary spherocytosis is usually established by a combination of clinical history and examination, family history, and RBC indices and morphology.[86] In unclear or atypical cases, initial screening tests (cryohemolysis test and eosin-5-maleimide–binding test) are performed, followed by confirmatory tests (gel electrophoresis analysis of RBC membranes).[87]

TREATMENT

In severe cases, splenectomy generally will reverse the anemia,[83,88] except in the unusual cases of autosomal recessive variants. After splenectomy, spherocytes are still present. Patients with severe anemia may need blood transfusions.[84]

Acknowledgment: We would like to acknowledge Dr. Susanna Bortolusso Ali (TMRI-University of the West Indies Jamaica) for her contribution to this chapter.

REFERENCES

The complete reference list is available online at www.TintinalliEM.com.

Acquired Hemolytic Anemia

Laurie Ann Dixon
Robin R. Hemphill

INTRODUCTION

Acquired hemolytic anemias are a group of disorders characterized by hemolysis of red blood cells (RBCs) not due to congenital or inherited disorders of hemoglobin synthesis or of the RBC membrane. Hemolysis of RBCs can take place within the intravascular space or in the extravascular spaces of the spleen and liver and can produce a spectrum of disease from mild, asymptomatic illness to severe hemodynamic compromise leading to critical ED encounters.

Presenting symptoms and signs of hemolytic anemia include those common to anemia in general: weakness, fatigue, dizziness, shortness of breath, dyspnea on exertion, tachycardia, palpitations, chest pain, new or accentuated cardiac murmur, and pallor. RBC destruction generates free hemoglobin that is then broken down into bilirubin. When bilirubin production exceeds the liver's ability to conjugate it for biliary and fecal excretion, jaundice and darkened urine may develop. Splenic enlargement may promote the storage and extravascular breakdown of RBCs.

The laboratory findings characteristic of acquired hemolytic anemia demonstrate hemolysis of RBCs, hemoglobin breakdown, and compensatory RBC production (**Table 237-1**). The peripheral blood smear displays abnormal RBC morphology consistent with hemolysis: schistocytes generated by intravascular shearing of RBCs and spherocytes produced by extravascular phagocytosis of RBCs within the liver and spleen.

Intravascular hemolysis of RBCs releases hemoglobin into the bloodstream that then binds to haptoglobin and other serum proteins. The hemoglobin–haptoglobin complex travels to the liver for processing, thus decreasing the amount of free haptoglobin in the serum—an important laboratory finding of intravascular hemolysis. Breakdown of RBCs releases lactate dehydrogenase and potassium, leading to elevation of both in serum. With excessive hemoglobin breakdown comes increased bilirubin production that cannot be conjugated by the liver for biliary and fecal excretion. Laboratory findings associated with excess bilirubin production include elevated total bilirubin; elevated indirect or unconjugated bilirubin; and increased urinary urobilinogen, a by-product of bilirubin breakdown formed by the intestine and passed into the urine. Excess free hemoglobin may escape binding by serum haptoglobin as well as reabsorption by the renal tubules, creating hemoglobinuria and darkened urine.

TABLE 237-1 Basic Tests and Findings in the Evaluation of Hemolytic Anemia

Purpose	Test	Finding
Confirm anemia/blood loss	Hemoglobin	Decreased
	Hematocrit	Decreased
Confirm compensatory RBC production	Reticulocyte count	Increased
Confirm hemolysis	Peripheral smear	Schistocytes—intravascular hemolysis, RBCs fragmented by shear mechanism
		Spherocytes—extravascular hemolysis, RBC phagocytosis by macrophages
Confirm hemolysis	Lactate dehydrogenase	Increased, released by RBCs
	Potassium	Increased, released by RBCs
Confirm hemolysis	Haptoglobin	Decreased, indicative of intravascular hemolysis
	Free hemoglobin	Increased, indicative of intravascular hemolysis
	Hemoglobinuria	Present
Confirm hemoglobin breakdown	Total bilirubin	Increased
	Indirect (unconjugated) bilirubin	Increased (hepatic conjugation of bilirubin overwhelmed)
	Urinary urobilinogen	Increased

Abbreviation: RBC = red blood cell.

IMMUNE-MEDIATED ACQUIRED HEMOLYTIC ANEMIA

Immune-mediated acquired hemolytic anemia encompasses three main categories: autoimmune, alloimmune, and drug induced.

AUTOIMMUNE HEMOLYTIC ANEMIA

Individuals with autoimmune hemolytic anemia make antibodies against their own RBCs.[1] Diagnosis requires evidence of an antibody on the patient's RBCs, usually accompanied by an autoantibody in the plasma. The direct antigen test, also known as the **direct Coombs test**, is performed by combining the patient's anticoagulated, washed RBCs with anti–immunoglobulin G and anti-C3d (complement) antibodies to detect the presence of immunoglobulin G and/or complement on the RBC surface. A positive direct antigen test consists of the detection of either immunoglobulin G or complement on the RBC surface; it does not require the detection of both.[2] A positive direct antigen test is not specific for a diagnosis of autoimmune hemolytic anemia (**Table 237-2**), nor does the presence of immunoglobulin G and/or complement on a patient's RBCs indicate the severity of disease; the direct antigen test is, however, a critical confirmatory screen. The **indirect Coombs test** looks for the presence of autoantibodies in the patient's serum, testing against a panel of RBCs bearing specific surface antigens. Hemolysis can take place within the vascular space or extravascularly within the liver or spleen.

Autoimmune hemolytic anemia can be divided into primary and secondary disease; primary, or idiopathic, disease occurs without a known underlying etiology, whereas secondary disease is associated with an underlying disorder.[1] Primary disease is more common in women, with peak incidence during the fourth and fifth decades. Many cases initially designated as primary are later found to be associated with lymphoproliferative, autoimmune, or infectious diseases. In children, the disorder is commonly associated with viral or respiratory infections and can cause acute, fulminant hemolysis. Pregnancy can increase the risk of autoantibody development fivefold, but significant RBC destruction is not common. Autoimmune hemolytic anemia is further divided into autoantibody type: warm type, cold type, and mixed type (**Table 237-3**).[1]

Warm Antibody Autoimmune Hemolytic Anemia Warm autoantibody–mediated hemolysis is predominantly extravascular, with antibody-coated RBCs consumed mostly by splenic macrophages

TABLE 237-2 Differential Diagnosis of Positive Direct Antigen (Direct Coombs) Test

Autoimmune hemolytic anemia
Hemolytic transfusion reaction, acute or delayed
Hemolytic disease of newborn
Transplantation
Drug-related hemolytic anemia
IV immunoglobulin therapy
Rh(D) immunoglobulin therapy
Antilymphocyte globulin therapy
Antithymocyte globulin therapy
Sickle cell disease
β-Thalassemia
Renal disease
Multiple myeloma
Hodgkin's disease
Systemic lupus erythematosus
Human immunodeficiency virus/acquired immunodeficiency syndrome

TABLE 237-3 Categories of Autoimmune Hemolytic Anemia (AIHA)

Warm antibody AIHA: Autoantibodies adhere most strongly to RBCs at 37°C (98.6°F).	70%–80% of AIHA cases 2:1 female predominance 50% primary (idiopathic) disease 50% secondary disease: lymphoproliferative, autoimmune disease, postinfection (transient) Usually immunoglobulin G (IgG) autoantibody against Rh(D) antigen Hemolysis usually extravascular Steroid responsive: 70%–80%
Cold antibody AIHA: Autoantibodies adhere most strongly to RBCs at 0–4°C (32–39.2°F).	**Cold agglutinin disease: IgM autoantibody against I antigen** Primary disease: older females Secondary disease: lymphoproliferative disorders, postinfection (transient) Raynaud's phenomenon, livedo reticularis, vascular occlusion Attacks precipitated by cold exposure Rarely intravascular hemolysis Not steroid responsive **Paroxysmal cold hemoglobinuria: IgG autoantibody against P antigen** Primary disease: rare, in adults Secondary disease: usually in children after upper respiratory infection Intravascular hemolysis during cold weather Usually not steroid responsive
Mixed-type antibody AIHA: Autoantibodies have variable temperature-dependent RBC adherence.	Primary disease: more common in older females Secondary disease: lymphoproliferative and autoimmune disorders Usually chronic course with severe exacerbations Usually steroid responsive

Abbreviation: RBC = red blood cell.

and, to a lesser degree, by hepatic macrophages known as *Kupffer cells*. Partial phagocytosis of the original RBC membrane structure leads to the formation of the more rigid, fragmentation-prone spherocyte. Increased spherocytosis found on peripheral blood smear correlates positively with severity of extravascular hemolysis.

Autoimmune hemolytic anemia is initially treated with high-dose corticosteroids, typically oral at 1 to 2 milligrams/kg per day for 3 to 4 weeks, with improvement expected in 80% to 85% of patients but complete remission in only up to 30% of patients.[3]

Monoclonal antibodies (e.g., rituximab), immunosuppressive agents (e.g., azathioprine, mycophenolate mofetil, cyclosporine, cyclophosphamide), or semisynthetic androgens (e.g., danazol) can be used to decrease autoantibody production.[3,4] Splenectomy removes both the main site of extravascular hemolysis in IgG-mediated disease and a major site of general autoantibody production. Splenectomy shows clinical benefit in up to 60% of patients, with potential for long-term remission or a complete cure. A serious complication of splenectomy is overwhelming postsplenectomy infection due to sepsis with encapsulated bacteria.[5] Such **patients should receive regular pneumococcal and meningococcal vaccinations** and may benefit from daily penicillin prophylaxis.

Severe hemolysis in cases of warm antibody autoimmune hemolytic anemia may be treated with plasma exchange as a transient stabilizing measure while waiting for steroids or immunosuppressive agents to take effect. IV immunoglobulin has been used as an adjunctive treatment in children who cannot tolerate the side effects of chronic high-dose steroids or immunosuppressive agents.[6]

For a patient with life-threatening anemia, the goal is to transfuse allogeneic RBCs without producing potentially harmful transfusion reactions. Laboratory personnel must determine whether the patient's blood contains alloantibodies against RBC antigens, but first, autoantibodies—usually directed against more commonly occurring or higher prevalence RBC antigens, and thus typically panreactive against RBC panels—must be identified and sifted out because the presence of autoantibodies can hide the existence of alloantibodies.[7] The testing process can be both labor and time intensive, sometimes requiring 6 hours or longer. Once completed, however, antigen-free, compatible RBC units can then be selected in hopes of providing safe and effective transfusion for the patient. If emergently needed, transfusion of the *least incompatible* units may be administered slowly and in the smallest amounts necessary with close monitoring.[8]

Cold Antibody Autoimmune Hemolytic Anemia Cold autoantibodies lead to clumping or agglutination of RBCs on peripheral smear at cooler temperatures. Cold antibody autoimmune hemolytic anemia is associated with complement fixation on the RBC surface and triggering of the complement cascade. Hemolysis occurs in both the extravascular and intravascular spaces. Instead of splenic macrophages, the hepatic macrophages known as *Kupffer cells* are responsible for most of the extravascular RBC destruction. The two major cold antibody disorders are **cold agglutinin disease** and **paroxysmal cold hemoglobinuria**. Fifty percent of secondary cold antibody cases are associated with lymphoproliferative disorders, with underlying infection as the next leading cause.

Cold agglutinin disease is exacerbated by the cold, so more episodes of acute hemolysis are seen during winter.[9] Because the peripheral circulation is typically cooler than the central circulation, secondary Raynaud's phenomenon and vascular occlusion can complicate cold agglutinin disease, leading to acrocyanosis and tissue necrosis/gangrene. Painful discoloration and mottling of the skin consistent with livedo reticularis may be seen.[10] Less commonly, cold urticaria and hemorrhagic vesicles may develop.[11]

Primary cold agglutinin disease causes chronic, recurrent hemolysis in older adults, particularly females, with a peak incidence at age 70 years old. As with all of the idiopathic autoimmune hemolytic anemias, an associated underlying disease process may be discovered well after initial presentation of cold agglutinin disease; in particular, an occult lymphoproliferative disorder may be the source of the aberrant cold autoantibodies.

Secondary cold agglutinin disease may present after infection with *Mycoplasma pneumoniae*, Epstein-Barr virus, or infectious mononucleosis, adenovirus, cytomegalovirus, influenza, varicella-zoster virus, human immunodeficiency virus, *Escherichia coli*, *Listeria monocytogenes*, or *Treponema pallidum*. Hemolysis typically begins 2 to 3 weeks after the onset of illness, corresponding with peak antibody development against the infectious agent, and resolves about 2 to 3 weeks after resolution of the infectious illness. Many patients with *Mycoplasma* pneumonia and infectious mononucleosis will have measurable cold agglutinin titers, but far fewer will develop symptoms and signs of hemolytic anemia. Conversely, cold agglutinin disease associated with lymphoproliferative diseases such as chronic lymphocytic leukemia and lymphoma produces high autoantibody levels with the potential for significant hemolysis.

Agglutination of RBCs can confound an automated CBC device; the mean corpuscular volume may be falsely elevated, whereas the hemoglobin registers spuriously low. Holding the blood tube in warm hands may decrease RBC clumping for more reliable CBC results. A CBC with confusing or bizarre results should undergo peripheral smear examination. Peripheral smear findings of cold agglutinin disease include spherocytosis, anisocytosis, poikilocytosis, polychromasia, and agglutination.[12] The direct antigen test demonstrates adherence of complement to patient RBCs, but cold autoantibodies are typically washed off the RBCs during the elution process and thus are not identified. Other laboratory findings correspond with those routinely seen in cases of hemolytic anemia, including findings consistent with intravascular hemolysis in some cold agglutinin disease cases (Table 237-1).

An important principle in treating cold agglutinin disease is keeping the extremities and appendages, particularly the nose and ears, warm in cold weather. Patients should take a daily folate supplement for healthy RBC production. Cold agglutinin disease is less likely to respond to steroids, with response rates as low as 35%.[9] Splenectomy is less effective in treating cold agglutinin disease because splenic macrophages play a lesser role in IgM-mediated cold antibody disease. Severe hemolysis has been treated successfully with immunosuppressive agents such as chlorambucil, cyclophosphamide, interferon-α, fludarabine, or rituximab.[9] Because immunoglobulin M autoantibodies have an intravascular distribution, plasmapheresis may assist by removing autoantibodies from the circulation when combined with immunosuppressive agents.

Infection-related cold antibody disease does not require immunosuppressive therapy because the hemolytic anemia is usually self-limited. RBC transfusion can be performed for patients at risk for significant cardiac or cerebrovascular ischemia, but transfused blood should be infused at 37°C (98.6°F) using a blood warmer. Transfusions should be limited as they may worsen ongoing hemolysis because most cold antibodies act against the I/i group antigens that are found on most donor RBCs. Donor complement in the transfused product also may exacerbate ongoing hemolysis.

Paroxysmal cold hemoglobinuria is caused by a biphasic hemolysin immunoglobulin G autoantibody called the *Donath-Landsteiner (D-L) antibody* that is directed against the P antigen system found on most RBCs.[13] This potent autoantibody binds to RBCs and fixes early complement cascade proteins at low temperatures, whereas terminal complement components adhere and produce intravascular lysis of RBCs at warmer, physiologic temperatures.

Bursts of cold weather–induced intravascular hemolysis lead to bouts of dark urine or hemoglobinuria for which the disease is named. Other presenting symptoms include attacks of high fever, chills, headache, abdominal cramps, nausea and vomiting, diarrhea, and leg and back pain, all exacerbated by cold weather. Cold urticaria may develop as well as extremity paresthesias and Raynaud's phenomenon.

Primary paroxysmal cold hemoglobinuria is a rare, idiopathic, chronic condition occurring in adults, characterized by cold-induced episodes of massive hemolysis. Secondary disease occurs predominantly in children, usually seen after a preceding upper respiratory infection. Most pediatric cases are self-limited and nonrecurring, but severe cases may take weeks to resolve. With severe hemolysis, hemoglobinuria is common, and methemoglobinemia may be seen. Acute renal failure may develop as a complication. Pediatric paroxysmal cold hemoglobinuria may occur after infections with measles, mumps, Epstein-Barr virus, cytomegalovirus, varicella, adenovirus, influenza A, *M. pneumoniae*, *Haemophilus influenzae*, and *E. coli*. Adult patients with chronic, relapsing disease should be tested for syphilis, because cold-provoked hemolysis has been associated with tertiary or late syphilis as well as with congenital syphilis.

During an attack of paroxysmal cold hemoglobinuria, acutely low hemoglobin may be seen on CBC due to sudden, severe hemolysis. The peripheral smear may demonstrate erythrophagocytosis, the engulfment of RBCs by neutrophils.[12] Presence of the biphasic D-L immunoglobulin G antibody on laboratory testing is pathognomonic. Patient serum is added to two tubes containing human type O RBCs. The first tube, the control, is incubated at 37°C (98.6°F) or physiologic temperature, whereas the second tube is incubated first at 0°C (32°F) and then at 37°C (98.6°F). The D-L test is positive if hemolysis is present in the second tube, indicating presence of the biphasic D-L antibody, while absent in the control tube.[14] The direct antigen test is usually positive for complement just before or after a paroxysm but often negative in between paroxysms in patients with chronic, relapsing disease.

Patients with paroxysmal cold hemoglobinuria should be kept warm. Steroids can be considered in children with severe hemolytic anemia, but because infection-related disease tends to be self-limited, benefit is uncertain. Disease secondary to syphilis responds to effective antibiotic treatment. Splenectomy is not helpful, and plasmapheresis should be used only as a temporizing measure in life-threatening cases. RBC transfusion using a blood warmer should be limited to cases of severe hemolysis because most donor units are P antigen positive and may stimulate further production of antibodies. Rituximab can successfully treat primary paroxysmal cold hemoglobinuria in adults.[15]

Mixed-Type Autoimmune Hemolytic Anemia Mixed-type autoimmune hemolytic anemia, with both warm and cold autoantibodies to RBCs, presents as primary or secondary disease, most commonly associated with lymphoproliferative and autoimmune diseases, particularly systemic lupus.[1] The course of illness is usually chronic with severe exacerbations. Like the warm antibody disorder, the mixed type is usually steroid responsive, can be treated with splenectomy, and responds to immunosuppressive therapy.

ALLOIMMUNE HEMOLYTIC ANEMIA

Alloimmune hemolytic anemia requires exposure to allogeneic RBCs with subsequent alloantibody formation. In the laboratory, alloantibodies react specifically with the allogeneic RBCs that triggered their production; these antibodies do not react against a patient's own RBCs. A well-known example of this is when the Rh(D)-negative maternal immune system develops immunoglobulin G alloantibodies on exposure to Rh(D)-positive fetal RBCs. The maternal alloantibodies can then cross the placenta, leading to fetal RBC destruction in a condition known as *hemolytic disease of the newborn*.[16] Anemia can range from mild to potentially fatal, producing intrauterine fetal death. The term *hydrops fetalis* has been used to describe the anasarca seen in severe cases. Transplacental or fetomaternal hemorrhage, the inciting stimulus for maternal alloantibody formation, may occur during amniocentesis, chorionic villus sampling, delivery, or abortion (threatened or otherwise) or even during external cephalic version. Administration of anti-D immunoglobulin G with any fetomaternal hemorrhage event and soon after delivery will suppress maternal alloantibody formation and prevent hemolytic disease of the newborn. Treatment of established hemolytic disease of the newborn employs intrauterine and intravascular fetal transfusion and may include plasma exchange and/or IV immunoglobulin therapy.

Most adults who develop alloimmune hemolytic anemia have a history of RBC transfusion, which sensitizes patients to allogeneic RBC antigens. A subsequent transfusion can result in immediate alloantibody production, resulting in the fever, chest and flank pain, tachypnea, tachycardia, hypotension, hemoglobinuria, and oliguria seen in the hemolytic transfusion reaction (see chapter 238, "Transfusion Therapy"). In patients with high alloantibody titers, the hemolytic reaction can be immediate. Delayed alloantibody-mediated hemolysis is possible, with hemolytic transfusion reaction symptoms presenting 3 to 7 days after transfusion (see chapter 238).

DRUG-INDUCED HEMOLYTIC ANEMIA

Drug-induced hemolytic anemia is rare, estimated at 1 in 1,000,000 patients, where drug exposure induces antibody formation leading to the destruction of RBCs.[17] More than 100 drugs are known to induce autoantibody production against patient RBCs (**Table 237-4**).[18]

TABLE 237-4 Most Often Cited Drugs Inducing Hemolytic Anemia

Cephalosporins	Cefotetan
	Ceftriaxone
	Cephalothin
Chemotherapeutic agents	Fludarabine
	Interferon
	Oxaliplatin
Nonsteroidal anti-inflammatory drugs	Diclofenac
	Mefenamic acid
	Phenacetin
	Tolmetin
Penicillins	Penicillin G
	Piperacillin
Miscellaneous	Catechin (antidiarrheal)
	Levodopa (antiparkinsonian)
	Methyldopa (antihypertensive)
	Nomifensine (antidepressant)
	Quinidine (antiarrhythmic)
	Rifampin (antibiotic)

Drug-induced hemolytic anemia can result in either a positive or negative direct antigen test and can be difficult to distinguish from autoimmune hemolytic anemia, so a careful review of current medications is important in patients with a new hemolytic anemia.

Patients with severe hemolysis and anemia require hospitalization and further evaluation. In all cases, stop the offending drug immediately. In the event that medications are required for treatment of patients in the ED who have evidence of ongoing hemolysis, refrain if possible from using listed agents (Table 237-4). Steroids can be used in cases of drug-related severe hemolysis.

MICROANGIOPATHIC SYNDROMES

The two classic syndromes associated with microangiopathic hemolytic anemia are thrombotic thrombocytopenic purpura (TTP) and hemolytic-uremic syndrome (HUS).[19,20] Both syndromes involve platelet aggregation in the microvascular circulation via mediation of von Willebrand factor. Microangiopathic hemolytic anemia or schistocyte-forming hemolysis occurs from fragmentation of RBCs during travel through these partially occluded arterioles and capillaries. Although TTP and HUS are clinical syndromes with characteristic features, overlap does occur, sometimes making differentiation difficult. TTP is more common in adults, whereas HUS is more common in children. TTP typically induces more prominent neurologic effects, with deposition of platelet aggregates in a broader distribution, whereas HUS more specifically affects the renal system.

THROMBOTIC THROMBOCYTOPENIC PURPURA

The classic pentad for TTP includes CNS abnormalities, renal pathology, fever, microangiopathic hemolytic anemia, and thrombocytopenia. Untreated TTP carries a high mortality rate, but plasma exchange therapy can achieve remission of disease in >80% of patients.[20-22] Groups at higher risk for TTP include women, patients age 30 to 50 years old, individuals of African descent, and Hispanics.

Pathophysiology The pathophysiology of TTP is connected to a specific metalloprotease ADAMTS-13 (*a d*isintegrin *a*nd *m*etalloproteinase with a *t*hrombo*s*pondin type 1 motif, member 13, also known as *von Willebrand factor–cleaving protease*). ADAMTS-13 is made by hepatic stellate cells, glomerular podocytes, and vascular endothelial cells. Its function is to cleave von Willebrand factor that has been unfolded by shear stress within the microvasculature of arterioles and capillaries. Without this cleavage function, unfolded von Willebrand factor monomers can form large multimers that lead to formation of intravascular microthrombi. TTP has been associated with ADAMTS-13 activity at levels <10% of normal.[23] Severely deficient ADAMTS-13 activity alone does not reliably trigger TTP; often other precipitating or contributing factors are important, including pregnancy, infection, inflammation, and medication use.

ADAMTS-13 activity levels typically decrease by up to 30% during pregnancy, although not usually to the severely low levels associated with TTP.[23] It is hypothesized that the hypercoagulable state of pregnancy combined with the decreased ADAMTS-13 activity level may set the stage for TTP in pregnancy. TTP is rare during pregnancy, seen in <1 per 100,000. Published literature offers conflicting opinions as to when TTP most commonly occurs during pregnancy—either during the second trimester or early in the third trimester,[24-26] or at term or postpartum.[27] TTP shares many clinical and laboratory features with pre-eclampsia–eclampsia, HELLP syndrome (*h*emolysis, *e*levated *l*iver enzymes, *l*ow *p*latelet count), and acute fatty liver of pregnancy.[20] Still, symptoms of severe pre-eclampsia or HELLP before 24 weeks of gestation should raise suspicion for TTP.

Human immunodeficiency virus infection, particularly with progression to acquired immunodeficiency syndrome, is associated with the microangiopathic anemia and thrombocytopenia that characterize TTP. On testing, some human immunodeficiency virus patients with TTP-like illness have severely deficient ADAMTS-13 activity levels and thus may benefit from plasma exchange therapy. However, others with microangiopathic hemolytic anemia and thrombocytopenia in the setting of human immunodeficiency virus/acquired immunodeficiency syndrome have normal ADAMTS-13 activity levels, questioning whether the TTP label and plasma exchange therapy should be applied.[28,29]

Influenza vaccination has been implicated as a TTP trigger, leading to production of autoantibody against ADAMTS-13.[30] Acute pancreatitis, capable of inducing a systemic inflammatory response, has also been associated with TTP, although moderately rather than severely low ADAMTS-13 activity levels lead to uncertainty about a TTP diagnosis versus some other thrombotic microangiopathic process.[31,32]

Drugs associated with TTP include ciprofloxacin, ofloxacin, levofloxacin, quinine, sirolimus when used with calcineurin inhibitors such as cyclosporine, risperidone, clopidogrel, lansoprazole, valacyclovir, mitomycin, infliximab, and ticlopidine.[20] Ticlopidine in particular is thought to induce autoantibody formation against ADAMTS-13 as well as microvascular endothelial cell injury in genetically susceptible individuals within 2 to 12 weeks of starting the medication. Clopidogrel use can also incite microvascular endothelial cell injury within 2 weeks of use. Ticlopidine has been associated with more severe thrombocytopenia and microangiopathic hemolysis than clopidogrel, whereas clopidogrel has produced more significant renal insufficiency not readily responsive to plasma exchange therapy.[33] Days to weeks may be required to achieve remission in ticlopidine/clopidogrel-associated TTP cases.

Clinical Features Shearing of RBCs across these microthrombi produces the microangiopathic hemolytic anemia. Platelet aggregation in TTP leads to systemic platelet depletion or thrombocytopenia. When these microthrombi are concentrated in the CNS and renal arterioles and capillaries (though notably not found in venules), they promote tissue ischemia and necrosis, with resultant end-organ damage such as seizure, stroke, other focal neurologic deficits, coma, and acute renal injury.

Along with findings of severe anemia and thrombocytopenia of <20,000/mm^3 (<20 × 10^9/L), serum and urine tests may corroborate ongoing intravascular hemolysis (Table 237-1) with renal injury or failure. Because TTP thrombi do not incorporate fibrin, TTP can be distinguished from disseminated intravascular coagulation by normal coagulation studies.

Treatment Plasma exchange therapy is very effective in TTP with the goal to achieve a normal platelet count.[20,21] Daily plasmapheresis (plasma exchange) of 40 mL/kg or up to 1.0 to 1.5 times a patient's plasma volume is performed and then either weaned in frequency or stopped once normal counts are reached for 2 to 3 consecutive days. Infusion of plasma replaces defective or insufficient ADAMTS-13, and removal of plasma rids the body of defective ADAMTS-13, autoantibodies against the metalloprotease, and large von Willebrand factor multimers.

If plasmapheresis cannot be performed immediately, fresh frozen plasma infusion can be initiated, with pheresis occurring later.[20] Infusion with factor VIII concentrate containing ADAMTS-13 activity can be considered for patients with plasma allergy after specialist consultation and review.

Severe TTP may require additional interventions such as RBC transfusion, anticonvulsants, antihypertensives, and hemodialysis. **Avoid platelet transfusions**, except in life-threatening bleeding or intracranial hemorrhage, because acutely worsened thrombosis can lead to renal failure and, potentially, death. **Aspirin** can exacerbate hemorrhagic complications in the setting of severe thrombocytopenia but can still be used for cerebrovascular and cardiovascular indications in patients with adequate platelet counts. Heparin is not beneficial in TTP. Corticosteroids, rituximab, and cyclosporine may play a role in the treatment of autoimmune TTP.[20,21] Discontinue the inciting drug in all cases of drug-associated TTP.

Outcome TTP relapse, defined as a new case onset >30 days after completion of remission-achieving plasma exchange therapy, is seen in 20% to 50% of cases, most often within 2 years after the initial episode. Patients with ADAMTS-13 activity levels <10% are at increased risk for relapse.[23] Triggers for relapse may be the same as those inciting original cases. Relapses may present with milder symptoms and less severe hematologic findings. Patients with multiple relapses may experience them farther and farther apart, and total volume and duration requirements for plasma exchange therapy are lessened in subsequent cases.[34]

The maternal mortality rate from TTP has been reduced significantly with the use of plasma exchange therapy, but fetal mortality has remained high secondary to placental microvascular occlusion, ischemia, and infarction. TTP may relapse with subsequent pregnancy, so affected women should be counseled accordingly. Because of this association, females of child-bearing age presenting with microangiopathic hemolytic anemia and thrombocytopenia should be assessed for an unsuspected pregnancy.

HEMOLYTIC-UREMIC SYNDROME

HUS, a common cause of acute renal failure in childhood, consists of microangiopathic hemolytic anemia, acute nephropathy or renal failure, and thrombocytopenia.[19,20,35] HUS can be classified as typical or atypical, with prognosis favoring typical cases.[34] Typical HUS occurs in children about 1 week into a case of infectious diarrhea, often bloody and without associated fever. The causative agent of typical HUS is Shiga toxin–producing *E. coli*, with serotype O157:H7 predominating in North America.[35,36] Shiga toxin is sometimes alternatively labeled *verocytotoxin* in the literature. Other less common causes of diarrhea-associated HUS include *Shigella*, *Yersinia*, *Campylobacter*, and *Salmonella*. Atypical HUS occurs in older children and adults; may be difficult to distinguish from TTP because of extrarenal involvement; is caused by other infectious organisms, such as *Streptococcus pneumoniae* and Epstein-Barr virus; or may have a noninfectious source, such as bone marrow transplantation or the administration of immunosuppressant or chemotherapeutic agents.[35]

Store-bought refrigerated ground beef and frozen ground beef patties, frozen pepperoni pizza, bagged fresh spinach, prepackaged raw cookie dough, as well as lettuce, cheddar, and ground beef found in fast food have been implicated in multistate *E. coli* O157:H7 infection outbreaks with HUS occurring as a complication of each of the outbreaks.[36] HUS has also occurred after drinking water from a municipal source contaminated by *E. coli* O157:H7.

Pathophysiology Ingested via contaminated food or water, Shiga toxin–producing *E. coli* O157:H7 possesses potent virulence factors that allow invasion of intestinal epithelial cells and subsequent transmural intestinal migration.[35] The ensuing colonic inflammation produces the characteristic hemorrhagic colitis associated with *E. coli* O157:H7 and other Shiga toxin–producing bacteria. Shiga toxin, once absorbed into the systemic circulation, binds with greatest affinity to receptors found on the surfaces of glomerular and renal tubular epithelial and endothelial cells and, to a lesser extent, to receptors lining cerebral and colonic epithelial and endothelial cells and pancreas. Molecular mimicry may exist between human CD36, an antigen found on endothelial cells and platelets, and Shiga toxin, so that antibody formed against the toxin may bind to CD36 and incite the pathologic processes leading to HUS.[37]

Toxin-mediated microvascular injury promotes platelet aggregation (and therefore, systemic depletion, leading to thrombocytopenia) and thrombus formation at the injury site. Further upregulation of epithelial and endothelial cell receptors with high affinity for Shiga toxin creates a vicious cycle of thrombosis, and microangiopathic hemolytic anemia via shearing of RBCs over microthrombi contributes to tissue ischemia and necrosis. Microthrombi within the pancreas have been postulated to cause pancreatic β-cell death and subsequent deficits in insulin secretion. Thus, patients with HUS may present with hyperglycemia consistent with new-onset diabetes mellitus. Some may even go on to have chronic insulin requirements with increased morbidity and mortality rates.[38]

Clinical Features Onset of HUS is typically 2 to 14 days after diarrhea develops, so patients may present during the diarrheal illness phase, with abdominal cramps, with or without bloody diarrhea, and, often, without fever. For the patient with nonbloody diarrhea, testing stool for fecal leukocytes can reveal occult inflammatory colitis, thereby prompting stool culture, specifically for *E. coli* O157:H7.[35] For the patient with bloody diarrhea, the results of stool testing for Shiga toxin–producing bacteria, including *E. coli* O157:H7, can guide medical treatment, alert providers that the complication of HUS should be anticipated, and aid in the cause of public health disease monitoring and outbreak prevention. In addition to the studies required for diagnosing hemolytic anemia, electrolyte and renal function panels should be obtained to detect nephropathy and associated electrolyte disturbances, while urinalysis should be examined for RBCs, RBC casts, protein, and other evidence of acute nephropathy.[35]

Treatment Typical HUS is treated with supportive care, with focus on hydration, pain control, and RBC or platelet transfusion in cases of significant anemia or profound thrombocytopenia associated with active bleeding.[39] Should acute renal failure develop, hemodialysis may be required. Infection with *E. coli* O157:H7 should not be treated with antimotility drugs because these agents appear to increase the risk of developing HUS.[40] Antibiotics for the treatment of *E. coli* O157:H7 diarrhea is controversial because in vitro studies have found that antibiotics may increase Shiga toxin expression from the bacteria, and case-control human studies have found that antibiotic treatment of the diarrheal illness may increase the risk of developing HUS.[40,41] Atypical HUS is treated with eculizumab.[42]

Outcome Acute renal failure occurs in 55% to 70% of patients with typical HUS, but most, up to 85%, recover kidney function.[35] Mortality in typical HUS is about 5% to 15%. Historically, patients with atypical HUS had a poor outcome, with permanent renal failure or neurologic damage occurring in about half of patients and a morality rate approaching 25%. Aggressive treatment, including eculizumab, appears to significantly reduce the incidence of permanent renal failure and lower the death rate in atypical HUS.[42]

MACROVASCULAR HEMOLYSIS

A **prosthetic heart valve** may create turbulent blood flow with high shear stress across the valve. Older generation mechanical heart valves were subject to deterioration that produced subsequent hemolysis, but hemolysis associated with current prosthetic heart valve models is most often attributed to paravalvular leak. Such leaks may occur at the time of valve placement or develop later in the life of the prosthetic valve if infection or calcification promotes dehiscence.[43] Particularly after mitral valve replacement, hemolysis may occur at both clinically insignificant and significant levels.

Macrovascular hemolysis can also occur after **intracardiac patch repair** or **aortofemoral bypass**; in patients with **coarctation of the aorta, severe aortic valve disease, or ventricular assist devices**; and in patients requiring the use of extracorporeal circulation such as during cardiopulmonary bypass, plasma exchange, or hemodialysis.[44-46] Although the mechanics and shear stress applied to blood through extracorporeal circulatory interventions may drive hemolysis, the composition or contamination of diluents and dialysates may also contribute.[45]

RBCs hemolyzed in the macrocirculation bear the characteristic fragmented appearance of schistocytes seen on peripheral smear. Increased schistocytosis correlates with more severe hemolysis.[43] Other laboratory findings are consistent with intravascular hemolysis (Table 237-1).

Patients with ongoing mild macrovascular hemolysis should receive supplemental iron and folate to promote healthy reticulocytosis. By reducing the heart rate, β-blocker therapy may decrease RBC shear stress in the presence of a prosthetic valve and thereby mitigate hemolysis. Pentoxifylline, a xanthine derivative that reduces blood viscosity and improves RBC flexibility and deformability, can reduce hemolysis associated with prosthetic heart valves.[43] Hemolysis associated with extracorporeal circulation typically begins during the procedure, but such patients may or may not exhibit symptoms until hours afterward. In particular, dialysis patients treated in the outpatient setting may present to the ED for evaluation and treatment of symptoms caused by hemolysis. Severe macrovascular hemolysis may necessitate blood transfusion, whether during an isolated episode or repeat episodes.

ADDITIONAL CAUSES OF HEMOLYSIS

Infection, envenomation, chemical exposure, and trauma can also result in hemolysis (**Table 237-5**).

TABLE 237-5 Additional Causes of Hemolysis

Cause	Disorder	Comments
Infection		
	Malaria	Blackwater fever or hemoglobinuria
	Babesiosis	Protozoan infects and damages with RBC
	Clostridium perfringens	Toxin lyses RBCs
	Leptospirosis	Weil's syndrome; toxin lyses RBCs
Envenomation		
	Hymenoptera stings	Requires massive venom injection
	Brown recluse spider	Part of systemic loxoscelism
	Pit viper; Crotalinae; Elapidae; Viperinae	Intravascular RBC destruction
Chemical exposure		
	Arsine	Hemolysis can present 24 h after exposure
	Naphthalene	Mothballs; well water contaminated by toxic dumps; can affect fetus in utero and neonates; patients with G6PD deficiency at higher risk[47,48]
Direct impact trauma		
	March hemoglobinuria	Runners, soldiers, karate, conga drummers[49,50]; hemoglobinuria but usually not anemia

Abbreviations: G6PD = glucose-6-phosphate dehydrogenase; RBC = red blood cell.

REFERENCES

The complete reference list is available online at www.TintinalliEM.com.

CHAPTER 238 Transfusion Therapy

Clinton J. Coil
Sally A. Santen

INTRODUCTION

Modern transfusion practice uses blood that has been separated into specific components (**Table 238-1**). Coagulation factors, either derived from human plasma or manufactured with recombinant technology, are used treat hemorrhage associated with a deficiency of one or more factors (**Table 238-2**). Transfusion in the ED typically is done for acute blood loss and/or circulatory shock. As medical care is moved to outpatient settings, emergency physicians may be responsible for transfusion therapy or complications previously relegated to inpatient settings.[1]

Blood products are provided using standardized preparations as "units" (Table 238-1). Provide information to patients about the risks, benefits, and alternatives to transfusion prior to the initial infusion of red blood cells, plasma, or platelets.[2,3] Obtain informed consent or document that the patient was unable to consent if a medical emergency exists.[2] Use great care to assure that the correct blood product is delivered to the correct patient because of the consequences of transfusing the wrong unit; use two individuals to verify the identification of the patient and the unit before transfusion. Bar-code identification along with verification by one individual is an alternative to two-person verification.[4]

TRANSFUSION OF BLOOD PRODUCTS

PACKED RED BLOOD CELLS

Adult total blood volume is approximately 2.5 L/m^2, 75 mL/kg, or about 5 L in a 70-kg person. Whole blood transfusion would seem ideal to replace acute blood loss; however, storage of whole blood inactivates platelets and other factors. Therefore, whole blood is fractionated to its components for storage and transfusion. Packed red blood cells (PRBCs) are prepared by the centrifugation of whole blood to remove approximately 80% of the plasma; then a preservative solution is added (most commonly, citrate-phosphate-dextrose) with the additional nutrients adenosine, and mannitol (Table 238-1).

The primary reason for PRBC transfusion is to increase oxygen-carrying capacity.[1,4] Emergency PRBC transfusion is usually performed for acute blood loss or, occasionally, profound anemia with impaired oxygen delivery. Transfusion thresholds assist the physician in assessing whether PRBC transfusion will benefit the patient. Current evidence is substantial that a restrictive threshold for PRBC transfusion is appropriate for most patients.[5-9] In previously healthy adults, transfusion should be considered at hemoglobin concentrations less than 7 grams/dL (70 grams/L), and for patients with sepsis or ischemic heart or brain injury, transfusion should be considered at a hemoglobin concentration less than 8 to 9 grams/dL (80 to 90 grams/L).[10-13] Transfusion threshold values for children may be higher and depend on the etiology of their anemia.[14] Some patients with severe sepsis receiving early, goal-directed therapy may benefit from transfusion up to a hemoglobin of 10 grams/dL (100 grams/L) when the central venous oxygen saturation is less than 70%.[15]

For actively bleeding patients, transfusion is based on clinically estimated blood loss rather than hemoglobin levels, because the fall in measured hemoglobin will lag behind the clinical impact of acute blood loss. A loss of about 30% blood volume (1500 mL in an adult) generally produces symptoms and signs, but young, healthy patients can tolerate this degree of loss when treated with crystalloid. However, patients with chronic illness such as underlying anemia, cardiac diseases, or pacemakers or those on β-blockers or similar medications may not tolerate blood loss. Consider emergency PRBC transfusion for unstable trauma patients based on an inadequate response to an initial 2-L bolus of IV crystalloid or 40 mL/kg in children. The anticipated clinical course also guides the decision to transfuse the patient with acute hemorrhage; the transfusion threshold is lower if the source of bleeding cannot be controlled immediately compared to a patient whose acute hemorrhage has stopped.

Use the minimum amount of PRBCs to accomplish the desired clinical outcome.[7,12] **A single PRBC unit will raise the hemoglobin by 1 gram/dL (10 grams/L) and hematocrit by 3% in adults. In children, 10 to 15 mL/kg of PRBCs will raise the hematocrit by 6% to 9% and the hemoglobin level by approximately 2 to 3 grams/dL (20 to 30 grams/L).**[14]

One unit of PRBCs, approximately 250 mL in volume, is generally transfused over 1 to 2 hours. PRBCs should be transfused more rapidly in patients with hemodynamic instability. Single-unit PRBC transfusions should not exceed 4 hours to prevent contamination. If a slow transfusion is desired (e.g., in a patient at risk for volume overload), the blood bank should be asked to split a unit so that the first half can be transfused over 4 hours while the second half waits in the blood bank refrigerator. During standard transfusions, the initial infusion rate is slower over the first 30 minutes so that if there is a transfusion reaction, the infusion may be stopped.

Type and Cross-Match PRBC transfusion requires matching the recipient's and donor's red blood cells according to blood type (ABO and Rh) and screening the recipient's plasma for antibodies to the minor red blood cell antigens. Screening is done using a mixture of commercially available red blood cells that have all of the important minor antigens.[12] If the screen is positive, then the recipient's plasma is cross-matched against the specific PRBC unit intended for transfusion. Blood type can be determined in approximately 15 minutes, whereas it takes about 45 to 60 minutes to perform a serologic cross-match. If an anti–red blood cell antibody is found in the recipient's plasma, cross-matching may take longer and require additional blood specimens from the patient. For most patients with no antibodies detected on the screen, serologic cross-matching can be foregone and ABO-Rh–compatible PRBC units can be released by the blood bank using a process termed *electronic* (or *computerized*) *cross-match*. This process has computer-based verifications to ensure the patient receives ABO-Rh–compatible blood.[12] Electronic cross-matching typically takes 5 minutes or less to perform.

Type O Rh-negative (universal donor) blood may be used in critical circumstances because these transfused red cells do not contain major

TABLE 238-1 Characteristics of Blood Products

Component	Shelf Life	Volume/Unit (mL)	Approximate Content/Unit*	Initial Dose	Dosage Effect
Packed red blood cells (PRBCs)	21–42 d	250–350	Red cells 65%–80% Plasma 10–20 mL	Adult: 2 units Pediatrics: 10–15 mL/kg	Raises hemoglobin concentration approximately 2 grams/dL (20 grams/L) or hematocrit by 6% in adults (2–3 grams/dL [20–30 grams/L] or 7%–9% in children)
Platelets (apheresis-collected single-donor platelet concentrate)	5 d	250–300	Platelets 3–6 × 10^{11}	1 unit or 5 mL/kg	Raises platelet count by up to 50,000/mm^3 (50 × 10^9/L), but less in many cases
Platelets (pooled donor platelet concentrate, rarely used in the United States)	5 d	50–60	Platelets 8–9 × 10^{10}	6 units or 5 mL/kg	Raises platelet count by up to 50,000/mm^3 (50 × 10^9/L), but less in many cases
Fresh frozen plasma (FFP)	1 y frozen and up to 5 d after thawing	200–250	Each coagulation factor about 200–250 units Fibrinogen 400–500 milligrams	Four units or 15 mL/kg	Raises most coagulation factors levels approximately 20%; volume issues may make factor correction difficult; benefits are transient
Cryoprecipitate	1 y frozen and 4 h thawed	20–50	Factor VIII 80–140 units Fibrinogen 225–420 milligrams von Willebrand factor in variable amounts Factor XIII and fibronectin in some amounts	0.2 units/kg or 10–15 units in an adult	Increases fibrinogen 50–100 milligrams/dL (0.5– 1.0 grams/L)

*Unless specifically prepared, most blood-derived products contain some small amount of WBCs, red blood cells, platelets, and plasma in addition to the specific component.

blood group antigens (A or B). Type O Rh-positive blood may be used if type O Rh-negative is not available, but should be avoided in girls and women of childbearing potential. Approximately 20% of Rh-negative patients transfused with 1 unit of Rh-positive PRBCs will develop anti-Rh(D) antibodies, creating the risk for hemolytic disease of the newborn with subsequent pregnancies. This is usually clinically inconsequential for men or postmenopausal women.

Treated Red Blood Cells PRBCs may be further treated for specific clinical applications: leukocyte-reduced PRBCs, irradiated PRBCs, washed PRBCs, and frozen PRBCs.[16] Leukocyte-reduced PRBCs have 70% to 85% of the white cells removed. Leukocyte-reduced PRBCs are used (1) to decrease the occurrence of nonhemolytic febrile reactions due to cytokines from transfused white cells, (2) to prevent sensitization to human leukocyte antigen antibodies found on white cells in patients who may be eligible for bone marrow transplantation, and (3) to minimize the risk of intracellular virus transmission, such as cytomegalovirus. Leukocytes can be reduced by filtration or other methods before storage of the PRBCs or during transfusion. Irradiation of PRBCs eliminates the capacity of T lymphocytes to proliferate, thereby preventing the donor's T lymphocytes from reacting to the recipient's cells and causing graft-versus-host disease. Irradiated cells are used in transplant patients, neonates, and immunocompromised patients, and with directed donations from relatives of the patient. Washed PRBCs are indicated in patients who have a hypersensitivity to plasma, such as immunoglobulin A deficiency or persistent febrile reactions. For rare blood types, red cells may be frozen and saved for up to 10 years for later use. Freezing red blood cells is more expensive than normal storage, and once thawed, the blood must be washed and transfused within 24 hours.

TABLE 238-2 Coagulation Factor Products

Type of Product*	Initial Dose	Comments and Approved Indications
Fibrinogen concentrate (human) RiaSTAP® (CSL Behring)	Dosed to increase fibrinogen level from baseline to over 150 milligrams/dL (1.5 grams/L) If baseline fibrinogen level unknown, administer 70 milligrams/kg	Each vial contains 900–1300 milligrams of fibrinogen Acute bleeding episodes in patients with congenital fibrinogen deficiency
Three-factor prothrombin complex concentrate (human) Profilnine SD® (Grifols Biologicals) Bebulin VH® (Baxter Healthcare Corporation)	Dosed according to desired factor IX increase	Contains factors II, IX, and X Treat hemophilia B (factor IX deficiency)
Four-factor prothrombin complex concentrate (human) Kcentra® or Beriplex® P/N (CSL Behring) Octaplex® (Octapharma)	Dosed in factor IX units according to pretreatment INR	Contains factors II, VII, IX, and X Urgent reversal of bleeding due to vitamin K antagonist (e.g., warfarin)–induced coagulation factor deficiency in adult patients
Anti-inhibitor coagulant complex FEIBA NF® (Baxter)	50–100 units/kg	Contains factors II, IX, and X, mainly nonactivated, and factor VII mainly in activated form Bleeding in patients with hemophilia A or B with inhibitors
Coagulation factor VIIa (recombinant) NovoSeven® RT (Novo Nordisk)	90 micrograms/kg	Bleeding episodes and perioperative management in adults and children with hemophilia A or B with inhibitors Congenital factor VII deficiency Glanzmann's thrombasthenia with refractoriness to platelet transfusions Bleeding episodes and perioperative management in adults with acquired hemophilia

*Commercial trade names provided for ease of specific identification.

MASSIVE TRANSFUSION

Massive transfusion is the replacement of one blood volume or approximately 10 units of PRBCs in an adult within a 24-hour period. If only PRBCs are used, platelets and coagulation factors lost or consumed will not be replaced, potentially producing increased bleeding. The military medical experience during the past decade finding good results with using fresh whole blood transfusion for trauma patients[17] has led to the concept of incorporating the platelets and plasma in addition to PRBCs to closer mimic whole blood during a massive transfusion.[18,19] Studies routinely using platelets and fresh frozen plasma (FFP) with PRBCs during massive transfusion have yielded mixed results on reducing mortality.[20,21]

Institution-specific massive transfusion protocol is recommended to guide the clinician in correct ordering of the individual products and facilitate release from the blood bank.[22] The best ratio of PRBCs to platelets to FFP during a massive transfusion is controversial.[23] **Some experts advocate a 1:1:1 ratio**, although lower ratios of platelets and FFP have been used without clear evidence of inferiority.[24] Including cryoprecipitate,[20] fibrinogen concentrate,[24] or coagulation factor VIIa (recombinant)[20,24] during a massive transfusion has produced mixed results, depending on the outcome measured.

If fixed ratios of platelets or FFP are not used, suggested indications for their administration during massive transfusion include the following: (1) when the platelet count is <50,000/mm^3(<50 × 10^9/L), a platelet transfusion is warranted; (2) if the INR is >1.5, FFP may be given; and (3) if the fibrinogen level is <100 milligrams/dL (<1 g/L), it may be replaced with cryoprecipitate or fibrinogen concentrate.

Draw sufficient specimens early in the course from massive transfusion patients because once the patient has received close to one blood volume of transfused products, new blood specimens will contain so much donor blood that it will confuse further cross-matching of subsequent units. Hypothermia is a risk during massive transfusion, so blood and crystalloid should be warmed, in addition to instituting warming measures for the patient. Hypocalcemia from the preservative citrate chelating calcium may occur with a massive transfusion.[22]

PLATELET TRANSFUSION

Platelet transfusions are used either prophylactically to prevent bleeding in thrombocytopenia or therapeutically when patients with thrombocytopenia are actively bleeding.[25,26] One apheresis-collected, single-donor platelet concentrate is the standard product in developed countries (Table 238-1). Platelets collected from six different donors (a "six pack") can be combined for transfusion but are not recommended because this increases the risk of disease transmission and transfusion reaction.

One apheresis single-donor platelet unit will increase the platelet count by up to 50,000/mm^3 (50 × 10^9/L), an amount sufficient to stop most spontaneous and minor traumatic bleeding. Check platelet levels at 1 and 24 hours after transfusion completion because the response is variable. Failure of platelets to rise appropriately may be due to increased consumption of platelets from an underlying process, active thrombosis due to ongoing hemorrhage, destruction due to platelet antibodies, or sequestration due to hypersplenism. Transfused platelets should survive 3 to 5 days unless there is a platelet-consumptive process.

The decision to transfuse platelets depends on the severity of thrombocytopenia and clinical circumstances (**Table 238-3**).[13,25-27] Patients with comorbid conditions, such as infection, fever, medications, and CNS involvement, may be more likely to bleed or be at higher risk if they bleed; therefore, the threshold for platelet transfusion is more liberal.[13,28]

There are no clear recommendations concerning platelet transfusions in patients with nonfunctioning platelets (antiplatelet medications, uremia, von Willebrand's disease, or hyperglobulinemia) and active bleeding. In von Willebrand's disease, normal platelets may help deliver von Willebrand factor to the bleeding site. Conversely, in uremic patients, the transfused platelets may not function any better than native platelets. In these complex cases, consult with a hematologist or transfusion medicine specialist for recommendations.

Relative contraindications to the transfusion of platelets are disorders associated with platelet activation, such as thrombotic thrombocytopenic purpura or heparin-induced thrombocytopenia, in which transfusion may worsen thrombosis. In these conditions, ongoing bleeding or the need to perform procedures may necessitate platelet transfusion in consultation with the appropriate specialist.

Platelet transfusions are usually ABO-type specific because the platelets are bathed in plasma, although a serologic cross-match is usually not done. As a result, patients receiving platelets are subject to many of the same complications described for plasma transfusion. Depending on availability, non–type-specific platelets may sometimes be transfused. This practice is usually avoided in children or patients receiving multiple transfusions because they are at higher risk for complications. Transfusing non–type-specific platelets may also shorten the half-life of the transfused platelets.

As with PRBCs, platelets can be leukocyte reduced or washed. Patients who have had repeated transfusions may become alloimmunized and refractory to platelet transfusion, noted by the lack of expected rise in platelet count after transfusion. Such patients need human leukocyte antigen–matched or cross-matched platelets. Other factors may affect the efficacy of platelet transfusion, including bacterial sepsis in the recipient, antibiotics forming an antigen complex epitope with the platelet, disseminated intravascular coagulation, and splenomegaly.

FRESH FROZEN PLASMA TRANSFUSION

FFP is plasma obtained after the separation of whole blood from erythrocytes and platelets and then frozen within 8 hours of collection.[29] FFP takes approximately 20 to 40 minutes to thaw, and this process cannot be sped up through artificial heating. Once thawed, FFP can be transfused up to 5 days later. Trauma centers and other specialty hospitals may keep prethawed units of FFP available.

Transfused FFP should be ABO-type compatible, and Rh compatibility is unnecessary. A common misconception is that type O plasma is the universal FFP donor, as it is for PRBCs. This is not the case, because type O plasma contains antibodies to A and B blood group antigens. **Type AB is the universal donor for FFP, and in emergencies, universal donor FFP can be given minutes after thawing.** Each unit of FFP has a volume of 200 to 250 mL and contains approximately 1 unit of each coagulation factor and 2 milligrams of fibrinogen per milliliter (Table 238-1). FFP is used for replacement of multiple coagulation deficiencies in cases such as liver failure, warfarin-induced overanticoagulation, disseminated intravascular coagulation, and massive transfusion in bleeding patients, although evidence of benefit is weak (**Table 238-4**).[30] FFP is also used with bleeding due to an individual coagulation factor deficiency when a specific replacement factor is not available. FFP is unlikely to reverse anticoagulation from oral anticoagulants such as dabigatran and rivaroxaban, which are specific inhibitors of thrombin and factor Xa, respectively (see chapter 239, "Thrombotics and Antithrombotics" and the "Prothrombin Complex Concentrate" section, below).[31]

TABLE 238-3 General Indications for Platelet Transfusion
Platelet count <5000/mm^3 (<5 × 10^9/L)
Platelet count <20,000/mm^3 (<20 × 10^9/L) with a coagulation disorder, low-risk procedure, or during outpatient treatment
Platelet count <50,000/mm^3 (<50 × 10^9/L) with active bleeding or invasive procedure within 4 h
Platelet count <100,000/mm^3 (<100 × 10^9/L) with neurologic or cardiac surgery
As part of a massive transfusion protocol

TABLE 238-4 General Indications for Fresh Frozen Plasma Transfusion
Reversal of warfarin overanticoagulation (not the primary agent)
Bleeding with multiple coagulation defects
Correction of coagulation defects for which no specific factor is available
As a component of a massive transfusion protocol
As part of plasma exchange when treating thrombotic microangiopathies or neurologic disorders

Response to FFP treatment is monitored by tests of the coagulation system: the prothrombin time, INR, and activated partial thromboplastin time. Using fresh frozen plasma to achieve complete normalization of coagulation studies is neither necessary nor realistic in most circumstances. Clinically adequate hemostasis is generally present with functional coagulation factor levels of 30% to 40% of normal, which corresponds to an INR of about 1.7. Although it is common to administer FFP before a procedure when the INR exceeds 1.5,[13,27] there is little evidence to support this practice,[32] and it will likely have little effect on patients with an INR less than 1.85.[33] If rapid reversal of a vitamin K antagonist coagulopathy is needed, prothrombin complex concentrate or coagulation factor VIIa (recombinant) is faster and more reliable.[34]

Administering FFP prophylactically to nonbleeding patients is not indicated, and prophylaxis is not needed before procedures in patients with a coagulopathy.[32] Procedures such as abdominal paracentesis[35] or endoscopy with variceal banding[36] can be performed safely with a coagulopathy. If correction is desired, the effect of FFP is transient, dose dependent, and may subject the patient to volume overload.

Other possible indications for FFP include hereditary angioedema if C1 esterase inhibitor is not available (see chapter 14, "Anaphylaxis, Allergies, and Angioedema").[37,38] FFP is used during plasma exchange for treatment of diseases such as thrombotic thrombocytopenic purpura and Guillain-Barré syndrome.[39,40]

For isolated factor deficiencies, specific factor replacement is preferred over FFP for major bleeding, with fresh frozen plasma sometimes used for minor bleeding episodes (**Table 238-5**).

The increase in individual coagulation factors seen after FFP infusion varies depending on the specific factor. In general, 1 unit of FFP will increase most coagulation factors by 3% to 5% in a 70-kg adult. Administering 2 units of FFP to an adult (approximately 7 to 8 mL/kg) will increase coagulation factors up to 10%, a clinically inconsequential benefit in most circumstances. For clinically relevant correction of coagulation factor deficiencies, a dose of 15 mL/kg (or 4 units in a 70-kg adult) is often required (Table 238-1). After transfusion, coagulation studies should be repeated and further FFP transfusion guided by the results.

TABLE 238-5 Replacement Therapy for Congenital Factor Deficiencies

Coagulation Factor	Approximate Incidence*	Replacement Therapy
Factor I (fibrinogen)	1 per million	Cryoprecipitate Fibrinogen concentrate
Factor II (prothrombin)	1 per 2 million	3- or 4-factor PCC for major bleeding
Factor V	1 per million	FFP
Factor VII	1 per 500,000	4-factor PCC for major bleeding Coagulation factor VIIa (recombinant)
Factor VIII†	1 per 5000–10,000 males	Recombinant factor VIII Desmopressin for mild hemophilia
Von Willebrand's disease‡	Up to 1 per 100 persons	Desmopressin or factor VIII concentrates (or cryoprecipitate if either unavailable)
Factor IX†	1 per 30,000 males	Recombinant factor IX 3- or 4-factor PCC
Factor X	1 per million	FFP for minor bleeding episodes 3- or 4-factor PCC for major bleeding
Factor XI‡	3 per 10,000 Ashkenazi Jews 1 per million in general population	FFP
Factor XII	25 per 1000	No bleeding manifestations, replacement not required
Factor XIII	1 per million	FFP or cryoprecipitate

Abbreviations: FFP = fresh frozen plasma; PCC = prothrombin complex concentrate.

*Source van Herrewegen F, Meijers JC, Peters M, van Ommen CH: Clinical practice: the bleeding child. Part II: disorders of secondary hemostasis and fibrinolysis. *Eur J Pediatr* 171: 207, 2012.

†See chapter 235, "Hemophilias and von Willebrand's Disease."

‡Factor XI levels correlate poorly with bleeding complications; many patients have low levels but no bleeding complications.

TABLE 238-6 General Indications for Cryoprecipitate Transfusion

Bleeding with a fibrinogen level of <100 milligrams/dL (< 1 g/L)
Dysfibrinogenemia
Bleeding in some subtypes of von Willebrand's disease that are unresponsive to desmopressin, and factor VIII concentrates are unavailable

CRYOPRECIPITATE

Cryoprecipitate is the cold-insoluble protein fraction of fresh frozen plasma.[34] With the development of recombinant factor VIII products for use in hemophilia, the current role for cryoprecipitate is as replacement of fibrinogen.[41] Cryoprecipitate may be used in bleeding patients with fibrinogen levels <100 milligrams/dL (< 1 g/L) due to severe liver disease, uremia, disseminated intravascular coagulation, and dilutional coagulopathy, although there is controversy over dosing and efficacy (**Table 238-6**).[42,43] Five units of cryoprecipitate are typically pooled for use, with adults receiving one to three pooled infusions. Cryoprecipitate may also be included in some massive transfusion protocols.[20,24]

FIBRINOGEN CONCENTRATE

Fibrinogen concentrate is derived from pooled human plasma and used to treat bleeding episodes in patients with congenital fibrinogen deficiency.[44] Fibrinogen has been investigated for benefit in other hemorrhagic conditions with an observed ability to reduce bleeding and transfusion requirements, but without a measurable effect on mortality.[45] Four products are commercially available. The advantages over cryoprecipitate are minimal risk of disease transmission due to viral inactivation, accurate dosing because each vial is assayed for fibrinogen content, a lower volume for infusion, no need for thawing, no requirement of ABO testing and compatibility, and a rapid reconstitution for infusion.

Fibrinogen is dosed according the patient's baseline fibrinogen level, the target level (in most circumstances >150 milligrams/dL),[46] volume of distribution, and body weight. If the baseline fibrinogen level is unknown, the initial dose is 70 milligrams/kg. The most common adverse reactions include allergic reactions, fever, chills, nausea, and vomiting.

PROTHROMBIN COMPLEX CONCENTRATE

Prothrombin complex concentrates are blood-derived concentrations of three or four vitamin K–dependent clotting factors: prothrombin and factors VII, IX, and X.[47] Some prothrombin complex concentrate formulations may also contain the anticoagulant proteins C, S, and antithrombin, as well as heparin. Three-factor prothrombin complex concentrate is approved for treatment of hemophilia B (factor IX deficiency) (Table 238-2). Four-factor prothrombin complex concentrate is approved for urgent reversal of overanticoagulation from vitamin K antagonists (such as warfarin),[48,49] resulting in a more reliable reduction in the elevated INR than three-factor prothrombin complex concentrate.[50,51] The four-factor prothrombin complex concentrate dose in this circumstance is administered using factor IX units and adjusted according to the pretreatment INR value. Off-label use of three- or four-factor prothrombin complex concentrate includes bleeding in patients with congenital factor II, IX, or X deficiency.

Prothrombin complex concentrate does not require thawing, does not necessitate ABO-compatibility testing, and does not carry the risk of volume overload, all of which can hinder fresh frozen plasma use. Because prothrombin complex concentrate's effects are transient, vitamin K should usually be co-administered for sustained warfarin reversal. Prothrombin complex concentrate is part of some protocols for reversal of rivaroxaban and dabigatran in the setting of life-threatening bleeding, despite limited evidence for their effectiveness.[31,52,53] Thrombosis is the major complication of prothrombin complex concentrate, observed in about 5% of treated patients, although this incidence is not much higher than in similar patients treated with fresh frozen plasma.

COAGULATION FACTOR VIIa (RECOMBINANT)

Coagulation factor VIIa (recombinant) is primarily used for treatment of hemophilia A and B in patients who have developed inhibitor antibodies to factors VIII or IX, respectively. Other uses for this agent have been investigated, such as coagulation support in liver failure, multisystem trauma, intracranial hemorrhage, and postpartum bleeding, but evidence for overall safety and efficacy in these expanded indications is lacking.[54-58] The major drawbacks to this product are risk of thrombosis (up to 4% in patients with acquired hemophilia) and the high cost.

COMPLICATIONS OF BLOOD TRANSFUSIONS

Up to 20% of all transfusions may result in some type of adverse reaction.[4,59] Most reactions are minor; serious reactions are uncommon, and life-threatening ones are rare (**Table 238-7**).[60] In critically ill patients, transfusion reactions may be difficult to identify; therefore, watch for unexpected changes in patient status during a transfusion. **Two important first steps in any confirmed or suspected transfusion reaction are to (1) immediately stop the transfusion, and (2) contact the blood bank that issued the transfusion product.**[12,16] The blood bank physician is an important resource for managing the suspected transfusion reaction.

Although stopping the transfusion at the first sign of complications is an important step, a common error in management of a confirmed or possible transfusion reaction is to abandon all transfusion. Typically, transfusion reactions, such as hemolytic reactions or transfusion-related acute lung injury, are due to the interaction between a particular unit and a particular patient. Even patients with severe reactions can still safely receive future blood products if they are appropriately matched to the patient. In fact, a patient who had clinical indications for transfusion may need that product even more if a transfusion reaction has caused deterioration. One of the first steps in management of a transfusion reaction is to draw a new specimen to retype and cross-match new units so that transfusion can resume as soon as possible.[12,16]

Premedication with diphenhydramine and acetaminophen is a widespread practice to prevent febrile and/or allergic transfusion reactions[61]; however, the effects are limited,[62,63] and routine prophylactic premedication is not recommended. Premedication may be used for patients with previous febrile or allergic transfusion reactions.

HEMOLYTIC TRANSFUSION REACTIONS

Hemolytic transfusion reactions occur when the recipient's antibodies recognize and induce hemolysis of the donor's RBCs.[1,12,16,64] The reaction is usually acute when antibodies already exist as anti-A or anti-B immunoglobulin M antibodies or immunoglobulin G antibodies in very high titer. Reactions can be delayed when there is an amnestic response to a transfused red blood cell antigen to which the recipient has been previously sensitized.[16,64,65] Immediate transfusion reactions are caused by ABO incompatibility and usually are the result of technical errors made during the collection of blood, in pretransfusion testing, or in patient identification. The majority of transfusion fatalities are acute hemolytic reactions due to human error of incorrect cross-matching or inadvertent administration of the wrong blood to the wrong patient. The risk of acute hemolytic transfusion reaction due to incompatible blood is 1 to 4 per million units transfused.

With acute hemolytic reaction, most of the transfused cells are destroyed, which may result in activation of the coagulation system, disseminated intravascular coagulation, and release of anaphylatoxins and other vasoactive amines. Clinical features of an acute hemolytic reaction include back pain, pain at the site of the transfusion, headache, alteration of vital signs (fever, hypotension, dyspnea, tachycardia), chills, bronchospasm, pulmonary edema, bleeding due to developing coagulopathy, and evidence of new or worsening renal failure.

Ongoing transfusion should be stopped immediately on first indication of potential problems. While laboratory confirmation is being performed, the sequelae of hemolysis are treated supportively. Check renal function, electrolytes, and coagulation status. Maintain renal blood flow and urine output with fluids, mannitol, and furosemide, as needed. Treat circulatory shock with intravenous infusions and vasopressors to support blood pressure.

The remaining donor blood should be sent, along with a posttransfusion blood specimen from the recipient, to the blood bank. Diagnosis is

TABLE 238-7 Transfusion Reactions

Reaction Type	Signs and Symptoms	Management	Evaluation
Acute intravascular hemolytic reaction	Fever, chills, low back pain, flushing, dyspnea, tachycardia, shock, hemoglobinuria	Immediately stop transfusion. IV hydration to maintain diuresis; diuretics may be necessary. Cardiorespiratory support as indicated.	Retype and repeat cross-match. Direct and indirect Coombs test. CBC, creatinine, prothrombin time, activated partial thromboplastin time. Haptoglobin, indirect bilirubin, lactate dehydrogenase, plasma free hemoglobin. Urine for hemoglobin.
Delayed extravascular hemolytic reaction	Often have low-grade fever but may be entirely asymptomatic	Usually presents days to weeks after transfusion. Rarely causes clinical instability.	Hemolytic workup as above to investigate the possibility of intravascular hemolysis.
Febrile nonhemolytic transfusion reaction	Fever, chills	Stop transfusion. Initially manage as in intravascular hemolytic reaction (above) because one cannot initially distinguish between the two. Can treat fever and chills with acetaminophen. Usually mild but can be life threatening in patients with tenuous cardiopulmonary status. Consider infectious workup. Premedication with acetaminophen can mask this reaction.	Hemolytic workup as above because may not be able to initially distinguish febrile from hemolytic transfusion reactions.
Allergic reaction	Mild: urticaria, pruritus Severe: dyspnea, bronchospasm, hypotension, tachycardia, shock	Stop transfusion. If mild, reaction can be treated with diphenhydramine; if symptoms resolve, can restart transfusion. If severe, may require cardiopulmonary support; do not restart transfusion.	For mild symptoms that resolve with diphenhydramine, no further workup is necessary, although blood bank should be notified. For severe reaction, do hemolytic workup as above because initially may be indistinguishable from a hemolytic reaction.

confirmed by evidence of hemolysis (hemoglobinuria or hemoglobinemia) and by blood incompatibility. In rechecking the blood type and cross-match, the patient's serum is tested for blood group alloantibodies, and the donor's plasma is tested for the presence of antibodies that react with the patient's blood. In intravascular hemolytic transfusion reactions, serum haptoglobin will be decreased, serum lactate dehydrogenase will be elevated, and a direct antigen (Coombs) test usually will be positive. The blood bank will be able to test the blood, review records, confirm blood types, and determine if the patient's syndrome is from a transfusion reaction.

Extravascular delayed hemolytic reactions occur in approximately 1 per 1000 to 6000 PRBC units transfused.[16] Hemolysis most commonly occurs in the spleen and occasionally in liver and bone marrow. This type of reaction is less serious and rarely fatal. It may be identified by a positive Coombs test, elevated unconjugated (indirect) bilirubin level, and less than expected increase in hemoglobin from the transfusion.

FEBRILE TRANSFUSION REACTIONS

Febrile transfusion reactions are characterized by fever during or within a few hours of a blood transfusion.[1,12,16] A febrile reaction occurs in approximately 1 per 300 units of PRBCs infused. Febrile transfusion reactions are more common in patients who have been exposed to foreign blood antigens, such as multiparous women or multiply transfused patients. Febrile transfusion reactions result from a combination of recipient antibody against donor leukocytes and the release of cytokines that are produced during storage. Clinical presentation can range from a mild elevation in temperature to a high fever along with rigors, headache, myalgias, tachycardia, dyspnea, and chest pain. A febrile reaction may be difficult to initially differentiate from the more serious hemolytic transfusion reaction or sepsis.

For a febrile reaction during a patient's first-time transfusion, or in any severe reaction, the transfusion should be stopped and the product returned to the blood bank for testing. Laboratory investigation similar to that done for possible hemolytic transfusion is done and blood cultures should be obtained. The febrile transfusion reaction is usually self-limited and will respond to antipyretics. A mild fever in a patient who has been transfused before is usually not serious. In most cases, the transfusion can be restarted after consultation with the blood bank physician. For patients with recurrent febrile reactions, the use of leukocyte-reduced blood products may be helpful, as well as pretreatment with antipyretics.

ALLERGIC TRANSFUSION REACTIONS

Allergic transfusion reactions typically manifest with urticaria and pruritus during the infusion.[1,12,16] A small percentage of patients will have more severe reactions, such as bronchospasm, wheezing, and anaphylaxis. These reactions are caused by an immune response to transfused plasma proteins. The incidence of allergic transfusion reactions varies widely.[66]

Antihistamine therapy usually will control the symptoms. The transfusion should be stopped but can usually be restarted after evaluation. For severe symptoms, the transfusion should be stopped and treatment with epinephrine or bronchodilators initiated. Patients with immunoglobulin A deficiency may experience severe anaphylactic reactions in response to exposure from immunoglobulin A in donor products. Washing the plasma from the red blood cells minimizes this type of reaction.

INFECTIOUS COMPLICATIONS OF BLOOD TRANSFUSION

Improved blood donor screening, serologic testing, safer handling of blood products, and viral inactivation of blood products have reduced the risk of infection from transfusion.[67-70] Despite screening donor blood for antibodies to most concerning viral agents, there is still a small risk of viral transmission (**Table 238-8**). Most cases of transmission are thought to occur during the window period between infection and antibody production in the donor. This window can be reduced by antigen testing of donated blood for known viral antigens.

Prevalence for cytomegalovirus antibodies in the general population is between 50% and 80%; therefore, a transfusable unit is not tested routinely for cytomegalovirus unless the recipient is seronegative and either pregnant, a potential or present transplant candidate, immunocompromised, or a premature infant. Leukocyte-reduced blood components further decrease the risk of cytomegalovirus transmission to susceptible populations because most of the virus resides in the leukocytes.[68]

TABLE 238-8 Risk of Infections from Transfusion of Blood Products

Etiology	Estimated Frequency: One Infection per Number of Units Transfused
HIV-1	1 per 6 million
HIV-2	Unknown, but extremely low
Human T-cell lymphotropic virus types 1 and 2	1 per 640,000
Hepatitis B	1 per million
Hepatitis C	1 per 100 million
Parvovirus B19	1 per 10,000

Abbreviation: HIV = human immunodeficiency virus.

Other infections transmitted by blood transfusion include West Nile virus, variant Creutzfeldt-Jakob, babesiosis, and dengue.[66,67,69] Additionally, blood can become contaminated with bacteria during storage or processing. Transfusion-associated bacterial infection was more commonly reported with platelet concentrates than PRBC or fresh frozen plasma. Bacterial screening and inactivation procedures have dramatically reduced the incidence of transfusion-associated bacterial sepsis.[60] Response to a possible septic reaction involves immediate discontinuation of the transfusion, blood cultures from the patient, therapy with broad-spectrum antimicrobials, and examination of material from the blood container by Gram stain with cultures of specimens from the container and the administration set.[12,16]

TRANSFUSION-RELATED ACUTE LUNG INJURY

Transfusion-related acute lung injury is an uncommon but complex process that is thought to be due to granulocyte recruitment and degranulation within the lung.[65,71,72] Transfusion-related acute lung injury is usually a complication of fresh frozen plasma or platelet transfusion and is rare after PRBC transfusion alone. This syndrome presents with respiratory distress and the appearance of bilateral pulmonary infiltrates due to noncardiogenic pulmonary edema, during or within 6 hours of transfusion. By itself, transfusion-related acute lung injury is self-limiting and generally resolves spontaneously with only supportive care, although severe, fatal reactions can occur. Because the pulmonary edema is noncardiogenic, use care to distinguish this situation from volume overload and avoid aggressive diuresis, which can cause rapid deterioration.

OTHER COMPLICATIONS

Hypervolemia Transfusion of blood products can cause rapid volume expansion when compared to similar volumes of crystalloid fluids, leading to transfusion-associated cardiovascular overload.[65] Patients with limited cardiovascular reserve, such as infants, those with severe chronic compensated anemia, and the elderly, are at the highest risk. Clinical features include dyspnea, hypoxia, and pulmonary edema. Recognize the potential for volume overload so that blood can be transfused slowly, the patient can be monitored carefully, and treatment with diuretics can be initiated when necessary. The usual rate of PRBC or fresh frozen plasma transfusion is 2 to 4 mL/kg per h, but it can be slowed to 1 mL/kg per h in more delicate patients. Blood product units may also be split, as described earlier.

Electrolyte Imbalance Electrolyte imbalances of hypocalcemia, hypokalemia, or hyperkalemia due to large-volume transfusions or altered elimination are uncommon. The anticoagulant citrate is a component of many blood preservatives and chelates calcium. The effect of infused citrate is clinically insignificant because patients with normal hepatic function metabolize the citrate to bicarbonate. Rarely with massive transfusions, hepatic metabolism is overwhelmed, and hypocalcemia can develop and/or the excess bicarbonate generated causes alkalemia, driving potassium into the cells and causing hypokalemia.[22] The potassium content in stored blood products increases during storage, and uncommonly, patients with renal insufficiency or neonates can develop hyperkalemia from transfusion.

Acknowledgment: We would like to acknowledge Holli Mason, MD, and William Robb, RN, BSN, for their review of the material in this chapter.

REFERENCES

The complete reference list is available online at www.TintinalliEM.com.

Thrombotics and Antithrombotics

David E. Slattery
Charles V. Pollack, Jr.

INTRODUCTION

Antithrombotic therapy (i.e., **anticoagulants, antiplatelet agents, and fibrinolytics**) is used to treat arterial and venous thromboembolic conditions, including acute coronary syndrome, deep venous thrombosis, pulmonary embolism, transient ischemic attack, and ischemic stroke. Moreover, antithrombotic agents help prevent occlusive vascular events in patients at risk for thrombosis due to atherosclerotic arterial disease, atrial fibrillation, medical illness with immobility, or surgical insult. These agents, however, can cause life-threatening complications, primarily serious hemorrhage. Detailed management strategies for thromboembolic disorders are discussed in their respective chapters (see chapter 49, "Acute Coronary Syndromes"; chapter 56, "Venous Thromboembolism"; and chapter 167, "Stroke Syndromes").

Hemostasis—whether physiologic after accidental injury or pathologic after rupture of an atherosclerotic plaque—is initiated by platelet interaction with the vascular subendothelium and continues with a series of reactions among plasma coagulation proteins that generate the final product of cross-linked fibrin incorporated into the initial platelet plug (see chapter 232, "Tests of Hemostasis"). Arterial thrombi, composed primarily of platelets bound by thin fibrin strands, develop under high-flow conditions, especially at sites of ruptured plaques. **Both anticoagulants and platelet-inhibiting drugs may effectively prevent and treat arterial thrombosis.** In contrast, venous thrombi form in areas of sluggish blood flow and are composed mainly of red blood cells and large fibrin strands. **Anticoagulant drugs are more effective than antiplatelet drugs in preventing venous thromboembolism.**

Antithrombotic agents are classified by their mechanism of action. **Anticoagulants** block the synthesis or activation of clotting factors, interfering with the coagulation cascade at one or more steps. **Antiplatelet agents** interfere with platelet activation or aggregation. **Fibrinolytic agents** (often but inaccurately referred to as thrombolytic agents) stimulate the enzymatic dissolution of the fibrin component.

Thrombotic agents are used to diminish bleeding due to either an anithrombotic agent or and acquired or genetic bleeding disorder (see chapters 233 and 235, "Acquired Bleeding Disorders" and "Hemophilias and von Willebrand's Disease", respectively).

ORAL ANTICOAGULANTS

Oral anticoagulants are used to (1) stop further thrombosis when the condition already exists (e.g., venous thrombosis), (2) reduce the risk of embolism in patients with thrombotic disease (e.g., venous thrombosis or left ventricular mural thrombus), and (3) prevent thrombi from forming in patients with risk factors for their development (e.g., atrial fibrillation, prolonged immobilization, or prosthetic heart valve) (**Table 239-1**).

WARFARIN

Warfarin, a hydroxy coumarin compound, is the most widely used oral anticoagulant.[1,2] Warfarin is readily absorbed after ingestion, reaching peak blood concentrations in 2 to 4 hours, and has a circulating half-life of 20 to 60 hours. Warfarin is bound to albumin, metabolized by the liver, and excreted in the urine. Warfarin blocks activation of vitamin K and thereby interferes with hepatic carboxylation of coagulation factors II, VII, IX, and X. The decrease in these vitamin K–dependent cofactors impairs the extrinsic and common coagulation pathway. Warfarin also blocks the synthesis of proteins C and S. Activated protein C (with protein S and phospholipid as cofactors) proteolyses factors Va and VIIIa, thereby inhibiting the coagulation cascade. Thus, warfarin has both an antithrombotic effect (by inhibiting the synthesis of factors II, VII, IX, and X) and a prothrombotic effect (through inhibition of proteins C and S production), but during maintenance therapy, the overwhelming effect is one of anticoagulation.

Warfarin dosing is guided by measurement of the International Normalized Ratio (INR), a standardized measurement of prothrombin time, with a desired therapeutic range of 2.0 to 3.0 in most cases.[2] Drugs and food that interfere with warfarin absorption, bind to albumin, or alter hepatic metabolism can have a profound effect on warfarin activity (**Table 239-2**). Warfarin is generally contraindicated in pregnancy because it is teratogenic (especially during the 6th to 12th week of gestation) and can cause fetal hemorrhage.

Protein C has a short half-life (8 hours), and plasma levels quickly fall after starting warfarin. The vitamin K–dependent coagulation factors have half-lives that range from approximately 7 hours for FVII to approximately 60 hours for prothrombin (FII). **The phase delay between the fall in levels of protein C (an antithrombotic protein) and the fall in levels of the four affected coagulation factors (prothrombotic proteins) results in a transient state of increased thrombogenesis at the start of warfarin therapy that persists for 24 to 36 hours.** This hypercoagulable state is mitigated by providing sufficient overlap with a parenteral anticoagulant (e.g., heparin) during the first 3 to 5 days of warfarin treatment[1,2] and during any interruption of warfarin therapy for surgery or an invasive procedure.[3-5] Because factors X and II have relatively long half-lives, the parenteral anticoagulant should not be discontinued until the INR is in the desired therapeutic range for 2 consecutive days. **Thus, a noncompliant patient with the risk for catastrophic complications from sudden intravascular thrombosis—such as a patient with a mechanical prosthetic heart valve who has stopped oral anticoagulants—should be treated with a parenteral anticoagulant in addition to restarting warfarin.**

There is also a prothrombotic rebound during the first 4 days after cessation of warfarin therapy. However, there is no increased incidence of clinical episodes of thrombosis with termination of warfarin therapy, and thromboembolic events that occur in patients after warfarin discontinuation are most-likely related to the underlying condition.

The two major complications of warfarin therapy are bleeding and skin necrosis. The most important factor influencing the risk of bleeding is the intensity of anticoagulant therapy. The risk of clinically significant bleeding is increased when the INR is >4.5 to 5.0.[1,2] Skin necrosis occurs primarily (but not exclusively) in patients with protein C deficiency. This complication usually develops 3 to 8 days after starting treatment and is caused by thrombosis of small cutaneous vessels. Treatment includes discontinuation of warfarin, administration of a parenteral anticoagulant to maintain desired anticoagulation, vitamin K_1 administration, and screening for protein C and S deficiencies.

Patient-specific risk factors for increased risk of bleeding during warfarin treatment include hypertension, anemia, prior cerebrovascular disease, GI lesions, and renal disease. The relationship between advanced age and warfarin-associated bleeding is controversial. Elderly individuals who are otherwise appropriate candidates for anticoagulant therapy should not have warfarin withheld solely because of their age, although elderly patients require more frequent and careful monitoring. Medications that increase warfarin activity and antiplatelet medications increase bleeding risk during warfarin therapy (**Table 239-2**).

TABLE 239-1 Options for Antithrombotic Therapy

Clinical Indication	Comments
Treatment of Deep Venous Thrombosis and Pulmonary Embolism	
Unfractionated heparin 80 units/kg IV bolus followed by 18 units/kg per h continuous IV infusion, with the aPTT checked after 6 h and the infusion adjusted to maintain the aPTT 1.5–2.5 times control *with* concurrent institution of warfarin	In most cases, heparin and warfarin are started simultaneously, with an overlap of 3–5 d. Warfarin is monitored and dose adjusted to a target INR of 2.0–3.0 in most patients.
Enoxaparin 1 milligram/kg SC every 12 h or 1.5 milligrams/kg SC once a day	Monitoring not routinely required
Dalteparin 200 units/kg SC once daily or 100 units/kg SC twice daily	Not FDA approved for this indication
Fondaparinux weight-tiered regimen	Monitoring not routinely required
<50 kg: 5 milligrams SC once a day	—
50–100 kg: 7.5 milligrams SC once a day	—
>100 kg: 10 milligrams SC once a day	—
Rivaroxaban 15 milligrams PO twice daily for 21 d, followed by 20 milligrams PO once daily	Avoid use in patients with CrCl <30 mL/min
Dabigatran 150 milligrams PO twice daily (after 5 to 10 d of parenteral anticoagulation)	Avoid in patients with CrCl <30 mL/min or on hemodialysis
Apixaban 10 milligrams PO twice daily for 7 d, followed by 5 milligrams twice daily	Reduce dose by 50% if patient taking dual strong VYP3A4 and P-glycoprotein inhibitors
Streptokinase 250,000 units IV bolus, followed by 100,000 units/h continuous IV infusion for 1–3 d OR Alteplase 100 milligrams IV infused over 2 h OR Tenecteplase weight-tiered single IV bolus <60 kg: 30 milligrams 60–70 kg: 35 milligrams 70–80 kg: 40 milligrams 80–90 kg: 45 milligrams >90 kg: 50 milligrams	Fibrinolytic treatment of deep venous thrombosis and pulmonary embolism is recommended only in carefully selected patients.
Prophylaxis of Deep Venous Thrombosis and Pulmonary Embolism	
Unfractionated heparin 5000 units SC every 8–12 h	Highest-risk patients for venous thromboembolism should receive every 8 h dosing.
Dalteparin 2500 to 5000 IU SC once a day	—
Enoxaparin 40 milligrams SC once daily (normal renal function), 30 milligrams SC twice daily (trauma) or 40 milligrams twice daily (obese patients)	—
Fondaparinux 2.5 milligrams SC once a day	—
Rivaroxaban 10 milligrams PO once a day	—
Apixaban 2.5 milligrams PO twice daily	For prophylaxis after hip and knee replacement surgery, initial dose taken 12–24 h after surgery
ST-Segment Elevation Myocardial Infarction	
Aspirin (non–enteric coated) 162–325 milligrams PO once a day Clopidogrel 300 milligrams PO loading dose (consider 600 milligrams if PCI is planned) followed by 75 milligrams PO once a day OR Ticagrelor 180 milligrams PO loading dose, followed by 90 milligrams PO twice daily	All post–myocardial infarction patients should receive aspirin, 162–325 milligrams PO once a day, for an indefinite period (unless contraindicated or if on warfarin).
Unfractionated heparin 60 units/kg IV bolus (maximum, 4000 units according to the ACC/AHA guidelines or 5000 units according to the ESC guidelines) followed by 12 units/kg per h (maximum, 1000 units) continuous IV infusion adjusted to keep aPTT 1.5–2.5 times control OR Enoxaparin 30 milligrams IV bolus, followed by 1 milligram/kg SC every 12 h for patients <75 years of age or 0.75 milligrams/kg SC every 12 h of patients >75 years of age OR Bivalirudin 0.75 milligram/kg IV bolus followed by 1.75 milligrams/kg per h continuous IV infusion (FDA approved for use in cardiac catheterization laboratory only)	Optimal anticoagulation strategies are not completely defined.

(*Continued*)

TABLE 239-1 Options for Antithrombotic Therapy (*Continued*)

Clinical Indication	Comments
Streptokinase 1.5 million units IV over 60 min OR Alteplase 15 milligrams IV bolus over 1–2 min followed by 0.75 milligram/kg IV over 30 min (maximum, 50 milligrams) and 0.50 milligram/kg IV over 60 min (maximum, 35 milligrams) OR Reteplase 10 units IV bolus, then a second 10-unit dose at 30 min OR Tenecteplase weight-tiered single IV bolus <60 kg: 30 milligrams 60–70 kg: 35 milligrams 70–80 kg: 40 milligrams 80–90 kg: 45 milligrams >90 kg: 50 milligrams	Early administration is more important than choice of specific fibrinolytic agent.
Unstable Angina and Non-ST-Segment Myocardial Infarction	
Aspirin (non–enteric coated) 162–325 milligrams PO once a day	Optimal antiplatelet strategies are not completely defined.
Clopidogrel 300 milligrams PO loading dose (consider 600 milligrams if PCI is planned) followed by 75 milligrams PO once a day OR Prasugrel 60 milligrams loading dose followed by 10 milligrams PO once daily OR Ticagrelor 180 milligrams PO loading dose, followed by 90 milligrams PO twice daily	Dual therapy—aspirin plus another antiplatelet agent—is common.
Unfractionated heparin 60 units/kg IV bolus (maximum, 4000 units according to the ACC/AHA guidelines or 5000 units according to the ESC guidelines) followed by 12 units/kg per h (maximum, 1000 units/h) continuous IV infusion adjusted to keep aPTT 1.5–2.5 times control Enoxaparin 1 milligram/kg SC every 12 h Glycoprotein IIb/IIIa inhibitor, depending on risk and whether PCI is planned Bivalirudin 0.75 milligram/kg IV bolus followed by 1.75 milligrams/kg per hour continuous IV infusion (FDA approved for use in cardiac catheterization laboratory only)	Optimal anticoagulation strategies are not completely defined.
Peripheral Artery Disease	
Aspirin 162–325 milligrams PO once a day	—
Cilostazol 100 milligrams PO twice a day	—
Acute Ischemic Stroke	
Alteplase 0.9 milligram/kg (maximum, 90 milligrams) with 10% of total dose given as an IV bolus over 1 min followed by the remainder as an IV infusion over 60 min	Use of fibrinolytics in acute ischemic stroke requires *strict* adherence to recommended guidelines and should be done with informed consent. Adjunctive use of anticoagulants should be avoided for 48 h.
Postischemic Stroke	
Aspirin 81 milligrams PO once a day	—
Clopidogrel 75 milligrams PO once a day	Use clopidogrel if aspirin allergic.
Dipyridamole 200 milligrams extended-release PO twice a day	Usually combined with aspirin 25–50 milligrams PO twice a day.
Transient Ischemic Attack	
Aspirin 81 milligrams PO once a day	Use clopidogrel if "aspirin failure" or aspirin allergic.
Clopidogrel 75 milligrams PO per day	—
Stroke Prevention in Atrial Fibrillation	
Warfarin dose monitored and adjusted by INR	Target INR is 2.0–3.0 in most patients.
Dabigatran 75–150 milligrams PO twice daily	Dosing guided by renal function; not routinely monitored.
Rivaroxaban 15–20 milligrams PO once a day	Dosing guided by renal function; not routinely monitored.
Apixaban 2.5–5.0 milligrams PO twice daily	Dose adjustment in patients with any two of the following characteristics: Age >80 years Weight <60 kg Serum creatinine >1.5 mg/dL

Abbreviations: ACC = American College of Cardiology; AHA = American Heart Association; aPTT = activated partial thromboplastin time; ESC = European Society of Cardiology; FDA = U.S. Food and Drug Administration; PCI = percutaneous coronary intervention.

TABLE 239-2 Warfarin Interactions

Consideration	Effect on PT or INR*
Major	
Vitamin K malabsorption or dietary deficiency	↑
Excess vitamin K	↓
Reduced gut bacteria (antibiotics)†	↑
Decreased warfarin absorption	↓
Altered warfarin metabolism (cytochrome P-450)	Variable
Drug effects†	Variable
Other	
Decreased clotting factor production (liver disease)	↑
Increased metabolism of clotting factors (fever)	↓
Confounding technical or laboratory factors (e.g., phlebotomy, handling in transport, thromboplastin reagents)	Variable

*↑ = prothrombin time (PT) or INR prolonged; ↓ = PT or INR decreased.

†Consult drug-interaction reference for new medications.

Drug interactions with warfarin are numerous and complex. Emergency physicians should carefully review medications prescribed on ED discharge, and **it is recommended that drug–drug interaction references be utilized whenever adding a new medication to a patient on warfarin.** Drugs frequently prescribed upon ED discharge should generally be avoided in patients on warfarin because of the increased risk of bleeding, including nonsteroidal anti-inflammatory drugs, sulfa-containing drugs (e.g., sulfamethoxazole), macrolides (with the exception of azithromycin), and fluoroquinolones. Drugs that induce hepatic cytochrome P-450 activity may increase the metabolism and reduce the effect of warfarin. Because the effect may take several days to manifest, the following agents should only be prescribed upon ED discharge after careful review and with close follow-up: barbiturates, anticonvulsants (e.g., phenytoin, carbamazepine, primidone), antibiotics (e.g., dicloxacillin, nafcillin, rifampin), and antipsychotics or sedatives (e.g., haloperidol, trazodone).

The two important principles when warfarin-treated patients bleed with a prolonged INR are (1) attempt to identify and attenuate the cause of bleeding, and (2) lower the intensity of the anticoagulant effect. In patients with a modestly elevated INR without clinically evident bleeding, cessation of warfarin, careful observation, and periodic monitoring comprise the safest course (**Figure 239-1**).[2,6,7] Conversely, reversal is recommended when the INR is markedly elevated or there is clinically significant bleeding.[2,7] The speed and extent of reversal should be balanced against the risk of recurrent thromboembolism in patients who require therapeutic anticoagulation. For example, an over-anticoagulated patient with a prosthetic mitral valve may develop fatal thrombosis if supratherapeutic anticoagulation is rapidly and fully reversed.

Three approaches used to reverse warfarin-induced coagulopathy are as follows: (1) stop warfarin therapy; (2) administer **vitamin K_1** (PO or IV); and (3) replace deficient coagulation factors using either **fresh frozen plasma, 3- for 4-factor prothrombin complex concentrate**, or **recombinant activated factor VII (Figure 239-1)**.[2,8-11] In asymptomatic patients with an elevated INR of 4.5 to 10 due to warfarin, oral vitamin K_1 1.0 to 2.0 milligrams will produce a measurable reduction in INR by 16 hours, with a therapeutic level by the second day.[6,7] In asymptomatic patients with an INR >10, oral vitamin K_1 2 milligrams is also effective, although the reduction in INR takes longer. Although low-dose oral vitamin K_1 carries a small risk for patients who require therapeutic anticoagulation, it is recommended that the emergency physician consult an appropriate specialist before using vitamin K_1 to reverse anticoagulation in stable patients.

IV vitamin K_1 carries a rare but serious, non–dose-dependent risk of anaphylaxis and should not be used for routine reversal of therapeutic

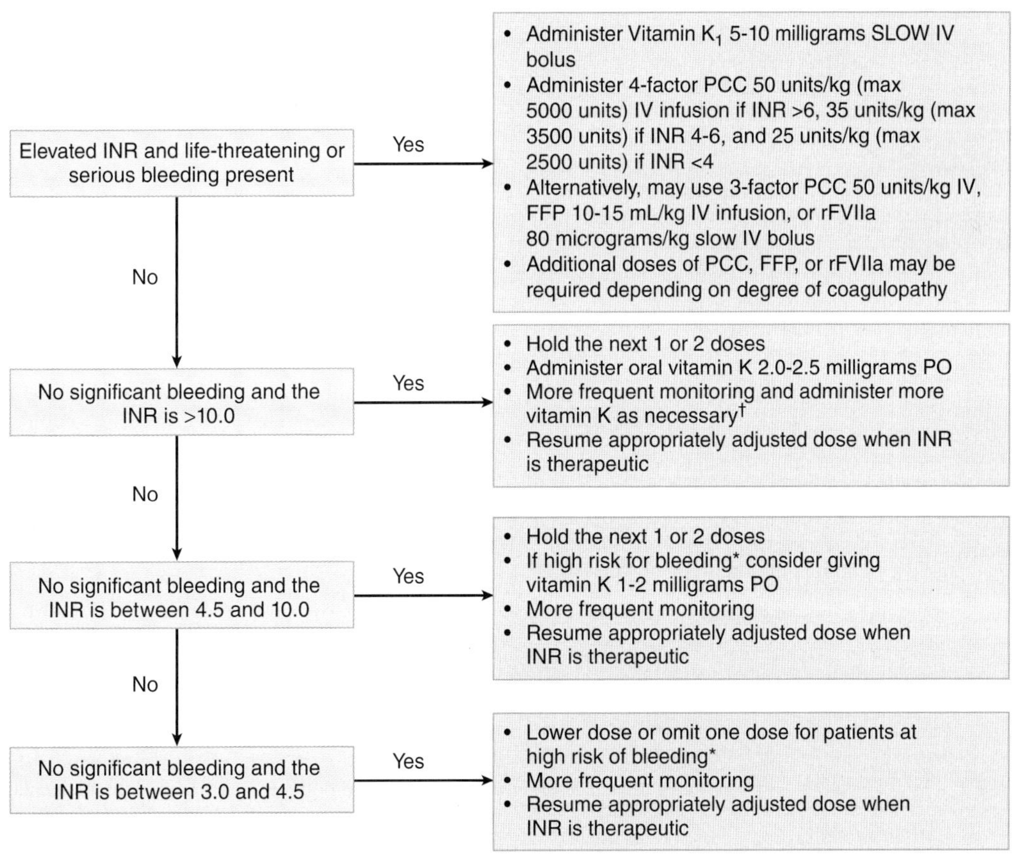

FIGURE 239-1. Management of prolonged INR (warfarin-induced coagulopathy). *High risk of bleeding: age >75 years, concurrent antiplatelet drug use, polypharmacy, liver or renal disease, alcoholism, recent surgery, or trauma. †There are no validated tools to predict risk of short-term major bleeding in patients with severe over-anticoagulation. The decision to admit for observation relies on physician judgement. FFP = fresh frozen plasma; 4-factor PCC = Prothrombin Complex Concentrate containing coagulation factors 2, 7, 9, and 10; 3-factor PCC = Prothrombin Complex Concentrate containing coagulation factors 2, 9, and 10; rFVIIa = recombinant activated factor VII.

over-anticoagulation. For patients who require continued anticoagulation, IV administration also carries the risk of overcorrection not associated with oral use. IV vitamin K_1 should be restricted to those patients with life-threatening bleeding[2] and to symptomatic patients poisoned by an excessive ingestion of warfarin (e.g., suicidal overdose). Generally, overdose patients do not require long-term therapeutic anticoagulation, and reversal does not carry the risk of recurrent thrombosis.

The fastest method of reversing therapeutic over-anticoagulation is with coagulation factor infusion, using either fresh frozen plasma, prothrombin complex concentrates, or recombinant activated factor VII.[8-11] For patients with intense anticoagulation (INR >10) who require only partial reversal, fresh frozen plasma 10 to 15 mL/kg would be expected to restore coagulation factors to about 30% of normal, corresponding to an INR of 1.7 to 1.8. Disadvantages of fresh frozen plasma include potential fluid overload, which can be difficult to reverse with furosemide. Some institutions provide **"universal donor" fresh frozen plasma**, which is derived from AB+ donors and thus contains no AB antibodies. If available and indicated, it can be given without a type and cross-match of blood of the recipient and as soon as it is defrosted (20 to 30 minutes).

For patients with life-threatening hemorrhage who require rapid, complete reversal, such as warfarin-associated intracranial hemorrhage, **prothrombin complex concentrates** or recombinant activated factor VII are preferred.[12-14] Four-factor prothrombin complex concentrate is preferred over the 3-factor product, and dosing is according to the patient's INR level; expert consultation is advised prior to administration. Additional doses of these products may be required depending on the degree of coagulopathy.

DIRECT THROMBIN INHIBITORS

Dabigatran etexilate, an oral direct thrombin inhibitor, is used to reduce the risk of stroke and systemic embolism in patients with nonvalvular atrial fibrillation, and the risk of recurrent DVT or PE after treatment of the acute episode.[1,15-18] After ingestion, dabigatran etexilate is converted to the active agent dabigatran by esterase, achieving peak serum concentrations in 2 hours with a terminal elimination half-life of 12 to 17 hours. Dabigatran is a reversible inhibitor of both circulating and clot-bound thrombin. Dabigatran has more predictable pharmacologic activity than warfarin, a broad therapeutic window, low interpatient variability, and no significant drug–drug (except for rifampin) or drug–diet interactions. Monitoring with standard coagulation tests during therapeutic use is not required. In routine use in patients with atrial fibrillation, dabigatran is generally safer than warfarin, with the notable exception of a higher risk of major GI bleeding. As with warfarin, the concomitant use of nonsteroidal anti-inflammatory drugs and other antiplatelet medications greatly increases the risk of bleeding for patients taking dabigatran.

Prothrombin time and the aPTT are insensitive to the activity of dabigatran, whereas the thrombin clotting time is typically overly sensitive.[1,19] The ecarin clotting time has a linear dose response through the range of dabigatran concentrations seen during clinical use, but this test is not commonly available. **For practical purposes, a normal thrombin clotting time excludes a significant coagulopathy due to dabigatran.**[1]

Only about 15% to 20% of absorbed dabigatran is metabolized, and the remainder is excreted unchanged in the urine. It is therefore important to maintain urinary output in patients with active bleeding while taking dabigatran to enhance drug elimination. **If emergency measures are required to reverse the anticoagulant effect of dabigatran, hemodialysis can be effective with removal of 60% or more of the drug within 2 hours.**[1,11,20]

Idarucizumab, a monoclonal antibiotic fragment that binds dabigatran, is in development to reduce serious bleeding or reverse anticoagulation in patients who require an urgent procedure in patients taking dabigatran.[20] Until idarucizumab is available, observational experience suggests that both recombinant activated FVII (rFVIIa) or activated prothrombin complex concentrate (aPCC) can reverse the anticoagulative effect of dabigatran,[21,22] whereas fresh frozen plasma does not.[1]

FACTOR Xa (FXa) INHIBITORS

Rivaroxaban and apixaban, oral direct FXa inhibitors, are used for the prevention of venous thromboembolism in adult patients undergoing elective hip or knee replacement surgery and for the reduction of the risk of stroke and systemic embolism in patients with nonvalvular atrial fibrillation.[1,23] Edoxaban, a third orally active direct FXa inhibitor is likely to become available soon for similar indications.[24] These FXa inhibitors have predictable pharmacologic properties and do not require routine laboratory monitoring.

The effect of rivaroxaban or apixaban on blood clotting is not easy to reliably measure. Although FXa inhibitors demonstrate a dose-dependent increase in prothrombin time, the sensitivity of this assay varies according to the thromboplastin reagent used. The activated partial thromboplastin time is less sensitive than the prothrombin time for measuring effects of FXa inhibitors. The currently available anti–FXa activity assays must be adjusted for the specific FXa inhibitor used.

Rivaroxaban and apixaban are metabolized by the liver, with about two thirds of the drug and metabolites excreted by the kidneys with an elimination half-life of 5 to 12 hours in healthy individuals. Discontinuation of the drug for at least 24 hours could be sufficient when there is no imminent need for reversal, as in elective or nonurgent procedures. However, in patients with renal impairment and the elderly, additional time for clearance would be required before any surgical procedures are undertaken. There is an increased risk of stroke or other thrombotic event when rivaroxaban is suddenly discontinued in patients with nonvalvular atrial fibrillation.[25] When possible, another anticoagulant should be substituted.

Andexanet alfa, a recombinant modified FXa, is in development for treatment of major bleeding due to FXa inhibitors, but is currently not available for clinical use. Due to high plasma protein binding, rivaroxaban or apixaban are not readily removed by dialysis. Current options for the emergency reversal include transfusion of blood products such as fresh frozen plasma, prothrombin concentrate complex, or recombinant activated factor VII.[1,23,26]

Administration of **activated charcoal** within 2 hours of taking an oral anticoagulant may adsorb the drug from the intestines before it reaches the plasma. It would be reasonable to administer activated charcoal to a patient who has deliberately or accidentally ingested an inappropriate amount of dabigatran, rivaroxaban, or apixaban, and likewise in a patient with significant bleeding who has recently ingested even a therapeutic dose.

HEPARINS AND POLYSACCHARIDES

UNFRACTIONATED HEPARIN (UFH)

Unfractionated heparin (UFH) is a heterogeneous mixture of polysaccharides ranging in molecular weight from 3 to 30 kD, with most commercial preparations possessing a mean molecular weight of about 15 kD, corresponding to about 45 saccharide units.[27,28] The anticoagulant effect of UFH requires binding to antithrombin (previously named antithrombin III), and heparins are therefore "indirect" anticoagulants.[27,28] Although the UFH–antithrombin complex interferes with several activated factors in both the extrinsic and common coagulation pathways (Xa, IXa, XIa, and XIIa, and thrombin), the primary anticoagulant effect of heparin is due to thrombin and FXa inhibition. The majority of heparin's anticoagulant effect is dependent on a unique pentasaccharide sequence found in only about one third of heparin molecules. Variations in polysaccharide chain lengths found in UFH likely contribute to the unpredictable nature of heparin's dose-response relationship.

UFH is given parenterally with a half-life (30 to 150 minutes) that depends on the dose and route. Weight-based IV UFH dosing protocols are the most reliable approach for achieving a therapeutic effect and preventing further thrombosis during acute thromboembolic events.[28] Subcutaneous UFH heparin is not recommended for the treatment of acute thromboembolic disease because the bioavailability via this route of administration ranges from 10% to 90%, depending on the dose. However, subcutaneous UFH can be used to prevent thromboembolism (**Table 239-1**). **Because UFH interferes with most laboratory investigations for hypercoagulable states, these tests should ideally be ordered before the patient is anticoagulated.** Neither UFH nor low-molecular-weight heparin crosses the placenta; consequently, both are safe to use in pregnancy.

UFH has an unpredictable anticoagulation effect, requires frequent monitoring, binds nonproductively to vascular endothelium and ubiquitous plasma proteins, and actually activates platelets by interacting with platelet factor 4. The unpredictable inhibition of thrombin by heparin is attributable to a low bioavailability from extensive nonspecific binding to serum proteins, macrophages, and endothelial cells. The anticoagulant effect of UFH is generally monitored with the activated partial thromboplastin time (**Table 239-1**).[28] For most purposes, a therapeutic range for UFH can be either an activated partial thromboplastin time of 1.5 to 2.5 times the "normal" value, a heparin level of 0.2 to 0.4 units/mL when assayed by protamine titration, or a level of 0.3 to 0.7 units/mL when measured for anti–FXa activity. UFH can increase the prothrombin time by a variable amount, typically 1 to 5 seconds depending on the heparin concentration and the thromboplastin reagent used in the assay.

LOW-MOLECULAR-WEIGHT HEPARIN (LMWH)

Low-molecular-weight heparins (LMWH) are polysaccharide chains ranging in molecular weight from 2 to 9 kD, with commercial preparations (enoxaparin, dalteparin, and tinzaparin) possessing a mean molecular weight of approximately 4 to 5 kD, corresponding to about 15 saccharide units. LMWH possesses many clinical advantages compared to the parent compound (**Table 239-3**).[27] Both UFH and LMWH exert their anticoagulant effect by binding to and enhancing the activity of antithrombin. This interaction is mediated by a unique pentasaccharide sequence that induces a conformational change in antithrombin, enhancing binding to and inaction of thrombin and factors Xa, IXa, XIa, and XIIa. Inhibition of thrombin is facilitated by an additional 13-saccharide group that brings the key binding regions of antithrombin and thrombin into contact. However, only the specific pentasaccharide sequence is necessary to bind to antithrombin for effective inhibition of FXa. UFH inhibits FXa and thrombin in roughly equal proportions (anti–FXa to anti-thrombin activity ratio about 1) because chains of at least 18 saccharide units predominate. In contrast, more than half of LMWH molecules are smaller than 18 saccharide units, resulting in a reduced ability to inactivate thrombin and an enhanced affinity for inactivating FXa (anti–FXa to anti-thrombin activity ratio between 2:1 and 4:1).[28]

LMWH is cleared by the kidneys, and bleeding complications due to accumulation of the agent can occur in patients with significant renal impairment. Appropriate dosing of LMWH in patients with severe renal insufficiency (creatinine clearance <30 mL/min) is unclear. In patients with severe renal insufficiency, it is suggested that either a reduced dose of enoxaparin (50% of the usual amount) be used or UFH be administered instead.[28] Obese patients (body mass index >30) should receive weight-based LMWH dosing.[28]

The plasma half-life of LMWH is two to four times longer than UFH, allowing for once- or twice-daily dosing. LMWH has a decreased binding affinity for plasma proteins, endothelial cells, and macrophages, thus yielding a more predictable anticoagulant and dose-response relationship, allowing for SC administration at fixed dosages. There are greatly reduced interactions with the platelet factor 4 receptor, resulting in a much lower incidence of heparin-induced thrombocytopenia than that seen with UFH. Laboratory monitoring of the activity of LMWH is unnecessary in most patients. If required, anti–FXa activity obtained 4 hours after drug administration is recommended, with a therapeutic range of 0.6 to 1.0 units/mL for enoxaparin.

TABLE 239-3 Advantages of Low-Molecular-Weight Heparin over Unfractionated Heparin

Pharmacologic Effects	Clinical Benefit
Quick and predictable SC absorption	More reliable level of anticoagulation
More stable dose response	Eliminates need for monitoring
Resistance to inhibition by platelet factor 4	Decreased incidence of thrombocytopenia
Decreased antiheparin antibody production	Greater antithrombotic effects
Greater anti–FXa activity	Potential for reduced bleeding
Less anti-thrombin activity	Absence of "rebound"
Ease of administration	Outpatient therapy

FONDAPARINUX

Fondaparinux is a synthetic pentasaccharide that binds to antithrombin and enhances its affinity for FXa, but not thrombin.[15,28] Fondaparinux is administered by SC injection using fixed doses stratified according to the indication and body weight (**Table 239-1**). The drug has a terminal half-life of about 17 hours, which allows for once-daily dosing. Laboratory monitoring of the activity of fondaparinux is unnecessary in most patients. If required, a fondaparinux-specific anti–FXa activity assay measured 3 hours after drug administration is recommended, but a therapeutic range has not been established.

COMPLICATIONS AND MANAGEMENT

The two major complications of heparin are bleeding and heparin-induced thrombocytopenia.[28-30] Up to one third of patients receiving UFH develop some form of bleeding complication, with a 2% to 6% incidence of major bleeding.[28] An increased risk of up to 20% for major bleeding is associated with concomitant conditions, such as recent surgery or trauma, renal failure, alcoholism, malignancy, liver failure, and GI bleeding, as well as the concurrent use of warfarin, fibrinolytics, steroids, or antiplatelet drugs.

Bleeding in patients being treated with UFH is managed according to the clinical severity and less by activated partial thromboplastin time level (**Table 239-4**).[2,28] Heparin-associated bleeding is not always reflected by a supratherapeutic activated partial thromboplastin time, so if bleeding develops during UFH therapy, heparin administration should be stopped immediately. **Although UFH half-life is dose dependent (30 to 150 minutes), its anticoagulation effect can last up to 3 hours.** Observation may be appropriate in less severe cases, with serial activated partial thromboplastin time used to determine when therapy may be resumed. Although **protamine** can reverse the anticoagulant effect of UFH, the adverse effects of protamine are significant. Protamine should be given slowly IV over 1 to 3 minutes and should not exceed 50 milligrams in any 10-minute period. However, because the half-life of protamine is shorter (7 minutes) than heparin, an anticoagulant rebound may occur, requiring a second treatment. Reversal of subcutaneously administered heparin may require repeated or prolonged protamine administration. Allergic reactions are possible, and approximately 0.2% of patients receiving protamine develop anaphylaxis. Thus, protamine should be reserved for major bleeding complications.

Platelet count may fall in 10% to 20% of patients 2 to 3 days following initiation of UFH treatment due to nonimmunologic direct platelet aggregation. This process is sometimes termed "heparin-associated thrombocytopenia" and was previously termed "type I heparin-induced thrombocytopenia." The platelet nadir is typically no lower than 100,000/mm^3 (100×10^9/L), there is no risk for associated thrombosis, and platelet count recovers within 4 days despite continued heparin treatment.

Heparin-induced thrombocytopenia (previously termed type II heparin-induced thrombocytopenia or HIT) is a syndrome due to the formation of immunoglobulin G or immunoglobulin M autoantibodies directed against both heparin and platelet factor 4 that activates platelets, producing both thrombocytopenia and a tendency for thrombosis.[30] Thrombosis may involve the skin (similar to warfarin-induced cutaneous necrosis), major arteries (e.g., ischemic limbs), or the veins (e.g., recurrent venous thrombosis or pulmonary embolism). The onset of HIT is usually 5 to 10 days after heparin treatment is started but may be sooner for patients who developed an antibody from a previous heparin exposure. Although rare, one of the earliest clues is an anaphylactoid reaction within 30 minutes of receiving an IV bolus of heparin, often while the patient is in the ED. Patients who exhibit acute systemic reactions such as fevers, chills, hypertension, tachycardia, dyspnea, or chest pain should be evaluated for HIT by obtaining an immediate platelet count. Because a decrease in platelet count may be transient and under these circumstances heparin is often stopped, the diagnosis can be missed if there is a delay in obtaining the platelet count.[30]

The incidence of HIT is variable and influenced by the specific heparin preparation used, dose, duration, and patient characteristics. In

TABLE 239-4 Emergency Treatment of Bleeding Complications of Antithrombotic Therapy

Agent	Management
Heparins	
Minor bleeding	Immediate cessation of heparin administration. Supratherapeutic aPTT not always present. Anticoagulation effect lasts up to 3 h from last IV dose. Observation with serial aPTT may be sufficient.
Major bleeding	Protamine 1 milligram IV per 100 units of total amount of IV UFH administered within the past 3 h. Protamine is given slowly IV over 1–3 min with a maximum of 50 milligrams over any 10-min period. Protamine has an anaphylaxis risk. Protamine does not completely reverse low-molecular-weight heparin. Enoxaparin: Protamine 1 milligram IV (maximum dose, 50 milligrams) for every 1 milligram of enoxaparin given in the previous 8 h. If 8–12 h since last enoxaparin dose, give protamine 0.5 milligram IV for every 1 milligram of enoxaparin given. Dalteparin and tinzaparin: Protamine 1 milligram IV per every 100 units of dalteparin or tinzaparin given. If aPTT (measured 2–4 h after the protamine infusion) remains prolonged, give a second dose of protamine 0.5 milligram IV per 100 units of dalteparin or tinzaparin.
Pentasaccharides	
Fondaparinux	Antithrombotic effect of fondaparinux is 24–30 h. For life-threatening bleeding, anecdotal evidence suggests rFVIIa 90 micrograms/kg IV is effective.
Oral Direct Thrombin Inhibitors	
Dabigatran	Oral activated charcoal if recent or excessive ingestion. Maintain urine output. Consider hemodialysis or charcoal hemoperfusion For life threatening bleeding, consider in descending order: aPCC, rFVIIa, or PCC. For severe bleeding or urgent reversal, Idarucizumab (when available), dose not established.
Oral Factor Xa Inhibitors	
Rivaroxaban	For major bleeding, experimental evidence suggests PCC can reverse the antithrombotic effect of rivaroxaban.
Apixaban	For major bleeding, andexanet alfa (when available), dose not established.
Oral Antiplatelet Agents	
Aspirin	Desmopressin 0.3–0.4 microgram/kg IV over 30 min. Platelet transfusion to increase count by 50,000/mm^3 (typically requires one single donor apheresis-collected platelet concentrate or 6 units of random donor platelets). Aspirin-induced platelet inhibition may last for 7 d, so repeat platelet transfusions are sometimes required.
Other antiplatelet agents: clopidogrel, prasugrel, ticagrelor	Platelet transfusion to increase count by 50,000/mm^3 (typically requires one single donor apheresis-collected platelet concentrate or 6 units of random donor platelets). Desmopressin 0.3–0.4 microgram/kg IV over 30 min. NSAID-induced platelet inhibition typically lasts <1 d. Clopidogrel-, prasugrel-, or ticagrelor-induced platelet inhibition may last up to 5–7 d.
Fibrinolytics	
Minor external bleeding	Manual pressure
Significant internal bleeding	Immediate cessation of fibrinolytic agent, antiplatelet agent, and/or heparin. Reversal of heparin with protamine as above. Typed and cross-matched blood ordered with verification of aPTT, CBC, thrombin clotting time, and fibrinogen level. Volume replacement with crystalloid and packed red blood cells as needed.
Major bleeding or hemodynamic compromise	All measures listed for significant internal bleeding. Fibrinogen concentrate 70 milligrams/kg IV, and recheck fibrinogen level; if fibrinogen level <100 milligrams/dL, repeat fibrinogen concentrate dose. If bleeding persists after fibrinogen concentrate or despite fibrinogen level >100 milligrams/dL, administer FFP 2 units IV. If bleeding continues after FFP, administer an antifibrinolytic such as aminocaproic acid 5 grams IV over 60 min followed by 1 gram/h continuous IV infusion for 8 h or until bleeding stops, or tranexamic acid 10 milligrams/kg IV every 6–8 h. Consider platelet transfusion.
Intracranial hemorrhage	All measures listed for significant internal and major bleeding with hemodynamic compromise. Immediate neurosurgery consultation.

Abbreviations: aPCC = activated prothrombin complex concentrate (not available in the United States); aPTT = activated partial thromboplastin time; FFP = fresh frozen plasma; NSAID = nonsteroidal anti-inflammatory drug; PCC = prothrombin complex concentrate; rFVIIa = recombinant activated factor VII; UFH = unfractionated heparin.

general, between 1% and 3% of postoperative patients treated with UFH for 4 to 14 days will develop HIT, compared with only 0.1% to 1.0% of medical or obstetric patients who receive UFH for a similar duration. In general, HIT is approximately 10 times less frequent in patients treated with LMWH products. With HIT, the platelet count nadir is variable, typically 20,000 to 150,000/mm^3 (20 to 150 $\times$ 10^9/L). During treatment with UFH, it is recommended that a baseline platelet count be obtained and the count be repeated at 24 hours and every 2 to 3 days thereafter during the duration of therapy. A drop of 50% or more from baseline is considered evidence of HIT, even if the platelet count is within a normal range. It is recommended to assess for recent use of UFH or LMWH before instituting heparin therapy for a new venous thrombosis that may, in fact, be a thrombotic complication of HIT.

With HIT, all heparin therapy (including "heparin lock" IVs and heparin-coated catheters) should be stopped. Protamine is not effective against the immune-mediated response. Platelet transfusion is not indicated because bleeding is not usually a manifestation of HIT and may precipitate thrombosis. The platelet count generally returns to normal in 4 to 6 days after heparin discontinuation. During the recovery phase, the risk of arterial or venous thrombosis is substantially elevated, and the potential complications include gangrene, stroke, and myocardial infarction. LMWH is not recommended to prevent thrombosis during this recovery period because of cross-reactivity between LMWH and the antiplatelet antibody. Additionally, warfarin should not be started until the platelet count has normalized and the patient is sufficiently anticoagulated by an alternative measure to avoid precipitating arterial or venous thrombosis or producing skin necrosis. Anticoagulation with a non-heparin anticoagulant, such as danaparoid, lepirudin, fondaparinux, or bivalirudin, is recommended for strongly suspected or confirmed cases of HIT, even in the absence of symptomatic thrombosis.[30,31]

In general, LMWH preparations cause less bleeding than UFH. Other reported side effects of LMWH include local skin reaction, pruritus, and rarely skin necrosis. Protamine will neutralize the inhibitory effect of LMWH on thrombin but not the inhibitory effect on FXa. Thus, protamine will not completely reverse the anticoagulant effect of LMWH (**Table 239-4**).

For fondaparinux-associated bleeding, limited data suggest that activated recombinant factor VII and activated prothrombin complex concentrates can reverse the coagulopathy.[22,32,33]

HIRUDINS

Hirudins (hirudin and lepirudin) and hirudin analogues (bivalirudin and argatroban) are parenteral direct thrombin inhibitors, possessing several potential advantages over heparin.[17,28] Unlike heparin, direct thrombin inhibitors are capable of inhibiting both circulating and clot-bound thrombin, do not inhibit other coagulation pathway or fibrinolytic enzymes, do not require antithrombin as a cofactor for activity, and do not interact with platelet factor 4 or plasma proteins. Therefore, direct thrombin inhibitors have a more predictable anticoagulant effect than UFH. Hirudin, lepirudin, and argatroban are used for anticoagulation in patients with heparin-induced thrombocytopenia.[30,31] Bivalirudin and argatroban are potential alternatives to UFH and LMWH for the treatment of acute coronary syndrome with percutaneous coronary intervention.[34,35]

The primary adverse effect of direct thrombin inhibitors is bleeding, and the majority of bleeding events occur at invasive sites. Because the half-life of hirudin and its analogues is relatively short (<2 hours), and an antidote is not currently available, management of hemorrhage may require only stopping the IV infusion and waiting. Coagulation factor replacement with fresh frozen plasma or prothrombin complex concentrates can be used if bleeding persists.

ANTIPLATELET AGENTS

ASPIRIN

Aspirin irreversibly blocks cyclooxygenase, an enzyme that in platelets catalyzes the conversion of arachidonic acid to thromboxane A_2, and in the blood vessel wall promotes prostacyclin synthesis (**Table 239-5**).[36,37] The net effect of aspirin in ischemic arterial beds depends on the balance between reduction in thromboxane A_2 (a vasoconstrictor and platelet-aggregation inducer) and reduction in prostacyclin (a vasodilator and platelet-aggregation inhibitor). Aspirin's antithrombotic effect can be seen with doses as low as 30 milligrams, but for reliable antiplatelet effect, an initial dose of 162 to 325 milligrams is recommended (**Table 239-1**).

Aspirin is quickly absorbed in the upper GI tract (unless consumed in an enteric-coated formulation), reaches peak blood concentrations in 20 to 40 minutes, and circulates with a half-life of 3 to 4 hours. However, cyclooxygenase inactivation is irreversible and lasts for the life span of the platelet. Only non–enteric-coated aspirin should be administered when prompt onset of action is necessary, as in patients with acute coronary syndrome.[38,39]

Side effects of aspirin use are mainly GI and are dose-related. The side effects may be reduced in the maintenance therapy setting with concomitant use of antacids, enteric coating, and buffering agents. Aspirin should be avoided in patients with known hypersensitivity and used cautiously in those with bleeding disorders or severe hepatic disease. Active GI hemorrhage (e.g., bleeding peptic ulcer) is a contraindication to aspirin use. However, in acute coronary syndrome with occult GI bleeding (e.g., guaiac-positive stool), most experts favor aspirin use with careful monitoring. Daily aspirin therapy is advocated in the prevention of cardiovascular events in patients with known cardiovascular disease.

TABLE 239-5 Oral Antiplatelet Agents

	Class/Mechanism of Action	Type of Inhibition	Time to Peak Effect	Half-Life	Duration of Antiplatelet Effect	Typical Dose
Aspirin	Nonselective cyclooxygenase inhibitor	Irreversible	20–40 min	3–4 h	Up to 7 d	162–325 milligrams PO once per day
Clopidogrel	ADP receptor inhibitor Prodrug, requires production of active metabolite	Irreversible	2–4 h	7–8 h	Up to 7 d	300 milligrams PO loading dose (consider 600 milligrams if PCI is planned) followed by 75 milligrams PO once per day
Prasugrel	ADP receptor inhibitor Prodrug, requires production of active metabolite	Irreversible	1–2 h	7–8 h	5–7 d	60 milligrams PO loading dose, followed by 10 milligrams (5 milligrams if <60 kg) PO once per day
Ticagrelor	ADP receptor inhibitor	Reversible	2–3 h	7–9 h	3–5 d	180 milligrams PO loading dose, 90 milligrams PO twice per day
Dipyridamole	Multiple: reduces platelet aggregation, vasodilator, weak phosphodiesterase inhibitor	Reversible	N/A	Biphasic: 40 min and 10 h	1–2 d	200 milligrams extended-release PO twice per day (usually combined with low-dose aspirin)
Cilostazol	Phosphodiesterase inhibitor: reduces platelet aggregation, vasodilator	Reversible	N/A	11–13 h	3–4 d	100 milligrams PO twice per day

Abbreviations: ADP = adenosine diphosphate; N/A = not applicable; PCI = percutaneous coronary intervention.

The benefits of patients without cardiovascular disease are modest and almost offset by the risk of hemorrhagic stroke and major bleeding.[40,41] In general, daily aspirin therapy does reduce the incidence of myocardial infarction, ischemic stroke, and sudden cardiovascular death, with an increased risk of major bleeding events, primarily GI, and cerebral hemorrhage. The overall effect tends to be beneficial, although the magnitude of change with individual outcomes does vary with indication and between genders.

Nonsteroidal anti-inflammatory drugs reversibly inhibit platelet cyclooxygenase and have the potential to reduce the antiplatelet efficacy of aspirin. Myocardial infarction patients have an increased risk of mortality, reinfarction, heart failure, and shock if taking nonsteroidal anti-inflammatory drugs within 7 days of presentation[42] and up to 90 days after the acute event.[43] Current acute coronary syndrome guidelines contain admonitions against the use of nonsteroidal anti-inflammatory drugs.[44-47]

Upper GI irritation is the most common side effect of aspirin therapy.[37] Some patients are markedly sensitive to aspirin, such that even low doses lead to markedly prolonged bleeding times and risk of severe clinical hemorrhage, particularly related to surgery or trauma. Uremia or the combination of ethanol and aspirin are two circumstances where patients are especially sensitive to bleeding induced by aspirin.

Management of acute aspirin-induced or nonsteroidal anti-inflammatory drug–induced hemorrhage involves the transfusion of enough normal platelets to increase the platelet count by 50,000/mm^3 (50×10^9/L), a level that will halt most bleeding. Alternatively, desmopressin alone or combined with platelet transfusion can reverse the effect of aspirin on platelet function.[22] Because of the irreversible effect of aspirin on platelets, the hemostatic compromise might last for up to 7 days after aspirin has been discontinued, and platelet transfusions may have to be repeated daily.

ADENOSINE DIPHOSPHATE RECEPTOR AGENTS

Clopidogrel, prasugrel, ticagrelor, and ticlopidine inhibit platelet activation by blocking the adenosine diphosphate receptor.[37,47] These agents are also termed "membrane-deforming" agents because by inhibiting the adenosine diphosphate receptor, the adjacent region of the platelet membrane containing the fibrinogen receptor is deformed and the fibrinogen receptor is rendered ineffective.

Clopidogrel is a prodrug that is metabolized into an irreversible adenosine diphosphate receptor inhibitor. Rapidly absorbed from the GI tract, oral doses of 600 milligrams result in a full antiplatelet effect by 2 hours that is sustained for up to 48 hours. Platelet function typically returns to normal 7 days after the last clopidogrel dose. Clopidogrel is used for the treatment of acute coronary syndrome[46,47] and established peripheral artery disease,[48] as well as for secondary prevention of myocardial infarction[49] and ischemic stroke.[50] Although clopidogrel is generally well tolerated, adverse effects include dyspepsia, rash, and diarrhea. Clopidogrel can also be used in patients who have a history of aspirin hypersensitivity or major GI intolerance.

The active metabolite is produced by the cytochrome P-450 system, principally isoenzyme 2C19 (CYP2C19). Patients with a diminished CYP2C19 metabolizer status have a lessened antiplatelet response to clopidogrel. The reported frequency for poor CYP2C19 metabolizer status varies by ethnic background: approximately 2% for whites, 4% for blacks, and 14% for Chinese. A patient's CYP2C19 metabolizer status can be determined with genotype testing, and a higher dose regimen (600-milligram loading dose followed by 150 milligrams once daily) is suggested in poor metabolizers, although this dose regimen has not been validated in clinical outcome trials.[51] Omeprazole is an inhibitor of CYP2C19 and reduces the antiplatelet activity of clopidogrel if both drugs are given within 12 hours of each other. While the effect on clinical outcome from this interaction is variable according to the patient's risk for cardiovascular events, it is prudent to not give omeprazole in the ED to patients receiving clopidogrel for acute coronary syndrome.[52]

Prasugrel, like clopidogrel, is a prodrug that is converted to the active metabolite that is an irreversible inhibitor of the adenosine diphosphate receptor on platelets.[47] Prasugrel is used in the treatment of acute coronary syndrome.[49] Compared to clopidogrel, prasugrel has an increased risk of bleeding and is less effective in patients with a history of a stroke or transient ischemic attack, patients >75 years of age, and patients with a body weight of <60 kg.

Ticagrelor is a reversible adenosine diphosphate receptor antagonist that does not need to be converted by the liver into an active metabolite.[47] Ticagrelor is used in a broad range of acute coronary syndrome patients.[47,53] Compared with clopidogrel, ticagrelor reduces the subsequent deaths from all cardiovascular causes or myocardial infarction.[54] There is a modest increase in the risk of major bleeding not related to coronary artery bypass graft surgery with ticagrelor and a trend toward more intracranial bleeding.

Ticlopidine is associated with significant risk for hematologic problems, such as neutropenia and thrombotic thrombocytopenic purpura. Therefore, ticlopidine is now rarely used in the United States.

Antiplatelet therapy is a risk factor for increased intracranial bleeding and worse outcome in closed head injury.[55] The observed risk is highest with clopidogrel.[55] Uncontrolled bleeding in patients on adenosine diphosphate receptor antagonist therapy should be treated with supportive therapy, platelet transfusion, and possibly desmopressin.[22]

PHOSPHODIESTERASE INHIBITORS

Dipyridamole is both a vasodilator and antiplatelet agent.[37,56] The specific antiplatelet effects are multiple and include reversible phosphodiesterase inhibition. Clinical efficacy of dipyridamole appears to be enhanced by formation into an extended-release preparation.[56] Current recommendations highlight the use of dipyridamole when combined with aspirin for the secondary prevention of stroke or transient ischemic attacks.[50,57] A fixed combination of aspirin, 25 milligrams, and extended-release dipyridamole, 200 milligrams PO twice a day, is commonly used for this indication. Dipyridamole is occasionally used in the standard formulation (not extended release) for angina prophylaxis and the prevention of prosthetic cardiac valve thrombosis when combined with warfarin or aspirin where doses of 50 to 100 milligrams PO three or four times a day are typical. Common adverse side effects include headache, dizziness, flushing, and abdominal pain.

Cilostazol is a strong reversible phosphodiesterase inhibitor in addition to having other effects on platelet metabolism.[56] Cilostazol is used to increase walking distance in patients with peripheral arterial disease[58] and reduce the incidence of stroke in patients with cerebrovascular disease.[50]

GLYCOPROTEIN IIB/IIIA ANTAGONISTS

During platelet aggregation, fibrinogen binds to the glycoprotein platelet-surface IIb/IIIa receptor. Thus, fibrinogen attached to glycoprotein IIb/IIIa receptors connecting adjacent platelets represents the final common pathway for platelet aggregation. Three parenteral glycoprotein IIb/IIIa receptor inhibitors are currently available (**Table 239-6**).[28,59] These agents are all administered as an initial IV loading dose (bolus for abciximab and eptifibatide, and 30-minute infusion for tirofiban) followed by a continuous IV infusion. Abciximab is a noncompetitive glycoprotein IIb/IIIa inhibitor with a much longer platelet effect than its plasma half-life of 10 minutes; platelet function will take up to 48 hours to return to normal after discontinuing the infusion. Conversely, eptifibatide and tirofiban are competitive glycoprotein IIb/IIIa inhibitors, with a plasma half-life of approximately 2.5 and 2.0 hours, respectively, and functional platelet recovery is usually seen 3 to 5 hours after stopping either eptifibatide or tirofiban infusion.

Glycoprotein IIb/IIIa inhibitors produce the greatest benefit in acute coronary syndrome patients undergoing percutaneous coronary intervention.[60,61] Delaying initiation of eptifibatide to the time of percutaneous coronary intervention results in less bleeding with otherwise similar outcomes, suggesting that the preferred time for administration of glycoprotein IIb/IIIa inhibitors is in the cardiac catheterization laboratory, not in the ED.[62]

Patients receiving glycoprotein IIb/IIIa inhibitors have an increased risk for bleeding complications (often related to catheterization or coronary artery bypass surgery) but have no increased risk of intracranial hemorrhage. Treatment of major hemorrhage in patients on glycoprotein IIb/IIIa inhibitors requires red cell and platelet transfusions and replacement of coagulation factors as needed.

TABLE 239-6 Glycoprotein IIb/IIIa IV Antagonists

	Type	Mechanism of Action	Half-Life	Duration of Antiplatelet Effect	Loading Dose	Continuous Infusion
Abciximab	Monoclonal antibody fragment	Noncompetitive inhibition	10 min	24–48 h	0.25 milligram/kg IV bolus	0.125 micrograms/kg per min (maximum 10 micrograms/min) IV
Eptifibatide	Cyclic heptapeptide	Competitive inhibition	2.5 h	3–5 h	180 micrograms/kg IV bolus over 1–2 min (maximum 22.6 milligrams)	2 micrograms/kg per min (maximum 250 micrograms/min) IV
Tirofiban	Nonpeptide	Competitive inhibition	2 h	3–5 h	25 microgram/kg per min IV for 30 min	0.15 micrograms/kg per min

FIBRINOLYTICS

Although mechanisms vary, each fibrinolytic agent enhances the conversion of plasminogen to plasmin, which then enzymatically breaks apart the fibrin component of thrombi. Currently approved fibrinolytic agents include streptokinase, anistreplase, alteplase, reteplase, and tenecteplase.[63,64]

STREPTOKINASE AND ANISTREPLASE (FIRST GENERATION)

Streptokinase, derived from β-hemolytic streptococci, binds to and activates circulating plasminogen, converting it to plasmin, which in turn attacks fibrin. Circulating fibrinogen also undergoes plasmin-induced lysis, producing a state of "systemic fibrinolysis." Streptokinase is administered as a slow infusion (usually 1.0 to 1.5 million units IV over 60 minutes) and has a serum half-life of approximately 23 minutes, but in most patients, the fibrinolytic effect persists for up to 24 hours. Because of the prolonged systemic fibrinolytic state and increased risk of hemorrhage, anticoagulation with heparin is usually delayed following treatment with streptokinase.

Anistreplase, a modified active plasminogen-streptokinase complex, has an effect similar to that of streptokinase, but its chief advantage is that it can be administered as a slow bolus (usually 30 units IV over 5 minutes) and has a serum half-life of approximately 90 minutes. Anistreplase has similar benefits and adverse effects compared to streptokinase.

Both streptokinase and anistreplase are antigenic, with allergic reactions occurring in approximately 6% of patients treated with streptokinase. Antibodies to streptokinase develop approximately 5 days after treatment and persist for 6 months, so retreatment with streptokinase or anistreplase is not advised during this interval. In addition, streptokinase or anistreplase should not be administered within 12 months of a streptococcal infection.

ALTEPLASE, OR TISSUE PLASMINOGEN ACTIVATOR (SECOND GENERATION)

Alteplase, or tissue plasminogen activator, is a naturally occurring enzyme in vascular endothelial cells that directly cleaves a specific peptide bond in plasminogen, converting it to active plasmin. Alteplase has binding sites for fibrin, which would suggest specificity for activity in the thrombus and less systemic fibrinolysis.[65] Despite the in vitro clot specificity of alteplase, its clinical side effect profile is comparable to that of other fibrinolytics. The serum half-life of alteplase is 4 to 8 minutes, and it produces a shorter fibrinolytic state than streptokinase. Heparin is commonly administered shortly after the completion of alteplase infusion.[46,64] Unlike streptokinase and anistreplase, alteplase is not antigenic; allergic reactions occur in <2% of patients treated with alteplase and IV heparin. Depending on the indication, alteplase is given as a weight-based dose via an IV infusion over 60 to 90 minutes.

RETEPLASE AND TENECTEPLASE (THIRD GENERATION)

Both reteplase and tenecteplase are derived from modifications of the parent alteplase molecule, with the intent of improving both efficacy and safety.[65] Reteplase is a deletion mutant in which the fibronectin finger (high-affinity fibrin binding), epidermal growth factor, and kringle-1 (receptor binding) regions of the wild-type alteplase molecule have been deleted. These modifications prolong the half-life of reteplase to 15 minutes, nearly fourfold longer than alteplase, allowing for bolus administration of reteplase as opposed to infusion administration of alteplase.[46,64,65]

Tenecteplase is created using amino acid substitutions in four different regions of the alteplase molecule, with the intention of producing a product with a longer half-life, higher level of fibrin specificity, and extended duration.[65] The long half-life of tenecteplase (approximately 20 minutes) allows for weight-tiered bolus dosing. The specific amino acid substitutions produce a 14-fold greater fibrin specificity than alteplase and reduced systemic plasmin generation. Tenecteplase has a plasminogen activator inhibitor 1 resistance 80 times greater than alteplase, thus allowing for a longer association of tenecteplase with the fibrin-rich clot. In addition, tenecteplase does not stimulate an increase in thrombin-antithrombin complexes, in contrast to a fourfold increase following administration of streptokinase and a twofold increase after administration of alteplase, with the potential for reduced bleeding complications.

Despite theoretical advantages associated with genetic modification, neither reteplase nor tenecteplase demonstrates an absolute mortality or safety benefit in the treatment of ST-segment elevation myocardial infarction. Although bolus-dose fibrinolytics result in fewer medication errors, when compared with more complicated regimens, this has not translated into improved patient outcome.[66,67]

CONTRAINDICATIONS TO FIBRINOLYTIC THERAPY

All available fibrinolytic agents have systemic antithrombotic effects and possess the potential for serious hemorrhage. Fibrinolytic-induced bleeding can be minor (such as oozing at IV sites), major (defined as hemodynamic compromise or significant drop in hemoglobin), or catastrophic (intracranial hemorrhage). The prevalence with which bleeding occurs varies according to the condition being treated. For example, intracranial hemorrhage typically occurs in <1% of patients treated with fibrinolytics for acute myocardial infarction[46] but is seen in approximately 6% of patients treated with alteplase for acute ischemic stroke.[68] Also, the risk of hemorrhage is increased according to patient characteristics and the use of concomitant drugs that also vary according to the condition under treatment.[68] General contraindications to fibrinolytic therapy are designed to reduce the risk of major and catastrophic bleeding (**Table 239-7**).

COMPLICATIONS AND MANAGEMENT

The most significant complications of fibrinolytic therapy are hemorrhagic, and the most catastrophic complication is intracranial hemorrhage. Allergic reactions and anaphylaxis from streptokinase and anistreplase should be treated with diphenhydramine 50 milligrams IV and methylprednisolone 125 milligrams IV. Hypotension occurs in up to 10% of patients treated with either streptokinase or alteplase and is treated by slowing the fibrinolytic infusion rate and administering IV crystalloid, paying close attention to the patient's volume status.

To minimize the bleeding risks associated with fibrinolytic therapy, the following precautions should be observed: (1) avoid all unnecessary needle sticks; (2) avoid any arterial punctures; (3) limit venous access to easily compressible sites (e.g., avoid central venous lines, especially the jugular or subclavian veins); and (4) avoid both nasogastric tubes and nasotracheal intubation.

TABLE 239-7 General Contraindications to Fibrinolytic Therapy

Absolute

- Active or recent (<14 d) internal bleeding
- Ischemic stroke within the past 2–6 months
- Any prior hemorrhagic stroke
- Intracranial or intraspinal surgery or trauma within the past 2 months
- Intracranial or intraspinal neoplasm, aneurysm, or arteriovenous malformation
- Known severe bleeding diathesis
- Current anticoagulant treatment (e.g., warfarin with INR >1.7 or heparin with increased aPTT)
- Current use of a direct thrombin inhibitor or direct factor Xa inhibitor with evidence of anticoagulant effect by laboratory tests
- Platelet count <100,000/mm^3 (<100 × 10^9/L)
- Uncontrolled hypertension (i.e., blood pressure >185/110 mm Hg)
- Suspected aortic dissection or pericarditis
- Pregnancy

Relative*

- Active peptic ulcer disease
- Cardiopulmonary resuscitation for longer than 10 min
- Hemorrhagic ophthalmic conditions
- Puncture of noncompressible vessel within the past 10 d
- Significant trauma or major surgery within the past 2 wk to 2 months
- Advanced renal or hepatic disease

Abbreviation: aPTT = activated partial thromboplastin time.

*Concurrent menses is not a contraindication.

Careful monitoring of the patient is crucial. The hemoglobin level should be checked every 4 to 6 hours after fibrinolytic therapy is initiated. A fall in hemoglobin >1 to 2 grams/dL (0.6–1.2 mmol/L) should prompt a search for the source of blood loss. Most bleeding episodes (>70%) occur at vascular puncture sites, but intracranial, intrathoracic, retroperitoneal, GI, urologic, or soft tissue extremity hemorrhage may occur.

External bleeding at any site should be controlled with prolonged manual pressure (**Table 239-4**). Significant bleeding, especially from an internal site, mandates discontinuation of the fibrinolytic agent along with any antiplatelet agents and heparin. Volume replacement should be provided as necessary and supplemented with red blood cell transfusions if clinically indicated. The thrombin clotting time, activated partial thromboplastin time, platelet count, and fibrinogen level should be checked. Heparin administered within 4 hours of the onset of bleeding can be reversed with protamine.

Massive bleeding with hemodynamic compromise necessitates empiric coagulation factor replacement with cryoprecipitate (rich in fibrinogen) and/or fresh frozen plasma. If bleeding persists after appropriate cryoprecipitate and fresh frozen plasma replacement, an antifibrinolytic agent (e.g., aminocaproic acid or tranexamic acid) with or without platelets should still be administered. Fibrinolytic-associated intracranial hemorrhage requires an aggressive response with protamine (if the patient received heparin), cryoprecipitate, fresh frozen plasma, platelet transfusion, and an antifibrinolytic agent.

ANTIFIBRINOLTYIC AGENTS

Two agents are used clinically to inhibit the enzymatic degradation of fibrin by plasmin; tranexamic acid and aminocaproic acid (**Table 239-8**). Both agents are derivatives of the amino acid lysine, have low-molecular weight, can be administered both orally and IV, attach to several sites on plasminogen, prevent plasminogen from binding to fibrin, are minimally metabolized, and are primarily excreted by the kidney, but tranexamic acid has roughly 8 times the antifibrinolytic activity of aminocaproic acid.

These agents are used in hemorrhagic disorders to stop excessive bleeding and reduce perioperative blood transfusion requirements (**Table 239-9**).[69-72] Both agents had minimal use in emergency practice until a randomized clinical trial of the effect of TXA on mortality and vascular thrombotic events in 20,211 adult trauma victims was published in 2010.[73] This study found that TXA (1 gram IV over 10 minutes followed by 1 gram infused over 8 hours) reduced death due to bleeding and all-cause mortality, assessed at 4 weeks, with no observed increase in vascular thrombotic complications.[73] Mortality reduction was dependent on timing; efficacy was seen if administered within 3 hours, but not afterwards.[74,75] Based on this study and additional analysis,[76] the World Health Organization added TXA to its List of Essential Medications in 2011. There is ongoing debate about the role of TXA in trauma care with questioning about its value in the modern trauma care systems found in heavily-resourced counties as opposed to the resource-limited hospitals that provided the bulk of patients in the CRASH-2 study.[77]

Both drugs have potential to cause vascular thrombosis, with reported rates that vary according to the condition being treated.[86] The observed incidence of limb ischemic and myocardial infarction is low, less than 1%.[86] The incidence of DVT and PE is highest with patients with subarachnoid hemorrhage, 2% and 3%, respectively.[86] In adult trauma, the observed incidence of DVT or PE after treatment with IV TXA was not significantly increased in the control group, about 1% for each thrombotic event.[73]

TABLE 239-8 Antifibrinolytic Agents

Agent	Suggested Initial Adult IV Dose for Emergent Indications*	Excretion	Elimination half-life
Tranexamic acid (TXA)	10 milligrams/kg IV over 10 min (max 1 g), repeat doses every 6–8 h	95% by kidney	3 h
Aminocaproic acid (ACA)	4–5 g IV over 1 h, then 1 g/h for 8 h or until bleeding stops (max 30 g/d)	65% by kidney	2 h

*Doses vary between indications and route, consult prescribing information for specifics.

TABLE 239-9 Emergent Conditions Where Antifibrinolytic Agents Have Been Used

Condition	Comment*
Adult trauma with significant hemorrhage (BP <90 mm Hg or HR >110 bpm) or considered at risk for significant hemorrhage	TXA IV reduces death from bleeding and all-cause mortality if administered within 3 h[74,76]
Postpartum hemorrhage	TXA IV may prevent and treat excessive postpartum hemorrhage[78]
Hemoptysis	TXA IV or PO may reduce the duration and volume of bleeding[79,80]
UGI bleeding	TXA IV may reduce mortality and rebleeding rate, no effect on transfusion requirement[81]
Aneurysmal subarachnoid hemorrhage	No proven benefit[82]
GI and nasal bleeding due to hereditary hemorrhagic telangiectasia	ACA PO may reduce bleeding and transfusion requirements[83,84]
Dental bleeding in hemophilia	FDA approved indication for TXA PO
Prevent bleeding in hemophilia patients during surgery	TXA and ACA reduces bleeding and transfusion requirements[71]
Traumatic hyphema	FDA approved indication for TXA PO; both TXA and ACA prevent secondary hemorrhage[85]
Heavy menstrual bleeding	FDA approved indication for TXA PO; TXA available without prescription in Europe for menstrual bleeding
When fibrinolysis contributes to bleeding	FDA approved indication for ACA IV

Abbreviation: bpm = beats per minute.

*Not a U.S. Food and Drug Administration (FDA) approved indication unless otherwise noted.

REFERENCES

The complete reference list is available online at www.TintinalliEM.com.

CHAPTER 240

Emergency Complications of Malignancy

J. Stephan Stapczynski

INTRODUCTION

The incidence of cancer is increasing as the general population ages and individual longevity grows. More patients with active malignancy are likely to come to the ED for care because of this increase, coupled with more intensive and varied treatments being applied in the outpatient setting.[1] Many conditions that prompt these patients to come to the ED will not be due to cancer.[2,3] Conversely, there are disorders often or uniquely related to malignancy that collectively are termed *oncologic emergencies*.[4-7] These malignancy-related emergencies are broadly categorized as: (1) those due to local physical effects, (2) those secondary to biochemical derangement, (3) those that are the result of hematologic derangement, and (4) those related to therapy (**Table 240-1**).

EMERGENCIES RELATED TO LOCAL TUMOR EFFECTS

MALIGNANT AIRWAY OBSTRUCTION

Malignancy-related airway compromise is usually an insidious process that results from a mass originating in the oropharynx, neck, or superior mediastinum progressively obstructing air flow.[6,8] Acute compromise may occur with supervening infection, hemorrhage, or loss of protective mechanisms, such as muscle tone. Iatrogenic factors, such as radiation therapy, may create additional difficulties by producing local inflammation with tissue breakdown. It is helpful to classify airway impairment due to malignant tumor obstruction in two manners, as to location—from the lips and nares to the vocal cords (**upper airway**) versus those from the vocal cords to the carina (**central airway**)—and, as to nature of the obstruction—**endoluminal**, **extraluminal**, or **mixed**. Almost regardless of the cause, airway obstruction usually presents with symptoms of shortness of breath and signs of tachypnea and stridor. The physical examination may show evidence of a mass in the pharynx, neck, or supraclavicular area.

Patients with airway obstruction due to a malignant tumor are evaluated with a combination of plain radiographs, CT, and endoscopic visualization.[6,8] Direct laryngoscopy is discouraged because injudicious manipulation of the upper airway may convert a partial obstruction into a complete one by provoking bleeding or edema.[9]

Emergency management includes the administration of supplemental humidified oxygen and maintenance of the best airway possible through patient positioning. Heliox—typically a 50:50 mixture of helium and oxygen—may provide symptomatic improvement in upper airway obstruction due to cancer when combined with other therapy.[10]

Mechanical intervention for critical airway obstruction from a tumor is rarely required in the ED. For patients with critical upper airway obstruction, emergency transtracheal jet ventilation or cricothyroidotomy could be lifesaving if the obstruction is above the vocal cords (see chapter 30, "Surgical Airways"). However, the presence of an overlying tumor or swelling may render such procedures technically difficult. Alternatively, passage of the endotracheal tube beyond the area of obstruction is a consideration when the patient is progressing to complete airway occlusion.[6,9] This is best done using awake fiberoptic intubation with a 5-0 or 6-0 endotracheal tube, wire reinforced, if possible. Placement of such a tube can provide symptomatic relief and time until procedures with more sustained benefit can be performed.

The two procedures that provide sustained relief of airway obstruction are neodymium-yttrium-aluminum-garnet laser photoradiation for vaporization of obstructing tissue and placement of a self-expanding stent at the stenotic site; these two modalities are often combined.[11,12] Alternatively, variations of radiotherapy—endobronchial brachytherapy, photodynamic therapy, and external-beam radiation therapy—can be directed to the obstructing tumor, but the time for symptomatic response is longer than the mechanical approaches of laser photoradiation and stenting.

TABLE 240-1 Emergency Complications of Malignancy

Related to local tumor effects	Malignant airway obstruction
	Bone metastases and pathologic fractures
	Malignant spinal cord compression
	Malignant pericardial effusion with tamponade
	Superior vena cava syndrome
Related to biochemical derangement	Hypercalcemia
	Hyponatremia due to inappropriate antidiuretic hormone secretion
	Adrenal insufficiency
	Tumor lysis syndrome
Related to hematologic derangement	Febrile neutropenia and infection
	Hyperviscosity syndrome
	Thromboembolism
Related to therapy	Chemotherapy-induced nausea and vomiting
	Chemotherapeutic drug extravasation

BONE METASTASES AND PATHOLOGIC FRACTURES

Anatomic disruption of bone weakened by preexisting conditions is termed a *pathologic fracture*. Pathologic fractures due to malignancy most commonly affect the axial skeleton (calvarium included) and the proximal aspect of the limbs. Most pathologic fractures are due to metastases from solid tumors (e.g., breast, lung, prostate) that localize in areas of bones with high blood flow, identified as containing red marrow.[13] Most patients with pathologic fractures have a known malignancy. Patients with bone metastases usually present with localized pain and a benign outward appearance of the involved area.

Malignancy alters the normal radiographic appearance of bone, including loss of trabeculae with indistinct margins (osteolytic, or "moth eaten"), poorly demarcated areas of increased density (osteoblastic), and/or a periosteal reaction. Plain radiographs may identify only about half of metastatic bone lesions.[14] Advanced imaging is often required; CT with IV contrast, particularly when using reconstruction software, can visualize three-dimensional bone integrity and soft tissue extension, whereas MRI best delineates soft tissue and bone marrow involvement. A total-body radionuclide bone scan can be used as a screening tool to identify areas of increased bone activity that could represent additional metastatic spread.[14] However, areas of radionuclide localization on the bone scan are not specific for cancer, and additional imaging studies of these areas are necessary for confirmation.

Treatment priorities are pain relief and restoration or salvage of function. For acute pain or fracture, parenteral analgesics are recommended for rapid treatment. Patients with bone metastases often require long-acting oral opioids and other adjunctive medications for pain relief (see chapter 38, "Chronic Pain"). Approximately 80% of painful bone metastases can be helped with palliative radiotherapy, although it may take several weeks after completion of a typical 5-day course of treatment to experience maximal benefit. The majority of pathologic fractures require open surgical repair.

MALIGNANT SPINAL CORD COMPRESSION

Up to 20% of cancer patients will develop neoplastic involvement of the vertebral column, and 3% to 6% will develop spinal cord compression.[4-6,15] Most cases of malignant spinal cord compression are due to metastases to vertebral bodies from solid organ tumors. with the thoracic vertebrae being the most common location for such metastases. Spinal cord compression occurs when these metastases enlarge, erode through the vertebral cortex into the spinal canal, and compress on the spinal cord. Less common causes of malignant spinal cord compression include local spread from paraspinal tumors through the intervertebral foramen or tumors (primary or metastatic) directly involving the spinal cord or meninges.

TABLE 240-2	Malignant Spinal Cord Compression
Suspect	Patient with known cancer: especially lung, breast, prostate
	Thoracic location: 70%
	Progressive pain and worse when supine
	Motor weakness: proximal legs
	Sensory changes: initially radicular, later distal anesthesia
	Bladder or bowel dysfunction: late findings
Imaging	Plain radiographs: may detect vertebral body metastases but less sensitive and specific for malignant spinal cord compression
	MRI: modality of choice, image entire vertebral column
	CT myelography: used when MRI not available or accessible
Corticosteroids	Dexamethasone, 10 milligrams IV followed by 4 milligrams PO or IV every 6 h
	Consider starting in ED if imaging is delayed
Radiotherapy	Standard approach, beneficial in approximately 70%
	No specific radiotherapy regimen proven superior
	Prognosis highly dependent on pretreatment neurologic function
Surgery	Consider in highly selected cases, such as
	Patient in good general condition and able to undergo extensive surgery
	Appropriate prognostic life expectancy
	Rapidly progressive symptoms
	Clinical worsening during radiotherapy
	Unstable vertebral column

Approximately 90% of patients with malignant spinal cord compression will have back pain (**Table 240-2**). Such pain is often described as unrelenting, progressive, worse when supine, and located in the thoracic vertebral area. Approximately 80% of patients with malignant spinal cord compression have a prior diagnosis of cancer, so individuals with known cancer and back pain should undergo radiographic imaging. Other symptoms of malignant spinal cord compression may include muscular weakness, radicular pain, and bladder or bowel dysfunction. Weakness is most apparent in the proximal extremity musculature and may progress to complete paralysis. Sensory changes initially may be confined to a band of hyperesthesia around the trunk at the involved spinal level and that eventually becomes anesthetic distal to the level. Urinary retention (with overflow incontinence), fecal incontinence, and impotence are late manifestations.

MRI is the imaging modality of choice to define the site and degree of cord compression and to identify the presence of additional vertebral lesions. The entire spinal column is usually imaged due to the potential for multiple level involvement, although because cervical metastases are unusual, it may be reasonable to not image the cervical spine if there are no symptoms referable to that region. CT with or without myelography is used when MRI is contraindicated or inaccessible. Plain radiography may identify an abnormality in approximately 80% of patients with painful vertebral metastases. However, plain radiographs are less useful in patients with suspected malignant spinal cord compression, because radiographic findings do not always correlate with the level of spinal cord compression, and causes of malignant spinal cord compression other than vertebral body metastases will not produce visible changes in vertebral body radiographic appearance.

Use opioid analgesics for initial pain control. Consider administration of corticosteroids in the ED, especially if there will be a delay in MRI or CT myelography.[4-6,15] Typically dexamethasone, 10 milligrams IV bolus, followed by 4 milligrams PO or IV every 6 hours, is used. Further treatment, with continued corticosteroids, radiation therapy, surgery, or a combination of modalities, will depend on the life expectancy of the patient, extent of disease, and degree of motor impairment. Radiation therapy has been the typical treatment for patients with malignant spinal cord compression, and a beneficial response is seen in approximately 70% of those treated.[16] The overall prognosis for those treated with radiotherapy is highly dependent on pretreatment functional ability; approximately 90% of those who can walk at the time of diagnosis remain ambulatory after radiation treatment, about half of those who have motor function but cannot walk will recover ambulatory ability with radiotherapy, but few patients with complete paraplegia at the time of diagnosis will recover lower extremity motor function. Therefore, **malignant spinal cord compression is considered a radiotherapy emergency.** Select patients with malignant spinal cord compression may benefit from surgical tumor resection, including those with neurologic impairment (Table 240-2).[15] Because of the complex decision making from among the therapeutic options, specialists in oncology, radiotherapy, and spinal surgery should be consulted early.

MALIGNANT PERICARDIAL EFFUSION WITH TAMPONADE

Pericardial involvement, often with effusion, occurs in up to 35% of patients with all types of cancer, although the effusions are often small and remain undiagnosed.[4-6] Symptomatic pericardial effusions occur less frequently and usually result from lung or breast cancer. Other etiologies for pericardial effusions in patients with malignant disease include other tumor types (such as melanoma, leukemia, or lymphoma) and a complication of treatment (radiotherapy or chemotherapy).

Symptoms and physical examination findings are a function of pericardial fluid accumulation rate and volume (see chapter 55, "Cardiomyopathies and Pericardial Disease"). Large effusions can develop gradually and are surprisingly well tolerated. Symptoms of a pericardial effusion include dyspnea, orthopnea, chest pain, dysphagia, hoarseness, and hiccups. Physical findings include distant cardiac sounds, jugular venous distention, and a pulsus paradoxus.

A sudden increase in fluid between the nondistensible pericardium and compressible heart creates a cardiac tamponade: the low-pressure right heart is unable to accept vena caval return or pump forward to the pulmonary arteries, and the left ventricle cannot fill or produce a sustainable ejection fraction. Signs and symptoms include accentuation of those noted with pericardial effusion with additional manifestations of circulatory shock. There is usually tachycardia, hypotension, and a narrowed pulse pressure.

The ECG may demonstrate reduced voltage in the QRS complex throughout all leads, a reflection of the insulating characteristics of the effusion. Electrical alternans is a classic, although infrequent, finding with a large pericardial effusion. The cardiac silhouette on chest radiography may appear large, reflecting the gradually accumulated effusion in the stretched pericardial sac. **Echocardiography is the diagnostic tool of choice, being noninvasive, portable, and highly accurate in trained hands.** Echocardiography can not only detect the presence of a significant pericardial effusion but also assess cardiac function and identify physiologic changes associated with cardiac tamponade.

Asymptomatic pericardial effusions do not require specific treatment. Patients with symptomatic effusions should undergo pericardiocentesis, ideally with echocardiographic guidance. See chapter 34, "Pericardiocentesis." Most often, this procedure can await the arrival of the specialist and transport of the patient to the appropriate procedural area. If patients with cardiac tamponade require emergent pericardiocentesis in the ED, use a portable US device to guide needle direction during the procedure.

Malignant pericardial effusions are treated depending on the tumor type and overall patient condition. Reduction in fluid production can be done by treating the tumor with appropriate systemic chemotherapy or radiotherapy. Intrapericardial chemotherapy may be useful in tumors sensitive to these agents. A pericardial window or partial pericardial resection can be done to prevent accumulation of fluid within the pericardial space. A percutaneous indwelling intrapericardial catheter can also prevent accumulation of fluid, but with the risks associated with percutaneous devices. Malignant pericardial effusion typically indicates the presence of advanced disease, and most patients die within 1 year after diagnosis.

SUPERIOR VENA CAVA SYNDROME

The term *superior vena cava (SVC) syndrome* describes the clinical effects of elevated venous pressure in the upper body that result from obstruction of venous blood flow through the SVC.[4-6,17,18] This syndrome is most commonly caused by external compression of the SVC by an extrinsic malignant mass. The most common tumors associated with malignant SVC syndrome are lung cancer in 70% and lymphoma in approximately 20%. Benign conditions and intravascular thrombosis (precipitated by indwelling vascular catheters or pacemaker leads) currently account for about one third of all SVC syndrome cases. SVC syndrome rarely constitutes an emergency; the vast majority of patients do not materially deteriorate during the initial 1 to 2 weeks after diagnosis. The exception is when neurologic abnormalities are present due to increased intracranial pressure.

Symptom development correlates roughly with the severity of obstruction and the rate of narrowing. If compression occurs over weeks, collateral vessels dilate to compensate for impaired flow through the SVC. Most patients will describe symptoms developing a few weeks before seeking medical attention. Clinical manifestations correlate with a jugular venous pressure of 20 to 40 mm Hg (2.7 to 5.4 kPa), as compared with a normal range of 2 to 8 mm Hg (0.3 to 1.0 kPa). The most common symptoms are facial swelling, dyspnea, cough, and arm swelling.[18] Less common symptoms include hoarse voice, syncope, headache, and dizziness. In rare but extreme cases, venous obstruction can lead to increased intracranial pressure that produces visual changes, dizziness, confusion, seizures, and obtundation. Physical examination findings may show swelling of the face and arm, sometimes with a violaceous hue or plethora, and distended neck and chest wall veins.

The plain chest radiograph will usually show a mediastinal mass in cases of malignant SVC syndrome. CT of the chest with intravascular contract is the recommended imaging modality to assess the patency of the SVC.[17,18] MRI is useful for patients who cannot receive IV contrast. Contrast venography is rarely needed, except in uncertain cases or as part of an intravascular interventional procedure. In patients with a known diagnosis of lung cancer, biopsy for pathologic confirmation of a malignancy is usually not required. For patients without a known intrathoracic cancer, tissue confirmation of a malignant cause is highly desirable before initiation of radiotherapy and required before initiation of chemotherapy.[17,18]

Initial management is with head elevation to decrease venous pressure in the upper body and supplemental oxygen to reduce the work of breathing. Corticosteroids and loop diuretics are commonly used, but there is no evidence that they contribute to clinical improvement, with the exception that corticosteroids would be expected to be helpful when the cause of the obstruction is lymphoma.

Radiation therapy is effective in reducing symptoms in approximately 75% of patients with SVC syndrome, reflecting the approximate incidence of radiosensitive tumors producing this disorder.[18] Many patients will experience a reduction in symptoms within 3 days after the start of radiation treatment. The mechanism by which radiotherapy reduces symptoms in SVC syndrome is unclear, because the majority of patients receiving such treatment do not achieve complete relief of the obstruction. It is likely that continued development of collaterals contributes to the reported benefit seen during radiotherapy.

Intravascular stents, with or without angioplasty, can be used to reduce obstruction to SVC flow.[17,18] These stents appear to produce a more rapid improvement in symptoms and signs compared with radiotherapy or chemotherapy, suggesting a preferential benefit in patients with severe manifestations who require urgent treatment.[18] Stent placement should also be considered for malignant causes that do not respond well to radiotherapy or chemotherapy (like mesothelioma), for benign causes (like fibrosing mediastinitis), or for intravascular thrombosis associated with an indwelling catheter.[17,18]

Chemotherapy is effective in producing symptomatic relief from SVC syndrome in approximately 80% of patients with lymphoma, 80% of patients with small-cell lung cancer, and 40% of patients with non–small-cell lung cancer. For these chemotherapy-sensitive cancers, there is no evidence of benefit from additive radiotherapy, again indicating that dilation of venous collaterals may play a role in clinical improvement.

Patients with SVC syndrome due to intravascular thrombosis can be treated with catheter-directed fibrinolytics.[18] Removal of an inciting intravascular object, such as a central venous catheter, should be considered. Postfibrinolytic anticoagulation is generally recommended to prevent recurrence, although there is no firm supporting evidence.[18] For cancer patients with an indwelling central venous catheter, there is no proven role for prophylactic anticoagulation to reduce the risk of venous thromboembolism.[19]

Recurrence of SVC syndrome is seen in approximately 20% of lung cancer patients treated with radiotherapy and/or chemotherapy and 10% treated with intravascular stents.[18] For patients with malignant SVC syndrome, survival is dependent in the causative cancer; with lung cancer, median survival is approximately 6 to 12 months.

EMERGENCIES RELATED TO BIOCHEMICAL DERANGEMENT

HYPERCALCEMIA

Hypercalcemia is seen in 5% to 30% of patients with advanced cancer at some time during their disease course.[20] Breast cancer, lung cancer, and multiple myeloma are the malignancies most commonly associated with hypercalcemia. The three key mechanisms whereby malignancy produces hypercalcemia are: (1) by production of a parathyroid hormone–related protein that is structurally similar to parathyroid hormone, (2) by extensive local bone destruction associated with osteoclast-activating factors, and (3) by production of vitamin D analogues. The most common mechanism with solid tumor–associated hypercalcemia is the production of the parathyroid hormone–related protein that binds to parathyroid hormone receptors, thereby mobilizing calcium from bones and increasing renal reabsorption of calcium.[20] Hypercalcemia from enhanced osteoclastic activity is associated with bone metastases from lung and breast cancer, and multiple myeloma. Production of vitamin D analogues is generally seen in lymphomas, usually Hodgkin's disease.

Classic symptoms of hypercalcemia include lethargy, confusion, anorexia, and nausea (see chapter 17, "Fluids and Electrolytes"). Because most patients with hypercalcemia due to malignancy have advanced cancer, symptoms of general debility due to tumor may be difficult to distinguish from those caused by hypercalcemia. Hypercalcemia reduces intestinal motility, so constipation is common, although that symptom can be produced by concomitant opioid therapy for pain. Hypercalcemia produces an osmotic diuresis, so some of the nonspecific symptoms can be due to relative hypovolemia. **Clinical symptoms of hypercalcemia are most correlated with the rate of rise in the serum calcium level, as opposed to the actual calcium level. Therefore, slow increases in serum calcium may be relatively asymptomatic until reaching high levels.**

Hypercalcemia does not always require treatment, especially if the patient is asymptomatic and well hydrated and the total serum calcium is less than 14 milligrams/dL (3.5 mmol/L). The initial treatment of symptomatic hypercalcemia is with IV isotonic saline at a rate adjusted to the ability of the patient's cardiovascular system to tolerate a volume load.[7] A typical dose would be normal saline, 1 to 2 L bolus, to restore intravascular volume, followed by an infusion at a rate of 200 to 250 mL/h.[7] Such treatment will result in clinical improvement and a modest decrease in the plasma calcium over 24 to 48 hours but rarely normalizes the level. Furosemide is useful in patients with heart failure or renal insufficiency to prevent volume overload from normal saline infusion but has little additive effect to the use of IV saline alone in the treatment of hypercalcemia in patients with normal cardiac and renal function. **Therefore, furosemide is not routinely recommended in the treatment of hypercalcemia due to malignancy.**

Because the initial priority is restoration of intravascular volume with IV saline, pharmacologic treatment of hypercalcemia is usually not initiated in the ED.[7] **Bisphosphonates** are the recommended agents to treat malignancy-associated hypercalcemia.[7,20] Bisphosphonates are potent inhibitors of bone resorption and produce a sustained decrease in calcium 12 to 48 hours after administration, with the effect lasting for approximately 2 to 4 weeks. Bisphosphonates, such as pamidronate, etidronate, or zoledronic acid, are given by slow IV infusion to prevent precipitation of bisphosphonate-calcium complexes in the kidney and subsequent renal failure.

Other agents have a limited role in the treatment of malignancy-induced hypercalcemia. Calcitonin, 4 units/kg SC or IV every 12 hours, lowers plasma calcium within 2 to 4 hours, but it may cause a hypersensitivity response, and tachyphylaxis develops within 3 days, so the beneficial effect is short lived. Glucocorticoids, such as prednisone 60 milligrams PO per day, may be helpful with steroid-sensitive tumors, such as lymphomas and multiple myeloma.[7] Gallium nitrate, mithramycin, and plicamycin are used infrequently due to their toxicity. Hemodialysis can be used to treat hypercalcemia and is indicated for those with profound mental status changes or renal failure or for those unable to tolerate a saline load.

HYPONATREMIA DUE TO INAPPROPRIATE ANTIDIURETIC HORMONE SECRETION

Inappropriate secretion of antidiuretic hormone is most commonly associated with bronchogenic cancer but may be seen in other malignancies and can also occur from chemotherapy, opioids, carbamazepine, and selective serotonin reuptake inhibitors.[21] Regardless of the etiology, the syndrome of inappropriate antidiuretic hormone consists of hyponatremia, decreased serum osmolality, and less than maximally dilute urine, all in the presence of euvolemia, absence of diuretic therapy, and normal renal, adrenal, and thyroid function (see chapter 17). **Syndrome of inappropriate antidiuretic hormone secretion should be suspected if a patient with cancer presents with normovolemic hyponatremia.**

Signs and symptoms of hyponatremia are primarily neurologic and correlate with severity and with rapidity of development. Anorexia, nausea, and malaise are the earliest findings, followed by headache, confusion, obtundation, seizures, and coma. Seizures are usually generalized tonic-clonic in nature; focal seizures are uncommon from hyponatremia, and their occurrence suggests focal CNS lesions. Life-threatening symptoms are almost invariably associated with sodium concentrations <110 mEq/L (<110 mmol/L).

Water restriction is the mainstay of treatment in euvolemic asymptomatic patients. Patients with sodium levels >125 mEq/L (>125 mmol/L) are generally asymptomatic and can be managed with water restriction of 500 mL/d and close follow-up. More severe hyponatremia—serum sodium between 110 and 125 mEq/L with mild to moderate symptoms—may require furosemide 0.5 to 1.0 milligram/kg PO with concomitant IV normal saline to maintain euvolemia and affect a net free water clearance. **For severe hyponatremia—serum sodium <110 mEq/L, usually with coma or repetitive or sustained seizures—use 3% hypertonic saline (510 mEq/L). Infuse carefully, usually at a rate of 25 to 100 mL/h, to avoid volume overload or too rapid correction in sodium level,** with subsequent osmotic demyelination syndrome (central pontine myelinolysis). The rate of correction of hyponatremia is controversial, but serum sodium increasing at a rate of 0.5 to 1.0 mEq/L per hour, with not more than a total increase of 12 to 15 mEq/L in the first 24 hours, is recommended (see chapter 17).

ADRENAL INSUFFICIENCY

Adrenal insufficiency associated with malignancy may be secondary to adrenal tissue replacement by metastases but is more commonly due to abrupt physiologic stress in the face of chronic glucocorticoid therapy with pharmacologic adrenal suppression (see chapter 230, "Adrenal Insufficiency"). The subsequent vasomotor collapse may be sudden and severe.[22] Clues for acute adrenal insufficiency include mild hypoglycemia, hyponatremia, and hypotension refractory to volume loading and vasoconstrictor therapy.

Along with rapid IV rehydration, the stressed and steroid-dependent patient should be given hydrocortisone, 100 to 150 milligrams IV, followed by an infusion of an additional 100 to 200 milligrams IV over 6 hours.[22] If possible, obtain a serum cortisol level before steroid treatment. While results will generally not be available to the ED, values can help future management.

TUMOR LYSIS SYNDROME

Tumor lysis syndrome is a metabolic crisis resulting from massive cytolysis and release of intracellular contents into the systemic circulation.[7,23] Of particular concern are the individual ions (potassium, phosphate, calcium), nucleic acids (which metabolize to uric acid), and intracellular proteins. Tumor lysis syndrome most commonly occurs with treatment of hematologic malignancies because of rapid cell turnover and growth rates, bulky tumor mass, and high sensitivity to antineoplastic agents. Tumor lysis syndrome is uncommon with solid tumors or without prior therapy ("spontaneous tumor lysis syndrome").

The manifestations of tumor lysis syndrome can be categorized by clinical effects (acute kidney injury, seizure, cardiac dysrhythmia or arrest) and laboratory abnormalities (hyperuricemia, hyperkalemia, hyperphosphatemia, hypocalcemia). Renal failure is the strongest predictor of morbidity in tumor lysis syndrome and usually results from uric acid precipitation within the renal tubules. Phosphorus released from tumor cells may combine with calcium and precipitate in renal tubules and parenchyma as well. Hypovolemia may contribute to the renal impairment seen with tumor lysis syndrome. The release of intracellular potassium can produce acute hyperkalemia and provoke or contribute to cardiac dysrhythmias or cardiac arrest. Because malignant cells can contain fourfold the amount of phosphorus as normal cells, the abrupt release of extensive phosphate into the circulation may produce a drop in serum calcium. The resultant hypocalcemia may induce tetany and seizures and contribute to dysrhythmias.

Recognize the potential for tumor lysis syndrome with treatment of hematologic malignancies. Prophylactic allopurinol and maintaining good hydration can reduce the risk of tumor lysis syndrome developing. Patients with established tumor lysis syndrome may experience sudden electrolyte changes and life-threatening complications, so admission to an intensive care unit with cardiac rhythm monitoring is indicated. Aggressive IV fluid administration to increase urinary excretion of the released intracellular solutes is the cornerstone for treatment of tumor lysis syndrome. Increased urine flow will counteract the precipitation of urate and calcium phosphate crystals in the renal tubules.

Hyperkalemia is the most immediate life-threatening element with tumor lysis syndrome because of induced cardiac dysrhythmias and cardiac arrest.[7,23] Treatment is identical to other causes of hyperkalemia: β-adrenergic agonists, sodium bicarbonate, and dextrose-insulin therapy (see chapter 17). Avoid calcium administration unless there is cardiovascular instability (ventricular dysrhythmias or wide QRS complexes) or neuromuscular irritability (seizures) because supplemental calcium may cause metastatic precipitation of calcium phosphate. Hyperphosphatemia is managed with phosphate binders (limited effect) or by the administration of dextrose and insulin. Hemodialysis can correct all biochemical abnormalities of tumor lysis syndrome, although a large phosphate burden may require repeat frequent and prolonged dialysis sessions or continuous renal replacement therapy.[7,23]

EMERGENCIES RELATED TO HEMATOLOGIC DERANGEMENT

FEBRILE NEUTROPENIA AND INFECTION

Infections are a common source of morbidity and mortality in patients with malignancies.[24] A common feature associated with the increased risk of infection in these patients is the presence of impaired immunity, especially neutropenia.[24,25] The absolute neutrophil count normal range is 1500 to 8000/mm^3 (1.5 to 8.0 × 10^9/L). For clinical decision making, neutropenia is defined as an absolute neutrophil count <1000/mm^3 (<1.0 × 10^9/L), severe neutropenia is defined as an absolute neutrophil count <500/mm^3 (<0.5 × 10^9/L), and profound neutropenia is defined as an absolute neutrophil count <100/mm^3 (<0.1 × 10^9/L).[25,26] Fever, the most consistent finding in bacterial infection, is defined for the purposes of clinical decision making as a temperature of 38.3°C (100.9°F) on one occasion or 38.0°C (100.4°F) persisting >1 hour.[25,26]

Neutropenia in cancer patients is most commonly caused by chemotherapy, with the lowest neutrophil count typically seen 5 to 10 days after the last chemotherapeutic dose and recovery usually seen within 5 days afterward.[25-27] The risk of developing an infection primarily depends on the severity and duration of neutropenia. Comorbid conditions and other circumstances, like indwelling devices, also contribute to the risk.[4,5,7,25,26]

Fever is the most common finding seen with bacterial infections in the neutropenic patient. Common symptoms and signs that usually localize the infectious source are often absent or muted in the neutropenic patient because the lack of neutrophils impairs the inflammatory response and diminishes the occurrence of expected findings.[25] Thus, a pulmonary infection may have minimal cough, have no productive phlegm, and lack radiographic infiltrates. A kidney infection may not produce pyuria.

Perform a careful physical examination, with attention to three areas typically overlooked in routine examination: the oral cavity, the perianal area, and entry sites of intravascular catheters. **Digital rectal examination is relatively contraindicated in neutropenic patients—withhold until after initial antibiotic administration. Evaluate the entry sites of IV and tunneled catheters for evidence of infection.** Clotted catheters represent a high risk of infection due to bacterial colonization, and central venous catheters may cause endocarditis.

Localizing signs and symptoms of a specific infection are often lacking, and an evaluation for an occult infection is indicated.[25-28] Obtain two blood culture samples, one from a peripheral vein and the other from a central catheter, if present. A urinalysis, urine culture, and chest radiograph should be performed. Sputum, stool, and wound drainage Gram stain and culture should be obtained if productive cough, diarrhea, or wound drainage, respectively, are present. Assess serum electrolyte levels, renal function, and hepatic function.

Risk Factors If an infectious source is found, therapy and disposition are guided by the presumed pathogens and the expected clinical course. If, after assessment, no localized infection can be found, the two major clinical decisions are: (1) Does this patient require hospitalization, and (2) should empiric antibiotics be started? To assist in addressing both these questions, consult with the patient's oncologist.

Although hospitalization enhances the ability to reassess the patient and intervene early if a severe infection or clinical deterioration develops, hospitalization exposes the immunocompromised patient to hospital flora that is often drug resistant. Patients who appear well, have no abdominal pain, have no physical signs of infection, have a normal chest radiograph, and are expected to resolve their neutropenia within 7 days have a low risk of severe infection and can be considered for outpatient care.[25,26] Scoring systems, such as the Multinational Association for Supportive Care in Cancer Risk Index[29,30] or the Clinical Index of Stable Febrile Neutropenia[31] can be used to determine if the febrile neutropenic patient is at low risk for serious complications and eligible for outpatient care. High-risk febrile neutropenic patients for whom hospitalization is recommended are defined by one or more of the following features: profound neutropenia expected to last >7 days, comorbid medical conditions, acute liver or renal injury, or non–low-risk scores by the Multinational Association for Supportive Care in Cancer Risk Index or Clinical Index of Stable Febrile Neutropenia tool.[25,26,29-31]

Treatment Empiric broad-spectrum antibiotics are used in febrile neutropenic patients when the benefits of early treatment are greater than the adverse side effects associated with such drugs.[25-28] **Clinical evidence consistently supports the benefits of empiric antibiotics when the absolute neutrophil count is ≤500/mm³** ($<0.5 \times 10^9$/L) . There is little convincing evidence for empiric antibiotics when the absolute neutrophil count is >1000/mm³. For neutrophil counts between 500 and 1000/mm³ (0.5 and 1.0×10^9/L), other risk factors for bacterial infection are used to make a decision regarding empiric antibiotics.[25-27]

Gram-positive bacteria currently account for 60% of microbiologically confirmed infections in febrile neutropenic patients, although gram-negative bacteria are undergoing resurgence in some institutions.[25] Bacteremia is most frequently due to aerobic gram-positive cocci (*Staphylococcus aureus*, coagulase-negative staphylococci, *Viridans* streptococci, or *Enterococcus faecalis/faecium*) or aerobic gram-negative bacilli (*Escherichia coli, Klebsiella* species, or *Pseudomonas aeruginosa*).

Administer the initial empiric antimicrobial therapy to cover the range of potential bacterial pathogens (**Table 240-3**).[25-28,32,33] No specific antibiotic regimen has proven consistently superior in clinical trials, and monotherapy with an appropriate broad-spectrum agent is as effective as dual-agent treatment in most circumstances. Add vancomycin in the following situations: hemodynamic instability, radiographic pneumonia, catheter-related infection, skin or soft tissue infection, known colonization with resistant gram-positive organism, or severe mucositis when fluoroquinolone prophylaxis was recently used.[26]

TABLE 240-3 Empiric Antibiotic Therapy in Febrile Neutropenia

Circumstance	Drug and Adult Dose	Comments
Outpatient	Ciprofloxacin 500 milligrams PO every 8 h or 1000 milligrams twice daily *or* Levofloxacin 750 milligrams PO daily *plus* Amoxicillin/clavulanate 500/125 milligrams PO every 8 h or 1000/62.5 milligrams PO twice daily *or* Moxifloxacin 400 milligrams PO daily	For low-risk patients with daily assessments by a medical provider for the initial 3 d
Monotherapy	Cefepime 2 grams IV every 8 h *or* Ceftazidime 2 grams IV every 8 h *or* Imipenem/cilastatin 1 gram IV every 8 h *or* Meropenem 1 gram IV every 8 h *or* Piperacillin/tazobactam 4.5 grams IV every 6 h	Monotherapy with these broad-spectrum agents is as good as dual-drug therapy in most circumstances
Dual therapy	One of the monotherapy agents *plus*	Increased risk of adverse effects
	Vancomycin 1 gram IV every 12 hours	If hemodynamic instability, catheter-related infection, cellulitis, pneumonia, or known colonization with resistant organism
	or	
	Metronidazole 1 gram IV, followed by 500 milligrams IV every 6 h	If abdominal symptoms are present

The median duration of fever after initiation of empiric antibiotics is 2 days in low-risk patients and 5 to 7 days in high-risk patients. Therefore continue initial empiric antibiotic therapy for 2 to 4 days before assessing clinical response and making therapeutic adjustments. Adjustments may be made earlier if clinical deterioration occurs or culture results become available. Continue empiric antibiotics until either a documented infection has clinically resolved and/or the absolute neutrophil count is >500/mm³ ($>0.5 \times 10^9$/L).[25,26]

HYPERVISCOSITY SYNDROME

Hyperviscosity syndrome is a pathologic condition in which blood is "thicker" than normal and its flow is impaired.[34,35] Blood viscosity depends on its plasma and cellular contents. Abnormal plasma contents that most commonly produce hyperviscosity are Waldenström's macroglobulinemia and immunoglobulin A–producing myeloma.[34] Hyperproduction of any cell line can lead to hyperviscosity. Polycythemia (with a hematocrit >60%) and leukemia (with a WBC count >100,000/mm³ ($>100 \times 10^9$/L) or a leukocrit >10%) are often are associated with clinically significant hyperviscosity.[35] Dehydration exacerbates hyperviscosity.

Initial symptoms are vague and may include fatigue, abdominal pain, headache, blurry vision, or, most commonly, altered mental status.[32-36] Cutaneous or mucosal bleeding is common. Intravascular thrombosis may occur, with the creation of focal or unusual findings. Patients with hyperleukocytosis often report dyspnea and fever. Funduscopic findings include retinal venous engorgement appearing as linked sausages, along with exudates, hemorrhages, and papilledema.

Laboratory findings suggesting hyperviscosity include rouleaux formation (red cells stacked like coins) on a peripheral blood smear and being unable to perform chemical testing due to serum stasis in the laboratory analyzers. Laboratory testing of blood viscosity is usually done on plasma or serum, and specific analytic methodology varies.[36] A common approach is to report the viscosity of the sample as a ratio to that of water; normal plasma viscosity is 1.7 to 2.1 and normal serum viscosity is 1.4 to 1.8, compared with water. Symptomatic patients usually have a serum viscosity >4.[36] **Laboratory measurement of plasma or serum viscosity will not identify hyperviscosity from polycythemia or leukemia.**

Initial therapy is intravascular volume repletion, early involvement of a hematologist, and emergency plasmapheresis or leukapheresis.[34-36] If coma is present and the diagnosis established, a temporizing measure can be a 2-unit (1000-mL) phlebotomy with concomitant volume replacement using 2 to 3 L of normal saline.[35] Transfusion of red blood cells should be done with caution because such treatment may increase blood viscosity. Long-term management is appropriate chemotherapy.

THROMBOEMBOLISM

Thromboembolism occurs with all tumor types and is the second leading proximate cause of death in cancer patients.[37-39] Symptomatic deep venous thrombosis occurs in approximately 15% of all patients with cancer and up to 50% of those with advanced malignancies.[37-39] Multiple factors contribute to an increased risk for thromboembolism. The tumor may release procoagulant factors or inflammatory cytokines that directly activate the coagulation system. Large tumors may cause venous obstruction and promote thrombosis. Impaired production of proteins C and S and antithrombin can produce a hypercoagulable state. Surgery with attendant postoperative immobilization or long-term central venous catheterization can incite thrombosis. Chemotherapy or hormonal therapy for breast cancer increases the risk for thromboembolism. The angiogenesis inhibitors thalidomide, sunitinib, and bevacizumab are associated with significant thrombotic risks.[37-39]

Low-molecular-weight heparin (LMWH) is recommended as the initial treatment for 5 to 10 days in cancer patients with venous thromboembolism, both deep venous thrombosis and pulmonary embolism.[40,41] Continued treatment with low-molecular-weight heparin for at least 6 months is also recommended because of better efficacy in preventing recurrent thromboembolic events compared to vitamin K antagonists.[41,42] There is little experience with the novel oral anticoagulants, so their use is not recommended.[41]

EMERGENCIES RELATED TO THERAPY

CHEMOTHERAPY-INDUCED NAUSEA AND VOMITING

Nausea and vomiting can be debilitating to an already compromised patient. Because most IV chemotherapeutic agents are emetogenic, antiemetics are commonly administered on the day of therapy and for 2 to 4 days afterward.[43] Guidelines recommend specific antiemetic regimens based on the emetogenic potential of the chemotherapeutic agent.[43,44] Recommended antiemetics include neurokinin-1 receptor antagonists, serotonin receptor antagonists, and corticosteroids (**Table 240-4**).[45] For refractory nausea and vomiting, benzodiazepines, dopamine receptor antagonists, or antipsychotic agents are added.[43]

Chemotherapy-induced vomiting can be anticipatory, acute, or delayed.[45] Anticipatory vomiting is a conditioned reflex where vomiting occurs prior to administration of the chemotherapeutic agent. Acute vomiting occurs during the first 24 hours with maximal intensity at 5 to 6 hours after administration. Delayed vomiting has maximal intensity 48 to 72 hours after administration and can last up to 7 days.

EXTRAVASATION OF CHEMOTHERAPEUTIC AGENTS

Most chemotherapeutic agents cause local tissue reaction when extravasated, but the agents associated with significant tissue damage are the vesicants primarily in the anthracycline, taxane, platin salt, and vinca alkaloid classes.[46-48] Clinical manifestations of chemotherapeutic drug extravasation include pain, erythema, and swelling, usually within hours of the infusion. Occasionally, clinical signs may be delayed if only a small amount of highly cytotoxic drug is extravasated. Serious injury produces blistering, induration, ulceration, and necrosis over a few days to weeks.

If extravasation happens to occur through an active peripheral line, the infusion is stopped and aspiration through the line is attempted and continued while the catheter is removed.[48] Aspirate palpable cutaneous blebs containing the extravasated chemotherapeutic agent. Elevate and

TABLE 240-4 Antiemetic Agents for Chemotherapy-Induced Vomiting

Class and Agent	Initial Adult Dose	Comments
Neurokinin-1 (NK1) Receptor Antagonists		
Aprepitant	125 milligrams PO	Expensive, use restricted to highly emetogenic chemotherapy agents, half-life 9–14 h
Fosaprepitant	150 milligrams IV	
Serotonin Receptor Antagonists		
Granisetron	1 milligram (10 micrograms/kg) IV	Common reactions: headache, abdominal pain
Ondansetron	8 milligrams (0.15 milligrams/kg) IV	Serious reactions: serotonin syndrome, QT interval prolongation
Palonosetron	0.25 milligram IV	Half-lives vary from 5 h for ondansetron, 9 h for granisetron, and 40 h for palonosetron
Tropisetron*	5 milligrams IV	
Ramosetron*	0.3 milligram IV	
Corticosteroids		
Dexamethasone	8–12 milligrams IV	Mechanism unknown
Benzodiazepines		
Lorazepam	1–2 milligrams IV	Sedation, half-life 14 h
Midazolam	1 milligram IV or 5 milligrams IM	Sedation, half-life 2–3 h
Dopamine Receptor Antagonists		
Metoclopramide	10 milligrams IV or IM	Dose-related extrapyramidal side effects, half-life 5–6 h
Prochlorperazine	5–10 milligrams IV or IM	Extrapyramidal side effects, half-life 7 h
Antipsychotics		
Olanzapine	10 milligrams PO or IM	Not FDA approved for this indication, half-life 21–54 h

Abbreviation: FDA = U.S. Food and Drug Administration.

*Not available in the United States.

TABLE 240-5 Antidotes for Selected Extravasated Chemotherapeutic Drugs

Drug	Antidotes	Comments
Anthracyclines (daunorubicin, doxorubicin, epirubicin, and idarubicin)	Dry cooling	Initially 1 h, then 15 min several times per day Hold during dexrazoxane therapy
	Dexrazoxane	IV infusion within 6 h, repeat doses at 48 and 72 h
	Dimethyl sulfoxide	Apply over involved area, repeat 4–6 times per day for 7 or more days
Vinca alkaloids (vincristine and vinblastine)	Dry warming	Do not press or rub area
	Hyaluronidase	Inject in and around extravasated area
Mitomycin, cisplatin, mechlorethamine	Dry cooling	Initially 1 h, then 15 min several times per day
	Dimethyl sulfoxide	Apply over involved area, repeat 4–6 times per day for 7 or more days
Paclitaxel	Hyaluronidase	Inject in and around extravasated area

immobilize the affected limb. Cooling or warming is beneficial for some agents (**Table 240-5**). Consult with the oncologist for treatment recommendations. Early referral to a plastic surgeon is suggested for anthracycline and vinca alkaloids.

Antidotes vary according to the specific agent (Table 240-5).[48] Dexrazoxane is used for anthracycline extravasation at dose of 1000 milligrams/m^2 IV infused over 1 to 2 hours within 6 hours of the extravasation event, with additional doses of 1000 milligrams/m^2 at 48 hours and 500 milligrams/m^2 at 72 hours.[49] Dimethyl sulfoxide and hyaluronidase are used to enhance absorption of the extravasated agent.[48] Dimethyl sulfoxide is applied as a generous trickle of the 99% solution over the involved area without pressing or rubbing and then covered with dry pads.[48] Hyaluronidase is reconstituted with normal saline to a concentration of 150 units/mL and then injected in and around the extravasation area via multiple punctures.[48] Inject about 0.2 mL per puncture site with a typical total dose of 1 mL, but up to 10 mL may be required. There is limited data supporting the use of sodium thiosulfate for reversal of alkylating agent toxicity.[48] Intralesional injections of corticosteroids or bicarbonate are not effective.

REFERENCES

The complete reference list is available online at www.TintinalliEM.com.

SECTION 19

Eye, Ear, Nose, Throat, and Oral Disorders

CHAPTER 241

Eye Emergencies

Richard A. Walker
Srikar Adhikari

INTRODUCTION AND EPIDEMIOLOGY

The breadth of ocular emergencies seen in the ED requires solid examination skills and an understanding of basic differential diagnosis. A recent review[1] of 1400 ED ocular emergencies identified the following conditions: ocular trauma in 27%, of which 73% involved corneal abrasions, 6% involved blunt eye trauma, and 5% involved a corneal foreign body; the second most common condition was conjunctivitis (15%), and retinal problems and glaucoma involved 6%.

This chapter reviews eye anatomy, the essential skills needed for the ED eye examination, and common ophthalmic medications. Common causes of the red eye, ocular infections and inflammation, trauma to the eye, acute visual reduction or loss, and acute cranial nerve palsies are discussed. The principles and advantages of ocular US are summarized.

EYE ANATOMY

The **orbit** is a pyramid of bony walls that converge to an apex posteriorly. The orbit is bordered superiorly by the frontal sinus, medially by the ethmoid sinus, inferiorly by the maxillary sinus, and laterally by the zygomatic bone. The ethmoid bone (lamina papyracea) is paper thin and is the most likely sinus wall to break in blunt eye trauma or to be perforated due to sinusitis with subsequent spread of infection to the orbit. The orbital contents include the ocular muscles, retroseptal fat, and the optic nerve, whereas the globe is considered a separate entity.

The anterior limit of the orbital cavity is the **orbital septum**, which is a layer of fascia extending from the periosteum along the orbital rim to the levator aponeurosis of the upper eyelid and to the edge of the tarsal plate of the lower eyelid. Abnormalities, such as the accumulation of blood or infection, are referred to as "preseptal" or "postseptal." Postseptal conditions are extremely serious. **The septum is generally impervious to bacteria, which serves to limit spread of infection from the facial skin into the orbit (Figure 241-1).** All nerves and vessels of the eye enter through the apex of the orbit, which is also the site of origin for the extraocular muscles. The optic nerve is subject to compression from mass effect due to tumors, abscesses, or hematomas.

The arterial blood supply of the eye and orbit is the ophthalmic artery, the first major branch of the intracranial portion of the internal carotid artery, which enters the orbit beneath the optic nerve. The **central retinal artery** is the first intraorbital branch of the ophthalmic artery and courses through the optic nerve. The venous drainage of the eye and orbit is through the ophthalmic veins, which drain into the central retinal vein. The ophthalmic veins communicate directly to the cavernous sinus. This venous system has no valves, and this fact is the basis for the spread of facial and periorbital infections to the cavernous sinus.

The eye itself is composed of several different layers (**Figure 241-2**). The outermost layer is a thin, transparent mucous membrane (the **bulbar conjunctiva**) that continues onto the posterior surface of the eyelids (the **palpebral conjunctiva**). Deep to the conjunctiva is the **episclera**, a layer of thin, elastic tissue containing blood vessels that nourish the next deepest layer, the sclera. The **sclera** is the collagenous protective coating of the eye, which is the thinnest (and prone to rupture) at the insertion of the rectus muscles.

The **cornea** forms the anterior surface of the eyeball and is attached to the sclera at the limbus. From anterior to posterior, the cornea has five separate layers: epithelium, Bowman layer, stroma, Descemet membrane, and endothelium. The epithelium is five or six cell layers thick and is subject to damage from minor mechanical forces, resulting in corneal abrasion (**Figure 241-3**).

The iris, ciliary body, and choroid (the vascular pigmented layer of the eye between the sclera and retina) make up the **uveal tract**. The uveal tract supplies nutrition to the eye and assists in accommodation and pupillary constriction. The lens separates the aqueous humor in the anterior chamber from the vitreous humor in the remainder of the globe. (See the section **Acute and Painful Vision Reduction or Loss, Acute Angle-Closure Glaucoma** in this chapter for discussion of the production and flow of aqueous humor.) The retina is the sheet of neural tissue containing the rods and cones that lines the posterior two thirds of the inner surface of the globe, extending anteriorly as far as the ciliary body.

EYE EXAMINATION

HISTORY

A detailed history is as important in the patient with an eye complaint as it is for a complaint related to any other organ system. History should first categorize the symptom as vision loss, change in appearance of the eye, eye pain/discomfort, or trauma. The onset (gradual or sudden) of symptoms, duration of the symptoms, and circumstances surrounding the onset are important. For example, a history of sudden, painless monocular vision loss associated with a history of atrial fibrillation or carotid stenosis would suggest a central retinal artery occlusion, but a history of eye pain occurring while hammering metal on metal would suggest a projectile causing corneal abrasion or intraocular foreign body. Eye discomfort should be characterized as pain (aching, burning, throbbing, etc.), pruritus (associated with allergy), or a foreign body sensation as seen with corneal foreign bodies, abrasions, or ulcers. "Flashing lights" and a "curtain or veil" obstructing a portion of the visual field suggest a retinal detachment. In the case of trauma, ask about onset (traumatic iritis occurs 1 to several days after blunt trauma to the eye) and mechanism (globe penetration may occur in association with hammering, grinding, or use of other high-speed machinery). Document tetanus status and give tetanus toxoid as appropriate.

Past medical history is always important and can focus the physical examination and narrow the differential diagnosis. Previous surgery may be the cause of an irregular pupil. Absence of corrective lenses may account for decreased visual acuity and will require modification of the method for testing visual acuity. Use of contact lenses, especially the extended wear type, may be associated with bacterial corneal ulcers. Chronic use of certain ophthalmic medications may cause chemical conjunctivitis and inflammatory changes of the cornea. A history of diabetes or chronic hypertension and acute isolated sixth-nerve palsy suggests an ischemic cranial neuropathy. Monocular diplopia following trauma in a patient with an intraocular lens implant suggests dislocation of the intraocular lens. Always ask about previous instances of similar **symptoms** and the associated diagnosis.

EXAMINATION

The eye examination typically proceeds in a sequential fashion unless the circumstances require otherwise (e.g., **chemical ocular injuries**

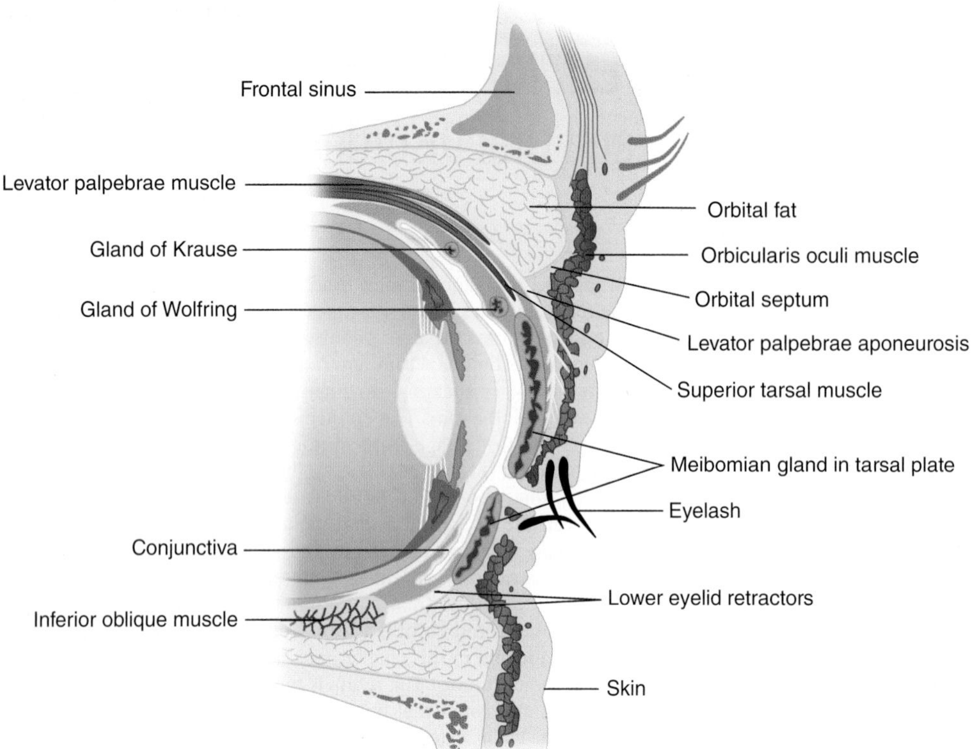

FIGURE 241-1. Cross-section of the eyelids. [Reproduced with permission from Riordan-Eva P, Whitcher J: *Vaughn & Asbury's General Ophthalmology,* 17th ed. New York: Lange Medical Books/McGraw-Hill, 2008.]

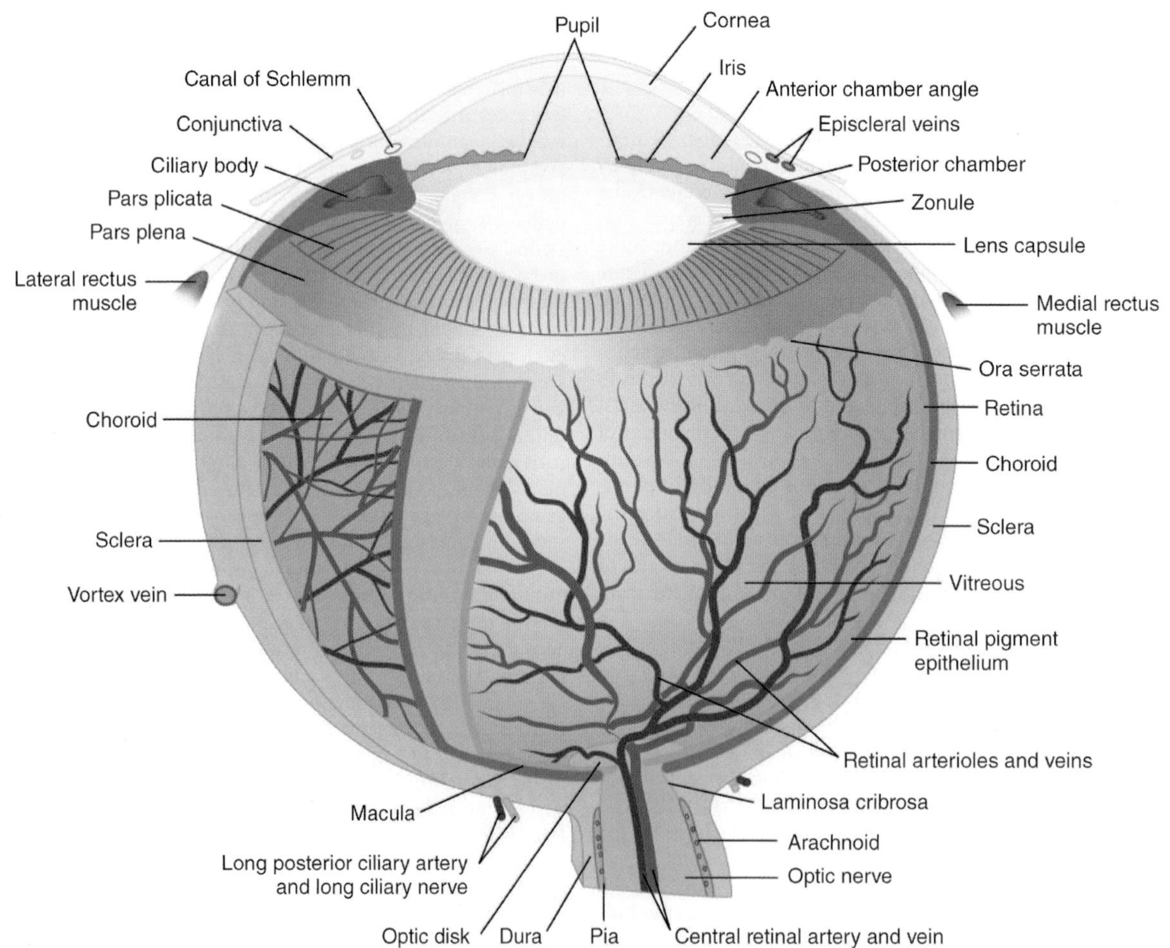

FIGURE 241-2. Internal structures of the human eye. [Reproduced with permission from Riordan-Eva P, Whitcher J: *Vaughn & Asbury's General Ophthalmology,* 17th ed. New York: Lange Medical Books/McGraw-Hill, 2008.]

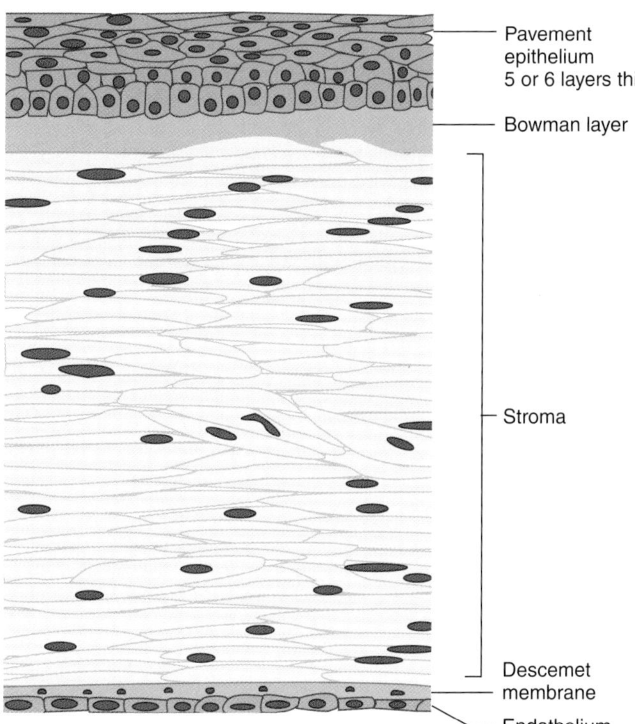

FIGURE 241-3. Transverse section of cornea. [Reproduced with permission from Riordan-Eva P, Whitcher J: *Vaughn & Asbury's General Ophthalmology*, 17th ed. New York: Lange Medical Books/McGraw-Hill, 2008.]

require irrigation *before* assessment of visual acuity). The glossary of terms and abbreviations in **Table 241-1** is helpful when communicating with the ophthalmologist.

Full examination should include the following, generally in the order listed: visual acuity, confrontational visual fields, extraocular movements, pupillary reactions, lids and adnexa, conjunctiva and sclerae, cornea, anterior chamber, iris, lenses, vitreous, intraocular pressure, and funduscopic examination. Measurement of intraocular pressure is done toward the end of the examination because physical touching of the cornea is more irritating and invasive than the rest of the examination. Performance of a thorough funduscopic examination requires dilatation of the pupil, so this part of the examination is performed last. Not all parts of the examination need to be done on every patient. For example, testing visual fields adds little to the evaluation of a corneal foreign body but is essential to the evaluation of acute vision loss.

Visual Acuity Most vision-threatening disorders present with decreased visual acuity. **Visual acuity testing is the vital sign of the eye** and is the first step in any eye examination, even before shining a light in the eye; bright light can temporarily decrease visual acuity. The only exception to this rule is for chemical burns to the eye, where irrigation takes precedence above all else. Test visual acuity with contact lenses or glasses in place if possible. If the patient's glasses or contacts are unavailable, use **pinhole testing** of visual acuity. A commercial pinhole occluder may be used, although a perforated metal eye shield or a note card perforated with an 18-gauge needle are acceptable substitutes. The pinhole allows only parallel light rays to fall on the macula, thereby reducing the refractive error and allowing an estimate of the person's corrected visual acuity. Visual acuity testing is ideally done with a standard wall-mounted visual acuity chart (**Snellen chart**) with the patient standing 20 ft (6 m) from the chart. Record the visual acuity as 20/x, where the numerator is the distance from which the patient can read the line (always 20) and the denominator is the distance from which a person with normal vision can read the same line. **The visual acuity is determined by the smallest line a patient can read with one half of the letters correct.** The number of incorrect letters is listed after the visual acuity as follows: 20/x-y (e.g., 20/40-2). Document best acuity in each eye and whether prosthetic devices were used in testing (glasses, pinhole).

Visual acuity can also be tested with a near card (**Rosenbaum chart**) held 14 in. (36 cm) from the patient. Patients in their mid-40s or older may require reading glasses or bifocals to read a near card because of presbyopia. If the bifocals are not available, use a pinhole occluder.

For patients with visual acuity <20/200, figure counting at a distance (e.g., figure counting at 3 ft or 1 m), perception of hand motion

TABLE 241-1 Glossary of Terms, Abbreviations, and Notations

AC	Anterior chamber, the first portion of the anterior segment.	IOP	Intraocular pressure (mm Hg).
Anisocoria	Unequal pupil size under equal lighting conditions.	Limbus	Circumferential border where clear cornea ends and white sclera begins.
Anterior segment	Consists of the anterior chamber and posterior chamber. Aqueous humor is produced in the posterior chamber of the anterior segment and circulates through the pupil into the anterior chamber of the anterior segment.	NLP	No light perception (blind).
		OD	Oculus dexter (right eye).*
		OS	Oculus sinister (left eye).
APD	Afferent pupillary defect (see **Figure 241-8**).	OU	Oculus uterque (each eye).*
CF	Counting fingers (visual acuity assessment).	PH	Pinhole visual acuity.
CVF	Confrontation visual fields.	RD	Retinal detachment.
EOM	Extraocular muscle. Extraocular movements.	Tono-Pen® (Reichert, Inc., Depew, NY)	A hand-held, pen-shaped device for measuring IOP.
HM	Hand motion (visual acuity assessment).		
Hyphema	RBCs in the anterior chamber.	T_{tono}	Tension (IOP) with subscript representing method used: (tono = Tono-Pen®; S = Schiötz; A = applanation).†
Hypopyon	WBCs in the anterior chamber.		
INO	Internuclear ophthalmoplegia.	V_{Ac}	Visual acuity with correction (glasses or contact lenses).†
IOFB	Intraocular foreign body.	V_{As}	Visual acuity without correction.

*By convention, in documenting the visual acuity (V_A) or IOP, the right eye is listed above the left, as follows:

$T_{tono} <$ 14 / 15 — †This represents an IOP of 14 mm Hg in the right eye and 15 mm Hg in the left eye measured by Tono-Pen®.

$V_{Ac} <$ 20/20 / 20/30 — †This represents a visual acuity *with* glasses/contacts of 20/20 right eye and 20/30 left eye.

$V_{As} <$ 20/400 → 20/30 / CF at 8 ft → 20/40 — This represents a visual acuity *without* glasses/contacts of 20/400 in the right eye, improving to 20/30 with pinhole testing; counting fingers at 8 ft (2.4 m) in the left eye, improving to 20/40 with pinhole testing.

at 1 to 2 ft (0.3 to 0.6 m), and ultimately light perception can be used to document visual acuity. If the patient is unable to detect hand motion, turn off all the lights in the room, fully occlude the contralateral eye, and test for light perception. Illiterate patients can be tested using the direction of the letter **E** on the chart, and a verbal child may be tested with an **Allen chart** (pictures). Corneal abrasions or foreign bodies can cause severe photophobia, pain, and tearing, so a topical anesthetic can reduce discomfort sufficiently to allow a more accurate assessment of visual acuity. In recording the results of visual acuity testing, refer to **Table 241-1.**

When alternating black-and-white lines are passed from one side to another in front of a patient's eyes, **involuntary horizontal nystagmus (optokinetic nystagmus)** will occur. The presence of optokinetic nystagmus excludes blindness in a patient with an otherwise normal examination who claims he or she cannot see (hysterical blindness). The test can be performed by placing thick black lines approximately 1 in. apart on a 2-ft strip of cardiac monitor paper, which is passed back and forth at eye level a distance of 1 ft from the patient.

Confrontation Visual Fields Test all four quadrants of the visual fields by having the patient cover one eye and look at the physician's nose. The examiner closes the opposite eye and holds a finger halfway between the patient and himself or herself. The finger is wiggled as it is moved medially toward the patient. The normal patient should see movement at approximately the same time as the physician does. A visual field defect may represent pathology anywhere from the occipital cortex to the optic nerve (**Figure 241-4**). Bitemporal hemianopia can occur in pituitary adenoma; homonymous hemianopia is associated with some cerebrovascular accidents; and monocular field cuts are sometimes seen with large retinal detachments.

Ocular Motility The normal patient can move the eye through the six cardinal positions of gaze, and the eye movements are controlled by the six extraocular muscles attached to each eye (**Figures 241-5** and **241-6**). Extraocular muscles are innervated by cranial nerves III, IV, and VI. **Cranial nerve IV controls the superior oblique muscle, cranial nerve**

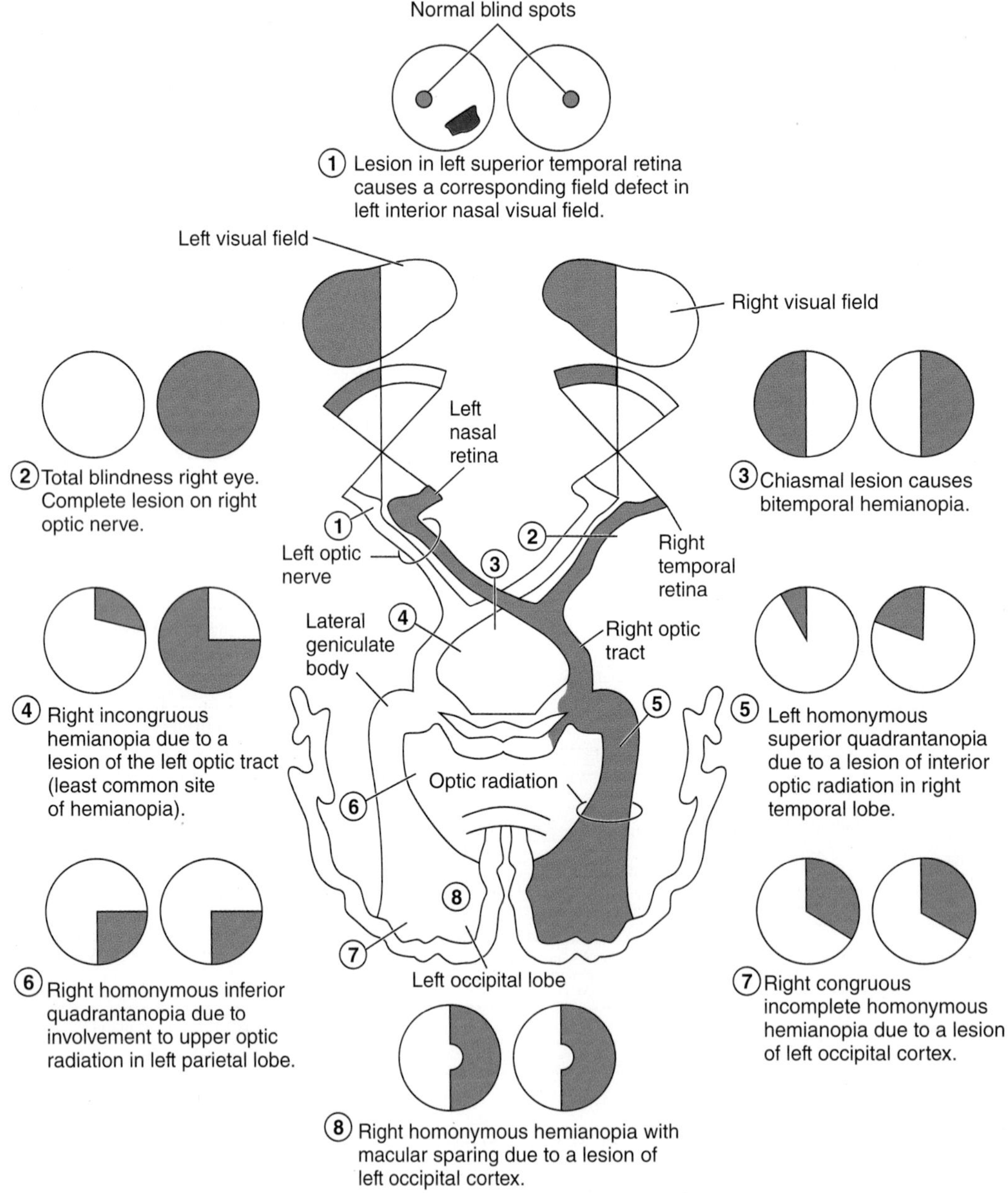

FIGURE 241-4. Visual field defects produced by lesions at various points along the optic pathways: (*1*) field defect caused by retinal lesion, (*2*) total blindness right eye, (*3*) bitemporal hemianopia, (*4*) right incongruous hemianopia, (*5*) left homonymous superior quadrantanopia, (*6*) right homonymous inferior quadrantanopia, (*7*) right congruous incomplete homonymous hemianopia, and (*8*) right homonymous hemianopia with macular sparing. [Reproduced with permission from Riordan-Eva P, Whitcher J: *Vaughn & Asbury's General Ophthalmology*, 17th ed. New York: Lange Medical Books/McGraw-Hill, 2008.]

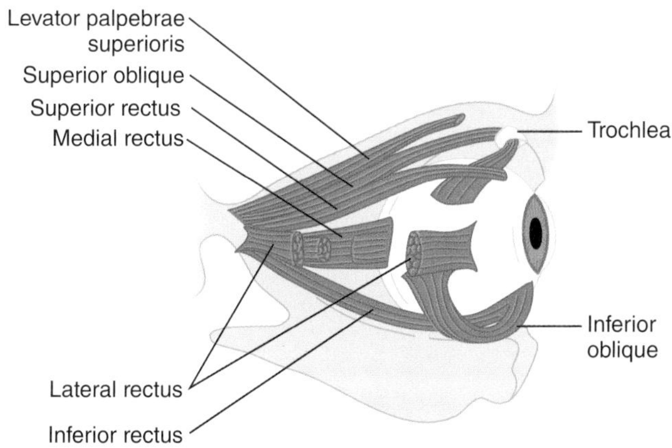

FIGURE 241-5. Extraocular muscles of the eye.

VI controls the lateral rectus muscle, and all other extraocular muscles are controlled by cranial nerve III. Extraocular movement can be impaired by restriction, interrupted or decreased innervation, or trauma. Examples of restriction include thyroid orbitopathy, myositis, and mechanical entrapment of a muscle secondary to an orbital blow-out fracture. Cranial nerve palsies or paresis may be caused by stroke, myasthenia gravis, diabetes, hypertension, tumors, aneurysms, infections, and trauma. Penetrating or blunt traumatic injury to an extraocular muscle also can result in motility disturbance.

Evaluate ocular alignment initially in *primary gaze* (looking straight ahead), and then test eye movements in all fields of gaze. Always ask the patient about diplopia, which may be a subtle sign of problems with extraocular muscles. Diplopia is usually worse when the patient is attempting to look in the direction of the malfunctioning muscle. Ask patients if diplopia persists when one eye is covered (monocular diplopia). **Monocular diplopia** can be caused by corneal irregularity, lens problems, or intraocular lens dislocation, or can be a sign of malingering. Resolution of diplopia when one eye is covered represents pathology of an extraocular muscle or its innervation. Patients with lesions of the superior oblique muscle or the fourth cranial nerve may tilt their head to compensate for the diplopia.

Pupils Note the pupil size in millimeters and test shape and reaction to light. An irregular pupil may occur from prior surgery or remote trauma. The patient will usually be able to relate a previous history of irregular pupil. The classic irregular teardrop-shaped pupil may also be seen in acute blunt or penetrating trauma with rupture of the iris (**Figure 241-7**).

Assess pupils under slightly dim light to test for an afferent pupillary defect (**Figure 241-8**). **A positive afferent pupillary defect indicates an optic nerve disorder.** Any pathology that prevents light from getting to the CNS, such as opacification of the vitreous with blood, retinal pathology, or optic nerve pathology, will cause an afferent pupillary defect, also known as a ***Marcus-Gunn pupil***. The pupils will be equal in size *before* testing because of the consensual light response. Therefore, an afferent pupillary defect does *not* cause a baseline anisocoria and will be discovered only if specifically tested for. Perform the "swinging flashlight test" to detect an afferent pupillary defect. Shine a light in the pupil. The light causes constriction of the ipsilateral pupil and consensual constriction of the opposite pupil. The light is then shined/swung to the opposite pupil. The opposite pupil will dilate if an afferent pupillary defect is present, because the effect of light is not getting through to the CNS.

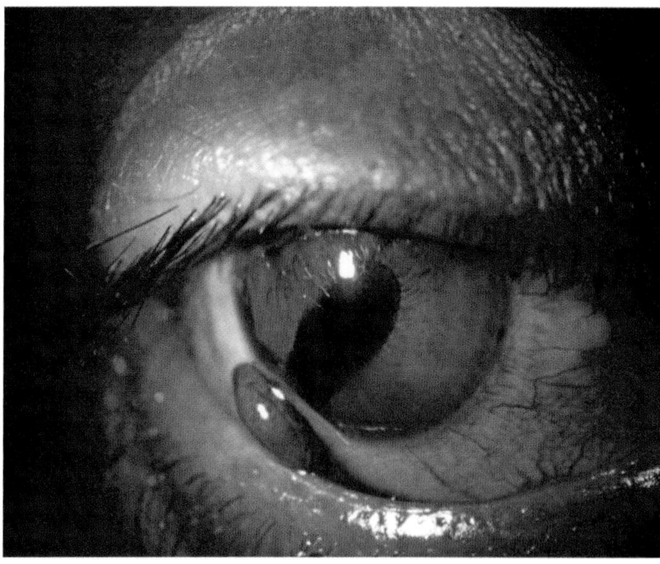

FIGURE 241-7. Prolapse of the iris with the classic teardrop-shaped pupil after penetrating trauma. [Courtesy of Allen R. Katz, Department of Ophthalmology, University of Nebraska Medical Center.]

Causes of unequal pupils (**anisocoria**) can range from an acute emergency (posterior communicating artery aneurysm) to chronic baseline conditions such as previous intraocular trauma or surgery, or they can be idiopathic. **Physiologic anisocoria (difference in pupil size) is the most common cause of asymmetric pupils.** The difference in size is usually <1 mm, and both pupils react normally by constricting to light and dilating in darkness. A single dilated pupil may represent impending **uncal herniation** (from pressure on the third nerve), but uncal herniation is accompanied by an altered level of consciousness and other focal neurologic signs. A single nonreactive dilated pupil may result from a topical cycloplegic agent (scopolamine, cyclopentolate, or atropine) for uveitis or if an anticholinergic medication (such as ipratropium from a nebulization treatment for bronchospasm) is splashed into the eye. A careful history is important to determine whether anisocoria is preexisting. **It is not worthwhile to attempt to "reverse" a suspected chemically altered pupil in the ED as a diagnostic test because the results are not reliable.**

External Eye: Periorbital Skin, Lids, and Adnexa The ocular adnexa include the eyebrows, eyelids, and lacrimal apparatus. Examine the periorbital skin and lids for trauma, infection, dysfunction, deformity, crepitus, or proptosis. Subcutaneous emphysema can be found with blow-out fractures of the medial orbital wall (ethmoid). Palpate the orbital rims for step-off deformities in trauma. Evert the upper eyelid to check for foreign bodies. Use of a cotton applicator is often recommended; however, this technique will only visualize the lower half of the inner upper eyelid (**Figure 241-9**). The edge of an eyelid retractor may be used to tent the upper lid while a second examiner looks under the lid from a caudal direction, so-called *double eversion of the eyelid*. This will allow visualization of the upper half of the inner eyelid. A large

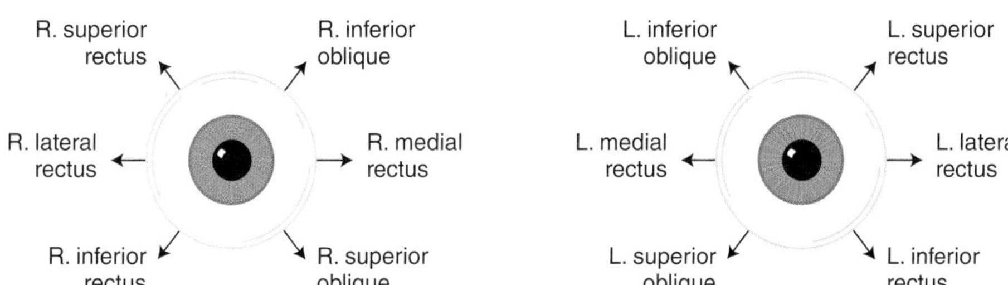

FIGURE 241-6. Arrows indicate direction of ocular movement by each muscle. Cranial nerve IV, superior oblique muscle; cranial nerve VI, lateral rectus muscle; cranial nerve III, superior rectus, inferior rectus, inferior oblique, and medial rectus muscles.

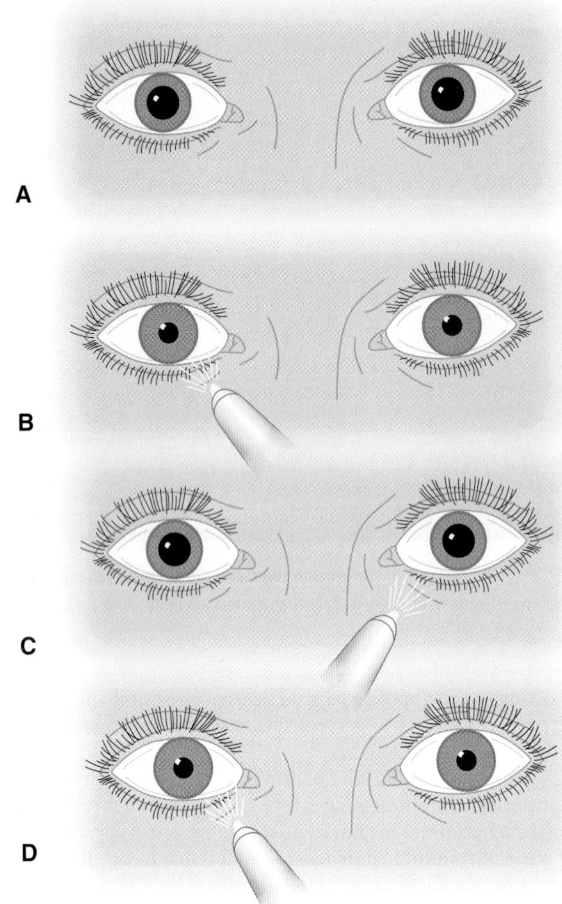

FIGURE 241-8. **A** and **B.** "Swinging flashlight test" revealing an afferent pupillary defect (Marcus-Gunn pupil) of the left eye. **A.** Pupils are normal and equal before light testing. **B.** Both pupils constrict when light is shined into the normal (right) eye. **C** and **D.** The test is positive when the affected pupil (left pupil) dilates in response to light. Conditions with an afferent pupillary defect include optic neuritis and central retinal artery occlusion.

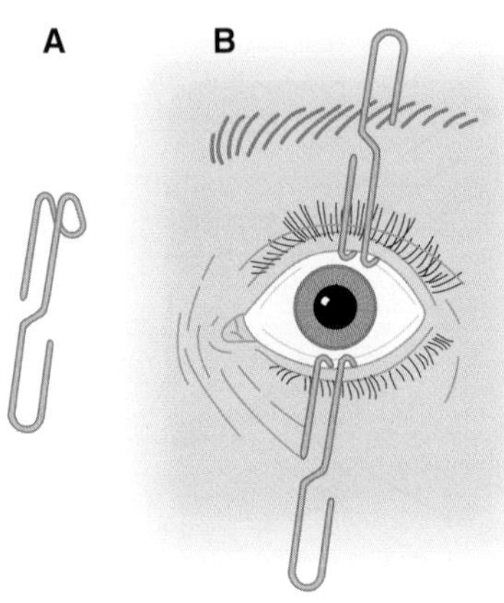

FIGURE 241-10. An alternative to an eyelid retractor. **A.** Unfold a paper clip and bend it into shape with a hemostat. **B.** Paper clips used to retract the eyelids. [Reproduced with permission from Reichman EF, Simon RR: *Emergency Medicine Procedures*. © 2004, Eric F. Reichman, PhD, MD, and Robert R. Simon, MD. McGraw-Hill Professional, Inc.]

paperclip may be bent into the shape of an eyelid retractor for this purpose (**Figure 241-10** and see **Figure 241-38**).

Anterior Segment and the Slit Lamp Examination The palpebral and bulbar conjunctiva, sclerae, cornea, anterior chamber, and iris and ciliary body make up the anterior chamber, and all except the ciliary body may be examined with the slit lamp (**Figure 241-11A**).

The slit lamp is a binocular microscope that affords a highly magnified three-dimensional view of ocular structures. Use the slit lamp to assess eye complaints whenever possible. The patient and examiner should both be seated on adjustable stools so that the examiner's and patient's eyes are at the same level. Cover the chin rest with tissue paper or a washcloth. Adjust the slit lamp height so the patient can lean forward and comfortably place the forehead against the upper plastic bar and the chin on the chin rest. Adjust the height of the chin rest so the patient's lateral canthus is even with the black line on the vertical bar. The oculars and light source are generally straight ahead for the general eye evaluation. Focus is adjusted by the anterior-posterior movement of the ocular and light source in relation to the patient. The joystick generally controls focus by moving the slit lamp closer to or farther away from the patient's eyes. Rotation of the joystick usually controls vertical movement of the light source and oculars. When one looks through the oculars, the focus should be close to correct if a narrow slit of light falls on

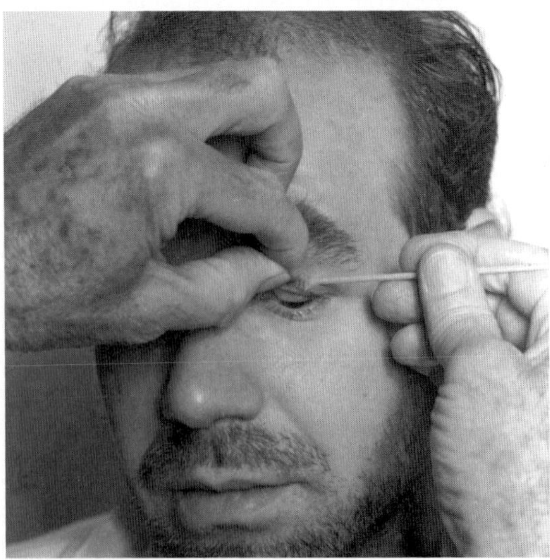

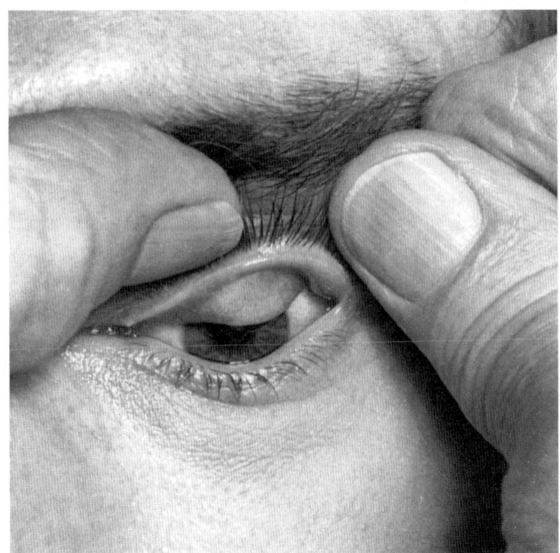

FIGURE 241-9. Single eversion of eyelid when a cotton applicator is used. [Reproduced with permission from Riordan-Eva P, Whitcher J: *Vaughn & Asbury's General Ophthalmology*, 17th ed. New York: Lange Medical Books/McGraw-Hill, 2008.]

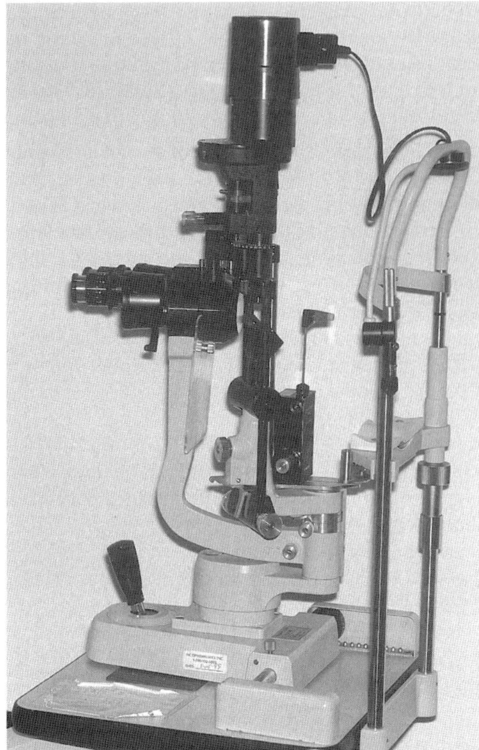

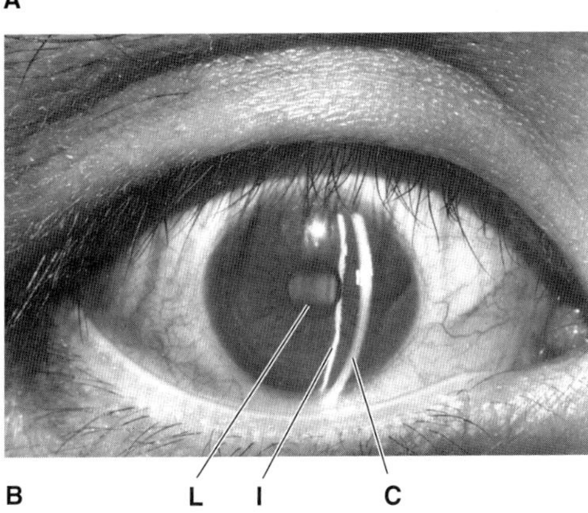

FIGURE 241-11. **A.** The slit lamp provides a magnified view of the eye. **B.** A thin slit can demonstrate the cornea (*C*), iris (*I*), and lens (*L*).

the structures to be examined. Fine adjustments in focus are then made with the joystick. Adjust the vertical light beam to the full height of the cornea with a width of approximately 1 mm (**Figure 241-11B**).

Examine the palpebral and bulbar conjunctivae for follicles (seen with allergic and viral conjunctivitis), chemosis (subconjunctival edema fluid), injection/inflammation, discharge, trauma, and foreign bodies.

To examine the cornea, rotate the light source to a 45-degree angle. The slit lamp can be brought close to the proper focus by looking at the slit of light on the cornea with the naked eye and moving the slit lamp in an anterior-posterior direction to obtain the thinnest and sharpest slit possible. The cornea is assessed by narrowing the light source to produce a slit beam that optically sections the cornea (**Figure 241-12**). Inspect the corneal epithelium for abrasions, ulcers, edema, and foreign bodies. Examine the corneal stroma for edema, scars, and lacerations, and examine the endothelium for precipitates (WBCs on the endothelium characteristic of iritis) and lacerations.

Assess the depth of the anterior chamber by adjusting the angle of the light source on the slit lamp or by shining a penlight onto the iris from a lateral direction. If the iris is bowed forward, as with a shallow anterior chamber, a shadow will be cast on the medial (nasal) iris (**Figure 241-13**).

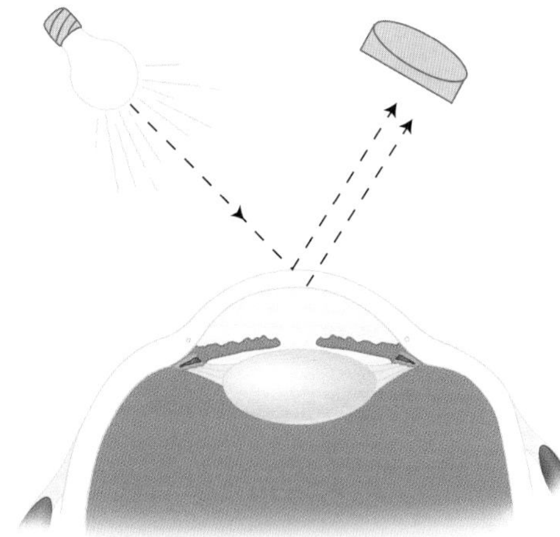

FIGURE 241-12. Optical sectioning. By creating an angle of 45 to 60 degrees between the slit-beam light source and the observer's biomicroscope objective, the cornea can be optically "sectioned" obliquely. This allows a cross-sectional view of the cornea and is helpful in ascertaining the depth of penetration of corneal foreign bodies and injuries.

Assess the anterior chamber for flare and cells as follows: shorten the slit beam to approximately 1 mm, and shut off the room lights. Select the high-magnification position of the oculars. The incident light source should create an angle of 45 to 60 degrees with the objective (similar to optical sectioning). Focus the light beam on the pupillary margin and pull the joystick back to focus on the cornea. One may see keratitic precipitates that are white spots on the undersurface of the corneal epithelium, representing deposits of inflammatory cells in iritis.

Now move the focus inward halfway between the iris and cornea, with the pupillary aperture as a dark backdrop. This will place your focus in the center of the aqueous humor, and the light beam will illuminate WBCs and red blood cells (if present) slowly drifting up and down in the aqueous convection currents, sometimes likened to snowflakes floating through the beam from a car's headlight at night. Iritis may result in WBC layers in the anterior chamber (hypopyon) (**Figure 241-14**). Trauma to the eye may cause red blood cells in the anterior chamber (hyphema or microhyphema). **Hyphema** is layering of the red cells in the anterior chamber visible to the naked eye (**Figure 241-15**). A hyphema may occasionally be clotted (**Figure 241-16**). Flare is described as the appearance of "headlights in a fog" and represents the ability to see the course of the normally transparent light beam through the aqueous humor. **Flare** is caused by increased aqueous protein in the anterior chamber, which is common with inflammatory conditions such as iritis.

Examine the iris for pupil irregularity and pupillary dysfunction. Irregularity of the pupil will occur whenever one portion of the iris is

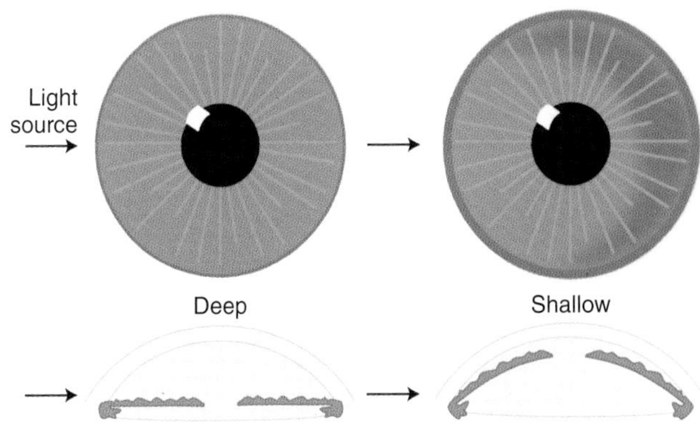

FIGURE 241-13. Estimation of depth of the anterior chamber by oblique illumination. Note the shadow cast in the shallow chamber. [Reproduced with permission from Riordan-Eva P, Whitcher J: *Vaughn & Asbury's General Ophthalmology,* 17th ed. New York: Lange Medical Books/McGraw-Hill, 2008.]

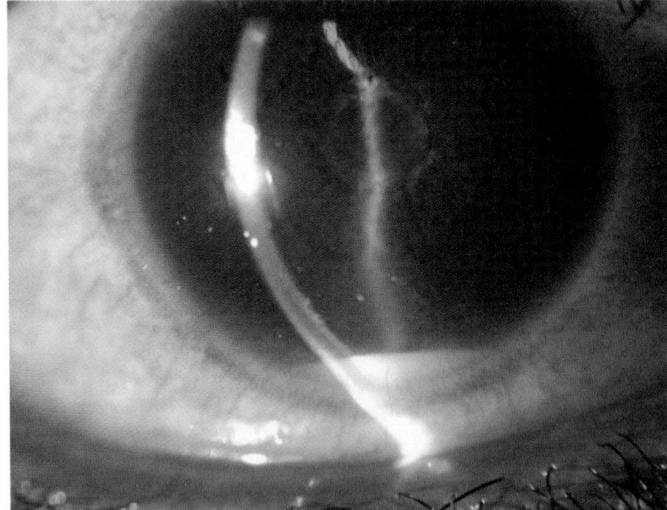

FIGURE 241-14. Hypopyon: a layering of WBCs in the inferior portion of the anterior chamber. [Courtesy of Allen R. Katz, Department of Ophthalmology, University of Nebraska Medical Center.]

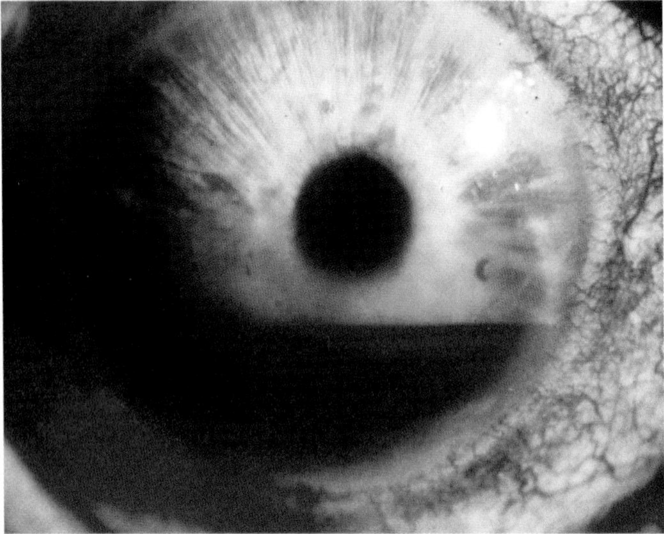

FIGURE 241-15. Hyphema secondary to blunt trauma. Note the blood filling the lower half of the anterior chamber and hazy appearance of cornea suggesting increased intraocular pressure. [Courtesy of Allen R. Katz, Department of Ophthalmology, University of Nebraska Medical Center.]

tethered into place and may occur from posterior synechiae, where the iris is adhesed to the anterior lens capsule as seen in uveitis, or when any portion of the iris plugs a corneoscleral laceration causing a peaked pupil. Trauma may also cause the iris to tear at the root, termed *iridodialysis*. Assess the lens for opacities, lacerations, and subluxation.

Fluorescein Examination The final part of the slit lamp examination is done after fluorescein is instilled into the eye. Fluorescein binds to damaged corneal epithelium and fluoresces green under a **Wood's lamp** or light through a cobalt-blue filter. **Always remove contact lenses, as fluorescein will cause permanent staining of the lenses.** Touching the fluorescein strip directly to the cornea will cause staining mimicking a linear abrasion. The best way to apply fluorescein dye is to apply several drops of eye-irrigating solution or saline onto a paper fluorescein strip, and then lightly apply the moistened end of the fluorescein strip into the inferior conjunctival fornix. Ask the patient to blink several times to distribute the fluorescein. Then examine the cornea for streaming of fluorescein-tinged aqueous humor (positive Seidel test) seen in full-thickness laceration of the cornea (**Figure 241-17**). **The Seidel test can be negative (no streaming) with a small or spontaneously sealing corneal laceration.** Ask the patient to blink to wash out the fluorescein, and then examine the cornea with the cobalt blue filter on the slit lamp. A corneal abrasion will fluoresce bright green. A Wood's lamp (ultraviolet light) may also be used to look grossly (without the slit lamp) for corneal abrasions, but microscopic/punctate abrasions will be missed without use of a slit lamp.

Funduscopic Examination Note the size, shape, and sharpness of the borders of the optic disk, the cup-to-disk ratio, the size ratio of the arteries to veins (normal 2:3), any nicking where the arteries and veins cross, the texture and color of the retina as well as the presence of lesions (e.g., hemorrhages or exudates) of the retina or vessels (e.g., aneurysms), and the color and size of the macula. To locate lesions of the retina note the direction (e.g., superonasal) and distance from the disk in terms of disk diameters. Opacities of the lens may obscure the view of the retina, and lens opacities appear as black spots of various shapes. Lesions in the vitreous, such as vitreous hemorrhage, will also obscure the view. Vitreous hemorrhage will have an irregular shape and may have a reddish hue.

The **direct hand-held ophthalmoscope** is used to examine the fundus. Pharmacologic dilatation will greatly enhance the view of the disk, macula, and proximal retinal vessels. Dilation is achieved by using one drop of 1% tropicamide in Caucasian patients and one drop each of 1% tropicamide and 2.5% phenylephrine in all others. An **indirect ophthalmoscope** provides an excellent three-dimensional view of the optic nerve and retina but requires extensive practice to use and generally is not a tool for the nonophthalmologist.

The Welch Allyn Panoptic™ direct ophthalmoscope allows a five times larger view of the fundus than the standard direct ophthalmoscope and provides a better view of the fundus with an undilated pupil (**Figure 241-18**). It also allows for more distance between the patient

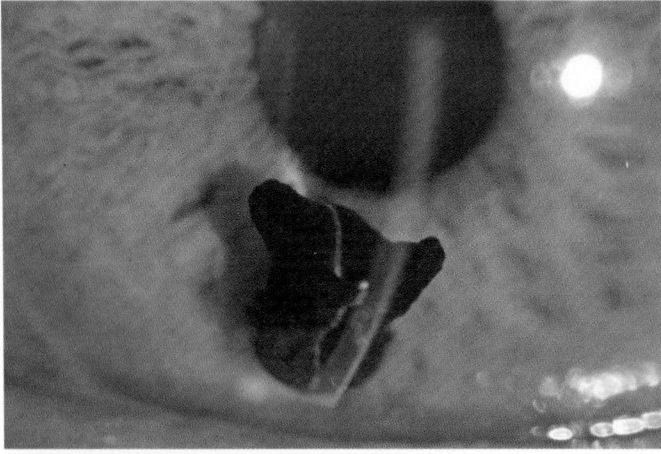

FIGURE 241-16. Hyphema appearing as a clot rather than layering out. [Courtesy of Allen R. Katz, Department of Ophthalmology, University of Nebraska Medical Center.]

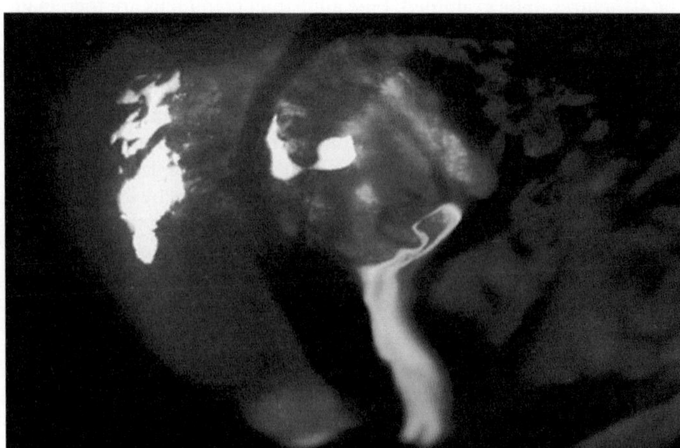

FIGURE 241-17. Positive Seidel test showing aqueous humor leaking through a full-thickness corneal wound. Aqueous humor will turn fluorescein lime-green under a cobalt-blue light as it oozes through the wound while being observed through the slit lamp.

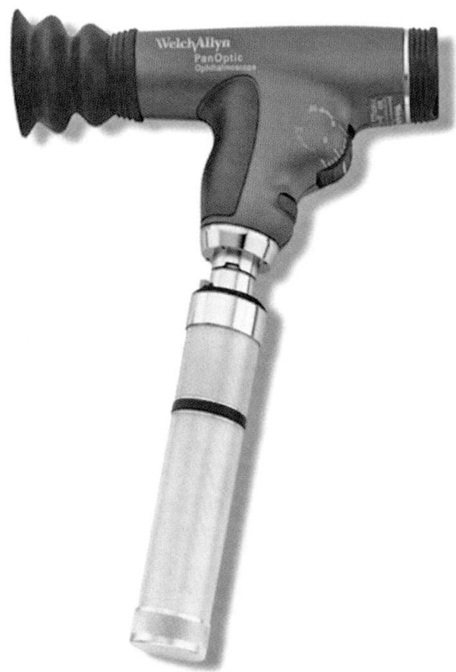

FIGURE 241-18. Welch Allyn Panoptic™ direct ophthalmoscope. Copyright © Welch Allyn, Inc. All rights reserved.

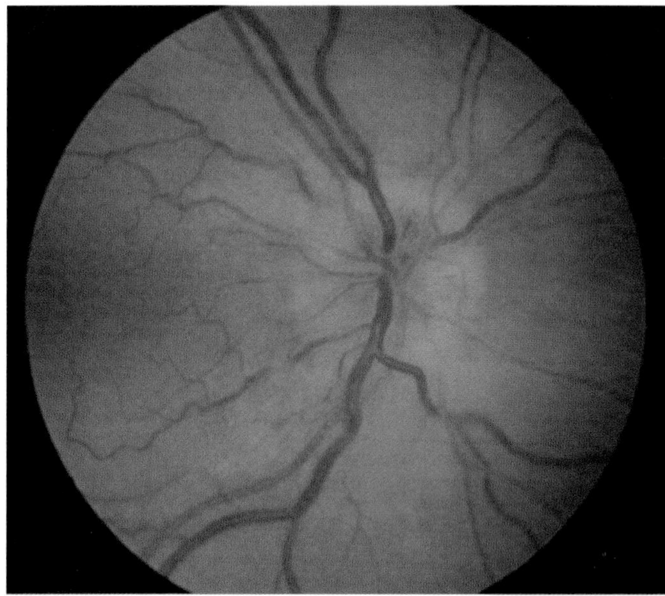

FIGURE 241-19. Optic nerve head edema. Vascular congestion, elevation of the nerve head, and blurred disk margins are characteristically seen in papilledema, papillitis, and compressive lesions of the optic nerve. [Reproduced with permission from Knoop K, Stack L, Storrow A: *Atlas of Emergency Medicine,* 2nd ed. © 2002, McGraw-Hill, New York.]

and examiner, for the comfort of both. The Panoptic™ device attaches to a standard Welch Allyn handle.

Use the Panoptic as follows:

1. Remove your and the patient's glasses; seat the patient upright or with the patient's stretcher set as upright as possible. Position yourself in a direct line of vision to the patient's eyes.
2. With the scope turned off, focus on an object at least 10 ft away.
3. Set the aperture dial to small ("home" position—green line).
4. Turn on the scope and adjust to maximum brightness.
5. Ask the patient to be still and look straight ahead, and tell him or her that the eyecup will touch the brow.
6. Place your hand on the patient's forehead, and position the scope 6 in. away at a 15- to 20-degree angle to the temporal side.
7. Locate the red reflex, and move the scope toward the patient keeping the red reflex in view.
8. Maximum view should be obtained when the eyecup is compressed by half.
9. If you have a dominant eye and prefer to use that for the examination, you may examine the opposite eye without switching your eye on the scope.
10. Make sure you wipe off the eyepiece with antiseptic/antibacterial solution after use, or change eyepieces between patients.

Papilledema **Papilledema** is bilateral edema of the head of the optic nerve due to increased intracranial pressure. Any disease process that increases the intracranial pressure and inhibits vascular or axoplasmic flow in the optic nerve causes congestion and edema of the nerve head. Bilateral papilledema is a common finding in malignant hypertension, pseudotumor cerebri, intracranial tumors, and hydrocephalus. The disk margins are blurred, the cup is diminished or absent, and the nerve head is elevated with vascular congestion (**Figure 241-19**). Frequently, flame-shaped hemorrhages are seen on or adjacent to the nerve head. A distinguishing feature of papilledema is prolonged preservation of visual acuity (frequently patients are visually asymptomatic).

Intraocular Pressure The eye remains consistently "inflated" because of a delicate balance between intraocular aqueous fluid production and outflow. Intraocular pressure can decrease due to reduced ciliary body production (some cases of iritis and uveitis) or loss of globe integrity (perforating injury). Intraocular pressure increases when intraocular fluid production exceeds outflow (glaucoma, hyphema). Measure intraocular pressure in all cases of vision loss, eye pain (suspected glaucoma), and acute or remote trauma. **Do not attempt to measure intraocular pressure if globe rupture from blunt or penetrating trauma is suspected**, as the pressure placed on the globe during pressure measurement may cause extrusion of intraocular contents. **The normal intraocular pressure is 10 to 20 mm Hg.** Digital palpation of the globe may give a rough estimation, using the examiner's eye or tip of the nose as control. Provide topical eye anesthetic when devices are used to measure pressure. To measure pressure, the lid must be open, and the patient must look straight ahead. Hold the lids open, with your fingers compressing the patient's lids against the bony rims of the orbit. Avoid placing any pressure on the globe with your fingers when holding the lids open, because this will cause a falsely high reading. Document the method used for determining intraocular pressure. In recording the pressure, refer to **Table 241-1**.

Schiötz Tonometer The **Schiötz tonometer** is a device using a plunger to indent the cornea. Counterweights are placed on top of the plunger, and the reading off the tonometer scale is correlated to numbers on a chart supplied with the tonometer to give a pressure reading. **The direct Schiötz scale reading is *not* the intraocular pressure.** Schiötz tonometry is inaccurate and not well tolerated by patients, and the instrument is difficult to sterilize, leading to potential spread of infection (**Figure 241-20**). The Tono-Pen® XL (Reichert, Inc., Depew, NY), Goldman® applanation tonometer, and pneumatonometer have supplanted the use of the Schiötz tonometer.

Tono-Pen® The **Tono-Pen® XL** and similar electronic devices have disposable latex covers and measure pressure by indentation of the cornea. The Tono-Pen® XL is touched to the cornea 4 to 10 times and will read out an average pressure reading (**Figure 241-21**).

Applanation Tonometer Use of the **Goldman® applanation tonometer** requires training and practice and is a method used by optometrists and ophthalmologists. **The cone must be sterilized between patients.** The cone of the tonometer is touched to the cornea after topical anesthesia, and fluorescein is instilled into the eye (without irrigation). When looking through the slit lamp, two half circles are seen and properly aligned by

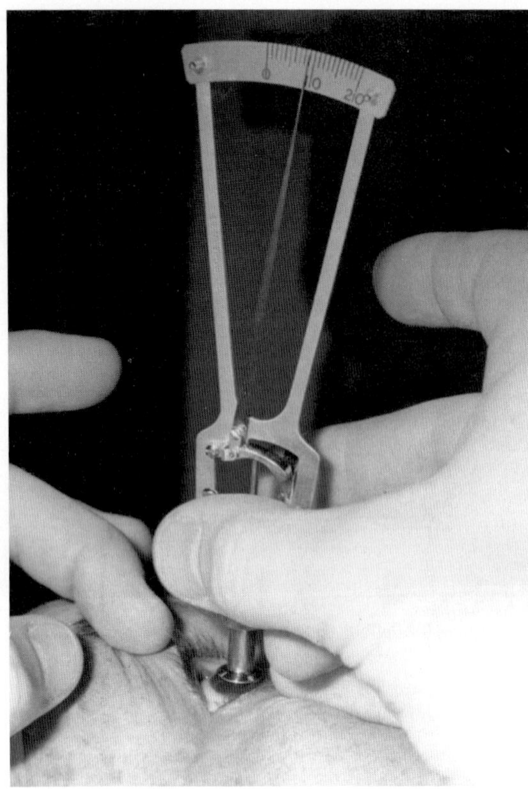

FIGURE 241-20. Schiötz tonometry. [Reproduced with permission from Riordan-Eva P, Whitcher J: *Vaughn & Asbury's General Ophthalmology,* 17th ed. New York: Lange Medical Books/McGraw-Hill, 2008.]

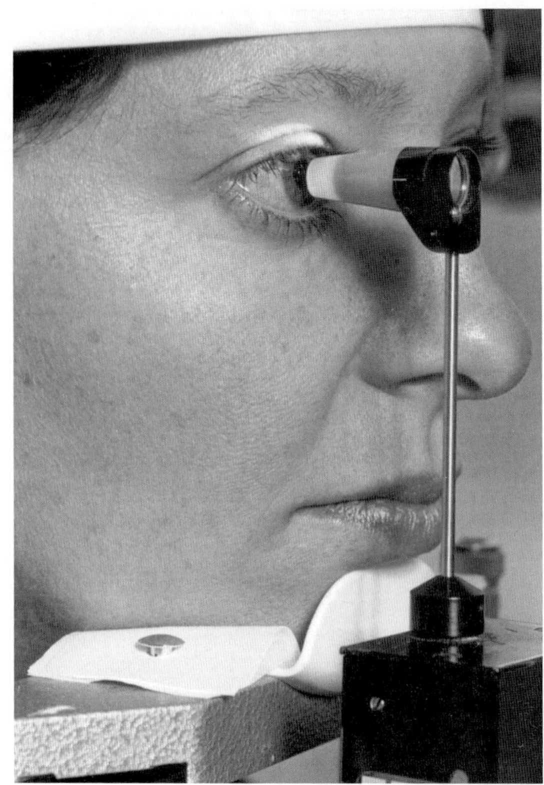

FIGURE 241-22. Goldman® application tonometry. [Reproduced with permission from Riordan-Eva P, Whitcher J: *Vaughn & Asbury's General Ophthalmology,* 17th ed. New York: Lange Medical Books/McGraw-Hill, 2008.]

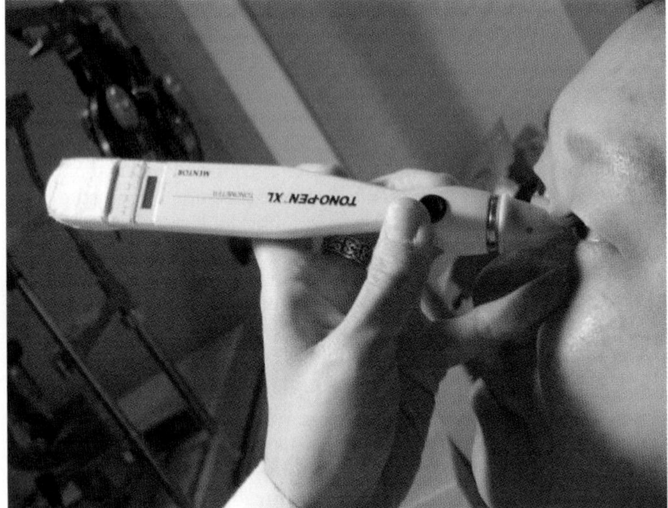

FIGURE 241-21. Tono-Pen® XL (Reichert, Inc., Depew, NY). [Reproduced with permission from Rhee J: *Glaucoma: Color Atlas and Synopsis of Clinical Ophthalmology*. New York: McGraw-Hill, 2003.]

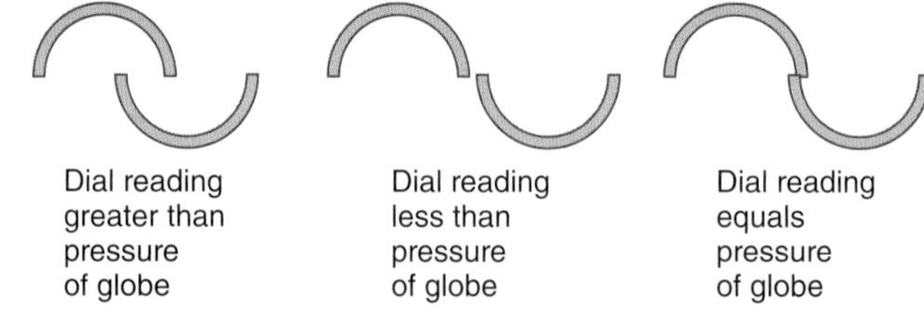

FIGURE 241-23. Appearance of fluorescein semicircles using applanation tonometry under the slit lamp. [Reproduced with permission from Riordan-Eva P, Whitcher J: *Vaughn & Asbury's General Ophthalmology,* 17th ed. New York: Lange Medical Books/McGraw-Hill, 2008.]

adjusting the dial on the tonometer, from which the pressure is read (**Figures 241-22** and **241-23**).

COMMON OPHTHALMIC MEDICATIONS USED IN THE ED

Topical anesthetics are needed for eye examination, intraocular pressure measurement, and corneal foreign body removal. Mydriatics and cycloplegics are needed for a more thorough eye examination. Ophthalmic antibiotics are prescribed for conjunctivitis and corneal abrasions. Antiviral medications are used for herpes simplex. Glaucoma may be treated with various combinations of topical nonselective and β_1-blockers, selective α_2-agonists, carbonic anhydrase inhibitors, cholinergic agents, and prostaglandin analogs. Allergic conjunctivitis is treated with topical nonsteroidal anti-inflammatory drugs, mast cell stabilizers, selective H_1 antagonists, or corticosteroids.

Table 241-2 lists common agents used in the ED and those that the consulting ophthalmologists may ask the emergency medicine physician to prescribe.

THE RED EYE

The differential diagnosis of the red eye is extensive. Key differentiating factors are the presence or absence of pain, itching, photophobia, systemic symptoms, discharge and injections, visual loss, and changes in the cornea, pupils, and intraocular pressure. **Table 241-3** lists various causes of the red eye with key differentiating features. Many of these conditions are discussed more extensively in the text.

TABLE 241-2 Ophthalmic Medications Used in the ED

Type	Generic Name	Trade Name	Indication	Cautions	Usual Dose
Mydriatic-cycloplegic					
Sympathomimetic	2.5% phenylephrine	Mydfrin® AK Dilate®	Pupil dilation, no cycloplegia, usually adjunctive to an anticholinergic	Hypertension, glaucoma; do not use after chemical injury to the eye	1 drop, onset 20–30 min, duration several hours
Anticholinergic	Cyclopentolate	Cyclogyl®	Short-term mydriasis and cycloplegia for examination	Glaucoma; higher concentrations in children can cause agitation	0.5% in children, one drop; 1% in adults, one drop; onset 30 min, duration ≤24 h
Anticholinergic	Tropicamide	Mydriacyl® Tropicamide Ophthalmic Solution	Short-term mydriasis and cycloplegia for examination	Glaucoma	One to two drops of 0.5% or 1% solution, onset 20 min; duration of action 6 h
Anticholinergic	Homatropine	Isopto Homatropine®	Intermediate-term pupil dilation, cycloplegia, treatment of iritis	Glaucoma, avoid in children	One to two drops of 2% solution; onset 30 min; duration of action 2–4 d; for iritis one to two drops twice a day
Antihistamine/ decongestant	Naphazoline and pheniramine	Naphcon-A® Visine A®	Conjunctival congestion/itching	Do not use >72 h; avoid in narrow angle glaucoma; hypertension; do not use with contact lenses in place	One drop three to four times a day
Antihistamine	Olopatadine	Patanol®	Allergic conjunctivitis	Do not administer while contact lenses are present	0.1% solution, one drop twice daily, onset of action 30–60 min, duration 12 h
Topical anesthetics	Tetracaine ophthalmic solution	—	Anesthetic for eye examination, foreign body removal	Sensitivity to ester-type anesthetics; no prolonged use; delays healing	0.5% solution, one to two drops; onset of action 1 min, duration 30 min
	Proparacaine ophthalmic solution	Alcaine® Ophthetic®	Anesthetic for eye examination foreign body removal		0.5% solution, one to two drops; onset of action 20 s, duration 15 min
Antibiotics	Erythromycin ophthalmic ointment	—	Conjunctivitis Do not use for corneal abrasion if a contact lens wearer	Not agent of choice for contact lens wearers	1/2 in. applied to lower eyelid two to four times a day
	Ciprofloxacin	Ciloxan® Ophthalmic Solution and Ointment	Conjunctivitis, corneal abrasion if a contact lens wearer	—	Solution: one to two drops when awake every 2 h for 2 d; ointment, 1/2 in. applied to lower eyelid three times a day for 2 d
	Tobramycin	Tobrex® Ophthalmic Solution and Ointment	Conjunctivitis, corneal abrasions if a contact lens wearer	—	0.3% solution, one to two drops every 4 h; 0.3% ointment, 1/2 in. applied to lower lid two to three times/d
	Gentamicin	Garamycin® Genoptic®	Conjunctivitis, corneal abrasion if a contact lens wearer	—	0.3% solution, instill one to two drops every 4 h; 0.3% ointment, 1/2 in. applied to lower lid two to three times/d
	Sulfacetamide sodium	Bleph-10 Ophthalmic Solution 10%®	Conjunctivitis	Do not use for corneal abrasion if a contact lens wearer or if allergic to sulfa	One to two drops four times/d
	Besifloxacin	Besivance Ophthalmic Suspension®	Conjunctivitis, corneal abrasion if a contact lens wearer	—	One drop three times a day for 7 d

(*Continued*)

TABLE 241-2 Ophthalmic Medications Used in the ED (*Continued*)

Type	Generic Name	Trade Name	Indication	Cautions	Usual Dose
Antibiotics (continued)	Levofloxacin	Iquix Ophthalmic Solution® Quixin Ophthalmic Solution®	Conjunctivitis, corneal abrasion if a contact lens wearer	Corneal ulcer	One to two drops every 30 min to 2 h while awake and every 4–6 h at night
	Moxifloxacin hydrochloride	Moxeza Ophthalmic Solution® Vigamox Ophthalmic Solution®	Conjunctivitis, corneal abrasion if a contact lens wearer		One drop twice a day for 7 d
	Ofloxacin	Ocuflox Ophthalmic Solution®	Conjunctivitis, corneal abrasion if a contact lens wearer		Conjunctivitis: one to two drops every 2–4 h for 2 d, then one to two drops four times a day for 5 d. Corneal ulcer: one to two drops every 30 min while awake and one to two drops every 4–6 hours after retiring for 2 d, then one to two drops every hour while awake for 5–7 days, then one to two drops four times a day for 2 d or until treatment completion
	Polymyxin b sulfate, trimethoprim sulfate	Polytrim Ophthalmic Solution®	Conjunctivitis	Do not use for corneal abrasion if a contact lens wearer	One drop every 3 h
	Gatifloxacin	Zymaxid Ophthalmic Solution®	Conjunctivitis, corneal abrasion if a contact lens wearer		
Antivirals	Idoxuridine	Dendrid Sterile Ophthalmic Solution®	Herpes simplex keratitis		One drop every hour
	Trifluridine	Viroptic Ophthalmic Solution®	Herpes simplex keratitis		One drop every 2 h
	Ganciclovir	Zirgan Ophthalmic Gel®	Herpes simplex keratitis		One drop five times per day
Antibiotic–steroid combination	Prednisolone acetate, sulfacetamide sodium	Blephamide Ophthalmic Suspension® Brimonidine Tartrate Ophthalmic Solution®	Conjunctivitis	Do not use for corneal abrasion if a contact lens wearer or if sulfa allergy	Suspension: instill two drops into conjunctival sac every 4 h during the day and at bedtime Ointment: apply ½-in. ribbon into conjunctival sac three to four times a day and two to four times a night
	Dexamethasone, neomycin sulfate, polymyxin b sulfate	Maxitrol Ophthalmic Ointment® Maxitrol Ophthalmic Suspension®	Conjunctivitis	Do not use for corneal abrasion if a contact lens wearer	Ointment: ½ inch in conjunctival sac(s) up to three to four times a day Suspension: instill one to two drops four to six times a day up to every hour
	Neomycin sulfate, polymyxin b sulfate, prednisolone acetate	Poly-Pred Ophthalmic Suspension®	Conjunctivitis	Do not use for corneal abrasion if a contact lens wearer	One to two drops every 3–4 h
	Dexamethasone, tobramycin	TobraDex Ophthalmic Ointment® TobraDex Ophthalmic Suspension® TobraDex ST Ophthalmic Suspension®	Conjunctivitis	Do not use for corneal abrasion if a contact lens wearer	Suspension: one to two drops every 4–6 h ST: one drop every 4–6 h Ointment: ½-in. ribbon three to four times a day
	Loteprednol etabonate, tobramycin	Zylet Ophthalmic Suspension®	Conjunctivitis	Do not use for corneal abrasion if a contact lens wearer	One to two drops every 4–6 h

Nonsteroidal anti-inflammatory drugs	Ketorolac	Acular Ophthalmic Solution® Acular LS Ophthalmic Solution® Acular PF Ophthalmic Solution® Acuvail Ophthalmic Solution®	Allergic conjunctivitis, corneal abrasions, UV keratitis		One drop four times a day for 3–4 d
	Bromfenac	Bromday Ophthalmic Solution®	Allergic conjunctivitis, corneal abrasions, UV keratitis		One drop every day
	Nepafenac	Nevanac Ophthalmic Suspension®	Allergic conjunctivitis, corneal abrasions, UV keratitis		One drop three times a day
	Diclofenac sodium	Voltaren Ophthalmic Solution®	Allergic conjunctivitis, corneal abrasions, UV keratitis		One drop four times a day
Mast cell stabilizers	Nedocromil sodium	Alocril Ophthalmic Solution®	Allergic conjunctivitis		One to two drops twice a day
	Pemirolast potassium	Alamast Ophthalmic Solution®	Allergic conjunctivitis		One to two drops four times a day
	Lodoxamide tromethamine	Alomide Ophthalmic Solution®	Allergic conjunctivitis		One to two drops four times a day
	Cromolyn sodium	Cromolyn Sodium Ophthalmic Solution®	Allergic conjunctivitis		One to two drops four to six times a day
Selective H_1 antagonist	Bepotastine besilate	Bepreve Ophthalmic Solution®	Allergic conjunctivitis		One drop two times a day
	Epinastine hydrochloride	Elestat Ophthalmic Solution®	Allergic conjunctivitis		One drop two times a day
	Emedastine difumarate	Emadine Ophthalmic Solution®	Allergic conjunctivitis		One drop up to four times a day
	Alcaftadine	Lastacaft Ophthalmic Solution®	Allergic conjunctivitis		One drop every day
	Azelastine hydrochloride	Optivar Ophthalmic Solution®	Allergic conjunctivitis		One drop two times a day
Combination mast cell stabilizers–H_1 antagonists	Olopatadine hydrochloride	Pataday Ophthalmic Solution® Patanol Ophthalmic Solution®	Allergic conjunctivitis		One drop two times a day
Nonselective β-blocker	Levobunolol hydrochloride	Betagan Ophthalmic Solution®	Glaucoma		0.5%: one to two drops once a day; twice a day for more severe or uncontrolled glaucoma 0.25%: one to two drops twice a day
	Timolol hemihydrate	Betimol Ophthalmic Solution®	Glaucoma		One drop 0.25% twice a day; may increase to maximum of one drop 0.5% twice a day
	Timolol maleate	Istalol Ophthalmic Solution® Timoptic Sterile Ophthalmic Solution® Timoptic-XE Sterile Ophthalmic Gel Forming Solution®	Glaucoma		One drop once a day
	Carteolol hydrochloride	Carteolol Hydrochloride Ophthalmic Solution® Ocupress Ophthalmic Solution®	Glaucoma		One drop twice a day
	Metipranolol	OptiPranolol Ophthalmic Solution®	Glaucoma		One drop two times a day

(*Continued*)

TABLE 241-2 Ophthalmic Medications Used in the ED (*Continued*)

Type	Generic Name	Trade Name	Indication	Cautions	Usual Dose
Selective β_1-blocker	Betaxolol hydrochloride	Betaxolol Hydrochloride Ophthalmic Solution® Betoptic S Ophthalmic Suspension®	Glaucoma		One to two drops twice a day
Selective α_2-agonists	Brimonidine tartrate	Alphagan P Ophthalmic Solution® Brimonidine Tartrate Ophthalmic Solution®	Glaucoma		One drop every 8 h
	Apraclonidine hydrochloride	Iopidine 0.5% Ophthalmic Solution® Iopidine Ophthalmic Solution®	Glaucoma		One to two drops three times a day
Combination α_2-agonist–nonselective β-blocker	Brimonidine tartrate, timolol maleate	Combigan Ophthalmic Solution®	Glaucoma		One drop every 12 h
Carbonic anhydrase inhibitors	Brinzolamide	Azopt Ophthalmic Suspension®	Glaucoma		One drop three times a day
	Dorzolamide hydrochloride	Trusopt Sterile Ophthalmic Solution®	Glaucoma		One drop three times a day
Combination carbonic anhydrase inhibitor–selective β-blocker	Dorzolamide hydrochloride, timolol maleate	Cosopt Sterile Ophthalmic Solution®	Glaucoma		One drop every 12 h
Cholinergic agents	Pilocarpine hydrochloride	Isopto Carpine Ophthalmic Solution®	Glaucoma; contraindicated in pupillary block glaucoma		Two drops three to four times a day
Prostaglandin analog	Bimatoprost	Lumigan Ophthalmic Solution®	Glaucoma		One drop once a day
	Travoprost	Travatan Z Ophthalmic Solution®	Glaucoma		One drop once a day
	Latanoprost	Xalatan Ophthalmic Solution®	Glaucoma		One drop once a day
	Loteprednol etabonate	Alrex Ophthalmic Suspension®	Allergic conjunctivitis, uveitis		One drop four times a day
	Difluprednate	Durezol Ophthalmic Emulsion®	Allergic conjunctivitis, uveitis		One drop four times a day
	Fluorometholone acetate	Flarex Ophthalmic Suspension® FML Forte Ophthalmic Suspension® FML Ophthalmic Ointment® FML Ophthalmic Suspension®	Allergic conjunctivitis, uveitis		One to two drops four times a day
	Loteprednol etabonate	Lotemax Ophthalmic Ointment® Lotemax Ophthalmic Suspension®	Allergic conjunctivitis, uveitis		Ointment: ½ inch four times a day Suspension: one to two drops four times a day
	Prednisolone acetate	Omnipred Ophthalmic Suspension® Pred Forte Ophthalmic Suspension® Pred Mild Ophthalmic Suspension®	Allergic conjunctivitis, uveitis		Two drops four times a day
	Rimexolone	Vexol 1% Ophthalmic Suspension®	Allergic conjunctivitis, uveitis		One to two drops every hour while awake

Note: Blue-eyed individuals are sensitive to mydriatics and cycloplegics and tend to have a longer duration of action, whereas brown-eyed individuals may require a double dose for adequate mydriasis.

Abbreviation: UV = ultraviolet.

TABLE 241-3 Differential Diagnosis of the Red Eye

Diagnosis	Pain	Itching	Photophobia	Systemic Symptoms	Visual Acuity	Discharge	Injection	Cornea	Pupils	IOP
Chalazion	Mild-moderate lid	No	No	No	Normal	No	Minimal localized	Normal	Normal	Normal
Hordeolum	Mild-moderate lid	No	No	No	Normal	No	Minimal localized	Normal	Normal	Normal
Blepharitis	Mild – foreign body sensation	Yes	Yes	No	Normal	Morning crusting, tearing	Diffuse	Normal	Normal	Normal
Dacryocystitis	Mild-moderate medial canthus	No	No	Fever if severe	Normal	No	Localized	Normal	Normal	Normal
Ectropion	Irritation	No	No	No	Normal	Watery	Lid margin and diffuse	Normal	Normal	Normal
Corneal abrasion	Yes	No	No unless associated iritis (after several hours)	No	Normal unless central or with associated iritis	Watery	Diffuse	Visible abrasion	Normal or constricted with associated iritis	Normal
Ultraviolet keratitis	Severe	No	No unless associated iritis (after several hours)	No	Decreased	Watery	Diffuse	Punctate lesions	Normal or constricted with associated iritis	Normal
Superficial keratitis	Mild	No	No	No	Normal	Watery	Diffuse	Punctate lesions	Normal	Normal
Corneal ulcer	Moderate	No	No	No	No unless central or with associated iritis	Watery	Diffuse	Visible ulcer	Normal	Normal
Corneal foreign body	Moderate	No	No	No	Normal unless central	Watery	Diffuse	Visible foreign body	Normal	Normal
Chemical burn	Moderate-severe	No	No	No	Normal unless central	Watery	Diffuse—none with severe alkaline burn	Cloudy if severe	Normal	Normal
Bacterial conjunctivitis	None or irritation	No	No	No	Normal	Purulent	Diffuse bulbar and palpebral	Normal, punctate lesions if associated keratitis	Normal	Normal
Viral conjunctivitis	None or irritation, severe with EKC	No	No	Occasional URI symptoms, fever with EKC	Normal	Watery	Diffuse bulbar and palpebral	Normal, punctate lesions if associated keratitis	Normal	Normal
Allergic conjunctivitis	None	Yes	No	Sneezing, rhinorrhea	Normal	Watery	Diffuse bulbar and palpebral	Normal	Normal	Normal
Stevens-Johnson syndrome	Foreign body sensation, burning	Yes	Yes	Fever, tachycardia, hypotension, skin and mucous membranes involved	Decreased	Watery	Diffuse	Punctate lesions, corneal ulcer, neovascularization, hazy, perforation	—	—
Orbital cellulitis	Pain with eye movement	No	No	Fever	Normal, decreased late	No	Yes	Normal	Normal	Occasionally increased
Preseptal cellulitis	Mild—no pain with eye movement	No	No	Fever	Normal	No	Yes	Normal	Normal	Normal
Episcleritis	Mild	No	No	Usually none; occasional rheumatologic symptoms	Normal	Watery	Focal	Normal	Normal	Normal
Scleritis	Severe, tender to palpation	No	No	Usually none; occasional rheumatologic symptoms	Decreased with advanced disease	Watery	Diffuse, occasionally violaceous color	Normal	Normal	Normal, may be increased

(Continued)

TABLE 241-3 Differential Diagnosis of the Red Eye (*Continued*)

Diagnosis	Pain	Itching	Photophobia	Systemic Symptoms	Visual Acuity	Discharge	Injection	Cornea	Pupils	IOP
Subconjunctival hemorrhage	None	No	No	No	Normal	No	No	Normal	Normal	Normal
Iritis/uveitis	Yes	No	Yes	Occasional rheumatologic or GI symptoms	Decreased	Watery	Perilimbal (ciliary) flush	Normal, flare and cells in anterior chamber	Constricted, poorly reactive	Usually normal, may be low
Acute angle closure glaucoma	Severe	No	No	Headache, nausea, vomiting	Decreased	Watery	Diffuse	Cloudy or hazy	Midpoint, poorly reactive	Increased
Endophthalmitis	Mild-moderate "ache"	No	Yes	Fever	Decreased	Purulent if present	Diffuse	Hazy, flare and cells anterior chamber, hypopyon	—	—

Abbreviations: EKC = epidemic keratoconjunctivitis; IOP = intraocular pressure; URI = upper respiratory infection.

OCULAR INFECTIONS AND INFLAMMATION

PRESEPTAL (PERIORBITAL) AND POSTSEPTAL (ORBITAL) CELLULITIS

Orbital and periorbital infections exist in a spectrum of increasing severity: preseptal (periorbital) cellulitis, postseptal (orbital) cellulitis, subperiosteal abscess, orbital abscess, and cavernous sinus thrombosis, from least to most severe. Preseptal cellulitis and postseptal cellulitis, although both of an infectious etiology and involving periocular tissues, are very different entities with different morbidities. **Preseptal cellulitis (periorbital cellulitis)** is an infection of the eyelids and periocular tissues that is anterior to the orbital septum. It is generally benign and may be treated in the outpatient setting. **Postseptal cellulitis (orbital cellulitis)** is an infection of the orbital soft tissues posterior to the orbital septum. It may be life- and vision-threatening and must be treated as an inpatient with IV antibiotics and occasionally surgical drainage. **Endophthalmitis** is an infection of the globe and is a completely separate entity.

The outward appearance of the patient with postseptal cellulitis may be very similar to that of the patient with preseptal cellulitis. Preseptal and postseptal cellulitis may both display excessive tearing, fever, erythema, edema, warmth, and tenderness to palpation of the lids and periorbital soft tissues. Laboratory studies do not discriminate between the two conditions, and blood cultures are not helpful. **CT scan differentiates the two conditions.** Differentiation of preseptal and postseptal cellulitis is essential. A misdiagnosis can result in significant neurologic disability and death. The differential diagnosis for preseptal and postseptal cellulitis is listed in **Table 241-4**.

TABLE 241-4 Differential Diagnosis of Preseptal and Postseptal Cellulitis

Preseptal cellulitis
Postseptal cellulitis
Subperiosteal abscess
Orbital abscess
Cavernous sinus thrombosis
Dacryoadenitis
Dacryocystitis
Hordeolum
Bacterial and viral conjunctivitis
Contact dermatitis
Herpes zoster
Herpes simplex

Preseptal Cellulitis **Preseptal cellulitis** is usually associated with upper respiratory tract infections, especially paranasal sinusitis, and may result from eyelid problems such as hordeolum, chalazion, insect bites, and trauma. Preseptal cellulitis is primarily a disease of childhood, with most patients <10 years of age. The most common organisms are *Staphylococcus aureus* and *S. epidermidis*, *Streptococcus* species, and anaerobes. Since the introduction of the *Haemophilus influenzae* type B vaccine, *H. influenzae* has become a rare cause of preseptal cellulitis in children.

Upper respiratory symptoms, low-grade fever, redness and swelling of the eyelid, and excessive tearing (epiphora) are signs and symptoms of preseptal cellulitis. **The eye itself is not involved, and visual acuity and pupillary reaction are maintained, and full painless ocular motility is preserved.**

CT scan of the orbit is not necessary for uncomplicated cases of preseptal cellulitis; however, when there is decreased ocular motility or other signs of orbital involvement, or in the young child in whom examination may be unreliable, or if there is any concern for postseptal cellulitis, obtain a CT scan of the orbit with contrast. MRI is also an option.

The nontoxic, adult patient and older child with mild preseptal cellulitis may be managed as outpatients with oral antibiotics (amoxicillin/clavulanic acid or a first-generation cephalosporin), hot packs, and close follow-up in 24 to 48 hours. For the young child and more severe cases of preseptal cellulitis, consider hospitalization; treatment with a third-generation cephalosporin such as ceftriaxone and vancomycin is often added for the possibility of methicillin-resistant *S. aureus*. Obtain ophthalmology consultation in young children (see Chapter 119, Eye Emergencies in Infants and Children).

Postseptal or Orbital Cellulitis **Postseptal cellulitis** occurs most frequently from the spread of paranasal sinusitis. The ethmoid sinus is most frequently implicated, probably due to perforation of the thin lamina papyracea. Trauma, intraorbital foreign body, spread of periorbital skin infection, seeding from bacteremia, and ocular surgery are also predisposing factors. The infection is often polymicrobial, with *S. aureus*, *S. pneumoniae*, and anaerobes being most common; however, *H. influenzae* should be considered in unimmunized young children and mucormycosis in diabetics and immunocompromised patients.

Orbital cellulitis is characterized by an insidious onset with preceding upper respiratory symptoms, including rhinitis, facial pressure, and fever. The patient will often complain of pain when moving the eyes. There may be a decrease in visual acuity. On examination, signs referable to orbital involvement are present, including limitation of extraocular muscle movement, chemosis, proptosis, abnormal pupillary response, and decreased visual acuity. **Involvement of cranial nerves 3, 4, or 6 suggests cavernous sinus thrombosis.**

Postseptal cellulitis may lead to vision loss and requires an aggressive approach with hospitalization and institution of IV antibiotics (see Chapter 119, Eye Emergencies in Infants and Children). Any patient suspected of having postseptal cellulitis clinically or by CT scan of the orbit should have immediate ophthalmologic consultation. Antibiotics should be broad spectrum with both aerobic and anaerobic coverage. Choices include second- or third-generation cephalosporins, ampicillin-sulbactam, ticarcillin-clavulanate, and carbapenems. A fluoroquinolone is used for penicillin-allergic patients, and metronidazole or clindamycin is added for anaerobic coverage. Adjuvant therapy includes a topical nasal decongestant such as oxymetazoline. Consider emergent **lateral canthotomy** if the intraocular pressure is elevated or an optic neuropathy is present. Patients with orbital abscess require operative drainage and debridement in addition to antibiotics. Complications include cavernous sinus thrombosis, frontal bone osteomyelitis, meningitis, subdural empyema, epidural abscess, and brain abscess that should be evident on CT or MRI scan.

LIDS

Stye (External Hordeolum) A **stye** is an acute bacterial infection (usually *Staphylococcus*) of the follicle of an eyelash and adjacent sebaceous glands (Zeis) or sweat glands (Moll). It is located at the lash line and has the appearance of a small pustule at the margin of the eyelid (**Figure 241-24**). An **internal hordeolum** is an acute bacterial infection of the meibomian glands associated with the eyelashes. Signs and symptoms are similar to a stye except that the pustule occurs on the inner surface of the tarsal plate. Signs and symptoms include pain, edema, and erythema of the eyelid. Warm compresses and erythromycin ophthalmic ointment twice daily for 7 to 10 days are usually sufficient treatment. Removal of the offending eyelash could be considered. Systemic antibiotics may be necessary if there is significant surrounding cellulitis. Should incision and drainage be considered, refer to an ophthalmologist.

Chalazion A **chalazion** is an acute or chronic inflammation of the eyelid secondary to blockage of one of the meibomian or Zeis oil glands in the tarsal plate (**Figure 241-25**). The condition tends to be subacute to chronic and is associated with a (usually) painless lump that develops in the lid or at the lid margin, occasionally with mild erythema. Clinical differentiation of an acute chalazion from an internal hordeolum may be impossible, but treatment is the same. Treatment of chronic or recurrent chalazia may require injection of corticosteroids into the lesion or incision and curettage/drainage depending on the size. Refer to an ophthalmologist in 1 to 2 weeks.

Blepharitis **Blepharitis** is a common cause of prolonged red eye due to inflammation of the eyelash follicles along the edge of the eyelid. The most common cause is overgrowth of *S. epidermidis*, and the inflation is

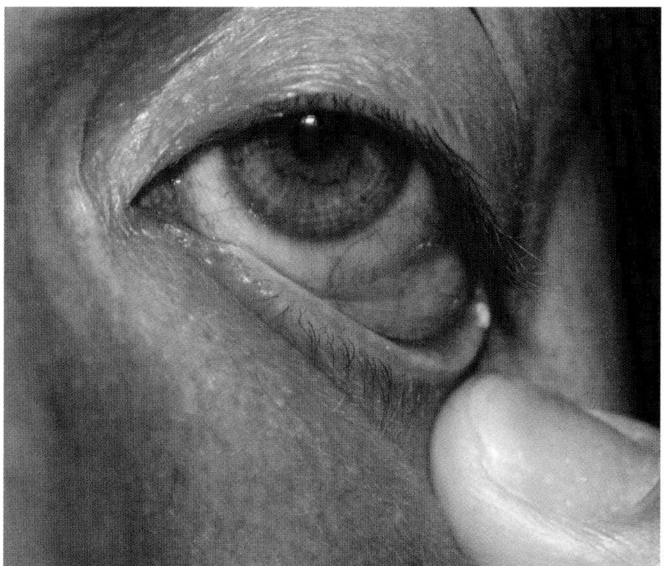

FIGURE 241-24. External hordeolum. [Courtesy of Allen R. Katz, Department of Ophthalmology, University of Nebraska Medical Center.]

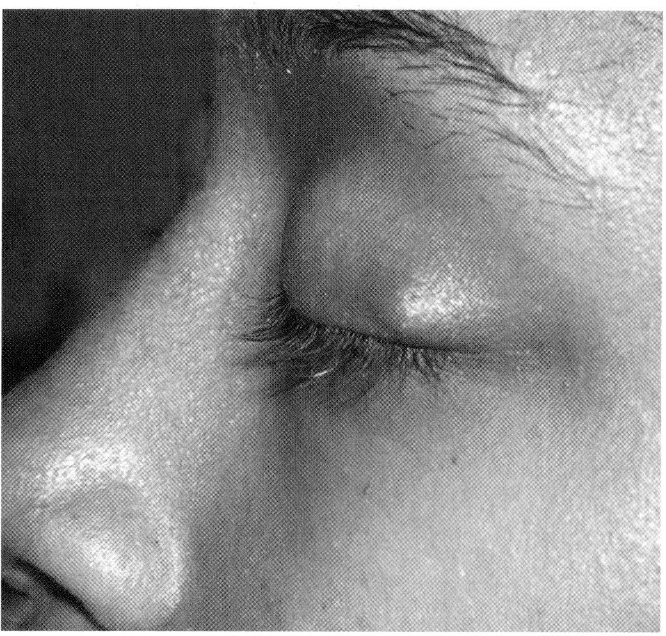

FIGURE 241-25. Chalazion. [Courtesy of Allen R. Katz, Department of Ophthalmology, University of Nebraska Medical Center.]

largely a reaction to the deltalike toxin produced by the bacteria. The disorder is associated with seborrheic dermatitis, atopic dermatitis, and occasionally eyelash infestation with lice or infection with *S. aureus*. Typical symptoms include conjunctival injection; crusting, swollen, pruritic eyelids; and occasional complaint of eye pain. It is most commonly treated with careful daily cleansing of the edges of the eyelids and eyelashes. In severe cases, antibiotic drops or ointment at night may be required.

Conjunctivitis **Conjunctivitis** is an inflammatory condition of the conjunctiva and is a common cause of the red eye. It is usually viral in etiology and is a benign self-limited condition. **The task is to sort out the occasional case of serious bacterial infection or corneal herpetic involvement that may result in vision loss without aggressive treatment.** Causes of conjunctivitis are viral, bacterial (including gonococcal and chlamydial), parasitic, or fungal infections and allergic, toxic, or chemical irritation. **Keratoconjunctivitis** is the term used to indicate corneal involvement, usually in the form of punctuate ulcerations.

Bacterial Conjunctivitis Symptoms of **bacterial conjunctivitis** are painless, unilateral, or bilateral mucopurulent discharge (**Figure 241-26**), frequently causing adherence of the eyelids on awakening. The conjunctiva is injected, and the cornea is clear *without* fluorescein staining. Chemosis (edema of the conjunctiva) is common, and preauricular lymphadenopathy is usually absent, except in gonococcal infections. Typical pathogens are *Staphylococcus* and *Streptococcus* species. Perform fluorescein stain of the cornea (especially in infants) to avoid missing a corneal abrasion, ulcer, or herpetic dendrite. Consider culture and sensitivity of the discharge in severe cases. Treatment consists of a topical ocular antibiotic four times daily for 5 to 7 days. Treatment with a broad-spectrum agent is safe for patients 2 months of age and older. Trimethoprim–polymyxin B is very effective and avoids potential allergies to sulfa and neomycin preparations. Wearers of soft contact lenses should be treated with a fluoroquinolone (besifloxacin, gatifloxacin, levofloxacin, moxifloxacin, or ofloxacin) or aminoglycoside (tobramycin) to treat *Pseudomonas*. Gentamicin is seldom used because of the high incidence of ocular irritation.

Gonococcal conjunctivitis is a cause of ophthalmia neonatorum, and **chlamydial conjunctivitis** is also a disease of the newborn (see Chapter 119, Eye Emergencies in Infants and Children, for discussion of ophthalmia neonatorum and chlamydia conjunctivitis).

Viral Conjunctivitis The most common cause of **viral conjunctivitis** is adenovirus, which generally resolves spontaneously with only symptomatic

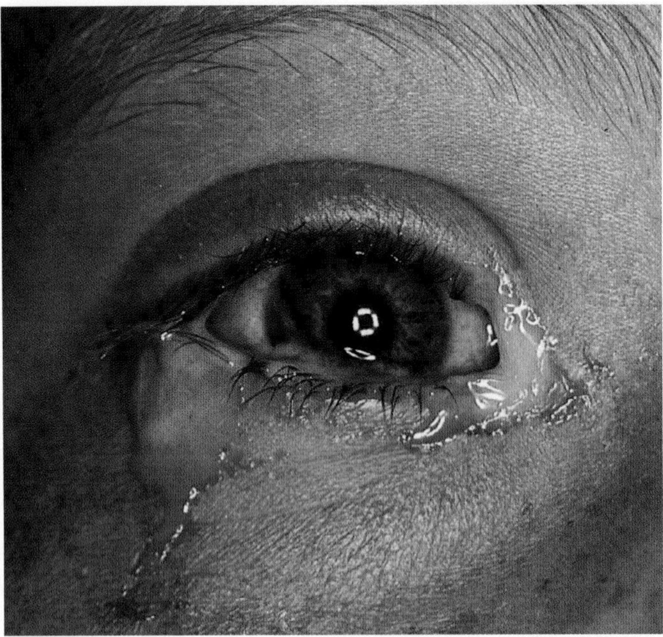

FIGURE 241-26. Bacterial conjunctivitis. Note the mucopurulent discharge, conjunctival injection, and lid edema in a pediatric patient with *Haemophilus influenzae* conjunctivitis. [Reproduced with permission from Knoop K, Stack L, Storrow A: *Atlas of Emergency Medicine,* 2nd ed. © 2002, McGraw-Hill, New York.]

treatment. Several systemic viral diseases, such as measles, influenza, and mumps, may also cause conjunctival injection. Viral keratoconjunctivitis may be caused by **herpes simplex** and **herpes zoster**, and, if left untreated, may result in corneal scarring and loss of vision. **Epidemic keratoconjunctivitis** (**Figure 241-27**) is a more severe type of adenovirus infection that is highly contagious and tends to occur in epidemics. It is often preceded by cough, high fever, malaise, and myalgias. Symptoms are marked eye redness, photophobia, foreign body sensation, and tearing. Physical examination findings are similar to viral conjunctivitis, except they are more severe.

Viral conjunctivitis is often preceded by an upper respiratory infection. Symptoms include a complaint of "red eye" and mild to moderate watery discharge. There is no eye pain unless there is some degree of keratitis. Generally, one eye will be involved initially, with the other eye becoming involved within days. Physical examination reveals unilateral or bilateral conjunctival injection, occasional chemosis and small subconjunctival hemorrhages, and preauricular lymphadenopathy. Slit lamp examination demonstrates follicles (small, regular, translucent bumps) on the inferior palpebral conjunctiva (**Figure 241-27**). Punctate fluorescein staining represents keratitis (**Figure 241-28**). Make sure to examine the cornea with fluorescein to avoid missing a herpetic dendrite.

Treatment consists of cool compresses; ocular decongestants such as Naphcon-A®, one drop three times daily as needed for redness and conjunctival congestion; and artificial tears five or six times a day. Viral conjunctivitis can take 1 to 3 weeks to run its course and is very contagious. Instruct the patient to wash hands frequently and use separate towels. The examiner should wear gloves to avoid self-contamination, and the slit lamp, exam table, and exam chair should be disinfected after patient contact. If, after a history and physical examination, it is still uncertain if the conjunctivitis is viral or bacterial, prescribe ocular antibiotics until the patient is reexamined by an ophthalmologist.

Allergic Conjunctivitis Allergens can cause watery discharge, redness, and itching. Physical findings may include erythematous swollen eyelids and injected and edematous conjunctiva with papillae (irregular mounds of tissue with a central vascular tuft) on the inferior conjunctival fornix (**Figure 241-29**). Try to identify and eliminate the offending allergen. Treatment is cool compresses four times daily and topical drops, depending on the severity of symptoms. Mild symptoms may be treated with artificial tears alone. Moderate symptoms may additionally require a topical antihistamine/decongestant, mast cell stabilizers, or nonsteroidal anti-inflammatory drugs, and severe symptoms may justify the use of topical steroids. We generally recommend against the use of ocular steroids except by an ophthalmologist because occult herpetic infection is always a possibility (see following section on herpes simplex virus infection of the cornea). **Should ocular steroids be chosen as a treatment option, consult an ophthalmologist first.**

Subconjunctival Hemorrhage The fragile conjunctival vessels can rupture from trauma, sudden increased venous pressure related to Valsalva maneuvers (sneezing, coughing, vomiting, straining), hypertension, or spontaneously (**Figure 241-30**). The eye examination is normal other than the presence of the subconjunctival hemorrhage. Reassurance is the only treatment necessary, and the hemorrhage usually resolves within 2 weeks. If multiple recurrent episodes occur, coagulation studies and further investigation are warranted.

CORNEA

Herpes Simplex Keratoconjunctivitis Herpes simplex virus can affect the eyelids, conjunctiva, and cornea. The patient may give a history of oral or genital herpes infection and complain of photophobia,

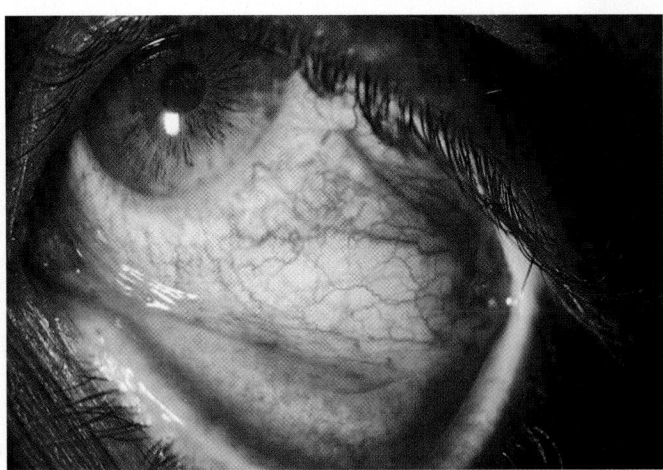

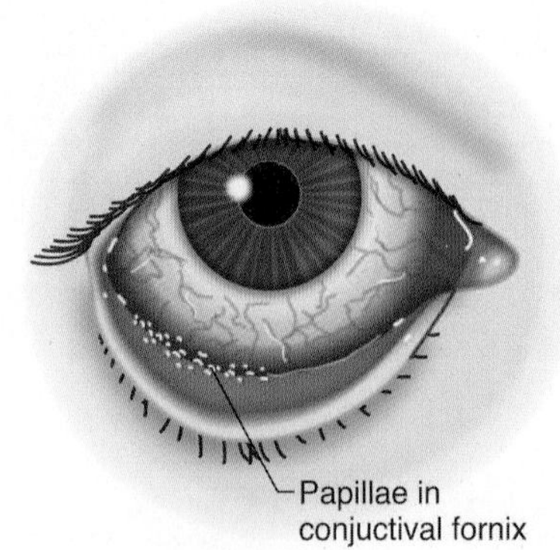

FIGURE 241-27. Epidemic keratoconjunctivitis (EKC). Diffuse bulbar conjunctival injection and inferior palpebral papillae as seen in EKC. The erythema is usually much more intense than in this photo. [Reproduced with permission from Knoop K, Stack L, Storrow A: *Atlas of Emergency Medicine,* 2nd ed. © 2002, McGraw-Hill, New York.]

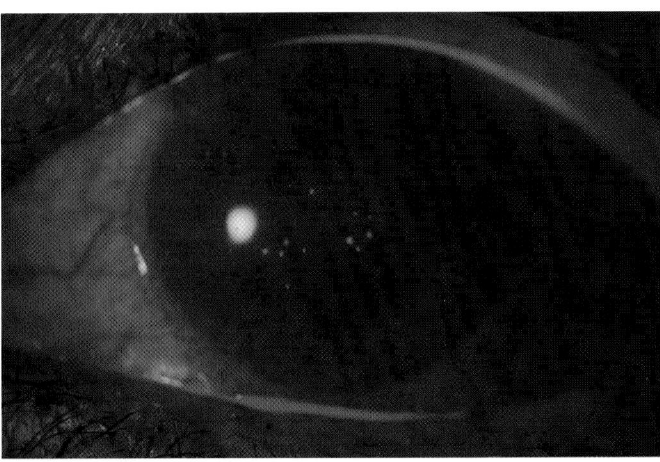

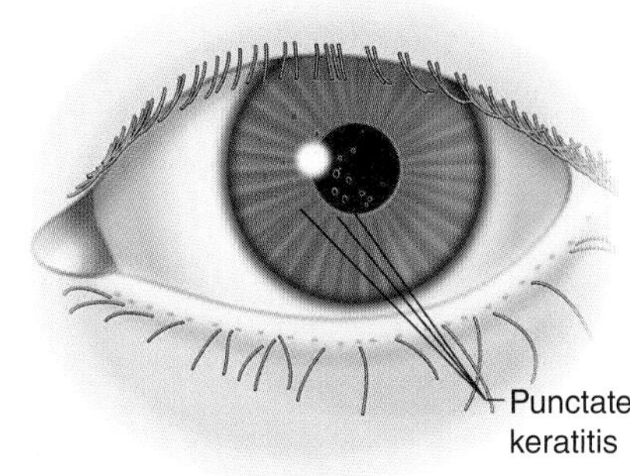

FIGURE 241-28. Fluorescein stain demonstrating punctate staining as seen with epithelial keratitis in epidemic keratoconjunctivitis. The keratitis is usually much more widespread than demonstrated here. [Reproduced with permission from Knoop K, Stack L, Storrow A: *Atlas of Emergency Medicine,* 2nd ed. © 2002, McGraw-Hill, New York.]

pain (which may be mild), eye redness, and decreased vision. The eyelid may have the typical herpetic vesicular eruptions. The infection tends to be unilateral with a palpable preauricular node. The conjunctiva can be injected, but ocular herpes simplex frequently presents with only corneal findings on physical examination. The findings can be subtle and are easily missed. The dendrite of herpes keratitis is an epithelial defect that can be seen with fluorescein staining and classically has a linear branching pattern with terminal bulbs (**Figure 241-31**), or may be a "geographic ulcer," which is an amoeba-shaped ulceration with dendrites at the edge. **Herpetic infection may be very difficult to diagnose**, as infection may present as involvement of the cornea with a neurotrophic ulceration, which is a smooth-edged ulcer over an area of underlying stromal disease; as stromal edema and/or white infiltrates with intact epithelium and an associated mild iritis with keratitic precipitates; or as an isolated uveitis, without epithelial or stromal involvement and with an elevated intraocular pressure. Corneal sensation may be decreased and should be checked before instillation of anesthetic drops. The diagnosis of herpes simplex is usually clinical, but check with the ophthalmologic consultant to see if cultures are desired.

Herpes simplex keratitis can progress to corneal scarring and requires prompt treatment with topical antiviral agents. **An initial outbreak of herpes simplex virus involving the lids is treated with an oral acyclovir derivative such as acyclovir (Zovirax®) or famciclovir (Famvir®). For conjunctival involvement, prescribe topical trifluridine (Viroptic®), one drop nine times a day.** Idoxuridine (Dendrid®), one drop every 1 hour during the day and every 2 hours at night, can be substituted for those who are allergic. Erythromycin ophthalmic ointment can be added to prevent secondary infection.

Oral acyclovir or other derivative agents do not prevent progression of corneal epithelial disease to deeper involvement of the stroma or uveal tract. Do not prescribe topical steroids, and refer patients to an ophthalmologist in 24 to 48 hours.

Herpes Zoster Ophthalmicus **Herpes zoster ophthalmicus** is shingles involving the first division (V1) of the trigeminal nerve distribution with ocular involvement. The rash usually does not cross the midline and involves only the upper eyelid, although rarely the cheek (V2) and mandible (V3) may be affected. **Involvement of the nasociliary nerve is associated with cutaneous lesions on the tip of the nose (Hutchinson sign) and predicts a high likelihood of ocular involvement.** Symptoms that may precede the rash are pain and paresthesias in a dermatomal distribution; fever, headache, and malaise; and red eye, blurred vision, and eye pain/photophobia. Eye involvement may take the form of epithelial keratitis, stromal keratitis, uveitis, retinitis, and choroiditis. Optic neuritis and other cranial nerve palsies may occur, as well as elevated intraocular pressure. The cornea can have a pseudodendrite, which is a poorly staining mucous plaque with no epithelial erosion (unlike herpes simplex virus, which has a true dendrite with epithelial

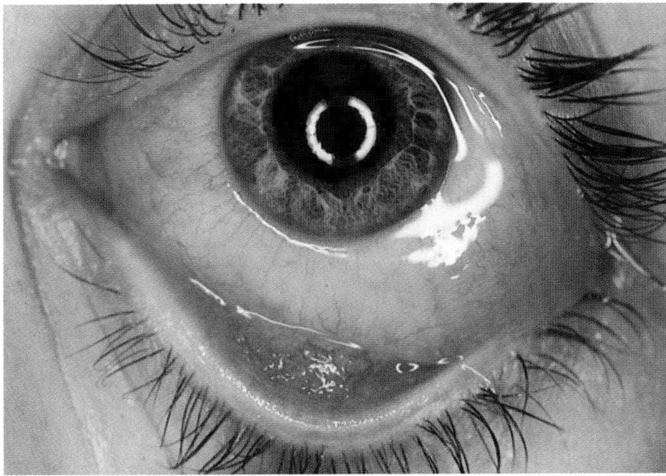

FIGURE 241-29. Prominent chemosis may be seen in allergic conjunctivitis. [Reproduced with permission from Knoop K, Stack L, Storrow A: *Atlas of Emergency Medicine,* 2nd ed. © 2002, McGraw-Hill, New York.]

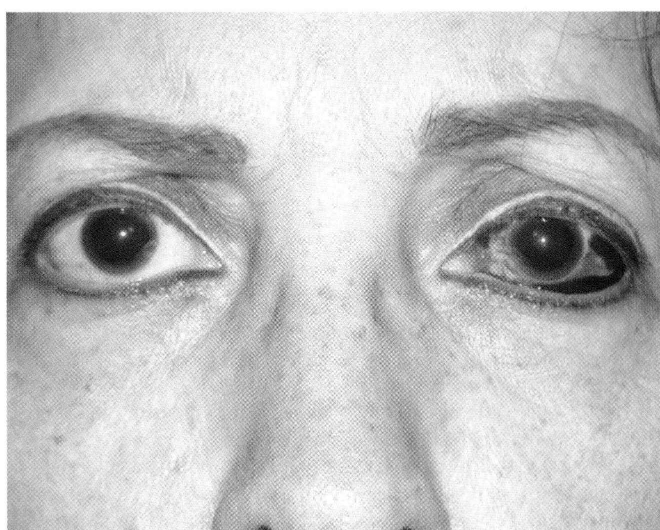

FIGURE 241-30. Spontaneous subconjunctival hemorrhage. [Courtesy of Allen R. Katz, Department of Ophthalmology, University of Nebraska Medical Center.]

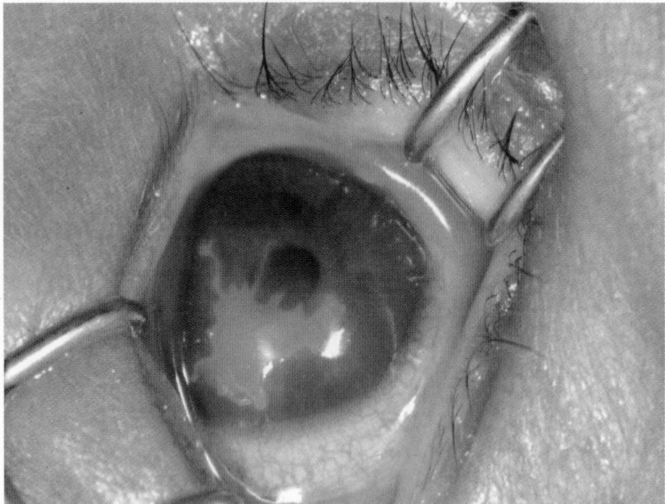

FIGURE 241-31. Herpes simplex corneal dendrite in an infant seen with fluorescein staining. [Courtesy of Allen R. Katz, Department of Ophthalmology, University of Nebraska Medical Center.]

erosion and staining). The anterior chamber on slit lamp examination can show the cells and flare of iritis. Consider the possibility of associated immunocompromise in patients <40 years old.

Skin involvement is treated with cool compresses, and patients presenting with a rash for <1 week should be treated with oral antiviral medications for 7 to 10 days. Choices include acyclovir, 800 milligrams five times a day; famciclovir, 500 milligrams three times a day; or valacyclovir, 1000 milligrams three times a day. Cutaneous lesions are treated with bacitracin or erythromycin ointment to prevent secondary bacterial infection. Conjunctivitis is treated with erythromycin ophthalmic ointment twice a day. Iritis can be treated with topical steroids such as prednisolone acetate 1%, one drop four to five times a day, but consultation with an ophthalmologist is recommended first. Pain reduction can be achieved with topical cycloplegic agents (cyclopentolate 1%, one drop three times daily). If herpes zoster ophthalmicus is diagnosed, in particular, when the orbit, optic nerve, or cranial nerves are involved, or if the patient is immunocompromised or systemically ill, consider admission and IV acyclovir.

Corneal Ulcer A **corneal ulcer** is a serious infection involving multiple layers of the cornea and develops secondary to breaks in the epithelial barrier, so that infectious agents invade the underlying corneal stroma. The initial disruption of the epithelial layer can be due to desquamation, trauma, or direct microbial invasion. Exposure keratitis from incomplete lid closure secondary to **Bell's palsy** can cause corneal desiccation and sloughing of the epithelium, allowing bacteria to gain access to the underlying stroma and create an ulcer. Trauma can also breach the epithelium and inoculate the cornea. *S. pneumoniae* and *S. aureus* are common causes of corneal ulceration. Contact lens users can develop *Pseudomonas* infection (**Table 241-5**). Wearing of soft contact lenses is a very common cause of corneal ulcers, and the incidence increases dramatically in those who use extended-wear lenses and wearers who sleep with them in place. Fungi and viruses have also become a more common cause of corneal ulcer due to the widespread use of both topical and systemic immunosuppressant medications.

The history should include an inquiry into the use of contact lenses, previous ocular surgery or injury, recent trauma, and presence or history of genital herpes. Medication history should include questions about the use of topical or systemic steroids or other immunosuppressants.

Patients may complain of redness and swelling of lids and conjunctivae, discharge from the eye, ocular pain or foreign body sensation, photophobia, or blurred vision. Visual acuity is decreased if the ulcer is located in the central visual axis or if uveal tract inflammation is present. The eyelids and conjunctiva may be erythematous with a mucopurulent discharge. Associated iritis may cause a miotic pupil and consensual photophobia due to ciliary spasm. Examination of the cornea reveals a round or irregular ulcer with a white, hazy base extending into the underlying stroma due to WBC infiltration, or with heaped-up edges (**Figure 241-32**). Slit lamp examination reveals flare and cell from iritis and occasionally a hypopyon.

TABLE 241-5 Causative Organisms in Corneal Ulcer

Bacteria
Pseudomonas aeruginosa
Streptococcus pneumoniae
Staphylococcus species
Moraxella species
Viruses
Herpes simplex
Varicella zoster
Fungi
Candida
Aspergillus
Penicillium
Cephalosporium

Diagnosis is made by the clinical appearance. The organism is identified by scraping of the ulcer and culture of the offending organism, generally done by the ophthalmologist. The differential diagnosis as to causative organisms is listed in **Table 241-5**.

Corneal ulcers need to be treated aggressively with topical antibiotics. Emergent ophthalmologic consultation for culture of the ulcer and institution of appropriate antibiotics should be considered. Once cultures are obtained, topical antibiotics are started. A fluoroquinolone such as ciprofloxacin (Ciloxan®) or ofloxacin (Ocuflox®), one drop every hour in the affected eye, is the current recommended treatment. If the suspicion is high for viral or fungal infection, a topical antiviral medication (e.g., natamycin, amphotericin B, or fluconazole) should be given.

Cycloplegic drops such as cyclopentolate 1% are often used due to pain from accompanying iritis. Topical steroids are relatively contraindicated in viral infections but may decrease the incidence of scarring and perforation. Steroid eye drops should not be initiated by the emergency physician unless advised to do so by the ophthalmologist. **Do not patch the eye because of the risk of *Pseudomonas* infection, which can cause rapid, aggressive ulceration with corneal melting and perforation.** All corneal ulcers should be referred to an ophthalmologist to be seen within 12 to 24 hours. Complications of corneal ulcers include corneal scarring, corneal perforation, development of anterior and posterior synechiae, glaucoma, and cataracts.

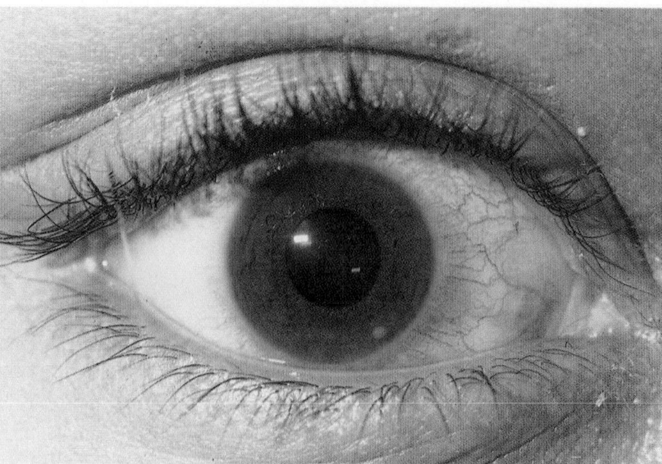

FIGURE 241-32. Corneal ulcer is seen at 5 o'clock. [Courtesy of Allen R. Katz, Department of Ophthalmology, University of Nebraska Medical Center.]

Ultraviolet Keratitis Light in the ultraviolet range can cause death of corneal epithelial cells. Classically described as "snow blindness," **ultraviolet keratitis** is also caused by unprotected exposure to arc welders and tanning beds and is often called "*welder's flash*." Ultraviolet keratitis may occur if protective glasses are not applied tightly to the face, allowing light to hit the cornea obliquely. Effects are cumulative, so multiple short exposures are the same as one long exposure. Corneal cells do not die immediately, so symptoms develop after a delay of up to 6 to 12 hours with slow onset of foreign body sensation and mild photophobia, progressing to severe pain and photophobia. Patients sometimes are awakened from sleep after midnight by pain. Physical examination may reveal blepharospasm, conjunctival injection, and prominent tearing. Topical anesthetic drops are often required to complete the eye examination. Slit lamp examination reveals diffuse punctate corneal edema, and instillation of fluorescein reveals diffuse punctate corneal abrasions. Treatment may include double patching of both eyes if the patient requests, and the use of cycloplegics, topical antibiotics (erythromycin), and oral analgesics. Healing occurs in 24 to 36 hours.

UVEAL TRACT

Uveitis/Iritis Iritis is inflammation of the anterior segment of the uveal tract. It is not a true ocular emergency, but does require follow-up by an ophthalmologist. Iritis is caused by inflammation of various local and systemic etiologies. Pain in iritis is caused by irritation of the ciliary nerves and ciliary muscle spasm. Ciliary spasm irritates the trigeminal nerve and can cause photophobia. Keratitic precipitates are deposits of inflammatory cells on the corneal endothelium. A proteinaceous transudate from uveal vessels occurs in the anterior chamber and causes flare seen with the slit lamp. WBCs released from the uveal vessels may be seen in the anterior chamber with the slit lamp and are termed *cells* (as in "flare and cells"). Cells appear as snowflakes in a headlight beam at night.

The patient will complain of unilateral pain, although the pain may be bilateral with systemic disease. There may be complaints of conjunctival injection, photophobia, and decreased vision. There is usually no discharge. Complaints of systemic symptoms, including arthritis, urethritis, and recurrent GI symptoms, are not unusual. Past medical history should include exposure to tuberculosis, history of genital herpes, or history of previous similar symptoms, and the associated diagnosis. Ask about recent trauma or exposure to welding without protective goggles.

Inspection of the eye may reveal a perilimbal flush (injection is greatest around the limbus) or diffuse conjunctival injection without mucopurulent discharge. Photophobia is usually present. **Consensual photophobia (shining light on the unaffected eye causes pain in the affected eye) is highly suggestive of iritis.** The pupil is usually miotic and poorly reactive. Visual acuity may be decreased with severe inflammation and clouding of the aqueous humor. Slit lamp examination will reveal flare and cells in the anterior chamber, culminating in a hypopyon with severe disease. Intraocular pressure may be decreased if the ciliary body is involved secondary to decreased production of aqueous humor. Fluorescein staining of the cornea may show abrasions, ulcerations, or dendritic lesions.

The diagnosis of iritis is based on the typical history and the finding of flare and cells in the anterior chamber on slit lamp examination. The differential diagnosis is listed in **Table 241-6**.

Blocking the pupillary sphincter and ciliary body with a long-acting cycloplegic agent, such as homatropine (duration 2 to 4 days) or tropicamide (duration 24 hours), will decrease pain. Refer the patient to an ophthalmologist in 24 to 48 hours.

TABLE 241-6 Differential Diagnosis of Iritis

Systemic diseases	Malignancies
Juvenile rheumatoid arthritis	Leukemia
Ankylosing spondylitis	Lymphoma
Ulcerative colitis	Malignant melanoma
Reiter syndrome	Trauma/environmental
Behçet's syndrome	Corneal foreign body
Sarcoidosis	Post-traumatic (blunt trauma)
Infectious	Ultraviolet keratitis
Tuberculosis	
Lyme disease	
Herpes simplex	
Toxoplasmosis	
Varicella zoster	
Syphilis	
Adenovirus	

VITREOUS HUMOR

Endophthalmitis Endophthalmitis is inflammation (usually infectious) of the aqueous or vitreous humor that frequently leads to loss of vision. The most frequent cause is postsurgical, followed by penetrating ocular injuries and, rarely, hematogenous spread. History may include ocular surgery, hammering with steel, working with high-speed machinery such as grinders or weed whackers, or ocular trauma. Symptoms may include headache, eye pain, photophobia, vision loss, and ocular discharge. Physical examination may reveal erythema and swelling of the lids, conjunctival and scleral injection, chemosis, hypopyon, and evidence of uveitis. If suspected, immediate ophthalmologic consultation is required. Treatment may include aspiration of the vitreous or pars plana vitrectomy, and administration of intravitreal antibiotics and steroids, in addition to systemic antibiotics. Admission is required except for postoperative cases.

Vitreous Detachment and Hemorrhage The vitreous is avascular and attached firmly to the anterior eye at the ora serrata, posteriorly at the optic nerve head, and along the major retinal vessels. Liquefaction of the vitreous can cause detachment from the retina, with or without accompanying hemorrhage. Symptoms are sudden onset of floaters, especially with eye movement. Traction at vascular areas due to trauma or pathologic neovascularization can cause vitreous hemorrhage. The most common causes of vitreous hemorrhage are proliferative diabetic retinopathy, posterior vitreous detachment in the elderly, and ocular trauma such as shaken baby syndrome in infants. An unusual cause is subhyaloid hemorrhage associated with subarachnoid hemorrhage. **History includes sudden painless vision loss and sudden appearance of black spots, cobwebs, or generalized unilateral hazy vision.** Past medical history may include diabetes or sickle cell disease. Examination of the retina of the affected eye may be impossible due to the hemorrhage. Examination of the contralateral retina may give clues to the diagnosis. Important differential diagnoses include sickle cell disease, diabetic retinopathy, retinal detachment, central retinal vein occlusion, subarachnoid hemorrhage, and lupus erythematosus. Consult ophthalmology if the diagnosis is suspected. Check the INR of patients receiving warfarin (Coumadin®) and withhold antiplatelet therapy. Ocular US can rule out retinal detachment.

TRAUMA TO THE EYE

CONJUNCTIVAL ABRASION, LACERATION, AND FOREIGN BODY

The conjunctiva has less innervation than the cornea, so **conjunctival abrasions** are far less symptomatic than corneal abrasions. The patient may complain of a scratchy foreign body sensation, mild pain, tearing, and, rarely, photophobia. Vision should not be affected unless there is a full-thickness conjunctival laceration with globe penetration. Physical examination may reveal mild conjunctival injection or subconjunctival hemorrhage. A conjunctival abrasion is seen with fluorescein staining.

Conjunctival lacerations may bleed, the edges of the bulbar conjunctiva may retract with underlying sclera visible to the naked eye, and fluorescein stain may pool in the defect. Perform the Seidel test to exclude globe perforation. **The Seidel test can be negative if a full-thickness laceration is small or has spontaneously closed.** Inspect the conjunctiva for a foreign body. Conjunctival foreign bodies usually can be removed with a moistened, cotton-tipped applicator after anesthetizing the eye with a topical anesthetic. Evert the upper eyelid and inspect under the highest magnification available to avoid missing any additional foreign bodies. Frequently, small wooden particles such as sawdust will blend into the conjunctiva when moistened by the tears and be difficult to find without slit lamp magnification.

Superficial conjunctival abrasions and lacerations without any other associated ocular injury only require erythromycin ophthalmic ointment 0.5% four times a day for 2 to 3 days or no treatment if very small. Suturing of lacerations is almost never required. Any suspicion of globe laceration requires immediate ophthalmologic referral.

CORNEAL ABRASION, LACERATION, AND FOREIGN BODY

The corneal epithelium is fragile and easily damaged. It is richly innervated and therefore very painful when injury occurs. Corneal epithelium regenerates quickly, so healing time for abrasions is short, usually within 24 to 48 hours. Intact corneal epithelium is resistant to infection, but damaged epithelium is a portal of entry for bacteria, viruses, and fungi. Most abrasions not treated immediately will develop an associated inflammatory iritis.

Corneal Abrasion Abrasions may be caused by contact lens wear, fingernails, makeup brushes, and foreign objects blown into eyes while driving or on windy days or that drop into the eye while working overhead (construction) or under a car (mechanics). Injury to the cornea causes intense pain that may be delayed several hours after the inciting event. Initial symptoms are a foreign body sensation, photophobia, and tearing. Ask about the work environment and the mechanism of injury if known, because corneal abrasions sustained using high-speed machinery, such as grinders, lawn mowers, or weed whackers, and hammering metal against metal are associated with corneal laceration and perforation of the globe.

Inspection of the eye may reveal conjunctival injection, tearing, and lid swelling. Blepharospasm may occur with severe pain, requiring a topical anesthetic to accomplish the examination and obtain the visual acuity. Relief of pain with topical anesthesia is virtually diagnostic of corneal abrasion. Photophobia may be evident when shining a light into the affected or the opposite eye. Decreased visual acuity may occur if the abrasion is in the central visual axis or if there is an associated iritis, but otherwise vision should be normal. The corneal abrasion is often visible to the naked eye as an irregular area of light reflection off the cornea.

Slit lamp examination may show flare and cells from iritis if the abrasion is large and >24 hours old, but there is no corneal infiltrate. Examine the entire thickness of the cornea for full-thickness laceration, and the Seidel test should be negative. The abrasion usually appears as a superficial, irregular corneal defect appearing bright green under the cobalt blue light after instillation of fluorescein (**Figure 241-33**). A series of small, fine-lined vertical corneal abrasions seen with fluorescein staining suggests the presence of a foreign body embedded in the tarsal conjunctiva of the upper lid. Multiple linear corneal abrasions or punctuate keratitis also suggest a retained foreign body under the upper lid.

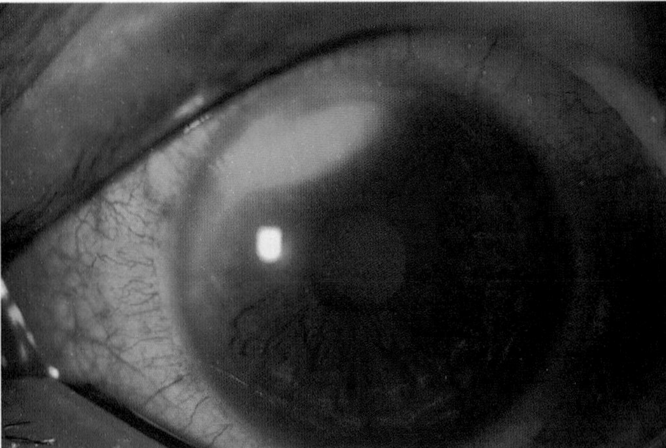

FIGURE 241-33. Corneal abrasion. [Reproduced with permission from Knoop K, Stack L, Storrow A: *Atlas of Emergency Medicine,* 2nd ed. © 2002, McGraw-Hill, New York.]

Some slit lamps (Haag-Streit) have a measuring dial attached to the mechanism that varies the length of the slit beam. If your slit lamp is equipped with this feature, you can vary the length of the slit beam on the cornea until it corresponds to the length or width of the abrasion. The reading on the wheel equals the length of the slit beam in millimeters. This additional feature allows you to document the dimensions of the abrasion precisely, thereby enabling subsequent examiners to evaluate the wound's healing response objectively.

Because the majority of corneal abrasions heal spontaneously, treatment is aimed at relieving pain and preventing infection. Cycloplegics relax the ciliary body and relieve pain from spasm as well as decreasing secondary iritis. Patching the eye does not promote healing, but some patients feel better with the eye patched. Loss of depth perception results from patching one eye, so patients should not drive a car. Abrasions from fingernails, vegetable matter, or a contact lens should not be patched, as they are at higher risk of infection.

If an abrasion is >2 mm or very painful, prescribe a **cycloplegic agent** (cyclopentolate 1% or homatropine 5%), one drop three to four times a day at home, to help control discomfort. The duration of action for each agent is much shorter in the inflamed eye, so a several times a day dosing schedule is recommended. **Cyclopentolate** 1%, one drop three times daily, wears off within 24 hours. Homatropine should be reserved for very large, painful abrasions and lasts several days. **Avoid atropine because the effect lasts for approximately 2 weeks.** Topical nonsteroidal anti-inflammatory drugs such as ketorolac and diclofenac give some degree of pain relief and do not impair healing in patients with corneal abrasions. Topical antibiotics can be provided (**Table 241-7**).

Large abrasions or abrasions in the central visual axis should be checked by an ophthalmologist in 24 hours; small abrasions should be checked in 48 to 72 hours. **Never prescribe topical anesthetics, as they inhibit corneal healing and obliterate the normal corneal protective mechanism** (blinking when material gets into the eye).

Applying an Eye Patch An eye patch may be preferred for comfort for some patients with corneal abrasions or may be needed to prevent keratitis in a patient with Bell's palsy. When an eye patch is properly applied, the eyelid will not move under the eye patch. Assemble supplies—two cotton oval eye pads and multiple pieces of tape pretorn to approximately 5 in. (13 cm). To properly apply an eye patch, have the patient sit with both eyes closed. Have the patient keep both eyes closed until the patch is applied and secure. Take one cotton oval eye pad, fold it in half, and hold the eye pad gently but firmly over the closed lid of the eye to be patched. Then take another eye patch, do not fold it in half, and place it over the first patch. Very deep set eyes may require a third patch. Keep holding firmly but gently. Then tape the patch in place, applying the tape in an X-fashion over the eye pad. Now have the patient open his or her eyes. If the patch is properly placed and taped, the lid under the patch will remain closed. If the patient says the lid can open, remove the patch and try again.

Corneal Laceration Full-thickness **corneal lacerations** can be identified by a misshapen iris, macro- or microhyphema, decrease in visual acuity, and shallow anterior chamber. The Seidel test should be positive. **However, small corneal lacerations can close spontaneously, the**

TABLE 241-7 Suggested Ophthalmic Antibiotics for Corneal Abrasions

Situation	Antibiotic
Not related to contact lens wear	Erythromycin ophthalmic ointment three to four times a day
Related to contact lens wear	Ciprofloxacin, ofloxacin, or tobramycin ointment three to four times a day
Organic source	Erythromycin ointment three to four times a day

Seidel test will be negative, and there may be no gross distortion of globe anatomy (see Figure 241-48). Corneal lacerations occur in young children from a wide variety of objects—sharp sticks, fingernails, thorns, broken glass, or sharp toys.[2] Objects as diverse as bungee cords and eyelash curlers[3,4] can cause globe perforation. A history of eye irritation while working with metal fragments or high-speed machinery suggests the possibility of a corneal laceration. Pain out of proportion to physical findings, decrease in visual acuity, or other unexplained ocular symptoms may be the only symptoms or signs of a small full-thickness corneal laceration. Evaluate the entire thickness of the cornea during slit lamp examination to identify a corneal laceration.

If there is any suspicion of penetrating injury, obtain a CT of the orbit to identify changes in globe anatomy or contour or a foreign body within the globe, and consult ophthalmology. The sensitivity of CT for the detection of occult globe perforation is reported as 56% to 68%,[5] further emphasizing the need for a high index of suspicion. Unrecognized corneal lacerations can quickly result in endophthalmitis or traumatic cataract. Once endophthalmitis develops, vision is at great risk.

Corneal Foreign Bodies Corneal foreign bodies are usually superficial and benign, but penetration of a foreign body into the globe can cause loss of vision. Foreign bodies are generally small pieces of metal, wood, or plastic that become embedded in the cornea. The presence of a corneal foreign body causes an inflammatory reaction, dilating blood vessels of the conjunctiva and causing edema of the lids, conjunctiva, and cornea. When the foreign body is present for >24 hours, WBCs may migrate into the cornea and anterior chamber as a sign of iritis.

The patient will usually complain of a "foreign body" sensation during blinking. Tearing, blurred vision, and photophobia are common. Ask about details surrounding the onset of symptoms, including patient activity. If a cause is not obvious, ask about all activities in the previous 24 hours, especially activities that cause high-velocity projectiles. High-velocity globe penetration injuries include grinding, hammering metal on metal, or operation of other high-speed machinery. Visual acuity should be normal. Inspection of the eye may reveal edema of the eyelid and diffuse or focal/perilimbal conjunctival injection.

Occasionally, the foreign body may be visible with the naked eye. Evert the lid to identify and remove other foreign bodies that may be present. When a metallic foreign body is present for more than a few hours, a **rust ring** (**Figure 241-34**) develops around the metal. Foreign bodies present for >24 hours may be surrounded by a white ring representing a WBC infiltrate. Anterior chamber flare and cells and a corneal foreign body are identifiable on slit lamp examination (**Figure 241-35**). **The presence of a gross hyphema or a microhyphema evident in the anterior chamber on slit lamp examination suggests globe perforation.** If the foreign body has penetrated the cornea, the tract of the projectile *may* be seen. The Seidel test *may* be positive with penetration of the globe.

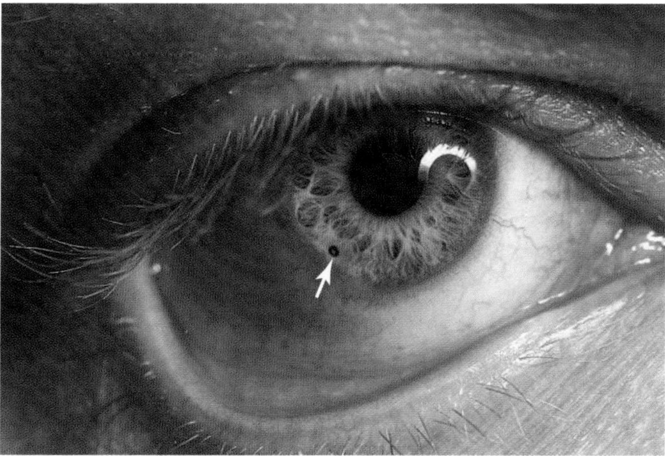

FIGURE 241-34. Rust ring. [Reproduced with permission from Knoop K, Stack L, Storrow A: *Atlas of Emergency Medicine,* 2nd ed. © 2002, McGraw-Hill, New York.]

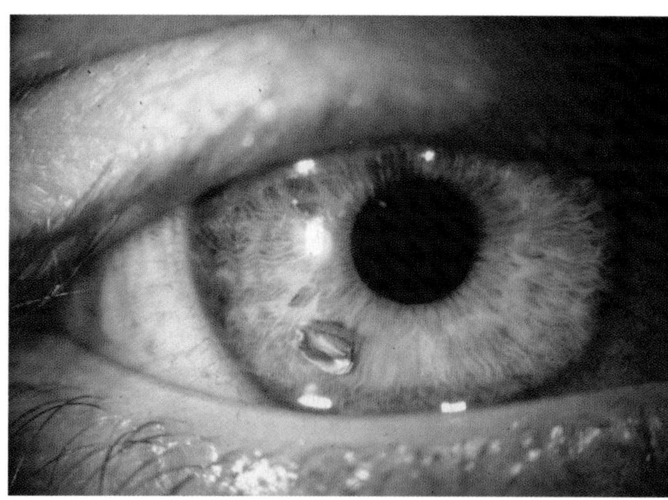

FIGURE 241-35. Corneal foreign body. [Courtesy of Allen R. Katz, Department of Ophthalmology, University of Nebraska Medical Center.]

Corneal Foreign Body Removal Corneal foreign bodies should be removed carefully, with the patient and physician seated at each other's eye level, and under the best magnification available. Anesthetize the cornea with a local anesthetic such as 0.5% proparacaine. Sometimes, anesthetizing both eyes is helpful, because that can eliminate reflex blinking during attempts at foreign body removal. Irrigate with normal saline first, as a very superficial foreign body may be irrigated off the cornea. Next, try to dislodge the foreign body with a moistened cotton applicator. Efforts at removal may themselves cause corneal abrasion.

If the foreign body is tightly adherent to or embedded in the cornea, inspect the cornea using optical sectioning to assess the depth of penetration (**Figure 241-12**). **Full-thickness corneal foreign bodies should be removed by an ophthalmologist.**

For superficial foreign bodies, a 25-gauge needle (using needle bevel up) or a sterile foreign body spud (1 mm diameter) on an **Alger brush** (a low-speed, low-torque, battery-operated hand-held drill) can be used to remove the foreign body. Use slit lamp magnification to ensure safe foreign body removal. Before the removal, prepare a moistened cotton applicator and set it aside on the slit lamp table. The upper lid can be held open by an assistant or by the clinician's nondominant hand. Many slit lamps have an attached "fixation light" that can be moved in front of the unaffected eye to give the patient a steady target to concentrate on. Using either the 25-gauge needle or the Alger brush, place the tip into the slit lamp beam using the naked eye. With the tip close to the cornea, look through the slit lamp and move the tip into contact with the cornea. Using the bevel-up edge of the tip of the 25-gauge needle, hook the edge of the foreign body and dislodge it. You may then lift it off the cornea using the previously moistened cotton applicator. Alternatively, using the spinning tip of the Alger brush, the foreign body may be dislodged and removed with the cotton applicator as above.

After successful foreign body removal, discharge the patient with a prescription for topical antibiotics, cycloplegics, and oral analgesics. Administer tetanus toxoid as appropriate. Provide ophthalmology follow-up the next day if the foreign body is in the central visual axis or if there is a residual rust ring. Otherwise, after complete removal of the foreign body, advise follow-up if symptoms persist at 48 hours.

Rust Ring Removal Metallic foreign bodies can create rust rings that are toxic to the corneal tissue (**Figure 241-34**). If a rust ring is present, the spud or an ophthalmic burr can remove superficial rust, but rust often reaccumulates by the next day, requiring additional burring. **It is therefore not necessary to remove a rust ring in the ED if the patient can be seen by an ophthalmologist the next day.** Once the metallic foreign body is removed, the rust ring area softens overnight and can be more easily removed in the office the next day. The deeper the stromal involvement, the higher is the risk of corneal scarring, so if rust ring removal is done in the ED, only perform superficial burring. **No ED drill burring should take place if the rust ring is located in the visual**

axis (pupil) owing to the risk of causing visually significant scarring. Such conditions require that an ophthalmologist remove the stromal rust in the office within 24 hours.

LID LACERATIONS

Eyelid lacerations that involve the lid margin, those within 6 to 8 mm of the medial canthus or involving the lacrimal duct or sac, those involving the inner surface of the lid, wounds associated with ptosis, and those involving the tarsal plate or levator palpebrae muscle need repair by an oculoplastic specialist. Lacerations medial to the lacrimal puncta are at high risk of canalicular involvement. Suspect involvement of the levator palpebral muscle in the presence of a horizontal laceration with ptosis or when orbital fat is seen protruding through the laceration, indicating a breach of the orbital septum.

Consider the possibility of corneal laceration and globe rupture in all full-thickness lid lacerations. Ocular injuries such as corneal abrasion, traumatic hyphema, and globe rupture are seen with lid lacerations in up to two thirds of cases. Lid lacerations require a thorough examination using a slit lamp to exclude other associated ocular injuries.

Deep lacerations medial to the punctum potentially can transect the canalicular system. These injuries need to be seen by an ophthalmologist for evaluation of the nasolacrimal duct system's integrity. Instillation of fluorescein dye in the eye with subsequent appearance in the wound indicates loss of canalicular integrity. If a canalicular laceration is discovered, the patient will need to go to the operating room within 24 to 36 hours for repair and Silastic® tube stenting. Because a meticulous repair by an experienced eye surgery team is preferable, it is not unreasonable for the ophthalmologist to discharge a patient seen late in the evening or on the weekend with arrangements for surgical repair to take place within the next 36 hours. Patients discharged pending repair should be placed on oral and topical antibiotics and told to use cold compresses. Oral cephalexin (Keflex®), 500 milligrams twice or four times daily, and topical erythromycin ophthalmic ointment four times daily are reasonable choices.

Partial-thickness lid lacerations not meeting the preceding criteria can usually be repaired in the ED, with referral for ophthalmologic evaluation in 2 to 3 days. Use a soft, absorbable or nonabsorbable 6-0 or 7-0 suture. Have the suture ends closest to the cornea tucked under more distant sutures to avoid corneal irritation (**Figure 241-36**). Cut the ends of each suture 1 cm long. When the second suture is tied, take the long ends of the first suture into the loop of the knot of the second suture. This keeps the ends of the first suture secure. Do this for every successive suture. Do not incorporate the ends of the suture into the wound itself, but make sure the suture ends are kept to the side of the wound margin. Sutures are removed from the bottom.

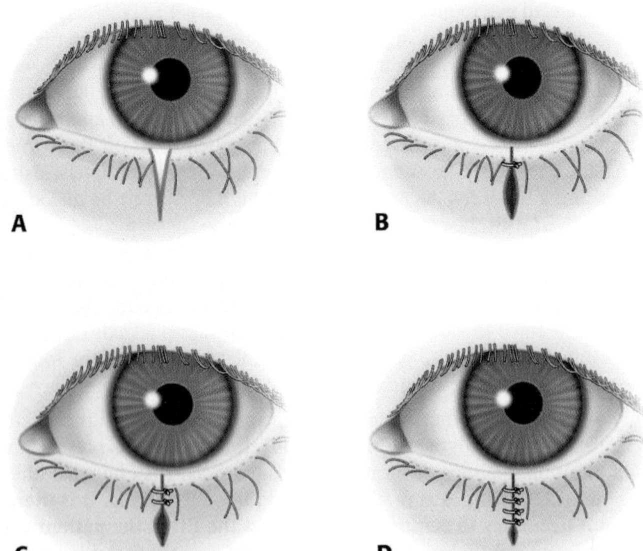

FIGURE 241-36. A through D. Each suture holds down the ends of the adjacent suture to prevent corneal irritation or abrasion. On this drawing, the lighter shade sutures are above the skin. Note that this illustration shows a laceration at the lid margin. Lid margin lacerations >1 mm need repair by an oculoplastic specialist.

Lacerations at the Lid Margin **Very small lacerations (<1 mm) at the lid edge only do not need suturing and can heal spontaneously.** Any laceration >1 mm at the lid edge needs repair by a specialist. Proper alignment of the lid margin during repair under magnification (loupe or microscope) is essential to preserve proper lid function and even corneal wetting with each blink. Notching of the lid can result in improper lid closure.

If there is no opportunity for the patient to see an ophthalmologist, repair should be performed as in **Figure 241-37**. Soft (gut or chromic) sutures 6-0 or smaller should be used for all repairs. One vertical mattress suture, using the meibomian gland orifices as a landmark, or two 6-0 soft sutures (one approximating the anterior and the other the posterior lamella) are used to repair the lid margin. The initial suture can be used for traction to extend the lid and facilitate the repair. The tarsus should be repaired with 6-0 absorbable suture (polyglactin) from the external side so as to approximate the wound without the need for sutures on the conjunctival side of the lid (which would abrade the cornea with each blink). Skin closure can be performed with 6-0 or smaller soft nonabsorbable suture.

BLUNT EYE TRAUMA

The first steps are assessment of the visual acuity, anterior chamber, and integrity of the globe. The eyelids frequently swell shut, making visualization of the globe difficult. Prying the eyelids open with the fingers is difficult, usually yields an unsatisfactory view of the globe, and can raise intraocular pressure. Insertion of a paperclip bent in an appropriate shape (**Figure 241-38**) or an eyelid speculum (**Figure 241-39**) provides a significantly improved view of the cornea and anterior chamber. Use of an eyelid retractor allows your hands to remain free for examination of the globe using the slit lamp.

If the anterior chamber is flat, a ruptured globe is certain, so stop the examination, place a metal shield over the injured eye, and consult ophthalmology. A **hyphema** is also evidence of significant ocular trauma and necessitates an ophthalmology consult. If the globe appears intact and vision is preserved, check ocular motility. Restricted upgaze or lateral gaze suggests a **blow-out fracture** with entrapment (see later section, Orbital Blow-Out Fractures), and a CT scan of facial bones should be obtained. A head CT scan may be indicated to assess for associated intracranial injury. Feel the orbital rim above and below for step-off deformities. Test for cutaneous sensation along the distribution of the inferior orbital nerve (below the eye and ipsilateral side of the nose). **Perform a slit lamp examination with fluorescein staining to check for abrasions, lacerations, foreign bodies, hyphema, iritis, and lens dislocation.** Measure intraocular pressure if there are no signs of a ruptured globe. Traumatic iritis is common, causing cell and flare to be seen on slit lamp examination. The pupil can be constricted or dilated after sustaining trauma. It is important to look for pupillary irregularity because the pupil often will peak toward the site of a penetration or rupture. If the anterior chamber is of normal depth and not shallow, apply a mydriatic. Nonwhite, brown-eyed individuals frequently will require an additional drop of a mydriatic to achieve adequate dilation. If vision and ocular anatomy and function are preserved, outpatient follow-up by an ophthalmologist in the next 48 hours should be planned. If a ruptured globe is suspected due to loss of visual acuity, flat anterior chamber, obvious full-thickness laceration, or intraocular foreign body, do not manipulate the eye or measure intraocular pressure. Consult ophthalmology immediately.

Hyphema A **hyphema** is blood or blood clots in the anterior chamber (**Figures 241-15** and **241-16**). Hyphemas are traumatic or spontaneous. A traumatic hyphema usually results from bleeding from a ruptured iris root vessel. Spontaneous hyphemas frequently are associated with sickle cell disease. In addition to standard ophthalmologic history, inquire as to the use of any anticoagulant or antiplatelet medications or history of a bleeding diathesis. **A hyphema may layer out posteriorly when the patient is**

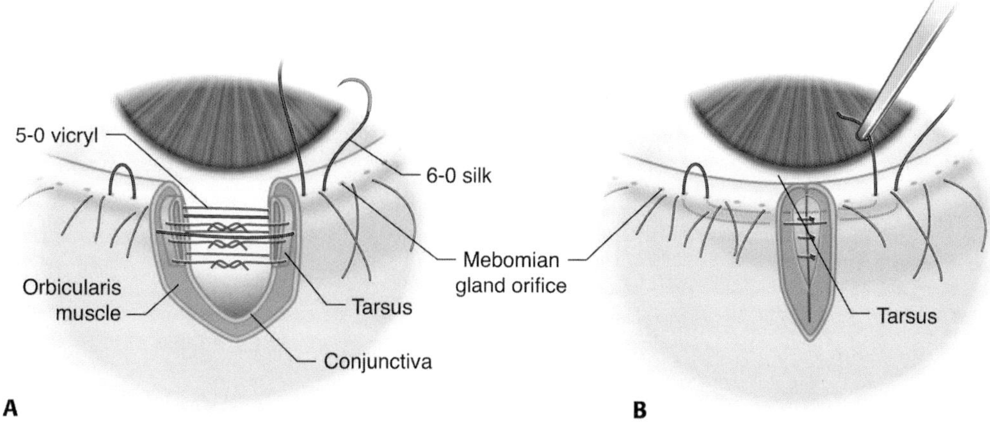

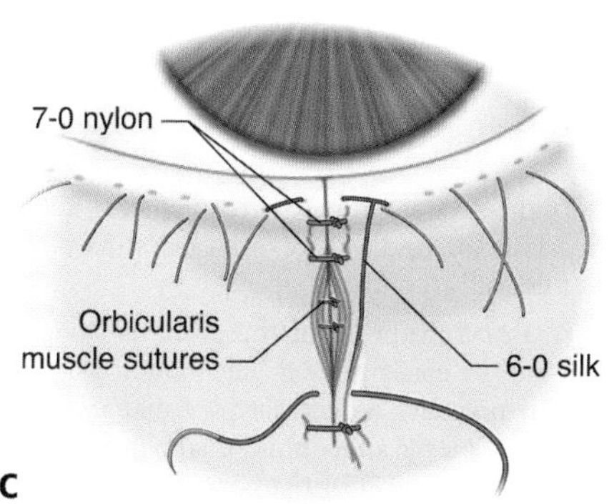

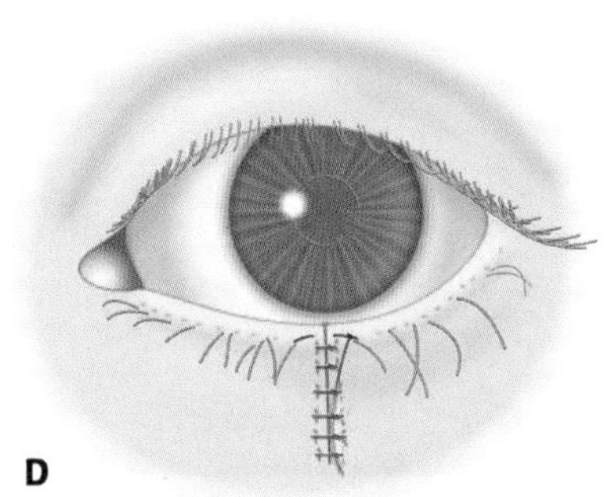

FIGURE 241-37. **A** through **D.** Full-thickness lid repair. 6-0 silk is used for lid margin. 5-0 Vicryl® is used to approximate the tarsal plate. The Vicryl® sutures should not pass through the conjunctiva on the inside of the eyelid to avoid mechanical abrasion of the cornea during blinking. 7-0 nylon is used for skin closure, and the lid margin silk suture tail can be incorporated into these sutures to avoid corneal irritation.

lying flat and may only become grossly evident when the patient is sitting upright. The complications of hyphema include increased intraocular pressure, rebleeding, peripheral anterior synechiae, corneal staining, optic atrophy, and accommodative impairment. Patients with large hyphemas, sickle cell disease, and bleeding tendency are more likely to develop vision loss. A **microhyphema** is suspension of red blood cells in the anterior chamber without the formation of a layered blood clot. It is generally seen with a slit lamp and can progress into a hyphema. The most significant complications of microhyphema include rebleeding and intraocular pressure elevation. Patients with sickle cell disease are more likely to develop these complications. The treatment of microhyphema is somewhat controversial, but the principles of management are the same as those for the hyphema.

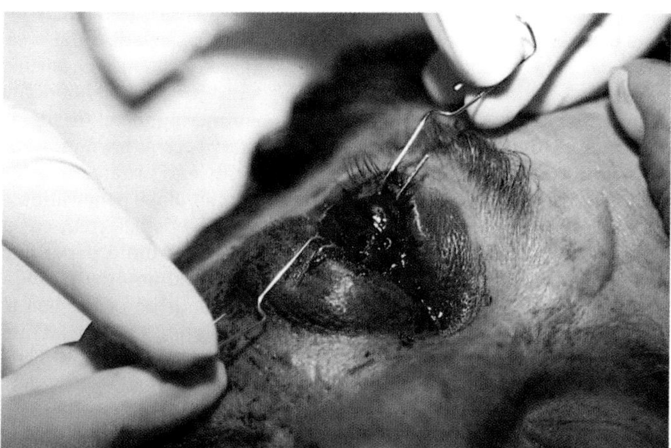

FIGURE 241-38. Eyelid retractors fashioned from paperclips. [Reproduced with permission from Knoop K, Stack L, Storrow A: *Atlas of Emergency Medicine*, 2nd ed. © 2002, McGraw-Hill, New York.]

Hyphemas should be evaluated by an ophthalmologist in the ED. Patients at high risk for complications include those with suspected ruptured globe, those with sickle cell disease, those taking anticoagulants, or those with a bleeding diathesis.

Treatment consists of the prevention of rebleeding and intraocular hypertension. Elevate the patient's head to 45 degrees to promote settling of suspended red blood cells inferiorly to prevent occlusion of the trabecular meshwork. After consultation with the ophthalmologist, dilate the pupil to avoid "pupillary play" (constriction and dilation movements of the iris in response to changing lighting conditions), which can stretch the involved iris vessel, causing additional bleeding. Pupillary dilation *does not* compromise the angle and aqueous outflow in normal individuals, and some ophthalmologists choose to dilate hyphemas to prevent pupillary activity. Control of intraocular pressure consists of topical β-blockers, IV mannitol, topical α-adrenergic agonists (apraclonidine), and oral, topical, or IV carbonic anhydrase inhibitors such as Diamox®. **Do not give carbonic anhydrase inhibitors to patients with sickle cell disease.** Carbonic anhydrase inhibitors lower the aqueous pH in the anterior chamber, causing the red blood cells to sickle and become less flexible, thereby clogging outflow through the trabecular meshwork and increasing intraocular pressure.

Rebleeding can occur 3 to 5 days later in up to 30% of cases, sometimes causing severe elevation of intraocular pressure and necessitating surgical anterior chamber "washouts." Because of this risk, some

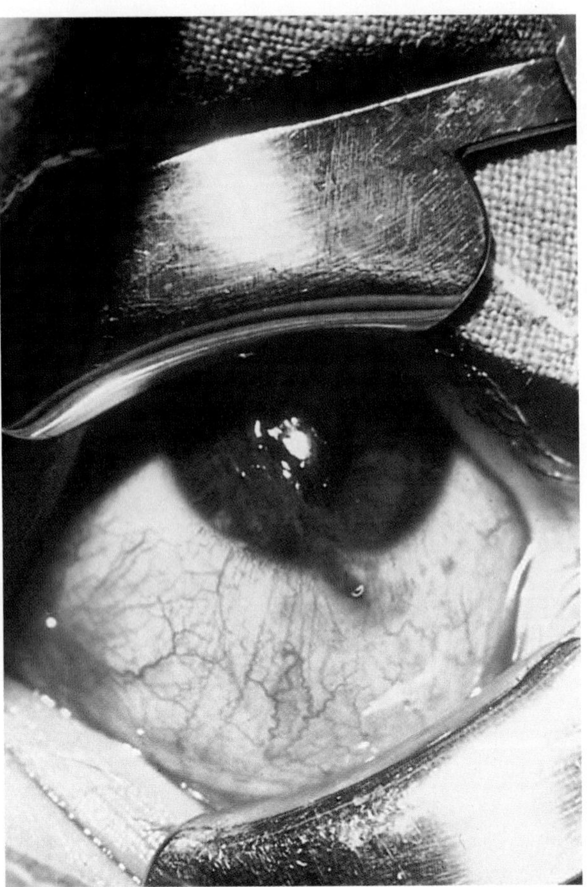

FIGURE 241-39. Commercial eyelid retractors. [Reproduced with permission from Knoop K, Stack L, Storrow A: *Atlas of Emergency Medicine*, 2nd ed. © 2002, McGraw-Hill, New York.]

ophthalmologists believe in admitting all patients with hyphemas, whereas others will choose to follow them closely as outpatients. Generally, patients with hyphemas occupying one third or less of the anterior chamber can be followed closely as outpatients. The disposition decision should be made by the ophthalmologist after examining the patient. Lower risk of rebleeding has been reported in patients who receive topical glucocorticoids. Additionally, topical steroids may prevent posterior synechiae and treat iridocyclitis. Close follow-up and serial examinations by an ophthalmologist are recommended in patients receiving topical ocular steroids to ensure no infection or corneal perforation occurs.

Orbital Blow-Out Fractures The most frequent sites of **orbital blow-out fractures** are the inferior wall (maxillary sinus) and medial wall (ethmoid sinus through the lamina papyracea). Fractures of the medial wall can be associated with subcutaneous emphysema, sometimes exacerbated by sneezing or blowing the nose. Fractures of the inferior wall with entrapment of the inferior rectus muscle can cause restriction of upgaze and diplopia (**Figure 241-40**). Orbital wall fractures are suspected on clinical examination and confirmed by CT scanning. About one third of blow-out fractures are associated with ocular trauma (abrasion, traumatic iritis, hyphema, lens dislocation/subluxation, retinal tear, or detachment); therefore, a careful eye examination in the ED is necessary. **All blow-out fractures with normal initial eye examination in the ED should be referred to an ophthalmologist for an outpatient fully dilated examination to rule out any unidentified retinal tears or detachments.** Orbital blow-out fractures without any evidence of serious eye injury do not require admission.

Isolated blow-out fractures with or without entrapment and without any eye injury do not require immediate surgery and can be referred to ophthalmology, plastic surgery, oral maxillofacial surgery, or otolaryngology (depending on the local referral patterns) for repair within the

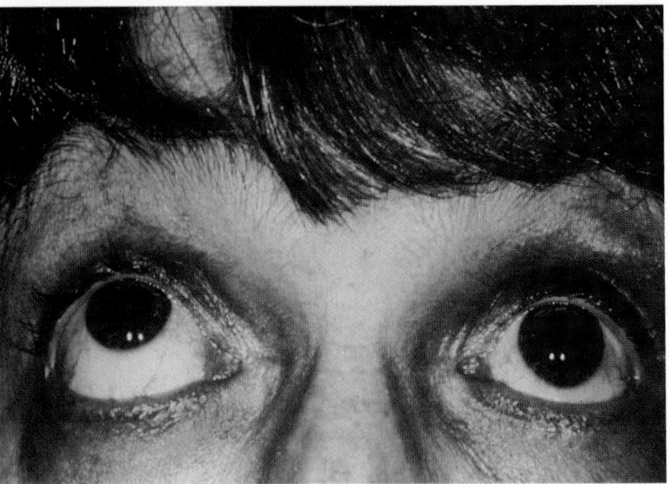

FIGURE 241-40. Inferior wall blow-out fracture of the left eye with entrapment of the inferior rectus muscle. The patient's right eye is unable to look upward, causing diplopia on upward gaze. [Courtesy of Allen R. Katz, Department of Ophthalmology, University of Nebraska Medical Center.]

next 3 to 10 days. Oral antibiotics (cephalexin, 250 to 500 milligrams PO four times daily for 10 days) are often recommended because of the presence of sinus wall fractures.

Ruptured Globe Rupture of the globe is a vision-threatening emergency that may be easily missed. The patient will usually complain of eye pain but may not have a decrease in visual acuity. Rupture of the globe presenting with a large subconjunctival hemorrhage is easily recognized, but a penetrating wound of the cornea caused by a tiny piece of metal launched from a grinder may be easily overlooked and requires a high index of suspicion to detect. Periorbital ecchymosis and maxillofacial fractures, including blow-out fracture with limitation of extraocular muscle movement , should raise one's suspicion for globe rupture.

Scleral rupture may occur from blunt or penetrating trauma. Blunt trauma directly to the eyeball (for example, a blow by a fist) will cause a sudden elevation of intraocular pressure, with the globe tending to rupture at the thinnest points of the sclera, the limbus, and at the insertion of the extraocular muscles. Any object that impacts the orbital rim at a high velocity and causes a seal around the orbit (tennis balls, racquetballs, etc.) will also cause a sudden peak in intraocular pressure and may result in rupture. A history of ocular surgery or previous ocular injury may predispose to globe rupture. Penetrating trauma may occur from bullets, BB pellets, knives, sticks, darts, needles, hammering, and lawn mower projectiles. **Any projectile injury has the potential for penetrating the eye.** The bony canal protects the globe from posterior and oblique injuries, but the eyelids afford little protection anteriorly. **Suspect globe penetration with any puncture or laceration of the eyelid or periorbital area,** and make sure to conduct a thorough slit lamp examination. The smaller the diameter of the offending object, the higher is the likelihood of occult injury. **Corneal abrasions occurring when hammering metal on metal; associated with the use of high-speed machinery such as lawn mowers, line trimmers (weed whackers), grinders, or drills; and sustained during explosions should always be investigated for occult globe penetration.**

Whenever globe rupture is obvious or strongly suspected, cover the eye with a metal eye shield or make a shield from a paper cup (Figures 241-41 and 241-42), and consult ophthalmology immediately without further manipulation. Elevate the head of the bed to 45 degrees. Administer broad-spectrum IV antibiotics, and give tetanus toxoid as appropriate. Provide sedation and analgesia, and administer antiemetics to prevent increased intraocular pressure and extrusion of intraocular contents from vomiting. Avoid any topical eye solutions. Give the patient nothing by mouth, anticipating surgery.

Most cases, however, will require an initial eye examination to determine the type and extent of injury before consulting ophthalmology. **If at any step of the examination globe rupture is suspected, stop the examination, place a protective shield over the eye, and consult**

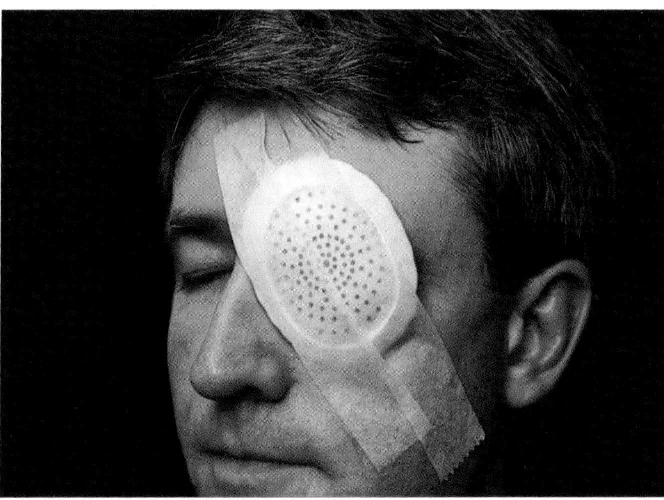

FIGURE 241-41. Metal eye shield placed in suspected globe rupture to prevent inadvertent pressure on the eye. [Reproduced with permission from Knoop K, Stack L, Storrow A: *Atlas of Emergency Medicine,* 2nd ed. © 2002, McGraw-Hill, New York.]

ophthalmology. Do not measure intraocular pressure as this may result in extrusion of globe contents.

Eye examination must be careful and gentle. Manufactured or homemade eyelid retractors should be used to gently retract the lids to examine the eye and to avoid increasing intraocular pressure during examination.

Examination of the eye may reveal decreased visual acuity, an irregular or teardrop-shaped pupil, an afferent pupillary defect, shallow anterior chamber, hyphema, positive Seidel test, and lens dislocation (**Figure 241-43**). Presence of a large subconjunctival hemorrhage involving the entire sclera or hemorrhagic chemosis (bullous, raised subconjunctival hemorrhage) is very suspicious for rupture of the globe (**Figures 241-44** and **241-45**). Uveal prolapse through a scleral wound may appear as a brownish-black discoloration against the white sclera (**Figure 241-46**). One may occasionally visualize a corneal laceration (**Figure 241-47**) or an intraocular foreign body on slit lamp examination (**Figure 241-48**). The Seidel test may or may not be positive with a small corneal laceration. Funduscopic examination may reveal a poor view of the optic nerve and posterior pole due to vitreous hemorrhage. **Unfortunately, the examination may be nearly normal after globe rupture from a tiny high-speed projectile.**

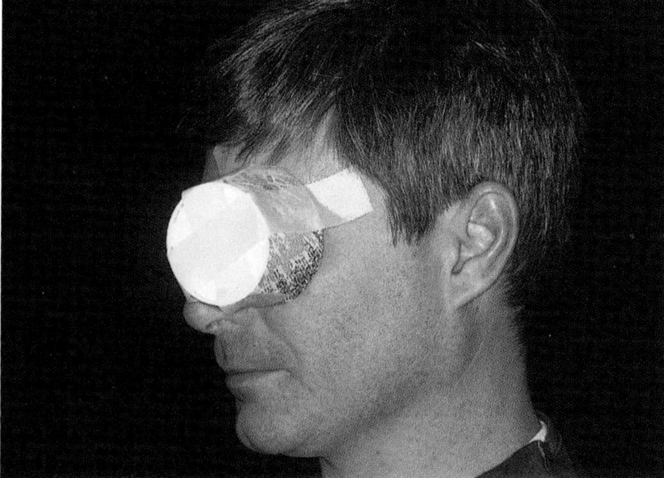

FIGURE 241-42. Protective eye shield fashioned from a paper cup. [Reproduced with permission from Knoop K, Stack L, Storrow A: *Atlas of Emergency Medicine,* 2nd ed. © 2002, McGraw-Hill, New York.]

The diagnosis is made based on a combination of history, physical examination, and selected radiologic studies. CT scan of the eye is the preferred imaging modality to detect occult open globe rupture and associated optic nerve injury. CT scan of the orbit using 2- to 3-mm cuts in both the axial and coronal planes will also localize small intraocular foreign bodies. US and both direct and indirect ophthalmoscopy after pupillary dilatation may assist in the diagnosis and can be helpful in locating and confirming the presence of orbital and intraocular foreign bodies. MRI is contraindicated if a metallic foreign body is possible.

For patients in the ED with multiple trauma and a possible ruptured globe who require rapid-sequence intubation, there is no clear consensus on the best agent to use because quick airway stabilization takes priority. Although a depolarizing agent like succinylcholine is associated with an increase in intraocular pressure, the underlying mechanism is not clear. Some studies suggest that intraocular pressure increases because of extraocular muscle contraction, although others suggest it increases because succinylcholine has a cycloplegic effect on the ciliary muscle. Pretreatment with a nondepolarizing muscle relaxant or a pretreatment dose of succinylcholine does not necessarily attenuate the increase in intracranial pressure. Use of a nondepolarizing agent like rocuronium can mitigate increases in intraocular pressure, but disadvantages are a longer onset and longer duration of action[6] (see Chapter 29, Intubation and Mechanical Ventilation).

Orbital Hemorrhage: Preseptal and Postseptal Severe blunt trauma to the orbit can occasionally cause an orbital hemorrhage. **Preseptal hemorrhage** is dramatic in appearance, but not as vision threatening as a **postseptal hemorrhage** (often called **retrobulbar hematoma**), which can cause an **orbital compartment syndrome**. A postseptal hematoma can cause an abrupt increase in intraocular pressure, resulting in decreased blood flow to the optic nerve and its blood supply and loss of vision.

Traumatic periorbital hematomas (black eyes) are common, but the extension of bleeding into the postseptal compartment is a true emergency. Differentiation of preseptal versus postseptal hematoma depends on the examination and noncontrast orbital CT findings. Clinical findings of postseptal hemorrhage are eye pain, proptosis, impaired extraocular movements, decreased vision, possibly an afferent pupillary defect, and elevated intraocular pressure. An intraocular pressure >40 mm Hg is a consideration for emergency lateral canthotomy. No matter what the intraocular pressure, if postseptal hematoma is suspected or confirmed, request emergency ophthalmology consultation. Preseptal hematomas can be observed to make sure that the hematoma is not expanding.

Lateral Canthotomy The goals of **lateral canthotomy** are to release pressure on the globe and to reduce intraocular pressure to reestablish retinal artery blood flow. To perform the procedure, place the patient in the supine position and anesthetize the lateral canthus area with 1% to 2% lidocaine with epinephrine. Place a straight Kelly clamp horizontally across the lateral canthus for about 1 to 2 minutes to crush the tissues and minimize bleeding. Remove the clamp, and with sterile scissors, make a 1- to 2-cm lateral incision in the compressed tissue at the clamp site. Then retract the lower lid to expose the lateral canthus tendon. With the scissors directed inferoposteriorly toward the lateral orbital rim, cut the inferior crus of the lateral canthus tendon. This critical incision is generally 1 to 2 cm in depth and length. If the procedure is successful, the intraocular pressure should be less than 40 mm Hg and the visual acuity should improve. If the intraocular pressure continues to remain elevated, the superior crus of the lateral canthus tendon can be cut in a similar fashion. The complications of lateral canthotomy include hemorrhage, infection, and mechanical injury. These complications generally respond to treatment better than does retinal injury from prolonged ischemia. Lateral canthotomy incisions usually heal well without suturing or significant scar formation.

Ocular Hemorrhage and Antithrombotic Therapy The use of anticoagulant and antiplatelet agents is very common in current clinical practice and can complicate the management of ocular hemorrhage from trauma. Spontaneous ocular hemorrhage has also been reported in patients taking these agents. Ocular complications in patients on oral anticoagulant therapy include subconjunctival hemorrhage, hyphema, vitreous hemorrhage, subretinal

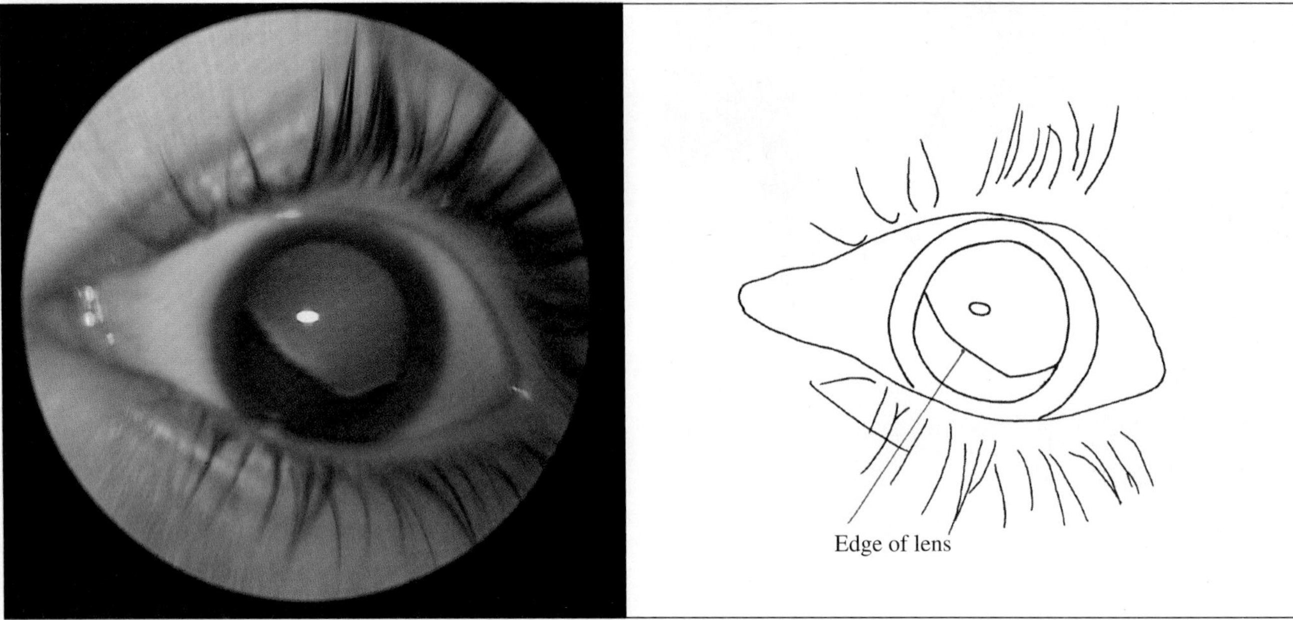

FIGURE 241-43. Lens dislocation. [Reproduced with permission from Knoop et al., *The Atlas of Emergency Medicine*, 3rd edition © 2010 McGraw-Hill Inc.; Photo contributed by Department of Ophthalmology, Naval Medical Center, Portsmouth, VA.]

hemorrhage, and choroidal hemorrhage. A higher incidence of hemorrhagic complications has been reported in patients with macular degeneration using anticoagulants or other antithrombotic drugs. Ocular hemorrhages in patients taking warfarin can potentially be vision-threatening events, but frequently they are benign and resolve without any sequelae.

There are no clear guidelines to guide treatment of ocular hemorrhage in patients taking anticoagulant and antiplatelet therapy. The severity of bleeding, INR levels, and benefits of using these agents should be taken into consideration when managing these patients. Ophthalmologic and hematology consultations should be obtained. These medications should be stopped in patients with active bleeding. Prothrombin complex concentrate, fresh frozen plasma, and vitamin K should be considered in patients taking warfarin (see chapter 239 for detailed discussion). Platelet transfusions might be beneficial to stop active bleeding in patients with thrombocytopenia or taking antiplatelet drugs. Currently, no specific reversal agent for dabigatran is available. Activated prothrombin complex concentrates, recombinant factor VIIa, or concentrates of coagulation factors II, IX, or X and dialysis should be considered in patients taking dabigatran with active hemorrhage.

CHEMICAL OCULAR INJURY

Chemical burns to the eye are a true ocular emergency. Complications of chemical burns to the eye include scarring of the cornea with permanent loss of vision and loss of the eye due to corneal perforation. Irrigation of the eyes with 1 to 2 L of normal saline must be done immediately and before any examination, including testing of vision.

Alkali and Acid Injuries **Alkali injuries** occur more frequently than acid injuries, due to the presence of alkaline substances in household cleaning agents and in building materials. The most serious alkali injuries are associated with ammonia, found in many household cleaners, and lye, a common ingredient in drain cleaners. Lye is also a component of concrete. Alkali injuries tend to be much more serious than acid injuries because they cause a liquefaction necrosis, characterized by denaturing of proteins and saponification of fats, allowing deep penetration into tissue. Acid, on the other hand, causes coagulation necrosis, with denaturing of protein forming a coagulum that acts as a barrier to further tissue penetration.

Irrigation should begin at the scene and continue in the ED. Instill a topical anesthetic and continue irrigation for at least 30 minutes. Then

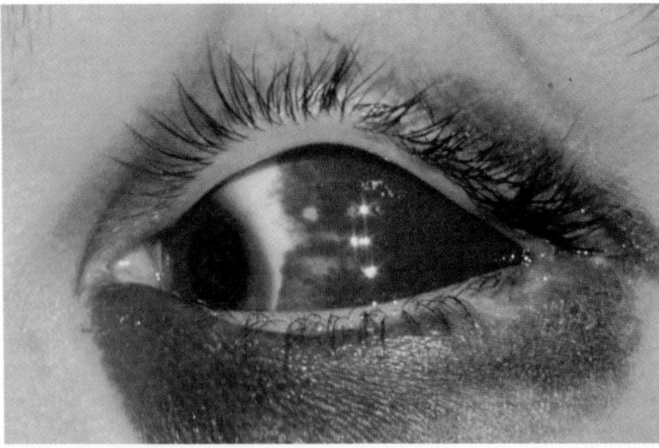

FIGURE 241-44. Large subconjunctival hemorrhage. Note that it is flat, not raised. [Reproduced with permission from Knoop K, Stack L, Storrow A: *Atlas of Emergency Medicine*, 2nd ed. © 2002, McGraw-Hill, New York.]

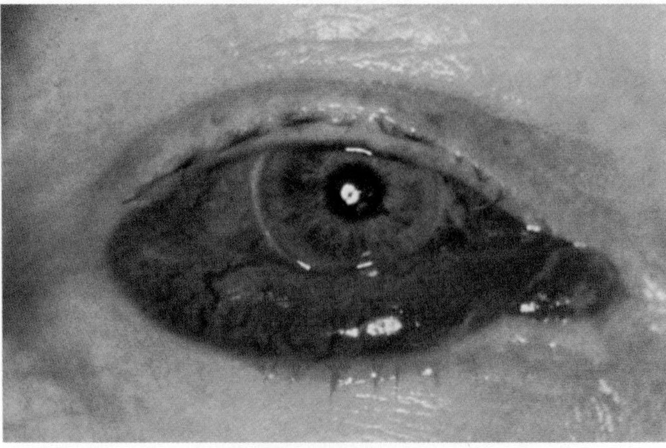

FIGURE 241-45. Bloody chemosis. Note the raised or bullous appearance. [Reproduced with permission from Knoop K, Stack L, Storrow A: *Atlas of Emergency Medicine*, 2nd ed. © 2002, McGraw-Hill, New York.]

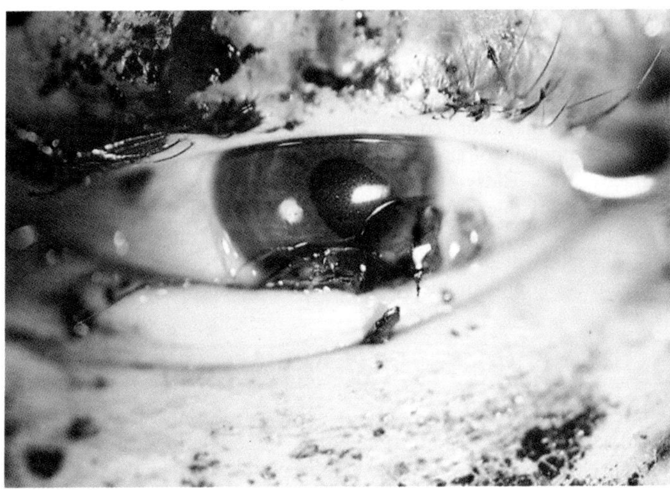

FIGURE 241-46. Uveal prolapse with globe rupture and teardrop pupil. [Reproduced with permission from Knoop K, Stack L, Storrow A: *Atlas of Emergency Medicine,* 2nd ed. © 2002, McGraw-Hill, New York.]

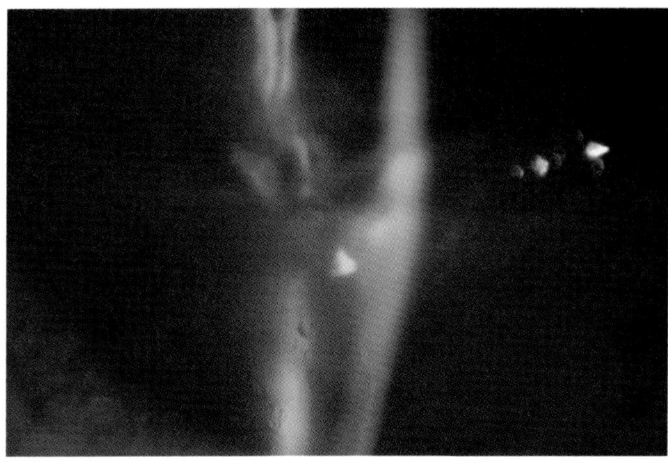

FIGURE 241-48. Intraocular foreign body associated with laceration in Figure 241-47 as seen on slit lamp examination. [Courtesy of Allen R. Katz, Department of Ophthalmology, University of Nebraska Medical Center.]

check pH by touching a strip of litmus paper to the inferior conjunctival fornix. **If the pH is >7.4, continue irrigation until the pH remains neutral 30 minutes after the last irrigation.** Irrigation should be with sterile normal saline or other isotonic solution and may be instilled into the eye by hand, using bottles of eye-irrigating solution, or by a Morgan Lens® (MorTan Inc., Missoula, MT) (**Figure 241-49**) attached to a bag of an isotonic IV solution.

After irrigation and maintainance of ocular pH >7.4, perform the eye examination. Inspect the facial skin and eyelids for burns. Evert the eyelids and remove any particulate matter with a cotton applicator.

Exposure to chemical agents can cause conjunctival injection and chemosis, but severe chemical burns can cause scleral whitening, secondary to ischemia and blood vessel injury. Document visual acuity and measure intraocular pressure. Intraocular pressure may be increased if the trabecular meshwork has been damaged. Use the slit lamp to evaluate corneal injury and to detect for cells and flare in the anterior chamber. Injury to the cornea may range from punctuate defects to complete loss of epithelium. The cornea may become cloudy with severe burns (**Figure 241-50**).

After irrigation, and once time permits, identify the substance. The pH is usually listed on bottles of household cleaners. The U.S. Occupational Health and Safety Administration requires the patient's workplace to maintain Material Data Safety Sheets, a list of all the physical properties, including pH, of chemicals used at the site. Data on the pH of

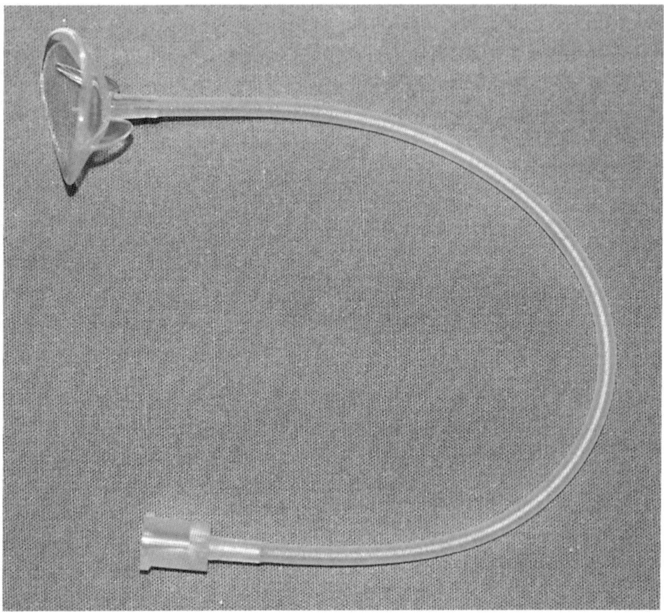

FIGURE 241-49. Eye irrigation with a Morgan Lens® (MorTan Inc., Missoula, MT). [Reproduced with permission from Reichman EF, Simon RR: *Emergency Medicine Procedures*. © 2004, Eric F. Reichman, PhD, MD, and Robert R. Simon, MD. McGraw-Hill, Inc.]

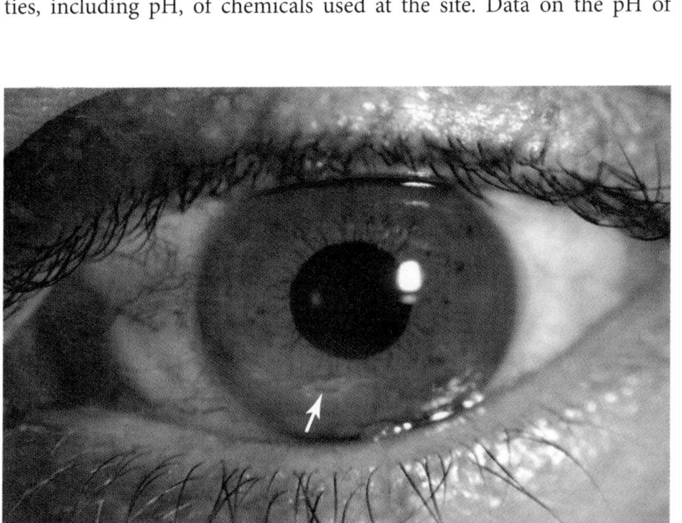

FIGURE 241-47. Corneal laceration due to hammering concrete. [Courtesy of Allen R. Katz, Department of Ophthalmology, University of Nebraska Medical Center.]

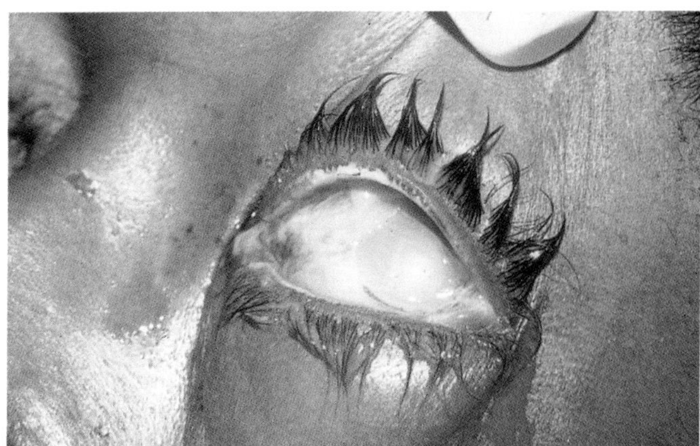

FIGURE 241-50. Severe lye burn with corneal opacification. [Reproduced with permission from Knoop K, Stack L, Storrow A: *Atlas of Emergency Medicine,* 2nd ed. © 2002, McGraw-Hill, New York.]

known chemicals can also be obtained from a poison control center or from Poisindex®. Alkaline substances with pH <12 or acidic substances with pH >2 are thought not to cause serious injury, but duration of exposure can increase severity of injury. Circumstances surrounding the injury (e.g., battery explosion) should be determined to identify any other associated ocular or facial injuries.

Obtain ophthalmology consultation for all but minor burns: Any patient with corneal clouding or an epithelial defect after irrigation should receive prompt ophthalmology referral.

Patients with chemosis (edema of the bulbar conjunctiva overlying the white sclera) and no corneal or anterior chamber findings should be treated after irrigation with erythromycin ointment four times daily and referred for an ophthalmologic examination in 24 to 48 hours. These patients are considered to have "**chemical conjunctivitis**."

A topical cycloplegic agent should be used three times daily for pain reduction if an epithelial defect is present. **Avoid phenylephrine as a cycloplegic**, as it will constrict blood vessels, causing further ischemia to the limbus. Apply erythromycin ophthalmic ointment four times daily to affected eyes. Administer tetanus toxoid as appropriate. Consider prescribing topical corticosteroids after consultation with an ophthalmologist to control inflammation.

CYANOACRYLATE (SUPER GLUE/CRAZY GLUE)

Accidental instillation of cyanoacrylate adhesives into the eye and adnexa can cause adherence of the lids and clumps of adhesive to form on the cornea. Medicinal-grade cyanoacrylates are occasionally used to seal corneal perforations and are not toxic to the cornea, so there is rarely permanent damage to the eye. The mechanical abrasive effect of hard, irregular glue aggregates rubbing against the cornea with eye movement and blinking may cause corneal abrasions. To remove crazy glue, instill generous amounts of **erythromycin ointment** onto the eye and on the surface of the eyelids to moisten, lubricate, and provide antibiotic coverage. Clumps of glue on the surface should begin to loosen. Remove only those pieces that are easily removable. Gentle traction may separate the lids. The glue will loosen and become easier to remove in a few days.

Refer to an ophthalmologist within 24 hours for complete removal.

ACUTE VISUAL REDUCTION OR LOSS

Acute visual loss is usually divided into painful and painless visual loss for diagnostic categorization. Other differentiating features include presence or absence of a relative afferent pupillary defect, the rapidity of onset, funduscopic exam, and various physical exam and historical features. The differential diagnosis of visual loss is listed in **Table 241-8**. Many of the diagnoses are discussed in further detail in the text.

ACUTE AND PAINFUL VISION REDUCTION OR LOSS

Acute Angle-Closure Glaucoma • *Pathophysiology* Glaucoma is a group of ocular disorders characterized by increased intraocular

TABLE 241-8 Differential Diagnosis of Visual loss

Diagnosis	Eye Pain	Relative Afferent Pupillary Defect	Onset	Fundoscopic Exam	Other Findings
Central retinal artery occlusion	No	Yes	Sudden	Pale retina, cherry red spot	
Central retinal vein occlusion	No	+/−	Sudden	"Blood and thunder"/"ketchup" fundus	
Acute ischemic optic neuropathy	No	Yes	Gradual	Swollen pale disk	Signs of temporal arteritis
Acute angle-closure glaucoma	Yes	+/−	Sudden	Difficult to visualize the fundus due to corneal edema	Painful red eye, hazy cornea, midpoint pupil, narrow anterior chamber, firm globe
Optic neuritis	Yes	Yes	Gradual	Papilledema	Painful EOM, young female patient
Giant cell arteritis	Possible retro-orbital headache/pain	Yes	Gradual	Normal	Headache, myalgias
Cataract	No	+/−	Gradual	Often unable to visualize fundus	Opacity in the lens
Uveitis	Yes	No	Gradual	Normal	Flare and cells in anterior chamber, ciliary flush, consensual photophobia
Vitreous hemorrhage	No	+/−	Sudden	Opacity in the vitreous	Floaters, cobwebs
Amaurosis fugax	No	No	Sudden	Normal	Transient monocular vision loss
Transient ischemic attack	No	No	Sudden	Normal	Transient binocular vision loss
Cortical blindness	No	+/−	Sudden or gradual	Possible papilledema	Complete visual loss or homonymous hemianopsia, headache
Migraine headache	Possible retro-orbital headache/pain	No	Sudden	Normal	Visual scotomata, nausea, vomiting
Retinal detachment	No	+/−	Sudden	Retina may be difficult to visualize (portion of retina out of focus)	Possible localized visual field defect, "cloudy veil," "window shade"; suspect by history
Diabetic retinopathy	No	+/−	Gradual	Neovascularization, retinal hemorrhages	History of diabetes mellitus
Macular degeneration	No	+/−	Gradual	Drusen, macular pigment clumps	Spots in visual field
Cytomegalovirus retinitis	No	+/−	Sudden or gradual	"Tomato and cheese" pizza (retinal necrosis), retinal hemorrhages	History of human immunodeficiency virus or other immunosuppression
Methanol	No	No	Gradual	Normal	Headache, nausea, vomiting, history of ingestion
Functional visual loss	No	No	Sudden or gradual	Normal	Optokinetic nystagmus

Abbreviation: EOM = extraocular muscle movement.

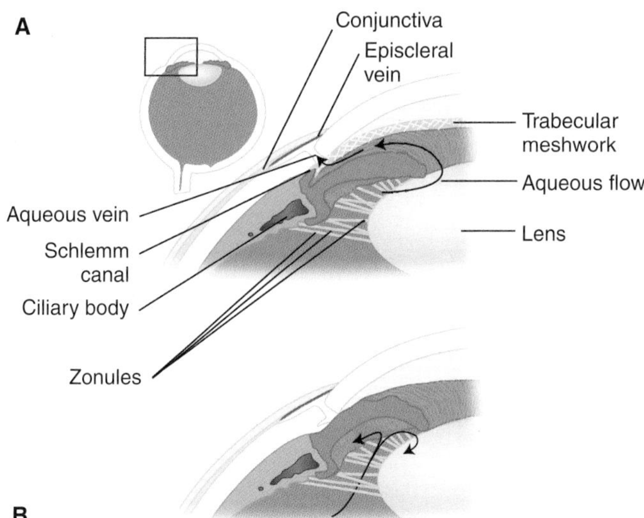

FIGURE 241-51. **A.** Normal flow of aqueous from ciliary body, through the pupil, and out through the trabecular meshwork and Schlemm canal located in the anterior chamber angle. **B.** Angle-closure glaucoma with pupillary block. Iris leaflet bows forward, blocking the chamber angle and prohibiting aqueous outflow. Meanwhile, aqueous production continues, and intraocular pressure rises.

pressure causing optic neuropathy and vision loss if left untreated. Obstruction to aqueous humor outflow is the basic underlying problem in glaucoma. In acute angle-closure glaucoma, the lens or the peripheral iris blocks the trabecular meshwork, obstructing the outflow of aqueous humor. This occurs more easily in persons whose eyes have shallow anterior chambers where the angle between the cornea and iris is reduced. A shallow anterior chamber results in a greater area of contact between the lens and iris, impeding flow of aqueous humor from the posterior to anterior chamber. This results in a pressure differential between the posterior and anterior chamber (referred to as *pupillary block*) and causes forward bowing of the iris, further narrowing the angle (**Figure 241-51**).

An acute attack is usually precipitated by pupillary dilation. Dilation increases contact between the iris and lens as the iris becomes thicker. When the pupil is mid-dilated, relative pupillary block and peripheral laxity of the iris are maximal. This increases the degree of pupillary block, increasing pressure in the posterior chamber and causing the iris to bulge forward (iris bombe). The angle between the peripheral iris, trabecular meshwork, and cornea becomes acutely closed, resulting in a precipitous increase in intraocular pressure. Intraocular pressure eventually exceeds the capacity of the corneal pump mechanism, causing the cornea to become edematous and less transparent, thus explaining the foggy vision or halos patients complain of and the hazy appearance of the cornea on physical examination.

As people age, the lens becomes less elastic and thicker, or cataracts may develop. These events can push the iris forward into greater contact with the lens, increasing the degree of pupillary block. Hypermetropic (farsighted) eyes have a shorter anterior to posterior length, a flatter cornea, and a narrower angle, increasing the risk of acute angle-closure glaucoma.

Anything causing pupillary dilatation can trigger an acute attack. The use of topical or systemic parasympatholytic agents (mydriatics, antihistamines) or sympathomimetics (epinephrine, pseudoephedrine), dim illumination, and emotionally upsetting events have all been implicated. Precipitation of acute angle-closure glaucoma has been reported with therapeutic use, and abuse of, intranasal cocaine, as well as therapeutic use of nebulized β-sympathomimetic and anticholinergic medications (e.g., albuterol and ipratropium).

Clinical Features Acute angle-closure glaucoma is abrupt in onset, painful, and may result in severe visual impairment if not treated quickly. Patients complain of sudden onset of severe eye pain or frontal or supraorbital headache. Associated symptoms include blurred vision, nausea,

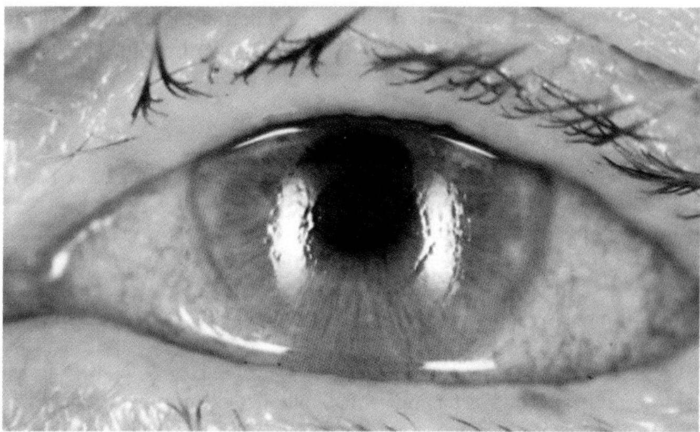

FIGURE 241-52. Acute angle-closure glaucoma. The cornea is cloudy, and there is marked conjunctival injection. [Reproduced with permission from Knoop K, Stack L, Storrow A: *Atlas of Emergency Medicine,* 2nd ed. © 2002, McGraw-Hill, New York.]

and vomiting. Rarely, acute angle-closure glaucoma may result in painless monocular vision loss. Acute angle-closure glaucoma may be misdiagnosed as migraine, temporal arteritis, subarachnoid hemorrhage, or intra-abdominal emergency.

Examination reveals a fixed, midposition pupil and a hazy (cloudy/steamy) cornea with conjunctival injection (**Figure 241-52**), most prominent at the limbus. The affected eye is rock hard. Measure the intraocular pressure to establish the diagnosis (see earlier section, Intraocular Pressure), although the presence of the characteristic symptom complex—a cloudy cornea, fixed midposition pupil, and rock hard globe—is diagnostic. Normal intraocular pressure is 10 to 20 mm Hg, and may exceed 60 to 80 mm Hg in an acute attack.

Treatment There have been no controlled studies regarding medical treatment for acute angle-closure glaucoma. Treatment of acute angle-closure glaucoma involves lowering the intraocular pressure by blocking production of aqueous humor, facilitating outflow of aqueous humor, and reducing the volume of vitreous humor (**Table 241-9**). IV mannitol quickly lowers intraocular pressure and should be given if there are no contraindications. Pilocarpine frequently will not cause the iris to constrict during the acute attack until the pressure is reduced, due to pressure-induced ischemic paralysis of the iris. Topical steroids are frequently recommended. Pilocarpine 1% or 2% should be instilled into the affected eye once the pressure is lowered (usually not effective until the intraocular pressure is <50 mm Hg) to make the pupil miotic, thereby pulling the peripheral iris away from the angle. Begin treatment immediately, simultaneously with consulting ophthalmology. Definitive treatment is laser iridectomy.

Concern exists regarding precipitation of acute angle-closure glaucoma in patients with shallow anterior chambers who undergo diagnostic mydriasis, but the incidence is low. Some clinicians believe that, if

TABLE 241-9 Treatment of Acute Glaucoma

Treatment	Effect
Topical β-blocker (timolol 0.5%), one drop	Blocks production of aqueous humor
Topical α_2-agonist (apraclonidine 1%), one drop	Blocks production of aqueous humor
Carbonic anhydrase inhibitor (acetazolamide), 500 milligrams IV or PO	Blocks production of aqueous humor
Mannitol, 1–2 grams/kg IV	Reduces volume of aqueous humor
Recheck IOP hourly	—
Topical pilocarpine 1%–2%, one drop every 15 min for two doses once IOP is below 40 mm Hg, then four times daily	Facilitates outflow of aqueous humor

Abbreviation: IOP = intraocular pressure.

necessary, it may be wise to dilate these patients in the ED because precipitation of an acute attack would ideally occur when the patient can get acute care.

ACUTE PAINLESS VISUAL LOSS

Optic Neuritis Acute optic neuritis is often painless but can be painful, especially with eye movement. Visual acuity can range from mildly reduced to profound loss with no light perception. Reduction of vision occurs most commonly over days, but occasionally over hours. Visual loss is usually unilateral, but can be bilateral. Color vision is affected more commonly than visual acuity, and there may be visual field deficits.

The red desaturation test is helpful in identifying optic neuropathies. This test is performed by having the patient look with one eye at a dark red object and then testing the other eye to see if the object looks the same color. The affected eye often will see the red object as pink or lighter red. An afferent pupillary defect (**Figure 241-8**) is commonly present. Funduscopic examination will reveal a swollen and edematous optic disk (papillitis) in approximately 30% of patients. If the head of the optic nerve is normal in appearance, the patient is said to have retrobulbar neuritis.

Optic neuritis can be idiopathic or an initial presentation of multiple sclerosis. Other causes of optic neuritis include postchildhood vaccination; viral infections such as measles, mumps, chickenpox, encephalitis, herpes zoster, and mononucleosis; inflammation of structures contiguous with the optic nerve such as the meninges, orbit, and sinuses; and other infections, including syphilis, tuberculosis, *Cryptococcus*, and sarcoidosis. The differential diagnosis includes ischemic optic neuropathy (sudden onset and painless), papilledema (bilateral, painless with preserved visual acuity), hypertensive retinopathy, orbital tumor compressing the optic nerve (proptosis frequent), intracranial tumor compressing the visual pathway (seen on CT), and toxic or metabolic optic neuropathy from alcohol or various toxins such as the heavy metals or chloroquine.

Neurology and ophthalmology consultation is needed to establish a diagnosis. MRI results are important prognosticators for optic neuritis.

Central Retinal Artery Occlusion The first branch off the internal carotid artery is the ophthalmic artery, which supplies the central retinal artery, which, in turn, provides the blood supply to the inner retina. The ciliary arteries also originate from the ophthalmic artery distal to the central retinal artery and supply the outer retina by the choriocapillaries of the choroid. If the central retinal artery becomes occluded, the inner retina will infarct and become pale, less transparent, and edematous. The macula is the thinnest portion of the retina, and the intact underlying choroidal circulation remains visible through this section of retina, creating the illusion of a "**cherry red spot**." The macular area maintains its normal color, and the surrounding ischemic retina turns pale, thus causing this classic finding on funduscopy (**Figure 241-53**). Causes include carotid or cardiac embolus, retinal artery thrombosis, giant cell arteritis, vasculitis (lupus, polyarteritis nodosa), sickle cell disease, trauma, vasospasm (migraine), elevated intraocular pressure (glaucoma), hypercoagulable states, and low retinal blood flow (carotid stenosis or hypotension).

Sudden (occurring over seconds), profound, painless, monocular loss of vision is characteristic of a central retinal artery occlusion. The event is often preceded by episodes of amaurosis fugax. Physical examination will often reveal an afferent pupillary defect in addition to the pale retina and cherry red macula. **Evidence-based treatment and information about the course of the disease are lacking.** Central retinal artery occlusion is rare, thought to account for 1/10,000 ophthalmic visits.[7] There are no data on ED visits. There is no evidence supporting or refuting the success of maneuvers such as digital massage, intraocular pressure–lowering drugs, and breathing into a paper bag to increase partial pressure of arterial carbon dioxide.[8,9] There are reports discussing the use of intra-arterial tissue plasminogen activator within 20 hours of onset of symptoms.[7] **Consult an ophthalmologist and neurologist immediately when suspecting the condition, and follow institutional protocols for treatment.** Irreversible loss of visual function usually occurs after 4 hours of ischemia.

Central Retinal Vein Occlusion Thrombosis of the central retinal vein causes retinal venous stasis, edema, and hemorrhage. Risk factors include diabetes, hypertension, cerebrovascular disease, cardiovascular disease, dyslipidemia, hypercoagulable states, vasculitis, glaucoma, and compression of the vein in thyroid disease and orbital tumors. Loss of vision is variable, ranging from vague blurring to rapid, painless, and monocular loss of vision. Funduscopic examination typically reveals optic disk edema and diffuse retinal hemorrhages in all quadrants ("blood-and-thunder fundus") (**Figure 241-54**). The contralateral optic nerve and fundus generally are normal, which helps distinguish central

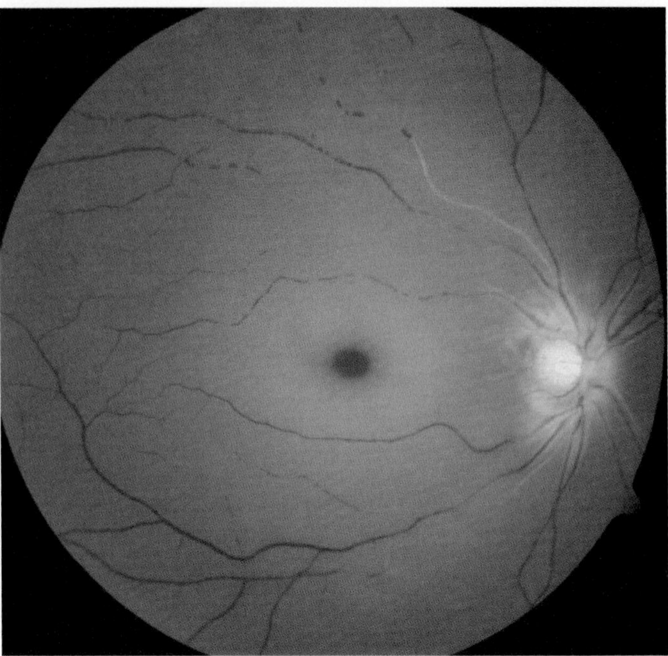

FIGURE 241-53. Central retinal artery occlusion. Note macular "cherry red spot" and retinal pallor as well as the plaques visible in the retinal vessels. [Courtesy of Allen R. Katz, Department of Ophthalmology, University of Nebraska Medical Center.]

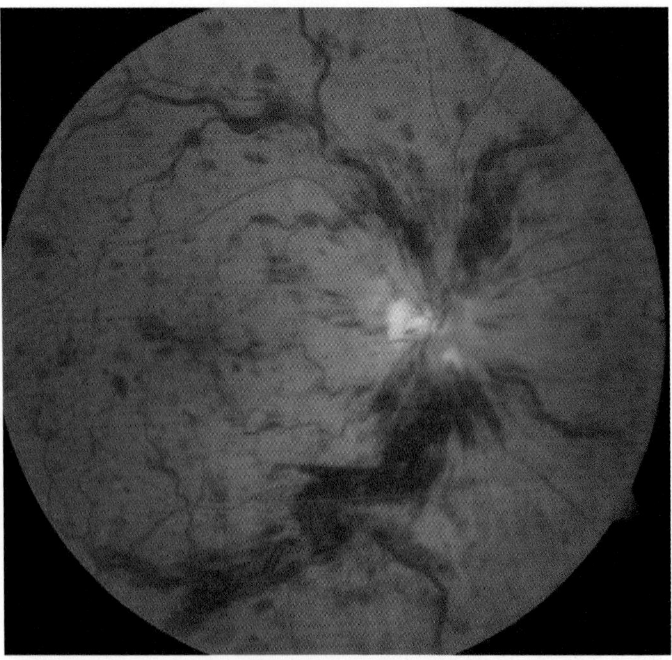

FIGURE 241-54. Central retinal vein occlusion. The disk margin is blurred, the veins are dilated and tortuous, and there is a large amount of hemorrhage typical of the "blood-and-thunder fundus." [Courtesy of Allen R. Katz, Department of Ophthalmology, University of Nebraska Medical Center.]

retinal vein occlusion from papilledema, and the diffuse retinal hemorrhages help distinguish it from optic neuritis (the peripheral retina is normal in optic neuritis). No specific treatment is available. Consult neurology and ophthalmology.

Flashing Lights and Floaters/Retinal Detachment Complaints about new-onset flashing lights and/or floaters commonly cause patients to seek urgent medical attention. The first distinction to make is if the symptoms are monocular or binocular. **Binocular complaints are almost always intracranial (i.e., ophthalmic migraines), whereas monocular complaints are almost always related to the symptomatic eye.**

The posterior segment of the eye is a large cavity filled with vitreous gel. As a person ages, this gel eventually contracts centrally and separates from the posterior wall of the eye. The vitreous is very sticky and tugs on the retina before separation, stimulating the retina, which the brain perceives as light. The average age of onset is 55 years old, but it can occur as early as the 20s in severely nearsighted people. If the vitreous gel separates successfully, then floaters occur, which may persist for years until the gel liquefies enough for the floaters to sink below the visual axis. If the gel creates enough traction on the retina before separation that it tears a hole in the retina, then fluid can go through the retinal hole and start to peel the retina off like wallpaper.

Symptoms may include flashes of light, floaters, a dark veil or curtain in the field of vision, and decreased peripheral and/or central visual acuity. This is an emergent condition requiring a retina specialist to evaluate and treat the patient. **Diagnosing a retinal detachment or tear or vitreous detachment requires a dilated indirect ophthalmoscopic evaluation by an ophthalmologist within 24 hours.** Most tears occur in the peripheral retina, which is not visualized on the direct funduscopic examination. A large retinal detachment will appear as a pale billowing parachute on dilated funduscopic examination. The diagnosis is mainly by history and confirmed by the ophthalmologist.

Temporal Arteritis **Temporal arteritis**, also called **giant cell** or **cranial arteritis**, is a systemic vasculitis involving medium-sized and large arteries. The temporal artery is the most common vessel involved. The disease causes a painless ischemic optic neuropathy with profound visual loss and contralateral ocular involvement in days to weeks if not diagnosed and treated promptly. Patients are generally >50 years of age and frequently have a history of polymyalgia rheumatica. Symptoms may include headache, jaw claudication, myalgias, fatigue, fever, anorexia, and temporal artery tenderness. Many patients may have associated symptoms of transient ischemic attacks or stroke. The physical examination frequently will reveal an afferent pupillary defect if the optic nerve circulation is involved. An elevated sedimentation rate is usually present, with the majority of biopsy-proven cases in the range of 70 to 110 mm/h. The added presence of an elevated C-reactive protein also suggests the diagnosis. Treatment consists of several doses of IV steroids followed by oral steroids. Steroids should not be delayed while waiting for a temporal artery biopsy to be performed. Biopsies will still be positive a week after initiation of steroid therapy.

CRANIAL NERVE PALSIES

BELL'S PALSY AND GENU VII BELL'S PALSY

Bell's palsy is a dysfunction of peripheral cranial nerve VII commonly of viral origin. It is palsy of the ipsilateral upper and lower face. The orbicularis muscles are involved, resulting in incomplete closure of the eyelids on the affected side and leading to corneal exposure keratitis. Prescribe viscous topical wetting agents to keep the corneal epithelium from breaking down, and patch the affected eye. Ophthalmology referral for outpatient monitoring of the cornea is warranted.

Treatment of Bell's palsy remains controversial. As of this writing, the most recent Cochrane review seems to conclude that antivirals provide no benefit over placebo in the treatment of Bell's palsy. Corticosteroids alone and antivirals with corticosteroids confer treatment benefit.[10] Consequently, the best evidence at present is to consider the administration of both antivirals and steroids, but not antivirals alone.[10]

Genu VII Bell's palsy is a stroke, masquerading as a peripheral seventh-nerve Bell's palsy, involving cranial nerve VI and the ipsilateral cranial nerve VII as it "genuflects" around the sixth-nerve nucleus. **This results in a cranial nerve VII palsy identical to a typical Bell's palsy (affecting the upper and lower face ipsilaterally) but with the added finding of the patient's inability to abduct the ipsilateral eye (cranial nerve VI palsy).** This underscores the importance of extraocular muscle testing in all Bell's palsy patients.

DIABETIC/HYPERTENSIVE CRANIAL NERVE PALSIES

Chronic diabetes and hypertension eventually can create vascular compromise to the vasa nervorum of any cranial nerve. **The pupil is spared in acute diabetic cranial nerve III palsy** due to vascular compromise of the central nerve fibers (the efferent pupillomotor fibers run in the periphery of the nerve) (**Figure 241-55**). Extraocular muscle testing will reveal an inhibition of ipsilateral medial gaze, upward gaze, and downward gaze as well as ptosis in an acute cranial nerve III palsy. Lateral gaze (abduction) will be preserved, and diplopia will be worse when the patient attempts to look toward the contralateral side due to the inability to adduct the eye (medial rectus dysfunction). In an acute cranial nerve VI palsy, lateral gaze will be diminished (abduction) on the ipsilateral side, and diplopia will be worse when the patient is trying to look to the affected side (lateral rectus dysfunction). Neuroimaging is needed in the ED to rule out an intracranial lesion.

If no other associated neurologic symptoms or findings are present, the blood sugar and blood pressure are under control, and neuroimaging does not suggest an alternative diagnosis, the patient can be discharged with ophthalmology and/or neurology follow-up.

POSTERIOR COMMUNICATING ARTERY ANEURYSM

Acute cranial nerve III palsy with ipsilateral pupillary dilatation is a posterior communicating artery aneurysm until proven otherwise. Concomitant headache is a frequent but not absolute finding. Expansion of an aneurysm of the posterior communicating artery frequently causes compression of the outer fibers of cranial nerve III. The pupillomotor fibers are located in the outer portion of cranial nerve III; therefore, the pupil becomes dilated on the affected side (**Figure 241-55**). Treatment is emergent blood pressure reduction if hypertensive, neuroimaging, and neurosurgical consultation.

HORNER'S SYNDROME

The physical findings of ipsilateral ptosis and miosis and anhydrosis are characteristic of Horner's syndrome (Figure 241-56). Interruption of the sympathetic nerve impulses controlling the Mueller muscle in the upper eyelid and the iris dilators causes these classic findings. Interruption can occur anywhere along the pathway from the brainstem to the sympathetic plexus surrounding the carotid artery (**Figure 241-57**). ED

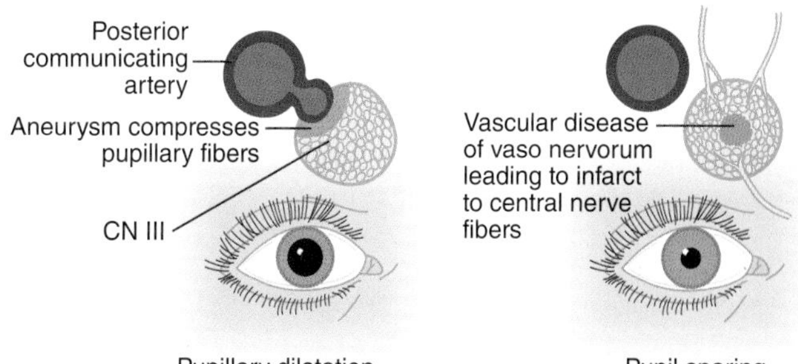

FIGURE 241-55. Posterior communicating artery aneurysm compresses the peripherally located pupillomotor fibers of cranial nerve (CN) III, causing a nerve palsy and pupillary dilatation. Diabetes and hypertension can cause microvascular compromise of the central nerve fibers, causing a nerve palsy with pupil sparing.

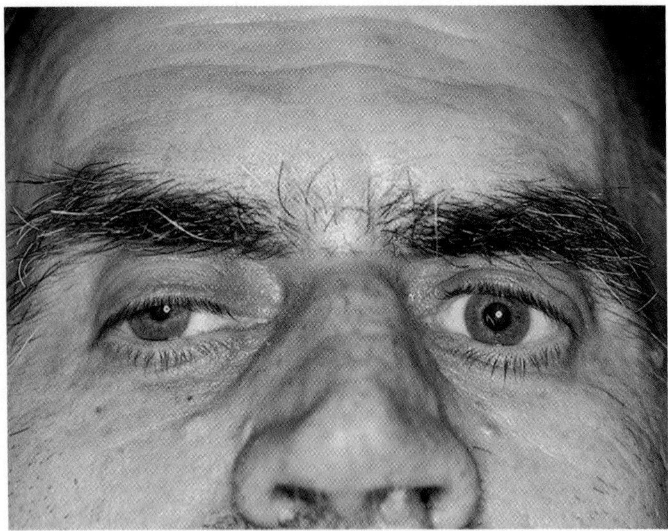

FIGURE 241-56. Horner's syndrome. Note the ptosis and miosis of the right eye. [Reproduced with permission from Knoop K, Stack L, Storrow A: *Atlas of Emergency Medicine*, 2nd ed. © 2002, McGraw-Hill, New York.]

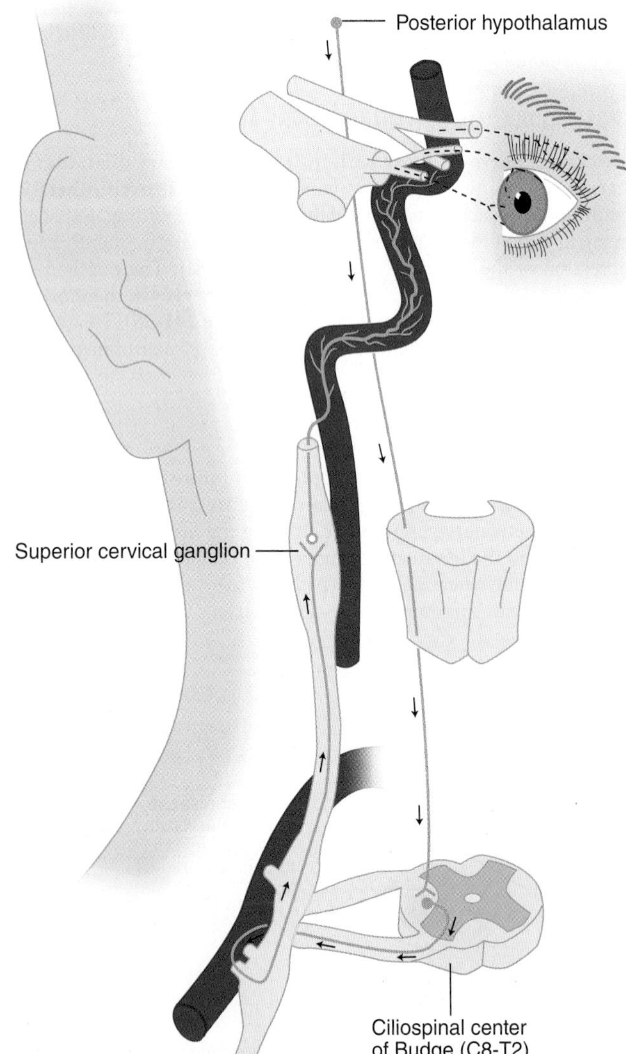

FIGURE 241-57. Sympathetic nerve pathway of the eye. An interruption anywhere along this pathway can cause Horner's syndrome.

evaluation includes a chest x-ray, CT scan of the brain and cervical region, and CT angiogram or magnetic resonance angiography of the head and neck vessels for carotid dissection. Institutional protocols determine if CT angiogram or magnetic resonance angiography is preferred.

In adults, causes of Horner's syndrome include cerebrovascular accidents, tumors, internal carotid artery dissection, herpes zoster, and trauma. In children, the causes include neuroblastoma, lymphoma, and metastasis. **Neck pain and acute Horner's syndrome suggest carotid dissection and can occur spontaneously (usually >30 years old) or as a result of blunt or penetrating neck injury.**

PSEUDOTUMOR CEREBRI (IDIOPATHIC INTRACRANIAL HYPERTENSION)

Increased intracranial pressure, papilledema, normal cerebrospinal fluid, and normal CT/MRI characterize pseudotumor cerebri. This condition can occur at any age. Patients complain of nausea, vomiting, headaches, and blurring of vision. **Patients can develop cranial nerve VI paresis, causing horizontal diplopia (double vision on lateral gaze).** A key component of examination is the identification of **visual field defects**. If CT/MRI is normal, perform lumbar puncture and record opening pressure; send cerebrospinal fluid for routine diagnostics. Consult neurosurgery for the treatment plan. Initial treatment is acetazolamide, 500 milligrams PO twice daily, and outpatient visual field monitoring.

OCULAR ULTRASONOGRAPHY

Direct visualization of intraocular structures can be limited by periorbital edema, corneal abrasions, hyphema, and cataracts. The superficial location of the eye and its cystic composition make US ideal in the assessment of a variety of ocular disorders. Ocular ultrasonography can expedite the diagnosis and management of several ocular emergencies, including retinal detachment, retrobulbar hematoma, globe perforation, lens dislocation, vitreous hemorrhage, and intraocular foreign body.[11-13] The indications for ocular ultrasonography include loss of vision/decreased vision, eye pain, eye trauma, suspected intraocular foreign body, and head injury. The ability of emergency physicians to accurately diagnose ocular pathology using bedside ocular ultrasonography has been well documented in emergency medicine literature.[11,12]

SCANNING TECHNIQUE AND NORMAL ANATOMY

Use a 7.5-to 10-mHz linear array transducer and set the unit to 'Ocular' for lower energy. Place the patient in a supine or partially upright position and have the patient keep the eyes closed (**Figure 241-58**). Apply a large amount of standard water-soluble US gel to the patient's closed eyelid so that the transducer does not touch the eyelid. US gel is not detrimental to the eye. Without applying any pressure, and asking the patient to look straight ahead with the eyes closed, scan the globe in sagittal and transverse planes. Stabilize the scanning hand over the bridge of the nose or on the forehead. Scan both eyes through closed eyelids for comparison. Examine the eyes in the neutral position and during gentle eye movements from side to side and up and down to thoroughly evaluate the orbit. Dynamic examination is crucial to identify adhesions, detachments, and membranes. The probe can also be moved side to side in both scanning planes to demonstrate the full extent of the structures in the eye. Adjust the depth so that the image fills the screen. The gain also needs to be adjusted multiple times during the examination to identify subtle abnormalities and avoid artifacts. Because the eye is a fluid-filled organ, it provides a perfect acoustic window for scanning and obtaining excellent images.[14-16]

The normal eye appears as a circular hypoechoic organ. The cornea is seen as a thin hyperechoic layer parallel to the eyelid attached to the sclera at the periphery. The iris is identified as a linear echogenic line extending from the periphery toward the lens on both sides. The anterior chamber contains anechoic fluid and is bordered by the cornea, iris, and anterior reflection of the lens. The normal lens has anterior and posterior boundary echoes with an anechoic center and is biconvex in

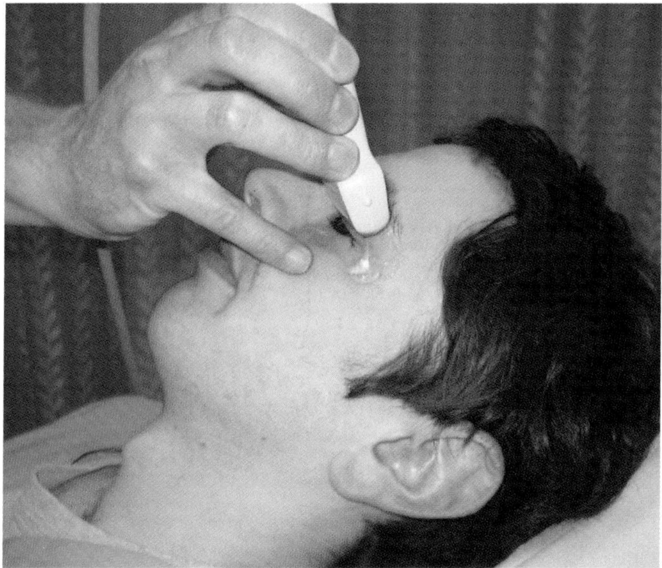

FIGURE 241-58. A high-resolution linear array US transducer is being applied to the closed eyelid. [Courtesy of Allen R. Katz, Department of Ophthalmology, University of Nebraska Medical Center.]

shape. The normal vitreous chamber is filled with anechoic fluid. Vitreous is relatively echo free in a young, healthy eye. Sonographically, the normal retina cannot be differentiated from the other posterior layers such as choroid and sclera (**Figure 241-59**). The evaluation of the retrobulbar space includes optic nerve, extraocular muscles, and bony orbit. The retro-orbital fat appears very echogenic. The optic nerve is visible as a hypoechoic linear region extending away from the globe posteriorly. Minor manipulations in the angulation of the probe are necessary to visualize the optic nerve. The central retinal artery and central retinal vein can be identified using Doppler.[14,15]

OCULAR TRAUMA

Assessment of patients with ocular trauma by US is of particular value when pain, soft tissue edema, and abnormalities like corneal edema, hyphema, or cataract make direct visualization of the posterior segment of the eye difficult. Ultrasound can detect a wide variety of ocular pathology

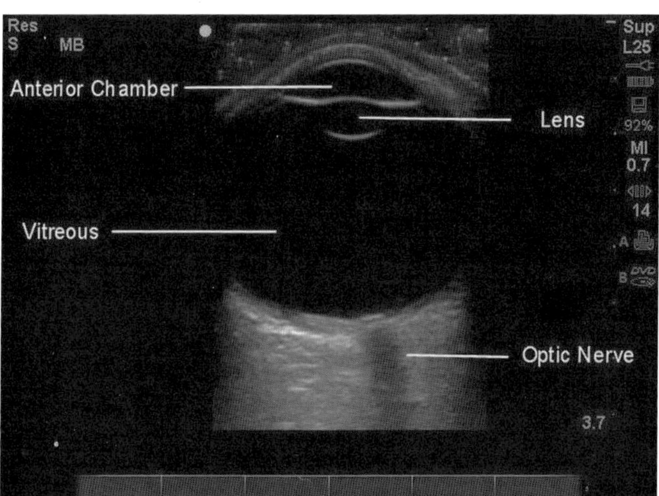

FIGURE 241-59. Normal eye in transverse view showing the anterior chamber, lens, vitreous, and optic nerve. [Courtesy of Allen R. Katz, Department of Ophthalmology, University of Nebraska Medical Center.]

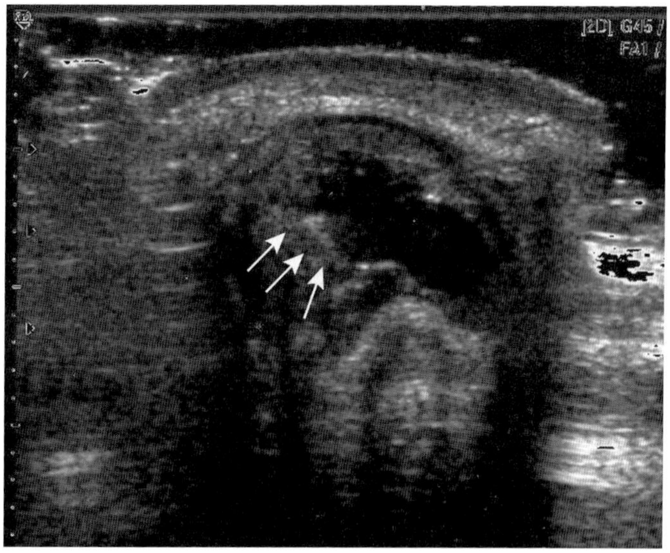

FIGURE 241-60. Extensive globe rupture from trauma. US shows abnormal, irregular shape of the eye with ocular contents displaced posteriorly (*arrows*). [Courtesy of M. Blaivas and Allen R. Katz, Department of Ophthalmology, University of Nebraska Medical Center.]

from trauma including dislocated lens, globe disruption, vitreous hemorrhage, hyphema, retinal detachment, orbital emphysema, and retrobulbar hemorrhage. **Suspected ruptured globe is a relative contraindication to US examination, due to the risk of extruding globe contents associated with direct pressure on and around the eye.**[12]

US findings of globe rupture include distortion of the normal shape of the globe, decrease in the size of the globe, anterior chamber collapse, and vitreous hemorrhage.[11] Ocular trauma can lead to buckling of the sclera and scleral folds, which appear sonographically as irregularities in globe contour, highly reflective at their top and shadowing the orbital tissues (**Figure 241-60**). Sonographically, **lens dislocation** is seen as a highly reflective oval mass moving independently of the surrounding structures with eye movements. The dislocation is more readily visualized if it is complete or a cataract has formed. **Hyphema** can be identified on US as an echoic structure of variable echogenicity depending on the age of the bleed. Fresh hyphema will have low echogenicity and becomes more echogenic as it becomes organized. A **retrobulbar (pre- or postseptal) hematoma** is visualized as an echoluceny posterior to the globe.[17]

INTRAOCULAR FOREIGN BODY

The presence of an intraocular foreign body may not always be apparent on clinical examination. US is a useful adjunct for detecting and localizing intraocular foreign bodies, but visualization of intraocular foreign bodies depends on their intrinsic echogenicity. Metallic objects are especially visible because of their bright echogenic acoustic profile and associated shadowing or reverberation artifacts in the echolucent vitreous, whereas materials such as wood are more difficult to detect (**Figure 241-61**). Sonographic patterns of shadowing and comet tail artifacts may help distinguish different foreign body materials. The dynamic nature of the US examination is also helpful in anatomic localization, determination of the size, and analysis of the composition of the foreign body.[18-20] With penetrating ocular injuries, a track of hemorrhage may be seen outlining the route of passage of a foreign body.

RETINAL DETACHMENT

Retinal detachment can be difficult to detect on physical examination, especially when the detachment is small. Bedside US reliably detects retinal detachment and is particularly useful when the examiner's view to the retina is obscured by periorbital edema, blood, or other opacities. For the detection of retinal detachment, ultrasonography performed by

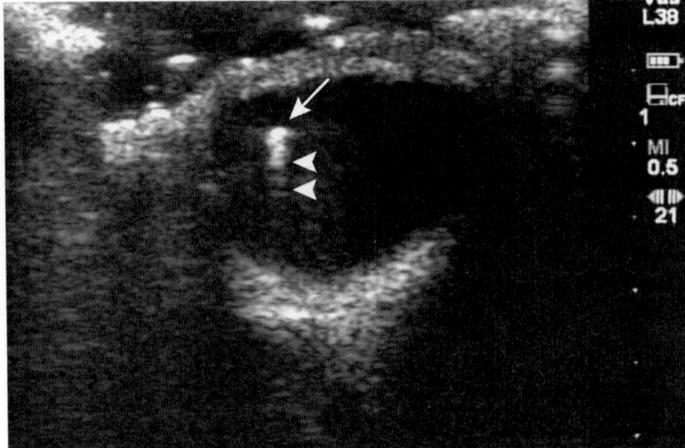

FIGURE 241-61. A hyperechoic foreign body (*arrow*) in the eye. Note the bright echogenic reverberation artifact (*arrowheads*). [Courtesy of M. Blaivas and Allen R. Katz, Department of Ophthalmology, University of Nebraska Medical Center.]

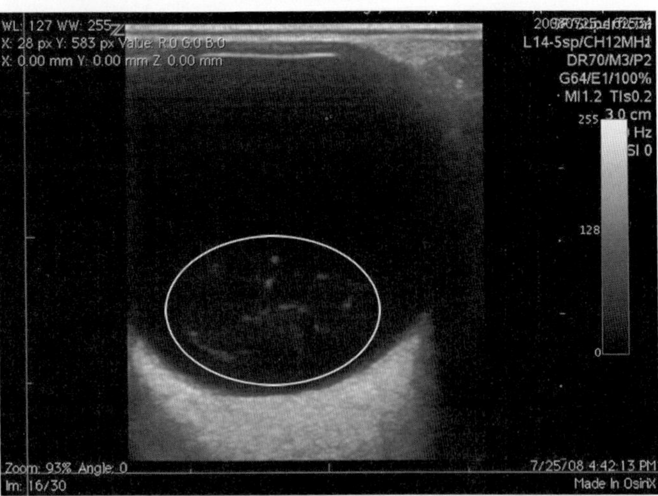

FIGURE 241-63. Bright echoes (enclosed in oval) in the posterior chamber demonstrating vitreous hemorrhage. [Courtesy of D. Chandwani and Allen R. Katz, Department of Ophthalmology, University of Nebraska Medical Center.]

an emergency physician has a sensitivity of 97% to 100% and a specificity of 83% to 92%.[21,22]

A retinal detachment is seen as an echogenic undulating membrane in the posterior to lateral globe, protruding into vitreous (**Figure 241-62**). Even in complete retinal detachments, the typically folded surface remains bound to the ora serrata anteriorly and the optic nerve head posteriorly. Unlike choroidal detachment that doesn't change with ocular movements, retinal detachment moves with eye movements.[16] A shallow cuff of subretinal fluid may also be seen along with the detachment. On occasion, retinal detachments are also accompanied by vitreous hemorrhages.

Vitreous Hemorrhage Vitreous hemorrhage can be spontaneous or associated with trauma. Vitreous hemorrhage can interfere with vision and, if it is large, can potentially cause blindness. It appears as echogenic material in the posterior chamber. The sonographic appearance of vitreous hemorrhage depends on its age and the severity of the bleed. Increasing gain is helpful for detecting acute hemorrhages because they are often minimally echogenic. Early mild hemorrhages are seen as small dots or scattered low-amplitude reflective mobile opacities in the vitreous. As the hemorrhage matures and organizes, thick mobile membranes are formed in the vitreous. Sonographically, this is seen as vitreous filled with multiple large echoes (**Figure 241-63**). Due to gravitational forces, these opacities may also layer inferiorly. Echogenic stranding and scarring of the vitreous occurs as time progresses.[16,23,24] As vitreous hemorrhage becomes more echogenic, it can mimic the appearance of a retinal detachment. The main characteristics that can help in differentiating vitreous hemorrhage from retinal detachment are as follows: (1) Retinal detachment moves with eye movements unlike vitreous hemorrhage, which will remain horizontal; and (2) vitreous hemorrhages are frequently seen in the middle portion of the posterior chamber and retinal detachments almost always occur at the posterior-most portion of the eye, adjacent to the optic disk and macula.[21]

Elevated Intracranial Pressure—Optic Nerve Sheath Measurement Another novel use of bedside ocular US is the evaluation of the optic nerve sheath diameter to assess possible elevated intracranial pressure. Multiple studies have shown good correlation between intracranial pressure and sonographic optic nerve sheath diameter.[25-32] On US, a normal optic nerve sheath measures up to 5.0 mm in diameter in adults, 4.5 mm in children, and 4.0 mm in infants.[33] The measurement is obtained 3 mm posterior to the globe for both eyes. A position of 3 mm behind the globe is selected because the US contrast is greatest at this point, and the measurements are more reproducible (**Figure 241-64**). Typically, three measurements are

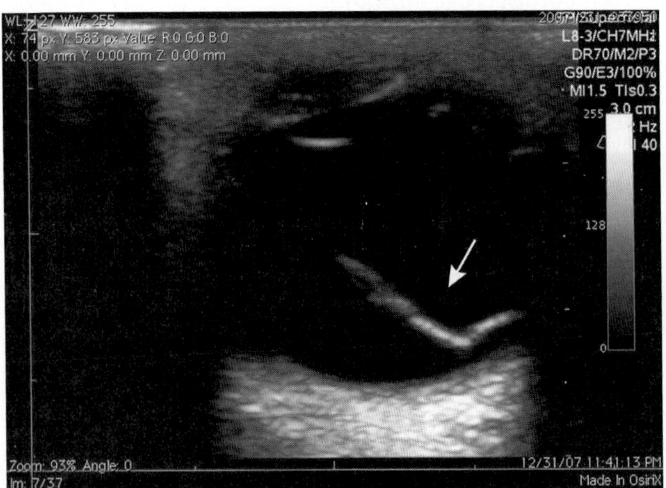

FIGURE 241-62. Retinal detachment is seen as a hyperechoic membrane in the posterior aspect of the globe (*arrow*). [Courtesy of D. Chandwani and Allen R. Katz, Department of Ophthalmology, University of Nebraska Medical Center.]

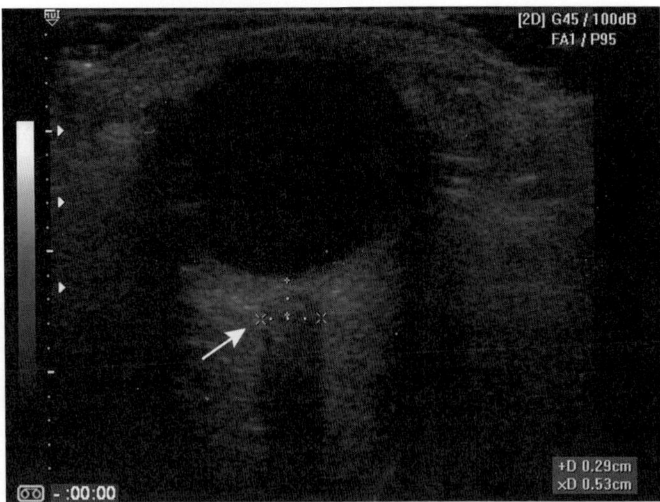

FIGURE 241-64. An optic nerve sheath measuring 5.3 mm in a patient with head injury is shown. One set of calipers measures 3 mm behind the globe, and the second measures the optic nerve sheath diameter (*arrow*). [Courtesy of M. Blaivas and Allen R. Katz, Department of Ophthalmology, University of Nebraska Medical Center.]

averaged. Current literature suggests that the cut-off value that provides the best accuracy for the prediction of intracranial pressure >20 mm Hg is 5.7 to 6.0 mm, and increased intracranial pressure should be suspected with values above this threshold. The sensitivity and specificity in detecting increased intracranial pressure using a cut-off value of 5.7 to 6.0 mm are in the range of 87% to 95% and 79% to 100%, respectively.[34]

CAUTIONS WITH OCULAR US

- **If globe rupture is suspected, avoid any manipulation or pressure upon the globe or eyelid.**
- Limit the duration of ocular US examination, especially when using spectral and color Doppler, and **set the US unit for 'ocular imaging'**. The recommended exposure limits are half that of fetal imaging.
- Various artifacts may interfere with ocular ultrasound examination. Orbital emphysema can make it difficult to visualize contents of the orbit.
- Air bubbles within the vitreous, which may appear in the setting of trauma to the globe, may resemble an intraocular foreign body.

Acknowledgment: The authors gratefully acknowledge the contributions of John D. Mitchell, the author of this chapter in the previous edition.

REFERENCES

The complete reference list is available online at www.TintinalliEM.com.

Ear Disorders

Kathleen Hosmer

This chapter discusses common nontraumatic conditions affecting the external, middle, and inner ear. Selected traumatic conditions include auricular hematoma, burns, and frostbite. Lacerations to the ear are discussed in the chapter 40, "Face and Scalp Lacerations." Ear disorders in children are discussed in chapter 115, "Ear and Mastoid Disorders in Infants and Children."

ANATOMY

EXTERNAL EAR

The auricle, or pinna, is the visible external portion of the ear, whose trumpet shape enables it to collect air vibrations. It consists of a thin plate of elastic cartilage with a tightly adherent covering of skin. The external auditory canal is an S-shaped skin-lined tube that extends from the auricle to the tympanic membrane (TM). The outer one third of the external auditory canal is composed of an incomplete cartilaginous tube. Its thick skin supports hair follicles plus apocrine and sebaceous glands. The inner two thirds of the canal is composed of bone covered by a thin layer of tightly adherent skin, which is easily torn by minimal trauma.

The blood supply to the external ear is derived from the posterior auricular, superficial temporal, and deep auricular arteries. Venous drainage of the external ear is into the superficial temporal and posterior auricular veins, which then drain into the external jugular vein. The posterior auricular vein frequently connects to the sigmoid sinus, providing a route for extension of infected material into the intracranial cavity.

MIDDLE EAR

The middle ear is an air-containing cavity in the petrous temporal bone. It contains the auditory ossicles, which transmit vibrations of the TM to the perilymph of the internal ear. It communicates with the nasopharynx anteriorly via the eustachian tube and with the mastoid air spaces posteriorly via the aditus ad antrum (**Figure 242-1**).

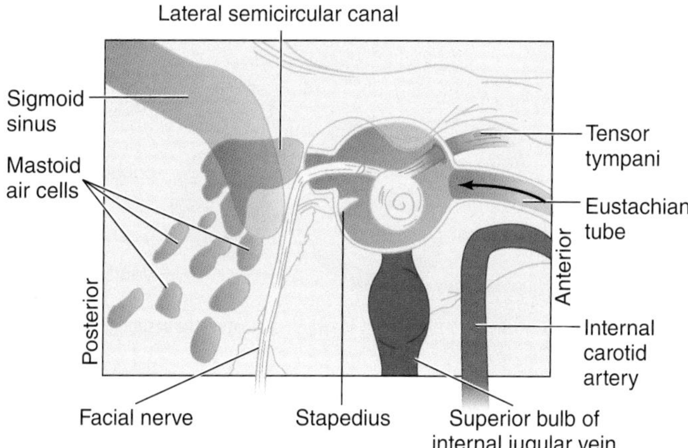

FIGURE 242-1. Sagittal section of the middle ear and related structures.

The TM is a thin, pearly gray, fibrous membrane that produces a cone-shaped light reflex anteroinferiorly when illuminated. Superiorly, the pars flaccida is the relatively slack portion of the membrane between the malleolar folds; the remainder of the membrane is tense and is called the pars tensa. The auditory ossicles are the malleus, incus, and stapes. Both the incus and the handle and lateral processes of the malleus are typically visible through the TM (**Figure 242-2**). Figure 242-1 shows the relationships of the facial nerve, sigmoid sinus, and internal carotid artery to the middle ear.

INNER EAR

The inner ear consists of the cochlea, which contains the auditory sensory receptors, and the vestibular labyrinth, which contains balance receptors. Cristae in the semicircular canals detect angular acceleration, and macules detect linear acceleration. Afferent nerves from the vestibular labyrinth connect to brainstem nuclei to maintain smooth movement of the eyes during head movement and to the cerebellum to control oculomotor and postural functions. Blood supply is from the vertebrobasilar system (**Figure 242-3**). The otolithic organs (utricle and saccule) lie in the vestibule. The internal auditory artery divides into the common cochlear artery and the anterior vestibular artery. The anterior vestibular artery provides the blood supply to the anterior and horizontal semicircular canals but not to the cochlea. Isolated occlusion of the anterior vestibular artery may therefore cause acute vestibular syndrome without hearing loss.

OTALGIA

Primary otalgia is caused by auricular and periauricular disease, whereas referred otalgia is caused by disease originating from remote structures.[1] Referred otalgia is common because the ear and several structures of the

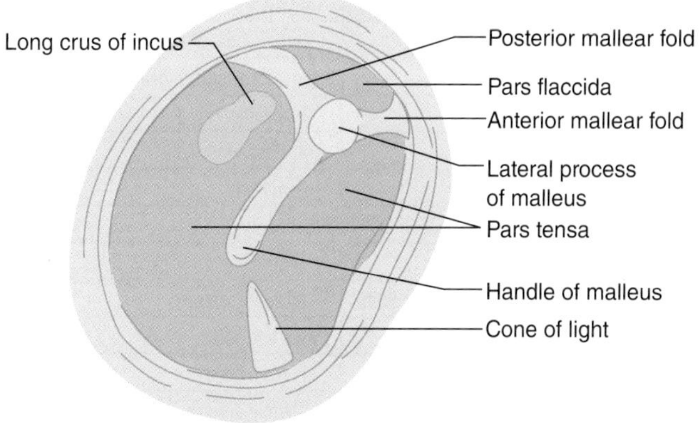

FIGURE 242-2. Right tympanic membrane as seen through the otoscope.

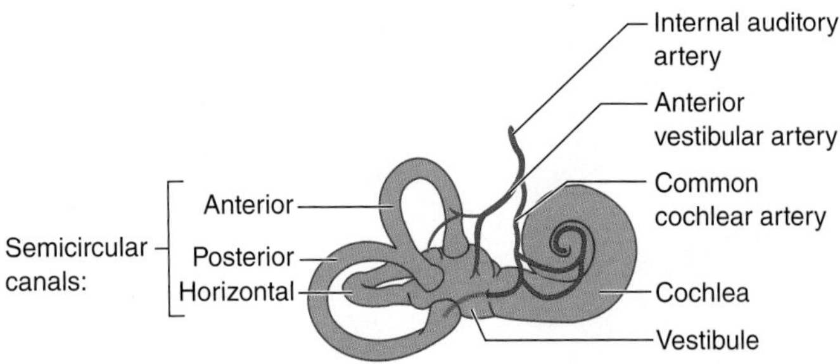

FIGURE 242-3. Schematic of the bony labyrinth containing the vestibular and auditory sensory organs.

head and neck share sensory innervation from the fifth, seventh, ninth, and tenth cranial nerves, as well as by the cervical plexus. **Table 242-1** lists common causes of primary and referred otalgia, including related neuralgias.[1]

TABLE 242-1 Causes of Otalgia

Primary	Referred
Trauma	Temporomandibular dysfunction syndrome
Infection	Dental
Otitis externa	Abscessed teeth/dental carries
Otitis media	Malocclusion
Mastoiditis	Bruxism
Bullous myringitis	Eustachian tube dysfunction
Pinna cellulitis	Retro- and oropharyngeal
Cerumen impaction	Tonsillitis
Cholesteatoma	Abscess
Neoplasms	Neoplasm
Foreign bodies	Nasal cavity
	Sinusitis
Facial Neuralgias with Periauricular Pain	Deviated septum
Trigeminal neuralgia	Throat and neck
Ramsay Hunt syndrome	Foreign body
Great auricular neuralgia	Thyroid disease
	Neoplasm

TINNITUS

Tinnitus is the perception of sound without external stimulation. It may be constant, pulsatile, high- or low-pitched, hissing, clicking, or ringing. It is most prevalent between the ages of 40 and 70 years old.[2]

Tinnitus is divided into two types: objective and subjective. Objective tinnitus may be heard by the examiner. Subjective tinnitus is more common. Its exact origin is unknown, although it is believed to result from damage to cochlear hair cells. **Table 242-2** outlines causes of tinnitus.[2]

A number of drugs are associated with tinnitus, and some also cause hearing loss[2] (**Table 242-3**).

Accurate diagnosis usually requires referral to an otolaryngologist. Many medications have been suggested as therapies; antidepressants may help patients tolerate their tinnitus but do not change the course.

TABLE 242-2 Common Causes of Tinnitus

Objective	Subjective
Vascular	Sensorineural hearing loss
Arteriovenous malformations	Hypertension
Arterial bruits	Conductive hearing loss
Mechanical	Head trauma
Enlarged eustachian tube	Medication side effects
Palatal myoclonus	Temporomandibular joint disorders
Stapedial muscle spasm	Anxiety, depression,
	Neurologic
	Acoustic neuroma
	Multiple sclerosis
	Benign intracranial hypertension
	Ménière's disease
	Cogan's syndrome

SUDDEN HEARING LOSS

Sudden hearing loss occurs over 3 days or less and is divided into sensorineural (cochlea, auditory nerve, or central auditory processing) and conductive (external ear, TM, and ossicles). Conductive hearing loss is more likely due to a reversible cause, such as otitis media, serous otitis, or a cerumen impaction. Indicators of poor prognosis include more severe hearing loss on presentation and the presence of vertigo. **Table 242-4**[3] lists causes of sensorineural hearing loss.

Viral infections, most typically mumps, have long been associated with sudden hearing loss.[4] Because of the terminal branches and interosseous location of the blood supply to the inner ear, the ear is uniquely vulnerable to a variety of vascular and hematologic diseases. Cogan's syndrome is an autoimmune disorder that presents with a bilateral hearing loss classically associated with tinnitus and vertigo.[5] Sudden hearing loss may also be caused by rupture of the TMs. Many common medications are implicated (Table 242-3).[3,5]

The evaluation begins with a complete history and physical examination. Differentiate conductive hearing loss from sensorineural hearing loss with a tuning fork. To perform the Weber test, place a vibrating tuning fork on the forehead and ask the patient where it is heard: it is normal to hear it equally in both ears; if the sound lateralizes to one ear, there is conductive hearing loss in that ear, or there is sensorineural loss in the opposite ear. To perform a Rinne test, place the vibrating tuning fork on skin over the mastoid bone of one ear, and then move the tuning fork to the entrance of the ear canal on the same side; the sound is normally heard better through air conduction at the entrance of the ear. If the sound is heard better over the mastoid bone, there is conductive hearing loss in that ear. Sudden conductive hearing loss may result from obstruction of the external auditory canal or from disturbances (or infection) of the TM or ossicles. Evaluate all current medications for possible ototoxic agents. A history of trauma or recollection of a "popping" noise preceding the hearing loss may indicate perforation of the

TABLE 242-3 Ototoxic Agents Causing Tinnitus and/or Hearing Loss

Loop diuretics	Chemotherapeutic agents
Ethacrynic acid	Cisplatin
Furosemide	Carboplatin
Bumetanide	Vinblastine
Salicylates and salicylate-containing compounds*	Vincristine
Nonsteroidal anti-inflammatory drugs*	Topical agents
Quinine	Solvents
Antibiotics	Propylene glycol
Aminoglycosides*	Antiseptics
Erythromycin	Ethanol
Vancomycin	Polymyxin B
	Neomycin

*Most commonly implicated agents.

TABLE 242-4 Causes of Sudden Sensorineural Hearing Loss

Idiopathic (71.0%)	**Trauma (4.2%)**
Infectious disease (12.8%)	Head injury
Unspecified respiratory infection (viral)	Acoustic trauma
Meningitis*	Barotrauma
Group A *Streptococcus*	**Vascular or hematologic (2.8%)**
Epstein-Barr virus	Cardiovascular disease
Toxoplasma gondii	Neurovascular disease
Syphilis	Hemorrhage (brain)
Herpes simplex virus	**Neoplastic (2.3%)**
Otologic disease (4.7%)	Vestibular schwannoma
Meniere's disease	Cerebellar angioma
Skull base or otologic surgery	**Other causes (2.2%)**
Autoimmune inner ear disease	Pregnancy related
Drug toxicity†	Nonotologic surgery

*Decreased incidence of hearing loss due to meningitis in the postimmunization era.
†See list of drugs in Table 3.

TM or ossicle dislocation. Coexistent tinnitus or vertigo may point to Ménière's disease. Also consider systemic illness.

The differential diagnosis includes both potentially reversible and potentially ominous causes (Table 242-4). If the physical examination does not identify the cause, consult otolaryngology. Treatment of idiopathic sudden sensorineural hearing loss is 60 milligrams of prednisone daily for 7 to 14 days or until follow-up, which is usually arranged within 2 weeks.[5-7]

ACUTE DIFFUSE OTITIS EXTERNA

Otitis externa includes infections and inflammation of the external auditory canal and auricle. It is divided into acute diffuse and malignant types. Acute diffuse disease is simply called *otitis externa* or *swimmer's ear.*

PATHOPHYSIOLOGY AND MICROBIOLOGY

Predisposing factors for the development of otitis externa are trauma to the skin of the external auditory canal and elevation of the local pH. Factors include frequent contact with water from swimming or bathing in hot tubs, pools, or freshwater lakes, and living in a humid environment. Trauma is most commonly due to scratching or overzealous disimpaction of cerumen. Cerumen is an acidic mixture of sebaceous and apocrine gland secretions and desquamated epithelial cells. It forms a physical barrier that protects the skin of the external auditory canal, whereas the acidic pH has antimicrobial properties.

The most common organisms are *Pseudomonas aeruginosa*, *Staphylococcus aureus*, Enterobacteriaceae, and *Proteus* species.[8] Otomycosis, or fungal otitis externa, is found in tropical climates and in the immunocompromised or after previous long-term therapy with antibiotics. Most cases are caused by *Aspergillus* or *Candida*.[9] Noninfectious causes include contact dermatitis from topical medications or resins in hearing aids, seborrhea, and psoriasis.

CLINICAL FEATURES

Acute diffuse otitis externa is characterized by pruritus, pain, and tenderness of the external ear. Physical signs include erythema and edema of the external auditory canal, which may spread to the tragus and auricle. Other signs are clear or purulent otorrhea and crusting of the external canal. As the disease progresses, the pain may become intolerable and occur with mastication or any movement of the periauricular skin. Increasing edema may eventually narrow the canal lumen and can lead to hearing impairment. In severe cases, infection may spread to the periauricular soft tissues and lymph nodes, and there may be lateral protrusion of the auricle secondary to inflammation.

TABLE 242-5 Topical Agents for Acute Diffuse Otitis Externa

Constituents	Comments
Ofloxacin 0.3%	Safe with perforations; one or two times per day
Ciprofloxacin 0.3%/dexamethasone 0.1%	Safe with perforations; two times per day
Acetic acid 2% solution	pH 4.5–6.0 (not safe with perforation)
Acetic acid 1%, hydrocortisone 2%	pH 3.0 (not safe with perforation)
Neomycin/polymyxin B/hydrocortisone	Ototoxic; higher risk of contact hypersensitivity; avoid in chronic otitis externa

TREATMENT

The treatment consists of analgesia, cleansing of the external auditory canal, acidifying agents, topical antimicrobials with or without steroids, and, in certain cases, adding an ear wick.[10,11] Cleansing may be done with gentle irrigation using hydrogen peroxide or saline, or gentle suction under direct visualization.[10] For the immunocompromised, atraumatic cleaning with aural suctioning under microscopic guidance can be done by an otolaryngologist.[10] Nonototoxic ototopical antibiotics are first-line therapy, particularly when the integrity of the TM is unknown or in the presence of a known TM perforation or tympanostomy tubes. Recommended topical agents are listed in **Table 242-5**.[11] Although there are few established cases of ototoxicity, there is a theoretical risk of both auditory and vestibular toxicity with the use of aminoglycosides, polymyxin, and acetic acid preparations.[10]

If cost is a factor and there are no known contraindications, acetic acid drops may be used because they are less expensive than the quinolones. In this case, a suspension should be used and not a solution; theoretically, a suspension has less chance of middle-ear penetration and resultant ototoxicity.

Instill the medication into the cleansed ear with the ear facing up, with this position held for 3 minutes. If edema of the external canal obstructs the lumen, insert a commercial wick to enhance delivery of topical drops throughout the full length of the canal.

For cases unresponsive to initial treatment, obtain bacterial and fungal cultures. Oral antibiotics are not routinely recommended[10] and should be reserved for febrile patients and those with periauricular extension (consider malignant otitis externa, discussed below). Instruct patients with otitis externa to avoid predisposing factors to eliminate recurrences. Strategies include ear plugs while swimming or bathing (cotton wool impregnated with petroleum jelly or commercial ear plugs), brief use of a hair dryer to remove water from the ear canal, and avoiding cotton-tipped applicators or other devices to remove cerumen.

In countries where otomycosis is more common, topical agents, such as clotrimazole 1% solution, are used.[12] Topical clotrimazole is available in the United States but not made specifically for otomycosis, and safety with ruptured TM has not been established. Fluconazole can be started (200 milligrams for one dose, then 100 milligrams daily for 3 to 5 more days);[13] however, the patient will need follow-up to determine the need for extended therapy. Patient growing *Aspergillus* in culture should be treated with voriconazole, 4 milligrams/kg PO two times daily.[9,13]

Instruct patients to follow up with their primary physician or an otolaryngologist in 1 week to be reevaluated; they should return to the ED for sudden worsening with fever or marked swelling.

MALIGNANT OTITIS EXTERNA

Malignant otitis externa is a potentially life-threatening infection of the external auditory canal involving the pinna and soft tissues with variable extension to the skull base, called *skull-base osteomyelitis*.

PATHOPHYSIOLOGY AND MICROBIOLOGY

Malignant otitis externa begins as a simple otitis externa that then spreads to the deeper tissues of the external auditory canal and infects cartilage, periosteum, soft tissue, and bone, with the normal anatomy of the ear serving as the conduit for the spread of infection. Previously, >90% of cases were caused by *P. aeruginosa*,[13] but methicillin-resistant *Staphylococcus aureus* now accounts for 15% of cases.[14] Fungal disease occurs in diabetics and patients with immunocompromise.[15] Acquired immunodeficiency syndrome patients tend to be younger, have etiologic organisms other than *Pseudomonas*, and have a worse prognosis than patients without acquired immunodeficiency syndrome. The cerumen of diabetic patients has a higher pH than that of normal controls and represents an additional breakdown in local defense mechanisms. Small blood vessel disease of diabetics may lead to cartilaginous degeneration, further promoting the spread of infection.

CLINICAL FEATURES AND DIAGNOSIS

An individual with persistent otitis externa despite 2 to 3 weeks of topical antimicrobial therapy should be suspected of having malignant otitis externa. The typical presentation is severe otalgia (90%) and edema of the external auditory canal with otorrhea (70%).[16] Granulation tissue may be evident on the floor of the external auditory canal.

Examine both ears, inspecting both pinnas from the anterior, lateral, and posterior aspects. The infected ear will be erythematous, edematous, and more prominent than the unaffected ear. Assess nearby structures. Parotitis may be present, and trismus indicates involvement of the masseter muscle or temporomandibular joint. Cranial nerve involvement is a serious sign. The seventh cranial nerve is usually the first nerve affected by cranial extension, and the presence of dysfunction of the 9th, 10th, or 11th cranial nerve implies even more extensive disease. Lateral or sigmoid sinus thrombosis and meningitis are more serious possible complications.

Blood counts are typically normal. Erythrocyte sedimentation rate and C-reactive protein are frequently elevated but not essential for diagnosis[16] Clinical diagnosis and staging are confirmed by contrasted CT of the head or MRI.

TREATMENT

Institute antibiotics in the ED using imipenem in children; in adults, use an aminoglycoside and antipseudomonal penicillin or a cephalosporin or quinolone.[13] If fungal disease has grown from a prior culture, start voriconazole, 6 milligrams/kg IV every 12 hours. Selected cases of early infection may be managed as outpatients with oral quinolones. Mild cases are likely to completely resolve with a single course of antibiotic therapy, whereas more advanced stages may require IV antibiotics and possibly surgical debridement.

OTITIS MEDIA

Otitis media (OM) is primarily a disease of infancy and childhood (see chapter 118 for management of OM in children). While the management of OM in children and adults is similar, there are important differences in adults, highlighted below, especially for the management of OM with effusion.

PATHOPHYSIOLOGY AND MICROBIOLOGY

Viral upper respiratory tract infections precede or coincide with 70% of acute OM cases.[17] The most common associated viral pathogens are respiratory syncytial virus, adenovirus, and cytomegalovirus.[18] The most common bacterial pathogens recovered in acute OM are *Streptococcus pneumoniae* (43% to 49%), nontypable *Haemophilus influenzae* (29% to 70%), and *Moraxella catarrhalis* (15% to 28%).[17,19] The *H. influenzae* type b vaccine has no effect on nontypable *H. influenzae*. Most adults have never received this vaccine and thus remain unprotected from all *Haemophilus* flu strains. The predominant organisms involved in chronic OM are *S. aureus* (35%), *P. aeruginosa* (22%), *Aspergillus* (13%), and less commonly, anaerobic bacteria.[20] OM with effusion is differentiated from acute OM. In adults, OM with effusion is frequently associated with significant pathology: acute or chronic sinusitis in 66%, smoking-induced nasopharyngeal lymphoid hyperplasia and adult-onset adenoidal hypertrophy in 19% of cases, and head and neck tumors (mainly nasopharyngeal carcinomas) in 4.8%.[21] Adult patient with OM with effusion may also have symptoms of gastroesophageal reflux.[22]

CLINICAL FEATURES AND DIAGNOSIS

The typical ED presentation is a prodrome of an upper respiratory tract infection followed by sudden increase in otalgia, with or without fever. Otorrhea and hearing loss are variably present, while tinnitus, vertigo, and nystagmus are uncommon but possible findings. Diagnosis is clinical. The TM may be retracted or bulging. It may be red in color, indicating inflammation, or it may be yellow or white, as a result of middle-ear fluid. Pneumatic otoscopy almost uniformly demonstrates impaired mobility. Pain and new otorrhea (in the absence of external otitis) helps to confirm the diagnosis. **Always assess facial nerve function because of the nerve's proximity to the middle ear.** Guidelines are available for the diagnosis and management of OM in children,[23] but none have been published for adults. In adults, OM with effusion presents with ear discomfort or fullness or may present with decreased hearing without discomfort. OM with effusion is diagnosed based on physical exam findings of middle-ear effusion with little inflammatory changes, including pneumatic otoscopy showing an immobile TM. In adults, there will typically be other physical exam findings such as sinusitis or enlarged adenoids behind the uvula. Coexistent symptoms of reflux should be elicited.

TREATMENT

There are no treatment guidelines specifically for adults. The "wait-and-see" method recommended in children[24] has not been evaluated in adults. The preferred adult initial treatment is amoxicillin.[11] The dose in adults (weighing >40 kg) is 875 or 1000 milligrams every 12 hours, or 500 milligrams every 8 hours, for 7 to 10 days. Alternative agents include amoxicillin-clavulanate, cefdinir, or cefpodoxime. For OM unresponsive to initial therapy after 72 hours, consider changing to amoxicillin-clavulanate, levofloxacin, or moxifloxacin.

Provide pain control with acetaminophen or ibuprofen or with narcotics for severe pain. Topical agents such as antipyrine/benzocaine otic may also be given.[25] OM with effusion requires treatment with the same antimicrobials, but for 3 weeks, and prednisone may be added at follow-up. Patients with OM with effusion and coexisting symptoms of reflux should be treated with appropriate antireflux medications (see chapter 74, "Esophageal Emergencies").

Adults with OM should receive follow-up to assess treatment efficacy and to ensure that there is no anatomic obstruction to the eustachian tube, as, for example, from occult neoplasm. Any patient who presents with complications of OM or who appears septic should have urgent consultation for diagnostic and therapeutic tympanocentesis and admission for IV antibiotics.

COMPLICATIONS OF OTITIS MEDIA

Complications of OM are intratemporal and intracranial. Perforation of the TM is a common intratemporal complication and most often occurs in the pars tensa from the increased pressure of middle-ear secretions, with resultant otorrhea. Healing usually occurs in 1 week, although a chronic perforation may result. A temporary conductive hearing loss may occur from fluid in the middle ear. Hearing loss should resolve as the fluid is resorbed. Acute serous labyrinthitis may occur when bacterial toxins enter the inner ear through the round window. **Facial nerve paralysis** is an uncommon complication but requires emergent otolaryngology consultation.

Acute Mastoiditis and Cholesteatoma **Acute mastoiditis** results from spread of infection from the middle ear to the mastoid air cells by the aditus ad antrum. When this opening becomes blocked, the mastoid cavity becomes a closed space, and the mastoid air cells become inflamed and fill with fluid. The most common pathogens are *S. pneumoniae* (38%), *Streptococcus pyogenes* (11%), and *P. aeruginosa* (11%).[26] In addition to otalgia, fever, and otorrhea (especially in patient with *Pseudomonas*), patients with mastoiditis will have postauricular erythema, swelling, and tenderness, with protrusion of the auricle and obliteration of the postauricular crease. Diagnosis is suspected based on the history and physical examination and confirmed on IV contrast CT scan. Mastoiditis requires admission for IV antibiotics, tympanocentesis, and myringotomy. For first episode, treat with ceftriaxone, 1 gram IV every 24 hours, or levofloxacin, 750 milligrams every 24 hours.[13] For recurrent episodes, treat with vancomycin, 1000 milligrams IV, and piperacillin-tazobactam, 3.375 gram initial dose IV, or imipenem. Incision and drainage of subperiosteal abscess or mastoidectomy may ultimately be required.

Aural **cholesteatomas** are collections of epidermis and exfoliated keratin within the middle ear or mastoid. As the cholesteatoma expands, it may erode the ossicular chain, bony labyrinth, or facial nerve canal. Cholesteatomas are often infected, and their intracranial extensions may be life threatening. Treatment requires otolaryngolic evaluation.

Intracranial Complications Intracranial complications of OM are more likely with chronic than with acute OM and are, in general, decreasing with the widespread use of antibiotics in the treatment of OM. However, suppurative intracranial extension is a severe complication, and suggestive signs and symptoms should be investigated appropriately. Meningitis and brain abscess are the most common intracranial complication of OM with an incidence of 0.42 per 100,000 per year.[27] The most prevalent causative organisms are *S. pneumoniae* (33%) and *Neisseria meningitidis* (23%).[27] Extradural abscess and subdural empyema are also potential complications.

Lateral Sinus Thrombosis Lateral sinus thrombosis is another ominous complication of acute OM. It arises from extension of infection and inflammation in the mastoid, with eventual inflammation of the adjacent lateral or sigmoid sinus. Reactive thrombophlebitis with mural clot formation, intraluminal empyema, or perforation of the venous wall may occur.

Headache is the most common symptom, with papilledema, sixth-nerve palsy, and vertigo being less frequently present. Angiography with venous phase and MRI are more sensitive than CT in diagnosing lateral sinus thrombosis. The employed antibiotic regimen should cover *Staphylococcus*, *Streptococcus*, and upper respiratory anaerobes, and have good penetration of the blood–brain barrier. A combination of IV penicillin or nafcillin, ceftriaxone, and metronidazole is one initial empiric regimen.[28]

BULLOUS MYRINGITIS

Bullous myringitis is a painful condition of the ear characterized by bulla formation on the TM and deep external auditory canal. The blisters are believed to occur between the highly innervated outer epithelium and the inner fibrous layer of the TM, explaining the severe otalgia. The blisters may be blood filled, serous, or serosanguineous. Reactive middle-ear effusions may accumulate. Otorrhea as a result of ruptured bullae is short lived. A reversible hearing loss is commonly associated with the condition and may be conductive, sensorineural, or mixed. This disorder is not caused by *Mycoplasma pneumoniae*, as commonly believed, but is a severe manifestation of the typical organisms that cause OM.[29] Treatment is as above for acute OM.

EAR HEMATOMA

An auricular hematoma can develop from almost any type of trauma to the ear. As a result of the lack of subcutaneous fat on the anterior surface of the auricle, blunt force applied to this area tends to shear the perichondrium from the underlying cartilage and tear the adjoining blood vessels. The cartilage depends on the perichondrial blood vessels for viability. Any interruption of the nourishing blood supply can result in necrosis. In addition, a subperichondrial collection can lead to stimulation of the overlying perichondrium, which can result in an asymmetric formation of new cartilage growth and deformity of the appearance of the external ear anatomy. The resultant deformed auricle has been referred to as "*cauliflower ear*," which is commonly seen in boxers or wrestlers secondary to repeated head/ear trauma. The auricular hematoma itself is a painful swelling that obscures the normal contour of the ear. The hematoma may accumulate immediately or several hours following an injury. Aspiration alone does not completely evacuate the clot and therefore leads to deformity and increased morbidity. The goal of treatment is to remove the fluid collection and maintain pressure in the area for several days to prevent reaccumulation of fluid.

ASPIRATION OF AND DRESSING FOR HEMATOMA OF THE EAR

Using sterile technique after local anesthesia, make a semicircular incision through the skin, and be careful not to incise the underlying perichondrium. The incision should be the minimal necessary to drain the underlying hematoma and positioned in an area with the least chance of cosmetic deformity. This is usually accomplished by incising the skin inside the inner curvature of the helix or anthelix. The hematoma can then be removed by gentle suction or curettage. Suture the incision after hematoma removal.

There are a few ways to prevent the hematoma from recurring. Place a dental roll or a firm sterile pledget coated with antibiotic ointment over the resutured site with through-and-through sutures connected to a similar bolster on the opposite side of the ear. Apply a light nonpressure dressing and reevaluate the ear within 24 hours to assure there has been no reaccumulation of the hematoma. A pressure dressing can also be employed if you do not want to suture a dental roll though the cartilage. Simply pack the helix with petroleum jelly–impregnated gauze and then place regular gauze both in front of and behind the ear. Lastly circle the head with a compressive wrap (**Figure 242-4**). Prophylactic antibiotics can be reserved for immunocompromised patients and should cover *P. aeruginosa* and *S. aureus*, the two likely participants in posttraumatic chondritis.

EAR FOREIGN BODIES

Cerumen loops/scoops, a right-angle hook, and alligator forceps are the instruments of choice for foreign body removal (**Figure 242-5**). Live objects should be drowned with a 2% lidocaine solution or viscous lidocaine, which immediately paralyzes the offending insect and provides modest topical anesthesia. The liquid can then be suctioned out with butterfly tubing and the insect removed with gentle suction or forceps under direct visualization. Remove all insect debris from the canal.

Irrigation with room-temperature water is adequate for small particles such as hard sand or cerumen and can mobilize distally positioned objects. Irrigation should not be used unless the TM is completely visualized and free of perforation. Organic matter that can expand when moistened is also a relative contraindication to irrigation.

Inspect the ear canal after removal of the foreign body to exclude injury to the canal skin, TM, and ossicles caused by the foreign body or its extraction. Small abrasions heal spontaneously. Topical antibiotics should be considered in cases where there was more serious cutaneous damage or where the foreign body consisted of organic material or generated a local inflammatory reaction (Table 242-5).

CERUMEN IMPACTION

Symptoms of cerumen impaction are decreased hearing, a sensation of pressure or fullness in the ear, dizziness, tinnitus, or otalgia. These symptoms are often precipitated by the use of cotton-tipped applicators. Most of the time, cerumen loops/scoops can be used to remove impacted cerumen (Figure 242-5). In particularly difficult cases or when the canal is completely occluded, softening of the material can be accomplished using half-strength hydrogen peroxide, sodium bicarbonate, mineral oil, or an over-the-counter preparation such as Debrox® (carbamide peroxide otic). Left in place for 30 minutes, such preparations soften the cerumen and facilitate its removal. If irrigation is the treatment of choice, it can usually be accomplished with an ear syringe, a flexible 18-gauge IV catheter, or a syringe attached to the tubing of a butterfly infusion catheter. Pretreatment with triethanolamine polypeptide oleate (Cereuminex®) improves success rates.[30] Use body-temperature irrigant to minimize the development of vertigo. Insert the catheter into the cartilaginous canal (external third) and gently irrigate along the superior portion of the external auditory canal. Using this technique, the pressure of the stream is directed toward the wall of the canal and not the TM.

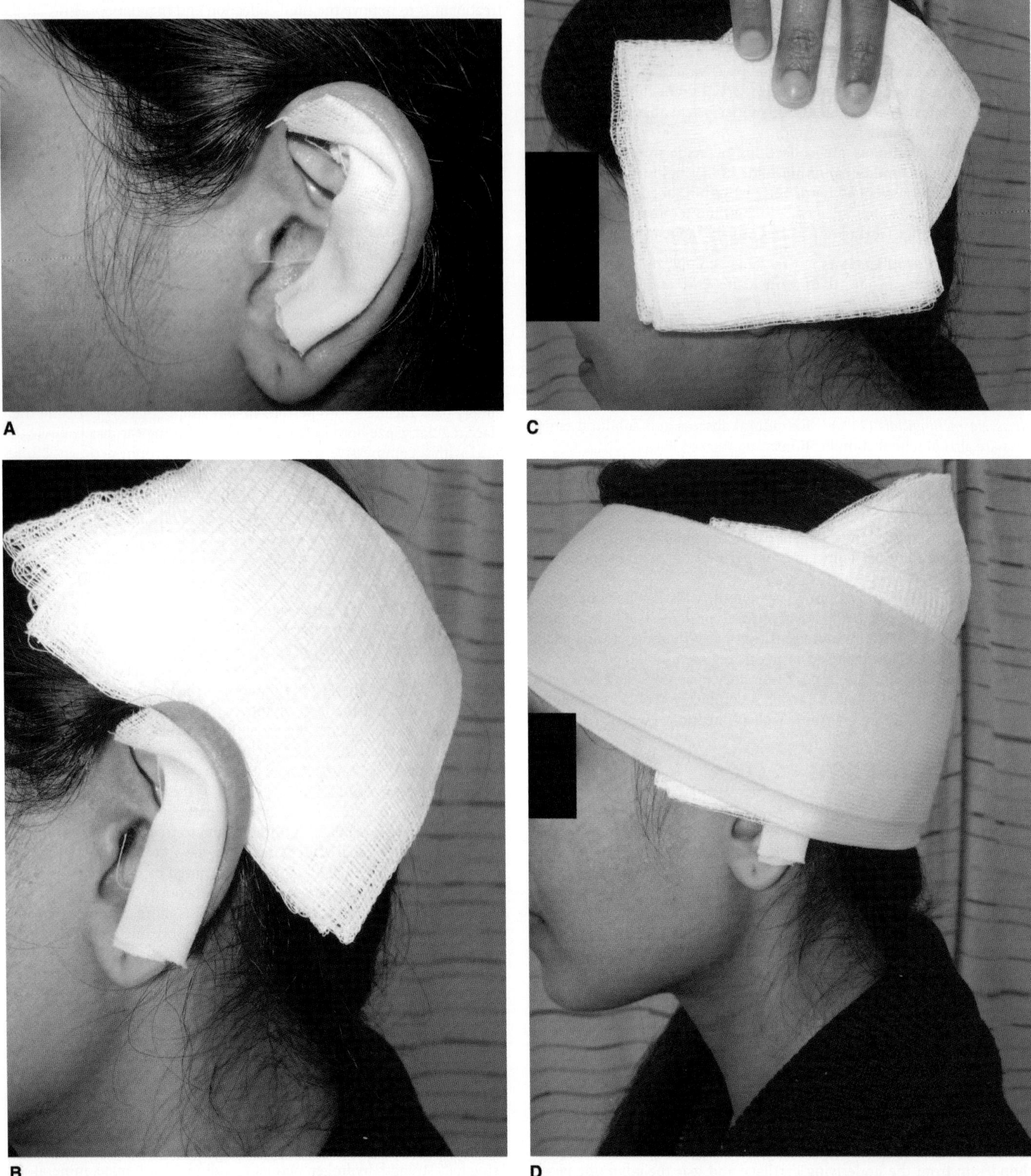

FIGURE 242-4. Stepwise progression to build an auricular bandage to help compress a drained hematoma in the auricle of the ear. Use a petroleum jelly–impregnated gauze inside the helix of the ear (**A**) and then add dry gauze to both the back (**B**) and front (**C**) of the ear. **D.** Wrap it lightly to add slight compression to hold the perichondrium to the auricular cartilage.

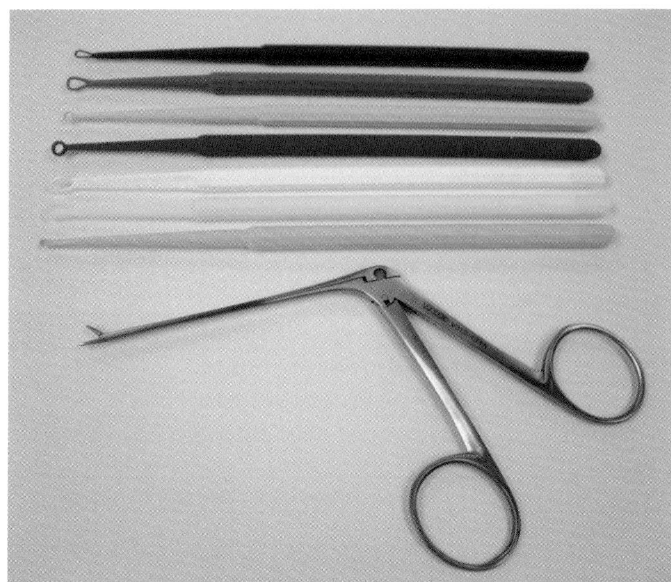

FIGURE 242-5. Different-shaped ear scoops and loops are useful to remove cerumen from an impacted ear. Miniature alligator forceps can be used to extricate foreign bodies from the external ear canal.

Irrigation of the canal when the middle ear is not infected often causes a temporary redness of the TM.

The most common iatrogenic injury associated with syringing of the ear is traumatic TM perforation. Predisposing factors for perforation include previous ear surgery, a previous or current history of OM, and severe otitis externa. When in doubt, it is safer to defer irrigation to an otolaryngologist. When determining if a perforation has occurred, it is important to rely on symptoms (sudden hearing loss, severe otalgia, or vertigo) rather than signs, because visualization of the TM may be impaired by the irrigating fluid and debris. In case of suspected perforation, reassurance, analgesia, and otolaryngology referral in 1 to 2 weeks are indicated. Prophylactic antibiotics are not necessary. If injury to ossicles is suspected, emergency ear, nose, and throat consultation is warranted.

TYMPANIC MEMBRANE PERFORATION

TM perforations can occur secondary to middle-ear infections or as a result of barotrauma, blunt/penetrating/acoustic trauma, or, on rare occasions, lightning strikes. Perforation is also discussed in the chapter 7, "Bomb, Blast, and Crush Injuries." When perforation is secondary to blunt or noise trauma, the perforation almost always occurs in the pars tensa, usually anteriorly or inferiorly. The pars tensa, the largest area of the TM, is only a few cell layers thick and thus is easily torn.

Symptoms are acute onset of pain and hearing loss, with or without bloody otorrhea. There may also be associated vertigo or tinnitus, but this is usually transient unless there has been injury to the inner ear or rupture of the round or oval windows. The TM should be completely visualized and the canal must be cleared of blood and debris.

Most TM perforations heal spontaneously. Patients with perforations secondary to blunt or noise trauma that are isolated injuries can be safely discharged and referred to a specialist for further evaluation and a formal audiogram as soon after the injury as possible. Patients should be instructed not to allow water to enter the canal of the ear. Topical or systemic antibiotics are not needed unless foreign material is suspected of remaining in the canal or in the middle ear. Perforations in the posterosuperior quadrant or those secondary to penetrating trauma have a greater likelihood of ossicular chain damage and should be referred to an otolaryngologist within 24 hours.

REFERENCES

The complete reference list is available online at www.TintinalliEM.com.

CHAPTER 243 Face and Jaw Emergencies

Stephanie A. Lareau
Corey R. Heitz

FACIAL CELLULITIS, ERYSIPELAS, AND IMPETIGO

Cellulitis and erysipelas are discussed in detail in the chapter 147, "Soft Tissue Infections." Impetigo is discussed in the chapter 136, "Rashes in Infants and Children." The differential diagnosis of facial infections is provided in **Table 243-1**.[1]

Cellulitis is a superficial soft tissue infection that lacks anatomic constraints.[2-4] Facial cellulitis is caused most commonly by *Streptococcus pyogenes* (group A β-hemolytic) and *Staphylococcus aureus*,[4] with an increasing predominance of methicillin-resistant *S. aureus*.[5] Less commonly, cellulitis may represent extension from deep space infections (see "Masticator Space Infection" section below). In children, buccal cellulitis from *Haemophilus influenzae* is now very uncommon if children have received the *H. influenzae* type b vaccine.[6]

Bedside US can exclude or identify facial abscess (**Figure 243-1**). CT can identify deep-seated, extensive infections that involve the soft tissues of the neck or pharynx.

Treatment is provided in **Table 243-2**. Duration of therapy is not well studied, but recommendations range from 7 to 14 days.[3,5,7,8] Treatment failures range from 15% to 20% for β-lactams (cephalexin, dicloxacillin, and amoxicillin-clavulanate) as well as for the anti–methicillin-resistant *S. aureus* therapies[9] due to the failure to cover methicillin-resistant *S. aureus* and streptococcal species, respectively. Cephalexin appears to be the most cost-effective therapy based on a probability of 37% for infection with *S. aureus* and a 27% methicillin-resistant *S. aureus* prevalence.[10] In selected cases, traditional β-lactam therapy may be added to anti-methicillin-resistant *S. aureus* therapy, but this strategy increases cost and potential for adverse effects of the medication.

Erysipelas is most common in the lower extremities (66% to 76%)[11-13] but is classically described as a disease of the face (see Figure 152-3). The nasopharynx is typically the source of bacteria.[14] In the majority of cases, erysipelas is caused by *S. pyogenes*.[3,4] Bullous erysipelas is a more severe form of the disease, and half of the infections reported in a 2004 case series were due to methicillin-resistant *S. aureus*.[15] Penicillin is the antibiotic treatment of choice[3,13] but is chosen as empiric therapy in a minority of cases.[11,12,16,17] If the suspicion exists of a staphylococcal infection (i.e., bullae, trauma, or the presence of a foreign body), alternatives include dicloxacillin, amoxicillin-clavulanate, or a cephalosporin[3] (Table 243-2). One randomized, prospective trial compared the use of a macrolide, roxithromycin, with penicillin and found no difference in efficacy.[18]

Impetigo is a discrete, superficial bacterial epidermal infection, characterized by amber crusts (nonbullous) or by fluid-filled vesicles (bullous) (see Figures 141-14 and 141-15). It is most common in children. *S. aureus* alone or in combination with *S. pyogenes* (group A β-hemolytic) is the most common cause of nonbullous impetigo. Bullous impetigo is always caused by *S. aureus*.[3,19,20] Treatment should cover streptococcal and staphylococcal species. Topical therapy is sufficient for uncomplicated patients with only a few nonbullous lesions.[21] Mupirocin, retapamulin, or fusidic acid ointment is recommended; however, some resistance is developing.[3,20,22,23] Consider oral antibiotics for extensive lesions or lesions that do not respond to topical therapy alone. Erythromycin and cloxacillin are superior to penicillin, but there is no clear preference between macrolides, β-lactamase–resistant penicillins, and cephalosporins.[3,19] Preferred choices are penicillinase-resistant penicillins (cloxacillin, dicloxacillin, amoxicillin-clavulanic acid) or first-generation cephalosporins (cephalexin).[3] For methicillin-resistant *S. aureus*, treat with trimethoprim-sulfamethoxazole or clindamycin[3] (**Table 243-3**).

SALIVARY GLAND INFECTIONS

There are three groups of salivary glands: the parotid, submandibular, and sublingual. The facial nerve passes through the superficial portion of the parotid gland, and the parotid (Stensen's) duct opens into the

TABLE 243-1 Differential Diagnosis of Superficial Facial Infection

	Historical Features		
	Onset/Timing	Risk/Inciting Factors	Physical Findings
Infectious			
Cellulitis	Gradual	Skin breaks, foreign bodies, prostheses, immunosuppression	Diffuse erythema without clear borders, pain
Impetigo	Acute	Infants, children	Discrete vesicles or bullae; patches of crusty skin
Erysipelas	Gradual	Elderly, infants and children, immune deficiency, diabetes, alcoholism, skin ulceration, impaired lymphatic drainage	Well-defined, raised area of erythema, pain
Viral exanthem	Often acute	Preceding or concurrent viral illness, fever	Variable
Parotitis	Gradual	Dehydration, diabetes, immunosuppression	Swollen angle of mandible, potentially visible sialolith
Necrotizing fasciitis	Rapid	Trauma, may be minor or not apparent	Crepitus, skin necrosis, may be subtle
Cutaneous anthrax	Gradual	Animal contact	Black eschar with surrounding erythema
Herpes zoster	Acute	Elderly, immunosuppression	Exquisitely tender erythematous or vesicular rash following a dermatome
Malignant otitis externa	Gradual	Diabetes, water exposure	Ear pain with drainage, facial swelling, tragal tenderness
Trauma			
Soft tissue contusion	Acute	Associated trauma	Tender swelling
Burn	Acute	Occupational, recreational exposure	May be difficult to distinguish from cellulitis
Inflammatory			
Insect envenomation	Acute	Environment supporting insect life	Diffuse, red, puffy
Apical abscess with secondary buccal swelling	Gradual	Usually associated dental pain/caries	Similar to cellulitis; may have intraoral/gingival findings
Contact dermatitis	Gradual or acute	Often identifiable exposure	Variable; maculopapular, itchy rash
Immunologic			
Systemic lupus erythematosus	Gradual	Female-to-male ratio, 9:1	Erythema in classic "malar" distribution
Angioneurotic edema	Acute	Exposure to angiotensin-converting enzyme inhibitor, allergen	Lip, oral mucosal swelling, sometimes facial
Vancomycin flushing reaction	Acute	Recent exposure to vancomycin	Facial erythema, warmth

mouth opposite the upper second molar. The submandibular and sublingual glands lie below the plane of the tongue. The submandibular ducts open into the mouth at either side of the frenulum of the tongue. The multiple sublingual ducts open into the sublingual fold or directly into the submandibular duct.[24]

Signs of salivary gland infections are unilateral or bilateral facial swelling. Recurrent symptoms, dry mouth and eyes, or joint symptoms suggest etiologies such as immunologic or collagen vascular disorders. Other medical conditions, such as nutritional disorders, toxic exposures, diabetes, dehydration, medication usage (i.e., phenothiazines), pregnancy, and obesity, can result in salivary gland enlargement. On physical examination, determine the location of the swelling to identify the gland involved. Multiple gland involvement suggests infection. A palpable tender mass may be a sign of tumor or obstruction by a stone. The differential diagnosis of salivary gland swelling is provided in **Table 243-4**.[24]

VIRAL PAROTITIS (MUMPS)

Viral parotitis is an acute infection of the parotid glands, characterized by unilateral or bilateral parotid swelling. It is most often caused by the paramyxovirus and may be caused less commonly by influenza, parainfluenza, coxsackie viruses, echoviruses, lymphocytic choriomeningitis virus, and even human immunodeficiency virus.[25] It is most common in children under the age of 15 years old, but since November 2014, clusters of mumps have been reported in adult members of professional hockey teams. The virus is spread by airborne droplets, incubates in the

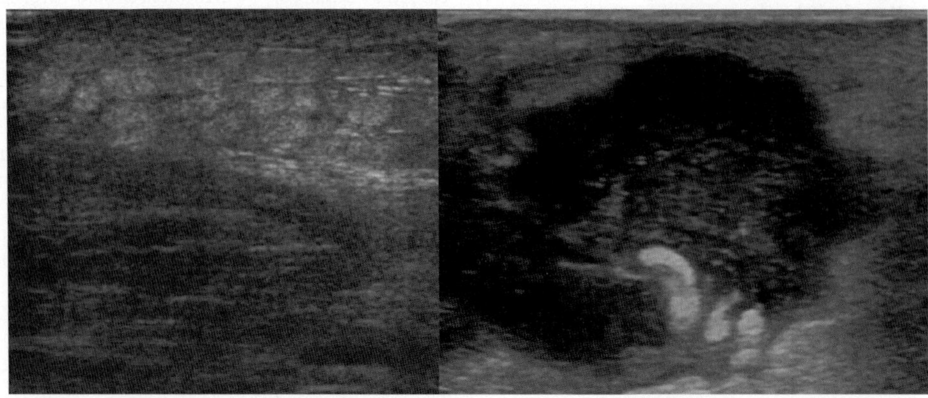

FIGURE 243-1. Cellulitis versus abscess. The image on the left shows the cobblestoned appearance of cellulitis, while the one on the right shows a heterogenous fluid collection of abscess. [Photo contributed by R. Gordon, MD.]

TABLE 243-2 Antibiotic Therapy for Facial Infections

Cellulitis	Oral therapy: dicloxacillin, cephalexin, clindamycin; vancomycin and cephalosporins are alternatives Suspected MRSA: trimethoprim-sulfamethoxazole, clindamycin, doxycycline, minocycline, linezolid Parenteral therapy: nafcillin, vancomycin, clindamycin Total duration 7–10 d
Erysipelas	Oral therapy: penicillin (only if MRSA is unlikely) Methicillin-sensitive *Staphylococcus aureus* suspected: amoxicillin-clavulanate, cephalexin, dicloxacillin Bullous erysipelas (or MRSA suspected): trimethoprim-sulfamethoxazole, clindamycin, doxycycline, or minocycline Parenteral therapy: vancomycin, nafcillin, clindamycin Total duration 7–10 d
Impetigo	Topical: mupirocin or retapamulin ointment alone or with oral therapy Oral therapy: dicloxacillin, amoxicillin-clavulanate, cephalexin Alternative: azithromycin MRSA suspected: clindamycin or trimethoprim-sulfamethoxazole Total duration 7 d[3]
Suppurative parotitis	Parental therapy: nafcillin, amoxicillin-clavulanate or ampicillin-sulbactam; if penicillin allergic, clindamycin or the combination of cephalexin with metronidazole, or vancomycin with metronidazole Hospital acquired or nursing home patients: consider vancomycin Total duration: 10–14 d
Masticator space infection	Parenteral therapy: IV clindamycin is recommended; alternatives include ampicillin-sulbactam, cefoxitin, or the combination of penicillin with metronidazole Oral therapy: clindamycin or amoxicillin-clavulanate Total duration: 10–14 d

Abbreviation: MRSA = methicillin-resistant *Staphylococcus aureus.*

TABLE 243-3 Antibiotic Doses for Facial Infections

Antibiotic	Dosage
Oral Antibiotics	
Amoxicillin/clavulanate	875/125 milligrams twice per day
Azithromycin	500 milligrams first day, 250 milligrams 4 more days
Cephalexin	500 milligrams four times per day
Clindamycin	300–450 milligrams three times per day
Dicloxacillin	500 milligrams four times per day
Doxycycline	100 milligrams twice per day
Metronidazole	500 milligrams every 8 h
Minocycline	100 milligrams twice per day
Penicillin V	500 milligrams four times per day
Trimethoprim-sulfamethoxazole	1 double-strength tablet twice per day
Parenteral Antibiotics	
Antibiotic	**Dosage**
Ampicillin-sulbactam	1.5–3.0 grams every 6 h
Clindamycin	600 milligrams every 8 h
Cefazolin	1 gram every 8 h
Metronidazole	1 gram loading dose, then 500 milligrams every 8 h
Nafcillin	1–2 grams every 4 h
Penicillin G	2–3 million units every 6 h
Vancomycin	1 gram every 12 h

upper respiratory tract for 2 to 3 weeks, and then spreads systemically. Vaccine protection is not 100%, and outbreaks occur in settings of close contact, such as schools, colleges, sports teams, and camps.[26]

After a period of incubation, one third of patients experience a prodrome of fever, malaise, headache, myalgias, arthralgias, and anorexia during a 3- to 5-day period of viremia.[25] The classic salivary gland swelling then follows. Unilateral swelling is typically followed by bilateral parotid involvement. The gland is tense and painful, but erythema and warmth are notably absent. Stensen's duct may be inflamed, but no pus can be expressed.[25]

Diagnosis is clinical and treatment is supportive. Salivary gland swelling typically lasts from 1 to 5 days. The patient is contagious for 9 days after the onset of parotid swelling, and children with mumps should be excluded from school or day care for this interval.

Mumps is usually benign in children but can be severe in adults. Unilateral **orchitis** affects 20% to 30% of males (with a predisposition of ≥8 years of age), whereas **oophoritis** affects only 5% of females. Other complications of the mumps virus include mastitis, pancreatitis, aseptic meningitis, sensorineural hearing loss, myocarditis, polyarthritis, hemolytic anemia, and thrombocytopenia.[25] Immunocompetent patients with isolated viral parotitis or orchitis can be managed as outpatients. Admit patients with systemic complications.

SUPPURATIVE PAROTITIS

Suppurative parotitis is a serious bacterial infection of the parotid gland that occurs in patients with compromised salivary flow. It is caused by the retrograde migration of oral bacteria into the salivary ducts and parenchyma.[25] Predisposing factors include recent anesthesia, dehydration, prematurity or advanced age, sialolithiasis, oral neoplasms, salivary duct strictures, tracheostomy, and ductal foreign bodies.[25] Medications that cause either systemic dehydration or decreased salivary flow specifically can cause parotitis. These include diuretics, antihistamines, tricyclic antidepressants, phenothiazines, β-blockers, and barbiturates.[25] Several chronic illnesses also predispose patients to suppurative parotitis, such as human immunodeficiency virus, hepatic or renal failure, diabetes mellitus, hypothyroidism, malnutrition, Sjögren's syndrome, depression, anorexia, bulimia, hyperuricemia, and cystic fibrosis.[25]

Most cases of suppurative parotitis are caused by *S. aureus*, with *S. pneumoniae*, *S. pyogenes*, and *H. influenzae* as more infrequent pathogens.[3,25] Anaerobes such as *Bacteroides* species, peptostreptococci, and fusobacteria may be found in up to 43% of isolates. In the immunocompromised host, gram-negative organisms such as *Escherichia coli* and *Pseudomonas* may be seen.

The onset of suppurative parotitis is rapid, and the skin over the parotid gland is red and tender. Pus may be expressed from the Stensen's duct. There is often fever and trismus.

Suppurative parotitis is diagnosed clinically, with evidence of purulent drainage from Stensen's duct. Cultures of Stensen's duct drainage can guide therapy in the patient not responding to first-line antibiotics.[27] Imaging is not helpful unless an abscess is suspected, in which case US or CT is diagnostic.

Because suppurative parotitis is caused by states of decreased salivary flow, treatment should optimize salivary flow. Hydrate the volume-depleted patient. Massage and apply heat to the affected gland. Stimulate salivation using sialagogues, such as lemon drops. When possible, discontinue drugs that cause dry mouth, and attempt to correct underlying medical problems.[27]

Treat patients with oral antibiotics if they can tolerate oral liquids and have no evidence of systemic illness. Admit for parenteral antibiotics patients who have trismus and cannot tolerate oral liquids, are immunocompromised or incapable of complying with an outpatient treatment regimen, or have not shown improvement after 48 hours of outpatient treatment.[27]

Antimicrobial therapy consists of agents that cover both staphylococcal and streptococcal species (Tables 243-2 and 243-3). The initial choice for oral therapy includes amoxicillin-clavulanate; in penicillin-allergic patients, use clindamycin or a combination of cephalexin with metronidazole.[3,27] When parenteral therapy is indicated, choices include nafcillin, ampicillin-sulbactam, or a combination of vancomycin with

TABLE 243-4 Differential Diagnosis of Salivary Gland Swelling

	Historical Features		
	Onset	Risks/Inciting Factors	Clinical Features
Infectious			
Viral parotitis (mumps)	Gradual	Nonimmunized	Prodromal illness, unilateral tense swelling, absent warmth/erythema
Buccal cellulitis	Gradual	*Haemophilus influenzae* infection in nonimmunized	Erythematous, tender
Suppurative parotitis	Rapid	Dehydration, immunosuppression, chronic illness, recent anesthesia	Painful buccal swelling, fever, pus expression from Stensen's duct
Masseter space abscess	Gradual	Dental infection, post trauma	Trismus, posterior inferior facial swelling
Tuberculosis	Gradual	Exposure, immunosuppression	Chronic crusting plaques
Immunologic			
Sjögren's syndrome	Gradual	—	Dry mouth, eyes, sclerosis
Systemic lupus	Gradual	Female sex, Asian or African American race	No signs of infection
Sarcoidosis	Gradual	Female sex, African American race	No signs of infection
Other			
Neoplasm	Gradual	—	No erythema, warmth
Sialolithiasis	Gradual	Dehydration, chronic illness	Swelling, tenderness, no signs of infection

metronidazole. In hospitalized or nursing home patients, the possibility of methicillin-resistant *S. aureus*, for which vancomycin is appropriate,[27] must be considered. In neonates, treat with gentamicin and antistaphylococcal antibiotics combined with hydration. If there is no improvement in 24 to 48 hours, surgical drainage is required.

SIALOLITHIASIS

Sialolithiasis is the development of a calcium carbonate and calcium phosphate stone (sialolith) in a stagnant salivary duct. Salivary calculi can develop in any age group but usually are symptomatic in men between the third and sixth decades.[28] More than 80% of stones occur in the submandibular gland, with most of the remainder in the parotid.

The symptoms of pain, swelling, and tenderness may resemble those of parotitis. It may be hard to distinguish parotitis from sialolithiasis, and the two conditions may coexist. Sialolithiasis is typically unilateral. The pain and swelling of sialolithiasis are colicky and exacerbated by meals.

The diagnosis is clinical. A stone may be palpated within the duct, and the gland is firm.[28] Intraoral radiographs are more sensitive than extraoral films in identifying salivary calculi. The calculi are radiopaque in about 70% of cases. US and thin-cut CT also will identify sialoliths but are usually obtained only if abscess is in the differential diagnosis. ED bedside US has been shown in a case report to be a useful diagnostic tool to determine number, size, and location of stones (**Figure 243-2**).[29] A conservative course of treatment should precede imaging studies. Occasionally on CT, the diagnosis of sialolithiasis is made by the typically glandular swelling and inflammatory changes (signifying ductal obstruction) without an obvious stone seen in the duct (**Figure 243-3**).

Treatment is outpatient therapy with analgesics, antibiotics if there is concurrent infection, massage, and sialagogues, such as lemon drops.[28] Palpable stones in the distal duct may be digitally "milked" from the duct. Complications of salivary duct obstruction include recurrent or persistent obstruction, strictures, infection, and gland atrophy.[28]

MASTICATOR SPACE INFECTION

The masticator space consists of four potential spaces bounded by the muscles of mastication (**Figure 243-4**). These spaces include the masseteric (or submasseteric), superficial temporal, deep temporal, and pterygomandibular spaces.[30] The spaces are all contiguous. Masticator space infections occur when one or more bacterial agents invade all of these spaces. Bacteria may gain entry to the space from dental infections, trauma, surgery, or injections. Infections of the masticator space are polymicrobial and generally anaerobic, although aerobic oral streptococcal species may predominate briefly.[4,30] Typical organisms include species of *Streptococcus, Peptostreptococcus, Bacteroides, Prevotella, Porphyromonas, Fusobacterium, Actinomyces, Veillonella*, and anaerobic spirochetes.[4,30]

The most frequent acute clinical findings are facial swelling, pain, erythema, and trismus. When infection occurs in the masseteric space, there is facial swelling posteriorly and inferiorly, with mild to moderate trismus. If the temporal space is infected, there is soft tissue swelling over the temporalis muscle and trismus. Trismus without swelling suggests pterygomandibular space abscess. In chronic infection, the patient can be afebrile but may complain of intermittent trismus.[31] Constitutional signs may include fever, malaise, dehydration, dysphagia, nausea, or vomiting. In more advanced cases, systemic signs of sepsis are present. The differential diagnosis includes other sources of lateral facial pain and swelling (Table 243-4).

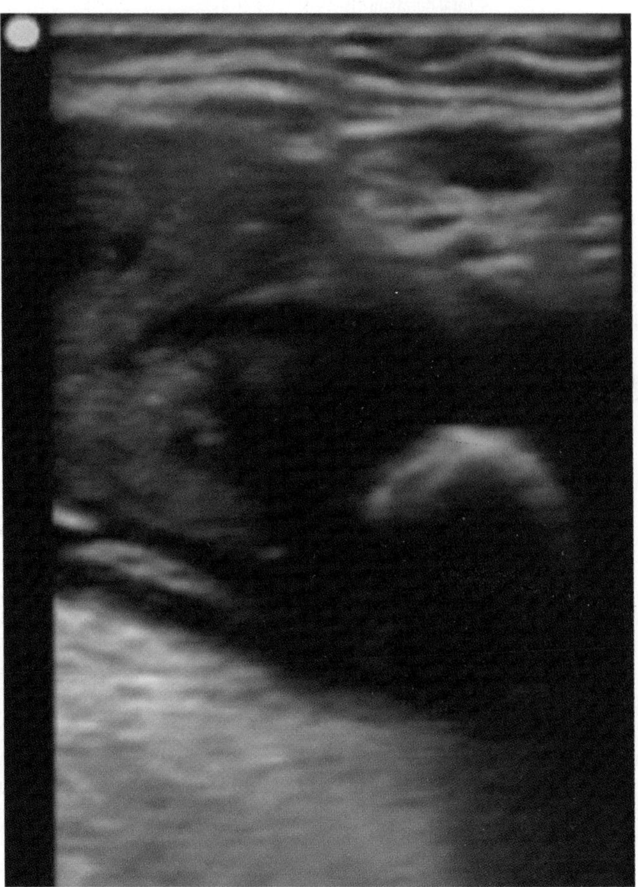

FIGURE 243-2. US image of sialolithiasis. [Photo contributed by R. Gordon, MD.]

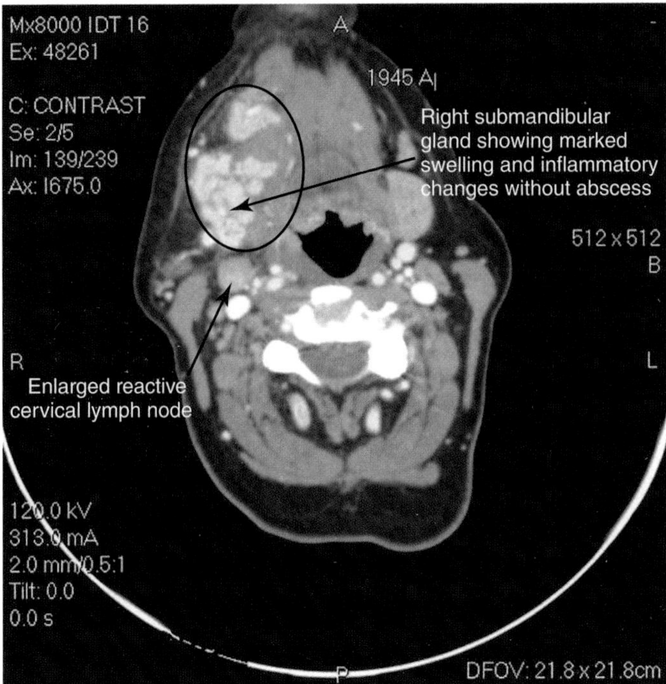

FIGURE 243-3. Marked enlargement of the right submandibular gland. This contrasted CT image shows marked enlargement of the right submandibular gland and surrounding inflammatory changes without an obvious stone or abscess formation. [Image used with permission of John Wightman, MD.]

Ultrasonography is helpful in differentiating abscesses from cellulitis (Figure 243-1), for the diagnosis of lymphadenitis, and to identify internal jugular thrombosis.[29] Contrast-enhanced CT is the preferred diagnostic tool for masseteric and related deep space infections.[30-32] CT can define the extent of the abscess and distinguish cellulitis from abscess in all spaces except the retropharyngeal.[30] MRI can be considered if infection is thought to reach the skull base.[29]

The patient's condition determines therapy. Because all the subordinate spaces of the masticator space communicate with each other and ultimately with the tissue planes that extend down the neck to the mediastinum, the extent of the infection should be defined efficiently and treatment begun promptly. Airway compromise is rare in unilateral masticator space infection. Treatment is airway control, stabilization, and treatment of infection. Administer antibiotics in the ED (Table 243-3), and admit the patient. IV clindamycin is recommended, with alternatives including ampicillin-sulbactam, cefoxitin, or the combination of penicillin with metronidazole.[4,30] Antibiotics are continued for 10 to 14 days. The macrolides (e.g., erythromycin) are generally no longer used for masticator space infections.[30] Otolaryngology consultation is recommended.

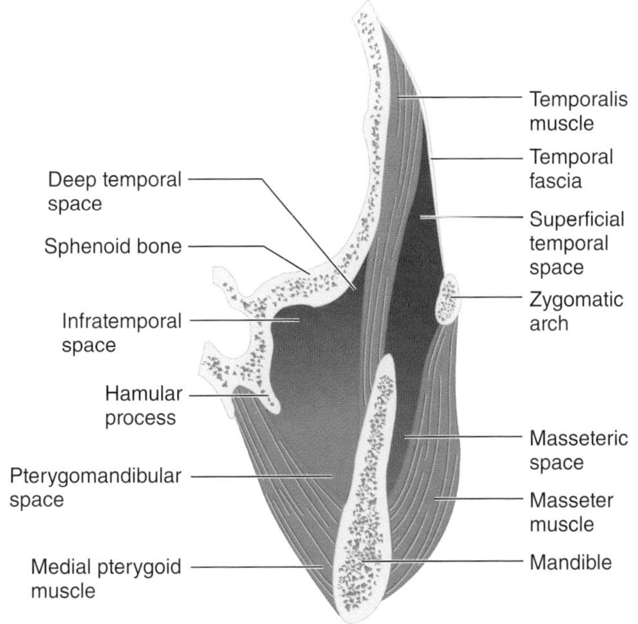

FIGURE 243-4. Masticator space.

TEMPOROMANDIBULAR JOINT DISORDERS

The temporomandibular joint combines both a hinge and gliding action. The articular surfaces of the joint are separated by the articular disk, or meniscus, which assists in the hinge action between the mandibular condyle and the disk and in the gliding action between the disk and temporal bone.[33]

TEMPOROMANDIBULAR JOINT DYSFUNCTION

Temporomandibular joint dysfunction causes pain of the joint and its surrounding anatomic structures. Assess for temporomandibular joint injury when evaluating direct jaw trauma or acute dental injury.[34] Most studies have found no significant correlation between occlusal parameters or bruxism and signs or symptoms of temporomandibular joint disorders.[35,36] Over time, degenerative joint disease (osteoarthritis) may result from chronic internal derangement or occur secondary to systemic disease such as rheumatoid arthritis or systemic lupus erythematosus.[34]

The chief complaint is usually pain localized to one of the muscles of mastication or pain with chewing in one or both temporomandibular joints. The masseter muscle is the most frequently identified painful area, followed by the temporalis, sternocleidomastoid, splenius capitis, and trapezius muscles.[35] Physical findings may include limitation in the range of motion of the mandible. Palpate the muscles of mastication to find areas of sensitivity, induration, rigidity, and swelling. Palpate the condylar heads with the teeth together and then with the teeth apart. The differential diagnosis of temporomandibular joint dysfunction includes jaw trauma, including fracture and dislocation; odontogenic pain, including from abscess, carie, or trauma; otologic referred pain, including from otitis media, otitis externa, and foreign body; and temporal arteritis.

Temporomandibular joint dysfunction is diagnosed by history and physical examination. Isolated temporomandibular joint clicking without pain or other dysfunction is not diagnostically sufficient.[35] For acute trauma, the panoramic x-ray view (Panorex) of the mandible is usually the initial imaging of choice. Panorex also provides information about the teeth and other parts of the jaw that may be contributing to pain.[37] CT is appropriate in the assessment of potentially complex fractures, infections, and neoplastic disease.

The oral maxillofacial surgeon manages fractures and should be consulted for trismus and significant mandible displacement. Otherwise, for uncomplicated fractures and nontraumatic conditions, give simple analgesics, including nonsteroidal anti-inflammatory drugs and, if necessary, narcotics. Advise the patient to eat soft foods until definitive treatment is provided. The management of chronic temporomandibular dysfunction may ultimately require referral to a dentist, maxillofacial surgeon, or pain specialist.

TRIGEMINAL NEURALGIA

Trigeminal neuralgia, or **tic douloureux**, is characterized by facial pain in the distribution of cranial nerve V. The cause is not known. Some postulate there is peripheral nerve injury or disease that increases afferent firing or a failure of central inhibition. Compression of the nerve by vessels, tumors, or inflammation is also a potential cause.[38]

Trigeminal neuralgia is characterized by paroxysms of severe unilateral pain in the trigeminal nerve distribution lasting only seconds, with normal findings on neurologic examination. There is no pain between paroxysms. Trigeminal neuralgia is divided into two categories. **Classic trigeminal neuralgia** includes idiopathic cases and cases due to microvascular compression. **Secondary, or symptomatic, trigeminal neuralgia** is due to tumor, multiple sclerosis, or other structural abnormalities.

The history is key for diagnosis. Pain is a severe, shocking or stabbing, and brief, lasting seconds to minutes. Complete resolution occurs between episodes. Pain is clearly in the distribution of cranial nerve V. Classically, the pain is unilateral, although it can be bilateral. Triggers include light touch, chewing, or a light breeze. Pain can be accompanied by facial spasms. Physical exam is unremarkable.

Treatment is most often medical, but severe cases may require surgical intervention. Carbamazepine, started at 100 milligrams PO twice a day and then increased in dosage as needed, is an effective treatment. Baclofen has also been shown to be successful.[39] Patients with trigeminal neuralgia may present to the ED because symptoms are of recent onset or recurrent and should be started or restarted on carbamazepine. Pain control is rarely an issue because the paroxysms are so brief. Refer patients to a neurologist.

BELL'S PALSY

Bell's palsy is the most common cause of unilateral facial paralysis. The cause, however, is not clear. A leading theory is that as the facial nerve exits the temporal bone, edema and ischemia result in compression of the nerve. Inflammatory, demyelinating, or compressive processes have all been suggested, including infections (herpes simplex virus, herpes zoster, Lyme disease, syphilis, Epstein-Barr virus, cytomegalovirus, human immunodeficiency virus, mycoplasma), microvascular disease (diabetes and hypertension), and medications, including chemotherapeutics.[40]

Symptoms of Bell's palsy include acute onset of unilateral upper and lower facial paralysis, posterior auricular pain, decreased tearing, hyperacusis (oversensitivity to certain frequency and volumes), and otalgia. Some of these symptoms may develop prior to the classic facial paralysis. Onset is typically sudden, with a peak of symptoms in 48 hours.[40]

Diagnosis is confirmed by thorough history and physical exam. Examination reveals **weakness and/or paralysis of both the upper and lower portion of the face on the affected side.** Flattening of the forehead and nasolabial folds on the affected side is present. Careful neurologic exam is useful in ruling out other conditions, such as stroke. In addition, examine the ear to ascertain presence of cranial herpes zoster, which along with stroke and Guillain-Barré syndrome accounts for >85% of misdiagnoses.[41] Laboratory studies are not needed.

There is much controversy surrounding the treatment for Bell's palsy. Goals of emergency care include increasing the chances of recovery of facial nerve function and protection of the eye. The American Academy of Neurology guidelines state that steroids are highly likely to be effective and increase the likelihood of recovery.[42] When initiated within the first 72 hours of symptom onset, steroids improve chances of full recovery. The recommended dosing is 1 milligram/kg up to 60 milligrams/d for 6 days, followed by a 10-day taper. Use of antivirals, such as acyclovir or valacyclovir, is controversial. According to the American Academy of Neurology's 2012 guidelines, benefits from antivirals have not been established and are thought be modest at best.[41] A variety of other therapies including physical therapy, acupuncture, and surgical decompression have also been used with variable success. Cessation of the offending agent is indicated if the medications or chemotherapy is implicated. Apply ocular lubricants to protect against corneal abrasions, and it may be necessary to tape the patient's eyelid, especially during sleep.

MANDIBLE DISLOCATION

The mandible can be dislocated in an anterior, posterior, lateral, or superior direction. **Anterior dislocation is most common and occurs when the mandibular condyle is forced in front of the articular eminence.** Muscular spasm then traps the mandible in anterior dislocation, and the mandible is elevated before retraction. Factors that predispose patients to symptomatic anterior dislocation include a shallow glenoid fossa, increased muscle tone (such as during a seizure), and a loss of joint capsule tone from previous trauma. Spasm of the temporalis and lateral pterygoid muscles tends to prevent reduction once dislocation has occurred. Dislocations are usually bilateral but can be unilateral.[33] Posterior dislocations are rare. They follow a blow that may or may not break the condylar neck. In posterior dislocation, the mandibular condyle is thrust backward against the mastoid, and the condylar head may prolapse into the external auditory canal.[33] Lateral dislocations are often associated with mandibular fracture. With a lateral dislocation, the condylar head is forced laterally and then superiorly into the temporal space. Superior dislocations occur from a blow to the partially open mouth that forces the condylar head upward. Associated injuries include cerebral contusions, facial nerve palsy, and deafness.

Acute jaw dislocation causes severe pain, difficulty in speaking or swallowing, or malocclusion after a blow to the jaw or a seizure or, sometimes, spontaneously. There may be loose or missing teeth and areas of sensory deficit at the chin or mouth. With anterior dislocation, pain is localized anterior to the tragus. Symptoms may develop after extreme mouth opening from laughing, yawning, vomiting, taking a large bite, or trauma, or iatrogenically during dental extraction, general anesthesia, and tonsillectomy.[33] With anterior dislocations, the lower jaw is prominent appearing, and there is visible and palpable preauricular depression from the displacement of the mandibular condyle. There also will be difficulty with jaw movement. If the dislocation is unilateral, there is deviation of the jaw away from the dislocation. **When a posterior dislocation is considered, examine the external auditory canal.** Confirm that hearing is at baseline. With lateral dislocations, the condylar head is palpable in the temporal space, and there are always signs of jaw fracture (e.g., malocclusion). **Posterior, lateral, or superior dislocations result from severe trauma.** The differential diagnosis includes mandibular fracture, traumatic hemarthrosis, acute closed locking of the temporomandibular joint meniscus, and temporomandibular joint dysfunction.[33]

In the cooperative patient with a **spontaneous atraumatic anterior dislocation**, the diagnosis is clinical. In other dislocations, including any traumatic dislocation, obtain radiographs. The panoramic (Panorex) view usually demonstrates the pathology and excludes other mandibular injury. In patients with more serious trauma, where there may be a superior dislocation or intracranial injury, CT will provide more information.

Perform reduction in the ED for closed anterior dislocations without fracture.[33] A short-acting IV muscle relaxant (e.g., midazolam) may help to decrease muscle spasm. Appropriate airway and hemodynamic monitoring is required. Procedural sedation has been used successfully.[43] Alternatively, local anesthetic can be placed into the joint space. Using aseptic technique, place a 21-gauge needle into the preauricular depression just anterior to the tragus and inject 2 mL of 2% lidocaine[44] (**Figure 243-5**).

REDUCTION OF ANTERIOR TEMPOROMANDIBULAR JOINT DISLOCATION

The most commonly used technique requires the patient to be firmly seated with the head against the wall or chair back, positioned so that the examiner's flexed elbow is at the level of the patient's mandible. Apply a

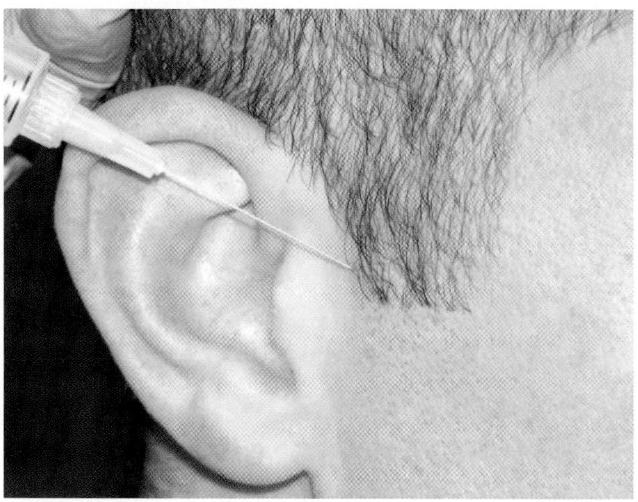

FIGURE 243-5. Site for injection of local anesthesia for reduction of dislocated mandible. Place a 21-gauge needle into the preauricular depression just anterior to the tragus and inject 2 mL of 2% lidocaine.

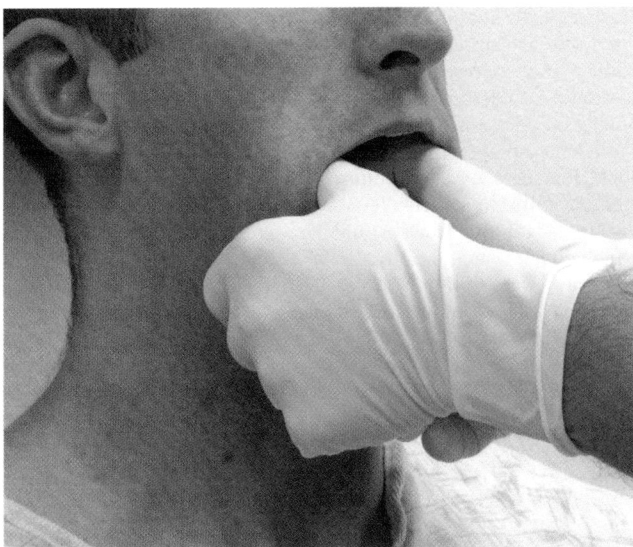

FIGURE 243-6. Reduction of dislocated mandible technique in a seated patient. The thumbs are placed over the molars, and pressure is applied downward and backward.

few layers of gauze over gloved thumbs for protection, in case the mandible snaps closed after reduction.[33]

Facing the patient, place gloved thumbs in the patient's mouth, over the occlusal surfaces of the mandibular molars, as far back as possible. Curve your fingers beneath the angle and body of the mandible. Using the thumbs, **apply pressure downward and backward (toward the patient)**. Slightly opening the jaw may help disengage the condyle from the anterior eminence (**Figure 243-6**). When the dislocation is bilateral, it may be easier to relocate one side at a time.

In the second technique, with the patient recumbent and supine, stand at the head of the bed, place the thumbs on the molars, and apply downward and backward pressure (toward the stretcher) (**Figure 243-7**).[33]

In addition to the above common methods, other approaches include the ipsilateral, in which the thumb is externally used to apply downward pressure on the displaced condyle; the wrist pivot method, in which the healthcare provider's thumbs are placed on the mentum, applying

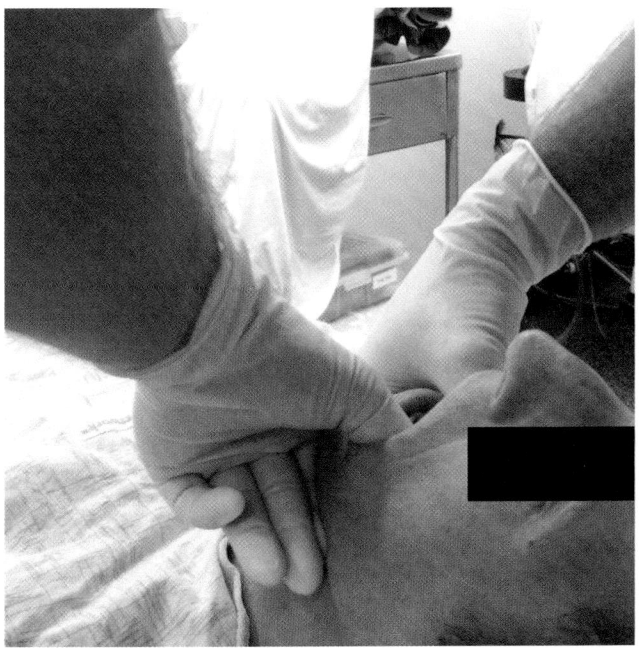

FIGURE 243-7. Alternate mandibular reduction technique, with the examiner behind and above the reclined patient. Place the thumbs on the molars and apply downward and backward pressure (toward the stretcher).

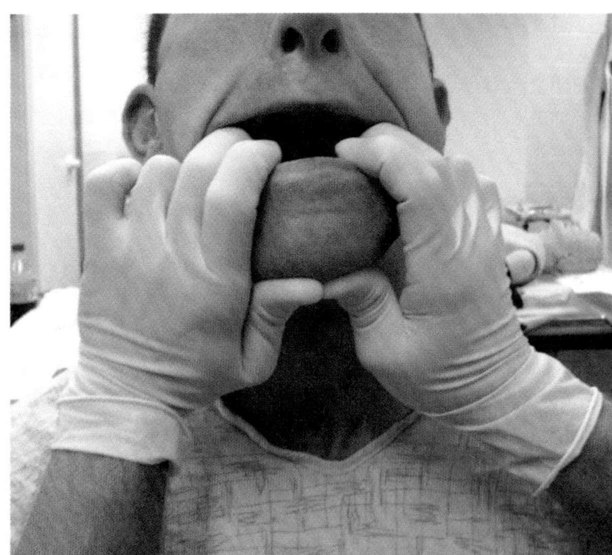

FIGURE 243-8. Wrist pivot method for mandibular reduction. The operator's thumbs are placed on the mentum, applying upward force, while the fingers apply downward force on the body of the mandible.

upward force, while the fingers apply downward force on the body of the mandible (**Figure 243-8**); and the gag reflex approach. In the gag reflex method, the provider stimulates the patient's soft palate with a tongue blade or dental mirror, thereby producing muscle relaxation and descent of the mandible, resulting in relocation of the condyle.[33]

After successful reduction, the patient should be able to close his or her mouth immediately. Postreduction radiographs usually are not needed unless the procedure was difficult or traumatic or there is significant postreduction pain. Complications from the reduction itself are unusual but can include iatrogenic fracture or avulsion of the articular cartilage.

Dislocations that are open, superior, associated with fracture, have any nerve injury, or are irreducible by closed technique should be referred urgently to an otolaryngologist or maxillofacial surgeon.

Following successful reduction of an acute dislocation, patients may be discharged home, placed on a soft diet, and cautioned against opening their mouths >2 cm for the following 2 weeks.[33] Advise patients to support the mandible with a hand when they yawn. Nonsteroidal analgesics may help the initial discomfort. Elective referral to an oral maxillofacial surgeon is recommended. In severe cases, intermaxillary fixation may be required to control jaw motion during healing. Chronic dislocations may require operative intervention.

REFERENCES

The complete reference list is available online at www.TintinalliEM.com.

CHAPTER 244 Nose and Sinuses

Henderson D. McGinnis

EPISTAXIS

EPIDEMIOLOGY

Epistaxis occurs most frequently in children under 10 years old and in those over 70 years old.[1] Local causes of epistaxis include digital trauma, a deviated septum, dry air exposure, rhinosinusitis, neoplasia, or chemical

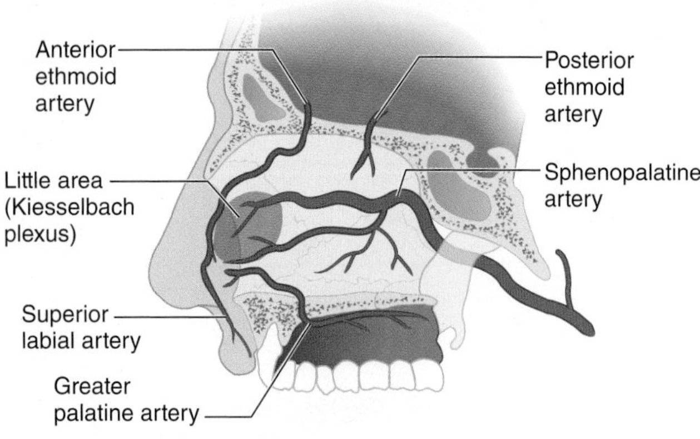

FIGURE 244-1. Arterial blood supply to the nasal cavity. The most common site of nasal hemorrhage is at Little's area of the nasal septum. The most common origin of posterior epistaxis is from the sphenopalatine artery.

irritants such as inhaled corticosteroids or chronic nasal cannula oxygen use. Systemic factors that increase the risk of bleeding include chronic renal insufficiency, alcoholism, hypertension, vascular malformations such as hereditary hemorrhagic telangiectasia, or any kind of coagulopathy, including warfarin administration, von Willebrand's disease, or hemophilia.[2]

ANATOMY AND PATHOPHYSIOLOGY

The superior labial branch of the facial artery joins the anterior ethmoidal and terminal branch of the sphenopalatine artery to form Kiesselbach plexus on the anterior nasal septum, which is the source of 90% of nosebleeds and can usually be visualized with anterior rhinoscopy (**Figure 244-1**). The most likely source for posterior bleeds is the sphenopalatine artery, which is a terminal division of the internal maxillary artery (branch of the external carotid system). Endoscopic or open surgical techniques are needed to visualize the vessel.[2,3] Sensory innervation is detailed in **Figure 244-2**.

CLINICAL FEATURES

A directed history and physical examination is usually sufficient to identify the source of acute epistaxis. Ask about prior or recurrent epistaxis, duration and severity of the current episode, and laterality.

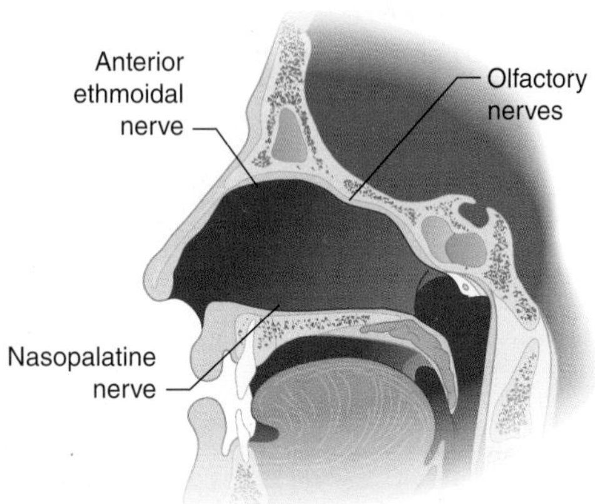

FIGURE 244-2. Sensory innervation of the external nose. [Reproduced with permission from Reichman EF, Simon RR: *Emergency Medicine Procedures.* © 2004, Eric F. Reichman, PhD, MD, and Robert R. Simon, MD.]

Ask specifically about nonsteroidal anti-inflammatory drugs, warfarin, heparin, or aspirin use. Alcohol or cocaine abuse, trauma, prior head and neck procedures, and a personal and family history of coagulopathy should be assessed.

Make preparations for nasal examination and tamponade. The ED should have a preprepared, readily available epistaxis kit or cart. The kit should include a nasal speculum, bayonet forceps, headlamp, suction catheter, cotton pledgets, 0.05% oxymetazoline and 4% lidocaine solutions, silver nitrate swabs, and some combination of absorbable and nonabsorbable materials for anterior and posterior packing.

Assemble a good light source, suction, and a nasal speculum. Have the patient seated and in the "sniffing" position. The sniffing position is achieved by having the patient flex and extend the head while keeping the base of the nose straight ahead. With the patient in this position, brace the speculum by resting the index finger on the tip of the nose and insert the speculum with the handle parallel to the floor. Open the blades in a cephalad-to-caudad direction to visualize the bleeding site and facilitate the performance of direct hemostatic techniques.

DIAGNOSIS

Differentiating an anterior versus posterior source of bleeding is important for treatment and disposition; failure to identify the source of bleeding is associated with rebleeding and return for treatment.[4] The division between anterior and posterior bleeding in the ED is often based on the ability to visualize the site of bleeding with a light source and a nasal speculum.[5] Generally, the diagnosis of posterior hemorrhage is only made in the ED once measures to control anterior bleeding have failed. Clinical features suggestive of a posterior source include elderly patients with either inherited or acquired coagulopathy, a significant amount of hemorrhage visible in the posterior nasopharynx, hemorrhage from bilateral nares, or epistaxis uncontrolled with either anterior rhinoscopy or an anterior pack.[6] Laboratory evaluation or other ancillary studies are not required unless management of comorbid illness requires it or the hemorrhage is poorly controlled. In the latter case, collect blood for CBC, type and cross-match, and coagulation studies if coagulopathy is suspected.

TREATMENT

Initial ED management for epistaxis begins with a rapid primary survey addressing potential airway or hemodynamic compromise. Obtain IV access in patients with severe bleeding, and request cross-matched blood if there is hemodynamic instability. The need for transfusion is more common in patients with posterior epistaxis and those on anticoagulants.[7] Reversal of coagulopathy with blood products can be considered based on clotting studies and individual patient context. Rapid reduction of blood pressure during an episode of acute epistaxis is generally not advised.[8] For uncontrolled epistaxis requiring packing or surgical intervention, gentle reduction of persistent hypertension reduces hydrostatic pressure and thereby may aid clot formation.[8]

DIRECT NASAL PRESSURE

First, ask the patient to blow the nose to expel clots to prepare mucosa for topical vasoconstrictors. Instill a topical vasoconstrictor such as oxymetazoline or phenylephrine. The patient should lean forward in the "sniffing" position and pinch the soft nares between the thumb and the middle finger for a full 10 to 15 minutes, breathing through the mouth. If the patient is uncooperative, fashion a hands-free pressure device made from two tongue depressors that are taped together between halfway and two thirds of the way up the depressors. Place the device on the nose and leave it undisturbed for 10 to 15 minutes. These initial measures are often sufficient to achieve hemostasis and facilitate further examination by anterior rhinoscopy.

CHEMICAL CAUTERIZATION

If two attempts at direct pressure have failed, chemical cauterization with silver nitrate is the next appropriate step for mild bleeding. Before cautery, anesthetize the nasal mucosa using three cotton pledgets soaked in a 1:1 mixture of 0.05% oxymetazoline and 4% lidocaine solution.[2] Do not attempt chemical cautery unless the bleeding vessel is visualized. Electrical cautery should be left to the otolaryngologist due to the risk of septal perforation.

After visualizing the (anterior) bleeding site, silver nitrate sticks may be judiciously placed just proximal to the bleeding source on the anterior nasal septum. Silver nitrate requires a relatively bloodless field, as the chemical reaction leading to precipitation of silver metal and tissue coagulation cannot proceed in the setting of active hemorrhage due to washout of substrate. Once a relatively bloodless field is achieved, gently and briefly (a few seconds) apply silver nitrate directly to the bleeding site. Chemical cautery should never be attempted on both sides of the nasal septum. Subsequent attempts on the same side of the nasal septum should be separated by 4 to 6 weeks to avoid perforation.[9]

THROMBOGENIC FOAMS AND GELS

Thrombogenic foams and gels are a good option, and they may be considered after attempts at chemical cautery have failed and before insertion of nasal tampons. Gelfoam® and Surgicel® (oxidized cellulose) are effective hemostatic agents that can be placed simultaneously on visualized bleeding mucosa, and they are bioabsorbable, so removal is not needed. FloSeal®, a hemostatic gelatin matrix that is mixed in a syringe with thrombin and injected into the nasal cavity, may decrease episodes of rebleeding and the need for specialty follow-up compared to other agents.[10] A 2013 randomized controlled trial involving 216 patients demonstrated that 5 mL of the injectable form of tranexamic acid, equal to 500 milligrams, applied topically to the nasal mucosa using a 15-cm piece of cotton pledget, stopped anterior epistaxis in 70% of patients, compared to a 31% success rate in those who received anterior packing alone.[11] There were no adverse events. Topical use of injectable tranexamic acid may prove to be a valuable procoagulant.

ANTERIOR NASAL PACKING

Anterior nasal packing can be placed if direct pressure, vasoconstrictors, or chemical cautery are unsuccessful in controlling epistaxis and if thrombotic foams and gels are not available. A variety of nasal balloons or sponges are available, or an anterior pack created by layering ribbon gauze in the nasal cavity can be used.

ANTERIOR EPISTAXIS BALLOONS

Anterior epistaxis balloons (Rapid Rhino®) are easy to use and more comfortable for the patient than layered strip gauze or nasal sponges. Anterior epistaxis balloons are available in different lengths and are coated with cellulose or other materials that promote platelet aggregation. Soak the balloon with water, insert it gently along the floor of the nasal cavity, and inflate slowly with air until the bleeding stops. Stop inflation if the patient develops discomfort. Do not inflate with saline; if a saline-filled balloon ruptures, aspiration could result. Read specific insertion instructions for each product before use. If there is a drawstring at the distal end, tape the drawstring to the face to secure the balloon in place.

PREFORMED NASAL TAMPONS OR SPONGES

Preformed nasal tampons or sponges are made of synthetic material that expands after hydration (**Figure 244-3**). These devices are commercially available in 5- and 10-cm lengths, for anterior and posterior packing, respectively. One product is Merocel®, a compressed dehydrated polyvinyl acetate sponge. Coat the sponge with water-soluble antibiotic ointment and insert it gently along the floor of the nasal cavity. If the tampon has not expanded within 30 seconds of placement, gently irrigate it (while in place) with 5 mL of normal saline to promote expansion. An alternative method is to cut the Merocel® pack lengthwise in two equal halves, and coat each half with lubricating ointment. Insert the two halves parallel to each other and parallel with the nasal septum; irrigate each half with about 2 mL of normal saline. This method may provide better compression of septal bleeding.[12] Whichever method is used, tape the drawstring to the face (Figure 244-3) to secure the tampon in place and prevent inadvertent aspiration. Merocel® nasal packs work effectively but sometimes cause more pain than balloons with removal.[13]

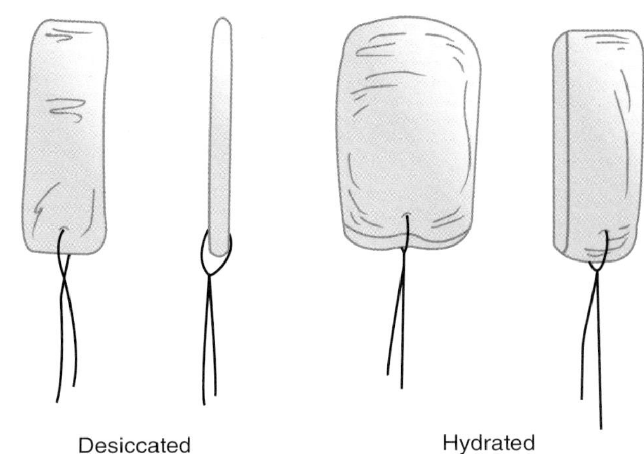

FIGURE 244-3. The Merocel® nasal sponge in its desiccated (*left*) and hydrated (*right*) forms.

RIBBON GAUZE PACKING

If the preceding devices are unavailable, ribbon gauze packing can be placed to control epistaxis (**Figure 244-4**).

POSTERIOR NASAL PACKING

Failure to control hemorrhage after direct pressure, optimal use of vasoconstrictors, cautery, and anterior packing suggests (but is not diagnostic of) posterior bleeding. Bilateral anterior packing may help augment tamponade of the nasal septum. If that is not successful, the previously mentioned devices are usually available in longer lengths to provide posterior packing. If longer posterior-length packs do not work, ear, nose, and throat (ENT) consultation and assistance are needed. Posterior packing is associated with higher complication rates, including pressure necrosis, infection, hypoxia, and cardiac dysrhythmias, especially in patients with underlying cardiopulmonary disease, and thus, posterior packing is generally applied as a temporizing measure while awaiting ENT support. A formal nasal block may be required for analgesia, as posterior packing is often quite uncomfortable for the patient, but topical anesthesia may be sufficient if applied properly. The Rapid Rhino® has both an anterior (5.5 cm) and posterior (7.5 cm) balloon that can be inflated as required to tamponade bleeding. **Figure 244-5** shows the placement of a dual balloon catheter. All posterior packing should be accompanied by an anterior pack.

If resources are limited, a satisfactory posterior pack can be achieved using a 14-French Foley catheter. The procedure is as follows. Place the patient in "sniffing position," and anesthetize the nasal mucosa by placing three cotton pledgets soaked in a 1:1 mixture of 4% lidocaine solution and 0.05% oxymetazoline intranasally for 5 minutes. Consider cutting off the Foley tip beyond the balloon as the tip may stimulate the gag reflex. Lubricate the distal third of the catheter with lidocaine gel, and advance the Foley catheter along the floor of the nasal cavity until the end is visualized in the posterior oropharynx. Inflate the balloon with 7 mL of air, and gently retract the catheter approximately 2 to 3 cm until it is lodged in the choanal arch of the posterior nasopharynx. Do not use saline for balloon insufflation because rupture could result in aspiration. If the balloon slides back into the nasal cavity, deflate the balloon, and advance the catheter as before. Inflate with 10 mL of air in total, and retract to secure the balloon. Avoid using more than 10 mL

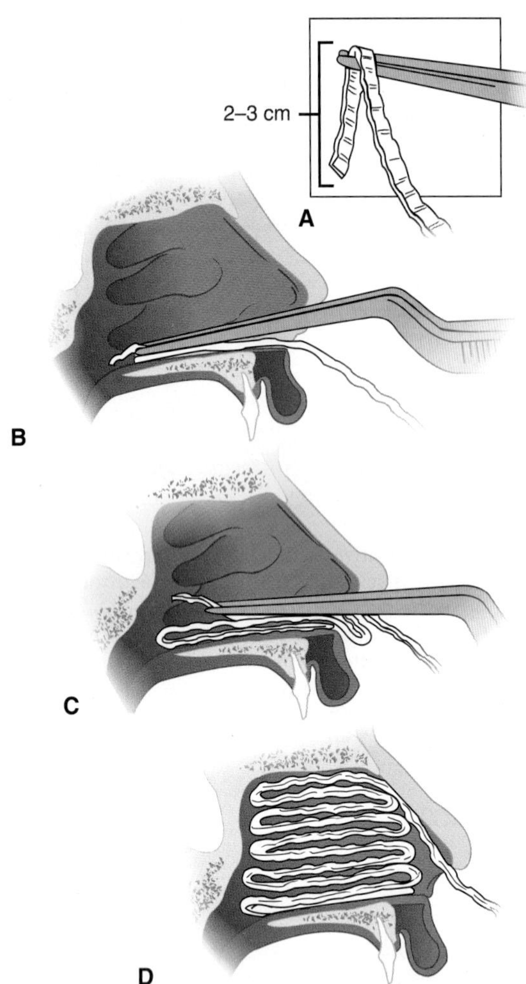

FIGURE 244-4. The key to placement of an anterior nasal pack that will control epistaxis adequately and stay in place is to lay the packing into the nasal cavity in an accordion-like manner so that part of each layer of packing lies anteriorly, preventing the gauze from falling posteriorly into the nasopharynx. **A.** The first layer of $^1/_4$-inch petrolatum-impregnated gauze strip is grasped approximately 2 to 3 cm from its end. **B.** The first layer is then placed on the floor of the nose through the nasal speculum (not pictured here). The bayonet forceps and nasal speculum are then withdrawn. **C.** The nasal speculum is reintroduced on top of the first layer of packing, and a second layer is placed in an identical manner. After several layers have been placed, it is often useful to reintroduce the bayonet forceps to push the previously placed packing down onto the floor of the nose, making it tighter and more secure. **D.** A complete anterior nasal pack can tamponade a bleeding point anywhere in the anterior nasal cavities and will stay in place until removed by the provider or patient.

of air to prevent risk of pressure necrosis. Secure the pack by taping the catheter to the patient's cheek.

In patients requiring posterior packing or in cases of uncontrolled anterior epistaxis, early ENT intervention reduces charges and length of stay.[14] Approximately 10% of patients admitted for epistaxis require invasive therapy; success is similar for arterial ligation or embolization, but cost and risk of stroke are higher for patients receiving embolization.[15]

DISPOSITION AND FOLLOW-UP

If hemorrhage is controlled and hemodynamic stability is ensured over a period of observation (1 hour or more in the ED), patients with anterior epistaxis can be discharged home with ENT follow-up within 48 hours ideally. Provide patients with instructions for simple techniques to control repeat hemorrhage, and consider prescription of inhaled vasoconstrictors such as oxymetazoline for rebleeding. Patients

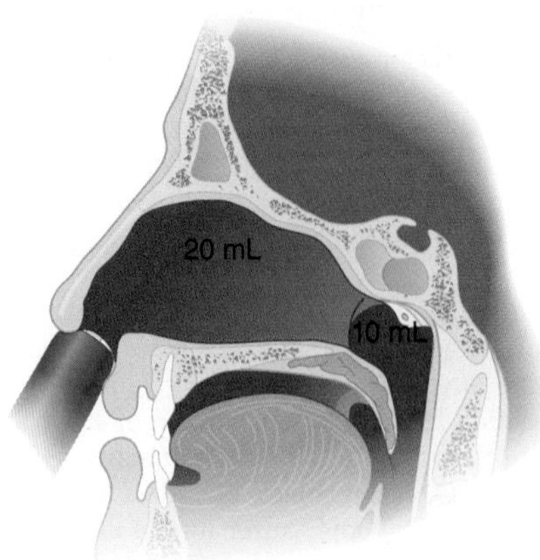

FIGURE 244-5. A dual balloon epistaxis catheter providing anterior and posterior compression. Overinflation of the posterior balloon may cause pressure necrosis; avoid using more than 10 mL.

on warfarin with INR levels in the desired range may continue medication. Discontinue nonsteroidal anti-inflammatory drugs for 3 to 4 days. If anterior packing with either absorbable or nonabsorbable material is going to be in place for more than 48 hours, an antibiotic with staphylococcal coverage such as amoxicillin-clavulanic acid has been traditionally recommended to prevent infection with *Staphylococcus aureus* and possible associated toxic shock syndrome.[16] However, benefit is not clear.[17,18] If the packing will be removed in 24 to 36 hours, prophylactic antibiotics may not be needed.[16] Consider potential drug interactions that may increase bleeding.[19] Instruct the patient to follow-up with ENT or return to the ED in 2 to 3 days for removal of nonbiodegradable packing. If the patient requires posterior packing, admission is strongly advised to monitor for complications.

NASAL FRACTURES AND SEPTAL HEMATOMA

ANATOMY

The nasal pyramid is formed by two rectangular-shaped bones that articulate with the frontal bone, the frontal process of the maxilla, and the perpendicular plate of the ethmoid to form a "tent-like" configuration (**Figures 244-6 and 244-7**). A large proportion of the structural integrity is maintained by a cartilaginous framework of the nasal septum, lateral processes, and medial and lateral crura of the alar cartilages (**Figure 244-8**).

CLINICAL FEATURES

Determine the mechanism of injury to evaluate the potential location of displaced bony fragments and to assess other associated pathology, especially head and neck injury. Assess the midface, zygomatic arch, orbits, sinuses, teeth, and cervical spine. Naso-orbital-ethmoid injuries are characterized by a broad, flattened nasal bridge with increased intercanthal distance (**Figure 244-9**). Malocclusion and palatal instability suggest Le Fort's fracture (see chapter 255, "Trauma to the Face").

NASAL EXAMINATION

After a general exam, perform an examination of the nose to include an external assessment for bony crepitus, deformity, and edema (**Figure 244-10**). Periorbital ecchymosis in the absence of other findings of orbital injury is suggestive of nasal fracture.[6] Profuse epistaxis may also suggest nasal fracture. Nasal bone mobility, which is virtually diagnostic of fracture, is appreciated by grasping the dorsum of the nose between the thumb and index finger and attempting to rock the nasal

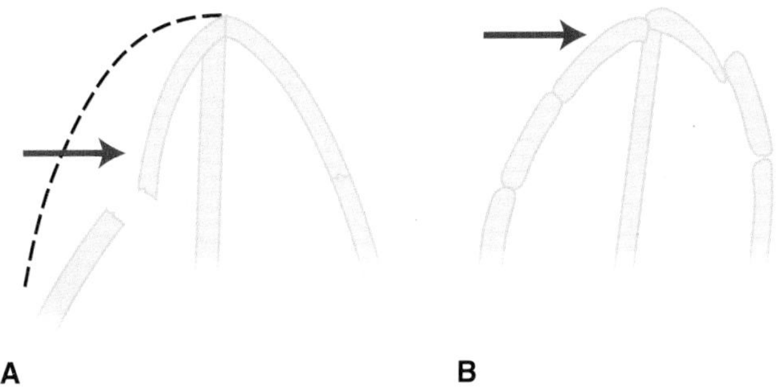

FIGURE 244-6. **A and B.** Lateral impact nasal injury. [Reproduced with permission from Reichman EF, Simon RR: *Emergency Medicine Procedures*. © 2004, Eric F. Reichman, PhD, MD, and Robert R. Simon, MD.]

pyramid back and forth.[6] Perform anterior rhinoscopy after obtaining a relatively bloodless field with topical vasoconstrictors and evacuation of clots. Key components of the internal examination should include assessment for mucosal lacerations, septal fractures or deviation, and septal hematoma.

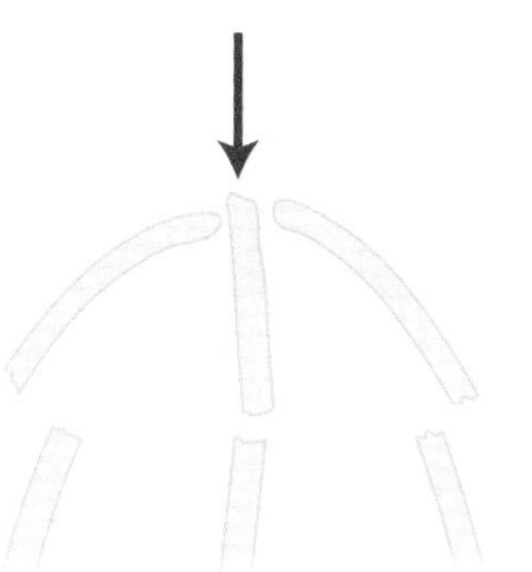

FIGURE 244-7. Frontal impact nasal injury. [Reproduced with permission from Reichman EF, Simon RR: *Emergency Medicine Procedures*. © 2004, Eric F. Reichman, PhD, MD, and Robert R. Simon, MD.]

DIAGNOSIS AND IMAGING

The diagnosis of nasal fracture is clinical, and radiologic confirmation of isolated nasal fracture is not required. The results of plain films rarely change management.[20,21] The indications for closed reduction are limited to alleviation of nasal obstruction and correcting deformity to improve cosmesis. These indications are best evaluated clinically at the bedside and usually are not emergency procedures.[20] Ultrasonography is an alternative to plain radiographs for the diagnosis of nasal fractures and has sensitivities and specificities similar to plain radiography[22-24] (**Figures 244-11 and 244-12**). CT scanning is not needed for isolated nasal fractures and is best reserved when there is concern for intracranial injury or other facial fractures.[25]

TREATMENT

The main priority is the exclusion of other associated traumatic injuries (see chapter 255) and nasal septal hematoma (see septal hematoma section below). Nasal fractures with overlying lacerations should be treated similarly to other open fractures. Concern for cerebrospinal fluid rhinorrhea or otorrhea requires further imaging and otolaryngologic or neurosurgical consultation. Nasal fractures in children should be referred to an ENT specialist within 2 to 4 days to account for rapid healing in children.[6]

Once serious injury is excluded, the management of uncomplicated nasal fractures is dictated by the timing of the examination in relation to the injury and ability to evaluate for significant displacement of the nasal pyramid. Early in the course, significant soft tissue swelling may obscure an adequate physical examination. If the patient presents immediately after the injury event, there may be opportunity to reduce a displaced nasal fracture before edema distorts the landmarks. Otherwise, it is prudent to recommend ENT consultation for an elective closed reduction within 6 to 10 days of the initial insult. Because of the development of fibrous connective tissue along the fracture line, failure to perform an adequate reduction within this time frame may result in an unacceptable cosmetic outcome and may ultimately require rhinoseptoplasty.[26] Most nasal fractures do not require immediate intervention and can be managed at ENT follow-up within the specified time frame of 6 to 10 days. Closed reduction is best left to the ENT specialist.

NASAL SEPTAL HEMATOMA

Vascular supply to the septal cartilage is provided through the perichondrium. A hematoma lifts the perichondrium, disrupting blood

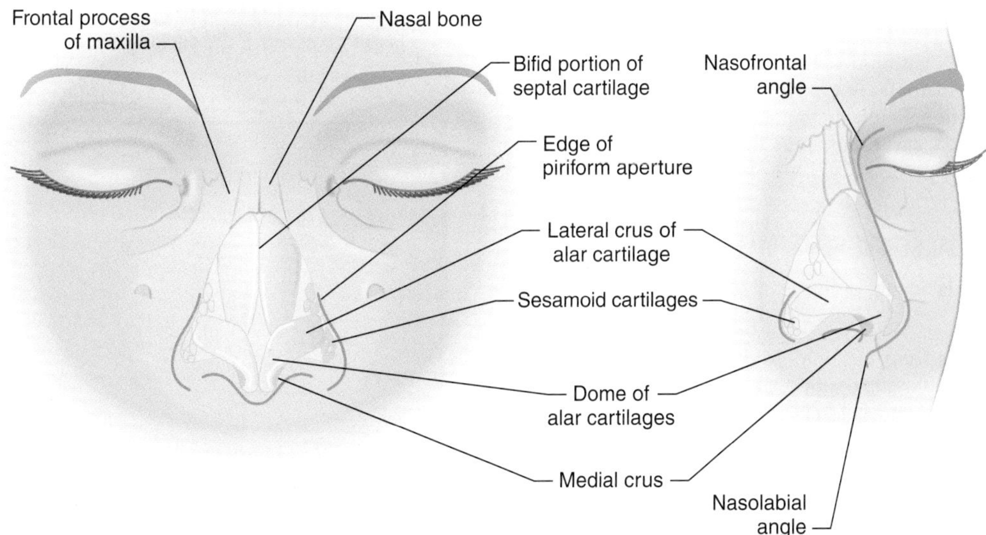

FIGURE 244-8. The nasal cartilages and the keystone area where they articulate with the nasal bones. [Reproduced with permission from Reichman EF, Simon RR: *Emergency Medicine Procedures*. © 2004, Eric F. Reichman, PhD, MD, and Robert R. Simon, MD.]

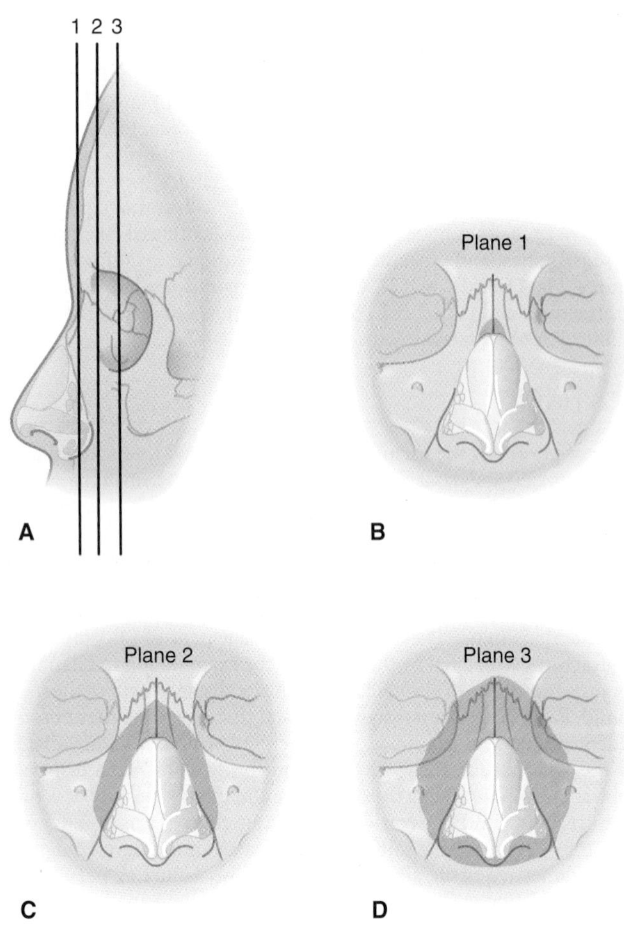

FIGURE 244-9. A through D. Stranc and Robertson classification of frontal impact injury. Plane 3 injury results in naso-orbital-ethmoid disruption.

supply to the cartilage. If a septal hematoma is identified, incise and drain the hematoma urgently to avoid ischemic necrosis of the nasal septum (**Figures 13 and 14**). Necrosis can lead to saddle deformity and nasal obstruction, ultimately requiring rhinoseptoplasty. Because pooled, clotted blood is a nidus for infection, unidentified septal hematomas can develop into abscesses. Systemic symptoms developing after facial trauma should prompt investigation for nasal septal abscess, and any suspicion should prompt ENT referral, urgent surgical drainage, and IV antibiotics to avoid serious complications. Untreated infected hematomas not only increase risk for saddle deformity and a poor functional outcome but can also spread contiguously, leading to osteomyelitis, cavernous sinus thrombosis, meningitis, and intracranial abscesses.[27]

DRAINAGE OF NASAL SEPTAL HEMATOMA

The procedure for incision and drainage of a nasal septal hematoma is as follows:

1. Place patient in "sniffing position," and be prepared to perform adequate anterior rhinoscopy with a nasal speculum, light source, suction, irrigation, and packing materials.
2. Properly anesthetize the nasal mucosa by placing three cotton pledgets soaked in a 1:1 mixture of 4% lidocaine solution for 5 minutes, followed by infiltrative anesthesia if required.
3. Although sterile technique cannot be fully achieved in the nasal cavity, use sterile instruments, and keep the operative area as clean as possible with irrigation of foreign debris.

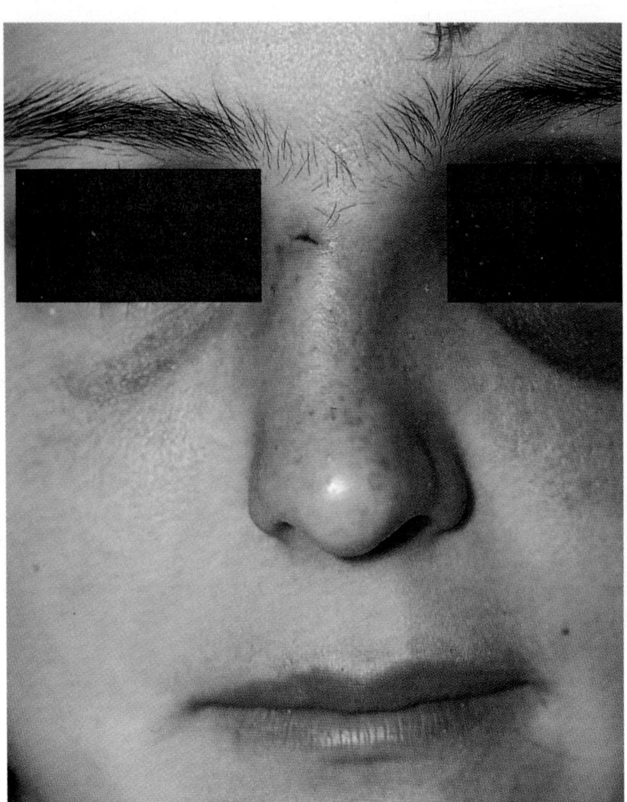

FIGURE 244-10. Nasal fracture clearly identifiable on physical examination with deformity and periorbital ecchymosis. [Photo contributed by David W. Munter. Reproduced with permission from Knoop K, Stack L, Storrow A, Thurman RJ: *Atlas of Emergency Medicine,* 3rd ed. © 2010, McGraw-Hill, New York.]

4. While obtaining adequate visualization of the hematoma with the nasal speculum, make a small horizontal incision superficially through the mucosa, making sure you do not incise the cartilaginous septum.
5. Evacuate the clot with Frazier suction or with forceps.
6. Perform bilateral anterior nasal packing with nasal tampons coated in topical antibiotic ointment to prevent reaccumulation of the clot and keep the septum midline.
7. Discharge with 24-hour ENT of ED follow-up.[28] Some recommend the use of prophylactic antibiotics for patients with packing in place, but this is not necessary if the packing will be removed in 24 to 36 hours.

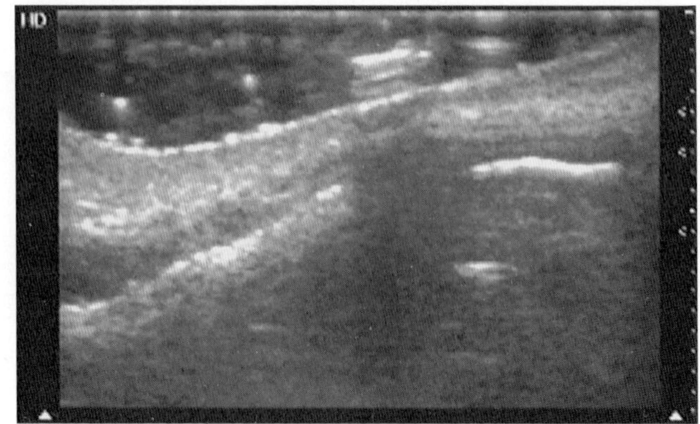

FIGURE 244-11. US still image of nasal fracture demonstrating cortical disruption. A large gap is seen between bone fragments. [Reproduced with permission from Ma OJ, Mateer JR, Blaivas M: *Emergency Ultrasound,* 2nd ed. © 2008, McGraw-Hill, New York.]

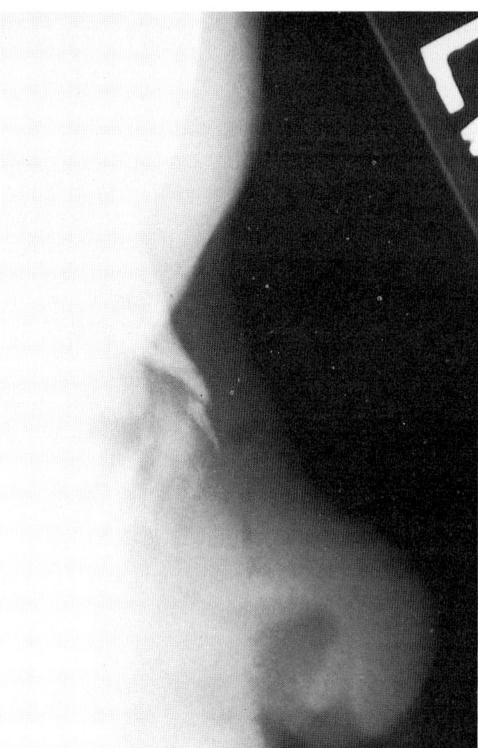

FIGURE 244-12. Nasal radiograph lateral view demonstrating depressed nasal fracture with cortical disruption. [Photo contributed by Lorenz F. Lassen, MD. Reproduced with permission from Knoop K, Stack L, Storrow A, Thurman RJ: *Atlas of Emergency Medicine*, 3rd ed. © 2010, McGraw-Hill, New York.]

NASAL FOREIGN BODIES

Although nasal foreign bodies are most common in children (see chapter 117, "Nose and Sinus Disorders in Infants and Children"), they should also be considered in psychiatric and mentally retarded adults.[29,30] Morbidity of undiagnosed nasal foreign bodies includes aspiration, infection, pressure necrosis, or perforation. Consider a nasal foreign body in patients with purulent unilateral nasal discharge or recurrent unilateral epistaxis. It is important to recognize button battery impaction because it may cause liquefaction necrosis and septal perforation.[31] Plain radiography is a potential tool for foreign body identification, but many objects are not radiopaque.[32] Nasal foreign body removal is discussed in the Pediatric Section, "The Nose and Sinuses."

SINUSITIS AND RHINOSINUSITIS

Sinusitis is inflammation of the mucosal lining of the paranasal sinuses. There are six nasal sinuses: two maxillary and two frontal sinuses, and a single ethmoid and frontal sinus. Rhinosinusitis is defined as an inflammation of the paranasal sinuses and the nasal cavity. The term *rhinosinusitis* is preferred because sinusitis is almost always accompanied by rhinitis.[33] Depending on the duration of the disease, rhinosinusitis is classified into acute (<4 weeks), subacute (4 to 12 weeks), or chronic (>12 weeks).[34-36]

PATHOPHYSIOLOGY

All six paranasal sinuses are coated by respiratory mucociliary epithelium, and the sinuses drain through the ostia into the nose. Any type of acute inflammation of the mucosa leads to obstruction of the ostia, accumulation of secretions within the sinuses, and reabsorption of air, resulting in negative pressure in the sinuses and clinical symptoms. Acute rhinosinusitis, like otitis media, is usually viral. *Haemophilus influenzae* and *Streptococcus pneumoniae* are the usual organisms in acute bacterial rhinosinusitis.[37] Chronic infections are usually due to anaerobes, gram-negative bacteria, *Staphylococcus aureus*, and, occasionally, fungi, especially in the immunocompromised.[35]

CLINICAL FEATURES

Acute rhinosinusitis is defined by two or more of the following symptoms: blockage or congestion of the nose, facial pain or pressure, diminished ability to smell or detect odors, and either anterior or posterior nasal discharge, for 7 days to 4 weeks. Additional symptoms can include tooth pain, fever, or sinus pressure while bending forward or changing head position.[35] On physical examination, the patient may have pain and tenderness over the sinuses with percussion. Inspect the face for swelling and redness, and inspect the nose for mucosal swelling, anatomic abnormality, and foreign bodies. Also perform a neurologic examination, and examine the ears, eyes, and

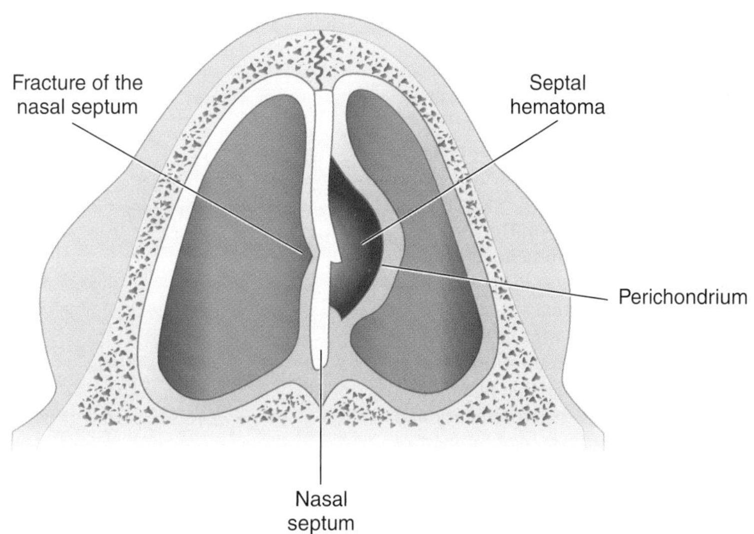

FIGURE 244-13. Graphic depiction of nasal septal hematoma. [Reproduced with permission from Reichman EF, Simon RR: *Emergency Medicine Procedures*. © 2004, Eric F. Reichman, PhD, MD, and Robert R. Simon, MD.]

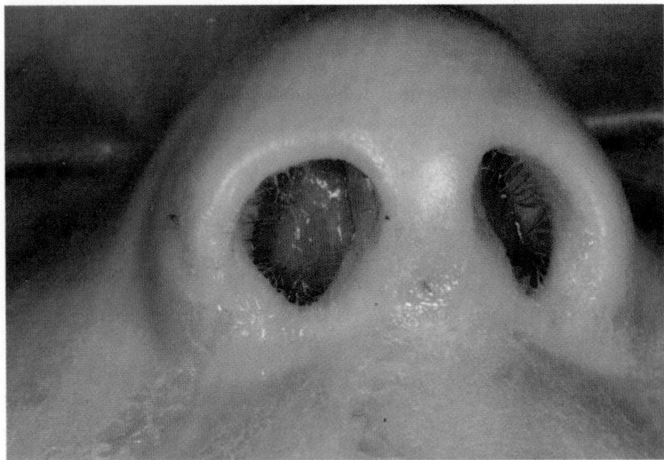

FIGURE 244-14. Trauma patient with nasal septal hematoma in the right nares. [Photo contributed by Lawrence B. Stack, MD. Reproduced with permission from Knoop K, Stack L, Storrow A, Thurman RJ: *Atlas of Emergency Medicine*, 3rd ed. © 2010, McGraw-Hill, New York.]

teeth to evaluate for extension of disease. Subacute and chronic sinusitis persist for 4 weeks or more.

DIAGNOSIS

The diagnosis of uncomplicated **acute rhinosinusitis** is clinical.[37] Plain sinus radiographs or CT scans are not needed. The symptoms of acute rhinosinusitis are similar to a common cold or viral upper respiratory infection, but symptom duration ranges from 7 days to up to 12 weeks.[37] CT scans are helpful to diagnose complications in a toxic patient or to evaluate for intracranial extension. The differential diagnosis of rhinosinusitis includes migraine headache, craniofacial neoplasm, foreign body retention, and dental caries.

TREATMENT

The treatment for **acute uncomplicated rhinosinusitis** is generally supportive. Nasal saline irrigation alone, or in conjunction with other adjunctive measures like nasal decongestants, may decrease symptom severity.[34] Restrict the use of topical decongestants like oxymetazoline to approximately 3 days to avoid rebound mucosal congestion or edema (rhinitis medicamentosa). Topical (intranasal spray) corticosteroids may shorten the duration of illness.[38]

In a 2014 Cochrane database systematic review analyzing the efficacy of antibiotic therapy, the authors concluded that antibiotics may provide a small treatment effect in patients with symptoms of rhinosinusitis lasting >7 days.[33] However, because 80% of patients treated with placebo also improved within 2 weeks, it is unclear whether the treatment effect is clinically significant. In general, **antibiotics should be reserved for patients with purulent nasal secretions and severe symptoms for ≥7 days.** If antibiotics are prescribed, amoxicillin is recommended as first-line therapy for most adults,[37] at a dose of 500 milligrams PO three times per day. Patients with penicillin allergies may receive macrolide antibiotics or trimethoprim-sulfamethoxazole.[37] For patients who have received antibiotics within the past 4 to 6 weeks, consider a fluoroquinolone or high-dose amoxicillin-clavulanate.[34] Use caution in selection of antibiotics in patients who are on oral anticoagulation.[19] In the aforementioned Cochrane review, comparisons between different classes of antibiotics showed no significant difference.[33] Follow-up with a primary care provider is advised.

Patients with **subacute, chronic or recurrent rhinosinusitis** should be evaluated for conditions that modify management, such as allergy, cystic fibrosis, or immunocompromise. Outpatient noncontrasted CT of the sinuses can evaluate for invasion of neighboring tissues and neoplasms.[34] Bacterial cultures may be helpful to tailor therapy in outpatients who are at risk for multidrug-resistant organisms. ENT follow-up is advised.[37,39]

COMPLICATIONS

Complications of rhinosinusitis are mostly related to extension of the infection beyond usual anatomic boundaries. Meningitis, cavernous sinus thrombosis, and intracranial abscesses are rare but important complications associated with contiguous spread of sinus disease. Up to 75% of cases of orbital cellulitis, which can lead to blindness through venous congestion and ischemia of the optic nerve, are attributable to disease of the sinuses.[37] Frontal sinusitis can lead to osteomyelitis of the frontal bone with a doughy swelling of the forehead called *Pott's puffy tumor*, and can also be associated with an extradural or subdural empyema. In general, patients with these deeper infections usually appear systemically ill or have focal neurologic signs and require admission and IV antibiotics.

REFERENCES

The complete reference list is available online at www.TintinalliEM.com.

Oral and Dental Emergencies

Ronald W. Beaudreau

ORAL AND DENTAL ANATOMY

The normal adult dentition consists of 32 permanent teeth. The adult dentition has four types of teeth: 8 incisors, 4 canines, 8 premolars, and 12 molars. The primary or deciduous dentition consists of 20 teeth of three types: 8 incisors, 4 canines, and 8 molars. **Figure 245-1** shows the

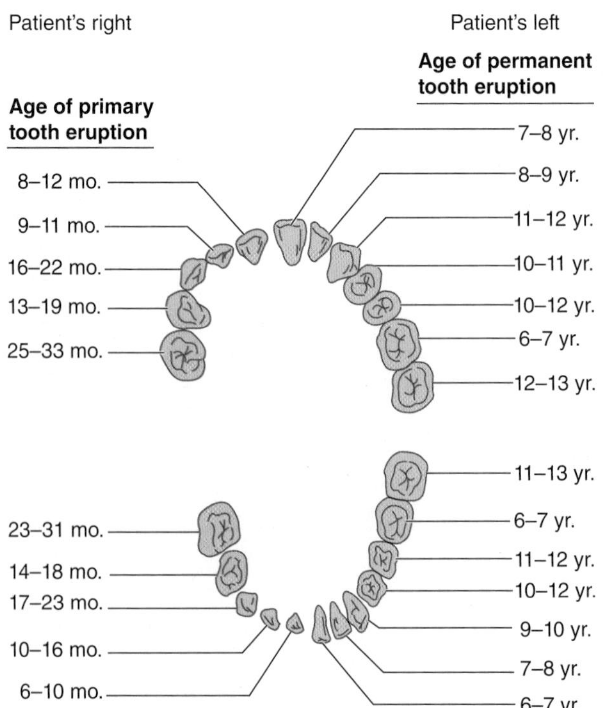

FIGURE 245-1. Normal eruptive patterns of the primary and permanent dentition. mo. = month; yr. = years.

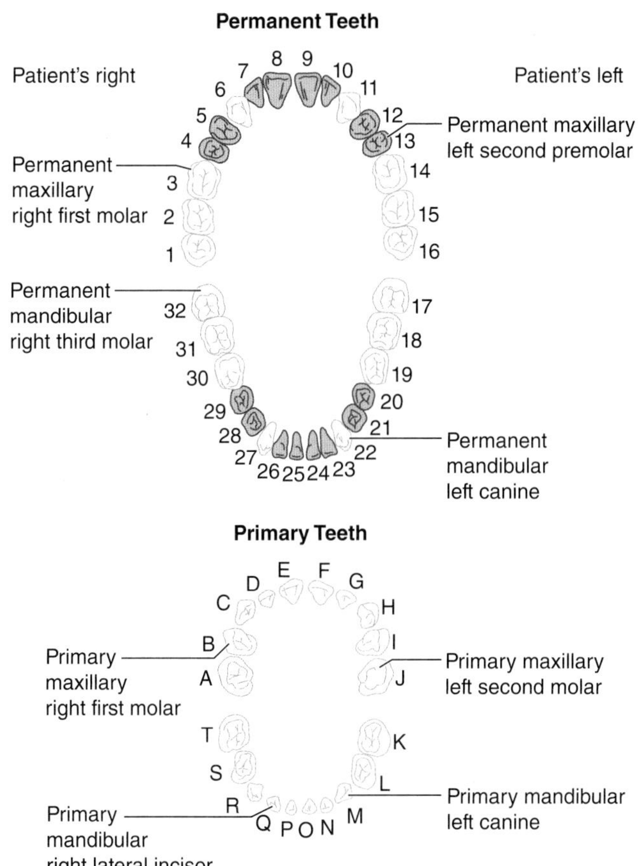

FIGURE 245-2. Identification of teeth.

eruptive pattern of both the primary and permanent dentition. **Figure 245-2** illustrates the most commonly used tooth numbering system; however, description of the tooth type and location is also appropriate.

ANATOMY OF THE TEETH

A tooth consists largely of *dentin,* which surrounds the *pulp*, the tooth's neurovascular supply (**Figure 245-3**). Dentin is a homogeneous material produced by pulpal odontoblasts throughout life. Dentin is deposited as a system of microtubules filled with odontoblastic processes and extracellular fluid. The *crown*, or the visible portion of tooth, consists of a thick *enamel* layer overlying the dentin. Enamel, the hardest substance in the human body, consists largely of hydroxyapatite and is produced by ameloblasts before eruption of the tooth into the mouth. The *root* portion of the tooth extends into the alveolar bone and is covered with a thin layer of *cementum.*

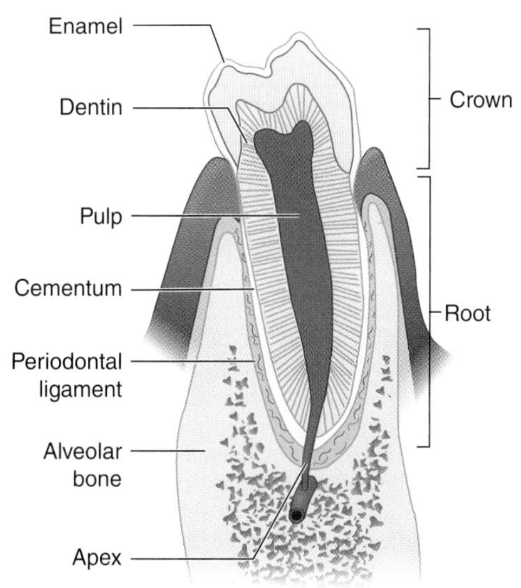

FIGURE 245-3. The dental anatomic unit and attachment apparatus.

THE NORMAL PERIODONTIUM

The periodontium, or attachment apparatus, is essential for maintaining the integrity of the dentoalveolar unit. The attachment apparatus consists of a gingival component and a periodontal component. The gingival component includes the junctional epithelium, gingival tissue, and gingival fibers and primarily functions to maintain the integrity of the periodontal component. The periodontal component includes the periodontal ligament, alveolar bone, and cementum of the root of the tooth and forms the majority of the attachment apparatus. Disease states such as gingivitis and periodontal disease weaken and destroy the attachment apparatus, resulting in tooth mobility and tooth loss.[1]

Gingival tissue is keratinized stratified squamous epithelium. It can be divided into the free gingival margin and the attached gingiva. The free gingiva is the portion that forms the 2- to 3-mm-deep *gingival sulcus* in the disease-free state. The attached gingiva adheres firmly to the underlying alveolar bone. The nonkeratinized alveolar mucosa extends from the attached gingiva to the vestibule and floor of the mouth. The mucosal tissue of the cheeks, lips, and floor of the mouth is also comprised of nonkeratinized squamous epithelium.

OROFACIAL PAIN

Table 245-1 lists common causes of orofacial pain. Pain of dental origin may be diffuse in nature, presenting as a headache, sinus pain, eye pain, or jaw or neck pain, or may be localized to a single tooth. Remember to consider myocardial infarction as a cause of jaw pain.

Examine the soft tissue using a tongue depressor to expand your view looking specifically at the inner lips, the buccal and labial mucosa, the hard and soft palate, and the tongue and floor of the mouth. Ask the patient to extend the tongue, and gently grasp it with a piece of dry gauze, further extending it to the right and to the left, to expose each base. The floor of the mouth should be palpated with a finger in the mouth and one externally under the chin to check for a mass or lesion. Examine the teeth visually, and then gently percuss the suspected teeth with a firm clean object to determine if a specific tooth is the source of pain. After trauma, test for mobility and tenderness with gentle pressure and percussion. Assure that all the teeth occlude as normal for the patient. The degree of opening of the mouth should be evaluated. Palpate for potential fractures of the mandible of maxilla. Finally, the temporomandibular joint should be evaluated by placing your index fingers in the ears and feeling for crepitance or popping while the mandible is fully opened and closed.

PAIN OF ODONTOGENIC ORIGIN

Tooth Eruption and Pericoronitis Discomfort is commonly associated with the eruption of primary or deciduous teeth in infants. Irritability, drooling, and decreased intake are commonly associated findings. Approximately 11% to 12% of teething infants will have a mildly elevated temperature when examined in a doctor's office, but a cause-and-effect relationship between teething and fever has never been demonstrated.[2] Eruption of permanent teeth, especially third molars, or *wisdom teeth,* may cause pain. Gingival irritation and inflammation associated with tooth eruption are common and must be distinguished from *pericoronitis.* Pericoronitis is inflammation of the *operculum*, or the gingival tissue, overlying the occlusal surface of an erupting tooth. Impaction of food and debris beneath the operculum results in a severe inflammatory response. Without intervention, this progressive inflammatory process

TABLE 245-1 Differential Diagnosis of Orofacial Pain

Nontraumatic Causes of Potential Dental Pain	
Odontogenic origin	
Tooth eruption	Cracked tooth syndrome
Pericoronitis	Periradicular periodontitis
Dental caries	Periapical abscess/facial space infection
Dentinal sensitivity/cervical erosion	Postextraction discomfort
Reversible pulpitis	Postextraction alveolar osteitis
Irreversible pulpitis	Post-restorative pain
Periodontal pathology	
Gingivitis	Periodontal abscess
Periodontal disease	Acute necrotizing gingivostomatitis
Gingival abscess	Peri-implantitis
Neurogenic/neurophysiologic syndromes	
Trigeminal neuralgia	Bell's palsy
Other cranial neuralgias	Temporomandibular disorder
Nondental infections	
Oral candidiasis	Hand-foot-and-mouth disease
Herpes simplex types 1 and 2	Sexually transmitted infections
Varicella-zoster, primary and secondary	Herpangina
Mumps	Sinusitis
Sialadenitis	Parotitis
Malignancies	
Squamous cell carcinoma	Leukemia
Kaposi's sarcoma	Melanoma
Lymphoma	Graft-versus-host disease
Other etiologies	
Aphthous ulcers	Pyogenic granuloma
Traumatic ulcers	Lichen planus
Stomatitis and mucositis	Cicatricial pemphigoid
Uremia	Pemphigus vulgaris
Vitamin deficiency	Erythema multiforme
Radiation/chemotherapy related	Crohn's disease
Benign migratory glossitis	Behçet's syndrome
Orofacial Trauma	
Dental fractures	Alveolar ridge fractures
Subtle enamel cracks/infractions	Facial bone fractures
Dental crown and/or root fractures	Oral soft tissue lacerations
Dental luxations and avulsions	

will result in localized infection. Because of the close proximity of the masticator space (comprised of the masseteric space, pterygomandibular space, and the superficial and deep temporalis space) to third molars, this infection can cause trismus. If the infection spreads into the connecting parapharyngeal spaces, it can be life threatening. Treatment of mild to moderate pericoronitis without associated systemic symptoms consists of appropriate antibiotic therapy such as penicillin VK, 500 milligrams PO four times a day, or clindamycin, 300 milligrams PO four times a day; local irrigation of food and debris from underneath the operculum; saline mouth rinses; and analgesia with nonsteroidal anti-inflammatory drugs (NSAIDs) and opiates as appropriate. More severe cases may require IV antibiotics and admission. If pericoronitis is related to trauma from an opposing tooth during mastication, as is frequently the case with third molars, antibiotics and extraction of the opposing tooth will bring marked relief within 24 hours. For outpatient management, referral to a general dentist or an oral and maxillofacial surgeon within 24 to 48 hours is appropriate.[3]

Dental Caries and Pulpitis *Dental caries* is the loss of integrity of the tooth enamel from hydroxyapatite dissolution by prolonged exposure to the acidic metabolic by-products of plaque bacteria. Caries most commonly occurs in areas where plaque accumulates such as pits and fissures of the occlusal surface, interproximally, and along the gingival margins. When a sufficient breach of enamel integrity occurs and the dentin is involved, caries spreads along dentinal microtubules. Direct communication between the oral environment and the vital dental pulp is established, and sensitivity to cold or sweet stimulus may result.

The pulpal inflammatory process is initially reversible, but with continued stimuli, the pulp's ability to respond and repair is compromised. *Irreversible pulpitis* can be distinguished from *reversible pulpitis* by the duration of symptoms. In reversible pulpitis, the duration of pain is short, lasting seconds, as compared with irreversible pulpitis, in which the pain may last for minutes to hours. The most common stimulus is heat or cold, although sweet or sour stimuli also can elicit pain. Spontaneous tooth pain usually represents *pulpal necrosis* and is treated with analgesia; penicillin VK, 500 milligrams PO four times a day, or clindamycin in penicillin-allergic patients; and referral to a general dentist. Antibiotics for dental pain are controversial; two systematic reviews have concluded there is there is insufficient evidence to determine whether antibiotics for irreversible pulpitis reduce pain[4,5] if there is no obvious infection. The use of local anesthetics as discussed in this chapter's section on dental local anesthesia techniques can greatly reduce symptoms and should be considered for short-term pain management. The definitive treatment for irreversible pulpitis and pulpal necrosis is root canal therapy or dental extraction.

Cracked Tooth Syndrome *Cracked tooth syndrome* is an incomplete fracture of a tooth that may extend into the vital pulp. Molars are most commonly affected. The patient experiences sharp pain on chewing that resolves when chewing ceases. Cold and sweet stimuli may also evoke pain. NSAIDs are frequently effective at temporarily controlling pain.[3] The patient should avoid chewing on the affected side and see a dentist for definitive treatment.

Periradicular Periodontitis Acute *periradicular periodontitis* is the extension of pulp disease, inflammation, or necrosis into the tissues surrounding the root and apex of the tooth (deepest portion of the tooth socket). Occasionally it can be due to occlusal trauma. Periradicular lesions appear as a slight widening of the periodontal ligament space, a thinning of the lamina dura, or a radiolucent area associated with the root apex on a periapical dental radiograph. A Panorex is rarely useful for identification of all but the most extensive periradicular lesions, but can be important in identifying other painful osseous pathology (**Figure 245-4**).

Pain on percussion of the suspected tooth with a light metal instrument, such as a handle of a dental mirror, helps to identify the offending tooth. Radiographically and clinically indistinguishable from periradicular periodontitis, a *periapical abscess* by definition contains a collection of pus. A small swelling of the gingiva with a draining fistula adjacent to the affected tooth is known as a *parulis*, and can help identify the involved tooth (**Figure 245-5**). If a dental abscess erodes through the cortical bone but does not drain spontaneously, then subperiosteal extension results in intraoral or facial swelling and fluctuance that should be incised and drained. Treat dental abscesses or other periapical lesions with penicillin VK, 500 milligrams PO four times a day, or clindamycin, 300 milligrams PO four times a day, and analgesia with an NSAID or opiate. Refer to a dentist for definitive treatment.

Facial Space Infections Spread of odontogenic infections into the various facial spaces is relatively common. Buccal extension of a periapical infection of the mandibular teeth will involve the buccinator space. Maxillary labial extension of infection primarily will involve the infraorbital space. Perforation through the lingual cortical bone of mandibular molars, particularly the second and third molars, usually occurs below the mylohyoid ridge and involves the submandibular space. Lingual spread of periapical infections associated with mandibular anterior teeth will affect the lingual space. The submandibular space and lingual space communicate with each other at the posterior border of the mylohyoid muscle. Cellulitis of bilateral submandibular spaces and the lingual space is called **Ludwig's angina** and is potentially life threatening. As

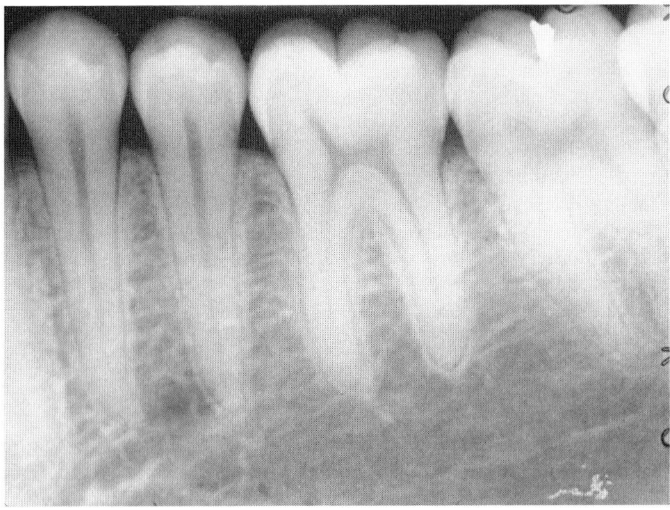

A

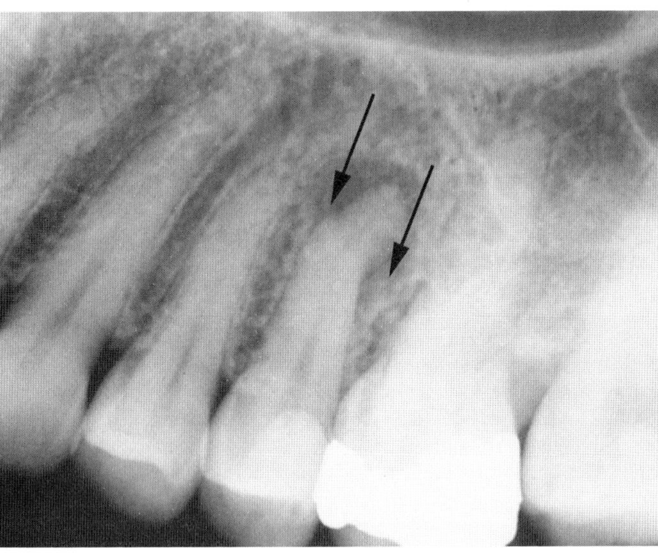

B

FIGURE 245-4. The radiographic appearance of a healthy tooth with a normal periodontal ligament space and distinct lamina dura (**A**) compared with the radiographic appearance of periapical radiolucency (*arrows*) consistent with periradicular periodontitis, a periapical abscess, or periradicular cyst (**B**). [Image used with permission of Gary M. Beaudreau.]

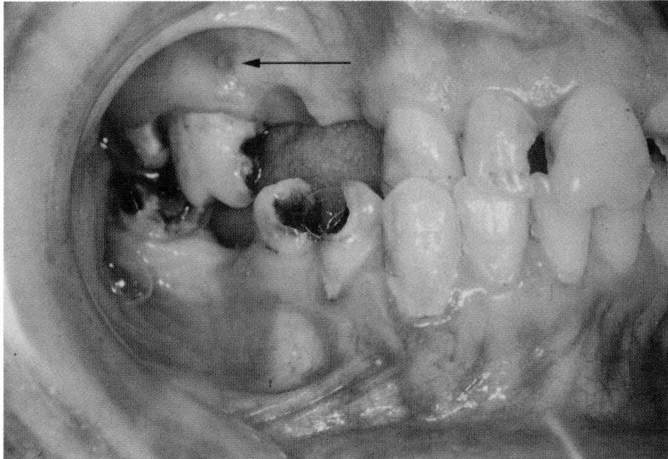

FIGURE 245-5. A parulis (*arrow*) superior to the maxillary molar. [Image used with permission of David E. Beaudreau.]

these spaces and the masticator space communicate directly with the parapharyngeal space, airway compromise is the immediate concern. For detailed discussion, see chapters 243, "Face and Jaw Emergencies" and 246, "Neck and Upper Airway."

Infection of the infraorbital space may have a potentially devastating outcome if retrograde spread through the ophthalmic veins occurs and the cavernous sinus becomes involved. **Cavernous sinus thrombosis** presents as an infraorbital or periorbital cellulitis with rapidly developing meningeal signs, sepsis, and coma. Early recognition and treatment with a high-dose IV antibiotic, as above, are essential in decreasing morbidity and mortality.

Postextraction Pain Immediate postoperative pain is most commonly related to the trauma of surgery. Postoperative edema, such as with extraction of third molars, peaks within the first 24 to 48 hours and is best managed with ice packs, elevation of the head of the bed to 30 degrees, NSAIDs, and oral narcotics. Trismus, common immediately after extraction, can result from direct injury to the temporomandibular joint, injury to the muscles of mastication during administration of the inferior alveolar nerve block or during the surgery, and, most commonly, normal perioperative inflammation. Trismus peaks in the first 24 hours and usually decreases thereafter unless infection develops. Progressively worsening trismus is concerning for a postoperative infection.

Postextraction Alveolar Osteitis (Dry Socket) *Postextraction alveolar osteitis*, or **dry socket**, usually occurs on the second or third postoperative day and is associated with exquisite oral pain. Total or partial displacement of the clot from the socket or fibrinolytic dissolution of the clot results in exposure of the alveolar bone and initiates a localized osteomyelitis of the exposed bone. Risk factors for developing postextraction alveolar osteitis include smoking, preexisting pericoronitis or periodontal disease, a traumatic extraction, a prior history of alveolar osteitis, and hormone replacement therapy.[6] The incidence of postextraction alveolar osteitis is 1% to 5% of all extractions but is considerably higher (up to 30%) among impacted third molar extractions.[6,7]

Treatment is gentle irrigation of the socket with warmed normal saline or chlorhexidine 0.12% oral rinse.[6-9] Local dental anesthesia (see the section on dental local anesthesia techniques) or topical anesthesia may be needed. Management of pain with NSAIDs or opiate medication is necessary. Antibiotic therapy with penicillin VK, 500 milligrams PO four times a day, or clindamycin, 300 milligrams PO four times a day, is reserved for the most severe cases. Refer for dental follow-up.[6-9]

Postextraction Bleeding Postextraction bleeding is not uncommon. Displacement of the clot may result in recurrent or continued bleeding. Generally, firm pressure applied to the extraction site is adequate to control bleeding. This is best accomplished by folding a 2 × 2-inch gauze pad and placing it over the extraction site and applying firm pressure by clenching with the opposing teeth. Pressure must be held firmly, not a chewing action, for 20 minutes or until hemostasis is complete. If direct pressure is not successful, then apply an absorbable gelatin sponge (Gelfoam®, Pfizer Inc., New York, NY), microfibrillar collagen (Avitene®, Davol, Inc., Warwick, RI), or regenerated cellulose (Surgicel®, Ethicon, Inc., Somerville, NJ) into the socket to provide a matrix for clot formation. Sutures can be used for holding such agents in place or to loosely close the gingiva over the socket. **Do not suture the gingiva tightly because this may cause necrosis of the gingival flap.** If this is not successful, careful injection of the soft tissue surrounding the extraction with lidocaine with epinephrine may control the bleeding. Careful cautery with silver nitrate can also be useful. If these methods are unsuccessful, then oral and maxillofacial surgical consultation is necessary.

Postrestorative Pain Postrestorative pain can result from normal trauma from mechanical instrumentation of the tooth or direct exposure of the pulpal tissue during instrumentation. Pain associated primarily with mastication may be the result of improper occlusion of the new dental restoration or filling. After endodontic therapy, buildup of pressure in the pulpal chamber can cause severe pain. Provide NSAIDs or narcotic analgesia and refer to the patient's dentist. Temporary prolonged pain relief can also be obtained using 0.5% bupivacaine with epinephrine and the appropriate dental anesthetic block as discussed in the dental local anesthesia technique section of this chapter. Follow-up with the dentist the next day then should be possible.

Orthodontic Appliances The most common emergency is a broken or bent wire that is irritating or lacerating the cheek or lip. This wire needs to be bent back away from soft tissue. This can easily be accomplished with dental instruments, or something soft like a pencil eraser can be used to gently bend the wire. Cutting the wire is generally not indicated as it makes the end sharper. The broken portion of the wire can be removed in its entirety by removing the rubber ligatures from each orthodontic bracket, but this generally is not necessary. The patient should follow up as soon as possible with the orthodontist.

PERIODONTAL PATHOLOGY

Periodontal Disease Periodontal disease is a continuum of disease that begins with gingival inflammation and bleeding, or gingivitis, and can progress to destruction of the periodontal attachment apparatus, deepening of the normal gingival sulcus, periodontal pocket formation, bone loss, tooth mobility, and ultimately loss of teeth.[1] Besides oral hygiene, many factors including hormonal variations, medications, and systemic disease can also influence periodontal health.

Periodontal disease usually progresses painlessly but may present as swollen gingival tissue or gingival bleeding. Treatment is directed at slowing or arresting the progression of disease primarily by the removal of plaque and its by-products.[1] Antibiotics may play a role in treatment. Referral to a dentist for definitive treatment is indicated because the treatment involves extensive dental cleaning, instruction and improvement in oral hygiene, and in some cases, periodontal surgery.

Gingival and Periodontal Abscess A *gingival abscess* is an acutely painful swelling confined to the margin of the gingiva or interdental papilla. It usually rapidly enlarges over 24 to 48 hours, and purulent exudate can frequently be expressed from the orifice. The most common etiology is the entrapment of foreign matter such as a popcorn kernel, piece of meat, toothbrush bristle, or piece of food in the gingiva. Treatment includes identifying and removing the embedded foreign body and irrigating with normal saline. Continued home irrigation is beneficial, and symptoms resolve quickly.[3]

When plaque and debris are entrapped in the periodontal pocket, a *periodontal abscess* may form, resulting in severe pain. Small periodontal abscesses respond to local therapy with warm saline rinses and antibiotics such as penicillin VK, 500 milligrams PO four times a day, or clindamycin, 300 milligrams PO four times a day. Larger periodontal abscesses require incision and drainage. Chlorhexidine 0.12% mouth rinses twice daily are useful in the short term. Provide analgesia with NSAIDs or narcotics as indicated.[3]

Acute Necrotizing Ulcerative Gingivitis *Acute necrotizing ulcerative gingivitis* is an aggressively destructive process (**Figure 245-6**). Also known as *Vincent's disease* or *trench mouth*, it is part of a spectrum of disease ranging from localized ulceration of the gingiva to often fatal noma, in which localized ulceration and necrosis spread to the adjacent tissues of the cheeks, lips, and underlying facial bones.[10] The diagnostic triad includes pain, ulcerated or "punched out" interdental papillae, and gingival bleeding. Secondary signs include fetid breath, pseudomembrane formation, "wooden teeth" feeling, foul metallic taste, tooth mobility, lymphadenopathy, fever, and malaise.[3,10]

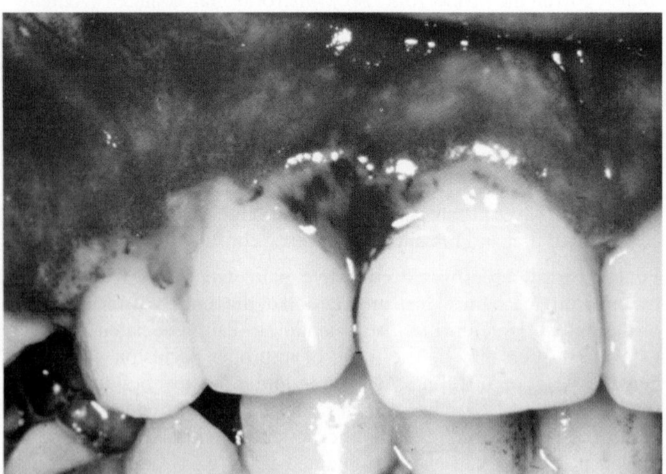

FIGURE 245-6. Acute necrotizing ulcerative gingivitis. [Image used with permission of Philip J. Hanes.]

The differential diagnosis for acute necrotizing ulcerative gingivitis is quite extensive, but herpes gingivostomatitis is the most difficult to differentiate. Herpes gingivostomatitis usually has smaller vesicular eruptions, less bleeding, more systemic signs, and lack of interdental papilla involvement.[10]

The cause is still poorly understood. Acute necrotizing ulcerative gingivitis appears to be an opportunistic infection in a host with lowered resistance. Anaerobic bacteria such as *Treponema*, *Selenomonas*, *Fusobacterium*, and *Prevotella* invade otherwise healthy tissue, resulting in an aggressively destructive disease process.[10,11] The most important predisposing factor is human immunodeficiency virus infection. A previous episode of necrotizing gingivitis is the second most important predisposing factor. Other contributing factors include poor oral hygiene, unusual emotional stress, poor diet and malnutrition, inadequate sleep, Caucasian descent, age <21 years old, poor socioeconomic status, recent illness, alcohol use, tobacco use, acatalasia, and various infections such as malaria, measles, and intestinal parasites.[10,11]

Treatment consists primarily of bacterial control. Chlorhexidine 0.12% oral rinses twice a day, professional debridement and scaling, and adjunctive antibiotic therapy with metronidazole, 500 milligrams PO three times a day, are the mainstay of treatment. Reduction in pain can be expected within 24 hours of institution of this regimen. Identification and resolution of the predisposing factors and supportive therapy with a soft diet rich in protein, vitamins, and fluids are important in establishing and maintaining a disease-free state.[10,11]

Peri-Implantitis Osseointegrated dental implants have become common over the last 30 years, allowing for a dental implant to replace a tooth. However, as with any procedure, complications do occur, and problems related to implants may present to the ED. Pathologic changes around an implant are all given the general term of *peri-implant disease*. Patients who present with *peri-implantitis* present with a similar presentation to that of a periodontal abscess and require similar treatment. Gentle removal of the plaque and debris from around the implant and irrigation with normal saline or 0.12% chlorhexidine solution should be done. Antibiotic treatment with metronidazole, 500 milligrams PO three times a day for 10 days, or amoxicillin, 500 milligrams PO three times a day for 10 days, is indicated. Give analgesia as needed, and refer to a dentist for definitive care.[3]

NEUROGENIC AND NEUROPHYSIOLOGIC SYNDROMES

Craniofacial Neuralgias *Trigeminal neuralgia* is the most common of the craniofacial neuralgias. Other significantly less common neuralgias of the craniofacial region include *glossopharyngeal neuralgia*, *vagal neuralgia*, and *superior laryngeal neuralgia* involving the respective nerve distributions. Post–herpes zoster–related neuralgia is also a cause of acute facial pain and may become chronic in nature. See chapter 165, "Headache" for further discussion.

Bell's Palsy (Idiopathic Facial Nerve Palsy) *Bell's palsy* is a peripheral unilateral weakness of the facial nerve of unknown etiology. As part of the differential diagnosis for orofacial pain, patients with a facial nerve palsy related to herpes zoster may present with nonspecific facial pain prior to the onset of weakness or the onset of any visible vesicles. In such cases, this diagnosis must be considered. See chapter 243 for a more extensive discussion on facial nerve palsy.

Temporomandibular Disorder *Temporomandibular disorder* is a common cause of facial pain and headache representing a group of signs and symptoms that involve the muscles of mastication or the temporomandibular joint. See chapter 243 for a more extensive discussion.

SOFT TISSUE LESIONS OF THE ORAL CAVITY

APHTHOUS STOMATITIS

Aphthous stomatitis, or ulceration, is one of the most common oral lesions, affecting 20% of the normal population (**Figure 245-7**). The cause appears to be a cell-mediated immune response to a yet unidentified triggering agent. Multiple factors predispose to aphthous ulcer formation: local trauma, stress, poor sleep, a hormonal imbalance, smoking, and certain foods such as chocolate, coffee, peanuts, cereals, almonds, strawberries, cheese, tomatoes, and gluten. Aphthous ulceration involves the nonkeratinized epithelium, especially the labial and buccal mucosa, and begins as an erythematous macule that ulcerates and forms a central fibropurulent eschar. Aphthous stomatitis occurs in a major and minor form. *Minor aphthae* usually measure from 2 to 3 mm to several centimeters in diameter, are painful, and frequently are multiple. They usually resolve spontaneously in 10 to 14 days. *Major aphthae* have larger, deeper ulcers that take significantly longer to heal. A third form, called *herpetiform aphthae*, has up to 100 ulcers, each 1 to 2 mm in diameter. They tend to coalesce, creating much larger ulcers that require 10 to 14 days to heal. Treatment is symptomatic but, in severe cases, may consist of topical corticosteroids such as Orobase® (Colgate Oral Pharmaceuticals, Canton, MA) or 0.01% dexamethasone elixir as a mouth rinse. Resolution typically occurs quickly after onset of therapy. Major aphthae are more resistant to therapy and may require intralesional steroid injection or systemic steroid therapy.[12,13]

HERPES ZOSTER AND OTHER INFECTIONS

Herpes zoster (see chapter 153, "Serious Viral Infections") frequently occurs along the distribution of the trigeminal nerve. Herpes zoster typically begins as a 1- to 4-day prodrome of exquisite pain in the area innervated by the affected nerve and may be mistaken for a simple headache or toothache. Vesicular eruptions characteristically occur unilaterally, do not cross the midline, and last 7 to 10 days. Isolated intraoral lesions can occur but are not common. Involvement of the ophthalmic branch of the trigeminal nerve requires urgent ophthalmologic consultation.

Other common infections such herpes simplex type 1 and 2, herpangina, hand-foot-and-mouth disease, and varicella-zoster cause painful ulcerative lesions of the oral cavity and perioral region. These conditions are adequately discussed in chapter 121, "Mouth and Throat Disorders in Infants and Children." Many sexually transmitted infections can affect the oral cavity. In general, the appearance of oral lesions is similar in appearance to that of their genital counterpart. Treatment of sexually transmitted diseases of the oral cavity is the same as for genital involvement. See chapter 149, "Sexually Transmitted Infections," for detailed discussion.

TRAUMATIC ULCERS

Traumatic ulcers are a result of direct trauma to epithelial tissue. Common sources of trauma include rough or jagged edges on teeth or restorations, ill-fitting dentures, oral hygiene mishaps, and burns to the hard or soft palate secondary to hot foods. Removal of persistent sources of trauma is essential; otherwise, treatment is palliative.

MEDICATION-RELATED SOFT TISSUE ABNORMALITIES

Gingival hyperplasia is associated with many commonly used medications (**Figure 245-8**). Approximately 50% of patients on phenytoin will develop significant gingival hyperplasia. Many other medications, such as cyclosporine and calcium channel blockers, especially nifedipine, cause gingival hyperplasia. Concomitant use of two such medications results in accelerated gingival proliferation. Enlargement begins in the interdental papillae. The clinical and histologic characteristics of gingival hyperplasia related to phenytoin, cyclosporine, and calcium channel blockers appear to be identical. The clinical appearance of the gingival tissue depends on oral hygiene and secondary inflammation. In the absence of inflammation, gingival proliferation results in dense tissue, normal in coloration, with a smooth, stippled, or granular texture. Inflammation causes edematous changes and an erythematous coloration. Inflamed tissue bleeds readily. Histologically, an increase in collagen fibers, fibroblasts, and glycosaminoglycans is seen. Epithelial acanthosis also occurs. Although the cause of drug-related gingival hyperplasia is unclear, poor oral hygiene clearly increases its likelihood and severity. Treatment includes fastidious oral hygiene to slow the hyperplasia and gingivectomy in advanced cases.

Many other medications are known to cause abnormalities of the oral mucosa or dental structures. Allergic mucositis, erythema multiforme, and fixed drug-type reactions are examples. Xerostomia and associated mucosal alterations are a side effect of many medications such as anticholinergics, antidepressants, and antihistamines.[1] Stomatitis and mucosal ulcerations from chemotherapeutic agents are also common.

LESIONS OF THE TONGUE

Many systemic conditions and local stimuli affect the appearance of the tongue. Many systemic conditions, various vitamins deficiencies, and iron-deficiency anemia cause atrophy of the filiform papillae, resulting in a smooth erythematous appearance. Occurrence of ectopic thyroid tissue on the midline posterior portion of the tongue is called a *lingual thyroid* and is a common finding. Some common conditions affecting the tongue are discussed below.

Benign Migratory Glossitis Geographic tongue, or benign migratory glossitis, is a common benign finding on oral examination, occurring in

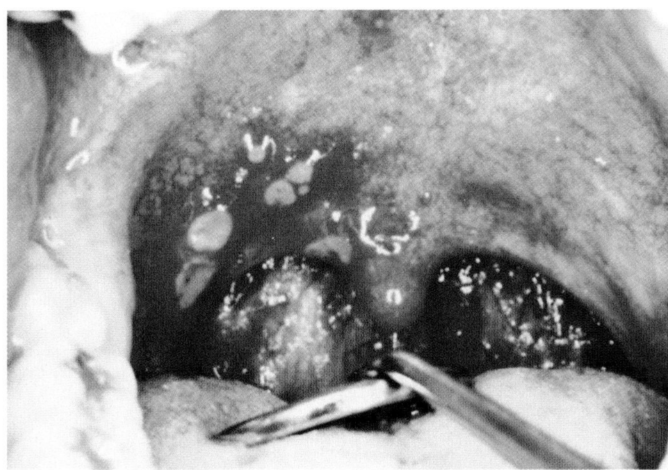

FIGURE 245-7. Aphthous stomatitis. [Image used with permission of Baldev Singh.]

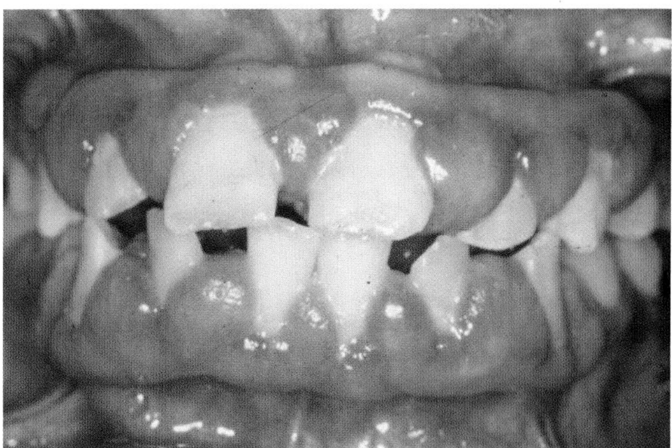

FIGURE 245-8. Gingival hyperplasia (overgrowth) secondary to phenytoin (Dilantin). [Used with permission of Philip J. Hanes.]

1% to 3% of the population. Females are affected twice as often as males. The typically multiple, well-demarcated zones of erythema on the tongue are caused by atrophy of the filiform papillae. The lesions concentrate on the tip and lateral borders of the tongue and heal in several days, only to quickly reappear in other areas. These lesions usually are asymptomatic; however, a burning sensation or sensitivity to hot or spicy foods has been described. The cause is unknown, but fluctuations with stress and menstrual cycle occur. Generally, treatment is not indicated because this entity is benign. Reassurance of patients is usually sufficient. In patients in whom discomfort is a major factor, oral topical steroids such as fluocinonide gel applied several times daily may provide relief.[14]

Strawberry Tongue Strawberry tongue is associated with erythrogenic, toxin-producing *Streptococcus pyogenes*. Clinically, the tongue has prominent red spots on a white-coated background. Microscopically, the fungiform papillae are hyperemic with a smooth glossy surface. Treatment is with antibiotics directed at group A streptococci.

LEUKOPLAKIA AND ERYTHROPLAKIA

Leukoplakia is a white patch or plaque that cannot be scraped off and cannot be classified as any other disease. Leukoplakia is the most common oral precancer; however, only 2% to 4% of leukoplakic lesions show dysplastic changes. The cause is unknown, but tobacco, alcohol, ultraviolet radiation, candidiasis, human papillomavirus, tertiary syphilis, and trauma have all been implicated. The most common intraoral site involved is the buccal mucosa. Other sites of involvement include the hard and soft palates, maxillary gingiva, and lip mucosa. Biopsy is mandatory for all persistent leukoplakic lesions. Leukoplakic lesions of the floor of the mouth, tongue, and vermilion border are most likely associated with malignancy. Lesions demonstrating dysplastic changes warrant removal.[15]

Erythroplakia is defined as a red patch that similarly cannot be clinically or pathologically characterized as any other disease. Although erythroplakia is far less common than leukoplakia, it has a greater potential for dysplastic changes.

ORAL CANCER

Oral cancer accounts for 2% to 4% of the cancers in the United States. More than 90% of all oral malignancies are squamous cell carcinoma (**Figure 245-9**).[15] Lymphomas, Kaposi's sarcoma, and melanoma comprise most of the remainder. Several intrinsic and extrinsic etiologic factors for oral squamous cell carcinoma have been identified. Extrinsic factors include tobacco use, especially chewing tobacco or snuff; excessive alcohol consumption; and sunlight exposure. Intrinsic factors include general malnutrition and chronic iron-deficiency anemia. Oral candidiasis, especially the hyperplastic form, immunosuppressive states such as human immunodeficiency virus infection, and oncogenic viruses such as human papillomavirus, herpes simplex virus, and various adenoviruses and retroviruses may play some role in the etiology of oral cancer.

Oral squamous cell carcinoma has four common morphologic presentations. It can be exophytic, with an irregular surface, or ulcerative, with irregular depressions and rolled borders. Malignant leukoplakic and erythroplakic lesions are believed to represent squamous cell carcinomas that have yet to form a mass or ulcerate.

The most common site involved in oral cancer is the tongue, particularly the posterolateral border, accounting for 50% of the oral cancers in the United States.[15] Cancer of the floor of the mouth accounts for nearly 35%. Cancer of the lips is common and usually secondary to sunlight exposure. Oral cancer is generally painless, and patients are often unaware of the presence of a mass until it is advanced. Oral cancer is usually firm, may bleed from ulceration, and have a history of poor healing. There may be associated firm lymphadenopathy. Early diagnosis is the key to successful treatment of oral squamous cell carcinoma. All ulcers, erythroplakic lesions, and leukoplakic lesions of the oral cavity that do not respond to palliative treatment in 10 to 14 days warrant biopsy. Treatment depends on site of involvement and staging of disease.

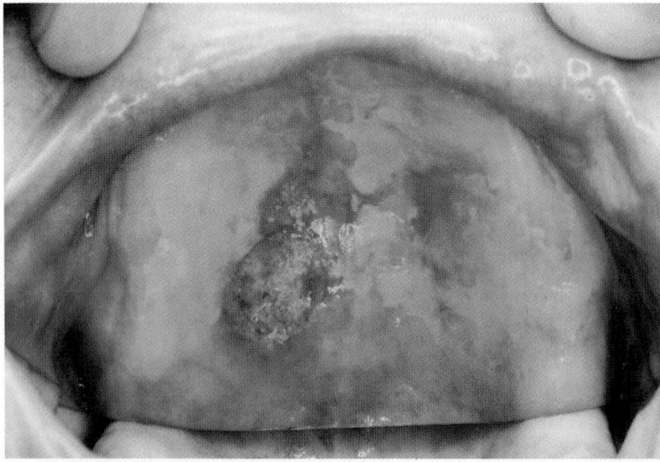

FIGURE 245-9. Oral squamous cell carcinoma of the hard palate. [Image used with permission of H. Anthony Neal.]

DENTOALVEOLAR TRAUMA

Management of dentoalveolar trauma depends on the extent of tooth and alveolar involvement, the degree of development of the apex of the tooth, and the age of the patient. In injuries in younger patients, especially those who are <12 years of age, the pulp of anterior teeth is quite large, and dental fractures involving the pulp are common. Fortunately, in this age group, the apex of the root also is usually incompletely formed, allowing for a greater pulpal regenerative capability. As one ages, more dentin is formed. Thus, in older patients, the pulp chamber may be very small and pulpal exposure highly unlikely. Involvement of the root of the tooth compromises the attachment apparatus and makes it difficult to restore the tooth to function.

DENTAL FRACTURES

The International Association of Dental Traumatology system divides dental trauma into eight categories: enamel infraction, enamel fracture, enamel-dentin fracture, enamel-dentin-pulp fracture, crown-root fracture without pulp exposure, crown-root fracture with pulp exposure, root fracture, and alveolar bone fracture (**Figure 245-10**). The International Association of Dental Traumatology has developed guidelines to aid dentists and other healthcare professionals in the management of each these categories.[16]

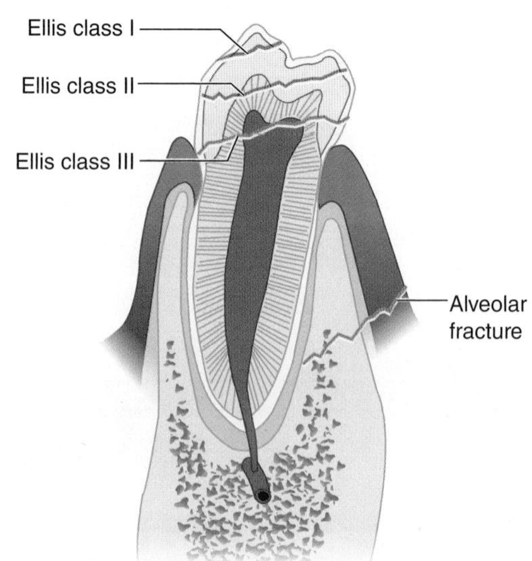

FIGURE 245-10. The International Association of Dental Traumatology classification of dental fractures.

The goal of the emergency treatment of a fractured tooth is maintaining pulpal vitality and completion of the formation of the root and apex of the tooth. The proximity of the fracture to the pulp and the length of time before treatment, as well as other associated injuries, are most important in determining outcome. Treatment is aimed at sealing the dentinal tubules and creating a barrier between the dental pulp and the oral environment. In properly treated uncomplicated dental fractures, 1% to 3% of the affected pulps undergo necrosis. Because pulpal necrosis is a process, it can occur at any time after trauma, and serial follow-up with a dentist is recommended.[16]

A fracture of the crown of the tooth can involve any part of the enamel, dentin, and pulp of the tooth. *Infraction* is the least serious type dental injury and essentially is a crack in the enamel of the tooth without loss of structure. This can be obvious or quite subtle. No emergency treatment is needed.

Enamel fractures do not extend into the dentin of the tooth (**Figure 245-11**). Generally, no emergency treatment is indicated, except to smooth sharp corners that may irritate the tongue or mucosa. If the enamel fragment is recovered and kept moist, the patient's dentist can bond it back in place. If the fragment was not recovered, soft tissue radiographs of any oral lacerations are necessary to rule out foreign bodies. Referral to a general dentist for aesthetic repair depends on the degree of cosmetic concern of the patient.[16]

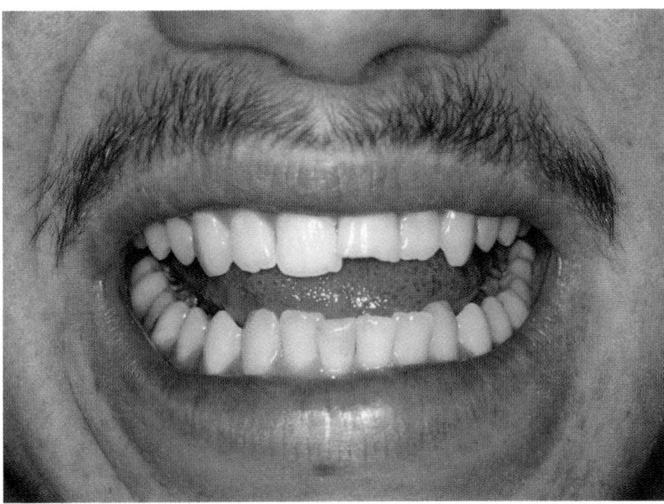

A

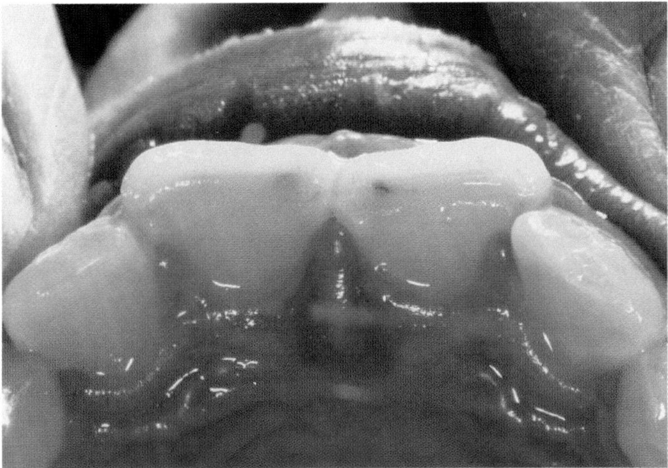

B

FIGURE 245-11. International Association of Dental Traumatology classification for fractures of teeth (clinical). **A.** Enamel fracture. **B.** Enamel-dentin fracture of the central incisor on the left in the photograph (notice the pink blush of the pulp through the thin layer of dentin), and an enamel-dentin-pulp fracture of the central incisor on the right in the photograph. [Image used with permission of Felicity K. Hardwick.]

Enamel-dentin fractures involve the dentin of the tooth and require intervention (Figure 245-11). These fractures account for 70% of tooth fractures. Generally, patients experience sensitivity to hot or cold stimuli as well as air passing over the exposed surface during breathing. The enamel-dentin fracture can be identified both by the patient's symptoms and visualization of exposed dentin, which is a creamy yellow color compared with the whiter enamel. Because dentin is microtubular in structure, communication with the oral environment or desiccation from mouth breathing initiates an inflammatory response in the dental pulp. The thickness of remaining dentin determines the rate of pulpal contamination. Greater than 2 mm of remaining dentin is felt to offer some protection to the pulpal tissue. A delay in treatment of more than 24 to 48 hours increases the likelihood of pulpal necrosis. The ED goal is the identification of a fracture. If definitive treatment cannot be assured in 1 to 2 days, then cover the exposed dentin to decrease likelihood of pulpal injury. This is best achieved using glass ionomer dental cement that is easily mixed according to the manufacturer's instructions and carefully applied to the dried exposed dentin (DenTemp®, Majestic Drug Co., South Fallsburg, NY; and others). If the dentin layer is less than 0.5 mm and the pulp can be seen as a pink area without bleeding, then first place a thin layer of calcium hydroxide base (Dycal®, Dentsply International, York, PA) followed by glass ionomer, as described above, to further protect the dental pulp. Referral to a dentist for definitive treatment is important.[16]

In *enamel-dentin-pulp* fractures, exposure of the pulp has occurred (Figure 245-11). On wiping the fractured surface dry with sterile gauze, blood originating from the pulp of the tooth is easily identified. After carefully controlling pulpal bleeding with sterile gauze or a cotton pellet, cover the exposed pulp with a calcium hydroxide base (Dycal®, Dentsply International, York, PA), and then cover this and the remaining exposed dentin with glass ionomer cement as in enamel-dentin fractures until urgent dental evaluation can occur. If the pulpal exposure is extremely small, placing a calcium hydroxide base and glass ionomer is adequate until dental evaluation. For all but the smallest pulpal exposures, definitive treatment is some kind of endodontic or root canal therapy. Oral analgesics should be prescribed and topical analgesics avoided.[16]

Crown-root fractures and *root fractures* are an uncommon consequence of dental trauma. The coronal segment of the tooth may be displaced or simply mobile. Tenderness to percussion is usual. With any dental trauma, careful attention must be paid to identifying fractures of the root, as they can be clinically obscure and dental radiographs from several angles may be necessary to identify these fractures. This, however, is beyond the scope of most EDs. Crown-root fractures may or may not involve the pulp. Emergency treatment consists of stabilizing the coronal segment until definitive treatment can be arranged. In isolated root fracture, the pulp is always involved. Healing of stabilized root fractures has been reported; thus, current recommendations are to reposition the coronal segment to its original position, confirm that position by radiograph, if available, and then stabilize with a flexible splint as described below for luxation injuries. Dental follow-up within 24 to 48 is important, as splinting for a minimum of 4 weeks is required. In the ED, where oral surgical or dental consultation may not be readily available, extraction of an extremely mobile coronal segment of the tooth may be required to prevent possible aspiration. If less than one third of the root is involved, a dentist can perform root canal therapy, and restoration of the tooth may be possible.[16,17]

LUXATION INJURIES

The same forces that cause dental fractures may result in loosening of a tooth from the attachment apparatus. Careful evaluation of the teeth for tenderness, malpositioning, or mobility must be performed. Luxations account for nearly 50% of injuries to teeth. There are six types of luxations: concussion, subluxation, extrusive luxation, lateral luxation, intrusive luxation, and avulsion.[16]

Concussion is injury to the supporting structures of a tooth with clinical tenderness to percussion but no mobility. *Subluxation* is injury resulting in mobility without clinical or radiographic evidence of dislodgment of the tooth. *Extrusive luxation* is partial or total disruption of the periodontal ligament resulting in a partial dislodgment of a tooth from the alveolar bone. *Lateral luxation* is displacement of a tooth labially (toward the lip) or lingually (toward the tongue) with concomitant fracture of the alveolar bone. *Intrusive luxation* is displacement of a tooth into its socket with associated periodontal ligament damage and alveolar bone contusion and fracture. Treatment of luxations depends on the tooth involved, the severity of injury, and the presence of associated root fracture and/or significant associated alveolar fracture.[16]

Concussions A concussive injury to a tooth is minor. The degree of tenderness to percussion determines the treatment. Stabilizing the tooth by splinting it to adjacent teeth is not indicated. Management of pain with NSAIDs, soft diet, and referral to a dentist to confirm the diagnosis and exclude more severe injury is the most appropriate course of action for the emergency physician.[16]

Luxations *Subluxation* represents a more significant injury and is associated with a higher incidence of subsequent pulpal necrosis. Clinically, tooth mobility and some bleeding along the gingiva may be noted. A subluxed tooth generally does not require splinting.[16]

An *extrusive luxation* requires repositioning the tooth to its original position and splinting to stabilize the tooth during healing. Ideally, dental radiographs should be obtained prior to repositioning the tooth to ensure that there is not a fracture of the root of the tooth, but in most EDs, this may not be possible, and repositioning and stabilizing should be attempted regardless. Repositioning the tooth may require local anesthesia. Firm, gentle pressure usually will reposition the tooth. If a clot has formed apical to the tooth, then more aggressive manipulation may be required. A flexible wire splint placed by a dentist provides ideal stabilization.[16] In the ED, a temporary splint with a noneugenol zinc oxide periodontal dressing (Coe-Pak™, GC America Inc., Alsip, IL; or ZONE Periopak®, DUX Dental, Oxnard, CA) (**Figure 245-12**) is acceptable. Avoid excess material placement, especially on the occlusal surface, because interference in occlusion will place stress on the tooth during mastication. Other treatment options include wire splinting, bondable reinforcement ribbon, calcium hydroxide paste, and light cured composite.[18] The patient should see a dentist or oral and maxillofacial surgeon within 24 hours.

A *lateral luxation* represents a more extensive injury and is associated with fracture of the surrounding alveolar bone. Repositioning of the tooth is generally more difficult. It usually can be accomplished by manipulating the displaced tooth with the thumb and forefinger. Once the apex has been dislodged from its locked-in position labially, apically directed axial pressure will reposition the tooth. Intra-arch stabilization is necessary for a minimum of 4 weeks. Temporary splinting with a periodontal dressing is acceptable if a minimal associated alveolar fracture occurred. Otherwise, splinting by an oral and maxillofacial surgeon or general dentist in the ED is mandatory.[16]

Intrusive luxations are the most serious because significant damage to the alveolar socket and periodontal ligament occurs. Root resorption is common as a result of damage to the periodontal ligament. Recommended treatment is allowing the tooth to erupt on its own or to orthodontically extrude the tooth if no eruption is noted by 3 weeks.[16]

All patients who sustain luxation injuries should be instructed to maintain a soft diet for at least 2 weeks. Meticulous oral hygiene is essential. Twice daily rinsing with chlorhexidine 0.12% mouth rinse is helpful. Referral to a dentist for close follow-up is indicated.

Avulsions

Tooth Replantation and Care at the Scene **Total displacement of a tooth from its socket, or *avulsion*, represents up to 16% of all dental injuries and is a true dental emergency.[19]** Replantation at the scene is the treatment of choice because the long-term prognosis for the replanted tooth is highly time dependent. Ideally, the patient or a healthcare provider at the scene should perform this procedure. Handling only the crown portion

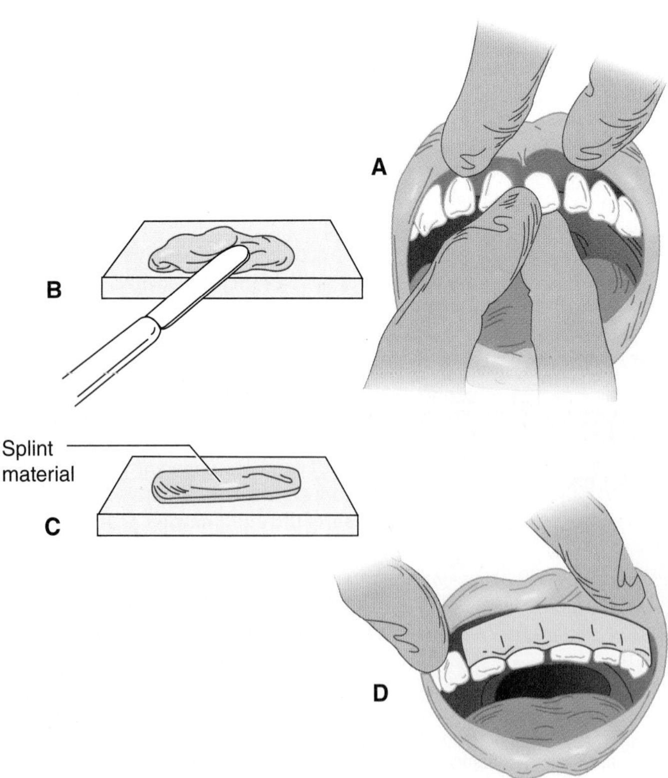

FIGURE 245-12. Temporary stabilization of a replanted or repositioned tooth. **A.** Tooth is repositioned back into its original position in the socket. **B.** Splint material is mixed thoroughly. **C.** Splint material is shaped and made ready for application. **D.** Packing is molded over repositioned tooth and two adjacent teeth to each side.

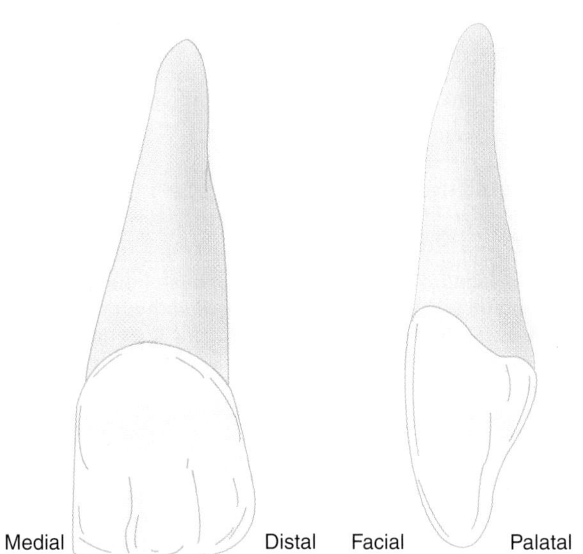

FIGURE 245-13. Illustration of a maxillary left central incisor. Note that the part of the tooth facing medially comes to more of a right angle at the incisal edge (biting edge) than occurs distally. The facial portion of the tooth is more convex.

of the tooth, gently rinse the tooth for a maximum of 10 seconds with sterile normal saline or tap water to remove debris. Then replace it immediately into the socket. Anterior teeth are most commonly affected, and **Figure 245-13** illustrates the morphology of the maxillary central incisor to assist replantation in the proper orientation. Early improper replantation holds a higher success rate for tooth salvage than delayed replantation resulting from waiting for arrival at the ED or for an oral and maxillofacial surgeon.[19]

If immediate replantation is not possible, or if the risk of aspiration is high, such as in a child or a patient with a decreased level of consciousness, then transport the tooth with the patient to the ED. Acceptable transport media include isotonic solutions such as Hank's balanced salt solution, sterile saline, milk, and saliva. Commercial preparations of Hank's balanced salt solution such as Save-A-Tooth® (Phoenix-Lazerus, Inc., Pottstown, PA) and EMT Tooth Saver™ (Smart Practice, Phoenix, AZ) are available and come with a useful transport container as part of the system. If the avulsed tooth was not recovered, obtain radiographs to ensure that the tooth was not aspirated.[19]

Survival of the periodontal ligament fibers that remain attached to the root of an avulsed tooth is key to successful replantation. Milk is an acceptable storage medium because of its osmolarity and essential concentration of calcium and magnesium ions. Hank's balanced salt solution, a pH-balanced cell culture medium, is the best transport medium and maintains periodontal ligament cell viability for up to 4 to 6 hours. Hank's solution can help to restore cell viability in a tooth that has been avulsed longer than 20 minutes.[19]

Tooth Replantation in the ED In the ED, before replantation, rinse the tooth root clean of dirt and debris with sterile saline or, preferably, Hank's balanced salt solution. Do not scrub the root of the tooth, and do not disrupt existing periodontal fibers. Handle only the crown of the tooth. If an avulsed tooth with an open apex has been dry for <20 minutes, then the prognosis for reestablishing a vital pulp is good. If the apex is completely closed and cannot be opened with saline irrigation, then revitalization is not possible. If the tooth has been dry from 20 to 60 minutes regardless of apices, soak the tooth in a physiologic solution while preparing to replant the tooth. Physiologic solution decreases the chance of ankylosis (fixation of the tooth to the underlying bone). For an avulsed tooth that has been dry for >60 minutes, the periodontal cells are dead, and the goal is to maintain alveolar bone contour and aesthetics; however, ankylosis, root resorption, and eventual tooth loss are the expected outcome. **Table 245-2** provides specific recommendations.[19]

Preparation of the dental socket plays little role in the success or failure of the replanted tooth. Prepare the socket by carefully removing the clot and gently irrigating with sterile normal saline. Avoid socket manipulation if possible. However, any fracture of the socket wall should be carefully repositioned with an appropriate instrument. Local anesthesia is usually required. Replantation is accomplished with firm pressure.

TABLE 245-2 Specific Recommendations for Replantation of Avulsed Teeth

Clinical Scenario	Treatment
Open apex	1. Gently irrigate the tooth root clean with sterile saline.
Moist tooth stored in acceptable media, and/or <60 min extra oral dry time	2. If available, cover root with minocycline hydrochloride microspheres (Arestin™, OraPharma, Inc.) or soak for 5 min in doxycycline solution (doxycycline, 1 milligram/20 mL saline). 3. Administer local anesthesia. 4. Remove coagulum from the socket with a stream of saline. Examine the socket. If there is a fracture of the socket wall, reposition it with an appropriate instrument. 5. Firmly replant tooth and verify the tooth position clinically and radiographically, if possible. 6. Flexible splint for up to 2 wk.
Open apex	1. Remove from tooth attached necrotic soft tissue carefully with gauze.
Extra oral dry time >60 min or other reason suggesting nonviable cells	2. If available, immerse tooth in 2% stannous fluoride solution for 20 min. 3. Administer local anesthesia. 4. Remove coagulum from the socket with a stream of saline. Examine the socket. If there is a fracture of the socket wall, reposition it with an appropriate instrument. 5. Firmly replant tooth and verify the tooth's position clinically and radiographically, if possible. 6. Flexible splint for up to 4 wk.
Closed apex	1. Gently irrigate the tooth root clean with sterile saline.
Moist tooth stored in acceptable media, and/or <60 min extra oral dry time	2. Administer local anesthesia. 3. Remove coagulum from the socket with a stream of saline. Examine the socket. If there is a fracture of the socket wall, reposition it with an appropriate instrument. 4. Firmly replant tooth and verify the tooth's position clinically and radiographically, if possible 5. Flexible splint for up to 2 wk.
Closed apex	1. Remove from tooth attached necrotic soft tissue carefully with gauze.
Extra oral dry time >60 min or other reason suggesting nonviable cells	2. If available, immerse tooth in 2% stannous fluoride solution for 20 min. 3. Administer local anesthesia. 4. Remove coagulum from the socket with a stream of saline. Examine the socket. If there is a fracture of the socket wall, reposition it with an appropriate instrument. 5. Firmly replant tooth and verify the tooth's position clinically and radiographically, if possible. 6. Flexible splint for up to 4 wk.

Having the patient bite on gauze until more permanent stabilization can be arranged is acceptable. Some form of stabilization of the tooth in the ED such as a periodontal dressing (Figure 245-12) is necessary until follow-up with an oral and maxillofacial surgeon.[18,19]

All patients need antibiotics. Doxycycline, 100 milligrams PO twice a day, is the preferred antibiotic choice. For children <12 years old, penicillin VK PO four times a day (12.5 milligrams/kg/dose) is acceptable. Tetanus prophylaxis is necessary if the tooth has been contaminated by soil and the tetanus status is uncertain. Posttreatment instructions for most dental trauma are essentially the same. Patient should be instructed to maintain a soft diet for 2 weeks, brush carefully with a soft toothbrush after each meal, and use chlorhexidine 0.12% mouth rinse twice a day.[19]

Sequelae of Luxation Injuries Posttraumatic sequelae are variable. Pulp canal obliteration, pulpal necrosis, internal and external resorption of the root, and ankylosis may occur. The severity of luxation or avulsion is the most important determining factor in sequela occurrence. Transient apical breakdown occurs with all type of luxations but is especially common with extrusive and lateral luxations and avulsions. More than 50% of extrusively luxated teeth undergo pulpal necrosis within 1.5 years of the traumatic event. Close dental follow-up is essential for early identification of these sequelae.

Significant force must occur to dislodge or fracture teeth; consequently, associated **alveolar ridge fracture** is common. Care to ensure the integrity of the maxilla and mandible is also important. Stabilization of repositioned alveolar segments and associated teeth is essential for optimal results. This is best accomplished with flexible fixation placed by a general dentist or oral surgeon. Stabilization is maintained for up to 4 weeks depending on the severity of the involvement of alveolar bone. With significant alveolar ridge fracture, segments may require intermaxillary stabilization for up to 6 weeks in order to ensure adequate healing.[19]

Luxation Injuries of Primary Teeth Avulsion or luxation injuries of primary teeth are treated differently from those of permanent teeth. In patients age 6 to 12 years old, dentition is mixed, so it is very important to distinguish primary from permanent teeth. Avulsed primary teeth are never replanted. Most luxation injuries in children require no treatment and heal spontaneously. However, severe luxations of primary teeth generally require extraction of the tooth. Repositioning or replanting primary teeth risks injuring the underlying permanent teeth and thus is avoided. Intruded primary teeth are generally left alone to re-erupt into normal position. Because of the risk of damage to the permanent dentition, unless there is occlusal interference or the risk of aspiration, a dentist should manage most complicated luxation injuries of primary teeth. Referral to a general dentist for follow-up is essential to ensure optimal long-term outcome.[20]

SOFT TISSUE TRAUMA

ORAL CAVITY MUCOSAL LACERATIONS

Traumatic injuries to the soft tissue of the oral cavity are common and can involve any of the soft tissues of the mouth. Appropriate treatment remains an area of controversy. Generally, because of the vascularity of the oral tissue, lacerations of the mouth heal quickly. See the "Intraoral Mucosal Laceration" section of chapter 42, "Face and Scalp Lacerations" for management recommendations. Lacerations involving the cheek or buccal mucosa must be examined carefully for involvement of Stensen's duct, which drains the parotid salivary gland (the duct opens into the mouth opposite the upper second molar). If Stensen's duct is compromised, repair by an oral and maxillofacial surgeon or otorhinolaryngologist is indicated. Likewise, lacerations to the floor of the mouth require careful evaluation for involvement of Wharton's duct of the submandibular salivary glands.

LIP LACERATIONS

Lip lacerations are a potential cosmetic problem, so careful closure is essential. (see chapter 42 for management recommendations).[21]

FRENULUM LACERATIONS

Laceration of the maxillary labial frenulum, unless unusually large, does not require repair. These lacerations can be very painful, so provide adequate analgesia. Because of the vascularity of adjacent tissue, lacerations to the lingual frenulum of the tongue usually do need to be repaired. An absorbable suture such as 4-0 chromic gut or Vicryl® is appropriate.

TONGUE LACERATIONS

Lacerations of the tongue require special consideration because bleeding and delayed swelling can compromise the airway. **Simple linear lacerations less than 1 cm involving the central portion of dorsal surface of the tongue and that do not gape open heal well without repair.** Except for the most extensive tongue lacerations, suturing does not necessarily improve outcome or reduce morbidity. All lacerations that bisect the tongue require repair. Partial amputations can be successfully replanted with the appropriate microsurgical techniques.[21]

Local anesthesia can be obtained by local infiltration or topically by placing 4% lidocaine-soaked gauze for 5 minutes on the laceration. Bilateral lingual nerve blocks can be used for lacerations of the anterior two thirds of the tongue that cross the midline. Repair of the tongue, especially in children, presents a special challenge, and many adjuncts such as a dental bite block or a Molt mouth prop can be helpful in keeping the mouth open. A piece of 4 × 4 gauze can be used to grasp the tongue, or a surgical towel clamps or a large caliber suture such as 0-silk or nylon placed through the anterior portion of the anesthetized tongue can facilitate retraction and control the tongue.[21]

When laceration repair is warranted, absorbable sutures such as 4-0 chromic gut or Vicryl should be used. Sutures should be placed so as to include the muscular layer and the superficial mucosal layers of the tongue. Wound edges should be approximated and closed very loosely to allow for swelling of the tongue, which can be significant. Placing a closed hemostat between the suture and the tongue while tying can help prevent overtightening of the suture. The constant motion of the tongue quickly unties sutures in the mouth so sutures should be tied with at least four square knots. If feasible, the sutures can also be placed so that the knots are buried into the wound. All patients should be instructed rinse several times daily with a saline or chlorhexidine 0.12% mouth rinse.[21]

DENTAL LOCAL ANESTHESIA TECHNIQUES

Competence in dental local anesthesia is a useful skill for the emergency provider. The maxillary teeth can be anesthetized using local infiltrative or supraperiosteal techniques, which are easily learned by reading.

ANATOMY

The trigeminal nerve is the largest cranial nerve, and although it has important motor function, it is primarily a sensory nerve (**Figure 245-14**). It divides into three main braches: the ophthalmic nerve, maxillary nerve, and mandibular nerve. The maxillary nerve provides sensory innervation to the maxilla and associated structures including the maxillary teeth and gingiva and oral mucous membranes. The third division, or mandibular nerve, is the largest of the three branches. The mandibular nerve has three main divisions. The first is the long buccal nerve that provides sensory innervation to the mucosa of cheek and buccal gingiva of the mandibular molars. The second is the lingual nerve that runs superficial to the internal pterygoid muscle and innervates the anterior two thirds of the tongue, lingual gingiva, and floor of the mouth. Finally, the largest branch is the inferior alveolar nerve, which accompanies the inferior alveolar vein and artery in a neurovascular bundle passing between the ramus of the mandible and the sphenomandibular ligament to enter the mandibular canal. It divides at the region of the premolars with the mental nerve exiting the mental foramen to innervate the soft tissue of the lip and chin, and the incisal nerve continuing within the mandibular canal to innervate the teeth and gingiva.

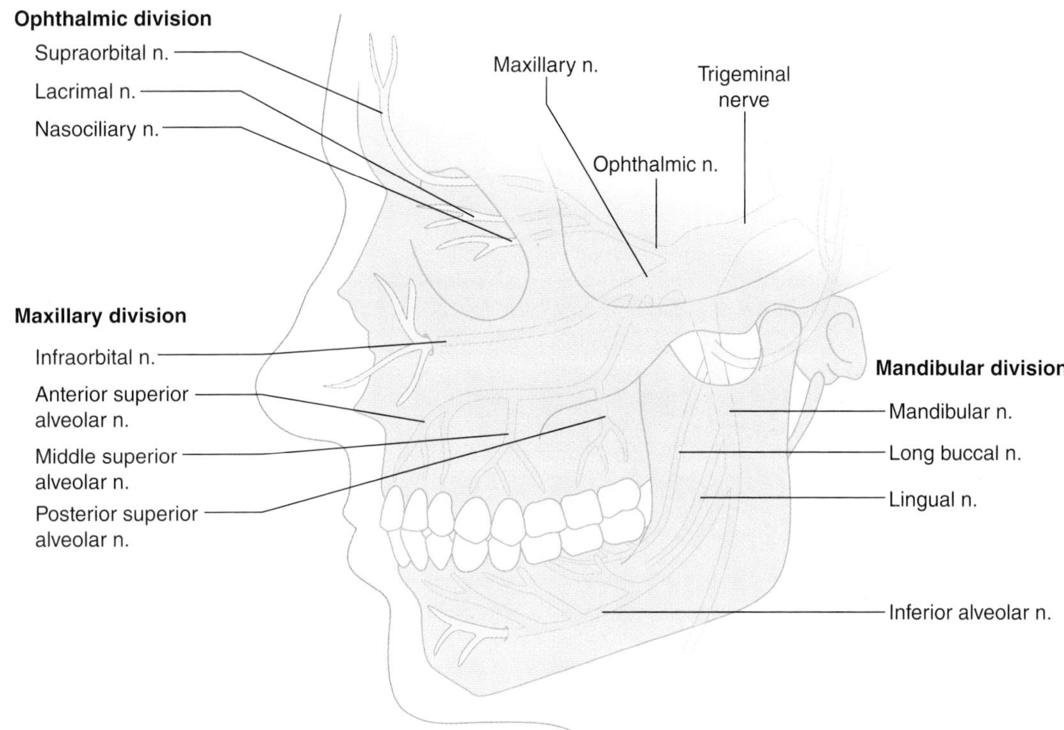

FIGURE 245-14. The trigeminal nerve and its three main divisions.

EQUIPMENT

Specialized equipment is useful when giving dental injections, especially the inferior alveolar nerve block. Equipment includes:

1. A monojet aspirating dental syringe
2. Dental cartridges of anesthetic solution
3. Disposable 27-gauge, 32-mm needle
4. Topical anesthetic, if possible

If an aspirating dental syringe is not available any 3-mm aspirating syringe can be used. With larger syringes, the inferior alveolar nerve block is difficult because the syringe barrel interferes with the proper positioning of the needle.

Position the patient in a dental chair or stretcher in a semi-reclined position with the head firmly against the headrest. Anticipate sudden movement of the patient. An overhead light is essential because dental injections require good visibility and control at all times to ensure safety of both the patient and the physician.

MAXILLARY INJECTIONS

Supraperiosteal Infiltration Maxillary cortical bone is thin and porous enough to allow the diffusion of anesthetic solution to reach the apex of the root and effectively anesthetize the tooth. **Figure 245-15** illustrates the supraperiosteal infiltration technique. The upper lip or cheek, depending on which tooth you are anesthetizing, is pulled up and taut. With the bevel facing toward the bone, the needle is inserted at the height of the buccal fold adjacent to the tooth. The needle should be directed along the long axis of the tooth and inserted to height of or slightly above the apex of the tooth. In most cases, the needle only needs to be inserted a few millimeters. Aspirate, and if negative, then slowly inject 0.5 to 1 mL of anesthetic solution. It is important to remember that the root of the canine is significantly longer than that of other teeth and that, in general, the roots of teeth are inclined in a distal direction. The goal is to deposit the anesthesia at or above the apex of the desired tooth.[22-24]

Palatal Injection

Supraperiosteal infiltration of the maxillary teeth provides adequate anesthesia for pain control for a toothache, but not for procedures such as management of a dry socket or avulsed tooth. This may also require anesthesia of the palatal tissue, which can simply be accomplished by local infiltrative anesthesia. With a fine-gauge needle, puncture the palatal mucosa about half way up the palate adjacent to the target tooth (**Figure 245-16**). Inject 0.1 mL of anesthetic solution. Blanching of the surrounding tissue is common, and this injection is usually quite uncomfortable. If a larger area of anesthesia is required, anesthesia of the anterior portion of the palate can be obtained by injecting anesthesia over the incisive foramen. The landmark is the incisive papilla. Anesthesia to the unilateral posterior portion of the palate can be obtained by injecting a small amount of anesthesia over the greater palatine foramen.[22-24]

MANDIBULAR INJECTIONS

In contrast to the maxilla where the cortex of overlying bone is relatively thin and infiltrative anesthesia is usually effective, the mandibular boney cortex is relatively thick and the inferior alveolar nerve block is usually required to gain adequate anesthesia of the mandibular molars and premolars. A mental nerve block, as described in chapter 36, "Local and Regional Anesthesia," can provide anesthesia for the premolars, canines, and incisors, as well as soft tissue of the lip and chin, when properly administered. The bone adjacent to the canines and incisors is thinner and more amenable to infiltrative anesthesia. Also, soft tissue anesthesia of the tongue can be obtained using the basics of the inferior alveolar nerve block. Injection of the long buccal nerve may be necessary for incision and drainage of dental abscesses in the mandibular molar region, and this technique will be described.

Inferior Alveolar Nerve Block (Direct Technique) The patient should be instructed to open the mouth widely to ensure good visualization of anatomic landmarks (**Figure 245-17**). First, the physician needs to palpate the greatest depth of the anterior border of the ramus or coronoid notch with the index finger or thumb. Then with that

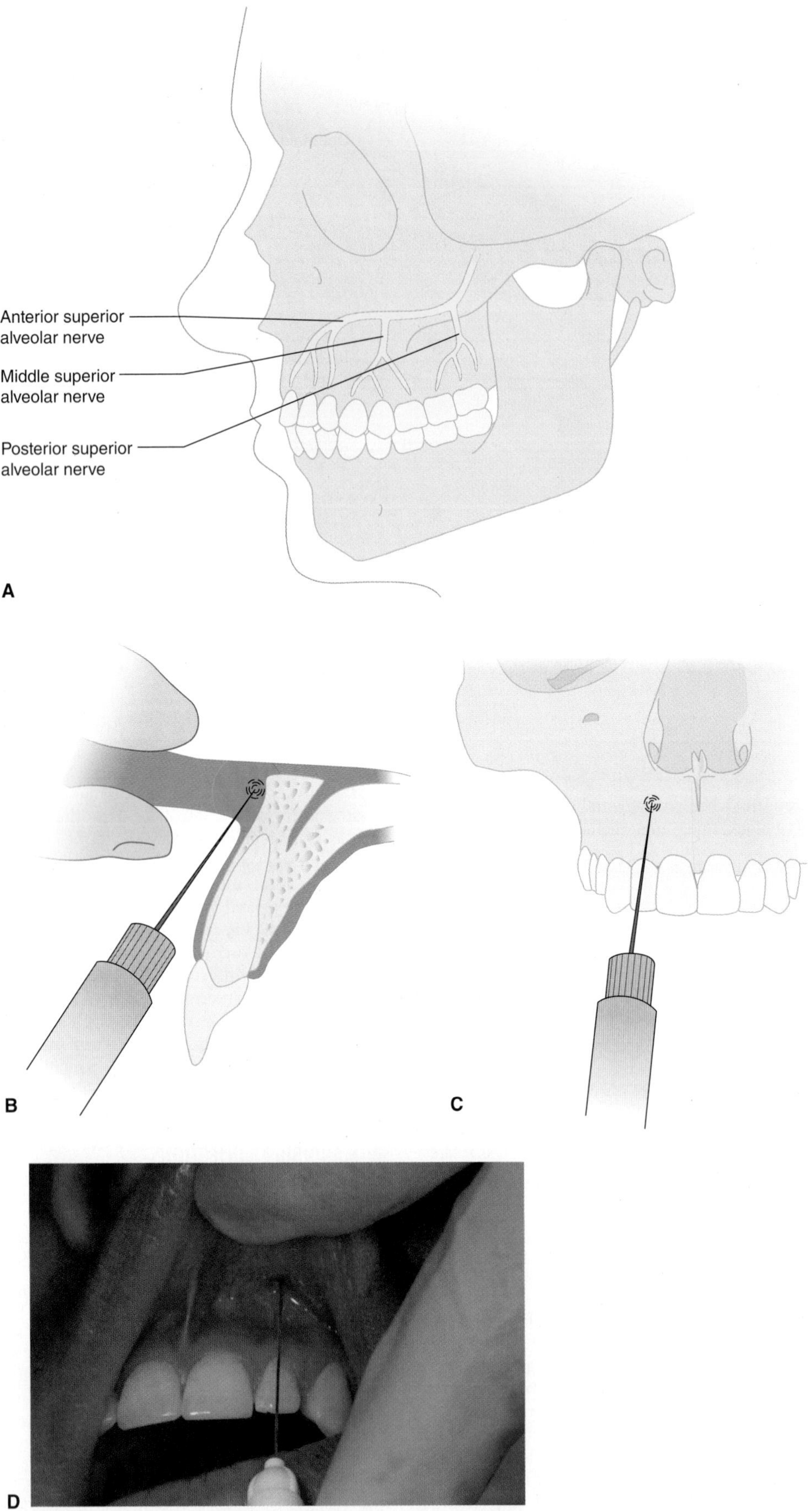

FIGURE 245-15. The supraperiosteal infiltration. **A.** The maxillary nerve and innervation of the maxillary teeth by the posterior superior alveolar nerve, the middle superior alveolar nerve, and the anterior superior alveolar nerve. **B.** With the lip or cheek pulled taught, the needle is inserted at the height of the buccal fold. Note: the 2-3 concentric circles of dotted lines around the needle tip indicate the area where the anesthesia is deposited. **C.** The needle is directed along the long axis of the tooth, and anesthesia is deposited just superior to the area of the root apex. **D.** Clinical photograph depicting a supraperiosteal infiltration of the maxillary lateral incisor.

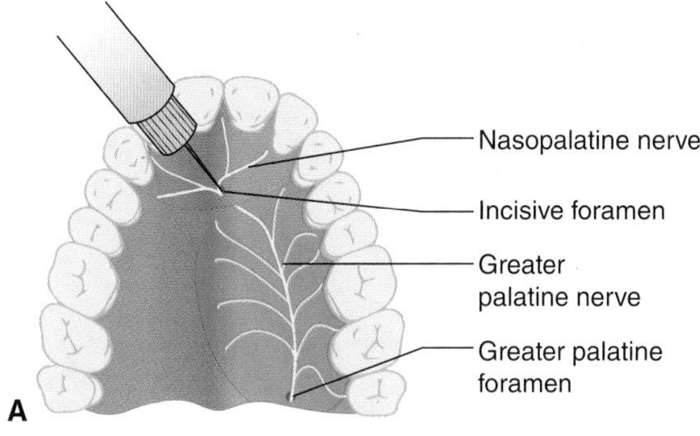

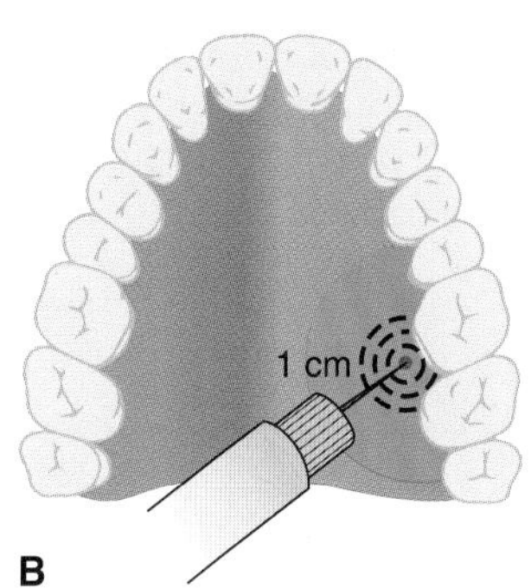

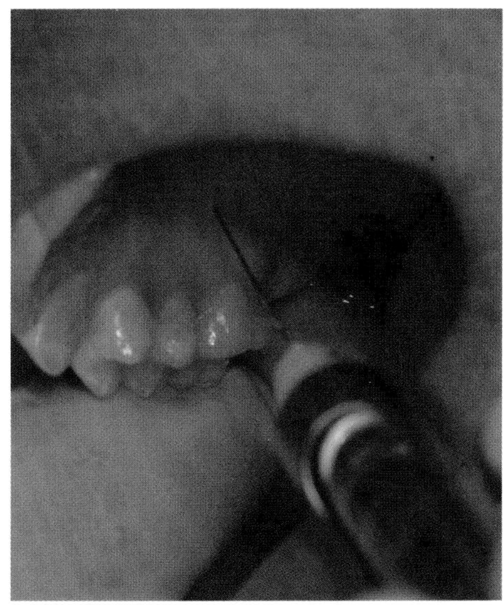

FIGURE 245-16. Palatal Infiltration. **A.** The innervation to the soft tissue of the hard palate. The posterior portion of the palate is innervated by bilateral greater palatine nerves after they each exit their respective greater palatine foramens (see blue shaded area). The anterior portion of the hard palate is innervated by the nasopalatine nerve after exiting the incisive foramen. Injection over the incisive foramen (shown) will result in anesthesia to the purple shaded area. **B.** A fine-gauge needle is inserted into the palatal tissue about 1 cm below the gingival margin, and a small amount of anesthesia is injected. Blanching of the palatal tissue surrounding the injection site is noted. This will provide anesthesia to the tissue adjacent to area injected as shown. A similar injection over the area of the greater palatine foramen or the incisive foramen will provide anesthesia to their respective zones. **C.** Clinical photograph depicting a palatal infiltration.

finger or thumb, the tissue is retracted toward the cheek revealing the pterygotemporal depression that is between the raised ridge of mucosa (pterygomandibular raphe) medially and coronoid notch laterally. With the syringe directed from the opposite premolar area, the needle is inserted into the pterygomandibular depression at a point 1 to 1.5 cm above the occlusal plane. This is approximately at the level of index finger or thumb. The needle is then slowly advanced until bone is contacted (about 20 to 25 mm). Once bone has been contacted, the needle should be withdrawn about 1 to 2 mm and then aspirated. If no blood is aspirated, then about 1.5 mL of anesthetic solution should be slowly injected. The needle then should be withdrawn about half of the distance, and the remainder of the dental carpule injected. This will ensure the anesthesia of the lingual nerve.[22-24] With experienced operators, the direct technique has about a 20% to 25% failure rate. Most commonly, failure is due to using too low of a point of injection. This places the anesthesia below the sphenomandibular ligament, which impedes its flow toward the inferior alveolar nerve. Repositioning the syringe higher above the occlusal plane will usually result in a successful injection.

Lingual Nerve Block If only lingual nerve anesthesia is desired, then the above technique can be followed except the needle need only be initially inserted about 10 mm, aspirated, and then the anesthetic agent instilled. This will provide anesthesia to the ipsilateral half of the anterior two thirds of the tongue (**Figure 245-18**).[22-24]

Long Buccal Injection If buccal soft tissue anesthesia is required, then this injection should be used. The needle is inserted into the mucosa in the buccal vestibule adjacent to the second or third mandibular molars (Figure 245-18).[22-24]

Injection Complications The normal vasovagal symptoms including syncope that can occur with any injection may occur during or after a dental injection. Flushing and elevation of the heart rate can also occur. Mild to severe allergic reactions are possible. Due to the close proximity of the inferior alveolar artery and vein and the pterygoid plexus, a potential complication of inferior alveolar nerve block is traumatic hematoma formation. These are usually self-limiting and treated with ice to the face but can be quite uncomfortable and an aesthetic issue for more than a week. Due to the superficial nature of the lingual nerve relative to the inferior alveolar nerve, inadvertent injury to the lingual nerve with subsequent temporary or permanent paresthesia can occur. This not only can affect sensation to the anterior two thirds of the affected side but also may affect taste because taste fibers run with the lingual nerve. Postinjection trismus, due to local trauma to the muscles of mastication, can occasionally occur. Needle breakage, although uncommon, has been reported, especially with improper technique such as bending the needle prior to use or redirecting the needle while injecting. Finally, unintentional injection too posteriorly may result in injection into the parotid region and can cause temporary facial nerve palsy.[24]

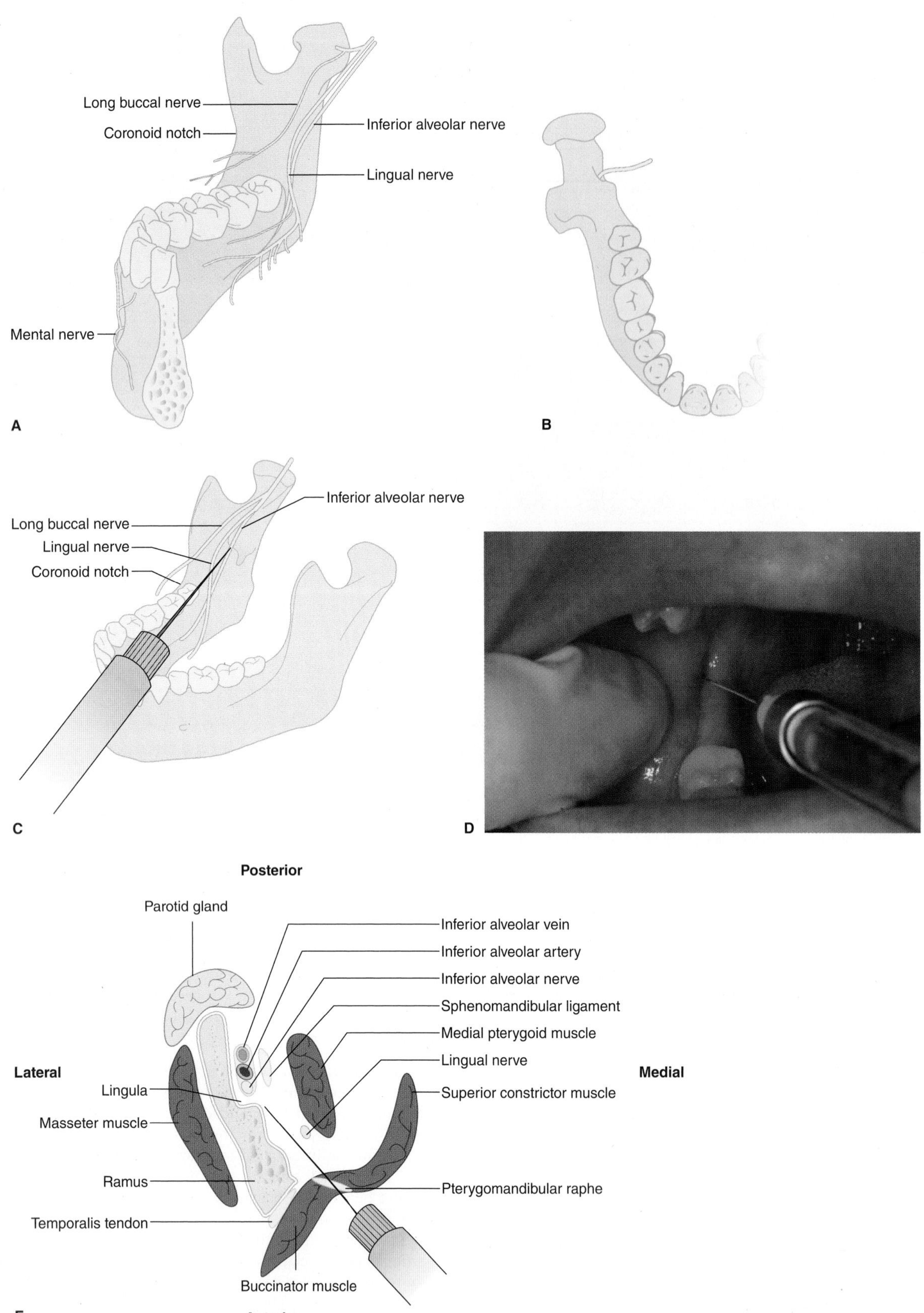

FIGURE 245-17. Inferior alveolar nerve block (direct technique). **A.** Shows the anatomy of the inferior alveolar nerve as it enters the mandibular foramen in the pterygomandibular space. The lingual nerve lies superficial and medial to the inferior alveolar nerve. The coronoid notch is noted. **B.** The area of anesthesia obtained with a successful inferior alveolar nerve block. Usually the lingual nerve is also blocked, which provides anesthesia to the floor of the mouth, lingual gingiva, and the anterior two thirds of the tongue. **C.** The syringe should be directed from the contralateral premolar area about 1 to 1.5 cm above the mandibular plane. It is inserted about 20 to 25 mm until bone is touched in an area above the lingula. The needle should then be withdrawn 1 to 2 mm and aspirated for blood before injecting anesthesia. The sphenomandibular ligament attaches to the lingula and prevents the anesthesia from reaching the inferior alveolar nerve if the injection is too low. **D.** Clinical photograph of the direct technique. Note the point of injection in the pterygomandibular depression just lateral to the pterygomandibular raphe. **E.** A diagram of a transverse section of the pterygomandibular fossa at the level of an inferior alveolar nerve injection. Note that the needle passes through the buccinator muscle to an area just superior to the lingula.

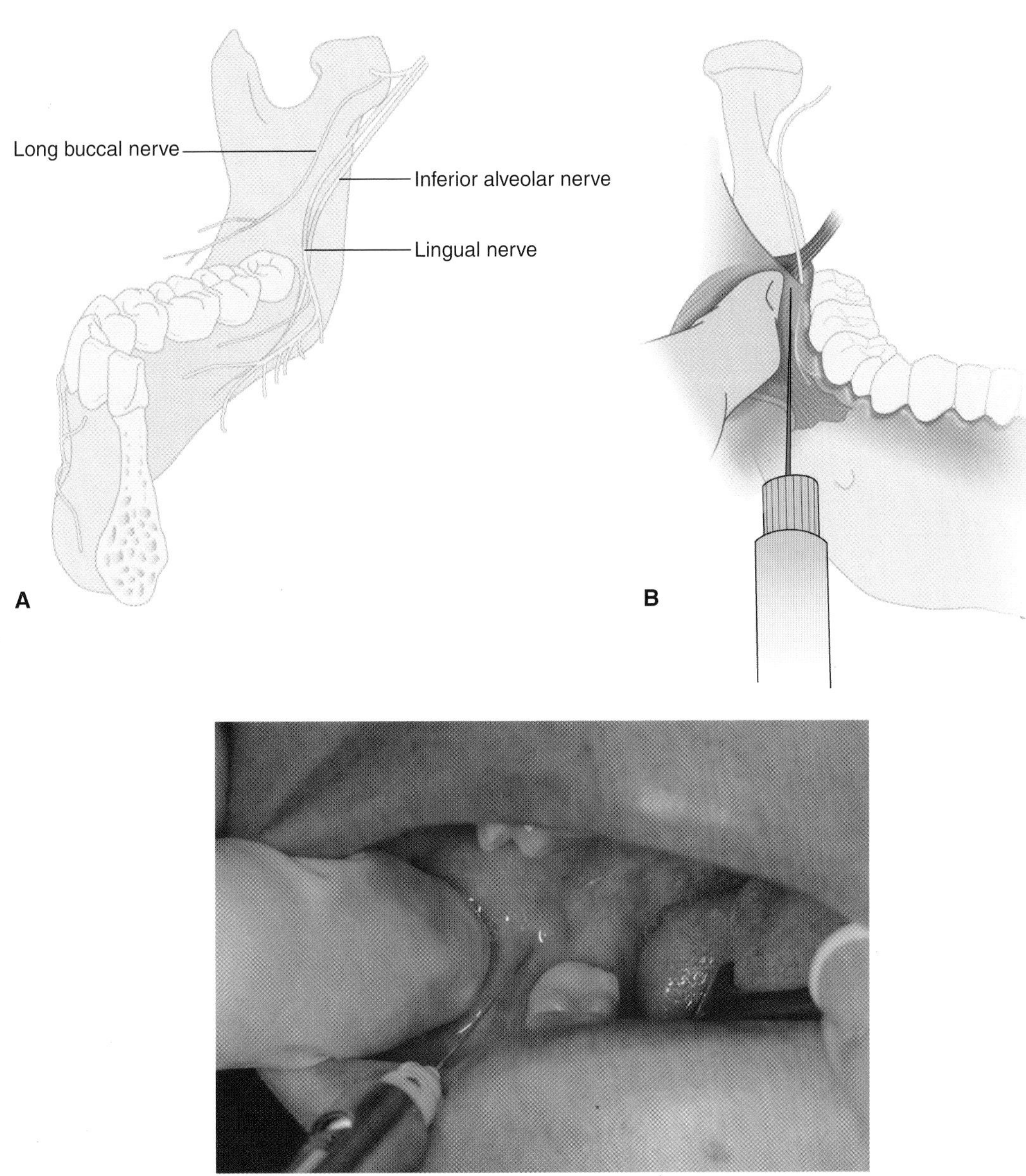

FIGURE 245-18. The lingual nerve block and the long buccal nerve block. **A.** The shaded areas represent the area in which anesthesia should be deposited for their respective blocks. The lingual nerve runs superficial and medial to the inferior alveolar nerve and can be easily anesthetized as part of the inferior alveolar nerve block. The lingual nerve block can be performed by depositing anesthesia about half the depth of the inferior alveolar nerve block. **B.** A diagrammatic representation of the long buccal nerve block. The long buccal nerve requires a separate injection of a small quantity of anesthetic just lateral to the molars in the buccal mucosa. **C.** Clinical photograph of the long buccal nerve block.

REFERENCES

The complete reference list is available online at www.TintinalliEM.com.

CHAPTER 246 Neck and Upper Airway

Nicholas D. Hartman

This chapter reviews infectious and noninfectious conditions that can obstruct the upper airway. These disorders must be recognized quickly because early airway management may be lifesaving. Neck trauma is discussed in the chapter 260, "Trauma to the Neck," and angioedema is discussed in the chapter 14, "Anaphylaxis, Allergies, and Angioedema."

NECK AND UPPER AIRWAY INFECTIONS

PHARYNGITIS/TONSILLITIS

Viruses account for the majority of cases of pharyngitis or tonsillitis. Acute viral pharyngitis is most commonly caused by rhinovirus but can be caused by multiple other viral agents (**Table 246-1**).[1]

VIRAL PHARYNGITIS

Viral pharyngitis generally displays a vesicular or petechial pattern on the soft palate and tonsils and is associated with rhinorrhea. However, in

TABLE 246-1 Microbial Causes of Acute Pharyngitis

Pathogen	Syndrome/Disease	Estimated % of Cases*
Viral		
Rhinovirus (100 types, 1 subtype)	Common cold	15–20
Coronavirus (3+ types)	Common cold	>5
Adenovirus (types 3, 4, 7, 14, 21)	Pharyngoconjunctival fever, acute respiratory disease	6
Herpes simplex virus (type 1, 2)	Gingivitis, stomatitis, pharyngitis	4
Parainfluenza virus (types 1–4)	Common cold, croup	2
Influenza virus (types A, B)	Influenza	2
Respiratory syncytial virus	Bronchiolitis, pharyngitis	1–2
Coxsackievirus A (types 2, 4, 5, 6, 8, 10)	Herpangina	<1
Epstein-Barr virus	Infectious mononucleosis	<1
Cytomegalovirus	Infectious mononucleosis	<1
Human immunodeficiency virus type 1	Acute retroviral syndrome	<1
Bacterial		
Streptococcus pyogenes (GABHS)	Pharyngitis, tonsillitis, scarlet fever	10–22
Fusobacterium necrophorum	Pharyngitis, tonsillitis, Lemierre's syndrome	5–10
Streptococcus dysgalactiae subspecies *equisimilis* (formerly group C β-hemolytic streptococci)	Pharyngitis, tonsillitis	3–5
Neisseria gonorrhoeae	Pharyngitis	<1
Corynebacterium diphtheriae	Diphtheria	<1
Arcanobacterium haemolyticum	Pharyngitis	<1
Chlamydial		
Chlamydia pneumonia	Pneumonia, bronchitis, pharyngitis	<1
Mycoplasmal		
Mycoplasma pneumonia	Pneumonia, bronchitis, pharyngitis	<1

Abbreviation: GABHS = group A β-hemolytic *Streptococcus*.

*Estimates of percentage of all cases of pharyngitis due to the indicated organism.

patients with nonstreptococcal pharyngitis (mostly viral), 16% have tonsillar exudate, 55% have cervical adenopathy, and 64% lack cough.[2] Most cases of viral pharyngitis require no specific diagnostic testing. There are three notable exceptions where testing may be indicated: suspected influenza, infectious mononucleosis, and acute retroviral syndrome. See Centers for Disease Control and Prevention influenza Web site for testing and treatment recommendations (http://www.cdc.gov/flu/). Infectious mononucleosis, influenza herpesvirus, and cytomegalovirus infections are discussed in the chapter 153, "Serious Viral Infections." The acute retroviral syndrome of early human immunodeficiency virus infection can also mimic mononucleosis. Symptoms of pharyngitis develop 2 to 4 weeks after exposure and resolve within 2 weeks. See the chapter 154, "Human Immunodeficiency Virus Infection" for recommendations on testing and treatment. Non–human immunodeficiency virus, noninfluenza viral pharyngitis should be treated symptomatically with oral hydration, antipyretics, analgesics, and rest. Patients unable to tolerate oral fluids or who become dehydrated should be given IV fluids.

BACTERIAL PHARYNGITIS

Group A β-Hemolytic *Streptococcus* **Group A β-hemolytic *Streptococcus* (GABHS) pharyngitis,** Lancefield group A species of *Streptococcus pyogenes*, is responsible for 5% to 15% of pharyngitis in adults.[1,2] After an incubation period of 2 to 5 days, patients develop the sudden onset of sore throat, painful swallowing, chills, and fever. Headache, nausea, and vomiting are common. Signs and symptoms of GABHS pharyngitis include marked erythema of the tonsils and tonsillar pillars (found in 62% of cases); tonsillar exudate (32%); and enlarged, tender cervical lymph nodes (76%).[2] A 2012 epidemiologic study found that only 6% of GABHS cases had fever and 28% had cough.[2] Patients may have uvular edema, myalgias, and malaise but are less likely to have rhinorrhea or conjunctivitis compared to viral pharyngitis.

Uvula edema, sometimes referred to as *Quincke's edema*, can be associated with upper airway infections such as GABHS pharyngitis, peritonsillar abscess, or epiglottitis. It can also be idiopathic. If it is an isolated finding and symptoms are uncomfortable to the patient, dexamethasone, 4 milligrams IV or PO, can be given as a single dose in the ED.

The original Centor criteria listed four clinical indicators of GABHS pharyngitis: (1) tonsillar exudates, (2) tender anterior cervical adenopathy, (3) absence of cough, and (4) history of fever.[2] The Centers for Disease Control and Prevention reversed its prior recommendation for empiric treatment based on clinical findings in 2012 in concert with the Infectious Diseases Society of America.[3] The Centers for Disease Control and Prevention and Infectious Diseases Society of America recommend using two or more Centor criteria as a threshold for selecting patients for rapid strep testing and treating only those with positive tests.[3,4] Guidelines do not recommend throat cultures in adult patients with one or fewer Centor criteria or routine throat culture for those with negative rapid strep tests, unless considering other bacterial pathogens.[3]

Untreated, GABHS infection lasts 7 to 10 days. Antibiotic therapy of GABHS hastens resolution by 1 to 2 days if initiated within 2 to 3 days of symptom onset and prevents suppurative complications and rheumatic fever, although not glomerulonephritis.[3] **GABHS has never been resistant to penicillin, so penicillin remains the recommended first-line drug for GABHS.**[5,6] Adults should receive a single IM dose of 1.2 million units of benzathine penicillin G, 500 milligrams of penicillin VK PO two times daily for 10 days, or amoxicillin 500 milligrams PO two times daily or 1000 milligrams one time daily. A first-generation cephalosporin antibiotic or clindamycin may be used for penicillin-allergic patients.[5] A single dose of PO or IM dexamethasone in immunocompetent adults with moderate to severe pharyngitis can achieve an earlier onset of pain relief and a shorter duration of pain.[7]

Other Causes of Bacterial Pharyngitis Several other bacteria can cause pharyngitis, although these infections are less common (Table 246-1). ***S. dysgalactiae* subspecies *equisimilis***, previously known as β-hemolytic groups C and G streptococci, are important pathogens causing pharyngitis, skin infections, and more serious infections such as meningitis or toxic shock syndrome in the elderly or immunocompromised.[8] *S. dysgalactiae* subspecies *equisimilis* frequently colonizes the upper respiratory tract (60% who are culture positive are asymptomatic),[8] so distinguishing acute infection from a carrier state may be difficult;[9] treatment is recommend for patients with acute symptoms.[8] *S. dysgalactiae* subspecies *equisimilis* pharyngitis is almost uniformly susceptible to penicillin.[8] Clindamycin and fluoroquinolones are alternatives.[8]

Fusobacterium necrophorum, a gram-negative anaerobe,[10] is the causative agent in **Lemierre's syndrome**, a complication of pharyngitis causing suppurative thrombophlebitis of the internal jugular vein, with or without bacteremia and septic emboli. Suspect *F. necrophorum* in adolescents or young adults with worsening symptoms and neck swelling.[11] Treatment is with penicillin, clindamycin, or third-generation cephalosporins; *F. necrophorum* resistance to macrolides is high.[11]

Gonococcal pharyngitis is usually associated with genital infection and is treated by the same antibiotics. **Diphtheria** is caused by *Corynebacterium diphtheriae* and is rare in well-immunized populations. It is characterized by a slow onset of mild to moderate pharyngeal discomfort and low-grade fever. On physical examination, a gray membrane is seen adherent to the tonsillar or pharyngeal surface and may extend to the uvula, soft palate, pharynx, and larynx. Treatment is with diphtheria antitoxin and metronidazole to prevent transmission to others.

PERITONSILLAR ABSCESS

A peritonsillar abscess is a collection of purulent material between the tonsillar capsule, the superior constrictor, and palatopharyngeus muscles. Risk factors include periodontal disease, smoking, chronic tonsillitis, multiple trials of antibiotics, and previous peritonsillar abscess.[12] Peritonsillar abscess develops primarily in adolescents and young adults without seasonal variation as previously thought.[12,13] Although peritonsillar abscesses are typically polymicrobial infections, in patients 15 to 24 years of age, *Fusobacterium necrophorum* has been the most common organism in many communities.[13,14]

CLINICAL FEATURES AND DIAGNOSIS

Patients with peritonsillar abscess (adolescents and adults) appear ill and present with sore throat (99%), fever (54%), malaise, odynophagia, dysphagia, and/or otalgia.[15] Physical signs include inferior and medial displacement of the infected tonsil(s) (46%), contralateral deflection of the swollen uvula (43%), tender cervical lymphadenopathy (41%), trismus (32%), muffled voice ("hot potato voice"), palatal edema, and dehydration[15] (**Figure 246-1**). The differential diagnosis of a peritonsillar abscess includes peritonsillar cellulitis, mononucleosis, lymphoma, herpes simplex tonsillitis, retropharyngeal abscess, neoplasm, and internal carotid artery aneurysm. In peritonsillar cellulitis, erythema and edema of the tonsillar pillar and soft palate are evident, but pus has not yet formed. Diagnosis of a peritonsillar abscess is often made by history and physical examination alone. When the diagnosis is in question, intraoral US has a sensitivity of 89% to 95% with a specificity of 79% to 100% for peritonsillar abscess.[16] CT scan with contrast is indicated if there is concern for spread beyond the peritonsillar space or lateral neck space complications.[16]

TREATMENT

Treatment options include drainage of the abscess by needle aspiration, incision and drainage, or, rarely, immediate tonsillectomy. Choice of treatment depends on clinical symptoms, degree of patient cooperation, history of previous tonsil disease, and healthcare personnel experience. There is no difference in outcome when comparing needle aspiration with incision and drainage.[16] Abscess tonsillectomy ("quinsy tonsillectomy") should only be considered when patients have strong indication for tonsillectomy, such as sleep apnea, recurrent tonsillitis, or recurrent peritonsillar abscess.[16] Needle aspiration is minimally invasive, less painful than incision and drainage, and may be performed by general or specialized medical personnel. Approximately 90% of patients will be treated effectively after a single needle aspiration.[16]

Needle aspiration should be performed by an individual trained in the technique. First, apply lidocaine spray or gel or benzocaine-tetracaine spray to the overlying mucosa. Then inject 1 to 2 mL of lidocaine with epinephrine into the mucosa of the anterior tonsillar pillar using a 25-gauge needle **The drainage needle should penetrate no more than 1 cm because the internal carotid artery usually lies laterally and posterior to the posterior edge of the tonsil.** The plastic sheath of the needle can be cut 1 cm from its tip to serve as a guard. If the internal carotid artery lies more medial and anterior, it can usually be palpated in this area. Once adequate anesthesia is achieved, introduce an 18-gauge needle just lateral to the tonsil, approximately halfway between the base of the uvula and the maxillary alveolar ridge, until the abscess cavity is encountered and pus is aspirated. Often, multiple aspirations may be required to find the abscess. If not done previously, a contrast CT scan of the neck is recommended when the results of needle aspiration are negative and a parapharyngeal or retropharyngeal space process is suspected.

Initial therapy should include a 10-day course of antimicrobials effective against group A *Streptococcus* and oral anaerobes (including *F. necrophorum*). Proven agents are penicillin VK plus metronidazole[15] or clindamycin for penicillin-allergic patients. Toxic patients or patients unable to take medicine PO should receive piperacillin-tazobactam, 3.375 grams IV, or similar agent. Single IV use of high-dose steroid (methylprednisolone, 125 milligrams, or dexamethasone, 10 milligrams) in addition to antibiotics and drainage improves severity and duration of pain.[15,17] Provide follow-up within 24 to 36 hours of aspiration, with instructions to return to the ED if worse. If the patient is not improving, consider repeating the aspiration, otolaryngologic consultation for incision and drainage or tonsillectomy, or obtaining a CT scan to confirm or reject the diagnosis. Complications of a peritonsillar abscess include airway obstruction, rupture of the abscess with aspiration of the contents, hemorrhage secondary to erosion of carotid sheath, retropharyngeal abscess, mediastinitis, and poststreptococcal sequelae.

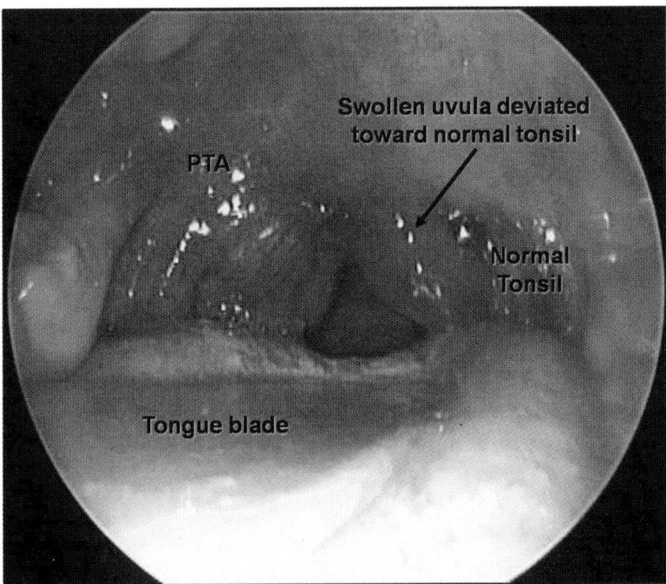

FIGURE 246-1. Right peritonsillar abscess (PTA) displacing right tonsil medially and the uvula toward the normal left tonsil. Abscess is between the right tonsil and the superior constrictor muscles.

ADULT EPIGLOTTITIS (SUPRAGLOTTITIS)

Epiglottitis is an inflammatory condition, usually infectious, primarily of the epiglottis but often including the entire supraglottic region (many prefer the term *supraglottitis*). It can lead to rapid airway obstruction. Prior to the introduction of a conjugate vaccine for *Haemophilus influenzae* type b in the 1980s, most cases of epiglottitis affected children age 1 to 5 years. In the postvaccine era, the dramatic decline in pediatric cases has confined the disease primarily to adults, with an estimated mean age of 45 years.[18,19] Most cases in adults are caused by *Streptococcus* species, *Staphylococcus* species, viruses, and fungi, although most frequently, no organism can be isolated.[19] Risk factors for mortality in patients with epiglottitis are advanced age and male sex.[20]

CLINICAL FEATURES AND DIAGNOSIS

Symptoms are typically a 1- to 2-day history of worsening dysphagia, odynophagia, and dyspnea, particularly in the supine position. The clinical triad of the "three Ds" (drooling, dysphagia, and distress) is a classic but infrequent presentation. Other symptoms are fever, tachycardia, cervical adenopathy, and anterior neck tenderness with pain on gentle palpation of the larynx and upper trachea. Stridor is primarily inspiratory. Patients often position themselves sitting up, leaning forward, mouth open, head extended, and panting.

Diagnosis is clinical and confirmed by radiographs or transnasal fiberoptic laryngoscopy. Lateral cervical soft tissue radiographs demonstrate obliteration of the vallecula, swelling of the aryepiglottic folds,

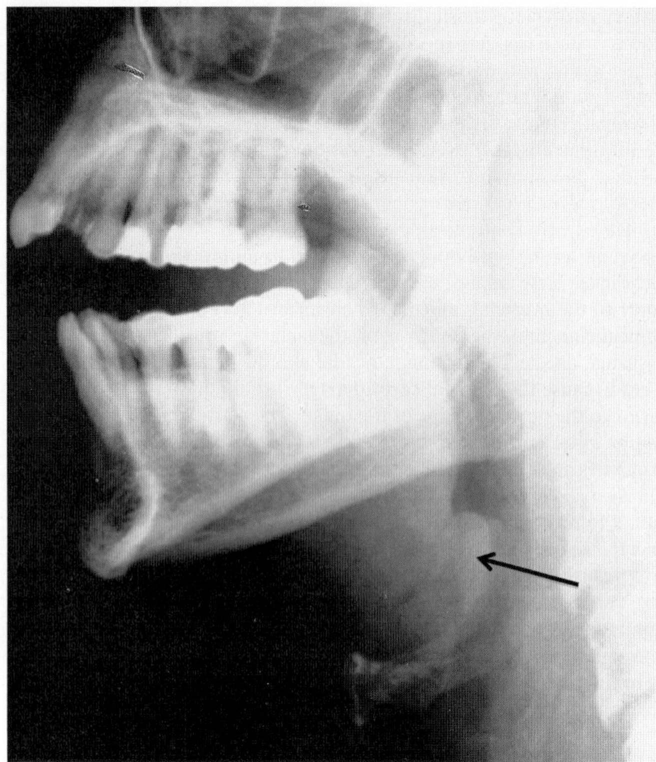

FIGURE 246-2. Acute epiglottitis. *Arrow* points to thickened epiglottis resembling a thumb print on a soft tissue lateral radiograph.

edema of the prevertebral and retropharyngeal soft tissues, and ballooning of the hypopharynx (**Figure 246-2**). The epiglottis appears enlarged and thumb-shaped. Direct laryngoscopy examination can confirm the diagnosis in adults if necessary but should be done carefully to avoid sudden, unpredictable airway obstruction. **Patients with worsening dyspnea in the supine position should *not* be sent to the CT scanner; CT of the neck is not needed to make the diagnosis.**

TREATMENT

Obtain immediate otolaryngologic consultation for suspected epiglottitis. Be prepared to establish a definitive airway. Patients should not be left unattended, and they should remain sitting up. Initial treatment consists of supplemental humidified oxygen, IV hydration, cardiac monitoring, pulse oximetry, and IV antibiotics. Humidification and hydration can help decrease the risk for sudden airway blockage. Steroids are often given to decrease airway inflammation and edema (methylprednisolone, 125 milligrams IV).

In adults, the need for intubation usually can be determined by transnasal fiberoptic examination of the supraglottis. Intubation is generally accomplished by "awake" fiberoptic intubation in the operating room, with preparations for immediate awake tracheostomy or cricothyrotomy. In cases of airway obstruction in the ED, be prepared for a very difficult intubation secondary to the swollen, distorted anatomy. In the case of intubation failure, the last resorts for preserving the airway are cricothyrotomy and needle cricothyrotomy.

Current antibiotic recommendations are cefotaxime 50 milligrams/kg IV every 8 hours plus vancomycin 15 milligrams/kg every 12 hours.[21] Alternative antibiotics include ampicillin-sulbactam, ceftriaxone, or piperacillin-tazobactam.[21] Respiratory fluoroquinolones are an option for patients with severe penicillin allergies.

RETROPHARYNGEAL ABSCESS

The retropharyngeal space is a potential space anterior to the prevertebral fascia that extends from the base of the skull to the tracheal bifurcation. In adults, a retropharyngeal abscess is usually due to intraoral procedures, trauma, foreign bodies such as a fishbone, or extension from odontogenic infection.[22] Cultures from retropharyngeal abscesses are usually polymicrobial: group A β-hemolytic streptococci, *Staphylococcus aureus* (including methicillin-resistant *S. aureus*), *H. influenzae*, and *Bacteroides*, *Peptostreptococcus*, and *Fusobacterium* species.

CLINICAL FEATURES AND DIAGNOSIS

The most common symptoms in adults are sore throat, dysphagia, neck pain, and less commonly, stridor. In addition, patients may also have complaints of cervical lymphadenopathy, poor oral intake, muffled voice, and respiratory distress. Visible neck swelling is not common.

A lateral soft tissue radiograph of the neck taken during inspiration with moderate cervical extension can demonstrate thickening and protrusion of the retropharyngeal wall, classically with 5 to 7 cm of prevertebral widening at the second cervical vertebra.[23] However, contrast-enhanced CT scan of the neck is the test of choice for diagnosis of a retropharyngeal abscess.[24] Early CT findings may reflect reactive, nonsuppurative edema, mild fat stranding with discernible tissue planes, linear fluid, minimal mass effect, and no associated enhancement. Necrotic nodes with central low attenuation and ring enhancement reflect an abscess (**Figure 246-3**). A patient with airway distress should not be sent unobserved for CT scanning.

TREATMENT

Obtain immediate otolaryngologic consultation. Provide IV hydration and antibiotic treatment with either clindamycin or cefoxitin IV; alternatively, piperacillin-tazobactam or ampicillin-sulbactam may be used.[21] Although a few patients with small abscess cavities may be managed with IV antibiotics alone, most patients will require surgical intervention. Catastrophic complications from retropharyngeal abscess include extension of

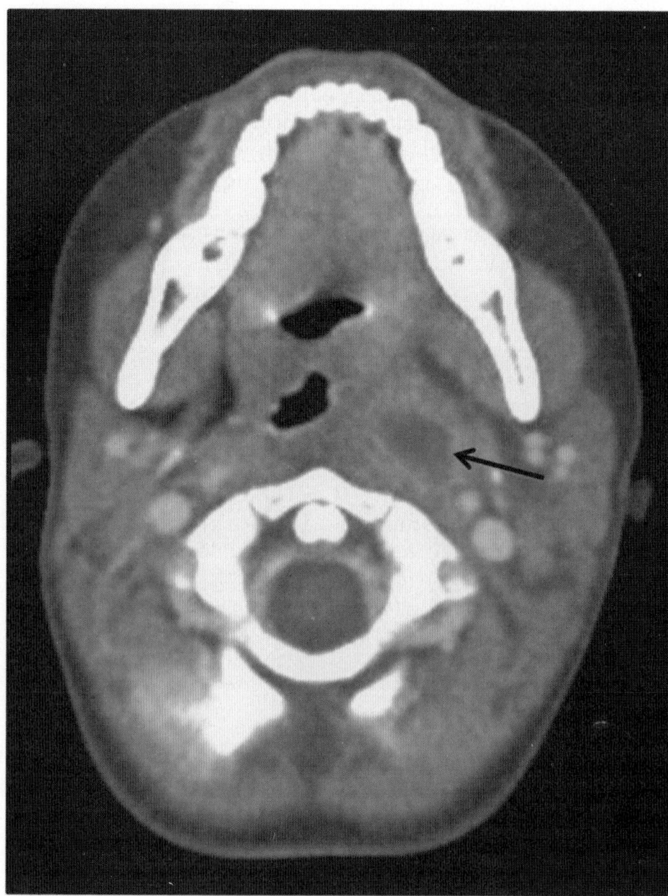

FIGURE 246-3. Contrasted CT of a left retropharyngeal abscess (*arrow*).

the infection into the mediastinum and upper airway asphyxia from direct pressure or aspiration after sudden rupture of the abscess.[25]

ODONTOGENIC ABSCESS

Odontogenic infections can arise from an infected tooth or after a tooth extraction. Development of the infection varies from <1 day to up to 1 to 3 weeks after the onset of tooth pain and may occur despite oral antibiotics. Odontogenic infections are polymicrobial; the most common bacteria are *Streptococci viridians*, *Peptostreptococcus*, *Prevotella*, and staphylococci.[26] **Most deep neck infections originate from an odontogenic source, usually the mandibular teeth.** Dental abscesses may spread into the parapharyngeal and retropharyngeal spaces. Presenting features include neck mass, trismus, fever, leukocytosis, dysphagia, and dyspnea. Potential complications include necrotizing fasciitis, descending necrotizing mediastinitis, orbital infections, and hematogenous dissemination to distant organs.

CLINICAL FEATURES

See chapter 245,"Oral and Dental Emergencies" for management of dental infections isolated to the mandible or maxilla. Soft tissue extension from odontogenic infection ranges from diffuse cellulitis to abscess formation in labial or buccal gingiva. In some cases, intraoral or dentocutaneous fistula formation may occur. Fascial layers of the head and neck produce planes or potential spaces for infectious spread. Infections associated with maxillary teeth tend to spread into potential spaces in the face. Infections of maxillary molars tend to involve the masticator space, which can extend into the parapharyngeal space and downward into the neck and mediastinum. Infections of anterior mandibular teeth tend to spread into the neck. Infections of anterior teeth, bicuspids, and first molars of the mandible tend to enter the sublingual space, with edema of the floor of the mouth with little extraoral swelling. Involvement of the submandibular space is typically the result of second and third mandibular molar infections.

DIAGNOSIS AND TREATMENT

Superficial odontogenic abscesses can be diagnosed with US at the bedside.[27] For diagnosis of suspected deep space infections, contrast-enhanced CT scan is recommended to identify the need for surgical management.[27] Treatment of odontogenic infections includes appropriate antibiotic therapy (aerobic and anaerobic coverage) and surgical drainage of abscesses. Penicillin VK and amoxicillin remain appropriate options for outpatient treatment; amoxicillin-clavulanate, clindamycin, cefuroxime, and levofloxacin are second-line choices.[28,29] Patients with deep-neck infections require IV antibiotics; ampicillin-sulbactam with clindamycin and ciprofloxacin is one recommended regimen. Other useful agents include piperacillin-tazobactam, imipenem-cilastatin, and ertapenem.

COMPLICATIONS

Ludwig's angina is infection of the submental, sublingual, and submandibular spaces. Patients usually present with poor dental hygiene, dysphagia, and odynophagia. Clinical examination reveals trismus and edema of the entire upper neck and floor of mouth. Infection progresses rapidly and can posteriorly displace the tongue, causing airway compromise. Definitive airway management should be considered early in the course, including awake fiberoptic intubation or awake tracheostomy.[30] Stridor, difficulty managing secretions, and cyanosis are late signs and require emergent airway management. Systemic antibiotics are not a substitute for definitive airway management because it may take >1 week for edema resolution with antibiotic therapy.

Patients with **necrotizing infections** are critically ill, with overlying skin discoloration, crepitus of the subcutaneous tissue, and systemic signs, including fever, tachycardia, hypotension, and confusion. CT reveals subcutaneous emphysema, deep tissue gas, and pockets of suppuration (**Figure 246-4**). Aerobic and anaerobic cultures are necessary for identification of causative organisms. Therapy of necrotizing fasciitis is immediate surgery with fasciotomy with wide local debridement and broad-spectrum IV antibiotics. Mediastinal extension places the patient at risk for great vessel erosion, retroperitoneal extension, pleural abscess, pericardial effusion, and sepsis; mortality ranges from 10% to 40%.[31] Tracheostomy should be performed if airway obstruction develops. Surgery can be lifesaving, and immediate surgical consultation is required for this rapidly progressing disease.[31]

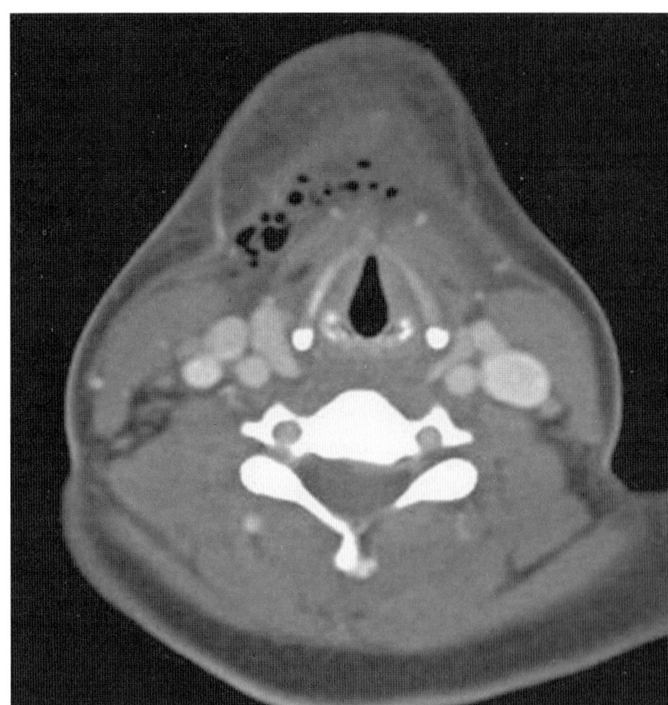

FIGURE 246-4. CT demonstrating necrotizing fasciitis with gas in the deep tissue of the anterior neck.

NECK AND UPPER AIRWAY MASSES

CLINICAL FEATURES

Neck masses (**Figures 246-5 and 246-6**) can result from congenital, infectious, glandular, or neoplastic disorders. Enlargement may lead to airway compromise, dehydration secondary to dysphagia and odynophagia, or secondary infected. Age of the patient and characteristics including location of the mass may aid in the diagnosis (**Tables 246-2 and 246-3**).[32] Neck masses in children are discussed in the chapter 122, "Neck Masses in Infants and Children," in the Pediatrics section. **In adults >40 years old, up to 80% of lateral neck masses persistent for >6 weeks are malignant.**[33]

DIAGNOSIS AND MANAGEMENT

The urgency for evaluation of a neck mass depends on patient acuity.[33] Patients with airway compromise or significant dysphagia and odynophagia should be evaluated by flexible nasopharyngolaryngoscopy **before** CT scan. CT scan will delineate the extent of the mass and likely will be required for surgical intervention. If no airway compromise or dehydration is present, the patient should follow up with primary care for outpatient imaging and further evaluation. The final diagnosis for a neck or upper airway mass will not be made in the ED. All neck masses should have follow-up for diagnosis and treatment.

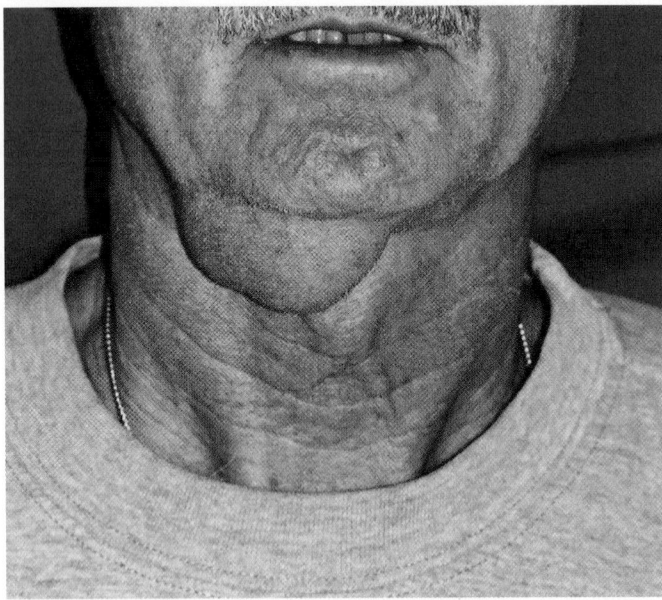

FIGURE 246-5. Right plunging ranula presenting as a painless ballotable submandibular mass.

Empiric antibiotic therapy should be initiated for inflammatory lymph nodes, usually with cephalexin, 250 to 500 milligrams PO three to four times daily; amoxicillin, 250 to 500 milligrams PO three times daily; or clindamycin, 300 milligrams three to four times daily. Resolution is expected in 2 weeks for those lesions that are due to infection alone. Empiric therapy of sialoadenitis should include staphylococcal coverage most commonly, clindamycin[34] (see chapter 118, "Neck Masses in Children").

TABLE 246-2 Neck Masses in Young and Older Adults

Young Adult	Adult
Reactive lymphadenopathy	Metastatic aerodigestive tract carcinoma
Mononucleosis	Salivary gland infection or neoplasm
Lymphoma	
Branchial cleft cyst	Lymphoma
Thyroglossal duct cyst	Thyroid disorder Tuberculosis

POSTTONSILLECTOMY BLEEDING

Tonsillectomy is the second most common reason for care in pediatric hospitals in the United States.[35] Postoperative bleeding is a well-known complication of tonsillectomy that can, rarely, lead to death from airway obstruction or hemorrhagic shock. Rate of secondary hemorrhage varies according to the method used for the procedure. The incidence of post-tonsillectomy bleeding ranges from 1% to 8.8%, with approximately half requiring surgical intervention for control of bleeding.[36]

Although bleeding can be seen within 24 hours of surgery, most significant hemorrhage occurs between postoperative days 5 and 10. There is a significantly higher incidence of bleeding in patients between 21 and 30 years of age, as well as those over age 70.[36] Posttonsillectomy bleeding can be fatal and requires prompt intervention with control of the airway. An otolaryngologist should be consulted early.

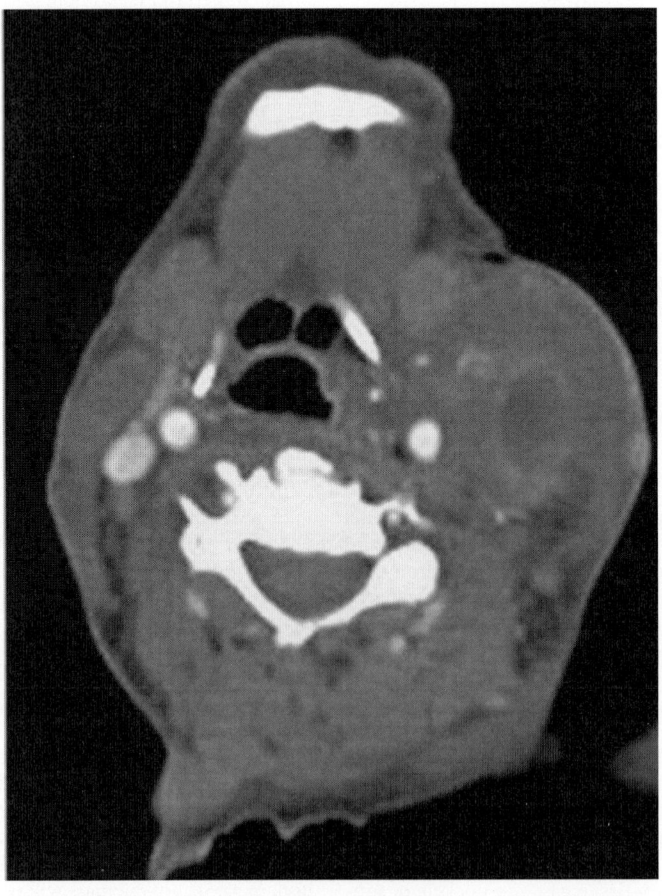

FIGURE 246-6. Hypopharyngeal squamous cell carcinoma metastatic to left cervical lymph nodes. Note the thrombosis of the left jugular vein with displacement of the airway to the right.

TABLE 246-3 Common Causes of Neck Masses in Adults

Disorder	Physical Finding	Pathology	Management
Ranula	Sublingual area swelling	Mucus retention cyst due to ductal obstruction of the sublingual gland	Surgical excision
Laryngeal papillomas	Sessile, warty-appearing lesions on the soft palate or tonsillar pillars	Human papillomavirus type 6 or 11 infection	Surgical excision
Palatine torus	Boney smooth painless mass of the hard palate	Exostoses of the palate	No treatment needed in most cases
Mandibular torus	Boney smooth painless growth of the mandible under the tongue	Exostoses of the mandible	No treatment needed in most cases
Branchial cleft cysts	Painless, fluctuant masses close to the angle of the mandible	Incomplete obliteration of the branchial apparatus during development	Antibiotics if infected, surgical excision
Thyroglossal duct cysts	Soft, mobile, subhyoid bone midline mass	Remnant of the thyroid anlage	Antibiotics if infected, surgical excision
Lymphoma	Multiple, rubbery low-neck masses, night sweats, fever, malaise	Malignant process	Biopsy, referral to ENT and oncology
Acute retroviral syndrome	Generalized adenopathy, unprotected sex by history	Human immunodeficiency virus infection	Antiretroviral medication
Squamous cell carcinoma	Firm, possibly fixed cervical lymph node	Oral lesion metastatic to cervical node	Biopsy, referral to ENT and oncology
Parotid tumors	Nonpainful masses under or anterior to the ear	Benign or malignant process	Biopsy, referral to ENT and oncology as needed
Sialoadenitis	Tender swelling in area of parotid, submandibular, or sublingual salivary gland	Salivary gland infection	Antibiotics, salivary stimulants, also see chapter 122, "Neck Masses in Children"
Thyroid enlargement	Diffuse nodular thyroid enlargement or solitary nodular thyroid	Benign or malignant process	See chapters 228, "Hypothyroidism," and 229, "Hyperthyroidism"

Abbreviation: ENT = otolaryngology.

TREATMENT

Keep the patient NPO (nothing by mouth) and sitting upright, monitor with pulse oximetry, and maintain IV access. Obtain a CBC and coagulation studies, and type and cross-match blood. Examine the oropharynx to see if bleeding can be visualized. A grayish-white eschar is normal following a tonsillectomy. **Apply direct pressure to the bleeding tonsillar bed using a tonsillar pack or a 4×4 gauze on a long clamp, moistened with either thrombin or lidocaine and epinephrine.** To prevent loss of the pack into the airway, place a suture through the pack and tape the suture to the face. Place pressure on the lateral pharyngeal wall, avoiding midline manipulation, to decrease stimulation of the gag reflex. Massive bleeding is rare, but when it occurs, intubation may be the only means of protecting the airway. This is always difficult, with oropharyngeal edema from recent surgery and blood obscuring visualization of the cords. Plans should be made for an emergent cricothyrotomy prior to attempting intubation.

Pressure alone can be adequate for control of posttonsillectomy hemorrhage until the otolaryngologist arrives. Alternatively, if a bleeding site can be visualized, bleeding may be cauterized with silver nitrate after local infiltration with 1% lidocaine with epinephrine. Otolaryngologic consultation in the ED is always needed because patients may have a second or even third posttonsillectomy hemorrhage,[37] and surgery or endovascular embolization may be necessary for definitive control.[38]

REFERENCES

The complete reference list is available online at www.TintinalliEM.com.

CHAPTER 247 Complications of Airway Devices

John P. Gaillard

TRACHEOSTOMY TUBES AND CANNULAS

A tracheostomy is an opening between cartilaginous rings in the trachea and the skin, with a tracheostomy tube placed into the stoma to facilitate ventilation. Tracheostomy is usually performed by an otolaryngologist as an elective or semi-elective procedure and is not an emergency procedure. Most tracheostomies are performed on chronically ill patients requiring prolonged mechanical ventilation.

There are many types of tracheostomy tubes available, including those made of plastic, silicone, nylon, and metal. Most hospitals stock only a few types of tracheostomy tubes, and one must be familiar with the types available. Tracheostomy tubes vary in diameter, total length, the length before and after the curve, and the presence or absence of a cuff (**Figure 247-1**). The size of the tracheostomy tube is usually defined by the inner diameter, ranging in adults from 5 to 10 mm and in pediatric patients from 2.5 to 6.5 mm. Most pediatric and adult tracheostomy tubes have a 15-mm standard respiratory connection that may be used with ventilator tubing or a bag-valve device.

Fenestrated tracheostomy tubes have an opening along the dorsal surface of the body of the tube. The fenestration allows the passage of air through the tracheostomy tube to the vocal cords so the patient can speak. Irritation from the fenestration may promote growth of granulation tissue, which may extend into the fenestration, leading to bleeding, obstruction, and difficulty removing the tracheostomy tube. If any difficulty is encountered removing a fenestrated tracheostomy tube, obtain surgical or ear, nose, and throat consultation.

Most adult tracheostomy tubes have a removable inner cannula, which allows secretions to be cleared from the lumen without removing the entire tube from the trachea. In assessing an adult tracheostomy patient, remove and examine the inner cannula for crusting or obstruction. Both disposable and reusable inner cannulas may be cleaned by using a small brush dipped in a solution of hydrogen peroxide and then

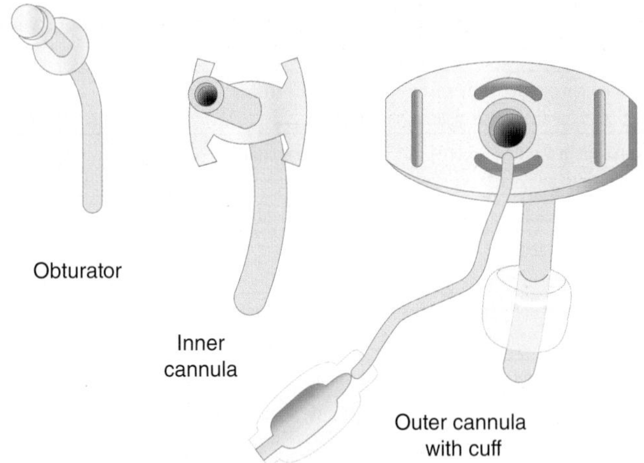

FIGURE 247-1. Common components of most tracheostomy tube sets.

rinsing the cannula with warm tap water. If the correct size of disposable inner cannula is not available in the ED, use the existing inner cannula temporarily, or change the entire tracheostomy tube. **Pediatric tracheostomy tubes never have an inner cannula because of the small inner diameter, so the entire tube must be removed for cleaning.**

COMPLICATIONS OF TRACHEOSTOMIES

Complications due to the surgery are grouped according to the timing since the tracheostomy and the technique. Summed complication rates from randomized controlled trials show 10.0% for percutaneous technique and 8.7% for open tracheostomy.[1] Bleeding, obstruction, dislodgement, and infection are all potential early complications, occurring within the first week. Late complications are those that occur after 1 week. Granulation, tracheal stenosis, a fistula (tracheocutaneous, tracheoesophageal, or tracheoinnominate) plus any of the early complications may be late complications.[1-4] Risk factors for tracheal stenosis are intubation duration of more than 1 week and having an endotracheal tube larger than 7.5 mm.[4]

Patients with tracheostomy tubes can develop respiratory distress. **Figure 247-2** is a step-by-step approach to assess and treat respiratory distress. In the ED, the provider must be proficient in the following skills (as outlined in the sections that follow): replacement of an uncuffed with a cuffed tracheostomy tube for mechanical ventilation, replacement of a tracheostomy tube after accidental decannulation, correction of a tube obstruction, and control of bleeding or infection at the tracheostomy site. It is important to determine a few key elements about the tracheostomy: when and why was the procedure performed, what type of tracheostomy tube is the patient using currently, and can the patient be orally intubated if needed? **Patients who have undergone a laryngectomy or who have tumors or scarring that occlude the upper airway cannot be orally intubated.**

Tracheostomy Tube Obstruction Consider mucus plugging of the trachea or mainstem bronchi distal to the tube. If the tracheostomy is patent and is in the airway, leave it in place. If the tracheostomy tube is obstructed, mucous plugging is commonly the cause. Secretions may act as a ball-valve mechanism, allowing air in but restricting exhalation. Suctioning may relieve the obstruction. Preoxygenation and placement of sterile saline solution into the trachea will aid in suctioning. Prolonged use of large suction catheters without preoxygenation will cause hypoxemia. If mucous plugging cannot be relieved by suctioning, the inner cannula of the tracheostomy tube and, occasionally, the entire tracheostomy tube may need to be removed and cleaned.

Tracheostomy Dislodgement It is possible for the tracheostomy tube to become dislodged from the trachea but still be in the neck. In this case, a suction catheter cannot be passed through the tube, and on x-ray, the tracheostomy tube may be seen to extrinsically compress the trachea (**Figure 247-3**). In this circumstance, remove the entire tracheostomy tube. It may be difficult to accurately identify the actual tracheal stoma when replacing the tube (see "Changing a Tracheostomy Tube" section below). A nasopharyngoscope or flexible bronchoscope should be inserted into the visible stoma in an attempt to identify the tracheal opening. If the opening still cannot be identified, obtain ear, nose, and throat or surgical consultation. If the patient cannot maintain the airway, oral intubation will be necessary.

Tracheostomy Site Infection Indwelling tracheostomy tubes are contaminated with normal or pathogenic flora. Surgical site infection is more common in patient post open tracheostomy (7%) than percutaneous insertion (3.4%).[5] Stomal skin infection, tracheitis, and bronchitis can be a recurring problem. Infection may be polymicrobial, including *Staphylococcus aureus*, *Pseudomonas*, and *Candida*. Antibiotics are indicated in the setting of clinical disease. Stable patients can be treated with amoxicillin-clavulanate, 875 milligrams PO twice daily.[6] Unstable patient should receive piperacillin-tazobactam, 3.375 grams IV, plus vancomycin, 1000 milligrams IV. Use a fluoroquinolone for *Pseudomonas*. Dressing changes with gauze soaked in 0.25% acetic acid are effective for local wound infections.

Tracheostomy Site Bleeding Bleeding can occur at any time after a tracheostomy. Granulation tissue in the stoma, trachea, or thyroid or erosion of the thyroid vessels, the tracheal wall (frequently from suction trauma), or the innominate artery are all sources of hemorrhage. Slow bleeding originating from the stoma may be controlled by packing the site with saline-soaked gauze. If this is ineffective, remove the tube and examine the stoma and tracheal wall. Local bleeding can be controlled with silver nitrate. Electrocautery should be done by a surgeon. If bleeding is brisk, replace the tracheostomy tube with a cuffed endotracheal tube with the cuff below the bleeding site.

Tracheoinnominate artery fistula is a rare but life-threatening complication of tracheostomy. Cuff pressure >25 mm Hg, tracheostomy below the third tracheal ring, and deformed neck or chest are all risk factors.[7] Bleeding results from vessel erosion caused by either direct pressure of the tip of the tracheal cannula against the innominate artery or from a cuff with inappropriately high pressures due to overinflation. Most patients with a tracheoinnominate artery fistula present within the first 3 weeks after tracheostomy, with the peak incidence between the first and second week. Some patients may have a sentinel arterial bleed or hemoptysis. Bleeding may be mild or severe and should be thoroughly investigated because of the potential for sudden massive hemorrhage.[8] Immediate otolaryngologic and thoracic surgery consultation is required, and operative repair is lifesaving.

If patients present with massive bleeding, the first maneuver is to hyperinflate the cuff to control brisk bleeding while planning operative intervention. If bleeding persists, slowly withdraw the tube while exerting pressure against the anterior trachea. If these interventional maneuvers do not control the bleeding, then place a cuffed endotracheal tube from above to prevent pulmonary aspiration of blood. Passing the endotracheal tube past the tracheoinnominate fistula will require direct visualization with a flexible nasopharyngoscope or bronchoscope through the tube and an assistant to withdraw the tracheostomy tube as the endotracheal tube passes.[5] **Stomal hemorrhage is then controlled with digital pressure of the innominate artery against the manubrium.** This is known as the Utley maneuver.[9] Tamponade of the hemorrhage should be maintained during transport to the operating room, as the patient will need emergent surgery with rigid bronchoscopy.

Tracheal Stenosis Tracheal stenosis may present weeks to months after decannulation and results from mucosal necrosis and subsequent scarring. Signs and symptoms include dyspnea, wheezing, stridor, and the inability to clear secretions. A chest radiograph may demonstrate the narrowed tracheal airway. Medical treatment includes humidified oxygen, nebulized racemic epinephrine, and steroids. Operative treatment involves rigid bronchoscopy with laser excision of the scar bands, and stenting or tracheal reconstruction in more severe cases.

MECHANICAL VENTILATION WITH A TRACHEOSTOMY TUBE

If the patient requires mechanical ventilation, an uncuffed tracheostomy tube will result in a large air leak, and it will be difficult to ventilate the patient. In this case, the uncuffed tube should be exchanged for a cuffed tube. If a tracheostomy tube is not readily available, an endotracheal tube may be inserted into the stoma to maintain airway security. If the

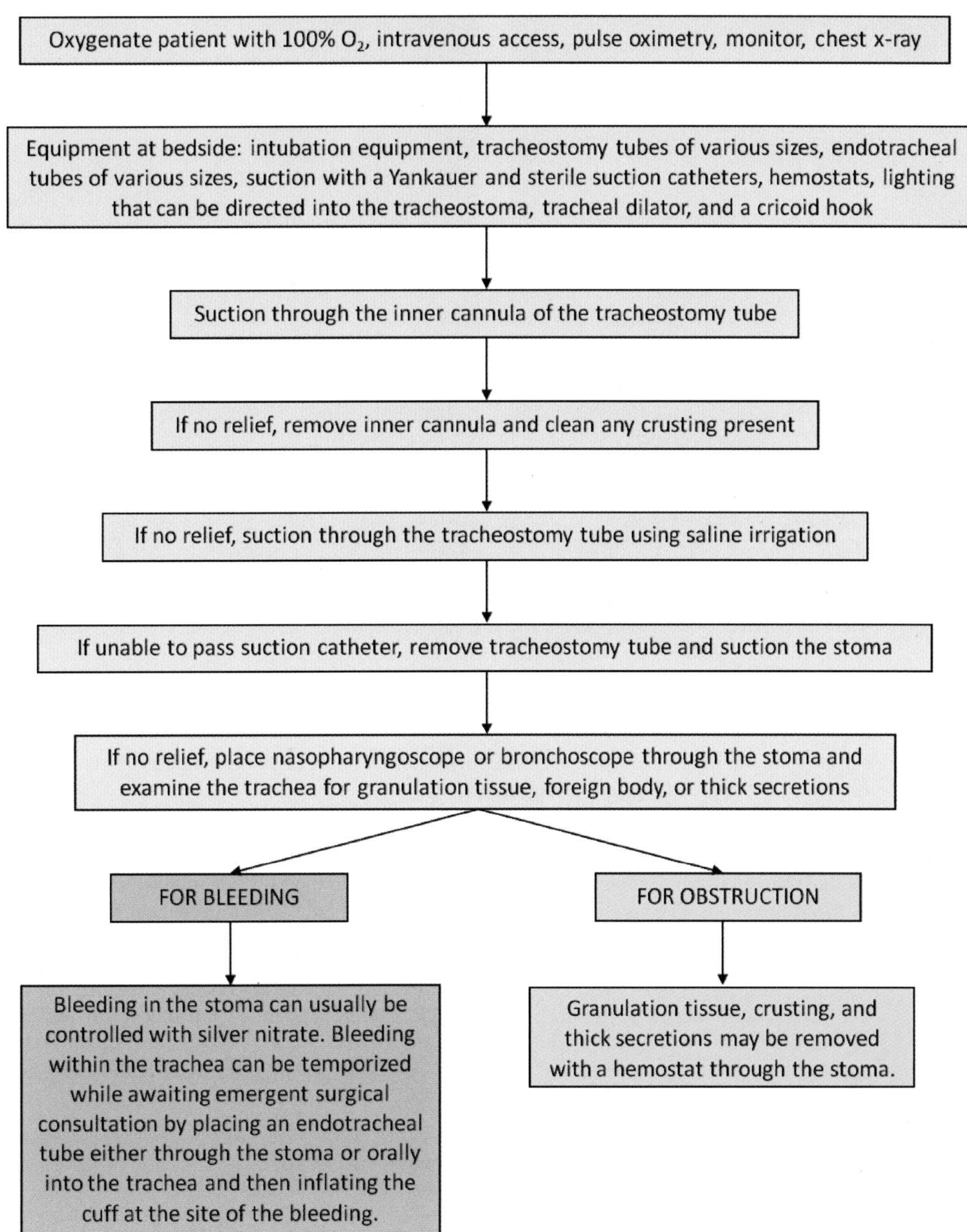

Oxygenate patient with 100% O_2, intravenous access, pulse oximetry, monitor, chest x-ray
Equipment at bedside: intubation equipment, tracheostomy tubes of various sizes, endotracheal tubes of various sizes, suction with a Yankauer and sterile suction catheters, hemostats, lighting that can be directed into the tracheostoma, tracheal dilator, and a cricoid hook
Suction through the inner cannula of the tracheostomy tube
If no relief, remove inner cannula and clean any crusting present
If no relief, suction through the tracheostomy tube using saline irrigation
If unable to pass suction catheter, remove tracheostomy tube and suction the stoma
If no relief, place nasopharyngoscope or bronchoscope through the stoma and examine the trachea for granulation tissue, foreign body, or thick secretions
FOR BLEEDING
FOR OBSTRUCTION
Bleeding in the stoma can usually be controlled with silver nitrate. Bleeding within the trachea can be temporized while awaiting emergent surgical consultation by placing an endotracheal tube either through the stoma or orally into the trachea and then inflating the cuff at the site of the bleeding.
Granulation tissue, crusting, and thick secretions may be removed with a hemostat through the stoma.

FIGURE 247-2. Steps in assessing a tracheostomy patient with respiratory distress.

stoma cannot be cannulated, the patient may be orotracheally intubated to secure the airway—unless the patient has a laryngectomy (see the following "Larnygectomy Patients" section).

CHANGING A TRACHEOSTOMY TUBE

The amount of difficulty encountered when changing a tracheostomy tube depends on when the procedure was performed and on patient anatomy. **If the tracheostomy is <7 days old, the tract will not be mature and manipulation may easily create a false passage within the soft tissue of the neck. In addition, a tract may easily collapse at any time in patients with obese necks or neck masses. If the situation is not emergent and the tracheostomy is <7 days old, tracheostomy tubes should be changed by a surgeon familiar with the procedure.**

An uneventful tracheostomy change depends on adequate preparation and is best accomplished with an assistant. The spontaneously breathing, stable patient can easily breathe through a patent stoma without the tube in place, so there is no reason to rush through this procedure. The needed equipment is listed in **Table 247-1**. If a cuffed tube is used, test the balloon before use and make sure the balloon is completely deflated before insertion. A cricoid hook can be inserted just under the cricoid and used to lift and stabilize the trachea. The dilator is particularly useful if a larger tube is to be inserted, but if dilation is needed and time permits, obtain surgical consultation. Dilation may require injection of local anesthesia. Become familiar with the cricoid hook and tracheal dilator before using them. To minimize soft tissue damage, use an obturator whenever a tracheostomy tube is replaced. When the obturator is placed within the outer cannula, the tube presents a solid, rounded end that is less likely to damage the neck soft tissue during tube insertion (Figure 247-1). **After placement, quickly remove the obturator and place the inner cannula, because the patient cannot breathe through the tracheostomy tube when the obturator is in place.**

Once the equipment is ready, place the patient supine with a shoulder roll to extend the neck. Remove the old tube and gently suction and examine the stoma. In most cases, the opening in the trachea and the posterior tracheal wall can be seen. Gently direct the fresh tube with the balloon deflated into the opening, curving it downward into the trachea (**Figure 247-4**). The movement should be smooth and gentle. If resistance

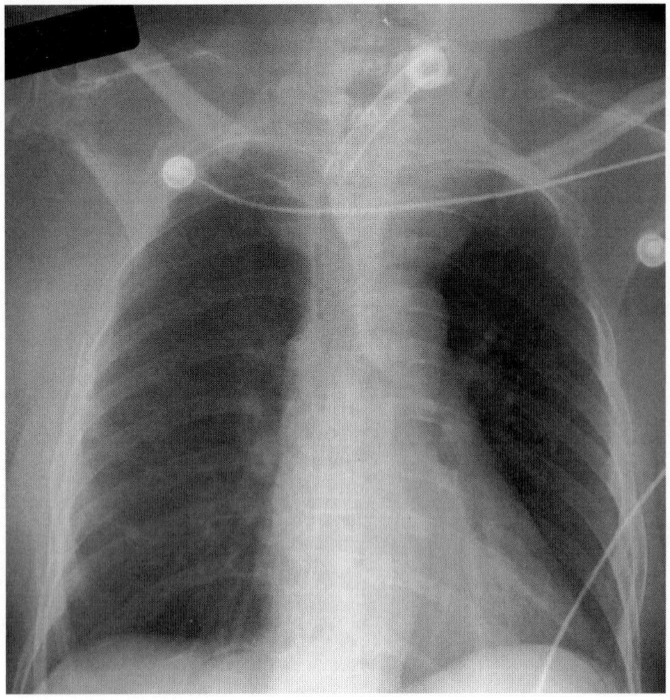
A

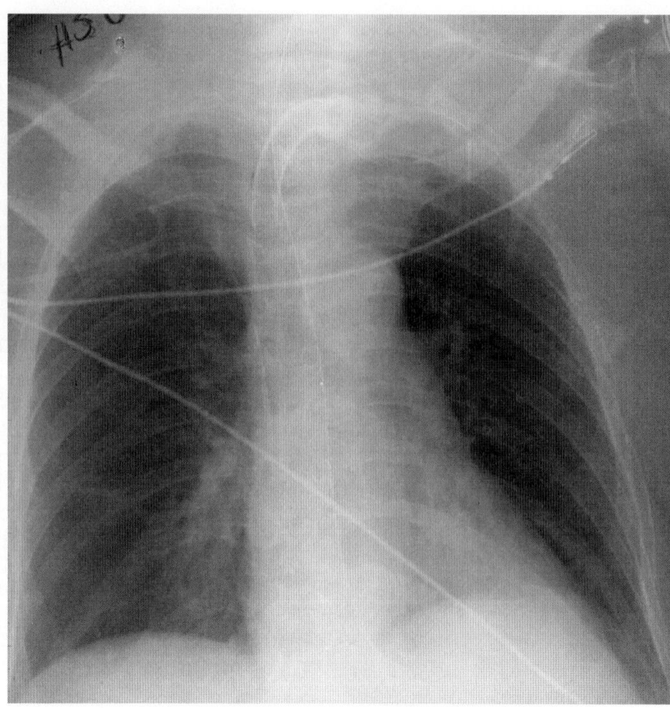
B

FIGURE 247-3. **A.** Patient with a large goiter and a No. 4 Shiley tracheostomy tube with the tip of the tube outside the trachea and compressing the tracheal wall. **B.** Same patient with a longer No. 6 Shiley tracheostomy tube with the tip of the tube correctly placed inside the trachea.

is met, the tube is likely caught on the cartilaginous tracheal wall. Remove the tube and reexamine the stoma, and again place the tube directly into the tracheal opening. If the tube still cannot be placed, consider placing a smaller tracheostomy tube. **However, a smaller tube will also be shorter and may not be long enough for the patient's neck.** Another helpful method is to place a small suction catheter or nasogastric tube into the trachea and thread the tracheostomy tube over the catheter using a modified Seldinger technique.

Once the tube is in place, verify correct tube position by inserting a suction catheter into the tube or attaching an end-tidal carbon dioxide detector. It should easily pass beyond the length of the tracheostomy tube without resistance. If there is a question about placement, pass a nasopharyngoscope or flexible bronchoscope through the tube for direct visualization of placement or obtain an x-ray.

Patients with accidental decannulation who are not in distress can have the tracheostomy tube replaced as described. **If the tube has been out for several hours, the stoma may begin to close and dilation may be needed before tube insertion.** In these cases, and if the stoma is small or the tracheostomy is the patient's only airway, ear, nose, and throat or surgical consultation is recommended for tube replacement.

LARYNGECTOMY PATIENTS

It is impossible to orally intubate patients who have had a laryngectomy. The only access to the tracheobronchial tree is through the tracheostoma in the neck. Occasionally, laryngectomy patients will have a laryngectomy tube in the stoma, similar in appearance to a tracheostomy tube. Laryngectomy patients can be distinguished from tracheostomy patients by history and physical examination and by the fact that laryngectomy patients are unable to vocalize (or breathe) when the laryngectomy tube is occluded. **Laryngectomy patients can be emergently intubated by placing an endotracheal tube into the tracheostoma.** Do not advance the tube too far, as the carina may be only 4 to 6 cm from the tracheostoma.

TABLE 247-1 Equipment Needed to Change a Tracheostomy Tube
Suction device with both a Yankauer tip and suction catheters that fit inside the tracheostomy tube
Good lighting directed into the tracheostoma
An appropriate size tracheostomy tube with obturator in place
Another tracheostomy tube one size smaller than planned
Tracheostomy tube tie
Cricoid hook and tracheal dilator (if physician is familiar with their use)

LARYNGEAL STENTS

The surgical management of severe laryngotracheal stenosis often employs the insertion of tracheal stents for various periods of time. Placement of an endolaryngeal stent renders a patient tracheostomy dependent until the stent is removed because the solid stent blocks the airway at the level of the larynx (**Figure 247-5**). **Stents and their associated tracheostomy tubes should only be removed by a surgeon familiar with the devices and their placement.** There are many different endolaryngeal stent designs and materials, including silastic molds secured by cutaneous buttons (a stent secured by a strap that exits the tracheal stoma and is attached to the skin), the Aboulker stent complex (a metal tracheostomy tube wired to a silastic stent used in pediatric airway reconstruction), and the Montgomery T-tube stent (**Figure 247-6**). Although endolaryngeal stents are secured by buttons or straps, dislodgement is a known complication of these devices. If a stent becomes dislodged but the tracheostomy tube remains in position, airway security is usually not an issue. Consult the otolaryngologist for extrusion or dislodgment of a stent.

The Montgomery T-tube configuration is commonly used in adult laryngotracheal reconstruction.[10] It is a modification of a tracheostomy tube that does not have an inner cannula. Humidification and suctioning of the T-tube is essential to prevent mucous plugging. These tubes are also used in tracheal stenosis as a bridge to surgery, a treatment for those patients who are not surgical candidates, and in cases where there is a long segment of stenosis.[10] Airway obstruction should be addressed by first suctioning both the upper and lower limbs of the T-tube (**Figure 247-6**). If suctioning both limbs of the T-tube does not

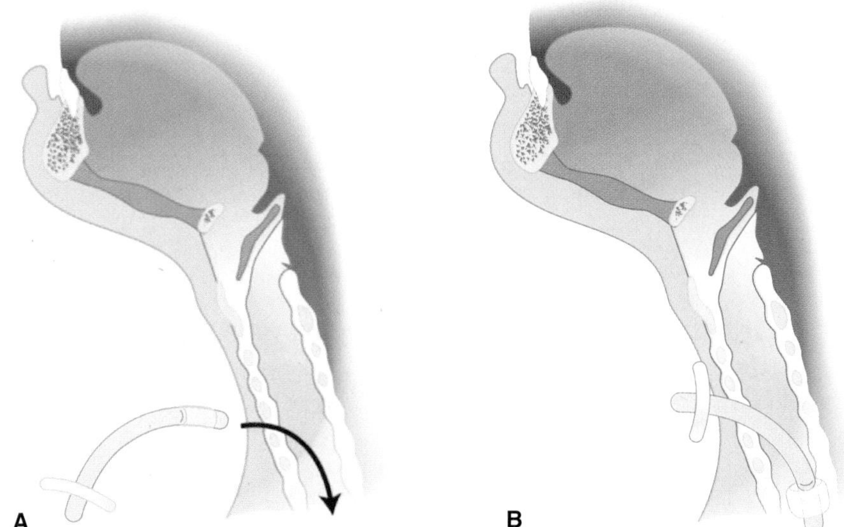

FIGURE 247-4. Insertion (**A**) and placement (**B**) of the tracheostomy tube. Cuffed tubes should be inserted with the cuff deflated.

relieve the obstruction, the T-tube should be removed and the trachea cannulated with an appropriately sized tracheostomy tube or an endotracheal tube. Do not try to use a bag-valve device through the T-tube because most tubes do not take a standard 15-mm connector.[11] Removal requires a strong, steady pull on the T-tube and should only be attempted if the operating surgeon is unavailable or the patient is in airway distress.

SPEECH DEVICES

The Passy-Muir valve is a one-way valve that fits directly over the opening of an uncuffed tracheostomy tube and allows the patient hands-free speech. When the patient inhales, the valve opens and allows air to pass into the trachea and lungs. Speech is created when the patient exhales with enough force to close the Passy-Muir valve. The exhaled air is directed around the tracheostomy tube and through the vocal cords (**Figure 247-7**). Because the patient exhales around the tracheostomy tube, **a Passy-Muir valve should never be used with a cuffed tube.** If a patient with a Passy-Muir valve develops signs of airway obstruction or an inability to speak, the speaking device should be removed from the tracheostomy tube so that air can pass freely during both inhalation and exhalation. If this does not relieve symptoms, check the tracheostomy tube itself for obstruction.

A tracheoesophageal prosthesis allows speech in postlaryngectomy patients. This one-way valve is surgically placed between the posterior wall of the tracheal stoma and the anterior wall of the cervical esophagus. To speak, patients exhale while occluding the stoma with their thumb or finger, thus forcing the exhaled air into the esophagus. The air vibrates the esophagus (as a belch does), and the resultant tone is used to provide speech (**Figures 247-8 and 247-9**).

The most common complication associated with tracheoesophageal prosthetic valves is leakage, either around the valve or through the valve lumen. Both types of leakage may be confirmed by looking at the prosthesis while the patient drinks a colored liquid (e.g., grape juice). Leakage commonly occurs due to enlargement of the tracheoesophageal fistula.[12]

Leakage increases the risk of aspiration pneumonia. A temporary solution to a leaking valve begins with removal of the entire prosthesis and replacement with a larger Foley catheter into the tracheoesophageal fistula. This will prevent the tracheoesophageal fistula from closing completely as the fistula contracts in size. Leakage through a voice prosthesis

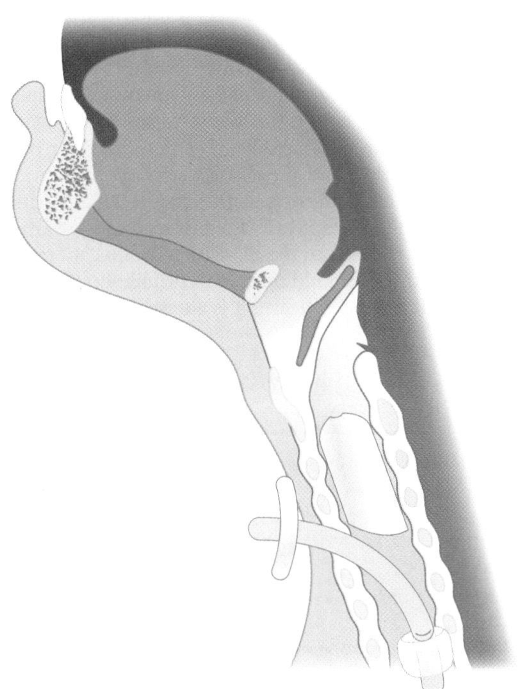

FIGURE 247-5. Relation of the tracheostomy tube to the laryngeal stent. The stent lies within the lumen of the trachea, superior to the tracheostomy tube.

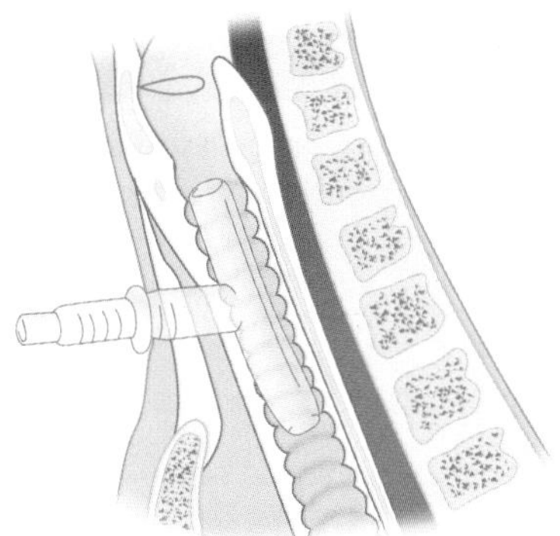

FIGURE 247-6. Suctioning is required of both the upper and lower limbs of the Montgomery T-tube. If necessary, the entire T-tube can be removed.

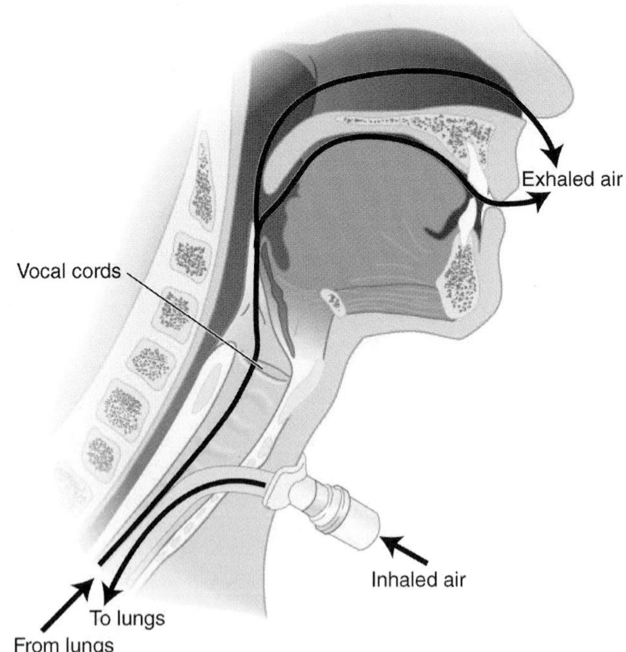

FIGURE 247-7. The Passy-Muir valve is a one-way valve that fits directly on the opening of the tracheostomy tube. Speech is created when the patient exhales as air is passed up through the vocal cords and out of the mouth.

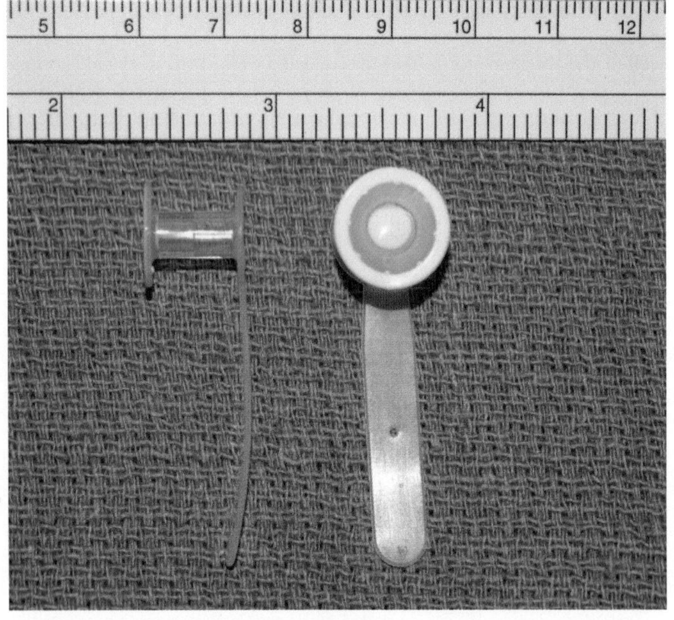

FIGURE 247-8. Tracheoesophageal prosthesis. The bobbin-shaped device is placed with the smaller flange in the esophagus and the tagged flange in the posterior tracheostoma.

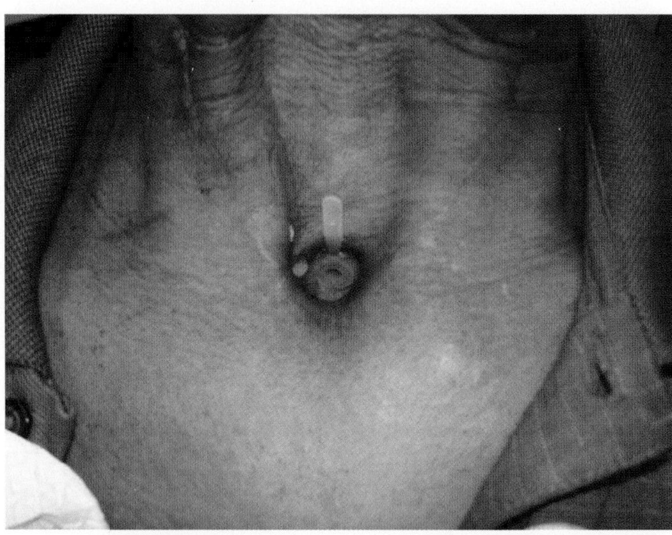

FIGURE 247-9. Tracheoesophageal prosthesis in place in a laryngectomy patient. The prosthesis is in place, and the tag is usually held with tape. Finger occlusion of the tracheostoma with exhalation leads to increased airway pressure, which opens the one-way valve and allows air to enter the esophagus. This vibrates and allows the patient to speak.

is predominantly due to valve damage caused by fungal colonization or contact of a duckbill-style device against the posterior esophageal wall and is treated by replacement of the prosthesis with a temporary tube (usually a Foley catheter). Once a Foley catheter is placed and secured, the patient is unable to speak. Arrange otolaryngologist follow-up the next day. Do not inflate the balloon on the Foley catheter, as this will interfere with swallowing.

Another common complication with tracheoesophageal prostheses is valve aspiration or valve extrusion. A loose valve or coughing while changing a valve can result in aspiration of the valve into the airway. Aspiration results in persistent cough, dyspnea with discomfort, and even respiratory distress. If there is suspicion of aspiration or if the prosthesis is dislodged, obtain a chest x-ray to visualize the radiopaque valve and consult an otolaryngologist. The tracheoesophageal puncture tract will close quickly, typically within 24 to 48 hours after the tube is dislodged. A Foley or red rubber catheter inserted into the tract will maintain its patency. **Do not attempt temporary catheter placement if the tract is <2 weeks old, as a false passage may result.**

Pharyngeal stricture and stomal stenosis are other complications associated with tracheoesophageal prosthetic valves.[13] Granulation tissue and polyp formation around the valve prosthesis may also occur and dislodge or obstruct airflow and prevent speech. Application of silver nitrate cauterization will treat the granulation tissue, but it is critical that a portion be sent to pathology to verify the histopathology of the tissue.

Whenever a patient presents to the ED with a complication due to an airway device, the provider should be able to troubleshoot many of the common problems. If there is concern, it is advisable to consult an otolaryngologist.

REFERENCES

The complete reference list is available online at www.TintinalliEM.com.

SECTION 20
Dermatology

CHAPTER 248 Initial Evaluation and Management of Skin Disorders

William Rushton
Joseph M. Grover
William J. Brady

INTRODUCTION

Most ED chief complaints involving skin lesions are due to infections, irritants, and allergies.[1] Visual pattern recognition is the key to diagnosis. The recommended approach for the diagnosis of a skin disorder in the ED (assuming resuscitation or stabilization is not required) is to:

1. Determine the chief complaint.
2. Obtain a brief history (duration, rate of progression, and location of lesions).
3. Perform the dermatologic examination (morphology and extent of distribution).
4. Formulate the age-appropriate differential diagnosis based on lesion morphology and distribution.
5. Elicit additional concerns from the history (associated complaints, comorbidity, medications, or exposures), and include or exclude syndromes in the differential diagnosis based on this information.
6. Evaluate for systemic involvement, and consider ancillary investigations, if necessary.
7. Obtain dermatologic consultation, if necessary, and arrange for appropriate referral (primary care or dermatologic).

DIAGNOSTIC APPROACH

HISTORY

Determine the chief complaint and obtain a brief history (discomfort, duration, rate of progression, percentage of body surface involvement, and location of lesions). The secondary history should include issues relating to the lesion: morphology, evolutionary nature, rate of progression, and distribution. Associated systemic complaints and mucosal systems must be identified. Ask about exposures, immunizations, toxins, chemicals, foods, animals, insects, plants, and ill contacts. Sexual history, if appropriate, and medical and family histories should be reviewed. If applicable, a detailed occupational history should be obtained; industrial exposure may be the causative etiology. Asking about medication use, sun exposure, travel history, or particular food ingestion also may yield helpful information. Be sure to include any other housemates or partners in your history of exposures; contact dermatitis can occur from exposure to fragrances or other products that a partner is using.[2] The patient should also be asked about the degree of discomfort of the dermatoses; a painful dermatitis is often a red flag and is not usually associated with a self-limiting lesion.[3]

A detailed medication history is important and particular attention should be paid to recently started drugs or dosage increases. Erythema multiforme, exfoliative dermatitis, photosensitivity reactions, toxic epidermal necrolysis, and vasculitis are common medication-induced drug reactions. Dermal necrosis should prompt consideration of anticoagulant use, whereas a diffuse rash in a patient on sulfa drugs, anticonvulsants, or some antimicrobials may aid the clinician in diagnosing Stevens-Johnson syndrome or toxic epidermal necrolysis.

EXAMINATION

The patient should be gowned and in a room with adequate lighting and appropriate privacy to allow entire skin examination. Inspect all skin and mucosal surfaces, including hair, nails, scalp, and mucous membranes. Then evaluate the specific skin lesions. A magnifying lens and a portable light are helpful aids.

Examine the skin systematically. Determine the **distribution, pattern, arrangement, morphology, extent, and evolutionary changes** of the lesions. **Distribution** is the location of the skin findings, and the **pattern** is their anatomic, functional, and physiologic arrangement. For example, a unilateral band-like arrangement of lesions on the thorax suggests varicella-zoster virus infection. Skin diseases often present with a predilection for certain body areas; the distribution of lesions will assist in narrowing the diagnostic possibilities. From the anatomic perspective, the skin surfaces that are usually considered as separate areas of distribution are generalized body; face and scalp; trunk and axillae; groin and skin folds; and hands, feet, and nails. The extremities may be further subdivided into upper versus lower, proximal versus distal, wrists versus ankles, and hands versus feet.

In a patient with diffuse erythema in whom toxic shock syndrome is suspected, the presence of a foreign body such as a retained tampon should be investigated. Petechia should prompt the investigation of meningococcemia or Rocky Mountain spotted fever. Rashes on exposed portions of the skin should prompt inquiries about sun exposure, jewelry, topical agents, or exposures. See **Table 248-1** for a differential diagnosis of skin lesions as a function of location, including both distribution and pattern considerations.

Use the burn **rule of nines** (see chapter 216, "Thermal Burns") to estimate the degree of skin involvement in disorders with widespread distribution. This calculation also may be used to determine the amount of topical medication required for a specific treatment course or whether an oral medication might be more appropriate. Extensive erythroderma (often >90% of body surface area) is a dermatologic emergency.[3,4] Severe erythroderma can represent underlying severe infectious dermatitis, toxic shock syndrome, cutaneous T-cell lymphoma, drug reaction, psoriasis, or seborrheic dermatitis.

TABLE 248-1 Differential Diagnosis Relative to Lesion Distribution and Pattern

Distribution and Pattern	Differential Diagnosis
Flexor surfaces	Atopic dermatitis, candidiasis, eczema, ichthyosis
Sun exposure (face, upper thorax, distal extremities)	Sunburn, photosensitive drug eruption, photosensitive dermatitis, systemic lupus erythematosus, viral exanthem, porphyria
Distal extremities	Viral exanthem, atopic or contact dermatitis, eczema, Rocky Mountain spotted fever, gonococcemia
Front and back of chest	Pityriasis rosea, secondary syphilis, drug eruption, atopic or contact dermatitis, psoriasis
Clothing covered (thorax and distal lower extremities)	Contact dermatitis, psoriasis, folliculitis
Acneiform (face and upper thorax)	Acne, drug-induced acne, irritant dermatitides

Lesion arrangement refers to the symmetry and configuration. Bilateral symmetry suggests a systemic internal event or symmetric external exposure, as seen in erythema multiforme, with plaque-like lesions on the flexor surfaces of the extremities, or contact dermatitis related to a lotion application. An asymmetric arrangement supports a localized process. *Configuration* may apply to a single lesion with reference to its individual features or, alternatively, to multiple lesions and their relation to one another. For instance, internal configuration is illustrated by the relation between the central papule relative to the erythematous ring in the target lesion of erythema multiforme; on the total-body scale, configuration is demonstrated by clustering of lesions in a herpesvirus infection or by a linear arrangement as with a reaction from poison ivy or oak. Other terms used to describe the lesion configuration are listed in **Table 248-2**.

Recognition of the primary lesion is vital in establishing the diagnosis; the use of the primary lesion's **morphology** is very important regarding the generation of an appropriate differential diagnosis and ultimately the correct dermatologic diagnosis. The primary lesion is the one that has not been altered by secondary issues, including healing, complicating infection, medication application, or scratching. Examples of primary skin lesions are macules, papules, nodules, tumors, cysts, plaques, wheals, vesicles, bullae, and pustules. Careful attention should be paid to a nonblanching lesion. Secondary lesions have had their appearance altered due to disease evolution or various external factors, as noted earlier, and include crusts, scales, fissures, erosions, ulcerations, excoriations, atrophy, scarring, and lichenification. See **Table 248-3** for a listing and descriptions

TABLE 248-2 Lesion Configuration Descriptors

Descriptor	Configuration
Annular	Ring-like or pertaining to the outer edge
Arcuate	Curved or pertaining to the curve
Circinate	Circular
Confluent	Blending together
Dermatomal	Belt-like or limited to one side of the body in anatomic dermatome
Discoid	Solid, round, slightly raised, or pertaining to a disk
Discrete	Separate or individual
Grouped	Clustered
Guttate	Scattered
Gyrate	Coiled or winding
Herpetiform	Creeping
Iris	Concentric circles
Linear	In a line
Polycyclic	Overlapping circles or borders of irregular curves
Retiform	Net-like
Serpiginous	Snake-like

TABLE 248-3 Lesion Morphology

Descriptor	Morphology	Lesion Nature	Height Relative to Adjacent Skin	Image
Excoriation	Linear marks from scratching	Secondary	Flat	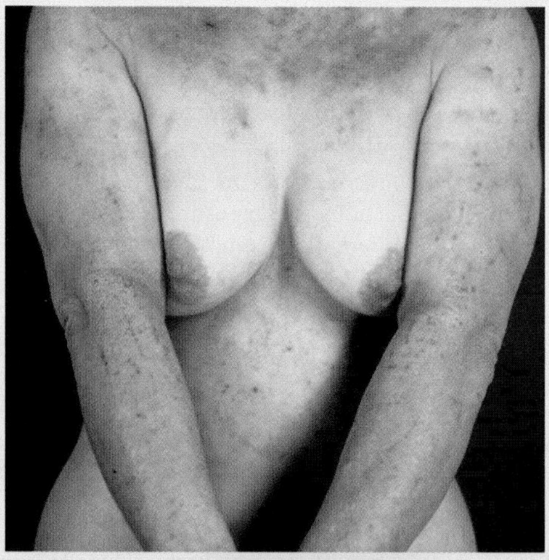
Erosion	Ruptured vesicle or bulla with denuded epidermis	Secondary	Depressed	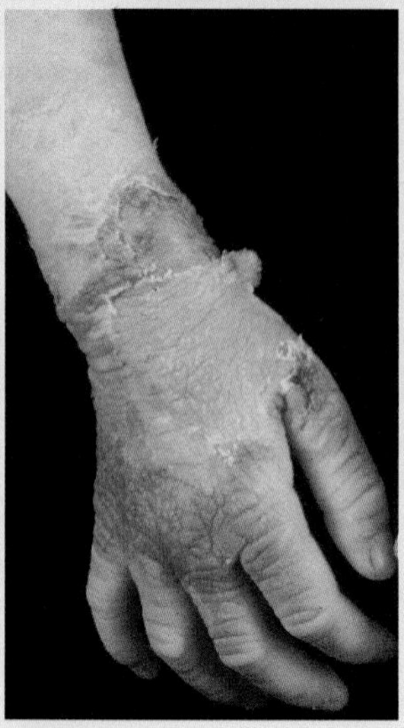

(*Continued*)

TABLE 248-3 Lesion Morphology (*Continued*)

Descriptor	Morphology	Lesion Nature	Height Relative to Adjacent Skin	Image
Fissure	Linear cracks on skin surface	Secondary	Flat	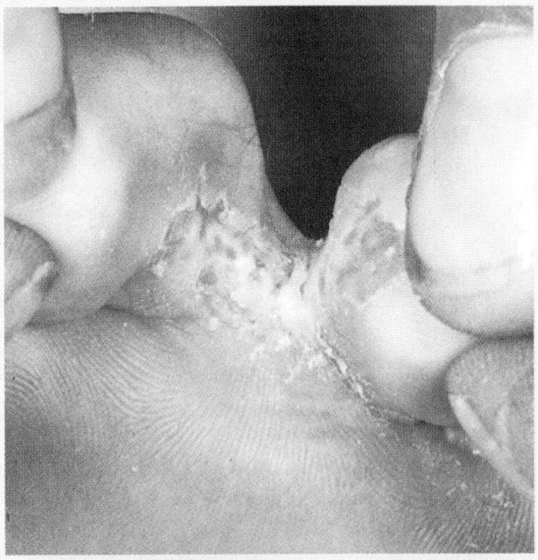
Ulcer	Epidermal or dermal tissue loss	Secondary	Depressed	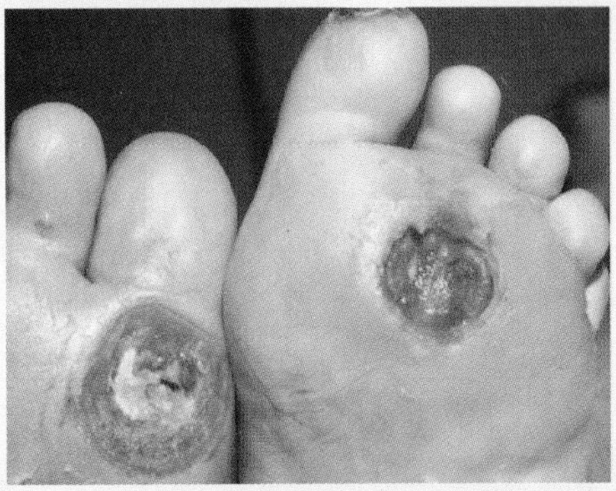
Macule	Flat, circumscribed discoloration ≤1 cm in diameter; color varies	Primary	Flat	
Petechiae	Nonblanching purple spots <2 mm in diameter	Primary	Flat	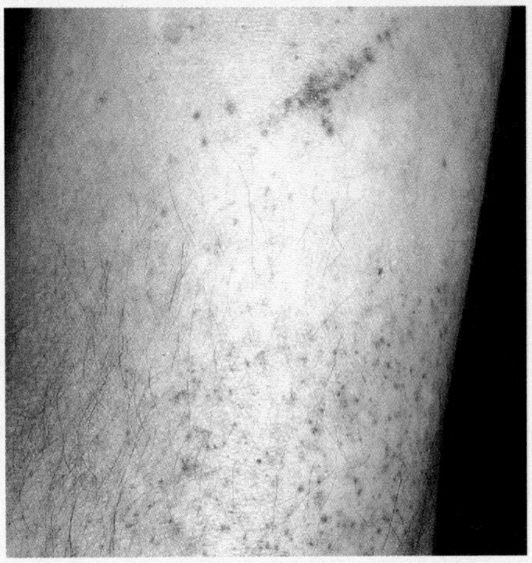

(*Continued*)

TABLE 248-3 Lesion Morphology (*Continued*)

Descriptor	Morphology	Lesion Nature	Height Relative to Adjacent Skin	Image
Sclerosis	Firm, indurated skin	Secondary	Flat or elevated	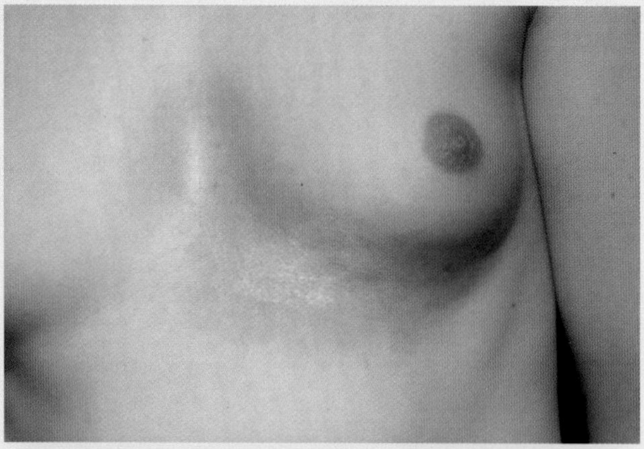
Telangiectasia	Small, blanchable superficial capillaries	Primary	Flat	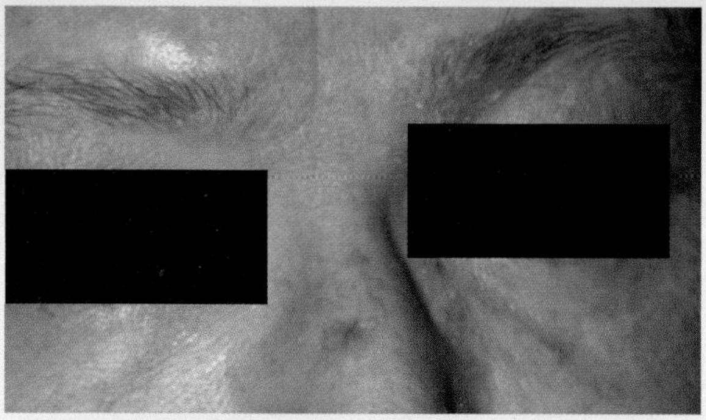
Purpura	Nonblanching purple discoloration of the skin	Primary	Flat	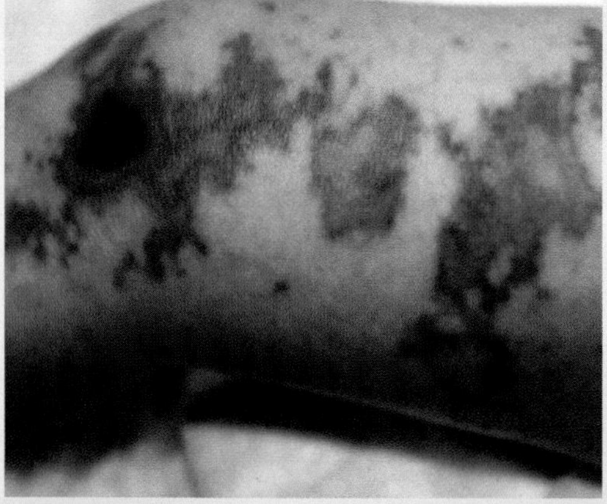
Abscess	Tender, erythematous, fluctuant nodule	Primary	Elevated	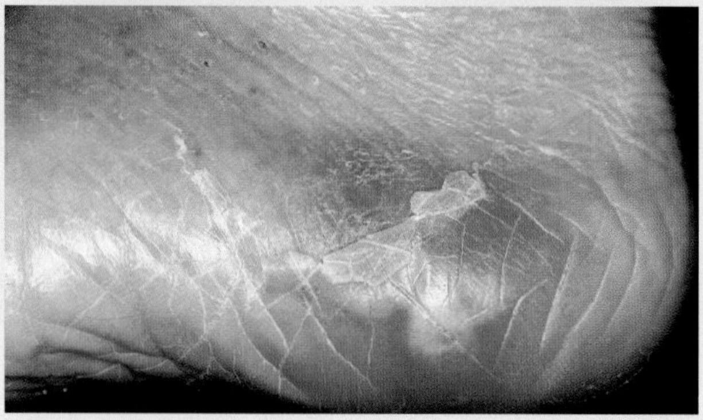

(*Continued*)

TABLE 248-3 Lesion Morphology (*Continued*)

Descriptor	Morphology	Lesion Nature	Height Relative to Adjacent Skin	Image
Cyst	Sack containing liquid or semisolid material	Primary	Elevated	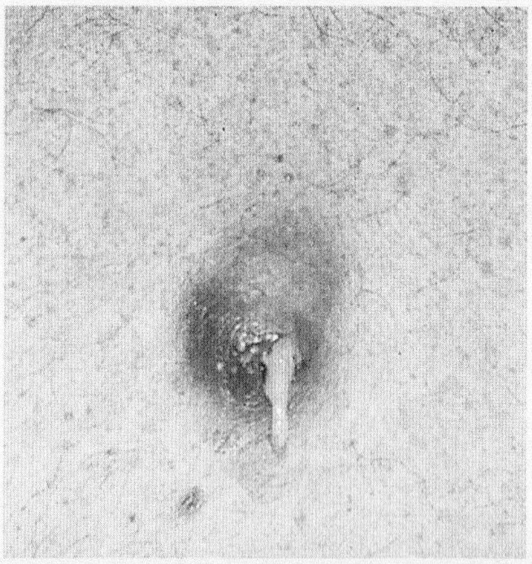
Nodule	Palpable solid lesion <1 cm in diameter	Primary	Elevated	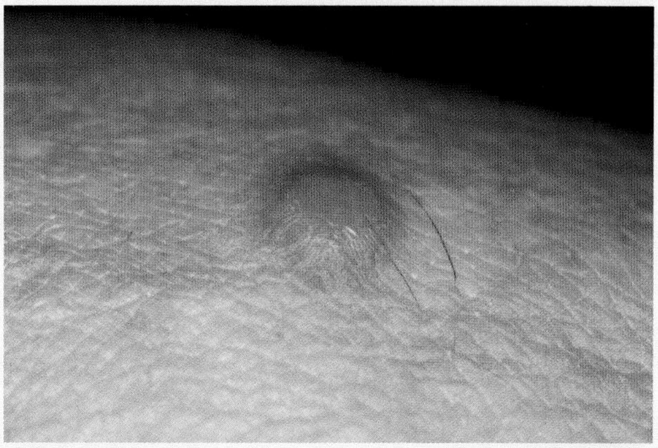
Tumor	Palpable solid lesion >1 cm in diameter	Primary	Elevated	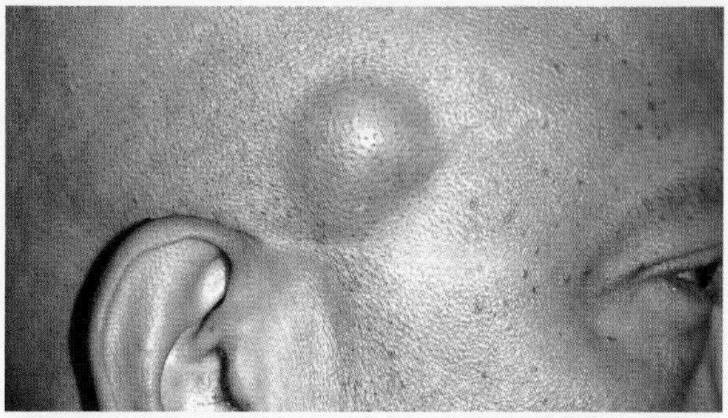 A 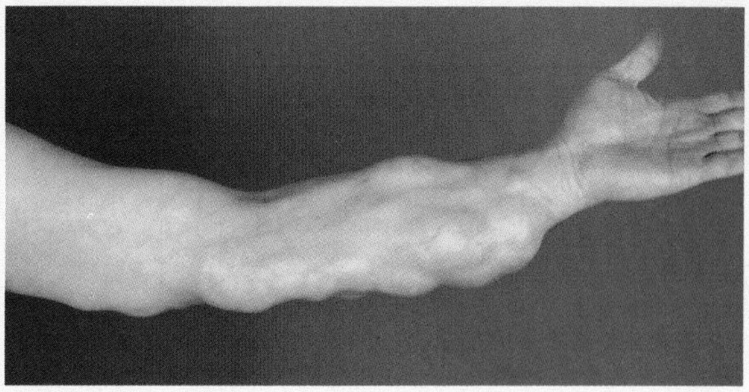 B

(*Continued*)

TABLE 248-3 Lesion Morphology (*Continued*)

Descriptor	Morphology	Lesion Nature	Height Relative to Adjacent Skin	Image
Scar	Sclerotic area of skin	Secondary	Flat or elevated	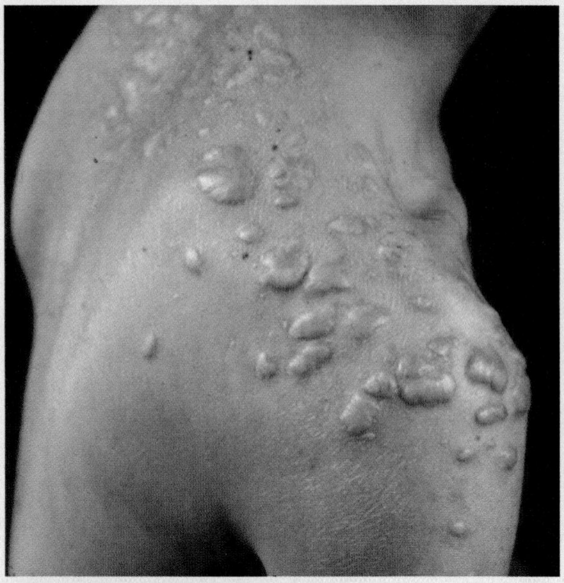
Wheal	Transient, edematous papule or plaque with peripheral erythema	Primary	Flat or elevated	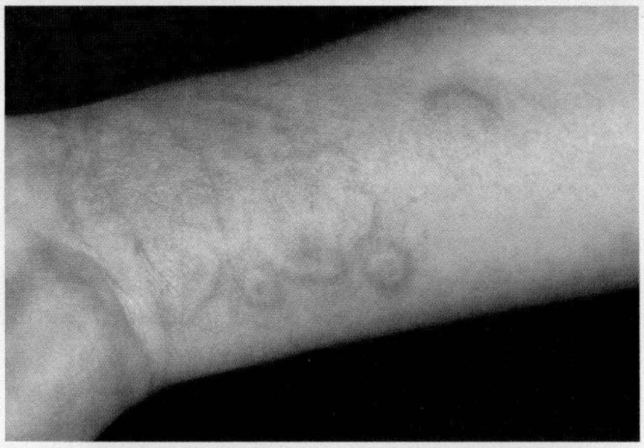
Vesicle	Circumscribed, thin-walled, elevated blister <5 mm in diameter	Primary	Elevated	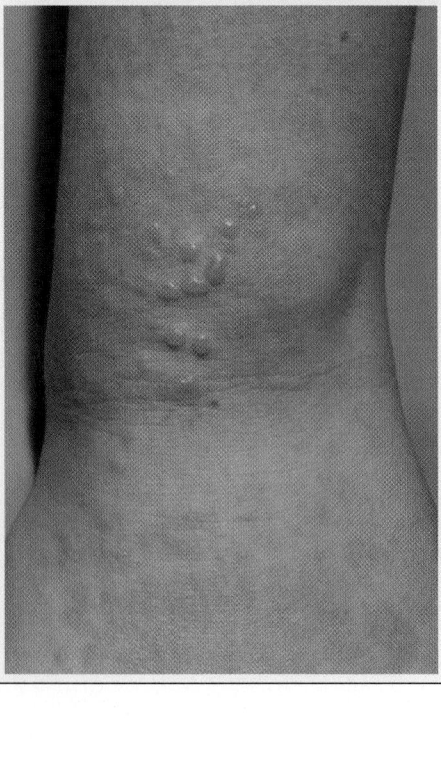

(*Continued*)

TABLE 248-3 Lesion Morphology (*Continued*)

Descriptor	Morphology	Lesion Nature	Height Relative to Adjacent Skin	Image
Bulla	Circumscribed, thin-walled, elevated blister >5 mm in diameter	Primary	Elevated	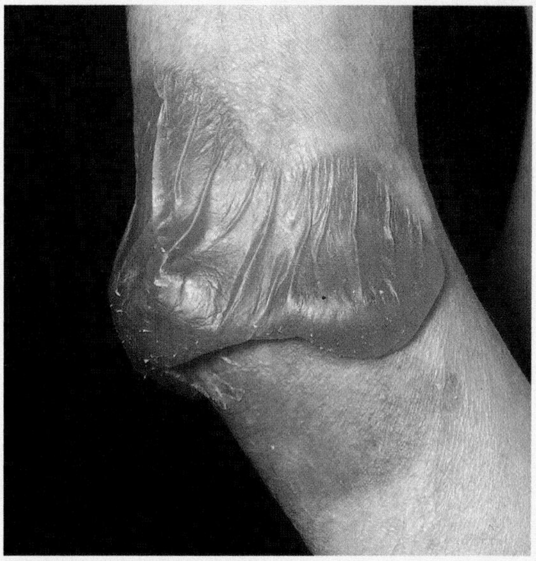
Pustule	Vesicle containing purulent fluid	Primary	Elevated	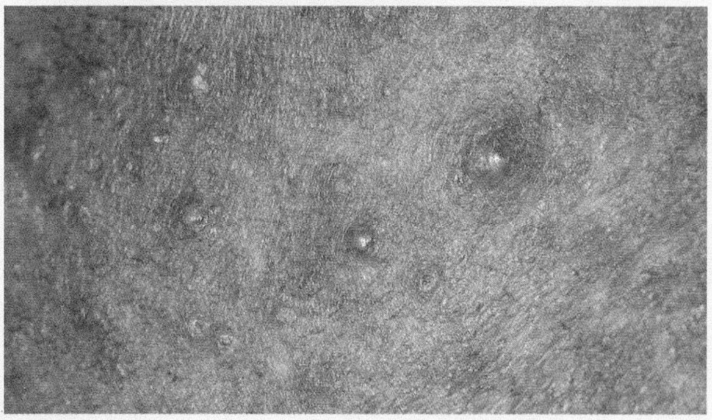
Papule	Elevated, solid, palpable lesion <1 cm in diameter; color varies	Primary	Elevated	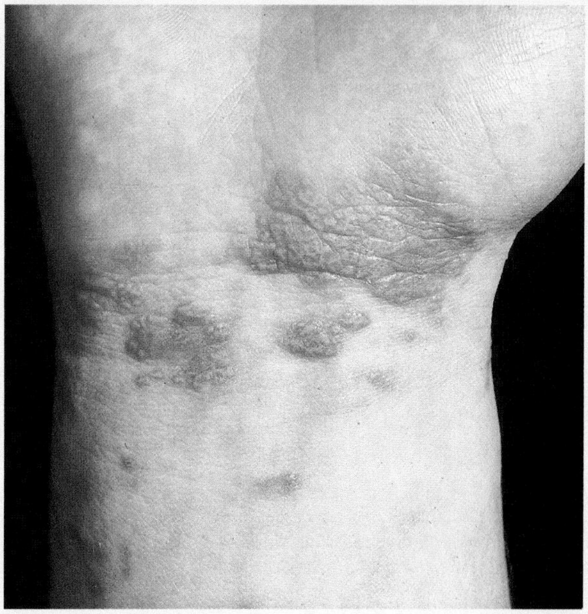

(*Continued*)

TABLE 248-3 Lesion Morphology (*Continued*)

Descriptor	Morphology	Lesion Nature	Height Relative to Adjacent Skin	Image
Plaque	Flat-topped elevation formed by confluence of papules >0.5 cm in diameter	Primary	Elevated	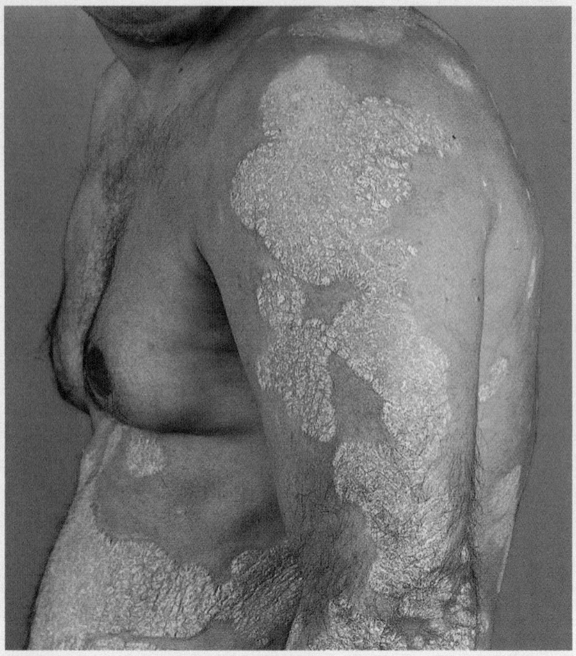
Comedo	Papule with an impacted pilosebaceous unit	Primary	Elevated	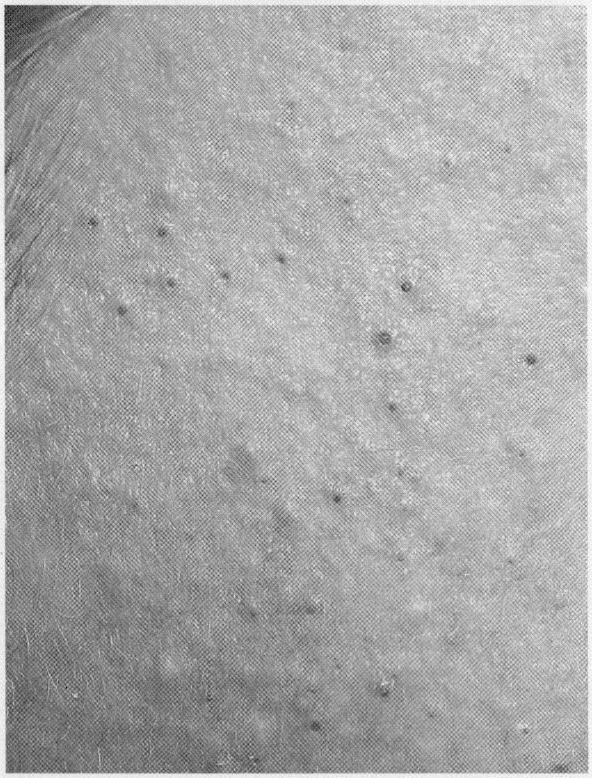

Source: Images reproduced with permission from Wolff KL, Johnson R, Suurmond R: *Fitzpatrick's Color Atlas & Synopsis of Clinical Dermatology*, 5th ed. © 2005, McGraw-Hill, New York; and Fleischer AB Jr, Feldman SR, McConnell CF, et al: *Emergency Dermatology: A Rapid Treatment Guide*. © 2002, McGraw-Hill, New York.

of the various morphologic descriptors of dermatologic lesions; see **Tables 284-4 and 284-5** for a differential diagnosis of the various skin disorders relative to primary and secondary lesion morphologies.

DIAGNOSTIC TECHNIQUES

A potassium hydroxide preparation is used in patients with suspected molluscum contagiosum and dermatophytic infections. The test is performed on loose skin scales, nail parings, subungual debris, short residual hairs, or small pearly globules (from a molluscum body). Test steps are in **Table 248-6**.

The material is then viewed under a microscope at low power, with the condenser and light at low levels. As the slide is scanned, rapidly focus up and down. True hyphae (**Figure 248-1**), seen in dermatophytic infections, are long, branching, green rods of constant width that cross the borders of epithelial cells. Molluscum bodies are oval

TABLE 248-4 Differential Diagnosis of Selected Skin Disorders Relative to Primary Lesion Morphology*

Lesion Morphology	Differential Considerations	Images
Macule	Drug eruption (fixed or photosensitive), nevus, tattoo (ink), rheumatic fever, syphilis (secondary), viral exanthema, toxic or infectious erythemas, meningococcemia (early), external trauma (ecchymosis), vitiligo, tinea versicolor, cellulitis (early)	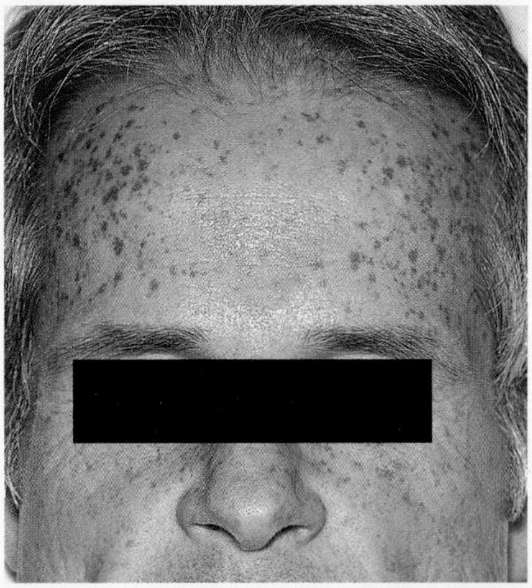
Papule	Acne, basal cell carcinoma, melanoma, nevus, warts, molluscum contagiosum, skin tags, atopic dermatitis, urticaria, eczema, folliculitis, insect bites, vasculitis, psoriasis, scabies, *Toxicodendron* dermatitis (poison ivy, oak, sumac), erythema multiforme, varicella (early), gonococcemia	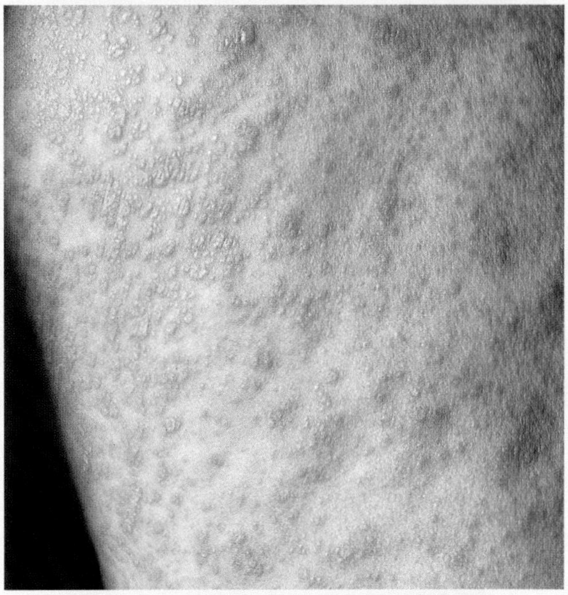
Plaque	Eczema, pityriasis rosea, tinea corporis and versicolor, psoriasis, seborrheic dermatitis, urticaria, syphilis (secondary), erythema multiforme	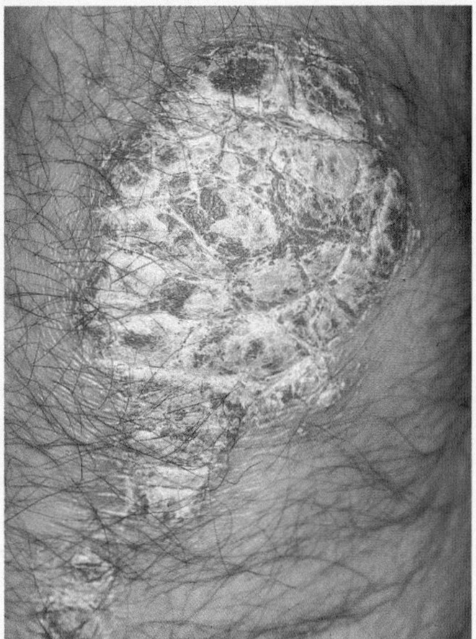

(*Continued*)

TABLE 248-4 Differential Diagnosis of Selected Skin Disorders Relative to Primary Lesion Morphology* *(Continued)*

Lesion Morphology	Differential Considerations	Images
Nodule	Basal cell, squamous cell, or metastatic carcinoma; melanoma; erythema nodosum; furuncle; lipoma; warts	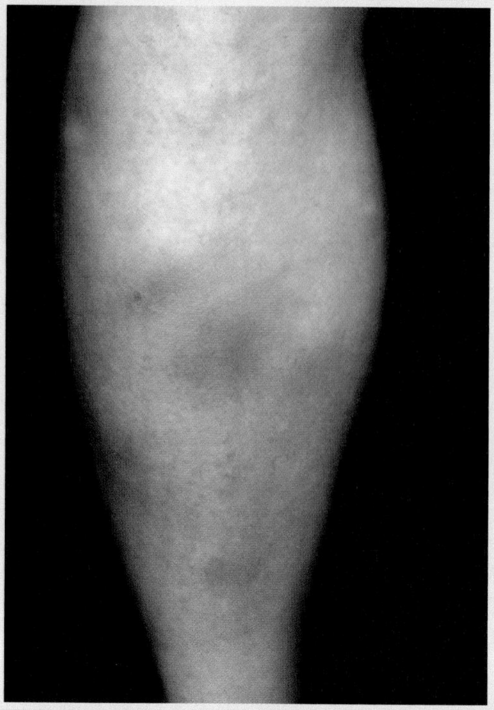
Wheal	Urticaria, angioedema, insect bites, erythema multiforme	
Pustule	Acne, folliculitis, gonococcemia, hidradenitis suppurativa, herpetic infection (herpes simplex, herpes zoster, varicella), impetigo, psoriasis, rosacea, pyoderma gangrenosum	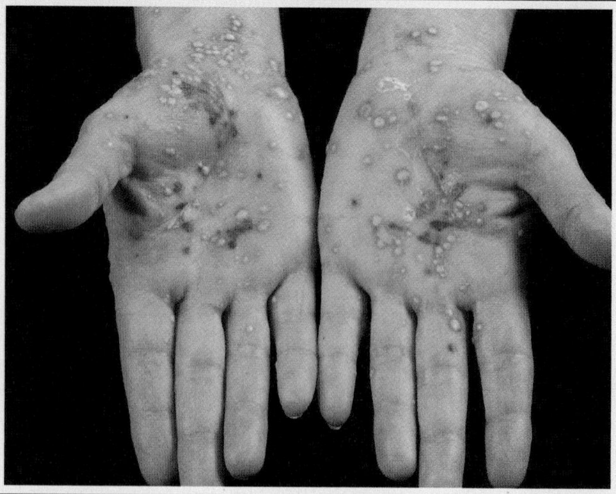

(Continued)

TABLE 248-4 Differential Diagnosis of Selected Skin Disorders Relative to Primary Lesion Morphology* (*Continued*)

Lesion Morphology	Differential Considerations	Images
Vesicle	Herpetic infection (herpes simplex, herpes zoster, varicella), impetigo, *Toxicodendron* dermatitis (poison ivy, oak, sumac), thermal burn, friction blister, toxic epidermal necrolysis, bullous pemphigoid, pemphigus vulgaris	
Bulla	Bullous impetigo, *Toxicodendron* dermatitis (poison ivy, oak, sumac), thermal burn, friction blister, toxic epidermal necrolysis, bullous pemphigoid, pemphigus vulgaris	

*This list is not exhaustive, but it represents the more common syndromes likely to be encountered by the emergency physician.

Source: Images reproduced with permission from Wolff KL, Johnson R, Suurmond R: *Fitzpatrick's Color Atlas & Synopsis of Clinical Dermatology*, 5th ed. © 2005, McGraw-Hill, New York; and Fleischer AB Jr, Feldman SR, McConnell CF, et al: *Emergency Dermatology: A Rapid Treatment Guide.* © 2002, McGraw-Hill, New York.

discs with homogeneous cytoplasm (**Figure 248-2**). In hair fragments, the organisms appear as small, round spores packed closely within the hair shaft.

Scabies and lice preparations are useful in patients with possible infestation. In scabies infestations, the rash itself may resemble other dermatologic syndromes; microscopic analysis will confirm the diagnosis. The donor site for skin specimen selection is very important. The best sites include burrows (10 mm, elongated papule with a pustule or vesicle) and papules on the fingers, wrists, and elbows (**Figure 248-3**). Within the vesicle or pustule, a small black dot is noted, which is the mite. The point of the scalpel is scraped across the lesion while holding the skin taut; the mite is then removed. A single drop of mineral oil may be applied to the blade to ensure that the scrapings adhere to the instrument. The material is then placed on the microscope slide with an additional drop of mineral oil; gentle pressure on the coverslip will flatten thick specimens. Using low power, the slide is scanned for presence of the mite, eggs, or feces. Mites are eight-legged creatures that are easily identified on thin smears; thick specimens may require additional viewing to look for the mite. Additional findings supportive of the diagnosis include eggs (smooth ovals) and feces (clusters of red-brown pellets; **Figure 248-4**). Lice are usually found on the scalp, eyelashes, and pubic areas and may be visible to the unaided eye (**Figure 248-5**).

TABLE 248-5 Differential Diagnosis of Selected Skin Disorders Relative to Secondary Lesion Morphology*

Lesion Morphology	Differential Considerations	Images
Scales	Psoriasis, pityriasis rosea, toxic and infectious erythemas, syphilis (secondary), dermatophytic infection (tinea), tinea versicolor, xerosis (dry skin), thermal burn (first degree)	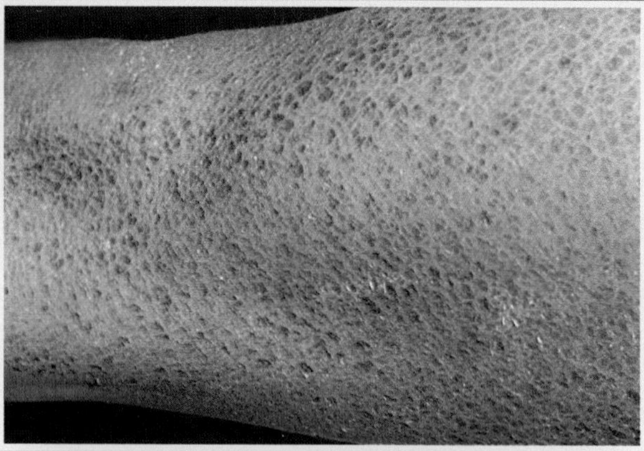
Crusts	Eczema, dermatophytic infection (tinea), impetigo, contact dermatitis, insect bite	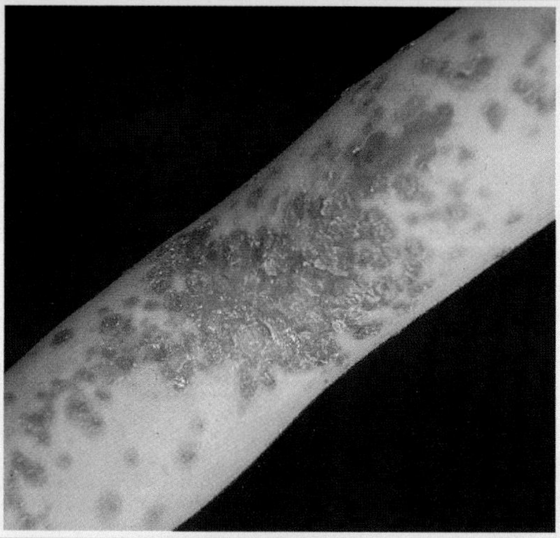
Erosions	Candidiasis, dermatophytic infection (tinea), eczema, toxic epidermal necrolysis, toxic-infectious erythemas, erythema multiforme, primary blistering disorders (bullous pemphigoid and pemphigus vulgaris), brown recluse spider envenomation	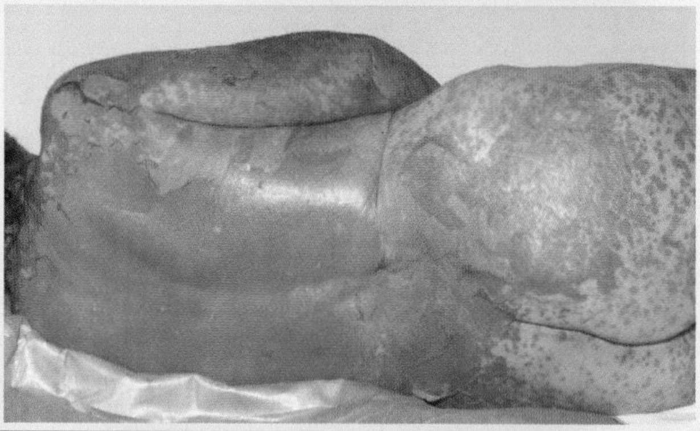
Ulcers	Aphthous lesions, chancroid, decubitus ulcer, thermal or friction injury, subacute or chronic ischemia, malignancy, chancre (primary syphilis), primary blistering disorders (bullous pemphigoid and pemphigus vulgaris), brown recluse spider envenomation, pyoderma gangrenosum, stasis ulcer, factitial ulcer	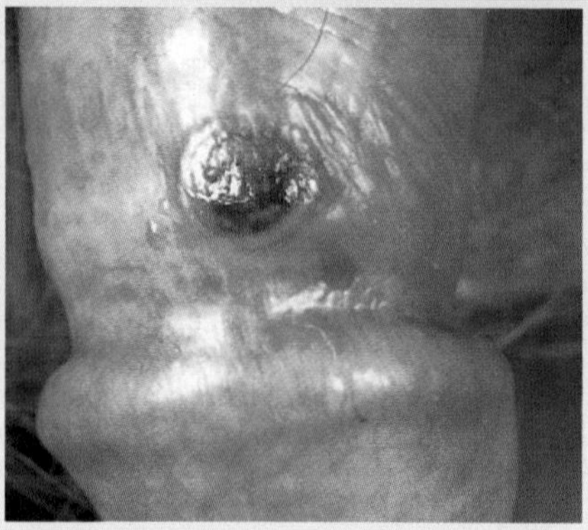

*This list is not exhaustive, but it represents the more common syndromes likely to be encountered by the emergency physician.

Source: Images reproduced with permission from Wolff KL, Johnson R, Suurmond R: *Fitzpatrick's Color Atlas & Synopsis of Clinical Dermatology*, 5th ed. © 2005, McGraw-Hill, New York; and Fleischer AB Jr, Feldman SR, McConnell CF, et al: *Emergency Dermatology: A Rapid Treatment Guide.* © 2002, McGraw-Hill, New York.

TABLE 248-6 Potassium Hydroxide (KOH) Examination

1. Collect scale with a scalpel edge, place in small heap on slide, cover with coverslip.
2. Apply KOH 10%–40% solution to edge of coverslip; it will be drawn under coverslip.
3. Apply heat to underside of slide (match or lighter) until bubbles appear under coverslip.
4. Visualize under 10× magnification.

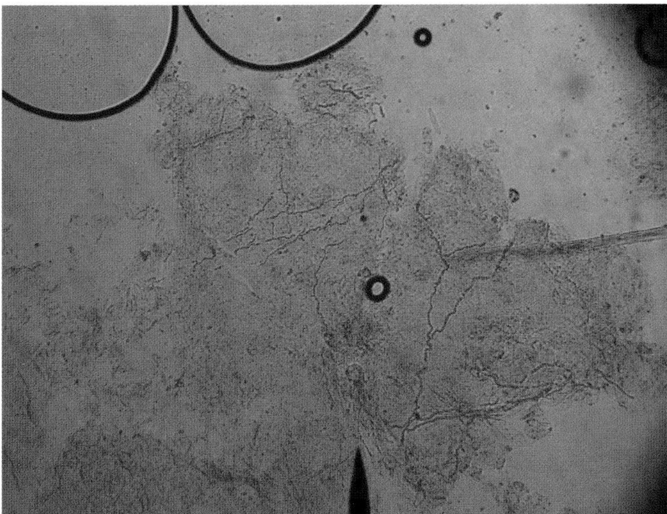

FIGURE 248-1. Hyphae in scraping from tinea pedis. [Photo contributed by University of North Carolina Department of Dermatology.]

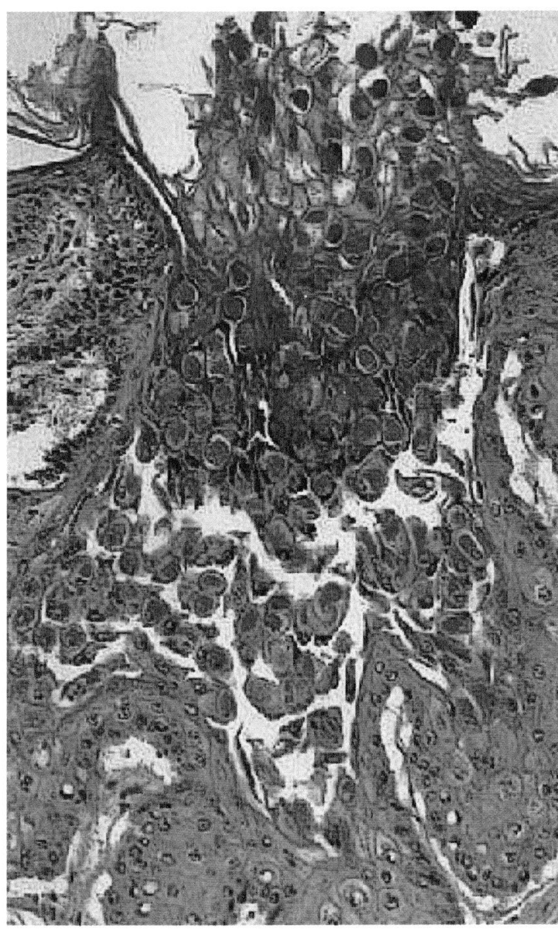

FIGURE 248-2. Molluscum bodies. [Reproduced with permission from the Centers for Disease Control and Prevention Public Health Image Library: http://phil.cdc.gov/phil/home.asp.]

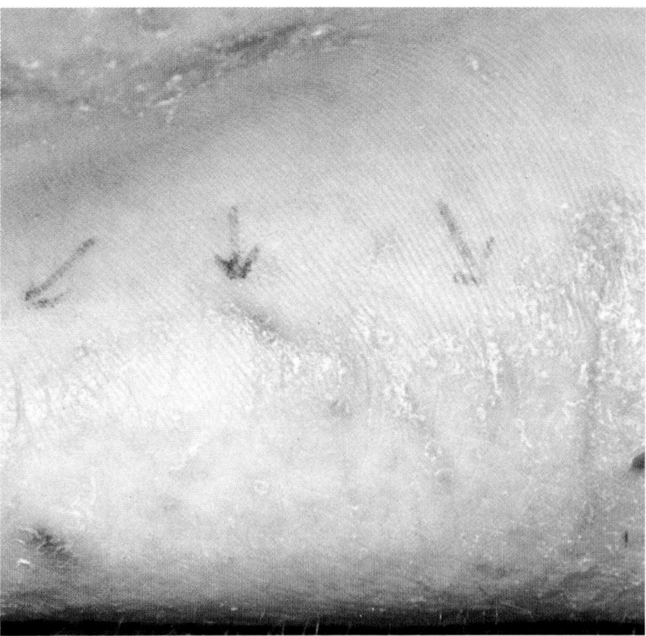

FIGURE 248-3. Classic burrows of scabies. [Reproduced with permission from Fleischer AB Jr, Feldman SR, McConnell CF, et al: *Emergency Dermatology: A Rapid Treatment Guide.* © 2002, McGraw-Hill, New York.]

The **Tzanck smear**, useful in blistering disorders, assists in establishing the diagnosis of a herpes infection: herpes simplex, herpes zoster, and varicella. The choice material for examination is obtained from the base of a recently unroofed lesion; purulent fluid at the base of the lesion is removed with a scalpel and placed on a microscope slide. The material is allowed to air dry and then is stained with Giemsa or Wright stain. Using low power, the slide is scanned for epithelial cells. Multinucleated giant cells (**Figure 248-6**), indicative of a herpes infection, are a syncytium of epidermal cells with multiple overlapping nuclei. The presence of the multinucleated giant cell does not distinguish between herpes simplex, herpes zoster, and varicella syndromes.

Wood's light examination is helpful in several different situations, including erythrasma (a superficial *Corynebacterium* infection of moist skin in the groin, axilla, and web spaces), fungal infections caused by *Malassezia* species or *Microsporum* species, certain pseudomonal skin infections, and porphyria cutanea tarda. Wood's light is an ultraviolet source that emits light at a wavelength of 365 nm. The following fluorescent findings are noted in these conditions: erythrasma, red or pink; tinea, green or yellow; *Pseudomonas*, yellow or green; and porphyria cutanea tarda, urine fluoresces orange or red (**Figure 248-7**).

Ancillary studies may also be required to assess for systemic involvement. Fever and leukocytosis may be indicative of an underlying infectious disorder or an underlying autoimmune reaction. In patients on anticonvulsants, elevated transaminases may represent underlying DRESS syndrome (drug reaction with eosinophilia and systemic symptoms). Furthermore, disseminated intravascular coagulation, thrombocytopenia, and acute kidney injury may alert the astute clinical to underlying bacteremia or toxic shock syndrome.[3] Imaging may be required to rule out foreign bodies or to assess to depth of tissue involvement in conditions such as Fournier's gangrene.

ED TREATMENT

SYSTEMIC CORTICOSTEROIDS

Systemic corticosteroids are the treatment of choice for some generalized conditions and are discussed in the chapters dealing with specific diagnoses. Some severe widespread dermatologic syndromes, such as erythema multiforme, toxic epidermal necrolysis, and vasculitis, are best

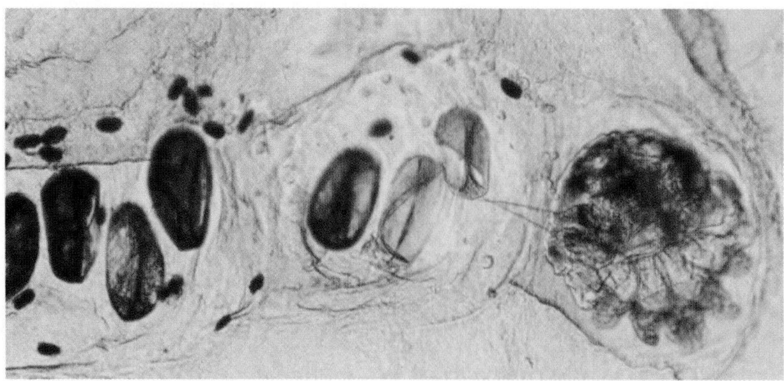

FIGURE 248-4. Microscopic view of a scabies mite with visible eggs and feces. [Reproduced with permission from Wolff KL, Johnson R, Suurmond R: *Fitzpatrick's Color Atlas & Synopsis of Clinical Dermatology*, 5th ed. © 2005, McGraw-Hill, New York.]

treated with systemic steroids only after consultation with a dermatologist. Other disorders, including urticaria, angioedema, *Toxicodendron* dermatitis (rhus, poison ivy, or poison oak), and other contact or allergic disorders are potential indications for systemic corticosteroids when an extensive area of skin (>20%) is involved. Patients with severe disease can see significant relief with oral corticosteroids within 12 to 24 hours.[5] In one study, small bursts of prednisone (40 milligrams daily for 4 days) markedly reduced the pruritus and hastened the clinical improvement of urticaria.[4,6] Patients with poison ivy or oak eruptions who require systemic steroids should be treated with oral prednisone (1 milligram/kg body weight) with a slow 2- to 3-week taper to avoid rebound dermatitis. Other contact or allergic dermatitides may benefit from an abbreviated course (4 days) of oral prednisone. However, oral corticosteroids are relatively contraindicated, or must be used with great care, in those with diabetes, hypertension, active peptic ulcer disease, psychiatric disease, and immunodeficiency. Follow-up within 2 to 3 days with the primary care physician or a dermatologist is needed if oral corticosteroids are prescribed to patients with these comorbidities.

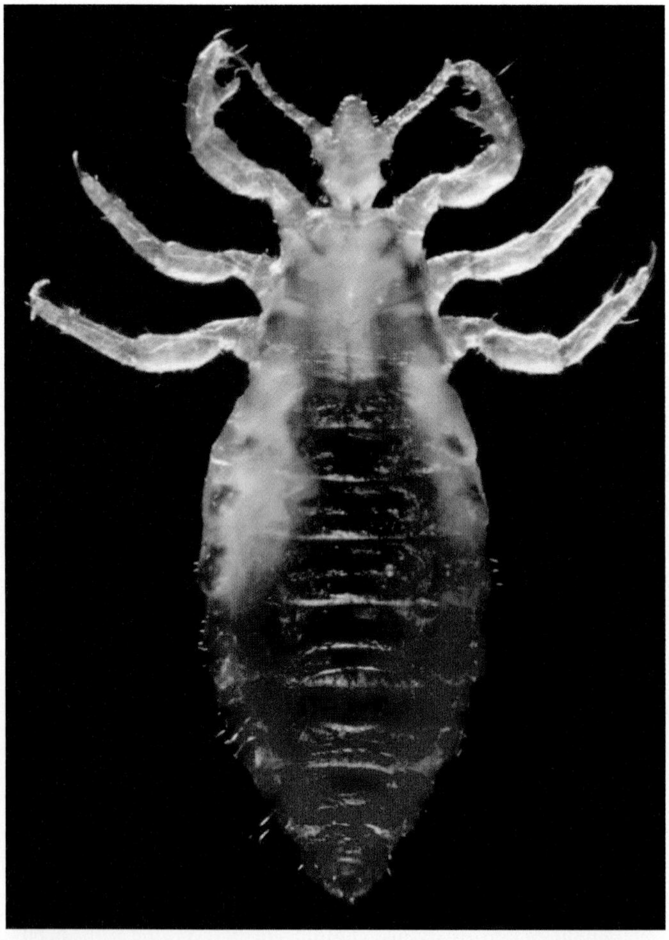

FIGURE 248-5. Adult head lice. [Reproduced with permission from the Centers for Disease Control and Prevention Public Health Image Library: http://phil.cdc.gov/phil/home.asp.]

TOPICAL CORTICOSTEROIDS

Topical corticosteroids are powerful and useful tools in the management of dermatologic disease. Numerous agents are available for use. They differ in concentration, base components, and cost. Familiarity with a single agent in each potency class is sufficient to treat any steroid-responsive skin ailment safely and effectively. Corticosteroid potency or strength (i.e., the anti-inflammatory property) is measured by the agent's ability to induce vasoconstriction. Agents' strengths are rated by vasoconstricting ability on a scale of 1 to 7 group 1 agents are the most powerful corticosteroids, and group 7 medications are the least potent (**Table 248-7**). In general, ointments are more potent than creams or lotions.

Topical Corticosteroid Strength Marked variation in potency is seen across various corticosteroids, whereas much smaller differences in strength are encountered for different concentrations of individual agents. Many corticosteroids are fluorinated. Fluorination greatly increases the potency but also increases the risk of adverse reactions, and **fluorinated formulations should not be used in pregnancy**.

Use of the appropriate-strength topical steroid is strongly encouraged at the start of therapy. Starting with a less powerful agent is not likely to spare the patient from potential adverse effects or to produce adequate control of the disease. **Hydrocortisone**, perhaps the most frequently used topical corticosteroid in the outpatient setting, is available over the counter in strengths up to 1% and by prescription in strengths to a maximum of 2.5%. Hydrocortisone is safe and may be used on most body surfaces, including the face, genitalia, flexure creases, and intertriginous zones. It also is safe for use in infants and children. For the treatment of diseases involving the palms and soles, hydrocortisone is a poor choice, because the thickened skin does not allow adequate penetration of this relatively low-potency steroid. Corticosteroids of moderate potency, including **triamcinolone acetonide and fluocinolone acetonide**, are useful in treating severely inflamed skin and the thicker skin of the scalp, trunk, extensor surfaces, palms, and soles. These agents should not be applied to the face or genitals or used in infants because of the risk of skin atrophy. See **Table 248-8** for recommendations on the potency of corticosteroid to use in treating various dermatologic diseases. When using agents found in group 6 or 7, consultation with a dermatologist may be advised.

Different skin surfaces respond differently to topical corticosteroid therapy; this differential response relates to the absorption of the steroid into the deeper tissues. The relatively thin skin surfaces of the face respond very rapidly to the use of group 7 agents, whereas the thicker

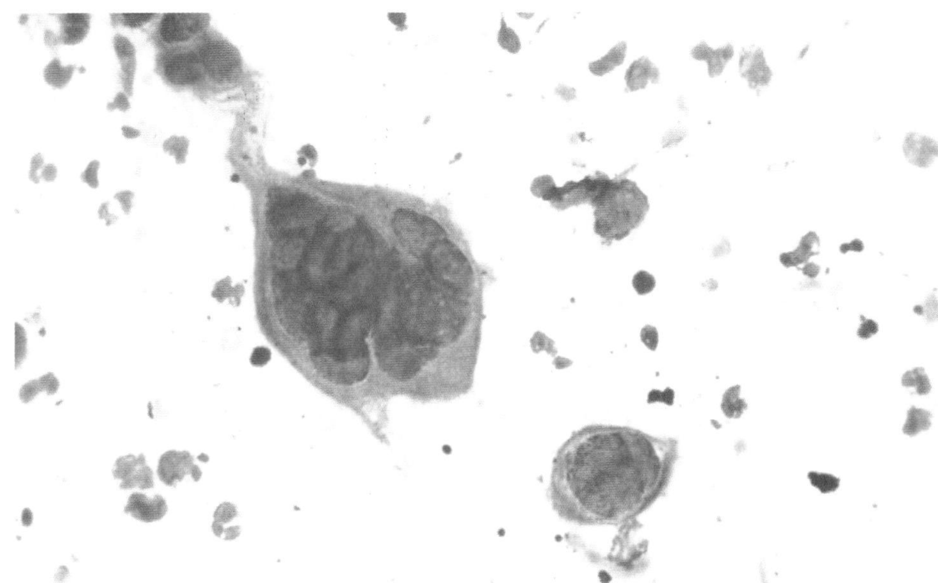

FIGURE 248-6. Tzanck smear under microscopy showing a multinucleated giant cell, indicative of a herpetic infection. [Reproduced with permission from Wolff KL, Johnson R, Suurmond R: *Fitzpatrick's Color Atlas & Synopsis of Clinical Dermatology*, 5th ed. © 2005, McGraw-Hill, New York.]

skin of the palms and soles requires a highly potent steroid. Irritations for which a low-potency agent may provide the same treatment effectiveness as a higher potency agent include those involving raw, inflamed skin (such skin absorbs medication more rapidly and readily); treatment regions with skin surfaces in frequent contact, such as intertriginous areas (the apposition of two skin surfaces produces enhanced absorption of drug, similar to the effect of an occlusive dressing); and areas of skin under tight clothing, such as the diaper area (absorption of the agent is enhanced due to the occlusive effect of the garment). In general, lower potency agents are acceptable in these situations.

Application of Topical Steroids The application of creams, ointments, gels, and lotions is relatively straightforward. The medication is applied in a thin layer and should be massaged daily into the skin, as directed. Washing the skin before corticosteroid application is unnecessary. Advise patients to follow directions closely both early and late in the treatment course. Using extra medication per dose or applying medication more frequently early in the treatment period is not desirable; likewise, reducing the frequency of application or decreasing the amount of medication as the disease process responds to therapy can cause relapse. Optimal application regimens have not been determined for topical corticosteroids in most dermatologic syndromes. The more potent agents are best applied two to three times daily for 1 to 2 weeks followed by a drug-free week; additional therapy may be required as determined by the disease and by the particular patient's response to the initial therapy. Agents from the less potent steroid groups may be applied three times daily for 2 to 4 weeks followed by a 7-day steroid-free period.

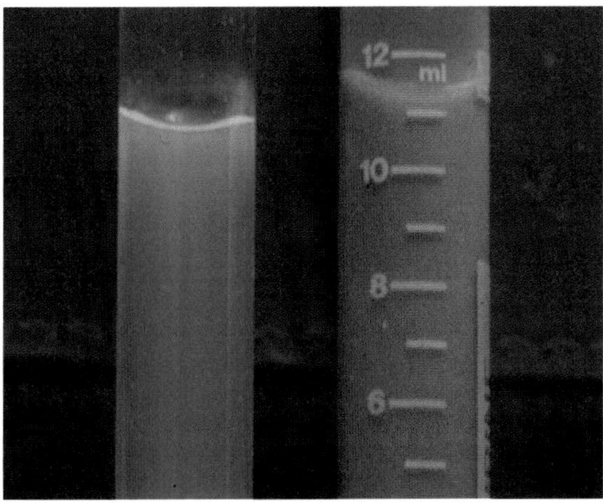

FIGURE 248-7. Pink coloration of the urine of a patient with porphyria cutanea when exposed to the light of a Wood's lamp. [Reproduced with permission from Wolff KL, Johnson R, Suurmond R: *Fitzpatrick's Color Atlas & Synopsis of Clinical Dermatology*, 5th ed. © 2005, McGraw-Hill, New York.]

Prescribing the Correct Amount of Topical Steroid Determining the correct amount of topical steroid to prescribe is at times difficult. The burn rule of nines may be used to estimate the amount of topical corticosteroid to prescribe. Calculate the percentage of body surface area requiring therapy and then multiply the percentage by a correction factor of 30. This calculation provides the amount of topical corticosteroid in grams for a single application. Next, determine the number of administrations required in the treatment course. For example, a three-times-daily regimen for a duration of 10 days requires 30 applications. The number of applications is multiplied by the grams required for a single dose to yield the total amount to be prescribed (**Table 248-9**). In general, 9 grams of topical steroid cover 9% of the body surface area for 1 day with a thrice-daily application. See **Table 248-10** for a description of the amount of topical corticosteroid to be dispensed relative to the coverage area and duration of therapy.

Avoid Tachyphylaxis *Tachyphylaxis* refers to the decrease in responsiveness to a drug as a result of enzyme-mediated events. The term is used in relation to topical corticosteroids to describe the early development of tolerance to vasoconstricting ability. In general, vasoconstriction has been demonstrated to decrease progressively over time after a topical steroid has been applied. Such reductions in strength due to tolerance are encountered as soon as 4 days into the treatment course in all potency groups but are thought to be more important for corticosteroids in groups 1 and 2. A reasonable strategy to counter the development of tachyphylaxis is the use of interrupted application schedules. An interrupted treatment course might include an initial three-times-daily application for 2 weeks, followed by 1 week without use of the drug, and then a repeat of the cycle.

ANTIHISTAMINES

Antihistamines (histamine-1 antagonists) are useful to control pruritus. These agents include the first-generation antihistamines such as diphenhydramine and hydroxyzine. These histamine-1 antagonists may be used PO, IM, or IV. The second-generation antihistamine agents, including astemizole, cetirizine, fexofenadine, and loratadine, are newer

TABLE 248-7 Examples of Topical Corticosteroid Agents by Potency Group*

US Classification	British Classification	Representative Topical Agent	Formulation
1: Superpotent	1: Very Potent	Clobetasol (Temovate, Clobex) Halobetasol (Halonate, Ultravate) Betamethasone (Diprolene)	0.05% cream or ointment
2: Potent	2: Potent	Fluocinonide (Lidex,Vanos) Halcinonide (Halog) Mometasone (Elocon)	0.05% ointment 0.1% cream 0.1% ointment
3: Upper mid-strength		Betamethasone (Diprolene) Fluticasone (Cutivate) Triamcinolone (Kenalog)	0.05% lotion 0.005% ointment 0.1% ointment
4: Mid-strength		Mometasone (Elocon)	0.1%cream, lotion
5: Lower mid-strength	3: Moderate	Betamethasone (Diprolene) Fluocinolone (Synalar) Fluticasone (Cutivate)	0.1% cream 0.025% cream 0.05% cream
6: Mild		Alclometasone (Alclovate) Desonide (Desonate, Desocort) Triamcinolone (Kenalog)	0.05% cream or ointment 0.05% cream 0.025% cream
7: Least Potent	4: Mild	Hydrocortisone	1% or 2.5% cream, lotion or ointment

Note: Trade names vary. Strength classification can vary. Strength also depends upon the product itself, amount applied, and nature of skin at the application site.

*Preparations are listed by US and British potency groups: Group 1 is most potent, group 7 (British 4) is least potent.

TABLE 248-8 Recommended Corticosteroid Potency for Treatment of Various Dermatologic Diseases

Groups 1 and 2	Groups 3 to 5	Groups 6 and 7
Psoriasis	Atopic dermatitis	Nonspecific dermatitis of face, eyelids, and perineum
Eczema of hand (severe)	Stasis dermatitis	
Poison ivy dermatitis (severe)	Seborrheic dermatitis Tinea	
Atopic dermatitis (severe)	Scabies Nonspecific dermatitis of face (severe)	

TABLE 248-9 Determination of the Correct Amount When Prescribing Topical Steroids

1. Use burn rule of nines to determine percentage of body surface area affected.
2. Percentage of body surface area × 30 = grams of topical corticosteroid per application.
3. Application times per day × number of days of treatment = total number of applications.
4. Total Grams to Prescribe = [% BSA x 30] x [times per day x number of days].

TABLE 248-10 Amount of Corticosteroid Cream to Dispense*

Body Area	Suggested Potency	Amount to Dispense (grams)
Face	Low	45
Arm	Intermediate or low	90
Leg	Intermediate or low	180
Hand or foot	Intermediate or low	45
Forearm	Intermediate or low	45
Chest or back	Intermediate or low	180

*Based on application three times a day for 10 days of therapy.

agents that may be used in certain circumstances. In general, the newer antihistamines offer the advantages of reduced dosing frequency and less sedative effect, but they are more costly. Comparisons of these new medications with hydroxyzine are generally favorable, but differences are not dramatic; comparisons of the various second-generation agents do not demonstrate significant differences among them.[7,8] Increasing the dosage of these antihistamine medications above their recommended dosages may increase the sedative effect but does not provide greater reduction in itching.[9] The use of topical antihistamine preparations is discouraged, because these agents are readily absorbed and dosing is difficult to predict. Accidental overdosage may result in patients who aggressively apply the preparation or are also using similar oral agents. See **Table 248-11** for suggested dosing, administration schedules, and

TABLE 248-11 Antihistamines Useful in the Management of Dermatologic Disease

Medication (trade name)	Adult Dosage	Pediatric Dosage
Diphenhydramine (Benadryl)	25–50 milligrams PO/IV/IM four times a day	5 milligrams/kg/d PO/IV/IM in four divided doses; maximum dose, 300 milligrams/d
Hydroxyzine (multiple trade names)	25–100 milligrams PO three or four times a day	2 milligrams/kg/d PO in four divided doses
Cetirizine* (Zyrtec)	5–10 milligrams PO once a day	For children ≥6 y, 5–10 milligrams PO once a day†
Fexofenadine* (Allegra)	60 milligrams PO twice a day	For children ≥6 y, 30 milligrams PO twice a day
Loratadine* (Claritin)	10 milligrams PO once a day	For children ≥6 y, 10 milligrams PO once a day†
Famotidine	20 milligrams PO twice daily	0.5 milligram/kg/d in two divided doses; maximum dose, 40 milligrams/d
Ranitidine	150 milligrams PO twice daily	5–10 milligrams/kg/d PO in two divided doses; maximum dose, 300 milligrams/d

*Indication limited to chronic idiopathic urticaria (see package inserts for details).

†Pediatric use is recommended only in children ≥6 y (see package inserts for details).

routes of therapy for these antihistamines. Histamine-2 antagonists (ranitidine or famotidine) also have demonstrated some benefit in patients with an allergy-mediated event, in particular urticaria, and therefore are recommended in combination with histamine-1 antagonists in the more severe allergic reactions.[10,11]

Numerous other antipruritic therapies are recommended, including Domeboro solution (aluminum sulfate diluted 1:10 with water) soaks and oatmeal baths.

ANTIMICROBIAL AGENTS

Topical antibacterial agents are used primarily as adjuncts to wound dressing and are rarely useful as primary therapy for superficial bacterial infections of the skin. The exception to this statement is topical mupirocin, which is as effective as oral antimicrobial agents in the management of impetigo. For wound dressing, the agents commonly used include polymyxin B, bacitracin, neomycin, and silver sulfadiazine. **Do not use silver sulfadiazine on the face because it will stain.** When reapplying silver sulfadiazine, thoroughly wipe off the prior medication before applying a new dose to avoid silver staining of the skin. Benefits of topical antibacterial agents include reduced adherence of bandaging material to the wound, reduced coagulum, and decreased bacterial colonization. The impact on the rate of wound healing and the prevention of wound infection is less well characterized. Another application of topical antibacterial agents is in the treatment of aphthous stomatitis, for which oral tetracycline rinses are used.

Other disorders treated with topical agents include *Candida* infections, dermatophyte infections, herpes simplex, and lice infestations and scabies. Diagnostic features and specific treatment are discussed in other chapters by the specific diagnosis.

NONANTIMICROBIAL TOPICAL AGENTS

In general, the maxim "If it's dry, wet it, and if it's wet, dry it" applies to the initial treatment of many rashes. Water, protein, and lipid losses characterize dry skin diseases. Emollient creams and lotions restore water and lipids to the epidermis, hasten the healing process, and reduce pruritus and pain. Emollients are moisturizers that reduce skin dryness and decrease skin friction and the sensation of tightness. In patients with chronic drying dermatitides, ointments are best, particularly in the winter months. In warm climates, less viscous, less oily preparations, such as a cream, are better tolerated. Open wet dressings using tap water or normal saline not only reduce discomfort due to the drying but also cleanse the skin by painlessly loosening crusts and exudates. The various wet cutaneous syndromes involve similar protein and lipid losses due to excessive flow of transudative or exudative fluid from the diseased skin with leaching of the complex macromolecules of the epithelial cells. Drying agents retard this flow of fluid and associated biologic materials from the body, thus assisting in the curative process.

Topical Agent Medication Base (Vehicle) The **vehicle,** or medication base, is the substance in which the active ingredient is dispersed. The base determines the rate at which the active ingredient is absorbed through the skin. Components of some bases may cause irritation or allergy.

Creams, a mixture of oils, water, and preservative, are white and greasy in texture. Creams are the most versatile vehicle and can be applied to any body surface area. They are particularly useful in the intertriginous areas. Creams are best used for acute therapy only; chronic application may cause excessive drying. Some patients are allergic to the preservatives in creams; in these patients, consider switching to an ointment preparation of the medication.

Ointments are composed of greases such as petroleum jelly and are free of preservative. Little water is added to this vehicle. Ointments are translucent and, when applied to the skin, remain greasy. This greasy consistency lubricates particularly dry lesions. In general, ointment vehicles allow deeper tissue penetration compared with cream bases. Ointments also are occlusive, providing very thorough coverage with deep tissue penetration and allowing little movement in moisture and other material into and out of the skin. Acute exudative syndromes and intertriginous areas of the body should not be treated with topical steroids formulated using an ointment vehicle.

Gels are greaseless mixtures of propylene glycol and water and at times contain alcohol. Gels have a translucent appearance and are described as "sticky." Alcohol-containing gels are best for acute exudative lesions, such as poison ivy dermatitis, whereas alcohol-free combinations should be used for dry, scaling conditions. In denuded areas, the alcohol component may cause discomfort. Gels are sometimes preferred for the scalp, because they do not alter the hair style and are cosmetically tolerable.

Solutions or lotions may contain water or alcohols in addition to other agents. They are clear or milky in appearance and are most useful for the scalp and other dense hair-bearing areas because they leave no significant residue on the hair. In denuded areas, the alcohol component may cause discomfort.

Some topical steroids are available as *foams*. Clobetasol (a very potent topical steroid) is safe and effective as a foam.[12] It is important to note that the absorption rate of clobetasol is greater for the foam vehicle formulation than for the topical solution.[13]

Topical Agent Toxicity Topical agents with certain active ingredients must be used with caution. These ingredients are often very effective, but the delivery is uncontrolled. Although the patient can control the amount and frequency of application, the actual amount of systemic absorption is not easily managed. For instance, certain agents are well absorbed through normal skin and mucous membranes, whereas other medications are absorbed only through irritated skin or mucosa. Topical formulations containing agents absorbed through irritated skin include the Lidoderm patch (containing lidocaine), Caladryl lotion (containing pramoxine, a local anesthetic), Bengay (containing methyl salicylate), and Icy Hot (containing menthol and methyl salicylate). Reports of significant toxicity, including death, have been reported with these and similar agents when excessively applied topically.

SMELLY FEET SYNDROME ("TOXIC SOCK SYNDROME")

A common secondary problem encountered in the ED is that of severely malodorous feet. This issue is often much more urgent from the perspective of the staff than from that of the patient, but may require attention for the benefit of everyone involved. The most extreme cases are seen in patients with poor hygiene who rarely remove or change their socks and shoes, primarily the indigent population. Because the perspiration and moisture collect around the foot, there is no opportunity for the area to dry. This moisture combines with the bacteria present on the skin and results in bacterial proliferation in the area of the poorly cared for feet. The bacteria produce a very strong-smelling compound (isovaleric acid) that can be quite overwhelming in certain circumstances. Isovaleric acid is the same compound that is produced by bacteria during the ripening of Swiss cheese.[14] To improve the odor and neutralize the acidic environment that allows the bacteria to thrive, an antacid solution can be applied directly to the feet. Application of HCO_3 spray to the contaminated skin or the direct applications of oral antacid solutions (such as Mylanta or Maalox) to the patient's feet are two methods that have been used with success.[13,15] Clean socks, disposable foot booties, or any type of foot wrap may be used to keep the medication in place to allow the acidic environment to be neutralized and the odor to be controlled. The key to permanent resolution of the problem is proper foot hygiene, regular changing to clean socks, and avoidance of a prolonged moist environment around the foot.

REFERENCES

The complete reference list is available online at www.TintinalliEM.com.

CHAPTER 249 Generalized Skin Disorders

Mark Sochor
Amit Pandit
William J. Brady

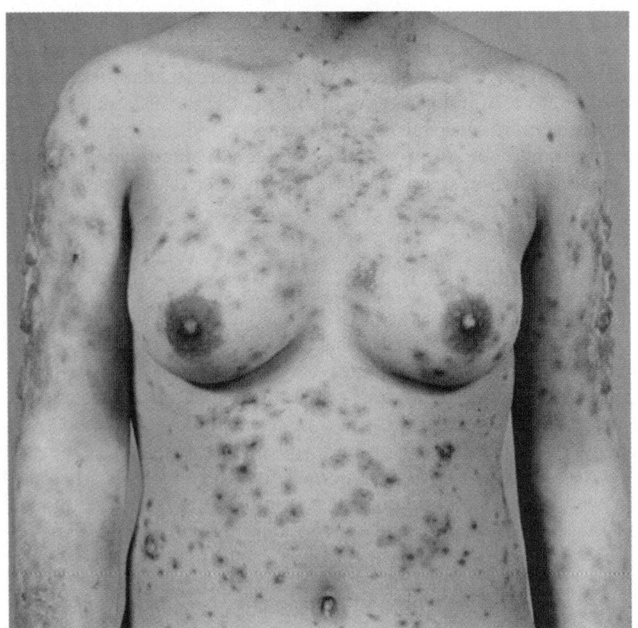

FIGURE 249-1. Erythema multiforme.

INTRODUCTION

This chapter describes selected serious generalized skin disorders in adults and discusses their dermatologic diagnosis and treatment. Covered are erythema multiforme, toxic epidermal necrolysis, exfoliative erythroderma, the toxic infectious erythemas, disseminated viral infections, Rocky Mountain spotted fever, disseminated gonococcal infection, purpura fulminans, and pemphigus vulgaris. Staphylococcal scalded skin syndrome and meningococcemia are discussed in the pediatric section, in chapter 141, "Rashes in Infants and Children." Staphylococcal and streptococcal toxic shock syndrome are also discussed in chapter 150, "Toxic Shock Syndromes." Disseminated viral infections are discussed in chapter 153, "Serious Viral Infections" and in chapter 141.

The disorders erythema multiforme, toxic epidermal necrolysis, exfoliative erythroderma, staphylococcal and streptococcal toxic shock syndrome, and staphylococcal scalded skin syndrome share some features in common. **Table 249-1** can help in differentiating these disorders.

ERYTHEMA MULTIFORME

Erythema multiforme is an acute inflammatory skin disease ranging from a localized papular eruption of the skin (erythema multiforme minor) to a severe, multisystem illness (**Figure 249-1**) with widespread vesiculobullous lesions and erosions of the mucous membranes, known as **Stevens-Johnson syndrome**. The spectrum is defined by the amount of epidermal detachment present, with erythema multiforme minor having no epidermal detachment, Stevens-Johnson syndrome having <10% of the body surface area with epidermal detachment, overlapping of Stevens-Johnson syndrome and toxic epidermal necrolysis having 10% to 30% epidermal detachment, and toxic epidermal necrolysis having >30% epidermal detachment.[1] Morbidity and mortality rise with the amount of epidermal detachment.[2] The highest incidence is in young adults (age range, 20 to 40 years), and erythema multiforme occurs commonly in the spring and fall. Common precipitating factors are infection, especially with *Mycoplasma* and herpes simplex virus; drugs, especially antibiotics and anticonvulsants; and malignancies. However, the cause is often unknown.[3] Most likely, erythema multiforme is the result of a hypersensitivity reaction, with immunoglobulin and complement components demonstrated in the cutaneous microvasculature on immunofluorescent studies of skin biopsy specimens, circulating immune complexes found in the serum, and mononuclear cell infiltrate noted on histologic examination.[3,4]

Symptoms include malaise, fever, myalgias, and arthralgias. Diffuse pruritus or a generalized burning sensation can occur before the skin lesions develop. The morphologic configuration of the lesions is variable, hence the descriptor *multiforme*. Maculopapular (**Figure 249-2**) and target, or iris (**Figure 249-3**), lesions are the most characteristic. Erythematous papules appear symmetrically on the dorsum of the hands and feet and on the extensor surfaces of the extremities. The maculopapule evolves into the classic target lesion during the next 24 to 48 hours. As the maculopapule enlarges, the central area becomes cyanotic,

TABLE 249-1 Comparison of Inflammatory and Infectious Generalized Skin Disorders

Disorder	Appearance	Special Features
Erythema multiforme	Erythematous macules, papules Target lesions Urticaria or vesiculobullous lesions	Cutaneous reaction to drugs or infectious agents. Stevens-Johnson syndrome is the most severe form.
Toxic epidermal necrosis	Painful, tender erythroderma Vesicles and bullae Exfoliation	Nikolsky sign present. Stevens-Johnson syndrome is most severe form. Drugs most common cause.
Exfoliative erythroderma	Nontender erythema Skin flaking and scaling Thickening of skin	Often preexisting eczema or psoriasis; can be drug induced.
Staphylococcal or streptococcal toxic shock syndrome	Staphylococcal: fine punctuate erythematous lesions that become confluent; blanching erythroderma; desquamation first of trunk and face, then extremities Streptococcal: can be indistinguishable from staphylococcal toxic shock; scarlatiniform erythroderma with sheet-like desquamation of skin	Colonization or infection with *Staphylococcus aureus*; menstruation associated with tampon use; nonmenstrual associated with burns, cellulites, sinusitis, wounds, etc. Group A streptococcal cellulitis, puerperal sepsis, any group A β-hemolytic *Streptococcus* infection source.
Staphylococcal scalded skin syndrome	Scarlatiniform rash or erythema Bullae or bullous impetigo Sloughing of skin	Usually seen in neonates or children <5 years of age. Nikolsky sign present.

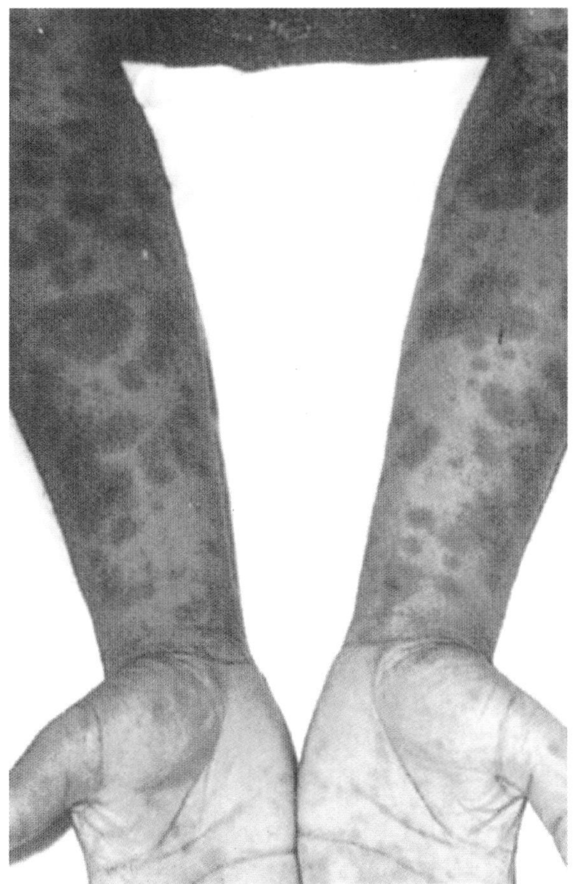

FIGURE 249-2. Maculopapular erythema multiforme.

occasionally accompanied by central purpura or a vesicle. Urticarial plaques also may occur with or without the iris lesion in a similar distribution. Vesiculobullous lesions, which may be pruritic and painful, develop within preexisting maculopapules or plaques, usually on the extensor surface of the arms and legs and less frequently on the trunk. Vesiculobullous lesions are found most often on mucosal surfaces, including the mouth, eyes, vagina, urethra, and anus; they may also be seen on the trunk. Ocular involvement occurs in approximately 9% of patients with erythema multiforme minor, whereas ophthalmologic lesions are seen in almost 70% of patients with Stevens-Johnson syndrome.[5] The various

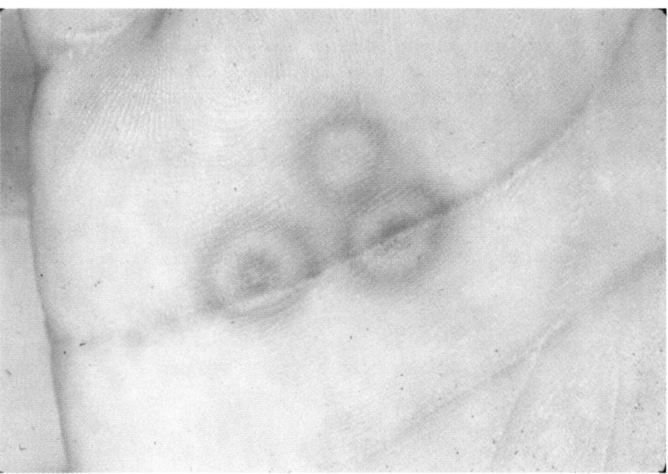

FIGURE 249-3. Target, or iris, lesions of erythema multiforme. [Photograph used with permission of Kenneth Greer, MD, University of Virginia Dermatology.]

TABLE 249-2 Erythema Multiforme and Toxic Epidermal Necrolysis

Lesions of Erythema Multiforme	Lesions of Toxic Epidermal Necrolysis
Erythematous maculopapules	Warm, tender erythroderma
Iris or target lesions	Vesicles and bullae
Urticaria	Exfoliation
Mucous membranes involved	Mucous membranes involved

lesions (**Table 249-2**) develop in successive crops during a 2- to 4-week period and heal over 5 to 7 days. The **differential diagnosis of erythema multiforme** includes herpetic (herpes simplex virus and varicella-zoster virus) infection, vasculitis, toxic epidermal necrolysis, various primary blistering disorders (pemphigus and pemphigoid), urticaria, Kawasaki's disease, and the toxic and infectious erythemas.

Recurrence may be noted on repeat exposure to the etiologic agent, a special concern in cases associated with herpes simplex virus infection or medication use.[6] **The rate of erythema multiforme recurrence is very high in children with herpes simplex virus infection.** For example, 75% of children with a history of herpes simplex virus–related erythema multiforme developed erythema multiforme recurrence after herpes simplex virus reactivation.[6] Fluid and electrolyte disorders and secondary infection from cutaneous sites are the most frequent complications.

Systemic steroids are commonly used for localized disease and provide symptomatic relief but are of unproven benefit in influencing the duration and outcome of erythema multiforme.[7] Many authorities recommend a short, intensive steroid course of prednisone, 60 to 80 milligrams PO once a day, particularly in drug-related cases, with abrupt cessation in 3 to 5 days if no favorable response is noted. Systemic analgesic agents and antihistamines provide symptomatic relief. Stomatitis is treated with diphenhydramine and viscous lidocaine mouth rinses. Do not swallow oral viscous lidocaine because it causes neurotoxicity. Treat blisters with cool compresses of Burow solution (5% aluminum acetate). Ocular involvement should be monitored by an ophthalmologist. Unfortunately, burst steroid therapy does not reduce the chance of development or significance of existing ocular lesions.

Disposition is admission to an intensive care or burn unit. Acyclovir may reduce recurrence of herpes simplex virus infection and therefore lessen the potential for another bout of erythema multiforme; prolonged prophylactic acyclovir therapy may reduce the chance of recurrent erythema multiforme related to herpes simplex virus.[6]

TOXIC EPIDERMAL NECROLYSIS

Toxic epidermal necrolysis (**Figure 249-4**) is an explosive dermatosis characterized by tender erythema, bullae formation, and subsequent exfoliation. Patients are systemically ill. Many authorities consider the Stevens-Johnson syndrome variant of erythema multiforme and toxic epidermal necrolysis to be the same process.[4] Toxic epidermal necrolysis is found in all age groups without predilection for either sex. The syndrome has multiple causes, with medications being the most common cause.[3,4,8] Sulfa and penicillin antibiotics, anticonvulsants, and oxicam nonsteroidal anti-inflammatory drugs are the most frequent drug triggers for toxic epidermal necrolysis.[9,10] Other causes include malignancy and human immunodeficiency virus infection.[8] In many cases, a cause is not found. The pathogenesis is poorly understood and may be partly immunologic and partly genetic.[11]

Symptoms include a 1- to 2-week prodrome of malaise, anorexia, arthralgias, fever, or symptoms of upper respiratory tract infection. Skin tenderness, pruritus, tingling, or burning may be found at this time. Skin signs (Table 249-2) begin with a warm erythema, initially involving only the eyes, nose, mouth, and genitalia, but later becoming generalized. The erythematous areas become tender and confluent within hours. Flaccid, ill-defined bullae then appear within the areas of erythema. Lateral pressure with a finger on normal skin adjacent to a bullous lesion dislodges the epidermis, producing denuded dermis and demonstrating **Nikolsky sign**. Nikolsky sign is slippage of the epidermis from the dermis when slight rubbing pressure is applied to

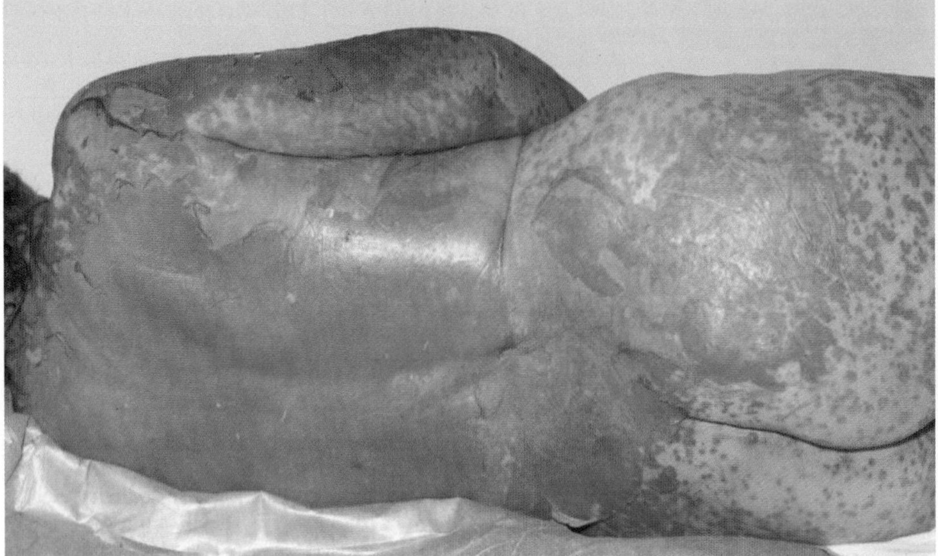

FIGURE 249-4. Toxic epidermal necrolysis.

the skin. The bullae form along the cleavage plane between the epidermis and the dermis. The epidermis is then shed in large sheets, which leaves raw, denuded areas of exposed dermis. The average time until onset after exposure to the inciting agent is 2 weeks. Cutaneous extension follows an unpredictable time course, ranging from 24 hours to 15 days, with some severe cases demonstrating rapid, extensive involvement within 24 hours.

Perilabial blistering and erosive lesions are disfiguring and often impair adequate oral intake, contributing to hypovolemia. Ocular complications include purulent conjunctivitis, painful erosions, and potential blindness. Anogenital lesions are common. Additional mucous membrane involvement includes the GI, urinary, and respiratory tracts. The two major complications and leading causes of death in toxic epidermal necrolysis are infection and hypovolemia with electrolyte disorders. A broad range of pathogens is usually found, with staphylococcal and pseudomonal species predominating. The mortality rate has been reported as being between 25% and 35%.[8,11] The clinical characteristics associated with poor prognosis include advanced age, extensive disease, idiopathic nature, use of multiple medications, steroid therapy, azotemia, hyperglycemia, leukopenia, and thrombocytopenia.[9] The differential diagnosis of toxic epidermal necrolysis is presented in Table 249-1 and also includes primary blistering disorders (pemphigus and pemphigoid) and Kawasaki's disease in children.

Management of toxic epidermal necrolysis requires hospitalization in an intensive care or burn unit.[9] Immediate concerns center on the airway, because sloughing of airway and respiratory epithelium can occur. Hypovolemia and electrolyte abnormalities should be corrected. Prompt, aggressive antibiotic administration is necessary in suspected or documented infection; initial prophylactic antibiotics are not recommended by most. Solicit the advice of the burn center regarding any topical dressings that are applied before transfer.

PEMPHIGUS VULGARIS

Pemphigus vulgaris is a generalized, mucocutaneous, autoimmune, blistering eruption with a grave prognosis characterized by intraepidermal acantholytic blistering (**Table 249-3**). The primary lesions of pemphigus vulgaris are vesicles or bullae (**Figure 249-5**) that vary in diameter from <1 cm to several centimeters. They commonly first affect the head, trunk, and mucous membranes. The blisters are usually clear and tense, originating from normal skin or atop an erythematous or urticarial plaque. Within 2 to 3 days, the bullae become turbid and flaccid. Rupture soon follows, producing painful, denuded areas. These erosions are slow to heal and prone to secondary infection. The Nikolsky sign is present in pemphigus vulgaris. Mucous membranes are affected in most patients, and in some, the mucous membranes are the primary sites of involvement. Blisters on mucous membranes are more transitory than blisters on the skin in that they are more vulnerable to rupture; this is particularly true in the mouth, where ragged ulcerative lesions readily develop after inadvertent biting of the tissues.

Limited oral intake and accelerated protein, fluid, and electrolyte losses through the involved skin can rapidly lead to hypovolemia and electrolyte disturbances. Admission and aggressive fluid and electrolyte resuscitation, as well as treatment with corticosteroids and immunosuppressive agents, are needed to prevent mortality. Plasmapheresis and IV immunoglobulins may also be needed.

EXFOLIATIVE DERMATITIS

Exfoliative dermatitis is a condition in which most or all of the skin surface is involved with a scaly erythematous dermatitis. It is a cutaneous reaction in response to a drug or a chemical agent or to an underlying systemic or cutaneous disease, Most patients are >40 years old. The cause is unknown.

Exfoliative dermatitis can have an abrupt onset, particularly when related to a drug, contact allergen, or malignancy; exacerbations related to an underlying cutaneous disorder usually evolve more slowly. Exfoliative dermatitis tends to be a chronic condition, with a mean duration of 5 years, when related to a chronic illness; the course is often shorter after suppression of the underlying dermatosis, discontinuation of causative drugs, or avoidance of allergen. Idiopathic and chronic disease–related exfoliative dermatitis can continue for ≥20 years; death is rare.

Generalized erythema and warmth are noted, but skin tenderness is usually lacking. Erythema is accompanied by scaling or flaking, and the patient often complains of pruritus and skin tightness (**Figure 249-6**). The process generally begins on the face and upper trunk with progression to other skin surfaces. The patient usually has a low-grade fever. Excessive heat loss and hypothermia can complicate exfoliative dermatitis.

TABLE 249-3 Characteristics of Lesions of Pemphigus Vulgaris
Large, flaccid bullae
Nikolsky sign present
Skin ulcerations
Exfoliation
Mucous membrane involvement

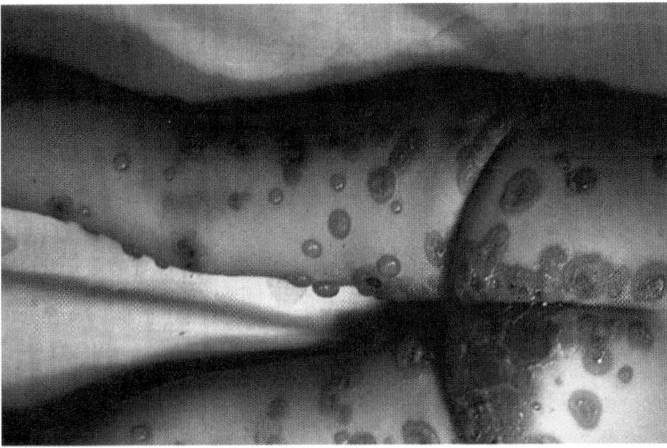

FIGURE 249-5. Scattered bullous lesions intermixed with erosions and painful inflammatory plaques in a patient with pemphigus vulgaris.

Widespread cutaneous vasodilation may result in high-output congestive heart failure. The disruption of the epidermis results in increased transepidermal water loss, and continued exfoliation can result in significant protein loss and negative nitrogen balance. Chronic inflammatory exfoliation produces many changes, such as dystrophic nails, thinning scalp and body hair, and patchy or diffuse pigmentation changes.

The differential diagnosis of exfoliative dermatitis in adults is found in Table 249-1. Patients generally require admission. Correct hypothermia and hypovolemia. Obtain dermatology consultation before giving systemic corticosteroids.

DRESS: DRUG RASH WITH EOSINOPHILIA AND SYSTEMIC SYMPTOMS SYNDROME

Drug rash with eosinophilia and systemic symptoms (DRESS) syndrome is a severe adverse drug reaction that usually develops within 8 weeks of initiation of drug therapy. Aromatic anticonvulsants (such as phenytoin and phenobarbital), allopurinol, and sulfa medications are the most common culprits; however, other causes include nonsteroidal anti-inflammatory drugs, antiretroviral medications, angiotensin-converting enzyme inhibitors, calcium channel blockers, and other antibiotics.[12]

It is believed that there is a genetic predisposition if exposed to the appropriate medication.[12] Because of the potential genetic risk, DRESS syndrome should be discussed with the family members of any patient in whom it is diagnosed.

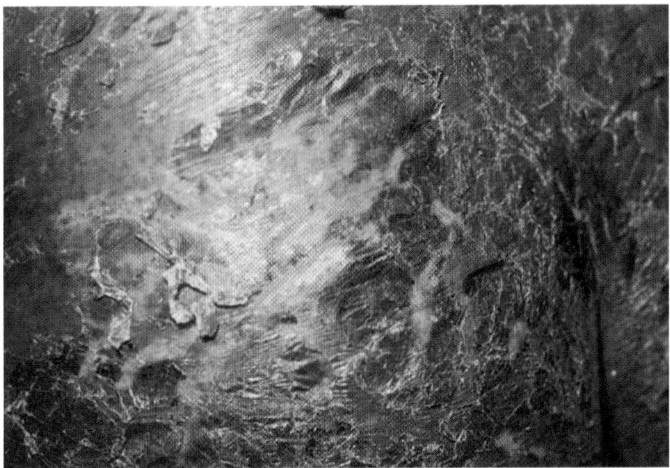

FIGURE 249-6. Exfoliative dermatitis demonstrated by generalized, warm erythema accompanied by scaling or flaking.

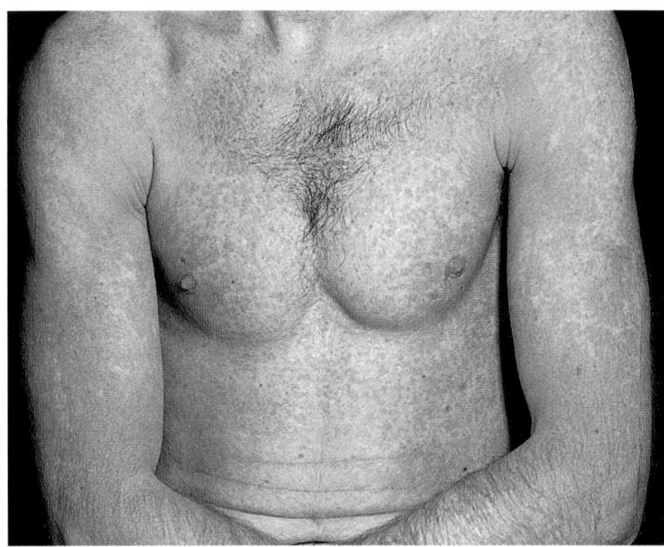

FIGURE 249-7. Drug rash with eosinophilia and systemic symptoms (DRESS) syndrome caused by phenytoin.

DRESS syndrome is defined by fever, rash, and internal organ involvement, with the liver, kidneys, and hematologic system being most commonly affected.[12] Rash and fever are typically the first signs of the syndrome, and they may have associated lymphadenopathy (**Figure 249-7**). The rash itself can take multiple forms, ranging from an erythematous scaly rash similar to that of exfoliative dermatitis, to a blistering/bullous rash similar to that of Stevens-Johnson syndrome, with varying degrees of severity. Abnormal laboratory findings include eosinophilia, which occurs in about 30% of DRESS syndrome patients,[13] and hepatic and renal dysfunction. Because of the variety of clinical presentations, early diagnosis of DRESS syndrome is difficult and requires a high level of clinical suspicion. The current standard of care involves immediate stoppage of the suspected culprit medication, administration of systemic steroids in severe cases (those with evidence of hepatitis, pneumonitis, or extensive exfoliative dermatitis), supportive care including antipyretic and antipruritic medications, and hospital admission.[13,14]

PURPURIC DISORDERS

MENINGOCOCCEMIA

Meningococcemia is a potentially fatal infectious illness caused by the gram-negative diplococcus *Neisseria meningitidis*. Meningococcal disease presents across a wide clinical spectrum in the acute and chronic forms. The acute entities include pharyngitis, meningitis, and bacteremia. Meningococci are present in mucosal samples from approximately 5% to 10% of the general population (the carrier state).[15,16] In high-risk populations, such as military recruits, the organism may be found in almost half of people without evidence of active disease.[17]

The illness usually strikes patients <20 years of age, with the vast majority of cases occurring in children and infants <5 years old. A rash is frequently noted on presentation and is an invaluable clue to the correct diagnosis early in the disease course. The dermatologic manifestations include petechiae, urticaria, hemorrhagic vesicles, macules, and/or maculopapules (**Figure 249-8**). The classic petechial lesions are found on the extremities and trunk but also are noted on the palms, soles, head, and mucous membranes. The petechiae evolve into palpable purpura with gray necrotic centers, a pathognomic finding for meningococcal infection. The skin findings result from the organism's invasion and destruction of the endothelium. Histopathologic analysis shows an infectious vasculitis. For further discussion, see chapters 141, "Rashes in Infants and Children," and 117, "Meningitis in Infants and Children."

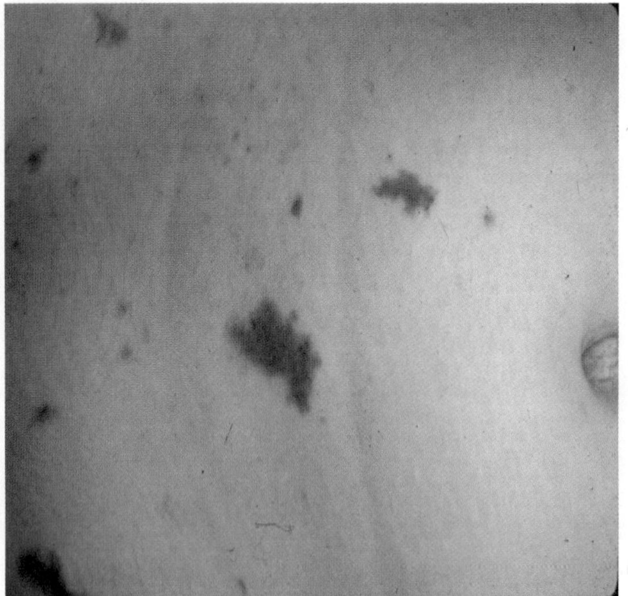

FIGURE 249-8. Early findings of meningococcemia with petechiae evolving into pruritic lesions. [Photograph used with permission of Kenneth Greer, MD, University of Virginia Dermatology.]

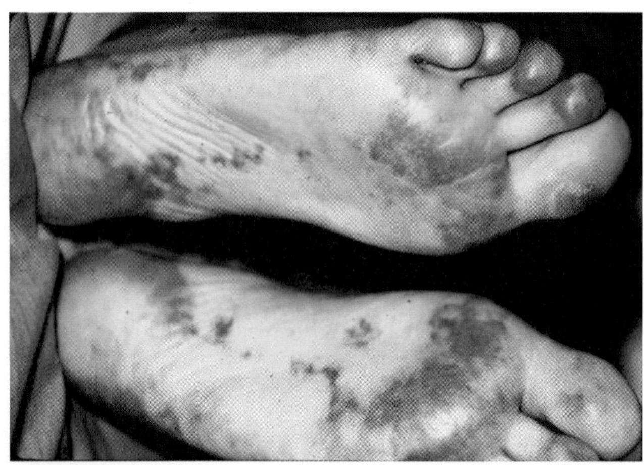

A

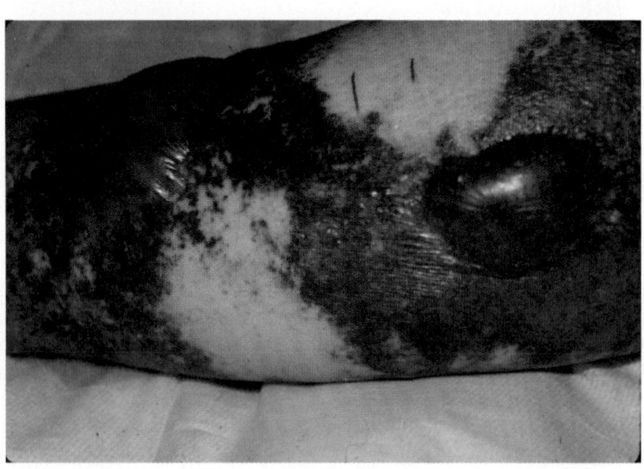

B

FIGURE 249-9. Purpura fulminans (**A**) with early skin necrosis and (**B**) later with hemorrhagic bullae. [Photographs used with permission of Kenneth Greer, MD, University of Virginia Dermatology.]

PURPURA FULMINANS

Purpura fulminans is a rare vascular disorder characterized by fever, shock, multiorgan failure, and the rapid development of hemorrhagic skin necrosis. It is associated with dermal vascular thrombosis, vascular collapse, and disseminated intravascular **coagulation**. Purpura fulminans can result from hereditary or acquired protein C deficiency, activated protein C resistance, or protein S deficiency. It may also result from any condition that causes disseminated intravascular coagulation.

Purpura fulminans presents with the dermatologic triad of widespread ecchymoses, hemorrhagic bullae (**Figure 249-9**), and epidermal necrosis. Cyanosis with initial ecchymoses and ultimate necrosis of the tip of the nose, ears, and genitalia frequently occur; in general, distal tissue areas with end circulation are affected. Large confluent ecchymoses can develop, often on the extremities, from distal to proximal, and on the perineum, buttocks, and abdomen. The extremities are often involved symmetrically. Treatment is directed at the underlying cause.

REFERENCES

The complete reference list is available online at www.TintinalliEM.com.

CHAPTER 250

Skin Disorders: Face and Scalp

Dean S. Morrell
Kevin W. Dahle

INTRODUCTION

Many generalized dermatologic conditions can affect the face and scalp. This chapter discusses the acneiform eruptions, seborrheic dermatitis, erysipelas and facial cellulitis, herpes zoster, herpes simplex, tinea capitis and barbae, head lice, allergic contact dermatitis, and photosensitivity/sunburn. Impetigo and bullous impetigo are discussed in chapter 141, "Rashes in Infants and Children."

ACNEIFORM ERUPTIONS

The acneiform eruptions include acne vulgaris, rosacea fulminans, dissecting cellulitis of the scalp, and acne keloidalis nuchae. Pathophysiology of these disorders is similar. Sebum secretion is increased within the sebaceous follicle by androgen stimulation. Keratin accumulates in the hair follicle as well as sebum. Host inflammation occurs, and the bacteria *Propionibacterium acnes* (gram-positive rods) proliferate and accumulate, intensifying inflammation. At this stage, an inflammatory papule or pustule occurs with an influx of neutrophils and helper T cells. In addition, marked inflammation can cause a nodule or cyst, and scarring can occur.

Acne fulminans is the most severe form of nodulocystic acne and may prompt patients to seek emergency medical attention. It usually affects males between the ages of 13 and 16 years. Clinical features include acute onset of suppurative cysts and nodules with ulcerations and hemorrhagic crusting on the face, chest, and back (**Figure 250-1**). Ulcerating lesions can lead to severe scarring. Systemic symptoms also occur and include osteolytic bone lesions of the clavicle and sternum, fever, arthralgias, myalgias, and hepatosplenomegaly. Diagnosis is clinical. Acute treatment includes administration of 40 to 60 milligrams of prednisone once daily. If the patient is already taking isotretinoin, continue the medication in conjunction with corticosteroids. **Isotretinoin should not be started in the acute care setting.** Refer to a dermatologist.

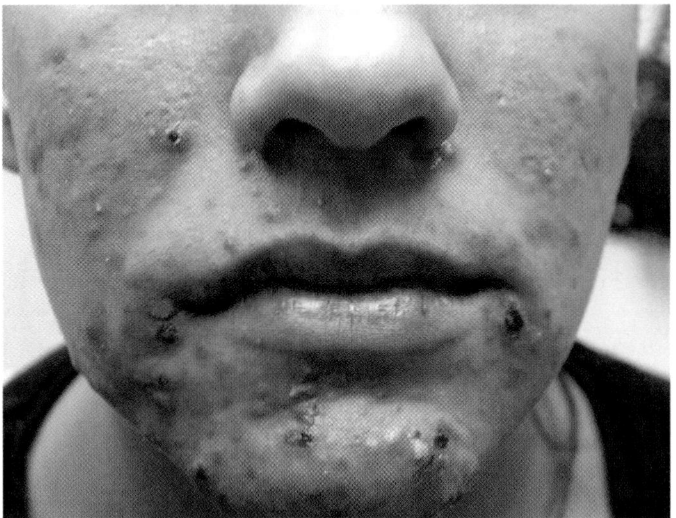

FIGURE 250-1. Nodulocystic acne. [Photo contributed by University of North Carolina Department of Dermatology.]

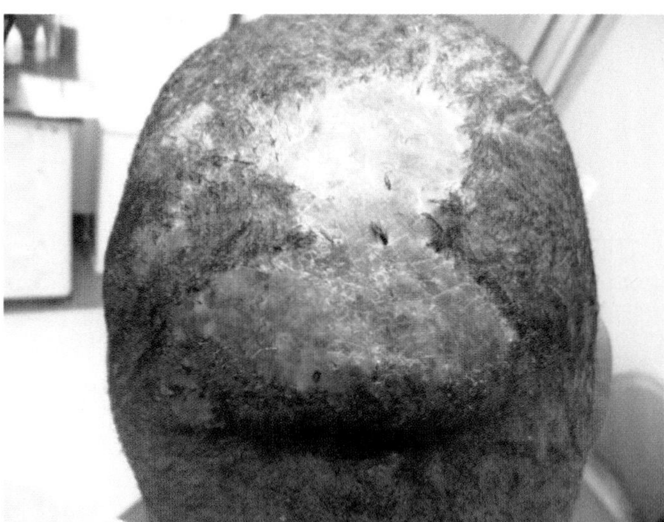

FIGURE 250-3. Acne keloidalis nuchae. [Photo contributed by University of North Carolina Department of Dermatology.]

Rosacea fulminans, or pyoderma faciale, is an inflammatory cystic acneiform eruption on the central face of young women. The eruption may occur with or without a history of rosacea. Inflamed papules and pustules are present on the centrofacial region and can coalesce into large plaques. Diagnosis is clinical. Severe scarring can occur without treatment. Treatment is similar to that of acne fulminans—oral prednisone, 40 to 60 milligrams once daily, and referral to a dermatologist for consideration of isotretinoin.

Dissecting cellulitis of the scalp, also called *perifolliculitis capitis abscedens et suffodiens*, is an inflammatory and scarring disease of the scalp and neck. It occurs most commonly in young men of African descent. It consists of boggy tender nodules in multiple areas of the scalp and the neck (**Figure 250-2**). It is not a true cellulitis but is an intense inflammatory condition of the scalp. The nodules suppurate and develop interconnecting sinus tracts. Hair loss develops over these nodules, and permanent scarring, alopecia, and keloids can occur. If associated with acne conglobata, hidradenitis suppurativa, and pilonidal cysts, the disease is referred to as the *follicular occlusion tetrad*. Osteomyelitis of the skull has developed under lesions of dissecting cellulitis.[1] **ED therapy** includes antibacterial washes, such as chlorhexidine, which is available without prescription, and oral antibiotics, such as doxycycline and minocycline. Refer to a dermatologist. Dapsone, intralesional corticosteroids, and prednisone can be initiated at follow-up but are often unsuccessful. Treatment with isotretinoin has been successful. Surgical excision, laser treatment, and tumor necrosis factor-α blockers have also been used successfully.[2]

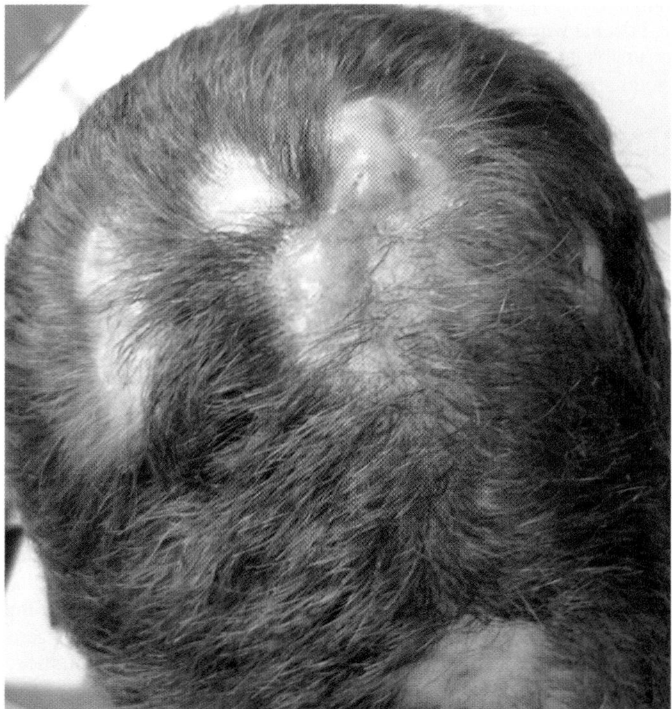

FIGURE 250-2. Dissecting cellulitis of the scalp. [Photo contributed by University of North Carolina Department of Dermatology.]

Acne keloidalis nuchae is a perifollicular inflammation (**Figure 250-3**) consisting of follicular-based papules and pustules on the nuchal region. The individual keloidal papules enlarge and coalesce to form keloidal plaques with an associated scarring alopecia. At the edges of the plaque, hair that is tufted often resembles hair on a "doll's head." The area may also have a bad odor, which may be the patient's primary complaint. **Treatment** includes topical application of clindamycin solution, topical corticosteroids such as fluocinonide or clobetasol solution, and oral doxycycline or minocycline. Refer to a dermatologist for intralesional corticosteroids.

SEBORRHEIC DERMATITIS

Seborrheic dermatitis has both infantile and adult forms. The infantile form is called "cradle cap" and peaks in the first 3 months of life. See chapter 141 for further discussion in infants. Adults with acquired immunodeficiency syndrome and Parkinson's disease are predisposed to severe disease. Common dandruff is a mild form of seborrheic dermatitis. The cause is not known. The disorder occurs in areas of active sebaceous glands. *Malassezia* yeasts and underlying inflammation are implicated[3] and may explain why seborrheic dermatitis responds to both antifungal and anti-inflammatory agents. In adults, the condition is chronic and without any systemic symptoms. Pruritus can be variable but is usually mild. Dandruff may be present. Lesions can extend onto the central upper chest and intertriginous regions. Erythema and scaling are present on the vertex and parietal regions diffusely. On the face, there is symmetric involvement of the eyebrows, nasolabial folds, and retroauricular areas (**Figure 250-4**). The skin is sensitive to sun and heat.

Treat adults with an antidandruff shampoo containing zinc pyrithione, selenium sulfide 2.5%, salicylic acid, or tar. Ketoconazole shampoo can also be used and is available over the counter at 1% and by prescription at 2%. The shampoo should be lathered into the scalp and left on

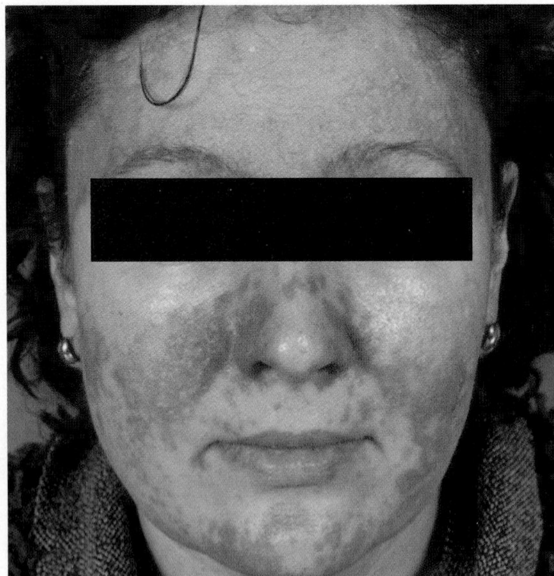

FIGURE 250-4. Adult seborrheic dermatitis. Erythema and scaling on face and facial skin folds. [Reproduced with permission from Wolff K, Johnson R, Suurmond R: *Fitzpatrick's Color Atlas & Synopsis of Clinical Dermatology*, 5th ed. New York, McGraw-Hill, 2005, p. 51.]

briefly before rinsing. Ketoconazole 2% cream can also be used. A topical corticosteroid such as fluocinonide solution may be applied to the scalp in severe cases. For the face, hydrocortisone 2.5% or desonide 0.05% cream or lotion applied twice per day should be the initial management. **The use of higher potency topical corticosteroids on the face can lead to the development of perioral dermatitis or steroid rosacea and should be avoided.** Treatment continues until the dermatitis is cleared. Re-treatment is needed for recurrences.

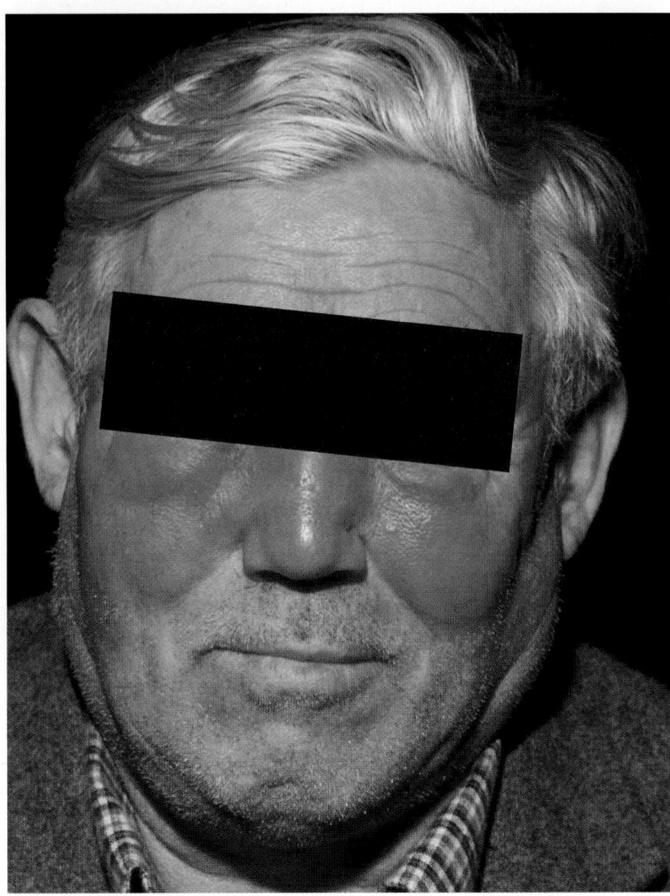

FIGURE 250-5. Facial erysipelas. [Reproduced with permission from Wolff K, Johnson R, Suurmond R: *Fitzpatrick's Color Atlas & Synopsis of Clinical Dermatology*, 5th ed. New York, McGraw-Hill, 2005, p. 605.]

ERYSIPELAS AND FACIAL CELLULITIS

Erysipelas and cellulitis are infections of the dermis and subcutis, respectively. Erysipelas is most often caused by group A *Streptococcus*, specifically *Streptococcus pyogenes*. It usually affects the very young or elderly. Episodes increase in the summer. Bacterial inoculation into the skin may be caused by trauma. Cellulitis extends deeper than erysipelas, although treatment is the same. The two main causes of cellulitis in immunocompetent patients are *S. pyogenes* and *Staphylococcus aureus*.

Erysipelas and cellulitis of the face present as hot, bright red, tender, edematous, indurated plaques that can be unilateral or bilateral (**Figure 250-5**). The area of involvement is sharply demarcated and expands peripherally. There is no central clearing. Vesicles or bullae may be present. Systemic symptoms include fever, chills, regional lymphadenopathy, and malaise. The infection resolves with desquamation and possibly pigmentary change. In children, *Haemophilus influenzae* is a rare cause of erysipelas due to widespread use of the *H. influenzae* type b vaccine.

If unilateral, erysipelas and cellulitis must be distinguished from early herpes zoster infection. When bilateral, these diseases may be mistaken for the malar eruption of systemic lupus erythematosus. If there is eye involvement, consider periorbital cellulitis and obtain a CT scan to exclude orbital cellulitis. Bacterial cultures from the portal of entry should be done when possible for directed therapy. Anti-DNase and anti-streptolysin O titers can be done to confirm group A streptococcal infections. Skin biopsies are not usually helpful.

Unless history is suggestive of an unusual organism, direct **treatment** toward *Staphylococcus* and *Streptococcus* species in adults. Typically, if there is no clinical toxicity, cephalexin is initially prescribed with follow-up in 24 hours. In children, coverage should include these organisms and *H. influenzae*. If the patient does not respond to conventional therapy, other causes should be considered such as *Moraxella* species.[4] If bullous lesions are present, suspect methicillin-resistant *S. aureus* infection and add appropriate antibiotics.[5]

Patients who are toxic, immunocompromised, very young or elderly, or unable to complete the outpatient antibiotic regimen require admission for IV antibiotics.

HERPES ZOSTER INFECTION

Herpes zoster, or "shingles," usually involves the thoracic dermatomes. Eruptions on the face are due to trigeminal nerve involvement, which can have serious sequelae. Herpes zoster results from reactivation of latent varicella-zoster virus. The initial eruption of varicella-zoster virus is chickenpox.

Pain or dysesthesia precedes herpes zoster by 3 to 5 days. Erythematous papules progress to clusters of vesicles with an erythematous base in a dermatomal distribution (**Figure 250-6**). The vesicles evolve to pustules and then crust in about 1 week. Generalized eruptions may occur in immunocompromised patients. Any of three branches of the trigeminal nerve may be involved on the face. Involvement of the ophthalmic branch (V1), especially with vesicles on the tip of the nose indicating involvement of the **nasociliary branch**, raises concern for keratitis and other ocular complications. Emergency ophthalmologic consultation is needed. The virus may spread to motor root ganglia, resulting in motor weakness or paralysis. **Ramsay Hunt syndrome** results from reactivation of varicella-zoster virus in the geniculate ganglion and may present with ear pain, vesicles in the external auditory canal, facial nerve paralysis, and vestibulocochlear dysfunction.[6]

Differential diagnosis includes other blistering disorders, such as herpes simplex infection, bullous impetigo, and contact dermatitis. The key to diagnosis is the unilateral distribution and pronounced pain in the

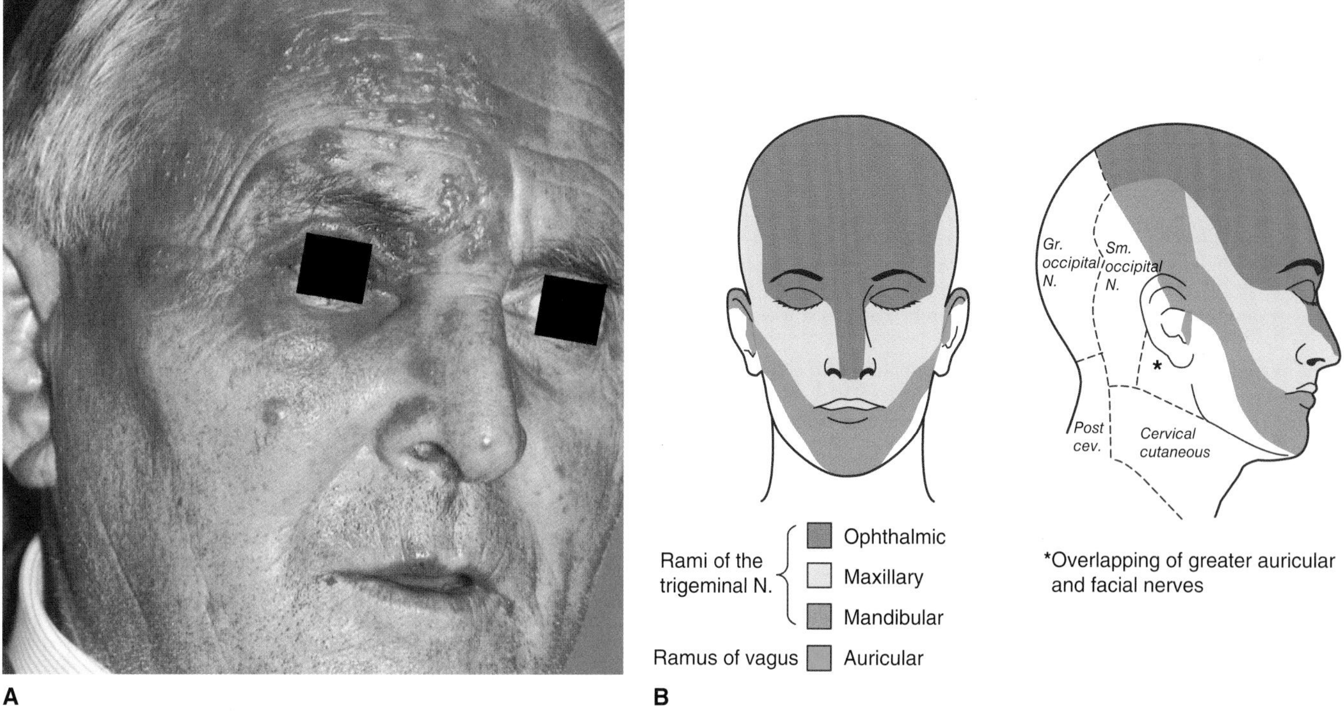

FIGURE 250-6. **A.** Herpes zoster in trigeminal nerve distribution. Note lesion on the tip of the nose, which suggests nasociliary branch involvement. **B.** Dermatomes of the head and neck. cev. = cervical; Gr. = greater; N. = nerve; Sm. = smaller. [**A.** Reproduced with permission from Fleischer A Jr, Feldman S, McConnell C, et al: *Emergency Dermatology: A Rapid Treatment Guide*. New York, McGraw-Hill, 2002, p. 157. **B.** Reproduced with permission from Wolff K, Johnson R, Suurmond R: *Fitzpatrick's Color Atlas & Synopsis of Clinical Dermatology*, 5th ed. New York, McGraw-Hill, 2005.]

area of involvement. Diagnosis can be confirmed by a Tzanck preparation showing multinucleated giant cells. However, Tzanck preparations have largely been replaced by polymerase chain reaction analysis of swabs taken from the base of a vesicle. Polymerase chain reaction results are generally available within 24 hours and can differentiate between varicella-zoster virus, herpes simplex 1, and herpes simplex 2.

Treatment is most effective if it is initiated within the first 72 hours of symptoms—this shortens healing time, decreases new lesion formation, and decreases the risk of postherpetic neuralgia. Treatment in an immunocompetent patient is acyclovir, 800 milligrams PO five times a day for 7 days, or valacyclovir, 1 gram PO three times a day for 7 days. In immunocompromised patients, treatment with acyclovir, 10 milligrams/kg IV every 8 hours for 7 to 10 days, is indicated. Valacyclovir should not be prescribed in patients with human immunodeficiency virus/acquired immunodeficiency syndrome due to risk of hemolytic-uremic syndrome. Local care can be provided with aluminum acetate compresses three times daily followed by antibiotic ointment. Narcotic analgesics may be needed. The zoster vaccine markedly reduces morbidity from herpes zoster and postherpetic neuralgia among older adults, reducing the burden of illness by 61.1%, the incidence of postherpetic neuralgia by 66.5%, and the incidence of herpes zoster by 51.3%.[7]

Patients with herpes zoster are contagious to individuals who have not had chickenpox. In the ED, isolation is needed for patients suspected of the disease at triage. In follow-up instructions, patients should be told to cover all open areas when visiting the physician.

HERPES SIMPLEX VIRUS INFECTIONS

Herpes simplex virus (HSV) type 1 most commonly occurs on the face. Initial infection occurs during childhood or adolescence and varies in its presentation. Many individuals experience mild symptoms, whereas a few experience a debilitating eruption. Recurrences tend to be mild and occur primarily on the lips, nose, and oral cavity.

The typical lesions of HSV are painful, grouped vesicles on an erythematous base (**Figure 250-7**). The primary eruption may be preceded by constitutional symptoms. The characteristic primary eruption is a gingivostomatitis with herpetic lesions on the lips and in the oral cavity. It may persist for weeks. Recurrent herpes simplex virus is typically seen as herpes labialis ("fever blisters" or "cold sores"). Individuals often experience a prodrome of localized tingling or burning several hours before the onset of the eruption. The herpetic lesion usually occurs along the lip margin and completely heals within 10 days. Ultraviolet light, fever, or local trauma can induce these eruptions.

In patients with underlying atopic dermatitis, a severe form of herpes infection can occur called *eczema herpeticum* in which herpes simplex virus or varicella-zoster virus can infect active atopic dermatitis lesions (see chapter 141).

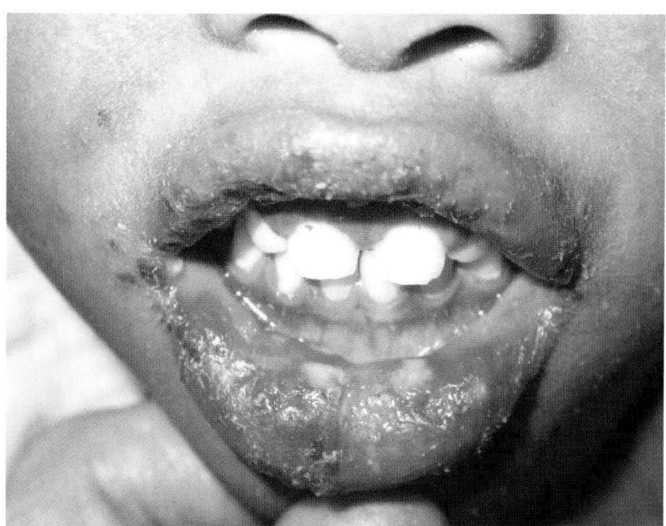

FIGURE 250-7. Herpetic gingivostomatitis. [Photo contributed by University of North Carolina Department of Dermatology.]

TABLE 250-1 Treatment of Herpes Simplex Virus (HSV) Gingivostomatitis (Herpes Labialis)

Condition	Acyclovir Treatment	Valacyclovir Treatment
First episode	400 milligrams PO three times a day for 7 d *or* 200 milligrams PO five times a day for 7 d	1 gram PO twice a day for 7 d
Recurrent episode	400 milligrams PO five times a day for 5 d *or* 800 milligrams PO twice a day for 5 d	2 grams PO twice a day for 1 d
Suppression	400 milligrams PO twice a day	500 milligrams PO daily

Treatment for primary HSV gingivostomatitis works best when given within the first 24 hours (**Table 250-1**).[8] Treatment can continue for up to 10 days if lesions have not crusted. Immunocompromised patients with severe involvement require hospitalization for IV acyclovir. Suppressive treatment with acyclovir or valacyclovir has been shown to decrease outbreaks of herpes labialis.[8] Patients with recurrent disease should be instructed to avoid triggers, especially the sun, by using sunscreen and a lip balm with ultraviolet light protection.

TINEA CAPITIS

Tinea capitis is a dermatophyte infection of the scalp. Causative agents are usually from the genus *Trichophyton*. The fungi invade the hair shaft and stratum corneum of the skin.

Clinically, there are nonscarring areas of alopecia with broken-off hairs and scale at the periphery (see Figure 141-13). Occasionally, there is intense inflammation, with a boggy, tender, indurated plaque with superficial pustules and overlying alopecia. This reaction, referred to as a *kerion*, may result in permanent scarring and alopecia. Cervical and/or occipital lymphadenopathy may be present. In some cases of tinea capitis, especially after initiation of oral antifungal therapy, patients will mount an immune response to the dermatophyte called an "id reaction" at distant sites. This id reaction appears as widespread, symmetric, and monomorphic eczematous papules and responds to topical steroids.

Diagnosis is based on a positive potassium hydroxide preparation or positive fungal culture. Scraping only the scalp rarely gives a positive potassium hydroxide examination because *Trichophyton* species invade the hair shaft. If fungal culture is necessary to establish or confirm the diagnosis, it usually takes 3 to 4 weeks for the culture to grow. Wood's lamp examination (**Table 250-2**) is becoming less helpful, because the most common types of dermatophyte infections fail to fluoresce. **More than 90% of dermatophyte cultures are due to *Trichophyton*, which do not fluoresce**. A positive culture will help to exclude other conditions such as atopic dermatitis or seborrheic dermatitis.

Topical treatment alone is not effective for tinea capitis. **The current first-line therapy is oral griseofulvin.** Higher doses of griseofulvin are needed to treat *Trichophyton* species, which represent the most common cause of tinea capitis. Liquid microsize griseofulvin, 20 to 25 milligrams/kg/d (maximum, 1 gram/d), is an effective treatment. Ultramicrosize griseofulvin (tablets only), 10 to 15 milligrams/kg/d (maximum, 750 milligrams/d), can also be used if patients are able to swallow pills. Individuals should be treated for a minimum of 8 weeks. At that point, patients should be reevaluated to determine whether therapy should be continued. Alternative treatment is with terbinafine granules, which are given at 125 milligrams/d for patients weighing <25 kg, 187.5 milligrams/d for patients weighing 25 to 35 kg, and 250 milligrams/d for patients weighing >35 kg for 6 weeks. To decrease contagiousness and scale, patients should also wash hair with antifungal shampoo (ketoconazole 2% or selenium sulfide 2.5%) three times per week for the first 2 weeks of therapy.

TABLE 250-2 Fluorescence with Wood's Lamp

Nits
Lice
Microsporum
Malassezia

Other family members, especially children, and other close contacts, such as classmates at school or day care, should be evaluated. Other affected members should be treated simultaneously to prevent reinfection. If *Microsporum* is diagnosed by culture, pets (cats and dogs) should be examined by a veterinarian. Follow-up with a primary care provider or dermatologist is crucial, because persistent infection may only be manifest as scale and go unrecognized by caregivers.

TINEA BARBAE AND SYCOSIS BARBAE

Tinea barbae is a dermatophyte infection involving the beard area of the face and neck and occurs in postpubertal males. Etiology usually involves the genus *Trichophyton*. Predisposing factors to tinea barbae include use of topical steroids, contact with infected pets, and diabetes mellitus.[9] Sycosis barbae is a deep folliculitis within the beard area. Perifollicular inflammation also occurs. The causative agent is usually *S. aureus*.

In tinea barbae, severe inflammatory plaques and follicular pustules occur in the beard area (**Figure 250-8**). A kerion-like lesion can develop as well as abscess and sinus tracts. Hairs are usually loosened or broken off.

In sycosis barbae, discrete pustules, usually involving *S. aureus*, with perifollicular inflammation are evident (**Figure 250-9**). Unlike tinea barbae, the hairs are usually not loosened or broken off.

The diagnosis is clinical, but tinea barbae sometimes can resemble acne vulgaris or bacterial folliculitis. A potassium hydroxide preparation or fungal culture can be done to confirm the diagnosis. Permanent alopecia and scarring can result if left untreated.

Treatment of tinea barbae requires oral antifungals. Microsize griseofulvin, 500 milligrams PO daily, or ultramicrosize griseofulvin, 375 milligrams PO daily, for 4 to 6 weeks can be used. Terbinafine can also be used, but baseline liver function studies should be drawn in adults prior to starting the medication. Supportive care is done with shaving or depilating the hair along with warm compresses to remove the crust.

For sycosis barbae, initial treatment with warm compresses and mupirocin ointment may be sufficient. If lesions are chronic, treatment usually requires systemic antibiotics with adequate *S. aureus* coverage.

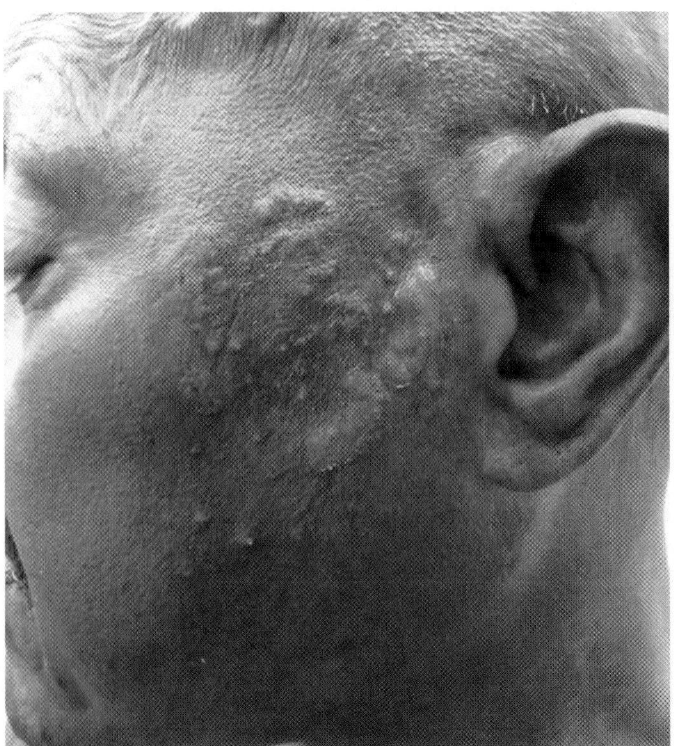

FIGURE 250-8. Tinea barbae. [Photo contributed by University of North Carolina Department of Dermatology.]

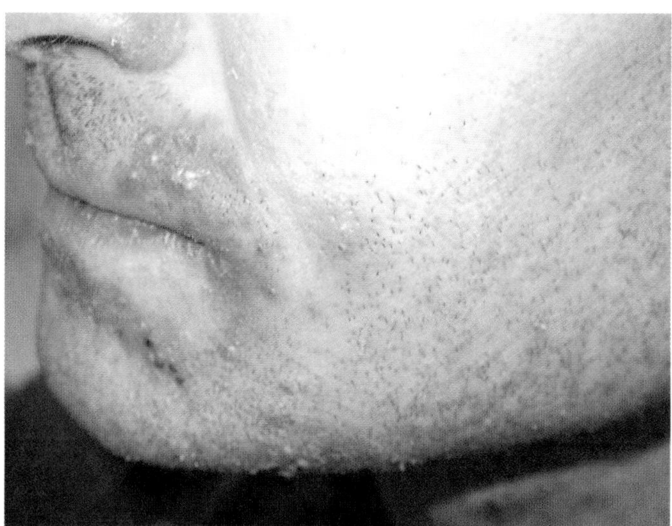

FIGURE 250-9. Sycosis barbae. [Photo contributed by University of North Carolina Department of Dermatology.]

HEAD LICE (PEDICULOSIS CAPITIS)

Head lice, or pediculosis capitis, is a common worldwide infestation that usually occurs in children age 3 to 11 years but can occur at any age. It is caused by the head louse, *Pediculus capitis*, which is approximately 2 to 3 mm in size. Lice need a blood meal every 4 to 6 hours and live for 30 days while laying numerous eggs. Adults cannot survive more than 24 hours without a blood meal. The eggs are cemented to the hair by a proteinaceous matrix (**Figure 250-10**). Transmission occurs by head-to-head contact and by brushes and combs.

Head lice are limited to the scalp, behind the ears, and on the back of the neck. Intense pruritus is a feature. Diagnosis is made by identification of nits and/or adult lice in the scalp hair. Nits are oval, gray-white egg capsules. If all nits are located >7 mm from the scalp surface, active infestation is unlikely. Nits and lice fluoresce with a Wood's lamp.

Topical application of permethrin cream is the first-line treatment and should be repeated 1 week later to kill any surviving active nits. Apply 1% or 5% permethrin cream to the hair and leave it on overnight. The next morning, follow with a shampoo. Or, apply pyrethrin cream or ivermectin lotion for 10 minutes and then rinse out. Malathion 0.5% cream is another alternative and is applied to the scalp overnight, but malathion is flammable, so be careful in application. Do not use malathion in children <6 years old. Application of thick moisturizing creams to hair followed by drying with a blow dryer has also been used for resistant cases. Children with head lice do not need to be removed from school, because "no-nit" policies have been shown to be excessive.[10]

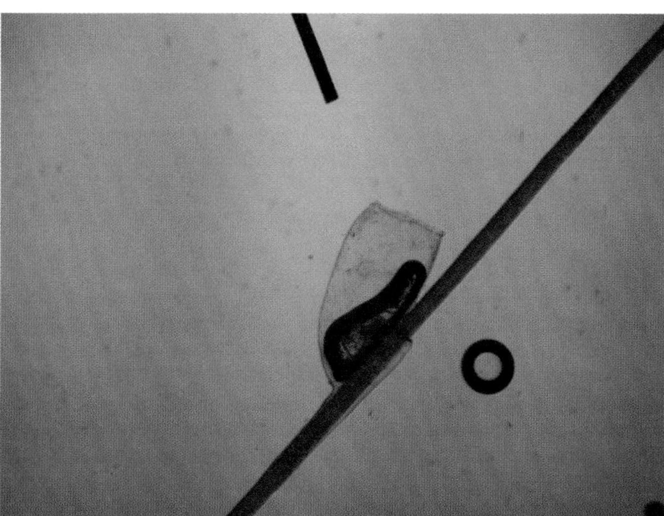

FIGURE 250-10. Empty nit attached to hair shaft. [Photo contributed by University of North Carolina Department of Dermatology.]

ALLERGIC CONTACT DERMATITIS

Two types of contact allergies are likely to result on the face. The first is the result of an aerosolized allergen. The second is direct physical contact that is most prominent on the sensitive parts of the face. Examples of aerosolized contactants include poison ivy and poison oak when the plant has been burned. Examples of common direct contactants affecting the face include nickel, nail polishes, toothpaste, preservatives in makeup, contact lens solutions, eyeglasses, and hair care products. Chemical-splash injuries are a common cause of facial irritant contact dermatitis. A thorough history is necessary to uncover the offending agent. Referral to a dermatologist or allergist may be necessary if the history is unrevealing.

Clinically, allergic contact dermatitis from an aerosolized allergen presents as erythema and scale with or without vesiculation (**Figure 250-11**). The involvement is diffuse, with upper and lower eyelids affected. This distribution is in contrast with photosensitive eruptions in which non–sun-exposed areas, such as the upper eyelids and the upper lip, are spared. Direct allergic contact dermatitis tends to be most prominent on the most sensitive skin, such as the eyelids.

Medical treatment is of little value if the offending agent is not removed from the patient's environment. Depending on the severity, topical or oral corticosteroids and oral antihistamines are used in medical management. Aluminum acetate (Burow solution, available

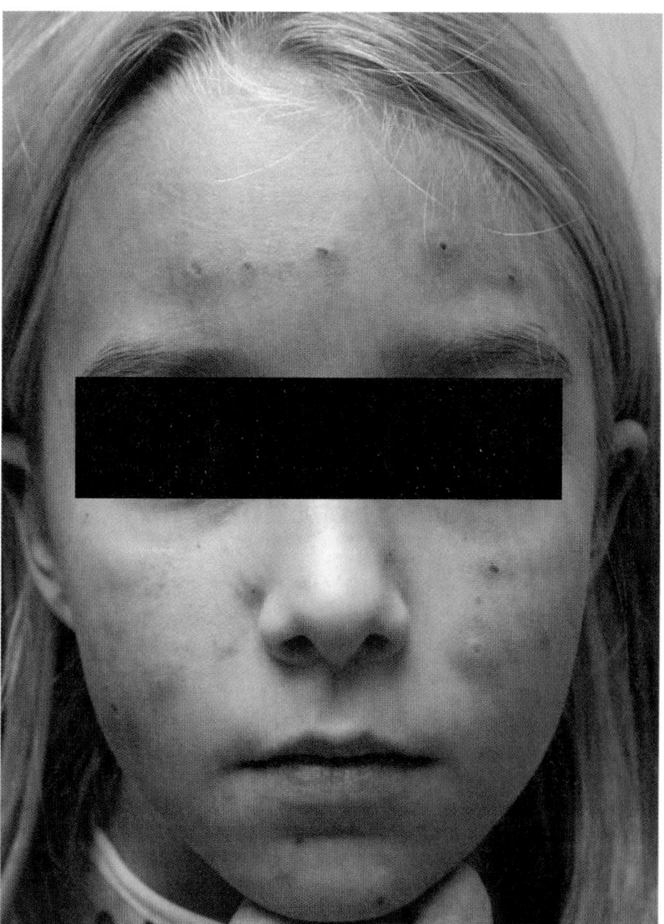

FIGURE 250-11. Poison ivy—a typical allergic contact dermatitis. [Photo contributed by University of North Carolina Department of Dermatology.]

commercially as Domeboro®) compresses can be beneficial as well. Short duration (3 to 5 days) of medium- to high-potency topical corticosteroids can be used on the face. Often, extensive and severe periocular involvement requires oral prednisone. See chapter 253, "Skin Disorders: Extremities" for further discussion of treatment of rhus, or poison ivy or oak.

SUNBURN AND PHOTOSENSITIVITY

Reactions to ultraviolet light are varied. In many disorders, ultraviolet light aggravates but does not cause disease. Examples of this type of reaction include lupus erythematosus, dermatomyositis, porphyria cutanea tarda, dermatitis of niacin deficiency (pellagra), and recurrences of herpes simplex virus. Other disorders are caused by the sun, the most common of which is a sunburn reaction. A sunburn reaction is the inflammatory response to skin injury as a result of ultraviolet radiation. Individuals with fair skin, light eyes, and naturally light hair color are more susceptible to sunburns; however, darker pigmented skin can develop skin injury with sufficient ultraviolet light exposure.

Exogenous photosensitivity disorders result from topical application or ingestion of an agent that causes the skin to be more sensitive to ultraviolet light. Photosensitivity disorders may be phototoxic or photoallergic. Phototoxic drug reactions occur quickly and appear as a sunburn. Photoallergic reactions occur later and exhibit eczema-like changes in the skin with vesiculation (**Figure 250-12**).

Topical photosensitizers usually result in a cutaneous eruption at the sites of application. Ultraviolet exposure is necessary for the eruption to occur. Furocoumarins are the most common group of agents causing topical photoeruptions. Lime juice, fragrances, figs, celery, and parsnips contain furocoumarins. **Table 250- 3** lists some ingested substances that can result in a photosensitivity eruption.

The sunburn reaction begins 2 to 6 hours after exposure and peaks in 1 to 3 days. It may be minimal with little discomfort to the patient, or it may be severe with extensive blistering. Erythema and warmth in sun-exposed areas occurs. Vesiculation is equivalent to a second-degree burn.

The diagnosis of sunburn is clinical and typically self-reported by the patient. For phototoxic and photoallergic reactions, history and distribution of the eruption can assist in differentiation. Often a linear or spray pattern suggests that an externally applied substance is the culprit. Because photosensitizing medications are ingested and distributed throughout the body, the eruption can involve all sun-exposed areas. The characteristic distribution of a photosensitivity eruption is the face, posterior neck, dorsal hands, and extensor arms. Certain areas, including the creases of the eyelids, upper lip, submental anterior neck, and posterior auricular neck, are spared.

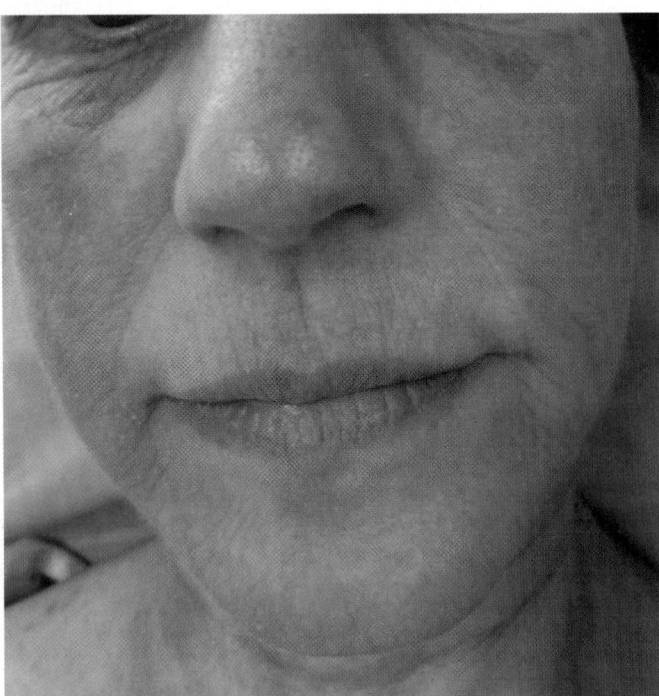

FIGURE 250-12. Photosensitivity reaction. [Photo contributed by University of North Carolina Department of Dermatology.]

TABLE 250- 3 Medications Commonly Causing Photosensitivity Eruptions

Phototoxic	Photoallergic
Chlorpromazine	Nonsteroidal anti-inflammatory drugs
Furosemide	Griseofulvin
Tetracyclines (demeclocycline > doxycycline)	Sulfonamides
Thiazides	Para-aminobenzoic acid and most sunscreens
Psoralen	Promethazine
Coal tar	Psoralen
Amiodarone	Sulfonylureas (glipizide, glyburide)
Isotretinoin	Fragrances
Fluoroquinolones	Dapsone

The diagnosis is based on identifying the offending agent. Photopatch testing performed by a dermatologist or allergist may be helpful in identifying the photosensitizing agent. If the diagnosis is unclear, other photosensitivity disorders, such as lupus erythematosus, dermatomyositis, and polymorphous light eruption, should be excluded.

The most important part of treatment of sunburn and photosensitivity is prevention. Avoid the midday sun, apply sunscreen liberally and frequently (ultraviolet A and B protection with sun protection factor of at least 30), wear protective clothing, and seek shade. Manufactured clothing with a sun protection factor of 50+ is available and helpful. Sunburns can be treated symptomatically with nonsteroidal anti-inflammatory drugs and tepid baths and by application of topical antibiotics to areas of vesiculation. Emollients may be soothing but will not prevent eventual exfoliation. Individuals should also be advised to avoid the sun until the eruption resolves.

In cases of photosensitivity, discontinue the causative agent. Initial management includes topical corticosteroids and management similar to a sunburn reaction. The patient should avoid the sun until the eruption has cleared completely.

REFERENCES

The complete reference list is available online at www.TintinalliEM.com.

Skin Disorders: Trunk

Dean S. Morrell
Kara Luersen Brooks

INTRODUCTION

There are many conditions that can have truncal involvement. This section focuses on some common eruptions that frequently affect the trunk: papulosquamous disorders; urticarial and morbilliform disorders; blistering disorders; and miscellaneous disorders. Urticaria and angioedema are discussed in chapter 14, "Anaphylaxis, Allergies, and Angioedema." Although the truncal location of an eruption can be a helpful clue for diagnosis, the clinical appearance of the lesions and overall assessment of the patient are needed to make the correct diagnosis.

PAPULOSQUAMOUS DISORDERS

Scaling conditions include psoriasis, seborrheic dermatitis, tinea corporis, pityriasis ("tinea") versicolor, eczema/atopic dermatitis, lichen planus, secondary syphilis, and scabies. **Table 251-1** lists common features distinguishing these eruptions.

PSORIASIS

Psoriasis is discussed in detail in chapter 253, "Skin Disorders: Extremities." Stress or alcohol ingestion can be associated with a flare of psoriasis. The following medications can also be related to an exacerbation: steroid withdrawal, lithium, β-blockers, interferon, and antimalarials.[1] The differential diagnosis is listed in Table 251-1.

Diagnosis is clinical. The disorder is characterized by well-demarcated erythematous papules and plaques with a silvery white scale (**Figure 251-1**). Removal of the scale typically reveals minute bleeding points referred to as **Auspitz sign**. Chronic plaque psoriasis is the most common variety, and localization to the sacrum, gluteal cleft, or umbilicus can occur. In the skin folds, psoriasis often lacks the characteristic silvery scale and is present only as well-demarcated, red- to salmon-colored plaques. Involvement of the scalp and nails is not uncommon. Lesions of psoriasis tend to be symmetric with a predilection for the extensor surfaces. Localized physical trauma can cause new lesions to form (**Koebner phenomenon**—scratching causes new lesions to form in linear distribution of the scratch). Scattered discrete lesions, like water droplets, represent a distinctive form of psoriasis called **guttate psoriasis** (**Figure 251-2**). This can be seen on the trunk as an abrupt eruption following an infection such as streptococcal pharyngitis. Generalized pustular psoriasis (**Figure 251-3**) should be included in the differential diagnosis of the acutely ill patient.

Topical treatment for localized plaques includes moisturization with plain petroleum jelly or topical steroids. Ointment-based products have the highest hydration efficacy. High-potency steroids, such as clobetasol foam, spray, ointment, or cream, can be used on the trunk. Prolonged use may result in atrophy, steroid acne, pyoderma, or rebound with abrupt discontinuation. **Do not prescribe systemic steroids due to the great risk of rebound or induction of pustular psoriasis.**

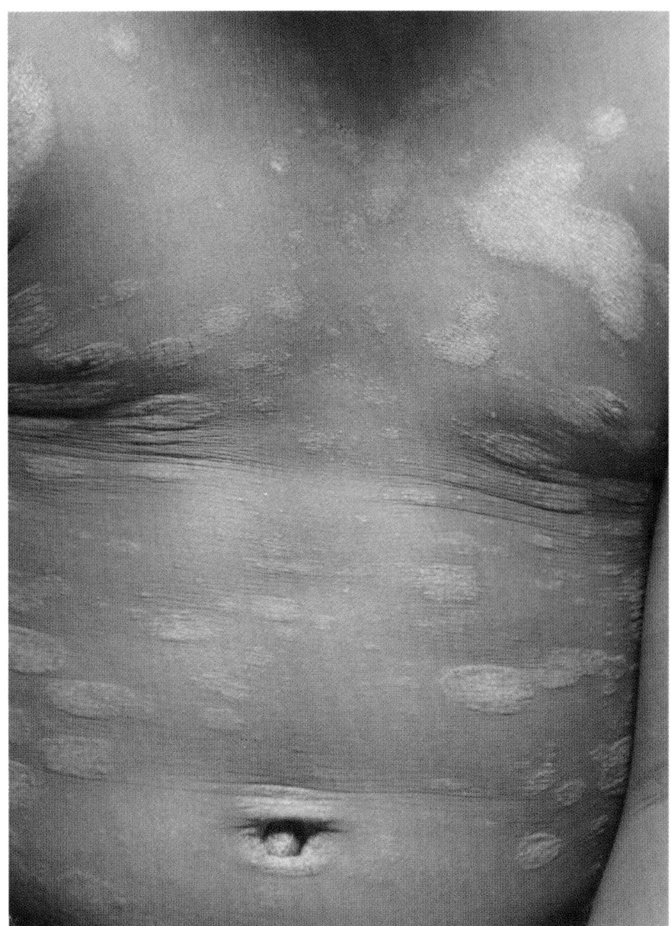

FIGURE 251-1. Psoriasis. Large, well-marginated scaling plaques. [Photo contributed by University of North Carolina Department of Dermatology.]

TABLE 251-1 Comparison Features of Common Papulosquamous Eruptions

Condition	Distinguishing Clinical Features	Location	Special Signs	Comments
Psoriasis	Erythematous, well-marginated papules and plaques with silvery scale	Trunk, extensor surfaces, scalp	Auspitz sign; Koebner phenomenon, nail pitting	Hereditary predilection; onset in early 20s
Seborrheic dermatitis	Greasy, yellow scales	Midchest, suprapubic, scalp, facial creases	Can overlap with psoriasis, "sebopsoriasis"	Debilitated, elderly, or infants (cradle cap)
Atopic dermatitis	Ill-defined vesicles forming plaques with scale; chronic lesions lichenified	Flexures > trunk	Spares the nose	Pruritus "itch that rashes"; atopic individuals
Lichen planus	5 P's: purple, pruritic, polygonal, planar papules	Any skin, mucous membranes, hair follicles	Wickham striae; Koebner phenomenon	Age 20–60 y old
Pityriasis rosea	Lines of skin tension, collarette of scale	Trunk, in Christmas tree pattern following skin lines	Herald patch 1–2 wk before general eruption	Spring and fall, age 15–40 y old; viral exanthem, herpes 6 and 7
Tinea corporis	Sharply demarcated, erythematous, scaly annular plaques; may coalesce into gyrate patterns	Trunk, legs, arm, neck	May need KOH/culture to diagnose; septate branching hyphae on KOH	All ages; from pets, soil, or autoinoculation from hands/feet; incubation days or months
Pityriasis (tinea) versicolor	Versicolored—red, salmon, light brown, dark brown, hypopigmented; well-demarcated scaly patches	Central upper chest and back	Spaghetti and meatballs on KOH; nonseptate pseudohyphae and budding yeast	Young adults, summer, hot humid environments
Secondary syphilis	At 2–10 wk, macular erythema on trunk, abdomen, inner extremities; followed by papular or papulosquamous lesions	Palms, soles, trunk	Serology	Great masquerader—can take any form; can be confused with pityriasis rosea
Scabies	Pruritic papules and burrows with crusting	Finger webs, wrists, axillae, areolae, umbilicus, abdomen, waistband, genitals	Scrapings show mites, feces, eggs	Can be chronic "7-year itch"; intensely pruritic, especially at night

Abbreviation: KOH = potassium hydroxide.

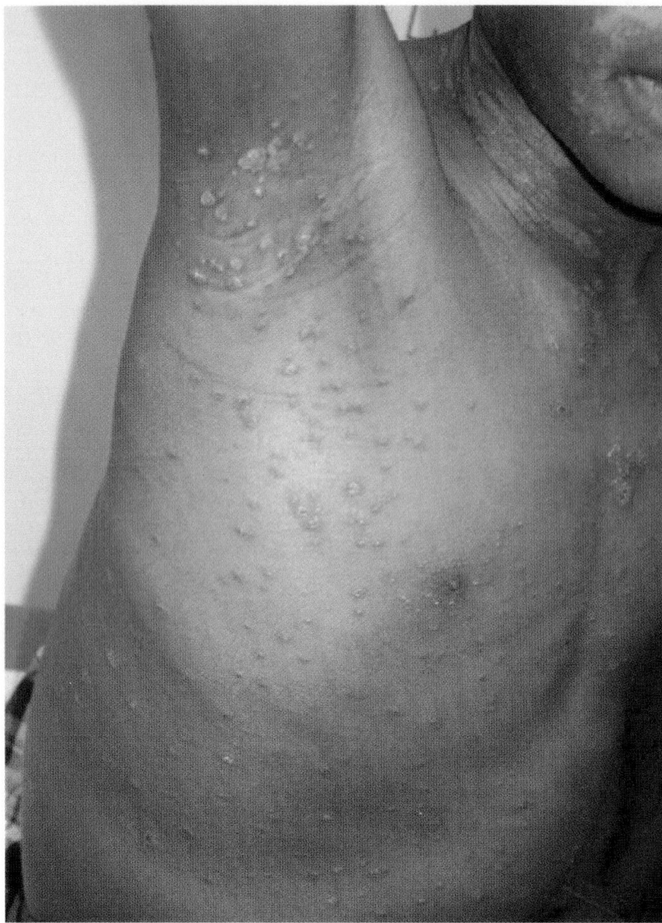

FIGURE 251-2. Guttate psoriasis. Note discrete erythematous scaly papules resembling raindrops on the trunk. [Photo contributed by University of North Carolina Department of Dermatology.]

SEBORRHEIC DERMATITIS

Seborrheic dermatitis is a chronic inflammatory disease with a predilection for areas of increased sebaceous gland activity. Incidence increases with age and in specific disease states.[2] Erythema with a greasy yellowish scale is seen in the sebum-producing areas, such as the scalp, eyebrows, ears, beard, midchest, and groin (**Figure 251-4**). The lesions are often well marginated and symmetric. Weeping and crusting may occur, especially in the body folds and ears. Pruritus may be present. Severe involvement may occur in debilitated patients such as those with Parkinson's disease, Down's syndrome, or acquired immunodeficiency disease.

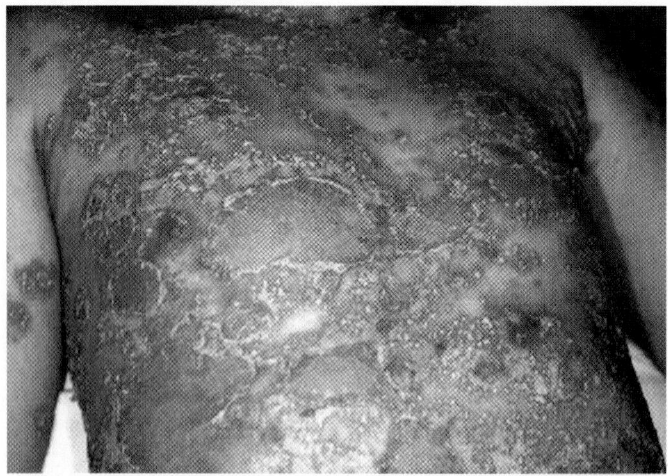

FIGURE 251-3. Pustular psoriasis. [Photo contributed by University of North Carolina Department of Dermatology.]

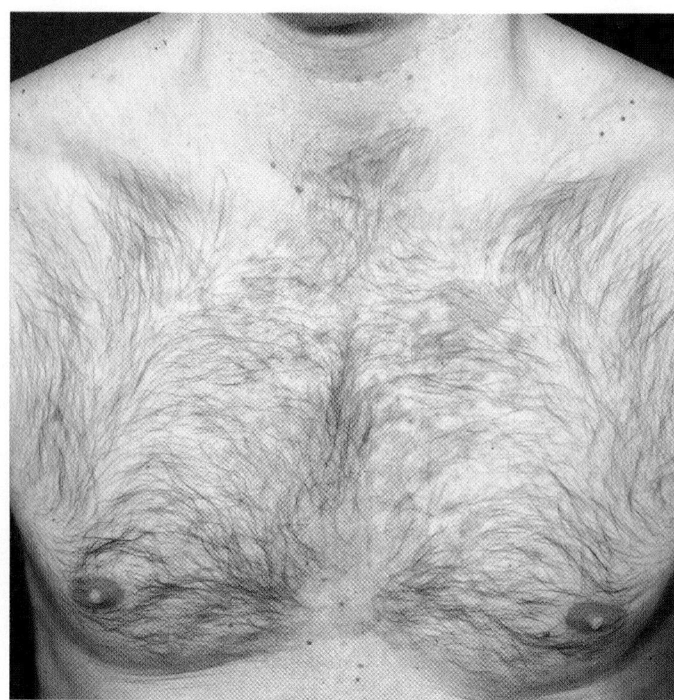

FIGURE 251-4. Seborrheic dermatitis. [Reproduced with permission from Wolff KL, Johnson R, Suurmond R: *Fitzpatrick's Color Atlas & Synopsis of Clinical Dermatology*, 5th ed. © 2005, McGraw-Hill, New York.]

The presternal area, axillae, and groin are common sites for truncal involvement. The axillary involvement typically starts in the apices, similar to a contact dermatitis to deodorants, whereas clothing dermatitis involves the periphery but spares the axillary vault. The inframammary regions and umbilicus may also be involved. The differential diagnosis is presented in Table 251-1.

Treatment is aimed at controlling disease. Mild cases may respond to over-the-counter shampoos containing ketoconazole 1%, selenium sulfide, zinc pyrithione, or salicylic acid. These can be lathered into any affected area on the scalp or body. Prescription-strength ketoconazole 2% shampoo can be used several times weekly, or ketoconazole cream for the face can be used twice daily. Hydrocortisone 1% cream or lotion, or 2.5% cream or lotion for more difficult cases, can be used twice daily in combination with antifungals.

PITYRIASIS ROSEA

Pityriasis rosea is a viral exanthema associated with herpesvirus 6 and 7. It may be a reactivation of the latent herpesvirus that triggers a viremia and subsequent eruption.[3] It most frequently affects those between 15 and 40 years old, most often in spring and fall. Pityriasis typically begins with a single, or "herald," patch, which is a fine scaling, erythematous- to salmon-colored discrete oval patch 2 to 5 cm in size (**Figure 251-5**). In 1 to 2 weeks, a generalized eruption occurs on the trunk and proximal arms, with a characteristic "Christmas tree" pattern of macules and plaques, with the long axis of the lesions oriented along skin tension lines (**Figure 251-6**). A collarette of scale with the open edge of scale on the inside of the lesion is a helpful diagnostic finding. Rarely, the face, palms, soles, or oral cavity can be involved. Pruritus can be moderate to severe. Mild constitutional symptoms may also occur at the onset of the eruption. Spontaneous resolution occurs within 4 to 16 weeks. Relapses or recurrences are uncommon.

Table 251-1 lists the major differential diagnoses. In addition, several medications can cause a pityriasis-like eruption: captopril, barbiturates, lisinopril, ketotifen, arsenicals, interferon, imatinib mesylate, gold, and

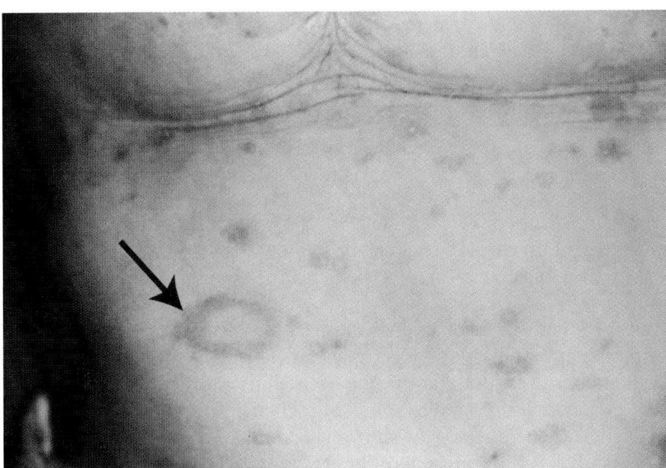

FIGURE 251-5. Herald patch in pityriasis rosea (*arrow*). [Courtesy of the Centers for Disease Control and Prevention.]

clonidine. Guttate psoriasis can mimic pityriasis rosea but does not have the characteristic collarette of scale.

Treatment is symptomatic. Oral antihistamines by mouth and topical steroid creams (triamcinolone 0.1% in adults or hydrocortisone 1% in children) with emollients (petroleum jelly–based preparations) can help the pruritus. Ultraviolet B phototherapy from a dermatologist or natural sunlight may speed the resolution of the lesions. Macrolides are not indicated.[4,5]

TINEA CORPORIS

All superficial dermatophyte infections of the trunk, neck, arms, and legs are referred to as *tinea corporis*. Specific names are used for eruptions involving the groin (tinea cruris), feet (tinea pedis), hands (tinea manuum), face (tinea faciei), and scalp (tinea capitis); see associated chapters in this book for more detailed information about these specific locations. All ages can be affected, and lesions can spread by autoinoculation from other parts of the body. *Trichophyton rubrum* and *Trichophyton mentagrophytes* are the most common organisms that can spread from involvement of the feet. Occupational or recreational exposure (gyms, locker rooms) occurs from contaminated clothing, furniture, and/or equipment. Exposure to animals or contaminated soil may also cause tinea corporis. Pets may harbor *Trichophyton verrucosum* or *Microsporum canis*, whereas *T. mentagrophytes* from Southeast Asia

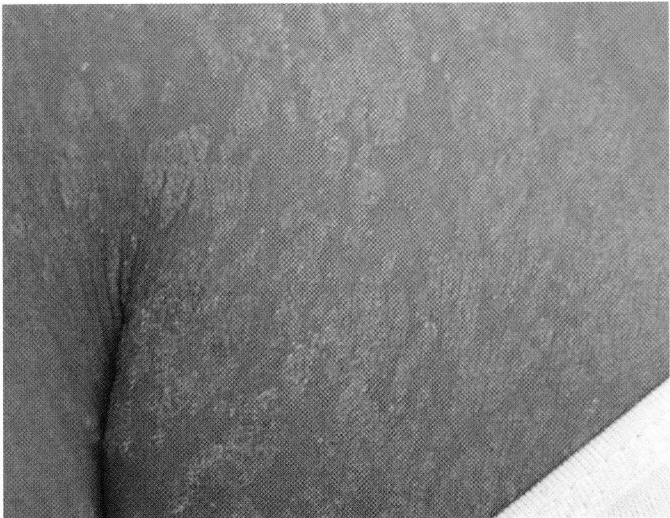

FIGURE 251-6. Pityriasis rosea. Fine scaly plaques along skin tension lines. [Photo contributed by University of North Carolina Department of Dermatology.]

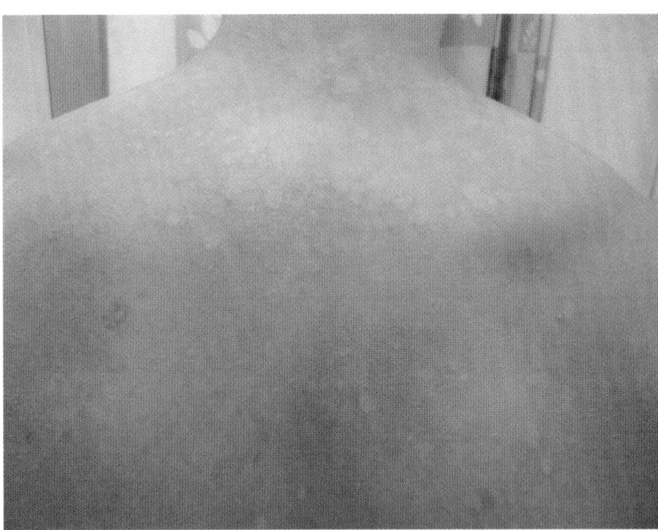

FIGURE 251-7. Tinea versicolor. Hypopigmented macules with fine scale. [Photo contributed by University of North Carolina Department of Dermatology.]

bamboo rats can cause a very inflamed and highly contagious widespread eruption. The incubation period is variable and may be days or months after exposure.[6] The eruption may be chronic with mild pruritus as the only symptom. Tinea corporis is characterized by one or more sharply demarcated, mildly erythematous, annular scaling plaques (**Figure 251-7**). Central clearing gives the name "**ringworm**." The advancing scaling border is a characteristic finding, and the border is an excellent area to demonstrate long branching hyphae with a potassium hydroxide preparation (see Figure 248-1 and Table 248-6). Abrupt onset of widespread tinea may be associated with acquired immunodeficiency syndrome or other immunosuppressive disorders or use of topical steroids. Occlusion, shaving, or topical steroid use may result in a deep, purulent, boggy folliculitis. The differential diagnosis is provided in Table 251-1.

Treatment of limited lesions is with topical antifungal preparations (**Table 251-2**). Apply twice a day and **extend the application to at least 3 cm beyond the advancing margin**. Treat for at least 4 weeks and continue for 1 week after resolution. If tinea pedis or unguium is also present, apply the antifungal to the feet and nails. Widespread tinea corporis or involvement of the follicles warrants oral therapy (Table 251-2).[6] Oral agents may be expensive and can have interactions and contraindications in specific patient populations. Refer to a drug reference manual for specific details. **Terbinafine** requires baseline liver function tests before administration. **Itraconazole** is contraindicated in congestive heart failure and in patients taking lovastatin or simvastatin. **Griseofulvin** will cause a disulfiram (Antabuse®)-like effect with alcohol consumption in some patients and can be photosensitizing (caution patients to avoid intense light). Safety profiles in children are similar to adults.[7] Provide scheduled follow-up to assess treatment response.

"TINEA" PITYRIASIS VERSICOLOR

Pityriasis versicolor is caused by the overgrowth of the yeasts *Malassezia furfur* (previously *Pityrosporum ovale*) and *Malassezia globosa*. *Malassezia* species are part of the normal cutaneous flora and reside in keratin of skin and hair follicles. They require oil to grow, so the disease is more prevalent in young adults when sebaceous gland activity is highest. Predisposing factors include high temperature/humidity, oily skin, and steroid treatment.

Asymptomatic, hypo- or hyperpigmented, and coalescing scaly macules are seen on the trunk or proximal extremities. The central upper chest and back are the most common areas of involvement (**Figure 251-7**). Facial lesions may be present in infants and the immunocompromised. The "versicolor" refers to the varying shades of erythema and pigmentation. In untanned individuals, the lesions may be salmon or light brown. On darkly pigmented skin, the lesions may be hypopigmented. The fine scale is best appreciated by gently abrading the lesions with a glass slide or blade. The condition may be present for months or years and is

TABLE 251-2 Treatment of Tinea Corporis

Condition	Method	Agent(s)	Dosage
Limited involvement	Topical	Clotrimazole	Twice a day, extend ≥3 cm beyond edges; treat ≥4 wk and 1 wk after clearing
		Terbinafine	
		Ciclopirox cream	
		Sulconazole cream	
		Oxiconazole cream	
		Ketoconazole cream	
		Econazole cream	
		Naftifine cream	
		Butenafine cream	
Widespread	Oral*	Terbinafine	250 milligrams PO daily for 2 wk
		Itraconazole	200 milligrams PO daily for 2 wk
		Griseofulvin	500 milligrams twice a day for 4 wk; 20 milligrams/kg/d in children
		Fluconazole	200 milligrams PO daily for 4 wk; 3–5 milligrams/kg/d in children

*Costs vary; primary care or dermatology follow-up needed; baseline chemistries needed for some; check detailed references for adverse effects and drug interactions.

usually asymptomatic. Patients usually present due to cosmetic concerns regarding the inconsistent pigmentation.

The hyperpigmented, scaling pink macules of pityriasis versicolor may appear similar to those found in tinea corporis, psoriasis, pityriasis rosea, seborrheic dermatitis, or nummular eczema. Hypopigmented lesions should be differentiated from pityriasis alba, leprosy, or postinflammatory conditions. A potassium hydroxide preparation obtained by gently scraping the surface of the lesion and examining under the microscope (see Table 248-6) will reveal the characteristic short chopped hyphae and yeast forms termed "spaghetti and meatballs" (**Figure 251-8**).

Treat with ketoconazole 2% shampoo, applied daily for a week, washing off after 10 to 15 minutes. Other topical options include econazole, miconazole, clotrimazole, or ketoconazole cream (Table 251-2). Widespread involvement usually makes these less cost effective and more difficult to apply. Extensive or refractory pityriasis versicolor can be treated with oral ketoconazole, 400 milligrams, itraconazole, 400 milligrams, or fluconazole, 300 milligrams, in weekly doses.[6,8]

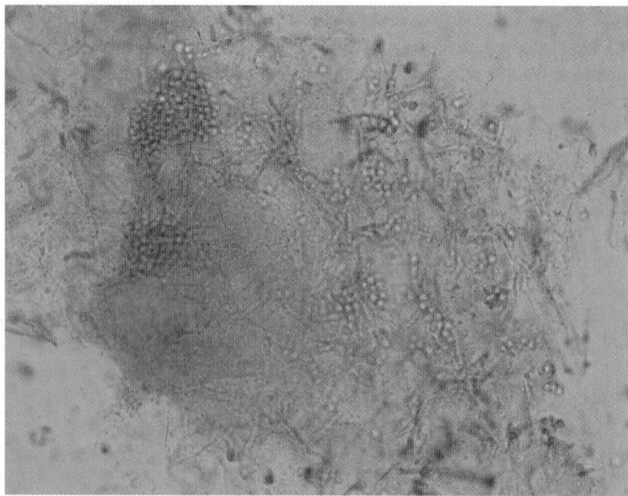

FIGURE 251-8. Potassium hydroxide preparation with pseudohyphae, showing "spaghetti and meatballs" pattern. [Photo contributed by University of North Carolina Department of Dermatology.]

Discoloration may take months to resolve after treatment and is not a sign of treatment failure. Relapses are frequent, and instructions on prophylactic regimens should be given to include once-weekly selenium sulfide 2.5% or ketoconazole 2% shampoo.

ECZEMA/ATOPIC DERMATITIS

The terms *eczema* and *atopic dermatitis* are often used interchangeably and have a variety of presentations. This section focuses on truncal involvement. In chronic eczema, the hallmark is the "itch that rashes," in which an itch–scratch cycle perpetuates the condition. Itching is common and often worse at night and is aggravated by heat and sweat. Atopic individuals have a personal or family history of asthma, allergic rhinitis, nasal polyps, or "sensitive" skin. The acute stage demonstrates erythematous plaques that may be edematous and with miniature vesicles. Subacute lesions have more scale. The chronic stage presents with thickened (lichenified) skin showing accentuation of the normal skin markings caused by chronic rubbing (**Figure 251-9**). Scratching causes excoriations.

Chronic contact dermatitis may be misdiagnosed as eczema or atopic dermatitis (Table 251-1) or may actually be a factor in the flare of eczema. See chapter 253 for further discussion. The acute stage is typically limited to the area of contact with well-marginated erythema and edema. Papules and vesicles may be present, and bullae may occur in severe reactions with secondary crusting and erosions. Linear (such as from poison ivy) or geographic lesions (such as nickel allergy; **Figure 251-10**) are typical. Pruritus can be severe. Subacute lesions have mild erythema, dry scale, and fine papules. Chronic eruptions will be lichenified with accentuation of the skin markings and show postinflammatory pigmentary changes. The subacute and chronic stages are frequently confused with endogenous eczema. The distribution is initially confined to the site of exposure but later can spread to sites beyond.

Treatment is directed at disease control.[9] Avoid harsh soaps and other irritants or contactants. Moisturize within 2 minutes of bathing with

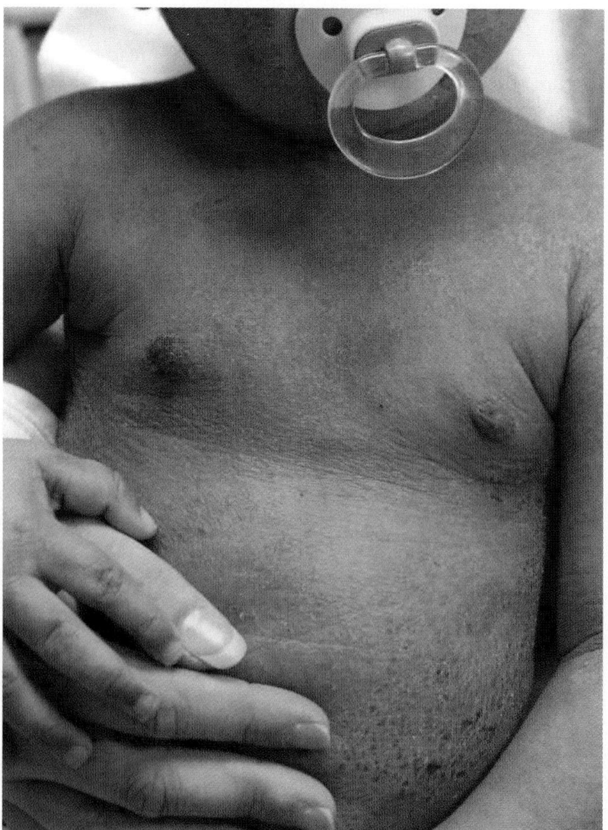

FIGURE 251-9. Atopic dermatitis. Lichenification, excoriations, and ill-defined scaling erythema. [Photo contributed by University of North Carolina Department of Dermatology.]

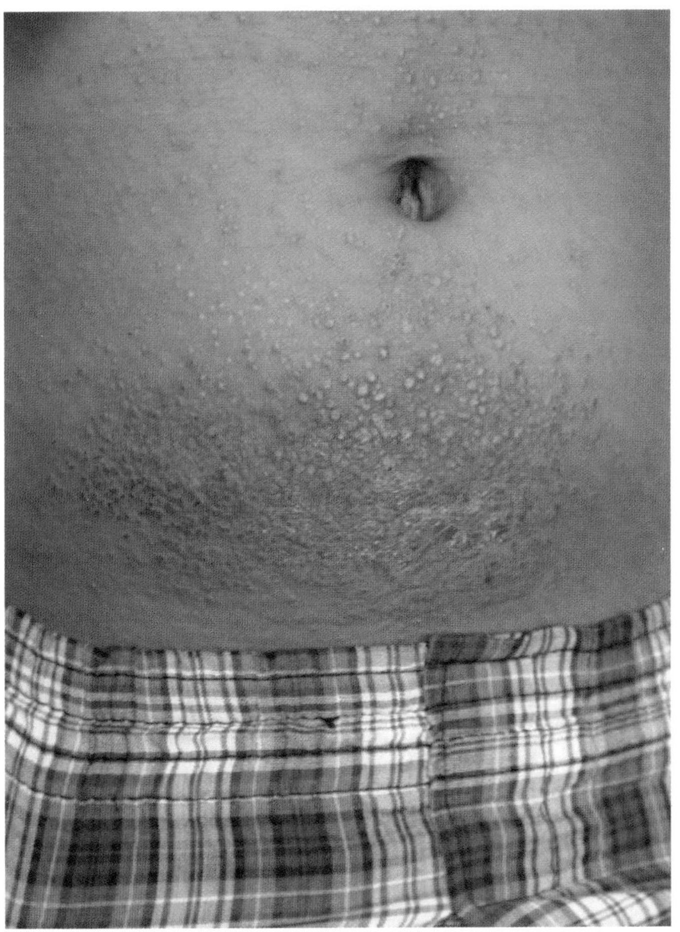

FIGURE 251-10. Allergic contact dermatitis. Erythematous scaly papules and lichenified plaques on the lower abdomen (contact with belt buckles). [Photo contributed by University of North Carolina Department of Dermatology.]

plain petroleum jelly, Aquaphor®, or Eucerin® cream. Use topical steroids, such as 1% hydrocortisone ointment, for mild disease or intertriginous sites; medium-potency preparations, such as triamcinolone 0.1%, for moderate involvement; or higher potency steroids, such as clobetasol, for more severe eruptions. Ointments are the most effective vehicle, but foam delivery systems are effective and more cosmetically elegant. Severe contact reactions may require an oral prednisone taper over 3 weeks. The usual dose in a child is prednisone, 1 to 2 milligrams/kg PO, up to 40 milligrams/d. Adults respond well to a tapering dose of prednisone, 40 to 60 milligrams/d PO each morning. Oral antihistamines, such as diphenhydramine or hydroxyzine, can control nighttime pruritus and scratching. Staphylococcal or streptococcal superinfections typically present with crusting and exudates. Prescribe cephalexin or dicloxacillin because antibiotic resistance is common with erythromycin. Treat for community-acquired methicillin-resistant *Staphylococcus aureus* based on cultures or local patterns of bacterial resistance.

LICHEN PLANUS

Lichen planus may affect the skin, mucous membranes, and hair follicles. It is idiopathic in most cases, although cell-mediated immunity and human leukocyte antigen genetic susceptibility probably play a role. Age of onset is usually between 20 and 60 years old, and there is a 1% to 2% familial incidence.[10]

The hallmark of lichen planus is the constellation of the "5 P's": purple, polygonal, pruritic, planar papules. The onset may be abrupt or over several weeks. The course is variable and may last months to years. Spontaneous resolution may occur, but recurrences are also common. The violaceous flat-topped papules may be discrete or generalized

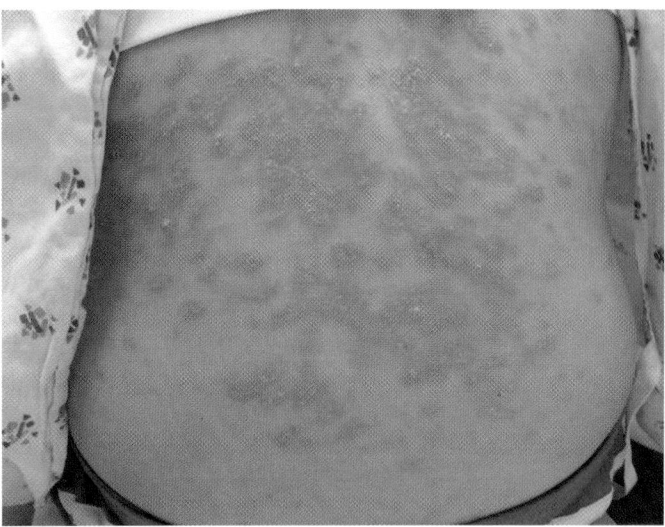

FIGURE 251-11. Lichen planus. Violaceous, flat-topped polygonal papules on the back. [Photo contributed by University of North Carolina Department of Dermatology.]

(**Figure 251-11**). Common sites of involvement include the lumbar region, flexor wrists, pretibia, scalp, and penis. **Koebner phenomenon**, caused by scratching, may result in a linear array of papules. In pigmented skin, a deep brown hyperpigmentation may occur. **Wickham striae** are fine white lacy reticulate lines that adhere to the papules and are pathognomonic for this condition (**Figure 251-12**). Involvement of the mucous

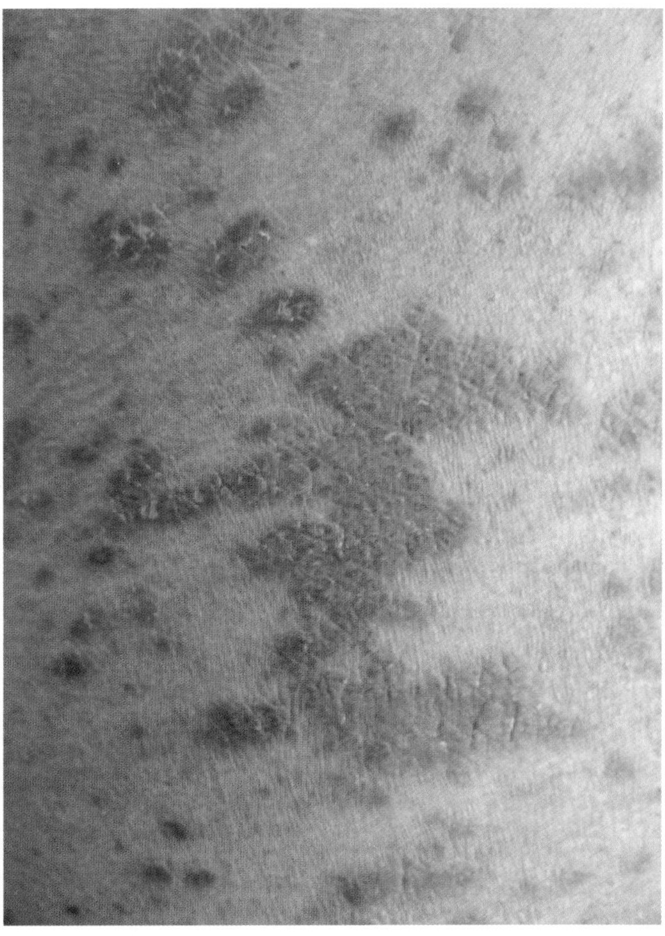

FIGURE 251-12. Wickham striae, lace-like striations. [Photo contributed by University of North Carolina Department of Dermatology.]

membranes occurs in approximately half of those with the disease, and it is not uncommon to have only oral involvement. The posterior buccal mucosa is most commonly affected; however, gingiva, tongue, and lips may also be involved. Painful erosions may be present, and these patients have a 2% to 3% lifetime risk of squamous cell carcinoma developing in these areas. About 70% of patients with mucosal vulvovaginal lichen planus also have oral involvement, so it is important to ask about genital symptoms.[10]

There are many other variants of lichen planus, with the most common being hypertrophic, which presents with thick, hyperkeratotic plaques on the shins. Annular lichen planus is more common in men and typically involves the axillae, penis, or groin. This variant presents with asymptomatic ringed lesions approximately 1 cm in diameter. Follicular involvement of the scalp can result in a scarring alopecia. Nail changes can result in destruction of the nail fold and nail bed, with longitudinal splintering (pterygia).

Other papulosquamous diseases are included in the differential diagnosis of lichen planus (Table 251-1). The oral mucosal involvement and Wickham striae are helpful in distinguishing lichen planus from psoriasis. Chronic discoid lupus and fungal infections may have similar cutaneous findings.

Lichenoid drug eruptions can be identical to lichen planus, except they tend to be more generalized and photodistributed and there is a history of drug ingestion. The latent period can be months to years, with an average of 12 months, and it may take years to resolve after withdrawal of the offending agent. Common medications are listed in Table 251-3 in the later section "Drug Reactions." Chronic graft-versus-host disease, dermatomyositis, and malignant lymphomas may also have lichenoid eruptions.

Treatment is with topical or intralesional steroids. Mid- to high-potency preparations, such as triamcinolone 0.1% ointment or fluocinonide 0.05% ointment twice a day, are helpful, although treatment does not cure the disease. Intralesional triamcinolone, 3 milligrams/mL, can be used for very symptomatic cutaneous or mucous membrane lesions. Fluocinonide, 0.05% gel four times a day, can be used in the mouth. Oral analgesics, such as lidocaine jelly 2%, can be applied to the erosions three times a day before meals. Severe erosions or oral involvement may require PO prednisone, 40 to 60 milligrams every morning for 1 to 2 weeks. Other systemic treatments include cyclosporine, retinoids, azathioprine, methotrexate, and mycophenolate mofetil.

SECONDARY SYPHILIS

Although the lesions are transient and often clinically unimpressive, the inclusion of secondary syphilis in the differential diagnosis of papulosquamous conditions in the ED is important.

Secondary syphilis exhibits skin manifestations in most patients and consists of early and later manifestations. The early eruption appears 2 to 10 weeks after the appearance of the primary chancre and is an evanescent macular rash lasting only a few hours or days. The macular erythema commonly appears on the sides of the trunk, midabdomen, and inner extremities. The discrete round macules are of varying shades from light pink to rose or even brownish red. It may be faint and difficult to appreciate on darkly pigmented skin. This phase of the disease is often asymptomatic, although associated symptoms can include fever, sore throat, fatigue, headache, meningismus, and shotty, firm, nontender lymphadenopathy of the posterior cervical, axillary, and epitrochlear regions. Pruritus may be present. The macular eruption resolves spontaneously and may leave postinflammatory hyperpigmentation.[11]

Later eruptions may present in a variety of forms, hence the referral to syphilis as the *great imitator*. This phase typically lasts 2 to 6 weeks and resolves spontaneously. Multiple recurrences over a period of 1 year can occur before infection enters the latent stage. The later eruptions of secondary syphilis are often papular lesions 2 to 5 mm in size, may be generalized, and are reddish to copper in color. The papules may be subtle or deeply infiltrated and firm. The surface may be smooth and shiny or have a thick, adherent scale (**Figure 251-13**). Palmar-plantar involvement is a helpful finding and is characterized by tender copper-colored discrete macules with a collarette of scale. Postinflammatory hyperpigmentation can be prominent and persist for weeks to months. Psoriasiform, follicular, lichenoid, or acneiform lesions can occur. Vesiculobullous lesions of the palms and soles are seen in neonatal syphilis. Patients with human immunodeficiency virus may have atypical presentations, including very large infiltrated, scaling, and crusted plaques. Annular lesions may occur, most frequently around the mouth, and may mimic sarcoidosis. Patchy nonscarring "moth eaten" alopecia may be present. Split papules at the corners of the mouth, asymptomatic white plaques on mucous membranes, and condyloma lata in the genitals are highly infectious stigmata.

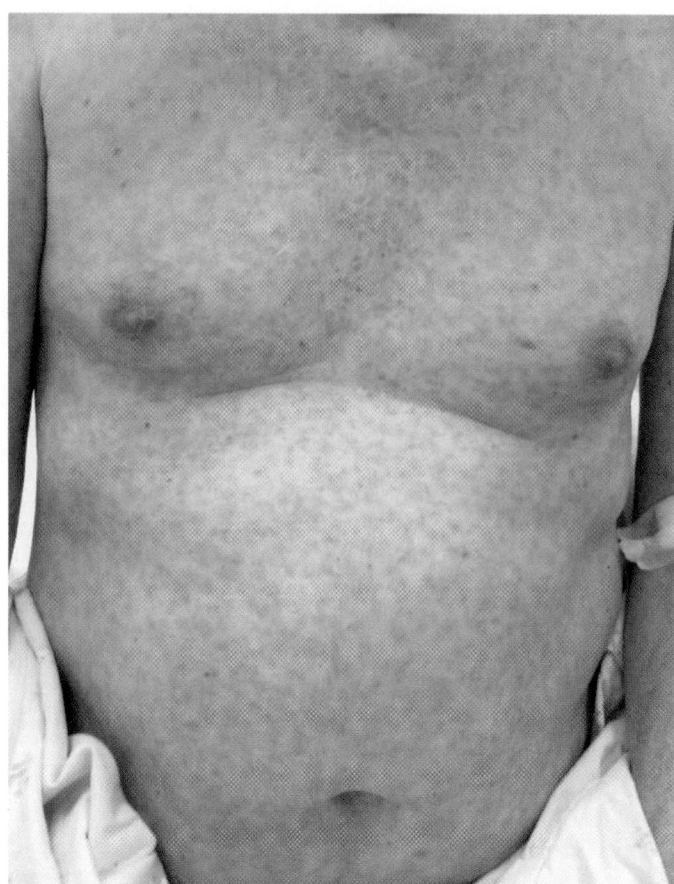

FIGURE 251-13. Secondary syphilis. Papulosquamous eruption. [Photo contributed by University of North Carolina Department of Dermatology.]

In secondary syphilis, the nontreponemal serologic tests are strongly reactive. Exceptions include the prozone phenomenon, in which a false-negative result occurs with high antibody titers, and rarely, in patients with acquired immunodeficiency syndrome, seronegative syphilis may occur. Histologic stains of affected tissues can be performed to confirm the diagnosis in seronegative patients.

The various cutaneous manifestations of syphilis may resemble many other cutaneous diseases (Table 251-1). **Pityriasis rosea** is the most common condition to consider and can have very similar cutaneous findings. However, the lesions of syphilis tend to be more circular and randomly arranged on the trunk, not with the oval "Christmas tree" distributed findings in pityriasis rosea. Pityriasis rosea also lacks palmoplantar and mucous membrane lesions and lymphadenopathy.

Treatment is benzathine penicillin G (single dose of 2.4 million units IM, 1.2 million units in each buttock). Doxycycline, 100 milligrams PO twice a day for 2 weeks, can be used in penicillin-allergic patients. Further discussion is provided in chapter 149, "Sexually Transmitted Infections."

SCABIES

Scabies is infestation by the *Sarcoptes scabiei* mite and should be considered in any patient with complaints of severe generalized pruritus. The mite burrows and multiplies within the upper layer of the skin. In classic scabies, there are 6 to 10 live mites present on the skin. In immunocompromised patients, there may be more than 1 million mites present.

Scabies is usually spread by skin-to-skin contact and can occur in any age group. The mite can also remain alive for >48 hours on inanimate objects, such as clothing and linens. The eruption can vary, ranging from minimal findings to extensive secondary excoriations and eczematous lesions. Hypersensitivity to the mite occurs before the development of symptoms. The initial exposure may not produce symptoms for several weeks. Reinfestation may produce pruritus within 1 to 3 days. Previous sensitization, inadequate treatment, and the host's immune status can alter the appearance of the condition. Chronic, undiagnosed scabies is referred to as *the 7-year itch*.

Intense pruritus is common, especially at night, although immunosuppressed patients may be asymptomatic. Women frequently complain of nipple itching, whereas men most frequently note the penile or scrotal pruritic lesions. Pruritic papules, secondary excoriations, and burrows are the classic findings. Secondary infection with crusting may occur. The head and neck are typically spared, although they may be involved in infants and the immunocompromised. Common sites of involvement include the finger webs, wrists, axillae, areolae, umbilicus, lower abdomen, waistband, and genitals (**Figure 251-14, A and B**).

Red-brown papules and nodules may occur on the penis and scrotum. Crusted scabies occurs in immunosuppressed or debilitated patients. The lesions can be generalized and include the face and scalp, with marked crusting and heavy scaling. Pressure-bearing sites, such as the buttocks, elbows, and feet, are common areas of hyperkeratotic lesions. The tips of the fingers can be swollen, crusted, and have a psoriasiform scaling under the nails.

Atypical lesions can be seen in infants with involvement of the face and scalp, as well as vesicles or pustules on the palms and soles. An autosensitization-type reaction ("id") can occur with widespread urticarial papules predominantly on the trunk and proximal extremities. Other pruritic disorders, including eczema, atopic dermatitis, contact dermatitis, urticarias, dermatitis herpetiformis, pediculosis infestation, lichen planus, and metabolic disorders such as uremia or hypo- or hyperparathyroidism, should be considered in the evaluation. The presence of pruritus in other family members or close contacts is a helpful clue to scabies. A #15 blade can be gently scraped across a typical burrow and placed on a slide with mineral oil for microscopic confirmation. Diagnosis is made by the presence of the mite, feces, or ova (**Figure 251-15**).

Treat with **permethrin 5% cream** applied overnight to the patient and all family members and close contacts. It should be applied from the neck down, covering all areas of the body, including under the nails, in the umbilicus, around the nipples, and the genitals. The face and scalp should be treated in affected infants and young children. It is washed off in 8 to 12 hours. A second application administered 1 week after the first is recommended. **Lindane® is no longer recommended** because of potential neurotoxicity and resistance.[12]

Ivermectin, 200 micrograms/kg PO single dose, is a very effective therapy for common and crusted scabies. Once-a-week dosage for two treatments is recommended. Three or more treatments may be required in the heavily infested or immunocompromised patient. This is also a convenient treatment for institutions or large groups.

Equally important in the treatment is the decontamination of the clothing, bed linens, and towels by hot water washing and machine drying. Items that cannot be washed should be sealed in plastic bags for 10 days. Itching may last for several weeks after treatment and is a sensitivity reaction to the remaining dead mites and mite products in the skin. Cortisone creams, such as triamcinolone 0.1%, or oral antihistamines can be given for the pruritus.

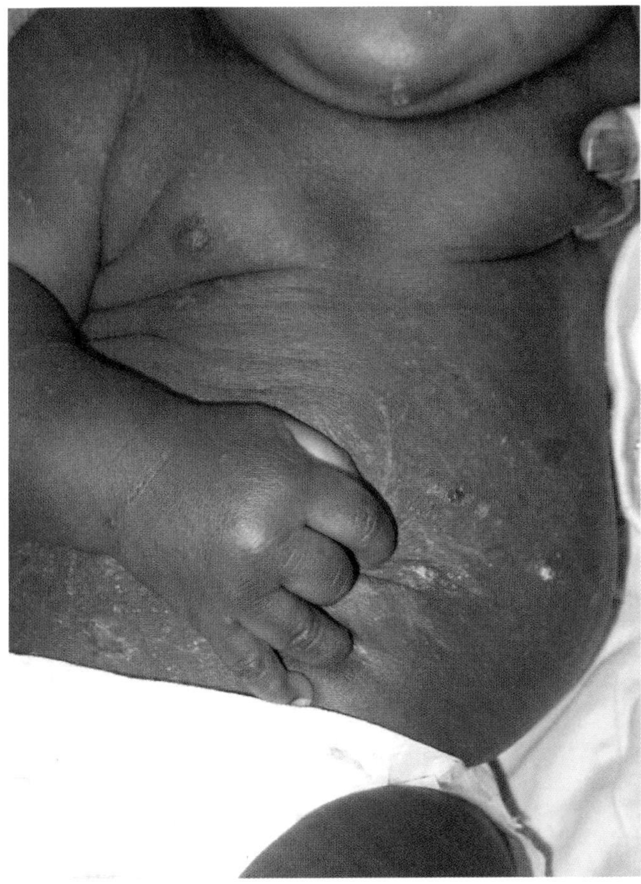
A

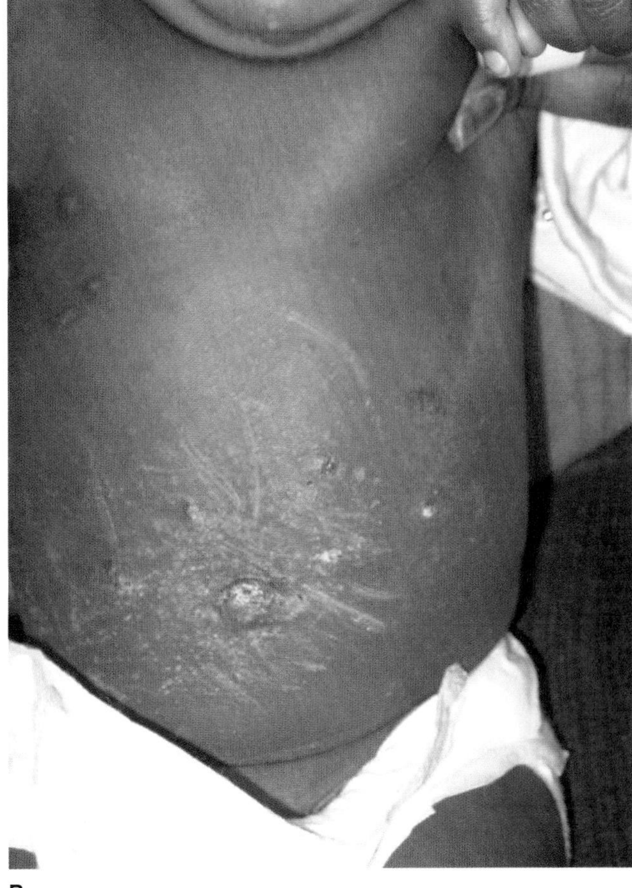
B

FIGURE 251-14. A and B. Scabies. Erythematous scaling papules with excoriation. [Photos contributed by University of North Carolina Department of Dermatology.]

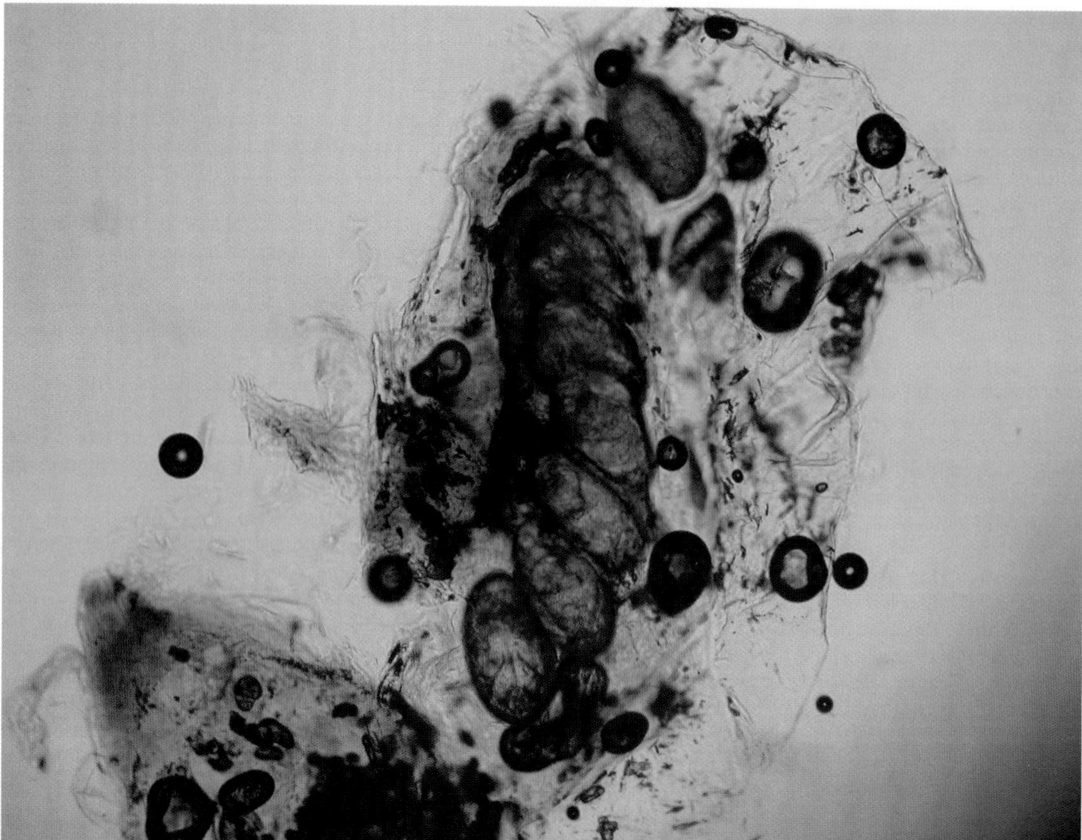

FIGURE 251-15. Scabies eggs and feces. [Photo contributed by University of North Carolina Department of Dermatology.]

MORBILLIFORM/URTICARIAL ERUPTIONS

This section discusses the common morbilliform and urticarial eruptions: urticaria, pruritic urticarial papules and plaques of pregnancy, erythema migrans, and drug eruptions.

URTICARIA AND ANGIOEDEMA

Urticaria is a vascular leak in the superficial dermis of the skin characterized by transient pruritic wheals and welts. **Angioedema** is the presence of larger edematous areas that involve the deeper dermis and the subcutaneous tissue. Both of these conditions may be acute or chronic. The lesions come and go within 24 hours, and the course is <6 weeks.

Urticaria can be immunologically mediated (immunoglobulin E dependent), triggered by penicillins, sulfa drugs, minocycline, food allergies, stings or bites, and infections. Nonimmunologic causes include nonsteroidal anti-inflammatory drugs and radiocontrast material.

Angioedema occurring in the absence of urticarial wheals can occur in hereditary and nonhereditary forms. C1 esterase inhibitor deficiency is a hereditary cause of recurrent angioedema without wheals. Nonhereditary, non–immunologic-mediated triggers include nonsteroidal anti-inflammatory drugs, angiotensin-converting enzyme inhibitors, radiocontrast material, penicillins, and monoclonal antibodies. **In the case of angiotensin-converting enzyme inhibitors, an angioedema reaction can occur more than a year after starting the medication and is a reason for discontinuation of the medication.**[13,14]

Chronic urticaria consists of recurring lesions over a minimum of 6 weeks. Intolerance to nonsteroidal anti-inflammatory drugs, benzoates, contrast dye, and opiates is common, but the cause is often unknown. Physical stimuli such as cold, pressure, and extreme exercise may produce urticarial reactions.[14]

Pruritic edematous papules coalescing into plaques can affect any area of the skin. The urticarial wheals are white, pink, or erythematous nonscaling lesions that range in size from <1 cm to >10 cm. The pattern can be annular, serpiginous, or confluent (**Figure 251-16, A and B**). Lesions wax and wane over 24 hours. Angioedema consists of deeper, less well-demarcated edematous plaques and can be associated with bronchospasm and hypotension. The diagnosis is clinical. **Atypical erythema multiforme** can resemble urticaria, but the lesions of erythema multiforme are not pruritic or transient. Contact urticaria can develop from specific allergies (latex) or chemicals.

Treatment consists of H_1 blockers taken daily. Long-acting, nonsedating (second-generation) antihistamines such as fexofenadine (Allegra®, 180 milligrams/d), loratadine (Claritin®, 20 milligrams/d), or cetirizine (Zyrtec®, 10 to 20 milligrams/d) can lessen new lesions and control pruritus. The short-acting (first-generation) H_1 blockers diphenhydramine and hydroxyzine are helpful for breakthrough and nighttime pruritus. H_2-blocking agents such as ranitidine can be used in chronic urticaria along with H_1-blocking agents, but not as a monotherapy. Doxepin (10 to 25 milligrams), which has H_2-blocking effects, can be used at night, but it is also sedating.

Prednisone may be required for angioedema and widespread urticaria. The dose is 40 to 60 milligrams daily for 5 to 7 days. Reassure patients that acute urticaria nearly always resolves within several weeks. Refer refractory cases to a dermatologist or allergist.

PRURITIC URTICARIAL PAPULES AND PLAQUES OF PREGNANCY

Pruritic urticarial papules and plaques of pregnancy (PUPP) are intensely pruritic eruptions that usually begin in the third trimester of pregnancy. Primiparous women and women with multiple-gestation pregnancies are most often affected, but it rarely recurs in subsequent pregnancies.[15] It does not affect fetal or maternal outcomes. The cause is unknown.

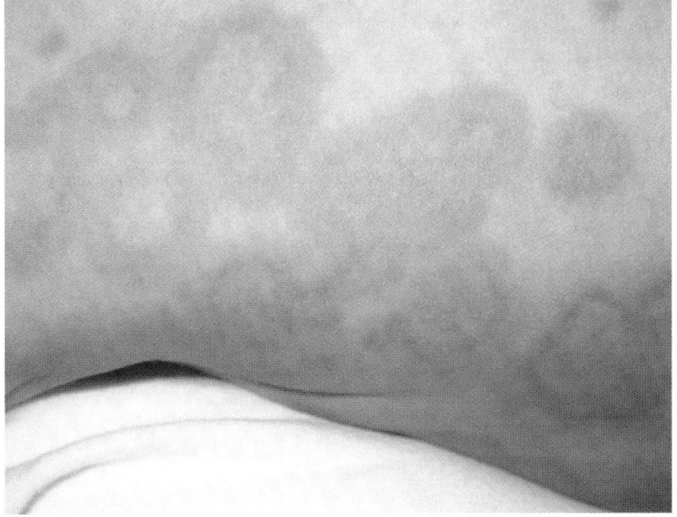

A

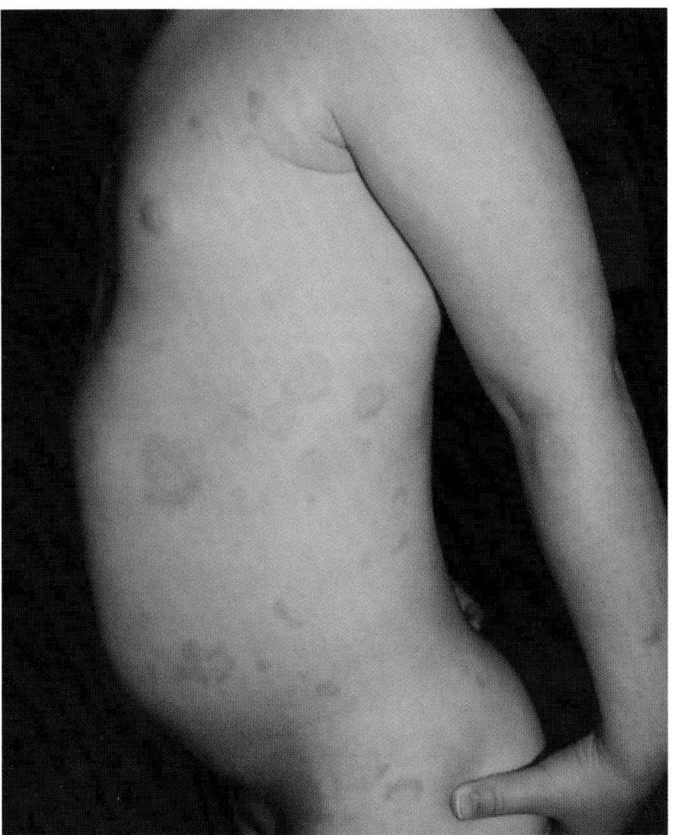

B

FIGURE 251-16. A and B. Urticaria. Characteristic wheals. [Photos contributed by University of North Carolina Department of Dermatology.]

Intensely pruritic, erythematous, 1- to 2-mm papules begin in the abdominal striae and quickly spread into plaques over several days. The abdomen, buttocks, proximal thighs, and, in some cases, arms can be involved (**Figure 251-17**). The face, mucous membranes, palms, and soles are spared. Urticarial plaques can be polycyclic or figurate and can sometimes have discrete tiny vesicles present. Most cases resolve within 10 days of delivery.

Conditions to consider in the differential diagnosis include drug reactions, erythema multiforme, cholestasis of pregnancy, atopic dermatitis, and the rare autoimmune condition pemphigoid gestationis.[15]

Treatment with topical **nonfluorinated** high-potency steroids can be useful for the pruritus. **Fluorinated steroids are contraindicated in pregnancy.** Some patients require PO prednisone, 20 to 40 milligrams/d, for relief of the symptoms. Oral antihistamines are generally not effective.

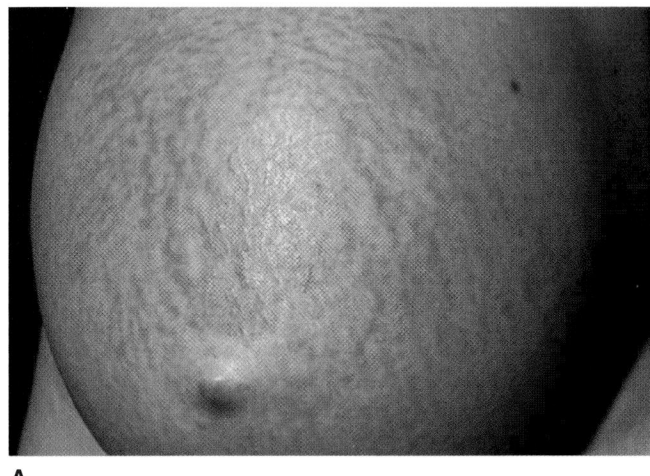

A

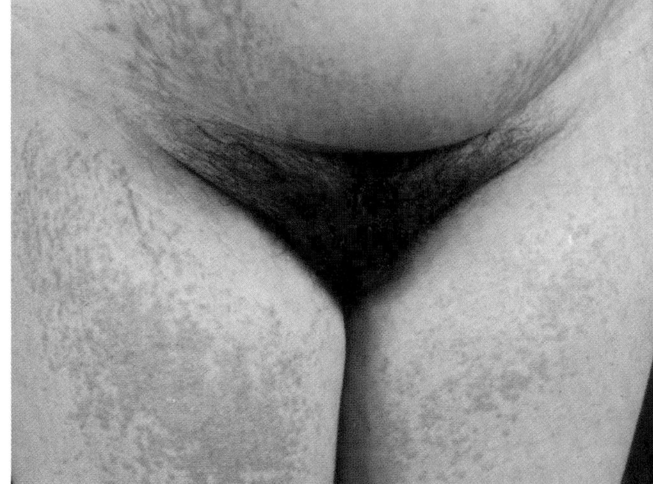

B

FIGURE 251-17. A and B. Pruritic urticarial papules and plaques of pregnancy (PUPP). Urticarial papules accentuated in the striae. [Reproduced with permission from Fleischer AB Jr, Feldman SR, McConnell CF, et al: *Emergency Dermatology: A Rapid Treatment Guide.* © 2002, McGraw-Hill, New York.]

ERYTHEMA MIGRANS

Lyme borreliosis is caused by spirochetes in the genus *Borrelia*, and the Ixodidae tick is the vector. It is a complex multisystem disease and can present with cutaneous findings of erythema migrans in the localized stage 1 disease (**Figure 251-18**). Stage 2 is disseminated infection involving multiple organ systems and can have numerous skin lesions. Stage 3 is persistent infection that can develop months to years later with lesions of acrodermatitis chronica atrophicans.

Early **Lyme disease** begins with a red macule or papule at the site of the tick bite. Disease transmission is more likely if the tick was attached for >24 hours. Slow expansion of nonscaling erythema occurs over 3 to 32 days after the bite. It may become annular with central clearing around the bite site. Varying shades of red in concentric rings may be seen, and, less commonly, the central portion may be indurated, blistering, or necrotic. There is usually no pain or itching. Patients may develop 2 to 100 multiple smaller lesions, sparing the palms and soles; this reflects disseminated infection. Most lesions fade within 1 month, but recurrences can occur over the following months.[16] Other cutaneous findings include diffuse urticaria, malar rash, or conjunctivitis.

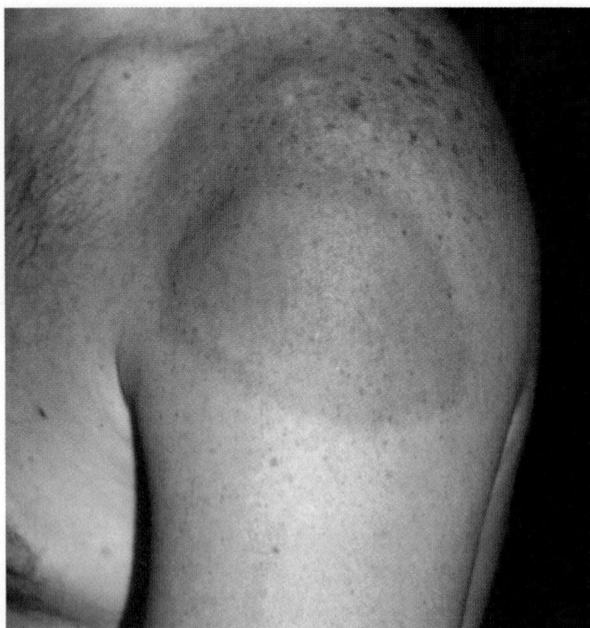

FIGURE 251-18. Erythema migrans. Well-defined erythematous plaque. [Reproduced with permission from Wolff KL, Johnson R, Suurmond R: *Fitzpatrick's Color Atlas & Synopsis of Clinical Dermatology*, 5th ed. © 2005, McGraw-Hill, New York.]

Mild flu-like symptoms of malaise, fever, headaches, arthralgias, GI symptoms, and lymphadenopathy may be present.

Early Lyme disease diagnosis is clinical, due to poor test standardization and variable results of testing methods.[16,17] Approximately 50% of biopsies may demonstrate spirochetes if obtained from the center of the lesion.[16] Culture and polymerase chain reaction testing are specific, but are neither sensitive nor widely available. Serologic testing is variable. Immunoglobulin M and G titers can be measured, with immunoglobulin M peaking between the third and sixth weeks of infection and immunoglobulin G developing over months. Enzyme-linked immunosorbent assay testing should be followed by Western blot testing if the results are equivocal or positive.[16] The lesions of erythema migrans can resemble urticaria, cellulitis, insect bites, dermatophytoses, granuloma annulare, early morphea, erythema multiforme, or even annular subacute cutaneous lupus.

Avoid exposure by applying tick repellents containing *N,N*-diethyl-*m*-toluamide (DEET) to clothing and exposed skin. Check the skin after possible exposure, and promptly remove ticks.[15,16] Antibiotic prophylaxis is not routinely recommended unless the tick was engorged at time of removal or if the *Ixodes* tick was identified in a hyperendemic region, or if in a pregnant patient, or in an immunocompromised patient. In nonpregnant patients, a single dose of doxycycline, 200 milligrams, after a known tick bite (with above risk factors) is recommended.[16,17] Further information regarding treatment of tickborne diseases is found in chapter 160, "Zoonotic Infections." Most recommend at least 3 weeks of therapy for erythema migrans.

DRUG REACTIONS

Adverse cutaneous drug eruptions (**Table 251-3**) are a potential complication of nearly all medications. They can be immunologically mediated or nonimmunologic. Nonimmunologic reactions can be due to enzyme deficiencies, cumulative ingestion, photosensitivity, or topical irritants. Risk factors may include age, gender, dose, and the type of medication.

Cutaneous drug eruptions can mimic almost any other skin disease. Most reactions occur within 1 to 3 weeks of exposure, but hypersensitivity reactions may take longer to develop, so obtain a careful drug history when evaluating any type of rash.[18] Patients may have taken the drug in the past without any problems.

TABLE 251-3 Drug Reactions and Common Causative Agents

Type of Reaction	Common Drugs	Comments
Morbilliform exanthem	Penicillins/cephalosporins, sulfonamides, minocycline, anticonvulsants	Usually <14 d of exposure, resolves within 2 wk; trunk first then extremities
Urticaria or angioedema	Aspirin, NSAIDs, opiates, iodinated contrast material	Usually <36 h since exposure, or within minutes of exposure
Photosensitivity eruption	**Toxic:** tetracyclines, NSAIDs, fluoroquinolones, amiodarone, psoralens, phenothiazides **Allergic:** thiazides, sulfonamides, antimalarials, quinidine, quinine, tricyclic antidepressants, NSAIDs	Sun-exposed areas; exaggerated sunburn responses
Lupus erythematosus–like	Procainamide, phenytoin, minocycline, hydralazine, penicillamine	Photodistributed eruption
Acneiform eruption	β-Lactam antibiotics, steroids, contraceptives, phenytoin, halogens, lithium, phenobarbital, haloperidol, ethambutol, isoniazid	No comedones; monomorphic papules and pustules on back, shoulders, and chest; within 5 d of exposure
Pigmentation	Zidovudine, heavy metals, phenytoin, oral contraceptives, minocycline, amiodarone, clofazimine, antimalarials	Chronic drug ingestion
Fixed drug eruption	Tetracyclines, sulfas, NSAIDs, barbiturates, phenolphthalein	Reexposure causes recurrence in same location
Vesiculobullous eruption	Penicillamine, captopril, sulfas, thiols	Hard to distinguish from bullous disorder
Lichenoid eruption	ACE inhibitors (captopril enalapril), β-blockers (labetalol, propranolol), methyldopa, antimalarials, quinidine, TNF inhibitors (etanercept, infliximab), hydrochlorothiazide, gold and other metals, penicillamine, NSAIDs	May occur months after exposure, oral lesions, slow resolution up to 2 y
Anticoagulant necrosis	Coumadin, heparin	Onset in 3–5 d, well-demarcated painful area of fatty tissue

Abbreviations: ACE = angiotensin-converting enzyme; NSAIDs = nonsteroidal anti-inflammatory drugs; TNF = tumor necrosis factor.

The most common presentation is the **morbilliform exanthem** (**Figure 251-19**). Diffuse, symmetric, pruritic, erythematous macules and papules appear first on the trunk and then spread to the extremities. The initial eruption is usually within 7 to 14 days of exposure, usually resolves within 2 weeks after discontinuation, and resembles a viral exanthem. **Pruritus is common with a drug eruption but absent with a viral exanthem.** Common offending agents are the semisynthetic penicillins, trimethoprim-sulfamethoxazole, and anticonvulsants. Ampicillin or amoxicillin given to patients with Epstein-Barr virus infection and sulfonamides administered to patients with human immunodeficiency virus have a high incidence of exanthems.

Frequent offenders causing **urticaria or angioedema** are aspirin, nonsteroidal anti-inflammatory drugs, opiates, and iodinated contrast material. The eruptions usually occur within 36 hours of initial exposure or within minutes of rechallenge. Few to hundreds of lesions can be present, pruritus is prominent, and respiratory symptoms and serum sickness–like symptoms (fever, arthralgias, lymphadenopathy, and myalgias) can occur.[14]

Photosensitivity eruptions are characterized by confluent erythema, macules, papules, or even vesicles in sun-exposed areas such as the chest, neck, face, and arms[18] (Table 251-3). Photosensitivity can be divided into photoallergic and phototoxic reactions based on the mechanism. When prescribing drugs with a propensity for photosensitivity, advise patients to use skin protection and proper clothing to avoid sun exposure.

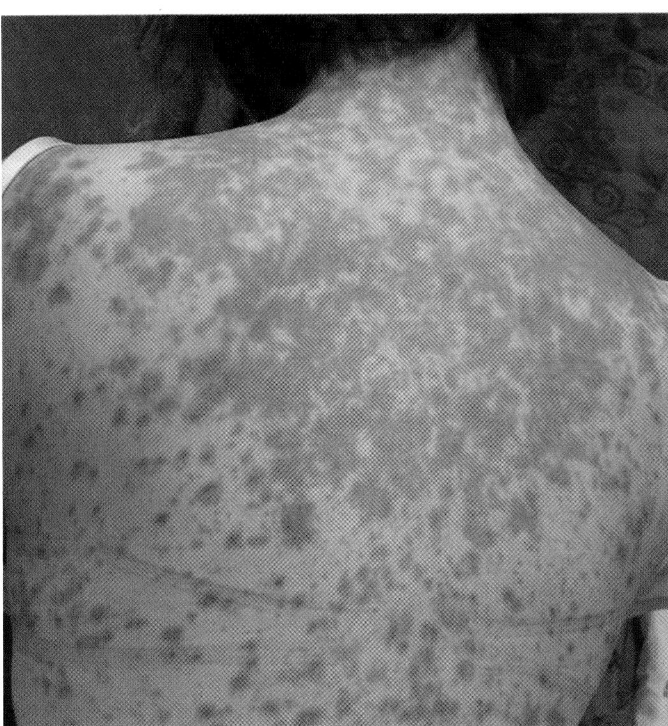

FIGURE 251-19. Drug eruption. [Photo contributed by University of North Carolina Department of Dermatology.]

Pigmentation from drug ingestion can be striking in appearance. It may be related to postinflammatory changes, increased melanin production, or actual deposition of the drug or metabolites in the skin. Zidovudine is associated with both nail and generalized hyperpigmentation. Heavy metals, phenytoin, or oral contraceptives may cause pigmentation. Minocycline or amiodarone may give a gray-blue coloration. Clofazimine can cause a diffuse red hue and also blue-gray discoloration, especially in leprosy lesions. Antimalarials may produce gray or yellow discoloration.

Fixed drug eruptions (**Figure 251-20**) occur as solitary or occasionally multiple, discrete, round to oval erythematous patches that eventually turn dusky red or violaceous. Although the trunk may be involved, most cases occur in the oral mucosa or genitals. Lesions may become edematous, forming vesicles or bullae, and then erode. Reexposure to the causative drug results in recurrence of lesions in the identical location of the primary eruption within hours.

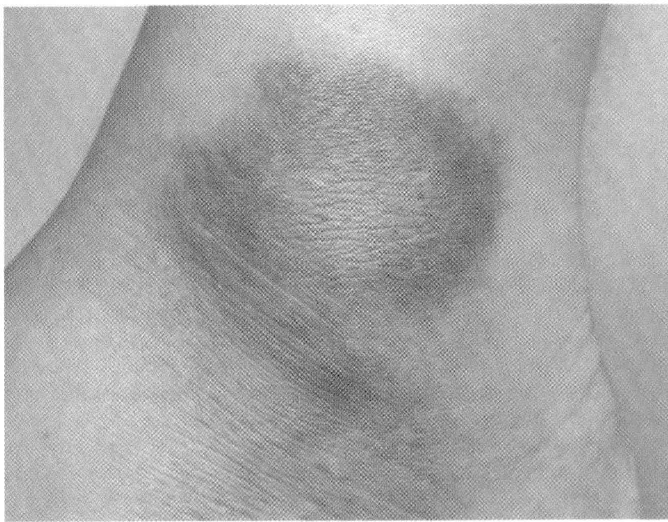

FIGURE 251-20. Fixed drug eruption. [Photo contributed by University of North Carolina Department of Dermatology.]

Anticoagulant necrosis may occur within 3 to 5 days of initiation of warfarin or heparin. It typically begins with a single painful area, followed by erythema that rapidly turns blue-black with subsequent necrosis of the skin. The lesion is very well demarcated. Common sites of involvement are regions of high subcutaneous fat distribution, including the buttocks, thighs, or breasts. Risk factors include high doses, obesity, female gender, and deficiency of protein C, S, or antithrombin III.

Some drugs produce **vesiculobullous eruptions** that can be difficult to distinguish from pemphigus or bullous pemphigoid. Penicillamine, captopril, sulfas, and thiol drugs can cause a blistering eruption. A pseudoporphyria-like reaction with tense small blisters and vesicles on the extensor arms and dorsal hands is associated with furosemide, nonsteroidal anti-inflammatory drug, tetracycline, and penicillamine exposure.

Drug Reaction with Eosinophilia and Systemic Symptoms (DRESS) and erythema multiforme, Stevens-Johnson syndrome, and toxic epidermal necrolysis are most commonly caused by the aromatic amines, phenytoin, carbamazepine, and phenobarbital, as well as sulfonamides. These reactions are discussed in chapter 249, "Generalized Skin Disorders."

For diagnosis, exclude exanthems triggered by infections, and then obtain a thorough history of exposure to prescription and over-the-counter agents. The pattern of the eruption and the likelihood of particular agents associated with the clinical findings can be found in drug reference manuals.[9]

Treatment is discontinuation of the suspected agent. When the patient is on multiple medications, simplify drugs and discontinue unnecessary agents. Rechallenge, even at reduced dosages, may produce rapid recurrence of the reaction. Oral antihistamines can be helpful for pruritus. Severe symptoms may require topical or oral steroids. Patients may be referred for skin testing in evaluation of type 1 immunoglobulin E–mediated reactions, such as penicillin, anesthetics, or vaccines. Radioallergosorbent tests for immediate reactions and lymphocytotoxicity assays can also be performed to identify anticonvulsant or sulfonamide hypersensitivity reactions.

BLISTERING DISEASES

Blistering diseases can be divided into vesicular, bullous, and pustular. A small blister <1 cm is termed a *vesicle*. Primary vesicular diseases that may affect the trunk include herpes infection (both simplex and varicella), insect bites, and allergic contact dermatitis. Larger blisters, >1 cm, are called *bullae* and may actually begin as vesicles. The most common bullous disease to affect the trunk is bullous pemphigoid. Severe allergic contact dermatitis, Stevens-Johnson syndrome/toxic epidermal necrolysis, and bullous impetigo may also present with bullae. Blood-filled, or hemorrhagic, bullous diseases include necrotizing fasciitis, vasculitis, and bite reactions to brown recluse spiders or rattlesnakes. Cloudy, whitish fluid within a blister is termed a *pustule*. Any blistering condition can become pustular as the lesion ages or becomes secondarily infected. Life-threatening blistering conditions are discussed in chapter 249. **Varicella** is discussed in chapter 141, "Rashes in Infants and Children."

HERPES ZOSTER

Reactivation of the latent varicella virus produces the unilateral, painful, localized, vesicular eruption of herpes zoster. It primarily affects one dermatome, although overlap to adjacent areas can be seen. It is more common in the elderly or immunosuppressed but can affect an individual of any age who has had prior varicella. After exposure, the virus remains latent in the sensory dorsal root ganglia until it later begins to replicate and spreads down the sensory nerve to the skin.[19]

Herpes zoster is more common with increasing age. One in 1000 persons <45 years old will experience zoster. After the age of 75, the incidence is four times greater. The lifetime risk of developing the condition is 10% to 30% for persons >80 years old. Human immunodeficiency virus infection, lymphoma, and immunosuppression are risk factors for reactivation of the latent virus and recurrent infections.[19]

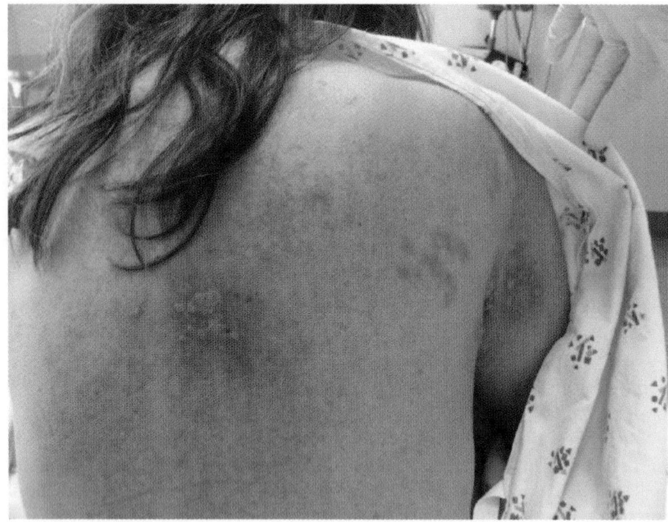

FIGURE 251-21. Herpes zoster. [Photo contributed by University of North Carolina Department of Dermatology.]

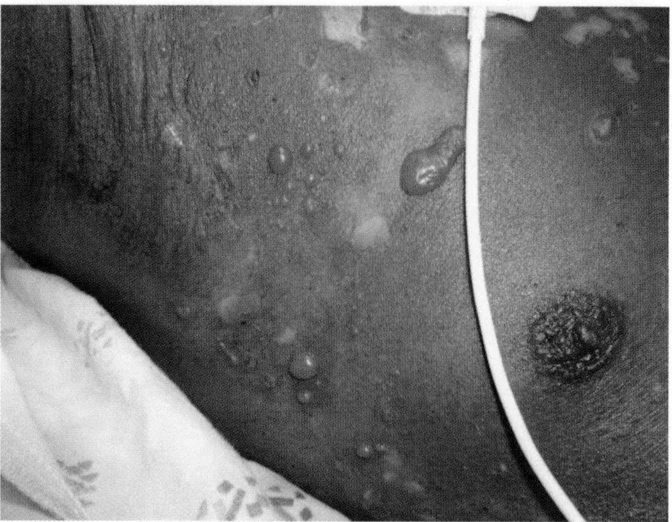

FIGURE 251-22. Bullous pemphigoid. [Photo contributed by University of North Carolina Department of Dermatology.]

Herpes zoster is most frequently a unilateral condition involving a spinal or cranial sensory nerve with some overlap into the surrounding dermatomes. More than half of cases affect the thoracic nerves, 20% affect the cranial or trigeminal region, 15% affect the lumbar region, and 5% affect the sacral region.[19] Pain in the affected area may precede the eruption by several days or even weeks. The pain can be severe, with a stabbing or deep boring sensation, or the patient may present with an area of increased sensitivity, tingling, burning, or pruritus.

The initial lesions are erythematous papules coalescing into plaques within a dermatome. Vesicles or bullae develop within 24 to 48 hours (**Figure 251-21**). Single lesions in varying stages resemble varicella. Lesions may become pustular, hemorrhagic, or necrotic over the following days. New lesions may develop for up to 1 week. Crusting of the lesions occurs within 7 to 10 days. Contiguous dermatomes may be involved but usually have fewer than 20 lesions present.

Mucous membrane lesions involving the mouth, vagina, or bladder can occur, depending on the dermatome affected. Involvement of the lower thoracic dermatomes may present with symptoms of colonic pseudo-obstruction. Hematogenous dissemination can occur and is more common in patients with low serum antibodies against varicella-zoster virus (VZV), the elderly, the immunosuppressed, or the debilitated. Constitutional symptoms include headache, malaise, lymphadenopathy, and fever.

Herpes zoster infection can be difficult to distinguish from herpes simplex. Definitive differentiation can be done by polymerase chain reaction or viral cultures. Herpes simplex more commonly involves the perioral, lumbosacral, or external genital areas, and a history of recurrent lesions with typical prodromal symptoms is helpful. Other diseases to include in the differential diagnosis of the dermatomal eruption are allergic contact reactions, erysipelas, and impetigo.

Diagnosis is clinical. A Tzanck test (see Figure 248-6) can be performed. The Tzanck test is also positive in varicella. Definitive diagnosis can be made by polymerase chain reaction studies or viral cultures on the vesicle fluid or biopsy specimen.

Treatment is with oral acyclovir, valacyclovir, or famciclovir. Dose adjustment is required for patients with renal impairment. Combined treatment with gabapentin and acyclovir at the time of outbreak may be more effective at reducing postherpetic neuralgia than antivirals alone.[20] In severe cases, such as ophthalmic zoster or disseminated disease, IV acyclovir should be given at a dose of 10 milligrams/kg three times a day. Topical antiviral therapy or antibiotics are not useful in the treatment of zoster. Application of moist dressings (Burrow solution or petroleum jelly) may be soothing. Rest and nonsteroidal anti-inflammatory drugs are recommended. Pain management may require narcotic analgesics. Herpes zoster is contagious several days before the lesions appear and until all the lesions have crusted over. Exposure may result in varicella infection in those without previous infection or in immunocompromised individuals.

BULLOUS PEMPHIGOID

Bullous pemphigoid is the most common autoimmune blistering disease in the elderly. It mostly affects individuals between 60 and 80 years old and has equal incidence in males and females. Bullous pemphigoid is generally self-limited and typically resolves over 5 to 6 years. Relapses occur in 10% to 15% of patients.

Autoantibodies to the basal keratinocyte hemidesmosomal antigens cause blisters at the basement membrane zone between the epidermis and dermis. Circulating basement membrane zone immunoglobulin G antibodies can be detected in most patients, and blood eosinophilia is present in about half of patients.

Bullous pemphigoid often begins with pruritic urticarial plaques and papules. These are not transient like urticaria. Bullae evolve over weeks to months. The bullae are tense and firm-topped, appearing on normal or erythematous skin (**Figure 251-22**). They do not extend when lateral pressure is applied. Sites of predilection include the axillae, abdomen, inner thighs, flexural forearms, and lower legs. The eruption may be localized or generalized. Bullae eventually rupture, leaving a thin blister roof overlaying the lesion, crusts, and erosions.

Bullous pemphigoid can be confused with urticaria or urticarial reactions in the early phase. Dermatologic consultation, with histopathology and immunofluorescence studies, is required for diagnosis and treatment.

Treatment is typically provided by a dermatologist. High-potency topical steroid (clobetasol) ointment can be used for localized disease. The mainstay of treatment for extensive disease is PO prednisone, 1.0 to 1.5 milligrams/kg/d. This dose can be gradually tapered when the disease is in remission. Dapsone, azathioprine, mycophenolate mofetil, cyclophosphamide, and methotrexate are useful steroid-sparing agents.

INSECT BITES

Bites can produce an inflammatory or allergic reaction. Sensitive individuals can develop an intensely pruritic papule, vesicle, or bulla within hours to days after the bite. The lesions can last for days to weeks. Patients are often unaware of exposure. Systemic symptoms may occur in some individuals, ranging from mild to severe, including anaphylactoid reactions. Spiders, centipedes, millipedes, shellfish, fleas, mosquitoes, and fire ants are responsible for most bites.

Each type of bite can cause a different type of reaction, and individuals will differ in their local response. Transient red macules may occur at the site of the bite. Urticarial papules and vesicles can form, and secondary excoriations are frequent (**Figure 251-23**). A central punctum may be noted at the site of the bite. Large bullae may occur, particularly in patients with chronic lymphocytic leukemia. Necrosis can develop and

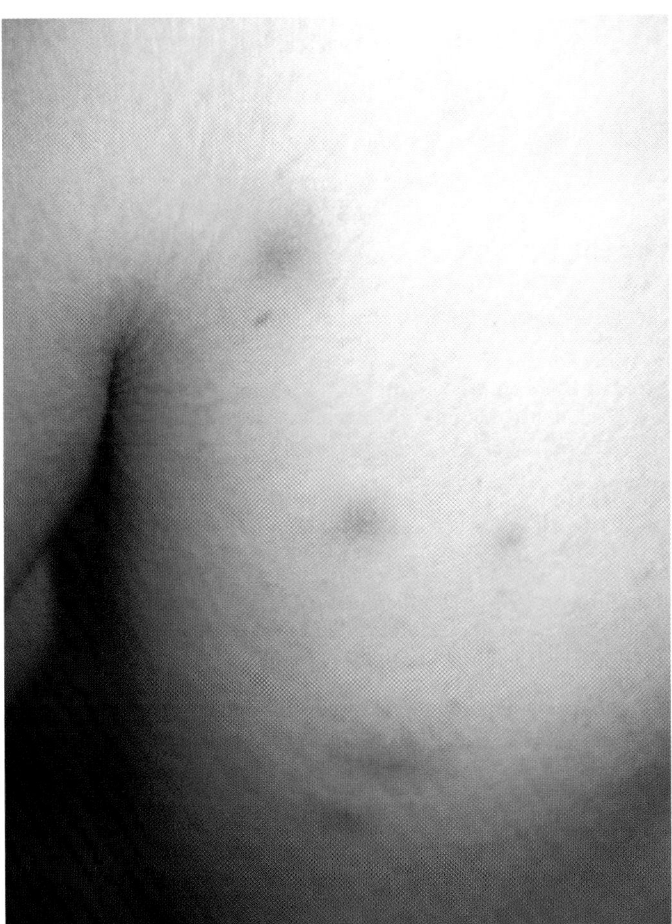

FIGURE 251-23. Bug bites. [Photo contributed by University of North Carolina Department of Dermatology.]

may be associated with systemic symptoms, including fever, headache, malaise, and arthralgias. **Flea bites** most commonly occur on the lower extremities, although children are more likely to have generalized bites. Mosquito bites occur on any exposed areas. **Bedbugs** will bite in linear groups ("**breakfast, lunch, dinner**") on sites exposed during sleep. **Fire ants** produce a brisk inflammatory reaction that forms a sterile pustule and can be quite painful. Other causes of blistering reactions include the **blister beetle**, which contains the chemical cantharidin and, when crushed, can produce vesicles and blisters on exposed areas. The **caterpillar** family can cause an immunoglobulin E–mediated allergic contact dermatitis. Clinical features and treatment of bites with envenomation are discussed in chapter 211, "Bites and Stings."

Treat with nonsteroidal anti-inflammatory drugs to relieve pain and reduce the local reaction. Remove any stingers. Deflea animals and the house. Topical corticosteroids can be used, such as fluocinonide 0.05% or clobetasol 0.05% cream or ointment. Severe reactions may require a short course of oral steroids: prednisone, 40 to 60 milligrams once a day (adults) or 1 to 2 milligrams/kg once a day (children) each morning for 3 to 5 days. Antihistamines can help control pruritus. Provide an EpiPen® to any patient who has had a severe bite reaction.

Botfly Bite One unusual bite is that of botfly or furuncular myiasis, caused by *Dermatobia hominis*. The condition is endemic to Mexico and Central America. Botfly larvae are deposited onto the surface of a mosquito or fly. When an individual is bitten, the botfly larva painlessly penetrates the skin. Bites most commonly affect the trunk, followed by the head, legs, and arms—any exposed skin areas. The initial lesion is usually felt to be a generic "insect bite." In 3 to 4 weeks, the lesion evolves into a furuncle with a central pore, which clinically appears as an infected bite, inflamed cyst, or cellulitis. There may be a sensation of movement within the furuncle. Diagnosis is typically made when the furuncle is drained, and the larva is seen. Completely extract the larva, or infection or a foreign body reaction will develop. There are no systemic complications, and no specific prevention exists, other than the application of insect repellents.

SELECTED COMMON MISCELLANEOUS DISORDERS OF THE TRUNK

MOLLUSCUM CONTAGIOSUM

Molluscum contagiosum is a common viral infection of the epidermis occurring in children, sexually active adults, and immunosuppressed individuals (especially patients with human immunodeficiency virus). It is caused by poxvirus variants molluscum contagiosum virus 1 to 4, with the most common being molluscum contagiosum virus 1 in children and molluscum contagiosum virus 2 in human immunodeficiency virus infections. Transmission is by direct skin-to-skin contact.

There can be a single skin-colored, pearly, umbilicated papule (1 to 2 mm) or multiple, scattered papules or nodules and plaques (5 to 10 mm) (**Figure 251-24**). Autoinoculation is evident by the clustering of lesions in areas of rub or friction, some with a linear array from scratching. The lesions may become crusted, inflamed, or pustular if irritated. An inflammatory reaction may precede the spontaneous resolution of the lesions. In children, the lesions may range in number from a few to >100. The face, trunk, and extremities are commonly affected. Generalized involvement may occur in atopic dermatitis. If the lesions are isolated to the genital region, consider sexual abuse. In sexually active adults, there are 20 or fewer lesions on the lower abdomen, thighs, and genital region. Other sexually transmitted diseases may coexist. In immunosuppressed patients, hundreds of lesions may be present, and involvement of the face, with lesions being spread by shaving, is common. In human immunodeficiency virus, this occurs when CD4 counts are less than 100 cells/mm^3. Giant molluscum lesions, involvement of the oral and genital mucosa, and facial disfigurement may occur (CD4 <50 cells/mm^3).

Diagnosis is clinical. If necessary, a Giemsa stain of the expressed keratotic core demonstrates intracytoplasmic inclusion bodies ("molluscum bodies") (see Figure 248-2). In the immunocompromised, if diagnosis is unclear, obtain a biopsy to exclude fungal infection.

Most patients require no **treatment** because spontaneous resolution of molluscum occurs within 6 months to 4 years. Avoid shaving the affected area. For bothersome cases, application of topical cantharidin (blister beetle fluid) will produce good resolution of lesions, although multiple treatments may be necessary.[21] Curettage, cryotherapy, or

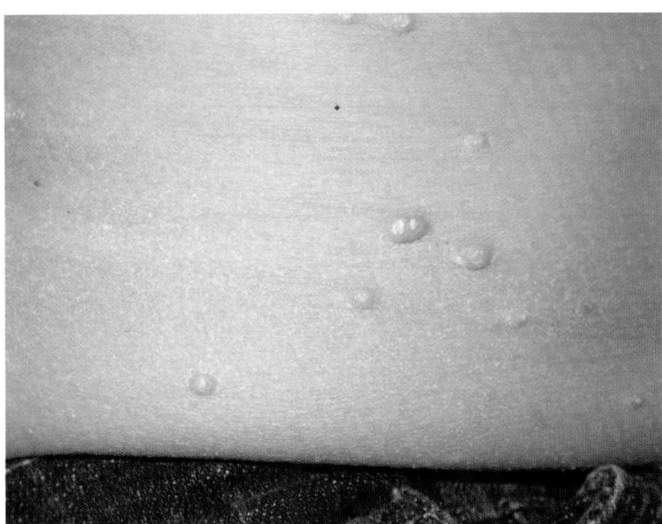

FIGURE 251-24. Molluscum contagiosum. Centrally umbilicated papules. [Photo contributed by University of North Carolina Department of Dermatology.]

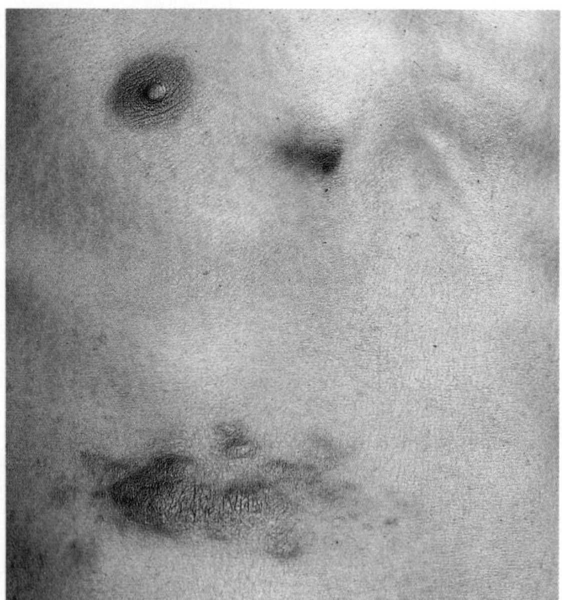

FIGURE 251-25. Kaposi's sarcoma. [Reproduced with permission from Wolff KL, Johnson R, Suurmond R: *Fitzpatrick's Color Atlas & Synopsis of Clinical Dermatology*, 5th ed. © 2005, McGraw-Hill, New York.]

electrodesiccation can also be done. In individuals infected with human immunodeficiency virus, treatment of the underlying human immunodeficiency virus infection may lead to resolution.

KAPOSI'S SARCOMA

Kaposi's sarcoma is a vascular neoplasia characterized by endothelial cell proliferation with multisystem involvement. Human herpesvirus 8 has been identified in all variants of the lesions, although it is not known how this virus induces the proliferation of the microvasculature. Individuals infected with human immunodeficiency virus are at high risk for Kaposi's sarcoma. The use of highly active antiretroviral therapy has reduced the incidence by 10-fold. The clinical presentation of Kaposi's sarcoma is different from the classic form seen in elderly males of eastern European heritage. Patients with human immunodeficiency virus can present with widespread, numerous lesions. The lesions may be erythematous or violaceous macules that can progress to tumors or nodules. The lesions on the trunk may be arranged parallel to the skin tension lines and can occur in areas of trauma (**Figure 251-25**). Erosions, ulceration, crusting, and hyperkeratosis may be secondary changes seen. The trunk is an area of predilection, as are the hard palate, penis, and lower extremities.

Classic or European Kaposi's sarcoma occurs in elderly males of Mediterranean or Ashkenazi Jewish heritage. This variant predominantly arises on the lower extremities and can be associated with edema. It can also affect the lymph nodes and abdominal viscera.

Treatment depends on the extent and severity of the disease and underlying cause. Referral to infectious disease and hematology/oncology specialists is necessary in most cases.

REFERENCES

The complete reference list is available online at www.TintinalliEM.com.

CHAPTER 252

Skin Disorders: Groin and Skinfolds

Dean S. Morrell
Edith V. Bowers

INTRODUCTION

The skinfolds of the body include the groin, intergluteal cleft, axilla, inframammary, and pannus regions. The skinfolds have unique characteristics that set them apart from other regions of the body. For one, these areas are almost continuously occluded. As a result, scale does not develop; maceration and fissuring develop instead. This situation alters the appearance of papulosquamous diseases and inflammatory processes. The occlusion also allows for the development of a warm, moist environment favorable to the growth of fungi, yeast, and bacteria. Although many skin diseases can affect the skinfolds to some degree, this chapter focuses on common disorders where skinfold eruptions are the main finding. This chapter discusses common infections, infestations, and inflammatory and reactive conditions that involve the groin and skinfolds. Sexually transmitted infections are discussed in chapter 149. Molluscum contagiosum is discussed in chapter 251.

An important point for treatment of intertriginous diseases is avoiding combination corticosteroid/antifungal products. Although processes in the groin folds can be confusing and complicated by secondary change, using combination products may further cloud the clinical picture. If improvement is seen, it is difficult to ascertain which medication prompted the change. And, finally, the corticosteroid component of these medications is too strong to be used in the occluded intertriginous skin and may produce irreversible striae with long-term use.[1]

INFECTIONS

TINEA CRURIS

Tinea cruris is a fungal infection of the groin commonly called *jock itch*. It is very common in males, uncommon in females, and exceedingly rare in children. Tinea cruris results from invasion of the stratum corneum by the dermatophyte types of fungi (see Table 253-4). It is transmitted via direct contact (person to person, or animal [usually kittens or puppies] to person) or fomites.

Examination is significant for symmetric erythema with a peripheral annular slightly scaly edge (**Figure 252-1**). The groin is typically involved, and the process may extend onto the inner thighs and even the buttocks. The penis and scrotum are typically spared, a distinguishing feature of tinea cruris because most other eruptions will affect the scrotum. Frequently, tinea pedis is also found and the dermatophyte infection may be spread from the feet to the groin through putting on clothes.

Scraping the leading edge and performing a potassium hydroxide examination (see Table 252-6) will demonstrate branching hyphae (see Figure 252-1), unless the patient has recently applied topical antifungal preparations. If a potassium hydroxide examination is negative, consider one of the other disorders discussed in this chapter (**Table 252-1**).

Treatment is with antifungal creams, such as clotrimazole, ketoconazole, or econazole, twice a day (**Table 252-2**). Clotrimazole is often suggested initially because it is a low-cost treatment and is available without a prescription. Econazole also has antibacterial properties and is preferred if maceration is present. Treatment also includes keeping the affected area as cool and dry as possible, which is facilitated by wearing loose-fitting clothing. Use an antifungal powder daily to prevent recurrences. Recommend follow-up with a primary care provider or dermatologist if the eruption has not resolved in 4 to 6 weeks.

CUTANEOUS CANDIDIASIS

Candidal infections of the skin favor moist, occluded areas of the body. Although any skinfold may be involved, superficial *Candida* infections

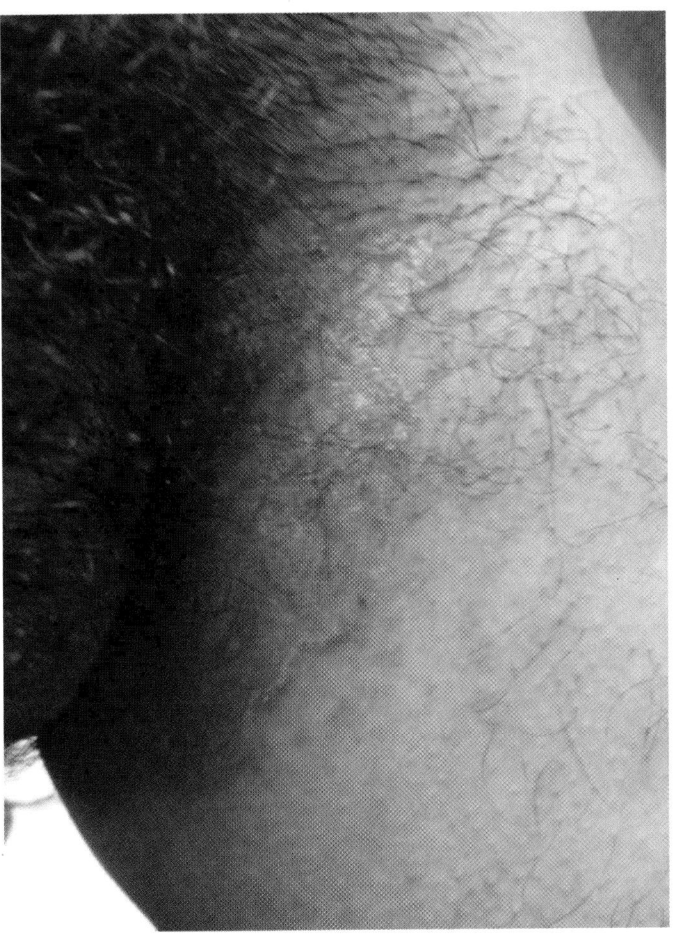

FIGURE 252-1. Tinea cruris. Note raised, sharp-edged margins. [Photo contributed by University of North Carolina Department of Dermatology.]

TABLE 252-1 Inflammatory Disorders of the Skinfolds

Infection
Tinea cruris
Cutaneous candidiasis
Erythrasma
Lymphogranuloma venereum
Granuloma inguinale
Infestation
Scabies
Pediculosis pubis
Dermatitis
Seborrheic dermatitis
Intertrigo/irritant contact dermatitis
Allergic contact dermatitis
Atopic dermatitis
Lichen simplex chronicus
Psoriasis
Neoplasia
Bowen disease (squamous cell carcinoma in situ)
Extramammary Paget's disease
Langerhans cell histiocytosis X
Miscellaneous disorders
Hidradenitis suppurativa
Cutaneous Crohn's disease
Hailey-Hailey disease (benign familial pemphigus)

are commonly seen in the diaper area of infants, vulva and groin of women, glans penis (balanitis) of uncircumcised males, and inframammary and pannus folds of obese patients. Antibiotic therapy, systemic corticosteroid therapy, urinary or fecal incontinence, immunocompromised states, poorly controlled diabetes mellitus, and obesity are predisposing factors. Women with vulvar or inner thigh involvement will often have vaginal candidiasis as well. Frequently, *Candida* infection may complicate other inflammatory intertriginous disorders.

The typical presentation is erythema and maceration with peripheral small erythematous papules or satellite pustules (**Figure 252-2**). **The rim of satellite pustules helps to distinguish *Candida* infection from other eruptions of the skinfolds.** Patients will often complain of burning or itching. The other inflammatory disorders listed in Table 252-1 should be considered in the differential diagnosis.

A potassium hydroxide preparation of the pustules or of the leading edge scale may demonstrate short hyphae and spores, but these may be difficult to find in cases with just erythema and maceration. If *Candida* is suspected but not visualized on potassium hydroxide preparation and the diagnosis is in question, a skin swab should be performed and submitted for fungal culture.

Treatment involves keeping the affected area dry and cool. After bathing, air drying or drying with a hair dryer should be encouraged. Clothing should be loose and lightweight. Astringent solutions (such as aluminum acetate [Burow solution]) aid in drying weepy inflammatory eruptions. After compress application and drying, a topical antifungal cream, such as clotrimazole, ketoconazole, or econazole, should be applied. Once the infection is controlled, drying powders should be used on a daily basis to minimize recurrences. Patients with vulvar candidiasis should be evaluated for *Candida* vaginitis and treated appropriately (see chapter 102, "Vulvovaginitis"). Patients with *Candida* balanitis often have a female sexual partner with *Candida* vaginitis; therefore, partners should be evaluated and treated as well. In infants or in adults with urinary or fecal incontinence, diapers or sanitary pads should be changed frequently. Zinc oxide paste applied over the antifungal agent provides a protective barrier to the irritation of urine and feces.

INFESTATIONS

SCABIES

Infestation of the skin by *Sarcoptes scabiei*, or scabies mite, produces an intensely pruritic eruption. Symptoms manifest approximately 30 days following exposure to the organisms as a result of the host immune response to the mites and their excrement. Typically, history will elicit an encounter with another person, or with a new environment, approximately 4 to 6 weeks before the initiation of symptoms.

The main presenting feature is intense, intractable pruritus, most notable at night. In adults, the typical findings are slightly longitudinal erythematous or brown papules, predominantly on the lateral feet, wrists, ankles, and interdigital spaces of the fingers and toes. Involvement may be evident within the axillae, groin, and extensor extremities (**Figure 252-3**). The head and neck are characteristically spared. In immunocompromised hosts, or persons with significant psychiatric compromise, lesions may appear as thick, crusted, confluent plaques on the hands, feet, and scalp, with or without a generalized distribution. In such patients, the condition is termed *crusted scabies*.

Sampling of a longitudinal burrow by scraping with a scalpel blade is typically most helpful in establishing the diagnosis. Light microscopy of the sample, which is transferred to a glass slide and covered with a drop of mineral oil followed by a coverslip, may reveal intact scabies organisms, ova, or excrement (see Figure 252-4). However, sensitivity of this test is limited, and a negative result does not rule out the diagnosis.

Treat with 5% permethrin cream (pregnancy category B), apply from the neck down, leave on for 12 hours, and then bathe with soap and water. Treatment should be repeated in a similar fashion in 1 week. Treat all resident family members and household and intimate contacts.

Lindane should be avoided in children and pregnant women secondary to neurotoxicity.

TABLE 252-2 Comparison of Commonly Used Antifungal Preparations

Generic	Trade	Formulations	Pregnancy Category	Sizes (grams)	Cost (U.S. $)	Status
Clotrimazole	Lotrimin	1% cream or solution	B	Cream (15, 30)	Cream (8–16)	OTC
	Mycelex			Solution (10, 30)	Solution (12–22)	
Ketoconazole	Nizoral	2%	C	Cream (15, 30, 60)	Cream (15–36)	Prescription
	Kuric gel			Gel (15)		
	Xolegel					
Econazole	Spectazole	1%	C	Cream (15, 30, 85)	Cream (15–50)	Prescription
Miconazole	Zeasorb AF	2%	C	Powder (56)	Powder (9)	OTC

Abbreviation: OTC = over the counter (no prescription required in United States).

Oral ivermectin (pregnancy category C) is an alternative treatment to permethrin cream and is easier to administer; however, it may have a slightly lower cure rate.[2] **Ivermectin should be avoided in pregnant and lactating women.**

Supportive care involves use of oral antihistamines and topical corticosteroids after use of the appropriate scabicidal agent. Patients should be told to expect resolution of symptoms gradually over 1 to 2 weeks, although pruritus can sometimes persist for several weeks. Return of new lesions after initial improvement signifies incomplete treatment or reinfestation.

PEDICULOSIS PUBIS

Pediculosis pubis is infestation of the groin with *Phthirus pubis*. Rarely, the eyebrows, eyelashes, chest, or axillary hair may also be involved.

Close examination of the hair-bearing areas reveals multiple small flesh-colored or slightly reddish organisms grasping the hairs close to the skin surface (**Figure 252-4**). In severe infestations, small bluish-gray macules may be noted, called *maculae caerulea*. Secondary infection and excoriations may also be present. Diagnosis of pediculosis pubis in children should prompt evaluation for potential sexual abuse. Diagnosis is based on physical examination findings.

Treatment is the same as for scabies. Topical treatments should be applied liberally to all affected hair-bearing areas, including the perirectal

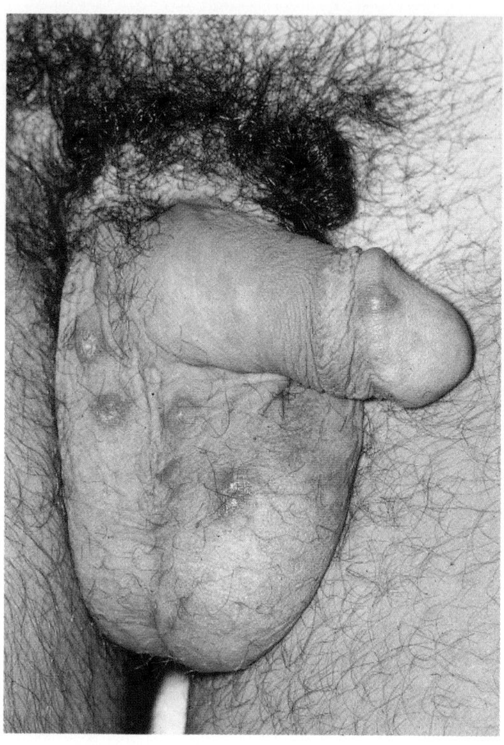

FIGURE 252-3. Scabetic papules and burrows. [Reproduced with permission from Wolff KL, Johnson R, Suurmond R: *Fitzpatrick's Color Atlas & Synopsis of Clinical Dermatology*, 5th ed. © 2005, McGraw-Hill, New York.]

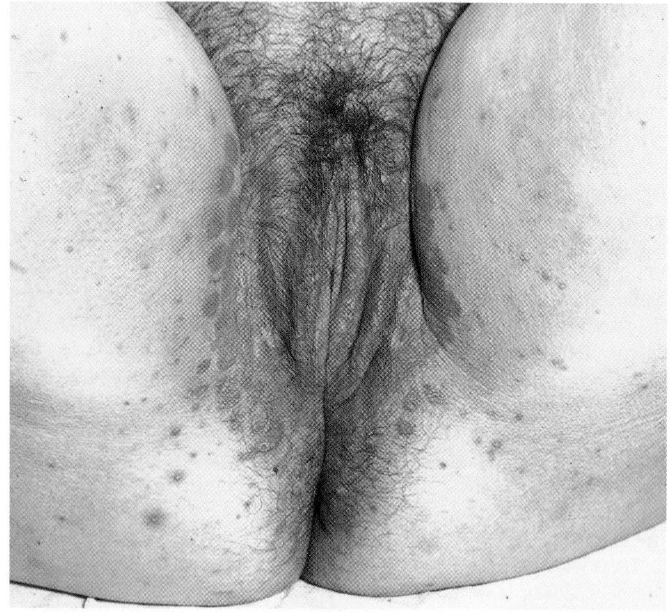

FIGURE 252-2. Cutaneous candidiasis with satellite papules and pustules. [Reproduced with permission from Wolff KL, Johnson R, Suurmond R: *Fitzpatrick's Color Atlas & Synopsis of Clinical Dermatology*, 5th ed. © 2005, McGraw-Hill, New York.]

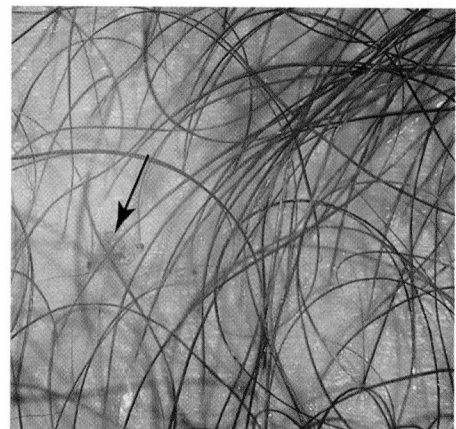

FIGURE 252-4. *Arrow* points to louse on the skin. [Reproduced with permission from Wolff KL, Johnson R, Suurmond R: *Fitzpatrick's Color Atlas & Synopsis of Clinical Dermatology*, 5th ed. © 2005, McGraw-Hill, New York.]

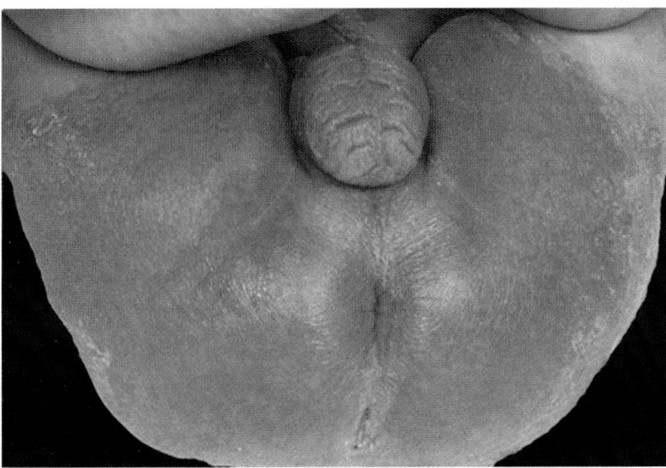

FIGURE 252-5. Seborrheic dermatitis involving the diaper area of an infant. [Reproduced with permission from Wolff KL, Johnson R, Suurmond R: *Fitzpatrick's Color Atlas & Synopsis of Clinical Dermatology*, 5th ed. © 2005, McGraw-Hill, New York.]

hairs.[3] Attempts to identify the source of the infestation are important because reexposure may continue to occur.

INFLAMMATORY AND REACTIVE CONDITIONS

Seborrheic Dermatitis Seborrheic dermatitis is one of the most common skin disorders. It most notably affects the scalp ("dandruff") and creases of the face and ears; however, other skinfolds, such as the intergluteal cleft, groin, axilla, inframammary folds, and umbilicus, can be affected (see chapters 250 and 251).

Seborrheic dermatitis of the scalp and skinfolds of the face presents as erythema with a greasy yellow scale (see Figure 250-4). When seborrheic dermatitis affects other skinfolds, erythema and maceration are evident (**Figure 252-5**).

Diagnosis is clinical and based on typical findings of seborrheic dermatitis on the face and scalp. By itself, groin or other skinfold involvement is hard to differentiate from the other inflammatory disorders such as cutaneous candidiasis, inverse psoriasis, allergic contact dermatitis, or streptococcal infection.

Treatment can relieve signs and symptoms, but there is no cure. The eruption will return after treatment ceases. Shampoos containing zinc pyrithione, selenium sulfide, salicylic acid, or tar preparations are used. Ketoconazole shampoo can be effective and is available by prescription (2%) or over the counter (1%). Hydrocortisone 1% cream can be used in mild cases, whereas hydrocortisone 2.5% cream or desonide cream or lotion may be required initially in more severe cases. Patients should be cautioned against long-term regular use of corticosteroids on facial or intertriginous skin, which may result in irreversible skin thinning and striae formation.

INTERTRIGO

Intertrigo is an irritant dermatitis of the skinfolds resulting from moisture, heat, friction, and irritating substances like urine and feces. Intertrigo presents as erythema, maceration, and fissures in the occluded area of skinfolds, especially the groin and inframammary folds (**Figure 252-6**). **Satellite papules and pustules are absent**, and the affected areas are pruritic and may burn. **Streptococcal superinfection** should be considered if there is marked erythema and tenderness, especially in the extremes of age and the immunocompromised.

Intertrigo is a diagnosis of exclusion (Table 252-1). Bacterial infection, especially with *Streptococcus*, is common. Differentiating cutaneous candidiasis from inflammatory intertrigo can be difficult. A diagnosis of cutaneous candidiasis is supported by the presence of satellite pustules and a positive potassium hydroxide examination. However, a negative

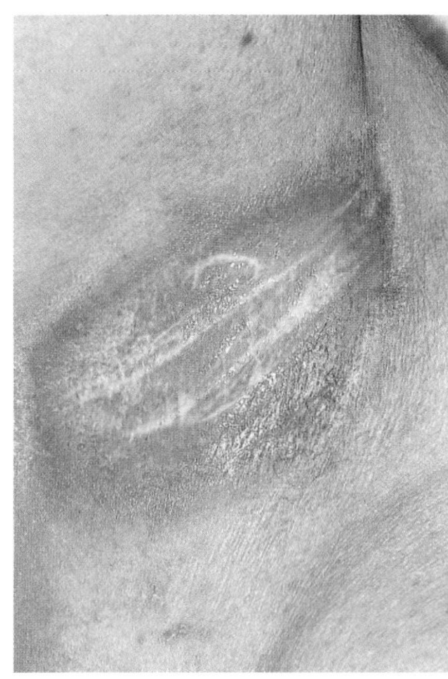

FIGURE 252-6. Intertrigo with possible streptococcal superinfection. [Reproduced with permission from Wolff KL, Johnson R, Suurmond R: *Fitzpatrick's Color Atlas & Synopsis of Clinical Dermatology*, 5th ed. © 2005, McGraw-Hill, New York.]

potassium hydroxide examination does not exclude this possibility because yeast is difficult to obtain and visualize with this procedure. Scraping of peripheral scale or a pustule to send for fungal culture may help clarify the diagnosis.

Clinically, irritant dermatitis cannot always be distinguished from allergic contact dermatitis. A history should be taken to uncover any possible contact allergens or irritants such as neomycin-containing ointments, anesthetic creams, diphenhydramine cream, deodorants, feminine hygiene sprays, or other lotions, solutions, or home remedies.

Treat by keeping the affected areas dry and cool. All potential irritants should be avoided. Zinc oxide paste provides an excellent barrier to urine and fecal material.

For moist, weepy intertrigo, aluminum acetate (Burow solution) compresses can be used. Secondary bacterial infection should be treated with oral antibiotics with staphylococcal and streptococcal coverage. Topical antiyeast preparations, such as ketoconazole, may be helpful. If significant inflammation is present, a short course of 1% hydrocortisone cream or lotion may be helpful.

HIDRADENITIS SUPPURATIVA

Hidradenitis suppurativa is an inflammatory condition, typically affecting the apocrine gland–bearing areas of the skin with recurrent, painful, draining nodules. The inciting event is follicular occlusion, prompting rupture of the follicular contents and resulting intense inflammation.[4]

Axillary and inguinal skin demonstrates varying numbers of inflammatory nodules, many of which may form connecting tracts, with resultant drainage onto the skin surface (**Figure 252-7**). Lesions may heal with characteristic icepick scarring, which may facilitate diagnosis.

Diagnosis is clinical. **Treatment** is clindamycin 1% lotion twice daily and use of antibacterial soaps, such as chlorhexidine, once to twice weekly. Incision and drainage should be minimized because it may increase scarring. Further systemic treatments, such as acitretin, finasteride, or prednisone, may work in some cases and are best coordinated by a specialist. In severe cases, systemic biologics or surgical excision of apocrine-bearing skin has been attempted.

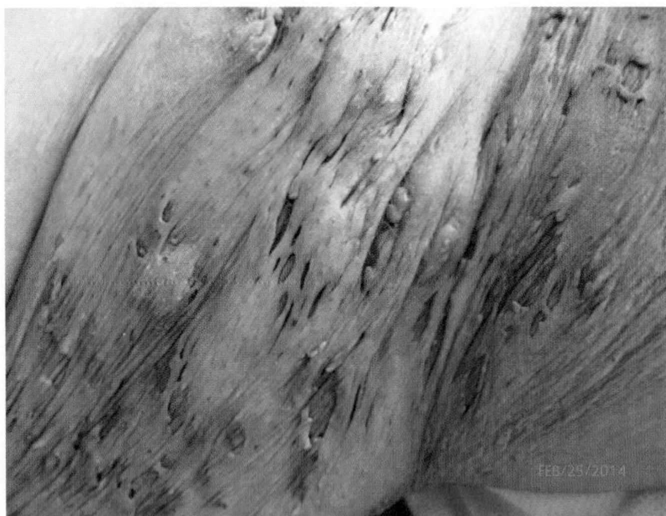

FIGURE 252-7. Hidradenitis suppurativa involving the buttock region. [Photo contributed by University of North Carolina Department of Dermatology.]

REFERENCES

The complete reference list is available online at www.TintinalliEM.com.

CHAPTER 253 Skin Disorders: Extremities

Rachna A. Bhandari
Dean S. Morrell

INTRODUCTION

This chapter focuses on common disorders of the hands, feet, and extremities and is organized into the following subgroups: ulcers, inflammatory conditions, cutaneous infections, and vascular cutaneous conditions.

ULCERS

VENOUS STASIS DERMATITIS AND VENOUS LEG ULCERS

The vast majority of leg ulcers are venous stasis ulcers resulting from chronic venous insufficiency.[1] Chronic venous insufficiency is usually caused by episodes of phlebitis or varicose veins, both of which damage venous valves. This results in poor venous return from the lower extremities, leading to increased hydrostatic pressure and lower extremity edema and stasis dermatitis.

Dependent edema, erythema, and orange-brown hyperpigmentation characterize early stasis dermatitis. The medial distal legs and the pretibial leg are the areas most frequently affected. More chronic and severe cases may have bright weepy erythema and even ulceration (**Figure 253-1**). Pruritus is common. Cellulitis and lymphangitis may complicate stasis dermatitis. The presence of honey-colored crust and pustules suggests secondary bacterial infection.

Stasis ulcers often begin within areas of stasis dermatitis. The bilateral malleoli and the medial aspect of the calf are the most common sites of involvement. Diagnosis is clinical. With acute exacerbation, secondary infection is common. **Table 253-1** lists the differential diagnosis of leg ulcers. Certain disorders, such as arterial ulcerations, pyoderma gangrenosum, and polyarteritis nodosa require immediate attention. If peripheral pulses are diminished or absent, obtain vascular blood flow studies to exclude arterial ulcers. If the patient reports a rapidly developing ulcer that began as a pustule or erythematous nodule and has violaceous overhanging borders, suspect pyoderma gangrenosum. If the diagnosis is in question, consult with a dermatologist.

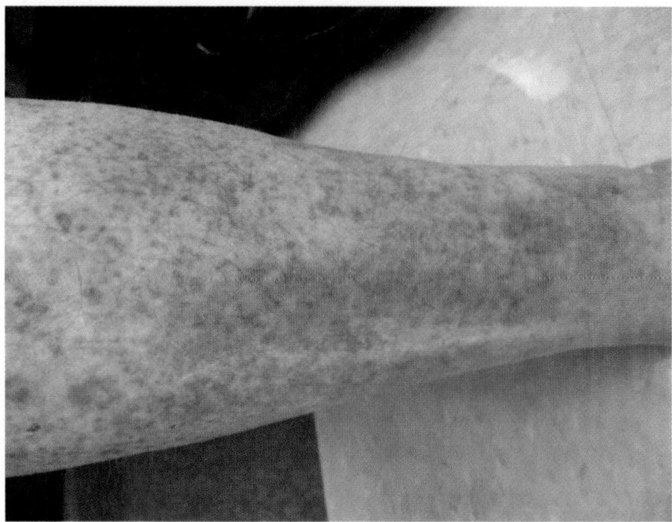

FIGURE 253-1. Venous stasis. [Photo contributed by University of North Carolina Department of Dermatology.]

TABLE 253-1 Differential Diagnosis of Extremity Ulcers

Trauma
Injuries, burns, injections, decubitus, chilblains (pernio), neuropathic ulcers
Infections
Viral: herpes simplex virus, cytomegalovirus
Bacterial: gangrene, ecthyma gangrenosum, ecthyma secondary to *Staphylococcus aureus* and/or group A *Streptococcus*; osteomyelitis, methicillin-resistant *S. aureus*
Mycobacterial: Buruli ulcer (West Africa, *Mycobacterium ulcerans*), Bairnsdale ulcer (Australia, *M. ulcerans*), tuberculosis, leprosy
Fungal: blastomycosis, coccidioidomycosis, paracoccidioidomycosis, chromomycosis, mucormycosis
Spirochetal: syphilis, yaws
Parasitic: leishmaniasis, amebiasis, schistosomiasis
Bites
Spiders, scorpions, snakes
Metabolic
Diabetes, gout, calciphylaxis (cutaneous necrosis from small- and medium-sized vessel calcification in diabetes, end-stage renal disease, or hyperparathyroidism)
Vascular
Venous: varicose veins, venous insufficiency
Arterial: hypertension, arterial insufficiency, thrombosis, embolism
Vasculitis
Polyarteritis nodosa, vasculitis, collagen vascular disease, Behçet's syndrome
Malignancy
Cutaneous: squamous cell carcinoma, basal cell carcinoma
Lymphoma: T-cell or B-cell lymphoma
Hematologic
Polycythemia, sickle cell anemia
Dermatologic
Bullous pemphigoid, necrobiosis lipoidica
Drugs
Hydroxyurea

Treatment of venous stasis dermatitis and ulcers begins with leg elevation and the use of support stockings. Weeping eruptions should be treated with an astringent compress. A low- to mid-potency topical steroid, such as fluocinolone acetonide 0.025% or hydrocortisone 2.5% ointment, should be applied twice a day until erythema, scale, and pruritus resolve. Oral antihistamines, such as diphenhydramine or hydroxyzine, should be used for pruritus and for nighttime sedation. Secondary bacterial infection should be treated with cephalexin, dicloxacillin, or ciprofloxacin for 7 to 10 days. **Topical neomycin, antihistamine creams, and anesthetic creams should be avoided because they may complicate the condition with allergic contact dermatitis.** Cellulitis or lymphangitis may require hospitalization for IV antibiotics. Otherwise, follow-up should be arranged with a chronic wound care team.[1]

PYODERMA GANGRENOSUM

Pyoderma gangrenosum is a recurrent cutaneous, necrotizing, and non-infective ulceration of the skin that most commonly occurs in women between 30 and 50 years of age.[2] Most cases are associated with underlying disease, such as inflammatory bowel disease, rheumatoid arthritis, and myeloproliferative disorders.[3]

The classic lesion of pyoderma gangrenosum begins as a superficial pustule or erythematous nodule that expands into a large painful ulcer on the lower extremity with a purulent base and irregular, undermined borders and gun metal gray hue (**Figure 253-2**). There is no associated lymphadenopathy. Up to 50% of patients develop lesions at the sites of trauma, such as surgery sites or injection sites, or after blood drawing.[2] A history of multiple surgical debridements with sterile cultures should suggest a potential diagnosis of pyoderma gangrenosum.

The diagnosis is clinical and one of exclusion. Search for associated conditions, such as inflammatory bowel disease and myeloproliferative disorders. The onset of new skin lesions or ulcers at previous sites of trauma can also be helpful in identifying pyoderma gangrenosum.[4]

Treatment of the underlying disorder and corticosteroids, either topical, intralesional, or combined local and systemic, are the standard therapy for pyoderma gangrenosum. Resistant disease may require adjunctive systemic therapy with immunosuppressive or cytotoxic agents.[4]

DIABETIC AND NEUROPATHIC ULCERS

Most patients with diabetic foot ulcers have coexistent diabetic neuropathy.[5] Other causes of neuropathic leg ulcers are much rarer and include leprosy, tabes dorsalis, medications, and spinal cord lesions. In most patients with foot ulcers, one will note a triad of neuropathy, deformity, and trauma. Neuropathy leads to atrophy of the intrinsic muscles of the foot, collapse of the arch, and loss of stability of the metatarsal-phalangeal joints. The musculoskeletal alterations result in abnormal pressure points and greater friction on the foot during ambulation. Lack of sensation allows for repeat injury. The most common source of trauma is inappropriate footwear.[6]

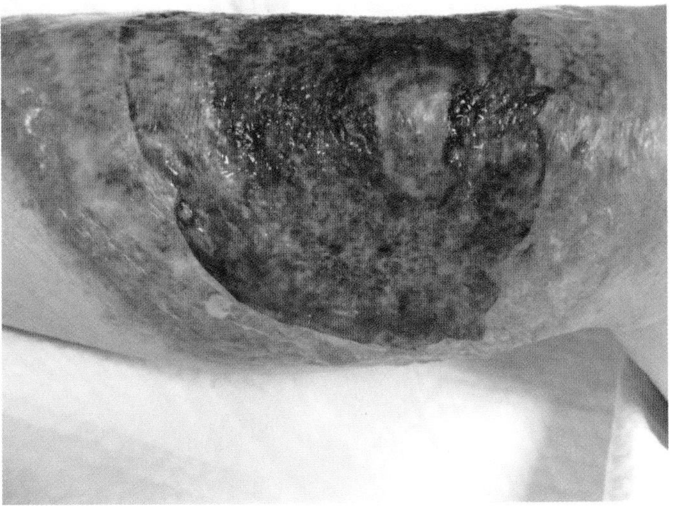

FIGURE 253-2. Pyoderma gangrenosum. [Photo contributed by University of North Carolina Department of Dermatology.]

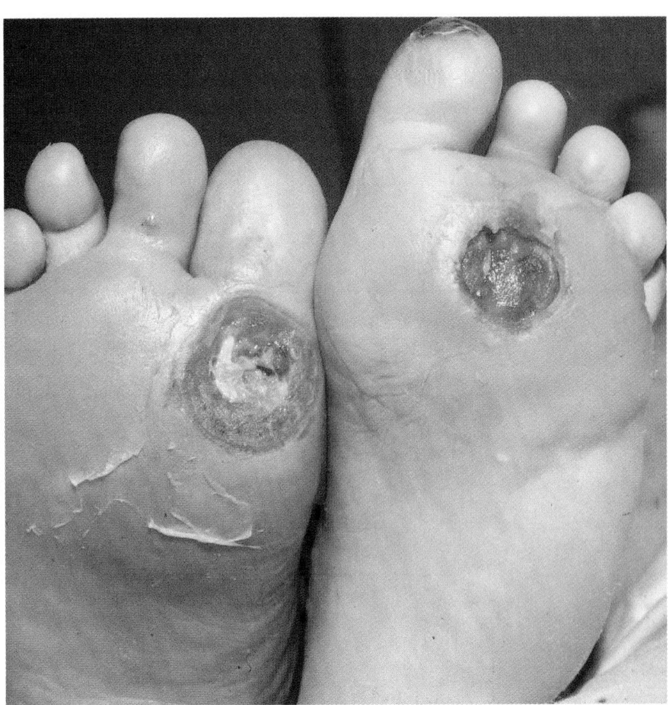

FIGURE 253-3. Diabetic foot and diabetic neuropathy. [Reproduced with permission from Wolff KL, Johnson R, Suurmond R: *Fitzpatrick's Color Atlas & Synopsis of Clinical Dermatology*, 5th ed. © 2005, McGraw-Hill, New York.]

Classic locations for neuropathic ulcers are the plantar surface underlying the first and fifth metatarsal heads, great toe, and heel. Ulcers are usually asymptomatic and "punched out" with a thick rim of surrounding callous (**Figure 253-3**). However, patients may complain of burning, numbness, itching, or paresthesias. The architecture of the foot is also altered, with flexed toes and prominent metatarsal heads secondary to neuropathy of the intrinsic muscles of the foot. Hypo- or anhidrosis from autonomic impairment may lead to dryness and fissuring of the surrounding skin. The diagnosis is clinical.

Patients with vascular insufficiency should be referred to a vascular specialist for further evaluation. A diabetic foot infection is diagnosed clinically when there are systemic signs of infection, purulence, or multiple signs of local inflammation (redness, warmth, pain, tenderness, or edema).[6] Osteomyelitis is suggested by the ability to probe bone with a blunt, sterile, stainless-steel probe and should be confirmed with imaging.

Treatment includes offloading or redistributing the pressure off the wound, maintenance of a moist wound environment, debridement of nonhealing tissue, and treatment of infection. Soft tissue infections can be treated for 7 to 14 days in an outpatient setting with oral cephalosporin, clindamycin, amoxicillin/clavulanate, or fluoroquinolones.[7]

More severe ulcers or those with associated cellulitis or osteomyelitis require admission and treatment with IV antibiotics for 4 to 6 weeks, such as cefotetan, ampicillin/sulbactam, or clindamycin and a fluoroquinolone. Vancomycin should be given if methicillin-resistant *Staphylococcus aureus* is suspected. Further discussion is provided in chapter 224, "Type 2 Diabetes Mellitus"; Table 224-4 lists the various cutaneous manifestations of diabetes.

BURULI ULCERS

Buruli ulcer is a new emerging disease and the third most common chronic mycobacterial infection in humans after tuberculosis and leprosy.[8] Buruli ulcers are rapidly growing ulcers caused by the acid-fast bacillus,

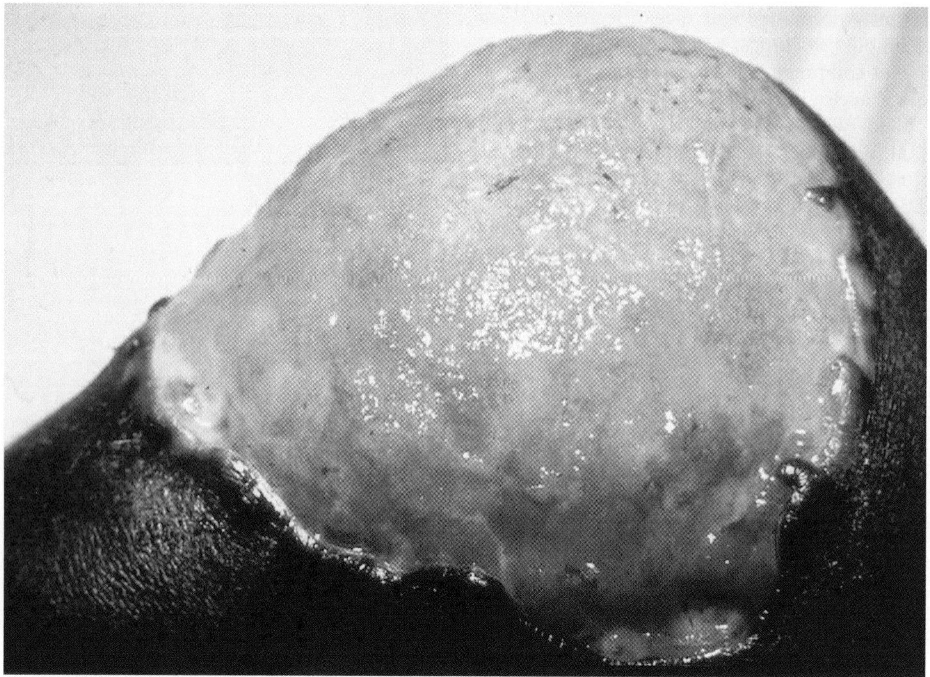

FIGURE 253-4. Buruli ulcer. [Reproduced with permission from Wolff KL, Johnson R, Suurmond R: *Fitzpatrick's Color Atlas & Synopsis of Clinical Dermatology*, 5th ed. © 2005, McGraw-Hill, New York.]

Mycobacterium ulcerans. It is usually confined to the tropical areas, with the highest rate in sub-Saharan Africa, but reports have come from subtropical and nontropical nations, including Australia, China, and Japan.[9]

M. ulcerans is an environmental saprophyte that is present on lush vegetation in swampy areas.[10] It infects humans after abrasions come into contact with contaminated soil, water, or vegetation.[10] *M. ulcerans* produces mycolactone, a cytotoxic lipid and necrotizing immunosuppressive polypeptide toxin that induces both apoptotic and necrotic changes in fibroblasts, lipid cells, macrophages, and keratinocytes.[11] Buruli ulcers are painless, and it is thought mycolactone damages the peripheral nerves.[12]

The Buruli ulcer begins as an erythematous nodule approximately 8 weeks after inoculation that eventually ulcerates. The lesions develop on exposed parts of the body, especially on the extremities and face. The resulting painless ulcer has a deep white or yellow necrotic base and undermined edges, as well as edematous surroundings (**Figure 253-4**). Regional lymphadenopathy and systemic symptoms are minimal to absent. Without treatment, ulcers may spontaneously heal within 6 to 9 months, or they may spread rapidly, causing extensive deformity.

Smears from the base of the ulcer or biopsy specimens should be cultured and examined for acid-fast bacilli. Visible growth by culture requires 6 to 8 weeks, and its success rate is low. Polymerase chain reaction performed on a fresh biopsy is the best method for early diagnosis. Surgical excision is the treatment of choice. Local heating and hyperbaric oxygen also promote healing.[13] Antimycobacterial treatment is often ineffective.[13] The World Health Organization recommends rifampin and streptomycin dual therapy for 8 weeks. New skin lesions may develop during antimicrobial therapy, and this is known as "paradoxical reactions."[8]

CUTANEOUS LEISHMANIASIS

Cutaneous leishmaniasis is transmitted by the bite of the sand fly, which is infected by protozoan parasites of the genus *Leishmania*. In tropical and subtropical regions, leishmaniasis is one of the most common and serious infectious diseases. It is endemic in North Africa, the Mediterranean, the Middle East, India, Central Asia, and Central and South America. Reactivation of latent leishmaniasis can occur in immunosuppressed, human immunodeficiency virus, malnourished, or organ transplant patients.[14] There are many varieties of cutaneous leishmaniasis. The typical cutaneous ulcer usually occurs on unclothed skin, is painless, varies in size from 0.5 to 3.0 cm in diameter, and is covered with an exudative crust (**Figure 253-5**). Diagnosis is clinical but can be confirmed with culture, biopsy, or polymerase chain reaction test. Most lesions heal spontaneously over several months.[15]

INFLAMMATORY CONDITIONS

HAND AND FOOT DERMATITIS

Hand and foot dermatitis simply means inflammation of the skin of the hands and/or feet. This nonspecific term is used for several more

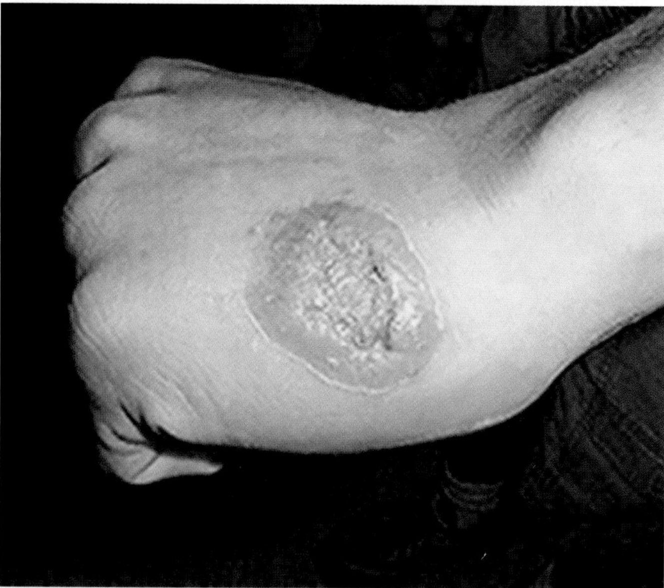

FIGURE 253-5. Cutaneous leishmaniasis. [Reproduced with permission from Walter Reed Army Institute of Research.]

TABLE 253-2 Differential Diagnosis of Hand and Foot Dermatitis
Allergic contact dermatitis (poison ivy, poison oak, etc.)
Irritant contact dermatitis (soaps, detergents, shoe/glove leather, etc.)
Dyshidrosis
Atopic dermatitis
Dermatophytosis (see Table 253-4)
Psoriasis
Lichen planus
Pityriasis rubra pilaris
Palmoplantar keratoderma
Autoimmune bullous disease
Dermatomyositis
Scabies

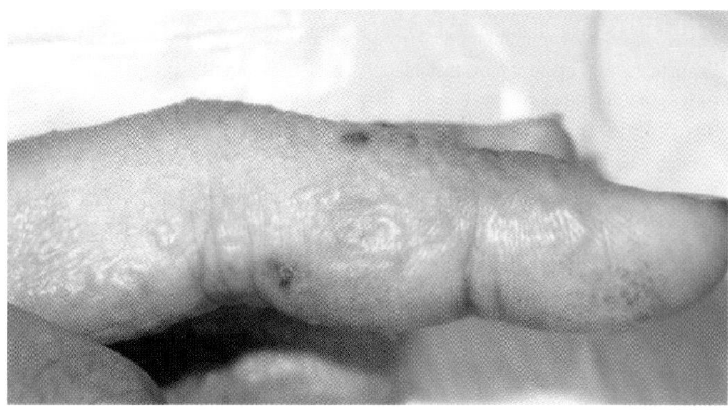

FIGURE 253-7. Dyshidrosis. Clear, tapioca-like lesions with secondary encrustation. [Photo contributed by University of North Carolina Department of Dermatology.]

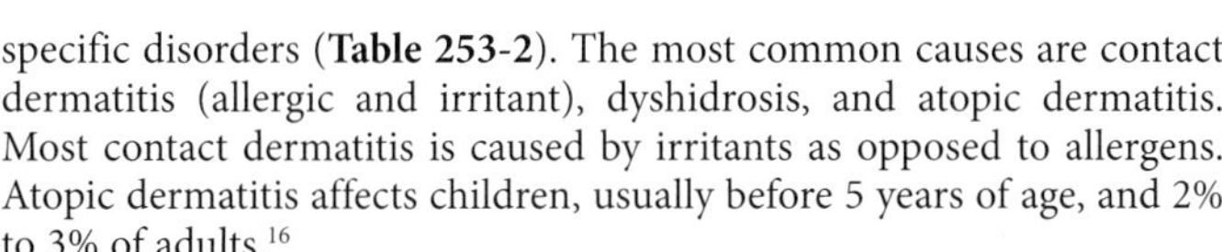

specific disorders (**Table 253-2**). The most common causes are contact dermatitis (allergic and irritant), dyshidrosis, and atopic dermatitis. Most contact dermatitis is caused by irritants as opposed to allergens. Atopic dermatitis affects children, usually before 5 years of age, and 2% to 3% of adults.[16]

Common irritants include soaps, detergents, friction, frequent hand washing, and cold, dry air, resulting in erythema, scaling, and fissuring. Strong irritants like an acid or alkali cause immediate burning, followed by erythema, vesiculation, and bullae formation.

Common allergens include poison ivy/poison oak, nickel, chromate, rubber components of gloves and shoes, dyes in leather and socks, and dichromates used in tanning leather. In acute allergic contact dermatitis, erythema with papules, vesicles, and/or bullae is present. Pruritus is intense, and excoriations are present. Distribution is the most helpful clue to aid in diagnosis. When the hands or feet are involved in allergic contact dermatitis, the eruption tends to be present on the dorsal surfaces, sparing the palms, soles, and web spaces. The thick stratum corneum of the palms and soles prevents penetration of potential allergens. Distribution with linear streaks suggests a plant allergy such as rhus (poison ivy or oak) hypersensitivity (**Figure 253-6**). Sharp demarcation of footwear indicates a reaction to a component of the patient's shoes.

Dyshidrosis initially begins as very small, deep-seated, pruritic vesicles on the lateral aspects and the volar surfaces of the palms and soles (**Figure 253-7**). The dorsal surface of the distal phalanges may also become involved. There is no erythema. Over time, the vesicles may form pustules or desquamate to leave small collarettes of scales. In chronic cases, erythema and scales become more prominent and may be difficult to distinguish from other forms of hand and foot dermatitis.

Atopic dermatitis is part of the "atopic triad" consisting of dermatitis, asthma, and allergic rhinitis.[17] Atopic dermatitis of the hands and feet often presents as erythematous, pruritic, scaly patches with prominent involvement of the dorsal surfaces as well as the palms and soles. Chronic atopic dermatitis will also have hyperpigmentation and lichenification and fissuring. Often, other areas of the body are involved. Common areas of involvement include the antecubital and popliteal fossae, posterior neck, and wrists and ankles (**Figure 253-8**).

The diagnosis is clinical. Differentiating contact dermatitis (allergic and irritant) from dyshidrosis and atopic dermatitis can be extremely difficult. More than one disorder may be present at a time, such as atopic dermatitis complicated by irritant dermatitis. Always consider a fungal infection (see later section "Tinea Pedis and Tinea Manuum"), and a potassium hydroxide preparation can exclude this possibility. A biopsy cannot differentiate between the different types of dermatitis. See **Table 253-3** for definitions of terms in superficial cutaneous fungal infections and **Table 253-4** for causes of superficial cutaneous fungal infections. Dermatologic consultation is often necessary for specific diagnosis.

Treatment is the removal of offending agents. Antihistamine, anesthetic, antibiotic, and anti-itch creams should be stopped because they may cause a second allergy. Lubricate with petroleum jelly, or thick ointments with a petroleum base, frequently and liberally.

For acute eruptions with vesiculation, use **aluminum acetate**, two to three times per day. Mix one aluminum acetate powder packet or tablet with 1 pint of water, and then apply with a towel or gauze to the affected

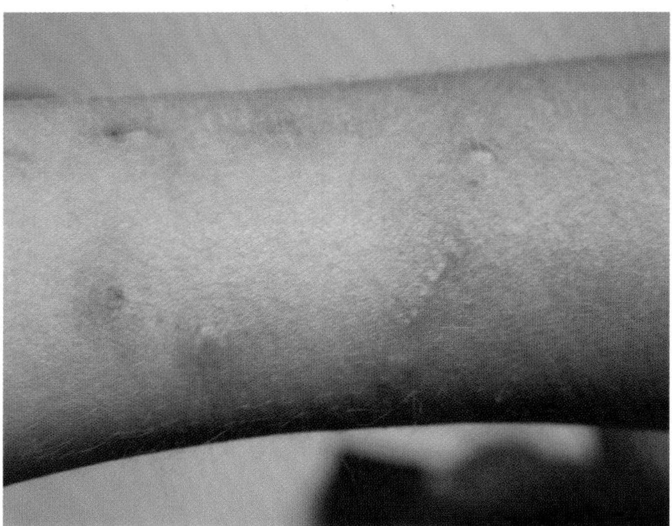

FIGURE 253-6. Allergic contact dermatitis secondary to poison ivy. [Photo contributed by University of North Carolina Department of Dermatology.]

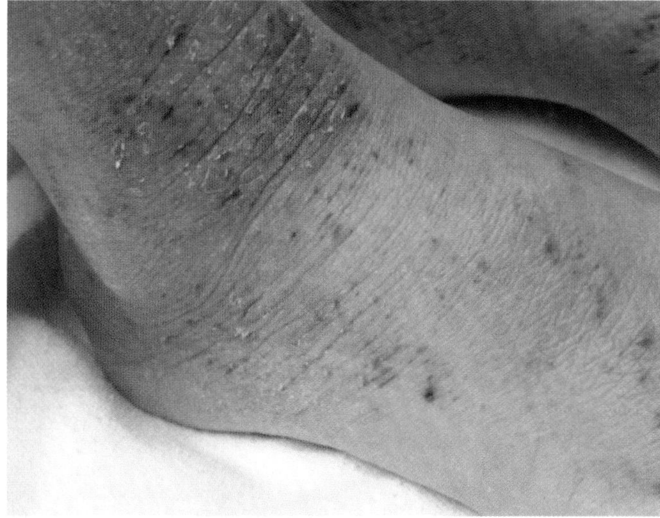

FIGURE 253-8. Atopic dermatitis with lichenification. [Photo contributed by University of North Carolina Department of Dermatology.]

TABLE 253-3 Definitions of Terms for Superficial Cutaneous Fungal Infections

Dermatophytes: a group of fungi that infect nonviable keratinized cutaneous structures such as stratum corneum, nails, and hair. They most commonly include *Trichophyton* species, *Microsporum* species, and *Epidermophyton* species.
Dermatophytosis: an infection caused by dermatophytes
Tinea: a term used for specific clinical manifestations of dermatophyte or dermatophyte-like infections, with the addition of a term that usually indicates the anatomic area affected (tinea pedis, tinea manuum, etc.)
Malassezia species: a yeast causing tinea versicolor or pityriasis versicolor

area for 15 to 20 minutes. Use a high-potency topical corticosteroid, such as clobetasol ointment, twice a day, after the compress. Hydroxyzine, 25 to 50 milligrams up to four times a day, can relieve itching.

In severe cases with debilitating eruptions, systemic glucocorticoids are indicated. For **poison ivy or oak**, give oral prednisone, 60 milligrams/d, for 2 to 3 weeks. Shorter courses of prednisone can result in relapse.

Treat chronic eruptions with high-potency topical corticosteroids two to three times a day. Ointments are preferred because they help with lubrication. Systemic glucocorticoids should be avoided in chronic cases and atopic dermatitis. Although systemic steroids may provide temporary relief, rebound activity after cessation is common.

PSORIASIS

Psoriasis vulgaris or plaque-type psoriasis may involve only the palms and soles but often extends to other areas, especially the elbows, knees, scalp, umbilicus, and gluteal cleft (see chapter 251 for more discussion). If pustules are present, the disorder is called *pustular psoriasis.* Peak ages of onset are between 20 and 30 years old and between 50 and 60 years old.

Psoriasis is an inherited disease in which the principal abnormality is believed to be an abnormal T lymphocyte–driven immune process. These altered T cells are believed to secrete cytokines that shorten the keratinocyte cell cycle and produce arthropathy.

Psoriasis is characterized by discrete plaques of erythema, scales, and fissures on the extremities (**Figure 253-9**). Extensive disease may extend over the entire palms, soles, and dorsal surfaces of the hands or feet (**Figure 253-10**). Onycholysis (separation of the nail plate from the nail bed), nail pits, and yellow discoloration of the nails help support the diagnosis of psoriasis (**Figure 253-11**).

In pustular psoriasis of the palms and soles, erythema, minimal scale, and numerous sterile pustules are seen. The pustules are in various stages of evolution from small pustules to larger confluent "lakes of pus" to crusts to rings of scale (**Figure 253-12**). Pustules are most commonly seen bilaterally on the instep of the foot and the thenar and hypothenar eminences of the hands.

Complete examination of the skin focusing on the sites commonly affected by psoriasis, including the elbows, knees, scalp, lower back, gluteal cleft, umbilicus, and nails, may reveal other areas of involvement to aid in diagnosing psoriasis. If no other psoriatic plaques are noted, differentiation from hand and foot dermatitis can be difficult (**Table 253-5**). A biopsy may be helpful in this instance. A potassium hydroxide examination should be performed to exclude a dermatophyte infection. Bacterial and viral cultures should be obtained when disease is pustular and localized to one area.

Initial treatment includes the use of a high- or ultrahigh-potency topical corticosteroid such as fluocinonide, clobetasol propionate, or betamethasone dipropionate ointment. Encourage liberal use of white petrolatum-based topical emollients. **Do not prescribe systemic steroids because of the risk of rebound or induction of pustular psoriasis.** The disease is chronic and slow to respond to treatment. Arrange follow-up with a dermatologist.

TABLE 253-4 Causes of Superficial Cutaneous Fungal Infections

Dermatophytes
Trichophyton species (cause most superficial cutaneous fungal infections)
Microsporum species
Epidermophyton species
Candida
Malassezia species

TABLE 253-5 Differential Diagnosis of Psoriasis

Psoriasis vulgaris
Hand and foot dermatitis
Lichen simplex chronicus
Reiter's syndrome
Pustular psoriasis
Tinea pedis and tinea manuum
Staphylococcus aureus infection
Herpes simplex infection
Dyshidrosis

ERYTHEMA NODOSUM

Erythema nodosum is an inflammatory eruption of the subcutaneous fat. It has many possible causes (**Table 253-6**) and is idiopathic in nearly half of cases. All age groups can be affected.

Tender, warm, ill-defined erythematous nodules characterize erythema nodosum (**Figure 253-13**). Nodules are most commonly seen on the pretibial area of the lower extremities, although the extensor aspects of the arms and torso can occasionally be involved. Ulceration is not a feature and suggests another diagnosis. Nodules can persist for weeks.

The diagnosis is clinical and should include evaluation for possible causes (Table 253-6). If the diagnosis is unclear (**Table 253-7**), refer for a biopsy.

Treatment is symptomatic, with leg elevation and nonsteroidal anti-inflammatory drugs. Treat the underlying cause. Refer refractory cases to a dermatologist.

LICHEN SIMPLEX CHRONICUS, CORNS, AND CALLUSES

Lichen simplex chronicus, corns, and calluses are all thickenings of the upper layer of the skin (stratum corneum) in response to chronic friction and scratching. Most commonly, ankles, lower extremities, neck, scrotum, and vulva are involved. When friction occurs in the absence of pruritus and is distributed over a large area, a callus is formed. When the

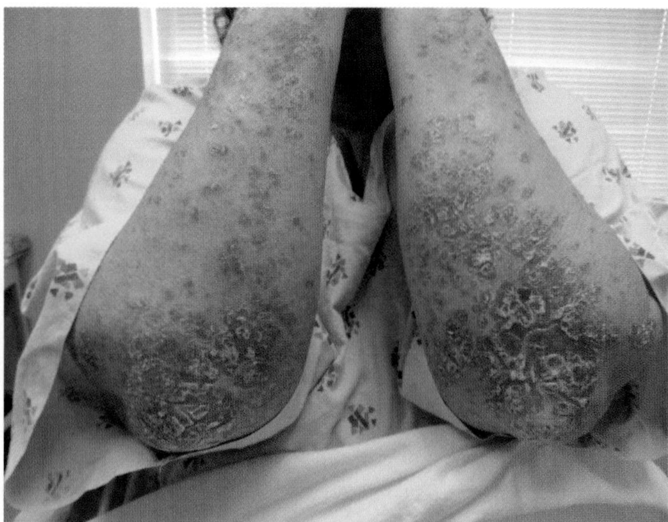

FIGURE 253-9. Psoriasis vulgaris. [Photo contributed by University of North Carolina Department of Dermatology.]

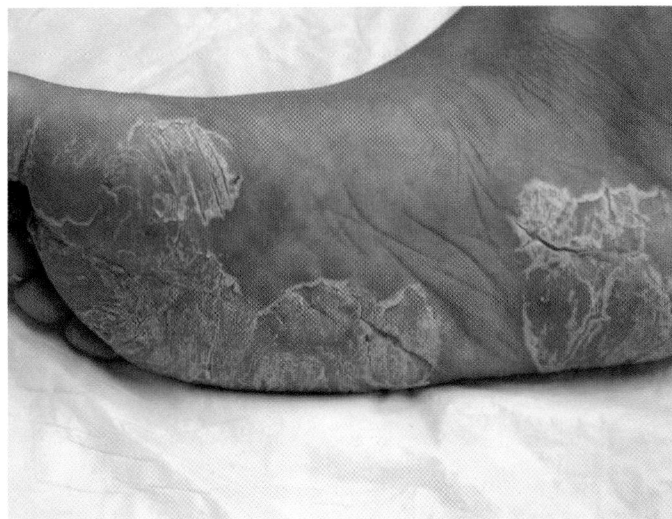

FIGURE 253-10. Psoriasis vulgaris of the plantar foot. [Photo contributed by University of North Carolina Department of Dermatology.]

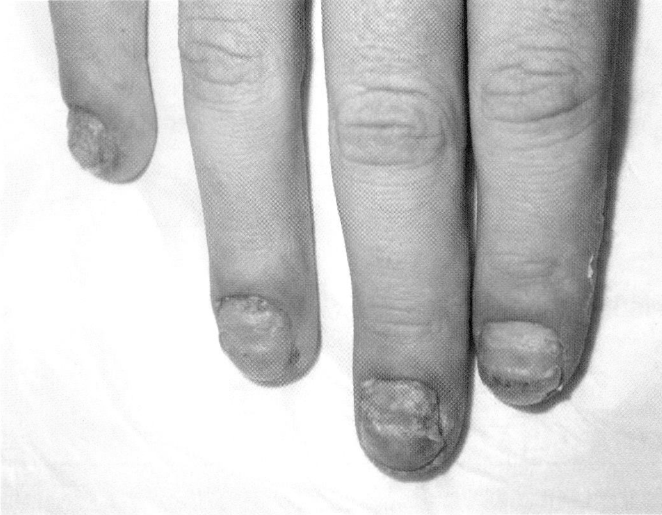

FIGURE 253-11. Psoriasis nails. [Photo contributed by University of North Carolina Department of Dermatology.]

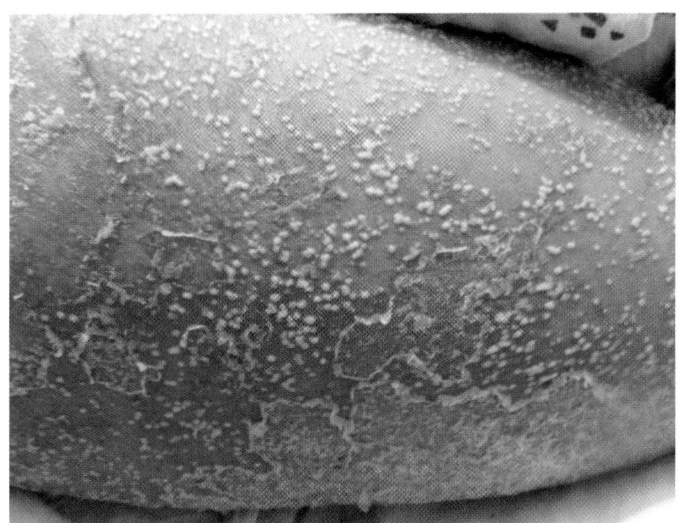

FIGURE 253-12. Pustular psoriasis. [Photo contributed by University of North Carolina Department of Dermatology.]

TABLE 253-6 Causes of Erythema Nodosum

Infectious	Pharmacologic
Fungal	Sulfonamides
Blastomycosis	Oral contraceptive pills
Coccidioidomycosis	Penicillin
Histoplasmosis	Bromides
Dermatophyte	Vaccines
Bacterial	Sarcoidosis
Streptococcal infections	Inflammatory bowel disease
Campylobacter	Pregnancy
Yersinia species	Behçet's syndrome
Tuberculosis	Leukemia and lymphoma
Leprosy	Idiopathic
Parasitic	
Leishmaniasis	
Toxoplasmosis	
Viral	
Herpes simplex	
Infectious mononucleosis	

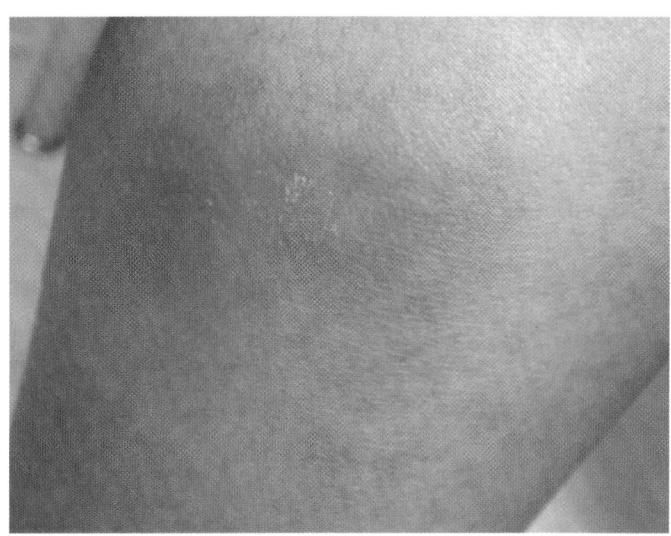

FIGURE 253-13. Erythema nodosum—painful palpable erythematous nodules. [Photo contributed by University of North Carolina Department of Dermatology.]

TABLE 253-7 Differential Diagnosis of Erythema Nodosum

Erythema induratum (nodular vasculitis)
Pancreatic panniculitis
Lupus profundus
Connective tissue panniculitis
Cold panniculitis
Malignant subcutaneous infiltrates
Cytophagic histiocytic panniculitis
Hematoma
Infection (fungal, bacterial, or mycobacterial)

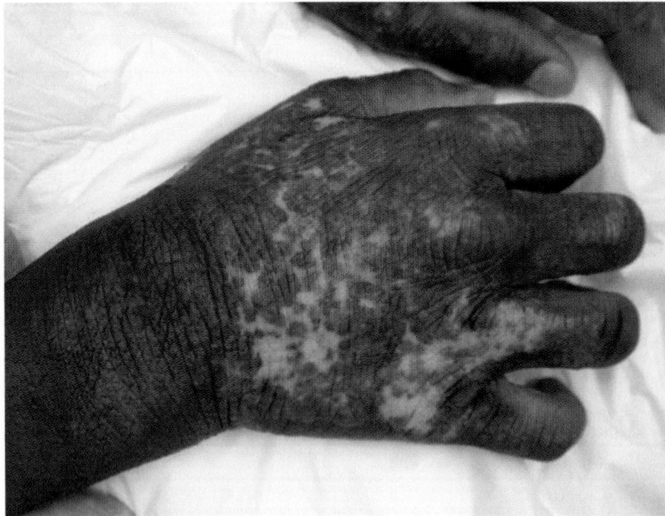

FIGURE 253-14. Lichen simplex chronicus. [Photo contributed by University of North Carolina Department of Dermatology.]

same frictional forces occur over a localized area of the foot, a corn is formed. Calluses and corns are most commonly located on the feet.

Lichen simplex chronicus presents as one or several intensely pruritic, well-demarcated plaques, with lichenification because of chronic scratching and rubbing (**Figure 253-14**). Erythema, hyperpigmentation, and excoriations are also present. Scale is minimal. The ankles, shins, dorsal feet, and hands may be affected.

Calluses and corns present as thickened plaques at areas of repetitive trauma. Corns form firm, dome-shaped papules with translucent central cores on the dorsal, lateral, and interdigital toes (**Figure 253-15**).

Diagnosis is clinical (**Table 253-8**). A potassium hydroxide examination can be helpful to rule out a dermatophyte infection. If the diagnosis is uncertain, refer for a skin biopsy. Paring of warts reveals punctuate thrombosed capillaries, which are not found in calluses or corns.

For lichen simplex chronicus, interrupting the scratch–itch cycle is the most important aspect of treatment. High-potency topical corticosteroids such as fluocinonide or clobetasol ointment should be applied to the plaque two to three times a day. Oral antihistamines help for pruritus.

Paring and keratolytics, such as salicylic acid, are first-line treatments for corns and calluses, as well as proper footwear and medical management.[18] For further treatment, refer to a podiatrist or dermatologist.

DERMATITIS HERPETIFORMIS

Dermatitis herpetiformis is a cutaneous manifestation of **gluten sensitivity**. It is most common in individuals of northern European descent.[19] Often, there is familial involvement, and there is almost universal association with HLA-DQ2 or HLA-DQ8, located on chromosome 6, with close relatives being affected by either dermatitis herpetiformis or celiac disease.[20]

Granular deposits of immunoglobulin A are found at the dermal–epidermal junction of all patients with dermatitis herpetiformis. These deposits are believed to attract neutrophils, which induce vesicle formation. The presence of immunoglobulin A antibodies to tissue transglutaminase is also highly sensitive and specific for the disorder.[21]

Extremely pruritic vesicles, papules, or urticarial plaques are symmetrically distributed on extensor surfaces of the extremities, back, and buttocks (**Figure 253-16**). Chronic scratching may result in excoriations and lichenification in these locations. Approximately 20% of patients will have clinical evidence of malabsorption.[22]

The diagnosis is supported by clinical, biopsy, and laboratory findings (**Table 253-9**). Diagnosis and treatment require dermatology referral.

Treatment for dermatitis herpetiformis includes oral dapsone and a gluten-free diet. Oral dapsone relieves pruritus within 72 hours of beginning therapy. Systemic steroids are ineffective.

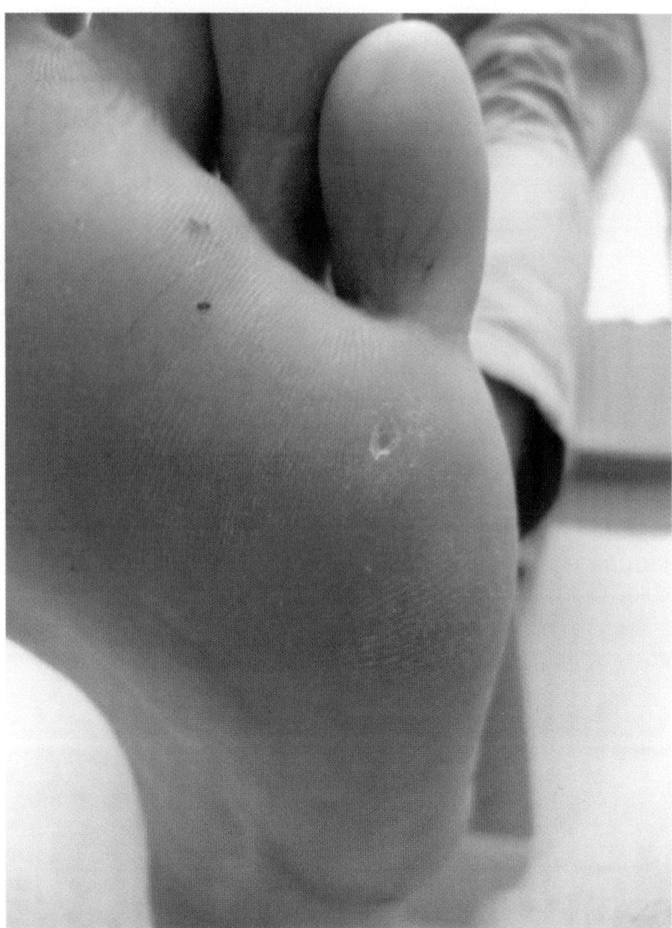

FIGURE 253-15. Corn. Painful, hyperkeratotic lesion. [Photo contributed by University of North Carolina Department of Dermatology.]

CUTANEOUS INFECTIONS

FISH TANK GRANULOMA

Fish tank granuloma is an infection by *Mycobacterium marinum* that classically presents as an ulceration or suppurating abscess with a line of nodules along the corresponding lymphatic drainage. It most commonly affects individuals frequenting swimming pools or who clean fish tanks.[23] *M. marinum* is found in all aquatic environments, including fresh, salt,

TABLE 253-8 Differential Diagnosis of Lichen Simplex Chronicus, Corns, and Calluses
Lichen simplex chronicus
Dermatophyte infection
Nummular eczema
Psoriasis
Squamous cell carcinoma
Corns and calluses
Plantar wart
Arsenical keratosis
Squamous cell carcinoma
Palmoplantar keratoderma
Punctuate palmoplantar keratoses
Punctuate porokeratosis
Poroma (benign hair follicle tumor)

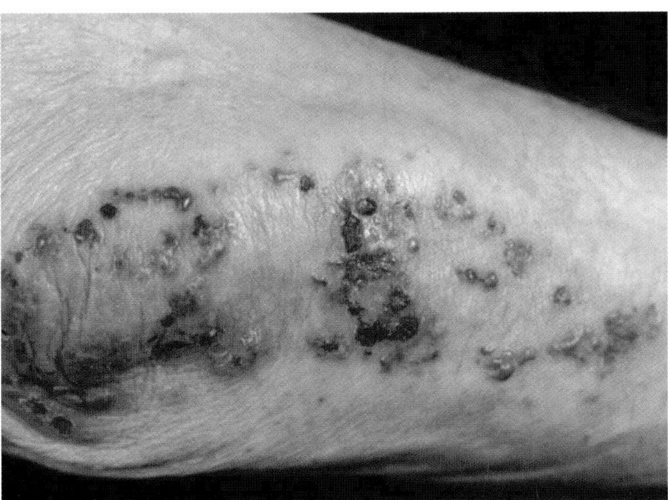

FIGURE 253-16. Dermatitis herpetiformis. Papules and vesicles are grouped together, not in a dermatomal distribution, and are symmetrically distributed on extensor areas of elbows and knees. [Reproduced with permission from Wolff KL, Johnson R, Suurmond R: *Fitzpatrick's Color Atlas & Synopsis of Clinical Dermatology*, 5th ed. © 2005, McGraw-Hill, New York.]

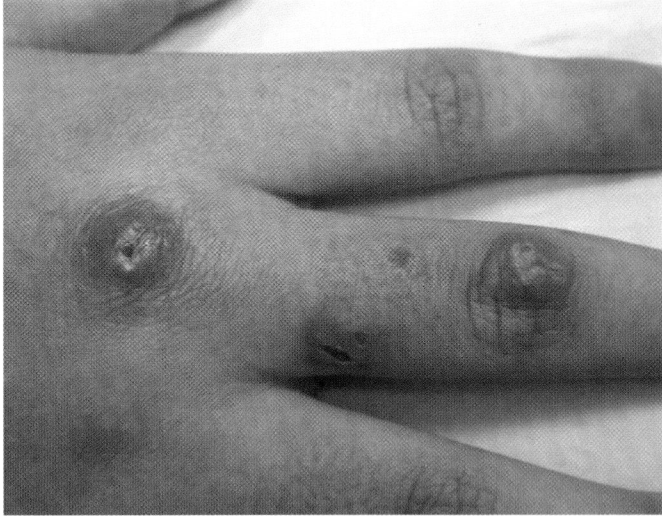

FIGURE 253-17. Fish tank granuloma. Red-violet papules and plaques at sites of abrasion. [Photo contributed by University of North Carolina Department of Dermatology.]

and brackish water, swimming pools, and lakes. Infection requires exposure of abraded or traumatized skin to a contaminated environment.[23]

Two to three weeks after exposure, a solitary nodule or pustule forms. The skin breaks down into a crusted ulcer, suppurative abscess, or verrucous nodule (**Figure 253-17** and **Table 253-10**). Often, multiple lesions will form along the course of the draining lymphatics, with minimal lymphadenopathy.[24]

The history and clinical features should evoke suspicion, which should be confirmed by culture. A clinical distinction can also be made from cat-scratch fever and primary inoculation tuberculosis by noting an absence of significant lymphadenopathy in patients infected with *M. marinum*. Other diagnoses can be excluded by a skin biopsy.

M. marinum is sensitive to rifampicin, clarithromycin, tetracyclines, and trimethoprim-sulfamethoxazole.[24,25] After sensitivity testing, antibiotic therapy is usually continued for approximately 6 weeks, typically under direction of an infectious disease specialist.

CUTANEOUS LARVA MIGRANS

Cutaneous larva migrans is a cutaneous eruption caused by the migration of **hookworm larvae** within the epidermis. The disease is most commonly found in tropical and subtropical climates where people walk barefoot in environments contaminated with animal feces.

Erythematous and serpiginous tracts are formed as the larva migrates within the skin (**Figure 253-18**). The patient will often complain of pruritus. A CBC may demonstrate peripheral eosinophilia; patients are otherwise well. Diagnosis is clinical. A single oral dose of **albendazole** or **ivermectin** is usually effective.[26]

TABLE 253-9 Differential Diagnosis of Dermatitis Herpetiformis
Erythema multiforme
Bullous lupus erythematosus
Linear immunoglobulin A bullous dermatosis
Bullous pemphigoid
Atopic dermatitis (eczema)
Papular urticaria
Chronic prurigo
Scabies

PLANTAR WARTS

Plantar warts are a common infection of children caused by the human papillomavirus. They may be acquired through direct contact with infected individuals or indirectly through contaminated surfaces. Most warts will spontaneously regress within 1 to 2 years.

Plantar warts occur on the sole of the foot, especially over pressure points, as thickened papules and plaques that disrupt normal skin lines (**Figure 253-19**). Black dots, representing thrombosed capillaries, will often cover the surface or become evident upon superficial paring. Diagnosis is clinical (**Table 253-11**).

Initial treatment is topical salicylic acid. Cryotherapy and electrodesiccation are other options.

TINEA PEDIS AND TINEA MANUUM

Tinea pedis, or athlete's foot, is a fungal infection of the feet, and tinea manuum involves the hand. Tinea manuum is often unilateral and associated with tinea pedis. Often, if one hand is involved, both feet are involved as well. It is unclear why the other hand is spared in this "two foot, one hand" type of fungal infection. Tinea pedis is very common and usually begins in early adulthood. It is rare in children. Predisposing factors include hot, humid weather, excessive sweating, and occlusive footwear. *Trichophyton rubrum*, *Trichophyton mentagrophytes*, and *Epidermophyton floccosum* are the most common organisms involved. *T. mentagrophytes* is most likely to cause inflammatory bullous tinea pedis. Infections are transmitted from person to person or from animal to person via fomites or direct contact.

There are three main clinical types: interdigital, hyperkeratotic (scaling), and bullous. Interdigital tinea pedis is the most common and is characterized by maceration and scale in the web spaces between the toes. Ulceration may even be present in severe cases that have a secondary infection with bacteria or yeast (**Figure 253-20**).

Hyperkeratotic, chronic, dry scales involve palms and soles, with little, if any, inflammation. When involving the medial and lateral aspects of

TABLE 253-10 Differential Diagnosis of Fish Tank Granuloma
Cat-scratch fever
Primary inoculation tuberculosis
Inoculation leishmaniasis
Sporotrichosis
Other mycobacterial infections
Deep fungal infections

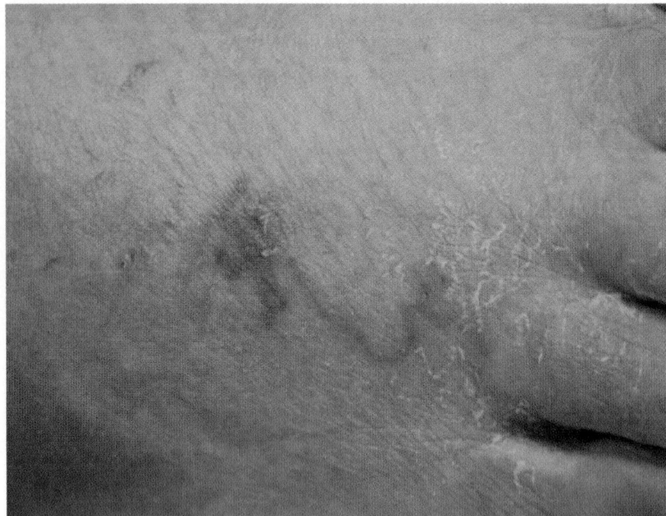

FIGURE 253-18. Cutaneous larva migrans with elevated serpiginous tracks caused by migration of the larva under the skin. [Photo contributed by University of North Carolina Department of Dermatology.]

the feet, it is called "moccasin" tinea (**Figure 253-21**). Nails may be affected.

Bullous tinea consists of an acute, painful, erythematous and pruritic vesicular eruption on the palms or soles (**Figure 253-22**). Toenails and web spaces are usually not involved.

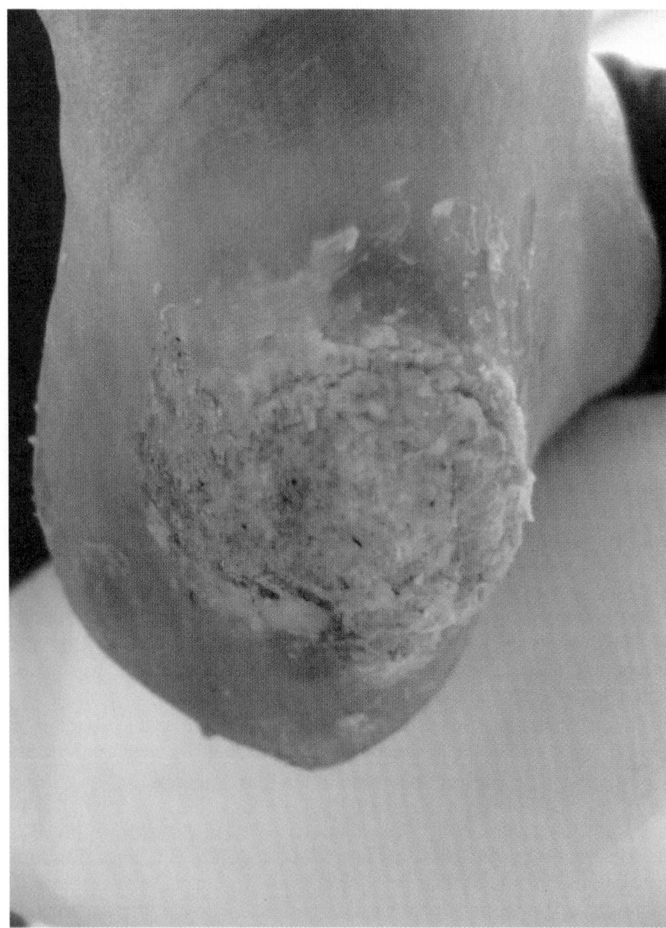

FIGURE 253-19. Plantar warts. Painless papules with red-black dots of thrombosed capillaries. [Photo contributed by University of North Carolina Department of Dermatology.]

TABLE 253-11 Differential Diagnosis of Plantar Warts

Callus
Corn
Epithelioma cuniculatum
Squamous cell carcinoma
Arsenic keratoses
Palmoplantar keratoderma
Punctuate palmoplantar keratoses
Punctuate porokeratosis
Verrucous carcinoma
Benign hair follicle tumor (poroma)

Diagnosis is based on clinical examination and identification of fungal elements on a potassium hydroxide preparation or with fungal culture. If the clinical examination is highly suspicious for a fungal infection, empiric therapy is reasonable. If the diagnosis is uncertain, obtain scrapings for fungal cultures before beginning therapy because culture results (whether positive or negative) can help the follow-up physician choose the most appropriate therapy.

Although a potassium hydroxide examination appears to be a simple test, it is often difficult for clinicians to perform and interpret (see Table 248-6). Scraping of scale can also be sent to the laboratory for potassium hydroxide examination and fungal culture. Hyphae appear as light-green, thin strands that cross over cells and have branches (see Figure 248-1).

Treat interdigital and hyperkeratotic (nonbullous) tinea with topical antifungals, such as clotrimazole, miconazole, ketoconazole, or econazole cream. Apply to affected areas twice a day and continue for 1 week after clearing. Although econazole cream is expensive, it is preferred for interdigital tinea pedis because it has antibacterial properties to treat secondary bacterial (often *Corynebacterium*) infection. Topical **terbinafine cream** is a nonprescription alternative and is applied once a day. Topical agents do not treat nail infections. For treatment of onychomycosis, an oral agent such as itraconazole, fluconazole, or terbinafine is needed, but this treatment is best managed by the primary care physician or dermatologist.

Bullous tinea pedis often does not respond to topical treatment. For mild cases, a topical agent can be tried initially. In more severe cases, oral antifungal treatment is necessary. Itraconazole, 200 milligrams PO each day for 14 days, or terbinafine, 250 milligrams PO each day for 14 days, is effective. **The prescribing physician should be familiar with the potential drug interactions and the uncommon, but serious, side effects (hepatotoxicity and erythema multiforme/toxic epidermal**

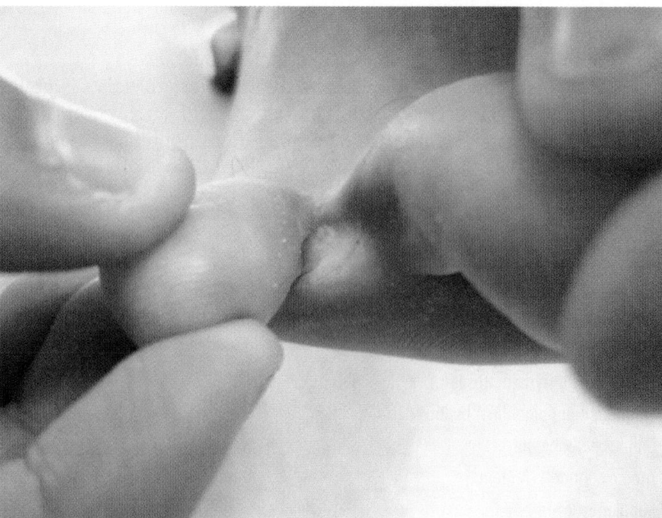

FIGURE 253-20. Interdigital tinea pedis. [Photo contributed by University of North Carolina Department of Dermatology.]

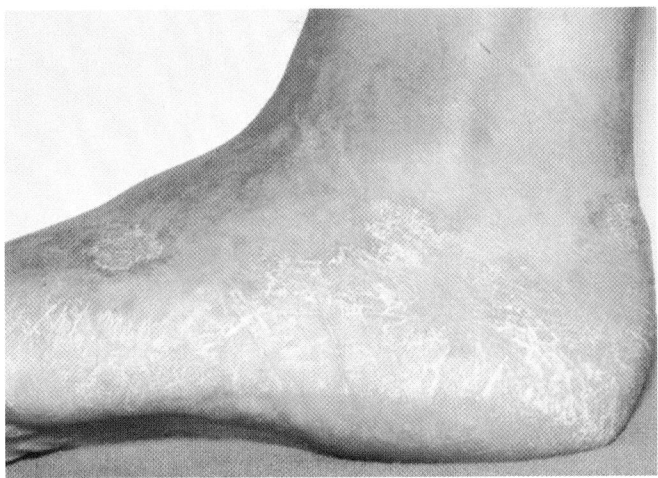

FIGURE 253-21. Moccasin-type tinea pedis. [Reproduced with permission from Fleischer AB Jr, Feldman SR, McConnell CF, et al: *Emergency Dermatology: A Rapid Treatment Guide.* © 2002, McGraw-Hill, New York.]

necrolysis) before prescribing these medications. Baseline liver function studies should be obtained when prescribing terbinafine.

Hands and feet should be kept as dry as possible. After bathing, web spaces should be thoroughly dried. Socks should be changed any time they become wet with sweat. If the eruption is not clear in 4 to 6 weeks, dermatology referral is needed. The disease is chronic, and recurrences are common.

VASCULAR CUTANEOUS CONDITIONS

ROCKY MOUNTAIN SPOTTED FEVER

Rocky Mountain spotted fever is a potentially fatal multisystem illness caused by *Rickettsia rickettsii*. Symptoms begin 2 to 14 days after an infected tick bite. The organism disseminates through the bloodstream and invades the vascular endothelium, causing a necrotizing vasculitis. Fever, headache, and myalgias develop about 1 week after exposure. The rash in classic Rocky Mountain spotted fever is evident 2 to 5 days after the onset of fever and other symptoms. In most patients, some type of rash develops during the illness, but about 10% never develop a rash.[27]

The rash first appears on the wrists and ankles and rapidly spreads to the palms and soles (**Figure 253-23, A and B**). As the rash moves centrally, the proximal extremities, trunk, and face become involved. The skin lesions at the onset are described as discrete macules or maculopapules that blanch with pressure. The initial lesions evolve into petechiae over 2 to 4 days, fade slowly over 2 to 3 weeks, and heal occasionally with hyperpigmentation. Rarely, the petechiae may coalesce into ecchymotic areas with eventual gangrene of the distal extremities, nose, ear lobes, scrotum, and vulva—purpura fulminans. Treatment for adults is doxycycline, 100 milligrams PO twice a day; for children under 45 kg with permanent teeth, treatment is doxycycline, 2.2 milligrams/kg twice a day. Doxycycline does not cause staining of permanent teeth. For further discussion of the treatment of this and other tickborne diseases, see chapter 160, "Zoonotic Infections."

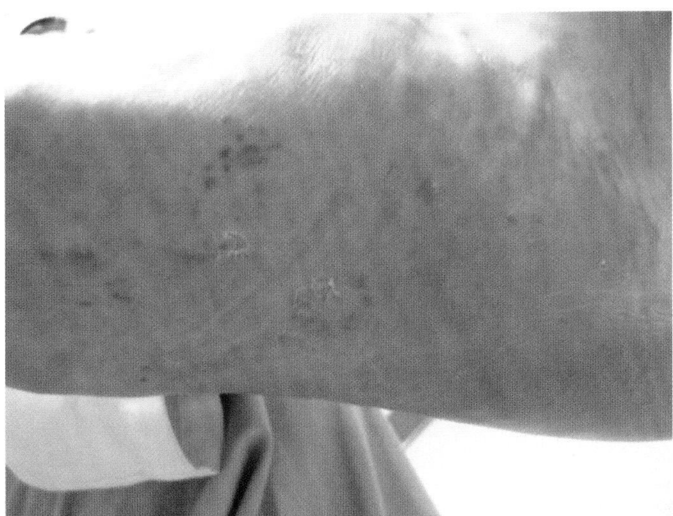

FIGURE 253-22. Bullous tinea pedis. [Photo contributed by University of North Carolina Department of Dermatology.]

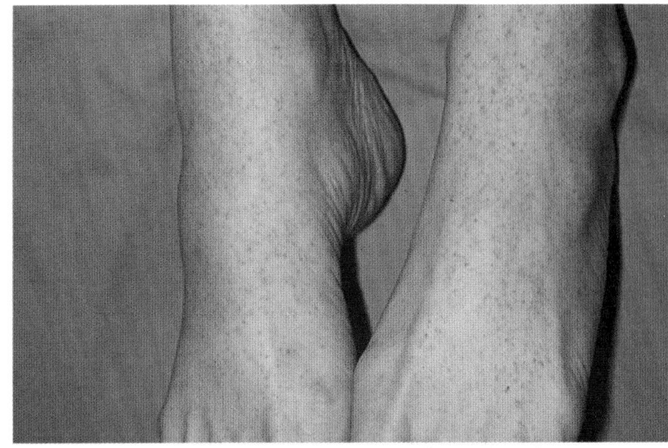

A

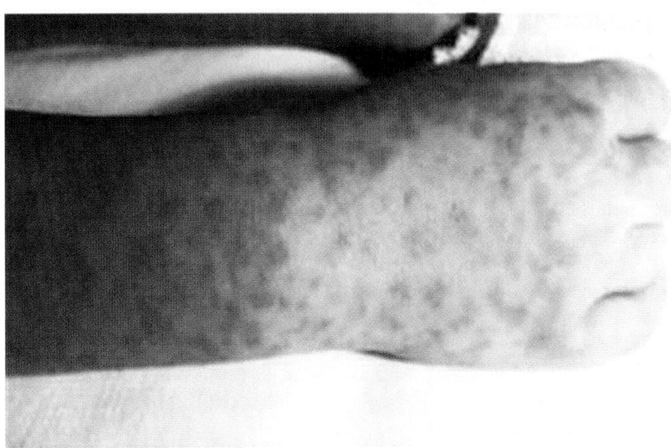

B

FIGURE 253-23. A. Petechiae on the ankles of a patient with Rocky Mountain spotted fever. **B.** Petechiae involving hand, wrist, and forearm. [From the Centers for Disease Control and Prevention; National Center for Emerging and Zoonotic Infectious Diseases; Division of Vector-Borne Diseases: Rocky Mountain Spotted Fever. www.cdc.gov/rmsf/symptoms/. Updated September 5, 2013.]

PURPURA

Purpura is visible hemorrhage into the skin or mucous membranes. Small, flat lesions are petechiae, and large, flat lesions are ecchymoses. Palpable purpura has a physically palpable elevation. Diverse abnormalities of coagulation and blood vessel function lead to hemorrhage into the skin. These include abnormalities of platelet number or function, procoagulant defects, poor dermal support of vessels, increased pressure within vessels, trauma, vascular inflammation, and vascular occlusion.

The cutaneous and systemic causes of purpura are broad. Nevertheless, some broad generalizations can be made. Large ecchymoses generally signify coagulation defects or trauma and may be associated with signs of external or internal bleeding. Petechiae are often associated with thrombocytopenia and bleeding in other locations. Palpable purpura

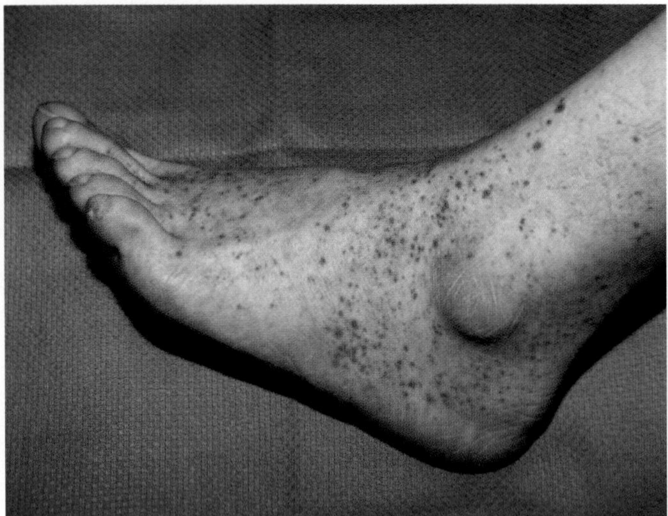

FIGURE 253-24. Purpura from cutaneous vasculitis. [Photo contributed by University of North Carolina Department of Dermatology.]

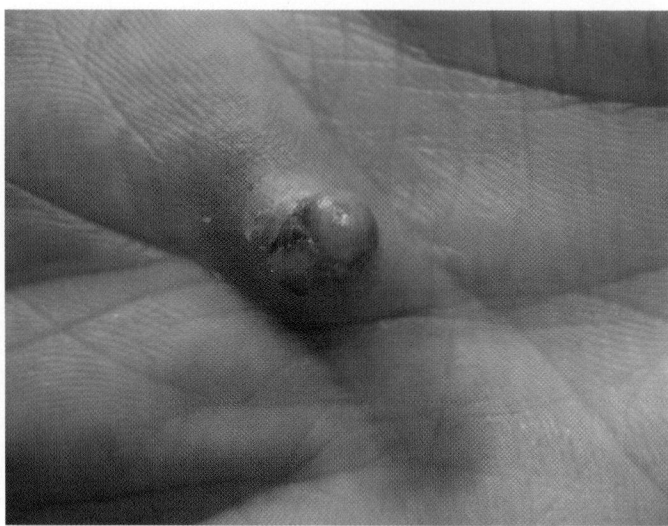

FIGURE 253-25. Pyogenic granuloma. Solitary vascular nodule that develops after minor trauma. [Photo contributed by University of North Carolina Department of Dermatology.]

and persistent, localized purpura suggest vasculitis (**Figure 253-24**). Because vasculitis can affect any organ system, a complete history and physical examination and a detailed laboratory investigation are required.

Major coagulation defects and platelet disorders can be diagnosed through coagulation studies. Cutaneous vasculitis is diagnosed by skin biopsy. Systemic vasculitis is diagnosed by laboratory investigation. Treatment and disposition are based on the underlying diagnosis. For additional discussion, see chapters 141, "Rashes in Infants and Children" and 249, "Generalized Skin Disorders."

PYOGENIC GRANULOMA

A pyogenic granuloma is a benign proliferation of immature capillaries occurring at the site of minor skin trauma. The name is a misnomer because it is neither an infection nor a granuloma. It most commonly occurs in children, young adults, and pregnant women. In pregnant women, it is called *granuloma gravidarum*. A pyogenic granuloma initially presents as a bright red, shiny papule with a surrounding thin collarette of hyperkeratosis (**Figure 253-25**). It may be ulcerated and tends to bleed profusely with minor injury. Later, the lesion reepithelializes and becomes a dull red to purple color. Although lesions can occur anywhere on the body, the extremities, especially hands, are the most common sites of involvement. If the lesion is bleeding profusely, obtain hemostasis with pressure or suturing. Refer for a biopsy of the lesion to exclude other disorders, especially an amelanotic melanoma (**Table 253-12**). Lesions do not resolve without specific treatment by laser therapy or electrodesiccation.

TABLE 253-12 Differential Diagnosis for Pyogenic Granuloma
Amelanotic melanoma
Squamous cell carcinoma
Bacillary angiomatosis
Cutaneous metastasis
Kaposi's sarcoma

REFERENCES

The complete reference list is available online at www.TintinalliEM.com.

SECTION 21 Trauma

CHAPTER 254 Trauma in Adults

Peter Cameron
Barry J. Knapp

INTRODUCTION AND EPIDEMIOLOGY

Trauma accounts for 41 million annual ED visits and 2.3 million hospital admissions across the United States. Trauma is the number one cause of death for Americans between age 1 and 44 years and is the number three cause of death overall.[1] In all countries, the incidence of death from injury increases more than threefold with increasing poverty. For the 90% of patients who survive the initial trauma, the burden of ongoing morbidity from traumatic brain injury, loss of limb function, and ongoing pain is even more significant.

The major causes of death following trauma are head injury, chest injury, and major vascular injury. Trauma care should be organized according to the concepts of rapid assessment, triage, resuscitation, diagnosis, and therapeutic intervention.[2] Worldwide, there are few countries or regions that have comprehensive systems of trauma care, from roadside to rehabilitation, and that incorporate effective injury prevention strategies.

TRAUMA SYSTEMS AND TIMELY TRIAGE

A systematic approach is required to reduce morbidity and mortality that occur after traumatic injury (**Figure 254-1**).

Recognizing the need to establish a system to triage injured patients rapidly to the most appropriate setting and the importance of promoting collaboration among emergency medicine, trauma surgery, and trauma care subspecialists, the U.S. Congress passed the Trauma Care Systems Planning and Development Act of 1990.[3] This act provided for the development of a model trauma care system plan to serve as a reference document for each state in creating its own system. Each state must determine the appropriate facility for treatment of various types of injuries. Trauma centers are certified based on the institution's commitment of personnel and resources to maintain a condition of readiness for the treatment of critically injured patients. Some states rely on a verification process offered by the American College of Surgeons for the designation of certain hospitals as trauma centers.[2] In a well-run trauma center, the critically injured patient undergoes a multidisciplinary evaluation, and diagnostic and therapeutic interventions are performed with smooth transitions between the ED, diagnostic radiology suite, operating room, and postoperative intensive care setting. **Table 254-1** details the requirements for designation as a Level 1 trauma center. A complete list of trauma center requirements is available at the American College of Surgeons website (http://www.facs.org/trauma/verificationhosp.html).

A well-functioning trauma system defines trauma centers with specific triage criteria, so that patients can be initially transported by EMS to these centers or transferred to trauma centers from other hospitals after stabilization (**Table 254-2 and Figure 254-2**). In accordance with the principles of advanced trauma life support, injured patients are assessed and treated based on their presenting vital signs, mental status, and mechanism of injury.[4]

PRIMARY SURVEY

Prior to the patient's arrival at the hospital, EMS providers should inform the receiving ED about the mechanism of trauma, suspected injuries, vital signs, clinical symptoms, examination findings, and treatments provided. In preparation for the patient's arrival, ED staff should assign tasks to team members, prepare resuscitation and procedural equipment, and ensure the presence of surgical consultants and other care team members. For patients transported to EDs that are not trauma centers, consider immediately whether transfer to a trauma center is appropriate and what resuscitation or stabilization can or should be performed prior to transfer.

A focused history obtained from the patient, family members, witnesses, or prehospital providers may provide important information regarding circumstances of the injury (e.g., single-vehicle crash, fall from height, environmental exposure, smoke inhalation), ingestion of intoxicants, preexisting medical conditions (e.g., diabetes, depression, cardiac disease, pregnancy), and medication use (e.g., steroids, β-blockers, anticoagulants) that may suggest certain patterns of injury or the physiologic response to injury.

ED care of the trauma patient begins with an initial assessment for potentially serious injuries. A primary survey is undertaken quickly to identify and treat immediately life-threatening conditions, with simultaneous resuscitation and treatment. Specific injuries that should be immediately identified and addressed during the primary survey include airway obstruction, tension pneumothorax, massive internal or external hemorrhage, open pneumothorax, flail chest, and cardiac tamponade. After assessing the patient's airway, breathing, and circulation, perform a more thorough head-to-toe examination (the **secondary survey**) (**Table 254-3**). Follow the secondary survey with appropriate diagnostic testing, further therapeutic interventions, and disposition. When derangements are identified in any of the systems assessed in the primary survey, undertake treatment immediately.

AIRWAY MANAGEMENT WITH CERVICAL SPINE CONTROL

Determine airway patency by inspecting for foreign bodies or maxillofacial fractures that may result in airway obstruction. Perform a jaw thrust maneuver (simultaneously with in-line stabilization of the head and neck) and insert an oral or nasal airway as part of the first response to a patient with inadequate respiratory effort. Insertion of an oral airway may be difficult in patients with an active gag reflex. Avoid nasal airway insertion in patients with suspected basilar skull fractures. **Whenever possible, use a two-person spinal stabilization technique in which one provider devotes undivided attention to maintaining in-line immobilization and preventing excessive movement of the cervical spine while the other manages the airway.** If the patient vomits, logroll the patient and provide pharyngeal suction to prevent aspiration. Perform endotracheal intubation in comatose patients (Glasgow coma scale score between 3 and 8) to protect the airway and to prevent secondary brain injury from hypoxemia. Agitated trauma patients with head injury, hypoxia, or drug- or alcohol-induced delirium may be at risk for self-injury. Trauma patients are frequently difficult to intubate due to the need for neck immobilization, the presence of blood or vomitus, or upper airway injury. Video laryngoscopy devices are beneficial because they aid in vocal cord visualization while minimizing

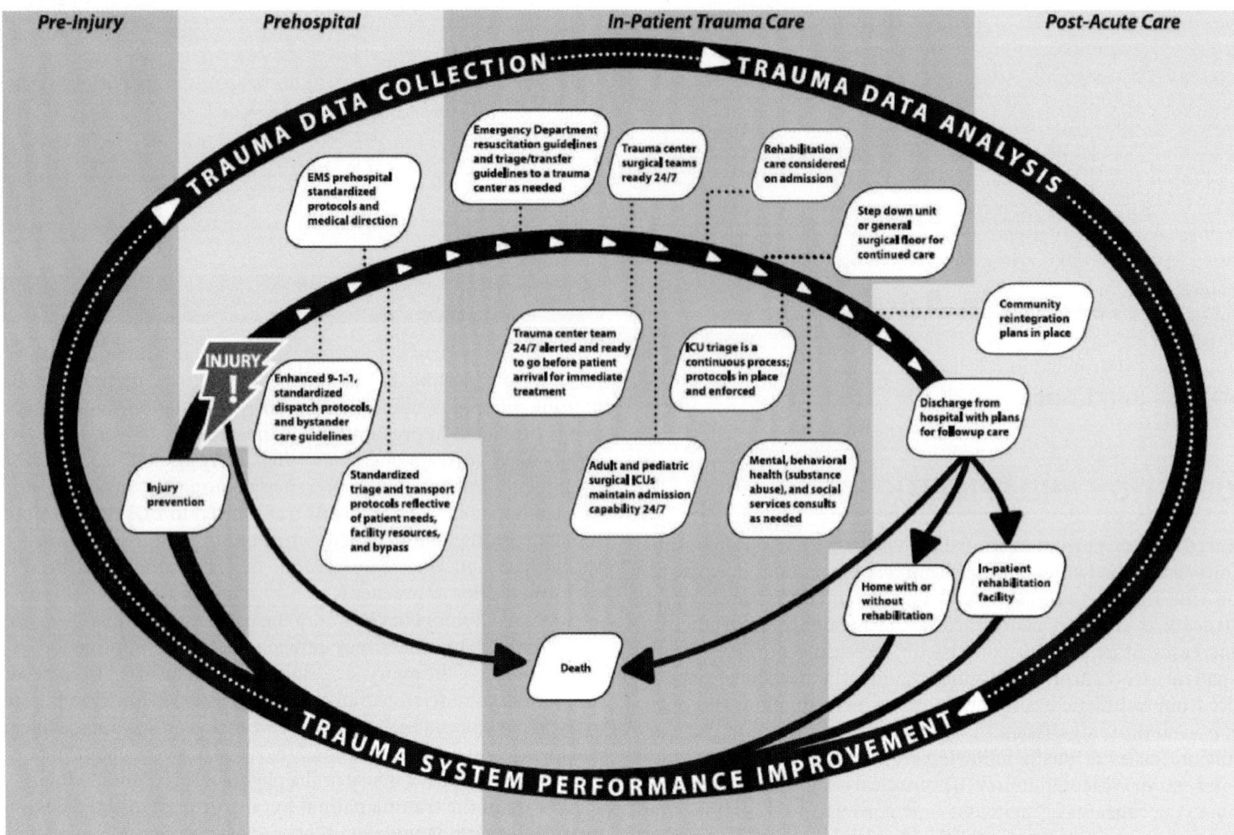

FIGURE 254-1. Phases of a preplanned trauma care continuum. [From U.S. Department of Health and Human Services, Health Resources and Services Administration. Model Trauma System Planning and Evaluation. Rockville, MD: U.S. Department of Health and Human Services; 2006. Available at: www.facs.org/trauma/tsepc/pdfs/mtspe.pdf. Accessed June 17, 2014.]

cervical spine manipulation. If anatomy or severe maxillofacial injury precludes endotracheal intubation, cricothyroidotomy may be needed. **Use a rapid-sequence intubation technique for intubation** (see chapter 29, "Intubation and Mechanical Ventilation").

Clearance of the cervical spine from serious injury involves careful clinical assessment, with or without radiologic imaging. Not all patients require cervical spine radiographs. The **National Emergency X-Radiography Utilization Study (NEXUS) criteria (Table 254-4)**[5] and the **Canadian cervical spine rule (Table 254-5)**[6] are useful only in awake and alert patients and are not a substitute for good clinical judgment. Patients meeting NEXUS or Canadian criteria for low risk of cervical spine injury should undergo full examination of the cervical spine, including active range-of-motion testing in all directions along with a thorough neurologic examination.

If the patient is obtunded, assume a cervical spine injury until proven otherwise. Even when plain radiographs or CT images show normal findings, it is possible for a patient to have unstable ligamentous injuries. Therefore, maintain spinal immobilization during the resuscitation. Imaging of the spine should not delay urgent operative procedures because imaging results will not change the immediate management. CT of the cervical spine is the preferred initial imaging modality. For full discussion of cervical spine imaging and management in trauma, see chapter 258, "Spine Trauma."

TABLE 254-1 Essential Characteristics of Level 1 Trauma Centers

24-h availability of surgeons in all subspecialties (including cardiac surgery/bypass capability)
24-h availability of neuroradiology and hemodialysis
Program that establishes and monitors effect of injury prevention and education efforts
Organized trauma research program

BREATHING

Once the airway is controlled, inspect, auscultate, and palpate the thorax and neck to detect abnormalities such as a deviated trachea (tension pneumothorax); crepitus (pneumothorax); paradoxical movement of a

TABLE 254-2 Triage and Trauma System Entry Criteria

Physiologic abnormalities
Systolic blood pressure <90 mm Hg
Glasgow coma scale score <14
Inadequate airway or need for immediate intubation
Injury pattern
Penetrating wound to head, neck, or torso
Gunshot wound to extremities proximal to elbow or knee
Extremity with neurovascular compromise
Amputation proximal to wrist or ankle
CNS injury or paralysis
Flail chest
Suspected pelvic fracture
Mechanism of injury
MVC with intrusion into passenger compartment >12 in
MVC with major vehicular deformity >20 in
Ejection from vehicle
MVC with entrapment or prolonged extrication of >20 min
Fall of >20 feet
MVC with fatality in same passenger compartment
Auto–pedestrian or auto–bicycle collision at >5 mph
Motorcycle crash >20 mph

Abbreviation: MVC = motor vehicle crash.

chest wall segment (flail chest); sucking chest wound; fractured sternum; and absence of breath sounds on either side of the chest (simple or tension pneumothorax, massive hemothorax, or right mainstem intubation). Any of these findings warrants immediate intervention, including needle thoracostomy for tension pneumothorax (see the section "Needle Decompression" in chapter 68, "Pneumothorax"); insertion of large-bore chest tubes (36-F) to relieve hemopneumothorax (see chapter 261, "Pulmonary Trauma"); and application of an occlusive dressing to a sucking chest wound. For asymmetric or absent breath sounds in the intubated patient, partially withdraw the endotracheal tube from the right mainstem bronchus or reintubate. If no breath sounds are heard, and if massive hemothorax or vascular injury is suspected (initial chest tube output of >1000 mL, or >200 mL/h), a thoracotomy or video-assisted thoracic surgery is indicated to identify and control the source of bleeding.

CIRCULATION AND HEMORRHAGE CONTROL

Assessment of the patient's overall hemodynamic status is critical. This assessment includes evaluation of level of consciousness, skin color, and presence and magnitude of peripheral pulses. Note the heart rate and pulse pressure (systolic minus diastolic blood pressure), particularly in young, previously healthy trauma patients.

As part of the primary survey in the prehospital and hospital settings, identify and control external hemorrhage. Apply direct pressure, a compression bandage, or a hemostatic dressing to control active external bleeding. QuikClot Combat Gauze is a kaolin-impregnated rayon and polyester hemostatic dressing that is safe and effective for arterial or venous bleeding.[2,7] For exsanguinating extremity injury, apply a tourniquet (see "Tourniquets"). Prehospital use of tourniquets on the battlefield has become commonplace. With aggressive tourniquet use, death rates from isolated limb exsanguination in Iraq dropped to 2% compared to 9% in the Vietnam War.[8]

Tourniquets

Robert L. Mabry

More than a decade of combat operations in Afghanistan and Iraq have provided the opportunity to evaluate methods for minimizing morbidity and mortality from traumatic injury. One of the greatest advances in the prevention of death on the modern battlefield is the rediscovery of the tourniquet.[9] During the war in Vietnam, tourniquet application was generally felt to be a technique of last resort.[10] The myth arguing against tourniquet use was primarily based on World War I and II experiences when evacuation to definitive care took many hours, and tourniquets were felt to increase ischemia in an already vulnerable extremity.

However, proper tourniquet application, coupled with rapid transport times to definitive care, can be life- and limb-saving in military and civilian settings.[7] Tourniquets saved lives at the Boston Marathon bombing, and as a result, the Boston Police Department and Boston EMS now carry tourniquets.[11-13]

Civilian tourniquet use is based on the military Tactical Combat Casualty Care guidelines for first responder care in the battlefield. Tourniquet use is a key component to Tactical Combat Casualty Care.

The Tactical Combat Casualty Care guidelines currently recommend three different tourniquets[14]: the Combat Application Tourniquet (C-A-T®), the SOF Tactical Tourniquet (SOF TT®), and the Emergency and Military Tourniquet (EMT®). The C-A-T® (**Figure 1**) is a lightweight windlass tourniquet, which can be applied with one hand. The SOF TT® (**Figure 2**) is another windlass tourniquet. The EMT® (**Figure 3**) is a pneumatic device, which carries the disadvantage of potential tourniquet failure if it were to be damaged or punctured by debris. Do not use narrow, elastic, or bungee-type tourniquets.[7]

If direct pressure is ineffective or impractical in controlling external bleeding, apply the tourniquet directly to the skin or over clothing, 2 to 3 inches above the wound. Tighten the tourniquet to eliminate the distal pulse. Do not release the tourniquet until the patient reaches definitive care and there is a positive response to resuscitation efforts.

The Tactical Combat Casualty Care guidelines recommend the application of a junctional tourniquet (SAM JT®) (**Figure 4**) if the bleeding site is appropriate (groin or axilla, where the torso meets the extremities) and the application of a hemostatic dressing with pressure has no effect.[14] However, as of this writing, the American College of Surgeons Committee on Trauma has not provided recommendations for the application of junctional tourniquets in the civilian environment.[7]

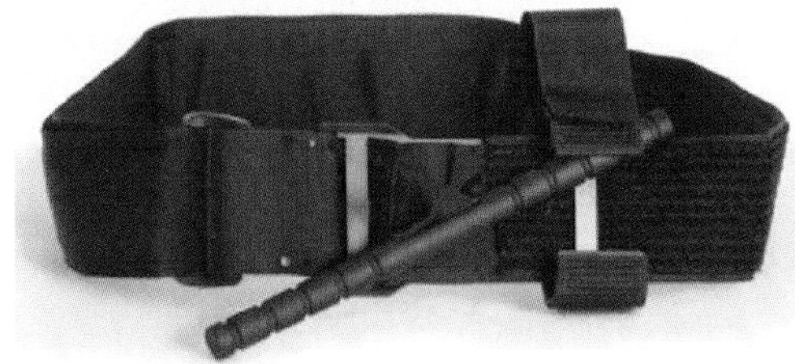

FIGURE 1. C-A-T®.

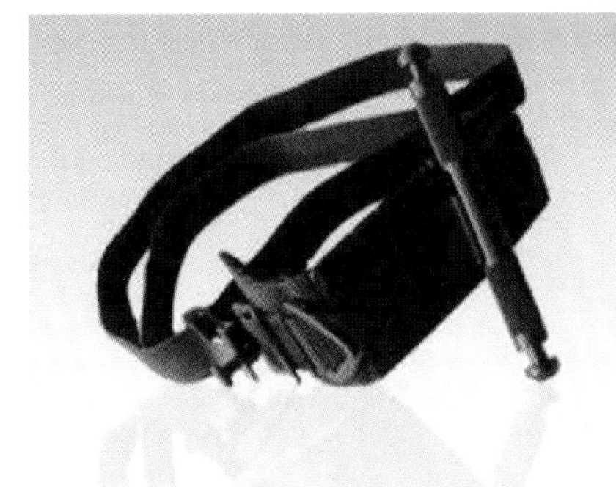

FIGURE 2. SOF TT®.

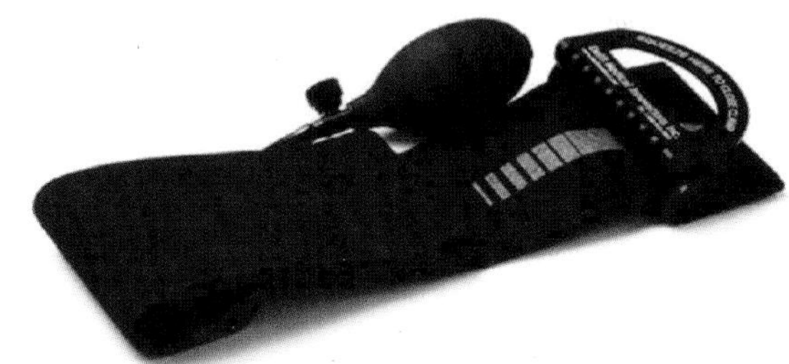

FIGURE 3. EMT®.

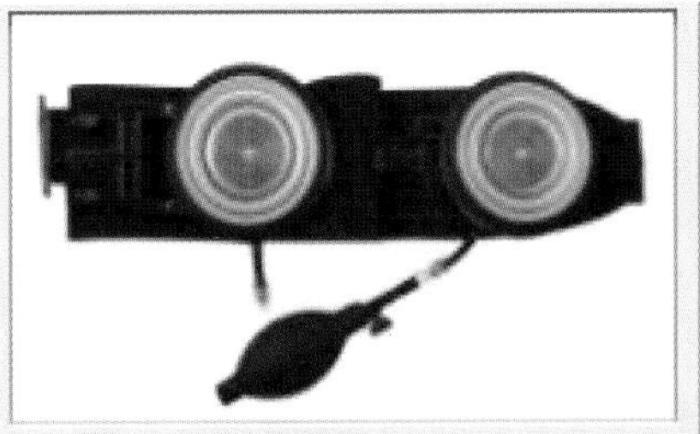

FIGURE 4. SAM-JT junctional tourniquet (internal view).

Pre-Hospital Trauma Triage Criteria
Adult/Pediatrics

Indications: Trauma patients who meet any of the following criteria shall be transported to the closest appropriate trauma center within a 30-minute ground transport time. Trauma patients who are not within 30 minutes ground transport time of a trauma center should be transported to the closest hospital if they cannot be delivered to an appropriate facility more rapidly by air ambulance.

Physiologic Criteria
- Glascow Coma Scale less than 14, or
- Systolic blood pressure of less than 90 mm/Hg, or
- Respiratory rate of less than 10 or greater than 29 breaths per minute (less than 20 breaths per minute in infants less than 1 year old)

Anatomic Criteria
- Penetrating injuries to head, neck, torso and extremities proximal to elbow or knee
- Flail Chest
- 2 or more proximal long bone fracures
- Crushed, degloved or mangled extremity
- Amputation proximal to wrist or ankle
- Pelvic fractures
- Open or depressed skull fractures
- Paralysis

Mechanism of Injury
- **Falls**
  - Adults – greater than 20 feet
  - Children less than 15 years old – greater than 10 feet, or 2-3 times the child's height
- **High-risk auto crash**
  - Intrusion- more than 12 inches to the occupant site or more than 18 inches to any site
  - Ejection (partial or complete) from automobile
  - Death in the same passenger compartment
  - Vehicle telemetry data consistent with high risk of injury
- **Auto versus pedestrian / bicyclists**- thrown, run over or with significant (greater than 20 mph) impact
- **Motorcycle crash** at speed greater than 20 mph
- **Special Considerations**
- **Burns** (with or without other trauma) – absent other trauma, burns that meet Burn Center criteria should be transported to a burn center
- **Pregnancy**- Injured women who are more than 20 weeks pregnant should be considered for transport to a trauma center or a hospital with obstetrical resources
- **Age** – greater than 55 years of age
- **Anticoagulation and Bleeding Disorders** – EMS should contact medical control and consider transport to trauma center
- **Time- Sensitive Extremity Injury** – open fracture(s) or fracture(s) with neurovascular compromise
- **EMS Provider Judgment** – EMS provides, based on experience and expertise, may always exercise clinical judgment regarding atypical patient presentations

FIGURE 254-2. Current Tidewater EMS (Norfolk, VA) prehospital trauma triage guidelines. [Photo contributed by Current Tidewater EMS (Norfolk, VA) Prehospital Trauma Triage Guidelines.]

CIRCULATION

Any hypotensive trauma patient is at risk for development of hemorrhagic shock, a common cause of postinjury death. One system is commonly used for classifying the degree of hemorrhage (**Table 254-6**), although it has not been validated and there is wide variability in individual patient response to hypovolemia. Hemorrhage and shock are on a continuum, and some patients can compensate for significant blood loss better than others. Hemorrhage of up to 30% of total blood volume may be associated with only mild tachycardia and a decrease in pulse pressure, but may quickly progress to profound hypoperfusion and decompensated shock if not recognized early. Be aware that medications, such as β-blockers, can mask early hemodynamic indicators of shock.

Establish two large-bore IV lines (18 gauge or larger), infuse lactated Ringer's or normal saline, and obtain blood samples or specimens for laboratory studies, particularly blood type and screen. In patients who are in unstable condition or in whom upper extremity peripheral veins are not easily cannulated, establish central venous access via the subclavian, internal jugular, or femoral vein. Avoid placement of a central venous line distal to a potential venous injury. Intraosseous access is an alternative technique for providing rapid vascular access in difficult clinical situations. Most medications including blood products can be administered through the interosseous route. Use a pressure bag to maximize flow rates. Decades of study have failed to demonstrate an advantage of colloid therapy over crystalloid infusion. Therefore, a balanced salt crystalloid (normal saline or lactated Ringer's) is the fluid of choice for initial resuscitation. There is some theoretical advantage of lactated Ringer's over saline when large volumes are given in order to avoid hyperchloremic acidosis, although this is unlikely to be significant for most patients during initial resuscitation.

Reassess hypotensive patients without an obvious indication for surgery after rapid infusion of 2 L of crystalloid solution (lactated Ringer's or normal saline). If there is no marked improvement, then transfuse type O blood (O-negative for females of childbearing age). Aggressive volume resuscitation is not a substitute for definitive hemorrhage control. A full discussion of the long-standing controversies over volume, timing, and composition of fluid resuscitation is beyond the scope of this chapter. One major study demonstrated higher mortality in patients receiving immediate IV fluid resuscitation than in those from whom fluid was

TABLE 254-3 Primary and Secondary Survey in Trauma Resuscitation

Primary Survey (rapid identification and management of immediately life-threatening injuries)

A. Airway and cervical spine

Assess, clear, and protect airway: jaw thrust/chin lift, suctioning.

Perform endotracheal intubation with in-line stabilization for patient with depressed level of consciousness or inability to protect airway.

Create surgical airway if there is significant bleeding or obstruction or laryngoscopy cannot be performed.

B. Breathing

Ventilate with 100% oxygen; monitor oxygen saturation.

Auscultate for breath sounds.

Inspect thorax and neck for deviated trachea, open chest wounds, abnormal chest wall motion, and crepitus at neck or chest.

Consider immediate needle thoracostomy for suspected tension pneumothorax.

Consider tube thoracostomy for suspected hemopneumothorax.

C. Circulation

Assess for blood volume status: skin color, capillary refill, radial/femoral/carotid pulse, and blood pressure.

Place two large-bore peripheral IV catheters.

Begin rapid infusion of warm crystalloid solution, if indicated.

Apply direct pressure to sites of brisk external bleeding.

Consider central venous or interosseous access if peripheral sites are unavailable.

Consider pericardiocentesis for suspected pericardial tamponade.

Consider left lateral decubitus position in late-trimester pregnancy.

D. Disability

Perform screening neurologic and mental status examination, assessing:

- Pupil size and reactivity
- Limb strength and movement, grip strength
- Orientation, Glasgow coma scale score

Consider measurement of capillary blood glucose level in patients with altered mental status.

E. Exposure

Completely disrobe the patient, and inspect for burns and toxic exposures.

Logroll patient, maintaining neutral position and in-line neck stabilization, to inspect and palpate thoracic spine, flank, back, and buttocks.

Secondary Survey (head-to-toe examination for rapid identification and control of injuries or potential instability)

Identify and control scalp wound bleeding with direct pressure, sutures, or surgical clips.

Identify facial instability and potential for airway instability.

Identify hemotympanum.

Identify epistaxis or septal hematoma; consider tamponade or airway control if bleeding is profuse.

Identify avulsed teeth or jaw instability.

Evaluate for abdominal distention and tenderness.

Identify penetrating chest, back, flank, or abdominal injuries.

Assess for pelvic stability; consider pelvic wrap or sling.

Inspect perineum for laceration or hematoma.

Inspect urethral meatus for blood.

Consider rectal examination for sphincter tone and gross blood.

Assess peripheral pulses for vascular compromise.

Identify extremity deformities, and immobilize open and closed fractures and dislocations.

withheld until operative intervention. The study speculated that aggressive fluid resuscitation before operative control of bleeding was harmful.[15]

Patients requiring massive transfusions generally require urgent surgical intervention to control hemorrhage. A well-defined source of bleeding may be evident on external examination, assessment of chest tube output, extended FAST examination (**Figure 254-3**), or conventional or

TABLE 254-4 NEXUS (National Emergency X-Radiography Utilization Study) Criteria for Omitting Cervical Spinal Imaging*

No posterior midline cervical spine tenderness

No evidence of intoxication

Alert mental status

No focal neurologic deficits

No painful distracting injuries

*Failure to meet any one criterion indicates need for cervical spine imaging.

TABLE 254-5 Canadian Cervical Spine Rule

Any high-risk factor that mandates radiography? (Age >64 y or dangerous mechanism or paresthesias in extremities) **No**	**If Yes, radiography indicated**
Any low-risk factor that allows safe assessment of range of motion? (Simple rear-end collision or sitting position in the ED or ambulatory at any time or delayed onset of neck pain or absence of midline cervical spine tenderness) **Yes**	**If No, radiography indicated**
Able to rotate neck actively? (45 degrees left and right) **Yes**	**If No, radiography indicated**
No radiography indicated	

TABLE 254-6 Classification of Hemorrhage Based on Estimated Blood Loss at Initial Presentation

	Class I	Class II	Class III	Class IV
Blood loss (mL)*	Up to 750	750–1500	1500–2000	>2000
Blood loss (% blood volume)	Up to 15	15–30	30–40	40
Pulse rate (beats/min)	<100	100–120	120–140	>140
Blood pressure	Normal	Normal	Decreased	Decreased
Pulse pressure	Normal or increased	Decreased	Decreased	Decreased

*Assumes a 70-kg patient with a preinjury circulating blood volume of 5 L.

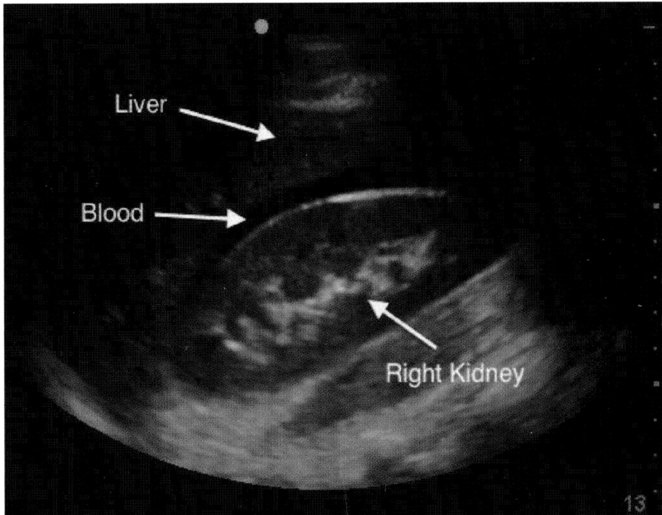

FIGURE 254-3. Positive extended FAST exam with blood identified in Morison's pouch. [Photo contributed by Barry Knapp, MD.]

CT imaging of the chest or abdomen. There may also be considerable blood loss from blunt trauma to the pelvis and limbs without a discrete source. Immobilize open pelvic fractures in a pelvic wrap or sling and reduce and immobilize limb fractures to tamponade bleeding from fractured bone ends.

Major trauma patients may develop a bleeding diathesis almost from the time of injury, which results in defective clotting and platelet function. Data from both military and civilian experience reveal that patients receiving >10 units of packed red blood cells showed decreased mortality when they simultaneously receive fresh frozen plasma in a ratio of packed red blood cells to fresh frozen plasma of 1:1 rather than 1:4 (26% vs 87.5% mortality, respectively).[16] Another consensus article examining use of blood products worldwide supported the administration of platelets in massive transfusion protocol in a 1:1:1 ratio with packed red blood cells and fresh frozen plasma.[17] Both acidosis and hypothermia contribute to the coagulopathy and should be corrected as quickly as possible.

TRANEXAMIC ACID

Tranexamic acid is an antifibrinolytic agent that reduces blood loss after surgery and may reduce blood loss after traumatic injury. It prevents cleavage of plasmin and degradation of fibrin. It is on the World Health Organization list of essential medications affecting coagulation.[18] Studies involving >20,000 patients reported a risk reduction of death from bleeding of 10% to 15%. There was no reported difference in risk of death from myocardial infarction, vascular occlusion, stroke, pulmonary embolism, mutiorgan failure, or head injury.[19] Criticism of CRASH-2 was that the patient populations studied were heterogeneous in terms of injury and were in low- to middle-income countries with basic and very limited resources for major trauma management.[20] For these and other reasons, major Western nation trauma centers have not rushed to adopt the use of tranexamic acid in trauma management algorithms.[21] Nevertheless, the evidence to date indicates that tranexamic acid may reduce mortality without significant adverse side effects when given as early as possible after injury, with administration within 1 hour of injury reported to decrease the relative risk of death from bleeding by 32% and within 1 to 3 hours by 21%.[22] Administration of tranexamic acid more than 3 hours after injury is less effective and potentially harmful.[19] Tranexamic acid must be given before transfer/arrival to a trauma center in order to meet the time requirement of early administration.[20] The dose is 1 gram of tranexamic acid IV bolus over 10 minutes, followed by 1 gram IV over 8 hours.

DISABILITY

Once airway, breathing, and circulation have been addressed and stabilized, perform a focused neurologic evaluation to assess level of consciousness, pupillary size and reactivity, and motor function. Assess the Glasgow coma scale (see chapter 257, "Head Trauma"). A search for the cause of depressed level of consciousness should include measurement of capillary blood glucose level and consideration of possible intoxicants. Despite the concomitant use of drugs and alcohol in many trauma patients, do not simply attribute altered mental status in the setting of trauma to intoxication. Assume that a patient with an appropriate mechanism for head trauma and with altered mental status or a Glasgow coma scale score of <15 has a significant head injury until proven otherwise. **The Glasgow coma scale assessment can be insensitive in patients with normal or near-normal scores, and a Glasgow coma scale score of 15 does not completely exclude the presence of traumatic brain injury.** However, patients with a persistent Glasgow coma scale score of ≤8 generally have a graver prognosis; secure a definitive airway to protect against aspiration or asphyxia. Direct efforts toward resuscitating brain-injured patients in order to maintain normal cerebral perfusion. Monitor serum glucose levels and maintain euglycemia. Mild hyperventilation may reduce intracranial pressure, although at the expense of cerebral vasoconstriction and hypoperfusion. Avoid hyperventilation during the first 24 hours after injury when cerebral blood flow is often critically reduced. **Prophylactic hyperventilation (partial pressure of arterial carbon dioxide of 25 mm Hg or less) is not recommended.**[23]

EXPOSURE

No primary survey is complete without completely disrobing the patient and examining carefully for occult bruising, lacerations, impaled foreign bodies, and open fractures. After completing the primary survey, logroll the patient, with one team member assigned to maintain in-line cervical stabilization. **Palpate the spinous processes of the thoracic and lumbar spine for tenderness or deformity, and then carefully logroll the patient back to a neutral position.** The utility of routine rectal examination is debated, but it is useful to identify gross rectal bleeding or loss of rectal tone in patients with suspected spinal injury. Examine the perineum for bruising, laceration, or bleeding. Cover the patient with warm blankets to prevent heat loss. Some have advocated the use of hypothermia in cases of severe brain injury. However, as of this writing, there is no conclusive evidence in favor of this therapy. Potential therapeutic benefits must be weighed against the coagulopathy and increased bleeding that hypothermia also causes in trauma patients.

SPECIFIC INJURIES OF IMPORTANCE

Place special emphasis on identifying the injuries described in the following sections during the primary survey, because they can be rapidly fatal if not recognized and treated.

SEVERE HEAD AND SPINAL TRAUMA

Rapidly assess neurologic status in patients with suspected traumatic brain injury. **To quickly identify patients with intracranial injuries who may benefit from operative treatment, defer any procedures that do not correct a specific problem discovered during the primary survey until after the head CT is performed.** In patients requiring intubation, provide in-line immobilization when the cervical collar is removed during intubation, and then reapply after intubation. Obtain a chest radiograph to assess endotracheal tube placement and exclude pneumothorax. The use of US to rapidly confirm endotracheal tube placement and exclude large pneumothorax is also an option.

TENSION PNEUMOTHORAX, OPEN PNEUMOTHORAX, AND MASSIVE HEMOTHORAX

Tension pneumothorax, open pneumothorax, and massive hemothorax all should be readily apparent during the primary survey. If tension pneumothorax is clinically suspected, immediately perform tube thoracostomy. If equipment is not immediately available, needle thoracostomy can be a temporizing measure. Delays in diagnosis and treatment (including awaiting confirmatory chest x-ray) can result in complete hemodynamic collapse. In equivocal cases, US can confirm the presence of pneumothorax and prompt emergent intervention. Perform tube thoracostomy in a timely manner in patients with a significant pneumo- or hemithorax, as determined by US, chest x-ray, or CT (see chapter 261).

PENETRATING ABDOMINAL TRAUMA

Abdominal tenderness or distention on palpation, coupled with hypotension, indicates the emergent need for exploratory laparotomy in a patient who has sustained a penetrating abdominal injury; this should prompt immediate transport to the operating room. Early operative intervention in patients experiencing penetrating trauma who are in shock results in better outcomes. Placement of nasogastric, urinary, and

IV catheters may proceed in the ED only if they do not delay definitive operative intervention. Otherwise, these procedures should take place in the operating room as the patient is being prepared for general anesthesia. In the setting of a penetrating gunshot wound to the abdomen, diagnostic imaging (US, CT) is rarely indicated because almost all cases undergo emergent exploratory laparotomy.

IMPALED OBJECTS

Objects deeply impaled in the chest and abdomen should be left in place and the patient emergently transported to the operating room for surgical removal under direct visualization to ensure vascular control and hemostasis. The impaled object may be cut or shortened outside the skin to facilitate transport.[24]

TRAUMATIC CARDIAC ARREST

Unless obvious signs of death are present in the field, providers in most emergency medical systems continue to transport patients without pulse or respiration to a hospital once cardiopulmonary resuscitation has been initiated. For patients in traumatic arrest upon arrival to the ED, a critical decision must be made regarding the appropriate level of intervention and, specifically, the use of emergent thoracotomy. One study analyzing 862 patients undergoing ED thoracotomy at a regional trauma center showed that the proportion of neurologically intact survivors was 3.9%. The best outcomes were in patients with stab wounds to the chest. Further analysis revealed that the survival rate was 23% among thoracic stab wound victims who showed breathing or pulse in the field and 38% among those who were moribund but had some indication of respiration or pulse on arrival to the ED. Therefore, **the strongest recommendation for performing ED thoracotomy can be made for patients with penetrating chest trauma with witnessed signs of life during transport to or in the ED and at least cardiac electrical activity upon arrival.**[25-27] There were no survivors among patients with blunt trauma and no respiration or pulse in the field. ED thoracotomy for this group is not indicated (including in the presence of myocardial electrical activity) (**Table 254-7**).[4]

An extended FAST examination performed upon arrival can be useful in identifying cardiac tamponade or the absence of ongoing cardiac activity and can prevent an unnecessary ED thoracotomy.

SECONDARY SURVEY

The secondary survey is a rapid but thorough head-to-toe examination for injuries (Table 254-3). Do not start the secondary survey until basic functions have been corrected in conjunction with the primary survey (airway, breathing, circulation, disability, exposure) and resuscitation has been initiated. The secondary survey can help set priorities for ongoing evaluation and management. Frequent reassessment of the patient's blood pressure, pulse rate, and response to interventions should continue during this period.

Scalp lacerations can bleed profusely. Bleeding can be controlled with plastic Raney clips (see chapter 42, "Face and Scalp Lacerations") or staples that grasp the full thickness of the scalp. Inspect the tympanic membranes for hemotympanum and repeat the pupil examination. Repeat the examination of the neck and thorax for any changes. When there is facial trauma or evidence of basilar skull fracture, insert the gastric tube through the mouth rather than the nose.

Inspect the urinary meatus, scrotum, and perineum for the presence of blood, hematoma, or laceration. Perform a rectal examination, noting sphincter tone, gross blood, and prostatic bogginess or displacement. The rectal examination is no longer routinely performed in alert patients without evidence of pelvic or spinal injury. If the prostate is normal and there is no blood at the urethral meatus, a urinary catheter can be placed in the bladder. **If meatal blood is present or the prostate is displaced, which suggests a urethral injury, perform retrograde urethrography before inserting a Foley catheter.** If there is vaginal bleeding, perform a manual and speculum examination to identify a possible vaginal laceration in the presence of a pelvic fracture. Evaluate the extremities for fracture and soft tissue injury, with attention to peripheral pulses. Perform a more thorough neurologic examination, carefully checking motor and sensory function.

Certain conditions are typically not evident during the secondary survey unless specifically sought. Injuries to the esophagus, diaphragm, and small bowel often remain undiagnosed, even with diligent examination, and further imaging and hospital observation for delayed presentation may be required. The most frequently missed conditions are orthopedic. Careful consideration of orthopedic extremity injuries is essential in patients with multisystem trauma. A tertiary survey has been recommended in patients with multisystem trauma within the first 24 hours to lessen the risk of missed injury.[28]

TABLE 254-7 Indications for ED Thoracotomy upon Arrival to ED

Penetrating Thoracic Trauma	
CPR (pulseless) with signs of life (Signs of life include reactive pupils, spontaneous movement, or myocardial electrical activity)	Consider ED thoracotomy
CPR (pulseless) without signs of life	No further resuscitative efforts indicated
Blunt Trauma	
CPR (pulseless) with myocardial electrical activity	No further resuscitative efforts indicated

IMAGING AND LABORATORY TESTING

For patients who are not rapidly transported to the operating room or CT suite after the initial assessment, standard radiographic imaging may include cervical spine, chest, and pelvic radiographs. The chest and pelvic radiographs image regions outside the peritoneal cavity that can accommodate volumes of blood sufficient to produce hypotension and shock. In patients with gunshot wounds to the torso, a chest radiograph is required, with or without abdominal films, depending on the site of injury.

The **extended FAST** examination is a rapid and effective screening tool for the identification of major intraperitoneal bleeding, pericardial tamponade, pneumothorax, and hemothorax as the source of hypotension or shock.[29] It should be performed to identify causes of shock immediately after the primary survey (Figure 254-3). Perform a CT scan with IV contrast for definitive imaging of the abdomen. Obtain appropriate extremity radiographs to exclude fractures as directed by the physical examination findings.

In obtunded patients or those with multisystem trauma, consider imaging of the **entire spine** if the mechanism of injury warrants it. In patients undergoing head CT, most EDs perform cervical spine CT at the same time. If chest and abdominal CTs are performed, CT images of the thoracic and lumbar spines can be reconstructed.

The liberal use of CT scanning in the setting of traumatic injury has the potential to detect injuries that are not clinically apparent. In one study of cooperative patients with no obvious signs of chest or abdominal injury, this "pan scan" method identified clinically significant abnormalities in 4% of head CT scans, 5% of cervical spine CT scans, 20% of chest CT scans, and 7% of abdominal CT scans. Overall treatment was changed in 19% of patients.[30] This approach should be balanced by the estimation that approximately 29,000 future cancers could be related to CT scans performed in the United States in 2007 alone.[31] Children represent a subgroup that deserve special consideration because exposure to radiation in childhood significantly increases the incidence of cancer later in life.[32] **In younger patients in whom the clinical indication for CT scan may be equivocal, avoid the use of ionizing radiation whenever possible.** In general, use clinical judgment to direct focused application of diagnostic imaging.

Routine laboratory studies often include blood type and screen, hemoglobin level, urine dipstick testing for blood, and ethanol level. In women of childbearing age, always perform a pregnancy test. Check capillary blood glucose level in patients with altered mental status or a history of diabetes mellitus. In patients older than 55 years, consider obtaining an ECG and measuring levels of markers for cardiac ischemia, such as troponin I.

DISPOSITION AND FOLLOW-UP

Expeditiously transport patients with hemodynamic instability and ongoing bleeding to the operating room or transfer the patient to another facility with appropriate surgical or critical care resources. Complete a rapid but thorough primary and secondary survey prior to transfer. In most urban Level 1 trauma centers, the trauma surgeon will have been present for the primary and secondary surveys. In rural hospitals that transfer the most severely injured trauma patients, the resuscitating physician should relate all the physical findings discovered during the primary and secondary surveys to the physician receiving the patient. Laboratory results, imaging studies, and the chronologic record of the patient's blood pressure, pulse, fluids infused, urine output, gastric output, and neurologic findings should accompany the patient. Personnel capable of performing ongoing resuscitation of the patient should accompany a patient transported to another facility.

Serial examinations are essential for patients without clear indications for surgery identified on initial assessment. Patients may be admitted to the hospital or an ED observation unit. Blunt abdominal injuries such as those involving the pancreas and bowel may not be readily apparent on initial CT. These injuries may become clinically apparent upon serial examinations. In addition, consider admission or observation for patients with closed head trauma who have normal levels of consciousness and require repeat neurologic examinations as well as patients at risk for delayed pneumothorax or pulmonary contusion that require repeat chest radiography.

REFERENCES

The complete reference list is available online at www.TintinalliEM.com.

CHAPTER 255 Trauma in the Elderly

Ross J. Fleischman
O. John Ma

INTRODUCTION AND EPIDEMIOLOGY

The elderly have worse outcomes following trauma because of physiologic changes that occur with aging. They are more susceptible to serious injury from low-energy mechanisms, less able to compensate from the stress of injury, and more likely to suffer complications during treatment and recovery. Emergency physicians should have a higher suspicion for injury and lower threshold for diagnostic testing and admission than in younger patients.

Studies have variously defined the lower limits of the geriatric age group to be as young as 55 years and as old as 80 years. Some have shown mortality to increase with individuals as young as 45 years of age.[1] Regardless of the definition, caring for injured elders constitutes a large and growing portion of emergency medicine practice. The U.S. Census Bureau projects that those ≥65 years old will increase from 13% to 16% of the population by 2020 and to 20% by 2040.[2,3] Geriatric patients represented 12% of the population in the Major Trauma Outcomes Study.[4] Although the elderly are less likely to be involved in trauma, they are more likely to have fatal outcomes when injured, with a mortality rate twice that of younger patients. Those age 65 years and older consumed a disproportionate share of trauma hospitalizations (23%) and trauma costs (28%) relative to the 12% of the U.S. population they comprised in 1985.[5]

PATHOPHYSIOLOGY

Part of the difficulty in describing the elderly population derives from the discrepancy between chronologic and physiologic age. Chronologic age is the actual number of years the individual has lived, whereas physiologic age describes the functional capacity of the patient's organ systems. Studies have shown a clear association between age and mortality. Comorbid diseases have been shown to be associated with increased mortality after minor and moderate injuries in all age groups.[6]

The physiologic changes of aging complicate recovery from injury and make assessment of injury more difficult. With age, myocytes are lost and replaced by collagen. This results in decreased contractility and compliance for any given preload.[7] An 80-year-old person will have approximately 50% of the cardiac output of a 20-year-old, even without significant atherosclerotic coronary artery disease. Maximal heart rate and cardiac output decrease with age. Aging myocardium has a decreased chronotropic response to catecholamines and is dependent on preload (intravascular volume); hypovolemia can easily result in shock. Deterioration of the cardiac conduction system leads to atrial fibrillation and bundle-branch blocks. Medications, especially digoxin, β-blockers, and calcium channel blockers, impair the tachycardic response to catecholamines, both impairing the body's inability to compensate for hemorrhage and making heart rate an unreliable predictor of hypovolemia.

Chest wall compliance, respiratory muscle strength, and the capacity for oxygen exchange all decrease with age. The response to hypoxia may decline by 50% and that to hypercarbia by 40%, such that the patient may not appear to be in respiratory distress despite impending respiratory failure.[8] Because of weakened respiratory muscles and degenerative changes in the chest wall, maximum inspiratory and expiratory force may be decreased by up to 50% compared with younger patients. Age-related reductions in vital capacity, functional residual capacity, and forced expiratory volume can limit older patients' ability to compensate for chest injuries.

Renal function declines with age, predisposing patients to dehydration, requiring medication dose adjustments based on calculated creatinine clearance, and making them susceptible to contrast-induced nephropathy.

COMMON MECHANISMS OF INJURY

Falls Falls are the most common cause of fatal and nonfatal injury in people ≥65 years of age.[9,10] One third of older adults fall annually, and the rate of falls increases with age. Hip fractures are the most common fracture in elders hospitalized for injury, but the overall incidence of nonhip, nonspine fractures in women >55 years old is five times greater than hip fractures.[11,12] There are age-related changes in postural stability, balance, motor strength, coordination, and reaction time that make the elderly more prone to tripping and falling. Other causes of falls in the elderly are listed in **Table 255-1**. Bathroom falls are concerning because hard bathroom surfaces can result in head and spinal injuries, and slippery surfaces can cause falls. Falls on stairs involve higher energy and potential for injury than those on flat ground. Falls in which an individual is unable to get help for a prolonged period should prompt investigation for rhabdomyolysis and dehydration with a check of the creatinine kinase and electrolytes.

Motor Vehicle Crashes Motor vehicle crashes are the second most common cause of injury in the elderly and are the leading cause of death, with a case fatality rate twice that of those under 65 years.[4] The elderly make up 17% of U.S. traffic fatalities.[13]

Pedestrian–Motor Vehicle Collisions The elderly are second only to children as victims of pedestrian–motor vehicle collisions. Those ≥65 years old account for 19% of pedestrian–automobile fatalities in the United States.[14] Pedestrian–motor vehicle collisions are one of the most lethal mechanisms of injury in this age group, with a 53% case fatality rate.

Burns There is a direct relationship between age and burn mortality, as evidenced by the traditionally taught **Baux score**, in which the sum of age and body surface area burned yield the percentage likelihood of mortality. Although the Baux score still has prognostic value, advances in

TABLE 255-1 Common Causes of Falls in the Elderly

Associated with syncope/loss of consciousness
Dysrhythmias
Seizures
Acute coronary syndrome
Hypoglycemia
Pulmonary embolism
Associated with near-syncope, positional change, vasodilation (e.g., hot water)
Antihypertensive medications (especially β-blockers, calcium channel blockers)
Dehydration, diuretic medications
Hemorrhage (GI bleed, abdominal aortic aneurysm)
Hot bath or shower
Sepsis
Anemia
Nonsyncopal, "mechanical" causes
Deconditioning
Decreased visual acuity
Unsafe home conditions (e.g., poor lighting, loose rugs)
Alcohol
Sedating medications (narcotics, benzodiazepines, antihistamines, sleep aids)
Neurologic disease (cerebrovascular attack, Parkinson's disease)

critical care and burn treatment have raised the point of futility of treatment to a Baux score of 160 (rather than 100) and a 50% risk of mortality to a Baux score of 110.[15] In patients >65 years old, a 50% mortality is anticipated with a body surface area of burn of 28%. The presence of inhalation injury adds the equivalent of 17 years or points of body surface area burned to the predictive score.[16]

Elder Abuse Maintain a high suspicion for intentional injuries and injuries caused by neglect. Warning signs include poor hygiene, untreated decubitus ulcers, injuries not explained by the reported mechanism, and subacute injuries in various stages of healing.

CLINICAL FEATURES

HISTORY

Treat injured elders as both trauma and medical patients. Ask the patient, family, and prehospital care providers about the exact events leading up to the injury. Avoid skipping the review of systems, past medical history, and medications list. **Investigating the cause of a fall may uncover serious underlying medical causes or prevent future trauma.**

PRIMARY SURVEY

Avoid feeling reassured by "normal" vital signs. A tachycardic response to pain, hypovolemia, or anxiety may be absent or blunted in the elderly trauma patient. Medications such as β-blockers may mask tachycardia and hinder the evaluation of the elderly patient. One study demonstrated that eight of 15 geriatric blunt trauma patients initially considered to be hemodynamically "stable" had cardiac outputs <3.5 L/min, and none had an adequate response to volume loading. Of seven patients with normal cardiac outputs, five had inadequate oxygen delivery.[17] Another study reported that 39% of patients with a systolic blood pressure >90 mm Hg and heart rate <120 beats/min had occult hypoperfusion, defined by lactate >2.2 or base deficit less than −2.[18] The elderly also have blunted responses to hypoxia, hypercarbia, and acidosis, which can mask the signs of respiratory failure.

Blood pressures are also misleading in the elderly patient. Because of the high incidence of underlying hypertension approaching 90%, the clinician must use a higher cutoff for hypotension than in younger patients. **In blunt trauma patients ≥65 years old, there is an association between hypotension and mortality starting with systolic blood pressures below 110 mm Hg and heart rates above 90 beats/min.** Therefore, it is reasonable to use these more conservative cutoffs as markers of abnormal vital signs.[19] A decrease in blood pressure of 30 mm Hg below a known baseline or a falling trend is also a marker of instability.

Remain highly concerned about the elderly patient with abnormal vital signs. One study found that geriatric trauma patients with a respiratory rate <10 breaths/min had 100% mortality.[20] Likewise, a systolic blood pressure <90 mm Hg in the elderly blunt trauma patient is associated with a mortality between 82% and 100%.[21]

Anatomic variations may complicate airway management. These include the presence of dentures (which may occlude the airway and make laryngoscopy more difficult), cervical arthritis (which adds danger to extending the neck), or temporomandibular joint arthritis (which may limit mouth opening).

SECONDARY SURVEY

A thorough secondary survey is essential to uncover less serious injuries. **Patients with no apparent life-threatening injuries can have potentially fatal injuries if there is some degree of limited physiologic reserve.** Seemingly stable geriatric trauma patients can deteriorate rapidly and without warning. Undertake a medication review early in the patient's evaluation, paying particular attention to medications that affect heart rate, blood pressure, and coagulation.

DIAGNOSIS

HEAD INJURY

Head injuries in the elderly cause almost 142,000 United States ED visits resulting in discharge, 82,000 survivable hospitalizations, and 14,000 deaths annually.[22] Age is an independent predictor for morbidity and mortality in patients with moderate or severe head trauma. When evaluating the patient's mental status, it would be a grave error to assume that alterations in mental status are due solely to dementia or senility.

Elders are less prone to develop **epidural hematomas** than the general population because of the denser fibrous bond between the dura mater and the inner table of the skull. There is, however, a higher incidence of **subdural** and **intraparenchymal hematomas** in the elderly than in younger patients. As the brain mass decreases with age, there is greater stretching and tension of the bridging veins that pass from the brain to the dural sinuses. Bridging veins are more susceptible to traumatic tears. Diagnosis of intracranial bleeding may be delayed because brain atrophy increases intracranial free space, allowing blood to accumulate without initial signs or symptoms.

One study of blunt head trauma patients taking warfarin who were experiencing no or minimal symptoms found a rate of injury on head CT that changed disposition in 7%.[23] Therefore, **immediate noncontrast head CT is recommended for patients who take warfarin and have a mechanism of injury concerning for even a minor head injury**. Check the INR, because the degree of anticoagulation correlates with the risk of adverse outcomes.[24] The risk conferred by other anticoagulant medications is less known. Some studies have shown the antiplatelet medication clopidogrel to confer an increased risk of intracranial bleeding after head injury.[25] There is insufficient evidence to delineate the risk conferred by aspirin, low-molecular-weight heparins, or the newer oral anticoagulants.[26,27]

CERVICAL SPINAL INJURIES

The incidence of cervical spine injury is about twice as great in elders as in a younger cohort of blunt trauma patients. Odontoid fractures are particularly common in geriatric patients, accounting for 20% of geriatric cervical spine fractures, as compared with 5% of nongeriatric fractures.[28] Preexisting cervical spine pathology, such as osteoarthritis, bulging discs, and osteoporosis, may predispose elderly patients to spinal cord injuries. With hyperextension injuries, elderly patients may develop a **central cord syndrome**, which causes motor deficits in the upper extremities more often than the lower extremities, variable sensory loss, and bladder dysfunction. The **Canadian Cervical-Spine Rule**, but not the **National Emergency X-Radiography Utilization Study** criteria, excludes patients age ≥65 years from being considered low risk for cervical spine injury.[29,30]

Thus, liberal imaging of the cervical spine in geriatric trauma patients is warranted. **Because of the higher pretest probability of injury, as well as the difficulties in interpreting plain radiographs in a patient with age-related degeneration, CT scan is the preferred initial modality for assessing the geriatric cervical spine.** Many fractures in one section of the spine are accompanied by fractures in another section, **so identification of one fracture should prompt imaging of the entire spinal column.**[31]

THORACOLUMBAR SPINAL INJURIES

Thoracic and lumbar spine fractures account for almost half of all osteoporotic fractures.[32] They are most common at the thoracolumbar junction (T12-L1) and midthoracic areas (T7-T8).[33] Anterior wedge compression fractures are the most common. Because of the low sensitivity of plain films for identifying thoracolumbar fractures in trauma patients, CT scan is the first-line imaging modality for adult patients.[34] This is even more significant in elders, in whom osteoporosis and degenerative changes make plain radiographs more difficult to interpret. See chapter 258, Spine Trauma, for more information on specific fracture types and management.

CHEST TRAUMA

The elderly are more susceptible to chest injuries from blunt trauma and have a decreased ability to compensate for these injuries. In blunt trauma, rib fractures are the most common injury found. Rib fractures in the elderly often lead to morbidity, pneumonia, and death. The adjusted odds of death in the elderly with rib fractures is about five times that of a younger cohort.[35] Rates of pneumonia and mortality in patients ≥65 years old are twice that of younger patients, with the rates increasing with each additional fractured rib.[36] In young adults, a chest radiograph to exclude complications such as pneumothoraces may be sufficient evaluation for suspected rib fractures, as isolated fractures may be treated conservatively at home. Because of the significant mortality associated with rib fractures in elders, a CT may be necessary to assess the extent of injuries that might not be seen on plain radiographs.

ABDOMINAL TRAUMA

The abdominal examination in elderly patients is unreliable. The FAST examination is an ideal imaging study to detect free intraperitoneal fluid. Even with an initially benign physical examination, maintain a high suspicion for intra-abdominal injuries in those with associated pelvic and lower rib cage fractures. As in younger patients, many solid organ injuries can be managed nonoperatively. Rates of successful nonoperative management of splenic injuries in elderly patients range from 62% to 85%.[37] Therefore, CT with contrast is a valuable diagnostic test for evaluating the extent of injury and ongoing hemorrhage; however, the risk of contrast-induced nephropathy increases with age, hypovolemia, diuretic and nephrotoxic medications, diabetes, and preexisting renal disease. **The risk can be reduced by volume expansion with isotonic crystalloids.** Oral *N*-acetylcysteine does not appear to prevent contrast-induced nephropathy in patients undergoing coronary angiography.[38] Other strategies, including sodium bicarbonate, ascorbic acid, and use of iso-osmolar versus low osmolar contrast, have had mixed results in studies.[39-43]

ORTHOPEDIC INJURIES

Pelvic Fractures While pelvic fractures in the young are generally caused by high-energy mechanisms, the elderly, especially women, frequently suffer pelvic fractures from low-energy falls to the ground from standing or from a seated position. Pubic ramus fractures are the most common injuries, and lateral compression is the most common mechanism.[44]

CT of the pelvis should be ordered in stable patients with pelvic tenderness after an injury if plain radiographs are negative.[45,46] Plain radiography is especially insensitive for posterior fractures involving the sacrum and iliac wings, so tenderness of the posterior pelvis strongly suggests the need for cross-sectional imaging.[47] Plain radiography may be omitted in stable patients who will be going promptly to CT.[48] Even CT may be only 77% sensitive for pelvic fractures in the elderly, particularly with nondisplaced posterior fractures in osteoporotic bone. Therefore, consider MRI for patients with pelvic pain or pain on weight bearing with negative CT imaging.[49]

Studies have been contradictory on whether age is an important predictor of the need for angiographic assessment for bleeding in pelvic fractures.[50] One study found that 94% of patients 60 years of age and older taken to angiography required embolization, which is significantly higher than the 52% in younger patients.[51] Therefore, these authors advocate liberal use of angiography in elderly patients with significant pelvic fractures, even in the absence of hemodynamic instability or need for transfusion. Other studies have not demonstrated an association between age and the need for angioembolization.

Hip Fractures Hip fracture is the single most common injury diagnosis that leads to hospitalization in the elderly. Hip fractures are a significant cause of morbidity and mortality, with about 25% of elderly patients dying within a year of injury.[54] The vast majority of hip fractures are caused by falls to the ground. The age-adjusted incidence of hip fractures in women is approximately twice that of men. Hip fractures in men occur at older ages than in women. Femoral neck (intracapsular) and intertrochanteric fractures are about equally common, with subtrochanteric fractures comprising the remaining 5% to 10%.[55] Bleeding from closed pelvic and long-bone fractures can cause hypovolemia in elderly patients.

Obtain anteroposterior radiographs of the pelvis, as well as dedicated anteroposterior and cross-table lateral radiographs of the affected hip. Because plain radiographs are only 90% sensitive for hip fractures, and delay in operative repair is associated with an increase in morbidity and mortality, **normal plain radiographs should be followed by more definitive imaging in patients in whom suspicion of hip fracture persists.**[56] MRI has higher sensitivity than CT for detecting hip fractures, with one study finding that 17% of hip fractures that were occult on plain radiographs were seen by MRI but not CT.[57] The sensitivity of CT is likely lower in patients with risk factors for osteoporosis (older age, female sex, chronic steroid use, alcoholism, inactivity, poor calcium intake, endocrine disorders) and a lower energy mechanism of injury, in which fractures are less likely to be displaced. If MRI is difficult to obtain, CT may yield a diagnosis, but should be followed by MRI if nondiagnostic. Nuclear medicine scintigraphy is highly sensitive for fractures but has the disadvantages of low specificity, difficulty obtaining the study from the ED, and limited ability to delineate the full nature of the fracture. Consider admitting patients with hip fractures to a multidisciplinary team of geriatricians, orthopedists, and rehabilitation specialists.

Upper Extremity Injuries Distal radius fractures (**Colles' fractures**) are the most common fractures in women up to age 75, with a lifetime risk of about 15%.[58,59] Such fractures are often caused by a fall onto an outstretched hand and are associated with low bone mineral density or osteoporosis. Assess median nerve function before and after reduction, as a deficit will require immediate orthopedic consultation for possible nerve decompression. Unstable or displaced fractures require closed reduction with a hematoma block for anesthesia. A systematic review of unstable distal radius fractures in the elderly reported that functional outcomes were similar with nonoperative and operative management, even though nonoperative management was associated with a less satisfactory radiographic appearance.[60] So while elderly patients with active lifestyles and good functional statuses may benefit from surgical treatment, many can do as well with conservative treatment.

Fractures of the proximal humerus and humeral shaft are also common after falls from standing. Carefully assess for axillary nerve injury by checking sensation at the area of deltoid muscle insertion and deltoid muscle engagement with shoulder abduction. Note that the initial 18 degrees of shoulder abduction are generated by the supraspinatus muscle, so movement in this range may still be possible with an axillary nerve injury.

LABORATORY TESTING

Elderly trauma patients should receive more intensive laboratory evaluation than younger patients (**Table 255-2**). This may be helpful to identify comorbid diseases (e.g., creatinine for renal dysfunction) or acute causes of syncope (e.g., troponin for myocardial infarction) or to uncover occult

TABLE 255-2 Useful Laboratory Studies to Guide Management in Geriatric Trauma Patients

CBC
Electrolytes
Renal function
Serum glucose
Coagulation profile
Disseminated intravascular coagulation panel
Base deficit
Lactate
Troponin
Ethanol
Creatine kinase

physiologic insults (e.g., lactate, INR, and base deficit). As discussed earlier, vital signs are an unreliable marker of shock in the elderly. **Base deficit and lactate levels are useful initial indicators of shock, and serial measurements can guide resuscitation progress.** Elevated lactate levels correlate with systemic hypoperfusion, intensive care unit and hospital length of stay, and mortality.[61,62] A "normal" or mild base deficit of −3 to −5 correlates with 24% mortality, a moderate base deficit of −6 to −9 correlates with 60% mortality, and a severe base deficit of ≤−10 correlates with 80% mortality.[63] Check creatine kinase levels to assess for rhabdomyolysis in patients who have fallen and been unable to receive assistance for a prolonged period.

TREATMENT

OUT-OF-HOSPITAL CONSIDERATIONS

EMS providers should recognize that seemingly minor trauma mechanisms, such as ground-level falls and low-speed motor vehicle crashes, may result in significant injury to older persons. For these reasons, the threshold for scene triage or transfer to a trauma center should be lower for elderly patients than for younger patients.[64]

Rates of prehospital undertriage are higher in older than in younger patients, with significant associated mortality.[65,66] For the reasons discussed earlier, traditional triage criteria of physiology (e.g., heart rate and blood pressure), anatomical injury, and mechanism are unreliable in elderly patients. Therefore, the 2011 U.S. Centers for Disease Control and Prevention National Expert Panel on Field Triage recommended a lower threshold for triage of injured elderly patients, giving three key recommendations: **"Risk of injury/death increases after age 55 years. Systolic blood pressure < 110 mm Hg might represent shock after age 65 years. Low impact mechanisms (e.g. ground level falls) might result in severe injury."**[67] The American College of Surgeons recommends that EMS providers consider contacting medical control and transporting injured patients ≥55 years old to a trauma center regardless of apparent injury severity.[68]

The elderly can rapidly develop tissue damage leading to decubitus ulcers. Consider padded backboards or vacuum splints for prolonged transports. Patients with cervical kyphosis may need firm padding placed behind the head when in spinal immobilization in order to prevent forcing the spine into an abnormal position.

BLEEDING AND HEAD INJURY

The volume of intracranial blood and hematoma expansion are the most important determinants of morbidity and mortality in head injury.[69] Rapidly reverse anticoagulation in patients taking warfarin with intracranial bleeding on CT scan. Despite a lack of sufficient positive or negative evidence, it is reasonable to reverse other forms of anticoagulation (e.g., aspirin, clopidogrel, heparin) in patients with diagnosed intracranial hemorrhage. Studies have not shown a benefit to platelet transfusion in patients on aspirin.[70,71]

Admit patients with bleeding on CT scan to an intensive care unit. The disposition of patients taking warfarin but with a normal initial CT scan is challenging because such patients have a reported rate of delayed intracranial hemorrhage between 1% and 8%.[72,73] Admission for a repeat head CT at 24 hours will catch most, but not all, delayed hemorrhages. Discharge after an initial negative head CT may also be reasonable in patients with lower INRs, with caregivers to watch them closely at home, and who are reliable to return if they develop symptoms and who have a plan for next-day follow-up by telephone or in person.

RIB FRACTURES AND RESPIRATORY FAILURE

Maintain a low threshold for admitting elderly patients with rib fractures for a period of observation until good pain control and pulmonary toilet are assured. More severe thoracic injuries, such as hemopneumothorax, pulmonary contusion, flail chest, and cardiac contusion, can quickly lead to decompensation in the elderly, especially those with baseline respiratory insufficiency. Pain control after chest wall trauma is vital to encourage ventilation in order to reduce atelectasis and the risk of infection. Pain control is challenging because the elderly may have decreased tolerance for opioid analgesics, which can have profound respiratory (hypoventilation), hemodynamic (hypotension), and CNS effects.

Continuous pulse oximetry and capnometry are helpful to assess oxygenation and ventilation. Administer supplemental oxygen to maintain oxygen saturation at >95%. Serial arterial blood gas analysis may provide early insight into respiratory function and reserve. Consider prompt tracheal intubation and use of mechanical ventilation in patients with more severe injuries, respiratory rates >40 breaths/min, or when the partial pressure of arterial oxygen is <60 mm Hg or the pressure of arterial carbon dioxide is >50 mm Hg.

SHOCK

One study of elderly trauma patients showed a marked increase in survival from 7% to 53% with early placement (within 2.2 hours) of a pulmonary artery catheter followed by goal-directed volume resuscitation and inotropic support.[17] This study also identified a subset of patients with occult shock despite "stable vital signs." Given the complications associated with pulmonary artery catheters, research on the assessment of shock by serum lactate and central or mixed venous oxygen saturation, and ongoing advances in less invasive hemodynamic monitoring and echocardiography, the optimal approach to recognizing and treating occult hypoperfusion is uncertain. A general strategy is to perform the initial imaging necessary to identify life-threatening injuries (e.g., chest radiograph, CT of the head, spine, chest, abdomen, and pelvis) and then transport to the intensive care unit for aggressive optimization of hemodynamics, after which nonessential imaging and interventions (e.g., extremity radiographs and suturing) can be performed.

Resuscitate the elderly trauma patient with small volumes of isotonic crystalloid (normal saline or lactated Ringer's), watching for a response, to avoid underresuscitation or volume overload. Strong consideration should be made for early and liberal use of red blood cell transfusion, which may enhance oxygen delivery, minimize tissue ischemia, and prevent volume overload. Depending on the type of injury and severity of blood loss, consider switching to blood transfusion after 1 to 2 L of crystalloid resuscitation.

ENVIRONMENTAL AND IATROGENIC INJURY

The decreased lean muscle mass and impaired peripheral circulation associated with aging makes the elderly patient more susceptible to pressure sores and hypothermia. Patients with prolonged extrications or transport in cool climates may be hypothermic. Expose the patient as needed for a thorough examination, but keep the patient covered as much as possible to maintain body heat. Hypothermia not explained by environmental factors may be a sign of sepsis or endocrine abnormalities. Log-roll patients onto a padded surface as soon as possible.

DISPOSITION AND FOLLOW-UP

Have a low threshold for admitting geriatric trauma patients. Admit elderly patients with polytrauma, significant chest wall injuries, abnormal vital signs, or evidence of overt or occult hypoperfusion to the intensive care unit.

Even in patients without the need for inpatient treatment or observation, consider whether the patient is immediately ready to return home. In patients whose preinjury mobility was already tenuous, pain, decreased mobility, and medications may make a return to home dangerous. While opioid analgesics may be necessary, they may also cause delirium, decrease balance, and impair ambulation. Observation for establishment of a safe and effective pain regimen, consultation with physical therapy, and assurance of a safe home environment may be advisable to prevent a secondary injury.

OUTCOME

The ultimate goal is to return the elderly trauma patient to the preinjury state of function. Immediately after discharge, about half of survivors return home, and half go to skilled nursing or rehabilitation facilities.[74] The general consensus is that elderly trauma patients benefit from preferential triage to trauma centers and from aggressive and thoughtful resuscitation. In light of investigations showing that elderly patients often return to preexisting health status after trauma and the value of early invasive monitoring, it appears that **aggressive resuscitation efforts for geriatric trauma patients are warranted**.

PRACTICE GUIDELINES

Jacobs DG, Plaisier BR, Barie PS, et al: Practice management guidelines for geriatric trauma: the EAST Practice Management Guidelines Work Group. *J Trauma* 54: 391, 2003. [PMID: 12579072]

Jagoda AS, Bazarian JJ, Bruns JJ, et al: Clinical policy: neuroimaging and decision making in adult mild traumatic brain injury in the acute setting. *Ann Emerg Med* 52: 714, 2008. [PMID: 19027497]

Sasser SM, Hunt RC, Faul M, et al: Guidelines for field triage of injured patients: recommendations of the National Expert Panel on Field Triage, 2011. *MMWR Recomm Rep* 61: 1, 2012. [PMID: 22237112]

REFERENCES

The complete reference list is available online at www.TintinalliEM.com.

CHAPTER 256 Trauma in Pregnancy

Nicole M. Delorio

INTRODUCTION AND EPIDEMIOLOGY

Trauma remains the leading cause of nonobstetric morbidity and mortality in pregnant women.[1] The severity of maternal injuries may be a poor predictor of fetal distress and outcome after a traumatic event (even minor ones). Trauma during pregnancy is associated with an increased risk of preterm labor, placental abruption, fetomaternal hemorrhage, and pregnancy loss. Achieving successful outcomes for both mother and fetus requires a collaborative effort by the prehospital provider, emergency physician, trauma surgeon, obstetrician, and neonatologist.

Trauma during pregnancy is common. One study estimated that 32,810 pregnant women sustain injuries in motor vehicle crashes every year in the United States, a rate of 9 per 1000 live births.[2] **Motor vehicle crashes** are the most common cause of blunt abdominal trauma, accounting for up to 70% of acute injuries. This is followed by **falls** and **direct assault** in decreasing order of frequency.[3] The incidence of falls appears to increase with the advancement of pregnancy, presumably due to alterations in maternal balance and coordination. Penetrating injuries are less common than blunt trauma during pregnancy.

PHYSIOLOGY OF PREGNANCY

Physiologic changes in pregnancy are discussed in detail in chapter 25, "Resuscitation in Pregnancy." In addition to normal physiologic changes, conditions such as pregnancy-induced hypertension, placenta previa, preeclampsia, and eclampsia may significantly alter the presentation and complicate evaluation and treatment in the setting of trauma (see chapter 100, "Maternal Emergencies after 20 Weeks of Pregnancy and in the Postpartum Period").

Table 25-1 summarizes important physiologic changes in pregnancy that affect resuscitation. Maternal blood volume expands at approximately week 10 of gestation and peaks at about a 45% increase from baseline at week 28. Because plasma volume increases more than red cell mass, mild physiologic anemia may be evident. Cardiac output increases by 1.0 to 1.5 L/min at week 10 of pregnancy and remains elevated until the end of pregnancy. Heart rate in the mother is generally increased by 10 to 20 beats/min in the second trimester, accompanied by decreases in systolic and diastolic blood pressures of 10 to 15 mm Hg.

The relative hypervolemic state can mislead the clinician during maternal resuscitation after trauma and make clinical findings difficult to interpret. **A pregnant patient may lose 30% to 35% of circulating blood volume before manifesting hypotension or clinical signs of shock.** Uterine blood flow is directly proportional to maternal mean arterial pressure, so maintain and replace maternal blood volume aggressively and adequately.

After week 12 of gestation, the uterus becomes an intra-abdominal organ, removing it from the relative protection of the maternal pelvis and making it susceptible to direct injury. The bladder moves anteriorly into the abdomen in the third trimester of pregnancy, increasing its vulnerability to injury. Uterine blood flow may increase to upward of 600 mL/min; severe maternal hemorrhage from uterine injury enters the equation at this point. The gravid uterus also causes passive stretching of the abdominal wall and peritoneum as it enlarges, and this may lead to diminished sensitivity to injury and irritation from intraperitoneal blood. **At approximately weeks 18 to 20 of gestation, the expanding mass of the gravid uterus may put the mother at risk for the "supine hypotension syndrome," in which venous return and cardiac output are diminished by compression of the maternal inferior vena cava in the supine position.** The enlarging uterus may also cause engorgement of lower extremity and lower abdominal vessels, which predisposes the patient to severe retroperitoneal injury. Avoid placing IV lines in the femoral region and lower extremity because of inferior vena cava compression by the uterus and the possibility of pooling in engorged or injured pelvic veins.

As pregnancy progresses, the diaphragm elevates by as much as 4 cm, and tidal volume increases by 40% as residual volume diminishes by 25%. These changes may significantly impair the ability of a pregnant trauma patient to compensate for respiratory compromise and can result in rapid development of hypoxia from pulmonary disorders or during intubation. **Consider diaphragmatic elevation when thoracostomy tube placement is indicated during maternal resuscitation.**

Gastric emptying is delayed, increasing the likelihood of gastroesophageal reflux and the potential for aspiration from acute injuries or endotracheal intubation. The small bowel is moved upward in the abdomen by the enlarging uterus, which increases the chance of complex bowel injuries in penetrating trauma of the upper abdomen.[4] The liver is typically unaffected by pregnancy, and the most common cause of abdominal hemorrhage remains splenic injury, as in nonpregnant patients.

CLINICAL FEATURES

Rapidly assess gestational age by palpating uterine fundal height. At week 12 of gestation, the uterine fundus is at or about the level of the pubic symphysis, and at week 20, it is at the umbilicus. The uterus then expands approximately 1 cm beyond the umbilicus per additional week of gestation. Assessing fetal age helps determine fetal viability. **Gestation ≥24 weeks is compatible with fetal viability.** Examine the abdomen and uterus for evidence of injury as well as for uterine tenderness or contractions. Placental abruption may be suggested by a rigid, boardlike uterus, or no signs may be evident at all.

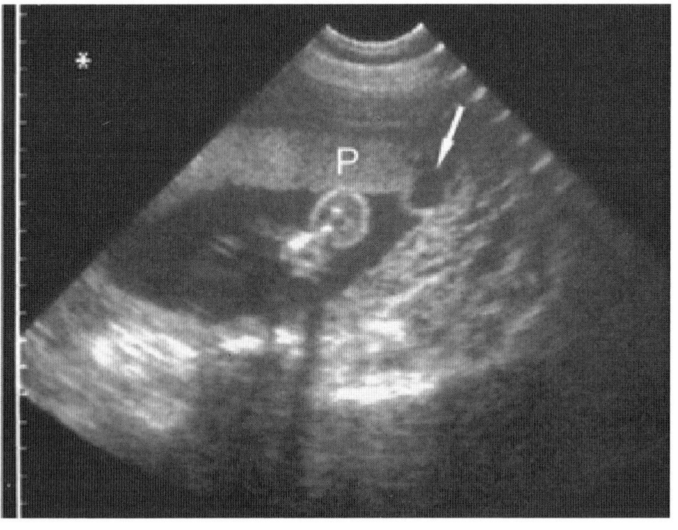

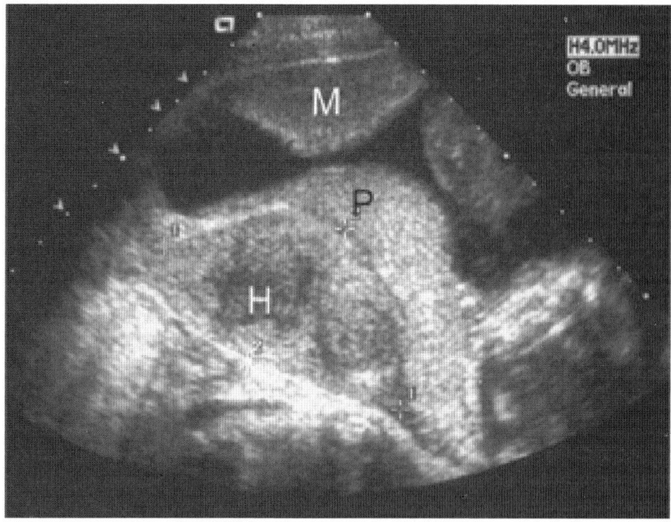

A B

FIGURE 256-1. **A.** Placental abruption. Transabdominal long-axis scan shows an anterior placenta with a contained marginal abruption (arrow). [Image used with permission of L. Sens and L. Green, Gulfcoast Ultrasound.] **B.** Placental abruption. Transabdominal scan, sagittal plane, demonstrating retroplacental hematoma (H) in an 18-week pregnancy. The placenta (P) is located on the posterior wall. A myometrial contraction (M) of the anterior wall is evident.

MATERNAL AND FETAL INJURIES

Direct fetal injury is relatively rare in blunt abdominal trauma during the first trimester. When fetal injuries do occur, they are typically seen later in gestation and tend to involve the fetal skull and brain. Such injuries can be sustained in association with fractures to the maternal pelvis when the fetal head is engaged. When the uterus is penetrated by a sharp object or projectile, the fetus can be injured.

Uterine rupture accounts for <1% of all injuries in pregnancy and is more likely to occur during the late second and third trimesters and when there is direct and forceful impact on the uterus.[3] The fetal mortality rate is high. The clinical presentation of uterine rupture is quite nonspecific, but loss of the palpable uterine contour, ease of palpation of fetal parts, or radiologic evidence of abnormal fetal location suggests the diagnosis.

Uterine irritability and the onset of preterm labor may be precipitated by acute abdominal trauma during pregnancy. The use of tocolytic agents to manage premature labor in pregnant trauma patients is not generally recommended, so consult an obstetrician before considering tocolytics. Tocolytic agents have numerous adverse side effects, such as fetal and maternal tachycardia, that may complicate trauma evaluation.

Placental abruption is second only to maternal death as the most common cause of fetal death (**Figure 256-1**). Placental abruption complicates 1% to 5% of minor injuries during pregnancy and up to 40% to 50% of major traumatic injuries. During direct abdominal or deceleration injury, intrauterine pressures increase, the relatively elastic uterus deforms at the relatively inelastic placenta, and the placenta shears from the uterine wall. Even "minor" maternal injuries such as minor motor vehicle crashes, falls, and assaults can be associated with placental abruption and sudden fetal demise.[5] The most sensitive clinical finding for placental abruption after trauma is uterine irritability (more than three contractions per hour), most evident immediately after trauma, on initial presentation to the ED.[5,6] Other clinical findings of placental abruption include abdominal pain, painful vaginal bleeding, and tetanic uterine contractions. Placental abruption may also lead to the introduction of placental products into the maternal circulation, stimulating **disseminated intravascular coagulation** or **amniotic fluid embolism.**

Fetomaternal hemorrhage is the entry of fetal red blood cells into the maternal blood stream and should be assumed in the setting of maternal trauma. If the mother is Rh negative and the fetus is Rh positive, if as little as 0.1 μL of fetal blood enters the maternal circulation, it can sensitize the mother[7] and endanger the pregnancy and subsequent pregnancies. This is the basis for administering Rho(D) immunoglobulin to Rh-negative mothers after maternal trauma.

PREHOSPITAL CARE

Prehospital care providers should ask about the possibility of pregnancy when evaluating injured women of childbearing age. Prioritize attention to the fundamentals of resuscitation (airway, breathing, circulation) in the mother. Administer supplemental oxygen because compensation for hypoxia is limited in pregnancy. Similarly, consider early endotracheal intubation when indicated by the nature or severity of injuries. Establish peripheral IV lines, and provide 50% more volume than would be given to the nonpregnant patient.

For patients at >20 weeks of gestation who must be transported in the supine position or in whom spinal immobilization is indicated, place a wedge under the right hip area, tilting the patient approximately 30 degrees to the left, to prevent hypotension from inferior vena cava compression by the gravid uterus. Triage to a hospital with trauma, obstetric, and neonatal services if at all possible.[4,8]

MATERNAL DIAGNOSIS

Follow the traditional airway, breathing, circulation, disability, and exposure assessment for maternal injury, and simultaneously stabilize and resuscitate the mother. After completing the primary survey and performing resuscitative steps, proceed with secondary assessment.

ULTRASOUND

Begin with bedside expanded focused assessment with sonography for trauma to identify intra-abdominal or thoracic injury, and identify fetal activity and fetal heart rate. Transvaginal US can be performed once the mother is stabilized to complete the fetal survey and identify placental location. The sensitivity and specificity of abdominal US for the detection of intraperitoneal fluid are similar in pregnant and nonpregnant patients.[9]

RADIOGRAPHS

Carefully select imaging studies to minimize fetal exposure to the potential adverse effects of ionizing radiation. **Do not withhold imaging needed for appropriate maternal trauma management.** The greatest risk to fetal viability from ionizing radiation is within the first 2 weeks after conception, and the highest potential for malformation is during embryonic organogenesis from 2 to 8 weeks after conception. The risk of CNS teratogenesis is highest when exposure occurs between weeks 8 and 15 (see Table 99-9). **A dose <5 rad is the threshold for human teratogenesis.**[9] Fetal exposure can be decreased by shielding the maternal abdomen and pelvis during many studies and by performing modified studies and using dose-reducing techniques, such as decreasing the number of imaging slices obtained.

Standard trauma plain radiographs, such as cervical spine, chest, and pelvis films, deliver <1 rad (10 mGy) each. Abdominopelvic CT and pelvic angiography result in the highest delivered doses of radiation. The amount is typically 2.5 to 3.5 rad (25 to 35 mGy), with some variation due to equipment quality, techniques used, and duration of study. If abdominal-pelvic CT scanning is necessary to evaluate maternal status, CT also detects placental abruption, with a reported sensitivity of 86% and specificity of 98% for abruption.[10] Table 99-10 provides the estimated amounts of fetal radiation exposure for some common trauma imaging studies.[11]

Potential effects of contrast agents employed in CT scanning are not well studied, and their use requires individualization, because iodinated agents can potentially cause neonatal hypothyroidism.

PELVIC EXAMINATION

Perform pelvic examination only after US to determine placental location and exclude placenta previa.[6] **Do not perform pelvic examination if placenta previa is identified.** A sterile pelvic examination can identify injuries of the lower genital tract, vaginal bleeding, and rupture of amniotic membranes.

To assess for amniotic membrane rupture, test vaginal fluid with pH paper. **Fluid in the vagina with a pH of 7 is suggestive of amniotic fluid, whereas fluid with a pH of 5 is consistent with vaginal secretions.** A branchlike pattern, or "ferning," seen upon drying of vaginal fluid on a microscope slide, also suggests amniotic fluid.

LABORATORY TESTING

Obtain a CBC, serum chemistries, blood type and Rh status, coagulation profiles with fibrin degradation products and fibrinogen to assess for disseminated intravascular coagulation, and additional laboratory studies as clinically indicated. An Apt test or Kleihauer-Betke test can be performed by the laboratory. The Apt test is a qualitative determination of the presence of fetal hemoglobin in maternal blood. The Kleihauer-Betke test applies acid elution to an aliquot of maternal blood, and then maternal and fetal red blood cells are counted under the microscope. An extrapolation is then made regarding the volume of fetomaternal hemorrhage.

Serial Kleihauer-Betke testing can assess ongoing fetomaternal transfusion. If there is doubt whether the woman is pregnant or not, confirm pregnancy at the bedside with qualitative urine testing or with point-of-care US.

FETAL DIAGNOSIS

For pregnant trauma patients >20 weeks gestation (clinically identified by uterus at or above the umbilicus), obtain bedside US to assess fetal size, heart rate, gestational age, amniotic fluid volume, placental location, and fetal activity or demise. **Fetal viability is ≥24 weeks' gestation. Normal fetal heart rate is 120 to 160 beats/min. US may not detect uterine rupture or fetal-placental injuries, does not monitor for fetal distress, and is not sensitive for placental abruption.**[5,12] US sensitivity for placental abruption is about 25%, although specificity is >90%.[12]

Even for women ≥20 weeks, gestation with "minor" direct or indirect abdominal trauma, **as soon as possible apply cardiotochodynamometry** to monitor uterine contractions and fetal heart rate pattern. Decelerations, tachycardia, and bradycardia are signs of fetal distress. **The most sensitive clinical finding for placental abruption after trauma is uterine irritability, which is frequent uterine contractions (more than three uterine contractions in an hour).**[5,6] Fetal distress and demise can occur quickly and abruptly, so vigilant monitoring is necessary. If fetal heart tones are confirmed to be absent, then direct the remainder of treatment efforts solely at maternal resuscitation.[11]

TREATMENT

Develop a protocol involving the ED, trauma service, obstetrician, and obstetrics nurse for major trauma. For minor direct or indirect abdominal trauma (such as minor motor vehicle accident, simple fall, or assault), a simpler protocol involving ED and the obstetrics team is effective. Because most emergency physicians are unfamiliar with the patterns of early, late, and variable decelerations, the labor and delivery nurse is an essential part of the ED monitoring team. In case of fetal deterioration, the labor and delivery nurse can identify the need for emergency cesarean section.

Follow the standard steps for trauma resuscitation. **Maternal resuscitation is the best fetal resuscitation.** Manage the airway, ensure adequate ventilation, and provide supplemental oxygen. Place a nasogastric tube early, because delayed stomach emptying and diminished lower esophageal sphincter tone increase the risk of aspiration of gastric contents. **Keep the patient in the semi-left lateral decubitus position to the extent possible to minimize vena caval compression.** Identify and control sources of hemorrhage since maternal blood loss and hypovolemia exacerbate fetal hypoperfusion. Increase crystalloid infusions by 50% to account for the patient's additional plasma volume. Do not administer vasopressors until volume and blood are replaced to minimize risk of uteroplacental hypoperfusion. If vasopressors are needed for maternal resuscitation, however, do not restrict their use (see chapter 25 for further discussion).

Table 256-1 summarizes critical ED interventions for trauma in pregnancy. Do not withhold critical maternal interventions or diagnostic procedures out of concern for potential adverse fetal consequences.

Administer Rho(D) immunoglobulin to Rh-negative pregnant women with abdominal trauma. Two dose options are acceptable: 50 micrograms IM for gestation of ≤12 weeks and 300 micrograms IM for gestation of ≥13 weeks, or 300 micrograms IM for all gestational ages. The rationale for the lower dose for ≤12 weeks gestation is that the total fetal blood volume at 12 weeks gestation is about 4.2 μL, and a 50-microgram dose is effective for up to 5 μL of fetomaternal hemorrhage. A 300-microgram dose will protect for up to 30 μL of fetomaternal hemorrhage. The obstetrician can best determine if doses of >300 micrograms should be administered. Because the 72-hour window for Rho(D) immunoglobulin therapy established for postpartum administration has been extrapolated to apply after abdominal trauma, serial fetomaternal hemorrhage testing may be performed in the hospital.[7,13]

Provide **tetanus prophylaxis** as needed. Although tetanus toxoid is a category C drug for all trimesters of pregnancy, it is commonly accepted as safe. Tetanus antibody crosses the placenta, so it can also reduce the incidence of neonatal tetanus.

Continue to carefully monitor fetal heart rate patterns and frequent uterine contractions with cardiotochodynamometry. If fetal distress develops, consult obstetrics if not already at the bedside. Treat maternal hypovolemia, hemorrhage, and hypoxia and continue assessment for

TABLE 256-1 Checklist for Trauma in Pregnancy

Before arrival: Assemble ED, obstetrics, and trauma team, as appropriate for >20 wk gestation
Attend to maternal airway, breathing, and circulation as a priority for both mother and fetus. Increase volume resuscitation 50% above that given to nonpregnant patients.
Maintain patient in the semi-left lateral decubitus position, or manually deflect the uterus to the left.
Bedside US: FAST for intraperitoneal fluid and to determine fetal heart rate and estimate fetal age to determine viability.
Initiate fetal cardiotocographic monitoring as soon as possible and continue for at least 4–6 h even if the patient is apparently uninjured and > 20 weeks gestation.
Perform needed imaging.
Include blood typing and Rh status in laboratory studies.
Administer Rho(D) immunoglobulin to Rh-negative mothers. Give tetanus as indicated.
Screen for potential intimate partner violence.

Abbreviation: FAST = focused assessment with sonography for trauma.

placental abruption. In a viable gestation, the presence of fetal tachycardia, lack of beat-to-beat or long-term variability, or late decelerations on tocodynamometry indicate fetal distress and may be indications for emergency cesarean delivery.[6]

A minimum of 4 to 6 hours of external tocodynamometric monitoring of the potentially viable fetus appears sufficient to predict immediate adverse pregnancy outcomes and is indicated for all pregnant patients evaluated for trauma, even those without obvious abdominal injury. In patients demonstrating persistent contractions or uterine irritability, extend tocodynamometry to a minimum of 24 hours. Although no uniform standards exist, many obstetricians believe that patients with fewer than three contractions per hour during an initial 4-hour observation period can be safely discharged.

LAPAROTOMY

The indications for emergent laparotomy in the management of pregnant trauma patients remain unchanged from those for nonpregnant patients. The fetus appears to tolerate surgery and anesthesia well if adequate oxygenation and uterine perfusion are maintained. Do not withhold surgery out of concern for fetal compromise. Emergency cesarean delivery in the setting of trauma results in a fetal survival rate as high as 75% when gestation is ≥26 weeks, fetal heart tones are present on admission, and the procedure is performed at the earliest indication of fetal distress (see "Perimortem Cesarean Section" in chapter 25).[14]

DISPOSITION AND FOLLOW-UP

Disposition of a pregnant trauma patient after the emergency assessment and management is based on the nature and severity of presenting injuries and the gestational length of the pregnancy. Manage patients with multisystem trauma or with minor but potentially serious injuries jointly with trauma surgeons and obstetricians. Women at ≥20 weeks of gestation require observation or admission for fetal monitoring. If there is evidence of fetal distress or uterine irritability during the initial assessment, then immediately consult an obstetrician. When the patient needs transfer to other facilities for definitive care, stabilize the patient's condition as much as possible prior to transfer, with provisions for an appropriate level of care during transport. Adhere to transfer policies that comply with federal regulations. If the patient can be discharged, ensure adequate follow-up obstetrical care.[15]

SPECIAL CONSIDERATIONS

AUTOMOBILE RESTRAINT

Motor vehicle seat belt use during pregnancy helps protect both the mother and the fetus, and pregnant drivers and passengers should wear safety belts throughout pregnancy. The best predictors of fetal loss or adverse outcome are crash severity and lack of, or improper use of, seat belts.[16] The lap belt should be placed as low as possible under the gravid uterus (across both the anterior superior iliac spines and the pubic symphysis), and the shoulder harness should be positioned snugly between the breasts but off to the side of the uterus.[17,18] Pregnant women should use both seat belts and air bags. **Do not disconnect air bags for pregnant women.**[17] Although there is a risk of injury to the more proximally located gravid uterus, as long as the pregnant woman is properly seated and uses properly placed seat belts, the benefits of air bags appear to outweigh the risks.[19]

INTERPERSONAL VIOLENCE

Assaults are the third most common mechanism of injury for pregnant women after falls and motor vehicle crashes.[3] To screen for the possibility of interpersonal violence, encourage a social services evaluation or referral in all but the most obvious cases of accidental injury (**Table 256-2**).[1]

TABLE 256-2 Special Considerations Regarding Mechanism of Injury (in order of prevalence)

Motor vehicle crash	Fetus most at risk during third trimester
Intimate partner violence	Prevalence increases during pregnancy Increased risk of multiple adverse fetal outcomes not just due to fetal injury
Falls	More common in pregnancy due to changing center of gravity, ligamentous laxity Most indoors, due to stairs
Toxic exposure	Most reported events due to deliberate ingestion Fetal risk highest during first weeks due to birth defects
Burns	Can increase risk of spontaneous abortion Risks to fetus due to maternal sepsis, smoke inhalation Maternal-fetal risks from carbon dioxide intoxication

REFERENCES

The complete reference list is available online at www.TintinalliEM.com.

Head Trauma

David W. Wright
Lisa H. Merck

INTRODUCTION AND EPIDEMIOLOGY

Traumatic brain injury is brain function impairment that results from external force.[1] The clinical manifestations represent a broad constellation of symptoms from brief confusion to coma, severe disability, and/or death. The underlying pathology ranges from temporary shifts in cellular ionic concentrations to permanent structural damage.

Traumatic brain injury (TBI) is classified as mild, moderate, and severe based on the Glasgow Coma Scale (GCS) score. Over 80% of TBI is defined as **mild** (GCS 14 to 15) (**mTBI**) and is often called "concussion."[2] The label of mild, however, is a misnomer. mTBI may lead to significant, debilitating short- and long-term sequelae. **Moderate** TBI (GCS 9 to 13) accounts for approximately 10% of head injuries. Mortality rates for patients with isolated moderate TBI are <20%, but long-term disability can be higher. Overall, 40% of patients with moderate TBI have an abnormal finding on CT scan, and 8% will require neurosurgical intervention. In **severe** TBI (GCS 3 to 8), mortality rate approaches 40%, with most deaths occurring in the first 48 hours after injury. Fewer than 10% of patients with severe TBI experience good recovery.[2,3]

The prevalence of TBI is twice as high in males as in females. Distribution of age at injury is trimodal, with peaks at 0 to 4 years, 15 to 24 years, and >75 years of age. Mortality rate increases with age at time of injury.[4,5] Motor vehicle collisions are the primary cause of blunt head injury in young adults and children, and falls are more common in the elderly.[2] TBI has been called the "signature injury" of the conflicts in Iraq and Afghanistan.[6]

PATHOPHYSIOLOGY

CEREBRAL BLOOD FLOW

Autoregulation, cerebral perfusion pressure (CPP), mean arterial pressure (MAP), and intracranial pressure (ICP) are interrelated factors that affect cerebral blood flow (**Table 257-1**). Under normal circumstances,

TABLE 257-1 Factors that Affect Cerebral Blood Flow

MAP = DBP + [(SBP – DBP)/3]
CPP = MAP – ICP

Abbreviations: CPP = cerebral perfusion pressure; DBP = diastolic blood pressure; ICP = intracranial pressure; MAP = mean arterial pressure; SBP = systolic blood pressure.

TABLE 257-2 Intracranial Pressure by Age Group

Age Group	Intracranial Pressure (mm Hg)
Adults	<10–15
Young children	3–7
Infants	1.5–6.0

autoregulation regulates local cerebral blood flow to maintain equilibrium between oxygen delivery and metabolism.[7] Other systemic factors, such as hypertension, hypocarbia, and alkalosis, can affect cerebral blood flow by causing vasoconstriction.

Under normal situations, autoregulation can adjust to CPPs from 50 to 150 mm Hg to maintain local cellular oxygen demands and regional cerebral blood flow. In brain injury, autoregulation is often impaired, so even modest drops in blood pressure can decrease brain perfusion and result in cellular hypoxia. A CPP <60 mm Hg is considered the lower limit of autoregulation in humans, below which local control of cerebral blood flow cannot be adjusted to maintain flow adequate for function.[8] Traumatic hypotension leads to ischemia within low flow regions of the injured brain, so aggressive fluid resuscitation may be required to prevent hypotension and secondary brain injury. In the absence of an ICP monitor, it is important to maintain a MAP of **≥80 mm Hg**, because **low blood** pressure in the setting of elevated ICP will result in a low CPP and brain injury.

The cranium is an enclosed space with a fixed volume. Any changes to the volume of the intracranial contents (such as bleeding) affect the **ICP**, and an increase in ICP can decrease the CPP. ICP is determined by the volume of the three intracranial compartments: the brain parenchyma (<1300 mL in the adult), cerebrospinal fluid (100 to 150 mL), and intravascular blood (100 to 150 mL). When one compartment expands, there is a compensatory reduction in the volume of another, and/or the baseline ICP will increase (**Figure 257-1**). Elevations in ICP are life threatening and may lead to a phenomenon known as the **Cushing reflex** (hypertension, bradycardia, and respiratory irregularity). Hypertension is an attempt to maintain cerebral perfusion. Normal values for ICP vary with age (**Table 257-2**).

PRIMARY BRAIN INJURIES

The initial insult associated with moderate and severe TBI imparts mechanical forces that produce high levels of direct damage and strain to the brain parenchyma. The **primary injuries** include contusions (bruises to brain parenchyma), hematomas (subdural, epidural, intraparenchymal, intraventricular, and subarachnoid), diffuse axonal injury (stress or damage to axons), direct cellular damage (neurons, axons, and other supportive cells), loss of the blood–brain barrier, disruption of the neurochemical homeostasis, and loss of the electrochemical function.

SECONDARY BRAIN INJURIES

A wave of secondary damage is unleashed by the impact that results in a series of deleterious cellular and subcellular events (also known as the **secondary neurotoxic cascade**).[10,11] The secondary neurotoxic cascade causes ongoing damage to the brain and ultimately results in a poorer neurologic outcome than might have occurred based on the original mechanism.

The secondary neurotoxic cascade should not be confused with the term **secondary insults**, a term used in the clinical literature to describe conditions or circumstances (e.g., hypotension, hypoxemia, hyperglycemia) that accelerate neurotoxic damage and worsen long-term outcome.[12,13] Mediation of secondary insults reduces morbidity and mortality and is discussed in the treatment section.

The **secondary neurotoxic cascade** is a massive release of neurotransmitters, such as glutamate, into the presynaptic space, with activation of *N*-methyl-D-aspartate, α-amino-3-hydroxy-5-methyl-4-isoxazole propionic acid, and other receptors.[10] Ionic shifts activate cytoplasmic and nuclear enzymes, induce mitochondrial damage, and lead to cell death and necrosis.[10,14,15] Proinflammatory cytokines and other enzymes are released in an attempt to clean and repair the damage. Secondary injury, however, is indiscriminant and produces extensive neuronal loss. Additionally, many survivable cells undergo apoptosis, or programmed cell death, during secondary injury.[16] Apoptosis has been reported to occur longer than a year after injury.[16,17]

BRAIN EDEMA

Brain edema results from two distinct processes and can be fatal in TBI.[18] Cellular swelling, or **cytotoxic edema**, results from large ionic shifts and the loss of cellular membrane integrity from mitochondrial damage (loss of adenosine triphosphate, ion pump productivity, and

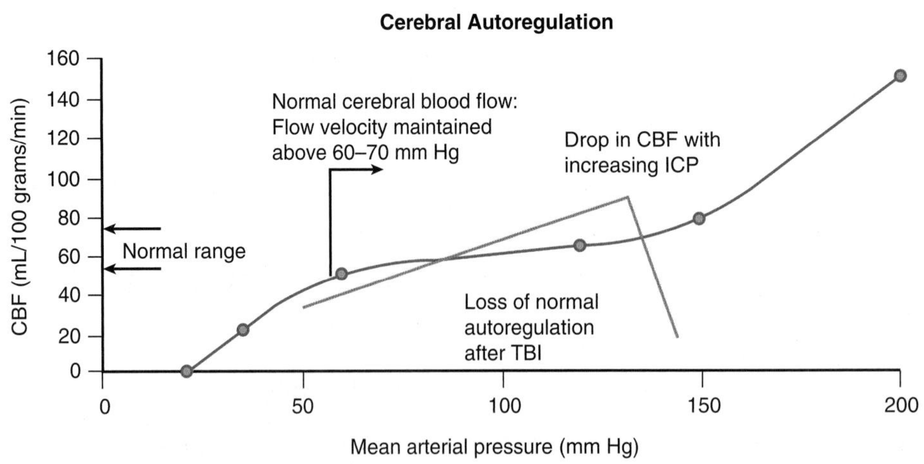

FIGURE 257-1. Pressure–volume relationship in brain injury. Normal cerebral blood flow autoregulation curve and the abnormal curve with traumatic brain injury (TBI). Normal autoregulatory control (*blue line*) maintains a relatively constant cerebral blood flow over a broad range of mean arterial pressure (MAP).9 Loss of autoregulation results in a more linear relationship between cerebral blood flow (CBF) and MAP. Elevated intracranial pressure (ICP) can dramatically decrease CBF when autoregulation is impaired (*inflection point of red line*). Increases in ICP may result in a net loss in CBF.

increased free radical production). **Extracellular edema** results from direct damage to, or the breakdown of, the blood–brain barrier, ionic shifts, and alteration of water exchange mechanisms (e.g., aquaporins).[19,20] As intracellular and extracellular water content rises, the brain swells and the ICP increases, leading to direct compressive tissue damage, vascular compression-induced ischemia, brain parenchyma herniation, and brain death.

BRAIN HERNIATION

There are four major brain herniation syndromes: uncal transtentorial, central transtentorial, cerebellotonsillar, and upward posterior fossa. The most common is uncal herniation, which occurs when the uncus of the temporal lobe is displaced inferiorly through the medial edge of the tentorium. This is usually caused by an expanding lesion in the temporal lobe or lateral middle fossa. **Uncal transtentorial herniation leads to compression of parasympathetic fibers running with the third cranial (oculomotor) nerve, causing an ipsilateral fixed and dilated pupil due to unopposed sympathetic tone. Further herniation compresses the pyramidal tract, which results in contralateral motor paralysis.** In some cases, the pupillary changes can be contralateral, whereas the motor changes are ipsilateral.

Central transtentorial herniation is less common and occurs with midline lesions, such as lesions of the frontal or occipital lobes, or vertex. **The most prominent symptoms are bilateral pinpoint pupils, bilateral Babinski's signs, and increased muscle tone.** Fixed midpoint pupils follow along with prolonged hyperventilation and decorticate posturing.

Cerebellotonsillar herniation occurs when the cerebellar tonsils herniate through the foramen magnum. **This may lead to pinpoint pupils, flaccid paralysis, and sudden death.** Upward transtentorial herniation results from a posterior fossa lesion and leads to a conjugate downward gaze with absence of vertical eye movements and pinpoint pupils.

THE GLASGOW COMA SCALE

TBI severity is classified using the GCS (Table 257-3). The scale is composed of three components: eye opening (1 to 4 points), verbal response (1 to 5 points), and motor response (1 to 6 points) (Table 257-3). The sum of these components defines the TBI severity classification into **severe** (GCS score of 3 to 8), **moderate** (GCS score of 9 to 13), and **mild** (GCS score of 14 or 15). The motor score independently correlates with outcome, almost as well as the full score.[21]

The GCS is an objective measurement of clinical status, correlates with outcome, is a reliable tool for interobserver measurements, and is effective for measuring patient recovery or response to treatment over time. However, the scale has several limitations. It measures behavioral responses, not the underlying pathophysiology. Patients with similar GCS scores may have dramatically different underlying structural injuries and require different clinical interventions (**Figure 257-2**). It is not as useful as a single acute measure of severity as it is as a tool to measure disease progression over time. The GCS may additionally be affected by drugs, alcohol, medications, paralytics, or ocular injuries. Finally, the scale lacks the granularity necessary to assess mTBI.

TABLE 257-3 Glasgow Coma Scale for All Age Groups

	4 y to Adult	Child <4 y	Infant
Eye opening			
4	Spontaneous	Spontaneous	Spontaneous
3	To speech	To speech	To speech
2	To pain	To pain	To pain
1	No response	No response	No response
Verbal response			
5	Alert and oriented	Oriented, social, speaks, interacts	Coos, babbles
4	Disoriented conversation	Confused speech, disoriented, consolable, aware	Irritable cry
3	Speaking but nonsensical	Inappropriate words, inconsolable, unaware	Cries to pain
2	Moans or unintelligible sounds	Incomprehensible, agitated, restless, unaware	Moans to pain
1	No response	No response	No response
Motor response			
6	Follows commands	Normal, spontaneous movements	Normal, spontaneous movements
5	Localizes pain	Localizes pain	Withdraws to touch
4	Moves or withdraws to pain	Withdraws to pain	Withdraws to pain
3	Decorticate flexion	Decorticate flexion	Decorticate flexion
2	Decerebrate extension	Decerebrate extension	Decerebrate extension
1	No response	No response	No response
3–15			

Note: In intubated patients, the Glasgow Coma Scale verbal component is scored as a 1, and the total score is marked with a "T" (or tube) denoting intubation (e.g., 8T).

CLINICAL FEATURES

The results of history, examination, and diagnostic imaging will allow the distinction into two categories of injury: moderate-severe brain injury and mild brain injury. Treatment and disposition are quite different in the two categories and are detailed below.

HISTORY

Obtain an accurate history from the patient, witnesses, and EMS crews to gain important insight into the mechanism of injury and overall severity of TBI (e.g., height of fall, impact surface condition, damage sustained to vehicle, airbag deployment, seat belt use, history of ejection from the vehicle, or report of fatalities at the scene). Premorbid medical history, medications (especially anticoagulants), drug use, and/or alcohol intoxication are also important in the assessment and treatment of acute TBI. **Initial clinical findings and physical exam as reported by EMS are an essential component of triaging and managing TBI.** The presence of a focal neurologic deficit, seizures, emesis, or depressed level of consciousness increases concern for underlying brain injury.

PHYSICAL EXAMINATION

Follow Advanced Trauma Life Support principles to perform the trauma-focused examination, with simultaneous lifesaving procedures as needed. Protect the cervical spine during evaluation, treatment, and imaging.

Obtain the GCS. Classify the injury as **severe (GCS score of 3 to 8), moderate (GCS score of 9 to 13), or mild (GCS score of 14 or 15). If emergency intubation is necessary, obtain a preintubation GCS and record the patient's best score.**

Determine **pupillary response.**[22] In an unresponsive patient, a single fixed and dilated pupil may indicate an intracranial hematoma with uncal herniation that requires rapid surgical decompression. **Bilateral fixed and dilated pupils** suggest increased ICP with poor brain perfusion, bilateral uncal herniation, drug effect (such as atropine), or severe hypoxia. Bilateral pinpoint pupils suggest either opiate exposure or central pontine lesion.

Altered **motor function** can indicate brain, spinal cord, or peripheral nerve injuries. Assess movement in a coma patient by observing the patient's reaction to noxious stimuli, such as pressure to a nail bed. **Decorticate posturing** (upper extremity flexion and lower extremity extension) indicates severe intracranial injury above the level of the midbrain. **Decerebrate posturing** (arm extension and internal rotation with wrist and finger flexion and internal rotation and extension of the

6 Different Examples of Severe TBI

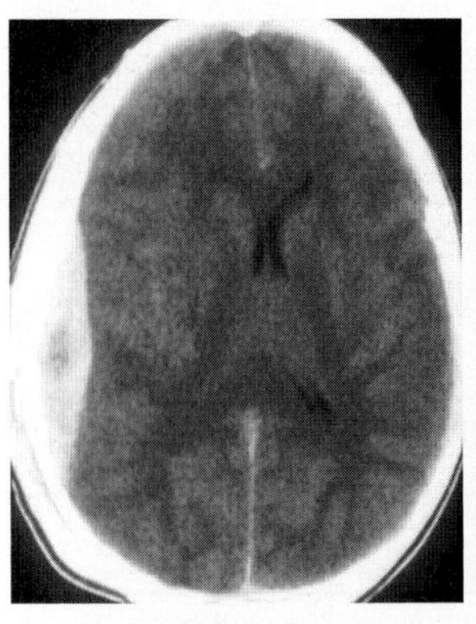

Epidural hematoma

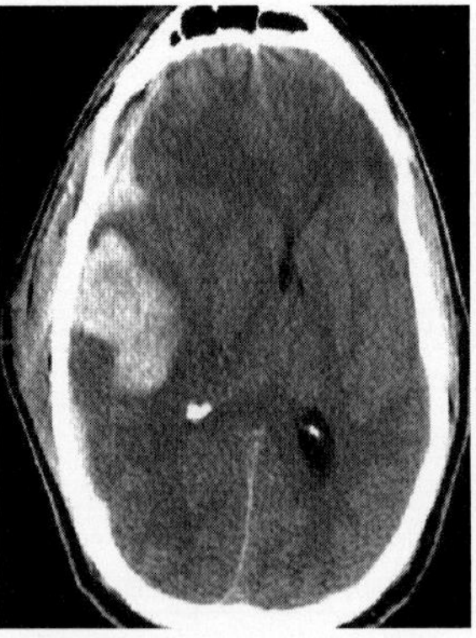

Contusion/Hematoma

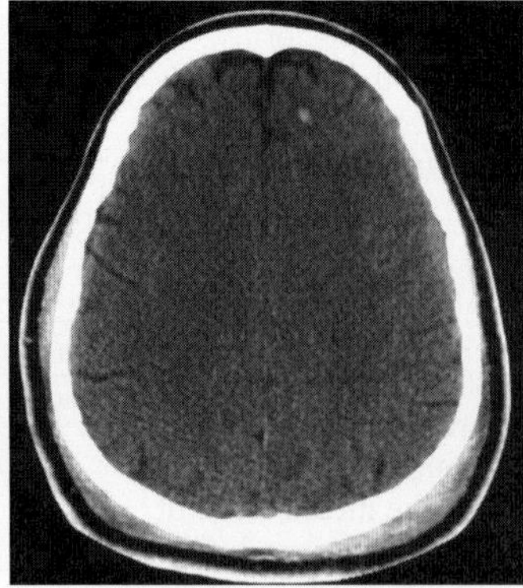

Diffuse axonal injury

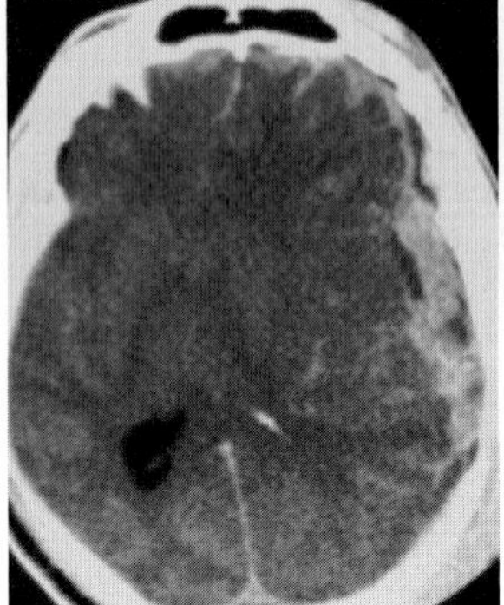

Subdural hematoma

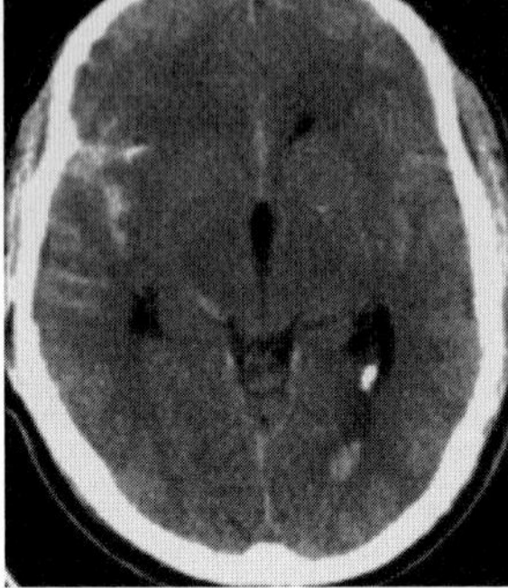

Subarachnoid hemorrhage

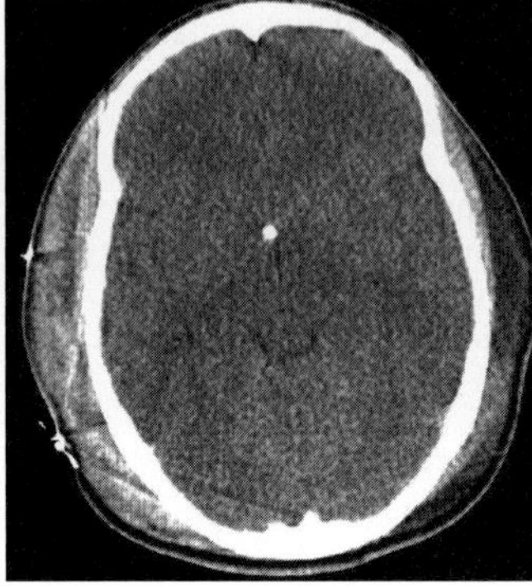

Diffuse swelling

FIGURE 257-2. Each of these CT images shows a distinct trauma-induced pathophysiologic abnormality, yet all patients had a Glasgow Coma Scale score of 4. [Image used with permission of Alisa Green, MD, University of California, San Francisco.]

lower extremities) indicates a more caudal injury. For completely unresponsive patients, respiratory pattern and eye movements can provide information regarding brainstem function. Remember, do not assess oculovestibular (cold caloric) and oculocephalic (doll's eyes) responses in a patient under cervical spine precautions.

IMAGING

Individually assess each patient's mechanism of injury, history, comorbidities, and signs and symptoms when determining the need for CT imaging of the head and cervical spine.

Head CT is exquisitely sensitive to the presence of blood and guides ED management. Do not delay head CT, because expanding hemorrhagic lesions need emergency neurosurgical intervention. Therefore, **if the patient is uncooperative or combative, intubation and sedation are often the best options to enable rapid CT imaging.** Other means to control agitated patients with TBI include midazolam (1 to 2 milligrams IV) and propofol (20 milligrams every 10 seconds to desired effect).

Several decision rules have been developed to minimize unnecessary head CT imaging.[23-27] The guidelines strive to identify patients with surgical emergencies. These studies do not specifically address the relationship between minor CT findings (which may place the patient at risk for the development of seizures), the duration of postconcussive symptoms, and progressive changes on CT during the course of a patient's evaluation. Adults with mTBI and a GCS score of 14 or 15 will have an intracranial lesion on CT about 15% of the time, but <1% will require neurosurgical intervention.[28]

The prevalence of **cervical fractures** in comatose TBI patients is approximately 8%, and an estimated 4% of injuries are missed on the initial assessment of the trauma patient.[23] Cervical imaging is a vital component in the care of the brain-injured patient. Perform CT imaging of the cervical spine in patients with altered mental status and who were injured by a mechanism that increases the risk of cervical spine injury. CT is superior to plain radiography in patients with altered mental status and can be performed at the same time as the head CT.

The **NEXUS** and **Canadian Cervical Spine Rules** are discussed in detail in chapter 258, "Spine Trauma."

MRI can detect subtle lesions missed by CT imaging and can better define the extent of contusions. However, MRI may not detect subtle lesions, cannot be performed if the patient is unstable, and is not always available.

DECISION RULES FOR HEAD CT IMAGING IN ADULTS

Decision rules can guide clinical practice, but each patient must be assessed individually, and none of the rules described below address short- or long-term nonoperative sequelae of TBI. See chapter 110, "Pediatric Trauma," for a discussion of the role of head CT imaging in children with minor head injury.

The two most commonly used evidence-based clinical decision rules for head CT in adults are the **New Orleans Criteria**[29] and the **Canadian CT Head Rule.**[23] Both rules have been validated and are 100% sensitive in detecting patients who will need neurosurgical intervention, but they have limited specificity (5% versus 37%, respectively). The Canadian CT Head Rule is less sensitive (83%) if intracranial lesion is the defined end point. *A negative feature of these two decision rules is that loss of consciousness or amnesia is required as the entry point.* **Most minor brain injury events do not result in loss of consciousness, and loss of consciousness is not the best predictor of intracranial pathology (Table 257-4). Do not apply these rules to patients taking anticoagulants or antiplatelet agents, or to children, because these variables were not included in the validation studies.**

The *National Institute for Clinical Excellence* and the *Neurotraumatology Committee of the World Federation of Neurosurgical Societies* have evaluated clinical signs and symptoms associated with TBI in adults and adolescents and adults, respectively.[27,30] The resultant decision rules for head CT have been applied to large data sets and shown to be relatively sensitive (National Institute for Clinical Excellence: 94% for neurosurgical lesions, 82% for intracranial lesions; Neurotraumatology Committee: 100% for neurosurgical lesions and intracranial injuries). One study evaluated 1101 patients with mTBI who had GCS scores of 14 or 15;

TABLE 257-4 New Orleans Criteria and Canadian CT Head Rule Clinical Decision Rules

New Orleans Criteria—GCS 15*	Canadian CT Head Rule—GCS 13–15*
Headache	GCS <15 at 2 h
Vomiting	Suspected open or depressed skull fracture
Age >60 y	Age ≥65 y
Intoxication	More than one episode of vomiting
Persistent antegrade amnesia	Retrograde amnesia >30 min
Evidence of trauma above the clavicles	Dangerous mechanism (fall >3 ft or struck as pedestrian)
Seizure	Any sign of basal skull fracture
Identification of patients who have an intracranial lesion on CT	
100% sensitive, 5% specific	83% sensitive, 38% specific
Identification of patients who will need neurosurgical intervention	
100% sensitive, 5% specific	100% sensitive, 37% specific

Abbreviation: GCS = Glasgow Coma Scale.

*Presence of any one finding indicates need for CT scan.

TABLE 257-6 CT Scanning for Adults with Brain Injury (American College of Emergency Physicians Guidelines)

Adults with a Glasgow Coma Scale score of <15 at the time of evaluation should undergo CT imaging

Mild traumatic brain injury with or without loss of consciousness: if one or more of the following is present:

- Glasgow Coma Scale score <15
- Focal neurologic findings
- Vomiting more than two times
- Moderate to severe headache
- Age >65 y
- Physical signs of basilar skull fracture
- Coagulopathy
- Dangerous mechanism of injury (e.g., fall >4 ft)

Mild traumatic brain injury with loss of consciousness or amnesia: if one or more of the following is present:

- Drug or alcohol intoxication
- Physical evidence above the clavicles
- Persistent amnesia
- Posttraumatic seizures

approximately 2% of these patients without loss of consciousness had intracranial lesions and 0.6% required surgery (rates similar to patients with loss of consciousness).

One of the most important findings from these studies is the relative significance of certain elements of the history and physical examination. For example, nausea and vomiting after concussion has an odds ratio comparable to that of loss of consciousness for a positive CT finding (**Table 257-5**). Importantly, the predictive value of individual clinical signs and symptoms differs between adults and children (see chapter 138, Head Injury in Infants and Children).

A summary of the American College of Emergency Physicians recommendations[28] is given in **Table 257-6**. A combination of rules helps identify patients *at risk* and determine the possible need for a head CT (**Tables 257-4, 257-5 and 257-6**).

TREATMENT

PREHOSPITAL CARE

Early appropriate management can have a profound impact on the patient's final outcome. For patients with moderate to severe head injury, provide stabilization and rapid transport to a facility with experience in the management of brain injury. The most important prehospital interventions are airway and blood pressure management. If the patient needs prehospital intubation, avoid hyperventilation (which causes cerebral vasoconstriction and can negatively affect outcome), and use **capnometry** to keep P_{CO_2} at 35 to 45 mm Hg. Treat hypotension aggressively. If transport times are short, do not give mannitol or hypertonic saline for elevated ICP. Guidelines for prehospital care are available at http://www.braintrauma.org.

TABLE 257-5 Odds Ratio (OR) for Head CT and Clinical Features

	Smits et al[30]	Ibanez et al[26]	Fabbri et al[27,70]
	OR (95% CI)	OR (95% CI)	OR (95% CI)
Glasgow Coma Scale score of 14	2 (1–3)	7 (4–14)	19 (14–26)
Neurologic deficits	2 (1–3)	7 (2–25)	19 (13–28)
Signs of basilar skull fracture	14 (8–22)	11 (6–23)	10 (6–16)
Loss of consciousness	2 (1–3)	7 (4–11)	2 (2–3)
Posttraumatic amnesia	1.7 (1–2)	3 (2–5)	8 (6–12)
Headache	1.4 (1–2)	3 (2–6)*	—
Vomiting	3 (2–4)	4 (2–7)	5 (3–8)
Posttraumatic seizure	3 (1–10)	2 (0.25–17)	3 (2–5)
Intoxication	1 (0.6–2)	1 (0.3–3)	—
Antithrombotics	2 (1–4)	4 (3–7)	8 (3–9)
Age >65 y	—	2 (1–3)	2 (1–3)
Dangerous mechanism of injury	2 (1–4)	—	3 (2–4)

Abbreviation: CI = confidence interval.

*For severe headache.

ED TREATMENT

Principles for ED care of moderate/severe brain injury are provided at http://www.braintrauma.org and are discussed in the following section. The primary goals of treatment are to maintain cerebral perfusion and oxygenation by optimizing intravascular volume and ventilation; prevent secondary injury by correcting hypoxia, hypercapnia, hyperglycemia, hyperthermia, anemia, or hypoperfusion; recognize and treat elevated ICP; arrange for neurosurgical intervention to evacuate intracranial mass lesions; and treat other life-threatening injuries.

Systolic blood pressure of <90 mm Hg and hypoxemia (Pa_{O_2} <60) are associated with a 150% increase risk in mortality.[31]

Observe for the **signs/symptoms of elevated ICP**: change in mental status, pupillary irregularities, focal neurologic deficits, decerebrate or decorticate posturing, or CT pathology. Some CT signs of intracranial hypertension are attenuation of the visibility of sulci and gyri, because the brain is compressed against the skull; compressed lateral ventricles; and poor grey/white matter distinction. Papilledema may not be evident if pressure rises rapidly. **Sedation and analgesia** may decrease baseline ICP and prevent transient rises in ICP from agitation, coughing, or gagging from the endotracheal tube. Prevent and control **seizure activity**.

Treat hypotension, hypoxemia, hypercarbia, and hyperglycemia. A single occurrence of hypotension and hypoxia after brain injury is associated with a 150% increase in mortality.[22] TBI is progressive, so appropriate early management will have a greater impact on outcome than treatments initiated after neuronal cell death and the development of secondary injury, such as cerebral edema. Jointly develop and apply goal-directed protocols with emergency medicine, trauma, neurosurgery, and intensive care teams. An example of early goal-directed therapy is provided in **Table 257-7**.

Airway and Breathing Treat any condition that compromises ventilation (e.g., altered mental status, facial/neck trauma, pneumothorax). **Patients with severe injury (GCS score of ≤8) require intubation.** Use short-acting induction agents that have limited effect on blood pressure

TABLE 257-7 Checklist for ED Treatment of Brain Injury

	Treatment	Comments
Cervical spine	Spinal precautions	
Airway	Maintain airway, intubate for GCS <8 or as needed	
Oxygenation and ventilation	Oxygen saturation >90; Pco_2 35–5	No prophylactic hyperventilation
BP	Systolic BP >90 mm Hg, MAP 80 mm Hg; give NS, blood products, or transfuse as needed	No permissive hypotension; pressors may be required if fluids not sufficient
Exam and GCS	GCS before paralytics if possible; treat life-threatening injuries and active bleeding	Serial GCS is helpful in identifying change; keep goal of "brain resuscitation" as top priority
Stat head CT and cervical spine CT	Identify mass lesions and signs of increased ICP	Protect cervical spine until cleared
Repeat exam	Check GCS for changes and for signs of impending herniation/deterioration	Change of more than 2 points should prompt further workup
Check glucose	Treat hypoglycemia *and* hyperglycemia	Hyperglycemia is bad for the brain
Control temperature	Maintain between 36°F and 38.3°F	Aggressive cooling: Tylenol, cooling blanket, etc.
Seizure prophylaxis	Give antiepileptic drug if GCS ≤10, acute seizure with injury, or abnormal head CT scan	Phenytoin (Dilantin)/fosphenytoin/levetiracetam
Identify and treat elevated ICP, herniation	Keep head of the bed at 30 degrees; ensure good BP, ventilation, and temperature control; give mannitol 1 gram/kg IV bolus; urgent NS consult	Consider adding hypertonic saline (3% NaCl 250 mL/30 min) for refractory elevations in ICP; monitor BP and electrolytes
Neurosurgery referral/transfer for advanced care	ICP monitoring, ventriculostomy for ICP management, aggressive tiered approach to management, emergency surgery	ICP monitoring and CSF diversion in GCS ≤8

Abbreviations: BP = blood pressure; CSF = cerebrospinal fluid; GCS = Glasgow Coma Scale; ICP = intracranial pressure; MAP = mean arterial pressure; NS = normal saline.

or ICP (**Table 257-8**). Avoid nasotracheal intubation if facial trauma or basilar skull fracture is evident or suspected. Monitor blood pressure throughout the procedure. Preinduction agents such as low-dose succinylcholine, vecuronium, pancuronium, and lidocaine do not improve outcome, but can be used as adjuncts if they do not delay airway control.[32] Maintain in-line cervical spine stabilization during intubation.

Maintain oxygenation and use capnometry to control Pco_2 and avoid hyperventilation. Prolonged (>6 hours) hypocapnia causes cerebral vasoconstriction and worsens cerebral ischemia. **Keep oxygen saturation >90, Pao_2 >60, and Pco_2 at 35 to 45.**

Circulation Traumatic hypotension leads to ischemia within low flow regions of the injured brain. Ischemia amplifies the neurotoxic cascade and increases cerebral edema. Provide aggressive fluid resuscitation to prevent hypotension and secondary brain injury. **Maintain systolic blood pressure at >90 mm Hg and MAP >80 mm Hg.** A blood pressure within "normal" range may be inadequate to maintain adequate flow and CPP if ICP is increased. **Permissive hypotension worsens outcome in patients with brain injury.**

Isolated head injury rarely produces hypotension, except as a preterminal event. Hypovolemic shock may be seen with polytrauma, massive blood loss from scalp lacerations, or in small children from subgaleal hematoma. If fluid and blood resuscitation is not effective, use vasopressors to preserve cerebral perfusion.

Pain and increased ICP can cause hypertension. Treat pain, and assess for impending herniation (*Cushing reflex*). For management, see discussion within this chapter under "Increased Intracranial Pressure Management" section.

TABLE 257-8 Intubation Agents in Brain Injury

Agent	Comments
Induction agent	
Etomidate, 0.3 milligram/kg IV	May be neuroprotective; may lower intracranial pressure; adrenal suppression unlikely with single use
Propofol 1–3 milligrams/kg IV	Rapid onset and offset; antiseizure properties; can cause hypotension if inadequate fluid resuscitation
Paralytics	
Succinylcholine 1–1.5 milligrams/kg IV	Short acting; avoid in burns, extensive muscle injury, etc.
Rocuronium, 0.6–1.0 milligram/kg IV	Short acting, safe in hyperkalemia

Patient Positioning Raising the head of the bed may improve cerebral blood flow by lowering ICP. However, the interaction between ICP, MAP, and tissue oxygenation is complex and highly variable. Response to position change depends on many factors such as degree of intact autoregulation, brain compliance, and individual patient variability. There is still uncertainty as to whether this procedure is beneficial, but in the setting of suspected elevated ICP, it is currently recommended as a simple maneuver to improve cerebral blood flow. One must ensure that the patient's blood pressure is maintained above the minimum recommended level (MAP 80 mm Hg), because elevation of 30 degrees can drop the mean pressure within the brain by up to 10 to 15 mm Hg and improve CPP (remember CPP = MAP − ICP, so lowering the ICP improves CPP, but lowering MAP in the setting of hypotension could be counterproductive and lower CPP). Elevating the head of the bed to 30 degrees can be safely accomplished even when the spine has not been cleared, as long as neck movement is secured.[33]

Glucose Control Hyperglycemia in the setting of neurologic injury (both stroke and TBI) is associated with worse outcome. Tight hyperglycemic control is recommended in patients with moderate to severe TBI. Insulin drips may be required to achieve adequate control (glucose 100 to 180 milligrams/dL or 5.55 to 9.99 mmol/L).

Temperature Control Elevated temperature is associated with an increased metabolic demand and excessive glutamate release. Elevated temperature elevates ICP and worsens outcome in many neurologic critical care conditions including TBI. Treat fever with the goal of normothermia. The evidence for hypothermia in TBI is not sufficient to recommend its use.

Seizure Treatment and Prophylaxis Seizures after head injury can change the neurologic examination, alter oxygen delivery and cerebral blood flow, and increase ICP. Prolonged seizures can worsen secondary injury. Treat acute seizures with IV lorazepam, and if seizures continue, treat as for status epilepticus. Give prophylactic phenytoin/phosphenytoin if the GCS is ≤10, if the patient has an abnormal head CT scan, or if the patient has had an acute seizure after the injury. The dose is 18 milligrams/kg IV at 25 milligrams/minute. Prophylactic anticonvulsants reduce the occurrence of posttraumatic seizures within the first week. Phenytoin/phosphenytoin is the agent most studied. Levetiracetam can be used, but there are less data supporting its use. Steroids have no role.

Cerebral Herniation Develop a team approach to ICP management between emergency medicine, neurosurgery, intensive care unit, and trauma teams.

Use patient history and physical examination to identify signs and symptoms of impending herniation. Indicators of rising ICP include severe headache, visual changes, numbness, focal weakness, nausea, vomiting, seizure, change in mental status, lethargy, hypertension, coma, bradycardia, and agonal respirations. Signs of impending transtentorial herniation include unilateral or bilateral pupillary dilation, hemiparesis, motor posturing, and/or progressive neurologic deterioration.

Measure neurologic deterioration by comparing sequential GCS scores. In a patient with a rapidly deteriorating GCS, if time permits, obtain a repeat head CT to identify an expanding intracranial hematoma.

Mannitol and/or hypertonic saline can lower ICP. Mannitol is an osmotic agent that can reduce ICP and improve cerebral blood flow, CPP, and brain metabolism. Mannitol is also a free radical scavenger. It generally has an effect within 30 minutes. Mannitol expands plasma volume and can improve oxygen-carrying capacity. Administer mannitol by repetitive bolus (0.25 to 1 gram/kg), and not by constant infusion. Because no dose-dependent effect is seen with mannitol, some clinicians advocate beginning at the lower range of the suggested dose. Mannitol results in a net intravascular volume loss because of its diuretic effect. Monitor the patient's input and output. Osmotic diuresis is *relatively contraindicated* in hemorrhage and hypotension. However, in the setting of acute herniation, mannitol has been demonstrated to effectively reduce life-threatening elevations of ICP.

Hypertonic saline may be used as an alternative to mannitol in the patient who is not adequately fluid resuscitated or hypotensive. The Brain Trauma Foundation indicates that at this time, data support the primary use of mannitol for the acute treatment of ICP. Most EDs have 3% NaCL available; the dose for adults is 250 mL over 30 minutes. Intensive care units may stock 23.4% sodium chloride solution; the dose for adults is 30 mL over 30 minutes. Monitor serum osmolality and serum sodium.

Mannitol and hypertonic saline may be given serially and in conjunction with one another.

ADVANCED TREATMENT OF BRAIN INJURY

Advanced treatment of brain injury requires invasive and close monitoring (**Table 257-9**).

Cerebral Perfusion Pressure Management If the GCS is ≤8, arrange for placement of an intracranial bolt or extraventricular drain with monitoring capabilities as soon as possible to monitor ICP and to direct treatment. Maintain CPP at 55 to 60 mm Hg to adequately perfuse brain tissue.[8] Increasing CPP >70 mm Hg may result in injury to other organs (e.g., acute respiratory distress syndrome from lung tissue trauma).

Consider ICP monitoring for patients with a normal admission brain CT scan if two or more of the following criteria are met: age over 40 years, unilateral or bilateral motor posturing, and systolic blood pressure <90 mm Hg. In addition, provide ICP monitoring in patients undergoing emergency surgery (e.g., orthopedic repair). Management of CPP is essential intraoperatively, where the patient with elevated ICP may experience large shifts in central volume status due to surgical blood loss.

Increased Intracranial Pressure Management An ICP of >20 mm Hg increases morbidity and mortality. Early consultation with neurosurgery for direct ICP monitoring, cerebrospinal fluid diversion, or surgical intervention is highly recommended in moderate and severe TBI. In certain circumstances, an ICP monitor will be placed in the ED by neurosurgery to help guide medical management of ICP, as well as for direct cerebrospinal fluid diversion to lower ICP.

TABLE 257-9 Goal-Directed Therapy of Brain Injury

Goal-Directed Therapy—Suggested Targets		
Pulse oximetry ≥90%	CPP ≥60 mm Hg	Physiologic sodium 135–140 mEq/L
SBP ≥90 mm Hg	ICP <20 mm Hg	INR ≤1.4
MAP ≥80 mm Hg	$PbtO_2$ ≥15 mm Hg	Platelets ≥75 × 10^3/μL
$Paco_2$ 35–45 mm Hg	pH 7.35–7.45	Hemoglobin ≥8 grams/dL
Temperature 36.0–38.3°C	Glucose 80–180 milligrams/dL	

Abbreviations: CPP = cerebral perfusion pressure; ICP = intracranial pressure; MAP = mean arterial pressure; $PbtO_2$ = brain tissue oxygen tension monitoring; SBP = systolic blood pressure.

SPECIFIC HEAD INJURIES

SCALP LACERATIONS

Scalp lacerations can lead to massive blood loss, so control bleeding as rapidly as possible. If direct pressure is not effective, locally infiltrate lidocaine with epinephrine and clamp or ligate bleeding vessels. Before closure, carefully examine wounds to identify foreign bodies, underlying fractures, and galeal lacerations. Large galeal disruptions should be repaired. For discussion of repair of scalp lacerations, see chapter 42, "Face and Scalp Lacerations."

SKULL FRACTURES

Patients who have or are suspected of having a skull fracture require a head CT scan (see Table 257-4). Skull fractures are usually categorized by location (basilar versus skull convexity), pattern (linear, depressed, or comminuted), and whether they are open or closed (**Figures 257-3 and 257-4**). A linear skull fracture with an overlying laceration is an open fracture. Explore wounds gently to avoid driving bone fragments into the brain.

Fractures that cross the middle meningeal artery, a major venous sinus, or linear occipital fractures have high intracerebral complication rates. Patients with skull fractures that are open or depressed, involve a sinus, or are associated with pneumocephalus should be given antibiotics (vancomycin, 1 gram IV, and ceftriaxone, 2 grams IV). A skull fracture that is depressed by more than the thickness of the skull usually requires operative repair.

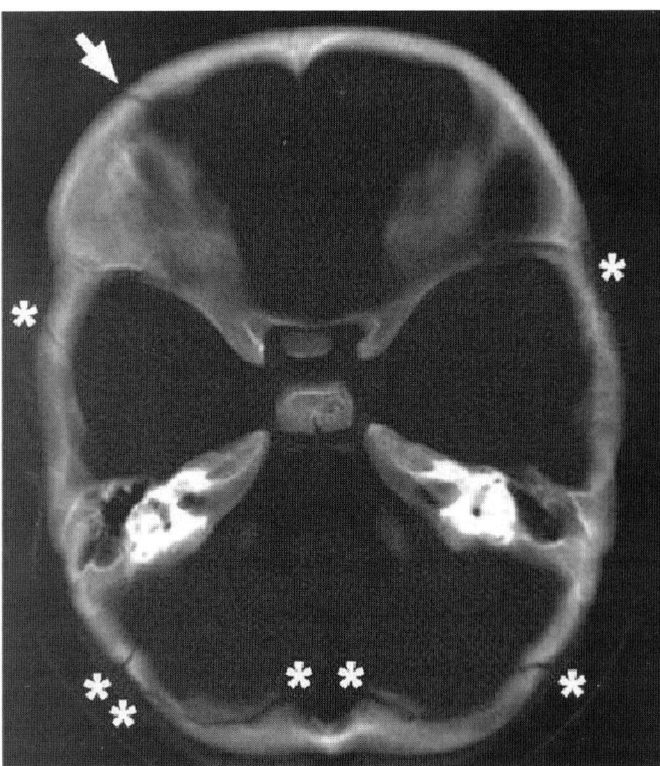

FIGURE 257-3. Linear fracture seen on CT. *Arrow* indicates skull fracture; *asterisks* indicate normal cranial suture lines. [Image used with permission of Joseph Piatt, Jr., MD, Division of Neurosurgery, A. I. duPont Hospital for Children, Wilmington, Delaware; Departments of Neurological Surgery and Pediatrics, Thomas Jefferson University, Philadelphia, Pennsylvania.]

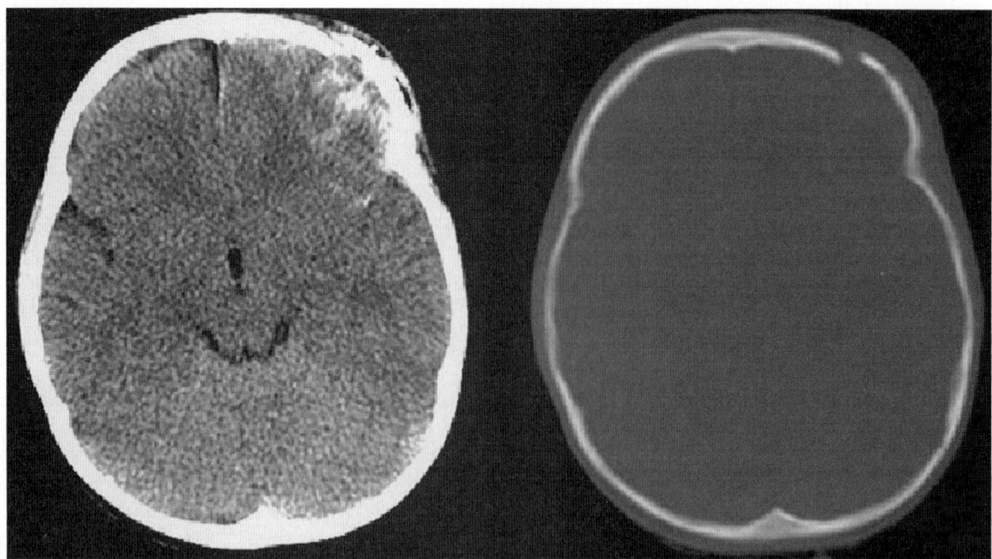

FIGURE 257-4. Open skull fracture with underlying cerebral contusion. This injury was sustained from a fall of two stories. [Image used with permission of Joseph Piatt, Jr., MD, Division of Neurosurgery, A. I. duPont Hospital for Children, Wilmington, Delaware; Departments of Neurological Surgery and Pediatrics, Thomas Jefferson University, Philadelphia, Pennsylvania.]

BASILAR SKULL FRACTURE AND CEREBROSPINAL FLUID LEAKS

The presence of a basilar skull fracture is a significant risk factor for intracranial injury. The most common basilar skull fracture involves the petrous portion of the temporal bone, the external auditory canal, and the tympanic membrane. It is associated with dural tearing, which often leads to otorrhea or rhinorrhea. Basilar skull fractures may occur anywhere along the skull base, from the cribriform plate through the occipital condyles. Do not place a nasogastric tube through the nares if cribriform plate fracture is suspected; this can lead to direct intracranial injury. **Signs and symptoms associated with basilar skull fractures include cerebrospinal fluid leak, mastoid ecchymosis (Battle sign), periorbital ecchymoses (raccoon eyes), hemotympanum, vertigo, decreased hearing or deafness, and seventh nerve palsy.** Periorbital and mastoid ecchymoses develop gradually over hours after an injury and are often absent in the ED. Cerebrospinal fluid leaks (otorrhea or rhinorrhea) are difficult to diagnose; however, the patient often complains of discharge of clear fluid from the nose or ears. Fluid may be collected and sent for analysis (identification of β transferrin). The β2 transferrin isoform of transferrin is found only in cerebrospinal fluid, and not in blood, mucus, or tears.

Patients with acute cerebrospinal fluid leaks are at risk for meningitis. Antibiotic prophylaxis is often recommended to reduce the incidence of infection.[30] Administration of antibiotics should be done in consultation with the neurosurgeon who will be following the patient. If prophylactic antibiotics are instituted, the drugs selected should have broad coverage with good penetration into the meninges, such as ceftriaxone, 2 grams IV, and vancomycin, 1 gram IV. The head of the patient's bed should be elevated to 30 degrees. A lumbar drain is often placed by the neurosurgical team. Cerebrospinal fluid leaks may require repair by a neurosurgeon or otolaryngologist.

CEREBRAL CONTUSION AND INTRACEREBRAL HEMORRHAGE

Contusions most commonly occur in the subfrontal cortex, in the frontal and temporal lobes, and, occasionally, in the occipital lobes (**Figure 257-5**). They are often associated with subarachnoid hemorrhage. Contusions may occur at the site of the blunt trauma or on the opposite side of the brain, known as a *contrecoup* injury.

Intracerebral hemorrhage can occur days after significant blunt trauma, often at the site of resolving contusions. This complication is more common in patients with coagulopathy. CT scan findings immediately after injury may be normal. Obtain serial CTs if any change in mental status occurs in a patient with coagulopathy until the clot is stable.

SUBARACHNOID HEMORRHAGE

Traumatic subarachnoid hemorrhage results from the disruption of the parenchyma and subarachnoid vessels and presents with blood in the cerebrospinal fluid (**Figure 257-6**). Patients with isolated traumatic

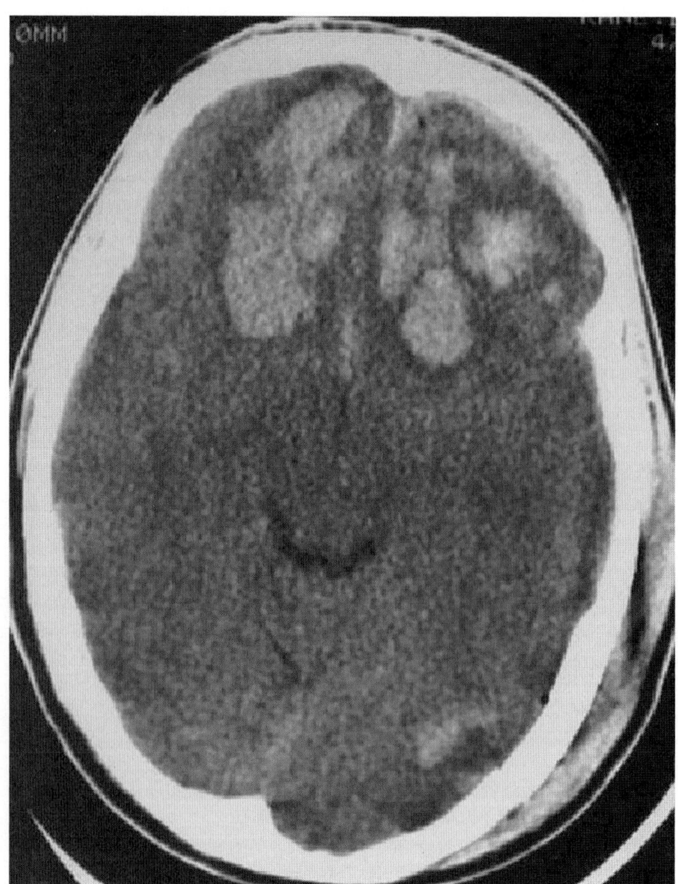

FIGURE 257-5. CT scan demonstrating delayed intraparenchymal hemorrhages from a traumatic contusion. [Image used with permission of Jack Fountain, Jr., MD, Emory University and Grady Memorial Hospital.]

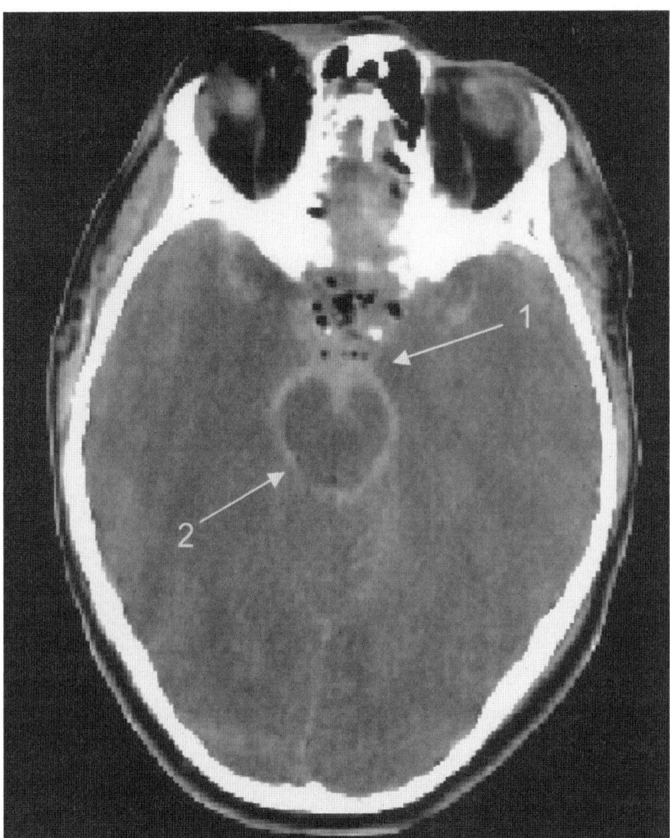

FIGURE 257-6. CT scan demonstrating subarachnoid hemorrhage. *Arrow 1* indicates prepontine cisternal blood, and *arrow 2* identifies blood in the ambient cistern. [Image used with permission of Jack Fountain, Jr., MD, Emory University and Grady Memorial Hospital.]

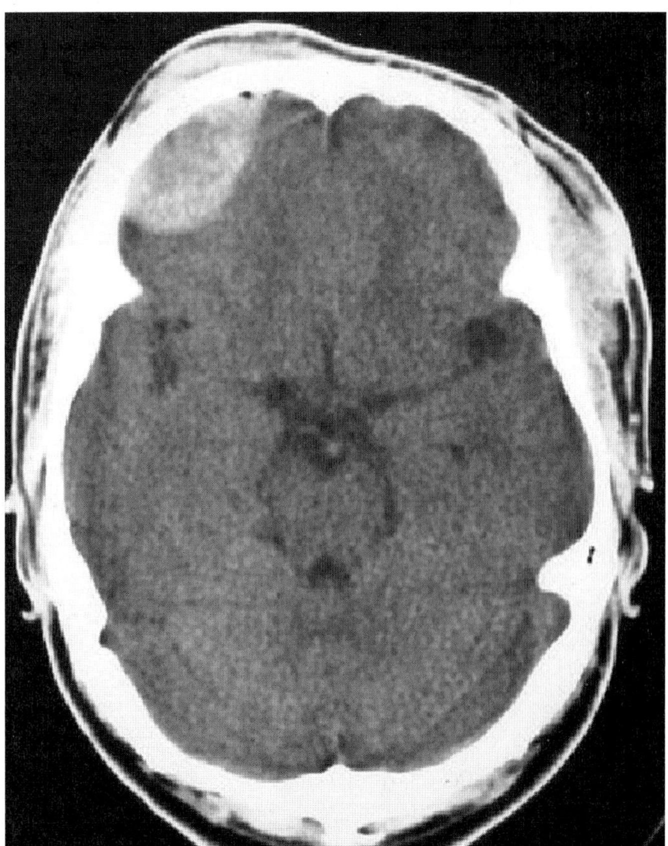

FIGURE 257-7. Epidural hematoma. Note the convex shape and focal location. [Image used with permission of Jack Fountain, Jr., MD, Emory University and Grady Memorial Hospital.]

subarachnoid hemorrhage may present with headache, photophobia, and meningeal signs. **Traumatic subarachnoid hemorrhage is the most common CT abnormality in patients with moderate to severe TBI.** Patients with early development of traumatic subarachnoid hemorrhage have a threefold higher mortality risk than those without traumatic subarachnoid hemorrhage (42% versus 14%, respectively).[34] Some traumatic subarachnoid hemorrhages can be missed on early CT scans. Generally, CT scans performed 6 to 8 hours after injury are sensitive for detecting traumatic subarachnoid hemorrhage.

EPIDURAL HEMATOMA

An epidural hematoma results when blood collects in the potential space between the skull and the dura mater (**Figure 257-7**). The anatomic relationships of the branches of the middle meningeal artery and the sequelae of fracture and laceration of the artery are shown in Figure 257-2.

Blunt trauma to the temporal or temporoparietal area with an associated skull fracture and middle meningeal arterial disruption is the primary mechanism of injury. Occasionally, trauma to the parieto-occipital region or the posterior fossa causes tears of the venous sinuses with epidural hematomas.

The classic history of an epidural hematoma involves a significant blunt head trauma with loss of consciousness or altered sensorium, followed by a lucid period and subsequent rapid neurologic demise. This clinical presentation occurs in a minority of cases. Traumatic blows to the thin temporal bone over the lateral aspect of the head carry the highest risk (e.g., baseball or pool stick injury). The diagnosis of an epidural hematoma is based on CT scan and physical examination findings. The CT appearance of an epidural hematoma is a biconvex (football-shaped) mass, typically found in the temporal region.

The high-pressure arterial bleeding of an epidural hematoma can lead to herniation within hours after an injury. Early recognition and evacuation reduces morbidity and mortality. Underlying injury of the brain parenchyma is often absent; full recovery may be expected if the hematoma is evacuated prior to herniation or the development of neurologic deficits.

SUBDURAL HEMATOMA

Subdural hematoma is caused by sudden acceleration-deceleration of brain parenchyma with subsequent tearing of the bridging dural veins. This results in hematoma formation between the dura mater and the arachnoid (**Figures 257-8 and 257-9**). Subdural hematoma tends to collect more slowly than epidural hematoma because of its venous origin. However, subdural hematoma is often associated with concurrent brain injury and underlying parenchymal damage. **Brains with extensive atrophy, such as in the elderly or in chronic alcoholics, are more susceptible to the development of acute subdural hematoma.** Even seemingly benign falls from standing position can result in subdural bleeding in the elderly. Children <2 years old are also at increased risk of subdural hematoma.

Traditionally, subdural hematomas have been classified as acute, subacute, or chronic depending on the length of time from onset and occurrence of active hemorrhage. Acute symptoms usually develop within 14 days of the injury. After 2 weeks, the term *chronic subdural hematoma* is used. There is no specific clinical syndrome associated with a subdural hematoma. Acute cases usually present immediately after severe trauma, and often the patient is unconscious. In the elderly or in alcoholics, chronic subdural hematomas may result in vague complaints or mental status changes. Often, there is no recall of injury. On CT scan, acute subdural hematomas are hyperdense (white), crescent-shaped lesions that cross suture lines. Subacute subdural hematomas are isodense and are more difficult to identify. CT scanning with IV contrast or MRI can assist in identifying a subacute subdural hematoma. A chronic subdural hematoma appears hypodense (dark) because the iron in the blood has been metabolized.

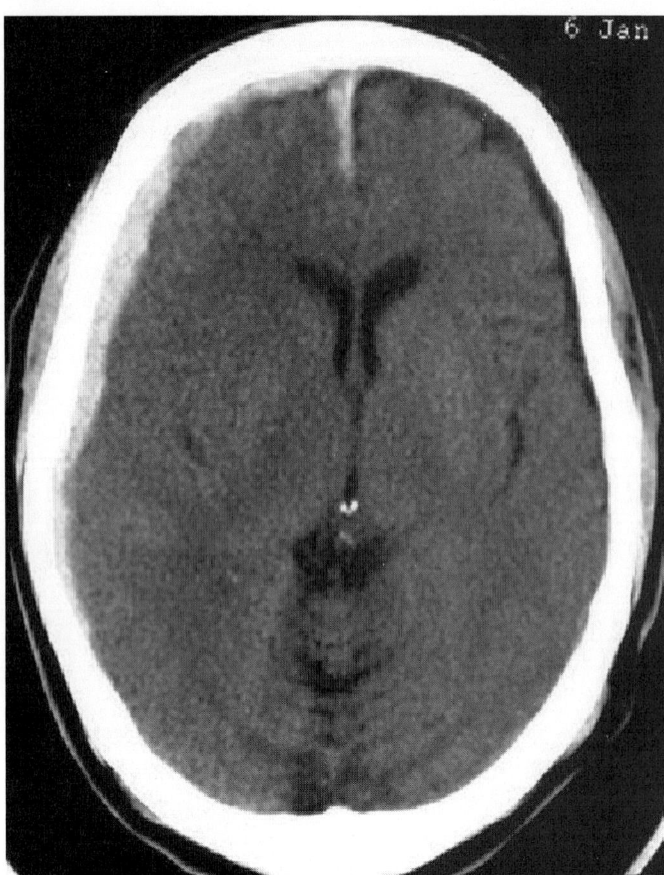

FIGURE 257-8. Small subdural hematoma in the right frontotemporal region in an adult. [Image used with permission of Jack Fountain, Jr., MD, Emory University and Grady Memorial Hospital.]

The definitive treatment depends on the type, size, effect on underlying brain parenchyma, and the associated brain injury. Mortality and the need for surgical repair are greater for acute and subacute subdural hematomas. Chronic subdural hematomas can sometimes be managed without surgery depending on the severity of the symptoms. **Table 257-10** compares intracranial injuries.

DIFFUSE AXONAL INJURY

Diffuse axonal injury is the disruption of axonal fibers in the white matter and brainstem. Shearing forces on the neurons generated by sudden deceleration cause diffuse axonal injury. The condition is seen after blunt trauma, such as from a motor vehicle crash. In infants, shaken baby syndrome is a well-described cause.[35]

In severe diffuse axonal injury, edema can develop rapidly. The underlying injury can result in devastating and often irreversible neurologic deficits. A CT scan of a patient with diffuse axonal injury may appear normal, but classic CT findings include punctuate hemorrhagic injury along the grey-white junction of the cerebral cortex and within the deep structures of the brain (**Figures 257-10 and 257-11**). Treatment options are very limited, but an attempt should be made to prevent secondary damage by reducing cerebral edema and limiting pathologic increases in ICP.

PENETRATING INJURY

As a bullet passes through the brain, it creates a cavity three to four times larger than its diameter. Direct penetration of the bullet through the brain substance and the transfer of kinetic energy cause the majority of the destruction (**Figure 257-12**). The GCS can be used to predict the prognosis for nonintoxicated patients with a gunshot wound to the brain.

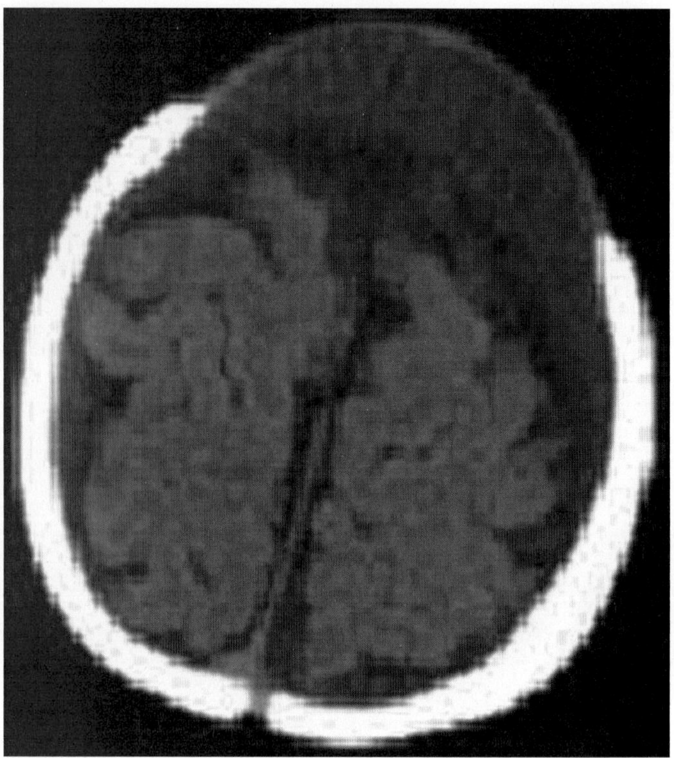

A

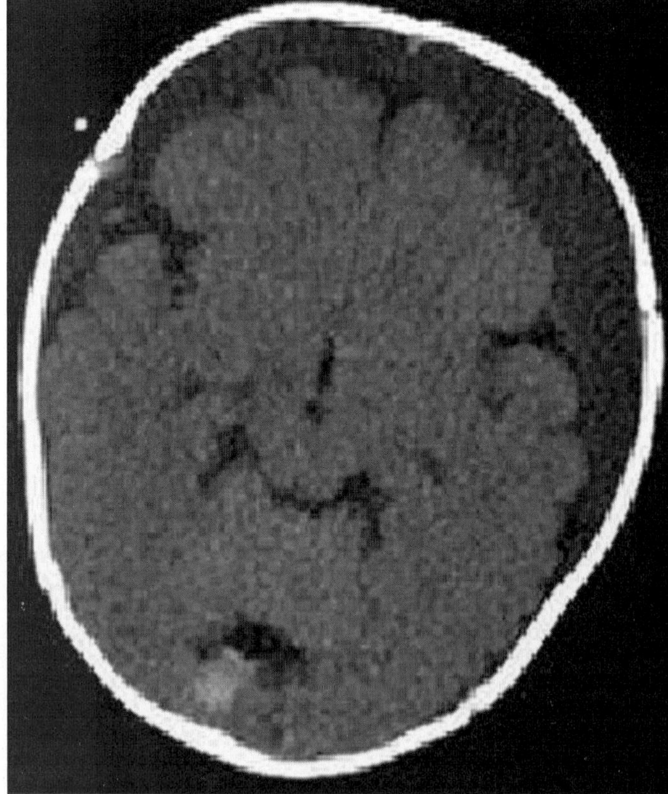

B

FIGURE 257-9. **A.** Bifrontal chronic subdural hematoma extending through the anterior fontanelle in a 1-month-old child. **B.** Second image in the same child showing bifrontal chronic subdural hematoma, as well as small, acute intraparenchymal hemorrhage in the posterior fossa.

TABLE 257-10 Comparison of Intracranial Injuries

	Type of Patient	Anatomic Location	CT Findings	Common Cause	Classic Symptoms
Epidural	Young, rare in the elderly and those age <2 y	Potential space between skull and dura mater	Biconvex, football-shaped hematoma	Skull fracture with tear of the middle meningeal artery	Immediate LOC with a "lucid" period prior to deterioration (only occurs in about 20%)
Subdural	More risk in the elderly and alcoholic patients	Space between dura mater and arachnoid	Crescent- or sickle-shaped hematoma	Acceleration-deceleration with tearing of the bridging veins	Acute: rapid LOC, lucid period possible Chronic: altered mental state and behavior with gradual decrease in consciousness
Subarachnoid	Any age group after blunt trauma	Subarachnoid	Blood in the basilar cisterns and hemispheric sulci and fissures	Acceleration-deceleration with tearing of the subarachnoid vessels	Mild, moderate, or severe traumatic brain injury with meningeal signs and symptoms
Contusion/ intracerebral hematoma	Any age group after blunt trauma	Usually anterior temporal or posterior frontal lobe	May be normal initially with delayed bleed	Severe or penetrating trauma; shaken baby syndrome	Symptoms range from normal to LOC

Abbreviation: LOC = loss of consciousness.

Patients with a GCS score of >8 and reactive pupils have a 25% mortality risk, whereas mortality approaches 100% in those with a GCS score of <5. Patients with a penetrating gunshot wound to the brain should be intubated and treated with prophylactic antibiotics, such as vancomycin, 1 gram IV, and ceftriaxone, 2 grams IV.

Stab wounds have very low energy and impart only direct damage to the area contacted by the penetrating object. Patients with penetrating injury require admission, broad-spectrum antibiotics, and operative intervention. **Leave impaled objects in place until controlled surgical removal is facilitated.**

MILD TRAUMATIC BRAIN INJURY

mTBI (often called a concussion) is impairment in brain function without overt hemorrhage or other gross lesions, is caused by an external force, and results in a GCS score of 14 or 15 (also see chapter 110 and **Table 257-3**).[1] The diagnosis is made by a history of any alteration in consciousness at the time or shortly after the inciting event (acceleration-deceleration or blunt force). Alteration in consciousness includes the individual's account of "getting his/her bell rung," "seeing stars," or being dazed or confused as a result of the force. The presence of amnesia further supports the diagnosis and is often associated with more significant injury.

Signs and symptoms such as vomiting, headache, loss of consciousness, focal neurologic deficit, age >65 years, coagulopathy, and/or dangerous mechanism of injury are factors that increase risk of serious injury (see Tables 257-4, 257-5, and 257-6).[26,27,30,36] The presence of alcohol, distracting injuries, and other barriers to obtaining a clear history of the event confound the signs and symptoms of mTBI.

PATHOPHYSIOLOGY

In its mildest form, mTBI is an ionic shift that causes a momentary disruption in function. Symptom recovery is rapid, and the concussive injury results in no obvious structural damage. However, mild insults can also cause a temporary upregulation of ion channels, especially along axons.[37,38] After a single injury, the ion channel density returns to normal over time. Repeated exposure to injury, however, greatly increases the resting number of channels. An increase in the density of ion channels leaves the brain vulnerable to overactivation, neuronal toxicity, and cell death.

In addition to ion channel upregulation, large shifts of balance in ion concentrations may lead to mitochondrial dysfunction and depletion of

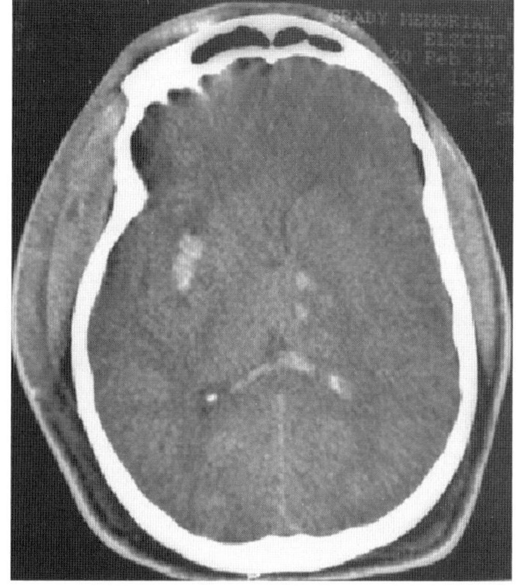

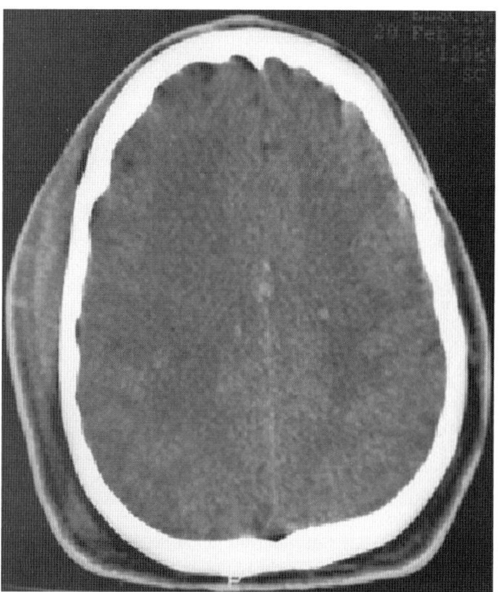

FIGURE 257-10. Diffuse axonal injury with intraventricular blood. [Image used with permission of Jack Fountain, Jr., MD, Emory University and Grady Memorial Hospital.]

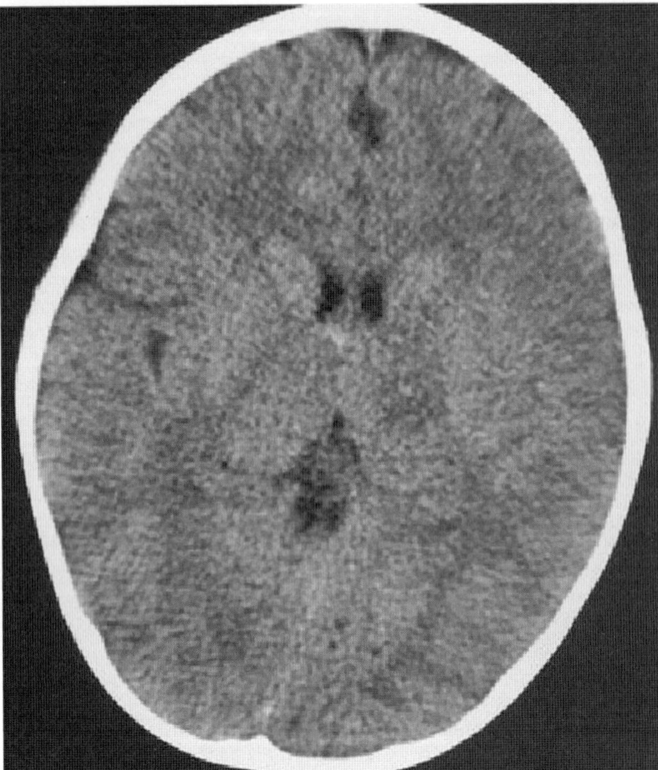

FIGURE 257-11. Diffuse axonal injury with loss of the grey matter–white matter interface. [Image used with permission of Daniel Curry, MD, PhD, Texas Children's Hospital and Baylor College of Medicine.]

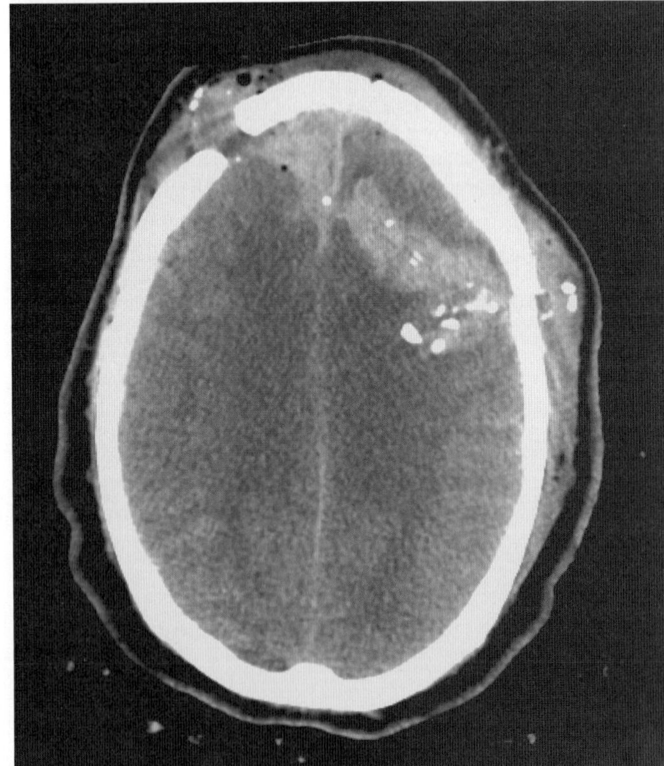

FIGURE 257-12. Gunshot wound traversing through frontal lobes bilaterally; note bone fragments. [Image used with permission of Thomas Egglin, MD, Director of Emergency Radiology and an Associate Professor of Diagnostic Imaging at the Warren Alpert Medical School of Brown University, Providence, RI.]

intracellular energy stores in mTBI.[14,39-41] This state creates a metabolic "mismatch" during which neuronal dysfunction persists until recovery occurs. This pathway is a recognized pattern of injury in moderate/severe TBI and is thought to also play a role in mTBI.

Metabolic insults, electrochemical imbalances (calcium influx and sodium and potassium shifts), and mitochondrial dysfunction also result in damage to axonal transport systems. Structural abnormalities are not always identified on MRI or CT. However, histopathology shows microscopic injury. Indeed, evidence of damage on diffusion tensor imaging has been demonstrated in high school athletes after a single football season, even without clinical signs or symptoms of a concussion.[42,43] Chronic traumatic encephalopathy[44] is hypothesized to occur as a result of repeated exposure to TBI in sports.[45-47]

Repetitive concussions can result in long-term cognitive deficits and structural damage to the brain.[48-51] In extreme cases, when a second concussion occurs prior to recovery from the first, rapid onset of cerebral edema and death can occur, particularly in athletes prematurely returning to play (**second impact syndrome**).[52]

DIAGNOSIS

The physical examination findings in isolated mTBI are often normal. Currently, there are no reliable tests that can confirm the diagnosis of concussion. The GCS lacks the detail to assess the full spectrum of signs and symptoms. Head CT scans are usually normal, and a normal scan only eliminates the concern for an underlying lesion requiring surgery.

Perform a thorough neurologic examination and obtain the GCS. Focal findings suggest potential intracranial pathology or a postictal state. Assess for signs of global impairment, such as confusion, perseveration, or amnesia.[53] Observe gait and test balance. **The most consistent abnormalities in mTBI are subtle impairments in cognitive function (see Table** 257-7**).** The gold standard written neuropsychological examination is impractical to perform in the ED setting. However, perform some assessment of cognition.

Clinical symptoms (**Table 257-11**) may begin immediately after the insult or may be delayed for days to weeks. Therefore, **the lack of obvious signs and symptoms at the time of evaluation does not exclude mTBI if the historical account is consistent with such injury**. Another complicating factor is that many of the signs and symptoms are nonspecific and overlap with those of other conditions.

The practice of grading concussions is widely employed but is not evidence based. There are >20 different classification systems in existence.[54]

Biomarkers Serum markers specific to neurologic injury may improve future diagnosis and management.[36,55,56]

Of the biomarkers currently under study, S100B (calcium binding protein B antibody) is the only one that is relatively sensitive (94% to 99% sensitive) for detecting the presence of injury, but only under specific conditions. S100B serum levels rise and fall rapidly, so time

TABLE 257-11 Signs and Symptoms of mTBI

Cognitive Symptoms	Physical Signs and Symptoms	Behavioral Changes
Attention difficulties	Headaches	Irritability
Concentration problems	Dizziness	Depression
Amnesia and perseveration	Insomnia	Anxiety
Short-term and long-term memory problems	Fatigue Uneven gait	Sleep disturbances Emotional lability
Orientation problems	Nausea, vomiting	Loss of initiative
Altered processing speed	Blurred vision	Loneliness and helplessness
Altered reaction time Calculation difficulties and problems with executive function	Seizures	Problems related to job, relationship, home, or school management

Note: At 3 months after injury, <30% are symptomatic; at 1 year, 15% are symptomatic.

from injury determines the relevance of a negative finding. S100B is also not currently approved by the U.S. Food and Drug Administration for mTBI. The American College of Emergency Physicians provides the following guidance: "***Level C recommendations.*** *In mTBI patients without significant extracranial injuries and a serum S-100B < 0.1 μg/L measured within 4 hours of injury, consideration can be given to not performing a CT.*"[57]

Cognitive Screening and Psychometrics Cognitive testing in the ED is currently limited to the use of brief memory screens such as the **Mini-Cog** (see Figure 288-2) or the **Quick Confusion Scale** (see Table 286-7). Other tools, primarily developed for sports, such as the Sports Concussion Assessment Tool, the Standardized Assessment for Concussion, and other similar instruments, have not been validated for ED use.

Neuropsychological testing[58-61] consists of a battery of individual tests that evaluate a number of domains required for normal brain function, including memory, attention, concentration, executive function, and reaction time. Several of these tests are used by sports programs to assess recovery from concussion. They are most valuable when baseline scores are available for comparison.

TREATMENT AND DISPOSITION

The primary treatment for mTBI is rest. Make sure the patient avoids aspirin and nonsteroidal anti-inflammatory drugs after acute injury. ED treatment objectives are to identify patients who have intracranial lesions requiring neurosurgical intervention; to admit patients whose condition might deteriorate over time; and for those discharged, to provide instructions for cognitive and physical rest and provide follow-up for reassessment before return to normal activities.

When the patient is safe for discharge, one of the most important "interventions" is to provide thorough concussion discharge instructions. A template is available at http://www.cdc.gov/ncipc/tbi/Physicians_Tool_Kit.htm. Physical and neurologic rest is needed until symptoms abate fully. Discharge the patient to the care of a responsible individual and provide instructions to both the patient and that individual. Patients with mTBI may not comprehend or remember detailed discharge instructions. Have the patient return to the ED for increasing symptoms, headaches, altered mental status, nausea, or vomiting. Refer patients for further evaluation and follow-up care. Patients at an increased risk for reinjury, such as athletes, should undergo a formal graduated return-to-activity program (**Table 257-12**).

Return to Activity Symptoms reflect underlying metabolic dysfunction and are currently the only reliable guide to brain health.[40,54] Return to play or work decisions are based on symptoms and a graduated evaluation program.

Assessments incorporate serial symptom checklists, neuropsychological tests (memory and reaction time assessment), and a balance evaluation (see Table 257-12).[54,62] **Because this type of assessment is not practical in the ED, ED clinicians should not provide definitive return-to-activity directions.**

TABLE 257-12 Return-to-Activity Program

Sports Related	Non–Sports Related
No activity (rest until symptom-free)	No activity (rest until symptom-free)
Light aerobic exercise	Light aerobic exercise
Sport-specific training (noncontact)	Moderate aerobic exercise
Noncontact drills	Return to normal activities
Full-contact drills	
Game play	

Note: Patient must remain asymptomatic for 24 hours between each step. Development of symptoms at any level requires return to the previous symptom-free level.

SPECIAL CONSIDERATIONS

POSTCONCUSSIVE SYNDROME

Patients often report a series of physical, emotional, and cognitive symptoms in the days and weeks after mTBI. The estimated prevalence of postconcussive syndrome varies widely, with about 20% to 40% of patients reporting symptoms at 3 months and about 15% at 1 year.[63,64] The most commonly reported postconcussion symptoms are headache, dizziness, decreased concentration, memory problems, sleep disturbances, irritability, fatigue, visual disturbances, judgment problems, depression, and anxiety.[65] When a cluster of symptoms becomes chronic after mTBI, they are often called **persistent postconcussive symptoms** or **postconcussion syndrome**. Clinical findings at the time of the injury do not reliably predict the development of postconcussive syndrome. Postconcussive syndrome symptoms can overlap those of posttraumatic stress disorder. Neuropsychological testing and use of a symptom checklist are the cornerstones of diagnosis and management. Treatment is symptomatic. Refer patients to a neuropsychologist or mTBI clinic.

RECURRENT CONCUSSIONS

Three or more concussions pose a risk for long-term sequelae, especially in adolescents and young children.[48,49,66] Almost all cases of **second impact syndrome** have occurred in young athletes. **Chronic traumatic encephalopathy**,[44] characterized by early onset of memory loss and depression, is a concern in professional athletes. Pathologically large deposits of tau protein are seen in the brains of deceased chronic traumatic encephalopathy patients.[47] Tau protein deposits have recently been discovered even in youth football players who died from other causes.

SECOND IMPACT SYNDROME

Second impact syndrome is a rare disorder that results in rapid cerebral edema and high mortality (60% to 80%).[52] The pathophysiology and the predictors are not well understood. It is hypothesized that occurrence of a second impact before the brain has reset or recovered from a first mTBI causes a loss of autoregulation and ion imbalance, and leads to rapid cerebral edema. This explanation fits well with the concept of enhanced vulnerability due to metabolic disturbances, energy-demand mismatch, and ion channel upregulation after a concussion.[67,68]

ANTICOAGULATION

Anticoagulants and antiplatelet agents increase the risk of intracranial hemorrhage after injury, especially in the elderly.

Intracranial hemorrhage in patients taking warfarin and who have an elevated INR is associated with a high mortality rate (89%).[69] In general, patients with head trauma, who are taking anticoagulants or antiplatelet agents, should undergo emergent head CT. The OR for the risk of intracranial lesions after mild head injury in patients taking any antiplatelet therapy is 2.6.[70] Clopidogrel seems to be a potent risk factor.[71] The effect of low-dose aspirin (162 mg or less taken daily) on post-head injury bleeding has not been determined.

Patients with intracranial hemorrhage need immediate anticoagulant reversal. Patients taking Warfarin who have an elevated INR are optimally treated with plasma or 4-factor concentrate. See chapters 239, "Thrombotics and Antithrombotics" and 166, "Spontaneous Subarachnoid and Intracerebral Hemorrhage" for further discussion.

A negative initial CT finding in an asymptomatic TBI patient receiving anticoagulation or antiplatelet therapy is reassuring, but delayed hemorrhage may occur and is not easily predicted. [71]

REFERENCES

The complete reference list is available online at www.TintinalliEM.com.

CHAPTER 258 Spine Trauma

Steven Go

INTRODUCTION AND EPIDEMIOLOGY

Trauma to the spine can cause a vertebral spinal column injury, a spinal cord injury, or both. A few studies have tried to estimate the annual incidence of spinal column injury in the general population with results ranging from 11.8 to 64 cases per 100,000,[1,2] but no current figures are available for the U.S. population. In contrast, the estimated annual incidence of spinal cord injury in the United States is 40 cases per million or 12,000 new cases per year, with 81% male victims, a mean age of 42.6 years, and a 67% Caucasian predominance.[3] Since 2010, the leading causes of spinal cord injury are vehicular (37%), falls (29%), and violence (14%). Lifetime costs for spinal cord injury victims vary according to age at time of injury, severity of injury, and socioeconomic status; however, estimates range in millions of dollars per patient.[3]

FUNCTIONAL ANATOMY

VERTEBRAL COLUMN

The vertebral column is composed of 33 vertebrae: 7 cervical, 12 thoracic, 5 lumbar, 5 fused sacral, and 4 (usually fused) coccygeal. The axial vertebrae (C1 and C2) are anatomically unique in that they are designed for rotary motion. The odontoid (dens) of the axis (C2) is held against the atlas (C1) by the strong transverse ligament. The remaining vertebrae share some common anatomical features (**Figure 258-1**). A typical subaxial vertebra is composed of an anterior body and a posterior vertebral arch. The vertebral arch is comprised of two pedicles, two laminae, and seven processes (one spinous, two transverse, and four articular). These articulations enable the spine to engage in flexion, extension, lateral flexion, rotation, or circumduction (combination of all movements). The orientation of these articular facet joints changes at different levels of the spine and accounts for variations in motion of specific regions of the vertebral column. Due to its inherent flexibility, the cervical spine is the most commonly injured region of the spinal column, with most injuries occurring at the C2 level and from C5 to C7.[4] The second most common region of injury is in the thoracolumbar transition zone.

A series of ligaments serves to maintain alignment of the spinal column. The anterior and posterior longitudinal ligaments run along the vertebral bodies. Surrounding the vertebral arch are the ligamentum flavum and the supraspinous, interspinous, intertransverse, and capsular ligaments. Between adjacent vertebral bodies are the intervertebral disks, consisting of a peripheral annulus fibrosus and a central nucleus pulposus. The intervertebral disks act as shock absorbers to distribute axial load. When compressive forces exceed the absorptive capacity of the disk, the annulus fibrosus ruptures. This allows the nucleus pulposus to protrude into the vertebral canal, and this may result in spinal nerve or spinal cord compression.

SPINAL CORD

The spinal cord is a cylindrical structure that begins at the foramen magnum, where it is continuous with the medulla oblongata of the brain and extends down the spinal canal to the first and second lumbar vertebrae. The spinal cord gives rise to 31 pairs of spinal nerves: 8 cervical, 12 thoracic, 5 lumbar, 5 sacral, and 1 coccygeal. Each spinal nerve emerges through the intervertebral foramen corresponding to the appropriate spinal cord level. The lower nerve roots form an array of nerves called the *cauda equina*.

PATHOPHYSIOLOGY

SPINAL COLUMN INJURIES

Given their multiple axes of motion, the bony vertebrae can be injured via several mechanisms and present with a number of different injury patterns (**Table 258-1**).[5-10]

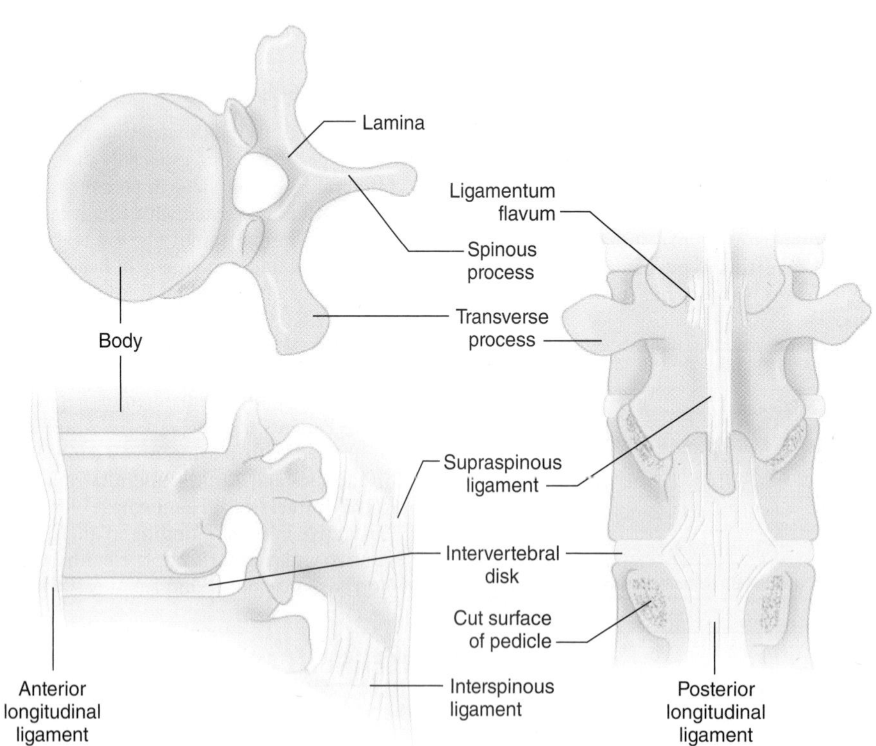

FIGURE 258-1. Vertebral anatomy. Each vertebra consists of a vertebral body and posterior element. Vertebrae are stabilized by an anterior longitudinal ligament, posterior ligament, and interspinous ligament.

TABLE 258-1 Major Spinal Column Injuries

Mechanism of Injury	Injury	Spinal Column Regions Typically Affected	Image	Notes
Flexion	Anterior subluxation (hyperflexion sprain) (usually stable, but depends on the integrity of posterior ligaments)	Cervical	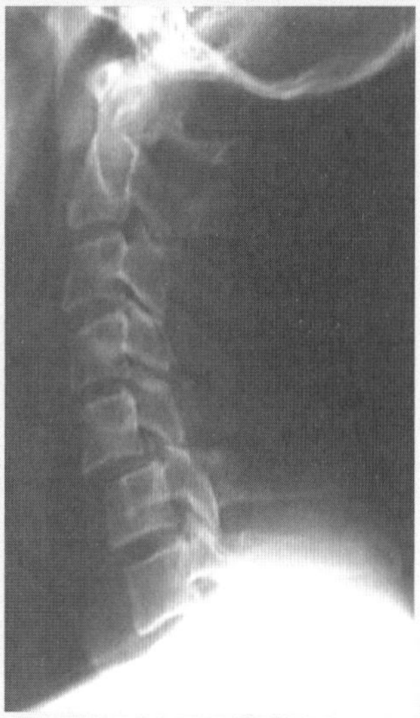 [Photo contributors: Mark Silverberg, MD/Steven Pulitzer, MD. Reproduced with permission from Shah BR, Lucchesi M, Amodio J (eds): *Atlas of Pediatric Emergency Medicine*, 2ed, © 2013, McGraw-Hill Education, New York, NY. Figure 20-57.]	Anterior subluxation produces ligamentous failure and may have no associated fractures. Plain films can be normal. However, significant ligamentous injury can display anterior soft tissue swelling, a widening of the spinous processes at the level of injury ("fanning"), posterior widening of the intervertebral space, and cervical disk space alignment ≥11 degrees between adjacent spaces.
	Atlantoaxial dislocation (unstable)	Cervical	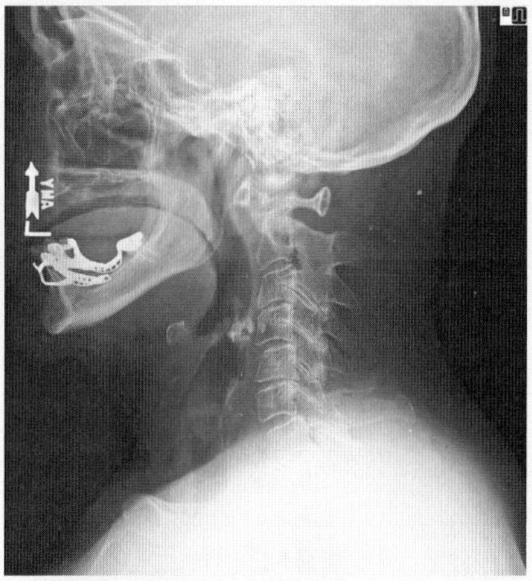 [Used with permission of Jake Block, MD.]	Transverse ligament **rupture** without an associated fracture can occur in older patients from a direct blow to the occiput. Radiographic diagnosis relies on measuring the *predental space*, which is the space between the posterior aspect of the anterior arch of C1 and the anterior border of the odontoid. A predental space of >3 mm on a lateral radiograph (2 mm for CT images) implies damage to the transverse ligament; >5 mm implies rupture of the transverse ligament.
	Bilateral interfacetal dislocation (unstable)	Cervical	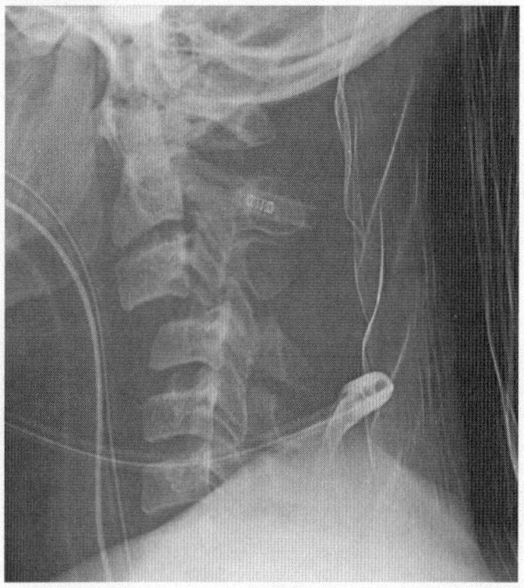	Bilateral interfacetal dislocation (*locked facets*) occurs when the articular masses of one vertebra dislocate anteriorly and superiorly from the articular surfaces of the adjacent vertebra below. Disruption of all ligamentous structures occurs. On radiographs, the vertebral body is dislocated anteriorly ≥50% of its width. These injuries usually present with neurologic deficits due to compromise of the intervertebral foramen, unless the dislocation is only partial (*perched facets*).

(Continued)

TABLE 258-1 Major Spinal Column Injuries (*Continued*)

Mechanism of Injury	Injury	Spinal Column Regions Typically Affected	Image	Notes
	Simple wedge (compression) fracture (usually stable)	Cervical; TL	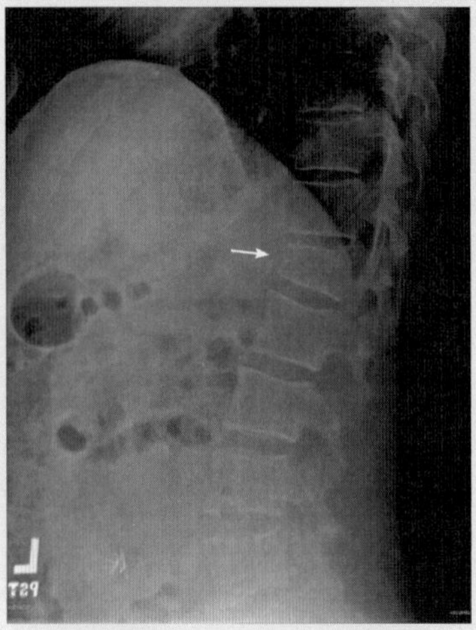 [Reproduced with permission from Block J, Jordanov MI, Stack LB, Thurman RJ (eds): *The Atlas of Emergency Radiology*. McGraw-Hill, Inc., 2013. Fig 11-22 Part A.]	Most common thoracic fracture (52%).[5] A vertebral wedge fracture typically involves a fracture of the superior end plate of the vertebral body while sparing the inferior end plate. An isolated simple wedge fracture is stable, but the presence of significant posterior ligamentous disruption can make the injury unstable. A simple wedge fracture is differentiated from a burst fracture by the absence of a vertical fracture of the vertebral body and lack of bulging of the posterior vertebral border.
	Spinous process avulsion (clay shoveler's) fracture (stable)	Cervical	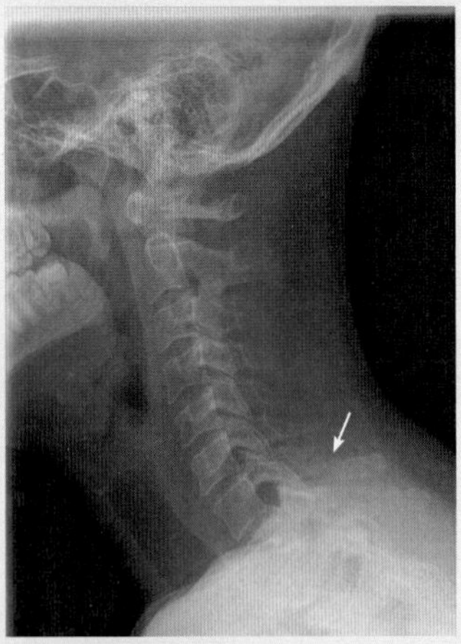 [Reproduced with permission from Block J, Jordanov MI, Stack LB, Thurman RJ (eds): *The Atlas of Emergency Radiology*. McGraw-Hill, Inc., 2013. Fig 11-10 Part A.]	This is an avulsion off the end of one of the lower cervical spinous processes (classically C7). It is thought to be caused by strong muscle contractions pulling on the bone via the ligamentous complex. It is not associated with neurologic compromise.
	Flexion teardrop fracture (highly unstable)	Cervical	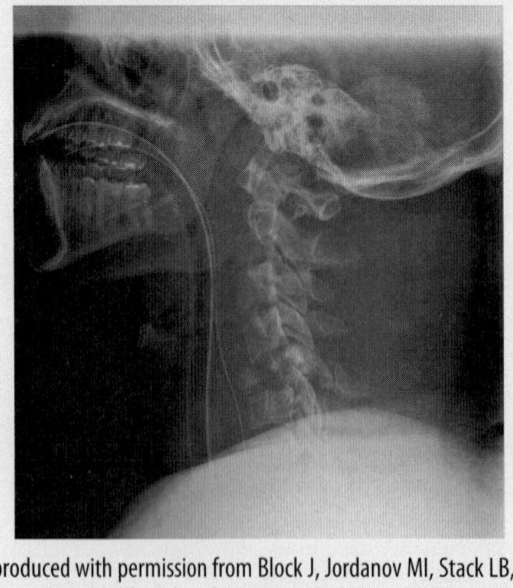 [Reproduced with permission from Block J, Jordanov MI, Stack LB, Thurman RJ (eds): *The Atlas of Emergency Radiology*. McGraw-Hill, Inc., 2013. Fig 11-1.]	Extreme hyperflexion causes complete disruption of the spinal ligaments at the level of injury. The "teardrop" is the anteroinferior portion of the vertebral body that is separated and displaced from the vertebral body by the anterior spinal ligament. "Fanning" of the spinous processes may be present, with or without fracture. A sagittal fracture through the vertebral body may be seen on CT. Anterior spinal cord syndrome is associated with this injury

(*Continued*)

TABLE 258-1 Major Spinal Column Injuries (*Continued*)

Mechanism of Injury	Injury	Spinal Column Regions Typically Affected	Image	Notes
Flexion-rotation	Unilateral facet dislocation (stable unless associated with an articular mass fracture)	Cervical	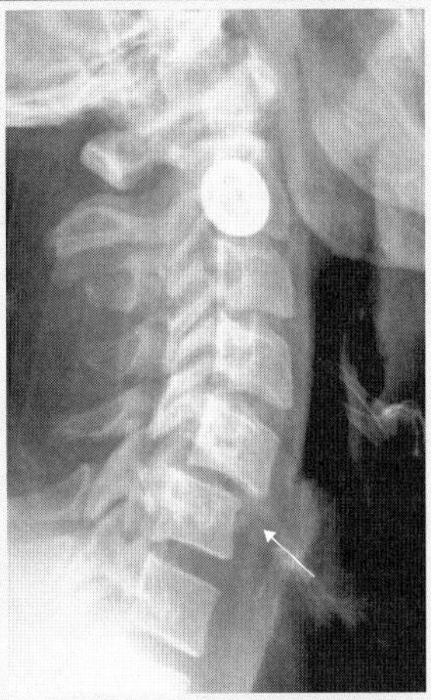 [Reproduced with permission from Simon RR, Sherman Scott C (eds): *Emergency Orthopedics*, 6th ed. McGraw-Hill, Inc., 2011. Fig 9-21B.]	A unilateral facet dislocation occurs when the articular mass and inferior facet on one side of the vertebra are anteriorly dislocated. On a lateral radiograph, the involved vertebral body will be displaced <50% of its width. On the anterior view, the spinous process at the level of the rotation will be pointing toward the side that is dislocated.
	Fracture of lateral mass (can be unstable)	Cervical	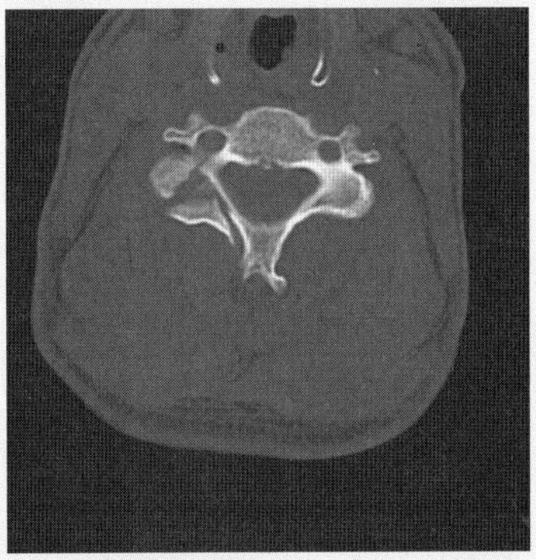 Comminuted fracture of the lateral mass of C4 extending into the right lamina.	Typically presents with severe neck pain and sometimes radicular symptoms. May be associated with Brown-Séquard syndrome or vertebral artery injury; therefore, some experts feel that magnetic resonance angiography should be done in all patients with this lesion.[6] A *pillar fracture* is a type of lateral mass fracture that consists of an isolated vertical or oblique fracture through the lateral mass. The adjacent lamina and pedicle remain intact. The fractured articular mass is displaced posteriorly and may be visible as a double outline on the lateral radiograph.
Flexion-distraction	Anterior compression with associated transverse fracture through vertebral body (unstable)	TL	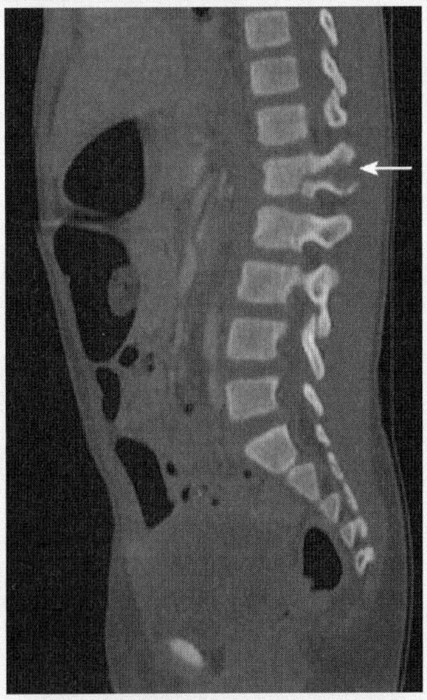 *Arrow* points to splaying of the posterior elements. [Reproduced with permission from Block J, Jordanov MI, Stack LB, Thurman RJ (eds): *The Atlas of Emergency Radiology*. McGraw-Hill, Inc., 2013. Fig 11-27C.]	These injuries are associated with seat-belt injuries, especially when lap belts alone are used. Radiographic findings include posterior vertebral wall fracture, increased height of the posterior vertebra, and "fanning" of the spinous processes. The **Chance fracture** variant presents with minor anterior vertebral compression and significant distraction of the middle and posterior ligamentous structure. It often occurs from T11 to L2 (TL transition zone). These injuries are often misdiagnosed as an anterior compression fracture. They may require CT to visualize and are often associated with intra-abdominal injuries.

(*Continued*)

TABLE 258-1 Major Spinal Column Injuries (*Continued*)

Mechanism of Injury	Injury	Spinal Column Regions Typically Affected	Image	Notes
Vertical compression	Jefferson burst fracture of atlas (potentially unstable)	Cervical	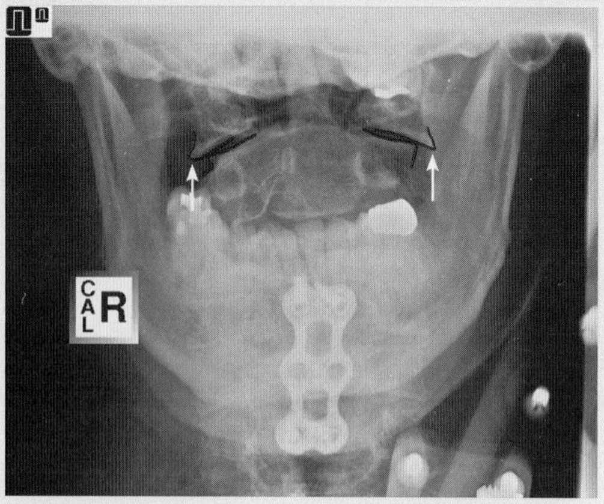 [Reproduced with permission from Block J, Jordanov MI, Stack LB, Thurman RJ (eds): *The Atlas of Emergency Radiology*. McGraw-Hill, Inc., 2013. Fig 11-13.]	Vertical compression forces the occipital condyles downward and produces a burst fracture by driving the lateral masses of C1 apart. This is best seen as outward displacement of the lateral masses on the open-mouth odontoid radiograph or on CT. If displacement of both lateral masses (measured as offset from the superior corner of the C2 vertebral body on each side) is >7 mm when added together, rupture of the transverse ligament is likely, and the spine is unstable.
	Burst fracture (unstable)	Cervical; TL	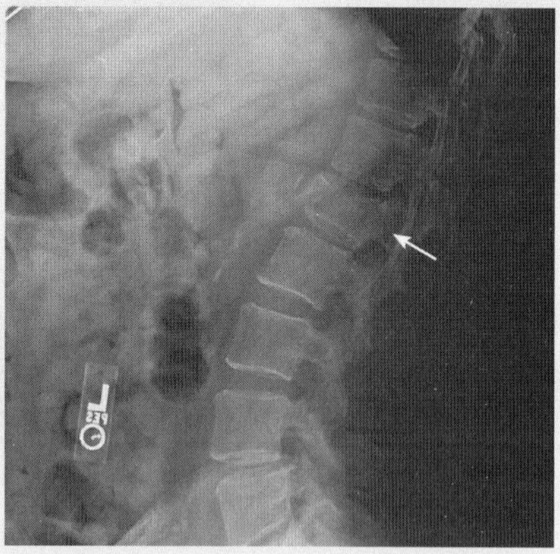 *Arrow* shows posterior displacement of posterior vertebral body cortex. [Reproduced with permission from Block J, Jordanov MI, Stack LB, Thurman RJ (eds): *The Atlas of Emergency Radiology*. McGraw-Hill, Inc., 2013. Fig 11-31B.]	A burst fracture occurs when a vertebra is crushed by an axial load, causing fragments to displace in all directions. The lateral radiograph may show an obvious fracture of the end plates, but sometimes all that is seen is a bowing or disruption of the posterior cortex of the affected vertebra. The anterior radiographic view may show a vertical fracture through the vertebral body and widening of the interpedicular distance. The burst fracture is usually obvious on CT. The spinal cord may be injured if a retropulsed fragment enters the spinal canal.
Extension	Hyperextension dislocation (unstable)	Cervical	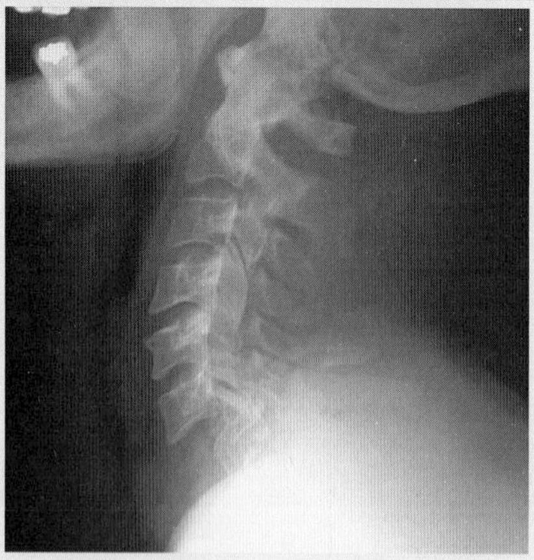 [Reproduced with permission from Schwartz DT (ed): *Emergency Radiology: Case Studies*. McGraw-Hill, Inc., 2008. Sect V: Cervical Spine Radiology; Fig 6.]	Extreme hyperextension can cause a complete tear of the anterior longitudinal ligament and intervertebral disk, with disruption of the posterior ligamentous complex. On the lateral radiographic view, the vertebrae may appear normal if the dislocation spontaneously reduces or if the injury is masked by a cervical immobilization collar. **Prevertebral soft tissue swelling may be the only radiographic finding present.** Anterior disk space widening or fracture of the anteroinferior end plate of the vertebral body may occur. Patients usually present with a central cord syndrome.

(*Continued*)

TABLE 258-1 Major Spinal Column Injuries (*Continued*)

Mechanism of Injury	Injury	Spinal Column Regions Typically Affected	Image	Notes
	Hyperextension teardrop fracture or extension corner avulsion fracture (unstable in extension)	Cervical	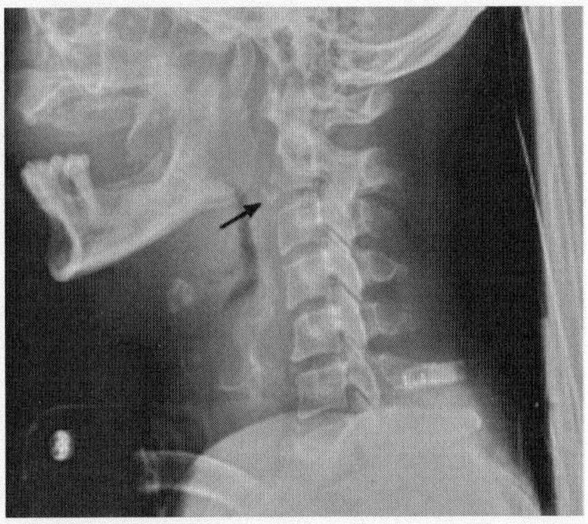	Hyperextension may cause the anterior longitudinal ligament to avulse a fragment off the anteroinferior corner of the vertebral body. The height of the avulsed fragment usually exceeds its width. This fracture is more common in older patients with osteoporosis.
	Fracture of posterior arch of atlas (stable)	Cervical	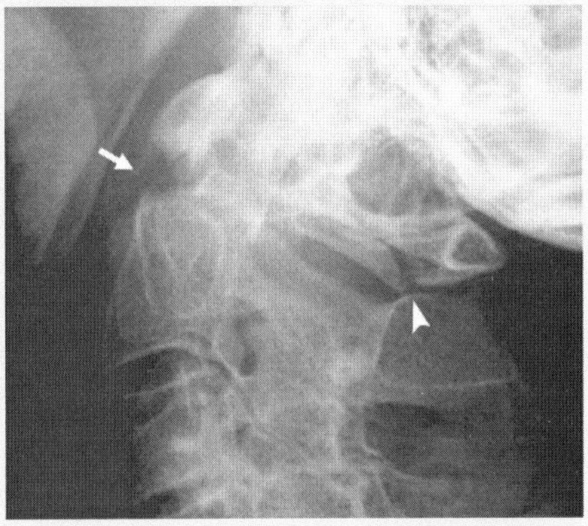 *Arrowhead* indicates the posterior arch fracture. There is also a displaced dens fracture (*arrow*). [Reproduced with permission from Galli, et al: *Emergency Orthopedics: The Spine*. New York, NY: McGraw-Hill;1989]	Fracture occurs from wedging of the posterior arch between the occipital bone and the C2 vertebra. A CT is indicated to rule out an associated Jefferson fracture or a dens fracture.
	Laminar fracture (usually stable)	Cervical	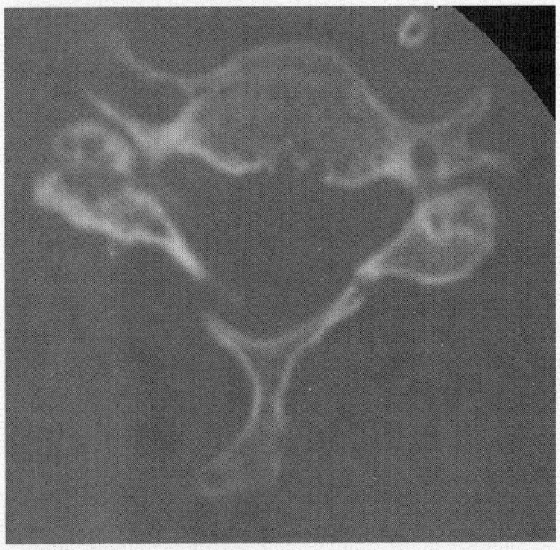 Bilateral laminar fractures. [Reproduced with permission from Simon RR, Sherman SC (eds): *Emergency Orthopedics*, 6th ed. McGraw-Hill, Inc., 2011. Fig 9-26B.]	Laminar fractures may be associated with spinous process fractures. They may not be evident on plain radiographs and usually require CT for diagnosis.

(*Continued*)

TABLE 258-1 Major Spinal Column Injuries (*Continued*)

Mechanism of Injury	Injury	Spinal Column Regions Typically Affected	Image	Notes
	Traumatic spondylolisthesis (hangman's fracture) (unstable)	Cervical	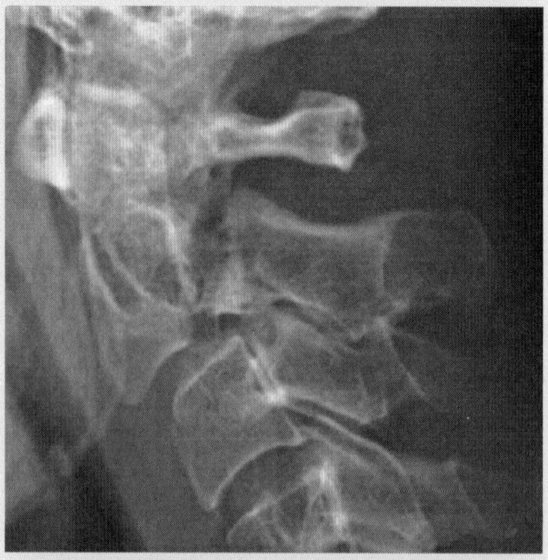	The hangman's fracture is a fracture of both pedicles of C2, with the anterior displacement of C2 on C3. This was associated with the neck hyperextension from judicial hangings, where the noose knot is placed under the subject's chin and snaps the head backward. Suicidal hangings do not usually cause extreme hyperextension and are not associated with the hangman's fracture. Because the spinal canal at the level of C2 is large, a hangman's fracture does not cause neurologic injury.
Injuries caused by a combination of mechanisms or poorly understood mechanisms	Occipital condyle fractures (usually stable)	Cervical	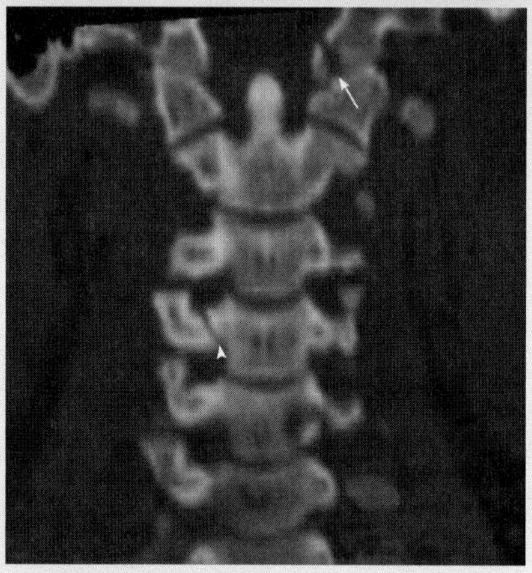 [Reproduced with permission from Block J, Jordanov MI, Stack LB, Thurman RJ (eds): *The Atlas of Emergency Radiology*. McGraw-Hill, Inc., 2013. Fig 11-11B.]	Occipital condyle fractures are rarely visible on plain radiographs and usually require CT imaging for detection. Presentation is rather variable due to proximity of multiple neurovascular structures.[7] Neurologic impairment is common and usually involves lower cranial nerve deficits and/or limb weakness.
	Atlanto-occipital dissociation (AOD) (highly unstable)	Cervical	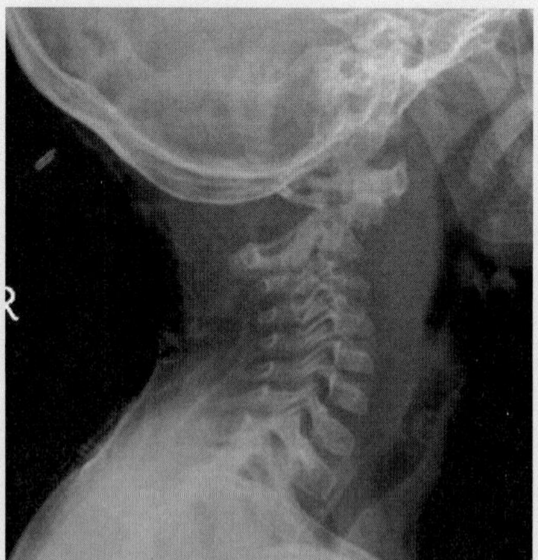 [Photo contributors: Konstantinos Agoritsas, MD/Steven Pulitzer, MD. Reproduced with permission from Shah BR, Lucchesi M, Amodio J (eds): *Atlas of Pediatric Emergency Medicine*, 2nd ed. © 2013, McGraw-Hill Education, New York, NY. Fig 20-52.]	Secondary to high-energy impact. Historically, strongly associated with mortality[8]; however, modern patients may survive due to better prehospital care/transport. The classic presentation is paralysis of upper extremities with lack of lower extremity paralysis or weakness (cruciate paralysis).[9] However, presentation can be variable with a common presentation being lower cranial nerve deficits. CT may be required for detection. In radiographs in the normal patient, the distance between the basion and the superior cortex of the dens (basion-dental interval [BDI]) should be ≤10 mm in adults (≤8.5 mm on CT). In addition, the distance from the basion to the posterior border of the body of C2 (basion-atlantal interval [BAI]) should be ≤12 mm anterior displacement or ≤4 mm posterior displacement on a lateral radiograph. If there are abnormalities in both the BDI and BAI, this strongly suggests the existence of AOD.[10]

(*Continued*)

TABLE 258-1 Major Spinal Column Injuries (*Continued*)

Mechanism of Injury	Injury	Spinal Column Regions Typically Affected	Image	Notes
	Odontoid (dens) fractures (type II and III are unstable)	Cervical	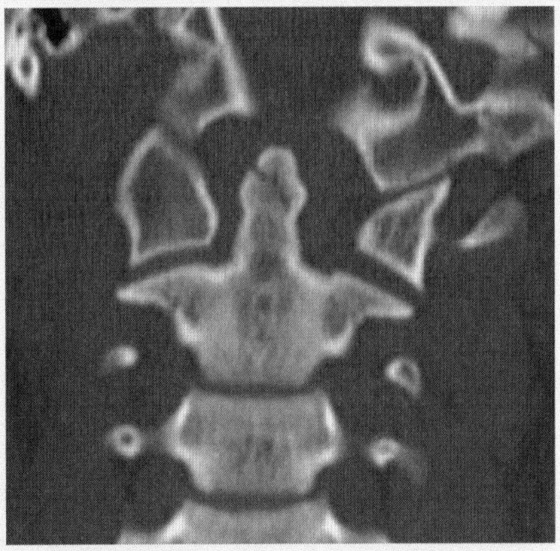 Type 1 odontoid fracture. [Reproduced with permission from Block J, Jordanov MI, Stack LB, Thurman RJ (eds): *The Atlas of Emergency Radiology*. McGraw-Hill, Inc., 2013. Fig 11-18.] 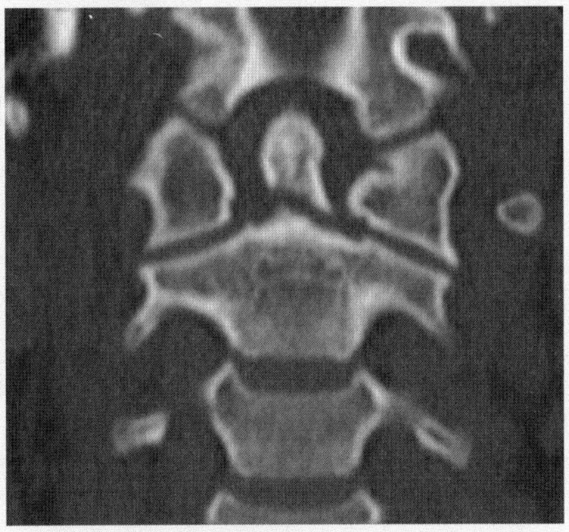 Type 2 odontoid fracture. [Reproduced with permission from Block J, Jordanov MI, Stack LB, Thurman RJ (eds): *The Atlas of Emergency Radiology*. McGraw-Hill, Inc., 2013. Fig 11-19C.] 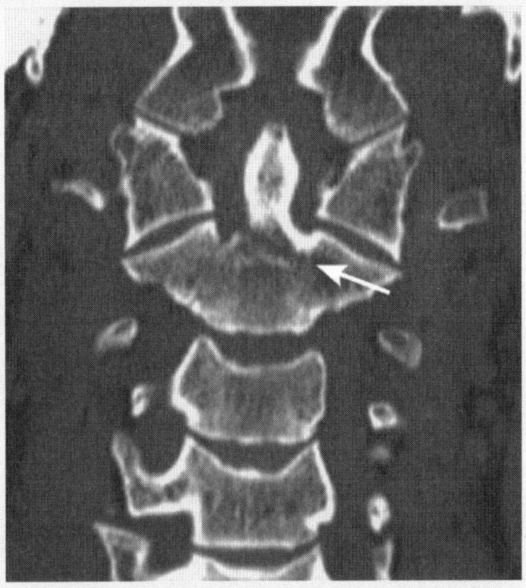 Type 3 odontoid fracture. [Reproduced with permission from Block J, Jordanov MI, Stack LB, Thurman RJ (eds): *The Atlas of Emergency Radiology*. McGraw-Hill, Inc., 2013. Fig 11-20C.]	Frequently involves other injuries to the cervical spine and multisystem trauma. Conscious patients will usually describe immediate and severe high cervical pain with muscle spasm. The pain may radiate to the occiput. Neurologic injury is present in 18% to 25% of cases with odontoid fractures, ranging from minimal sensory or motor loss to quadriplegia. Odontoid fractures are classified according to the level of injury. CT can miss odontoid fractures if the fracture line is aligned with the cut of the CT (*en face*).

(*Continued*)

TABLE 258-1 Major Spinal Column Injuries (*Continued*)

Mechanism of Injury	Injury	Spinal Column Regions Typically Affected	Image	Notes
	Translational fracture-dislocation (unstable)	TL	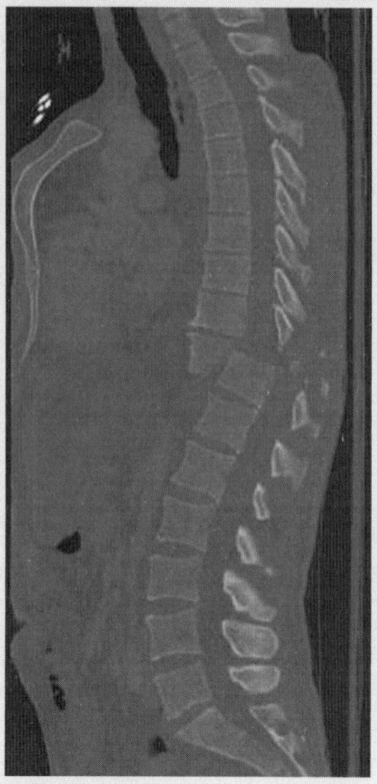 T10-T11 fracture-dislocation.	This is a high-energy disruption of all three columns of spine and is readily apparent both on radiographs and CT. Patients commonly present with severe neurologic findings. These fractures are most often unstable; however, in the absence of destabilizing rib cage fractures, lesions above T7 can be stable.
Sacrum and coccyx fractures	Sacral fracture		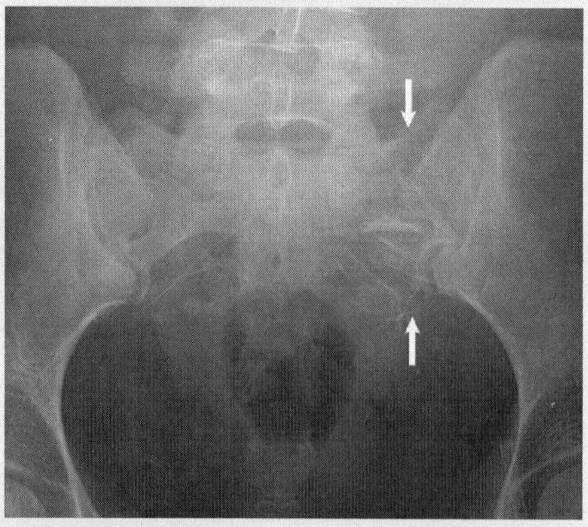 [Reproduced with permission from Block J, Jordanov MI, Stack LB, Thurman RJ (eds): *The Atlas of Emergency Radiology*. McGraw-Hill, Inc., 2013. Fig 8-16A.]	Usually associated with pelvic fracture(s). Transverse fractures through the body can injure the cauda equina. Longitudinal fractures can cause radiculopathies. Central sacral fracture can present with bowel/bladder incontinence.
	Coccyx fracture		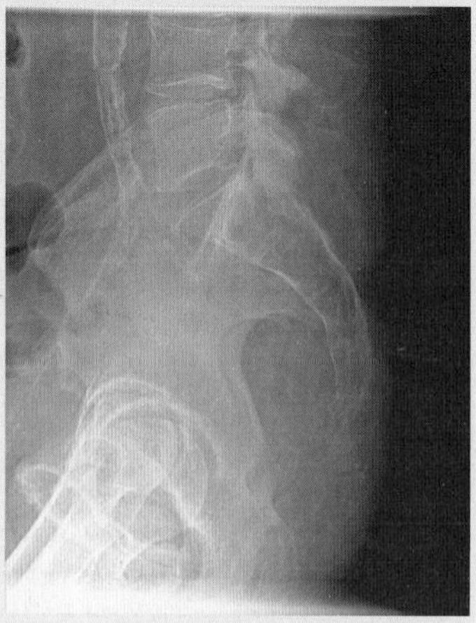 [Reproduced with permission from Block J, Jordanov MI, Stack LB, Thurman RJ (eds): *The Atlas of Emergency Radiology*. McGraw-Hill, Inc., 2013. Fig 8-24.]	Coccygeal injuries are usually associated with a direct fall onto the buttocks, with resultant coccyx pain exacerbated by sitting or straining. Localized tenderness can be elicited with coccyx palpation during a rectal exam, but this is not required for diagnosis. Imaging is not needed to diagnose coccygeal fractures. Treatment is symptomatic with analgesics and use of a rubber doughnut pillow.

Abbreviations: C1 = first cervical vertebra; C2 = second cervical vertebra; C3 = third cervical vertebra; C7 = seventh cervical vertebra; T1 = first thoracic vertebra; T7 = seventh thoracic vertebra; TL = thoracolumbar.

The variable anatomic qualities of the regions of the spinal column cause characteristic injury patterns in each region. The exposure and extreme mobility of the **cervical spine (C1-C7)** make it particularly vulnerable to injury, because it is the most flexible and mobile portion of the spinal column. The **cervicothoracic junction (C7-T1)** is one of the **transitional zones** of the spinal column, which are locations where the vertebral morphology changes. This designation is important because transitional zones sustain the greatest amount of stress during motion and are most vulnerable to injury. In contrast to the cervical spine, the **thoracic spine (T1-T10)** is a rigid segment, with its stiffness enhanced by articulation with the rib cage. Therefore, not only is injury to the thoracic spine less common than in other regions, but this also means that the presence of a thoracic vertebral injury indicates the patient was subjected to severe traumatic forces and is at high risk for intrathoracic injuries. Moreover, the spinal canal in the thoracic region is also narrower than in other regions. This increases the risk of cord injury, which is often complete when it occurs. The **thoracolumbar junction (T11-L2)** is a transitional zone between the highly fixed thoracic and relatively mobile lumbar spine. In addition to this change in bone anatomy, the thoracolumbar junction serves as the level of transition from the end of the spinal cord (about L1) to the nerve roots of the cauda equina. Relative to the thoracic spine, the width of the spinal canal in the thoracolumbar region is greater. Therefore, despite a large number of vertebral injuries at the thoracolumbar junction, most do not have neurologic deficits, or, if present, they are partial or incomplete. Relative to the thoracic and thoracolumbar regions, the **lower lumbar spine (L3-L5)** is more mobile. Because of the width of the spinal canal in the lumbar region and the ending of the spinal cord at the L1 level, isolated fractures of the lower lumbar spine rarely injure the spinal cord or result in neurologic injury. The **sacrum** and **coccyx** form the lower portion of the spinal column. The vertebral foramina of the sacrum together form the sacral canal that contains the nerve roots of the lumbar, sacral, and coccygeal spinal nerves and the filum terminale. The coccyx, which articulates with the sacrum, consists of four vertebrae fused together. When neurologic injuries occur, they are usually complete cauda equina lesions or isolated nerve root deficits. **Sacral fractures that involve the central sacral canal can produce bowel or bladder dysfunction.**

FRACTURE STABILITY

Much has been written regarding determining whether or not a particular injury is "stable." Spinal stability is defined as the ability of the spine to limit patterns of displacement under physiologic loads so as not to damage or irritate the spinal cord or nerve roots. Several paradigms have been created, including the Denis column system, which splits the spinal column into anterior, middle, and posterior elements.[11] A spine injury is considered unstable if at least two columns of a particular region are involved. Although this schema and other instability scoring systems have been published,[12-14] determining spinal stability after an acute injury in the ED is particularly difficult. This is because these injuries often occur in the setting of polytrauma, altered mental status, and severe pain, which may result in suboptimal initial imaging. In addition, many EDs lack quick access to emergent MRI to evaluate the spinal ligaments. Therefore, **assume any spine fracture is unstable and maintain appropriate precautions until expert consultation can be obtained from a spine surgeon**.

SPINAL CORD INJURIES

Damage to the spinal cord is the result of two types of injury. First is the **primary injury** from mechanical forces from traumatic impact. This insult sets into motion a series of vascular and chemical processes that lead to **secondary injury**. The initial phase is characterized by hemorrhage into the cord and formation of edema at the injured site and surrounding region. Local spinal cord ischemia ensues secondary to vasospasm and thrombosis of the small arterioles within the gray and white matter. Extension of edema may further compromise blood flow and increase ischemia. A secondary tissue degeneration phase begins within hours of injury. This is associated with neural membrane dysfunction, driven by a pathologic excitation of sodium ion channels, an influx of calcium ions, and the release of glutamine.[15] Cell death ensues from a combination of mechanisms including electrolyte imbalances, cell edema, and the formation and release of oxidative substances.[15]

SPINAL CORD LESIONS

The severity of spinal cord injury determines the prognosis for recovery of function, so it is important to distinguish between complete and incomplete spinal cord injuries. The American Spinal Injury Association defines a **complete neurologic lesion as the absence of sensory and motor function below the level of injury**. This includes loss of function to the level of the lowest sacral segment. In contrast, **a lesion is incomplete if sensory, motor, or both functions are partially present below the neurologic level of injury**. This may consist only of sacral sensation at the anal mucocutaneous junction or voluntary contraction of the external anal sphincter upon digital examination. Complete lesions have a minimal chance of functional motor recovery. Patients with incomplete lesions are expected to have at least some degree of recovery. The differentiation between complete and incomplete spinal cord damage may be complicated by the presence of spinal shock. **Patients in spinal shock lose all reflex activities below the area of injury, and lesions cannot be deemed truly complete until spinal shock has resolved.**

A significant number of descending and ascending tracts have been identified in the spinal cord (**Figure 258-2**). The three most important of these in terms of neuroanatomic localization of cord lesions are the corticospinal tracts, spinothalamic tracts, and dorsal (posterior) columns.

The corticospinal tract is a descending motor pathway. Its fibers originate from the cerebral cortex through the internal capsule and the middle of the crus cerebri. The tract then breaks up into bundles in the pons and finally collects into a discrete bundle, forming the pyramid of the medulla. In the lower medulla, approximately 90% of the fibers cross to the side opposite that of their origin and descend through the spinal cord as the lateral corticospinal tract. These fibers synapse on lower motor neurons in the spinal cord. The 10% of corticospinal fibers that do not cross in the medulla descend in the anterior funiculus of the cervical and upper thoracic cord levels as the ventral corticospinal tract. **Damage to the corticospinal tract neurons (upper motor neurons) in the spinal cord results in ipsilateral clinical findings such as muscle weakness, spasticity, increased deep tendon reflexes, and a Babinski's sign**.

The two major ascending pathways that transmit sensory information are the *spinothalamic tracts* and the *dorsal columns*. The spinothalamic tract transmits pain and temperature sensation. As the axons of the first neurons enter the spinal cord, most ascend one or two levels before entering the dorsal gray matter of the spinal cord, where they synapse with the second neuron of the spinothalamic tract. The second neuron immediately crosses the midline in the anterior commissure of the spinal cord

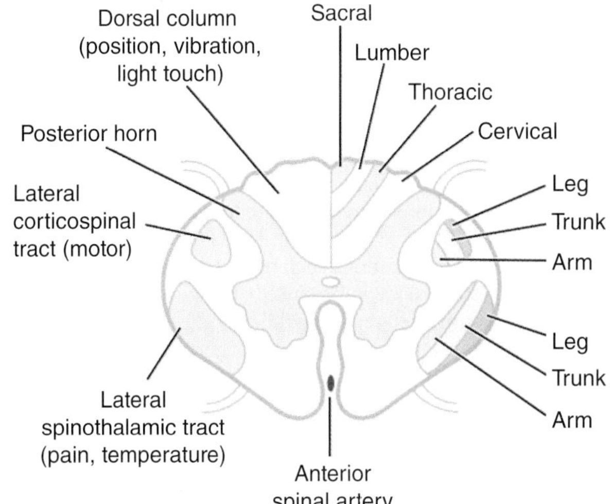

FIGURE 258-2. The anatomy of a cross section of cervical spinal cord. [Reproduced with permission from Simon RR, Sherman SC (eds): *Emergency Orthopedics*, 6th ed. McGraw-Hill, Inc., 2011. Fig 9-5.]

and ascends in the anterolateral funiculus as the lateral spinothalamic tract. **When the spinothalamic tract is damaged, the patient experiences loss of pain and temperature sensation in the contralateral half of the body.** The (pain and temperature) sensory loss begins one or two segments below the level of the damage.

The dorsal columns transmit vibration and proprioceptive information. Neurons enter the spinal cord proximal to pain and temperature neurons. They differ from pain and temperature neurons in that they do not immediately synapse in the spinal cord. Instead, these axons enter the ipsilateral dorsal column and do not synapse until they reach the gracile or cuneate nuclei of the medulla. From these nuclei, fibers cross the midline and ascend in the medial lemniscus to the thalamus. **Injury to one side of the dorsal columns will result in ipsilateral loss of vibration and position sense**. The sensory loss begins at the level of the lesion. Light touch is transmitted through both the spinothalamic tracts and the dorsal columns. Therefore, **light touch is not completely lost unless there is damage to both the spinothalamic tracts and the dorsal columns.**

Each spinal nerve is named for its adjacent vertebral body (see Figure 258-3). In the cervical region, there is an additional pair of spinal nerve roots compared to the number of vertebral bodies. The first seven spinal nerves are named for the first seven cervical vertebrae, each exiting through the intervertebral foramen above its corresponding vertebral body. The spinal nerve exiting below C7, however, is referred to as the C8 spinal nerve, although no eighth cervical vertebra exists. All subsequent nerve roots, beginning with T1, exit below the vertebral body for which they are named.

During fetal development, the downward growth of the vertebral column is greater than that of the spinal cord. Because the adult spinal cord ends as the conus medullaris at the level of the lower border of the first lumbar vertebra, the lumbar and sacral nerve roots must continue inferiorly below the termination of the spinal cord to exit from their respective intervertebral foramina. These nerve roots form the cauda equina. A potential consequence of this arrangement is that injury to a single lower vertebra can involve multiple nerve roots in the cauda equina. For example, an injury at the L3 vertebra can involve the L3 nerve root as well as the lower nerve roots that are progressing to a level caudal to the L3 vertebra.

PREHOSPITAL CARE

The prehospital treatment of patients with spinal injury involves recognition of patients at risk, appropriate immobilization, and triage to an appropriate facility (see chapters 1, "Emergency Medical Services" and 2, "Prehospital Equipment"). Presume that patients with an appropriate traumatic mechanism who have complaints of neck or back pain, tenderness on prehospital exam, neurologic complaints, significant injury above the clavicles, or altered sensorium that precludes accurate evaluation of the spine to have a spinal cord injury, and take appropriate spinal precautions. Transport of the patient to a center that is capable of rapid diagnostics and therapeutics is important to optimize outcome following spinal injury.

Prehospital care for spinal injuries traditionally involves immobilization of the entire spine at the scene with a rigid cervical collar (or similar devices) plus a long backboard. However, there is little evidence that cervical collars and/or long spine boards reduce neurologic injury, spinal instability, or mortality.[16,17] In contrast, cervical collars and long backboards can induce complications such as pressure sores,[18,19] patient discomfort,[20] and respiratory compromise.[21] In light of these data, some experts have recommended retaining the cervical collar but transporting the patient on a gurney with a scoop stretcher[22] or other soft, padded devices[23] to avoid the rigid spine board. Some authors have even proposed abandoning the routine use of cervical collars.[24] Nevertheless, in the absence of controlled data regarding the safety of such measures, current neurosurgery guidelines[25] still recommend usage of the rigid cervical collar and long spine board. In contrast, **spinal immobilization is no longer recommended for fully conscious, neurologically intact patients with isolated *penetrating* neck injury** because collars can delay resuscitation and obscure neck injuries.[26,27]

INITIAL ED STABILIZATION

AIRWAY

ED evaluation of the patient with potential spinal injury should not differ substantially from that of any patient with multiple injuries, with the first priority being the airway. **The higher the level of spinal injury, the more likely is the need for early airway intervention.** For example, unstable spine lesions above C3 can cause immediate respiratory arrest, and lesions affecting C3-C5 can affect the phrenic nerve and diaphragm function. For this reason, some experts recommend that **any patient with an injury at C5 or above should have the airway secured by endotracheal intubation**. Delayed respiratory compromise can occur if spinal cord edema from more caudal lesions progresses rostrally to cause phrenic nerve paralysis. Many patients can initially support ventilatory function using intercostal muscles or abdominal breathing, but they eventually tire and subsequently develop respiratory failure. Therefore, be vigilant for respiratory compromise in patients with high cervical injuries. If safety allows, perform a brief focused neurologic assessment before sedation and intubation.

Maintain in-line spinal stabilization while intubating, because human cadaver studies demonstrate less cervical motion and glottis visualization with in-line stabilization than with cervical collars in place, and movement of an unstable cervical spine can worsen or produce spinal cord injury.[28] Video-assisted intubation improves intubation success over direct laryngoscopy, but manual in-line stabilization is still necessary to minimize cervical extension.[28]

HYPOTENSION

Hypotension in patients with spinal cord injuries may be due to neurogenic shock, blood loss, cardiac injury, tension pneumothorax, or other injuries. Although hypotension and relative bradycardia are classic signs of neurogenic shock, bradycardia can also be associated with intraperitoneal bleeding or prior medication with calcium channel blockers or β-blockers. In one study,[29] 74% of hypotensive patients with penetrating spinal cord injury had major blood loss causing hypotension. Therefore, presume **blood loss as the cause of hypotension in spinal injury patients until proven otherwise.** Hypotension is initially treated with IV crystalloid.

SPINE IMMOBILIZATION

Long spine boards are associated with pressure sores, so remove them as soon as possible. Log rolling is the traditional method for board removal, because it requires only a few staff and allows visualization of the patient's back and performance of a rectal examination. Some experts recommend the "6+ lift and slide maneuver" because it produces less spine motion than log rolling.[30] The 6+ maneuver consists first of unstrapping the patient from the board. Next, one person maintains in-line stabilization at the head, while six others positioned at the chest, pelvis, and lower extremities levels lift the patient as a unit 10 to 20 cm above the board. Another person slides the board out from under the patient, and the patient is then lowered to the bed, maintaining spinal alignment. Disadvantages are the need for many staff members to perform this maneuver and inability to visualize the patient's back.[31]

Hard cervical collars are associated with patient discomfort and pressure sores of the neck.[32] Therefore, promptly clear the cervical spine if possible (see "Clinical Decision Rules in Cervical Spine Imaging" and "Cervical Spine Imaging" below). Do not overtighten the cervical collar on head-injured patients, because jugular venous compression can raise intracranial pressure,[33] although Stifneck® and Miami J® collars may be better than other rigid collars in this regard.[34]

CLINICAL FEATURES

HISTORY

If the patient is able to give a history, focus on key historical points as they pertain to spine injury. Specifically, seek the presence or absence of the historical elements included in imaging decision rules (see Tables 4,[35] 5,[36] and 6[37]). Evaluate for symptoms of midline spine pain, painful distracting injury, paresthesias, loss of function, change in mental status (including loss of consciousness), or other neurologic symptoms (especially urinary or fecal incontinence or priapism). **Pay particular attention to any symptoms indicating present or impending respiratory compromise, including dyspnea, palpitations, abdominal breathing, and anxiety, which may indicate a high cervical spine injury**.

PHYSICAL EXAMINATION

Once the patient is stabilized and other life-threatening injuries have been excluded or treated, perform a detailed neurologic assessment. An appropriately detailed initial neurologic examination is important to allow for comparison later should the patient deteriorate. Assess the patient's mental status and note any clinical evidence of intoxication. Physical examination should focus on delineating the level of the spinal cord injury (**Figure 258-3**). Document the presence or absence of midline neck or back tenderness. Test motor function for muscle groups (**Table 258-2**). Determine the level of sensory loss (**Figure 258-4**), and investigate proprioception or vibratory function to examine posterior column function. Test for "saddle anesthesia," which is sensory deficit in the region of the buttocks, perineum, and inner aspect of the thighs. Test deep tendon reflexes along with **anogenital reflexes because "sacral sparing" with preservation of anogenital reflexes denotes an incomplete spinal cord level, even if the patient has complete sensory and motor loss.** To test the bulbocavernosus reflex, squeeze the penis to determine whether the anal sphincter simultaneously contracts. Assess rectal tone at the same time. Test the cremasteric reflex by stroking the medial thigh with a blunt instrument. If the scrotum rises, some spinal cord integrity exists. Document rectal tone and sensation around the anus. An "anal wink reflex" (contraction of the anal musculature when the perianal region is stimulated with a pin) indicates some sacral sparing. Conversely, priapism implies a complete spinal cord injury. In 2013, the American Spinal Injury Association published a revised version of the International Standards for Neurological Classification of Spinal Cord Injury.[38] This scoring system is used by spine surgeons to document their initial examination and

TABLE 258-2 Motor Grading System

Grade	Movement
0	No active contraction
1	Trace visible or palpable contraction
2	Movement with gravity eliminated
3	Movement against gravity
4	Movement against gravity plus resistance
5	Normal power

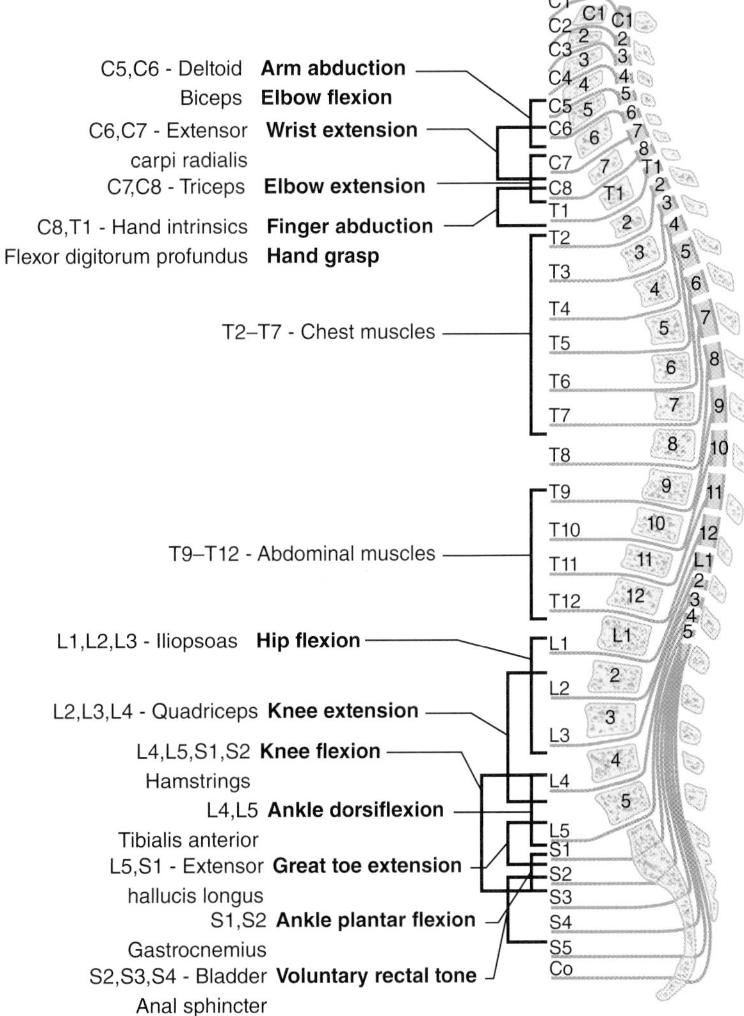

FIGURE 258-3. Spinal cord level. The spinal cord level of injury can be delineated by physical examination, including a detailed neurologic examination.

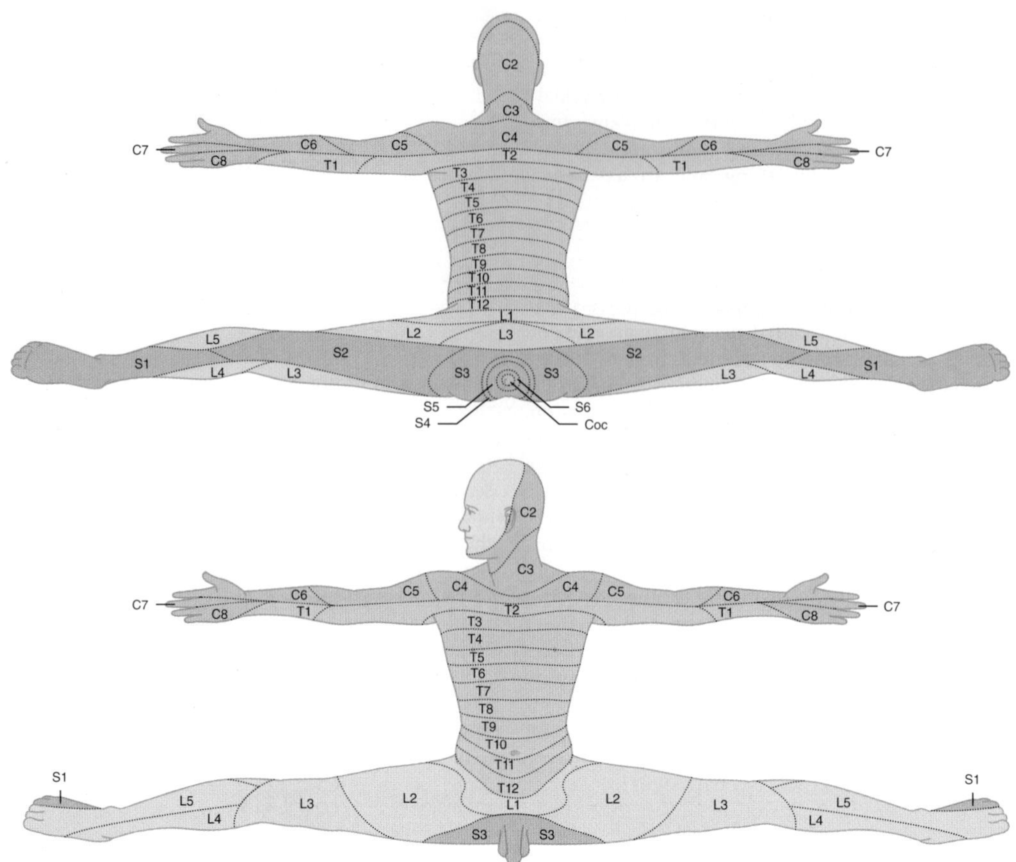

FIGURE 258-4. Dermatomes for sensory examination.

has prognostic value[39]; however, the scale is rather lengthy and is not practical for ED initial assessment.

INCOMPLETE SPINAL CORD SYNDROMES

There are three major incomplete spinal cord syndromes identified by predictable physical examination findings, although overlap in findings may occur (**Table 258-3**).

TABLE 258-3 Four Major Incomplete Spinal Cord Syndromes

Syndrome	Mechanisms	Symptoms	General Prognosis*
Anterior cord	Direct anterior cord compression	Complete paralysis below the lesion with loss of pain and temperature sensation	Poor
	Flexion of cervical spine		
	Thrombosis of anterior spinal artery	Preservation of proprioception and vibratory function	
Central cord	Hyperextension injuries	Quadriparesis—greater in the upper extremities than the lower extremities. Some loss of pain and temperature sensation, also greater in the upper extremities	Good
	Disruption of blood flow to the spinal cord		
	Cervical spinal stenosis		
Brown-Séquard	Transverse hemisection of the spinal cord	Ipsilateral spastic paresis, loss of proprioception and vibratory sensation, and contralateral loss of pain and temperature sensation	Good
	Unilateral cord compression		

*Outcome improves when the effects of secondary injury are prevented or reversed.

ANTERIOR CORD SYNDROME

The anterior cord syndrome results from damage to the corticospinal and spinothalamic pathways, with preservation of posterior column function. **This is manifested by loss of motor function and pain and temperature sensation distal to the lesion. Only vibration, position, and tacticle sensation are preserved.** This syndrome may occur following direct injury to the anterior spinal cord. Flexion of the cervical spine may result in cord contusion or bone injury with secondary cord injury. Alternatively, thrombosis of the anterior spinal artery can cause ischemic injury to the anterior cord. Anterior cord injury can also be produced by an extrinsic mass that is amenable to surgical decompression. The overall prognosis for recovery of function is poor.

CENTRAL CORD SYNDROME

The central cord syndrome is usually seen in older patients with preexisting cervical spondylosis who sustain a hyperextension injury. As named, this injury preferentially involves the central portion of the cord more than the peripheral. The centrally located fibers of the corticospinal and spinothalamic tracts are affected. The neural tracts providing function to the upper extremities are most medial in position compared with the thoracic, lower extremity, and sacral fibers that have a more lateral distribution. Clinically, **patients with a central cord syndrome present with decreased strength and, to a lesser degree, decreased pain and temperature sensation, more in the upper than the lower extremities**. Vibration and position sensation are usually preserved. Spastic paraparesis or spastic quadriparesis can also be seen. The majority will have bowel and bladder control, although this may be impaired in the more severe cases.

BROWN-SÉQUARD SYNDROME

The Brown-Séquard syndrome results from hemisection of the cord. It is manifested by **ipsilateral loss of motor function, proprioception, and vibratory sensation, and contralateral loss of pain and**

temperature sensation. The most common cause of this syndrome is penetrating injury.[40] It can also be caused by lateral cord compression secondary to disk protrusion, hematomas, spine fractures, infections, infarctions, or tumors.

CAUDA EQUINA SYNDROME

Cauda equina syndrome is not a true spinal cord syndrome because the cauda equina is composed entirely of lumbar, sacral, and coccygeal nerve roots; therefore, injuries to this region produce peripheral nerve injuries. **Symptoms and signs may include bowel and/or bladder dysfunction, decreased rectal tone, "saddle anesthesia" (sensory deficit over the perineum, buttocks, and inner thighs), variable motor and sensory loss in the lower extremities, decreased lower extremity reflexes, and sciatica.** Bowel or bladder incontinence is **not** a universal finding, because rectal tone can be spared,[41] and if the patient presents early, the patient's bladder may not yet be full enough to cause overflow incontinence. Careful history and physical examination, including identification of saddle anesthesia,[42] are helpful to suggest the diagnosis, but no one symptom or sign has 100% predictive value for this entity.[42] Therefore, perform an MRI of the lumbosacral spinal cord if clinical suspicion warrants. See the section "Epidural Compression Syndrome" in chapter 279, "Neck and Back Pain," for further discussion of cauda equina syndrome.

NEUROGENIC SHOCK

Neurogenic shock is a type of distributive shock that can occur with CNS or spinal cord injury that probably occurs in less than 20% of spinal cord–injured patients.[43] Loss of peripheral sympathetic innervation results in extreme vasodilatation secondary to loss of sympathetic arterial tone. This causes blood pooling in the distal circulation with resultant hypotension. If the T1 through T4 cord levels are compromised, loss of sympathetic innervation to the heart leaves unopposed vagal parasympathetic cardiac innervation. This results in bradycardia or an absence of reflex tachycardia. In general, **patients with neurogenic shock are warm, peripherally vasodilated, and hypotensive with a relative bradycardia**. Patients tend to tolerate hypotension relatively well, because peripheral oxygen delivery is presumably normal. Loss of sympathetic tone and subsequent inability to redirect blood from the periphery to the core may cause excessive heat loss and hypothermia.

The diagnosis of neurogenic shock is one of exclusion. Certain clues, such as bradycardia and warm, dry skin, may be evident, but **hypotension in the trauma patient can never be presumed to be caused by neurogenic shock until other possible sources of hypotension are excluded**.[29]

SPINAL SHOCK

Spinal shock is **not** neurogenic shock; the two terms have very different meanings and are not interchangeable. **Spinal shock is the temporary loss or depression of spinal reflex activity that occurs below a complete or incomplete spinal cord injury.** The typical presentation involves flaccidity, loss of reflexes, and loss of voluntary movement.[44] The lower the level of the spinal cord injury, the more likely it is that all distal reflexes will be absent. Loss of neurologic function that occurs with spinal shock can cause an incomplete spinal cord injury to mimic a complete cord injury. Therefore, cord lesions cannot be called complete until spinal shock has resolved. The delayed plantar and bulbocavernosus reflexes are among the first to return as spinal shock resolves.[45] The duration of spinal shock is variable; it generally lasts for days to weeks but can persist for months.[46]

DIAGNOSIS

Although spinal column and spinal cord injuries can sometimes be diagnosed clinically, diagnostic imaging is necessary to confirm the diagnosis and direct definitive care. However, judicious use of imaging is desirable to avoid unnecessary costs and ionizing radiation exposure to patients. Therefore, the challenge is identifying the appropriate patients to image and selecting the appropriate imaging modality.

CLINICAL DECISION RULES IN CERVICAL SPINE IMAGING

In some cases, it is obvious who needs cervical spine imaging. For example, patients with head or neck trauma who are not fully alert (Glasgow coma scale score of <15) should undergo imaging of their cervical spine because the frequency of cervical spine injury in association with traumatic brain injury ranges from 1.7% to 8%.[47] However, in less obvious cases, the decision to perform imaging is not quite so clear cut.

An unstructured clinical exam is not adequately sensitive for the detection of cervical spine injuries,[48] so guidelines can assist clinical judgment in deciding whom to image. In alert, stable adult trauma patients who have no neurologic deficits (i.e., low-risk trauma patients), two major clinical decision rules have been defined to avoid unnecessary radiography.

The first decision rule was derived by the **National Emergency X-Radiography Utilization Study (NEXUS)**, which determined that plain cervical spine imaging is unnecessary in patients who lack any one of five clinical criteria (**Table 258-4**).[35] In the study population of 34,069 patients, the NEXUS criteria were 99.6% sensitive (95% confidence interval [CI], 98.6% to 100%) for detecting prospectively defined clinically significant cervical spine injuries, but only 12.9% specific (95% CI, 12.8% to 13.0%), with a negative predictive value of 99.9% (95% CI, 99.8% to 100%). The original NEXUS trial excluded patients >60 years old, but the criteria were subsequently shown to be 100% sensitive (95% CI, 97.1% to 100%) and 14.7% specific (95% CI, 14.6% to 14.7%) for clinically significant injuries in 2943 patients ≥65 years of age.[49] In a subsequent prospective trial (n = 2785) investigating NEXUS's performance in patients ≥65 years of age, NEXUS was only 65.9% sensitive (vs 84.2% in younger patients) for cervical spine injuries detected on CT.[50] However, this trial contained several sources of bias (use of convenience sample, a very high incidence of cervical spine injuries in the elderly group [12.8% vs 4.6% in the previous trial], and every elderly patient included was a trauma team activation). This latter study did not clarify whether the fractures detected on CT were clinically significant or if any intervention was required.

The **Canadian Cervical Spine Rule for Radiography (CCR)** was developed for alert, stable trauma patients to reduce practice variation and inefficiency in the ED use of plain cervical spine radiography.[36] The Canadian rule consists of three assessments, which are asked **in sequential order** (**Table 258-5**).[36] To proceed to the next assessment, the answer to the previous assessment must be "Yes." If the answer to any assessments is "No," then imaging is immediately performed. In the original study sample of 8924 patients, the CCR was 100% sensitive (95% CI, 98% to 100%) and 42.5% specific (95% CI, 40% to 44%) for identifying patients with "clinically important" cervical spine injuries.[36] The CCR has also been validated in both larger hospital-based studies[51] and prehospital studies,[52] but has been criticized for its complexity relative to NEXUS.[53]

There is one published direct prospective comparison of NEXUS and CCR (n = 8283) that reported that CCR was more accurate for detecting cervical spine injury compared to NEXUS, with superior sensitivity (99% vs 91%), specificity (45% vs 37%), positive likelihood ratio (1.81 vs 1.44), and negative likelihood ratio (0.01 vs 0.25).[54] However, some have questioned the methodology of this comparison as being biased in favor of CCR.[55,56] A meta-analysis of 15 studies (79,526 patients) concluded that the CCR appeared to have better diagnostic accuracy than NEXUS[57]; however, the quality of methods of the included studies were termed "modest," and further more rigorous studies were suggested to be done. In both rules, the more subjective parts ("absence of painful distracting injury" and "no evidence of intoxication" for NEXUS; "dangerous

TABLE 258-4 NEXUS Criteria

NEXUS Criteria
Absence of midline cervical tenderness
Normal level of alertness and consciousness*
No evidence of intoxication
Absence of focal neurologic deficit
Absence of painful distracting injury†

*Defined as Glasgow coma scale score <15; disorientation to person, place, time, or events; inability to remember three objects at 5 minutes; delayed or inappropriate response to external stimuli.

†Any injury thought "to have the potential to impair the patient's ability to appreciate other injuries."

TABLE 258-5 Canadian Cervical Spine Rule for Radiography: Cervical Spine Imaging Unnecessary in Patients Meeting These Three Criteria

Assessment	Definitions
Assessment #1:	High-risk factors include:
There are no high-risk factors that mandate radiography.	Age 65 years or older A dangerous mechanism of injury* The presence of paresthesias in the extremities
Assessment #2:	Low-risk factors include:
There are low-risk factors that allow a safe assessment of range of motion.	Simple rear-end motor vehicle crashes Patient able to sit up in the ED Patient ambulatory at any time Delayed onset of neck pain Absence of midline cervical tenderness
Assessment #3: The patient is able to actively rotate his/her neck (regardless of pain).	Can rotate neck 45 degrees to the left and to the right

*Defined as fall from a height of >3 feet; an axial loading injury; high-speed motor vehicle crash, rollover, or ejection; motorized recreational vehicle or bicycle collision.

mechanism of injury" and assessment of range of motion for CCR) are the most common misinterpretation of the rules, which obviously affects their performance.[57]

Both NEXUS and CCR were developed in an era prior to the routine use of CT as a primary tool to evaluate the cervical spine in blunt trauma patients. Consequently, studies have been done to compare both decision rules using CT scan as the gold standard. In a 2011 study of 2606 blunt trauma patients, NEXUS was found to only be 82.8% sensitive and 45.7% specific for spine injury. Of the 26 missed injuries, 19 patients required further intervention, including 2 who went to the operating room and 1 needing a Halo.[58] The same group compared CCR to CT scan (3201 blunt trauma patients), finding excellent sensitivity of 100% but only 0.60% specificity.[59] Nevertheless, the use of NEXUS has been recommended for use in several national guidelines and trauma societies.[60,61]

In summary, many experts feel that **because both NEXUS and CCR have been widely validated and have demonstrated adequate sensitivity, either rule may be used to determine which low-risk patients should undergo plain or CT cervical spine imaging.**[57]

CERVICAL SPINE IMAGING

Plain Radiography Standard radiography for the identification of bony cervical injury includes three views of the cervical spine: lateral, anterior-posterior, and odontoid. A single lateral cervical spine film will identify only about 90% of injuries to bone and ligaments.[24] The anterior-posterior and open-mouth odontoid views will identify many of the remaining abnormalities. **It is important to image all seven cervical vertebrae, along with the superior border of the first thoracic vertebra**, given the propensity for injuries at the cervical-thoracic junction. Therefore, a "swimmers view" may be necessary to visualize this junction clearly, but this often requires an assistant to pull down the shoulders during the radiograph. The main advantages of plain radiography are that it can be done at the bedside, exposes the patient to only small amounts of ionizing radiation, and has a relatively low cost. One of the main disadvantages of plain films is that they are poor for imaging C1 and C2. In addition, visualization of the entire cervical spine by plain films is often problematic in obese, elderly, or extremely muscular patients, especially with a cervical collar in place.

Cervical Spine CT The practice in many trauma centers is to obtain CT as the initial imaging modality to evaluate the cervical spine. **Multidetector CT is more sensitive and specific than plain radiography for evaluating the cervical spine in trauma patients and can be performed quickly.**[62,63] CT can be used to visualize the entire cervical spine and is particularly useful at the craniocervical and cervicothoracic regions, where the sensitivity of plain films is most limited. In addition, a 3-year retrospective review found that plain radiography did not add any clinically useful information to a cervical spine CT.[64] Furthermore, a cost analysis showed CT to be cost-effective to screen for cervical spine injuries in moderate- to high-risk patients.[65] The Eastern Association for the Surgery of Trauma recommends CT as the primary diagnostic tool for suspected cervical spine injury.[60] In addition, if plain radiography is chosen as the primary imaging modality, a CT should be ordered if an injury is detected or suspected or if the initial plain radiograph is inadequate.

Imaging for Cervical Ligamentous Injury In patients with pure ligamentous injuries, the ligaments are disrupted, but the spine spontaneously reduces to a normal position. The resulting instability risks subsequent neurologic injury if the spine moves. Signs and symptoms include persistent neck pain/midline tenderness, extremity paresthesias, or focal neurologic findings despite normal plain radiographs and/or CT.

Although flexion and extension radiographs have been traditionally used to try to detect ligamentous instability, numerous studies have demonstrated their lack of sensitivity and inefficiency (30% to 80% of flexion and extension radiographs are inadequate), and they provide no further information beyond a CT.[66-70] Therefore, flexion and extension radiographs should not be ordered when more advanced imaging is available.

MRI is the imaging modality of choice if a ligamentous injury is strongly suspected because MRI has excellent sensitivity for soft tissue injuries.[71,72] However, there are practical limitations on its use, including the requirement for the patient to be stable, availability, cost, and patient tolerance for the procedure. If emergent MRI is not feasible, reliable patients with persistent pain but normal CT can be discharged in a firm foam collar with outpatient follow-up in 3 to 5 days. Most patients' symptoms will resolve over a few days. A patient with persistent pain at follow-up will likely require additional imaging. Unreliable patients with severe persistent pain and normal CT images should be considered for an MRI study, although this is rarely indicated as part of the initial investigation. In fact, some data have suggested that newer-generation CTs are sufficient to detect significant injuries without MRI even in obtunded patients.[73,74] However, the results of these studies cannot currently be externally generalized to awake, symptomatic patients.

Thoracic and Lumbar Spine Imaging As of this writing, there are no well-validated clinical decision rules for imaging in possible thoracolumbar spine injuries. However, **Table 258-6** provides practice guidelines for imaging in blunt trauma victims who are suspected of having thoracolumbar injuries.[37,75]

TABLE 258-6 Eastern Association for the Surgery of Trauma Guidelines for Thoracic and Lumbar Imaging after Trauma

Level I (convincingly justifiable based on scientific evidence)	When imaging is deemed necessary, CT scans with axial collimation should be used to screen for and diagnose injury, because CT scans are superior to plain films in identifying thoracolumbar spine fractures.
Level II (reasonably justifiable based on scientific evidence and expert opinion)	Patients with back pain, thoracolumbar spine tenderness on examination, neurologic deficits referable to the thoracolumbar spine, altered mental status, intoxication, distracting injuries, or known or suspected high-energy mechanisms should be screened for thoracolumbar spine injury with CT scan.
	In blunt trauma patients with a known or suspected injury to the cervical spine, or any other region of the spine, thorough evaluation of the entire spine by CT scan should be strongly considered due to a high incidence of spinal injury at multiple levels within this population.
	Patients without complaints of thoracolumbar spine pain who have normal mental status, as well as normal neurologic and physical examinations, may be excluded from thoracolumbar spine injury by clinical examination alone, without radiographic imaging, provided that there is no suspicion of high-energy mechanism or intoxication with alcohol or drugs.
Level III (supported by available data, but scientific evidence lacking)	MRI should be considered in consultation with the spine service for CT findings suggestive of neurologic involvement and of gross neurologic deficits.

Abbreviation: CT = multidetector CT.

As with the cervical spine, CT has largely supplanted plain radiography in the imaging of thoracic and lumbar injuries with significant blunt trauma. CT scanning is indicated in almost all patients with proven bony spinal injury, subluxations, neurologic deficits (but no apparent abnormalities on plain films), or severe neck or back pain (with normal plain films) and when the thoracic and lumbar spine should be examined to define the anatomy of a fracture and the extent of impingement on the spinal canal. Rather than obtaining separate plain radiographs or dedicated CT images, the thoracic and abdominal CT scans obtained to evaluate the multiple trauma patient can be used to reconstruct images of the thoracic and lumbar spine, although some authors have suggested that spinal image reconstruction is not necessary because the spine can be seen on the visceral CT scans.[76,77] CT can reveal the anatomy of an osseous injury, grade the extent of spinal canal impingement by bone fragments, and assess the stability of an injury. If an associated spinal cord or nerve root injury is suspected, MRI is the imaging study of choice.

It is less clear how to screen for thoracolumbar injuries in patients who have less severe mechanisms of injuries. Although it has been shown repeatedly that CT is more sensitive for thoracolumbar injuries in severely injured patients,[37] there has been no prospective controlled comparison between plain radiography and CT in more mildly injured patients. Nevertheless, some published guidelines suggest CT should be considered the standard screening modality for thoracolumbar injuries.[37]

Spinal Cord and Neural Tissue Imaging MRI is not as sensitive as CT for detecting or delineating bone injuries but is superb at defining neural, muscular, and soft tissue injury. **MRI is the diagnostic test of choice for describing the anatomy of nerve injury. Entities such as herniated disks or spinal cord contusions can also be delineated on MRI.** MRI is indicated in patients with neurologic findings with no clear explanation after plain films and/or CT scanning. If the patient is stable and MRI is unavailable, transfer to a tertiary care facility with MRI capabilities is appropriate.

Concurrent Spine Injury Imaging The determination of a spinal column injury at one level should prompt imaging of the entire remainder of the spine with CT because approximately 20% of patients with a spine fracture in one segment will have a noncontiguous second fracture at another segment.[78,79]

Spine Imaging in Obtunded Patients While experts recommend that all obtunded patients with significant blunt trauma should have their entire spine imaged, consensus does not yet exist on what imaging is necessary to clear the spine in obtunded patients. Specifically, **it is controversial whether a negative CT of the spine is adequate or if a subsequent MRI needs to be done,**[80] although at this writing, the trend in the literature suggests that a negative CT is sufficient.[73,74] In the absence of definitive data, maintain spinal precautions in the obtunded trauma patient in the ED, and defer any spine clearance to local expert consultants.

TREATMENT AND DISPOSITION OF SPINAL COLUMN INJURIES

The goals of treatment are to prevent secondary injury, alleviate cord compression, and establish spinal stability. Maintain spinal immobilization and keep movement to a minimum. **Obtain emergent consultation with a spine surgeon (neurosurgeon or orthopedic surgeon depending on the particular facility) on all spinal column fractures or ligamentous injuries, regardless of neurologic compromise**.

CERVICAL SPINE FRACTURES

The majority of cervical spinal fractures will require admission for definitive treatment or for the care of associated injuries. Until transfer of care to a surgeon, spine precautions should be maintained, associated injuries stabilized, and the patient carefully monitored for respiratory or neurologic deterioration.

THORACIC AND LUMBAR SPINE FRACTURES

Thoracolumbar fractures are also high risk for associated spinal cord or other traumatic injuries, such as aortic, intrathoracic, or intra-abdominal visceral injuries. Although many of these injuries will require admission, there are two types of thoracolumbar factures that may be amenable to outpatient therapy.

Compression fractures, also known as "wedge" or "anterior" compression fractures, comprised approximately 52% of thoracolumbar fractures in one published series.[81] These fractures occur as a result of a hyperflexion during an axial load that crushes the anterior portion of the vertebra. If the percentage of loss of vertebral height is <40%, the patient may be a candidate for outpatient therapy, and this should be discussed on a case-by-case basis by the spine surgeon. However, if the loss of vertebral height is ≥50% or if the angle between the damaged vertebra and the rest of the spinal column is >25% to 30%, the compression fracture is generally considered unstable.

In addition, make certain that an apparent compression fracture seen on plain radiographs is not a **burst fracture**, which is a compression-type fracture that involves the posterior half of the vertebrae. Burst fractures may result in retropulsed fragments that can impinge on the spinal canal and cause neurologic injury. In two studies, the incidence of misdiagnosis of burst fractures on plain radiographs ranged from 20% to 23%.[82,83] Another fracture that is sometimes misdiagnosed as a wedge compression fracture on plain radiograph is the **Chance fracture**. This fracture occurs via a flexion-distraction mechanism and involves minor anterior vertebral compression and significant distraction of the middle and posterior ligamentous structures. Typical radiographic findings reveal a transverse fracture lucency in the vertebral body, an increased height of the posterior vertebral body, fracture of the posterior wall of the vertebral body, and posterior opening of the disk space. Finally, minor to moderate trauma can cause **pathologic fractures** secondary to preexisting neoplastic, infectious, or osteoporotic processes in the spine. Because the above mentioned fractures can be easily misdiagnosed with plain radiography alone, **some experts recommend that compression fractures of the thoracolumbar spine on plain radiographs be further evaluated with CT**.[84]

If, after a thorough evaluation, a stable wedge compression fracture with no neurologic compromise is diagnosed, the patient may be treated as an outpatient with analgesia, heat, massage, rest, and appropriate follow-up for consideration of physical therapy.

SACRUM AND COCCYX FRACTURES

Injuries of the sacral spine and nerve roots are very unusual. When they occur, they are frequently associated with fractures of the pelvis. In general, transverse fractures through the body are most significant in that they cause injury to part or all of the cauda equina. Longitudinal fractures may cause radiculopathy. **Sacral fractures that involve the central sacral canal can produce bowel or bladder dysfunction.**

One notable exception to the need for emergent consultation is an **isolated coccyx fracture.** Coccygeal injuries are usually associated with a direct fall onto the buttocks, with resultant coccyx pain exacerbated by sitting or straining. Imaging is not needed to diagnose coccygeal fractures. Treatment is symptomatic with analgesics and use of a rubber doughnut pillow.

SPECIAL CONSIDERATIONS

CORTICOSTEROIDS

High-dose methylprednisolone remains a controversial treatment in acute blunt spinal cord injury and should not be given routinely. The major neuroprotective mechanism by which high-dose methylprednisolone is believed to work is in its inhibition of free radical–induced lipid peroxidation. Other proposed beneficial actions include its ability to increase levels of spinal cord blood flow, increase extracellular calcium, and prevent loss of potassium from injured cord tissue. Methylprednisolone is advocated in preference to other steroids because it crosses cell membranes more rapidly and completely.

In the 1990s, the National Acute Spinal Cord Injury Study (NASCIS) group published three prospective, double-blind studies to evaluate the efficacy of methylprednisolone in blunt spinal cord injury: NASCIS I, II, and III.[85-87] NASCIS I compared high-dose methylprednisolone and a lower-dose methylprednisolone regimen (n = 330). NASCIS I showed no evidence in recovery of function between the groups. NASCIS II compared a higher dose of methylprednisolone (**Table 258-7**), naloxone, and

TABLE 258-7	The National Acute Spinal Cord Injury Study II High-Dose Methylprednisolone Protocol
Indications	Blunt trauma
	Neurologic deficit referable to the spinal cord
	Treatment must be started within 8 h of injury
Treatment	Methylprednisolone, 30 milligrams/kg IV bolus over 15 min
	Followed by a 45-min pause
	Methylprednisolone, 5.4 milligrams/kg/h IV is then infused for 23 h

placebo (n = 427). This trial was also negative, but based on post hoc subgroup analysis, NASCIS II showed modest improvements in motor function when steroids were administered within 8 hours of injury. NASCIS III compared high-dose methylprednisolone for 24 hours, high-dose methylprednisolone for 48 hours, and tirilazad mesylate for 24 hours (n = 499). NASCIS III was also a negative trial, but post hoc analysis found that patients who received the 48-hour methylprednisolone regimen within 3 to 8 hours of their injury showed motor improvement. In all three trials, patients who received high-dose methylprednisolone and longer duration protocols were more likely to develop complications such as severe sepsis, severe pneumonia, wound infection and delayed healing, pulmonary embolism and deep vein thrombosis, GI bleeding, and death. A recent Cochrane systematic review (written by the lead author of the NASCIS trials) essentially confirmed the conclusions of NASCIS II and III that high-dose methylprednisolone was beneficial when administered within 8 hours of injury, but these patients were also more likely to develop complications.[88] The systematic review also recommended that more randomized trials be done urgently.

The results of the NASCIS clinical trials have been criticized as not providing sufficient clinical evidence to support the use of steroids in acute spinal cord injury. Examples of bias cited include the use of post hoc subgroup analysis, the artificiality of the 3- and 8-hour time limits, and a difference in the severity of injury in particular treatment groups. Reassessment, meta-analysis, and studies by other authors have questioned the validity of the NASCIS trials and the effectiveness of high-dose steroid therapy in these patients.[89-91] Consequently, the 2013 updated guidelines for the management of acute spinal cord injuries endorsed by the American Association of Neurological Surgeons and the Congress of Neurological Surgeons stated that "there is no consistent or compelling medical evidence of any class to justify the administration of methylprednisolone for acute spinal cord injury," and that "methylprednisolone should not be routinely used in the treatment of patients with acute spinal cord injury."[92] Moreover, the U.S. Food and Drug Administration has not approved corticosteroids for acute spinal cord injury.[93]

Nevertheless, the use of methylprednisolone persists in some centers. Therefore, given the continued controversy over its use,[94,95] **the decision to start corticosteroids should only be made in conjunction with the surgeon who will ultimately be caring for the patient, and *not* given routinely**.

It is important to realize that the NASCIS trial protocol was evaluated only in patients with **blunt** spinal cord injury, while penetrating injuries were excluded from these studies. In fact, **high-dose methylprednisolone therapy has not been found to be efficacious in penetrating spinal cord injury**.[96] In addition, because corticosteroids worsen outcomes in brain-injured patients, they should be avoided in this population as well.[97]

CARDIOVASCULAR COMPLICATIONS

If neurogenic shock is present, initiate an infusion of IV crystalloid to correct this relative hypovolemia. **If IV fluids are not adequate to maintain organ perfusion, positive inotropic pressor agents may be beneficial adjuncts to improve cardiac output and raise perfusion pressure.** In terms of target systolic blood pressure and mean arterial pressure, the evidence in the literature is limited at best. However, it has been recommended that systolic blood pressure should be kept greater than 90 mm Hg, with the mean arterial pressure kept at 85 to 90 mm Hg.[98] The aggressive use of fluids in neurogenic shock should be performed with careful monitoring, because there is danger of excessive fluid replacement, resulting in heart failure and pulmonary edema. There is no definitive evidence that any particular vasopressor is superior to another for this indication.[99]

Bradycardia, when present, usually occurs within the first few hours or days after spinal cord injury because of a predominance of vagal tone to the heart. In cases of hemodynamically significant bradycardia, atropine may be needed. Rare occurrences of atrioventricular conduction block with significant bradycardia require a pacemaker.

PENETRATING INJURY

Penetrating injuries to the neck are discussed in chapter 260, "Trauma to the Neck." For spinal gunshot wounds with a transabdominal or transintestinal trajectory, administer prophylactic broad-spectrum IV antibiotics in the ED. **Corticosteroids are contraindicated in patients with any type of penetrating spinal injuries,** and emergent consultation with a spine surgeon is indicated.

Acknowledgments: The author gratefully acknowledges the prior contributions of Bonny J. Baron, Kevin J. McSherry, James L. Larson, Jr., and Thomas M. Scalea, the authors of this chapter in the previous edition. The author would also like to thank Lawrence R. Ricci, DO, for his invaluable assistance with locating images.

REFERENCES

The complete reference list is available online at www.TintinalliEM.com.

CHAPTER 259 Trauma to the Face

John Bailitz
Tarlan Hedayati

INTRODUCTION AND EPIDEMIOLOGY

Assaults, motor vehicle crashes, falls, sports, and gunshot wounds account for the majority of facial fractures (in descending order of incidence), with motor vehicle crashes and gunshot wounds resulting in a higher severity of injury.[1] The lack of a seat belt or airbag increases the risk of facial fractures and panfacial fracture.[2] The most common fractures are to the nasal bone, followed by orbital floor, zygomaticomaxillary, maxillary sinuses, and mandibular ramus.[1] Mechanisms and injury patterns vary with geography. In the urban setting, penetrating trauma and assaults result in midface and zygomatic fractures. In the rural setting, motor vehicle crashes and recreational injuries result in fractures of the mandible and nose. Males are more frequently affected than females, but domestic violence and elder and child abuse must always be considered in any patient presenting with facial trauma. The majority of abused women and children will have injuries to the head, face, and neck.[3,4]

PATHOPHYSIOLOGY

The facial skeleton is designed to create effective mastication. Vertical and horizontal buttresses are formed by bony arches joined at suture lines. Stronger vertical buttresses are formed by the zygomaticomaxillary buttress laterally and the frontal process of the maxilla medially. Weaker horizontal buttresses are formed by the superior orbital rims, orbital floor, and hard palate. The orbit itself is comprised of seven different bones, with the inferior and medial walls being particularly fragile. Therefore, frontal, lateral, and oblique forces often result in facial fractures.

The identification of facial injury and the restoration of normal appearance, sight, mastication, smell, and sensation are all essential tasks,[5] but the principal focus should be on protecting the patient's airway during the primary survey and the other initial considerations described in **Table 259-1**.

Up to 44% of patients with severe maxillofacial trauma require endotracheal intubation due to mechanical disruption or massive hemorrhage into the airway.[6] The incidence of associated injury to the brain, orbit, cervical spine, and lungs is directly related to the mechanism of injury and severity of facial fractures.[6-8] Evaluate facial injuries as part of the secondary survey only after managing life-threatening injuries. Because up to 6% of patients with maxillofacial trauma will develop vision loss, a detailed eye examination is essential, especially in patients with high-energy mechanisms, orbital fractures, significant head injury, and abnormal pupillary findings.[8,9]

CLINICAL FEATURES

The mechanism of injury helps estimate the extent of injury. Exact details of motor vehicle crashes and assaults are often incomplete due to associated traumatic brain injury, intoxication, or other factors. Always address the possibility of abuse. When reported mechanisms do not match the injury, ask patients, especially women and the elderly, about interpersonal violence. Contact pediatricians and local child protective services when considering child abuse. It is better to report all suspected abuse than allow violence to continue and escalate. Obtain history of allergies, medications (especially cardiovascular and antithrombotic agents), comorbidities, tetanus immunization status, and time of last meal from the trauma patient or other available sources.

The secondary survey begins with three screening questions to help localize injuries while simultaneously examining the patient from the upper to the lower face. Important clinical findings in facial trauma are presented in **Table 259-2**.

(1) How is your vision? Any patient with visual complaints or evidence of periorbital injury requires a thorough eye examination. (2) Is your face numb? Ask this question while checking for anesthesia of the forehead, lower eyelid, cheek and upper lip, or chin, suggesting injury to the supraorbital, infraorbital, or mental nerves. (3) Do your teeth fit together normally? Malocclusion typically occurs in patients with mandibular or maxillary fractures. Pain and tenderness near the ear indicate mandibular condyle injury. With zygomaticomaxillary complex fractures, patients often report pain over the cheek and trismus from masseter spasm or mechanical impingement of either the temporalis muscle or coronoid process of the mandible.

Inspect the face from the front, sides, feet, and above to detect subtle asymmetry in facial structure from zygomatic, orbital, and Le Fort injuries (**Figures 259-1 to 259-3**). Palpate the entire orbital rim for tenderness and step-off deformities, which suggest fracture, and for crepitus, which suggests sinus involvement.

Examine the eyes before significant swelling occurs, or use lid retractors to better inspect the globe. Begin with corrected visual acuity using a wall, pocket, or phone app Snellen eye chart, name tag, or finger counting. In patients with loss of visual acuity, note light perception and color perception. **Loss of vision implies injury to the optic nerve or globe.** Subconjunctival hemorrhage and bloody chemosis occur with orbital fractures.

TABLE 259-1 Initial Considerations in Facial Trauma

Primary survey
Airway—endotracheal intubation for mechanical disruption or severe hemorrhage.
Circulation—early packing of nasal and oral cavity. Apply direct pressure to external wounds. Avoid blind clamping.
Evaluate and manage emergent life-threatening conditions before facial injuries.
Secondary survey
Early meticulous facial and ocular examinations.
History
Mechanism predicts severity of facial and associated brain, cervical spine, and pulmonary injury.
Screen for abuse, especially in women, children, and elders.

TABLE 259-2 Important Clinical Issues in Facial Trauma

History
How is your vision?
Do any parts of your face feel numb?
Does your bite feel normal?
Inspection
Lateral view for dish face with Le Fort III fractures.
Frontal view for donkey face with Le Fort II or III fractures.
Bird's eye view for exophthalmos with retrobulbar hematoma.
Worm's view for enophthalmos with blow-out fractures or flattening of malar prominence with zygomatic arch fractures.
Raccoon eyes (bilateral orbital ecchymosis) and Battle's sign (mastoid ecchymosis) typically develop over several hours, suggesting basilar skull fracture.
Palpation
Palpating the entire face will detect the majority of fractures.
Intraoral palpation of the zygomatic arch, palpating lateral to posterior maxillary molars to distinguish bony from soft tissue injury.
Assess for Le Fort fractures by gently rocking the hard palate with one hand while stabilizing the forehead with the other.
Eye
Examine early before swelling of lids, or use retractors. Document visual acuity. Systematically examine the eye from front to back. Specifically, check the pupil for teardrop sign pointing to globe rupture; hyphema; and swinging flashlight test for afferent papillary defect.
Fat through wound indicates orbital septal perforation.
Check intraocular pressure for evidence of orbital compartment syndrome only in absence of globe injury.
Nose
Crepitus over any facial sinus suggests sinus fracture.
Nasal septal hematoma appears as blue, boggy swelling on nasal septum.
Cerebrospinal fluid leak.
Ears
Auricular hematoma.
Hemotympanum.
Cerebrospinal fluid leak.
Oral
Jaw deviation due to mandible dislocation or condyle fracture. Malocclusion occurs in mandible, zygomatic, and Le Fort fractures.
Missing or injured tooth.
Lacerations and mucosal ecchymosis suggest mandible fracture.
Place finger in external ear while the patient gently opens and closes jaw to detect condyle fractures.
Tongue blade test: Patient without fracture can bite down on a tongue blade enough to break blade twisted by examiner.

Assess extraocular motion and pupils. **Binocular double vision suggests entrapment of the extraocular muscles, whereas monocular double vision suggests lens dislocation.** Limitation on upward gaze occurs with fractures of the inferior and medial orbital wall from entrapment or injury to the inferior rectus, inferior oblique, or oculomotor nerve (**Figure 259-4**). Examine the pupils for shape, position, symmetry, and reactivity. Teardrop-shaped pupil indicates globe injury. Note the distance between the medial canthi; normal is the width of the patient's globe. **Telecanthus, widening of this distance with normal interpupillary distance, occurs with naso-orbito-ethmoid injuries.** Widening of the interpupillary distance, or hypertelorism, results from a "blow-out" injury to the orbits, often resulting in blindness.

Check the swinging flashlight test for evidence of an afferent papillary defect (Marcus Gunn pupil) (see chapter 241, "Eye Emergencies"). With normal function, the swinging light results in brief dilation during movement followed by constriction when the light is directly over the eye. With injury to the optic nerve or retina, the affected pupil will not constrict

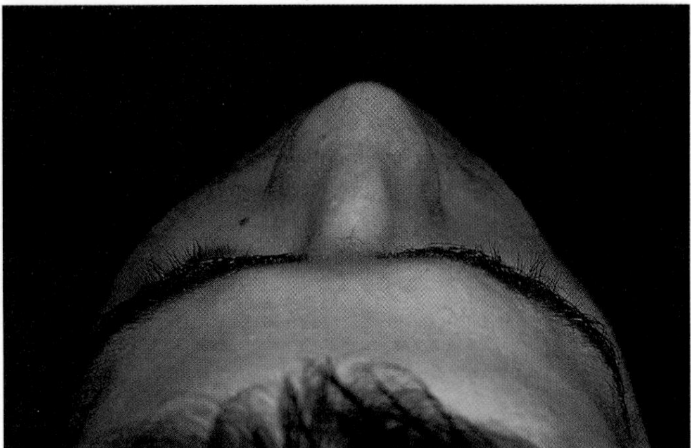

FIGURE 259-1. Zygomatic arch fracture. Note flattening of the right malar eminence on bird's eye. [Reproduced with permission from Knoop K, Stack L, Storrow A, Thurman RJ: *Atlas of Emergency Medicine,* 3rd ed. © 2010, McGraw-Hill, New York.]

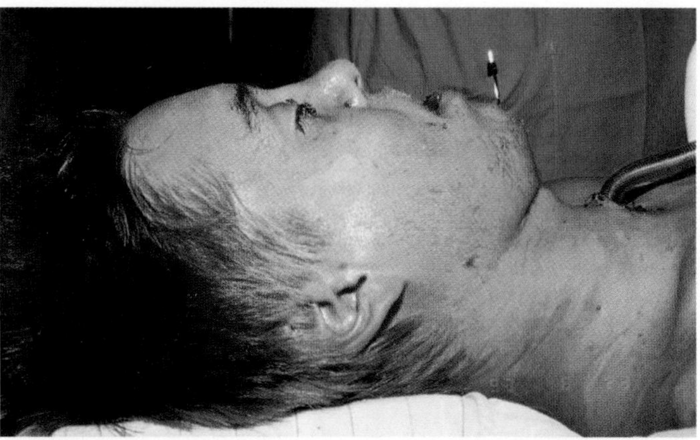

FIGURE 259-3. Le Fort III fracture has a classic dish face deformity on lateral view. [Reproduced with permission from Knoop K, Stack L, Storrow A, Thurman RJ: *Atlas of Emergency Medicine,* 3rd ed. © 2010, McGraw Hill, New York.]

until the light is again moved to the unaffected eye. The test is sensitive but not specific for optic nerve injury because an afferent papillary defect may result from pathology anywhere along the visual pathway.

Finish the physical examination of the eye by completing funduscopic, slit-lamp, and fluorescein examinations, as well as checking intraocular pressures when indicated. Flashes of light and floaters may be reported in patients with retinal detachments and vitreous hemorrhage. Foreign-body sensation and photophobia suggest corneal abrasions. Check for hyphema after having the patient sit upright for several minutes. In patients without evidence of globe rupture, check intraocular pressure in patients with significant exophthalmos, afferent nerve defects, or other evidence of retrobulbar hematoma.

Check carefully for globe injury with any penetrating injury to the periorbital area. Consult ophthalmology for suspected hyphema or vitreous hemorrhage. Fat herniating through the wound suggests an injury through the orbital septum. Through-and-through injuries, tarsal plate injuries, and injuries to the medial quadrant involving the lacrimal duct require repair by an ophthalmologist.

Begin the examination of the nose by checking for deformity from multiple angles while asking the patient about prior nose injury. Check for tenderness, crepitus, septal hematoma, and cerebrospinal fluid rhinorrhea. A septal hematoma appears as a blue, boggy, and tender area of swelling along the nasal septum (**Figure 259-5**). Incision and evacuation are required to prevent destruction of cartilage resulting in a saddle nose deformity. Ensure that simple nasal fractures are not associated with complex naso-orbito-ethmoid injuries. Perform the bimanual nasal palpation test with tenderness over the medial canthus. Begin by anesthetizing the nose. Then insert a cotton tip applicator inside the nose along the lateral nasal wall to the area behind the medial orbital wall and canthus. Palpate the area of the medial canthus externally with the opposite hand to check for movement from fracture of the medial wall of the orbit. Obtain a CT scan for suspected injury to the medial canthus or when telecanthus is present. Isolated nasal fractures and septal hematoma evacuation are reviewed in chapter 244, "Nose and Sinuses."

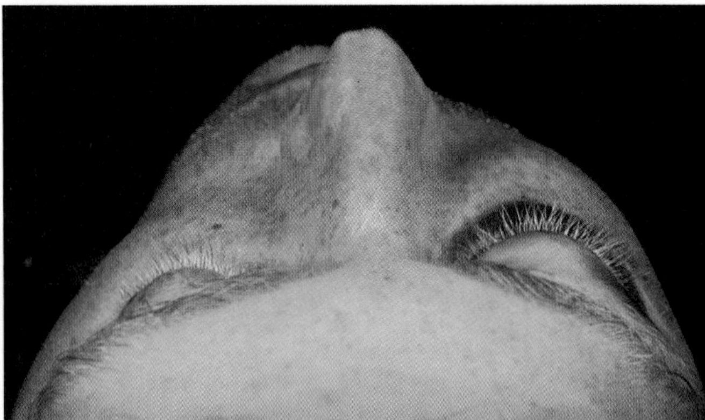

FIGURE 259-2. Traumatic exophthalmos. Note significant right exophthalmos on bird's eye view due to retrobulbar hematoma. [Reproduced with permission from Knoop K, Stack L, Storrow A, Thurman RJ: *Atlas of Emergency Medicine,* 3rd ed. © 2010, McGraw-Hill, New York.]

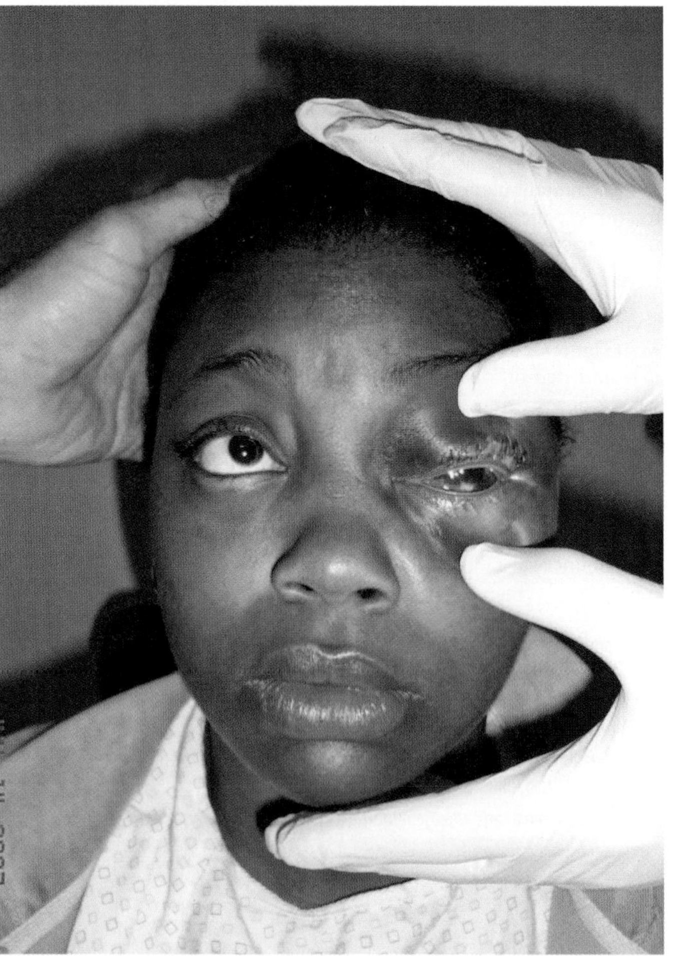

FIGURE 259-4. Orbital blow-out fracture causes limitation of upward gaze due to entrapment of inferior rectus.

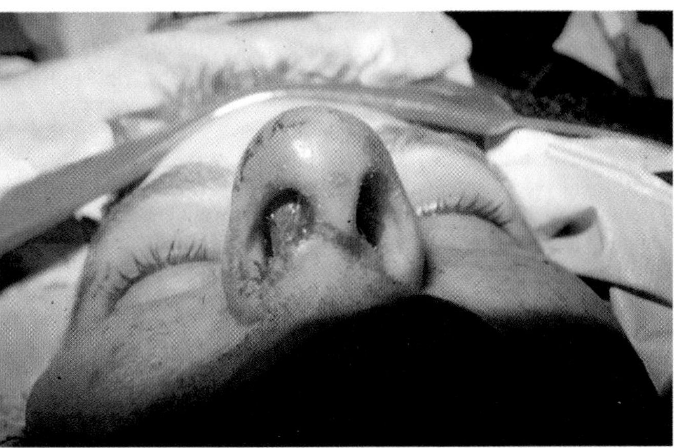

FIGURE 259-5. Septal hematoma presenting as a grapelike mass on left nasal septum. [Reproduced with permission from Knoop K, Stack L, Storrow A, Thurman RJ: *Atlas of Emergency Medicine,* 3rd ed. © 2010, McGraw-Hill, New York.]

Classic tests for cerebrospinal fluid rhinorrhea are not accurate in distinguishing cerebrospinal fluid from serous nasal discharge in the presence of nasal bleeding. The double ring or halo sign occurs when clear cerebrospinal fluid diffuses past blood when dropped on a paper towel. Trauma-related serous nasal discharge will also diffuse past blood. The glucose test is likewise not reliable. Nasal discharge does not contain glucose, whereas cerebrospinal fluid does. Bleeding may create a false-positive glucose test.

Begin the inspection of the ear by checking the mastoid process for Battle's sign (suggesting a basilar skull fracture) and the ear for auricular hematoma. Incision and drainage are required to prevent destruction of cartilage resulting in a cauliflower deformity. Traumatic injury to the ear, including auricular hematoma evacuation, is reviewed in chapter 242, "Ear Disorders." Check the external auditory canal for lacerations, cerebrospinal fluid leak (temporal bone or middle cranial fossa injury), and hematotympanum (a purple and often bulging tympanic membrane). Insert a finger into the external auditory canal and ask the patient to gently open and close the mouth to check for a mandibular condyle fracture.

Inspect the jaw for deviation resulting from a fracture or dislocation. Malocclusion occurs in mandibular fractures, Le Fort fractures, and zygomatic fractures. Check the mouth carefully for missing or subluxed teeth, fractures of the alveolar ridge, sublingual hematoma, or breaks in the oral mucosa (**Figure 259-6**). Be sure to inspect the tongue for lacerations that may result in significant swelling later on. The tongue blade test has been reported to be 96% sensitive in identifying clinically significant mandibular fracture injuries in facial trauma patients.[10-12] The patient without a mandible fracture bites down forcefully enough on a tongue blade to allow the physician to snap the tongue blade with a twisting motion. Patients who open the mouth and cannot break the blade require further imaging. The tongue blade test is best used in conjunction with other clinical findings because test sensitivity may be as low as 85%.[12]

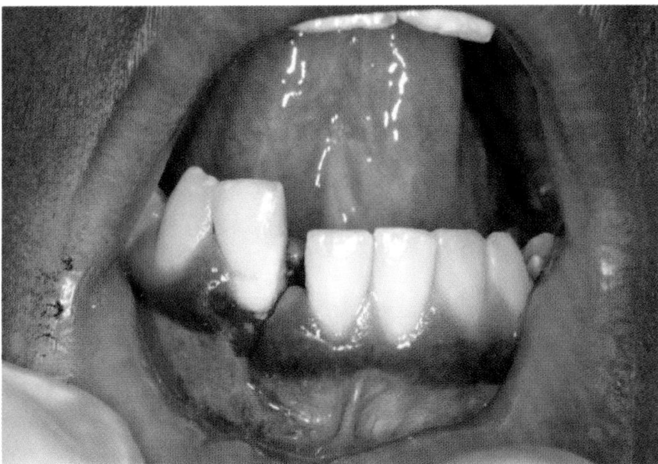

FIGURE 259-6. Open mandible fracture with a fracture line through gingiva into oral cavity. [Reproduced with permission from Knoop K, Stack L, Storrow A, Thurman RJ: *Atlas of Emergency Medicine,* 3rd ed. © 2010, McGraw-Hill, New York.]

DIAGNOSIS

IMAGING

Noncontrast CT is the imaging modality of choice. Plain radiographs remain helpful when CT is not available or to exclude injury in the low-risk patient. Recommendations for imaging based on level of injury and clinical findings are summarized in **Table 259-3**.

Subtle fractures of the frontal bone require head CT with bone windows for optimal evaluation. Because fracture of the frontal bones requires a significant force, head CT is also required to evaluate for associated traumatic brain injury. With involvement of the supraorbital ridge, include a facial CT with axial and coronal sections to better define often complex orbital fracture anatomy.

The Waters' view safely replaces the multiple views in traditional facial series for midfacial fractures.[13,14] One study suggested that at least two views be obtained due to recalculated sensitivities as low as 87% and the lack of comparison of the Waters' view to CT.[15] Not included in this analysis was a study of 730 patients demonstrating a sensitivity of 100% for Waters' view read by emergency physicians versus facial series read by specialists.[16]

Head CT has been reported to be 90% sensitive in excluding injury found on facial CT. **An additional Waters' view is unnecessary with a low clinical suspicion for facial fracture in patients undergoing a head CT for suspected traumatic brain injury.**[17] Using this strategy avoids additional radiation from unnecessary Waters' view or facial CT, and prevents additional trips to CT after cervical spine clearance required for facial CT coronal positioning.

Facial CT with coronal and axial sections is the imaging study of choice for patients with an abnormal Waters' view or as the initial study with significant clinical findings.[16] Computer-generated three-dimensional reconstructions are helpful to better identify complex fractures but do not add additional information in minimally displaced fractures.[18] Head and cervical spine CT scans are recommended in addition to facial CT in patients with high-energy mechanisms or significant clinical findings.

Panorex (orthopantomogram) remains the imaging study of choice for mandible fractures. However, mandible CT is 92% to 100% sensitive

TABLE 259-3 Recommendations for Imaging Based on Level of Injury and Clinical Findings

Level	Low Suspicion	Significant Clinical Findings	Additional Considerations
Frontal bone	Head CT	Head CT (skull windows)	Facial CT with orbital involvement.
			Cervical spine CT with significant clinical findings.
Midface	Waters' view	Face CT with coronal and axial sections; head CT as strong force causes midface fractures	Coronal face sections require cervical spine clearance for positioning.
			Computer-generated, three-dimensional reconstructions with complex injuries.
			Head CT can replace Waters' view.
Mandible	Panorex (orthopantomogram)	Mandible CT	Facial CT detects mandible fractures.

for detecting injury compared with 70% to 86% for Panorex in adults and children and has become the "gold standard" for diagnosing mandible fractures.[19,20] Mandible CT is easier to interpret with less interphysician variability compared with Panorex.[21] Mandible CT scans may miss fractures of the dental root.[19] Panorex is not often available in the ED, requires an upright patient, and may miss mandibular condyle fractures. Mandible CT is recommended in patients requiring head CT to evaluate for traumatic brain injury or when a Panorex is not available. The traditional mandible series (including posterior-anterior, Towne's view, and lateral oblique view) remains an option when Panorex and CT are not available.

TREATMENT

AIRWAY MANAGEMENT

During the primary survey of facial trauma patients, aggressively protect the airway from hemorrhage and mechanical obstruction. Significant hemorrhage into the airway can result from mandible and midfacial fractures. Loss of mechanical support resulting in airway obstruction can occur with bilateral posterior mandible fractures. Significant edema of the soft palate may result from midfacial injuries. Furthermore, the patient is often unable to maintain the damaged airway due to concomitant traumatic brain injury, intoxication, or other life-threatening injuries.

Reposition the airway as needed with a jaw thrust, or head tilt and chin lift after cervical spine clearance. Grasp an obstructing tongue with gauze, a towel clip, or suture, to pull anteriorly and out of the airway with mandible fractures. Remove avulsed teeth and foreign bodies. Use nasal trumpets very carefully to avoid worsening of the injury or intracranial placement in severe midfacial injuries. Bag-mask ventilation often requires a two-person technique because of loss of normal facial bony structures and the need to suction the airway secondary to significant hemorrhage. When the cervical spine has been clinically cleared, allow the alert patient without significant associated injury to remain in an upright position of comfort, with suction in hand, to better handle bleeding and secretions.

Each patient's unique clinical presentation and the physician's experience dictate the best method for establishing a definitive airway. Rapid-sequence intubation is the preferred method of airway management in trauma. The presence of mandible fractures occasionally makes intubation easier than expected. However, always plan for the difficult airway in patients with facial trauma. **To prevent the "can't intubate/can't oxygenate" failed airway, do not administer paralytics unless a patient can be bagged effectively or alternative airway devices or plans are in place.**

Awake intubation with sedation and local airway anesthesia may allow the emergency physician to quickly determine how difficult orotracheal intubation will be while preserving airway reflexes.[22] Etomidate and ketamine both provide sedation with preservation of respiratory drive. When oral endotracheal intubation appears more straightforward than expected on direct laryngoscopy, the endotracheal tube may be placed or paralytics administered followed by orotracheal intubation. When endotracheal intubation appears more difficult or impossible, primary cricothyrotomy or alternative airway management techniques may be performed (see chapters 22, "Basic Cardiopulmonary Resuscitation," 108, "Resuscitation of Neonates," and 109, "Resuscitation of Children").

The best approach to the difficult trauma airway involves planning ahead by having equipment ready for oral endotracheal intubation as well as the neck prepared and a cricothyrotomy kit ready. A laryngeal mask airway device may be a temporizing measure but does not protect the airway from aspiration of stomach contents and may not be possible with injuries involving the pharynx. Fiberoptic devices are an excellent option in the rare case when time, a lack of significant hemorrhage, and an experienced operator are present. Avoid nasal intubation to prevent worsening of injury, hemorrhage, or intracranial placement.[8]

HEMORRHAGE

Significant hemorrhage with severe midfacial or mandible injury can obstruct the airway and make attempts at intubation difficult. The blood supply to the face originates primarily from the sphenopalatine and greater palatine branches of the external carotid artery. Extensive anastomoses occur in the nasal cavity with the anterior and posterior ethmoidal branches of the internal carotid artery. Control posterior nasal epistaxis early with nasal tampon, dual balloon device, or traditional Foley catheter placement with anterior layered gauze packing. Be careful to avoid intracranial placement of nasal packing in severe midfacial fractures. After intubation, oral packing may be needed in a patient with significant mid- and lower facial bleeding. Reduction of significantly displaced nasal fractures and Le Fort injuries may be needed (although rarely) to stop arterial bleeding. Life-threatening hemorrhage can occur in up to 10% of patients with midface fractures.[23] With significant persistent bleeding, immediate operative intervention is required for ligation of injured vessels or better reduction of fractures. Arterial embolization may also be effective in controlling bleeding from branches of the external carotid artery but is associated with a small risk of stroke and other complications.[24] To date, there are no reports describing the use of tranexamic acid for control of massive bleeding from facial injury in the ED.

SPECIFIC FACIAL FRACTURES

FRONTAL BONE FRACTURES

Frontal bone fractures are uncommon injuries resulting from high-energy mechanisms such as unrestrained motor vehicle crashes or assaults with blunt objects. The significant amount of force needed to fracture the thick frontal bone likewise increases the immediate risk of traumatic brain injury, additional facial fractures, and cervical spine injury. Concomitant craniofacial injuries are present in 56% to 87% of patients with frontal sinus fractures.[25] Severe frontal fractures may extend to the temporal bones and require a hearing and facial nerve function evaluation. Otorrhea in this setting is a cerebrospinal fluid leak until proven otherwise.[26] Ocular injuries can occur in up to 25% of patients with frontal bone fractures. The most common finding is an afferent pupillary defect, occurring in about 10% of patients.[27]

Lacerations typically overlie frontal sinus fractures. Careful exploration is needed to identify all fractures. Crepitus is frequently palpable with any sinus fracture. In cases of suspected fracture, obtain a head CT to evaluate the anterior and posterior tables as well as the underlying intracranial structures (**Figures 259-7 and 259-8**).

Because the dura is adherent to the posterior table, operative repair of through-and-through frontal sinus fractures is necessary to prevent pneumocephalus, cerebrospinal fluid leak, and infection. Consider rhinorrhea in any patient with a frontal bone fracture to be a cerebrospinal

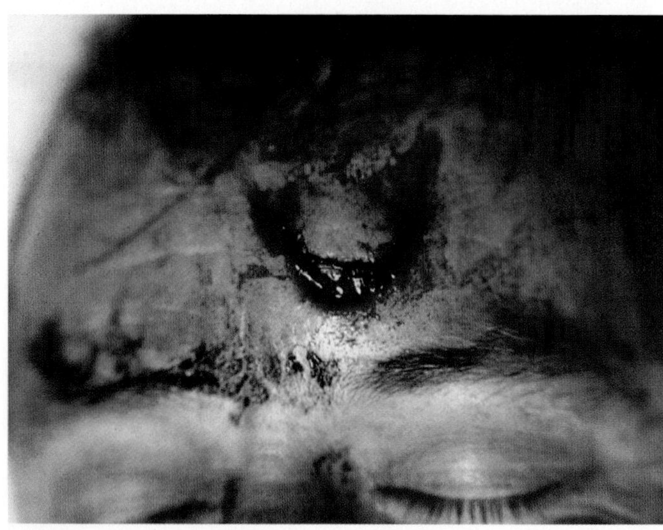

FIGURE 259-7. Forehead laceration overlying a frontal sinus fracture. [Reproduced with permission from Knoop K, Stack L, Storrow A, Thurman RJ: *Atlas of Emergency Medicine,* 3rd ed. © 2010, McGraw-Hill, New York.]

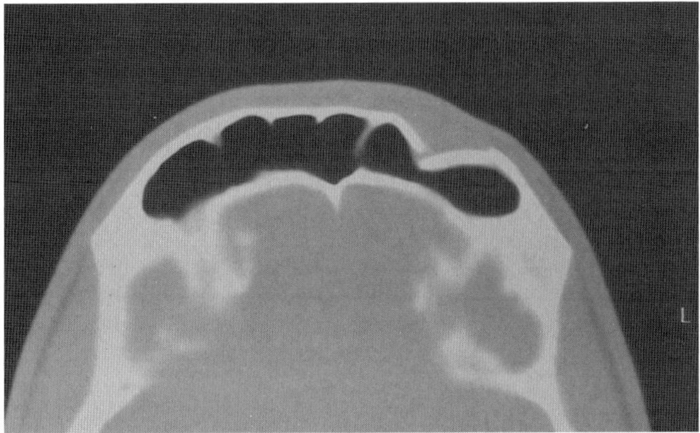

FIGURE 259-8. Frontal sinus fracture from patient in Figure 259-7. CT demonstrating fracture of the anterior table of the frontal sinus. [Reproduced with permission from Knoop K, Stack L, Storrow A, Thurman RJ: *Atlas of Emergency Medicine,* 3rd ed. © 2010, McGraw-Hill, New York.]

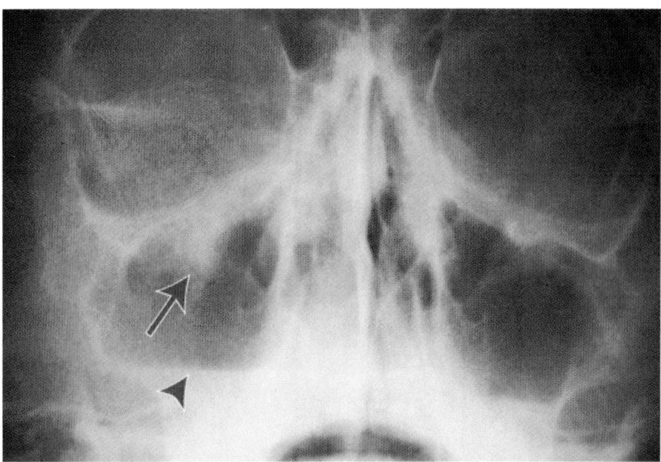

FIGURE 259-10. Blow-out fracture. Waters' view with teardrop sign (*arrow*) and fluid in right maxillary sinus (*arrowhead*). [Reproduced with permission from Knoop K, Stack L, Storrow A: *Atlas of Emergency Medicine,* 2nd ed. © 2002, McGraw-Hill, New York.]

fluid leak until proven otherwise.[26] Mucopyoceles, collections of pus that develop as a result from nasal ducts blocked by fracture, and cranial empyema can result. Oral antibiotics, such as first-generation cephalosporins or amoxicillin clavulanate, are recommended with any sinus fracture. The patient with an isolated anterior table fracture may be discharged with nasal and oral decongestants and appropriate follow-up with a facial surgeon (otolaryngologist, plastic surgeon, or ophthalmology). Admit patients with depressed fractures for IV antibiotics and operative repair.

ORBITAL FRACTURES

The orbit is traditionally thought of as a four-walled structure. It is made up of the frontal bone superiorly, the zygoma and sphenoid bones laterally, the zygoma and maxilla inferiorly, and the thin-walled lamina papyracea of the ethmoid bone medially. There are two categories of orbital fractures: pure, blow-out fractures and unpure, orbital fractures. The pure orbital blow-out fracture involves only the orbital walls and occurs when an object of small diameter strikes the globe without causing an orbital ridge or rim fracture. Force transmitted through the fluid-filled globe results in a fracture of the weaker inferior or medial orbital walls. Adipose tissue, the inferior rectus, or the inferior oblique can then herniate and become entrapped within the maxillary or ethmoid sinus (**Figure 259-9**). Lateral, inferior, and superior orbital ridge fractures typically occur with other facial fractures. **Significant force applied to the nasal bridge can result in naso-orbito-ethmoid fractures that are often accompanied by injury to the lacrimal duct, dural tears, and traumatic brain injury.**

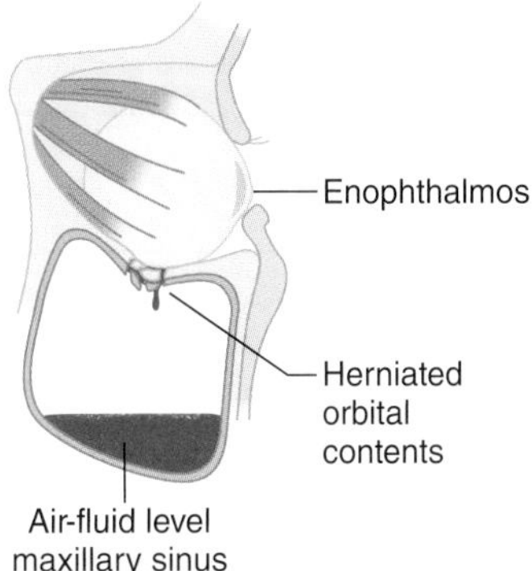

FIGURE 259-9. Blow-out fracture findings, including fluid in the maxillary sinus, herniated fat or muscle, and delayed enophthalmos, occur with orbital floor fracture. [Reproduced with permission from Scaletta TA, Schaider JJ: *Emergency Management of Trauma,* 2nd ed. © 2001, McGraw-Hill, Inc., New York.]

Several key physical examination findings suggest orbital fracture. Enophthalmos occurs with herniation of globe contents before significant edema. Carefully palpate the entire orbital rim to detect any step-off deformity or crepitus. Infraorbital anesthesia often occurs with fracture of the orbital floor. Diplopia on upward gaze occurs with entrapment of the inferior rectus, inferior oblique, or orbital fat, or from injury of muscles or the oculomotor nerve. Naso-orbito-ethmoid fractures result in pain on eye movement, traumatic telecanthus, epiphora (tears spilling over the lower lid), and cerebrospinal fluid leak.[28]

Radiographic findings consistent with orbital fracture are seen in **Figure 259-10**. Additional findings include air-fluid levels or opacification of the maxillary sinus. Obtain a facial or orbital CT with axial and coronal sections to plan surgical management in patients with positive findings on a Waters' view or as the initial study in patients with significant clinical findings (**Figure 259-11**).

The patient with an isolated orbital fracture requires treatment with oral amoxicillin-clavulanate to treat sinus pathogens, decongestants, and instructions to avoid nose blowing until the defect has been repaired. Specialty consultation before discharge is important because controversy continues regarding the best time and indications for operative repair. Repair may be delayed 1 to 2 weeks in adults, whereas children require a shorter time for follow-up and repair. Naso-orbito-ethmoid fractures require admission for specialty consultation with facial surgery and neurosurgery.

Emergent ophthalmology consultation is required for associated ocular injury. **Retrobulbar hematoma or malignant orbital emphysema may create an ocular compartment syndrome, resulting in an acute ischemic optic neuropathy (Figure 259-12).** Physical examination findings include exophthalmos, decreasing visual acuity, and increased intraocular pressure. Emergency lateral canthotomy reduces ocular pressure and ischemia. Orbital fissure syndrome results from a fracture of the orbit involving the superior orbital fissure with injury to the oculomotor and ophthalmic divisions of the trigeminal nerve. Physical examination findings include paralysis of extraocular motions, ptosis, and periorbital anesthesia. Orbital apex syndrome occurs when the optic nerve is also involved, resulting in the preceding physical examination findings and diminished visual acuity.

ZYGOMA FRACTURES

The prominent location of the zygoma results in frequent fractures. Zygomatic arch fractures occur when an anterior and lateral force is applied typically from a fist or blunt object. **The less common zygomaticomaxillary (or "tripod") fracture results classically from a**

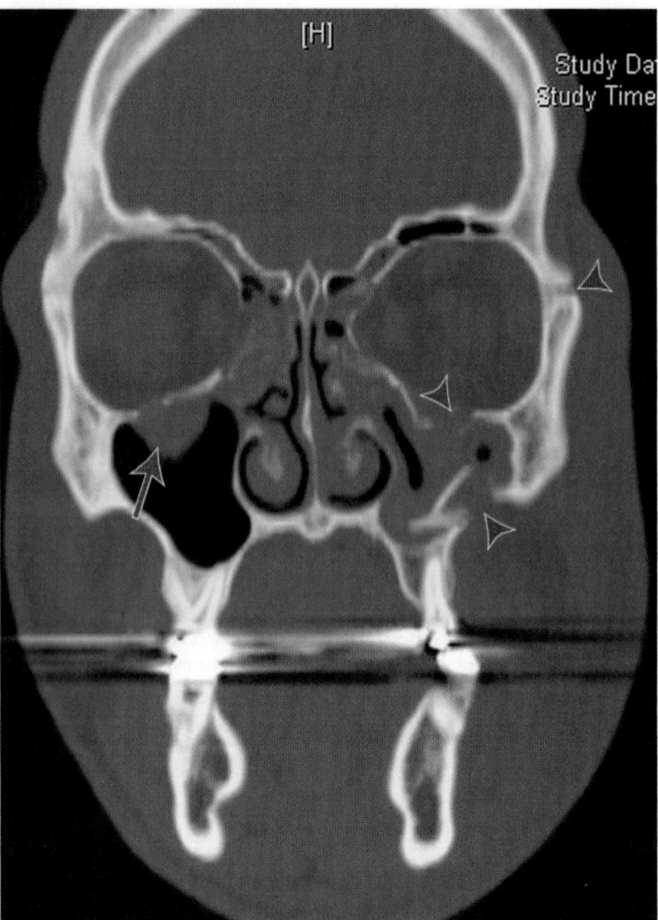

FIGURE 259-11. Left zygomatic maxillary complex and right blow-out fractures. Disruption of zygomatic frontal suture and maxillary sinus on left (*arrowheads*) with herniation of orbital contents into maxillary sinus on the right (*arrow*) on face CT coronal section.

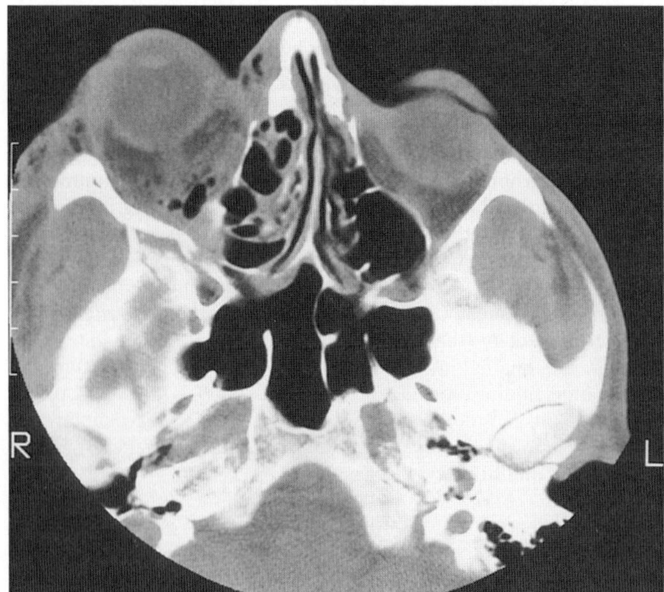

FIGURE 259-12. Retrobulbar hematoma. CT of patient in Figure 259-2 demonstrates right retrobulbar hematoma. [Reproduced with permission from Knoop K, Stack L, Storrow A, Thurman RJ: *Atlas of Emergency Medicine, 3rd ed.* © 2010, McGraw-Hill, New York.]

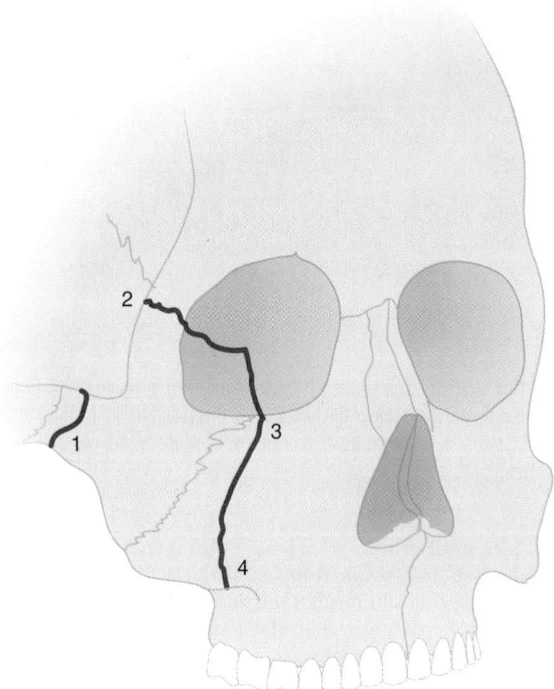

FIGURE 259-13. Tripod fracture locations. Zygomatic arch fracture (*1*), lateral orbital rim fracture (*2*), inferior orbital rim fracture (*3*), and lateral wall of maxillary sinus fracture (*4*). [Reproduced with permission from Schwartz DT: *Emergency Radiology: Case Studies.* © 2008, McGraw-Hill, New York.]

high-energy deceleration injury with disruption of the zygomaticofrontal suture, zygomaticotemporal junction, and infraorbital rim (Figures 259-13 and 259-14). Because the zygoma forms the inferior and lateral walls of the orbit and superior and lateral roof of the maxillary sinus, zygomaticomaxillary fractures are considered orbital and sinus fractures.

On physical examination, flattening of the malar eminence will be noted in the absence of often significant swelling (Figure 259-1). The eye may appear to tilt as the lateral canthus is pulled inferiorly, often with a large lateral subconjunctival hemorrhage. Trismus results from masseter spasm or mechanical impingement of either the temporalis muscle or coronoid process of the mandible. Place a finger adjacent to the maxillary molars and palpate the posterior surface of the arch for tenderness or loss of the space compared to the uninjured side. Diplopia, infraorbital anesthesia, and crepitus occur with significant orbital and sinus involvement. Facial CT is needed to define the extent of the injury.

Patients with isolated temporal arch fractures can be discharged with appropriate medications and follow-up. Patients with zygomaticomaxillary fractures with any loss of vision or significant displacement require admission for IV antibiotics and operative repair.

MIDFACIAL FRACTURES

Midfacial fractures can be caused by motor vehicle crashes, sports, assault, and falls due to seizures or intoxication or in the elderly. The incidence of midfacial fractures in motor vehicle crashes has declined significantly due to improvements in vehicle restraint systems.[29] Fractures of the maxilla require a significant force such as an unrestrained motor vehicle crash patient whose face strikes the dashboard or the severely battered patient.

Le Fort injuries often present dramatically, with significant hemorrhage, early swelling, bilateral orbital ecchymosis, and cerebrospinal fluid leaks in Le Fort II and III injuries. Each pattern results in a unique movement of the midface while gently rocking the hard palate with one hand and stabilizing the forehead with the other hand (**Figure 259-15**).

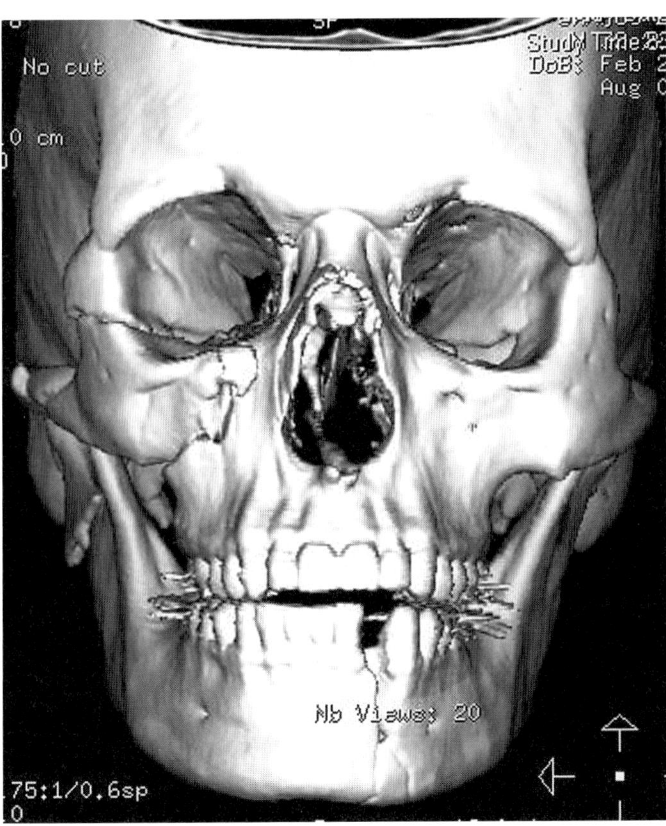

FIGURE 259-14. Zygomatic maxillary complex fracture. Face CT with three-dimensional reconstructions demonstrating right tripod fracture.

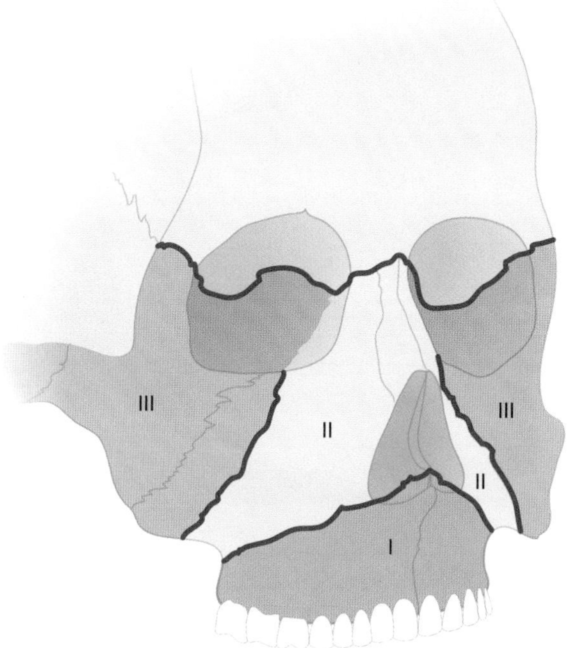

FIGURE 259-15. Le Fort injury patterns. Illustration of the fracture lines of Le Fort I (alveolar), Le Fort II (zygomatic maxillary complex), and Le Fort III (craniofacial dysjunction) fractures. [Reproduced with permission from Knoop K, Stack L, Storrow A, Thurman RJ: *Atlas of Emergency Medicine,* 3rd ed. © 2010, McGraw-Hill, New York.]

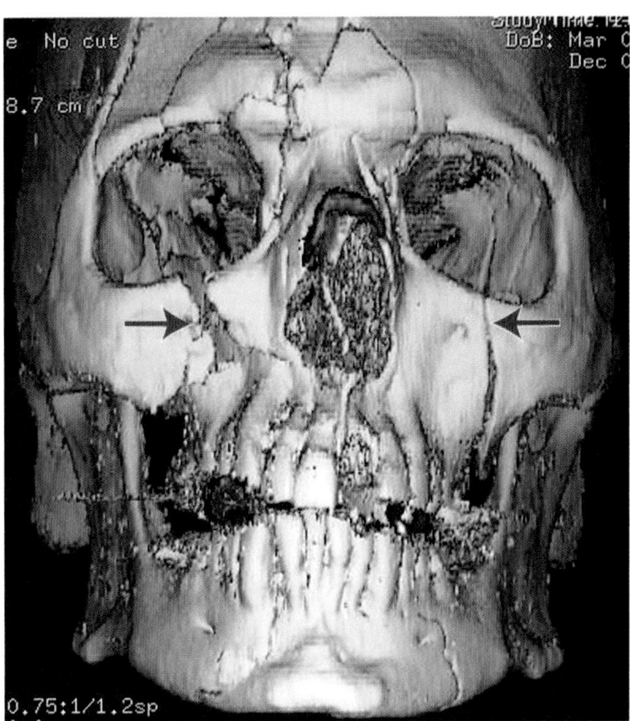

FIGURE 259-16. Bilateral Le Fort II fractures. Face CT with three-dimensional reconstructions demonstrating bilateral Le Fort II in a panfacial fracture patient (*arrows*).

Le Fort I is a transverse fracture separating the body of the maxilla from the pterygoid plate and nasal septum. Only the hard palate and teeth move, similar to a loose upper denture. **Le Fort II** is a pyramidal fracture through the central maxilla and hard palate. Movement of the hard palate and nose occurs, but not the eyes (**Figure 259-16**). **Le Fort III** is craniofacial dysjunction when the entire face is separated from the skull from fractures of the frontozygomatic suture line, across the orbit and through the base of the nose and ethmoids. The entire face shifts with the globes held in place only by the optic nerve. A **Le Fort IV** fracture includes characteristics of the Le Fort III and also involves the frontal bone. CT scan of the face with coronal and axial slices with three-dimensional reconstructions best defines these complex injuries.

Patients with Le Fort injuries often present with significant hemorrhage, requiring airway protection and nasal packing. Oral packing is often required for control of fractures involving the hard palate. Le Fort injuries require admission for management of significant associated injuries, IV antibiotics, and surgical repair.

MANDIBLE FRACTURES

Mandible fractures are the second most common facial fracture after nasal fractures. Assaults, motor vehicle crashes, and falls are the most commonly reported mechanisms.[30] One large trauma center reported 36% of fractures in the region of the angle, followed by 21% in body, and 17% in the parasymphyseal region.[31] Always look for multiple mandibular fractures with one injury at the site of impact and a second subtle injury on the opposite side of the ring. In fact, a mandibular fracture should be considered bilateral until proven otherwise. Comminuted mandible fractures could result in upper airway obstruction due to the tongue being unsupported anteriorly. Presume an open fracture until a thorough intraoral examination determines otherwise. Fractures are classified as either favorable or unfavorable, depending on whether the musculature reduces or opens the fracture.

Patients with mandible fractures usually complain of malocclusion with pain worsened by attempted movement. On inspection, the mandible may appear widened or displaced to one side. Patients may present with trismus due to pain and swelling. Palpation reveals loss of the smooth counters of the mandible, tenderness, and anesthesia in the

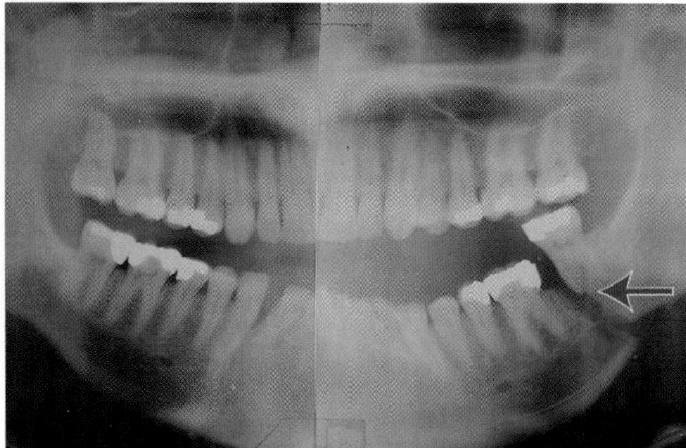

FIGURE 259-17. Mandible fracture. Panoramic view demonstrating an unfavorable mandibular fracture with obvious misalignment (*arrow*) due to the distracting forces of the masseter muscle. [Reproduced with permission from Knoop K, Stack L, Storrow A, Thurman RJ: *Atlas of Emergency Medicine,* 3rd ed. © 2010, McGraw-Hill, New York.]

distribution of the proximal inferior alveolar or distal mental nerve. **A careful intraoral examination is important to exclude small breaks in the mucosa seen with open fractures, sublingual hematoma or ecchymosis, and dental or alveolar ridge fractures and to identify missing teeth.** Examine the ears for evidence of tympanic membrane perforation, hematotympanum, or evidence of condyle displacement. Place a finger into the external auditory canal and ask the patient to open and close the mouth to palpate for injury to the condyle.

Panorex remains the initial imaging study in patients with a low clinical suspicion of injury (**Figure 259-17**). Order mandible or face CT with coronal and axial sections in patients suspected of having condyle fractures, complex fractures, or multiple facial fractures (**Figure 259-18**). A chest radiograph is necessary in the unconscious patient with missing teeth to exclude aspiration of the missing teeth.

In the patient with a stable airway, placement of a Barton's bandage, an ace wrap over the top of the head and underneath the mandible, will stabilize the fracture and help relieve pain. Administer pain control and antibiotics, such as penicillin G 2 to 4 million units IV (or clindamycin, 600 to 900 milligrams, in penicillin-allergic patients), for open fractures. Although studies question the utility of antibiotics, given the overwhelming number of potentially virulent oral anaerobes contaminating open mandible fractures, antibiotics remain a logical therapeutic agent.[32,33] Patients with closed fractures may be given urgent outpatient follow-up. Open fractures require admission for operative repair.

PEDIATRIC CONSIDERATIONS

Facial fractures in the pediatric population are typically due to falls, bicycle accidents, pedestrian accidents, and transport accidents. The nasal bones and mandible are most commonly fractured.[34] Several unique considerations must be made in the initial management of the pediatric patient with facial trauma. Cricothyrotomy is contraindicated in patients <8 years old because the cricothyroid membrane is not developed until age 8 and should be avoided in those between 9 and 12 years of age. In children with severe midfacial injury in whom oral endotracheal intubation is not possible, laryngeal mask airway placement or needle cricothyrotomy serves as a temporizing measure pending emergency tracheostomy. Facial trauma in children should always prompt the consideration of child abuse.

Skull development predisposes children to certain facial and associated injuries while making others less likely. The child's high center of gravity, relatively poor balance, explorative nature, and prominent forehead make the child more susceptible to frontal bone impact and underlying brain injury. Cervical spine injury in children occurs at higher levels and more often without bony radiographic injury (spinal cord injury without radiologic abnormality). The maxillary sinuses do not

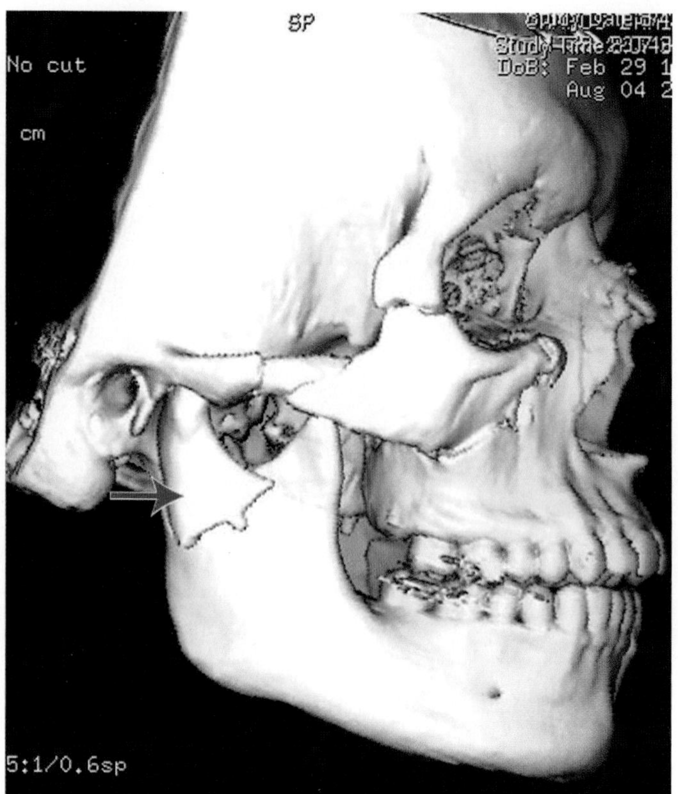

A

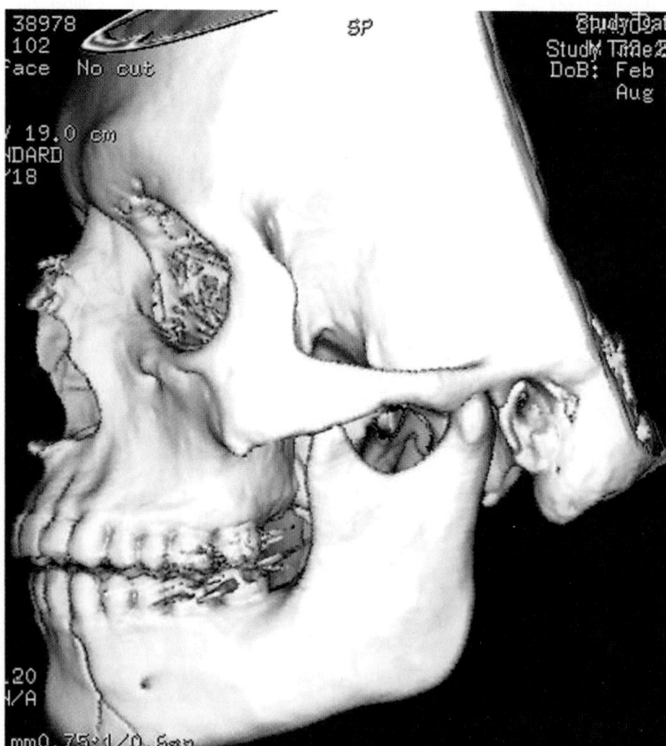

B

FIGURE 259-18. Mandibular condyle fracture—right (**A**) and left (**B**). Face CT with three-dimensional reconstructions demonstrating right mandibular condyle fracture (**A**) and left mandibular fracture (**B**) in patient with zygomatic maxillary complex fracture in Figure 259-14.

begin developing until age 6 years old, which reduces the incidence of midfacial fractures compared with adults.

The pliable pediatric orbital floor is more likely to bend and crack, forming a small "trapdoor" through which muscle and fat become entrapped and potentially ischemic.[35] Pediatric mandible fractures are more likely to be incomplete fractures and more irregular secondary to the underlying developing teeth.[36] Rapid bone remodeling in children with callous formation begins within 1 week and makes delayed reduction difficult. Children with mandible fractures require prompt diagnosis and 1- to 2-day referral to a pediatric facial surgeon to prevent long-term problems with asymmetrical facial growth, cosmetic deformities, and difficulty with mastication.[37]

REFERENCES

The complete reference list is available online at www.TintinalliEM.com.

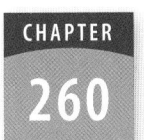

Trauma to the Neck

Ashley S. Bean

INTRODUCTION

The human neck contains numerous vital structures. Both blunt and penetrating injuries can damage structures from many organ systems. The challenge is to treat immediate, life-threatening complications of neck injury, such as airway compromise and hemorrhage, and also to recognize subtle signs of serious pathology.

ANATOMY

The neck is anatomically defined by triangles, zones, and fascial planes. Each sternocleidomastoid muscle separates the neck into two descriptive triangles, anterior and posterior (**Figure 260-1**). The posterior triangle is bordered by the anterior surface of the trapezius, posterior surface of the sternocleidomastoid muscle, and the middle third of the clavicle. The anterior triangle is formed by the borders of the sternocleidomastoid muscle, inferior mandible, and midline of the neck. Most vital structures are contained within the anterior triangle.

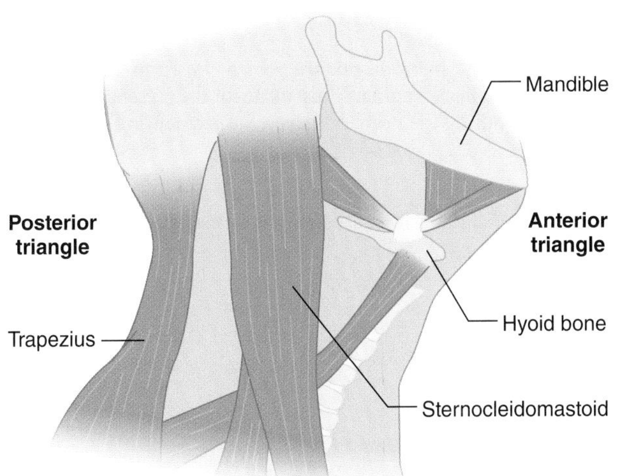

FIGURE 260-1. Triangles of the neck.

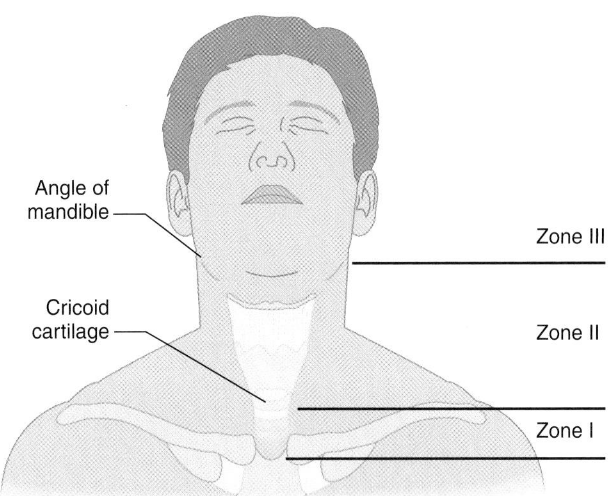

FIGURE 260-2. Zones of the neck.

The anterior triangle is further subdivided into three horizontal zones (**Figure 260-2**), which have historically determined whether a patient undergoes mandatory surgical exploration or further diagnostic evaluation.[1] Using this classification system, the index of suspicion for injury to a particular structure is dictated by the zone (**Table 260-1**). **Classically, zone II injuries undergo surgical exploration; zone I and III wounds undergo further evaluation.** This zone-based approach assumes a direct correlation between the site of the external wound and damage to deep structures; however, the trajectory of the penetrating object can be difficult to determine clinically, and nearly half traverse multiple zones.[2-4]

Finally, the neck is divided into fascial planes (**Figure 260-3**). The platysma is a thin muscle that stretches from the facial muscles to the thorax, demarcating superficial from deep wounds. **Wounds that do not penetrate the platysma are not life threatening.** The platysma muscle is enclosed within superficial fascia anteriorly and deep fascia posteriorly. The deep fascia is comprised of the investing, pretracheal, and prevertebral fascia and the carotid sheath.[5] These fascial layers compartmentalize neck structures and, thus, can prevent exsanguination by confining hematomas. Conversely, increased pressure from expanding hematoma or edema can compromise the airway. Further,

TABLE 260-1 Anatomic Zone and Structures of the Anterior Neck

Neck Zone	Anatomic Boundaries	Structures
Zone 1	Clavicles to the cricoid cartilage	Proximal carotid vertebral arteries Major thoracic vessels Superior mediastinum Lungs Esophagus Trachea Thoracic duct Spinal cord
Zone 2	Cricoid cartilage to the angle of the mandible	Carotid and vertebral arteries Jugular veins Esophagus Trachea Larynx Spinal cord
Zone 3	Angle of the mandible and the base of the skull	Distal carotid and vertebral arteries Pharynx Spinal cord

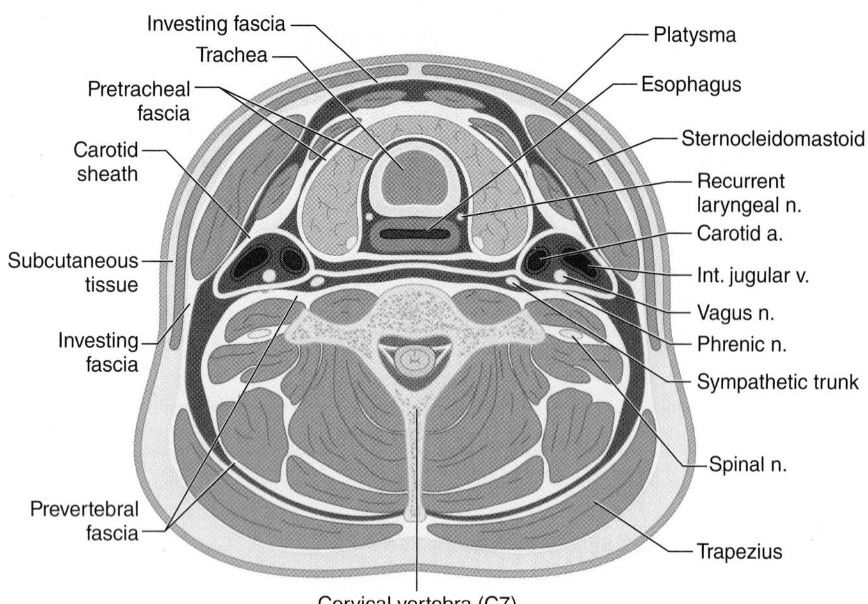

FIGURE 260-3. Fascial layers of the neck. a. = artery; Int. = internal; n. = nerve; v. = vein.

the layers can serve as a conduit for infection tracking from the neck into the mediastinum.[6]

INITIAL MANAGEMENT OF NECK INJURIES

The initial management of neck trauma follows the Advanced Trauma Life Support Guidelines with the systematic Airway, Breathing, Circulation, and Disability approach. Perform a primary survey to identify and treat immediate life-threatening injuries, followed by a secondary survey to discover further injuries.[7]

AIRWAY

Many patients with neck trauma have signs and symptoms of airway compromise.[8] Patients with shock, airway obstruction, impending airway collapse, or altered mental status require immediate airway control (**Table 260-2**). Although there is disagreement about the timing of definitive airway management in less emergent patients, airway anatomic distortion can progress rapidly. Promptly intubate any patient at risk for airway compromise (**Table 260-3**).[9] **Assume a difficult airway in a patient with neck trauma.** Keep all your adjuncts to intubation, as well as a secondary means of securing the airway, readily available.

Rapid-sequence orotracheal intubation is the preferred modality for securing the airway in patients with neck trauma and is successful in 98% of patients.[10,11] When bag-mask ventilation proves difficult due to airway distortion or physical characteristics, perform an awake, orotracheal intubation using a sedative without a paralytic. Anticipate difficulty with bag-mask ventilation in patients with facial hair precluding a seal; unstable mid-facial fractures; airway obstruction from blood, vomitus, or expanding hematoma; subcutaneous emphysema; or an open laryngeal injury that allows external passage of air.[6]

Video laryngoscope–guided intubation[12] and endotracheal intubation over a fiberoptic bronchoscope are useful techniques to secure the airway.[10,13,14]

The laryngeal mask airway is a bridging device but is contraindicated in patients with significant airway distortion. Even if effective, the laryngeal mask airway is only a temporary method for ventilating trauma patients, not a definitive airway.[7]

A surgical cricothyrotomy, or needle-cricothyrotomy if the patient is younger than 8 years of age, is generally the last step in the failed airway management. Patients with neck trauma are at increased risked for requiring a surgical cricothyrotomy due to disruption of the laryngotracheal anatomy.[13] Although there are no absolute contraindications to cricothyrotomy, relative contraindications include suspected or known tracheal transection, fractured larynx, or laryngotracheal disruption with retraction of the distal segment into the mediastinum. Tracheal transection can occur in patients with a "clothesline injury." In such patients, pharmacologic paralysis may cause loss of muscle tone with disruption of the proximal and distal tracheal segments.[6] If the patient has an open laryngeal disruption, you can perform direct intubation through the wound into the distal segment.[11] If other airway techniques are unsuccessful, however, tracheostomy is indicated.[10]

BREATHING

Pneumothorax and hemothorax are present in up to 20% of patients with penetrating neck trauma.[15] Auscultate for the presence or absence of breath sounds during the primary survey. Suspect tension pneumothorax

TABLE 260-2 Clinical Factors Indicating Need for Aggressive Airway Management
Stridor
Acute respiratory distress
Airway obstruction from blood or secretions
Expanding neck hematoma
Profound shock
Extensive subcutaneous emphysema
Alteration in mental status
Tracheal shift

TABLE 260-3 Relative Indications for Airway Management
Progressive neck swelling
Voice changes
Progressive symptoms
Massive subcutaneous emphysema of the neck
Tracheal shift
Alteration in mental status
Expanding neck hematoma
Need to transfer symptomatic patient
Symptomatic patient with anticipated prolonged time away from ED

in patients with unilateral breath sounds, hypotension, and respiratory distress, and treat with needle decompression and/or placement of a thoracostomy tube.[6] Provide continuous pulse oximetry monitoring and supplemental oxygen.

CIRCULATION

Exsanguination is the proximate cause of death in most penetrating neck injury victims,[8] and massive bleeding from trauma kills more rapidly than an unstable airway. Control hemorrhage by applying direct pressure to bleeding wounds. Be careful not to simultaneously occlude both carotid arteries or obstruct the patient's airway. Do not blindly clamp vessels in the ED because this practice can lead to cerebral ischemia or nerve injury.[6] If life-threatening hemorrhage is not controlled by simple pressure, you can insert a Foley catheter into the wound tract and inflate the balloon until bleeding stops or you encounter resistance.[16] Animal model and anecdotal tactical medicine experience suggests that topical hemostatic static agents may improve the survival of patients with bleeding not controlled by pressure. Although the ideal hemostatic agent has not been identified, hemostatic dressings combined with direct pressure appear to decrease blood loss and increase patient survival.[17] Hemostatic dressings may benefit patients with uncontrolled bleeding who need transfer to another hospital for definitive care. Patients with uncontrolled hemorrhage despite these attempts require immediate surgery.[18] If subclavian vessels are involved, uncontrolled hemorrhage in zone I injuries may require emergent thoracotomy.[19]

DISABILITY

Unstable cervical spine injury is uncommon in awake, neurologically intact patients with an **isolated penetrating neck injury**.[20] Vertebral fractures and spinal cord injury are exceedingly rare in patients with isolated stab wounds to the neck.[21] Therefore, cervical collar placement may, in fact, be detrimental by obscuring the injury and increasing the difficulty of hemorrhage control and intubation.[20] Cervical collars should not be maintained at the expense of monitoring the injury or life-saving procedures.

Spinal cord damage is more likely from gunshot wounds, and cord damage is sustained at the time of injury. Deficits, which are usually permanent, should be evident at time of presentation unless the patient has an altered sensorium. Place a cervical collar on patients with a neurologic deficit or altered mental status precluding exam, after checking the neck to identify any penetrating injuries, vascular thrills or bruits, or bleeding or hematoma.[22,23]

However, patients with blunt neck trauma frequently have cervical spine fractures, so maintain cervical spine immobilization in such injuries.[24]

INITIAL RADIOLOGIC EVALUATION

Although conventional radiographs of the chest and neck may suggest a variety of pathologies in the patient with neck trauma (**Table 260-4**),[7,18,25,26] most patients with penetrating or blunt neck trauma will require advanced imaging in the form of multidetector CT angiography (MDCTA), MRI, or magnetic resonance angiography. Obtain a chest radiograph to evaluate for pneumothorax and hemothorax in patients with neck trauma because there is a high incidence of these thoracic complications. In addition, pneumothorax and hemothorax can be detected rapidly by bedside ultrasound.[27] Do not delay transfer of patients between hospitals or to the operating room to obtain conventional radiographs of the neck.

DIAGNOSIS AND TREATMENT

Any wound deep to the platysma raises concern for damage to the vital structures of the neck. Simple diagnostic maneuvers add valuable information to the physical exam. Instruct awake and cooperative patients to cough (to check for hemoptysis), to swallow saliva (to assess for dysphagia from esophageal injury), and to speak (to evaluate for laryngeal fracture).[6] **In patients with penetrating neck trauma, a careful, structured physical exam is more than 95% sensitive for detecting clinically significant vascular and aerodigestive injuries.**[23] The physical exam is most accurate for identifying arterial injuries; conversely, esophageal and venous injuries may be missed. Assess the patient for "hard" and "soft" signs of injury (**Table 260-5**).[15,28] **Nine out of 10 patients with hard signs will have an injury requiring repair and should be rapidly transferred to the operating room or angiography suite.** If your institution does not have the requisite surgical or diagnostic capabilities readily available, transfer to an appropriate hospital. Presence of soft signs increases suspicion of structural damage and indicates the need for additional diagnostic evaluation; however, only a minority of patients with soft signs will have a clinically significant injury.[15,29-31]

TABLE 260-4 Pathologic Findings on Conventional Radiographs

Chest radiograph
Pneumothorax
Hemothorax
Mediastinal air
Widened mediastinum
Subcutaneous emphysema
Foreign body or bullet fragments
Pulmonary edema
Aspiration pneumonia
Soft tissue neck radiograph
Prevertebral air
Foreign body or bullet fragments
Tracheal narrowing or deviation
Subcutaneous or retropharyngeal emphysema
Cervical spine radiograph (anteroposterior, lateral, and odontoid)
Vertebral fracture
Hyoid bone fracture

TABLE 260-5 Signs and Symptoms of Neck Injury

Hard	Soft
Vascular injury	
Shock unresponsive to initial fluid therapy	Hypotension in field
Active arterial bleeding	History of arterial bleeding
Pulse deficit	Nonpulsatile or nonexpanding hematoma
Pulsatile or expanding hematoma	Proximity wounds
Thrill or bruit	
Laryngotracheal injury	
Stridor	Hoarseness
Hemoptysis	Neck tenderness
Dysphonia	Subcutaneous emphysema
Air or bubbling in wound	Cervical ecchymosis or hematoma
Airway obstruction	Tracheal deviation or cartilaginous step-off
	Laryngeal edema or hematoma
	Restricted vocal cord mobility
Pharyngoesophageal injury	
	Odynophagia
	Subcutaneous emphysema
	Dysphagia
	Hematemesis
	Blood in the mouth
	Saliva draining from wound
	Severe neck tenderness
	Prevertebral air
	Transmidline trajectory

PENETRATING NECK INJURY

Although penetrating neck wounds account for only 1% of traumatic injuries, the mortality rate is as high as 10%.[8] Gunshot wounds and stab wounds are the predominant mechanisms of injury, whereas flying debris and sharp object impalement are less frequent causes.[8,18,32] Patients often have significant concurrent wounds to the head, chest, or abdomen.[8,18,28,32]

Gunshot wounds are more likely than stab wounds to cause vascular and aerodigestive system damage. Transcervical gunshot wounds have at least a 70% chance of substantial associated injuries.[28,33] **Vascular injuries are the most common cervical injury and the leading cause of death from penetrating neck trauma.**[18] The remainder of associated neck injuries are split among spinal cord, aerodigestive tract, and peripheral nerve injuries.[15,28,32]

There is no debate regarding the treatment of unstable patients with clear evidence of vascular or aerodigestive injury—this group of patients should undergo invasive intervention.[2,8,29,32] Controversy arises in two areas concerning the management of stable patients:

1. Should all zone II injuries undergo mandatory exploration?
2. Should all zone I and III injuries undergo a specific, extensive battery of diagnostic testing?

GENERAL TREATMENT OPTIONS

Mandatory Operative Exploration Historically, all zone II injuries were surgically explored. This aggressive practice began during World War II as a response to a high incidence of missed injuries and mortality, but selective management is generally recommended today to minimize unnecessary surgery.[34] Zone II is the most commonly injured area and is easily accessed surgically.[29,32] Exposure and vascular control are more difficult for zone I and III injures, so most patients with zone I and III injuries undergo angiography and endoscopy to determine the need for operative intervention.[35]

Selective Management The movement toward selective management rather than mandatory exploration began in response to the high rate of negative neck explorations. Furthermore, advocates of a more conservative methodology cite the sensitivity of physical exam in detecting clinically significant injuries. Contrarians maintain concerns about missed lethal injuries when relying solely on the clinical exam.[36,37] Less invasive, selective protocols, which mandate rapidly obtained angiography, esophagography, and panendoscopy, have radically decreased nontherapeutic neck operations without increasing morbidity and mortality; however, the yield of angiography and endoscopic studies in asymptomatic patients is exceedingly low.[8,15,38]

No-Zone Targeted Diagnostic Workup A new iteration in selective management has evolved with the addition of information gleaned from MDCTA to the diagnostic process. MDCTA now permits fast, reliable information about injuries in all neck zones. Furthermore, physical examination plus MDCTA is up to 100% sensitive and 97.5% specific for detecting significant vascular or aerodigestive injury. Perhaps more importantly, the negative predictive value for arterial injury is 98% to 100%.[39,40] Unlike angiography, MDCTA also allows assessment of the aerodigestive tracts and the cervical spine.[5]

In addition to defining specific injuries, MDCTA can determine if the wound track approximates important structures. Wounds with a trajectory not concerning for injury do not need further invasive (angiographic or endoscopic) workup. Conversely, trajectories in close proximity to vital structures should prompt a targeted diagnostic workup.[4] Disadvantages of MDCTA include exposure to ionizing radiation, use of iodinated IV contrast, and image artifacts due to motion or metallic foreign bodies.[41] Furthermore, patients cannot undergo angiography, either for diagnosis or intervention, directly after MDCTA due to iodinated contrast exposure.[3]

A penetrating neck trauma protocol (**Figure 260-4**) that combines a -structured physical exam and MDCTA dramatically reduces formal neck explorations.[2,42] In this scheme, the zone of injury has little impact on the management of the patient because the neck is considered to be a single unit. Per this protocol (see Figure 260-4), symptomatic patients with hard signs of neck injury undergo emergent operative or angiographic intervention. Symptomatic patients with only soft signs of injury are at intermediate risk and should undergo MDCTA. Further diagnostic testing can be guided by MDCTA findings. Symptomatic patients with an indeterminate MDCTA artifact should undergo traditional testing.[2,6,18,43]

Although patients who are asymptomatic are at low risk for injury, it is unclear what their diagnostic algorithm should entail. Options include observation and/or targeted diagnostic testing including MDCTA. Specific concern for digestive tract injuries can be addressed via esophagoscopy or esophagram; potential laryngotracheal injuries can be evaluated with endoscopy. Trauma centers with a high volume of penetrating neck injuries may opt to observe patients with serial physical exams in lieu of advanced diagnostic testing. Hospitals that infrequently manage penetrating neck injuries may be more likely to order adjunctive screening testing.[29,44]

PENETRATING VASCULAR INJURIES

Vascular injuries are present in up to 40% of patients with penetrating neck trauma and are the most commonly associated cervical injury in this population. Arterial injuries, which predominately involve the carotid artery, account for 45% of penetrating neck vascular trauma and are the most frequent cause of death.[8,15,19,32] The morbidity and mortality of vascular injuries are related both to exsanguination and neurologic complications.[5] For instance, **carotid artery injury** leads to stroke in 15% of patients and death in up to 22%. **Venous injuries** are discovered in up to 20% of patients with penetrating neck wounds.[32] Signs of venous injury are often subtle and difficult to identify by physical exam; however, most asymptomatic venous injuries do not require repair.[30]

The overwhelming majority of patients with hard signs of vascular injury (Table 260-5) will require operative intervention. In contrast, while up to one quarter of patients with soft signs of vascular injury will have a vascular abnormality identified at angiography, only 3% of these patients will require vascular repair.[15]

Diagnosis Several imaging modalities are useful during the evaluation of vascular neck trauma (**Table 260-6**). Although angiography remains the gold standard for investigating penetrating neck vascular injuries, **MDCTA is now the first-line imaging modality**.[5] Angiography continues to be useful, however, in specific circumstances. MDCTA findings that are inconclusive or incongruent with the patient's clinical exam should be refined by angiography.[45] In addition, stable patients with injuries suitable for endovascular repair may undergo definitive angiographic intervention.[5]

Disadvantages of **angiography** include its inability to provide a comprehensive evaluation of nonvascular neck structures, limited availability, and mobilization of additional personnel.[3] Potential complications include contrast-induced nephropathy, puncture site hematoma, thrombosis, embolism, vascular spasm, ischemia, and arterial dissection.[32]

The advent of CT angiography and improvements in multidetector CT technology have revolutionized the diagnosis and treatment of penetrating neck injuries. MDCTA images the vascular, aerodigestive, and osseous structures of the neck. Furthermore, MDCTA is sensitive for the detection of injury, can be rapidly performed, and is noninvasive, accurate, and widely available.[3]

Color flow Doppler US is highly sensitive for detecting clinically important vascular injuries. Advantages of US include its portability, noninvasive nature, lack of ionizing radiation, and relatively decreased capital expense. Disadvantages include the inability to scan through subcutaneous emphysema, hematoma, marked operator variability, and limited availability. Additionally, US cannot penetrate bone and is thus unable to image intrathoracic or intracranial vessels.[3,26] Finally, it cannot evaluate the aerodigestive structures of the neck.[3]

MRI or MRI angiography in patients with metallic projectiles is contraindicated due to concern for ferromagnetic material.[5] Furthermore, the role of MRI in the diagnosis of aerodigestive injuries has not been evaluated. Thus, MRI cannot be used to comprehensively evaluate neck structures.[3] MRI may play a select role in the evaluation of nonprojectile penetrating trauma, which involves the cervical spine.[46]

Treatment Treatment of vascular injuries depends on the vessel involved and accessibility of the lesion. Options vary from observation to surgical repair to angiographic embolization or stenting. Patients with

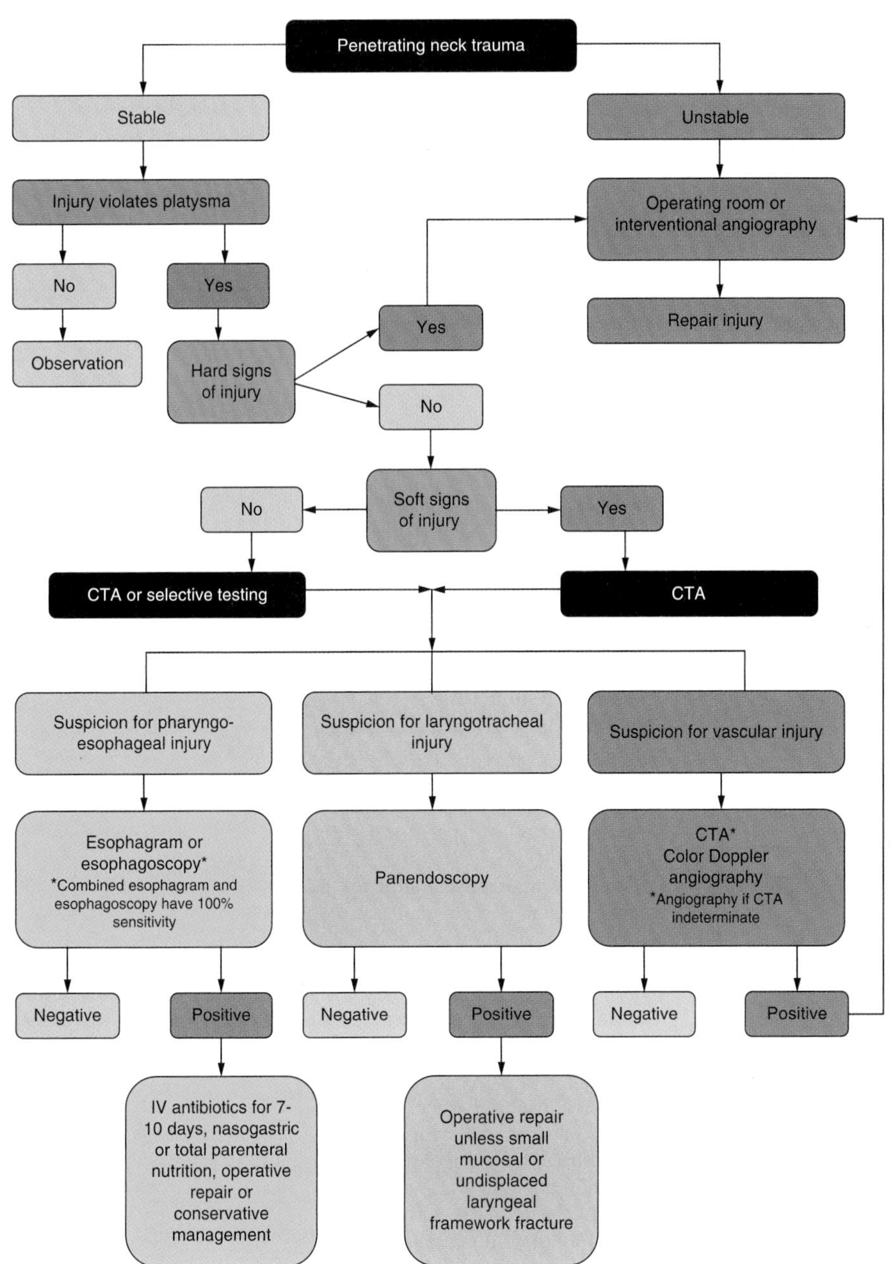

FIGURE 260-4. Penetrating neck trauma protocol.

carotid artery injuries that are asymptomatic, low-velocity injuries, or small intimal tears or pseudoaneurysms may not need repair if they have intact distal circulation and reliable surgical follow-up.[6]

BLUNT NECK INJURY

Blunt neck trauma comprises only 5% of traumatic injuries to the neck. Road traffic accidents are the most common cause of blunt neck trauma. Other causes of blunt neck injury include assault, pedestrians struck by vehicles, falls, and hanging.[47] While vascular injury occurs in approximately 1% of patients with blunt neck trauma,[48] cervical aerodigestive injuries are rare. As with penetrating neck trauma, patients with blunt neck injury frequently have significant associated injuries.[49] In contrast, airway occlusion rather than hemorrhage is the most rapidly fatal injury.[6]

BLUNT CAROTID AND VERTEBRAL DISSECTION

The mortality rate of symptomatic blunt cerebral vascular injury approaches 60%.[48] However, most patients with blunt cerebral vascular injury are initially asymptomatic and do not develop neurologic symptoms for hours to days.[49] Fortunately, angiographic screening of certain asymptomatic patients for blunt cerebral vascular injury can increase the likelihood of diagnosis 10-fold.[48] Moreover, early identification and treatment of blunt cerebral vascular injury significantly reduce the rate of stroke and death.[49] Numerous screening criteria can be used to increase blunt cerebral vascular injury detection in asymptomatic patients (**Table 260-7**).[24,50,51] Unfortunately, 20% of blunt cerebral vascular injuries occur without any established risk factor.[52]

The mechanism of injury for blunt cerebral vascular injury is cervical hyperextension and rotation or hyperextension during rapid deceleration, which can result in intimal dissections, thromboses, pseudoaneurysms, fistulas, and transections.[52] Intimal tears expose subendothelial collagen that acts as a substrate for platelet aggregation. The subsequent thrombus can embolize, cause stenosis, or create critical vessel occlusions. Furthermore, tears can provide a pathway for dissection.[53]

Diagnosis Diagnostic four-vessel cerebral angiography is the gold standard for the diagnosis of blunt cerebral vascular injury.[51] Unfortunately, MDCTA has a low sensitivity for the detection of blunt cerebral vascular injury. Even when scanners with 16 or more slices are used and the images are interpreted by a neuroradiologist, sensitivity of MDCTA

TABLE 260-6 Vascular Evaluation of Penetrating Neck Trauma

Imaging Modality	Advantages	Disadvantages
Catheter angiography	Gold standard Both diagnostic and therapeutic Access to zone I and III injuries where surgical repair is difficult	Invasive Expensive Labor intensive Requires skilled operators
Helical CT angiography	Readily available Fast Minimally invasive Visualization of missile trajectory High-resolution images of vascular, aerodigestive, and bone structures with single study	Only diagnostic, not therapeutic Requires IV contrast Image quality affected by technique of contrast injection Metallic streak artifact may obscure findings Limited evaluation of low zone I and high zone III injuries May miss small intimal flaps, pseudoaneurysms, and arteriovenous fistulas
Duplex ultrasonography	Noninvasive Inexpensive No contrast medium	Highly operator dependent Limited view of zones I and III Obscured by subcutaneous emphysema and hematomas May miss small lesions

remains less than 80%. However, because MDCTA has excellent specificity (97%), patients with blunt cerebral vascular injury identified by MDCTA do not require confirmatory angiographic evaluations.[54]

US has a low sensitivity for blunt cerebral vascular injury and should not be used as a screening test.[51]

Although MRI has been gaining acceptance in the evaluation of blunt cerebral vascular injury, the sensitivity and specificity of this imaging modality are lower than those of diagnostic four-vessel cerebral angiography. Therefore, do not use MRI as the sole screening study for blunt cerebral vascular injury.[51]

Treatment Antithrombotic agents (aspirin, clopidogrel, or heparin) and operative or interventional angiographic repair are blunt cerebral vascular injury treatment options. Specific therapy is determined by a grading scale (**Table 260-8**).[51,55]

TABLE 260-7 Compiled Screening Criteria for Blunt Cerebral Vascular Injury

Signs and symptoms
- Arterial hemorrhage from nose, neck, or mouth
- Cervical bruit in patients <50 y old
- Expanding cervical hematoma
- Focal neurologic deficit: transient ischemic attack, hemiparesis, vertebrobasilar symptoms, Horner's syndrome
- Stroke on secondary CT
- Neurologic deficit unexplained by head CT

Risk factors for blunt cerebral vascular injury
- High-energy transfer mechanism and one of the following:
  - Facial fractures: Le Fort II or III fracture, mandible fracture, frontal skull fracture, orbital fracture
  - Cervical spine fracture patterns: subluxation, fractures extending into the transverse foramen, fractures of C1–C3
  - Any basilar skull fracture or occipital condyle fracture
  - Petrous bone fracture
  - Diffuse axonal injury with Glasgow Coma Scale score ≤8
  - Concurrent traumatic brain and thoracic injuries
  - Neck hanging with anoxic brain injury
  - Clothesline type injury with significant swelling, pain, or altered mental status

TABLE 260-8 Blunt Carotid and Vertebral Artery Injury Grading Scale

Grade	Description	Treatment
Grade I	Luminal irregularity or dissection with <25% luminal narrowing	Antithrombotic agent
Grade II	Dissection or intramural hematoma with ≥25% luminal narrowing, intraluminal thrombus, or raised intimal flap	Antithrombotic agent or surgical repair if accessible
Grade III	Pseudoaneurysm	Antithrombotic agent or surgical repair if accessible
Grade IV	Occlusion	Antithrombotic agent or surgical repair if accessible
Grade V	Transection with free extravasation	Surgical repair if accessible Balloon occlusion or embolization

UPPER AIRWAY AND ESOPHAGEAL INJURIES FROM BLUNT AND PENETRATING TRAUMA

LARYNGOTRACHEAL INJURIES

Penetrating neck trauma causes laryngotracheal injury in 2% to 5% of penetrating trauma patients and has a 2% to 15% mortality rate.[2,15,32] **Significant laryngotracheal injuries should be detected by physical exam.** Patients with hard signs of laryngotracheal injuries (see Table 260-5) need urgent airway control and operative intervention. Soft signs of laryngotracheal injury (see Table 260-5) are present in approximately 18% of patients with penetrating neck injury, but only 15% of these patients will have a laryngotracheal injury diagnosed.[15]

Blunt laryngotracheal injuries occur in less than 0.5% of blunt trauma patients.[56] The majority of blunt laryngotracheal trauma is caused by car collisions. Such injuries are rare because the larynx is protected by the mandible and supported by muscles that deflect most external forces.[57] **Patients with laryngotracheal injuries due to blunt trauma may have a quiescent phase with progressively increasing subclinical airway edema or hematoma that can result in delayed airway obstruction.**[58]

Diagnosis Evaluate patients with a history of significant anterior neck trauma[59] or signs and symptoms of a laryngotracheal injury[57,58,60] with flexible fiberoptic laryngoscopy to define airway patency and the extent of intraluminal injury. CT imaging is critical in patients with suspected laryngotracheal injury without airway compromise and can impart information that influences management.[61]

Treatment Treatment of laryngotracheal injuries is based on the classification system developed by Schaefer and Brown (**Table 260-9**).[62] Patients with grade I and II injuries can be managed medically; grade III, IV, and V injuries typically require operative intervention.[63]

PHARYNGOESOPHAGEAL INJURIES

Up to 9% of patients with **penetrating neck trauma** have pharyngoesophageal injuries.[28] Whereas laryngotracheal injuries are usually apparent, **pharyngoesophageal injuries typically have more subtle**

TABLE 260-9 Laryngeal Injury Grading Scale

Grade	Description
Grade I	Minor endolaryngeal hematoma without detectable fracture
Grade II	Edema, hematoma, minor mucosal disruption without exposed cartilage, nondisplaced fractures
Grade III	Massive edema, mucosal disruption, exposed cartilage, vocal fold immobility, displaced fracture
Grade IV	Grade III with two or more fracture lines or massive trauma to laryngeal mucosa
Grade V	Complete laryngotracheal separation

signs resulting in diagnostic delays. In fact, there are no hard signs of pharyngoesophageal injury. Deaths from esophageal injury are usually due to mediastinitis and sepsis.[32] Soft signs and symptoms (see Table 260-5)[26] that portend injury may be present and signal the need for further evaluation.[28] Also suspect this injury if the trajectory of the bullet visualized by CT is in close proximity to the pharynx or esophagus.[5] Finally, in patients receiving conventional soft tissue neck radiographs, prevertebral air is suggestive of a pharyngoesophageal injury.[18]

Pharyngoesophageal injuries are exceedingly rare in patients with blunt neck trauma. Between 1970 and 2003, 11 cases of cervical digestive tract injury due to blunt forces were reported.[64] **Suspect esophageal injury in patients with a history of a sudden acceleration or deceleration event in which the neck was extended.** In this scenario, injuries occur as the esophagus is forced against the spine. However, the low incidence of injuries coupled with their subtle clinical presentation can lead to a delay in diagnosis, leading to morbidity and mortality. In patients with blunt trauma, the signs and symptoms of pharyngoesophageal injury are much more likely to result from laryngotracheal pathology.[6]

Diagnosis Patients with hard signs of vascular or laryngotracheal injuries should undergo intraoperative endoscopy if a pharyngoesophageal injury is identified or suspected during exploration. Symptomatic patients who do not meet criteria for neck exploration can be evaluated by either direct esophagoscopy or swallowing studies.[8] Esophagoscopy is more sensitive for detecting esophageal injuries with the added benefit of quantifying the size and extent of the injury. It can be performed intraoperatively and on unstable or intubated patients. The combination of these two studies achieves 100% sensitivity for detecting these injuries.[65]

Patients who are asymptomatic can be evaluated for digestive tract injuries with multidetector CT. Patients without evidence of injury by multidetector CT should either be observed or, if a high suspicion for injury exists, undergo direct esophagoscopy or swallowing studies using a water-soluble agent.[8]

Treatment Give patients with pharyngoesophageal injuries IV antibiotics and either parenteral or enteral nutrition via a nasogastric tube. Small pharyngeal perforations may be managed medically, whereas pharyngeal perforations larger than 2 cm and esophageal perforations require surgical repair.[28]

STRANGULATION

Strangulation is one form of blunt neck trauma. Mechanisms include hanging, postural strangulation, ligature strangulation, and manual strangulation.[66] Accidental, homicidal, and suicidal strangulations are frequent causes of death. In fact, 10% of violent deaths in the United States are due to strangulation,[25] and hanging is the second most common means of suicide death in the United States.[67] Accidental strangulation is more frequent in children, but also occurs in adults whose clothing or hair becomes entangled in machinery or who participate in the paraphilia of erotic asphyxiation.[66,68] In all forms of strangulation, death is ultimately due to cerebral anoxia and ischemia; obstruction of cerebral venous return rather than acute airway compromise is postulated to be the most common pathophysiologic mechanism of death.[6]

CLINICAL FEATURES

Although airway compromise is envisioned by most people to be the cause of strangulation deaths, **the major pathologic mechanism is neck vessel occlusion rather than airway obstruction**. There are numerous case reports of people with functioning tracheostomies committing suicide by hanging or strangulation. Only limited pressure is needed for venous compression. If both external and internal jugular veins are simultaneously occluded, cerebral vascular congestion, edema, and unconsciousness result.[66] Next, loss of muscle tone allows arterial compression with subsequent cerebral anoxia. Airway obstruction and carotid body reflex–mediated cardiac dysrhythmia are minor mechanisms of death in strangled patients.[69]

In addition to cerebral anoxia, strangulation injuries include laryngotracheal fractures, cervical spine fractures, pharyngeal lacerations, and carotid artery injuries.[70] Although hyoid bone fractures are classically associated with strangulation, they are found in a minority of these patients—even those with fatal injuries. Furthermore, with the exception of judicial hangings, cervical spine and cord injuries are not frequently seen in patients who survive strangling.[66] Carotid artery dissection is a rare complication, but should be suspected in a patient with a lateralizing neurologic exam or bruising or tenderness over the carotid artery. Moreover, consider unreported strangulation in young patients with acute neurologic deficits or a spontaneous carotid artery dissection.[69]

Physical signs of strangulation include petechiae and neck contusions; however, half of victims have no visible signs of neck trauma, and two thirds are asymptomatic.[25] In fact, patients with extensive laryngeal injury may have few external signs.[71] In those who are symptomatic, the most common complaints are neck pain, voice changes, swallowing difficulty, and breathing problems. Any of these symptoms can signal impending airway compromise and should be investigated.[69]

Patients presenting in cardiac arrest have a dismal prognosis.[66] Conversely, recovery of patients with neurologic symptoms is unpredictable. Patients with severe neurologic symptoms, such as a Glasgow Coma Score of 3, may recover without sequelae, whereas patients with normal initial exams may progressively deteriorate.[68] Most in-hospital, post-strangulation deaths occur due to laryngeal or pulmonary edema or cerebral anoxia.[66]

Perhaps the most difficult task in caring for strangled patients is evaluating the "walking and talking" victim who lacks physical signs of strangulation. Victims may be under the influence of alcohol or drugs or be hyperventilating. Physicians may be tempted to ascribe symptoms to anxiety and to discount the patient's story.[25] Furthermore, there is a subset of seemingly asymptomatic patients who die after developing delayed cerebral or pulmonary edema.[71]

DIAGNOSIS

The evaluation of patients with suspected strangulation is multifaceted and may involve radiologic imaging or endoscopy. Although pulmonary edema, aspiration pneumonia, larynx or hyoid bone fractures, or tracheal deviation caused by edema or hematoma may be visible on chest radiography, CT and MRI can provide more detailed information of soft tissue neck structures. Radiologically demonstrated intramuscular hemorrhage or edema, swelling of the platysma, subcutaneous bleeding, and hemorrhagic lymph nodes are indicative of strangulation injury.[25,72] To exclude carotid dissection, carotid artery imaging should be performed on patients with neurologic deficits discordant with brain CT findings.[25] Finally, patients with symptoms of laryngeal tracheal injury such as dyspnea, dysphonia, aphonia, or odynophagia should undergo laryngobronchoscopy, which may reveal petechiae, edema, or vocal cord paralysis.[25]

TREATMENT AND DISPOSITION

Unconscious patients and those with progressive symptoms such as odynophagia, hoarseness, neurologic changes, or dyspnea require aggressive respiratory management including intubation. Patients with pulmonary edema may benefit from positive end-expiratory pressure ventilation. Furthermore, patients may develop cerebral edema, requiring strategies to reduce intracranial pressure or seizure prophylaxis. Observe asymptomatic patients for delayed respiratory and neurologic dysfunction.[68]

Addressing the numerous psychosocial issues that are typically present in strangled victims is a critical element of their overall coordinated treatment plan. Victims of domestic violence may need social services. Only 5% of strangled domestic violence victims seek medical attention within 2 days of the strangulation.[73] Such patients are at high risk for subsequent harm and death from the same abuser.[25] Survivors are also at risk for posttraumatic stress disorder.[6] Patients who have attempted suicide require psychiatric evaluation. Hangings are often one component of a complex suicide attempt. When suicide is suspected, evaluate patients for other methods of self-harm such as wrist lacerations, self-stabbing, gunshot wounds, or ingestions.[68]

SPECIAL CONSIDERATIONS

CHILDREN

Children with blunt or penetrating trauma are susceptible to the same mechanisms and injuries as adults. Additional mechanisms of injury seen in childhood include child abuse, playground trauma, and handlebar injuries during bike falls.[74]

The initial management and indications for emergent intervention for children with penetrating neck trauma mirror those of adults. Children are at higher risk for complications from angiography, endoscopy, and ionizing radiation. Thus, the need for an extensive workup in the asymptomatic child must be critically evaluated.[75]

Children have the same incidence of injury and ischemic sequelae of blunt cerebral vascular injury. The 40% rate of ischemic symptom development in untreated children with blunt cerebral vascular injury is reduced to nearly zero when treatment is initiated during the quiescent phase.[76]

Children have certain anatomic characteristics that protect them from laryngeal injury. In addition to being more flexible, the larynx is located in a higher, more protected position.[77] Conversely, there are features that predispose children to developing symptomatic airway edema. During childhood, the diameter of the larynx is smaller and its mucosa is more loosely attached, allowing edema and hematomas to progress. Therefore, children are more likely to present with respiratory distress.[36]

As with adults, pharyngoesophageal injuries are rare and often have a subtle, delayed presentation. Maintain a high index of suspicion for these injuries.[78]

ANTICOAGULATED OR MASSIVELY BLEEDING PATIENTS

Correct coagulopathy in patients with neck trauma who are taking anticoagulants. See Table 166-5 for suggested protocols for anticoagulant reversal. The exception to this recommendation is for patients with blunt cerebral vascular trauma, because the majority of these injuries are treated with antithrombotic agents.

Finally, resuscitate massively bleeding patients with blood products in ratios as outlined by a **massive transfusion protocol**.[79] Also, consider administering tranexamic acid to bleeding trauma patients. The **CRASH-2 trial** demonstrated that this antifibrinolytic significantly reduces deaths from traumatic bleeding when given within 3 hours of the inciting injury.[80]

REFERENCES

The complete reference list is available online at www.TintinalliEM.com.

CHAPTER 261 Pulmonary Trauma

David Jones
Anna Nelson
O. John Ma

INTRODUCTION AND EPIDEMIOLOGY

Blunt thoracic injuries account for up to one fourth of all injury-related deaths.[1] The mechanism of injury and severity of tissue damage predict the clinical course and outcome.[2] Injuries that do not violate the pleura usually can be managed with conservative measures, such as wound management or observation. **Penetrating injuries** that violate the pleura typically result in pneumothorax, with an accompanying hemothorax in most cases. Treatment is generally supportive care after tube thoracostomy.

Blunt trauma produces damage by direct injury, compression, and forces of acceleration or deceleration. Patients with significant blunt injury may require intubation and mechanical ventilation and invasive procedures such as tube thoracostomy. In general, victims of penetrating injuries who survive to reach the hospital often have better outcomes than those who have sustained blunt injuries. Blunt chest trauma from blast injuries is discussed in chapter 7, "Bomb, Blast, and Crush Injuries." Penetrating chest injuries in the "cardiac box" (see Figure 262-1), an area bounded by the sternal notch, xiphoid process, and nipples, should be presumed cardiac or great vessel injuries until proven otherwise.

CLINICAL FEATURES

HISTORY

The most frequent symptoms of thoracic trauma are chest pain and shortness of breath. The pain is most often localized to the involved area of the chest wall, but sometimes it is referred to the abdomen, neck, shoulder, back, or arms. Dyspnea and tachypnea are nonspecific findings and may also be caused by blood loss or pain from other injuries or by anxiety.

PHYSICAL EXAMINATION

Rapidly perform the physical examination during the primary and secondary surveys to detect life-threatening injuries.

Inspect the chest wall for contusions, abrasions, and other signs of trauma, including a "seat belt sign" that can indicate deceleration or vascular injury. Examine the chest for signs of paradoxical segments or flail chest, intrathoracic bleeding, and open chest wounds. The patient must be making a reasonable ventilatory effort to demonstrate these injuries.

Distended neck veins may indicate the presence of pericardial tamponade, tension pneumothorax, cardiac failure, or air embolism; however, in the setting of hypovolemia, this sign may be absent. If the face and neck are cyanotic and/or swollen, then suspect severe injury to the superior mediastinum with occlusion or compression of the superior vena cava. Subcutaneous emphysema from a torn bronchus or laceration of the lung can also cause severe swelling of the neck and face.

A scaphoid abdomen may indicate a diaphragmatic injury with herniation of abdominal contents into the chest. Excessive abdominal movement during breathing may indicate chest wall damage that might not otherwise be apparent.

Breath sounds are most readily heard in the axillae. Unilaterally decreased breath sounds may indicate the presence of hemothorax or pneumothorax. If the patient has an endotracheal tube in place, assess the depth of the tube for mainstem bronchus intubation (the usual depth is no more than three times the inner diameter of the endotracheal tube—23 cm in adult males and 21 cm in adult females) before performing tube thoracostomy in these patients. Persistent decreased breath sounds on one side may also be due to a bronchial foreign body or ruptured bronchus. The presence of bowel sounds in the thorax usually indicates a diaphragmatic injury.

Palpate the neck to determine whether the trachea is midline or displaced. Palpation of the chest wall may reveal areas of localized tenderness or crepitus due to fractured ribs or subcutaneous emphysema. Localized and consistent tenderness over ribs should be attributed to rib fractures, even in the absence of findings on conventional chest radiography. Severe localized tenderness, crepitus, or a mobile segment of the sternum may be the only objective evidence of a sternal fracture. Palpation of the chest with the patient coughing or straining may detect abnormal motion of an unstable portion of the chest wall better than visual inspection.

Sensitivity of physical examination findings is not high enough to rule in or out common thoracic injuries. A study of hemodynamically stable chest trauma patients showed that the sensitivity of auscultation for the detection of a hemopneumothorax is only 50%.[3] Consider patient symptoms, vital signs, and physical examination findings together to detect significant injuries in stable chest trauma patients and to guide further investigation with imaging.

IMAGING

CHEST RADIOGRAPH

Plain chest radiographs are helpful to screen for abnormal mediastinal contours, hemothorax, pneumothorax, pulmonary contusions, diaphragmatic injury, and osseous trauma. Mark penetrating surface wounds before imaging. Most chest radiographs are initially taken in the supine position at the bedside due to concern for occult spinal cord injuries and to facilitate resuscitation. **Chest radiographs frequently underestimate the severity and extent of chest trauma and may fail to detect an injury.** Up to 50% of blunt chest trauma patients with normal initial chest radiography have multiple injuries on CT; however, some of these occult injuries do not change management or outcome.[4-8] Chest x-ray is obtained to identify findings such as pneumothorax, hemothorax, aortic or great vessel injury, multiple rib fractures, sternal fracture, diaphragmatic rupture, and pulmonary contusions or lacerations. The National Emergency X-Radiography Utilization Study (NEXUS) Chest Rules were developed in a manner similar to NEXUS Cervical Spine Imaging rules to identify patients with **blunt chest trauma** with very low risk of thoracic injury. The rules were developed and validated in a convenience sample of 9905 patients >14 years old. If all of the NEXUS Chest criteria were absent, chest imaging (plain radiography or CT) could be omitted (**Table 261-1**). Patients in this cohort were not evaluated with bedside US, and decision for plain chest radiography or chest CT was left to the discretion of the caring physician. Sensitivity and specificity were 98.8% and 13.3%, respectively, for thoracic injury. Only about half of the study group underwent CT, limiting any conclusions about plain radiography versus CT in patients with blunt chest trauma.

ULTRASOUND

Bedside US can quickly diagnose pneumothorax, hemothorax, and pericardial tamponade as part of the FAST examination. In trained hands, US has a greater sensitivity and equal specificity for detecting hemothorax in patients with chest trauma compared with chest radiography.[9] Likewise, the sensitivity of US for detecting pneumothorax approaches 92%, with near 100% specificity (as compared with 50% to 80% sensitivity and 90% specificity for chest radiographs)[10]; thus, US appears to have greater "diagnostic performance" than clinical exam and chest radiograph together.[11] **US in the ED can detect occult pneumothorax as accurately as CT.**[12] In addition, US has also been found helpful for describing small, medium, or large pneumothoraces with good agreement with CT (**Figure 261-1**).[13]

COMPUTED TOMOGRAPHY

CT can detect major and occult injuries and identify the need for additional interventions, but may demonstrate incidental findings that require follow-up and do not change acute care.[8] CT is more sensitive for detecting pulmonary contusion and hemothorax than plain radiography.[4] For penetrating lung injury, if the clinical condition allows, CT is performed to identify the extent of injury and involvement of the heart or great vessels.

TABLE 261-1 NEXUS Rules for Chest Radiography

Blunt trauma in patients >14 y old in whom chest imaging is considered to exclude intrathoracic injury	Presence of 1 or more criteria: cannot exclude intrathoracic injury and obtain chest imaging
	Age >60 y old
	Rapid deceleration: fall >20 ft (>6 m); motor vehicle crash >40 mph (>64 km/h)
	Chest pain
	Intoxication
	Abnormal alertness or abnormal mental status
	Distracting painful Injury
	Tenderness to chest wall palpation

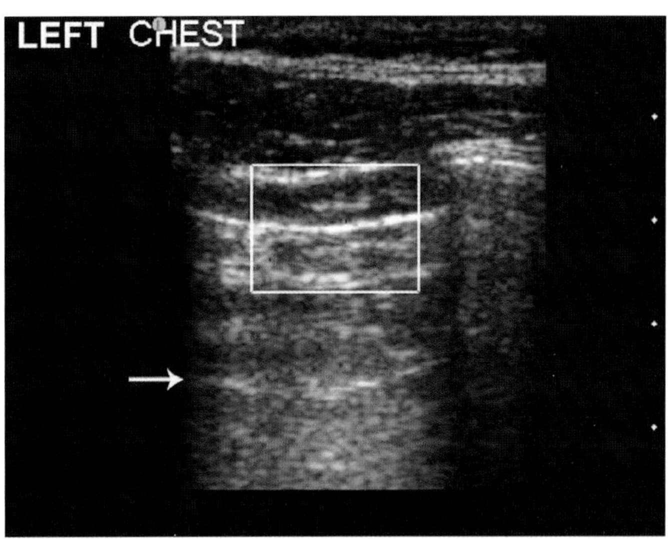

FIGURE 261-1. Pneumothorax (7.5–10 MHz). Power Doppler is activated and the gain adjusted correctly by comparison with the normal right hemithorax. The patient's left hemithorax showed a negative pleural sliding sign, no comet tail artifacts, and no power Doppler signal at the pleural interface. The specificity for pneumothorax is improved when an A-line is also visible (*arrow*). [Reproduced with permission from Ma OJ, Mateer JR, Reardon RF, Joing S (eds): *Emergency Ultrasound,* 3rd ed. McGraw-Hill, Inc., 2014. Fig 5-26, p. 82.]

OTHER DIAGNOSTIC STUDIES

Thoracic trauma often requires a contrast esophagogram to diagnose esophageal injury. **Water-soluble contrast is preferred over barium-containing contrast in patients with high suspicion for esophageal rupture.** Barium swallow imaging has fewer false positives, but may cause mediastinitis if there is leakage of contrast out of the esophagus.

In selected cases, such as in penetrating wounds of the chest or lower neck, bronchoscopy or esophagoscopy may be indicated to exclude an injury to the aerodigestive tract. Such studies may be deferred until the patient is resuscitated and hemodynamically stable.

GENERAL TREATMENT

INITIAL RESUSCITATION

Perform initial resuscitation and airway management according to established principles (see chapter 254, "Trauma in Adults"). If the patient is making little or no respiratory effort, consider CNS dysfunction due to head trauma, intoxication, or spinal cord injury. In patients with respiratory effort but with little or no air movement, suspect upper airway obstruction. Absent or abnormal breath sounds may indicate flail chest, hemopneumothorax, diaphragmatic injury, or parenchymal lung damage. Although each of these has unique therapies, respiratory distress that is not immediately relieved by specific intervention should prompt intubation and ventilation. Suspect, diagnose, and treat specific life-threatening pulmonary injuries during the primary survey. These include tension pneumothorax, massive hemothorax, and open pneumothorax.

VENTILATORY SUPPORT

The management of chest trauma patients with respiratory instability is challenging. Hypoxia and hypoventilation are two preventable causes of mortality; therefore, **maintaining adequate oxygenation and ventilation in the acute chest trauma patient is essential**. Monitor all trauma patients by continuous noninvasive pulse oximetry to assure adequate oxygen saturation. In patients with severe chest trauma or respiratory compromise, an arterial blood gas is helpful to monitor metabolic status and adequate oxygenation and ventilation. Metabolic acidosis with insufficient respiratory compensation is an indication for ventilatory

TABLE 261-2 Considerations for Early Ventilatory Assistance after Thoracic Trauma

Altered mental status
Hypovolemic shock
Multiple injuries
Multiple blood transfusions
Elderly patient
Preexisting pulmonary disease
Respiratory rate >30–35 breaths/min
Vital capacity <10–15 mL/kg
Negative inspiratory force <25–30 cm H_2O

support. Ventilatory support is indicated in chest trauma patients who continue to exhibit impaired ventilation despite measures to relieve chest wall pain and evacuate hemopneumothorax (**Table 261-2**).

CARDIAC ARREST ASSOCIATED WITH ENDOTRACHEAL INTUBATION

Decompensation leading to cardiac arrest may occur during or after endotracheal intubation for reasons related to the initial injury or the procedure (**Table 261-3**). If the patient has poor venous return due to hypovolemia, hyperventilation may increase intrathoracic pressure and decrease venous return to the heart. In the hypovolemic patient, the resultant reduction in cardiac output can lead to cardiac arrest. Ventilate hypovolemic patients with tidal volumes of no more than 5 to 8 mL/kg and at rates not exceeding 10 to 14 times per minute. Excessive hyperventilation can also cause severe alkalosis, which shifts the oxyhemoglobin saturation curve to the left, impairing oxygen unloading at the tissue level. **In the presence of pulmonary injury or preexisting bullous disease, vigorous positive-pressure ventilation can lead to tension pneumothorax, further reducing venous return.**

Unexplained bradycardia associated with assisted ventilation should prompt immediate verification of proper endotracheal tube position and exclusion of esophageal tube placement, as well as evaluation for tension pneumothorax.

LIFE-THREATENING PULMONARY INJURIES

TENSION PNEUMOTHORAX

Diagnose tension pneumothorax clinically, before the chest x-ray is obtained. Although the classic presentation includes distended neck veins, hypotension or evidence of hypoperfusion, diminished or absent breath sounds on the affected side, and tracheal deviation to the contralateral side (**Figure 261-2**), one or more of these elements may be absent in the presence of hypovolemia. **Perform immediate needle decompression.**

NEEDLE DECOMPRESSION

The most common approach to needle decompression is to introduce a 14-gauge IV needle and catheter into the pleural space in the midclavicular line just above the rib at the second intercostal space (**Figure 261-3**). An anterior midclavicular approach is important because this is the shortest distance from the skin to the pleura, avoids the internal mammary vessels that are located approximately 3 cm lateral to the sternal border, and avoids mediastinal vessels.[14-16] A standard needle and catheter may not be long enough for decompression, as the mean chest wall thickness in the United States is 4.5 cm.[15] An alternative site is the fourth to fifth intercostal space at the anterior axillary line.[16] A rush of air exiting the pleural space may be audible and is diagnostic of a pneumothorax. Needle depression converts the tension pneumothorax into an open pneumothorax; needle decompression is a temporizing measure and should be followed promptly with tube thoracostomy. If the patient's hemodynamics fail to improve following decompression, consider other causes of hypoperfusion, including pericardial tamponade.

TABLE 261-3 Potential Causes of Cardiac Arrest after Endotracheal Intubation

Inadequate preoxygenation
Esophageal intubation
Intubation of the right or left mainstem bronchus
Tension pneumothorax
Systemic air embolism
Decreased venous return due to excessive ventilatory rate or pressures
Vasovagal response

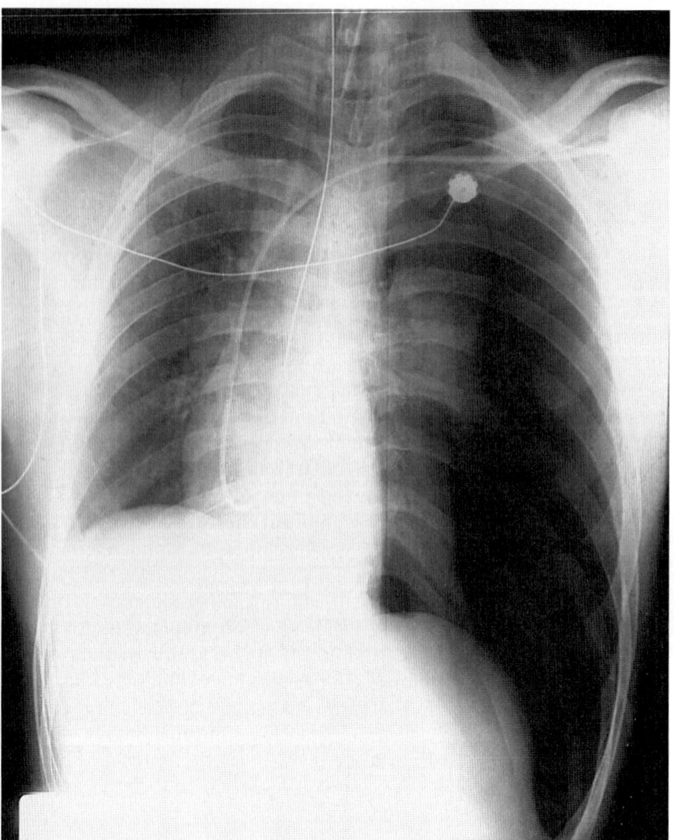

FIGURE 261-2. Tension pneumothorax. Supine chest radiograph of a tension pneumothorax. Note the deviation of the trachea and shifting of the mediastinal contents to the right. Tension pneumothorax should normally be diagnosed prior to chest radiograph. [Reproduced with permission from Schwartz DT (ed): *Emergency Radiology, Case Studies*. © 2008 McGraw-Hill Inc., Fig I-9-10.]

MASSIVE HEMOTHORAX

Common causes of massive hemothorax include injury to the lung parenchyma, intercostal arteries, or internal mammary arteries. Each hemithorax can hold 40% of a patient's circulating blood volume. A massive hemothorax is defined in the adult as at least 1500 mL. Massive hemothorax is life threatening by three mechanisms. First, acute hypovolemia does not allow for sufficient preload to sustain left ventricular function and adequate cardiac output. Second, the collapsed lung results in hypoxia by creating alveolar hypoventilation, ventilation–perfusion mismatch, and anatomic shunting. Third, the hydrostatic pressure of the hemothorax compresses the vena cava and the pulmonary parenchyma, further impairing preload and raising pulmonary vascular resistance, respectively. Although the clinical signs and symptoms of hemothorax in the chest trauma patient can vary, suggestive findings include decreased or absent breath sounds and no chest movement with respiratory effort.

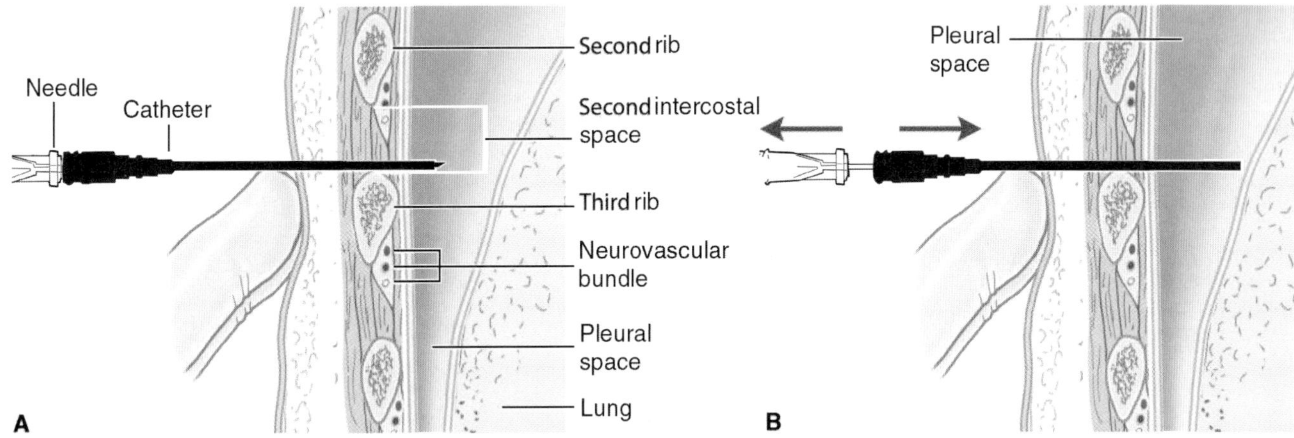

FIGURE 261-3. Decompression of a tension pneumothorax with a catheter-over-the-needle. **A.** The catheter-over-the-needle is inserted through the second intercostal space and into the pleural cavity. **B.** The catheter is advanced while the needle is removed. [Reproduced with permission from Reichman EF (ed): *Emergency Medicine Procedures*, 2nd ed. © 2013. McGraw-Hill Education, New York, NY. Fig 38-2A&B.]

The diagnosis is made by plain chest radiography when complete opacification of a hemithorax is observed. As an alternative to chest radiography in the unstable patient, point-of-care US may reveal a layer of fluid between the chest wall and lung (**Figure 261-4**). Lung collapse, due to intubation of the contralateral mainstem bronchus, can mimic the appearance of hemothorax; always verify proper endotracheal tube placement. Treatment is tube thoracostomy and replacement of blood products as clinically indicated.

OPEN PNEUMOTHORAX

Open pneumothorax is a communication between the pleural space and surrounding atmospheric pressure. This is sometimes referred to as a "sucking chest wound," but also may be due to small rents in the parietal pleura or small air passages without an obvious penetrating injury. Respiratory distress is due to lung collapse and subsequent inability to ventilate the affected lung. Air entry and breath sounds are often diminished on the affected side, and chest wall motion can be impaired. The initial therapeutic maneuver to treat a sucking chest wound is to cover the wound with a three-sided dressing such that air can exit but not enter the chest. Avoid complete occlusion, as this may convert the injury into a tension pneumothorax. Do not insert a chest tube through the trauma wound, as it is likely to follow the missile or knife tract into the lung or diaphragm.

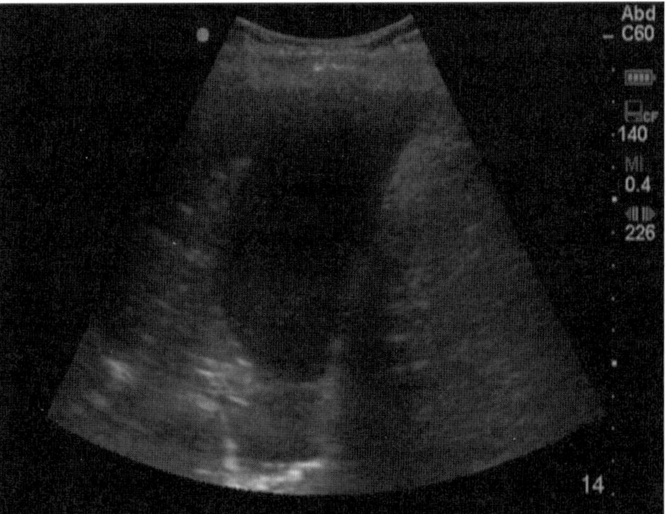

FIGURE 261-4. Hemothorax. US can evaluate for pleural fluid, which usually represents hemothorax. This is a view of the lung, diaphragm, and spleen. Pleural fluid (hemothorax) can be seen superior to the diaphragm.

SYSTEMIC AIR EMBOLISM

Systemic air embolism is an acute complication of severe chest trauma and presents with disastrous circulatory and cerebral complications. Patients with penetrating chest wounds who require positive-pressure ventilation are at risk for developing air embolus. High ventilatory pressures, especially >50 cm H_2O, may force air from an injured bronchus into an adjacent injured vessel. Air embolus may lead to severe dysrhythmias or CNS deficits. Patients presenting with hemoptysis in the setting of penetrating chest trauma are at particular risk for this serious complication.

If systemic air embolism is suspected or diagnosed, place the patient in a flat supine position with 100% oxygen applied, which may decrease air bubble size by displacing nitrogen and promoting resorption of the embolus. **There is no evidence to support the theoretical benefit of the Trendelenburg (head down) position in arterial air embolism.** Hyperbaric oxygen therapy, if available, helps to decrease size and increase resorption of air bubbles. Airway management of patients at risk for systemic air embolism should include maneuvers that can selectively ventilate each lung. In unilateral lung injury, isolating and ventilating the uninjured lung can, in theory, be used to prevent systemic air embolism. In the event of circulatory collapse, treatment begins with cardiopulmonary resuscitation protocols and an immediate thoracotomy to clamp the injured area of lung. This is followed by air aspiration from the heart and ascending aorta.[17,18] Open cardiac massage with clamping of the ascending aorta may help push air through the coronary arteries. Initiate cardiopulmonary bypass promptly, if available.

TUBE THORACOSTOMY

Evacuate large hemothoraces or hemopneumothoraces as rapidly as possible to decrease their negative effects on ventilation and perfusion. Double-check clinical and radiographic findings to make sure you are placing the chest tube on the proper side of the patient. Historically, a 24F or 28F (8.0 or 9.3 mm) chest tube was recommended for a simple pneumothorax and a >32F (>10.7 mm) chest tube for a suspected hemothorax. One study suggests there are no differences in efficacy of drainage, complication rate, pain, or need for additional procedures when using small or large chest tubes.[19]

INSERTION SITE

Perform tube thoracostomy for treatment of traumatic pneumothorax or hemothorax in the anterior axillary line at the level of the nipple in men or inframammary crease in women (corresponding to the fifth intercostal space) just behind the lateral edge of the pectoralis major.

Make an oblique skin incision at least 1 to 2 cm **below** the interspace through which the tube will be placed. Insert a large clamp through the skin incision and into the muscles in the next higher intercostal space, just **above** the rib, thus avoiding the neurovascular bundle (**Figure 261-5**). The resulting oblique tunnel through the subcutaneous tissue and intercostal muscles usually closes promptly after the chest tube is removed, thereby reducing the chances of recurrent pneumothorax.

Once the clamp is pushed through the internal intercostal fascia, open it to enlarge the hole to at least 2.0 cm. Insert a finger along the top of the clamp through the hole to verify the position within the thorax and to verify that the lung is not adhering to the chest wall (**Figure 261-6**).

CHEST TUBE INSERTION

Advance the tube at least until the last side hole is 2.5 to 5.0 cm (1 to 2 inches) inside the chest wall. For a pneumothorax, direct the tube toward the apex, away from the hilum and mediastinum. For a hemothorax, direct the tube posteriorly and laterally. However, do not reposition any tube position that functions effectively unless indicated by abnormal or suboptimal placement identified on the chest radiograph. In general, do not clamp the chest tube for any reason. Any continuing air leakage can rapidly collapse the lung or cause a tension pneumothorax. Importantly, loss of vital signs and clinical deterioration after chest tube placement may indicate exsanguinating injury and loss of the protective vascular tamponade effect as the hemothorax is evacuated. In this circumstance, clamp the chest tube and transport the patient directly to the operating room for an emergency thoracotomy.

CONNECT TO SUCTION

Attach the open end of the tube to a combination fluid-collection water-seal suction device, with 20 to 30 cm H_2O of suction. If a significant hemothorax is known to be present or if a large amount of blood starts to drain immediately, consider collecting the blood in a heparinized autotransfusion device so that it can be returned to the patient.

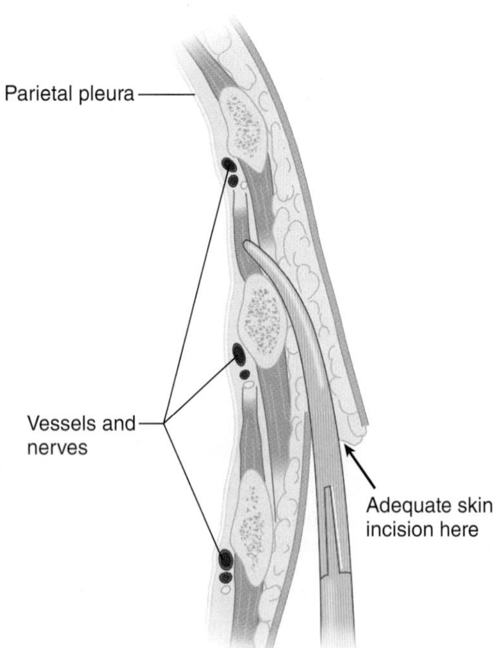

FIGURE 261-5. Chest tube insertion. The clamp is inserted through the incision and is tunneled up to the next intercostal space.

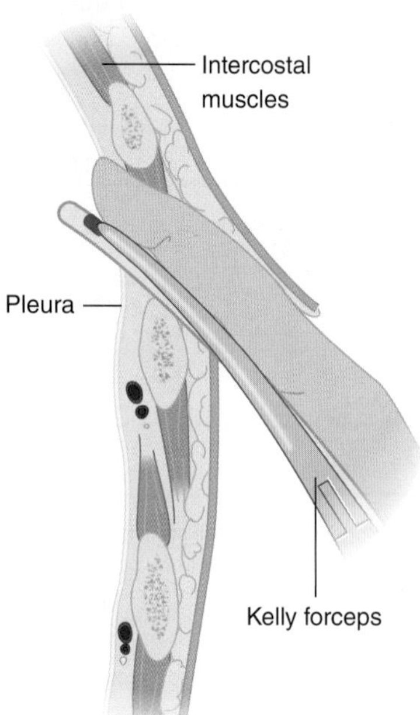

FIGURE 261-6. Chest tube insertion. Using the finger as a guide, place the tip of the clamp into the pleural cavity just above the rib to avoid intercostal vessels and nerves.

DOCUMENT TUBE PLACEMENT AND FUNCTION

Check the intrathoracic position of the chest tube and of its last hole and the amount of air or fluid remaining in the pleural cavity with a portable chest radiograph as soon as possible after the tube is inserted. Serial chest auscultation, chest radiographs, and careful recording of the volume of blood loss and the amount of air leakage are important guides to the functioning of chest tubes. If a chest tube becomes blocked and a significant pneumothorax or hemothorax is still present, replace the tube or place a second chest tube on the affected side. Irrigating an occluded chest tube or passing a Fogarty catheter through it in an effort to reestablish its patency is not advised.

Leave chest tubes in place on suction at least 24 hours after all air leaks have stopped (if placed for a simple pneumothorax) or until drainage is serous and <200 mL/24 h (if placed for hemothorax).[20] However, in intubated patients, maintain chest tubes throughout mechanical ventilation to prevent sudden development of a new pneumothorax.

The use of prophylactic broad-spectrum antibiotics in patients who require tube thoracostomy for a traumatic hemothorax or pneumothorax remains controversial.[21-23] Whether or not antibiotics are given, adhere to protocols for the placement, maintenance, and early removal of chest tubes to decrease the risk of infection.

SPECIFIC LUNG INJURIES

PULMONARY CONTUSION

Pulmonary contusions, defined as direct injury to the lung resulting in both hemorrhage and edema in the absence of a pulmonary laceration, are a source of severe morbidity and mortality following penetrating and blunt trauma. CT has shown this entity to be much more prevalent than previously recognized.[4] The most common cause of pulmonary contusions is a compression-decompression injury to the chest, such as seen in high-speed motor vehicle crashes.

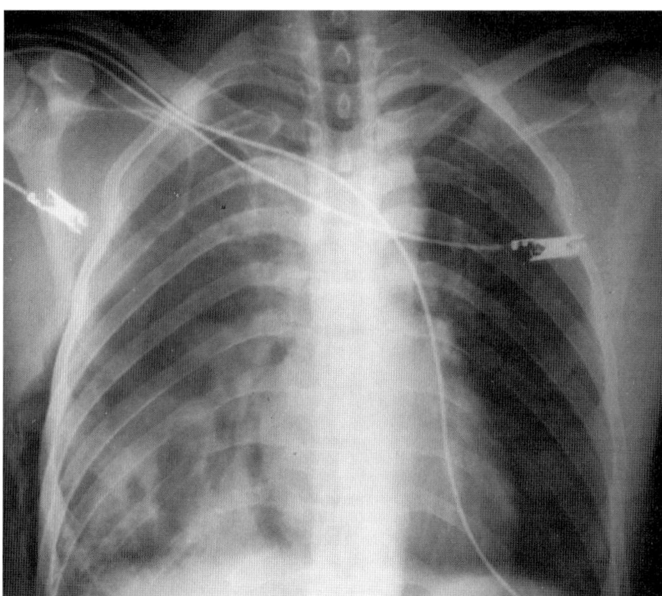

A

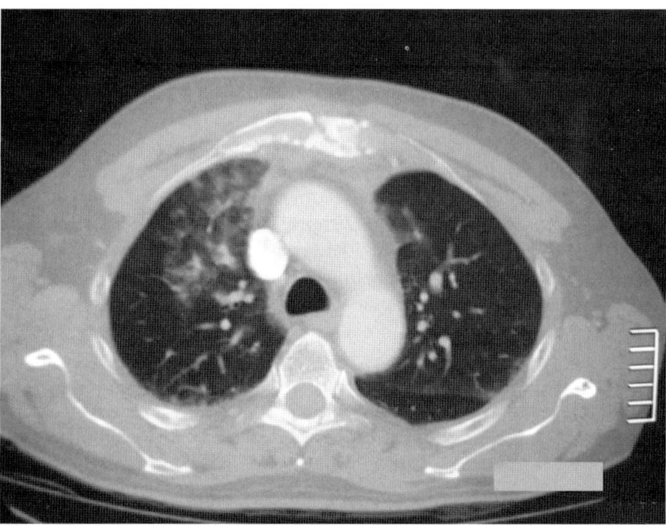

B

FIGURE 261-7. Pulmonary contusion. **A.** Chest radiograph shows pulmonary contusion from blunt chest trauma, along with 9th and 10th rib fractures. **B.** CT shows pulmonary contusions on the anterior part of the right lung and a sternal fracture with mediastinal hematoma.

There are two stages in the pathophysiology of pulmonary contusions. First, there is direct injury to lung parenchyma. Second, resuscitative measures, particularly IV crystalloid fluid administration directed at restoring intravascular volume loss due to hemorrhage, can precipitate cardiopulmonary decompensation. Fluid resuscitation in the setting of unilateral pulmonary contusion can cause extravasation of fluid into the contralateral (uninjured) lung. Increased capillary hydrostatic pressures result in leakage of blood and fluid into the interstitium and alveoli. Unfortunately, the process is self-perpetuating; as each proximate segment of lung sees the full force of the right heart activity, it becomes functionally congested and contused, and the process continues to the next uninjured segment of lung. This process results in increased intrapulmonary shunting and resistance to airflow, decreased lung elasticity, and increased work of breathing, leading to hypoxia, hypercarbia, and respiratory acidosis. Cardiopulmonary decompensation may quickly ensue.

Chest pain, tachypnea, chest wall contusions, and hypoxia suggest underlying pulmonary contusion. Physical examination may reveal decreased or coarse breath sounds over the affected lung field. Chest radiograph and CT may show patchy, ground-glass opacities in mild or moderate contusion and widespread consolidation in severe contusion.[5] Contusions are found in nonsegmental areas of the lung and across pleural fissures. Radiographic findings of pulmonary contusion may mimic those associated with aspiration pneumonia and fat embolism, but these entities are typically not seen for 12 to 24 hours and usually have a segmental distribution. **Areas of lung opacification on chest imaging within 6 hours of blunt trauma are usually considered diagnostic of pulmonary contusion (Figure 261-7).** CT is more sensitive for the detection of pulmonary contusions than plain radiographs, with as many as 70% of pulmonary contusions not visible on the initial radiograph.[4] In addition to the high diagnostic rate of CT scan for pulmonary contusion, it may also be possible to anticipate complications such as acute lung injury (also known as *acute respiratory distress syndrome* or *noncardiogenic pulmonary edema*), depending on the extent of the pulmonary contusion. Patients who have a contusion >20% of lung volume have up to an 80% risk of developing acute lung injury.[24]

Treatment primarily involves maintenance of adequate ventilation and pain control. Epidural analgesia is the preferred method of pain control; however, consider intercostal nerve blocks and paravertebral analgesia when an epidural is contraindicated.[25] The volume of contused lung influences the need for mechanical ventilation. Patients with less than one fourth of total lung volume involvement (about one lobe) usually do not require such support. If ventilatory assistance is required, avoid overinflation of normal alveoli. Placing the noninjured lung dependent by turning the patient to the decubitus position may improve ventilation–perfusion matching. Patients with extensive pulmonary contusion may be candidates for high-frequency oscillatory ventilation, a technique that can improve oxygenation, although it may not improve survival.[26] Guidelines for the management of pulmonary contusion and flail chest are listed in **Table 261-4**.[25]

Patients with severe unilateral lung injury who are not responding to conventional mechanical ventilation may benefit from synchronous independent lung ventilation provided through a double-lumen endobronchial catheter. This technique helps prevent overinflation of the normal lung and underinflation of the damaged, poorly compliant lung.

HEMOTHORAX

Bleeding from direct lung injury is the most common cause of hemothorax. The compressing effect of the blood within the pleural space, high concentration of lung thromboplastin, and low pulmonary arterial pressure help limit bleeding as a result of torn lung parenchyma. Bleeding into the hemithorax may arise from mediastinal, diaphragmatic, pulmonary, pleural, chest wall, or even abdominal injuries. Bleeding of venous origin usually tamponades without intervention. Damage to intercostal or internal mammary arteries or pulmonary vessels causes more severe bleeding and almost always requires invasive management.

Evacuate hemothoraces of >300 to 500 mL expeditiously to avoid complications. Large clots in the pleural space can act as a local anticoagulant by releasing fibrinolysins from their surface. Bleeding from multiple small intrathoracic vessels often stops fairly rapidly after the hemothorax is completely evacuated.

Fluid collections >200 to 300 mL can usually be seen on upright or decubitus chest radiographs. However, if the patient is supine, >1000 mL of blood may be missed due to posterior layering of blood, producing only diffuse haziness on that side (**Figure 261-8**). Point-of-care US may be used in the critically ill patient to detect hemothorax (**Figure 261-9**), showing a fluid density between visceral and parietal pleura normally occupied by lung tissue. **CT has the highest sensitivity and specificity for detecting hemothorax.**

If the hemothorax is judged large enough to drain (>200 to 300 mL), tube thoracostomy remains the standard of care.

INDICATIONS FOR OPERATIVE INTERVENTION

Most patients with intrathoracic bleeding can be treated adequately by IV administration of fluids and evacuation of the hemothorax with a chest tube. Fewer than 5% of patients will require operative management. **Consider surgical exploration in the following circumstances:**

TABLE 261-4 Eastern Association for Surgery of Trauma Practice Management Guideline for Pulmonary Contusion—Flail Chest

Level 1 recommendations (convincingly justifiable based on the available scientific information alone)	None.
Level 2 recommendations (reasonably justifiable by available scientific evidence and strongly supported by expert opinion)	Unnecessary fluid administration should be meticulously avoided; a pulmonary artery catheter may be useful to avoid fluid overload.
	Obligatory mechanical ventilation should be avoided.
	The use of optimal analgesia and aggressive chest physiotherapy should be applied to minimize the likelihood of respiratory failure and ensuing ventilatory support.
	Patients with pulmonary contusion requiring mechanical ventilation should be weaned from the ventilator at the earliest possible time.
	Positive end-expiratory pressure/continuous positive airway pressures should be included in the ventilatory regimen.
	Steroids should not be used in the therapy of pulmonary contusion.
Level 3 recommendations (supported by available data but adequate scientific evidence is lacking)	A trial of mask continuous positive airway pressure should be considered in alert, compliant patients with marginal respiratory status.
	Independent lung ventilation may be considered in severe unilateral pulmonary contusion.
	Diuretics may be used in the setting of hydrostatic fluid overload as evidenced by elevated pulmonary capillary wedge pressures in hemodynamically stable patients or in the setting of known concurrent congestive heart failure.
	Surgical repair may be considered in severe unilateral flail chest or in patients requiring mechanical ventilation when thoracotomy is otherwise required.

>1500 mL of blood is evacuated immediately after tube thoracostomy, chest tube drainage of blood occurs at 150 to 200 mL/h for 2 to 4 hours, or persistent blood transfusion is required to maintain hemodynamic stability.

PNEUMOTHORAX

To establish the diagnosis of a pneumothorax with upright plain chest radiography, identify a thin white pleural line usually seen best in the upper lateral aspect of the affected hemithorax in the **upright** patient (**Figure 261-10**). Avoid interpreting skinfolds or a scapular border as a pneumothorax. If the radiograph is obtained with the patient supine, small pneumothoraces may not be apparent as air migrates to the anterior chest, resulting in loss of the interface between the parietal pleura and the air-filled pleural space. Point-of-care US can also diagnose simple pneumothorax. Sonographic imaging of a *normal* lung with the high-frequency linear probe at the anterior superior aspect of the chest will reveal "marching ants" or the "sliding lung sign," a result of the movement of the pleural layers during the ventilatory phase. This movement is absent in the presence of pneumothorax.

Pneumothorax is found in approximately 20% of patients with significant chest trauma.[26] Traumatic pneumothorax can be open, closed, or occult. In an individual without preexisting cardiopulmonary disease, an isolated pneumothorax usually does not cause severe symptoms unless it occupies >40% of the hemithorax. Occult pneumothoraces may complicate the management of patients who are emergently taken to the operating room because intubation and positive-pressure ventilation may convert a small occult pneumothorax into a tension pneumothorax.

A pressure differential across the pulmonary pleura results in airflow down the gradient. Therefore, positive pulmonary pressure or negative intrapleural pressure during inspiration increases the tendency for air or blood to leak into the pleural cavity through any wound in the lung or chest wall. Any collection of air or blood within

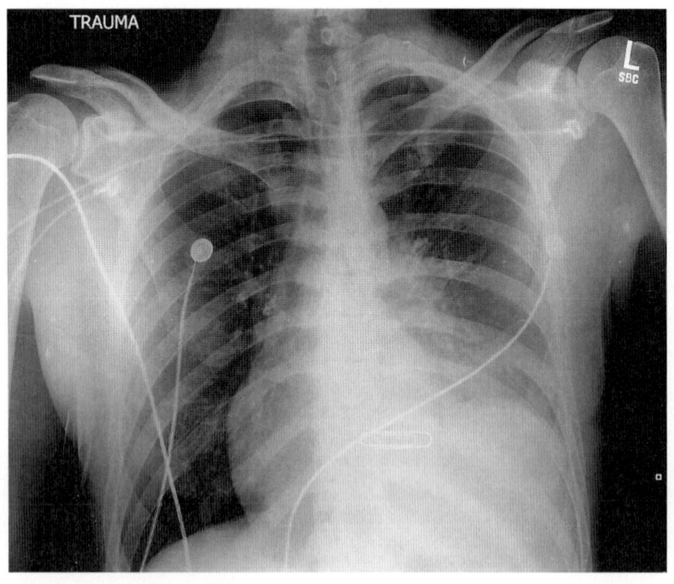

A

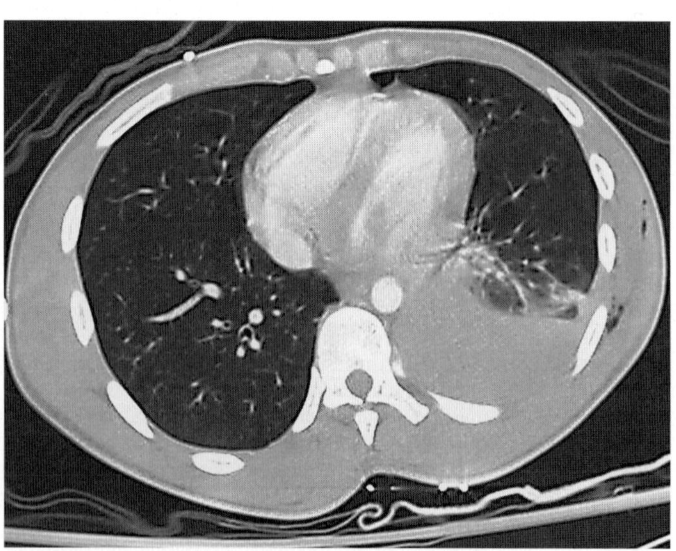

B

FIGURE 261-8. Hemothorax. **A.** Anteroposterior view of the chest in patient with penetrating knife injury to the posterior left thorax. The site of injury is marked by a paperclip. Hazy opacity on the left, with associated volume loss in the left lung, is indicative of posteriorly layering hemothorax and atelectatic change. **B.** CT image in the same patient showing large hemothorax layering dependently in the supine patient. [Reproduced with permission from Block J, Jordanov MI, Stack LB, Thurman RJ (eds): *The Atlas of Emergency Radiology*. McGraw-Hill, Inc., 2013. Fig 4.23 & 4.24.]

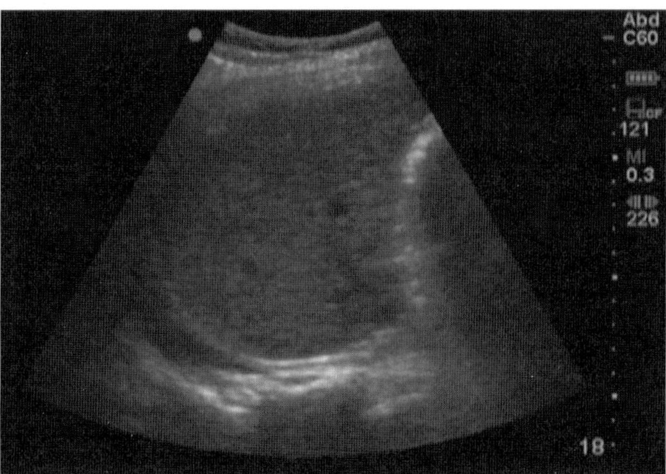

FIGURE 261-9. Hemothorax. US can evaluate for pleural fluid, which usually represents hemothorax. Pleural fluid (hemothorax) can be seen superior to the diaphragm.

the pleural cavity may reduce vital capacity, increase intrathoracic pressure, and decrease minute ventilation and venous return to the heart. Additional air may be forced into the pleural cavity during expiration in patients with outflow obstruction, such as in chronic obstructive lung disease or airway occlusion, thus increasing the likelihood of tension pneumothorax.

Maintain a high suspicion for occult pneumothoraces in patients with more subtle injuries. **Although chest radiography remains the most common diagnostic tool for detecting pneumothorax in the ED (Figure 261-11), it will miss between 17% and 80% of pneumothoraces for upright and supine chest radiographs, respectively.** US is more sensitive than a supine radiograph and is rapid and accurate for detecting pneumothorax.[10,11,13] Occult pneumothoraces are usually detected by CT (**Figure 261-12**).[26] Importantly, with the exception of patients who may require intubation and positive-pressure ventilation (which may convert a small occult pneumothorax into a tension pneumothorax), the detection of occult pneumothoraces using chest CT has minimal clinical significance and does not improve outcome.[7,8]

If pneumothorax is suspected despite normal initial chest radiography, repeat films or performing US or CT may be helpful. **Pneumothorax after a stab wound may be delayed for up to 6 hours.** Consequently, repeat chest imaging in 4 to 6 hours is indicated in these patients or at any time when symptoms worsen. Patients with initially asymptomatic stab wounds to the chest have a reported 12% incidence of delayed hemothorax or pneumothorax that required tube thoracostomy.[27] A common practice is to observe patients with asymptomatic thoracic stab wounds, repeat the chest radiograph in 4 to 6 hours, and discharge the patient if no delayed pneumothorax is seen in the absence of other concerns.

If the patient cannot be observed closely, requires intubation and mechanical ventilation, or will be transported by air or over a long distance, insert a chest tube or small pleural catheter. Small pneumothoraces (<1.0 cm wide, confined to the upper third of the chest) that are unchanged on two chest radiographs taken 4 to 6 hours apart in an otherwise healthy individual can usually be treated by observation alone.

Occult pneumothoraces (small pneumothoraces not apparent on conventional chest imaging, but seen on a CT scan of the chest or abdomen) usually do not require chest tube drainage unless the patient requires mechanical ventilation. Avoid unnecessary tube thoracostomy because there is a 22% risk of major insertional, positional, and infective complications.[28]

In general, small- or moderate-sized pneumothoraces, once treated, do not cause significant problems unless there is a continuing air leak or preexisting cardiopulmonary disease. Even a small air leak usually will not result in serious complications, provided the lung is completely expanded. However, the incidences of empyema and bronchopleural fistula are greatly increased in pneumothoraces with continued air leak persisting for >24 to 48 hours.

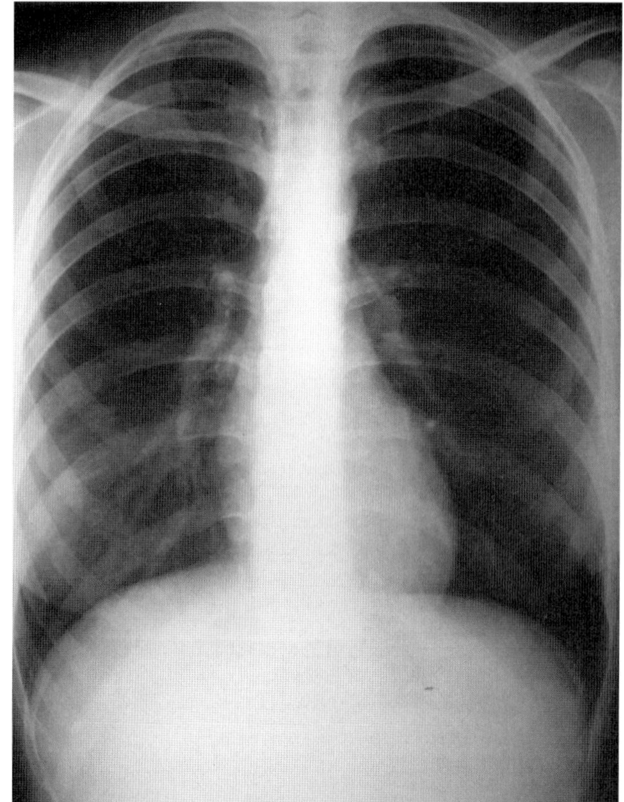

A

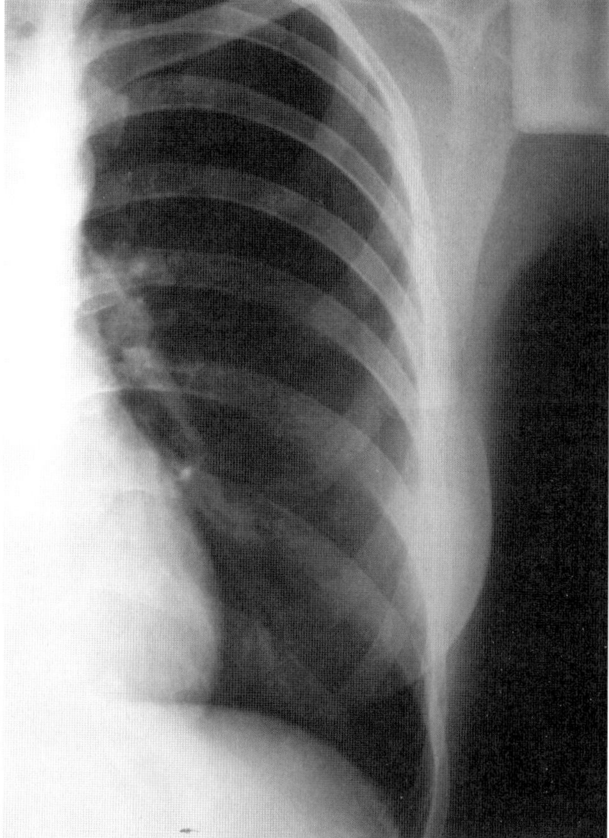

B

FIGURE 261-10. Pneumothorax. **A.** The pleural line is seen in the left hemithorax, but lateral to the pleura, there is increased lucency (air density) and an absence of lung markings. These findings should prompt concern for a pneumothorax. **B.** Enlarged area of the same image to further illustrate the increased lucency and absent lung markings lateral to the pleural line.

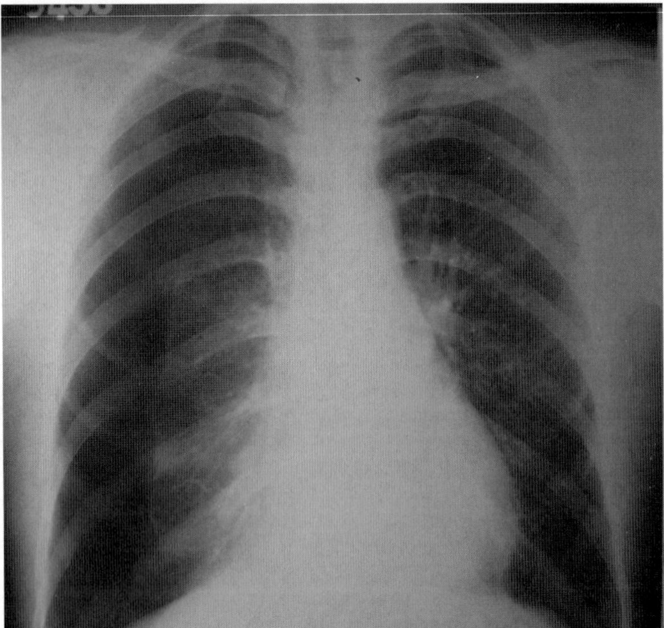

FIGURE 261-11. Pneumothorax. This right-sided pneumothorax can be diagnosed by the absence of lung markings and increased (air density) lucency lateral to the pleural line.

If the lung does not completely expand or the pneumothorax does not evacuate, then investigate potential causes (**Table 261-5**).

If a pneumothorax persists or there is a large air leak, perform emergency bronchoscopy to examine and clear the bronchi or to identify and repair any damage to the tracheobronchial tree. Continued large air leakage or failure of the lung to adequately expand, despite these measures, is an indication for early thoracotomy.

PNEUMOMEDIASTINUM

Subcutaneous emphysema in the neck or the presence of a crunching sound (Hamman's sign) over the heart during systole suggests the presence of a pneumomediastinum. This diagnosis can usually be made on chest radiography (**Figure 261-13A**) and is readily apparent on CT images of the chest (**Figure 261-13B**). Pneumomediastinum in blunt chest trauma is most commonly the result of alveolar rupture, followed by dissection along the bronchoalveolar sheath and subsequent spread of air to the mediastinum, a process known as the *Macklin effect*. Traumatic pneumomediastinum may be asymptomatic or can cause mild to moderate chest pain, voice change, cough, or stridor. **Pneumomediastinum alone does not require further diagnostic testing or intervention unless the patient is symptomatic,** in which case a search for other serious injuries to the larynx, trachea, major bronchi, pharynx, or esophagus is essential.

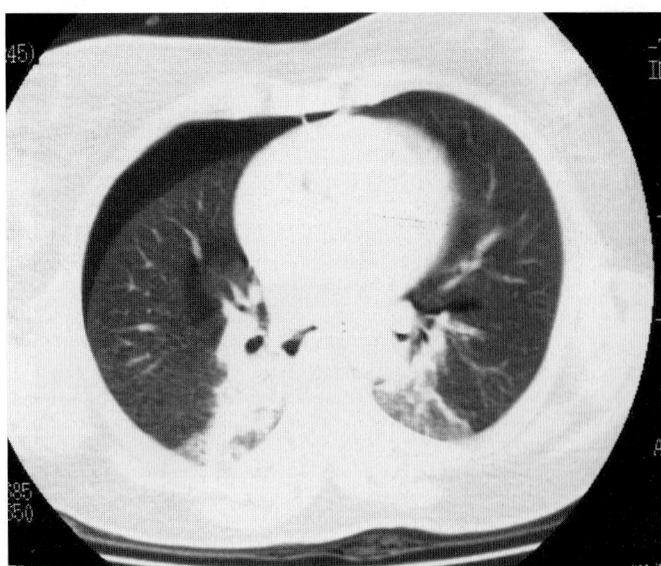

FIGURE 261-12. Pneumothorax. Pneumothorax of the right hemithorax, with small bilateral posterior pulmonary contusions.

TABLE 261-5 Causes for Failure of Complete Lung Expansion or Evacuation of a Pneumothorax
Improper connections or leaks in the external tubing or water-seal collection apparatus
Improper positioning of the chest tube
Occlusion of bronchi or bronchioles by secretions or foreign body
Tear of one of the large bronchi
Large tear of the lung parenchyma

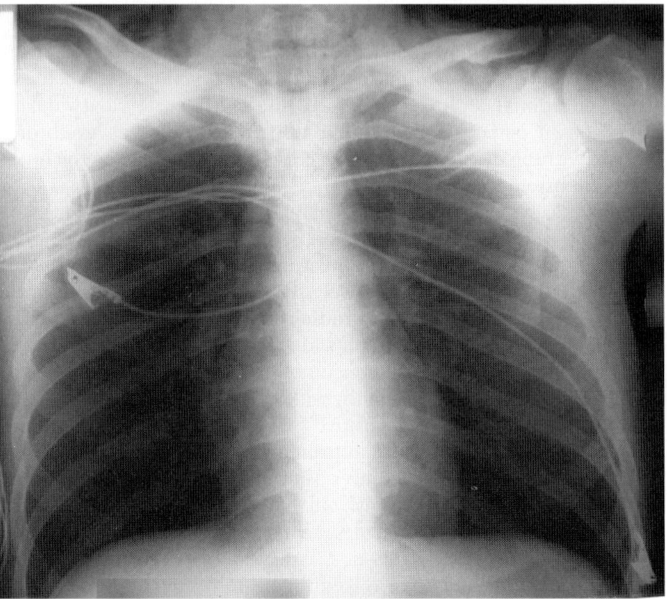

A

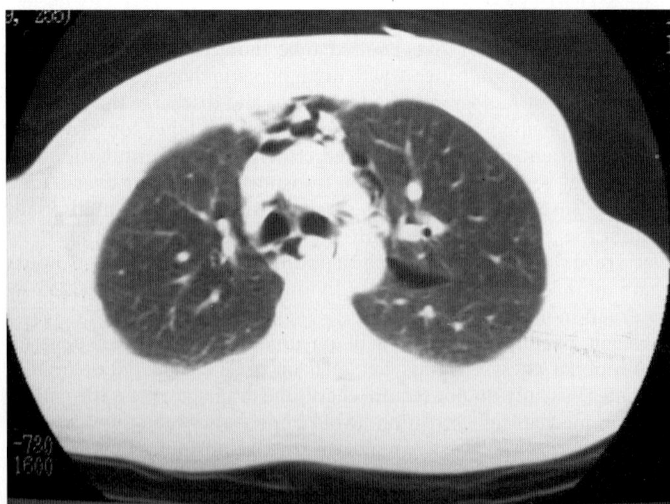

B

FIGURE 261-13. Pneumomediastinum. **A.** Blunt trauma to the chest while playing basketball. Patient had sudden onset of chest pain and shortness of breath. Subcutaneous emphysema was evident in the neck. Chest radiograph reveals mediastinal and subcutaneous air. **B.** In this same patient, a CT scan shows pneumomediastinum.

PULMONARY HEMATOMA

Pulmonary hematomas are parenchymal tears filled with blood. Although these generally resolve spontaneously over a few weeks, they sometimes can become infected and progress to lung abscesses. Infection is more likely in patients on a ventilator, who require prolonged chest tube drainage or who are post-thoracotomy.

PULMONARY LACERATION WITH HEMOPNEUMOTHORAX

Hemorrhage from pulmonary lacerations is most commonly seen in the setting of displaced rib fractures due to direct trauma from the exposed ends of bone. Hemorrhage may also be due to the effect of shear forces on preexisting pleural adhesions during rapid deceleration injuries or from penetrating chest injuries.

TRACHEOBRONCHIAL INJURY

INTRABRONCHIAL BLEEDING

Intrabronchial bleeding can lead to severe hypoxemia and rapid death. Hemorrhage into dependent alveoli hinders gas exchange in a mechanism similar to drowning. It is important to identify the involved lung and to keep the other lung as free of blood as possible. Bronchoscopy is often necessary to identify injury and control bleeding. Intubation with frequent tracheal suction may be effective. If the hemorrhage is severe, a double-lumen endotracheal tube can be used as a temporizing measure to confine the bleeding to one lung. If a double-lumen endotracheal tube is not available, a standard tube may be inserted over a flexible bronchoscope into the unaffected lung, or an endotracheal tube can be purposely passed into the right mainstem bronchus as a diagnostic measure and the patient placed with the affected lung in the dependent position.

ASPIRATION

Aspiration of gastric contents is common after severe trauma, especially if the patient was unconscious at any time. Radiologic changes may be delayed for up to 24 hours and can include consolidation virtually anywhere in the lungs, with the most common sites being the right middle and lower lung fields. This is the result of a chemical pneumonitis as lung parenchyma is exposed to gastric contents. Frequent suctioning is indicated, as well as continual assessment of the need for endotracheal intubation if the patient is at further risk for aspiration. **There is no evidence to support the use of prophylactic antibiotics to prevent pulmonary infection after gastric aspiration.**

Aspirated opaque foreign bodies in the tracheobronchial tree may be diagnosed on plain radiographs, but even teeth can be easily missed due to size, relative lucency, and the presence of overlying bone and soft tissue densities. Once recognized, prepare for urgent bronchoscopy to remove tracheal or bronchial foreign bodies.

Expiratory chest radiographs may help diagnose foreign bodies that act as a one-way valve, causing air trapping and hyperinflation on the affected side. Undiagnosed bronchial foreign bodies lead to recurrent or difficult-to-treat pulmonary infections, sometimes taking months to discover. Persistent or recurrent cough, atelectasis, and pneumonia after trauma are indications for bronchoscopy.

LOWER (INTRATHORACIC) TRACHEA AND MAJOR BRONCHI

Injuries to the major bronchi occur primarily due to rapid deceleration injuries, which cause shear forces to mobile distal bronchi relative to more fixed proximal structures. Forced expiration against a closed glottis and compressive forces on the pulmonary tree against the vertebral column may also cause injury to these structures. **Most tracheobronchial injuries occur within 2 cm of the carina or at the origin of lobar bronchi.**

The most common presenting signs and symptoms are dyspnea, hemoptysis, subcutaneous emphysema, Hamman's sign, and sternal tenderness. A large pneumothorax, pneumomediastinum, or deep cervical emphysema may also suggest tracheobronchial injury. On careful inspection, the endotracheal tube balloon may have a spherical rather than oval appearance on chest radiographs. Approximately 10% of patients present with very mild symptoms or are completely asymptomatic.

The air leak due to bronchopleural fistula following tube thoracostomy is continuous and massive. High-frequency oscillation is the ventilator modality of choice to maintain gas exchange and expand the alveoli in the face of the massive gas leak.

All lacerations of the bronchi involving more than one third of the circumference should be surgically repaired. Untreated tracheal tears may result in severe mediastinitis or can lead to severe bronchial stenosis with atelectasis and repeated pulmonary infections.

Intrathoracic tracheal transection is usually associated with two or more major injuries and is almost invariably fatal. Patients who survive a tracheal transection generally sustain an injury in the cervical trachea and have no other associated injuries. Concurrent esophageal injuries occur in almost 25% of penetrating tracheobronchial injuries and can be missed unless esophagoscopy or contrast studies are also performed.

CERVICAL TRACHEAL INJURIES

Blunt injuries to the upper (cervical) trachea are usually found at the junction of the trachea and cricoid cartilage. This most frequently occurs when the anterior neck strikes the steering wheel or dashboard in an automobile accident. **Evidence of direct trauma to the neck, including subcutaneous emphysema and inspiratory stridor, should raise suspicion for this injury as well as accompanying vascular and spinal injuries.** Cricotracheal separation may not be suspected until attempts to pass the endotracheal tube past the cricoid cartilage are unsuccessful. Treatment and diagnosis are discussed in chapter 260, "Trauma to the Neck."

DIAPHRAGMATIC INJURY

Diaphragmatic injuries are caused most frequently by penetrating trauma, particularly gunshot wounds of the lower chest or upper abdomen. Diaphragmatic rupture due to blunt trauma is much less common and occurs in <5% of patients hospitalized with chest trauma. If there is a fracture of the pelvis, the incidence of diaphragmatic hernia increases.

More diaphragmatic injuries following blunt trauma are diagnosed on the left hemidiaphragm compared to the right.[29] This left-sided predominance is likely the result of the protective effect of the liver on the right hemidiaphragm and the possible increased weakness of the left posterolateral diaphragm.

The initial signs and symptoms of diaphragmatic hernia are often masked by other injuries and have a delayed presentation unless the defect is large. Over time, the abdominal viscera can gradually migrate into the chest through even small diaphragmatic tears; patients may present years after the initial injury with a traumatic diaphragmatic hernia. The intrathoracic bowel may become obstructed or ischemic due to torsion or strangulation or cause severe compression of the adjacent lung, a phenomenon referred to as *tension enterothorax*.

If a penetrating wound of the abdomen is associated with intrathoracic injury or foreign body, it should be assumed that the injury traversed the diaphragm. Chest radiographs may display injury to the diaphragm in only approximately 25% of such patients.[30] With blunt trauma, any abnormality of the diaphragm or lower lung fields on chest images should arouse suspicion of a diaphragmatic tear (**Figure 261-14**).

Techniques for diagnosing diaphragmatic injuries include (1) orogastric tube placement with evaluation to see if the tube curves up from the abdomen into the chest; (2) upper GI series looking for displacement of viscera into the chest; and (3) CT of the chest and abdomen with contrast. **CT is the imaging standard for diaphragmatic injuries (Figure 261-15).**[31] Still, many diaphragmatic injuries are diagnosed only during a thoracotomy or laparotomy.

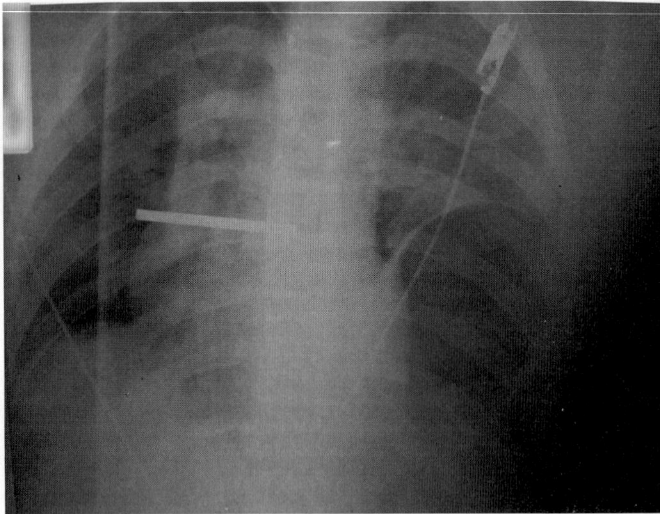

FIGURE 261-14. Diaphragmatic injury. Patient with diminished breath sounds of the left hemithorax after blunt thoracoabdominal injury. Chest radiograph shows left diaphragmatic injury.

Laparotomy is necessary to repair the diaphragm, and thoracotomy may be necessary for associated chest injury, resuscitation, delayed repair of the diaphragm, or management of thoracic complications.

ESOPHAGEAL AND THORACIC DUCT INJURIES

ESOPHAGEAL INJURIES

Injuries to the thoracic esophagus may occur through direct penetrating trauma and, less often, via blunt trauma. Mortality is high as a result of associated injuries to other organs in the chest. Lacerations of the esophagus also occur iatrogenically as a result of endoscopic biopsy or dilatation of a narrowed or obstructed esophagus. Swallowed foreign bodies can also traumatize the esophagus.

If esophageal injury is suspected, obtain an esophagogram using water-soluble contrast. It is recommended that a negative study with water-soluble contrast be repeated with barium due to the relatively high false-negative rate.

Flexible esophagoscopy is being increasingly performed for diagnosis but may miss occasional injuries, even if combined with an esophagogram. Some trauma surgeons prefer rigid esophagoscopy in combination with bronchoscopy to rule out associated tracheobronchial injuries. Neither barium nor water-soluble contrast will interfere with a subsequent esophagoscopy.

Despite the diagnostic and therapeutic advances, esophageal injuries are associated with significant morbidity and mortality, particularly if there is a delay in recognition and definitive management.

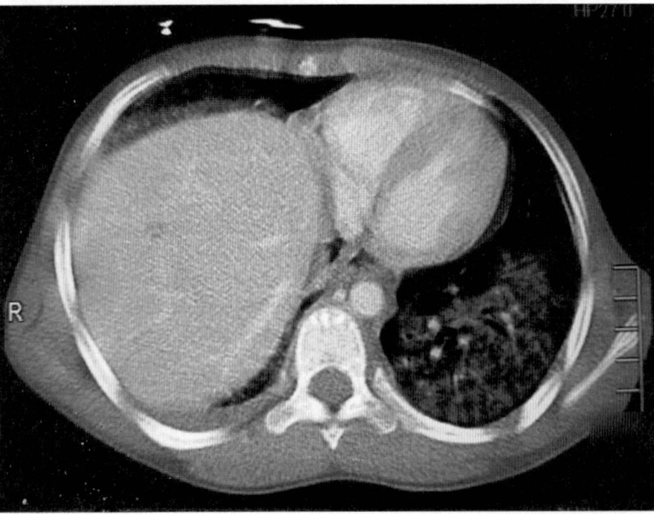

FIGURE 261-15. Diaphragmatic injury. Right diaphragmatic injury on CT.

THORACIC DUCT INJURIES

Suspect thoracic duct injuries in patients with penetrating trauma near the left proximal subclavian vein. Although the diagnosis is rarely made in the ED, the development of a chylothorax, accumulation of lymphatic fluid in the pleural space, is associated with a mortality rate of ~50% and should be considered in chest trauma patients.

INJURIES TO THE CHEST WALL

BLEEDING AND TISSUE LOSS

Probing of a penetrating chest wound to determine its depth or direction is not recommended and may not give an accurate picture of the depth of penetration. Such wounds, especially if there is continued bleeding, are better managed by local exploration in the operating room.

Injuries caused by high-powered rifles or close-range shotgun blasts may cause large tissue defects of the chest wall. In such patients, intubation and mechanical ventilation are required until the defect is definitively closed.

SUBCUTANEOUS EMPHYSEMA

Subcutaneous emphysema usually develops because air from lung parenchyma or the tracheobronchial tree gains access to the chest wall through an opening in the parietal pleura. The air may also reach the chest wall from an interstitial lung injury by dissecting back along the bronchi into the hilum and mediastinum and then into the extrapleural spaces. Extensive subcutaneous emphysema may also suggest an injury to the pharynx, larynx, or esophagus.

Presume patients with subcutaneous emphysema have an underlying pneumothorax, even if it is not visible on the chest radiograph. If the patient requires intubation and subsequent positive-pressure ventilation, insert a chest tube on the involved side. If subcutaneous emphysema is severe, suspect a major bronchial injury and investigate further by bronchoscopy.

RIB FRACTURES

Rib fractures are the most common bony injuries in chest trauma and are diagnosed in approximately 50% of patients admitted to the hospital following chest trauma.[26] Rib fractures are painful injuries, heal slowly, and are closely associated with mortality and morbidity.[32] Rib fractures can be markers of potential internal injury; the principal diagnostic goal with clinically suspected rib fractures is the detection of significant associated complications, such as hemopneumothorax, pulmonary contusion, intra-abdominal injury, or major vascular injury. In the patient with severe chest trauma or significantly displaced rib fractures or in the presence of other injuries, perform serial chest imaging to evaluate for developing pneumothoraces or other injuries.

Assume the presence of rib fractures in any patient with localized pain and tenderness over one or more ribs after chest trauma. Up to 50% of rib fractures (especially those involving the anterior and lateral portions of the first five ribs) are not be apparent on conventional radiography, particularly in the first few days after injury.[33] Furthermore, injuries to the cartilaginous portions of the ribs may never be appreciated on plain radiographs. US is a promising diagnostic tool for evaluating rib fractures and even for cartilaginous injury.[34]

The pain of rib fractures can greatly interfere with ventilation and cause splinting and atelectasis. Rib fractures can also prolong the time for weaning from ventilator support. Do not immobilize the chest wall with tape or binders. A combination of opioids, benzodiazepines, topical lidocaine patch, and nonsteroidal anti-inflammatory drugs provides the most effective analgesia for mild to moderate chest wall pain.

For patients admitted to the hospital, an intercostal nerve block with a long-acting agent such as bupivacaine will relieve pain associated with muscle spasm and ventilation for up to 12 hours. Epidural analgesia or intrapleural catheters for administration of local anesthetics also relieve chest wall pain.[35] Epidural analgesia for blunt chest trauma may be a better choice than IV opioid analgesia.[36]

With the exception of direct local trauma, **it takes great force to fracture the first and second ribs,** given their short length, relative immobility, and protection by other structures in the upper chest. Such fractures can be associated with significant injuries to underlying organs such as blunt myocardial injury, bronchial tears, or a major vascular injury, with 15% to 30% associated with poor outcome, usually from head injury or rupture of a major vessel.

In patients with multiple fractured ribs (especially ribs 9, 10, and 11), unexplained hypotension may be the result of intra-abdominal bleeding from the liver or spleen. Consider imaging of the abdomen by CT or US in any patient with lower rib fractures. Patients with multiple fractured ribs will often have difficulty coughing or adequately clearing secretions and should be considered for 24- to 48-hour observation unit admission, especially the elderly or those with preexisting pulmonary disease.

FLAIL CHEST

Segmental fractures of three or more adjacent ribs anteriorly or laterally often result in an unstable chest wall physiology known as *flail chest.* This injury is characterized by a paradoxical inward movement of the involved chest wall segment during spontaneous inspiration and outward movement during expiration. Although paradoxical motion can greatly increase the work of breathing, the primary cause of the hypoxemia is contusion to the underlying lung. These patients may fatigue rapidly as a vicious cycle of decreasing ventilation, increased work of breathing, and hypoxemia may develop, resulting ultimately in sudden respiratory arrest.

Patients with mild to moderate flail chest and, importantly, little or no underlying pulmonary contusion or associated injury can often be managed without a ventilator. Adequate pain relief by analgesics or intercostal nerve block and maintaining good ventilation and pulmonary toilet are important adjuncts when managing these patients. **Indications for early ventilatory support include shock, severe head injury, comorbid pulmonary disease, fracture of eight or more ribs, other associated injuries, age >65 years, or arterial partial pressure of oxygen (Po2) <80 mm Hg despite supplemental oxygen.** Early intubation and ventilatory assistance in patients with flail chest reduce mortality compared with delaying intubation until the onset of respiratory failure.

The role of surgical fixation in the management of rib or sternal fractures remains controversial. The aim of fixation is to reduce the need for ventilatory assistance; however, improved pain relief and ventilatory support may achieve a similar goal.[37,38] The Eastern Association for the Surgery of Trauma recommends consideration of surgical fixation in flail chest patients requiring mechanical ventilation when thoracotomy is undertaken to manage other injuries (Table 261-3).[25]

STERNUM FRACTURE

Tenderness over the sternum may indicate sternal fracture. Sternal fractures usually occur at the body.[39] Lateral chest radiography can detect a fracture (**Figure 261-16**), but diagnosis is usually made by CT (**Figure 261-17**).[24] US is more sensitive and specific than chest radiographs for sternal fractures.[40,41]

Fracture of the sternum has been historically considered a marker of serious life-threatening injury, particularly cardiovascular injury. However, in clinical practice, it is the type of associated injury that determines morbidity and mortality. Patients with isolated sternal fractures and otherwise negative workup (including chest CT, echocardiogram, cardiac US, and cardiac enzymes at the time of presentation and 6 hours afterward) can safely be discharged home.[42] Current experience with sternal fractures as a result of motor vehicle crashes notes a 1.5% incidence of cardiac dysrhythmias requiring treatment and a mortality rate of <1%.[43] Such data suggest that sternal fractures are not an indicator of significant blunt myocardial injury. Patients with sternal fractures presenting with normal vital signs and an initial normal ECG should have a repeat ECG in 6 hours and, if unchanged, require no further workup for cardiac injury.[44,45]

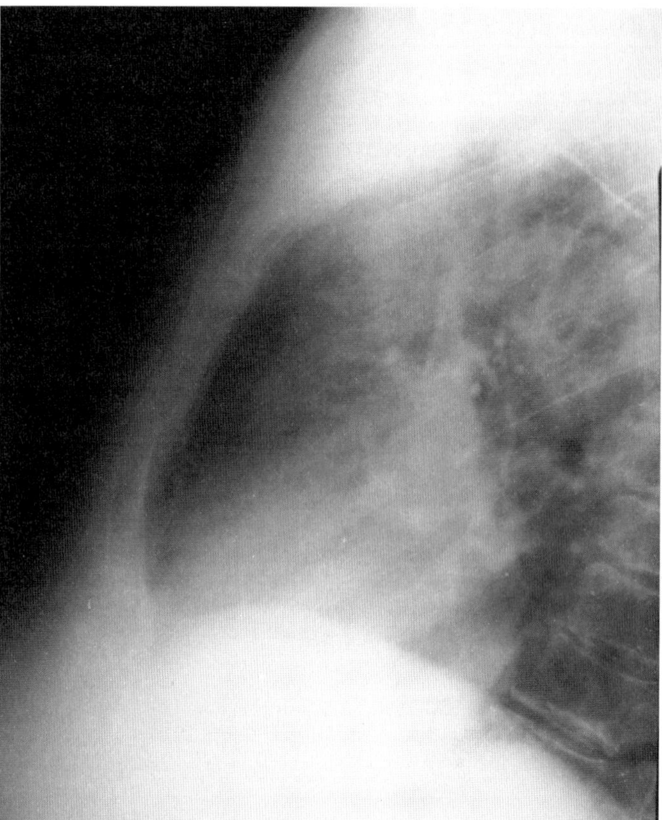

FIGURE 261-16. Sternal fracture. Lateral chest radiograph reveals a sternal body fracture after blunt chest injury.

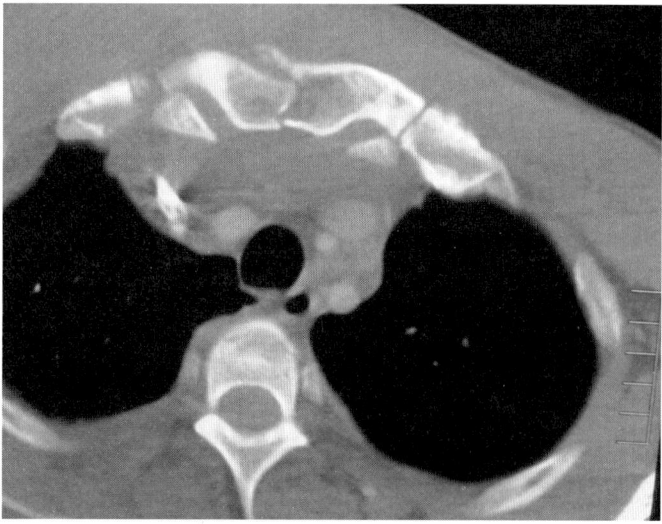

FIGURE 261-17. Sternal fracture. Patient presents with seat belt sign on the chest wall and tenderness over the sternum. CT shows vertical fracture of sternum and mediastinal hematoma under the fracture.

TRAUMATIC ASPHYXIA

Sudden, severe crush injury to the chest may be associated with subconjunctival hemorrhage, petechiae, vascular engorgement, facial edema, and cyanosis of the head, neck, and upper extremities. This clinical picture is likely due to an abrupt sustained rise in superior vena caval pressure and concurrent closure of the airway after deep inspiration. Although these patients often look moribund initially, neurologic impairment, if any, is usually temporary, and any long-term morbidity is due primarily to associated injuries.

Acknowledgments: We would like to acknowledge the seventh edition contributors—Patrick H. Brunett, Lalena M. Yarris, and Arif A. Cevik.

REFERENCES

The complete reference list is available online at www.TintinalliEM.com.

CHAPTER 262 Cardiac Trauma

Christopher Ross
Theresa Schwab

INTRODUCTION AND EPIDEMIOLOGY

Detection of cardiac injuries is critical for patient survival. Penetrating cardiothoracic injury causes 25% of deaths immediately following trauma, and the majority of these fatalities involve either cardiac or great vessel injury.[1] Cardiac injury may account for up to approximately 10% of deaths from gunshot wounds.[2] The incidence of blunt cardiac injury has been reported to range anywhere from 8% to 71%.[3] Suspect the diagnosis of cardiac and great vessel injury in a patient with chest, lower neck, epigastric, or precordial injury. Closely observe for evidence of hemodynamic instability, loss of circulating blood volume, electrocardiographic changes, cardiac tamponade, and hemothorax.

Penetrating cardiac injury results when a foreign object enters the body and pierces the pericardium or heart. Blunt cardiac injury results from physical forces acting externally on the body. Iatrogenic injuries to the heart are due to the invasive nature of procedures. All invasive cardiac procedures and therapies have the potential to cause trauma to both the pericardium and myocardium. Even noncardiac procedures like central lines placed into the internal jugular vein can lead to penetration of the pericardium, heart, and great vessels.[4]

PENETRATING CARDIAC TRAUMA

Most injuries occur from guns and knives.[5] The injury usually involves only the free cardiac wall, but other structures can be injured, such as cardiac valves, chordae tendineae, papillary muscles, atrial or ventricular septum, coronary arteries, and conduction system (**Table 262-1**).[6]

ANATOMY AND PATHOPHYSIOLOGY

Pericardial injury can result in acute tamponade. Rates of involvement of cardiac structures due to penetrating injuries to the right ventricle, left ventricle, right atrium, and left atrium are approximately 40%, 35%, 20%, and 5%, respectively.[7,8] The right ventricle is at greatest risk due to its large anterior exposure on the chest wall. The right and left atria are less frequently involved due to their smaller surface area. Knives tend to involve a single chamber, producing a single slit-like defect that is often more amenable to medical and surgical therapy than gunshot wounds. Gunshot wounds can leave a spectrum of injury from multiple-chamber perforation to gaping defects depending on the caliber and velocity of the missile. Patients with stab wounds to the heart are 17 times more likely to survive than those with gunshot wounds.[9] Atrial injuries are less common and generally less severe, whereas multichamber injuries are associated with higher mortality.

The anatomic "cardiac box" (Figure 262-1) is the area of the chest bounded by the sternal notch superiorly, the xiphoid process inferiorly, and the nipples laterally. Most stab wounds injuring the heart enter through this area. Gunshot wounds, however, may enter at regions well outside this area, so any penetrating injuries involving the thoracoabdominal region, back region, or any potential of transmediastinal trajectory place the heart at risk for injury.

TABLE 262-1 Penetrating Wounds of the Heart

Pericardial damage
Laceration or perforation
Hemopericardium with or without cardiac tamponade
Serofibrinous or suppurative pericarditis
Pneumopericardium
Constrictive pericarditis
Myocardial damage
Laceration
Penetration or perforation
Retained foreign body
Structural defects
Aneurysm formation
Septal defects
Aorticocardiac fistula
Valvular injury
Leaflet or cusp injury
Papillary muscle or chordae tendineae laceration
Coronary artery injury
Laceration or thrombosis with or without myocardial infarction
Arteriovenous fistula
Aneurysm
Embolism
Foreign body
Thrombus (septic or sterile)
Infective endocarditis
Rhythm or conduction disturbance

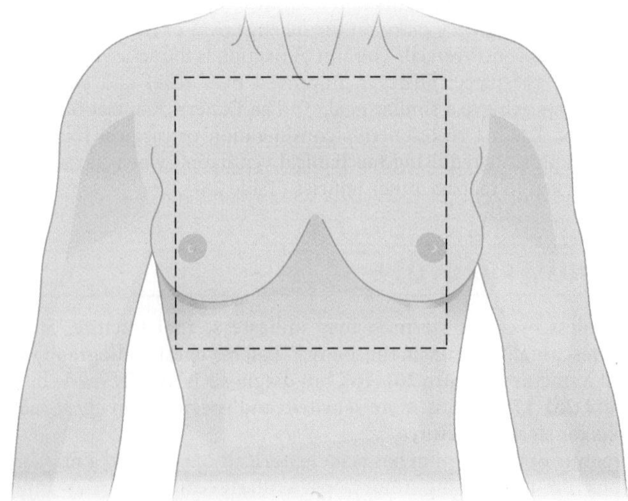

FIGURE 262-1. The cardiac box: chest area with potential for cardiac injury.

The two conditions that can occur after penetrating cardiac injury are exsanguinating hemorrhage and cardiac tamponade. Pericardial defects that are large or remain open may present with hemothorax and clinical signs of blood loss that may progress to rapid exsanguination and death. If the pericardial wound seals itself, which is common with the linear defect in a stab wound, the result is intrapericardial hemorrhage that may progress to cardiac tamponade. The location of the wound will also determine the rate of accumulation. Right ventricular wounds tend to seal themselves more readily than right atrial wounds due to the thicker, more muscular walls of the ventricle. Atrial injuries may have subtle or no clinical findings initially; however, rapid clinical deterioration can occur. Injury to the coronary arteries is manifested by tamponade or myocardial ischemia.

CARDIAC TAMPONADE

Cardiac tamponade, characterized by the accumulation of pericardial fluid under pressure, can be found in up to 2% of penetrating trauma to the thoracoabdominal region and very rarely in blunt trauma. Up to 80% of myocardial stab wounds may develop cardiac tamponade. Gunshot wounds leave defects in the pericardium that are larger and more irregular than stab wounds. Gunshot wounds are therefore less likely to develop tamponade because it is more difficult for the pericardium to seal the defect.[10]

Blood in the pericardial cavity may be defibrinated by the lytic activity normally present in the pericardium, resulting in a hematoma that may inhibit normal myocardial function. Intrapericardial blood accumulation eventually causes elevated intrapericardial pressure, which leads to decreasing right and left ventricular filling. Catecholamines are released in this state as a compensatory mechanism that results in tachycardia and further elevated right-sided filling pressures. Once the distensibility limits from intrapericardial fluid are reached by the pericardium, the myocardial septum shifts toward the left side, which further reduces left ventricular filling and subsequent cardiac output. This downward spiral eventually produces irreversible shock and death. Even small amounts of blood (65 to 100 mL) can lead to an acute rise in intrapericardial pressure. Hypovolemic shock from other injuries may partially or completely compensate for the elevated right-sided pressures, resulting in normal or even low central venous pressures.

Cardiac tamponade is identified by the FAST exam. Without bedside US, cardiac tamponade can be deceptively difficult to diagnose as the body compensates for the hemodynamic effects by various mechanisms. The reduced cardiac output is offset by the increase in heart rate and increase in systemic vascular resistance. Often, the only clinical finding of pericardial tamponade is sinus tachycardia. Hypotension may be a sign of ominous decompensation and emergent need for surgical intervention if due to pericardial tamponade or systemic hypovolemia from other injuries. The classic finding of Beck's triad of muffled heart sounds, hypotension, and distended neck veins is present in less than 10% of cases.[2] Pulsus paradoxus, a substantial fall in systolic blood pressure during inspiration, and Kussmaul's sign, an increase in jugular venous distention on inspiration, are not reliable signs and may only be found with moderate to severe tamponade.[11] A more reproducible sign of cardiac tamponade is a narrowing of the pulse pressure, which along with elevation of the central venous pressure, is cardiac tamponade until proven otherwise. The narrowed pulse pressure is not sensitive, and its absence should never be used to exclude tamponade. Usually the jugular venous pressure is elevated and may be associated with venous distention of the neck veins, forehead, and even scalp.

INTRACARDIAC MISSILES

The heart may have a retained missile from a direct injury or as a result of venous migration from another injury. These missiles, or the thrombus that may form as a result, may embolize into systemic or pulmonary arteries.[12] Many patients with a retained cardiac missile are hemodynamically stable. The patients may do well with prolonged observation and no operative intervention.[13] The treatment for missiles is highly variable, depending on missile size, shape, and location. Missiles that cause any hemodynamic instability or symptoms should be removed. A left ventricular missile that is free or partially exposed should be removed to prevent systemic embolization.[13] Right-sided missiles may be removed or left alone because embolization to the pulmonary vascular bed usually has minimal consequences.[14] Most intramyocardial and intrapericardial bullets and pellets are generally well tolerated and left in place. Embolized missiles need immediate removal because of the downstream ischemic effects of arterial occlusion. If a missile is embedded or adjacent to a coronary artery, it should be removed because of the potential for erosion and bleeding, which may lead to myocardial infarction and pericardial tamponade. Long-term effects of a retained missile may include bacterial endocarditis, thrombosis, embolization, and cardiac neurosis (many patients feel that they need any missile removed at all cost).[13]

IATROGENIC CARDIAC INJURY

Diagnostic and therapeutic percutaneous procedures may lead to many cardiovascular complications. Vascular (including extra- and intracardiac), valvular, and myocardial injuries are well-recognized complications of procedures such as central line placement, thoracentesis, chest tube placement, pericardiocentesis, percutaneous coronary catheterization, valvuloplasty, and electrophysiologic lab procedures.[15]

TREATMENT OF PENETRATING CARDIAC TRAUMA

Perform pericardiocentesis if cardiac tamponade is identified on the FAST exam. This may be an effective temporizing measure. Perform ED thoracotomy in unstable patients with cardiac tamponade who may not survive transfer to an operating room.

PERICARDIOCENTESIS

Pericardiocentesis is a prelude to formal thoracotomy if there are inevitable delays to definitive surgery (i.e., transport to trauma center). Use of US guidance of the needle increases accuracy and is a class I American College of Cardiology/American Heart Association recommendation for critically injured patients. Detailed discussion is provided in chapter 34, "Pericardiocentesis."

ED THORACOTOMY

Patients in extremis but with electrical cardiac activity should be rapidly transported to the ED. Resuscitative ED thoracotomy can be lifesaving in carefully selected patients. The decision to perform an ED thoracotomy or alternately determine that resuscitation is futile must be made in short order under highly stressful circumstances.

Candidates for ED thoracotomy include penetrating chest trauma patients who are hemodynamically unstable and those who demonstrated signs of life (palpable pulse, a blood pressure, pupil reactivity, any purposeful movement, organized cardiac rhythm, or any respiratory effort) either in the field or ED but subsequently lost these signs of life. Resuscitative ED thoracotomy is likely to be futile in patients under the following clinical scenarios: (1) no pulse or blood pressure in the field; (2) asystole is the presenting rhythm and there is no pericardial tamponade; (3) prolonged pulselessness (>15 minutes) at any time; (4) other massive, nonsurvivable injuries; or (5) blunt traumatic cardiac arrest.

Exposure to the heart is accomplished by a left anterolateral thoracotomy. No matter where the penetrating injury occurs, use the left-sided approach initially. This approach allows for quick access to the pericardium and heart and exposure for aortic cross-clamping if necessary. Identify the left fourth or fifth intercostal space, which corresponds to an intercostal space below the male nipple or at the inframamillary fold in a woman. Make the incision in a single stroke through all layers down through the intercostal musculature from sternum to posterior axillary line. Use Mayo scissors to cut the remaining intercostal muscles. Insert a Finochietto retractor with the crank positioned near the bed. Open the retractor to allow exposure of the left thorax. Remove blood and inspect for brisk bleeding. Control intrathoracic hemorrhage with direct pressure, the application of appropriate pulmonary or vascular clamps, and direct suture ligation. Gently push the lung out of the field to expose the pericardium. To minimize the left lung obscuring the field, a right mainstem bronchus intubation may be performed.

A distended, discolored, and often tense pericardial sac confirms cardiac injury. Perform a pericardiotomy by making a long incision from the apex of the heart to the root of the aorta just anterior to the phrenic nerve. Remove any blood and clot from the pericardial sac. Patients who do not have blood in the pericardium and do not exhibit cardiac activity may be declared dead at this point. If there is evidence of blood in the pericardium or cardiac activity, then expose the heart for inspection. After extruding the heart through the incision in the pericardium, identify the cardiac wound. One of several techniques may be used to control hemorrhage (**Figure 262-2**). Simple digital occlusion on top of the wound is the first maneuver to attempt initial hemostasis. Never insert a finger into the wound because this may extend the defect. The defect can then be stapled with regular skin staplers, which is a quick and easy method of temporary cardiac repair. Suturing of wounds is often technically difficult due to the dynamic nature of the myocardium, the slippery edges, the ease with which the sutures pull through the myocardium, inadequate lighting, and bloody field. Putting a Foley catheter into the defect and blowing up the balloon can fill a large circular defect. Gentle traction on the catheter will allow the balloon to seal the defect. A purse string suture can then be placed around the Foley catheter so that when the catheter is removed, tightening of the suture will seal the defect. Myocardial defects can be sutured with horizontal mattress sutures, but use pledgets to reinforce the repair and prevent cutting through the heart tissue.

Perform internal cardiac massage in the absence of coordinated cardiac function. Whatever type of repair is attempted, be careful and do not ligate major coronary vessels. If there is no evidence of injury to the left side or there is a high index of suspicion of right-sided injury, the ED thoracotomy incision can be extended to the right side. This is done by extending the incision across the sternum ("clam shelling") in the same manner as the primary left-sided incision to gain access to the right side of the chest and allow for better exposure of the right ventricle and atrium. Patients with suspected intra-abdominal hemorrhage should have the descending aorta cross-clamped.

After resuscitative ED thoracotomy, if vital signs are regained, transfer the patient to the operating room for definitive repair. The survival rate for patients who make it to the operating room is 70% to 80% for stab wounds and 30% to 40% for gunshot wounds.

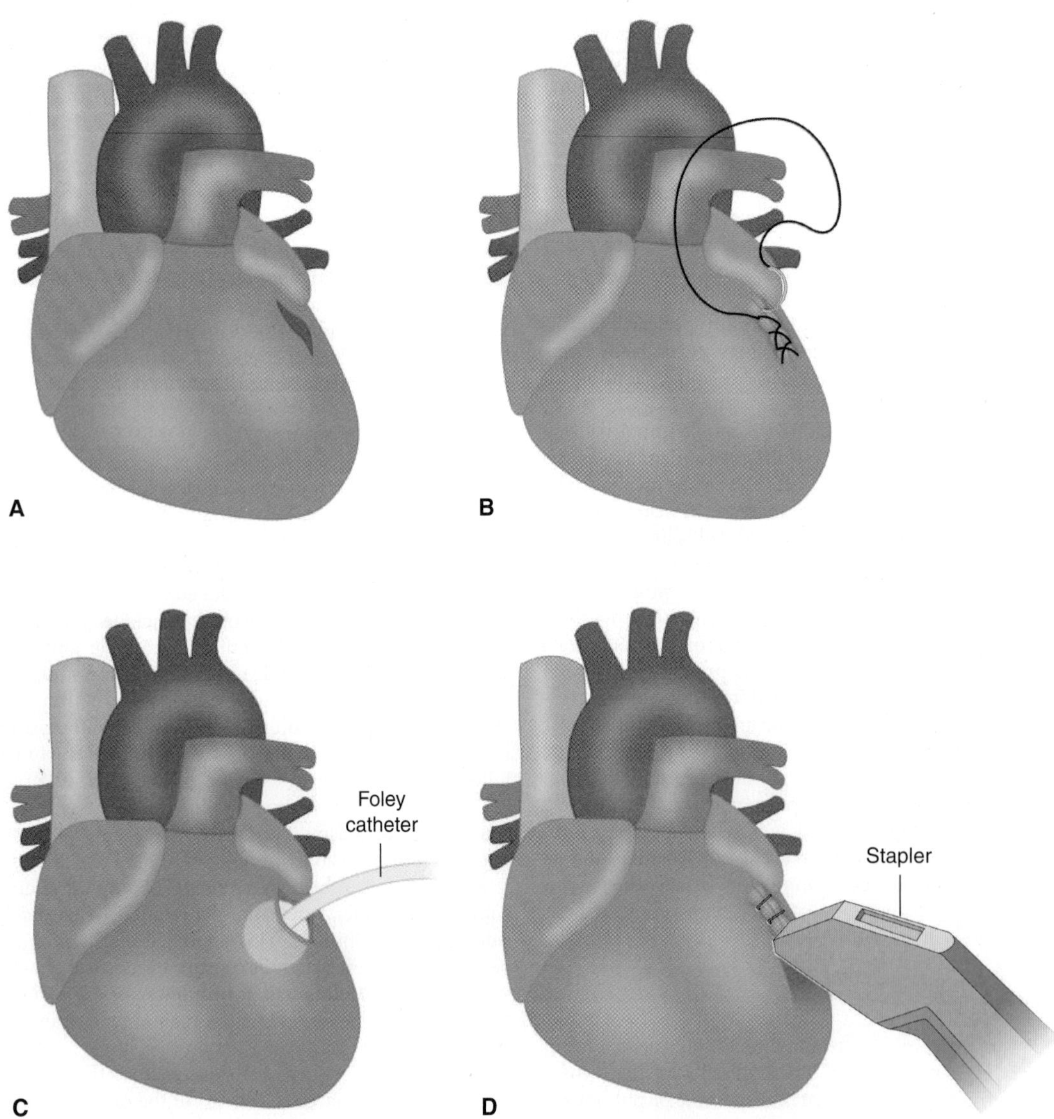

FIGURE 262-2. Temporary techniques to control bleeding of myocardial laceration. Emergency center management of injury to the epicardium. **A.** Stab wound to the left ventricle. **B.** Initially managed with either a continuous 4-0 polypropylene suture or interrupted sutures tied beneath the surgeon's finger. **C.** Injuries that are more complex and cannot be managed in the ED can be temporized using a Foley catheter for ventricular injuries and either a Foley catheter and/or partial occluding clamp for atrial injuries. **D.** Because of concerns about surgeon needle stick during cardiorrhaphy on the beating heart, hemostasis can initially be achieved with the skin stapler. Care must be observed in avoiding ligation of coronary arteries.

BLUNT CARDIAC TRAUMA

Up to 20% of all motor vehicle collision deaths are due to blunt cardiac injury, which can be sustained from any of the mechanisms listed in **Table 262-2**.[16] Rapid deceleration is the most common mechanism responsible for most blunt cardiac injury followed by a direct blow to the precordium. Blunt cardiac injury results in a range of conditions from clinically silent transient dysrhythmias to cardiac wall rupture

The most common reported injury is "myocardial or cardiac contusion." These terms are nonspecific and have been used to report a wide range of injuries. Further, there is not a clear definition or a gold standard for testing, which makes the diagnosis and treatment difficult. The term *blunt cardiac injury* has replaced the terms *cardiac contusion* and *myocardial contusion*. Blunt cardiac injury can encompass cardiac dysfunction (diminished contractility in the absence of dysrhythmia or hemorrhage), dysrhythmias, specific injuries (septal rupture, valvular injuries, myocardial infarction), and cardiac rupture, the most devastating blunt cardiac injury.[3,17,18]

PATHOPHYSIOLOGY

Blunt cardiac injury most often involves the right heart due to the anterior location of the right atrium and ventricle within the mediastinum. Injury often involves more than one chamber in over half of the reported cases.[19]

The pathologic changes seen in blunt cardiac injury typically include subendocardial hemorrhage and a much larger area of focal myocardial edema, interstitial hemorrhage, and myocytolysis with infiltrates of polymorphonuclear leukocytes. Additional myocardial injury may occur if there are concomitant intimal tears or compression from adjacent hemorrhage or edema. Myocardial injury may also be due to redistribution of coronary blood flow. Minor myocardial marker elevation or ECG abnormalities and dyskinesia or dysrhythmias resolve over time, usually within the first 24 hours.[16] Blunt cardiac injury can lead to death from complex dysrhythmias, acute heart failure, cardiac-free wall rupture, or laceration of a coronary artery that causes extracardiac hemorrhage. Most of these lethal mechanisms result in death at the scene of the injury.[20-22] Less severe injuries to the ventricular wall may lead to delayed necrosis and clinically manifest as delayed rupture days after admission. If a low-pressure chamber or coronary vein is injured, patients may survive until presentation to the hospital.[23]

Blunt cardiac injury can also result in rupture of an atrial or ventricular septum, resulting in shunting of blood and presentation similar to heart failure.[24] Similarly, blunt cardiac injury can result in regurgitation of blood from a high-pressure chamber or artery into a lower-pressure chamber, such as with an acute valve dysfunction or papillary muscle injury.[25,26] Valvular injury, as opposed to blunt myocardial injury, tends to worsen over time. The degeneration of the valve's function appears to depend on its location. High-pressure valves like the aorta and mitral valves tend to manifest symptoms immediately or within the first few weeks, whereas lower-pressure valves like the pulmonic and tricuspid can be asymptomatic for years.[16] Coronary arteries can have occlusion, dissection, or spasm that can manifest as immediate or delayed injury patterns. Coronary artery injury presents most often in a myocardial infarction pattern.[27]

Nonspecific signs and concomitant injuries will affect clinical presentation. These other findings in the trauma patient may make it difficult to determine whether symptoms stem from cardiac or other injuries. Specific signs of cardiac injury (e.g., distended neck veins or specific murmurs) may not be present if the patient is hypotensive from other injuries. Symptoms of cardiac injury may occur in a delayed fashion coincident with fluid resuscitation.

TABLE 262-2 Mechanisms for Blunt Cardiac Injury

Mechanisms for Blunt Cardiac Injury
Direct precordial impact
Crush injury from compression between the sternum and spine
Abrupt pressure fluctuations in the chest and abdomen
Shearing from rapid deceleration or torsion causing a tear in the heart at a point of fixation (right atrium and vena cava)
Injury from rib fracture fragments
Hydraulic effect resulting in cardiac rupture
Blast injury

COMMOTIO CORDIS

Commotio cordis, meaning "disturbance of the heart" in Latin, is sudden death as a result of blunt trauma to the chest wall. It often results from an innocent-appearing chest wall blow. It is the second most common cause of death in youth athletics following hypertrophic obstructive cardiomyopathy. Usually victims are young athletes who are struck in the chest by hard projectiles that are used in the particular sport. Sports using small dense projectiles like baseball, hockey, and lacrosse have the highest incidence of commotio cordis. The hardness of the impact object, location of impact, and velocity of the object impacts the risk of development of ventricular fibrillation. Commotio cordis blows are generally low impact, most of which are insufficient to cause any significant structural damage to the ribs, sternum, or heart. Commotio cordis is a primary electrical event resulting in the induction of ventricular fibrillation; it is a result of a blow that occurs 10 to 30 ms before the peak of the T wave, a time of vulnerability to ventricular fibrillation. Autopsy findings show normal cardiac anatomy with no evidence of injury. The overall survival rate is less than 15%, but due to increasing prevalence of automated external defibrillators being placed in sporting venues, survival rates may improve.[28]

CARDIAC DYSFUNCTION

The exact incidence of cardiac dysfunction (decreased contractility) in blunt cardiac injury is unknown. Further, the cause of dysfunction may be difficult to determine in the hypotensive, multiply injured trauma patient. Patients almost universally present with chest pain. The pain usually results from associated thoracic trauma (**Table 262-3**). Associated blunt injury to the lung can lead to a rise in pulmonary vascular resistance, which can result in a reduction in preload of the left ventricle. This, coupled with the reduced cardiac output of the involved right ventricle, can lead to hypotension.[18,29] The damaged myocardial tissue may be a focus for both atrial and ventricular dysrhythmias, which may further produce decreased contractility and hemodynamic deterioration.

Monitor for dysrhythmias. Persistent tachycardia, new bundle branch block, supraventricular tachycardia, atrial and ventricular fibrillation, and minor dysrhythmias (occasional premature ventricular contraction) can occur after blunt injury.

TABLE 262-3 Associated Injuries with Blunt Cardiac Trauma[3]

Associated Injuries	Incidence of Finding in Patients with Blunt Cardiac Injury
Thoracic injury	
Chest pain	18%–92%
Rib fracture	18%–69%
Aortic or great vessel injury	20%–40%
Hemothorax	7%–64%
Pulmonary contusion	6%–58%
Pneumothorax	7%–40%
Flail chest	4%–38%
Sternal fracture	0%–60%
Head injury	20%–73%
Extremity injury	20%–66%
Abdominal solid organ injury	5%–43%
Spinal injury	10%–20%

Source: With permission from Schultz JM, Trunkey DD. Blunt cardiac injury. *Crit Care Clin*. 2004;Jan;20(1):57-70. Copyright Elsevier.

INJURY TO THE PERICARDIUM

Direct impact or increased intra-abdominal pressure can cause pericardial tears. The tears usually occur on the left side of the pericardium parallel to the phrenic nerve. Herniation can occur through the defect leading to cardiac dysfunction and dysrhythmias. These tears in the pericardium often are missed and may have little clinical impact. Physical examination (pericardial rub), point-of-care US, or CT findings (pneumopericardium, displacement of the heart, abnormal bowel gas in chest or around heart, or evidence of intra-abdominal contents inside pericardium) may lead to the diagnosis. Patients with detectable pericardial rents are usually taken to the operating room for repair unless the tear is too large so that closure would lead to tension on the pericardium and potentially produce myocardial dysfunction.

INJURY TO CARDIAC VALVES, PAPILLARY MUSCLES, CHORDAE TENDINEAE, AND SEPTUM

Injury to cardiac valves occurs in approximately 10% of blunt cardiac injury. Isolated valvular injuries appear to be rare. The aortic valve is most often involved, followed by the mitral and tricuspid valves. Injury to the aortic valve can cause severe regurgitation with development of pulmonary edema. Presentation may vary from new murmur to acute valvular insufficiency with right- or left-sided cardiac failure. A widened pulse pressure can be seen with acute aortic valvular injuries. Septal injuries are also rare with variable presentations, ranging from insignificant tears to frank rupture. They may occur in isolation or with valvular injury. The muscular portion of the septum can rupture several days after blunt trauma. Suspect patients with new-onset murmurs of having valvular, septal, or papillary muscle pathology. Any patients with clinical or echocardiographic evidence of injury require emergent surgical consultation. Treatment for septal and valvular injury is generally surgical, and timing depends on the presenting signs and acuity. Acute heart failure resulting from elevated pulmonary pressure due to structural injury warrants rapid surgical intervention, whereas small septal injuries with minimal clinical effects can be treated conservatively because many eventually close spontaneously.[30]

INJURY TO CORONARY VESSELS/MYOCARDIAL INFARCTION

Although blunt cardiac injury rarely leads to injury of the coronary vessels, arteriovenous fistula, coronary artery dissection, and coronary thromboses have been reported.[31,32] The most common artery involved is the left anterior descending artery. Coronary artery injury presents in the same fashion as atherosclerotic heart disease, has similar treatment by percutaneous coronary intervention with stenting, and has a more favorable prognosis. Because of the possibility of other injuries, extreme caution must be taken in using anticoagulation therapy due to bleeding complications.[31,32] Fibrinolytic therapy is contraindicated.

CARDIAC RUPTURE

The most severe form of blunt cardiac injury is cardiac rupture. Most patients with cardiac rupture die at the scene of the trauma. The right-sided portion of the heart is much more prone to rupture due to its more anterior location, as are the thin-walled atria compared with the thicker-walled, stronger ventricles. In patients who survive to ED arrival, the physical examination may reveal a "splashing mill wheel" sounding murmur ("bruit de Moulin"), but this finding is rare. ECG may show conduction defects or, if herniation has occurred, axis deviation. A skilled sonographer can rapidly reveal the diagnosis, and immediate thoracotomy is required for survival.[22]

CLINICAL FEATURES OF BLUNT CARDIAC TRAUMA

HISTORY

The most common symptom of cardiac trauma is chest pain. All different qualities of chest pain occur, ranging from pleuritic to pressure-like. Even the classic crushing retrosternal pain of myocardial ischemia can occur if coronary arteries are involved. Patients with injuries on the chest wall such as rib fractures, sternal fractures, or clavicular fractures may have underlying cardiac injury. Be cautious about attributing symptoms only to superficial chest wall because pericardial and myocardial structures may be damaged as well. Patients may have shortness of breath due to overlying chest and pulmonary injury or due to myocardial dysfunction from cardiac tamponade or heart failure. Other nonspecific symptoms such as lightheadedness and palpitations are also common.[18] Clinical findings vary widely depending on the structures injured, the extent of the injuries, concomitant injuries, and the patient's body habitus and mental status.

PHYSICAL EXAMINATION

Close observation of heart rate and blood pressure and their associated trends is important. Listening to breath sounds and heart sounds may assist in diagnosing cardiac injury. Clear lungs with muffled heart sounds may be indicative of cardiac tamponade, but this finding is quite rare and difficult to detect in a noisy ED. Course crackles in the lungs, extra heart sounds, and elevated jugular venous pressure may be present if myocardial dysfunction leads to heart failure. Often, the presence of unexplained tachycardia may be the only finding of cardiac injury.

DIAGNOSIS

ELECTROCARDIOGRAM

Place the patient on a cardiac monitor, and obtain an ECG. The negative predictive value for cardiac injury in a patient with a normal ECG is about 80% to 90%, but using the ECG alone does not exclude cardiac injury.[18,33] A clinically significant cardiac event can occur over the first 24 hours following injury.[34] The ECG is more sensitive for left ventricular injury than right-sided injury and is poorly sensitive for the more common right-sided injuries. Nondiagnostic findings on ECG, such as sinus tachycardia and nonspecific ST-T wave changes, do not help diagnose blunt cardiac injury. A small subset of blunt cardiac injury patients may have symptoms and ECG findings consistent with myocardial infarction. In such patients, consider coronary artery disease or acute coronary artery dissection, which may manifest with thrombosis of a cardiac artery and typically develops 5 to 7 days after injury[17,35] (**Table 262-4**).

In patients in whom concern for blunt cardiac injury exists but in whom the ECG is normal, monitor for 4 to 6 hours with repeat examinations,

TABLE 262-4 Electrocardiographic Findings in Cardiac Injury[36]

Nonspecific abnormalities
Pericarditis-like ST-segment elevation
Prolonged QT syndrome
Myocardial injury
New Q wave
ST-T segment elevation or depression
Conduction disorders
Right bundle branch block
Fascicular block
Atrioventricular nodal conduction disorders (first-, second-, and third-degree atrioventricular block)
Dysrhythmias
Sinus tachycardia (most common)
Atrial and ventricular extrasystoles
Atrial fibrillation
Ventricular tachycardia
Ventricular fibrillation
Sinus bradycardia
Atrial tachycardia

Source: Reproduced with permission from Sybrandy KC, Cramer MJ, Burgersdijk C. Diagnosing cardiac contusion: old wisdom and new insights. *Heart*. 2003;May;89(5):485-489.

ECGs, and cardiac monitoring. If there are no new signs or symptoms and no abnormalities occur during this time period, patients can be safely discharged in absence of any other injuries.[37] If the ECG is abnormal but there is no hemodynamic instability, admit the patient to a monitored setting, with serial ECGs to monitor for disease progression.

CARDIAC BIOMARKERS

Although cardiac markers can be used to assist in the diagnosis of myocardial trauma, the utility of cardiac biomarkers in the setting of blunt cardiac injury remains unclear.[38] Creatine kinase has limited reliability in the trauma patient because it is elevated in cases of severe skeletal muscle, liver, diaphragm, or intestinal injury; the creatine kinase-MB fraction will therefore be elevated as well. Creatine kinase-MB fraction elevation has been shown to occur in this situation in the absence of clinical evidence of cardiac injury. The isolated elevation of creatine kinase-MB, with no other associated injury, is not predictive of complications and mortality.[39] Thus, obtaining creatine kinase-MB measurements is of no value.

Cardiac troponins, specifically troponin I and troponin T, are very specific to myocardial injury and can detect very small amounts of myocardial necrosis. Neither cardiac troponin I nor cardiac troponin T is released with skeletal muscle injury. Elevation of troponins occurs in all myocardial trauma, including both blunt and penetrating trauma, surgery, ablation, pacing, defibrillator shocks, cardioversion, and interventional cardiac procedures. The sensitivity and specificity of troponins for blunt cardiac injury vary from 12% to 23% and 97% to 100%, respectively.[33,40] Also, injuries remote from the chest from multisystem trauma and the presence of preexisting disease may result in dysrhythmia and elevated biomarkers, making their presence even less specific.[41]

Troponins in conjunction with a presenting ECG may increase the effectiveness of risk stratification. Patients with a normal ECG and normal serial measurements of serial cardiac troponin I had no significant blunt cardiac injury–related complications in one study.[42] The sensitivity of an abnormal ECG and elevated cardiac troponin I for clinically significant blunt cardiac injury (cardiogenic shock, dysrhythmias requiring intervention, or structural cardiac abnormalities related to trauma) was 100%, with a positive predictive value of 62%.[40] Clinically significant blunt cardiac injury can occur without elevation of troponins, but there is usually an abnormality of the ECG. Monitor any serum troponin elevation and follow serially. Increased troponin levels at admission or within 6 hours of arrival have correlated with increasing risk of dysrhythmia and decreased ejection fraction.[43] Troponin elevations have been associated with ventricular dysrhythmias and left ventricular dysfunction.[44]

Ultimately, the use of cardiac biomarkers may not affect the management of blunt trauma patients with hemodynamic instability, signs of severe injury, or an abnormal ECG. Such patients generally undergo echocardiography and are admitted regardless of biomarker elevation.

In rare blunt trauma patients with ECG findings of myocardial infarction, obtain cardiac biomarkers and immediately consult with cardiology and cardiac surgery.

ECHOCARDIOGRAPHY

The FAST examination includes a cardiac window using either the subxiphoid (**Figure 262-3**) or parasternal long-axis approach. This allows detection of free pericardial fluid and can give an estimation of general cardiac function. Point-of-care US has been shown to have a sensitivity of 100% and a specificity of 99% for detecting pericardial effusion.[45]

Point-of-care US is an invaluable tool for blunt trauma patients with unexplained, persistent shock out of proportion to apparent injuries and in any patients with signs consistent with blunt cardiac injury. Echocardiography provides information about global cardiac function, individual chamber function and wall motion, valvular function, and ejection fraction. It can also assist in alternative diagnoses for conditions such as aortic disruption/dissection, pericardial effusion, pleural effusion, and intracardiac thrombus.[46] Transesophageal echocardiography has been shown to be up to three times more sensitive in diagnosing blunt cardiac injury than transthoracic echocardiography.[47] Transthoracic echocardiography and transesophageal echocardiography, however, are not helpful in identifying patients at risk for developing blunt cardiac injury–related complications.[16] Order echocardiography for patients demonstrating elevated cardiac markers, dysrhythmias, or myocardial dysfunction.[48]

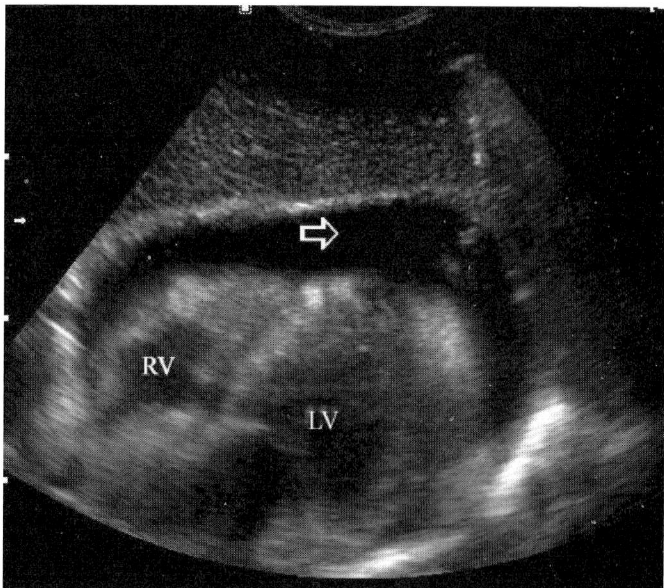

FIGURE 262-3. Traumatic pericardial effusion. Large pericardial effusion (*arrow*) after stab wound to chest visualized by subxiphoid approach of a FAST scan. The effusion can be seen outside the right ventricular (RV) and left ventricular (LV) walls.

TREATMENT OF BLUNT CARDIAC INJURY

Treat hypotension with boluses of crystalloid to optimize intravascular blood volume, which will also optimize preload. Trauma patients often have multiple injuries, especially in blunt injury, so the most common reason for hypotension is due to hypovolemia, not myocardial dysfunction.

Otherwise, the management of blunt cardiac injury (myocardial or cardiac contusion) is not standardized. The only universally accepted practice pattern is to observe patients with hemodynamic and continuous cardiac monitoring.[18] It is generally agreed that low-risk patients (minor injuries, no dysrhythmias, and normal ECG) usually will not develop complications so that further workup is not warranted. Moderate- to high-risk patients (evidence of associated injuries, dysrhythmias, abnormal ECG) should have an evaluation that includes myocardial markers and echocardiogram. Admission to ward telemetry is appropriate for the patient with minor ECG abnormalities (premature ventricular or atrial contractions), no significant concomitant injuries, and normal hemodynamics.[49,50] Telemetry monitoring criteria do not exist, but 24 to 48 hours of monitoring are reasonable for minor abnormalities.

Subsequent management depends on complications. After ruling out hypovolemia as the source of hypotension, inotropic support may be required to maintain cardiac output and blood pressure. Dysrhythmias that result in hemodynamic instability or are ventricular in origin are treated according to advanced cardiac life support algorithms. Evaluate patients who present in cardiogenic shock for a structural injury. Patients with cardiac rupture, valvular injury, papillary muscle or chordae tendineae rupture, or coronary thromboses or dissection require emergent surgery or percutaneous coronary intervention.

SPECIAL CONSIDERATIONS

PERICARDIAL INFLAMMATION SYNDROME

The cause of pericardial inflammation may be a delayed hypersensitivity reaction to the presence of damaged myocardium in the pericardial cavity. Consider this syndrome in individuals who develop chest pain, fever, and pleural or pericardial effusions 2 to 4 weeks after cardiac trauma (or surgery). Patients may also have friction rubs, arthralgia, and pulmonary infiltrates. The ECG will often show ST-T wave changes consistent with pericarditis. Treatment is primarily symptomatic. Nonsteroidal anti-inflammatory drugs and rest can often reduce symptoms dramatically within 12 to 24 hours, and glucocorticoids are occasionally required. Rarely, drainage of pleural or pericardial fluid may be required to relieve symptoms or to exclude other problems.

INJURY TO THORACIC GREAT VESSELS

The thoracic great vessels consist of the aorta and its brachiocephalic trunk and its branches; the left subclavian, left common carotid, and pulmonary arteries and veins; the superior and intrathoracic venae cavae; and the innominate and azygos veins. Injuries to these vessels occur in both penetrating and blunt trauma. The large blood volume flowing through these vessels leads to exsanguinating hemorrhage as the primary acute manifestation of trauma. Even if not immediately ruptured, injury to these vessels can produce aneurysm and pseudoaneurysm through fistula formation, which in turn can lead to massive hemorrhage. Most patients who present with thoracic great vessel injury have sustained penetrating trauma and have a dire prognosis; most die before they reach medical care.[51] Aortic injuries from blunt trauma are usually due to motor vehicle crashes. Over 90% of patients who sustain this injury die at the scene; of the remaining 10% who survive, 50% die within 24 hours and 90% die within 4 months.[52] The mortality for untreated patients is 1% per hour for the initial 48 hours.[53]

PATHOPHYSIOLOGY

BLUNT INJURY

Blunt trauma injury to the great vessels involves high-speed deceleration. Usually the chest strikes the steering wheel, which subsequently transmits the force across the mediastinum. There may also be vascular compression of the vessels between the sternum and vertebral bodies and subsequent marked increases in intraluminal pressure.[53] Consider blunt aortic injury when the mechanism involves sudden deceleration such as a fall over 10 ft (3 m) or a motor vehicle collision at speeds greater than 30 mph (50 km/h).

The proximal descending aorta is most commonly injured in blunt trauma because of the fixation of the vessels between the left subclavian artery and the ligamentum arteriosum. The aorta is mobile and continues to move forward as the tethered portions decelerate with the remainder of the chest, leading to shearing forces that produce aortic injury. The diagnosis of ascending aortic injury is rarely made since very few patients survive long enough to diagnosis and repair. Ascending aortic injuries are frequently associated with cardiac rupture or severe myocardial contusion, and the aortic tears are often multiple. Usually large amounts of energy are required to injure the ascending aorta. The distal descending aorta is also a less frequently injured structure. Patients may present with paraplegia, mesenteric ischemia, anuria, or lower extremity ischemia. The more distal the injury, the better is the anticipated outcome, provided the patient does not exsanguinate prior to repair.

Although the subclavian artery is occasionally avulsed at its origin because of sudden deceleration, direct trauma to the distal artery with intimal damage and occlusion associated with fractures of the first rib or clavicle is more likely. Shoulder restraints that are loose may be a major factor in causing this injury. Injuries to the innominate artery are second in frequency only to rupture of the aorta at the isthmus. This injury is difficult to diagnose because less than half of patients have any physical findings at all and those who do have some diminution of the right radial or brachial pulse, a systolic murmur, or distal ischemia (rarely).

The pulmonic veins and the venae cavae attach to the atria and can serve as a nidus for injury with shearing forces. Venous thoracic great vessel injury is extremely rare, and most are fatal. Suspicion of inferior vena caval injury should occur with major hepatic injury, and both the superior and inferior venae cavae should be considered a source if there is cardiac tamponade or arterial bleeding that cannot be identified.

The aorta is primarily involved in about 85% of cases, but branch vessels are involved in 15% of documented vascular injuries.[54] The branch injuries are potentially fatal so their identification is of the utmost importance as well. Concurrent vascular injuries should be identified because the definitive surgical approach may change depending on where the injuries occur.[55]

PENETRATING INJURY

The pathophysiology of penetrating trauma to the great vessels is straightforward: either there is direct vessel injury or the kinetic energy damages the vessels by propagation through the tissues. Patients with penetrating injuries rarely survive to reach the hospital. Iatrogenic injuries from central line placement and other invasive thoracic procedures can lead to great vessel injury.

Bullets entering large systemic veins or the right heart can embolize to the lungs, whereas bullets entering the pulmonary veins or left heart can embolize to major systemic arteries. Some of these embolized foreign bodies do not cause symptoms or signs and can be located only after taking multiple radiographs. Suspect embolization if the missile appears distant from the anticipated trajectory. The other explanation for missiles off trajectory is gravity: low-velocity bullets that violate the pleural space but are not trapped in lung parenchyma often fall to the lowest place in the hemithorax, namely the posterior costophrenic recess.

CLINICAL FEATURES

Blunt trauma involving motor vehicle crashes can injure the aorta with side-impact collisions just as often as head-on collisions. Any blunt trauma from significant force (falls from a significant height, blast injuries, high-speed motor vehicle crash, crush injuries, pedestrian versus automobile injuries) can lead to blunt aortic injury.

Half the patients with blunt thoracic vascular injury present without external physical signs of injury. Although the physical examination findings of great vessel injury can be minimal to nonexistent, several important clues should be investigated. Hypotension, hypertension in the upper extremity and hypotension in the lower extremity, unequal blood pressures in the extremities, external evidence of major chest trauma (seatbelt or steering wheel contusion on the chest), thoracic outlet expanding hematoma, intrascapular murmurs or bruits, palpable fractures of the sternum and ribs, or flail chest should increase suspicion of great vessel injury.

Proximity of a missile trajectory to the brachiocephalic vessels, even without any physical findings of vascular injury, is an indication for pursuing a diagnosis of vascular injury. Close inspection of a penetrating wound should look for evidence, by inspection only, of retained implement or foreign body. Under no circumstances should the wound be deeply probed to determine depth or trajectory. Perform a complete neurologic examination due to involvement of the spinal arteries from the initial trauma.

DIAGNOSIS

CHEST X-RAY

Many findings on the initial chest radiograph may be indicative of great vessel injury (**Tables 262-5 and 262-6**), but many of these findings are insensitive and nonspecific.

Widening of the mediastinum on chest radiograph (**Figure 262-4**) has classically been considered as being a very sensitive test for detection of major vascular injury. Definitions of a widened mediastinum have included a measured width greater than 8 cm or a clinician gestalt of mediastinal widening and chest width ratio of >0.38. Trauma patients have <20% probability of having major thoracic vascular injury with this finding on chest radiograph.[56] However, a normal mediastinum on chest

TABLE 262-5 Radiographic Findings Suggestive of a Great Vessel Injury

Fractures
Sternum
Scapula
Multiple ribs
Clavicle in multisystem-injured patients
First rib
Mediastinal Clues
Obliteration of the aortic knob contour
Widening of the mediastinum
Depression of the left mainstem bronchus >140 degrees from trachea
Loss of paravertebral pleural stripe
Calcium layering at aortic knob
Abnormal general appearance of mediastinum
Deviation of nasogastric tube to the right at T4
Lateral displacement of the trachea
Lateral Chest X-Ray
Anterior displacement of the trachea
Loss of the aortic/pulmonary window
Other Findings
Apical pleural hematoma (cap)
Massive left hemothorax
Obvious diaphragmatic injury

Source: Reproduced with permission from Mattox KL, Moore EE, Feliciano DV: *Trauma*, 7th edition. New York, NY: McGraw-Hill: 2013. Table 26-5.

radiograph does not rule out aortic injury. Therefore, the investigation of great vessel injury should occur if mechanism of injury, physical examination findings, or radiographic indicators are consistent with injury. One sensitive radiographic sign for traumatic aortic injury is deviation of the esophagus more than 1 cm to the right of the spinous process at T4.[57]

CT ANGIOGRAPHY

CT angiography is the diagnostic modality of choice for both penetrating and blunt trauma of the thorax. Because CT is widely used in the evaluation of multisystem trauma, incorporating CT imaging for vascular injury can be easily done. Newer-generation multidetector scanners are very sensitive and specific for injury to the great vessels. Three-dimensional reconstructions of high-resolution data sets produce extremely accurate representations of the vascular anatomy and may be the only diagnostic imaging studies required by vascular surgeons. Although CT does require the patient to leave an intensive monitoring area, the information it provides can lead to treatment avenues vital for patient survival. Full-body scans are relatively rapid, with image acquisition occurring in less than 5 minutes. In comparison to classical angiography, CT angiography is faster, less expensive, and eliminates complications related to vessel catheterization. Most institutions use multidetector CT scanners with CT angiography as the screening study of choice for aortic injury. Thin-slice multidetector CT with rapid scanning and contrast-bolus timing has shown great promise in detecting and localizing a variety of nonaortic vascular injuries, including active bleeding that can lead to early surgical or angiographic intervention to control blood loss.[55] Major CT angiography findings for blunt trauma can be seen in **Table 262-7**.

The major role of CT in penetrating trauma is determination of the presence or absence of mediastinal involvement along or near the course of the penetrating object (**Figure 262-5**). This can lead to direct finding

TABLE 262-6 Reliability of Selected Clinical and Radiographic Criteria in the Detection of Traumatic Rupture of the Aorta[*†]

Chest X-Ray Finding	Correlation with TAI (*P* value)	Sensitivity	Specificity	Accuracy
Widened mediastinum (<65 years old)	.001	0.95	0.82	0.84
Widened mediastinum (all ages)	.001	0.80	0.82	0.82
Murmur	.002	0.32	0.93	0.84
Pneumothorax/ pulmonary contusion	.07	0.22	0.67	0.51
Hemothorax	.21	0.25	0.88	0.81
First/second rib fracture	.39	0.36	0.73	0.68

Abbreviations: FN = false negative; FP = false positive; TAI = traumatic aortic injury; TN = true negative; TP = true positive.

*All other clinical and radiographic criteria were less useful in detecting TAI.

†Sensitivity = TP/(TP + FN); specificity = TN/(TN + FP); accuracy = (TP + TN)/All tests.

Source: Table 259-6 from Tintinalli, et al: *Emergency Medicine: A Comprehensive Study Guide*, 6th ed. © 2002, McGraw-Hill, New York.

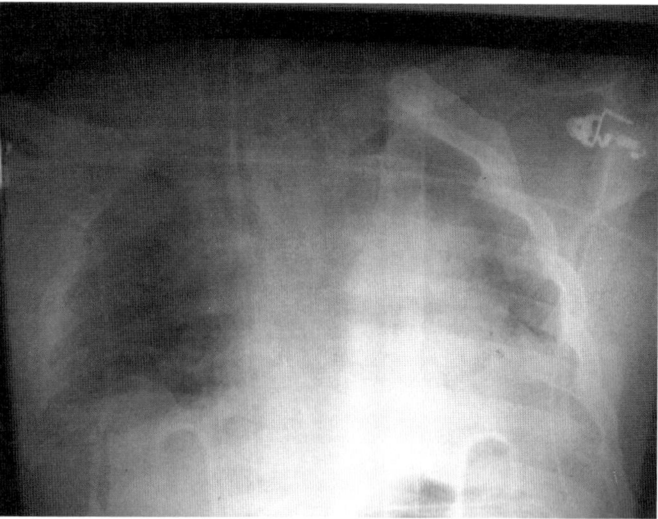

FIGURE 262-4. Portable chest radiograph of a patient with blunt thoracic trauma: chest x-ray shows widened mediastinum, obliteration of the aortic knob contour, and loss of visualization of the left hemidiaphragm, which are consistent with aortic injury.

TABLE 262-7 CT Signs of Traumatic Aortic Injury[55]

Common Signs
Aortic pseudoaneurysm
Periaortic hemorrhage
Displacement of the trachea and esophagus to the right by hematoma, an irregular shape to the aortic lumen
Intimal flaps projecting into the lumen
Uncommon Signs
Luminal clot at sites of intimal disruption
Sudden change in caliber of the aorta without intervening branch vessels (coarctation)
A small aortic caliber in the lower chest and abdomen
Peridiaphragmatic hemorrhage (from proximal intraluminal thrombus)
Rare Signs
Transection of the aorta
Active bleeding from the aorta into the mediastinum

Source: Reproduced with permission from Mirvis SE. Thoracic vascular injury. *Radiol Clin North Am*. 2006 Mar;44(2):181-197. Copyright Elsevier.

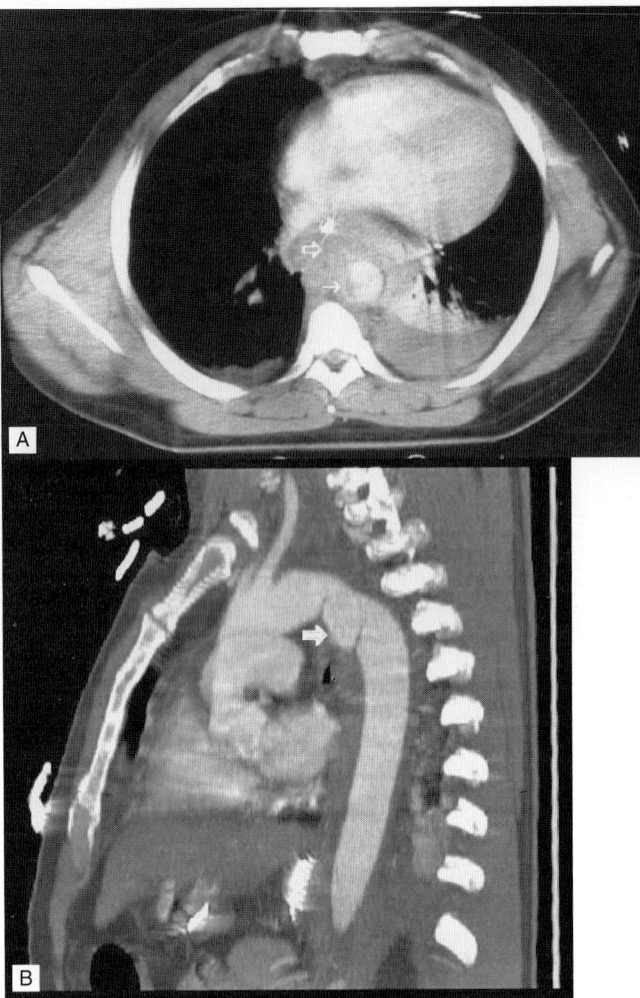

FIGURE 262-5. CT scan of traumatic aortic injury. **A.** Axial CT scan showing mediastinal hematoma (*open arrow*) and irregularity and thrombus in the aorta (*closed arrow*). **B.** Sagittal CT scan of same patient with pseudoaneurysm (*arrow*) from tear in aorta distal to left subclavian artery.

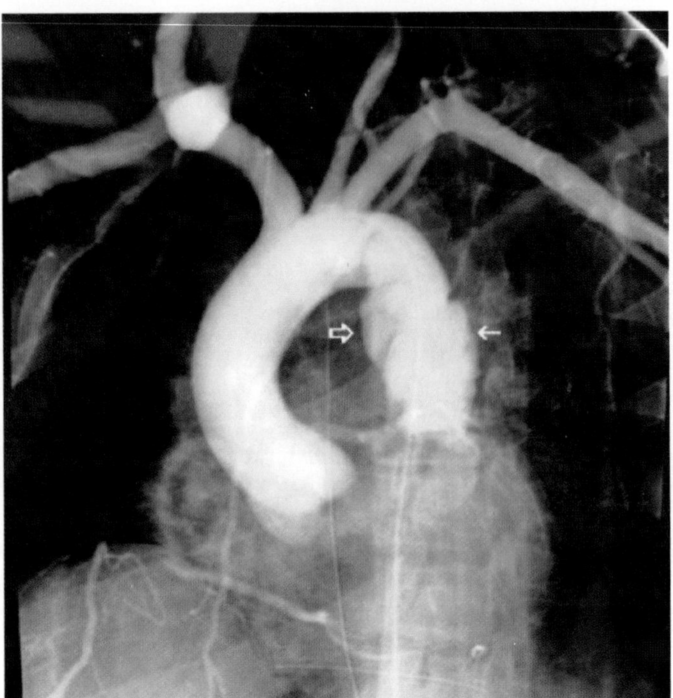

FIGURE 262-6. Angiogram of the same patient in Figure 262-5 showing pseudoaneurysm (*open arrow*) and irregular lumen (*closed arrow*) of injured aorta.

of injury to major mediastinal structures. Aortic or major arterial injuries can be detected and appear as irregular vascular contours, luminal narrowing or irregularity, pseudoaneurysms, dissections, and acute bleeding. CT angiography is also helpful in penetrating injury to the thoracic great vessels.[55] In some cases, the vessel lumen may appear completely normal on CT due to the external forces to the vessel. Damage surrounding the vessel, usually in the form of perivascular hemorrhage, is present. Following the tract of the missile on CT should also help in determining the likelihood of direct vascular involvement.[55]

OTHER IMAGING MODALITIES

MRI and magnetic resonance angiography provide similar detailed information. However, MRI and magnetic resonance angiography require lengthy study times, have limited emergent availability at most institutions, and require the transport of a potentially unstable patient away from a monitored environment. These limitations make MRI and magnetic resonance angiography impractical for most trauma patients presenting to the ED.

Transesophageal echocardiography remains a very attractive diagnostic option because of its advantages of speed, portability, immediate availability of results, and low cost. With recent advances in echocardiographic instrumentation and technology, it has evolved as a promising imaging technique that can provide comprehensive information of the location and extent of aortic injury. Transesophageal echocardiography allows diagnosis of limited intimal lesions frequently missed by other conventional methods and permits rapid diagnosis of complete rupture at the bedside hemodynamically unstable patients. One study demonstrated that despite significant blurring of the aortic outline in 20% of cases and intraluminal artifacts being observed in 36% of cases, the accurate diagnosis of traumatic aortic injury was made.[58] Transesophageal echocardiography is contraindicated in patients with potential airway problems or suspected cervical spinal injuries.

Aortography remains a viable imaging option for determining the location of aortic injury, which is paramount in operative management (**Figure 262-6**). Angiography is more time consuming to perform, invasive, and not as readily available as CT on an acute basis. It more expensive than CT as a screening study. Angiography is useful when CT results are indeterminate and may be required by surgeons for planning and guiding operative repair. Angiography may be used to pursue injury in the aorta or branch vessels in penetrating injuries that have only proximity to these vessels. Caution should be exercised with "negative" results because a clot or an intimal flap may close the luminal defect. The overall complication rate of angiography has remained at about 25%, but rates for serious complications, such as amputation and death, remain low at 0.1% and 0.3%, respectively.[59]

TREATMENT

Consult a trauma or vascular surgeon at the time of initial suspicion of great vessel injury or immediately upon diagnosis. Transport patients with great vessel injury who exhibit hemodynamic instability, profound hemorrhage from chest tubes, and radiographic evidence of a rapidly expanding mediastinal hematoma immediately to the operating room.

Immediate surgical repair may not be possible in all patients. Patients with instability from other injuries, such as from intra-abdominal injuries or severe closed head injuries, may have a delayed repair due to the severity of these other life-threatening issues. Some elderly patients may have comorbidities that require medical management prior to surgery. Pharmacologic control of blood pressure and heart rate is extremely important when delayed or nonoperative management is contemplated.[60] Avoid large swings in blood pressure that may increase vessel-shearing forces in patients who are hemodynamically stable. Administer sedatives, analgesics, vasodilators, and β-adrenergic blocking agents to keep the patient's systolic blood pressure at safe levels. Use autotransfusion devices in cases of large bleeding vessels.

Traumatic aortic injuries can be partial thickness (as in the classic intimal flap of aortic dissection) or full thickness with containment by surrounding structures. These histopathologic entities mandate a similar therapeutic approach as aortic dissection. Decreasing the slope of the dP/dT (change in pressure over the change in time) will decrease wall tension and shearing forces. This may lead to permissive hypotension and bradycardia as a treatment and temporizing measure in aortic disruption. **Maintain systolic blood pressure in the 100 to 120 mm Hg range with a heart rate around 60 beats/min.** This will decrease the shearing forces on the internal lumen. Patients should not perform any maneuver, like a Valsalva, that will increase intrathoracic pressure. Titrating a short-acting β-blocker, such as esmolol, can decrease the heart rate. Once the heart rate is controlled, an arterial vasodilator, such as sodium nitroprusside, can be added to help control the blood pressure. Do not use sodium nitroprusside alone due to the reactive tachycardia associated with its administration.

REFERENCES

The complete reference list is available online at www.TintinalliEM.com.

CHAPTER 263 Abdominal Trauma

L. Keith French
Stephanie Gordy
O. John Ma

INTRODUCTION

Abdominal trauma accounts for 15% to 20% of all trauma deaths.[1] Although the liver is the most frequently injured abdominal organ, the spleen is the most frequently injured intra-abdominal organ from sports accidents.[2] Death may occur as a consequence of massive hemorrhage and generally results in early demise soon after the injury. Patients who survive the initial traumatic insult are at risk for infection and suffer mortality or morbidity secondary to sepsis.

PATHOPHYSIOLOGY

BLUNT ABDOMINAL TRAUMA

The most common mechanism for blunt abdominal trauma is a motor vehicle collision.[1] All abdominal structures are at risk, and ultimately the biomechanics of the traumatic force determine which organs are affected. Compressive, shearing or stretching, and acceleration/deceleration forces impact the abdominal cavity differently. This potentially leads to abdominal wall, solid organ, or hollow viscous injuries. Abdominal organs may be relatively mobile or fixed. Injury is common in transition areas between these structures. The ligament of Treitz and the distal small bowel represent transition areas where mesenteric or small bowel injuries may occur.

Falls from significant heights produce injury as a function of the fall distance, the surface the victim lands on, and the manner of surface impact. Hollow viscous rupture is the typical intra-abdominal injury.[3] Retroperitoneal injury and hemorrhage may occur as force is transmitted along the axial skeleton.

Pedestrians struck by vehicles or motorcyclists and bicyclists who crash generally have no protection to their abdomen and are at high risk for intra-abdominal injuries.

PENETRATING ABDOMINAL TRAUMA

Stab and gunshot wounds produce injury as the foreign object passes through tissue. With gunshot wounds, there may be additional injury from the transmitted energy of the blast. Furthermore, gunshot wounds create secondary missiles such as fragmented bone that may increase the traumatic burden.

The length, trajectory, and fragmentation of the penetrating object will not necessarily be known during the evaluation. **Therefore, assume any penetrating injury to the lower chest, pelvis, flank, or back to have penetrated the abdominal cavity until proven otherwise.**

CLINICAL FEATURES

Clinical signs may be obvious (such as evisceration) or occult. Factors making the diagnosis of an abdominal injury challenging include concomitant injuries (particularly significant head injuries), referred pain, intoxication with alcohol or other toxicological substances, or language barriers. Young, healthy patients may be able to compensate for intra-abdominal hemorrhage before clinical signs become overt.

PHYSICAL EXAMINATION

Inspect the abdomen for external signs of trauma (e.g., abrasions, lacerations, contusions, seatbelt marks). A normal-appearing abdomen does not exclude serious intra-abdominal injury. **Cullen's sign** and **Grey Turner's sign** (periumbilical and flank ecchymosis) generally represent delayed findings of intraperitoneal bleeding. Following inspection, palpate the abdomen in all quadrants, making note of tenderness, tympany, or rigidity. For patients who are observed in the ED, serial assessments by the same provider are ideal.

Abdominal tenderness, rigidity, distention, or tympany may not be present during the initial examination and may take hours or days to develop. Reliance on physical exam alone, particularly with a worrisome mechanism of injury, may result in an unacceptably high misdiagnosis rate. As many as 45% of blunt trauma patients thought to have a benign abdomen on initial physical exam are later found to have a significant intra-abdominal injury.[4]

ABDOMINAL WALL INJURIES

Contusions of the abdominal wall musculature may result either from a direct blow or indirectly via a sudden muscular contraction. Symptoms include pain with flexion and rotation of the trunk as well as focal tenderness to percussion. Rectus abdominis hematomas may mimic intra-abdominal injury. Rectus hematomas occur from epigastric trauma or injury to the vessels of the abdominal wall. As a hematoma develops between the rectus sheath, the patient develops pain and often a palpable mass inferior to the umbilicus.[2]

SOLID ORGAN INJURIES

Signs and symptoms of a solid organ injury are generally due to blood loss. An increase in pulse pressure may be the only clue to loss of ≤15% of total blood volume. As blood loss continues, heart and respiratory rate increase. Hypotension may not occur until a 30% decrease in circulating volume occurs. At this point, urinary output drops and patients may become anxious and confused. With some injuries, pain and bleeding may be minimal and overlooked or dismissed. Delayed rupture can occur in splenic and hepatic injuries.

Splenic injuries may cause referred pain into the left shoulder or arm. Patients with liver injuries may complain of right shoulder pain. **Pregnancy and mononucleosis are conditions that may predispose a patient to splenic injuries.**

HOLLOW VISCOUS AND MESENTERIC INJURIES

In blunt abdominal trauma, the incidence of blunt bowel and mesenteric injuries varies (1% to 12%) but occurs in about 5% of patients.[5,6] Hollow viscus injuries produce symptoms from the combination of blood loss and peritoneal contamination by GI contents. Hemorrhage from a mesenteric injury may be minimal and not be obvious on physical exam. Chemical irritation of the peritoneum from gastric acid contents may produce immediate pain, although bacterial contamination of the abdominal cavity may result in delayed signs and symptoms. Delays in diagnosis and operative management are associated with an increase in mortality.[6]

RETROPERITONEAL INJURIES

The retroperitoneal structures discussed in this chapter include the pancreas (excluding the tail) and duodenum. See "Genitourinary Injuries" for a discussion of kidney, ureter, and bladder injuries.

Pancreatic injuries are present in approximately 4% of patients with abdominal trauma and are associated with significant morbidity and mortality.[7] There are no specific signs and symptoms of pancreatic injury, but mechanism of injury provides some clues to diagnosis. Pancreatic trauma often occurs from rapid deceleration. Unrestrained drivers who hit the steering column or bicyclists who fall against a handlebar are at risk for pancreatic injuries. Initial symptoms may be delayed if the injury is minor.

Duodenal injuries may be relatively asymptomatic on presentation, and a small hematoma of the duodenum may go undiagnosed. As a duodenal hematoma expands, however, signs and symptoms of gastric outlet obstruction develop (abdominal pain, distention, and vomiting). Duodenal rupture generally occurs following high-velocity deceleration events where the intraluminal pressure of the pylorus and proximal small bowel rapidly increases. The ruptured contents are generally contained within the retroperitoneum and may be missed with studies that investigate the peritoneum exclusively. For patients with a delayed presentation, fever and leukocytosis herald the development of an abscess or sepsis.

DIAPHRAGMATIC INJURIES

The diaphragm may spasm secondary to a direct blow to the epigastrium. The patient will experience difficulty breathing as the diaphragm loses its ability to relax and allow the lungs to expand. This process is sometimes referred to as "getting the wind knocked out." As the diaphragm relaxes, symptoms abate.

Diaphragmatic rupture may result from a penetrating injury or blunt force mechanism. The condition is uncommon (0.8% to 5% of patients with thoracoabdominal injury) and is almost exclusively a **left-sided** phenomenon.[8] Signs and symptoms are nonspecific and may be attributed to associated injuries. Failure to diagnose and treat diaphragmatic rupture may lead to delayed herniation or strangulation of abdominal contents through the diaphragmatic defect.

DIAGNOSIS

Although multiple diagnostic modalities exist to detect intra-abdominal injuries, no study is fail proof. Therefore, a combination of careful physical exam, attention to the mechanisms and circumstances of injury, and judicious selection of diagnostic studies is used for diagnosis. Hemodynamic instability may limit the utilization of some diagnostic testing before definitive treatment is initiated (such as laparotomy or transfer to a trauma center).

Not every patient with multisystem or isolated abdominal trauma will need a diagnostic evaluation beyond a physical exam. However, because the consequences of a missed intra-abdominal injury may be significant, augment an initial exam with laboratory analysis, imaging study, or repeat examination in several conditions (**Table 263-1**).

ULTRASONOGRAPHY

The focused assessment with sonography for trauma (**FAST**) examination is a widely accepted primary diagnostic study. The underlying premise of the FAST exam is that many clinically significant injuries will be associated with free intraperitoneal fluid (**Figure 263-1**). **The greatest benefit of FAST is the rapid identification of free intraperitoneal fluid in the hypotensive patient with blunt abdominal trauma.**

TABLE 263-1 Abdominal Injuries That Need Expanded Evaluation

Presence of abdominal pain, tenderness, distention, or external signs of trauma
Mechanism of injury with a high likelihood of causing an abdominal injury
Suspicious lower chest, back, or pelvic injury
Inability to tolerate a delayed diagnosis (e.g., patients who are elderly, on anticoagulants, or have liver cirrhosis/portal hypertension)
Presence of distracting injuries
Altered consciousness/sensorium (e.g., CNS injury, intoxicating substances)

Advantages of the FAST examination are that it is accurate, rapid, noninvasive, repeatable, and portable, and involves no nephrotoxic contrast material or ionizing radiation exposure to the patient. There is limited risk for patients who are pregnant, coagulopathic, or have had previous abdominal surgery. The average time to perform a complete FAST examination of the thoracic and abdominal cavities is 4 minutes or less.[9] Massive hemoperitoneum is quickly detected with a single view of Morrison's pouch in 82% to 90% of hypotensive patients,[10,11] and this maneuver required an average of only 19 seconds in one study.[10] One

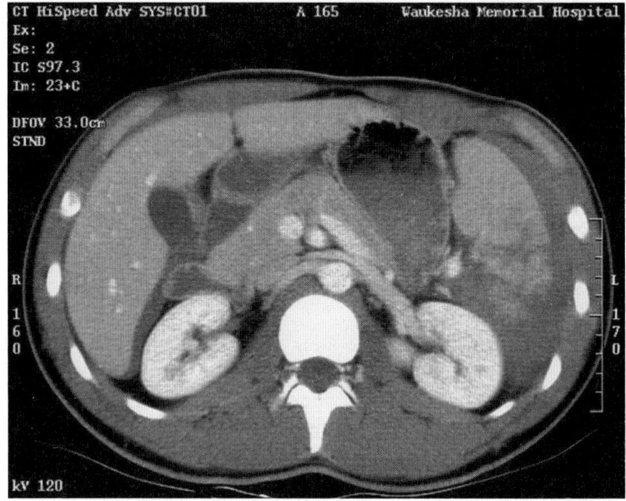

A

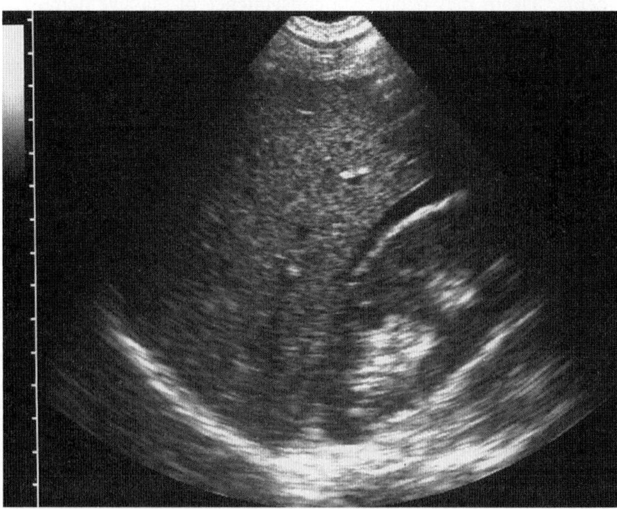

B

FIGURE 263-1. Hemoperitoneum. The abdominal IV contrast CT. **A.** A fractured spleen with surrounding hematoma is demonstrated, but a small stripe of fluid is also present above the right kidney in Morrison's pouch. **B.** A right intercostal oblique US view from the same patient reveals a thin stripe of fluid in Morrison's pouch. [Reproduced with permission from Ma OJ, Mateer JR, eds: *Ma and Mateer's Emergency Ultrasound,* 3rd ed. © 2014, McGraw-Hill, Inc. New York.]

major advantage of the FAST examination compared to diagnostic peritoneal lavage (DPL) is the ability of FAST to also evaluate for free pericardial or pleural fluid and for pneumothorax.

The main disadvantage of US compared to CT is the inability to identify the exact source of free intraperitoneal fluid. This limitation may change with the adoption of contrast-enhanced US for the identification and treatment of solid organ injuries.[12,13] Other potential disadvantages of the FAST examination are the operator-dependent nature of the examination, the difficulty in interpreting the images in patients who are obese or have subcutaneous air or excessive bowel gas, and the difficulty in distinguishing intraperitoneal hemorrhage from ascites. The FAST examination also cannot evaluate the retroperitoneum as well as CT. Therefore, US and CT are complementary rather than competing technologies when time permits and the potential benefits of CT outweigh the risks.

US has other useful applications in the trauma bay. For example, US may guide the placement of a suprapubic catheter when indicated. The inferior vena cava diameter of trauma patients, as measured on initial CT imaging, is a marker of intravascular volume and a predictor of mortality.[14,15] Although the best modality to measure inferior vena cava diameter is debated,[16] US can be a clinically helpful tool for trauma resuscitation.

Because the FAST examination can reliably detect small amounts of free intraperitoneal fluid and can estimate the rate of hemorrhage through serial examinations, US has essentially replaced DPL for blunt abdominal trauma in the majority of North American trauma centers. A positive DPL in isolation is no longer an absolute indication for exploratory laparotomy; the amount of hemorrhage and the hemodynamic status of the patient are important factors for determining further management steps.

COMPUTED TOMOGRAPHY

Abdominopelvic CT with IV contrast is the noninvasive gold standard study for the diagnosis of abdominal injury (unless the patient has allergy to iodinated contrast). The addition of PO contrast can result in aspiration and is too time-consuming to be practical in trauma management. Although most institutions use IV contrast CT for trauma assessment, there are still some institutions that use noncontrast CT or add PO contrast in the evaluation of trauma.[17] The major advantage of IV contrast CT over other diagnostic modalities is that the precise location(s) and grade of injury can be identified (Figure 263-1). CT can quantify and differentiate the amount and type of free fluid in the abdomen. Because CT can evaluate for retroperitoneal injuries, it is the ideal study for assessment of the duodenum and pancreas. The use of multiphasic CT (arterial, portal, and equilibrium phases) accurately identifies life-threatening mesenteric hemorrhage and transmural bowel injuries.[5] CT evidence of a flat inferior vena cava suggests hypovolemia.

Some patients with free intraperitoneal fluid seen on CT with IV contrast but without an obvious solid visceral injury may have a very small liver or splenic injury that is missed by CT, although mesenteric or small bowel injuries must also be considered. Often the safest course is surgical exploration to avoid late diagnosis of GI perforation or ischemia. Careful observation and repeat CT with the addition of oral contrast is also an option.

Two distinct disadvantages of CT are the ionizing radiation burden and the need to leave the trauma bay to obtain imaging. Radiation is of great concern in children and young adults. Although CT is the most sensitive modality, use it judiciously based on the clinical circumstances. Furthermore, limit the practice of repeat CT imaging following transfer to another facility whenever possible. Outcomes and time to definitive care are not significantly improved when imaging is repeated at the accepting trauma center.[18]

DIAGNOSTIC PERITONEAL LAVAGE

Despite the reproducibility and prospectively validated sensitivity of DPL to diagnose intraperitoneal injury, the advent and acceptance of other diagnostic modalities have reduced the frequency of DPL.[19] DPL can be performed using a closed (**Figure 263-2**) or open technique. However, the open DPL technique requires advanced training and

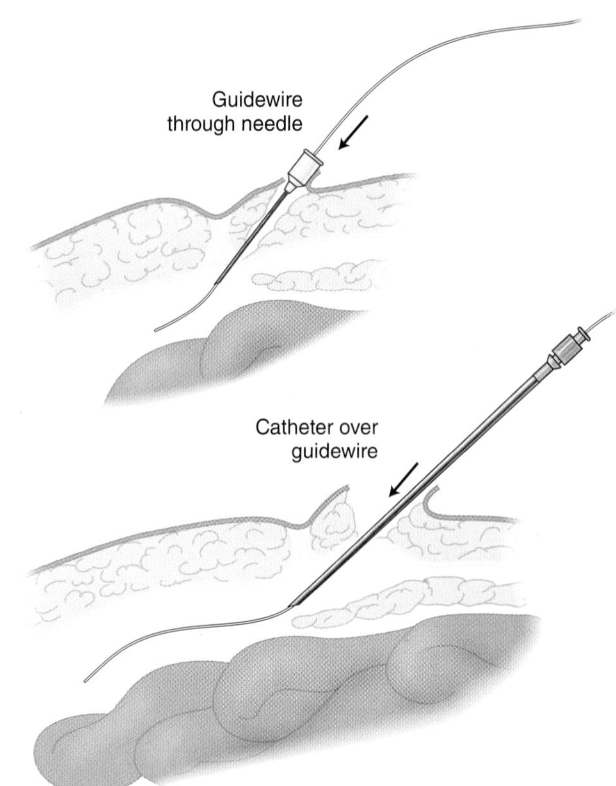

FIGURE 263-2. Closed diagnostic peritoneal lavage. Drain the urinary bladder. Infiltrate the area just below the umbilicus with lidocaine and epinephrine. Insert the needle two fingerbreadths below the umbilicus. Aspirate directly with a syringe attached to the needle, or insert a guidewire into the abdomen and place the peritoneal lavage catheter over the guidewire. Instill 1 L of normal saline through the catheter, and then aspirate.

expertise. Some advocate the use of DPL in the hemodynamically unstable patient with concern for intra-abdominal injury when the FAST exam is negative.[19] **Table 263-2** lists criteria for laparotomy based on DPL results.[20]

DIAGNOSIS IN PENETRATING TRAUMA

The same diagnostic tools are available for evaluation of intraperitoneal injury in the patient with penetrating trauma (CT, US, and DPL). Mandatory exploration for patients sustaining a stab wound to the abdomen has yielded unacceptably high rates of nontherapeutic laparotomy,[21] yet physical exam alone can miss important intra-abdominal injuries. **Locally explore anterior abdominal stab wounds** (**Figure 263-3**) to assess for violation of the peritoneum. Patients with transabdominal gunshot wounds almost always have intra-abdominal injuries. In the hemodynamically stable patient with penetrating trauma, CT can help guide the surgeon for operative versus nonoperative management.[22]

TREATMENT

LAPAROTOMY

Laparotomy remains the gold standard therapy for significant intra-abdominal injuries. It is definitive, rarely misses an injury, and allows for complete evaluation of the abdomen and retroperitoneum. **Table 263-3**

TABLE 263-2 Criteria for Positive Diagnostic Peritoneal Lavage
>10 mL free flowing blood immediately on aspiration
>15,000 RBC/mm^3 in abdominal wounds or >25,000 RBC/mm^3 in lower chest wounds

Abbreviation: RBC = red blood cell.

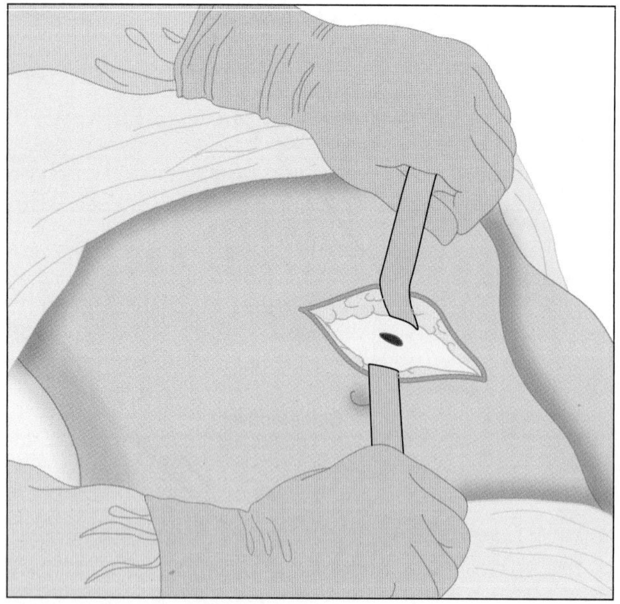

FIGURE 263-3. Local abdominal wound exploration for anterior abdominal stab wounds. This is a surgical procedure requiring expertise, proper instrumentation, and lights. Use only for anterior abdominal stab wounds. Widen the stab wound and explore down to the level of the fascia to determine if the anterior fascia and/or posterior fascia have been violated.

describes generally accepted indications for exploratory laparotomy. **All patients with persistent hypotension, abdominal wall disruption, or peritonitis need surgical exploration.** In addition, the presence of extraluminal, intra-abdominal, or retroperitoneal air on plain radiograph or CT should prompt surgical exploration. Some patients with positive DPL or FAST examination can be managed nonoperatively. In smaller medical centers or community hospitals, transfer to a trauma center may best serve such patients.

TABLE 263-3 Indications for Laparotomy

	Blunt	Penetrating
Absolute	Anterior abdominal injury with hypotension Abdominal wall disruption Peritonitis Free air under diaphragm on chest radiograph Positive FAST or DPL in hemodynamically unstable patient CT-diagnosed injury requiring surgery	Injury to abdomen, back, and flank with hypotension Abdominal tenderness GI evisceration High suspicion for transabdominal trajectory after gunshot wound CT-diagnosed injury requiring surgery
Relative	Positive FAST or DPL in hemodynamically stable patient Solid visceral injury in stable patient Hemoperitoneum on CT without clear source	Positive local wound exploration after stab wound

Abbreviations: DPL = diagnostic peritoneal lavage; FAST = focused assessment with sonography for trauma.

NONOPERATIVE MANAGEMENT OF BLUNT TRAUMA

Nonoperative management of trauma patients has been greatly advanced by the evolution of CT. CT can make the diagnosis of solid organ injury along with ruling out other injuries requiring surgery. Solid visceral injuries are graded according to their severity.

CT grading may not agree with intraoperative observation and does not always predict the success of nonoperative management. CT precisely reveals the condition of the internal parenchyma but not external injury anatomy. Operative grading provides an excellent external view of the organ, but may underestimate internal damage. **CT is a single snapshot in time, not a dynamic assessment.**

As patients age, the capsule of the spleen and liver weakens. Parenchymal changes may occur as well. The consequences of rebleeding increase and the failure rates of nonoperative management are much higher in the older population than in a younger population for some injuries. Accordingly, nonoperative management of even very severe injuries is the norm in children but not necessarily in adults.

Several technologic advances have increased the sophistication of nonoperative therapy. The increased resolution of helical CT can identify intraparenchymal vascular injuries (i.e., pseudoaneurysms or arteriovenous fistulae) and active extravasation of contrast. Patients without vascular injury can usually be managed nonoperatively. In patients in whom vascular injury is diagnosed, percutaneous transcatheter embolization with either stainless steel coils or Gelfoam pledgets can reliably arrest hemorrhage.

For patients with suspected abdominal trauma who present in extremis, **resuscitative endovascular balloon occlusion of the aorta** for end-stage shock is gaining attention as a way to quickly stop suspected intra-abdominal hemorrhage.[23] Resuscitative endovascular balloon occlusion of the aorta is a percutaneous method to achieve temporary occlusion of the aorta, to maintain or increase perfusion to the heart and lungs in the setting of shock from blunt and penetrating injury, and to avoid the morbidity of a thoracotomy for control of the proximal aorta. The femoral artery is accessed, typically percutaneously with US guidance. Using the Seldinger technique, a sheath is introduced, and a latex balloon is placed inside the sheath, with sheath length and balloon size based on the level of the aorta to be occluded. For resuscitative endovascular balloon occlusion of the aorta, the aorta is divided into the following three zones: I, descending thoracic aorta between the origin of the left subclavian and celiac arteries; II, between the celiac and lowest renal artery; and III, the lowest renal artery and the aortic bifurcation. The balloon is inflated to get inflow control of the aorta. For example, for massive bleeding from a pelvic fracture, the balloon can be inflated below the renal arteries providing control of bleeding until definitive surgical care or embolization is done.[24] Sixty minutes of resuscitative endovascular balloon occlusion of the aorta is tolerated and recoverable. Further studies are under way before widespread clinical application.

DISPOSITION AND FOLLOW-UP

Patients with significant intra-abdominal injury need admission to the surgical or trauma service for definitive surgical intervention or observation. Given the high rate of concomitant injuries, even patients who suffer minor abdominal injury may need hospitalization to manage other injuries. In patients in whom ED discharge is considered, discuss appropriate follow-up and careful instructions for return to the ED. Patients who develop fever, vomiting, increased pain, or symptoms suggestive of blood loss (e.g., dizziness, weakness, fatigue) should return promptly for reevaluation.

REFERENCES

The complete reference list is available online at www.TintinalliEM.com.

CHAPTER 264 Trauma to the Flank and Buttocks

Alicia Devine

INTRODUCTION AND EPIDEMIOLOGY

The number of serious retroperitoneal, intraperitoneal, or vascular injuries that can occur, many of which require operative repair, complicates the evaluation of penetrating injuries to the flank or buttocks. Imaging assists in diagnosis and can direct selective conservative management. The choice of management, conservative or operative, is based on the emergency evaluation, making the emergency physician's input essential to a correct decision and a clinically successful outcome.

PENETRATING FLANK TRAUMA

PATHOPHYSIOLOGY

The flank is located between the anterior and posterior axillary lines, bordered superiorly by the sixth rib and inferiorly by the iliac crest. Although a penetrating wound to the flank can produce intraperitoneal injury with the associated findings of peritonitis or hemoperitoneum, it is possible that a penetrating flank injury could injure only the retroperitoneal organs. A solitary injury to the retroperitoneum from a penetrating flank injury may not induce peritoneal signs initially, and reliance on physical exam findings alone could lead to a delay in diagnosis, resulting in septic or hemorrhagic shock. Essentially any intra-abdominal organ is at risk for injury from a penetrating flank wound, and injuries to the kidney, ureter, bladder, liver, spleen, gallbladder, pancreas, colon, adrenal gland, diaphragm, stomach, duodenum, lung, esophagus, heart, and vascular structures have all been reported.[1-4]

The path of a gunshot or stab wound to the flank could track in any direction. Once inside the abdominal cavity, bullets may ricochet off the bony structures of the spine and produce a unique bullet path and injury pattern. The extent of injury caused by a projectile depends on its velocity, with higher-velocity objects causing more injury than lower-velocity objects, as well as on the construction of the projectile, which affects the movement of the object once inside the abdominal cavity. The greater the surface area interface, the greater is the tissue damage. Stabbing injuries are low velocity and induce injury through direct contact with tissue.[5]

CLINICAL FEATURES

Obtain information about the mechanism of injury, how much time has passed since the event, and the nature of the weapon. In the case of a gunshot wound, determine the nature of the gun (e.g., shotgun, handgun, BB gun) and the distance between the gun and the patient at the time of the gun's discharge. **For gunshot wounds, attempt to identify an exit wound and reconstruct the bullet path.** For stab wounds, determine the size of the weapon and, if possible, estimate a measure of the depth of penetration. Perform a rectal examination because the presence of red blood in the stool may indicate bowel injury. Note any blood around the urinary meatus or blood in a Foley catheter drainage that would suggest bladder or urethral injury.

DIAGNOSIS

Patients with penetrating flank trauma who are hemodynamically unstable or who have peritoneal signs require emergent laparotomy. Patients who are not taken emergently to the operating room require further evaluation to ascertain the extent of injury and to determine if the wound has penetrated the peritoneum and caused intraperitoneal organ injury. Evaluation of flank trauma represents challenges related to its unique anatomic position and potential for retroperitoneal injury with late manifestations. Few data exist on isolated penetrating flank trauma, and most of the recommendations for management come from studies of both flank and back trauma or flank and abdominal trauma.[6] Several diagnostic modalities exist to further evaluate penetrating flank trauma, each with some degree of limitation in its ability to exclude injury. **Table 264-1** lists the diagnostic modalities available (see also chapter 263, "Abdominal Trauma"). Triple-contrast CT scan can detect the trajectory of the penetrating object and evaluate the retroperitoneum and is highly accurate in detecting injuries requiring laparotomy, but is less sensitive for the detection of injuries to the diaphragm or colon.[2,3,7,8] US has limited ability to detect hollow viscous or retroperitoneal injury and cannot be used alone in penetrating flank trauma to exclude occult injury.[9,10,11] Diagnostic peritoneal lavage can detect intraperitoneal penetration, but cannot evaluate the retroperitoneum, and has a high false-positive rate leading to nontherapeutic laparotomy. Local wound exploration has a false-positive rate of 14% to 45%.[7] Diagnostic laparoscopy is very sensitive for the detection of peritoneal violation and can help prevent the morbidity and mortality associated with unnecessary laparotomy.[11-13]

TABLE 264-1 Diagnostic Modalities for Evaluation of Flank Trauma
CT
Ultrasonography
Diagnostic peritoneal lavage
Local wound exploration
Laparoscopy

LABORATORY TESTING

Table 264-2 lists the baseline laboratory and imaging studies that should be obtained.

TABLE 264-2 Baseline Studies for Penetrating Flank or Buttock Trauma
Hematocrit
Type and screen
Chest radiograph
Urine pregnancy test (as appropriate)
Urinalysis

IMAGING

CT is the diagnostic modality of choice in hemodynamically stable patients with penetrating flank trauma.[2,3,6,7,14] Use double (PO and IV) contrast or triple (PO, IV, and PR) contrast; add rectal contrast if there is any likelihood of a rectal or sigmoid injury.[3,6,7] Fine cuts through the site of injury may be required (**Figures 264-1 and 264-2**). Free intraperitoneal fluid or air suggests peritoneal perforation. Bowel wall thickening with hematoma near the bowel or contrast extravasation from the bowel suggests bowel injury. The presence of a wound track near either the diaphragm or bowel mandates close scrutiny for injury to either of those organs.[3,6,15]

TREATMENT AND DISPOSITION

Evaluate and resuscitate patients with penetrating trauma to the flank according to standard protocols (see chapter 254, "Trauma in Adults"). Following stabilization, try to find an exit wound and reconstruct the bullet path. Obtain emergent surgical consultation. Administer broad-spectrum IV antibiotics to cover for gram-negative aerobic and anaerobic organisms for peritonitis.

Exploratory laparotomy is indicated for patients who are hemodynamically unstable or who exhibit peritoneal signs after sustaining a gunshot wound to the flank. Historically, all patients with gunshot wounds to the flank underwent exploratory laparotomy, but a more conservative approach should be taken at trauma centers when penetrating wounds are found to be tangential and there are no peritoneal signs.

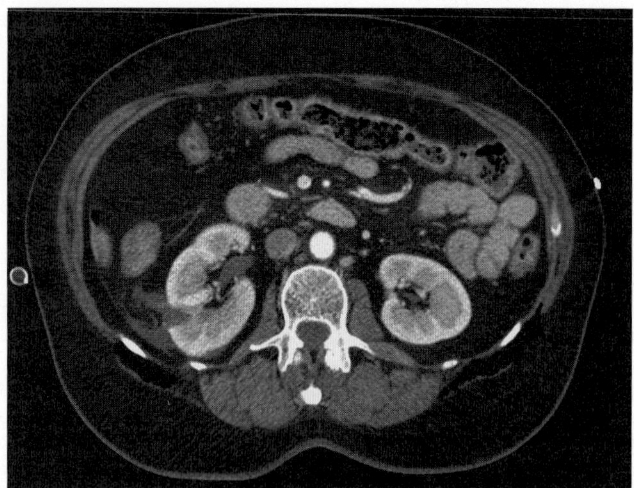

FIGURE 264-1. IV contrast abdominal CT demonstrating a renal laceration from a stab wound. [Reproduced with permission from Block J, Jordanov MI, Stack LB, Thurman RJ (eds): *The Atlas of Emergency Radiology*. New York: McGraw-Hill, Inc.; 2013, Fig. 6-21.]

In the case of high-velocity gunshot wounds, take into account the blast effect. Depending on the exact location and type of injury, consideration of the blast effect may lead to exploratory laparotomy if there is concern about bowel, bladder, or vascular integrity.

Patients with stab wounds to the flank who are hemodynamically stable and lack peritoneal signs or diffuse abdominal tenderness may be managed conservatively after triple-contrast CT scan or local wound exploration.[2,3,6,7,11,14] Patients with either gunshot or stab wounds who are managed nonoperatively will usually require admission to the hospital for observation and serial abdominal exams.

PENETRATING BUTTOCK TRAUMA

PATHOPHYSIOLOGY

The gluteal region extends from the iliac crest to the gluteal fold and is bordered by the greater trochanters. The gluteal region is divided into an upper zone and a lower zone by a line drawn at the level of the trochanters. Although any pelvic or intra-abdominal structure is susceptible to injury following a penetrating injury to the buttocks, the most common structures injured in a stab wound to the buttock are the rectum, superior gluteal artery, and iliac artery, and the most common structures injured in a gunshot wound to the buttock are the small bowel, colon, rectum, bony pelvis, and bladder. Most of the major pelvic vascular structures, the sciatic nerve, ilium, sacrum, lower colon, upper rectum, bladder, and female reproductive organs reside in the upper zone, and penetrating wounds in the upper zone have a higher risk of major injury compared to wounds in the lower zone. The lower zone contains the male bladder, prostate, urethra, and external genitalia as well as the lower part of the rectum.[1,16-18] An important component of the history is information regarding the weapon used and the patient's position at the time of injury, because this information will help determine the trajectory of the bullet or knife.

DIAGNOSIS AND TREATMENT

The evaluation of penetrating buttock wounds focuses on identification of potential injury to the lower GI and GU tract, as well as to pelvic vasculature. Perform a rectal examination to identify gross blood, and perform stool guaiac testing. Guaiac testing is not completely sensitive for GI injury; therefore, a negative guaiac test does not rule out rectal injury. Evaluate for the presence of hematuria. Assess the peripheral pulses in the lower extremities for decreased pulses or pallor as evidence of a more proximal injury. Perform a neurologic examination of the lower extremities searching for any injury to the sciatic or femoral nerve. Buttock wounds rarely cause direct damage to the sciatic plexus or femoral plexus. Injury could include transection, partial transection, or stretch injury secondary to the trauma. Table 264-2 lists the needed baseline laboratory and imaging studies.

Exploratory laparotomy is indicated for patients with hemodynamic instability or peritoneal signs. For peritonitis, obtain emergent surgical consultation and administer broad-spectrum IV antibiotics to cover for gram-negative aerobic and anaerobic organisms.

Patients with penetrating buttock injury who do not meet criteria for emergent laparotomy may be candidates for nonoperative management.[1] Selective nonoperative management uses a combination of serial exams and adjunctive modalities, including the focused assessment with sonography for trauma exam, CT, sigmoidoscopy, cystourethrogram, and angiography. Upper zone gluteal stab wounds can undergo local wound exploration to evaluate for muscle violation. Patients without muscle violation can be observed with serial exams, whereas those with muscle violation require CT and rigid sigmoidoscopy, plus cystography for hematuria.[19] Selective nonoperative management for lower zone gluteal stab wounds and all gluteal gunshot wounds is similar. CT scan, preferably with triple contrast, should be used to evaluate for injury in the stable patient (**Figure 264-3**). Obtain a cystourethrogram if there is blood on urinalysis or the wound is close to the GU tract. Perform a cystourethrogram either as a separate study or in conjunction with CT with rectal and IV contrast material, with clamping of the urethral catheter to obtain a CT cystogram.

In most cases, sufficient diagnostic workup may be obtained with CT, but rigid sigmoidoscopy is advised if there is any concern about injury to the rectum or because of the trajectory of the bullet. If the CT

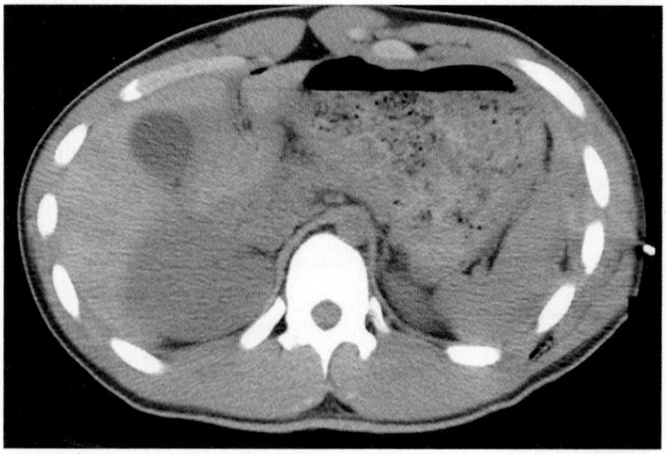

FIGURE 264-2. Noncontrast abdominal CT demonstrating splenic hematoma after a stab wound.

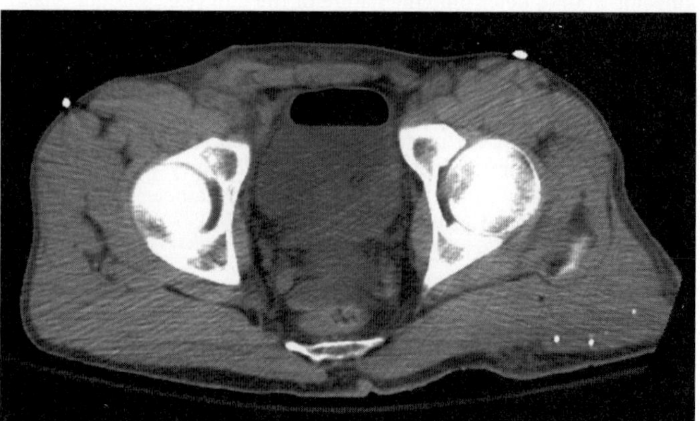

FIGURE 264-3. Noncontrast abdominopelvic CT scan after gunshot wound to the buttock. This CT scan shows bullet fragments in the gluteal muscles but no pelvic injury.

demonstrates a pelvic hematoma, angiography or venography may be indicated to document a significant vascular injury; in many centers, CT angiography has replaced these techniques, but interventional angiography may be required for extensive pelvic bleeding.[1]

REFERENCES

The complete reference list is available online at www.TintinalliEM.com.

CHAPTER 265 Genitourinary Trauma

Matthew C. Gratton
L. Keith French

INTRODUCTION

Falls, assaults, motor vehicle crashes, and sports injuries are the most common mechanisms for blunt genitourinary injuries, whereas gunshot wounds and stab wounds are the most common causes for penetrating injuries.[1] The majority of ureteral injuries are caused by penetrating trauma.[1,2] Bladder injuries are typically caused by pelvic fracture, with urethral injuries seen in 5% to 10% of pelvic fractures.[1,3] Children are more susceptible to genitourinary injury than the general population. Children lack periadipose tissue, and kidney size is large relative to overall body size.[4] Appropriate management will minimize or prevent complications such as renal function impairment, urinary incontinence, and sexual dysfunction.

CLINICAL FEATURES

HISTORY

Obtain a detailed history to determine the time and mechanism of injury and the magnitude of forces involved. In motor vehicle crashes, seat location, use of restraints, vehicle speed, and crash details provide information about forces applied to the victim. Sudden deceleration can cause major vascular disruption and parenchymal damage to the kidneys and bladder, even in the absence of symptoms and physical findings. For penetrating trauma, obtain information about the caliber of weapon or type of knife, its length, any contamination, and whether removed intact.

An inability to urinate may be due to an empty bladder or inability to void because of pain, but can also result from bladder perforation, urethral injury, or spinal cord injury.

PHYSICAL EXAMINATION

Inspect the perineum during the secondary survey. Blood on the underwear or pants is an important finding and may suggest genital trauma. Inspect the folds of the buttocks for ecchymoses, abrasions, or lacerations, which may be related to an open pelvic fracture. Do not deeply probe perineal injuries because probing could disrupt a clot.

Rectal examination identifies sphincter tone, position of the prostate gland, and presence of blood. If the prostate is "missing" or riding high or feels boggy, assume disruption of the membranous urethra until proven otherwise. In males, examine the scrotum for ecchymoses, laceration, and testicular disruption. Palpate and inspect the penis for ecchymoses, deformity, and blood at the meatus. In females, examine the vaginal introitus for lacerations and hematomas. Lacerations and hematomas can accompany pelvic fracture. Perform a speculum examination when vaginal bleeding or hematoma is present to exclude vaginal laceration. Complications of missed vaginal injuries include infection, fistula formation, and hemorrhage.

KIDNEY INJURIES

DIAGNOSIS

Renal injury is present in up to 10% of patients with abdominal trauma.[1,3] Because of the protected position of the kidneys, most injuries are associated with other intra-abdominal injuries.[5] Flank contusions or ecchymosis, palpable mass, lower rib fractures, and penetrating wounds in the flank mandate consideration of renal injury. Renal injuries consist of lacerations, avulsions, and hematomas to the kidney itself and renal pelvis. Renal vascular injuries (avulsion, laceration, occlusion) are uncommon but must be considered in the specific diagnosis of kidney injury.[6]

URINALYSIS

Although urinalysis is a commonly ordered laboratory study for suspected renal injury, **there is no direct relationship between the presence, absence, or degree of microscopic hematuria and the severity of injury**.[1,3,5] Microscopic and dipstick urinalysis are equally reliable for detecting the presence of hemoglobinuria.[5,7] However, **renal pedicle injuries and segmental arterial thrombosis may be present without hematuria**. In blunt trauma, there is some evidence suggesting that gross hematuria has predictive value for more severe renal injury.[1,5,7] In addition, patients with a systolic blood pressure of <90 mm Hg and microscopic hematuria have a higher likelihood of significant injury.[1,5] Children with <50 red blood cells per high-powered field have a low likelihood of significant renal injury.[5]

IMAGING

The main objectives of imaging are to (1) accurately stage the renal injury, (2) recognize preexisting pathology of the injured kidney, (3) document the function of the opposite kidney, and (4) identify associated injuries to other organs.[5] Imaging guidelines are listed in **Table 265-1**. An IV contrast-enhanced CT scan of the abdomen and pelvis is the imaging "gold standard" for the stable patient with suspected renal injury.[5,8,9] Contrast-enhanced CT detects contusion, lacerations, hematomas, and perfusion abnormalities (**Figure 265-1**). Early contrast extravasation is consistent with ongoing hemorrhage. However, urinary extravasation cannot be detected until the contrast-enhanced urine is excreted into the collecting system, which usually can take up to 10 minutes. Therefore, a delayed scan of the kidney, ureter, and bladder is recommended to exclude urinary extravasation from any source. If the

TABLE 265-1 Imaging for Genitourinary Trauma

Injury	Imaging	Comments
Multisystem trauma or suspected renal parenchymal or vascular injury	Abdominal-pelvic IV contrast CT scan	Include pelvis to view entire GU tract Delayed films needed to identify urinary extravasation
Any visceral injury resulting in free intraperitoneal fluid	FAST	Identifies free fluid, but does not specify type of visceral injury and does not identify renal vascular injury
Renal artery injury	Renal angiography	Details vascular injuries
Ureteral injury	Abdominal-pelvic IV contrast CT scan	Delayed films needed to identify extravasation; obtain IV pyelogram or retrograde pyelogram if still suspicious with negative CT
Bladder injury	Retrograde cystogram	Can use plain radiographs or CT scan
Urethral injury	Retrograde urethrogram	Discuss sequencing with radiologist, because if performed prior to abdominal-pelvic contrast CT scan, can interfere with diagnosis
Scrotal/testicular injury	Color Doppler US	Contrast-enhanced US or MRI if suspicion is high and initial US is negative

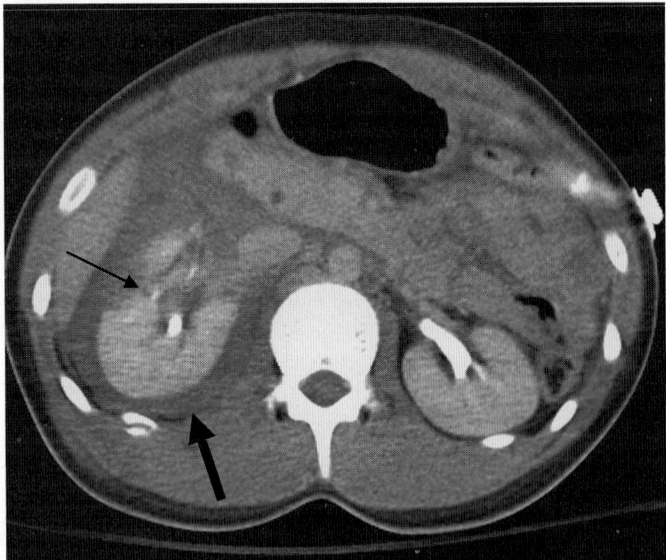

FIGURE 265-1. Renal laceration. Narrow arrow = renal laceration. Thick arrow = perinephric hematoma. [Image used with permission of Matthew C. Gratton, MD.]

kidney is normal and there is no abnormal fluid collection in the perinephric, retroperitoneal, or peripelvic areas, then the delayed scan can be omitted.

The focused assessment with sonography for trauma (FAST) examination is useful for identifying free intraperitoneal fluid, but does not specifically evaluate renal injury. FAST does not identify renal vascular injury. US examination may be useful for identifying and following postoperative fluid collections and for patients who are managed without operative intervention.[8,9]

Renal angiography can identify vascular injuries. Embolization of appropriate injuries can then be accomplished. Embolization can also be used to treat delayed traumatic arteriovenous fistulas.

GRADING OF RENAL INJURY

Grading of the renal injury is based on the American Association for the Surgery of Trauma organ injury scale (**Table 265-2**).[10] This grading system correlates with the need for operative repair and nephrectomy. In a study of 2467 patients with renal trauma, 86.5% were grade I, 3.5% grade II, 4.8% grade III, 4.0% grade IV, and 1.1% grade V. The rate of nephrectomy ranged from 0% for grades I and II to 82% for grade V.[11] Decreased kidney function is also directly correlated with renal injury grade.[12]

TREATMENT OF RENAL INJURIES

Absolute indications for renal exploration and intervention include life-threatening hemorrhage due to a renal injury; expanding, pulsatile, or noncontained retroperitoneal hematoma (thought to be from a renal avulsion injury); and a renal avulsion injury (grade V vascular injury) demonstrated on imaging studies.[5,7,8] High injury grade, high injury severity score, large blood transfusion requirement, and hemodynamic instability are predictive of the need for nephrectomy. Urinary extravasation alone is not an indication for exploration because it resolves spontaneously in the majority of cases. Extravasation from a renal pelvis or ureteral injury, however, does require repair.

TABLE 265-2 Renal Injury Scale

Grade	Description
I	Hematuria with normal anatomic studies (contusion) or subcapsular, nonexpanding hematoma; no laceration
II	Perirenal, nonexpanding hematoma or <1 cm renal cortex laceration with no urinary extravasation
III	>1 cm renal cortex laceration with no collecting system involvement or urinary extravasation
IV	Laceration through cortex and medulla and into collecting system or segmental renal artery or vein injury with hematoma
V	Shattered kidney or vascular injury to renal pedicle or avulsed kidney

Most authorities agree that grade I, II, and III renal injuries can be handled nonoperatively. Selected grade IV and V parenchymal injuries may be managed nonoperatively, although many of these patients have other indications for operative intervention.

If the trauma patient is hemodynamically stable and there is suspicion for renal injury with or without gross hematuria or if the patient has a penetrating injury, then CT imaging is indicated. If the CT scan reveals no renal pelvis, vascular, or ureteral injury and the patient remains clinically stable, then observe until the gross hematuria clears. If the CT scan reveals a renal pelvis, vascular, or ureteral injury, then surgical consultation is indicated.

Many gunshot and stab wounds to the kidneys can be treated nonoperatively. The absolute indications for operation remain those listed previously. Many patients with renal injuries have associated injuries that mandate operative intervention.

Renal Vascular Injury Renal vascular injury is identified on CT scanning and requires emergent surgical consultation in order to arrange treatment to minimize the time of renal ischemia. The optimal time to revascularization is not clear, with recommendations for timing of definitive treatment ranging from 4 to 20 hours.[6] Follow local institutional urology and trauma protocols once renal vascular injury is identified.

COMPLICATIONS

Complications that may result from renal trauma include delayed bleeding, urinary extravasation, urinoma, perinephric abscess, and hypertension and failure of the affected kidney. Delayed bleeding can occur up to a month after injury and is most commonly due to an arteriovenous fistula that has developed after a deep parenchymal laceration. Arteriovenous fistula occurs in up to 25% of cases of grade III or IV injuries that are managed conservatively.[5,13] Most can be managed with angiographic embolization, but renorrhaphy or nephrectomy may be necessary.[8,13] A urinoma may develop from a few weeks to many years after injury and may have no symptoms or may cause a feeling of abdominal discomfort, mass, or low-grade fever. Treatment is usually percutaneous drainage or ureteral stenting. A perinephric abscess can present similarly and can also be treated with percutaneous drainage. Hypertension may occur due to renal artery injury, devascularized tissue, renal parenchymal compression by clot, or by arteriovenous malformation, and may occur from days to many years after injury. Nephrectomy is the most common treatment, but medical management may be indicated.

DISPOSITION AND FOLLOW-UP

Most patients with significant renal injury are admitted on the basis of associated injuries. For patients with isolated renal trauma, few data support specific recommendations for disposition and follow-up.

Patients with isolated renal trauma and a class I injury can be separated into two groups after urology consultation. Those with a renal contusion (microscopic hematuria with normal imaging) can be discharged home as above. Patients with a subcapsular hematoma can be admitted for a short observation stay followed by a hematocrit and clinical reevaluation. Patients with gross hematuria usually need admission and require bed rest until the gross hematuria clears. Admit patients with grade II or higher injury to the hospital under the care of a trauma surgeon, general surgeon, or urologist as appropriate for the practice setting.

URETERAL INJURIES

DIAGNOSIS

Isolated ureteral injury is rare in trauma patients because the ureter is well protected in the retroperitoneum.[14,15] Approximately 80% of ureteral injuries occur from intraoperative, iatrogenic damage. Of the 20% of injuries due to external trauma, almost 90% occur as a result of

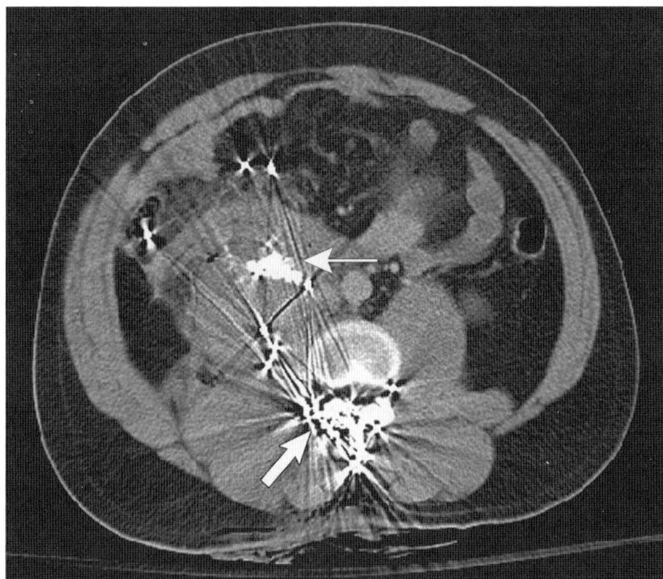

FIGURE 265-2. Ureteral injury. Narrow single arrow = contrast material that has leaked from a transected ureter. Thick arrow = multiple metallic foreign bodies with artifact (shotgun pellets).

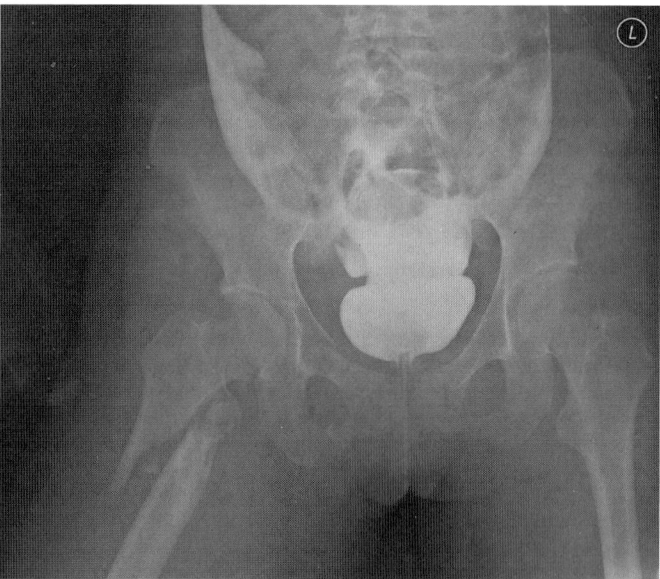

FIGURE 265-3. Bladder rupture. Retrograde cystogram demonstrates an intraperitoneal rupture of the bladder.

penetrating trauma (81% gunshot wounds, 9% stab wounds) and 10% occur due to blunt trauma.[14,15] Because there are no history or physical examination findings that are specific for ureteral injuries, these injuries can be easily missed.[7] Approximately 70% of patients with ureteral injuries have either gross or microscopic hematuria. The absence of hematuria does not exclude ureteral injury.[2,7,14]

In the stable patient with suspicion of ureteral injury, obtain a CT of the abdomen and pelvis with IV contrast with a delayed phase. Extravasation of contrast along the course of the ureter is diagnostic for ureteral injury (**Figure 265-2**).[2,7,15] If the CT is nondiagnostic and there remains a high index of suspicion for this injury, perform IV pyelography or retrograde pyelography. If there is intraoperative suspicion of ureteral injury from the course of a missile or stab wound, then further exploration is indicated.

TREATMENT AND DISPOSITION

Treatment of ureteral injuries is operative. Partial tears can be stented, and simple lacerations can be primarily repaired over a stent. More complex injuries can be reconstructed using a variety of techniques. Complications include urinary leakage, urinoma, periureteral abscess, peritonitis, ureteral stricture, and urinary fistula. All cases require urology consultation and admission for operative management.

BLADDER INJURIES

DIAGNOSIS

Bladder injury occurs in approximately 2% of blunt abdominal trauma cases, with 70% to 97% associated with pelvic fractures.[7,16] A direct blow to a distended bladder is associated with bladder rupture. Therefore, suspect bladder injury in alcohol-intoxicated patients (bladder often distended) who are in a motor vehicle crash (potentially high-energy transfer resulting in pelvic fracture).[16] Lower abdominal pain and tenderness and gross hematuria are commonly associated findings. Lower abdominal bruising, abdominal swelling from urinary ascites, perineal or scrotal edema from urinary extravasation, and inability to void are also common findings on examination of patients with bladder injury. Bladder injury also occurs secondary to penetrating trauma, and penetrating injuries to the rectum or buttocks may also have associated bladder injury.

Gross hematuria is present in most significant bladder injuries, and gross hematuria in the setting of pelvic fracture requires investigation of the bladder with a retrograde cystogram.[3,7,16] The presence of microscopic hematuria associated with a pelvic ring fracture can indicate a bladder injury, but the exact degree of microscopic hematuria warranting cystogram in this setting is undetermined and depends on clinical judgment.[16]

A retrograde cystogram is the "gold standard" imaging study for the diagnosis of bladder rupture.[16] The diagnosis is made when contrast material is seen spilling out of the bladder into the peritoneal cavity (intraperitoneal rupture) or into the retroperitoneal area surrounding the bladder (extraperitoneal rupture). This study can be performed with plain radiographs or with CT (**Figure 265-3**).[3,16] The bladder must be filled in a retrograde fashion (through an indwelling bladder catheter) by gravity feed with enough contrast material (at least 350 mL) to distend the bladder. Obtain a postvoid film. A contrast-enhanced CT with passive bladder filling, even with a clamped catheter, is not sensitive enough to exclude bladder rupture. Sonographic diagnosis of bladder rupture is not accurate.[16]

TREATMENT AND DISPOSITION

Extraperitoneal ruptures of the bladder are most common (55%), followed by intraperitoneal (38%) and combined intra-/extraperitoneal ruptures (5% to 8%).[7] Intraperitoneal ruptures always require surgical exploration and repair.[7] Extraperitoneal ruptures can usually be managed with bladder catheter drainage alone. Approximately 85% to 90% will heal within 10 days with simple drainage, and the remainder will likely heal within 3 weeks.[3,7,16] **Table 265-3** lists conditions when operative repair may be needed for extraperitoneal rupture.[7]

Missed intraperitoneal rupture can lead to urinary ascites, local abscess, peritonitis, or sepsis.[7] If bladder neck injuries or rectal or vaginal injuries are missed, then incontinence or fistula may result.[7] Associated injury to the sacral nerve roots or pelvic nerves can damage innervation of the bladder, resulting in a neurogenic bladder or impotence.[7] Simple ruptures are less likely to produce complications but may occasionally be

TABLE 265-3 Operative Repair May Be Needed for Extraperitoneal Rupture of the Bladder
Urinary catheter does not allow appropriate drainage
Associated rectal or vaginal injury
Associated bladder neck injury
Open fixation of a pelvic fracture (to avoid contamination of the hardware)

associated with persistent bladder diverticulum, decreased bladder volume, or urinary tract infection.

Because bladder rupture is frequently associated with other injuries, admitting the patient for either operative intervention or catheter drainage under the care of a trauma surgeon, general surgeon, or urologist is the general rule.

URETHRAL INJURIES

DIAGNOSIS

Timely diagnosis and effective treatment of urethral injury are paramount to limiting long-term adverse outcomes, including impotence, stricture, urinary retention, or incontinence. Urethral injuries are less common in women primarily due to differences in urethral length (4 cm in women vs. 20 cm in men).[1] Urethral injuries are classified anatomically as either anterior or posterior, an important distinction because comorbid injuries and treatment may vary.

POSTERIOR URETHRAL INJURIES

The posterior urethra consists of prostatic and membranous portions. Because the posterior urethra is relatively well insulated by bony and soft tissues, injuries here are generally the result of major blunt-force trauma from deceleration mechanisms such as motor vehicle collisions or falls from heights. Such mechanisms lead to shearing forces applied to the prostatic-membranous urethral junction. Posterior urethral injuries may occur in about 10% of patients with pelvic fractures.[17]

ANTERIOR URETHRAL INJURIES

The anterior urethra is divided into the relatively fixed bulbar segment and the pendulous (penile) segment. Anterior urethral injuries are generally the result of direct perineal trauma, either blunt or penetrating. Trauma to the anterior urethra may be missed initially, and patients may present years later with urethral stricture. Straddle injury is the classic mechanism, although strikes or kicks to the perineum may lead to the same injury. The bulbar rather than pendulous segment is typically affected.[18] Anterior urethral trauma can also occur as a result of penile fracture. Penetrating trauma to the urethra usually occurs to the penile urethra. Evaluate for female urethral injuries in association with extensive pelvic fractures.

CLINICAL FEATURES

Suspect urethral injury from common mechanisms (straddle or penetrating perineal injuries), comorbid injuries (pelvic fractures), or iatrogenic complications (traumatic catheterization). Symptoms may include hematuria, dysuria, or inability to void. Rectal and perineal examination may demonstrate a perineal hematoma or high-riding prostate. Posterior urethral injury is suggested by the triad of urinary retention, blood at the meatus, and a high-riding prostate.[19] Intuitively, hematuria should be a helpful clue; however, this is neither specific nor sensitive enough to be used alone to diagnose or exclude a urethral injury.[20] Difficulty passing a Foley catheter raises concern for a urethral injury; insertion should never be a forceful process. Most female urethral injuries present with vaginal bleeding. A careful vaginal inspection is important because this may reveal findings suggestive of urethral injury, such as blood at the vaginal introitus.[19] In women, no consensus exists on the best modality to detect urethral injury because cystography or urethrography may not be adequate.[21]

DIAGNOSIS

The diagnosis of urethral injury is made by retrograde urethrogram, which should be performed before catheterization to prevent further urethral injury. If there are any signs of possible urethral injury, such as high-riding prostate, meatal blood, perineal ecchymosis, scrotal hematoma, pelvic fracture, or gross hematuria, do not insert a Foley catheter until urethral injury is excluded.[22]

Perform retrograde urethrogram by gently injecting 20 to 30 mL of contrast into the urethra and obtaining a radiograph. Extravasation identifies the existence and location of the urethral tear. In partial anterior urethral lacerations, the retrograde urethrogram reveals contrast extravasation at the site of injury and contrast material outlining the urethra proximal to the site of injury (**Figure 265-4**). In complete anterior urethral lacerations, the retrograde urethrogram reveals contrast extravasation at the site of injury without contrast proximal to the site of injury. Extravasation of contrast along fascial planes of the perineum is another indication of urethral disruption. **Performing a retrograde urethrogram before completing a CT of the abdomen and pelvis to evaluate for other life-threatening injuries can interfere with CT diagnosis and embolization treatment of pelvic arterial extravasation from pelvic fractures, so discuss the sequencing of studies with the trauma surgeon, urologist, or radiologist.**[23,24] If a Foley catheter has

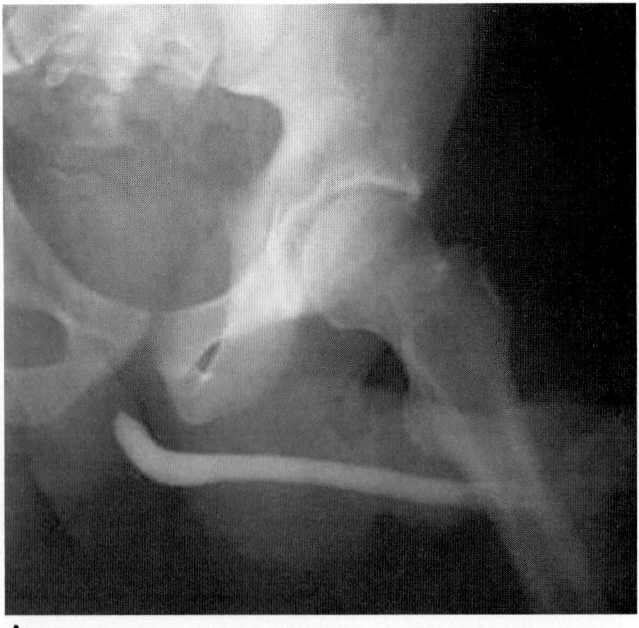

A

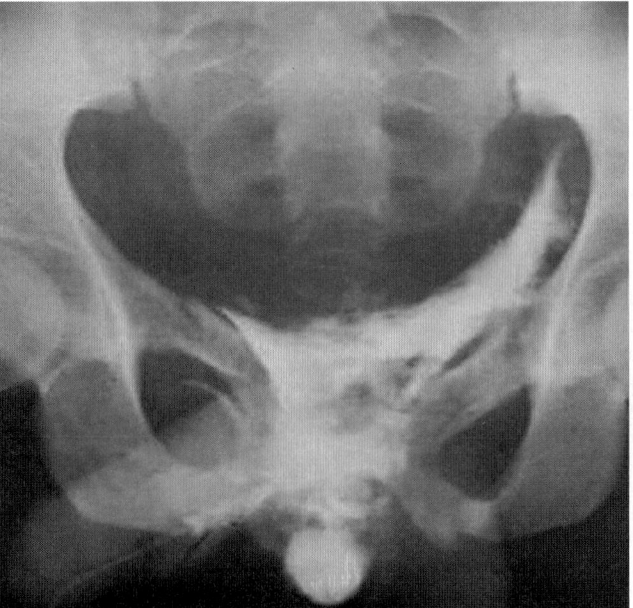

B

FIGURE 265-4. **A.** Normal retrograde urethrogram. **B.** Extravasation of contrast.

already been successfully inserted, and then a urethral injury is considered, keep the Foley catheter in place. Using a 16-gauge angiocatheter, inject contrast material at the meatus, around the urinary catheter, and then obtain radiographs in the standard fashion.[25] In males, the location and displacement of anterior pelvic fractures, if present, can predict the risk of urethral injury. For every millimeter of symphysis pubis diastasis or inferomedial pubic bone fracture displacement, the risk of urethral injury increases by 10%.[26]

TREATMENT AND DISPOSITION

Patients with urethral trauma often have multiple injuries, some of which take precedence over the urethra trauma. Prioritize treatment(s) according to standard Advanced Trauma Life Support guidelines. The treatment for male patients with posterior urethral injury secondary to pelvic fracture has generally been immediate placement of a suprapubic catheter (for bladder drainage) with delayed surgical repair (often weeks later). Suprapubic catheter placement allows for urinary drainage without urethral manipulation or disruption of a pelvic hematoma. The suprapubic catheter can be placed either percutaneously or by an open approach using a small incision. Use US guidance to aid in the percutaneous approach. Early endoscopic repair may lead to equally good potency and continence outcomes while reducing the rates of urethral stricture.[27-29]

Most penetrating injuries to the anterior urethra require surgical exploration and repair. Female urethra injuries are difficult to manage because the diagnosis is often clinical. It is more difficult to perform urethrography in women. Concomitant bladder injury needs to be excluded with CT cystography. Consider antegrade cystogram through a suprapubic tube and cystoscopy if the diagnosis remains uncertain. Because urethral injury is frequently associated with other injuries, admit the patient for either operative intervention or catheter drainage under the care of a trauma surgeon, general surgeon, or urologist.

INJURIES TO THE EXTERNAL GENITALIA

CLINICAL FEATURES

One study reported that 25% of patients sustaining injury to the external genitalia required red blood cell transfusion due to blood loss from genital injury alone, so carefully assess for signs of blood loss as well as evaluating for local injury.[30]

Penile fracture, with or without urethral injury, occurs when the corpus cavernosum ruptures after being forcibly bent, usually during sexual intercourse. A cracking sound may be heard, followed by penile pain, rapid swelling, discoloration, and visible deformity ("eggplant deformity").[31] Amputations are usually self-inflicted or result from clothing trapped by heavy machinery. Self-inflicted trauma to the penis can also result from vacuum cleaner injuries, which cause extensive injury to the glans penis and urethra. Strangulation from constricting penile rings used to enhance erections is another mechanism of injury. Penetrating injuries are less common and may also involve the urethra.

Injuries to the scrotum may occur from blunt or penetrating trauma, burns, and avulsions. More than half of all testicular trauma is a result of sporting activity.[31] Impingement of the testicles against the symphysis pubis is the primary cause of blunt testicular injuries. Resultant injury to the testicle ranges from contusion to rupture. In both conditions, the tunica vaginalis fills with blood, forming a hematocele. If the tunica albuginea is disrupted, a rupture has occurred. Traumatic dislocation of the testicle is a rare event and most commonly occurs following straddle injuries from motorcycle accidents.[32]

Symptoms after a direct scrotal blow are usually scrotal pain and swelling. Other signs may include scrotal discoloration and a tender, firm scrotal mass that fails to transilluminate, which indicates a hematocele. An empty hemiscrotum suggests testicular dislocation. An open wound to the scrotum suggests the possibility of testicular involvement. Many patients will be exquisitely tender, potentially limiting a thorough exam. Furthermore, the external signs of trauma may not correlate well with the degree of testicular injury; thus, there should be a low threshold for diagnostic imaging.[31]

DIAGNOSIS

Color Doppler US is the diagnostic modality of choice in the evaluation of scrotal/testicular trauma.[31] Although there is no advantage initially, contrast-enhanced US and testicular MRI may be useful adjuncts if the Doppler US results are inconclusive and clinical suspicion remains high for testicular injury.[32-35] CT plays an important role in the evaluation of concomitant abdominopelvic injuries. Penile injuries often result in urethral injuries; thus, consider retrograde urethrogram in this scenario. While the diagnosis of penile fracture is largely clinical, US may detect corpus cavernosum hematomas and can be an adjunct to both diagnosis and operative management.[36]

TREATMENT

Most closed testicular contusions are managed conservatively with narcotic analgesics, ice, elevation, scrotal support, and appropriate urologic follow-up. Testicular rupture requires immediate drainage and repair. The salvage rate following testicular rupture may be as high as 90% if treated promptly.[31] Any patient with penetrating scrotal trauma should undergo immediate scrotal exploration.[37] Obtain emergent urologic consultation for all confirmed or suspect penile fractures. With immediate surgical intervention, erectile function may be spared.[36]

Traumatic epididymitis is a noninfectious inflammatory condition that usually occurs within a few days after a blow to the testis. Treatment is similar to that for nontraumatic epididymitis.[38]

All penetrating trauma to the penis requires surgical consultation and, in most cases, exploration. Loss of penile skin by avulsion injury or burns is managed by split-thickness skin grafts after the denuded penis is clean and sterile. Do not reapply avulsed skin, because avulsed skin invariably becomes necrotic and infected and must be subsequently removed. Penile amputations require repair by microsurgical reimplantation if the amputated segment is deemed viable by the urologist.

Strangulation injuries can usually be managed simply by removing the constricting agent. Zipper injury to the penis is caused when the penile skin is trapped in the trouser zipper. Mineral oil and lidocaine infiltration are useful in freeing the penile skin from the zipper. Otherwise, wire-cutting or bone-cutting pliers are used to divide the median bar (or diamond) of the zipper, which causes the zipper to fall apart, freeing the penile skin. Contusions of the perineum or penis are treated conservatively with cold packs, rest, and elevation. Insert a Foley catheter if the patient is unable to void.

SPECIAL POPULATIONS

ELDERLY

As men age, they experience anatomic changes, including laxity of scrotal tissue, atrophy of the perineal muscles, and loss of collagen tissue. Changes in women are secondary to declining secretion of estrogen after menopause and include atrophy of the cervix and uterus, atrophy of the walls of the vaginal canal, decrease in vaginal length and width, and decrease in vaginal lubrication.[39] These changes predispose the elderly to complex injuries of the external genitalia even with a minor mechanism of injury. Compared to younger trauma patients, trauma to the genitourinary system in the elderly patient tends to be more common from blunt mechanisms and tends to result in higher rates of bladder and urethral injuries.[40]

The presence of a **penile prosthesis** can transform a minimal blunt trauma genital injury into a complicated surgical issue for the patient.[41] Extrusion and rupture of penile prostheses predispose patients to infection and complications of wound healing. This becomes a special concern in diabetic patients who are more likely to have prostheses. Obtain urologic consultation for any patient who has sustained trauma to the genitalia with a prosthesis in place (see chapter 95, Complications of Urologic Procedures and Devices).

PREGNANT WOMEN

With pregnancy, women experience physiologic changes that predispose them to more severe injury in both blunt and penetrating trauma to the genitalia. During pregnancy, venous outflow from the perineal area is slowed because of the pressure on the vena cava from the enlarging uterus. Slowed blood flow to the area can cause edema of the vulva. The increased level of progesterone during pregnancy also contributes to fluid retention and edema of the genitalia. Engorgement of the perineum predisposes pregnant patients to increased risk of hemorrhage from penetrating trauma to this anatomic region.

CHILDREN

Roughly 33% of males worldwide are circumcised.[42] The aim of circumcision is to excise sufficient foreskin (both penile shaft and inner preputial epithelium) to leave the glans uncovered. Complications of circumcision are more common in children than in neonates. Several different techniques and devices are employed to perform circumcision, each with its own complication profile. Early complications of circumcision include bleeding, infection, pain, and inadequate skin removal.[42] Bleeding is the most common complication, occurring in 1% of patients.[43] Direct pressure alone is adequate to stop bleeding in most scenarios, although in some instances, the application of pressure alone is insufficient to control local hemorrhage and other methods of hemostasis must be employed. Circumferential dressings may cause urinary retention and even necrosis of the distal penis if blood flow is compromised.

The clinical evaluation of prepubescent females with blunt urogenital trauma may underestimate the severity of injuries when compared with examination under anesthesia. Consider consultation for examination under anesthesia for accurate diagnosis and to minimize psychological sequelae of examination.[44] In boys, nonsexual trauma to the external genitalia most commonly occurs between ages 6 and 12 years. Sports accidents, kicks, and falls are the typical mechanisms, and scrotal and penile lacerations or testicular contusions are the most common injuries.[45]

REFERENCES

The complete reference list is available online at www.TintinalliEM.com.

CHAPTER 266 Trauma to the Extremities

James Heilman

INTRODUCTION AND EPIDEMIOLOGY

Isolated trauma to an extremity with associated vascular injury has nearly a 10% rate of mortality or limb loss.[1] Injuries involving the lower extremities are more common than injuries involving the upper extremities. The two most commonly injured blood vessels are the femoral and popliteal vessels.[2] Penetrating trauma with early shock from proximal arterial hemorrhage is more likely to lead to mortality. Blunt distal extremity trauma with associated distal vascular injury is more commonly involved in early limb loss and amputations.

Advances in diagnostic imaging[3] and surgical management have dramatically reduced the rate of limb loss and disability due to limb ischemia.[4] The extent of injury to extremity nerves, bones, and soft tissues now determines if the limb can be surgically salvaged. Identifying and detecting which injuries require surgical evaluation and/or imaging are essential skills for emergency physicians.

PATHOPHYSIOLOGY

Gunshot and knife wounds are the two most common causes of penetrating trauma. Stab wounds have a more predictable pattern of injury, making them more straightforward to manage. Gunshot injuries are more difficult to evaluate due to the extent of tissue damage and wider range of patterns of injury. More sophisticated vascular surgical repair techniques of arterial injuries,[5] advances made during military conflicts, improved imaging, and other factors have led to a decreased rate of limb amputations and limb disability associated with penetrating trauma.[6]

CLINICAL FEATURES

Perform the primary trauma survey, immediate resuscitation, and secondary survey before focusing on injuries to the extremities. Apply direct pressure, pressure dressings, or a tourniquet to any actively bleeding extremity (see chapter 254, "Trauma in Adults," and "Tourniquets"). Do not get distracted or deviate from the initial trauma management because associated injuries to other areas of the body are common with penetrating injuries. After identifying an injury during the secondary survey, thoroughly evaluate the affected extremity for vascular integrity, nerve function, skeletal injury, and soft tissue injury. The rapid evaluation of extremities for associated arterial injury is critically important for the management of these injuries. Note any hard or soft signs of vascular injury (**Table 266-1**). Use a Doppler flow device to detect a pulse if distal pulses cannot be palpated.

Thoroughly evaluate nerve, tendon, and muscle function during the physical exam (**Table 266-2**). Pain on palpation or movement of bony structures or obvious deformities suggests an underlying fracture. Note any intra-articular hematomas or other signs of joint injury. Measure soft tissue lacerations and other associated injuries with a tape measure or ruler. Accurately describe injuries to consultants because measurement of the injury may change management in some situations.[7]

ANKLE-BRACHIAL INDEX

In the absence of hard signs, determine the ankle-brachial index for any injured extremity along with the nonaffected extremity for comparison. An ankle-brachial index reading of <0.9 is considered abnormal and is concerning for associated arterial injury. The ankle-brachial index reliably detects occlusive arterial injury with accuracy as high as 95%, but the true sensitivity and specificity have varied in clinical studies.[8,9] Use caution in relying on a normal ankle-brachial index to rule out arterial injury, because it does not detect nonocclusive arterial injuries such as intimal flaps, focal narrowings, small pseudoaneurysms, and arteriovenous fistulas in up to 10% of cases.[10]

DIAGNOSIS

Diagnosis of associated injuries depends on a complete history and physical exam of the involved extremity. If any hard signs of vascular injury are present, then consult vascular surgery immediately. If there are any soft signs of vascular injury and/or if the ankle-brachial index is <0.9, then order imaging tests to evaluate for associated vascular

TABLE 266-1 Clinical Manifestations of Extremity Vascular Trauma

Hard signs
Absent or diminished distal pulses
Obvious arterial bleeding
Large expanding or pulsatile hematoma
Audible bruit
Palpable thrill
Distal ischemia (pain, pallor, paralysis, paresthesias, coolness)
Soft signs
Small, stable hematoma
Injury to anatomically related nerve
Unexplained hypotension
History of hemorrhage
Proximity of injury to major vascular structures
Complex fracture

TABLE 266-2 Clinical Examination of the Nerves of the Extremities

Nerve	Test of Motor Function	Test for Sensation
Axillary (C5-C6)	Arm abduction	Lateral aspect of shoulder
	Arm internal, external rotation	
Musculocutaneous (C5-C6)	Forearm flexion	Lateral forearm
Radial (C5-C8)	Forearm, wrist, and finger extension	Dorsoradial hand, thumb
Median (C6-T1)	Wrist flexion, finger adduction	Volar aspect of thumb and index finger
Ulnar (C7-T1)	Finger abduction	Volar aspect of little finger
Femoral (L1-L4)	Knee extension	
Obturator (L2-L4)	Hip adduction	
Superior gluteal (L4-S1)	Hip abduction	
Sciatic (L4-S3)	Knee flexion	
Deep peroneal (L4-S1)	Ankle and great toe dorsiflexion	
Superficial peroneal (L5-S1)	Foot eversion	
Tibial (L5-S2)	Ankle plantar flexion	
Posterior tibial (L5-S2)	Great toe plantar flexion	
Spinal L4		Medial calf
Spinal L5		Dorsal foot
Spinal S1		Lateral plantar foot

injuries, or transfer to an institution with vascular care capability (**Figure 266-1**).

DIFFERENTIAL DIAGNOSIS

The differential diagnosis for injuries associated with penetrating trauma to the extremities includes arterial or venous injury, nerve damage, tendon lacerations, fractures, soft tissue injury, degloving injuries, damage to joint capsule, bullet embolization of artery, or vein and compartment syndrome.[11]

LABORATORY TESTING

No specific laboratory testing is indicated for isolated penetrating extremity injuries; in certain cases, type and screening and a CBC may be indicated. If the patient has soft signs of vascular injury or an ankle-brachial index <0.9, then obtain a creatinine to determine renal function in patients with risk for preexisting renal disease. Underlying renal insufficiency creates potential for contrast-induced nephropathy when performing CT angiography. See chapter 88, "Acute Kidney Injury" for discussion of radiocontrast-induced nephropathy.

IMAGING

Plain Radiographs Obtain anteroposterior and lateral radiographs of extremities with suspected fracture, joint injury, or retained bullet or other foreign body fragments. Oblique views may add value if the physician has a strong clinical suspicion of retained foreign body and it is not shown on anteroposterior and lateral views. Obtain radiographs of the joint above and below the site of injury. Evidence of air in the joint or an intra-articular fracture on the radiograph demonstrates that joint involvement has occurred.

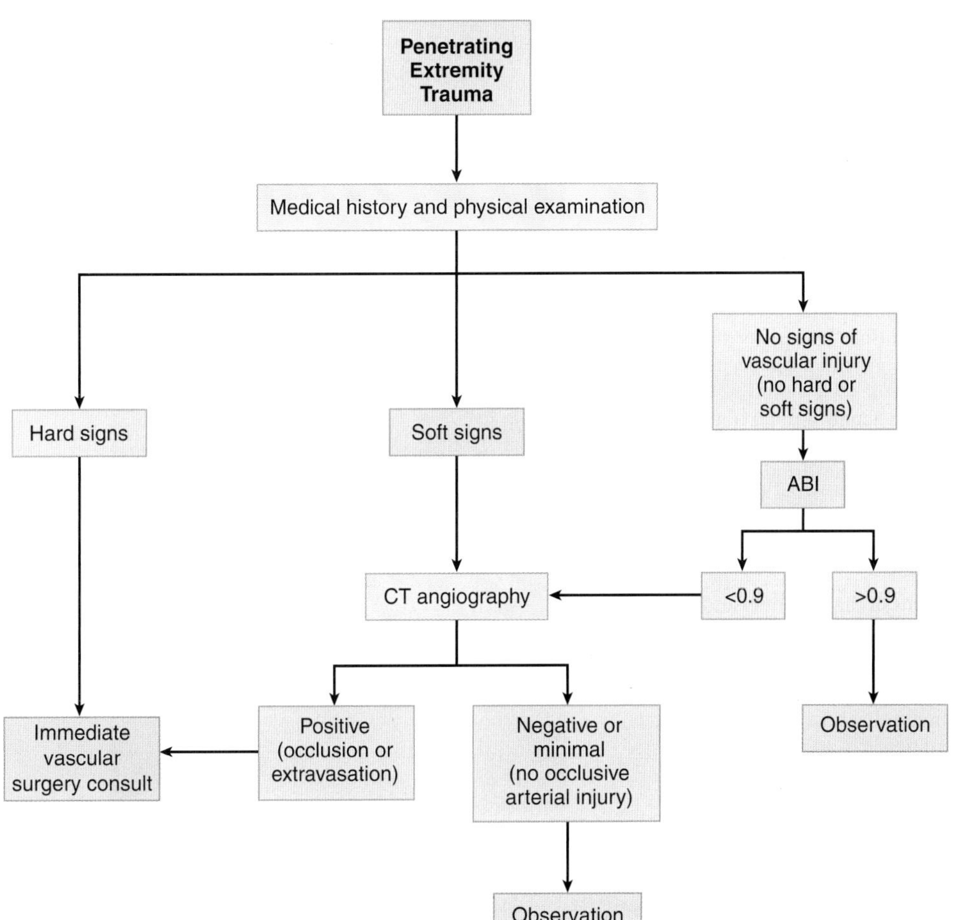

FIGURE 266-1. Algorithm for penetrating extremity trauma. ABI = ankle-brachial index.

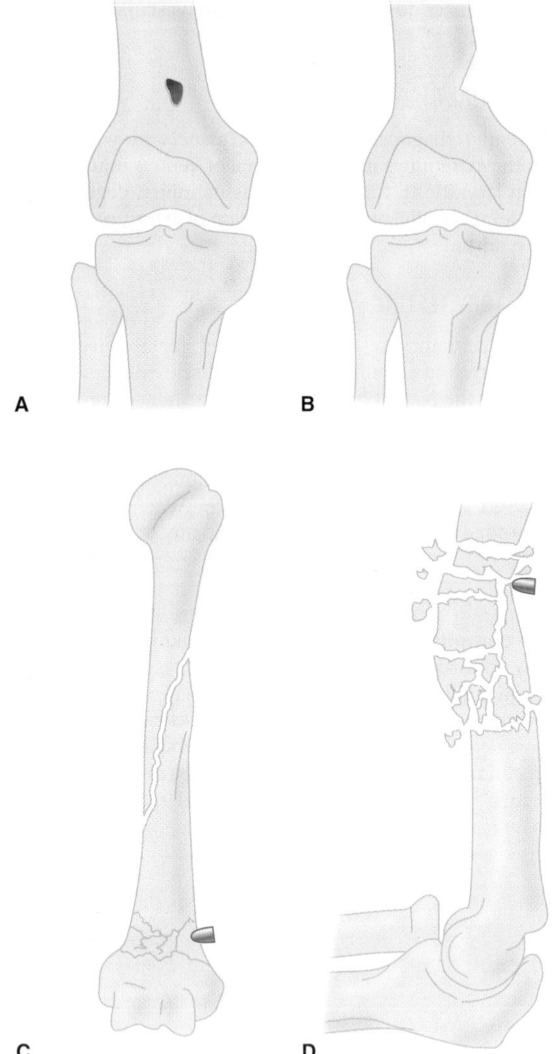

FIGURE 266-2. Fracture patterns created by bullets: drill-hole (A), unicortical (B), distant spiral (C), comminuted (D).

There are four types of fracture patterns associated with low-energy gunshots[12] (**Figure 266-2**). The drill-hole wound track pattern appears in the more porous and lower density cancellous bone. This pattern is most common in the distal femur, pelvis, and proximal humerus. Unicortical fractures appear in the metaphyses of long bones and occur only due to tangential impact with the bone. Comminuted fractures occur most frequently in diaphyseal bone; multiple bone fragments are common. The fourth type of fracture is the distal spiral fracture, and this occurs most commonly in the femur. There is controversy in the literature over whether this fracture is caused by the bullet itself or associated with falls that occur after the gunshot injury is sustained.[13]

For shotgun or blast injuries, obtain radiographs of the extremity and joint distal to the injury in order to detect any pellets that have embedded into the bone, remain in the soft tissues, or have potentially entered into a joint capsule (**Figure 266-3**).

CT Angiography CT angiography is the primary diagnostic study for the evaluation of vascular injuries to the extremities.[2] CT angiography is noninvasive, provides higher resolution images, and is less expensive when compared to catheter angiography. It provides three-dimensional reconstruction with minimal artifact. CT angiography also assists in the evaluation of extravascular injuries such as fractures, foreign objects, or joint involvement.[14] Studies comparing CT angiography to catheter angiography have demonstrated that the CT angiography sensitivity and specificity rates for identifying clinically significant arterial injuries are

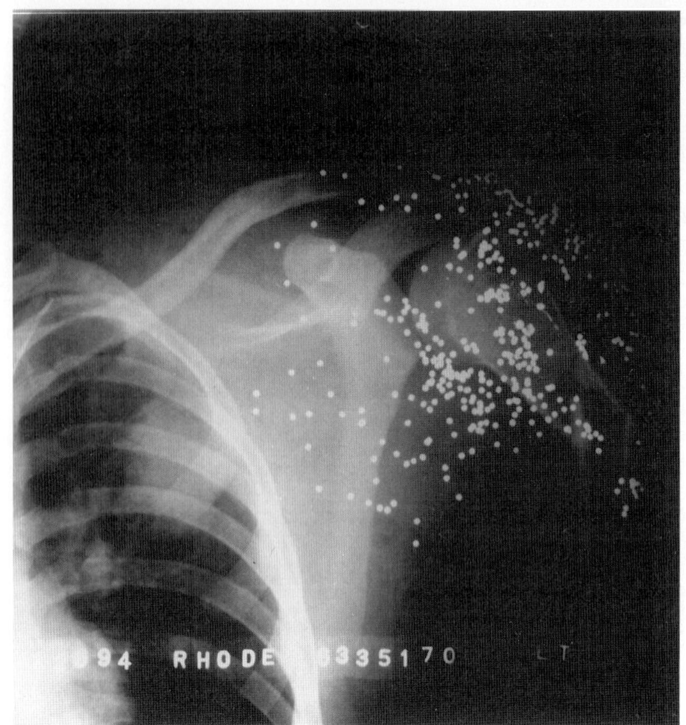

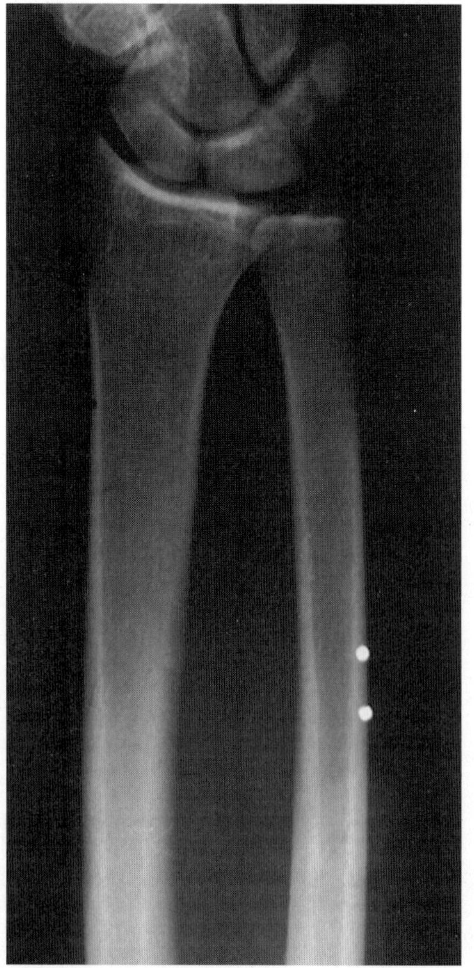

FIGURE 266-3. A. Gunshot wound to the shoulder and axilla. B. Embedded pellet of shotgun in the distal ulna, illustrating the importance of obtaining images of the extremity distal to such injuries.

equivalent to those with conventional catheter angiography.[15-18] Limitations of CT angiography include scatter artifact interference caused by bullets, poor visualization of tibial vessels, and the inability to perform any therapeutic interventions during the study.

Ultrasonography Color flow duplex ultrasonography has a sensitivity that ranges from 50% to 100% for evaluating vascular injuries.[19,20] Given this mixed evidence of accuracy, color flow duplex ultrasonography should not be used as the primary diagnostic study to rule out vascular injuries associated with penetrating trauma to extremities.[10]

TREATMENT

CONTROL OF BLEEDING

Patients with venous trauma can bleed profusely. Control bleeding with direct pressure, pressure dressing, or a tourniquet. Avoid clamping vessels in an attempt to control bleeding, as this risks nerve damage. Nerves are bundled with vascular structures and can be easily damaged by blind clamping or ligation during the initial trauma resuscitation.

ARTERIAL INJURY

Penetrating injuries to the extremities that involve any associated arterial injury are critically important to recognize early. Figure 266-1 outlines the approach to these injuries.

FRACTURES AND JOINT INJURIES

Penetrating trauma can cause joint sepsis and destruction, rapid chondrolysis, and loss of anatomic contours. These can lead to serious long-term consequences, including posttraumatic degenerative arthritis and partial or total loss of flexibility. Treat bone fractures from penetrating trauma as open fractures. Surgically debride the injury and admit the patient for IV antibiotics, such as a cephalosporin plus gentamicin. Synovial joint fluid is an organic acid, which causes lead bullets to become soluble in the joint and can cause systemic lead toxicity.[21] If a patient has an obvious bony or joint capsule injury, obtain consultation to evaluate the injury.

WOUND MANAGEMENT

Careful wound management is critical to prevent infection after penetrating injuries. The most important component of wound management is irrigation. Copiously irrigate with saline or tap water (500 to 1000 mL) at high pressures (15 to 20 pounds per square inch). Antiseptic solution does not decrease infection rate and may actually be harmful.[22]

Heavily contaminated wounds may require more fluid and/or more pressure. If the wound is older than 3 to 4 hours, gently scrub the wound. Despite the importance of irrigation and wound management, there are many other factors that play a role in infection risk and proper healing, including bacterial inoculum, tissue devitalization, blood supply, time to presentation and treatment, presence of foreign bodies, and host immune status.

WOUND CLOSURE

The decision to close associated open wounds depends on the time that has elapsed since the injury and the degree of contamination. If there is minimal contamination and the wound is well irrigated, it can be closed. It is important to arrange close follow-up in 24 to 48 hours in order to check for developing wound infection. Extremity wounds with retained foreign bodies, major tissue destruction, or contamination should be closed after a delay of 72 to 96 hours. Do not routinely administer antibiotics for uncomplicated extremity gunshot and knife wounds because there is an approximately 2% rate of infection in these injuries.[23] However, antibiotics may be beneficial for treating hand injuries, joint or bony involvement, immunocompromised patients, and wounds with significant contamination.[24]

SOFT TISSUE FOREIGN BODIES

Plain radiographs will detect glass, metal, bone, or gravel. Wood and other organic material may be missed on plain films, and US is better at identifying these objects. CT scanning is the best modality for identifying both radiolucent and opaque foreign bodies. Several factors impact whether the foreign body should be removed. The benefit of exploring the wound and removing the substance must be weighed against the associated damage to surrounding tissues and the increased risk of infection. Organic material is more reactive and has a higher rate of infection than metal or glass. A bullet generally should not be removed unless the bullet has potential to migrate into surrounding vital structures or if it is in the joint capsule.

DISPOSITION, FOLLOW-UP, AND DISEASE COMPLICATIONS

Hard signs of arterial injury require immediate surgical consultation, and such patients will need further imaging, surgery, and hospital admission. All other patients with penetrating extremity trauma should undergo a period of observation with associated serial examinations to detect any delayed or missed injuries. There is no consensus on the required observation time required, but a minimum of 24 hours is reasonable.[17]

Wound healing may be complicated by infections, missed nerve injuries, tendon or joint injuries, delayed vascular injury, and compartment syndrome. Discuss return precautions with patients before discharge. State these precautions as clearly as possible. Recommend that patients return to the ED for increasing pain, numbness, weakness, redness, or pus drainage from the wound site. Ensuring follow-up with the appropriate surgical service, a primary care provider, or the ED is essential, especially in uninsured patients or patients transported long distances from home, as well as for other high-risk populations.

SPECIAL CONSIDERATIONS/SPECIAL POPULATIONS

Uninsured, African American, and Latino populations have higher traumatic injury mortality when compared to the general population. Increased mortality has been demonstrated in the uninsured and the nonwhite populations for lower extremity vascular injuries.[25] Ensure appropriate follow-up and outline clear return precautions. If reliable follow-up cannot be arranged, then consider a longer period of ED or hospital observation.

PRACTICE GUIDELINES

- American College of Surgeons: *Advanced Trauma Life Support (ATLS®) Manual*, 9th ed. Washington, DC: American College of Surgeons, 2012.
- American College of Emergency Physicians (ACEP): Clinical policy for the initial approach to patients presenting with penetrating extremity trauma. 1999.
- Eastern Association for the Surgery of Trauma (EAST): Evaluation and management of penetrating lower extremity arterial trauma: An Eastern Association for the Surgery of Trauma practice management guideline. 2012.

REFERENCES

The complete reference list is available online at www.TintinalliEM.com.

SECTION 22

Injuries to Bones and Joints

CHAPTER 267 Initial Evaluation and Management of Orthopedic Injuries

Jeffrey S. Menkes

INTRODUCTION

Musculoskeletal trauma involves injury to one or more of the following structures:

Bone: A unit of the skeleton composed of the hardest variety of connective tissue. Bones give shape and support to the body. In addition to surrounding and protecting vital organs, they serve as points of attachment for the muscles of the limbs, making movement possible.

Joint: The area where two or more bones articulate with one another. Joints are usually classified in terms of the amount of motion permitted at the articulation. Most joints of the extremities are synovial joints, which allow the greatest amount of motion.

Ligament: A bundle of connective tissue forming part of the fibrous capsule surrounding a joint and attached to it. Every joint of the extremities is reinforced by two or more ligaments, whose purpose is to stabilize the joint by confining its movements to specific planes and preventing movement beyond physiologic limits.

Tendon: The fibrous structure connecting a voluntary muscle to bone, cartilage, or ligaments. Tendons enable muscles to effect motion in the joint or body area to which they are attached.

Orthopedic injuries to these structures include the following:

Fracture: A disruption of bone tissue. Fractures may be caused by: (1) an application of force exceeding the strength of the bone, (2) repetitive stress, or (3) an invasive process that undermines the bone's integrity.

Dislocation: Complete disruption of a joint, such that the articular surfaces of the bones that comprise the joint are no longer in contact with one another.

Subluxation: Partial disruption of a joint, in which some degree of contact between the articular surfaces remains.

Fracture-dislocation or fracture-subluxation: Disruption of a joint combined with fracture of at least one of the bones involved in the articulation.

Strain: A tearing injury to muscle fibers resulting from excessive tension or overuse.

Sprain: A tearing injury to one or more ligaments of a joint, which occurs when the joint is forced beyond the limits of its normal planes of motion.

PATHOPHYSIOLOGY OF FRACTURES

Properly assessing and treating bony injuries in the ED requires an understanding of the physiologic processes by which fractures are created and by which they heal. Practical knowledge of fracture pathophysiology may provide the index of suspicion needed to diagnose an injury that might otherwise be missed. It also may help prevent or minimize complications and sometimes may form the basis for advising the patient regarding the outlook for recovery of function.

TYPES OF FRACTURES

Although fractures are sometimes classified in terms of the mechanism that created them, they also may be described in terms of the physiology involved.

"Common" Fractures Most fractures are the result of significant trauma to healthy bone. The bony cortex may be disrupted by a variety of forces, including a direct blow, axial loading, angular (bending) forces, torque (twisting stress), or a combination of these.

Pathologic Fractures Fractures that result from relatively minor trauma to diseased or otherwise abnormal bone are termed pathologic fractures. In such cases, a preexisting process has weakened the bone and rendered it susceptible to fracture by forces that, under normal circumstances, would not disrupt the cortex. Common examples of such injuries are fractures through metastatic lesions, fractures through benign bone cysts, and vertebral compression fractures in patients with advanced osteoporosis. Numerous other disease processes may render an individual susceptible to pathologic fracture. Because these injuries often are not associated with a history of significant trauma, subtle pathologic fractures may go undetected unless there is a clinical index of suspicion.

Stress Fractures Bone may undergo a "fatigue" fracture by being subjected to repetitive forces before the bone and its supporting tissues have had adequate time to accommodate to such forces. An example is a metatarsal shaft fracture in unconditioned foot soldiers ("**march fracture**"). Radiographs often are negative early in the clinical course of stress fractures. The initial diagnosis may be presumptive, based solely on the history and findings of point tenderness or localized swelling. Days or weeks may pass before the fracture line or new bone formation becomes visible radiographically.

Salter (Epiphyseal Plate) Fractures Fractures involving the physis, the cartilaginous epiphyseal plate near the ends of the long bones of growing children, were originally classified by Salter and Harris[1] and are commonly called *Salter fractures*. New bony material needed for the elongation of bones during growth is provided by specialized cells within the physis. When growth is completed, the physis transforms from cartilage into bone, ultimately fusing with the bone surrounding it, and disappearing as a distinct entity. By definition, Salter fractures cannot occur in fully grown adults.

Damage to the epiphyseal plate during a child's growth may destroy part or all of its ability to produce new bone substance, resulting in aborted or deformed growth of the limb. The potential for growth disturbance from an epiphyseal plate injury is related to the number of years the child has yet to grow (the older the child, the less time remains for deformity to develop) and to the pattern of the fracture line through the epiphyseal area. Classification of Salter fractures and their clinical implications are discussed in the section Describing Radiographs in this chapter.

FRACTURE HEALING

An understanding of the short- and long-term aspects of bone healing helps decision making regarding fracture reduction, treatment modality, and the prognosis for regaining function or being left with residual deformity. Fracture healing consists of three phases: inflammatory, reparative, and remodeling, each of which blends into the next, with some degree of overlap between them.[2] When a fracture occurs, the microvessels crossing the fracture line are severed, depriving the damaged bone ends of their blood supply. As a result, the bone ends gradually necrose, triggering a classic inflammatory response in which neutrophils, macrophages, and lymphocytes migrate to the area. The proteins and peptides (collectively termed *cytokines*) released by these cells promote revascularization.[3] This early phase is brief but creates the tissue environment for the most predominant aspect of fracture healing, the reparative phase.

Granulation tissue soon begins to infiltrate the area.[4] Within the granulation tissue are specialized cells capable of forming collagen, cartilage, and bone—the ingredients of callus. Callus gradually surrounds the fractured ends and stabilizes them, becoming more densely mineralized with time.

Meanwhile, the necrotic edges of the fragments are removed by osteoclasts, cells whose function is to resorb bone. That is why some "hairline" fractures do not appear on a radiograph until days after injury. Invisible initially, the diagnostic fracture line appears only after necrotic bone has been resorbed from the area.

The final phase of bone healing, the remodeling phase, is the longest, sometimes lasting years. Remodeling is the tendency of bone gradually to regain its original shape and contour. During this phase, superfluous portions of callus are resorbed, and new bone is laid down along the natural lines of stress. These layers, easily visible on radiographs of normal bone, are the bony trabeculae. The formation of trabecular bone is a physiologically efficient process providing maximum strength relative to the amount of bone material used.

The anticipated degree of remodeling after a fracture is related to a number of factors. Predictors of satisfactory remodeling include youth, proximity of the fracture to the end of the bone (but not involving the epiphyseal plate), the amount of angulation, and the extent to which the direction of angulation coincides with the plane of natural joint motion.

Clinical decisions regarding the aggressiveness of fracture reduction are directly linked to knowledge of bone-healing physiology. Some angulation near the end of a long bone, for example, may be more acceptable than the same amount of angulation near the midshaft. In the wrist, dorsal or volar angulation has a better prognosis than does ulnar or radial angulation because the natural plane of wrist motion is dorsal to volar. Mild angulation in a 2-year-old child may be left to remodel on its own, whereas the same amount of angulation in an adult may require correction.

ORTHOPEDIC EMERGENCIES

OPEN FRACTURE

An open fracture is a fracture associated with overlying soft tissue injury, creating communication between the fracture site and the skin. Although this term may convey the image of grossly exposed bone, the term is equally applicable to any puncture wound extending to the depth of an underlying fracture. Such puncture wounds may be created by external forces or may occur from within, when a sharp bone fragment transiently protrudes through the skin before receding back beneath the surface.

A potential major complication of open fracture is osteomyelitis. Once established, osteomyelitis may result in months or years of pain, disability, medical therapy, surgical procedures, and, in some cases, amputation. Although osteomyelitis may sometimes be unavoidable, it is less likely when treatment is prompt and meticulous.

Open fractures are usually classified by their severity, based on the extent of overlying tissue disruption, lack of bone coverage, kinetic energy of the injuring force, and evidence or likelihood of significant contamination. Irrespective of these factors, any open fracture should be promptly and carefully treated.

SUBLUXATION AND DISLOCATION

Subluxation is a condition in which the articular surfaces of a joint are nonconcentric to any degree. Dislocation is the most extreme form of subluxation. A joint is dislocated when the articular surfaces of the bones that normally meet at the joint are completely out of contact with one another. The urgency of reducing a dislocation is based on several factors. One is the potential for neurologic or circulatory compromise. The neurovascular bundle passing close to the affected joint may become "kinked" around the dislocation. This may result in neurologic or vascular deficit that might be temporary if the deformity is reduced promptly but irreversible if treatment is delayed. Another consideration is that the longer a joint has been dislocated, the more difficult it may be to reduce and the less stable the reduction is likely to be. This is probably due, at least in part, to edema, muscle spasm, and other tissue changes that increase over time.

Dislocation of the hip also carries the potential for avascular necrosis of the femoral head. The necrosis occurs because much of the blood supply to the femoral head is delivered through vessels that emerge from the acetabulum. When the joint is dislocated, circulation to the femoral head is disrupted. At some point, the vascular insult becomes irreversible, and bony necrosis results. Although aseptic necrosis may occur despite the clinician's best efforts, its likelihood increases with the delay until reduction.

NEUROVASCULAR INJURY

Any injury associated with neurologic or vascular compromise should be addressed as soon as possible. The longer such a deficit goes untreated, the longer it is likely to persist and the greater the possibility that it will be irreversible. In some cases, reducing a deformity by means of longitudinal traction is all that is necessary to restore circulation or nerve function.

PREHOSPITAL CARE

PRELIMINARY SPLINTING

Effective splinting of an injured extremity is important for several reasons: (1) it reduces pain, (2) it reduces damage to nerves and vessels by preventing them from being compressed between the fracture fragments or being stretched by angulation at the fracture site, (3) it reduces the chance of inadvertently converting a closed fracture to an open one should a sharp bone fragment poke its way through the skin, and (4) it reduces the pain associated with patient transport by minimizing motion of the fracture fragments.

PREHOSPITAL SPLINTING DEVICES

Many splinting modalities are available to EMS personnel. These may range from sophisticated devices, such as vacuum splints containing small beads that conform to the extremity when air is removed, to simpler techniques such as cardboard or pillow splints, or padded IV boards.

Sling and Swath For injuries of the wrist or forearm, consider using a sling to supplement the splint, because optimal immobilization includes the joint above and the joint below the fracture, and a sling helps keep the elbow at rest.

For suspected injuries to the shoulder, humerus, or elbow, a sling-and-swathe arrangement works well. This method involves applying a sling, then binding the affected arm to the thorax with a gauze wrap. An exception to this principle is immobilization of patients with suspected anterior dislocation of the shoulder. Many patients with this injury have difficulty adducting the forearm, and forcibly binding it to the thorax may be painful. A simple sling is adequate in such cases. Injuries to the ankle may be immobilized in a pillow or well-padded cardboard splint. If a fracture of the tibial shaft or knee is suspected, the device should extend well above the knee to immobilize the joint above and the joint below the fracture.

Splints Some injuries warrant special splints, such as a winch-mechanism traction apparatus for femoral shaft fractures. Although such a device does not immobilize the hip (the joint above the fracture), the traction component makes this unnecessary. If a traction device is not available, then both the hip and knee should be immobilized. One method of accomplishing this is to bind the legs together, then bind the patient to a backboard from ankles to thorax with folded sheets or towels beneath the lower legs (but not the feet) to ease pressure on the heels.

Other types of splints exist, but their use is controversial. Inflatable plastic splints, for example, may be used for injuries to the ankle or wrist but sometimes are used inappropriately for fracture of the humerus or femur. Because these devices normally do not extend sufficiently proximally, they provide inadequate immobilization for such injuries. Also, overinflating the device may impair circulation. **If the inflatable splint cannot be dented by moderate thumb pressure, it is probably overinflated.** Inflatable splints should not be applied over clothing, because wrinkles in the clothing may cause pressure sores in swollen and vulnerable tissue.

Also controversial are nonmalleable aluminum splints, because they are based on the "one size fits all" principle, which some clinicians interpret as "this size fits none." Malleable aluminum splints are preferable, as they can be made to conform more closely to the contour of the extremity, even accommodating some degree of deformity. If used, aluminum splints of either type should be well padded, because their hard surface may cause pressure sores. Like any splint, they should immobilize the joint above and the joint below the fracture when used for long-bone injuries. For example, an above-knee splint is indicated for suspected fracture of the tibial shaft. Aluminum splints should be removed promptly once a fracture is diagnosed or ruled out. If a fracture is confirmed, replace the splint with an alternative immobilization dressing before the patient leaves the ED, because aluminum splints may cause pressure sores even when padded.

Military Antishock Trousers Another controversial device is military antishock trousers. This device may be used during ambulance transport of patients with already diagnosed pelvic ring fracture, or for patients with a clinically apparent femoral fracture when a traction device is not at hand, as the device immobilizes the joints above and below the fracture. Some EMS systems also advocate its use for patients with bilateral femur fractures even when traction is available, because of the anatomic difficulty of applying two traction splints. However, military antishock trousers are cumbersome to apply, their efficacy is not firmly established, and they can possibly contribute to compartment syndrome, fluid and electrolyte imbalance, and circulatory impairment.[5,6]

REDUCING DEFORMITY IN THE FIELD

Many EMS programs do not recommend prehospital reduction of deformity for an injured extremity, as injudicious manipulation may convert a pure dislocation to a fracture-dislocation. Even if a fracture had already existed, there would be no way to prove it was not caused by the manipulation. One circumstance in which prehospital reduction of obvious fracture to the shaft of a long bone may be justified is a nonpalpable distal pulse. In the absence of a common standard, the indications for reduction of deformity by prehospital personnel remain at the discretion of the supervising EMS program.

TABLE 267-1 Mechanisms Associated With Particular Orthopedic Injuries

Mechanism	Possible Injury
Bilateral compression of the shoulders	Anterior or posterior sternoclavicular dislocation
Direct blow to the medial clavicle	Posterior sternoclavicular dislocation
Fall, landing on the apex of the shoulder	Acromioclavicular separation
Direct blow to the anterior shoulder, fall on the outstretched arm, seizure or electroconvulsive muscular activity	Posterior dislocation of the shoulder
Sudden traction force to a toddler's arm	Subluxed radial head (sometimes misdiagnosed as brachial plexus injury because of pseudoparalysis of the arm)
Fall, landing on the outstretched arm or with the elbow beneath the body	Fracture of the radial head (may be occult on initial x-ray)
Forced dorsiflexion of the wrist	Fracture of the scaphoid, lunate dislocation, perilunar dislocation, Colles fracture
Striking the knee against the dashboard in a high-speed collision	Posterior dislocation of the hip
Landing flat on the feet from a height	Calcaneus fracture; tibial plateau fracture; acetabular fracture; vertebral compression fracture, usually lumbar
Ankle inversion force	Fracture of any of the three malleoli, fracture of the base of the fifth metatarsal
Rotatory ankle force	Fracture of any of the three malleoli, disruption of the anterior tibiofibular ligament with proximal fibular fracture (Maisonneuve's injury)
Inversion or medial or lateral stress to the forefoot; axial load on the metatarsal heads with the ankle plantarflexed	Midfoot dislocation (Lisfranc's injury)

CLINICAL FEATURES

The importance of a careful history and physical examination cannot be overstated. Orthopedic diagnosis is sometimes thought of as being as simple as taking a radiograph of the painful area. Although imaging is an important adjunct, it is not the ultimate diagnostic resource. **The pain of a fracture or a dislocation may be referred to another area.** For example, patients with disruption of the sternoclavicular joint or fracture of the humeral shaft may complain only of shoulder pain. If the radiograph is based solely on where the patient reports discomfort, then the injured part might not be included on the film. **Imaging decisions should be based not only on the chief complaint, but also on systematic palpation, observation of subtle deformity or significant point tenderness, and mechanism of injury.**

Some fractures or dislocations may be demonstrated only by special radiographic views, which are not part of the standard series for that body part. Such views will never be ordered unless the clinician has already formulated a presumptive diagnosis based on the history and physical findings.

Some injuries might not be radiographically apparent on the first day, regardless of what views are taken. Common examples are fracture of the scaphoid, nondisplaced fracture of the radial head, and stress fracture of a metatarsal. The classic radiographic signs accompanying these injuries, such as the fat-pad sign of the elbow, are not always conveniently present, but mechanism, history, and findings suggesting the injury often are. CT or MRI may allow early diagnosis of fractures that are not radiographically evident. However, such tests are not always available or feasible on the day of injury. In such cases, the diagnosis of fracture may be purely clinical until 7 to 10 days post-trauma, when enough bony resorption has occurred at the fracture site to reveal a lucency on plain radiographs.

HISTORY

The value of the history in cases of orthopedic trauma is often underestimated. Knowing the precise mechanism of injury may be the key to diagnosing some fractures or dislocations. For example, a history of shoulder injury combined with the complaint of dysphagia may be the only clue to the existence of posterior sternoclavicular dislocation. This entity, which causes pressure on mediastinal structures, often can be demonstrated only by CT and may result in severe complications if treatment is delayed. **Table 267-1** provides other examples of mechanisms that may lead the clinician to suspect, or presumptively treat for, specific injuries. This is by no means a definitive or exhaustive list. Some of the mechanisms described may produce injuries other than those mentioned. Conversely, the injuries may be produced by mechanisms in addition to those listed.

Some musculoskeletal injuries or conditions may not necessarily be associated with a history of direct trauma. Occult fracture of the hip in an osteoporotic individual, occult stress fracture of a metatarsal in someone who has recently done an unusual amount of walking, and slipped capital femoral epiphysis in a preteenager or young adolescent are examples of injuries in which symptoms may be gradual and insidious in onset, unrelated to an isolated traumatic event. **Exquisite tenderness to palpation or pain on weightbearing or passive range of motion suggests the possibility of an occult or easily missed fracture.** Depending on the index of suspicion, further studies, such as a bone scan or MRI, may be indicated to exclude significant pathologic conditions before the patient is allowed to resume weightbearing.

History taking should not necessarily be limited to orthopedic issues. Depending on the situation, a general medical history should be obtained because it may have implications for further workup, the potential for complications, or ultimate prognosis for recovery of function. Relevant issues may include a history of heart disease or neurologic disease, taking anticoagulant medication, falling due to syncope or transient hemiparesis, or an unsteady baseline gait that cannot withstand further impairment.

PHYSICAL EXAMINATION

Essential components of the examination for musculoskeletal trauma are (1) inspection for swelling, discoloration, or deformity; (2) assessment of active and passive range of motion of the joints proximal and distal to the injury; (3) palpation for tenderness or deformity; and (4) assessment of neurovascular status.

Inspection and Range of Motion Gross deformity along the shaft of a long bone is pathognomonic for fracture. Deformity at a joint, loss of range of motion, and severe pain at rest suggest the presence of a dislocation or fracture near the joint. An exception is posterior dislocation of the shoulder, which, although intensely painful, might not be accompanied by obvious deformity, although the humeral head may be palpable posteriorly.

Palpation When gross deformity is not present, presumptive diagnosis strongly depends on findings noted on palpation. Palpation may disclose areas of bony step-off and the precise location of point tenderness.

The palpation examination should be done systematically and consistently from one patient to the next. The area palpated should extend well beyond the location of pain described by the patient, as the pain may be referred. For example, when an injured patient complains of shoulder pain, palpation should begin at the sternoclavicular joint, then proceed along the clavicle onto the acromioclavicular joint, then onto the humeral head and along the entire humeral shaft. In addition, the scapula should be palpated for tenderness, and the posterior aspect of the shoulder should be palpated for any unnatural prominence or fullness that might suggest posterior dislocation of the humeral head. Injury to any of these areas may be reported by the patient as "pain in the shoulder." Only a meticulous palpation examination may protect the clinician from being misled by referred pain and missing a crucial diagnosis.

Neurovascular Assessment When injury involves an extremity, as opposed to the vertebral column, sensorimotor testing should be performed on the basis of peripheral nerve function, rather than nerve root and dermatomal distribution (**Figure 267-1**). In the upper extremity, the radial, median, and ulnar nerves should be tested. When the shoulder is anteriorly dislocated, two additional nerves, the axillary (supplying sensation to the lateral aspect of the shoulder) and the musculocutaneous (supplying sensation to the extensor aspect of the forearm), also should be checked. In the lower extremity, examination of the saphenous (sensory only), peroneal, and tibial nerves should be performed. Neurologic deficit is important to document early, particularly before the patient has undergone any significant manipulation or reduction maneuvers.

Assess vascular status early. **The sooner circulatory compromise is identified and addressed, the better the chance of avoiding tissue ischemia or necrosis.** Injuries such as dislocation of the knee (tibiofemoral joint), fracture-dislocation of the ankle, and displaced supracondylar fracture of the elbow in children may be associated with vascular disruption, with resulting circulatory impairment.

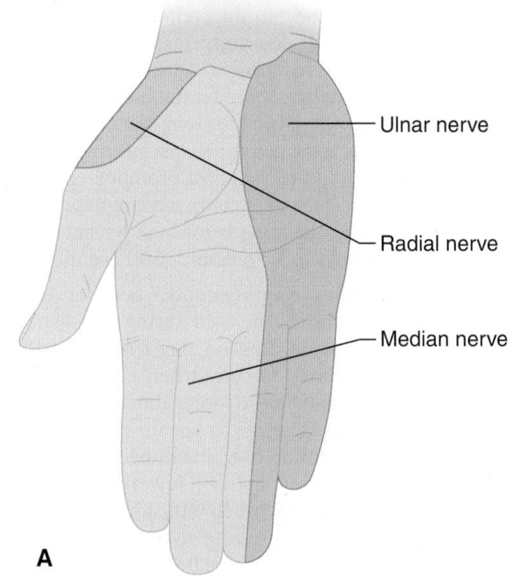

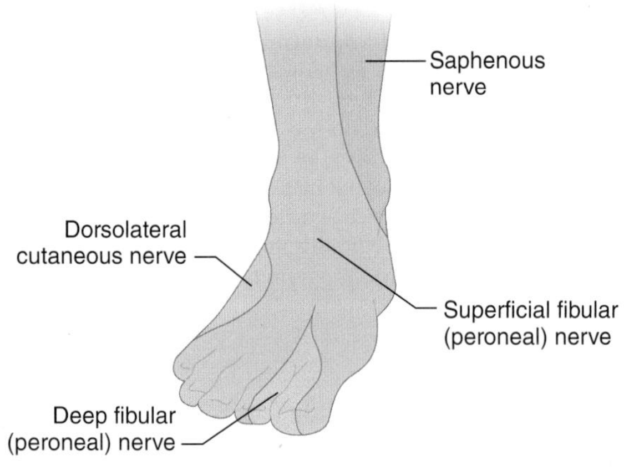

FIGURE 267-1. **A.** Peripheral sensory nerve distribution of the hand. **B.** Peripheral sensory nerve distribution of the foot.

DIAGNOSIS

IMAGING

The joints above and below a fracture should generally be imaged because injury at the proximal or distal joint may coexist with long-bone fractures. Injuries that may require special views or advanced imaging modalities in order to be visualized include acromioclavicular separation, fracture of the scaphoid, posterior shoulder dislocation, and sternoclavicular dislocation.

The use of bedside US has been reported for pediatric clavicle and forearm fractures and long-bone fractures. However, US for these purposes is operator dependent and has not replaced traditional diagnostic imaging.[7-10]

Children who have sustained trauma at or near a joint may need comparison studies of the opposite extremity to differentiate fracture lines from normal epiphyseal plates or ossifying growth centers. This is particularly true of the pediatric elbow, which typically exhibits six ossification centers sequentially as the child grows.

Although the clinician may be tempted to base diagnostic and treatment decisions on the radiologist's report, this is not advisable for at least two reasons. First, **a negative radiologic report does not exclude significant injury.** Fracture of the radial head, scaphoid, or metatarsal shaft, for example, may be undetectable on radiographs initially, even when special views are taken. Second, the terminology used by radiologists to describe malposition of fracture fragments or disrupted joints often differs from the terminology used by orthopedists. Because the emergency physician may confer with an orthopedist regarding the initial management of a patient, and because this interaction commonly involves describing the radiographic appearance of an injury, it is important that the two physicians "speak the same language."

DESCRIBING RADIOGRAPHS

As more hospitals convert from film-based to digital imaging, orthopedic consultants are increasingly likely to be able to examine a patient's imaging studies by remote access. In the absence of such technology, proper management of the patient may depend on the emergency physician's ability to convey the radiographic appearance of the injury to the consultant. In such cases, the narrative often will influence the orthopedist's decision regarding the need for hospital admission and whether surgical versus nonsurgical management is warranted. In essence, the emergency physician should be able to transmit a virtual copy of the radiograph by means of verbal description.

There are a number of ways to characterize the appearance of fractures. The method presented below is intended to be the most practical from the standpoint of communicating with an orthopedic consultant.

Open Versus Closed Although not a radiologic finding per se, whether a bony injury is open or closed is an important consideration and should be conveyed to the orthopedist at the outset. The implications of open fracture are of such significance that this factor alone may determine the patient's immediate care or ultimate disposition.

Location of the Fracture **Typical reference points used by orthopedists to describe the location of a fracture along the shaft of a long bone are the midshaft, the junction of the proximal and middle thirds, and the junction of the middle and distal thirds.** Any fracture more proximal or distal than these locations may be described in terms of its distance, in centimeters, from the bone end.

When a fracture extends into the adjacent joint, it is termed intra-articular. Intra-articular fractures have special significance because disruption of the joint surface may warrant surgery to restore the joint's contour and prevent subsequent traumatic arthritis. This feature of a fracture line, if present, constitutes important information.

Anatomic bony reference points should be cited when applicable. A fracture just above the condyles of the distal humerus or femur, for example, is termed a supracondylar fracture. A fracture running from the greater to the lesser trochanter of the proximal femur is an intertrochanteric hip fracture, whereas a fracture just below the trochanters is subtrochanteric, a fracture just above them is said to involve the femoral neck, and a higher fracture just below the femoral head is referred to as subcapital. The area at or proximal to the coronoid process of the ulna is the olecranon and should be referred to as such, rather than simply the "proximal ulna." Other bony landmarks include the radial head at the elbow, radial styloid at the wrist, and the greater tuberosity of the humeral head. Numerous additional examples exist.

Orientation of the Fracture Line The most common orientations of fracture lines are illustrated in **Figure 267-2**. Torus and greenstick fractures occur almost exclusively in young children, whose bones are more pliable than those of adults. Note the segmental fracture, which is commonly described incorrectly as a comminuted fracture. To an orthopedist, the term *comminuted* implies splintering or shattering. A single, large, free-floating segment of bone between two well-defined fracture lines is a segmental fracture.

Displacement and Separation The term *displacement* may be used in either of two ways. In the broadest sense, it pertains to any deviation from anatomic position or alignment. Used more precisely, displacement refers to the extent to which fracture fragments are nonconcentric or offset from each other. The magnitude of displacement may be expressed in terms of direct measurement (e.g., 4-mm displacement) or in terms of the percentage of the width of the bone (e.g., 50% displacement, complete displacement). The direction of displacement is based on the position of the distal fragment relative to the proximal fragment.

Displacement should not be confused with separation, which is the distance two fragments have been pulled apart. **Figure 267-3** illustrates principles of displacement and separation.

Shortening Shortening, expressed in millimeters or centimeters, is the amount by which a bone's length has been reduced. Shortening may occur by impaction (telescoping of the fragments into one another) or by the overlap of two completely displaced fragments (**Figure 267-4**). The latter is referred to by some orthopedists as *overriding*. Because a radiograph affords no depth perception, a fracture that appears impacted on one view needs to be visualized at an angle 90 degrees from the first to differentiate it from a fracture whose ends are completely displaced and overriding. Depending on the location of the fracture and the age of the patient, shortening may have long-range functional implications and may have to be corrected by closed manipulation or by surgery.

Angulation Angulation is described in terms of two parameters: degree and direction (**Figure 267-5**). Quantifying the angulation is relatively simple. One need only estimate the amount of "unbending" (expressed in degrees) that would be needed to make the fragments parallel.

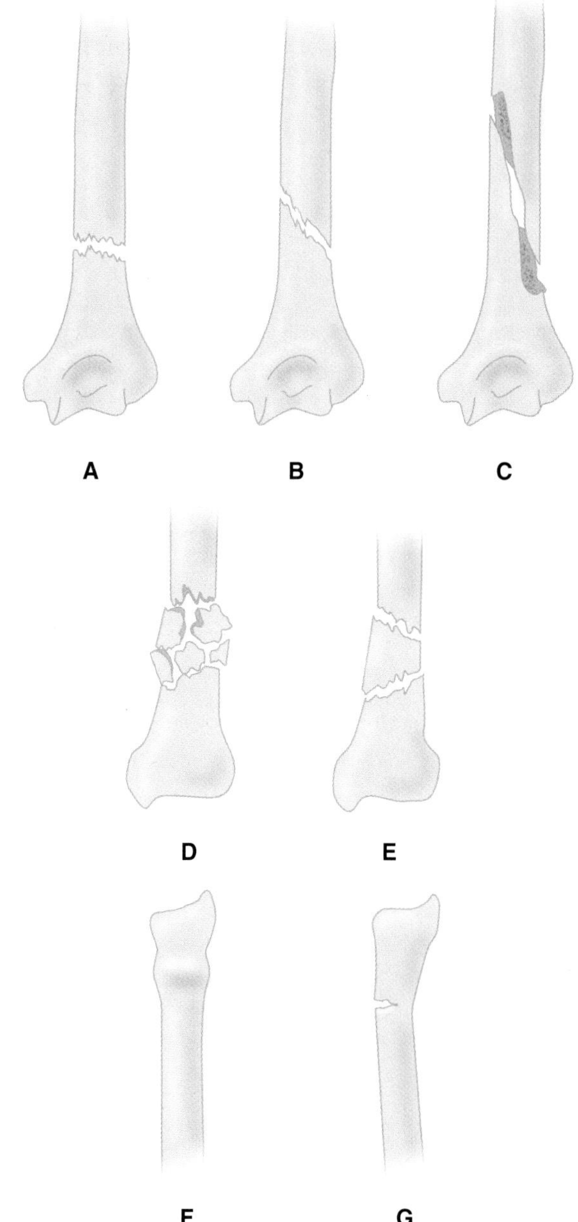

FIGURE 267-2. Fracture line orientation. **A.** Transverse. **B.** Oblique. **C.** Spiral. **D.** Comminuted. **E.** Segmental. **F.** Torus. **G.** Greenstick.

Conveying the direction of angulation may be more difficult because the terminology is less consistent among clinicians. In general, when a fracture is near the midshaft of a long bone, the direction of angulation is the direction of the apex of the angle formed by the two fragments. (**Figures 267-5A** and **267-5B** illustrate 30 degrees of dorsal angulation.) When a fracture is near the end of a bone, however, angulation is described in terms of the direction the terminal fragment is deviated. Thus **Figure 267-5C** also shows 30 degrees of dorsal angulation, even though the apex of the angle formed by the fragments is pointing in the opposite direction from that in the preceding figures. **If there is a possibility of ambiguity in the description, specifying the *direction of deviation of the distal fragment* usually can resolve it.**

Depending on the anatomic area involved, direction of angulation may be expressed as anterior or posterior, lateral or medial, radial or ulnar, or dorsal or volar.

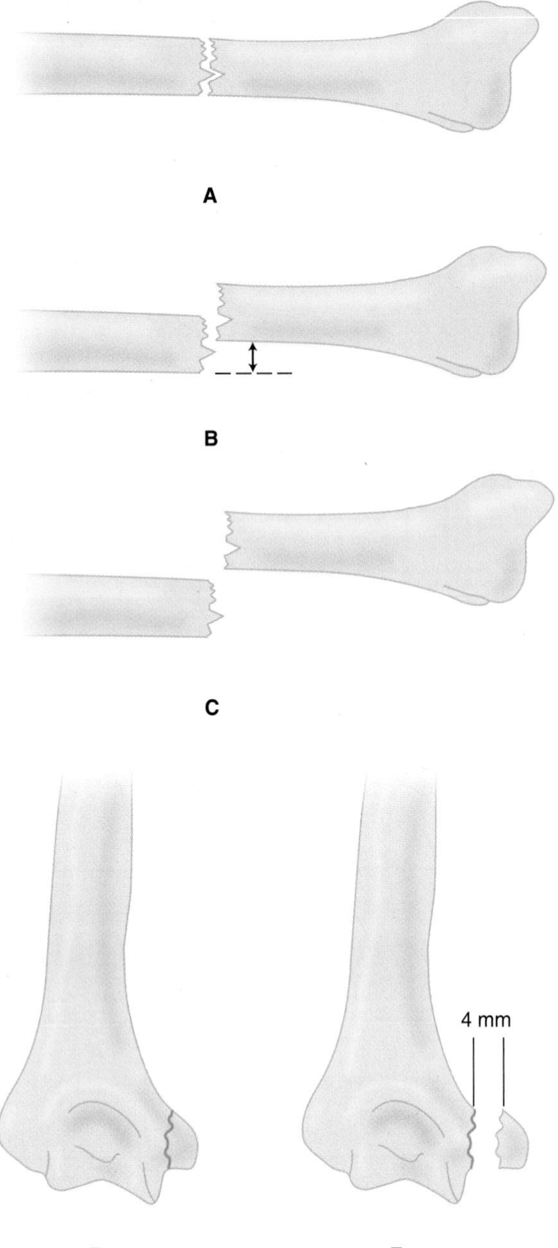

FIGURE 267-3. Fracture displacement and separation. **A.** No displacement, slight separation. **B.** Fifty percent dorsal displacement. **C.** Complete dorsal displacement. **D.** Nondisplaced, no separation. **E.** A 4-mm separation.

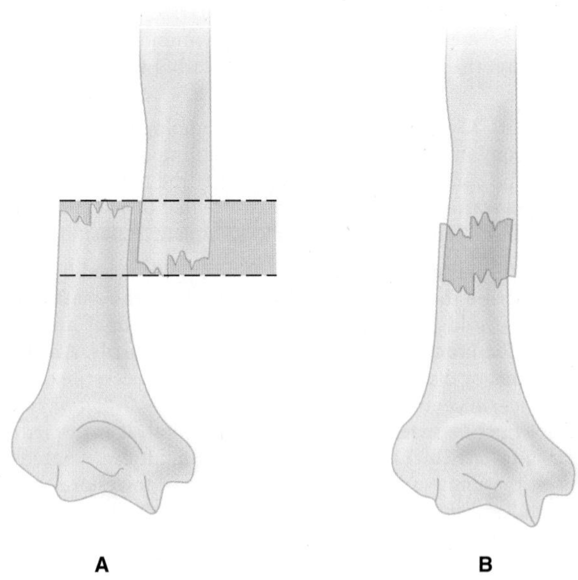

FIGURE 267-4. Shortening at fracture site. **A.** Complete displacement with overriding. **B.** Impaction. In both cases, the width of the shaded area represents the amount of shortening.

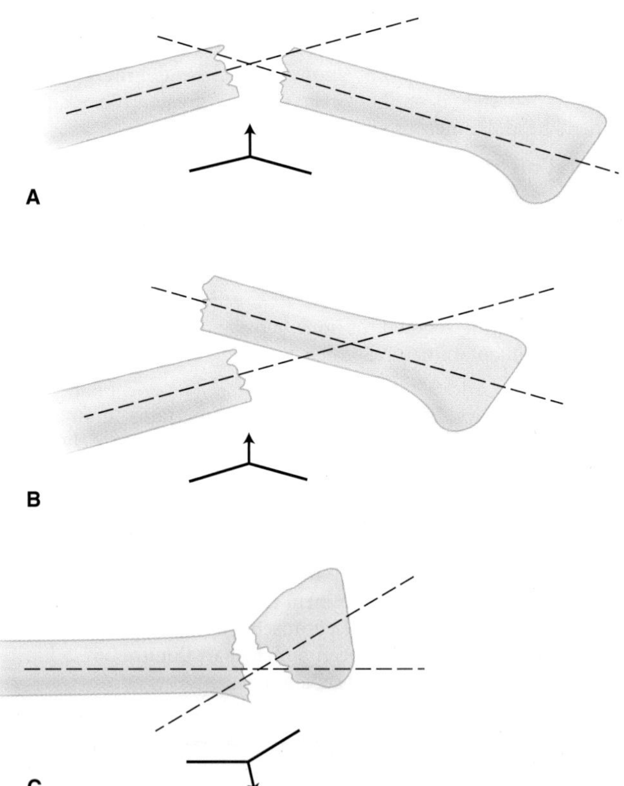

FIGURE 267-5. Fracture angulation. All figures depict 30-degree dorsal angulation. **A, B.** Direction is based on the apex of the angle drawn below the figures. **C.** Direction is based on the direction of the terminal fragment.

Rotational Deformity Rotational deformity—that is, the extent to which the distal fracture fragment is twisted on its own axis relative to the proximal fragment—is generally not apparent on radiographs. This element of fracture description depends on physical examination. Its detection is particularly important in the phalanges of the fingers, where, if rotational deformity goes unrecognized and uncorrected, the injured finger will permanently be malaligned when the hand is closed.

Fracture Combined With Dislocation or Subluxation Injuries near a joint may involve dislocation or subluxation combined with a proximate fracture. An example is fracture of one or more ankle malleoli, together with partial or complete displacement of the talus from beneath the tibia. These are significant injuries, often requiring surgical intervention. If, in describing the injury, the clinician emphasizes the fracture component but expresses the dislocation or subluxation as mere "displacement," then the full severity may not be appreciated by the orthopedist. Such injuries should be described as fracture-dislocations or fracture-subluxations.

Salter-Harris Fractures Salter and Harris classified fractures involving the epiphyseal plate at the end of the long bone of a growing child into

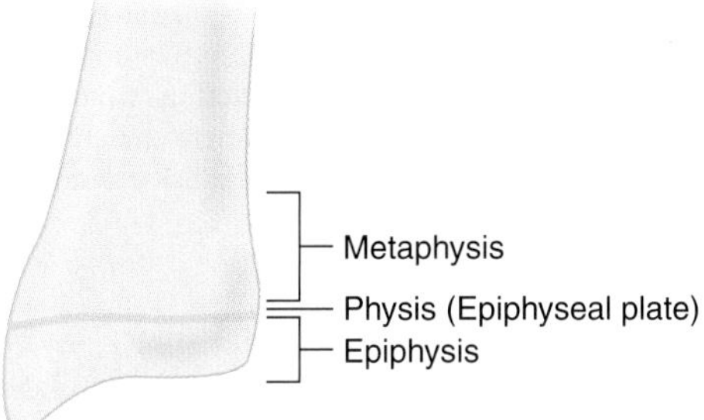

FIGURE 267-6. Epiphyseal anatomy in the growing child.

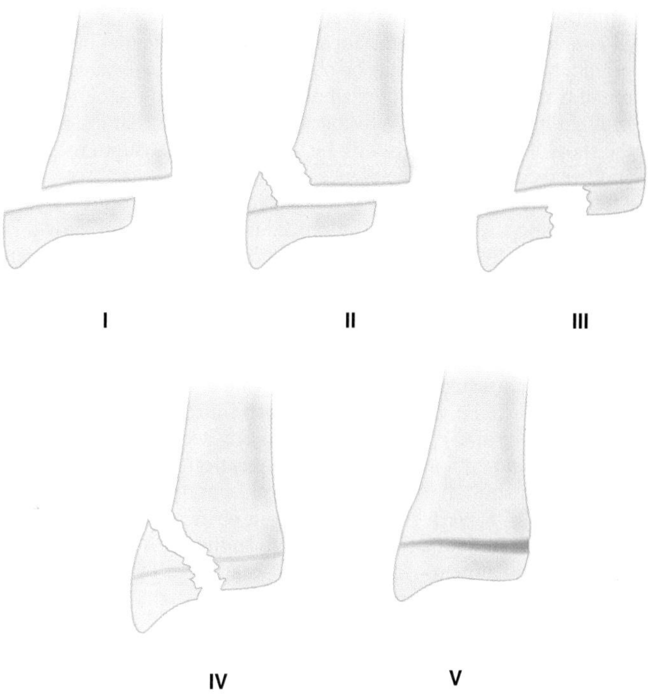

FIGURE 267-7. Epiphyseal plate fractures based on the classification of Salter and Harris.

five types based on the pattern of the fracture line. Because the type generally correlates with the potential for future growth disturbance (and, consequently, with the aggressiveness of the treatment warranted), the ability to identify the fracture type based on its radiographic appearance is important.

Perhaps the easiest way to remember the Salter-Harris classification system is to think of these injuries not in terms of where the fracture line runs, but in terms of what has been *broken off.* **Figure 267-6** illustrates the anatomy involved. **Table 267-2** lists the five types of Salter-Harris fractures, which are illustrated in **Figure 267-7**. The potential for growth disturbance is least for type I and increases with the classification number, with the worst prognosis being associated with type V injuries.

Type I and type V Salter fractures may be radiographically undetectable. Type I injuries usually involve no transverse displacement and little or no separation of the epiphysis from the rest of the bone. Also, the lucent fracture line is not visible within the equally lucent epiphyseal plate. Diagnosis of acute Salter type I fractures is usually presumptive, based on the presence of swelling and tenderness in the region of the physis.

Type V injuries may be evident only retrospectively, when growth disturbance first begins to appear. At the time of initial presentation, however, a history of a significant axial loading force, coupled with significant tenderness in the area of the epiphyseal plate, should suggest the possibility of a type V injury. Such injuries should be immobilized and referred for orthopedic follow-up.

TREATMENT

CONTROL PAIN AND SWELLING

Initiate measures to reduce swelling early. Severe swelling not only intensifies the pain of injury but also may delay the application of a definitive immobilization dressing and may make the skin more susceptible to pressure sores. Although sometimes regarded as trivial modalities, the application of cold and elevation are often quite effective in keeping swelling to a minimum or at least halting its progression. Jewelry, watches, or rings that may cause compression or constriction as an extremity swells should be removed.

Give analgesics as necessary. If the patient is relatively comfortable at rest, medication may not be required. **Even narcotic analgesics may have minimal effect on the pain of movement or manipulation unless combined with other CNS-acting agents.**

TABLE 267-2 Description of Salter-Harris Fractures

Salter Type	What Is Broken Off
I	The entire epiphysis
II	The entire epiphysis *along with* a portion of the metaphysis
III	A portion of the epiphysis
IV	A portion of the epiphysis *along with* a portion of the metaphysis
V	Compression injury of the epiphyseal plate (nothing is "broken off")

WITHHOLD ORAL INTAKE

Any patient who might be a candidate for prompt surgical fixation, manipulation, or any other procedure under general anesthesia or procedural sedation should not be allowed to eat or drink from the moment of arrival until the need for, and timing of, such a procedure has been ascertained.

REDUCE FRACTURE DEFORMITY

The long-term purpose of reducing significant deformity associated with fractures is restoration of normal appearance and function of the extremity. However, there are also short-term benefits to reducing deformity early: (1) alleviating pain, (2) relieving the tension on nerves or vessels that may be stretched as they pass along the deformity, (3) eliminating or significantly minimizing the possibility of inadvertently converting a closed fracture to an open one when the skin is tented by a sharp bony fragment, and (4) restoring circulation to a pulseless distal extremity.

After the patient has been appropriately sedated, deformity at or near the midshaft of a long bone is usually reduced with gradual, steady, longitudinal traction. Any rotational deformity should be corrected only after the angular component has been addressed and should be performed while traction is maintained.

The nearer a deformity is to a joint, the more difficult it may be to correct and the more specialized the reduction maneuver may have to be. **When deformity is associated with circulatory deficit, a true emergency exists, and the anticipated delay until reduction should be considered.**

REDUCE DISLOCATIONS

The techniques used to reduce specific dislocations are discussed in subsequent chapters. In general, prereduction radiographs are advisable when there has been significant trauma, unless time is crucial because circulation is threatened. Radiographs are needed because dislocations and fracture-dislocations may have a similar appearance on physical examination, but the techniques used to treat them may be very different.

Of course, there are circumstances in which the potential benefits of a prereduction radiograph may be outweighed by the associated expenditure of time and money. For example, a prereduction radiograph may be omitted in a patient with a history of multiple recurrent dislocations of the shoulder who presents with history, signs, and symptoms typical of another recurrence in the absence of significant trauma.

After a reduction maneuver, postreduction radiographs are valuable for confirming the success of the procedure, as well as for providing documentation, in the event that the joint redislocates after the patient is discharged from the ED.

INITIAL MANAGEMENT OF OPEN FRACTURES

Open fractures warrant prompt and meticulous attention. The most important elements in the treatment of open fractures, aside from tetanus prophylaxis that applies generally to any wound, are irrigation, debridement, and antibiotics as soon as is practical.[11]

Early administration of antibiotics can prevent or reduce the clinical consequences of bacterial contamination in open fractures.[12,13] Consequently, initiate antibiotic therapy promptly in the ED. There is no standard antibiotic regimen. An accepted approach, but by no means the only regimen in use, is a first-generation cephalosporin, with the addition of an aminoglycoside when the wound is >10 cm with severe soft tissue injury and loss of bone coverage.[14,15] Some studies advocate the use of ciprofloxacin as an alternative to a cephalosporin.[16] When there is significant contamination by plants or soil, consider the addition of penicillin (or metronidazole, clindamycin, or vancomycin for penicillin-allergic patients) for anaerobic coverage. Aerobic and anaerobic wound cultures may be obtained before antibiotics are administered, although the value of pretreatment cultures for open fractures is controversial.[17]

To lower the infection rate, not only antibiotics but also generous irrigation and adequate debridement are necessary to reduce bacterial contamination and colonization.[18] The purposes of debridement and irrigation are (1) to expose the wound in order to allow better identification of the limits of injury and facilitate inspection for foreign material; (2) to identify and remove clots, debris, and nonviable tissue; and (3) to reduce bacterial contamination and make the wound more resistant to the effects of any residual contamination. (See chapter 40, Wound Preparation, for complete discussion of wound irrigation.)

Debridement and irrigation of minor wounds overlying a fracture sometimes may be performed in the ED. When tissue damage is moderate or severe, debridement and irrigation are typically performed in the operating room.

ORTHOPEDIC CONSULTATION IN THE ED

In many cases, such as fracture of the hip, the need for hospital admission and/or orthopedic consultation in the ED is obvious. In some situations, however, differences of opinion may exist regarding whether the patient needs to be seen by an orthopedist in the ED or whether the patient may be treated in preliminary fashion and referred for definitive orthopedic management. Even patients with injuries that ultimately may require surgical repair, such as an unstable ankle fracture, sometimes may be immobilized and discharged with a referral for prompt orthopedic follow-up.

COMPARTMENT SYNDROME

In cases of known or suspected compartment syndrome, obtain prompt orthopedic consultation. Emergency surgical intervention may be required to try to avert permanent tissue damage and muscle contracture. The physiology and potentially catastrophic consequences of compartment syndrome are described in the section Complications later in this chapter and in chapter 278, Compartment Syndrome.

IRREDUCIBLE DISLOCATION

The emergency physician sometimes may be unable to reduce a dislocation, even with the aid of a nerve block or procedural sedation. Although technique is certainly a factor, there may be other reasons closed reduction cannot be accomplished, such as the interposition of soft tissues within the joint or the presence of an associated fracture. Orthopedic consultation should be sought in such cases. Timely reduction, which sometimes can be achieved only surgically, may help minimize the complications (and shorten the duration of pain) resulting from a dislocated joint.

CIRCULATORY COMPROMISE

Circulatory deficit due to musculoskeletal injury warrants prompt orthopedic consultation. Even if circulation has been restored by the emergency physician through the correction of deformity, the orthopedist may wish to investigate the integrity of the involved vessels and should at least be contacted to discuss the case.

OPEN FRACTURE

Some open fractures need to be treated aggressively in the operating room. Other types, such as those involving the phalanges, often may be irrigated in the ED and referred for follow-up. If there is any question, a discussion with the orthopedist may result in a mutually agreeable plan of care.

INJURIES REQUIRING SURGICAL INTERVENTION

Whereas some musculoskeletal injuries require operative intervention as soon as possible, others may be treated on a delayed basis. In many cases, orthopedists differ in their preferred approach to the timing of surgery. Orthopedic consultation, at least by telephone, is indicated in cases of musculoskeletal injury that the emergency physician believes may require operative fixation or repair. The orthopedist may then exercise the option to admit the patient or to see the patient in timely follow-up and schedule any necessary surgery at that time.

SPLINTING MATERIALS AND TECHNIQUES

Immobilization is indicated not only for fractures, but also for dislocated joints that have been reduced. When a joint becomes dislocated, the ligaments that had provided its stability are disrupted, and the joint is susceptible to redislocation until healing has occurred.

The materials most commonly used for orthopedic immobilization are plaster of Paris (calcium sulfate) and fiberglass fabric combined with a polyurethane resin. Fiberglass has the advantages of being lightweight, fast setting, and resistant to damage by moisture. However, it is not as malleable as plaster, so it might not conform as well to the contour of the limb. This may be an issue when the purpose of the dressing is not only to provide immobilization but also to maintain the position of the fragments once a displaced fracture has been reduced.

Whether plaster or fiberglass is used for immobilization depends on a number of factors, including the emergency physician's preference, the philosophy of the orthopedic community, the needs of the patient, and the hospital's resources.

PRINCIPLES OF SPLINTING

The chemical reactions that cause plaster or fiberglass to set are initiated by contact with water. The higher the water temperature, the faster the materials harden. However, these reactions are exothermic, meaning they liberate heat. The faster the setting process, the more heat is generated. Therefore, the temperature to which the skin ultimately is exposed will be the additive result of the water temperature and the heat released by the chemical reaction. For this reason, severe burns may occur when plaster or fiberglass has been immersed in mildly hot water, even though the temperature of the water itself would not be sufficient to cause such burns. Although there is no universally prescribed ideal water temperature, a safe practice is to make the water room temperature. If steam is visible, the water is certainly too hot.

To avoid irritation and to minimize the potential for pressure sores, plaster or fiberglass dressings should include several layers of padding over the skin. When non-prepadded longitudinal plaster splints are used, cast padding has to be applied separately. The padding does not necessarily have to be circumferential. Several layers of longitudinal padding will effectively protect the skin as long as they exceed the width and length of the splinting material. The best way to ensure this is to fashion the dry splint first, then measure the padding over it. Longitudinal splints may be fashioned from fixed-length plaster strips, from plaster rolls normally used to create circumferential casts, or from prepadded material with plaster or fiberglass enclosed. The splint should be long enough to provide the leverage needed to immobilize the injured joint. To immobilize the elbow, for example, a splint should begin distal to the wrist and extend high up the lateral arm, almost to the level of the humeral neck. To immobilize the ankle effectively, a splint should extend from beneath the metatarsal heads to the proximal calf. If the fracture is along the midportion of a distal extremity (i.e., the forearm or the lower leg) rather than at a joint, the splint should be long enough to immobilize the joint above and the joint below the fracture.

NON-PREPADDED PLASTER

When a splint is fashioned from plaster rolls, determine the length of the splint by measuring out a single layer along the extremity according to the principles described previously. Then, on a flat surface, unroll the plaster back and forth over itself to make a multilayered splint. If fixed-length plaster strips are used instead of rolls, the only way their length can be customized is to shorten them, so an adequate length should be selected at the outset and trimmed as necessary. In either case, the splint should be at least 12 layers thick for an adult. Even more layers should be used for children, who typically remain as active as possible and have little regard for protecting the dressing.

When the dry splint has been prepared, measure out several layers of padding over it, making the padding longer and wider than the plaster. After setting the padding aside, grip each end of the splint and immerse it in water, keeping it submerged until bubbling stops (indicating that water has been fully absorbed into the interstices of the material). Then withdraw the splint and remove the excess water by sliding the compressed thumb and index finger along the length of the plaster on each edge. (Use a stripping motion, rather than crumpling or wringing out the dressing, or much of the plaster may be lost.)

The next step, frequently overlooked, is to lay the splint on a flat surface and massage the layers into one another so that they fuse together. This creates a strong dressing that is solid on cross-section. A splint whose separate layers are still visible on cross-section is much weaker.

The padding should now be laid on the plaster and the dressing applied to the extremity, with the padded surface against the skin. When two plaster segments are used, as for a thumb spica or a posterior ankle mold with an additional transverse "sugar tong" component, no padding should be interposed between the segments. Rather, they should be molded into each other where they overlap. An assistant can hold the splint against the extremity while it is wrapped in place with gauze bandage. The assistant should use the palms, rather than the fingertips, when holding the splint in place. Hardened finger dents may cause irritation or even pressure sores. When a compressive effect is desired, an elastic bandage may be wrapped over the gauze. (If an elastic bandage is wrapped directly onto plaster without an interposed layer of gauze, it will set into the plaster and may lose most of its compressive function.)

While the plaster is setting, the affected joint may need to be held in a particular position. Again, use the palms, rather than the fingers, for reasons already described. Once the setting process is well under way, the position of a joint should not be changed, or the dressing may crack and become functionally useless. If the joint has gradually migrated from the desired position, the clinician must decide to accept the current position or remove the dressing and start over. There is no need to feel hesitant about the latter course. Patients generally appreciate a desire for perfection by their clinician.

PREPADDED MATERIAL

Some plaster or fiberglass splinting products are manufactured with the immobilization material already enclosed in padding, either as strips of predetermined length or as rolls from which splints may be cut to the desired length. Precut strips come packaged in air-tight foil. When a roll is used, the cut end is sealed with a tight clip to protect the exposed material. (Even when not immersed in water, fiberglass may set within 10 to 15 minutes, simply from exposure to moisture in the air.)

Prepadded material is fast and convenient to use because the layers are already in place and the padding need not be applied separately. However, the potential disadvantages are that the thickness of the dressing cannot be customized, and the material does not lend itself to applying two overlapping segments, because they cannot be molded into each other to create a sturdy dressing. If these issues are not a consideration, then prepadded material is a reasonable choice.

TYPES OF IMMOBILIZATION DRESSINGS

The more common immobilization dressings used in the ED are discussed next and are summarized in **Table 267-3**.

TABLE 267-3 Immobilization Devices and Uses

Immobilization Technique	Clinical Application
Shoulder immobilizer	Clavicle fracture
	Acromioclavicular separation
	Shoulder dislocation (postreduction)
	Humeral neck fracture
Sling	A variety of upper-extremity injuries, in conjunction with other immobilization techniques; may be used alone for nondisplaced or clinically suspected fracture of the radial head.
Long-arm gutter	Elbow fracture other than nondisplaced radial head fracture
	Reduced elbow dislocation
Sugar-tong	Wrist or forearm fracture
Short-arm gutter	Metacarpal or proximal phalanx fracture. (Ulnar gutter for fourth or fifth ray; radial gutter for second [index] or third [middle] ray.)
Thumb spica	Scaphoid fracture (proven or suspected)
	Thumb metacarpal or proximal thumb phalanx fracture
Knee immobilizer	Fracture or reduced subluxation of patella
	Knee dislocation, postreduction (temporary)
	Tibial plateau fracture
	Knee ligament injury
	Suspected meniscal tear (provided the knee can be fully extended)
Posterior ankle mold (consider above-the-knee extension and/or adjunctive use of ankle sugar-tong for unstable ankle injuries)	Ankle dislocation or fracture-dislocation
	Unstable ankle fracture (high distal fibular fracture or medial and/or posterior malleolar fracture)
	Widened medial mortise (indicates disruption of stabilizing medial structures)
	Metatarsal fracture (alternative immobilization dressings may be used)
Ankle stirrup	Simple ankle sprain
	Stable lateral malleolus fracture (below the superior border of the talus) without other ankle involvement (no medial swelling or tenderness, posterior malleolus intact)
Hard-soled shoe	Toe fracture
	Some metatarsal fractures (see the section Hard-Soled Shoe later in this chapter)
Short-leg walking boot	Some toe or foot contusions or fractures where weightbearing is allowed[19]

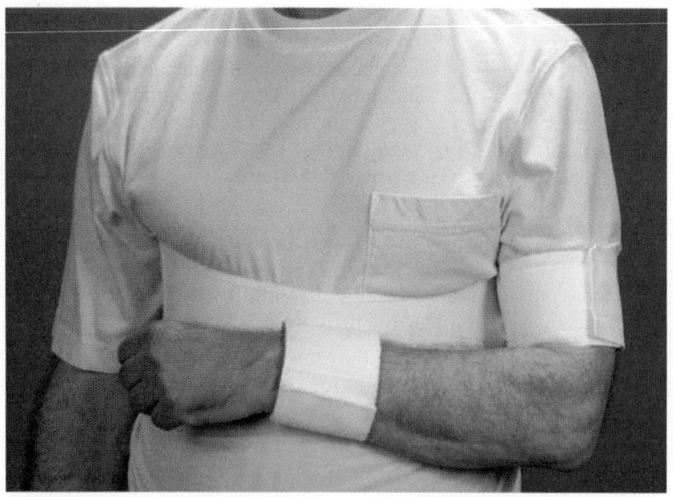

FIGURE 267-8. Shoulder immobilizer.

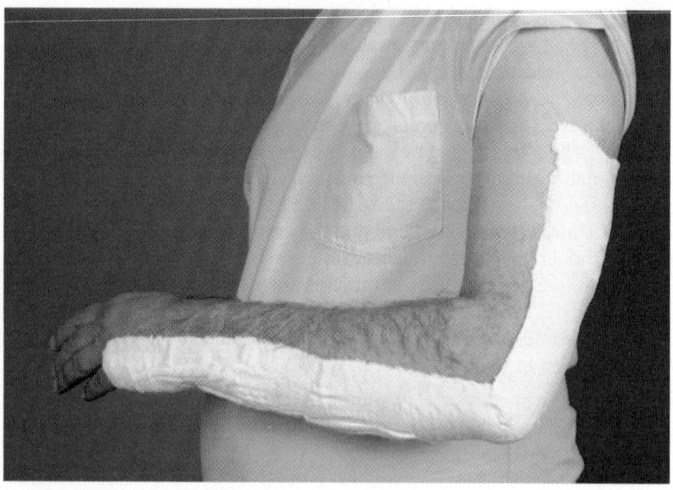

FIGURE 267-10. Long-arm gutter splint.

Shoulder Immobilizer This is a removable Velcro®-fastened device that keeps the arm in "sling position" but allows less mobility than a sling (**Figure 267-8**). A wide band wraps around the thorax. Two cuffs are attached to the thoracic piece: one on the lateral side, which grasps the upper arm, keeping the shoulder adducted; and one anteriorly, which holds the wrist to the chest, keeping the shoulder internally rotated. This dressing is suitable for fractures about the shoulder girdle, including clavicle and well-positioned humeral neck fractures, and for reduced shoulder dislocations.

A shoulder immobilizer is also commonly used for acromioclavicular separations, although from a mechanical standpoint, the ideal dressing for this injury is one that exerts upward pressure on the elbow and downward pressure on the clavicle to bring the clavicle and acromion back into alignment. Commercial versions of such dressings exist, but they are cumbersome to apply and uncomfortable to wear, leading to noncompliance. A shoulder immobilizer (or sling and swathe) is an acceptable alternative dressing.

Arm Sling Although it does not provide rigid immobilization, a sling (**Figure 267-9**) may be used as an adjunct to other splinting techniques for a variety of upper extremity injuries to enhance comfort, reduce motion, and provide some degree of support and elevation to the upper extremity. In some cases, as for nondisplaced fracture of the radial head, it may be used alone, without the need for supplementary immobilization.

Clavicle Strap (Figure-of-Eight Bandage) The figure-of-eight clavicle strap is mentioned only as a historical note. This dressing had long been considered the appropriate immobilization method for fracture of the clavicle, but in fact it is fairly ineffective at maintaining alignment of the fracture fragments and produces no difference in clinical outcome compared with a simple sling.[20] In addition, the clavicle strap may be awkward to apply, may require frequent readjustment, may cause problems related to pressure on the brachial plexus, and is often uncomfortable for the patient. A shoulder immobilizer or sling is a much better choice.

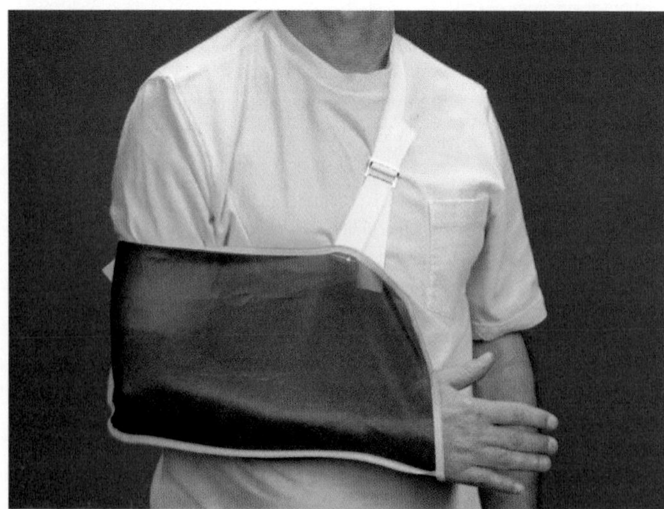

FIGURE 267-9. Arm sling.

Long-Arm Gutter Splint A long-arm gutter splint immobilizes the elbow (**Figure 267-10**). The upper extremity is placed in "sling position" (elbow flexed about 90 degrees and palm facing the abdomen). The splint begins on the ulnar surface of the hand at the metacarpal heads and extends along the ulnar surface of the forearm, past the elbow, to a spot high on the lateral surface of the upper arm just opposite and below the axillary crease. It should be supplemented with a sling.

The most common error associated with fashioning this dressing is insufficient length. If the splint is not carried far enough above the elbow, it will not exert enough leverage to prevent motion of that joint.

The long-arm gutter is useful for injuries about the elbow, including displaced radial head fracture, supracondylar humeral fracture, and reduced dislocation of the elbow.

Sugar-Tong Splint The sugar-tong is a splint that prevents motion of the wrist and elbow, including pronation-supination (**Figure 267-11**). The upper extremity is placed in "sling position," as described in the preceding section Long-Arm Gutter Splint. The splint begins on the extensor aspect of the hand at the level of the metacarpal heads and runs along the extensor aspect of the forearm, around the elbow and humeral condyles, onto the flexor aspect of the forearm, and ultimately to the palmar aspect of the hand, ending at the level of the metacarpal heads. It is wrapped in place with gauze and often topped off with an elastic compression bandage. It should be supplemented with a sling.

Proper length of the sugar-tong dressing is important. Too short a splint will fail to immobilize the wrist. If the dressing is too long, it will impair motion of the metacarpophalangeal joints, leaving them stiff and making the fingers more susceptible to swelling due to immobility.

The sugar-tong splint is appropriate for fractures about the wrist or distal forearm. Some orthopedists use it as a definitive dressing after reduction of wrist fractures.

Cock-Up Wrist Splint (to Be Avoided) A cock-up splint extends from the distal forearm to the proximal portion of the hand and maintains the wrist in a dorsiflexed position. **It should not be used for fractures of the wrist or carpals** because injuries to those areas usually are caused by forceful dorsiflexion, and a cock-up splint reproduces the position of injury, imposing considerable pain in the process. Generally, fractures about the wrist are immobilized in neutral position. Colles fractures may sometimes be immobilized in palmar flexion after reduction.

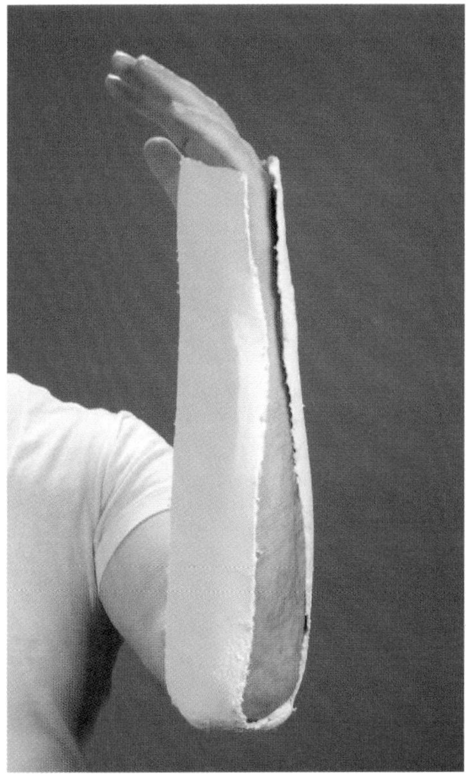

FIGURE 267-11. Sugar-tong splint.

Cock-up splints may be useful in some situations not related to trauma, such as to immobilize the wrist for tendinitis or to support it in the case of wrist drop due to radial nerve palsy. In such instances, passive dorsiflexion of the wrist is indicated to preserve grip strength.

Short-Arm Gutter Splint A short-arm gutter splint immobilizes the wrist and the ulnar or radial half of the hand (**Figure 267-12**). The ulnar gutter, for example, extends along the ulnar surface of the hand and forearm, beginning just proximal to the tip of the fifth finger and ending high on the forearm. It should be wide enough to encompass the fourth and fifth rays (phalanges and metacarpals) on the extensor and flexor aspects of the hand. The splint is wrapped in place so that the fourth and fifth fingers are bound together, with a thin layer of padding between them to prevent maceration of the skin. The metacarpophalangeal joints and interphalangeal joints are positioned in gentle flexion. The dressing may be supplemented with a sling.

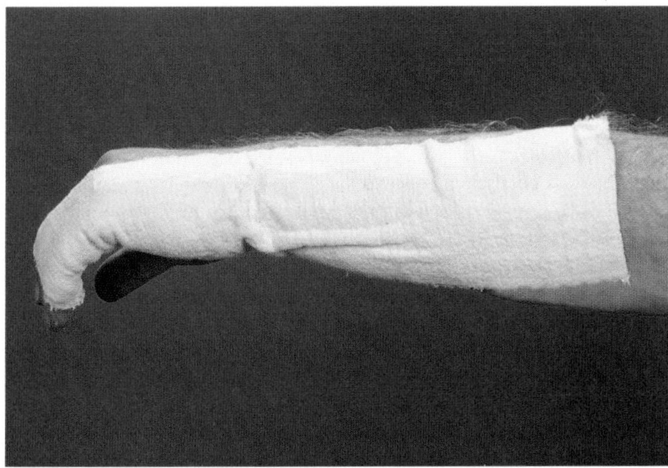

FIGURE 267-12. Short-arm ulnar gutter splint.

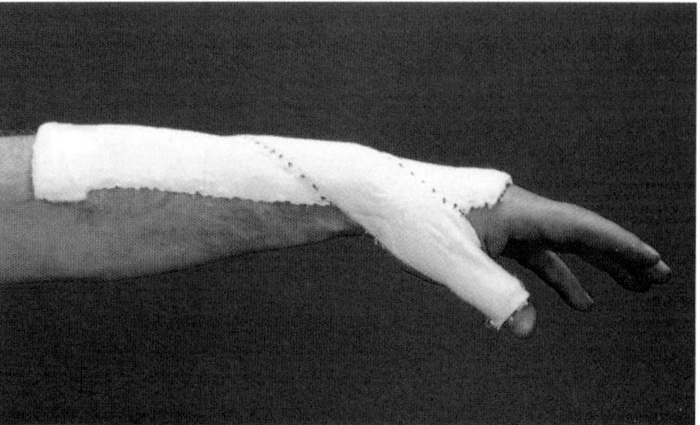

FIGURE 267-13. Thumb spica splint.

The short-arm ulnar gutter is useful for fracture of the proximal phalanx of the ring or little finger or for fracture of the fourth or fifth metacarpal (including the common "boxer's fracture"). The counterpart of this splint, the short-arm radial gutter, is designed in similar fashion but extends along the radial surface of the hand and forearm and is used for comparable injuries of the index or middle rays. It can be fashioned with a hole that allows the thumb to pass through, or by splitting the distal end so the two halves can be run along the extensor and volar aspects of the index and middle rays while the thumb remains free.

Thumb Spica Splint A thumb spica immobilizes the wrist and the thumb (**Figure 267-13**). The term *spica* applies to any dressing that encompasses a main trunk plus one or more of its branches—in this case, the forearm plus the thumb. It is used for fracture of the scaphoid or for fracture of the thumb metacarpal or proximal phalanx.

A thumb spica may be fashioned from one wide splint that runs along the thumb and radial aspect of the wrist and forearm, but an even more effective dressing can be made from two separate non-prepadded plaster splints. The wrist piece runs along the extensor aspect of the hand and forearm, beginning at the metacarpal heads and ending just short of the antecubital crease. The more narrow thumb piece, approximately 2 in. wide, extends from the tip of the thumb, along the outer aspect of the thumb metacarpal, and onto the extensor aspect of the forearm, well overlapping the first splint. Along their area of contact, the two splints are molded into each other, with no padding between them, to form a sturdy dressing. The plaster is wrapped in place with gauze, and a compression wrap may be added at the clinician's discretion. The dressing may be supplemented with a sling.

This technique is not suitable for prepadded splints with plaster or fiberglass already enclosed, as the two pieces cannot be molded into one another, which compromises the structural integrity of the dressing. When prepadded material is used, a single wide splint encompassing the thumb must suffice.

While the dressing is setting, optimal position may be achieved by keeping the wrist in neutral position and having the patient oppose the tips of the thumb and index finger in the form of an "OK" sign. This preserves thumb-to-index pinch function, so as to minimize the patient's incapacitation. The neutral position of the wrist also avoids reproducing the position of injury in the case of scaphoid fracture, which is typically caused by forced dorsiflexion.

Knee Immobilizer The knee immobilizer is a removable circumferential device that extends from the thigh to just above the ankle (**Figure 267-14**). The splint contains longitudinal struts that, in some cases, may be repositioned as needed, and is secured with Velcro® straps.

A knee immobilizer maintains the knee in extension, the position of maximum stability. The device is useful for a variety of injuries, including fracture of the lateral or medial tibial plateau, fracture of the patella, meniscal injuries (provided the knee is not locked in partial flexion), and ligamentous strains or tears.

Use of an immobilizer for more than a few days in the elderly or for more than a week or two in young patients may result in painful stiffness

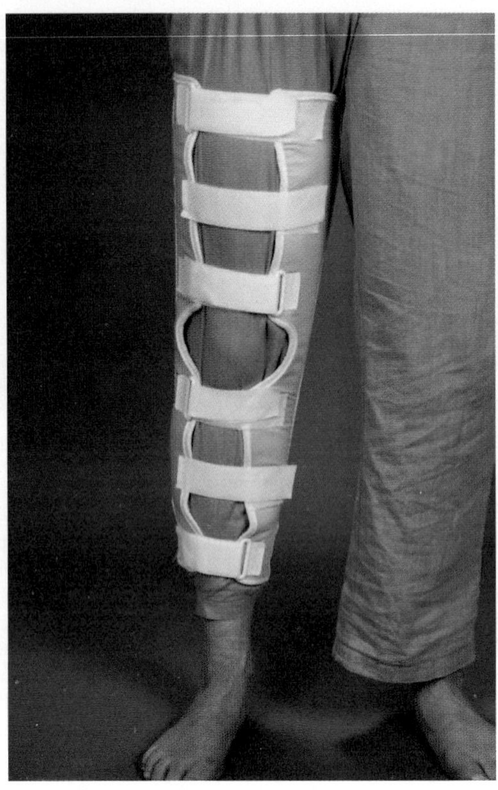

FIGURE 267-14. Knee immobilizer.

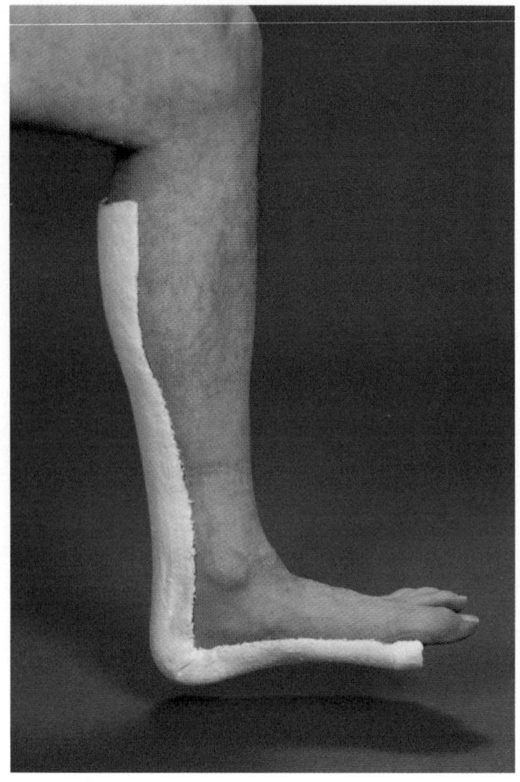

FIGURE 267-15. Posterior ankle mold.

of the knee joint. For that reason, orthopedic follow-up should occur within approximately 7 days. If immobilization is indicated beyond that point, the orthopedist may replace the original device with a cast brace or other orthosis that allows controlled and progressive range of motion.

Motion and Strength Exercises for the Knee Joint stiffness and instability due to quadriceps weakness may occur rapidly when the knee is immobilized. **Patients wearing an immobilizer should be encouraged to remove the device periodically and perform the following exercises:**

1. Passive flexion: While sitting on a flat surface, grasp the ends of a towel draped beneath the sole of the foot and pull upward, creating as much knee flexion as possible without undue pain.
2. "Gravity-assisted" flexion: While sitting on the edge of a bed or chair, support the knee in extension, with the well foot beneath the ankle of the injured extremity, then gradually lower the supporting foot so the injured knee "drops" into flexion. When tolerance is reached, bring the knee back into extension.
3. Quadriceps strengthening: While lying supine with a pillow beneath the knee, actively bring the knee to full extension in a straight leg raise, then relax.

Each of these exercises should be performed as multiple repetitions several times a day.

Posterior Ankle Mold The posterior ankle mold is used to immobilize the ankle (**Figure 267-15**). It begins beneath the metatarsal heads, runs along the plantar aspect of the foot, and continues up the back of the lower leg, ending at high calf. The splint is used for fractures or severe sprains of the ankle. Support may be supplemented by a transverse sugar-tong component running down the lateral side of the lower leg, beneath the heel, and up the medial side. Where the two components overlap, they are molded together. (Non-prepadded plaster should be used in this situation). The transverse component helps minimize inversion and eversion of the ankle. Even more stability is provided by continuing the posterior splint past the back of the knee to the high posterior thigh, using wider splinting material for this area. With the knee slightly flexed, rotational motion at the ankle also will be prevented.

While the dressing is setting, the ankle should be maintained in a position as close as possible to neutral dorsiflexion—that is, at 90 degrees to the leg. This may facilitate regaining range of motion after the dressing is removed. Because most patients with ankle injuries tend to keep the ankle plantarflexed, the clinician usually will have to counteract this by exerting gentle pressure with a palm beneath the metatarsal heads. An exception to the 90-degree principle is immobilization for rupture of the Achilles tendon. Patients with this injury should be immobilized in plantar flexion to reduce tension on the tendon.

Ankle Stirrup Easier to apply and less cumbersome for the patient than a posterior mold, the ankle stirrup (**Figures 267-16A** and **267-16B**) is useful for stable ankle sprains and for stable lateral malleolus fractures. The ankle stirrup is essentially an air-padded "sugar-tong" splint held in place by Velcro® straps. Unlike the posterior mold, this device is intended for use in conjunction with weightbearing. It limits inversion more effectively than taping but allows normal plantarflexion and dorsiflexion. This feature and the graduated compressive effect of the air-filled bladders may result in less swelling and edema, less joint stiffness, and a faster return to comfortable ambulation than is typically observed after rigid immobilization.[21]

The stirrup may be removed for purposes of bathing or when not bearing weight. If the patient does remove the splint temporarily, a common error when reapplying it is to fail to unwrap the straps completely—specifically, to leave the straps attached posteriorly, so that the splint is "hinged like a book" along its posterior aspect. This may result in the foot persistently slipping forward and out of the splint. The clinician may wish to instruct the patient that the proper way to reapply the splint is to unwrap the straps all the way around, so that the sides fall apart bilaterally, with the heel pad acting as the "hinge" on the plantar aspect (**Figure 267-17**). The foot may then be positioned on the lower pad, and the sides reapplied to the medial and lateral aspects of the ankle and lower leg. The final step is to rewrap the straps around the dressing.

Motion and Strength Exercises for the Ankle Exercises to restore range of motion, stability, and balance should be started as soon as possible after an ankle injury.

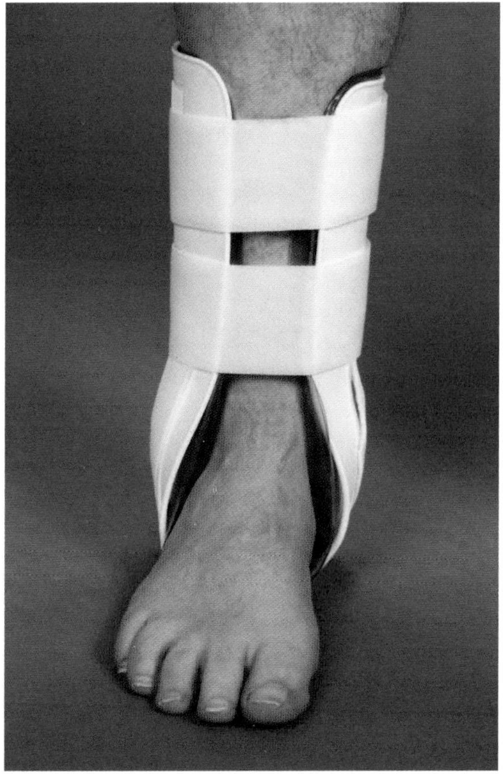

A

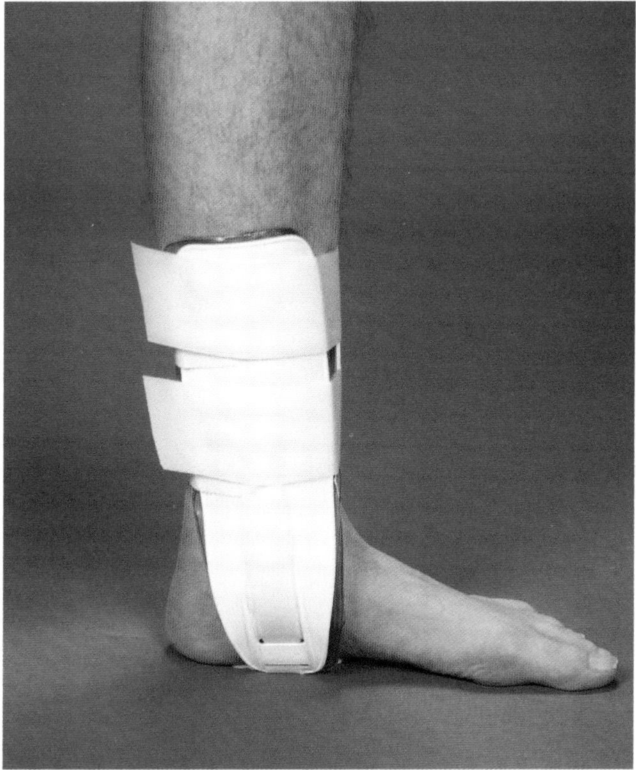

B

FIGURE 267-16. **A, B.** Ankle stirrup.

1. Active dorsiflexion and plantarflexion: When performed supine with the foot well elevated, this exercise may also enhance lymphatic drainage, thereby reducing swelling.
2. Passive dorsiflexion: One method for performing this exercise is to stand with the palms braced against the wall, then to bend the knee toward the wall while keeping the heel flat on the floor.

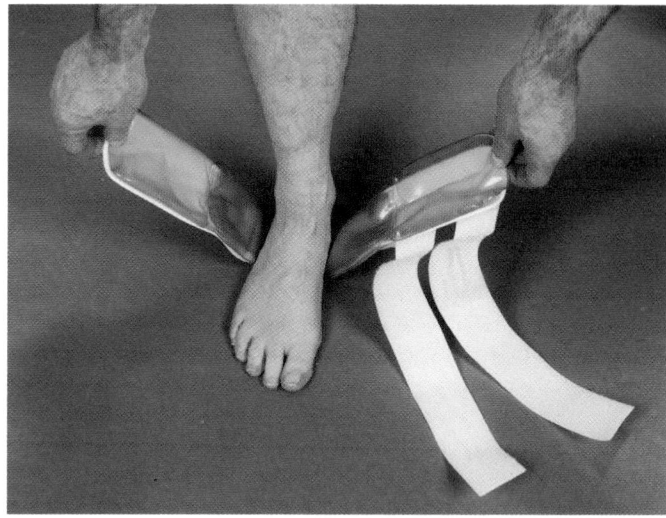

FIGURE 267-17. Technique for applying ankle stirrup.

3. Eversion, dorsiflexion, and plantarflexion against resistance: This exercise may be accomplished by manually applying a counterforce with a stretchable elastic cord (commercially available). Standing on the toes is another means of resistive plantarflexion.

Each of these exercises should be performed as multiple repetitions several times a day.

Hard-Soled Shoe A hard-soled shoe is a removable "sandal" with wraparound sides usually secured with Velcro® and a flat, nonflexible sole (**Figures 267-18A** and **267-18B**). This device is intended to allow weight-bearing by patients with toe fractures or certain types of metatarsal fractures. The firm sole prevents the toes from bending and provides support for the forefoot. Although immobilization dressings may be warranted for some metatarsal fractures, the hard-soled shoe is an accepted treatment modality for fracture of the second, third, fourth, or proximal fifth metatarsal.[22,23]

Pneumatic Walking Brace The pneumatic walking brace is a device that provides firm support about the foot, ankle, and lower leg. It is available in high-top or short-top varieties. The high-top walker (**Figure 267-18C**), which extends almost to the knee, is suitable for injuries such as moderate to severe ankle sprains or for stable fractures of the foot or ankle. Short-top walkers extend just above the ankle joint and may be used for phalangeal or stable metatarsal fractures.

The term *pneumatic* refers to the fact that the inner lining of the brace is inflatable. Though non-pneumatic models are available, the pneumatic component has at least two advantages. It provides added compression, which helps reduce swelling and pain, and allows the walker to conform more closely to the contour of the extremity, which enhances immobilization.

ADJUNCTS TO AMBULATION

CRUTCHES

Crutches should be used by patients who can bear little or no weight on an injured lower extremity. Ideal crutch height is one hand width below the axilla. The grip bar should be adjusted to a height at which the elbows are mildly flexed while supporting the body weight. The patient should be instructed to bear the pressure of the pads against the sides of the thorax rather than in the axillae, or brachial plexus injury (crutch palsy) might result.

Any of several crutch gaits may be prescribed. The most common is the three-point gait, in which the patient keeps the injured extremity off the ground, advances both crutches simultaneously, then brings the well leg to a point between the crutches ("swing-to" gait) or just past them ("swing-through" gait). Alternatively the patient may use a two-point gait, in which one crutch and the opposite extremity are advanced together followed by the other crutch and extremity, or a four-point gait, in which one crutch is

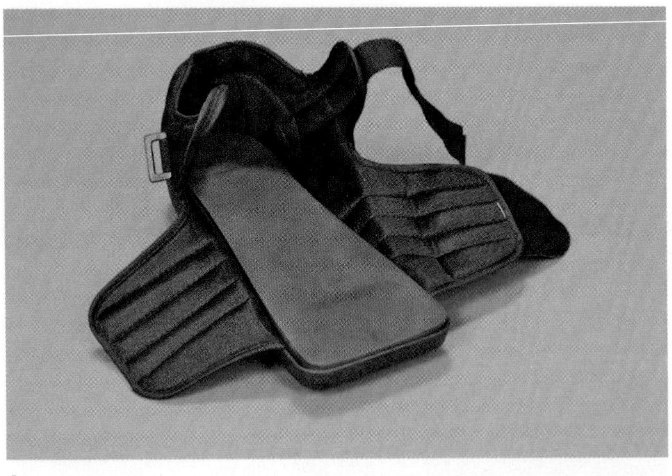

A

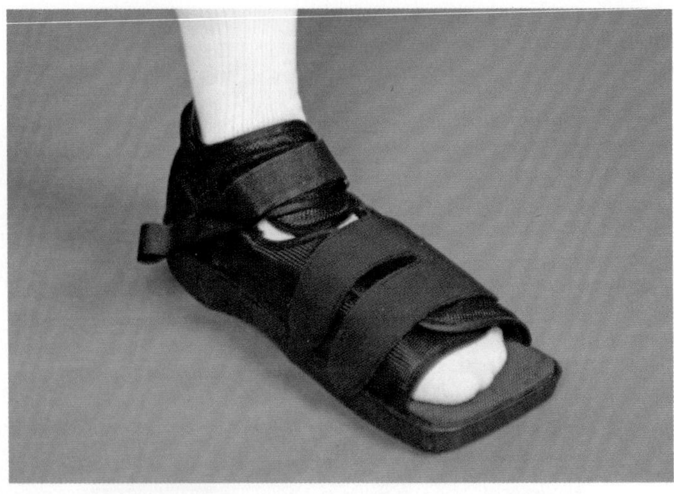

B

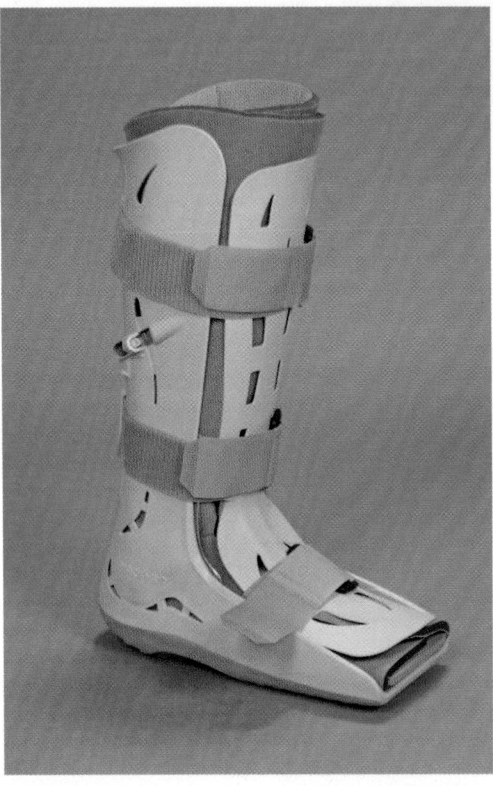

C

FIGURE 267-18. **A, B.** Hard-soled shoe. **C.** Pneumatic walking brace.

advanced, then the opposite extremity, then the other crutch, then the remaining extremity. The two- and four-point gaits are slower in forward progression than the three-point gait but require less arm and wrist strength. They should be used only for patients who are able to bear some weight on the injured extremity. To ascend stairs, the patient advances the well extremity up to the next step, followed by the crutches and the injured extremity. To descend stairs, the crutches are lowered first.

WALKERS AND CANES

Most elderly or infirm patients do not have the strength needed to use crutches safely. For them, a walker or a cane is more suitable. Unfortunately, these devices are more appropriate for partial weightbearing than for nonweightbearing conditions. Elderly patients who can bear no weight at all on an injured extremity may require initial bedrest or use of a wheelchair and subsequent rehabilitation.

The technique for using a walker is essentially intuitive, with the patient simply lifting it and placing it a short distance ahead and then advancing toward it. In contrast, the technique for using a cane tends to be counterintuitive. Many patients instinctively hold a cane on the same side as the injured extremity. In fact, when the cane is held in the hand on the well side, less strength is required to maintain balance, resulting in a less awkward gait. The patient should be instructed to advance the cane (held on the well side) and the injured extremity simultaneously, and then advance the noninjured extremity to meet them.

DISCHARGE INSTRUCTIONS

Elevation of the injured part usually helps minimize pain and swelling. Elevation must be above the level of the heart to be effective. Patients with an injured lower extremity often sit at home or at work with the foot resting on a stool or chair, thinking they are complying with instructions. The patient should understand that the benefits of elevating a lower extremity can be achieved only in a recumbent or near-recumbent position, with the leg supported higher than the rest of the body.

Patients discharged in a lower-extremity plaster dressing should be cautioned not to rest the heel on the floor or any other hard surface during the first day, as plaster takes about 24 hours to fully set. During this time, prolonged pressure on the heel might create an indentation that could cause significant discomfort or even a pressure sore. This is not a consideration with fiberglass, which sets almost immediately.

If an upper-extremity sugar-tong dressing has been applied, the patient should be instructed to work the fingers (wiggle or wave) as much as possible to minimize stiffness and swelling. The sugar-tong splint should extend to, but not beyond, the metacarpal heads, so as to allow full flexion of the metacarpophalangeal joints.

Patients should be advised to monitor the fingers or toes for excessive swelling, decreased sensation, or cyanosis and to be alert for a significant increase in pain. Any of these signs or symptoms warrants a return to the ED or prompt evaluation by the follow-up physician.

When crutches, a cane, or a walker is supplied, instruction for use should be provided, and the patient's ability to navigate with such aids should be verified.

COMPLICATIONS

Complications associated with musculoskeletal injury may be early or delayed and may occur minutes, days, weeks, or even months later.

NEUROLOGIC DEFICIT

Neurologic injury resulting from long-bone fracture or joint dislocation is usually due to traction or pressure on a peripheral nerve or a nerve plexus. Such complications usually manifest themselves early. Recovery may take hours, days, or weeks. Sometimes, the injury is irreversible. Prompt reduction of deformity often may prevent, eliminate, or mitigate the effects of neurologic involvement, but it is not a guarantee against permanent deficit.

VASCULAR INJURY

Peripheral vessels that run close to a joint sometimes may be compressed or disrupted when the joint becomes dislocated, as, for example, with dislocation of the ankle or knee (tibiofemoral joint). Loss of peripheral pulses or poor to absent capillary refill calls for expeditious reduction of deformity. Even after reduction, evidence of significant vascular injury may be delayed. Patients who experience tibiofemoral dislocation, for example, often undergo routine postreduction angiography to verify the integrity and patency of the popliteal vessels, regardless of whether a circulatory deficit has been observed clinically.

COMPARTMENT SYNDROME

After a fracture or a direct blow to an extremity, there may be extravasation of blood, swelling of muscle tissues, and impairment of venous flow within one or more fascial compartments. The resulting increase in pressure within the limb may lead to circulatory compromise, neurologic damage, and muscle necrosis, known collectively as *compartment syndrome*. This is a surgical emergency, and early recognition is crucial. Compartment syndrome is discussed further in chapter 278, Compartment Syndrome.

DELAYED AND LATE COMPLICATIONS

Patients who have sustained a fracture may be at risk for pulmonary fat embolus, usually originating from the marrow of a large bone, such as the femur. If fat embolism occurs, it is typically within the first few days after injury, rather than the first hours. This event may have a variable effect on pulmonary function, ranging from mild distress to severe or even fatal respiratory failure.

The most delayed complications of fracture include nonunion, malunion (healing with deformity), joint stiffness, traumatic arthritis, avascular necrosis of bone, and, in the case of open fracture, osteomyelitis.

DISPOSITION AND FOLLOW-UP

There is no universally prescribed follow-up interval for specific injuries. Orthopedists differ in their opinions regarding how soon patients should be seen. In general, patients with unreduced fractures or injuries that may require surgical intervention should be seen within a few days.

Sometimes the situation may be discussed with the follow-up physician and an appointment arranged while the patient is still in the ED. Alternatively, the emergency physician may instruct the patient to contact the follow-up physician or clinic as soon as possible. If the name of the injury is written on the discharge instruction sheet, the patient can convey it at the time of the call. This information may help the follow-up physician decide when the patient should be seen.

Acknowledgments: The author wishes to thank the following: Eleanore Denton Rhodes, AMI, for original artwork, and Joe Driscoll for original photography.

REFERENCES

The complete reference list is available online at www.TintinalliEM.com.

CHAPTER 268 Injuries to the Hand and Digits

Moira Davenport
Peter Tang

ANATOMY

The hand consists of 27 bones: 14 phalangeal bones, 5 metacarpal bones, and 8 carpal bones arranged in five rays of metacarpals and phalanges having its base at the carpometacarpal (CMC) articulation (**Figure 268-1**).

The carpal bones are made up of two rows, each with four bones. The bones are concave volarly and are bridged by the flexor retinaculum. This forms the carpal tunnel through which the median nerve and the nine long flexor tendons of the fingers pass (flexor pollicis longus [FPL]; flexor digitorum profundus [FDP] from the index, middle, ring, and small fingers; and flexor digitorum superficialis [FDS] from the index, middle, ring and small fingers) (**Figure 268-2**).

The index and middle finger CMC articulations have relatively little mobility, whereas the thumb, ring, and small finger CMC articulations have greater mobility at the CMC joint, which allows grasping and adaptive movements of the hand. More metacarpal deformity can be accepted in the great mobility CMC joints.

Multiple soft tissue structures support the bones and joints of the hand: capsules and ligaments provide stability, whereas muscles/tendons of the hand and forearm generate mobility (Figures 268-2, 268-3, and 268-4). The collateral ligaments of the metacarpophalangeal (MCP) joints are tightest in flexion in the index through small fingers (to allow stability in grasp), while the collateral ligaments of the MCP thumb are tight in flexion and extension (which also provide stability for the thumb in all positions) (Figure 268-3). The collateral ligaments of the interphalangeal (IP) joints are also tight throughout the entire range of motion.

INTRINSIC HAND MUSCLES

The intrinsic muscles of the hand are those that have both their origins and insertions within the hand. They consist of the thenar and hypothenar muscles, the adductor pollicis, the interossei, and the lumbricals (**Figures 268-3, 268-4, and 268-5**).

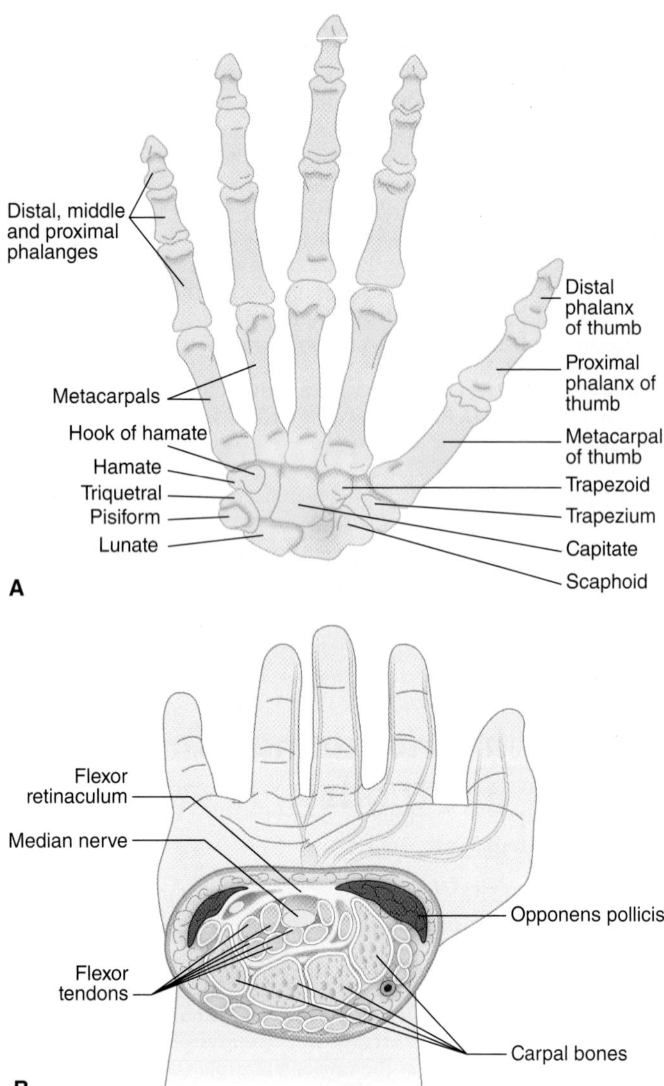

FIGURE 268-1. **A.** Bones of the hand and wrist. **B.** Carpal tunnel.

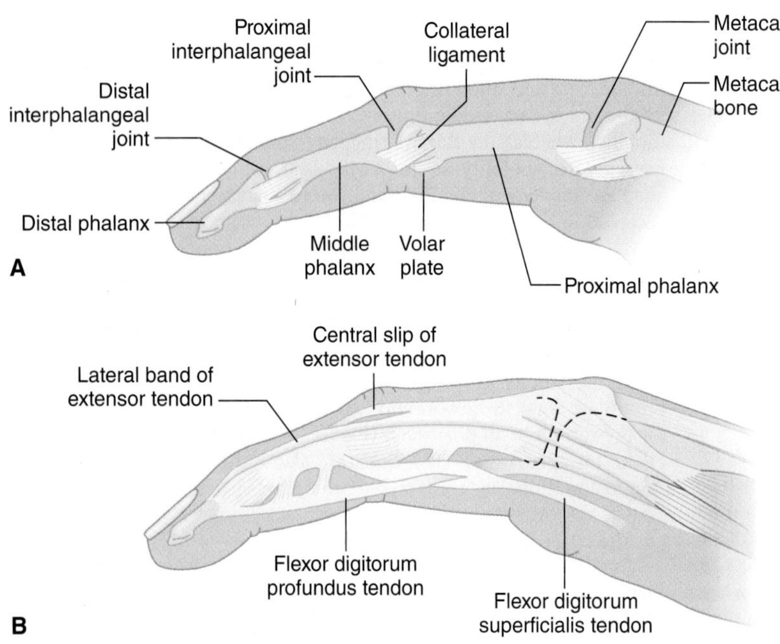

FIGURE 268-2. Joints, ligaments, and tendons of the digits.

The **thenar muscles** (from superficial to deep: abductor pollicis brevis, opponens pollicis, and flexor pollicis brevis) originate in the flexor retinaculum and carpal bones and insert on the radial base of the thumb proximal phalanx and the radial aspect of the first metacarpal. The motor branch of the median nerve innervates all three muscles except for the deep head of the flexor pollicis brevis, which is innervated by the ulnar nerve. The adductor pollicis is innervated by the ulnar nerve and originates from the capitate and second and third metacarpals and inserts on the ulnar base of the thumb proximal phalanx.

The **hypothenar muscles** include, from superficial to deep, the abductor digiti minimi, the flexor digiti minimi, and the opponens digiti minimi. These muscles, innervated by the ulnar nerve, originate in the flexor retinaculum and carpal bones and insert at the ulnar base of the small finger proximal phalanx and the ulnar aspect of the fifth metacarpal.

There are seven **interosseous muscles**, all innervated by the ulnar nerve (Figure 268-5). The three palmar and four dorsal interossei lie between the metacarpal bones and originate from them. The palmar interosseous muscle and the palmar portion of the dorsal interosseous muscle have an insertion into the extensor hood. The palmar interosseous muscle adducts the index, ring, and small finger to the midline, which is designated as the middle finger. The dorsal portion of the dorsal interosseous muscle has a tendinous insertion into the base of the proximal phalanx. The dorsal interosseous muscles abduct the fingers away from the midline.

The **lumbrical muscles** (Figure 268-3) do not attach to bone. They arise from the FDP tendons in the palm, course radially near the MCP joints, and attach to tendons or expansions, reinforcing the interosseous lateral band on the radial side of the digit. They flex the MCP joints while extending the IP joints.The median nerve innervates the radial two lumbricals, and the ulnar nerve innervates the ulnar two. The lumbricals flex the MCP joint and extend the IP joints of the index to the small fingers. Lumbrical muscles also play a critical role coordinating the flexor and extensor systems of the digits.

EXTENSOR AND FLEXOR TENDONS

The **extensor tendons** course over the dorsal side of the forearm, wrist, and hand (Figure 268-4). Nine extensor tendons pass under the extensor retinaculum and separate into six compartments. In the dorsum of the hand, the extensors digitorum communis are connected by juncturae (**Figure 268-6**). **Based on this anatomy, finger extension may still be possible with a complete tendon laceration that is proximal to the juncture.** In the finger, the extensor mechanism divides into a central slip that attaches to the middle phalanx and into two lateral bands that join with the tendons of the lumbrical and interosseous muscles, which then attach to the dorsal base of the distal phalanx as the terminal tendon.

The **flexor tendons** (flexor carpi radialis, flexor carpi ulnaris, and palmaris longus) course over the volar side of the forearm, wrist, and hand, and primarily flex the wrist. The remaining nine tendons (four FDP, four FDS, and the FPL) pass through the carpal tunnel (Figure 268-1). The FPL goes to the base of the distal phalanx of the thumb. The other four digits have two tendons each (Figure 268-2). The FDS inserts into the volar, proximal half of the middle phalanx and flexes all the joints it crosses, including the proximal interphalangeal (PIP) joint and MCP joints. The FDP runs deep to the FDS until the level of the MCP joint, at which point it bifurcates. The FDP inserts at the volar base of the distal phalanx and acts primarily to flex the distal interphalangeal (DIP) joint as well as all the PIP and MCP joints. Unlike the extensor tendons, the flexor tendons are enclosed in synovial sheaths, making them prone to deep space infections.

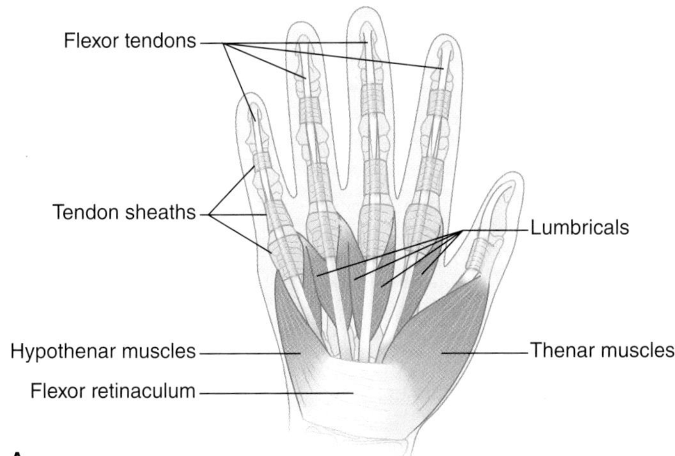

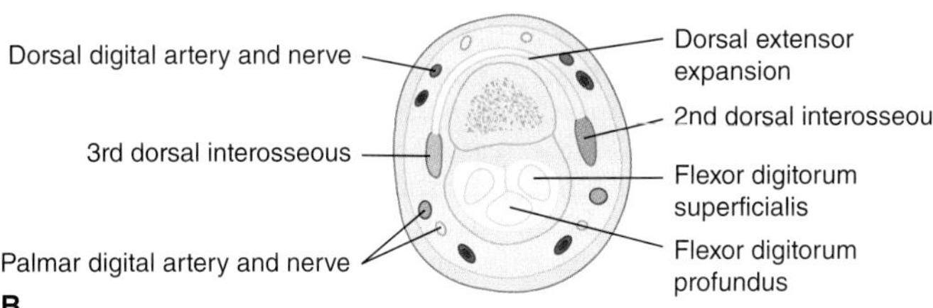

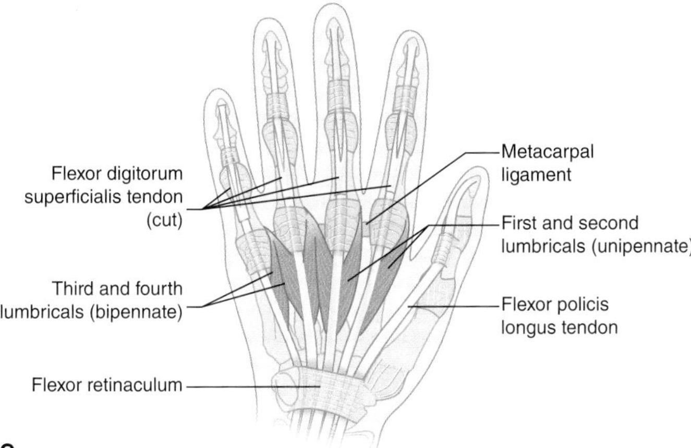

FIGURE 268-3. **A.** Palmar (volar) view of the hand showing the relationship of the some of the intrisic muscles, and flexor tendons and sheaths. **B.** Cross-sectional view of digit at the middle phalanx. **C.** Lumbricals.

VASCULAR SUPPLY

The hand and digits are perfused by the radial and ulnar arteries. The radial artery forms the deep palmar arch, whereas the ulnar artery forms the superficial palmar arch. The common digital arteries (in the second, third, and fourth web spaces) arise from the superficial palmar arch (**Figure 268-7**) and provide blood supply to the fingers. The blood supply to the thumb arises from the princeps pollicis, which is the radial artery as it turns into the palm. The radialis indicis, which is on the radial side of the index finger, arises from the radial artery or the princeps pollicis.

NERVE SUPPLY

The radial, ulnar, and median nerves innervate the hand (**Figure 268-8**). In the hand, the median and ulnar nerves have mixed motor and sensory function. The superficial radial nerve (C5-T1) provides sensation to the dorsal radial aspect of the hand. The ulnar nerve (C7-T1) supplies sensory function to the small finger and the ulnar volar half of the ring finger and motor function to the hypothenar muscles, ulnar two lumbricals, interossei, adductor pollicis, and deep head of the flexor pollicis brevis. The median nerve (C5-T1) supplies sensory function to the thumb, index, middle, and radial volar half of the ring fingers, and motor function to the abductor pollicis brevis, opponens pollicis brevis, and superficial head of flexor pollicis brevis. As the digital nerves course across the palm, they are superficial structures and thus are easily injured. Digital nerve sensation and two-point discrimination should be routinely assessed when evaluating lacerations of the palm (**Figure 268-8**). **Normal two-point discrimination is 5 mm.** Consult a hand specialist if the extent of injury is uncertain. In the digits, the digital nerves divide into volar and dorsal branches to supply sensation to the fingers. Knowing the location of these nerves is important to properly perform a digital block (Figure 268-3, cross-sectional view).

CLINICAL FEATURES

Do not allow a visually striking hand injury to delay the identification and treatment of other potentially life-threatening injuries. After hemorrhage control, assessment involves a detailed history, general hand examination, testing of nerves and tendons, anesthesia, and direct wound inspection. Compare with the uninjured hand, especially to identify partial motor or sensory deficits.

HISTORY

The history should include the time and cause of injury as well as the position of the hand at the time of injury. Ask about the possibility of associated crush, burn, injection, or chemical exposure. When applicable, determine the type and amount of chemical to which the patient was exposed. Document the patient's occupation, avocations, prior hand injuries, and hand dominance to determine the functional impact of the injury.

PHYSICAL EXAMINATION

Detail the extent of injury by documenting the vascularity, status of the skin, posture of the fingers, and presence of deformity or active bleeding. Ask the patient to demonstrate the hand position at the time of injury. **Injuries with the digits in flexion may result in retraction of the cut end of the tendon when the digit is examined in extension.** Check bilateral grip strength. Compare motor, sensory, and tendon function of both hands to assess baseline function. Test range of motion and strength against resistance. Have the patient make a clenched fist to observe the orientation and rotation of the middle and distal phalanxes. All phalanges should be oriented parallel to each other with the nails positioned in the same plane and be pointing toward the scaphoid when the fist is clenched. Circulation is assessed by regional pulses and capillary refill.[1] Doppler assessment can also help assess digital artery flow.

NERVE TESTING

To test the **median nerve**, have the patient flex the IP joint of the thumb against resistance, which tests FPL function. Alternatively, hold the index or middle finger PIP and MCP joints in extension and have the patient flex the DIP joint, which tests FDP function of the index and middle fingers. **The "OK" sign** will reveal the ability to flex the IP joint of the thumb and the DIP joint of the index finger. To test the motor branch of the median nerve, position the thumb in palmar abduction with the palm up. Have the patient resist a force directing the thumb toward the palm, and assess the motor power while palpating the belly of the abductor pollicis brevis muscle to ensure it is contracting. It is important to note that a laceration at the level of the wrist or distal forearm may have intact FDP function of the index and middle fingers and FPL function to the thumb because these muscles have been innervated at the proximal forearm. A median nerve injury at the level of the wrist or distal forearm can only be determined by examining two-point

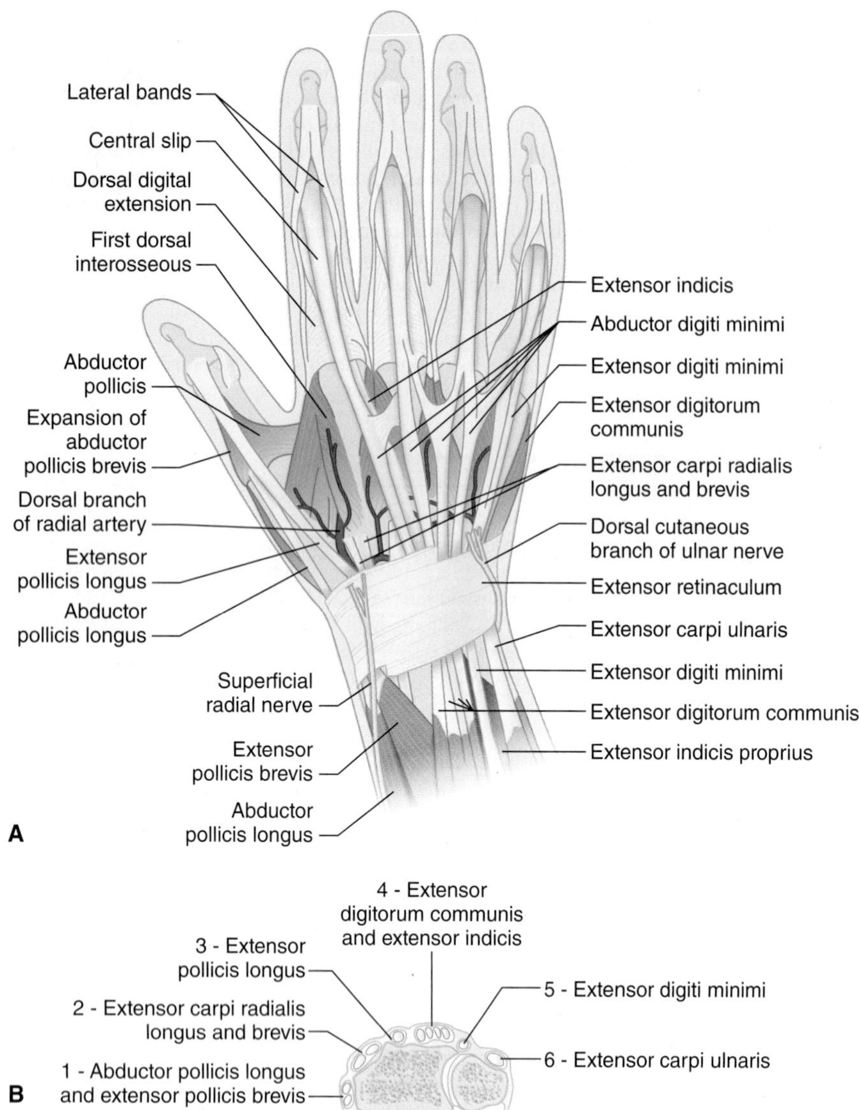

FIGURE 268-4. **A.** Dorsal view of the hand showing the extensor tendons and retinaculum, and intrinsic musculature. **B.** Cross-sectional view with the six extensor compartments.

discrimination in the three and a half radial digits or motor branch integrity to the thenar muscles.

To assess ulnar nerve integrity, have the patient spread the fingers apart (finger abduction) and assessing the motor power by resisting a force pushing the index and small fingers to midline. Alternatively, have the patient cross the fingers. To test thumb adduction (**the ulnar nerve innervates the adductor pollicis muscles**), have the patient hold a piece of paper with the volar pulp of the thumb against the radial side of the PIP joint of the index finger. If the patient can maintain the key pinch of the paper against resistance then the adductor pollicis is relatively strong. If the patient cannot hold the paper and uses the FPL and flexes the IP joint to compensate for the weak adductor pollicis this is a positive Froment's sign and indicates ulnar nerve pathology. All these reviewed maneuvers for the ulnar nerve test intrinsic muscles so that an ulnar nerve injury at the level of the wrist would be revealed by these test maneuvers.

To test the **radial nerve**, have the patient hyperextend the finger MCP joints against resistance, which will test the extensor digitorum communis tendons. One way to test this is to have the patient put the palm on a table, with fingers flat and hyperextended, and then lift each digit straight up and extend up from the table while keeping the palm flat. Finger resistance can also be checked in this extended, upright position. During this maneuver, it is important to keep the finger MCP joints in hyperextension because the interossei extend the IP joints of the fingers (but flex the MCP joints), and failure to keep the digit in full extension can mislead the examiner into believing the radial nerve is intact. The interossei cannot hyperextend the finger MCP joints. By extending the thumb against resistance, the extensor pollicis longus integrity is confirmed. If a patient has a posterior interosseous nerve (which innervates the majority of the extensor muscles) palsy, the patient will be unable to hyperextend his or her fingers, but may be able to extend the wrist in a radial direction because the extensor radialis longus and extensor radialis brevis are innervated by the radial nerve proper before the posterior interosseous nerve branches.

Sensation is determined by two-point discrimination. **Normal two-point discrimination is 5 mm at the volar fingertips. Older patients may have 6 mm of two-point discrimination.** Compare both injured and contralateral fingers to establish a reasonable baseline, because patients may have preexisting compressive neuropathies such as carpal and cubital tunnel syndrome or previous nerve injuries. Examine the radial and ulnar sides of each finger to determine which digital nerve is injured. Hand specialists recommend repeating two-point discrimination testing two to four times on each side of the digit, because patients can guess sensation correctly by chance. At least 80% accuracy is considered acceptable. Less than 80% or indeterminate accuracy suggests the possibility of digital nerve injury. **A sensory deficit also implies a potential digital artery laceration because of the close proximity of the two.**

TESTING OF TENDONS

Assess full range of motion of each tendon against resistance and compare with the uninjured side. It is important to test resistance because **up to 90% of a tendon can be lacerated with preservation of range of motion without resistance.** In addition, the juncturae tendinum contributes to digital extension, so patients with lacerations to the extensor digitorum communis may be able to extend the digit but may not have the same motor power. **Pain along the course of the tendon during resistance testing suggests a partial laceration even if strength appears adequate.** Test FDP function by checking flexion of the DIP joint against resistance while holding the PIP and MCP joints in extension. Test the FDS by having the patient flex the PIP joint against resistance while the remaining fingers are held in full extension. When the rest of the fingers are in extension, the FDP of the tested finger cannot fire and the FDS function is isolated. If the test is not performed this way, PIP joint flexion may be due to the FDP because this tendon also traverses the PIP joint, whereas the FDS does not.

To determine whether the central slip is intact, perform the **Elson's test**. Hold the PIP joint of the affected finger in flexion (therefore tightening the central slip and loosening the lateral bands) and ask the patient to extend the finger at the PIP. The examiner should resist extension; if the DIP is loose, then Elson's test is negative, meaning the central slip is intact and the extension force is being transmitted to the central slip. If the DIP is rigid and the PIP does not extend, Elson's test is positive, meaning the central slip is not intact and the extension force is being transmitted through the lateral bands to the terminal tendon to the DIP joint. The contralateral finger should be examined.

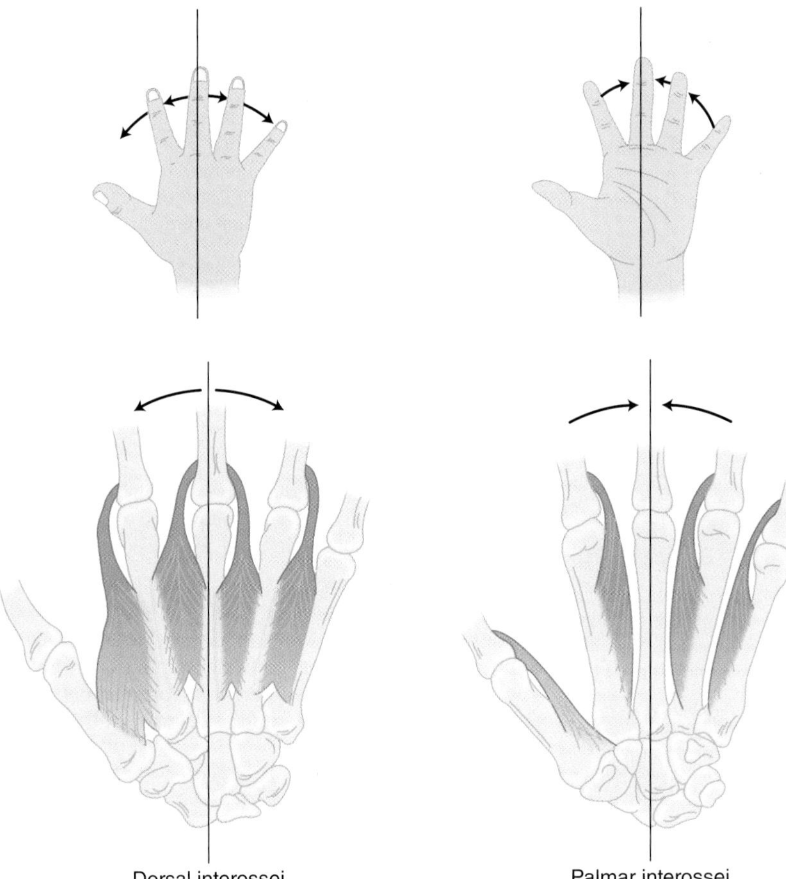

FIGURE 268-5. Origins, insertions, and actions of the palmar and dorsal interossei.

Sometimes the patient can overpower the examiner and should be asked to decrease the extension force on the finger. Lastly, if the patient resists PIP flexion due to pain, a digital block can be placed and the test repeated.

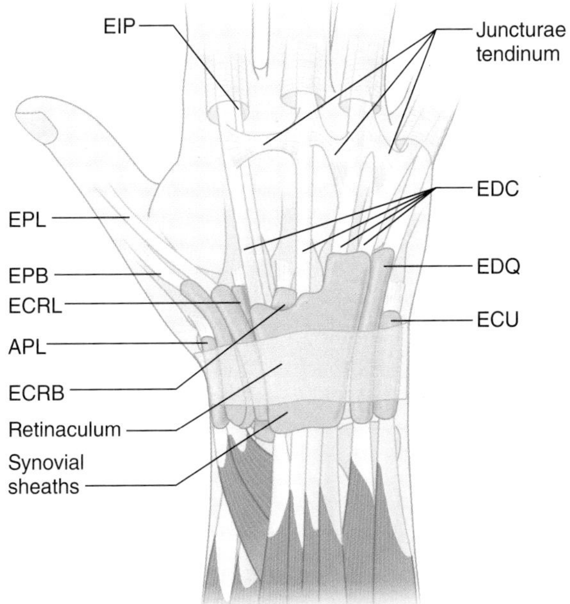

FIGURE 268-6. Dorsal view of the hand showing juncturae tendinum. EPL, extensor pollicis longus; EPB, extensor pollicis brevis; ECRL, extensor carpi radialis longus; APL, abductor pollicis longus; ECRB, extensor carpi radialis brevis; EIP, extensor indicis proprius; EDC, extensor digitorum communis; EDQ, extensor digitorum quinti; ECU, extensor carpi ulnaris.

ANESTHESIA AND DIRECT WOUND EXAMINATION

Anesthesia and direct wound inspection are necessary because partial tendon lacerations or intra-articular injuries are not always readily apparent. Perform the initial motor and sensory exam before anesthesia. **If pain limits the motor exam, a digital block can be performed and then motor function reassessed.** A bloodless field can be facilitated by milking the digit proximally and then applying a local tourniquet or Penrose drain around the base of the digit. The tourniquet should not be stretched to more than 150% of its length and can be held in place with a hemostat. The digit can be milked by wrapping another Penrose drain circumferentially around the entire digit, going from distal to proximal, or by reconfiguring a 4 × 4-inch gauze dressing into a narrow band and wrapping that circumferentially around the entire digit. Only moderate compression should be used to avoid compression injury to the digit. **Do not leave the tourniquet in place for >20 minutes.** Irrigate contaminated wounds copiously with normal saline, and administer antibiotics. Cephalosporins are often the first choice, but tailor antibiotic selection to the particular contaminant. Administer tetanus toxoid as needed.

RADIOGRAPHS, CONSULTATION, AND DISPOSITION

Radiologic evaluation should include at a minimum posteroanterior (PA), lateral, and oblique projections of the hand. Similar projections are used for the digits, except that the radiographic beam is centered over the affected digit(s), so that true PA and lateral views should be obtained of the affected digit. Actual or suspected injuries of tendons and nerves should be referred to a hand specialist. Whether consultation is provided in the ED or in follow-up (1 to 3 days) depends on local resources. Injuries requiring immediate and delayed follow-up by a hand surgeon are listed in **Tables 268-1 and 268-2**, respectively.

Table 268-3 provides guidelines for immobilization and follow-up for specific hand injuries referred for delayed hand surgery evaluation. Often, the skin can be closed and the hand splinted in the position of function. The wound can be extended and explored at follow-up, with definitive repair performed by the hand specialist. **Most hand specialists prefer to do definitive repair of the acute injuries as soon as possible so patients should be informed to seek evaluation immediately and *not* in 2 weeks, as is often instructed.** Also, some diagnoses may be missed in the acute stage when patients are in pain and a thorough exam is difficult. Thus, early referral to a hand specialist verifies the diagnosis and can detect other injuries. Although most injuries involving <20% of the tendon are not surgically repaired, hand specialist follow-up and rehabilitation are still necessary to accurately determine the extent of injury, minimize scarring and tendon contraction, and minimize neuroma formation.

For patients with hand or digit lacerations that are sutured in the ED, and when there is no suspicion of neurovascular or tendon injury, follow-up evaluation and suture removal in the ED should always include repeat hand examination to make sure that significant injuries have not been missed.

FLEXOR TENDON INJURIES

The most common cause of flexor tendon injury is laceration. Flexor tendon lacerations can be subtle. A hand surgeon should repair all flexor tendon lacerations. Temporary stabilization and loose closure may be performed in the ED but should occur within 12 hours. Definitive treatment can occur up to 4 weeks after the injury but as soon as possible is best. In general, flexor tendon lacerations of <25% do not

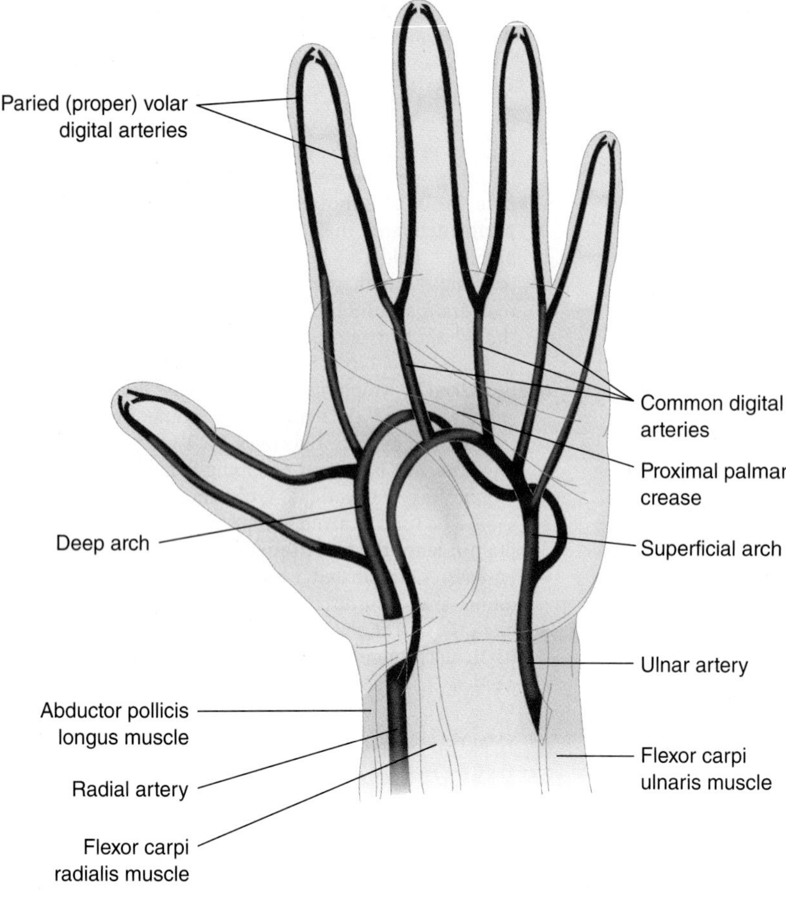

FIGURE 268-7. The dual blood supply to the hands and digits.

need to be repaired, but it is difficult to make this assessment in the ED. A distal-to-proximal five-zone (I to V) classification system for flexor tendon injuries has been developed based on location, treatment considerations, and prognosis (**Figure 268-10**).[2]

ZONE I

Zone I is distal to the insertion of the FDS so that injuries involve the FDP alone. Patients with such injuries lose flexion at the DIP joint.

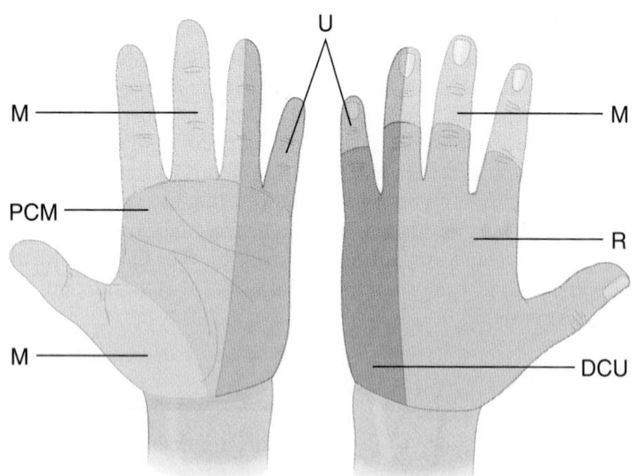

FIGURE 268-8. The cutaneous nerve supply in the hand. DCU = dorsal cutaneous branch of ulnar nerve; M = median nerve; PCM = palmar cutaneous branch of median nerve; R = superficial radial nerve; U = ulnar nerve.

ZONE II

Zone II involves the portion of the digital canal occupied by both FDS and FDP tendons (Figure 268-5). This zone is known as *no man's land* because injury in this zone has historically resulted in poor outcomes. This is due to the narrow fibro-osseous tunnel that consists of the metacarpals/phalanges. Lacerations in this zone are common, and partial lacerations are more common than complete injuries.

ZONE III

Zone III extends from the distal edge of the carpal tunnel to the proximal edge of the flexor tendon pulley system. The lumbrical muscles originate from the FDP tendons in this region. Outcomes are generally favorable.

ZONE IV

Zone IV is at the level of the carpal tunnel. The area must be explored carefully because many vital structures traverse this region. Isolated injuries are the exception.

ZONE V

Zone V involves injuries to tendons proximal to the carpal tunnel. Injuries here tend to be severe and often involve multiple tendons as well as the median or ulnar nerve (i.e., "spaghetti wrist"). Examine and test all major structures.

EXTENSOR TENDONS

The extensor tendons are the most common site of tendon injuries because of the superficial nature of the tendons on the dorsum of the hand. A separate zone classification system (I to VIII) for extensor tendon injuries has been developed for assessing injury patterns, repair techniques, and rehabilitation[3] (**Figure 268-11**). There is growing opinion that extensor tendon injuries should now be repaired operatively as well, although ED repair has often been the standard of care. In general, extensor tendon lacerations <25% do not need repair.

EXTENSOR ZONE I

Zone I involves the area over the distal phalanx and DIP joint. Injury can occur from blunt or sharp trauma. Complete laceration or rupture

TABLE 268-1 Immediate Hand Surgery Consultation Guidelines
Vascular injury with signs of tissue ischemia or poorly controlled hemorrhage
Irreducible dislocations
Grossly contaminated wounds
Severe crush injury
Open fracture
Compartment syndrome
High-pressure injection injury
Hand/finger amputation

TABLE 268-2 Delayed Hand Surgery Consultation Guidelines
Extensor/flexor tendon laceration (if not repaired in ED)
Flexor digitorum profundus rupture (closed) (Jersey finger) or extensor digitorum rupture (mallet finger)
Nerve injury
Closed fractures
Dislocations
Ligamentous injuries with instability

TABLE 268-3 Immobilization for Common Hand Injuries

Injury	Splint
Ligamentous injuries	
Thumb MCP ulnar collateral ligament rupture	
Partial tears	Thumb spica, IP free to flex
Complete or equivocal	Thumb spica (presurgical repair)
Tendon injuries	
Mallet finger	Dorsal splint, full extension at DIP
Flexor tendon laceration	Dorsal splint, 30-degree wrist flex, 70-degree MCP flexion, 30- to 45-degree PIP flexion (presurgical repair)
Dislocations	
DIP joint	Dorsal splint, full extension
PIP joint	
Stable/postreduction	Dorsal splint, 30-degree PIP flexion
Unstable/postreduction	Dorsal splint, 30-degree PIP flexion
MCP joint	Buddy-taping
Carpometacarpal joint	Dorsal-volar splint
Thumb IP joint	Dorsal splint, full extension
Thumb MCP joint	Thumb spica
Fractures	
Distal phalanx	Volar or hairpin splint not immobilizing PIP
Middle/proximal phalanx	
Stable/nondisplaced	Buddy taping/dynamic splinting
Unstable/displaced	Radial/ulnar gutter, 90-degree MCP flexion, <15- to 20-degree PIP flexion, <5- to 10-degree DIP flexion
Thumb proximal phalanx	Thumb spica
Metacarpal	
Index, middle	Radial gutter, 20-degree wrist flexion, 90-degree MCP flexion, PIP left mobile
Ring, small	Ulnar gutter, 20-degree wrist flexion, 90-degree MCP flexion, PIP left mobile
Thumb metacarpal	
Extra-articular	Thumb spica
Intra-articular	Thumb spica for initial immobilization (presurgical repair)

Abbreviations: DIP = distal interphalangeal; IP = interphalangeal; MCP = metacarpophalangeal; PIP = proximal interphalangeal.

Note: Hairpin splint: metal backed splint with foam padding; dynamic splint: spring-loaded splint that allows some motion at unaffected joints while protecting the injured joint, usually available from a hand surgeon or occupational therapist.

of the tendon at this level will result in the inability to extend the DIP joint. This injury is often called a **mallet finger** (**Figure 268-12**), and it is the most common tendon injury in athletes. This injury has been classified as type I if there is tendon-only rupture, type II if there is a small avulsion fracture, and type III if >25% of the articular surface is involved. Type I can be treated with the DIP joint immobilized in continuous full extension for 6 to 10 weeks. For the best outcome, **no** flexion of the DIP joint is permitted for the duration of splinting. Thus, instruct patients not to take off the splint. If they do remove the splint to clean the finger and the splint, the DIP should be held in extension. The DIP **cannot** be allowed to fall into flexion. Splints for the mallet finger can be a Stax or aluminofoam splint as long as the splint holds the DIP in full extension (**Figure 268-13**).

Type II injuries can be treated the same way if on x-ray the splinted finger in extension shows congruency with the rest of the noninjured articular surface of the distal phalanx on the distal articular surface of the middle phalanx. Other indications for surgery include an open injury and >30% to 50% articular fracture involvement. Chronic untreated mallet finger may result in a **swan-neck deformity** (**Figure 268-14**). This occurs when the lateral bands are displaced dorsally, resulting in increased extension forces on the PIP joint.

EXTENSOR ZONE II

Zone II involves the area over the middle phalanx. Injuries are usually a result of laceration. Injuries to this area are treated similarly to zone I injuries.

EXTENSOR ZONE III

Zone III involves the area over the PIP joint. The central tendon is the most commonly injured structure. Complete disruption of the central tendon may result in the volar displacement of the lateral bands, causing them to be flexors, along with the unopposed FDP. Additionally, the extensor hood retracts, causing extension of the DIP joint, resulting in the **boutonnière deformity** (**Figure 268-15**). Controversy exists regarding whether treatment of zone III injuries should be conservative or operative. Closed injuries are initially treated with the PIP joint immobilized in continuous extension for 5 to 6 weeks and should be followed closely by a hand specialist.

EXTENSOR ZONE IV

Zone IV involves the area over the proximal phalanx. These injuries have clinical findings similar to zone III injuries. These injuries are often less likely to have long-term morbidity because the joint is not involved and the tendon at this level is broad and flat.

EXTENSOR ZONE V

Zone V involves the area over the MCP joint. Open injuries to this area should be considered human bites until proven otherwise. Wounds from human bites should have delayed repair following hospital admission for a course of broad-spectrum IV antibiotics. This injury may require operative washout. Clean, nonbite wounds can be repaired primarily using mattress sutures to reapproximate tendon edges.

EXTENSOR ZONE VI

Zone VI involves the area over the dorsum of the hand. Because the tendons in this area are so superficial, even minor-appearing lacerations may be associated with one or more tendon injuries. If the laceration is proximal to the juncturae tendineae, the patient may be able to extend the involved MCP joint, because extensor forces are transmitted to the juncturae from adjacent extensor tendons. Injuries to zones VI, VII, and VIII typically require advanced suture techniques.[4]

EXTENSOR ZONE VII

Zone VII involves the area over the wrist. Repair can be difficult because of the presence of the extensor retinaculum. This thick, fibrous structure on the dorsum of the wrist contains 12 extensor tendons and six synovial-lined retinacular compartments. Due to the anatomic complexity of this region, operative repair is needed.

EXTENSOR ZONE VIII

Zone VIII involves the area of the distal forearm. Injuries to this area require a thorough exploration to identify all injured structures. The tendons frequently retract into the forearm and must be retrieved and repaired. After repairs in zones V through VII, splinting should occur with the wrist in 15-degree extension, the MCP joint in 15-degree flexion, and the IP joint in 15-degree flexion in the involved and adjacent digits.

LIGAMENTOUS INJURIES AND DISLOCATIONS

Soft tissue injuries to the hand are extremely common. Accurate diagnosis and treatment are important to avoid complications such as joint luxation, loss of motion, chronic pain, and deformity.

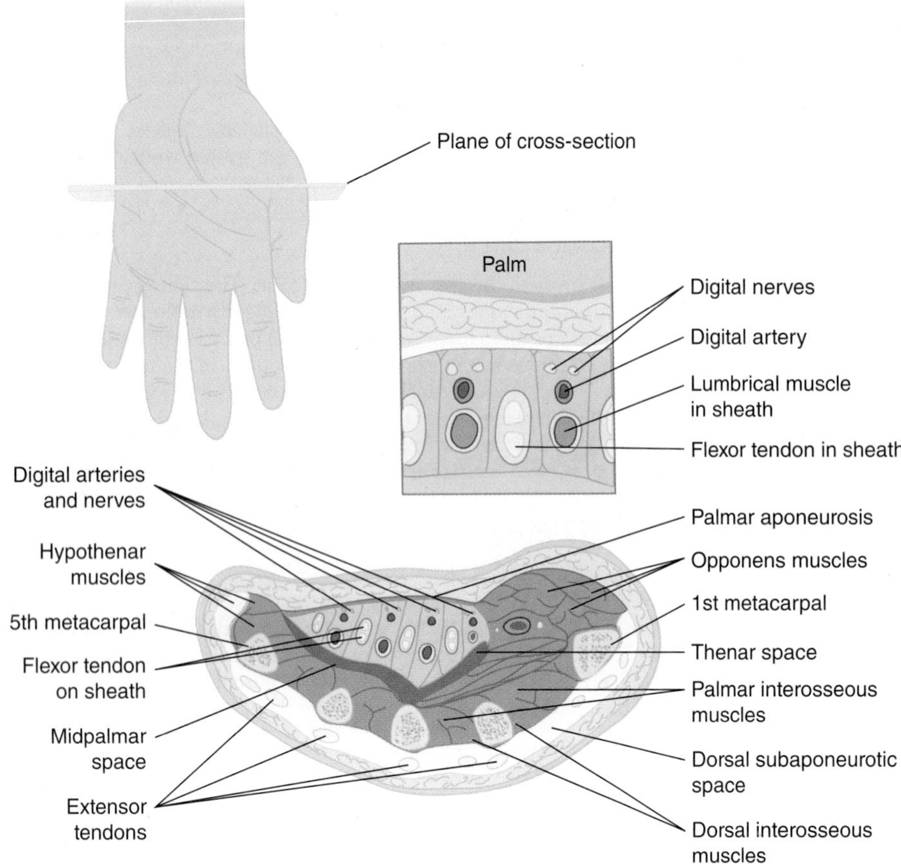

FIGURE 268-9. Relationship of nerves, arteries, tendons, and muscles at the level of the metacarpals.

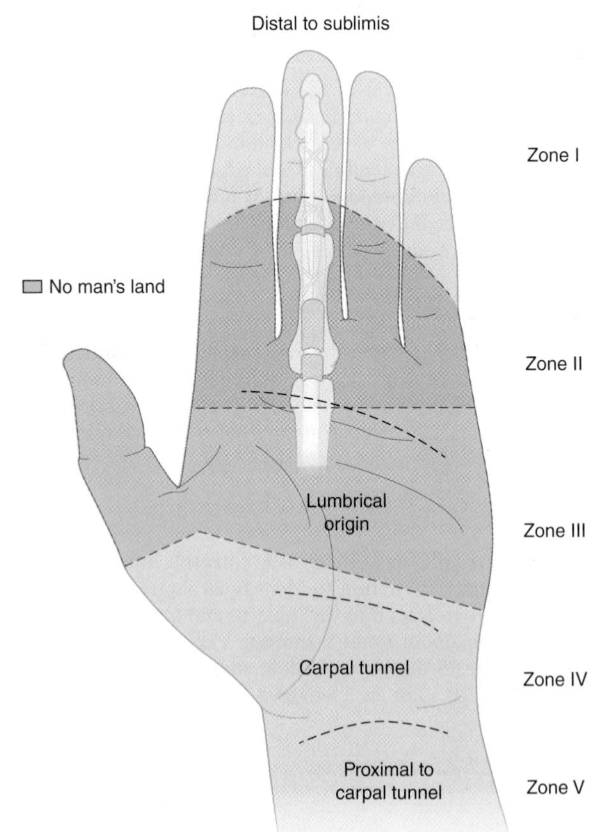

FIGURE 268-10. Flexor tendon zones and no man's land.

DISTAL INTERPHALANGEAL JOINT

Dislocations of the DIP joint are uncommon because of the firm attachments of the skin and subcutaneous tissue to the underlying bone by osteocutaneous fibers. Additional stability is provided by the flexor and extensor tendons. When dislocations do occur, they are usually dorsal. Longitudinal traction and hyperextension followed by direct dorsal pressure to the base of the distal phalanx usually accomplish reduction. Attempts at reduction should be made after a digital nerve block or other means of anesthesia has been performed. **Irreducible cases may be due to the entrapment of an avulsion fracture, the profundus tendon, or volar plate.**

PROXIMAL INTERPHALANGEAL JOINT

Dislocations of the PIP joint are common hand injuries. The mechanism is usually due to axial load and hyperextension. Dorsal dislocation occurs when the volar plate ruptures. Lateral dislocations occur when one of the collateral ligaments ruptures with at least a partial avulsion of the volar plate from the middle phalanx. The digit is usually ulnarly deviated because the radial collateral ligament is six times more likely than the ulnar collateral ligament to rupture. Volar dislocations are rare. Dorsal dislocations are reduced in the same manner as dorsal DIP joint dislocations. Active motion and strength should be tested following reduction. If testing is normal, splint the joint at 30-degrees of flexion for 3 weeks. **If the joint is irreducible or there is evidence of complete ligamentous disruption, operative repair is required.**

METACARPOPHALANGEAL JOINT

Dislocations of the MCP joint are usually due to hyperextension forces that rupture the volar plate, causing dorsal dislocation. Subluxation is more common than dislocation. In subluxation, the joint appears to be hyperextended 60 to 90 degrees, and the articular surfaces are still in contact. Reduction here does not involve hyperextension because it might convert a subluxation into a complete dislocation. **Reduction is performed by flexing the wrist to relax the flexor tendon and then applying pressure over the dorsum of the proximal phalanx in a distal and volar direction.** After reduction, splint the MCP joint in flexion. Multipart dislocations appear less deformed because of the number of disrupted structures. Because the volar plate is interposed in the MCP joint space, closed reduction is usually not possible. Volar dislocations are rare and usually require operative reduction.

CARPOMETACARPAL JOINT

Dislocations of the CMC joint are uncommon because the joint is supported by strong dorsal, volar, and interosseous ligaments and is reinforced by the broad insertions of the wrist flexors and extensors. The cause is usually a result of high-speed mechanisms such as motor vehicle crashes, falls, crushes, or clenched fist trauma. If a dislocation occurs, it is usually dorsally oriented and associated with fracture(s). **Reduction of dorsal CMC joint dislocations can be attempted after regional anesthesia is administered. Traction and flexion with simultaneous longitudinal pressure on the metacarpal base should reestablish normal anatomic alignment.** Early referral after reduction is needed to determine if further fixation is needed. Volar CMC joint dislocations are exceedingly rare and should be referred to a hand specialist.

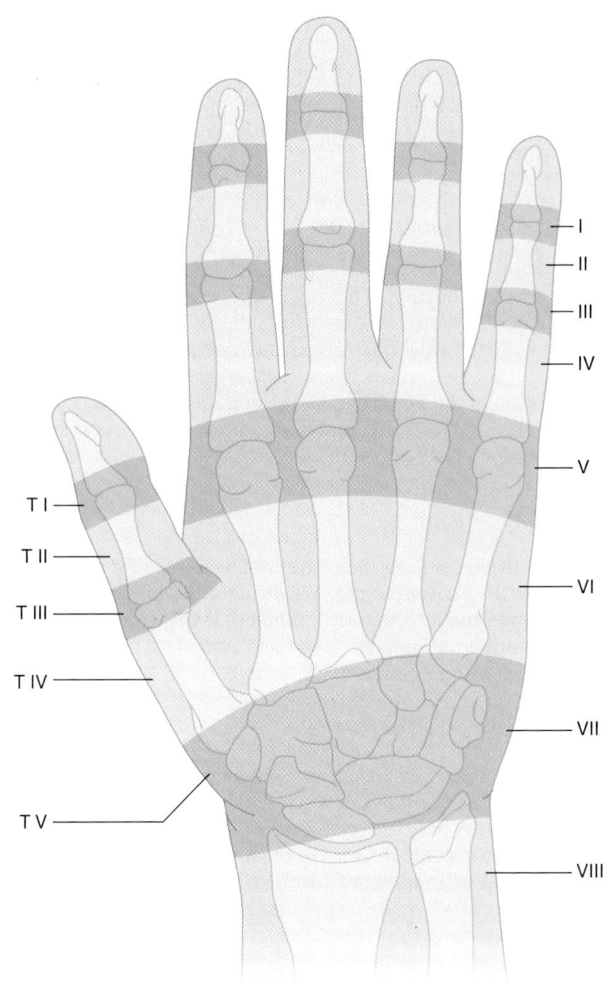

FIGURE 268-11. Extensor tendon zones of the hand. T = thumb.

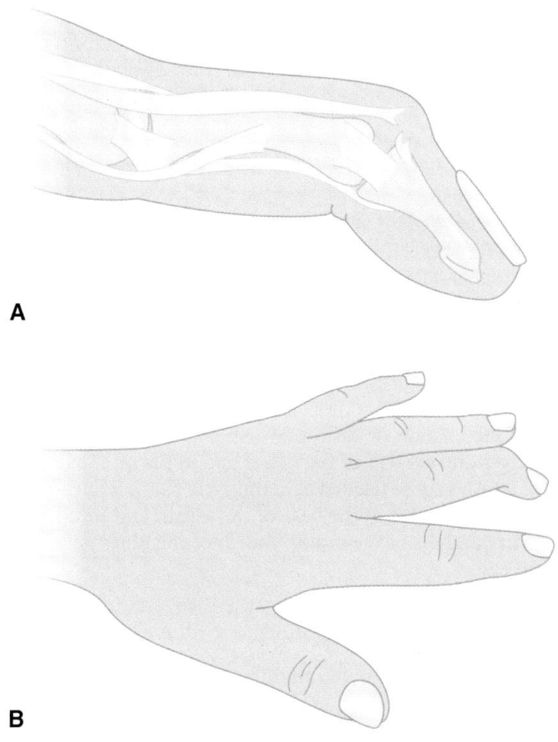

FIGURE 268-12. A. Mallet finger. B. Clinical appearance.

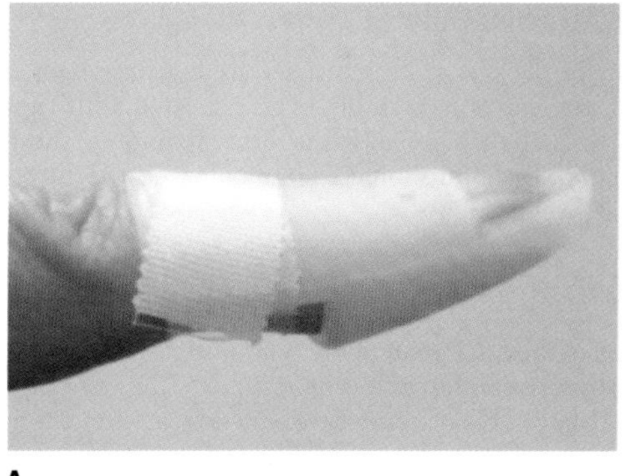

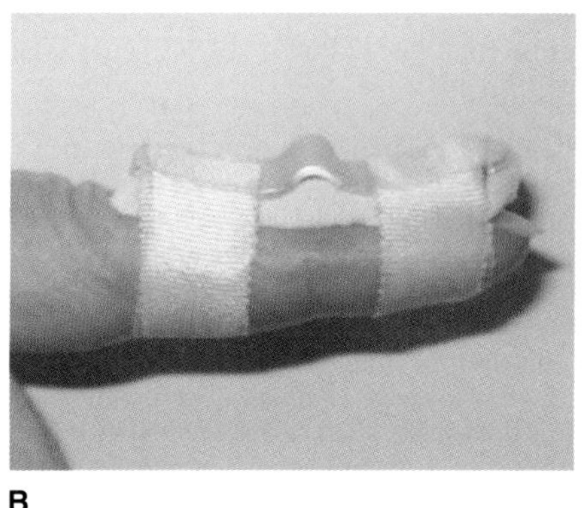

FIGURE 268-13. A and B. Splinting for mallet finger.

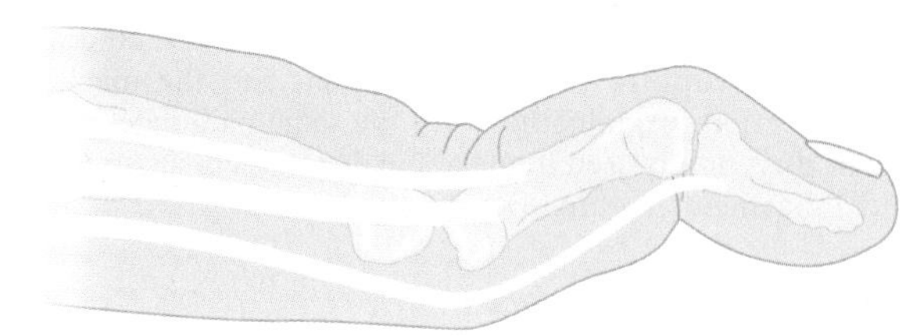

FIGURE 268-14. Swan neck deformity.

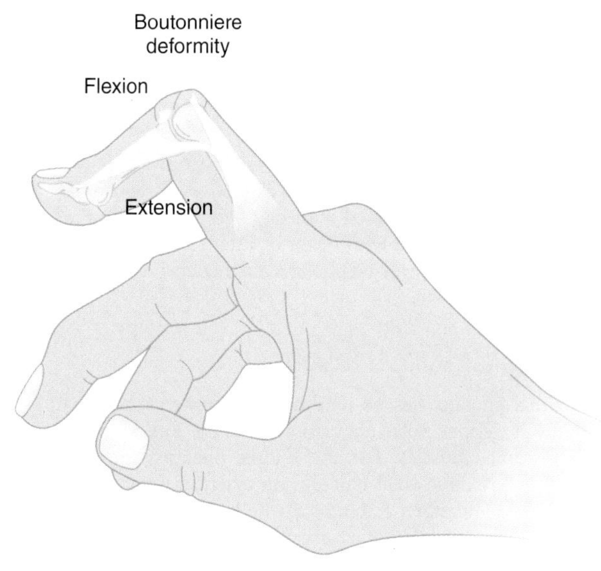

FIGURE 268-15. Boutonnière deformity.

THUMB INTERPHALANGEAL JOINT

Dislocations of the thumb IP joint are rare but, if present, are usually open. The mechanism is typically hyperextension with rupture of the volar plate. Reduction is similar to that of the IP joints of the other digits. After reduction, the joint should be immobilized in 15 to 20 degrees of flexion for 3 weeks.

THUMB METACARPOPHALANGEAL JOINT

Dislocations of the MCP joint of the thumb are usually dorsal and result from a hyperextension force causing rupture of the volar plate. The dislocation may be simple or complex. Reduction, after radial nerve block, is accomplished with pressure directed distally on the base of the proximal phalanx with the metacarpal flexed and abducted.

THUMB METACARPOPHALANGEAL (ULNAR) COLLATERAL LIGAMENT RUPTURE

Rupture of the ulnar collateral ligament (**gamekeeper's thumb**, **skier's thumb**) occurs when the mechanism causes radial deviation (abduction) of the MCP joint. The tear usually occurs at the insertion into the proximal phalanx. Often significant injury to the dorsal capsule and volar plate occurs. **Hand surgery referral is recommended for all patients with suspected complete tears of the ulnar collateral ligament of the thumb,** signs of which are pain, ecchymosis of the thumb MCP, and weakness of pinch. The diagnosis is made with stress testing of the ulnar collateral ligament. The examiner tests the thumb MCP joint, both in full extension and 30-degree flexion, by stabilizing the metacarpal with one hand while applying lateral (radial) stress on the proximal phalanx with the other. **More than 30 to 35 degrees of radial angulation or 10 to 15 degrees more than the contralateral thumb indicates complete rupture and requires surgical consultation.** If patients are discharged from the ED, a thumb spica splint should be applied and urgent orthopedic follow-up arranged. Repair is best accomplished within 1 week. **Radial collateral ligament rupture** is not as common, and the mechanism is forced adduction. Examination with the same parameters applied in the ulnar direction is used to make the diagnosis of a complete radial collateral ligament rupture.

THUMB CARPOMETACARPAL JOINT

Isolated thumb CMC joint dislocation is rare compared with the more common Bennett's fracture dislocation (see below). These are easy to reduce but unstable after reduction. After reduction, a thumb spica splint should be applied. These injuries should have a surgical referral for a decision on operative repair.

FRACTURES

DISTAL PHALANX

Fractures of the distal phalanx usually result from crush or shearing forces. The fractures can be classified as tuft, shaft, or intra-articular. Tuft fractures can be associated with nail bed lacerations. Fractures at the base may be associated with flexor or extensor tendon involvement. Generally, fractures of the distal phalanx are treated as soft tissue injuries with protective splinting.

PROXIMAL AND MIDDLE PHALANX

The proximal phalanx has no tendinous attachments, so fractures frequently result in apex volar angulation from the forces of the extensor and interosseous muscles. For the middle phalanx, the FDS tendon inserts on the proximal volar half and the extensor tendon inserts at the proximal base. Therefore, fractures at the base of the middle phalanx demonstrate apex dorsal angulation, and fractures at the neck result in apex volar angulation. A direct blow mechanism usually causes a transverse or comminuted fracture, whereas a twisting mechanism will more often result in a spiral fracture. Most often, such fractures are stable and nondisplaced and can be treated with early protected motion by buddy taping. Unstable fractures amenable to closed reduction can be splinted from the MCP to the DIP joint with the MCP joint in 70 degrees of flexion and the IP joints in extension. Midshaft transverse fractures, spiral fractures, and intra-articular fractures often require internal fixation.

METACARPAL (SECOND TO FIFTH) FRACTURES

The second and third metacarpals are relatively immobile, and fractures require anatomic reduction. The ring and fifth metacarpals have 15- to 20-degree anteroposterior motion, which allows for some compensation for malunion. Metacarpal fractures are categorized as head, neck, shaft, or base fractures.[5] The presence of a metacarpal fracture should prompt close evaluation of the associated CMC joint, because CMC joint dislocation often accompanies these fractures and is often missed at the initial presentation.[6]

METACARPAL HEAD FRACTURES

Fractures of the metacarpal head are usually caused by a direct blow, crush, or missile. These fractures are distal to the insertion of the collateral ligaments and are often comminuted. If a laceration is present, a human bite must be considered. Treatment consists of ice, elevation, and immobilization with referral to a hand surgeon.

METACARPAL NECK FRACTURES

Fractures of the metacarpal neck are usually caused by a direct impaction force. A fracture of the fifth metacarpal neck is often referred to as a **boxer's fracture**. These fractures are usually unstable with volar angulation. **Angulation of ≤20 degrees in the fourth and ≤40 degrees in the fifth metacarpal will not result in functional impairment. If greater angulation in these metacarpals occurs, reduction should be attempted.** To perform the reduction, flex the wrist and the MCP joint. Apply slight force to the volar aspect of the affected metacarpal while distracting the phalanx away from the palm. Following splinting, patients may have residual cosmetic deformity (not prominent metacarpal head), but in most cases regain full function. The amount of angulation at the time of injury does not correlate with resultant cosmetic defects.[7] **With second and third metacarpal fractures, angulation of <15 degrees is acceptable.** Splint metacarpal neck fractures with the wrist in 20-degree extension and the MCP joint flexed at 70 degrees. Fractures of the second or third metacarpal that are significantly displaced or angulated require anatomic reduction and surgical fixation.

METACARPAL SHAFT FRACTURES

A direct blow usually results in fractures in the metacarpal shaft region. Rotational deformity and shortening are more likely in shaft fractures than in neck fractures. If manipulative reduction is necessary, operative fixation is usually indicated.

METACARPAL BASE FRACTURES

Fractures at the base of the metacarpal are usually caused by a direct blow or axial force. They are often associated with carpal bone fractures. CMC joint subluxation or dislocation should be suspected with these injuries. Given the overlap of the bones and joints on the lateral radiograph, a CT scan may be needed to definitively rule out joint subluxation or dislocation. Fractures at the base of the fourth and fifth metacarpals can result in paralysis of the motor branch of the ulnar nerve, although this is rare.[8]

THUMB METACARPAL FRACTURES

Because of the mobility of the thumb metacarpal, shaft fractures are uncommon. Fractures usually involve the base.

Extra-Articular Fractures Extra-articular fractures are caused by a direct blow or impaction mechanism. The mobility of the CMC joint can allow for 30-degree angular deformity. Angulation greater than this requires reduction and a thumb spica splint for 4 weeks. Spiral fractures often require fixation.

Intra-Articular Fractures: Bennett's Fracture and Rolando's Fracture Intra-articular fractures are caused by impaction from striking a fixed object.

Bennett's fracture is an intra-articular fracture with associated subluxation or dislocation at the CMC joint. The ulnar portion of the metacarpal usually remains in place ("constant fragment"). The distal portion usually subluxes radially and dorsally from the pull of the abductor pollicis longus and the adductor pollicis. Treatment is application of a thumb spica splint and orthopedic referral.

Rolando's fracture is an intra-articular comminuted fracture at the base of the metacarpal. The mechanism of injury is similar to Bennett's fracture but less common. Treatment includes a thumb spica splint and orthopedic consultation.

COMPARTMENT SYNDROME

Crush injury of the hand, with or without associated fracture, may result in compartment syndrome. Iatrogenic causes of compartment syndrome of the hand include extravasation of IV fluids or contrast media or arterial punctures.[9,10] The involved compartments of the hand include the thenar, hypothenar, adductor pollicis, and four interossei muscles. Edema of tissues or hemorrhage within any of these compartments may lead to elevated pressures that result in tissue necrosis and subsequent loss of hand function due to contracture.[3] Classic signs and symptoms of compartment syndrome typically include pain and paresthesias early, with paralysis and pulselessness occurring later in the course of the ischemic injury. **Hand compartment syndromes, however, may not be associated with paresthesias, and the extremely subtle motor deficits and difficulty in assessing response to passive stretch make the diagnosis more elusive than at other anatomic sites.** Pain, the most consistent clinical sign, is often described as deep, constant, poorly localized, and disproportionate to clinical findings. Physical examination findings suggestive of hand compartment syndrome include extreme swelling, the intrinsic minus position at rest (MCP joint extended with PIP joint slightly flexed), pain with passive stretch of the involved compartment muscles (interosseous: performed with MCP joint extended and PIP joint fully flexed with slight radial and ulnar deviation; thenar, hypothenar: performed by extension of MCP joint), and tense swelling of the affected compartment. Compartment pressure measurement is difficult and inexact in the relatively small compartments of the hand. The diagnosis is typically made on a clinical basis, not on actual compartment pressures.[11]

In the setting of severe crush injury with signs and symptoms suggestive of compartment syndrome, immediately consult with a hand specialist to determine if emergency fasciotomy is indicated.

HIGH-PRESSURE INJECTION INJURY

The injection of certain substances under high pressures (often 2000 to 10,000 psi) into the soft tissues of the hand may initially appear benign but are actually true orthopedic emergencies. The operator of the high-pressure device typically attempts to test or clean the nozzle with the nondominant hand and inadvertently injects the substance. The initial dissipation of kinetic energy through the soft tissues of the hand and the subsequent chemical inflammation produce tissue edema and ischemia. The most commonly injected substances include grease, paint, hydraulic fluid, diesel fuel, paint thinner, and water. Paint, especially oil-based paint, triggers an intense inflammatory response that contributes to significant ischemic injury.[12] The benign appearance of the small injection site in the immediate postinjection period is misleading, and historical information must dictate treatment and disposition decisions. With time, the digit becomes edematous, pale, and severely tender to palpation, suggesting ischemic injury. Pressure to areas surrounding the wound may express the injected substance. Plain radiographs of the injected hand and forearm provide valuable information, as radiopaque substances, such as lead-based paints or grease, or subcutaneous emphysema may delineate the extent of the injection. **Definitive treatment of high-pressure injection injuries is early surgical decompression and debridement of injected areas.** Obtain immediate hand surgery consultation, immobilize and elevate the affected hand, administer tetanus prophylaxis and broad-spectrum antibiotics, and provide adequate analgesia.[13-15] Amputation rates following injection injury are as high as 30%,[16] highlighting the need for rapid identification and proper treatment of the injury.

REFERENCES

The complete reference list is available online at www.TintinalliEM.com.

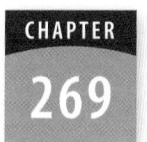

Wrist Injuries

Robert Escarza
Maurice F. Loeffel, III
Dennis T. Uehara

INTRODUCTION AND EPIDEMIOLOGY

The wrist is the area from the distal radius and ulna to the carpometacarpal joints. It is a complex unit with articulations among the eight carpal bones and the distal radius and ulna. Wrist injuries are common, accounting for 2.5% of ED visits annually.[1] Clinical diagnosis is often difficult, and even subtle injuries may lead to significant impairment if not properly diagnosed and treated. Management options vary from conservative to surgical, so an understanding of the functional anatomy, mechanisms of injury, and clinical evaluation is needed for proper diagnosis and treatment.

ANATOMY

DISTAL RADIUS AND ULNA

The distal radius is the only forearm bone that articulates directly with the carpal bones (scaphoid and lunate). The distal radius has three articular surfaces: radiocarpal, distal radioulnar, and the triangular fibrocartilage complex. The radiocarpal surface is concave and tilted in two planes. It has an ulnar inclination, or tilt, of 15 to 25 degrees in the frontal plane, and a volar tilt of 10 to 15 degrees in the sagittal plane[2] (**Figure 269-1**). The ulna is separated from the carpal bones by the triangular fibrocartilage complex, the main stabilizer of the distal radioulnar joint, on its distal end. The triangular fibrocartilage complex forms a smooth, continuous, ulnarly directed extension of the distal radial surface, and supports the lunate and triquetrum on the distal ulna. The distal radius has a concave sigmoid notch at its ulnar aspect that articulates with the curvature of the ulnar head, which permits wrist rotation during pronation/supination of the forearm.[3] The distal radioulnar joint is also supported by dorsal and volar radioulnar ligaments that merge with the triangular fibrocartilage complex.[4]

CARPAL BONES

Eight carpal bones are arranged in two rows. The distal carpal row (trapezium, trapezoid, capitate, and hamate) is joined tightly together and to the adjoining metacarpals. The distal row is quite stable and moves with the metacarpals as a unit in a relatively stable arch. The proximal carpal row (scaphoid, lunate, triquetrum, and pisiform) is also arranged in an arch between the distal radius and the distal carpal row. In this arrangement, the proximal row functions as a mobile link, or "intercalated segment," and is potentially unstable by virtue of this position. The scaphoid is critical to wrist stability, by acting as a stabilizing strut and linking the proximal and distal carpal rows at the radial aspect of the wrist. This position explains the scaphoid's greater propensity for injury.

Forearm muscles that insert onto the bases of the metacarpals produce wrist motion. Except for the pisiform, a sesamoid bone of the flexor

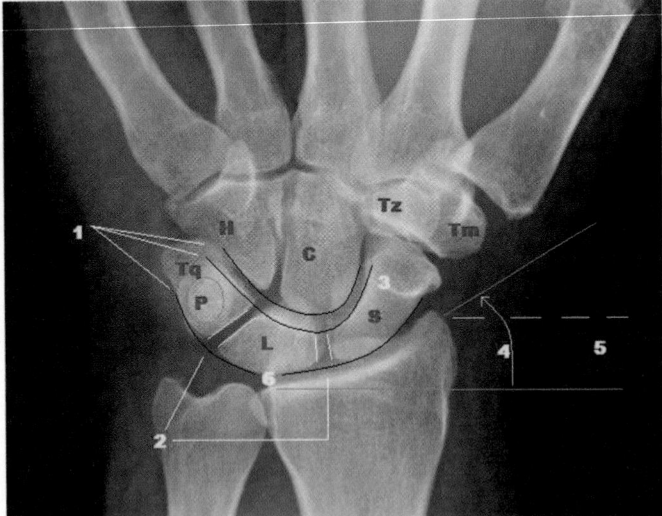

FIGURE 269-1. Wrist. Normal posteroanterior (PA) view. 1. The carpal bones are arranged in two rows forming three smooth arcs (Gilula lines). 2. The carpal bones are separated by a uniform 1- to 2-mm space. 3. The scaphoid (S) is elongated. 4. The radius has an ulnar inclination of 13 to 30 degrees. 5. The radial styloid projects 8 to 18 mm. 6. Half the lunate articulates with the radius, with equal length over the ulna (neutral ulnar variance). C = capitate; H = hamate; L = lunate; P = pisiform; Tm = trapezium; Tq = triquetrum; Tz = trapezoid.

carpi ulnaris, there are no direct tendon insertions on the carpal bones.[5] The carpal bones move passively in response to hand position. Often, the radiocarpal joint is referred to as the "*wrist joint*." However, wrist motion is divided almost equally between the radiocarpal and midcarpal joints.[6] This is best understood by viewing carpal movement from the sagittal view. During flexion and extension of the wrist, each row moves in the same direction with similar degrees of angulation.

The carpal bones are stabilized to one another by intrinsic ligaments and to the bones of the forearm by extrinsic ligaments. The key extrinsic ligaments are arranged in three arcades, two of which are volar and one dorsal. The two volar ligaments are arranged in two inverted V-shaped arches, and are thought to play a major role in stabilizing the wrist. The apex of one arch inserts on the lunate supporting the proximal carpal row, whereas the other arch reaches to the distal carpal row, inserting on the capitate. The area between these two palmar arches is inherently weak and is known as the *space of Poirier* (**Figure 269-2**). This space lies at the junction of the capitate and lunate and widens upon dorsiflexion

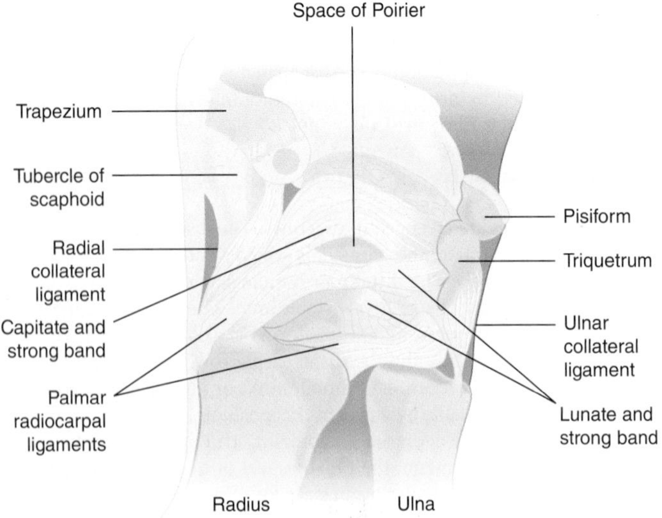

FIGURE 269-2. Ligaments of the wrist

of the wrist. Forceful dorsiflexion may tear the capsule here and produce a lunate or perilunate dislocation. The single dorsal arcade has its origins on the rim and styloid of the radius on one side and distal ulna/triangular fibrocartilage complex on the other. This ligament is less important for wrist stability, acting as a sling across the dorsum of the wrist.[6]

The space of Poirier is on the volar aspect of the wrist and is inherently weak. It is the site of disruption in perilunate and lunate dislocations. The intrinsic ligaments are largely responsible for holding the carpal bones together as a kinematic unit in their respective carpal rows. The intrinsic ligaments of the mobile proximal carpal row are particularly important because of their greater propensity for injury. The intrinsic ligaments of the proximal carpal row are named after the respective carpal bones they connect: the scapholunate and triquetrolunate. The palmar flexed posture of the scaphoid produces a flexion torque on the lunate that is counterbalanced by an extension torque from the triquetrum. This delicate balance is lost if either ligament is disrupted, producing a dorsal or volar tilt of the proximal carpal row and carpal instability.

PATHOPHYSIOLOGY

It is helpful to understand the mechanism of injury when assessing wrist injuries. Most injuries are caused by a fall creating an axial load on an outstretched arm and dorsiflexed wrist and hand. Impact on the thenar eminence is likely to injure the scaphoid and its supporting ligaments. An impact on the hypothenar eminence is likely to cause injury to the triquetrum, pisiform, and their supporting ligaments. Age affects the maturity of the bones and predisposes patients to certain types of injury.[7] **Children are likely to sustain injuries to the immature, weaker epiphyseal plate or metaphysis of the radius, sparing the still-cartilaginous carpal bones.**[8] Young adults, particularly those with active lifestyles, are likely to be injured with greater force and disrupt either the scaphoid, proximal row intrinsic ligaments, or distal radial metaphysis.[8] **In the elderly, especially with underlying osteoporosis, the weak point is the brittle distal radial metaphysis, resulting in a Colles fracture, often with intra-articular involvement.**[9]

CLINICAL FEATURES

Begin assessment by **looking at both wrists** to assess for symmetry and range of motion in dorsiflexion, palmar flexion, and radioulnar deviation, in addition to obvious deformities and soft tissue swelling. Pinpoint areas of tenderness and correlate them to anatomic landmarks of the wrist to determine which structure may be injured and the best way to evaluate it radiographically (**Figure 269-3**).

The most noteworthy landmark on the dorsum of the wrist is the anatomic snuffbox. **The anatomic snuffbox is a triangle formed by the bony radial styloid at tis proximal base, the extensor pollicis brevis tendon at its radial aspect, and the extensor pollicis longus tendon at its ulnar aspect. Palpate the scaphoid within this triangle.** Tenderness in this area may suggest a scaphoid fracture.[10] The extensor pollicis longus tendon wraps around a bony prominence of the distal radius, known as **Lister's tubercle**. The area immediately distal to this point marks the location of the scapholunate joint. Tenderness in this area suggests scapholunate ligamentous injury or lunate fracture.[11] The **scaphoid shift test** can further assess scapholunate ligament injury. To perform the scaphoid shift test, place the wrist in ulnar deviation and apply pressure with your thumb over the scaphoid tuberosity. Then move the wrist from ulnar to radial deviation; in the event of ligament injury, you will feel a palpable "clunk."

Immediately ulnar to the scapholunate joint is a palpable indentation in the center of the wrist. This is the location of the lunate and capitate, which are palpable as they rise out of this space during wrist flexion.[11] Tenderness here may indicate lunate or triquetrolunate joint injury. The ulnar styloid is the bony prominence on the ulnar aspect of the wrist. The triquetrum and triangular fibrocartilage complex are located just distal to this prominence. Tenderness over the ulnar styloid may indicate ulnar styloid or triangular fibrocartilage complex injury. The **ulnocarpal stress test** can further evaluate the triangular fibrocartilage complex; apply a compression load to the wrist in ulnar deviation.[7] Pain or clicking may indicate triangular fibrocartilage complex injury.

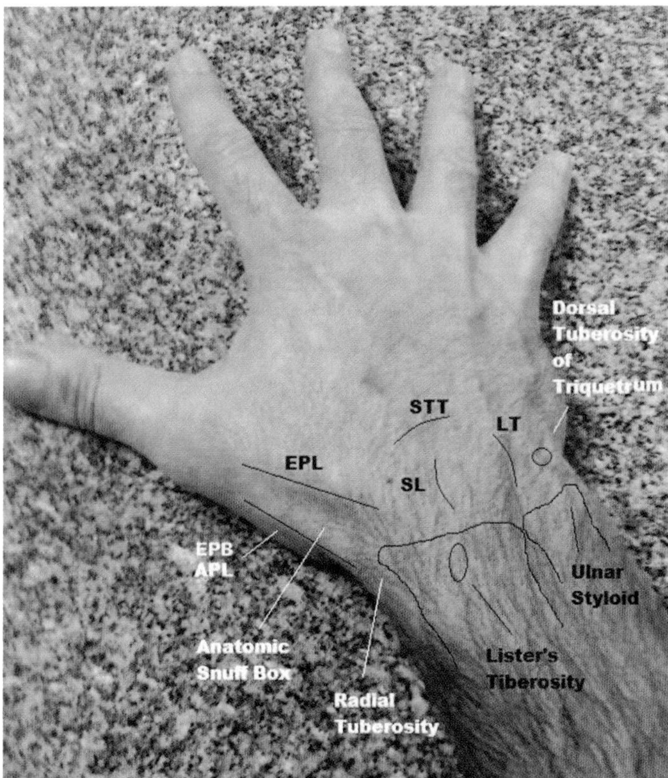

A

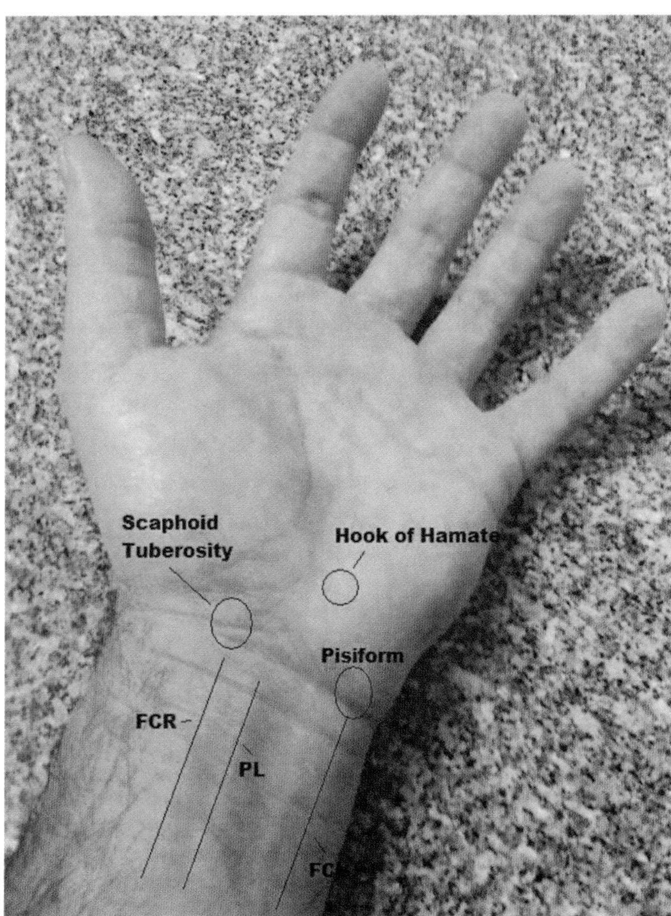

B

FIGURE 269-3. Surface anatomy of the wrist. A. Dorsal aspect. **B.** Palmar aspect. APL = abductor pollicis longus; EPB = extensor pollicis brevis; EPL = extensor pollicis longus; FCR = flexor carpi radialis; FCU = flexor carpi ulnaris; LT = lunotriquetral joint; PL = palmaris longus; SL = scapholunate joint; STT = scaphotrapeziotrapezoid joint.

Pain with pronation and supination of the forearm may indicate distal radioulnar joint injury. The **piano key sign**, which is the ulnar head springing back when depressed while supporting the forearm in pronation, suggests distal radioulnar joint injury.[11]

The crease noted on the volar aspect of the wrist marks the location of the proximal carpal row (Figure 269-3). The scaphotrapezial joint is palpable at the base of the thenar eminence. The pisiform is the palpable bony prominence at the base of the hypothenar eminence. The hook of the hamate is palpable in the soft tissue distal and radial to the pisiform. Tenderness in these areas may require further evaluation than standard radiographic views.[12]

IMAGING

Clinical examination determines which radiographic views will best support a diagnosis. Standard views of the wrist include posteroanterior, lateral, and oblique views. These views are adequate in most cases, but other projections may be necessary for specific injuries.[12,13]

The key to interpreting the radiograph is to first ensure proper hand positioning, then identify specific features on each projection. On a properly positioned posteroanterior view, the distal radius and ulna should not overlap at their distal articulation, and the axis of the third metacarpal should parallel that of the radius. In addition to looking for disruption of the bony cortex, key elements on the posteroanterior view are illustrated in Figure 269-1.

On the posteroanterior view, three smooth arcs (Gilula lines) outline the articular surfaces at the radiocarpal and midcarpal joints. Two of these arcs are formed by the proximal and distal surfaces of the scaphoid, lunate, and triquetrum. The third arc is formed by the proximal articular surface of the capitate and hamate in the midcarpal joint. Any distortion of these lines implies a fracture, dislocation, or subluxation at the site.

The carpal bones fit together much like a jigsaw puzzle, with the pieces separated by a uniform 1- to 2-mm space. This space is increased or obliterated with ligament disruption, carpal instability patterns, or fracture/dislocations. This occurs most often around the lunate at the scapholunate and capitolunate joints.

The **scaphoid** has an elongated shape in its normal, palmarly flexed position. Fractures or ligament disruption may cause further palmar rotation, causing the scaphoid to appear shortened on the posteroanterior view. Injuries to the scaphoid also may obscure the **scaphoid fat stripe**, a linear or triangular radiolucent collection of fat distal to the radial styloid and parallel to the radial border of the scaphoid.

Unfortunately, incorrect positioning can produce overlap patterns that can be misinterpreted as pathologic. For example, radial deviation of the wrist causes normal physiologic rotation of the proximal carpal row, obliterating the capitolunate space. At the same time, the scaphoid that should appear elongated on the posteroanterior view appears shorter as it rotates palmarly and can be confused with a rotary subluxation of the scaphoid.

The **radial styloid** should project 8 to 18 mm beyond the distal radioulnar joint and create an ulnar inclination of 13 to 30 degrees on the PA view. Distal radius fractures can alter these measurements. At the distal radioulnar joint, the ulna and adjacent portion of the radius should be of equal length, forming a smooth articular surface, and the distal radius generally should articulate with at least half the lunate. The extrinsic ligaments along with the triangular fibrocartilage complex prevent ulnar translocation (migration of the carpal bones down the ulnar tilt of the radiocarpal surface).[14] The lunate would have less contact and support from the radius if ulnar translocation were present. A shorter ulna (negative ulnar variance) also provides less support to the lunate and increases potential shear stress to the lunate, predisposing the lunate to injury.[15]

A properly positioned lateral radiograph is important for determining carpal alignment and degree of fracture angulation.[12] The radius and ulna should completely overlap one another, and the radial styloid should be centered over the distal radial articular surface. The key elements are illustrated in Figure 269-4A.

The axis of the radius, lunate, and capitate is collinear on the lateral view. If the articular surfaces of these bones were highlighted, they

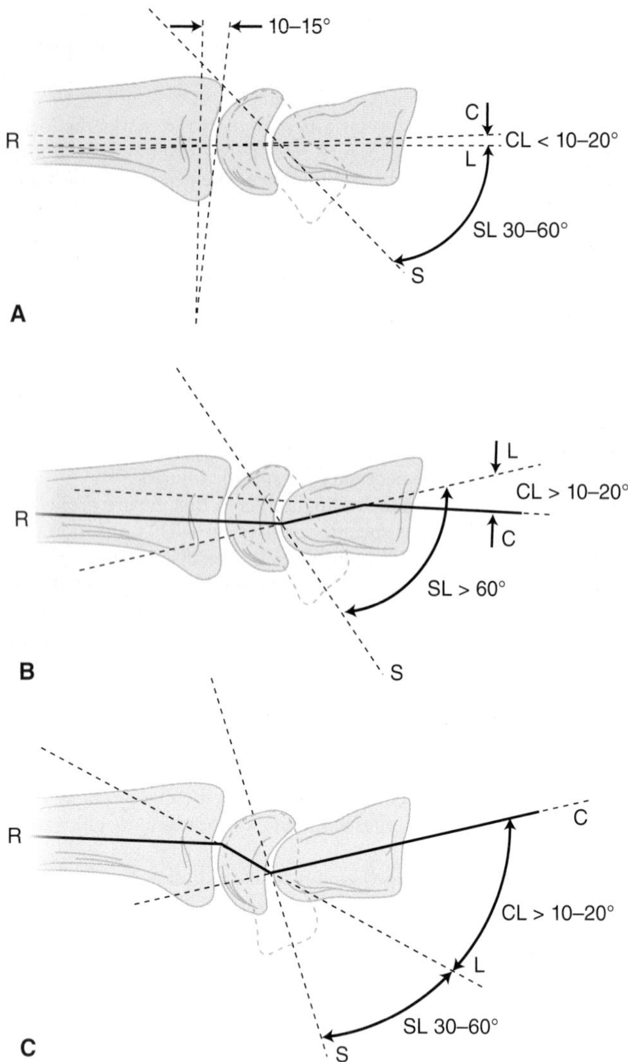

FIGURE 269-4. **A.** Normal wrist. Axis of the radius (R), lunate (L), and capitate (C) are collinear (three C's sign). The capitolunate (CL) angle is <10 to 20 degrees. The scapholunate (SL) angle is between 30 and 60 degrees. The radial volar tilt is 10 to 15 degrees. **B.** Dorsal intercalated segment instability. The lunate tilts dorsal and slides palmar, increasing the capitolunate angle. The scaphoid (S) tilts more palmar and increases the scapholunate angle. The axes of the radius, lunate, and capitate take on a zigzag pattern (yellow line). **C.** Volar intercalated segment instability. The lunate tilts palmar and the capitolunate angle increases, but the scapholunate angle is maintained. The zigzag pattern is in the opposite direction.

would appear as three consecutive C's. This provides a simple radiographic assessment of wrist dislocation. Measurement of the capitolunate and scapholunate angles is a more precise assessment of carpal alignment. The axis of the capitate, lunate, and scaphoid runs through the center of their proximal and distal articular surfaces. The axis of the lunate and capitate should nearly overlap and form an angle that is <10 to 20 degrees. **The scaphoid is normally palmar-flexed on the lateral view; its axis should form an angle between 30 and 60 degrees with the lunate.** Deviation from either of these angles suggests ligament disruption and carpal instability patterns (**Figure 269-4B** and **C**).[16]

Fracture of the distal radius is the most common fracture in the wrist.[14] Although a displaced fracture is the obvious deformity, the **alteration of the normal volar tilt of 10 to 15 degrees of the distal radial articular surface has greater long-term consequences for wrist function**, resulting in carpal misalignment and, subsequently, the instability patterns mentioned above.[15]

Other radiographic views profile specific areas of the wrist. Oblique views are performed in either partial pronation or supination, and project the scaphotrapezial joint or pisiform away from overlapping adjacent carpal bones. The scaphoid view is a cone-down posteroanterior view of the scaphoid in ulnar deviation. This position extends the normal flexed posture of the scaphoid so that the bone is projected lengthwise. This view may assist in detecting subtle fractures and is used whenever scaphoid injury is suspected.[13] The carpal tunnel view is a tangential view through the carpal tunnel and is helpful in visualizing the pisiform and hook of the hamate. Motion studies are dynamic views in flexion, extension, and radial and ulnar deviation. These views examine carpal movement relative to one another, and stress the intercarpal ligaments for laxity, characterized by widening of the intercarpal space.[17] Likewise, the grip compression or fist view is a stress view in the posteroanterior projection of the tightly clenched fist. The capitate is pushed into the proximal carpal row and forces the carpal bones apart if intrinsic ligaments are disrupted. CT is useful for defining fractures and dislocations, whereas MRI is useful for evaluation for both bony and soft tissue abnormalities such as occult fractures, avascular necrosis, and triangular fibrocartilage complex abnormality.[17] **Table 269-1** presents a summary of standard and supplemental wrist radiographs and the injuries they enhance.

TABLE 269-1 Wrist Radiography

View	Injuries to Identify
Posteroanterior	Distal radius/ulna fractures, carpal bone fractures, ligamentous disruptions
Lateral	Radius/ulna fractures, lunate/perilunate dislocation, dorsal intercalated segment instability, volar intercalated segment instability
Scaphoid	Scaphoid fracture, scapholunate dissociation
Carpal tunnel	Pisiform and hamate fractures
Motion studies	Scapholunate or triquetrolunate instability
Grip compression	Scapholunate or triquetrolunate instability
CT	All fractures and dislocations
MRI	Occult fracture, avascular necrosis, soft tissue abnormality

LIGAMENTOUS INJURIES

The lunate is located in the middle of the wrist, so it is not surprising that the majority of ligamentous injuries are centered on the **lunate**. Injuries usually result from forceful dorsiflexion of the wrist, most often from a fall on an outstretched hand. The various injuries occur sequentially depending on the degree of force and range from isolated tears to perilunate and lunate dislocations.[18,19]

SCAPHOLUNATE LIGAMENT INSTABILITY

The scapholunate ligament is the intrinsic ligament that binds the scaphoid and lunate. Because the scaphoid bridges the proximal and distal carpal rows, it is not surprising that the **scapholunate ligament has a marked propensity for injury and is the most commonly injured ligament of the wrist**. Injury most often is from a fall on an outstretched hand with impact on the thenar eminence.[18] Patients complain of pain and swelling on the radial side of the wrist and often a "clicking" sensation with wrist movement. Examination reveals localized tenderness on the dorsum of the wrist in the area immediately distal to Lister's tubercle. Ballottement of the scaphoid may also produce pain in this area.[16]

This injury is often referred to by the various radiographic appearances it may take. There are three different radiographic signs that may occur separately or in combination with one another (**Figure 269-5A**). **Scapholunate dissociation is a widening of the scapholunate joint space of >3 mm on the posteroanterior view.** If it is not apparent on routine views, a grip compression view or motion study may be necessary to demonstrate the abnormal gap (**Figure 269-5B**).[19] These maneuvers are particularly helpful in identifying an incomplete tear of the ligament. Rotary subluxation of the scaphoid is another radiographic finding that often accompanies scapholunate dissociation. A torn scapholunate liga-

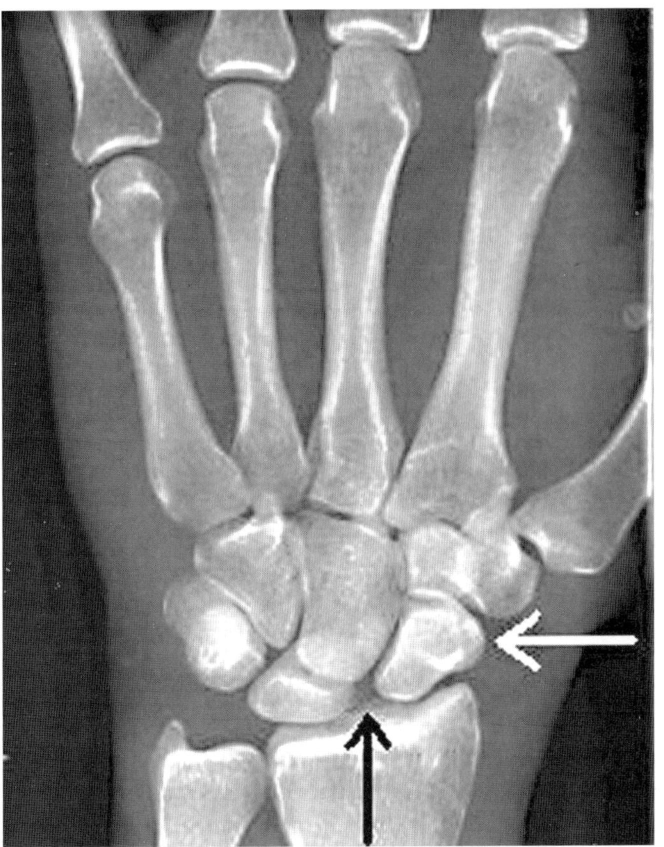

A

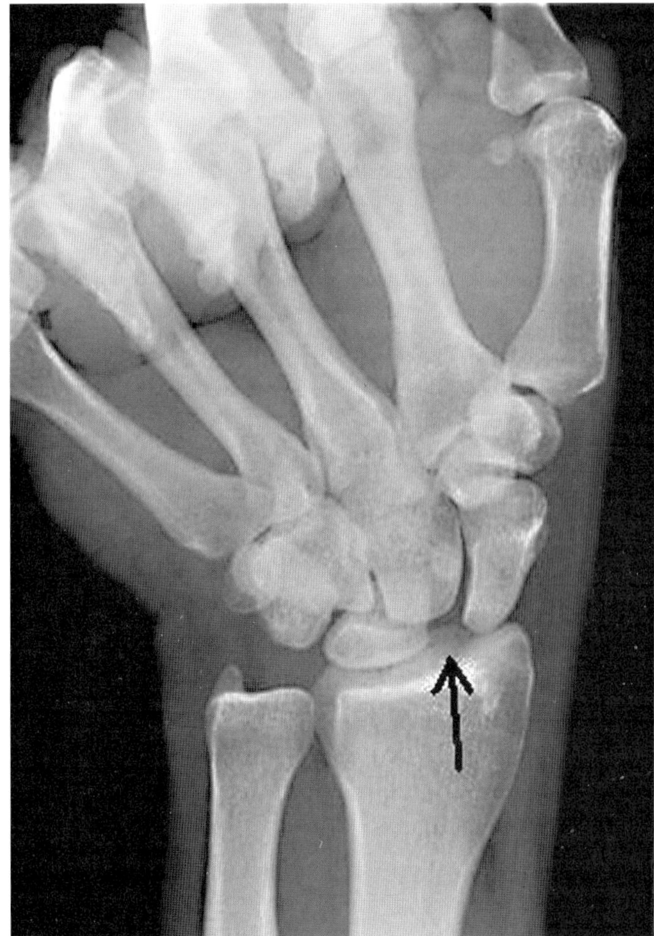

B

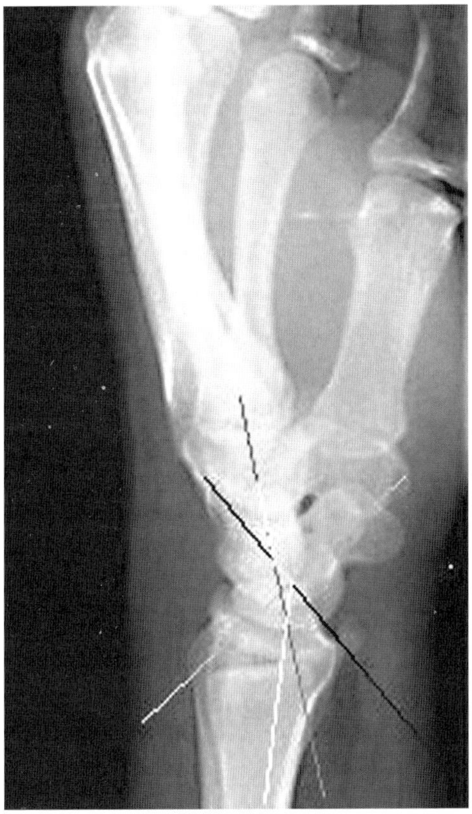

C

FIGURE 269-5. **A.** Scapholunate dissociation and rotary subluxation of the scaphoid. The scaphoid and lunate are separated by a gap of >3 mm (*black arrow*), and the scaphoid appears shorter from rotation with a dense ring, the "cortical ring sign" (*white arrow*). **B.** Grip compression view showing enhancement of scapholunate dissociation (*arrow*). **C.** Dorsal intercalated segment instability. Lateral view exhibiting dorsal intercalated instability with scapholunate dissociation. (See fig 269-4.)

ment can cause the scaphoid to tilt more palmar and increase the scapholunate angle to >60 degrees on the lateral view. On the posteroanterior view, the scaphoid tilts toward the observer so that it appears shorter as it is viewed more on its end. This causes the circular cortex of the bone to become more prominent and appear as a ring, known as the "cortical ring sign" (Figure 269-5A). A third radiographic abnormality is a carpal instability pattern known as **dorsal intercalated segment instability** (Figure 269-4B). The normal flexed posture of the scaphoid produces a flexion torque on the lunate that is counterbalanced by an extension torque from the triquetrum. When the scapholunate ligament is torn, this balance is disrupted. The lunate tilts dorsal from the unopposed extension torque from the triquetrum, whereas the scaphoid tilts more palmar (rotary subluxation of the scaphoid) because it has lost support from the lunate. The dorsal tilt of the lunate also causes a slight flexion tilt of the capitate. In the lateral view, the normal collinear arrangement of the axes of the capitate, lunate, and radius are replaced by a characteristic zigzag pattern. Both the scapholunate and capitolunate angles are increased. The concept of the proximal carpal row being the middle link or "intercalated segment" in this system, combined with the lunate's pathologic dorsal tilt and zigzag pattern (**Figure 269-5C**), is how this abnormality came to be named dorsal intercalated segment instability.

Refer to an orthopedist or hand surgeon. **ED treatment is with a radial gutter splint or short arm volar posterior mold.** Orthopedic referral is necessary because these injuries require either closed reduction with percutaneous pinning or open reduction and internal repair of the ligament.[18] Dorsal intercalated segment instability and subsequent early, severe degenerative arthritis can occur if left untreated.[15]

TRIQUETROLUNATE LIGAMENT INSTABILITY

The triquetrolunate ligament binds the triquetrum and lunate on the ulnar aspect of the wrist. Injury to this ligament is the ulnar equivalent of the scapholunate ligament injury. Triquetrolunate ligament injury occurs much less often than scapholunate ligament injury, is more stable, and can be confused with other causes of ulnar-sided wrist pain such as triangular fibrocartilage complex injury or distal radioulnar joint abnormality.[15,16] This injury most often results from falls on the outstretched, dorsiflexed hand with impact on the hypothenar eminence. There will be localized tenderness on the ulnar aspect of the wrist just distal to the ulna. Ballottement of the triquetrum may produce a painful clicking sensation.

Subtle injuries may have a normal radiographic appearance.[15] Complete disruption of the triquetrolunate ligament removes the ability of the triquetrum to counterbalance the flexion torque from the palmar-flexed scaphoid. The lunate then tilts palmar, and the capitate extends slightly in response. A zigzag pattern in the opposite direction of the scapholunate injury is produced. The capitolunate angle is increased >10 to 20 degrees; however, the scapholunate angle is unaffected because the scapholunate ligament is still intact. The lateral radiograph may reveal the "volar intercalated segment instability" pattern (Figure 269-4C and **Figure 269-6**). The posteroanterior view may reveal a widening of the triquetrolunate joint space and obliteration of the capitolunate joint space and the normal smooth arcs typically seen because of the volar tilt of the lunate.

Refer to an orthopedist or hand surgeon. **ED treatment is an ulnar gutter splint or short arm posterior mold** and referral to an orthopedist. Immobilization in a cast for 6 to 8 weeks, followed by a protective splint, is sufficient in most cases. Open reduction and internal fixation are generally reserved for chronic injuries.[15] Unrecognized injuries can cause early degenerative arthritis and chronic wrist pain.

PERILUNATE AND LUNATE DISLOCATIONS

Perilunate and lunate dislocations represent the final stages of midcarpal ligament disruption and are thought to account for 10% of all carpal injuries.[20] These injuries are the result of forceful dorsiflexion and impact on the outstretched hand, but usually with great force, such as a fall from height, impact from a motor vehicle collision, or a sporting event.[21]

Perilunate dislocation is the posterior dislocation of carpal bones while the lunate maintains its position with respect to the distal radius. This is a very rare dislocation. **Lunate dislocation** produces posterior dislocation of carpal bones with the concavity of the lunate facing anteriorly.

The injury can begin on either side of the lunate, but typically begins on the radial aspect, with either a tear of the scapholunate ligament or

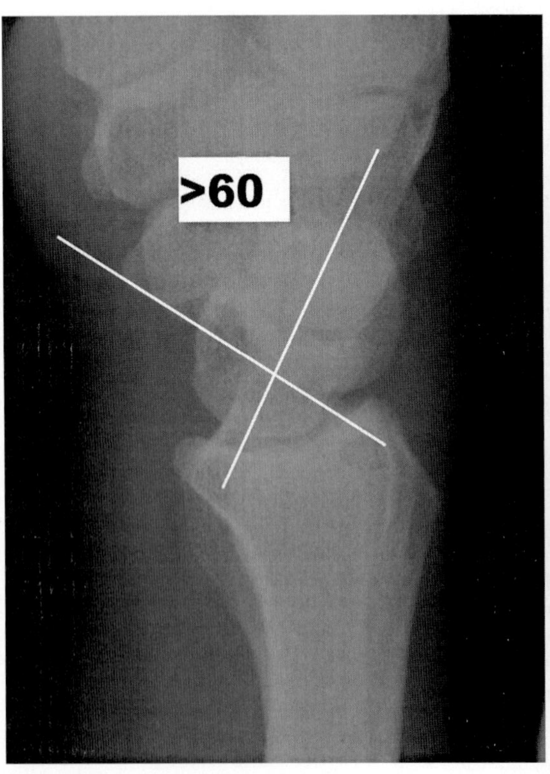

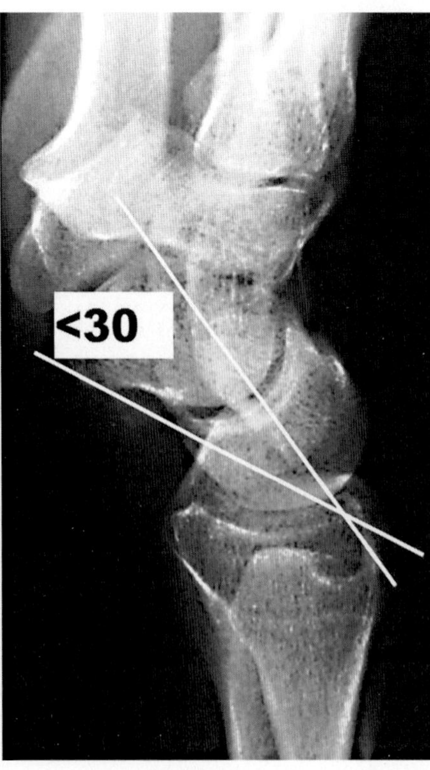

FIGURE 269-6. A. Volar intercalated instability. Note widened capitolunate angle. **B.** Dorsal intercalated instability.

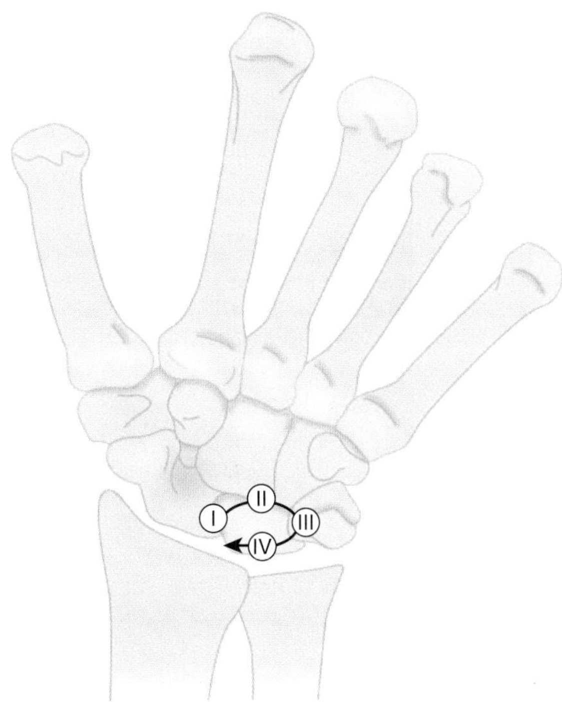

FIGURE 269-7. Four stages of perilunate instability. The first stage (I) is disruption of the scapholunate articulation (scapholunate dissociation). The second (II) and third (III) stages are separation of the capitolunate and triquetrolunate joints (perilunate dislocation). The fourth (IV) stage is a lunate dislocation.

a fracture of the scaphoid. Injury progresses around the lunate in a semicircular fashion, tearing the volar ligament arcade at the radiocapitate ligament. Remember that the extrinsic ligaments form two strong volar arcades with an inherently weak area between them that widens with dorsiflexion of the wrist (Figure 269-2). The **space of Poirier** lies at the junction of the lunate and capitate. This space opens further as heavy loading disrupts the lunatotriquetral ligament. Besides ligament disruption, any number of carpal bones may fracture along an arc around the lunate (Figure 269-7). If sufficient force is applied, the ligaments and carpal bones around the lunate are stripped away. The capitate is displaced dorsal to the lunate, producing a **perilunate dislocation**. If the capitate rebounds with sufficient force, it can push the lunate off the radius and into the palm, creating a **lunate dislocation**. These injuries are all part of a continuous spectrum of ligament disruption (**Figure 269-7**).[22]

On clinical examination, there is generalized swelling, pain, and tenderness of the wrist. However, a gross deformity, typical of many joint dislocations, is often absent. Radiographic interpretation is the key to diagnosis. **The perilunate dislocation is best appreciated on the lateral view. The linear arrangement of the three C's sign is disrupted with the capitate, represented by the third C, displaced dorsal to the lunate. The lunate retains its contact with the radius.** The scapholunate and capitolunate angles are increased. On the posteroanterior view, the three smooth arcs are disrupted, and the capitolunate joint space is obliterated as the bones overlap one another. The scapholunate and triquetrolunate joint space may either be increased because of torn ligaments or obliterated by rotation of the fractured carpal fragments. The scaphoid will appear shortened from rotary subluxation or fracture (**Figure 269-8**). A perilunate dislocation may also overshadow any associated carpal bone fracture. The scaphoid and capitate are most often involved, so carefully inspect these bones for fractures. Such fractures are designated by adding the prefix "trans-" to the carpal bone name (e.g., transscaphoid perilunate dislocation) (**Figure 269-9**).

A lunate dislocation has many similar and several distinct radiographic features when compared with a perilunate dislocation. On the posteroanterior view, the lunate has a triangular shape ("piece-of-pie" sign) that is suggestive of lunate dislocation (**Figure 269-10A**). On the lateral view, it also disrupts the three C's sign. **The lunate (represented by the middle C) is pushed off the radius into the palm. This has been called the "spilled teacup" sign because it resembles a cup spilling in the direction of the palm (Figure 269-10B).** The capitate may rebound back and even rest on the radius. The signs of ligament disruption

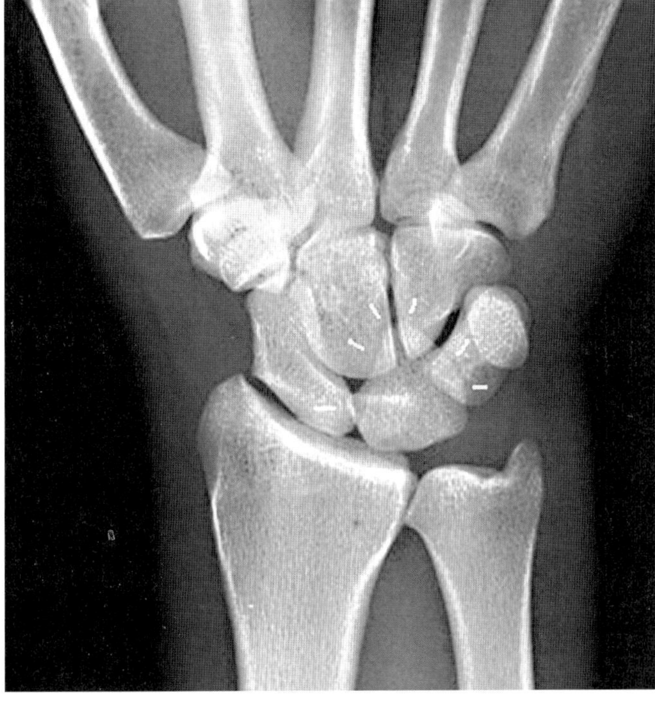
A

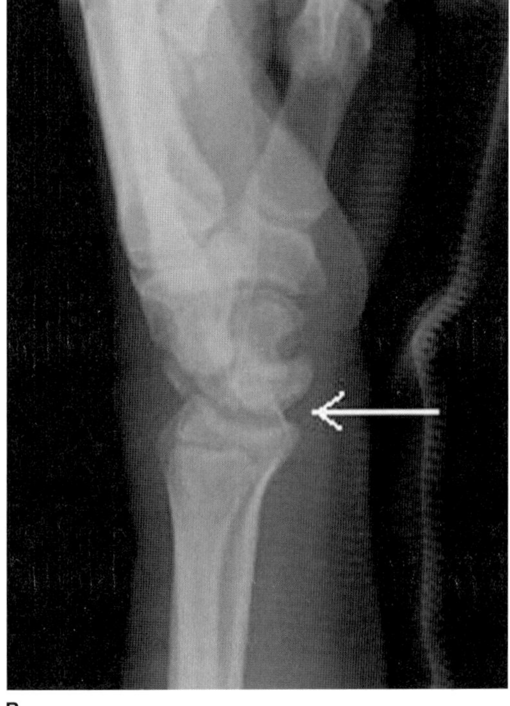
B

FIGURE 269-8. Perilunate dislocation. **A.** Posteroanterior view shows obliteration of the three smooth arcs as bones overlap one another (*white hash marks*). **B.** Lateral view shows capitate dorsal to lunate, disrupting the "three C's" (*arrow*).

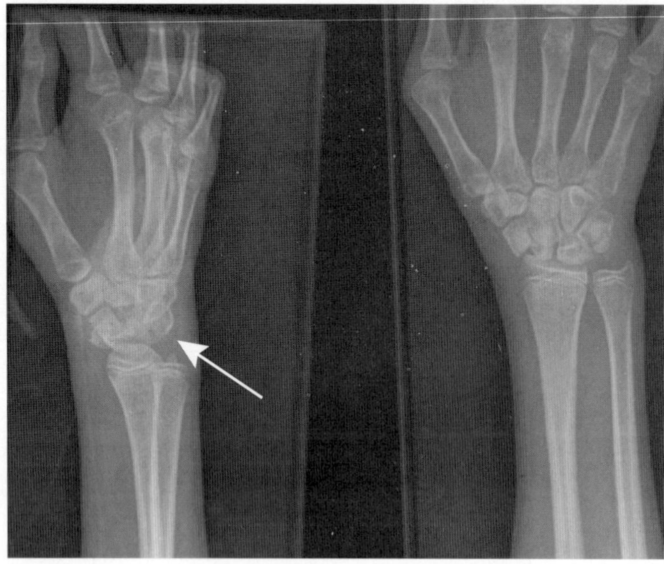

A

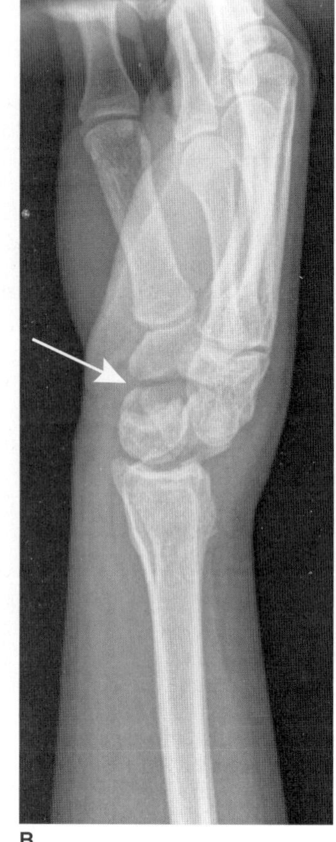

B

FIGURE 269-9. **A** and **B.** Transscaphoid perilunate dislocation. [Photos contributed by: Brooke Beckett, MD, Department of Radiology, Oregon Health & Science University, Portland, OR.]

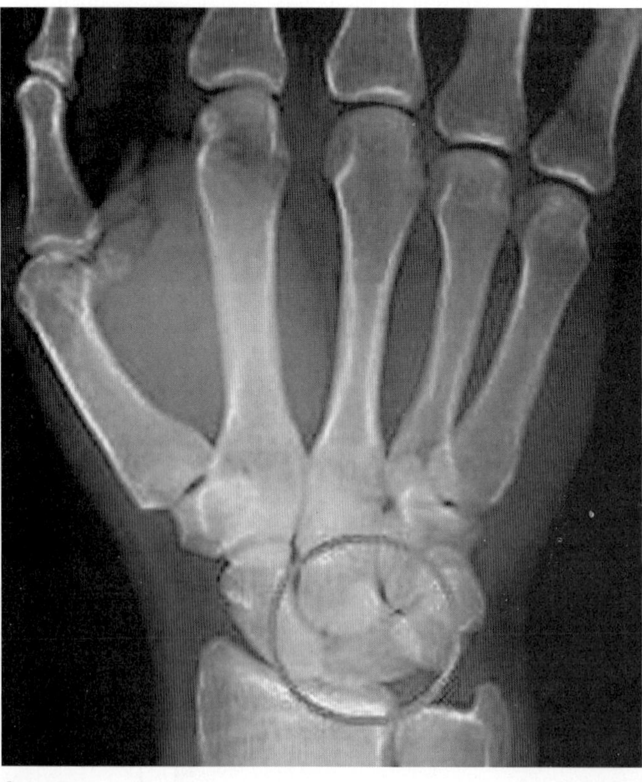

A

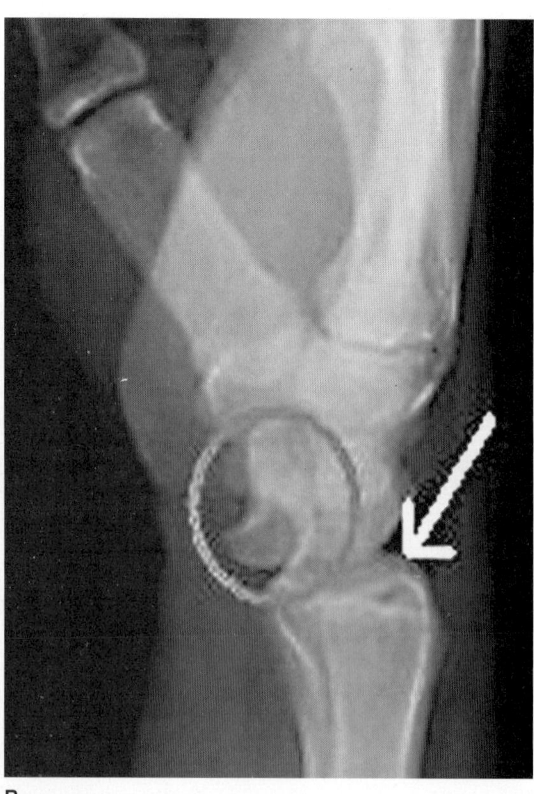

B

FIGURE 269-10. Lunate dislocation. **A.** Posteroanterior view demonstrates pathognomonic triangular shape of the lunate (piece-of-pie sign; *circle*). **B.** Lateral view exhibits the lunate tilting into the palm (spilled teacup sign; *circle*) and the capitate positioned dorsal to the lunate (*arrow*).

and the associated carpal bone fractures described with perilunate injuries may also be present.

Perilunate or lunate dislocations require emergency orthopedic/hand consultation.[22] Treatment is determined by the extent of the injury. Closed reduction and long arm splint immobilization is appropriate for reducible dislocations.[23] Open, unstable, and irreducible dislocations require open reduction and internal fixation, with repair of the ligaments and fractures. Some orthopedists operate on all perilunate and lunate dislocations.[15] **The complications include development of carpal instability patterns that lead to early degenerative arthritis, delayed union, malunion, nonunion, avascular necrosis, and, occasionally, median nerve compression from the volar dislocation of the lunate into the carpal tunnel.**[21]

CARPAL BONE FRACTURES

Carpal bone fractures are the most commonly missed wrist injuries. A careful examination is critical to recognize carpal bone fractures. The carpal fractures are in **Table 269-2** listed in descending order of occurrence.

SCAPHOID FRACTURE

The scaphoid is the most common carpal bone fractured. Injuries result from a fall on either an outstretched dorsiflexed hand or from an axial load directed along the thumb's metacarpal. There is pain along the radial aspect of the wrist and localized tenderness in the anatomic snuffbox.[24,25] Examination of the wrist in ulnar deviation exposes more of the scaphoid to direct palpation within the anatomic snuffbox. Eliciting pain in this area when the patient resists supination or pronation of the hand or pain with axial pressure directed along the thumb's metacarpal also suggests injury.

Radiographic evaluation includes both standard and scaphoid views for cortical disruption (**Figure 269-11**). The scaphoid view profiles the bone lengthwise and may assist in detecting subtle fractures. Distortion of a soft tissue fat stripe adjacent to the radial aspect of the scaphoid is suggestive of injury. Two thirds of the fractures occur at the waist or middle third of the bone, 16% to 28% in the proximal third, and 10% in the distal third. A scaphoid fracture may also have an associated injury in 12% of cases. Associated injuries may include the radius, neighboring carpal bones, a carpal instability pattern, or a dislocation. In patients with initial negative plain films, yet in whom a high index of suspicion remains for fracture, MRI is considered the gold standard for definitive diagnosis.[26]

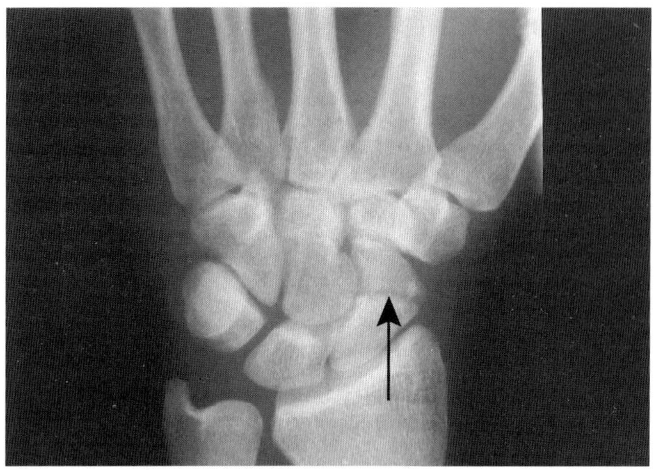

FIGURE 269-11. Scaphoid fracture in the middle third or waist (*arrow*).

A scaphoid fracture can develop avascular necrosis of the proximal fracture segment that can lead to disabling arthritis.[27] Because the vascular supply to the scaphoid enters the distal portion of the bone through small branches off the radial artery and palmar and superficial arteries, a fracture can easily disrupt the blood supply to the proximal segment. The more proximal, oblique, or displaced a fracture, the greater the risk of developing avascular necrosis. A scaphoid fracture is considered unstable if it is oblique, if there is as little as 1 mm of displacement, if there is rotation or comminution, or if a carpal instability pattern is present. Two thirds of the scaphoid's surface is articular. This only adds to the scaphoid's problems because articular fractures are more difficult to heal. Thus, the main complications of improperly healed scaphoid fractures are avascular necrosis, delayed union, nonunion, malunion, and subsequent early degenerative arthritis.

Up to 10% of initial radiographs fail to detect a fracture, so initial treatment should be directed by clinical suspicion. Nondisplaced fractures and those that are only clinically suspected can be treated in a short arm thumb spica splint. Splinting in dorsiflexion and radial deviation helps to compress the fracture fragments. Patients with unstable fractures should be placed in a long arm thumb spica splint and should be seen promptly by an orthopedic or hand surgeon for definitive treatment.

TABLE 269-2 Summary of Carpal Bone Fractures and ED Management

Carpal Bone	Mechanism of Injury	Examination	Initial ED Management
Scaphoid	Fall on outstretched hand	Snuffbox tenderness; pain with radial deviation and flexion	Short arm thumb spica splint, in dorsiflexion with radial deviation
Triquetrum	Avulsion fracture—twisting of hand against resistance or hyperextension Body fracture—direct trauma	Tenderness at the dorsum of the wrist, distal to the ulnar styloid	Short arm sugar tong splint
Lunate	Fall on outstretched hand	Tenderness at shallow indentation of the mid-dorsum of the wrist, ulnar and distal to Lister tubercle	Short arm thumb spica splint
Trapezium	Direct blow to thumb; force to wrist while dorsiflexed and radially deviated	Painful thumb movement and weak pinch strength Snuffbox tenderness	Short arm thumb spica splint
Pisiform	Fall directed on the hypothenar eminence	Tender pisiform, prominent at the base of the hypothenar eminence	Short arm volar splint in 30 degrees of flexion and ulnar deviation
Hamate	Interrupted swing of a golf club, bat, or racquet	Tenderness at the hook of the hamate, just distal and radial to the pisiform	Short arm volar wrist splint with fourth and fifth metacarpal joints in flexion
Capitate	Forceful dorsiflexion of the hand with radial impact	Tenderness over the capitate just proximal to the third metacarpal	Short arm volar wrist splint
Trapezoid	Axial load onto the index metacarpal	Tenderness over the radial aspect of the base of the index metacarpal	Short arm thumb spica splint

TRIQUETRUM FRACTURE

Triquetrum fractures are the second most common carpal bone injury, and occur as an avulsion or fracture through the body.[23] Avulsion fractures are produced when a twisting motion of the hand is suddenly resisted or a hyperextension shear stress pushes the hamate or ulnar styloid against the triquetrum. Fractures of the body occur from direct trauma and are found in association with perilunate and lunate dislocations (part of the arc fractures). Localized tenderness is found over the dorsum of the wrist in the area immediately distal to the ulnar styloid. **The dorsal avulsion fracture is best seen on the lateral radiograph or an oblique view in partial pronation.** The fracture appears as a tiny flake of bone on the dorsum of the triquetrum best seen on lateral view (**Figure 269-12**). Triquetrum body fractures are usually nondisplaced because numerous ligaments encase the bone; these are best seen on the posteroanterior view. Nonunion is possible, but avascular necrosis has not been reported.

Refer triquetrum fractures to an orthopedist or hand surgeon. Patients with a dorsal avulsion fracture have an excellent prognosis for full recovery. Symptomatic patients are treated with a wrist splint for 1 to 2 weeks. Asymptomatic or minimally symptomatic patients may be treated with early range of motion. Stable body fractures are treated in a cast for 6 weeks. Unstable body fractures (>1 mm displacement) and those associated with perilunate/lunate dislocations may require internal fixation.[28]

LUNATE FRACTURE

Lunate fractures tend to occur with other carpal injuries. Isolated lunate injuries are rare. The mechanism of injury is commonly the result of a fall on the outstretched hand. The lunate is present in the shallow indentation on the mid-dorsum of the wrist. The lunate is easily palpable as it rises out of the floor of this indentation when the wrist is in a flexed position. Examination reveals tenderness at this point. Axial compression applied along the third metacarpal ray may also elicit pain in this area and is suggestive of injury. **The lunate's blood supply enters through the distal end of the bone. A fracture subjects the lunate to risk for avascular necrosis of the proximal portion.**

The lunate is seated in the middle of the wrist, so overlap with other carpal bones may make it difficult to identify an injury on a plain radiograph. On the lateral radiograph, the lunate, capitate, and distal radius should lie in the same vertical plane.

Refer suspected or actual lunate fractures to an orthopedist or hand surgeon. Clinical suspicion dictates the acute treatment. A short arm thumb spica splint should be applied when the diagnosis is unclear. MRI and CT may be used to identify occult fractures. The major complication is avascular necrosis (Kienböck's disease), leading to lunate collapse, osteoarthritis, chronic pain, and decreased grip strength.

TRAPEZIUM FRACTURE

The trapezium is a saddle-shaped bone that articulates with the thumb metacarpal. Injuries are produced by a direct blow to the thumb or from a dorsiflexion and radial deviation force. Fractures occur either at the trapezial ridge or body and are often intra-articular. Vertical fractures occur and are analogous to a Bennett's fracture (an intra-articular proximal thumb metacarpal fracture) (**Figure 269-13**). Examination reveals painful thumb movement and a weak pinch. There is tenderness at the apex of the anatomic snuffbox and at the base of the thenar eminence. This injury is best profiled on a 20-degree pronated oblique view. The major complication is nonunion.

Refer to an orthopedist or hand surgeon. Initial ED stabilization of nondisplaced fractures is a short arm thumb spica splint. **Displaced fractures >1 mm or diastases >2 mm require surgery.**[29]

PISIFORM FRACTURE

The pisiform is a sesamoid bone within the flexor carpi ulnaris tendon. It is positioned immediately volar to the triquetrum and is the palpable bony prominence at the base of the hypothenar eminence. Injuries usually result from a fall directed on the hypothenar eminence. There will be localized tenderness on the pisiform itself. If the wrist is flexed, the pisiform can be grasped and palpated between the examiner's fingers. This should elicit pain. The pisiform and hook of the hamate form the bony walls of **Guyon's canal** that contains the ulnar nerve and artery; therefore, it is important to exclude injury to them.[30] Radiographs in partial supination, or the carpal tunnel view, are optimal because they remove the overlap with the triquetrum that is present on standard views (**Figure 269-14**).[31] The pisiform is the last carpal bone to ossify, and it is usually complete by age 12 years old. Before the age of 12, multiple ossification centers in the pisiform may be confused with a fracture. The ossification centers differ in that they will have smoother margins and lack the perfect jigsaw-puzzle fit seen with

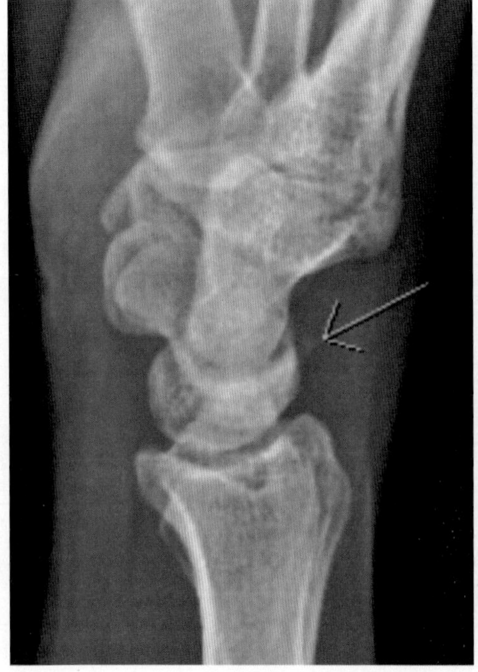

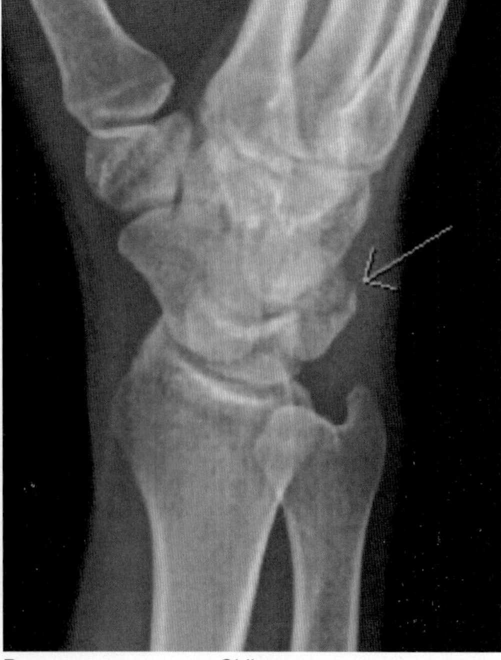

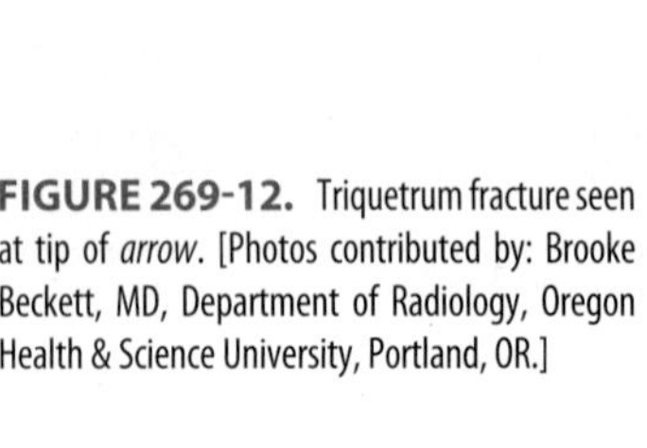

FIGURE 269-12. Triquetrum fracture seen at tip of *arrow*. [Photos contributed by: Brooke Beckett, MD, Department of Radiology, Oregon Health & Science University, Portland, OR.]

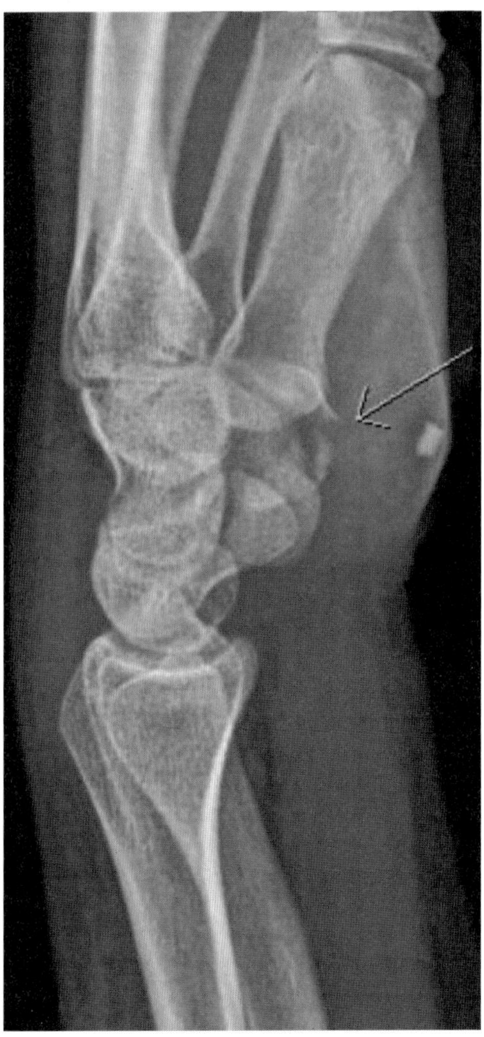

FIGURE 269-13. Trapezium fracture seen at tip of *arrow*. [Photo contributed by: Brooke Beckett, MD, Department of Radiology, Oregon Health & Science University, Portland, OR.]

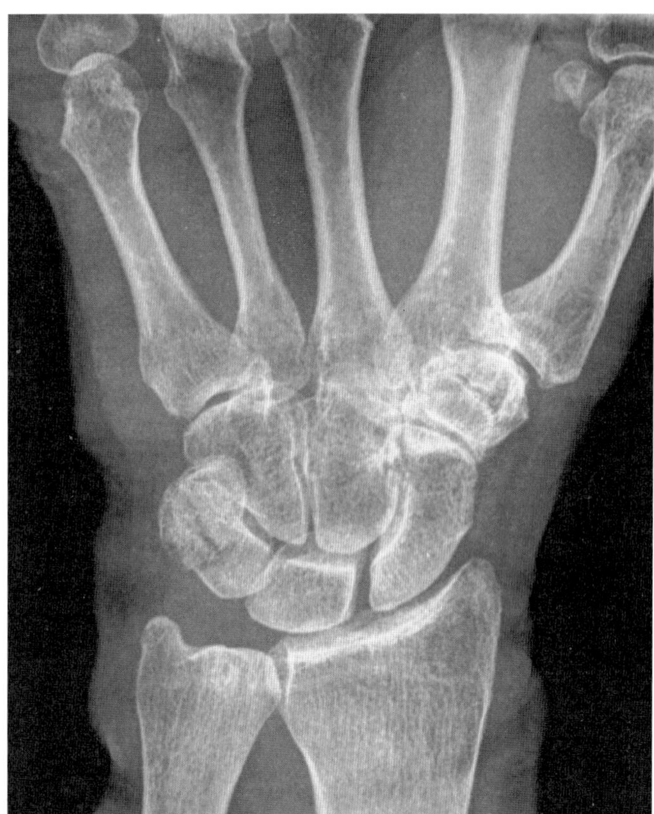

FIGURE 269-14. Pisiform fracture. [Photo contributed by: Brooke Beckett, MD, Department of Radiology, Oregon Health & Science University, Portland, OR.]

fracture fragments. After age 12, any radiographic line is suggestive of fracture.

Refer to an orthopedist or hand surgeon. ED treatment is either a compression dressing or a splint in 30 degrees of flexion with ulnar deviation that relaxes the tension from the flexor carpi ulnaris. Pisiform fractures have an excellent prognosis.

HAMATE FRACTURE

Hamate fractures may involve the body of the hamate, the hook of the hamate, or any of its articular surfaces. Body fractures are rare and are generally associated with fracture dislocations of the fourth or fifth metacarpals (**Figure 269-15**). Most hamate fractures involve the hamate hook, which is a small bony prominence on its volar aspect. The classic mechanism is an interrupted swing with a golf club, bat, or racquet. The handle impacts against the hypothenar eminence and compresses the bone. Localized tenderness over the hook of the hamate is found by palpating the soft tissue of the hypothenar eminence, distal and radial to the pisiform. **Standard and carpal tunnel views are necessary to visualize the fracture. Occult fractures may be identified by bone scan or CT.** Physical examination should assess for injury to **Guyon's canal (Figure 269-16)**, which houses the ulnar nerve and artery.

Refer to an orthopedist or hand surgeon. In the ED, treat hamate hook fractures with a compression dressing or splint. Nonunion is common, and excision of the bone may be necessary. Nondisplaced body fractures are treated by splint immobilization. Displaced body fractures or those with injury to Guyon's canal are surgically treated.

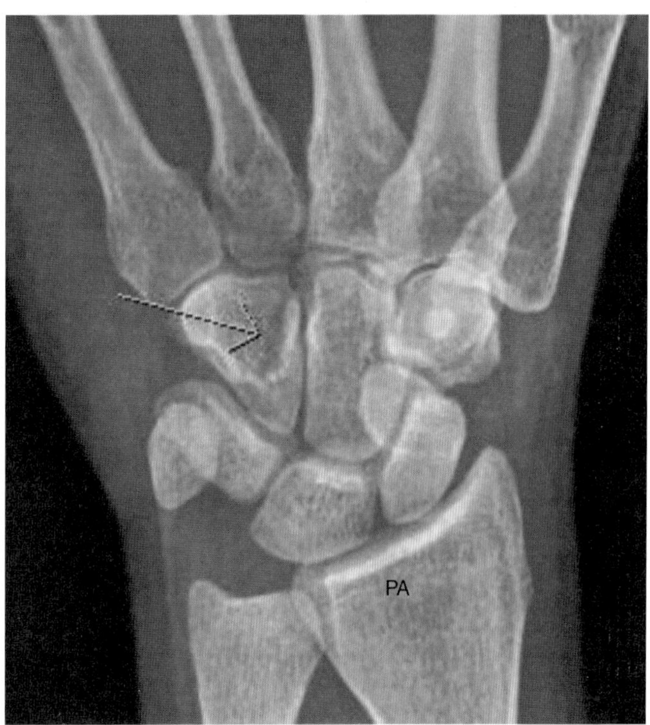

FIGURE 269-15. Hamate fracture (*arrow*) is best seen on posteroanterior view. [Photo contributed by: Brooke Beckett, MD, Department of Radiology, Oregon Health & Science University, Portland, OR.]

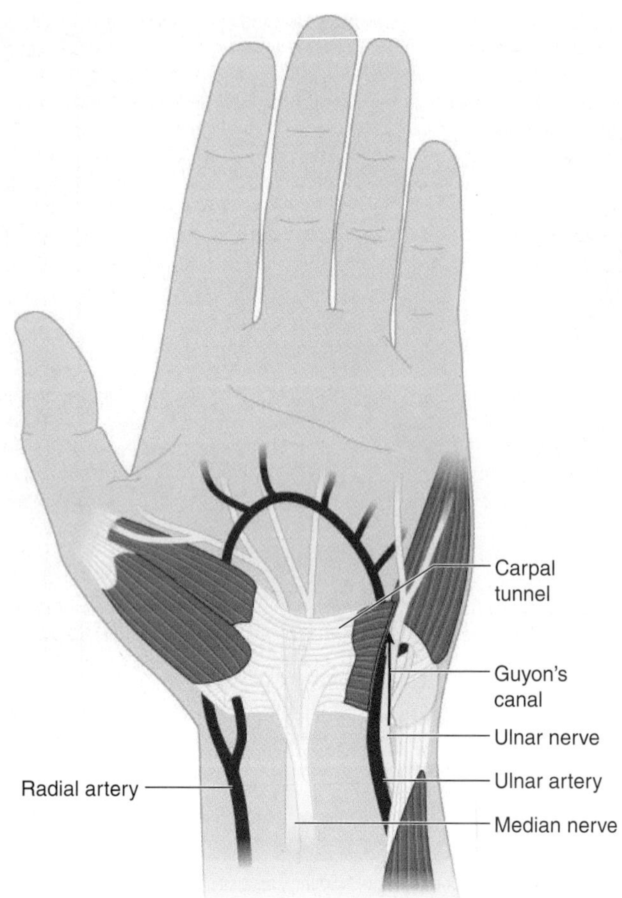

FIGURE 269-16. Guyon's canal.

CAPITATE FRACTURE

The capitate is the largest carpal bone. It is an elongated bone with a large proximal head that articulates with the lunate. The midportion of the bone is the neck, and the distal end, or body, articulates with the third metacarpal. Capitate fractures most often occur in the neck and usually occur in conjunction with a scaphoid fracture (**Figure 269-17**). The association of scaphoid and capitate fractures is called the **scaphocapitate syndrome**. Isolated capitate fractures are rare.[32] Capitate fractures result from forceful dorsiflexion of the hand with impact on the radial side. The scaphoid fractures first, and then the neck of the capitate fractures. The fracture can continue around the lunate, creating other so-called arc fractures, eventually resulting in perilunate or lunate dislocation. The capitate's blood supply enters through the distal end. Thus, capitate fractures also share the same potential avascular necrosis of the proximal fracture segment as the lunate and scaphoid.

Physical examination reveals diffuse swelling and tenderness over the capitate, just proximal to the third metacarpal. Capitate neck fractures are best seen on the lateral radiograph. The head of the capitate should be carefully identified because it can rotate as much as 180 degrees. A capitate fracture is often overlooked because of the accompanying scaphoid fracture or perilunate/lunate dislocation that overshadows it. Complications include avascular necrosis, delayed union, nonunion, and malunion.

ED treatment of undisplaced, isolated capitate fractures is splint immobilization and early orthopedic/hand surgeon referral. Most capitate fractures, however, are displaced or associated with the scaphocapitate syndrome and require surgical treatment.[33]

TRAPEZOID FRACTURE

Trapezoid fracture is extremely rare. The injury results from an axial load onto the index metacarpal. There will be tenderness on the radial aspect that is augmented by applying pressure along the index metacarpal ray. Fractures are difficult to visualize on standard radiographs, and CT or MRI may be necessary. ED treatment is with a thumb spica splint.

DISTAL RADIUS AND ULNA FRACTURES

Fractures of the distal metaphysis of the radius and ulna are among the most common injuries affecting the wrist. Among the factors that influence the type and amount of displacement of the fracture are the point and direction of impact, the degree of force, and the patient's age (**Table 269-3**).

In general, the thinner cortices of the elderly make them more likely to sustain extra-articular fractures, whereas younger adults often sustain more complicated intra-articular fractures.

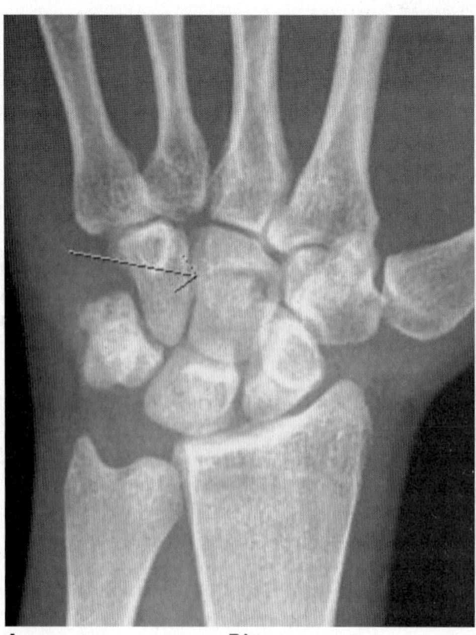

FIGURE 269-17. Capitate fracture (*arrow*) is seen best on posteroanterior view. [Photos contributed by: Brooke Beckett, MD, Department of Radiology, Oregon Health & Science University, Portland, OR.]

TABLE 269-3 Radiographic Appearance of Distal Radius Fractures

Colles' fracture
Dorsal angulation of the plane of the distal radius
Distal radius fragment is displaced proximally and dorsally
Radial displacement of the carpus
Ulnar styloid may be fractured
Smith's fracture
Volar angulation of the plane of the distal radius
Distal radius fragment is displaced proximally and volarly
Radial displacement of the carpus
The fracture line extends obliquely from the dorsal surface to the volar surface 1–2 cm proximal to the articular surface
Barton's fracture
Volar and proximal displacement of a large fragment of radial articular surface
Volar displacement of the carpus
Radial styloid may be fractured

COLLES' FRACTURE

Colles' fracture results most often from a fall on the outstretched hand. This mechanism produces a distal radial metaphysis fracture that is dorsally angulated and displaced proximally and dorsally (**Figure 269-18**). Compression forces on the dorsal side often produce dorsal comminution of bone. The fracture line may also comminute and extend into the radioulnar or radiocarpal joint ("die-punch" fracture). A fracture of the ulnar styloid is often present and may be suggestive of injury to the triangular fibrocartilage complex.

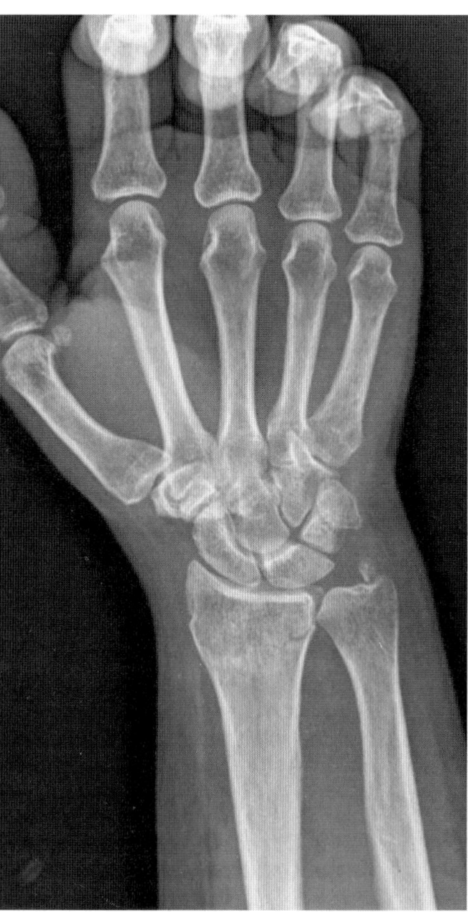
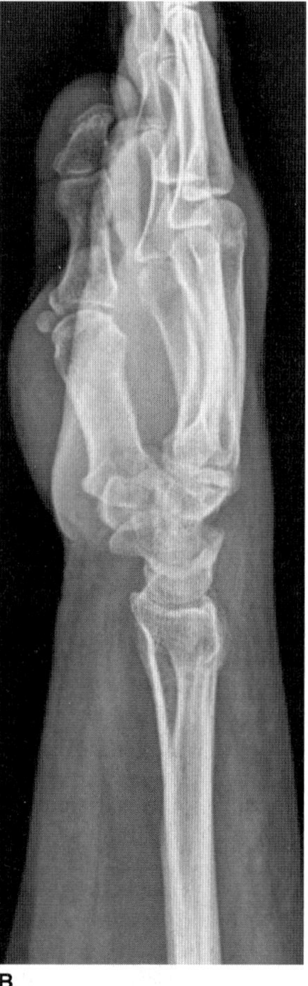

A B

FIGURE 269-18. Colles' fracture. A. Anteroposterior view. B. Lateral view. [Photos contributed by: Brooke Beckett, MD, Department of Radiology, Oregon Health & Science University, Portland, OR.]

The wrist has the characteristic dorsiflexion, or "dinner-fork," deformity. Patients may complain of palmar paresthesias from pressure on the median nerve. Posteroanterior radiographs reveal a distal metaphyseal fracture of the radius that often appears shortened from the angulation or comminution. **The lateral view provides the best view of the dorsal angulation and comminution. In general, unstable fractures have >20 degrees of angulation, intra-articular involvement, marked comminution, or more than a centimeter of shortening.** These injuries are more likely to develop loss of reduction, distal radioulnar joint instability, radiocarpal instability patterns, and subsequent arthritis.

Stable fractures may be treated with a compression dressing and splint until they can be evaluated by an orthopedic surgeon; otherwise, closed reduction is performed. After adequate local anesthesia (see chapter 36, "Local and Regional Anesthesia"), provide traction with finger traps while the fracture fragment is pushed distal and palmar and the patient's forearm is held firmly (**Figure 269-19**). The goal is to restore the volar tilt, radial inclination, and proper length to the radius. This is particularly important in younger patients. The volar tilt ideally should be restored to its normal position, but a minimum of neutral or zero degrees of angulation is acceptable.

Most Colles' fractures can be treated with closed reduction and application of a sugar tong splint. If a short arm cast is applied, it should be bivalved to allow for edema. Fractures that are unstable, severely comminuted, or intra-articular may require surgery. **All open and neurovascularly compromised fractures require prompt evaluation by an orthopedic surgeon.**

Complications include malunion, median nerve injuries, triangular fibrocartilage complex injuries, radioulnar and radiocarpal instability, and arthritis. These complications may result in a weak, stiff, and painful wrist.

SMITH'S FRACTURE

Smith's fracture, or **reverse Colles' fracture**, is a volar angulated fracture of the distal radius. This may result from a fall or direct blow on the dorsum of the hand and wrist, or from a fall on the outstretched hand in supination that then shifts into a pronated position. The hand is displaced palmar and produces a "garden-spade deformity" on physical examination. The posteroanterior radiograph looks much like the Colles' fracture, with a distal metaphyseal radius fracture that may be shortened and comminuted. **The lateral radiograph shows the volar angulated and displaced fracture (Figure 269-20).**

The treatment objectives and complications are much like those seen with the Colles' fracture. In this case, however, the angulation is volar rather than dorsal, and during reduction, pressure is applied in the opposite direction.

BARTON'S FRACTURE

Barton's fractures are dorsal or volar rim fractures of the distal radius. The dorsal rim fractures result from a dorsiflexion and pronation force, whereas the less common volar rim fracture is produced by a fall on the outstretched hand in supination. These injuries are often fraction-dislocations or subluxations, because the carpus is frequently displaced in the direction of the fracture. Accompanying ligamentous injuries create radiocarpal instability. This instability is not fully appreciated in the acute setting but may lead to various secondary carpal instability patterns and premature degenerative arthritis.

The posteroanterior radiograph often shows a comminuted fracture of the distal radial metaphysis. The lateral view reveals an intra-articular fracture of the volar or dorsal rim of the radius, which may be accompanied by carpal subluxation in the same direction (**Figure 269-21**).

Minimally displaced fractures can be treated acutely in a sugar tong splint until evaluation by an orthopedist. **Unstable fractures involving >50% of the radial articular surface or those with accompanying carpal subluxation require open reduction and internal fixation.**

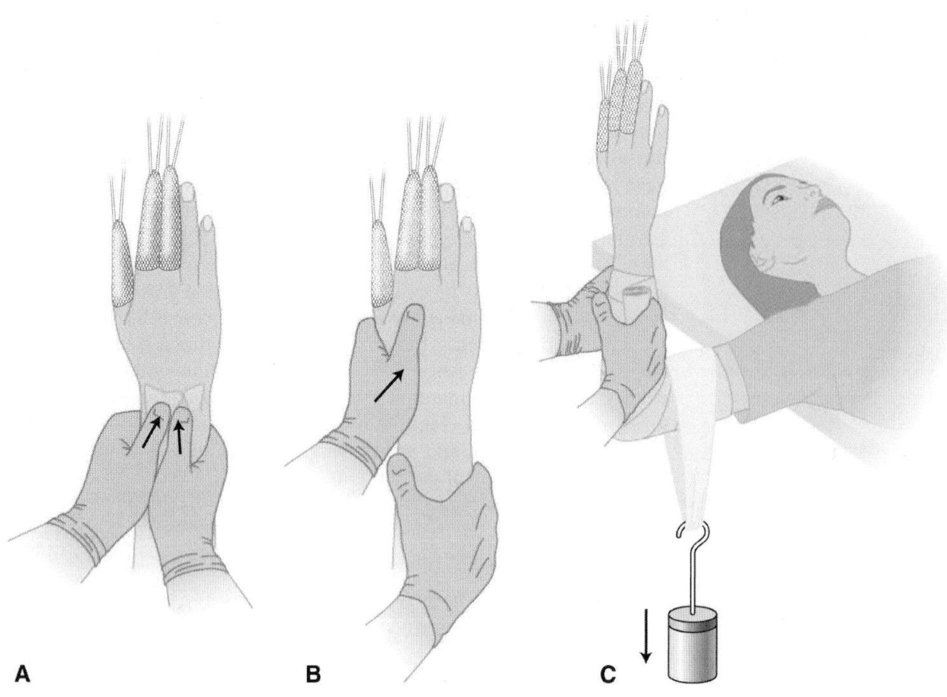

FIGURE 269-19. A and B. *Arrows* demonstrate application of force for proper reduction. C. Figure demonstrates proper patient position with the use of finger traps. [Reproduced with permission from Reichman EF, Simon RR: Emergency Medicine Procedures. © 2004, McGraw-Hill, New York.]

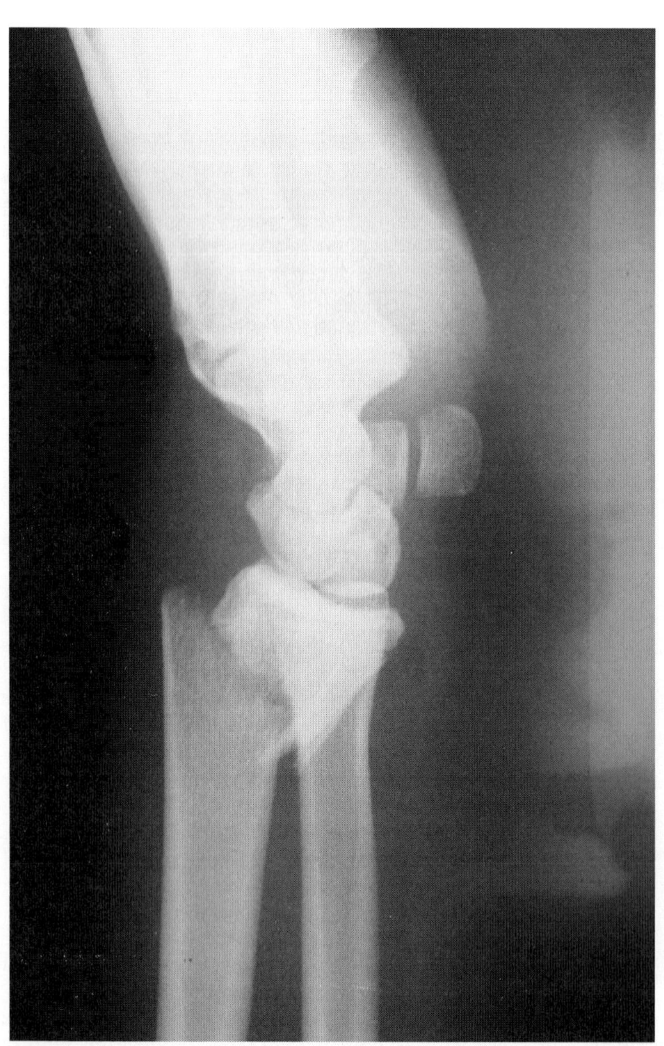

FIGURE 269-20. Smith's fracture.

RADIAL STYLOID FRACTURE

A force directed along the radial aspect of the hand can produce a transverse or oblique fracture that extends from the scaphoid fossa to the metaphysis of the radius (**Figure 269-22**). **Radial styloid fracture** is often accompanied by a dislocation of the lunate. It is best seen on the posteroanterior radiograph as a thin, lucent line beneath the radial styloid. Because the major carpal ligaments along the radial aspect of the wrist insert on the radial styloid, displacement of this fracture can produce carpal instability. This instability is aided by the extracarpal ligaments (i.e., wrist/finger flexors and extensors causing further displacement of the styloid). Displaced fractures often require open reduction and internal fixation. Displacement of as little as 3 mm is often associated with accompanying scapholunate dissociation. Failure to recognize intercarpal ligament tears adds to the potential for subsequent posttraumatic arthritis. Refer to an orthopedist. In the ED, place a short arm splint positioning the wrist in mild flexion and ulnar deviation.

ULNAR STYLOID FRACTURE

A forced radial deviation, dorsiflexion, or rotatory stress can fracture the **ulnar styloid**. The ulnar styloid fracture may be isolated or may accompany other injuries, such as a Colles' fracture. Clinically, avulsion fractures are rarely significant, with the major consideration being the associated radial soft tissue and bony injuries. Displaced ulnar base fractures can be intra-articular and be associated with tears of the triangular fibrocartilage complex, which is the main stabilizer of the distal radioulnar joint. Patients complain of a painful clicking or locking sensation in the wrist. If the distal radioulnar joint is stable, ulnar styloid fractures are treated acutely in an ulnar gutter splint in slight ulnar deviation and neutral positioning of the wrist. If there is any question about stability, these patients should be referred acutely for surgical evaluation. Arthrograms or MRI imaging may be necessary to delineate the full extent of injury.

DISTAL RADIOULNAR JOINT DISRUPTION

Distal radioulnar joint disruption is generally seen with intra-articular or distal radial shaft fractures (**Galeazzi fracture-dislocation**)[34] or with fractures of both bones of the forearm. These more apparent injuries often overshadow distal radioulnar joint disruption and, unfortunately,

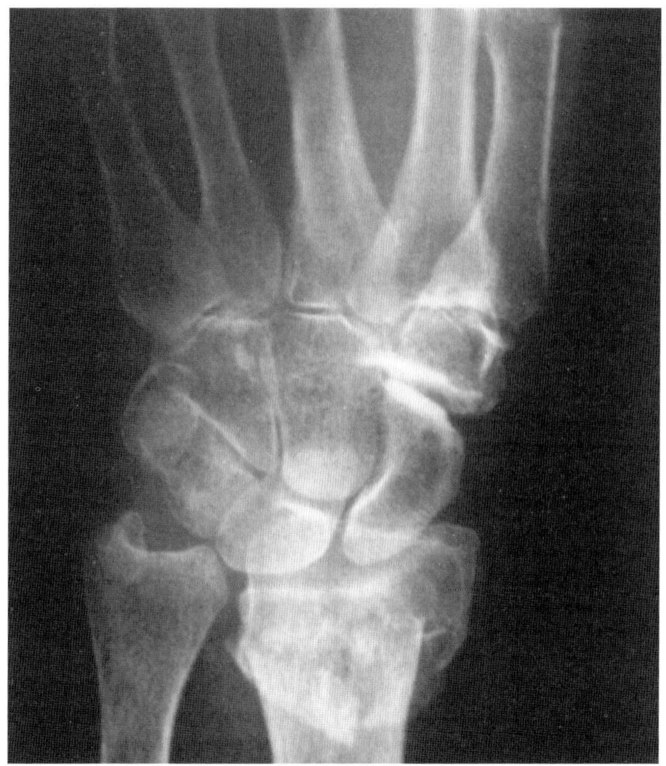

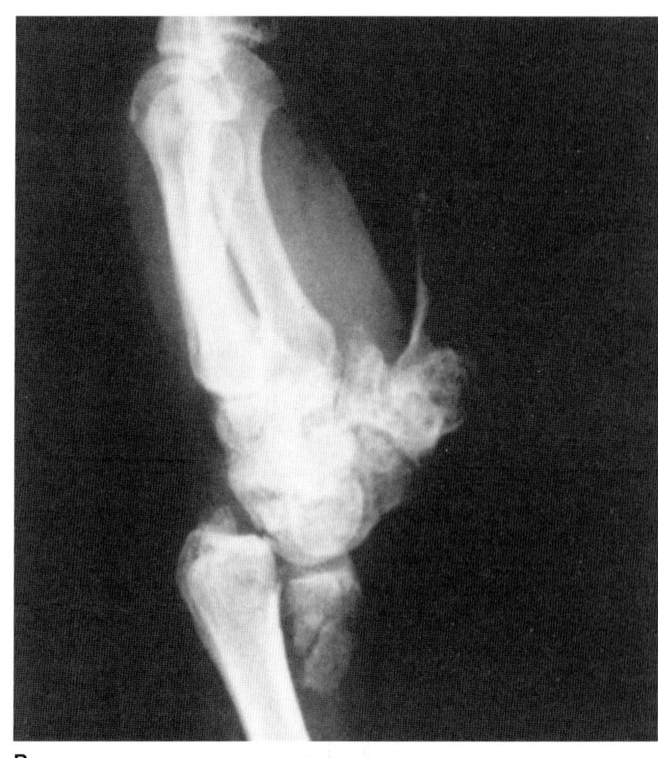

FIGURE 269-21. Volar Barton's fracture. **A.** Posteroanterior view. **B.** Lateral view.

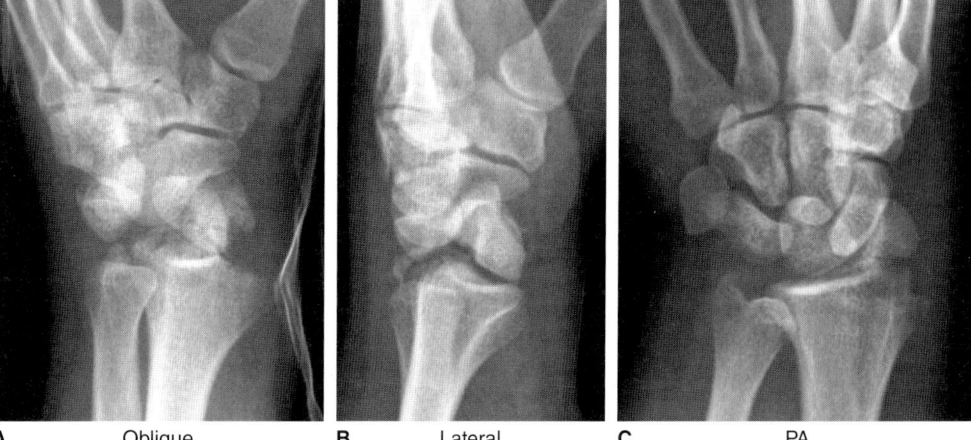

FIGURE 269-22. Radial styloid fracture (*arrow*) with lunate dislocation. [Photos contributed by: Brooke Beckett, MD, Department of Radiology, Oregon Health & Science University, Portland, OR.]

may remain unrecognized until subsequent pain and diminished wrist movement are appreciated.

Isolated radioulnar joint dislocations are uncommon and are often unrecognized acutely. Dorsal dislocation of the ulna results most often from falls on the wrist in hyperpronation. The rare volar dislocation results from forced hypersupination of the wrist. Patients with disruption of the distal radioulnar joint present with pain at the distal radioulnar joint, weak grip, and restricted range of motion, especially pronation and supination. The ulnar head is often prominent but may be subtle and easily overlooked.

The posteroanterior radiograph reveals narrowing and overlap of the distal radioulnar joint. **The lateral radiograph demonstrates either volar or dorsal displacement of the ulna, which is normally centered and overlapping the radius.** Because slight oblique positioning of the wrist can produce a misleading appearance of ulnar displacement, make sure to obtain a properly positioned lateral view. A true lateral view should have superimposition of the four ulnar metacarpals, superimposition of the proximal pole of the scaphoid with the lunate and triquetrum, and the radial styloid centered over its distal articular surface. CT scanning may be necessary to establish the diagnosis if plain films are inconclusive.

Immobilizing the wrist in supination reduces dorsal dislocations, whereas volar dislocations are placed in pronation. Patients with acute distal radioulnar joint disruption are referred acutely for orthopedic follow-up. These injuries have a high recurrence rate and may require reconstructive surgery, particularly if there is a delay in diagnosis.

Acknowledgments: The authors wish to acknowledge the contributions of Dean Wolanyk, MD, and Harold Chin, MD, to previous editions of this chapter.

REFERENCES

The complete reference list is available online at www.TintinalliEM.com.

CHAPTER 270 Elbow and Forearm Injuries

Yvonne C. Chow

ANATOMY

Articulations of the distal humerus and proximal ulna and radius form the elbow joint (**Figure 270-1**).

The epicondyles are nonarticulating surfaces that serve as sites of origin for forearm, wrist, and digit flexors and pronators (medial), and extensors and supinators (lateral). Medially, the trochlea articulates with the olecranon to form a uniaxial hinge joint. Laterally, the capitellum abuts the radial head to form a pivot joint. Between the condyles, the coronoid fossa is anterior, and the olecranon fossa is posterior. These allow for full flexion and extension of the ulna. The radial fossa lies proximal to the capitellum anteriorly and permits full flexion of the radius.

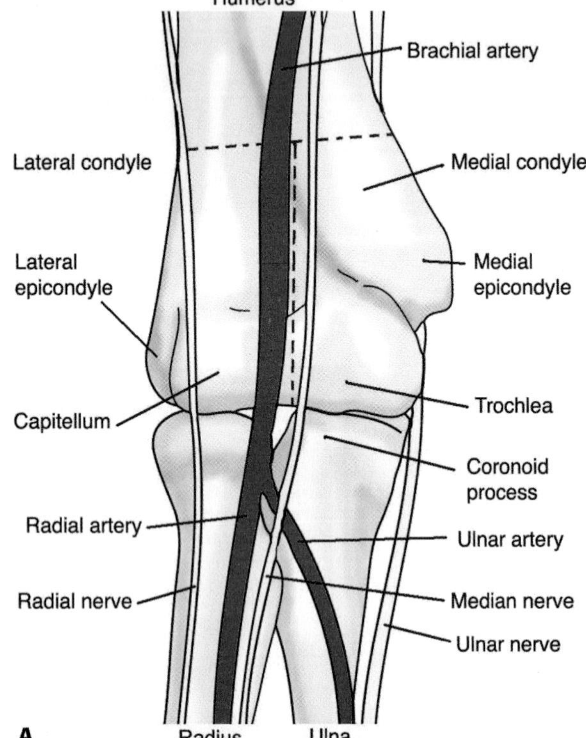

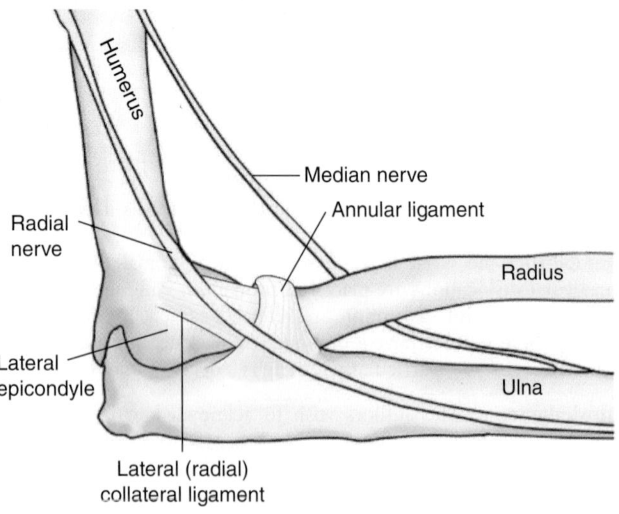

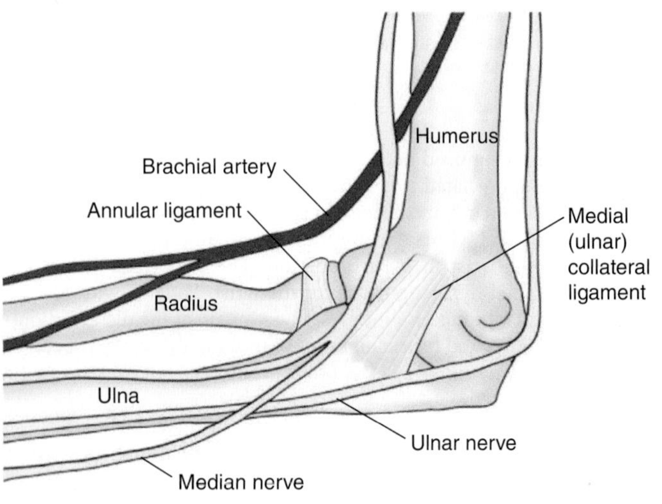

FIGURE 270-1. Elbow anatomy. **A.** Anterior view. **B.** Lateral view. **C.** Medial view.

TABLE 270-1 Sensory and Motor Function Testing of the Radial, Median, and Ulnar Nerves

	Radial	Median	Ulnar
Test for sensory function	Dorsum of the thumb index web space	Two-point discrimination over the tip of the index finger	Two-point discrimination over the little finger
Test for motor function	Extend both wrist and fingers against resistance	"OK" sign with thumb and index finger; abduction of the thumb (recurrent branch)	Abduct index finger against resistance

The radius and ulna are joined together along their entire length by a fibrous interosseous membrane, and articulate only at their ends to form the complex proximal and distal radioulnar joints. The ulna is a comparatively straight bone, whereas the radius has an important outward bowing. During the motions of supination and pronation, the radius rotates around the relatively fixed ulna. Because these bones have such a close relationship to one another, injury to one will have a direct impact on the other. A displaced or angulated fracture of one bone typically disrupts the other or causes a dislocation at the proximal or distal radioulnar joint.

Several important neurovascular structures lie in close proximity to the distal humerus, and evaluation of their function is essential. These include the brachial artery, palpable just medial to the distal biceps tendon in the antecubital fossa, and the radial, median, and ulnar nerves (**Table 270-1**).

The neuroanatomy is best understood by appreciating the neural control of basic wrist and finger movement (**Figure 270-2**). The radial nerve travels over the lateral epicondyle and supplies the muscles of wrist extension before it branches off into the posterior interosseous nerve. This deep branch travels around the proximal radius and through the supinator muscle and controls the muscles of finger and thumb extension. The remainder of the radial nerve lies adjacent to the radial artery. This superficial branch is purely sensory and innervates the dorsal aspect of the hand from the thumb to the radial half of the ring finger. Thus, the proximal portion of the radial nerve controls the more proximal function of wrist extension, the deep branch (posterior interosseous nerve) controls the more distal function of finger extension, and the superficial branch is purely sensory. Therefore, an isolated injury to the posterior interosseous branch affects finger extension but spares wrist extension and sensation to the dorsum of the hand.

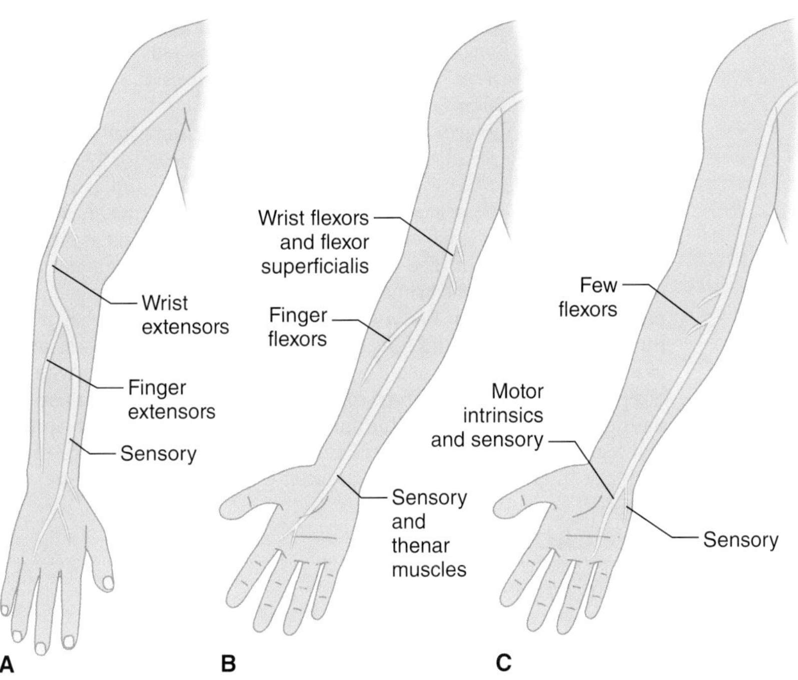

FIGURE 270-2. Neural innervation of the forearm, wrist, hand, and digits. **A.** Radial nerve innervation. **B.** Median nerve innervation. **C.** Ulnar nerve innervation.

The median nerve supplies the muscles of wrist and finger flexion and sensation over the volar surface of the hand from the thumb to the radial half of the ring finger, including the dorsal tips of the thumb and index and middle fingers. The proximal portion of the median nerve innervates the muscles that control wrist flexion and the flexor digitorum superficialis before it gives off the anterior interosseous nerve. This branch controls portions of the remaining deep finger flexors. The remaining portion of the median nerve provides sensation to most of the volar surface of the hand in addition to controlling the thenar muscles of the thumb via a separate motor branch (recurrent branch of the median nerve).

The ulnar nerve provides innervation to forearm muscles and controls the intrinsic muscles of the hand while providing sensation to the little finger and the ulnar half of the ring finger. Proximal to the elbow, the ulnar nerve courses under a ligamentous band called the arcade of Struthers prior to entering the cubital tunnel posterior to the medial epicondyle. These are two sites where the nerve can become entrapped, leading to ulnar neuropathy syndromes. The ulnar nerve is palpable as a cord in the cubital tunnel and is vulnerable to injury with trauma over this area.

The biceps muscle has two proximal heads (**Figure 270-3**). The long head originates at both the supraglenoid tubercle of the scapula and the superior labrum of the glenohumeral joint, and then travels through the capsule of the shoulder and along the intertubercular (bicipital) groove of the humerus. The short head originates at the coracoid process of the scapula. The distal attachments are to the radial tuberosity by the distal biceps tendon and the forearm by the bicipital aponeurosis. A bicipitoradial bursa lies adjacent to the radial tuberosity. The biceps muscle is innervated by the musculocutaneous nerve (C5 and C6) and functions to flex the supinated forearm and supinate the flexed forearm.

The brachialis muscle lies deep to the biceps muscle. It originates on the distal anterior humerus and inserts on the ulnar tuberosity of the proximal ulna. The brachialis muscle is innervated by both the musculocutaneous and radial nerves (C5, C6, C7, and C8) and is the primary flexor of the forearm.

The triceps muscle has three proximal heads (**Figure 270-4**): a long head originating from the infraglenoid tubercle of the scapula; a lateral head on the posterior surface of the humerus superior to the radial (spiral) groove; and a medial head inferior to the radial groove. The triceps inserts at the olecranon. A subtendinous bursa separates the triceps from the olecranon, and a subcutaneous bursa lies just distal to the tendinous insertion. The latter frequently becomes inflamed. The triceps

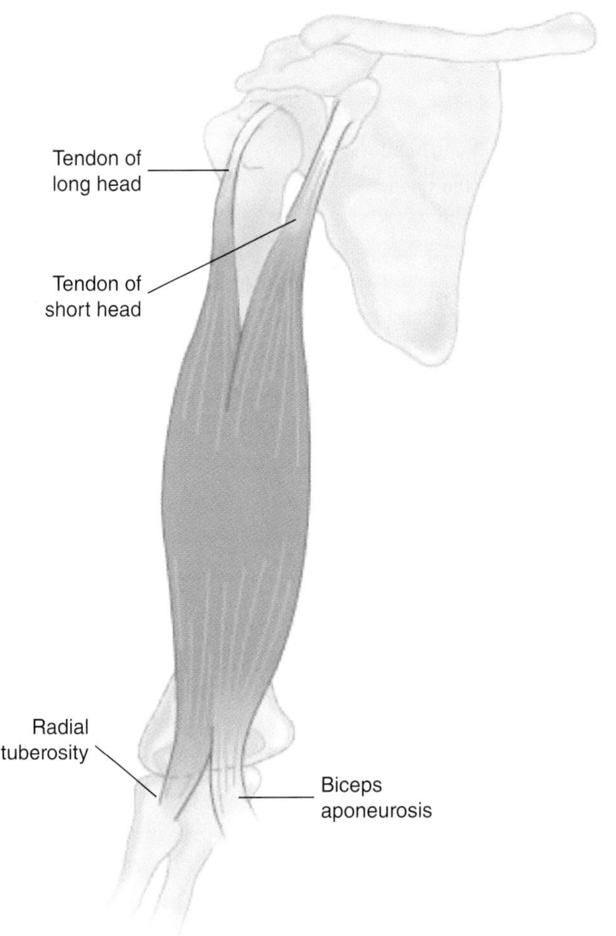

FIGURE 270-3. Biceps muscle anatomy.

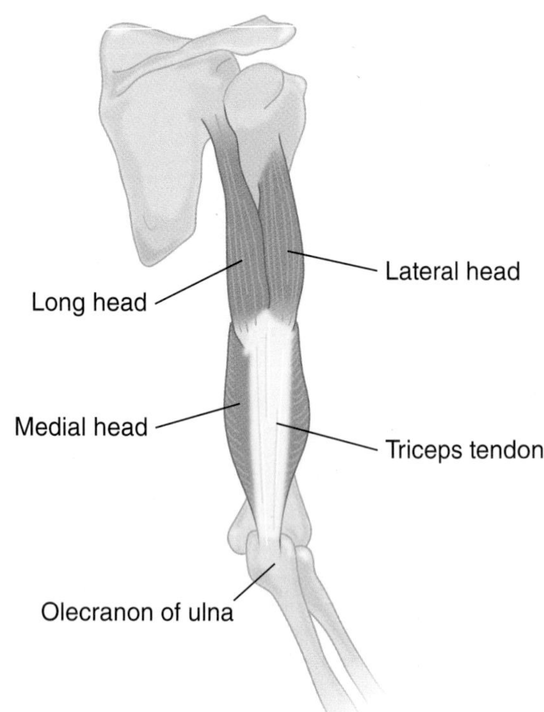

FIGURE 270-4. Triceps muscle anatomy.

muscle is innervated by the radial nerve (C6, C7, and C8) and is the sole extensor of the forearm. Additionally, the triceps aids extension and adduction of the arm, and the long head stabilizes the head of the humerus in abduction.

The intrinsic forearm muscles include the brachioradialis, pronator teres, pronator quadratus, anconeus, and supinator (**Figure 270-5**). The brachioradialis muscle originates at the lateral condyle and assists with forearm flexion. The pronator teres muscle has two proximal heads that originate from the medial epicondyle and the proximal ulna; it pronates and flexes the forearm. The pronator quadratus muscle originates from the distal ulna and is the primary pronator of the forearm. The anconeus muscle originates from the posterior lateral epicondyle and has trivial function in extending the forearm. Lastly, the supinator muscle originates from the posterior medial ulna and supinates the forearm with the biceps muscle. The deep branch of the radial nerve (posterior interosseous nerve) pierces the supinator muscle after branching off of the proximal segment of the radial nerve. Thus, a compression neuropathy to the posterior interosseous nerve can occur at this level (**Figure 270-6**).

CLINICAL FEATURES

HISTORY

A thorough history is essential for determining the correct diagnosis in a patient with elbow or forearm pain. Onset of symptoms, mechanism of injury, exact location of pain, and associated symptoms such as numbness, weakness, or distal wrist and hand complaints are important elements to obtain. Most acute traumatic injuries to the elbow and forearm occur due to a fall onto an outstretched hand or a direct blow. Chronic overuse injuries should correlate with preceding activity involving a repetitive motion. A history of arthritides may point to a systemic disorder such as lupus, rheumatoid arthritis, or gout.

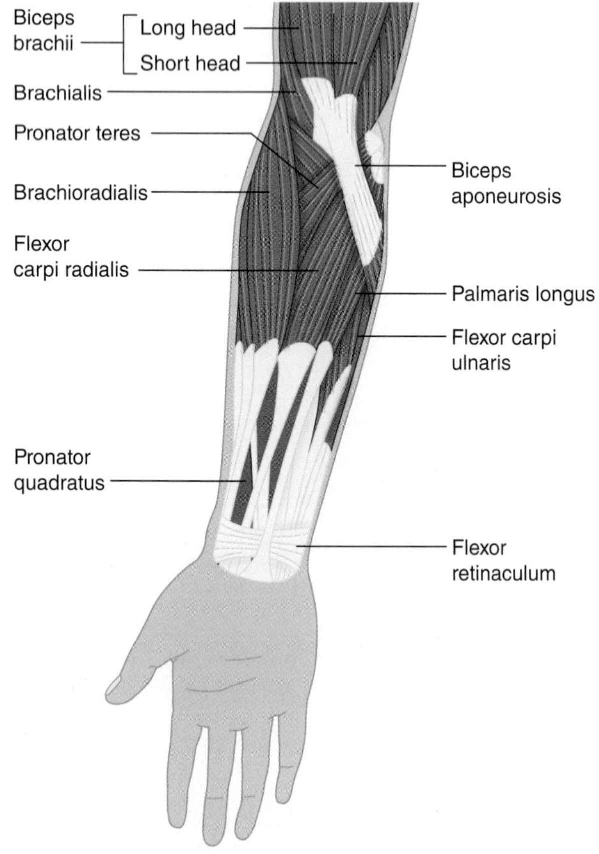

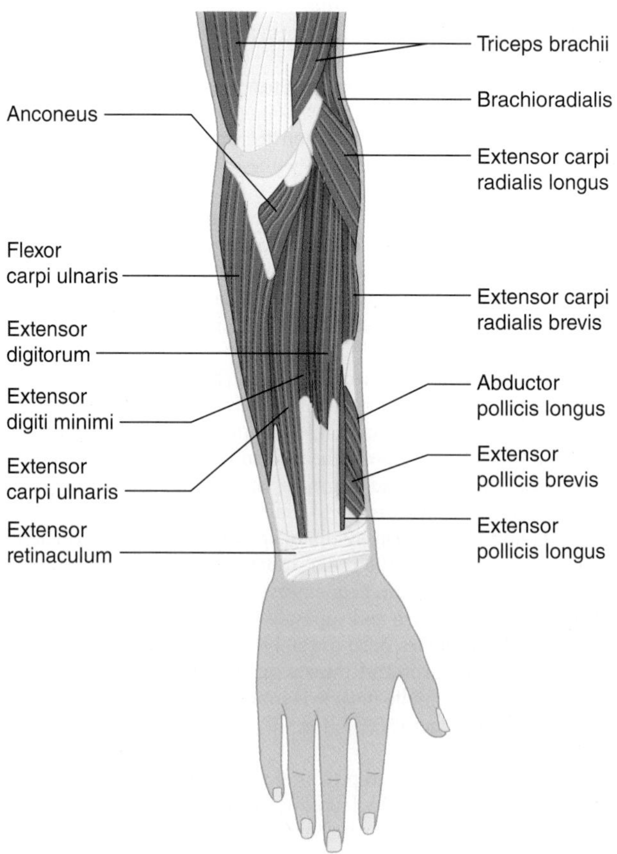

FIGURE 270-5. Intrinsic forearm muscles.

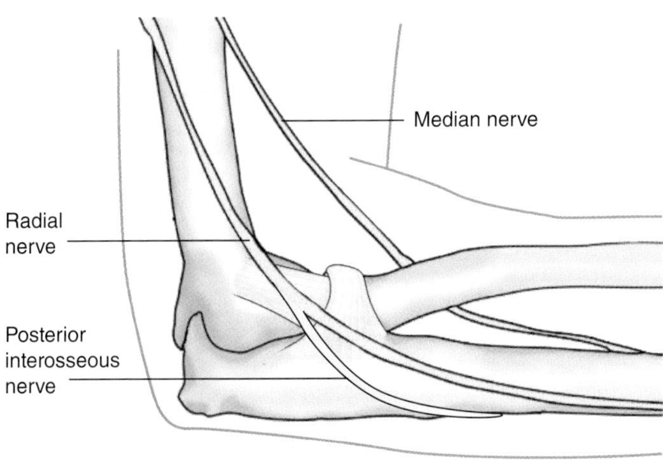

FIGURE 270-6. Posterior interosseous nerve.

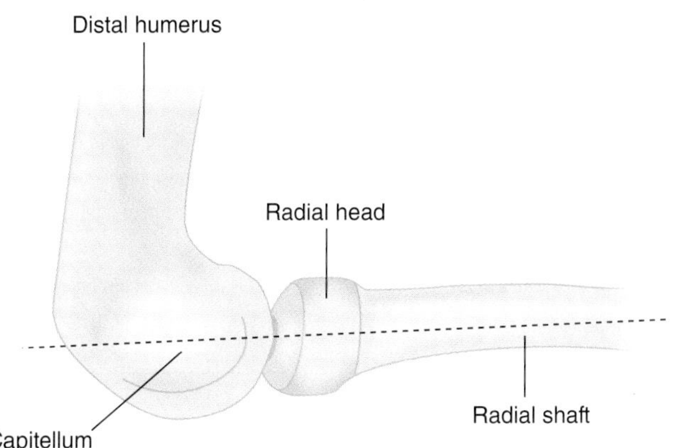

FIGURE 270-7. The radiocapitellar line. On lateral views, a line drawn through the center of the radius transects the radial head and middle third of the capitellum. This relationship is lost even in subtle fractures.

PHYSICAL EXAMINATION

General examination of the elbow and forearm should include inspection for gross deformity, soft tissue swelling such as bursitis, or open wounds. Assess range of motion of the elbow in flexion, extension, pronation, and supination. Inability to fully extend the elbow is correlated with the presence of a fracture.[1] Strength testing against resistance should also include wrist flexion and extension. Carefully assess radial, median, and ulnar nerve function. **The single best test of radial nerve motor function is to have the patient extend both the wrist and fingers against resistance** (Table 270-1). Test sensation with two-point discrimination over the dorsum of the thumb index web space. Evaluate the median nerve by assessing its distal branches. **A simple test of anterior interosseous nerve function is the ability to make a circle, or "OK" sign, with the thumb and index finger.** Abduction of the thumb against resistance (recurrent branch of the median nerve) and sensory testing over the tip of the index finger complete the evaluation of the median nerve**. The easiest way to test ulnar nerve function is to have the patient spread the fingers apart against resistance.** Sensation is tested over the tip of the fifth digit.

DIAGNOSIS

IMAGING

Initial imaging studies should include anteroposterior and lateral views of the elbow, and anteroposterior, lateral, and oblique views of the humerus and forearm. If a distal forearm injury is present, anteroposterior, lateral, and oblique views of the wrist instead of the humerus should be obtained. Attempts to derive a clinical decision rule to guide imaging decisions for the elbow, similar to published ankle and knee imaging rules, have so far produced conflicting data.[1-3]

On lateral films of the elbow, a line drawn straight through the center of the radial shaft should bisect the radial head and capitellum (radiocapitellar line) (**Figure 270-7**). Loss of this relationship should raise suspicion for an occult radius fracture or dislocation. A line drawn straight along the anterior border of the humerus should transect the posterior two thirds of the capitellum (anterior humeral line) (**Figure 270-8**). Abnormal extension of the line through the anterior one third of the capitellum suggests a distal humerus (in adults) or supracondylar fracture (in children). A small anterior fat pad may be a normal finding. Large anterior and any posterior fat pads are always abnormal and indicate the presence of a joint effusion (**Figure 270-9**).

CT imaging provides greater radiographic detail when evaluating certain elbow fractures, particularly coronoid and comminuted intra-articular fractures. MRI is useful in the evaluation of soft tissue injuries such as ligament or tendon ruptures but has limited value in the acute setting. Bedside US can demonstrate effusions and tendon injury but requires operator skill.[4,5]

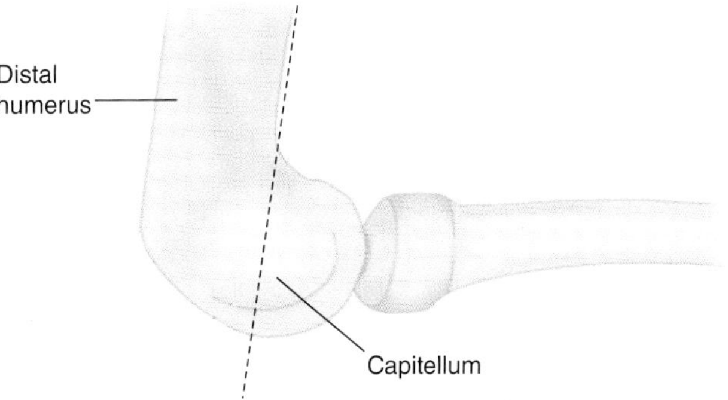

FIGURE 270-8. The anterior humeral line. On lateral views, a line drawn along the anterior cortex of the humerus transects the posterior two thirds of the capitellum. Transection of the line through the anterior one third of the capitellum suggests a fracture.

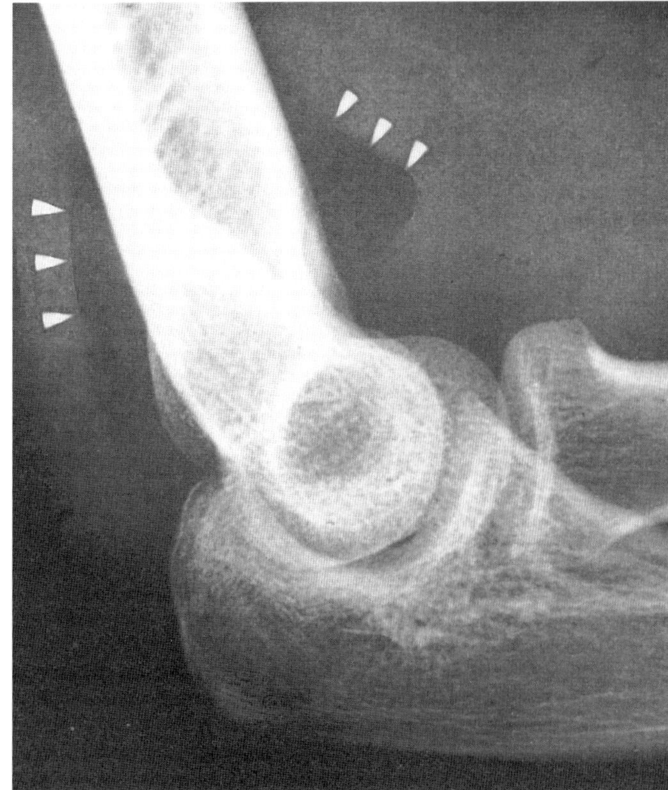

FIGURE 270-9. Anterior and posterior fat pad signs.

TABLE 270-2 Immobilization and Follow-Up Guidelines

Injury	Splint	Referral
Soft tissue injuries		
Biceps tendon rupture	Sling immobilization	1 wk
Triceps tendon rupture	Sling immobilization	1 wk
Lateral/medial epicondylitis	Forearm counterforce brace	2–4 wk PRN
Elbow dislocation		
Stable/postreduction	Long arm posterior splint, forearm in pronation	1 d
Unstable/postreduction	Long arm posterior splint (presurgical stabilization)	Immediate
Irreducible	Long arm posterior splint (presurgical stabilization)	Immediate
Elbow fractures		
Distal humerus nondisplaced	Long arm posterior splint, forearm neutral	1 wk
Supracondylar	Long arm posterior splint (presurgical stabilization)	Immediate
Intercondylar	Long arm posterior splint, forearm neutral	1–2 d
Lateral condyle/epicondyle		
Nondisplaced	Long arm posterior splint, forearm in supination, wrist extended	1–2 d
Displaced	Long arm posterior splint (presurgical stabilization)	Immediate
Medial condyle/epicondyle		
Nondisplaced	Long arm posterior splint, forearm in pronation, wrist flexed	1-2 d
Displaced	Long arm posterior splint (presurgical stabilization)	Immediate
Articular surface	Long arm posterior splint, forearm neutral	1–2 d
Coronoid		
Nondisplaced or minimally displaced	Long arm posterior splint, elbow past 90 degrees, forearm in supination	1–2 d
Markedly displaced or unstable	Long arm posterior splint (presurgical stabilization)	Immediate
Olecranon	Long arm posterior splint, forearm neutral	<24 h
Radial head		
Nondisplaced	Sling immobilization with early range of motion	1 wk
Displaced or range of motion block	Long arm posterior splint, forearm neutral	<24 h
Forearm fractures		
Both bones		
Pediatric		
Greenstick	Long arm posterior splint	1 wk
Displaced	Long arm posterior splint (prereduction stabilization)	Immediate
Adult		
Nondisplaced	Anteroposterior long arm splint	1 wk
Displaced	Long arm posterior splint (presurgical stabilization)	<24 h
Isolated ulna shaft	Long arm posterior splint, forearm neutral *or* sugar tong splint if stable and nondisplaced	1 wk
Proximal two thirds of radius	Long arm posterior splint, forearm neutral	1 wk
Monteggia's	Long arm posterior splint (presurgical stabilization)	Immediate
Galeazzi's	Long arm posterior splint (presurgical stabilization)	Immediate

TREATMENT

Consult an orthopedic surgeon immediately for open fractures, irreducible dislocations, injuries resulting in a grossly unstable elbow joint, or vascular injury with signs of ischemia or uncontrolled hemorrhage. All other injuries may be referred for follow-up within 1 to 2 days for operative planning or up to a week for nonoperative treatment. **Table 270-2** outlines guidelines for ED immobilization and appropriate orthopedic consult time frames for the conditions discussed in this chapter.

SOFT TISSUE INJURIES

BICEPS TENDON RUPTURE

Of all injuries to the biceps, the vast majority are proximal, and nearly all involve the proximal long head. Injuries are usually the result of repetitive microtrauma and overuse. Steroids, whether injected locally or used systemically, can accelerate the breakdown of tendons. Biceps tendon rupture usually occurs when there is sudden or prolonged contraction against resistance in middle-aged and older individuals with a history of chronic bicipital tenosynovitis. A snap or pop is usually described, and pain is present in the anterior shoulder. Examination of the anterior shoulder will reveal swelling, tenderness, and often crepitus over the bicipital groove. Ecchymosis may extend the entire length of the biceps. **Flexion of the elbow will elicit pain and may produce a midarm "ball," which represents the distally retracted biceps muscle.** Comparing arms for symmetry helps. Loss of strength is minimal due to the function of the brachialis and supinator. Avulsion fractures occasionally occur, so radiographs of the shoulder should be obtained.

ED treatment includes sling, ice, analgesics, and referral to an orthopedic surgeon for definitive care. Surgical repair is usually recommended for young, active patients. A conservative approach with immobilization may be adequate for elderly patients whose activities of daily living are not significantly compromised by the injury.

Distal biceps injuries are less common than proximal injuries.[6,7] Complete ruptures of the tendon are most common in middle-aged men and usually involve the dominant extremity. Partial tears are seen in men and women. Mechanism of injury is typically a sudden eccentric (extension) load applied to a flexed elbow. In ruptures of the distal biceps, pain is felt in the antecubital fossa, with swelling, ecchymosis, and tenderness to palpation noted on examination. A distal rupture is indicated by a palpable defect in the antecubital fossa and a midarm "ball." Strength loss, especially supination, is usually greater than with proximal ruptures. The **biceps squeeze test**, similar to the Thompson test for assessing Achilles tendon rupture, can detect biceps rupture.[8] With the patient seated and the forearm at 60 to 80 degrees of flexion, place one hand on the muscle belly of the biceps brachii and the other hand on the myotendinous junction, and squeeze with both hands. The squeeze should result in forearm supination, indicating an intact biceps. Lack of supination is considered a positive test, indicating rupture of the distal biceps brachii. To perform the **hook test**,[9] flex the patient's elbow to 90 degrees, and during active supination, if the biceps tendon is intact, the examiner can "hook" the index finger under the distal biceps tendon in the antecubital fossa. Obtain elbow radiographs to search for an associated avulsion fracture. Although most complete distal ruptures are diagnosed clinically, MRI and US can aid in confirming the diagnosis of partial tears.[10,11]

ED treatment includes sling, ice, analgesics, and referral to an orthopedic surgeon for definitive care. Without surgical repair of complete ruptures, supination strength is decreased by approximately 50% and flexion strength by almost 30%.[12,13]

TRICEPS TENDON RUPTURE

Injury to the triceps is rare and almost always occurs distally.[14] Ruptures result from either a fall on an outstretched hand causing a forceful flexion of an extended elbow or a direct blow to the olecranon. Spontaneous ruptures from systemic illnesses, particularly hyperparathyroidism and chronic renal failure requiring hemodialysis, have also been reported.[15,16] Triceps rupture usually causes pain in the posterior elbow. Examination of the elbow reveals swelling and tenderness posteriorly just proximal to the olecranon. A sulcus with a more proximal mass, representing the retracted triceps muscle, may be palpated. With partial tears, some degree of function remains; however, **with complete ruptures, the ability to extend the elbow is lost**. A modified Thompson test can be used to evaluate triceps function. The upper extremity is positioned such that the arm is supported and the forearm is hanging in a relaxed position with 90 degrees of flexion. Squeezing the triceps muscle should produce extension of the forearm unless a complete rupture is present. Radiographs of the elbow are needed because avulsion fractures of the olecranon are common. US and MRI may aid in diagnosis, especially of partial tears.

ED treatment includes sling, ice, analgesics, and referral to an orthopedic surgeon for definitive care. Complete ruptures require surgical repair, whereas most partial tears can be treated conservatively with immobilization.

LATERAL EPICONDYLITIS

The lateral epicondyle serves as the origin for wrist and digit extensors and forearm supinators. Lateral epicondylitis, or "tennis elbow," is an overuse syndrome affecting these soft tissues. Although the condition is often seen in tennis players, it can arise as a result of any repetitive movement involving these muscle groups. The diagnosis is made clinically by tenderness over the lateral epicondyle and pain with resisted wrist and digit extension and forearm supination. Treatment is usually conservative, with rest, ice, anti-inflammatory medications, and immobilization, often via a counterforce brace. Physical therapy consisting of forearm stretching and strengthening exercises has been proven to be a useful adjunct in addition to the above.[17,18] Corticosteroid injections can provide short-term relief of symptoms but have been shown to result in higher recurrence rates at 1 year compared to conservative measures.[17,18] Surgery may be indicated for refractory cases.

MEDIAL EPICONDYLITIS

The less common counterpart to lateral epicondylitis is medial epicondylitis ("golfer's elbow"). As with lateral epicondylitis, the diagnosis is made clinically, with tenderness over the medial epicondyle and pain with resisted wrist and digit flexion and forearm pronation, as these are the muscle groups affected. In addition, patients may develop an ulnar neuropathy, given the proximity of the ulnar nerve to the medial epicondyle. Treatment is similar to that of lateral epicondylitis, with rest, ice, anti-inflammatory medications, bracing, and physical therapy.

ELBOW DISLOCATION

The elbow is one of the more stable joints. The muscular attachments, lateral collateral ligament, and medial ulnar collateral ligament augment its inherent stability in the flexion-extension plane. Despite this, dislocations of the elbow are commonly seen and rank third in large-joint dislocations, after glenohumeral and patellofemoral dislocations. Possible fractures of the coronoid process, radial head, medial epicondyle, and olecranon complicate the treatment of elbow dislocations. **The "terrible triad" injury describes an unstable joint consisting of an elbow dislocation coupled with fractures of the radial head and coronoid.** This injury creates an unstable joint and requires surgical repair after initial reduction.

Elbow dislocations include five types: posterior, anterior, medial, lateral, and divergent (**Figure 270-10**). Some dislocations may involve a combination of the above based on the direction of force applied during the injury. **Approximately 90% of all elbow dislocations are posterolateral.**[19] The mechanism of injury is usually due to a fall on an outstretched hand.

Clinically, the patient presents with the elbow in 45 degrees of flexion. The olecranon is prominent posteriorly, and the deformity resembles a displaced supracondylar fracture. If the patient is seen immediately after the injury, the bony landmarks can be identified. Later, however, the swelling may be quite severe, with no possibility of evaluating the injury topographically. **The first priority of care is to assess the neurovascular status of structures most vulnerable to entrapment, namely the brachial artery and the ulnar, radial, and median nerves.** Perform neurovascular examination before and after manipulation, because neurovascular complications (most frequently the ulnar nerve) occur in 8% to 21% of patients. Vascular complications (most frequently the brachial artery) occur in 5% to 13% of elbow dislocations.[20] Absence of a radial pulse before reduction, an open dislocation, and systemic injuries (such as those of the head, chest, and abdomen) are associated with arterial injury.[21,22] If vascular injury is suspected, then angiography may be required to assess the extent of injury and need for repair.

On the lateral radiograph, both the ulna and radius are displaced posteriorly (**Figure 270-11**). In the anteroposterior view, there may be lateral or medial displacement, with the ulna and radius in their normal relationship to each other. Assess for associated fractures, particularly of the coronoid process and radial head. In a child, an associated fracture of the medial epicondyle is common.

Due to the amount of force that is necessary to reduce a dislocated elbow, success is often dependent on adequate analgesia and muscular relaxation. This may require the use of intravenous analgesics or procedural sedation, particularly in children. As an alternative to procedural sedation or intravenous analgesia, anecdotal success has been reported using intra-articular lidocaine to provide regional anesthesia for closed reduction of dislocated elbows, similar to the well-described use of intra-articular blocks for reduction of anterior glenohumeral shoulder dislocations.[23,24] In the elbow, intra-articular lidocaine is effective for postoperative pain control following arthroscopic procedures in adults and supracondylar fracture repairs in children.[25,26] Regardless of the type of analgesia used, ensure appropriate patient comfort prior to attempting closed reduction.

Closed reduction can be accomplished by several methods. In the first two-person reduction technique, position the patient supine and apply gentle longitudinal traction on the wrist and forearm with one hand while an assistant applies a stabilizing countertraction force on the upper

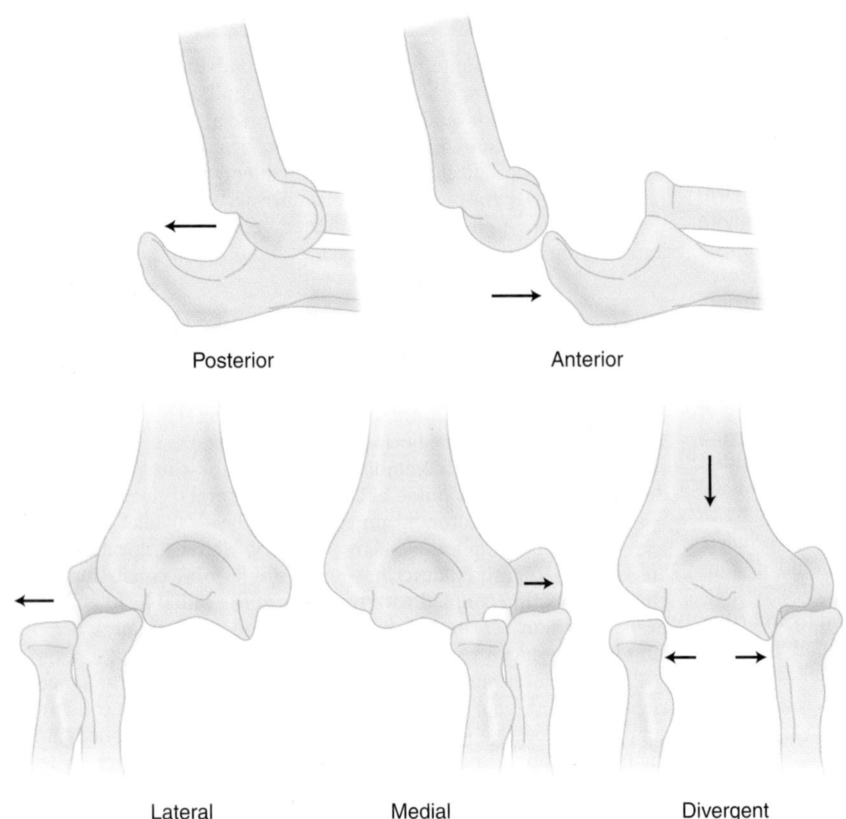

FIGURE 270-10. Elbow dislocations. [Reproduced with permission from Browner BD, Levine AM, Jupiter JB, et al: *Skeletal Trauma: Basic Science, Management, and Reconstruction*, 4th ed. Vol 1. © 2009, Saunders, an imprint of Elsevier Inc., Philadelphia, PA. Figure 42-40, p. 1533.]

arm (**Figure 270-12**). First, correct any medial or lateral displacement with the other hand. Then apply downward pressure to the proximal forearm with the other hand to help disengage the coronoid process from the olecranon fossa. Continue distal traction, and flex the elbow. In the second two-person technique, position the patient prone with the arm abducted and the elbow slightly flexed. The patient may also be positioned supine with the affected arm adducted across the torso and the elbow slightly flexed (**Figure 270-13**). Have an assistant apply longitudinal traction on the wrist and forearm. Then, grasp the elbow, positioning both thumbs on the olecranon, and apply firm pressure against the olecranon to push it up and over the trochlea and back into anatomic position. Apply countertraction with the fingers against the distal humerus. The last technique is a modification of the Stimson hanging technique used in shoulder reductions (**Figure 270-14**). One benefit of this technique is that it can be performed by a single provider. Place the patient prone with the elbow flexed over the edge of the stretcher. Support the humerus proximal to the elbow with a folded blanket or pillow. Suspend 5-lb weights from the wrist. The patient's elbow should reduce over a period of several minutes. Gentle manipulation may be applied to the olecranon to aid reduction.

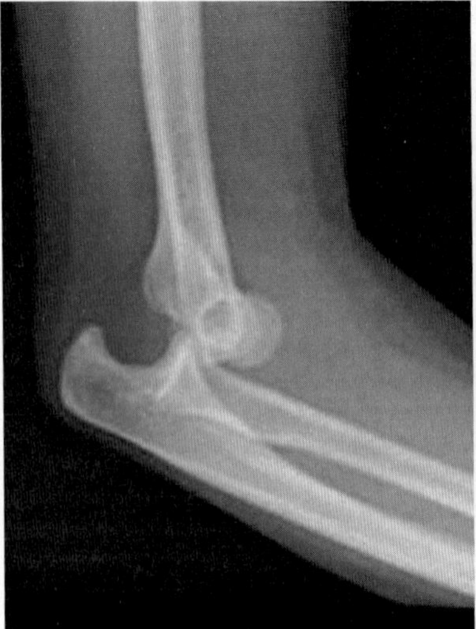

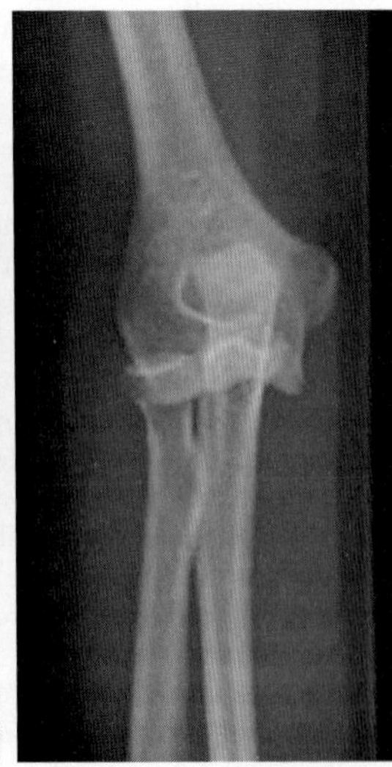

FIGURE 270-11. Posterior elbow dislocation.

With reduction, a palpable "clunk" is felt as the olecranon is seated in the humeral articular surface (trochlea). Then move the elbow through its full range of motion to assess stability. Inability to maintain reduction through full range of motion necessitates orthopedic consultation for surgical repair. If full and smooth passive range of motion is not possible, examine the postreduction radiograph for entrapment of the medial epicondyle, especially common in children, or other intra-articular fragments. If the elbow remains reduced through full range-of-motion testing, assess medial and lateral stability with gentle valgus and varus stress on the elbow in full extension. Valgus (medial) laxity is more common and suggests disruption of the medial (ulnar) collateral ligament complex, which is the primary stabilizing structure of the elbow joint against valgus forces. Medial instability that stabilizes with 90 degrees of flexion and maximal pronation of the forearm should be splinted in this position and referred for follow-up.[27] Instability that cannot be stabilized with flexion and pronation suggests associated fractures or more significant disruption of the capsule and ligaments. In this case orthopedic consultation for surgical repair is necessary.

After reduction, immobilize stable dislocations in a long arm posterior splint with the elbow in slightly less than 90 degrees of flexion and the forearm in mild pronation. Obtain a neurovascular follow-up examination the following day. Treatment with an early range-of-motion program after 1 week of splinting generally leads to favorable results.

Appropriate treatment of elbow dislocations requires adequate reduction and recognition of neurovascular complications, associated fractures, and postreduction instability. If there is any question of neurovascular

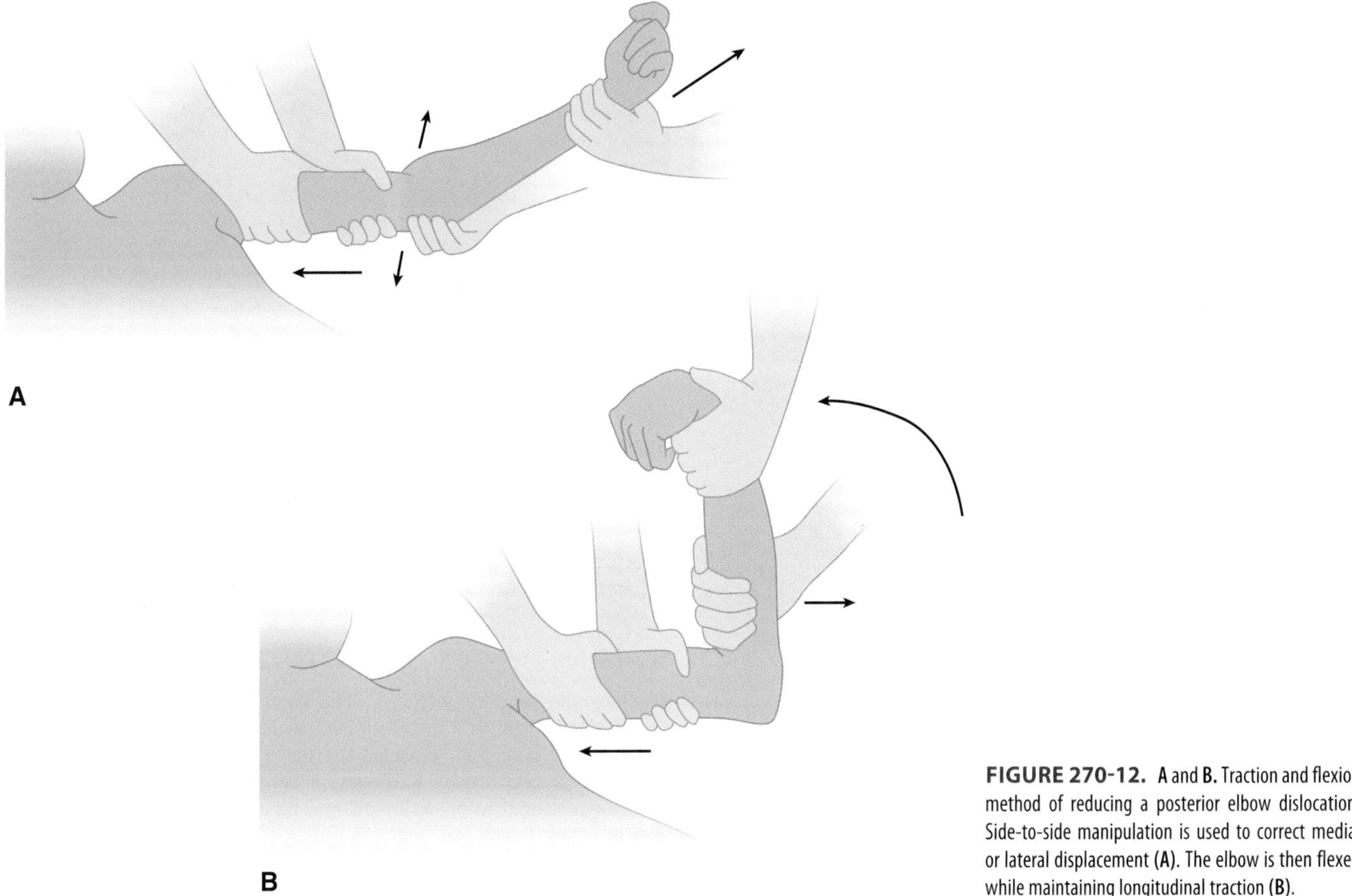

FIGURE 270-12. **A** and **B.** Traction and flexion method of reducing a posterior elbow dislocation. Side-to-side manipulation is used to correct medial or lateral displacement **(A)**. The elbow is then flexed while maintaining longitudinal traction **(B)**.

compromise, then consider admitting the patient for observation. Obtain emergency orthopedic consultation for irreducible dislocations, neurovascular compromise, postreduction instability, associated fractures, and open dislocations. Potential late complications include posttraumatic stiffness, posterolateral joint instability, ectopic ossification, and occult distal radioulnar joint disruption.

FRACTURES ABOUT THE ELBOW

Elbow fractures can be divided into those of the distal humerus, proximal ulna, and proximal radius. The distal humerus includes the condylar structures and the articular surface (trochlea and capitellum). The proximal ulna includes the coronoid process and olecranon, and the proximal radius is essentially the radial head.

Radiographs of fractures about the elbow may reveal abnormal fat pads (Figure 270-9).[28] Normally, a posterior fat pad is not visible, and an anterior fat pad may be visible as a thin lucent stripe. **With injury, fat from the olecranon fossa is displaced posteriorly (posterior fat pad), and the anterior fat pad may become quite prominent ("sail sign") due to hemarthrosis.** Abnormal fat pads may also be seen with nontraumatic joint effusions. Furthermore, they may be absent in severe trauma that disrupts the joint capsule and allows intra-articular fluid extravasation. In some nondisplaced fractures, the fracture line may not be seen, with the fat pad sign being the only evidence of injury. Treatment is initiated as though a fracture were identified, with splint immobilization and orthopedic consultation.

DISTAL HUMERUS FRACTURES

Routine ED care of nondisplaced distal humerus fractures with normal neurovascular function includes immobilization, ice, elevation, analgesics, and orthopedic referral. Displaced fractures or those with neurovascular compromise require immediate orthopedic consultation. See chapter 271, "Shoulder and Humerus Injuries," for a detailed discussion of shoulder and humerus injuries.

SUPRACONDYLAR FRACTURES

Supracondylar fractures are the most common fracture about the elbow in children between 5 and 10 years of age, but can occur in adults, especially as a result of high-velocity injuries. Fractures can be either extension type (>95%), which are displaced posteriorly, or flexion type (<5%), which are displaced anteriorly. Treatment largely depends on the degree of displacement of the distal fragment.

EXTENSION-TYPE SUPRACONDYLAR FRACTURES

Injuries most often occur with a fall on an outstretched hand with the elbow in full extension. The patient will have significant edema and tenderness at the elbow, a prominent olecranon, and a depression proximal to the elbow. The appearance may be easily mistaken for a posterior elbow dislocation. Nondisplaced fractures may be subtle and diagnosed only by the presence of a posterior fat pad, anterior "sail sign," or disruption to the normal path of the anterior humeral line. Initially treat with immobilization using a long arm posterior splint, keeping the elbow at 90 degrees of flexion and the forearm in neutral rotation, followed by outpatient referral for casting. The presence of >20 degrees of angulation necessitates orthopedic consultation for reduction under anesthesia and possible pin fixation.[29] In displaced fractures, the anteroposterior radiograph usually reveals a transverse fracture line. More severely displaced fractures may show medial or lateral displacement or rotation along the axis of the humerus (**Figure 270-15**). The lateral radiograph will reveal the fracture line extending obliquely from posterior proximal to anterior

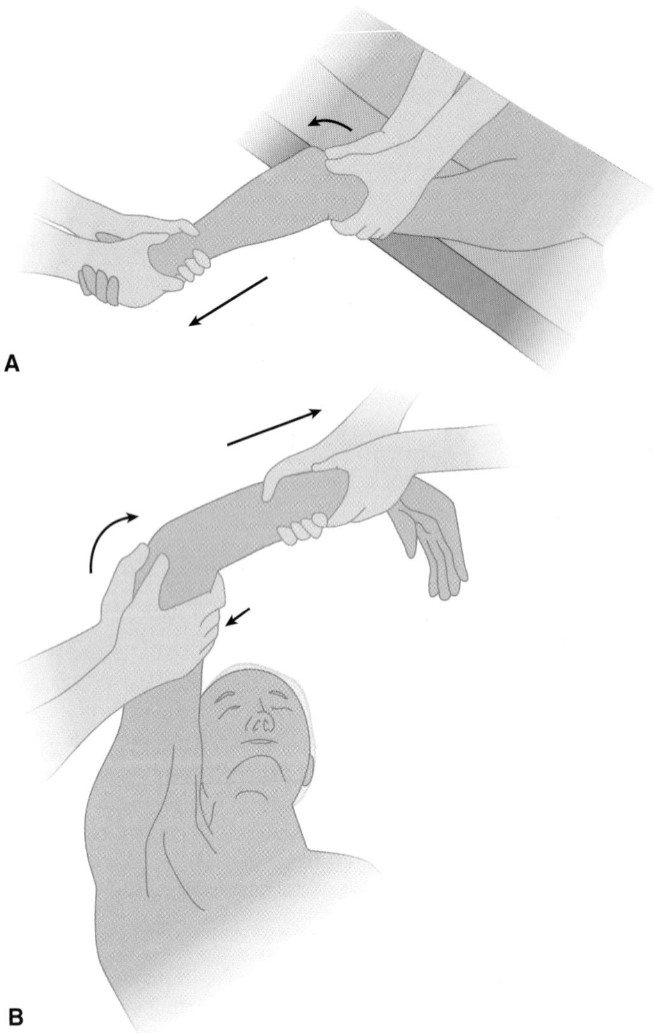

FIGURE 270-13. A and B. Olecranon manipulation method of reducing a posterior elbow dislocation with the patient positioned prone (A) or supine (B).

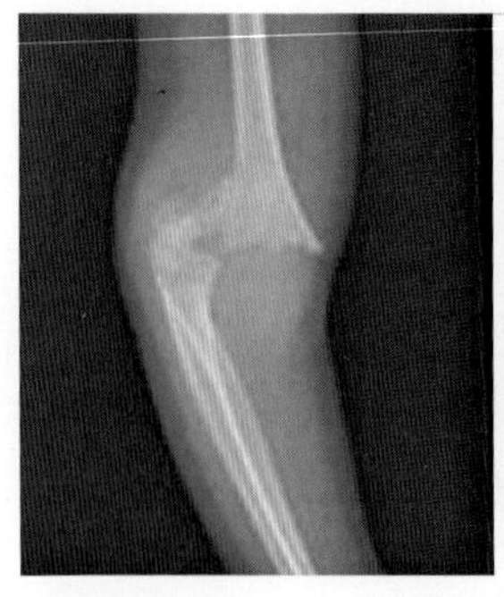

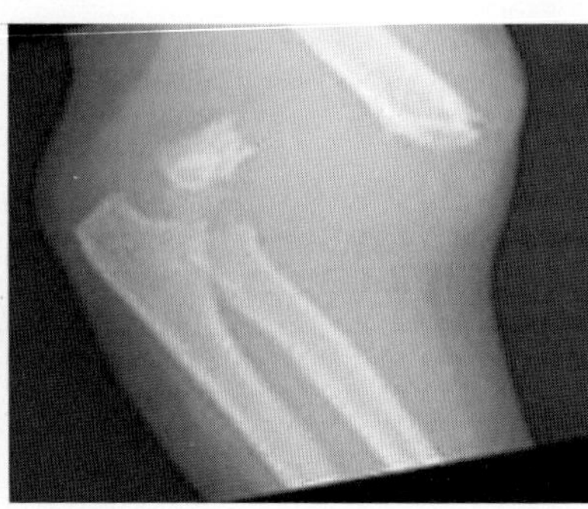

FIGURE 270-15. Extension-type, displaced supracondylar fracture.

distal. The distal fragment will be displaced proximally and posteriorly. **Displaced fractures must be reduced and require orthopedic consultation.** Indications for open reduction are vascular insufficiency with a probable entrapped brachial artery in the fracture site or an irreducible fracture. Admit patients with displaced fractures or significant soft tissue swelling for observation of neurovascular function.

FLEXION-TYPE SUPRACONDYLAR FRACTURES

Flexion-type fractures are rare. The mechanism of injury is a direct anterior force against a flexed elbow, resulting in anterior displacement of the distal fragment. Because the mechanism is direct force, these fractures are often open. Radiographs reveal an oblique fracture from anterior proximal to posterior distal. The distal fragment is anterior to the humerus. Displaced fractures must be reduced and require immediate orthopedic consultation. Indications for open reduction are vascular insufficiency with a probable entrapped brachial artery in the fracture site or an irreducible fracture. Admit patients with displaced fractures or significant soft tissue swelling for observation of neurovascular function.

COMPLICATIONS OF SUPRACONDYLAR FRACTURES

There are numerous potential complications of supracondylar fractures (**Table 270-3**). Neurologic complications—resulting from traction,

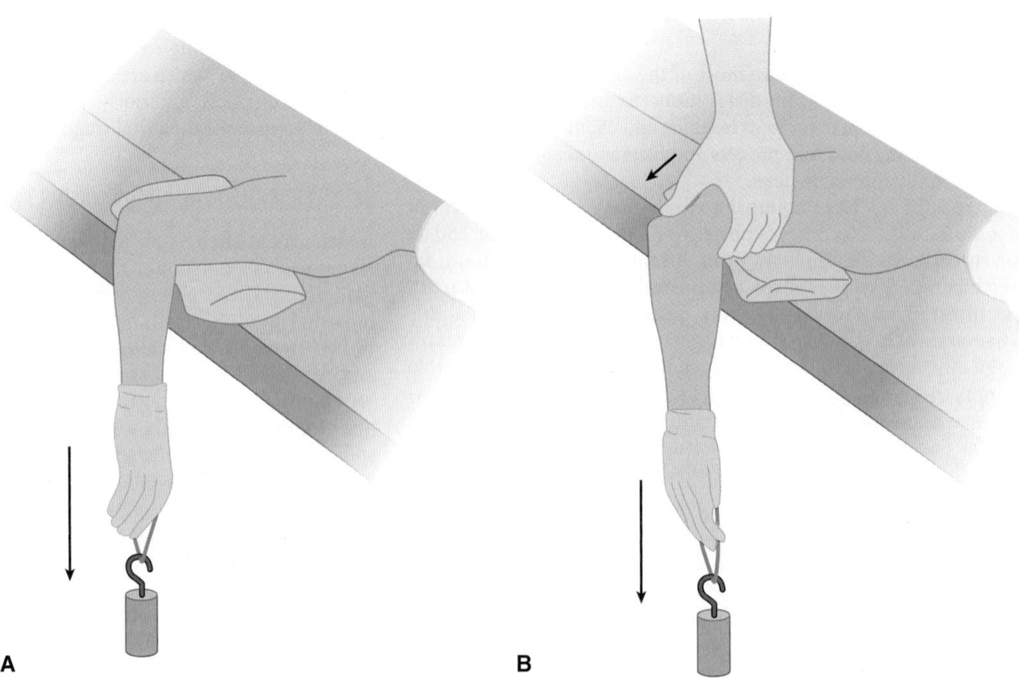

FIGURE 270-14. A. Hanging arm method of reducing a posterior elbow dislocation. B. Gentle manipulation can be applied to the olecranon if necessary.

TABLE 270-3 Complications of Supracondylar Fractures

Early complications	**Neurologic** Radial nerve Median nerve (anterior interosseous branch) Ulnar **Vascular** Volkmann's ischemic contracture (compartment syndrome of the forearm)
Late complications	Nonunion Malunion Myositis ossificans Loss of motion

direct trauma, or nerve ischemia—have an incidence of 7%. **Posteromedial displacement may involve the radial nerve, and posterolateral displacement usually affects the median nerve.** Ulnar nerve injuries are uncommon, with the highest incidence reported from pin placement. However, **a high incidence has been noted of anterior interosseous nerve injuries with supracondylar fractures**. This nerve arises from the median nerve. The mechanism of injury is usually traction or contusion. Complete transection is rare, and entrapment within the fracture occurs only occasionally. **Because there is no sensory component to the anterior interosseous nerve, identification of the injury can be made only by motor testing, which consists of flexion at the index finger distal interphalangeal and thumb interphalangeal joints (making the "OK" sign).** Patients usually regain full flexion and strength after 4 to 17 weeks.[30]

Acute vascular injuries must always be suspected in patients with supracondylar fractures. Absence of a radial pulse is common in children and, in the majority of published cases, is an indicator of brachial artery injury, even if the hand appears warm, pink, and well perfused.[31] Injury can be due to a partial or complete transection, an intimal tear and thrombosis, or entrapment within the fracture fragment of the brachial artery. Treatment of supracondylar fractures with absent radial pulse begins with closed reduction and percutaneous pinning. Extremities still without a pulse despite adequate reduction warrant more aggressive vascular exploration and repair.

The most serious complication is a compartment syndrome of the forearm, also known as *Volkmann's ischemic contracture*. This classically occurs following a supracondylar fracture. Postischemic swelling, producing increased pressure within the enclosed osteofascial forearm compartment, reduces capillary blood perfusion below the level necessary for tissue viability. If unrelieved, the end result is muscle and nerve necrosis and eventual replacement by fibrotic tissue, producing a contracture. Refusal to open the hand in children, pain with passive extension of the fingers, and forearm tenderness are signs of impending Volkmann's ischemia. **It is now well understood that the mere lack of a radial pulse does not indicate ischemia unless accompanied by these signs.** Extremities with signs of ischemia are taken emergently to the operating room for fasciotomy and brachial artery exploration.

INTERCONDYLAR FRACTURES

Intercondylar fractures, in which the condylar fragments are separated, are much more common in adults than in children. Assume any distal humerus fracture in an adult to be intercondylar rather than supracondylar. The mechanism of injury is a force directed against the posterior elbow, driving the olecranon against the humeral articular surface, separating the condyles and producing the typical fracture. Carefully search for a fracture line separating the condyles from each other and from the humerus. By definition, all intercondylar fractures involve the articular surface. CT imaging is useful for identifying comminuted fractures and for planning operative therapy for displaced fractures. Treatment is dependent on the amount of displacement of the fracture fragments.

Nondisplaced intercondylar fractures are stable and can be treated initially with immobilization in a long arm posterior splint with the elbow flexed at 90 degrees and the forearm in neutral position. Treatment of displaced, rotated, or comminuted fractures is often directed at reestablishing articular surface congruity. If this cannot be achieved by closed methods, then the integrity of the articular surface is restored by an open reduction and fixation. In older patients with severely comminuted injuries, elbow replacement may be considered.[32] As in supracondylar fractures, admit patients with severe edema or displaced fractures.

EPICONDYLE FRACTURES

Lateral epicondyle fractures almost never occur, because the anatomic position of the condyle reduces its exposure to direct blows, resulting instead in fractures of the lateral condyle. When they do occur, lateral epicondyle fractures are usually avulsion fractures and may be treated by long arm posterior mold, with the elbow flexed to 90 degrees and the forearm in supination, and orthopedic referral.

Isolated medial epicondyle fractures are considered extra-articular injuries and usually occur in children and adolescents. Mechanisms include a posterior elbow dislocation, repeated valgus stress, such as throwing a baseball (Little League elbow), or a direct blow. If there is an associated tear of the medial (ulnar) collateral ligament, the epicondyle itself may become entrapped in the joint space. Patients present with pain over the medial elbow that is exacerbated by supination of the forearm and flexion of the forearm, wrist, and digits. Edema and tenderness are noted in the same area. Standard radiographs are obtained with special attention to any intra-articular fragment. Carefully test ulnar nerve function. Nondisplaced or minimally displaced medial epicondyle fractures can be treated nonoperatively, with early range of motion. There is an increasing trend toward operative treatment for these fractures due to significantly increased odds of bony union with fixation.[33] Open fractures, unstable joints, fragment displacement >5 mm, and an intra-articular fragment are well-described indications for surgical treatment with internal fixation. ED treatment consists of long arm posterior splint immobilization, with the forearm in flexion and pronation, and orthopedic referral.

Complications of lateral and medial epicondyle fractures are frequent and include nonunion, cubitus valgus or varus deformity, ulnar nerve palsy, and avascular necrosis.[34] Careful neurovascular assessment is required for these injuries. Because surgical treatment is generally preferred, orthopedic consultation is recommended for both lateral and medial epicondyle fractures.

CONDYLE FRACTURES

Lateral condyle fractures occur in children and are more common than their medial counterpart.[35] Lateral condyle fractures result from a direct blow to the lateral elbow or from varus stress with the forearm extended, as in a fall on an outstretched hand. Patients complain of pain in the lateral elbow, and swelling is noted in the same area.

Medial condyle fractures are uncommon and are mostly limited to children. Mechanism of injury is from either a transmitted force from the ulna, such as a fall on an outstretched hand, or excessive valgus stress. Pain and swelling medially are prominent findings. The injury is often confused with the more common medial epicondyle fracture for two reasons. First, the mechanism and examination findings are similar. Second, because the trochlea ossification center does not appear until age 9 to 10 years old, it is often missed on radiographs.

ED care of nondisplaced lateral and medial condyle fractures with normal neurovascular function includes long arm posterior splint immobilization, ice, elevation, analgesics, and orthopedic referral. Follow-up imaging every 2 weeks is recommended due to the risk of late displacement, which is treated with surgical fixation. Displaced fractures or those with neurovascular compromise require immediate orthopedic consultation. Complications include malunion with resultant cubital valgus or varus deformity, delayed ulnar nerve injury, and arthritis.

ARTICULAR SURFACE FRACTURES

TROCHLEA FRACTURES

Isolated trochlea fractures are rare, and they are more often associated with other elbow injuries, such as posterior elbow dislocations. Physical findings usually include swelling, tenderness, and limited movement of the elbow joint. Radiographic findings can be subtle, and CT or MRI may be required for diagnosis. ED treatment includes long arm posterior splint immobilization and orthopedic consultation because this is an articular surface injury and surgical repair is usually indicated. Complications are common and include limited flexion and extension, elbow joint instability, avascular necrosis, nonunion, and arthritis.

CAPITELLUM FRACTURES

Isolated capitellum fractures are rare. They are usually associated with radial head fractures. Pain and tenderness are present over the lateral elbow, and examination reveals swelling, lateral tenderness, and limitation of flexion and extension. If pain and tenderness are present medially, then suspect injury to the medial collateral ligament. Radiographic findings may be subtle and are best seen on a lateral view. The capitellum has no tendinous or ligamentous attachments, so many fractures are nondisplaced. A radial head–capitellum view can be helpful in addition to standard anteroposterior and lateral views. CT imaging is useful for diagnosis. ED treatment is similar to that of trochlea fractures. Definitive care is surgical, and complications are similar to those of trochlea fractures.

PROXIMAL ULNA FRACTURES

The distal humerus articulates with the proximal ulna to form a uniaxial hinge joint, which allows flexion and extension of the forearm and provides some intrinsic stability. The trochlea of the humerus rests in the greater sigmoid (semilunar) notch of the ulna. The anterior projection of the notch is the coronoid, and the posterior prominence, which is easily palpable, is the olecranon. The brachialis muscle inserts at the coronoid, and the triceps muscle inserts at the olecranon. Nearly all proximal ulna fractures are considered intra-articular, with the exception of a proximal olecranon chip fracture.

CORONOID FRACTURES

Coronoid fractures are usually associated with posterior elbow dislocations as the trochlea is driven into the coronoid. A coronoid fracture can rarely occur as an isolated injury secondary to elbow hyperextension.[36] There is pain, swelling, and tenderness over the antecubital fossa. Radiographic visualization is best with lateral and oblique films. Often CT is needed to make the diagnosis.

ED treatment should include long arm posterior splint immobilization with the elbow in flexion and the forearm in supination, ice, elevation, analgesics, and referral to an orthopedic surgeon within 24 hours. Conservative treatment of nondisplaced coronoid fractures remains controversial, and early orthopedic referral is indicated. Displaced fractures or those associated with joint instability require open reduction and internal fixation and frequently have poor outcomes.

OLECRANON FRACTURES

The olecranon is usually fractured by direct trauma or by a fall with forced hyperextension of the elbow. Olecranon fractures are quite common and represent up to 10% of upper extremity fractures.[37] Associated injuries are common, including open fractures, dislocations, other fractures (especially of the radial head), and ulnar nerve injury. Pain is present over the posterior elbow, and examination reveals swelling, tenderness, and occasionally crepitus. Because the triceps muscle inserts at the olecranon, triceps function is usually compromised. It is important to test forearm extension against resistance, as the patient may falsely appear to have intact forearm extension by using gravity to draw the forearm down. Ulnar nerve injury is common; therefore, a careful neurologic examination is required. Lateral radiographs offer the best view of the olecranon. In adolescents, the epiphysis ossifies by age 11 years old and fuses by age 16 years old, so comparison films and the appearance of an abnormal fat pad can aid in the diagnosis. ED treatment includes long arm posterior splint immobilization with the elbow in flexion and forearm neutral, ice, elevation, analgesics, and referral to an orthopedist within 24 hours. Stable, nondisplaced fractures with intact extensor function can be treated conservatively with immobilization. Nonoperative treatment may also be considered for poorly functioning elderly patients who would not tolerate surgery. All other olecranon fractures require surgical repair.[38]

RADIAL HEAD FRACTURES

The radial head is located just distal to the lateral epicondyle. Pronating and supinating the forearm with the elbow flexed allows the examiner to palpate the radial head. It articulates with the capitellum and the lesser sigmoid notch of the ulna to form a pivot joint. The radial head serves as a stabilizer of the elbow against valgus stress, along with the medial collateral ligament, and against longitudinal forces.

Radial head fractures are the most common fractures of the elbow. They result from a fall on an outstretched hand causing the radial head to be driven into the capitellum. **Associated injuries are common and may include capitellum, olecranon, and coronoid fractures, medial collateral ligament injury, medial epicondyle avulsion fracture secondary to valgus stress, and elbow dislocation.** A specific associated injury, the Essex-Lopresti lesion, occurs when there is disruption of the triangular fibrocartilage of the wrist and the interosseous membrane between the radius and ulna, causing pain in the wrist and forearm. The result is a distal radioulnar joint dissociation, which can cause migration of the radius proximally if radial head excision is performed. Open reduction and internal fixation of the proximal radius fracture is indicated for this injury.

Radial head fractures cause pain in the lateral elbow, especially with pronation and supination of the forearm. On examination, there may be swelling laterally and tenderness with palpation of the radial head. On standard elbow radiographs, radial head fractures may be subtle (**Figure 270-16**). Additional images, including obliques and a radial head–capitellum view, may be helpful. Furthermore, two radiographic clues can aid in the diagnosis. The first is abnormal displacement of the radiocapitellar line away from the center of the capitellum (Figure 270-7). This is especially helpful in children whose epiphysis has not fused. The other clue is the appearance of an abnormal fat pad (Figure 270-9).

Nondisplaced fractures with no mobility restrictions can be treated conservatively with immobilization. For these, ED treatment consists of sling immobilization with the elbow in flexion, ice, elevation, analgesics, and referral to an orthopedic surgeon within 1 week. Consider aspiration of the joint hematoma in the ED to improve pain and facilitate early mobilization.[39] Additional pain control may be obtained with intra-articular injection of lidocaine or bupivacaine following aspiration, but this does not offer any long-term benefit over aspiration alone.[40] For displaced fractures or those with restricted range of motion, surgical repair is generally indicated, and orthopedic referral within 24 hours is needed. Complications of radial head fracture include chronic pain and restricted range of motion at the elbow.

FOREARM FRACTURES

In adults, solitary fractures of the forearm are uncommon due to the close relationship of the radius and ulna. The fibrous interconnection between the radius and ulna transmits traumatic energy above and below the injury. So, fractures usually occur at two or more sites or involve a fracture of one bone with a ligamentous injury, with or without an associated joint dislocation. Because distant structures are commonly injured, examine joints above and below the involved bones both clinically and radiologically. Be especially observant for associated injuries if there is significant angulation of the fracture.

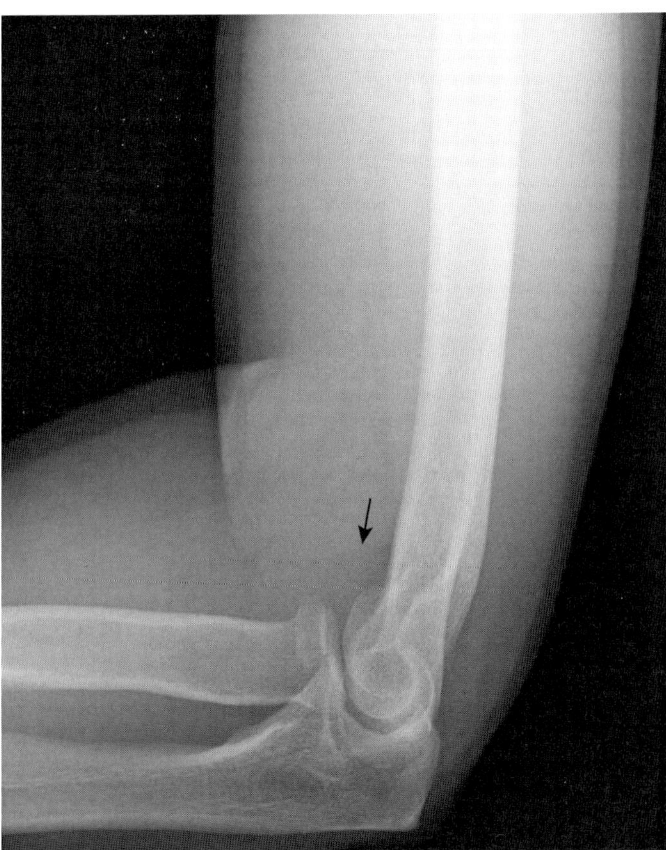

FIGURE 270-16. Subtle radial head fracture and anterior fat pad sign (*arrow*).

The radius and ulna are under the influence of numerous muscle groups, such as those that supinate and pronate (Figure 270-5). The biceps brachii and the supinator insert on the proximal radius and are the powerful supinators of the forearm. The pronator teres inserts on the radial shaft and exerts a pronating force. Radius fractures that are located between these muscle groups will result in marked displacement of the radius, with supination of the proximal segment and pronation of the distal portion. However, if the fracture is distal to the insertion of the pronator teres, these forces tend to neutralize one another and result in less rotational deformity. When considering treatment of these fractures, careful attention must be paid to the maintenance of length, alignment, and angulation. Also, the lateral bow of the radius must be preserved to allow full pronation and supination after healing.

FRACTURES OF BOTH RADIUS AND ULNA

A great amount of force is necessary to fracture both the radius and the ulna. This injury occurs most often from vehicular trauma, falls from a height, or a direct blow. Force magnitude determines injury type. Moderate forces produce transverse or mildly oblique fractures. High-impact forces produce comminuted and segmental fractures (often displaced).

Nondisplaced fractures of both bones are exceedingly rare because the force necessary to produce the injury is also sufficient to displace the bones. Examination of the forearm reveals swelling, deformity, and tenderness. Carefully assess the neurovascular status. Nerve injuries can be seen with severe open fractures but are uncommon with most closed injuries. Because of the excellent collateral circulation of the forearm, vascular compromise is generally not a major problem if either the radial or ulnar circulation is intact.

The fractures are clearly visible on the radiographs. Note the degree of angulation, displacement, and shortening. Changes in rotational alignment may be subtle. Noting the normal orientation of various bony prominences of these bones can make a rough estimate of rotational alignment. On the anteroposterior view, the radial styloid and radial (bicipital) tuberosity normally point in opposite directions, whereas the ulnar styloid and coronoid process do so on the lateral view. A change in this arrangement suggests rotation malalignment. Because these bones are also oblong rather than circular in their cross-sectional appearance, a sudden change in the bone's width at the fracture site is another clue to a rotational deformity. Obtain radiographs of the wrist and elbow because of the likelihood of an associated dislocation or articular fracture.

Treatment depends on the type of fracture. Torus or greenstick fractures with minimal angulation in children can be treated with immobilization in a long arm splint. Angulation >15 degrees warrants referral for closed reduction. In younger children, treat displaced fractures with closed reduction and cast immobilization due to the continued remodeling that occurs after fracture healing. Perform closed reduction urgently in the ED by an orthopedic consultant to ensure appropriate alignment. Surgical intervention is becoming increasingly popular, although there is a lack of evidence showing improved outcomes from surgery over conservative management.[41,42] Nondisplaced fractures in adults can be immobilized with a long arm splint and referred for urgent follow up. All other fractures in adults require operative reduction and internal or external fixation, ideally within 24 to 48 hours.

Complications include reduced ability to supinate and pronate, osteomyelitis, nonunion, malunion, neurovascular injury, and compartment syndrome. **Recognizing the development of a compartment syndrome is particularly important to prevent debilitating ischemic or Volkmann's contractures of the forearm.** The diagnostic findings are palpable induration of the area, pain with passive movement of the fingers, and pain disproportionate to the physical findings. Loss of radial pulse is often a late finding, and presence of a radial pulse does not exclude compartment syndrome. Direct measurements of elevated compartment pressures confirm the diagnosis. Urgent fasciotomy is required, ideally within 8 hours of the onset of symptoms.

ULNA FRACTURES

ISOLATED ULNA FRACTURE (NIGHTSTICK FRACTURE)

Isolated fractures of the ulna most often result from direct blows to the forearm. A fracture resulting from the natural response to raise the forearm in defense of a blow from a club is referred to as a *nightstick fracture*. Nondisplaced fractures are immobilized in a splint and closely followed for subsequent displacement. A short arm cast is preferable to a long arm cast for treatment.

Fractures with >50% displacement, with >10% angulation, or that involve the proximal third of the ulna are considered unstable.[43] Obtain orthopedic consultation for unstable fractures. Open reduction and internal fixation with a compression plate and screws are necessary to prevent angulation, loss of length, and rotational deformity. Assess injuries for any possible radius fracture or dislocation.

MONTEGGIA'S FRACTURE-DISLOCATION

Fracture of the proximal third of the ulna with a radial head dislocation is often referred to as *Monteggia's fracture-dislocation* (**Figure 270-17**). The associated radial head dislocation may be easily missed.[44] **Missing the radial head dislocation can lead to chronic pain, limited range of motion, and, possibly, radial head excision as treatment.** Monteggia's fractures can occur following a fall onto an outstretched hand or a direct blow. The most typical injury pattern seen is a diaphyseal fracture in the proximal third of the ulna with an anterior dislocation of the radial head (60% of cases). Clinically, there is considerable pain and swelling at the elbow. The radial head may be palpable in an anterolateral or posterolateral location. The forearm may appear shortened and angulated. The ulnar fracture is clearly visible and may overshadow the less obvious radial head dislocation. As a rule, the radial head normally points to the capitellum in all radiographic views of the elbow. In a Monteggia's fracture, the apex of the ulna fracture points in the direction of the radial head dislocation.

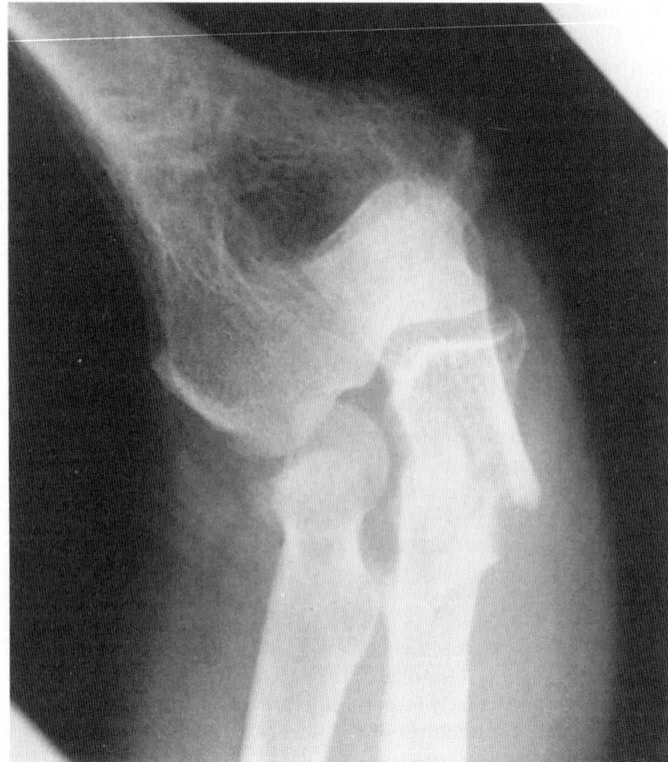

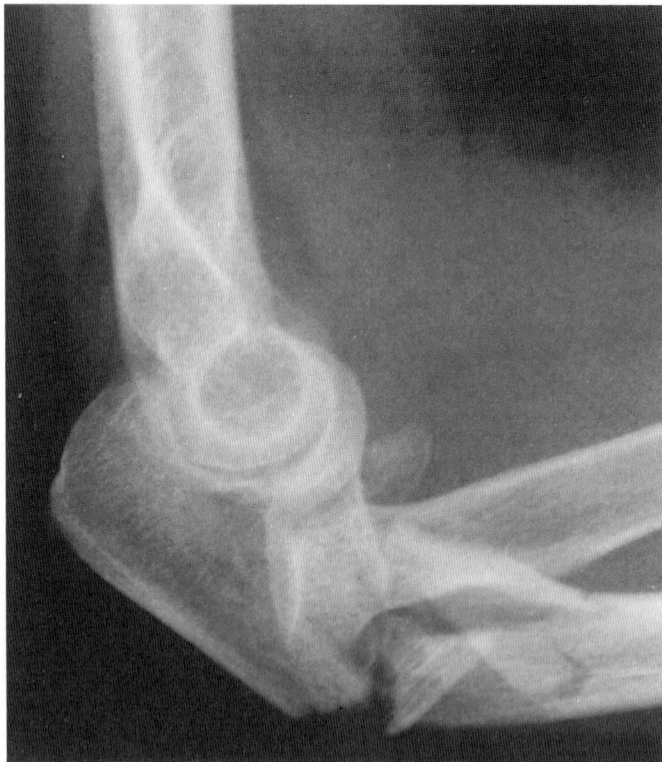

FIGURE 270-17. Monteggia's fracture-dislocation. The angulation of the comminuted fracture of the proximal ulna points in the direction of the radial head dislocation.

Obtain consultation with an orthopedic surgeon. Monteggia's fracture-dislocations are generally treated with open reduction and internal fixation of the ulna and closed reduction of the radial head dislocation. In children, the injury may be treated with closed reduction and long arm splinting. Complications include nonunion, recurrent dislocation, chronic pain, infection, and paralysis of the posterior interosseous nerve, a deep branch of the radial nerve.

RADIUS FRACTURES

FRACTURES OF THE PROXIMAL TWO THIRDS OF THE RADIUS

Radius fractures can be divided into those that are proximal and those that are distal to the junction of the middle and distal thirds of the bone. Excluding radial head fractures, isolated fractures of the proximal two thirds of the radius are uncommon because the radius is relatively well protected from direct blows by the ulna and surrounding forearm musculature. Nondisplaced fractures are rare and treated with cast immobilization. Fractures of the proximal two thirds of the radius are often displaced by both the force of the injury and the action of the supinators and pronators on the radius. They require internal fixation to prevent rotational deformity. Compartment syndrome is rare with these fractures. Most complications involve malunion or nonunion because of inadequate or lost reduction.

GALEAZZI'S FRACTURE-DISLOCATION

Fractures of the distal third of the radial shaft are produced by falls on the outstretched hand in forced pronation or by a direct blow. The radius, generally the distal third, is fractured along with a dislocation of the distal radioulnar joint. Galeazzi's fracture is often referred to as the *reverse Monteggia's fracture*. There is localized tenderness and swelling over the distal radius and wrist. The radius fracture is usually short oblique or transverse with dorsal lateral angulation. The distal radioulnar joint injury can be subtle. Radiographs may show only a slightly increased distal radioulnar joint space on the anteroposterior view. On the lateral view, the ulna is displaced dorsally. This injury is treated surgically by open reduction and internal fixation of the radius fracture. Complications include infection, nonunion, and malunion. Injuries to the ulnar nerve and anterior interosseous branch of the median nerve have been reported but usually heal spontaneously. If the radius heals with a rotational deformity, there may be pain at the distal radioulnar joint with extreme pronation and supination.

Acknowledgments: The authors wish to recognize the contributions of Harold Chin, MD, and Arthur F. Proust, MD, in previous editions of this chapter, and of Christopher Sullivan for his research and editorial assistance.

REFERENCES

The complete reference list is available online at www.TintinalliEM.com.

Shoulder and Humerus Injuries

Lars Petter Bjoernsen
Alexander Ebinger

STERNOCLAVICULAR SPRAINS AND DISLOCATIONS

ANATOMY

The sternoclavicular joint contains an intra-articular fibrocartilaginous disc and has the least amount of bony stability of any major joint because less than half of the medial end of the clavicle articulates with the upper sternum. However, it is remarkably stable, due to the strong surrounding ligaments, and as a result, most injuries are simple sprains, while dislocations and fractures are uncommon.[1-3]

The medial clavicular epiphysis is the last epiphysis of the body to appear radiographically (age 18 years old) and the last to close (age 22 to 25 years old). An apparent sternoclavicular joint dislocation in children and young adults is typically a Salter-Harris type I or II fracture, with either anterior or posterior displacement of the clavicular metaphysis that requires orthopedic consultation and follow-up for optimal healing and remodeling.[1,4]

CLINICAL FEATURES

A **posterior dislocation** results from a direct blow or from an indirect force to the shoulder, causing the shoulder to roll forward at the time of impact. An **anterior dislocation** may result from a similar indirect force if the shoulder is rolled backward at the moment of impact.

The major symptom is severe pain, exacerbated by arm motion and lying supine. The shoulder may appear shortened and rolled forward. On examination, anterior dislocations have a prominent medial clavicle end that is visible and palpable anterior to the sternum, although swelling and tenderness may impede diagnosis. In posterior dislocations, the medial clavicle end is less visible and often not palpable, and the patient may have signs and symptoms of impingement of the superior mediastinal contents, such as stridor, dysphagia, and shortness of breath (**Figure 271-1**).[3] Minor trauma, on the other hand, may result in a sprain to the sternoclavicular joint with only pain and swelling localized to the joint.

DIAGNOSIS

Routine radiographs have a low sensitivity for the detection of dislocation, but immediate chest x-ray is needed to exclude a pneumothorax, pneumomediastinum, and hemopneumothorax. Special views and comparison with the other clavicle may be helpful.[1] CT is the imaging procedure of choice (**Figure 271-2**) and is recommended in any posterior dislocation with concern for injury to the mediastinal structures. IV contrast may be administered to further delineate injury. US can identify sternoclavicular joint effusions.

STERNOCLAVICULAR SPRAIN

Sprains of the sternoclavicular joint are treated with ice, sling, and analgesics. In a nontrauma patient, pain at the sternoclavicular joint should raise suspicion for septic arthritis, especially in injection drug users. US can detect effusion and aid in joint aspiration.

ANTERIOR STERNOCLAVICULAR DISLOCATIONS

Patients with uncomplicated anterior dislocations may be discharged without an attempted reduction, because this injury has little or no impact on function. Clavicular splinting, ice, analgesics, sling, and orthopedic referral are required.

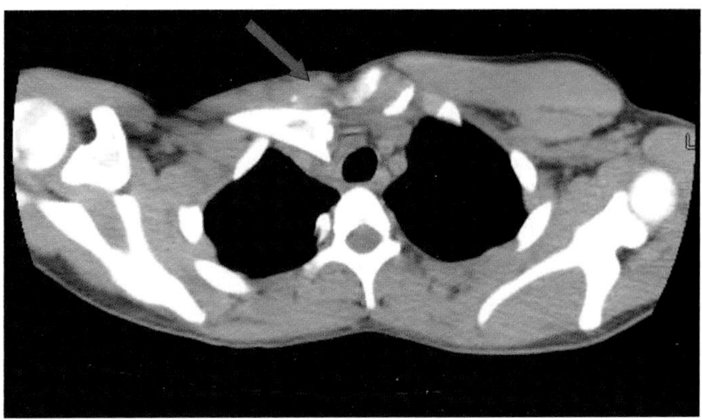

FIGURE 271-2. CT scan of right posterior sternoclavicular dislocation. Arrow indicates disrupted sternoclavicular joint with posterior displacement of clavicle and compression of adjacent lung.

For closed reduction, which can be performed within 10 days of the injury, the patient is placed supine with a towel roll or similar between the scapulae. The arm is abducted to 90 degrees, longitudinal traction is applied with slight extension by moving the arm toward the ground, and pressure is placed over the medial end of the clavicle.[5] Even with reduction, the joint is usually unstable and redislocates (50%) when pressure is released.

POSTERIOR STERNOCLAVICULAR DISLOCATIONS

Posterior dislocations may be associated with life-threatening injuries to adjacent structures, including pneumothorax or compression or laceration of surrounding great vessels, trachea, or esophagus.[1,2] Orthopedic consultation is necessary for closed or open reduction. Open reduction should be performed in the operating room with trauma or vascular surgery available.[1,3,5]

CLAVICLE FRACTURES

ANATOMY

The clavicle provides support and mobility for upper extremity tasks by functioning as a strut that connects the shoulder girdle to the trunk. It

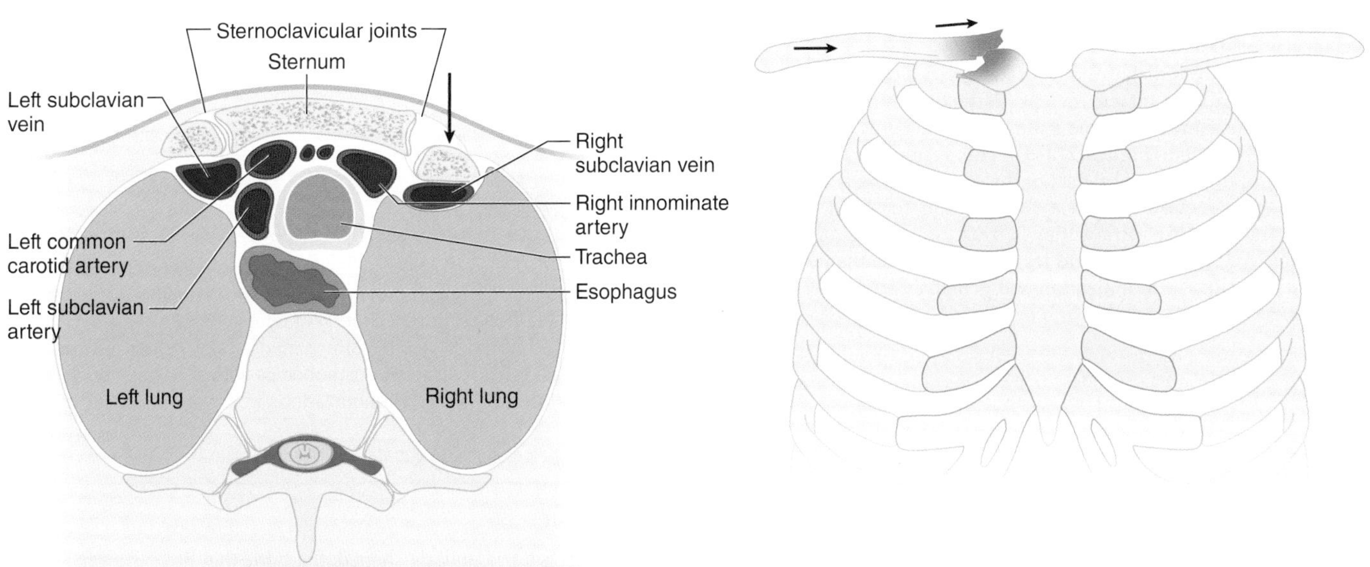

FIGURE 271-1. Posterior sternoclavicular joint dislocation impinging on the mediastinal structures.

articulates with the sternum proximally and the acromion distally. In addition, the clavicle protects the adjacent lung, brachial plexus, and subclavian and brachial blood vessels. The clavicle is S-shaped, and the mid-portion of the clavicle is the thinnest, having no accompanying ligamentous or muscular attachments. Fracture results from a direct blow to the shoulder, buckling the clavicle.

CLINICAL FEATURES

Clinical signs are swelling, deformity, and tenderness overlying the clavicle. The arm is slumped inward and downward, and range of motion is limited. The fracture can often be palpated, and crepitus may be present.

DIAGNOSIS

Most clavicle fractures can be diagnosed on standard shoulder and clavicle x-rays. Occasionally, routine clavicle radiographs may miss some fractures, particularly at either end of the bone, due to overlap of surrounding structures. If a fracture is clinically suspected but not initially diagnosed with standard radiographs, a 45-degree cephalad tilt view may be used for further assessment. Definitive diagnosis may require CT.

Obtain emergent orthopedic consultation for open fractures, fractures with neurovascular injuries, and fractures with persistent skin tenting.

MIDDLE THIRD CLAVICLE FRACTURES

Fractures of the middle third of the clavicle are most common. Although midclavicular fractures are often managed nonoperatively, operative fixation may result in improved functional outcome and a lower rate of malunion and nonunion.[6-8] Some fractures (**Table 271-1**), including severely comminuted or displaced fractures, benefit from referral and possible operative intervention.[9,10] Additional considerations for orthopedic referral include athletes, professional impact, and cosmetic concerns. Referral to an orthopedist within a few days of injury should be considered in the above instances. In cases where the patient does not want surgery or is a poor surgical candidate, conservative treatment is an appropriate strategy. Initial treatment of midclavicle fractures includes immobilization with either a sling or figure-of-eight brace. The length of immobilization is typically 4 to 8 weeks, until the fracture is no longer painful. Initial primary care or orthopedic follow-up should be in 1 to 2 weeks after injury in conservative treatment. The patient may use the arm as pain permits but should avoid repeat injury from direct contact. Encourage daily range of motion of the elbow immediately and of the shoulder as soon as pain allows (3 to 5 days).

DISTAL CLAVICLE FRACTURES

Distal clavicle fractures are divided into three subtypes. In type I fractures, the fracture is distal to the coracoclavicular ligaments, with the ligaments remaining intact. In type II fractures, the location of the fracture is the same as in type I; however, the coracoclavicular ligaments are disrupted (**Figure 271-3**). This results in an upward displacement of the proximal aspect of the clavicle. Type II distal clavicle fractures may require operative intervention to avoid nonunion.[11] Type III fractures are intra-articular fractures through the acromioclavicular (AC) joint. Type I and III fractures can be managed conservatively with sling immobilization and primary care follow-up in 1 to 2 weeks.[12]

TABLE 271-1 Middle Clavicle Fracture Nonunion Risk Factors

Initial shortening >2 cm
Comminuted fracture
Displaced fracture >100%
Significant trauma
Female
Elderly

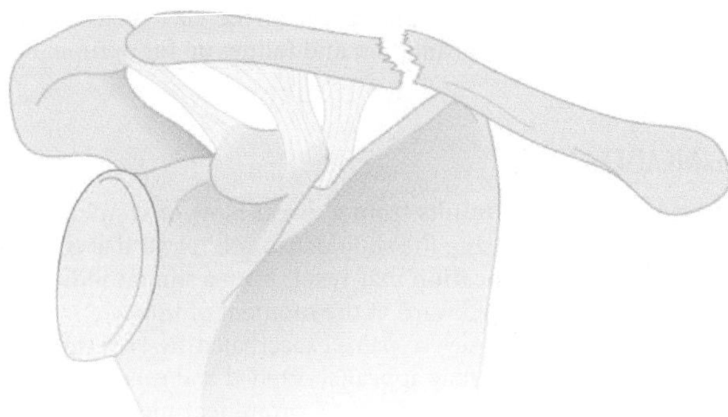

Type IIa

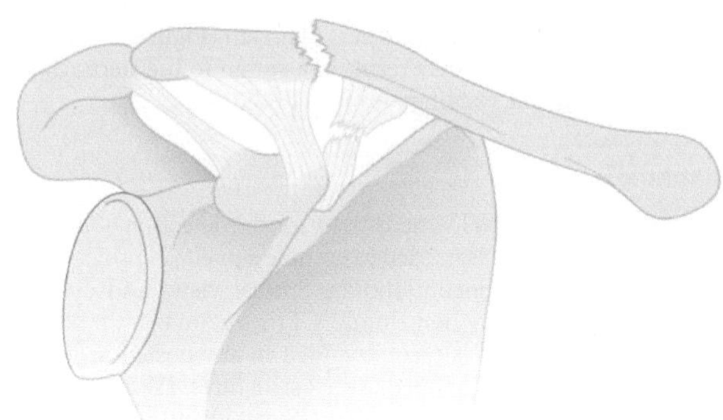

Type IIb

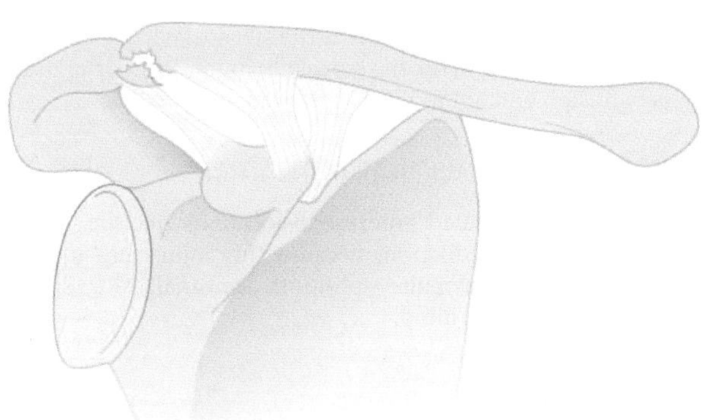

Type III

FIGURE 271-3. Classification of distal clavicular fractures. A-P = anteroposterior.

PROXIMAL THIRD CLAVICLE FRACTURES

Proximal third clavicle fractures are often high-mechanism injuries and can be associated with intrathoracic trauma. CT can diagnosis the fracture and identify additional injuries. Emergent referral is required when posteriorly displaced fragments compromise mediastinal structures. Refer all other proximal third fractures to orthopedics within 1 to 2 weeks. Initial management includes sling immobilization.

SCAPULA FRACTURES

ANATOMY

The scapula is a triangularly shaped, flat bone that links the axial skeleton to the upper extremity and stabilizes motion of the arm. It serves as the site of origin of the rotator cuff and muscles about the shoulder. The

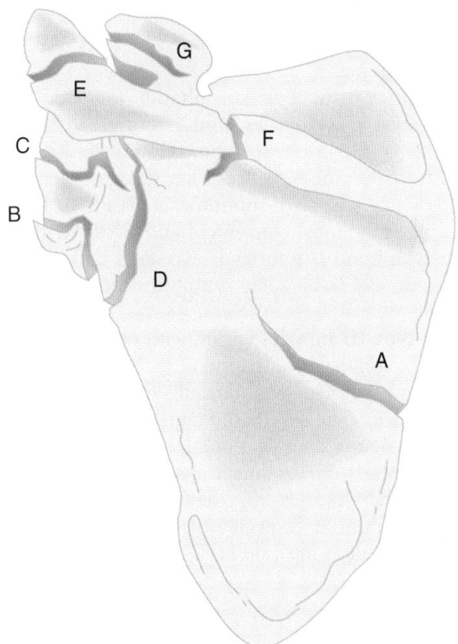

FIGURE 271-4. Sites of scapular fractures. **A.** Body. **B.** Glenoid rim. **C.** Intra-articular glenoid. **D.** Neck. **E.** Acromion. **F.** Spine. **G.** Coracoid.

mechanism of injury usually is from high-energy trauma to the shoulder area or from a fall on an outstretched hand. Scapular fractures are classified by their anatomic location (**Figure 271-4**),[13] with fractures of the body (**Figure 271-5**) and glenoid neck being most common.

CLINICAL FEATURES

Patients with isolated scapular fractures typically present with localized tenderness over the scapula and the arm held in adduction. Arm movement exacerbates pain. Due to the high energy typically required to fracture this protected bone, there is a high association of injuries to the ipsilateral lung, thoracic cage, and shoulder girdle, with fractures of the ribs being most common. Carefully determine the mechanism of injury to assist in diagnosis and raise suspicion for concurrent injuries. Assess the spine and pelvis, because scapular injuries often occur with high-impact trauma.[13,14] The indirect axial load transmitted by a fall on an outstretched arm may result in a scapular neck fracture or **glenoid fracture** through shoulder impaction or dislocation.

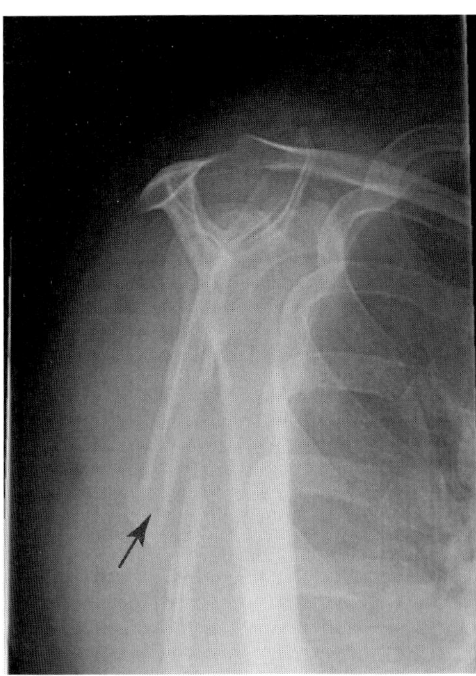

FIGURE 271-5. Scapular Y view demonstrating scapular body fracture. [Photo used with permission of Alexander Ebinger, MD.]

DIAGNOSIS

Overlying structures may obscure a scapular fracture on a single trauma anteroposterior chest radiograph. A dedicated scapular series, including anteroposterior, lateral, and axillary scapular views, will identify most fractures and will guide the need for a CT scan (Figure 271-4). Scapular fractures are often associated with other significant injuries, and hence, diagnosis may be delayed or initially missed entirely. CT scan of the chest can identify both scapular and associated pathology, and a dedicated CT of the scapula can also be obtained.

Most scapular fractures are treated nonsurgically, with sling, ice, analgesics, and early range-of-motion exercises. Surgery may be necessary for significant or displaced articular fractures of the glenoid, angulated glenoid neck fractures, acromial fractures associated with a rotator cuff tear, and some coracoid fractures.[13,15] Disability is more likely to be associated with fractures of the glenoid, acromion, or coracoid. Isolated scapular fractures should be referred to an orthopedic surgeon.

SCAPULOTHORACIC DISSOCIATION

Traumatic dislocation of the scapula from the thoracic wall results from severe massive traction force applied to the ipsilateral upper extremity and shoulder girdle. Associated disruption of the subclavian or axillary arteries and brachial plexus makes proper identification and treatment critical.[16,17]

Chest x-ray demonstrates significant lateral displacement of the scapula.[16,17] Associated radiographic abnormalities include distracted clavicle fracture, AC separation, and sternoclavicular dislocation. Perform a CT scan to identify intrathoracic injuries.

ACROMIOCLAVICULAR (AC) JOINT INJURIES

ANATOMY

The AC joint is a diarthrodial joint that, together with the sternoclavicular joint, connects the upper extremity to the axial skeleton (**Figure** 271-**6**).

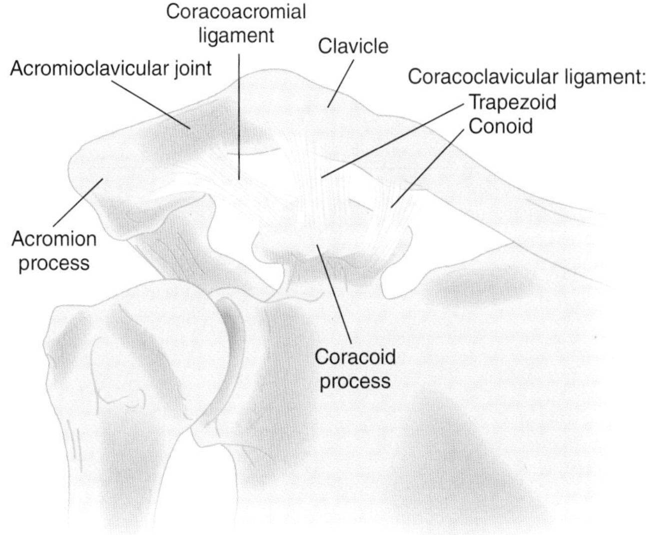

FIGURE 271-6. Anatomy of the acromioclavicular joint.

Support of the AC joint is through the AC and coracoclavicular ligaments and the attachment of the trapezius and deltoid muscles. Surrounding the AC joint is a thin capsule, which is reinforced by the AC ligaments. The AC ligaments provide horizontal stability to the joint. The strong coracoclavicular ligaments consist of two parts, the more lateral trapezoid and the medial conoid, and attach the distal inferior clavicle to the coracoid process of the scapula. The coracoclavicular ligament is the major suspensory ligament of the upper extremity and provides vertical stability to the AC joint.

AC joint injuries range from mild sprain to complete disruption of the ligaments that link the scapula and clavicle. The mechanism of injury is usually direct trauma to the joint from a fall with the arm adducted. The result is that the scapula and shoulder girdle are driven inferiorly while the clavicle remains in its normal position. An indirect mechanism is a fall on the outstretched hand with transmission of force to the AC joint.

CLINICAL FEATURES

The diagnosis of AC joint injuries is clinical. The mechanism of injury and tenderness and deformity at the AC joint, especially when compared with the contralateral AC joint, are confirmatory. Range of motion may be limited, depending on the severity of injury. Cross-arm abduction testing is often painful.

DIAGNOSIS

Radiographs are useful for identifying other fractures and determining the severity of injury. AC radiographs should specifically be ordered because they require only one-third to one-half of the penetration of standard shoulder films. Shoulder radiographs may overpenetrate the AC joint, and small fractures can be missed. Although standard AC radiographs are generally sufficient, an axillary view is required to identify posterior clavicular dislocation (type IV). Stress radiographs are no longer routinely obtained.[18]

Obtain emergency orthopedic consultation for open fractures, fractures with neurovascular injuries, and fractures with persistent skin tenting. **Table 271-2** describes specific AC joint injuries. Treatment of **type I and II injuries** consists of rest, ice, analgesics, and immobilization, followed by early range-of-motion exercises (7 to 14 days).[19]

A simple sling is the most convenient and effective initial treatment. Prognosis for type I and II injuries is excellent, with only a small percentage of patients developing late symptoms requiring excision of the distal clavicle.

Treatment of **type III injuries** varies, with most orthopedists recommending a trial of conservative treatment with sling immobilization.[20-22] Surgical strategies have yielded good results in selected patients, with the specific management being operator dependent. Treatment decisions are based on such factors as age, occupation, and activity level. **Types IV, V, and VI are severe injuries**, and most experts recommend surgical repair. Because other injuries are associated with these more severe forms of AC joint injuries (especially type VI), a careful clinical and radiographic examination must be performed.[20,21]

GLENOHUMERAL JOINT DISLOCATION

ANATOMY

The glenohumeral joint is a ball-and-socket joint, with the articulation between the glenoid fossa of the scapula and the articular surface of the humeral head. The socket of the shoulder is shallow. The glenoid labrum deepens the socket and helps provide joint stability. The capsule and tendinous attachments about the joint also provide stability. Anterior dislocations of the glenohumeral joint are the most common; posterior

TABLE 271-2 Classification and Physical Findings in Acromioclavicular Joint Injuries

Type	Injury	Mechanism	Radiograph/Exam
I	Sprained acromioclavicular ligaments	Type I	Radiograph: Normal Exam: Tenderness over acromioclavicular joint
II	Acromioclavicular ligaments ruptured; coracoclavicular ligaments sprained	Type II	Radiograph: Slight widening of acromioclavicular joint; clavicle elevated 25%–50% above acromion; may be slight widening of the coracoclavicular interspace Exam: Tenderness and mild step-off deformity of acromioclavicular joint

(Continued)

TABLE 271-2 Classification and Physical Findings in Acromioclavicular Joint Injuries (*Continued*)

Type	Injury	Mechanism	Radiograph/Exam
III	Acromioclavicular ligaments ruptured; coracoclavicular ligaments ruptured; deltoid and trapezius muscles detached	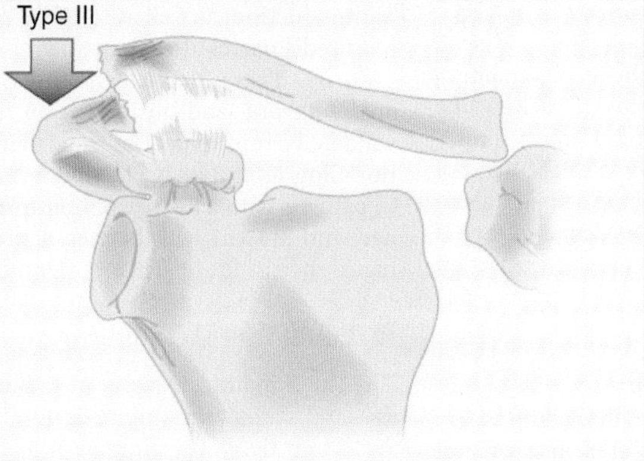 Type III	Clavicle elevated 100% above acromion; coracoclavicular interspace widened 25%–100% Exam: Distal end of clavicle prominent; shoulder droops
IV	Rupture of all supporting structures; clavicle displaced posteriorly in or through the trapezius	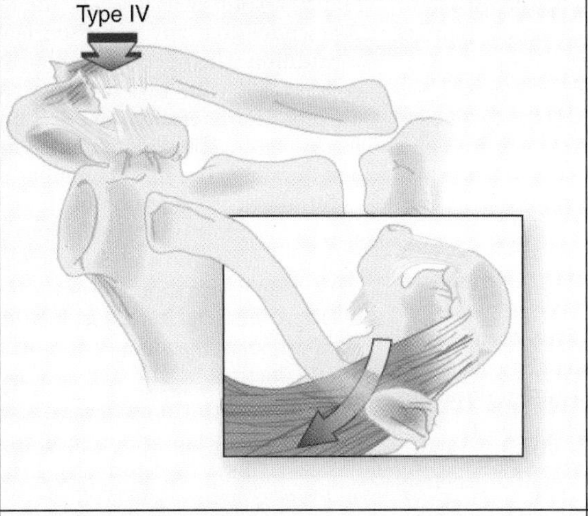 Type IV	Radiograph: May appear similar to type II and III; axillary radiograph required to visualize posterior dislocation Exam: Possible posterior displacement of clavicle
V	Rupture of all supporting structures (more severe form of type III injury)	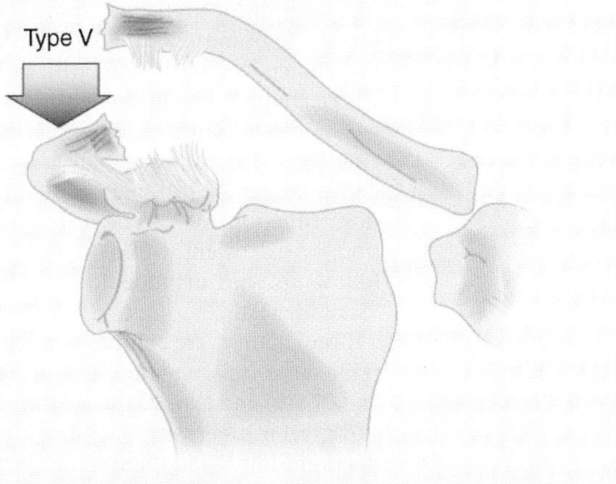 Type V	Radiograph: Acromioclavicular joint dislocated; generally 200%–300% disparity of coracoclavicular interspace compared to normal shoulder Exam: More pain; gross deformity of clavicle
VI	Acromioclavicular ligaments disrupted; coracoclavicular ligaments may be disrupted; deltoid and trapezius muscles disrupted	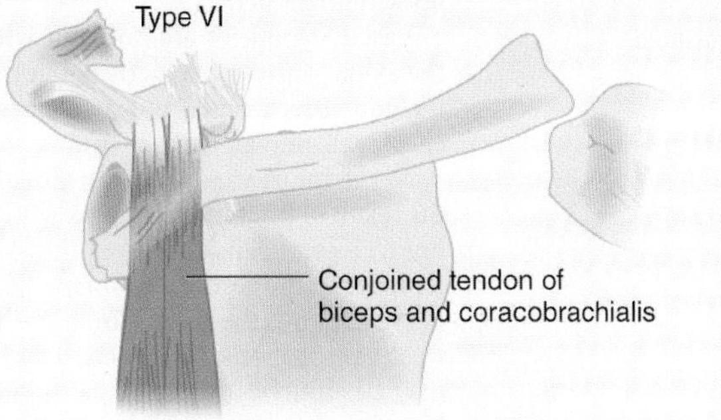 Type VI Conjoined tendon of biceps and coracobrachialis	Radiograph: Acromioclavicular joint dislocated; clavicle displaced inferiorly Exam: Severe swelling; multiple associated injuries

dislocations account for <1%. Other dislocations include inferior (luxatio erecta) and superior (very rare).

CLINICAL FEATURES

In an anterior dislocation, the associated arm is usually in slight abduction and external rotation. The shoulder is "squared off," lacking the normal rounded contour. The patient resists adduction and internal rotation and often cannot touch the contralateral shoulder with the hand of the affected extremity. The humeral head can often be palpated anteriorly. Perform a careful neurovascular examination. The axillary nerve is most commonly injured. This nerve may be tested by pinprick sensation over the skin of the deltoid muscle.

DIAGNOSIS

Obtain anteroposterior and scapular lateral or "Y" radiographs before reduction is attempted to confirm the anatomic type of dislocation and identify any associated fractures. Although the anteroposterior radiograph will reveal the dislocation, the scapular Y radiograph will indicate whether the dislocation is anterior or posterior.[23]

ANTERIOR GLENOHUMERAL DISLOCATIONS

The combination of abduction, extension, and external rotation with sufficient force will cause an anterior dislocation. There are multiple types of anterior glenohumeral dislocations (**Figure 271-7**). These include subcoracoid, which is the most common; subglenoid; subclavicular; and the very rare intrathoracic dislocation.

Prereduction radiographs are advisable when there has been significant trauma, unless time is crucial because circulation is threatened. Radiographs are needed because dislocations and fracture-dislocations may have a similar appearance on physical examination, but the techniques used to treat them may be very different. Shoulder dislocations or subluxations combined with proximal humerus fractures generally require orthopedic consultation and may need operative repair. Shoulder dislocations with associated proximal humerus fracture increase with age. Through the third decade, fracture-dislocations occurred less than 1% of the time. This percentage rises with each decade of life.[24] Postreduction radiographs are valuable for confirming the success of joint reduction, as well as for providing documentation, in the event the joint redislocates after the patient is discharged from the ED.

There is an expenditure of time, money, and radiation associated with pre- and postreduction films; however, there is currently no validated clinician decision rule that allows safe elimination of prereduction films after injury.[25] In clinical practice, films are sometimes omitted in patients with a history of multiple recurrent dislocations of the shoulder who present with history, signs, and symptoms typical of another recurrence in the absence of significant trauma.[23,25]

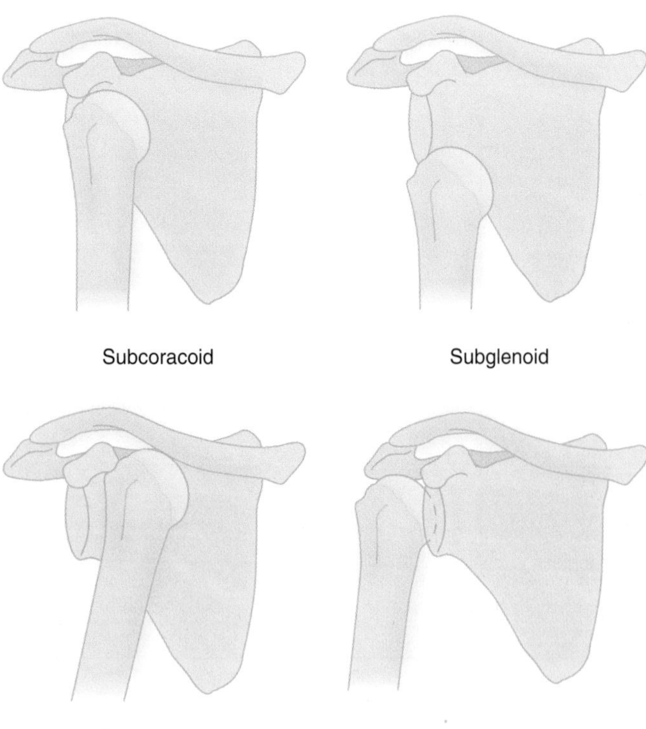

FIGURE 271-7. Types of anterior shoulder dislocations.

REDUCTION TECHNIQUES

The three main categories of reduction techniques are traction, leverage, and scapular manipulation.[26-29] Success rates are between 70% and 96% regardless of technique. It is essential to provide appropriate systemic narcotic analgesia. The use of procedural sedation is highly recommended, but any reduction technique may be attempted without medication when performed slowly and atraumatically. It is best to be comfortable with two or three techniques in case of a failed first attempt. Considerations in selection of a technique include ease of performance, effectiveness, requirement for sedation, number of assistants, and duration. The most common techniques are described below.

Intra-articular injection of 10 to 20 mL of 1% lidocaine (10 mL provides a total dose of 100 milligrams of lidocaine) reduces the pain associated with reduction and can complement procedural sedation.[30,31] After sterile skin preparation, introduce the needle at the hollow created by the displaced humeral head, just inferior to the acromion. US can facilitate intra-articular injection. Perform neurovascular examination before and after reduction.

Complications Complications associated with anterior glenohumeral dislocations include recurrence, rotator cuff tears, humeral head bony defects (Hill-Sachs deformity), glenoid labral defects (Bankart lesions), and rarely, neurovascular injuries.[32] The most common complication is recurrent dislocation, and children and young adults may have a recurrence rate of more than 90%.[32,33] Early surgical repair may decrease the recurrence rate, so patients with first-time shoulder dislocations should be referred for orthopedic evaluation.[34-36]

The rotator cuff weakens with advancing age, and in older patients, anterior dislocation is usually associated with rotator cuff tears. Rotator cuff tears can be difficult to identify on ED examination after dislocation reduction, but can be suspected with weakness upon external rotation.[32] Any patient with pain persisting for greater than 2 weeks should follow up with orthopedics. For further discussion, see chapter 280, "Shoulder Pain."

Bony injuries are common and include fractures of the humeral head (Hill-sachs lesions) and glenoid (bony Bankart lesion) (**Figures 271-8** and **271-9**) and tears of the anterior glenoid labrum (soft Bankart lesion) and greater tuberosity. Such fractures are often evident only on postreduction films,[23] and there is no specific ED treatment other than follow-up with orthopedics.

Vascular injuries are rare, but when they occur, they tend to involve the axillary artery in elderly patients. Clinical findings of vascular injury include absent radial pulse, axillary hematoma, bruising of the lateral chest wall, and an axillary bruit.

Nerve injuries, which occur in 10% to 25% of acute dislocations, are the result of traction neurapraxia. Most involve the axillary nerve, resulting in loss of sensation over the skin of the upper arm. This injury is temporary and resolves spontaneously. The motor portion of the axillary nerve supplies the teres minor and the deltoid, and injury can result in weakness of shoulder abduction and external rotation. Other nerves that may be injured are the radial, ulnar, median, musculocutaneous, and brachial plexus.[32]

Disposition After reduction, place the arm in a shoulder immobilizer or sling that maintains the shoulder in adduction and internal rotation (**Figure 271-10**). Provide instructions for orthopedic follow-up in 1 week for uncomplicated dislocations and within 1 to 2 days for dislocations complicated by bony or soft tissue injury.[37]

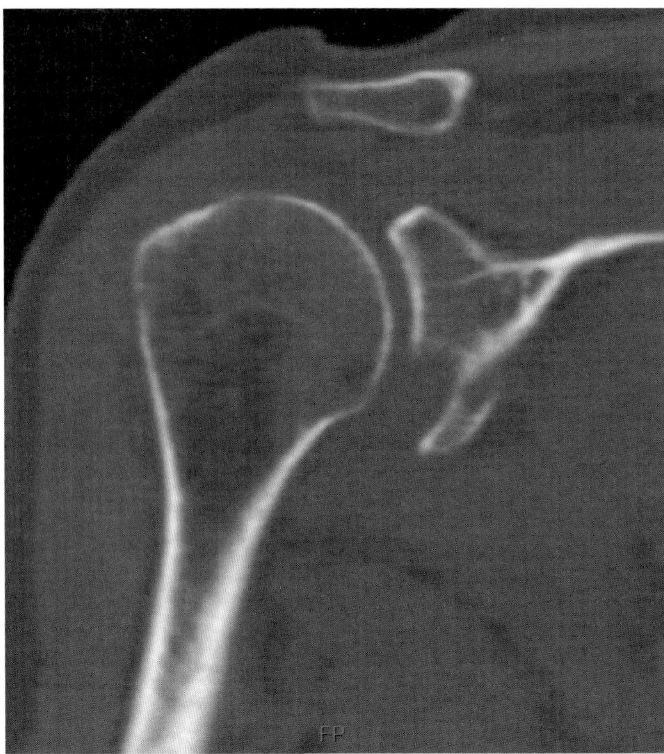

FIGURE 271-8. CT right shoulder showing a frontal view with fracture tear of the anterior-inferior glenoid bony cavity (Bankart lesion). [Photo used with permission of Erik Magnus Berntsen, MD, PhD, Department of Radiology, St. Olavs University Hospital, Trondheim, Norway.]

TRACTION-COUNTERTRACTION TECHNIQUE (MODIFIED HIPPOCRATIC)

A modification of the Hippocratic method uses traction-countertraction (**Figure** 271-**11**). The patient is supine with the arm abducted and elbow flexed at 90 degrees. A sheet is tied and placed across the thorax of the patient and then around the waist of the assistant. Another sheet is tied and placed around the forearm of the patient at the elbow and the waist

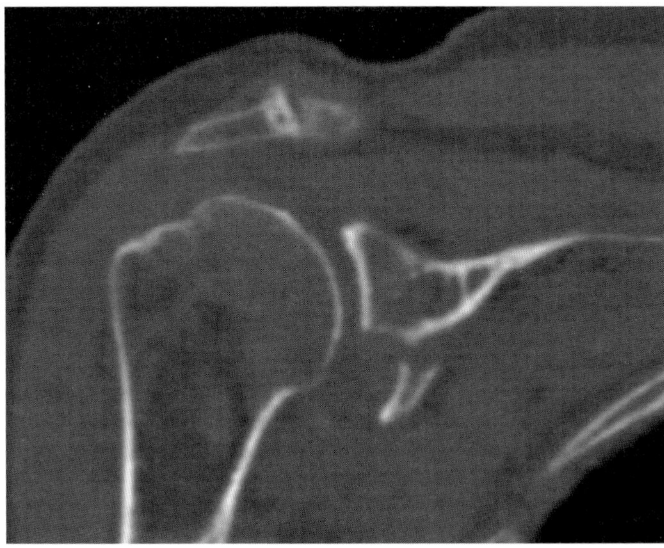

FIGURE 271-9. CT right shoulder, oblique coronal view, demonstrating both the bony Bankart lesion and the Hill-Sachs fracture of the humeral head. [Photo used with permission of Erik Magnus Berntsen, MD, PhD, Department of Radiology, St. Olavs University Hospital, Trondheim, Norway.]

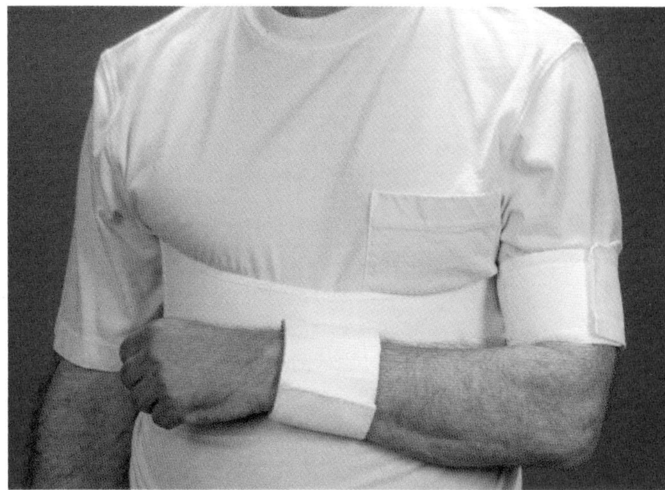

FIGURE 271-10. Arm sling.

of the physician. Gradually apply traction to the proximal forearm as the assistant provides countertraction. Gentle internal and external rotation or outward pressure on the proximal humerus may aid reduction.

SNOWBIRD TECHNIQUE

Another version of the traction-countertraction technique is the Snowbird technique.[28] The patient should sit upright in a chair or bed with the elbow flexed to 90 degrees. Place a belt or strap across the patient's proximal forearm, so the bottom of the belt can be used to apply downward pressure with the foot. Use an assistant to place a sheet across the patient's thorax to provide countertraction. Keep the patient's elbow at 90 degrees and apply traction to the extremity by stepping on the belt with the foot (**Figure 271-12**). Gentle external rotation will facilitate reduction.

STIMSON TECHNIQUE

Place the patient prone with the dislocated extremity hanging over the side of the stretcher and a 10-lb weight attached to the wrist. Inject intra-articular lidocaine. Complete muscle relaxation is required. Reduction occurs in 20 to 30 minutes. Although the time to reduction can be a drawback, this technique is safe, effective, and easy to learn.

SCAPULAR MANIPULATION TECHNIQUE

The patient is positioned with weights in the same manner as the Stimson technique (**Figure 271-13**). After adequate sedation, the physician pushes the tip of the scapula medially using the thumbs, while stabilizing the superior aspect with the cephalad hand. This technique reports a 96% success rate.[29]

EXTERNAL ROTATION TECHNIQUE (KOCHER'S TECHNIQUE)

Place the patient supine with the affected arm adducted to the patient's side. With the elbow at 90 degrees of flexion, slowly externally rotate the arm (**Figure 271-14**). No longitudinal traction is applied. Perform the movement slowly to allow time for spasm and pain to resolve. Reduction is usually complete before reaching the coronal plane and is often not noted either by the patient or physician. If needed, the elbow may be brought anteriorly and internally rotated to the opposite shoulder.[38]

MILCH TECHNIQUE

The maneuvers for the Milch technique are external rotation, arm abduction to 180 degrees with simultaneous pressure on the humeral head, and in-line longitudinal traction with continued pressure on the humeral head (**Figure 271-15**).

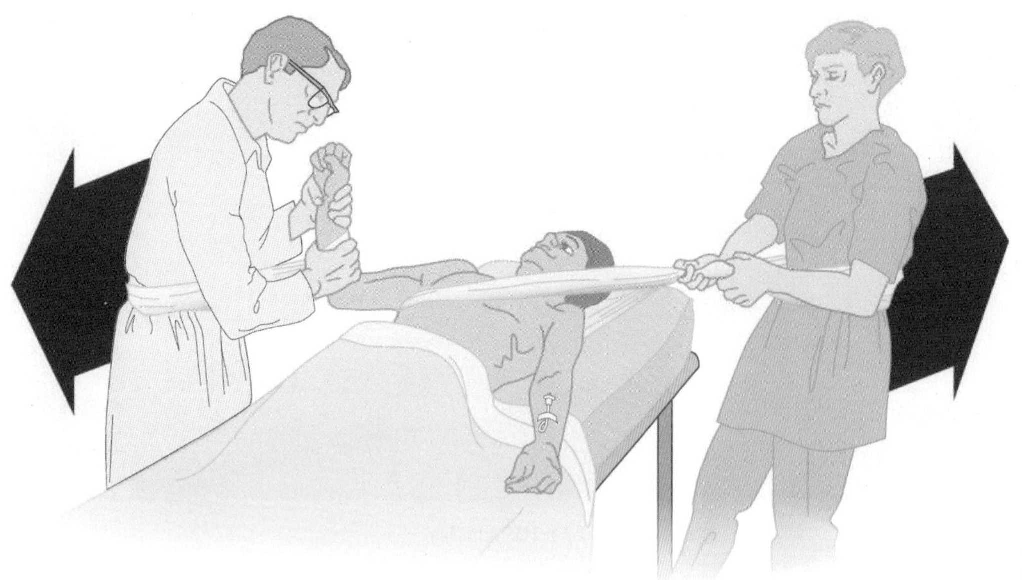

FIGURE 271-11. Modified Hippocratic technique.

CUNNINGHAM TECHNIQUE

The Cunningham technique is based on the combination of humerus and scapular positioning and specific massage of a spasming biceps muscle (**Figure 271-16**). Seat the patient comfortably, as upright as possible, with shoulders relaxed. Supporting the affected arm, slowly and gently move the humerus into full adduction with the elbow in flexion. Have the hand of the affected extremity resting against the physician's shoulder. Gently massage the trapezius and deltoids, which helps to relax the patient. Then, gently massage the biceps at the mid-humeral level. Ask the patient to elevate and shrug or retract the shoulders (attempting to touch the scapulae together) and continue the biceps massage. The goal is to wait for the patient to relax fully and have the humeral head slip back into place.[26]

POSTERIOR GLENOHUMERAL DISLOCATIONS

Posterior dislocation may occur with the humeral head in the subacromial, subglenoid, or subspinous position, but most often, it occurs with the humeral head posterior to the glenoid and inferior to the acromion (**Figure 271-17**). The subglenoid and subspinous positions are rare. The usual mechanism is an indirect force that produces forceful internal rotation and adduction or a direct blow to the anterior shoulder. On examination, there is a prominence of the posterior shoulder and anterior flattening of the normal shoulder contour on the affected side, especially when compared to the nonaffected side. The patient will be unable to externally rotate or abduct the affected arm.

The scapular Y radiograph is diagnostic (**Figure 271-18**).

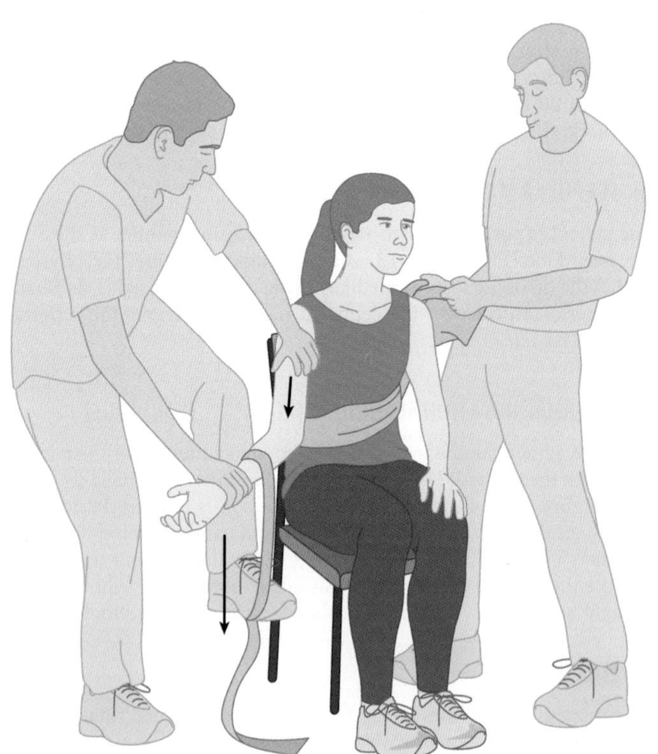

FIGURE 271-12. Snowbird technique.

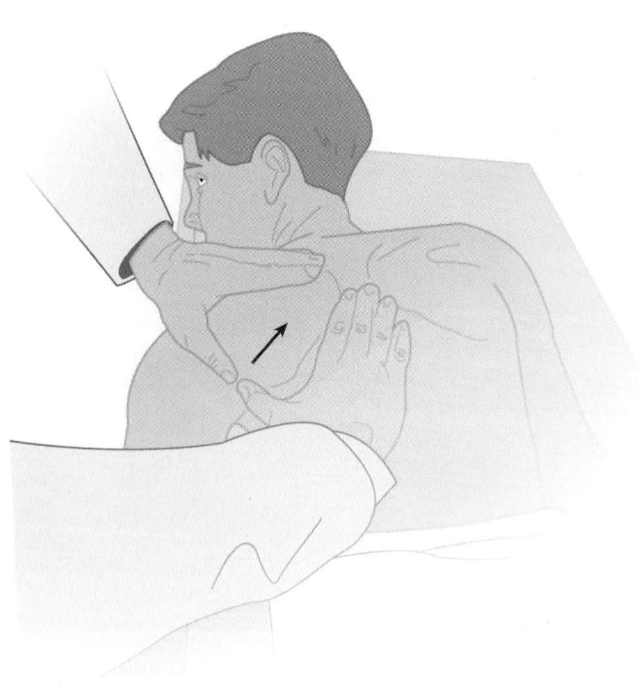

FIGURE 271-13. Scapular manipulation technique.

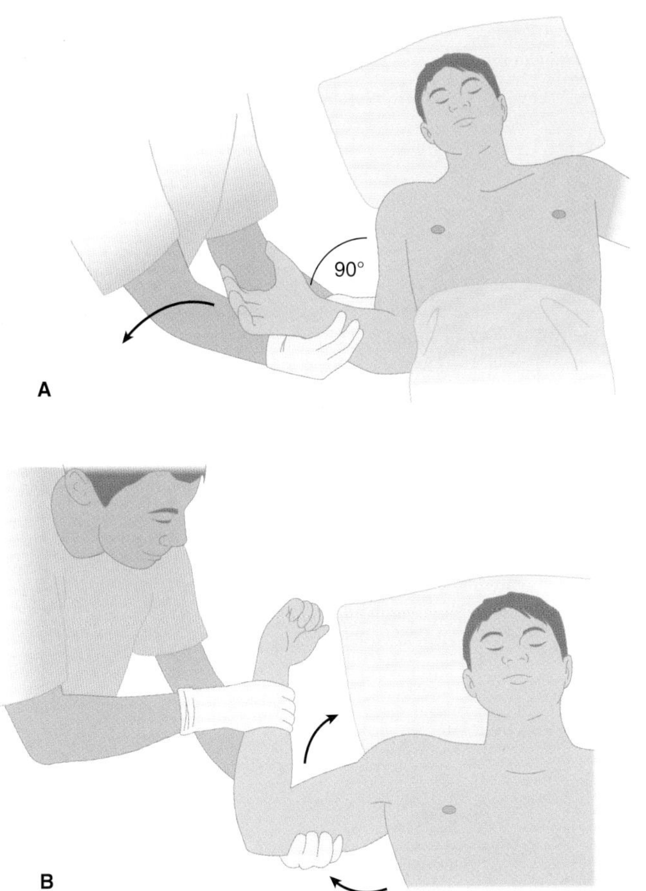

FIGURE 271-14. A and B. External rotation (Kocher's) technique. [Reproduced with permission from Simon RR, Sherman SC, Koenigsknecht SJ: *Emergency Orthopedics, The Extremities*, 5th ed. © 2007, McGraw-Hill Inc., New York.]

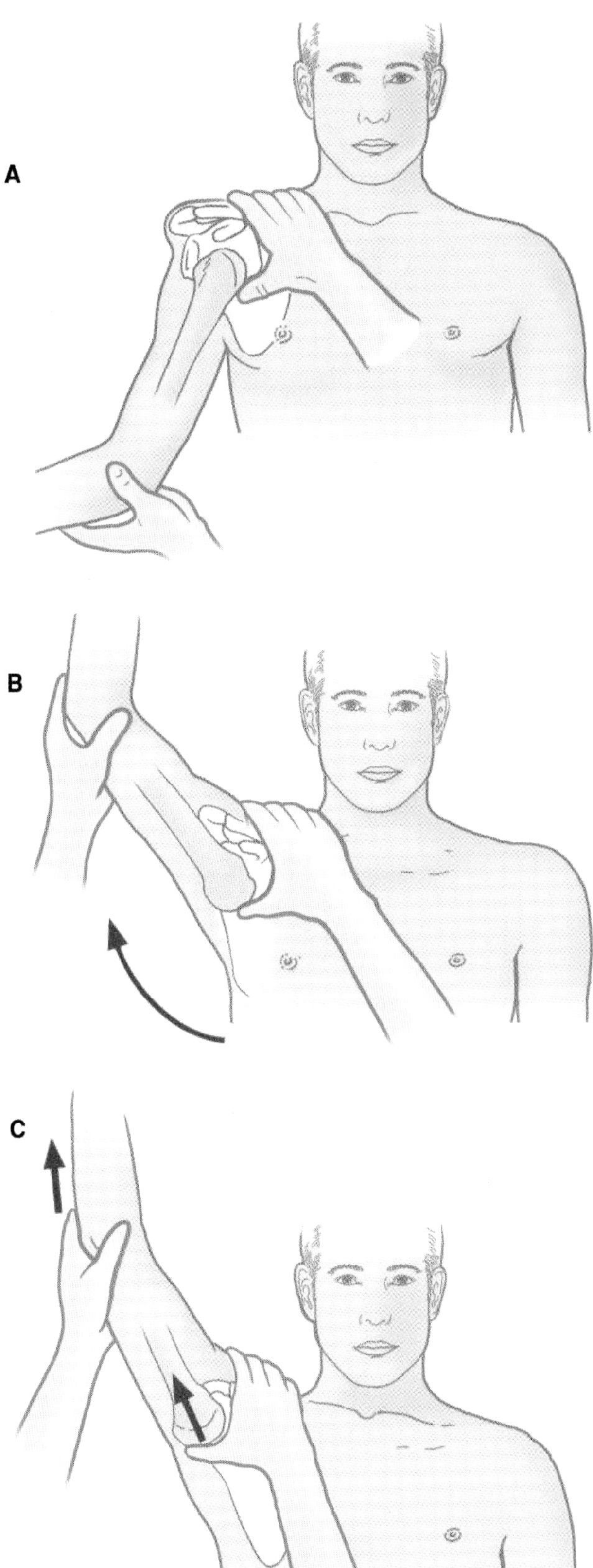

FIGURE 271-15. Milch technique. [Reproduced with permission from Reichman EF: *Emergency Medicine Procedures*, 2nd ed. Chapter 81. Shoulder Joint Dislocation Reduction. McGraw-Hill, Inc., 2013. Figure 81-7A-C.]

Reduction of a posterior dislocation is performed with the patient supine. Because severe pain and muscle spasms are common, muscle relaxation and analgesia are needed. Apply traction to the adducted arm in the long axis of the humerus. Have an assistant gently push the humeral head anteriorly into the glenoid fossa.[39] Fractures of the posterior glenoid rim, humeral head (reversed Hill-Sachs deformity), humeral shaft, or lesser tuberosity are common complications. Neurovascular and rotator cuff tears are less common than in anterior dislocations. Obtain postreduction radiographs to confirm successful reduction. Immobilize the shoulder with an arm sling, with follow-up with an orthopedist.

INFERIOR DISLOCATIONS (LUXATIO ERECTA)

Inferior dislocation is associated with significant soft tissue trauma or fracture. The mechanism of injury is a hyperabduction force, which levers the neck of the humerus against the acromion. As the force continues, the inferior capsule tears, and the humeral head is forced out inferiorly. The patient presents with the humerus fully abducted, the elbow flexed, and the patient's hand on or behind the head. The humeral head can be palpated on the lateral chest wall.

Reduction consists of traction in an upward and outward direction in line with the humerus (**Figure 271-19**). Have the assistant apply countertraction. Reduction is signaled by a "clunk." The arm is then brought to the patient's side and immobilized in a shoulder immobilizer.

Complications include severe soft tissue injuries and fractures of the proximal humerus. The rotator cuff, which usually becomes detached, requires orthopedic follow-up. Neurovascular compression injuries are usually found but almost always resolve after reduction. When the humeral head is buttonholed through the inferior capsule, the dislocation is irreducible, and operative reduction is required.

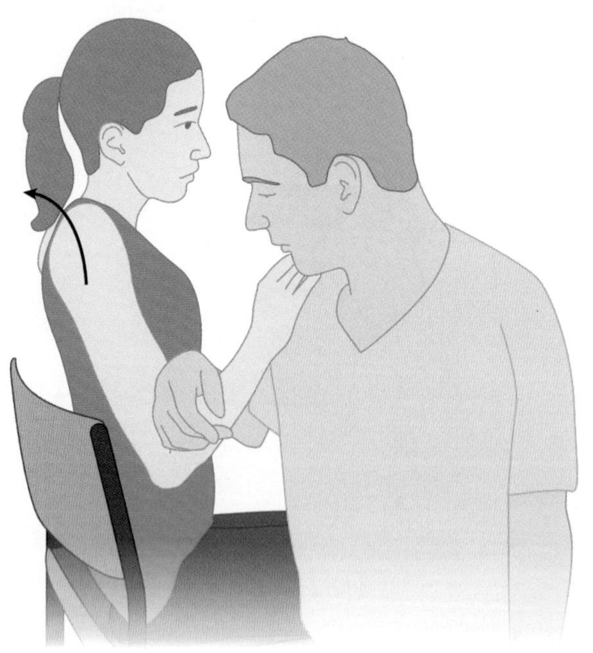
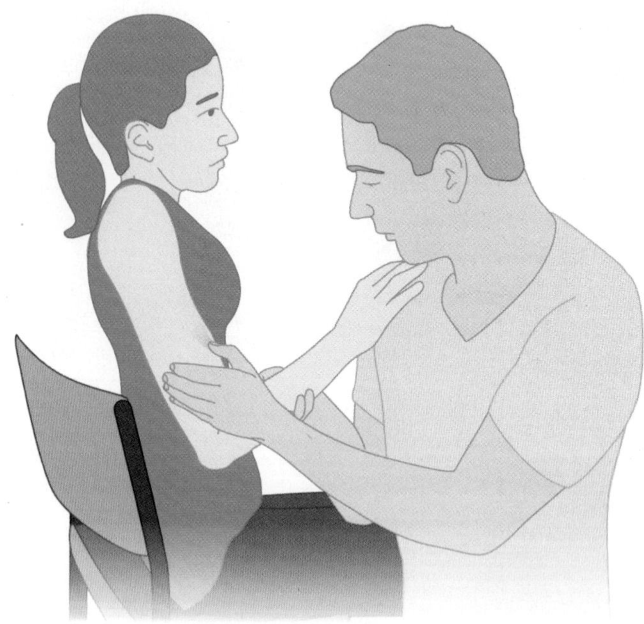

FIGURE 271-16. Cunningham technique.

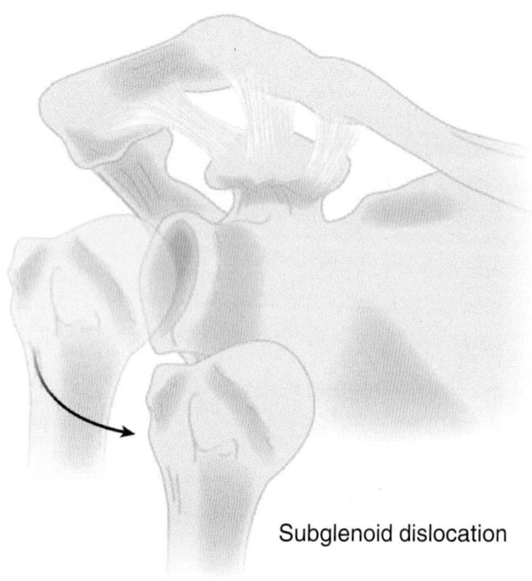

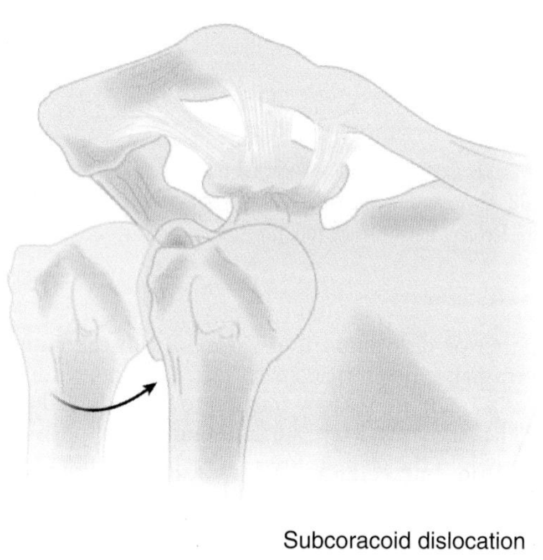

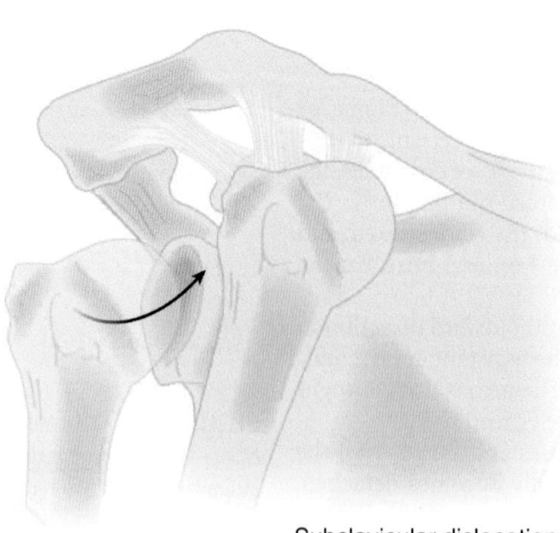

FIGURE 271-17. Posterior shoulder dislocations.

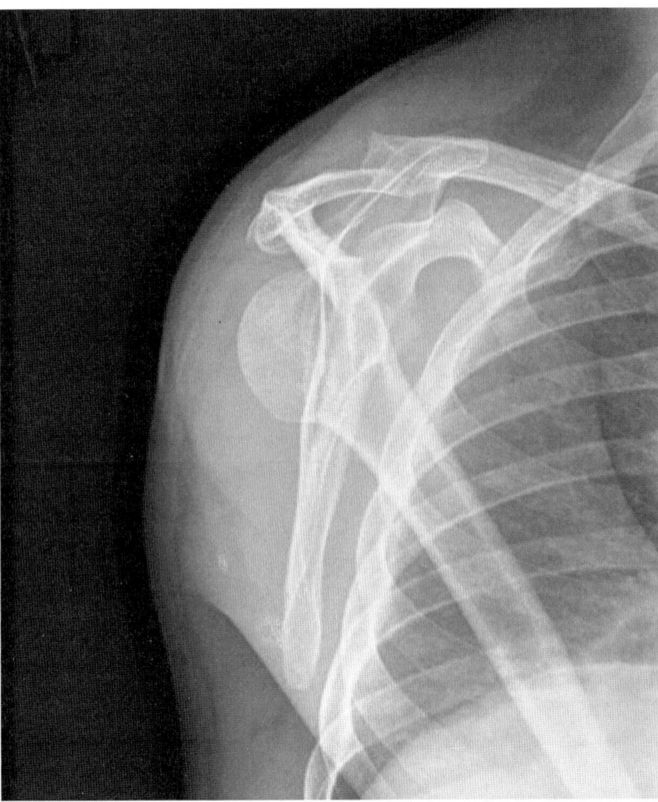

FIGURE 271-18. Scapular Y view of posterior dislocation, with the humeral head posterior. [Photo used with permission of Alexander Ebinger, MD.]

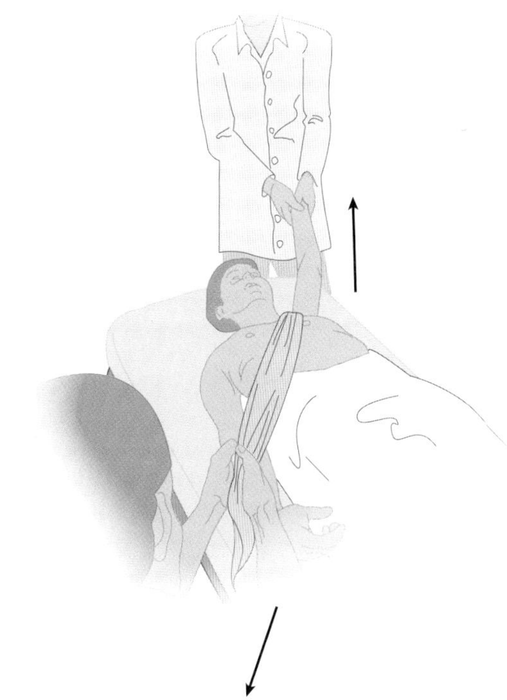

FIGURE 271-19. Reduction of luxatio erecta.

HUMERUS FRACTURES

ANATOMY

The proximal humerus is composed of the articular segment and anatomic neck, the greater and lesser tuberosities, and the proximal shaft (**Figure 271-20**). The supraspinatus, infraspinatus, and teres minor insert on the greater tuberosity, whereas the subscapularis inserts on the lesser tuberosity. The biceps tendon passes through the bicipital groove. The anterior and posterior humeral circumflex arteries branch off the axillary artery and course around the surgical neck.

CLINICAL FEATURES

Patients with fractures typically present with pain, swelling, and tenderness about the shoulder. Range of motion is often significantly limited, and the arm is held in adduction. Crepitus and ecchymosis may be present. Carefully perform the neurovascular examination. The most commonly injured nerve is the axillary nerve, and sensation overlying the deltoid muscle should be tested. The second most commonly injured nerve is the suprascapular nerve, which innervates the supraspinatus and infraspinatus.[40] Range of motion may be limited, but assessment of shoulder abduction should be performed. Vascular injuries may occur with even trivial trauma in atherosclerotic elderly patients. The most common vascular injury is to the axillary artery and may be suggested by weak distal pulses compared to the uninjured side, paresthesias, pallor, pulselessness, or an expanding hematoma. Neurovascular injuries can occur in nondisplaced and displaced fractures but are much higher (>50%) in displaced fractures.

DIAGNOSIS

Radiographs consisting of anteroposterior, lateral shoulder, and axillary views will diagnose most proximal humerus fractures and evaluate for accompanying glenohumeral dislocation.

Specific Injuries The most common fractures of the proximal humerus include the surgical neck and greater tuberosity. To guide treatment, the Neer system classifies fracture displacement into "parts." The proximal humerus is divided into four segments based on epiphyseal lines where fractures primarily occur: the articular surface of the humeral head; the greater tuberosity; the lesser tuberosity; and the shaft of the humerus (**Figure 271-21**). The displacement of a fracture fragment from the proximal humerus is called a "part." Parts are therefore not based on the number of fracture lines or segments. Rather, a "one-part" fracture is one in which the fragment is not displaced at all, is displaced <1 cm, or is not angulated >45 degrees. There can be multiple fragments, but if none of the fragments is displaced >1 cm or is angulated >45 degrees, the proximal humerus fracture is termed a "one-part" fracture. Approximately 50% of all proximal humerus fractures are one-part fractures.[41,42] Treatment of a one-part proximal humerus fracture generally consists of

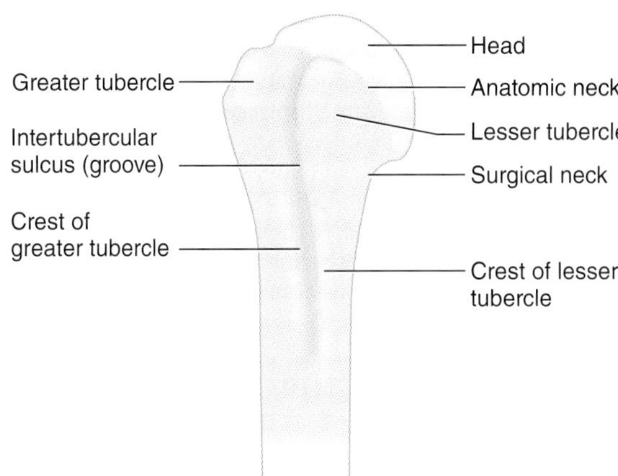

FIGURE 271-20. Proximal humerus. [Reproduced with permission from Pansky B: *Review of Gross Anatomy*, 6th ed. New York: McGraw Hill, 1995.]

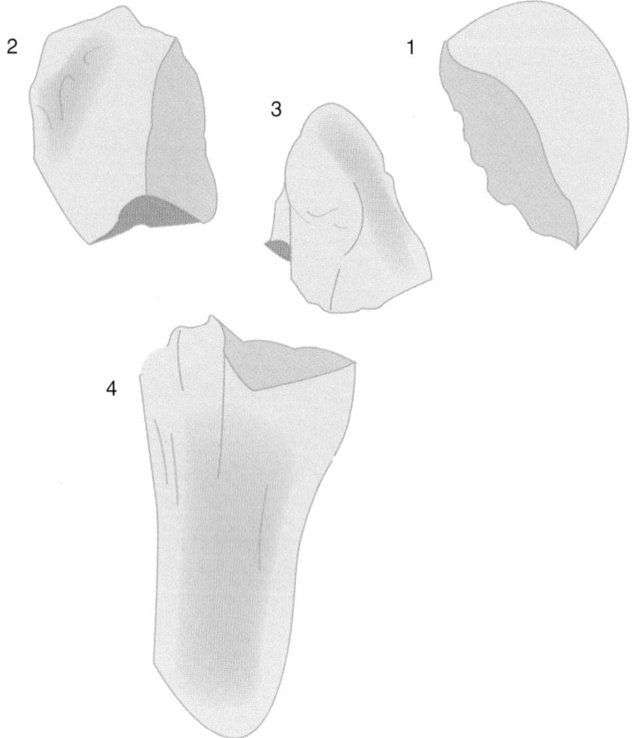

FIGURE 271-21. The four segments of the humerus according to the Neer classification: 1, articular surface of the humeral head; 2, greater tubercle; 3, lesser tubercle; 4, diaphysis or shaft of humerus. A one-part fracture is defined as a fracture fragment displaced by <1 cm or <45 degrees; two-, three-, and four-part fractures have more displacement and angulation.

immobilization (such as sling and swathe), ice, analgesics, and orthopedic referral. Early mobilization is important to avoid subsequent adhesive capsulitis and can be started when pain allows. The prognosis is generally good. All other proximal humerus fractures and fracture-dislocations require orthopedic consultation in the ED because they are more frequently associated with complications and are often difficult to manage. Closed reduction, operative treatment, or a combination of the two may be necessary.

Any fracture involving the anatomic neck or the articular surface may result in compromise of the blood supply to the articular segment of the humeral head. If ischemic necrosis of the articular segment occurs, insertion of a humeral head prosthesis may be required. Significantly angulated surgical neck fractures are a risk for neurovascular damage (axillary neurovascular structures as well as the brachial plexus) and should be immobilized and radiographed in the position of presentation.

Significant displacement of a greater tuberosity fracture implies a concomitant rotator cuff tear, with surgical repair often necessary for the active patient. Fracture of the lesser tuberosity should alert the examiner to a potential posterior shoulder dislocation.

Children may have significant displacement or separation of the proximal humeral epiphysis and need early orthopedic consultation for anatomic reduction if near skeletal maturity. Salter II injuries are most common after age 6 years old and will require closed reduction if >20 degrees of angulation is present. A shoulder spica is often used after reduction for unstable injuries, with sling and swathe immobilization for other injuries. If there is a question about the acceptability of angulation, consult the orthopedist.

HUMERAL SHAFT FRACTURES

ANATOMY

The humerus serves as the attachment site for the rotator cuff muscles, deltoid, pectoralis major, and coracobrachialis. Additionally, it is the site of origin of the biceps, triceps, and brachioradialis. The radial nerve courses along the spiral groove on the posterior aspect of the humerus.

Fractures of the humeral shaft occur in a bimodal age distribution, with peaks in the third and seventh decades of life, representing active young men and osteoporotic elderly women, respectively. Humeral shaft fractures may be caused by a direct blow that produces a bending force resulting in a transverse fracture. They may also be caused by an indirect mechanism, such as a fall on an outstretched hand that produces a torsion force, resulting in a spiral fracture. A combination of bending and torsion forces results in an oblique fracture, sometimes with comminution, producing the "butterfly" fragment. The humerus is also a common site of pathologic fractures, especially from metastatic breast cancer. Fractures in young children should raise suspicion of abuse.[43]

CLINICAL FEATURES

Clinical examination reveals localized tenderness, swelling, pain, and abnormal mobility or crepitus on palpation. Displaced fractures are associated with shortening of the upper extremity. Attention must be given to the initial neurovascular status. Complications may include injury to the brachial artery and vein, or the radial, ulnar, or median nerves. A radial nerve injury, which is the most common, may be manifested by weak wrist extension, wrist drop, or altered sensation at the dorsal thumb index web space. Fractures of the distal third are particularly prone to entrapment of the radial nerve, either as a result of the initial injury or after closed reduction. Neurovascular injuries require emergency orthopedic consultation.[44]

DIAGNOSIS

Radiographs should include two views of the humerus. Images of the shoulder and elbow should be obtained if additional injuries cannot be excluded.

FRACTURES OF THE MIDDLE THIRD OF THE HUMERUS

The most common site of fracture is the middle third of the humerus. Displacement of fracture fragments is the result of the insertions and actions of the various muscles (deltoid, biceps, triceps, supraspinatus, and pectoralis major) that act on the upper arm (**Figure 271-22**). Most closed fractures of the shaft of the humerus are managed nonoperatively, although treatment options vary. A 2012 Cochrane Review did not find any evidence to suggest outcome differences from surgery versus nonsurgical management.[45] Fractures with less than 20 degrees of angulation in the sagittal plane and less than 30 degrees of varus or valgus angulation and are shortened less than 2 to 3 cm often can be managed nonoperatively.[46] The treatment of uncomplicated fractures includes immobilization, ice, analgesia, and referral. Closed treatment options include the coaptation splint (sugar tong), hanging cast, and functional bracing. A simple sling and swathe are adequate for the emergency management of most such patients.

DISTAL HUMERUS FRACTURES

Distal humerus fractures require emergency orthopedic consultation. These fractures are complex given the anatomical relationship of the bony and neurovascular structures. Clinical examination should include evaluation of the radial, median, ulnar, and anterior and posterior interosseous nerves. See chapter 270 for a discussion of supracondylar fractures.

BRACHIAL PLEXUS INJURIES

ANATOMY

The brachial plexus (**Figure 271-23**) and its peripheral nerve branches are infraclavicular and lay anteromedial to the glenohumeral joint. Anatomically, the brachial plexus stems from the C4-T1 cervical roots and ultimately from the lateral, posterior, and medial cords. At the lateral border of the pectoralis minor, these cords ultimately form the five major peripheral nerves of the arm (musculocutaneous nerve, axillary nerve, radial nerve, median nerve, and ulnar nerve).[47] Traumatic brachial plexus lesions are the most common form of plexus injuries and can occur from

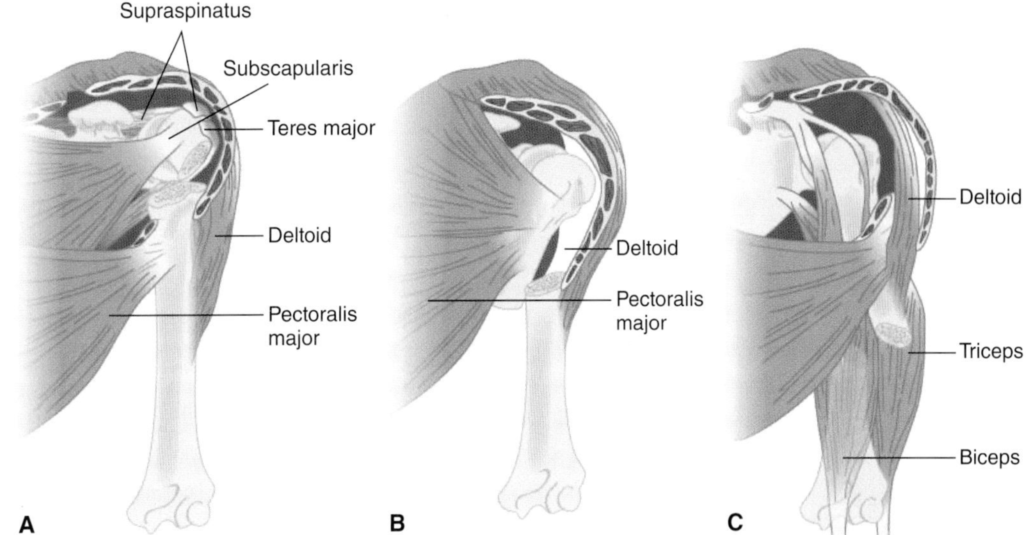

FIGURE 271-22. Humeral fractures anterior view. The actions of the muscles inserting on the humeral shaft determine fracture angulation and displacement. **A.** Angulation of fragments with fracture line distal to rotator cuff insertion. **B.** Angulation of fragments with fracture line distal to pectoralis major insertion. **C.** Angulation of fragments with fracture line distal to deltoid insertion.

penetrating, compression, or closed traction injuries. Injuries can be divided into supraclavicular (roots and trunks) or infraclavicular (cords and terminal nerves) injuries.

CLINICAL FEATURES

High-speed motor vehicle or motorcycle crashes result in traction injuries as nerves are stretched longitudinally, with simultaneous traction of the arm and opposite distraction of the head.[47,48] Penetrating trauma and surgical interventions can also lead to a disruption of the nerves. The initial identification of brachial plexus injuries is often overshadowed by the presence of other severe injuries to, for example, the head, chest, and vasculature. In addition to neurologic impairment, neuropathic pain in the arm is frequently present. Significant swelling and soft tissue injury to the neck and shoulder girdle suggest traumatic forces sufficient to injure the brachial plexus. The accumulation of cerebrospinal fluid from avulsed spinal roots may cause swelling in the posterior triangle. Horner's syndrome (ipsilateral ptosis, miosis, and anhidrosis of the face) may be present due to adjacent ganglion damage. However, brachial plexus injury may not be clinically apparent until a responsive patient can indicate the extent of motor and sensory deficits, days to weeks after initial stabilization and treatment. Arm pain that is constant and burning in character is common. The pain is usually worst in the distal parts of the arm and hand, typically in a nondermatomal distribution.

DIAGNOSIS

Upper limb and shoulder girdle motor and sensory deficits define the extent of damage to the brachial plexus. Adduction and internal rotation of the shoulder indicate weakness of the deltoid and infraspinatus

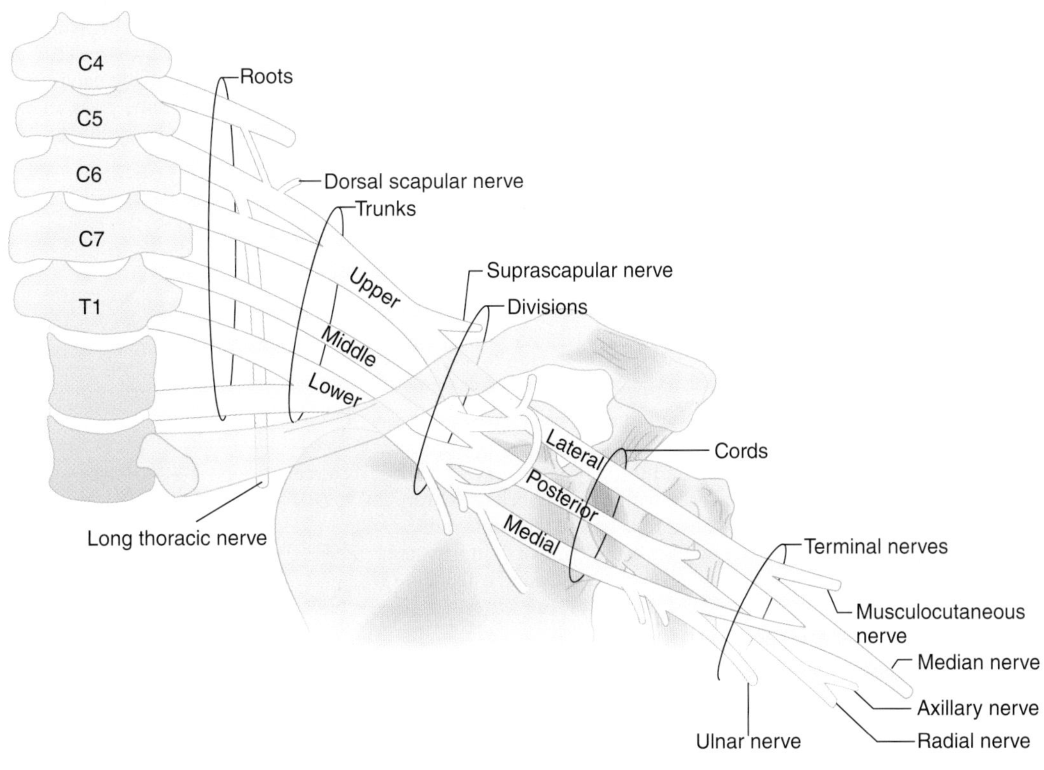

FIGURE 271-23. Brachial plexus.

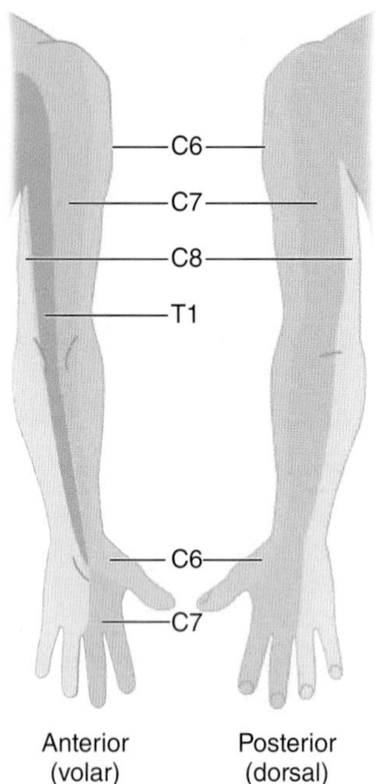

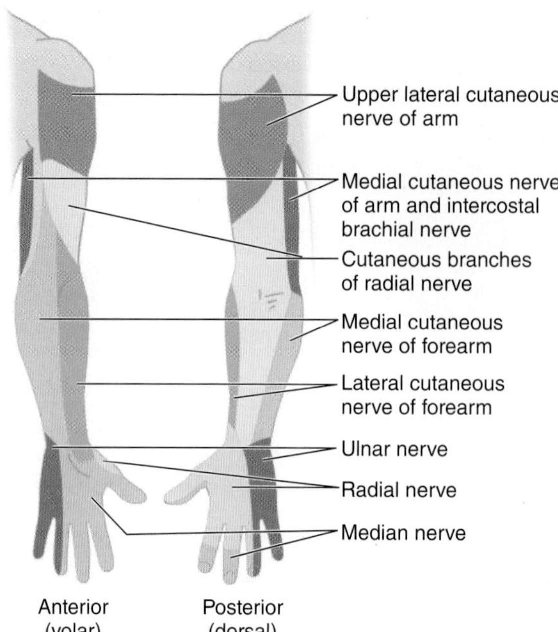

FIGURE 271-24. Sensory distribution of the brachial plexus.

muscles (C5), whereas elbow extension is due to weakness of the biceps (C6), and flexion of the digits and wrists is due to weakness of the extensors (C7). The sensory distributions of the cervical roots and the peripheral nerves are shown in **Figure 271-24**.

MRI and CT myelography are common radiographic imaging procedures. Electromyographic and nerve conduction velocity studies may aid in diagnosis, and surgical exploration of the area may be necessary. The delineation of pre- and postganglionic injury may not be possible until Wallerian degeneration is completed 2 weeks after injury. Treatment and prognosis will depend on the location and extent of nerve damage.

REFERENCES

The complete reference list is available online at www.TintinalliEM.com.

CHAPTER 272

Pelvis Injuries

Melissa A. Barton
H. Scott Derstine
Ciara J. Barclay-Buchanan

EPIDEMIOLOGY

Most pelvic fractures are secondary to automobile passenger or pedestrian accidents but are also the result of minor falls in older persons and from major falls or crush injuries. The mortality rate from all pelvic fractures is approximately 5%. However, with complex pelvic fractures, the mortality rate is about 20%.[1] Isolated fractures of the pubic rami are likely in the elderly who sustain a low-energy mechanism of injury, such as falling off a chair, and are due to underlying fragility and osteopenia.[2]

ANATOMY AND BIOMECHANICS

The major functions of the pelvis are protection, support, and hematopoiesis. The pelvis consists of the sacrum and coccyx as well as the bilateral "innominate bones," which are comprised of three separate bones: the ischium, ilium, and pubis. These bones provide pelvic stability that is further supported by the strong posterior sacroiliac (SI), sacrotuberous, and sacrospinous ligaments (**Figures 272-1 and 272-2**). A small amount of pelvic stability is also provided by the pubic symphysis. The bladder lies in close proximity to the symphysis, as does the rectum to the sacrum, putting each of the structures at risk for injury in a trauma patient.

Incorporated in the pelvic structure are five joints that allow some movement in the bony ring. The lumbosacral, sacroiliac, and sacrococcygeal joints, as well as the symphysis pubis, allow little movement. The acetabulum is a ball-and-socket joint that is divided into three portions: the iliac portion, or superior dome, is the chief weight-bearing surface; the inner wall consists of the pubis and is thin and easily fractured; and the posterior acetabulum is derived from the thick ischium. Any single break in the ring will yield a stable injury without significant risk of displacement, whereas the occurrence of two breaks in the ring is considered an unstable pelvis.

The pelvis is extremely vascular. The iliac artery and venous trunks pass near the sacroiliac joints bilaterally. The nerve supply through the

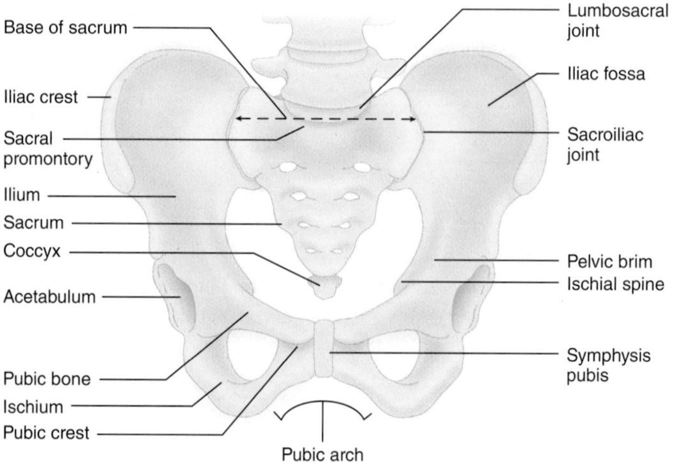

FIGURE 272-1. Bones and joints of the pelvis.

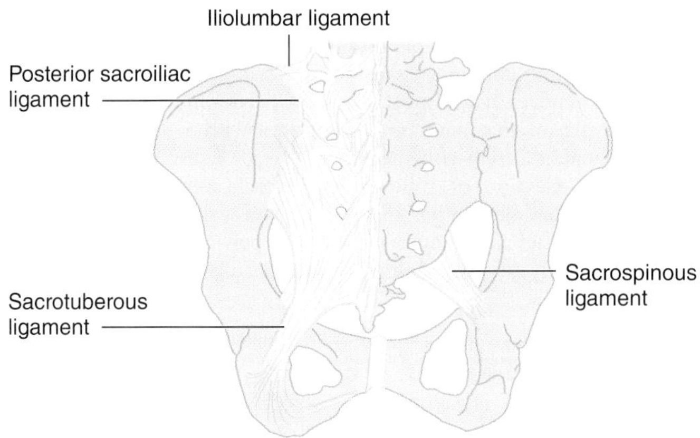

FIGURE 272-2. Pelvic ligaments.

pelvis is derived from the lumbar and sacral plexuses. Injury to the pelvis may produce deficits at any level from the nerve root to small peripheral branches (**Figure 272-3**). The lower urinary tract is contained in the pelvis (**Figure 272-4**). In the adult, the bladder lies behind the symphysis and pubic bones, and the peritoneum covers the dome and base posteriorly. The location of the bladder and the degree of peritoneal reflection are determined by urine content. The lower GI tract housed in the pelvis includes a small portion of the descending colon, the sigmoid colon, the rectum, and the anus. In women, the uterus and vagina are also housed in the bony pelvis.

CLINICAL FEATURES

HISTORY

Consider the possibility of pelvic fracture in every patient with serious blunt trauma (e.g., falls from a height, pedestrian hit by a motor vehicle, crush injury, individuals ejected from a vehicle). Determine the mechanism of injury and the prehospital evaluation and treatment. Ask the patient about areas of pain, last urination or defecation, present bladder sensation, and last solid and fluid intake. In addition, determine the time of the last menses or the presence of pregnancy, brief past medical history, current medications, and allergies.

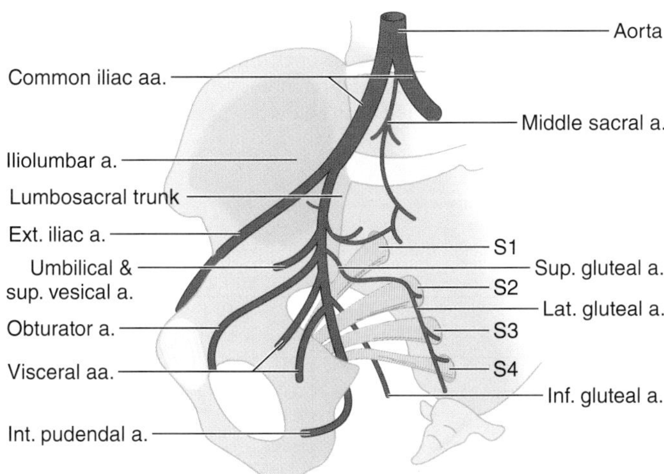

FIGURE 272-3. Arterial and nerve supply of the pelvis. a. = artery; aa. = arteries; Ext. = exterior; Inf. = inferior; Int. = interior; Lat. = lateral; sup. = superior. [Reproduced with permission from Pansky B: Review of Gross Anatomy, 6th ed. Copyright © 1995, McGraw-Hill, New York.]

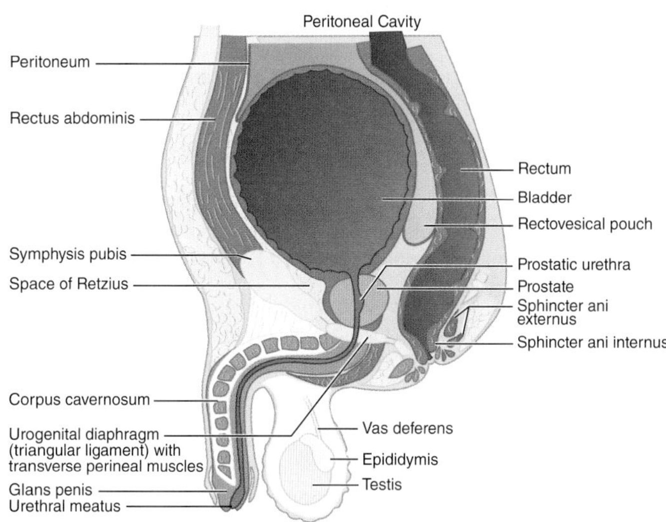

FIGURE 272-4. Sagittal section of the male pelvis showing the relation of the full bladder.

PHYSICAL EXAMINATION

In patients who are awake and alert, a careful physical examination is likely very sensitive (93% in one study) for the diagnosis of a pelvic fracture.[3] Symptoms and signs of pelvic injuries vary from local pain and tenderness, or inability to bear weight, to pelvic instability and severe shock. Unexplained hypotension may be the only sign of a major pelvic disruption.

Serious Injury For a patient with a serious or high-energy mechanism of injury, examine for abdominal tenderness, perineal and pelvic ecchymoses, lacerations, and deformities. Scrotal hematoma (Destot's sign) indicates a pelvic fracture. Leg length discrepancy or rotational deformity of the lower extremity without an obvious fracture suggests a pelvic fracture. Evidence of blood at the urethral meatus suggests a urethral injury.

Perform **focused abdominal sonogram for trauma** (FAST) examination as an adjunct to the physical examination during the primary trauma survey in any unstable patient or when the mechanism of injury could suggest a pelvic fracture. Fluid in the peritoneum can suggest solid organ injury, but fluid in the pelvis can also lead the clinician to suspect a pelvic fracture prior to radiologic confirmation.

Do not perform compressive pelvic maneuvers in a patient with shock or an obvious pelvis fracture because movement of unstable fractures could produce further injury and blood loss.

However, some type of assessment for pelvic instability should be done on every trauma patient, which could include only visual inspection in patients with obvious pelvic fractures, physical examination by pelvic rim compression, or radiologic survey. Gentle downward and medial manual compression of the pelvis over the iliac wings should be performed only **once** during the trauma survey. Repeated manipulation of the pelvic ring on any patient with a suspected pelvic fracture can increase the severity of injury, resulting in greater blood loss. Rectal examination may detect superior or posterior displacement of the prostate, rectal injury, or an abnormal bony prominence or large hematoma or tenderness along the suspected fracture line. Proctoscopic and/or bimanual pelvic examination may be required to fully assess mucosal tears in order to properly diagnosis open fractures. Such injuries increase the risk of infection at the fracture site and sepsis.[4] Decrease in anal sphincter tone may suggest neurologic injury. Carefully evaluate lower extremity pulses and sensation. If a pelvic fracture is found, assume intra-abdominal, retroperitoneal, gynecologic, and urologic injuries until proven otherwise.

Stable Patient and Low Mechanism of Injury In stable patients and those with a low-energy mechanism of injury, such as in the elderly patient who falls from a seated position, examine the entire spine and the abdomen. Palpate for tenderness along the pelvic bony structures—the iliac crests, pubic rami, sacrum, and coccyx. Compress the pelvis, lateral to medial, through the iliac crests as well as through the greater trochanters. Additionally, compress the pelvic ring from anterior to posterior through the symphysis pubis and iliac crests. Evaluate lower extremity pulses, motor function, and sensation.

IMAGING

The initial stabilization of the patient takes priority over obtaining radiographs. If not already done, perform a FAST scan to identify intraperitoneal bleeding.

In patients with suspected hip fracture, a standard anteroposterior pelvis radiograph is often used to evaluate for bony injury. If there is no tenderness to palpation in an otherwise stable, alert patient, then a plain pelvic radiograph is not indicated.[5,6] Indications for a pelvis radiograph include a hemodynamically unstable blunt trauma patient, pelvic tenderness, or other finding on physical examination concerning for pelvic fracture. With an ***unstable*** blunt trauma patient, a pelvic radiograph can be used to identify a pelvic fracture quickly, allow early stabilization maneuvers, and mobilize resources for emergent angiography. Routine pelvic radiographs are not needed in ***stable*** patients who will undergo an emergency CT scan of the abdomen and pelvis anyway.[7-10]

CT is the gold standard for evaluating pelvic injuries. **CT is more sensitive than plain radiographs for the detection of pelvic fractures; plain radiographs rarely change the management plan in stable patients. Compared with CT, pelvic radiographs have a sensitivity of ≤85% for identifying pelvic fractures in blunt trauma patients.**[2] CT is also superior to radiography in evaluating pelvic ring instability.[7-9,11] Therefore, indications for CT include a high clinical suspicion for pelvic fracture but negative pelvic radiographs, or pelvic fractures on plain films with need to evaluate for additional pelvic fractures and instability. Contrast-enhanced CT provides useful information about posterior pelvic ring ligamentous injuries, contrast extravasation, pelvic hematoma, and retroperitoneal bleeding. Contrast extravasation on CT scan is 80% to 90% sensitive for the identification of arterial bleeding.[12,13]

If additional radiograph views are needed for stable patients, obtain lateral views, anteroposterior views of either hemipelvis, internal and external oblique views of the hemipelvis, or inlet and outlet views of the pelvis. An inlet view shows anterior-posterior displacement of ring fractures. An outlet view shows superior-inferior displacement. Oblique views of the hemipelvis are true anteroposterior and lateral views of the acetabulum. Sacral fractures may be difficult to visualize on plain films, so obtain CT or three-dimensional reconstruction of CT images when there is concern.[14]

Extremes of age require different approaches for pelvic imaging. Up to half of elderly patients with a low-energy mechanism and pubic ramus fracture may have an associated posterior pelvic ring disruption demonstrated on CT scan.[15] Pain on sacral palpation may suggest posterior ring disruption and indicate the need for pelvic CT scan. This often overlooked finding may contribute to the fact that one third of the elderly with isolated rami fractures do not return to their previous living independence or may fail conservative treatment for pain management.[15] Most children with a low-energy mechanism and normal examination do not usually require even plain radiographs, because pelvic fractures are rare in young children. Avulsion/iliac wing fractures from sports injuries are reportedly the most common pelvic injuries in children.[16] Clinical scenarios that have been associated with a pelvic fracture in children include a high-risk mechanism (e.g., motor vehicle collision with/without ejection or rollover; automobile versus pedestrian or bicycle) combined with either a Glasgow coma scale score <14 or pelvic tenderness.[17] Other associations with serious pelvic fractures in children include medically complex children, preexisting bone disease, or developmental delay.[16]

PELVIC FRACTURE PATTERNS

Pelvic fractures include those that involve a break in the pelvic ring, fractures of a single bone without a break in the pelvic ring, and acetabular fractures. Pelvic fractures involving a break in the pelvic ring can be complex and difficult to classify.

The most clinically useful classification, the Young-Burgess Pelvis Fracture Classification System, is presented in a simplified version in **Table 272-1**. This system differentiates fracture patterns based on mechanism of injury and direction of causative force. Incidence of complications (i.e., urogenital and vascular) is correlated with the fracture pattern, making identification of the type more clinically significant and useful.

There are three main types of pelvic fracture patterns: lateral compression, anterior-posterior compression (open-book), and vertical shear. The different injury types may be suggested by history but may often be differentiated radiographically. The alignment of pubic rami fractures is a clue to the mechanism and direction of force. In general, horizontal fractures suggest lateral compression injury, whereas vertical fractures point to vertical shear force. Open-book fractures point to an anteroposterior injury. Based on the recognition of the fracture pattern, one can then predict the likelihood of severe hemorrhage or urogenital injury (Table 272-1).

LATERAL COMPRESSION FRACTURE

Lateral compression fractures are the most common mechanism, accounting for 60% to 70% of pelvic fractures with an overall mortality rate of 8%.[18] Motor vehicle crashes in which a car is broadsided or a pedestrian is struck from the side are examples. At a minimum, a pubic ramus will be fractured. As the pelvis is further compressed and the degree of injury progresses, the sacroiliac joint is crushed, leading to disruption of the posterior ligaments, fracture of the sacrum, and rotation of the contralateral hemipelvis. (**Figure 272-5**).

ANTERIOR-POSTERIOR COMPRESSION OR OPEN-BOOK FRACTURE

Anterior-posterior compression, or open-book fracture, accounts for about 25% of severe injuries. A head-on motor vehicle crash is the classic example. The force is delivered in an anteroposterior direction (arrow in

TABLE 272-1 Abbreviated Young-Burgess Classification System and Potential Incidence of Complications

Category	Characteristics	Severe Hemorrhage (%)	Bladder Rupture (%)	Urethral Injury (%)
Lateral compression fractures	Transverse fracture of pubic rami, ipsilateral or contralateral to posterior injury	60	20	20
Anterior-posterior fractures (open-book)	Symphyseal diastasis and/or longitudinal rami fractures *Secondarily injured structures vary based on severity of AP pelvic fracture*			
	Minimal widening of SI joint with intact posterior ligaments	1	8	12
	Complete SI joint widening with disruption of posterior ligaments	53	14	36
Vertical shear fractures	Separation of symphysis and/or SI joint with vertical displacement anteriorly or posteriorly, occasionally through iliac wing and/or sacrum	75	15	25
Mixed patterns	Combination of other injury patterns, LC/VS being the most common	58	16	21

Abbreviations: AP = anteroposterior; LC = lateral compression; SI = sacroiliac; VS = vertical shear.

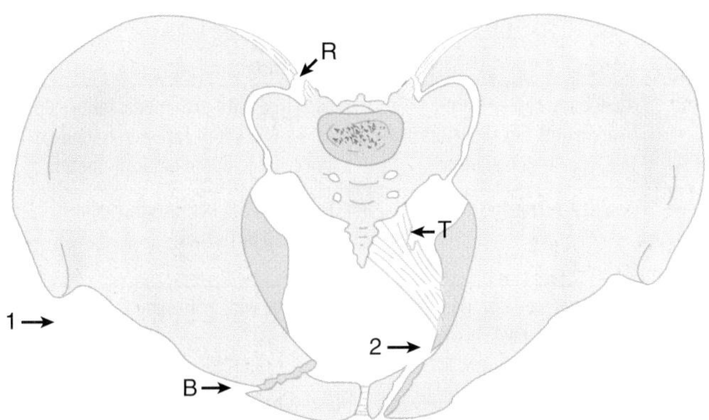

FIGURE 272-5. Lateral compression fracture (*arrows 1 and 2*) with rupture of posterior sacroiliac ligaments (R), sacrospinous/sacrotuberous complex (T), and rupture of pubic ramus (B).

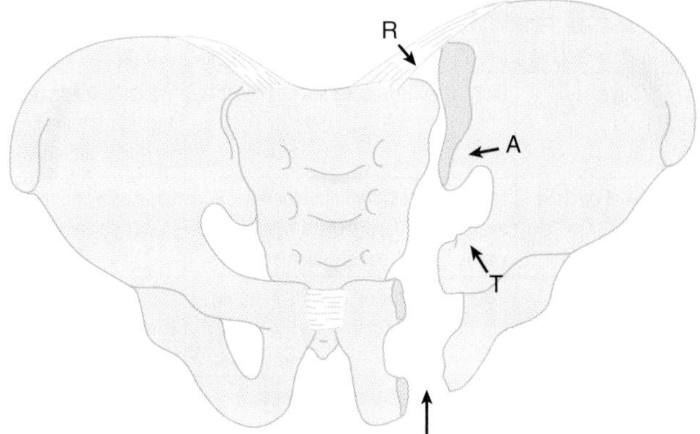

FIGURE 272-7. Vertical shear fracture. Injury vector is delivered in a vertical plane (*arrow*). There is injury to the posterior (R) and anterior (A) sacroiliac ligaments and sacrospinous/sacrotuberous (T) ligaments.

Figure 272-6), tending to "open" the pelvis. This splays the pubic symphysis and ruptures the sacral ligaments (**Figure 272-6**). Finally, total disruption of the sacroiliac joint will occur because of the wide "opening" of the pelvis. All supporting ligament groups, including the posterior sacroiliac ligaments, can be disrupted.

VERTICAL SHEAR FRACTURE

The least common mechanism is **vertical shear fractures**, which are typified by a fall or jump from a height, accounting for approximately 5% of fractures. Combinations of injury patterns can make up the other 20% to 25% of injuries. In vertical shear injury, the injury force vector is delivered in a vertical plane (**Figure 272-7**). Fractures of the pubic rami are usually seen anteriorly, whereas fractures of the sacrum, sacroiliac joint, or iliac wing are usually seen posteriorly. Any of the pelvic ligaments may be disrupted.

AVULSION AND SINGLE-BONE PELVIC FRACTURES

Isolated, closed avulsion fractures of the pelvis or single-bone, closed pelvic fractures are more commonly encountered in the ED than pelvic ring disruptions. It is important to know which of these subsets of fractures require further diagnostic testing, orthopedic consultation, or admission.

Isolated fractures of the anterior superior iliac spine, anterior inferior iliac spine, ischial tuberosity, pubic ramus, body of the ischium, iliac wing, sacrum, or coccyx typically do not disrupt the pelvic ring and, as a result, typically do not require surgical repair (**Figure 272-8** and **Table 272-2**). Most of these fractures require only appropriate analgesia, crutches, either bed rest or non–weight-bearing status, and orthopedic follow-up on an outpatient basis.

Simple fractures in the elderly may not be as benign as at first glance. If indicated by physical exam or mechanism of injury, obtain a CT scan of the pelvis with bone windows to detect occult posterior pelvic ring disruption that will alter management (**Figures 272-9** and **272-10**).[15] Although isolated pelvic ramus fractures are frequently due to low-impact trauma (e.g., fall from standing) in the elderly, isolated pelvic fractures still result in an increased rates of hospital admission, morbidity, need for living assistance after hospital discharge, and overall mortality at 1 year.[19]

Pay special attention to isolated fractures of either the sacrum or iliac wing due to the tremendous amount of force that has occurred. If there is concern for associated injuries, then a more extensive evaluation is mandated with admission for observation.

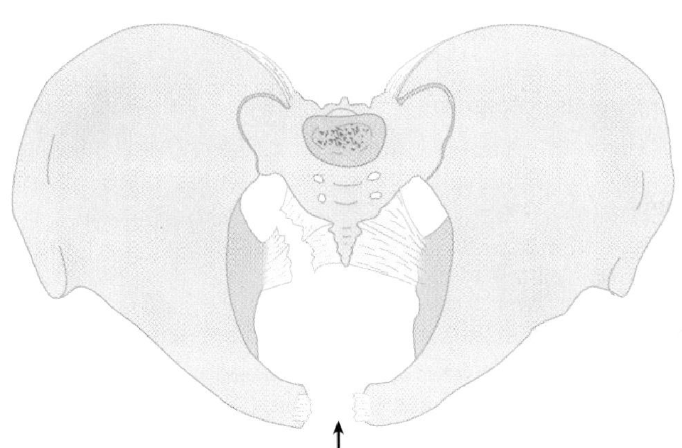

FIGURE 272-6. Open-book fracture, with opening of the anterior pelvis (*arrow*) and rupture of the sacral ligaments.

ACETABULAR FRACTURES

Acetabular fractures are usually secondary to motor vehicle crashes. The fracture force is either transmitted laterally through the hip or posteriorly through the femur as with a knee-versus-dashboard mechanism. Acetabular fractures are seen commonly with other injuries, including pelvic, femur, and hip fractures and dislocations (**Figure 272-11A**), and

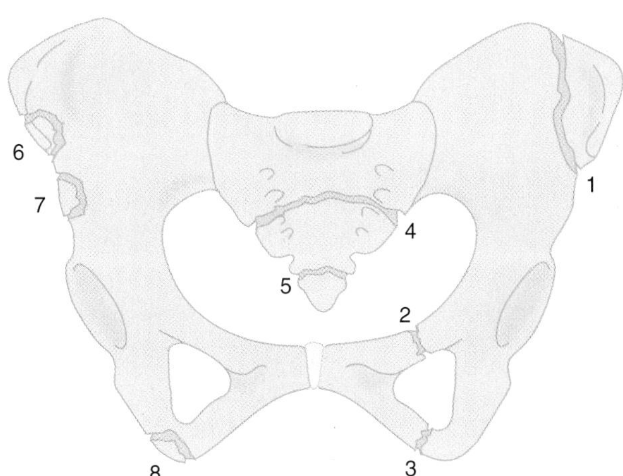

FIGURE 272-8. Avulsion fractures of the pelvis. (1) Iliac wing fracture (Duverney fracture). (2) Superior pubic ramus fracture. (3) Inferior pubic ramus fracture. (4) Transverse sacral fracture. (5) Coccyx fracture. (6) Anterior superior iliac spine avulsion. (7) Anterior inferior iliac spine avulsion. (8) Ischial tuberosity avulsion.

TABLE 272-2 Avulsion and Single Bone Fractures

Fracture	Description/Mechanism of Injury	Clinical Findings/Associated Injuries	Treatment	Disposition and Follow-Up
Iliac wing (Duverney) fracture	Direct trauma, usually lateral to medial	Swelling, tenderness over iliac wing; abdominal pain; ileus; acetabular fractures; serious injury infrequent	Analgesics, non–weight-bearing until hip abductors pain-free, usually nonoperative	Discharge with orthopedic follow-up in 1–2 wk; admit for open fracture or concerning abdominal examination
Single ramus of pubis or ischium	Fall or direct trauma in elderly; exercise-induced stress fracture in young or in pregnant women	Local pain and tenderness; may have inability to ambulate	Analgesics, crutches	Discharge with PCP or orthopedic follow-up in 1–2 wk
Ischium body	External trauma or from fall in sitting position; least common pelvic fracture	Local pain and tenderness; pain with hamstring movement	Analgesics, bed rest, donut-ring cushion, crutches	Discharge with orthopedic follow-up in 1–2 wk
Sacral fracture	Transverse fractures from direct anteroposterior trauma; upper transverse fractures from fall in flexed position	Pain on rectal examination; sacral root injury with upper transverse fractures; vertical fractures may transect the pelvic ring	Analgesics, bed rest, surgery may be needed for displaced fractures or neurologic injury	Discharge with orthopedic follow-up in 1–2 wk; orthopedic consultation for displaced fractures or neurologic deficits
Coccyx fracture	Fall in sitting position; more common in women	Pain, tenderness over sacral region; pain on compression during rectal examination	Analgesics, bed rest, stool softeners, sitz baths, donut-ring cushion	PCP or orthopedic follow-up in 2–3 wk; surgical excision of fracture fragment if chronic pain
Anterior-superior iliac spine	Forceful sartorius muscle contraction (e.g., adolescent sprinters)	Pain with hip flexion and abduction	Analgesics, bed rest for 3–4 wk with hip flexed and abducted, crutches	Discharge with orthopedic follow-up in 1–2 wk
Anterior-inferior iliac spine	Forceful rectus femoris muscle contraction (e.g., adolescent soccer players)	Pain in groin; pain with hip flexion	Analgesics, bed rest for 3–4 wk with hip flexed, crutches	Discharge with orthopedic follow-up in 1–2 wk
Ischial tuberosity	Forceful contraction of hamstrings	Pain with sitting or flexing the thigh	Analgesics, bed rest for 3–4 wk in extension, external rotation, crutches	Discharge with orthopedic follow-up in 1–2 wk

Abbreviation: PCP = primary care physician.

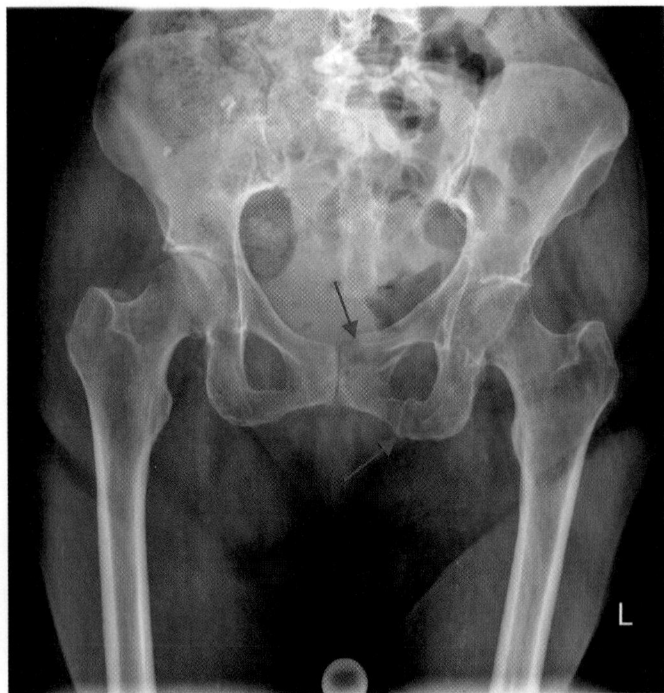

FIGURE 272-9. Fracture of superior ramus (top *arrow*) as the result of fall from standing. Healed fracture of the inferior ramus is noted as well (bottom arrow). [Photo used with permission of Patrick Studer, MD.]

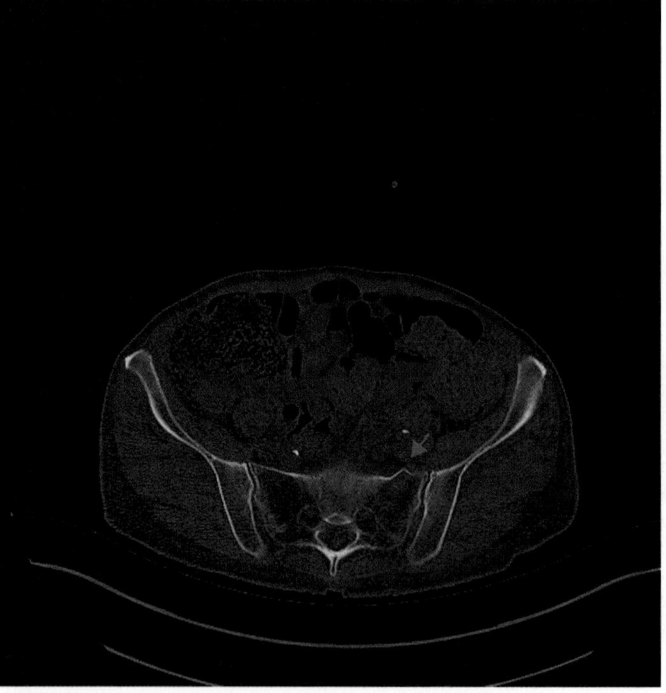

FIGURE 272-10. Same patient with fracture of left lateral sacral body discovered on CT scan. [Photo used with permission of Patrick Studer, MD.]

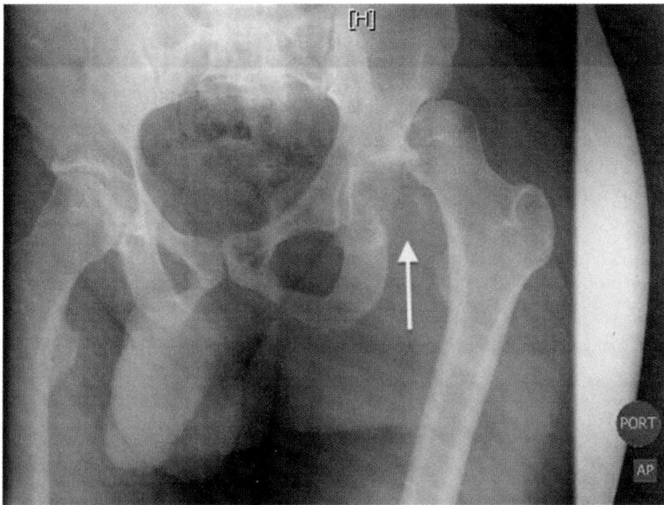

A

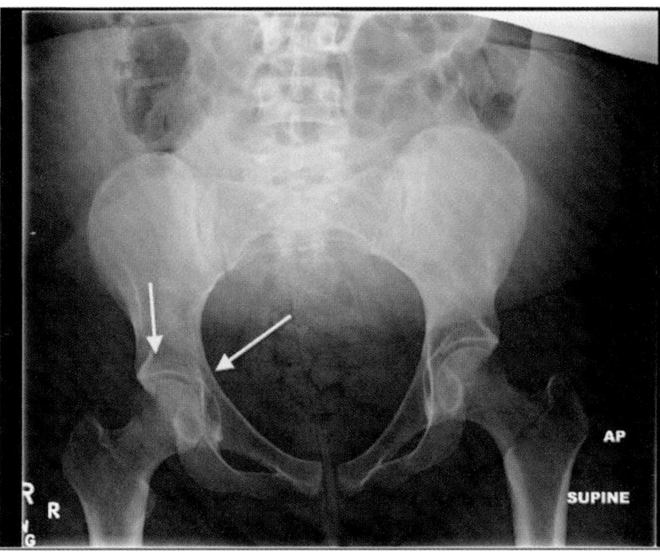

B

FIGURE 272-11. A. Left posterior hip dislocation with avulsed fracture fragments of the posterior acetabular rim. B. Multiple curvilinear lucencies demonstrating nondisplaced fractures (*arrows*) of the right acetabulum and right ischium. Pubic symphysis is also slightly widened.

knee injuries. However, these fractures may be subtle and, as a result, necessitate careful inspection on x-ray (**Figure 272-11B**). If an acetabular fracture is suspected, it can be evaluated with an anteroposterior film, a 45-degree iliac oblique, and a 45-degree obturator oblique view—together known as *Judet views*. **CT is more sensitive than radiography in detecting acetabular injury.**[20] Also, CT is able to give more detailed information about the displacement of fracture fragments, degree of comminution, and other information that is useful in preoperative planning.

Patients with acetabular fractures require hospital admission and orthopedic consultation. Look for associated visceral, neurovascular, and orthopedic injuries. Sciatic nerve injury is a common complication.

TREATMENT

Prevent movement of fracture segments, particularly in the hemodynamically unstable patient. The pelvis can be temporarily yet quickly stabilized with a bed sheet or other pelvic binding device to reduce pelvic volume and stabilize fracture ends.[21-23] The simplest technique is the application of either a folded bed sheet secured with towel clips or a commercially manufactured binder that is tightly wrapped around the pelvis at the level of the greater trochanters. A pelvic binder can decrease the volume of the pelvis and, in turn, help diminish blood loss for both open-book and vertical shear fractures. Lateral compression pelvic fractures would not benefit from the application of a pelvic binder because they are already rotated internally; in fact, these patients may be harmed from further lateral compression.[24]

Provide resuscitation as needed with crystalloid, blood, and blood products. **Retroperitoneal bleeding may complicate pelvic fractures. Up to 4 L of blood can be accommodated in the pelvis, until vascular pressure is overcome and tamponade occurs.** Most bleeding is due to low-pressure venous bleeding and bleeding from mobile bone edges. Predictors for the need for either a transfusion or a therapeutic intervention due to hemorrhage include: (1) initial hematocrit less than 30%, (2) presence of pelvic hematoma on CT scan, or (3) a systolic blood pressure of less than 90 mm Hg upon arrival.[25] Presence of any of these factors mandates close observation of the patient in an intensive care setting.[25] Moreover, a recent prospective study showed that base deficit <6 mmol/L or worsening base deficit >2 mmol/L while in the ED also significantly correlated with the need for either angiography or laparotomy.[26]

FAST, CT, AND PELVIC FRACTURE

In hemodynamically unstable trauma patients with pelvic fractures, carefully evaluate for other sources of blood loss. Patients who have sustained a pelvic fracture from a significant mechanism of injury should undergo a thoraco-abdomino-pelvic CT scan even if the FAST is negative. In the presence of pelvic fracture and serious mechanism blunt trauma, FAST-negative patients are still very likely to have concomitant visceral injury.[27]

If the FAST examination reveals free intraperitoneal fluid (**Figure 272-12**), then CT scan is also needed to determine the next treatment step. The FAST false-positive rate for intraperitoneal hemorrhage in patients with pelvic ring disruption can be up to 30%.[28,29] Distortion of the anatomy from fractures, retroperitoneal bleeding, urine from ruptured bladder, or pelvic hematomas may result in fluid collections that mimic free intraperitoneal fluid. The sensitivity and specificity of FAST for free peritoneal blood in major pelvic injury appear to be related to the severity of the pelvic fracture.[28,29]

One study reported the overall sensitivity and specificity of FAST to detect free peritoneal fluid in major pelvic injury to be 81% and 87%, respectively.[29] The fluid was blood in 76% and urine in 19%.[29] Moderate to large free fluid as evidenced by fluid noted in two or more regions of

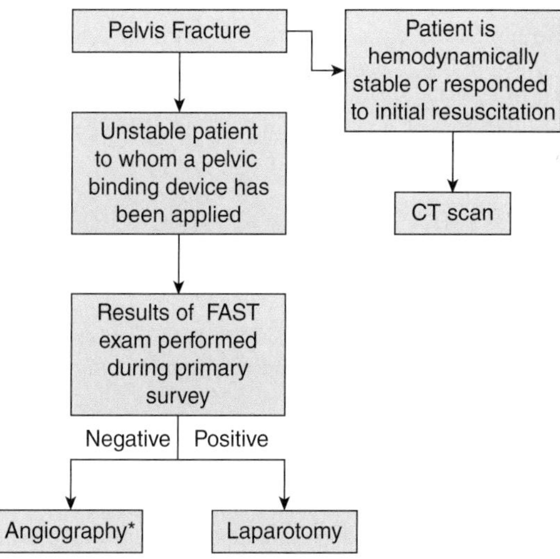

FIGURE 272-12. Suggested algorithm for pelvic fracture treatment. FAST = focused abdominal sonogram for trauma; OR = operating room.

the FAST exam is reported to be associated with the need for hemorrhage control, either by laparotomy or angiography.[30]

ANGIOGRAPHY, EMBOLIZATION, AND EXTERNAL FIXATION

If a patient with a pelvic fracture is hemodynamically unstable and other sources of bleeding (e.g., splenic or liver laceration) have been excluded through CT scan or laparotomy, treatment options include angiography with embolization, with or without external fixation of the pelvic fracture. Angiographic embolization is effective at controlling arterial bleeding, and external fixation is thought to be effective at controlling venous bleeding.[31,32] Both may be needed to control hemorrhage.

Shock and death are generally due to arterial rather than venous bleeding.[12,13,33,34] Arterial bleeding can occur in all types of pelvic fractures yet does so in only 10% to 15% of cases.[31] The arteries involved are typically branches of the internal iliac system, with the superior gluteal artery and the obturator artery being the most common (Figure 272-2). Hemorrhage from pelvic fractures refractory to resuscitation is more likely arterial than venous in origin; angiography and embolization can control arterial hemorrhage in most patients.[31-33] **Consider angiography early in a hemodynamically unstable patient with a pelvic fracture, after other sources of bleeding have been excluded.**

Contrast extravasation on CT is considered by many to be an indication for angiography to evaluate for an arterial source of bleeding that may be amenable to embolization.[12,13,32,35] Some protocols advocate angiography based on hemodynamic status, the need for ongoing blood transfusion, or in patients who meet certain blood transfusion amounts.[13,31] No intervention is needed for nearly half of all patients who demonstrate a pelvic blush on CT scan without clinical signs of ongoing bleeding.[36] The need for arterial embolization has a positive predictive value of 39% for death in open pelvis fractures, as noted in one recent study.[4]

Another hemorrhage control method used in the treatment of pelvic fractures is extraperitoneal packing. This technique involves surgically placing packing in the pelvis to reduce the potential space needed to tamponade bleeding. Consider this treatment option for an unstable patient who is bleeding secondary to a significant pelvis fracture in a hospital where angiography is not readily available, when a laparotomy is needed prior to angiography, or the patient is in extremis and needs quick stabilization prior to angiography.[25]

The definitive treatment of pelvic fractures occurs once the patient has been stabilized and after other associated injuries have been addressed. All pelvic fractures require orthopedic consultation and admission, even in the most stable of patients. Elderly patients with simple pubic ramus fractures typically require admission for pain control, observation for complications, and physical therapy for ambulation. The exact treatment of pelvic fractures is guided by fracture location and pelvic stability. Fractures that disrupt the pelvic ring need open reduction and internal fixation within 5 to 14 days of injury.[37] The decision as to which service to which to admit the patient will vary between hospitals and depend on multiple factors including the presence of a trauma surgery service, volume of orthopedic cases, comorbidities of the patient, and absence of other significant injuries.[38]

COMPLICATIONS OF PELVIC FRACTURES

Acute complications and associated injuries of pelvic fractures include urogynecologic injury, rectal injury, ruptured diaphragm, and nerve root injury. Pelvic fractures can also have long-term effects, including chronic pain, sexual dysfunction, and persistent functional disability.

UROGYNECOLOGIC INJURY

If a urethral injury is suspected clinically, perform retrograde urethrography before placing a Foley catheter. Urinary tract injuries are discussed in greater detail in chapter 265, "Genitourinary Trauma." Gynecologic injuries are uncommon with pelvic trauma. Vaginal laceration can occur with anterior pelvic fractures. Perform a bimanual pelvic examination on women with pelvic fractures. If blood is detected, a speculum examination is needed to identify vaginal hematoma, laceration, or urethral bleeding.

RECTAL INJURY

Rectal injuries are uncommon and are usually associated with urinary injuries and ischial fractures. Diagnosis is by careful rectal examination or by proctoscopy, during which gross blood is found in the rectum. Treatment includes early diverting colostomy with washout of the distal colon and presacral space drainage. Antibiotics that cover gram-negative organisms should be administered as soon as the injury is discovered.

NERVE ROOT INJURY

Nerve root or peripheral nerve injuries can occur because of traction, pressure from hemorrhage, callus or fibrous tissue, and impingement laceration by bone fragments. The onset of symptoms and signs may be delayed, but deficits usually follow a nerve root pattern. Lumbar nerve root injuries are associated with sacroiliac joint dislocation or fracture and longitudinal displacement of the fracture.[14] Sacral root injuries are associated with transverse fractures of S1 and S2 as can be seen secondary to trauma from a suicidal jump (Figure 272-4).[14]

REFERENCES

The complete reference list is available online at www.TintinalliEM.com.

CHAPTER 273 Hip and Femur Injuries

Mark Steele
Amy M. Stubbs

INTRODUCTION AND EPIDEMIOLOGY

Injuries to the hip and femur are common, occurring most often in the elderly population secondary to falls. Hip fractures are a significant and costly public health concern. Age, race, and gender are important risk factors for hip injuries; the incidence is more than two times greater in women than in men.[1]

Morbidity and mortality from hip and femur fractures are due to complications from prolonged immobilization, with venous thromboembolism being the most common complication. Patients with hip fracture have a five- to almost eightfold increased risk of all-cause mortality in the first 3 months after the injury, and increased mortality persists for years afterward. Another significant portion of patients will have markedly decreased functional capacity. Advanced age, male gender, and comorbidities all increase mortality risk following hip fracture.[2]

This chapter discusses the diagnosis and ED management of fractures of the hip and proximal femur, fractures of the femoral shaft, and anterior and posterior hip dislocations. Fractures involving the femoral condyles are discussed in chapter 274, Knee Injuries.

ANATOMY AND PATHOPHYSIOLOGY

For purposes of this chapter, we define the hip as the anatomic region including the head and neck of the femur to 5 cm distal to the lesser trochanter. The femoral shaft is the portion of the femur distal to the lesser trochanter, down to but not including the femoral condyles.

The hip is a ball-and-socket joint formed by the femoral head and the acetabulum. The fibrous capsule that surrounds the joint on all sides is quite strong, attaching proximally at the acetabulum and distally on the intertrochanteric line on the anterior surface. The joint capsule is weakest posteriorly where it attaches to the femoral neck. The femoral head and shaft are connected at the obliquely angled femoral neck. Blood is supplied to the femoral head mainly from the medial and lateral femoral circumflex arteries that form an extracapsular ring with branching retinacular arteries in the joint capsule. Therefore, intracapsular fractures can compromise blood supply to the femoral head. Less important blood

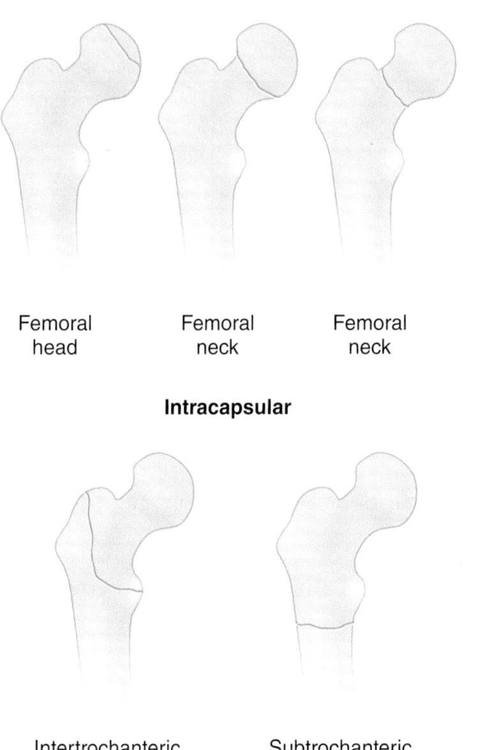

FIGURE 273-1. Fractures of the proximal femur are traditionally classified as intracapsular and extracapsular.

supply includes branches of the obturator and gluteal arteries, with a small contribution from the foveal artery at the ligamentum teres.

Hip fractures are classified as **intracapsular** (femoral head and neck) or **extracapsular** (trochanteric, intertrochanteric, and subtrochanteric). See **Figures 273-1** and **273-2** and **Table 273-1**. The prognosis for successful union and restoration of normal function varies considerably with the fracture type. Most fractures occur in older patients with osteoporosis or other bony pathology secondary to systemic disease. Younger patients are more likely to have femoral shaft fractures or hip dislocation secondary to high-energy trauma.

In intracapsular fractures with displacement, blood supply to the femoral head may be compromised due to direct injury to the blood vessels, tension from the fracture, or compression secondary to a hemarthrosis. Urgent reduction of the fracture may restore blood flow, although avascular necrosis occurs in 15% to 35% of patients unless some of the capsular vessels remain intact.[3] Extracapsular fractures less commonly cause vascular compromise.

CLINICAL FEATURES

HISTORY

History of a recent fall or motor vehicle crash suggests the possibility of hip fracture and other injuries. Falls should also prompt questioning about possible syncope, especially in the ill or elderly. Understanding the mechanism of injury can identify associated fractures, such as fractures of the pelvis or about the knee. Important historical factors, such as cancer, chronic kidney disease, or prolonged steroid use, increase the risk of osteoporosis, avascular necrosis, and pathologic fractures.

Patients with hip fracture or dislocation will typically have pain at the site of the injury, but may also report knee pain, groin pain, or pain at sites of other injuries. Determine the duration of immobilization to assess for dehydration, venous thrombosis, or rhabdomyolysis.

PHYSICAL EXAMINATION

After the primary survey and stabilization, carefully examine the patient for deformities, shortening, rotation, lacerations, bruising, or instability of the limbs or tenderness of the pelvis or sacrum. Note any focal tenderness or crepitance. If no significant abnormalities are found, evaluate range of motion of the hips. If rotation of the hip with the leg in extension is painful, avoid other hip maneuvers. Identification of a hip or pelvic injury in a trauma victim should raise suspicion for concomitant intra-abdominal, retroperitoneal, femoral shaft, knee, or urologic

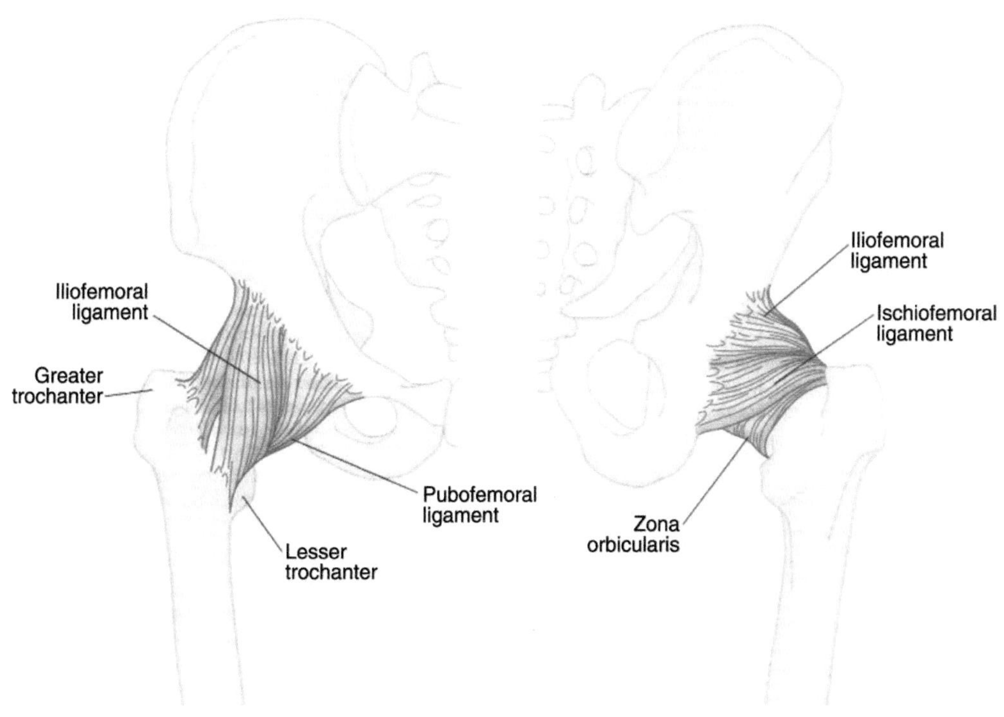

FIGURE 273-2. Hip and joint capsule.

TABLE 273-1 Proximal Femur Fractures: Demographics and Clinical Features

Fracture	Incidence/Demographics	Mechanism	Clinical Findings	Concomitant Injuries
Femoral head	Isolated fracture rare; seen in 6%–16% of hip dislocations	Usually result of high-energy trauma; dashboard to flexed knee most common	Limb shortened and externally rotated (anterior dislocation); shortened, flexed, and internally rotated (posterior dislocation)	Closed head injury; intrathoracic and/or intra-abdominal injuries; pelvic fracture, knee injuries
Femoral neck	Common in older patients with osteoporosis; rarely seen in younger patients	Low-impact falls or torsion in elderly; high-energy trauma or stress fractures in young	Ranges from pain with weight bearing to inability to ambulate; limb may be shortened and externally rotated	Ipsilateral femoral shaft fracture
Greater trochanteric	Uncommon; older patients or adolescents	Direct trauma (older patients); avulsion due to contraction of gluteus medius (young patients)	Ambulatory; pain with palpation or abduction	—
Lesser trochanteric	Uncommon; adolescents (85%) > adults	Avulsion due to forceful contraction of iliopsoas (adolescents); avulsion of pathologic bone (older adults)	Usually ambulatory; pain with flexion or rotation	—
Intertrochanteric	Common in older patients with osteoporosis; rare in younger patients	Falls; high-energy trauma	Severe pain; swelling; limb shortened and externally rotated	Anemia from blood loss into thigh; concomitant traumatic injuries
Subtrochanteric	Similar to intertrochanteric; 15% of hip fractures	Falls; high-energy trauma; may also be pathologic	Severe pain; ecchymosis; limb shortened, abducted, and externally rotated	Vascular injuries, anemia/hypovolemic shock from fracture itself or other traumatic injuries

injuries. Perform a rectal exam if concern exists for concurrent spinal or pelvic injuries, including evaluation of the prostate in males.

Injuries to the hip and femur should also raise concern for damage to adjacent nerves and vasculature, especially the femoral and sciatic nerves and femoral blood vessels. **Assess motor and sensory function of these nerves and their major branches (Table 273-2).** Evaluate pulses distal to the site of injury, including popliteal, dorsalis pedis, and posterior tibialis pulses. If concern exists for vascular injury, further testing should be performed and may include ankle-brachial indices, angiography, or duplex US.

DIAGNOSIS

IMAGING

Consider radiographic evaluation of the pelvis and hips in all unconscious patients who have sustained multiple injuries or have a concerning mechanism for pelvic, hip, or lower extremity injury.

Include anteroposterior and lateral views of the hip in the initial radiographic evaluation. An anteroposterior pelvis view is also useful as it allows comparison of both sides. Conventional radiographs are estimated to be 90% to 98% sensitive for hip fractures.[4] Other views may be requested by consulting orthopedists; in certain instances, additional views (e.g., Judet view) may allow better identification and detail of the acetabulum or femoral head and neck. Imaging of the femoral shaft or knee may also be necessary, following the adage to **assess the joint above and the joint below the injury**.

Pain with weight bearing in the face of normal radiographs should raise suspicion for occult fracture, especially at the femoral neck or acetabulum.[5] MRI is highly sensitive (nearly 100%) for occult fractures and is also useful in identifying other injuries that may explain the patient's symptoms. CT may be useful in identifying nondisplaced fractures not easily seen on conventional radiographs but is not as sensitive or accurate as MRI for occult fracture. Although bone scanning is sensitive for detecting occult fracture, neoplasm, and avascular necrosis, MRI has largely replaced it.[4-7]

TABLE 273-2 Motor and Sensory Evaluation of Sciatic and Femoral Nerves

Nerve	Motor	Sensory
Sciatic	Knee flexion	
Common peroneal	Dorsiflexion of foot and toes	Lateral lower leg, first web space of foot
Tibial	Plantarflexion of foot and toes	Posterior lower leg
Femoral		
Anterior branch	Hip flexion	Anterior and medial thigh
Posterior branch	Knee extension	Medial lower leg

HIP FRACTURES

FEMORAL HEAD FRACTURES

Isolated femoral head fractures are uncommon and are typically associated with dislocations of the hip (Table 273-1). The signs and symptoms are often from the dislocation rather than from the fracture itself. They are usually best seen on radiographs obtained after reduction of a hip dislocation.

The standard anteroposterior and lateral views usually demonstrate the fragment adequately. Judet views or thin-cut CT scans are often recommended for further evaluation of the acetabulum and fracture fragmentation.

Treatment is to reduce the associated dislocation and then attain anatomic reduction of the fracture fragment (**Table 273-3**). See subsequent section on dislocations for further discussion. Management of concomitant life-threatening injuries due to high-energy trauma must take priority.

Prognosis is related to the severity of the initial trauma resulting in the dislocation and associated injuries, delay to reduction, and repetitive unsuccessful reduction attempts.[8]

FEMORAL NECK FRACTURES

Femoral neck fractures are most commonly seen among older adults with osteoporosis and occur more frequently in women than in men. Falls are the most common cause (90%), but stress or traumatic femoral neck fractures may be seen in younger patients (Table 273-1).[9] There are multiple classification systems for femoral neck fractures, but it is most useful to describe them as displaced or nondisplaced. **Femoral neck fractures are intracapsular, and blood supply to the femoral head may be disrupted.**

The symptoms seen with femoral neck fractures range from complaints of mild pain in the groin or inner thigh in patients with an incomplete fracture, to moderate to severe pain in patients with displaced fractures. Patients with nondisplaced fractures may be somewhat ambulatory, whereas those with displaced fractures are typically unable

TABLE 273-3 Proximal Femur Fractures: Treatment Issues

Fracture	ED Management	Disposition and Follow-Up	Complications
Femoral head	Immediate orthopedic consultation; emergent closed reduction of dislocation; ORIF if closed reduction is unsuccessful	Admission to orthopedic or trauma service	AVN; posttraumatic arthritis; sciatic nerve injury; heterotopic ossification
Femoral neck	Orthopedic consultation; ranges from nonoperative to total hip arthroplasty	Admission to orthopedic service	AVN; infection; DVT and/or pulmonary embolus
Greater trochanteric	Analgesics; protected weight bearing	Orthopedic follow-up 1–2 wk; possible ORIF if displacement >1 cm	Nonunion rare
Lesser trochanteric	Analgesics; weight bearing as tolerated; evaluate for possible pathologic fracture	Orthopedic or PCP follow-up in 1–2 wk; admit or urgent follow-up for pathologic fracture	Nonunion rare
Intertrochanteric	Orthopedic consultation	Admit for eventual ORIF; may need preoperative testing and clearance by PCP or hospitalist	DVT and/or pulmonary embolism; infection
Subtrochanteric	Orthopedic consultation; consider Hare® or Sager® splint	Admit for ORIF	DVT and/or pulmonary embolism; infection; malunion (shortened limb); nonunion

Abbreviations: AVN = avascular necrosis; DVT = deep venous thrombosis; ORIF = open reduction and internal fixation; PCP = primary care physician.

to bear weight at all. Examination findings can be subtle in nondisplaced fractures, while displaced fractures are quite evident with the leg held in external rotation, abduction, and shortened (**Figure 273-3**).

Radiographic evaluation is essential in any patient suspected of having a femoral neck fracture. Ideally, the standard anteroposterior view should have the patient internally rotated as much as patient condition allows to best demonstrate the femoral neck. Nondisplaced fractures may be subtle. The anteroposterior view should be inspected for a fracture line starting on the superior surface of the neck (**Figure 273-4**). Disruption of **Shenton's line**, a smooth curvilinear line along the superior border of the obturator foramen and the medial aspect of the femoral metaphysis, may be appreciated on the anteroposterior view in some instances (**Figure 273-5**). Evaluate the **neck-shaft angle** in suspected fractures; normal is 120 to 130 degrees (**Figure 273-6**). The neck-shaft angle is measured at the intersection of lines drawn down the axis of the femoral shaft and the femoral neck.[10] Displaced fractures are obvious on the anteroposterior view, but a lateral view should also be obtained to ascertain the exact fracture position. Approximately 6% to 9% of patients with a femoral neck fracture will have an ipsilateral femoral shaft fracture.[11]

Treat pain, immobilize the extremity in a position of comfort, and obtain orthopedic consultation in the ED. **Skeletal traction is contraindicated for femoral neck fractures because it may further compromise femoral head blood flow.**

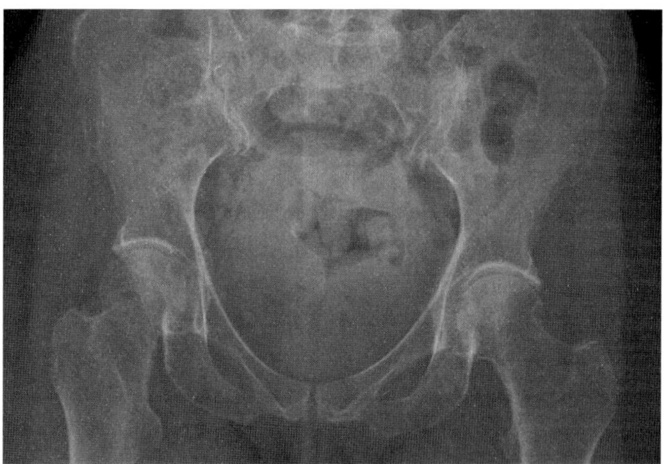

FIGURE 273-4. Radiograph of femoral neck fracture. The disruption of the bone is most visible when following the superior surface of the femoral neck. Also notice the shortening and impaction of the femoral neck.

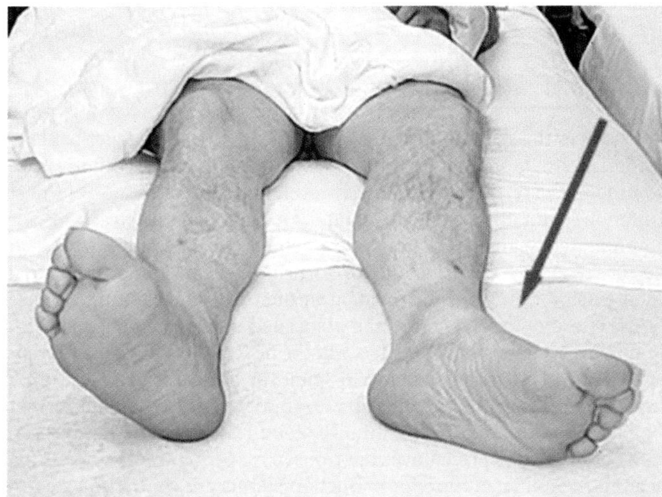

FIGURE 273-3. Shortened, abducted, externally rotated limb (*arrow*) seen in femoral neck fracture. [Image used with permission of Dr. Allan Mishra, http://www.emedx.com.]

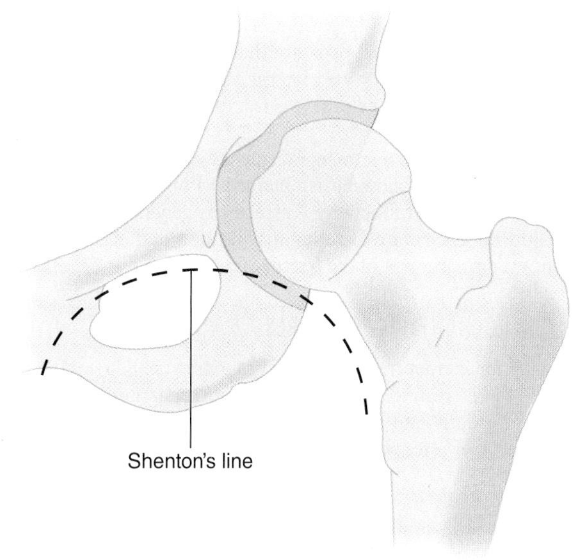

FIGURE 273-5. Shenton's line.

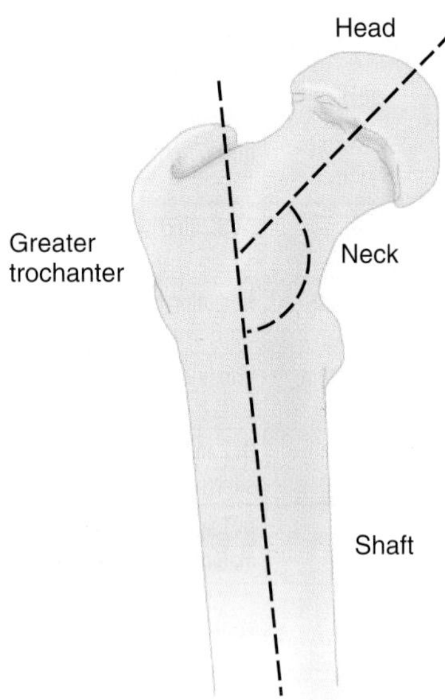

FIGURE 273-6. Neck-shaft angle.

For both displaced and nondisplaced fractures, outcomes are generally best with surgical fixation because this leads to earlier mobilization and less morbidity and mortality than with conservative management.[12,13] Decisions regarding the timing and type of operative intervention depend on the patient's physiologic age, activity level, and fracture severity.[14] Conservative treatment may be considered in those whose operative risk outweighs potential benefit or in patients who are not ambulatory.

The complications of femoral neck fractures are significant (Table 273-3). Prognosis is related to the number and severity of complications. A higher grade of fracture displacement also implies a worse prognosis for healing and repair.

ISOLATED TROCHANTERIC FRACTURES

Greater trochanteric fractures are usually caused by avulsions at the insertion of the gluteus medius. In the younger population (7 to 17 years of age), this is a true epiphyseal separation, in contrast to the adult population, in whom the cause is direct trauma (Table 273-1).

Lesser trochanteric fractures caused by an avulsion secondary to forceful contraction of the iliopsoas are commonly seen in children and young athletic adults, particularly gymnasts and dancers. Lesser trochanter fractures in older patients with minimal trauma should be considered pathologic until proven otherwise.[15]

Standard anteroposterior and lateral views reveal the displacement. CT of the pelvis may be helpful if a fracture is strongly suspected but difficult to visualize.

In most instances, the treatment is crutches with weight bearing as tolerated until orthopedic follow-up is obtained within 3 to 5 days, and then gradually increasing to full activity. Full recovery generally occurs in patients with healthy bone. Operative fixation may be indicated in cases where there is significant displacement of the fracture fragment (Table 273-3).

INTERTROCHANTERIC FRACTURES

Intertrochanteric fractures are defined as extracapsular fractures occurring in a line between the greater and lesser trochanters. They generally occur in the elderly and are more common in women, again due to the high incidence of osteoporosis. The mechanism of injury is usually a fall (**Table 273-1**).

Patients typically have marked pain and deformity on examination, and fractures are usually easily visualized on standard anteroposterior and lateral views. Intertrochanteric fractures should be classified as stable or unstable based on the number of fracture lines and the amount of displacement.[16]

After life-threatening injuries have been excluded, the consulting orthopedic physician can then admit the patient to the hospital and perform surgical fixation as soon as possible (Table 273-3). Skin traction is not recommended for either stabilization or pain control.[17,18]

The complications and prognosis are related to associated injuries and prior disease. **Blood loss into the leg can be significant, and some patients will require crystalloid or blood transfusion.**[19] Infection and pulmonary embolism are the main complications. Avascular necrosis and nonunion are uncommon complications.

SUBTROCHANTERIC FRACTURES

Subtrochanteric fractures may be seen in three different populations: older patients with osteoporosis who fall (Table 273-1), younger patients as a result of major trauma, or patients with bony metastases.

The symptoms and signs are similar to those of intertrochanteric or femoral shaft fractures: localized pain, deformity, swelling, and crepitance. Significant blood loss may develop. Evaluate for concomitant life-threatening injuries.

Standard anteroposterior and lateral views of the hip are typically sufficient to evaluate these fractures. Consider radiographic studies of the pelvis, femur, and knee to exclude associated fractures.

ED treatment consists of pain control, immobilization, and orthopedic consultation. Hare® (Dynamed, Westbury, Tasmania) or Sager® (Minto Research and Development, Inc., Redding, CA) splints (**Figures 2-7** and **2-8,** respectively) are commonly employed in the prehospital setting and infrequently in the ED (also see chapter 2, Prehospital Equipment and Adjuncts). Traction splinting may ease pain and provide some fracture reduction.[18] Do not apply a traction splint if there is open fracture, suspected pelvic fracture, hip dislocation, suspicion for neurovascular injury to the extremity, or injury about the knee, as a traction splint may exacerbate neurovascular or knee injury. Operative reduction/internal fixation is generally indicated for complicated fracture management.

OCCULT HIP FRACTURES

Symptoms suggestive of fracture, but with negative plain radiographs, are called occult hip fractures.[4] Anywhere from 3% to 38% of hip fractures are initially "occult."[6] Stress, incomplete, or nondisplaced fractures may not become evident on plain radiographs for days or weeks after injury. **Pain with axial loading, restricted mobility prior to the injury, and risks for osteoporosis should all raise suspicion for occult fracture.**[20] MRI is the imaging of choice because it is both sensitive and specific.[4] If clinical suspicion is high, obtain an MRI in the ED, or if that is not possible, obtain an MRI within the next 24 to 48 hours—with the patient non–weight bearing until diagnosis is confirmed and orthopedic follow-up is obtained.

FEMORAL SHAFT FRACTURES

Fractures of the shaft of the femur most often occur in younger patients secondary to high-energy trauma; associated traumatic injuries are common. Severe, direct trauma may result in transverse fractures (most common) with displacement, oblique or spiral oblique fractures, or comminuted segments. Pathologic fractures are uncommon but can occur secondary to metastases or to primary bone tumors. Femoral shaft fractures are generally evident in the prehospital setting because of the shortening, deformity, and associated swelling. Initial stabilization of the patient should take place in the field along with spinal immobilization. It is generally advised to splint the affected extremity with a traction splint at the time of injury, to minimize pain, prevent further fracture comminution, and minimize blood loss. Hare® or Sager® traction splints can be placed over the trousers, applying traction to a sling around the ankle and forefoot. Traction splints are contraindicated in cases of open fracture or in suspected sciatic nerve, knee, or vascular injury. For the latter, splint placement without application of traction is indicated.

Neurovascular examination of the affected extremity is important since sciatic nerve injury, though uncommon, can occur (Table 273-2). The fracture is typically evident on standard anteroposterior and lateral views of the femur. Evaluation, including a thorough exam and imaging, of the joints above and below (pelvis, hips, knees) is generally needed to assess for other orthopedic injuries. Open femur fractures require broad-spectrum antibiotics and copious irrigation. Further irrigation and debridement are accomplished in the operating room. Obtain early orthopedic consultation; most patients require surgical intervention. Blood loss can be significant from the fracture itself or from other injuries.

Intermedullary nailing is the preferred treatment for most femoral shaft fractures. In severely contaminated open fractures, external fixation may be the preferred method of treatment. Patients with severe concomitant injuries may benefit from early external fixation and delayed operative reduction and internal fixation.[21]

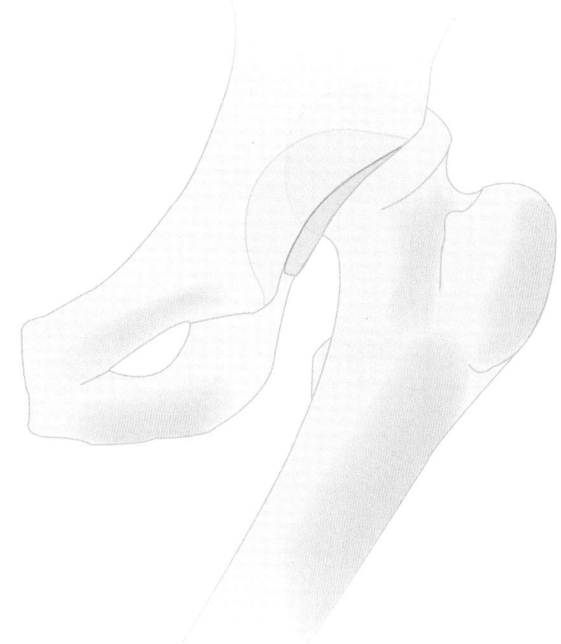

B

FIGURE 273-7. Posterior dislocation of the hip. **A.** Posterior dislocation of the hip. **B.** The clinical appearance of a posterior dislocation of the right hip.

HIP DISLOCATION

Dislocations of native hips typically result from high-energy trauma, and up to 95% of patients have other associated injuries.[22] Motor vehicle crash is the most common cause. **Posterior dislocations of native hips account for >90% of dislocations**; the remaining 10% are anterior and can be classified as superior or inferior.[23] Dislocations of prosthetic hips can occur with minimal trauma. This section discusses the diagnosis and management of posterior and anterior native hip dislocation and the ED management of prosthetic hip dislocation.

Hip dislocations (dislocations of native hips) are orthopedic emergencies and should be reduced as quickly as possible, preferably within 6 hours of the event, in order to reduce the risk of avascular necrosis to the femoral head. Dislocations with neurovascular compromise need reduction as soon as possible. Treatment options include closed reduction of posterior hip dislocations or prosthetic hip dislocations in the ED under procedural sedation, or in the operating room with general anesthesia. Anterior hip dislocations require reduction in the operating room. Open reduction by an orthopedic surgeon is indicated for irreducible fractures, unsatisfactory reductions, and complex fracture dislocations.[23]

POSTERIOR HIP DISLOCATION AND REDUCTION MANEUVERS

Posterior hip dislocations (**Figure 273-7**) are caused by posterior force applied to a flexed knee, most commonly a dashboard injury from high-speed motor vehicle crashes. Acetabular fractures often result; femoral neck, femoral shaft, and knee injuries are often seen as well. On examination, the extremity is shortened, internally rotated, and adducted. Perform a careful neurovascular examination to identify associated sciatic nerve injury or vascular injury (Table 273-2).

Anteroposterior and lateral radiographs of the pelvis and hip identify the posterior dislocation (**Figure 273-8**), but further assessment of the acetabulum and femur must be performed, either with Judet views or CT, to evaluate for associated fractures. Hip dislocations are difficult to recognize if there is an associated femoral shaft fracture, so routinely obtain radiographs of the pelvis and hips in such cases. **Complications of posterior dislocation include sciatic nerve injury in approximately 10% of patients and avascular necrosis of the femoral head that increases in direct proportion to the delay in anatomic reduction.**

Multiple techniques exist for closed reduction of posterior hip dislocations (Figures 273-9 to 273-12); it is advisable for the ED physician to be proficient with more than one technique. Nearly all of the techniques involve providing in-line traction while flexing the hip to 90 degrees, and then performing gentle internal-to-external hip rotation.

The **Allis maneuver** is the most commonly performed technique. In-line traction is performed with simultaneous hip flexion and internal

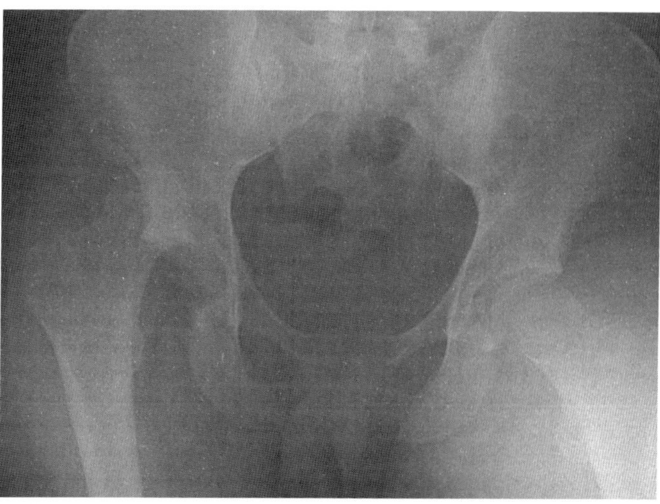

FIGURE 273-8. Radiograph of posterior hip dislocation. There is also a concomitant acetabular fracture visible.

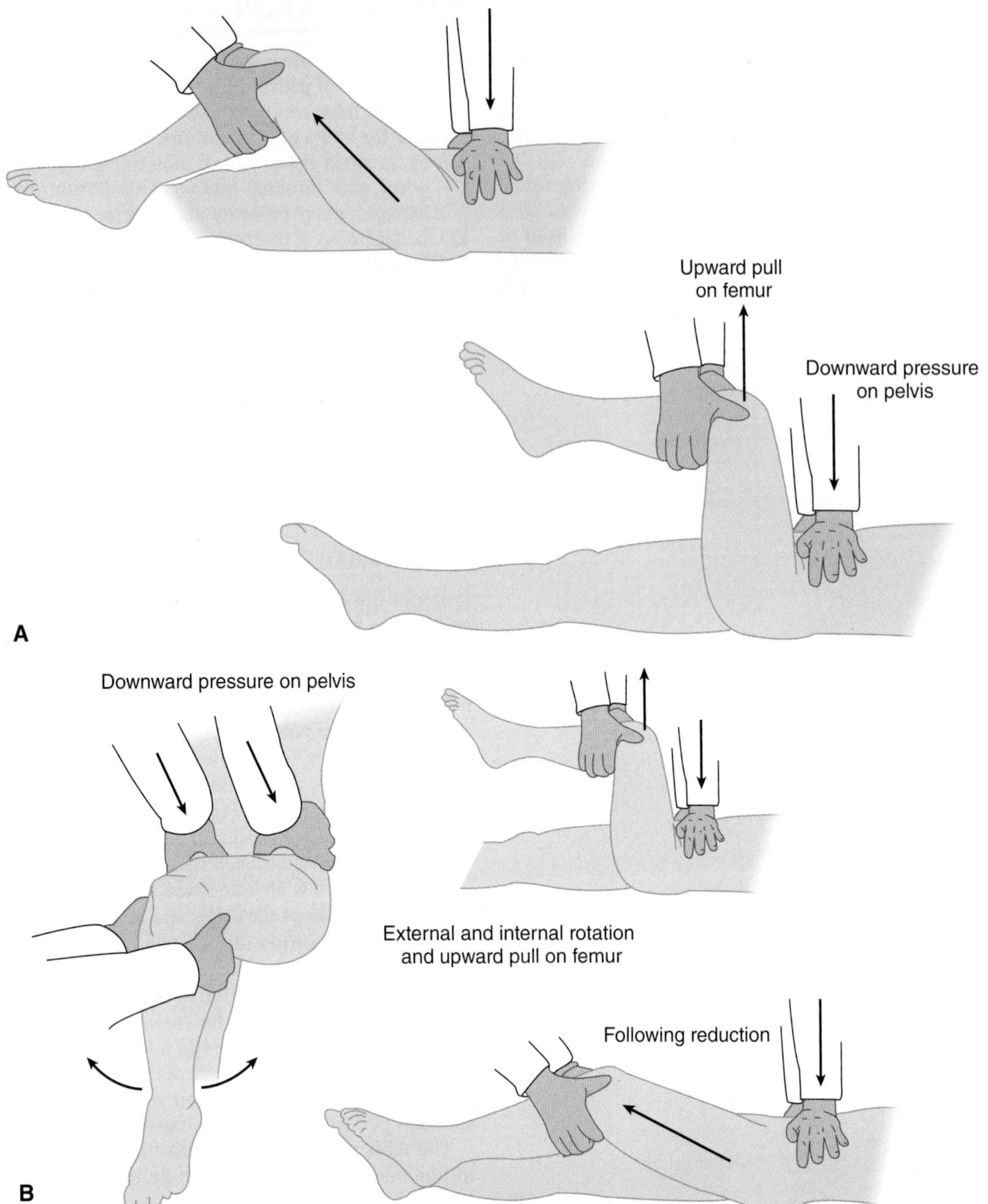

FIGURE 273-9. **A** and **B.** Allis maneuver for reduction of posterior hip dislocation.

rotation (**Figure 273-9**). Flex the patient's knee and hip to 90 degrees. An assistant should apply downward pressure to the anterior superior iliac spines. Grasp the knee with both hands. Pull and simultaneously rotate the femur laterally and medially.

With the **Bigelow maneuver**, the patient should lie supine with the affected hip and knee flexed 90 degrees (**Figure 273-10**). Secure the patient's knee with your flexed elbow, and grasp the patient's foot with the opposite hand. Have an assistant apply downward pressure to the anterior superior iliac spines. Now, using your flexed elbow, lift upward at the patient's knee to apply traction to the femur. Externally rotate and extend the hip while applying traction to the femur at the patient's knee. Another variation is represented in **Figure 273-11**.

Another method is the **Captain Morgan technique**, in which the physician's knee is used as a fulcrum (**Figure 273-12**).[24]

After reduction, gently take the hip through range of motion to ensure stability, repeat the neurovascular examination, and obtain postreduction imaging to ensure reduction is satisfactory. The patient may then be placed in an abduction pillow or brace, a hip binder, or a knee immobilizer based on the consulting orthopedist's preference. Most patients will require admission, because this injury is most often due to significant trauma.

If several attempts at reduction are unsuccessful, emergency orthopedic consultation is needed to provide reduction either in the ED or the operating room. Difficulties with reduction may be due to occult fracture or incarcerated tendon or capsule. A postreduction CT is generally recommended to specifically identify associated acetabular or femoral head fractures that were not evident on plain radiographs.[23]

ANTERIOR HIP DISLOCATION

In anterior hip dislocations (**Figure 273-13 A,B**), the femoral head rests anteriorly to the coronal plane of the acetabulum. Anterior dislocations can be superior (pelvic) or inferior (obturator) depending on the degree of hip flexion present at the time of injury. The mechanism of injury is forced abduction that causes the femoral head to be levered out through an anterior capsular tear. The affected extremity is in abduction and external

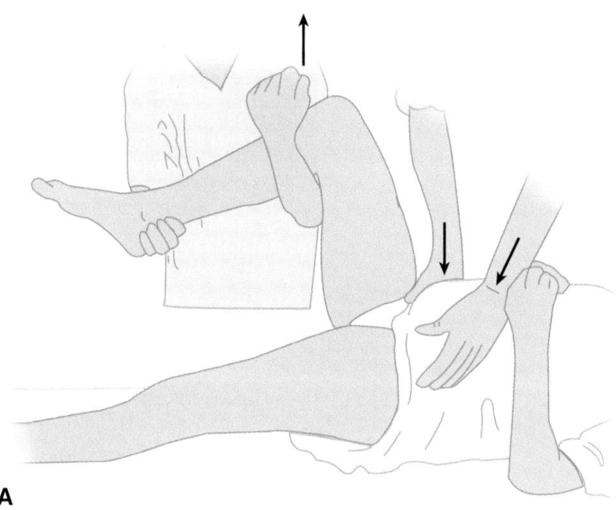

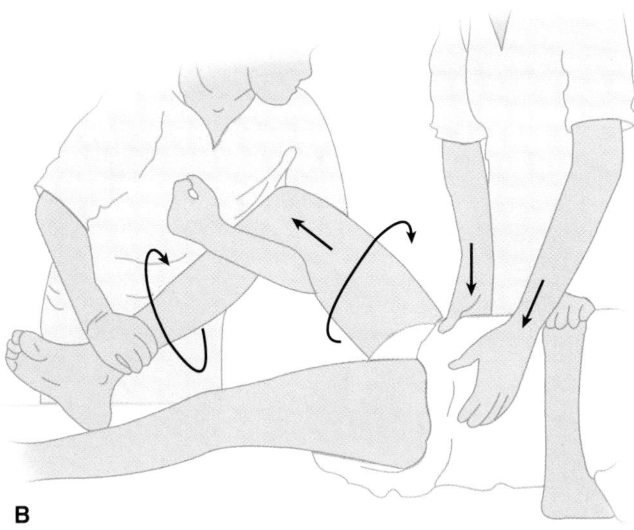

FIGURE 273-10. The Bigelow maneuver for reduction of posterior hip dislocation. **A.** The physician applies upward traction on the femur while an assistant stabilizes the pelvis. **B.** The hip is externally rotated and extended while the femur is distracted. [Reproduced with permission from Reichman EF, Simon RR: *Emergency Medicine Procedures*. © 2004, McGraw-Hill, New York.]

rotation. The clinical appearance of superior versus inferior dislocations is dramatically different (**Figure 273-13 C,D**). Neurovascular compromise is an unusual complication. However, a thorough exam is warranted to detect injury to the femoral artery or nerve (Table 273-2).

An anteroposterior view of the pelvis can easily demonstrate the femoral head to be anterior to the acetabulum. A lateral view illustrates the anterior dislocation more clearly, although it may be difficult to obtain secondary to patient discomfort. Anterior hip dislocations usually require reduction in the operating room.

DISLOCATIONS OF PROSTHETIC HIPS

Prosthetic hips may dislocate relatively easily from minor trauma or movements that place the hip past 90 degrees of flexion while adducted. Approximately 1% to 10% of prosthetic hips dislocate, the majority in the first few months after surgery.[25] Avascular necrosis of the femoral head is not a complication since there is no blood flow to the prosthetic joint capsule. However, sciatic nerve injury or damage to the prosthesis may occur.

Most dislocations of prosthetic hips are posterior and can be reduced using procedural sedation in the ED with the techniques described previously. A review of 410 prosthetic hip dislocations reported that

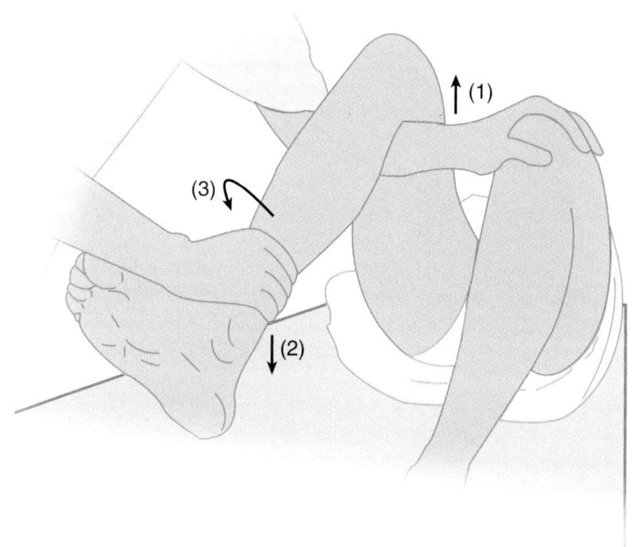

FIGURE 273-11. (*1*) Flex the patient's knee 90 degrees and place your flexed elbow under the patient's knee while placing your hand on the other knee to stabilize the pelvis. (*2, 3*) With the other hand, externally rotate the leg. [Reproduced with permission from Reichman EF, Simon RR: *Emergency Medicine Procedures*. © 2004, McGraw-Hill, New York.]

emergency physicians were successful at 79% of reductions in the ED, and orthopedists were successful at 71% of reductions in the ED—with no difference between emergency physicians and orthopedists in the proportion of successfully relocated hips in the ED and no difference in complications. The ED length of stay for ED-reduced prosthetic hip dislocations was about one third shorter than that for orthopedist-reduced dislocations. This study did not describe the types of prostheses reduced.[26] There are multiple types of implants, such as modular or constrained implants, which may not be amenable to closed reduction. **It is advisable to discuss the treatment plan with the consulting orthopedist prior to attempting any reduction maneuvers.**

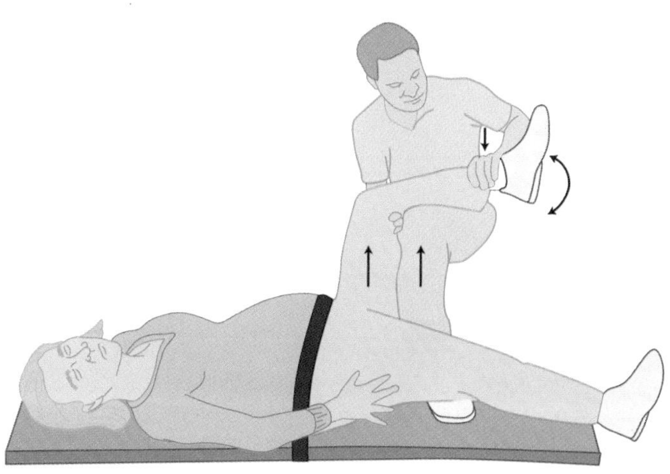

FIGURE 273-12. The Captain Morgan technique for reduction of posterior hip dislocation. (*1*) Stabilize the patient's pelvis by placing the patient on a backboard in the supine position and strapping the pelvis to the board, or have an assistant stabilize the pelvis on the stretcher by placing both hands on the patient's iliac crests and using pressure to keep the pelvis stable. (*2*) To reduce the dislocation, place your foot on the stretcher or board with your knee posterior to the patient's knee. (*3*) With the patient's knee in flexion, gently pull downward at the patient's ankle while applying an upward force to the patient's hip by lifting your heel by stepping on your toes and contracting your calf. Gently rotate the patient's hip while applying the upward traction behind the patient's knee.

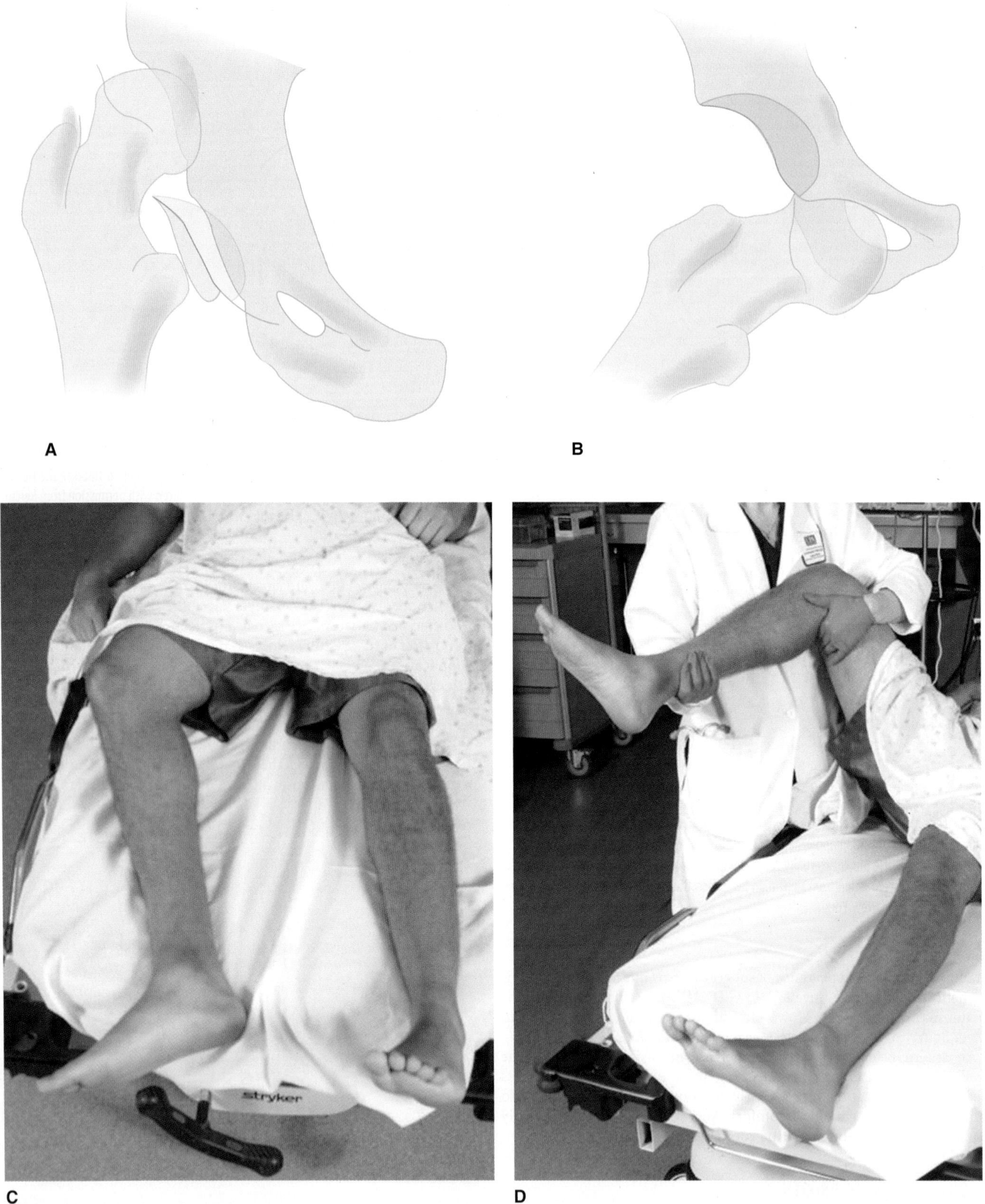

FIGURE 273-13. Anterior hip dislocation. **A.** Anterior superior dislocation of the hip. **B.** Inferior dislocation. **C.** Clinical appearance of a superior-type anterior dislocation of the hip. **D.** Clinical appearance of an inferior-type dislocation of the hip.

SPECIAL POPULATIONS

ATHLETES

Stress fractures of the femoral neck are a recognized cause of hip pain in athletes, especially runners and football players. The onset of pain is often insidious and may mimic other common conditions such as bursitis or muscle strain. Patients often report pain in the groin, medial thigh, or knee. Consider MRI if clinical suspicion is present for stress fracture in a high-risk patient.[27] If imaging is not readily available, then the patient should be made non–weight bearing and told to avoid all athletic activities until orthopedic evaluation can be obtained (optimally in the next 48 hours).[28]

ELDERLY PATIENTS

The majority of hip and femur injuries occur in the elderly. Most will have underlying comorbidities that also require evaluation. For this reason, it is often useful to employ a multidisciplinary approach, which may involve social services to follow up for home safety evaluation as well as early involvement of the patient's primary care physician or a hospitalist.[12] Admit patients with suspected fractures who have poor follow-up, no social support, or suboptimal living conditions. Consider the possibility of elder abuse in elderly patients with falls and fractures. See chapter 295, Abuse of the Elderly and Impaired, for a detailed discussion of elder abuse.

SPECIAL CONSIDERATIONS

PAIN CONTROL

Nearly all patients with hip or femur injuries will require analgesia. Patients with orthopedic injuries sometimes receive inadequate analgesia in the ED.[29] Use parenteral narcotics for pain control unless there is a contraindication. Femoral nerve block should be considered (see chapter 36, Local and Regional Anesthesia, for technique).

INJURY PREVENTION

The use of hip protection pads for the prevention of hip fractures in the elderly have yielded conflicting results, with no definitive reduction in fracture rates demonstrated.[30] The increasing use of bisphosphonates for osteoporosis prevention has coincided with the modest reduction in hip fracture incidence in the U.S.; however, there is no evidence for a directly causal relationship as of now. Calcium and vitamin D supplementation may also play a role.[1] The best current recommendations are finding strategies to reduce falls and preventing osteoporosis.

REFERENCES

The complete reference list is available online at www.TintinalliEM.com.

Knee Injuries

Rachel R. Bengtzen
Jeffrey N. Glaspy
Mark T. Steele

ANATOMY

The knee consists of two joints, the tibiofemoral joint and the patellofemoral joint. Within the tibiofemoral joint, the distal femur (comprised of the medial and lateral femoral condyles) articulates with the proximal tibia (comprised of the medial and lateral tibial condyles) (**Figure 274-1**). The medial and lateral menisci are situated between the articular surfaces, and the menisci provide cushion, lubrication, and resistance to articular wear (**Figure 274-2**). In the patellofemoral joint, the patella articulates with the distal femur along the anterior depression called the patellofemoral groove during flexion and extension of the knee. The patella is stabilized by the patellar tendon and medial retinaculum.

There are four ligaments in the knee: the anterior cruciate ligament, the posterior cruciate ligament, and the medial and lateral collateral ligaments (Figure 274-2). These ligaments provide strength and stability to the knee. The posterior aspect of the knee, the popliteal fossa, contains the popliteal artery and vein, the common peroneal nerve, and the tibial nerve (**Figure 274-3**).

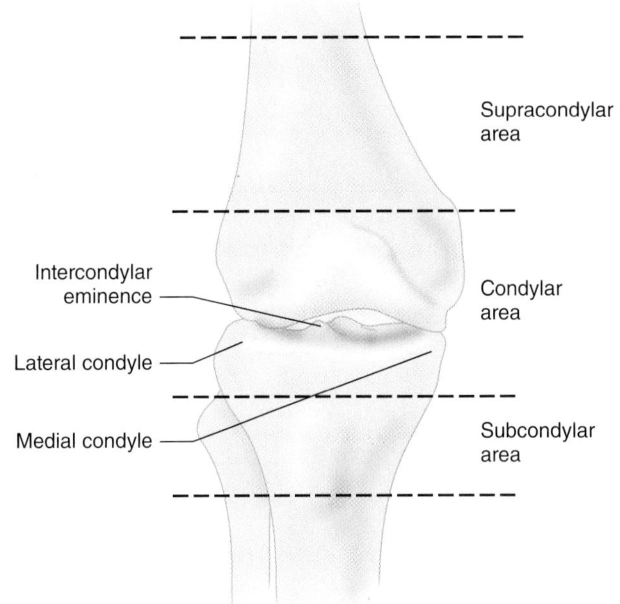

FIGURE 274-1. The supracondylar and condylar areas of the femur, and the medial and subcondylar areas of the tibia.

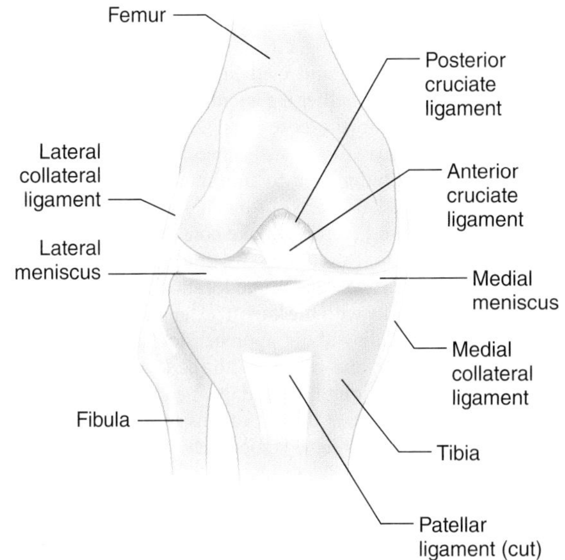

FIGURE 274-2. Ligaments of the right knee joint. The articular capsule and the patella have been removed.

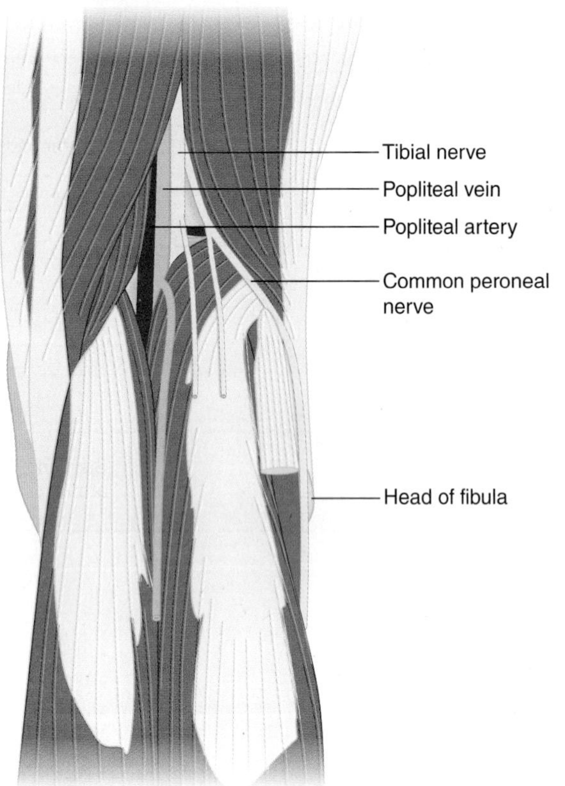

FIGURE 274-3. Posterior knee: popliteal fossa anatomy.

CLINICAL FEATURES

Determine the mechanism of knee injury and review all prior orthopedic injuries or surgical procedures. As with all orthopedic examinations, compare the noninjured or normal joint with the injured joint during all aspects of the examination, but especially during palpation and stress testing.

The first examination is usually the easiest to perform and may be the most valid, because the patient does not anticipate pain and may not guard against the examination, and because inflammation and effusion limiting the examination may have not yet developed.

Assess gait (if possible), functional range of motion, and the ability to perform a straight leg raise (evaluates the extensor complex). Evaluate the knee for ecchymoses, swelling, effusion, masses, patella location and size, muscle mass, erythema, and evidence of local trauma. With the patient supine, determine whether leg lengths are equal or unequal. Ask the patient to demonstrate the best possible active range of motion. Assess distal neurovascular function. Palpate the nontender areas first and work toward the tender area to minimize patient apprehension. Palpate the patella, patellar facets, proximal fibula, and femoral and tibial condyles for pain and crepitus. Make note of joint effusion, tenderness, increased temperature, strength, sensation, and location of pulses.

Examine the patella for size, shape, and location with the knee in flexion. Check patellar mobility with the knee in extension, making sure it can move laterally and medially without apprehension. Palpate the popliteal space for masses, swelling, and pulses. With the knee in flexion, palpate both the medial and lateral joint lines and the medial and lateral collateral ligaments, because tenderness at those locations suggests the possibility of a meniscal or ligamentous injury, respectively. The final phase of the examination of the knee is stress testing (see "Ligamentous and Meniscal Injuries" below). This is the most difficult aspect of the examination, although potentially the most informative. The patient must be relaxed and made as comfortable as possible. Testing is often easier if the patient sits up with the leg hanging over the side of the bed and with the bed supporting the posterior thigh. Examine the uninjured, presumably normal, opposite knee first to determine the patient's normal laxity.

NEUROVASCULAR INJURIES

Popliteal artery injury can occur from fractures about the knee, especially femoral condyle fractures or displaced tibial plateau fractures, and from ligamentous injuries such as isolated posterior cruciate ligament injuries, multiple ligamentous injuries, or knee dislocation.[1,2] Popliteal artery circulation must be restored within 8 hours to avoid amputation, because collateral circulation is insufficient to maintain blood flow to the leg. Measure distal pulses on ED admission and after any manipulation, and compare pulses to those in the noninjured leg. A diminished pulse raises concern for vascular injury and should not be interpreted as vascular spasm. An abnormal finding on pulse examination is reported to have a sensitivity of only 79% and a specificity of 91% for arterial injuries that require surgical intervention,[2] so it is important to remember that vascular injury can be present even in the presence of normal pulses. Ancillary studies include measurement of ankle-brachial index (<0.9 in a patient with peripheral vascular disease or vascular injury) and duplex US (reported to be 95% sensitive and 99% specific for arterial injury).[1] Vascular surgery consultation is required for any potential popliteal arterial injury to determine the need for angiography, as well to monitor for the development of compartment syndrome, venous injury, and arterial thrombosis.

Peroneal nerve injuries can result from severe ligamentous knee injuries and knee dislocations. Nearly half of fibular head fractures or avulsions are associated with peroneal nerve injury. The deep peroneal nerve provides sensation to the first dorsal web space of the toes and allows dorsiflexion of the foot and extension of the toes. Injury results in foot drop and gait difficulty. Prognosis is variable, depending on the severity of injury.

DIAGNOSIS

IMAGING

The **Ottawa Knee Rules** (**Table 274-1**) are sensitive in identifying fracture, and their use reduces ED waiting times and costs. The **Pittsburgh Knee Rules** (**Figure 274-4**) are similar and may have greater specificity.[3,4]

Both rules are applicable to children >2 years old and adults.[4] It would be reasonable to order radiographs on a higher number of patients with knee pain who are multisystem trauma patients, and thus immobilized and unable to undergo gait testing.

Anteroposterior and lateral radiographs are typically obtained if radiographs are needed.[5] Fat-fluid levels (lipohemarthrosis) suggest intra-articular fracture and may be identified on a lateral view of the knee.[6] Consider weight-bearing radiographs when tolerated, which allows for a functional assessment. Additional radiograph views can be very useful. Oblique views are particularly helpful for detecting subtle tibial plateau fractures (internal oblique view is best for visualizing the lateral plateau, and external oblique view is best for visualizing the medial plateau).[5,7] A tunnel or intercondylar view provides a clear image of the intercondylar region and is particularly useful in identifying tibial spine fractures. A sunrise (skyline, axial, or tangential) view is most useful in detecting nondisplaced vertical or marginal fractures of the patella, which may be missed with the conventional views. The sunrise view is indicated if patellar subluxation or fracture is suspected. CT may be necessary to fully delineate the extent of tibial plateau fractures. MRI is also helpful in this regard and has the added benefit of being able to assess soft tissue (i.e., ligamentous and meniscal) injury.[5]

TABLE 274-1 Ottawa Knee Rules: X-Ray if One Criterion Is Met
Patient age >55 y (rules have been validated for children 2–16 y of age)
Tenderness at the head of the fibula
Isolated tenderness of the patella
Inability to flex knee to 90 degrees
Inability to transfer weight for four steps both immediately after the injury and in the ED

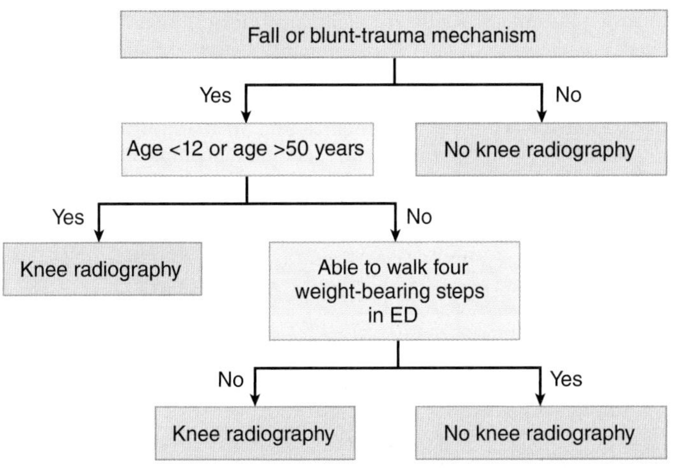

FIGURE 274-4. Pittsburgh Knee Rules for radiography. [Reproduced with permission from Seaberg DC, Yealy DM, Lukens T, et al: Multicenter comparison of two clinical decision rules for the use of radiography in acute, high-risk knee injuries. *Ann Emerg Med.* 1998;Jul;32(1):8-13. Copyright Elsevier.]

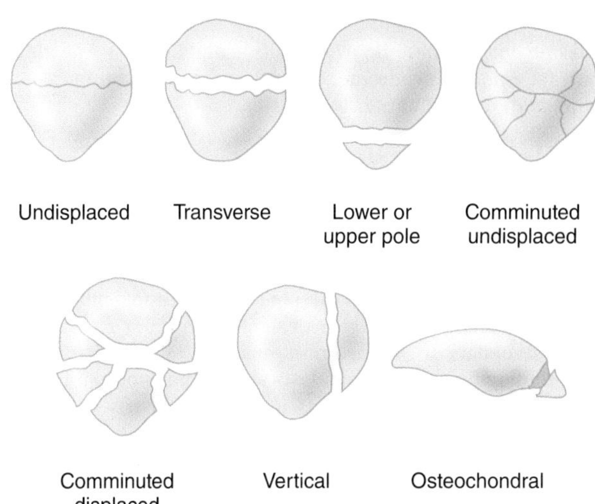

FIGURE 274-5. Classification of patellar fractures.

SPECIFIC INJURIES

PATELLA FRACTURES

Table 274-2 reviews the mechanisms of injury and treatment of patellar fractures. Patellar fractures may be transverse, comminuted, or of the avulsion type when the quadriceps or patellar tendon pulls off a small portion of the patella (**Figure 274-5**).

Transverse fractures of the patella are most common, followed by stellate and comminuted fractures. Patients with nondisplaced fractures may be ambulatory. On examination, there is focal patellar tenderness, swelling, and effusion. Check the integrity of the extensor mechanism of the knee by having the patient perform a straight-leg raise against gravity. Nonoperative management is indicated for fractures with an intact extensor mechanism and <2 mm of step-off and <3 mm of fracture displacement.[8,13] Transverse fractures are more likely to be displaced and to be associated with a disrupted extensor mechanism. Differential diagnosis of patellar fractures radiographically includes bipartite patella. This condition involves the superior lateral corner of the patella, is typically bilateral, and is differentiated from fracture by the smooth cortical margins.

FEMORAL CONDYLE FRACTURES

Fractures of the femoral condyles account for 6% of femur fractures and include supracondylar, intercondylar, condylar, and distal femoral epiphyseal fractures (Figure 274-1). Table 274-2 reviews the mechanisms of injury and treatment for femoral condyle fractures. Examination reveals pain, swelling, deformity, rotation, shortening, and an inability to ambulate. Although neurovascular injuries are uncommon, the potential for popliteal artery injury exists, so the status of distal sensation and pulses must be checked. Test the space between the first and second toes, innervated by the deep peroneal nerve, for sensation. In addition, search for associated injuries, including ipsilateral hip

TABLE 274-2 Mechanisms of Knee Injury and Treatment

Fracture	Mechanism	Treatment
Patella	Direct blow (i.e., fall, motor vehicle crash) or forceful contraction of quadriceps muscle	Nondisplaced fracture with intact extensor mechanism: knee immobilizer, rest, ice, analgesia. Follow-up for serial radiographs. Displaced >3 mm, articular incongruity >2 mm, or with disruption of extensor mechanism: above treatment plus early referral for ORIF.[8] Severely comminuted fracture: surgical debridement of small fragments and suturing of quadriceps and patellar tendons. Open fracture: irrigation and antistaphylococcal antibiotics in the ED; debridement and irrigation in the operating room.
Femoral condyles	Fall with axial load with valgus/varus/rotational forces, or a blow to the distal femur	Incomplete or nondisplaced fractures in any age group or stable impacted fractures in the elderly: long leg splinting and orthopedic referral. Displaced fractures or fractures with any degree of joint incongruity: splinting and orthopedic consult for ORIF.[9,10]
Tibial spines and tuberosity	Force directed against flexed proximal tibia in an anterior or posterior direction (i.e., motor vehicle crash, sporting injury)	Incomplete or nondisplaced fractures: immobilization in full extension (knee immobilizer) and orthopedic referral in 2–7 d. Complete or displaced fracture: early orthopedic referral, often requires ORIF.[11]
Tibial tuberosity	Sudden force to flexed knee with quadriceps contracted	Incomplete or small avulsion fracture: immobilization. Complete avulsion: ORIF.[8]
Tibial plateau	Valgus or varus forces combined with axial load that drives the femoral condyle into the tibia (i.e., fall, leg hit by car bumper)[12]	Nondisplaced, lateral fracture: knee immobilizer with non–weight bearing and orthopedic referral in 2–7 d. Depression of articular surface: early orthopedic consult for ORIF.[12]

Abbreviation: ORIF = open reduction internal fixation.

dislocation or fractures and damage to the quadriceps apparatus. The overall outcome of these injuries is fair. Complications include deep venous, fat embolus syndrome, delayed union or malunion, and the subsequent development of osteoarthritis.[9]

TIBIAL SPINE AND TUBEROSITY FRACTURES

Although isolated injuries of the tibial spine are uncommon, they usually result in cruciate ligament insufficiency. Table 274-2 reviews the mechanism of injury and treatment for tibial spine and tuberosity fractures. Fracture of the anterior tibial spine is about 10-fold more common than fracture of the posterior spine. Examination shows a painful, swollen knee secondary to hemarthrosis, inability to extend fully, and a positive finding on the Lachman test (see "Ligamentous and Meniscal Injuries" below).[11] The quadriceps mechanism inserts on the tibial tubercle. A sudden force to the flexed knee with the quadriceps muscle contracted may result in a complete or incomplete avulsion of the tibial tubercle. The fracture line may extend into the joint. Examination reveals pain and tenderness over the proximal anterior tibia with pain on passive or active extension.

TIBIAL PLATEAU FRACTURES

Fractures of the tibial plateau are seen more commonly in the older population and can be very difficult to detect. Table 274-2 reviews the mechanism of injury and treatment for tibial plateau fractures. Both medial and lateral plateaus may be fractured simultaneously, although the lateral plateau is more often fractured.[12] Direct trauma to the lateral aspect of the knee may account for the preponderance of lateral tibial plateau fractures. The patient may experience painful swelling of the knee and limitation of motion. Radiographs may demonstrate a fracture, but often show only a lipohemarthrosis on the lateral view. Consider adding an anteroposterior view in the plane of the plateau (10 to 15 degrees caudal) or oblique views to help assess for displacement. If the patient cannot tolerate the additional views, or there are negative radiographs but the patient cannot bear weight, consider obtaining a CT scan.[5] Soft tissue injuries associated with tibial plateau fractures may influence outcomes. Anterior cruciate ligament and medial collateral ligament injuries are associated with lateral plateau fractures, whereas posterior cruciate and lateral collateral ligament injuries occur with medial plateau fractures. A Segond's fracture (see below) is pathognomonic for an anterior cruciate ligament injury, and it is important recognize and treat the ligament injury, rather than just the plateau fracture.[12] Potential complications of tibial plateau fractures include popliteal artery injury with high-energy displaced fractures, the development of deep venous thrombosis, and osteoarthritis.

LIGAMENTOUS AND MENISCAL INJURIES

The knee joint depends on ligaments and muscles for support (Figure 274-2). It is frequently subjected to injuries from traumatic forces, including hyperextension, valgus and varus stresses, and anteroposterior displacement. By far the most common forces are valgus, which produce injuries to the medial side of the knee. Injuries to the lateral side of the knee are produced by varus stresses. Such forces may result in a strain or rupture of the medial or lateral collateral ligaments, the anterior or posterior cruciate ligaments, or the capsular structures, or a tear in the medial or lateral meniscus or both. Functional instability of the knee is determined by stress testing, which may demonstrate abnormal laxity when properly done. **Table 274-3** summarizes the reported sensitivity, specificity, and positive and negative likelihood ratios for diagnosis of ligamentous and meniscal injury.[14]

MEDIAL COLLATERAL LIGAMENT AND LATERAL COLLATERAL LIGAMENT INJURIES

The medial stabilizers of the knee are tested by applying a valgus stress (**Figure 274-6**) to the knee in approximately 30 degrees of flexion to determine the integrity of the medial capsular and ligamentous structures. The medial collateral ligament supplies the majority of restraint to valgus deformities of the knee in all stages of flexion. A varus force is then applied to the lateral aspect of the knee, again with approximately 30 degrees of flexion, to ascertain the integrity of the lateral structures. The lateral collateral ligament, analogous to the medial collateral ligament, is the major restraint to varus laxity on the knee at all positions of flexion. Injuries to these ligaments can include a strain, partial tear, or

TABLE 274-3 Reliability of Physical Examination for Diagnosis of Knee Ligamentous and Meniscal Injuries

Structure	Maneuver	Mean Sensitivity (range)	Mean Specificity (range)	Positive LR (95% CI)	Negative LR (95% CI)	Comments
Anterior cruciate ligament	Composite examination*	82% (62–100)	94% (56–100)	25 (2.1–306)	0.04 (0.01–0.48)	When limited to acute injury (one study), 62% sensitivity and 56% specificity.
	Anterior drawer test	62% (9–93)	67% (23–100)	3.8 (0.7–22.0)	0.3 (0.05–1.5)	Variability of studies may be due to small sample sizes.
	Lachman test	84% (60–100)	100% (100)	42 (2.7–651.0)	0.1 (0.0–0.4)	Only one study commented on specificity. Therefore specificity and LRs may be inaccurate.
	Lateral pivot shift	38% (27–95)	NA	NA	NA	No study commented on specificity.
Posterior cruciate ligament	Composite examination*	95.5% (91–100)	89.5% (80–99)	21 (2.1–205.0)	0.05 (0.01–0.50)	Results limited to two studies.
	Posterior drawer test	55% (51–86)	NA	NA	NA	No study commented on specificity.
Medial collateral ligament/lateral collateral ligament	NA	NA	NA	NA	NA	No study was identified that adequately examined diagnostic accuracy for these injuries.
Meniscal injury	Composite examination*	77% (64–82)	81% (78–84)	NA	NA	Only three of five studies commented on specificity.
	Joint-line tenderness	79% (76–85)	15% (11–43)	0.9 (0.8–1.0)	1.1 (1.0–1.3)	Only two of four studies included acute injuries, all four included chronic injuries; consequently, applicability to ED is limited.
	McMurray test	53% (29–63)	59% (29–100)	1.3 (0.9–1.7)	0.8 (0.6–1.1)	

Abbreviation: LR = likelihood ratio; NA = not applicable.

*These studies reported a "composite examination" without giving data on the specific examination maneuvers.

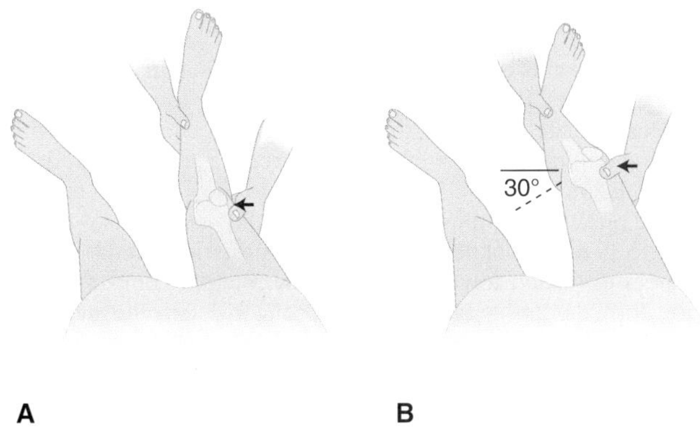

FIGURE 274-6. Valgus stress in full extension (**A**) and in 30 degrees of flexion (**B**).

complete rupture. If there is no demonstrated laxity but the valgus or varus test reproduces pain, a strain has likely occurred. If there is a laxity demonstrated without a firm end point compared with the other knee, this is concerning for a complete tear of the medial or lateral collateral ligament. If there is laxity with the varus or valgus test performed with 30 degrees of flexion, similar maneuvers should be applied with the leg in full extension, if possible. Laxity to valgus stress while in full extension indicates a significant lesion involving the entire medial collateral ligament complex and/or in association with a cruciate ligament and posterior capsule tear.[15] Laxity to varus stress in full extension likewise indicates a significant injury that may involve the posterolateral corner of the knee as well as the cruciate ligaments. Peroneal nerve injuries may also occur in lateral injuries. Although these tests may aid in the diagnosis of medial collateral ligament and lateral collateral ligament injuries, there are no adequate published reports to allow comment on their sensitivity and specificity.[14]

ANTERIOR CRUCIATE LIGAMENT INJURIES

The mechanism of injury to the anterior cruciate ligament is usually noncontact—a deceleration, hyperextension, or marked internal rotation of the tibia on the femur resulting in an injury to this ligament. Injury is often associated with a "pop," swelling that develops within hours, and a sense of instability. The pop is considered pathognomonic for anterior cruciate ligament injury.[16] The history of this mechanism of injury combined with the presence of a traumatic effusion is very suggestive of an anterior cruciate ligament disruption.

The diagnosis of an anterior cruciate ligament injury is made using the **Lachman test** (**Figure 274-7**), the anterior drawer sign (**Figure 274-8**), and the pivot shift (**Figure 274-9**). The Lachman test is the most sensitive and specific test (84% and 100%, respectively).[14] For this test the examiner places the knee in 30 degrees of flexion and stabilizes the femur above the knee with his or her nondominant hand. The dominant hand is placed grasping the lower leg at the level of the tibial tubercle, and the examiner introduces an anterior force, attempting to displace the tibia anteriorly on the femur. If a displacement compared with the opposite knee is found, or if there is a soft end point, then a tear in the anterior cruciate ligament has occurred. Although the **anterior drawer sign** has been used for a long time, its sensitivity is only approximately 62%. The maneuver is done with a 45-degree flexion at the hip and a 90-degree flexion at the knee. Then attempt to displace the tibia from the femur in an anterior direction. A displacement of >6 mm compared with the normal, opposite knee indicates an injury to the anterior cruciate ligament. False-negative findings may be associated with this maneuver. False-positive results may occur when there is a posterior cruciate ligament tear as the tibia will start out in a more posterior position, thus allowing for a perceived increase in translation when moved anteriorly. Although the Lachman test is more sensitive than the anterior drawer test and is able to identify partial tears in the anterior cruciate ligament when the examiner is skilled, it can be difficult to perform on patients with large legs. The **pivot shift** (Figure 274-9) is the third maneuver by which the examiner can determine the integrity of the anterior cruciate ligament. The pivot shift may be somewhat painful to the patient and is often most easily tested in the operating room. The pivot shift test

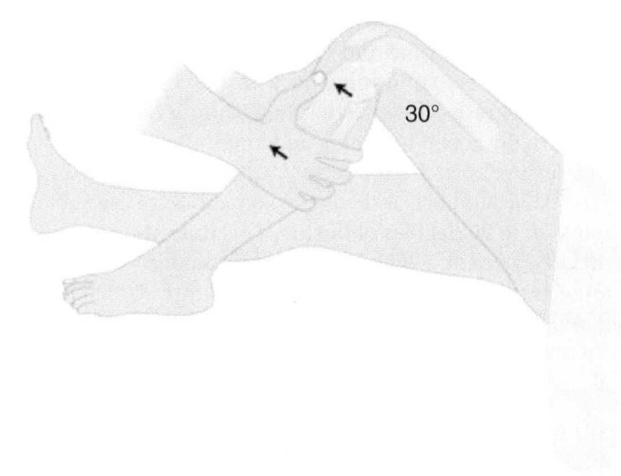

FIGURE 274-8. Anterior drawer test, performed with 45-degree flexion at the hip and a 90-degree flexion at the knee. Try to displace the tibia from the femur in an anterior direction.

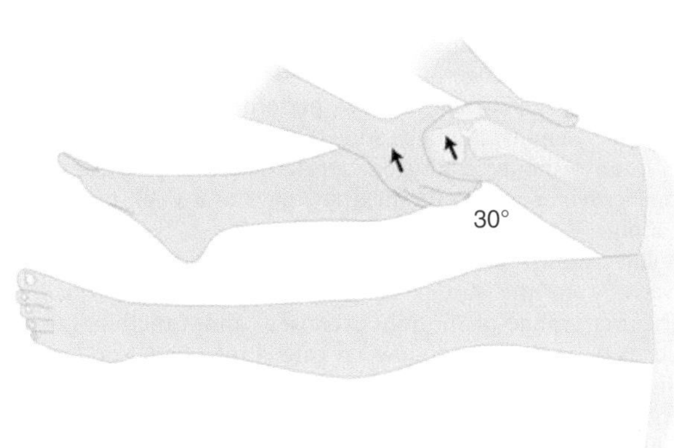

FIGURE 274-7. Lachman test, performed with the knee flexed between 15 and 30 degrees. One hand stabilizes the thigh while the other moves the tibia anteriorly.

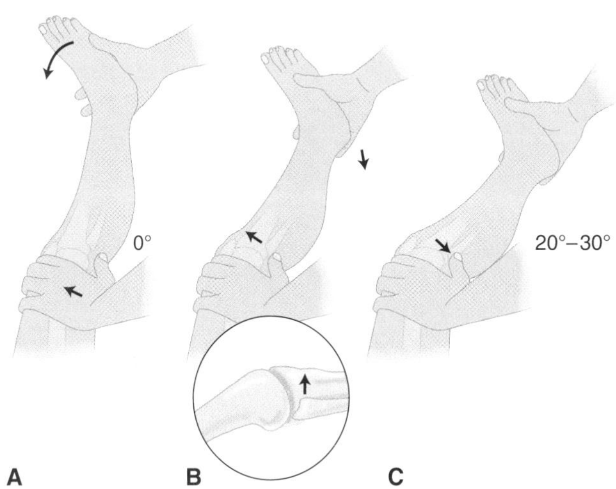

FIGURE 274-9. **A through C.** In the pivot shift of Galway and MacIntosh, the test is done with the knee in full extension with application of a valgus and internal rotation stress. The "clunk" of reduction is felt in the first 20 to 30 degrees of flexion.

without anesthesia was found to be only 24% sensitive but 98% specific.[17] With the patient supine and relaxed, lift the heel of the foot to approximately 45 degrees of hip flexion with the knee fully extended. The opposite hand grasps the knee with the thumb behind the fibular head. Then internally rotate the ankle and knee, apply a valgus force to the knee, and flex the knee. If an anterior subluxation of the tibia is present, a sudden visible, audible, and palpable reduction of the subluxation occurs at about 20 to 30 degrees of flexion. This indicates a deficit in the anterior cruciate ligament, which is required to stabilize the knee in this position. Other tests are described in the literature to determine the integrity of the anterior cruciate ligament, including the jerk test and dynamic extension testing.

POSTERIOR CRUCIATE LIGAMENT INJURIES

The posterior cruciate ligament can be injured in isolation or in combination with other ligamentous structures of the knee. In contrast to anterior cruciate ligament injuries, isolated posterior cruciate ligament injuries are much less common. The posterior cruciate ligament provides initial resistance to posterior translation at all angles of flexion of the knee. The mechanism of injury then is usually an anterior-to-posterior force applied to the tibia or lower leg. Posterior cruciate ligament injuries are seen in association with other ligamentous injuries when a serious injury has occurred to the knee. A deficit of this ligament is identified by the posterior drawer test (**Figure 274-10**) and the sag sign. The posterior drawer test is performed with the knee and hip in flexion as described for the anterior drawer test. The physician applies a posterior force to the tibial tubercle. If there is displacement posteriorly, then the examiner can diagnose an injury to this ligament. One might also notice a sag sign, where there is a posterior sag or drop back of the tibial tubercle because of loss of integrity of the posterior cruciate ligament when observing the knee with 45-degree flexion at the hip and 90-degree flexion at the knee. Results of this test can be misleading, however, if there is a straight anterior instability resulting in a subluxation of the knee forward. This abnormal position gives the false impression of too much posterior play when the posterior drawer test is performed, because the knee is reduced to its normal anatomic alignment from the forwardly subluxed position. Although the posterior drawer test has only a 55% sensitivity, the composite history and physical examination findings are much more accurate in the diagnosis of posterior cruciate ligament injuries.[14,18]

Combined ligamentous laxity of the knee is often seen, especially in acute athletic injuries. Combined anteromedial and anterolateral laxity occurs most frequently, but virtually any combination of medial and lateral laxity of the knee can occur.

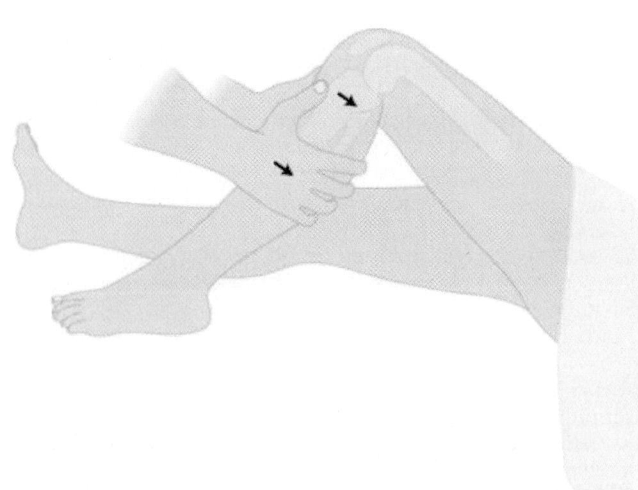

FIGURE 274-10. Posterior drawer test.

POSTEROLATERAL INJURY

One knee injury that is especially difficult to detect is injury to the posterolateral structures. Posterolateral instability usually involves a tear of the popliteus–arcuate complex, which may occur in combination with lateral ligament injury and possible anterior cruciate ligament or posterior cruciate ligament injury. Isolated injuries to the popliteus–arcuate complex are rare. Isolated posterolateral instability is demonstrated by testing at 0 to 30 degrees of flexion for maximal posterior translation and at 90 degrees of flexion for maximal external rotation compared with that of the normal opposite knee. Further testing to determine the integrity of the lateral collateral ligament and anterior or posterior cruciate ligaments must be done as well.

HEMARTHROSIS OR EFFUSION

The presence of a hemarthrosis can suggest an underlying ligamentous injury to the knee, most commonly the anterior cruciate ligament. Serious ligament injuries, however, may present with minimal pain and no hemarthrosis because of complete disruption of the ligamentous and capsular fibers, which allows leakage of the blood into the soft tissue spaces. Hemarthrosis can also be caused by osteochondral fractures or fractures that extend into the joint line, or peripheral meniscal tears. Traumatic hemarthroses usually occur within minutes to hours of injury, in contrast to chronic effusions of the knee due to synovial inflammation, which occur 1 to 2 days after strenuous use of the joint.

With ligamentous injuries, plain radiographs are typically normal or reveal only an effusion. An avulsion fracture at the site of attachment of the lateral capsular ligament on the lateral tibial condyle (Segond's fracture) is a marker for anterior cruciate ligament rupture.[7,12] Cortical avulsion of the medial tibial plateau (very uncommon) is associated with tears of the posterior cruciate ligament and medial meniscus.[19] Continued refinements in MRI have enabled this imaging method to produce high-quality images of the ligamentous and meniscal structures of the knee, which results in an accuracy rate of close to 90% to 95% in identifying meniscal and cruciate ligament disruption.[20] Such an MRI examination, however, is typically ordered by the patient's primary care provider, sports medicine physician, or orthopedist in follow-up.

TREATMENT OF SPECIFIC INJURIES

LIGAMENTOUS INJURIES

Injuries involving a single ligament with a minor strain can be managed with a knee immobilizer, ice packs, elevation, nonsteroidal anti-inflammatory drugs, and ambulation as soon as is comfortable for the patient.[21] When knee immobilizers are placed, instruct the patient to perform daily range-of-motion exercises to avoid contracture and maintain mobility. Contractures are more common in the elderly and can occur after only a few days of immobilization. Although there is no universally accepted regimen for range-of-motion exercise, one procedure is first to apply ice to relieve pain and then to perform 10 to 20 knee flexion-extensions (no weights should be added) three or four times a day. Refer patients to an orthopedic surgeon, sports medicine physician, or primary care provider within the next few days to a week for follow-up examination.

Complete rupture of an isolated ligament can initially be treated conservatively in the same fashion, with straight leg quadriceps strengthening, range-of-motion exercises, and functional bracing included as a part of the follow-up care. Professional athletes with single-ligament ruptures or patients with more than one torn ligament need urgent orthopedic consultation so that definitive surgical management can be planned.

Arthrocentesis may be of therapeutic benefit in patients with large, tense effusions of the knee; however, good evidence of its efficacy has not been reported. A systematic review to ascertain whether aspiration improves symptoms in patients with acute traumatic hemarthrosis found no conclusive data.[22] Furthermore, recurrence of the effusion following aspiration is common. Arthrocentesis may be of assistance diagnostically if the effusion is not clearly due to trauma. The presence of blood and glistening fat globules is pathognomonic of lipohemarthrosis, which indicates intra-articular knee fracture. The major complication of arthrocentesis is septic arthritis.

MENISCAL INJURIES

Meniscal injuries of the knee occur by themselves or in combination with ligamentous injuries. For example, anterior cruciate ligament injuries are commonly associated with meniscal injuries. Cutting, squatting, or twisting maneuvers may cause injury to the meniscus. The medial meniscus is approximately twice as likely as the lateral meniscus to be injured. Four fifths of the tears involve the peripheral posterior aspect of the meniscus.[23] Many maneuvers have been described in the literature to determine whether a meniscus has been injured. Most of these tests, however, have an unacceptable sensitivity and specificity (e.g., joint line tenderness has a sensitivity of 70% and specificity of 15% in the ED population).[14] Although the diagnosis of a meniscal tear is difficult to make in certain patients, the combination of a suggestive history and physical findings on examination should lead the emergency physician to consider the diagnosis. Ask if the patient experiences painful locking of the knee joint on either flexion or extension and if this limits further activity. This sign clearly points to the diagnosis of a torn meniscus. Effusions that occur after activity; a sensation of popping, clicking, or snapping; a feeling of instability in the joint, especially with activity; and tenderness in the anterior joint space after excessive activity suggest the diagnosis of a meniscal tear.

At physical examination, attempt to identify atrophy of the quadriceps muscle because of disuse and joint-line tenderness. Various maneuvers, such as the McMurray test or the grind test, have been described but yield positive results only about 50% of the time.[14,24] If a tentative diagnosis of a meniscal tear is considered, refer to an orthopedic surgeon or the patient's primary care provider and instruct partial weight bearing, as tolerated. Definitive diagnosis can be made by MRI or arthroscopy, with the latter also allowing for definitive surgical treatment (usually partial meniscectomy or meniscal repair).

LOCKED KNEE

The "locked knee" describes when a knee cannot actively or passively fully extend. A patient who presents to the ED with a locked knee can experience a great deal of pain along with loss of mobility. The most common cause of an acutely locked knee is a torn meniscus. The differential diagnosis also includes anterior cruciate ligament rupture, patella dislocation, loose bodies, or foreign body. Historically the treatment includes one attempt at closed reduction under procedural sedation. After procedural sedation is initiated, one can attempt to unlock the knee. Position the patient with the leg hanging over the edge of the table and the knee in 90 degrees of flexion. After a period of relaxation, apply longitudinal traction to the knee, along with internal and external rotation, in an attempt to unlock the joint. If this maneuver is unsuccessful, orthopedic consultation for operative arthroscopy is indicated. If the unlocking is successful, referral to an orthopedist for MRI and/or arthroscopy is appropriate.[25]

KNEE DISLOCATION

Knee dislocation (**Figure 274-11**) is a result of tremendous ligamentous disruption due to hyperextension or application of direct posterior force to the anterior tibia, force to the fibula or medial femur, force to the tibia or lateral femur, or rotatory force resulting in anterior, posterior, lateral, medial, or rotatory dislocation. This injury typically occurs following high-velocity mechanisms such as motor vehicle crashes or low-velocity mechanisms in sports; however, dislocations can also occur spontaneously in morbidly obese patients.[1,26] An anterior dislocation is most common, occurring about 40% of the time, with posterior dislocations (33%), lateral dislocations (18%), medial dislocations (4%), and rotary dislocations also occurring.[2,26] Because of severe ligamentous damage, spontaneous reduction occurs in up to 50% of knee dislocations.[2] Therefore, **a severely injured knee that is unstable in multiple directions raises suspicion of a spontaneously reduced knee dislocation.** Maintaining awareness of the possibility of this injury is important because of the high incidence of associated complications, including popliteal artery injury and peroneal nerve injury (mostly with posterolateral dislocations), in addition to ligamentous and meniscal injury.

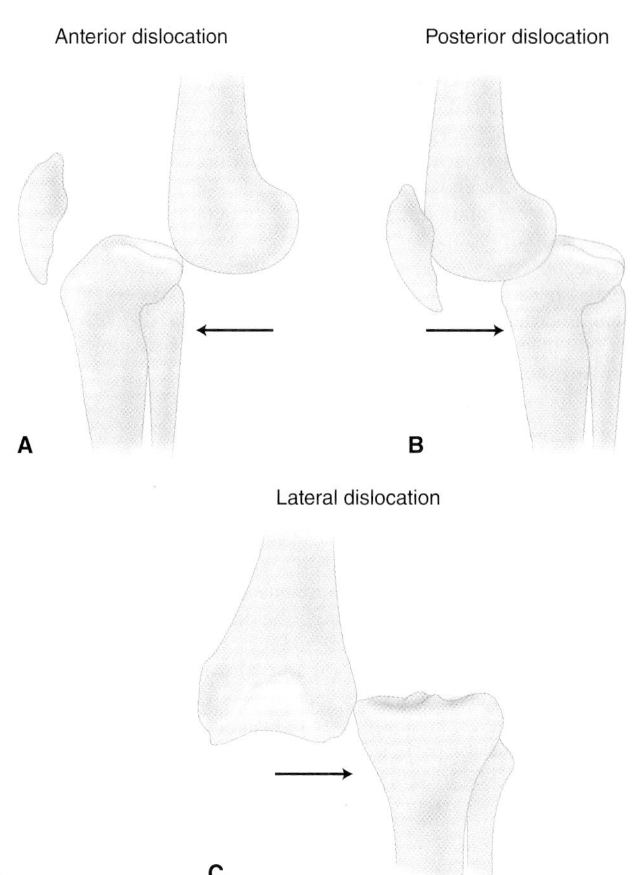

FIGURE 274-11. Types of knee dislocation: anterior (**A**), posterior (**B**), and lateral (**C**).

Timely reduction of the dislocated knee is essential. Apply longitudinal traction to the affected knee. Document neurovascular status of the extremity before and after reduction. **Splint the lower extremity with the knee at 20 degrees of flexion after dislocation reduction** to prevent redislocation. Reimage after splint application. Hospitalization is required along with emergent orthopedic and vascular surgery consultation. If the patient is neurovascularly intact and vascular and/or orthopedic surgery consultation is unavailable, then transfer the patient prior to reduction to the nearest hospital with those clinical services. Timely reduction can occur at that time.

There are no clear guidelines for arteriography in patients with knee dislocation. Because of the high incidence of popliteal artery injury (up to one third of patients) and poor outcomes associated with delays in vascular reconstruction, some authors recommend arteriography for all patients with confirmed knee dislocations.[1,27] Another option after reduction of a knee dislocation is to repeat the neurovascular exam and perform Doppler pressure indices[28] (ankle-brachial index; see chapter 61, "Arterial Occlusion"). Patients with distal pulses present before and after reduction and an ankle-brachial index >0.9 can be observed with serial neurovascular checks. The orthopedist may want a CT angiogram prior to ligamentous reconstruction. For patients in whom distal pulses are asymmetric, the ankle-brachial index is <0.9, or there is any other clinical concern of vascular injury (including ischemia, hemorrhage, or an expanding hematoma), proceed with CT angiogram or angiography. Patients with absent pulses before reduction with a return of a pulse after reduction need measurement of an ankle-brachial index and emergent vascular surgery consultation.[2] Patients with an open knee dislocation, absent distal pulses after reduction, or any other signs of vascular injury, as above, need emergent vascular surgery consultation for surgical exploration and possible angiography in the operating room.[2,26,28]

Close observation of patients with suspected knee dislocation is essential, because the presence of normal distal pulses does not rule out a popliteal artery injury. Splint the affected knee in 20 degrees of flexion, with care taken to construct the splint in a manner that allows for serial vascular examinations.

PATELLAR DISLOCATION

Dislocation of the patella usually occurs from a twisting injury to the extended knee. The patella is displaced laterally over the lateral condyle, which results in pain and deformity of the knee (**Figure 274-12**). Tearing of the medial knee joint capsule often occurs. Reduction is accomplished with the patient under conscious sedation by flexing the hip, hyperextending the knee, and sliding the patella back into place. This results in immediate relief of pain; however, caution patients that they will have residual soreness from the medial patellofemoral retinacular tissue injury. Obtain x-rays of the patella and knee to exclude a fracture, and place a knee immobilizer after reduction[10] and provide crutches. Give instructions for partial weight bearing and straight leg raises to strengthen the quadriceps. Arrange follow-up with an orthopedist within 1 week. Recurrent lateral dislocation of the patella occurs in approximately 15% of patients, and superior, horizontal, and intercondylar dislocations require referral to an orthopedic surgeon for possible surgical intervention.[29]

In the case of irreducible patellar dislocation, surgical correction is needed. Clues that a patient may have an irreducible patellar dislocation include older age, preexisting patellofemoral arthritis, flexion of <45 degrees, anterolateral (rather than pure lateral) patellar position, and internal rotation of the patellar axis.[30]

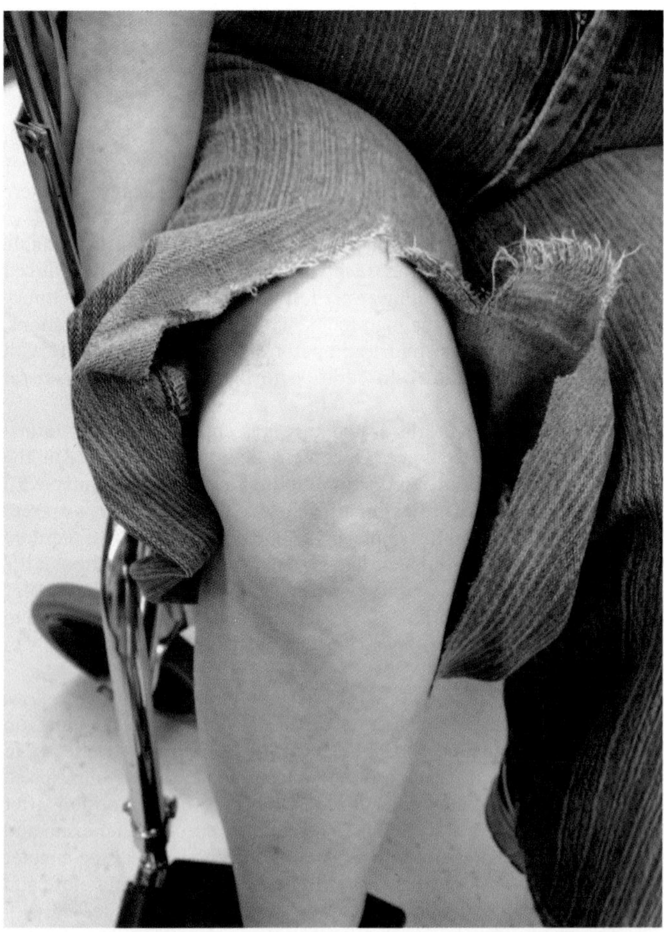

FIGURE 274-12. Lateral dislocation of the right patella. [Photo contributed by Rob Hendrickson, MD, and Michael Martinez, MD.]

QUADRICEPS OR PATELLAR TENDON RUPTURE

Rupture of the quadriceps or patellar tendons can occur from forceful contraction of the quadriceps muscle or falling on a flexed knee. Quadriceps tendon rupture is most frequent in those >40 years of age. Patellar tendon rupture occurs most commonly in individuals <40 years of age. A history of tendinitis or past oral or injected steroid can increase risk of rupture.[8] Quadriceps or patellar tendon rupture disrupts the extensor mechanism of the knee. There is severe pain and diffuse swelling, and the patient is unable to actively extend the knee or maintain a passively extended knee against gravity in both types of tendon rupture. Depending on the tendon ruptured, a defect may be palpable proximal or distal to the patella. **Figure 274-13** shows a quadriceps tendon rupture. A high-riding patella (patella alta) may be seen on a lateral radiograph of the knee in the setting of a patellar tendon rupture (**Figure 274-14**). The treatment of a complete tear is surgical repair of the involved tendon. Orthopedic consultation in the ED is indicated. Incomplete tears with an intact extensor mechanism can be treated with immobilization and close follow-up.[8]

PATELLAR TENDINITIS

Also known as jumper's knee, patellar tendinitis is primarily seen in runners, high jumpers, and basketball and volleyball players. Pain is located at the patellar tendon and is worsened when going from sitting to standing, jumping, or running up hills. Evaluate the extensor mechanism to rule out tendon rupture. Point tenderness can be found at the distal aspect of the patella or proximal part of the patellar tendon. Treatment consists of nonsteroidal anti-inflammatory drugs, eccentric quadriceps-strengthening exercises, and activity modification. Steroid injections predispose to tendon rupture and thus should be avoided.

POSTARTHROSCOPY PROBLEMS

Patients may present to the ED following arthroscopy because of pain and swelling. Effusions are common after arthroscopy, but joint infection

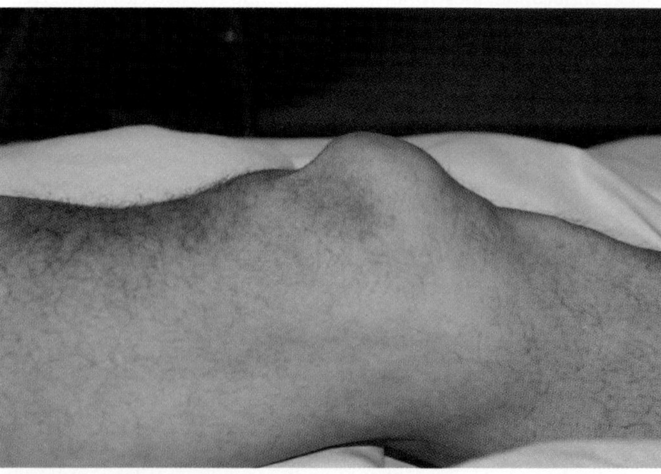

FIGURE 274-13. Quadriceps tendon rupture. Note the defect above the patella and prominence of the proximal edge of the patella. [Reproduced with permission of the Department of Emergency Medicine, Feinberg School of Medicine, Northwestern University.]

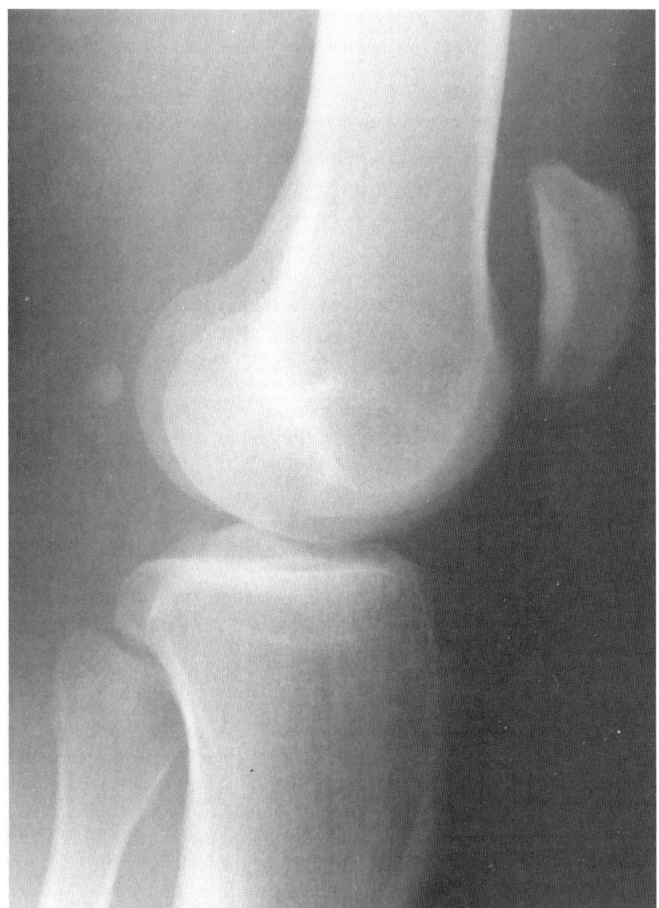

FIGURE 274-14. Patella alta.

is very uncommon. Perform diagnostic arthrocentesis if joint infection is suspected. Arthrocentesis and then injection of bupivacaine may be helpful therapeutically for large, tense effusions and may reduce the need for systemic analgesia.

PENETRATING KNEE INJURY AND JOINT FOREIGN BODIES

The history should elicit information to re-create the position of the knee when the penetrating injury occurred. Many occupational injuries occur with the knee flexed, and failure to appreciate the trajectory of injury with the knee flexed can lead to misdiagnosis and failure to anticipate joint penetration. Management of lacerations in proximity to joint spaces is discussed in chapter 44, "Leg and Foot Lacerations," in the section "Wound Management."

Radiopaque foreign bodies (i.e., metal, glass) can be visualized on conventional radiographs. In general, foreign bodies in the knee joint need to be removed. A bullet in the joint can destroy the cartilage, and lead poisoning can occur.[31] Antibiotics to cover streptococci and staphylococci are generally indicated for both penetrating knee wounds and foreign bodies. Administer tetanus prophylaxis as indicated.

REFERENCES

The complete reference list is available online at www.TintinalliEM.com.

CHAPTER 275 Leg Injuries

Paul R. Haller

ANATOMY

BONE

The tibia provides primary support for weight bearing. The tibia has a thick cortex, and significant force is required to fracture it. Proximally, the tibia splays out to form the medial and lateral plateaus that articulate with the femoral condyles. The lateral plateau is higher and smaller than the medial and is more susceptible to fracture. The distal tibia articulates with the fibula laterally and the talus inferiorly. A dense interosseous membrane connects the tibia and fibula. The distal tibial articulation is supported by the ankle syndesmosis, a series of ligaments inferior to the interosseous membrane. The fibula has a small diameter and lies lateral and posterior to the tibia. It bears little weight but is more easily fractured than the tibia.

COMPARTMENTS

The lower leg is divided into four compartments, each coursing parallel to the tibia (**Figure 275-1**). The compartments are enclosed by nonexpandable bones and connective tissue that limit the compartment size and prevent compartment expansion if its volume increases. Each compartment contains muscles and nerves that may sustain permanent damage with elevated tissue compartment pressure (**Table 275-1**). (See also chapter 278, "Compartment Syndrome.")

A cross-section at the midcalf level shows the anterior compartment enclosed by the tibia, interosseous membrane, and anterior crural septum (Table 275-1 and Figure 275-1). Muscles in the anterior compartment group dorsiflex the foot and ankle. The deep peroneal nerve courses within the anterior compartment and exits to provide sensation to the dorsal web space between the first and second toes.

The lateral compartment is bordered by the anterior crural septum, the fibula, and the posterior crural septum. Its muscles plantarflex and evert the foot. The superficial peroneal nerve in this compartment provides sensation to the dorsum of the foot. The superficial posterior compartment contains muscles that flex the knee and the tibiotalar joints. Its sural nerve provides sensation for the lateral aspect of the foot and the distal calf. The muscles of the deep posterior compartment plantarflex the foot and toes and invert the foot. The posterior tibial nerve that exits this compartment provides sensation to the sole of the foot.

CLINICAL FEATURES

The history may give clues about the mechanism of injury and nontraumatic soft tissue injuries. Evaluate the nerves by checking sensation in the web space, lateral heel, and sole of the foot. Plantarflex and dorsiflex the foot, and evert the foot to test motor function. Evaluate the extent of soft

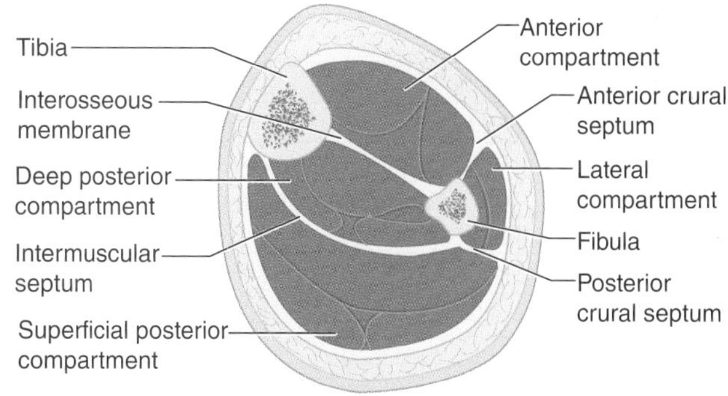

FIGURE 275-1. Lower leg anatomy.

TABLE 275-1 Lower Leg Anatomy

	Compartments			
	Anterior	Lateral	Superficial Posterior	Deep Posterior
Muscles	Dorsiflex foot and ankle	Plantarflex and evert foot	Flex knee and ankle	Plantarflex toes, inversion of foot
Nerve	Deep peroneal	Superficial peroneal	Sural	Posterior tibial
Sensation	First dorsal web space	Dorsum of foot	Lateral aspect of foot and distal calf	Sole of foot
Artery	Anterior tibial	—	—	Posterior tibial

tissue injury visually and by palpating the compartmental muscle groups. It is often the extent of soft tissue injury, rather than the fracture itself, that determines the outcome. Palpate the knee, and the tibia and fibula along their entire lengths. Palpate the popliteal, dorsal pedal, and posterior tibial pulses. An absent or decreased pulse may indicate the need for urgent fracture reduction and further vascular evaluation.

DIAGNOSIS

Anteroposterior and lateral radiographs of the leg that include the knee and ankle are sufficient to evaluate bony injuries. If ankle or knee injuries are suspected, then further imaging is needed. If a tibial shaft fracture is suspected, splint the leg with a radiolucent device to control pain and prevent further soft tissue damage before obtaining films. Check pulses, movement, and sensation before and after splinting the leg.

TREATMENT

Cleanse wounds and debride loose tissue and foreign material. Administer tetanus immunization as indicated. Splint fractures before obtaining radiographs; this will prevent further damage to soft tissue caused by movement of bone fragments. Irrigate open wounds and administer parenteral antibiotics (such as cefazolin, 1 gram IV) for open fractures. If compartment syndrome is suspected, measure compartment pressure (see chapter 278, "Compartment Syndrome"). Treatment of compartment syndrome is fasciotomy of the involved compartment. Details of suturing pretibial lacerations are provided in the chapter 44, "Leg and Foot Lacerations."

COMPLICATIONS

Wounds that are not adequately cleansed and debrided are prone to infection. Patients with compartment syndromes may develop permanent disability if elevated tissue pressures are not suspected or diagnosed in a timely fashion. Fractures that are not adequately aligned or immobilized heal poorly or not at all.

SPECIFIC INJURIES

TIBIAL SHAFT FRACTURES

The tibia is the most commonly fractured long bone. Fractures often result in open injuries because of the minimal amount of subcutaneous tissue between the tibia and the skin. The fracture pattern seen on radiographs will give a clue to the force that caused the injury. Transverse shaft fractures typically result from a direct blow to the bone. Spiral fractures are the result of rotational forces. A comminuted fracture suggests the mechanism had a very-high-energy impact. A force powerful enough to shatter the dense cortex of the tibial shaft will often be transmitted through the interosseous membrane to the fibula, fracturing that bone as well.

Open tibial shaft fractures have been classified (**Table 275-2**).[1] A grade 1 injury has minimal soft tissue contusion and a skin laceration that is 1 cm in length or less. A grade 2 injury involves a wound with a >1-cm laceration with moderate soft tissue injury and moderate contamination; the tibia is moderately comminuted. A grade 3 injury can involve segmental injury to the tibia, a vascular injury, a highly contaminated wound, or a >10-cm laceration. This classification system is prognostic in terms of healing time and rate of nonunion. The soft tissue injuries often are determinants of the immediate treatment plan.

The initial management of tibial fractures involves administration of analgesics. Promptly splint the leg with radiolucent material to avoid further soft tissue injury from the movement of the bony fragments. Assess for possible compartment syndrome. Some closed injuries may be treated simply by casting if reduction is able to achieve adequate alignment. Parameters for acceptable reduction include 50% or more of cortical contact, <10 to 15 degrees of angulation on the lateral film, <10 degrees of angulation on the anteroposterior film, and <5 degrees of rotational deformity.[2] Injuries with significant edema and spiral fractures often require surgical fixation. An intact fibula may make obtaining or maintaining reduction of the tibial fracture more difficult.

A *long leg splint* from high above the knee with the knee at 5 degrees of flexion and the foot in slight plantarflexion can be applied. **Tight-fitting splints or casts may increase the risk of compartment syndrome.** Injuries amenable to casting often heal in 4 to 5 months. Initiate weight bearing as soon as possible to facilitate bone union. Patients usually can achieve full weight bearing with crutches in 7 to 14 days.[2]

Patients who can be discharged home after splinting include those who suffered low-energy injuries, have their pain well controlled, and are not at risk of compartment syndrome.

The patient with an open tibial fracture requires orthopedic consultation. Injuries with type 1 soft tissue damage may be cleaned in the operating room and medullary nails inserted to maintain reduction. Those

TABLE 275-2 Gustilo Classification of Open Tibia Shaft Fractures

	Gustilo Grade				
	1	2	3A	3B	3C
Energy	Low	Moderate	High	High	High
Wound size	<1 cm	>1 cm	Often large zone of injury	Often large zone of injury	Often large zone of injury
Soft tissue damage	None	None	Extensive	Extensive	Extensive
Contamination	Clean	Moderate	Extensive	Extensive	Extensive
Fracture pattern	Simple fracture pattern with minimal comminution	Moderate comminution	Severe comminution or segmental fractures	Severe comminution or segmental fractures	Severe comminution or segmental fractures
Periosteal stripping	No	No	Yes	Yes	Yes
Skin coverage	Local coverage	Local coverage	Local coverage	Requires replacement of exposed bone with a free flap for coverage	Local coverage
Neurovascular injury	Normal	Normal	Normal	Normal	Exposed fracture with arterial damage that requires repair

with more extensive injuries may require external fixation or medullary nailing after debridement in the operative room.

SEVERELY INJURED TIBIAL SHAFT

Some patients suffer such extensive damage to their leg that they may be better served by amputation of the leg rather than an attempt to salvage the limb. There are four functional components of the leg: bone, vessels, nerves, and soft tissue. Severe injury to any three of these puts the limb at risk. Most severe injuries are caused by a crushing mechanism. Motor vehicle crashes or farm or industrial accidents are most common, followed by falls. Penetrating injuries caused by gunshot wounds or explosives may also put a limb at risk. There are about 3700 amputations per year performed due to these extensive injuries.

Initial management of the patient with a mangled extremity should include attention to life-threatening injuries, immobilization of the leg, diagnostic imaging, pain control, IV antibiotic administration, and tetanus prophylaxis as needed.

PILON FRACTURES

Pilon is a French word for pestle, a tool used to grind substance in a mortar. In the lower leg, an axial force on the foot can drive the talus into the articular surface of the tibia, grinding or crushing the distal tibia. This injury is also called a *tibial plafond fracture* (**Figure 275-2**).

The amount of energy involved in the accident often predicts the type of injury and is important in planning treatment. A high-energy mechanism (motor vehicle crash) often results in significant soft tissue damage with extensive fragmentation of the bone. By contrast, low-energy injuries (skiing) have minimal surrounding soft tissue damage and less comminution of the bone. Radiographs may show at least one fracture plane that extends proximally from the articular surface of the ankle. There are often several fracture planes present. Obtain a CT scan while the leg is in a splint or cast. The scan will help determine the direction of the fracture planes, reveal the amount of articular surface displacement that exists, and aid in the development of a treatment plan. **Pilon fractures may be accompanied by compartment syndrome or by vertebral body fractures, particularly a fracture of the first lumbar vertebrae (L1).**[3]

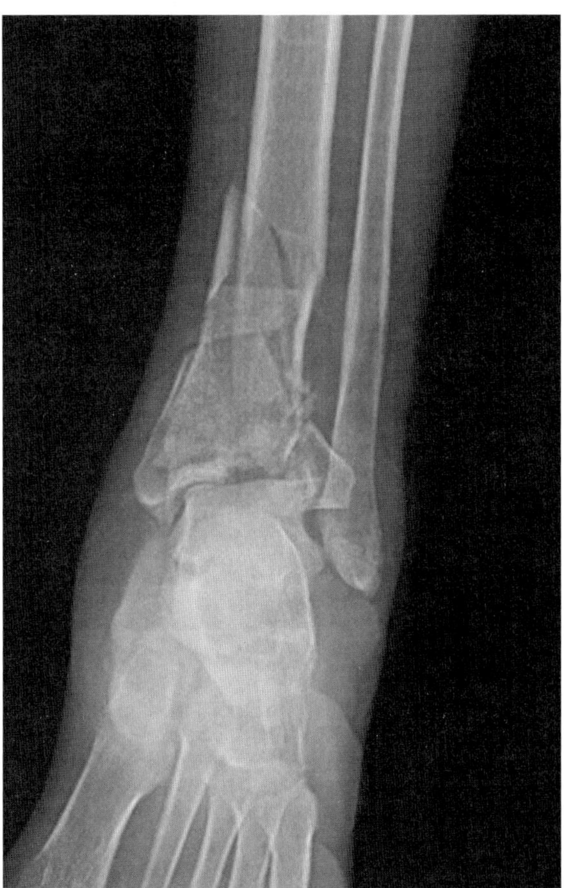

FIGURE 275-2. Plafond fracture. Tibial plafond fracture (pilon fracture) due to an axial compression force. [Reproduced with permission from Simon RR, Sherman SC, Koenigsknecht SJ: *Emergency Orthopedics: The Extremities*, 5th ed. © The McGraw-Hill Companies. All rights reserved. Part III: Lower Extremities, Chapter 17 Ankle, Fractures, Axial Compression, Imaging, Figure 17-24.]

The goal of treatment is reduction of the fracture fragment and optimal alignment of the articular surfaces. The extent of soft tissue damage may determine when surgical repair occurs. In the setting of significant soft tissue damage, an external fixation device may temporarily be used to allow this tissue time to heal before definitive surgery.

TRIPLANE FRACTURES

The distal tibial growth plate begins to fuse when adolescents are between the ages of 12 and 15 years old. The process takes about 18 months. The medial portion of the growth plate fuses before the lateral. It is this relatively weak lateral growth plate that makes them susceptible to a triplane fracture.

An external rotational force applied to the foot causes stress and a fracture of the tibia. The fracture plane extends from the lateral side of the tibia through the growth plate until it reaches the already fused medial aspect of the physis. At that point, the fracture planes are redirected into sagittal and coronal planes. The resulting injuries can appear to be a Salter III fracture on the anteroposterior radiographic view and a Salter II injury on the lateral view. **Evaluate this injury with a CT scan, which often can reveal further deformity of the articular surface.**

The treatment goal is producing good articular surface alignment, which can be obtained with closed reduction in most cases.[4] With a complex fracture pattern, some patients will require surgery to attain optimal joint surface alignment.

PROXIMAL FIBULA FRACTURE (MAISONNEUVE'S FRACTURE)

Maisonneuve's fracture results from an external rotation force applied to the foot. This creates a plane of injury that starts at the medial ankle as either a deltoid ligament rupture or a medial malleolus injury. The injury is then directed upward and laterally, tearing the interosseous membrane that tethers the distal tibia to the fibula. The third component of this injury is a fracture of the proximal fibula. The word *proximal* is relative; the fibula may be fractured at its head or as far down as 6 cm above the ankle joint (a Weber C ankle fracture).

The surgical treatment for this injury is to reduce and stabilize the fractured medial malleolus and to secure the fibula to the distal tibia, allowing the ruptured interosseous membrane to heal.

MIDSHAFT FIBULA FRACTURES

The shaft of the fibula is most often fractured by a force that has also fractured the tibia; in these cases, treatment is directed by the tibial injury. A direct blow to the fibula can result in an isolated injury to this bone. The patient typically presents with pain or tenderness over the fracture site. With the tibia intact, the patient is often able to bear weight and should be treated with a short leg cast and crutches. Patients with less intense pain may be immobilized with a knee immobilizer (proximal fibula) or elastic wrap (distal fibula) and directed to bear weight as tolerated.

STRESS FRACTURE

Stress fracture occurs when there is increased muscle activity on bones that are not able to tolerate the additional forces. Extrinsic causes may include a recent increase in activity, running over hard surfaces, or excessive wear on the athlete's shoes. Adolescent female athletes with eating disorders and military recruits are at high risk for stress fractures. As our population ages, the elderly are taking up activities that may result in stress fractures. The prototypical patient is the Caucasian woman with demineralized bone. Stress fractures are twice as common in women compared with men. About half of stress fractures in athletes occur in the tibia. Less common sites are the tarsals and fibula. Stress fractures may be bilateral. In adolescents, the site is often the proximal third of the tibia. Runners typically sustain fractures at the junction of the middle and distal third of the tibia. The distal fibula is another common site.

The history typically involves a change in the patient's training pattern. In an early stage of stress fracture, the patient notices activity-induced pain that is relieved by rest. This can progress to constant pain. On examination, there is pain on palpation over the fracture site, and there may be edema. The pain may be intensified by load bearing on the affected bone.

The radiographs of the site are often normal on initial presentation. They may reveal the fracture, which can have the appearance of sclerosed areas oriented linearly. Radiographs obtained 10 to 15 days later may show periosteal elevation or demineralization at the fracture line. Plain films that are initially normal do not exclude the diagnosis. More sensitive tests for stress fracture are the bone scan and MRI. Although these studies are typically ordered at follow-up and not in the ED setting, they can demonstrate the severity of the change and can be used to predict time to recovery.[5]

Treatment of a suspected stress fracture includes discontinuation of the activity. A cast can be applied if significant pain continues. It is not unusual to have pain lasting up to a year despite treatment.

ACHILLES TENDON RUPTURE

The Achilles tendon is the largest and strongest tendon in the human body. The gastrocnemius and soleus muscles of the calf have tendinous complexes that coalesce to the Achilles tendon that extends about 15 cm to where it inserts on the calcaneus. **Its vascular supply is the weakest in the area 2 to 6 cm above the calcaneus, and this is the area that is most frequently ruptured.** A typical patient is a 30- to 50-year-old man who participates in strenuous activities on an occasional basis ("weekend warrior"). **Risk factors for rupture include older age, prior quinolone use, and prior steroid injection.** The injury often occurs when eccentric force is suddenly applied to a dorsiflexed foot. The patient suffers sudden severe pain and is unable to run, stand on toes, or climb stairs. The most notable finding on examination is a palpable gap in the Achilles tendon 2 to 6 cm proximal to the calcaneus. The calf may be swollen. The patient will be unable to stand on toes. The Thompson test (see Figure 44-6 in chapter titled "Leg and Foot Lacerations") will help demonstrate the tendon rupture. The patient lays prone with the knee bent at 90 degrees. The examiner squeezes the calf: an intact Achilles tendon will transmit this force to the foot resulting in its plantarflexion. **If the Achilles tendon is ruptured, the foot will not plantarflex when the calf is squeezed.** The diagnosis of Achilles tendon rupture can be made without radiographs. When the diagnosis is not clear, an US or MRI of the Achilles tendon may be obtained. The reliability of US is largely dependent on the operator's skill. Initial care for Achilles tendon rupture involves immobilization from just below the knee to the metatarsals with the ankle in some plantarflexion. Crutches are necessary for non–weight-bearing status. Ice and analgesics are also used.

Subsequent therapy may involve either surgical repair of the ruptured tendon or immobilization and gradual physical therapy to regain range of motion. There has been controversy about whether surgery is superior to conservative management. In both treatment modalities, the rerupture rate is less than 5%, but there was some suggestion that conservative care was associated with a slightly higher rate of rerupture. Two studies have shown equivalent rates of rerupture in those treated surgically versus conservatively.[6,7] Refer patients with Achilles tendon rupture to an orthopedist or sports medicine specialist. They will typically be immobilized for 2 to 3 months and be able to return to their sport in 3 to 6 months.

MEDIAL GASTROCNEMIUS MUSCLE STRAIN

The medial gastrocnemius originates from the medial femoral condyle, crosses the knee, and joins the lateral gastrocnemius. The tendon complex of this muscle merges with that of the soleus muscle to form the Achilles tendon, which inserts on the calcaneus to act in plantarflexion of the foot. Injury to the medial gastrocnemius muscle usually occurs when a person forcefully plantarflexes the foot while the knee is extended, occurring when the gastrocnemius is at its maximal length. The typical patient is 40 to 60 years old and an intermittently active athlete. A sharp pain is suddenly felt in the calf as if a stick had struck the person. An audible "pop" may be heard. The pain is severe enough to cause an immediate cessation of the activity, as plantarflexion of the ankle is too painful.

On examination, there may be asymmetric calf swelling and tenderness of the calf. The Achilles tendon is intact. The patient's pain can be elicited by passive dorsiflexion of the ankle. Differential diagnosis can include deep vein thrombosis, ruptured Baker's cyst, and compartment syndrome. Radiographs are not necessary for making the diagnosis. Nonurgent MRI can be obtained to confirm the diagnosis. Treatment includes immobilization with the foot maximally plantarflexed. Rest, ice, and elevation may decrease swelling.

SHIN SPLINTS

Shin splints is a complex syndrome that may eventually be found to include several different injuries. The patient presents with exercise-induced pain over the medial aspect of the tibia. This is also referred to as a *medial tibial stress syndrome*. It may be caused by a repetitive trauma-induced periostitis of the tibia.

The population at risk includes runners, military recruits, and those with flat feet. It is uncommon before the age of 15 years old. The condition typically starts after a sudden increase in training, particularly running on hard surfaces. Physical examination findings may include tenderness over the medial or posterior tibia. Radiographs are normal. A bone scan may be needed to exclude the possibility of a stress fracture. The diagnosis is primarily a clinical one based on history and an examination that excludes other pathology. The mainstay of treatment is a several-week cessation of the activity that precipitated the pain.

REFERENCES

The complete reference list is available online at www.TintinalliEM.com.

CHAPTER 276 Ankle Injuries

Daniel A. Handel
Sarah Andrus Gaines

INTRODUCTION AND EPIDEMIOLOGY

Given the mobility of the ankle joint and our bipedal existence, ankle injuries are a common complaint. They represent 14.6% of all visits to the ED.[1] Fractures of the lateral malleolus are more prevalent in men younger than 50 years old and in women older than 50 years old.[2,3] Previous ankle sprain and participation in sports like soccer, basketball, rugby, and football are risk factors for ankle injuries.[4-7] A review of the National Electronic Injury Surveillance System in 2009 reported an incidence of ankle sprains of 206 per 100,000 people in the United States.[8]

ANATOMY

The proximal part of the ankle mortise is comprised of the distal fibula and tibia that fits on top of the talus. These bones are wider anteriorly than posteriorly. Joint stability is provided by medial and lateral malleoli extending on either side of the talus. The **medial deltoid ligament**, **lateral ligament complex**, and **syndesmosis** are the three distinct groups of ligaments that stabilize the ankle[9] (**Figure 276-1**). The deltoid ligament is the strongest of these ligaments and is a thick, triangular band of

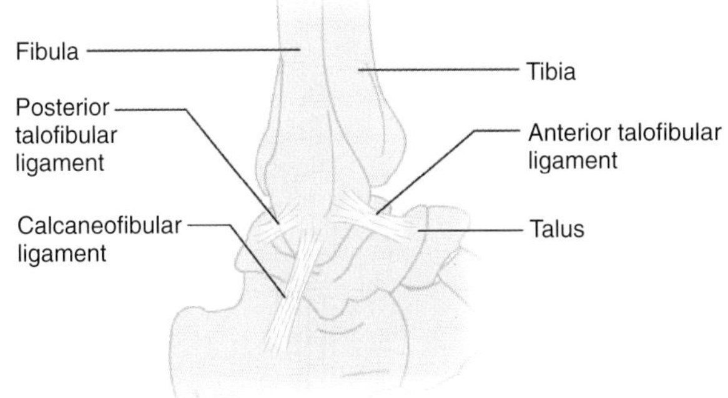

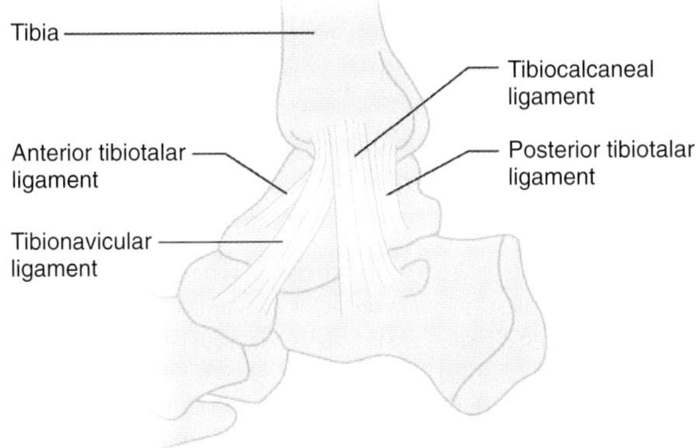

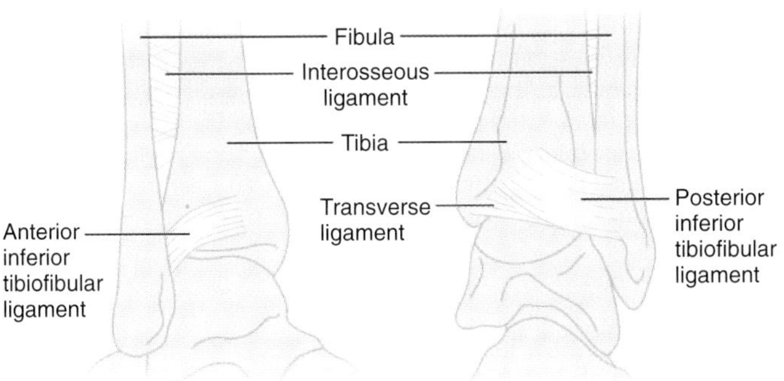

FIGURE 276-1. Ligaments of the ankle joint. **A.** The three lateral ligaments: the anterior and posterior talofibular ligaments and the calcaneofibular ligament. **B.** The four bands of the deltoid ligament: the anterior and posterior tibiotalar, the tibiocalcaneal, and the tibionavicular. **C.** Anterior and posterior view of the ankle syndesmosis. The ligaments of the syndesmosis are the anterior inferior tibiofibular ligament, the posterior inferior tibiofibular ligament, the transverse ligament, and the interosseous ligament, which connects the entire length of the tibia and fibula.

tissue originating from the medial malleolus. The lateral ligament complex consists of the lateral malleolus that attaches to the anterior and posterior aspects of the talus and calcaneus by the anterior talofibular, posterior talofibular, and calcaneofibular ligaments, respectively. This ligament complex, the anterior talofibular ligament in particular, is the weakest and most commonly injured in lateral sprains and represents 85% of all ankle sprains.[10] The syndesmosis, which holds the tibia and fibula together, is a group of four distinct ligaments attaching the distal tibia to the fibula just above the talus (Figure 276-1). The syndesmosis allows the fibula to rotate and carries approximately 16% of the axial load.[9]

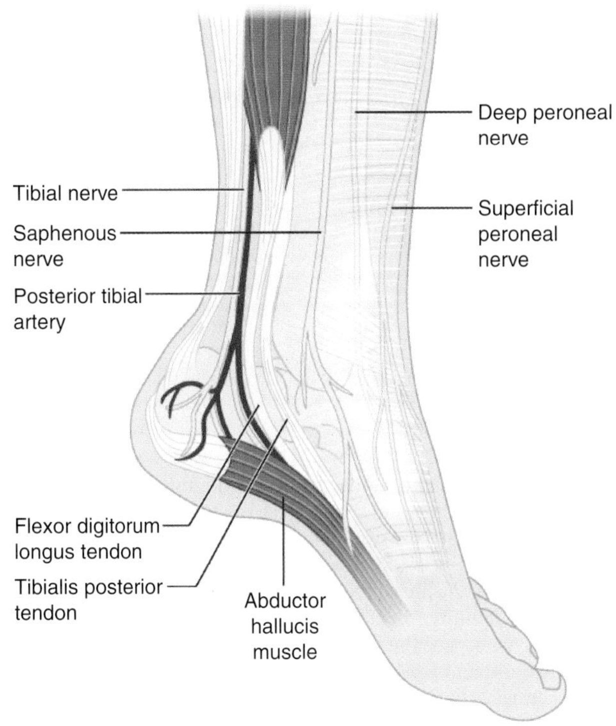

FIGURE 276-2. Neurovascular anatomy of ankle.

The ankle is considered a hinged joint, but ligamentous attachments allow for some rotation and translation within the mortise of the talar dome.[9] Branches of the sciatic nerve, the superficial peroneal, deep peroneal, peroneal, and tibial, innervate the four muscle groups of the ankle joint with branches of the popliteal artery serving as the blood supply (**Figure 276-2**). The tibialis anterior, extensor digitorum longus, and extensor hallucis longus muscles run over the anterior aspect of the joint and are responsible for dorsiflexion. Inversion is accomplished by the tibialis posterior, flexor digitorum longus, and flexor hallucis longus. The peroneus longus and brevis muscles, sharing a common synovial sheath held in place by a groove on the posterior aspect of the lateral malleolus and superior retinaculum, run laterally to evert and plantarflex the joint. Plantarflexion is primarily accomplished by the gastrocnemius and soleus muscles.

CLINICAL FEATURES

HISTORY

Understanding the mechanism and timing of the injury is important. Document these details along with any previous bony or soft tissue injuries. Patients with signs of neurovascular compromise, including coldness and numbness of the foot, a rapid onset of swelling, extreme pain, and complicating conditions such as diabetes, require urgent evaluation.[5] A normal-appearing ankle does not preclude the need for further inquiry. Due to the significant swelling typically present after acute injuries, examining the ankle is challenging but can be helped by elevation of the injured extremity and ice applied at triage. Peroneal spasms may mask any instability in the joint.[9]

PHYSICAL EXAMINATION

Place the patient on a stretcher to perform a thorough evaluation. A systemic approach to the examination decreases the chance of missed injuries. Starting with the skin and soft tissues, note any ecchymosis, abrasions, or swelling. Note the position, swelling, and skin integrity of the joint as well as any areas of tenderness or crepitus. Joints above and below the ankle need to be examined for any concomitant injuries. Suspect a **Maisonneuve fracture** (or fibulotibialis ligament tear) if

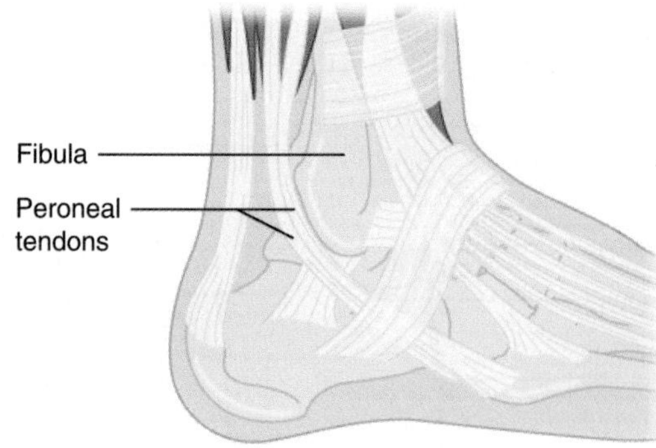

FIGURE 276-3. Peroneal tendon of the foot, lateral view.

there is tenderness of the fibular head or proximal fibular shaft. Palpate the area of obvious injury last. Test the functionality of the joint with both active and passive plantarflexion, dorsiflexion, and full range-of-motion exercises. **Peroneal tendon injuries** can occur from forced dorsiflexion, which presents as weakness on eversion (**Figure 276-3**). Check stability in external rotation, varus, and valgus. Palpate the posterior aspects of the lateral and medial malleoli, starting proximally to the joint and working distally. If there is a concern for isolated fibular fractures, check for evidence of injury to the syndesmosis or deltoid ligament.[9] A positive anterior drawer test (**Figure 276-4**) is indicative of a torn anterior talofibular ligament. A positive anterior drawer test, swelling, and a hematoma are signs of a grade III sprain. **Syndesmosis injuries** can be deceiving because the patient describes ankle pain, but there is typically little ankle edema or ecchymosis. The **crossed-leg test** (compressing the fibula toward the tibia just above the midpoint of the calf[11]) can detect a syndesmosis injury and is indicated if pressure to the medial aspect of the knee elicits pain in the syndesmosis (**Figure 276-5**). The **squeeze test** is performed by squeezing the calf just above the ankle joint. Pain indicates syndesmosis injury. Calcaneofibular ligament instability can be detected with the **inversion stress test** or **talar tilt**.[6] If the examination is uncomfortable for the patient, consider a hematoma block, sedation, or both to perform a more thorough examination.[11]

Examine areas in close proximity to the ankle as well. What may be described as an ankle injury may end up being an injury to the Achilles tendon or foot and cannot be excluded by ankle radiographic imaging. Assess the integrity of the **Achilles tendon**. Fluoroquinolones and corticosteroids increase the risk of such an injury.[12] Perform the **Thompson test** (see Figure 44-4 in chapter titled "Leg and Foot Lacerations") if there is tenderness or a defect. Place the patient prone on the stretcher and squeeze the calf. Loss of plantarflexion indicates a complete Achilles tendon rupture. Palpate the hindfoot and midfoot over the calcaneus, tarsals, and base of the fifth metatarsal to check for areas of tenderness that may require further investigation.

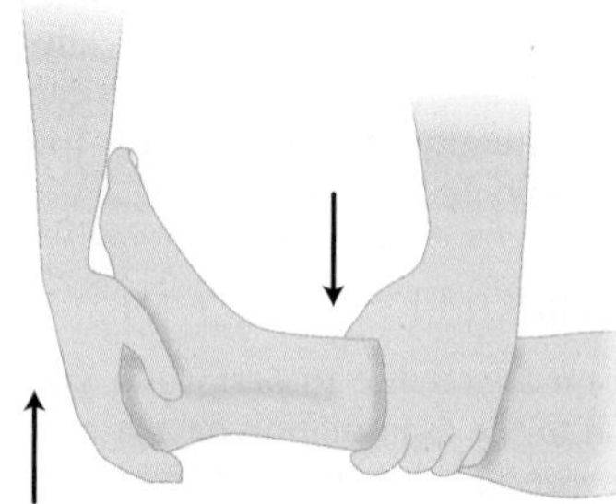

FIGURE 276-4. Technique for performing the anterior drawer stress test of the ankle. [Reproduced with permission from Simon RR, Sherman SC, Koenigsknecht SJ: *Emergency Orthopedics, The Extremities*, 5th ed. © 2007, McGraw-Hill Inc., New York.]

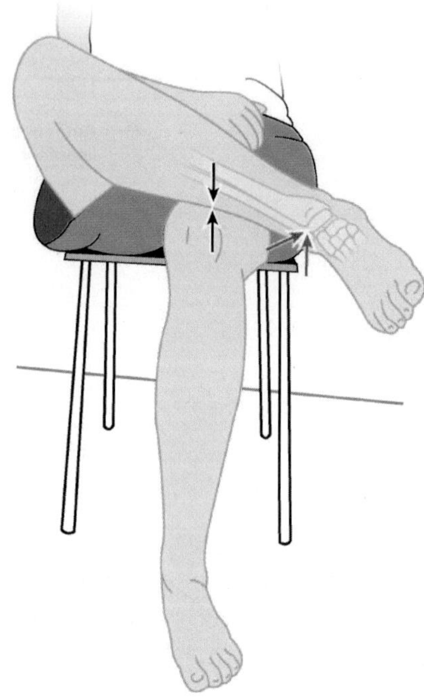

FIGURE 276-5. The crossed-leg test. The affected leg is crossed over the opposite leg as demonstrated. If pain results at the arrow sites when pressure is applied to the medial side of the affected knee, the test is positive and indicates syndesmosis injury. [Copyright © 2010 by the American Orthopaedic Foot and Ankle Society, Inc., originally published in *Foot & Ankle International* in Kiter E, Bozkurt M: The crossed-leg test for examination of ankle syndemosis injuries. *Foot Ankle Int* 2: 187, 2005, and reproduced here with permission.]

Perform a neurovascular examination. Check dorsalis pedis and posterior tibial pulses and document digital capillary refill. Inability to dorsiflex the toes suggests a tibial nerve injury. Inability to plantarflex the great toe is suspicious for peroneal nerve injury.

If there are any significantly displaced fractures or dislocations, immobilize the joint in a neutral position with a well-padded splint to reduce further soft tissue injury. Follow this with elevation and application of ice to reduce edema. Emergently reduce any displaced fractures or dislocations with neurovascular compromise (see later treatment section under "Dislocations").

DIAGNOSIS

IMAGING

The Ottawa Ankle Rules for Ankle and Midfoot Injuries[2,13-17] are easily applied by physicians and triage nurses.[18,19] The rules are summarized in **Figure 276-6**.

The rules were originally developed for patients older than age 18 years who were able to cooperate, were not intoxicated, and had no distracting injuries or decreased sensation. Assuming the patient does not have any bony tenderness, assess the ability to bear weight by having the patient take four steps, resulting in two transfers to and from the injured ankle. The initial studies demonstrated a 30% reduction for the need of ankle radiographs.[16,20]

The standard ankle trauma series consists of three views: anteroposterior, 15-degree internal oblique, and lateral views. See **Figure 276-7** for normal anatomy. About 95% of all ankle fractures can be detected with any two of these views.[9]

When there is an abnormal motion of the talus within the mortis, there is stress on the malleoli and ligaments, which causes the injury. Fractures above the talus and those that cause disruption of both sides of the joint have the potential to create an unstable injury. Instability of the joint is usually diagnosed based on plain radiographs because pain and swelling make it difficult to determine true stability of an acutely injured ankle. If radiographs are normal but there is concern about sta-

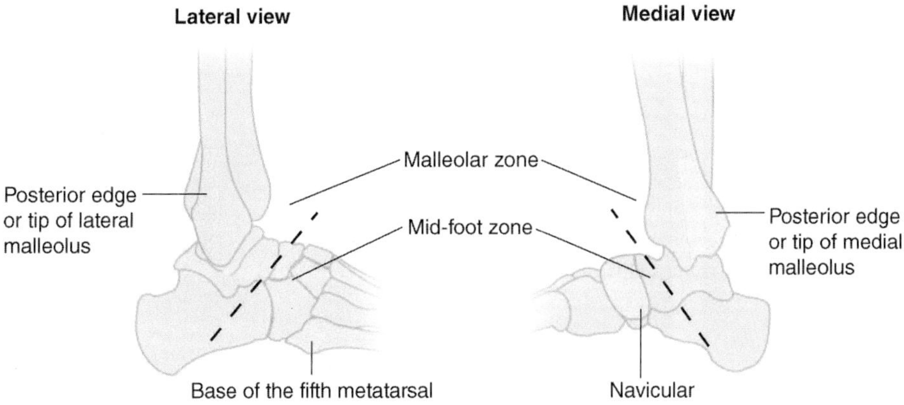

FIGURE 276-6. Ottawa Ankle Rules for Ankle and Midfoot Injuries. Ankle radiographs are required only if there is any pain in the malleolar zone or midfoot zone along with bony tenderness in any of these four locations or the inability to bear weight both immediately and in the ED.

bility, weight-bearing ankle films can be helpful. US can detect Achilles tendon injuries[21] and ankle fractures.[22]

CT and MRI may play a role in better delineating pathology. Ideal imaging for a CT includes both axial and direct coronal images with sagittal reformations. To obtain these images, keep the ankle between neutral and 20 degrees of plantarflexion when possible, similar to that for plain radiographs. CT can be used for operative planning by orthopedic surgeons and to evaluate comminuted fractures and complex bony injuries like pilon fractures and malunions.[7] MRI can help define soft tissue, muscle, ligamentous, and tendon injuries and is used more in the outpatient setting for subacute and chronic pain presentations.[9,23]

TENDON INJURIES

CLINICAL FEATURES

A **peroneal tendon** subluxation and dislocation occurs when there is a sudden hyperdorsiflexion of the foot in a position of eversion, as in skiing. The superior retinaculum, which holds the peroneal tendons in place, is torn from the posterolateral malleolus. This leads to a small avulsion fracture in more severe injuries with a dislocation or anterior subluxation of the peroneal tendon over the tip of the fibula. Consider this injury when there is ecchymosis or tenderness over the posterior edge of the lateral malleolus and no tenderness over the talofibular ligament.

Achilles tendon ruptures happen with sudden plantarflexion of the foot. A complete tendon rupture will become apparent with palpation of a defect over the Achilles tendon and is identified by the Thompson test (**Figure 276-8**). US can also identify Achilles tendon ruptures (**Figure 276-9**).

TREATMENT

The treatment for both types of tendon rupture is often operative repair, especially for those who wish to return to full activity.

LIGAMENT INJURIES

CLINICAL FEATURES

The most common type of ankle sprains is one to the **lateral ankle**. Typically, these are minor and are due to an inversion injury when the ankle is plantarflexed. Sprains are categorized into three grades. Grade I involves no tearing of the ligaments with minimal functional loss, pain, swelling, and ecchymosis. Weight bearing is tolerable. Grade II sprains occur with a partial tear and some loss of functional ability. Grade II sprains tend to be more painful, with swelling, ecchymosis, and difficulty bearing weight. Grade III sprains result from a complete tear, with significant functional loss, pain, swelling, and bruising, and almost a universal inability to bear weight.[6] It has been argued, however, that assigning a grade to the sprain is less important than the stability of the joint.[24] Joint stability is the primary determinant of a treatment plan for a sprain.

An isolated sprain of the medial deltoid ligament is rare. **Medial deltoid ligament** tears are usually associated with a fibular fracture or tear of the tibial-fibular syndesmosis from an eversion injury. If there is significant medial malleolus tenderness and swelling, suspect a Maisonneuve fracture of the proximal fibula and fibular shaft. Negative radiographs should suggest syndesmosis tears.

Injuries to the tibiofibular syndesmotic complex are associated with hyperdorsiflexion injuries when the talus moves superiorly and separates the tibia and fibula. This leads to a partial or complete tear of the syndesmosis with complaints of pain just above the talus.

If there is concern for an unstable ligamentous injury, weight-bearing views of the ankle can help diagnosis—an unstable ligamentous injury may demonstrate talar shift.

TREATMENT

The immediate goals are to decrease pain and swelling and protect ligaments from further injury. The **PRICE protocol** (protection, rest, ice, compression, elevation) involves elevating the ankle and protecting it with a compressive device along with applying ice and resting up to 72 hours to allow the ligaments to heal.[6] There is controversy as to whether or not early immobilization versus functional treatment results in the best outcomes. There is a trend toward favoring early functional treatment over immobilization.[7] Patients returned to mobility anywhere between 4.6 and 7.1 days sooner with functional treatment when compared with immobilization.[25] Functional treatment usually consists of three phases: (1) PRICE protocol within the first 24 hours of injury; (2) motion and strength exercises to begin within 48 to 72 hours; and (3) endurance training, focused toward specific sports when applicable, and training to improve balance after the second phase begins.[6]

In patients with a lateral ligament sprain, a stable joint, and the ability to bear weight, treatment consists of analgesics, an elastic bandage or ankle brace, and no sports involvement, with follow-up in a week if no improvement. Lace-up supports may reduce persistent swelling when compared to elastic bandages or rigid ankle supports.[26] For patients who are unable to bear weight but have a stable joint, provide an ankle brace and crutches and have them follow-up with either their primary care provider or orthopedic surgeon within 1 week for repeat evaluation. Given the trend for early immobilization, functional braces, such as semirigid (e.g., Aircast) and soft, lace-up braces, are commonly used. There is no consensus as to which leads to a more favorable outcome,[27] although early rehabilitation of low-grade ankle sprains results in a good outcome.[28] Another option is an inflatable cast boot (also called walking fracture boot or air cast boot) that molds to the foot with inflatable air bladders. This device can also be used for stable ankle fractures.

Treat medial ligament sprains with PRICE and early referral to an orthopedic surgeon given the risk for undetected underlying fractures. Consider early orthopedic referral for **syndesmotic complex sprains** given the expected prolonged recovery time.

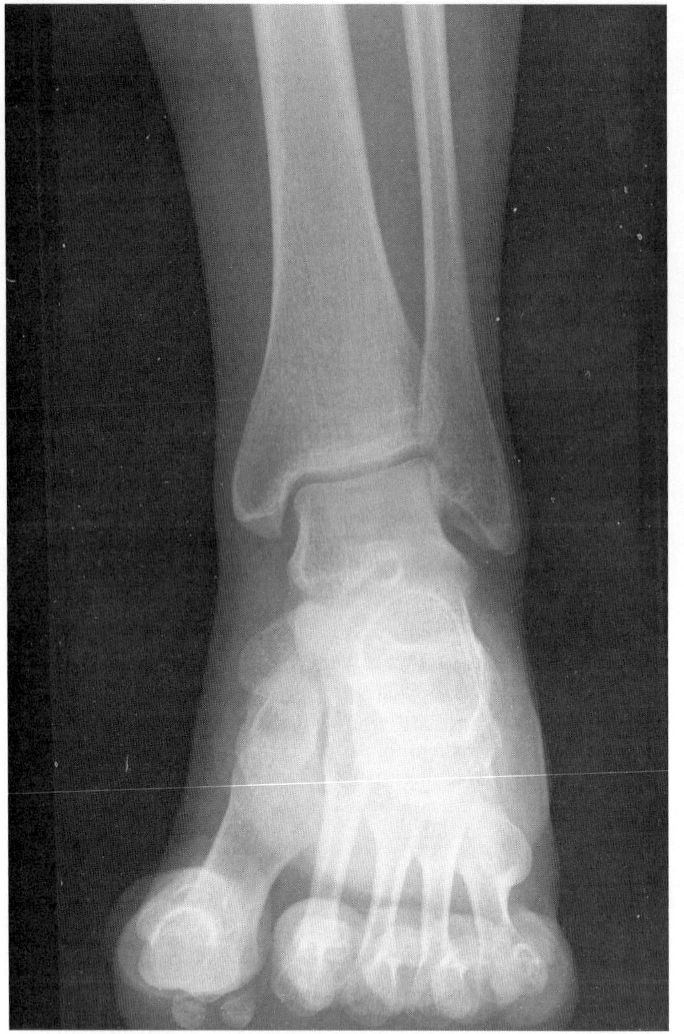

A

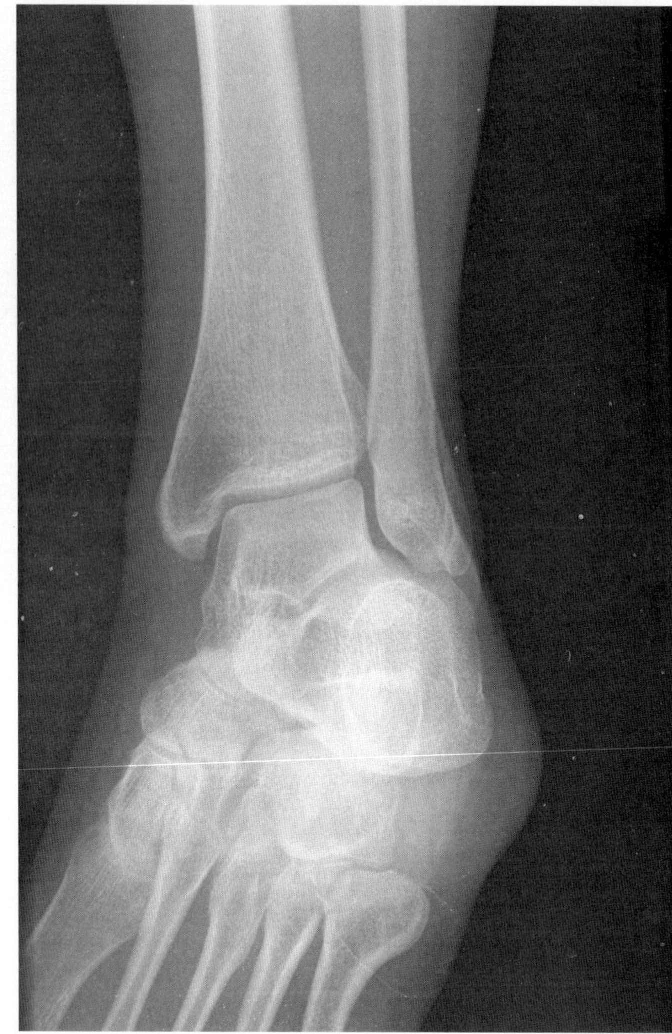

C

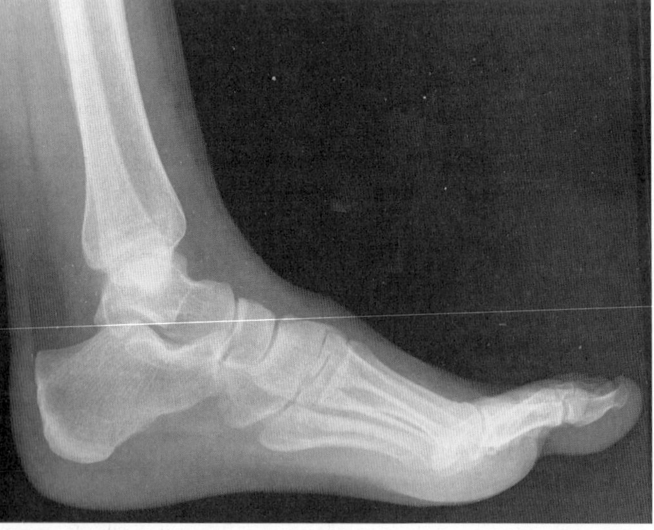

B

FIGURE 276-7. Normal ankle radiograph. **A.** Anteroposterior view. **B.** Lateral view. **C.** Oblique view. [Image used with permission of Robert DeMayo, MD.]

Refer patients with an unstable joint to an orthopedic surgeon after placement of a posterior splint for stabilization. Establish contact with the orthopedic surgeon early because the timing of treatment and follow-up is ultimately at his or her discretion.

There is no consensus as to whether surgery versus conservative treatment results in more favorable outcomes.[29] Cryotherapy with ice will help decrease pain and limit swelling and should be applied directly to the ankle or splint but not left on for >20 minutes at a time. Therapeutic ultrasonography is not helpful.[5]

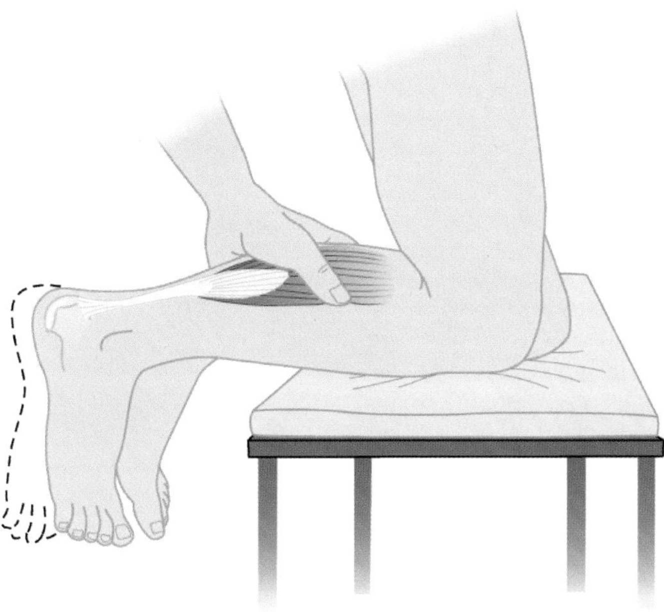

FIGURE 276-8. Thompson test. There is no plantarflexion with squeezing the calf of the affected leg, or less plantarflexion compared with the normal leg. [Adapted with permission from Stone CK, Humphries RL. *Current Diagnosis and Treatment Emergency Medicine*, 7th ed. Copyright @ The McGraw Hill Companies, 2011. Figure 28-20.]

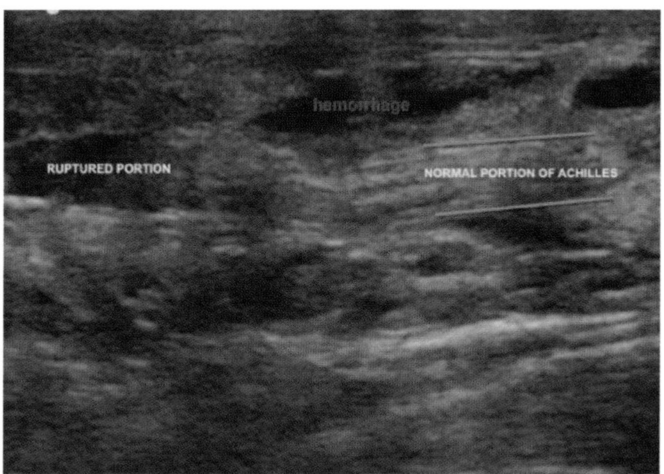

FIGURE 276-9. Ultrasound of ruptured Achilles tendon. [Used with permission from http://www.em.emory.edu/ultrasound/ImageWeek/achilles_tendon_rupture1.html; Drs. Backster and Ciardulli, Department of Emergency Medicine at Emory University.]

DISLOCATIONS

CLINICAL FEATURES

Most ankle dislocations are associated with a fracture and can occur in one of four planes. Posterior dislocations are the most common and occur with a backward force on the plantarflexed foot, usually resulting in rupture of the tibiofibular ligaments or a lateral malleolus fracture. The less common anterior dislocation results from a force on the dorsiflexed foot with an associated anterior tibial fracture. A lateral dislocation results in ligamentous disruption and fracture of one or both malleoli (**Figure 276-10**). An axial compression force can drive the talus upward with an associated fracture of the talar dome and disruption of the syndesmosis.

TREATMENT

There is a significant concern for neurovascular compromise. Check carefully for an open fracture in these instances. If the patient has intact pulses, dislocations associated with fractures should be reduced by an orthopedic surgeon. If vascular compromise is present, as evidenced by a dusky foot or absent pulses, or there is tenting of the skin, an immediate reduction by the emergency physician is warranted without any prereduction radiographs.

First provide appropriate sedation and analgesia before attempts at reduction. Grasp the heel and foot with both hands, and gently apply traction and rotation opposite to the direction of the mechanism of injury. Confirm pulses and distal perfusion, and then apply a splint and elevate the foot while waiting for orthopedic evaluation. Confirm and document distal perfusion again after splint application. Any dislocations that cannot be reduced using closed techniques will require open reduction.

MUSCULAR INJURIES

CLINICAL FEATURES

Strains are injuries to muscle or tendons not usually associated with a specific injury but due to repetitive stress and overuse. Common muscles and tendons involved include the extensor digitorum longus, extensor hallucis longus, peroneus brevis and longus, and anterior tibial tendon (**Figure 276-11**). Strains can be due to athletics or poorly fitting footwear. Contusions are usually caused by direct trauma from a projectile like a baseball or hockey puck. Fractures associated with contusions are rare and usually involve only the bony cortex.

TREATMENT

For overuse injuries, analgesics, especially nonsteroidal anti-inflammatory drugs, will help, along with rest and cessation of the activities that are causing the strain. Targeted exercises may help in the recovery as well. Contusions are treated symptomatically with analgesia and ice.

FRACTURES

CLINICAL FEATURES

Radiographically, ankle fractures are described as unimalleolar, bimalleolar (**Figure 276-12**), and trimalleolar (**Figure 276-13**). A bimalleolar fracture is fracture of the lateral and medial malleoli; trimalleolar fracture additionally involves the posterior malleolus.

The ankle consists of a ring of bone and ligaments around the talus. The ring is composed of the tibia, tibiofibular ligament, fibula, lateral and medial ankle ligaments, and calcaneus.[30] A single ring disruption is typically a stable injury. Injuries involving two or more components of the ring are unstable injuries and usually need surgical fixation.

The Danis-Weber and Lauge-Hansen schemes are used by orthopedic surgeons to classify ankle fractures and help determine surgical repair. The Danis-Weber system classifies fracture patterns based on the level of the fracture of the fibula.[31-33] The Lauge-Hansen system classifies fractures based on the position of the foot at the time of injury.[34]

Critical aspects of the examination for ankle fractures are summarized in **Table 276-1**.

TREATMENT

The goal is to restore the anatomic relationship of the ankle, maintain reduction during the healing, and mobilize the ankle early. Treat small fibular avulsion fractures as stable ankle sprains (see earlier section, "Ligament Injuries") if they are minimally displaced (<3 mm in diameter) and there is no sign of medial ligament injury.

Most other ankle fractures require immobilization by either cast alone or surgical repair and casting.[35,36] Severe comminuted fractures are at risk for compartment syndrome, fat emboli, and poor healing. Urgent orthopedic consultations in the ED is necessary. Until definitive fracture treatment can be provided, apply a posterior splint and keep the patient non–weight bearing (see Figure 267-15 in chapter 267,

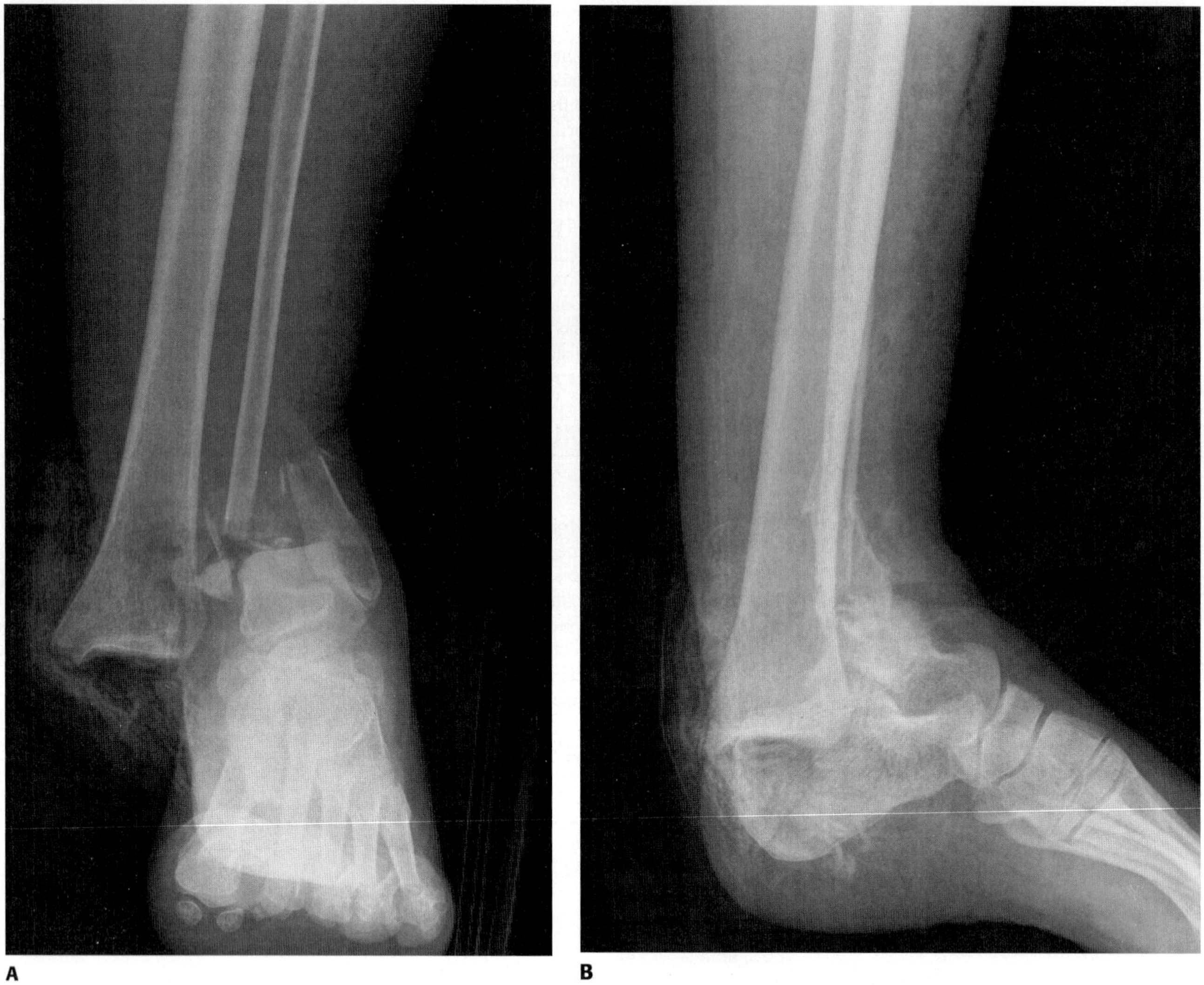

A

B

FIGURE 276-10. Open fracture with dislocation. **A.** Anteroposterior view. **B.** Lateral view. [Image used with permission of Robert DeMayo, MD.]

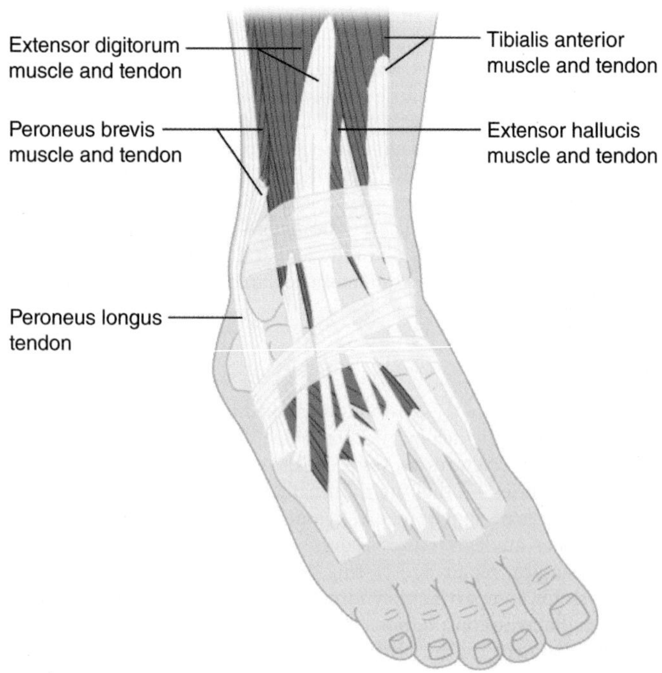

FIGURE 276-11. Muscles of the ankle.

TABLE 276-1 Associated and Occult Injuries of the Ankle

Injury	Clinical Suspicion	Confirmatory Test
Maisonneuve fracture	Examine proximal fibula and shaft, tenderness to palpation; proximal fracture and syndesmosis tear indicate unstable fracture[9]	Fibula radiograph
Peroneal tendon dislocation	Palpable anterior tendon dislocation or subluxation	Clinical examination
Usually identified in follow-up of ankle sprains		
Osteochondral injuries	Diffuse ankle swelling, passive plantarflexion	Ankle mortise view/CT
Syndesmosis tear	Significant ankle pain, positive squeeze test	Widened mortise with weight bearing
Anterior calcaneal process fracture	Tenderness more inferoanterior than a typical ankle sprain	Lateral ankle radiograph/CT
Lateral talar process fracture	Tenderness just distal to the tip of fibula	Ankle mortise view/CT
Os trigonum	Tenderness anterior to Achilles tendon	Lateral ankle radiograph

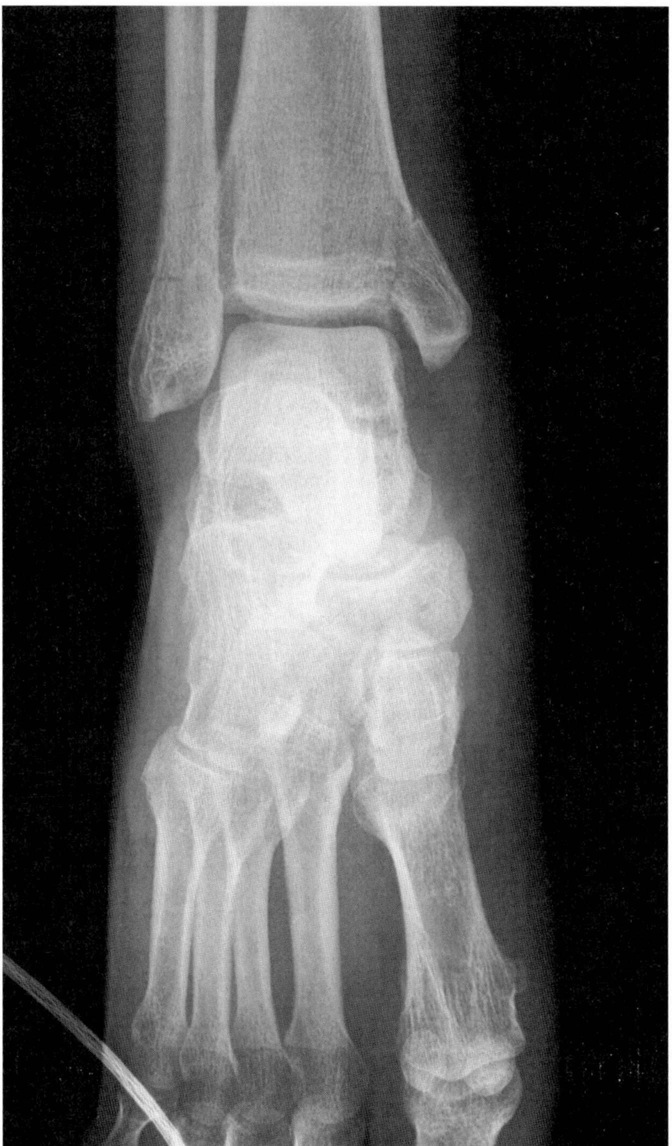

A

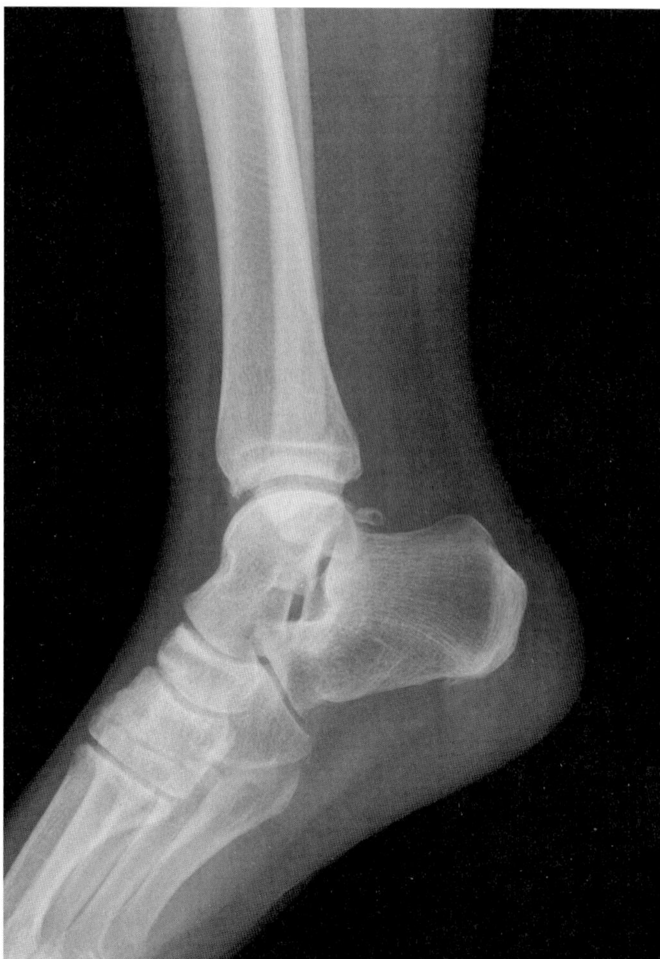

B

FIGURE 276-12. Bimalleolar fracture. A. Anteroposterior view. B. Lateral view. [Image used with permission of Robert DeMayo, MD.]

"Initial Evaluation and Management of Orthopedic Injuries, Posterior Ankle Mold). Provide analgesics, and remind the patient to elevate the leg and apply ice. **Table 276-2** provides guidelines for orthopedic consultation and follow-up.

OPEN FRACTURES

The most important prognostic factor in open ankle fractures is the amount of energy involved in the injury and amount of soft tissue damage involved. Open fractures require rapid surgical management that involves aggressive debridement of nonviable tissue and either internal or external fixation.[9] Administer empiric antibiotics, most commonly IV cefazolin, and add an aminoglycoside for contaminated wounds. Use clindamycin in patients with a penicillin allergy. Update the tetanus status of the patient as needed.

While waiting for the orthopedic surgeon, irrigate the wound with several liters of normal saline, then apply sterile gauze soaked in saline over the open wound, and secure it in place with a gauze roll. Do not use iodine solutions, as they are caustic to tissues. Splint the injury to stabilize it while obtaining radiographs and coordinating orthopedic care.

TABLE 276-2 Timing of Consultation

Immediate Consultation in ED	Deferred Consultation*	Within 1 Week
All open fractures	Stable unimalleolar fractures	Potentially unstable sprains
All fracture dislocations	Unstable ligamentous injuries	
All dislocations	Acute peroneal dislocations	
All trimalleolar fractures†		
All bimalleolar fractures†		
Unstable unimalleolar fractures†		
Maisonneuve fractures†		

*Implies that communication is established at time of diagnosis and specific time of consultation has been set.

†Consultation can be delayed in the ED in fractures without neurovascular compromise and appropriate splinting.

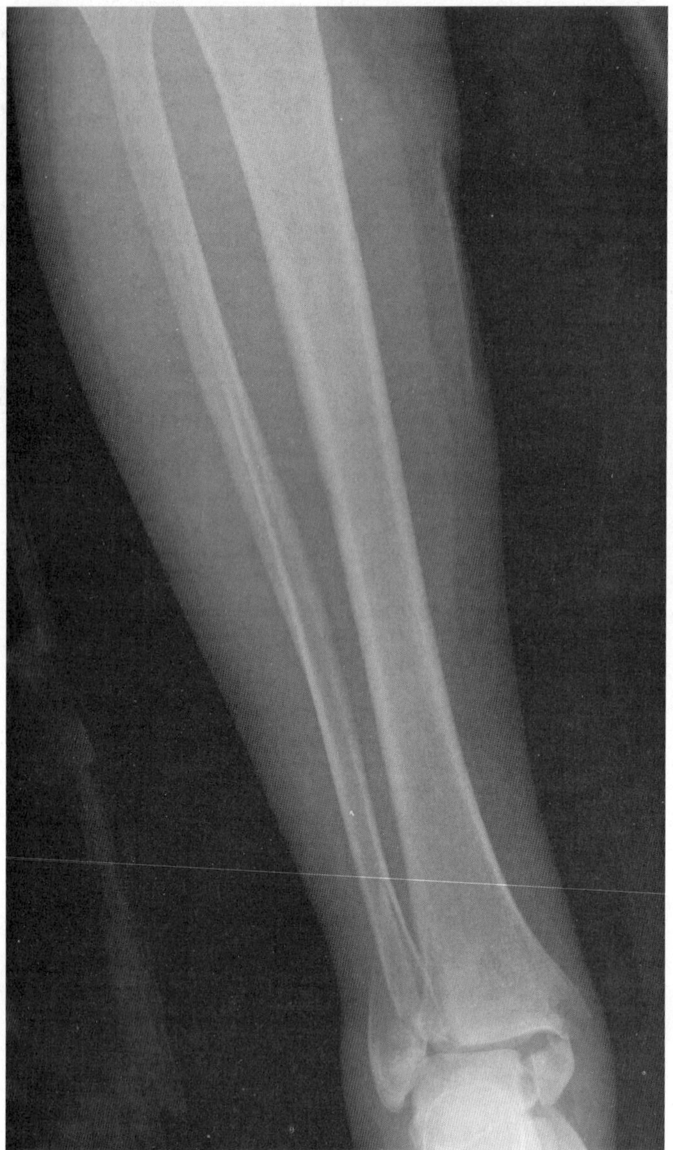

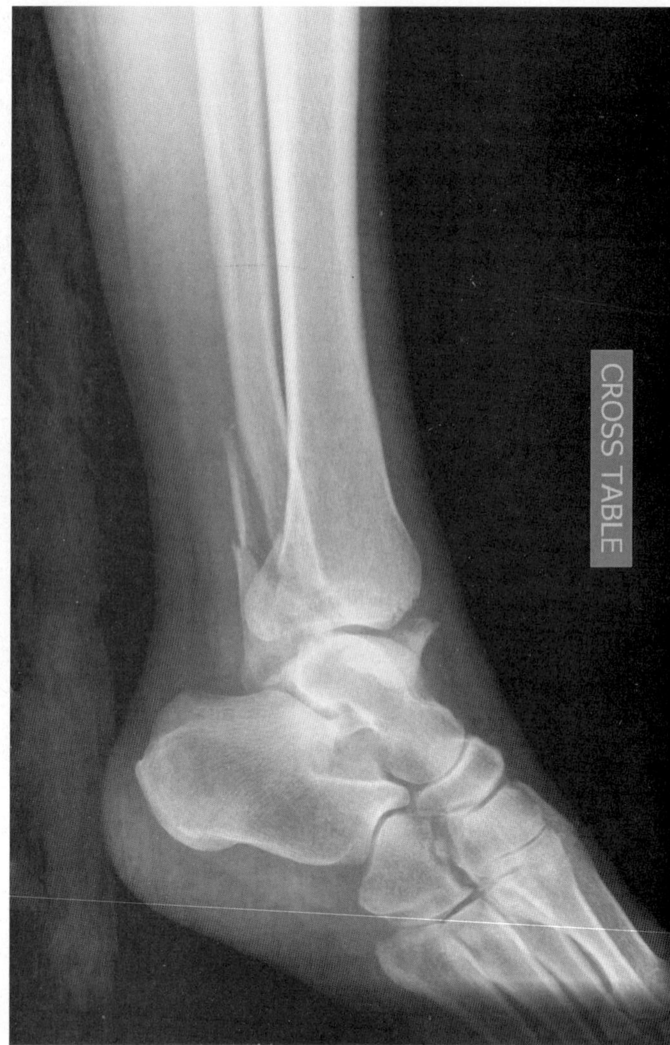

FIGURE 276-13. Trimalleolar fracture. **A.** Anteroposterior view. **B.** Lateral view. [Image used with permission of Robert DeMayo, MD.]

DISPOSITION AND FOLLOW-UP

To date, there is no established standard of care regarding the time of orthopedic consultation and follow-up. Whether or not an orthopedic surgeon sees the patient in the ED depends on the specialist resources available. Table 276-2 can serve as a general guideline for local practice standards and resources. Most severe fractures require orthopedic consultation in the ED.

Acknowledgments: The authors would like to thank Drs. John A. Michael and Ian G. Stiell for their contributions to previous editions of this chapter. We would also like to thank Drs. Esther Choo and Robert DeMayo for the radiology images.

REFERENCES

The complete reference list is available online at www.TintinalliEM.com.

CHAPTER 277

Foot Injuries

Sarah Andrus Gaines
Daniel A. Handel

INTRODUCTION

Foot injuries occur most commonly in work and athletic environments.[1] Work-related foot injuries can be associated with substantial medical costs and lost wages.[2] Sport-related foot and ankle injuries require care so the athlete can return to the demands of the sport as quickly as possible.[3] Motor vehicle crash patients with a foot or ankle injury typically have a higher injury severity score than those without such injuries.[4]

ANATOMY

The foot is divided into three sections: the hindfoot, the midfoot, and the forefoot. The **Chopart joint** separates the hindfoot from the midfoot.

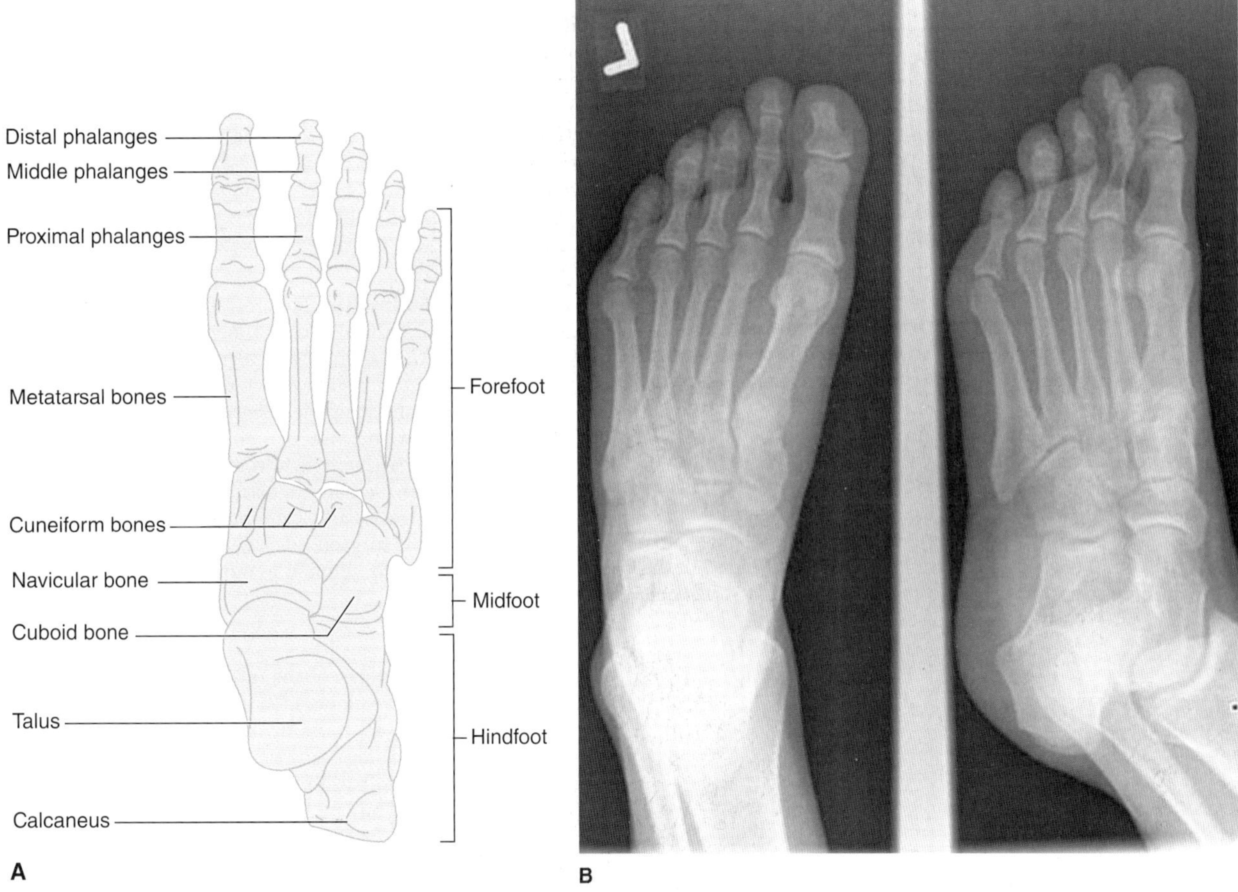

FIGURE 277-1. **A.** Diagram of normal bony anatomy of the foot. **B.** Radiograph of normal bony alignment of the foot. [Panel B image used with permission of Robert DeMayo, MD.]

The Lisfranc joint divides the midfoot and the forefoot. The hindfoot is comprised of the talus and the calcaneus. The midfoot encompasses the medial, middle, and lateral cuneiforms; the navicular; and the cuboid. The tarsus refers to the bones of the hind and midfoot. The forefoot includes the metatarsals and the proximal, middle, and distal phalanges (**Figure 277-1**). Ligaments and muscles enable foot movements of eversion, inversion, adduction, and abduction.

Vascular supply of the foot originates from branches of the popliteal artery: the anterior tibial artery, with its branch the dorsalis pedis supplying the dorsal aspect of the foot; and the posterior tibial and peroneal arteries supplying the sole (**Figure 277-2**).

The sural, saphenous, peroneal, and lateral plantar nerves innervate the foot for both motor and sensory function and originate in branches from the sciatic and femoral nerves.

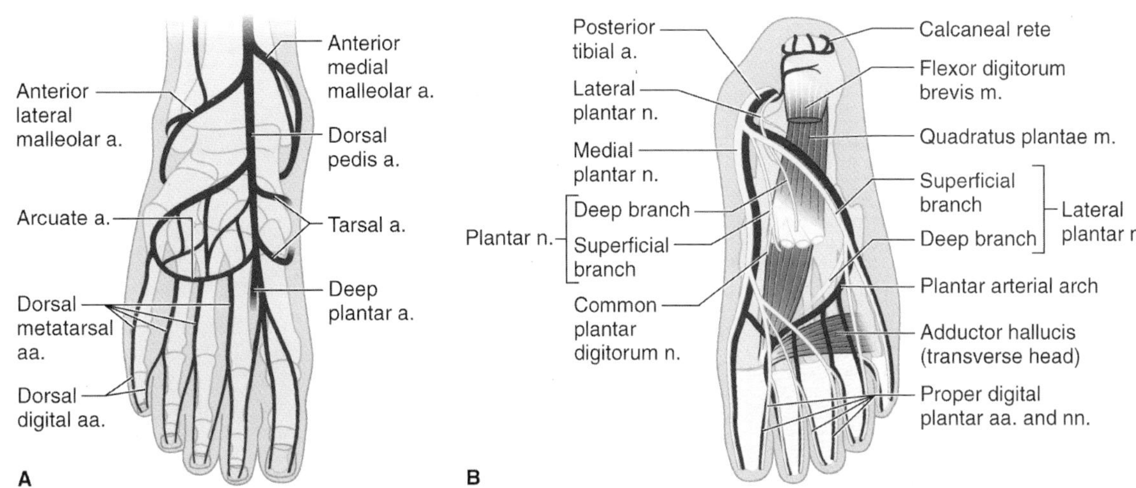

FIGURE 277-2. A. Arteries of the dorsum of the foot. B. Vessels and nerves of the sole of the foot. a. = artery; aa. = arteries; Abd. hall. = abductor hallucis; Ant. lat. = anterior lateral; Ant. med. = anterior medial; br. = branch; brev. = brevis; dig. = digitorum; Flex. = flexor; Lat. = lateral; Med. plant. = medial plantar; n. = nerve; nn. = nerves; Post. = posterior; Quad. = quadratus; Superf. = superficial; trans. = transverse.

CLINICAL FEATURES

HISTORY

Ask about the mechanism of injury and direction of force. Obtain key information, including ability to bear weight after the injury, prior injury or surgery to the area, and any other potential injuries. Because it requires great force to fracture the foot, other injuries can coexist, and foot pain can distract from other serious injuries.

PHYSICAL EXAMINATION

The foot examination does not necessarily begin with the foot, but with the entire lower extremity on the affected side. Examine the hip, knee, and ankle. Evaluate neurovascular integrity. Vascular compromise of the foot is identified with diminished pulses, a cool extremity, and mottled skin. Once the general examination is completed and the focused foot examination begins, start with the general appearance of the foot and compare it with the uninjured side. Look for obvious closed or open deformities. Ask the patient to identify painful areas. Palpate the foot for abnormal findings or tenderness. Pay particular attention to the base of the fifth metatarsal and the dorsal aspect of the base of the second metatarsal. Range the joint both passively and actively through all typical motions of the foot. Evaluate gait when possible.

HINDFOOT INJURIES

CALCANEUS INJURIES

Clinical Features The calcaneus is the most commonly fractured tarsal bone, whereas the talus is infrequently fractured.[5] Fractures in the hindfoot typically require a large force, like an axial load to the heel, to occur. Because of this force, associated injuries are common.

Calcaneal fractures are subdivided into intra-articular and extra-articular fractures, with intra-articular fractures being the more common of the two. A displaced intra-articular fracture is common and poses its own challenges for long-term care. Some surgeons advocate for open reduction and internal fixation; others prefer nonoperative closed reduction; and still others prefer primary arthrodesis.[6]

Diagnosis Plain radiographs, specifically the lateral view, are needed for fracture diagnosis. The Boehler angle is measured using the lateral view and represents the intersection of two lines: (1) the line drawn from the highest part of the anterior process of the calcaneus and the highest point of the posterior articular surface of this bone, and (2) the line between the highest point of the posterior articular surface of the calcaneus and the most superior part of the calcaneal tuberosity. The normal angle measures between 25 and 40 degrees. When the angle is <25 degrees, suspect a fracture (**Figure 277-3**). Because this angle varies widely between individuals, a comparison view is helpful if the diagnosis is in question. Although plain radiographs are helpful when the fracture is visible, a CT can provide detail and help clarify the management plan.

Treatment and Follow-Up For intra-articular fractures, obtain orthopedic consultation to determine the management plan. For nondisplaced fractures, treat an intra-articular fracture with immobilization, a well-padded posterior splint, strict elevation, non–weight-bearing status, and appropriate analgesia. Elevate the leg above the heart to minimize edema and the risk of compartment syndrome (see the chapter titled "Compartment Syndrome"). Displaced fractures may require surgical repair. Care for an extra-articular fracture is elevation, immobilization, analgesia, and orthopedic follow-up. Some of these will require outpatient surgical intervention, with less invasive, percutaneous approaches being adopted in more recent years.[7]

TALUS INJURIES

Clinical Features Fractures of the talus usually require a significant mechanism such as extreme dorsiflexion or a fall from a great height. "Major" talus fractures are those involving the head, neck, or body of the talus (**Figure 277-4**) and can result in avascular necrosis. "Minor" talus fractures are those that do not cross the central part of the talus (**Figure 277-5**). A lateral process talar fracture is sometimes called "snowboarder's ankle," and is commonly mistaken for a lateral ankle sprain.

Diagnosis, Treatment, and Follow-Up Diagnosis begins with plain radiography, but CT provides better visualization of the talus. Minor talus fractures can be treated on an outpatient basis with a posterior splint, non–weight-bearing status, analgesia, and orthopedic referral. Major talar fractures ideally require orthopedic consultation in the ED.

Dislocations of the talus, when the tibiotalar joint remains intact, are either peritalar or subtalar. The talocalcaneal and talonavicular joints are disrupted by a rotational-inversion force. Dislocations are rare but are orthopedic emergencies. Immediate orthopedic consultation and reduction are necessary to prevent neurovascular compromise to the foot.

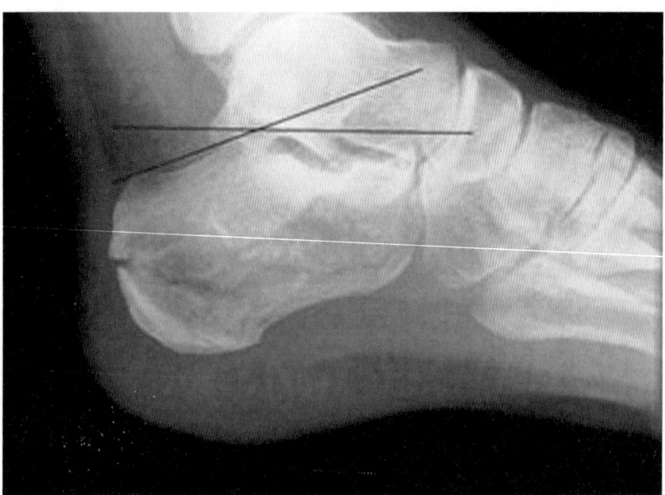

A

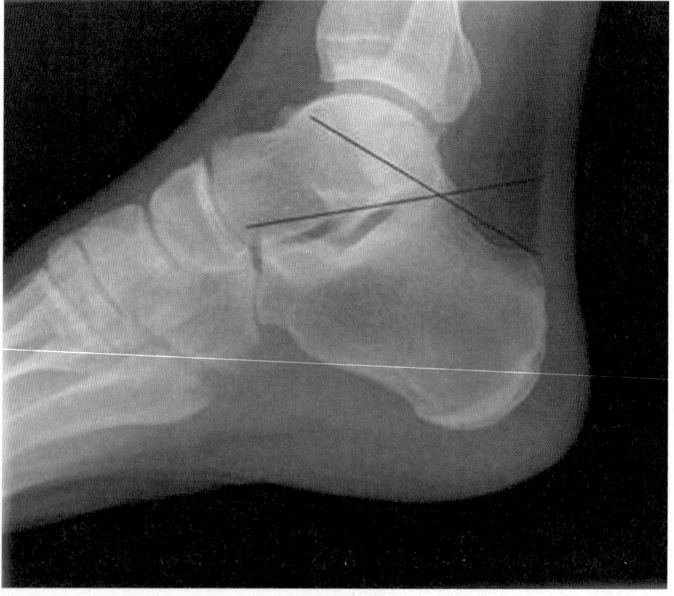

B

FIGURE 277-3. **A.** Calcaneal fracture with abnormal Boehler angle. **B.** Normal radiograph with normal Boehler angle. [Image used with permission of Robert DeMayo, MD.]

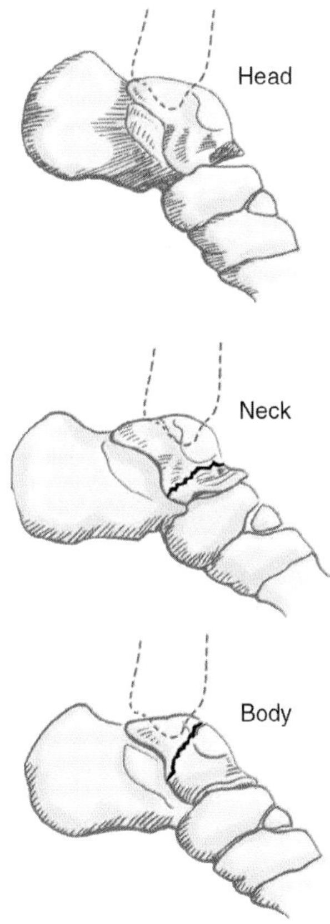

FIGURE 277-4. Major talus fractures. [Reproduced with permission from Simon RR, Sherman SC (eds): *Emergency Orthopedics*, 6th ed. New York: McGraw-Hill, 2011; Fig. 23-13, p. 525.]

MIDFOOT INJURIES

LISFRANC INJURIES

Clinical Features The midfoot is divided into two columns, with the medial column containing the navicular, cuneiforms, and the first three tarsometatarsal joints; the lateral column contains the cuboid and fourth and fifth tarsometatarsal joints (Figure 277-1). The midfoot is a vital bridge between the hindfoot and the forefoot. Injuries to the midfoot have the potential to dramatically affect an individual's daily function, including the ability to stand and walk. Untreated midfoot injuries in diabetics can lead to the development of **Charcot's foot** (collapse of the mid-foot arch) and lifelong complications with ambulating.[8]

The cornerstone of mechanism, diagnosis, and treatment of Lisfranc injuries lies in the anatomy of the second metatarsal and the Lisfranc ligament, which runs between the lateral base of the medial cuneiform and the medial base of the second metatarsal. Its strength exceeds that of the plantar ligament construct by severalfold.[9] Lisfranc injuries range from sprains to fracture-dislocations, with concurrent fractures of the hind and forefoot being relatively common, especially fractures of the second metatarsal. The usual mechanism of injury for sprains is a low-velocity indirect force, whereas plantar-flexion with an axial load (such as strenuous jumping over an obstacle) is seen in more significant injuries. Sports injuries (specifically football) and motor vehicle crashes are common situations for these injuries.[10,11]

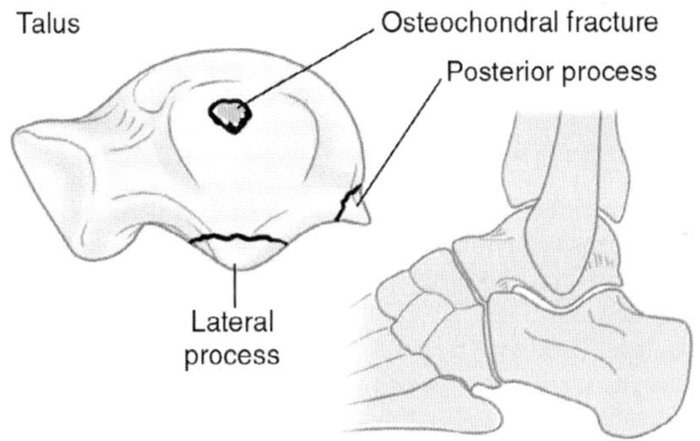

FIGURE 277-5. Minor talus fractures. [Reproduced with permission from Simon RR, Sherman SC (eds): *Emergency Orthopedics*, 6th ed. New York: McGraw-Hill, 2011; Fig. 23-14, p. 527.]

Diagnosis Pain elicited by torsion of the midfoot raises suspicion for a Lisfranc injury. Also, injuries about the tarsometatarsal joint, with pain on passive dorsi- or plantarflexion of the foot, should result in a specific evaluation of the midfoot for a Lisfranc injury. Radiographic studies should include at minimum bilateral weight-bearing anteroposterior (when tolerable), lateral, and 30-degree oblique views of the foot. Bony displacement of 1 mm or greater between the bases of the first and second metatarsals is considered unstable. CT imaging is the ideal imaging study for this injury.[12] It provides better delineation of bony structures and diagnoses occult fractures or subluxations that can be missed on plain radiographs (**Figure 277-6**).

Lisfranc injuries have multiple classification systems.[10] The Nunley classification groups low-energy ligamentous injuries by diastasis and preservation or loss of arch height: type I are nondisplaced, type II involve diastasis between the first and second metatarsal heads, and type III involve diastasis with loss of arch height.[11]

Treatment and Follow-Up Treatment of a nondisplaced injury (<1 mm between the bases of the first and second metatarsals) is with a non–weight-bearing splint, rest, ice, and elevation. Orthopedic reevaluation is usually scheduled within 2 weeks when repeat imaging will likely be obtained and a cast will likely remain on for an additional 4 weeks. At 6 weeks, gradual progressive weight bearing can be attempted.

Displaced Lisfranc injuries are unstable and require orthopedic consultant in the ED and anatomic reduction.[13] Whether the reduction is open or closed depends on the degree of the injury and is determined by the orthopedic consultant. Surgical options are variable and range from open reduction and internal fixation to primary arthrodesis.[14] Compartment syndrome is an acute complication of significant Lisfranc injuries (see the chapter titled "Compartment Syndrome").

NAVICULAR INJURIES

Navicular fractures are typically caused by a direct blow or axial loading. Avulsion injuries can also occur with a pulling or rotational force. On physical examination, tenderness and ecchymosis are found about the navicular. Imaging includes bilateral weight-bearing anteroposterior, lateral, and oblique radiographs. CT is best for evaluating the talonavicular joint surfaces. The goals of treatment are maintenance of anatomy and restoration of articular congruity. Nondisplaced fractures should be treated in a non–weight-bearing short leg cast for 6 to 8 weeks, with orthopedic reevaluation in approximately 2 weeks. Orthopedic consultation in the ED is usually required for displaced, and therefore unstable, fractures, to determine the management plan. Given that the central part of the navicular bone is avascular,[15] complications include avascular necrosis, nonunion, and instability, all of which can lead to a flatfoot deformity.

CUBOID INJURIES

The cuboid articulates with the calcaneus and the fourth and fifth metatarsals. Plantarflexion and abduction is the most common mechanism of injury. Imaging includes bilateral weight-bearing anteroposterior, lateral, and oblique radiographs. CT may be helpful. Nondisplaced fractures are treated with a short leg cast and initial non–weight-bearing status. Comminuted injuries are treated with surgery. Complications include foot instability and joint arthrosis.

CUNEIFORM INJURIES

The cuneiforms all articulate with the navicular. Isolated cuneiform injuries are very rare, but especially with a high-energy mechanism of injury, cuneiform fractures can coexist with other fractures of the foot.

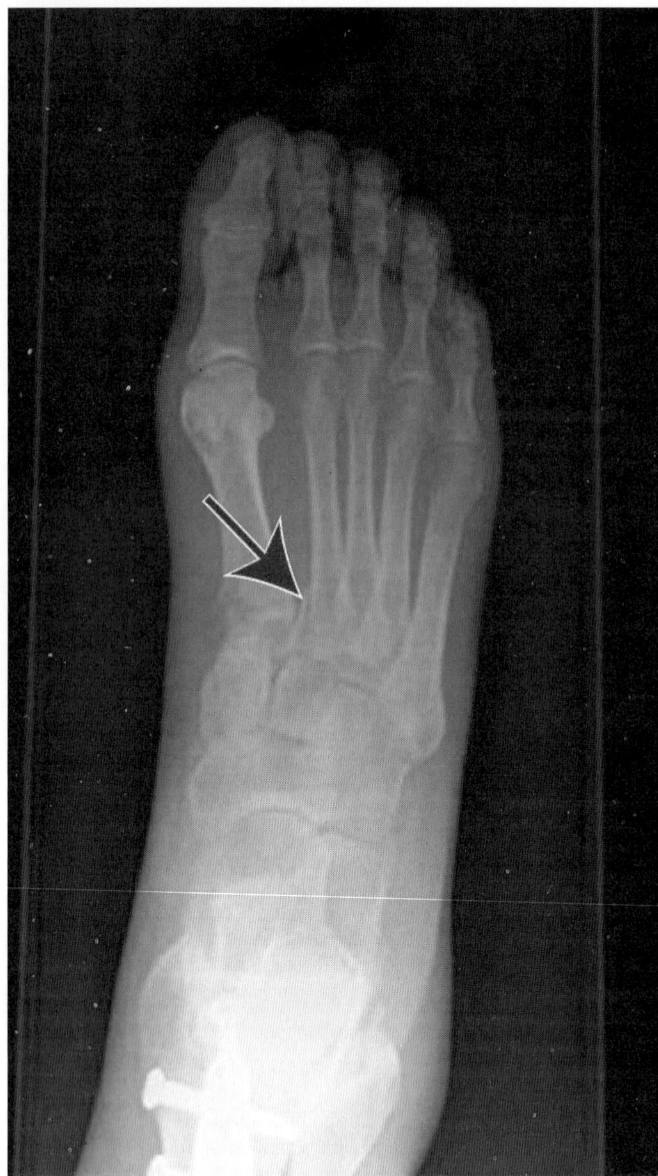

A

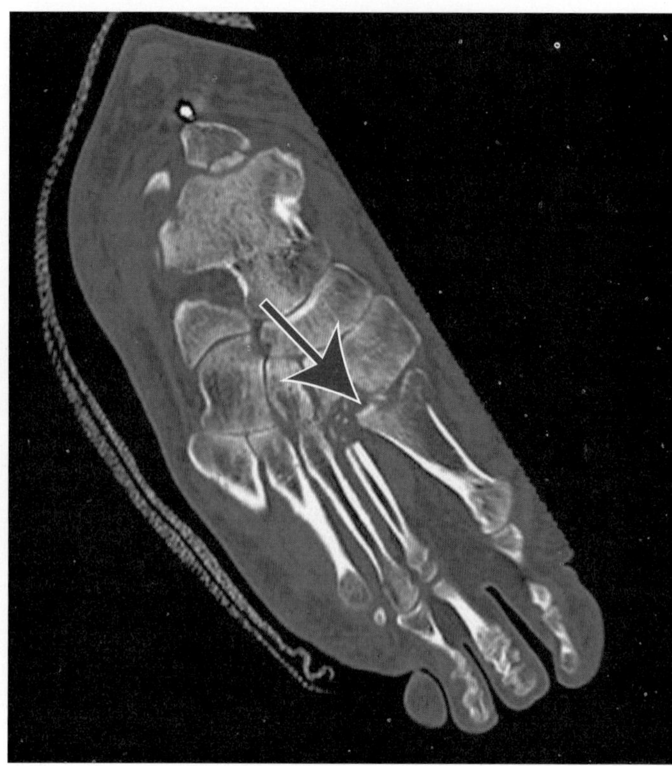

B

FIGURE 277-6. **A.** Radiograph of Lisfranc injury. **B.** CT of Lisfranc injury. Note the metatarsal bones are fractured (*arrow*) and displaced from the tarsus. [Image used with permission of Robert DeMayo, MD.]

Imaging studies are the same as for the other bones of the midfoot. Treatment depends on which bone is injured: medial cuneiform injuries are typically treated with surgery, whereas closed reduction usually suffices for the middle and lateral cuneiform bones.

FOREFOOT INJURIES

Forefoot injuries cover a broad range from those requiring minimal intervention to those requiring operative repair. Fractures range from the minimally displaced to open, comminuted fractures.

FIFTH METATARSAL INJURIES

Clinical Features Fractures of the proximal fifth metatarsal occur in three forms and can be identified using the joint between the proximal fourth and fifth metatarsal as a guide: (1) tuberosity or styloid fractures, which are proximal to the joint; (2) Jones fractures, which are also known as metaphyseal-diaphyseal junction fractures; and (3) diaphyseal stress fractures.

Diagnosis Plain radiographs are usually adequate. CT scans should be considered for more detailed imaging in the high-performance athlete[17] (**Figure 277-7**).

Treatment and Follow-Up Patients with nondisplaced Jones fractures should be non–weight bearing in a cast for 6 to 8 weeks. Complications of a Jones fracture treated nonoperatively include bony nonunion, which may later require intramedullary screw fixation. Shock wave therapy has also been reported for treatment of nonunion.[17] Some orthopedic surgeons are advocating for early surgical correction, especially in athletes, so posterior splinting and outpatient referral to an orthopedic surgeon are appropriate initial treatment.[18] Nondisplaced avulsion fractures of the tuberosity, also known as a pseudo-Jones fracture, can be treated with a walking cast and pain control with weight bearing as tolerated.

METATARSAL INJURIES

Proximal fractures of the first through fourth metatarsals are typically caused by a crush injury or direct blow. **Take care to exclude an associated Lisfranc injury**. An isolated proximal metatarsal fracture can be treated with a posterior splint and non–weight-bearing status. Orthopedic follow-up within 2 to 3 days is needed for the likely placement of a more definitive cast.

Nondisplaced isolated fractures of the shaft of a metatarsal, usually caused by an acute direct blow or twisting force, can typically be seen on oblique or lateral foot films. These can typically be treated with a posterior splint or orthopedic shoe or walking boot (see chapter titled "Initial Evaluation and Management of Orthopedic Injuries"). Repeat imaging can be performed 1 week after injury and then again at 6 weeks. Fractures with displacement of 3 to 4 mm or angulation >10 degrees usually require surgical reduction[13] (**Figure 277-8**).

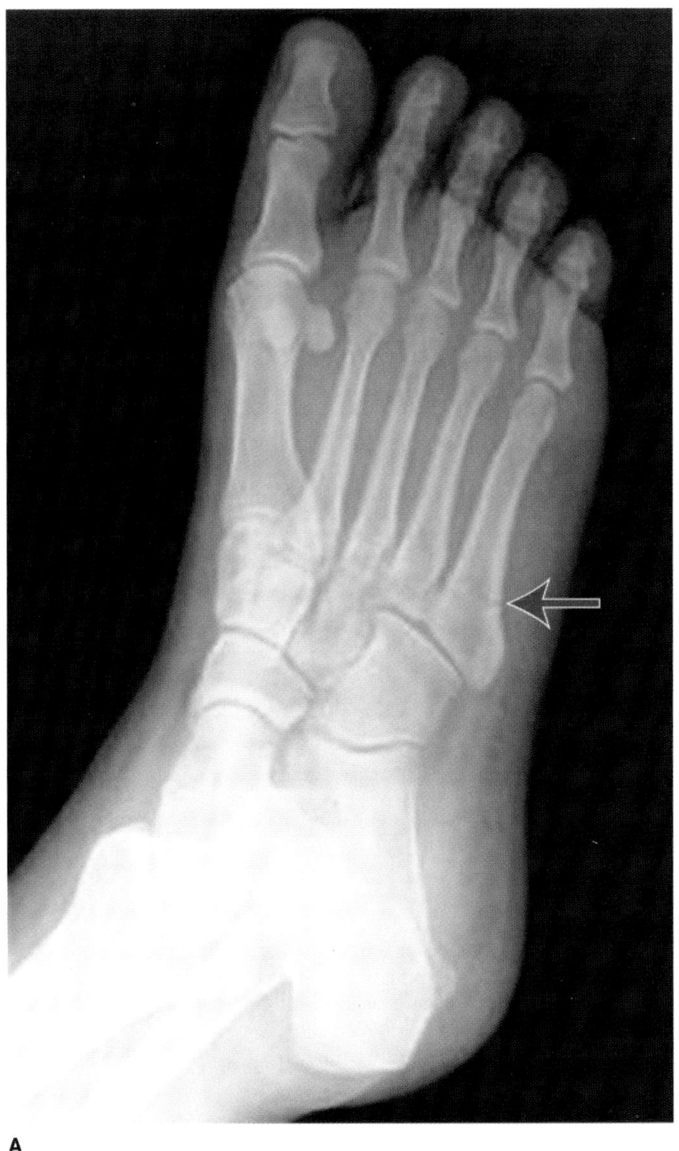

A

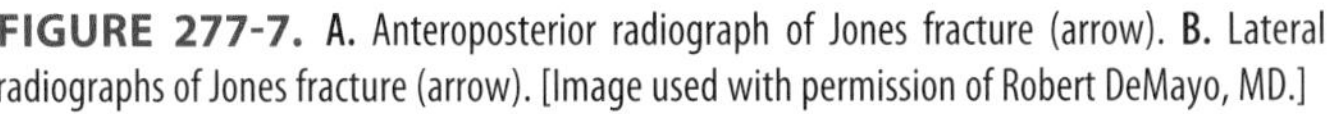

B

FIGURE 277-7. **A.** Anteroposterior radiograph of Jones fracture (arrow). **B.** Lateral radiographs of Jones fracture (arrow). [Image used with permission of Robert DeMayo, MD.]

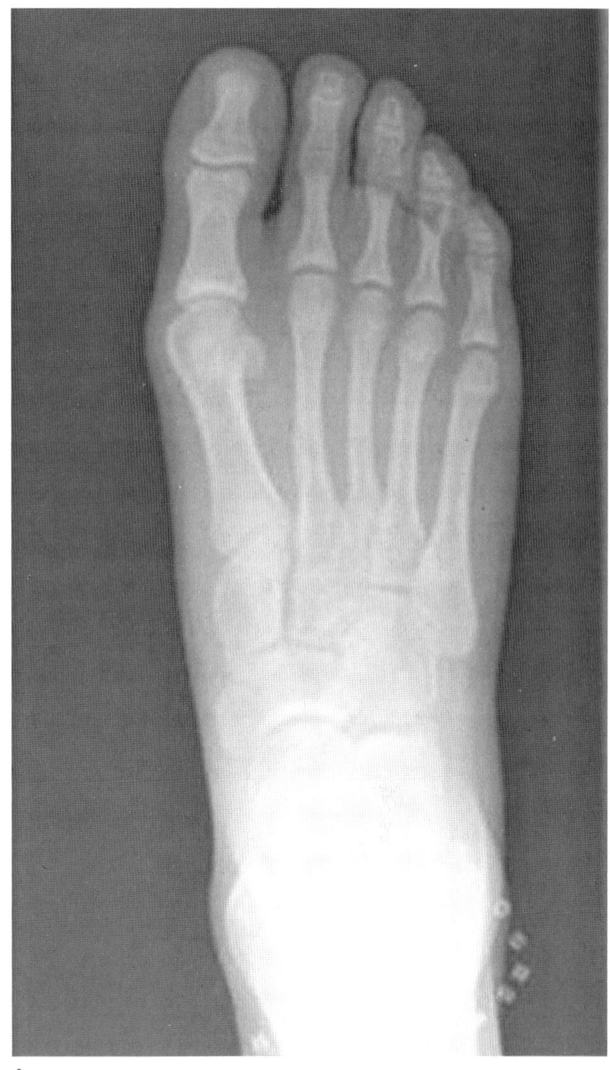

A

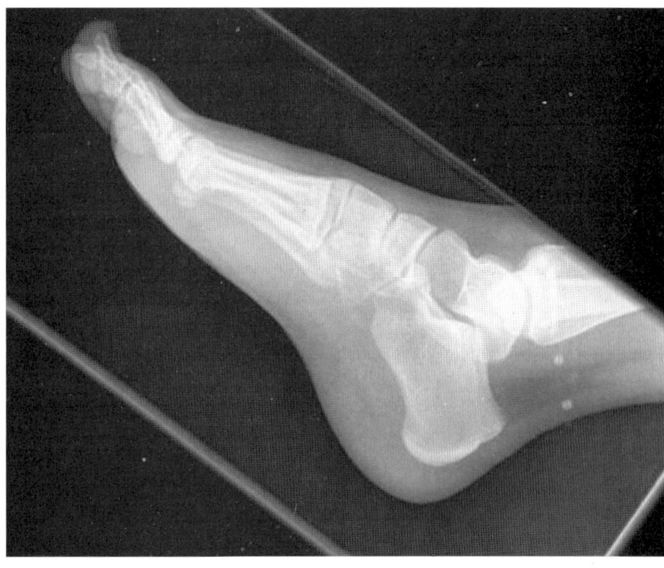

B

FIGURE 277-8. **A.** Anteroposterior radiograph of multiple metatarsal shaft fractures. **B.** Lateral radiograph of multiple metatarsal shaft fractures. [Image used with permission of Robert DeMayo, MD.]

TABLE 277-1 Summary of Emergent Care of Bony Foot Injuries

Fracture or Injury Type	ED Imaging	ED Care*	Orthopedic Referral (immediate: within 24 h; early: within 2 wk)	Home Care/Weight-Bearing Status	Advice on Long-Term Care and Management	Special Considerations
Calcaneal, intra- and extra-articular	Plain films, Boehler angle; CT for subtle findings	Posterior splint	Intra-articular: immediate; extra-articular: early	NWBS; RICE	Possible surgery	
Talus fracture	CT	Posterior splint	Major: immediate; minor: early	NWBS; RICE	Possible surgery	Risk of avascular necrosis
Lisfranc	CT	Splint	Displaced: ortho consult in ED; nondisplaced: early	NWBS; RICE	Possible surgery	Risk of compartment syndrome; arthritis
Navicular fracture	Plain films or CT	Splint	Nondisplaced: early; displaced: immediate	NWBS; RICE	Possible surgery	Risk of avascular necrosis; nonunion
Cuboid fracture	Plain films or CT	Splint	Early	NWBS; RICE	Comminuted: possible surgery	
Cuneiform fracture	Plain films or CT	Splint	Early	NWBS; RICE	Medial: possible surgery	
Jones	Plain films; CT for athletes	Splint	Early	NWBS; RICE	Athletes: possible surgery	
Metatarsal fracture	Plain films	Posterior splint	Within a week for a cast	NWBS; RICE	Surgery not likely	
Stress fracture	Clinical			Cessation of causative activity		
Phalange fracture	Plain films	Buddy taping		Hard-soled shoe and weight bearing as tolerated		
Open fractures of any kind	Consider antibiotics, Td	Pain control	Ortho consult in ED			

*All patients with fractures should receive adequate analgesia, and splints should be well padded.

Abbreviations: NWBS = non–weight-bearing status; ortho = orthopedist; RICE = rest, ice, compression, elevation; Td = Tetanus booster.

STRESS INJURIES

Chronic direct forces cause stress fractures. Stress fractures typically occur in the setting of increasing activity or chronic overuse and are sometimes called "march fractures." Stress fractures are rarely visible on plain radiographs; MRI can be used when pain is persistent. A clinical diagnosis typically suffices. Cessation of the causative activity usually results in good outcomes for recovery.[18]

METATARSOPHALANGEAL INJURIES

Metatarsophalangeal joint injuries are caused by multiple mechanisms and occur in various forms, including sprains, subluxations, and dislocations. **Turf toe** is a form of a sprain that results when there is acute or chronic hyperdorsiflexion of the first metatarsophalangeal joint while the foot remains in plantarflexion. History usually yields the diagnosis. When radiographs are obtained, a capsular avulsion, the hallmark of this injury, is seen. On physical examination, passive ranging results in a pathologically increased range of motion. Treatment is rest, ice, and elevation. Upon returning to sports, a reinforced shoe can be helpful and protective from further injury.[19] MRI is useful and can diagnose subtle associated injuries.[20]

Dislocations of the metatarsophalangeal joint, usually dorsal, can also occur. A high-energy mechanism is the usual cause, and this injury often accompanies other foot injuries. Treatment ranges from closed reduction to operative repair, depending on the severity of injury.

PHALANGE INJURIES

Fractures of the phalanges are the most common fractures of the forefoot, with a stubbing mechanism of the hallucal proximal phalanx being the most common injury.[19] Radiographs are obtained if there is extensive injury, suspicion of foreign body or open fracture, or if the great toe is injured. Radiographs are not necessarily obtained for the distal phalanges of the other toes if the only injury is a closed isolated injury of the distal phalanx. Crush mechanisms can lead to distal phalanx fractures. Treatment is with buddy taping to the adjacent toe or application of tape about the forefoot for greater stability (taking care to avoid undue pressure from the tape) and a hard-soled shoe.

For general guidance regarding the care of patients with acute bony foot injuries, see **Table 277-1**.

TENDON INJURIES

Lacerations to the foot may result in injury to the **extensor hallucis longus tendon**, with inability to dorsiflex the great toe, or **tibialis anterior tendon**, with loss of dorsiflexion of the foot. Consult with the orthopedist. Treatment is primary repair if the tendon edges are opposable; otherwise, tendon reconstruction is necessary.[21]

Lacerations of the **flexor hallucis longus** are typically repaired. Lacerations to the **flexor tendons of the other toes** are generally left unrepaired, as there is little if any functional impact.

Dislocation of the **posterior tibial tendon** is uncommon and is often misdiagnosed as ankle sprain. Mechanism of injury is forced dorsiflexion of the foot and ankle eversion when the posterior tibial tendon is contracted, as may occur in snowboarding or ice skating.[22] Treatment is surgical repair.

Achilles tendon injuries are discussed in the chapters titled "Leg Injuries" and "Soft Tissue Problems of the Foot." Repair of lacerations of the foot is discussed in the chapter titled "Lacerations of the Leg and Foot."

Acknowledgments: The authors would like to thank Drs. John A. Michael, Ian G. Stiell, and Peter Ramsey for their contributions to previous editions of this chapter. We would also like to thank Drs. Esther Choo and Robert DeMayo for the radiographic images.

REFERENCES

The complete reference list is available online at www.TintinalliEM.com.

CHAPTER 278

Compartment Syndrome

Paul R. Haller

INTRODUCTION

Compartment syndrome occurs when increased pressure within a limited space compromises the circulation and function of the tissues within that space. It was first described in 1881 by Richard Van Volkmann, a German physician who noted that paralysis and contractures were the late sequelae of an interruption of the blood supply to the muscles in the forearm. In 1924, it was shown that the result could be prevented by prompt surgical decompression of the compartment.

Today, a high degree of clinical suspicion, coupled with timely surgery, can be used to save function of the muscles and nerves that are at risk of permanent damage from elevated compartment pressures.

ANATOMY

The borders of a confined space are often made up of bone or tissue that offers minimal capacity to stretch. Any increase in volume within that compartment results in an elevated intracompartmental pressure. In the lower extremity, the most common site is at the level of the tibia and fibula, where 40% of compartment syndromes occur. The lower leg has four compartments: anterior, lateral, superficial posterior, and deep posterior (**Figure 278-1**). (Also see Figure 271-1 in chapter 275, Leg Injuries.)

The upper leg has three compartments: anterior, posterior, and medial. Due to the larger size of these compartments and their interconnectivity, they are less predisposed to elevated tissue pressures. The foot and buttock region of the leg also have a lower incidence of compartment syndrome.

In the upper extremity, the forearm has three compartments: flexor, extensor, and mobile wad (**Figures 278-2** and **278-3**). These are the high-risk areas in the arm. The hand (**Figure 278-4**) or upper arm (**Figure 278-5**) is less likely to develop a compartment syndrome.

PATHOPHYSIOLOGY

Muscle death and nerve damage in the setting of compartment syndrome are caused by prolonged elevation of tissue pressures. This can result from external forces, such as a cast or tight dressing, which compress a compartment. It can also result from an increase in the volume of a compartment that exceeds the limits of the surrounding fascia's ability to stretch. This may be the result of hemorrhage into a compartment or edema caused by reperfusion injury (**Table 278-1**). In effect, any mechanism that increases the volume of blood or tissue within the compartment has the potential to cause a compartment syndrome. Tissue perfusion is determined by the difference between the arterial blood pressure and the pressure of the venous return. As tissue pressure increases within a compartment, the normal gradient between arterial and venous pressure decreases.

The normal pressure within a compartment is <10 mm Hg. Anoxia and muscle death occurs with prolonged elevated pressure. Pressures up to 20 mm Hg can be tolerated without significant damage. The exact level of pressure elevation that causes cell death is unclear and may be related to the length of time that the pressure remains high. Tissue pressures exceeding 30 to 50 mm Hg have traditionally been thought to be toxic if left untreated for several hours.[1] However, the difference between the diastolic pressure and the measured tissue pressure may be a better determinant of potential for irreversible muscle damage.[2] This "delta pressure" is the diastolic blood pressure minus the intracompartmental pressure, and the critical level has been found to range between 10 and 35 mm Hg.[3] **The delta pressure that is most commonly used to diagnose acute compartment syndrome is 30 mm Hg.**[4] Using the delta pressure as a threshold for surgical intervention may help avoid unnecessary fasciotomies and can correctly classify patients with pressures sufficient to cause tissue compromise. In one study, none of the patients with a delta pressure >30 mm Hg suffered clinically significant complications related to acute compartment syndrome when fasciotomy was withheld, although such clinical parameters may not be sufficiently sensitive to exclude all sequelae that may result from a compartment syndrome.[4] For example, a hypotensive patient may be less able to tolerate the same degree of pressure elevation when compared to a normotensive patient.

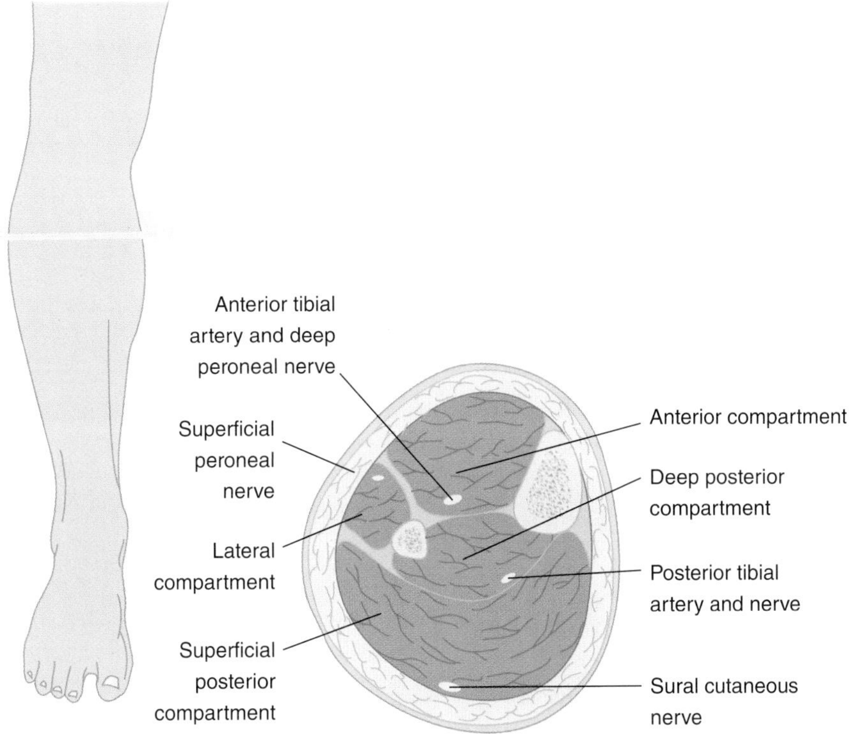

FIGURE 278-1. The four compartments of the lower leg.

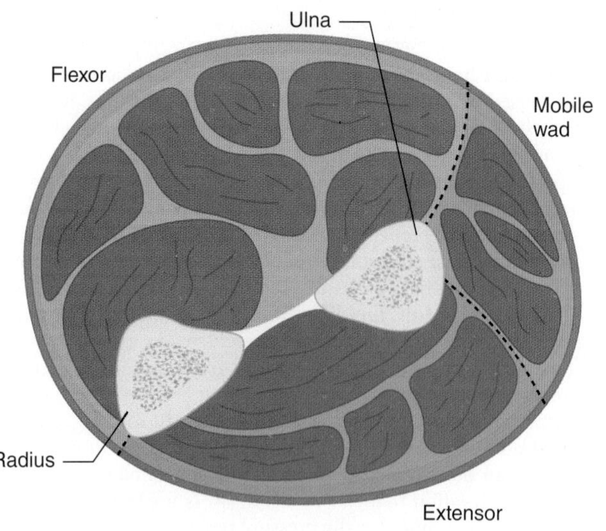

FIGURE 278-2. Forearm compartments.

Some tissues are more sensitive to the ischemic injury produced by elevated compartment pressures. Bone is relatively resistant to this ischemia. The muscles and nerves in the compartment are most susceptible to permanent damage. Short periods of elevated pressures may cause reversible damage, whereas longer periods lead to permanent deficits (see **Table 278-2**).

CLINICAL FEATURES

HISTORY

Compartment syndrome may occur with or without known trauma. For example, patients with hemophilia or rhabdomyolysis can develop compartment syndrome without direct trauma, and crush injury or tibial fracture can result in compartment syndrome to the affected extremity. In the post-trauma setting, symptoms usually develop within a few hours of the injury. The awake patient may initially complain of severe pain in the affected compartment; pain often may be refractory to opioids. The pain is due to elevated tissue pressures within a compartment. Thus the pain worsens when the muscle groups in that compartment are passively or actively stretched.

PHYSICAL EXAMINATION

This pain and the aggravation of pain by passive stretching of muscles in the compartment in question are the most sensitive (and often the only) clinical findings before the onset of ischemic dysfunction in the nerves and muscles.

When nerve conduction is affected, the patient will note numbness or dysesthesia in the sensory distribution of the nerve traversing that compartment. Motor nerve function may also be affected. Because tissue pressures do not become higher than arterial pressures, the distal pulse in the extremity will remain normal and there will not be a change in the color or warmth of the extremity. Squeezing or palpation of the muscle groups in the compartments will exacerbate pain. Firmness or fullness in the affected compartment is often detected.

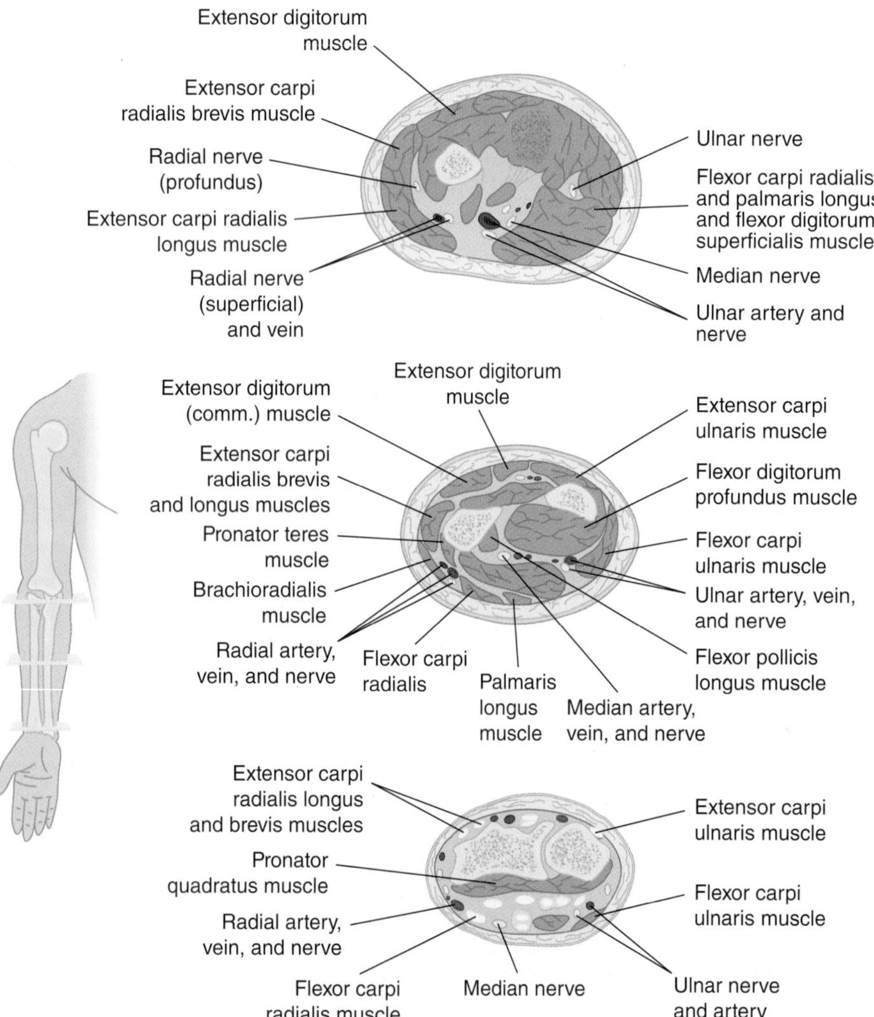

FIGURE 278-3. Forearm compartments: transverse sections through the right forearm at various levels.

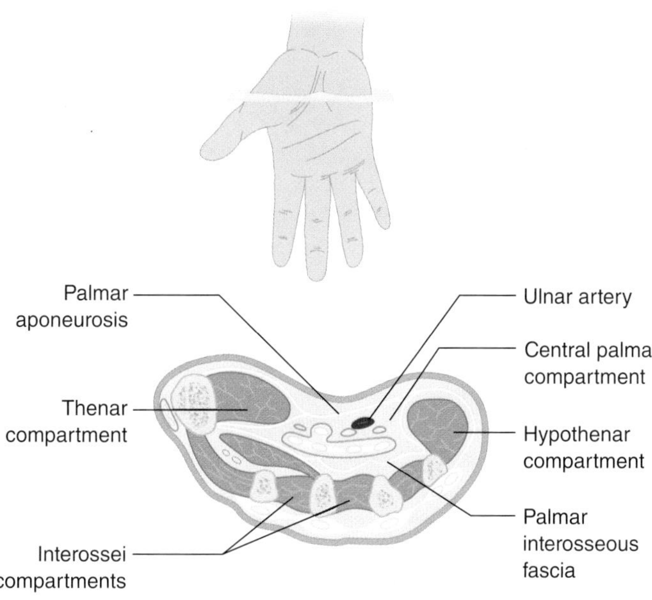

FIGURE 278-4. Hand compartments: transverse section through the right hand.

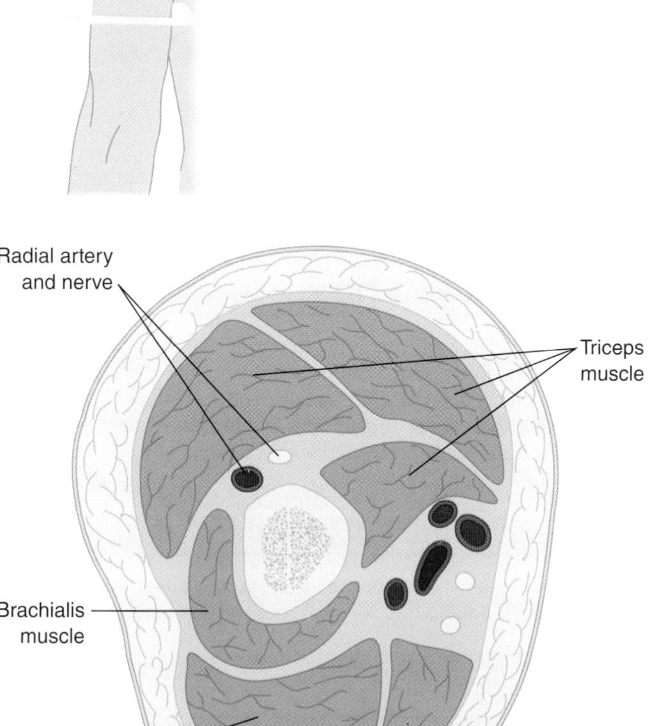

FIGURE 278-5. The biceps-brachialis (anterior) and triceps (posterior) compartments of the right arm.

TABLE 278-1 Causes of Compartment Syndrome

Orthopedic	Tibial fractures Forearm fractures
Vascular	Ischemic-reperfusion injury Hemorrhage
Iatrogenic	Vascular puncture in anticoagulated patients IV/intra-arterial drug injection Constrictive casts
Soft tissue injury	Prolonged limb compression Crush injury Burns
Hematologic	Hemophilia Adverse effects of anticoagulants (warfarin)

DIAGNOSIS

In the appropriate clinical setting, these exam findings alone may be sufficient to make the diagnosis and propel the patient in a timely fashion to the operating room for surgical treatment. At times, direct measurement of the tissue pressures in the compartment should be performed to help calculate the delta pressure, confirm the diagnosis, and determine patient disposition.

COMPARTMENT PRESSURE MEASUREMENT

Several commercial devices are available for measuring intracompartmental pressures. A Stryker Kit® is one such system. The kit consists of a saline-filled syringe, a manometer, and a needle with a side port. Connect the manometer between the syringe and the needle. Insert the needle into the compartment. Inject a few drops of saline to ensure that there are no air pockets and that the needle is not inserted into a tendon. The gauge gives the pressure reading in mm Hg. Check pressures twice in each compartment. Also check adjacent compartment pressures. Because pressures are highest near the injured area, obtain the measurements within 5 cm of a fracture site. Figure 278-1 demonstrates appropriate sites for pressure measurements in the lower leg, whereas **Figure 278-6** shows sites for the forearm. The hands and feet have many compartments within them, all too numerous and small to easily measure. If compartment syndrome is suspected in these sites, some specialists opt for surgical intervention without documentation of elevated pressures.

The measurement of compartment pressures may be helpful in certain settings. The patient may be obtunded, making clinical evaluation with suspected compartment syndrome difficult. Patients who are to go to the operating room for other procedures will be difficult to monitor clinically while under anesthesia.

It is not necessary to measure compartment pressures in a clinically obvious compartment syndrome.

LABORATORY TESTING

Laboratory testing is of no benefit in the setting of compartment syndrome. At times, the serum creatine phosphokinase may be elevated, as may myoglobin levels. Urinalysis may reveal myoglobinuria. Hemophiliacs or patients with clotting disorders need assay of coagulation parameters and factor levels.

TABLE 278-2 Tissue Survival of Ischemia

Muscle		Nerve	
3–4 Hours	Reversible change	2 Hours	Loss of nerve conduction
6 Hours	Variable damage	4 Hours	Neurapraxia
8 Hours	Irreversible damage	8 Hours	Irreversible damage

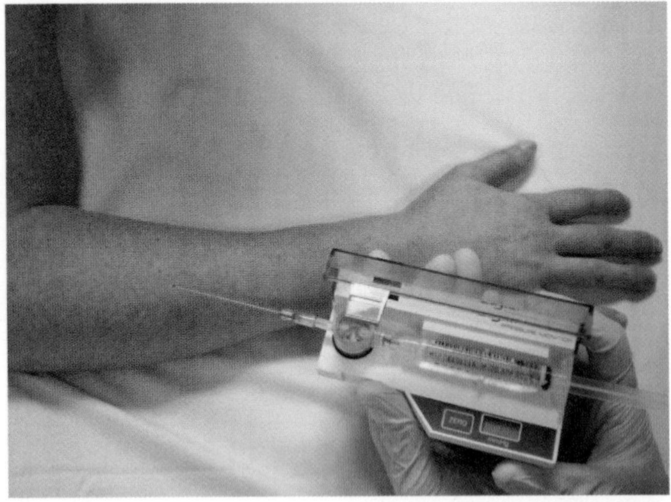

A

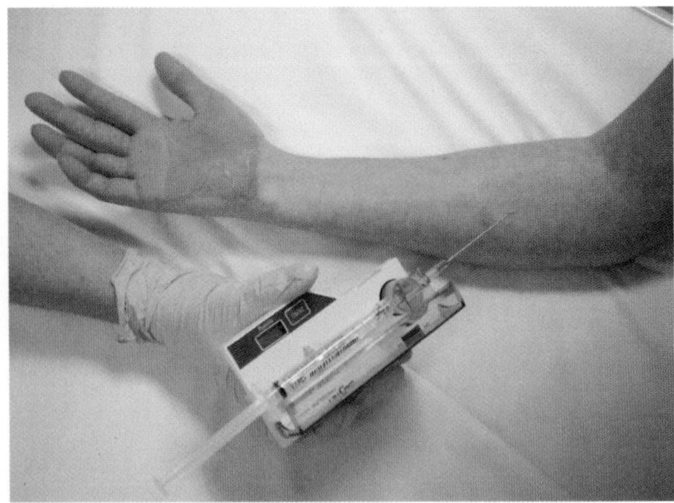

B

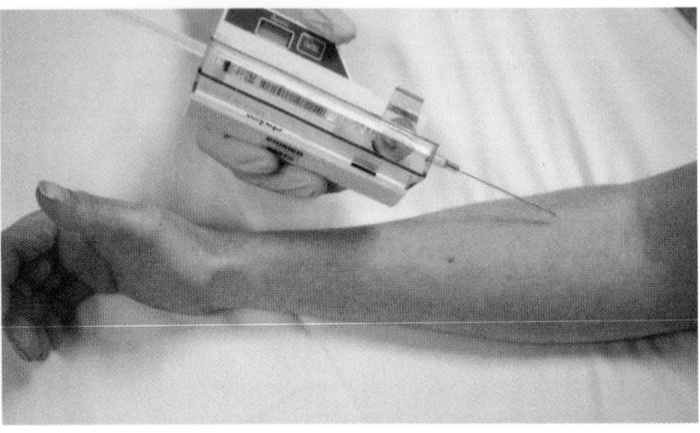

C

FIGURE 278-6. **A.** Forearm extensor compartment. **B.** Forearm flexor compartments. **C.** Mobile wad compartment.

TREATMENT

The initial medical management of these patients includes supplemental oxygen, if needed, and blood pressure support in the hypotensive patient. Immediately remove restrictive casts or dressings. This alone can markedly reduce tissue pressures. Place the affected limbs at the level of the heart; elevation higher than the heart increases the arteriovenous pressure gradient.

Hemophiliacs should have replacement of factor levels (see chapter 235, Hemophilias & von Willebrand Disease), and patients on anticoagulants should have reversal or factor replacement (see chapter 239, Thrombotics and Antithrombotics).

Surgical fasciotomy reduces intracompartmental pressure. Long incisions are necessary to release pressure in the affected compartment and simultaneously incise adjacent compartments. Tissue edema within the compartment will typically cause the muscle to bulge from the incision sites. The wounds should be initially left open and a second look procedure for debridement and possible closure scheduled for 48 to 72 hours after the initial intervention. Ideally, definitive wound closure is obtained within 7 to 10 days. This may require skin grafting.

A contraindication to fasciotomy is a missed timely diagnosis of compartment syndrome. Tissue pressures that have been elevated for 24 to 48 hours may have already caused permanent dysfunction and opening the compartments at this time may be futile.

DISEASE COMPLICATIONS

When fasciotomy is performed in a timely fashion, it can prevent death of the muscle within that compartment and the nerves that travel through it. When delayed, permanent neuropathy may occur, as can muscle death. Functional impairment is unlikely when compartment syndrome is diagnosed and treated within 6 hours of its onset.

DISPOSITION AND FOLLOW-UP

Admit all patients with compartment syndrome to the operating room or appropriate inpatient unit for serial observation and re-examination.

REFERENCES

The complete reference list is available online at www.TintinalliEM.com.

SECTION 23

Musculoskeletal Disorders

CHAPTER 279

Neck and Back Pain

David Della-Giustina
Jeffrey S. Dubin
William Frohna

EPIDEMIOLOGY

Low back pain alone accounts for approximately 3% of all ED visits in the United States.[1] Nearly one third of ED back pain patients receive x-rays, and 10% undergo CT or MRI imaging.[2] Analysis of the 2010 Global Burden of Disease study reveals a point prevalence of 5% for low back pain and 9% for neck pain. Back pain is the number one cause of disability in the United States; neck pain is number four.[3,4]

RISK FACTORS FOR SERIOUS CAUSES OF NECK AND BACK PAIN

There are many causes of neck and back pain, including trauma and biomechanical injuries, degeneration, inflammation (arthritides), infection (e.g., discitis, meningitis, and epidural abscess), infiltration (e.g., metastatic cancer and spinal cord tumors), and compression (e.g., epidural hematoma and abscess). In many cases of atraumatic neck and back pain, no specific cause can be identified. However, due to the high volume of ED patients with neck and back pain, clinicians can develop an indifference to this complaint and potentially overlook serious causes. Take care to perform a systematic evaluation based on risk factors in the history and physical examination, and let findings guide diagnostic testing and management (**Table 279-1**). Consider spinal anatomy while focusing on the presence or absence of neurologic signs to identify pathologic causes and prevent complications.

Radiculopathy and myelopathy are identified through pattern recognition of the motor and dermatome innervations and their associated spinal level (see Figure 164-1 and Tables 164-1 and 164-2 in chapter titled “Neurologic Examination”).

TABLE 279-1 Risk Factors for Serious Causes of Neck and Back Pain

Risk Factors	Concern
Historical Risk Factors	
Pain >6 weeks	Tumor, infection
Age <18, >50	Congenital anomaly, tumor, infection
Major trauma	Fracture
Minor trauma in elderly or rheumatologic disease	Fracture
History of cancer	Tumor
Fever and rigors	Infection
Weight loss	Tumor, infection
Injection drug use	Infection
Immunocompromised	Infection
Night pain	Tumor, infection
Unremitting pain, even when supine	Tumor, infection
Incontinence	Epidural compression
Saddle anesthesia	Epidural compression
Severe/progressive neurologic deficit	Epidural compression
Anticoagulants and coagulopathy	Epidural compression
Physical Risk Factors	
Fever	Infection
Patient writhing in pain	Infection, vascular cause
Unexpected anal sphincter laxity	Epidural compression
Perianal/perineal sensory loss	Epidural compression
Major motor weakness/gait disturbance	Nerve root or epidural compression
Positive straight leg raise test	Herniated disk

CLINICAL FEATURES OF NECK PAIN

In general, it is helpful to classify patients with neck pain into two groups: those with uncomplicated neck pain arising mainly from the joints and associated ligaments and muscles of the neck, and those with neck pain and *radiculopathy* (signs and symptoms attributable to a single nerve root) and/or *myelopathy* (signs or symptoms due to a spinal cord lesion, stenosis, or compression).

HISTORY IN PATIENTS WITH NECK PAIN

Ask about the onset, duration, and location of the neck pain; recent or remote trauma; associated symptoms; stiffness; deformity; neurologic complaints (e.g., weakness, changes in sensation, gait, or vision); constitutional symptoms such as fever, anorexia, and weight loss; and comorbid conditions such as arthritis, cancer, and infections. See Table 279-1 for clues to serious pathology to investigate in the history. Rheumatoid arthritis, ankylosing spondylitis, and psoriatic spondyloarthropathy may involve the C1-C2 joint, damage the transverse ligament, and erode the odontoid process, yielding instability of the atlantoaxial joint. Subluxation may occur spontaneously or following a trivial injury. Morning stiffness may signify arthritic joints. Identify precipitating and palliative factors, maneuvers, or activities. Inquire about prior episodes of neck pain, past diagnostic studies, and treatment. Determine the character of pain and its distribution. Patients with radiculopathy often complain of sharp, burning, intense pain that radiates to the trapezius, periscapular area, or down the arm. Weakness or paresthesias may develop weeks after pain onset. Patients with myelopathy may have neck pain that progresses insidiously and may complain of clumsy hands, gait disturbances, and sexual or bladder dysfunction. **Table 279-2** summarizes important differences in symptoms between uncomplicated mechanical neck pain and neck pain associated with radiculopathy or myelopathy.

PHYSICAL EXAMINATION IN PATIENTS WITH NECK PAIN

Begin with a general assessment of the patient, noting evidence of weight loss, pallor, adenopathy, and abnormalities of posture, movement, and facial expression.[5] Pain may cause splinting of the head on the shoulders during position change. Assess active and passive movement, including rotation (chin to shoulder), lateral flexion (ear to shoulder), and flexion-extension (chin down, then up). Most mechanical causes of neck pain result in asymmetric lesions and asymmetrically limited or painful movements, whereas inflammatory or neoplastic disorders are typically more widespread, with pain and movement restriction being more symmetric.[5] When localized ipsilateral neck pain is felt toward the side of head movement, suspect facet (zygapophyseal) joint irritability. Examine for **Spurling's**

TABLE 279-2 Differentiating Cervical Radiculopathy from Uncomplicated Musculoskeletal Neck Pain

Factors Favoring Cervical Radiculopathy or Myelopathy*	Factors Favoring Uncomplicated Musculoskeletal Neck Pain*
Pain from the neck radiates down the arm in dermatome pattern.	Tenderness of involved muscles, examiner may find a focal point of tenderness.
Sensory changes along dermatome distribution.	Atrophy or thinning of shoulder muscles (may occur after rotator cuff injury).
Pushing down on top of head, with neck in extension (chin up) and head leaning toward symptomatic side elicits pain, typically toward or down the arm (positive **Spurling's sign**); 90% specific, 45% sensitive.	Pain increases with shoulder abduction on the side of neck pain (increased pain could derive from rotator cuff–related pain; radicular pain may decrease with this maneuver).
Pain may worsen with Valsalva, which increases intrathecal pressure.	Repetitive movement of arm or shoulder at work or play; may be new activity.
Flex neck forward until chin meets chest or pain stops movement. An electric shock sensation radiating down spine into both arms is a positive result (**Lhermitte's sign**). Occasionally, paresthesias occur.	History of recent injury or recent event of awkward position (such as neck or head position during sleep in an unfamiliar setting) or awkward standing posture to accommodate a special situation.
Depressed reflexes or, uncommonly, increased reflexes (see also Table 279-3).	Pain is accompanied by "stiffness" of involved muscle group.

*Patient in either pain category is not expected to have all, or majority, of listed signs.

TABLE 279-3 Signs and Symptoms of Cervical Radiculopathy

Disk Space	Cervical Root	Pain Complaint	Sensory Abnormality	Motor Weakness	Altered Reflex
C1-C2	C2	Neck, scalp	Scalp		
C4-C5	C5	Neck, shoulder, upper arm	Shoulder	Infraspinatus, deltoid, biceps	Reduced biceps reflex
C5-C6	C6	Neck, shoulder, upper medial, scapular area, proximal forearm, thumb, index finger	Thumb and index finger, lateral forearm	Deltoid, biceps, pronator teres, wrist extensors	Reduced biceps and brachioradialis reflex
C6-C7	C7	Neck, posterior arm, dorsum proximal forearm, chest, medial third of scapula, middle finger	Middle finger, forearm	Triceps, pronator teres	Reduced triceps reflex
C7-T1	C8	Neck, posterior arm, ulnar side of forearm, medial inferior scapular border, medial hand, ring, and little fingers	Ring and little fingers	Triceps, flexor carpi ulnaris, hand intrinsics	Reduced triceps reflex

sign (see Table 279-2). The **abduction relief sign**, performed by having the patient place the hand of the affected upper extremity on the top of his or her head to obtain relief, may indicate soft disk protrusion causing radicular pain. When neck pain occurs on the side away from head movement, suspect a ligamentous or muscular source.

Palpate the posterior cervical triangle, the supraclavicular fossa, carotid sheaths, and the anterior neck. C5-C6 root lesions often elicit tenderness over the brachial plexus at Erb's point, 2 to 3 cm above the clavicle, midway up the posterior border of the sternocleidomastoid muscle in the posterior triangle of the neck. A C8-T1 root lesion may cause tenderness over the ulnar nerve at the elbow.

Pathology in the lymph nodes, salivary glands, or thyroid gland may cause neck pain. A bruit over the carotid may signal cerebral insufficiency; a bruit over the subclavian arteries may be associated with thoracic outlet or vascular steal syndrome. Examine the temporal artery for tenderness, because temporal arteritis may be the cause of neck and shoulder pain (see also chapter 165, "Headache").

Sensory symptoms of pain or dysesthesias are difficult to evaluate, particularly when motor signs are absent, which is often the case in cervical spinal radiculopathies. The discrete separation of the motor and sensory roots at the cervical neural foramina can explain motor sparing despite severe sensory symptoms. For example, C7 root irritability without motor weakness can present as aching at the medial to middle scapular border; aching in the myotome distribution to the chest, axilla, or triceps; or numbness or tingling in the middle finger.

Early detection of cervical spinal myelopathies requires a complete neurologic examination. Hyperreflexia, a positive Babinski's sign, clonus, gait disturbance, sexual or bladder dysfunction, lower extremity weakness, impaired fine hand movement, and upper and lower extremity spasticity may signal myelopathy. Examine for **Lhermitte's sign** (Table 279-2), which is indicative of possible cord compression. **Hoffman's sign** indicates an upper motor neuron lesion and is performed by flicking the tip of the middle finger as the hand is relaxed in a neutral position. A positive (abnormal) response is flexion of the thumb and index finger in a pinching motion.

Table 279-3 summarizes the sensory, motor, and reflex findings in cervical radiculopathy. This information should be used to determine the level of motor and sensory involvement and to compare findings in the affected and unaffected sides. Bilateral or multilevel involvement usually implies serious pathology.

DIAGNOSIS OF NECK PAIN

Laboratory testing is rarely helpful, unless considering infection. See the "Epidural Compression Syndrome," "Transverse Myelitis," and "Spinal Infection" sections later in this chapter, as well as chapter 246, "Neck and Upper Airway."

The need for **imaging studies** depends on the clinical condition suspected and the duration of neck pain. Acute (days to weeks), uncomplicated, nonradicular, nonmyelopathic, atraumatic neck pain typically requires no imaging because the cause is likely benign and the treatment is conservative.[5] Obtain three-view cervical spine films in patients with chronic (weeks to months) neck pain with or without a history of trauma, those with neck pain and a prior history of malignancy or remote neck surgery,[5] and those with neck pain and preexisting spinal disorders such as rheumatoid arthritis, ankylosing spondylitis, and psoriatic spondyloarthropathy. Flexion-extension films may be useful if instability is suspected, especially in patients with rheumatoid arthritis or other inflammatory arthritides.[6] Patients with normal radiographs, patients with radiographic evidence of degenerative changes without neck instability, or patients with radiographic evidence of previous trauma *and* no neurologic signs or symptoms require no further imaging.[5] **MRI is indicated for patients with chronic neck pain with neurologic signs or symptoms regardless of the plain radiographic findings.**[5] MRI is also indicated when plain radiographs reveal bone or disk margin destruction, if there is cervical instability, and (with intravenous contrast) if epidural abscess or malignancy is suspected.[5] CT myelography is recommended when contraindications to MRI exist.

DIFFERENTIAL DIAGNOSES OF NECK PAIN

Mechanical Neck Disorders Mechanical neck disorders are also called hyperextension strain, acceleration-deceleration injury, hyperextension-hyperflexion injury, neck strain, neck sprain, and whiplash. The most common precipitating events are motor vehicle collisions, falls, sports injuries, and work-related injuries (see chapter 258, "Spine Trauma" for discussion of acute injury). Strain injury, caused by an awkward position during sleep or prolonged abnormal head-neck positions during work or recreation, is another cause.

Cervical Disk Herniations Cervical disk herniations occur as the nucleus pulposus protrudes through the posterior annulus fibrosis, producing an acute radiculopathy or, occasionally, a myelopathy. Protrusions are usually confined by the posterior longitudinal ligament but can occasionally extrude through this ligament as free fragments. Direct posterior ruptures, although infrequent, can produce progressive myelopathy, whereas the more common posterolateral herniations can cause acute cervical radiculopathy. The levels of most frequent involvement are C5-C6 (C6 root) and C6-C7 (C7 root).

The symptoms of an acute cervical disk prolapse include neck pain, headache, pain distributed to the shoulder and along the medial scapular border, dermatome pain, and dysesthesia in the spinal root distribution to the shoulder and arm. Motor signs include fasciculations, atrophy and weakness in the dermatome distribution of the spinal root, loss of deep tendon reflexes, and, with cervical myelopathy, lower extremity hyperreflexia, Babinski's sign, and in rare cases, loss of sphincter control. Cervical hyperextension and lateral flexion to the symptomatic side (Spurling's sign; see Table 279-2) may replicate the symptoms, as can a Valsalva maneuver, whereas manual cervical distraction in flexion alleviates them. A thorough physical examination, including strength, sensory, and reflex testing, may delineate the level of root involvement (see Table 279-3). MRI is necessary for diagnosis.

Cervical Spondylosis and Stenosis Cervical spondylosis (or degenerative disk disease or osteoarthritis) is a progressive, degenerative condition resulting in a loss of cervical flexibility, neck pain, occipital neuralgia, radicular pain, or occasionally progressive myelopathy. There is progressive degeneration of the disks, ligaments, facet joints (zygapophyseal joints), and uncovertebral joints (joints of Luschka). From a radiographic standpoint, cervical spondylosis may be diagnosed if any one of three findings is present: osteophytes, disk space narrowing, or facet disease. However, there is a high prevalence of cervical spondylosis in asymptomatic individuals, and care must be taken in ascribing painful syndromes to findings on imaging. Degenerative disk disease predisposes a patient to progressive osteoarthrosis of the cervical spine, joint instability, and incongruous joint motion during neck movement. Spondylosis most commonly occurs at the C5-C6 and C6-C7 levels.

Osteophytic spurs can encroach posteriorly on the spinal canal, producing cervical myelopathy; laterally on the intervertebral foramen, producing cervical radiculopathy; and anteriorly on the esophagus, producing dysphagia. Spurious osteophytes may also produce Horner's syndrome, vertebrobasilar symptoms, severe radicular symptoms without associated neck pain, painless upper extremity myotome weakness, and chest pain mimicking angina. Neurologic findings (radiculopathy or myelopathy) may be gradual in onset unless there is a history of recent trauma.

The combination of a congenitally narrowed spinal canal, further compromised by a vertebral osteophytic bar anteriorly and a buckling ligamentum flavum posteriorly, increases the risk of myelopathy secondary to cervical spinal stenosis as the diameter of the spinal canal is reduced to less than 13 mm.

Cancer of the Cervical Spine Consider metastatic cancer in the differential diagnosis of chronic neck pain, especially unremitting night pain. Lung, breast, and prostate cancers and lymphoma and multiple myeloma may involve the cervical spine. Although most cases of epidural cord compression occur in the thoracic spine, involvement of the cervical spine and multiple levels are not unusual. Myelopathy, which is commonly caused by disk or degenerative disease, is rarely caused by metastatic tumors. Plain films have inadequate sensitivity (10% to 17% false-negative rate) in detecting spinal metastases but may reveal destruction of the vertebral bodies, lytic lesions of the pedicles, and pathologic compression fractures. MRI is the standard for the detection of spinal epidural metastatic disease and cord compression, and cancer patients with radiographic evidence of bone or disk margin destruction should undergo MRI.[5]

Cervical Myofascial Pain Syndrome Myofascial pain syndrome is a cause of chronic neck pain and is often confused with radiculopathy. Myofascial pain symptoms may present or exacerbate acutely, especially after trauma. Psychological distress and specific personality traits are risk factors. Typically, patients complain of pain in the neck, scapula, and shoulder with or without nondermatomal radiation into the upper extremity. Tender spots, "trigger points," may be evident on palpation of the head, neck, shoulder, and scapular region. Neurologic examination is normal. Because radiographic cervical spine abnormalities develop with age in the asymptomatic population, radiographic findings cannot be relied upon to verify the source of neck pain or upper extremity symptoms. Imaging reveals either nonspecific degenerative or disk changes that do not correlate with the clinically suspected site.

Other Conditions Epidural abscess, osteomyelitis, and transverse myelitis are infectious and inflammatory causes of neck pain (see related sections later in this chapter). Cervical spinal epidural hematoma often presents as neck pain followed by symptoms and signs of cord compression (see later section on epidural compression syndrome) and should be considered in the patient taking anticoagulants or in the patient with a bleeding diathesis. Pain from ischemic heart disease may radiate into the neck and shoulder. Peripheral nerve involvement, such as carpal tunnel syndrome, may present as a C6-C7 sensory radiculopathy, whereas multiple sclerosis, amyotrophic lateral sclerosis, subacute combined degeneration, and syrinx are in the differential of myelopathy.

TREATMENT AND DISPOSITION OF PATIENTS WITH NECK PAIN

Treatment issues can be divided into three categories: neck pain, neck and arm pain consistent with radiculopathy, and myelopathy. There is little evidence-based science to support many of the commonly recommended conservative treatment modalities (e.g., physiotherapy, acupuncture, electrotherapy, manipulation, traction, thermotherapy, medicinal and injection therapies, exercises).[7-11] Individual patients may indeed benefit from one or more of these therapies.

TREATMENT OF UNCOMPLICATED NECK PAIN

Most cases of neck pain without clear underlying pathology will improve with minimal intervention. The patient should be advised to "act as usual" and avoid activities that produce pain. Initial medications may include nonsteroidal anti-inflammatory drugs (NSAIDs), muscle relaxants, and for significant pain, a short course of oral opiates; no NSAID, muscle relaxant, or opiate is clearly superior to another in its class. Encourage follow-up with the primary physician to assess the need for physical or manual therapies or additional medications.

Patients with acute neck pain following an acceleration-deceleration (whiplash) injury may benefit from a similar pharmacologic regimen as that described earlier. In a Danish study of 458 patients, immobilization with a semi-rigid collar, advice to "act as usual," and active mobilization had similar effects in terms of preventing long-lasting pain and disability.[12] A soft collar reduces range of motion of the neck less than 20% and provides little immobilization or neck support.[13] If a soft collar is given, it should be used for no more than 10 days. Spinal manipulation therapy or home exercises after two 60-minute physical therapy sessions may each be more effective than medication therapy for short- and long-term pain relief.[14]

Therapy for neck pain from myofascial pain syndrome should address both muscular tension and psychobehavioral issues. See chapter 38, "Chronic Pain" for further discussion including recommendations for alternative therapies.

TREATMENT OF CERVICAL RADICULOPATHY

In the absence of myelopathy, first-line treatment is conservative activity modification to prevent symptom exacerbation or injury and oral medications. Immobilization with a soft or hard cervical collar is controversial without clear evidence for or against its use. Encourage follow-up with a primary physician for possible referral to a neurosurgical or orthopedic spine specialist, an electrodiagnostic evaluation, and additional rehabilitation interventions. Oral medications may include NSAIDs, opioid analgesics, and muscle relaxants. A 7- to 10-day course of oral steroids (e.g., methylprednisolone or prednisone) is commonly prescribed for acute radiculopathy, but steroid efficacy has been shown in only small low-quality studies of low back pain. Epidural steroid injections may be effective for chronic cervical radiculopathy when other treatments have failed. If the symptoms and signs of acute cervical root compression fail to respond to conservative treatment, or if they recur, and if imaging demonstrates concordant findings, surgery may be recommended. Indications for hospital admission include progressive upper extremity weakness, especially in the C7 distribution; acute or progressive symptoms or signs of myelopathy; and finally, in a small subset of patients, intractable radicular pain unresponsive to treatment.

TREATMENT OF CERVICAL MYELOPATHY

Treatment decisions for patients with symptoms and signs of cord compression should be made in conjunction with specialists. Cervical spondylotic myelopathy causes the greatest degree of impairment and disability in the continuum of spondylosis. Also, myelopathy is the most common cause of spastic paraparesis in patients older than 55 years of age, thus paralleling the time course of spondylosis. The patient with myelopathy should be referred to a neurosurgeon or orthopedic spine surgeon to discuss the possibility of decompressive surgery. Additional therapeutic considerations (e.g., steroids and radiation in spinal epidural metastases) will depend on the time course of symptoms and signs and etiology but should be addressed in conjunction with a neurosurgeon.

CLINICAL FEATURES OF THORACIC AND LUMBAR PAIN SYNDROMES

Back pain is categorized based on the duration of symptoms: acute back pain lasts <6 weeks, subacute pain lasts between 6 and 12 weeks, and chronic pain continues beyond 12 weeks.[15] Pain lasting >6 weeks is an indicator of more serious disease, since most episodes of nonspecific back pain (80% to 90%) resolve within 6 weeks. Risk factors for serious causes of back and neck pain are listed in Table 279-1; specific historical factors that help to identify benign verses serious causes of back pain are listed in the following sections.

HISTORICAL RISK FACTORS IN BACK PAIN

Patient Age In patients <18 years old and >50 years old, back pain is more likely to be caused by tumor or infection than in the 18- to 50-year-old age group. Patients <18 years old also have a higher incidence of congenital and bony abnormalities such as spondylolysis, spondylolisthesis, and Scheuermann's kyphosis. Patients >50 years old are more prone to fractures (age >65 years is more specific for fracture), spinal stenosis, and intra-abdominal processes such as an abdominal aortic aneurysm.

Pain Location and Radiation Pain that originates from muscular, ligamentous, vertebral, or disk disease without nerve involvement is located primarily in the back, possibly with radiation into the buttocks or thighs. *Sciatica*, radicular back pain in the distribution of a lumbar or sacral nerve root, is often accompanied by sensory or motor deficits.[15] Sciatica occurs in only 1% of patients with back pain and is associated with disk herniation or nerve root impingement below the L3 nerve root. Ninety-five percent of herniated disks occur at the L4-L5 or the L5-S1 lumbar disk spaces, impinging on the L5 or S1 nerve roots, respectively.[15]

Trauma History of major trauma is a risk factor for fracture in all patients. In the elderly, minor trauma, such as falling from standing or from sitting in a chair, may cause fracture due to associated osteoporosis. Risk factors for osteoporosis increase the incidence of compression fractures (i.e., female sex, steroid use, alcoholism).

Systemic Complaints Systemic symptoms such as fever, chills, night sweats, malaise, and an undesired weight loss suggest infection, systemic rheumatologic disease, or malignancy. These symptoms are more concerning for infection if the patient has any of the following risk factors: recent bacterial infection (including urinary tract infection, pneumonia, and especially skin abscesses), recent GU or GI procedure, immunocompromised status, injection drug use, alcoholism, renal failure, or diabetes.[16-18] Injection drug use is a substantial risk factor for spinal infection, so assume that back pain in a patient who is an injection drug user is due to spinal infection until proven otherwise.

A rupturing abdominal aortic aneurysm is the most immediately life-threatening extraspinal cause of back pain. Other potential causes of pain referred to the back include pancreatitis, a posterior lower lobe pneumonia, nephrolithiasis, and renal infarct.

Pain Features A dull, aching pain that generally worsens with movement but improves with rest and lying still is the typical description of benign back pain. Symptoms suggestive of tumor and infection include pain that occurs at night and often awakens the patient from sleep or that is unrelenting despite appropriate use of analgesics and rest.[15,19] Pain worsened by coughing, Valsalva maneuver, or sitting and that is relieved by lying in the supine position suggests herniation. Spinal stenosis is associated with bilateral sciatic pain that is worsened by activities such as walking, prolonged standing, and back extension and is relieved by rest and forward flexion. In the authors' experience, night pain and unrelenting pain are worrisome symptoms that should be specifically queried as part of the history, because these symptoms are risk factors for serious disease and such queries are often omitted in history taking.

Neurologic Deficit by History Neurologic complaints such as paresthesias, numbness, weakness, and gait disturbances must be further addressed in the history and delineated in the physical examination to determine whether the symptoms involve single or multiple nerve roots. Bowel or bladder incontinence is a serious symptom that raises concern for an epidural compression syndrome, such as spinal cord compression, cauda equina syndrome, or conus medullaris syndrome. If a patient has back pain and has a history of urinary incontinence (acute or chronic), but an otherwise completely normal history and evaluation, measure the postvoid residual volume with bedside US or by catheterization if US findings are in doubt. A large postvoid residual volume (e.g., >100 mL) indicates overflow incontinence, which, when combined with the presence of low back pain, suggests neurologic compromise and an epidural compression syndrome.[15,20]

Past Medical History History of cancer is a risk factor because back pain is the initial symptom in the majority of those with spinal metastases.[20] Malignant neoplasm is the most common systemic disease affecting the spine. Most patients with this diagnosis are >50 years old. However, only one third of patients diagnosed with spinal malignancy have a known history of cancer. Thus, symptoms such as unremitting pain, night pain, and weight loss require further diagnostic testing.

PHYSICAL EXAMINATION RISK FACTORS IN BACK PAIN

Although fever is a marker of infection, sensitivity for infection is low, varying from 27% for tuberculous osteomyelitis to 50% for pyogenic osteomyelitis, 60% to 70% for pyogenic discitis, and 66% to 83% for spinal epidural abscess.[16,19] Careful history, examination, and possibly diagnostic testing are needed for patients with back pain and fever. In patients with severe or excessive pain, consider acute spinal infection or abdominal aortic aneurysm. Examine the abdomen, listen for bruits, and palpate for masses, tenderness, and an enlarged aorta.

Examine the back for signs of erythema, warmth, skin abscesses, furuncles, and purulent drainage, which suggest an underlying spinal infection. Contusion and swelling suggest trauma. Palpate the back and percuss the vertebral bodies. Consider fracture or bacterial infection if there is point tenderness to vertebral percussion. Perform **straight leg raise testing**. With the patient lying supine, lift each leg separately to approximately 70 degrees in an attempt to produce radicular pain. A positive straight leg raise test causes a radicular pain radiating below the knee of the affected leg. This pain is worsened by ankle dorsiflexion and improved with ankle plantar flexion or decreasing leg elevation. Reproduction of the patient's back pain or pain in the gluteal or hamstring area when the leg is raised is **not** a positive result. The straight leg raise test can be easily replicated with the patient in the seated position with similar leg extension and foot dorsiflexion (**Figure 279-1**). Straight leg raise testing is a screening examination for a herniated disk. One third of those with positive straight leg raising test and a negative sitting knee extension test have an MRI-proven herniated disk.[21] **A positive straight leg raise test is 68% to 80% sensitive for a L4-L5 or L5-S1 herniated disk.**[21] Radicular pain down the affected leg when lifting the asymptomatic leg is called a positive **crossed straight leg raise test**. A positive result is highly specific but insensitive for nerve root compression by a herniated disk.

Neurologic Examination For Back Pain The neurologic examination is directed to detecting deficits in each of the specific spinal nerve roots. Sensation may be tested by using light touch initially, followed more formally by pinprick, temperature, proprioception, and vibration testing if there are any questions regarding diminished sensation. Next assess strength, with a focus on those muscle groups innervated by individual nerve roots (**Figure 279-2**). Individually test

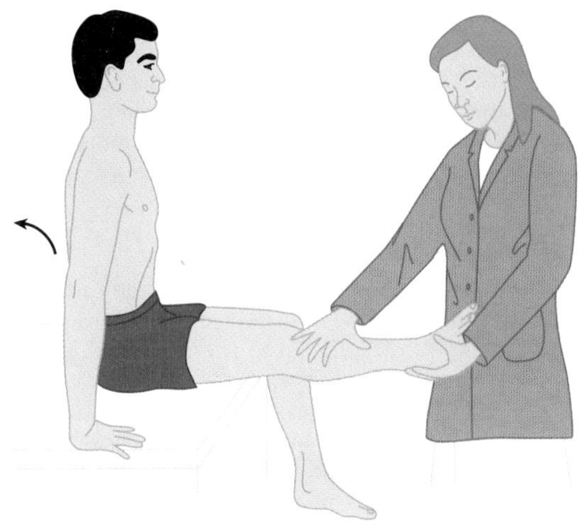

FIGURE 279-1. Sitting knee extension test. With the patient sitting on a table, both hip and knees flexed at 90 degrees, slowly extend the knee as if evaluating the patella or bottom of the foot. This maneuver stretches nerve roots as much as a moderate degree of supine straight leg raising.

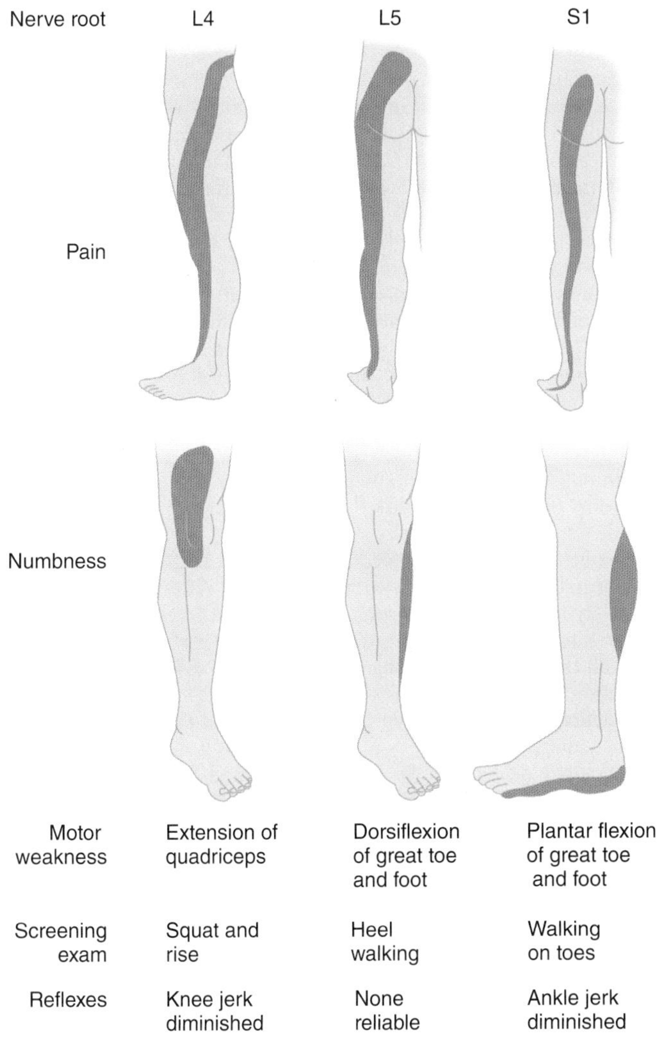

Nerve root	L4	L5	S1
Pain			
Numbness			
Motor weakness	Extension of quadriceps	Dorsiflexion of great toe and foot	Plantar flexion of great toe and foot
Screening exam	Squat and rise	Heel walking	Walking on toes
Reflexes	Knee jerk diminished	None reliable	Ankle jerk diminished

FIGURE 279-2. Testing for lumbar nerve root compromise.

the ankle dorsiflexors (L4), extensor hallucis longus (great toe dorsiflexion) (L5), and ankle plantar flexors (S1/S2). Finally, evaluate the patellar (L3-L4), Achilles (S1), and Babinski's reflexes. There is no easily obtainable reflex for the L5 nerve root.

It is not necessary to perform a digital rectal examination on all patients with back pain. However, perform rectal examination in patients with neurologic complaints or findings on physical examination and those with risk factors for serious disease. Evaluate rectal sphincter tone and perianal sensation and the presence of prostatic and rectal masses. Poor rectal tone in association with back pain and saddle anesthesia indicates an epidural compression syndrome.

DIAGNOSIS OF BACK PAIN SYNDROMES

For most patients, no testing is required. However, laboratory testing is indicated in the ED if there is concern for infection, tumor, or rheumatologic causes of the back pain. Order a CBC, erythrocyte sedimentation rate, and urinalysis. With infection, the WBC count may be normal or elevated. However, the erythrocyte sedimentation rate is typically elevated (>20 mm/h), even in immunocompromised patients, with a sensitivity of 90% to 98% for spine infection.[16,19,22] The erythrocyte sedimentation rate will also be elevated in patients with a rheumatologic or neoplastic disease of the spine.[15] The C-reactive protein will also be elevated with acute spinal infection.[15,19] Obtain a urinalysis to identify urinary tract infection or renal disease causing pain referred to the back.

IMAGING

Plain spinal radiographs can be considered when one suspects fracture, tumor, or infection, but sensitivity is only 83% for tumor and very poor for infection. Anteroposterior and lateral views are sufficient. The coned-down L5-S1 and oblique views rarely add clinically useful information while more than doubling gonadal radiation exposure and cost.

CT scanning is most useful for evaluating vertebral fractures, the facet joints, and the posterior elements of the spine. It shows good detail of the vertebral bodies but has poor resolution of the spinal canal and spinal cord in comparison with MRI. CT may be useful if MRI is unavailable or unsuitable, but CT myelography is the best substitute for conditions such as epidural abscess or cord compression when MRI is unavailable.

MRI provides the best resolution for lesions in the vertebral bodies, spinal canal, and spinal cord, and for disk disease. MRI is also the standard study in cases of suspected spinal infection, neoplasm, and epidural compression syndromes. MRI is also used to determine progression of neoplastic processes of the spine and disk disease and for continued back pain for 6 to 8 weeks.

DIFFERENTIAL DIAGNOSIS AND MANAGEMENT OF BACK PAIN SYNDROMES

ACUTE NONSPECIFIC BACK PAIN

Nonspecific back pain is a symptom complex that has countless names, including back strain/sprain, mechanical back pain, and lumbago. However, because strain and/or sprain have no histopathologic findings, a more accurate term to use is *idiopathic or nonspecific back pain*. Nonspecific back pain is the authors' choice of term, especially because most patients will never be given a more precise diagnosis.

Diagnosis is clinical. The pain is mild to moderate and is aggravated with movement and relieved with rest. Although the typical mechanism is usually minor exertion or lifting, the patient may not recall any remarkable etiology. There are no risk factors for serious disease on the history and physical examination, or if any risk factors are present, the diagnostic evaluation is normal.

Treatment focuses on restriction of activity, analgesia, manipulation, and other physical modalities. Monitor symptoms for 4 to 6 weeks before embarking on further diagnostics. In 80% to 90% of patients, symptoms will resolve on their own within this time period.[15] Watchful waiting avoids wasting time and money and eliminates exposure to unnecessary radiation. This course of action should be discussed with patients because they may expect diagnostic testing.

Patients who resume their normal activities to the furthest extent tolerable recover more rapidly than those on 2 or 7 days of bed rest or those who perform back-mobilizing exercises.[23] Thus, patients should continue daily activities using pain as the limiting factor.[15] Withhold exercise programs until the acute painful episode has resolved or improved significantly.

Medication is a combination of **acetaminophen and NSAIDs**. Acetaminophen is an excellent first-line agent, and there is little evidence that NSAIDs are more effective for symptomatic relief.[24,25] Most NSAIDs are equally efficacious for back pain. However, there are significant differences in the side effect profiles and toxicity. In one review, ibuprofen was the least toxic of the 12 NSAIDs studied, particularly with regard to upper GI bleeding. Because there is a linear relationship between dose and toxicity, the lowest dose possible should be used in patients at risk. In patients at risk for GI bleeding, the addition of a proton pump inhibitor or misoprostol can reduce the risk.[25]

We recommend using acetaminophen in combination with NSAIDs or as the sole initial agent when treating patients at higher risk for adverse effects of NSAIDs (the elderly and those with renal disease or peptic ulcers). One regimen is acetaminophen, 650 to 975 milligrams every 4 to 6 hours (do not exceed 4 grams in a 24-hour period), either alone or in conjunction with ibuprofen, 800 milligrams three times daily, or naproxen, 250 to 500 milligrams twice daily. If there is a concern for GI bleeding, then add a proton pump inhibitor such as omeprazole, 20 milligrams once daily.

Opioid analgesics should be offered to patients with moderate to severe pain, but for a limited (1 week) duration, as they are only effective in the short term.[15,24,26] When prescribing opioid analgesic combinations that include acetaminophen, warn patients not to combine them with other acetaminophen products.

Muscle relaxants are useful for treating back pain.[26] Muscle relaxants, such as diazepam, 5 to 10 milligrams every 6 to 8 hours, and methocarbamol, 1000 to 1500 milligrams four times a day, are effective. Although their efficacy appears equal to NSAIDs, there are no studies comparing muscle relaxants alone with NSAIDs in the treatment of nonspecific low back pain. Additionally, there does not appear to be any additional pain relief or synergistic benefit when these medications are used in combination.[27] Corticosteroids taken systemically or injected locally or into the epidural space have no role in the treatment of nonspecific back pain.[15,28]

Manipulative therapy, while not generally an ED treatment, is one of the more controversial treatment options for back pain. Clinical outcome of manipulation is no better than standard medical therapy according to a Cochrane review,[29] but is not harmful.[15]

Other physical modalities include traction, diathermy, cutaneous laser treatment, exercise, US treatment, and transcutaneous electrical nerve stimulation. None of these have any proven efficacy in the treatment of acute low back symptoms. The application of heat or ice may provide temporary symptomatic relief in some patients, with evidence favoring heat.[15]

CHRONIC NONSPECIFIC BACK PAIN

There is a higher concern for serious disease in patients with ongoing or intermittent symptoms for a time period of months to years. The best approach is to review the previous evaluations for completeness and to be sure that abnormalities were not overlooked. If the evaluation has been incomplete, then consider completing it in the ED at that visit, or facilitate referral for an outpatient evaluation, with urgency guided by the severity of symptoms. If the evaluation has been thorough but negative, then treat as described for nonspecific back pain. If opioid analgesics are needed, prescribe them for only a very limited time. Chronic back pain is a difficult condition to manage, and benefit of medications is small.[15,24,26,30] Further information on the management of chronic back pain can be found in chapter 38.

LOW BACK PAIN WITH SCIATICA

Although sciatica only affects a very small proportion of all patients with back pain, it is present in the vast majority of patients with a symptomatic herniated disk. Although disk herniation is the most common cause of sciatica, anything that compresses or impinges on the spinal nerve roots, cauda equina, or spinal cord can cause sciatica. Other important etiologies to consider in the ED include intraspinal tumor or infection, foraminal stenosis, extraspinal plexus compression, piriformis syndrome (see chapter 281, "Hip and Knee Pain"), and lumbar canal stenosis (spinal stenosis).

DISK HERNIATION

Diagnosis is suspected clinically and confirmed with nonurgent MRI (urgent MRI only in the setting of suspected spinal cord compression). Patients who present with sciatica due to a herniated disk generally complain more about the radicular symptoms than about back pain. Because the vast majority of disk herniations occur at the L4-L5 (L5 nerve root) or L5-S1 (S1 nerve root) level, the radicular pain extends below the knee in the dermatomal distribution of that nerve root. A small proportion (often the elderly) have disk herniation at the L2-L3 (L3 nerve root) and L3-L4 (L4 nerve root) levels. The physical examination generally demonstrates localization of pain and a neurologic deficit in a unilateral single nerve root, usually L5 or S1, and frequently includes a positive result on straight leg raise testing.

If the patient has no risk factors in the history and physical examination for serious disease other than sciatica, treat conservatively and do not perform any diagnostic tests in the ED.[15] If the patient has a demonstrable neurologic deficit, consider obtaining plain radiographs to look for other possible causes for symptoms such as tumor, fracture, spondylolisthesis, and infection. Guidelines recommend imaging (MRI preferred) in patients with severe or progressive neurologic deficits and those with serious underlying conditions suspected based on history or physical examination.[15] If the symptoms have not progressed rapidly or the symptoms are not severe, the MRI can be ordered routinely or urgently rather than emergently.

Treatment is as for nonspecific back pain. Routine daily activity is as good as 2 weeks of bed rest in terms of intensity of pain, distress associated with symptoms, and functional status.[23] Recommendations for analgesic (acetaminophen, NSAID, and opiates) and muscle relaxant therapy remain the same.[31] NSAIDs are less effective in treating the symptoms of a herniated disk than they are in treating nonspecific back pain.

Corticosteroid therapy for herniated disk has limited benefit. Specifically, epidural corticosteroid injection provides a minor reduction in leg pain and sensory deficits in comparison with placebo. However, the improvement in symptoms is not associated with any significant functional benefit, and it does not reduce the need for surgery. Although epidural steroid injection is not an ED procedure, it offers an alternative for the moderately to severely symptomatic patient in follow-up. Although oral steroids are used widely, they appear to have little measurable benefit in patients with sciatica.

Manipulation is not recommended for the routine management of symptoms from herniated disk.[29] Local application of heat or ice may provide temporary relief.

Most patients with a herniated disk may be treated and monitored by their primary care physician without specialist referral. Most patients ultimately improve with nonsurgical therapy, with over half recovering in 6 weeks. Most spine surgeons agree that surgery is appropriate only when all three of the following criteria are met: definitive evidence of herniation on imaging study; corresponding clinical picture and neurologic deficit; and conservative treatment for 4 to 6 weeks that fails to produce improvement.

Emergency decompressive surgery is required only in patients with acute epidural compression syndromes. Patients who underwent surgery had improved function and fewer symptoms at 1 and 2 years postoperatively, compared with those treated conservatively; however, by 4 and 10 years postoperatively, both groups had comparable results.[32,33]

SPINAL STENOSIS

Spinal stenosis is a narrowing of any part of the lumbar spine, including the spinal canal, nerve root canal, and intervertebral foramina, which may occur at single or multiple spinal levels. Degenerative disease causes narrowing and compression of vascular and neural structures. It is a cause of chronic back pain, with or without associated sciatica. The symptoms, which usually begin in the sixth decade, include low back pain that is aggravated by prolonged standing and spinal extension and is relieved by rest and forward flexion. Typically, symptomatic patients present with low back and lower extremity pain while walking that is symptomatically similar to vascular claudication. This symptom is termed *neurogenic claudication* or *pseudoclaudication* to distinguish it from vascular claudication. **Neurogenic claudication is relieved with rest and forward flexing the spine and worsened by extending the spine.**[34] Physical examination findings are often absent. The diagnosis is made principally by history with confirmation by CT scan or MRI. Symptomatic treatment is the same as chronic back pain with primary care follow-up.

ANKYLOSING SPONDYLITIS

Ankylosing spondylitis is an autoimmune arthritis that primarily affects the spine and pelvis. It is associated with human leukocyte antigen B-27, trauma, and infection. It most commonly occurs in patients <40 years old with a 3:1 male predilection. Patients complain of awakening with low back pain and stiffness that improves throughout the day with mild activity. The diagnosis is suspected by history and physical exam in individuals with symptoms longer than 3 months in duration and is confirmed by imaging and laboratory tests. Radiographic studies demonstrate sacroiliitis and squaring of the vertebral bodies, the so-called *bamboo spine*. Patients can be treated symptomatically with NSAIDs and should be referred to a rheumatologist for diagnostic confirmation and further management.

EPIDURAL COMPRESSION SYNDROME

Epidural compression syndrome is a collective term encompassing **spinal cord compression**, **cauda equina syndrome**, and **conus medullaris syndrome**.

Although the diagnosis of a complete epidural compression is obvious, the challenge is diagnosis in patients with early signs and symptoms. The initial differential diagnosis is broad and includes most conditions that cause weakness, sensory changes, or autonomic dysfunction of the lower extremities. The history and physical examination should narrow the differential diagnosis to a compressive lesion of the spinal cord or cauda equina.

Possible causes of epidural compression include spinal canal hemorrhage with hematoma, tumors of the spine or epidural space, spinal canal infections including spinal epidural abscess, and massive midline disk herniation. Transverse myelitis is a noncompressive condition that may present clinically like a compressive lesion of the spinal cord.

The history usually includes back pain with associated neurologic deficits. Specifically, it may include perianal sensory loss, fecal incontinence or urinary incontinence with or without retention, and sciatica in one or both legs. The duration of symptoms does not differentiate these syndromes from benign causes of back pain. In one small study, **urinary retention of >500 mL alone or in combination with two of the following characteristics—bilateral sciatica, subjective urinary retention, or rectal incontinence symptoms—is the most important predictor of MRI-confirmed cauda compressions.**[35] Also, a history of malignancy and a rapid progression of neurologic symptoms, especially bilateral symptoms, increase the likelihood of compression.

The physical examination findings vary depending on the level of compression and the amount and area of the spinal cord or cauda equina that is compressed. **The most common finding in cauda equina syndrome is urinary retention with or without overflow incontinence**, with a sensitivity of 90% and a specificity of about 95%.[35] Other common findings for epidural compression include weakness or stiffness in the lower extremities, paresthesias or sensory deficits, gait difficulty, and abnormal results on straight leg raise testing.[36] The most common sensory deficit occurs over the buttocks, posterosuperior thighs, and perineal regions and is commonly called *saddle anesthesia*. Anal sphincter tone is decreased in 60% to 80% of cases.

When one clinically suspects epidural compression, especially due to tumor, treat the patient with dexamethasone, 10 milligrams IV, before obtaining any confirmatory tests.[36] **After the patient has received dexamethasone, obtain an emergent MRI of the spine.** If investigating the possibility of epidural compression due to neoplasm, obtain an MRI of the **entire spine** because 10% of patients with vertebral metastases have additional silent epidural metastases that would be missed by a localized imaging study.[36] The presence of tumors remote from the symptomatic site may change patient management. Additionally, the neurologic examination may falsely localize the spinal lesion(s) and limited regional MRI may not detect the lesion. If one suspects a pure cauda equina syndrome from a herniated disk, then it is reasonable to obtain an MRI localized to the lumbosacral spine.

The functional clinical outcome for epidural compression from tumor depends on patient symptoms at presentation. Patients who cannot walk before treatment rarely walk again. Those who are too weak to walk without assistance but who are not paraplegic have a 50% chance of walking again. Those who are able to walk when treatment begins are likely to remain ambulatory.[36] Of those patients who require a catheter for urinary retention before treatment, 82% will continue to require the urinary catheter after treatment. The presence of cord compresion is an indication for urgent consultation with a spine surgeon for decompression and/or radiation therapy for a tumor mass, determined by MRI findings.[37,38]

TRANSVERSE MYELITIS

Transverse myelitis is an inflammatory disorder that involves a complete transverse section of the spinal cord. It usually presents with neck or back pain in association with neurologic complaints and findings on physical examination, depending on the level of the spinal cord that is involved. The typical clinical syndrome involves bilateral motor, sensory, and autonomic disturbances that may progress over a period of days to weeks. Fecal and urinary retention and incontinence are common.[39] Transverse myelitis may result from viral infection, after vaccination, or as part of a systemic disease such as systemic lupus erythematosus, cancer, or, more commonly, multiple sclerosis. The most important issue regarding transverse myelitis is recognition of the potential for a compressive lesion of the spinal cord and managing the patient as outlined under epidural compression syndromes. The MRI may demonstrate lesions of the spinal cord, but MRI findings may lag the clinical presentation, especially early in the disease process.[38] In those situations where the patient has definite neurologic findings that are consistent with epidural compression but has a normal MRI, transverse myelitis is one of the primary working diagnoses. In such cases, consult a neurologist for admission and consider performing a lumbar puncture to assist in the diagnosis. The spinal fluid most commonly demonstrates lymphocytosis and elevated protein.[38] Treatment includes corticosteroids and plasma exchange at the direction of a neurologist.[38]

SPINAL INFECTION

Spinal infections, such as *vertebral osteomyelitis, discitis,* and *spinal epidural abscess*, are uncommon but serious causes of back pain. Unfortunately, these infections are commonly missed on first assessment.[19,22] Risk factors for infection include the following: immunocompromised states (diabetes, HIV infection, and organ transplant recipients), alcoholism, recent invasive procedures, spinal implants and devices, injection drug use, and skin abscesses.[16,19,22]

Vertebral Osteomyelitis Patients with **vertebral osteomyelitis** usually have had prolonged symptoms, and in many cases, pain has been present for >3 months.[19,40] On physical examination, about half have fever and vertebral body tenderness to percussion.[19,40] The WBC may be normal, but the erythrocyte sedimentation rate and C-reactive protein are almost always elevated, although this is nonspecific.[16,17,19,40] Blood cultures are positive in approximately 40% of cases of vertebral osteomyelitis and should be routinely drawn as part of the management. In osteomyelitis, plain radiographs are normal until the bone demineralizes, which can take from 2 to 8 weeks. **The most common radiographic abnormalities with vertebral osteomyelitis are bony destruction, irregularity of vertebral end plates, and disk space narrowing.**[19] See the section on osteomyelitis in chapter 281 for further discussion.

Discitis In patients with discitis, >90% present with a complaint of unremitting back or neck pain, which awakens them at night and is relieved by neither rest nor analgesics.[19] Fever is present in 60% to 70% of patients, whereas the percentage of patients with neurologic deficits is highly variable, from 10% to 50%.[19] Elevation in the erythrocyte sedimentation rate occurs in >90% of patients, whereas elevated WBC count occurs in less than half of patients.[19]

Spinal Epidural Abscess The classic triad of symptoms suggesting spinal epidural abscess is severe back pain, fever, and neurologic deficits, but the triad occurs in only 8% to 13% of patients.[22] Spinal epidural abscess is commonly found in association with vertebral osteomyelitis and discitis, in 62% and 38% of cases, respectively.[16,22] Risk factors 98% sensitive for epidural abscess include injection drug use, immunocompromise, alcohol abuse, recent spine procedure, distant site of infection, diabetes, indwelling catheter, recent spine fracture, chronic renal failure, and cancer.[22] Erythrocyte sedimentation rate is elevated (>20 mm/h) in >95% of patients,[16,17,22] and the C-reactive protein is elevated in >90% of patients.[19] For all spinal infections, contrast-enhanced MRI is the gold standard imaging study. For detailed discussion, see chapter 174, "Central Nervous System and Spinal Infections."

Treatment of Spinal Infections Epidural abscess requires antibiotics and emergent evaluation and treatment by a spine surgeon. The treatment for discitis is long-term antibiotics, with surgery reserved for those with spinal cord compression or biomechanical instability. The treatment for vertebral osteomyelitis is primarily medical, consisting of 6 weeks of IV antibiotics followed by a 4- to 8-week course of oral antibiotics. For vertebral osteomyelitis, consult with a spine surgeon before antibiotic administration, because antibiotics may result in negative culture results from a bone biopsy. However, do not withhold antibiotics unless specifically directed by the spine surgeon. Empiric antibiotic therapy should be directed against *Staphylococcus aureus*. Parenteral piperacillin-tazobactam, 3.375 grams IV, and vancomycin, 1 gram IV, or similar agents with broad-spectrum coverage can be given until culture results are available.[17,18] The remainder of treatment is symptomatic.

REFERENCES

The complete reference list is available online at www.TintinalliEM.com.

Shoulder Pain

David Della-Giustina
David Hile

ANATOMY

The shoulder is designed for mobility in all directional planes, but stability is less than other joints. To meet the many demands placed on it, the shoulder uses three bones, four joints, and a specialized set of soft tissues consisting of muscles, tendons, ligaments, and bursae. The most common causes of nontraumatic shoulder pain in descending order of frequency are rotator cuff tendinopathy, acromioclavicular joint disease, adhesive capsulitis, and referred pain.[1]

BONES AND JOINTS

The humerus, clavicle, and scapula are the bones of the shoulder complex. The scapula consists of the body plus three bony extensions: the glenoid, the coracoid, and the acromion.

The four joints of the shoulder are the glenohumeral, acromioclavicular, sternoclavicular, and scapulothoracic. The glenohumeral joint is a ball-and-socket joint and is the central axis of shoulder motion. The glenohumeral joint is the most mobile and least stable joint in the body. Stability is derived from three components. The first is the glenoid labrum, which is a fibrous ring of tissue encircling the glenoid cavity. The glenoid labrum increases the surface contact area of the humeral head within the relatively shallow glenoid fossa. The second component consists of three glenohumeral ligaments, which aid stability by reinforcing the joint capsule. Finally, four specialized muscles, known as the *rotator cuff*, encompass the glenohumeral joint and provide stability during motion.

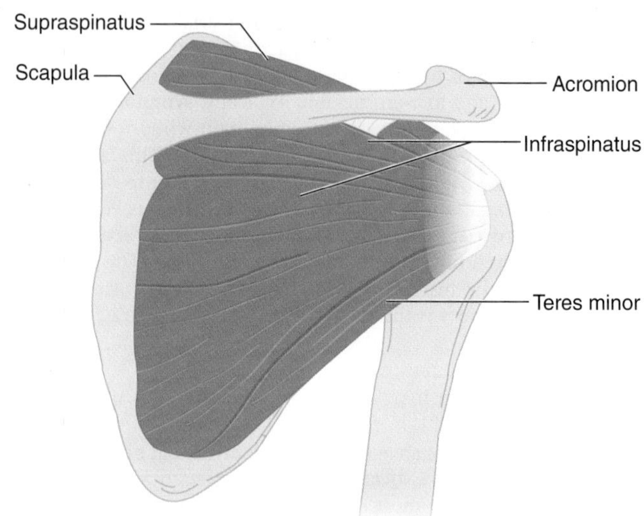

FIGURE 280-1. Posterior view of the shoulder illustrating rotator cuff muscles.

The sternoclavicular and acromioclavicular joints together contribute to glenohumeral motion, but their primary function is to suspend and stabilize the shoulder girdle. Rotation at the acromioclavicular joint and elevation at the sternoclavicular joint allow complete arm elevation. The scapulothoracic joint represents the articulation of the scapula on the posterior wall of the thorax. Scapular motion is essential for overall shoulder motion: every degree of scapulothoracic motion allows 2 degrees of glenohumeral motion.

SHOULDER MUSCLES

The deltoid, which drapes the shoulder complex and forms its contour, acts as a powerful and independent elevator of the arm. Along with the pectoralis, the deltoid is the primary source of movement of the upper extremity.

The **rotator cuff** consists of four muscles: supraspinatus, infraspinatus, teres minor, and subscapularis (**Figures 280-1 and 280-2**). All originate

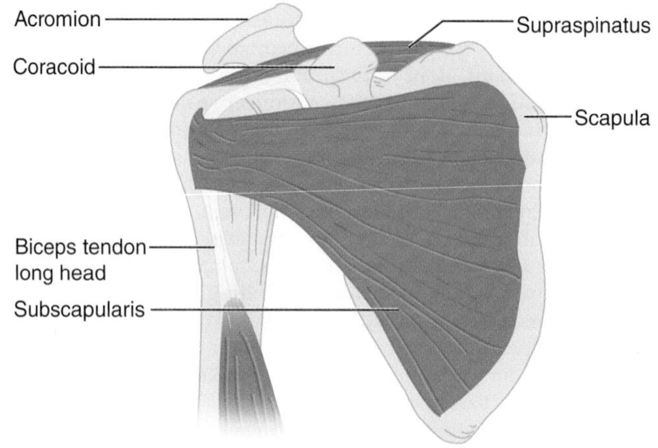

FIGURE 280-2. Anterior view of the shoulder illustrating the supraspinatus muscle and the long head of the biceps.

on the scapula, traverse the glenohumeral joint, and insert on the proximal humerus. The rotator cuff muscles also contribute to the power of the upper extremity, providing 30% to 50% of the power in abduction and 90% in external rotation.

The supraspinatus muscle originates on the posterior and superior aspect of the scapula and passes beneath the acromion, inserting onto the great tuberosity of the humeral head. It initiates arm elevation and abducts the shoulder. It also balances the power of the deltoid, keeping the humerus centered in the glenoid during deltoid contraction. The infraspinatus originates on the posterior scapula just inferior to the scapular spine. It inserts on the posterior aspect of the greater tuberosity and acts primarily as an external rotator of the arm (**Figure 280-1**). The teres minor originates on the lateral border of the scapula just inferior to the infraspinatus and inserts on the posterior aspect of the humerus. It works with the infraspinatus to provide external rotation (Figure 280-1). The subscapularis is the only rotator cuff muscle that arises from the anterior aspect of the scapula. It attaches to the lesser tuberosity of the humeral head and provides internal rotation of the arm (**Figure 280-2**).

The long head of the biceps tendon, although not part of the rotator cuff, assists in rotator cuff function. The long head of the biceps tendon courses superiorly in the bicipital groove of the humerus between the greater and lesser tuberosities, passes between the subscapularis and supraspinatus tendons, and penetrates the glenohumeral joint to insert on the labrum (Figure 280-2). During arm elevation, the tendon of the long head of the biceps depresses the humeral head, helping it remain centered in the glenoid.

BURSAE

The bursae facilitate frictionless motion between the components of the shoulder. Although there are eight bursae in the shoulder complex, only the extra-articular subacromial bursa is clinically significant. Its roof adheres to the undersurface of the deltoid, and its floor to the underlying rotator cuff. The bursa is lubricated by synovial fluid and surrounded by a layer of peribursal fat.

CORACOACROMIAL ARCH

The coracoacromial arch is formed by the coracoid posteriorly, by the acromion anteriorly, and by the coracoacromial ligament that forms the anterior roof of the arch (**Figure 280-3**). The humeral head provides the floor of the arch. This arch defines the space within which the tendons of the rotator cuff, the tendon of the long head of the biceps, and the subacromial bursa must function.

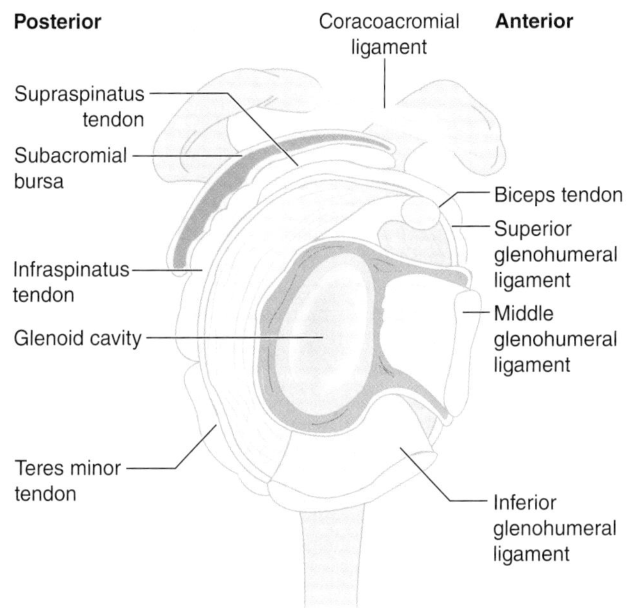

FIGURE 280-3. Lateral view of the shoulder illustrating the coracoacromial arch with the rotator cuff and subacromial bursa.

IMPINGEMENT SYNDROME (SUBACROMIAL BURSITIS, ROTATOR CUFF TENDINITIS, SUPRASPINATUS TENDINITIS, PAINFUL ARC SYNDROME)

PATHOPHYSIOLOGY

Repetitive overhead use of the arm or movement of the shoulder above the horizontal causes encroachment on the subacromial space by the humeral head (**Figure 280-4**).[2-4] Repetitive subacromial encroachment or "impingement" produces pathologic changes of the bursa, rotator cuff, and biceps tendon that result in a loss of the normal gliding mechanism between the rotator cuff and related soft tissues within the coracoacromial arch. *Impingement syndrome* is the encompassing term used for the conditions of subacromial bursitis, rotator cuff tendinitis, supraspinatus tendinitis, and painful arc syndrome.[2-5]

Repetitive impingement of the subacromial space evolves in a progressive pattern classified in three stages.[3,4] In stage 1, reversible edema and hemorrhage about the rotator cuff occur. Although possible at any age, it is classically seen in young athletes <25 years old who have excessive overhead use of the shoulder. During this stage, patients complain of a dull ache over the anterolateral shoulder that is aggravated by activity and improved by rest. The clinical course at this point is typically reversible.

Repeated mechanical trauma from the impingement can progress to stage 2, where tendinitis of the rotator cuff creates fibrosis and thickening of the tendons of the rotator cuff and bursa. This stage is typically seen in patients between the ages of 25 and 40, and the prolonged duration (weeks to months) or recurrence of symptoms is useful in making this diagnosis. During this stage, patients complain of a recurrent or chronic aching pain with daily activities, pain with vigorous activity, and night pain (caused by irritation triggered by a relaxed supporting muscle tone).

Continued overuse can lead to stage 3 with rotator cuff tears, rupture of the long head of the biceps, and subacromial spurs. Patients at this stage have progressive symptoms and disability, and they often require surgical decompression of the subacromial space.

CLINICAL FEATURES

The primary symptom with impingement syndrome is pain, developing insidiously over a period of weeks to months. The pain is located over the anterior to lateral shoulder and frequently radiates to the lateral midhumerus, but not below the elbow.[2,6] Patients usually complain of pain at night that is deep and aching and interferes with sleep. This pain occurs especially when the patient lies on that shoulder or sleeps with the arms

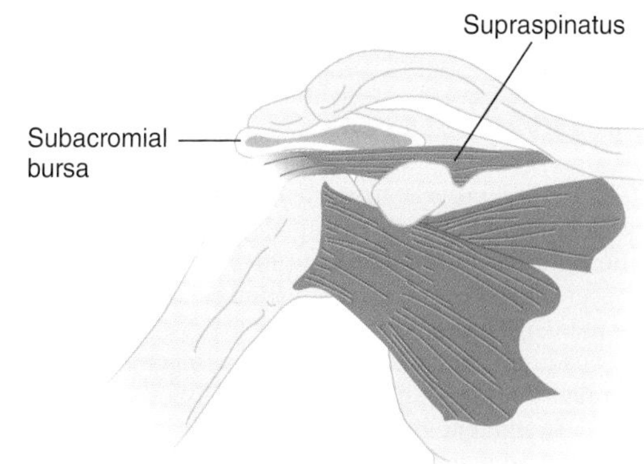

FIGURE 280-4. Impingement of the subacromial bursa and rotator cuff.

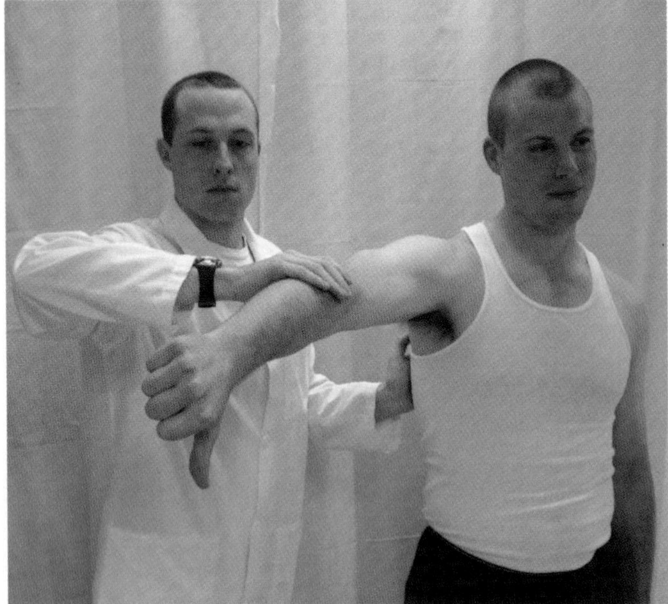

FIGURE 280-5. The "empty can" position, which isolates the supraspinatus tendon. Pain or weakness against resistance in this position suggests injury to the supraspinatus muscle.

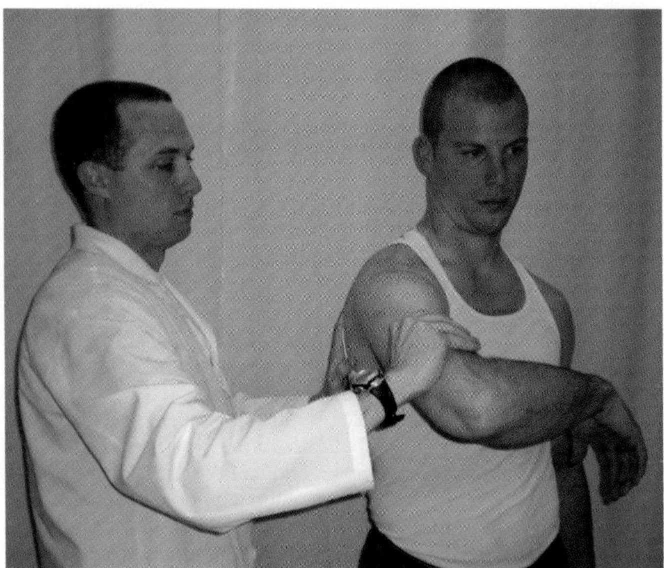

FIGURE 280-6. Hawkins impingement test. The examiner positions the patient's shoulder at 90 degrees of abduction and 90 degrees of elbow flexion. The examiner then rotates the shoulder internally and brings the patient's arm across the front of the patient.

overhead. The pain may be exacerbated by activities that require overhead arm use, such as brushing the hair or reaching into a cupboard. Patients also note weakness and stiffness of the shoulder that is usually secondary to pain.[2,6] Once the shoulder pain has resolved, any weakness should trigger a search for a rotator cuff tear or cervical radiculopathy.

Disuse atrophy of the shoulder musculature occurs when impingement or tendinitis symptoms are chronic (stages 2 and 3). Palpation of the rotator cuff insertion at the lateral aspect of the proximal humerus usually produces pain and tenderness. During range-of-motion maneuvers, fibrosis and scarring within the tendon can cause crepitus, but the patient should have a normal and full active and passive range of motion.[6] Pain with an active arc of abduction, especially between 60 and 100 degrees, is consistent with rotator cuff pathology.[2] A sensation of catching also may be present if scar tissue is trapped beneath the acromion. Rotator cuff strength testing usually reveals mild to moderate weakness secondary to pain. The pain is usually present when resistance is applied.

The individual muscles of the rotator cuff should be isolated and tested individually, looking for pain or weakness; **to isolate the supraspinatus**, abduct the arm to 90 degrees and forward flex it 30 degrees with the thumb pointed down in the "empty can" position (**Figure 280-5**). Either symptom against resistance (continued abduction) in this position suggests inflammation or injury to the supraspinatus muscle, the most likely to be involved in the impingement syndrome.[3]

To isolate the infraspinatus and the teres minor, externally rotate the shoulder with the patient's arm against the body and the elbow bent to 90 degrees and the forearm in neutral position. Stabilize the elbow against the patient's waist and instruct the patient to rotate the arm outward.

To isolate the subscapularis, have the patient place the hand behind the back and attempt to push the examiner's hand away by moving the dorsum of the hand away from the back (lift-off test).

Specific maneuvers on physical examination test for signs of impingement by compressing the rotator cuff and bursa between the humeral head and coracoacromial arch. In the classic impingement **maneuver of Neer**, the examiner prevents scapular rotation with one hand while raising the patient's straightened arm smoothly in full forward flexion to overhead. A positive sign is pain in the arc between 70 and 120 degrees. A second test, the **Hawkins impingement test** (**Figure 280-6**), requires the examiner to position the patient's arm (shoulder) in 90 degrees of abduction and 90 degrees of elbow flexion. Rotation of the arm inwardly across the front of the patient with internal rotation of the shoulder compresses the cuff and bursa between the humeral head and coracoacromial ligament. The Neer and Hawkins tests are 75% to 89% and 91% to 92% sensitive, respectively, but specificity is much lower at 30% to 40% and 25% to 44%, respectively.[7]

DIAGNOSIS

The diagnosis is based on a history of chronic shoulder pain with a full range of motion, with possible weakness of the rotator cuff muscles and positive responses to provocative maneuvers. Radiography is used to identify other causes like fracture or degenerative joint changes. Early nonspecific radiographic signs of rotator cuff syndromes include sclerosis and subchondral cyst formation of the greater tuberosity of the humerus or sclerosis or spur formation on the anterior edge of the acromion.[8]

TREATMENT

The goals of treatment of impingement syndrome are to reduce pain and inflammation and to prevent progression of the process. Therapy starts with a conservative treatment program that should include the following:

1. *Relative rest and activity modification.* Advise the patient to avoid the aggravating activity and minimize all overhead activities. Although brief periods of support with a sling help, **avoid complete immobilization and prescribe range-of-motion exercises** (see below) three to four times daily to minimize the chance of developing adhesive capsulitis.
2. *Anti-inflammatories and analgesics.* Nonsteroidal anti-inflammatory agents for 7 to 21 days are key, with short-term opioid analgesics added for moderate to severe pain, and acetaminophen may aid in lesser pain syndromes.
3. *Cryotherapy.* Apply ice to the affected shoulder for 10 to 15 minutes three to four times daily for analgesic effects and potential reduction of inflammation and edema.
4. *Range-of-motion exercises.* Two simple exercises can help the patient maintain glenohumeral motion. Pendulum swings are done with the patient slightly bent at the waist with the arm hanging freely in front of the body. The arms should be swung in gentle arcs of motion in both a clockwise and counterclockwise direction to the level of pain tolerance for 5 to 10 minutes three to four times daily. The size of the

arcs should increase daily as symptoms allow. Also, the patient should stand sideways an arm's length from a wall and walk the fingers up the wall to the level of pain tolerance, repeating the exercise three to four times daily.

5. *Stretching and strengthening.* Stretching and strengthening exercises are best carried out under the supervision of a physical therapist.
6. *Corticosteroid injections.* Although local corticosteroid injections into the subacromial space relieve pain, adverse effects include muscular atrophy, weakness, and further tissue degeneration. Injection directly into the tendon can lead to necrosis and rupture. Injection is not an emergency procedure and is best left to the primary care physician or orthopedist.
7. *Follow-up.* Ensure reassessment within 7 to 14 days with an orthopedist and/or a rehabilitation expert.

ROTATOR CUFF TEARS

PATHOPHYSIOLOGY

Patients with rotator cuff tears present with shoulder pain after acute traumatic injury, chronic injury, or an acute extension of a chronic impingement (stage 3) of the rotator cuff. Rotator cuff tears due to chronic impingement in patients >40 years of age account for most tears. In younger patients, rotator cuff tears are seen in laborers and athletes who participate in sports that require overhead activities like tennis, swimming, and baseball.[9] In general, healthy rotator cuff tendons are resistant to acute injury, with acute rotator cuff tears accounting for only 10% of all rotator cuff tears. These acute tears usually occur as a result of trauma, such as forced or extreme hyperabduction or hyperextension from falling on an outstretched arm, lifting a heavy object, or catching a heavy object as it falls. Glenohumeral dislocation is a common cause of acute rotator cuff tears. In patients >40 years of age with a first-time dislocation, there is a 57% incidence of acute rotator cuff tear; think of a rotator cuff tear in patients with weakness >3 weeks after an acute dislocation.[9]

In addition to being categorized by the acuteness of the injury, rotator cuff tears can be full or partial thickness, with either difficult to detect on the clinical evaluation. Partial-thickness tears are twice as common as full-thickness tears, and most commonly occur on the inferior aspect of the tendon. The type and extent of the tear have significant implications for the ultimate treatment and prognosis. The supraspinatus, due to its location within the coracoacromial arch, is the most commonly affected tendon of the rotator cuff.

CLINICAL FEATURES

The clinical features of a chronic rotator cuff tear differ from those of an acute tear. Only about half of patients with chronic rotator cuff tears can recall specific trauma or an event associated with the onset of pain, often seemingly insignificant in description. Patients more commonly report a history of gradual and progressive pain; while initially described as worse at night, the pain eventually becomes persistent. The pain may be diffuse, but is commonly localized to the lateral aspect of the upper arm. Often, initial therapy with rest, anti-inflammatory agents, and glucocorticoid injections helps. If the rotator cuff weakens, the frequency, intensity, and duration of the symptoms increase and are less responsive to the usual treatments. Shoulder dysfunction progressively worsens and interferes with work, recreation, and normal daily activities. Arm elevation, external rotation, and lifting of even light objects worsen the symptoms.

With acute injuries, such as those due to falling or catching a heavy object, the patient may report a "tearing" sensation in the shoulder followed by severe pain and inability to raise the arm. An acute rotator cuff tear produces immediate profound pain and disability, with asymmetry often present due to local swelling. Active motion is limited, with inability to abduct or externally rotate the arm against even minimal resistance. On examination, disuse atrophy is often present in patients with chronic rotator cuff tears. Palpation may produce discomfort at the lateral aspect of the upper arm or in the subacromial region. Most patients with rotator cuff tears have weakness and pain on abduction, elevation, and, most commonly, external rotation. The result of the **drop arm test** is positive if the patient is unable to hold or lower a fully extended arm at 90 degrees of shoulder abduction without dropping it. Crepitus and pain are usually present on range-of-motion testing.

DIAGNOSIS

It may be very difficult to distinguish a full-thickness tear from a partial-thickness tear or a rotator cuff injury from impingement syndrome. The diagnosis is primarily clinical based on a finding of rotator cuff weakness on examination in a patient with a history of chronic shoulder pain or acute shoulder pain after significant trauma. In patients with an acute injury, it may be difficult to diagnose the tear due to excessive pain from the injury. In these cases, assume a preliminary diagnosis of acute rotator cuff tear and treat conservatively, with appropriate follow-up in 1 week.

Routine shoulder radiographs occasionally give additional diagnostic information. The most specific radiographic sign for large rotator cuff tears is a narrowing of the acromiohumeral space (<7 mm).[8] **No radiographic findings are diagnostic of an acute rotator cuff tear, and the diagnosis should rely on clinical findings.** MRI, US, and arthrography are the most sensitive modalities for detecting rotator cuff tears, although all tend to underestimate the extent of the tear.

TREATMENT

The basic goals of emergency care for suspected rotator cuff injuries are the same as with impingement (see above), with analgesia, support, and prevention of further dysfunction and disability. An arm sling can provide support and comfort until the acute symptoms subside. However, avoid prolonged immobilization and prescribe range-of-motion exercises three to four times daily to minimize the development of adhesive capsulitis.

Any evidence or suspicion of neurovascular compromise requires immediate orthopedic consultation. Refer all patients with an acute rotator cuff tear (with or without a history of chronic symptoms) and those with significant disability to an orthopedist for follow-up within a week. Complete rotator cuff tears usually require surgical repair, and functional results are better if repair is carried out early, before retraction, fibrosis, tendon degeneration, and muscular atrophy have occurred. Partial-thickness or chronic tears may respond to conservative measures.

CALCIFIC TENDINITIS

PATHOPHYSIOLOGY

Calcific tendinitis is a self-limiting disorder characterized by calcium crystal deposition within one or more tendons of the rotator cuff. In time, the calcium undergoes painful spontaneous resorption with subsequent healing of the tendon. Middle-age patients are most commonly affected, and this process is rarely seen in patients >70 years of age. Females are slightly more likely to be affected than males, and calcification is often present bilaterally. Primary tendon degeneration as a result of chronic repetitive microtrauma, age, and tissue hypoxia are causes of this disorder. The supraspinatus is by far the most commonly affected tendon, with calcium deposition usually occurring near its origin on the humerus. Any of the rotator cuff tendons or the long head of the biceps may be affected.

CLINICAL FEATURES

Because calcification occurs over a period of time, patients are generally asymptomatic or have mild pain at rest or at night. Pain with abduction or a "catching" sensation may be present on movement. During the **resorptive phase**, incapacitating pain can occur from vascular proliferation, formation of granulation tissue, and calcium crystal extravasation into the subacromial bursa. Symptoms are usually self-limited, lasting 1 to 2 weeks in most cases. After the initially painful resorptive phase, patients can have variable levels of pain and shoulder dysfunction that may last for several months (**postcalcific period**). Adhesive capsulitis is the most common complication of calcific tendinitis and creates more chronic symptoms.

Symptomatic patients experience sudden onset of shoulder pain, usually at rest, and shoulder motion reproduces significant pain. The pain is often worse at night and interferes with sleep. During an acute attack with intense pain, the patient holds the arm across the body and often is reluctant to move it. A point of maximum tenderness may be palpated over the proximal humerus near the tendinous insertion of the rotator cuff. Both active and passive range of motion of the glenohumeral joint are usually limited to varying degrees. Flexion, extension, abduction, and internal and external rotation of this joint should be documented. Muscle atrophy and crepitus may also be present.

DIAGNOSIS

Obtain shoulder radiographs for patients with suspected calcific tendinitis to localize deposits and seek any signs of possible impingement. During the initial formative phase, calcium deposits are usually dense and well-defined if visualized. In patients who are experiencing intense pain in the resorptive phase, calcium deposits may appear hazy with poorly defined borders. The presence of visible calcifications is not necessarily specific for this disorder. US is unlikely to be helpful during the resorptive phase as the poorly defined calcifications produce little or no acoustic shadowing.[10,11]

TREATMENT

Treatment is similar to that for impingement syndrome, and nonoperative management is successful in 90% of cases. During an acute attack, nonsteroidal anti-inflammatory agents, opioid analgesics, and ice help calm the intense pain. The shoulder may be rested using a sling for brief periods of immobilization, but avoid prolonged immobilization. Instruct patients to rest the shoulder in abduction on the back of a chair as often as is tolerable. Sleeping with a pillow beneath the axilla can also help prevent restriction of motion. Local application of heat may be used once acute symptoms have diminished. Gentle and progressive range-of-motion exercises should be emphasized and encouraged. Physical therapy is indicated in patients with more chronic cases who have significantly limited range of motion of the shoulder.

Subacromial corticosteroid injection, oral steroids, platelet-rich plasma therapy, transcutaneous electrical nerve stimulation, and therapeutic US are sometimes used, but no strong supporting evidence exists for their use. Extracorporeal shockwave therapy appears to improve success rates.[12] A recent randomized controlled trial compared US-guided needle lavage with corticosteroid injection to corticosteroid injection alone, with modestly favorable clinical and radiographic results for the US group at 1 year.[13]

DISPOSITION AND FOLLOW-UP

Calcific tendinitis is a self-limited process in the vast majority of cases. For patients with new presentation of this disease, arrange follow-up with a primary care doctor within a week. For the 10% of patients in whom nonoperative methods are unsuccessful, arthroscopic or open surgery may be indicated. Refer patients who have progression of symptoms, constant pain interfering with daily activities, or absence of improvement after conservative therapy.[14]

ADHESIVE CAPSULITIS

PATHOPHYSIOLOGY

Adhesive capsulitis, commonly referred to as *frozen shoulder syndrome*, begins as painful inflammation of the glenohumeral joint, followed by eventual fibrosis of the joint capsule and restriction of shoulder motion. Primary or idiopathic adhesive capsulitis is associated with a wide variety of unrelated conditions, including diabetes, thyroid disease, postmenopausal, pulmonary neoplasm, and autoimmune disorders. Secondary adhesive capsulitis produces similar findings, but results from a known cause, such as prolonged immobilization after trauma, surgery, stroke, or a primary inflammatory condition of the shoulder such as impingement syndrome or bicipital tendinitis. The condition resolves with conservative therapy in most patients within 1 to 2 years, although some are left with residual pain or stiffness.

Four stages of this disorder exist, although patients do not necessarily follow these stages in a linear fashion. Stage 1, around the first 2 to 3 months, presents with acute synovial inflammation with limitation of shoulder movement due to pain. Stage 2 (**freezing stage**), about months 3 to 9, has decreased shoulder motion from capsular thickening and scarring, and chronic pain. Stage 3 (**frozen stage**), months 9 to 15, is characterized by less pain, but a more fibrotic and thick capsule and more limitation in range of motion. Stage 4 (**thawing stage**), usually after 15 months, has minimal pain and progressive improvement in the range of motion of the shoulder.[15]

DIAGNOSIS

Limited active and passive range of motion is the hallmark of adhesive capsulitis. Pain is typically diffuse and aching, poorly localized, accompanied by stiffness, and often extends down the upper arm. The pain is frequently worse at night and at rest, especially in earlier stages. Disuse atrophy may be present. Impingement testing is difficult due to the restriction of motion. Occasionally, posterior glenohumeral dislocation creates restricted motion of the shoulder; exam and imaging can help detect this condition. US may demonstrate increased vascular flow, thickening of rotator cuff structures, and bulging of the supraspinatus tendon. MRI or magnetic resonance angiography findings approach 70% sensitivity and 95% specificity for the condition.[15]

TREATMENT

The goals of treatment are to reduce pain and restore motion and function. Avoid shoulder immobilization; if a sling is used in patients in early stage 1 who have severe pain, limit it to days to prevent increased loss of motion due to further capsular restriction. Although physical therapy is difficult in the early, more painful stages of disease, it is key along with nonsteroidal anti-inflammatory drugs, analgesics, and ice.

Although it is not an ED procedure, intra-articular steroid injection is a potential option during follow-up to improve pain and function in the short term; the long-term effects are less clear.

Refer patients to an orthopedist if ongoing symptoms exist despite good therapy (usually after >6 months) or when the diagnosis is unsure. Closed manipulation under general anesthesia, arthroscopic capsular release, and open capsular release are surgical options.

DISORDERS OF THE BICEPS TENDON

PATHOPHYSIOLOGY

Disorders of the proximal aspect of the long head of the biceps tendon include tendinopathy, subluxation or dislocation, and partial or complete tears; these occur from inflammation, instability, or trauma.[16] The long head of the biceps tendon originates from the superior labrum and the supraglenoid tubercle on the scapula. As it exits the glenohumeral joint, it courses through the bicipital groove as it travels anterior and superior to the humeral head.[16] Approximately 50% of the long head of the biceps tendon originates from the superior labrum. Forces applied tend to pull the labrum off the glenoid rim. Due to this anatomic association, tears of the superior labrum, known as SLAP (superior labrum anterior to posterior) lesions, are frequently found in conjunction with long head of the biceps tendon pathology. Injuries of one or the other structure may be difficult to distinguish, both clinically and operatively.

The biceps tendon may also become inflamed, may become partially displaced out of the bicipital groove, or may rupture altogether. (See chapter 271, "Shoulder and Humerus Injuries" for the approach to traumatic ruptures of the distal bicipital tendon.)

CLINICAL FEATURES

Bicipital tendinopathy may be due to inflammation (tendinitis) or collagen tears in or around the tendon (tendinosis) and may be acute or chronic. Tendinitis and tendinosis are difficult to distinguish clinically. Bicipital tendinopathy triggers intense and localized pain at the anterior aspect of the shoulder. Repetitive overhead arm motion may result in inflammation chronically or an acute SLAP lesion, particularly in athletes. Pain at rest, night pain, and pain on rotation are common. Dislocation or subluxation of the biceps tendon from the bicipital groove is painful and occurs medially or laterally, while complete dislocation is seen only medially and is associated with a subscapularis tear. Posterolateral instability is associated with a supraspinatus tear. Concurrent injury to the biceps reflection pulley is necessary for tendon dislocation in either direction.[16]

Partial or complete rupture is almost always proximal and is due to micro-tears and other age-related degenerative changes in this area of the tendon. In younger patients, mild trauma may cause complete rupture of the biceps tendon, which is heralded by an audible snap or pop followed by severe pain and deformity.

DIAGNOSIS

Palpation of the tendon within the bicipital groove reproduces the intense pain. Forearm supination, one of the main actions of the long head of the biceps, also reproduces pain, especially when resistance is applied. In assessing for instability, resisted forearm supination may cause palpable subluxation or a painful popping sensation as the tendon undergoes subluxation; these findings are classic but not common.

Because biceps tendon pathology is frequently associated with pathology of adjacent structures, clinical testing is often inconclusive and inaccurate.[16] Many provocative tests to confirm the presence of pathology of the long head of the biceps or superior labrum have been described in the literature. **Speed's test** identifies tear or tendinitis of the long head of the biceps; flex the shoulder to 90 degrees with the patient's arm (elbow) fully extended and supinated. Provide downward resistance against shoulder flexion. Pain localized to the bicipital groove indicates a positive test. The Speed's test appears to have a sensitivity of 87% and a specificity of 80% for tear of the long head of the biceps.[17]

SLAP lesions or labral tears are complex, and a recent Cochrane review concluded that physical examination alone cannot be used as the sole basis by which to diagnose a SLAP lesion. The test most likely to help diagnose a SLAP lesion is the **active compression test**. To perform, have the standing patient flex his or her shoulder to 90 degrees, and then adduct 10 to 15 degrees medially and rotate fully, with elbow extended. The examiner stands behind the patient and applies a uniform downward force to the arm. This is repeated in full lateral position. A positive response is indicated by eliciting pain on the first maneuver, which is reduced or eliminated on the second maneuver; the test is 60% to 100% sensitive and 85% to 98% specific.[17]

In biceps tendon rupture, the classic finding is described as a "Popeye" deformity caused by distal contraction of the muscle belly. Supination is weak on muscle testing, but elbow flexion remains strong because of the presence of other intact elbow flexors (short head of the biceps and brachialis muscles).

Plain radiographs are generally unhelpful in diagnosing biceps tendon or SLAP lesions. MRI is also poor in diagnosing biceps tendon and SLAP lesions; magnetic resonance arthrography is preferable. In the hands of skilled operators, US is poorly sensitive but very specific in diagnosing disorders of the long head of the biceps. Arthroscopy is considered the gold standard, although recent studies have demonstrated poor intrarater reliability of arthroscopic diagnosis.[18]

TREATMENT

Manage tendinitis and subluxation with brief use of a sling as needed for support and comfort, aided by analgesics, anti-inflammatory agents, application of ice several times daily, and elevation to reduce swelling. Prescribe early mobilization with stretching exercises and follow-up within 7 to 14 days with a primary care provider.

Although not commonly administered by emergency physicians, intra-articular injections of local anesthetic and steroid can improve symptoms. Intra-articular injections can relieve bicipital symptoms but may be ineffective if adhesions or synovitis prevent dispersal into the bicipital groove. Direct injection into the bicipital groove with US guidance may be an option for specialists if previous intra-articular injections have not worked.[18] Bicipital tendinitis usually resolves with conservative therapy.

Reserve orthopedic consultation for those with tendinopathy associated with instability, partial rupture, or high-grade SLAP lesion or those failing to respond to a conservative treatment regimen. Surgical options include debridement, tenotomy, or tenodesis.[18] Bicipital tendon rupture often requires surgical repair, so orthopedic consultation in 24 to 48 hours is best. Patients with suspected SLAP lesions or other mechanical proximal biceps injuries generally require arthroscopic or other surgical intervention when symptomatic.

OSTEOARTHRITIS

Because the glenohumeral joint is non–weight bearing, primary osteoarthritis is rare. When it does occur, presentation is similar to that of degenerative disease in other joints: the patient experiences gradual and progressive onset of pain, worse with motion and better with rest. This usually occurs concurrently with degenerative disease of the acromioclavicular joint.

Secondary osteoarthritis is more common and is usually associated with a previous fracture, recurrent dislocations, or an underlying rheumatologic, metabolic, or endocrinologic disorder. ED care of both primary and secondary arthritis relies on analgesics, anti-inflammatory agents, and gentle exercises to preserve range of motion.

OTHER CAUSES OF SHOULDER PAIN

Although disorders of the rotator cuff and other intrinsic structures of the shoulder are the most common cause of shoulder pain, extrinsic conditions outside the shoulder complex can refer pain to the shoulder. The differential diagnosis includes disorders of the cervical spine, brachial plexus injuries, axillary artery thrombosis, suprascapular nerve injury, thoracic outlet syndrome, Pancoast's tumor, and miscellaneous thoraco-abdominal disorders.

The *neck* is the most common source of pain referred to the shoulder. Degenerative disease of the cervical spine, degenerative disk disease, and herniated nucleus pulposus can all refer pain to the shoulder. A patient with a C5-C6 herniated disk may present with pain very similar to that due to rotator cuff disease. Careful and thorough examination of the cervical spine and a complete neurovascular examination should be included in the evaluation of any patient with shoulder pain. (See chapter 279, "Neck and Back Pain").

Brachial plexus injury can cause pain referred to the shoulder and can produce weakness and atrophy in the muscles of the shoulder within weeks of injury. Radiographic evaluation of the cervical spine should be included in the ED evaluation of patients with suspected brachial plexus injury or involvement. **Brachial plexus neuritis** is uncommon but can be very painful. Its etiology is unknown, although inflammatory, postimmunization, and viral origins have been proposed. Inflammation of the brachial plexus can lead to weakness and atrophy of the muscles of the shoulder complex within weeks following the onset of pain.[19] Brachial plexus neuritis is usually self-limiting. Referral to a neurologist should be arranged if this disorder is suspected.

The most serious vascular injury that can cause shoulder pain is **acute thrombosis of the axillary artery**. Repetitive mechanical trauma or explosive stress from lifting heavy objects can compress and contuse the intimal lining of the axillary artery, predisposing the artery to thrombosis.

Compression of the suprascapular nerve can cause shoulder pain. This nerve originates from the brachial plexus distal C5-C6 nerve roots and courses posteriorly to the suprascapular notch. It can become entrapped beneath the transverse ligament at the level of the suprascapular notch. Traction injuries from explosive movements can also injure the nerve. On examination, active external rotation typically reveals infraspinatus atrophy and associated weakness. The initial treatment is conservative. Electromyography and nerve conduction velocity studies will reveal the extent and location of nerve injury. Surgery for decompression is considered if conservative measures fail.

Compression of the brachial plexus and blood vessels proximal to the shoulder, the **thoracic outlet syndrome**, can cause shoulder pain. Women in the childbearing years are affected three times more commonly than men. The medial trunk of the brachial plexus is most commonly involved, and the symptoms usually include pain that radiates through the shoulder to the medial forearm and occasionally to the small and ring fingers. Patients also complain of numbness and tingling of the fingers and a weak grip. Patients can usually identify motions that reproduce the symptoms. Plain radiographic evaluation is often nondiagnostic, although some will have evidence of a prior clavicular fracture with malunion or the presence of a cervical rib band that compress the brachial plexus. Conservative measures include activity modification, education, postural exercises, nonsteroidal anti-inflammatory drugs, and physical therapy. Referral to the primary care provider is important to allow for a thorough evaluation to differentiate between neurogenic, arterial, or venous thoracic outlet syndrome.[20,21]

Pancoast's tumor may compress the brachial plexus against the chest wall and cause shoulder pain. The patient may experience local or radicular shoulder pain or a sense of fullness in the supraclavicular fossa.

Finally, myocardial ischemia and infarction, pneumonia, pulmonary embolism, or any disorder that irritates the diaphragm can also cause referred shoulder pain. Abdominal disorders that can cause shoulder pain include biliary tract disease, splenic injury or inflammation, perforated viscus, and ruptured ectopic pregnancy.

Acknowledgment: The authors gratefully acknowledge the contributions of Dr. Benjamin Harrison, coauthor of this chapter in the previous editions.

REFERENCES

The complete reference list is available online at www.TintinalliEM.com.

CHAPTER 281 Hip and Knee Pain

Kelly P. O'Keefe
Tracy G. Sanson

INTRODUCTION AND EPIDEMIOLOGY

Every practicing emergency physician over his or her career will see hundreds of patients with complaints of hip or knee pain that are unrelated to major trauma or an acute fracture. Discomfort and limitations to normal use in these areas are typically related to the minor trauma that occurs on a repetitive basis from performing routine daily functions or exercising. Athletes of all varieties are especially prone to these maladies, where strenuous activity transmits forces that are equivalent to three to five times the body weight directly to these major joints. Conversely, the problem of obesity similarly contributes to joint and supporting structural stress and pain.[1]

However, be alert to the various catastrophic processes that can mimic more mundane etiologies, including ruptured abdominal aortic aneurysm, epidural abscess, and septic joint (among others). Pay close attention to historical points, specific risk factors, abnormal vital signs, and physical findings to avoid making a life- or limb-threatening misdiagnosis.

PATHOPHYSIOLOGY AND ANATOMY

The hip is a ball-and-socket joint (enarthrosis), allowing motion in all directions. The hip is similar to the shoulder in this capacity, but is much more stable and relatively resistant to dislocation. The bones of the joint (femoral head, pelvic acetabulum) are strongly reinforced with a fibrocartilaginous labrum, a joint capsule, overlying ligaments, and numerous muscles.

The knee is the largest synovial joint in the body and is relatively complicated in structure, comprising two distinct articulating groups: the tibiofemoral and patellofemoral joints. The patella floats above the main joint, attaching to the femur superiorly by the quadriceps tendon and inserting into the tibia inferiorly by the patellar ligament. The knee is stabilized internally by the anterior and posterior cruciate ligaments, and externally by the medial and lateral collateral ligaments. In addition, distal to the main joint, the fibular head attaches by ligaments to the proximal lateral tibia. The medial and lateral menisci are interposed between, and protect, the femoral and tibial condyles. Numerous muscles, tendons, bursa, and additional ligaments add to the complexity of the joint and serve as potential sources for pain and dysfunction (**Figures 281-1 and 281-2**).

NERVES OF THE UPPER LEG AND REFERRED PAIN

The femoral and sciatic nerves are the major nerves within the thigh (**Figure 281-3**). The femoral nerve is the largest branch of the lumbar plexus, and the sciatic is the longest nerve in the body, traveling posteriorly and supplying sensation to the hip joint through its articular branches. The femoral and obturator nerves also innervate the hip. The femoral nerve divides into anterior and posterior branches, with the posterior becoming the saphenous nerve and providing sensation to the lower leg. The anterior nerve supplies sensation to the anterior medial thigh by the medial and intermediate cutaneous nerves. The two major branches of the sciatic, the peroneal and tibial nerves, course through the posterior fossa of the knee, along with the popliteal artery and vein.

Pain in the area of the knee is not commonly referred to other sites, and knee pain is usually due to local pathology. However, referred pain from hip pathology is commonly felt in the buttocks, thigh, or groin; may extend to the knee; and may even travel to the foot. Pain felt in the hip and surrounding locations may be referred from pressure on the

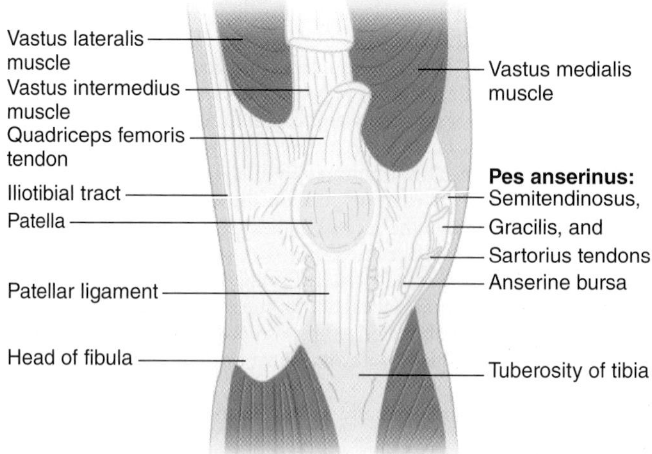

FIGURE 281-1. Anterior view of the knee. [Reproduced with permission from Simon RR, Sherman SC, Koenigsknecht SJ: *Emergency Orthopedics: The Extremities,* 5th ed. © 2007, McGraw-Hill Inc., New York.]

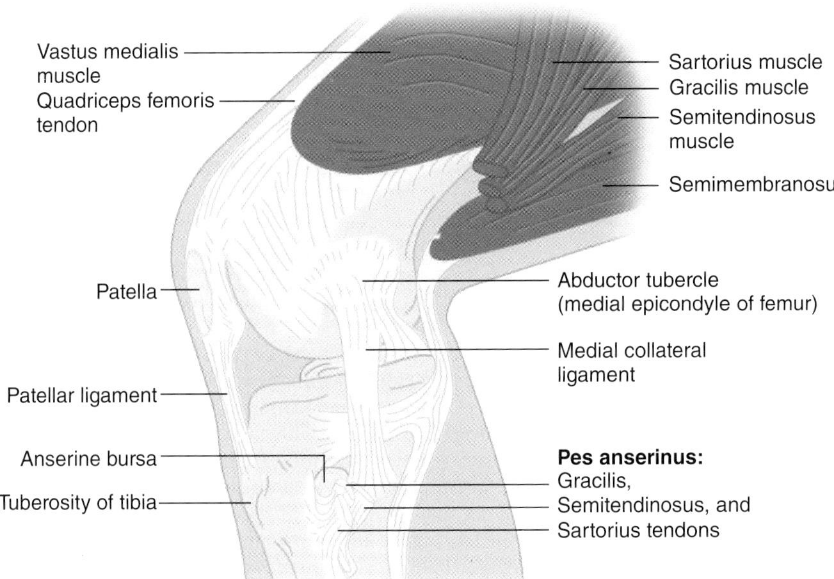

FIGURE 281-2. Medial view of the knee. [Reproduced with permission from Simon RR, Sherman SC, Koenigsknecht SJ: *Emergency Orthopedics: The Extremities,* 5th ed. © 2007, McGraw-Hill Inc., New York.]

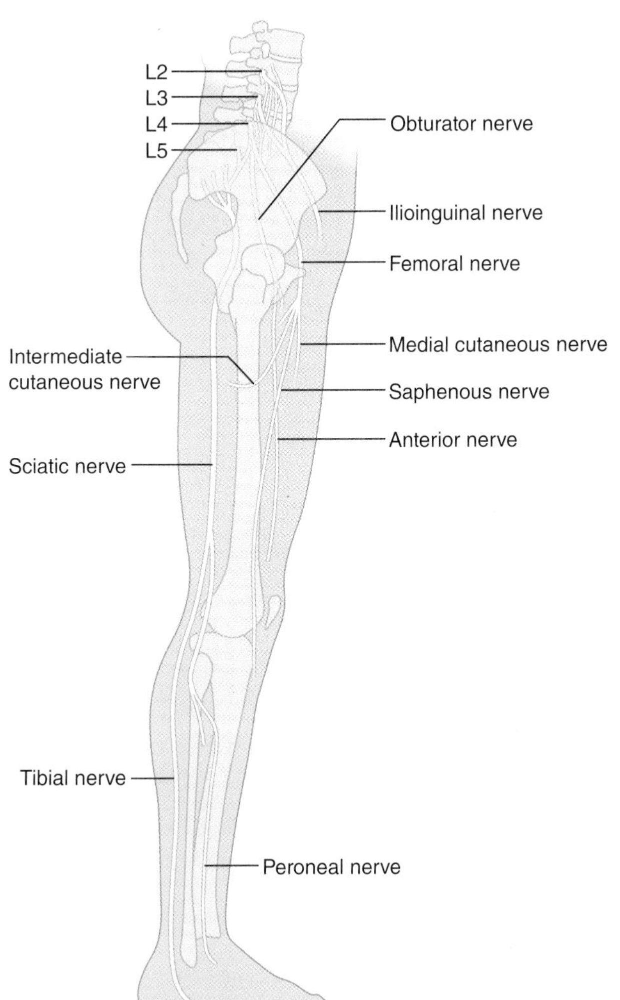

FIGURE 281-3. Nerves that innervate the thigh.

proximal nerve roots as they exit the lumbar and sacral spine. **In the patient with appropriate risk factors, consider expansion or rupture of an abdominal aortic aneurysm as the cause of hip pain that is not otherwise explained by the history or physical examination, especially when there are no preexisting joint issues.** Bedside US may exclude this life-threatening diagnosis. Other extra-articular sources of hip pain include intra-abdominal or pelvic tumors; diverticular, epidural, or psoas abscess; and the generally less worrisome diagnoses of herpes zoster or herniated lumbar disc.

DIAGNOSIS OF KNEE AND HIP DISEASES AND SYNDROMES

The majority of knee and hip problems can be diagnosed or excluded with a focused history and physical examination (**Table 281-1**).

IMAGING

A suspected diagnosis obtained via history and physical examination is confirmed or ruled out by imaging. For the majority of soft tissue injuries or overuse syndromes, radiographs are not particularly useful unless a history of significant trauma or cancer exists. More sophisticated imaging is typically not needed for evaluation in the ED but may

TABLE 281-1 Suggested Clues for the Differential Diagnosis of Hip and Knee Pain
Determine the location of the pain to narrow down the potential diagnosis.
Determine the activities that bring on the pain.
Complaints that the joint "gives out" or "buckles" generally are due to pain and reflex muscle inhibition rather than an acute neurologic emergency. This complaint may also represent patellar subluxation or ligamentous injury and joint instability.
Poor conditioning or quadriceps weakness generally causes anterior knee pain of the patellofemoral syndrome; therapy should address this weakness.
Locking of the knee suggests a meniscal injury, which may be chronic.
A popping sensation or sound at the onset of pain is reliable for a ligamentous injury.
A recurrent knee effusion after activity suggests a meniscal injury.
Pain at the joint line of the knee (palpable indentation between distal femur and proximal tibia) suggests a meniscal injury.

be indicated at follow-up or for selected ED patients on an individual basis. US can identify intra-articular or bursal effusions and soft tissue swelling and can localize muscle or tendon injuries. Normal comparison US views from the unaffected leg can be helpful. US is very helpful for the evaluation of popliteal cysts and arterial structures and will exclude deep venous thrombosis as a cause of pain and swelling.

Plain films are helpful in the evaluation of bony abnormalities such as severe arthritic changes and spurring, calcification derangements, and other inflammatory processes late in their courses. CT scan provides superior detail of osseous structures, will identify intra-articular loose bodies, and visualizes the early changes of osteonecrosis. Abnormalities of the labrum and joint capsule may also be seen. MRI, as the test of choice, precisely defines the anatomy of both the hip and knee and provides great detail for soft tissue and bony abnormalities. MRI is usually obtained on an outpatient basis. Although not frequently ordered from the ED, bone scans may be useful for the assessment of a variety of infectious and inflammatory processes, including avascular necrosis. Ultimately, arthroscopy of the knee and hip allows direct visualization of intra-articular lesions and simultaneous treatment.

SPECIFIC SYNDROMES AND DISEASES BY LOCATION

See **Table 281-2** for a summary of the most important conditions.

PSOAS ABSCESS

The psoas muscle is susceptible to the hematogenous spread of infection from distant sites because of its rich blood supply and proximity to overlying retroperitoneal lymphatic channels.[2] *Staphylococcus aureus* is the most common pathogen (80%); other less frequent pathogens include *Serratia marcescens*, *Pseudomonas aeruginosa*, *Haemophilus aphrophilus*, *Proteus mirabilis*, and enteric pathogens.

Symptoms include abdominal pain radiating to the hip, flank pain, fever, and limp. Presentation may be insidious. Other symptoms include nausea, weight loss, and malaise. To provoke pain, instruct the patient to perform forceful contraction of the psoas. Place your hand just proximal to the patient's ipsilateral knee, and have the patient raise his or her thigh against your hand. Confirm the diagnosis by CT scan. Treatment includes antibiotics and surgical consultation for percutaneous (most commonly) or open drainage.[2]

REGIONAL NERVE ENTRAPMENT SYNDROMES

Lateral Femoral Cutaneous Nerve Entrapment/Meralgia Paresthesia (Anterolateral Thigh Pain) *Meralgia paresthetica*, or compressive inflammation of the lateral femoral cutaneous nerve, is the best known of the lower extremity nerve entrapment syndromes. The nerve enters the thigh under the inguinal ligament near the anterior superior iliac spine and is subject to a variety of minor, reoccurring traumatic events. The syndrome can be triggered by (among other causes) wearing tight belts, heavy tool belts, car seat belts, or corsets; pregnancy; certain sitting positions (i.e., on a riding lawnmower); focal trauma, including surgical interventions such as appendectomy or hysterectomy; and obesity. It has been reported in women with muscular thighs performing activities that require repetitive flexion/extension of the leg, such as cheerleading, and in runners. Symptoms include pain to the hip area, thigh, or groin along the distribution of the nerve (proximal anterior lateral aspect of the leg; **Figure 281-4**), burning or tingling paresthesias, and hypersensitivity to light touch. Pain may be worsened or reproduced during physical examination by tapping over the area of the anterior superior iliac spine. Those affected should limit the exacerbating activity and eliminate the source of the irritation. Nonsteroidal anti-inflammatory drugs, local injections, weight loss, and (rarely) surgical excision of the nerve are other treatment options.[3,4]

Obturator Nerve Entrapment (Medial Thigh/Groin Pain) Obturator nerve entrapment is typically a sequela of pelvic fractures or abdominal/pelvic surgery. Obturator nerve inflammation is generally sensed in the groin and down the inner thigh (Figure 281-4) and aggravated by movement of the hip. Exercise-induced medial thigh pain may be the predominant symptom. The nerve is entrapped in athletes due to the presence of a fascial band at the distal obturator canal or may be compressed due to pelvic hematomas or other masses. Surgery may be required for pain relief. Imaging studies are of limited value, but needle electromyography reveals the characteristic findings of chronic denervation. Local injection of lidocaine into the area of the nerve relieves the pain and

TABLE 281-2 Selected Syndromes by Location

Diagnosis Category	Diagnosis	Pain Location
Nerve entrapment	Meralgia paresthetica	Anterolateral thigh pain or paresthesias
	Obturator nerve entrapment	Groin and inner thigh pain
	Ilioinguinal nerve entrapment	Groin pain
	Piriformis syndrome (sciatic nerve compression by piriformis muscle)	Buttocks and hamstrings pain
Hip bursitis	Trochanteric bursitis	Hip pain when lying on side or with hip abduction and adduction
	Ischiogluteal bursitis	Ischial pain
	Iliopectineal and iliopsoas bursitis	Anterior pelvis and groin, hip extension
Knee bursitis	Pes anserine bursitis	Anterior medial knee pain
	Prepatellar bursitis	Pain anterior to patella
Hip overuse syndromes	External snapping hip syndrome (coxa saltans)	Posterior lateral hip pain
	Fascia lata syndrome	Lateral thigh pain
Knee overuse syndromes	Patellofemoral syndrome (runner's knee)	Anterior knee pain, worse with prolonged knee flexion
	Medial plica syndrome	Anterior medial knee pain, knee snapping during repeated flexion/extension
	Iliotibial band syndrome or snapping knee syndrome	Pain over lateral epicondyles, or snapping when iliotibial band passes over femoral condyle
	Popliteus tendinitis	Posterior lateral knee pain, worse on downhill exercise
	Patellar tendinitis (jumper's knee)	Inferior patellar or proximal patellar tendon pain
	Quadriceps tendinitis	Proximal patellar pain
	Popliteal (Baker) cyst	Posterior knee pain

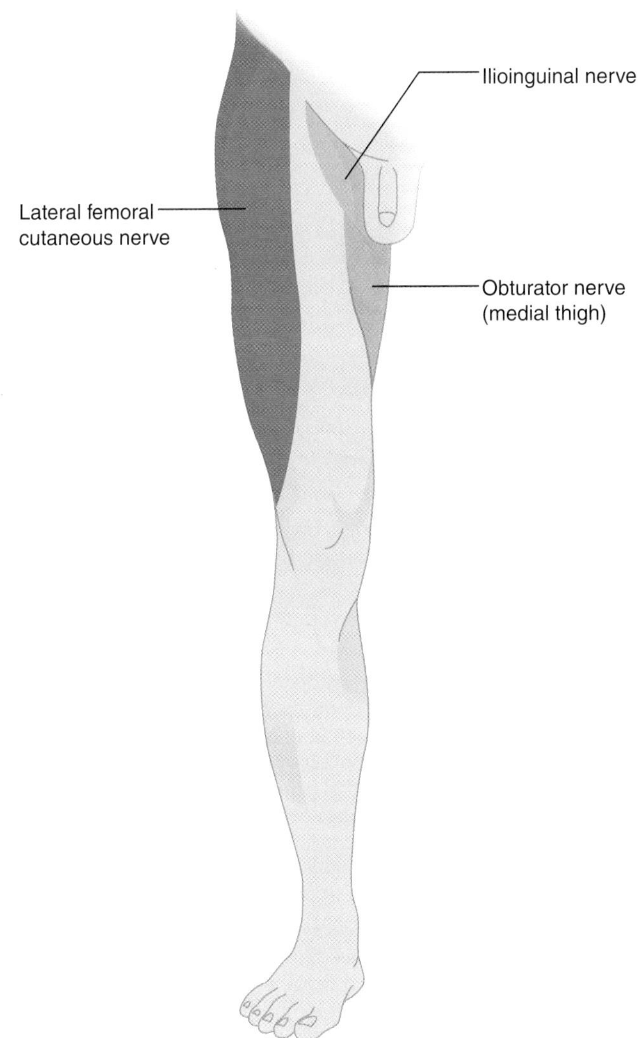

FIGURE 281-4. Local innervation and locations of pain for specific thigh and groin nerves.

associated reactive weakness and may make the diagnosis; however, the nerve block is both difficult to perform and rarely done in the ED.[5]

Ilioinguinal Nerve Entrapment (Groin Pain) The ilioinguinal nerve arises from the lumbar plexus and passes through the psoas muscle, the transverses abdominal muscle adjacent to the anterior superior iliac spine, and the abdominal oblique muscles into the inguinal canal to innervate the groin and scrotum or labrum. Entrapment occurs due to hypertrophy of the abdominal wall musculature or pregnancy. Hyperextension of the hip produces pain and hypoesthesia in the distribution of the nerve, yielding groin pain.[6]

Piriformis Syndrome (Buttock/Posterior Thigh Pain) Compression of the sciatic nerve generally produces pain in the distal extremity, but irritation of the sciatic nerve from the piriformis muscle, referred to as the piriformis syndrome, causes pain in the area of the buttocks and hamstring muscles that is worsened by sitting, climbing stairs, or squatting (**Figure 281-5**). The clinician may palpate a tender mass over the piriformis muscle and elicit pain in the region of the sacroiliac joint or gluteal musculature. Hip flexion and passive internal rotation will exacerbate the symptoms. Imaging is useful only to rule out other conditions. Treatment is conservative.

SPECIFIC BURSAL SYNDROMES OF THE HIP AREA

Bursae are self-contained flat sacs, lined with synovium, that reduce friction between tissues moving over each other in a repetitive fashion, such as ligaments, tendons, and bone. New bursae may form at any area

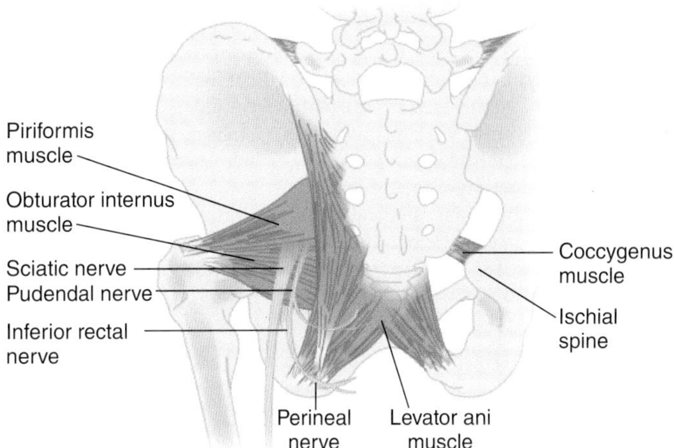

FIGURE 281-5. Proximity of the piriformis muscle and the sciatic nerve. [Reproduced with permission from Simon RR, Sherman SC, Koenigsknecht SJ: *Emergency Orthopedics: The Extremities,* 5th ed. © 2007, McGraw-Hill Inc., New York.]

that is subject to repeat irritation. Causes of bursal pain include inflammation (with repetitive minor trauma; rheumatologic disorders, such as psoriatic arthritis, rheumatoid arthritis, or ankylosing spondylitis; and crystalline disease, such as gout or pseudogout) and infection. Certain bursae are more prone than others to these insults, and these produce symptoms in specific locations that the practitioner should recognize.

Inflammation may be very difficult to distinguish from infection, because both disorders share common symptoms and signs, with a significant overlap in diagnostic cell counts when bursal fluid is aspirated. A Gram stain positive for bacteria and a culture growing pathogens are definitive for infection and septic bursitis, but infection may be present in the absence of these findings. Occasionally, with trauma or prolonged inflammation, a bursa may end up communicating with a joint. Arthrocentesis is required in these circumstances or any other when a septic joint is suspected. The development of a draining sinus tract favors septic bursitis (see chapter 284, "Joints and Bursae").

Trochanteric Bursitis (Posterolateral Hip Pain) The trochanteric bursae lie between the gluteus maximus and the posterolateral greater trochanter, with a deep and superficial component (**Figure 281-6**). Female

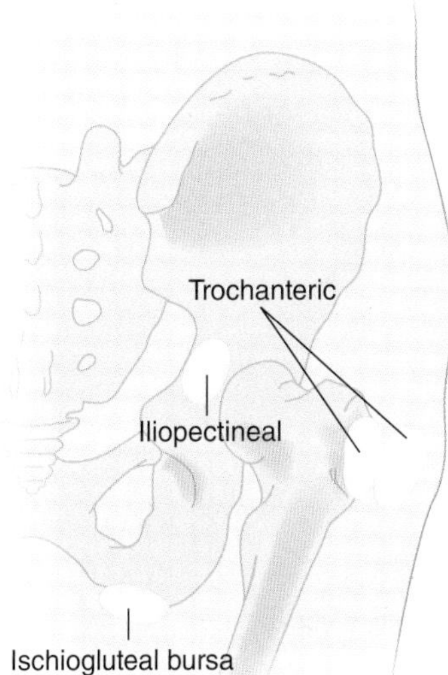

FIGURE 281-6. Selected bursae of the hip and pelvis. Proximity of the piriformis muscle and the sciatic nerve. [Reproduced with permission from Simon RR, Sherman SC, Koenigsknecht SJ: *Emergency Orthopedics: The Extremities,* 5th ed. © 2007, McGraw-Hill Inc., New York.]

runners with a broad pelvis are prone to inflammation in this location. Inflammation is commonly seen in older women and can be a complication of rheumatoid arthritis. The patient complains of pain due to direct pressure when lying on the involved side, with activities where the hip is abducted (involving the deep bursa), and when adducted for the superficial component. Simple walking and climbing stairs aggravate the pain as well. Pain is revealed by palpation over the greater trochanter and resisted abduction or adduction of the hip.[7,8]

Bursitis from abnormal calcification is uncommon, but may affect the trochanteric bursa. Calcific bursitis is identified on plain radiographs or CT as a poorly marginated line that is clearly separated from the femoral cortex. Calcification may also form around tendons.

ISCHIAL OR ISCHIOGLUTEAL BURSITIS (POSTERIOR/GLUTEAL PAIN)

Ischiogluteal bursitis presents with pain over the ischial prominence (Figure 281-5), which thus is increased in the sitting position. "Weaver's bottom" is a nickname for the inflammatory version of this bursitis, which is particularly exacerbated by sitting on a hard surface for long periods. As expected, this condition most often occurs in sedentary individuals. The bursa is also subject to focal, direct trauma. The bursa lies in close proximity to the sciatic nerve and the posterior femoral cutaneous nerve, predisposing to concomitant inflammation of these nerves and subsequent characteristic radicular pain.

Iliopectineal Bursitis (Anterior Hip, Pelvis/Groin Pain) The iliopectineal bursa is interposed between the hip joint and the iliopsoas muscle (Figure 281-6). Pain is located over the anterior pelvis and the groin on the affected side. The patient may reflexively assume a position of hip flexion and external rotation to aid in relief. On examination, extend the hip and palpate the area overlying the joint capsule to reproduce pain.[9]

Iliopsoas Bursitis (Groin Pain) The iliopsoas bursa lubricates movement of the iliopsoas tendon over the lesser trochanter and is the largest bursa in the hip region. The patient complains of pain to extension of the hip, which is reduced by hip flexion. There may be tenderness over the middle third of the inguinal ligament in the area of the femoral pulse (**Figure 281-7**). This process may be confused with iliopsoas tendinitis, hernias, femoral aneurysms, adenopathy, or psoas abscess.[10]

SPECIFIC BURSAL SYNDROMES OF THE KNEE

Pes Anserine Bursitis (Anterior Medial Knee Pain) The pes anserine (from the Latin for three-toed foot of the goose) bursa lies deep to the three tendons that insert on the medial aspect of the tibia below the knee joint—the gracilis, sartorius, and semitendinosus—and above the medial collateral ligament and medial femoral condyle (**Figure 281-8**). Pes anserine bursitis is commonly seen in obese women with osteoarthritis of the knee, in runners, and with other various overuse syndromes. The patient complains of anterior medial pain below the joint line, and focal swelling may be noted over the bursa, with increased tenderness to palpation. The symptoms are sometimes confused with the pain from a medial meniscal tear or a medial collateral ligament injury.[11]

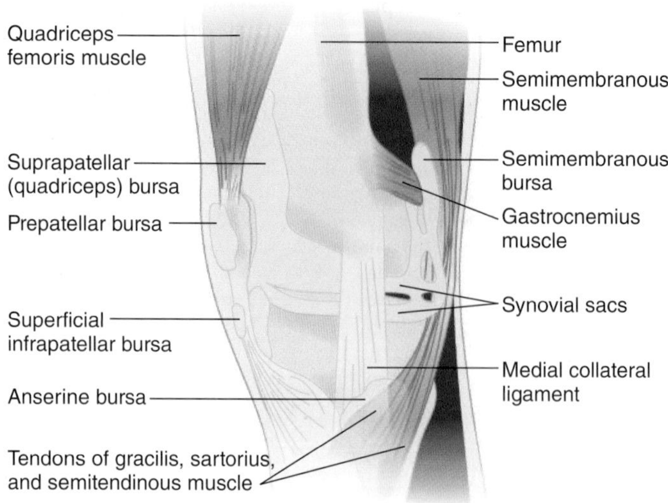

FIGURE 281-8. Medial view of the right knee, showing local bursa. [Reproduced with permission from Reichman EF, Simon RR: *Emergency Medicine Procedures*. © 2004, McGraw-Hill, New York.]

Prepatellar Bursitis (Pain Anterior to the Patella) Also known as *housemaid's knee*, *nun's knee*, or *carpet-layer's knee*, this bursa is commonly inflamed through repetitive kneeling on hard surfaces. Pain is frequently mild, with a restricted range of motion from the swelling, presenting as an effusion over the lower pole of the patella. This swelling may be so significant that one must differentiate it from a joint effusion (**Figure 281-9**). The area is tender to palpation, and bursal margins are often palpable. The prepatellar bursa is also one of the more common sites for septic bursitis, especially in children (see chapter 284).[12,13]

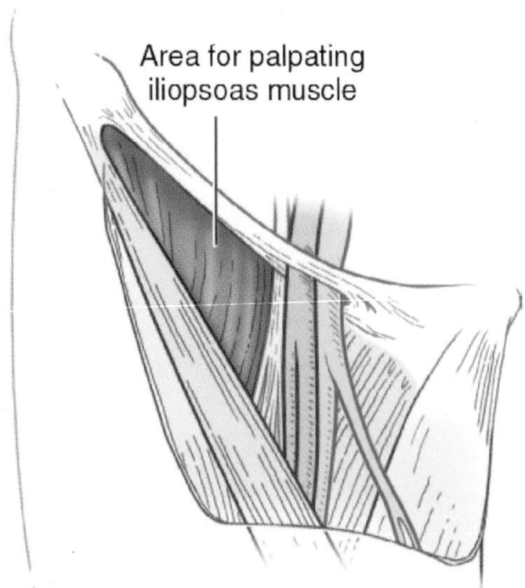

FIGURE 281-7. Iliopsoas bursitis. Area for palpating the iliopsoas muscle and bursa. [Reproduced with permission from Simon RR, Sherman SC, Koenigsknecht SJ: *Emergency Orthopedics: The Extremities*, 7th ed. © 2014, McGraw-Hill Inc., New York. Figure 18-21.]

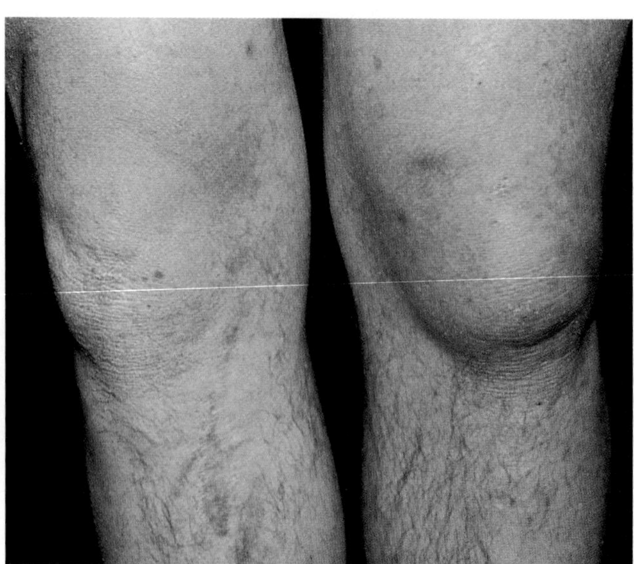

FIGURE 281-9. Prepatellar bursitis. Photograph reveals local bursal swelling of the left knee. [Reproduced with permission from Knoop K, Stack L, Storrow A, Thurman RJ: *Atlas of Emergency Medicine*, 3rd ed. © 2010, McGraw-Hill, New York.]

Other Knee Bursae The superficial infrapatellar bursa lies between the tibial tubercle and the overlying skin (Figure 281-8). The deep infrapatellar bursa is situated between the patellar tendon and the tibia. Neither bursa is commonly inflamed or infected. Consider infection when symptoms resemble septic arthritis or osteomyelitis of the proximal tibia, with swelling and loss of full extension of the knee.[14]

The tibial collateral ligament bursa lies between the ligament and the knee capsule. Calcification may occur here, and point tenderness accompanies fibrositis of the ligament. Consider this diagnosis in the patient with medial joint line pain, especially when there is no history of knee instability. Pellegrini-Stieda disease refers to the ossification of the proximal portion of the medial collateral ligament. This results from injury and presents as a palpable, tender mass. The fibular collateral ligament has a surrounding bursa; when inflamed, it produces lateral knee pain that is increased with varus strain.

TREATMENT OF BURSITIS

Treatment is aimed at the suspected cause. For inflammatory conditions, nonsteroidal anti-inflammatory drugs, rest, heat, and time are the basis of conservative treatment. Steroids may occasionally be required, and steroid injections into the more readily accessible bursa are useful only when it is clear that no infection exists. **Do not inject steroids into tendons, because this may weaken the tendon and lead to rupture.**

For bursal pain with an unclear cause, concomitant treatment for inflammation (rest, nonsteroidal anti-inflammatory drugs) and infection (antibiotics, most commonly for *S. aureus* and *Streptococcus* species) may be reasonable while awaiting culture results. See chapter 284 for recommendations concerning bursal aspiration and diagnosis. Serial aspiration and surgical drainage or removal of the afflicted bursa are indicated for refractory, chronic conditions. If infection is suspected in an immunosuppressed patient or if any patient presents with toxicity, admit for IV antibiotics in consultation with orthopedic surgery.

When fibrosis or synovial thickening leads to the development of painful nodules, surgical excision of the bursa is indicated. Inflammation of the bursa and the surrounding ligaments and tendons frequently coexists and is difficult to separate clinically.

MYOFASCIAL SYNDROMES/OVERUSE SYNDROMES

The diagnosis of these syndromes is largely clinical. Overuse syndromes are simply the result of repetitive stresses and microtrauma outpacing the body's ability to heal.

Hip Myofascial Syndromes/Overuse Syndromes • *External Snapping Hip Syndrome (Posterior Lateral Hip Pain)* Also known as *coxa saltans*, a snapping sound is heard and popping sensation felt as the iliotibial band (an extension of the fascia lata) slips over the greater trochanter (**Figure 281-10**). In athletes, the syndrome is usually associated with painful inflammation of the band and the involved bursa. The iliotibial band courses from the iliac crest, sacrum, and ischium to the lateral condyles and fibular head, separating the vastus lateralis from the hamstrings, the posterior thigh muscles (semitendinosus, semimembranosus, and biceps femoris). The patient will be able to voluntarily cause the snap with hip flexion and extension. Young women are predisposed to this syndrome, which occurs with activities such as dancing or stair climbing. Occasionally, the snap may be due to an intra-articular loose body. MRI may identify intra-articular causes or demonstrate inflammation of the local bursa, the iliotibial band, or the gluteal musculature. Dynamic sonography is also an aid for the diagnosis of extra-articular causes.[15,16]

Fascia Lata Syndrome (Lateral Thigh Pain) The fascia lata syndrome is a potential cause of pain in the lateral thigh region and is associated with pain to palpation and trigger points. Unilateral enlargement of the tensor fascia lata may occur with overuse or as a protective mechanism in injury. Athletes develop pain in the anterior groin and point tenderness over the anterior iliac crest. US is a useful aid to confirm the diagnosis.

Knee Myofascial Syndromes/Overuse Syndromes • *Patellofemoral Syndrome/Runner's Knee (Anterior Knee Pain)* This syndrome is a major cause of anterior knee pain, with three typical causes: focal trauma (least common), overuse, and abnormal patellar tracking as it glides and rotates in the patellar groove. A major contributor to abnormal patellar tracking is weakness of the quadriceps muscle. The syndrome is more common in females due to the presence of an abnormal Q angle (>20 degrees), resulting from a broader pelvis. The Q angle is measured at the junction of a line drawn from the anterior superior iliac spine to the central patella and a second line drawn from the central patella to the tibial tubercle (**Figure 281-11**). A normal angle is approximately 15 degrees. An increased Q angle increases the risk for patellar subluxation. Because of

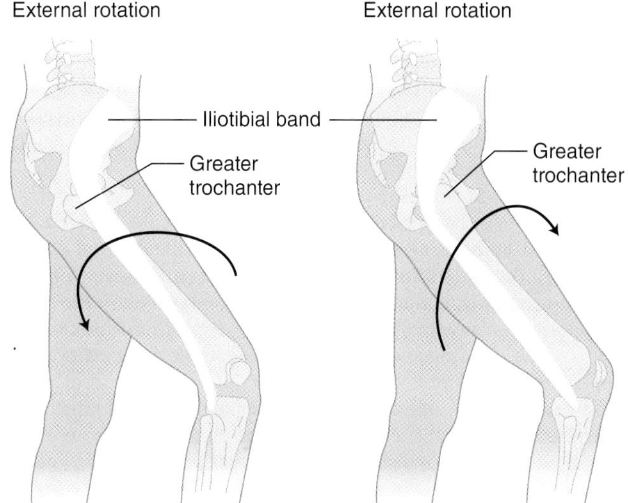

FIGURE 281-10. External snapping hip syndrome. In the snapping hip syndrome, the iliotibial band courses over the greater trochanter. [Reproduced with permission from Simon RR, Sherman SC, Koenigsknecht SJ: *Emergency Orthopedics: The Extremities*, 5th ed. © 2007, McGraw-Hill Inc., New York.]

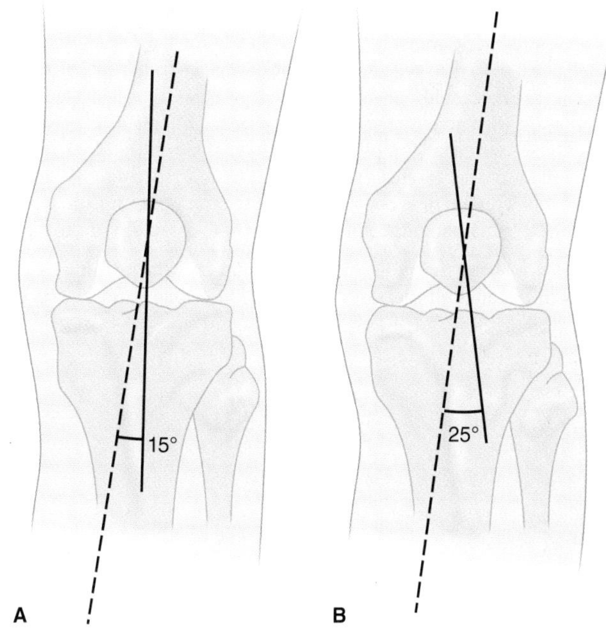

FIGURE 281-11. Measuring the Q angle. **A.** The normal Q angle is approximately 15 degrees. **B.** A Q angle of >20 degrees is considered to be abnormal. Patellar malalignment is determined clinically by measuring the *Q angle*. The Q angle is formed by a line drawn from the midpoint of the patella through the midpoint of the femoral shaft and a second line drawn from the midpoint of the patella through the tibial tuberosity. [Reproduced with permission from Simon RR, Sherman SC, Koenigsknecht SJ: *Emergency Orthopedics: The Extremities*, 5th ed. © 2007, McGraw-Hill Inc., New York.]

this relationship, females have a 50% to 100% greater incidence of knee injuries compared with males in both athletes and nonathletes.

The symptoms of anterior knee pain are gradual in onset, nonradiating, and typically unilateral. Pain is exacerbated by prolonged flexion of the knee, such as on air flights or at the movie theatre (moviegoer syndrome). Pain frequently occurs with activities of daily living, such as walking, and especially with stair climbing.

The presence of crepitus to palpation at the patella-femoral joint suggests degenerative changes but may be normal. The patellar grind test is accomplished by pressing the patella away from the femoral condyles while asking the patient to contract the quadriceps muscles. A positive test is represented by sudden patellar pain and relaxation of the muscle. The opposite test involves lifting the patella away from the knee joint while passively bending and straightening the knee. If this relieves pain, the patellofemoral joint is likely the source. Radiographic studies are of limited value but may detect arthritis of the patellofemoral joint.

Treatment involves the usual conservative measures, with an emphasis on physical therapy and strengthening. Brace support of the knee will also help correct the patellofemoral mechanism.[17,18]

Inflammatory pain to the knee may last for months to a few years following surgery or trauma and is based on a genetic predisposition to arthrofibrosis from these insults. Arthroscopy may cause the release of calcium pyrophosphate from tissue, resulting in a severe synovitis.

Chondromalacia Patellae (Anterior Knee Pain) *Chondromalacia patellae* refers to a softening of the cartilage on the posterior surface of the patella, most commonly occurring with the patellofemoral syndrome. Symptoms are pain on palpation of the patella (**Figure 281-12**).

This diagnosis is a surgical one, where the affected cartilage has a ragged appearance on arthroscopic visualization. Therefore, it is preferred that this term not be used for a new diagnosis in the ED, where the symptoms are more properly referred to simply as *anterior knee pain* or the *patellofemoral syndrome*.

Medial Plica Syndrome (Anterior Medial Knee Pain) The plica syndrome is uncommon and is difficult to distinguish from other causes of patellofemoral pain. Plicae are abnormal, redundant folds in the connective tissue of the knee, persisting from the normal embryologic septa that initially divide the knee into compartments and normally disappearing as the fetus matures. Plicae become symptomatic for unclear reasons. Reoccurring synovitis may result in a palpable, inelastic band that interferes with normal knee movement and leads to pain. This band-like structure is best palpated parallel to the medial border of the patella and produces pain in the area of the medial femoral condyle that radiates anteriorly. Pain may be brought on with activity or may occur at rest. Patients may also report a snapping sensation as the plica moves over the femoral condyle with repeated flexion and extension. Arthroscopy or MRI findings confirm the diagnosis. Treatment is conservative, with strengthening and stretching exercises; some patients require arthroscopic resection of the band.[19]

Iliotibial Band Syndrome (Lateral Knee Pain) Iliotibial band syndrome is most common in distance runners or cyclists. The iliotibial band inserts onto

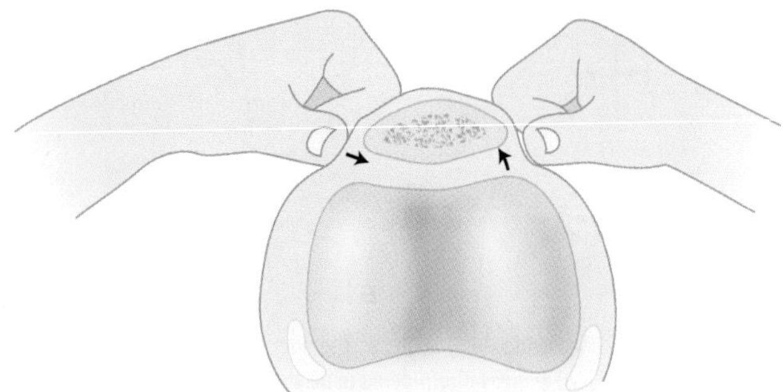

FIGURE 281-12. Patellar tenderness in chondromalacia. Palpation of the undersurface of the patella will elicit tenderness in chondromalacia of the patella. [Reproduced with permission from Simon RR, Sherman SC, Koenigsknecht SJ: *Emergency Orthopedics: The Extremities*, 5th ed. © 2007, McGraw-Hill Inc., New York.]

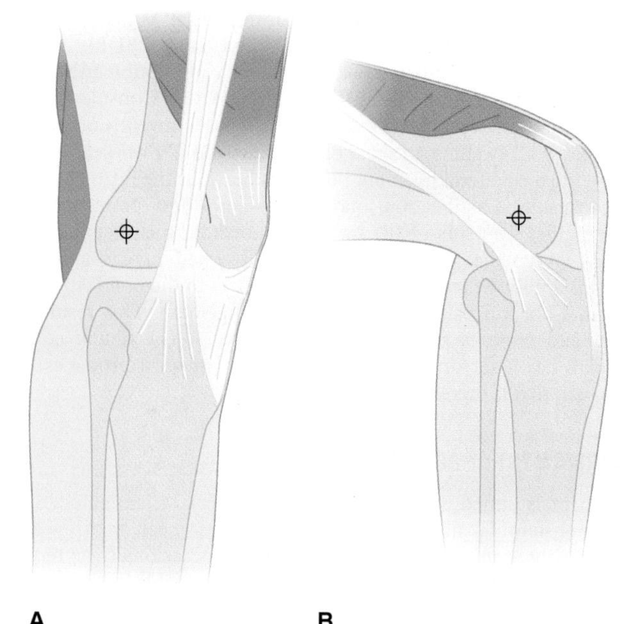

FIGURE 281-13. Iliotibial band site. **A.** The iliotibial band lies anterior to the lateral femoral epicondyle when the knee is in extension and passes posterior to it with flexion. **B.** The coursing back and forth over this bony prominence is the cause of a symptom complex referred to as the *iliotibial band syndrome*. [Reproduced with permission from Simon RR, Sherman SC, Koenigsknecht SJ: *Emergency Orthopedics: The Extremities*, 5th ed. © 2007, McGraw-Hill Inc., New York.]

the lateral femoral and tibial condyles (**Figure 281-13**). The thickened fascia serves as a ligament and stabilizes the joint in extension. With overuse, the bursa underlying the band becomes irritated. Pain is reproduced consistently after reaching a certain mileage during running or other physical exertion, and on examination, there is localized tenderness to palpation over the lateral epicondyles. Treatment involves rest, decreasing the distance in training, changing shoes to reduce stress on the structures, stretching exercises, and steroid injections locally.

Popliteus Tendinitis (Posterior Lateral Knee Pain) The small popliteus muscle passes under the lateral head of the gastrocnemius and inserts into the posterior tibia. It assists with internal rotation of the tibia, withdraws the meniscus during flexion to prevent impingement, and stabilizes the knee, preventing forward displacement. A bursa separates the tendon from the underlying structures in the area of the lateral femoral condyle. Overuse syndromes of the popliteus tendon and irritation of the bursa are associated with excessive use of the quadriceps muscle and are seen most commonly in athletes. Pain is localized over the posterior lateral aspect of the knee and is worsened by running downhill. Point tenderness may be appreciated over the insertion on the proximal posterior tibia or along the lateral joint line (palpable "soft" area between the lateral proportions of the "hard" femur and tibia). The Webb test assists in making the diagnosis: internally rotate the leg in the supine patient, flex the knee at 90 degrees, and ask the patient to force external rotation while the examiner provides resistance. A positive test produces pain with the maneuver. Treatment is rest and eventual quadriceps rehabilitation, aided by ice and nonsteroidal anti-inflammatory drugs.[20]

Patellar Tendinitis/Jumper's Knee (Anterior Superior Knee Pain) The patella tendon is subject to significant wear, with microtears and complete ruptures occurring in athletes and nonathletes alike (**Figure 281-14**). Any activity that involves jumping can result in focal pain, typically at the inferior pole of the patella or proximal portion of the tendon. Other activities that may exacerbate pain include running (especially uphill), squatting, cutting maneuvers, standing from a sitting position, or even simple walking. Symptoms may improve with activity early in the course or may progress to the point of significant discomfort at rest. Treatment involves

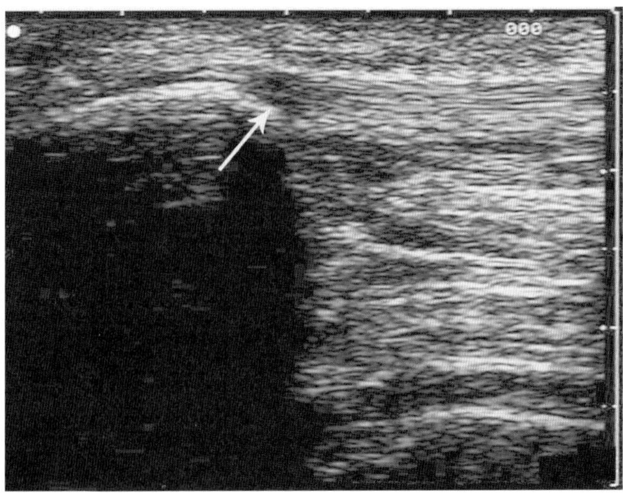

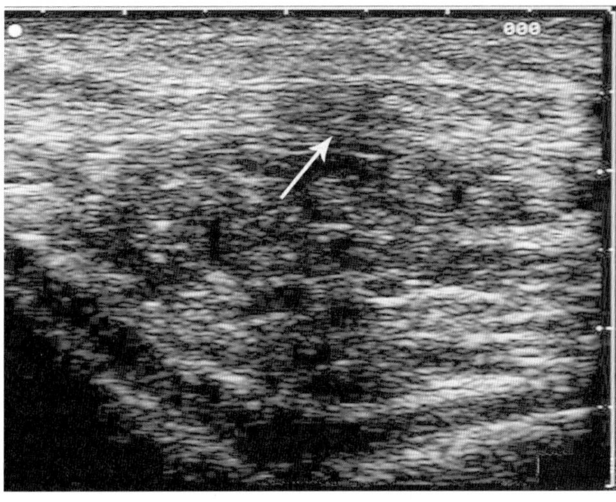

FIGURE 281-14. Patellar tendon defect. **A.** Long-axis sonogram of the proximal patellar ligament showing a hypoechoic tendon defect near the origin of the patellar tendon (*arrow*). The remainder of the tendon appears fibrillar and echogenic. A heel–toe insonating technique confirmed that a hypoechoic defect was present and that a tendinopathy ("jumper's knee") was present. **B.** Short-axis sonogram of the same patellar ligament. The ligament is seen as a somewhat echogenic horizontal structure approximately 5 mm beneath the skin surface and approximately 4 mm in width. In the central portion of the tendon, there is a focal area of hypoechogenicity that persists with careful imaging (*arrow*). This is the classic location and appearance of a "jumper's knee" or tendinopathy of the proximal patellar tendon. [Reproduced with permission from Ma OJ, Mateer JR, Blaivas M: *Emergency Ultrasound,* 2nd ed. © 2008, McGraw-Hill, New York.]

rest, nonsteroidal anti-inflammatory drugs, and cryotherapy. Steroid injections are contraindicated. Complete immobilization is not recommended, because this will reduce collagen production and stimulation of healing by loadbearing. Most recently, US-guided intratendinous injection of platelet-rich plasma has been suggested to allow rapid healing in the patellar tendon and other major tendons. However, insufficient evidence exists to support this modality definitively.[21,22] Further diagnosis and management of complete patellar tendon rupture are discussed in chapter 274, "Knee Injuries."

Infrapatellar Fat Pad Syndrome (Anterior Inferior Knee Pain) The infrapatellar fat pad location is suggested by its name: it fills the anterior part of the knee joint and is held in place by the patellar tendon, the retinaculum on both sides, and the infrapatellar synovial plica inferiorly. Due to its close anatomic relationship, the fat pad commonly becomes inflamed with patellar tendinitis.

Quadriceps Tendinitis (Anterior Superior Knee Pain) The quadriceps muscles and tendon are subject to significant forces in athletes, resulting in microtears and inflammatory changes, localized predominately at the insertion of the tendon into the proximal pole of the patella. Chronic recurrent injury or acute explosive trauma can result in complete tear of the tendon. Tendinitis is more likely to occur on a hard playing surface and with increased frequency of training. Diagnosis and management of complete quadriceps tendon rupture are discussed in chapter 274.

Semimembranosus Tendinitis (Posteromedial Knee Pain) Pain is elicited just distal to the joint line, where the tendon is easily palpated in most patients. In younger patients, the pain is associated with athletics and overuse. In older patients, it is seen secondary to degenerative changes of the knee joint, especially within the medial compartment. MRI will confirm the diagnosis if conservative therapy fails.

Snapping Knee Syndrome (Knee Pain) Snapping syndrome of the knee, similar to the same process in the hip, is a result of the iliotibial band passing over the lateral femoral condyle. The same effect may also result from the semitendinosus muscle passing over the medial condyle with the initiation of flexion and termination of extension of the knee. The snapping sensation and sound may be accompanied by pain in the location of the involved tendon. A third cause is the popliteal tendon snapping over the incisura poplitea extensoria on the lateral femoral condyle. Other causes of a snapping knee include intra-articular ganglion cysts, intra-articular loose bodies, and degenerative joint disease.[23,24]

POPLITEAL (BAKER) CYST (POSTEROINFERIOR KNEE PAIN)

A popliteal (Baker) cyst develops posteriorly and inferiorly to the knee as a distention of a local bursa, with several potential contributors existing in the areas of the hamstring tendons, the collateral ligaments of the knee, the condyles, and the heads of the gastrocnemius (**Figure 281-15**). The cyst frequently communicates with the knee (especially in adults),

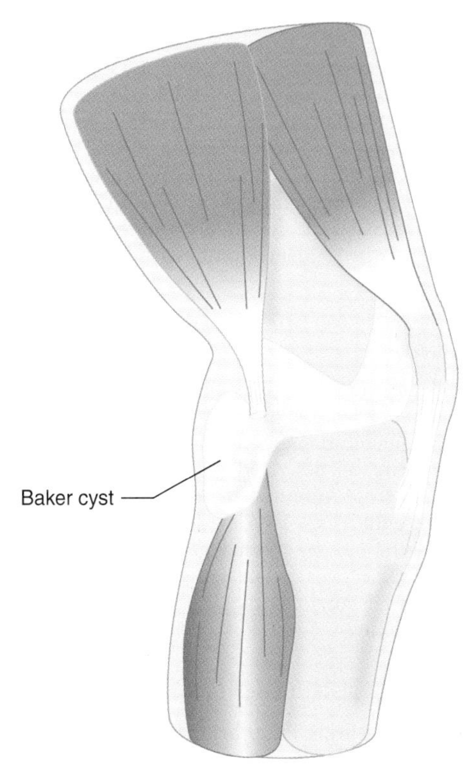

FIGURE 281-15. A Baker cyst (an extension of the semimembranosus bursa). [Reproduced with permission from Simon RR, Sherman SC, Koenigsknecht SJ: *Emergency Orthopedics: The Extremities,* 5th ed. © 2007, McGraw-Hill Inc., New York.]

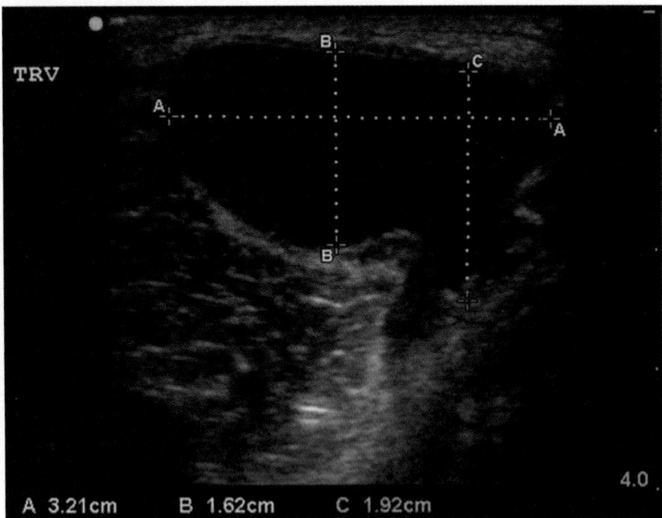

FIGURE 281-16. US of a Baker cyst. Transverse US view of Baker cyst, measuring approximately 3 cm by 2 cm.

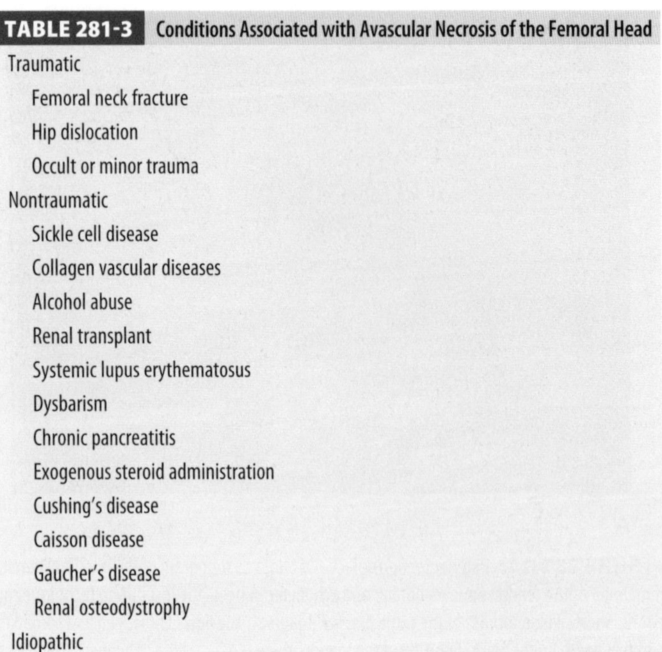

TABLE 281-3 Conditions Associated with Avascular Necrosis of the Femoral Head

Traumatic
Femoral neck fracture
Hip dislocation
Occult or minor trauma
Nontraumatic
Sickle cell disease
Collagen vascular diseases
Alcohol abuse
Renal transplant
Systemic lupus erythematosus
Dysbarism
Chronic pancreatitis
Exogenous steroid administration
Cushing's disease
Caisson disease
Gaucher's disease
Renal osteodystrophy
Idiopathic

and associated intra-articular pathology is common. The cyst may develop as a herniation of the synovial membrane through the posterior joint capsule. Giant synovial cysts of the calf may develop in patients with rheumatoid arthritis and will also communicate with the knee. Popliteal venous thrombosis can be confused with the pain and swelling produced by these posterior cysts or may exist concomitantly.[25] Other potential diagnoses include aneurysms, vascular tumors, fibrosarcoma, lipoma, and other tumors.

US is useful and readily available for cyst evaluation and for the identification of other conditions (**Figure 281-16**). Arthrography or MRI is suggested for complete evaluation. Excision may eventually be required for symptom relief.[26]

PIGMENTED VILLONODULAR SYNOVITIS

Pigmented villonodular synovitis is a proliferative synovitis, also referred to as *giant cell tumor of the tendon sheath*. The articular form can be present in many joints, including the hip and knee. The synovium and synovial fluid may appear red or brown, hence the name. Radiographs show specific findings, with erosions and cysts on both sides of the articular surface, usually with normal joint space and bone density. Typically only one joint is involved. Chronic discomfort may be present, or the radiographic findings may be incidental for the asymptomatic joint.[27]

GENERALIZED ARTHROPATHY OR TENDINOPATHY RELATED TO MEDICATIONS

An important source of generalized joint pain and swelling, as well as debilitating tendinopathy/tendinitis, including frank tendon rupture, is the use of specific medications and drugs.[28] In particular, the fluoroquinolone antibiotics are well described as causing these problems. In 2008, the U.S. Food and Drug Administration issued a black box warning to this effect for the quinolones. This issue occurs with enough frequency that providers should consider alternatives to the use of these antibiotics when possible.[29] Other agents that are associated with tendinopathy include corticosteroids, oral contraceptives, and the recreational drugs marijuana and cocaine.

BONE/ARTICULAR DERANGEMENTS (DIFFUSE/VARIED JOINT PAIN)

Septic arthritis, viral arthritis, the arthritis of Lyme disease, osteoarthritis, and the other arthritides such as rheumatoid arthritis, crystalline arthritis, and seronegative spondyloarthropathy are covered in chapter 284.

Osteonecrosis Other terms used to describe osteonecrosis include *avascular necrosis, aseptic necrosis*, and *ischemic necrosis*. Osteonecrosis is the result of bone infarction caused by a lack of blood supply. Osteonecrosis may occur as an idiopathic or primary disorder, secondary to a variety of systemic conditions, or following trauma (**Table 281-3**). The trauma may be major and obvious or occult and due to repetitive injury. Major trauma leads to sudden disruption of the blood supply, as commonly occurs following dislocation or fracture in the area of the joint. When the hip is involved, pain may be present anywhere in the region of the joint, the buttocks, thigh, or even the knee. Plain radiographs are helpful in establishing the diagnosis, with findings ranging from mottled densities and lucencies to severe collapse of the femoral head (**Figure 281-17**). With the knee, the weight-bearing medial femoral condyle is more commonly affected. Early in the disease process, CT or MRI will be more helpful in establishing the diagnosis (**Figure 281-18**). Joint replacement may be required.

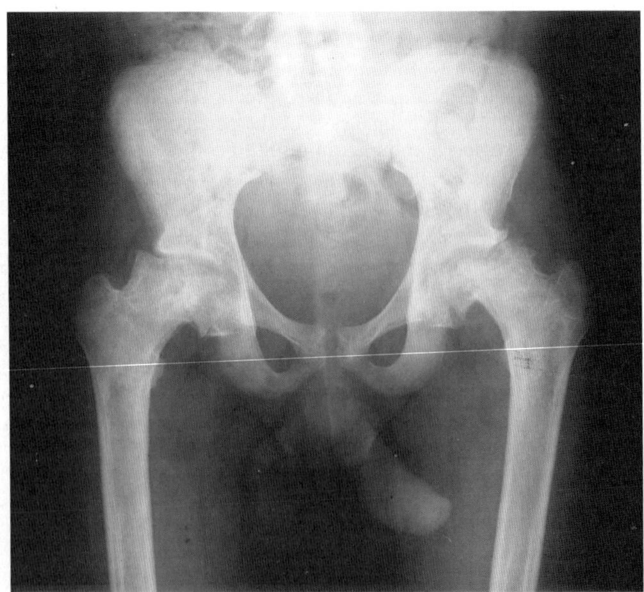

FIGURE 281-17. Avascular necrosis, bilateral hips (stage IV). [Reproduced with permission from Simon RR, Sherman SC, Koenigsknecht SJ: *Emergency Orthopedics: The Extremities*, 5th ed. © 2007, McGraw-Hill Inc., New York.]

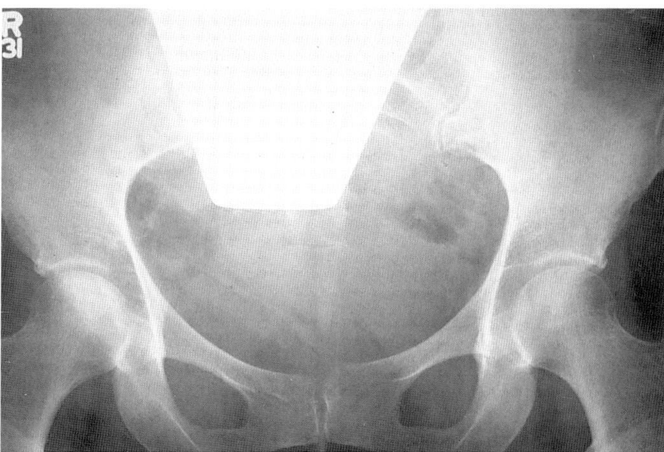

A

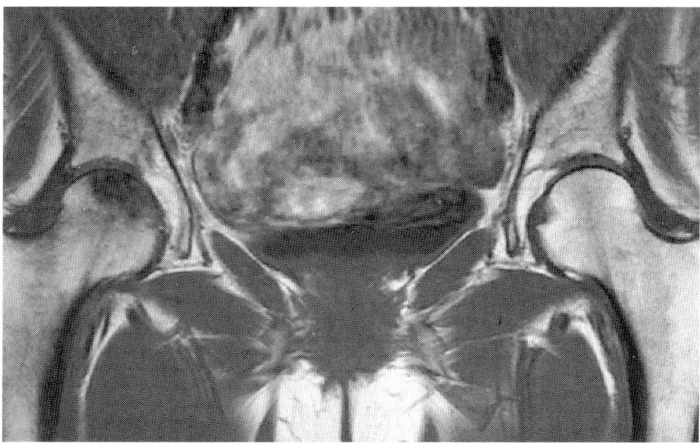

B

FIGURE 281-18. Osteonecrosis of femoral head: MRI versus plain films. A 45-year-old woman receiving high-dose glucocorticoids developed right hip pain. A. Conventional x-rays demonstrated only mild sclerosis of the right femoral head. B. T1-weighted MRI demonstrated low-density signal in the right femoral head, diagnostic of osteonecrosis. [Reproduced with permission from Fauci AS, Kasper DL, Braunwald E, et al: *Harrison's Principles of Internal Medicine,* 17th ed. © 2008, McGraw-Hill, New York.]

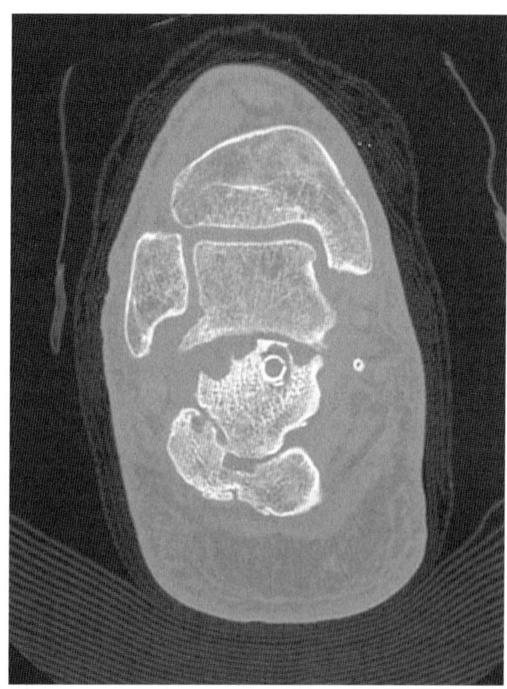

FIGURE 281-19. CT scan of the posterior ankle. Calcaneal osteomyelitis is seen after percutaneous fixation of a closed fracture with a large pin. Thermal necrosis of bone from drilling resulted in a ring sequestrum around the path of the pin, best shown on this CT scan. This sequestrum needed to be removed in order to control the infection. [Reproduced with permission from Slaven EM, Stone SC, Lopez FA: *Infectious Diseases: Emergency Department Diagnosis & Management.* © 2007, McGraw-Hill, New York.]

Osteomyelitis Osteomyelitis is an infection of the bone by bacteria or fungus, resulting in bony changes and destruction (**Figure 281-19**). It develops by spread of infection from contiguous structures (~80%) or by hematogenous spread (~20%). Hematogenous spread is more common to the long bones in children and to the spine in adults. Spinal epidural abscess is an important differential diagnosis to consider (see chapter 279, "Neck and Back Pain"). Risk factors for osteomyelitis are listed in **Table 281-4**. Pain at the site is a universal complaint and may be accompanied by warmth, swelling, and erythema. Radiographs are normal early in the course, but later will show bone demineralization, periosteal elevation, and lytic lesions. MRI is the preferred imaging modality, with approximately 95% sensitivity, but bone biopsy confirms the diagnosis with certainly. The urgency to make the diagnosis depends on the clinical situation. Osteomyelitis in diabetics is more common with skin ulcerations >2 cm, a positive probe-to-bone test result (sterile instrument reaches periosteum when probed into wound), an erythrocyte sedimentation rate >70 mm/h, or an abnormal radiograph. *S. aureus* is the most common causative agent overall. Other infectious agents and recommended therapies are listed in Table 281-4.

Blood cultures may identify the causative agent. When a blood culture is negative, bone biopsy is necessary to guide long-term antibiotic therapy. In acutely ill patients, begin presumptive treatment based on the clinical findings, with high-dose, broad-spectrum, parenteral antibiotics ensuring coverage for *S. aureus*. A 2009 Cochrane systematic

TABLE 281-4 Risk Factors, Likely Infecting Organism, and Recommended Initial Empiric Antibiotic Therapy for Osteomyelitis

Risk Factor	Likely Infecting Organism	Recommended Initial Empiric Antibiotic Therapy*
Elderly, hematogenous spread	*Staphylococcus aureus*, including MRSA, gram-negative bacteria	Vancomycin *plus* piperacillin-tazobactam, or imipenem
Sickle cell disease	*Salmonella*, gram-negative bacteria (*S. aureus* becoming more common)	Ciprofloxacin; consider vancomycin
Diabetes mellitus, or vascular insufficiency	Polymicrobial: *S. aureus, Streptococcus agalactiae,* and *Streptococcus pyogenes* plus coliforms and anaerobes	Vancomycin *plus* piperacillin-tazobactam, or imipenem
Injection drug user	*S. aureus*, including MRSA, and *Pseudomonas*	Vancomycin
Developing nations	*Mycobacterium tuberculosis*	See chapter 67, "Tuberculosis"
Newborn	*S. aureus* including MRSA, gram-negative bacteria, group B *Streptococcus*	Vancomycin *plus* ceftazidime
Children	*S. aureus* including MRSA	Vancomycin *plus* ceftazidime
Postoperative with or without retained orthopedic hardware	*S. aureus* and coagulase-negative staphylococci	Vancomycin
Human bite	Streptococci or anaerobic bacteria	Piperacillin-tazobactam or imipenem
Animal bite	*Pasteurella multocida, Eikenella corrodens*	Cefuroxime if known *P. multocida*, piperacillin-tazobactam or imipenem

Abbreviation: MRSA = methicillin-resistant *Staphylococcus aureus*.

*All patients require bone biopsy and debridement of infected/dead bone.

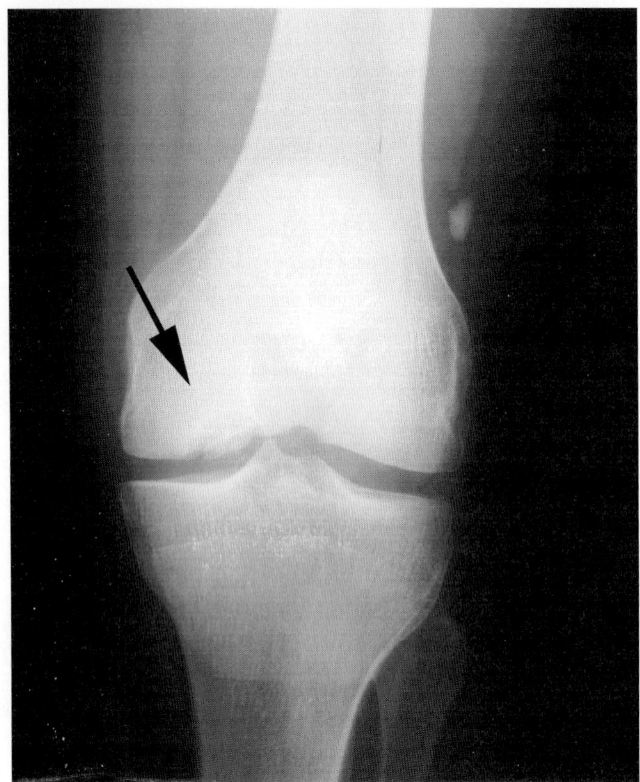

FIGURE 281-20. Osteochondritis dissecans (*arrow*) is shown at the lateral portion of the medial femoral condyle. [Reproduced with permission from Simon RR, Sherman SC, Koenigsknecht SJ: *Emergency Orthopedics: The Extremities,* 5th ed. © 2007, McGraw-Hill Inc., New York.]

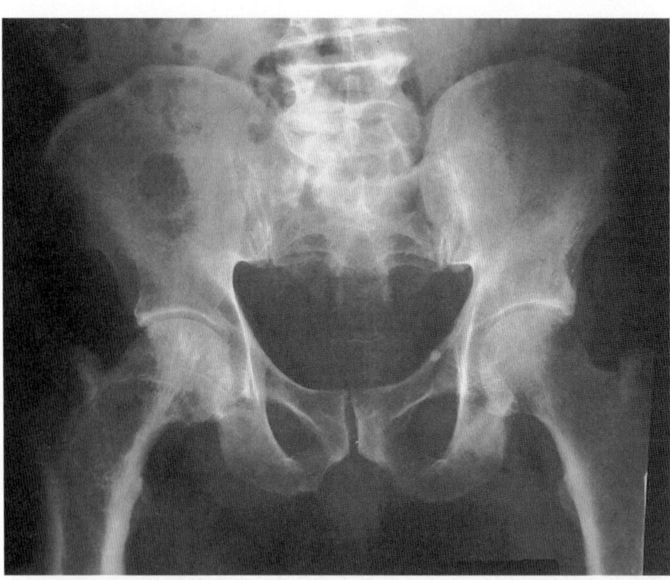

FIGURE 281-21. Radiograph of a 73-year-old man with Paget's disease of the right proximal femur. Note the coarsening of the trabecular pattern with marked cortical thickening and narrowing of the joint space consistent with osteoarthritis secondary to pagetic deformity of the right femur. [Reproduced with permission from Fauci AS, Kasper DL, Braunwald E, et al: *Harrison's Principles of Internal Medicine,* 17th ed. © 2008, McGraw-Hill, New York.]

review could not identify the optimal empiric antibiotic agent from randomized controlled trials in the literature.[30] Therefore, empiric therapy is based on the suspected organism(s) from risk factors, as listed in Table 281-4.

Osteochondritis Dissecans (Knee Pain) In osteochondritis dissecans, a portion of the joint surface cartilage separates from the underlying bone. It is rare, but seen most often in adolescents, and is of unclear origin. Occult trauma likely plays a role. The lateral portion of the medial femoral condyle is predominately involved, with unilateral occurrence. The patient experiences pain and swelling. Plain radiographs may reveal a thin rim of calcium separated from the underlying bone (**Figure 281-20**), with MRI showing much greater detail.[31] Arthroscopic repair of the lesion or removal of associated loose bodies is required if conservative therapy fails.[32]

Synovial Osteochondromatosis (Hip or Knee Pain) Synovial osteochondromatosis is characterized by idiopathic, nodular synovial membrane proliferation and subsequent calcification of the affected tissue. Eventually, multiple fragments of this growth (as large as 2 cm) break off and occupy the joint space or the area of the bursa and tendon sheaths. With time, degenerative changes and joint deterioration with secondary osteoarthritis occur. The disease is more common in males between the ages of 20 and 50 years old. Patients complain of chronic symptoms, with pain and joint swelling. There is a limitation in range of motion, and the joint may lock. The large joints are commonly involved. Radiographs will show the calcification and the intra-articular bodies and later the changes of osteoarthritis. Surgical excision of the proliferating synovium and removal of the ossified bodies from the joint space are required.[33]

Transient Osteoporosis of the Hip (Hip Pain) Transient osteoporosis of the hip occurs in middle-aged men and in pregnant women in the third trimester. The disease is uncommon, idiopathic, and characterized by sudden onset of hip pain, with the findings of osteoporosis on plain films. The disease spontaneously resolves within 6 to 12 months. Symptoms may abate before the associated radiographic findings have resolved. Take precautions against hip fracture while the disease remains active.[34,35]

Paget's Disease Osteitis deformans, or Paget's disease, is a chronic disorder resulting in enlarged, deformed bones from overactive breakdown and reformation. Paget's disease affects the hip joint in 50% of patients. The disease is familial and is suggested by an elevated serum alkaline phosphate level. Patients complain of pain, and radiographs reveal joint space narrowing with minimal hypertrophic changes (**Figure 281-21**). Treatment is symptomatic, and medications that slow the rate of bone turnover (calcitonin, alendronate, others) may be helpful to control the disease systemically. Surgery is required for complications of the disease, such as fracture and severe arthritis.[36,37]

Osteitis Pubis (Midline Pelvis and Groin Pain with Radiation to Hips) Osteitis pubis should be considered as a possible diagnosis in athletes with pain in the region of the pubis. It also occurs following pregnancy and after bladder and prostate surgery. In athletes, it is an inflammatory process related to overuse of the adductors and gracilis muscles. Bony changes with periostitis occur at the sites of the origins of the involved muscles. The disease is seen in runners, soccer players, weightlifters, fencers, and football players. Symptoms start off gradually and progress to severe pain with any movement of the legs. Rolling over in bed may be next to impossible due to excruciating pain, and there is a characteristic "duck waddling gait." The symptoms may resolve completely over a period of months with rest and nonsteroidal anti-inflammatory drug use. Rarely, arthrodesis of the pubic symphysis and local debridement are required.

Radiographs show symmetric bone reabsorption medially, widening of the pubic symphysis, and sclerosis along the pubic rami. These changes may take several weeks to develop. MRI more clearly details the changes, and bone scans show evidence of the inflammatory process.[38-40]

Diseases of Abnormal Calcification Myositis ossificans, or heterotrophic calcification, is the deposition of bone at a site where bone does not normally occur. The process is related to direct trauma, with the thigh and hip muscles frequently involved. Bleeding follows direct trauma to the muscle, and calcium deposits form inside the hematoma. A firm, palpable, painful mass will develop within 2 weeks and may persist for up to 1 year. Plain radiographs reveal an irregularly shaped mass around the joint or in the fascial planes (**Figure 281-22**). The appearance may be confused with a primary neoplasm, such as osteosarcoma or periosteal osteogenic sarcoma. Range of motion in the muscle

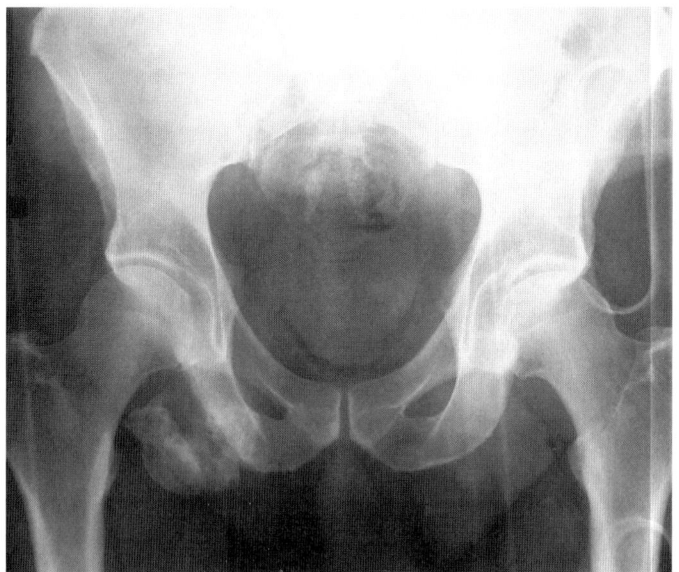

FIGURE 281-22. Myositis ossificans. This radiograph shows extraskeletal ossification of the medial proximal right thigh (immediately inferior to the head of the femur), approximately 3 weeks after a severe contusion to that area. [Reproduced with permission from Simon RR, Sherman SC, Koenigsknecht SJ: *Emergency Orthopedics: The Extremities,* 5th ed. © 2007, McGraw-Hill Inc., New York.]

TABLE 281-5 Treatment Caveats

Do not inject steroids in areas where infection is a concern, or where they may accidentally be injected into tendon sheaths and contribute to tendon rupture.
Use caution in the examination of the immunocompromised patient, because signs of infection may be subtle or altered.
Injuries in athletes should be referred to a sports medicine specialist to optimize therapy and decrease time to return to maximum activity levels.

or joint is limited due to pain or physical presence of the mass. Operative removal may be required.

Calcifying peritendinitis and bursitis are also traumatic in origin but are relatively uncommon. The trochanteric bursa of the hip is frequently affected. Radiographs reveal a thin, poorly marginated white line that is separated from the cortex of the hip.[41]

CORE TREATMENT

Treatment for the majority of inflammatory and overuse syndromes consists of nonsteroidal anti-inflammatory drugs, rest, heat, and time as the basis of conservative treatment (**Table 281-5**). "Rest" does not require full immobilization, which can lead to muscle atrophy and delayed return to normal function. Full knee immobilization, which is commonly prescribed from the ED, should therefore be used sparingly in the majority of these conditions. Appropriate rest is followed by gradual resumption of activities, physical therapy, and strengthening activities where appropriate. Steroids may occasionally be required, and steroid injections into the more readily accessible bursa are useful when it is clear that no infection exists but can be detrimental when infection is present. It is critical to avoid steroid injections into tendons, because steroids may weaken the tendon and lead to rupture. Athletes are best served by referral to a sports medicine specialist or an orthopedist.

REFERENCES

The complete reference list is available online at www.TintinalliEM.com.

Systemic Rheumatic Diseases

R. Darrell Nelson

INTRODUCTION

Systemic rheumatic diseases are chronic, inflammatory, autoimmune disorders, such as rheumatoid arthritis, systemic sclerosis (scleroderma), or systemic lupus erythematosus. ED patients with systemic rheumatic diseases have complex clinical and pharmacologic histories and multi-organ system pathology. Many extra-articular manifestations of rheumatic diseases can result in serious morbidity or mortality if not recognized and properly managed. This chapter discusses rheumatologic emergencies from an organ system perspective. **Table 282-1** categorizes emergencies associated with systemic rheumatic diseases.[1]

CLINICAL FEATURES AND DIAGNOSIS

Table 282-2 reviews clinical manifestations common to many of the systemic rheumatic diseases. **Table 282-3** lists typical clinical manifestations and complications specific to rheumatic diseases. The clinical descriptors may allow suspicion for a systemic rheumatic disease in a previously undiagnosed patient. However, the diagnosis cannot be confirmed during an ED visit. The diagnostic criteria and testing sequence, which are usually completed in the outpatient setting, are beyond the scope of this chapter. The need to admit a patient with a known or suspected systemic rheumatic illness depends on the severity of the patient's presentation. Complications of systemic rheumatic disease frequently require intensive care unit admission, and in 20% of patients with systemic rheumatic disease admitted to the intensive care unit, the diagnosis is made for the first time during the intensive care unit stay.[2] Rheumatoid arthritis is the most common rheumatic disease requiring intensive care unit admission, followed in decreasing frequency by systemic lupus erythematosus and systemic sclerosis.[2-4] Infection is the leading cause for intensive care unit admission, followed by rheumatic disease flare.

AIRWAY EMERGENCIES

Critical airway obstruction may develop (**Table 282-4**) at the level of the larynx, subglottic region, or trachea.

CRICOARYTENOID JOINT ARTHRITIS

In patients with rheumatoid arthritis, systemic lupus erythematosus, and relapsing polychondritis, arthritis or edema of the cricoarytenoid joints can lead to acute upper airway obstruction.[5] In addition, secondary infections such as bacterial epiglottitis or tracheitis can quickly

TABLE 282-1 Categories of Emergencies in Patients with Systemic Rheumatic Diseases

Category	Clinical Manifestations
Disease exacerbation	Flare-up of preexisting systemic rheumatic disease
Complication	Known complication of an acute systemic rheumatic disease (i.e., pulmonary hemorrhage, pericarditis, respiratory, or renal impairment)
Infection	Infection complicated by immunosuppressive therapy
Comorbidity exacerbation	Worsening or onset of a serious illness that is not a direct manifestation of the systemic rheumatic disease
Adverse drug reaction	Reaction to a systemic rheumatic disease drug treatment

TABLE 282-2 Clinical Signs and Symptoms Associated with Systemic Rheumatic Diseases

General manifestations	**Cardiovascular manifestations**
Fatigue	Chest pain
Fever	Hypertension
Lymphadenopathy	Pericarditis and Raynaud's syndrome
Malaise	Recurrent DVT
Splenomegaly	Recurrent thrombophlebitis
Syncope	Valvular diseases
Weight loss	**Neurologic manifestations**
Joint and muscle manifestations	Dizziness and gait disturbance
Arthralgias	Headache
Arthritis	Peripheral neuropathy
Back pain	Cognitive disturbances
Myalgias	Seizures
Morning stiffness	**Eye manifestations**
Muscle weakness	Corneal ulcers
Synovitis	Eye pain
Mucocutaneous manifestations	Red eye, tearing, photophobia
Alopecia	Episcleritis and scleritis
Nasal, or oral ulcers	Uveitis
Edema	**Renal manifestations**
Erythema nodosum	Microscopic hematuria, proteinuria
Palpable purpura	Renal failure
Rash	**GI manifestations**
Recurrent sinusitis	Abdominal pain
Sclerodactyly	Acute pancreatitis
Telangiectasias	Bowel dysmotility
Respiratory manifestations	Dysphagia
Airway disturbances	Esophageal reflux
Asthma	GI bleeding
Dyspnea	Xerostomia (dry mouth)
Hemoptysis	**Urogenital manifestations**
Interstitial lung disease	Acute scrotum
Pleurisy	Urogenital ulcers
Pneumonitis	**Nonspecific laboratory abnormalities**
Pulmonary hypertension	Thrombocytopenia
Restrictive pulmonary failure	Anemia, elevated creatinine

Abbreviation: DVT = deep vein thrombosis.

compromise the airway. Signs and symptoms of cricoarytenoid arthritis are throat pain or tenderness over cartilaginous structures (aggravated by swallowing or speaking), foreign body sensation or fullness in the throat, voice changes or hoarseness, and, in more severe cases, dyspnea, cough, or stridor.[1] Pain from cricoarytenoid arthritis is sometimes referred to the ear or to the neck.

CT scanning and fiber optic laryngoscopy can evaluate the cricoarytenoid joint. Initial treatment consists of systemic high-dose corticosteroids such as methylprednisolone 250 to 500 milligrams IV.[5]

TRACHEOMALACIA

Relapsing polychondritis can cause inflammation, destruction, and collapse of tracheobronchial cartilage, resulting in airway obstruction. Regions of segmental collapse due to tracheomalacia or refractory stenosis may be resected or treated with stents. The use of noninvasive ventilation may help to prevent airway collapse. Cartilaginous destruction results in a small glottis, so, when intubation is required, use a smaller endotracheal tube than normal.

SUBGLOTTIC STENOSIS

An acute upper airway obstruction can be observed in Wegener's granulomatosis, resulting from subglottic stenosis with inability to clear tracheobronchial secretions. Subglottic stenosis can be a presenting sign of Wegener's granulomatosis. Stenosis often requires surgical intervention.

INTUBATION IN PATIENTS WITH SYSTEMIC RHEUMATIC DISEASES

Endotracheal intubation is considered "difficult" in patients with systemic rheumatic diseases because of airway-related aspects of the disease. Anticipate the need for adjunctive airway techniques. Consider fiber optic intubation and fully prepare to perform an emergency cricothyrotomy. In cases where the airway is patent but intubation is anticipated and the patient can be transferred, it may be preferable to go to the operating room for a "double setup," with preparation for a formal tracheostomy if oral intubation is unsuccessful.

Patients with rheumatoid arthritis and ankylosing spondylitis can develop temporomandibular joint dysfunction with reduced mouth opening. Patients also have a high incidence (25%) of atlantoaxial instability, C1-C2 subluxation, or dislocation. Therefore, avoid neck hyperextension in patients with rheumatoid arthritis.

Neck hyperextension and cervical manipulation are also a hazard in ankylosing spondylitis. Patients with cervical ankylosis are at high risk for cervical fractures (even after minor trauma).

In patients with scleroderma, hardening of the skin of the face and neck can be severe, decreasing the ability to open the mouth and limiting neck mobility.

PULMONARY EMERGENCIES

Lung involvement, due to the underlying disease itself or secondary to infection, is a frequent cause of major morbidity and death (Table 282-4), particularly in systemic sclerosis, rheumatoid arthritis, systemic lupus erythematosus, Wegener's granulomatosis, and polymyositis/dermatomyositis. Pulmonary complications of systemic rheumatic disease manifest primarily as interstitial lung disease and vascular disease. Due to chronic lung injury, interstitial pulmonary fibrosis, or pulmonary hypertension, even mild infection in patients with systemic rheumatic disease can cause respiratory failure.[6,7] Respiratory arrest has been reported in systemic lupus erythematosus and dermatomyositis/polymyositis patients due to phrenic nerve involvement, in rheumatoid arthritis patients due to cervicomedullary compression associated with rheumatoid atlantoaxial dislocation, and in Sjögren's syndrome patients due to hypokalemic paralysis secondary to distal renal tubular acidosis.[6]

Symptoms can develop due to chronic manifestations of the underlying disease (i.e., interstitial lung disease), or new symptoms caused by an acute complication such as pneumonia or alveolar hemorrhage. Rheumatoid arthritis patients treated with methotrexate experience increased adverse respiratory events including pneumonia.[8] Several complications outside the pulmonary parenchyma cause respiratory symptoms: involvement of the joints of the thoracic cage (in ankylosing spondylitis), pleural effusion, respiratory muscle inflammatory disease (polymyositis/dermatomyositis), cardiac involvement, and anemia. Pulmonary embolism risk is higher in systemic rheumatologic diseases.[9,10]

ALVEOLAR HEMORRHAGE

Alveolar hemorrhage is an uncommon but catastrophic pulmonary emergency.[1,3] It is a complication of systemic lupus erythematosus (where it may be the presenting manifestation), antiphospholipid syndrome, systemic

TABLE 282-3 Common Features and Complications of Systemic Rheumatic Diseases

Disorder	Common and Characteristic Clinical Features	Complications
Antiphospholipid syndrome	Multiple and recurrent venous and arterial thromboses, recurrent abortions. Secondary form is associated with systemic lupus erythematosus, rheumatoid arthritis, systemic sclerosis, and Sjögren's syndrome. Thrombophlebitis and deep vein thrombosis, thrombocytopenia, hemolytic anemia, microangiopathic hemolytic anemia, livedo reticularis, stroke, transient ischemic attack, eye vascular complications. Coronary, renal, mesenteric, and cerebral vascular occlusion.	ARDS, pulmonary embolism, ischemic complications of vascular occlusion, bleeding, severe anemia, vision loss, catastrophic antiphospholipid syndrome.
Ankylosing spondylitis	Chronic inflammatory disease of the axial skeleton, with progressive stiffness of the spine. Young adults (peak at 20 and 30 years old). Back pain (improves with exercise), buttock, hip, or shoulder pain, systemic complaints (fever, malaise, fatigue, weight loss, myalgias), uveitis, and restrictive pulmonary failure due to costovertebral rigidity, ILD, renal impairment, fracture of the ankylosed spine, asymptomatic ileal and colonic mucosal ulcerations. Secondary amyloidosis.	Acute spinal cord or nerve compression, subluxation of the atlantoaxial joint, aortic regurgitation.
Adult Still's disease	Inflammatory disorder (similar to systemic onset juvenile rheumatoid arthritis). Systemic complaints (fever, malaise, fatigue, weight loss, myalgia), arthritis, myalgia, evanescent rash, pharyngitis, lymphadenopathy, splenomegaly, anemia, thrombocytopenia. Pericarditis, myocarditis, pleurisy.	ARDS, arrhythmias, heart failure, fulminant hepatic failure, red cell aplasia, disseminated intravascular coagulation, microangiopathic hemolytic anemia.
Behçet's disease	Chronic, relapsing, inflammatory disease. Systemic vasculitis involving arteries and veins of all sizes (carotid, pulmonary, aortic, and inferior extremity vessels are most commonly involved, with aneurysm, dissection, rupture, or thrombosis). Systemic complaints (fever, malaise, fatigue, weight loss, myalgia), recurrent painful skin and mucosal lesions; asymmetric, nondeforming arthritis of the medium and large joints; thrombophlebitis and deep vein thrombosis; ocular complications. Neuropsychiatric manifestations. Pericarditis, myocarditis.	Hypopyon, retinal vasculitis, optic neuritis, eye vascular complication. Dural sinus thrombosis, aseptic meningitis and encephalitis. Arrhythmias. Superior and inferior vena cava syndrome. Abdominal aorta or pulmonary artery emergencies. Bowel perforation.
Churg-Strauss syndrome	Vasculitis with a multisystemic involvement. Systemic complaints (fever, malaise, fatigue, weight loss, myalgia), myalgia, allergic rhinitis, nasal obstruction, recurrent sinusitis, asthma, and peripheral blood eosinophilia. Systemic hypertension, pericarditis, abdominal pain, peripheral symmetric neuropathy; skin lesions and rash.	Heart failure, acute myocardial infarction, acute and constrictive pericarditis, GI bleeding, bowel perforation.
Dermatomyositis/polymyositis	Idiopathic inflammatory myopathies. Muscle weakness, myalgia, and muscle tenderness. Elevated serum creatine kinase. Systemic complaints (fever, malaise, fatigue, weight loss, myalgia), Raynaud phenomenon, nonerosive inflammatory polyarthritis, esophageal dysfunction, ILD, aspiration lung infections.	ARDS. Respiratory failure and arrest due to diaphragmatic or chest wall muscle weakness, alveolar hemorrhage, and ILD. Heart failure, arrhythmias, and conduction disturbances.
Giant cell arteritis (temporal arteritis)	Chronic vasculitis of large- and medium-sized vessels. Elderly (mean age at diagnosis: 70 years old). Associated with polymyalgia rheumatica in 50% of cases. Localized headache of new onset, tenderness of the temporal artery, and biopsy revealing a necrotizing arteritis. Temporal artery may be normal on clinical examination. Gradual onset, systemic complaints, jaw or tongue claudication, eye complaints and visual loss. Aortic regurgitation and aortic arch syndrome. Neurologic complications due to carotid and vertebrobasilar vasculitis.	Ischemic optic neuropathy, eye vessel occlusion. Aortitis (especially the thoracic tract) and aortic emergencies. Stroke.
Henoch-Schönlein purpura	Systemic vasculitis associated with immunoglobulin A deposition, generally in children. Frequently, acute presentation follows an upper respiratory infection. Palpable purpura (in patients with neither thrombocytopenia nor coagulopathy), arthritis/arthralgia, abdominal pain, and renal impairment (adult), ILD.	Respiratory failure and alveolar hemorrhage. Seizures, intracranial bleeding, GI hemorrhage, bowel ischemia or perforation, acute pancreatitis, intussusception (children). Acute scrotum.
Microscopic polyangiitis	Small-vessel systemic vasculitis, characterized by rapidly progressive glomerulonephritis and pulmonary involvement. Lung complications differentiate microscopic polyangiitis from polyarteritis nodosa. Systemic complaints (fever, malaise, fatigue, weight loss, myalgia), arthralgias, skin lesions, hemoptysis, abdominal pain, renal impairment, systemic hypertension.	Rapidly progressive glomerulonephritis, severe lung hemorrhage, GI bleeding.
Polyarteritis nodosa	Systemic necrotizing vasculitis of the medium-sized muscular arteries. Systemic complaints (fever, malaise, fatigue, weight loss, myalgia), arthralgias, skin lesions, abdominal pain, renal impairment, systemic hypertension, peripheral mononeuropathy typically with both motor and sensory deficits, eye complications, leukocytosis, and normochromic anemia.	Acute scrotum, ischemic and hemorrhagic stroke, acute coronary syndrome, heart failure, peripheral artery ischemia, mesenteric ischemia and bowel perforation, GI bleeding, acute pancreatitis, malignant hypertension.
Relapsing polychondritis	Immune-mediated condition. Ears (violaceous and erythematous auricula), nose (saddle nose deformity), and other cartilaginous structures inflammation (especially joints and respiratory tract). One-third of cases associated with other systemic rheumatic diseases. Sternoclavicular, costochondral, and manubriosternal arthritis, upper airway involvement, aortic or mitral valvular regurgitation, pericarditis, renal impairment, peripheral neuropathies, ocular complications.	Airway obstruction. Acute renal failure, aortitis and aortic emergencies, heart block, ACS, scleritis, peripheral ulcerative keratitis, and acute scrotum.
Rheumatoid arthritis	Chronic, systemic, inflammatory disorder. Symmetric and potentially destructive arthritis. Systemic symptoms (fever, malaise, fatigue, weight loss, myalgia), skin lesions, splenomegaly. Cervical spine involvement, pleuritis, ILD, pericarditis, myocarditis, and aortitis. Cricoarytenoid arthritis with potential for airway obstruction, ocular involvement. Peripheral artery disease, Sjögren's syndrome, vasculitis, and renal impairment. Abdominal pain. Anemia, leukopenia, thrombocytosis, and Felty's syndrome. Increased risk of lymphoproliferative diseases, particularly non-Hodgkin's lymphoma.	Airway obstruction, obliterative bronchiolitis, acute respiratory failure. ACS, heart failure, thoracic aorta dissection, arrhythmias and conduction disturbances, subluxation of the atlantoaxial joints, bowel ischemia and perforation. Septic arthritis. Scleritis.

(*Continued*)

TABLE 282-3 Common Features and Complications of Systemic Rheumatic Diseases (*Continued*)

Disorder	Common and Characteristic Clinical Features	Complications
Systemic lupus erythematosus	Systemic autoimmune disease, characterized by relapses and remissions, and affecting virtually every organ. Systemic complaints (fever, malaise, fatigue, weight loss, myalgia), symmetric and polyarticular arthritis (small joints of the hands, wrists, and knees), butterfly rash, mucocutaneous manifestations, oral and/or nasal ulcers, Raynaud's phenomenon. Neuropsychiatric manifestations, pleurisy, lupus pneumonitis, shrinking or vanishing lung syndrome, ILD, and pulmonary hypertension. Libman-Sacks endocarditis, pericarditis, myocarditis, endocarditis. GI unspecific complaints. Renal impairment, leukopenia, mild anemia, and thrombocytopenia. Antiphospholipid syndrome. Ocular complications.	Airway obstruction, ARDS, respiratory failure and arrest, alveolar hemorrhage, ACS, cardiac tamponade, heart failure, arrhythmias, pulmonary embolism, stroke, acute renal failure, Guillain-Barré–like syndrome, transverse myelitis, seizures. Bowel ischemia and perforation, GI bleeding, acute pancreatitis. Hemolytic anemia, thrombotic microangiopathic hemolytic anemia.
Sjögren's syndrome	Autoimmune disease. May be primary; secondary form is mostly associated with rheumatoid arthritis, systemic lupus erythematosus, polymyositis, or dermatomyositis. Xerophthalmia and xerostomia, systemic symptoms, arthralgia, skin lesions, Raynaud's phenomenon. ILD, pulmonary hypertension, pericarditis, neuropsychiatric manifestations, peripheral neuropathy, hepatic abnormalities, renal impairment, increased risk of non-Hodgkin's lymphoma.	Hypokalemic respiratory arrest. Heart block, pulmonary embolism, ischemic stroke, transverse myelitis, optic neuritis, renal tubular acidosis, acute pancreatitis.
Systemic sclerosis (scleroderma)	Inappropriate and excessive accumulation of collagen and matrix in a variety of tissue; widespread vascular lesions with endothelial dysfunction, vascular spasm, thickening of the vascular wall and narrowing of the vascular lumen. Systemic complaints (fever, malaise, fatigue, weight loss, myalgia), skin lesions (fingers, hands, and face), carpal tunnel syndrome, Raynaud's phenomenon. ILD, renal impairment, GI dysmotility, gastroesophageal reflux (aspiration pneumonitis), chronic esophagitis and stricture formation. Vascular ectasia in the stomach ("watermelon stomach").	Scleroderma renal crisis. Respiratory failure, ARDS, aspiration pneumonitis, pulmonary hypertension, alveolar hemorrhage, heart failure, arrhythmias, and conduction disturbances.
Takayasu's arteritis	Chronic vasculitis, young women, predominantly Asians. Systemic complaints (fever, malaise, fatigue, weight loss, myalgia), arthralgias, skin lesions, abdominal pain and diarrhea. Aorta and its primary branches, and pulmonary artery involvement. Neurologic manifestations, syncope, subclavian steal syndrome, extremities ischemia. Renovascular hypertension. Normochromic normocytic anemia.	ACS, bowel ischemia and perforation, GI bleeding, stroke.
Wegener's (granulomatosis with polyangiitis)	Multiple organ system vasculitis and necrotizing granulomas. Respiratory tract manifestations in approximately of 100% cases, with nose, oral cavity, upper trachea, external and middle ear, and orbit inflammations. Upper airway and pulmonary manifestations. Constitutional symptoms, arthralgias, glomerulonephritis and small vessel vasculitis (scleritis and episcleritis, palpable purpura or cutaneous nodules, peripheral neuropathy, deafness). Systemic hypertension. Pericarditis, myocarditis. Renal impairment. Anemia, leukocytosis, and thrombocytosis.	Airway obstruction, subglottic stenosis, bronchiolitis obliterans organizing pneumonia, and alveolar hemorrhage. ACS, arrhythmias. Rapidly progressive glomerulonephritis.

Abbreviations: ACS = acute coronary syndrome; ARDS = adult respiratory distress syndrome; ILD = interstitial lung disease.

TABLE 282-4 Airway and Pulmonary Emergencies in Patients with Systemic Rheumatic Diseases

		Ankylosing Spondylitis	Adult Still's Disease	Antiphospholipid Syndrome	Behçet's Disease	Churg-Strauss Syndrome	Dermatomyositis/Polymyositis	Giant Cell (Temporal) Arteritis	Henoch-Schönlein Purpura	Microscopic Polyangiitis	Polyarteritis Nodosa	Rheumatoid Arthritis	Relapsing Polychondritis	Systemic Lupus Erythematosus	Sjögren's Syndrome	Systemic Sclerosis	Takayasu's Arteritis	Wegener's Granulomatosis
Airway	Obstruction											X	X	X				X
	Tracheobronchial stenosis and collapse												X					
Pulmonary	Acute respiratory distress syndrome		X	X			X							X		X		
	Acute respiratory failure in interstitial lung disease		X				X		X			X		X	X	X		
	Aspiration pneumonitis						X									X		
	Asthma				X													
	Obliterative bronchiolitis											X						X
	Pulmonary alveolar hemorrhage			X	X		X		X	X				X		X		X
	Pulmonary hypertension			X								X		X	X	X	X	
	Respiratory arrest due to phrenic nerve involvement						X							X				
	Respiratory arrest due to cervicomedullary compression	X										X						
	Respiratory arrest due to hypokalemic paralysis														X			
	Respiratory failure due to chest-wall joints or muscle impairment		X				X											
	Severe asthma					X												
	Shrinking lung													X				
	Spontaneous pneumothorax													X				

vasculitis, Wegener's granulomatosis, dermatomyositis/polymyositis, microscopic polyangiitis, and systemic sclerosis. Early recognition and aggressive management are critical for improved outcome.[3,11] Delay in treatment, age >60 years old, end-stage renal failure, and cardiovascular comorbidity worsen prognosis.[11] Patients with alveolar hemorrhage complain of acute shortness of breath, fever, and cough. Symptom onset is usually abrupt, with a progression to respiratory failure requiring mechanical ventilation in more than half of cases.

The classical triad of hemoptysis, pulmonary infiltrates on chest x-ray, and rapid fall in hemoglobin level supports the diagnosis, but the triad is not always present.[12,13] New lung infiltrates (83% to 100%) and anemia (75% to 100%) are more sensitive signs of alveolar hemorrhage; the most common initial diagnosis is "atypical" pneumonia.[12] If symptoms are accompanied by high fever, it is difficult to distinguish between alveolar hemorrhage, acute lupus pneumonia, and infectious pneumonia. The distinction is of utmost importance, because the therapeutic options are exactly the opposite (immunosuppressant vs antibiotics). Emergency bronchoscopy with bronchoalveolar lavage can confirm the diagnosis but is done after admission. Treatment is directed to the underlying condition and includes high-dose glucocorticosteroids, cyclophosphamide, local vessel embolization, or plasma exchange. [12]

INTERSTITIAL LUNG DISEASE

Interstitial lung disease is characterized by infiltration of the pulmonary interstitium by inflammatory cells and matrix, leading to fibrosis, pulmonary hypertension, and respiratory insufficiency. Rheumatoid arthritis, systemic sclerosis, polymyositis/dermatomyositis, and Henoch-Schönlein purpura are commonly associated with interstitial lung disease. Interstitial lung disease may be asymptomatic, may produce slowly progressive symptoms (cough and dyspnea), or, rarely, can cause acute respiratory failure. Treatment in the ED is ventilatory support, with oxygen, noninvasive ventilation, and intubation as needed.[14]

PULMONARY HYPERTENSION

Pulmonary arterial hypertension can be a complication of any rheumatic disease with associated pulmonary fibrosis and interstitial lung disease, but is especially common in systemic sclerosis and systemic lupus erythematosus. Pulmonary vasculitis and pulmonary thromboembolism (i.e., in antiphospholipid syndrome patients) may also lead to pulmonary arterial hypertension. Clinical symptoms reported by patients with pulmonary arterial hypertension range from cough or mild shortness of breath, to severe dyspnea, cardiac arrhythmias, chest pain, and right ventricular failure. For further discussion, see chapters 57 and 58, "Systemic Hypertension" and "Pulmonary Hypertension," respectively.

CARDIOVASCULAR EMERGENCIES

Heart disease develops through several pathophysiologic mechanisms, accounting for different manifestations: inflammation, fibrosis, infiltration, vasculitis, thromboembolism, and accelerated coronary atherosclerosis.[15] Pulmonary hypertension can lead to right heart failure. Coronary atherosclerosis can be due to an imbalance between the inflammatory and anti-inflammatory activity and the use of specific drugs, such as corticosteroids. **Table 282-5** provides a review of cardiac disorders in patients with systemic rheumatic diseases.[15-20]

ACUTE CORONARY SYNDROMES

Based on epidemiologic, clinical, laboratory, and experimental data, systemic lupus erythematosus, antiphospholipid syndrome, rheumatoid arthritis, and a few other rheumatic diseases promote accelerated coronary atherosclerosis and have an increased rate of cardiovascular morbidity and mortality.[15-17] The relative risks for atherosclerosis vary from about 1.6 in ankylosing spondylitis and psoriatic arthritis to 3.0 in rheumatoid arthritis (with a threefold increased adjusted risk of myocardial infarction) and 6.0 in systemic lupus erythematosus.[17] The risk of cardiovascular disease equals that of type 2 diabetes with coronary artery disease more prominent in rheumatoid arthritis and peripheral arterial disease more prevalent in type 2 diabetes.[21]

From a clinical point of view, it is useful to consider systemic rheumatic disease a "new" risk factor for coronary atherosclerosis. Patients with rheumatoid arthritis are less likely to undergo invasive evaluation and treatment.[19] Contributing factors may be low incidence of typical angina symptoms and attribution of chest pain to arthritis.

Coronary atherosclerosis is a major cause of cardiac mortality in young patients with systemic lupus erythematosus.[16] The risk of myocardial infarction in premenopausal women is more than twofold compared with women without lupus.[16] Medical management of acute coronary syndrome is the same as in the normal population. Coronary arteritis, fibrosis, and coronary artery vasospasm may occur in systemic sclerosis and vasculitis.

ACUTE HEART FAILURE

Acute heart failure may develop as a consequence of a myocardial disease (ischemia, cardiomyopathy, myocarditis, fibrosis), pericardial disease (tamponade or constrictive), valvular diseases (acute regurgitation), and/or conduction or rhythm disturbance.[15,16] Acute management of decompensated heart failure does not differ from the normal population, except when a flare of the underlying disease is responsible. In systemic sclerosis, diastolic dysfunction, malignant hypertension during a sclerodermal renal crisis, and decompensated pulmonary hypertension are important causes of acute heart failure.

CARDIAC ARRHYTHMIAS

Rhythm and conduction disturbances are common, especially in rheumatoid arthritis, systemic sclerosis, systemic lupus erythematosus, and polymyositis/dermatomyositis. The physiopathologic basis for these disorders is complex, involving reentry pathways, fibrosis, altered automaticity, conduction system injury, primary and/or secondary myocardial injury, and side effects of treatment. Population studies demonstrate a 40% higher risk for atrial fibrillation in patients with rheumatoid arthritis.[22] Arrhythmias and sudden cardiac death in systemic rheumatic disease have a higher incidence compared with the normal population.[19,20] Ventricular arrhythmias are a risk for sudden cardiac death, especially in patients with systemic sclerosis.[20]

MALIGNANT HYPERTENSION

Systemic hypertension may be a clinical manifestation of renal injuries or an adverse effect of disease treatment. Severe malignant hypertension is a complication of systemic sclerosis (usually observed during a "renal crisis"), but it can be also observed in catastrophic antiphospholipid syndrome, polyarteritis nodosa, and a few other rheumatic diseases.

VASCULAR AND VALVULAR DISEASE

Valvular heart disease is an extra-articular manifestation of spondyloarthropathies, particularly ankylosing spondylitis. Fibrotic changes of the aortic valve cusps lead to valvular insufficiency of the aortic and/or mitral valves. Arterial lesions can be aneurysmal (frequently complicated by fatal rupture) or, less commonly, occlusive. Aortitis may lead to aortic aneurysms in patients with giant cell arteritis (temporal arteritis), Takayasu's arteritis, and Behçet's disease, and aneurysms may rupture or dissect. In giant cell arteritis, great vessel involvement due to arteritis can result in aortic valve incompetence and aortic rupture as a late complication of the disease.

Any part of the arterial tree can be affected in Behçet's disease, but the abdominal aorta is the most frequently involved site. Pulmonary artery inflammation can be complicated by hemoptysis, aneurysm, thrombosis, hemorrhage, and pulmonary infarction. In Takayasu's arteritis, arterial narrowing and/or aortitis can produce neurologic symptoms or

TABLE 282-5 Cardiovascular Emergencies in Patients with Systemic Rheumatic Diseases

		Ankylosing Spondylitis	Adult Still's Disease	Antiphospholipid Syndrome	Behçet's Disease	Churg-Strauss Syndrome	Dermatomyositis/Polymyositis	Giant Cell (Temporal) Arteritis	Henoch-Schönlein Purpura	Microscopic Polyangiitis	Polyarteritis Nodosa	Rheumatoid Arthritis	Relapsing Polychondritis	Systemic Lupus Erythematosus	Sjögren's Syndrome	Systemic Sclerosis	Takayasu's Arteritis	Wegener's Granulomatosis
Cardiovascular	Acute coronary syndrome and acute myocardial infarction			X	X	X					X	X	X	X			X	X
	Acute pericarditis				X	X						X	X	X	X	X		X
	Aortic emergencies				X			X				X	X				X	
	Aortic valve regurgitation	X						X					X				X	
	Arrhythmias and conduction disturbances		X		X		X					X	X	X	X	X		X
	Heart failure		X			X	X				X	X				X		
	Cardiac tamponade					X						X		X		X		
	Deep vein thrombosis and pulmonary embolism			X	X									X	X	X		
	Catastrophic antiphospholipid syndrome			X			X					X		X		X		
	Endocarditis				X									X				X
	Malignant hypertension			X							X					X	X	
	Myocarditis		X		X		X					X		X		X		X
	Peripheral artery ischemia				X						X	X					X	
	Pulmonary artery injury				X												X	
	Artery inflammation and aneurysm				X													
	Budd-Chiari syndrome				X													
	Superior vena cava syndrome				X													
	Subclavian steal syndrome																X	
	Sudden cardiac death											X		X		X		

syncope related to the subclavian steal syndrome. Acute coronary syndrome, mesenteric artery ischemia, and peripheral arterial ischemia are other complications of Takayasu's arteritis.

THROMBOEMBOLISM

Superficial thrombophlebitis and deep vein thrombosis are common in Behçet's disease. After the veins of the lower extremities, other affected veins are the inferior and superior vena cavae, veins of the upper extremities, and hepatic and portal veins. Thrombosis is related to vascular inflammation and is not usually complicated by peripheral embolism. Deep venous thrombosis and pulmonary vasculitis can coexist. Hemoptysis, a sign of pulmonary artery inflammation, may mimic signs of pulmonary embolism. Treatment with anticoagulant or fibrinolytic may increase the risk of fatal hemorrhage.

Thromboembolic disease may also be observed in antiphospholipid syndrome and systemic lupus erythematosus. Vessel thrombosis can be venous and/or arterial, affect any vessel, and be recurrent and bilateral. Peripheral gangrene, acute coronary syndrome, renal artery thrombosis, sagittal sinus thrombosis, transient ischemic attack, and Budd-Chiari syndrome due to hepatic vein thrombosis are some examples of thromboembolism resulting from antiphospholipid syndrome and systemic lupus erythematosus.

CATASTROPHIC ANTIPHOSPHOLIPID SYNDROME

This uncommon vaso-occlusive process leads to multiorgan failure and is usually associated with systemic lupus erythematosus, but it may be observed in rheumatoid arthritis, systemic sclerosis, dermatomyositis, and other systemic rheumatic diseases.[23] Multiple simultaneous venous and/or arterial occlusive thromboses (involving mainly small vessels) and multiorgan failure develop suddenly and progress rapidly. In half of the cases, a precipitating factor may be identified (i.e., infection, surgery, trauma, cancer, drugs such as oral contraceptives). The kidney is the primary organ involved (acute renal failure), followed by the lungs (adult respiratory distress syndrome, embolism), CNS (stroke, seizures, venous occlusion), the heart (acute myocardial infarction and heart failure), and skin (necrosis). *Livedo reticularis* (lacelike purplish discoloration of the lower extremities due to vein engorgement) and thrombocytopenia are important diagnostic findings (a decrease in platelet count is observed in 60%), and occasionally, laboratory features of disseminated intravascular coagulation may be present.[23] This dramatic clinical scenario is frequently fatal, with a reported mortality rate approaching 50% despite therapy. Treatment is IV heparin and high-dose glucocorticosteroids with or without plasma exchange and IV immunoglobulins.[23]

NEUROLOGIC EMERGENCIES

Neurologic disease can result from accelerated atherosclerosis, direct involvement by the primary disease, vasculitis, arterial aneurysm, rupture or dissection, embolism, or infection[24] (**Table 282-6**). Libman-Sacks valvular endocarditis of lupus can result in embolism of valve vegetations. Vasculitis of the cerebral vessels, with vessel rupture or occlusion, may lead to ischemic or hemorrhagic stroke. Giant cell arteritis affects the extracranial vasculature, causing transient ischemic attacks, especially

TABLE 282-6 Neurologic and Ocular Emergencies in Patients with Systemic Rheumatic Diseases

		Ankylosing Spondylitis	Adult Still's Disease	Antiphospholipid Syndrome	Behçet's Disease	Churg-Strauss Syndrome	Dermatomyositis/Polymyositis	Giant Cell (Temporal) Arteritis	Henoch-Schönlein Purpura	Microscopic Polyangiitis	Polyarteritis Nodosa	Rheumatoid Arthritis	Relapsing Polychondritis	Systemic Lupus Erythematosus	Sjögren's Syndrome	Systemic Sclerosis	Takayasu's Arteritis	Wegener's Granulomatosis
Neurologic	Aseptic meningitis				X									X				
	Cerebral hemorrhage				X				X		X			X		X		
	Cerebral ischemia			X	X			X			X	X		X	X		X	
	Cord or spinal nerve compression due to spine involvement	X											X					
	Encephalitis				X													
	Hypertensive encephalopathy										X					X		
	Optic nerve injury							X							X			
	Psychosis/delirium				X									X	X			
	Seizures			X					X		X			X		X	X	
	Subclavian artery syndrome																X	
	Transverse myelitis													X	X			
	Venous cerebral thrombosis			X	X													
Ocular	Episcleritis											X	X					X
	Ischemic eye complications				X	X		X										X
	Scleritis					X						X	X	X				X
	Optic neuritis				X									X	X			
	Peripheral ulcerative keratitis					X					X	X	X	X				X
	Retinal vasculitis				X													X
	Scleromalacia perforans											X						
	Uveitis	X			X								X					

involving the vertebrobasilar circulation, with signs and symptoms of vertigo, hearing loss, gait disturbance, and other focal neurologic deficits involving the brainstem.

Neurologic disease can also manifest as a consequence of therapy for systemic rheumatic diseases. Medications such as infliximab and adalimumab, which block tumor necrosis factor-α, increase the risk for herpes zoster outbreaks, especially multidermatomal and zoster ophthalmicus.[25] Lupus and rheumatoid arthritis are independent risk factors for herpes zoster outbreaks.[26]

SPINAL CORD COMPRESSION AND SPINAL FRACTURES

Degenerative disease of the cervical spine may result in acute spinal cord compression, vertebral artery compression syndrome (with diplopia and dysphasia), gait abnormalities, paresthesias, or obstructive hydrocephalus in patients with rheumatoid arthritis and ankylosing spondylitis. Rigidity and osteoporosis of the spine in ankylosing spondylitis increase the risk for fracture and spinal cord injury. Occult fracture of the ankylosed spine may occur, even in the absence of trauma, and may result in acute radiculopathy, paraparesis, or tetraparesis. The most common symptom is severe and progressive pain. Cauda equina syndrome is a rare complication.

INSTABILITY OF THE CERVICAL SPINE

The atlantoaxial joint is a preferred target of rheumatoid arthritis. Instability of the cervical spine and spontaneous atlantoaxial subluxation can result in acute cervical myelopathy, even after minor trauma. The signs and symptoms that raise suspicion of an unstable cervical spine are severe neck pain with occipital radiation and paresthesias or motor weakness involving the upper extremities. Instability may produce vertigo or other signs of vertebral insufficiency. The patient may complain of an electric shock sensation radiating down the back during neck flexion, a change in bladder function, or progressive quadriparesis.

Atlantoaxial instability can be clinically silent, so avoid neck flexion in the patient with rheumatoid arthritis. After even mild trauma, or if neurologic symptoms as described above develop, keep the cervical spine stabilized. CT of the cervical spine will detect fracture, but MRI is needed to assess spinal cord integrity. Neurosurgical (or orthopedic spine specialist) consultation is needed for management.

TRANSVERSE MYELITIS

Transverse myelitis is a rare, devastating acute inflammatory process affecting a focal area of the spinal cord that may lead to rapid onset of irreversible paraplegia. It is clinically manifested with acute or subacute progressive symptoms and signs of neurologic dysfunction of the spinal cord. The clinical picture may be insidious at the beginning, with weakness, back or limb pain, urinary retention, and autonomic and sensory deficits.[27]

Transverse myelitis occurs more commonly in patients with Sjögren's syndrome and patients with systemic lupus erythematosus, in whom acute transverse myelitis may be the initial manifestation. The clinical picture of transverse myelitis may also be caused by vasculitis, arterial thrombosis, embolism, or artery dissection. An anterior spinal artery syndrome may be observed in other rheumatic diseases and is caused by the blood supply impairment secondary to dissection of the aorta, vasculitis, or embolism involving the anterior spinal artery. The clinical picture is indistinguishable from transverse myelitis.

OCULAR EMERGENCIES

The eye is a sensitive barometer for onset or flare of rheumatic diseases.[28] Ocular pain or discomfort, vision disturbances, red eye, tearing, photophobia, diplopia, or reduced visual acuity should lead to careful evaluation (Table 282-6). Optic neuritis and keratitis are complications of systemic rheumatic diseases and are discussed in brief in chapter 241, "Eye Emergencies."

Sudden and permanent blindness is also a concern in temporal or giant cell arteritis, a systemic disease that may lead to vasculitis and ischemia and that affects middle-aged to elderly individuals. The patient may report amaurosis fugax and complain of new headache, tender scalp, visual disturbance, or jaw, tongue, or upper extremity claudication. Frequently, vision loss is the presenting feature of giant cell arteritis. To prevent permanent vision loss, high-dose steroids are administered based on the clinical diagnosis, even before biopsy of the temporal artery (see chapter 241).

RENAL EMERGENCIES

The kidney is almost always involved in systemic rheumatic disease and is a major factor leading to morbidity and mortality (**Table 282-7**).

A decline in renal function should prompt careful observation and follow-up in any rheumatic disease patient. Kidney impairment may be related to the rheumatic disease itself, the results of therapy, or both. Acute nephritic syndrome, renal thrombotic events, renal artery lesions, and rhabdomyolysis are other possible causes of acute renal failure. In polyarteritis nodosa, rupture of arterial aneurysms can cause a perirenal hematoma.

Renal disease is the most common cause of death in systemic sclerosis, and a sudden catastrophic form of renal involvement, named *scleroderma renal crisis*, may be the cause. Scleroderma renal crisis typically develops early in the course of systemic sclerosis, and 75% of cases occur during the first 4 years after the onset of disease.[29] Scleroderma renal crisis presents with abrupt and rapid deterioration in renal function and is heralded by severe headache, visual disturbance, and hypertensive encephalopathy. Microangiopathic anemia with mild thrombocytopenia is another important but nonspecific diagnostic finding in scleroderma renal crisis.

The mainstay of therapy in scleroderma renal crisis is effective and prompt blood pressure control with angiotensin-converting enzyme inhibitors.[29] Start captopril, 6.25 to 12.5 milligrams PO three times daily, and increase as tolerated (during admission or follow-up).[29] Enalaprilat can be used if PO therapy is not possible. Consult nephrology for dialysis recommendations; dialysis is required in 50% of patients.[30] Avoid diuretics as they can exacerbate renal failure. For further discussion, see chapters 57 and 58.

Distal renal tubular acidosis occurs in 30% of patients with primary Sjögren's syndrome. This condition is characterized by hyperchloremic metabolic acidosis with low bicarbonate levels and hypokalemia. Consider hypokalemia as a cause of progressive weakness in patients with Sjögren's syndrome. Hypokalemia is corrected with standard treatment (see chapter 17, "Fluids and Electrolytes").

GI EMERGENCIES

GI emergencies are outlined in Table 282-7. GI complications include ischemia (primarily due to vasculitis), infarction, perforation, vascular rupture, infection (i.e., cholecystitis, diverticulitis), and hemorrhage. Vasculitis is the most common GI manifestation and may affect large vessels (giant cell arteritis), medium-sized vessels (polyarteritis nodosa), or small vessels (systemic lupus erythematosus). Lupus mesenteric

TABLE 282-7 Renal and GI Emergencies in Patients with Systemic Rheumatic Diseases

		Ankylosing Spondylitis	Adult Still's Disease	Antiphospholipid Syndrome	Behçet's Disease	Churg-Strauss Syndrome	Dermatomyositis/Polymyositis	Giant Cell (Temporal) Arteritis	Henoch-Schönlein Purpura	Microscopic Polyangiitis	Polyarteritis Nodosa	Rheumatoid Arthritis	Relapsing Polychondritis	Systemic Lupus Erythematosus	Sjögren's Syndrome	Systemic Sclerosis	Takayasu's Arteritis	Wegener's Granulomatosis
Renal	Acute renal failure								X		X	X		X		X		X
	Distal renal tubular acidosis														X			
	Ischemic renal complications			X	X													
	Renal crisis															X		
	Renal artery aneurysm										X							
	Rapidly progressive glomerulonephritis									X		X	X	X				X
Severe hypokalemia														X				
GI	Acute pancreatitis					X			X		X			X	X			
	Bowel perforation			X	X	X			X		X			X				X
	Esophageal necrosis with perforation			X														
	GI bleeding			X		X			X	X	X			X			X	
	Mesenteric vasculitis and ischemia			X		X			X		X	X		X			X	X
	Severe hepatic failure		X															

vasculitis is one of the most serious complications of systemic lupus erythematosus, with mortality of 13%.[31] Leukopenia, hypoalbuminemia, and elevated serum amylase are associated with poor outcome.[31] Bowel ischemia can be the result of the same pathophysiologic process that leads to acute coronary syndrome or the result of ischemic stroke or mesenteric artery vasculitis, as in lupus and other systemic rheumatic diseases. The patient may complain of symptoms consistent with "abdominal angina" prior to bowel infarction. Due to chronic or recurrent ischemia, the bowel may develop wall edema, strictures, and stenosis. These changes may account for colicky abdominal pain, diverticular disease, intestinal obstruction, or episodes of paralytic ileus. Acute pancreatitis is common in several systemic rheumatic diseases.

INFECTIOUS EMERGENCIES

Rheumatic diseases predispose to infection in several ways. The disease itself results in immunocompromise; treatment results in further immunosuppression (see "Adverse Drug Reaction" section below for infections associated with specific drugs used to manage systemic rheumatic diseases); the disease can result in anatomic changes that predispose to infection (see "Pulmonary Emergencies" above). Empiric antibiotics are indicated until infection can be clearly excluded. Using an elevated procalcitonin of 0.5 nanogram/mL is 90% specific for sepsis in patients with autoimmune diseases but is only 75% sensitive.[32] Isolated organisms may not differ from the normal population, but chronic immunosuppressive therapy may predispose patients with systemic rheumatic disease to opportunistic infections (i.e., *Candida*, *Pneumocystis jiroveci*, *Legionella*, *Mycobacterium tuberculosis*).

The prevalence of septic arthritis is doubled in patients with rheumatoid arthritis who are treated with glucocorticoids or tumor necrosis factor-α blockers.[33] The physical findings of severe pain and limited range of motion may be absent in cases of septic arthritis in patients with systemic rheumatic disease or may mimic a typical exacerbation of inflammatory arthritis.[34] Procalcitonin can help to differentiate septic from nonseptic arthritis, but using the standard cutoff of 0.5 nanogram/mL yields a sensitivity of only 46% to 67% with a specificity of 91%.[34] Using a lower cutoff of 0.25 nanogram/mL yields a sensitivity of 93% and a specificity of 75%.[34] Patients suspected of having septic arthritis should have arthrocentesis. See chapter 284, "Joints and Bursae" for further discussion of diagnosis and treatment.

OTHER EMERGENCIES

Several hematologic complications and other emergencies are encountered in patients with rheumatic diseases (**Table 282-8**).

Anemia, thrombocytopenia, leukopenia, and coagulation abnormalities are some of the important hematologic emergencies. Severe hemolytic anemia may develop in systemic lupus erythematosus (autoimmune) and in systemic sclerosis during renal crisis (microangiopathic). Thrombocytopenia is also observed in antiphospholipid syndrome patients and may present as thrombotic thrombocytopenic purpura. A low WBC count may also occur as a part of underlying disease or secondary to drug use. Pancytopenia can be observed when autoimmune rheumatic disorder affects all the cellular lines, in acute hemophagocytic syndrome, and in medullar suppression secondary to cytotoxic drugs. In autoimmune hematologic emergencies, transfusion of blood product may carry some risk of transfusion reaction.

Raynaud's phenomenon, digital ulcers, spontaneous finger ischemia, rash, and cellulitis are some examples of skin manifestations. In systemic lupus erythematosus, toxic epidermal necrolysis can be triggered by medication.

Patients with steroid-dependent rheumatic diseases are at risk for acute adrenal insufficiency either from unexpected stressors or from abrupt cessation of prescribed steroid medication.

Orchitis is one of the most characteristic manifestations of polyarteritis nodosa, and reports of scrotal involvement in boys with Henoch-Schönlein purpura range from 2% to 38%. Clinical findings include pain, tenderness, and swelling of the involved testicle and/or scrotum. The presentation may mimic testicular torsion. Ultrasonography confirms the correct diagnosis.

ADVERSE DRUG REACTIONS

Table 282-9 lists the more common clinical manifestations of adverse reactions associated with drugs used to manage systemic rheumatic diseases. When patients with systemic rheumatic diseases develop new

TABLE 282-8 Other Emergencies in Patients with Systemic Rheumatic Diseases

		Ankylosing Spondylitis	Adult Still's Disease	Antiphospholipid Syndrome	Behçet's Disease	Churg-Strauss Syndrome	Dermatomyositis/Polymyositis	Giant Cell (Temporal) Arteritis	Henoch-Schönlein Purpura	Microscopic Polyangiitis	Polyarteritis Nodosa	Rheumatoid Arthritis	Relapsing Polychondritis	Systemic Lupus Erythematosus	Sjögren's Syndrome	Systemic Sclerosis	Takayasu's Arteritis	Wegener's Granulomatosis
Other emergencies	Acute scrotum								X		X		X					
	Adrenal insufficiency			X														
	Disseminated intravascular coagulation		X	X														
	Hemolytic anemia			X										X				
	Microangiopathic hemolytic anemia		X	X										X		X		
	Pure red cell aplasia		X									X						
	Thrombotic thrombocytopenic purpura		X											X				
	Thyroiditis													X				

TABLE 282-9 Common Clinical Manifestations of Adverse Reactions to Drugs Used to Manage Systemic Rheumatic Diseases

	Abatacept	Anakinra	Azathioprine	Cyclophosphamide	Cyclosporine	Etanercept	Glucocorticoid	Gold	Hydroxychloroquine	Infliximab	Leflunomide	Methotrexate	Mycophenolate	NSAID	Rituximab	Sirolimus	Sulfasalazine	Tacrolimus	Thalidomide	Zileuton
Abdominal pain	X	X								X			X		X		X			
Acute/hemorrhagic cystitis				X	X					X										
Adrenal insufficiency							X													
Anaphylaxis	X																			
Anemia				X	X								X			X		X		
Creatine kinase increase										X										
Constipation																			X	
Chronic obstructive pulmonary disease exacerbation	X																			
Dermatologic manifestations								X		X				X						
Diarrhea	X							X					X		X	X	X			
Influenza-like syndrome										X		X								
GI bleeding							X	X						X						
Headache		X			X					X		X						X		X
Hyperglycemia					X		X											X		
Hyperkalemia					X											X		X	X	
Hypertension	X				X		X			X	X		X	X	X	X		X		
Immunosuppression, infection	X	X			X	X	X				X		X					X		
Leukopenia		X	X	X	X											X		X	X	X
Nausea and vomiting			X										X			X	X			
Ophthalmic impairment									X											
Orthostatic hypotension																			X	
Peripheral neuropathy																			X	
Psychiatric symptoms							X													
Pulmonary impairment												X								
Renal impairment					X			X				X		X				X		
Seizures					X													X		
Somnolence and sedation																			X	
Stomatitis								X				X								
Thrombocytopenia					X											X		X		
Thromboembolisms																			X	

Abbreviation: NSAID = nonsteroidal anti-inflammatory drug.

alarming and unexplained symptoms, a drug reference guide or similar resource should be consulted for a listing of rare adverse drug reactions.

IMMUNOSUPPRESSION

IMMUNOSUPPRESSION CAUSED BY DRUGS USED TO MANAGE SYSTEMIC RHEUMATIC DISEASES

Immunosuppressants and disease-modifying antirheumatic drugs are used to treat multiple types of systemic rheumatologic diseases with the aim to induce or maintain remission, to reduce exacerbations or relapse, and/or to allow tapering of glucocorticoids. These drugs have a variety of actions that are not completely understood but that modify critical pathways in the inflammatory process. They may cause immunosuppression primarily or as a side effect and lead to secondary diseases, infections, and reactivation of latent diseases or malignancies[35-43] (**Table 282-10**).

Risk factors for infection during immunosuppression include the drug, dose, duration of use, concomitant use of immunomodulators, the nature of the disease process, the functional status of the patient, health-care facility exposure, and older age.[44]

Glucocorticoids impact both the innate and acquired immune system through a variety of inhibitory mechanisms. Immediate effects on the innate immune system include decreased phagocyte migration, eosinophil apoptosis, decreased macrophage production and function, decreased degranulation of mast cells, decreased inflammatory cytokine production, and decreased proinflammatory mediators. Neutrophils are affected by decreased ability to bind to and exit the endothelium, increased release from bone marrow, and decreased apoptosis resulting in increased overall leukocytosis but decreased effectiveness.

Acquired immunity is also affected by a decrease in dendritic cells, rapid depletion of T cells, increased apoptosis of CD4 and CD8 cells, B-cell reduction (although to a lesser extent than T cells), and in chronic use, a decrease in immunoglobulin G and immunoglobulin A.[45] Glucocorticoid therapies are associated with a dose-dependent increase in risk of infection. In trials, infection occurs more often with steroid therapy (relative risk, 1.6). Infection rates increase in therapy doses greater than 10 milligrams/d or cumulative doses greater than 700 milligrams.

TABLE 282-10 Categories of Drugs Used to Treat Rheumatic Diseases and Common Infections Associated With Their Respective Use

	Biologic Agents	Conventional Agents	Cytoxic Agents	Other Agents	Common Infections Associated with Agent
Abatacept	x				Pneumonia, bronchitis, cellulitis, and UTI. Pharyngitis. Overall infection risk 54% in adults and 36% in children.
Adalimumab	x				URI. Sinusitis.
Anakinra	x				Nasopharyngitis. Cellulitis. Overall serious infection risk 2%–3%.
Azathioprine			x		Various due to leukopenia. Reactivation of latent viruses, bacteremia, interstitial pneumonia.
Belimumab	x				Viral gastroenteritis. UTI. Influenza. Bronchitis. URI. Sinusitis. Reactivation of polyoma viruses.
Canakinumab	x				URI. Pharyngitis. Bronchitis. Sinusitis. Influenza. Overall infection risk in children 30%–55%.
Certolizumab pegol	x		x		Pharyngitis. Sinusitis. Bronchitis. TB. UTI. Overall infection risk 38%. Serious infection risk 3%.
Chlorambucil			x		Interstitial pneumonia. Sterile cystitis.
Cyclophosphamide			x		Reactivation of latent viruses, sepsis (*Salmonella, Staphylococcus, Meningococcus*), URI, pneumonia, opportunistic infections.
Cyclosporine				x	Viral infections, CMV, bacterial pneumonia, fungal infection/sepsis. Reactivation of polyoma viruses. Hemorrhagic cystitis. Squamous cell cancer.
Etanercept	x				URI. Rhinitis. Pharyngitis. Overall infection risk 50%–81% in adults and 62% in children. Viral infections 4%.
Glucocorticoid					
Gold				x	Interstitial pneumonitis. Enterocolitis (rare with mortality rate of 50%).
Golimumab	x				URI. Pharyngitis. Sinusitis. Bronchitis. Overall infection risk 27%.
Hydroxychloroquine		x			Overall infection is low.
Infliximab	x				Overall infection risk 36%. URI. Pharyngitis. Sinusitis. Bronchitis.
Leflunomide				x	URI. Bronchitis. Pharyngitis. Pneumonia. Sinusitis. Skin abscess.
Methotrexate			x		Viral infections, CMV, EBV, reactivation of latent viruses. Reactivation of polyoma viruses.
Mycophenolate				x	Viral infections, CMV, reactivation of polyoma viruses.
NSAID				x	None
Rituximab	x				Pneumonia. Cerebral toxoplasmosis. Reactivation of latent viruses. Progressive multifocal leukoencephalopathy due to JC virus reactivation.
Sirolimus				x	Viral/bacterial pneumonias. Reactivation of polyoma viruses.
Sulfasalazine		x			Overall serious infection risk is low but increased in the setting of neutropenia.
Tacrolimus				X	Viral/bacterial pneumonias, fungal infection/sepsis. Squamous cell cancer.
Thalidomide			x		Pharyngitis. Rhinitis. Sinusitis. Overall infection risk 6%–8%.
Tocilizumab	x				Pharyngitis. Rhinitis. Sinusitis. Conjunctivitis. HSV.
Zileuton				X	URI. Sinusitis. Pharyngitis.

Abbreviations: CMV = cytomegalovirus; EBV = Epstein-Barr virus; HSV = herpes zoster virus; JC = John Cunningham; TB = tuberculosis; URI = upper respiratory infection; UTI = urinary tract infection.

REFERENCES

The complete reference list is available online at www.TintinalliEM.com.

CHAPTER 283 Nontraumatic Disorders of the Hand

Carl A. Germann

HAND INFECTIONS

PATHOPHYSIOLOGY

The most common pathogens causing hand infection are *Staphylococcus aureus, Streptococcus* species, and gram-negative species.[1] Polymicrobial infections are common, especially with inoculation of mouth flora. In most U.S. cities, community-associated methicillin-resistant *Staphylococcus aureus* is the most common pathogen cultured from patients with skin and soft tissue infections in EDs,[2] including 47% to 78% of hand infections.[3-8]

Injection drug users typically present with abscesses or deep space infections secondary to *S. aureus* and gram-negative organisms.[9] These infections are most commonly caused by direct introduction, but hematogenous spread from bacterial endocarditis is a possibility (see chapter 296, "Injection Drug Users").

Hand infections are also discussed in chapter 46, "Puncture Wounds and Bites."

Paronychia and felons are caused by minor trauma like chewing fingernails or exposing minor injuries to saliva. Most of these infections are polymicrobial including anaerobic bacteria.

Infections caused by animal bites reflect the oral flora of the involved species. Bites introduce a broad range of bacteria, including gram-positive, anaerobic, and gram-negative organisms. Common pathogens include streptococci, staphylococci, *Haemophilus, Eikenella, Fusobacterium*, peptostreptococci, *Prevotella*, and *Porphyromonas* species.[10] Cat and dog bites harbor *Pasteurella multocida*, which typically produces an aggressive, rapidly spreading cellulitis that becomes suppurative. (See chapter 46.)

Patients with diabetes or acquired immunodeficiency syndrome have common bacterial infection or develop atypical infections, including those caused by *Mycobacterium* or *Candida albicans*. Those who are immunocompromised or asplenic are at risk for rapid progression and require prompt source control and antibiotics.

PRINCIPLES OF EVALUATION AND MANAGEMENT

Hand infections are most commonly introduced by an injury to the dermis. The infection initially may remain superficial and broader, termed *cellulitis*, or be localized as seen in a paronychia or felon. Left untreated, infections may spread along anatomic planes or to adjacent compartments in the hand. Deeper injuries may directly seed underlying structures, creating rapidly spreading infections such as those seen with closed fist injuries or cat bites.

Obtain a directed history to delineate a likely cause of the infection. The physical examination should note the anatomic limits of the infection. Look for skin, subcutaneous tissue, fascial space, tendon, joint, or bone involvement. If deep structures of the hand are involved, emergently consult a hand specialist because treatment likely will involve inpatient care and operative drainage.

With the exception of superficial cellulitis, hand infections are managed using basic principles. **First**, incise and drain any collection of pus. Superficial and discrete infections, such as paronychia and felons, can be drained in the ED. Deep infections are better treated in the operating room by a hand surgeon. **Second**, immobilize and elevate the extremity. This will rest the hand, reduce inflammation, avoid secondary injury, and limit extension of the infection. Immobilize by applying a bulky hand dressing and splinting the hand in a position of function: the wrist at 15 to 30 degrees of extension, the metacarpophalangeal joints at 50 to 90 degrees of flexion, and the interphalangeal joints at 5 to 15 degrees of flexion (**Figure 283-1**). Elevate the hand on pillows or suspended using stockinet. **Third**, use broad-spectrum antibiotics initially targeting possible common and serious bacteria, altering only based on response and culture results (**Table 283-1**). **Fourth**, if the patient is not admitted to the hospital, ensure reexamination within 48 hours.

Empiric treatment for these infections is based on local antibiotic resistance patterns, using trimethoprim-sulfamethoxazole, doxycycline or minocycline (outpatient), or vancomycin or linezolid (inpatient) for methicillin-resistant *S. aureus* infections.[11] In some communities, clindamycin is effective,[11] whereas in other communities, fluoroquinolones are effective.[6]

CELLULITIS

Cellulitis is the most superficial of hand infections and is treated with oral antibiotics absent widespread or systemic signs. Diagnosis is made by documenting erythema, warmth, and edema in the affected portion of the hand without any involvement of deeper structures in the hand. Specifically, range of motion of the digits, hand, or wrist should not be painful, and palpation of the deeper structures of the hand should not produce any tenderness.

The most common offending organisms are *S. aureus* (**predominately methicillin-resistant**)[1-8] and *Streptococcus pyogenes*. Initial treatment is in Table 283-1. Methicillin-resistant *S. aureus* infections are more common in patients with diabetes mellitus, immunocompromised patients, intravenous drug users, prisoners, and the homeless.[3,4] Given the increasing rates of methicillin-resistant *S. aureus* and difficulty distinguishing among the types of *S. aureus* cellulitis, routine empiric treatment of methicillin-resistant *S. aureus* should be considered. In addition, choose an agent active against streptococci.[10] Empiric monotherapy with trimethoprim-sulfamethoxazole or other methicillin-resistant *S. aureus*–targeted antibiotic is not recommended given the limited published efficacy data and concerns about effectiveness against streptococci.[10,12] For more extensive involvement, start parenteral antibiotics, admit, and consult a hand surgeon. Consider admission for the immunocompromised, those with clinical toxicity, and those with rapidly spreading infections.

Hand infections following **injuries from handling fish** require different antibiotics and admission to the hospital. Infecting organisms include *Vibrio vulnificus*, *Klebsiella pneumoniae*, *Streptococcus* group A, *S. aureus*, and *Enterobacter* species.[13] Antibiotic coverage with ceftazidime and doxycycline was successful in a large case series of patients.[13]

For all cases of cellulitis, immobilize the hand in a position of function, and make sure the patient keeps the hand elevated as much as possible. Remove digit rings and give tetanus prophylaxis as needed. Finally, for those discharged, arrange reexamination within 48 hours.

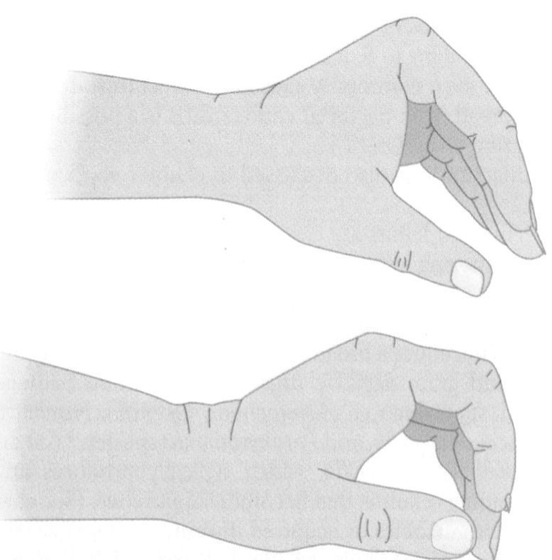

FIGURE 283-1. Positioning the hand during immobilization. Top position is used when splints are applied in fractures or severe sprains. Bottom position is the position of function used when applying a soft bulky dressing.

FLEXOR TENOSYNOVITIS

Flexor tenosynovitis is a surgical emergency. Failure to accurately diagnose and manage flexor tenosynovitis may result in adhesions, tendon vascular compromise and necrosis, or extension into adjoining deep spaces. This can lead to loss of function of the digit and eventually loss of function of the entire hand. The diagnosis is supported by the presence of the classic clinical signs described by Kanavel[1]; however, all four signs may not be present early in the course of infection (**Table 283-2**).

The infection usually is associated with penetrating trauma of the affected area, although the patient may be unaware of injury. *Staphylococcus* is the most common bacterium isolated; however, infections often harbor anaerobes or are polymicrobial. Suspect disseminated *Neisseria gonorrhoeae* in a patient with a recent history consistent with a sexually transmitted infection (see chapter 149, "Sexually Transmitted Infections").

Initiate treatment with parenteral antibiotics because the infection can spread rapidly through deep fascial spaces (Table 283-1). The use of vancomycin is recommended because of the high prevalence of methicillin-resistant *S. aureus* in most communities. Send any spontaneous exudate for Gram stain and culture with sensitivities.

Immobilize and elevate the hand, and consult the hand surgeon in the ED. If the infection is identified early in its course, nonoperative therapy with parenteral antibiotics, immobilization, elevation, and reevaluation is a common path.

DEEP SPACE INFECTIONS

The hand has compartments where infections may propagate and migrate. Infection of the spaces also occurs by direct inoculation or spread from surrounding structures. These areas include the thenar space, midpalmar space, radial bursa, and ulna bursa (see Figures 268-3 and 268-8 in chapter titled "Injuries to the Hand and Digits").

The volar aspect of the hand is covered by the tough and fixed tissues. The veins and lymphatics course through the softer tissues on the dorsum of the hand. Therefore, the dorsum of the hand often swells whenever there is an inflammatory or infectious process. For this reason, a deep space infection initially may be misdiagnosed as a cellulitis over the dorsum of the hand. An ideal **examination includes palpation of the volar surface of the hand to elicit tenderness, induration, or fluctuance.**

TABLE 283-1 Initial Antibiotic Coverage for Common Hand Infections

Infection	Initial Antimicrobial Agent(s)	Likely Organisms	Comments
Cellulitis	*For mild to moderate cellulitis*: TMP-SMX double strength, 1–2 tablets twice per day PO for 7–10 d.* *Plus/minus* cephalexin, 500 milligrams PO four times per day for 7–10 d, *or* dicloxacillin, 500 milligrams PO four times daily for 7–10 d. *For severe cellulitis:* Vancomycin, 1 gram IV every 12 h.	*Staphylococcus aureus* (MRSA) *Streptococcus pyogenes*	Clindamycin is an option, but increasing MRSA resistance to clindamycin has been reported. Consider vancomycin for injection drug abusers.
Felon/paronychia	TMP-SMX double strength, 1–2 tablets twice per day PO for 7–10 d.* *Plus/minus* cephalexin, 500 milligrams PO four times per day for 7–10 d,* *or* dicloxacillin, 500 milligrams PO four times daily for 7–10 d.* *Consider* addition of clindamycin or amoxicillin-clavulanate to TMP-SMX (rather than cephalexin) if anaerobic bacteria are suspected.	*S. aureus* (MRSA), *S. pyogenes*, anaerobes, polymicrobial	Antibiotics indicated for infections with associated localized cellulitis, otherwise drainage alone may be sufficient, culture recommended by hand surgeons.[4-7]
Flexor tenosynovitis	Ampicillin-sulbactam, 1.5 grams IV every 6 h, *or* cefoxitin, 2 grams IV every 8 h, *or* piperacillin-tazobactam, 3.375 grams IV every 6 h. *Plus:* vancomycin, 1 gram IV every 12 h, if MRSA is prevalent in community.	*S. aureus*, streptococci, anaerobes, gram negatives	Parenteral antibiotics are indicated; consider ceftriaxone for suspected *Neisseria gonorrhoeae*.
Deep space infection	Ampicillin-sulbactam, 1.5 grams IV every 6 h, *or* cefoxitin, 2 grams IV every 8 h, *or* piperacillin-tazobactam, 3.375 grams IV every 6 h. *Plus:* vancomycin, 1 gram IV every 12 h, if MRSA is prevalent in community.	*S. aureus*, streptococci, anaerobes, gram negatives	Inpatient management.
Animal bites (including human)	If no visible signs of infection: amoxicillin/clavulanate, 875/125 milligrams PO twice daily for 5 d. For signs of infection: ampicillin-sulbactam, 1.5 grams IV every 6 h, *or* cefoxitin, 2 grams IV every 8 h, *or* piperacillin-tazobactam, 3.375 grams every 6 h. For penicillin allergy, use clindamycin plus moxifloxacin or TMP-SMX and metronidazole.	*S. aureus*, streptococci, *Eikenella corrodens* (human), *Pasteurella multocida* (cat), anaerobes, and gram-negative bacteria	All animal bite wounds should receive prophylactic oral antibiotics.
Herpetic whitlow	Acyclovir, 400 milligrams PO three times daily for 10 d.	Herpes simplex	No surgical drainage is indicated.

Abbreviations: MRSA = methicillin-resistant *Staphylococcus aureus*; TMP-SMX = trimethoprim-sulfamethoxazole.

*While many sources recommend 7-10 days of therapy, the Infectious Disease Society of America recommends 5 days of therapy if symptoms resolve, continue therapy if symptoms persist.

Range of motion of the digits often produces marked pain for the patients with deep space infection.

Occasionally, infections will arise in the web space. These "collar button" abscesses present with pain and swelling of the web space causing separation of the affected digits. Examination reveals induration or fluctuance in the dorsal and/or volar web space, along with erythema, warmth, and tenderness.

Deep space infections arise from penetrating inoculation, contiguous spread, and rare, hematogenous seeding.[1] *S. aureus* and *Streptococcus* species are the most common organisms isolated.[1]

Give parenteral antibiotics (Table 283-1) and opioid analgesia, and immobilize and elevate the hand. Operative draining is often needed, requiring emergent hand surgeon consultation.

INFECTIONS FROM CLOSED FIST INJURIES

The most common human bite infection of the hand is the result of striking another individual's teeth with a clenched fist (**Figure 283-2**). Often termed "fight bite infections," these injuries usually occur over the dorsal aspects of the third, fourth, and fifth metacarpophalangeal joints. Although these injuries may at first appear innocuous, morbidity can result from late presentation or inadequate initial management

TABLE 283-2 Kanavel's Four Cardinal Signs of Flexor Tenosynovitis

Percussion tenderness	Tenderness over the entire length of the flexor tendon sheath
Uniform swelling	Symmetric finger swelling along the length of the tendon sheath
Intense pain	Intense pain with passive extension
Flexion posture	Flexed posture of the involved digit at rest to minimize pain

Because of the force and the penetrating nature of the human incisor, closed fist infections tend to occur in multiple planes and spread rapidly to adjacent compartments. Skin, extensor tendons, joint space, bone, and surrounding deep spaces often are involved because the inoculum may traverse all these structures.

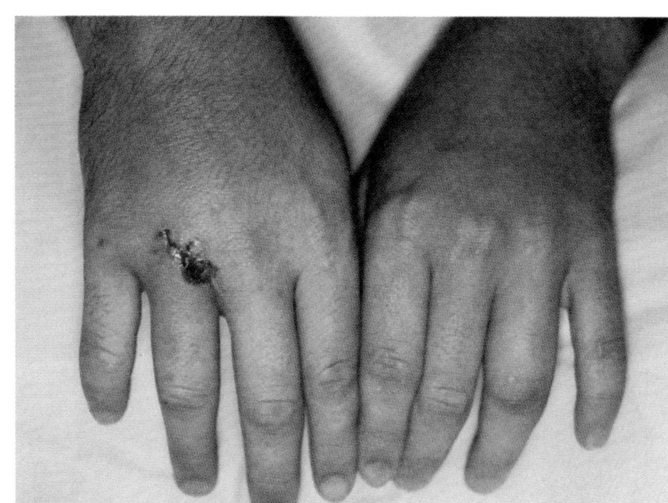

FIGURE 283-2. Clenched fist injury. The lacerations in this photograph were sustained from teeth during a fight. Note the subtle black ink stamp across the proximal metacarpals possibly revealing a clue about the wound's etiology. [Photo contributor: Lawrence B. Stack, MD. Reproduced with permission from Knoop KJ, Stack LB, Storrow AB, Thurman RJ (eds): *The Atlas of Emergency Medicine*, 3rd ed. New York: McGraw-Hill; 2010, Fig 11-30.]

On examination, document the extent of the infection. Plain radiographs will detect fractures or foreign material including tooth fragments. The most common organisms reflect the natural flora of the mouth and include *Streptococcus* species, *S. aureus, Eikenella corrodens, Fusobacterium, Peptostreptococcus,* and *Candida* species; polymicrobial sources are common. If you suspect any deep space, palmar space, joint, or tendon infection, give broad antibiotics and consult a hand surgeon for open debridement and irrigation in the operating room. Treat all infections with hand elevation and splinting in the position of function. Unless very superficial, use prophylactic antibiotics for wounds caused by a clenched fist (Table 283-1).

PARONYCHIA

Paronychia is an infection of the lateral nail fold or perionychium, occasionally extending to the cuticle or eponychium. It is usually caused by minor trauma such as nail-biting, manicures, or embedded lateral nails ("hangnails"). The infection often starts as a small area of induration that progresses to eponychial swelling, tenderness, erythema, and drainage. Most paronychia contains both aerobic and anaerobic bacteria, with *S. aureus* and *Streptococcus* species the most common aerobic bacteria cultured. Chronic paronychia occurs, particularly in patients who are immunocompromised, and may include usual pathogens or atypical bacteria and fungi such as with *C. albicans.*[14]

Absent fluctuance, treat the paronychia with warm soaks, elevation, and antibiotics (Table 283-1). Suppuration leads to either fluctuance or identifiable pus requiring drainage. Minor infections can be treated with elevation of the perionychium or eponychium with a flat probe to encourage drainage (**Figure 283-3**). If drainage is successful, use warm soaks for days after care. In general, only nonviable tissue can be incised without provoking pain.

More extensive infections that do not communicate directly with the nail fold require digital block and incision directly into the area of greatest fluctuance. Severe infections with pus beneath the nail require removal of a portion of the lateral or proximal nail to ensure adequate drainage. Rarely, a free-floating nail will be encountered on a bed of pus, necessitating removal of the entire nail.

Following incision and drainage, keep the hand elevated and immobilized. Warm soaks may be initiated to keep the wound open and clean. Routine antibiotics are not needed unless cellulitis, immunocompromise, or vascular insufficiency exists; when used, a 7-day course is common or until resolution of the infection.[13] In complicated or drained cases, reassess the wound within 48 hours.

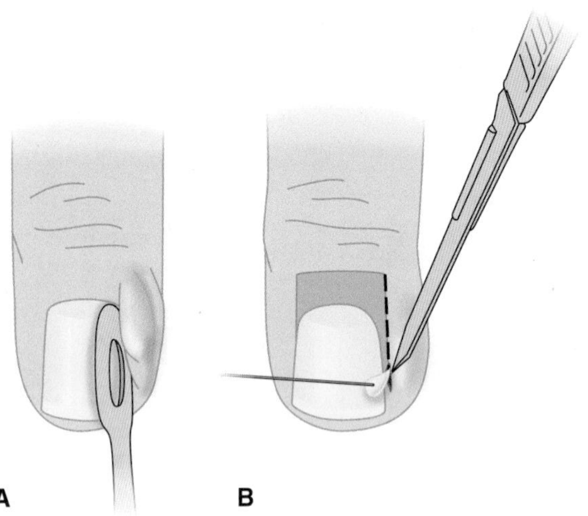

FIGURE 283-3. Paronychia. **A.** The eponychial fold is elevated using a flat probe or a #11 blade to allow the wound to drain. **B.** Alternatively, for more extensive infections, a #11 blade may be used to incise the area of greatest fluctuance directly into the eponychium. The wound may then be gently probed with a small clamp to ensure drainage.

FELON

A felon is a subcutaneous pyogenic infection of the pulp space of the distal finger or thumb. The septa of the finger pad produce multiple individual compartments and confine the infection under pressure. This results in a red, tense, and markedly painful distal pulp space. Infection typically begins with minor trauma to the dermis overlying the finger pad. The infection can start and spread between septae, forming multiple compartmentalized abscesses. Left untreated, the infection may spread to the flexor tendon sheath, causing flexor tenosynovitis, or to the underlying periosteum, resulting in osteomyelitis.

S. aureus is the most common organism (primarily methicillin-resistant *S. aureus*),[3] but *Streptococcus* species, anaerobes, and gram-negative organisms are frequent. If possible, obtain a Gram stain and culture since these infections may be difficult to eradicate, and chronic infections may be caused by atypical organisms. If osteomyelitis occurs, identification of the offending organism guides long-term antibiotic therapy.

Drain the infection if the finger pad is swollen and tense or if there is any palpable fluctuance. A digital block using a long-acting anesthetic is ideal for comfort (see chapter 36, "Local and Regional Anesthesia"). A unilateral longitudinal approach spares the sensate volar pad and achieves adequate drainage (**Figure 283-4A**). Do not incise the distal end of the finger pad because this can cause instability and loss of sensation to the fingertip. Dissect the septa using a small clamp to ensure complete drainage. A small wick encourages continued drainage.

If the felon is pointing toward the volar fat pad, an option is a longitudinal volar approach, depicted in **Figure 283-4B**. Avoid extending the incision to the flexor crease of the distal interphalangeal joint. **More extensive incisions such as the "fishmouth," "hockey stick," and through-and-through incisions are not indicated** as these can alter sensation to the fingertip or compromise pulp vascularity.

Following drainage, irrigate the wound and place a dry, sterile dressing; ask the patient to keep the extremity elevated. Reevaluate the wound within 48 hours, and use warm soaks to keep the wound clean and promote continued drainage.

Most felons have associated cellulitis that should be treated with oral antibiotics (Table 283-1). Refer chronic felons or felons not responding to the above treatments to a hand specialist for more definitive management and long-term follow-up.

HERPETIC WHITLOW

Herpetic whitlow is a viral infection of the distal finger caused by the herpes simplex virus, usually from contact with oral herpetic infections. Herpetic whitlow in children tends to be associated with gingivostomatitis and herpes simplex virus type 1, whereas adults most commonly harbor herpes simplex virus type 2. Healthcare workers, often nurses and respiratory and dental technicians, are at increased risk of this infection given their exposure to orotracheal secretions.

The patient develops a burning, pruritic sensation similar to all herpes simplex infections. On examination, the lesion is erythematous and tender, with vesicular bullae (**Figure 283-5**). The infection occurs 2 to 14 days after contact, usually maturing in 14 days.[1] The finger may be indurated, but is not tense, as is seen in a felon. **Do not mistake herpetic whitlow for a felon because incision and drainage may result in a secondary bacterial infection and prolonged failure to heal.** If there is any question concerning the diagnosis of herpetic whitlow, a vesicle may be unroofed, and the drainage fluid may be used for a Tzanck smear to confirm the diagnosis.

Herpetic whitlow usually resolves without treatment within 3 weeks.[15] Treatment consists of immobilization, elevation, and pain medication. Antiviral agents such as acyclovir or valacyclovir may abort recurrent infections and decrease the course of protracted cases[1] (Table 283-1). The finger should be kept in a clean dressing to prevent autoinoculation or spread of the herpes infection to other individuals.

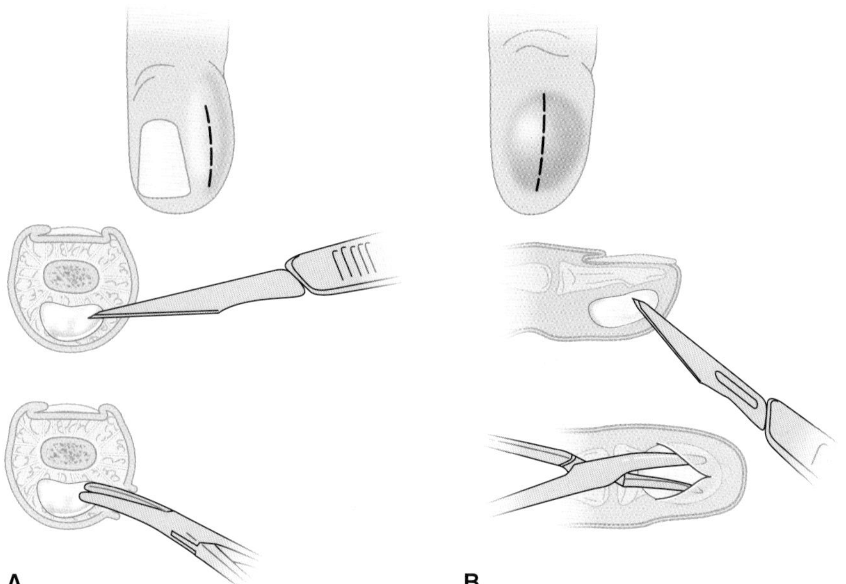

FIGURE 283-4. Felon. **A.** The unilateral longitudinal approach is the most frequently used method for draining felons. This approach minimizes interference with sensate areas of the finger pad. **B.** If the felon is pointing toward the volar surface of the finger pad, the longitudinal volar approach may be used.

NONINFECTIOUS INFLAMMATORY STATES OF THE HAND

Noninfectious inflammatory states of the hand often present as an acute exacerbation of symptoms related to recent overuse. Inflammatory states of joints and tendons are painful and difficult to distinguish from acute septic arthritis or suppurative tenosynovitis. If the diagnosis is in doubt, treat for infection, and consult a hand specialist.

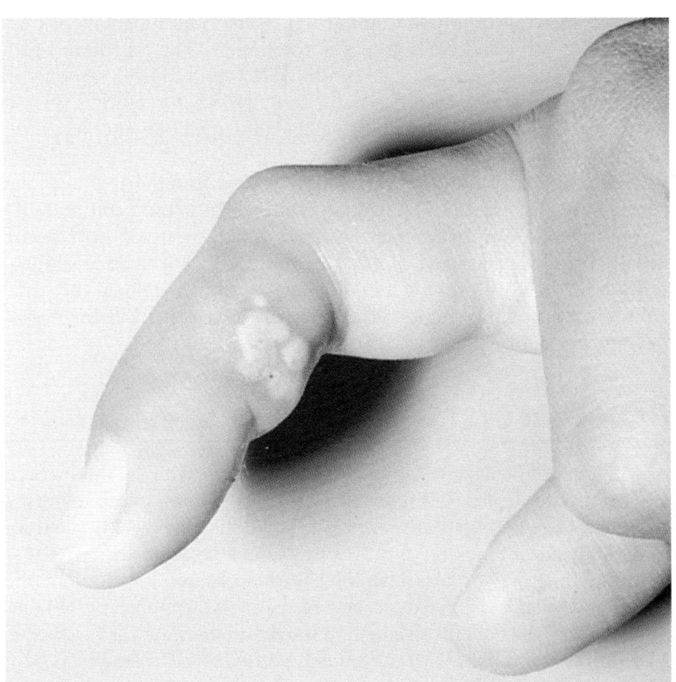

FIGURE 283-5. Herpetic whitlow. Note the cluster of vesicles on an erythematous base located at the distal finger. Tzanck smear is positive. [Photo contributor: Lawrence B. Stack, MD. Reproduced with permission from Knoop K, Stack L, Storrow A, Thurman RJ: *Atlas of Emergency Medicine,* 3rd ed. New York, NY: McGraw-Hill; 2010.]

If an inflammatory state is diagnosed, treat with rest, immobilization, elevation, and anti-inflammatory agents.

TENDINITIS AND TENOSYNOVITIS

Inflammatory tendinitis may involve the flexor or extensor tendons of the hand. Most often, the patient is able to recount a history of repetitive motion directly affecting the inflamed tendon. Palpation of the tendon produces tenderness. Active or passive movement of the tendon produces significant pain.

Treatment is splinting in the position of function with elevation of the affected area and prescribing nonsteroidal anti-inflammatory drugs, with referral for care from the primary care physician or a hand surgeon. Remind patients to return to the ED for worsening pain, increased swelling, or any signs of infection, including fever and erythema.

TRIGGER FINGER

Tenosynovitis can develop in the flexor sheaths of the fingers and thumb as a result of repetitive use. Scarring or inflammation may cause the tendon to become nodular, which results in friction and catching between the tendon and its sheath, usually in the vicinity of the A1 pulley at the volar crease at the base of each digit. The A1 pulley is the proximal portion of the tendon sheath. This is referred to as *stenosing tenosynovitis* or "*trigger finger*." The patient experiences binding of the tendon, usually as the finger extends, relieved by a painful "snap" as the tendon clears the obstruction. Occasionally, this condition may progress to the point that the finger locks, usually in flexion. Conservative treatment includes rest, anti-inflammatory medications, and immobilization (buddy tape or finger split) to reduce inflammation and swelling of the flexor tendon sheath. Early stages of trigger finger have been treated successfully with corticosteroid injection into the tendon sheath,[16] although recurrence occurs in over half of patients.[17] Surgical release of the A1 pulley is curative.

DE QUERVAIN'S STENOSING TENOSYNOVITIS

De Quervain's tenosynovitis is a common condition that occurs in patients who have experienced excessive use of the thumb or wrist. Often, no plausible cause is found. This is a tenosynovitis of the extensor

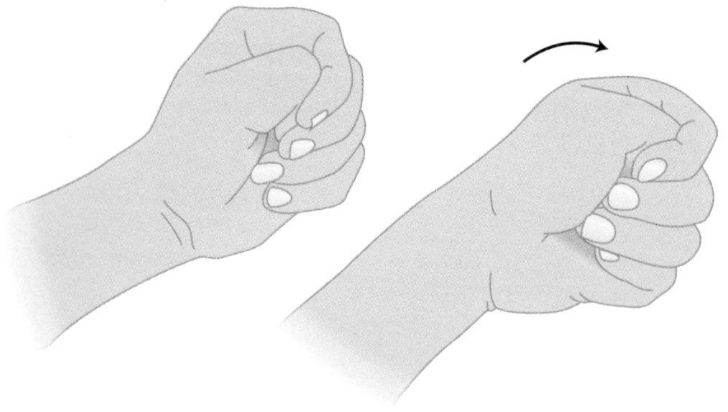

FIGURE 283-6. The Finkelstein test. The thumb is cupped in the closed fist, and ulnar deviation reproduces pain along the extensor pollicis and abductor pollicis.

pollicis brevis and abductor pollicis tendons, where the tendons lie in the groove of the radial styloid.

The patient presents with pain along the radial aspect of the wrist that may radiate to the thumb or extend into the forearm. The diagnosis of De Quervain's tenosynovitis is supported by a history of pain in this location along with a painful range of motion of the thumb and local tenderness over the distal portion of the radial styloid. Further confirmation of the diagnosis may be provided by a positive Finkelstein test (**Figure 283-6**), in which the patient grasps the thumb in the palm of the hand and the examiner ulnar deviates the thumb and hand. This stretches the tendons over the radial styloid and produces sharp pain along the involved tendons.

Immobilize the thumb and wrist with a splint. Instruct the patient to remove the splint briefly each day and perform range-of-motion exercises to prevent joint stiffness. Also, start an anti-inflammatory medication for 10 to 14 days. Recurrence of this condition is common, particularly when related to occupational stress. Persistent cases may benefit from local corticosteroid injection or surgical decompression.[17]

CARPAL TUNNEL SYNDROME

Carpal tunnel syndrome is a peripheral mononeuropathy involving entrapment of the median nerve in the carpal canal or tunnel, which is covered by the tense transverse carpal ligament. Whenever a condition causes swelling in the carpal tunnel, the median nerve is compressed, causing paresthesias extending into the index and long fingers, the radial aspect of the ring finger, and along the palmar aspect of the thumb. Pain may also radiate proximally into the forearm or shoulder. The patient often complains of awakening at night with burning pain and tingling in the hand, or numbness when driving a car or maintaining the wrist in prolonged flexion.

Carpal tunnel syndrome may develop from traumatic, hematologic, rheumatologic, anatomic, and infectious causes. A common scenario is overuse, in which the patient recounts a history of repeated flexion and extension of the wrist. Also, edematous conditions such as pregnancy and congestive heart failure may acutely exacerbate symptoms in patients with a predisposition for carpal tunnel syndrome. The final common pathway consists of a space-occupying lesion that increases intracanal pressures. As the pressure increases, perfusion of the epineurium decreases, causing ischemia and nerve conduction block.

Pain or paresthesia in the median nerve distribution suggests carpal tunnel syndrome and may be confirmed by electrodiagnostic testing. The median nerve sensory distribution is illustrated in chapter 36. Two-point discrimination in this distribution is described as one of the most useful physical examination maneuvers for diagnosing carpal tunnel syndrome.[18] In addition, Tinel's sign supports the diagnosis and involves tapping the volar aspect of the wrist over the median nerve. A positive sign produces paresthesias that extend into the index and long finger. Phalen's sign is more sensitive and specific, and involves flexing the wrist maximally and holding it in this position for at least 1 minute. A positive test occurs when the patient complains of tingling and numbness along the median nerve distribution. Both tests are subject to false-positive and false-negative results.

The presence of median nerve motor deficit requires emergency hand consultation. Otherwise, initial treatment is a volar splint to maintain the wrist in neutral position coupled with anti-inflammatory medications for 10 to 14 days. Refer those with persistent symptoms to a hand surgeon for surgical decompression. Most patients have complete resolution of their symptoms following surgical decompression, with around 5% requiring revision.[19]

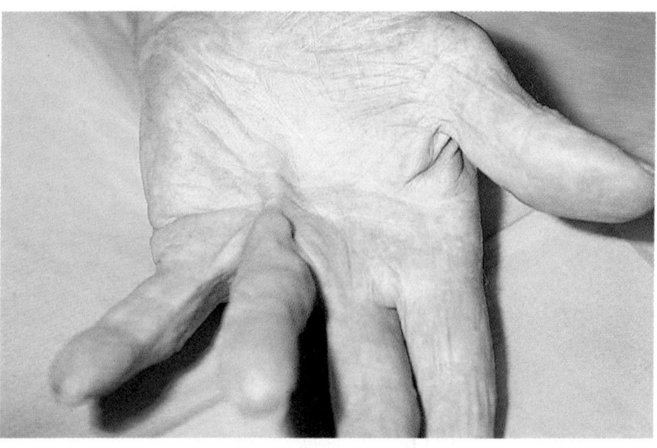

FIGURE 283-7. Dupuytren's contracture. This chronic problem is seen at the most common site: the ring finger. [Photo contributor: Alan B. Storrow, MD. Reproduced with permission from Knoop KJ, Stack LB, Storrow AB, & Thurman RJ (eds): *The Atlas of Emergency Medicine*, 3rd ed. New York: McGraw-Hill; 2010, Fig. 12-36.]

DUPUYTREN'S CONTRACTURE

Dupuytren's contracture is a relatively common yet poorly understood disorder characterized by fibroplastic changes of the subcutaneous tissues of the palm and volar aspect of the fingers. The fourth and fifth fingers are affected earliest. The condition is found most commonly in men of northern European descent. Dupuytren's contracture is seen in those with tobacco use, alcoholism, diabetes mellitus, and repetitive handling or overuse.[20]

This progressive fibrosis eventually may lead to tethering and joint contracture (**Figure 283-7**). Firm longitudinal thickening and nodularity of the superficial tissues over the distal tendon sheath of the palm are usually readily appreciated as the scarring process advances. The diagnosis is made by identifying a nodule in the palm, usually at the distal palmar crease of the ring or small finger, which is held in the classic flexion contracture. Refer to a hand specialist for excision.[21]

GANGLION CYSTS

A ganglion or synovial cyst is a cystic collection of synovial fluid within a joint or tendon sheath (**Figure 283-8**). It is common, often following an injury. Ganglion cysts arise from a herniation of synovial tissue from a joint capsule or tendon sheath. The patient presents with a tender cystic swelling over or near a tendon sheath. Common locations are the dorsal and volar wrist, flexor surface of the metacarpophalangeal joint, or the base of the nail. Involvement of the thumb may appear as generalized thumb pain, pain with movement, and edema. Treatment is pain control and anti-inflammatory medications. About one third of cysts resolve spontaneously, with referral to a hand surgeon for those with persistent or recurrent pain or cosmetic deformity. Treatment options include cyst aspiration, corticosteroid injection, or surgical excision. Surgery is generally effective; however, ganglion cysts may recur in up to 39% of patients.[22]

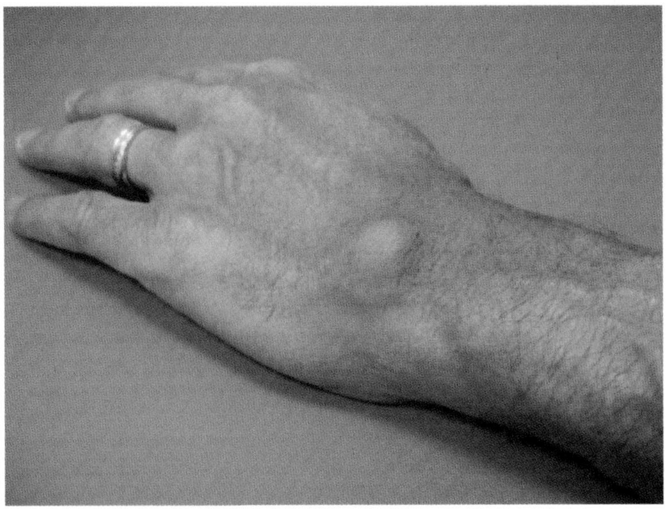

FIGURE 283-8. A dorsal ganglion cyst. [Reproduced with permission from Simon RR and Sherman SC (EDS). *Simon's Emergency Orthopedics*, 7th ed. New York, NY: McGraw-Hill, Inc., 2014.]

REFERENCES

The complete reference list is available online at www.TintinalliEM.com.

CHAPTER 284 Joints and Bursae

John H. Burton
Timothy J. Fortuna

INTRODUCTION

Many mechanisms provoke acute joint symptoms: degradation and degeneration of articular cartilage (osteoarthritis), deposition of immune complexes or immune system–related phenomena (rheumatoid arthritis, rheumatic fever and possibly, a component of gonococcal arthritis), crystal-induced inflammation (gout and pseudogout), seronegative spondyloarthropathies (ankylosing spondylitis [see chapter 282, "Systemic Rheumatic Diseases"] and reactive arthritis [postinfectious with HLA-B27 susceptibility]), and bacterial invasion (gonococcal and nongonococcal septic arthritis, including Lyme arthritis) or viral invasion (viral arthritis). These processes impact joint capsules and surfaces, resulting in a cascade of reactive and inflammatory events. S*eptic arthritis* is invasion of a joint by an infectious agent with organism proliferation and associated inflammation; bacterial arthritis is a subset of septic arthritis. Under ideal conditions, the infectious agent is recoverable from the joint fluid in septic arthritis, but in clinical practice, this is often not the case. This chapter reviews the common causes and treatments of acute nontraumatic joint pain. Joint injuries are discussed in section 22, "Injuries to Bones and Joints," and disorders due to repetitive use syndromes are discussed in section 23, "Musculoskeletal Disorders," by anatomic site.

CLINICAL APPROACH TO ACUTE JOINT PAIN

Septic arthritis is the most important consideration in the evaluation of a swollen, warm, and painful joint. Urgent treatment may prevent both joint destruction and mortality (11% with treatment).[1,2] The diagnosis of septic arthritis is clinical and is supported by diagnostic tests.[1,2] **No single diagnostic parameter is sufficiently sensitive to screen patients for septic arthritis including synovial WBC counts.**[3]

TABLE 284-1 Risk Factors for Nongonococcal and Gonococcal Septic Arthritis

Nongonococcal	Gonococcal
Injection drug use*	HIV infection*
Diabetes mellitus*	Injection drug use*
Rheumatoid arthritis*	Pregnancy
Prosthetic joint, knee,* or hip*	Menses
Immunosuppression, HIV*	Systemic lupus erythematosus
Age: >80 y old*	Complement deficiency
Skin ulceration and/or infection*	
Hemophilia	
Hypogammaglobulinemia	
Malignancy	
Hemodialysis	
Liver disease	
Alcoholism	
Steroid therapy	

Abbreviation: HIV = human immunodeficiency virus.
*Risk factors supported by epidemiologic study.

CLINICAL FEATURES AND RISK FACTORS

Risk factors (**Table 284-1**),[3,4] the number of joints involved (**Table 284-2**), and the migratory pattern (**Table 284-3**), if one exists, aid in the differential diagnosis. Approximately 85% of patients with nongonococcal septic arthritis present with a single joint infected; *Staphylococcus aureus* and *Streptococcus pneumoniae* are more likely to infect two or more joints simultaniously.[5-8] Septic arthritis involving more than one joint can occur in rheumatoid arthritis (50%), immunocompromise, gout, diabetes, and/or renal disease; the morality rate is significantly higher in patients with polyarticular septic arthritis (11% vs 30%).[5,7] Recent joint surgery and cellulitis overlying a prosthetic hip or knee are the only

TABLE 284-2 Differential Diagnosis of Arthritis by Number of Affected Joints

Number of Joints	Differential Considerations for Typical Presentations
1 = Monoarthritis	85% of nongonococcal septic arthritis*
	Crystal-induced (gout, pseudogout)
	Gonococcal septic arthritis
	Trauma-induced arthritis
	Osteoarthritis (acute)
	Lyme disease
	Avascular necrosis
	Tumor
2–3 = Oligoarthritis†	15% of nongonococcal septic arthritis, more common with *Staphylococcus aureus* and *Streptococcus pneumoniae*
	Lyme disease
	Reactive arthritis (Reiter's syndrome)
	Gonococcal arthritis
	Rheumatic fever
>3 = Polyarthritis†	Rheumatoid arthritis
	Systemic lupus erythematosus
	Viral arthritis
	Osteoarthritis (chronic)
	Serum sickness
	Serum sickness–like reactions

*Involvement of more than one joint does not rule out septic arthritis.
†The distinction between oligoarthritis and polyarthritis varies in the literature with a cut point of either three or four joints.

TABLE 284-3 Common Joint Disorders with a Migratory Distribution Pattern
Gonococcal arthritis
Acute rheumatic fever
Lyme disease
Viral arthritis
Systemic lupus erythematosus

findings on history or physical examination that significantly alter (both increase) the probability of nongonococcal septic arthritis.[3]

SYNOVIAL FLUID ANALYSIS

When septic arthritis is suspected, aspirate joint fluid, and obtain analysis and culture of the aspirate to direct treatment.[1,2] Table 284-4 provides diagnostic guidance based on synovial fluid results in the context of different patient characteristics.[1-12]

Analyze joint fluid for Gram stain, leukocyte count with differential, and a wet preparation for crystals.[4,6] Glucose, protein, and lactate dehydrogenase levels do not direct treatment decisions.[4] Synovial lactate levels may prove an aide in identifying septic arthritis if future studies confirm preliminary reports.[3] Culture for gonococci and anaerobes, in addition to typical gram-positive and -negative organisms.[1,2,4]

SERUM LABORATORY STUDIES

Serum erythrocyte sedimentation rate and C-reactive protein levels are commonly elevated in several acute inflammatory and reactive arthritides (gonococcal and nongonococcal septic arthritis, crystal-induced, spondyloarthropathies, and rheumatoid and Lyme arthritis) but are not helpful for establishing a specific diagnosis in adults. However, erythrocyte

TABLE 284-4 Septic Arthritis: Joint Aspiration Results in Different Patient Groups*

Key Factor	Patient Status	Joint Aspiration	Diagnostic Considerations/Management
Positive Gram stain	Acute joint pain and swelling	Gram stain positive for bacteria	Initiate empiric IV antibiotics, admit to the hospital, monitor culture and patient course (positive Gram stain is found in <50% of patients with septic arthritis).
Classic synovial WBC count	Acute joint pain and swelling	>50,000 WBC/mm^3 or >90% PMNs	Synovial fluid with >50,000 WBC/mm^3 is 56% sensitive and 90% specific for septic arthritis. Initiate empiric IV antibiotics and hospital admission.
Increased sensitivity of lower synovial WBC counts	Acute joint pain and swelling in a patient with risk factors for septic arthritis or systemic signs of infection	>25,000 WBC/mm^3 or >90% PMNs	Synovial fluid with >25,000 WBC/mm^3 is 73% sensitive and 77% specific for septic arthritis. Consider empiric IV antibiotics and admission to the hospital for monitoring of patient course and cultures.
Acute gout with coexisting septic arthritis	Acute joint pain and swelling; patient with acute gout or history of gout with systemic signs of infection	Crystals, >2000 WBC/mm^3, or >90% PMNs	Crystal-induced arthritis may coexist with septic arthritis; cell counts are <6000 WBC/mm^3 in 10% of infected joints; more than one joint is involved in 10%–45%. Look for infected tophi. Consider empiric IV antibiotics and admission to the hospital for monitoring of patient course and cultures.
Prosthetic joint	Acute pain and swelling in patient with prosthetic joint	>10,000 WBC/mm^3, >90% PMNs	Consult operating orthopedic surgeon before aspiration if possible. AAOS definition for acute periprosthetic infection is 3 of the following: (1) CRP elevated above 100 milligrams/L *and* ESR elevated above local norm, (2) synovial WBC >10,000/mm^3, (3) synovial PMNs >90%, (4) positive culture, and (5) positive histologic analysis of periprosthetic tissue.
Immunocompromise	Joint swelling in an immunocompromised patient or systemic signs of infection in a patient with immunocompromise	>200 WBC/mm^3, >25% PMNs	Immunocompromised patients sustain septic arthritis with diminished immune response; cell counts and percent PMNs are frequently lower than in immunocompetent patients with similar infections. Consider empiric IV antibiotics and admission to the hospital for monitoring of patient course and cultures.
Gonococcal arthritis	Monoarticular or polyarticular joint pain in a patient with history of unprotected sex (primarily in young patients)	10,000–80,000 WBC/mm^3	Positive culture in <50% of infected joints; collect urogenital cultures plus pharynx and rectum cultures as determined by history. Consider empiric IV antibiotics and admission to the hospital for monitoring of patient course and cultures.
Rheumatoid arthritis with coexisting septic arthritis	Joint pain and/or swelling in a patient with rheumatoid arthritis	2000–120,000 WBC/mm^3	Severe pain and limited range of motion may be absent in patients on immunosuppression. Look for infected rheumatoid nodules or ulcerated foot calluses; source in 76% of cases. Consider empiric IV antibiotics and admission to the hospital for monitoring of patient course and cultures.
Lyme disease	Acute joint pain in a patient living in a Lyme disease–endemic area or with a history of rash or tick bite	200–300,000 WBC/mm^3	Consider empiric antibiotics and close follow-up to monitor culture and patient course; admit if clinical picture is indistinguishable from septic arthritis. Arthralgia appears months after initial symptoms. Joint effusion (moderate to large) may be out of proportion to the patient's pain (mild to moderate). Knee is the most common affected joint.
Post trauma	Joint trauma several days prior, initial swelling, now increasing pain	0–2000 WBC/mm^3, <25% PMNs, 0–500 RBC/mm^3	Posttraumatic effusions may become infected in patients with skin infections or bacteremia. Aspiration of the joint reduces pain for approximately 1 week, but has no effect on long-term disability.
Dry tap	Patient with acute joint pain and suspected swelling, with or without other symptoms or signs to suggest septic arthritis	"Dry tap"	Major causes of dry tap are mistaken physical diagnosis of effusion; blockage of the needle by plica, fat, or debris; or synovial fluid with high viscosity or true lipoma arborescens (benign replacement of subsynovial tissue by fat cells). Use US to determine true effusion and direct needle to largest collection of fluid.
Normal synovial cell counts	Patient with sufficient joint pain and swelling to warrant arthrocentesis, no comorbidities, absent signs and symptoms of sepsis	<200 WBC/mm^3, <25% PMNs	Normal WBC cell counts and differential percentages make the diagnosis of septic arthritis unlikely in a patient without comorbidities or objective signs of infection. A mechanism should be in place for timely follow-up of culture results if they turn positive.

Abbreviations: AAOS = American Academy of Orthopedic Surgeons; CRP = C-reactive protein; ESR = erythrocyte sedimentation rate; PMNs = polymorphonuclear leukocytes.

*All patients who received joint aspiration for suspected septic arthritis should have cultures of synovial fluid, blood, and any nonjoint source clinically suspected of infection (e.g., skin, urine).

sedimentation rate and C-reactive protein are recommended as an aid to monitor response to therapy by the British Society of Rheumatology Guidelines,[2] and the American Academy of Orthopedic Surgeons guidelines include erythrocyte sedimentation rate and C-reactive protein as part of their minor criteria for the diagnosis of acute periprosthetic joint infection (Table 284-4).[11] The American Academy of Orthopedic Surgeons also recommends that an elevation of either erythrocyte sedimentation rate or C-reactive protein be used as criterion to aspirate a painful prosthetic joint with increased warmth.[11] The sensitivity of the serum WBC count in adults for the diagnosis of nongonococcal bacterial septic arthritis is approximately 60%.[3] Blood cultures should be obtained before antibiotic therapy for presumptive or possible septic arthritis. However, the sensitivity for identifying the causative organism in adults and children with nongonococcal bacterial septic arthritis is 23% to 36%.[3] Elevated procalcitonin levels provide 90% specificity to help rule in the diagnosis of septic arthritis but are only 67% sensitive in screening for the diagnosis.[3,13]

Laboratory studies can aid in the diagnosis at follow-up. Possible studies include Lyme titer, rheumatoid factor, antinuclear antibodies, antineutrophil cytoplasmic antibodies, HLA-B27 tissue typing, lupus anticoagulant, and repeat synovial fluid analysis.

IMAGING

Bedside US is useful to identify joint effusion and aids successful joint aspiration.[14,15] Obtain radiographs of an inflamed joint if trauma, tumor, avascular necrosis, and osteomyelitis are diagnostic considerations. Radioisotope scanning is not usually required for ED diagnosis but can be useful to detect osteomyelitis, occult fracture, avascular necrosis, or tumor. MRI is not recommended for routing assessment of septic arthritis but may be helpful for difficult diagnostic cases. MRI is more sensitive to identify joint effusion than specific for the diagnosis of septic arthritis.[16]

ARTHROCENTESIS

Prepare the site to avoid bacterial contamination. The skin overlying the affected joint should be free of cellulitis or impetigo to avoid contamination of the joint space during arthrocentesis. Orthopedics should be consulted before aspiration of a prosthetic joint for direction in diagnostic workup and interpretation of results.[11] Other relative contraindications to joint aspiration are coagulopathy, including hemarthrosis in hemophiliac patients before factor replacement.[17]

Cleanse a large area overlying and adjacent to the affected joint with povidone-iodine solution. After air drying, clean the skin with an alcohol wipe to remove the povidone-iodine solution from the skin surface. Removal of the overlying povidone-iodine prevents the introduction of the povidone-iodine antiseptic into the joint, which can result in chemical irritation or sterilization of the aspiration sample. Next place sterile drapes over the site and maintain sterile technique throughout the procedure.

Anesthetize the skin and soft tissues overlying the joint with a 25- to 30-gauge needle. Avoid intra-articular injection of anesthetic because the anesthetic can inhibit bacterial growth and may result in a spuriously negative culture in an early septic joint.

Use a large-bore needle (18 or 19 gauge) for aspiration of fluid from large joints. Use smaller-bore needles for small joints (no smaller than 22 gauge). Choose a syringe large enough to accommodate the anticipated volume of fluid within the joint space. Remove as much synovial fluid as possible to obtain a good diagnostic sample and to relieve pain from joint capsule distention. Promptly send aspirated fluid to the laboratory for culture, Gram stain, leukocyte count with differential, and crystal analysis. US should be used in the event of a dry tap (see Table 284-4).

SHOULDER JOINT ASPIRATION

US can facilitate shoulder aspiration. The anterior or posterior approach can be used.

Anterior Approach Have the patient sit upright, facing you, and externally rotate the humerus. Insert the needle just lateral to the coracoid process, between the coracoid process and the humeral head (**Figure 284-1A**). Direct the needle posteriorly. If it is difficult to locate the coracoid process, the posterior approach to the glenohumeral joint may be easier.

Posterior Approach Sit the patient upright with the back facing you. Palpate the spine of the scapula to its lateral limit: the acromion. Identify the posterolateral corner of the acromion. Use a 1.5-inch needle. The point for needle insertion is 1 cm inferior and 1 cm medial to the posterolateral corner of the acromion (**Figures 284-1B and 284-2**). Direct the needle anterior and medial toward the presumed position of the coracoid process. The glenohumeral joint is located at a depth of approximately 1.0 to 1.5 inches.

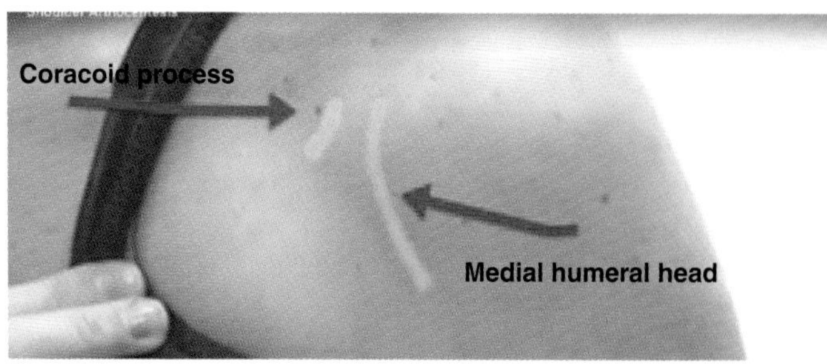

A

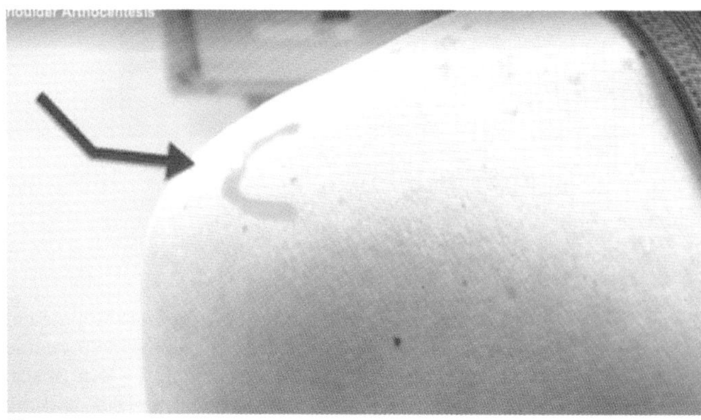
B

FIGURE 284-1. Shoulder arthrocentesis. **A.** anterior approach. **B.** Shoulder Arthrocentesis posterior approach.

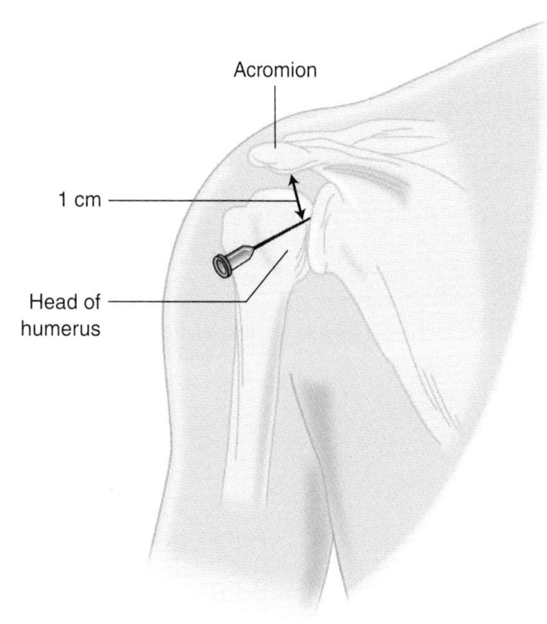

FIGURE 284-2. Shoulder arthrocentesis, posterior approach.

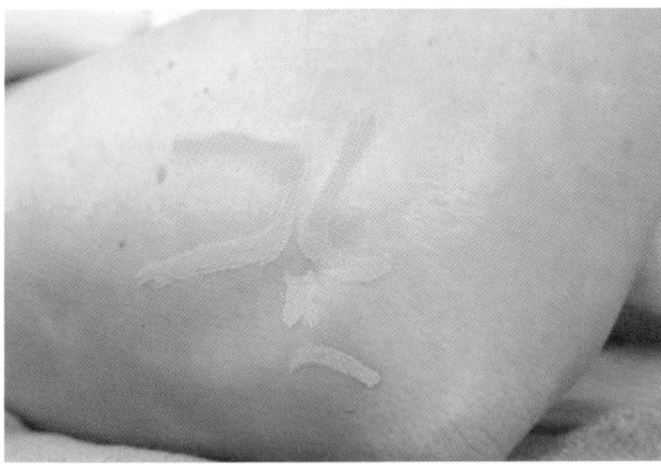

FIGURE 284-3. Arthrocentesis of the elbow.

ELBOW JOINT ASPIRATION

Use a lateral or posterior approach to the elbow joint. Do not use a medial approach to avoid neurovascular structures. Place the elbow in 90-degree flexion, resting on a table, with the hand prone to widen the joint space. Locate the radial head, lateral epicondyle of the distal humerus, and the lateral aspect of the olecranon tip. These three landmarks form the anconeus triangle. The center of this triangle is the site for needle entry into the skin. Using the tip of the gloved index finger of the nondominant hand, palpate a sulcus just proximal to the radial head. The sulcus is the needle entry point. Direct the needle medial and perpendicular to the radius toward the distal end of the antecubital fossa (**Figure 284-3**).

WRIST JOINT ASPIRATION

Landmarks for wrist arthrocentesis are palpable with the wrist in a neutral position. The landmarks are the radial tubercle of the distal radius, the anatomic snuffbox, the extensor pollicis longus tendon, and the common extensor tendon of the index finger (**Figure 284-4**). Insert the needle perpendicular to the skin, ulnar to the radial tubercle and the anatomic snuffbox, between the extensor pollicis longus (just ulnar to the extensor pollicis longus) and the common extensor tendons.

HIP JOINT ASPIRATION

Hip arthrocentesis may be performed by an anterior or medial approach. If local practice dictates open surgical assessment and drainage, an orthopedic consultant will often perform this procedure. US-guided arthrocentesis by an emergency physician or radiologist is also acceptable if local practices and training are in place to support this approach (**Figure 284-5).** Controversy exists regarding the utility of US or MRI as a screening test before open surgical evaluation.[15,18] Immediate consultation with an orthopedic surgeon is therefore desirable when a diagnosis of septic hip arthritis is considered.

KNEE JOINT ASPIRATION

The knee joint can be entered either medial or lateral to the patella. With the patient supine, fully extend the knee and make sure the quadriceps muscle is relaxed. Identify the midpoint of the patella. The insertion point of the needle is located approximately 1 cm inferior to the patellar edge, either lateral (**Figure 284-6**) or medial (**Figure 284-7**) to the middle of the patella. Direct the needle posterior to the patella and horizontally toward the joint space. Compression or "milking" applied to both sides (proximal and distal) of the joint space by an assistant who is using sterile technique may facilitate aspiration of small amounts of fluid. In patients with obese or large knees, it may be necessary to use a needle longer than 1.5 inches to enter the joint space. **Figure 284-8** demonstrates the use of US to visualize a knee joint effusion.

ANKLE JOINT ASPIRATION

Ankle arthrocentesis may be performed at either the tibiotalar joint (medial approach) (**Figure 284-9**) or the subtalar joint (lateral approach) (**Figure 284-10**). The medial approach is generally preferred.

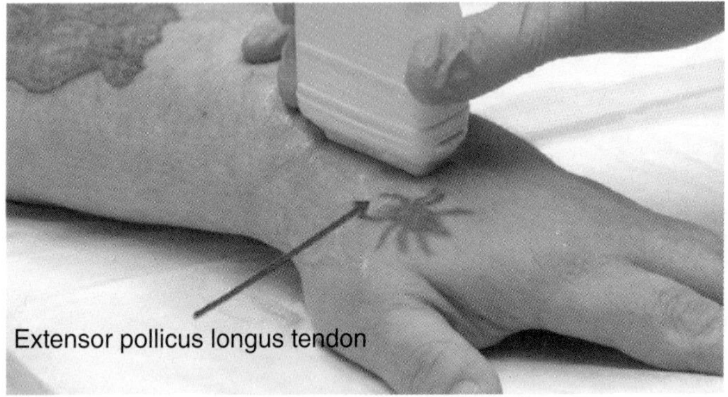

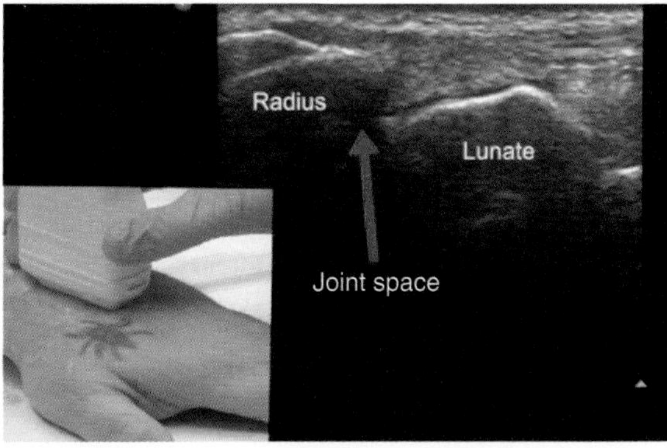

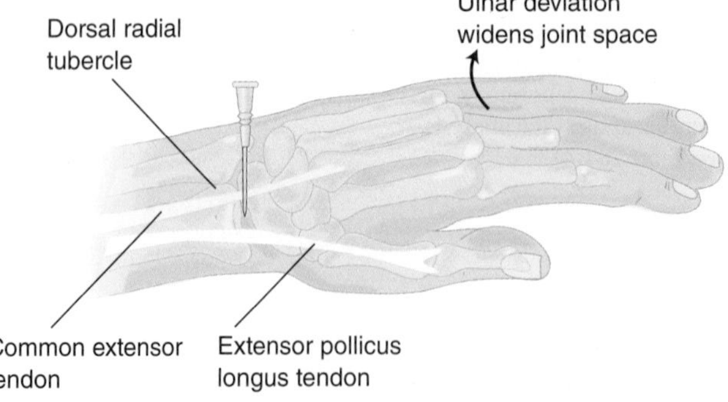

FIGURE 284-4. Arthrocentesis of the wrist. [Images used with permission of Sandra Werner.]

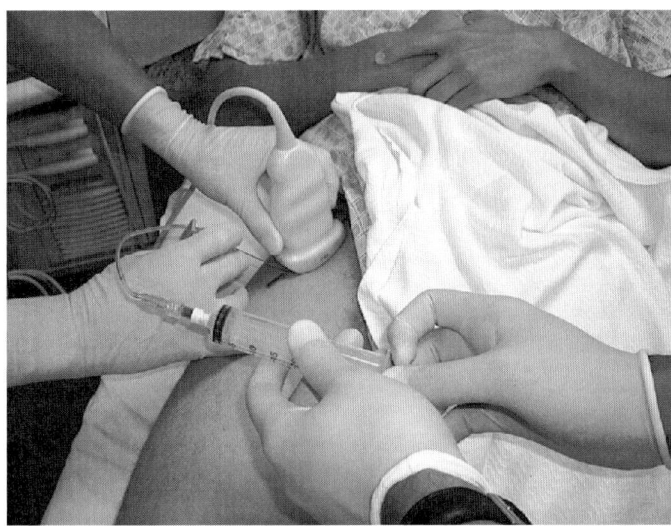

FIGURE 284-5. Demonstration of US-guided hip arthrocentesis with transducer orientation marker angled superomedially and drape and probe cover omitted for purpose of demonstration. [Reproduced with permission from Freeman K, Dewitz A, Baker WE: Ultrasound-guided hip arthrocentesis in the ED. *Am J Emerg Med 25: 80, 2007.* Copyright Elsevier.]

Medial (Tibiotalar) Approach Have the patient supine with the foot initially perpendicular to the leg. This position facilitates the location of a sulcus lateral to the medial malleolus and medial to the tibialis anterior and extensor hallucis longus tendons (Figures 284-9 and **284-11A and B**). Then plantar flex the foot with the needle entering the skin overlying the sulcus. Angle the needle slightly cephalad as it passes between the medial malleolus and the tibialis anterior tendon.

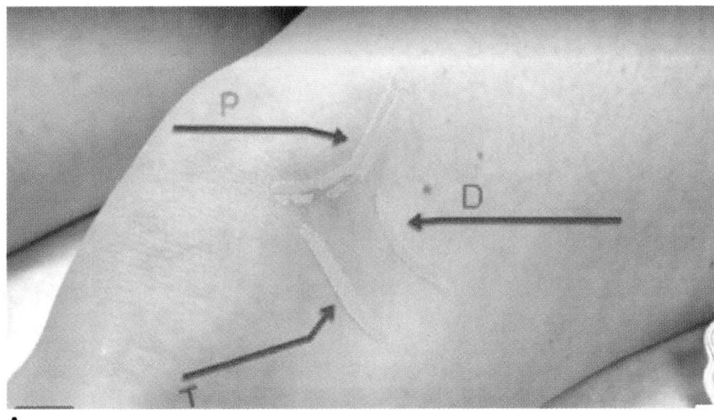

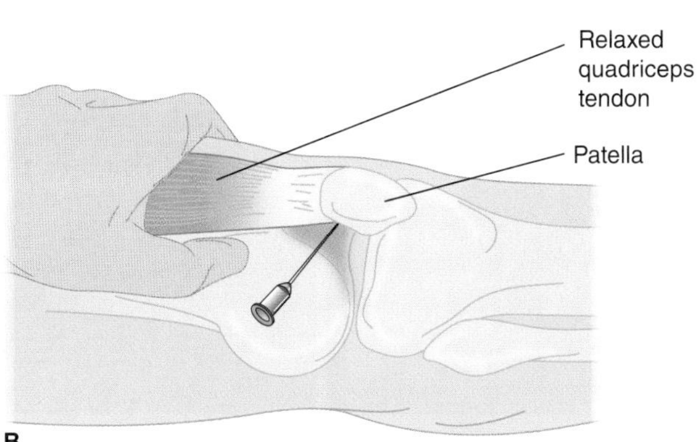

FIGURE 284-6. **A.** Landmarks for knee arthrocentesis. D = distal femur; P = patella; T = tibia. **B.** Arthrocentesis of the knee, lateral approach.

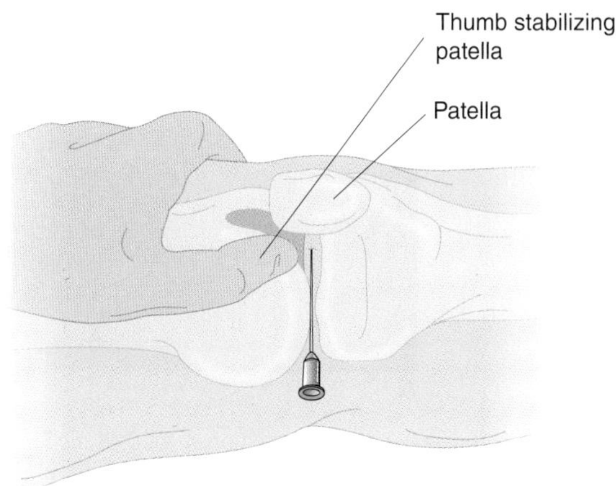

FIGURE 284-7. Arthrocentesis of the knee, medial approach.

Lateral (Subtalar) Approach Keep the patient's foot perpendicular to the leg. Enter the subtalar joint just below the tip of the lateral malleolus (Figure 284-10). Direct the needle medially toward the joint space.

SEPTIC ARTHRITIS

An acute hot, swollen, and tender joint (or joints) with restriction of movement is bacterial nongonococcal septic arthritis until proven otherwise.[1] Clinical features, risk factors, and treatment differ for bacterial, nongonococcal septic arthritis and gonococcal arthritis (Tables 284-1 through 284-4). For management of septic arthritis in infants and children, see chapter 140, "Musculoskeletal Disorders in Children." In young adults, sexual activity increases the prevalence of gonococcal arthritis and reactive arthritis (formerly known as Reiter's syndrome) associated with chlamydial urethritis.

BACTERIAL NONGONOCOCCAL SEPTIC ARTHRITIS

Although no clinical pattern is diagnostic of bacterial nongonococcal septic arthritis, certain general observations are helpful. Joint pain (85%), a history of joint swelling (78%), and fever (57%) are the only findings that occur in >50% of patients with bacterial nongonococcal septic arthritis.[4] Sweats (27%) and rigors (19%) are less common findings.[4]

The involved joint can become exquisitely painful over a few hours. The patient may splint the affected joint to relieve pain with movement. Joint effusion may be small or large. Resistance to passive and active movement and limitation of full joint movement are notable findings but are common with gout without infection and may be absent in immunosuppressed patients. Although joint aspiration and analysis are essential to the diagnosis, the sensitivity of any one finding for the diagnosis of nongonococcal septic arthritis is only moderate. For example, the sensitivity of joint fluid WBC to make the diagnosis of nongonococcal septic arthritis using the commonly quoted cutoff of 50,000 cells/mm^3 is only 56%.[3] The sensitivity of erythrocyte sedimentation rate for nongonococcal septic arthritis using a cutoff of 30 mm/h ranges between 76% and 96%,[3] but this test is nonspecific.

If a septic arthritis diagnosis cannot be reliably excluded after clinical evaluation, including arthrocentesis, admit the patient for parenteral antibiotics and pain control until synovial fluid culture results are available. Antibiotic coverage is directed at staphylococcal and streptococcal species including methicillin-resistant *S. aureus*. Vancomycin plus a third-generation cephalosporin is the preferred therapy (**Table 284-5**).[1,2,19]

Consult orthopedic surgery for possible joint irrigation in the operating room if the joint aspiration is positive for infection. Repeat closed-needle aspiration, arthroscopic irrigation, or less commonly, open surgical drainage may be required, depending on a number of factors, including consultant preference, patient age, affected joint,

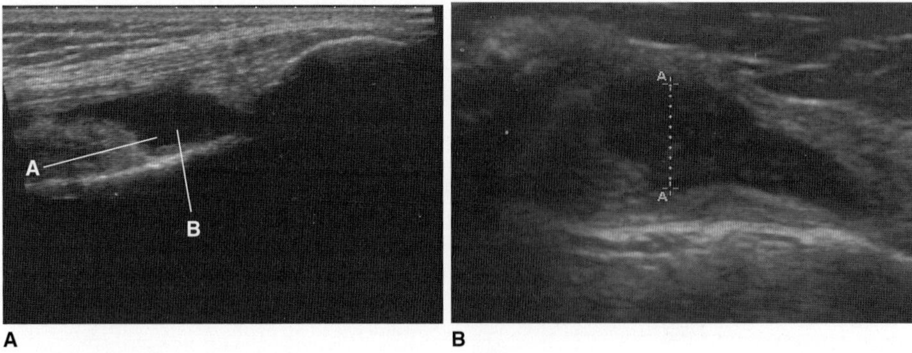

FIGURE 284-8. Bedside US of the knee in long axis (A) and short axis (B) demonstrating joint effusion.

comorbid illnesses, and likelihood of septic source.[1,20] Consultation with infectious disease may be required to determine ideal antibiotic choice in select patients.[2]

GONOCOCCAL SEPTIC ARTHRITIS

Gonococcal arthritis is the most common cause of septic arthritis in young sexually active adults.[21,22] Joint infection will typically have a prodromal phase in which migratory arthritis and tenosynovitis predominate before pain and swelling settle on one or more septic joints. Vesiculopustular lesions, especially on the fingers, may be found (see Figure 149-33 in chapter titled "Sexually Transmitted Infections").

Synovial fluid cultures are often negative in gonococcal arthritis, with only 25% to 50% of cases yielding positive identification of the organism.[4] Cultures of the posterior pharynx, urethra, cervix, and rectum (as directed by history of sexual contact) before antibiotic treatment

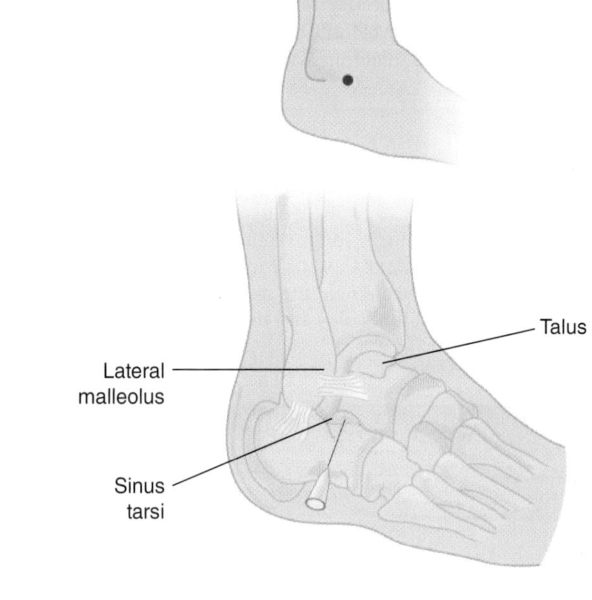

FIGURE 284-10. Arthrocentesis of the ankle, lateral approach.

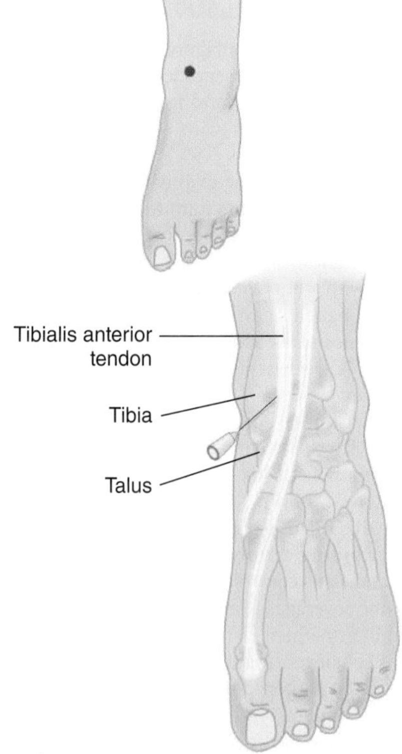

FIGURE 284-9. Arthrocentesis of the ankle, medial approach.

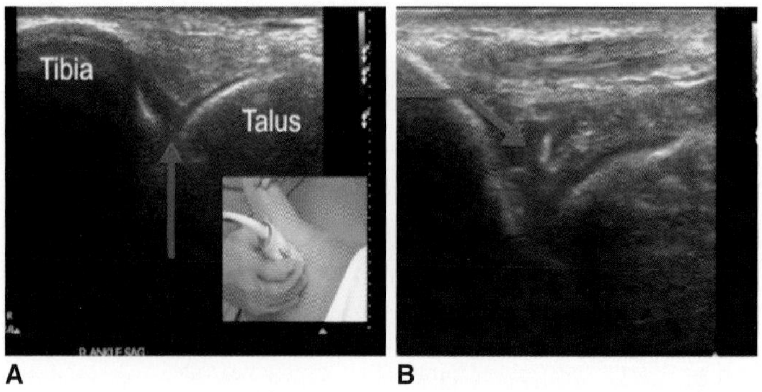

FIGURE 284-11. A. US-guided approach to medial ankle arthrocentesis. *Arrow* points to the ankle effusion. B. *Arrow* points to needle in the tibiotalar joint, medial approach with transducer in the sagittal plane. [Images used with permission of Sandra Werner.]

TABLE 284-5 Commonly Encountered Organisms in Septic Arthritis in Adolescents and Adults*

Patient/Condition	Expected Organisms	Antibiotic Considerations
Young healthy adults, or patients with risk factors for *Neisseria gonorrhoeae*	*Staphylococcus, N. gonorrhoeae, Streptococcus,* gram-negative bacteria	Vancomycin, 15 milligrams/kg IV load, if Gram stain reveals gram-positive organisms in clusters. Ceftriaxone, 1 gram IV, or imipenem, 500 milligrams IV, should be used/added if either gram-negative organisms are present or no organisms are present on Gram stain and *N. gonorrhoeae* is suspected (also culture urethra, cervix, or anal canal as indicated).
Adults with comorbid disease (rheumatoid arthritis, human immunodeficiency virus, cancer) or injection drug users	*Staphylococcus*, gram-negative bacilli	Vancomycin, 15 milligrams/kg IV load, plus cefepime, 2 grams IV, or imipenem, 500 milligrams IV. Meropenem 1 gram IV may be used as an alternative agent.
Sickle cell patients	*Salmonella* (increasingly *Staphylococcus*)	Vancomycin, 15 milligrams/kg IV load, plus ciprofloxacin, 400 milligrams IV. Imipenem, 500 milligrams IV, may be used as an alternative agent.

*Recommendations differ from the 2006 British Society of Rheumatology treatment guidelines due to the rising incidence of methicillin-resistant *Staphylococcus aureus* septic arthritis.

increase the culture yield.[21,23] Cases of gonococcal arthritis suspected clinically should be treated despite negative initial results while waiting for all culture results to return.

Treatment for gonococcal arthritis follows the same general principles as treatment for nongonococcal septic arthritis (see Table 284-5 for details). However, gonococcal arthritis does not yield joint destruction with the frequency of nongonococcal arthritis, and therefore, surgical intervention is rarely needed.[23,24] Daily joint aspiration is routinely done until there is clinical improvement.[21,23,24] *Neisseria gonorrhoeae*, in the setting of arthritis, remains sensitive to third-generation cephalosporin therapy (see chapter 149).

CRYSTAL-INDUCED SYNOVITIS (GOUT AND PSEUDOGOUT)

Crystal-induced synovitis is primarily an illness of middle-aged and elderly adults. Uric acid (gout) and calcium pyrophosphate (calcium pyrophosphate deposition, or pseudogout) are the two most common crystalline agents, with gout representing the most common form of inflammatory joint disease in men >40 years old.[25,26] The classic description of gout is monoarthritis involving the great toe or knee joint in a man >40 years old.[25] Gout is less common in women during their reproductive years but may occur in association with periods of increased insulin resistance such as gestational diabetes.[27]

CLINICAL FEATURES

Joint pain develops over hours. An acute gout or pseudogout attack often follows trauma, surgery, a significant illness, or change in medication. Gout results from precipitation of urine acid crystals in the joint, and pseudogout results from calcium pyrophosphate crystals. Crystalline involvement of joints has a predilection for the foot and knee. Although the first metatarsophalangeal joint is a classic focus for acute gout, no joint is the exclusive site of involvement for either crystal.

DIAGNOSIS

The diagnosis of a crystal-induced synovitis is by joint aspiration and identification of crystals through a polarizing microscope. Uric acid crystals (gout) appear needle shaped and blue when the source of light is perpendicular to the crystal (negative birefringence). Calcium pyrophosphate (pseudogout) is yellow in this alignment (positive birefringence), with a rhomboid shape. Crystals are located within phagocytes from aspirates of synovial fluid, or within inflamed tissues adjacent to the affected joint.

Serum uric acid levels are not generally useful for diagnosis, as up to 30% of patients will have normal uric acid levels during an acute gout attack.[25] There is no elevation of serum uric acid, calcium, or phosphate in pseudogout. The joint aspirate WBC can be elevated with gout and pseudogout.[25,26] However, the presence of crystals, the absence of bacteria on Gram stain or culture, and frequently, the dramatic response to nonsteroidal anti-inflammatory drugs (NSAIDs) clarify the diagnosis. When the diagnosis of a septic joint cannot be excluded, hospital admission until cultures and/or clinical response clarify the diagnosis is the safest course of action.[1,2]

TREATMENT

When the diagnosis of gout or pseudogout is established, treatment is an NSAID for 5 to 7 days. First-line treatment is indomethacin (or naproxen).[25,26] **Do not give NSAIDs to patients with renal insufficiency.** For patients with normal renal function, the initial dose of indomethacin is 50 milligrams. Therapy is continued three times a day for 3 to 7 days as needed. Substantial pain relief typically occurs within 2 hours of NSAID administration.[25,26] **Colchicine** is an alternative agent to treat acute gout and pseudogout in patients with normal renal and hepatic function. Oral colchicine is typically administered at a dose of 0.6 milligram/h until intolerable side effects (vomiting or diarrhea) or efficacy ensues. IV administration of colchicine can be associated with serious side effects, with risks such as bone marrow suppression, neuropathy, myopathy, and death.[25] For patients with renal insufficiency, narcotic analgesics are needed for pain relief because NSAIDs and colchicine are generally avoided. **Prednisone** is a first-line treatment option provided the patient is not diabetic.[25,26]

Discharge is typical unless pain is not controlled or if septic arthritis is a consideration. Once acute symptoms have resolved, long-term control may be achieved with reduction or elimination of gout-inducing agents (diuretics, aspirin, or cyclosporine) and treatment with prophylactic drugs, such as allopurinol or probenecid. There is no effective prophylaxis for pseudogout.

VIRAL ARTHRITIS

The most common causes of viral arthritis in the United States are parvovirus B19, rubella, and hepatitis B (**Table 284-6**).

PARVOVIRUS ARTHRITIS

Parvovirus B19 causes **erythema infectiosum** in children. In adults, this rash occurs in less than half of patients. Joint involvement is more common in adults, with morning stiffness, swelling, erythema, and a presentation similar to acute presentations of rheumatoid arthritis.[28,29]

HEPATITIS VIRUS ARTHRITIS

The most commonly involved joint with hepatitis B is the knee. Signs and symptoms are fever and lymphadenopathy, followed by joint pain, and then jaundice. Immune complexes in the synovium are responsible for synovial inflammatory changes. Hepatitis C causes a polyarticular arthritis, which may become chronic.[29]

RUBELLA ARTHRITIS

The arthritis of rubella is uncommon in children and adult males, but occurs in 50% of adult females with acute rubella, appearing soon after the emergence of the classic rash. The arthritis is polyarticular, most frequently involving the wrist, hand, knee, ankle, and elbow.

TABLE 284-6 Common Causes of Viral Arthritis

Virus	Prevalence of Arthritis	Findings	Duration	Additional Features
Parvovirus B19	Children 10% Adults 50%–70%	Polyarticular Symmetric	2–8 wk or chronic	Causes erythema infectiosum in children, rarely causes aplastic crisis
Rubella	Adults 50%	Polyarticular	5–7 d	Relapse
Epstein-Barr virus	1%–5%	Poly- or monoarticular	1–12 wk	Autoantibodies
Hepatitis B	10%–25%	Migratory	1–3 wk	Vasculitis
Hepatitis C	10%	Polyarticular	Chronic	Vasculitis
HIV	10%–50%	Mono- or oligoarticular	Chronic	Viral load >10,000 copies of HIV RNA, CD4 count <350 cells
Alphaviruses*	>50%	Oligoarticular	1–4 wk	More common in Asia, Africa; fever, myalgias

Abbreviation: HIV = human immunodeficiency virus.

*Alphaviruses include: Sindbis virus, Mayaro virus, Ross River virus, Semliki Forest virus, O'nyong-nyong virus, Chikungunya virus, and Barmah Forest virus.

ALPHAVIRUS AND HUMAN IMMUNODEFICIENCY VIRUS ARTHRITIS

Alphaviruses are common causes of arthritis in Africa, Asia, Australia, the West Pacific, and South America. Human immunodeficiency virus may cause an associated arthralgia/arthritis, a reactive arthritis, or psoriatic arthritis. In human immunodeficiency virus, CD4 counts below 350 cells/mm^3 increase the likelihood of bacterial arthritis. Counts below 200 cells/mm^3 are associated with an opportunistic cause of arthritis.[29] Overall management is discussed in chapter 154, "Human Immunodeficiency Virus Infection."

LYME DISEASE

The arthritic manifestations of Lyme disease occur weeks, months, or years after primary, stage I infection. Symptoms include monoarticular or oligoarticular asymmetric joint involvement. Large joints are most often affected, particularly the knee.[30] A migratory pattern of oligoarthritis may be noted in addition to brief attacks of bursitis and tendonitis.

The diagnosis of Lyme arthritis is initially suspected in patients residing in, or with a recent visit to, an endemic area. A history of tick bite or erythema chronicum migrans rash (see Figure 160-1 in chapter titled "Zoonotic Infections") is helpful but often absent. Arthrocentesis yields an inflammatory synovial fluid, usually with negative cultures. For detailed discussion of the diagnosis and treatment of Lyme disease, see chapter 160. Given the difficulty of making a definitive diagnosis in many patients, treatment of suspected Lyme arthritis is often initiated on the grounds of high clinical suspicion. Treatment is administered for 4 weeks, with a number of antibiotics recognized as effective, including ceftriaxone, 1 gram IV twice daily, switching to PO after clinical improvement; doxycycline, 100 milligrams PO twice daily; amoxicillin, 500 milligrams three times daily; or cefuroxime, 500 milligrams twice daily.[30]

HEMARTHROSIS

TRAUMATIC HEMARTHROSIS

Traumatic hemarthrosis has a high association with ligamentous injury or an intra-articular fracture. Effusions following trauma may range from small minor effusions to large painful fluid collections that impede range of motion. Aspiration of very large traumatic effusions will provide pain relief for approximately 1 week and increase range of motion but has no effect on long-term outcome.[12] Treatment of traumatic hemarthrosis consists of immobilization, ice, and elevation of the affected joint. In the absence of a fracture or significantly unstable joint requiring immediate orthopedic evaluation, follow-up is needed for possible ligamentous and articular injuries.

SPONTANEOUS HEMARTHROSIS

Spontaneous hemarthrosis usually indicates underlying systemic illness and should prompt consideration for primary or secondary coagulopathies. Hemophiliacs should receive specific clotting factor replacement for hemarthrosis (see chapter 235, "Hemophilias and von Willebrand's Disease"). Joint aspiration for acute hemarthrosis in hemophilia is controversial but recommended by some for a large hemarthrosis that can be aspirated during the first 12 hours of symptoms. **Joint aspiration should only be performed after factor replacement.**[17] Follow-up and/or consultation should be provided with hematology and orthopedics.

RHEUMATOID ARTHRITIS

Rheumatoid arthritis is typically a progressive disease, with polyarticular involvement of symmetric joints and sparing of the distal interphalangeal joints. Women are affected more commonly than men. Patients describe stiffness of the joints occurring after prolonged periods of inactivity (morning stiffness). A "boggy," slightly edematous synovium may be palpated. Arthrocentesis of synovial fluid is typically noted for an inflammatory profile. For further discussion of systemic clinical features of rheumatoid arthritis, see chapter 282.

Salicylates or other NSAIDs are the cornerstone of treatment for an acute exacerbation. Corticosteroids may be used for brief periods, with long-term therapy using agents such as methotrexate, leflunomide, sulfasalazine, and other nonbiologic and biologic disease-modifying antirheumatic drugs.[31] Consider septic arthritis in patients with an acute episode of arthritis who are also receiving immunosuppressives.

OSTEOARTHRITIS

Osteoarthritis is distinguished from rheumatoid arthritis by a lack of constitutional symptoms and/or multisystem involvement. Destruction of joints in osteoarthritis may involve the distal interphalangeal joints, with less dramatic symmetric, polyarticular exacerbations. Although osteoarthritis is a chronic, polyarticular disease, patients may present with an acute monoarthritis exacerbation, typically of the knee. Effusions are small and difficult to aspirate. If fluid is aspirated, it is noninflammatory.

Radiographs demonstrate characteristic joint space narrowing due to destruction of articular cartilage. Treatment is joint rest and NSAIDs or acetaminophen in the setting of GI complications.[32] Systemic corticosteroids are not indicated, although intra-articular corticosteroids may be administered by a primary care physician or orthopedist.

REACTIVE ARTHRITIS

Reactive arthritis (formerly known as *Reiter's syndrome*) is a seronegative spondyloarthropathy characterized by an acute, asymmetric oligoarthritis occurring 2 to 6 weeks after an infectious illness.[33-35] **The classic triad of Reiter's syndrome is arthritis, urethritis, and conjunctivitis. A history of all three components is not necessary for diagnosis.** *Chlamydia* or *Ureaplasma* are common inciting infectious agents (postvenereal reactive arthritis). Enteric infections may precipitate a reactive arthritis (postdysentery reactive arthritis). Implicated agents of postdysentery reactive arthritis are *Salmonella*, *Shigella*, *Yersinia*, and *Campylobacter*, and possible agents include *Escherichia coli* and *Clostridium difficile*.[33,34]

Conjunctivitis occurs in one third of postvenereal and >50% of post-dysentery forms of reactive arthritis.[34]

Joint involvement in reactive arthritis typically involves the lower extremities, including the feet. Back and buttock pain may occur. A diffuse swelling of an entire digit (sausage digit) may be found as well but is not specific to reactive arthritis.[33,34] Synovial fluid aspirates demonstrate an inflammatory profile. Treatment has traditionally been supportive, with emphasis on pain control with NSAID therapy. Antibiotics were previously thought to be of no benefit, but now long-term combination antibiotic therapy is being used for *Chlamydia*-induced reactive arthritis, using rifampicin combined with either doxycycline or azithromycin.[35] Arthroscopic synovectomy may also provide benefit.[36] Suspected cases should be referred to rheumatology for confirmation of diagnosis and management.

BURSITIS

NONSEPTIC BURSITIS

Bursitis is an inflammatory process involving one of the >150 bursae in the body, but most commonly the bursa overlying the elbow or the knee (see also chapter 281, "Hip and Knee Pain").[37] Bursitis can be caused by repetitive trauma or can be associated with gout, pseudogout, or rheumatoid arthritis. Repetitive activities that can precipitate bursitis are identified by the typical names given: "carpet layer's or housemaid's knee" (prepatellar bursitis) or "student's elbow" (olecranon bursitis). The affected bursa is easily palpated but is not tender and not erythematous. Bursal enlargement is usually chronic or progressive but not acute. If bursitis is acute, consider septic bursitis (see "Septic Bursitis" below). In nonseptic bursitis, there is no limitation of, or pain upon, joint movement. The skin over the bursa may be thickened and calloused, indicating chronic repetitive trauma or pressure. Treatment is NSAIDs and elimination of activities that produce symptoms. Aspiration and drainage of bursal fluid is controversial (if infection is not suspected), because bursal fluid often reaccumulates after aspiration.

SEPTIC BURSITIS

Unlike septic arthritis, septic bursitis is more likely secondary to bacterial spread from a skin lesion or local cellulitis to an injured or inflamed bursa. Therefore, cultures more closely reflect skin flora.[37] Septic bursitis is characterized by acute pain, tenderness, erythema of the affected bursa, and overlying warmth when compared with the unaffected side.[37,38] The most common sites for septic bursitis are the prepatellar bursa (50% to 53%) and the olecranon bursa (40% to 45%).[38-40]

Fever occurs in <50% of patients with septic bursitis.[38] Pain can occasionally be mild (10%) but is usually moderate or severe.[39] Associated cellulitis of the surrounding skin may be evident.

Most authors recommend the aspiration of bursal fluid if septic bursitis is considered.[37,39] Bursal aspiration can be diagnostic and therapeutic. Bursal fluid demonstrates characteristic findings in infection (**Table 284-7**).[37] Culture is the definitive test for presence or absence of infection. Diagnosis is presumed by one of the following criteria based on bursal fluid results: positive Gram stain, >3000 WBC/mm^3, >50% polymorphonuclear cells, glucose <31 milligrams/dL, or bursal to serum glucose ratio of <50%.[37]

S. aureus accounts for the majority of infections, but *Staphylococcus epidermidis* and *Streptococcus* species are also encountered.[37-39] Septic bursitis generally responds well to oral antibiotics, with emphasis on coverage of *Staphylococcus* and *Streptococcus* species. With the high prevalence of methicillin-resistant *S. aureus,* adjust antibiotic choice according to local sensitivities. Conditions that require hospital admission for incision and debridement and IV antibiotics include sepsis, extensive purulent bursitis, extensive surrounding cellulitis, suspected joint involvement, immunocompromise, or failure to respond to a course of oral antibiotics.[37] See specific treatment recommendations below.

OLECRANON BURSITIS

The olecranon bursa overlies the olecranon process on the extensor surface of the elbow. The bursa is tense and edematous. Pain elicited with range of motion at the elbow is minor until the motion tightens and compresses the distended overlying bursa. Gouty tophi on the extensor surface of the elbow may be palpable or visible if the cause of bursitis is crystal-induced bursitis. If bursal fluid is aspirated, uric acid crystals are evident on microscopy.

To aspirate the olecranon bursa, prepare the bursal skin and use antiseptic technique. The patient's arm can be extended to allow for maximal bursal distention. Use a lateral approach to the affected bursa. Remove as much fluid as possible, and send the aspirate to the laboratory for analysis for WBC, Gram stain, crystals, glucose, and culture.

Treatment depends on patient condition; if septic, the patient should be treated with vancomycin, 15 milligrams/kg, plus piperacillin/tazobactam, 4.5 grams IV, or meropenem, 500–1000 milligrams IV. Most patients can be treated as outpatients with a 14-day course of oral antibiotics.[37-39] Common antibiotics chosen include clindamycin, 300 milligrams three times per day for 10 days, or dicloxacillin, 500 milligrams four times per day.[39] Trimethoprim-sulfamethoxazole is an alternative.[38] Steroids are not indicated in the ED because infection cannot be definitively excluded by negative culture results. Admission is indicated for clinical toxicity, extensive surrounding cellulitis, failure of outpatient treatment, or immunocompromise. Some patients benefit from surgical excision of the bursa sac.[40]

PREPATELLAR BURSITIS

Bursitis may affect any of the four bursae surrounding the extensor aspect of the knee (see Figure 281-6). A history of overuse or repetitive trauma to the prepatellar area is typical.[37] The noninfected or aseptic bursa is enlarged and taut but nontender and not warm. There is full range of motion of the knee. If septic patellar bursitis is a consideration (**Figure 284-12**), aspirate the prepatellar bursa to obtain fluid for analysis. Prepare the skin overlying the bursa and use aseptic technique. Use either a lateral or medial approach. Fluid analysis and treatment are the same as for septic olecranon bursitis (see "Olecranon Bursitis" above).

TABLE 284-7 Characteristics of Bursal Fluid in Patients with Septic and Nonseptic Olecranon and Prepatellar Bursitis

	Septic	Traumatic and Idiopathic	Crystal Induced
Appearance	Purulent or serosanguineous	Straw colored, serosanguineous, or bloody	Straw colored to bloody
Leukocytes/mm^3	Range, 350–392,000; mean, 54,3300 ± 34,197; >3000 is considered diagnostic	Range, 0–11,700; mean, 2475 ± 1988	Range, 1000–6000; mean, 2900
Differential count	>50% polymorphonuclear cells is considered diagnostic	Predominantly mononuclear	Highly variable
Ratio of bursal fluid to serum glucose	<50% in 90% of cases (diagnostic)	>50%, 70%–80% in 98% of cases	Unknown
Gram stain	Positive in 70% (diagnostic)	Negative	Negative
Crystals present	No*	No	Yes
Culture results	Positive (diagnostic)	Negative	Negative

*The presence of crystals does not rule out infection.

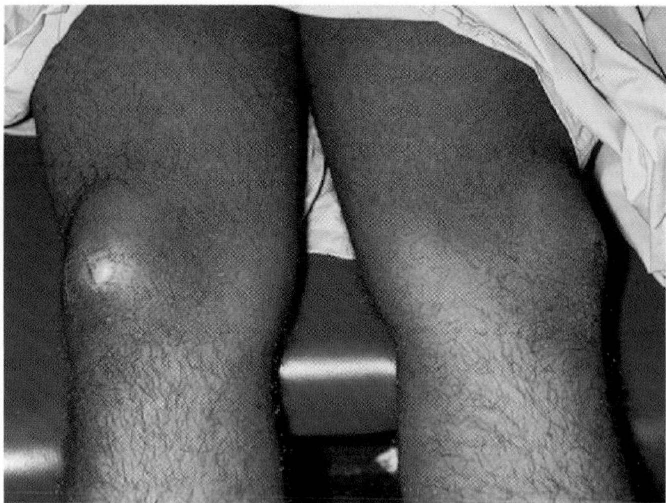

FIGURE 284-12. Septic prepatellar bursitis. This patient presented with obvious purulence of his right prepatellar bursal sac. Aspiration confirmed septic bursitis. [Courtesy of Alan B. Storrow, MD. Reproduced with permission from Knoop K, Stack L, Storrow A, Thurman RJ: *Atlas of Emergency Medicine*, 3rd ed. © 2010, McGraw-Hill, New York.]

REFERENCES

The complete reference list is available online at www.TintinalliEM.com.

CHAPTER 285

Soft Tissue Problems of the Foot

Mitchell C. Sokolosky

INTRODUCTION

This chapter discusses the common foot disorders that are likely to present to the ED. Patients with chronic or complicated foot problems generally should be referred to a dermatologist, orthopedist, general surgeon, or podiatrist, depending on the disease and local resources. Tinea pedis, foot ulcers, and onychomycosis are discussed in Section 20, "Skin Disorders," in chapter 253, "Skin Disorders: Extremities." Puncture wounds of the foot are discussed in Section 6, "Wound Management," in chapter 46, "Skin Disorders: Extremities.", "Puncture Wounds and Bites." Foot ulcers and osteomyelitis are discussed in Section 17, "Endocrine Disorders," in chapter 224, "Type 2 Diabetes Mellitus."

CORNS AND CALLUSES

Calluses are a thickening of the outermost layer of the skin and are a result of repeated pressure or irritation. Corns (clavus) develop similarly, but have a central hyperkeratotic core that is often painful. The causes can be external (poorly fitted shoe) or internal (bunion).

Calluses are protective and should not be treated if they are not painful. Calluses grow outward but may be pushed inward by continued pressure and become corns. Corns also develop in areas of scarring and between toes. Corns are classified as hard or soft. Hard corns are seen over bony protuberances where the skin is dry. Soft corns are seen between toes where the skin is moist. Corns may be painful or painless, but pressure on the corn usually produces pain. Diagnosis is based on clinical appearance. Corns interrupt the normal dermal lines and can thus be differentiated from calluses, which do not interrupt the normal dermal lines. Hard corns may resemble warts. However, when warts are pared, warts contain black seeds, which are thrombosed capillaries and may bleed, while corns do not bleed. Soft corns resemble tinea, and identifying tinea is important for proper treatment (see chapter 253).[1,2]

Keratotic lesions may indicate more severe underlying disease, deformity, local foot disorder, or mechanical problem. Differential diagnosis of keratotic lesions includes syphilis, psoriasis, arsenic poisoning, rosacea, lichen planus, basal cell nevus syndrome, and, rarely, malignancies.[2]

TREATMENT OF CORNS

Treatment of symptomatic corns often necessitates referral to a podiatrist because the treatment may involve repeated paring, use of keratolytic agents, and possibly surgery to correct any underlying source of pressure (bunion).[1-4] Salicylic acid treatments are more effective than paring with a scapel.[5] Recurrence can be prevented by weekly gentle trimming with a pumice stone or emery board after soaking in warm water for 20 minutes. Placing a pad on or around the lesion relieves pressure, and avoiding constrictive footwear also provides benefit.

PLANTAR WARTS

Plantar warts are caused by the human papillomavirus. Plantar warts are most common in children, young adults, and butchers or fishmongers. Infection occurs by skin-to-skin contact, with maceration or sites of trauma. The incubation period is 2 to 6 months. Spontaneous remission may occur in up to two thirds of patients within 2 years.[6] Recurrence is common. Single lesions are endophytic and hyperkeratotic. A mother-daughter wart is similar to a single lesion except for a small vesicular satellite lesion. Mosaic warts are often painless, closely grouped, and may coalesce. Diagnosis is clinical. The wart will obscure normal skin markings. If in doubt, use a #15 scalpel blade to pare down the lesion to expose thrombosed capillaries, called seeds. The only two effective treatments for warts are salicylic acid and liquid nitrogen (cryotherapy).[7,8] Some salicylic acid preparations are available without a prescription. Duct tape (silver or clear) as an adjunct provides no benefit.[8] Adequate paring is required for larger lesions.[7] Plantar warts may require prolonged treatment (several weeks or months) as well as cryotherapy, so refer to a dermatologist or podiatrist for follow-up.[8] Nonhealing lesions require referral to a specialist because they may represent undiagnosed melanoma.[7,9] Instruct patients to avoid touching warts on themselves or others, to wear slippers in public showers, and to not use paring down tools (pumice stone, file) on normal skin or nails.

INGROWN TOENAIL

Normal nail function requires maintenance of a small space between the nail and the lateral nail folds. Ingrown toenails occur when irritation of the tissue surrounding the nail causes overgrowth, obliterating the space.[10-12] Causes include improper nail trimming, using sharp tools to clean the nail gutters, tight footwear, rotated digits, and bony deformities.[10,12] Curvature of the nail plate is another predisposing factor.[12] Symptoms are characterized by inflammation, swelling, or infection of the medial or lateral aspect of the toenail. The great toe is the most commonly affected. In patients with underlying diabetes or arterial insufficiency, cellulitis, ulceration, and necrosis may lead to gangrene if treatment is delayed.

TREATMENT OF INGROWN TOENAILS

If infection or significant granulation is absent at the time of presentation, acceptable treatment is daily elevation of the nail with placement of a wisp of cotton or dental floss between the nail plate and the skin.[13] Daily foot soaks and avoidance of pressure on the nail help.[13] Another option, if no infection is present, is to remove a small spicule of the nail (**Figure 285-1**).[12]

A digital nerve block is placed (see Section 5, "Analgesia, Anesthesia, and Procedural Sedation," and chapter 36, "Local and Regional

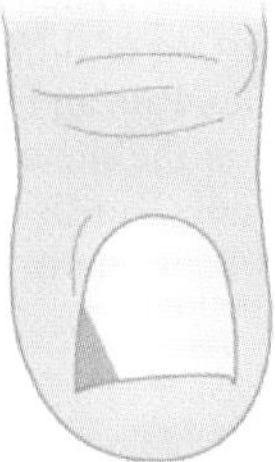

FIGURE 285-1. Partial toenail removal. This method is used for small nail fold swellings without infection. After antiseptic skin preparation and digital nerve block, an oblique portion of the affected nail is trimmed about one to two thirds of the way back to the posterior nail fold. Use scissors to cut the nail; use forceps to grasp and remove the nail fragment.

Anesthesia"). Cleanse the area and prepare the skin for an antiseptic procedure. Trim an oblique portion of the affected nail about one to two thirds of the way back to the posterior nail fold. The nail groove should then be debrided and a nonadherent dressing placed.[10,11]

If granulation or infection is present, a larger partial removal of the nail plate is indicated (**Figure 285-2**). Preprocedure antibiotics are not needed unless the patient is systemically ill.[14] First, perform a digital nerve block and prepare the area for antiseptic technique. Longitudinally, cut the entire affected area, base-to-tip, cutting about one fourth of the nail plate, including the portion of the nail beneath the cuticle. Cutting the nail is made easier by first sliding mosquito forceps or small scissors between the nail and nail bed on the affected side, freeing the nail from the bed below. Rotate the forceps, turning up the portion of the nail on the affected side. A nail splitter is the optimal instrument for cutting the nail; however, sturdy scissors are a reasonable alternative. Then grasp the affected cut portion of the nail with a hemostat and, using a rocking motion, remove it from the nail groove. Then debride the nail groove.[10] Once the procedure is completed, place a nonadherent gauze or antibiotic ointment on the wound and a bulky dressing over that, covering the toe. Check the toe in 24 to 48 hours.[10,12] If phenol is used for chemical matricectomy, massage the involved nail matrix vigorously with a cotton-tipped swab dipped in an aqueous solution of phenol 88%, with a rotation directed toward the lateral nail fold, for 1 minute. Irrigate the nail matrix using isopropyl alcohol to neutralize completely the phenol solution.[15,16] Do not expose normal skin or tissues to the phenol solution. Postprocedure antibiotics are not needed unless cellulitis is proximal to the toe.[11]

For recurrent ingrown toenails, refer to a podiatrist for permanent nail ablation, which may require a combination of surgical excision plus chemical matricectomy (phenol ablation).[15,16]

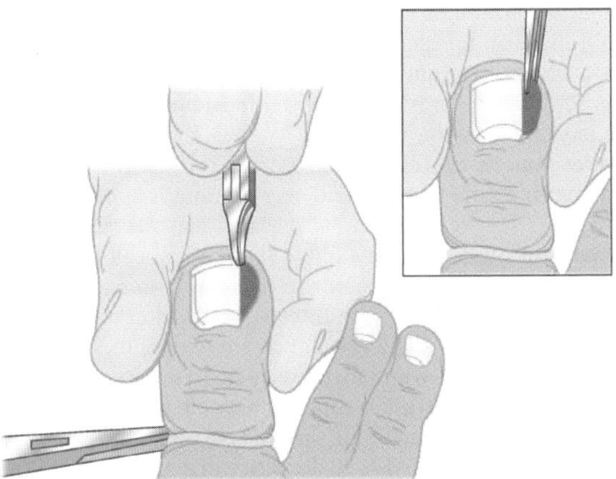

FIGURE 285-2. Partial toenail removal (infection present). This method is used for onychocryptosis in the setting of significant granulation tissue or infection. See "Treatment of Ingrown Toenails" for a description of the procedure.

OTHER NAIL LESIONS

Other common toenail afflictions include paronychia (see Section 23, "Musculoskeletal Disorders," chapter 283, "Nontraumatic Disorders of the Hand") and subungual hematoma (see Section 6, "Wound Management," chapter 43, "Arm and Hand Lacerations"), which are treated similarly to when they occur in the fingers. Hyperkeratotic toenails can be a problem in the elderly. These may become so severe as to affect gait and cause ulcerations and infections. Refer such patients to podiatry for repeated trimming or nail plate removal.

BURSITIS INVOLVING FEET

Calcaneal bursitis causes posterior heel pain that is similar to Achilles tendinopathy[17,18]; however, the pain and local tenderness are located at the posterior heel at the Achilles tendon insertion point. In contrast, Achilles tendinopathy causes symptoms 2 to 6 cm superior to the posterior calcaneus. Pathologic bursae can be divided into noninflammatory, inflammatory, suppurative, and calcified. Noninflammatory bursae are usually pressure induced and are found over bony prominences. Inflammatory bursitis is commonly due to gout or rheumatoid arthritis. Suppurative bursitis is due to bacterial invasion of the bursae (primarily staphylococcal species), usually from adjacent wounds. Acute bursitis can lead to the formation of a hygroma or calcified bursae. Diagnosis can be aided by the use of US and MRI[17] but is not indicated for evaluation in the ED. Treatment of the bursitis depends on its cause. For nonseptic bursitis, symptoms usually resolve with simple measures including heel lifts, comfortable footwear, rest, ice, and nonsteroidal anti-inflammatory drugs.[19] Management of septic bursitis is discussed in Section 23, "Musculoskeletal Disorders," in chapter 284, "Joints and Bursae." Diagnosis of these lesions is dependent on analysis of bursal fluid, which can be obtained by large-bore needle aspiration.[17]

PLANTAR FASCIITIS

Plantar fasciitis, inflammation of the plantar aponeurosis, is the most common cause of heel pain.[20-22] Peak age incidence is usually between 40 and 60 years old, but it has a younger peak in runners.[23,24] Plantar fasciitis is common among ballet dancers and those performing aerobics. The plantar fascia anchors the plantar skin to the bone and provides support to the foot during gait. The cause is usually overuse. Other causes of heel pain include abnormal joint mechanics, tightness of the Achilles tendon, shoes with poor cushioning, abnormal foot position and anatomy, and obesity.[17,20] In the younger patient, autoimmune and rheumatic diseases can be considered.

The symptom of plantar fasciitis is pain on the plantar surface of the foot that is worse when initiating walking. Examination usually reveals a point of deep tenderness at the anterior medial aspect of the calcaneus, the point of attachment of the plantar fascia. Pain and tenderness tend to be increased upon dorsiflexion of the toes. Diagnosis is clinical. Radiographic studies are not indicated unless other causes are being considered. The presence of heel spurs is of no diagnostic value because many patients without plantar fasciitis have this finding on imaging. For resistant cases, US and MRI may aid in diagnosis but are not indicated for evaluation in the ED.[17]

Plantar fasciitis is generally a self-limited disease. Eighty percent of cases resolve spontaneously within 12 months. Initial treatment consists of rest, ice, nonsteroidal anti-inflammatory drugs, heel and arch support shoe inserts, taping or strapping of the foot, and dorsiflexion night splints (molded ankle-foot orthotics that holds the plantar fascia and Achilles tendon stretched). Plantar-specific stretch exercises are the most beneficial treatment in the acute phase: with the ankle dorsiflexed, the patient uses one hand to dorsiflex the toes and with the other hand palpates the plantar surface of the foot, confirming tension.[25] Patients should be taught Achilles tendon stretching exercises and be told to avoid the use of flat shoes and barefoot walking.[17] In severe cases, a short-leg walking boot may be useful to unload and rest the plantar fascia. Corticosteroid injections provide short-term benefit, up to 1 month,[25] but are associated with plantar fascia rupture,[17] and are best left to the orthopedist.[20,21] Refer patients to a podiatrist, orthopedist, or primary care physician for follow-up care.[20,21]

NERVE ENTRAPMENT SYNDROMES

TARSAL TUNNEL SYNDROME

Tarsal tunnel syndrome is an uncommon source of foot pain and numbness in runners due to compression of the posterior tibial nerve as it courses behind the medial malleolus.[26,27] The cause is usually from prior injury (scar tissue, bone or cartilage fragments, or bony spurs) and overpronation during running.[26,27] Overpronation (inward rotation) makes the nerve more vulnerable both to direct trauma from stretch and to indirect trauma from inflammation of the surrounding structures, resulting in compression.[26,27] Other causes include activities requiring restrictive footwear (ski boots, skates), edema from pregnancy, ganglion cysts, and tumors, but frequently, no inciting event is known.[28]

Symptoms include numbness or burning pain of the sole and may be limited to the heel, mimicking plantar fasciitis. Distal calf pain may be due to retrograde radiation (Valleix phenomenon). Weakness is uncommon. Pain is often worse with running, at night, and after standing, and often leads to the desire to remove the shoes. **Tinel sign** is positive with percussion inferior to the medial malleolus yielding pain radiating to the medial or lateral plantar surface of the foot. Simultaneous dorsiflexion and eversion of the ankle exacerbates symptoms. Diagnosis is aided by nerve conduction studies or MRI,[26,27] but these are not routinely ordered from the ED.

The differential diagnosis includes plantar fasciitis and, if limited to the heel, Achilles tendinitis. Plantar fasciitis will cause point tenderness over the plantar heel, and pain is worse upon morning standing. Tarsal tunnel syndrome causes greater medial heel and arch pain due to involvement of the abductor hallucis muscle. Tarsal tunnel pain worsens with ambulation throughout the day. In addition, tarsal tunnel syndrome may produce distal calf pain, whereas plantar fasciitis does not.

Initial treatment includes avoidance of the exacerbating activities, nonsteroidal anti-inflammatory drugs, shoe modification, and occasionally orthotics. If there is no improvement or symptoms recur after a few weeks, then orthopedic evaluation is recommended.[26,27]

DEEP PERONEAL NERVE ENTRAPMENT

Deep peroneal nerve entrapment occurs most commonly at the location where the nerve courses under the inferior extensor retinaculum[29] (**Figure 285-3**). Recurrent ankle sprains, soft tissue masses, trauma (both acute and repetitive),[30] chronic biomechanical misalignment, edema, and tight-fitting footwear (ski boots) are the most common causes. Symptoms are dorsal and medial foot pain and sensory hypoesthesia at the first toe web space. There may be loss of the ability to hyperextend the toes due to wasting of the extensor hallucis brevis and extensor digitorum brevis muscles. Pain and tenderness can be elicited on palpation of the peroneal nerve at the site of entrapment and by plantar flexion with inversion of the foot. Pain is exacerbated by activity and relieved by rest. Nighttime pain is common. Treatment is the same as for tarsal tunnel syndrome.

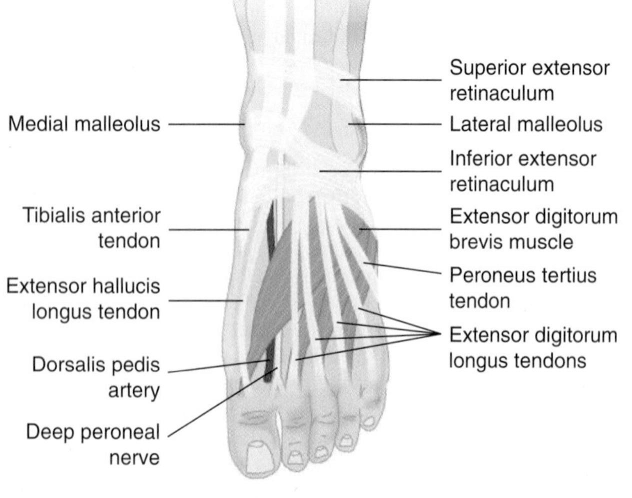

FIGURE 285-3. Tendons of the foot, anterior view, including deep peroneal nerve.

GANGLIONS OF THE FOOT

A ganglion is a common benign synovial cyst. Ganglions are 1.5 to 2.5 cm in diameter and are often attached to a joint capsule or tendon sheath. Although ganglions typically occur in the wrist or hand, they may also occur in the foot. Ganglions typically arise in the anterolateral aspect of the ankle, but can occur in many areas of the foot. The cause is unknown. Ganglions may appear suddenly or gradually, may enlarge and diminish in size, and may be painful or asymptomatic. On examination, a ganglion is a firm, cystic lesion. Diagnosis is usually made clinically, although US or MRI may exclude other causes when serious pathology is suspected. Aspiration and instillation of glucocorticoids by an orthopedist lead to the complete resolution of ganglions in some cases,[31] with surgical excision required for persistence.[32,33]

TENDON LESIONS OF THE FOOT

TENOSYNOVITIS AND TENDINITIS

Tenosynovitis and tendinitis may occur in the foot, usually due to overuse. Patients present with pain over the involved tendon (Figure 285-3). The flexor hallucis longus, posterior tibialis, and Achilles tendon are most commonly involved.[34] Treatment consists of rest, ice, and oral nonsteroidal anti-inflammatory drugs.[34]

Flexor hallucis longus tenosynovitis classically affects ballet dancers, but can also be seen in runners and nonathletes. Presentation is similar to plantar fasciitis and tarsal tunnel syndrome. Posteromedial ankle pain, medial arch pain, and a positive Tinel sign (see earlier description in "Tarsal Tunnel Syndrome") are seen. Conservative management (rest, mobilization, orthotic shoe implant, nonsteroidal anti-inflammatory drugs) is usually successful. Surgery is reserved for refractory cases.

TENDON LACERATIONS

Tendon lacerations can result from penetrating injuries to the dorsal or plantar aspect of the foot. Tendon repairs in the foot are complex, and orthopedic consultation is needed for repair.[34]

The foot should be casted in dorsiflexion after the repair of extensor tendons and in equinus after repair of flexor tendons.

TENDON RUPTURES

Spontaneous rupture of the Achilles tendon is common. Rupture of the anterior tibialis and posterior tibialis tendons may also occur.[34] Age and chronic corticosteroid and fluoroquinolone use are risk factors for spontaneous rupture. Diagnosis is usually clinical but is aided by US or MRI studies in difficult cases.

Achilles tendon rupture occurs when a sudden shear stress, such as sudden pivoting on a foot or rapid acceleration, is applied to an already weakened or degenerative tendon. Many patients report immediate sharp pain, and some hear an audible "pop." The peak age for rupture is 30 to 40 years, and rupture is four to five times more common in men than women.[35] Over 80% of ruptures occur during recreational sports ("weekend warrior"). Patients often present with pain, a palpable defect in the area of the tendon, and inability to stand on tiptoes. A minority of patients with complete tendon ruptures are able to ambulate and may be misdiagnosed as having an ankle sprain. Squeezing the calf of the prone patient whose knee is flexed at 90 degrees will normally cause the foot to plantar flex (calf squeeze or Thompson test. The absence of plantar flexion indicates a positive test indicative of rupture. Initial ED treatment consists of ice, analgesics, immobilization of ankle/foot in plantar flexion, crutches, and referral to an orthopedic surgeon. Definitive treatment is generally surgical in younger patients and conservative (casting in equinus or plantar flexion) in older patients.[34,36,37] For further discussion, see chapter 44, "Leg and Foot Lacerations," and Figure 44-1 (Thompson test) in that chapter, in Section 6, "Wound Management."

Ruptures of the **anterior tibialis tendon** are rare. Ruptures usually occur after the fourth decade and are not excessively painful. Patients present with varying degrees of foot drop and a palpable defect distal to the ankle joint in the area of the tendon. In most cases, disability is minimal, and surgery is not necessary.[34]

Spontaneous ruptures of the **posterior tibialis tendon** also occur after the fourth decade. Two thirds of these cases occur in women. The presentation is usually chronic and insidious. Patients notice a gradual flattening of their arch, with modest discomfort and swelling over the medial ankle. Examination reveals absence of the tendon's normal prominence and weakness on inversion of the foot. Patients find it impossible to stand on tiptoes. Treatment may be conservative or surgical, depending on the duration of the tear and activity of the patient.[22]

Flexor hallucis longus rupture presents as a loss of plantar flexion of the great toe. The need for surgery will depend on the patient's occupation and lifestyle.[34]

Disruption of the **peroneal retinaculum** can occur as a result of direct trauma during dorsiflexion of the foot. Besides pain localized to the peroneal tendon behind the lateral malleolus, the patient complains of a clicking when walking as the tendon subluxes. Peroneal tendon injuries may lead to lateral ankle instability. Treatment is generally surgical repair.[34]

PLANTAR INTERDIGITAL NEUROMA (MORTON'S NEUROMA)

Neuromas may form in a plantar digital nerve, usually proximal to its bifurcation. Neuromas may occur in any of the digital nerves but are most common in the third interspace. The cause is thought to be local irritation of the nerve due to entrapment, usually from tight-fitting shoes. Women between the ages of 25 and 50 years old are the most commonly affected group. Patients present with pain located in the area of the metatarsal head. The pain is described as burning, cramping, or aching. Pain is worsened by ambulation and resolved by rest and removal of shoes. The pain may radiate to the affected toes, and patients may note numbness in the toes. Pain is usually easily reproduced upon palpation of the area, and at times, a mass is felt. Diagnosis is usually made clinically, but nerve conduction studies, electromyograms, US, and MRI may be helpful at times. Conservative treatment consists of wearing wide shoes with good metatarsal head supports and metatarsal head off-loading inserts.[38] Local glucocorticoid injections can sometimes be curative. Surgical removal may be necessary for refractory symptoms.

COMPARTMENT SYNDROMES OF THE FOOT

The foot has up to nine compartments. Compartment syndrome occurs when an elevation of tissue pressure within one of these nonyielding fascial compartments impedes vascular flow. The cause of compartment syndrome is a high-energy injury (crush injury)[39] associated with multiple fractures. Compartment syndromes have been reported in association with foot and ankle fractures (especially calcaneal and Lisfranc's fracture/dislocation), burns, contusions, bleeding disorders, postischemic swelling after arterial injury or thrombosis, venous obstruction, snakebites, exercise, and prolonged pressure to the affected area (e.g., cast immobilization, prolonged abnormal positioning).[40] Diagnosis begins with a high index of clinical suspicion based on the mechanism of injury. Pain out of proportion to injury is one of the early findings. Additional symptoms include pain that is worsened on active or passive movement, paresthesias, and neurovascular deficits. An absent pulse and complete anesthesia are late findings and may be difficult to assess due to underlying swelling. The only reliable objective method to diagnose compartment syndrome is by obtaining compartment pressures using an intracompartmental pressure monitoring system (Stryker STIC Device [Stryker, Kalamazoo, MI] or similar equipment). A difference between diastolic blood pressure and intracompartmental pressure of <30 mm Hg is an indication for fasciotomy.[41] Once the diagnosis is made, fasciotomy should be performed emergently. In the ED, elevate the extremity to the level of the heart pending fasciotomy. The sequelae of compartment syndrome range from transient neurologic compromise to complete myoneural necrosis, fibrosis, and ischemic contractures. The prognosis of compartment syndrome is directly related to the time delay in diagnosis and treatment (see Section 22, "Injuries to Bones and Joints," chapter 278, "Compartment Syndrome").[41]

Chronic exertional compartment syndrome is due to overuse.[42] Symptoms occur with exertion and are relieved by rest. Patients should be instructed to avoid overexertion and be referred for further investigation and treatment.

MALIGNANT MELANOMA

Malignant melanoma of the foot accounts for up to 15% of all cutaneous melanomas. Melanomas can present as an atypical, pigmented, or nonhealing lesion of the foot, including the nail. These malignancies often imitate more common foot disorders such as fungal infections, foot ulcers, and plantar warts. Because prognosis is directly related to early diagnosis, maintain a high index of suspicion for the diagnosis. Acral lentiginous melanoma is an aggressive malignant tumor that more commonly affects nonwhites. This tumor has a predilection for the plantar surface of the foot. It may present with atypical features leading to a delay in diagnosis and poor outcome. All skin lesions that are either atypical or not healing despite treatment should be referred for biopsy.[43]

PRACTICE GUIDELINES

For heel pain, the *Journal of Foot and Ankle Surgery* published a guideline, "The Diagnosis and Treatment of Heel Pain: A Clinical Practice Guideline–Revision." This can be found online at http://www.acfas.org/Research-and-Publications/Clinical-Consensus-Documents/Clinical-Consensus-Documents/.

REFERENCES

The complete reference list is available online at www.TintinalliEM.com.

Mental Health Disorders: ED Evaluation and Disposition

Leslie Zun

INTRODUCTION AND EPIDEMIOLOGY

Over the last two decades, the rate of ED mental health–related visits increased 38%, from 17.1 to 23.6 per 1000 U.S. population.[1] Mental health and/or substance abuse accounts for about one of every eight ED visits in the United States, and covert mental health problems may be present in over 40% of all ED patients.[2] ED visit increases are especially notable for older persons and those living in urban areas, and with visits related to mood and anxiety disorders, suicide attempts, and substance abuse. Behavioral disorders in children account for at least 1.6% of ED pediatric visits, of which nearly 20% are admitted. ED visits in children are often related to substance use, anxiety and attention deficit disorders, disruptive behavior, and psychosis.[3]

Because there are about 4000 general hospital EDs in the United States but <200 psychiatric EDs, the vast majority of acute behavioral problems are assessed and treated in general hospital EDs.[4,5] Patients with behavioral health problems often provide vague and nonspecific symptoms, and obtaining collateral information as part of the assessment is difficult and time-consuming.

ED disposition decisions can be especially challenging for homeless patients and for those with repeated ED visits. Given the complexities of assessment, diagnosis, and disposition, it is important to maintain a positive and nonjudgmental attitude toward patients with mental health disorders.

A decision strategy for emergency assessment of patients with mental health disorders should follow the sequence of actions in **Table 286-1**.

TABLE 286-1 Emergency Psychiatric Assessment Steps

Step	Comment
Safety and stabilization	Contain violent and dangerously psychotic persons to provide a safe environment for staff, patients, family, and visitors while simultaneously attending to airway, breathing, and circulation.
Identification of homicidal, suicidal, or other dangerous behavior	Determine whether the patient needs to be forcibly detained for emergency evaluation.
Medical evaluation	Determine the presence of any serious organic medical conditions that might cause or contribute to abnormal behavior or thought processes (e.g., hypoglycemia, meningitis, drug withdrawal, or other causes of delirium).
Psychiatric diagnosis and severity assessment	If the behavior change is not due to an underlying medical condition, it is primarily psychiatric or functional, requiring a psychiatric diagnosis and assessment of the severity of the primary psychiatric problems.
Psychiatric consultation	Determine the need for immediate psychiatric consultation.

This chapter presents an overview of the care of adult patients with mental health disorders from ED entry to departure—triage, patient and staff safety, medical and psychiatric evaluation, admission and disposition decisions, and the care of patients with prolonged ED stays. Diagnostic criteria of the psychiatric disorders are summarized. Behavioral and psychiatric disorders in children are discussed in chapter 147, "Behavioral Disorders in Children."

TRIAGE

Paramedics or police often provide advance notice to the ED, especially of the severely agitated patient, so preparations can be made for patient arrival. The best preparation includes assembly of an ED "psychiatric code" team, designation of an appropriate room, and having medications on hand. Team members may consist of an ED physician and nurse, hospital nurse manager, psychiatric clinical nurse, and security staff who can respond to threats of harm to others, patients with altered mental status, and patients trying to leave against medical advice.[6]

In most Western countries, psychiatric patients are triaged in the same manner as medical patients using the Emergency Severity Index, Canadian Triage Acuity Scale, Manchester Triage System, or Australasian Triage Scale/National Triage Scale. These triage tools were originally designed for medical patients. For psychiatric patients, behavior descriptors determine acuity. The most acute behaviors are actively dangerous (e.g., violent, possession of a weapon), with decreasing acuity as the likelihood of dangerousness to self or others declines.

THE PRECAUTIONARY PRINCIPLE

Agitated or distressed patients, those expressing suicidal or homicidal ideation, or patients who raise concern about harm to self or others should not be allowed to leave the ED before medical or psychiatric evaluation is completed, even if departure is formalized as "against medical advice."[7] Many institutions have a formal process to make sure staff are aware that the patient cannot leave. Processes include the writing of an order (e.g., "sitter with patient," "precautionary hold," "suicide precautions"), but while the process varies by institution, the goal is to ensure patient and staff safety during the time-consuming process of evaluation. The foundation of such action is called the "Precautionary Principle," which is the need to prevent or minimize harm before it occurs.[8]

SAFETY FIRST

Fragmented mental health care and mass deinstitutionalization of the severely mentally ill have ensured that many psychotic, violent, and chronically mentally unwell patients now visit the ED on a regular basis. Mental health emergencies include situations in which patients are highly distressed, suicidal, and/or homicidal. Patients with suicidal or homicidal ideation, suicide or violence plans, or suicide or homicide attempts require measures to minimize the possibility of harm to themselves or others. Mental health disorders coexisting with substance abuse are also a recipe for violence.[9] In one study of psychiatric patients in a veteran's hospital, about one third of patients who committed violence during hospitalization did so in the ED. Violent incidents have been associated with dementia, court-ordered admission, and mood disorder.[10] Violent and aggressive behavior frequently demands immediate chemical or physical restraint to protect the patient, other patients, staff, and visitors.[11]

Although hospital security forces and police are often available to subdue violent patients and reduce risks of staff or patient injury, ED staff must be educated and equipped with a range of skills to protect themselves. These skills include enhanced awareness of risk factors and warning signs of violent behavior, verbal de-escalation techniques, quick access to rapidly tranquilizing or neuroleptic medications, and emergency strategies for getting help quickly in explosive circumstances.

Approach patients with potentially dangerous behavior cautiously and with a nonthreatening attitude, with adequate security nearby. If necessary, isolate and restrain threatening patients before they are disrobed, gowned, and searched for weapons. **Medical and nursing staff should stay distant from the patient; avoid excessive eye contact; maintain a calm, controlled posture and tone of voice; and stand in a location that neither threatens the patient nor blocks the exit of the healthcare worker from the room.**

A number of techniques can help de-escalate aggressive patient behaviors. Allow patients to verbally ventilate feelings. Provide an environment that decreases stimulation. Place the patient alone in a room designed for patient safety, but with close monitoring by staff. Offer food or drink. Set limits on acceptable behavior and respond with neutral comments. Adequate force nearby should be visible to the patient, and tell the patient that uncontrolled behavior will result in restraint.

EXAMINATION ROOMS AND SECLUSION

Waiting rooms and examination rooms need to be designed to ensure safety. Steps that promote safety include security staff, metal detectors, rooms with doors that permit rapid and easy exit, panic buttons, and the removal of any objects that could be used in violent attacks or suicide attempts (including neckties of both staff and patient, large earrings, patient belts or belt buckles, shoes, shoelaces, stethoscopes, blood pressure cuffs, and cutting instruments).

Seclusion rooms may be used to protect patients and staff. Remove or carefully secure any objects that could be used for self-injury or against staff. Austere seclusion rooms may be useful for some agitated patients by providing relief from external stimuli. Search patients before entry, and remove potentially dangerous objects, clothing, or weapons. Make sure staff are aware of the location of exits and of panic buttons. Initially, leave the door open, but if the patient remains agitated, lock the door. Keep the patient advised of each action and the expected duration, and explain the consequences of violent behavior. Monitor the patient in a seclusion room with a personal guard or nurse-monitor, by closed-circuit television, or by individual checks about every 10 minutes. Give the patient opportunities to comply with staff demands for acceptable behavior that can lead to release from seclusion. If violent behavior persists, physical restraint is justified. Document all steps in the use of seclusion and medical and physical restraints.

CHEMICAL RESTRAINT

Pharmacologic/chemical restraint of violent or agitated patients is discussed in detail in chapter 287, "Acute Agitation." The Sedation Assessment Tool score (SATS) is one method of grading behavior and assessing medication options.[12] Treatment options can be selected based on behavior (**Table 286-2**).

Ketamine has been used for acute agitation or depression, but concerns about hypoxia or oversedation, and lack of large clinical ED studies, limit its use in the ED at the present time.[13-15]

PHYSICAL RESTRAINTS

In many cases, there is no substitute for the application of physical limb restraints. Restraints should be applied rapidly and safely by individuals trained and skilled in their use. A team of five staff members is recommended: one team leader and one person for each limb. Sometimes, the show of force and the presence of many staff may in itself be sufficient to subdue the patient without recourse to restraints. The team leader oversees and orchestrates the procedure. The patient and any family members present should be provided with clear, ongoing explanations of all procedures. Place the patient on a bed or stretcher, and secure all four limbs with leather restraints. Be careful to avoid injury. Elevate the patient's head, if possible, to minimize risk of aspiration. Once the patient is restrained, offer medications, and if refused, administer medications involuntarily.[11]

TABLE 286-2 Sedation Assessment Tool Score (SATS) and Treatment Suggestions

Sedation Assessment Tool Score	Description	Treatment
3+	Combative, violent, out of control with continual loud outbursts	Physical restraint Lorazepam 1–2 milligrams IM AND Haloperidol 5–10 milligrams IM OR Olanzapine (Zyprexa®) 5–10 milligrams IM OR Droperidol 2 milligrams IM
2+	Very anxious and agitated with loud outbursts	As above, or if will take PO, lorazepam 1 milligram PO and haloperidol 5 milligrams PO OR Olanzapine ODT 5 milligrams
1+	Anxious and restless with normal to talkative speech	If will take PO, lorazepam 1 milligram PO and haloperidol 5 milligrams PO OR Olanzapine ODT 5 milligrams
0	Awake and calm, cooperative with normal speech	
−1*	Asleep but rouses if name is called with prominent slowing/slurred speech	
−2*	Responds to physical stimulation with few recognizable words	
−3*	No response to stimulation	

*Repeat Sedation Assessment Tool score 40–60 minutes after medication; goal score is 0 or −1. May repeat treatment if Sedation Assessment Tool score is >1+.

Abbreviation: ODT = orally disintegrating tablet.

Hospital policies dictate the frequency and type of observation (e.g., vital signs, pulses, range of motion, skin integrity, toileting) with written orders that limit the time in restraint and require renewal as needed. Once the patient is calm and compliant, restraints can be removed one at a time, while staff carefully monitor the patient to ensure the safety of all concerned.

MEDICAL EVALUATION OF PSYCHIATRIC PATIENTS

The initial steps include simultaneous medical and psychiatric evaluation while maintaining patient and staff safety.[16] Obtain vital signs including pulse oximetry, and perform point-of-care blood glucose determination. Simultaneously assess the patient's potential for dangerous behavior, such as harming self or others or leaving the ED without medical advice; stabilize the behavior; and evaluate the chief complaint. Then, obtain a focused history; perform physical examination and mental status/neurologic testing to identify comorbid or primary medical issues; and assess the need for hospitalization. Formulating a specific diagnosis is not as important as determining whether the patient is harmful to self or others or is unable to take care of self and needs hospitalization. Determining that an individual is suicidal and in need of protection and hospitalization, for instance, is more important than deciding whether that person has schizophrenia or psychotic depression.

The medical evaluation of patients with apparent psychiatric symptoms should be the same as for those with medical conditions[17] (**Table 286-3**). The findings of the history and physical examination should guide laboratory testing and diagnostic inquiry. The combined findings from history, physical examination, laboratory testing, and diagnostic inquiry form the basis of the medical description of the patient.

The evaluation of the patient with psychiatric symptoms in the ED is commonly termed "**medical clearance**." This term is a misnomer because many patients have medical problems and the term does not really mean that the patient's medical problems have been "cleared." Rather, this process identifies medical problems and their relationship to the patient's presentation. One alternative to the term "medically clear" is a discharge note that includes key features of the history, physical examination, and mental status and neurologic examination; laboratory results; discharge instructions; and follow-up plans.[18] Alternatively, the term "**medically stable**" could be used if a specific term is required.

The **medical evaluation** is used to determine whether the patient has a medical condition that causes or exacerbates the psychiatric illness. The medical evaluation process is also used to identify medical illnesses or injuries that are coincident to the psychiatric illness and that need to be identified and treated prior to a psychiatric admission. The determination of a medical versus psychiatric cause for psychiatric illness or behavioral change is difficult because many psychiatric patients have medical comorbidities and some with medical illness have undiagnosed psychiatric disorders. The most frequent medical comorbidities include diabetes, cardiovascular disease, and pulmonary disease.[17] If the patient with medical comorbidities needs hospitalization, be sure the psychiatric facility can provide care for concurrent medical illnesses.

MEDICAL AND BEHAVIORAL HISTORY

Medical comorbidities may produce changes in behavior. Ask specifically about fever, head trauma, immunocompetence (including malignancies and risk factors for human immunodeficiency virus infection), diabetes, pulmonary diseases, and toxic ingestions or overdose.

TABLE 286-3 Medical Evaluation of Psychiatric Patients

Document behavioral changes through history.
Identify medical symptoms.
Determine medical comorbidities.
Obtain medication and drug history.
Perform physical examination.
Perform neurologic examination.

Obtain information about recent changes in behavior from the patient, as well as from caregivers and family members. Obtain the history of previous psychiatric illness and treatment to identify patterns of relapse. Family and social history may identify stressors in the patient's environment that are a direct cause of changes in behavior or that accentuate any responses to underlying disease. Whenever possible, corroborate all history provided by the patient, with information from family members, care providers, or law enforcement. Compare direct observations of the patient's behavior with reports from the patient's family and caregivers. This is especially important for institutionalized or group home patients whose baseline mental capacity is often unclear to ED staff.

MEDICATION/DRUG HISTORY

Mental health disorders and substance abuse disorders frequently coexist.[19] The syndromes associated with alcohol and substance abuse that can result in altered behavior include intoxication, withdrawal, delirium, hallucinosis, paranoid behavior, and dementia. Identify any initiation of substance abuse, changes in the patterns of abuse, and medication compliance.

Behavioral changes may be due to prescription or over-the-counter drugs, especially sedatives-hypnotics, stimulants, psychotropic agents, anticonvulsants, anticholinergic agents, angiotensin-converting enzyme inhibitors, β-blockers, corticosteroids, fluoroquinolone antibiotics, histamine-2 receptor blockers, opioids, salicylates, selective serotonin reuptake inhibitors, thiazide diuretics, and antiparkinsonian agents.[20] The increasing use of serotonergic agents makes it important to check drug interactions (e.g., linezolid, tramadol) to identify serotonin syndrome as a cause of behavioral change.[21] Over-the-counter analgesics or herbals and alternative medications containing salicylates, anticholinergics, antihistamines, or bromides may produce delirium or toxic psychosis.[20] Alcohol and street drugs, such as phencyclidine, lysergic acid diethylamide, mescaline, amphetamines, and cocaine, can produce a toxic psychosis. Hypnosedatives, such as barbiturates and benzodiazepines, may produce a confusional state or delirium in both intoxication and withdrawal. Ask about alcohol and substance use in psychiatric presentations, even when the odor of ethanol or evidence of substance use is absent.

Psychoactive drugs are associated with a variety of hematologic and metabolic abnormalities. Clozapine, olanzapine, phenothiazines, and carbamazepine can cause neutropenia/agranulocytosis.[22] Hyponatremia (sodium level <136 mmol/L) can occur with typical and atypical antipsychotics.[23] Hepatotoxicity, manifested as transaminitis, obstruction, or hepatic failure, has been reported with norepinephrine-selective reuptake inhibitors more than with selective serotonin reuptake inhibitors, and also with tricyclics/tetracyclics, monoamine oxidase inhibitors, and typical and atypical antipsychotics.[24] Of the herbal medications, kava-kava can cause serious hepatotoxicity, while St. John's wort has been indirectly associated with hepatotoxicity due to its effects on the P450 system of other medications.[25]

PHYSICAL EXAMINATION

Perform a physical examination on every patient.[25-27] Measure vital signs, including temperature, and oxygen saturation by pulse oximetry. Investigate abnormal vital sign values, and do not dismiss them as due to anxiety or stress. Fever is especially important, because both local and systemic infections can cause altered mental status, as can meningitis, encephalitis, and brain abscess. Neuroleptic malignant syndrome and serotonin syndrome are causes of psychoactive drug-related fever.[28]

Patients with abnormal vital sign values, abnormal mental status examination results, psychosis, mental retardation, or advanced age usually require a complete head-to-toe physical examination, with street clothing removed and dressed in a hospital gown. Look for signs of trauma to the head, face, and neck, and reconstruct any mechanisms of injury. In the homeless, or in those with exposure, assess for hypothermia and check the extremities for frostbite. Examine for skin rash, extremity trauma, and needle tracks. Neurologic examination typically includes an assessment of most cranial nerves, gait, mental status, and general motor function and strength. For more focused neurologic examinations, test for apraxias, agnosias, right-left disorientation, aphasias, visual field cuts, and inability to follow complex spoken and written commands. Such

TABLE 286-4 Signs and Symptoms Suggesting Medical Cause of Behavioral Abnormalities

Abnormal vital sign values
Disorientation with clouded consciousness
Abnormal mental status examination findings
Recent memory loss
Age >40 y without a previous history of psychiatric disorder
Focal neurologic signs
Visual hallucinations
Important abnormalities on physical examination

signs may or may not occur in association with other localizing neurologic signs, such as asymmetric reflexes, paralysis, or hemiparesis.

Table 286-4 lists signs and symptoms associated with medical causes of behavioral abnormalities. Sudden onset of major changes in behavior, mood, or thought in a previously normal patient, or definite deterioration in a patient with a chronic behavioral disorder should stimulate evaluation for an underlying medical or neurologic disorder. A sudden change in behavior, especially in a patient >45 years old, is an important indicator of a possible medical disease process. Evaluate neurologic symptoms such as fainting, dizziness, disorientation, impairment of speech, confusion, loss of consciousness, headaches, difficulty performing routine tasks, new cognitive deficits, and focal weakness.

MENTAL STATUS EXAMINATION

The mental status examination is conducted to understand the patient's mental state and, when combined with the history and physical examination, aids the formulation of a diagnosis and disposition. A mental status examination can help identify delirium, medical disorders, and psychiatric disorders; identify patients who are dangerous to themselves or others; and help assess patient disposition (**Tables 286-5** and **286-6**). A great deal of the information obtained in mental status examinations becomes evident through observing the patient's appearance, behavior, language, comprehension, and affect during the initial patient interview. However, cognitive assessment and determination of suicidal or homicidal ideation or hallucinations and delusions generally require additional questioning.

Important components of the mental status examination include ability to provide historical information, attention, speech patterns, language comprehension, affect and mood, hallucinations and delusions, level of cognitive functioning, degree of insight and capacity for introspection, and ability to establish a therapeutic relationship. Abnormal findings in any of the above components may suggest a medical basis for abnormal thought or behavior. Liability of affect, the need for simple questions to be repeated, irritability, disorientation, and lack of cooperation are some additional signs of medical dysfunction.

During the examination, the patient's affect or outward display of emotion should be evaluated for sadness, euphoria, and anxiety, and whether such emotions are appropriate to the current situation. This may help distinguish between cognitive disturbance induced by depressive disorders and dementia due to cerebral pathology. An examiner can draw some conclusions regarding a patient's thought processes during the patient's telling of his or her personal history. Disordered thought processes include paranoid or grandiose delusions, fixed false beliefs, and delusional denial of illness. Such beliefs should be compared with reports from family and friends. **Visual hallucinations** can occur in psychiatric illnesses (schizophrenia or affective disorder) but most often result from medical disease; assume medical pathology until proven otherwise. Judgment can be gained by asking the patient to describe how he or she would deal with day-to-day problems, such as finding the way home from the hospital. Judgment may be impaired in medical disease, so ask about historical evidence of faulty judgment.

TABLE 286-5 Mental Status in the ED: An Outline

Behavior	What is the patient doing?
Affect	What feelings is the patient displaying?
Orientation	Does the patient know what is happening, where, and when?
Language	Is the patient understanding and being understood?
Memory	Can the patient recall historical details, recent and remote?
Thought content	Is the patient reporting beliefs that make little sense?
Perceptual abnormalities	Is the patient experiencing unusual sensory phenomena?
Judgment	Is the patient able to make rational decisions?

COGNITIVE ASSESSMENT

Assess cognitive impairment to identify the presence of dementia or delirium. Cognitive impairment often is not detected in ED patients, despite estimates suggesting that from 26% to 40% of older ED patients are cognitively impaired.[29] There are many tests of cognitive function, from simple to complex, but few have been investigated in the ED.

The **Quick Confusion Scale** consists of seven items and takes about 3 minutes to administer (**Table 286-7**; see also **Table 168-3**). A cut-off of ≤11 points has a sensitivity of 64% and specificity of 85% for identifying cognitive impairment.[30]

Another self-administered screening test for cognitive function is the **clock test**. Give the patient a piece of paper with a circle drawn on it, and ask the patient to "place the numbers on it to make it look like a clock." After completing this task, then ask the patient to place the hands of the clock to read a time such as "10 past 11." Although there are various methods for scoring the clock drawing test, the easiest for ED use is the simplest: correct or not correct. Using a more complex 10-point scoring system, the sensitivity for dementia detection was reported as 76% and specificity was 81%. Clock test results do not appear to be affected by depression.[31]

The **Mini-Mental State Examination** is a widely used tool for assessing cognitive impairment and to follow changes in cognition over time[32] but is not practical for general ED use.

LABORATORY EVALUATION

Obtain laboratory testing based on abnormalities in the history and the physical examination. There is no unanimity between specialties about the need for extensive laboratory testing for all ED psychiatric patients.[33,34] The psychiatric literature reports that 46% to 80% of psychiatric patients have undiagnosed medical illness,[35,36] whereas the emergency medicine literature supports a selective approach to laboratory testing in the ED.[37,38] Often, routine testing is a requirement of the psychiatric consultant or is part of the admission process of the psychiatric hospital.[39,40] The best approach is to collaboratively establish standards for testing on a local level.

For adults with new psychiatric complaints, obtain a through laboratory evaluation including a CBC, electrolytes, liver and renal function studies, urinalysis, and possibly chest radiograph, neuroimaging, or drug and alcohol testing depending on the patient and the circumstances.

Many institutions require drug and alcohol testing for all patients with psychiatric complaints whether the patient admits to substance abuse or not. However, specific drug and alcohol testing is not clinically necessary if the patient admits to using alcohol and drugs when asked and is awake and cooperative.[41] Urine drug testing and blood alcohol concentrations do not correlate with the degree of intoxication. The patient's cognitive abilities, rather than a specific blood alcohol level, should be the basis for assessment. On the other hand, patients with altered mental status without known cause need a complete evaluation including alcohol and drug testing.

One guide for the discretionary use of testing is provided in **Table 286-8**.[41,42] Documenting items in **Table 286-8** can also be used as a communication tool to psychiatrists about the ED evaluation process.

Advanced testing such as radiographs, electrocardiograms, and electroencephalograms should be based on the patient's clinical condition and suspicion for medical illness. CT and related brain imaging should be considered for a clear change in behavior or if an intracranial cause is suspected.

TABLE 286-6 Features of Delirium, Dementia, and Psychiatric Disorder

Clinical Feature	Delirium	Dementia	Psychiatric Disorder*
Onset	Acute, over days	Slow	Varies
Course over 24 h	Fluctuates	Stable	Varies
Consciousness	Reduced or hyperalert	Alert	Alert or distracted
Attention	Disordered	Normal	May be disordered
Cognition	Disordered	Impaired	Rarely impaired
Hallucinations	Visual and/or auditory	Often absent	Usually auditory
Delusions	Transient, poorly organized	Usually absent	May be present
Body movements	Tremor, asterixis, jerks	Often absent	Varies

*Features vary with the type of psychiatric disorder.

The type of diagnostic imaging depends on findings from the history, mental status examination, physical examination, and differential diagnosis.

DIAGNOSIS

Provisional psychiatric diagnoses can be made in the ED to facilitate treatment and disposition. Recognition of specific behavioral syndromes can assist in evaluating the presenting complaint, pursuing associated symptoms, and determining treatment and disposition. Emergency physicians should be sufficiently familiar with commonly seen psychiatric illnesses to describe their predominant clinical features.

The current official diagnostic nomenclature, most recently published in 2000 by the American Psychiatric Association, is the *Diagnostic and Statistical Manual of Mental Disorders*, fourth edition (text revision), commonly known as DSM-IV-TR.[43] A copy of DSM-IV-TR should be available for reference in the ED, because it contains a list of criteria for each disorder and additional material on demographics, associated symptoms and syndromes, and differential diagnoses. As of this writing, the fifth edition of the DSM is in preparation, and publication is anticipated later in 2013.

The DSM-IV-TR diagnoses are structured on a multiaxial system in which each axis refers to a different domain of information (**Table 286-9**).[43] This system aids in making a comprehensive assessment, organizing complex clinical information, and communicating with other professionals. **More details concerning selected psychiatric diagnoses are found at the end of this chapter, in the Overview of Axis I to V Disorders section.**

A useful strategy for making a DSM-IV-TR diagnosis is to classify the primary feature into a major category, consider possible nonpsychiatric causes for the complaint, and then use the decision trees in the appendix of DSM-IV-TR to identify the appropriate diagnosis. The decision trees guide the clinician who is unfamiliar with the intricacies of the criteria within a category to identify the features that distinguish closely related conditions. An example of the decision tree for evaluating acute psychosis to determine the diagnosis is shown in **Figure 286-1**. There are five other decision trees that aid in the differential diagnosis and demonstrate the hierarchical nature of the DSM-IV-TR: mental disorders due to a general medical condition, substance-induced disorders, mood disorders, anxiety disorders, and somatoform disorders.

GENERAL CRITERIA FOR DISPOSITION DETERMINATION

The determination to admit a patient with psychiatric illness from the ED is based on an assessment of danger to self or others and the ability to care for oneself. Some authorities also use additional criteria, such as desire and ability to cooperate with treatment and available support systems.

Many patients may benefit from outpatient or community resources instead of admission.[44,45] Knowledge of the specific options available in one's community helps determine disposition. The web site of the **Substance Abuse and Mental Health Services Administration (www.samhsa.gov)** is an excellent reference for local and community services. Once at the Substance Abuse and Mental Health Services Administration home page, select the "Topics" tab and query the Substance Abuse Treatment Services Locator or the Mental Health Treatment Services Locator. Resources can be identified by state, city, county, or zip code location and insurance status.

Psychiatric services available to the ED can reduce voluntary hospitalizations and increase patient compliance with outpatient visits.[46]

The determination for psychiatric admission is based on the ED psychiatric assessment, sometimes with limited information and most often within a short time frame for assessment. A study involving psychiatrists in four urban psychiatric emergency services identified five variables, in declining order of importance, that predicted admission: level of danger to self, severity of psychosis, ability for self-care, impulse control, and severity of depression.[47]

There are no currently validated tools that help determine the need for admission from the ED. The **Crisis Triage Rating Scale** (**Table 286-10**)[48] was developed by a community hospital's crisis intervention service but has not been validated for ED use. The scale ranks elements from three categories: dangerousness, support system, and ability to cooperate. A clinical scale/score cannot predict future behavior by a patient, but the scale items help in assessment of various factors to determine disposition.

Psychiatric consultation, by psychiatrists or psychiatric social workers, can be very helpful in determining patient disposition, especially when assessing danger to self or need for hospitalization.[49] Telepsychiatry

TABLE 286-7 The Quick Confusion Scale (abnormal ≤11 points)

Item	Score
What year is it?	2
What month is it?	2
State short key phrase to remember; have patient repeat it immediately	
What time is it?	2
Count backward from 20 to 1	2
Say months in reverse	2
Repeat key phrase	5

TABLE 286-8 A Suggested Medical Clearance Checklist*

Does the patient have a new psychiatric condition?	Yes	No
Is there a history of an active medical illness requiring evaluation?	Yes	No
Are there any abnormal vital signs?	Yes	No
Are there any abnormal findings on physical examination (conducted with the patient disrobed and in hospital gown)?	Yes	No
Are there any mental status abnormalities indicating medical illness?	Yes	No

*If the answer to any of the five questions is "Yes," follow with additional testing.

TABLE 286-9 Multiaxial Psychiatric Assessment

Axis I	Mental disorders: schizophrenia and other psychotic disorders; substance-related disorders; malingering; mood disorders; anxiety disorders; sleep disorders; eating disorders; factitious disorders; somatoform disorders; and dissociative disorders Delirium, dementia, and amnestic disorders; mental disorders due to a medical condition
Axis II	Personality disorders and mental retardation
Axis III	General medical conditions Medical conditions that impact mental health
Axis IV	Psychosocial and environmental problems
Axis V	Global assessment of functioning

TABLE 286-10 Crisis Triage Rating Scale

Ranking	Element
	Dangerousness
Most severe	Active SI or HI; current serious SI or HI attempt; unpredictable
	History of violent or impulsive behavior but no current signs
	Ambivalent SI/HI but ineffective gestures
	SI or HI but wants to control behavior
Least severe	No SI or HI and no history of violent or impulsive behavior
	Support System
Worst	None
	Some but limited effectiveness
	Some but not easy to mobilize
	Yes but limited
Best	Yes and good support
	Cooperation
Worst	Not able or refuses
	Little interest in cooperating
	Passive acceptance of help
	Wants help but desire limited
Best	Strong desire for help and will cooperate

Abbreviations: HI = homicidal ideation; SI = suicidal ideation.

can provide psychiatric consultations to facilities that do not have psychiatric resources. It is useful for rural, remote, and isolated populations and for a wide variety of diagnoses, ages, and mental health complaints. This resource can provide consultations, diagnostic assessment, medication management, and family and patient psychotherapy. It can aid in the determination of admission and care for psychiatric boarders.[50]

In the absence of medical indications for admission, refer to a psychiatrist or a psychiatric facility. Provide results of the ED medical and psychiatric evaluation to the consultant. For patients who can safely leave the ED, provide clear discharge instructions, and schedule specific follow-up.

ASSESSMENT OF HARM TO SELF OR OTHERS

The most difficult determination and highest risk is the assessment of self-harm. Assessment of suicide risk requires attention to diagnosis and treatment and to immediate and long-term safety. The interests of other people must be considered, because homicide may be a risk, especially when partner or family conflict exists. A full history is needed, a diagnosis must be reached, and a plan of management must be instituted, all with the patient's involvement insofar as that is possible. Establishing rapport and a therapeutic alliance is critical. The key points in initial assessment and management are summarized in **Table 286-11**.

Arrange privacy for an assessment and show respect and courtesy. Carefully elicit any symptoms of psychological and physical illness. Assess especially for evidence of depression, psychosis, or substance abuse. Identify predisposing and triggering risk factors. Avoid challenging or critical questions. Empathic comments like "You must have been pretty upset" encourage patients to share their difficulties. An open-ended question like "Can you tell me more about it?" is particularly useful. Some patients may resist. When the interviewer stresses the need to understand the story and displays willingness to listen actively, most patients respond and rapport increases. Direct questions may be necessary to elucidate events leading to suicidal ideation and behavior. A

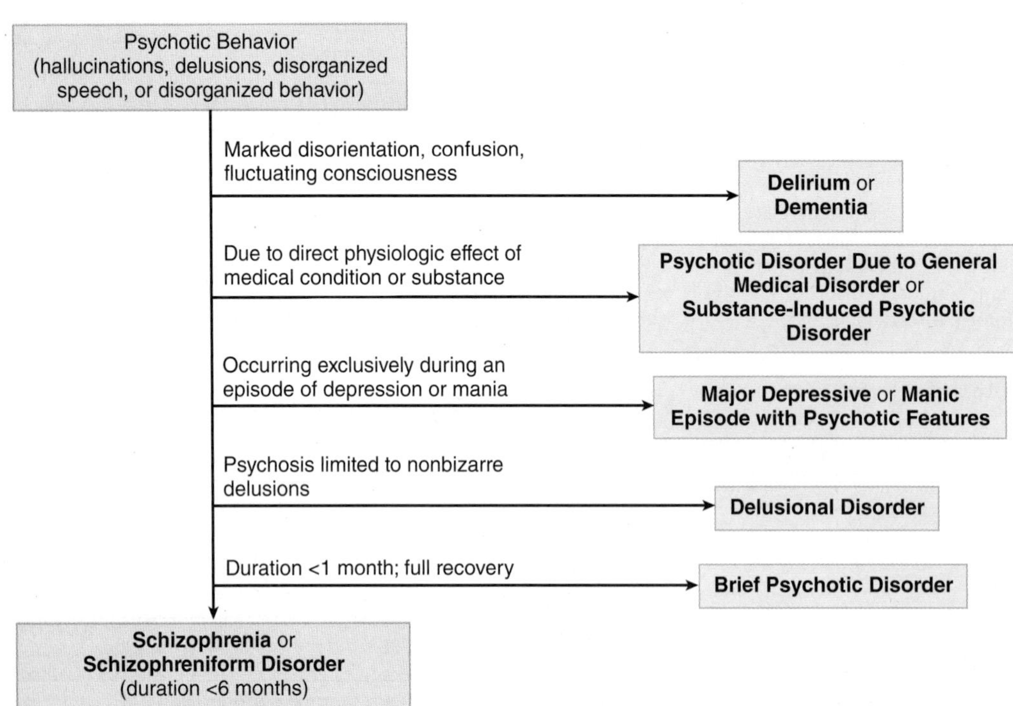

FIGURE 286-1. Decision tree for evaluating psychosis.

TABLE 286-11 Key Points in Assessment and Management of Suicidal Patients

Establish rapport.
Assess suicidal intent.
Determine access to means of suicide.
Assess current mental state.
If no evidence of a mental disorder, offer a safety plan, including help-seeking and problem-solving strategies.
If interpersonal or family issues, allow catharsis and offer problem-solving strategies; consider psychosocial referral.
If a mental disorder is present, arrange appropriate referral or management.
Ensure that a safety plan is in place before discharge.
Arrange follow-up before discharge.

systematic inquiry into stressful life events, relationships with family and other relevant people, and available social supports is always required.

After these are mapped out, decisions about future risk and treatment can be made. In general, risk of further suicidal behavior increases exponentially with increased number of health, mental health, and psychosocial risk factors.

SUICIDE RISK

A useful aid to assessing suicide risk is provided by the acronym **SAD PERSONS**, which is based on the first letters of 10 literature-identified suicide risk factors (**Table 286-12**).[51] Clinical rating scales cannot predict suicide in the individual. Strict cut-off scores should not be used to dictate admission to the hospital. There are at least 31 tests of risk of suicidal intent, but few were designed or validated for ED use. None of these tools have sufficient sensitivity and specificity to predict discharge from the ED. Rather, these tools are components in the determination of suicidal risk and can serve as guides to document the reasons for admission or discharge.

Suicidal intent can be determined based on the degree of planning, the lethality of the method considered, and the existence (and content) of any suicide notes. If patients are asked open-ended questions such as "What were your feelings about living and dying?" or "I guess you had mixed feelings about living and dying" instead of "Did you really want to live or die?" they are better able to verbalize their motivations, including ambivalence. When appropriate tact is used, the question, "What has stopped you from killing yourself so far?" may reveal protective factors and also remind patients of reasons to continue living.

Patients who are single, divorced, separated, widowed, or recently unemployed are at higher risk than those who are married and employed. Recently widowed older white males with access to lethal

TABLE 286-12 SAD PERSONS*

S	Sex
A	Age
D	Depression
P	Previous attempt
E	Ethanol use
R	Rational thinking loss
S	Social supports lacking
O	Organized plan
N	No spouse
S	Sickness

*Each factor is assigned 1 point, and patients who score ≥5 points should be considered at high risk of suicide.

Source: Reproduced with permission from Patterson WM, Dohn HH, Bird J, Patterson GA: Evaluation of suicidal patients: The SAD PERSONS Scale. *Psychosomatics* 24: 343, 1983. Copyright Elsevier.

means (e.g., a firearm) form the population at highest risk for completing suicide in the United States and thus should elicit a very careful evaluation. A psychotic patient who attempts suicide requires careful observation, with whatever restraint is necessary, and evaluation by a psychiatrist. A psychotic patient may respond unpredictably to distorted perceptions in a fearful or driven manner.

An important opportunity to assess future suicide risk is provided by asking patients their thoughts and feelings during the interview immediately after the suicide attempt.[52,53] For some patients, self-injury or suicide attempts appear to serve as a form of catharsis or emotional release, similar to weeping, talking to a friend, or becoming inebriated. Such patients did not undertake the attempt to die and do not identify the event as an attempt to do so. Often such patients may describe the attempts as being made when they were feeling angry, hurt, humiliated, ashamed, or vengeful and wanted to hurt others or extract a reaction from others. Patients who indicate remorse, shame, or embarrassment at having made a suicide attempt generally appear to have a lower risk of further suicidal behavior than those who do not show these responses. A patient who sits quietly; engages poorly with the physician; voices regret at surviving; expresses feelings of hopelessness, helplessness, or exhaustion; and refuses to provide additional information should be considered at high risk.

Secondary Gain *Secondary gain* is a term that indicates that although the primary motive for a suicide attempt appears to be death, the attempt may meet another need, such as a desire to gain attention or receive emotional help. When such needs are met by the attempt, a secondary gain is achieved, and the risk of subsequent suicide attempt is lessened momentarily. It is dangerous, however, to assume that secondary gain is the cause of a suicide attempt during an initial evaluation in an ED. All suicide behaviors should be taken seriously.

SUICIDE RISK AND DISPOSITION

Patient disposition can be assessed by estimating the lethality of the attempt and the likelihood of rescue, with the patient's perceptions and understanding of these taken into account. When there is a high likelihood of rescue and low lethality, there may be a lower risk of further suicidal behavior than if the possibility of rescue was remote and the patient believed the lethality of the agent or method was high. A patient who attempted suicide by hanging in an isolated area of the woods is at greater risk than a person who swallowed a few tablets of a substance of relatively low toxicity in front of witnesses.

Patients who have made previous suicide attempts are at greater risk for further suicide attempts and for suicide. Prior attempts are a particularly significant warning if the intensity and apparent lethality of the suicide attempts escalate with each subsequent attempt. **Table 286-13** provides details of assessment.

Table 286-13 also provides high-risk and low-risk suicide profiles. **High-risk patients** with strong, pervasive suicidal intent require psychiatric hospitalization. **Moderate-risk patients** are those who present in a serious suicidal crisis but who, because of a positive response to initial intervention and favorable social support, may not be in immediate danger. Hospitalization can often be avoided for such patients, provided outpatient treatment can be established immediately and the patient engages with treatment. Such disposition decisions are most often made in concert with a psychiatric consultant. Before discharge, develop a safety plan with the patient and the patient's family, remove available means of suicide (such as firearms or drug supplies), prescribe conservative amounts of psychotropic medication (usually no more than a 2-week supply), and provide help-seeking advice and problem-solving strategies. It is important to have a family member take responsibility for managing a patient's medications.

Low-risk patients frequently present with suicidal ideation, threats, plans, or minor attempts that occur in the context of a clearly definable external crisis. Family and social support is usually readily available, caring, and sympathetic. Low-risk patients with the following stipulations may be discharged from the emergency department: medical treatment not needed, no prior suicidal attempt, not actively suicidal, adult in house with good relationship, adult agrees to monitor, adult will remove guns and medications, contact for deterioration available, follow-up

TABLE 286-13 Evaluation of Suicide Risk in Adults

Demographic, Health, and Social Profile	High Risk	Lower Risk
Gender	Male	Female
Marital status	Separated, divorced, or widowed	Married
Family history	Chaotic, conflictual Family history of suicide	Stable No family history of suicide
Job	Recently unemployed	Employed
Relationships	Recent conflict or loss of a relationship	Stable relationships
School	In disciplinary trouble	No disciplinary problems
Religion	Weak or no suicide taboo	Strong taboo against suicide
Health Physical Mental	Acute or chronic, progressive illness Excessive drug or alcohol use Depression (SIG E CAPS + MOOD)* History of schizophrenia or bipolar disorder Panic disorder Antisocial or disruptive behavior Feelings of helplessness or hopelessness Few, weak reasons for living Unstable, inappropriate affect	Good health Little or no drug or alcohol use No depression No psychosis Minimal anxiety Directable, oriented Has hope, optimism Good, strong reasons for living Appropriate affect
Suicidal ideation	Frequent, intense, prolonged, pervasive	Infrequent, low intensity, transient
Suicide attempts	Repeated attempts Realistic plan, including access to means Previous attempt(s) planned Rescue unlikely Lethal method Guilt Unambiguous or continuing wish to die	No prior attempts No plan, lacks access to means Previous attempt(s) impulsive High likelihood of rescue Method of low lethality Embarrassment about suicide ideation No previous or continuing wish to die; large appeal component
Relationship with health professional	Lacks insight Poor rapport	Insight Good rapport
Social support	Unsupportive family, friends Socially isolated	Concerned family, friends Socially integrated

*SIG E CAPS + MOOD is a mnemonic for the eight symptoms of depression plus depressed mood: S = sleep disturbance; I = loss of interest in usual pleasurable activities; G = guilt; E = loss of energy; C = inability to concentrate; A = loss of appetite; P = psychomotor slowing; S = suicidal thoughts; MOOD = depressed mood (i.e., "Have you felt blue, down, or depressed most of the day for most days in the last 2 weeks?"). Fulfillment of five or more of the eight items from the list of eight symptoms indicates the presence of major depression. Symptoms must be present nearly every day for 2 weeks and must include depressed mood or loss of interest or pleasure in activities. Symptoms must represent a change from previous functioning resulting in social, occupational, or other life impairment, and they cannot be the direct result of substance use, a medical condition, or bereavement.

arranged, and patient and support group agreement to plan and recommendations.[54]

Before discharge, ensure that good social support is available to the patient. Social support includes a place to live and family or friends who will support the patient emotionally. Obtain agreement that a supportive individual can spend the next 24 hours with the patient.

However, because many attempts that appear trivial on first glance are found to have more serious implications on closer examination, carefully assess all patients coming to the ED after a suicide attempt. If there are any concerns about the safety of discharging a suicidal patient and psychiatric consultation is not immediately available, hospitalize the patient involuntarily.

No-Harm Contracts "**No-harm contracts**" or "suicide prevention contracts" have sometimes been used as a method to lower suicidal risk. Typically, the no-harm contract is a verbal or written agreement initiated by the physician or psychiatrist in which the suicidal patient agrees not to harm or kill himself or herself and to adopt agreed-upon help-seeking behaviors if a crisis arises. Although proponents argue that the no-harm contract can be therapeutic by helping to reveal the intent of the patient and reduce it, and diagnostic by eliciting the nature and severity of a patient's suicidality, there is little evidence that such contracts prevent further suicidal behavior.[54] Currently, the use of no-harm contracts is not supported. Rather, the preparation of a joint safety plan with the patient and the patient's family or a commitment by the patient to treatment is more likely to be of therapeutic benefit.

Self-Injury Behaviors Young adult and adolescent patients may present to the ED because of self-harm behaviors that are not dangerously suicidal but nonetheless require both medical and mental health care.[29] Typically, such patients cut or scratch their arms to "relieve tension" or burn themselves in an effort to feel a certain way. Females tend to more often cut themselves, while young men tend more often to burn themselves. Such acts are usually heralded by a state of mounting tension with depersonalization, followed by relief after the self-mutilating behavior. Self-injury is usually not suicidal behavior but rather a poorly learned coping mechanism that is used to reduce tension, self-soothe, and communicate feelings. For most young patients, self-injurious behavior appears to be time-limited and linked to problems with parents and is not associated with severe clinical symptoms or suicidality. However, some self-injuring patients do have clinical symptoms including high anxiety and active suicidality. In addition to tetanus prophylaxis and wound care, assess patients for suicidal ideation and further plans for self-harm. Nonsuicidal self-harm or self-mutilatory behaviors are seen in patients who may insert foreign bodies into their bladder, rectum, nose, or other orifices and may require GI or surgical intervention. Outpatient psychiatric follow-up and evaluation are usually appropriate for this type of behavior.

VIOLENCE TOWARD OTHERS

Potential victims who are clearly identified may need to be warned.[55] This can be done through the psychiatric consultant or hospital or local police. Clues that suggest potential violence include hostile behavior; homicidal ideas, fantasies, or preoccupations; verbal aggressiveness; statements about violent intent; weapons skill and access; motives for violence; and preattack planning and preparation.[55] Patients need immediate hospitalization.

ED TREATMENT

Treatment of acute agitation is discussed in detail in chapter 287, "Acute Agitation."

Psychiatric patients who are noncompliant to their psychotropic medications need to be restarted on their medications. Mental health patients with a new psychiatric diagnosis also need to start treatment. For schizophrenic patients, haloperidol 2 to 5 milligrams IM and lorazepam 1 to 2 milligrams IM have the quickest effect. Oral risperidone (Risperdal®) 3 to 6 milligrams per day or olanzapine (Zyprexa®) 15 milligrams daily also may be useful. Do not given benzodiazepines with olanzapine, because the two drugs coadministered can result in hypotension an hour later. Historically, it takes weeks to months for antidepressant medications to have a clinical effect, and so medications are not typically started in the ED unless in close consultation with the follow-up psychiatric provider.

Ketamine is proposed as a quick treatment for depression and suicidal ideation. Ketamine results in improvement within 2 hours and has an effect after 24 hours.[56] In a small trial of suicidal patients, 15 suicidal patients received a subanesthetic IV dose of ketamine. Thirteen of 14 patients were completely free of suicidal ideation at 10-day follow-up.[57]

Some advocate for treatment of suicidal patients in the ED. Techniques include a brief intervention, enhanced follow-up, video patient education, and family therapy, with a rapid ED response team consisting of a psychiatrist and psychiatric nurse or social worker. Such programs depend on sufficient ED resources and the ability to arrange solid follow-up.[58-60]

PSYCHIATRIC BOARDERS IN THE ED

Unfortunately, a nationwide scarcity of inpatient psychiatric beds has led to the phenomenon of "psychiatric boarders," patients staying for days in the ED before psychiatric admission. Psychiatric boarders have also increased because some patients are sent to the ED for conflict resolution or respite from family, group home, or nursing home. The ED becomes the arbitrator in social issues that are better handled by police, counselors, or social workers. Boarding psychiatric patients is thought to result in premature ED discharge,[61] increased complications while in the ED, escalated medical and psychiatric problems, and reduced ED efficiency. Psychiatric boarders in the ED stay longer in the ED than other patients.[62]

Protocols for appropriate use of the ED for these patients and alternative care sites need to be explored, such as mobile crisis teams, expanded use of social workers, and police training in crisis intervention.[63] Community treatment consisting of supportive services, case management, emergency care, medications, and assistance of daily living can reduce ED use. Mobile crisis units can provide crisis stabilization in patient homes.

PSYCHIATRIC OBSERVATION UNITS

The best option for reducing psychiatric admissions is the acute psychiatric stabilization unit, which is similar to medical observation units. Acute psychiatric stabilization units are usually managed by psychiatric services, whereas medical observation units are often managed by the emergency service. Psychiatric stabilization units provide psychiatric assessment, crisis stabilization and drug treatment, and linkage with community resources before discharge. Acute stabilization of psychiatric patients allows time for diagnostic clarity, development of alternatives to admission, and a respite for the patient and family.[64]

OVERVIEW OF AXIS I TO V DISORDERS

Axis I disorders include the clinical syndromes of mental disorders (**Figure 286-2**). For more than one axis I diagnosis, list the most important diagnosis first. **Axis II** includes personality disorders and developmental disorders, including mental retardation (**Figure 286-3**). The presence of axis II disorders complicates management of all other axis disorders. **Axis III** encompasses general medical conditions that are or could be relevant to the understanding or management of the patient's psychiatric illness. **Axis IV** consists of psychosocial and environmental stressors or problems. Axis IV conditions relate to primary support group, social environment, and educational, occupational, housing, economic, healthcare access, and legal issues. **Axis V** relates to the patient's current overall functioning using the global level of functioning scale. This scale ranges from 0 to 100, with 0 representing persistent danger to self or others and 100 indicating superior functioning in a wide range of

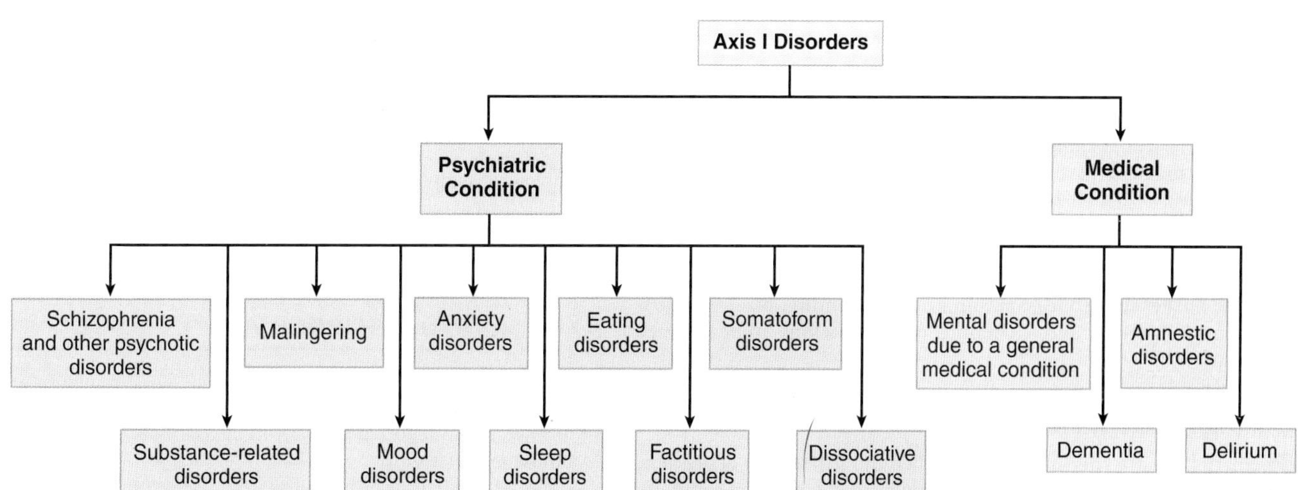

FIGURE 286-2. Axis I disorders (psychiatric syndromes).

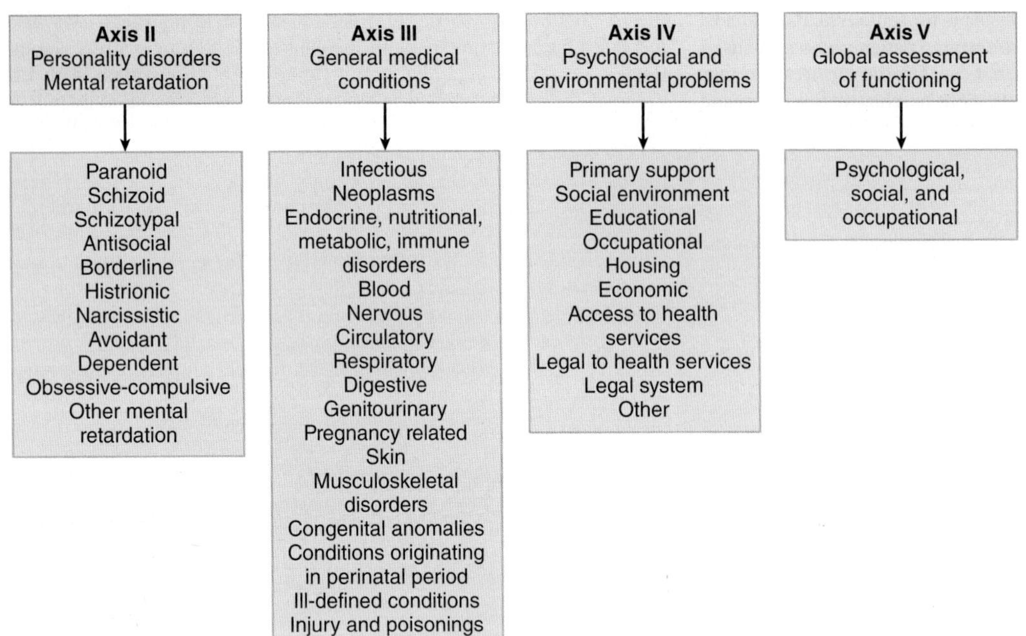

FIGURE 286-3. Axis II to V disorders.

activities. The axis I disorders most clinically relevant to ED practice are summarized below.

AXIS I: PSYCHOSES

SCHIZOPHRENIA

Schizophrenia is the most prevalent psychosis. The essential features of schizophrenia are a deterioration in functioning, characteristic positive symptoms (hallucinations, delusions, disorganized speech, disorganized behavior, and catatonic behavior), negative symptoms (blunted affect, emotional withdrawal, lack of spontaneity, anhedonia, and attentional impairment), cognitive impairment manifested by loose associations or incoherence for at least 1 month, and the relative absence of a mood disorder. Schizophrenia is most likely a group of disorders with different causes that share a final common pathway. There is no evidence that psychosocial stressors or poor parenting is responsible for causing the illness, although these may have a profound effect on the patient's adaptation to this usually chronic disorder.

Symptoms of schizophrenia usually begin in late adolescence or early adulthood, although the onset can occur at any age. The childhood history of schizophrenics often is marked by shyness, odd or eccentric behavior, school difficulties, or paranoid behaviors, but such features are not always present. A prodromal phase, in which a gradual deterioration of function is noted, usually precedes the development of active delusions or hallucinations. Such deterioration usually includes the worsening of social withdrawal or the new onset of social withdrawal, odd behavior or speech, and difficulty in functioning at school or work. Patients or their families rarely seek care until the onset of the active phase of psychosis. Schizophrenic individuals seldom seek care at all because they lack insight; they do not realize that their perceptions, thoughts, and behavior are abnormal.

Disorganization of thinking and behavior characterizes schizophrenia. Disheveled appearance and poor grooming, bizarre behavior, poor judgment, and loosening of associations indicate such disorganization.

SCHIZOAFFECTIVE DISORDER

Schizoaffective disorder is diagnosed when the patient has depression, mania, or mixed episode together with classic schizophrenic symptoms such as delusions, hallucination, disorganized speech, disorganized or catatonic behavior, and affect flattening. Delusions or hallucinations need to occur for at least 2 weeks after the mood symptoms have ceased. The mood symptoms should be present for a substantial portion of time and not be due to drug use or medical conditions.

BRIEF PSYCHOTIC DISORDER

Some individuals may become acutely psychotic after exposure to an extremely traumatic life experience. If such a psychosis lasts for <4 weeks, it is termed a brief psychotic disorder. Precipitants include the death of a loved one or a life-threatening situation such as combat or a natural disaster. Emotional turmoil, confusion, and extremely bizarre behavior and speech are common in this disorder.

AXIS I: SUBSTANCE-RELATED DISORDERS

Substance-related disorders are due to ingestion of a drug of abuse or alcohol, side effects of a prescribed or over-the-counter medication, toxic exposure, or substance withdrawal.[43] The specific features of intoxication syndromes commonly seen in the ED are described in chapters on specific agents in the Toxicology section (Chapters 176 to 207) and Chapter 292, Substance Use Disorders.

The diagnosis of withdrawal is made by identifying the withdrawal toxidrome and evidence of recent use of the substance in a pattern sufficient to produce withdrawal when the amount ingested is decreased or stopped. Specific withdrawal patterns depend on the agent.

AXIS I: MALINGERING

Malingering is the intentional invention or exaggeration of physical or psychological symptoms for external gain. The external gain may be maladaptive to avoid work or obtain drugs, or adaptive in response to being an enemy combatant in wartime. Malingering is distinguished from factitious disorders by the presentation of symptoms for a known secondary gain.

AXIS I: MOOD DISORDERS

The mood disorders are the most prevalent of the major psychiatric disorders. The lifetime prevalence of mood disorders in the age group of 17 to 39 years was reported as 11.5% in the National Health and Nutrition Examination Survey III.[65]

Mood, or affective, disorders differ from the normal extremes of sadness and happiness in that characteristic clusters of psychological and vegetative symptoms (depressive or manic syndrome) are present, and functioning is impaired. Depressive disorders are the major cause of completed suicide.

Mood disorders tend to be episodic, with periods of remission and normal function. Any of the features of schizophrenia such as delusions, hallucinations, or disorganization may be present, but if a full depressive or manic syndrome exists, the diagnosis is likely psychotic mood disorder. The more common mood disorders are briefly discussed in the following sections.

MAJOR DEPRESSION

The essential features of major depression are a persistent sad or depressed (dysphoric) mood or pervasive loss of interest in usual activities lasting for at least 2 weeks. Associated psychological symptoms include guilt over past deeds, self-reproach, feelings of worthlessness or hopelessness, inability to experience pleasure, and recurrent thought of death or suicide. Vegetative symptoms involve physiologic functioning and include weight loss or gain, sleep disturbance, fatigue, inability to concentrate, and psychomotor agitation or retardation. Depression may begin gradually or rapidly but is usually present for several weeks before the patient seeks help.

Major depression is often superimposed on other mental disorders, such as substance abuse, personality disorders, and anxiety disorders, and such conditions are frequently comorbid conditions. Major depression is often recurrent, so certain patients must be maintained on long-term treatment to prevent relapse.

DYSTHYMIC DISORDER

Dysthymic disorder is a more chronic and less severe form of depressive illness and was previously termed depressive neurosis. Depressed mood must have been present most of the day, more days than not, for at least 2 years. Psychotic features are not seen, and patients with this disorder often have a lifelong gloomy, pessimistic outlook. Women are affected more often than men, and the onset is typically in childhood, adolescence, or early adulthood.

BIPOLAR DISORDER

Bipolar disorder, previously termed manic-depressive illness, is characterized by periods of mania cycling with periods of depression. A full manic syndrome is one of the most striking and distinctive conditions in clinical practice. The essential disturbance in mood is one of elation or irritability. Manic patients feel "on top of the world," expansive, and energetic. The state is precarious, however, and patients may quickly become argumentative, hostile, irritable, and sarcastic, especially when their plans are thwarted. Bipolar disorders are classified into types I and II based on the presence of mania, which is found in bipolar I disorder and not found in bipolar II.

The disorder is equally common in men and women, and the onset is usually in the third and fourth decades. Complications include suicide, substance abuse (excessive alcohol use is common during the manic phase), and marital and occupational disruptions. The course of bipolar disorder is episodic, with the duration, frequency, and regularity of the episodes varying greatly. Depressive episodes are more frequent than manic episodes.

AXIS I: ANXIETY DISORDERS

The anxiety disorders are mental disorders in which apprehension, fears, and excessive worry dominate the psychological life of the individual. Pathologic degrees of anxiety are accompanied by different degrees of autonomic activity (sweating, tachycardia, or dizziness) out of proportion to any real danger or threat. Because anxiety is a ubiquitous condition and frequently associated with medical illness, depression, neurologic syndromes, and psychoses, a diagnosis of a primary anxiety disorder is made after exclusion of other causes.

PANIC DISORDER

Patients who experience recurrent attacks of severe anxiety are said to suffer from panic disorder. A panic attack consists of a sudden extreme surge of anxiety and dread accompanied by autonomic signs, including palpitations, tachycardia, shortness of breath, chest tightness, dizziness, sweating, and tremulousness. The symptoms develop over a few minutes at most and may be unprovoked or stimulus related.

GENERALIZED ANXIETY DISORDER

When anxiety attacks are absent but the patient complains of persistent worry, tension, or free-floating anxiety, a diagnosis of generalized anxiety disorder should be considered. This condition lasts at least 6 months and is characterized by apprehensive worrying, muscle tension, insomnia, irritability, restlessness, jumpiness, or distractibility. Associated autonomic symptoms include the cardiopulmonary, GI, and neurologic symptoms that are seen in panic attacks.

POSTTRAUMATIC STRESS DISORDER

Posttraumatic stress disorder is an anxiety reaction to a severe psychosocial stressor, such as military combat, fire, rape, a terrorist event, or natural disaster. Symptoms involve repetitive and intrusive memories of the event, nightmares, emotional numbing, survivor guilt, and different degrees of depression and anxiety. Substance abuse is a frequent complication.

OBSESSIVE-COMPULSIVE DISORDER

Obsessive-compulsive disorder is a mental disorder in which the patient experiences intrusive thoughts or images that cannot be eliminated from the mind. Typical thoughts involve images of graphic violence to self or others, contamination, or perverse sexual behavior that the patient would not carry out but nevertheless obsessively fantasizes about. To control the obsessive thoughts, the individual may engage in compulsive behavior or rituals, such as excessive washing, repetitive checking, or counting. When the obsessions and compulsions occupy a great deal of time, the patient may become significantly disabled and seek psychiatric attention.

AXIS I: SLEEP DISORDERS

Sleep disorders include hypersomnia, insomnia, and narcolepsy. Hypersomnia and insomnia can occur in association with other mental disorders. Narcolepsy is a neurologic sleep disorder, not caused by a mental disorder.

AXIS I: EATING DISORDERS

The eating disorders anorexia nervosa and bulimia nervosa are discussed in chapter 291, "Eating Disorders."

AXIS I: FACTITIOUS DISORDERS

Factitious disorders are characterized by physical or psychological symptoms that are exhibited in order to assume a sick role. Patients may fabricate complaints, falsify vital sign values, self-inflict an illness, or exaggerate a preexisting medical condition. A factitious disorder demonstrates a psychological need to be in the sick role without external incentives. Munchausen syndrome is an extreme form of this disorder. Munchausen by proxy, or factitious disorder by proxy, is inducing or fabricating disease in a child to get medical attention.

AXIS I: SOMATOFORM DISORDERS

Many patients have particular complaints or symptoms for which no medical explanation can be identified. These symptoms must cause the patient significant distress or impairment in social, occupational, or other areas of functioning. When a physical cause has been clearly eliminated and the complaint is not delusional or occurring in the context of a depression or anxiety disorder, somatoform disorders may be considered in the differential diagnosis. When the complaint involves a loss of function, usually in the neurologic system (e.g., paralysis, blindness, or numbness) and psychological factors are deemed etiologic, a conversion disorder may be present. **Conversion disorders** are much more common in culturally and psychologically unsophisticated persons. This diagnosis should be made with extreme caution, if at all, in the ED, because studies indicate that many patients (up to 50%) diagnosed with conversion disorder eventually develop signs of a physical disorder that explains the symptom.

Some patients have a wide variety of complaints and long, complicated histories of medical problems that have no apparent medical cause. Such individuals may have somatization disorder, a disorder beginning in the teens and twenties, usually in women, and leading to considerable unnecessary diagnostic and surgical intervention. The prototypical patient is a middle-aged woman who describes a "positive review of systems" in a dramatic and confusing way. As with conversion disorder, a diagnosis of somatization disorder should not be made on the basis of an ED visit, but the identification of somatizing behavior is useful for future reference, because patients frequently make repeated contacts with medical providers.

AXIS 1: DISSOCIATIVE DISORDERS

The dissociative disorders comprise a group of uncommon and poorly understood conditions in which the central feature is a sudden alteration in the normal integration of identity and consciousness. The dissociation often occurs under severe stress and may or may not be recurrent, although it is rarely permanent. The forms of dissociative state relevant to emergency practice are dissociative amnesia, a temporary loss of memory for important personal details related to a traumatic or stressful situation that is not due to a medical cause, and dissociative fugue, in which a similar loss of memory and assumption of a new identity are accompanied by travel away from home. Dissociative disorders are difficult to distinguish from malingering, in which an individual in pursuit of a clear goal, such as avoiding incarceration or military duty, may consciously feign amnesia. As always, medical illnesses and drug intoxication that may cause loss of memory, such as that resulting from transient global amnesia, must be ruled out.

AXIS I DISORDERS: MEDICAL CONDITIONS

This group of syndromes includes dementia, delirium, amnestic disorders, and other cognitive disorders characterized by a clinically significant deficit in cognitive or memory function due to a general medical condition. Dementia and delirium are also discussed in chapter 288, "Mental Health Disorders of the Elderly." Refer to **Tables 286-6** for features of delirium and dementia.

DEMENTIA

Dementia is a pervasive disturbance of cognitive functioning in several areas, including memory, abstract thinking, judgment, personality, and other higher cortical functions such as language. If clouding of consciousness is present, then the patient does not have solely a dementing illness but has delirium, intoxication, or withdrawal. The presence of global cognitive impairment may be detected through the use of a bedside cognitive examination (see **Table 286-7** and the **clock test**). Early in the course of dementia, anxiety, depression, or psychosis may dominate the clinical picture and obscure cognitive dysfunction. Maintain a high degree of clinical suspicion for dementia when evaluating an elderly patient with no prior psychiatric history who develops new psychiatric problems. Dementia is discussed in more detail in chapter 288, "Mental Health Disorders of the Elderly."

DELIRIUM

Delirium is characterized by global impairment in cognitive function but is distinguished from dementia in two major ways. In delirium, the patient has clouding of consciousness, a reduction in the awareness of the external environment (manifest as difficulty sustaining attention), varying degrees of alertness ranging from drowsiness to stupor, and sensory misperception. In most patients, an underlying general medical condition, substance intoxication, or withdrawal or medication use is the cause of the delirium. Delirium must be distinguished from psychiatric illnesses such as psychotic, mood, anxiety, and stress disorders. There is a long list of causes of delirium, including intoxicants, withdrawal syndromes, infections, trauma, seizures, endocrinopathies, inflammatory processes, shock, organ failure, and neoplasia.

The primary distinguishing feature of delirium is a typical acute course, with rapid deterioration in hours or days, rather than in months as with dementia. Also, the severity of delirium fluctuates over the course of hours; the patient may appear normal at one time and wildly agitated a few hours later. Hallucinations, often visual, are common. Delirium is discussed in more detail in chapter 288.

AMNESTIC DISORDERS

Amnestic patients typically are unable to learn new information or to recall information that is already learned. Amnestic disorders cause a problem in carrying out social and occupational functions and are not part of delirium or dementia. Causes of amnestic disorder include brain trauma, stroke, carbon monoxide poisoning, substance abuse, and chronic nutritional deficiency. Acute onset of amnesia needs to be carefully investigated.

MENTAL DISORDERS DUE TO A GENERAL MEDICAL CONDITION

When there is evidence that a psychiatric disturbance is a direct physiologic consequence of a general medical condition or substance, the mental disorder is specified as "due to" the medical problem, for example, "major depression due to hypothyroidism." The mental condition cannot be caused by another mental disorder, and it cannot be part of the course of delirium.

The diagnostic features of mental disorders due to a general medical condition rely on evidence from patient history, physical examination, and laboratory results indicative of a causative medical condition. Sometimes the cause cannot be determined in the ED, and the patient may need admission for further evaluation. General medical conditions may cause amnestic, psychotic, mood, and anxiety disorders.

REFERENCES

The complete reference list is available online at www.TintinalliEM.com.

CHAPTER 287 Acute Agitation

Shauna Garris
Caitlin Hughes

INTRODUCTION AND EPIDEMIOLOGY

EDs are the portal of access to the healthcare system for most patients with acute agitation and acute behavioral or mental health disorders.[1] Agitation is one of the most common manifestations of mental health and behavioral disorders, dementia, and intoxication and withdrawal syndromes. The last consensus updates for acute agitation were published in 2006,[2] prior to the release of newer therapeutic agents and prior to the recognition of QT_c prolongation with acutely administered psychotropics. This review provides a general pharmacotherapeutic approach for acute agitation and acute behavioral emergencies.

GENERAL THERAPEUTIC APPROACH

Try to obtain vital signs, obtain a patient history and perform a physical examination, and obtain baseline laboratory data. Psychosis, mania, withdrawal syndromes, drug intoxication, delirium, or even depression and anxiety can cause psychomotor agitation, aggressive behaviors, or disorientation. Other causes of acute agitation include adverse effects of medications, pain, substance abuse, or worsening of a chronic underlying illness.

TABLE 287-1 Comparison of Important Adverse Effects of Agents for Acute Agitation

	Benzodiazepines	Typical or First-Generation Antipsychotics	Atypical or Second-Generation Antipsychotics
Somnolence	++	+	+
Postural hypotension	+	+/−	+/−
Extrapyramidal symptoms	−	++	+
Respiratory depression	+	−	+/−
Neuroleptic malignant syndrome	−	+	+
QT_c prolongation/ torsades de pointes	−	+	+
Paradoxical CNS disinhibition	+	−	−

The most important goal in the care of the agitated patient is ensuring the safety of the patient and staff involved. Management of the patient's undifferentiated agitation ensures immediate safety and allows a more thorough evaluation for serious acute pathology.

Provide a sitter and try to address patient comfort needs. Decrease external stimuli by placing the patient in a quiet room. Remove potentially dangerous objects from the immediate environment. Use physical restraints if there is imminent harm to healthcare workers, other patients or visitors, or the patient him/herself.[1-4]

When considering pharmacologic treatment options, assess the underlying diagnosis, presenting signs and symptoms, and potential risks/benefits of specific agents (**Tables 287-1** and **287-2**), and determine the proper dose and easiest mode of administration. Because the oral and parenteral routes are equivalent for some agents,[5-8] offer oral agents first, if appropriate and feasible. If repeated dosing is needed, try to wait 1 hour before the next dose to adequately assess patient behavior and medication effect. Generally, all antipsychotics have similar efficacy at comparable dosages and may be used to treat acute agitation.

The FDA recommends evaluating the QT_c interval prior to the use of many of these agents, because all antipsychotic agents carry a bolded warning for altered cardiac conduction and risk of fatal arrhythmias. In clinical situations in which rapid tranquilization is necessary, prior determination of the QT_c interval is usually impractical and often impossible. If an electrocardiogram is available from a prior hospital visit, review it for evidence of QT_c prolongation.

The QT interval is used as a surrogate marker for the potential development of abnormal cardiac conduction. In general, the QT_c interval is considered prolonged when it is ≥450 milliseconds in men and 460 milliseconds in women.[9] **Medication-induced QT_c prolongation is considered highly significant at ≥500 milliseconds.**[9-12] Unfortunately, **QT_c prolongation does not directly correlate with clinical risk of dysrhythmias or the development of the malignant arrhythmia torsade de pointes.**

PHARMACOLOGY OF AGENTS FOR AGITATION

BENZODIAZEPINES

Of the benzodiazepines, **lorazepam** is the agent with the highest level of guideline and literature support for acute use and is considered first-line therapy in the treatment of undifferentiated agitation. Much of this preference is due to its availability for administration by the PO, IM, PR, or IV route; relatively quick onset of action; and lack of active hepatic metabolites. Benzodiazepines bind to benzodiazepine-1 receptors on the postsynaptic γ-aminobutyric-A receptor, which results in increased influx of chloride ions into the postsynaptic neuron, leading to hypoexcitability and neuronal stabilization.[13]

The initial dose of lorazepam for acute agitation is 2 milligrams, with repeated dosing, if needed, given at least 30 minutes after the initial dose. Cumulative studied dosage is 4 milligrams over 2 to 4 hours; however, dosage regimens of up to 8 milligrams have been described.[14-16] Onset of action is 0.5 to 1 hour, with a duration of 6 to 8 hours and a terminal half-life of 12.9 hours in adults that is extended to 15.9 hours in the elderly and up to 72 hours in patients with renal failure.

Lorazepam is effective in both undifferentiated and psychotic agitation, and 2 milligrams may be as effective 5 milligrams of haloperidol, with additive benefits when given in combination with other agents (except olanzapine).[5,14,17] The most common adverse effect of lorazepam or other benzodiazepines is sedation, and sedation is greater than that with haloperidol alone.[5,14] Lorazepam can cause respiratory depression and hypotension, particularly with repeated and high-dose administration. Another notable adverse effect is paradoxical agitation, or activation or worsening of confusion, most commonly seen in patients with delirium and in the elderly.

TYPICAL, OR FIRST-GENERATION, ANTIPSYCHOTICS

Typical antipsychotics are also called first-generation or conventional antipsychotics, classic neuroleptics, or major tranquilizers. This class of drugs blocks dopamine receptors and is strongly associated with extrapyramidal symptoms, such as dystonias, akathisia or restlessness, and parkinsonism, and anticholinergic blockade (dry mouth,

TABLE 287-2 Considerations When Treating Acute Agitation

Subgroup of Patients	Special Considerations
Agitation caused by alcohol/substance abuse Agitation of unknown origin	Consider benzodiazepine for added benefits of preventing potential withdrawal symptoms.
Agitation caused by psychosis/mania	Consider typical/atypical antipsychotic over benzodiazepine to concomitantly treat underlying psychosis; also beneficial when conversion to PO required.
Agitation caused by dementia	Consider atypical antipsychotic (especially if elderly) and use lowest effective dose.
Elderly	If using a benzodiazepine, use lorazepam, oxazepam, or temazepam ("LOT") because these are metabolized via glucuronidation and are safest. Consider atypical antipsychotic over typical antipsychotic, but use lowest effective dose and be aware of FDA Black Box warning in elderly.
History of seizures	Avoid haloperidol and atypical antipsychotics (lower seizure threshold); consider benzodiazepine.
Recent history of MI	Ziprasidone is contraindicated.
Prolonged QT_c	Benzodiazepines first choice; atypical antipsychotics second choice; typical antipsychotics last choice.
Concern for bradycardia or hypotension	Avoid olanzapine (and especially avoid olanzapine + benzodiazepine because this increases risk).
Uncooperative patient requiring rapid tranquilization	Consider IV or IM route.

Abbreviations: FDA = U.S. Food and Drug Administration; MI = myocardial infarction.

TABLE 287-3 Potency of Typical Antipsychotics Commonly Used for Agitation

Generic Name	Brand Name	D_2 Receptor Potency	FDA Warning or Concern	Available Routes of Administration
Chlorpromazine	Thorazine®	Low	QT_c prolongation	PO, IM
Fluphenazine	Prolixin®	High		PO, IM
Haloperidol	Haldol®	High	QT_c prolongation with high-dose or IV administration	PO, IM, IV
Droperidol	Inapsine®	High	QT_c prolongation, even with no risk factors Not approved by FDA for treatment of agitation	PO, IM, IV

Abbreviation: FDA = U.S. Food and Drug Administration.

hypotension, glaucoma exacerbation, delirium). Typical antipsychotics are classified as low, intermediate, or high potency when compared to 100 milligrams of chlorpromazine (Thorazine®). Low-potency typical antipsychotics tend to be more sedating and are associated with hypotension, dizziness, and anticholinergic symptoms. High-potency medications are less sedating but are associated with extrapyramidal symptoms (**Table 287-3**).

Agents commonly used for acute agitation within this class include haloperidol, fluphenazine, and chlorpromazine because these agents are available in multiple dosage forms and have decades of clinical and anecdotal data supporting their efficacy. Droperidol has historically been commonly used for agitation; however, U.S. Food and Drug Administration concerns of QT_c prolongation have limited its use for this purpose.

Adverse effects limiting the use of these medications in acute agitation include sedation, hypotension, risk of extrapyramidal symptoms, and QT_c prolongation and the risk of torsades de pointes. While all antipsychotics can increase the QT_c interval and risk of torsades de pointes, several agents within this first-generation subclass have been implicated for adverse outcomes. Among antipsychotics used for acute agitation, **haloperidol** and **droperidol** carry additional Food and Drug Administration warnings regarding QT_c prolongation, torsades de pointes, and sudden cardiac death.[18,19]

Neuroleptic malignant syndrome, though rare, is a potentially life-threatening adverse effect that consists of a constellation of signs including altered mental status, hyperthermia, muscular rigidity, autonomic instability, and elevated creatinine phosphokinase. Contributing factors for neuroleptic malignant syndrome may include high dose, rapid dose escalation, use of a high-potency first-generation agent, history of previous neuromuscular malignant syndrome, agitation, or dehydration.[20]

Common extrapyramidal symptoms encountered with the acute administration of first-generation agents include akathisia and the parkinsonian symptoms of tremor and gait disturbances. Acute dystonias, which occur less frequently but can be severe, include torticollis, laryngeal spasm, and oculogyric crisis. Acute dystonia is associated more frequently with the high-potency agents (e.g., fluphenazine, haloperidol, and droperidol). The mechanism of extrapyramidal symptoms is thought to be related to secondary acetylcholine dysregulation in response to decreased dopamine in the nigrostriatal pathway. **Treat acute dystonias with anticholinergic agents such as IM or IV diphenhydramine (25 to 50 milligrams) or benztropine (2 milligrams).** Coadministration of these agents with a typical IM antipsychotic to prevent dystonia and other extrapyramidal symptoms is also common practice. Be aware that diphenhydramine and benztropine carry their own risks of adverse reactions including sedation, constipation, and blurred vision.

Droperidol Despite strong clinical evidence supporting efficacy in acute agitation, **droperidol** is no longer U.S. FDA–approved for this use.[18] The FDA warning includes reports of death from QT_c prolongation even with use at low dosage and in patients with no cardiac risk factors. These risks led to removal of the drug from the European markets. Droperidol is still available in the United States and is Food and Drug Administration–approved for perioperative nausea and vomiting and is to be used only when other treatment methods fail. The maximum initial dosage is 2.5 milligrams given IV or IM, with repeat doses of 1.25 milligrams given until desired effect is achieved.

Haloperidol **Haloperidol** also carries an additional warning from the U.S. FDA regarding QT_c prolongation, specifically related to IV administration, and by any route at dosages higher than recommended,[21] most commonly defined as >35 milligrams/d or single doses of 20 milligrams or greater. Data supporting this warning include 73 cases of torsades de pointes, including 11 fatalities.[19] It is also important to note that, while used in common practice, haloperidol is not Food and Drug Administration–approved for IV administration. If used IV, doses of 2 to 10 milligrams have been studied, with repeat dosing every 15 to 30 minutes as needed to achieve calming effects, and subsequent administration of 25% of the required bolus dosing. Use the lowest effective single and cumulative dose. Continuous cardiac monitoring should be maintained after IV dosing.

IM haloperidol is often used for acute agitation and is considered second only to lorazepam as standard-of-care therapy.[22] Doses between 2.5 and 10 milligrams have been evaluated in clinical trials as either the primary medication or active comparator, with the most common dosage of 5 milligrams initially, with repeated dosing in 1 to 2 hours as needed. Coadministration with lorazepam has additive calming effects but a higher incidence of sedation.

Fluphenazine **Fluphenazine** IM is an additional injectable, high-potency, first-generation antipsychotic option. Its efficacy is generally considered interchangeable with haloperidol.[23] The average dosing of IM fluphenazine is 2.5 to 5 milligrams per injection, with a recommended dosing range of 1.25 to 10 milligrams per injection.[22]

Chlorpromazine **Chlorpromazine**, a low-potency, first-generation antipsychotic agent, may also be administered PO or IM at doses of 12.5 to 25 milligrams initially, with repeat doses of 25 to 50 milligrams given if necessary to calm agitation.[24] Chlorpromazine may also be given IV, although this is seldom done in clinical practice for the treatment of acute agitation. While this agent does not carry a formal bolded U.S. FDA warning, its label still advises cardiac monitoring, because QT_c prolongation is a concern.[25] Additionally, frequent monitoring of vital signs and orthostatic blood pressure is recommended with acute administration because hypotension, tachycardia, and sedation are common and can be profound. These adverse effects limit the usefulness of this agent in acute agitation.

ATYPICAL, OR SECOND-GENERATION, ANTIPSYCHOTICS

Atypical antipsychotics are also called **second-generation antipsychotics**. These agents block dopamine receptors, but their precise action is not known. Atypical antipsychotics are less likely than typical antipsychotics to cause extrapyramidal symptoms or neuroleptic malignant syndrome and have lower rates of tardive dyskinesia. These features have served to propel them to first-line therapy within the field of psychiatry. Another advantage of atypical antipsychotics is the decreased need for coadministration of medications to combat adverse anticholinergic effects. Less need for concomitant benzodiazepines is also an advantage, especially in the elderly.

Several agents in this class can be given orally or IM. Oral disintegrating tablets of olanzapine and risperidone, oral solution of risperidone, and IM preparations of olanzapine, ziprasidone, and aripiprazole have all been studied specifically for use in acute agitation. Additionally, **quetiapine** is effective for agitation in delirious critical care patients.[26] **Table 287-4** outlines dosage forms for the available options in this class.

TABLE 287-4 Dosage Form Availability for Selected Antipsychotic Agents

Antipsychotic	Oral Solution	Orally Disintegrating Tablet	IM Injection	Tablets or Capsules	IV
Chlorpromazine (Thorazine®)			X	X	X*
Fluphenazine (Prolixin®)	X		X	X	
Haloperidol (Haldol®)	X		X	X	X†
Risperidone (Risperdal®)	X	X		X	
Olanzapine (Zyprexa®)		X	X	X	
Ziprasidone (Geodon®)			X	X	
Aripiprazole (Abilify®)	X	X	X	X	
Quetiapine (Seroquel®)				X	

*not recommended due to hypotension

†IV is unlabeled use

Risperidone **Risperidone** (Risperdal®) has been studied in both ED and psychiatric settings for the treatment of acute agitation. It is not available as an IM preparation, but the oral liquid or rapid oral dispersible tablet (M-Tab®) is comparable to IM haloperidol with and without concomitant lorazepam. It is effective beginning 30 to 60 minutes after administration and has lower rates of extrapyramidal symptoms and sedation than haloperidol.[6,7] It also has comparable efficacy to olanzapine PO and IM, but with a longer time to onset of effect.[8,27]

Olanzapine **Olanzapine** (Zyprexa®) is available as a rapidly dissolving oral tablet (Zydis®) and an IM preparation. It is as effective as haloperidol or risperidone, with less extrapyramidal symptoms than haloperidol, but with more hypotension than risperidone.[8,27,28] Olanzapine given either orally or IM has a faster onset of action than IM haloperidol or oral risperidone, with effect beginning within 15 minutes after administration.[8]

Hypotension with IM olanzapine is a serious adverse effect and has led to fatalities in patients coadministered benzodiazepines or chlorpromazine.[29] **The product information for olanzapine warns against coadministration with benzodiazepines, because life-threatening sedation and hypotension can occur 1 hour after administration of lorazepam 2 milligrams IM.**[30] While recommendations differ, it is best to wait 1 to 2 hours between administering benzodiazepines with IM olanzapine, and if coadministering with oral olanzapine, monitor blood pressure frequently.

Ziprasidone **Ziprasidone** (Geodon®) is available in an IM preparation and has been compared with haloperidol for the treatment of patients with bipolar disorder or schizophrenia. Doses of 20 milligrams IM are comparable to 5 milligrams of IM haloperidol.[31,32] A potential barrier to use for ziprasidone is its effects on QT_c prolongation. In a direct-comparative study, IM ziprasidone was found to increase QT_c approximately 9 to 14 milliseconds longer than four other antipsychotic agents, including haloperidol.[33] As a result, ziprasidone is contraindicated in patients with a known history of QT_c prolongation, recent myocardial infarction, or uncompensated heart failure, or who are taking other medications known to prolong the QT_c interval. If possible, magnesium and potassium levels should be obtained and corrected prior to administration of ziprasidone, and the drug should be discontinued in patients with a QT_c >500 milliseconds.[31-33] This warning has limited its use for acute agitation in the ED.

Aripiprazole **IM aripiprazole** (Abilify®) is effective for acute agitation when compared with IM haloperidol, with onset of response within 1 hour. Patients treated with aripiprazole had lower rates of extrapyramidal symptoms when compared with patients treated with haloperidol, but a higher incidence of headache.[34,35] No studies have researched the utility of oral aripiprazole in the management of acute agitation. The dose of IM aripiprazole is 9.75 milligrams per injection, with a maximum dose of 30 milligrams per day. Aripiprazole is not recommended for use in children or adolescents with acute agitation due to an increased rate of akathisia in this patient group.[36]

Quetiapine **Quetiapine** is an atypical antipsychotic that has shown benefits for agitation associated with delirium in a critical care population.[37] Dosing ranges from 12.5 to 200 milligrams twice daily, and the most common adverse effects include somnolence and hypotension. Quetiapine has not been studied specifically for the treatment of undifferentiated or psychotic agitation in adults. Dosage forms are limited to oral tablets.

ANTIHISTAMINES

The most commonly used antihistamines for the treatment of agitation include diphenhydramine and hydroxyzine. Diphenhydramine is available in both liquid and parenteral dosage forms, but carries a higher rate of sedation and anticholinergic burden than hydroxyzine or other agents for agitation. Efficacy most supports the use of antihistamines in the treatment of anxiety in pediatric and adolescent patients, but antihistamines may be used as a single agent or adjunctive therapy in a generally agitated patient, particularly if the symptoms are anxiety driven.[38]

ANTICONVULSANTS

Anticonvulsants have been studied as agents for agitation, particularly in the acutely aggressive patient, as well as for anxiety. **Gabapentin** has shown some efficacy as adjunctive therapy of agitation in patients with major mental illnesses,[39] as well as some benefits in anxiety or agitation associated with dementia. Overall efficacy, however, is considered to be modest.[40] In patients with bipolar disorder, it is reasonable to consider **valproic acid/divalproex** as a treatment option for agitation because it can be "loaded" (i.e., dosed in a fashion that promotes efficacy for bipolar agitation quickly) and often produces calm and sedation as adverse effects.[41] Other anticonvulsants indicated for bipolar disorder such as **carbamazepine** or **lamotrigine** must be titrated to effect to avoid Stevens-Johnson syndrome and other adverse effects, therefore limiting their use in acute agitation associated with bipolar disorder. The same limitation applies for lithium as well, rendering it ineffective in acute symptom management.

α_2-AGONISTS

Clonidine, a centrally acting α_2-agonist, has historically been tried to combat acute agitation. Unfortunately, hypotension and bradycardia, along with mixed data for efficacy in this patient group, limit its use. However, the sedative agent **dexmedetomidine**, also an α_2-agonist, has gained attention for use in acute agitation in the intensive care unit setting.[42] It is currently under investigation for use in alcohol detoxification in intensive care unit patients as well. It is further hypothesized that the potential benefits of quetiapine and risperidone may be, in part, due to their alpha-agonist effects.[37] Although clonidine and dexmedetomidine are potentially of benefit, the current literature supports limiting them to adjunctive or alternative strategies.

TREATMENT

Acute agitation is acutely treated with either benzodiazepines or antipsychotic medications, or both. For children and adolescents or for adjunctive use, consider antihistamines. Agent-specific information is found in **Tables 287-3** to **287-6**.

SPECIAL POPULATIONS

Table 287-2 provides guidelines for pharmacotherapy in special circumstances and special populations.

TABLE 287-5 IM Atypical Antipsychotic Comparison to Haloperidol

Medication	IM Dose	Maximum IM Dose	Maximum IM Dose per 24 Hours	Time to Onset	Time to Repeat Dose	Half-Life (hours)
Haloperidol	2.5–10 milligrams	10 milligrams	30 milligrams	15 min	0.5–1 h	20
Lorazepam	2 milligrams	4 milligrams	10 milligrams	15 min	0.5–1 h	13
Chlorpromazine	12.5–25 milligrams	50 milligrams	200 milligrams	15 min	1 h	2
Fluphenazine	1.25–2.5 milligrams	5 milligrams	10 milligrams	≤60 min	4 h	15
Ziprasidone	10–20 milligrams	20 milligrams	40 milligrams	60 min	4 h	2–5
Olanzapine	5–10 milligrams	10 milligrams	30 milligrams	15–60 min	2–4 h	21–54
Aripiprazole	9.75 milligrams	15 milligrams	30 milligrams	45 min	2 h	75

THE ELDERLY PATIENT

No pharmacologic therapy has proven optimal for agitation in the elderly patient presenting to the ED with or without dementia. Nonpharmacologic therapies such as reorientation to surroundings; offering food, water, and bathroom facilities; and making sure the patient has his or her hearing aids and glasses are important. If medication is needed, select an agent based on its adverse effect profile at the lowest effective dose and least invasive route of administration. For delirium, treat the underlying disease processes.

Most atypical antipsychotics have not been investigated in the elderly for treatment of agitation in the ED setting, but small studies have investigated the safety and efficacy of IM ziprasidone and IM olanzapine in this group. Data for 15 patients aged 65 to 87 who received at least one dose of 20 milligrams of IM ziprasidone showed outcomes similar to those in patients treated with lorazepam and haloperidol together, or with physical restraints, with no spontaneous reports of adverse effects or changes in electrocardiogram parameters.[43,44] In a single study of agitated inpatients or nursing home residents with comorbid Alzheimer's disease, acute agitation decreased from 2 to 20 hours after a dose of 2.5 or 5 milligrams of IM olanzapine, with somnolence reported as the predominant adverse effect.[44] However, systematic evaluation of specific atypical antipsychotics in elderly patients with dementia showed minimal efficacy, even when used for up to 27 weeks.[45]

Overall, elderly patients are more susceptible to extrapyramidal symptoms, sedation, and confusion than younger populations, and, **if treatment with an antipsychotic agent is warranted, initial dosing should be lower than that in the general adult population. Suggested dosing ranges are described in Table 287-7** based on the data available for treatment of agitation (acute or chronic) in elderly patients.

Unfortunately, all antipsychotic agents carry a Black Box warning because their use increases all-cause mortality in the elderly, especially in those with dementia. Benzodiazepines should be used with caution, because they can cause paradoxical disinhibition and increased agitation in elderly patients, even at doses as low as 1 milligram of lorazepam.[45] If a benzodiazepine is used, consider a short-acting, glucuronidated agent such as **lorazepam, oxazepam, or temazepam** to minimize prolonged benzodiazepine effects. **Antihistamines have strong anticholinergic effects and can induce or worsen delirium in this patient group, and thus are generally avoided.**[45]

CHILDREN

The mainstays of therapy in children are antihistamines and benzodiazepines. If an antipsychotic regimen is needed, chlorpromazine, haloperidol, risperidone, olanzapine, or IM ziprasidone may be used.[36,38] Dosing information from these guidelines is presented in **Table 287-8** for patients aged 6 to 18 years.[36,38]

ACUTE WITHDRAWAL OR INTOXICATION SYNDROMES

Withdrawal or intoxication from substances can often lead to acute agitation, resulting in the potential for violence. History is often lacking, so it is necessary to treat without knowing the offending substance.

Benzodiazepines are considered the preferred treatment of agitation for the patient with alcohol or substance abuse. Benzodiazepines are beneficial for short-term sedation and cessation of agitation. They are associated with fewer cardiac and extrapyramidal side effects; however, be cautious of sedation and respiratory depression in an intoxicated patient. **Of the benzodiazepines, lorazepam is the favored agent** due to its lack of hepatic metabolites, rapid and complete IM absorption, and quick onset of action. Lorazepam may be given PO, IV, or IM. For agitation, using lorazepam "as needed" is as effective as a scheduled regimen. A typical starting dose is lorazepam 1 milligram PO, IV, or IM and repeating as needed. Higher doses may be required in a very agitated patient. In an elderly patient, considering a lower starting dose of lorazepam (0.5 milligram PO, IV, or IM once) and assessing efficacy is appropriate.

Acute Withdrawal Syndromes Withdrawal syndromes may result from the abrupt discontinuation of various substances including alcohol, opiates, benzodiazepines, and other prescription medications or illicit drugs. Intoxicated patients often present to the ED confused, agitated, combative, and disoriented. The goals of therapy are rapid reduction in agitation, maintaining patient and staff safety, and avoiding excessive sedation. Try to decrease external stimuli by providing a quiet room. The ED staff should communicate a safe and respectful attitude and remove any potentially dangerous objects from the patient's room.

Alcohol Withdrawal The abrupt discontinuation of alcohol can lead to delirium tremens and withdrawal seizures, which may be fatal. The **Clinical Institute Withdrawal Assessment Scale for Alcohol, Revised**

TABLE 287-6 PO Atypical Antipsychotic Comparison to Haloperidol

Medication	PO Dose	Maximum PO Dose	Maximum PO Dose per 24 Hours	Time to Onset	Time to Peak (hours)	Half-Life (hours)
Haloperidol	2.5–10 milligrams	10 milligrams	40 milligrams	30–60 min	2–6	20
Lorazepam	1–2 milligrams	4 milligrams	10 milligrams	30–60 min	2	13
Chlorpromazine	25–50 milligrams	100 milligrams	2000 milligrams	30–60 min	2.8	30
Fluphenazine	2.5–5 milligrams	20 milligrams	20 milligrams	≤60 min	0.5	15
Olanzapine (Zyprexa®, Zydis®)	5–10 milligrams	10 milligrams	30 milligrams	≤60 min	5–8	30
Risperidone (M-Tab®, PO solution)	1–2 milligrams	2 milligrams	8 milligrams	60–120 min	1–2	20
Quetiapine	12.5–50 milligrams	200 milligrams	800 milligrams	≤90 min	90 min	6

TABLE 287-7 Acute Agitation in the Elderly: Dosing Considerations

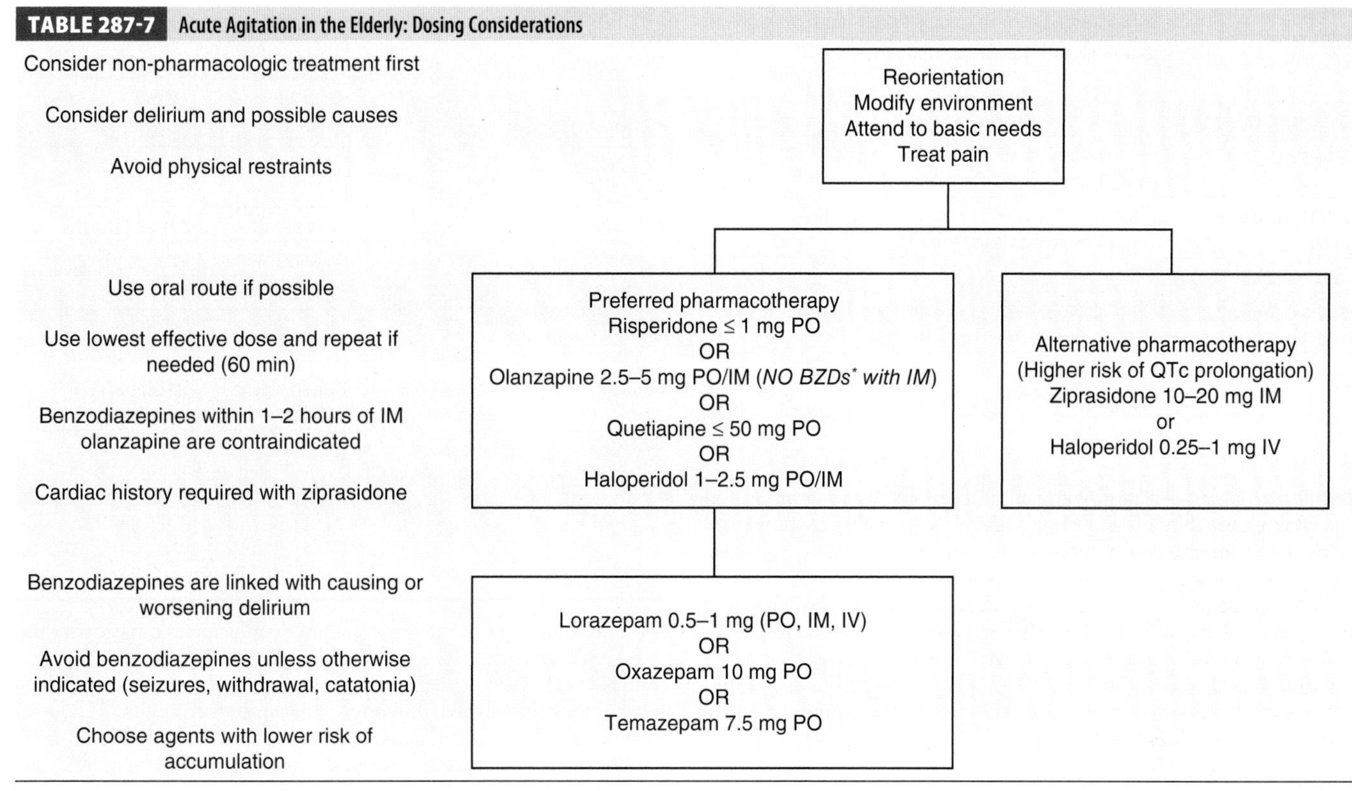

Consider non-pharmacologic treatment first
Consider delirium and possible causes
Avoid physical restraints
Reorientation
Modify environment
Attend to basic needs
Treat pain
Use oral route if possible
Use lowest effective dose and repeat if needed (60 min)
Benzodiazepines within 1–2 hours of IM olanzapine are contraindicated
Cardiac history required with ziprasidone
Preferred pharmacotherapy
Risperidone ≤ 1 mg PO
OR
Olanzapine 2.5–5 mg PO/IM (NO BZDs* with IM)
OR
Quetiapine ≤ 50 mg PO
OR
Haloperidol 1–2.5 mg PO/IM
Alternative pharmacotherapy
(Higher risk of QTc prolongation)
Ziprasidone 10–20 mg IM
or
Haloperidol 0.25–1 mg IV
Benzodiazepines are linked with causing or worsening delirium
Avoid benzodiazepines unless otherwise indicated (seizures, withdrawal, catatonia)
Choose agents with lower risk of accumulation
Lorazepam 0.5–1 mg (PO, IM, IV)
OR
Oxazepam 10 mg PO
OR
Temazepam 7.5 mg PO

*BZDs = benzodiazepines

is often used to assess symptom severity.[46] The severity of alcohol withdrawal syndrome and history of complications will determine whether the patient can be managed with "symptom-triggered" or "as-needed" medication administration or a fixed-schedule detoxification (**Table 287-9**).

Benzodiazepine Withdrawal Treatment of agitation secondary to benzodiazepine withdrawal is very similar to the treatment of alcohol withdrawal. A slow taper of the benzodiazepine is recommended. Consider switching short or intermediate half-life drugs to an equivalent dose of diazepam (multiply triazolam dose by 20, alprazolam dose by 10, and lorazepam dose by 5), and then taper. **A recommended tapering strategy is to decrease the dose by 25% the first week, by 25% the second week, and then by 12.5% every 7 days.**[47]

Opiate Withdrawal Opiate withdrawal is not fatal but can result in agitation and combative behavior. **Benzodiazepines are the treatment of choice in patients with acute agitation from opiate withdrawal.** Because patients often have polysubstance abuse, benzodiazepines will provide a sedative effect as well as prevent possible withdrawal seizures from alcohol or benzodiazepine withdrawal. Other options for managing symptoms of opiate withdrawal are discussed in chapters 186 and 292.

Acute Intoxication Syndromes Intoxication can occur from alcohol, prescription medications, hallucinogens, synthetic drugs, and a variety of drugs of abuse. Stimulants include prescription medications (e.g., methylphenidate, dextroamphetamine) and illicit substances (e.g., cocaine, methamphetamine). Hallucinogens, as categorized by the Substance Abuse and Mental Health Services Administration, include lysergic acid diethylamide (LSD or "acid"), phencyclidine (PCP), peyote, mescaline, psilocybin mushrooms, and methylenedioxymethamphetamine (MDMA or "ecstasy"). Synthetic drugs are easily obtained and are not detected on traditional drug screens.

TABLE 287-8 Pediatric Dosing of Drugs for Acute Agitation

Medication	Dose and Maximum Dosing	Time to Repeat Dose	Prepubertal Dosing	Pubertal Dosing
Diphenhydramine	1 milligram/kg/dose for 2–4 doses	20 min	25–50 milligrams PO/IM	50–100 milligrams PO/IM
Lorazepam	0.05 milligram/kg/dose until sedated	20 min	0.5–2 milligrams PO/IM	1–2 milligrams PO/IM
Chlorpromazine	0.5–1 milligram/kg PO 0.5 milligram/kg IM	30 min	25 milligrams PO (max, 100 milligrams/24 h) 12.5 milligrams IM (max, 75 milligrams/24 h)	50 milligrams PO (max, 200 milligrams/24 h) 25 milligrams IM (max, 100 milligrams/24 h)
Haloperidol	0.025–0.075 milligram/kg	60 min PO 30 min IM	0.5–2 milligrams PO/IM	1–2 milligrams PO/IM
Risperidone	0.025–0.05 milligram/kg for 2–4 doses until sedated	60 min	0.25–0.5 milligram	0.5–1 milligram
Olanzapine	0.1 milligram/kg for two doses	30 min	2.5 milligrams PO/IM	5–10 milligrams PO/IM
Ziprasidone			5 milligrams IM (≥6 years old)	10 milligrams IM

TABLE 287-9 Benzodiazepine Dosages for Fixed-Schedule Detoxification in Patients with Alcohol Withdrawal Syndrome[7]

Benzodiazepine	Dosage
Long-acting (12–24 h)	
Diazepam (Valium®)	10 milligrams every 6 hours for four doses, followed by 5 milligrams every 6 hours for eight doses
Chlordiazepoxide (Librium®)	50 milligrams every 6 hours for four doses, followed by 25 milligrams every 6 hours for eight doses
Short-acting (2–12 h)	
Lorazepam (Ativan®)	2 milligrams every 6 hours for four doses, followed by 1 milligram every 6 hours for eight doses
Oxazepam	30 milligrams every 6 hours for four doses, followed by 15 milligrams every 6 hours for eight doses

Herbal marijuana, commonly known as K2 or Spice, is a combination of synthetic cannabinoids and plant material. Marijuana alternatives are often sold as incense and potpourri and may induce anxiety, paranoia, agitation, delusions, and psychosis. Synthetic cathinones, or "bath salts," produce amphetamine-like euphoria, increased talkativeness, increased energy, and sexual arousal. **Supportive care and benzodiazepines are first steps in the management of agitation from suspected acute intoxication. However, for severe agitation impacting patient and staff safety that is not controlled with benzodiazepines, antipsychotics such as haloperidol or droperidol may be the only effective therapeutic options.**

REFERENCES

The complete reference list is available online at www.TintinalliEM.com.

Mental Health Disorders of the Elderly

Kristen Barrio
Kevin Biese

INTRODUCTION

This chapter discusses the diagnosis and differentiation of delirium and dementia in the elderly and provides an overview of selected common mental health disorders in the aging population.

The proportion of ED visits by older adults continues to increase with the exponential growth of the geriatric population.[1] Delirium, dementia, and depression can affect older adults, and the disorders are often interrelated. It can be difficult to identify delirium in patients with dementia, particularly because individuals with dementia are more likely to develop delirium.[2] Patients who develop delirium are more likely to develop dementia later in life.[3-6] Distinguishing between dementia and delirium is an important aspect of caring for older patients.

It can also be difficult to diagnose depression in patients with dementia given that both can present with similar symptoms such as apathy.[7] Also, depression in late life has been associated with increased risk of developing dementia, further demonstrating that dementia, delirium, and depression are interconnected, increase the risk of each other, and are all associated with increased risk of mortality and morbidity.[8-14] **Table 288-1** provides distinguishing features of delirium, dementia, and psychiatric disorders. Chapters 168, "Altered Mental Status and Coma," and 286, "Mental Health Disorders: ED Evaluation and Disposition," also discuss the distinctions between delirium, dementia, and psychiatric disorders.

TABLE 288-1 Features of Delirium, Dementia, and Psychiatric Disorder

Characteristic	Delirium	Dementia	Psychiatric Disorder
Onset	Over days	Insidious	Varies
Course over 24 h	Fluctuating	Stable	Varies
Consciousness	Reduced or hyperalert	Alert	Alert or distracted
Attention	Disordered	Normal	May be disordered
Cognition	Disordered	Impaired	Rarely impaired
Orientation	Impaired	Often impaired	May be impaired
Hallucinations	Visual and/or auditory	Often absent	May be present
Delusions	Transient, poorly organized	Usually absent	Sustained
Movements	Asterixis, tremor may be present	Often absent	Varies

DELIRIUM

Delirium is an acute change in cognition that fluctuates rapidly over time and is often reversible.[15] Delirium is frequently the first sign of underlying acute medical illness. Patients demonstrate altered levels of consciousness, inattention, disorganized thinking, and altered perception.[15] There are three main types of delirium: hypoactive, hyperactive, and mixed.[16] By far, the most common types are hypoactive and mixed delirium, which also have the highest potential to be missed.[17-23] Hypoactive delirium has been called "quiet delirium" because patients have decreased psychomotor activity and can appear somnolent. If hypoactive delirium is confused for depression, the underlying medical disorder causing the delirium can be missed.[24-26] Hyperactive delirium, in contrast, is characterized by increased psychomotor activity, and patients are often agitated, anxious, and sometimes combative. Mixed type can present with a combination of both hyperactive and hypoactive states that fluctuate over time.

Delirium is thought to be present in 7% to 10% of older patients presenting to the ED.[17,27,28] Environmental risk factors for delirium include functional dependence, living in a nursing home, and hearing impairment.[17,29] Delirium is an independent marker for mortality and is associated with a longer length of hospital stay than the median, increased hospital complications, discharge to long-term care facilities, and lasting cognitive deficits.[30-37] Even though delirium is a common disorder in the elderly, the diagnosis is missed by providers in 57% to 83% of cases.[27,38-41] If delirium is missed in the ED, it is likely to be missed on the inpatient services as well.[17]

CLINICAL FEATURES

The differential diagnosis of delirium includes dementia, depression, or another underlying psychiatric disorder. Such conditions can also be comorbidities of each other. However, first assess for delirium and then consider the possibility of the other disorders.

History Focus history taking on identifying the patient's baseline mental status and level of functioning and the time course of changes. Ask about past medical history and recent illness. Obtain an accurate medication list, and ask about over-the-counter medications, medications with anticholinergic properties, or any new medications.[42] Ask about substance abuse to assess the likelihood of intoxication or withdrawal. Any past psychiatric history requires close investigation of prior diagnoses, hospitalizations, and medications. Determine the patient's ability to make informed medical decisions, and determine whether another individual has legal power of attorney for medical decision making.

When attempting to differentiate delirium from dementia, consider several key factors. An acute change in mental status is more consistent with delirium than with dementia, and a fluctuating course over time is also more likely due to delirium.[43] Altered level of consciousness, inattention, and disorganized thinking are all more common in delirium than in dementia.[43]

TABLE 288-2 Mental Status Examination

Appearance, behavior, and attitude
Is dress appropriate?
Is motor behavior at rest appropriate?
Is the speech pattern normal?
Disorders of thought
Are the thoughts logical and realistic?
Are false beliefs or delusions present?
Are suicidal or homicidal thoughts present?
Disorders of perception
Are hallucinations present?
Mood and affect
What is the prevailing mood?
Is the emotional content appropriate for the setting?
Insight and judgment
Does the patient understand the circumstances surrounding the visit?
Sensorium and intelligence
Is the level of consciousness normal?
Is cognition or intellectual functioning impaired?

Physical Examination The physical examination should be thorough. Vital signs must be complete, to include oxygen saturation and temperature. Determine the blood glucose level. Baseline blood pressures may be higher than in younger age groups, and tachycardia can be masked by pharmacologic and/or physiologic limitations. Older patients have lower basal temperatures, with means of 97.3 to 97.8°F depending on the time of the day, so the threshold for a fever is lower than the assumed "normal" of 98.6°F.[44] Look for evidence of trauma, as patients may not recall falling or injuring themselves. Examine the entire body, making sure to look at the patient's back and heels for evidence of decubitus ulcers. Perform a complete neurologic exam, checking for focal findings, abnormal posturing, or difficulty with gait, coordination, or vision. A normal physical examination does not exclude the diagnosis of delirium.

Mental Status Examination Mental status examination is performed to identify delirium and differentiate it from other conditions.[27,35,38-41,45,46] The examination consists of an assessment of six mental-behavioral components (**Table 288-2**).

Two of the most common screening tests used to detect delirium are the **Confusion Assessment Method** for general use and the **Confusion Assessment Method–Intensive Care Unit** for intubated patients who are not heavily sedated.[47,48] **Figure 288-1** demonstrates the components of the Confusion Assessment Method. Inattention is characterized by an easily distracted patient who has difficulty keeping track of the conversation. Disorganized thought processes are rambling, unclear, or illogical. An altered level of consciousness is lethargy, lack of responsiveness, or coma—essentially anything other than alert. The diagnosis of delirium requires features 1 and 2 and either 3 or 4. See **Table 288-3** for further details about using the Confusion Assessment Method and the Confusion Assessment Method–Intensive Care Unit.[47,48]

Laboratory Testing and Imaging Laboratory testing and imaging are obtained to identify the treatable causes of delirium (**Tables 288-3 and 288-4**).[46]

In geriatric patients, infections, such as urinary tract infections and pneumonia, are associated with nearly half of cases of delirium,[49] and medications may account for another 40%.[50-52]

Laboratory Testing **Check point-of-care glucose as soon as possible after patient arrival in the ED.** Obtain CBC and basic metabolic studies, including calcium, phosphorus, and hepatic enzymes. Urinalysis is necessary because urinary tract infections are a frequent cause of delirium. Obtain cardiac markers. Consider an arterial blood gas analysis, especially in patients with chronic lung disease, because hypercarbia can cause delirium.[42] Obtain thyroid function studies.[53] Urine or serum

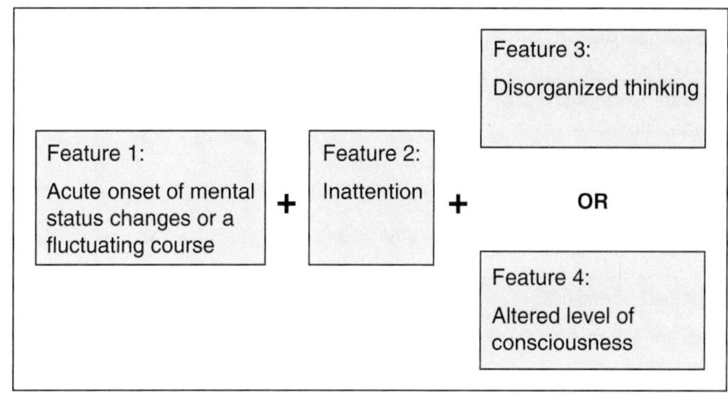

FIGURE 288-1. Confusion Assessment Method (CAM). To make a diagnosis of delirium, the patient must have features 1 and 2 and either 3 or 4.

toxicologic studies may be in order. Lumbar puncture may be necessary (after CT scan) if there is suspicion for meningitis or encephalitis or if the patient has had a new-onset seizure.[43] Further studies may be needed depending on the results of history, examination, and basic tests.

Imaging/Ancillary Tests Electrocardiogram and chest radiograph are essential.[54] Head CT scan is advised for patients with signs of, or a history of, trauma, focal neurologic deficits, impaired level of consciousness, or an otherwise unrevealing evaluation.[55,56]

TREATMENT

Medical Treatment Direct treatment to the underlying cause of delirium. Withhold or remove medications that are responsible for delirium. Treat infection, provide IV fluids for dehydration, correct hypoglycemia, and treat pain. Select doses of analgesics and narcotics for each individual patient and monitor for adverse effects.

The Medical Environment Provide the patient with his/her glasses or hearing aids, allow family or caregivers at the bedside, provide frequent reorientation about surroundings and course of care, and make sure there is access to a bathroom.[57] The Multicomponent Intervention to Prevent Delirium in Hospitalized Older Patients identified six risk factors (cognitive impairment, sleep deprivation, immobility, visual impairment, hearing impairment, and dehydration) for the development of delirium and targeted each risk factor with specific interventions carried out by a multidisciplinary team.[57] Precipitating factors in the development of delirium in the hospital include the use of physical restraints, malnutrition, use of a bladder catheter, more than three medications added, and any iatrogenic event.[58] Preventing and minimizing these factors are especially important when long ED stays are unavoidable.

Agitation If the patient is agitated, begin with a nonpharmacologic approach by addressing patient needs (such as using the restroom and, if possible, allowing the patient to eat or drink), providing comfortable surroundings, and having the family close by.[57,59] Avoid bladder catheters. Physical restraints should be an absolute last resort. If basic interventions are not successful, consider medication (**Figure 288-2**). **We recommend the avoidance of benzodiazepines in the elderly if at all possible, unless alcohol withdrawal is the cause of delirium.**[60] Benzodiazepines can cause paradoxical disinhibition and increased agitation in the elderly. If a benzodiazepine is used, consider a short-acting, glucuronidated agent such as **lorazepam, oxazepam, or temazepam** to minimize prolonged benzodiazepine effects. **Avoid antihistamines**, because this drug class has strong anticholinergic effects and can induce or worsen delirium in the elderly.

DISPOSITION AND FOLLOW-UP

The vast majority of patients with delirium should be hospitalized. Criteria for possible discharge include identification and treatment

TABLE 288-3 Confusion Assessment Method and Confusion Assessment Method (CAM)–Intensive Care Unit*

	Confusion Assessment Method	Confusion Assessment Method–Intensive Care Unit Version
Feature 1. Acute Onset and Fluctuating Course	Is there evidence of an acute change in mental status from the patient's baseline? Did the (abnormal) behavior fluctuate during the day, that is, tend to come and go, or increase or decrease in severity? Sources: Family or nurse	Is there evidence of an acute change in mental status from the baseline? Did the (abnormal) behavior fluctuate during the past 24 h, that is, tend to come and go or increase and decrease in severity? Sources of information: Serial Glasgow Coma Scale or sedation score ratings over 24 h, as well as readily available input from the patient's bedside critical care nurse or family
Feature 2. Inattention	Did the patient have difficulty focusing attention, for example, being easily distractible or having difficulty keeping track of what was being said?	Did the patient have difficulty focusing attention? Is there a reduced ability to maintain and shift attention? Sources of information: Attention screening examinations by using either picture recognition or Vigilance A random letter test. Neither of these tests requires verbal response, and thus they are ideally suited for mechanically ventilated patients.
Feature 3. Disorganized Thinking	Was the patient's thinking disorganized or incoherent, such as rambling or irrelevant conversation, unclear or illogical flow of ideas, or unpredictable switching from subject to subject?	Was the patient's thinking disorganized or incoherent, such as rambling or irrelevant conversation, unclear or illogical flow of ideas, or unpredictable switching from subject to subject? Was the patient able to follow questions and commands throughout the assessment? "Are you having any unclear thinking?" "Hold up this many fingers." (examiner holds two fingers in front of the patient) "Now, do the same thing with the other hand." (not repeating the number of fingers)
Feature 4. Altered Level of Consciousness	Is the patient's mental status anything other than alert, for example, vigilant, lethargic, stuporous, or comatose?	Any level of consciousness other than "alert." Alert—normal, spontaneously fully aware of environment and interacts appropriately Vigilant—hyperalert Lethargic—drowsy but easily aroused, unaware of some elements in the environment, or not spontaneously interacting appropriately with the interviewer; becomes fully aware and appropriately interactive when prodded minimally Stupor—difficult to arouse, unaware of some or all elements in the environment, or not spontaneously interacting with the interviewer; becomes incompletely aware and inappropriately interactive when prodded strongly Coma—unarousable, unaware of all elements in the environment, with no spontaneous interaction or awareness of the interviewer, so that the interview is difficult or impossible even with maximal prodding

*To diagnose delirium, the patient must have features 1 and 2 and *either* 3 or 4.

TABLE 288-4 DELIRIUM: Mnemonic for Reversible Causes of Delirium

Drugs	Any new additions, increased dosages, or interactions Consider over-the-counter drugs and alcohol Consider high-risk drugs*
Electrolyte disturbances	Dehydration, sodium imbalance, thyroid abnormalities
Lack of drugs	Withdrawals from chronically used sedatives, including alcohol and sleeping pills Poorly controlled pain (lack of analgesia)
Infection	Especially urinary and respiratory tract infections
Reduced sensory input	Poor vision, poor hearing
Intracranial	Infection, hemorrhage, stroke, tumor Rare; consider only if new focal neurologic findings, suggestive history, or diagnostic evaluation otherwise negative
Urinary, fecal	Urinary retention: "cystocerebral syndrome" Fecal impaction
Myocardial, pulmonary	Myocardial infarction, arrhythmia, exacerbation of heart failure, exacerbation of chronic obstructive pulmonary disease, hypoxia

*High-risk drugs: anticholinergics, anticonvulsants, antidepressants, antihistamines, antiparkinsonian agents, antipsychotics, barbiturates, benzodiazepines, H_2-blocking agents, zolpidem, opioid analgesics.

Reproduced with permission from: Marcantonio ER: Delirium. In: Pacala JT, Sullivan GM, eds. *Geriatrics Review Syllabus: A Core Curriculum in Geriatric Medicine*, 7th ed. New York, NY: American Geriatrics Society; 2010:297.

of the source of delirium; the patient returns to baseline function and mentation in the ED; the patient is discharged to the care of an active, capable individual or to a responsible facility; and the patient has access to follow-up in 24 hours or has the ability to return immediately to the ED if conditions deteriorate. Patients with unrecognized delirium who are discharged home are less apt to understand discharge instructions and less likely to seek further treatment, underscoring the importance of screening for delirium in geriatric patients.[61]

DEMENTIA

Dementia is a general term used to describe several types of disorders that gradually cause loss of cognitive functioning in two or more aspects of a person's life. The *Diagnostic and Statistical Manual of Mental Disorders*, fourth edition, definition of dementia requires memory impairment and at least one of the following: aphasia, apraxia, agnosia, or disturbance in executive functioning.[15] The diagnosis cannot be made in the setting of delirium, and the patient must show a decline in previous level of functioning that impacts social, functional, or occupational activities.[15] The most common form of dementia is Alzheimer's dementia, which affects approximately 5 million people in the United States.[62] Alzheimer's dementia is reported in 6% to 8% of those >65 years old and in ≥30% of those >85 years old.[63] Some other common types of dementia are vascular dementia, Lewy body dementia, frontotemporal dementia, dementia associated with Parkinson's disease, and mixed dementia.

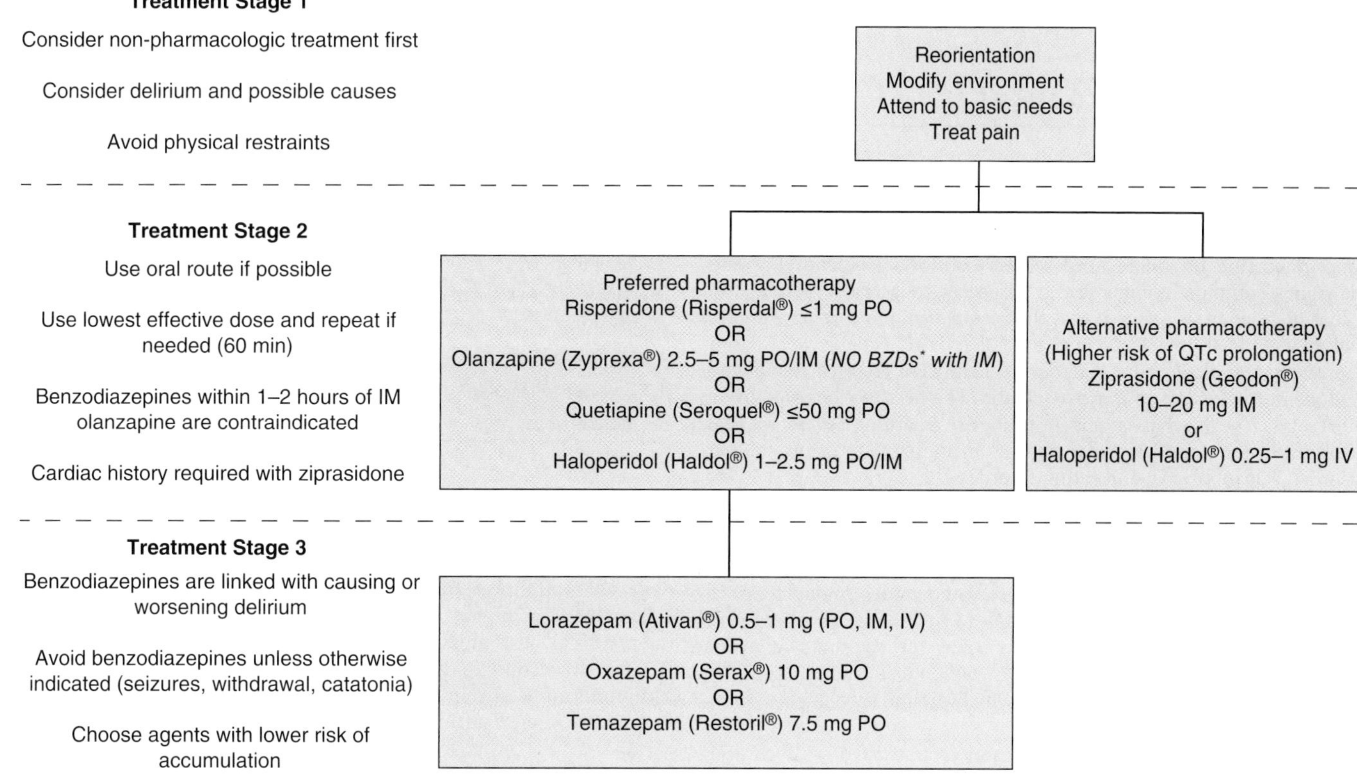
Treatment Stage 1
Consider non-pharmacologic treatment first
Consider delirium and possible causes
Avoid physical restraints
Reorientation
Modify environment
Attend to basic needs
Treat pain
Treatment Stage 2
Use oral route if possible
Use lowest effective dose and repeat if needed (60 min)
Benzodiazepines within 1–2 hours of IM olanzapine are contraindicated
Cardiac history required with ziprasidone
Preferred pharmacotherapy
Risperidone (Risperdal®) ≤1 mg PO
OR
Olanzapine (Zyprexa®) 2.5–5 mg PO/IM (NO BZDs* with IM)
OR
Quetiapine (Seroquel®) ≤50 mg PO
OR
Haloperidol (Haldol®) 1–2.5 mg PO/IM
Alternative pharmacotherapy
(Higher risk of QTc prolongation)
Ziprasidone (Geodon®)
10–20 mg IM
or
Haloperidol (Haldol®) 0.25–1 mg IV
Treatment Stage 3
Benzodiazepines are linked with causing or worsening delirium
Avoid benzodiazepines unless otherwise indicated (seizures, withdrawal, catatonia)
Choose agents with lower risk of accumulation
Lorazepam (Ativan®) 0.5–1 mg (PO, IM, IV)
OR
Oxazepam (Serax®) 10 mg PO
OR
Temazepam (Restoril®) 7.5 mg PO

FIGURE 288-2. Acute agitation in the elderly: dosing considerations. *BZDs = benzodiazepines.

PATHOPHYSIOLOGY

Alzheimer's disease has a gradual onset and primarily affects memory. The disease can also result in personality changes and visual-spatial problems.[62] Vascular dementia characteristically has a sudden or stepwise onset, and symptoms typically correlate with the area of brain ischemia.[62] Lewy body dementia has a gradual onset and presents with deficits in memory, and patients will also frequently have hallucinations and parkinsonian-like features.[62] **Patients with Lewy body dementia do very poorly when given typical antipsychotics, so avoid them in these patients.**[64,65] Patients with Lewy body dementia also frequently resemble patients with delirium given that patients can have a rapid decline, fluctuating course, and perceptual disturbances.[43] Frontotemporal dementia often presents in patients <60 years old and is associated with disinhibition, apathy, language difficulties, and atrophy in the frontal and temporal lobes.[62]

CLINICAL FEATURES

The main pharmacologic therapy for patients with dementia is cholinesterase inhibitors. The side effects of these medications include GI upset, anorexia, urinary incontinence, bradycardia, dizziness, and abdominal cramps; patients may come to the ED secondary to such complaints.[62]

Behavioral disturbances are frequently encountered in patients with dementia and are common reasons for ED presentation, especially when caregivers are feeling overwhelmed. The first steps are to screen for delirium and to identify the presence of a comorbid medical disorder (see earlier discussion and **Tables 288-1**, **288-3**, and **288-4**, and **Figure 288-1**). Subsequent management strategies for agitation are listed in **Figure 288-2**.

Mental Status Examination Perform a mental status exam on all geriatric patients because patients with dementia can often appear intact if formal evaluation is not performed. The Mini-Mental State Examination can be used to assess for dementia when there is appropriate time to administer the exam, but it is lengthy, and copyright restrictions sometimes limit access.[66] In the ED, short screening tests such as the **Mini-Cog**, which takes 3 minutes to complete, are more efficient. The Mini-Cog (**Figure 288-3**) combines a three-word recall with a **clock drawing test**.[67] Ask patients to remember three words (e.g., apple, table, penny). Then ask them to immediately repeat the words and remember them. Three minutes later, ask for the three words again. If patients can recall all three words, they do not need to complete the clock drawing test and do not have signs of cognitive impairment. If patients are not able to recall *any* of the words, assume cognitive impairment, and the clock drawing test is not needed. If patients recall one or two words, they will need to perform the clock drawing test. Ask the patient to draw a specific time, indicating hour and minute. The test is graded as either normal (negative for cognitive impairment) or abnormal (positive for cognitive impairment).[67] Alternatively, while waiting the 3 minutes to test

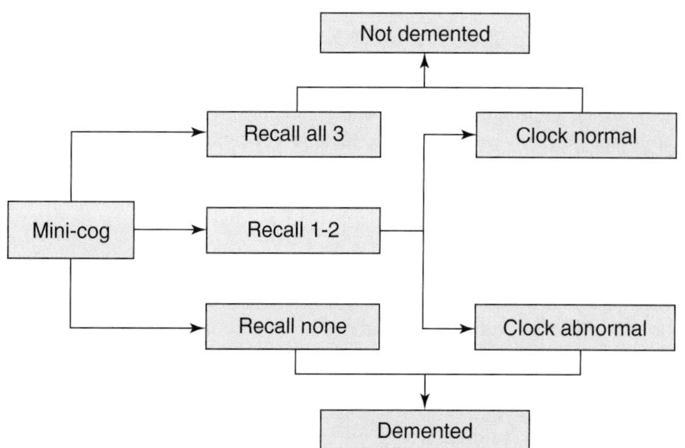
Not demented
Recall all 3
Clock normal
Mini-cog
Recall 1-2
Recall none
Clock abnormal
Demented

FIGURE 288-3. MINI-COG Screening Test. Scoring is as follows: 1 point for each word recalled and clock drawing test is rated as either normal or abnormal. If the patient scores a 0 in word recall or can recall one or two words but has an abnormal clock drawing test, this is consistent with cognitive impairment.

the patient's recall, ask the patient to draw the clock, as valuable information can be obtained from that exercise alone.

MENTAL HEALTH DISORDERS

As the population of older adults continues to increase, so will the number of geriatric patients with mental health disorders. One estimate predicts that the number of geriatric patients with mental illness will increase by 275% from 4 million in 1970 to 15 million in 2030.[68] Emergency medicine providers need to feel comfortable identifying and managing common mental health disorders in geriatric patients. A recent meta-analysis revealed that the mental health disorders with the highest estimated prevalence rates among geriatric patients were major depression and alcohol use disorders.[69] Significant research remains to be done in the field of geriatric psychiatry. The next sections will give a short overview of what is currently known regarding several mental health disorders found in older patients including depression, bipolar disorder, schizophrenia, and eating disorders.

DEPRESSION AND SUICIDE

Although the prevalence of major depressive disorder among community-dwelling older adults is low (1.4% to 4.4%), the proportion of patients with symptoms of depression below the threshold of major depressive disorder can be quite high, with most studies reporting around 8% to 16%.[7,70,71] Older patients with overt and subclinical depression can benefit from treatment.[72]

Depression in the geriatric population is associated with chronic medical illness, disability, increased use of health services, and poor health outcomes.[7,72,73] Risk factors associated with development of depression in older adults include lack of social support, living alone, being unmarried, cognitive impairment, bereavement, and lower socioeconomic status.[7,73]

Depression presents differently in older adults compared to younger age groups. Older adults with depression frequently report loss of appetite or sexual interest, rather than crying spells, feeling sad, or feeling like life is a failure.[7] They are more likely to be irritable and withdrawn than appear sad.[74] Older patients may also present with somatic or cognitive complaints when they are actually suffering from depression, which can make the diagnosis difficult.[7] Caregivers and patients themselves may attribute depressive symptoms to normal aging, again making the diagnosis difficult.[7] Comorbid anxiety is common with depression, and generalized anxiety disorder is frequently seen in the elderly population, with a reported lifetime prevalence of 15% in older adults.[75]

There are several screening tests for depression currently available to practitioners. Many are lengthy and would be difficult to use in the ED setting. The Patient Health Questionnaire-2 and Patient Health Questionnaire-9 are two- and nine-item self-administered questionnaires that have been developed to screen for depression based on *Diagnostic and Statistical Manual of Mental Disorders*, fourth edition, criteria.[76] The Patient Health Questionnaire-9 assesses nine features of depression: anhedonia, depressed mood, trouble sleeping, feeling tired, change in appetite, guilt or worthlessness, trouble concentrating, feeling slowed down or restless, and suicidal thoughts. The Patient Health Questionnaire-2 has two questions addressing anhedonia and low mood.[76] See **Table 288-5** for the Patient Health Questionnaire-2.[77] Both questionnaires can easily be located and have been found to be comparable to longer scales used to screen for depression with more evidence supporting the use of the Patient Health Questionnaire-9.[78] Several sources recommend starting with the Patient Health Questionnaire-2 and, if positive, then administering the Patient Health Questionnaire-9. It is important to find a screening test that you are familiar with and use it to screen for depression.

Screening for **suicide** is vital in the assessment of geriatric patients with depression.[79] People >65 years old have the highest rates of completed suicide of any age group.[80]

Older adults may give fewer warning signs of suicidal intent, and they are more successful in attempting suicide.[81] **Depression is the largest risk factor for suicide. Other risk factors include perceived poor health status, poor sleep quality, alcohol abuse, absence of a confidant, physical illness, functional decline, and presence of a firearm.**[79]

TABLE 288-5 Patient Health Questionnaire-2

Scores range from 0 to 6. A score of 3 or greater indicates the need for further screening.
Over the past 2 weeks, how often have you been bothered by any of the following problems?
Feeling down, depressed, or hopeless?
0 = Not at all
1 = Several days
2 = More than half the days
3 = Nearly every day
Have you often been bothered by little interest or pleasure in doing things?
0 = Not at all
1 = Several days
2 = More than half the days
3 = Nearly every day

Treatment combines both nonpharmacologic and pharmacologic interventions.[7] It is unlikely that new medications will be started in the ED for depression in geriatric patients, but recognizing depressive symptoms and assuring that the patient has appropriate follow-up are important. Review antidepressant doses, side effects, and drug interactions, as ED visits may be precipitated by symptoms from side effects or interactions. Selective serotonin reuptake inhibitors and selective norepinephrine reuptake inhibitors are some of the most frequently prescribed and effective antidepressants, but they can be associated with serotonin syndrome.[7]

SUBSTANCE ABUSE

Substance abuse is relatively common in the geriatric population and may increase with the baby-boomer cohort.[82] One estimate is that the number of older adults who will need substance abuse treatment is expected to increase from 1.7 million in 2000–2001 to 4.4 million in 2020.[82] Although the vast majority of substance abuse in the elderly is related to alcohol and prescription medications, there are reports of increased illicit drug use as well, highlighting the need to ask all patients about drug use.[83]

Alcohol abuse in geriatric patients specifically is frequent. In a cross-sectional study of 12,000 geriatric primary care patients, 15% of patients were felt to be at risk for, or were affected by, problem drinking.[84] Other community surveys estimate the prevalence of at-risk or problem drinking to be between 1% and 15%.[85-87] The current recommendation is that older adults consume no more than one standard drink per day or seven standard drinks per week.[88] Alcohol-related problems, such as falls, confusion, and malnutrition, may be attributed to normal aging, and thus alcohol abuse may be missed.[88] Physiologic changes from advancing age may also change alcohol tolerance, increasing risk for complications.[88] If at-risk drinking is identified, refer the patient to an inpatient or outpatient treatment facility. Also, if the plan is to admit a patient with known alcohol or substance abuse, notify the admitting physician so plans can be made to mitigate withdrawal.

BIPOLAR DISORDER

Bipolar disorder is a spectrum of illness that affects an individual's ability to regulate mood. There are four types: type I, which requires a manic episode for the diagnosis; type II, which requires one or more depressive episodes and a hypomanic episode; cyclothymia (cycling moods that do not meet criteria for depression or mania); and bipolar not otherwise specified.[89] Research regarding bipolar disorder in older adults is limited. The prevalence of bipolar disease in older adults is reported to be approximately 0.08% to 0.5%.[89] Given this low rate, older adults who present with new-onset mania require a complete medical evaluation before a new diagnosis of bipolar disorder should be made. Even though the prevalence rate of older adults in the community with bipolar disorder is low, one study found that 17% of patients >60 years old presenting to a psychiatric ED carried a diagnosis of bipolar disorder.[90] There are some differences between younger and older patients with bipolar disorder. Older people with bipolar disorder are more likely to be female. Late-onset bipolar disorder (onset between age 30 and 50 years) is associated with fewer genetic associations and more neurologic illnesses.[91] The frequency of psychotic features is essentially the same in young and old patients with bipolar disorder.[91] Older patients with bipolar disorder can have either early- or late-onset disease.

The treatment and adverse effects of treatment of bipolar disorder have implications in the elderly. One of the most customary treatments for bipolar disorder is lithium, which is a mood stabilizer.[92,93] Older patients can demonstrate beneficial effects at lower serum levels of lithium than younger patients. The renal clearance of lithium decreases with age, increasing the elimination half-life and predisposing to lithium toxicity.[94] Neurotoxicity can develop at serum levels that are therapeutic in younger adults.[94] Frequently reported side effects of lithium include tremor, muscle twitches, GI symptoms, and CNS effects such as sedation.[94] Many common medications interact with lithium, including thiazide diuretics, nonsteroidal anti-inflammatory agents, and angiotensin-converting enzyme inhibitors, which can increase serum lithium concentrations and the risk of toxicity.[94] **An older patient taking lithium can display signs of toxicity even if the level is in the therapeutic window.** See chapter 181, "Lithium," for further details of toxicity and treatment. Three anticonvulsants have also been approved to treat bipolar disorder: valproate, carbamazepine, and lamotrigine. The literature regarding their use in older adults is sparse.[89]

PSYCHOSIS (SCHIZOPHRENIA)

Several disorders, such as schizophrenia, psychosis associated with dementias, and more acute processes such as delirium, can present with symptoms of psychosis (hallucinations and delusions) in geriatric patients. This section provides a brief discussion of schizophrenia in older adults (please see earlier discussion regarding delirium and behavioral disturbances in dementia).

The estimated prevalence rate of schizophrenia in geriatric patients ranges from 0.1% to 0.5%.[95-97] The majority of patients with schizophrenia develop the disease in the second or third decade of life (considered early-onset schizophrenia), meaning that most geriatric patients with schizophrenia have had the disorder since they were much younger.[98] There are two other groups of patients with schizophrenia: late-onset schizophrenia (>40 years old) and very-late-onset schizophrenia-like psychosis (>60 years old).[98] Individuals with late-onset schizophrenia have many of the same attributes as patients with early-onset schizophrenia, but late-onset patients have fewer problems with learning, abstraction, and flexibility.[99] The diagnosis of very-late-onset schizophrenia-like psychosis is rare, but patients >60 years old can develop a late-life primary psychosis disorder.[98] Very-late-onset patients tend to have a lack of negative symptoms, greater risk of tardive dyskinesia, and evidence of a neurodegenerative process rather than a neurodevelopmental process.[98]

Schizophrenia in geriatric patients represents complexity in the psychiatric, medical, and social realms. Nonadherence to medical therapy is common.[100] Mortality secondary to cardiovascular disease is more than twice as common as in the general population, likely due to high rates of smoking, diabetes mellitus, hypertension, and obesity in schizophrenic patients. Older patients with schizophrenia typically have a sedentary lifestyle and poor diet.[100] Atypical antipsychotics used for treatment increase the risk of metabolic syndrome and weight gain, which in turn increase the risk of cardiovascular diseases.[101] The use of typical antipsychotics is limited because the risk of tardive dyskinesia is elevated in geriatric patients.[102] One study noted that the cumulative annual incidence of tardive dyskinesia in patients >45 years old treated with low-dose typical antipsychotics was 26%, which is five to six times greater than in younger patients.[102] Antipsychotic medications should be carefully selected and doses titrated upward slowly with close monitoring for side effects. Older patients with schizophrenia can also benefit from adjunctive psychosocial interventions. For example, Functional Adaptation Skills Training, a group therapy targeting everyday life skills, improves the functional adaptation of older patients with schizophrenia.[103-105]

EATING DISORDERS

There is little information regarding eating disorders such as anorexia nervosa and bulimia nervosa in older adults. One recent study examined women >50 years old for the presence of eating disorders and found that about 13% reported some form of core current eating disorder symptoms. Current binge eating, and purging in the absence of binge eating, were the most common symptoms.[106] Approximately 71% of women in the study were currently trying to lose weight.[106] Another review identified 48 cases of eating disorders in adults >50 years old. In this article, 88% were female and 60% were >65 years old. The most frequent diagnosis was anorexia nervosa (81% of cases).[107] Of the 48 cases, 79% had the onset of eating disorders later in life.[107] Importantly, this study identified a strong connection between eating disorders and other psychiatric conditions (60% of cases), with major depression being the most important. Eating disorders were often preceded by a stressful event, such as widowhood, bereavement, and marriage difficulties.[107] Of the 48 patients reviewed, 21% of the patients died from complications of the eating disorder.[107]

Diagnosis is difficult and is made by excluding any physical or medical cause of unexplained weight loss. Eating disorders in older patients are treated similarly to those in any other age group, with a combination of cognitive-behavioral treatment and pharmacotherapy.[107]

Acknowledgments: Special thanks to members of the Academy of Geriatric Emergency Medicine, Dr. Timothy Platts-Mills, and Dr. Debra Bynum for their contributions to this chapter.

REFERENCES

The complete reference list is available online at www.TintinalliEM.com.

Mood and Anxiety Disorders

Tracy M. DeSelm

MOOD DISORDERS

Mood disorders are divided into **depressive** and **bipolar disorders**. Worldwide, depressive disorder affects approximately 10% of the population,[1] whereas bipolar disorder has a lifetime prevalence of 2.4%.[2] In the United States, there is a 21% lifetime prevalence of any mood disorder.[3] One urban study showed that 32% of ED patients screened positive for depressive disorder, and 7% screened positive for bipolar disorder.[4,5] Depressive disorder affects women twice as often as men, whereas bipolar disorder affects men and women equally. **Bipolar disorder** is characterized by mania cycling with periods of depression. The depressive periods tend to last longer that the manic periods.

Although mood disorders may occur at any age, the average onset of depressive disorder is about 40 years of age, and that of bipolar disorder is about 30 years of age. There are no differences in prevalence regarding race.[6]

DEPRESSIVE DISORDER

Depressive disorder is often unrecognized, as the investigation of somatic complaints usually takes priority during patient evaluation.[7,8]

Adolescents[9] and the elderly (especially nursing home patients)[10] appear to be particularly vulnerable populations for depression. Increased rates of depressive disorder are seen in many chronic illnesses including CNS diseases,[11,12] cardiovascular disorders,[13] and cancer.[14] Also, patients with depressive disorder have increased risk of certain medical diseases, such as diabetes and coronary artery disease.[15]

The most common type of depressive disorder is **major depressive disorder** (also called **unipolar or major depression**). Diagnosis requires at least 5 of the 10 following symptoms: depressed mood, anhedonia (loss of pleasure in things that used to give pleasure), suicidal ideation with or without a specific plan, significant weight loss or gain, insomnia or hypersomnia, feelings of restlessness, agitation or psychomotor retardation, feelings of worthlessness or inappropriate guilt, fatigue or loss of energy, and difficulty with concentration. At least one of the symptoms must be depressed mood or anhedonia. Symptoms must be present for at least 2 weeks, cannot be due to substance abuse or a medical condition, and must cause significant impairment in normal functioning.[16]

PATHOPHYSIOLOGY

The pathophysiology of depressive disorder is likely multifactorial including genetic, biological, and psychosocial factors. A genetic predisposition, as evidenced by a 37% concordance rate in twin studies,[17] heightens susceptibility. Malfunctioning monoamine neurotransmitters (especially serotonin, norepinephrine, and dopamine)[18-20] are implicated and may explain the effectiveness of some current medical therapies. Abnormal γ-aminobutyric acid and glutamate levels in various areas of the brain have been noted.[21] Early childhood stress may alter corticotropin-releasing hormone cells in the hypothalamus to heighten future stress responses.[22,23] Four areas of the brain involved in normal emotional responses (the prefrontal cortex, anterior cingulate cortex, hippocampus, and amygdala) appear to be altered in patients with depressive disorder. Finally, psychosocial factors including isolation, lack of family support, stressful life events,[24,25] and substance abuse are risk factors for development of depression.

CLINICAL FEATURES

The most important part of evaluation is the assessment of suicide risk. The acronyms **SAD PERSONS**[26] (**Table 289-1**) and **SIG-E-CAPS** (**Table 289-2**) are helpful tools to assess suicide risk and identify depressive disorder, respectively. The easiest method is using straightforward, nonthreatening questions regarding the patient's suicide or homicide thoughts or intent, but seek corroborative information from family members, friends, law enforcement, EMS, or outside providers.

If the patient is at potential risk for harm to self or others, perform a thorough search for weapons, medicines, and potentially harmful items, and place the patient in a safe environment with monitoring. Follow with appropriate history taking, physical examination, and laboratory studies. Detailed evaluation of patients with mental health disorders is provided in chapter 286, "Mental Health Disorders: ED Evaluation and Disposition" and Table 286-1 of that chapter.

TABLE 289-1 SAD PERSONS (Assessment Tool for Suicide Risk)

S	Sex (male > female risk)
A	Age (older white men greatest risk)
D	Depression
P	Previous attempt
E	Ethanol/other substance abuse
R	Rational thinking loss
S	Social support lacking
O	Organized suicide plan
N	No spouse
S	Sickness (medical or psychiatric comorbidities)

Note: Each factor assigned 1 point; ≥5 points considered high risk of suicide.

Source: Reproduced with permission from Patterson WM, Dohn HH, Bird J, Patterson GA: Evaluation of suicidal patients: The SAD PERSONS Scale. Psychosomatics April:24(4): 343-345, 1983. Copyright Elsevier.

TABLE 289-2 SIG-E-CAPS (Prescribe Energy Capsules) (Assessment Tool for Depressive Disorder)

S	Sleep (too much or too little)
I	**Interest (lack of interest or pleasure and depressed mood)***
G	Guilt (excessive or inappropriate, or feeling worthless)
E	Energy (low)
C	Concentration (poor)
A	Appetite (increased or decreased weight)
P	Psychomotor (slowed or agitation)
S	Suicide (ideation/plan)

*Must include "I (lack of interest or pleasure and depressed mood)" to make diagnosis of depressive disorder.

Consider depressive disorder in a patient with vague, general complaints with unclear medical etiologies and multiple ED visits.[27] Two simple questions that have only been validated for depressive disorder assessment in primary care[28] but may prove useful in the ED setting are as follows:

1. During the past month, have you been bothered by feeling down, depressed, or hopeless?
2. During the past month, have you been bothered by little interest or pleasure in doing things?

Ask about substance abuse, because alcohol and drug abuse are important comorbidities.[29] Alcohol abuse is associated with an increased risk of suicide, and many of those with completed suicide demonstrate positive alcohol levels at autopsy. **Patients cannot be adequately evaluated for depression or suicidal intent until they are no longer intoxicated.** This does not necessarily mean an alcohol level of 0, but rather a return to normal (or baseline) cognition.

DIFFERENTIAL DIAGNOSIS

A large number of medical disorders, as well as many medications and substances of abuse, may cause symptoms of depression. Important medical mimickers include neurologic (CNS infection, cerebrovascular accident), endocrine (hypo- and hyperthyroid, hypoglycemia), and infectious disorders (especially in the elderly). Opiates, barbiturates, benzodiazepines, alcohol abuse, and corticosteroids may all cause depressive symptoms. A thorough history, examination, and appropriate laboratory studies will help differentiate the disorders. Consider medical causes of depression in patients with new symptoms of depression, in the elderly, and in those with complex medical problems.

TREATMENT OF DEPRESSIVE DISORDERS

Antidepressants are usually prescribed by primary care physicians or psychiatrists for conditions such as depression, neurogenic pain, or smoking cessation. The side effect profiles, potential serious adverse effects, and toxicities of common antidepressants are reviewed in **Table 289-3** and in the Toxicology section of this text. Antidepressant therapy is typically not initiated in the ED, although resumption of a well-tolerated, recently stopped medication may be considered. Antidepressants take about 2 to 3 weeks to have clinical effects. Ideally, any antidepressant prescribed from the ED should be done in conjunction with the follow-up practitioner, and the patient should be seen in follow-up within a week. Antidepressants may pose fetal risk, so the risks and benefits during pregnancy must be weighed carefully under the guidance of a psychiatrist and obstetrician. Sertraline and paroxetine are safe to use while breastfeeding (see **Table 289-3**).

The major categories of antidepressants in use today are the **heterocyclic antidepressants** (HCAs), **monoamine oxidase inhibitors**

TABLE 289-3 Commonly Used Antidepressants in the United States

Class of Antidepressant	Generic Name	Brand Name	Mechanism of Action for Class	Most Common Side Effects/Adverse Effects for Class	Starting Dose	Comments
Selective serotonin reuptake inhibitors (SSRIs)	Citalopram	Celexa	Blockage of presynaptic serotonin uptake	N/V, drowsiness, HA, dizziness, insomnia, agitation, precipitation of mania, paresthesias, sexual dysfunction, cognitive dysfunction, weight gain	10 milligrams once a day	
	Fluoxetine	Prozac			10 milligrams once a day	
	Fluvoxamine	Luvox			50 milligrams once a day	
	Paroxetine	Paxil			10 milligrams once a day	
	Sertraline	Zoloft			25 milligrams once a day	OK for breastfeeding
	Escitalopram	Lexapro			10 milligrams once a day	OK for breastfeeding
Serotonin norepinephrine reuptake inhibitors (SNRIs)	Duloxetine	Cymbalta	Blockage of presynaptic uptake of serotonin and NE	Same as for SSRIs, except less sexual dysfunction, elevated BP, urinary hesitancy/retention	30 milligrams once a day	
	Venlafaxine	Effexor			37.5 milligrams once a day	
Atypical	Bupropion	Wellbutrin Zyban	DA and NE reuptake inhibitor	Increase seizure risk, dry mouth, nausea, restlessness, insomnia, HA, pharyngitis, constipation	150 milligrams twice a day	Less sexual dysfunction, less weight gain, also used for smoking cessation
	Bupropion SR	Wellbutrin SR			150 milligrams twice a day	
	Bupropion XL	Wellbutrin XL			150 milligrams twice a day	
	Mirtazapine	Remeron	DA and NE reuptake inhibitor Increase release of NE, serotonin by antagonizing inhibitor receptors	Increase seizure risk, dry mouth, nausea, restlessness, insomnia, HA, pharyngitis, constipation, dizziness, somnolence, weight gain, malaise	15 milligrams once a day	Less sexual dysfunction, less weight gain, also used for smoking cessation Quicker onset of action by 1 week, low therapeutic index
	Trazodone	Desyrel	Serotonin antagonist and reuptake inhibitor	Marked sedation, priapism, orthostatic hypotension, ventricular dysrhythmias in patients with known cardiac disease	50 milligrams once a day	Also used in insomnia, anxiety disorders
Heterocyclic	Amitriptyline	Elavil	Blockage of presynaptic reuptake of NE, serotonin	Cardiotoxic: prolonged QTc/AV block Anticholinergic: sedation, dry mouth, tachycardia, constipation	75 milligrams once a day for pain control	Also used for chronic/neurogenic pain control, low therapeutic index

Abbreviations: AV = atrioventricular; BP = blood pressure; DA = dopamine; HA = headache; NE = norepinephrine; N/V = nausea and vomiting.

(MAOIs), **selective serotonin reuptake inhibitors** (SSRIs), the **selective serotonin norepinephrine reuptake inhibitors** (SNRIs), and the **atypical antidepressants**.

Heterocyclic Antidepressants HCAs, once commonly used for depression, are prescribed less often now due to low therapeutic index, many possible side effects at prescribed doses, and dangerous overdose potential. The side effects are mainly anticholinergic related and cardiotoxic, including prolonged QT_c interval and atrioventricular block. One agent in this category, **amitriptyline**, is commonly prescribed for chronic or neurogenic pain.

Monoamine Oxidase Inhibitors MAOIs are rarely used first line in treating depression because of potentially lethal drug–drug and dietary interactions. MAOIs block oxidative deamination of tyramine and may precipitate a sometimes fatal hypertensive crisis when certain drugs **(sympathomimetic amines, levodopa [L-dopa], narcotics, and heterocyclic antidepressants)** or **tyramine-containing foods or beverages** (aged cheese, beer, and wine) are co-ingested.

Selective Serotonin Reuptake Inhibitors and Selective Serotonin Norepinephrine Reuptake Inhibitors The mainstays of current antidepressant therapy are the SSRIs and SNRIs, which increase the amount of intrasynaptic serotonin or serotonin and norepinephrine, respectively. A significant advantage of SSRIs and SNRIs over other classes of antidepressants is their high therapeutic index and favorable side effect profile.

Common side effects for the **SSRIs** include nausea and vomiting, drowsiness, headache, changes in sleep patterns, sexual dysfunction, cognitive dysfunction, and precipitation of mania in bipolar patients. SSRIs may increase suicidal ideation, and the U.S. Food and Drug Administration currently requires that all antidepressants carry a black box warning that antidepressants may increase suicide risk in patients <25 years old. **When SSRIs are abruptly stopped, a withdrawal syndrome may occur**, characterized by a flulike symptoms, including nausea, vomiting, fatigue, myalgias, vertigo, headache, insomnia, and paresthesias. Although these symptoms are not life threatening, they may be very uncomfortable.

Serotonin syndrome, a potentially life-threatening adverse drug reaction, may occur in patients taking SSRIs (or any other antidepressant) when used in combination with another agent that has serotonergic activity such as MAOIs, opiates (including **tramadol**), CNS stimulants, serotonin agonists, St. John's wort, lithium, dextromethorphan, risperidone, olanzapine, ondansetron, and metoclopramide. The syndrome is manifest by neuromuscular hyperactivity (tremor, myoclonus, clonus, hyperreflexia, seizures), altered mental status (restlessness, agitation, excitement, confusion), autonomic hyperactivity (tachycardia, tachypnea, fever, diaphoresis), and GI irritability (nausea, vomiting, diarrhea). Treatment consists of discontinuation of the affecting agents, administering benzodiazepines, and supportive care.

SNRIs are very similar to SSRIs in side effect profile, although they may cause elevated blood pressure and less sexual dysfunction. Withdrawal may also occur several days after discontinuation of an SNRI.

Atypical Antidepressants Atypical antidepressants include **bupropion, mirtazapine, and trazodone**. Bupropion, a dopamine reuptake inhibitor, is also used for smoking cessation. It typically causes less weight gain and less sexual dysfunction than other antidepressants. Trazodone is a serotonin antagonist and reuptake inhibitor that is more sedating than other antidepressants with less anticholinergic effects and is also commonly used for anxiety or as a sleep aid. Mirtazapine is related to the HCAs, tends to cause weight gain, and has an onset of action of about 1 week. As with the other antidepressants, these medications may cause withdrawal when abruptly stopped.

DISPOSITION

The disposition of the depressed patient is based on the assessment of harm to self or others, the ability to care for one's self, level of supportive environment at home, and complicating medical or substance abuse problems. Any of the above may require psychiatric consultation for admission evaluation. Patients who may safely go home need specific follow-up plans with a primary care provider, psychiatrist, or other appropriate counselor. One helpful resource for patients and providers is the **Substance Abuse and Mental Health Services Administration** Web site at www.samhsa.gov.

SPECIAL CONSIDERATIONS

Mental disorders in the elderly are discussed in chapter 286 and mental disorders in children are discussed in chapter 147, "Behavioral Disorders in Children."

Postpartum Depression Postpartum depression affects 10% to 15% of women within 1 year of delivery,[30] but usually occurs within the first month. Symptoms are extreme fatigue, ambivalent feelings about caring for the newborn, guilt about those feelings, as well as the other classic depressive disorder symptoms. Low energy is in excess of the normal fatigue felt by most women postpartum. Risk factors for postpartum depression are prior depression, young age, low socioeconomic status, and partner abuse.[31] In one urban pediatric ED, one third of postpartum patients screened positive for depression.[32] Recognition in the ED is important to identify infant vulnerability.

Cross-Cultural Issues Surveys of depressive disorder show a wide range of prevalence across diverse cultures, although it is unclear how much of this difference is due to each culture's definition and expressions of depressive disorder. Non-Western cultures may emphasize somatic symptoms of depression, whereas in Western cultures, it may be more acceptable to express psychological complaints. Avoid stereotyping, but acknowledge the possibility of cultural influence in symptom description.

BIPOLAR DISORDER

Bipolar disorder, previously called **manic-depressive disorder**, is the other major type of mood disorder and is characterized by mania, usually cycling with periods of depression. The depressive periods tend to last longer than the manic periods. Mania can be diagnosed if there is a distinct period of elevated, expansive, or irritable mood for at least 1 week.[16] Mania may exist with or without psychotic features. Bipolar disorder is divided into several subtypes including bipolar I (mania, with or without major depressive episodes), bipolar II (intermittent hypomania with depressive episodes), and cyclothymic (recurrent dysthymic and hypomania episodes). A "mixed" state is one in which the patient meets the criteria for a manic episode plus depressive disorder symptoms for at least 1 week. It is not necessary for the emergency physician to delineate between the different subtypes of bipolar disorder, but rather understand that different types exist.

PATHOPHYSIOLOGY

The pathogenesis of bipolar disorder is likely multifactorial. There is a strong genetic component, with about 50% of all bipolar patients having a parent with a mood disorder.[6] The concordance rate is 40% in monozygotic twins compared with 6% in dizygotic twins.[33] Areas of the brain involved in normal emotional responses, ventral prefrontal networks and limbic regions, demonstrate decreased connectivity on functional MRIs.[33] Environmental factors, such as negative life events, increase the likelihood of developing bipolar disorder in predisposed persons.[34]

CLINICAL FEATURES

The manic patient may seem "fun," energetic, and expansive, but beware; the patient may quickly become irritable or even hostile if plans are antagonized by providers or family members. Manic patients may experience grandiose or delusional ideas and loss of cognitive abilities, with little insight. The initial evaluation of the manic patient is similar to that of patients with other psychiatric disorders and is discussed in chapter 286. Consider nonpsychiatric causes of agitation, such as thyroid disease, acute toxic ingestions (cocaine, stimulants), and drug withdrawal (antidepressants, alcohol, benzodiazepines). Consider other psychiatric diseases, such as schizophrenia and attention deficit disorder, because features may mimic the manic phase of bipolar disorder. Patients exhibiting mania should be questioned about a previous history of depressive disorder, because most bipolar disorder patients are initially diagnosed with depressive disorder.

TREATMENT OF BIPOLAR DISORDER

Treatment for bipolar disorder is complex, often requires more than one medication, and thus should not be initiated by the emergency physician, except for treatment of acute agitation (see chapter 287, "Acute Agitation") or to restart lithium or an anticonvulsant medication that has been recently stopped. Medications to treat the acutely manic patient include "**mood stabilizers**," such as **lithium, valproic acid, or carbamazepine**, with or without the addition of an antipsychotic, such as **haloperidol or a benzodiazepine** (**Table 289-4**). The same mood stabilizers may also be used for maintenance therapy. Lithium and valproic acid may be combined with an atypical antipsychotic medication for bipolar maintenance therapy. Lithium has a narrow therapeutic index and requires frequent monitoring. Patients taking lithium must avoid dehydration to prevent toxic levels from accumulating. The efficacy of antidepressant use in bipolar disorder is unclear because there is possible risk of precipitating mania.[35]

DISPOSITION

Disposition of the bipolar disorder patient is similar to that of the depressive disorder patient. Lack of insight to the loss of cognitive abilities and delusional ideas may put the patient at risk for self-harm. Bipolar disorder patients who are exhibiting psychotic features or are at risk for harm to self or others need psychiatrist evaluation for admission.

ANXIETY DISORDERS

Anxiety is a very common presenting symptom in the ED. Psychological, physical, or substance abuse disorders may all cause anxiety symptoms,

TABLE 289-4 Medications Used for Bipolar Disorder

Generic Name	Brand Name	Mechanism of Action	Side Effects (BLACK BOX WARNING IN CAPS)	Usual Starting Dose	Comments
Lithium carbonate	Eskalith, Lithonate, Lithotabs	? increase NE function ? increase serotonin function	Initially: nausea, dry mouth, excessive thirst, tremors, polyuria, peripheral edema, cognitive impairment Long-term: polyuria, diabetes insipidus, goiter, hypothyroidism, rashes, leukocytosis	300 milligrams 2 or 3 times a day	Effective for both acute and maintenance therapy Narrow therapeutic window; toxicity common; symptoms may be delayed up to 48 h in acute overdose
Valproic acid	Depakene, Depakote, Depacon	Antiepileptic; enhances transmission of GABA	Weight gain, nausea, vomiting, hair loss, bruising, tremor, thrombocytopenia, hepatic failure	250 milligrams 2 or 3 times a day	Effective for both acute and maintenance therapy Can monitor drug levels Monitor liver and platelet function May be used alone to treat BD, or in combination with antipsychotic or lithium
Carbamazepine	Tegretol	Antiepileptic; stabilizes sodium channels, potentiates GABA receptors	AGRANULOCYTOSIS, nausea, vomiting, hyponatremia, rash, leukopenia	100–200 milligrams 1 or 2 times a day	Effective for acute or maintenance therapy Can monitor drug levels Monitor LFTs May be better in rapid cycling disorder Do not use with antipsychotics Many drug interactions with similarly liver-metabolized medications
Lamotrigine	Lamictal	Antiepileptic; sodium channel blockade	STEVENS-JOHNSON SYNDROME/ TOXIC EPIDERMAL NECROLYSIS—rare complications but potentially fatal; nausea, vomiting, fatigue, dizziness	25 milligrams once a day	Used with more severe depressive symptoms
Olanzapine	Zyprexa	Antipsychotic; muscarinic; dopamine and serotonin antagonist	Sedation, constipation, dry mouth, glucose intolerance, orthostatic hypotension, hyperlipidemia	10–15 milligrams 1 or 2 times a day	May be used in combination with lithium or valproic acid
Quetiapine	Seroquel	Antipsychotic; dopamine, serotonin, and adrenergic antagonist	Headache, dry mouth, weight gain, sedation, dizziness, orthostatic hypotension	100–200 milligrams 1 or 2 times a day	May be used in combination with lithium or valproic acid
Risperidone	Risperdal	Antipsychotic; serotonin and dopamine antagonist	Extrapyramidal side effects, prolactin elevation, sedation, dyspepsia, nausea, weight gain	1–2 milligrams 1 or 2 times a day	May be used with lithium or valproic acid
Aripiprazole	Abilify	Antipsychotic; partial agonist of dopamine/ serotonin receptors; antagonist of other serotonin receptors	Headache, nausea, vomiting, extrapyramidal symptoms	10–30 milligrams once a day	May be used with lithium or valproic acid

Abbreviations: BD = bipolar disorder; GABA = γ-aminobutyric acid; LFTs = liver function tests; NE = norepinephrine.

alone or in combination. Patients with anxiety disorders seek medical care about twice as often as nonanxiety patients and are high users of the ED.[36,37] This is partly due to the fact that anxiety disorders, especially panic disorder, may mimic life-threatening conditions. **Anxiety disorders are characterized by excessive fear or worry about real or imagined events.** Fears often adversely impact both physical and psychological health.

Anxiety disorders are a heterogeneous group. Generalized anxiety disorder, panic disorder, and posttraumatic stress disorder are discussed here.

PATHOPHYSIOLOGY

The pathophysiology of anxiety disorder is multifactorial. Certain neurotransmitters, such as γ-aminobutyric acid, norepinephrine, and serotonin, may play a role, as evidenced by the utility of SSRIs and benzodiazepines to treat anxiety disorder. Areas of the brain that are involved in processing anxiety, such as the limbic system, and specifically the amygdala, have been implicated. There appears to be a genetic role, especially in panic disorder,[6] although it does not seem to be as strong a predictor as in other psychological illnesses. Exposure to stressful events, especially in childhood, is a risk factor for development of anxiety disorder.[38] A specific stressful event precedes the development of posttraumatic stress disorder.

CLINICAL FEATURES

The various types of anxiety disorders share many common somatic and cognitive symptoms (**Table 289-5**). Common physical symptoms include chest pain, palpitations, tachycardia, smothering feeling, shortness of breath, lightheadedness, abdominal pain, fatigue, trembling, numbness or tingling, and generalized vague pain. Psychological symptoms may include fear of impending death, feelings of depersonalization, irritability, inability to concentrate, obsessions and compulsions, and feeling "ill at ease."

Generalized Anxiety Disorder Patients with generalized anxiety disorder have chronic excessive anxiety and worry about real or imagined events, occurring more days than not for at least 6 months.[16] The symptoms cause significant impairment in daily functioning and are generally recognized by the patient as excessive and inappropriate. The anxiety and worry are associated with three or more of the following symptoms: restlessness or being keyed up or on edge, irritability, muscle tension, being easily fatigued, difficulty concentrating or "mind going blank," and sleep disturbance. General anxiety disorder is often accompanied by other psychiatric illness, most commonly mood disorders and other anxiety disorders. Patients may also have interspersed more intense panic attacks.[39]

Panic Disorder Panic disorder is a common, often chronic illness characterized by recurrent, spontaneous panic attacks. **Panic attacks are short-lived episodes of anxiety or intense fear accompanied by a range of somatic symptoms** (commonly cardiac, GI, or neurologic), usually peaking within 10 minutes and lasting up to an hour. The criteria for panic disorder also stipulate that the panic attack must be followed by 1 month of persistent concern about having additional attacks, or worry about the implications of the attack or its consequences, or a significant change in behavior related to the attacks. It cannot be better accounted for by another psychiatric or medical disorder.[16] Panic disorder is closely associated with other anxiety disorders, mood disorders, substance abuse and dependence, and personality disorders. Panic disorder may occur with or without agoraphobia (irrational fear of crowded spaces); panic disorder with agoraphobia may be severely disabling both socially and occupationally. Because of the often debilitating symptoms, panic disorder patients are high users of the ED. In one Canadian study, 25% of patients presenting to the ED with chest pain were ultimately diagnosed with panic disorder.[40] Underrecognition of anxiety disorders, which are treatable, continues the cycle of overutilization of medical resources. Panic disorder may have an association with several medical disorders, including asthma,[41] hypertension,[42] interstitial cystitis,[43] migraine headaches,[44] and cardiovascular disease.[45] The long-held association between mitral valve prolapse is less clear.[46]

Posttraumatic Stress Disorder/Acute Stress Disorder Posttraumatic stress disorder patients have all experienced or witnessed an intense traumatic event, such as rape, combat, natural disaster, child abuse, chronic exposure to an extreme stressor, or even vehicular trauma. The prevalence of posttraumatic stress disorder within the first several months after vehicular trauma is 25% to 40%, and in 15% of patients, posttraumatic stress disorder will persist.[47]

Diagnostic criteria state that the patient has to be exposed to the stressor and that the response involved intense fear, hopelessness, or horror.[16] This is followed by "intrusive recollection," which would include one or more of the following: recurrent distressing dreams of the event, acting or feeling as if the event were recurring ("flashbacks"), and intense psychological distress with or without physiologic reactivity upon exposure to internal or external cues that symbolize the traumatic event. There may also be avoidance of stimuli associated with the trauma and a numbing of general responsiveness. Hyperarousal demonstrated by hypervigilance or exaggerated startle may occur. The symptoms have to be present for at least a month and cause significant impairment in functioning and cannot be better explained by another psychiatric or medical cause.[16] Acute stress disorder is diagnosed when the same symptoms of posttraumatic stress disorder last between 2 days and 1 month. Patients often return to the ED after serious trauma for a variety of reasons (i.e., inadequate follow-up or pain control) and should be questioned about persistent pain, coping strategies, and general well-being, so as to possibly intervene and avert development of acute stress disorder or posttraumatic stress disorder.

TABLE 289-5 Symptoms of Anxiety Disorder

Somatic Symptoms	Cognitive Symptoms
Palpitations, pounding heart, or tachycardia	Fear of losing control Fear of dying
Sweating Sensations of shortness of breath or smothering	Derealization (feeling of unreality) or depersonalization (feeling detached from oneself)
Trembling or shaking	Inability to concentrate
Feeling of choking	Obsessions and compulsions
Chest pain or discomfort	Feeling ill at ease
Nausea or abdominal distress	
Feeling dizzy, unsteady, light-headed, or faint	
Paresthesias	
Chills or hot flashes	

DIAGNOSIS

Patients with anxiety disorder often go for many years to EDs and primary care settings, experiencing expensive workups and using health-care resources, before the diagnosis is established.[48] Assess patients with anxiety for life-threatening conditions, self-harm and harm to others, and patient and staff safety. There is about a 10-fold greater suicide risk among patients with anxiety disorders compared with the general population.[49] When a patient has both an anxiety disorder and a mood disorder, suicide risk is greater than for either disease alone.[50]

Through history taking, try to identify current stressful situations that may have precipitated symptoms. First consider serious medical conditions (such as myocardial infarction, pulmonary embolus, hypoglycemia, hypoxia, tachyarrhythmias, thyroid storm, and cerebrovascular accident). Comorbid psychiatric illnesses are common with anxiety; about half of the patients diagnosed with anxiety have comorbid depression.[51]

Anxiety symptoms may also be caused by certain medications or substances of abuse, including corticosteroids, neuroleptics, bronchodilators, decongestants, caffeine, nicotine, cocaine, and amphetamines. Withdrawal from benzodiazepines, opiates, SSRIs/SNRIs, and alcohol

TABLE 289-6 Pharmacotherapy for Anxiety Disorder

	Class of Drug	Drug and Dosage	FDA Approved for Which AD
Acute medication treatment	Benzodiazepines	Lorazepam (Ativan), 0.5–1.0 milligrams 3 times a day	All
		Clonazepam (Klonopin), 0.5–1.0 milligrams twice a day	All
		Alprazolam (Xanax), 0.25–1.0 milligrams 3–4 times a day	All
		Diazepam (Valium) 2–10 milligrams 2–4 times a day	All
Ongoing medication treatment	Selective serotonin reuptake inhibitor	Sertraline (Zoloft), 50–200 milligrams daily (initial dose, 25 milligrams)	PD, PTSD, SAD
		Paroxetine (Paxil), 40–70 milligrams daily (initial dose, 10–20 milligrams)	GAD, PD, PTSD, SAD
		Escitalopram (Lexapro), 10–20 milligrams daily	GAD
		Fluoxetine (Prozac) 20–60 milligrams daily (initial dose 10 milligrams)	PD
	Serotonin norepinephrine reuptake inhibitor	Venlafaxine (Effexor), 75–300 milligrams daily (initial dose, 37.5 milligrams) (Venlafaxine XR preferred in anxiety.)	GAD, PD, SAD
		Duloxetine (Cymbalta) 20–120 milligrams daily (initial dose, 20 milligrams)	GAD

Abbreviations: AD = anxiety disorder; FDA = U.S. Food and Drug Administration; GAD = generalized anxiety disorder; PD = panic disorder; PTSD = posttraumatic stress disorder; SAD = seasonal affective disorder.

may cause agitation and anxiety. One useful screening question is: "Have you experienced brief periods for seconds or minutes of an overwhelming panic or terror that was accompanied by racing heart, shortness of breath, or dizziness?"[52] Take care to identify victims of domestic violence or sexual abuse or assault, because such past or present experiences can provoke panic attacks.

TREATMENT OF ANXIETY DISORDERS

The two main classes of drugs are benzodiazepines for acute treatment and antidepressants for long-term treatment.

Consider initiating short-term benzodiazepine pharmacotherapy in the ED (**Table 289-6**) for acute panic attack, especially for patients who need rapid control of panic symptoms or who are unable to fulfill expected major obligations (e.g., work, school). The limitation of benzodiazepines is their potential for abuse and dependence. Use with caution in patients with a respiratory disorder or a history of substance abuse or dependence. Use caution in the elderly because common concerns include falling, cognitive slowing, paradoxical agitation, and drug interactions due to polypharmacy.

Initiating antidepressants for anxiety is ideally done in conjunction with a primary care or psychiatric practitioner with a follow-up plan in place. SSRIs and SNRIs are the antidepressants of choice. The TCAs and MAOIs are used primarily for treatment failures. Doses tend to be lower than used in treating depression and may take longer to be effective.

DISPOSITION

Once a diagnosis of AD is considered, the next step is to educate patients and provide reassurance that they are not dying or "going crazy." Emphasize that this is an illness that can be treated effectively. Although the different anxiety disorders vary somewhat in their specific treatments, generally, cognitive behavioral therapy and pharmacotherapy are effective. Choice of treatment is based on an individual assessment of risks, benefits, efficacy, availability, acuity, and patient preference. Although cognitive behavioral therapy is not practiced in the ED, education regarding it is worthwhile. It consists of patient education about a disorder, symptom and thought records, and learning anxiety management skills (e.g., breathing retraining) with the guidance of a trained therapist.

The need for admission is rare, except to exclude a life-threatening condition. Medication changes or initiation of antidepressants should be done in conjunction with the primary care provider or psychiatrist.

REFERENCES

The complete reference list is available online at www.TintinalliEM.com.

Psychoses

Adam Z. Tobias

INTRODUCTION & EPIDEMIOLOGY

Psychosis has been defined as a "fundamental derangement of the mind characterized by defective or lost contact with reality."[1] The *Diagnostic and Statistical Manual of Mental Disorders*, Fifth Edition (DSM-V),[2] defines psychotic disorders as those that include abnormalities in one or more of five domains: hallucinations, delusions, disorganized or abnormal motor behavior, disorganized thinking, and negative symptoms. The hallmark of these psychoses, schizophrenia, has a worldwide prevalence of 0.5% to 1%[3] and affects approximately 2.4 million adults in the United States.[4] Considered one of the leading causes of chronic incapacity, the term schizophrenia, meaning "split mind," was coined by Eugene Bleuler in 1911.[5] The economic burden of schizophrenia in the United States in 2002 was estimated at $62.7 billion[6] and typically accounts for 1.5% to 3% of the total national healthcare expenditure, with a high incidence of ED utilization.[7]

The assessment of the psychotic patient presenting to the ED can be challenging, because patients may be agitated, combative, uncooperative, or unable to provide any history. The goals of evaluation are multiple. First, minimize any potential harm to the patient and ensure the safety of the ED staff and other patients. In the case of an aggressive or violent patient, this may require the use of verbal de-escalation techniques or physical or chemical restraints. Second, assess for any coexisting or confounding medical or traumatic conditions. Emergency physicians are gatekeepers to the psychiatric world, because once the patient is funneled into the psychiatric treatment realm, organic conditions may become more difficult to identify and treat. Psychiatric conditions contribute to increased mortality from comorbid medical conditions as compared to the general population.[8] Finally, aim to optimize the treatment of the patient's underlying psychiatric illness, either by connecting him or her with the appropriate inpatient or outpatient resources, or, when possible, by contacting his or her psychiatrist.

PATHOPHYSIOLOGY

Both environmental and genetic factors contribute to the schizophrenia spectrum of disorders. The incidence of schizophrenia is higher in those growing up in urban areas[9] and in certain minority ethnic groups,[10] and the disorders have been linked to a spectrum of risk alleles. There is also overlap between the alleles associated with schizophrenia and those associated with other disorders such as autism and bipolar disorder.[11]

Traditionally, the *dopamine hypothesis*, wherein excessive dopamine leads to the pathophysiology of schizophrenia, has been the dominant theory.[12] Now, it is thought that dopamine acts as the common final pathway of a wide variety of predisposing factors, either environmental, genetic, or both, that lead to the disease. Other neurotransmitters, such as glutamate and adenosine, may also collaborate with dopamine to give rise to the entire picture of schizophrenia.[13]

CLINICAL FEATURES

HISTORY

Features of psychoses include hallucinations, delusions, disorganized thinking, and negative symptoms.

A **hallucination** is an "apparent, often strong subjective perception of an external object or event when no such stimulus or situation is present."[2] Although hallucinations may occur in any sensory modality, they are most commonly auditory in schizophrenia and other psychotic disorders. Typically these are experienced as voices distinct from the individual's own thoughts. Not all hallucinations are considered to be pathologic; they may be a normal part of certain religious and cultural experiences.

A **delusion** is "a false belief or wrong judgment, sometimes associated with hallucinations, held with conviction despite evidence to the contrary."[14] Delusions may be classified based on various themes, including *grandiose* (i.e., "when an individual believes that he or she has exceptional abilities, wealth, or fame"), *persecutory*, *erotomanic* (i.e., "when an individual believes falsely that another person is in love with him or her"), and *referential* (i.e., "belief that certain gestures, comments, environmental cues, and so forth are directed at oneself"). Delusions are considered bizarre if they are clearly implausible. In the ED, a nonbizarre delusion may be difficult to distinguish from a strongly held idea.[2]

Typically, **disorganized thinking** is inferred from a patient's speech. Commonly encountered patterns may include *derailment or loose associations*, wherein the individual switches from one topic to another; *tangentiality*, wherein answers to questions may be unrelated or loosely related; and *word salad*, wherein the individual's speech becomes so disorganized that it becomes nearly incomprehensible.[2]

Negative symptoms associated with psychotic disorders include *avolition* (decreased motivation), *diminished emotional expression*, *anhedonia* (decreased ability to experience pleasure), *asociality* (decreased interest in social interaction), and *alogia* (decreased speech).

PHYSICAL EXAMINATION

Aside from grossly disorganized or abnormal motor behavior (discussed below), there are no specific physical findings associated with the psychotic disorders. The goal of physical examination is the exclusion of coexisting medical or traumatic conditions. For agitated patients, be particularly vigilant to assess for any self-inflicted injuries, environmental injuries such as frostbite, or injuries occurring during the restraint process.

Grossly disorganized or abnormal motor behavior may take on various forms, although it is likely most familiar to emergency practitioners as unpredictable agitation. Catatonia, a "marked decrease in reactivity to the environment" is not frequently encountered in the ED. Catatonic features may range from *negativism*, which is a resistance to instructions, to maintenance of a rigid or inappropriate posture, to complete lack of motor or verbal response. Catatonic behavior may occur in association with a variety of psychiatric and medical conditions.[2]

DIAGNOSIS AND DIFFERENTIAL DIAGNOSIS

Psychotic symptoms may be caused by numerous medical conditions, including infections such as encephalitis, meningitis, or cystitis; CNS conditions such as stroke, seizure, Parkinson's disease,[15] or brain tumor; and metabolic derangements such as hypoglycemia or hepatic encephalopathy. Additionally, various medications and illicit substances may give rise to psychotic symptoms (**Table 290-1**).[16-19]

The DSM-V, delineates specific diagnostic criteria for the schizophrenia spectrum and other psychotic disorders (see discussion below).

TABLE 290-1 Common Medications and Drugs of Abuse Causing Psychosis

Medications	Drugs of Abuse
Corticosteroids	Ethanol*
Fluoroquinolones	Cocaine
Atropine and other anticholinergics	Amphetamines and other stimulants (including "bath salts")
Dextromethorphan	LSD and other hallucinogens
Benzodiazepines*	Marijuana
	Phencyclidine (PCP)
	MDMA (ecstasy)

*Psychosis is more commonly seen in benzodiazepine withdrawal; can occur with ethanol intoxication or withdrawal

However, such granular distinctions are typically not necessary or relevant for emergency assessment and treatment. Rather than making a specific psychiatric diagnosis, the ED provider's focus should be on emergency treatment and stabilization, identification of comorbid conditions, and appropriate disposition. Assignment of a specific diagnosis should be left to the purview of those with specialized psychiatric training. Diagnostic testing is directed by the history and physical examination. Routine laboratory testing for otherwise stable and cooperative psychiatric patients is of low yield and need not be performed in most cases. Similarly, urine toxicologic screening rarely affects ED management and need not be routinely obtained.[20]

Many psychotic patients presenting to the ED have been previously diagnosed with a psychiatric condition. In such cases, determine whether there has been an acute change from the patient's baseline and whether the current presentation is confounded by another condition that requires medical treatment. In cases where the patient is unable to aid with providing history, use other resources, including past medical records, medication lists, family members, and case workers.

For patients with new-onset psychosis, the ED is a common point of first contact with the healthcare system.[21] It is then incumbent on the provider to determine whether the patient's psychosis is the by-product of an acute medical condition, a reaction to a medication or illicit substance, or truly the new onset of a primary psychiatric illness. Newly symptomatic patients often warrant a more extensive medical evaluation than those with known underlying psychotic disorders.

DISPOSITION AND FOLLOW-UP

Psychotic patients may present anywhere along a spectrum ranging from high functioning to completely disabled. Guide disposition decisions by considerations of patient safety and optimization of treatment. Patients thought to be violent, at risk of self-harm, or unable to care for themselves typically require emergent psychiatric evaluation and possible inpatient psychiatric care. Patients with new-onset psychosis (not thought to be due to a medical cause) or those with worsening of underlying psychotic symptoms should have psychiatric consultation in the ED, if available, or be transferred to a psychiatric facility. Patients with known psychoses under apparent good control may be referred for outpatient management. Ideally, such referrals should be made in consultation with the patient's treating psychiatric provider.

Finally, patients with psychosis secondary to a medical condition or those with comorbid illness should be managed accordingly. Give special consideration to a patient's functional level and ability to manage the medical condition as an outpatient. For example, a schizophrenic patient with an infection that might otherwise be treated with oral antibiotics at home might benefit from hospitalization if there is doubt about the patient's ability to comply with treatment and follow-up instructions.

PHARMACOTHERAPY

Antipsychotic (neuroleptic) medications are typically used in the treatment of schizophrenia and the other psychoses. The exact mechanism of

TABLE 290-2 Typical Antipsychotics

Generic Name	Brand Name	Relative Potency	U.S. Food and Drug Administration Warnings
Phenothiazines			
Chlorpromazine	Thorazine	Low	
Mesoridazine	Serentil	Intermediate	QT_C prolongation
Thioridazine	Mellaril	Intermediate	QT_C prolongation
Perphenazine	Trilafon	Intermediate	
Trifluoperazine	Stelazine	High	
Fluphenazine	Prolixin	High	
Thioxanthenes			
Loxapine	Loxitane	Intermediate	
Thiothixene	Navane	High	
Dihydroindolones			
Molindone	Moban	Intermediate	
Butyrophenones			
Haloperidol	Haldol	High	QT_C prolongation and torsades de pointes
Droperidol	Inapsine	High	QT_C prolongation and torsades de pointes

action of the antipsychotics is not known. The majority of antipsychotics block the D_2 dopamine receptors and $5\text{-}HT_{2A}$ serotonin receptors in the brain to a varying degree. Antipsychotics are classified as either *typical* or *atypical*.

The typical antipsychotic medications are often categorized as being of low, medium, or high potency. The "potency" of these drugs does not refer to their effectiveness, but rather to the dosing of the drug for effective clinical response. In general, **low-potency medications** tend to be more sedating and are more often associated with hypotension, dizziness, and anticholinergic symptoms. **High-potency medications** are generally less sedating, but are more frequently associated with extrapyramidal effects such as tremors, rigidity, muscle spasms, and akathisia. **Table 290-2** reviews the common typical antipsychotics.

The U.S. Food and Drug Administration (FDA) has placed black box warnings on a number of the typical antipsychotics, due to concerns about possible cardiac dysrhythmias associated with their use. In particular, several of these medications have been associated with QT_c prolongation and the FDA recommends evaluation of the QT_c interval prior their use. In clinical situations in which rapid tranquilization is necessary, a priori determination of the QT_c interval is impractical and usually impossible. If ECG data are available from the ED visit, these should be reviewed for evidence of QT_c prolongation. Similarly, if prior ECG data are available, incorporate them into clinical decision making. Haloperidol remains a popular and effective agent for rapid tranquilization, and despite aggressive marketing claims to the contrary, its effectiveness is better supported by evidence than newer agents such as aripiprazole or ziprasidone.[22] Unfortunately, QT_c prolongation does not directly correlate with the clinical risk of dysrhythmias or the development of the malignant arrhythmia torsades de pointes. The black box warnings have led to apprehension in the use of highly effective medications.

The atypical antipsychotics (**Table 290-3**) are generally newer medications that more specifically target the dopamine receptors or inhibit the reuptake of serotonin. They also offer increased efficacy in the treatment of the negative symptoms of psychosis. Based on this improved receptor specificity, adverse effects such as sedation, extrapyramidal effects, QT_c prolongation, and tardive dyskinesia are generally reduced but are not completely eliminated. The incidence of hypotension does not appear to have been significantly altered. The FDA has placed a black box warning on both typical and atypical psychotics for their off-label use in managing agitation and psychosis in elderly patients with dementia. Increased rates of cerebrovascular accidents, cardiovascular events, and mortality have been associated with chronic use.[23,24]

TABLE 290-3 Atypical Antipsychotics

Drug	U.S. Food and Drug Administration–Approved Indications	Warnings and Common Side Effects (BLACK BOX WARNINGS IN CAPS)
Clozapin (Clozaril)	Treatment-resistant schizophrenia Reduction in the risk of recurrent suicidal behavior in schizophrenic or schizoaffective disorders	Sedation, dizziness, hypotension, tachycardia, salivation, weight gain, hyperthermia. AGRANULOCYTOSIS, SEIZURES, MYOCARDITIS, OTHER ADVERSE CARDIOVASCULAR AND RESPIRATORY EFFECTS
Olanzapine (Zyprexa)	Schizophrenia Bipolar disorder Agitation associated with schizophrenia and bipolar I mania	CVAE, sedation, postural hypotension, hyperglycemia, weight gain, dizziness
Quetiapine (Seroquel)	Bipolar mania Schizophrenia	NMS, hyperglycemia, sedation, hypotension, headache, weight gain CATARACT FORMATION
Risperidone (Risperdal)	Schizophrenia Bipolar mania	Extrapyramidal effects, hyperglycemia, hypotension, hyperprolactinemia, weight gain
Ziprasidone (Geodon)	Schizophrenia Bipolar mania Acute agitation in schizophrenic patients	Sedation, rash, dizziness, hypotension, hyperglycemia, extrapyramidal effects QT PROLONGATION AND RISK OF SUDDEN DEATH
Aripiprazole (Abilify)	Schizophrenia Bipolar disorder	NMS, CVAE, hyperglycemia, seizure, hypotension, headache, akathisia
Asenapine (Saphris, Sycrest)	Schizophrenia Bipolar mania	Blood dyscrasias, cerebrovascular effects, dyslipidemia, extrapyramidal symptoms, NMS, hyperglycemia, QT_c prolongation, orthostatic hypotension, increased mortality with chronic use in dementia patients
Iloperidone (Fanapt)	Schizophrenia	
Paliperidone (Invega, Sustenna)	Schizophrenia Schizoaffective disorder	

Abbreviations: CVAE = cerebrovascular adverse event; NMS = neuroleptic malignant syndrome.

ADVERSE EFFECTS

The following side effects are more commonly associated with the typical antipsychotics but may also occur with medications in the atypical class: acute dystonia, akathisia or restlessness, parkinsonism, anticholinergic effects, cardiovascular effects, and neuroleptic malignant syndrome.

Acute Dystonia Acute dystonias are probably the most common side effect of antipsychotic medications seen in the ED. Muscle spasms of the neck, face, and back are the most common dystonias, but oculogyric crisis and even laryngospasm may also occur. Treatment with either benztropine, 1 to 2 milligrams IV, or diphenhydramine, 25 to 50 milligrams IV, rapidly corrects the dystonia. For persistent reactions, both medications may be used, and benzodiazepines may be added for treatment failures. Dystonias often recur despite dosage reduction or discontinuation of the offending antipsychotic.

Akathisia (Motor Restlessness) Akathisia, a sensation of motor restlessness with a subjective desire to move, can begin several days to several weeks after initiation of antipsychotic treatment. Management can be difficult. If possible, decrease the dosage of the antipsychotic after psychiatric consultation. The best treatment is probably administration of β-blockers such as propranolol.

Antiparkinsonian or anticholinergic drugs such as benztropine, 1 milligram PO two to four times daily, may also afford some relief. In refractory cases, the antipsychotic may need to be changed to an atypical agent.

Antipsychotic-Induced Parkinson's Syndrome A complete Parkinson's syndrome, including bradykinesia, resting tremor, cogwheel rigidity, shuffling gait, masked facies, and drooling, can occur, but often only one or two features of the syndrome are obvious. Antipsychotic dosage reduction and/or anticholinergic medication is usually effective.

Anticholinergic Effects Anticholinergic effects range from mild sedation to delirium. Peripheral manifestations may include dry mouth and skin, blurred vision, urinary retention, constipation, paralytic ileus, cardiac dysrhythmias, and exacerbation of angle-closure glaucoma. The central anticholinergic syndrome is characterized by dilated pupils, dysarthria, and an agitated delirium. Treatment is discontinuation of the antipsychotic and supportive measures.

Cardiovascular Effects Cardiovascular side effects, such as orthostatic hypotension and tachycardia, are commonly encountered with use of the antipsychotics. These effects are likely related to anticholinergic and adrenergic blockade and occur at therapeutic dosages. Typically, hypotension can be easily managed with IV fluids. In severe cases, vasopressor support may be required. Additional effects caused by blockade of sodium, calcium, and potassium channels in the central nervous and cardiac systems are less well delineated. However, effects on specific potassium channels in the myocardium have been linked to the drug-induced prolongation of the QT_c interval associated with several of the antipsychotics.[25,26] It is this mechanism of action by which the antipsychotics are believed to induce torsades de pointes.

Neuroleptic Malignant Syndrome Neuroleptic malignant syndrome is an uncommon idiosyncratic reaction to neuroleptic drugs manifested by rigidity, fever, autonomic instability (tachycardia, diaphoresis, and blood pressure abnormalities), and a confusional state. Although high-potency antipsychotics may be more likely to cause the disorder, all antipsychotics are potential offenders. Neuroleptic malignant syndrome is a medical emergency and has a mortality rate as high as 20%. Management includes immediate discontinuation of the antipsychotic medication, hydration, and meticulous supportive treatment in an intensive care setting. Anticholinergic medications are not helpful and may worsen the condition by further impairing centrally mediated temperature regulation. Medications such as dantrolene sodium or bromocriptine are sometimes used to relieve the rigidity.

SCHIZOPHRENIA SPECTRUM OF DISORDERS

The schizophrenia spectrum of disorders is listed in **Table 290-4**. Some of the more commonly encountered conditions are discussed in detail below.

Schizophrenia is the most common form of psychosis. It typically involves a wide range of impairments in functioning and may affect all areas of a patient's life, including occupational and social aspects. It usually begins to manifest between the late teens and the mid-30s and is often preceded by a prodromal phase. Its course is characterized by acute episodes and periods of partial or full remission. There is a male-to-female rate ratio of 1.4, and the incidence varies significantly based on socioeconomic, racial, and geographic factors, with a higher incidence among migrants, urban populations, and ethnic minorities.[27-29] Patients with schizophrenia have high rates of medical comorbidity and concomitant substance abuse.[30,31]

TABLE 290-4 The Schizophrenia Spectrum of Disorders

Schizophrenia
Brief psychotic disorder
Substance/medication-induced psychotic disorder
Schizotypal personality disorder
Unspecified catatonia
Unspecified schizophrenia spectrum and other psychotic disorder
Catatonia associated with another mental disorder
Delusional disorder
Schizoaffective disorder
Schizophreniform disorder
Psychotic disorder due to another medical condition
Catatonic disorder due to another medical condition
Other specified schizophrenia spectrum and other psychotic disorder

TABLE 290-5 Diagnostic Criteria for Schizophrenia[2]

Criterion A*	Other Selected Criteria
Hallucinations	Disturbance present for at least 6 months
Disorganized speech	Significant deficiencies in major areas of function (work, self-care, interpersonal relations)
Delusions	Depression, bipolar disorder, schizoaffective disorder ruled out
Negative symptoms	Not attributable to another medical condition or substance
Grossly disorganized or catatonic behavior	

*Must have two or more criteria and at least one must be delusions or disorganized speech.

Signs of the disturbance must be present for at least 6 months for a formal diagnosis, and symptoms cannot be attributable to another medical condition or the effects of a substance. Diagnostic criteria are listed in **Table 290-5**.

Schizophreniform disorder differs from schizophrenia only in its duration of symptoms (1 to 6 months) and in the absence of impaired social and occupational functioning as a diagnostic criterion. In contrast, **brief psychotic disorder** lasts between 1 day and 1 month and involves the sudden onset of at least one of the following: delusions, hallucinations, disorganized speech, or grossly disorganized or catatonic behavior.[2]

Schizotypal (personality) disorder is considered part of the schizophrenia spectrum but is classified as a personality disorder, and its treatment is generally more similar to that of other personality disorders than to that of the other psychoses. The disorder is characterized by eccentricities of behavior, a reduced capacity for close relationships, and a pattern of social and interpersonal deficits.

Delusional disorder is diagnosed in the absence of schizophrenia and involves the presence of one or more delusions for at least 1 month. Risk factors include low socioeconomic status, family history of psychiatric disorders, older age, immigration, and exposure to stressful events, with persecutory delusions being the most common.[32] The central theme of the *somatic type*, and a potential trigger for an ED visit, is a preoccupation with health and organ function. For example, individuals may be convinced that they have an infestation of insects on their skin or that a part of their body is not functioning.[2]

Schizoaffective disorder is about one-third as prevalent as schizophrenia.[33] It is characterized by Criterion A of schizophrenia (see **Table 290-5**) occurring concurrently with a major mood episode (major depressive or manic). Furthermore, delusions or hallucinations must be present for at least 2 weeks in the absence of the mood symptoms. Patients may have problems with self-care, restricted social contact, and poor insight.[34,35] Patients with schizophrenia and schizoaffective disorder have a 5% lifetime risk of suicide, with higher risk in patients with depressive symptoms.[36]

Catatonia may occur in the context of various conditions and is categorized as either *catatonia associated with another mental disorder*, *catatonic disorder due to another medical condition*, or *unspecified catatonia*. Medical conditions associated with catatonia include encephalitis, head trauma, hepatic encephalopathy, and neoplasms. The acute presentation of catatonia often includes stupor, and therefore patients often have their first clinical contact in the ED. **It is therefore important to recognize that catatonia is frequently associated with an organic cause.**[37]

REFERENCES

The complete reference list is available online at www.TintinalliEM.com.

CHAPTER 291 Eating Disorders

Gemma C. Lewis

INTRODUCTION AND EPIDEMIOLOGY

Eating disorders, such as anorexia nervosa, bulimia nervosa, and binge-eating disorder, are psychological pathologies characterized by disordered relationships with food. Eating disorders are challenging to diagnose in the ED because physical manifestations may be subtle and historical features may not be elicited unless the disorder is suspected from medical complications or comorbidities. It is important for the emergency physician to recognize these conditions, however, because they are among the most deadly of psychiatric illnesses.[1] The fifth edition of the *Diagnostic and Statistical Manual of Mental Disorders* refines the diagnostic criteria of eating disorders from the previous edition (**Table 291-1**).[2]

There are two subtypes of anorexia, restrictive and binge/purge, with crossover between the two subtypes.[3] Patients with a predominantly restrictive pattern simply minimize their food intake. Patients with a predominantly binging/purging subtype make up for unacceptable food intake with diuretics, laxatives, enemas, or vomiting. There are also two subtypes of bulimia: purging and nonpurging. Those who purge do so by the above methods; those classified as nonpurging may use compensatory methods such as fasting or excessive exercise. There is a moderate amount of crossover between anorexia and bulimia, with up to 50% of anorexia patients eventually developing bulimia.[4] Binge eating disorder is characterized by habitual, recurrent binge consumptions that cause significant distress and is distinct from simple episodic overeating.

Anorexia nervosa has an overall incidence rate of 8 per 100,000 person-years,[5] with an estimated lifetime prevalence of 0.9% in women and 0.3% in men.[6] There is no significant difference in prevalence of anorexia between different races or ethnicities.[7] **Bulimia nervosa** has an overall incidence rate of 12 per 100,000 person-years,[5] with an estimated lifetime prevalence of 1.5% in women and 0.5% in men.[6] Bulimia is more common in Latinos (lifetime prevalence of 2.03%) and African Americans (1.31%) than in whites (0.51%).[7] **Binge eating disorder** is relatively more common in older individuals and males than both anorexia and bulimia.[5] It is also more prevalent in minority groups than in non-Latino whites.[7] In the United States, the incidence rate for those ≥14 years old is 1010 per 100,000 person-years in females and 660 per 100,000 person-years in males,[8] with a lifetime prevalence of 3.5% in women and 2.0% among men.[6] Although it is often associated with obesity, binge eating disorder is a distinct disorder.[9]

PATHOPHYSIOLOGY

There are several biologic and psychosocial factors that predispose toward disordered eating. There is evidence that eating disorders run in families,[10] possibly related to both genetic influences and similar underlying temperaments and behaviors.[11] Development of eating disorders has historically been associated with dysfunctional reward processing in relation to food,[12] but the pathogenesis of this abnormal response is not well understood.[13] MRI studies detect altered subcortical and cortical brain behavior as well as structural brain differences in patients with eating disorders compared to normal controls. Some of these studies implicate differences in brain regions involved in reward processing, but results are inconsistent.[14-16] Patients with eating disorders also demonstrate differences in certain peripheral and central chemical modulators involved in eating behavior and energy homeostasis compared to controls, but it is not known if such changes are causal or correlative.[17]

CLINICAL FEATURES

HISTORY

Patients with eating disorders often present to the ED with vague signs and symptoms, such as weakness, fatigue, pallor, dizziness, syncope, confusion, bloating, edema, or persistent nausea.[18] Alternatively complaints may be due to medical complications, such as chest pain and hematemesis caused by a Mallory-Weiss tear from purging; palpitations from electrolyte-induced dysrhythmias; dysmenorrhea from disruption of the hypothalamic-pituitary axis; or fractures from osteoporosis or extreme exercise. Depression, anxiety, substance abuse, self-injurious behavior, or suicidality may coexist.[19,20] A meta-analysis of 36 studies reviewing mortality rates for patients with eating disorders reported that one in five individuals with anorexia who died had committed suicide.[21] Data on patients with bulimia or binge eating disorder are confounded

TABLE 291-1 *Diagnostic and Statistical Manual of Mental Disorders*, **Fifth Edition, Criteria for Eating Disorders**

Anorexia Nervosa	Bulimia Nervosa	Binge Eating Disorder
Restriction of caloric intake relative to requirements, leading to a lower than expected body weight in the context of age, sex, development, and physical health (<85% predicted)	Recurrent episodes of binge eating characterized by both: 1. Eating in a discrete time period an amount of food that is larger than most people would eat in the same period under the same circumstance 2. A feeling of lack of control over eating during an episode	Recurrent episodes of binge eating characterized by both: 1. Eating in a discrete time period an amount of food that is larger than most people would eat in the same period of time under the same circumstance 2. A feeling of lack of control over eating during an episode
Fear of weight gain or becoming fat, despite lower than predicted body weight	Recurrent, inappropriate compensatory behaviors to prevent weight gain including self-induced emesis; abuse of laxatives, diuretics, or other medications; caloric restriction; or excessive exercise	The episodes are associated with three of the following: 1. Eating much more quickly than normal 2. Eating until feeling uncomfortably full or overfull 3. Eating large amounts of food even when not feeling hungry 4. Eating alone because of embarrassment about how much one is eating 5. Feeling disgusted, depressed, or guilty afterward
Derangement in the way the patient's body weight or appearance is experienced, undue effects of body weight on self-evaluation, or denial of the dangerousness of the current low body weight	Binging and purging at least 1 time a week for 3 weeks	The patient exhibits marked distress regarding binge eating.
	Self-evaluation is unduly influenced by body weight and appearance	The binge eating occurs at least 1 time a week for 3 months.
	The disturbance does not occur exclusively during episodes of anorexia	The binge eating is not associated with inappropriate compensatory behavior and does not occur exclusively during the course of anorexia, bulimia, or avoidant/restrictive food intake disorder.

by crossover diagnoses. **Therefore, if an eating disorder is suspected, consider screening for depression and suicidality.**

If clinical suspicion is raised for an eating disorder based on complaint cluster, physical examination, or family report, explore a more focused history. Important data points to elicit include eating and dieting behavior; desire for weight loss; typical daily dietary intake; presence or absence of calorie counting; compensatory exercise behavior; guilt patterns following eating; menstruation pattern; and use of over-the-counter dietary supplements or laxative agents. Certain sensitive history points may be difficult to elicit in the ED, such as early childhood GI issues or picky eating or obesity, self-esteem issues, societal thinness pressures, teasing, propensity toward perfectionism, or sexual abuse. Certain physical activities raise risk for eating disorders, such as gymnastics, ballet and other dance, wrestling, swimming, and cross-country running.[22-24] Because eating disorders are characterized by denial of symptoms and behaviors, when eliciting history, take a nonjudgmental approach to encourage trust and truthful disclosure.[19]

PHYSICAL EXAMINATION

Patients with **anorexia** are typically easily identifiable based on a very thin body habitus. Other possible signs include hypotension (resting or orthostatic); bradycardia or tachydysrhythmia; or hypothermia. Patients may also exhibit signs of vitamin deficiencies such as brittle, flaking, or ridged nails (nonspecific malnutrition); stomatitis or cheilitis (B vitamin deficiency); or perifollicular petechiae (scurvy). They may also develop fine, long hair on the arms and face, acral cyanosis (impaired thermoregulation), and/or pretibial edema secondary to malnutrition.[19]

Patients with **bulimia or binge eating disorder** can be difficult to detect in the ED because they tend to be normal weight or even slightly overweight. **Consider eating disorder diagnoses in the presence of other physical indicators, even in normal weight or overweight patients.** Self-induced vomiting can cause painless hypertrophy of the parotid glands, dental erosion, and trauma or callous formation to the dorsal hands (**Russell's sign**),[25] as well as pharyngeal erythema or abrasions, gingivitis, facial petechiae or subconjunctival hemorrhage, and halitosis. Laxative abuse may cause peripheral edema, anal fissures, hemorrhoids, perianal dermatitis, and rectal bleeding. Binge eating disorder may have no abnormalities apparent on physical examination.

DIAGNOSIS

The **SCOFF questionnaire** (**Table 291-2**) is useful for screening for anorexia and bulimia in a brief ED encounter and can be remembered by its acronym: Sick, Control, One stone, Fat, Food.[26] Other screening tools are more extensive and are more useful in a primary care setting. For reference, the Eating Disorder Diagnostic Scale is a 22-point questionnaire that is self-administered and can identify risk for all three major eating disorders.[27] The Eating Attitudes Test is nonspecific and can identify need for referral to a mental health professional for further evaluation.[28] The Questionnaire on Eating and Weight Patterns-Revised is specific for binge eating disorder and displays a reasonable level of concordance between its scores and diagnostic interviews.[29]

DIFFERENTIAL DIAGNOSIS

Consider organic pathology in the assessment of a patient with a potential eating disorder (**Table 291-3**).

TABLE 291-2 SCOFF Questionnaire

Do you make yourself sick because you feel uncomfortably full?
Do you worry you have lost control over how much you eat?
Have you recently lost more than 1 stone (14 lb) in a 3-month period?
Do you believe yourself to be fat when others say you are too thin?
Would you say that food dominates your life?

Note: A score of 2 or more indicates probable anorexia or bulimia nervosa with sensitivity of 88% and specificity of 88%.

TABLE 291-3 Differential Diagnosis of New-Onset Eating Disorders

Endocrine	Adrenal insufficiency Hyperthyroidism Diabetes
GI	Hepatitis Pancreatitis Celiac disease Inflammatory bowel disease Superior mesenteric artery syndrome
Infectious disease	Mononucleosis Human immunodeficiency virus Tuberculosis
Cancer	Nervous system malignancy Ovarian malignancy Intra-abdominal malignancy
Pregnancy	Hyperemesis gravidarum
Psychiatric	Substance abuse Major depressive disorder Bipolar disorder Schizophrenia
Inborn error of metabolism	Mitochondrial disorders Enzyme deficiency

LABORATORY TESTING

Initial testing should include a full chemistry panel including magnesium, calcium, and phosphorus, CBC, blood glucose, urinalysis, pregnancy test, hepatic function panel, serum albumin, lipase and amylase, and thyroid-stimulating hormone. Electrolyte derangements and other lab abnormalities are more common in purging-type eating disorders. Patients with restrictive-type anorexia may not demonstrate any laboratory abnormalities. Purging results in a metabolic alkalosis and may cause hypokalemia and hypochloremia. Purging and binge eating both may cause elevation of liver and pancreatic enzymes. Habitual vomiting can result in hyperamylasemia. Hyponatremia and hypochloremia are often seen in patients who vomit. Laxative and diuretic abuse and vomiting can lead to potassium depletion. Hyponatremia may develop in patients who abuse diuretics. Laxative abuse may cause a positive fecal occult blood test. Dehydration can lead to hemoconcentration. Malnutrition can cause low albumin. Starvation ketosis may cause spilling of ketones in the urine, and dehydration may cause increased urine specific gravity and urea concentration. In patients with very severe anorexia, anemia, leukopenia, hypoglycemia, and hypophosphatemia can develop.[19,30,31]

IMAGING

Obtain imaging to rule out an underlying organic cause of presenting symptoms or to exclude medical complications; for example, obtain chest films to exclude Boerhaave's syndrome or abdominal radiographs to diagnose paralytic ileus or acute gastric dilatation. Radiographic findings in anorexia include decreased muscle mass, paucity of subcutaneous fat, mild small bowel dilatation,[32] and osteoporosis.[33] These findings are reversed upon refeeding and appropriate weight gain. There are no specific radiographic findings diagnostic of binge eating disorder or bulimia, but a swallowed toothbrush or similar item suggests purging by induced vomiting.[34]

DISEASE COMPLICATIONS

Medical complications of eating disorders are many and varied. Medical complications of anorexia are typically more severe than bulimia or binge eating and are directly related to the starvation state. Bulimia medical complications are usually related to purging behaviors and are often the result of chemical derangements or structural damage to the GI tract.[35] The most common medical complication of binge eating is obesity, but acute structural complications such as gastric dilatation may also be seen.

CARDIOPULMONARY COMPLICATIONS

Among the most deadly of the eating disorder complications are changes to the cardiovascular system. Malnutrition in eating disorders leads to decreased muscle mass, including cardiac muscle mass, specifically in the interventricular septum and the left ventricle, as well as increased vagal tone. These effects lead to decreased contractility and cardiac output, and therefore result in hypotension, bradycardia, and orthostasis. Relative decreases in cardiac muscle mass compared to valve cross-sectional area can lead to the development of mitral valve prolapse.[36] Rarely, patients with anorexia nervosa can develop pericardial effusion, which in a few cases has led to cardiac tamponade requiring urgent pericardiocentesis.[37] Purging behavior leading to electrolyte abnormalities can cause cardiac arrhythmias. Syrup of ipecac, used as an emetogenic, is directly cardiotoxic and can cause an irreversible cardiomyopathy.[38] Prolongation of the QT interval on ECG has been described in patients with all types of eating disorders relative to controls. QT prolongation is a marker for risk of ventricular tachyarrhythmia, specifically *torsades de pointes*, and risk of sudden death. QT prolongation as a result of eating disorders is reversed by adequate refeeding and is associated with normalization of heart rate, heart rate variability, and exercise tolerance.[39] Therefore, QT normalization has been used as a marker to guide refeeding and rehabilitation.[40] Most cardiac sequelae are reversible with appropriate weight gain, but there is increased risk of cardiac complications during the first week of refeeding after severe nutrient depletion.[39,41] There are also case reports of pneumothorax and pneumomediastinum as complications of severe anorexia.[42]

NUTRITIONAL COMPLICATIONS

The proportion of eating disorder patients with vitamin deficiencies is difficult to determine, because many patients take supplementary vitamins. Decreased bone mineral density was reported in 18% of patients age 15 to 54 years old admitted to a specialized eating disorders unit but was not associated with decreased vitamin D levels.[43] Deficiencies of other vitamins are rare, and typically merit case reports. Iron and vitamin B_{12} deficiency can lead to anemia in severely food-restrictive patients. Skin erythema and pruritus with sun exposure, glossitis, epidermal desquamation, and diarrhea should raise suspicion of pellagra.[44] Confusion, confabulation, ataxia, ophthalmoplegia, and/or nystagmus suggest Wernicke-Korsakoff encephalopathy. Other vitamin deficiencies reported in association with eating disorders include wet beriberi and scurvy, although these are extremely rare.[45,46]

Refeeding following prolonged nutrient depletion can cause electrolyte abnormalities, most commonly hypokalemia, hypophosphatemia, and hypomagnesemia, due to redistribution of electrolytes from the extracellular to the intracellular space triggered by insulin release and from depletion of phosphorus during protein synthesis. This can lead to arrhythmias, congestive heart failure, pericardial effusions, and cardiac arrest.[41]

GI COMPLICATIONS

Patients with anorexia are at increased risk of constipation, gastroparesis, gastric dilatation, and gastroesophageal reflux.[19,47] Gastroesophageal reflux and laryngopharyngeal reflux commonly occur in patients with bulimia and may result in hoarseness or dysphagia.[19,48] Chronic stimulant laxative abuse can lead to development of rectal prolapse, melanosis coli, or the cathartic colon syndrome.[49-51] Other very rare GI complications include superior mesenteric artery syndrome; gastric dilatation, necrosis, and rupture; necrotizing colitis; and gastric bezoar.[42,52-55]

ENDOCRINE COMPLICATIONS

Profound food restriction affects the hypothalamic-pituitary axis. Low levels of gonadotropins, loss of the normal pulsatile waves of luteinizing hormone, and estrogen deficiency lead to hypothalamic amenorrhea.[56]

TABLE 291-4 Society of Adolescent Medicine Criteria for Hospital Admission

Anorexia Nervosa	Bulimia Nervosa
Body weight <75% of ideal for age, sex, and height	Potassium <3.2 mmol/L
Daytime heart rate <50 beats/min or night-time heart rate <45 beats/min	Chloride <88 mmol/L
Body fat <10% of body weight	Esophageal trauma and hematemesis
Dehydration	Vomiting unresponsive to antiemetics
Cardiac arrhythmia including QT prolongation	Dehydration
Temperature <96°F	Cardiac arrhythmia including QT prolongation
Orthostasis and syncope	Temperature <96°F
Acute psychiatric emergencies such as hallucinations or suicidality	Orthostasis and syncope
Systolic blood pressure <90 mm Hg	Acute psychiatric emergencies such as hallucinations or suicidality
Ongoing weight loss despite outpatient treatment	Ongoing purging despite outpatient treatment

Anorexia is also associated with the **"euthyroid sick syndrome"** in which thyroid-stimulating hormone is normal or slightly low, T_3 is low, and sometimes T_4 levels are also decreased. Thyroid deficiencies likely contribute to the bradycardia, orthostasis, and hypothermia in anorexia. High cortisol levels and low levels of insulin-like growth factor 1 (somatomedin C), T_3, estradiol, and testosterone contribute to loss of bone mass.[57] Refeeding and recovery from illness do not fully return bone mass to normal levels, and patients with anorexia remain at an increased risk of fracture for as many as 40 years following initial diagnosis.[58] The endocrine effects of bulimia and binge eating disorder are less well studied, more variable, and less predictable. Endocrine abnormalities in these disorders may be more related to comorbid obesity than to the eating disorder itself.

TREATMENT AND DISPOSITION

The ED treatment of eating disorders is limited to stabilization of urgent medical complications, followed by hospital admission or outpatient referral to a mental health specialist. **Tables 291-4 and 291-5** list guidelines for hospital admission.[59,60] Treatment requires a multidisciplinary approach, including medical management with pharmacotherapy, dietary interventions, and psychotherapy.[59] If pharmacotherapy is indicated, it should be initiated by a psychiatrist or primary care provider. Selective serotonin reuptake inhibitors may alleviate comorbid psychiatric symptoms including depression and anxiety, but are not associated with improved weight gain or longer times to relapse in patients with anorexia.[61] Fluoxetine is approved by the U.S. Food and Drug Administration for use in bulimia, and other antidepressants show some benefit in bulimia.[62] Avoid bupropion in all patients with eating disorders

TABLE 291-5 American Psychiatric Association Criteria for Hospital Admission

Medical instability (bradycardia or tachycardia, orthostatic hypotension, hypothermia, metabolic or electrolyte abnormality, dehydration, or evidence of organ compromise)
Weight <85% of ideal or acute decline despite outpatient or partial hospitalization treatment
Acute decline in oral intake despite outpatient or partial hospitalization treatment
Comorbid psychiatric conditions or acute stressors including suicidality
Poor motivation or high resistance to treatment interventions unless highly structured
Absence of treatment options of medium intensity, i.e., partial hospitalization treatment programs

because it can potentiate weight loss and reduce seizure threshold in patients with electrolyte abnormalities.

SPECIAL POPULATIONS

PREGNANT WOMEN

Pregnancy can be a particularly stressful time for a woman with an eating disorder, particularly with respect to maintaining adequate and appropriate weight gain for the pregnancy. There are conflicting data on whether the presence of eating disorders increases the risk of complications of pregnancy; certain studies have documented increased risk of miscarriage, lower birth weights, and lower Apgar scores, whereas others have reported no increase in medical complications and normal birth weights. However, the broadest study of its kind to date revealed that the majority of patients with anorexia and bulimia have normal pregnancies and healthy babies. There is, however, an increased risk of birth by cesarean section and an increased risk of postpartum depression following delivery, and these differences remained between groups who had active symptoms of their disease and those with a history of an eating disorder who were asymptomatic during pregnancy.[63]

MEN

Do not neglect the possibility of eating disorders in males. Men may account for between 10% and 25% of cases of anorexia and bulimia,[64] but the exact proportion of men with eating disorders is unknown, because men are less likely to be diagnosed and appropriately treated than women. Of the eating disorders, binge eating disorder is more common in men than is anorexia or bulimia. Excessive exercise is a common compensation in men for overeating. Eating disorders in males are typically characterized by the drive to add muscle bulk and increase lean mass. Eating disorders in men are often associated with antecedent obesity, athletic performance concerns, bullying, and occasionally, but not always, sexual abuse. Men with eating disorders are also more likely to abuse steroids and growth hormones, particularly when muscle dysmorphia is present.[65]

REFERENCES

The complete reference list is available online at www.TintinalliEM.com.

CHAPTER 292

Substance Use Disorders

Edward Bernstein
Judith A. Bernstein
Scott G. Weiner
Gail D'Onofrio

INTRODUCTION AND EPIDEMIOLOGY

In EDs around the world, on every shift, patients present for medical conditions related to the consequences of unhealthy drinking or drug use. Sometimes the cause of the presenting problem is obvious, but just as often, the connection of substance use with its medical consequences remains undiscovered. Emergency physicians are experts in stabilization, rapid diagnosis, and treatment of *acute* alcohol and drug emergencies and their secondary complications but often fail to identify and discuss drinking and drug use as a component of medical care. Factors that often accompany unhealthy alcohol and drug use, such as psychiatric illness, trauma, homelessness, low level of health literacy, inability to pay for medications, criminal justice involvement, absence of family support, and limited availability of treatment and recovery support services, make patient management and disposition difficult.

The scope of substance use disorders includes unhealthy use of alcohol, use of illicit drugs, and nonmedical use of prescription drugs. Severe substance use disorders (addictions) resemble asthma, diabetes, hypertension, and other chronic diseases in that they have genetic components and patients have problems with adherence to medication, loss to follow-up, repeat visits to the ED, and hospital admissions, yet only a small fraction of those needing alcohol or drug treatment are actually receiving indicated therapy, compared with a much higher fraction of patients with chronic medical conditions.[1]

Substance use is a significant global problem. The World Health Organization reports worldwide 185 million illicit drug users, 2 billion alcohol users, and 1.3 billion smokers. In 2000, tobacco, alcohol, and illicit drugs accounted for about 12% of all deaths worldwide.[2]

Those who begin drinking before age 15 have a fourfold increased risk of developing dependence than those who begin drinking later.[3] Underage drinking and drug use have a profound impact on the developing nervous system, so early intervention is needed to mitigate life-altering consequences.[4]

UNHEALTHY ALCOHOL USE

The term *unhealthy alcohol use* describes a spectrum of alcohol consumption ranging from "risky" or hazardous use (no consequences experienced), to harmful use (experience of consequences), to what was previously called *alcohol dependence* but is now termed *alcohol use disorders*.[5] The National Institute on Alcohol Abuse and Alcoholism defines low-risk drinking as follows[6]: for men, no more than 14 drinks per week and no more than four drinks over a 2-hour occasion. Women of all ages and men >65 years old are advised to drink no more than seven drinks per week and no more than three drinks over a 2-hour occasion because of gender and age differences in volume distribution and concentrations of alcohol dehydrogenase in the liver. Binge drinking (drinking too much too fast) is alcohol consumption that results in a blood alcohol level over the U.S. legal limit of 0.08 gram/dL, which for the average male is the result of more than four drinks in 2 hours and for the average female is more than three drinks in 2 hours. Abstinence is advised for pregnant women and underage drinkers, and a lower limit or abstinence is advised for patients with chronic conditions exacerbated by alcohol or who are taking medications with an alcohol interaction.[6]

SUBSTANCE USE DISORDERS

The *Diagnostic and Statistical Manual of Mental Disorders, Fifth Edition*, groups *substance abuse* and *dependence* into categories from mild to severe substance use disorders.[7] The diagnosis of substance use disorder requires two or more of the following 11 criteria: (1) tolerance; (2) withdrawal; (3) recurrent use in greater quantities or for a greater duration than intended; (4) failed attempts to cut back or quit substance use; (5) spending a great deal of time obtaining, using, or recovering from the substance; (6) persistent or recurrent use despite physical and or psychological consequences; (7) giving up important activities in order to use; (8) failure to fulfill responsibilities in work, school, and/or home because of recurrent use; (9) recurrent use resulting in physically hazardous behavior, such as driving under the influence; (10) persistent use despite social or interpersonal problems; and (11) craving alcohol or other drugs. Severity is based on the number of criteria: two or three of the criteria constitute mild substance use disorder, four to five constitute moderate, and six or more constitute severe.[7]

ALCOHOL WITHDRAWAL SYNDROMES

ALCOHOL WITHDRAWAL

Alcohol withdrawal symptoms develop in individuals with a history of heavy and prolonged consumption of alcohol who abruptly stop or reduce their drinking. The spectrum of alcohol withdrawal symptoms includes hand tremors, headache, loss of appetite, nausea and vomiting, diaphoresis, insomnia, tachycardia, hypertension, fever, psychomotor agitation, hyperarousal, craving, and anxiety, as well as the more serious manifestations of seizures, hallucinations, and delirium. The abrupt withdrawal of alcohol from the brain of chronic heavy drinkers is thought to reduce inhibitory neurotransmission through γ-aminobutyric acid and enhance excitatory neurotransmission through glutamate, but not all heavy drinkers experience withdrawal when stopping or cutting back their consumption.[8-10]

Alcohol withdrawal symptoms exist on a continuum from uncomplicated to moderate and severe, may begin as early as 2 to 6 hours after reduction in alcohol consumption, and can persist for up to 2 weeks. Up to 5% of patients in withdrawal progress to delirium tremens; those with a prior history are at greatest risk. Convulsions occur in 5% to 15%, and delirium tremens occurs in less than 5%. Deaths from delirium tremens among patients receiving early and aggressive treatment have declined from 35% in the early twentieth century to 5% in the current period.[8-10]

The first step in successful treatment is to identify alcohol withdrawal early and distinguish withdrawal from mimics. The most common mimics include toxic-metabolic abnormalities (hyponatremia, hypoglycemia, hypomagnesemia, diabetic ketoacidosis, Wernicke's encephalopathy), toxic alcohol ingestions (ethylene glycol, methanol), prescription or illicit drug ingestions (opioids, sedative-hypnotics, antihistamines), neurologic abnormalities (primary generalized seizures, withdrawal seizures), subdural or epidural hematoma, hypovolemic trauma, infection, and sepsis.

Gastritis, peptic ulcer disease, and pancreatitis are comorbidities with symptoms that often require abrupt cessation of alcohol consumption, leading to withdrawal. The gathering of collateral history, thorough serial examinations of the undressed patient, repeated monitoring of vital signs, measurement of oxygen saturation and bedside finger stick for blood glucose, laboratory assessment of metabolic conditions, and imaging as clinically indicated can detect most comorbidities.

ALCOHOL WITHDRAWAL SEIZURES

Alcohol withdrawal seizures are diffuse tonic-clonic seizures. According to the landmark observations by Victor and Brausch,[11] alcohol withdrawal seizures occur as early as 6 hours after the decrease in intake or the last drink, and 90% occur within 48 hours. Approximately 40% of patients have a single seizure, and 60% have multiple generalized seizures. Victor and Brausch reported that one-third of patients with alcohol withdrawal seizures develop delirium tremens, with the seizures terminating before the development of delirium. An alcohol withdrawal seizure may be brief, with a short or no postictal period.[10] The diagnosis of alcohol withdrawal seizures requires the exclusion of traumatic brain injury, hypoxia, hypoglycemia, structural lesions, infections, use of illicit drugs, idiopathic epilepsy, withdrawal from other recreational drugs, and withdrawal from prescription medications. Focal seizures suggest a focal cerebral lesion. Also consider noncompliance with antiseizure medications (in those with idiopathic or posttraumatic seizures).[12]

ALCOHOL WITHDRAWAL HALLUCINATIONS (ALCOHOL-INDUCED PSYCHOTIC DISORDER)

Alcohol-induced withdrawal hallucinations or alcohol-induced psychotic disorder may develop as an isolated finding 12 to 48 hours after decreasing or abstaining from alcohol. Auditory hallucinations predominate over visual and tactile hallucinations. Psychosis, paranoia, and agitation may last from days to weeks. Alcohol-induced psychotic disorder has a high risk for suicide and co-occurs with other psychiatric diagnoses. Patients with hallucinations lasting for >6 months have the worst prognosis; however, the prognosis is more favorable if abstinence can be maintained.[13]

ALCOHOL WITHDRAWAL DELIRIUM TREMENS

Alcohol withdrawal delirium tremens is characterized by acute and fluctuating disturbances in consciousness, confusion, psychomotor agitation, inattention and impairment in cognitive and perceptual function (hallucinations) unrelated to preexisting or established dementia.[8-10] Patients often develop life-threatening fluid, metabolic, and electrolyte imbalances. Among the risk factors associated with alcohol withdrawal delirium are past withdrawal seizure and delirium, severe dependence and prior detoxification history, high and long duration of alcohol intake, older age, use of other drugs, genetic polymorphism, and comorbidity.[8-10]

TREATMENT OF ALCOHOL WITHDRAWAL SYNDROMES

The goals of therapy for alcohol withdrawal are to alleviate autonomic hyperactivity and agitation, halt progression to delirium tremens, and if possible, provide motivation for and access to detoxification to promote long-term abstinence.[5,8-10] General therapy is the substitution of a benzodiazepine for alcohol (**Table 292-1**).[5,8-10] **Benzodiazepine equivalents are lorazepam 1 milligram = midazolam 2 milligrams = diazepam 5 milligrams = chlordiazepoxide 25 milligrams.** Oral diazepam has a rapid onset of action, and the onset of action of IV diazepam is almost immediate. IM diazepam absorption is erratic, so do not give it IM. Duration of action of diazepam is 20 to 50 hours, and metabolism is hepatic, with the major metabolite (desmethyldiazepam) having a half-life of 20 to 50 hours. Chlordiazepoxide is only available as an oral medication, has a long half-life of up to 28 hours, and has extensive hepatic metabolism with its major active long-acting metabolite, desmethyldiazepam. Lorazepam can be given PO, IM, or IV. Onset of action when given IV is within minutes, and duration of action is 8 hours.

TABLE 292-1 Treatment of Alcohol Withdrawal Syndromes

Condition	Treatment
Uncomplicated alcohol withdrawal (no seizures, no hallucinations, no delirium)	Lorazepam 2 milligrams PO *or* Diazepam 10–20 milligrams PO (hepatic metabolism with long-acting metabolite) *or* Chlordiazepoxide 50–100 milligrams PO (hepatic metabolism with long-acting metabolite) to maximum of 300 milligrams/day *or if vomiting* Diazepam 5–10 milligrams IV every 2–4 h *or* Lorazepam 1–2 milligrams IV every 1–2 h *and* Ondansetron 4 milligrams IV
Alcohol withdrawal seizures	Lorazepam 2 milligrams IV
Alcohol-induced psychotic disorder	Abstinence from alcohol Antipsychotics until symptoms remit
Alcohol withdrawal delirium tremens	Lorazepam 1–4 milligrams IV every 5–15 min PRN[9] *or* Midazolam 0.02–0.1 milligram/kg/h[14] *or* Diazepam 5 milligrams IV, @ 2.5 milligrams/min; repeat in 5–10 min, then 10 milligrams for third and fourth dose; 20 milligrams for fifth and subsequent doses until light somnolence, then 5–20 milligrams every hour PRN[9] *or if refractory to benzodiazepines* Phenobarbital 65 milligrams IV every 15–30 min to maximum 260 milligrams[10] (respiratory depression more common than with benzodiazepines, typically requires intubation) *or if refractory to benzodiazepines* Propofol 5 micrograms/kg/min (or 0.3 milligram/kg/h) titrated to effect; typically requires intubation (unlabeled use, primarily case reports of effectiveness)[10] Haloperidol 0.5–5.0 milligrams IV or IM every 30–60 min for severe agitation[9]

Lorazepam is metabolized rapidly by the liver with inactive metabolites excreted by the kidneys and recognized as the benzodiazepine most tolerated by patients with advanced liver disease.[8-10] Midazolam can be given IV or IM, but for delirium tremens, it is typically given IV. IV onset of action is 3 to 5 minutes.

Give individualized symptom-triggered therapy rather than fixed-schedule dosing. Symptom-triggered regimens result in less drug and shorter duration of treatment than fixed-drug dosing.[15] The Clinical Institute Withdrawal Assessment for Alcohol–Revised (CIWA) is the most commonly used validated, structured instrument for guiding continuing treatment once a diagnosis of alcohol withdrawal is established.[16] It has not been validated specifically for ED use, and comorbid conditions and medications make it difficult to score the Clinical Institute Withdrawal Assessment accurately. The CIWA score ranges from 0 to 67 and tracks 10 variables, with a 0 to 7 ranking for nine variables and a 0 to 4 ranking for the last variable (orientation and clouding of sensorium), where 0 is none and 7 (or 4) is the most severe manifestation of the variable. The variables are nausea/vomiting; tremor; paroxysmal sweats; anxiety; agitation; tactile disturbance; auditory disturbance; visual disturbance; headache; and orientation and clouding of sensorium (0 to 4 rank). A score <8 represents mild withdrawal; score of 9 to 15 moderate withdrawal, and score >15 severe withdrawal.[17]

Drug Therapy for Uncomplicated Alcohol Withdrawal For patients meeting criteria for uncomplicated alcohol withdrawal without seizures, hallucination, or delirium, the recommended first-line treatment is a benzodiazepine (**Table 292-1**).[8-10] Because no specific benzodiazepine is more effective than the others, physician choice, institutional availability, cost, and patient factors are taken into consideration.[10]

Drug Therapy for Alcohol Withdrawal Seizures Benzodiazepines are effective in protecting against seizures and reducing recurrent seizures in alcohol withdrawal.[18,19] A prospective randomized ED trial demonstrated a 3% seizure recurrence rate with a single dose of IV lorazepam, 2 milligrams, compared with 24% among patients receiving placebo.[20] Phenytoin is not recommended for prevention of further alcohol-related seizures and should not be used unless the patient has an underlying structural lesion. Repeated loading of phenytoin may, in fact, lower the seizure threshold.[20,21]

Drug Therapy for Alcohol Withdrawal Hallucinosis (Alcohol-Induced Psychotic Disorder) Antipsychotic therapy with alcohol abstinence is the recommended treatment. There is no long-term need for antipsychotic medication for abstinent patients once symptoms remit. Because patients with alcohol-induced psychotic disorder could be at risk for suicide, admission is recommended.[13]

Drug Therapy for Alcohol Withdrawal Delirium Alcohol withdrawal delirium develops within 3 to 5 days of the last drink and generally lasts 48 to 72 hours, but may last longer. The current practice guideline published by the American Society of Addiction Medicine recommends the use of sedative-hypnotics in high enough doses to quickly control agitation, minimize adverse events, and achieve light somnolence with arousal when stimulated.[9] A benzodiazepine is the initial treatment of choice (**Table 292-1**). If symptoms are unresponsive to adequate doses of benzodiazepines, additional agents include phenobarbital, propofol, or haloperidol.[22-24] Phenobarbital or propofol typically requires intubation. Propofol's central nervous system mechanism of action is thought to be similar to that of ethanol. Adverse effects of propofol include hypotension, and prolonged use >48 h and >5 milligrams/kg/h can cause propofol infusion syndrome,[25,26] with dysrhythmias, heart failure, hyperkalemia, lipemia, metabolic acidosis, and rhabdomyolysis. Antipsychotics such as haloperidol, droperidol, or ziprasidone should be reserved for psychosis or continued agitation (see chapter 287, "Acute Agitation") only after adequate benzodiazepines are administered.

Patients with delirium require thorough diagnostic assessment, aggressive treatment of co-occurring illnesses, supportive care, prevention of aspiration, and treatment of hyperthermia, dehydration, hypoglycemia, and electrolyte imbalance. Thiamine, 100 milligrams, and folate, 1 milligram, should be considered. Treat hypomagnesemia with IV magnesium. A benefit from magnesium therapy in the absence of hypomagnesemia is not established.[27] Physical restraints may be temporarily needed until chemical restraint is achieved; a quiet, calm, supportive environment with low stimuli contributes to successful management.[8-10]

DISPOSITION

Patients with mild or moderate uncomplicated alcohol withdrawal that responds well to initial ED treatment, without trauma or major medical comorbidities, with no suicidal or homicidal ideation, and without a seizure disorder can be managed successfully in a detoxification unit or discharged to a supportive family with referral to an outpatient program. Indications for admission include advanced age, mild or moderate withdrawal that does not respond well to ED treatment, the presence of active medical comorbidities, a prior history of delirium tremens, and alcohol withdrawal seizures. Consider intensive care unit admission for moderate withdrawal with comorbid conditions or severe withdrawal in which sedative requirements necessitate intubation or close monitoring to prevent respiratory compromise.

OPIOID WITHDRAWAL

Symptoms of opioid withdrawal include dilated pupils and tearing, sneezing and running nose, nausea, vomiting, diarrhea and abdominal cramps, yawning, piloerection (goose bumps), and myalgias. **Heroin** or short-acting opioid withdrawal symptoms appear within 36 to 72 hours after decreasing or stopping the agent and may last for 7 to 10 days.[8] Of the opioids, **withdrawal symptoms are most severe with heroin but most prolonged with methadone.**[9] Oxycodone or crushed and injected OxyContin® withdrawal resembles heroin in this regard. **OxyContin® (long-acting oxycodone) and buprenorphine are intermediate-acting opioids, and peak withdrawal symptoms occur in a time frame between heroin and methadone.** Methadone is used for pain control and also to transition patients from other narcotics as medication-assisted treatment for opioid addiction. Methadone has been associated with QT prolongation on the ECG and possibly torsade de pointes, so review the ECG prior to initiating the medication.[28,29] However, methadone withdrawal symptoms can be protracted, because methadone is firmly bound to tissue protein and there is slow release over time from tissue-binding sites. Methadone withdrawal symptoms appear at 72 to 96 hours and may last for 2 weeks or more. For methadone cessation, typically 10% of the maintenance dose is reduced every 2 weeks.

Buprenorphine is a partial opioid agonist and a weak antagonist. It has a high affinity for μ-receptors, displacing other opioids from the receptor, causing acute withdrawal in patients who have recently used opioids. The antagonist effects of buprenorphine block respiratory depression and provide a good margin of safety to treat withdrawal or to provide opioid substitution therapy. The U.S. Food and Drug Administration approved two sublingual formulations of buprenorphine in 2002 for the treatment of opioid dependence. The preferred preparation is a combination of buprenorphine combined with naloxone in a ratio of 4:1, as a sublingual tablet or film (brand name Suboxone® or Zubsolv®) to prevent diversion and overdoses.[30,31] The naloxone component is rapidly bioavailable and will precipitate withdrawal symptoms in opioid users. Overdoses can be managed with naloxone.[30]

OPIOID WITHDRAWAL TREATMENT

There are few options for treating opioid withdrawal. Clonidine in doses of 0.2 milligram three times a day can reduce autonomic symptoms to some degree, but it is not very effective with other symptoms. Patients who stop clonidine abruptly may develop severe rebound hypertension. Symptomatic relief of anxiety and muscle spasms can be achieved with muscle relaxants or benzodiazepines, and GI symptoms can be managed with antispasmodics, antiemetics, and antidiarrheals.[8]

Buprenorphine/naloxone can be used to treat mild withdrawal, but when symptoms are moderate or severe, the high affinity of the drug for the μ-receptor will displace the other opioid and precipitate severe withdrawal. It can be given approximately 12 hours after short-acting opioid use, 24 hours after long-acting opioid use, and up to 48 to 96 hours after high-dose methadone use (30 to 60 milligrams/d). Patient on methadone ideally should be tapered to <30 milligrams/d, and at this low dose, patients can be transitioned to buprenorphine/naloxone in 24 hours.

The starting dose for treatment of opioid withdrawal is sublingual buprenorphine/naloxone, 4 to 8 milligrams buprenorphine/2 milligrams naloxone, with a first-day maximum of 8 milligrams.[32] In an outpatient setting, the dose is titrated to control symptoms, usually 16 to 32 milligrams/d. Buprenorphine withdrawal is slower in onset and milder than withdrawal from opioids.[31] Patients taking buprenorphine who develop conditions associated with severe pain, may require large doses of potent opioids such as fentanyl to override buprenorphine's antagonist properties, with close observation for respiratory depression.

OPIOID ADDICTION MANAGEMENT

The Drug Addiction Treatment Act of 2000 established office-based opioid treatment in an effort to integrate treatment options into comprehensive clinical care practice and reduce stigmatization of medication-assisted treatment. The prescription of methadone for treatment of addiction is limited by the Federal Narcotics Act to inpatient units or outpatient facilities licensed by the U.S. Drug Enforcement Administration, and buprenorphine is limited to certified clinicians in office- or clinic-based practices. However, there is a "3-day rule" (Title 21, Code of Federal Regulations, Part 1306.07b) that allows a practitioner who is not separately registered as a narcotic treatment program or certified as a "waivered Drug Addiction Treatment Act of 2000" physician to administer (but not prescribe) narcotic drugs to a patient to relieve acute withdrawal symptoms while arranging for referral to treatment (http://www.buprenorphine.samhsa.gov/faq.html). Only one day's supply may be administered or given to a patient, and this may be done for 72 hours only, which cannot be extended. The intent of Title 21, Code of Federal Regulations, Part 1306.07b is to provide flexibility in emergency situations and is especially relevant to emergency physicians. This offers patients options for relief of withdrawal symptoms to bridge the patient for follow-up to either a specialized treatment program or an office-based physician program in the community.

The rise in opioid overdose hospitalizations and deaths has contributed to the White House Office of National Drug Control Policy[33] partnering with the Substance Abuse and Mental Health Services Administration and Centers for Disease Control and Prevention to address the epidemic. The four pillars of their national strategy are to (1) educate prescribers about opioid painkiller prescribing[34]; (2) expand prescription drug monitoring programs and promote links among state systems and to electronic health records[35]; (3) increase prescription return/take-back and disposal programs; and (4) assist states to address doctor shopping and pill mills via law enforcement. Additional national strategies include reducing social stigma and expanding access to medication-assisted treatment,[33,36] and implementing innovative policies to increase availability of naloxone to first responders and the lay public together with ED and community-based programs to train the public in overdose prevention education, calling 911, rescue breathing, and the proper use of bystander naloxone.[33,37,38]

BENZODIAZEPINE WITHDRAWAL

Symptoms of withdrawal may develop up to 7 to 10 days after stopping chronic benzodiazepine use. Patients may develop withdrawal seizures. The clinical picture resembles alcohol withdrawal with symptoms of hypertension, tachycardia and tachypnea, tremulousness, anxiety, agoraphobia, insomnia, altered mental status, delirium, and hallucinations. Mild withdrawal can be managed by a gradual taper over 10 weeks of the benzodiazepine that has been abused.[39]

COCAINE AND OTHER STIMULANT WITHDRAWAL

Stimulant withdrawal can produce symptoms often associated with depression such as disturbances in sleep, appetite, and mood. The duration is from 8 to 48 hours. Co-occurring opioid and sedative dependency may complicate withdrawal. There is no effective evidence-supported treatment currently available for cocaine and stimulant withdrawal.

MARIJUANA/CANNABIS WITHDRAWAL

Marijuana dependence has been associated with low energy, sleep and memory disturbances, deterioration in job and family function, and financial difficulties, but dependence is less likely than for other drugs. Marijuana withdrawal begins after 24 to 48 hours, usually lasts for 1 to 3 weeks after abstinence, and peaks within 4 to 6 days. Among the symptoms associated with withdrawal are difficulty sleeping, cravings, mood swings, depression and irritability, and decreased appetite. Withdrawal symptoms are considerably less severe than for heroin or alcohol, but nevertheless, like other drugs, withdrawal symptoms can interfere with efforts to quit or seriously cut back on use.[40]

ED SCREENING, BRIEF INTERVENTION, AND REFERRAL TO TREATMENT

Alcohol Screening in the ED (Revised and approved by the American College of Emergency Physicians [ACEP] Board of Directors April 2011)

ACEP believes alcohol abuse is a significant public health problem. Further, ACEP believes emergency medical professionals are positioned and qualified to mitigate the consequences of alcohol abuse through screening programs, brief intervention, and referral to treatment. ACEP encourages wide availability of resources necessary to address the needs of patients with alcohol-related problems and those at risk for them

Screening, brief intervention, and referral to treatment were established in 2003 by the U.S. Substance Abuse and Mental Health Services Administration to address the gap in preventive services for unhealthy alcohol and drug use, to stem the progression to addiction by early intervention, and to address the treatment gap by promoting help seeking and facilitating access to addiction treatment and recovery support services. Screening, brief intervention, and referral to treatment in the ED setting may have short-term benefits.[41-49]

SCREENING FOR UNHEALTHY DRINKING AND DRUG USE

Brief standardized screening questions have a higher sensitivity for identifying heavy and dependent drinkers and illicit drug–using patients than smell of alcohol on breath, patient self-report, or profiling based on demographics or presenting complaint. Brief screening instruments are easy to administer and may help match an individual to the most appropriate treatment resource. Validated brief screening questions useful for ED providers include the National Institute on Alcohol Abuse and Alcoholism Quantity/Frequency/Questions[6] and the Single Screening Questions for Alcohol[50] and Drug Use (**Table 292-2**).[51] Questions can be integrated into the triage electronic medical record.[52] Screening for heavy smoking is also important since there is an association between heavy smoking and poly drug use.[52]

As part of the social history, physicians can integrate questions that reflect their concern for the patient's overall health and safety. Substance use disorder screening questions could be embedded among other preventive health

TABLE 292-2 Single Screening Questions

"Would it be okay with you if I ask you some very personal questions that I ask all my patients to improve the care I give? You do not have to answer them if you are uncomfortable."

1. Single Screening Question for Alcohol: "Do you drink beer, wine, liquor, or distilled spirits? How many times in the past year have you had 5 or more (for men)/4 or more (for women) drinks in a day?"[6,50] Clarify that a standard drink is 1.5 oz of spirits, 6 oz of wine, and 12 oz of beer.[6]
2. Single Screening Question for Drug Use: "How many times in the past year have you used an illegal drug or used a prescription medication for nonmedical reasons?" You can add something like ". . . for instance, for the experience or feeling it gives you?"[51]

TABLE 292-3 Identifying Substance Abuse Risk

When assessing a prescription drug monitoring program (PDMP) profile, it is important to look at the following factors:

1. From how many providers did the patient receive prescriptions?
   — Patients who used 4 or more prescribers or 4 or more pharmacies in 6 months may have risk of death from overdose.[59,60]
2. Is the patient taking both opioids and benzodiazepines?
   — Patients who use combinations of medications may be at increased risk for overdose.[61]
3. How many morphine milligram equivalents of opioids is the patient taking per day?
   — Patients who take 50 to 100 morphine milligram equivalents per day are at greater risk of overdose death.[62-64]
4. Is the patient taking long-acting/extended-release (LA/ER) opioids?
   — Patients taking LA/ER may be at increased risk for overdose.[65]
5. How often did the patient fill another prescription before the previous one was scheduled to finish?
   — Early refills indicate nonmedical use or noncompliance with treatment plan.[65]
6. Is the patient taking buprenorphine?
   — Patients taking buprenorphine are likely under the care of a pain specialist who should be contacted prior to prescribing a scheduled medication.
7. Is the patient taking psychiatric medications, such as methylphenidate?
   — Psychiatric comorbidities are associated with increased risk of overdose.
8. If reported by the PDMP, how often did the patient self-pay?
   — Patients may pay out of pocket for a prescription without involving an insurer to avoid detection of nonmedical use.

issues to reduce stigma and patient resistance and encourage veracity and trust. Questions asked in a nonjudgmental, matter-of-fact fashion are well accepted by patients.[53]

Patients who are above the "low-risk" drinking guidelines could benefit from a brief intervention and primary care referral to motivate reducing consumption. For moderate to severe alcohol use, provide referral to a specialized treatment center.

The Centers for Disease Control and Prevention recommends screening for illicit drug use or nonmedical use of prescription drugs before writing an opioid prescription.[54] Screening may not detect all patients with an abuse problem. As an additional tool, nearly all states have implemented prescription drug monitoring programs,[55] which track the prescribing and dispensing of controlled substances at the retail pharmacy level. States with prescription drug monitoring programs appear to have lower rates of substance abuse treatment admission and lower rates of increase in abuse/misuse compared to states that do not have them.[56] Prescription drug monitoring program data can change prescribing behavior, because providers do not have a very good sensitivity (63%) or positive predictive value (41%) in determining drug-seeking behavior without the aid of a prescription drug monitoring programs.[57,58] There are still no evidence-based consensus guidelines for identifying possible drug-seeking activity or patients at risk for prescription drug abuse. Prescription drug monitoring programs do not detect medications that are diverted or purchased illegally, report prescriptions filled in another state (unless there is a data-sharing program in place), or identify residents writing prescriptions under a hospital's Drug Enforcement Administration number. Use prescription drug monitoring program data along with history, physical examination, and clinical impression. Do not use prescription drug monitoring program data as a reason to withhold adequate and necessary analgesia. Several factors from prescription drug monitoring program data may suggest concerning substance abuse risk (**Table 292-3**).

THE BRIEF NEGOTIATED INTERVIEW FOR SUBSTANCE USE INTERVENTION

The *brief negotiated interview*[41,43,48,49,66,67] has four key elements: establish rapport, provide feedback, enhance motivation, and negotiate plan of action. The first principle of promoting health behavior change is that the argument for change needs to come from the patient, not the healthcare provider. Begin a respectful, nonjudgmental conversation by recognizing the patient as the decision maker and asking the patient's permission to talk about alcohol or drug use and health concerns. The best time for early intervention may be during a medical, social, or criminal justice crisis.[69] The entire interaction often can be accomplished in 5 to 7 minutes,[66] and the conversation can take place at any point in care, such as at discharge or while suturing or casting or performing an incision and drainage of an abscess.

The brief negotiated interview algorithm incorporates key elements of motivational interviewing: open-ended questions, affirmations, reflective listening, and summaries (**Figure 292-1**) (see SBIRT for drug use).

Establish rapport *and ask the patient's permission to discuss his or her use of alcohol and drugs.* Establish an atmosphere of trust through respect. The patient is not the problem but is a person who has a problem.

Provide feedback. Elicit patient's thoughts on low-risk or safe alcohol and drug use. Provide information by reviewing current drinking and drug use and guidelines. Express concern that by drinking in excess of safe limits, the patient is at risk for injury or illness. Elicit/solicit the reaction to the guidelines. Ask patients to make a connection between alcohol and/or drug use and quality of life; possible negative consequences related to health, family, legal system, and employment; and, if applicable, the current ED visit or injury. If appropriate, discuss physical dependence, withdrawal, and the cycle of behaviors to obtain more alcohol and/or drugs.

Enhance motivation. *Assess readiness to change on a readiness ruler.* Ask patients to mark on a drawing of a ruler, with a scale of 1 to 10, how ready they are to change, cut back, or quit their alcohol and/or drug use. If they say 5, give affirmation and say that "You are 50% on the way," and ask, "Tell me why you didn't mark a 2 or 3, a lesser number?" Here is when we try to elicit change talk/reasons and motivation for change. Repeat what the patient has shared with you and follow up with, "It sounds like you have some important reasons to change, so what small steps can you take to stay healthy and safe?" If the patient shows resistance to the readiness ruler or the score is <2, then *explore the pros and cons of current use. A discussion of the pros and cons* promotes self-questioning and draws attention to the patient's own reasons for tipping the scale toward change. Use open-ended questions such as, "Help me to understand (or see it through your eyes) what you like and dislike about your use of alcohol?" Explore the importance to the patient of the issues that emerge. *Use reflective listening* to summarize what you think the patient said to verify your interpretation, for example: "On the one hand, you like the taste, how it helps you to loosen up and forget your problems, and it is something to do when you're bored. On the other hand, you said you don't like how you feel the next day and that wrecking your car in a crash and ending up in the ED is no fun. You also told me you are spending a lot of money on drinking and are concerned about not meeting some responsibilities. So then, in the balance, where does that leave you?"

Negotiate and advise. Negotiate an action plan. Explore with patients what life might be like if they made these changes. What would be the benefits of change, and what would be the challenges? Add the steps they would need to take to address challenges and explore and support confidence in ability to make a change. *Offer a menu of options and resources* to assist with the change plan, including, if appropriate, referrals to primary care providers and substance use disorder treatment. *Document the plan.* Ask the patient to state in her or his own words the agreed-on steps and document them on a piece of paper or discharge instructions as a reminder of goals (a prescription for change). Reflect back to the patient and reinforce reasons for, and steps toward, change. End the conversation by thanking the patient for being honest and spending time talking with you.

Afterward, take a minute for self-assessment. To what degree did you provide *f*eedback? Did you *l*isten carefully? Did you ask *o*pen-ended questions? Did you offer *a*ffirmations and *a*lternatives? (FLOAT) Did the patient have enough *t*ime to talk, or did you do the majority of talking? Did you negotiate a concrete action plan?

BNI Steps	Dialogue/Procedures
1. Raise subject	Hello, I am _______. Would you mind taking a few minutes to talk with me about your alcohol use? <<PAUSE and LISTEN>>
2. Provide feedback	
• Review screen	From what I understand you are drinking [insert screening data]... We know that drinking above certain levels can cause problems, such as [insert facts]...I am concerned about your drinking.
• Make connection	What connection (if any) do you see between your drinking and this ED visit? *If pt sees connection:* reiterate what pt has said *If pt does not see connection:* make one using facts
• Show NIAAA guidelines and norms	These are what we consider the upper limits of low risk drinking for your age and sex. By low risk we mean that you would be less likely to experience illness or injury if you stayed within these guidelines.
3. Enhance motivation	
• Readiness to change	[Show readiness ruler] On a scale from 1–10, how ready are you to change any aspect of your drinking?
• Develop discrepancy	*If patient says:* ≥2 *ask* Why did you choose that number and not a lower one?
• Explore pros and cons	*<2 or resistance ask pros and cons* Help me to understand what you enjoy about drinking? <<PAUSE AND LISTEN>> Now tell me what you enjoy less about drinking. <<PAUSE AND LISTEN>>
• Use reflective listening	On the one hand you said, <<RESTATE PROS>> On the other hand you said, <<RESTATE CONS>> So tell me, where does this leave you?
4. Negotiate and advise	
• Negotiate goal	What's the next step?
• Give advice	What do you think you can do to stay within the safe drinking guidelines? If you can stay within these limits you will be less likely to experience [further] illness or injury related to alcohol use.
• Summarize	This is what I've heard you say...Here is a drinking agreement I would like you to fill out, reinforcing your new drinking goals. This is really an agreement between you and yourself. Provide drinking agreement [pt keeps 1 copy]
• Provide handouts and suggest PC f/u	Suggest Primary Care f/u to discuss drinking level/pattern
• Thank patient	Thank patient for his/her time

FIGURE 292-1. Screening, brief intervention, and referral to treatment algorithm as taught in the standardized ED curriculum.[43,66] BNI = brief negotiated interview; f/u = follow-up; NIAAA = National Institute on Alcohol Abuse and Alcoholism; PC = primary care; pt = patient. [Reproduced with permission from D'Onofrio G, Pantalon MV, Degutis LC, Fiellin DA, O'connor PG: Development and implementation of an emergency practitioner-performed brief intervention for hazardous and harmful drinkers in the emergency department. *Acad Emerg Med* 12: 249, 2005. Copyright John Wiley & Sons.[43,66,70]]

REFERRALS FOR TREATMENT

Train ED staff in screening, brief intervention, and referral to treatment. Develop an ED collaborative team with staff such as social workers, care managers, psychologists, nurse specialists, peer alcohol and drug counselors, volunteers from Alcoholics Anonymous or Narcotics Anonymous, or health promotion advocates to enhance the efforts of existing staff and motivate and assist patients with identifying and accessing treatment options.[45,67,68]

Build and maintain a referral/resource service network.[45,67,68] Current practice in most EDs is to provide patient and family members with a list of detoxification or treatment resources in the community (see "Useful Web Resources" below). The Center for Substance Abuse Treatment at the U.S. Department of Health and Human Services also has an online resource locator (http://dasis3.samhsa.gov). The resource list includes specialized treatment facilities for patients with co-occurring medical, traumatic, and psychiatric illnesses; inpatient and outpatient detoxification, acupuncture, and medication-assisted treatment such as methadone maintenance programs, buprenorphine, and naltrexone for opioid and alcohol addiction; outpatient individual and group counseling; intensive outpatient or partial hospitalization; recovery residents; residential communities; Alcoholics and Narcotics Anonymous meetings; and programs focused on the needs of women, culture-specific programs, and programs designed for gay, lesbian, and transgender clients.

If patients are not ready to enter specialized treatment or attend Alcoholics Anonymous or Narcotics Anonymous, then try to provide information and negotiate a safety plan such as the identification of a designated driver or use of a taxicab when drinking heavily, or avoiding drinking while taking medications. The injecting drug user who is not ready to accept a treatment referral may accept a referral to a syringe exchange program or overdose education, a nasal naloxone rescue kit program, or a prescription for naloxone.

THE MEDICAL CLEARANCE EXAMINATION

EDs often function as sources for the medical clearance examination before patient transfer to a substance or psychiatric treatment facility. There is considerable variability in the levels of medical care provided in such facilities, ranging from facilities that manage an array of chronic health problems to those with minimal nursing support only for very stable patients. Medical clearance does not mean that the patient has no medical problems, but it does mean that "within reasonable medical certainty there is no medical emergency."[71] Criteria include the following: patients are stable for transfer (in the short term rather than long term), are ambulatory, can take oral medications, and are not suicidal or likely to seize. Patients on medications should bring them to the treatment facility or be given prescriptions or provided with several doses. Psychiatrically stable patients with dual diagnoses who are not suicidal or acutely psychotic can be medically cleared for transfer, as long as they have a supply of necessary nonpsychiatric medications and can be expected to be reliable in taking their medications correctly.

REFERENCES

The complete reference list is available online at www.TintinalliEM.com.

CHAPTER 293 Female and Male Sexual Assault

Lisa Moreno-Walton

INTRODUCTION AND EPIDEMIOLOGY

Sexual assault is a crime of violence, intended to dominate and humiliate the victim through the use of intimidation and fear.[1] In many parts of the world, sexual assault is a tool for oppression, a weapon of war, and an act of genocide. Psychological trauma is a universal consequence of rape and sexual assault, but the absence of physical injury does not indicate that an assault did not take place. Sexual assault remains a major public health problem throughout the world, with case rates of police-recorded incidents as high as 92.9 per 100,000 in Botswana to a first time record of 0.0 in Liechtenstein in 2010.[2] In the United States, the case rate is 27.3 per 100,000,[2] with nearly one in five (18.3%) women reporting being raped at some time during their lives.[3]

Although males are less commonly victimized, studies estimate that between 0.6% and 22.2% of males have experienced sexual assaults.[4-6] According to the National Electronic Injury Surveillance System (NEISS), sexual assaults accounted for over 150,000 ED visits in 2001 in the United States.[7] However, many sexual assault survivors do not report the assault to police or seek medical care.[8] Women are likely to seek treatment earlier for more severe assaults and injuries, and they are more likely to delay seeking assistance if assaulted by a known perpetrator.[8]

In most cases of rape in the United States, a single assailant is involved, and most often the perpetrator is known to the victim.[9] Force or coercion is used in most assaults, but a weapon is reported in only 11% of cases.[3]

About half of female[10] and male[11] assault survivors have genital or rectal trauma on examination, and about two thirds have some evidence of bruising elsewhere.[10] Injuries are more often found in female patients <20 years old or >49 years old, those who have experienced anal assault, and those who present within 24 hours of assault. Survivors age 12 to 17 years were more likely to have anogenital injuries than those age 18 to 49 years.[12]

HEALTHCARE RESPONSIBILITIES

Care of the sexual assault victim is complex and can be time-consuming. Responsibilities include obtaining the medical and forensic history; performing and documenting results of the medical examination; collecting forensic evidence and ensuring that material follows the proper chain of custody; treating potential sexually transmitted infections; treating other acute medical problems and injuries; assessing pregnancy risk and providing treatment options; providing referral for crisis intervention and medical follow-up; coordinating care with sexual assault advocates; and testifying in court if needed.[13] Although some hospitals provide **sexual assault nurse examiners** (see below) to aid in medical and forensic evaluation, in many institutions, emergency physicians will be expected to provide most of the care for sexual assault victims.

Sexual assault nurse examiners (SANEs) provide expert assistance for sexual assault evaluation. SANEs are certified by examination through the Commission for Forensic Nursing Certification. Requirements before examination include an unrestricted RN license, 2 years of nursing experience, 40 hours of coursework, and competency in supervised sexual assault examination.[14] Physicians, physician assistants, and nurses can also complete a separate course of training and receive certification as a **sexual assault forensic examiner (SAFE)**. The Department of Justice established national training standards for SAFEs in 2006.[15] Individuals, most often physicians and physician assistants, who complete the proscribed training and pass a standardized exam receive certification as a SAFE. There is little difference between SANE and SAFE training, but only registered nurses are eligible to train as SANEs, and the Commission for Forensic Nursing maintains authority over the certification of SANEs.

Because SAFEs and SANEs are specially trained to perform the precise and sensitive history, physical, and forensic examination, and preserve evidence in a chain of custody, many U.S. hospitals have designated these individuals as part of **sexual assault treatment teams (SARTs)**. Local EMS personnel can transport survivors of sexual assault to SARTs as a matter of protocol.

CULTURAL DIFFERENCES AND MINORITIES

Appropriate cultural competency skills often set the tone for the first steps toward healing. Some cultures consider rape a punishment or a consequence of aberrant sexual behavior.[16] Societies characterized by gender-based power disparities are often less likely to define sexual coercion and threats of violence as rape. Women from such cultures often present for care with other chief complaints or will give inconsistent histories if they feel they are culpable or could have offered more resistance.[17] In countries with a history of slavery, indentured servitude, human property laws, and rigid caste or class systems, policies, traditions, and biases affect the treatment and adjudication of sexual assault. Survivors may be reluctant to report victimization if they fear a biased criminal justice system, do not think police will help, or anticipate being blamed by their family or community.[9,18,19]

Fear of deportation may impact the decision of illegal aliens regarding evidence collection, police reporting, and testifying in court. Before encouraging patients to make a police report, learn your state's laws about illegal aliens who are crime victims.

Women of color face more challenges than white women obtaining assistance after rape. Services for victims of diverse backgrounds are limited, and minority victims are often reluctant to contact rape crisis centers.[9] Although most large cities have good referral services and resources for providers, smaller communities may not have support services for minority and ethnically diverse patients. For black women survivors of sexual assault, poverty is a positive predictor of increased life-long risk of depression and posttraumatic stress disorder.[9,20,21] **The Substance Abuse and Mental Health Services Administration National Council for Trauma-Informed Care** provides excellent resources for institutions, providers, and patients,[22] especially for referrals for continuing care.

THE SEXUAL ASSAULT EVALUATION

TRIAGE

Triage sexual assault patients as a high priority, in accordance with Department of Justice recommendations.[13] Notify the SAFE or SANE on call, and place the patient in a private room, ideally one reserved for the care of sexual assault victims. If a SAFE or SANE examiner is not in-house or if the hospital does not have a SART program, the triage nurse should notify the emergency physician of the patient's presence in the department. Make sure the patient does not undress or change into a hospital gown, as all clothing must be properly removed and stored for forensic evaluation. Tell the patient not to wash, drink, or rinse the mouth. Provide appropriate medical care whether or not patients agree to evidence collection, police reporting, or assisting with criminal prosecution.

TABLE 293-2 Medical History

Last menstrual period? Birth control method?
Last consensual intercourse?
If the patient has had consensual intercourse within the last 3 to 4 days, it may confuse laboratory analysis for sperm and acid phosphatase and genetic typing.
Allergies, medication history, and possible pregnancy?

HISTORY

Begin the interview with introductions, express regret about the assault, and provide reassurance that medical and psychological needs will be addressed. Maintain a professional, caring attitude. A patient's response is affected by the physician's attitude. A physician's shock or outrage may increase the patient's concern about physical injuries or cause her to feel marginalized. Questions perceived as critical or judgmental result in feelings of guilt and shame and interfere with the survivor's ability to provide a thorough history. Calm reassurance will facilitate the history, examination, and collection of evidence.

Ask open-ended questions about sexual history. For some women, sexual assault is the first sexual encounter, and for some lesbian patients, it may be the first sexual encounter with a male.

Obtain a thorough past medical history and general assault description, and ask the patient about injuries. In some instances, the triage nurse will have obtained the past medical history. In EDs with SANE services, a detailed assault history, to help guide the evidentiary examination, will be obtained by the SANE. If there are no SANE services, but a sexual assault advocate, police representative, or social worker is available, have those individuals in the room during the history taking so that the patient does not have to repeat information.

Details to gather about the assault and medical history are listed in **Tables 293-1 and 293-2**. Most authorities caution that the chances of finding forensic evidence >72 hours after the assault are slim, so **a forensic examination is not necessary if >72 hours have elapsed since the assault, unless the specific state allows evidence collection up to 96 hours after the assault**. Verify the policy in your state well in advance of the need to know.

TABLE 293-1 Assault History

Who?
Did the assault survivor know the assailant?
Was it a single assailant or multiple assailants?
Can the survivor recall any identifying features of the assailant (height, build, age, race, tattoos, scars, birthmarks, etc.)? (Document in the medical records.)
What happened?
Was the patient physically assaulted?
With what (e.g., gun, bat, or fist) and to what part of the body?
Was there actual or attempted vaginal, anal, or oral penetration?
Did ejaculation occur? If so, where?
Was a foreign object used?
Was a condom used?
When?
When did the assault occur?
(Emergency contraception is most effective when started within 72 h of the assault.)
Where?
Where did the assault occur?
(Corroborating evidence may be found based on the location of the assault.)
Suspicion of drug-facilitated rape?
Was there a period of amnesia?
Is there a history of being out drinking and then suddenly feeling very intoxicated?
Is there a history of waking up naked or with genital soreness?
Douche, shower, or change of clothing?
Did the patient douche, shower, or change clothing after the assault? (Performing any of these activities prior to seeking medical attention may decrease the probability of sperm or acid phosphatase recovery, as well as recovery of other bits of trace evidence.)

CONSENT FOR FORENSIC EXAMINATION

Have the patient sign the consent form for the forensic examination, collection of evidence, photography, and transfer of evidence to law enforcement authorities. Most hospitals have a prepackaged rape kit with equipment and directions. However, check with the police if you are unsure about the utility of your hospital's kit, because some police departments may require use of a specific kit for their precincts. Hospitals will usually allow the storage of a rape kit for a specified period of time while the patient decides whether or not she wishes to make a police report. In such a case, encourage the patient to consent to the forensic exam. **Not every part of the forensic evidence kit needs to be used every time. Tailor the collection of evidence to the specifics of the assault.**

If >72 hours (or 96 hours, according to your hospital's policy) have elapsed or the patient does not want an evidentiary examination, still perform a full history and physical examination, provide pregnancy and sexually transmitted disease prophylaxis, and refer for follow-up medical care and rape crisis counseling.

PHYSICAL EXAMINATION

General Examination Record general information such as vital sign values and alertness and orientation. After clothing is properly removed and stored, perform a head-to-toe inspection, and look for injuries. Focus on defensive injury areas such as the extremities, and carefully check potential areas of injury such as the oral cavity, strangulation signs at the neck, breasts, thighs, and buttocks. Describe all injuries, and record all areas of tenderness, even if there is no outward sign of injury. Injuries, predominantly bruises, are often located on limbs (32%), face (23%), and torso (7%), with most assault survivors sustaining light (44%) or moderate (18%) injuries.[23] Other nongenital injuries include abrasions (40%), lacerations (4%), and bites and burns (1%).[10]

FORENSIC EXAMINATION

The forensic examination includes collection of head and pubic hair and buccal swabs for DNA comparison, photographs of injuries, and vaginal and perineal examination, often with colposcopy. Tell the patient what the examiner is doing at each stage of the process. Tell the patient she can take a break at any point during the examination.

Assemble all of the needed equipment for forensic examination. Throughout the examination, keep the patient's body covered as much as possible. Have several pairs of gloves available for different parts of the examination—change gloves between the physical and the genital exam, and again between the genital and the anal exam. A detailed list of equipment and a demonstration of the examination and evidence collection is available. Take photographs of abrasions, bruises, contusions, lacerations, bite marks, burns, areas of erythema, hematomas, incisions, petechiae, and swelling. Document location, position of patient, and position of injury, using a clock face reference. Traditionally, when the patient is in lithotomy position, the pubic bone is at 12 o'clock, the left hip is at 3 o'clock, and the right hip is at 9 o'clock. Begin the photographic series with a photograph of the patient's face and end with a photograph of the patient's hospital wrist band. If photography is not available, describe signs of trauma and areas of tenderness in detail using a body map.

Begin the genital exam with combing of the pubic hair and extraction of hair samples. Patients can pluck their own hair, but make sure that the hair root is included. Examine the genital and rectal areas for injuries and signs of trauma. Note any vaginal discharge, vaginal abrasions, cervical abrasions, and cervical lacerations. In some institutions, a topical application of **toluidine blue dye** is used to highlight microtrauma. Toluidine is a dye with affinity for DNA and RNA.[24] When placed on an area where the topical nonnuclear layer has been removed (as by abrading by injury), toluidine dye will be taken up by underlying cellular tissue. It is typically mixed for use by the hospital pharmacy. Toluidine is applied to the external vulva, especially the posterior fourchette, but not onto mucous membranes. If toluidine dye is used, do not perform a speculum examination until after the toluidine dye examination is completed, because the speculum examination itself may induce small abrasions that can be confused with injuries from the assault.[25] After examination, remove excess dye with a water-soluble lubricant. If the solution is not used soon after it is mixed, cover the bottle with aluminum foil, store at 4°C (39.2°F), and bring to room temperature before use.[26] An alternative to bottles of toluidine blue dye is the commercially available **Forensic Blue Swabs®**.

Colposcopy detects injuries not visible to the naked eye.[11] In one study, only 34% of genital lesions were seen with the naked eye, 49% were seen with a colonoscopy, and 52% were seen with toluidine blue dye.[25] If the colposcope is used to photograph injuries, document magnification. If the patient reports anal penetration, examine the anus and rectum for abrasions or lacerations.

Finally, darken the room and scan the entire body surface with a **Woods lamp** to detect traces of semen. Swab areas where the perpetrator made any oral contact, and swab areas that illuminate with the Woods lamp. Dry and label all swabs and add to the rape kit.

After all evidence is collected, make sure to maintain chain of custody. Do not leave the kit unattended. Each party that releases and accepts the evidence kit must sign, date, and time the chain of evidence form. If the police are not present to receive the evidence, store the kit in a locked cabinet specifically designated for this purpose. Many rape kits contain elements which require refrigeration. In this case, when police are not available to accept the kit, store the entire kit in a locked refrigerator only used to store rape kits.

LABORATORY TESTING

Obtain ancillary tests as clinically indicated. If there is high suspicion of **drug-facilitated rape**, a urine sample can be sent to a laboratory for toxicologic testing. Drugs that are typically thought of as "date rape" drugs, such as ketamine, Rohypnol, and gamma hydroxybutyric acid (GHB), are not detected on routine ED toxicology screening tests, and special "send out" tests must be ordered. Rohypnol can be detected in the urine for up to 72 hours, and GHB can be detected for 12 hours. Results, however, are not available for days.[27] Most SANEs typically send these tests when indicated and assume responsibility for checking the results. In some hospitals with SART programs, consent forms give the right to the prosecuting attorney in the Special Victims Unit to receive the results. If these "send out" tests are ordered by the ED physician, develop a protocol for checking results and documenting results in the patient's record. Guidance for appropriate ordering can be obtained from womenshealth.gov or by calling 800-994-9662.

Obtain a urine or serum pregnancy test before giving emergency contraception. Testing for gonorrhea, chlamydia, and bacterial vaginosis is not necessary, because treatment is provided at the ED encounter. However, **do test for syphilis, hepatitis B and C, and human immunodeficiency virus (HIV)**. Obtain serum chemistry, liver function studies, and CBC for patients who will receive HIV postexposure prophylaxis (PEP).[28] Follow baseline HIV testing with repeat testing at 6 weeks and 3 and 6 months.

TREATMENT

Follow standard care protocols and also individually assess the needs of the survivor.[29,30] Treat physical injuries and provide immediate crisis intervention if needed. Offer emergency contraception, sexually transmitted disease prophylaxis, tetanus and hepatitis B vaccination if needed, and prophylaxis against HIV infection (**Table 293-3**).[28]

TABLE 293-3 Centers for Disease Control and Prevention Guidelines for Postassault Prophylaxis

Postexposure hepatitis B vaccination, if not previously vaccinated. Subsequent doses at 1–2 months and 4–6 months after first dose[28]; no hepatitis B immune globulin
Empiric antibiotics for chlamydia, gonorrhea, and trichomoniasis (see Table 4)
Tetanus prophylaxis if needed
Offer emergency contraception if the assault could result in pregnancy[28]
Baseline testing for syphilis, hepatitis C, and HIV
Obtain serum chemistries and liver function studies if HIV postexposure prophylaxis given

SEXUALLY TRANSMITTED INFECTION PROPHYLAXIS

The prevalence of sexually transmitted infections in an adolescent urban population varies as follows by causative organism: *Neisseria gonorrhoeae*, 0.0% to 26.3%; *Chlamydia trachomatis*, 3.9% to 17%; *Treponema pallidum*, 0.0% to 5.6%; *Trichomonas vaginalis*, 0.0% to 19.0%; and human papillomavirus, 0.6% to 2.3%.[31] The regimens currently recommended by the Centers for Disease Control and Prevention are provided in **Table 293-4**.

EMERGENCY CONTRACEPTION

Obtain a pregnancy test on all women unless there is a history of hysterectomy. Offer pregnancy prevention to those who are not pregnant.[32-37] Also prescribe an antiemetic for nausea and vomiting.[36,37] Offer meclizine 50 milligrams, metoclopramide 10 milligrams, or ondansetron 4 milligrams.[37] **Three common emergency contraceptive regimens are listed in Table 293-5.** A fourth method of emergency contraception recommended by the Centers for Disease Control and Prevention but not commonly used after sexual assault or in the ED is the insertion of a copper intrauterine device. Provide emergency contraception as soon as possible following exposure; the Centers for Disease Control and Prevention states it can be provided within 5 days of unprotected intercourse.[38] Pregnancy after emergency contraception is 3.6 times more likely for obese women than for women with a normal body mass index. Failure of emergency contraception is more likely to occur with levonorgestrel than with ulipristal acetate; however, in all women, regardless of body mass index, the most significant factor predicting failure is the cycle day of intercourse.[39] Because rape poses a risk of sexual disease transmission and because rape may have resulted in trauma, oral contraceptive pills are the preferred form of ongoing contraception.

Breastfeeding is not contraindicated following emergency contraception. Advise women that emergency contraception does not protect against HIV infection, other sexually transmitted infections, or subsequent unprotected intercourse. Recommend follow-up with a healthcare provider for all women and especially those with abnormal bleeding after cessation of emergency contraception.[37] Advise women who use emergency contraception to follow up with a regular provider to begin use of ongoing contraception in the form of oral contraception pills or

TABLE 293-4 Centers for Disease Control and Prevention Recommended Regimens for Infection Prophylaxis

Ceftriaxone, 250 milligrams IM, single dose; *or* cefixime 400 milligrams PO, single dose
Plus
Metronidazole, 2 grams PO, single dose
Plus
Azithromycin, 1 gram PO, single dose
Or
Doxycycline, 100 milligrams PO, twice a day for 7 d

Source: From Centers for Disease Control and Prevention: Sexually transmitted diseases: treatment guidelines 2010. http://www.cdc.gov/std/treatment/2010/sexual-assault.htm. Accessed April 11, 2013.

TABLE 293-5 Emergency Contraception

Drug	Dose	Comments
Levonorgestrel (Plan B)	1.5 milligrams once *or* 0.75 milligrams at 1 and 12 h	Prescribe antiemetics; less nausea than combined estrogen-progestin
Combined estrogen-progestin[40]	100 micrograms ethinyl estradiol *plus* 0.50 milligrams levonorgestrel, at 1 and 12 h	Prescribe antiemetics
Ulipristal acetate (Ella/Fibristal)	30 milligrams PO in a single dose	Prescribe antiemetics

copper intrauterine device to ensure successful prevention of pregnancy from subsequent unprotected intercourse.[38,39]

HIV POSTEXPOSURE PROPHYLAXIS

Viral load in the assailant is the most significant factor determining infectivity.[41] HIV seroconversion has occurred in persons whose only known risk factor was sexual assault or sexual abuse.[42] HIV transmission risk increases when bleeding occurs with vaginal, anal, or oral penetration; if viral load in the ejaculate is high; and if genital lesions are present in the assailant or the survivor.[28] Assistance in determining the advisability for PEP can be obtained by calling the toll-free 24-hour National HIV/AIDS Post Exposure Hotline at 1-888-448-4911 or by accessing their website at www.nccc.ucsf.edu/home. The Centers for Disease Control and Prevention recommendations for postexposure assessment of adolescents and adults are listed in **Table 293-6**.

If PEP is administered, follow the standard protocol recommended by your hospital's infectious disease specialists. When prescribing HIV PEP, ask about sulfa allergy. Truvada includes tenofovir which has a sulfa moiety.

DISPOSITION AND FOLLOW-UP

Excellent care for survivors of sexual assault requires the coordination of clinical medicine with forensic science, law enforcement, and survivor advocacy. Once injuries are assessed and managed, offer counseling. This can be done by a dedicated rape counselor or trained social worker. If injuries are not severe, a rape counselor may be present prior to the physician's assessment. Gaps in service and patient care have largely involved lack of treatment of sexually transmitted infections and lack of availability of pregnancy-related services.[43]

TABLE 293-6 Recommendations for Postexposure Assessment of Human Immunodeficiency Virus (HIV) Infection Risk for Adolescent and Adult Survivors within 72 Hours of Sexual Assault

Assess risk for HIV infection in the assailant.

Evaluate characteristics of the assault event that might increase risk for HIV transmission.

Because recommendations vary with time and between institutions, consult with a specialist in HIV treatment for specific postexposure prophylaxis (PEP).

If the survivor appears to be at risk for HIV transmission from the assault, discuss antiretroviral prophylaxis, including toxicity and lack of proven benefit.

If the survivor chooses to start antiretroviral PEP, provide enough medication to last until the next return visit. Reevaluate the survivor 3–7 d after initial assessment and assess tolerance of medications.

If PEP is started, perform CBC and serum chemistry panel at baseline. Do not delay PEP while awaiting laboratory results.

Perform HIV antibody test at original assessment; repeat at 6 weeks, 3 months, and 6 months. Repeat serologic assessment for syphilis can also be repeated at these times.[28]

Source: From Centers for Disease Control and Prevention: Sexually transmitted diseases: treatment guidelines 2010: sexual assault and STDs. http://www.cdc.gov/std/treatment/2010/sexual-assault.htm#adults. Accessed April 10, 2013.

Prior to discharge, make sure that the patient has a safe place to go, a safe way to get there, and a plan for addressing absence from home or work. This conversation should include a discussion of if, to whom, and how she will reveal her assault for the present time. Cultural competency of the caregivers is essential throughout the delivery of healthcare services to the survivors of sexual assault, but is critical at this juncture. If the team is not familiar with the cultural attitudes and practices surrounding sexual assault in the survivor's religious, ethnic, or social group, ask the patient how his or her family, religious community, or social network may respond.

Prior to discharge, provide the opportunity for bathing and oral care. Because clothing has been sequestered as part of the evidence kit, hospitals should provide fresh, packaged underwear and outerwear for the patient. Sweat suits are customarily provided at most SART hospitals. This is an appropriate time to raise the issue of returning to the home environment, since the patient will return in clothing that is not customary dress. Provide a headscarf for women who customarily wear head coverings in public.

Arrange follow-up appointments according to Centers for Disease Control and Prevention recommendations. Patients receiving PEP should be seen in 3 to 7 days following initial assessment, and all patients should be seen in 1 to 2 weeks.[28] This ensures the effectiveness of pregnancy prophylaxis and sexually transmitted infection treatment.

Male sexual assault survivors should follow up with a urologist or proctologist. Special populations, such as children, should be referred to a pediatrician or a pediatric abuse clinic.

SPECIAL POPULATIONS

ADOLESCENTS AND CHILDREN

Consider sexual abuse in children if no definitive explanation for nonsexual transmission of a sexually transmitted infection can be identified.[28] For extensive discussion, see chapter 148, "Child Abuse and Neglect." The most experienced examiner available should examine children to minimize pain or further trauma. Today, there are over 600 pediatric SANE programs in the United States.[44-46]

ELDERLY PATIENTS

Most elder assaults take place at the patient's home, and most assaults are by an unknown assailant.[47] In the case of an elderly assault survivor, the forensic interview and examination present unique challenges. The patient not only may resist the pelvic examination because of injury or pain, but the pelvic area may be difficult to visualize because of hip contractures or vaginal atrophy. It is also difficult to explain the examination to a patient with dementia or cognitive impairment. Further challenges include obtaining an accurate and reliable history of the details of the assault, the injuries sustained, and regions of pain or discomfort.[47,48] Special adjustments may be needed for the interview and sexual assault examination.[47,48]

TRANSGENDER AND LESBIAN PATIENTS

Information about sexual assault of lesbian and transgendered women has mostly relied on data from informal surveys.[49] A London clinic reported that transgender sex workers self-reported higher rates of violence and sexual assault than did biological female sex workers, but that rate was not specified.[50] **FORGE** (www.forge-forward.org) is a Wisconsin-based group for the support of the transgender population. The group has a Web site with printable handouts for lesbian and transgendered patients who are sexual assault survivors, survivor first-person narratives, and resource links for both patients and providers.

MEN

Male sexual assault is less common than sexual assault of women.[51] Assaults on males generally result in more severe injuries,[52,53] with 40% to 60% of males sustaining anogenital injuries,[53,54] and assaults on men are likely to involve multiple assailants.[55] At least a third of males who are sexually assaulted have a history of psychiatric or cognitive disability.[54] One major factor that complicates the care of male survivors is the fact

Global Issues in Sexual Assault

Lisa Moreno-Walton

In the 1990s, during the conflicts in Bosnia, Rwanda, the Democratic Republic of the Congo, and Liberia, rape became weaponized as a form of torture,[1] genocide,[2] and a means of humiliating and demoralizing the opponent.[3] Although women are subjected to sexual torture far more often than men,[4] sexual assault is calculated to destroy not only the man or woman who is raped, but entire families and communities. Rape of men is meant to be the ultimate humiliation of conquest, and the rape of women highlights the inability of men to perform their role as protectors of women and children. In the Congo, for example, over half of the victims of military rapes are children, 10% of them less than 10 years of age. In the ultimate depravity, fathers are forced to rape their daughters and sons their mothers in the presence of the entire community as a means of achieving total submission through fear.[5]

Systematic, repeated rape is now an adjunct to genocidal extermination camps and has been used in Sudan, Guatemala, the Congo, Rwanda, and Bosnia.[2] During the Bosnian War (1992 to 1995), the Serbian paramilitary created rape camps to imprison women and adolescent girls, and torture and gang rape them over months with the "assistance" and compliance of the local authorities.[6] There are reports, out of Liberia specifically, describing the dual role of combatants who are commanded to torture, rape, and murder and then to gratify the sexual desires of their superior officers in order to keep their jobs.[7] Societies demoralized by war, fearful of torture and death, hungry and poor, and knowing that there are no consequences for their assailants, often come to regard violence and the expectation of violence as customary and acceptable.[2,4-8]

Plagued by both poverty and concerns for their daughters, many parents coerce young girls into early marriages as a way of fetching a good bride price for a virgin daughter, who has not yet been raped by the military or paramilitary combatants. Instances of girls as young as 11 or 12 years being given in marriage to men in their 60s have been reported.[8,9] Girls who run away are beaten by their families and returned to their husbands either to protect the family's reputation or because some of the money from the bride price has already been spent. In many such traditional cultures, victims of rape are blamed for their assault and bring shame upon their families. Women may not access medical care without the permission of their husbands, increasing the likelihood that rape will never be reported.[9] And although sexual assaults by strangers are widely acknowledged as crimes, rape in marriage, sexual coercion in schools, demands for sex in return for a job, and forced marriage are tolerated or socially condoned in many countries. Women are expected to be submissive and sexually available to their husbands at all times, and it is considered both a right and an obligation for men to use violence in order to "correct" or chastise women for perceived transgressions.[10]

When rape is used as a weapon of war, the consequences to women are severe. Many women suffer fistulas, incontinence, infertility, depression, suicidal ideation, suicide, abandonment by family, and exile by the community.[2,4,5,11,12] Women who have been raped are more likely to be sexually abused again[2] and are more likely to engage in high-risk sexual behavior, such as exchanging sex for food and money, having sex with military personnel for perceived benefits of association with the powerful, and having unprotected sex with individuals known to be human immunodeficiency virus positive.[13] Both rape and high-risk sexual behavior in exchange for food, money, and/or cosmetics are reported to be frequent among internally displaced persons living in refugee camps.[12-14]

However disturbing these reports may be, investigation of the literature reveals that physicians and scientists still do not have a comprehensive understanding of the dynamics of sexual violence, that methods of data collection remain understandably flawed, and that methodology, including single-site studies of self-reports by small populations, may indeed not represent the scope of the actual problem. Although some countries' medical associations have issued guidelines to clinicians, global clinical standards of care need further development.[15] Journalists with an incomplete understanding of biostatistics often report inaccurate information that remains as fact in the minds of the general public, as evidenced by a media report that 75% of Liberian women were raped during the country's civil war. Peer-reviewed studies have set the estimated number at 9.2% to 15%, with 77% of women who were assaulted reporting sexual violence.[16] Overreporting of such sensitive data may make good news, but ultimately, it damages the credibility of future reports. Underreporting may trivialize a major human rights violation and the suffering of its victims.

Human rights organizations, national governments, physicians, and physician organizations must continue to take firm steps to ensure sanctions against governments, societies, and individuals who tolerate such practices.

REFERENCES

1. McLean IA: The male victim of sexual assault. *Best Pract Res Clin Obstet Gynecol* 27: 39, 2013. [PMID: 22951768]
2. Stark L, Wessells M: Sexual violence as a weapon of war. *JAMA* 308: 677, 2012. [PMID: 22893163]
3. Bullock CM, Beckson M: Male victims of sexual assault: phenomenology, psychology, physiology. *J Am Acad Psychiatry Law* 39: 197, 2011. [PMID: 21653264]
4. Sanders J, Schuman MW, Marbella AM: The epidemiology of torture: a case series of 58 survivors of torture. *Forensic Sci Int* 189: 1, 2009. [PMID: 19428203]
5. Brown C: Rape as a weapon of war in the Democratic Republic of the Congo. *Torture* 22: 24, 2012. [PMID: 23086003]
6. http://www.amnesty.org/en/library/info/EUR63/012/2012/en. (When everyone is silent: reparation for survivors of wartime rape in Repblika Srpska in Bosnia and Herzegovina.) Amnesty International. October 31, 2012. EUR 63/012/2012.
7. Johnson K, Asher J, Rosborough S, Raja A, Panjabi R, Beadling C, Lawry L: Association of combatant status and sexual violence with health and mental health outcomes in post-conflict Liberia. *JAMA* 300: 676, 2008. [PMID: 18698066]
8. McDuie-Ra D: Violence against women in the militarized Indian frontier: beyond Indian culture in the experiences of ethnic minority woman. *Violence Against Women* 18: 322, 2012. [PMID: 22615121]
9. Amowitz LL, Kim G, Reis C, Asher JL, Iacopino V: Human rights abuses and concerns about women's health and human rights in Southern Iraq. *JAMA* 291: 1471, 2004. [PMID: 15039414]
10. Oram S, Stock H, Busza J, Howard LM, Zimmerman C: Prevalence and risk of violence and the physical, mental, and sexual health problems associated with human trafficking: systematic review. *PLoS Med* 9: 5, 2012. [PMID: 22666182]
11. Trenholm JE, Olsson P, Ahlberg BM: Battles on women's bodies: war, rape, and traumatisation in eastern Democratic Republic of Congo. *Global Public Health* 6: 139, 2011. [PMID: 19787519]
12. Tankink MT: The silence of South-Sudanese women: social risks in talking about experiences of sexual violence. *Cult Health Sex* 15: 391, 2013. [PMID: 23298150]
13. Mahwezi WW, Kinyanda E, Mungherera M, et al: Vulnerability to high risk sexual behavior (HRSB) following exposure to war trauma as seen in post-conflict communities in eastern Uganda: a qualitative study. *Conflict Health* 5: 1, 2011. [PMID: 21310092]
14. Amowitz LL, Reis C, Lyons KH, et al: Prevalence of war-related sexual violence and other human rights abuses among internally displaced persons in Sierra Leone. *JAMA* 287: 513, 2002. [PMID: 11798376]
15. Mason F, Lodrick Z: Psychological consequences of sexual assault. *Best Pract Res Clin Obstet Gynaecol* 27: 27, 2013. [PMID: 23182852]
16. Palermo T, Peterman A: Undercounting, overcounting and the longevity of flawed estimates: statistics on sexual violence in conflict. *Bull World Health Organ* 89: 924, 2011 [PMID: 22271951]

that physiologically, the stimulation of anal penetration can lead to involuntary erection and sometimes to ejaculation. Furthermore, many assailants manually stimulate their victims to cause ejaculation. Numerous cases of male sexual assault have been determined to be consensual by judges and defense attorneys who fail to understand the involuntary nature of this physiologic response.[55] The survivors themselves can be confused and distressed by this response and may hesitate to offer this information. Use a short, simple explanation of the physiology using lay language to assist in history taking.

Hospitals have male rape kits available, and the same guidelines should be followed for history, physical exam, collection of forensic evidence, and maintaining chain of custody as have already been described. SANEs and SAFEs are all trained in the sexual assault forensic examination of males. Resources for counseling may be more difficult to find for the male survivor, especially in small communities. The **Rape, Abuse & Incest National Network** does have special resources for men. Their victim hotline can be reached at 1-800-656-HOPE, and their Web site can be accessed at www.rainn.org

PRACTICE GUIDELINES AND SOCIETY POSITION STATEMENTS

The American Academy of Pediatrics, American College of Obstetrics and Gynecology, American College of Emergency Physicians, and Centers for Disease Control and Prevention all have issued recommendations regarding the acute management of rape survivors.[28,56-59] The American College of Emergency Physicians issued a policy statement on the treatment of the patient with a complaint of sexual assault.[58] As an adjunct to this policy, the American College of Emergency Physicians Emergency

Medicine Practice Committee prepared a handbook, *Evaluation and Management of the Sexually Assaulted or Sexually Abused Patient*, to assist in developing a community or ED plan.[59]

Acknowledgment: The author would like to thank Sheryl L. Heron, MD, and Debra E. Houry, MD, for writing the prior edition of this chapter, which has been updated and revised for this edition.

REFERENCES

The complete reference list is available online at www.TintinalliEM.com.

CHAPTER 294 Intimate Partner Violence and Abuse

Mary Hancock

INTRODUCTION AND EPIDEMIOLOGY

Intimate partner violence is defined as a pattern of assaultive, coercive behaviors that may include inflicted physical injury, psychological abuse, sexual assault, progressive social isolation, stalking, deprivation, intimidation, and threats. Such behaviors are perpetrated by someone who is, was, or wishes to be involved in an intimate or dating relationship with an adult or adolescent individual and are aimed at establishing control by one partner over the other.[1]

Intimate partner violence and abuse is the preferred alternative for previously used terms such as *spousal abuse*, *wife battering*, and *domestic violence*. This term more accurately reflects the fact that this type of abuse occurs not only in adult heterosexual married relationships but also in relationships between cohabiting, separated, gay and lesbian, bisexual, and transgendered individuals as well as in adolescent dating relationships.[2,3]

Intimate partner violence and abuse occurs in every racial, ethnic, cultural, geographic, and religious group, and it affects individuals of all socioeconomic and educational backgrounds worldwide. Men are affected, but the overwhelming burden of victimization from intimate partner violence is borne by women.[2,4,5] Risk factors for intimate partner violence and abuse include female sex, age between 18 and 24 years, low income level of the household, and relationship status of separated rather than divorced or married.[2] Sexual and/or physical abuse during childhood and adolescence is a frequent predictor of future victimization.[2,6] Presence of weapons in the home and threats of murder are associated with increased risk of homicide.

Effects extend to family members, friends, coworkers, other witnesses, and the community at large.[2] Children who grow up in violent homes may be physically or emotionally abused or neglected, and witnessing violence can have short- and long-term adverse health consequences.[7] In families in which *either* child maltreatment or spousal abuse is identified, it is likely that both forms of abuse exist. Children may be incidentally injured or killed when they try to intervene in a struggle.[7] Children exposed to violence in the home may develop behavioral difficulties, including depression, abusive behaviors, and drug abuse. Frequent exposure to violence in the home may teach children that violence is a normal way of life. Perpetrators of violence, in particular severe violence, may be at risk for suicide, committing murder, or being murdered by a family member.[7,8]

Ask about a history of intimate partner violence or abuse during healthcare encounters. Failure to recognize and intervene in situations of intimate partner violence may have serious consequences for the survivor and family. Such consequences may include continued violence, physical and psychological health problems, and injury or even death.[2,9,10]

CLINICAL FEATURES

Intimate partner violence is most often cyclical in nature. The cycle begins with a period of tension building, which may include arguing, blaming, or controlling behaviors or jealousy. The next phase is escalation and may include verbal threats, physical and sexual abuse, or assault. Weapons may be used at this point. Subsequently, there is a "honeymoon" phase in which the perpetrator may apologize or make excuses for inappropriate behavior. Over time, the abusive behavior tends to increase in severity, and the intervals between abusive episodes become shorter.

There are no "usual" features by which a person who has experienced intimate partner violence may be identified in the ED. Often it is one of a number of health-related consequences of violence or abuse that causes persons who have experienced intimate partner violence to seek medical attention (**Table 294-1**). Therefore, screening and assessment for elements of the history and physical examination suggestive of intimate partner violence are needed to identify victims. Signs suggestive of intimate partner violence and abuse are summarized in **Table 294-2**.[1,2,4,11]

TABLE 294-1 Consequences of Intimate Partner Violence

Adults	Adolescents	Children
Injuries	Same as for adults	Low birth weight
Alcohol and substance abuse	*plus*	Prematurity and associated complications
Sexually transmitted infections	Victimization as an adult	Failure to thrive
Human immunodeficiency virus infection	Fertility problems	Parental neglect syndrome
Unplanned/unwanted pregnancy	Poor school performance and school dropout	Speech disorders
Headaches	Unwanted pregnancy and associated complications of pregnancy, frequent pregnancies	Bedwetting
Chronic pelvic pain		Headaches
Urinary tract infections	Eating disorders	Cognitive functioning problems—lower verbal and quantitative skills
Vaginal bleeding	Behavioral disorders	Psychological and emotional problems—aggression, hostility, withdrawal, acting out
Back pain	Involvement with the legal system and courts	
Eating disorders	Prostitution	
GI disorders	Increased suicide risk	
Depression	Smoking and substance abuse	
Panic disorders		
Suicide		
Posttraumatic stress disorder		
Homelessness		
Social isolation		

TABLE 294-2 Signs Suggestive of Intimate Partner Violence

Findings	Comments
Injuries characteristic of violence	Fingernail scratches, broken fingernails, bite marks, dental injuries, cigarette burns, bruises suggesting strangulation or restraint, and rope burns or ligature marks may be seen.
Injuries suggesting a defensive posture	Forearm bruises or fractures may be sustained when individuals try to fend off blows to the face or chest.
Injuries during pregnancy	Up to 45% of women report abuse or assault during pregnancy.[12] Preterm labor, placental abruption, direct fetal injury, and stillbirth can occur.
Central pattern of injury	Injuries to the head, neck, face, and thorax and abdominal injuries in pregnant women may suggest violence.
Extent or type of injury inconsistent with the patient's explanation	Multiple injuries at different anatomic sites inconsistent with the described mechanism of injury. The most common explanation of injury is a "fall." Embarrassment, evasiveness, or lack of concern with the injuries may be noted.
Multiple injuries in various stages of healing	These may be reported as "accidents" or "clumsiness."
Delay between the time of injury and the presentation for treatment	Victims may wait several days before seeking medical care for injuries. Victims may seek care for minor or resolving injuries.
Visits for vague or minor complaints without evidence of physiologic abnormality	Frequent ED visits for a variety of injuries or illnesses, including chronic pelvic pain and other chronic pain syndromes.
Suicide attempts	Women who attempt or commit suicide often have a history of intimate partner violence.[12]

A defensive, hostile, or aggressive partner accompanying the patient may provide clues to the diagnosis by exhibiting controlling or abusive behavior. Overly solicitous behavior by the partner may occur. The patient may appear frightened of the partner or refuse to answer questions and instead defer all responses to the partner. In situations raising concern, and if the patient agrees, hospital police can prevent the alleged perpetrator from visiting the patient in the ED and hospital. **Ask abused individuals if they have suicidal or homicidal ideation. Such ideation, particularly if accompanied by a concrete plan of action, should trigger immediate consultation with a mental health provider.**

SCREENING AND ASSESSMENT

Many experts, including the American Medical Association and The Joint Commission, recommend routine screening for intimate partner violence for all adolescent and adult women who present to the ED and for mothers of children brought to the ED. National screening consensus guidelines are available online at http://www.futureswithoutviolence.org.[13] Because of the known adverse long-term impacts of intimate personal violence on health, when time permits, consider screening for lifetime exposure.

The responsibilities of the ED team include identification of intimate partner violence; validation of the abused individual's experience; assessment of immediate risk and safety planning; referral to experts for care; and documentation in the medical record.[12]

Screening should be conducted by providers educated about the dynamics of intimate partner violence. Provide a safe and private environment for the interview. Take into account cultural differences and expectations. If translators are required, use individuals who have no connection to the patient and, if possible, who have education in the dynamics of abuse. Document screening results, safety assessment, and any interventions, including referrals and required reporting. Screening guidelines for adolescent and adult patients are summarized in **Table 294-3**.[13] Sample verbal screening questions are listed in **Table 294-4**.

Abused individuals want providers to be nonjudgmental, sensitive, and direct. They also want to be assured of confidentiality. They want the provider to have an understanding of the complexity of intimate partner violence and the difficulty of achieving a "quick fix." Women value the reassurance that their experiences with intimate partner violence and abuse are unacceptable and undeserved (it is not their fault). They also value a nonpressured encounter and a provider who respects their decisions and works with them to determine an appropriate course of action.[14]

TREATMENT AND DISPOSITION

Ensuring the safety of the abused individual and children is the foremost goal. "Placing the patient in a shelter" or "having the attacker arrested" may not be congruent with the individual's goals. Ultimately, the abused individual must make the determination of whether it is safe to return home. By providing information about intimate violence, risks, and options, the physician can help the patient decide what is best for themselves and their family members. The patient's decision making may be very complex, because depression, lack of self-esteem, lack of support, social isolation, financial dependence on the perpetrator, and fear make it difficult to leave the relationship.

Patients must be told that violence, abuse, and intimidation are not a part of normal, healthy relationships. For some, this may be the first

TABLE 294-3 Summary of National Consensus Guidelines for Screening for Intimate Partner Violence and Abuse in the ED[13]

Screening	Assessment	Intervention	Documentation	Referral and Follow-Up
Routinely screen at every visit. Screen for current abuse, and if time allows, screen for history of abuse. Screen privately (one on one) or with nonrelated trained interpreter. Ask: What happened? When did it happen? Where did it happen? Who did this? Respect patient decision to disclose or not. Discuss any required reporting. Include screening questions on intake forms.	Assess immediate safety. Assess health impact of abuse. Assess pattern of abuse. Assess for danger and potential lethality. If the danger assessment findings are positive, assess potential for suicide and homicide.	Listen carefully and provide support. "I'm concerned for your health and safety." "You are not alone." "Help is available." "It is not your fault." "You don't deserve it." "What happened to you can affect your health." Provide information and materials. "What can I do for you?" Provide a safety plan. Offer services, including an advocate, social worker, police, shelter, etc.	Legible, full signature; maintain confidentiality of records Abuse history: Subjective information: patient states... Objective information: detailed description of patient's appearance, behavioral indicators, injuries, and health complaints Use of rape kits where appropriate Results of physical examination Use of body maps Photographs (with patient's consent) Radiologic, laboratory findings, collection of forensic evidence: clothes, debris, etc. Any materials and referrals offered Results of health and safety assessments	Refer to primary care physician, mental health provider, social worker, or intimate partner abuse advocate. Obtain permission to notify provider. Know current phone numbers for: Abuse and assault prevention programs Legal services Children's programs Mental health services Law enforcement Substance abuse programs Transportation Local clergy or other community organizations

TABLE 294-4 Sample of Domestic Violence Screening Questions

The healthcare worker should explain the following in his or her own words:

We are concerned about your health and safety, so we ask all women the same questions about violence at home.

Violence is very common, and we want to improve our response to families experiencing violence.

The healthcare worker may ask the following questions of ALL patients:

1. Are you ever afraid of your partner?
2. In the last year, has your partner hit, kicked, punched, or otherwise hurt you?
3. In the last year, has your partner put you down, humiliated you, or tried to control what you can do?
4. In the last year, has your partner threatened to hurt you?

If domestic violence has been identified in any of the above questions, ask if the individual would like assistance today. Be prepared to offer resources, assess for safety, and discuss a safety plan with the individual.

time they have heard such information. The abused individual's reports and experiences should be acknowledged and believed. Let the patient know that you take the situation seriously and that you are concerned about the health and safety of her (or him) and the children. Emphasize that he or she has done nothing to warrant violence and abuse. It is the perpetrator whose behavior is unacceptable. Clarify that ED personnel can help patients contact trained social workers or intimate violence advocates, who can then help develop logistical plans either for safety or for ending the relationship. Respect the abused individual's wishes about the future of the relationship. Screening and validation may be the stimulus needed by the patient to begin planning for change.

Indicators of a high-risk and potentially lethal situation include escalation in the frequency or severity of violence; the threat or actual use of weapons, in particular firearms; obsession with the abused individuals; hostage taking; stalking; and homicide or suicide threats or attempts and evidence of violent behavior outside the home. Another risk factor for serious injury or death is substance abuse by the perpetrator, which can increase violent behaviors.[2,11]

The most dangerous periods for abused individuals are during the time of abuse disclosure and during attempts to leave the relationship. Some patients feel safer remaining in the violent relationship than leaving without adequate planning for a safe departure.[13]

Refer survivors to intimate violence experts, such as hospital social workers or community-based advocates, who can help the victim assess the situation, understand options, plan for safety, and arrange safe shelter. Community advocates are typically on call or available by telephone. If the patient can be safely discharged from the ED and personal contact with an advocate cannot be made before discharge, give the patient up-to-date information about available services in the community. **Intimate personal violence advocates should not be asked to call the patient directly unless the patient agrees, because calls to the home could jeopardize the patient's safety.**

Resources for healthcare providers to assist in preparing their practices for optimal response to victims of intimate personal violence are available from a number of organizations (**Table 294-5**).

If lethality risk is high, consult with experts before ED discharge. Hospital admission of the abused individual or children is an option in high-risk situations in which there is no other way to ensure safety. Use of a 24-hour safe room, a location established by some hospitals and communities to provide a safe place for the patient to stay while arrangements for safe disposition of the patient and family members are made, is another option. Use of an alias name on admission and screening of incoming phone calls may also be of benefit.

TABLE 294-5 Resources for Healthcare Providers

Futures Without Violence (formerly Family Violence Prevention Fund)	http://www.futureswithoutviolence.org
National Domestic Violence Hotline	800-799-SAFE (7233)
National Coalition Against Domestic Violence	http://www.ncadv.org

ED RECORD DOCUMENTATION

Documentation in the ED should be clear and legible. Voluntary descriptions of intimate personal violence should be quoted and described in the patient's own words. Do not use the word *alleged* because it implies that the person recording the incident does not believe the complaint. A complaint of "sexual assault" is no more alleged than is a complaint of "ear pain" or a "sore throat."

Record past and current abuse, with details of date, time, location, witnesses, and specific injury. Describe the patient's health complaints, injuries, appearance, and demeanor. Annotated body maps and photographs can supplement written notes.

Obtain relevant forensic evidence, and follow the appropriate chain of custody of evidence. If sexual assault has occurred, document ED testing and treatment.

Record safety assessment and disposition. A safety assessment form or referral notes from an expert are helpful adjuncts. Discussion of a safety plan with the patient is an important discharge function and also requires documentation.

LEGAL CONSIDERATIONS

Most states in the United States have laws that require healthcare providers to report injuries resulting from firearms, knives, or other weapons. Twenty-three states have reporting requirements for injuries resulting from crimes (intimate personal violence is a crime in all 50 states); seven states have statutes that specifically require health providers to report injuries resulting from intimate personal violence. The specifics of the reporting requirements vary from state to state, and the adequacy of response by the police to reporting varies by jurisdiction.[15] Inadequate or inappropriate response to the reports (e.g., informing the perpetrator of the report without providing for the safety of the abused individual) can increase the risk of harm to abused individuals. ED personnel should be aware of reporting requirements and police response in their area. Patients must be informed if there is an obligation to make a police report and should also be told about possible ramifications.

ED PREPARATION FOR OPTIMAL RESPONSE

The Joint Commission requires, and the Institute of Medicine recommends, that staff receive initial and ongoing training about intimate partner violence and abuse. This should include education related to cultural competency, victim perspective, and consequences of violence, as well as how to assess, intervene in, support, and document care. Employees should also be informed of their options for assistance if they or someone they know is in an abusive relationship.

A routine screening protocol should be implemented that addresses training of ED personnel, confidential interviewing, and appropriate interventions, including validation and referral.

Multicultural and multilingual information about interpersonal violence and effects on abused individuals and family members should be made available to the public and employees. This may consist of posters and/or brochures in areas of the hospital such as public areas, examination rooms, and restrooms. Community resources that provide services to victims should be a part of the shared information.

Implement a continuous quality improvement program that assesses adherence to recommended screening and intervention strategies.

Form professional relationships with hospital- and/or community-based experts to ensure appropriate referral practices.

SPECIAL POPULATIONS

PREGNANCY

Prevalence during pregnancy ranges from 6% to 22%.[5,11] Women who report intimate partner violence and abuse during pregnancy are at increased risk of postnatal abuse. Approximately half of female murder

TABLE 294-6 Strategies for Violence Prevention—World Health Organization

Increase safe, stable, and nurturing environments between children and their parents or caregivers.
Reduce availability and misuse of alcohol.
Reduce access to lethal means.
Improve life skills and enhance opportunities for youth.
Promote gender equality and empower women.
Change cultural norms that support violence.
Improve criminal justice systems.
Improve social welfare systems.
Reduce social distance between conflicting groups.
Reduce economic inequality and concentrated poverty.

Reproduced with permission from World Health Organization: *Preventing Violence and Reducing Its Impact: How Development Agencies Can Help*. Geneva: World Health Organization; 2008.

TABLE 294-7 Hotlines for Patients

National Domestic Violence Hotline: 24 h; links caller to help in her (or his) area—emergency shelter, domestic violence shelters, legal advocacy and assistance programs, social services	800-799-SAFE (7233) 800-787-3224 (TTY)
Rape, Abuse, and Incest National Network: 24 h; automatically transfers caller to nearest rape crisis center anywhere in the nation	800-656-HOPE (4673) http://www.rainn.org

victims are killed by a current or previous intimate.[2,11] Women assaulted during pregnancy are three times more likely to be admitted to the hospital than nonpregnant women.[11]

GLOBAL ISSUES

Globally, death from interpersonal violence is ranked as the 20th most common cause of death.[16] The World Health Organization's Violence Against Women Survey demonstrates that intimate partner violence and abuse not only are substantial health problems due to direct injury and mortality, but also contribute to other serious health problems because of an increased burden of disease. The associations between reported ill health in women and intimate partner violence and abuse are consistent within and across countries.[8,16] This effect persists even if the violence was in the past.[16]

In May 2014, the 67th World Health Assembly requested that the World Health Organization prepare a global plan of action to strengthen the health system to address interpersonal violence, especially against women, girls, and children (http://www.who.int/violence_injury_prevention).

Ten key strategies for violence prevention have been developed for international use[17] (**Table 294-6**).

For resources for patients (hotlines), see **Table 294-7**.

PRACTICE GUIDELINES

The *National Consensus Guidelines on Identifying and Responding to Domestic Violence Victimization in Health Care Settings*, revised in 2004, is available from Futures Without Violence (formerly Family Violence Prevention Fund) (http://www.futureswithoutviolence.org). Preparation of this report was funded by the Conrad N. Hilton Foundation and the U.S. Department of Health and Human Services.

Acknowledgment: The author gratefully acknowledges the contributions of Patricia R. Salber, the author of this chapter in the previous edition.

REFERENCES

The complete reference list is available online at www.TintinalliEM.com.

Abuse of the Elderly and Impaired

Jonathan Glauser
Frederic M. Hustey

INTRODUCTION

Elder abuse is an act or omission resulting in harm to the health or welfare of an elderly person. Three key groups have published definitions of elder abuse.[1-3] Although the incidence of elder neglect and abuse is unknown and widely felt to be underreported, the rate of different types of abuse among the elderly has been estimated to be in the mid-single digits, or between 500,000 and 1 million U.S. adults.[4,5] **Table 295-1** summarizes the categories of elder abuse.

CLINICAL FEATURES

PHYSICAL ABUSE

Physical abuse is the most easily recognized form of elder abuse. It is defined as the use of physical force that might result in bodily injury, physical pain, or impairment. Pushing, slapping, burning, striking with objects, and improper use of restraint are all examples of physical abuse. Chemical restraint (such as intentional overmedication or administration of tranquilizers) is a more subtle form. Regardless of mechanism, physical abuse is carried out with the intention of causing suffering, pain, or other physical impairment to the abused person.

CAREGIVER NEGLECT

Elder neglect is the most common form of elder maltreatment, accounting for more than half of all elder maltreatment cases reported to adult protective services agencies annually.[6] Elder neglect is defined as the failure of a caregiver to provide basic care to a patient and to provide goods and services necessary to prevent physical harm or emotional discomfort.[7,8] Examples of neglect include deprivation of food, clothing, hygiene, medical care, shelter, or supervision that a prudent person would consider essential for the well-being of another.[7,8]

Elder neglect is both underrecognized and potentially lethal. It likely accounts for the majority of cases of unreported abuse.[9] It is also an independent risk factor for mortality, even taking into account that the

TABLE 295-1 Categories of Elder Abuse

Categories of Abuse	Example
Physical abuse	Pushing, slapping, burning, striking with objects, improper use of restraint (physical or chemical)
Caregiver neglect	Deprivation of food, clothing, hygiene, medical care, shelter, or supervision
Sexual abuse	Unwanted touching, indecent exposure, unwanted innuendo, rape
Financial or material exploitation	Forcible transfer of property or other assets, including changing elderly person's will
Emotional or psychological abuse	Verbal threats (such as threats of violence, institutionalization, or deprivation), humiliation, intimidation, harassment, social neglect, and isolation
Abandonment	Desertion of an elder in the home or a hospital, nursing facility, shopping mall, or other public location by a caregiver or caretaker
Self-neglect	Failure or unwillingness to provide adequate food, clothing, shelter, medical care, hygiene, or social stimulation to self in individuals with diminished capacity to perform essential self-care tasks

Source: Reproduced from U.S. Department of Health and Human Services, Administration on Aging and Administration for Children and Families: *The National Elder Abuse Incidence Study*. Washington, DC: National Center on Elder Abuse, 1998.

deaths themselves may not be immediately ascribed to injury.[6] Elder neglect may be difficult to diagnose. Although some cases may be obvious (such as in a patient with multiple deep pressure ulcers), it is often more subtle and difficult to detect.

SEXUAL ABUSE

Sexual abuse is broadly defined as nonconsensual sexual contact of any kind with an elderly person. The spectrum of sexual abuse ranges from unwanted touching, indecent exposure, or unwanted innuendo, to rape itself. Although sexual abuse is underreported across all age groups, in the elderly, sexual abuse is even less likely to be reported. Fear of retaliation and shame on the part of patients, as well as stereotyping of older patients as asexual or not sexually desirable by clinicians, police, and others, may be factors in underrecognition and underreporting of sexual abuse.[10]

FINANCIAL OR MATERIAL EXPLOITATION

Financial abuse is estimated to be the second most common form of elder abuse, accounting for approximately 20% to 30% of abuse cases.[11] Financial or material exploitation is the illegal or improper use of an elder's funds, property, or assets.[12] It occurs when family members, caregivers, or friends take control of the elder person's resources. Coercion or outright theft may occur, with or without the awareness of the elder person experiencing abuse. An elderly person may unwittingly sign over access to savings accounts and other assets when he or she is in an incapacitated state. Social Security checks or pensions may be used by caregivers for personal gain. Theft may be blatant or coerced, with forcible transfer of property, including changing of the elder's will. Abuse may result in a decrease in the standard of living and an inability to pay bills, purchase food, or obtain medications.

EMOTIONAL OR PSYCHOLOGICAL ABUSE

Emotional or psychological abuse is defined as the infliction of anguish, emotional pain, or distress. Examples of psychological and emotional abuse include verbal threats (such as threats of violence, institutionalization, or deprivation), humiliation, intimidation, and harassment. Social neglect and isolation are also forms of abuse. Psychological and emotional abuse can contribute to the development and worsening of mental health problems such as depression, which is common in many older victims.[12]

ABANDONMENT

Abandonment constitutes the desertion of an elderly person by an individual who is that person's custodian or who has assumed responsibility for providing care to the elder. Desertion of an elder in the home, hospital, nursing facility, shopping mall, or other public location may occur.

SELF-NEGLECT

Self-neglect includes those behaviors of an elderly person that threaten his or her own safety. Such behaviors include failure or unwillingness to provide adequate food, clothing, shelter, medical care, hygiene, or social stimulation for oneself. It is the result of an adult's inability, due to diminished capacity, to perform essential self-care tasks. By definition, this applies to one who understands the consequences of his or her choices and makes a conscious decision to engage in acts that threaten his or her own health or safety.[13] Patients who have cognitive impairment or who are living in poverty are at greater risk of self-neglect and may have increased mortality.[9]

DIAGNOSIS

RISK FACTORS

An awareness of risk factors is important for the recognition of potential victims of elder abuse or neglect. Risk factors can be divided into two categories: factors associated with the elders and factors associated with the perpetrators (**Table 295-2**).[7,13-17]

TABLE 295-2 Risk Factors for the Occurrence of Elder Abuse

Risk Factors for Elders	Risk Factors for Perpetrators
Cognitive impairment	History of mental illness
Physical dependency	History of substance abuse
Lack of social support	Excessive dependence on elder for financial support
Alcohol abuse	History of violence within or outside the family
History of domestic violence	
Female gender	
Developmental disability	
Difficult behavior (such as aggression or verbal outbursts)	
Special medical or psychiatric needs	
Limited experience managing finances	
Institutionalization	

Patient characteristics associated with a higher risk for elder mistreatment are cognitive impairment, physical dependency, lack of social support, alcohol abuse, female sex, and a history of domestic violence.[14] In addition, developmental disabilities, special medical or psychiatric needs, and difficult behavior (such as aggression or verbal outbursts) also increase the risk for abuse. Individuals with limited experience in managing finances are at increased risk for financial or material exploitation. Although elder abuse is more common in residential than institutional settings, institutionalization is also recognized as a risk factor for neglect and abuse.[7,16]

Three characteristics of perpetrators have been identified as risk factors: a history of mental illness and/or substance abuse, excessive dependence on the elder for financial support, and a history of violence within or outside of the family.[17] Abusers are most often the primary caregiver. Adult children tend to be more inclined to abuse than are spouses, and males engage in abuse more often than females.[13] Caregivers may be well intentioned but simply overwhelmed by the amount of care required. They may themselves be impaired by mental or physical problems that serve as barriers to the provision of adequate care.

HISTORY

The approach to the patient interview is important. Potential sufferers of abuse should be interviewed in private. The presence of caregivers, family, or friends may cause the patient to feel intimidated or embarrassed, which limits the amount and accuracy of information obtained. Try to put the patient at ease by making the assessment seem like a routine part of the evaluation.[12] Separately interview individuals accompanying the patient. Screening tools are available to aid in the detection of elder abuse.[18-20] The use of lengthier tools is not feasible in a busy ED, but the American Medical Association has proposed a list of nine screening questions that may be more practical to implement (**Table 295-3**). An affirmative answer to any of the questions in this screening tool raises concern and mandates further exploration.

TABLE 295-3 Screening Questions for Elder Abuse

1. Has anyone ever touched you without your consent?
2. Has anyone ever made you do things you didn't want to do?
3. Has anyone taken anything that was yours without asking?
4. Has anyone ever hurt you?
5. Has anyone ever scolded or threatened you?
6. Have you ever signed any documents you didn't understand?
7. Are you afraid of anyone at home?
8. Are you alone a lot?
9. Has anyone ever failed to help you take care of yourself when you needed help?

TABLE 295-4 Clues during the Medical Interview That May Suggest Elder Abuse

The patient appears fearful of his or her companion.
There are conflicting accounts of an injury or illness from the patient and caregiver.
The caregiver displays an attitude of indifference or anger toward the patient.
The caregiver is overly concerned with the costs of treatment needed by the patient.
The caregiver denies the patient the chance to interact privately with the physician.
The caregiver appears overly concerned and attentive.

During the interview, be prepared to recognize behavioral signs and symptoms that suggest elder abuse. These include depression, fear, withdrawal, confusion, anxiety, low self-esteem, and helplessness. Other history-related indicators that suggest abuse or neglect include a pattern of "physician shopping," unexplained injuries inconsistent with medical findings, and recurrent visits for similar injuries. Additional history taking should explore risk factors for abuse as outlined earlier in "Risk Factors."

Information can be obtained by the physician prior to conducting the private interview or by other members of the healthcare team, such as nurses, who are likely to have more frequent interaction with the patient and caregivers. Observing the interaction between the accompanying individuals can yield valuable clues (**Table 295-4**).

PHYSICAL EXAMINATION

Physical examination findings range from subtle and nondiagnostic to highly suspicious. Abuse is often detected when examination findings prompt further history taking with results suggesting elder mistreatment. Psychological abuse and financial abuse are especially hard to diagnose in the ED setting because physical examination findings are uncommon. Nonetheless, it is important to perform a detailed evaluation, including obtaining adequate exposure of the body to evaluate for trauma and pressure ulcers. Common physical findings in sufferers of elder abuse are bruising or trauma, poor general appearance and hygiene, malnutrition, and dehydration.[19]

Although not the most common form of elder abuse, physical abuse is the most easily recognized. Evidence of injury to normally protected areas of the body is highly suspicious for physical abuse.[14] Examples include contusions or lacerations on the inner arms or inner thighs and injury to the mastoid area. It is important to expose these areas when examining the patient to avoid missing significant findings. Contusions on the palms, soles of the feet, and buttocks also raise concern for elder abuse.[14] Multiple injuries in various stages of healing can suggest abuse, but may also be seen in patients with recurrent falls. Taking a thorough history is especially important in differentiating these two causes. Although older patients may sustain burns through accidental injury (such as coming too close to an open flame while cooking), unusual burns or multiple burns in various stages of healing should also raise concern. Traumatic alopecia is highly suspicious, although not necessarily diagnostic (because it may be seen in patients with some psychiatric conditions). Rope or restraint marks on wrists or ankles[13] occur when elders are inappropriately restrained. Midshaft ulnar fractures (nightstick fractures) can occur from attempts to shield blows by raising the forearm. Fractures of the head, spine, and trunk may be more indicative of abuse, although these can occur by other mechanisms.[21] Spiral fractures of long bones and fractures with rotational components also raise suspicion of abuse.[21]

Findings resulting from caregiver neglect or self-neglect are less specific. Perhaps the most identifiable finding is that of multiple or deep pressure ulcers. Ulcers that are uncared for (such as open ulcers lacking appropriate dressings or packing) or those not in lumbar or sacral areas raise suspicion even further. Incapacitated patients should be turned as part of the examination to evaluate for skin breakdown. Poor personal hygiene, inappropriate or soiled clothing, dehydration, malnutrition, contractures, fecal impaction, and excoriations suggest neglect.[8]

Sexually transmitted diseases or findings of genital trauma, especially in an incapacitated patient, raise concern for sexual abuse. Patients may complain of genital or anal pain, itching, bruising, or bleeding. Torn or stained underwear, with unexplained difficulty walking or sitting, may be present. Oral trauma can also be a manifestation of sexual abuse.

Depression, anxiety, and fear can be manifestations of psychological abuse, although they are nondiagnostic. Observation of interactions with caregivers and companions can provide further important clues to this type of abuse.

Although elder abuse is widely underrecognized and underreported, remember that underlying medical disorders are often associated with findings that could otherwise be identified with abuse. Advanced neurologic disorders such as multiple sclerosis, amyotrophic lateral sclerosis, and Parkinson's disease may lead to immobilization and severe disability. Individuals with such conditions are at risk for pressure ulcers, pneumonia, or venous thromboembolism, even with adequate care.[13]

TREATMENT, DISPOSITION, AND FOLLOW-UP

Treatment of elder abuse in the ED involves three key components:

1. Addressing associated medical and psychological needs
2. Ensuring patient safety
3. Complying with local reporting requirements (http://www.ncea.aoa.gov)

Medical problems, including injuries, should be stabilized and treated, and may be best managed through hospital admission. In addition to physical injury, metabolic derangements may be present. Patients with dehydration or malnutrition can have a variety of electrolyte abnormalities and may also have coexisting renal failure. Elders left in the same position for an extended period of time may be at risk for rhabdomyolysis. Additional problems may exist due to failure to administer usual medications at home. These issues should all be addressed during the ED visit, including the ability to conduct activities of daily living, such as meal preparation, housework, bathing, dressing oneself, toileting, and managing finances.

Psychological problems brought on by abuse, as well as preexisting psychiatric conditions and substance abuse, should also be addressed. The severity of the problem and planned disposition can affect the extent to which treatment is completed in the ED. For patients requiring hospitalization, concerns and findings should be communicated to the admitting service and documented in the medical record. For patients who are discharged to home, arrangements should be made for appropriate follow-up. Follow-up must be arranged for the patient's medical and psychiatric needs, and arrangements must also be made for monitoring and assessment of home safety and assessment of caregiver stress or substance abuse. A variety of resources are available to assist with these issues (**Table 295-5**). Social work consultation can be helpful in finding local resources.

Patients in immediate danger should be hospitalized, transferred to the care of a friend or reliable family member, or placed in an emergency shelter. Suspected abuse should be reported to the appropriate state agency (http://www.ncea.aoa.gov) or local adult protective services agency in order to ensure a follow-up investigation and a thorough long-term assessment. Although all 50 states have adult protective services and long-term care ombudsman programs, reporting is not mandated by law in every state. Elderly who live in the community are protected in all states by adult protective services agencies. Elders in institutional settings are protected in all states by long-term care ombudsman programs. Violations specific to nursing home residents might include the following: failure to respond to calls for help, unattended symptoms, injury of unknown origin or falls, physical abuse, poor staff attitudes related to respect or dignity, inappropriate medications or dosages, stolen or lost property, or abuse by other residents. Much long-term facility abuse occurs between residents; many facilities have younger psychiatric patients who are more mobile and aggressive than the older debilitated residents.[22] Become familiar with requirements pertaining to your own practice area (http://www.ncea.aoa.gov).

In cases of unintentional neglect, education of the caregiver may be the only intervention necessary. Other support options include home

TABLE 295-5 Resources for Elder Abuse

Who to Contact	Services Provided	Who to Contact	Services Provided
Clinical Justice Services Public Policy Institute American Association of Retired Persons 601 E St., NW Washington, DC 20049 202-434-2222	Provides self-instruction training program, pamphlets, and brochures on elder abuse prevention	National Training Library for Adult Protective Services National Center on Elder Abuse and Elder Abuse http://www.ncea.aoa.gov/NCEAroot/Main_Site 302-831-3525	An ongoing project that gathers training materials from around the country for loan and referral. The library has >140 holdings, including printed materials, PowerPoint presentations, and CDs. Materials are available on loan at no charge.
National Center of Elder Abuse 1201 15th St., NW, Suite 350 Washington, DC 20005-2842 202-898-2586 http://www.ncea.aoa.gov	One of the main information sites for elder abuse; provides a variety of resources, both nationally and by state	Family Caregiver Alliance 690 Market St., Suite 600 San Francisco, CA 94104 415-434-3388 http://www.caregiver.org	Lead agency in Link2Care, a program designed to provide Internet services to caregivers of adults with cognitive impairments
National Organization for Victim Assistance 510 King St., Suite 424 Alexandria, VA 22314 800-TRY-NOVA or 703-535-6682 http://www.trynova.org	Provides referrals, resources in every state	AARP 601 E St., NW Washington, DC 20049 202-434-AARP http://www.aarp.org	Leading organization representing people over age 50. Provides publications on caregiving issues, financial planning, durable power of attorney, trusts, and insurance.
National Coalition Against Domestic Violence P.O. Box 18749 Denver, CO 80218 303-839-1852 http://www.ncadv.org	Provides training and education on domestic violence, publications, and programs	**Other resources:** Administration on Aging 330 Independence Ave., SW Washington, DC 29201 202-245-0641	
National Domestic Violence Hotline Toll free: 800-799-SAFE TTY: 800-787-3224 (for hearing impaired)	Provides intervention; cannot take reports; confidential; available 24 h	Commission on Legal Problems of the Elderly American Bar Association 1800 M St., NW Washington, DC 20036 202-331-2297	
National Long-Term Care Ombudsman Resource Center http://www.ltcombudsman.org	Provides background information on support, technical assistance	National Committee for the Prevention of Elder Abuse 1730 Rhode Island Ave., NW, Suite 1200 Washington, DC 20036 202-464-9481 http://www.preventelderabuse.org	
National Council on Aging 409 Third St., SW, Suite 200 Washington, DC 20024 800-424-9046 http://www.ncoa.org	Addresses many aging issues through various programs		
Commission on Law and Aging American Bar Association 750 N. Lake Shore Dr. Chicago, IL 60611 312-988-5000 http://www.abanet.org/aging	Provides information on laws pertinent to elders; has contact information by state and other law-related services for legal assistance providers; provides mandatory reporting requirements for each state. Makes available Domestic Violence and Sexual Assault in Later Life, a resource packet of information and materials accessible online.	National Committee for the Prevention of Elder Abuse c/o Institute on Aging 119 Belmont St. Worcester, MA 01605 508-793-6166	
		Elder Care Locator U.S. Administration on Aging 1-800-677-1116	

health aide visits, respite services, day programs, accessible transportation, support groups, adult day care, and church activities or pastoral visitations.[16,23] When mistreatment results because the caregiver is overburdened, interventions to decrease stress and anxiety may be welcomed by all parties. Spouses are most likely to be primary caregivers; most of these are women. Lack of sleep and inadequate exercise and nutrition are commonly expressed by caregivers, perhaps leading to anger and risk of abuse. Services for caregivers may be publicly funded or community based with support groups. Some programs provide home-delivered meals, respite care, counseling, and assistance with advance directives and estate planning.[24]

If available, medical case management teams can provide consultation and support by assisting in the multidisciplinary evaluation of suspected abuse cases and developing treatment plans. Team members generally are composed of a physician, nurses, and social workers.[25] Teams may make house calls, arrange physical and occupational therapy, and provide for nutritional improvement and management of disease states. Legal intervention teams can also be used to address financial management, probate and guardianships, and other legal and housing issues. Civil courts can issue protective orders, create guardianships, and issue emergency removal orders.

PRACTICE GUIDELINES

Recommendations for ED management of cases of elder abuse and neglect are provided in **Table 295-6**.

TABLE 295-6 American College of Emergency Physicians Policy on Domestic Family Violence[30]

Emergency personnel assess patients for intimate partner violence, child and elder maltreatment, and neglect.
Emergency physicians are familiar with signs and symptoms of intimate partner violence, child and elder maltreatment, and neglect.
Emergency medical services, medical schools, and emergency medicine residency curricula should include education and training in recognition, assessment, and interventions in intimate partner violence, child and elder maltreatment, and neglect.
Hospitals and EDs encourage clinical and epidemiologic research regarding the incidence and prevalence of family violence as well as best practice approaches to detection, assessment, and intervention for victims of family violence.
Hospitals and EDs are encouraged to participate in collaborative interdisciplinary approaches for the recognition, assessment, and intervention of victims of family violence. These approaches include the development of policies, protocols, and relationships with outside agencies that oversee the management and investigation of family violence.
Hospitals and EDs should maintain appropriate education regarding state legal requirements for reporting intimate partner violence and child and elder maltreatment.

SPECIAL CONSIDERATIONS

BARRIERS TO THE DETECTION OF ELDER ABUSE

Sufferers of elder abuse often have low self-esteem and may blame themselves for the abuse. They may not want to admit vulnerabilities and feel disgraced for having raised a child who would betray them.[23,26]

Elder abuse victims may also be unwilling to press charges against a family member. Abused older adults are frequently unaware of available resources.[26] In addition, they may harbor a fear of being removed from the home or placed in a nursing institution, of implicating family members, or of experiencing further abuse in retaliation for having divulged information. They may worry about not being believed. Abusers may control access to others and prevent encounters with outsiders to ensure that secrecy is maintained. There may also be differing perceptions as to what constitutes abuse based on cultural background.[27]

Physicians may fail to report abuse for a variety of reasons. They may not be familiar with reporting laws or adequately understand reporting mechanisms.[4] They may fear offending patients or their family members. Time constraints in the ED can also be a barrier to recognition and reporting. There are no published studies of physical markers of mistreatment to distinguish preventable injury from intentional, inflicted, or avoidable trauma.[28] In addition, some physicians may have the misperception that the law requires them to obtain the patient's permission before reporting suspected abuse.[29] Hospitals may also lack protocols for identifying or addressing elder abuse.

ABUSE IN LONG-TERM CARE FACILITIES

Elder abuse in nursing homes is well documented. In one study, 36% of nurses and nursing aides working in long-term care facilities reported witnessing at least one act of physical abuse in the previous year.[31] A study of 2400 deaths in Arkansas nursing homes found 50 cases of suspected abuse or neglect, which indicates that forensic studies need to play a larger role in the investigation of unexplained deaths of older adults in long-term care facilities.[32] Abuse in institutional settings manifests in similar ways to abuse in residential settings: theft of money or personal property, unsanitary conditions, poor personal hygiene, sexual assault, physical abuse or unexplained injury, bed sores, physical or chemical restraint, and malnutrition and dehydration. Nursing homes participating in Medicare and Medicaid programs must comply with certain quality-of-care requirements.[33] Suspicion of abuse or neglect among patients in nursing homes should be reported to the state nursing home ombudsman program (http://www.ltcombudsman.org) or to an adult protective services agency.

LEGAL CONSIDERATIONS

Circumstances may occur in which hospital admission is advised, but the patient refuses. If the patient is competent, his or her wishes must be honored, even if those wishes do not appear to be in the patient's self-best interest. Decisional capacity by the patient depends on his/her ability to understand all of the relevant information in order to make a choice, to communicate that choice, and to appreciate the current situation and treatment options. In these cases, it is especially important to interview the patient alone and to explain in detail the concerns of the healthcare provider. The physician should also attempt to explore reasons for the patient's reluctance to stay.

Patients who refuse admission but who lack decision-making capacity should not be discharged back to an unsafe environment. Contact with an adult protective services agency should be initiated. ED social workers can help locate contact information for the local adult protective services agency. If the agency determines that the victim of abuse lacks decision-making capacity, an emergency order for protective services may need to be sought from the courts.

REFERENCES

The complete reference list is available online at www.TintinalliEM.com.

SECTION 26

Special Situations

CHAPTER 296 Injection Drug Users

Thomas Grosheider
Suzanne M. Shepherd

INTRODUCTION AND EPIDEMIOLOGY

Illicit drug use is a major health issue globally. It is estimated that in 2011 between 167 and 315 million people worldwide used illicit substances.[1] In 2012, an estimated 23.9 million Americans ≥12 years of age used an illicit drug within the previous month, and of these, 669,000 used heroin, nearly triple the prevalence in 2008.[2] Between 2006 and 2011, heroin-related ED visits increased from 189,780 to 258,482, with the majority of visits made by men (69%) and patients age 35 to 44 years.[2] More recently, ED visits due to severe overdoses have been precipitated by drug distributor substitution of the synthetic opiate fentanyl for heroin as a "super high."[3]

The practice of injection drug use and the lifestyle and culture of the injection drug user place the individual at risk for a wide variety of complications, including human immunodeficiency virus (HIV) infection, hepatitis, tetanus, sexually transmitted diseases, trauma, and intimate partner violence.[4] The high incidence of migration, incarceration, homelessness, nutritional deficiencies, coincident smoking and alcohol use, and mental illness further compromises this population's health.[5]

PATHOPHYSIOLOGY

Injection drug use is associated with immune dysregulation. Exaggerated and atypical lymphocytosis, diminished lymphocyte responsiveness to mitogenic stimulation and depressed chemotaxis, hypergammaglobulinemia, increased opsonin production, decreased T-cell and natural killer cell activity, high levels of circulating immune complexes, and reticuloendothelial abnormalities have been found in injection drug users. False-positive results on nontreponemal syphilis serologic tests, positive results on Coombs tests, low measured antibody response to vaccination, and thrombotic thrombocytopenic purpura are some described abnormalities. HIV-infected patients who inject drugs are found to be less likely to suppress HIV-1 RNA than those who do not inject drugs. Given the immune dysfunction, febrile injection drug users should be suspected of having infections, even when the fever is low grade and WBC counts and erythrocyte sedimentation rates are normal.

CLINICAL FEATURES

To adequately evaluate the histories of injection drug users, be aware of the drugs used locally and regionally, drug street names (e.g., "smack," "H," "Mexican mud," "junk," "bud light," "theraflu"), and drug adulterants. Ask about drug type(s) and amount, preparation of materials for injection (e.g., crushing capsules in the mouth, licking needles, blowing on injection sites or blowing out clots in needles, or using saliva, lemon juice, or tap or toilet water for drug reconstitution), reuse of needles, needle sharing, use of antibiotics, and coincident medical and mental illness. Consider socioeconomic issues, such as the ability to purchase medications and access to outpatient follow-up, in patient disposition.

Complications of injection drug use may be obvious, such as a painful, erythematous, fluctuant skin abscess. However, subtle constitutional symptoms such as weakness, anorexia, body pains, myalgias and arthralgias, weight loss, and fever are common and may be the only signs of serious underlying disease (**Table 296-1**).

FEVER

Fever is associated with infection in more than two thirds of patients. Noninfectious causes of fever include acute toxic reactions to substances of abuse, reactions to injected adulterants, and withdrawal syndromes. Cocaine and amphetamines can cause acute fever, occasionally in excess of 40°C (104°F). Adulterants used to dilute active substances may also cause dramatic febrile reactions accompanied by alteration in mental status and leukocytosis. "**Cotton fever**" is a flulike syndrome developing within hours of injection, after the use of cotton balls as filters for drug suspensions. Physical findings may include tachypnea, tachycardia, abdominal pain, and inflammatory retinal nodules. Chest radiographs typically show normal findings but may demonstrate inflammatory pulmonary granulomata. This syndrome spontaneously resolves within 24 hours.[6] Drug withdrawal from benzodiazepines, barbiturates, or heroin also may cause acute illness with chest and abdominal pain, diaphoresis, tachycardia, and fever.

Because no reliable markers are available to exclude serious illness in the febrile injection drug user, common practice has been to obtain specimens for blood culture and admit such patients for observation while culture results are awaited (also see "Infective Endocarditis" section below). In clinically well patients for whom follow-up can be ensured, outpatient evaluation is reasonable as long as appropriate culture specimens are obtained.

DYSPNEA

A wide range of both infectious and noninfectious entities may produce dyspnea and cough in injection drug users. Pneumonia is typically community acquired (see "Pulmonary Infections" section below). However, dyspnea may have other infectious causes, including infections related to aspiration during drug intoxication, tuberculosis, opportunistic infections, and septic pulmonary emboli complicating right-sided endocarditis. The febrile injection drug user with dyspnea, cough, or abnormal findings on chest radiograph should be placed in respiratory isolation until tuberculosis has been excluded and/or an alternative diagnosis is found.[7]

Noninfectious causes of dyspnea include pneumothorax, hemothorax, toxic reaction to injected substances, and hypersensitivity reaction. Pneumothorax and hemothorax are seen most commonly in association with the practice of "pocket shooting," in which drug users, or their drug-injecting partners, inject into veins in the supraclavicular fossa to access the subclavian, jugular, or brachiocephalic vein. "Talc lung" is a syndrome of progressive respiratory distress and diffuse interstitial infiltrates caused by the injection of adulterant talc. Hypersensitivity reactions, associated with both heroin and cocaine injection, cause cough and wheezing and typically respond to inhaled β-agonist therapy. Noncardiogenic pulmonary edema is associated with both heroin and cocaine use. Signs and symptoms include dyspnea, hypoxia, and diffuse alveolar infiltrates on chest x-ray. Treatment is supportive. Finally, septic, air, or needle fragment emboli can produce dyspnea.

TABLE 296-1 Evaluation of Injection Drug Users in the ED

Presenting Symptom	Potential Findings	Possible Diagnoses	Ancillary Tests
Fever alone	Needle and track marks Heart murmur Rales and rhonchi Hypoxia	Pneumonia Endocarditis Occult bacteremia	Chest radiography Blood cultures Urinalysis Erythrocyte sedimentation rate Echocardiography
Fever with nausea and vomiting, rigors, abdominal pain	Diaphoresis Recent injection	Drug withdrawal "Cotton fever" Hepatitis	CBC count Blood cultures Hepatitis serologic testing Liver panel
Fever with dyspnea and cough	Rales and rhonchi Purulent sputum Hypoxia	Bacterial pneumonia Atypical pneumonia Tuberculosis Pneumonia due to opportunistic organisms Septic pulmonary emboli	Chest radiography Blood cultures Sputum culture and Gram staining Chest CT
Fever with weakness, weight loss, anorexia, night sweats, diarrhea	Cachexia Oral thrush	HIV infection Tuberculosis Hepatitis B and C	HIV serologic testing Blood cultures Chest radiography Sputum staining for acid-fast bacillus, sputum culture Hepatitis serologic testing
Fever with back pain	Heart murmur Focal neurologic signs Flank tenderness	Osteomyelitis Epidural abscess Endocarditis Renal abscess	Blood cultures Erythrocyte sedimentation rate Bone radiography CT or MRI Urinalysis
Dyspnea and cough	Expiratory wheezes Rales and rhonchi Fever Pleuritic chest pain	Hypersensitivity reaction Noncardiogenic pulmonary edema Pneumonia Septic pulmonary emboli Talc reaction	Chest radiography Spirometry Echocardiography Consider blood cultures
Painful limb	Localized erythema Tenderness Localized bruit Muscle pain and swelling Fever	Cellulitis Abscess Pseudoaneurysm Myositis Fasciitis Retained foreign body	Wound specimen cultures Soft tissue radiography CT Doppler US Consider blood cultures
Altered mental status	Obtundation Focal neurologic signs Meningismus Seizure	Drug overdose or intoxication Drug withdrawal CNS lesion Meningitis Tetanus	CT Drug screen Lumbar puncture Consider blood cultures
Eye pain and vision loss	Periorbital vesicles Subconjunctival lesions Keratitis Iridocyclitis Retinitis Poorly reactive pupil Vitreous exudates	Herpes zoster Kaposi sarcoma Keratoconjunctivitis sicca Herpes simplex Cytomegalovirus infection Varicella zoster Toxoplasmosis Syphilis Fungal infection	Viral and fungal cultures Serology for syphilis

Abbreviation: HIV = human immunodeficiency virus.

ALTERED MENTAL STATUS AND NEUROLOGIC ABNORMALITIES

Drug intoxication or withdrawal, stroke syndromes, hypoxia, delayed leukoencephalopathy, infectious diseases, mycotic aneurysms, and secondary trauma from either loss of consciousness and fall or drug-related violence may all produce altered mental status or other neurologic impairment in the injection drug user. CNS infections may result from contiguous spread of overlying soft tissue infection, embolic complications of distant infections (e.g., endocarditis), or extension of local infections (e.g., vertebral osteomyelitis). Infections that affect the nervous system and commonly occur in this population include epidural abscess, bacterial and fungal meningitis, and brain abscess. Meningococcus, pneumococcus, and *Staphylococcus aureus* bacteremia from primary endocarditis are the common causes of bacterial meningitis. Both tetanus and botulism are reported, with cranial nerve involvement, altered mental status, and progressive symmetric paralysis.[8]

Infections caused by opportunistic organisms, such as *Toxoplasma*, are common in patients with coincident HIV infection who have low CD4 counts (especially <100). Stroke syndromes may occur secondary to low-flow states during heroin intoxication; hypertensive hemorrhage from amphetamines, phencyclidine, or cocaine; and embolized vegetations associated with infectious endocarditis. Delayed leukoencephalopathies, both hypoxic and nonhypoxic, have been reported in injection drug users, but are rare.

BACK PAIN

Back pain may result from an epidural abscess, vertebral osteomyelitis, or complications from trauma. In patients with coincident HIV infection, opportunistic infections may present with a more indolent course, and the only symptom may be local pain. Nontraumatic focal back pain usually requires imaging studies such as CT and MRI to evaluate for possible infection.

SPECIFIC INFECTIONS IN INJECTION DRUG USERS

HUMAN IMMUNODEFICIENCY VIRUS INFECTION

The use of IV drugs continues to play a major role in the acquisition and transmission of HIV; however, data from the United States and Central and South America have demonstrated a gradual decline in the prevalence of HIV infection due to injection drug use. From 2003 to 2009, the prevalence decreased from 19% to 16%.[9] See chapter 154, "Human Immunodeficiency Virus Infection" for further management.

INFECTIVE ENDOCARDITIS

The incidence of endocarditis in injection drug users is rising,[10] and this patient group appears to be driving the increased incidence of infective endocarditis in North America.[11] Prior incidence estimates of endocarditis in injection drug users presenting with fever to the ED (13% in general[12,13] and 40% in an inner-city population[14]) were based on data two to three decades old. Two studies published since 2011 based on 485 patients reveal that 7.8% of febrile injection drug users hospitalized with "fever without a source" have evidence of endocarditis on echocardiography.[15,16] Unlike endocarditis in the general population, endocarditis in injection drug users involves the right side of the heart (57% to 86% of cases).[15,17] The most common causative organism for infective endocarditis in injection drug users is *S. aureus* (70%), and one third of those cases involve methicillin-resistant *S. aureus*.[17,18] Licking needles prior to injection has been implicated in infections with *Eikenella corrodens*, *Haemophilus parainfluenzae*, *Bacteroides* species, and *Neisseria* species. Up to 20% of cases of injection drug use–related endocarditis are polymicrobial infections.[8]

Clinical features of endocarditis in injection drug users are dominated by right-side heart involvement with respiratory complaints, including dyspnea, cough, and hemoptysis. Multiple opacities on chest radiograph, consistent with septic pulmonary emboli, are common (**Figures 296-1 and 296-2**). Other findings include pyuria (22%) and hematuria (35%) and are due to glomerulonephritis from immune complex deposition, embolic renal infarction, and perinephric abscess.[16,19] A clinical prediction rule to identify endocarditis in febrile injection drug users has been derived[15] and internally validated[16] and assesses sequentially for the presence of a pulse rate >100, absence of skin infection, and presence of murmur. The rule was 100% sensitive (95% confidence interval, 84% to 100%) in the derivation and validation cohorts, but specificity was only 13%,[16] and the scoring system used is complex, requiring comparison to a nomogram. The prediction rule has not been externally validated and cannot be recommended at this time. For further direction regarding diagnosis of endocarditis, treatment with antibiotics, and management of complications see chapter 155, "Endocarditis."

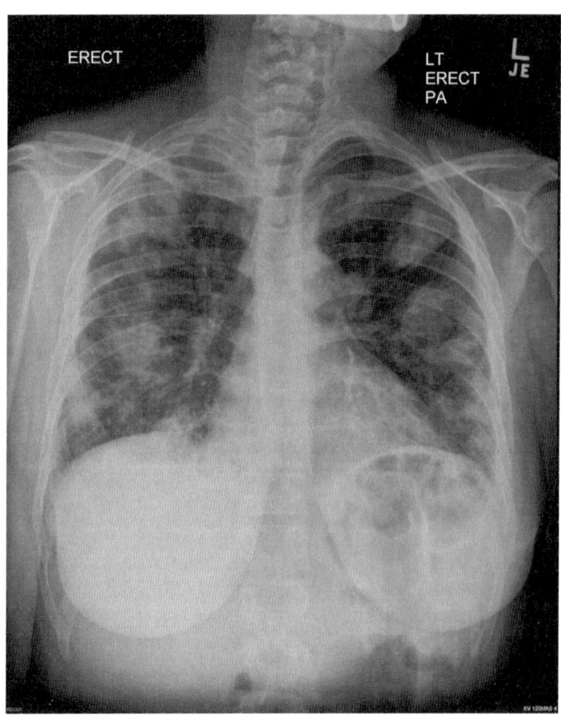

FIGURE 296-1. Chest radiograph showing septic emboli. Multiple opacities are seen in this chest radiograph of an injection drug–using female patient who was found to have bacterial endocarditis.

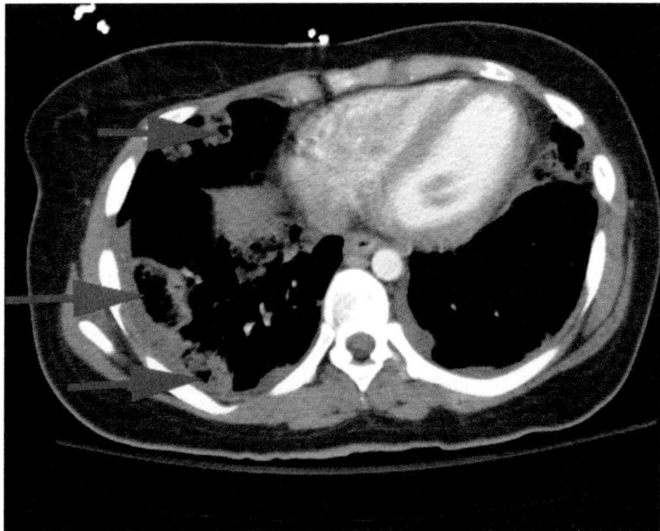

FIGURE 296-2. CT image showing multiple peripheral cavitary lesions (*arrows*) consistent with septic pulmonary emboli.

PULMONARY INFECTIONS

Community-acquired pneumonia caused by *Streptococcus pneumoniae* and *Haemophilus influenzae* remains the most common pulmonary infection in injection drug users, with a 10-fold increased risk for community-acquired pneumonia in the injection drug user population.[8] Patients are also at high risk for pneumonia due to *S. aureus*, including methicillin-resistant *S. aureus*; *Klebsiella pneumoniae* infection; aspiration pneumonia; tuberculosis; and, in HIV-positive patients, opportunistic infections caused by *Pneumocystis jiroveci*, cytomegalovirus, and atypical mycobacteria.[8] Results of the purified protein derivative (tuberculin) skin test may be negative in these patients. Patients may present with atypical clinical and radiographic findings of tuberculosis[20] (see chapter 67, "Tuberculosis").

Because of the risk of atypical infection, coincident bacteremia, and potential for endocarditis in patients with multiple infiltrates on chest radiograph, admission to the hospital is recommended, and respiratory isolation should be maintained until tuberculosis is excluded.[8,14] In patients without risk for *Pseudomonas* infection, IV quinolone and IV ceftriaxone or cefotaxime provide reasonable empiric coverage until culture results are available. In those at risk for *Pseudomonas* infection (structural lung disease, malnutrition, current or recent corticosteroid use or antibiotic use), a preferred regimen is an IV antipseudomonal β-lactamase agent (cefepime, imipenem, meropenem, or piperacillin/tazobactam) and an IV antipseudomonal fluoroquinolone or an antipseudomonal β-lactamase agent, IV aminoglycoside, and fluoroquinolone.[21] For further discussion, see chapter 65, "Pneumonia and Pulmonary Infiltrates."

SKIN AND SOFT TISSUE INFECTIONS

Skin and soft tissue infections are some of the most common infections among injection drug users and include cellulitis, subcutaneous abscesses, septic phlebitis, necrotizing fasciitis, Fournier's gangrene, gas gangrene, and pyomyositis. Most are caused by the user's own commensal flora, with *S. aureus* and streptococcal species remaining the most common pathogens. Because these infections are often self-treated and reporting is not required, the prevalence is difficult to determine but is estimated to be as high as 32%.[22]

Tap water, toilet water, lemon juice, or saliva may be used to dissolve narcotics or cocaine, and each has been implicated as a source of causative organisms, such as *Pseudomonas* and *Candida*, in both skin and blood-borne infections.[8] In 2013, an outbreak (43 individuals, 13 deaths in Scotland) of cutaneous anthrax in heroin users was reported from the United Kingdom.[23] The recent use of desomorphine (street name **Krokodil**), an extremely addictive morphine derivative that typically contains large amounts of toxic synthesis components, including iodine and phosphorus, demonstrates the serious damage to skin, blood vessels, bone, and muscles that illegal drug injection can produce. Many long-term desomorphine users have required limb amputation, which has given this drug the nickname "the flesh-eating drug."[24]

CLINICAL FEATURES AND DIAGNOSIS

Presenting signs and symptoms of cutaneous infections, including pyomyositis, are fever, pain, localized erythema, and edema. Carefully inspect the painful area for fluctuance, crepitus, and lymphangitis. Diagnosis is primarily clinical, except when evaluating an abscess where pulsations are present. Cellulitis and abscesses are typically caused by *S. aureus* (primarily community-acquired methicillin-resistant *S. aureus*) and *Streptococcus* species.[25] Cultures of specimens from cutaneous abscesses may also demonstrate polymicrobial growth, with aerobic gram-negative rods, anaerobic cocci, and bacilli.[8] Increased rates of *Clostridium botulinum* infection have also been found in injection drug users who engage in skin popping, particularly those using Mexican black tar heroin. Mortality rates due to tetanus are highest in older, unvaccinated patients. Other concerns include retained portions of broken needles, which act as a nidus for infection and, in addition, pose an increased risk to the examining healthcare provider. Needles may be identified by radiograph prior to exploration. Individuals may have already attempted to treat abscesses before coming to seek medical care by incision and drainage, illegally purchased antibiotics, or some form of homeopathic care. This is particularly prevalent in Latino populations and those who do not have a usual place of health care.[26]

Infections overlying venipuncture sites may produce thrombophlebitis and infected pseudoaneurysms. Femoral vein injection ("groin hit") has been associated with the development of local gangrene as well as rapidly progressive and fatal Fournier's gangrene. Injection into the jugular vein ("pocket shot") may lead to cutaneous abscess formation involving the carotid triangle and produce airway obstruction, vocal cord paralysis, and laryngeal edema.[8]

IMAGING

For nonpulsatile areas of induration, bedside US can define an underlying abscess. Pulsatile masses, however, must be imaged with Doppler US prior to incision and drainage, because attempts to aspirate or incise and drain an infected pseudoaneurysm can result in severe hemorrhage (see section titled "Vascular Infections" below). CT angiography may identify vasospasm, thrombosis, emboli, or mycotic aneurysms. Plain radiographs can demonstrate air in the soft tissues as well as radiopaque foreign bodies. CT delineates the involvement of other structures and the extent of deep abscesses, especially in complex areas such as the neck.

TREATMENT

Uncomplicated abscesses, large furuncles, and carbuncles should be incised, drained, and packed. Injection drug users with superficial cellulitis without evidence of systemic involvement can be managed as outpatients with oral antibiotics to cover streptococci and methicillin-resistant *S. aureus*. See chapter 152, "Soft Tissue Infections," for discussion of antibiotic choices, abscess drainage, care for the septic patient, and disposition decision making.

VASCULAR INFECTIONS

Distal vascular injury and endovascular infections associated with injection drug use include inadvertent arterial injection with resultant vasospasm or thrombosis, septic thrombophlebitis, venous and arterial pseudoaneurysms, and infected hematomas. Arterial injection rarely results in major vessel occlusion; instead, pain, edema, and patchy mottling of the affected limb occur due to ischemia. Tissue necrosis and gangrene are the consequence of persistent focal ischemia, the cause of which is thought to be a combination of vasospasm, embolization of particulate matter, and endothelial injury leading to thrombosis and vasculitis.[27]

When limb ischemia is suspected, a vascular surgeon should determine whether surgical intervention or intra-arterial thrombolysis is indicated. However, the majority of cases involve distal vessels, and treatment is limited to anticoagulation and supportive care. Limb edema can progress to compartment syndrome, which may require fasciotomy, or may be complicated by rhabdomyolysis.

Infected pseudoaneurysm is a commonly reported vascular complication in injection drug users due to accidental or intentional intra-arterial drug injection and is most often reported in the femoral artery, followed by the radial and brachial arteries.[27] **Figure 296-3** shows a radial artery pseudoaneurysm. Venous pseudoaneurysms are relatively rare and are usually secondary to septic phlebitis, with the femoral vein most often involved. Signs are typically fever and a painful mass. This is a severe complication that can result in life-threatening hemorrhage and sepsis, chronic claudication, chronic skin and soft tissue infections and post-traumatic ulcers, and limb loss. A 23% amputation rate is reported with involvement of the femoral bifurcation. Although the lesion is similar in gross appearance to an abscess, the presence of pulsations and a bruit suggest this diagnosis. Because of the disastrous hemorrhagic consequences of attempted incision and drainage, all painful masses, particularly in the groin, should be expeditiously imaged with US or contrast CT.

In all cases of suspected endovascular infection, antibiotic therapy should be initiated and may be guided by the therapeutic recommendations for endocarditis given above (see "Infective Endocarditis").

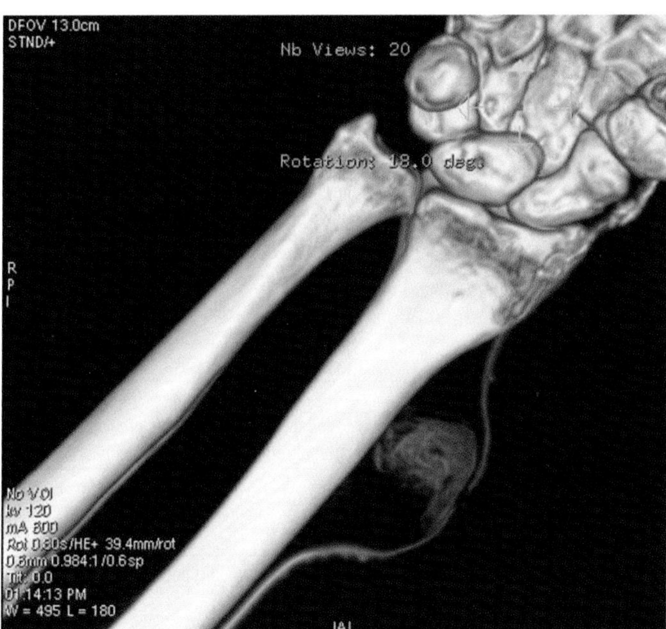

FIGURE 296-3. Volume-rendering CT of the wrist showing a radial artery pseudoaneurysm in the inferior portion of the image. The pseudoaneurysm has displaced the radial artery away from the bony radius.

Surgical treatment options for infected femoral artery pseudoaneurysm are limited due to infection of the surgical field, lack of available autologous graft materials because of deep and superficial venous thromboses from long-term injection, and a high likelihood of continued injection drug use, which increases the risk of postoperative infection and other complications. One therapeutic option is the ligation and resection of the infected pseudoaneurysm without revascularization. Initial outcomes may be favorable; however, long-term morbidity includes claudication, which can become severe, leading to eventual limb amputation.[28,29] A second option is ligation of the common femoral artery without revascularization, accompanied by excision and drainage of the internal femoral artery pseudoaneurysm and routine selective revascularization via either arterial reconstruction with an autologous greater saphenous vein graft or synthetic graft in situ or extra-anatomically.

BONE AND JOINT INFECTIONS

EPIDEMIOLOGY AND PATHOLOGY

Musculoskeletal infections usually occur either through contiguous spread from an overlying skin or soft tissue infection or, more commonly, through hematogenous spread from a distant site. Infecting microorganisms in injection drug users may be unusual, with *Candida* and gram-negative organisms seen, especially *Pseudomonas aeruginosa*. Likely organisms include *S. aureus* (including methicillin-resistant *S. aureus*), *Staphylococcus epidermidis*, *P. aeruginosa*, and *Streptococcus* species.[30] Because of the high incidence of sexually transmitted diseases in this population, also consider gonococcal arthritis and tenosynovitis. *E. corrodens* osteomyelitis is reported in those who lick their needles prior to injection.

CLINICAL FEATURES AND DIAGNOSIS OF OSTEOMYELITIS

Osteomyelitis can develop in the axial skeleton, with another common location being the tibia, often in association with hardware from treatment of a prior fracture.[30] Contiguous septic arthritis can coexist with osteomyelitis.[30] Candidal infections are postulated to be hematogenous in origin and have been related to the use of contaminated reconstituted lemon juice to mix drugs before injection.[8] Some patients report an initial flulike syndrome lasting 3 to 4 days, followed by the appearance of metastatic lesions involving the skin, eye (chorioretinitis and endophthalmitis; see "Ophthalmologic Infections" section below), and the bones and joints several days to weeks later. Rarely, *Aspergillus* species may cause osteomyelitis of the sternum in injection drug users.

Vertebral osteomyelitis usually presents with localized pain and tenderness to palpation over the involved bone, and a soft tissue mass may be palpable. Osteomyelitis may coexist with spinal epidural abscess.[31] Symptoms may be present for days in the case of bacterial infections to weeks in the case of fungal or mycobacterial infections. The presence of both fever and leukocytosis and an elevated erythrocyte sedimentation rate and C-reactive protein level are helpful, if present, but their absence does not exclude these infections. Drainage from contiguous abscesses should be cultured. Biopsy or needle aspiration of joint spaces and bony infections may be necessary, especially in the case of infection with unusual or fastidious organisms, such as *Mycobacterium*, *Candida*, or *Eikenella*.

Imaging for Osteomyelitis Imaging for patients with suspected osteomyelitis varies by institution, but MRI is generally the imaging modality of choice. CT may reveal disk space narrowing and bony lysis suggesting osteomyelitis, but it is neither as sensitive nor as specific as MRI.[31] Patients with osteomyelitis warrant admission, and unless the patient appears septic or has focal neurologic complaints or coincident endocarditis is a concern, antibiotic therapy should be withheld until culture results are obtained.

Treatment of Osteomyelitis Early consultation with the orthopedist or neurosurgeon should guide the timing of antimicrobial coverage, because blood culture results may not be sufficient, and a CT-guided needle biopsy for epidural abscess or a bone sample for culture for osteomyelitis may be required.[25] Antimicrobial choice should be based on culture results (for a biopsy specimen), and therapy is typically required for 4 to 6 weeks. Injection drug use patients in unstable condition who are suspected of having osteomyelitis should receive vancomycin to cover *S. aureus* and ceftazidime to cover *Pseudomonas* (see chapter 281, "Hip and Knee Pain," for further discussion).

SEPTIC ARTHRITIS

Septic arthritis in injection drug users usually involves the knee or hip but may coexist with osteomyelitis in approximately 16% of cases.[30] Sternoclavicular septic arthritis strongly suggests injection drug use.[32] For further discussion of diagnosis and treatment of septic arthritis, see chapter 284, "Joints and Bursae."

OPHTHALMOLOGIC INFECTIONS

Ophthalmologic infections in injection drug users are usually the result of hematogenous seeding from a primary source of infection, such as endocarditis, or of opportunistic infections associated with HIV disease. Bacterial endophthalmitis often presents acutely, with pain, redness, lid swelling, and decrease in visual acuity. Inflammation is usually present in both the anterior and posterior chambers. White-centered, flame-shaped embolic hemorrhages (Roth spots), cotton-wool exudates, and macular holes may be present. *S. aureus* is the most commonly isolated organism, followed by *Streptococcus* species. Treatment involves subconjunctival and systemic antibiotic therapy, most commonly vancomycin and ceftazidime.[33] Surgical intervention may be needed. Visual prognosis is poor.[33]

Fungal organisms, usually *Candida*, are an important cause of endophthalmitis among injection drug users. Such fungal infections were considered rare until Mexican black tar heroin arrived in the 1980s, and lemon juice was used to dissolve this relatively water-insoluble compound.[34] Symptoms include blurred vision, pain, poorly reactive pupil, and decreased visual acuity and can progress over days to weeks. White cotton-like lesions are seen on the choroid retina, with vitreous haziness. Uveitis, papillitis, and vitreitis also have been reported. Presumptive diagnosis is defined as the presence of typical ocular lesions in an injection drug user. Microbiologic diagnosis is made from the results of blood and vitreous culture. Treatment includes amphotericin B and voriconazole.[33] Aspergillosis is the second most common fungal cause of endophthalmitis in injection drug users, producing ocular symptoms and signs without cutaneous or musculoskeletal involvement. The visual prognosis for fungal endophthalmitis depends on prompt diagnosis and treatment but frequently is poor.[33] Immediate consultation with an ophthalmologist is necessary to ensure appropriate management and a positive outcome. In injection drug users co-infected with HIV, cytomegalovirus infection, toxoplasmosis retinitis, and choroidal *Cryptococcus* and *Mycobacterium avium-intracellulare* complex infections must also be considered.

REFERENCES

The complete reference list is available online at www.TintinalliEM.com.

The Transplant Patient

J. Hayes Calvert

INTRODUCTION

As of the beginning of 2013, there were 76,047 active candidates waiting for solid-organ transplants in the United States, with the kidney transplant waitlist being the largest at 57,903 candidates.[1] The kidney is the most commonly transplanted organ (58%), followed by liver (21%), heart (8%), lung (5%), pancreas (5%), and, less commonly, combined organ transplants and intestine transplants. Annually, there are around 18,000 hematopoietic stem cell transplants in the United States, with about one third of these transplants being allogenic transplants and two thirds being autologous transplants.[2]

Most transplant patients require lifelong immunosuppression. Transplant patients can develop a number of acute to life-threatening emergencies, including (1) transplant-related infection, (2) medication side effects, (3) rejection, (4) graft-versus-host disease, and (5) postoperative complications or complications of altered physiology secondary to the transplanted organ. Transplant patients may also have common medical problems that require unique management. Adverse outcomes often are directly proportional to increasing age of the recipient and the donor organ.[3]

The most common acute disorders prompting ED visits are infection (39%) followed by noninfectious GI/GU pathology (15%), dehydration (15%), electrolyte disturbances (10%), cardiopulmonary pathology (10%) or injury (8%), and rejection (6%).[4-7] Acute graft-versus-host disease is an important complication, especially in those with hematopoietic stem cell transplantation.[8] Coronary artery disease, sudden cardiac death, and heart failure are results of premature cardiovascular disease in solid-organ recipients, due to underlying comorbidities and metabolic effects of immunosuppression.[9] Preoperative and regular postoperative cardiovascular assessment identifies risk factors and enables treatment to mitigate risk effects.[10]

GENERAL APPROACH TO EVALUATION

HISTORY AND COMORBIDITIES

Key historical elements for the management of transplant patients are listed in **Table 297-1**.

PHYSICAL EXAMINATION

Direct the physical examination to the chief complaint, present illness, and evidence of complications of the transplant or immunosuppressive medications (**Table 297-2**).[4-8,11,12]

TABLE 297-1 Key Historical Elements Specific to Transplant Patients

Historical Item	Significance
Recent temperature increase or decrease from baseline	Potential clue to onset of infection or rejection.
Changes from baseline function	Decreased urine may signify rejection in renal transplant patients or acute dehydration. Decreased exercise tolerance may signify rejection in heart transplant patients. Change in skin color (jaundice specifically) may signify rejection in liver transplant patients or graft-versus-host disease.
Date of transplant surgery	The date from transplant helps to predict typical infections and types of posttransplant complications (i.e., graft-versus-host disease).
Graft source for solid-organ transplant, special features of graft if any, prior infections; donor living related vs cadaveric	These details predict the potential for certain infections and rejection.
Graft source for hematopoietic stem cell transplant: autologous, degree of match, related donor	These details predict potential graft-versus-host disease.
Rejection history	May predict current rejection if similar presentation and difficulty in controlling a current episode of rejection.
Recent changes in dosages of antirejection and other medications	Although a planned part of transplant management, rejection is very common when immunosuppression doses are reduced.
Chronic infections (CMV, Epstein-Barr virus, hepatitis B and C, other viruses)	History of chronic infections increases the chances that current presentation is an exacerbation.
Recent exposure to infections (chickenpox, CMV, tuberculosis)	Increases the chance of current infection.
Recent history of compliance with immunosuppressive medications	Noncompliance increases chance of rejection.
Recent travel, exposure to persons arriving from countries with endemic infections, exposure to potential foodborne illness or insect vectors	Exposure may predict unusual infections not commonly considered.
Complete list of all medications, including over-the-counter medication	Complex drug interactions are common causes of symptoms in transplant patients and must be evaluated.
Baseline: blood pressure, body weight, serum creatinine (for renal transplants), and expected levels of immunosuppressive medication	Changes in these parameters may predict rejection or acute illness.

Abbreviation: CMV = cytomegalovirus.

DIFFERENTIAL DIAGNOSIS

Consider complications of immunosuppressive medication, infection, solid-organ rejection, and graft-versus-host disease (**Tables 297-3 and 297-4**). Chronic immunosuppressant medications, including corticosteroids, cause a wide range of physical changes evident on physical examination. Medication changes should be made by, or in consultation with, the patient's transplant team. Outpatient or inpatient management depends on the severity of illness; the need for ongoing immunosuppression often requires admission when symptoms interrupt maintenance of medication.

Solid-organ rejection and graft-versus-host disease are immune-medicated inflammatory reactions that may present with fever, signs and symptoms, and laboratory and radiographic findings that resemble infection. Infection and rejection (or an exacerbation of graft-versus-host disease) can occur simultaneously, and treatment should be started for

TABLE 297-2 Physical Examination in Transplant Patients

Examination	Comments
Volume status	Check static vital signs, orthostatic blood pressures, and pulse. Use US to assess inferior vena cava diameter as a measure of intravascular volume status.
Head, ears, eyes, nose, and throat	Periorbital edema (glomerulonephritis), retina (CMV or toxoplasmic chorioretinitis, *Listeria* endophthalmitis), sinuses (*Staphylococcus aureus*, mucormycosis, and invasive fungal disease), mouth (*Candida*, HSV), neck (meningismus, retropharyngeal abscess), lymphadenopathy (CMV, EBV, hepatitis, posttransplant lymphoproliferative disorder).
Lungs	Pneumonia is a common source of infections in transplant patients. *Streptococcus pneumoniae* and other community-acquired agents are still common sources, but opportunistic infections, such as *Pneumocystis jiroveci* pneumonia, *Aspergillus*, tuberculosis, coccidioidomycosis, and viral pneumonias should be suspected. Noninfectious pulmonary infiltrates may also cause dyspnea.
Heart	Pericardial friction rubs as a complication of uremia and a wide range of viral infections. New heart murmur can represent infection.
Abdomen	Peritonitis without a defined source is one of the most common sites for infection in transplant patients. Right upper quadrant tenderness associated with hepatitis B and C, CMV, and EBV. Varicella-zoster virus causes pancreatitis. If left in place, peritoneal dialysis catheters can be sources of infection.
Flank and suprapubic area	The urinary tract was the most common site of infection identified.
Graft	Renal graft usually placed in abdominal flap; inspect (look for signs of wound infection), palpate (graft tenderness and swelling are often seen in acute rejection, outflow obstruction, and pyelonephritis), and auscultate (bruits suggest renal artery stenosis and AV malformation or AV fistula). Deep tenderness over liver graft could indicate abscess.
Rectal	Perirectal abscess is a common, yet often overlooked, source of infection in transplant patients.
Extremities	Access sites for hemodialysis can be sources of infection. Peripheral edema in the transplant patient can represent a number of different etiologies: recurrent versus de novo glomerulonephritis, renal graft failure, liver graft failure, cirrhosis, nephrotic syndrome (from native kidneys), renal vein thrombosis, malnutrition, hypoalbuminemia, and heart failure.
Skin	Rashes are commonly seen in graft-versus-host disease, viral syndromes (hepatitis B and EBV), cellulitis from indwelling catheter sites, nocardial cutaneous lesions, and drug reactions.
Mental status/neurologic examination	Cyclosporine/tacrolimus neurotoxicity, steroid psychosis, HSV encephalitis, *Listeria* meningitis/encephalitis, and cryptococcal meningitis.

Abbreviations: AV = atrioventricular; CMV = cytomegalovirus; EBV = Epstein-Barr virus; HSV = herpes simplex virus.

both. When suspecting acute rejection or acute graft-versus-host disease, consult the transplant team about treatment. Typically, high-dose corticosteroids are given, but the steroid, the dose, and the duration of therapy should be confirmed.

POSTTRANSPLANT INFECTIONS

Infections account for a large number of deaths in transplant patients, with many undiagnosed until autopsy. Viral and bacterial illnesses may occur concurrently. Febrile episodes in the early phase after allogenic stem cell transplantation are likely related to infections secondary to neutropenia. Immunosuppression-induced blunting of the inflammatory response may mask the classic signs, symptoms, and laboratory markers of infection if the patient presents early in the course of the illness. Later in the course of infection, patients may present with more advanced ominous signs such as seizure, obtundation, coma, and cardiac arrest.

TABLE 297-3 Adverse Reactions to Immunosuppressant Medications

Body System	Adverse Effects
Constitutional	Fever, rigors, malaise, dizziness, anorexia
Ophthalmologic	Blurred vision, conjunctivitis, cataracts, papilledema, blindness
Mouth/ears	Gingival hyperplasia, stomatitis, hearing loss, tinnitus
Respiratory	Cough, dyspnea, interstitial lung disease, pneumonitis, pleural effusion, noncardiogenic pulmonary edema
Cardiovascular	Hypertension, tachycardia, bradycardia, cardiomyopathy, congestive heart failure, hypotension, syncope
GI	Nausea, vomiting, diarrhea, epigastric pain, esophagitis, gastritis, hiccups, constipation, hepatotoxicity, ascites, pancreatitis, colonic necrosis, bleeding
Musculoskeletal	Myopathy, osteoporosis, tendon rupture
Hematologic	Neutropenia, lymphopenia, anemia, thrombocytopenia, bleeding, thrombosis
Renal	Nephrotoxicity, oliguria, dysuria, renal failure
Neurologic	Headache, vertigo, paresthesias, tremors, convulsions, agitation, neuropathy, confusion, generalized weakness, leukoencephalopathy, encephalopathy, cerebral edema
Skin	Alopecia, hirsutism, thickening, thinning, necrosis, edema
Metabolic	Electrolyte disturbances (sodium, potassium, calcium, magnesium, phosphorus), fluid retention, hypercholesterolemia, hyperlipidemia, hyperglycemia, hypoglycemia
Endocrine	Adrenal suppression
Immunogenic	Susceptibility to infection, acute allergic reactions, anaphylaxis

CLINICAL FEATURES

The most common reason for an ED visit by a transplant recipient is fever.[4-7] Fever may be masked by immunosuppressive agents and other factors such as steroids, uremia, and hyperglycemia, and may be absent in half of those with infection.[5] Fever may be due to factors other than infection, such as drug effects, hypersensitivity reaction, rejection, or malignancy. Fever in a transplant patient should prompt an aggressive workup, even if low grade.

TABLE 297-4 Physical Examination Clues to Complications of Medications and Graft-versus-Host Disease

Concern	Signs and Symptoms
Edema and other swelling	Assess symmetry, pain, color, temperature, and active range of motion. Suspect infection, orthopedic conditions, deep vein thrombosis (due to immobility).
Skin breakdown	The back, pressure points, heels, elbows, and leg ulcers (due to corticosteroid-induced weakness).
Joint range of motion	Shoulders, elbows, fingers, wrists, and knees (may be limited due to steroid-induced weakness or sclerodermatous skin changes).
Thoracic constriction	Relatively noncompliant edema like swelling on the chest wall. If present, ask about associated dyspnea on exertion.
Abdominal constriction	Firm skin. History of bloating, gas, constipation, diarrhea, nonspecific pains.
Sclerodermatous skin	Sclerodermatous skin changes can affect joint mobility and GI and respiratory function. Note the firmness of edema and skin, especially on the thorax and around joints. A firm, soft leather consistency of swelling, tougher than cardiogenic pitting edema, can be a serious problem. Assess for recent-onset dyspnea on exertion.
Dehydration	Increased thirst, loss of appetite, chills, fatigue, weakness, skin flushing, dark or decrease volume of urine, dry mouth, tachycardia, weight loss.
Electrolyte disturbance	Signs and symptoms of dehydration above, hypotension, headache, bradycardia or tachycardia, irregular heartbeat, tremor, muscle weakness, increased urination, constipation, altered tendon reflexes, mood changes, abdominal pain, weight loss, muscle cramping.

TABLE 297-5 Infections Stratified by Posttransplant Period

Period after Transplant/Conditions	Infection	Comments
<1 mo: resistant organisms	MRSA Vancomycin-resistant *Enterococcus faecalis* *Candida* species (including non-*albicans*)	Opportunistic infections are generally absent during this period as full effect of immunosuppression not complete. MRSA important in HSCT patients.
<1 mo: complications of surgery and hospitalization	Aspiration Catheter infection Wound infection Anastomotic leaks and ischemia *C. difficile* colitis	*Clostridium difficile* common during this period. Early graft injuries may abscess. Unexplained early signs of infection such as hepatitis, encephalitis, pneumonitis, or rash may be donor derived.
<1 mo: colonization of transplanted organ or HSCT neutropenia	*Aspergillus* *Pseudomonas* *Klebsiella* *Legionella*	Microbiologic analysis of aspirates or biopsy from surgery essential for therapeutic decisions.
<1 mo: HSCT-specific infections	Additional bacterial pathogens: *Streptococcus viridans* and enterococci Viral infections include respiratory syncytial virus and HSV	Neutropenia and mucocutaneous injury increase risk for HSCT patients. Lungs, bloodstream, and GI tract most commonly affected sites.
1–6 mo: in patients with *Pneumocystis jiroveci* pneumonia and antiviral (CMV, HBV) prophylaxis	Polyomavirus BK infection, nephropathy *C. difficile* colitis HCV infection Adenovirus infection, influenza *Cryptococcus neoformans* infection *Mycobacterium tuberculosis* infection Anastomotic complications	Activation of latent infections, relapse, residual, and opportunistic infections occur during this period. Viral pathogens and allograft rejection cause the majority of febrile episodes during this period. Polyomavirus BK, adenovirus infections, and recurrent HCV are becoming more common.
1–6 mo: in patients without prophylaxis	*Pneumocystis* Infection with herpesviruses (HSV, varicella-zoster virus, CMV, Epstein-Barr virus) HBV infection Infection with *Listeria, Nocardia, Toxoplasma, Strongyloides, Leishmania, Trypanosoma cruzi*	Discontinuation of prophylaxis at the end of this period may prompt active infection, especially CMV. Graft-versus-host disease and mucocutaneous injury increase risk for HSCT patients.
>6 mo: general	Community-acquired pneumonia and urinary tract infections Infection with *Aspergillus*, atypical molds, *Mucor* species Infection with *Nocardia, Rhodococcus* species	Community-acquired organisms dominate during this period. Transplant recipients have a persistently increased risk of infection due to community-acquired pathogens.
>6 mo: late viral infections	CMV infection (colitis and retinitis) Hepatitis (HBV, HCV) HSV encephalitis Community-acquired viral infections (severe acute respiratory syndrome, West Nile) JC polyomavirus infection (progressive multifocal leukoencephalopathy) Skin cancer, lymphoma (PTLD)	In some patients, chronic viral infections may cause allograft injury (e.g., cirrhosis from HCV infection in liver transplant recipients, bronchiolitis obliterans in lung transplant recipients, accelerated vasculopathy in heart transplant recipients with CMV infection) or a malignant condition such as PTLD or skin or anogenital cancers.

Abbreviations: CMV = cytomegalovirus; HBV = hepatitis B virus; HCV = hepatitis C virus; HSCT = hematopoietic stem cell transplant; HSV = herpes simplex virus; MRSA = methicillin-resistant *Staphylococcus aureus*; PTLD = posttransplantation lymphoproliferative disorder.

Signs and symptoms of infection depend on the type of infection and can, in part, be predicted by the time frame since the transplant (**Table 297-5**).[13] Combining all posttransplant period groups, urinary tract infections (43%) and pneumonia (23%) are likely to be the most common infections.[11] In contrast, a study of 238 ED presentations of febrile pediatric heart transplant patients found pneumonia in 24%, bacteremia in 3%, cellulitis in 2%, and urinary tract infection in 1%; the majority had a negative workup.[12]

DIAGNOSIS AND TREATMENT

The evaluation should include routine testing as well as additional tests based on complaint, history, and physical examination (**Table 297-6**).[14]

Leukopenia can represent acute bacterial infection,[5] and leukopenia with an increase in atypical lymphocytes is commonly seen with viral infections, especially cytomegalovirus. Pulmonary infections that are encountered frequently include *Pneumocystis jiroveci*, *Nocardia*, *Legionella pneumophila*, and *Aspergillus*; these require special stains and studies for accurate diagnosis.

Treatment recommendations should be determined by careful analysis of each individual patient for potential atypical infections requiring specific coverage. Empiric antimicrobial therapy for transplant patients is outlined in **Table 297-7**.[15-17] Empiric treatment prior to confirmatory studies centers first on antibacterial agents, and then, especially if there is concern for meningitis/encephalitis, on antiviral agents such as acyclovir. Discuss treatment of suspected fungal infections or atypical infections with the transplant team.

TABLE 297-6 Diagnostic Tests to Consider in the Evaluation of Infections in the Transplant Patient

Test	Comments
CBC	Leukocytosis or left shift of the WBC count may be blunted by immunosuppressive agents.
Renal function tests: BUN, creatinine	Essential in the evaluation of renal transplant patients, may help determine dosing of antibiotics in all transplant patients.
Liver function tests	May show mild transaminase elevations with cytomegalovirus and Epstein-Barr virus infections, and much higher elevations with hepatotropic viruses such as hepatitis B and C viruses. May be elevated in *Legionella* infections.
C-reactive protein	Significant elevations more likely in infections versus noninfectious infiltrates.
Procalcitonin level	Significant elevations more likely in infections versus noninfectious infiltrates.
CT of the brain	Focal infections in the brain are much more common in this population, but CT should be used only as clinically indicated.
Cyclosporine or tacrolimus level or other levels of immunosuppressants	These levels may be deliberately low depending on the desired level of immunosuppression. Bioavailability may be variable.
Cultures of mouth, sputum, urine, blood, stool, vascular access, and wound sites	Collect as indicated by history and physical. Urine *Legionella* antigen should be considered before treatment of patients with pneumonia with GI complaints. Bacterial and fungal cultures of blood and urine should be obtained on all patients.
Cerebrospinal fluid cultures and antigen tests	Collect as indicated by history and physical.
Serology: cytomegalovirus, Epstein-Barr virus, hepatitis, toxoplasmosis, cryptococcosis	Because viral and fungal cultures are not very sensitive, clinicians should rely on their acumen to order organism-specific antigen assays and antibody titers. When contemplating viral or parasitic infections, these tests should be obtained to allow identification of bacterial, fungal, and viral pathogens.
Chest radiograph	Infiltrates on chest radiograph may reflect infectious or noninfectious complications of hematopoietic stem cell transplant or organ transplant.
CT of the chest	Patients with evidence of pulmonary infiltrates on chest x-ray or high-resolution CT, but without productive sputum, may ultimately require bronchoscopy with bronchoalveolar lavage and transbronchial biopsy for definitive diagnosis.
CT or US to include the graft	These scans can be used to identify likely abscess formation or possible anastomotic leaks.
Tests after admission	Beyond the scope of this chapter, but may include biopsy of the transplanted organ, bronchoalveolar lavage on bronchoscopy, and focused imaging of suspected sites of infection.
Creatine kinase	May have increased levels in infections with certain organisms, such as *Legionella*.

GRAFT-VERSUS-HOST DISEASE

Graft-versus-host disease is a major cause of morbidity and mortality affecting approximately 50% of allogeneic hematopoietic stem cell transplantation patients,[18] but it also occurs after small bowel or liver transplantation.[19] Hyperacute graft-versus-host disease is an unusual and severe form of acute graft-versus-host disease. Onset occurs in the first week after hematopoietic stem cell transplantation and is characterized by fever, generalized erythroderma, severe hepatitis, fluid retention, widespread inflammation, and shock.[20]

Acute graft-versus-host disease is classified as appearance of the disease up to 100 days after transplant. A well-appearing hematopoietic stem cell transplantation recipient with a nonspecific **rash** (most common symptom) or **diarrhea** (second most common symptom) should be suspected of having new-onset or an exacerbation of graft-versus-host disease.[20] The most widely used graft-versus-host prophylaxis includes a combination of a calcineurin inhibitor (e.g., cyclosporine, tacrolimus) with methotrexate.[20] In patients who recover from acute graft-versus-host disease, later long-term complications from chronic graft-versus-host disease are common.

Chronic graft-versus-host disease is a late complication characterized by immune dysregulation.[21] It results in severe morbidity, with complications affecting skin (sclerodermatous contractures), muscles (myopathy), bone (osteoporosis), nerves (peripheral neuropathy), and the cardiopulmonary system (physical deconditioning).[22]

ACUTE GRAFT-VERSUS-HOST DISEASE

Consider graft-versus-host disease in any patient with a rash. Rash is often misattributed as a drug reaction. The typical rash is maculopapular, frequently demonstrating a brownish hue and slight scaling (**Figure 297-1**). The rash can be pruritic and painful. The distribution varies greatly but often affects palms and soles initially, and later progresses to cheek, ears, neck, trunk, chest, and upper back. In the more severe forms, erythroderma or bullae develop.[8] Mucositis has been reported to occur in 35% to 70% of patients.

Diarrhea, GI bleeding, or hepatic dysfunction can occur. Diarrhea, with or without upper GI symptoms such as anorexia, nausea, and emesis, is common. Symptoms include painful cramping, ileus, and, sometimes, life-threatening hemorrhage from the colon. Hepatic involvement is characterized by increase in liver function studies. GI hemorrhage in the early posttransplant period may be a result of coagulation abnormalities, especially thrombocytopenia. The differential diagnosis of GI bleeding in this setting includes all the usual causes of GI bleeding in addition to bleeding due to acute graft-versus-host disease–related damage to colonic tissues and infection (viral, fungal, or bacterial).[18,23] Diagnosis requires endoscopy.

Treatment is directed by the transplant team, typically PO prednisone or IV methylprednisolone, at 1 to 2 milligrams/kg daily, and possibly adjustment of other immunosuppressant doses.[8]

Disposition and interval for follow-up are also determined by the transplant team.

TRANSFUSION-ASSOCIATED GRAFT-VERSUS-HOST DISEASE

Most living cells that are in transfused blood survive for no more than a few days or weeks. However, in some patients, transfused cells engraft, expand, and circulate. When immunocompetent T lymphocytes engraft in an immune-suppressed patient, transfusion-associated graft-versus-host disease may occur and is almost always fatal.[24,25] It is possible to avoid transfusion-associated graft-versus-host disease by irradiating blood products before transfusion. Patients with immunocompromise or other risk factors (**Table 297-8**) should receive irradiated blood products.

SPECIFIC TYPES OF TRANSPLANTATION

RENAL TRANSPLANTATION

Renal transplantation is the preferred treatment for end-stage renal disease. Vascular complications that occur following renal transplantation include renal artery stenosis, allograft infarction, arteriovenous fistulas, pseudoaneurysm, and renal vein thrombosis. Nonvascular complications include ureteral obstruction, urine leak, periallograft fluid collections (hematomas, lymphoceles, and abscesses), neoplasms, GI complications, and posttransplant lymphoproliferative disease.[26] The major causes of renal transplant loss are death from vascular, malignant, or infectious disease, and loss of the allograft from chronic renal dysfunction associated with the development of graft fibrosis and glomerulosclerosis.

TABLE 297-7 Empiric Antimicrobial Therapy

Condition	Antimicrobial Agent	Comments*
All patients	Discuss agent(s) with transplant team.	The transplant team caring for the patient should always be consulted as soon as possible; however, in certain life-threatening situations, empiric broad-coverage therapy may be indicated immediately.
Suspected infection site based on history and physical examination	Site-specific agents are preferable if predicted by initial findings, balanced by known pathogens as listed in Table 297-5.	The urgency for treatment should be based on the patient's presenting condition; bacterial infections are the most aggressive organisms requiring coverage, but some fungal infections may yield sepsis. In general, broad coverage for any suspected site infection is recommended initially pending cultures and further workup to define noninfectious causes of fever.
Neutropenia in the absence of symptoms suggesting site-specific infection	Third-generation cephalosporin such as ceftazidime or a carbapenem plus coverage for MRSA below.	Multiple alternative agents used, including an aminopenicillin plus a β-lactam inhibitor such as piperacillin-tazobactam or cefepime. Monotherapy has fewer complications, but concern for MRSA remains high. Addition of antiviral and antifungal agents should be at the discretion of the transplant team.
Suspected MRSA	Vancomycin	In the majority of patients, MRSA infection should be seriously considered as a potential cause of infection, pending cultures. Linezolid is an alternative antibiotic.
Parasitic infections	Trimethoprim-sulfamethoxazole after discussion with transplant team	Consider *Toxoplasma gondii, Pneumocystis jiroveci.*
Viral infections	Ganciclovir or valganciclovir for CMV, acyclovir for herpes simplex and varicella-zoster	Consider treatment for CMV pneumonia, CMV chorioretinitis, CNS or disseminated herpes simplex or varicella-zoster.
Fungal infections	Discuss with transplant team; agent depends on site and severity of illness	Consider *Aspergillus, Candida albicans, Cryptococcus neoformans.*

Abbreviations: CMV = cytomegalovirus; MRSA = methicillin-resistant *Staphylococcus aureus.*
*Standard doses apply but may be altered by transplant team recommendations.

Medication changes, as well as imaging contrast agent use that may affect renal function (including gadolinium-based contrast agents), should be discussed with the patient's transplant team.

DIAGNOSTIC TESTING

Table 297-6 lists recommendations on diagnostic testing in transplant patients, including renal transplant patients. The serum creatinine level is the most valuable prognostic marker of graft function at all times after transplantation and should be obtained whenever renal failure or infection is suspected. The urinalysis provides important clues to acute changes in graft viability. Red blood cell casts and proteinuria are commonly seen in recurrent or de novo glomerulonephritis. The presence of WBCs, bacteria, and nitrites is helpful in diagnosing urinary tract infections. Proteinuria may signal rejection, drug toxicity, glomerular disease, or other graft nephropathy, although proteinuria from a remaining native kidney should also be considered. Obtain cyclosporine or tacrolimus blood levels for all patients on these medications. Contact the patient's transplant team regarding abnormal drug levels, because low drug levels are sometimes deliberately used to reduce side effects.

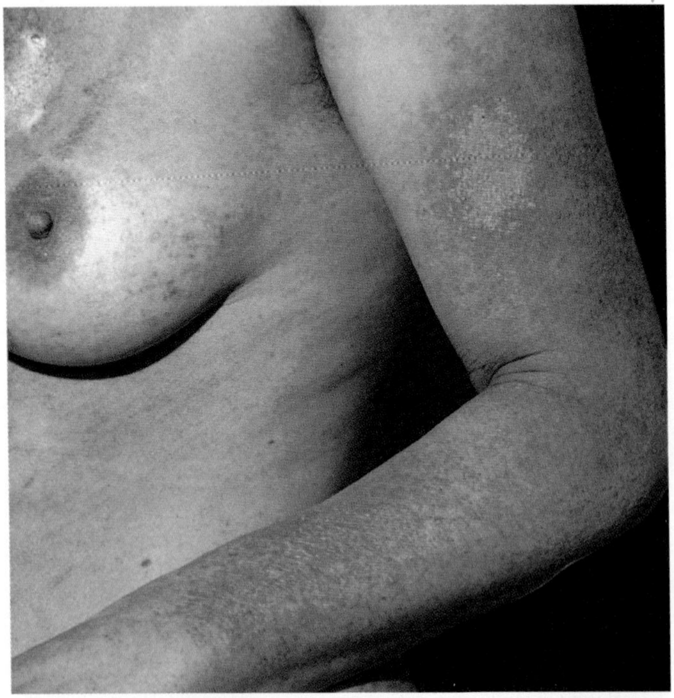

FIGURE 297-1. Rash of acute cutaneous graft-versus-host disease. The maculopapular lesions have acquired a brownish hue, and there is slight scaling. [Reproduced with permission from Wolff KL, Johnson R, Suurmond R: *Fitzpatrick's Color Atlas & Synopsis of Clinical Dermatology,* 6th ed. © 2009, McGraw-Hill, New York.]

IMAGING

Ultrasonography is the best test to detect urinary obstruction. Renal graft ultrasonography can also be useful in patients suspected of having pyelonephritis, vascular abnormalities (stenosis, thrombosis, pseudoaneurysm, and arteriovenous fistula), perinephric abscess, urine leak, wound infection, or an episode of rejection.

MRI can be helpful in evaluating hematomas and other fluid collections, vascular abnormalities, and small infarcts caused by medication-induced vasculitis. Magnetic resonance angiography has the advantage of requiring either no contrast material or a gadolinium chelate that is less nephrotoxic than other agents. However, gadolinium-based contrast agents

TABLE 297-8 Significant Risk Factors for the Development of Transfusion-Associated Graft-versus-Host Disease

Congenital and acquired immunodeficiency syndromes
History of bone marrow (stem cell) transplantation, whether allogeneic or autologous
Transfusions from blood relatives ("directed donation")
Transfusions with fresh whole blood
Premature infants receiving any sort of transfusion
Human leukocyte antigen–matched platelet transfusions
Hodgkin's disease, even when in remission
Leukemia not in remission
Patients treated with purine analogs; the effects of fludarabine and cladribine (2-CdA) persist for a year

TABLE 297-9 Differential Diagnosis of Renal Allograft Dysfunction

Deferential Disorder	Comments
Mechanical	At ultrasonography, a urine leak (i.e., urinoma) appears as a well-defined, anechoic fluid collection with no septations that increases in size rapidly.
Complications of surgery	
Ureteral obstruction	
Urine leak: urinoma, ascites, or abscess	
Vascular	The transplanted kidney is usually placed extraperitoneally in the right iliac fossa. End-to-side anastomosis to the external iliac vasculature provides circulation. Color duplex imaging of the renal artery and vein is helpful in assessing renal vascular stenosis or thrombosis.
Renal artery stenosis or thrombosis (12%)	
Renal vein thrombosis	
Renal artery and renal vein thrombosis are uncommon; they usually occur in the first month after transplant.	
Glomerulonephritis	
Infection	Urinary tract infections are the most common source of bacteremia in renal transplant recipients, and infectious diseases are the second leading cause of death in this population. See "Posttransplant Infections" section.
Urinary tract infection	
Interstitial nephritis from polyoma BK virus, cytomegalovirus, herpes viruses 1 and 2, and adenovirus	
Rejection	Most common presentation of rejection in renal transplant patients is hypertension and falling urine output. Comparison of creatinine at the time of presentation to prior levels is critical. Fever may be a presentation for rejection.
Hyperacute	
Acute	
Late (recurrent acute)	
Chronic cellular	
Chronic humoral	
Recurrent pyelonephritis/vesicoureteral reflux	—
Nephrotoxic agents	Drug serum levels do not correlate well with the degree of renal damage. Nonsteroidal anti-inflammatory drugs are contraindicated in this group. Avoid contrast agents if possible.
Aminoglycosides, fluoroquinolones, cidofovir, foscarnet, sulfonamides, calcineurin inhibitors (cyclosporin A and tacrolimus), nonsteroidal anti-inflammatory drugs, gadolinium-based and some other contrast agents, herbal preparations	
Noncompliance with	Diabetes often follows transplantation; marked exacerbations in hypertension are frequently associated with graft failure.
Medications	
Management of risk factors such as diabetes and hypertension	
Chronic allograft nephropathy	—

can cause acute renal failure in up to 3.5% of patients with underlying chronic renal insufficiency.[27] Therefore, the patient's transplant team should be consulted before using gadolinium-based contrast agents.

GRAFT DYSFUNCTION AND FAILURE

Chronic renal dysfunction precedes the majority of graft failures. Acute renal failure in transplant patients is defined as a 20% rise from baseline serum creatinine levels, as opposed to a 50% rise in other patients with acute renal failure. Consider the conditions described in **Table 297-9** when evaluating possible graft dysfunction or even a small increase in serum creatinine.[28,29]

LIVER TRANSPLANTATION

The most common reasons for ED visits are fever and abdominal pain.[6] Complications include bleeding, rejection, and infection, as well as biliary, vascular, and wound complications. Bacterial infection may accompany acute rejection.[30] Specific complications of liver transplantation are listed in **Table 297-10**. Obtain a CBC with platelet count and differential; serum chemistries, including electrolytes, BUN, creatinine, basic coagulation studies, liver function tests, amylase, and lipase levels; and cultures of blood, urine, bile, and ascites. Radiographic testing as indicated may include chest x-ray and abdominal ultrasonography with Doppler flow studies. US with Doppler can identify fluid collections, thrombosis of the hepatic artery or portal vein, and dilatation of the biliary tree (although the absence of biliary dilatation does not exclude obstruction or other posttransplantation pathology). With partial obstruction, the intrahepatic ductal system often does not appear to be dilated appreciably by US. With complete obstruction, duct dilation is usually seen. Patients often require cholangiography for complete evaluation. Patients with choledochocholedochostomy may be best evaluated by endoscopic retrograde cholangiopancreatography because it permits both a radiographic diagnosis and the potential for nonoperative intervention. Patients with a Roux-en-Y hepaticojejunostomy or those who cannot have endoscopic retrograde cholangiopancreatography must undergo percutaneous cholangiography. Early, broad-spectrum prophylactic antibiotics should be administered before any biliary tract manipulation. Discuss treatment and disposition with the transplant team.

TABLE 297-10 Complications of Liver Transplantation

Complication	Comments
Bleeding complications	GI bleeding should be managed in the usual fashion but may signal graft dysfunction.
Biliary complications	Bile leaks present early and biliary strictures present late (>2 mo from transplant). In both cases, cholestatic liver enzymes are elevated, typically with right upper quadrant pain (more pronounced with bile leak).
Bile leak	
Biliary stricture	
Hepatic artery complications	CT with contrast (if renal function adequate) or US is helpful in the evaluation of these conditions.
Hepatic artery thrombosis	
Hepatic vein thrombosis	
Portal vein complications	
Rejection	Early alkaline phosphatase and bilirubin levels rise, followed by a rise in aspartate aminotransferase and alanine aminotransferase.
Neurologic complications	Causes include hemorrhage, cerebrovascular infarct, cerebral abscess, hypertensive encephalopathy, osmotic demyelination syndrome, and sinus thrombosis. MRI is best for evaluation.
Malignancy	Increased risk for squamous cell carcinoma, lymphomas, and posttransplant lymphoproliferative disorder.

LUNG TRANSPLANTATION

Fever, cough, and increasing dyspnea are common reasons for ED visits in lung transplant patients. Important clinical features to note are the respiratory rate, pulse oximetry measurement, and physical findings of cyanosis, diaphoresis, use of accessory muscles, signs of congestive heart failure, and adequacy of peripheral perfusion. Obtain a chest radiograph and arterial blood gas analysis when adequacy of ventilation is in question. Give β_2-agonists and anticholinergics as indicated. Signs of infection often overlap with the signs and symptoms of rejection, and the management of infection is quite different from that of rejection. A drop in the forced expiratory volume in 1 second of >10% warrants clinical investigation, but pulmonary function testing cannot distinguish between acute rejection, infection, and nonimmunologic causes of respiratory dysfunction such as airway stenosis.[31] Therefore, bronchoscopy is required for specific diagnosis. Lung transplant patients can deteriorate very quickly in the absence of the proper therapy. Thus, it is common practice to cover both infection and rejection until additional histopathologic and culture results are obtained.[32]

TABLE 297-11 Time Course of Lung Transplant Complications

Days after Transplant	Complications Most Commonly Seen in Each Time Period
0–3 d	Hemorrhage from technical/mechanical problems Reperfusion injury Dysrhythmia
3 d–1 mo	Infection: bacterial, mycoplasma, community respiratory viruses Rejection Anastomotic failure Pulmonary embolism Muscle weakness Dysrhythmia
Starting at 1 mo	Rejection Obliterative bronchiolitis Infection Bacterial, fungal, community respiratory viral (can occur at any later time) Mycoplasma 0–4 mo Mycobacteria after 4 mo
Other	Cytomegalovirus infection and *Pneumocystis jiroveci* pneumonia may occur any time, but are more common when prophylaxis is not being given, especially when such treatment has been recently discontinued.

COMPLICATIONS OF LUNG TRANSPLANTATION

Complications occur most frequently in the first year but can occur at any time starting from the first few weeks after transplant and continue throughout the lifetime of the patient (**Table 297-11**).[32,33] Indications for hospital admission are listed in **Table 297-12**.

Acute rejection is common and may occur three to six times in the first postoperative year. After the first year, the frequency of acute rejection decreases, but it can occur for several years after transplant. Signs of rejection include cough, chest tightness, increase or decrease in temperature from baseline of >0.28°C (0.5°F), hypoxemia, decline in forced expiratory volume in 1 second (10% or more), and infiltrates on the chest radiograph. Radiographic abnormalities are less common >6 weeks after transplant, and an acute rejection episode actually may be "radiographically silent" after this. Discuss treatment with the transplant team. If the maintenance immunosuppressant regimen has been tapered, it can be very helpful to return to pretaper dosages. In addition, high-dose corticosteroids are often used to treat acute rejection. The usual dosing regimen is 15 milligrams/kg of IV methylprednisolone each day for 3 consecutive days. After the corticosteroid bolus, if the maintenance prednisone had been tapered, increasing the prednisone to 1 milligram/kg/d and tapering over the next 10 days may be helpful.[31] Clinical response to treatment is gauged by improvements in oxygenation, spirometry, and radiographic appearance and typically occurs within 24 to 48 hours after treatment is initiated. Failure to improve should suggest infection as an alternative diagnosis. After clinical improvement, the maintenance dose of prednisone is increased, with a slow taper back to baseline.

Pulmonary infections from bacteria, fungi, or viruses are the most common causes of morbidity and mortality in lung transplant patients[34,35] (Tables 297-5 and 297-11). Lung transplant patients are at risk for pneumonia because of colonization of the recipient's airway in the setting of transplantation for bronchiectasis and cystic fibrosis and at risk of aspiration in the presence of gastroesophageal reflux disease.[33] Antibiotic selection is best left to the lung transplant specialist.

TABLE 297-12 Indications for Hospital Admission for Lung Transplant Patients

Pretransplant patients
Respiratory failure
Infiltrate
Systemic infection
Decompensated congestive heart failure or pulmonary edema
Pneumothorax
Posttransplant patients
Respiratory failure
Acute rejection
Rapidly progressive airflow limitation (forced expiratory volume in 1 second decreases >10% over 48 h)
Infiltrate
Systemic infection
Febrile neutropenia
Pneumothorax

CARDIAC TRANSPLANTATION

Cardiac transplantation has been applied successfully to patients of all ages, from newborns through persons in their late 60s. Heart transplantation is indicated for patients with end-stage heart failure not remediable by standard medical or surgical therapy. Many in the latter group will have undergone previous coronary artery bypass or valve surgery or been bridged on mechanical assist devices. The leading causes of death in those age 60 to 69 are graft failure and infection.[36]

The success of a heart transplantation operation depends on the ability of the denervated heart to support the normal circulation. The lack of sympathetic and parasympathetic innervation does, however, induce an altered physiologic state. The denervated heart has a normal sinus rhythm with a heart rate between 90 and 100 beats/min. Denervation results in the absence of the initial centrally mediated tachycardia in response to stress or exercise, but the heart remains responsive to circulating catecholamines. Thus, the cardiac response to stress or exertion is blunted. With proper conditioning, patients are able to resume normal activity levels, including vigorous exercise, following transplantation.

The donor heart is implanted with its own sinus node intact to preserve normal atrioventricular conduction. The technique of cardiac transplantation also results in preservation of the recipient's sinus node at the superior cavoatrial junction, and the two sinus nodes remain electrically isolated from each other. Thus, ECGs frequently will have two distinct P waves (**Figure 297-2**). The sinus node of the donor heart is easily identified by its constant 1:1 relationship to the QRS complex, whereas the native P wave marches through the donor heart rhythm independently. The presence of the two separate P waves may lead to confusion about the patient's rhythm, mistakenly interpreting sinus rhythm as second-degree heart block. The ECGs may also be interpreted erroneously as showing atrial fibrillation, atrial flutter, or frequent premature atrial complexes. Some patients may have evidence of "cardiomegaly" related to the transplantation of a heart from a donor who was larger than the recipient (**Figure 297-3**). Clinical evaluation is based on the reason for the ED visit. Chest x-ray, ECG, and further evaluation are based on complications of cardiac transplantation (**Table 297-13**) and underlying patient comorbidities, especially in elderly transplant recipients.

CORNEAL TRANSPLANTATION

Corneal transplantation (penetrating keratoplasty) is the most common form of human solid tissue transplantation. Unlike other tissue and organ transplants, corneal allotransplantation usually does not require systemic or permanent immunosuppression. Reasons for graft failure include corneal graft rejection (30.9%), corneal endothelial cell failure (21.0%), glaucoma (8.5%), and other causes (26.2%).[37,38] **Ophthalmology consultation is required for any change in visual acuity or other ocular signs or symptoms in a patient with a corneal transplant.**

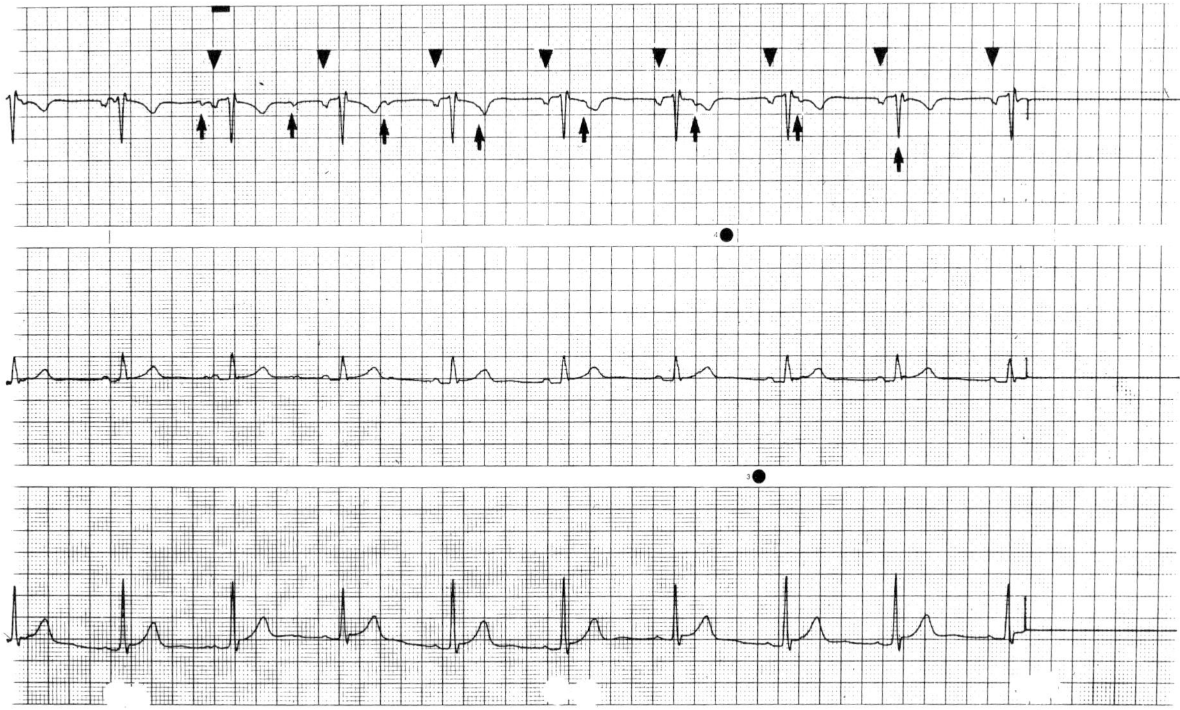

FIGURE 297-2. ECG in a heart transplant patient. ECG demonstrates donor and recipient P waves (*arrowhead* = donor P wave; *arrow* = recipient P wave).

Corneal graft rejection is a specific process in which a graft that has been clear suddenly develops graft edema with anterior segment inflammatory signs. Rejection can occur at any time starting at 10 days after transplant. The inflammatory process starts at the graft margin nearest to the most proximal blood vessels and then moves toward the center to involve the entire graft.[37] Signs and symptoms include eye pain, photophobia, corneal or scleral injection, or decreased visual acuity. Examination may reveal unilateral anterior chamber reaction with keratic precipitate or corneal edema in a previously clear graft. Late graft failure can present with gradual onset of graft edema with no associated inflammation or keratic

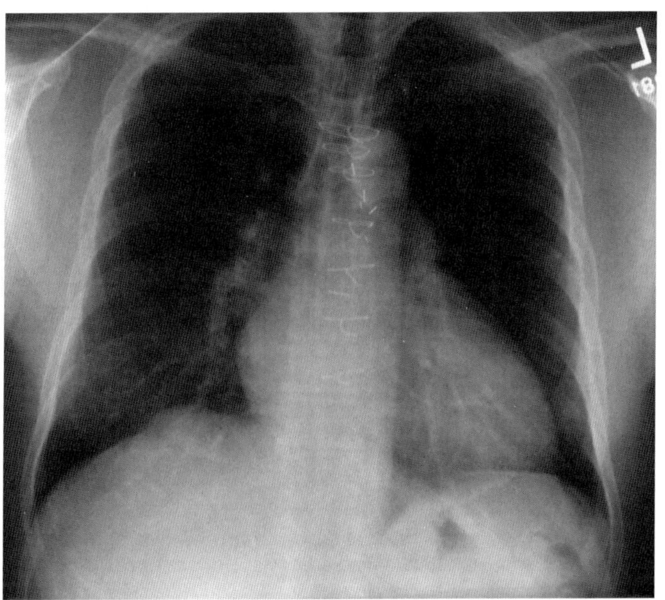

FIGURE 297-3. Chest radiograph of healthy post–heart transplant patient with typical postoperative changes, including "cardiomegaly" due to transplantation of a heart from a donor who was larger than the recipient.

TABLE 297-13 Complications after Cardiac Transplant

Complication	Comments
Altered physiology	See text in Cardiac Transplantation section.
Dysrhythmias	Dysrhythmias after transplantation are frequently due to rejection. Treat the unstable patient presenting in extremis with 1 gram of methylprednisolone IV; delay rejection therapy in the stable patient for consult with the transplant team and biopsy. Atropine has no effect due to denervation.
Sinus node dysfunction	Pacemaker usually required.
Pulmonary complications	Diagnosis may require CT or more invasive diagnostic procedures.
Pneumonia	
Thromboembolic disease	
Exercise-induced hypoxemia	
Pneumothorax	
Interstitial fibrosis	
Cardiac ischemia	Patients do not experience pain due to denervation; symptoms typically occur with complications such as congestive heart failure.
Rejection	Treat the patient presenting in extremis; withhold treatment for biopsy if possible.
Infection	See section "Posttransplant Infections"
Congestive heart failure	Echocardiography can help to determine etiology and therefore ideal treatment.
Ischemic stroke and intracranial hemorrhage	Increased risk after heart transplant.
Complications specific to ventricular assist devices	Increased risk of infection and thromboembolism.
Cardiac allographic vasculopathy	Pediatric heart transplant recipients are at risk for graft coronary artery disease and ischemia. May require retransplantation.

precipitates. Treatment includes topical or systemic steroids, cycloplegics, and immunosuppressive drugs such as local and systemic cyclosporine A and tacrolimus.

Wound dehiscence can occur early or late after corneal transplantation, as a result of infection or after eye trauma. Trauma may be unrecognized or be a result of events such as motor vehicle airbag deployment or a fall with the patient's glasses impacting the eye. There may be globe rupture, slight separation of part of the suture line, or just broken sutures.

Viral,[37] bacterial,[39] or fungal[40] infection can threaten the transplanted cornea. In patients with a history of herpetic keratitis, consider recurrence and examine with fluorescein for characteristic corneal staining and signs of anterior chamber inflammation.[37] Ophthalmology consultation is needed for diagnosis and treatment.

REFERENCES

The complete reference list is available online at www.TintinalliEM.com.

CHAPTER 298 The Patient With Morbid Obesity

Joanne Williams

INTRODUCTION AND EPIDEMIOLOGY

Since 1980, worldwide obesity has more than doubled. In 2008, more than 1.4 billion adults, 20 and older, were overweight. Of these, over 200 million men and nearly 300 million women were obese. Sixty-five percent of the world population resides in countries where overweight and obesity kill more people than underweight. In 2010, more than 40 million children under the age of 5 were overweight.[1]

In children, an age- and sex-specific percentile for body mass index (BMI) determines weight status rather than the BMI categories used for adults, because children's body composition varies as they age and varies between boys and girls.

The Centers for Disease Control and Prevention defines overweight as a BMI at or above the 85th percentile and lower than the 95th percentile for children of the same age and sex.[2] Obesity is a BMI at or above the 95th percentile for children of the same age and sex.[2] The World Health Organization definition is as follows: a BMI ≥25 is overweight, whereas a BMI ≥30 is obesity.[1]

PATHOPHYSIOLOGY

Obesity is an independent risk factor for acute coronary syndrome, especially in those <40 years old.[3,4] Atypical symptoms may pose a problem with acute coronary syndrome diagnosis.[5,6] About 11% of cases of congestive heart failure are attributable to obesity alone.[7] The physical deconditioning of obesity manifest by orthopnea, dyspnea, and lower extremity swelling is very similar to symptoms of acute congestive heart failure, making diagnosis problematic. Plain chest x-ray findings of congestive heart failure may be obscured by redundant overlying soft tissue and hypoventilation. Brain natriuretic peptide levels are lower in the obese patient than in the nonobese.[8,9] Cardiomyopathy may affect up to 10% of patients with a BMI >40 kg/m² and those with a long duration of significant obesity.[10] Obesity is a risk factor for venous thromboembolism[11] and its recurrence once anticoagulation therapy is withdrawn.[12]

The increase in the prevalence of type 2 diabetes is closely linked to the upsurge in obesity. About 90% of type 2 diabetes is attributable to excess weight.[13] Obesity has been strongly associated with insulin resistance in normoglycemic persons and in individuals with type 2 diabetes.[14]

TABLE 298-1 Diagnostic Criteria for Obesity Hypoventilation Syndrome

Body mass index 30 kg/m²
Daytime Pa_{CO_2} >45 mm Hg
Associated sleep-related breathing disorder (obstructive sleep apnea–hypopnea syndrome or sleep hypoventilation or both)
Absence of other known causes of hypoventilation

Abbreviation: Pa_{CO_2} = partial pressure of arterial carbon dioxide.

The accumulation of fat impairs the function of ventilation in obese children and adults.[15,17] Reductions in forced expiratory volume in 1 second, forced vital capacity,[15,16] total lung capacity, functional residual capacity, and expiratory reserve volume are associated with increasing BMI.[18]

Obesity is a well-recognized risk factor for obstructive sleep apnea. Forty percent of people who are obese have obstructive sleep apnea, and approximately 70% of people with obstructive sleep apnea are obese.[19]

Increased fat deposition in the pharyngeal area along with reduced operating lung volumes associated with obesity reduce upper airway caliber, modifying airway configuration, which in turn increases upper airway collapsibility. Thus, airways are predisposed to repetitive closure during sleep.[20] Daytime sleepiness increases and may be associated with accidental trauma.[19]

Cor pulmonale and hypercapnic respiratory failure are common. Obesity hypoventilation syndrome (**Table 298-1**) was first described over 50 years ago.[21,22] The most common symptoms are (1) respiratory failure, (2) severe hypoxemia, (3) hypercapnia, and (4) pulmonary hypertension.[22,23,24]

ESTIMATING PATIENT WEIGHT

The Broselow tape inaccurately predicts actual weight in one third of children.[25] The significance of this inaccuracy has not been studied in depth. A weight-estimation formula based on mid-arm circumference is reliable for use in school-age children and may be an alternative to the Broselow tape.[26] The formula is as follows: weight (kg) = (mid-arm circumference [cm] − 10) × 3. When compared to the Argal, Advanced Pediatric Life Support, and Best Guess formulas, Krieser et al[27] found that parental estimation of weight was more accurate.[27]

The concern for equipment weight capacity in the adult patient with obesity is an important determination for imaging. Scales in most EDs have a maximum weight capacity of 150 kg. Mechanized beds that weigh patients are not common in the ED but might be a consideration. Patients with obesity tend to significantly underestimate their own weight. A variety of formulas are available to estimate weight in adults who are obese using height and waist, hip, and arm circumference. The formula developed by Crandall et al[28] seems to require the least amount of time and patient manipulation. Two distinct formulas for nonpregnant females and males have been developed as follows:

$$\text{Nonpregnant females: Weight} = 64.6 + 2.15\ (\text{arm circumference in cm}) + 0.54\ (\text{height in cm})$$

$$\text{Males: Weight} = 93.2 + 3.29\ (\text{arm circumference in cm}) + 0.43\ (\text{height in cm})$$

SPHYGMOMANOMETRY

Improper blood pressure cuff width and circumference will artificially elevate pressure readings. The standard adult blood pressure cuff is too short for patients with an arm circumference of 32 cm or larger. Patients who are overweight or obese will require cuffs larger in size.

The American Heart Association recommends the following cuff widths when evaluating blood pressure in patients who are obese: (1) for arm circumferences ranging from 35 to 44 cm, a bladder measuring 16 cm in width is needed; (2) for circumferences from 45 to 52 cm, the bladder width should be 20 cm; and (3) in patients with short upper arm length, a 16-cm-wide cuff should be used.[29,30]

TABLE 298-2 Dosing of Select Drugs

Dosing	Drugs
Ideal body weight	Penicillins, cephalosporins, linezolid, corticosteroids, H_2-blockers, digoxin, β-blockers, atracurium, vecuronium, fentanyl*, midazolam*, lorazepam*, phenytoin, propofol
Total body weight	Succinylcholine, rocuronium, unfractionated heparin, enoxaparin, vancomycin
Dosing weight	Aminoglycosides, fluoroquinolones

*Initial dose based on total body weight.

MEDICATION DOSING

Little evidence-based literature is available for appropriate dosing in obesity, and nearly none is available in the obese child. Fortunately, many drugs used in resuscitation are not lipophilic, and lean body mass is a reasonable dosing guide. Altered physiology is characterized by an increased clearance of hydrophilic drugs, a larger volume of distribution for lipophilic drugs, and a decrease in lean body mass and tissue water content, as compared to their lean counterparts.[31] Altered mechanics can predispose the morbidly obese to systemic toxicity due to either overdosing or lack of efficacy from underdosing.[32,33]

A weight-based medication schedule uses ideal body weight, total body weight, or dosing weight to avoid systemic side effects and lack of clinical efficacy by underdosing. Ideal body weight according to the Devine formula is as follows[34]:

$$\text{Ideal body weight (male)} = 50.0 \text{ kg} + 2.3 \text{ kg (each inch} > 5 \text{ feet)}$$

$$\text{Ideal body weight (female)} = 45.5 \text{ kg} + 2.3 \text{ kg (each inch} > 5 \text{ feet)}$$

Dosing weight is an adjusted body weight of overweight or obese patients and is used only for drugs for which there are recommendations specifying that the actual body weight should be adjusted to use in the dose calculation.

$$\text{Dosing weight} = \text{Ideal body weight} + [0.4 \times (\text{Actual} - \text{Ideal body weight})]$$

$$\text{Exception: If actual} < \text{ideal body weight, then the dosing weight} = \text{actual}$$

Table 298-2 divides select drugs into ideal body weight, total body weight, and dosing weight dosing.[35] **Fentanyl and the benzodiazepines are lipophilic and have a prolonged half-life in obese patients.** With these drugs, the initial dose based on total body weight may be needed, but subsequent doses should be based on ideal body weight.[36] It is best to check with a pharmacist for specific dosage regimens.

VASCULAR ACCESS

Vascular access is problematic. Patients who are critically ill and morbidly obese patients require fluid administration often guided by central venous pressure and urine output.[37] Central venous pressure placement is extremely challenging even for the most skilled physician. In the obese patient, the distance from skin to vessel is much further than normal, anatomic landmarks are obscured (**Figure 298-1, A and B**), and the angle of approach may be too steep to allow cannulation even after reaching the vessel. There is no clear consensus as to the preferable site and approach to central venous catheterization. In general, there is an increased incidence of infection and deep venous thrombosis when using the femoral approach.[38] If this proves to be the only option, then use this site.

The internal jugular vein can be accessed with equal success to the subclavian approach in patients who are obese. The success rate might be increased with the head maintained in the neutral position, thereby reducing the risk of overlap of the internal jugular vein over the carotid artery.[39]

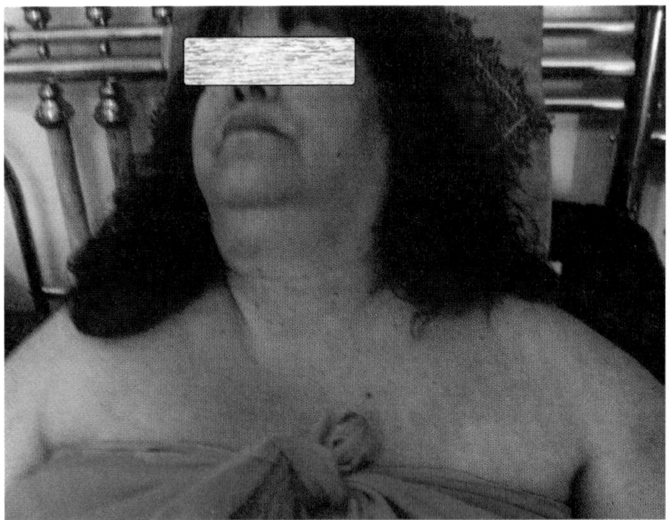

A

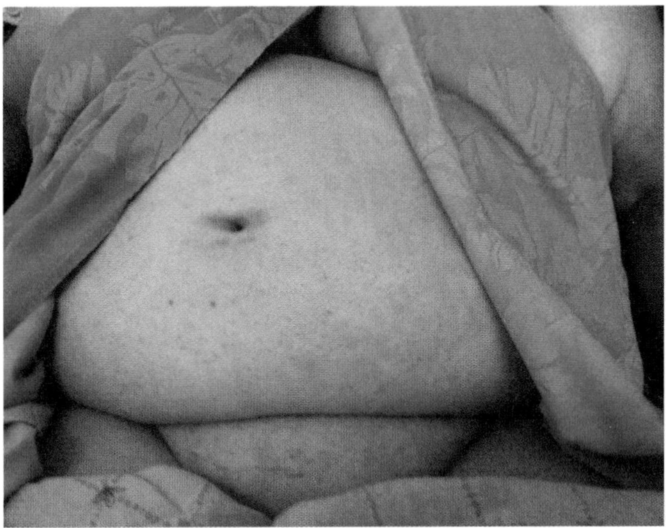

B

FIGURE 298-1. A and B. Difficulties in landmark identification.

A US-guided 15-cm catheter can be used to cannulate the brachial or basilic vein.[40] Another approach is the use of a pediatric central venous catheter placed into the basilic vein. The pediatric central venous catheter is 8 cm (3.15 in) in length, is a double-lumen catheter, and has 18- and 20-gauge lumens.[41] Longer catheters can also be considered to guard against inadvertent dislodgement.

IMAGING

Attenuation severely limits the image quality of plain radiographs (**Figure 298-2**). Increasing exposure time can improve the image but at the expense of increased radiation. Motion artifact increases with increased exposure time. Multiple cassettes may be required if the patient is too large for a single 14 × 17–inch film. Patients may be able to stand for plain radiography if too large for the tables.[42]

Newer CT scanners can accommodate up to 660 lbs. If the patient outweighs equipment capacity, veterinary schools and the local zoo are options.

In the patient with obesity and blunt abdominal trauma who is too large for imaging equipment, consider diagnostic peritoneal lavage.[43] Most standard MRIs have a maximum shoulder-to-shoulder width of 52 inches (137 cm) and weight limits of 300 to 350 lb (136 to 159 kg).

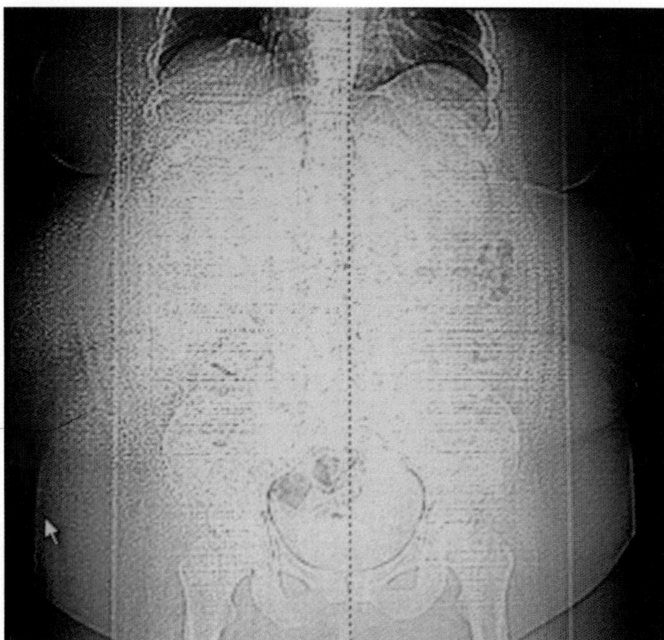

FIGURE 298-2. Attenuation can blur findings on plain radiographic films.

PROCEDURAL SEDATION

Give procedural sedation drugs and pain medications cautiously. Select doses at the lower end of the range, and titrate to effect. Local and regional anesthesia might be considered for complicated or prolonged procedures.[44]

AIRWAY MANAGEMENT

Difficulty with mask ventilation, rapid oxygen desaturation, and altered pharmacokinetics can make airway management challenging.[45] Impedance to airway management is caused by excess fatty tissue externally on the breast, neck, thoracic wall, and abdomen and internally in the mouth, pharynx, and abdomen. The respiratory compromise that is associated with morbid obesity leaves little room for error.

Patients who are obese have increased intra-abdominal pressure and increased incidence of hiatal hernia and gastroesophageal reflux disease. These characteristics render patients more prone to aspiration during airway management.[46]

Patients who are obese will desaturate more rapidly after preoxygenation than their lean counterparts. When no cervical spine injury is suspected, desaturation may be partially prevented by keeping the patient in a 25-degree head-up position during preoxygenation.[47]

Two-person bag-valve mask (BVM) with a two-handed bilateral jaw thrust is recommended in patients who are morbidly obese. If tolerated, an oral airway may be used to prevent the tongue from occluding the airway. The early use of noninvasive positive-pressure ventilation may abate the need for endotracheal intubation. High expiratory positive pressures may be needed.

Obesity is not a contraindication for rapid sequence intubation. Advance preparation is critical, and assessment for a potential difficult airway is of utmost importance.[48]

The "sniffing" position results in suboptimal positioning for laryngoscopy in patients who are obese, and this may also confound results and falsely worsen graded views.[49] The "ramping" position (**Figure 298-3A**) offers improved intubation conditions in patients who are morbidly obese compared to the "sniffing" position (**Figure 298-3B**). This position is achieved by placing multiple folded blankets under the upper body, head, and neck until the external auditory meatus and the sternal notch are horizontally aligned.[50]

First give consideration to awake intubation, given that patients who are obese may be difficult to mask ventilate and rapid oxygen desaturation may occur after the ablation of spontaneous ventilation, especially

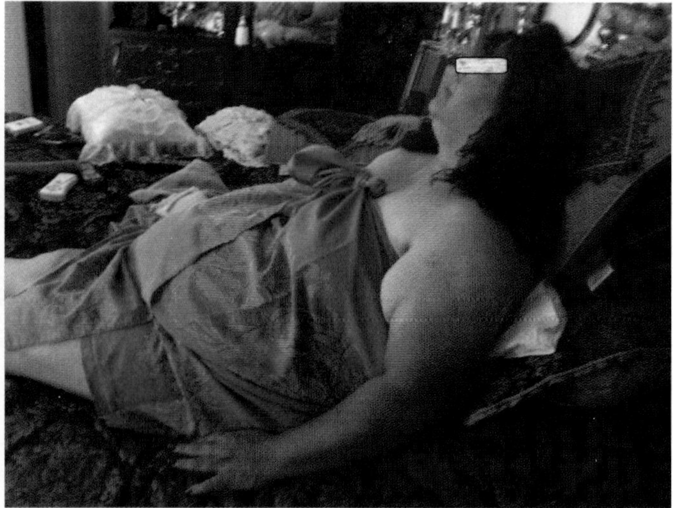

A

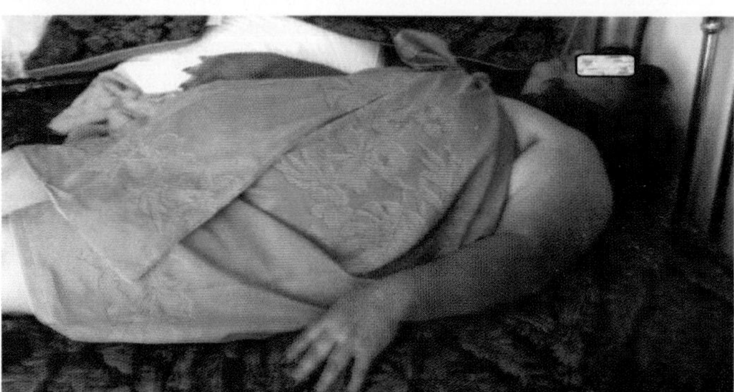

B

FIGURE 298-3. The ramping position (**A**) is more effective for intubation than the sniffing position (**B**) in patients with morbid obesity.

in patients with a BMI greater than 40 kg/m^2.[51-53] The awake intubation may be performed either by the nasotracheal or orotracheal routes.

The relative benefits and risks of the awake intubation approach must be weighed against the merits of rapid sequence intubation, which reduces risk of aspiration, improves intubating conditions, and results in easier insertion of advanced and rescue airway devices. During rapid sequence intubation, the chance for first-pass success can be optimized by video laryngoscopy. The intubating laryngeal mask airway is effective in obesity and should be readily available because surgical access to the airway may be difficult. The bougie is a good rescue device.[54]

Percutaneous and open surgical access to the airway may be difficult when landmarks are obscured by excess soft tissue and a short neck in the "cannot intubate, cannot ventilate" scenario.[55] Obesity and a short neck are associated with difficult transtracheal needle ventilation and retrograde tracheal intubation.[56,57] However, in the elective surgical airway management setting, cricothyroidotomy is technically feasible even in patients with difficult neck anatomy caused by obesity.[58] Unfortunately, the luxury of a controlled environment is often not an option for the emergency physician.

Until the proper size tracheostomy tube is located, a 6-mm-inner-diameter endotracheal tube passed through a cricothyroidotomy incision may serve as a temporizing measure.[59] There is limited literature concerning the success rates of surgical airways in patients in the emergency setting. Even in an ideal setting, cricothyroidotomy requires more than 100 seconds to achieve ventilation,[57] and the procedure is rarely performed in the ED.[60]

With respect to ventilator management, adjust tidal volume as per body weight and initially keep it at 8 mL/kg of ideal body weight in patients in whom mechanical ventilation is necessary, but patients with acute respiratory distress should be ventilated with much lower tidal volume. Lower tidal volumes can be compensated for by increasing the respiratory rate to maintain normal minute ventilation and thus avoiding hypoxemia and hypercarbia.[61] During prolonged ventilation, ventilatory settings are determined by serial measurements of arterial blood gasses and peak airway pressures.[62]

LUMBAR PUNCTURE

In the patient who is obese, lumbar puncture is best performed in the sitting position. US may help identify vertebrae.[63] A formula for predicting the required lumbar puncture depth was developed by Abe et al.[64] The formula is as follows:

Lumbar puncture depth (cm) = 1 + 17 (weight [kg]/height [cm])

Success rate can increase with the awareness of the predicted depth.[65]

A 22- to 24-gauge needle allows adequate flow and easier passage and may also decrease the likelihood of postpuncture headache. Fluoroscopy may be required in extreme, technically difficult, or unsuccessful cases.

TRAUMA

Victims of motor vehicle accidents who are obese (BMI >31 kg/m^2) have significantly more rib fractures, pelvic fractures, pulmonary contusions, and extremity fractures and fewer head and liver injuries.[66]

Mildly overweight patients, not the morbidly obese, are less prone to intra-abdominal injury because of the protective effect of the abdominal fat, known as the "cushion effect."[67]

REFERENCES

The complete reference list is available online at www.TintinalliEM.com.

Palliative Care

Robert J. Zalenski
Erin Zimny

INTRODUCTION

The goal of palliative care is to relieve the suffering of patients with serious illness. Regardless of the patient's prognosis, relief of suffering should be a primary goal for both emergency medicine and palliative care.[1] **Palliative care** is defined by specialty advocates as the physical, spiritual, and psychosocial care given by multiple disciplines to patients and their families who are living with life-threatening illness.[2] Although these principles are applicable to all stages of a patient's illness, a palliative care consultation from the ED is generally considered in the context of previously predicted end-of-life care. **Hospice care**, a branch of palliative care, is a comprehensive program of palliative treatment that is appropriate when patients with chronic, progressive, and eventually fatal illness are determined to have a life expectancy of 6 months or less. Palliative care is patient centered rather than disease centered. It strives to ensure that the patient or his or her (formal or informal) representatives have chosen realistic goals of care after the patient's diagnosis, prognosis, and therapeutic options have been considered. This discussion and decision making should take place during a meeting that includes the patient's healthcare team, surrogate decision maker(s), and those loved ones who are privileged to receive confidential information.

Palliative care is guided by the axiom that distressing symptoms should be treated. It thus provides expert assessment and treatment of symptoms, including pain, dyspnea, and vomiting. Pain is the most common reason for seeking care in the ED, accounting for 58% to 78% of visits in the United States.[3-5] Unfortunately, only 60% of patients reporting pain receive pain medications, and 74% of patients who present in pain are discharged in moderate to severe pain.[6] Dyspnea is the sixth most common chief complaint and vomiting the ninth most common chief complaint of patients presenting to the ED[7]; statistics are not available to document the success or failure of the emergency physician's attention to alleviating these symptoms.

Palliative care also trains healthcare professionals to compassionately communicate diagnosis, prognosis, and treatment alternatives and guide the formulation of a therapeutic plan. Palliative care clinicians work to coordinate caregivers and interventions for the patient and family, to make care more effective, and to lessen the stress and obstacles for achieving satisfactory outcomes. Standards for compassionate care spelled out by the Institute of Medicine[8] and numerous professional societies require that distressing symptoms be alleviated concurrently with all treatments directed toward the pathology of the medical disorder. The patient or surrogate must play a key role in decisions regarding care.

The subspecialty of hospice and palliative medicine was co-sponsored by the American Board of Emergency Medicine, recognized by the American Council of Graduate Medical Education, and officially approved by the American Board of Medical Specialties in 2006. In the spring of 2007, the American Board of Emergency Medicine approved the seating of duly qualified emergency physicians for the new Palliative Care Specialty. The first American Board of Medical Specialties board exam, administered in 2008, qualified the first emergency medicine physicians for practice of the subspecialty of hospice and palliative medicine.[9]

In June 2008, the American College of Emergency Physicians issued the policy statement, **Ethical Issues and End-of-Life Care (Table 299-1)**.[10] In March 2008, the Emergency Nurses Association published a position statement, **End-of-Life Care in the Emergency Department**, spelling out practice and leadership roles for nurses in the ED. And most recently, on November 10, 2011, The Center to Advance Palliative Care (the primary advocate for palliative care in the United States), released its **Improving Palliative Care in Emergency Medicine (IPAL-EM)** project. This project informs and enables EDs to develop thoughtful, creative, and streamlined programs to integrate palliative care into the day to day operation of the ED.[11]

TABLE 299-1 The American College of Emergency Physicians Board of Directors: Ethical Issues at the End of Life

The American College of Emergency Physicians believes that:
Emergency physicians play an important role in providing care at the end of life (EOL).
Helping patients and their families achieve greater control over the dying process will improve EOL care.
Advance care planning can help patients formulate and express individual wishes for EOL care and communicate those wishes to their healthcare providers by means of advance directives (including state-approved advance directives, do not attempt resuscitation orders, living wills, and durable powers of attorney for health care).
To enhance EOL care in the ED, the American College of Emergency Physicians believes that emergency physicians should:
Respect the dying patient's needs for care, comfort, and compassion.
Communicate promptly and appropriately with patients and their families about EOL care choices, avoiding medical jargon.
Elicit the patient's goals for care before initiating treatment, recognizing that EOL care includes a broad range of therapeutic and palliative options.
Respect the wishes of dying patients including those expressed in advance directives.
Assist surrogates to make EOL care choices for patients who lack decision-making capacity, based on the patient's own preferences, values, and goals.
Encourage the presence of family and friends at the patient's bedside near the end of life, if desired by the patient.
Protect the privacy of patients and families near the end of life.
Promote liaisons with individuals and organizations in order to help patients and families honor EOL cultural and religious traditions.

TABLE 299-2 Description of Palliative Care in Emergency Medicine

Who: Patients with serious, potentially life-threatening illness and their families.

What: From potentially curable conditions in the presence of chronic devastating disease when standard treatment impedes the patient's remaining quality of life, to incurable conditions like stage IV heart failure, metastatic lung cancer, or advanced dementia.

When: After a lifespan-limiting prognosis has been defined, or when requested by patients and their families to enhance the patient's quality of life. Late-stage palliative care for incurable illnesses with a prognosis estimated of six months or less is provided in the United States under the hospice benefit of Medicare.

Where: In the ED and every other setting in which the patient receives care, or wishes to receive care, such as at home.

Why: Because the relief of suffering is the primary goal of medicine, and there are few places with greater patient suffering than in the ED.

How: The patient/family decide the goals of care after a realistic discussion based on diagnosis, prognosis, and effectiveness of potential therapies. An interdisciplinary team consisting of at least the doctor and nurse provides care measures, such as symptom relief, and initiates the coordination of care needed to reach the patient's goals. Most commonly this occurs in consultation with a palliative care service, unless the emergency physician is trained in palliative care.

Who Decides: The patient, provided he/she retains decision-making capacity, or the surrogate decision maker, the legally appointed Durable Power of Attorney for Healthcare or closest family relative who speaks for the patient.

By implementing principles of palliative care (**Table 299-2**), emergency physicians will become better skilled at assessing patients' preferences and health status to determine whether initiating aggressive therapy is both concordant with the patients'/surrogates' preferences and potentially beneficial. Patients already receiving a palliative care approach will be able to have their existing care plan continued in a coordinated fashion when presenting to the ED for worsening symptoms, although they would be more optimally managed as outpatients.[12]

EPIDEMIOLOGY

In 2006 in the United States, 36% of people who died were receiving hospice care at the time of death, and a total of 1.3 million people received hospice care in 2006. Although hospice was initially designed for cancer patients, 53.6% of patients enrolled in hospice in 2005 had a noncancer diagnosis. About 58% of U.S. residents die in an acute hospital setting.[13]

In 2002, there were 12.7 million people aged >65 years in the U.S.[14] In 2030, there will be over 72 million elderly people. The **Hospitalized Elderly Longitudinal Project** study found that the very elderly (>80 years) are most likely to want and to consider comfort care as the best option when facing serious chronic illness.[15] The surge in growth in the aging population will increase the demand for quality palliative care.

The U.S. healthcare enterprise is facing a large crisis due to the high cost of health care, particularly Medicare. Approximately 30% of healthcare costs occur in the last 6 months of life. Data from the Health and Retirement Study showed that 51% of those over age 50 visit the ED during their last month of life, 77% of those are admitted to the hospital, and 68% of those admitted die during their hospital stay.[16] A meta-analysis published in 1999 found that the use of hospice saved as much as 40% of healthcare costs during the last month of life, and 17% over the last 6 months of life.[17] A subsequent study found that hospice care reduced Medicare costs during the last year of life by an average of $2309 per hospice user.[18] Admitting eligible patients to hospice is one promising route for addressing the quality/cost chasm.[19]

Currently, only 4% to 7% of hospitalized patients are referred to palliative care or hospice directly from the ED.[20-22] The average time in the hospital before transfer to a palliative care bed is 5 to 9 days.[21,22]

IDENTIFYING PATIENTS FOR PALLIATIVE CARE

In 2011, the Center to Advance Palliative Care released its Improving Palliative Care in Emergency Medicine program, a program that provides a thoughtful approach to palliative care practice in the ED, formulated for and by emergency clinicians. The program covers all aspects of palliative care in the ED.[11] Emergency physicians have enthusiastically received the Improving Palliative Care in Emergency Medicine program,[11] despite expressing concerns about the challenges facing them when discussing palliative or hospice care with patients such as interruption of workflow, lack of long-term relationships with patients, and lack of training to facilitate interactions.[23]

Palliative care needs include the management of a cluster of technologies associated with diagnoses of advanced, frequently incurable conditions.[24] Patients whose long-term care needs are complex and require skilled nursing care for transfusions, tracheostomy care, or infusions of antibiotics or inotropes are likely in need of palliative care, especially if the disease is progressive.

FUNCTIONAL DECLINE

Functional decline is the loss of the ability to care for oneself. This ranges from the loss of complex abilities, like driving, shopping, and managing finances, to basic activities like ambulating to the bathroom and getting safely out of bed. The loss of activities of daily living is the cardinal feature of decline, especially if accompanied by unintentional weight loss, and indicates the need for increased care assistance and suggests a short life expectancy.

PROGNOSIS

Space in this textbook does not allow for a comprehensive discussion of formulating a prognosis and how to share it with patients and families. There are several key diagnoses and prognostic findings that are extraordinarily helpful to understand. Patients with chronic, progressive, life-threatening diagnoses will almost always benefit from palliative care. Those with extensive disease, be it metastatic cancer, organ failure, or neurologic deterioration (with anorexia/cachexia and decreased self-care) are frequently on a dying trajectory.[25] Examples of diagnoses of patients who may benefit from palliative care are listed in **Table 299-3**. A predictive instrument known as the **Palliative Prognostic Score** correlates with prognosis.[26] Elements of the Palliative Prognostic Score include ability to ambulate, provide self-care, and maintain oral intake,

TABLE 299-3 Common Diagnoses and Key Findings of Patients Who May Benefit from Palliative Care

Diagnosis	Key Findings
Solid organ neoplasm	Widespread metastasis unresponsive to treatment
End-stage heart failure	Significant symptoms at rest despite therapy
End-stage COPD	Significant symptoms at rest despite therapy
Advanced dementia	Impaired mobility and inability to communicate health needs
Degenerative neurologic disease	Inability to complete ADLs or communicate health needs
End-stage AIDS	Multiple opportunistic infections and/or AIDS dementia
End-stage renal disease	Patient no longer willing or able to undergo dialysis
End-stage liver disease	Repeated episodes of hepatic encephalopathy, bleeding, or symptomatic ascites resistant to medical therapy
End-stage rheumatologic disease	Inability to complete ADLs without significant discomfort
Multisystem trauma	Nonsurvivable injury
Burn	When age plus percent burn exceeds or nears 140
Multiorgan failure	When two or more key body systems fail
Any chronic, progressive, debilitating disease	Whenever symptom burden exceeds resources and the ability of the patient and/or family to cope with medical condition

Abbreviations: ADLs = activities of daily living; AIDS = acquired immunodeficiency syndrome; COPD = chronic obstructive pulmonary disease.

and level of consciousness. A bed-bound patient completely dependent for all care with reduced oral intake and a diminished level of consciousness has a Palliative Prognostic Score of 10% and a 1-week median expected survival.[26]

REFRACTORY AND COMPLEX CONDITIONS

Multiple visits to the ED for the same condition generally indicate that the plan of care is failing. There may be many reasons for this, but the overall indication is that the patient is becoming resistant to physician-led interventions, and this suggests the potential benefit of palliative therapy.

DISCUSSING PROGNOSIS; SETTING THE PLAN OF CARE

DETERMINING PATIENT DECISIONAL CAPACITY AND IDENTIFYING SURROGATE DECISION MAKERS

The ED team should immediately identify the decision makers when a debilitated patient arrives in crisis to the ED. **A patient with decisional capacity is one who has the mental ability to grasp and retain information about his or her condition, weigh risks and benefits, and demonstrate these abilities by verbalizing a medical decision**[27] (see chapter 303, "Legal Issues in Emergency Medicine," for a more detailed discussion of patient capacity). **Table 299-4** lists phrases to aid meaningful communication with patients and families.[28] If the patient lacks decisional capacity, then the patient's advance directive should be accessed and the named surrogate decision maker should be contacted as soon as possible. If none of these resources are available, then the closest family member(s) should be consulted regarding the plan of care. If no one is available to speak for the patient, then the treating physician should act in the patient's best interest. This may include an order to "do not resuscitate" the patient if it is clear that aggressive therapy would not be beneficial.

TABLE 299-4 Key Communication Phrases[28]

Determining Decision-Making Capacity
Will you describe your current condition?
Tell me about the treatment options we have just discussed.
Explain to me why you feel that way.
Quality of Life
What symptoms bother you the most? What concerns you the most?
Prognosis
Has anyone talked to you about what to expect?
Do you have any sense of how much time is left? Is this something you would like to talk about?
Talking with Surrogate Decision Makers
These decisions are very hard; if [the patient] was sitting with us today, what do you think [he/she] would say?
Can you tell me why you feel that way?
It is not a question of whether we *will* care for your [loved one], but *how* we will care for them.
Then we will do everything possible to keep your [loved one] comfortable, but we won't be providing ineffective and burdensome therapies such as CPR or intubation.
Discussing Palliative Care or Hospice Referral
To meet the goals we've discussed, I've asked the palliative care team to visit with you; they are experts in treating the symptoms you are experiencing. They can help your family deal with the changes brought on by your illness.
Breaking Bad News—Death Pronouncement
I wish there is more we could have done; I'm very sorry for your loss. This has to be really difficult for you. Is there anyone I can call to be with you now?

FAMILY MEETING

Once the physician has determined the patient's decision-making capacity, chronic health status, a clinical diagnosis for the current visit, and a general understanding of the patient's care preference, the doctor and team are prepared to have an abbreviated family meeting with the decision maker(s) to discuss the approach to care. The physician must be clear in his/her own mind whether there is any available therapy that will restore the patient's health; have access to the advice of consultants, specialists, and the patient's primary care physician; and be prepared to issue honest, compassionate, and helpful recommendations based on his/her own assessment.

A productive approach to start such meetings is to ask the surrogate decision maker what he or she understands about the patient's past health and current condition (see **Table 299-4**). After patiently listening, the physician should share his or her insight into the patient's condition and prognosis while monitoring the family's reaction to determine whether the ED team and the family are in agreement. An example of a physician's opinion in a particular case follows: "Your mother's advanced medical condition cannot be cured, and her illness has made her defenseless against the bacteria in her own body. Treating her again and providing another round of intensive care will not bring her health or immune system back to normal, but may only prolong her suffering."

The next step is to ask the surrogate decision makers whether they know about the patient's values and preference for care, for example, how their mother would wish to be treated in the current circumstances. If the answer to that is unknown, ask how the surrogate decision makers would wish to be treated if they were in the same condition.

Based on the response to these questions, the plan of care should be negotiated and jointly affirmed. If the patient decision maker(s) indicate that they must have full resuscitative efforts despite your reservations, you can explore that thinking with them, although it would be best to provide symptom-blunting treatment (such as opiates) along with intubation or central line insertions.

Cultural difference should be taken into account when discussing treatment options with patients and families, including religious preferences. African Americans are more likely to select aggressive treatment options and less likely to select hospice care than non-Hispanic whites.[29] Reasons cited for end-of-life preferences among African Americans facing these decisions include historical mistrust toward the healthcare system and the importance of spirituality.[29]

CODE STATUS

Do not resuscitate (DNR) is a medical order, like intubation, oxygen, or IV fluids. Although a DNR order can be written by the physician without the agreement of a surrogate or family member, the order must be in accord with state law and hospital policy. However, DNR status or other limitations of resuscitation should evolve directly from harmonious decisions reached at the family meeting. Code status orders should be written on every patient justifying the particular approach recommended. There is no ethical obligation to provide ineffective and burdensome care.[30] Families are often grateful when a physician compassionately recommends treating a patient with comfort measures rather than prolonging his or her suffering with nonbeneficial interventions.

The Center for Ethics in Health Care at Oregon Health & Science University developed the **Physician Orders for Life-Sustaining Treatment** in 1995.[31] Since then, the program has expanded to 13 states, with 21 more states currently developing similar programs. This brightly colored form allows a patient to effectively communicate his or her wishes and have those wishes documented as a transportable medical order that is valid across all healthcare settings (ED, nursing home, community). The Physician Orders for Life-Sustaining Treatment form is helpful in initiating conversations about treatment preferences and can prevent unwanted resuscitations by EMS.[31]

CONSULTATION OPPORTUNITIES

Palliative care consultation services are likely available at your hospital and should be used just as you would any specialist consultation. ED consultation can provide assistance when conducting a family meeting or when access to an inpatient hospice or palliative care unit is needed. When symptom relief, medical decision making, or disposition and coordination of care are beyond your expertise or available time, a consult is appropriate. Notify the patient's attending physician of the consultation if time allows.[32]

TREATMENT/SYMPTOM MANAGEMENT

The most common targets of symptom management are pain control, dyspnea, nausea/vomiting, constipation, and agitation.

PAIN CONTROL

Acute and chronic pain are addressed elsewhere in detail (chapters 35 and 38, respectively). The biggest obstacle to aggressive pain management with opiates has been the fear of respiratory depression. Opioid dosing is reviewed in chapter 35, "Acute Pain Management," and is an essential skill in the practice of emergency medicine. It is also important to understand the progression of side effects from opioids, because these will serve as warnings to reduce the dose or delay the next dose of opioids. Respiratory depression is not a sudden occurrence, but instead is part of a progression that starts with sedation, somnolence, and then respiratory depression.[33] The safety of patient-controlled analgesic devices is predicated on this concept. A patient can be safely dosed and redosed until the pain is palliated, as long as level of consciousness is monitored. IV opiates reach maximum therapeutic levels and have peak effects/side effects at 6 to 10 minutes. **Therefore, IV pain medications can be safely redosed every 15 minutes until relief is reached if potential adverse effects are monitored.**

DYSPNEA

While identifying the cause of dyspnea and treating the underlying pathology may bring definitive relief, treatment should also be offered to palliate the symptoms. Although opioids have traditionally been withheld due to concerns about respiratory depression, opioids are beneficial in treating the agitation and anxiety provoked by dyspnea.[34] When treating breathlessness/dyspnea in an opioid-naïve patient, start with a dose of morphine 0.05 milligrams/kg IV, and monitor for sedation and hypoventilation. This is half of the starting dose of morphine when it is used to treat pain. Use a goal of maintaining a respiratory rate of at least 10 to 12 breaths per minute.

NAUSEA/VOMITING

Understanding the underlying cause of nausea can help identify the class of antiemetic drugs most likely to be therapeutic. Chemotherapy-induced nausea often responds to high doses of serotonin 5-hydroxytryptamine-3 antagonists such as ondansetron. Corticosteroids such as dexamethasone also may improve nausea from chemotherapy. Steroids can also improve symptoms caused by increased intracranial pressure and bowel obstruction from cancer. Dopamine antagonists such as haloperidol or droperidol are used for refractory nausea in the palliative care setting. Metoclopramide is excellent for the symptoms of diabetic gastroparesis or compression of the stomach due to tumor or ascites.

CONSTIPATION

Constipation is a commonly seen side effect in patients on opiates for pain control. Patients prescribed opiates need a concurrent bowel regimen, such as an osmotic agent (i.e., polyethylene glycol) or stimulant laxatives. A digital rectal exam is also important to rule out a suspected fecal impaction. When evaluating a patient for constipation, an abdominal radiograph can help to evaluate the amount of stool and lower the index of suspicion for bowel obstruction.

AGITATION

Patients with terminal illness may become agitated, with or without delirium. The causes of this agitation are multifactorial, including pain, effects of the terminal illness, anxiety, terminal restlessness, breathlessness, and mental anguish. The indicated class of medications varies depending on the situation but includes antipsychotics such as haloperidol, anxiolytics such as midazolam, and opiates such as morphine. There is no evidence that these palliative interventions hasten death.[35]

DISPOSITION AND COORDINATION OF CARE

Although the majority of patients consulted to palliative care services from the ED will be admitted to the hospital, outpatient treatment is always an option, depending on the resources available and the patient's needs.

OUTPATIENT PALLIATIVE CARE REFERRALS

Many hospitals and medical groups are accelerating the fielding of outpatient palliative care teams. Such teams are a resource for you, your patient, and family caregivers for appropriate care and follow-up, including measures that will prevent return ED visits, by providing effective care at home or in a nursing facility.[36] It can take a hospice referral to prevent readmission from a nursing home for a patient with advanced dementia, persistent vegetative state, or disabling stroke, so consider recommending hospice admission to the admitting physician to facilitate instituting palliative goals and care plans for the patient.

HOSPICE REFERRALS

Patients who qualify for the hospice benefit should be aware of these outstanding programs of care for the physically declining patient. Inpatient hospice units, where patients can be directly admitted, provide a good option for care and rapid ED disposition if available at your hospital.[37] Not all families are eager to hear the word "hospice," but such a recommendation should be phrased in a way that sends a message about your concern for the patient and his or her health status.

Patients are eligible for hospice care by Medicare regulations if they wish to take a palliative approach to their condition and if they have a prognosis that, in the judgment of two physicians, is likely ≤6 months, given the usual and natural course of the illness. Hospice referrals can be made from the ED for patients with qualifying debilitating illnesses, such as dementia with sepsis or stage IV cancer with poor performance status. Referrals also can be made for patients with clearly expressed prior wishes for comfort care should they sustain a catastrophic acute illness, such as those with an intracerebral bleed, infarcted bowel, devastating neurotrauma, or renal failure in the advanced heart failure patient, leading to multiorgan failure.

SPECIAL TOPICS

IMMINENT DEATH

It is common in the ED to receive a patient whose death is likely imminent. Such a patient has entered the process of multiorgan failure due to a disease such as sepsis, vascular crisis, uremia, or metastatic cancer. Vital signs indicate a patient in extremis; breathing may be irregular with pauses; a Foley catheter finds an empty bladder or only a small amount of concentrated urine. The assessment that a patient's death is imminent should be communicated to family members and the primary care physician. Agreement should be sought to offer comfort measures only. Opiate infusions plus intermittent or infused midazolam should be initiated and titrated to patient comfort. Delirium therapy can be directed to underlying cause (pain, fever) or, if not known or reversible, treated with 0.5- to 5-milligram doses of intravenous haloperidol. A total dose of 5 milligrams can produce a calming effect on a patient and, by extension, his or her family.

OPIOID DOSING AND ROTATION

In the opioid-naïve (hydrocodone, oxycodone, morphine, hydromorphone, and methadone) patient, a 2-milligram dose of IV morphine or a 0.5- to 1-milligram dose of hydromorphone is a reasonable starting dose. This should be administered every 15 minutes until the pain is relieved by approximately 50%. Dose stacking will produce additional, cumulative effects when the doses have all been distributed to the μ-receptors. In the opioid-tolerant patient, the average 4-hourly dose of opioids already prescribed should be doubled for severe pain and increased by 50% for moderate pain (pain scale score of 4 to 6).[38] Smaller doses are required in elderly patients, those with a low body mass index, patients with unstable vital signs, or those with baseline severe cardiorespiratory compromise (e.g., chronic obstructive pulmonary disease) because such patients are at risk for hypoventilation.

CARE OF THE PREVIOUSLY DESIGNATED HOSPICE PATIENT IN THE ED

Occasionally, hospice patients may be directed to the ED. The three most common scenarios are (1) a hospice patient with an acute symptom crisis (2) a hospice patient who has a health concern unrelated to the hospice diagnosis; or (3) a patient who has previously revoked and signed out of hospice and presents to the ED.

A patient enrolled in hospice may be hospitalized under the care of hospice (general inpatient hospice) if there is an acute symptom crisis related to the hospice diagnosis. An inpatient setting can allow for more aggressive treatment of symptoms such as a pain crisis, new onset dyspnea, or other concerning symptoms. A patient may also be sent to the ED for a new medical issue unrelated to the hospice diagnosis. For example, a patient admitted to hospice for refractory heart failure may fall and fracture a bone. The fracture is unrelated to the hospice issue.

A patient may revoke hospice care at any time for any reason, and may present to the ED for aggressive treatment rather than a palliative approach. Occasionally a patient or family may panic and call 911 when there is a change in the patient's health status. The ED physician should care for the patient as appropriate. It can be very helpful to contact the patient's hospice agency. Someone should be available 24 hours a day and may be very useful in helping to clarify the patient's goals and disposition.

PRACTICE GUIDELINES

Clinical practice guidelines have been published by the Improving Palliative Care in Emergency Medicine project, and can be found at : http://ipal-live.capc.stackop.com/downloads/ipal-em-clinical-practice-guidelines.pdf

REFERENCES

The complete reference list is available online at www.TintinalliEM.com.

Death Notification and Advance Directives

Lindsay Weaver
Cherri Hobgood

DEATH NOTIFICATION

Death notification is perhaps the most difficult, emotionally laden communication that physicians must perform. In most situations, the notification of death occurs during the first meeting of the emergency physician with the deceased patient's family. The notification often comes after extensive resuscitation efforts, creating a upheaval of emotion for the physician and ED staff leaving the team emotionally and physically exhausted.[1,2]

For survivors, death notification is a life-altering event. The language used during the communication, the venue, and the characteristics of the individual delivering the news create indelible memories for the family.[3]

EFFECTS ON SURVIVORS

Because death that occurs in the ED is frequently sudden, unexpected, and often violent, survivors can develop complicated bereavement and/or posttraumatic stress disorder.[4-7] Death notifications that provide limited or incorrect information about the death or occur in chaotic settings with limited support may exacerbate the grief reaction.[6] When properly performed, death notifications may mitigate substantial negative effects on surviving family members.[8] A well-delivered death notification can reduce the incidence of posttraumatic stress disorder in the families of patients who died suddenly, particularly notifications involving the loss of a spouse or the death of a child.[9]

EFFECTS ON PHYSICIANS

Physicians find death notification physically and emotionally difficult, with evidence of increased heart rate, heart rate variability, and cortisol levels immediately after the event.[10-13] Common emotional reactions in emergency physicians faced with the task of death notification are sadness (60%) and disappointment (38%), resulting in insomnia in 37%.[13] The cause of death, the patient's age, the presence of family, and the similarity to self are the most common reasons cited by emergency physicians for powerful impact of a recent death notification experience.[13,14] The need to rapidly switch between the cool emotional state required to lead a resuscitation and that of a warm empathic informant bearing difficult and tragic news may exacerbate this situation for the physician. The following factors also increase the stress level for the physician: racial and ethnic differences between the physician and the family, lack of a clear family leader, a nontraditional family (e.g., broken or blended), and situations in which the physician is personally emotional or cannot control his or her own reaction.[15]

Skillful death notification is a priority in emergency medicine practice.[2,3] Protocols to enhance communication skills for delivering bad news in the ED improve satisfaction of survivors.[16] The use of successful methods to communicate effectively with families may also mitigate physician burnout and reduce stress on ED staff.[17] First, providers must seek to understand and anticipate their personal emotions. Second, providers must learn to use compassionate communication methods in the delivery of this information. Third, providers must provide precise and complete information to families. Understanding and using compassionate methods of information exchange are critical to success. Providers must learn to recognize emotions, even when they are indirectly expressed, and allow these to be aired and displayed without judgment.[18]

GRIEV_ING© A METHOD FOR DELIVERY OF DEATH NOTIFICATION

The **GRIEV_ING©** mnemonic is a method for delivering concise and accurate death notification. This mnemonic provides physicians with an organized, sequenced approach to deliver the news of death (**Table 300-1**).[19] The structured organization of communication elements provides a coherent sequence of information to the family that is easy for providers to remember and ensures complete information transfer to the family.

G (GATHER)

As early as possible during the resuscitation, instruct ED staff, nursing, social work, or chaplain services to "gather" the family. Place the group in a quiet, private environment with few distractions. Assist the family with outreach to other family members or friends. **Gathering** allows the physician to deliver the information a single time, ensuring that

TABLE 300-1 The GRIEV_ING Mnemonic

G	Gather	Assemble the family in a calm, considerate place for the discussion. Gather as many family members as time allows. This mitigates the need for multiple episodes of information delivery. This step may be done by ED support staff.
R	Resources	Ask for any additional support available to aid the family (e.g., hospital chaplain services, family ministers, additional family and friends [especially if the survivor is alone], and, if needed, an interpreter).
I	Identify	Upon entering the room with the family: Identify yourself Identify the deceased patient by name Identify the family's state of knowledge. Are they aware of the situation, or will news of the death be unexpected?
E	Educate	In a concise manner, educate the family about the events that have transpired since the patient entered care. EMS should be included in this description. Fire a "warning shot" by stating that you bring "very bad news." Tell them the current state of their loved one.
V	Verify	Confirm the news of death. State emphatically that their family member is dead. *Be clear!* Use the words dead or died. Express your sincere condolences.
_	Space	Stop talking. Allow the news to settle and give them time to process the information.
I	Inquire	After a brief interval, ask if they have any questions. Then take the time to answer all of them.
N	Nuts and bolts	Provide additional information on: Organ donation. Funeral service that will collect the body. The deceased's personal belongings. Be sure to offer the family the opportunity to view the body.
G	Give	Give the family your card and contact information. Offer to answer any questions that they may have later. Return their call if contacted. Express condolences.

Modified with permission from Hobgood C, Harward D, Newton K, Davis W: The educational intervention "GRIEV_ING" improves the death notification skills of residents. *Acad Emerg Med* 12: 296, 2005. Copyright John Wiley & Sons.

everyone hears the same information. This also allows the family to support each other during this most difficult time.

R (RESOURCES)

Ask if there are any needs, and work to collect any needed items. Ask about desires for a chaplain, minister, or priest who may provide support for the family. Obtain interpreter services if needed.

I (IDENTIFY)

Confirm that the deceased individual is properly identified. As the physician and staff join the family, they must clearly identify themselves and their role in the resuscitation. They must then clarify and confirm that the family is associated with the deceased individual. This can be done by saying the patient's full name, for example, *"Are you the family of Ellen Smith?"* Ask the family members to state their relation to the patient. Identify the next of kin. All discussion moving forward is between you and the next of kin. Face that person directly and ask permission to discuss the events of the day in the presence of the extended family and those gathered in the room.

Ask for a brief statement of the state of knowledge of the family regarding the patient's status. This final step is important because it allows you to begin your story of the day's events at the point their knowledge ends. This assists you in providing complete and essential information. Depending on the prior state of knowledge, the family will process information differently and at different rates. Your story will be very different for family members who witnessed a complete arrest versus those who last saw their family member healthy. The following is an example of an introductory narrative:

> *"Good Afternoon, my name is Dr. Hobgood. I am the attending physician taking care of Mrs. Ellen Smith. Are you the family of Mrs. Smith? Thank you for coming. Would you mind introducing yourselves and your relationship to Mrs. Smith? Thank you. Mr. Smith, do I have your permission to discuss Mrs. Smith's case in the presence of your family? Thank you.*
>
> *Before I begin, it would be helpful to understand what you already know about what is going on. Can you tell me what you know about what happened to Mrs. Smith today?"*

If possible, before you begin your discussion, ask the family to take a seat. You and your team should sit as well. Having the family sit reduces the risk of falling and sustaining injury during the notification. Position yourself across from the next of kin, preferably at eye level, and address the majority of the dialogue to that person. This posture creates open communication and allows you to assess understanding as you deliver the information. As a physician, a seated posture indicates that you are open to discussion and are willing to remain as long as needed.

E (EDUCATE)

From this point forward, your role is to educate. Your description of the event should begin at the conclusion of the family's knowledge of events. The narrative should be a focused summary of the scene, including any EMS response and the events in the ED. Communicate with nontechnical, nonmedical words; be thoughtful with your language and listen and watch for incomprehension. **Throughout your summary, on multiple occasions, provide the family with "warning shots," such as "this is difficult news," "the information that I am relating is bad news," or "the news that I am bringing may be difficult for you to hear."** These "warning shots" are a communication strategy intended to adjust the family toward the idea that they are about to learn something difficult and portend the disclosure of death. Carefully observe the family's reactions and those of the next of kin. If it appears that they do not understand the severity of events, reemphasize the finality of the news. Once the family appears to be following your story with clarity then you must disclose the death.

V (VERIFY)

Continuing your dialogue seamlessly, you will "verify" the death. You should unequivocally state that their family member has died. You must decisively affirm this fact clearly and say the words *death, died,* or *dead.* Provide your condolences on their loss. This may include language such as "I am sorry for your loss" or "I can see how difficult it is for you to learn of the death of your [mother, brother, sister, friend, etc.]." Without knowing the religious convictions of the patient and everyone present, it is inappropriate to say "they are in a better place" or that the events "were God's will."

_ (SPACE)

Now **stop talking.** Give the family some room to comprehend what you have just said. Even families who were anticipating the death will need a moment to register the information and compose themselves. Once you have allowed an adequate period of time to pass, you may move into the last three steps of notification.

I (INQUIRE)

The next phase, "inquire," is a very natural progression of the dialogue. Ask the family, "Are there any questions for me?" or "How can I help you?" In most cases, if the preceding steps have gone well and there has been complete information transfer, then there will be no major questions. The family may ask if there was pain or suffering. This is a difficult question to answer. Maintaining your credibility is important and you can never state with full certainty that the patient did not suffer. If you did everything possible to mitigate pain and suffering while the patient was in the ED, you can reassure the family with this fact.

N (NUTS AND BOLTS)

The "nuts and bolts" are the necessary practical things that require attention. The physician has several key tasks at this stage. Inform the family that they will need to complete documents before they leave the hospital. You should also ask the family's wishes regarding autopsy and **organ donation** (see sections below). You should also offer the family the chance to view the body after it is appropriately prepped. This preparation includes removal of blood and secretions, closing the eyes, and covering the body except for the hands and face. It is fine to remove tubes and catheters as long as it is not a medical examiner's case. If the patient is disfigured, cover the wound as best as possible with towels or bandages. Sometimes it is impossible to completely cover wounds, particularly if they are on the face. You should warn the family that there is trauma or if tubes must be left in place and that these sights may result in a lasting memory of their loved one. Let them know that you are willing to take them to the bedside but that these wounds will be difficult for them to see. In all situations, it is best to have the family members seated.

G (GIVE)

The concluding step in the notification process is "give." During this period, you give the family your name and, if possible, your business card. Inform them that if they call you may not be immediately available but that you will contact them after you receive the message. If they reach out to you, be sure to return the call. Typically, calls are made to provide additional clarity or to thank you. Express your condolences and then close the encounter.

WHAT REACTIONS TO EXPECT

Responses to loss vary greatly. Families often describe themselves as numb immediately after learning of the loss. They have difficulty processing information and making decisions. Following the initial shock, the family may experience denial, anger, and/or guilt.[20] Denial is most typically expressed as incredulity and is thought to be a defensive mechanism, because it permits additional time to comprehend the new situation. Your role is to understand this condition and allow time and, if needed, provide additional information to confirm death. Seeing the body of the deceased may help the family to accept the truth. Anger is not unusual. Be prepared to react in a supportive manner rather than responding with anger or becoming defensive. If the family or individuals react with charges of negligence or malfeasance on the part of the care team, keep calm and provide support in a nonjudgmental way. These are typically expressions of grief and misplaced guilt.

The survivors' culture is an important predictor of the types of emotional responses that may be exhibited. These may range from no expression of emotion to wailing and hysterical collapse. Allow these expressions and remain calm and respectful. If you want to touch the grieving individual, the shoulder is the most suitable location.

SPECIAL SITUATIONS

LONG-DISTANCE NOTIFICATION

Occasionally, death notification must be made to survivors over the telephone. The GRIEV_ING protocol steps are still appropriate. Ask the survivor to "gather" other family members to join on the phone. If the survivor is alone, ask the survivor to get "resources," such as friends, relatives, or personal clergy, and call you back. At that time, proceed with the rest of the steps of in-person notification. After notification, the survivors may wish to come to the hospital to attend to the "nuts and bolts." Recommend that they do not drive alone and assure them someone will be available to answer all of their questions.

AUTOPSY AND MEDICAL EXAMINER CASES

The Joint Commission requires that physicians ask families if an autopsy is desired. Autopsies are voluntary and serve to clarify premortem diagnoses or aid in the diagnosis of new diseases. Autopsies do not prevent an open-casket funeral. If there are religious concerns, a chaplain can help. Local and institutional policies regarding autopsy billing and payment vary; however, if the family will be charged for the autopsy, they should be informed.

Depending on state laws, certain deaths must be referred to the medical examiner or coroner for investigation and/or autopsy. Deaths the medical examiner may choose to investigate are death due to trauma, homicide, suicide, or medical procedures; death from a disease that is a public threat; death of a person in custody or incarcerated; pediatric and sudden infant death syndrome deaths; and deaths that are unexpected and unexplained. An autopsy may or may not be performed in these cases, but the family is not allowed to refuse investigation or autopsy by the medical examiner if that is necessary. Families are still permitted to view the body, but they are discouraged from removing mementos or disturbing the body until after the medical examiner investigation. **Do not remove resuscitative lines and tubes in a medical examiner case.** Designation or the death as a medical examiner case does not prevent organ donation, but the consent of the medical examiner is required before organ procurement.

ORGAN DONATION

Currently >123,000 patients are on the national transplant list, and 21 people die daily waiting for a transplant.[21] The Joint Commission requires physicians to contact an organ-procuring agency for all deaths in the ED. The kidney, heart, liver, lungs, pancreas, and intestines are the most needed organs by critically ill patients. Tissues such as cornea, bone, skin, tendon, fascia, cartilage, sphenoid veins, and heart valves are also harvestable.

Traditionally, the family consent process has been the largest single obstacle to obtaining organ donation. The best predictor of consent is the family's initial reaction to the request for donation. Currently, all 50 U.S. states have first-person consent and registry laws associated with the Department of Motor Vehicles.[22] These laws increase families' satisfaction and likelihood of consent for organ donation.[23] Trained organ procurement specialists should manage conflicts with the family disagreeing with the deceased's stated wishes. They are trained in this type of conflict resolution and are aware of each state's laws. Physicians can provide information while allowing the coordinator to initiate and lead the conversation about organ donation. The role of the ED physician is to notify the family of the grave prognosis or death of the patient and remain supportive and available to the family.

WITNESSED RESUSCITATION

Emergency physicians should consider developing programs to educate staff and develop procedures to routinely invite family members to observe resuscitation in the ED.[24-26] Family-witnessed resuscitation gives family members closure and comprehension of the patient's situation and grave condition.[24] Emergency medicine providers may be concerned about the family interfering with resuscitation efforts, patient confidentiality, increased litigation, distraction from resuscitation efforts, wrongly prolonging the code, and increased stress for the family and staff members.[24] However, many of these concerns have been found to be unwarranted. In one study, family members who witnessed CPR had fewer symptoms of posttraumatic stress disorder and less complicated grief 1 year after the death.[27] It is essential, however, to consider the safety of the healthcare team. Therefore, family members should be screened for appropriateness to attend the resuscitation and escorted out if safety becomes a concern.[28] A staff member should prepare the family members for what they may see during the resuscitation and then remain with them to offer support, answer questions, and explain procedures.[24] Involving the family in the resuscitation may allow the emergency medicine provider to establish a relationship with the survivors and facilitate in death notification.

PEDIATRIC DEATH

Recognizing that the death of a child in the ED is uniquely different from other ED deaths, the American College of Emergency Physicians and the American Academy of Pediatrics addressed challenges by developing a set of principles.[28] They recommend ED physicians provide "personal, compassionate and individualized" support through a "family-centered and team-oriented approach." [28] The family-centered approach begins with allowing the family to be with the child during the resuscitation. After the child's death, the family should be encouraged to stay with the child. The healthcare team should respect families' "social, religious, and cultural diversity."[28] Many pediatric deaths are medical examiner cases. Therefore, tubes and lines may need to be kept in place, which may affect what the family can do. The team-oriented approach provides appropriate resources, including organizations and individuals that may assist families, and a coordinated response to the child's death.[28] In more than one third of pediatric deaths, an autopsy provides information of undiagnosed findings and complications.[28] Knowledge of an organic, identifiable cause of death may help to alleviate guilt, offer a source of comfort to the family, and help with future family planning. It may also provide a sense of solace to the family to know that the information gained is useful to help prevent the future suffering of other children. Organ donation may also provide a source of comfort. The ED physician should notify the child's pediatrician concerning the circumstances of the child's death so that the pediatrician can follow up with the child's family and siblings.[29]

ADVANCE DIRECTIVES AND PHYSICIAN ORDERS FOR LIFE-SUSTAINING TREATMENT

Only 20% to 30% of American adults have an advance care directive.[30,31] The traditional "do not resuscitate" (DNR) form facilitates the patient's or surrogate decision maker's refusal of cardiopulmonary resuscitation should the patient sustain a cardiac or respiratory arrest. However, DNR forms generally do not outline the patient's treatment wishes for a life-threatening condition. [30] The inadequacy of DNR forms led to the development of Physician Orders for Life-Sustaining Treatment forms, including other states' iterations (e.g., Medical Orders for Life-Sustaining Treatment, Physician Orders for Scope of Treatment). The Physician Orders for Life-Sustaining Treatment form is meant to translate a patient's end-of-life wishes into actionable physician orders. Forms may include directives concerning the patient's code status; desire for further medical interventions including hospital transport, intubation, IV fluids, and comfort measures; desire for antibiotics; and desire for artificial nutrition. Forms are transportable (authority transferred from the patient's living situation to the ED) and may be brought into the ED from extended-care facilities, from patients' homes, and with EMS.[32] These directives should be honored in the ED.

WITHDRAWAL OF LIFE-SUSTAINING TREATMENT

At times, it is appropriate to move from aggressive life-sustaining treatment to comfort measures for patients who are in imminent death in the ED. The patient and family should agree that continued aggressive therapies are futile. Discuss possible symptoms and outcomes. For example, patients may display restlessness, dyspnea, or air hunger that can be upsetting to the family. Explain that medicine will be given to treat symptoms and alleviate suffering. Explain that the time course is unpredictable. Encourage the family to stay and care for the patient and to notify a nurse and physician for concerning symptoms.

When possible, move the patient to a room that is quiet, private, secluded from high-traffic areas, with low lighting, and of sufficient size to accommodate chairs for the family. Offer to call the chaplain. Turn off or silence all alarms in the room, and remove any unnecessary equipment from the patient, such as cardiac leads, blood pressure cuffs, cardiac pads, and oxygen saturation monitors. Comfort treatment is further discussed in chapter 299, "Palliative Care."

REFERENCES

The complete reference list is available online at www.TintinalliEM.com.

Prison Medicine

Stephen H. Boyce
Richard J. Stevenson

INTRODUCTION

An established principle in civilized societies is that prisoners are entitled to the same level of medical health care as the law-abiding community.[1] Other ethical considerations involve the issue of prisoners' human rights.[2] The exact medical service provided will vary between countries and, in the United States, varies between states.[2] The concept of prison health care in general is the subject of debate and outside the remit of this chapter.

EDs may have to provide emergency health care to prisoners. Prisoners could be inmates of a local prison or recently arrested and detained in police custody. Many prisons have internal medical services of varied capability. There may be a ward or bedded observation unit for the management of uncomplicated medical conditions. Nursing staff are on duty for the full 24 hours working on a shift pattern. Doctors are present mainly for normal working hours, providing night, weekend, and holiday coverage on an on-call basis. Facilities will vary from site to site but may include radiography, a minor surgical treatment room, and consulting rooms for ambulatory care visits by local specialists. On-site or frequent access medical specialties can include a general prison medical officer(s), psychiatrists, psychologists, alcohol and drug abuse counselors, and social workers.[3]

DEMOGRAPHICS OF THE PRISON POPULATION

The population of a prison is not representative of the general population; typical characteristics are listed in **Table 301-1**.[4,5]

Within the prison, there exists a pool of chronic disease and drug misuse that can lead to significant morbidity and acute medical problems.[3] Disease profiling of prison inmates exhibits higher prevalence rates of certain diseases than those reported for the general population. The most common disease groups are infectious diseases (hepatitis, tuberculosis, human immunodeficiency virus/acquired immunodeficiency syndrome), diseases of the circulatory systems (ischemic heart disease, hypertension), diseases of the respiratory system (asthma, chronic obstructive pulmonary disease), and musculoskeletal and psychiatric conditions.[6] A study

TABLE 301-1 Prisoner Characteristics
Male
Age 15–44 y
Racial or ethnic minority (~60%)
Poorly educated
Lower socioeconomic classes
Smoker
Alcohol and/or drug misuse
Mental health problems (~70% carry ≥2 mental health disorders)
Chronic disease

of prisoner mortality (while incarcerated) attributed the most common causes of death to ischemic heart disease, followed by cerebrovascular disease, neoplasms, and pneumonia.[7] Upon release, former prisoners are at significant risk for suicide or accidental drug overdose within the first year.[8] With the prison population increasing, in particular elderly prisoners and those from an ethnic minority group,[9,10] the prevalence of chronic disease rises, increasing the likelihood of acute medical problems.

Persons in police custody are often intoxicated with alcohol and/or drugs. Common presenting complaints are injuries (sustained prior to or during arrest), exposure to police incapacitants (handcuffs, tear gas or pepper spray, electronic weaponry, batons), complications of substance misuse, and acute behavioral disturbance.

The demographics of police detainees are similar to those in prison; important differences to note are a higher incidence of females, and around 30% of detainees are not registered with a primary care doctor.[11,12] Adherence to treatment for long-term medical and psychiatric illness is very poor among those in police custody.[12]

SPECIFIC MEDICAL ISSUES

ACUTE MEDICAL EMERGENCIES

Prison medical emergencies should be managed according to standard treatment guidelines and protocols. If the prisoner requires admission after treatment, the prison authorities must make the necessary security arrangements at the facility of presentation or the referral location (**Table 301-2**).[3]

TRAUMA

Prison is a violent place. Violence among inmates is common. Minor injuries may be treated at the prison medical center. In one study, 18% of prison-related visits to the ED were due to violence.[3] Penetrating stab wounds, head injuries, fractures, soft tissue injuries, and wounds may result from violence. In severe cases, trauma resuscitation, emergency surgery, and admission may be required.

Injuries Associated with Police Restraint Persons in police custody often attempt to resist arrest; the police then may deploy tactics and equipment to aide in restraint and control. As a result, a variety of injuries may occur, including skin wounds, minor head injury, and joint dislocation.[13] Injuries secondary to a handcuff application include neuropathy (in particular, the superficial branch of the radial nerve), and fractures of the ulna styloid. The use of a baton commonly results in soft tissue bruising; however, lacerations and fractures may occur.

Conducted electrical weapons (TASER®) have two methods of application: "drive-stun," whereby direct contact to the skin by the device is used, and "shooting," whereby two small darts attached to wires are fired into the skin to deliver the electric current. Complications associated with the use of such devices relate primarily to dart penetration (e.g., the trachea,[14] brain,[15] eye,[16] and chest wall), resulting in pneumothorax.[17] The proarrhythmogenicity of a conducted energy weapon is subject to debate[18,19]; however, there has been a report of atrial fibrillation following its use.[20] Clinical management of individuals subjected to such devices is aimed at treating any complications secondary to penetrating injury. Electrocardiograms are advised, and for patients with pacemakers or internal defibrillators, device interrogation is warranted. Finally, the predisposing condition necessitating the requirement for the use of a conducted energy weapon should be assessed and, if necessary, treated.

DRUG ABUSE

It is estimated that 70% to 80% of prison inmates have been involved in some form of drug abuse before detention, with one-fifth being injecting opiate abusers.[3,21] Many inmates are on drug rehabilitation programs and maintained on regular doses of methadone or a similar opiate substitute. The main problem for emergency care is the provision of adequate analgesia. Due to the high level of opiate tolerance, standard doses of opiates (morphine, hydromorphone) may produce no analgesic effect. This can lead to high doses of opiate being given before producing an adequate analgesic effect.[22] If a prisoner is placed on a controlled opiate detoxification program sustained by the use of naltrexone, a long-acting opiate receptor blocker, opiate analgesia will have no effect regardless of the dose given.[23] An alternative form of analgesia will be required (e.g., nonsteroidal anti-inflammatory drugs, which may or may not be effective). Ketamine is another option for pain relief.

Concealed Drugs A person detained in custody may be suspected of concealing drugs in the rectum or vagina. Within the United Kingdom, unless the patient consents to the examination and removal of any such substances, any action is against the policy of the British Medical Association, even if the practitioner is protected legally by a warrant issued from the appropriate jurisdiction.[24] Legal practice may differ between countries. If the patient's ability to make an informed decision regarding their health care is compromised, then removal of drugs from the body is warranted should signs of drug toxicity be evident.

PSYCHIATRIC CONDITIONS

Within the prison population, there is a high prevalence of psychiatric illness. The most common is a personality disorder, found in 65% of men and 42% of women.[6] The main ED contact with psychiatric problems will be related to deliberate self-harm and personality disorders, manifesting as manipulative behavior, fictitious illness, and Munchausen-type behavior. Other presentations include deliberate insertion of foreign bodies or alleged ingestion of objects or substances.

EXCITED DELIRIUM SYNDROME

Excited delirium is a condition that has been formally recognized by the American College of Emergency Physicians as "a unique syndrome which may be identified by the presence of a distinctive group of clinical and behavioral characteristics that can be recognised in the pre-mortem state."[25] Once the domain of the forensic literature, recognition of excited delirium in the premorbid state is increasing.

Attempts to apply strict diagnostic criteria are hampered by a lack of quality research. By the very nature of the presentation, patients are in extremis both mentally and physically. **Table 301-3**[25] reports the frequencies of the presenting signs and symptoms.

TABLE 301-2 Common Clinical Conditions Seen in the ED[3]

Myocardial infarction
Acute coronary syndrome
Cerebrovascular accident
Exacerbation of chronic obstructive pulmonary disease
Acute asthma
Pneumonia
Overdose
Diabetic ketoacidosis
Alcohol liver disease
Deep venous thrombosis
Acute abdomen

TABLE 301-3 Features of Excited Delirium

Features	Frequency, % (95% Confidence Interval)
Increased pain tolerance	100% (83–100)
Tachypnea	100% (83–100)
Sweating	95% (75–100)
Agitation	95% (75–100)
Tactile hyperthermia	95% (75–100)
Police noncompliance	90% (68–99)
Lack of tiring	90% (68–90)
Unusual strength	90% (68–90)
Inappropriately clothed	70% (45–78)

The pathophysiology underlying excited delirium has yet to be fully elucidated; a background of stimulant drug use (predominantly cocaine) or, rarely, psychiatric illness is a consistent feature. Individuals exhibit confusion and agitation. Attempts to reason with patients and transport to medical facilities are met with resistance and aggression, often necessitating physical restraint. It is then observed that the detainee has pronounced tactile hyperthermia, struggles violently, and suffers cardiac arrest, from which successful resuscitation is rare. Severe metabolic acidosis, bradycardia, asystole, and pulseless electrical activity are the predominant preterminal findings.[26]

Treatment of excited delirium syndrome is predominantly aimed at reducing agitation. This can prove problematic, with issues regarding the safety of medical and law enforcement personnel, administration of parental medications, and the relative urgency necessary to reduce mortality. Physical restraint should be for as short duration as possible to reduce agitation and muscle activity–driven heat production. Intravenous access may prove difficult, and the intramuscular route for sedation is a viable, although slower onset, alternative.

Pharmacologic sedation is recommended: benzodiazepines (first line), antipsychotics (should not be used if long QT syndrome is suspected), and the dissociative anesthetic ketamine.[27] The choice of drug used will depend on user experience and route available; combination therapy allows reduced doses of each class of drug, minimizing the side effect profile.

As with any sedation, the ability to manage sudden loss of the patient's airway and facilities for resuscitation must be available. In some cases, rapid sequence induction of anesthesia may be necessary due to the large doses of sedation required and for definitive airway protection.

Supportive treatment is vital for patients with excited delirium, including cooled IV fluids, whole-body cooling (antipyretics are ineffective), and treatment of any electrolyte disturbance. Hypoglycemia, hyperkalemia, and rhabdomyolysis may be encountered. Metabolic acidosis is invariably present and may improve with fluid administration and cooling.

HEPATITIS C

Hepatitis C prevalence in prisoners is higher than in the general population, with studies demonstrating a prevalence of 25% to 39%.[6,28,29] Contrasting the range of values for hepatitis C prevalence within the community against the prevalence of hepatitis C in prisons, there is a theoretical risk of a several hundred–fold greater chance that a prisoner may be a hepatitis C carrier compared with a member of the general public. This raises issues regarding possible needlestick injuries or contamination with infected body fluids. All emergency personnel must be aware of the increased risk of contracting hepatitis C infection when dealing with prisoners and exert extreme vigilance in their clinical procedures.

SPECIFIC CONSIDERATIONS

SAFETY OF STAFF AND PATIENTS

The management of even one prisoner, disruptive or otherwise, will interfere with the running of the ED. The hospital has a duty to ensure that members of staff are not placed in undue danger. If possible, the management of the prisoner should be expedited to minimize disruption. This, in turn, allows the responsible officers the opportunity to return the prisoner to a more secure environment as soon as possible. Staff may be exposed to the risk of violence, but this should be minimal due to the use of restraints by prison officers. The presence of a restrained prisoner may alarm other patients or relatives within the ED, as they may erroneously assume the prisoner is either violent or dangerous. Examining the patient in a quieter area of the ED can help minimize other patients' natural anxieties.

USE OF RESTRAINTS

Prisoners will be restrained when arriving at the ED by virtue of the fact that they are in state custody. The physical mechanism of restraint will be variable but can include handcuffs, hand and foot cuffs with connecting shackles, or handcuffs with a chain attached to the prison officer (escort chains). Many doctors feel uncomfortable in dealing with prisoners who are shackled and are either unaware of the ability or unwilling to approach this issue with the prison officers.[30]

Legislation regarding the shackling or restraint of prisoners will vary between states and countries. In Scotland, for example, the prisoner must remain restrained to two prison officers at all times in the ED and throughout the course of the hospital admission period. Law governs the situations where the removal of restraints is acceptable. Restraints can be removed if the patient is unconscious, anesthetized, being resuscitated, or for "other good medical reasons."[3]

Cases have been highlighted in which female prisoners have given birth while restrained with chains, raising issues regarding the welfare and human rights of prisoners. Even when restraints are removed, the prison officers must maintain a line of sight with the prisoner and must be present at clinical emergencies such as resuscitation. Staff may be uncomfortable working with prison officers in close proximity, and restraints can present a mechanical obstruction to treatment.

Prisoners are not restrained in all countries. With the issue of human rights being raised, the British Medical Association produced a set of guidelines for doctors dealing with prisoners in the hospital setting.[31] The main points raised in these guidelines include advising doctors that they can request the prison officers to remove restraints to examine a patient fully and facilitate treatment, unless there is a high risk of escape or violence. In hospitals that treat prisoners on a regular basis, an area of the department should be modified into a secure area for examination. No blanket policy can exist, and all prisoners should be managed on a case-by-case basis.

However, these concerns must be balanced with the state's public and legal responsibility to carry out a prison sentence and ensure the safety of the general public. Management of prisoner patients requires consultation at a local level between the hospital and prison authorities.

MEDICAL CONFIDENTIALITY

Prison officers will be present at the consultation and during treatment. This raises issues regarding the doctor–patient relationship and medical confidentiality. There is a difficult balancing act between confidentiality for the prisoner and the legal responsibility to protect the public. In cases of nonviolent or minor offenders, the police or prison officers may step outside the room to allow a private consultation to take place. However, in the case of serious criminal offenses, the need for public safety will override medical confidentiality. A prisoner may have the right to challenge this in court, an argument best reserved for the legal profession.

COMMUNICATION

If prisoners are referred to the ED by a prison medical officer, they should be accompanied by a referral letter detailing the nature of the complaint, past medical history, medication, and whether the prisoner is high risk for violence. A medical chart from the prison will occasionally accompany the patient. If insufficient information is delivered with the prisoner, contact the prison medical officer. Once the consultation is complete, the prison medical officer should be advised of the outcome and any investigation results with electronic, paper, or telephone communication, as appropriate. In certain situations, liaison between the medical teams may avoid admission because the prison ward may have the facilities to handle continuing care.

When discharging from the ED back to the prison or police custody suite, consideration for the safety of the detainee is warranted. Police custody is no substitute for observation or administration of treatment for individuals who would otherwise be admitted to a hospital.

REFERENCES

The complete reference list is available online at www.TintinalliEM.com.

CHAPTER 302

Military Medicine

Ricardo C. Ong
Sean W. Mulvaney
Robert H. Lutz
Gerald W. Surrett
Andre M. Pennardt
Ian S. Wedmore

INTRODUCTION

Care for combat casualties is somewhat different from care for civilian trauma casualties, even though many civilian trauma management principles apply, and conversely, some military techniques have been adapted to the civilian sector. The principles of military medical care are applicable to care in civilian mass casualties, in remote settings, for tactical medicine, and in bioterrorism incidents. Civilian emergency medicine should regularly follow military medical advances and adapt as appropriate.

Advanced trauma life support approaches are well applied in a hospital setting, but in combat, how do you function without ancillary staff? What do you do without ready access to a surgical team? How will you manage in the dirt, at night, while engaged with enemy forces? Simple tasks such as obtaining vital signs or auscultating lung sounds are very challenging. Chapters 7, "Bomb, Blast, and Crush Injuries," 8, "Chemical Disasters" and 9, "Bioterrorism," discuss many conditions relevant to the combat situation. **Table 302-1** lists the roles of medical care for combat casualties.

EQUIPMENT

Combat situations require a properly supplied aid bag. A blood pressure cuff and central-line kit have little use on the battlefield. Pack one item that serves multiple purposes, rather than two or three items with limited applications. For example, a cravat can be used as a standard field dressing, pressure dressing, or tourniquet or to hang an IV bag, cover a face as a dust mask, protect against sun exposure on head or neck, filter parasites from water, or even clean weapons.

See **Tables 302-2 and 302-3** for examples packing list for aid bags. Not all items will be needed or packed in one bag; the nature of the mission, duration, terrain, weather, and other factors guide the packing list. Consider maintaining two or more different packing lists for different purposes (i.e., one for battle injuries and one for nonbattle injuries).

Have a copy of the nine-line medical evacuation request secured to the radio, train on your personal equipment, maintain it, and pack smartly to ensure easy access to critical items.

TACTICAL COMBAT CASUALTY CARE

The body of highly developed, standardized, prehospital combat trauma guidelines designed to address preventable causes of death is known as Tactical Combat Casualty Care (TCCC), which is organized into three phases of care: care under fire, tactical field care, and casualty evacuation.

TABLE 302-1 Military Roles of Medical Care

Role 1: self/buddy aid, nonmedical unit level combat lifesaver, medic or corpsman aid up to battalion aid station
Role 2: brigade or division level, medical companies/battalions, support battalions, forward surgical teams, PRBCs, limited x-ray and lab capability, damage control care for evacuation to next role
Role 3: corps level, combat support hospitals, in-theater military treatment facility (MTF), comprehensive stabilizing care for evacuation out of theater
Role 4: definitive care, ultimate treatment capability, full rehabilitative care, tertiary care MTF, typically located in continental United States or comparable out-of-theater safe havens

Abbreviation: PRBCs = packed red blood cells.

TABLE 302-2 Trauma Pack Suggested Packing List

Combat Application Tourniquet (Composite Resources, Rock Hill, SC) or equivalent (× 4–5) or Delfi EMT tourniquet (Delfi Medical Innovations, Inc., Vancouver, Canada) (× 1)	3-inch self-adherent elastic roll dressing × 4 (open package and pre–dog-ear exposed end for rapid utilization)
Examination gloves, heavy duty, four pairs	Hemostatic bandage (4 × 4 bandage) × 4
Protective ballistic eye wear	Large abdominal dressing (can also be used to stabilize flail chest segments)
Cervical collar, adjustable	Surgical skin stapler† (for rapid hemostasis of scalp lacerations)
Nasopharyngeal airway with water-based lubricant packet × 2	IV fluid administration kits × 2–3
Hypothermia prevention and management kit	500 mL Hextend × 2
Cricothyrotomy kit*	500–1000 mL colloid or crystalloid IV solution (250–500 mL bags)
Betadine swab	16-, 18-, and 20-gauge IV catheters
No. 20 scalpel	IV administration set, 10 drops per mL
Tracheal hook	Penrose drain or other tourniquet
No. 5 or 6 Shiley tracheostomy tube	Betadine wipe × 2
Securing tape or strap	Benzoin swab × 2 (aids dressing adherence in the presence of sweaty or bloody skin)
Endotracheal intubation kit†	
AA battery laryngeal scope handle	1-inch tape, short roll
Physician's preference of laryngeal scope blade	Clear IV site dressing (Tegaderm)
7.5-mm endotracheal tube	2 × 2-inch gauze
Stylette	5-mL syringe (for external jugular vein placement)
10-mL syringe	Saline lock
Carbon dioxide colorimetric indicator or esophageal bulb indicator	1 m of string, 550 paracord or cravat prefolded and taped (to expediently hang IV bag)
Carabiners/D ring × 2	Thermal angel or equivalent fluid warmer
Benzoin swabs	IO infusion system (sternum IO device)
1-inch tape	Pressure infuser bag
Oropharyngeal airway	Combat wound prophylaxis kit (3 medication pack)
Skin marker (to mark centimeters at the teeth on cheek to confirm tube placement during transport)	Wound antibiotic of choice × 3 doses (see section on antibiotics for options)
	10-mL sterile water or normal saline vial × 3
Adult bulb suction device such as Suction Easy (Remote Medical International, Seattle, WA)	10-mL syringe × 3 21-gauge needle 1.5 inch long × 3
Adult bag-valve mask	Gatifloxacin, 400-milligram tablets × 6
3 inch long 12-gauge catheter × 2 (decompressing tension pneumothorax in large adults)	Rocephin, 1-gram vial × 1 (CNS wound prophylaxis) Combat wound pain control kit
Adhesive one-way flutter valve/seal × 2–4 with benzoin swabs (sucking chest wound dressing with valve)	Cartridge unit (syringe holder to create a drug delivery system) Morphine, 10-milligram cartridge ampules × 5–10
Finger pulse oximeter	Nalbuphine hydrochloride, 10-milligram cartridge ampules × 3†
Stethoscope	19-gauge filter needles × 3†
Trauma shears	1-mL syringes × 3†
Field tube thoracostomy kit†	21-gauge needle 1.5 inch long × 3†

(Continued)

TABLE 302-2 Trauma Pack Suggested Packing List (*Continued*)

1% lidocaine with epinephrine, 10-mL vial	Acetaminophen, 500-milligram capsules × 10
10-mL syringe	Narcotics accountability paperwork with pen
1.5-inch 21-gauge needle	Cravat bandage × 3
Sterile gloves	SAM (structural aluminum malleable) splint (SAM Medical Products, Portland, OR) × 2
Betadine swab × 3	4-inch elastic wrap × 2
No. 10 scalpel	Gastric sump tube with water-based lubricant packet
Large curved Kelly forceps	60- or 35-mL syringe
32F–36F thoracostomy tube	Light-emitting diode headlamp with green lens filter (red filter will "wash out" blood)
Heimlich chest drain valve (or Penrose drain)	Mass casualty patient cards
0 silk (30 inches long) on a straight needle (needle driver not required to secure tube)	Red, green, blue, yellow safety light sticks (five of each)
3 × 18-inch Vaseline gauze	Fine-point indelible marker
4 × 4-inch gauze × 2	Fox eye shield
Benzoin swabs	Small sharps container
3-inch 3M Soft Cloth Surgical tape (3M, St. Paul, MN), one roll (appears to stick to bloody, sweaty patients better than most)	Large burn dressing (consider a roll of plastic cling wrap) Compact casualty blanket
6-inch Israeli Battle Dressings (First Care Products, Lod, Israel) × 4	Folding litter[†]
Kerlix large roll dressing (Covidien, Mansfield, MA) × 4–8	Compact traction splint[†]

*"Kits" are packaged together as a functional unit in a resealable plastic bag or vacuum sealed with quick open tabs.
[†]Optional items.

PHASE 1: CARE UNDER FIRE

This first phase of care occurs when the patient and care provider are under effective enemy fire. The medical actions taken are extremely limited: protect the casualty and move him or her to safety. The urge to tend to a casualty must be tempered by situational awareness: return fire, and secure the site before tending to casualties. The application of a tourniquet for massive bleeding is the only intervention typically performed in this phase (also see "Tourniquets," in chapter 254, "Trauma in Adults"). Needle decompression, fluid resuscitation, and cervical spine immobilization are not performed when under fire.

TABLE 302-3 Drop-Down Leg Pouch Suggested Packing List

Light-emitting diode headlamp with green lens filter
Combat Application Tourniquet (Composite Resources, Rock Hill, SC) or equivalent × 2
Examination gloves heavy duty (one pair)
Nasopharyngeal airway 32F
Compact percutaneous cricothyrotomy device (Lifestat device; French Pocket Airway, Inc., New Orleans, LA)
Trauma shears or rescue knife
Adhesive one-way flutter valve/seal × 2 with benzoin swabs
12- or 14-gauge 3 inch long catheter
6-inch Israeli Battle Dressing × 2
Kerlix Large Roll dressing (Covidien, Mansfield, MA) × 2
3-inch 3M self-adherent elastic roll dressing (open package and pre–dog-ear exposed end)
1-inch medical tape, one roll
9-line medical evacuation card

TOURNIQUET APPLICATION

With massive hemorrhage in a combat setting, a tourniquet is the first-line intervention.

Casualties with tourniquets applied before the onset of shock have a survival rate of 94%, but those with tourniquets applied after shock develops have a survival rate of 17%.[1,2]

There are a number of basic considerations for tourniquet application.[3] A wide tourniquet (at least 1.5 inches wide) causes less soft tissue damage and is more comfortable for the patient. To control hemorrhage from a large vessel, a tourniquet must have a windlass to gain a mechanical advantage when tightening. Tourniquets without a windlass cannot attain sufficient force to stop arterial bleeding. In combat, we use a tourniquet that can be applied with one hand for self-treatment.

Place the tourniquet about 2 inches proximal to the wound. Tighten to greater than arterial pressure, because tightening that exceeds venous but not arterial pressure may increase bleeding. Apply the tourniquet until the distal pulse disappears. If no distal pulse is present on initial evaluation, apply the tourniquet with a force estimated to be greater than the systemic blood pressure. If placement of a single tourniquet does not control bleeding, place a second tourniquet immediately adjacent and proximal to the first.

The U.S. Army Institute of Surgical Research (http://www. usaisr.amedd.army.mil) has identified three 100% effective tourniquets[4]: the Combat Application Tourniquet® (CAT) (Composite Resources, Rock Hill, SC), the Delfi EMT Pneumatic Tourniquet (EMT) (Delfi Medical Innovations, Inc., Vancouver, Canada), and the Special Operations Forces Tactical Tourniquet (SOFTT). The CAT and SOFTT are both strap tourniquets that use a built-in windlass as the mechanism for tightening (see Figures 254-1 and 254-2). Of these two strap-type tourniquets, the CAT is less painful, easier to use, smaller, and lighter than the SOFTT (59 grams vs 160 grams). The EMT (see Figure 254-3) is wider, less painful, and less likely to induce nerve damage than the strap tourniquets. The EMT weighs 215 grams and, when packaged, is similar in size to the SOFTT. The CAT tourniquet is standard issue to U.S. military personal. The EMT tourniquet is issued for medical evacuation vehicles and role I to III medical facilities. All of these tourniquets are available through the military medical supply system (http://www.usamma.army.mil/).

POSTTOURNIQUET CARE

The safe time limit for tourniquet application and the point at which limb loss becomes inevitable have not been determined. Tourniquets are routinely left in place for up to 2 hours in the operating room, and this is the basis for the recommendation to remove a tourniquet within 2 hours, situation permitting. It is certain that for every minute of tourniquet application time, the greater is the chance for permanent damage.[5] At 6 hours with a tourniquet in place, it is probably best not to remove it; at this point, the release of potassium, lactate, myoglobin, and other toxins from a severely acidotic limb into the circulation would likely cause more systemic harm than benefit. There are, however, several cases of limb salvage with tourniquet times greater than 6 hours.[6] Additionally, keeping a limb with tourniquet cool, but not freezing, may extend the safe application time substantially.

A tourniquet is a temporizing measure. The next step is to convert the tourniquet to an effective pressure dressing, using direct pressure and a basic gauze roll and elastic wraps and/or hemostatic agents, if required. A knee or hand can apply additional pressure to the bleeding site. Once an effective pressure dressing is applied, release but **DO NOT REMOVE** the tourniquet. If no bleeding occurs, leave the tourniquet in place but with all pressure released. If bleeding recurs, retension the tourniquet to control bleeding.

PHASE 2: TACTICAL FIELD CARE: THE PRIMARY SURVEY

This phase begins once the patient and provider are no longer under effective enemy fire. Conduct a complete primary survey and perform life-saving interventions.

Combat medicine deviates from the universally accepted *a*irway, *b*reathing, and *c*irculation (ABC) algorithm. Massive hemorrhage is the most common correctable cause of death on the battlefield, and lethal exsanguination can occur in minutes. Airway compromise accounts for relatively few combat deaths, and respiratory difficulties typically progress over time. This is the reason that TCCC recommends the modified primary survey algorithm of **MARCH**:

- Massive hemorrhage
- Airway
- Respiratory
- Circulation
- Hypothermia prevention/Head injury

After hemorrhage control, the algorithm mirrors the ABC algorithm, with the additional consideration of a closed head injury and hypothermia prevention as primary survey responsibilities. If a problem is noted during any part of the algorithm, it is addressed before moving further down the algorithm.

In a tactical setting, simple parameters such as level of consciousness and pulse strength are indicators of peripheral perfusion. Is the casualty verbally responsive? If yes, you have already gathered critical information: the blood pressure is strong enough to provide a modest level of cerebral perfusion, and the airway is patent. If the soldier's peripheral pulse is weak or absent, level of consciousness is altered, or if not verbally responsive, then immediate intervention is needed before moving down the algorithm.

MASSIVE HEMORRHAGE

Topical Hemostatic Agents If the wound is not amenable to tourniquet use and a pressure dressing is inadequate, use a hemostatic agent (**Figure 302-1**). The TCCC Committee recommends the following agents: Combat Gauze, Celox Gauze, and ChitoGauze. Combat Gauze (Z-Medica Corporation, Wallingford, CN) uses a zeolite compound impregnated into surgical gauze, which can be easily shaped into any wound. Celox Gauze (Medtrade Products LTD, Electra House, Crewe, UK) is a chitosan-impregnated gauze, as is ChitoGauze (HemCon Medical Technologies, Portland, OR).

To apply any of these gauze-like hemostatic agents, prepare the wound by evacuating excess blood, taking care to preserve any clot that may have formed around the damaged vasculature; pack the hemostatic gauze directly over the site of the most active bleeding; repack or adjust the gauze for optimum placement; use additional hemostatic agent as required. Hold direct pressure for a minimum of 3 minutes, then reassess for bleeding and repack as needed. Secure the hemostatic agent in place with a pressure dressing.

Junctional Hemorrhage Junctional hemorrhage (from the "junctional" anatomic area between the limbs and intracavitary areas of the abdomen or thorax) is difficult to control. Hemorrhage in the axilla and groin is not amenable to tourniquet application and hemostatic agents.[7] Specialized junctional tourniquets may be beneficial in certain cases.

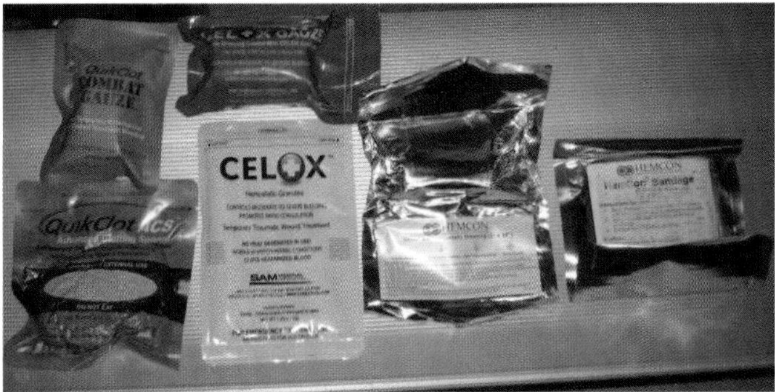

FIGURE 302-1. Examples of hemostatic dressings. [Image Reproduced with permission from COL Ian S. Wedmore, MD, FACEP, FAWN, DiMM.]

Presently these include the Abdominal Aortic Tourniquet,[8] the Combat Ready Clamp,[9] the Junctional Emergency Tourniquet Tool,[10] and the SAM Junctional Tourniquet. Each product has specific directions for application.

Systemic Hemorrhage Control: Tranexamic Acid Tranexamic acid decreases mortality in trauma.[11] It is recommended for use in all casualties that require significant fluid or blood products. Tranexamic acid is most effective when given within 1 hour of injury and must be given within the first 3 hours. The dose is 1 gram of tranexamic acid in 100 mL of normal saline.[12]

Prior to the Clinical Randomization of an Antifibrinolytic in Significant Hemorrhage (CRASH) study and introduction of tranexamic acid, recombinant factor VIIa was considered for use by some special operations forces.[13] The advent of tranexamic acid, with its ease of administration, efficacy, and improved safety profile (the risk of systemic hypercoagulability has always been a concern), has limited the use of recombinant factor VIIa to very specific intraoperative clinical scenarios.

AIRWAY

Airway intervention during the primary survey is similar for both combat and civilian casualties. Less than 1% of combat trauma requires lifesaving airway intervention in the prehospital setting.[14,15]

Lack of spontaneous respirations is a grievous prognostic sign. If there are no spontaneous respirations after opening the airway, the casualty is triaged to the expectant category (expected to die) in a mass casualty (MASCAL) situation (defined as more casualties than resources available); if the situation and resources allow, perform advanced airway techniques including cricothyrotomy,[16] supraglottic airway[17] intubation, and mechanical ventilation. If space is limited, cricothyrotomy equipment is the most important.[31] The threshold for performing a cricothyrotomy during combat should be low. It is critical to confirm placement and firmly secure the airway.

RESPIRATORY/BREATHING

Tension Pneumothorax The nearly universal use of body armor in present combat operations provides critical protection to the chest and upper abdomen, as evident in the 5% to 7% thoracic wound rate, the lowest in U.S. military conflicts.[18] Many combatants are alive today because of the proper use of body armor.

In a tactical setting, the threshold to perform a needle decompression is very low, as most casualties with penetrating chest trauma will have some degree of hemo-/pneumothorax, and even in the absence of tension pneumothorax, needle decompression is unlikely to cause harm. Use the largest and longest catheters available, because catheters are apt to kink or occlude, and the needle will have to penetrate through several inches of muscle and soft tissue to enter the thorax. The TCCC minimum standard is the 14-gauge 3 inch long needle, as any shorter length will often not penetrate through a muscular chest.[19] Also, there are 10- and 12-gauge catheters available in 3-inch lengths that are highly recommended over the standard, universally available 14-gauge catheters because they are even less likely to kink or occlude with patient movement. Two locations are recommended: (1) the second intercostal space, midclavicular line; or (2) the anterior axillary line at the fourth to fifth intercostal space (see chapter 68, "Pneumothorax," for further discussion).[20]

Penetrating Chest Trauma Penetrating chest trauma with open pneumothorax or sucking chest wounds is common with large injuries to the chest wall. There are many chest seals, including valved/vented and non-valved/vented chest seals. The updated TCCC standard is to use a valved/vented chest seal as the first choice. If not available, then an unvented seal can be used, but the patient will need to be continuously reassessed for the need for possible needle decompression.[21] Most casualties encountered in a combat setting are bloody and sweaty; applying a chest dressing that actually adheres to the chest is no small accomplishment and requires some skill and proper preparation of the skin. Wipe the skin as dry as possible. Consider using tincture of benzoin or Mastisol to facilitate dressing adherence if it is available and you have the luxury of time.

Chest Tubes Many physicians come into a field environment expecting to perform sophisticated interventions such as tube thoracostomy or thoracotomy at the point of injury. At this phase of tactical field care, do not expect to perform either of these procedures. The casualty is better served if you focus on basic, lifesaving procedures, prepare for immediate evacuation, and leave more sophisticated interventions for the next level of care. The lifesaving intervention for a chest injury is needle decompression; a chest tube is not immediately required. Needle decompression can be as effective as a chest tube in a patient for up to 4 hours if the patient is not subjected to much movement.[22] Needle decompression can be repeated as needed.

CIRCULATION

The TCCC mainstays of circulation management are the appropriate use of low-volume resuscitation (also known as **hypotensive or hypovolemic resuscitation**) and the selection of appropriate resuscitation fluids. The first step is vascular access.

IV Access Smaller-bore IVs (primarily 18-gauge catheters) are preferred in a tactical environment. Large-bore IVs are more appropriate to administer blood products, which typically are not an option at this phase of field care, and 18-gauge catheters are more than adequate to provide fluid resuscitation in a tactical setting. If blood products are available, then a larger-gauge catheter is indicated.

It is critical to firmly secure the catheter in the combat setting. Use a clear adhesive bandage first; then wrap enough tape to ensure that the catheter will hold in place if you were to throw the IV bag. There are also commercially available IV catheters with Velcro wraps that work very well. There is no one right way to secure a catheter, but give due attention to this because vascular access is the lifeline for severe combat casualties.

Intraosseous Access An intraosseous (IO) line is the alternative to IV access. There are a number of IO devices available commercially, designed for different osseous points of access. Nearly universal use of body armor in the modern tactical environment protects the sternum, so this site is ideal for IO access. Provide secure catheter fixation to prevent dislodgement during patient movement. Some devices may require a removal instrument, which you should secure to the patient; without this removal instrument, the catheter must be surgically removed at the next level of care.

Permissive Hypotension/Low-Volume Resuscitation Following the landmark 1994 Ben Taub study[23] and with subsequent extensive supporting research, permissive hypotension is the TCCC standard for treating noncompressible hemorrhage. **Noncompressible hemorrhage** is bleeding that occurs in any body part or area that cannot be controlled by a tourniquet or other method of compression. In combat injuries, this equates to penetrating wounds of the abdomen, thorax, and possibly junctional areas. This type of bleeding tends to decrease or even clot once the blood pressure has decreased significantly; however, at this low level of blood pressure and tissue perfusion, the casualty will eventually reach a state of irreversible shock. Providing large-volume resuscitation will initially raise blood pressure and perfusion, but it is also likely to "blow out" any formed clot, resulting in immediate rebleeding and further dilution of clotting factors as additional fluid is given to maintain blood pressure. This vicious cycle leads to rapid death.

We attempt to increase the survival time of casualties by maintaining a delicate balance between a blood pressure high enough to provide adequate tissue perfusion but low enough to avoid clot "blow-out" and clotting factor dilution. **Current recommendations are to maintain a mean arterial pressure of 60 mm Hg or a systolic blood pressure of approximately 80 to 90 mm Hg.**[24,25] A blood pressure of 80 to 90 mm Hg is clinically noted by a normal level of consciousness and a weakly palpable radial pulse.[26] Multitrauma patients with a head injury can be difficult to manage. If hypotensive resuscitation is required in a head-injured casualty, try to maintain a systolic blood pressure between 90 and 95 mm Hg.[27,28]

Resuscitation Fluid The prehospital resuscitation fluid of choice for combat trauma has changed over the last 10 years of U.S. military conflict. The goals of the TCCC Committee in recommending the appropriate resuscitation fluid are the following:

1. Enhance the body's ability to form clots with platelets, plasma, and red blood cells at sites of active bleeding.
2. Minimize adverse effects (edema and dilution of clotting factors) resulting from iatrogenic resuscitation injury.
3. Restore adequate intravascular volume and organ perfusion prior to definitive surgical hemorrhage control.
4. Optimize oxygen-carrying capacity as much as possible.

The current resuscitation fluid recommendations for a severe hypovolemic shock are as follows, in order of preference:

Fresh whole blood

Blood components in a 1:1:1 ratio of packed red blood cells (PRBCs):plasma:platelets

Blood components in a 1:1 ratio of PRBCs:plasma

Plasma: freeze-dried plasma or fresh frozen plasma appropriately reconstituted

PRBCs

Hextend

Lactated ringer's or Plasmalyte

Whole-Blood and Blood Component Infusions In the combat setting, prehospital blood transfusion is carried out under specifically approved theater protocols by specially trained and certified providers. For example, several special operations units can give European-produced freeze-dried plasma under an approved protocol.

Fresh whole blood is the TCCC primary resuscitation fluid of choice because it has all the required blood components in their natural state and provides a survival advantage to casualties with severe trauma and shock.[29,30] The use of whole blood in civilian institutions is rare. However, in a battlefield environment, whole blood is often obtained from fellow soldiers known as "walking blood banks" who are the only available blood source. During Operation Iraqi Freedom, 13% of blood transfusions used fresh whole blood.[28]

All U.S. combatants are tested for human immunodeficiency virus on a regular basis, but not for hepatitis. There is a U.S. Food and Drug Administration–approved rapid test (QuickVue; Quidel Corporation, San Diego, CA) for human immunodeficiency virus and hepatitis B and C that has been used for timely screening (manufacturer reports >98% sensitivity and specificity). All potential donors should be screened for risk, although perceived risk is often outweighed by potential benefit; additionally, all recipients and donors have blood samples sent to the Armed Forces Blood Program for retrospective analysis. The collection kits for fresh whole-blood transfusions are readily available through military medical supply channels. Because whole-blood transfusions are the treatment of choice for severe trauma and shock, we expect future developments in whole-blood storage to increase its availability for resuscitation.

If fresh whole blood is not available, the next preferred choice is plasma, PRBCs, and platelets in a 1:1:1 ratio.[31,32] A unit of plasma is given first, followed by the PRBCs, and then platelets. In addition to PRBCs, the military is now fielding frozen red blood cells and deglycerated red blood cells to augment current supplies of liquid-packed red blood cells.

The next preferred choice is PRBCs and plasma in a 1:1 ratio if platelets are not available.[33,34] Plasma is again given first followed by PRBCs. Advances in warm platelet storage will hopefully increase the availability of platelets in the near future.

If availability of blood products is limited, you may have to choose between PRBCs and plasma alone. There is some debate as to whether PRBCs or plasma alone is best, so product availability is more likely to drive this decision. Although availability of plasma is somewhat limited, some special operations combat medics now carry freeze-dried plasma as compared to PRBCs. The freeze-dried plasma concentrate currently carried by our medics is produced in France and available for use by North Atlantic Treaty Organization countries[35]; however, the French freeze-dried plasma should only be used to resuscitate casualties who have given prior informed consent, given the theoretical risk for transmission of certain viral diseases. Units that intend to use freeze-dried plasma typically arrange for consent of their soldiers prior to deployment and provide some method of identification for those who give consent and those who do not.

Colloids and Crystalloids If no blood products are available, **Hextend** (hetastarch in lactated ringer's solution) is recommended. There is no overwhelming evidence supporting the use of crystalloid over colloid in the young, healthy combat trauma casualty; additionally, colloid has a clear advantage from a weight/volume perspective in the prehospital environment, where the medic must carry the fluid on his back. Hetastarch 500 mL provides intravascular volume expansion of 600 to 800 mL. Hextend is potentially protective against multisystem trauma–induced acute respiratory distress syndrome, induces a favorable acid-base balance, and results in less severe coagulopathy.[36] Indiscriminate colloid use can have coagulopathic and immunologic effects, but these adverse effects typically do not occur with colloid administrations of <1500 mL.[37,38]

If fluid resuscitation requires >1500 mL of colloid, lactated ringer's solution is given next. Initial use of colloids to replenish intravascular volume during resuscitation must be balanced at some point with an appropriate volume of crystalloid to avoid extensive intracellular dehydration. Start with a 500-mL bolus, and repeat the bolus in 30 minutes if there is no clinical response, using pulse strength and level of consciousness to guide the volume infused. Maintain a systolic blood pressure of 80 to 90 mm Hg, but in head injury, a systolic blood pressure between 90 and 95 mm Hg is the goal.

One liter of infused lactated ringer's results in only 200 to 250 mL of intravascular volume expansion; normal saline is not recommended for resuscitation due to the hyperchloremic acidosis it produces.[39] Additionally, aggressive resuscitation with saline-based resuscitation strategies is associated with a number of adverse effects, including increased bleeding, acute respiratory distress syndrome, multiorgan failure, acute coronary syndrome, and increased mortality.[40-42]

Other Resuscitation Solutions Hypertonic saline (7.5% saline) has some benefits in the intensive care setting[43-45] but has not been evaluated in combat.[46] Hypertonic saline is neither commercially available nor Food and Drug Administration approved, and is not an option for use by U.S. Armed Forces.

Hemoglobin-based oxygen-carrying solutions are promising in theory, but at this time, clinical trials are ongoing and no hemoglobin-based, oxygen-carrying solutions are presently approved by the Food and Drug Administration or available on the commercial market.[47,48]

Oral Hydration Common practice in the civilian community is for patients to avoid any oral intake because of the risk of aspiration during anticipated surgery. In the combat setting, there are often limited IV fluids available and long waiting times for evacuation or surgical intervention. In the patient with a normal level of consciousness, the risk of aspiration is very low and outweighed by the benefit of maintaining adequate hydration and patient comfort if evacuation is delayed. As such, oral fluid hydration is acceptable for combat casualties in many situations, even if surgery is anticipated at the next level of care. The only contraindication is active vomiting or an altered level of consciousness that increases risk of aspiration. Time to surgery is not an issue in oral provision of clear liquids to combat casualties.[49]

HYPOTHERMIA AND HEAD INJURY

Rewarming a hypothermic casualty can be very difficult, so it is better to prevent than to treat. Under TCCC, we prevent hypothermia by wrapping the patient in a multilayer insulating wrap with a vapor barrier liner.

Closed head injury is one of the final considerations in this modified algorithm. If a casualty has an altered level of consciousness, it is either because of inadequate cerebral perfusion or cerebral injury. If hypovolemic shock has been ruled out or treated and the mechanism is consistent with closed head injury, then treat accordingly. Have the patient recline with the head elevated at 30 degrees. Give oxygen to maintain an oxygen saturation of at least 90%. Maintain a systolic blood pressure of at least 90 mm Hg.[26]

SECONDARY SURVEY

Expose the casualty as much as the tactical situation will allow. Be prepared to preserve body heat to avoid hypothermia. Stabilize fractures and treat less severe wounds. **Continually reassess the casualty.** This may seem obvious, but a tactical environment with multiple casualties is chaotic. Do not expect to have an assistant to monitor each casualty or call out periodic vital signs. Attend to the casualties who require intervention, but remember to reassess everyone. This can be as quick as asking a quick question to assess airway, hemodynamic status, and level of consciousness, or quickly palpate a radial pulse to determine rate and strength; obtain blood pressure if possible and if there are concerns about hemodynamic status. The character of the peripheral pulse and the Glasgow coma scale are reliable severity indicators.[50] Recheck dressings or bandages for continued bleeding.

PAIN CONTROL

Pain control is crucial for facilitating transport and patient comfort. Under TCCC, there are three primary pharmacologic modes of pain control. For lesser injuries with normal mental status, use a combat pill pack. This contains two 500-milligram acetaminophen tablets and a meloxicam tablet. This combination is effective for moderate pain control, does not affect mental status, and is administered orally. Because meloxicam has a favorable side effect profile and no effect on platelet function, it is the TCCC nonsteroidal anti-inflammatory drug of choice.

FENTANYL AND KETAMINE

For more severe pain, we recommended either **oral transmucosal fentanyl citrate lozenge**, informally known as the fentanyl "lollipop," or **ketamine**. Oral transmucosal fentanyl citrate provides rapid-onset, long-lasting pain relief for severe pain without the need for an IV. When placed into the buccal fold and slowly sucked on, 25% of the fentanyl is absorbed sublingually, with onset in 15 minutes. The remainder that is swallowed enters the GI tract and loses about 50% of its bioavailability through first-pass effect, but the remaining 50% is slowly absorbed, providing more extended pain relief for the next 4 to 6 hours.[51] An 800-microgram fentanyl lozenge is the recommended starting dose. Rapidly chewing and swallowing the lozenge will decrease the total amount of fentanyl received, because less is absorbed sublingually and more enters the digestive system, which is subject to first-pass effect. Should the casualty swallow the lozenge, he or she is generally not at risk of an uncontrolled fentanyl bolus. To avoid swallowing, the recommended technique is to tape the lozenge to the patient's finger, which will deter swallowing and prevent overdosing should the patient become somnolent (as the lozenge attached to the hand will fall from the mouth). If pain control is not achieved in 15 minutes, a second 800-microgram lozenge can be placed in the other cheek. Fentanyl can also be given intranasally with the use of a nasal atomizer.[52] If an IV is available, then IV fentanyl or IV ketamine can be used and titrated to effect.

Ketamine at subdissociative doses is an effective pain control agent. It can be given IM, IV, IO, or intranasally via nasal atomizer or syringe with rapid onset and good efficacy. The initial dose is 50 milligrams IM or intranasally repeated every 30 minutes and titrated to effect or 20 milligrams IV/IO by slow push repeated every 20 minutes and titrated to effect.

For treatment of nausea, the TCCC Committee now recommends ondansetron, oral dissolving tablets every six hours as needed.

ANTIBIOTICS

All war wounds are dirty and contaminated. Early antibiotic use with such wounds may decrease subsequent infection.[53] For those able to tolerate PO administration, a single 400-milligram dose of oral moxifloxacin, found in the combat pill pack, is recommended. For casualties with hypotension or an altered level of consciousness, administer either cefotetan, 2 grams, or ertapenem, 1 gram IV.

SPECIFIC INJURIES

BURN CARE: THE RULE OF 10S

TCCC has adopted the rule of 10s for burn management, which is clinically effective and easy to implement in a prehospital environment.[54] For burns >20% total body surface area, first estimate the total body surface area burned to the nearest 10%. Then, **for adults weighing 40 to 80 kg, give IV fluid as follows: 10 mL × % total body surface area burn per hour. For every 10 kg of patient weight above 80 kg, add another 100 mL of fluid per hour** (resuscitation for hemorrhagic shock takes precedence over resuscitation for burn shock).

For example, for a 90-kg patient with 40% total body surface area burns, the following would be given: 40% × 10 mL = 400 mL, plus 100 mL for 10 kg above the 40 to 80 kg range, giving a total of 500 mL of IV fluid per hour. Once the patient is at a higher level of care, the fluid rate can be adjusted based on clinical status and urinary output.

BLAST INJURIES

Injuries from explosions have historically been the leading cause of deaths in combat. This trend has continued, as we see approximately 50% of combat deaths and 77% of all injuries in the global war on terror caused by explosions. There is the tendency to rely on common clinical indicators to triage blast casualties. Tympanic membrane perforation and hypopharyngeal petechiae are common findings in blast casualties; however, no correlation has yet been shown between these findings and level of injury. There are many factors that contribute to a pattern of injury, such as body orientation relative to the blast and confined versus open space, so be wary of relying on a particular clinical finding to triage casualties.[55] If anything, the most reliable sign may be respiratory distress immediately after the blast. Casualties with clinically significant lung injury typically manifest as respiratory failure within minutes of the blast.[55,56] See chapter 7 for detailed discussion.

CERVICAL SPINE INJURY

As discussed earlier, the vast majority of penetrating injuries in the combat setting do not require cervical spine immobilization, unless there is direct injury to the neck with associated neurologic deficit.[57] In fact, cervical spine immobilization (particularly with a cervical collar) will impede the ability to manage the more immediate concerns of a penetrating neck injury. Therefore, cervical spine immobilization for penetrating injury in a combat casualty is not recommended. Blunt head trauma should be treated with cervical spine immobilization, situation permitting, as practiced in the civilian sector.[58]

ABDOMINAL TRAUMA

Although body armor does provide some protection to the upper abdomen, the lower abdomen is still relatively vulnerable. There is a groin attachment for the issued body armor that provides some protection to the lower abdomen, but it is not composed of a rigid Kevlar plate that is used to protect the chest and back; rather, this is a flexible Kevlar material that allows for movement at the hips, while providing some level of protection to the lower abdomen and groin region. Use of this additional piece of equipment has become more prevalent among our combat troops.

With a significant large-vessel (aorta, inferior vena cava, iliac vessels), liver, or splenic injury, there is not much a combat physician can do to save a casualty. In this situation, stabilize the casualty as best as possible, start an IV, administer antibiotics, and transport to a higher level of care with surgical capability immediately. For management of difficult-to-control, noncompressible massive hemorrhage, see the TCCC section on massive hemorrhage control.

If there is a bowel evisceration, replacing the contents will minimize insensible fluid and heat loss and allow for easier casualty movement. First remove any significant particulate matter or dirt; then attempt to replace the bowel contents intra-abdominally (this might not be possible if there is significant bowel edema and/or a small abdominal defect); cover exposed bowel and abdominal defect with a moist dressing; cover with plastic wrap or other fluid-impervious dressing to minimize insensible fluid loss; start an IV and administer IV fluids as needed; and administer IV antibiotics in preparation for evacuation.

PELVIC TRAUMA

The standard torso body armor does not provide any protection to the pelvis. A groin attachment protects the genital region and does provide some protection for the perineum, but the inguinal regions, containing large neurovascular bundles, are left largely unprotected. As such, the femoral vessels are vulnerable to penetrating injury, often resulting in life-threatening hemorrhage.

A tourniquet or pressure dressing to a proximal femoral artery or vein injury may be ineffective. For this type of injury, use of a hemostatic agent is imperative. Direct pressure should be applied to gain immediate control of the bleeding. Vessel clamping should only be attempted if an effective tourniquet or pressure dressing cannot be applied, a hemostatic dressing is not available, there is no device to control junctional hemorrhage, and there is no ability for immediate evacuation.

Pelvic fractures can result in significant hemorrhage that is difficult to control. Determination of a pelvic fracture, if not obvious, should be done from symptoms of pain and a clinical suspicion. The practice of "springing" or doing a "pelvic rock" is no longer recommended because this technique is likely more harmful than beneficial.[59] Past recommendations of improvised pelvic splinting with a sheet to produce needed compression for hemorrhage control can be used (if no other more effective options are available), but such splinting is inferior to more recent commercially manufactured pelvic splints and binders.[48,59]

EXTREMITY AMPUTATION

About 7% of wounded soldiers in Operation Iraqi Freedom and Operation Enduring Freedom had a major extremity amputation, and 50% of soldiers killed in action or who died of wounds had major amputations.[60] Field treatment of an amputation is focused primarily on hemorrhage control and preserving as much tissue as possible. Often the vessels of the limb have retracted from the initial force of the amputation, making it particularly difficult to identify and control hemorrhage. It may appear that hemostasis has been achieved with little effort; however, effective hemorrhage control may be necessary in the form of a hemostatic agent, pressure dressing, or tourniquet because delayed bleeding often occurs as the damaged vessels relax and dilate shortly after the patient appears stable. Constant reevaluation of the patient is essential. A partial amputation where the limb is still attached by substantial tissue or bone should be treated the same as an open fracture with hemorrhage control, wound debridement and irrigation, antibiotic administration, and splinting in an attempt to salvage the limb.

MASS CASUALTY TRIAGE

Mass casualty or MASCAL events are generally defined as situations in which the number and needs of the casualties exceed available resources (personnel and supplies). Three casualties might represent a MASCAL for one inexperienced physician, whereas 30 casualties might not represent a MASCAL for five well-prepared physicians.

Triage is a critical aspect of managing a MASCAL (**Table 302-4** provides one example of a simple triage algorithm). Another very effective method for handling a large number of casualties is the SALT mass casualty triage methodology (**Figure 302-2**). **SALT stands for sort, assess, lifesaving interventions, and treatment/transport,** which are the key activities that must be accomplished during the triage process.

THREE-TIER PRIORITIZATION

SALT begins with a global sorting of casualties, prioritizing them into three tiers for individual assessment. The triage physician directs casualties to walk to a designated area "if they need help." Those who follow the command to walk are the last priority for individual assessment, because they demonstrate an intact airway, breathing, circulation, and mental status and are therefore the least likely to have a life-threatening condition. The remaining casualties should then be asked to wave or be observed for purposeful movement. Those who remain still and do not move, as well as those with obvious life-threatening injuries, such as massive external hemorrhage, are assessed first. Those who wave are individually assessed next, followed by the ones who previously walked to a designated area. Although this initial sorting is not perfect, it is an attempt to organize numerous casualties.

TABLE 302-4 Mass Casualty Triage Algorithm

AIRWAY: *Is the casualty moving air?*
Yes—assess breathing
No—open airway, moving air now?
Yes—assess breathing
No—EXPECTANT
BREATHING: *Respiratory rate >30 breaths/min?*
Yes—IMMEDIATE, address cause
No—assess circulation
CIRCULATION: *Radial pulse weak/absent or heart rate >140 beats/min?*
Yes—IMMEDIATE, address cause
No—assess mental status
MENTAL STATUS: *Responds to simple commands?*
Yes—NOT an IMMEDIATE
No—IMMEDIATE, address cause

INDIVIDUAL CASUALTY ASSESSMENT

The second step of SALT is to perform individual assessments and apply lifesaving interventions, such as controlling massive external hemorrhage or opening an airway. Lifesaving interventions must meet all of the following criteria: can be provided quickly; can greatly improve a casualty's likelihood of survival; does not require the physician to stay with the casualty; are within the physician's scope of practice; and require only immediately available equipment. After appropriate interventions are performed, casualties are prioritized for treatment and assigned to one of the following triage categories: **immediate, delayed, minimal, and expectant** (includes the dead for the purpose of military triage), known in the military by the acronym **DIME**.

Colored triage tags or chemical light markers can mark casualties based on triage category. Colored triage tags typically are red for immediate, yellow for delayed, green for minimal, and black for expectant or deceased. If chemical light sticks are employed, red is typically used for immediate, green/yellow for delayed, and blue for expectant. Avoid using green and yellow chemical lights for different triage categories to mirror the markings on the triage tags, because it may be difficult to distinguish the two colors during night operations.

The **field triage score** is another easy, rapidly applicable method to identify casualties who are more seriously injured and expected to have a higher mortality. The field triage score is based on two variables: character of the radial pulse and the motor component of the Glasgow coma scale (GCS-M), namely the ability to follow commands. A weak or absent radial pulse, which correlates with a systolic blood pressure of ≤90 to 100 mm Hg, is assigned a score of 0, whereas normal pulse character (systolic blood pressure >90 to 100 mm Hg) is assigned a score of 1. Similarly, an abnormal GCS-M (<6) is assigned a score of 0, whereas the ability to follow simple commands (GCS-M of 6) receives a

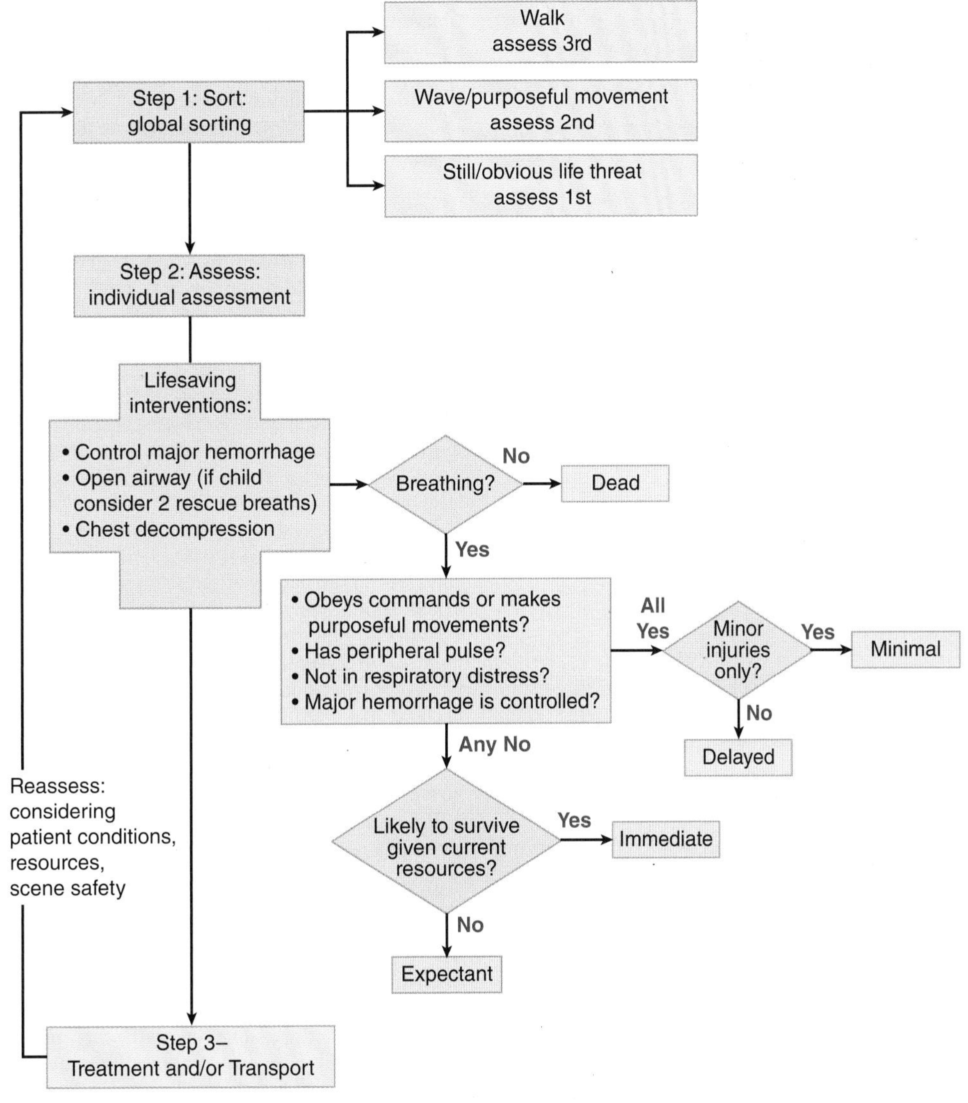

FIGURE 302-2. SALT (sort, assess, lifesaving interventions, treatment/transport) triage algorithm.

score of 1. A casualty can therefore receive an aggregate field triage score of 2, 1, or 0. A retrospective review of 4988 casualties in Iraq and Afghanistan from 2002 to 2008 demonstrated that those with a field triage score of 2 had a mortality of only 0.1% (5 of 4366), whereas those with a field triage score of 1 and 0 had a mortality of 10.8% (33 of 540) and 41.4% (34 of 82), respectively.[61]

Triage categories are not the same as evacuation categories. Triage identifies the severity of a casualty's injuries and determines a treatment priority based on the likelihood of survival, whereas evacuation is based on the urgency of transport to definitive care and the likelihood of deterioration over time. Triage is an ongoing, dynamic process, and triage categories may change if an intervention stabilizes a casualty or if a casualty deteriorates clinically. For example, a delayed casualty with second-degree burns over 30% of his body may become immediate if unrecognized inhalational injury leads to airway swelling and compromise.

CPR

Battlefield resuscitation of victims of blast or penetrating trauma who have no pulse, respiratory effort, or other signs of life will not be successful and should not be attempted because CPR on combat casualties has failed to show any benefit.[62,63] Therefore, CPR on the battlefield is not currently recommended. Even in the civilian setting, very few trauma arrest patients survive when prehospital CPR is performed.[64,65] In a tactical situation, CPR should only be considered as a last effort if the situation permits and appropriate resources are available, and in the case of nontraumatic disorders such as hypothermia, near-drowning, and electrocution. Casualties with torso trauma or polytrauma, who are pulseless and apneic, should receive bilateral needle decompression of the chest to ensure they do not have a tension pneumothorax prior to discontinuation of care. CPR may be initiated during evacuation for casualties that do not have obviously fatal injuries and will be arriving at a facility with surgical capability within a short period of time. CPR should not be done at the expense of mission compromise or denying lifesaving care to other casualties.[66]

REFERENCES

The complete reference list is available online at www.TintinalliEM.com.

CHAPTER 303 Legal Issues in Emergency Medicine

Jonathan E. Siff

INFORMED CONSENT

Informed consent is the legal standard under which providers educate patients (those who have the capacity to make medical decisions or their surrogates) about proposed treatments and alternatives.[1] The desirability of informed consent is based on the belief that it fosters the twin concepts of patient well-being and autonomy. Informed consent also provides a legal basis for autonomy.

Providers should act in their patients' best interests while preserving autonomy whenever possible. The American College of Emergency Physicians Code of Ethics[2] recognizes this dual obligation in stating that emergency physicians "serve the best interest of their patients by treating or preventing disease or injury and by informing patients about their condition." The code of ethics goes on to say, "Adult patients with decision-making capacity have a right to accept or refuse recommended health care, and physicians have a concomitant duty to respect their choices. This right is grounded in the moral principle of respect for patient autonomy and is expressed in the legal doctrine of informed consent."[2]

BASIC ELEMENTS OF INFORMED CONSENT

Most patients arriving at the ED sign a general consent for treatment. General consent for treatment is widely understood to cover history taking, standard examinations, and basic procedures such as venipuncture and blood analysis. General consent forms do not provide consent for more detailed, risky, or invasive procedures.

Informed consent requires two conditions: the patient possesses decision-making capacity, and the patient can make a voluntary choice free of undue influence. The process of informed consent begins with the delivery of information to the patient by the provider. The patient must then reach a decision and authorize the procedure or treatment. Each part of the process is considered individually.

Patient Capacity Decision-making capacity (hereafter called "capacity") is the ability of the patient to make informed medical decisions. It is the provider's task to determine the patient's capacity.[3] The definition of capacity varies among jurisdictions, but, in general, capacity describes an individual's ability to make a decision based on personal values and comprehension of the likely consequences of that decision.[4,5]

One definition of capacity as it relates to health care is from Illinois law and reads: "'Decisional capacity' means the ability to understand and appreciate the nature and consequences of a decision regarding medical treatment or forgoing life-sustaining treatment and the ability to reach and communicate an informed decision in the matter as determined by the attending physician."[6] The American College of Physicians Ethics Manual describes decision-making capacity as "the ability to receive and express information and to make a choice consonant with that information and one's values."[4]

Competence, which is often incorrectly used interchangeably with capacity, is a legal term indicating a ruling by a court that a person is able to manage his or her own affairs.[7]

The capacity to make a medical decision is based on several basic abilities: the ability to receive information; to process and understand information; to deliberate about a decision; and to make, articulate, and defend choices. Generally, the physician assesses the above-listed patient abilities informally, by taking a history from an alert patient with no barriers to communication. Any barriers to communication as a result of language should be removed through translation, when possible, by an impartial medical translator.

Patients with altered mental status may not possess the memory or attention to receive and process the information and thus lack capacity.[8,9] However, diagnoses often associated with altered mental status, such as stroke, psychiatric illness, or dementia, should not lead to a presumption of incapacity. Assess whether or not the disorder affects patients' cognitive abilities.[5] Disagreement with the physician's plan does not indicate a lack of capacity if the decision was made in a rational way, which the patient can defend based on their values and beliefs.[9] A patient's decision-making capacity may change over time in the ED based on changes in medical condition, for example, in patients recovering from intoxication, hypoglycemia, or hypoxia.

Capacity may depend on the complexity of the decision and consequences of accepting or rejecting the intervention. For example, a patient may be competent to make a minor decision but not a major decision at a given point in time.[10] The more important the decision, the more important is the assessment.[4,11]

Factors useful to assess capacity are summarized in **Tables 303-1**[1] **and 303-2.**[11]

If a patient has capacity to make a given decision, his or her wishes should be respected.

Free Choice Informed consent must be voluntary and free of coercion. The choice must be free of manipulation or threats by providers, family, or other outside influences, and free of emotional or physical coercion.[2]

Information Necessary for Patient Decision Making The physician must provide the patient with the information needed to make a reasoned, informed decision. Generally, the provider performing the procedure should be the one to obtain consent. A delegate such as a resident or nurse practitioner may obtain consent, but the supervisor is responsible to ensure that consent was truly informed.[12] The required

TABLE 303-1 Factors for Emergency Providers to Consider When Determining Capacity

Presence of conditions impairing mental function
Presence of basic mental functioning (awareness, orientation, memory, attention)
The patient has understanding of specific treatment-related information
Appreciation of the significance of the information for the patient's situation
Patient's ability to reason about treatment alternatives in light of values and goals
Complexity of the decision-making task
Risks of the patient's decision
Patient's ability to describe, and consistency in reporting, the basis of their decision

information for decision making is the diagnosis; the nature and purpose of treatment; risks and consequences of treatment; alternatives and their risks and benefits; and prognosis if treatment is or is not accepted.[12]

How much information is necessary to meet the above requirement depends on the standard of disclosure being applied. There are two standards, each used in a large number of states, that address the details of the disclosure for consent.[12] The "reasonable person standard" for informed consent requires providers to give the patient all the information a "reasonable person" would need to make the same decision under similar circumstances.[13] The alternate standard is the less stringent "professional standard" for informed consent, which requires disclosure to be the same as any reasonably prudent, similarly trained physician would provide in a similar circumstance.[12] Emergency providers are well served to give more, not less, information to the patient.

Discussion and Decision Give the patient the opportunity to ask questions while considering the decision. The patient can be made realistically aware of ED time constraints for decision making, but without using coercion. Patients willing to continue should then give explicit authorization for the treatment or procedure. If the patient agrees too easily, has no questions, or is not engaged in the process, review the situation for barriers to communication such as language issues. A patient who is unable or unwilling to express a preference for a particular course of action may be presumed to lack capacity.[14]

DOCUMENTATION OF CONSENT

When obtaining informed consent, it is the **process** that is most important. Some states have specific requirements regarding written consent.[12] Where specific requirements regarding written consent are not present, oral consent is generally as good as written consent except that written documentation signed by the patient can aid the provider should the consent process be challenged later on.[12] At a minimum, the chart or consent form (material forms are required by Medicare for all nonemergency surgical procedures) should reflect who obtained consent; the provider(s) authorized to perform the treatment; that information on risks, benefits, and alternatives were disclosed; and that the patient had the opportunity to ask questions.[12,13,15] Ideally, the chart will contain both a signed consent form and a well-documented recap of the consent process.[16]

TABLE 303-2 Common Errors in the Assessment of Capacity

Assuming that if the patient lacks capacity for one type of decision, he or she lacks capacity for all decisions
Assuming that legal competence is the same as medical decision-making capacity
Presuming that capacity is constant over time
Assuming that a blood alcohol level is related to competence
Presuming that psychiatric disorders preclude adequate capacity
Failing to ensure the patient has relevant and consistent information before making a decision
Assuming that capacity should only be considered for refusal of treatment
Failure to recognize that the capacity to make decisions varies with the risks and benefits inherent in the decision

EXCEPTIONS TO INFORMED CONSENT

There are a number of exceptions to the right to informed consent in response to specific healthcare situations. These exceptions include emergencies; therapeutic privilege; public health imperatives, such as the treatment of certain diseases; patient waiver of consent; and, rarely, emergency research.[12,17] Of these, only emergencies and public health imperatives are applicable to clinicians working in the ED on a day-to-day basis.

Emergencies **Emergency providers should render needed emergency treatment even in situations where consent cannot be obtained or ascertained in a timely fashion due to the nature of the illness. Implied consent**, the basis of this exception, is that a reasonable person would give consent to emergency or lifesaving treatment.[12,18] If treatment can be delayed without harm, obtain consent before treatment. Should the situation change during treatment, obtain consent before further treatment.

Public Health Imperatives Public health imperatives are situations where the public good may limit individual patient autonomy. Patients with high-risk communicable diseases,[19] such as severe acute respiratory syndrome and tuberculosis, and patients with mental illness who pose a danger to themselves or the public are examples. Each state has regulations regarding communicable diseases and mental health law, and providers should be familiar with rules in their practice location. When patients meet criteria for health department–mandated treatment and quarantine, yet do not give consent, consult hospital infectious disease staff and local health officials as soon as possible.

WHEN INFORMED CONSENT CANNOT BE OBTAINED

If a patient does not have the capacity to give informed consent for a condition where no exception exists or once an emergency has been stabilized and nonemergent decisions need to be made, providers should identify a surrogate decision maker or directive.[2,9] First, inquire about advance directives or healthcare powers of attorney that can provide guidance or specify a decision maker (see chapter 300, "Death Notification and Advanced Directives"). In the absence of a power of attorney, state law may determine the patient's decision maker. A typical decision-making progression would be: spouse, adult children, parents, adult siblings, and the nearest relative not previously described.[20] Surrogates are expected to help providers determine what the patient would want in a particular situation and should not substitute their values for the patient's. Should no person be available for treatment decisions, providers should proceed with the patient's best interest in mind and involve hospital counsel to begin a guardianship process if the patient's lack of capacity is likely to be of significant duration.[10]

INFORMED REFUSAL

Patients may refuse part of a treatment plan, refuse to be evaluated entirely, or wish to leave before the completion of the planned evaluation. In these situations, the physician should ensure there are no miscommunications or misunderstandings at the root of the refusal.[10] Often, when issues are clarified, an agreement can be reached. Second, correct issues that may prevent an open, noncontentious discussion—such issues may be a blanket, a call to the patient's personal physician, or additional pain medication.[10,21] Finally, try to develop an alternative to the original plan that does not significantly alter the risk to the patient. For instance, a patient may not want a certain procedure but would be willing to accept admission for further evaluation.[10]

When communication and negotiation between the patient and provider fail and the patient possesses decisional capacity, the patient may choose to refuse care or end the encounter "against medical advice."

ED DEPARTURE AGAINST MEDICAL ADVICE AND ED ELOPEMENT

Approximately 1.4 million patients left hospital EDs against medical advice in 2010, representing 1% of patients.[22] Studies have documented poor outcomes in patients leaving against medical advice.[23,24] Characteristics of patients who leave against medical advice include lack of insurance, male, younger age, alcohol or drug dependency, psychiatric illness, and low income.[23,24] Patients often have serious complaints such as chest pain, abdominal pain, or trauma. Patients give many reasons for their desire to leave, including outside obligations such as family or pets, the wish for treatment at another hospital, concerns for cost of treatment, fear of recommended treatment, a desire for tobacco, drugs, or alcohol, narcotic requests, or improvement in the condition that prompted the ED visit.[25]

To proceed with an against-medical-advice discharge, assess the patient's capacity, with special attention to barriers limiting capacity. Alcohol use and psychiatric diagnoses are not absolute barriers to discharge against medical advice, with the exception of suicidal and homicidal patients. Document the patient's behavior that clearly demonstrates there was no impairment of capacity by intoxication or mental illness. Educate the patient about the risks associated with refusing to complete evaluation and/or treatment. Discuss the patient's reasons for leaving, because these often present opportunities for negotiation and convincing the patient to continue care.[9] Use plain language and avoid medical terms. Given the medical-legal and patient risks of against-medical-advice discharge, make a substantial effort to convince the patient to remain but do not resort to threats. Incorrect statements such as "insurance will not pay for this visit if you leave against medical advice" may further damage the patient–provider relationship and discourage the patient from returning.[26,27] Model documentation of an against-medical-advice discharge should contain the following elements[21,28]:

- Documentation of capacity (ideally with examples and examination clearly noted)
- Discussion of the risks reviewed with the patient including what diagnoses were being considered
- Explicit documentation in the chart that the patient was leaving against medical advice and what treatments, procedures, and courses of actions were refused by the patient
- Offers made of alternative treatments or courses of action
- Efforts to involve family, friends, or clergy in the decision
- Explanation of any potentially problematic entries in the chart such as nursing notes or abnormal laboratory values—for example, if the patient has an elevated serum alcohol level, document that the patient is clinically sober and has capacity, if true
- Patient's signature on the against-medical-advice form, and if patient refuses to sign, document that fact
- Documentation of treatment and follow-up provided
- Documentation that the patient was told he or she is welcome to return at any time

While the most important part of documenting an against-medical-advice discharge is the discussion with the patient addressing the items above, having the patient sign an actual against-medical-advice form may help provide further liability protection in three ways: "1) it may terminate the providers legal duty to treat a patient; 2) creation of the affirmative defense of 'assumption of risk'; and 3) the creation of a record of evidence of the patient's refusal of care."[29]

When a patient leaves against medical advice, reasonable treatment should be provided as appropriate for the patient's medical condition and concordant with the patient's wishes. For example, provide antibiotics for infection, aspirin for chest pain, or stabilization for fractures. Tell the patient to return at any time. Provide a listing of resources for close follow-up and instruct the patient on signs and symptoms to prompt a return visit to the ED should the patient change his or her mind.[9,21]

It is also important to document situations when a patient leaves against advice or before treatment is completed without informing ED staff. Out of sight should not equal out of mind. Attempt to locate the patient within the facility and then check logical destinations. Often a phone call to the patient's home, cell phone, or emergency contact can provide an opportunity to encourage the patient to return to the ED. Document such communication attempts and their outcome.

The concepts of patient capacity and informed consent and refusal, their exceptions, and the moral obligations that underlie them should be integrated into daily ED practice.

ISSUES IN THE ED CARE OF MINORS

A minor is generally considered to be anyone less than 18 years of age, and parental consent is generally required for the treatment of minors. However, society and the legal system have determined that, in some circumstances, older children may be able to make many medical decisions independent of their parents.[30] Exceptions to parental consent for minors include emergencies, the treatment of certain diseases and conditions that are in the best interest of the minor or society, minors emancipated under law, and circumstances in which the best interests of the child are not being addressed by parents. State laws regarding minor care vary widely; providers caring for minors should review state regulations and call on legal counsel as needed.

TREATMENT OF MINORS IN EMERGENCIES

Minors often present to the ED without a parent or legal guardian in the care of an alternate caretaker such as a grandparent, school teacher, babysitter, camp counselor, or social worker.

In the United States under the Emergency Medical Treatment and Active Labor Act (EMTALA), EDs are legally obligated to evaluate all patients presenting with a medical condition and stabilize any emergency condition identified. There is no requirement for consent in this situation.[31,32] Providers have latitude in defining an emergency medical condition (EMC), especially if there is a delay in obtaining consent. It is always best to try to find parents or legal guardians while emergency care is being provided. Document all such efforts. Once the emergency condition is stabilized, the need for appropriate parental informed consent applies.

When an adult family member, such as a grandparent or adult sibling, brings the minor to the ED and has granted consent, care should be given while efforts are made to contact the parent or guardian. In the case of preplanned parental absence, not all U.S. states require a signed note from the parent authorizing treatment. In some U.S. states, laws authorize relatives to consent to medical treatment for minors under their care. However, if the treatment proposed carries a substantial risk and is not emergent, contact the parents or guardian before proceeding. Providers may obtain parental consent by telephone. In cases where no appropriate party can be reached to give consent, particularly in the case of invasive procedures, it is recommended that, when possible, the provider document a second opinion agreeing with the need to perform the procedure on an emergent basis.

EMANCIPATED MINORS

Minors who have become independent from the care and control of their parent or guardian are considered emancipated and may provide consent as adults. The definition of emancipation varies, and some states do not have specific emancipation statutes.[33] Common situations in which minors may be considered emancipated include minors who are married, enlisted in the U.S. armed services, pregnant or parents themselves, declared emancipated by a court, or self-supporting and not living at home.

Mature Minor Exception **The mature minor exception states that if a minor is sufficiently mature to understand the nature and consequences of a proposed medical treatment, then the minor should be able to consent or refuse treatment without parental involvement.** The mature minor exception is accepted under common law and, in some states, under specific legislation. Requirements for the mature minor exception are as follows: the child should generally be at least 14 or 15 years old; the treatment should be beneficial, not elective, and of low risk; and the minor must meet the requirements of informed consent.

Given the subjectiveness of this standard, it is prudent to carefully consider each individual case before treating a minor under the mature minor doctrine.[34]

If a minor is considered capable of providing informed consent for a given issue, then he or she should be considered equally capable of refusing that same treatment.

Sexually Transmitted Diseases Exemption All states allow minors to access testing and treatment for sexually transmitted diseases without parental consent. In most states, the minor must be at least 12 years old, but some states have a higher age requirement.[35,36] In some states, testing and/or treatment for human immunodeficiency virus may not be included in the exception.

Prenatal and Pregnancy Care Exemption Many states allow minors to consent to prenatal care and pregnancy-related care. In states lacking such statutes, minors are often provided prenatal care under the mature minor doctrine, particularly if the state allows minors to consent to other reproductive services.[35,36] About two-thirds of the states have laws allowing a minor to consent to treatment for their own child.[37]

Alcohol or Substance Abuse and Mental Health Treatment Exemption Nearly all states allow minors to access treatment for alcohol or substance abuse. A majority of states have no specific laws regarding access of mental health services, and of those that do, the range of services that can be accessed varies.[38]

Sexual or Physical Abuse Treatment Exemption The evaluation and treatment of sexual or physical abuse without parental consent is generally permitted. In many instances, these patients may be treated under the emergency exemption, because minors who have suffered physical or sexual abuse require prompt treatment. However, assuming that the parents are not the alleged perpetrators, seek parental involvement as early as possible.

PRACTICAL IMPLICATIONS OF TREATING MINORS UNDER STATUTORY EXCEPTIONS OR AS MATURE MINORS

The minor consenting to the treatment is generally responsible for the cost of treatment. Once a minor is treated under one of these statutes, the minor should be afforded the same confidentiality as an adult. In some states, certain exceptions exist if the provider feels that it is in the minor's best interest to have the parent notified. The Health Information Portability and Accountability Act of 1996 (HIPAA) Privacy Rule generally defers to state law or other applicable laws that expressly address a parent's ability to obtain health information about a minor including when a parent agrees to a confidential relationship between the physician and the minor.[39] The hospital bill may pose a potential risk for breach of confidentiality if charged to a parent's insurance carrier.

Assent and Refusal by the Older Minor Providers should seek the assent and cooperation of older or "mature" minors even when parents are granting permission for treatment. If the proposed treatment is nonemergent and the older minor refuses to give assent, the minor's decision should be strongly considered.

WHEN THE MINOR'S INTERESTS ARE NOT BEING PROTECTED

In almost all cases, parents make decisions they believe to be in their child's best interests. However, situations arise when the physician wishes to override or delay the decision making of the parent. For example, if the parent is intoxicated, carefully consider the parent's capacity to give informed consent or refuse care for the minor child. If parents disagree with a treatment plan based on religious or moral reasons, the court or child protective agencies may intervene if the disputed intervention is lifesaving. The American Academy of Pediatrics opposes religious doctrines that recommend opposition to medical attention for sick children and states that children who need medical care to prevent substantial harm or suffering should receive that care.[40]

PRIVACY, CONFIDENTIALITY, AND REPORTING

The ideas of privacy and confidentiality are important elements of ethics, religion, and law because they affirm the dignity and value of the individual.[41] Respect for these rights has been a cornerstone of medicine since ancient times. The Hippocratic Oath reads, "All that may come to my knowledge in the exercise of my profession . . . I will keep secret and will never reveal." The American College of Emergency Physicians Code of Ethics states that emergency physicians should "Respect patient privacy and disclose confidential information only with consent of the patient or when required by an overriding duty such as the duty to protect others or to obey the law."[42] The privacy of one's physical person and the privacy of one's personal information (confidentiality)[43] are considered together in this chapter. All states and the federal government have laws that govern privacy and confidentiality, including mandatory or voluntary reporting requirements that may override considerations of individual patient privacy and confidentiality.

BARRIERS TO PRIVACY AND CONFIDENTIALITY IN THE ED

ED barriers to privacy and confidentiality include ED physical design, operational issues, the presence of visitors, students, and other individuals, and video technology.

Design and operational issues that impact privacy and confidentiality include the triage area, frequent movement of patients between beds, open ED areas for documentation and work, and patient placement for close observation to minimize risk from falls or self-harm.[41,43] In addition, the growing problems of ED crowding and boarding lead to the use of hallway beds and nontraditional bed spaces, which greatly reduce the ability of staff to provide optimum privacy and confidentiality to patients.[44] ED staff should be vigilant when conducting interviews, teaching, or communicating to maximize patient privacy and confidentiality.

Students of various disciplines, law enforcement, and visitors should respect patient privacy and confidentiality.[45] Requests from patients to exclude healthcare students from observation or care should be considered, based on the patient's reasons for the request and the specific situation, but not guaranteed.[41,45] Obtain verbal consent from patients for the presence of students who do not participate in care, and accept refusals.

Law enforcement officials may engage in the collection of evidence and the interviewing of witnesses to crimes in the ED. Except where required by law, patients should have the option of whether or not to speak with law enforcement, and patient information releases, not expressly required by law, require the patient's consent.[46] Visitors should generally be allowed (as space permits), with consent from the patient.[41] Patients should be asked verbal permission for providers to discuss personal information in front of the visitor. In some cases, disclosure of certain diseases, such as human immunodeficiency virus, to a third party requires a written consent.[47] Providers should always consider the nature and gravity of the information being related to a patient and should try to give serious or very personal results and diagnoses in private, even if previously given permission to discuss in front of a visitor.

Patients brought to the ED in the custody of law enforcement pose unique challenges. The safety of staff and patients must be balanced with the privacy and confidentiality rights of the individual. The American College of Emergency Physicians recommends providing unbiased, attentive, and complete care to these patients and communicating instructions appropriate to the medical condition to correctional or law enforcement staff as indicated while maximizing patient privacy.[48]

Photography and video performed for the purposes of evidence collection, quality assurance, and documentation may be acceptable under certain circumstances, but patients should give consent except where not required under the law.[49] Photography and filming for educational and publication purposes always require patient consent. Images recorded for nonmedical or educational purposes without consent (especially with cell phones) are generally prohibited.[50,51] Obtain any necessary permissions from hospital administration and learn and follow all applicable policies and state laws surrounding filming and photography of patients in all circumstances. Cell phones, tablets, and laptop computers with identifiable patient information should be physically secured and protected with a password program, and images should never be sent via unencrypted email.

THE HEALTH INSURANCE PORTABILITY AND ACCOUNTABILITY ACT AND PROTECTED HEALTH INFORMATION

Definitions HIPAA is the most important U.S. law that protects the healthcare privacy and confidentiality of individuals. This legislation required the establishment of standards for the security, exchange, and integrity of electronic health information, and set rules for basic national privacy standards and fair information practices for health care.

The U.S. Department of Health and Human Services produced the "Standards for Privacy of Individually Identifiable Health Information," also called the *Privacy Rule*, in 2000. The rule has been amended several times with a major revision in January of 2013, commonly referred to as the *Omnibus Final Rule*.[52] These rules establish the obligations of "covered entities." Covered entities include "health plans, health care clearinghouses, and health care providers (broadly defined to include anyone who furnishes, bills, or is paid for health care in the normal course of business) and business associates of these entities, who transmit health information in electronic form when dealing with an individual's health information."[53] Only those parts of the privacy rule most applicable to emergency providers will be covered here.

Under HIPAA, health information (often referred to as *protected health information* [PHI]) is "any information, including genetic information, whether oral or recorded in any form or medium that (1) is created or received by a health care provider, health plan, public health authority, employer, life insurer, school or university, or health care clearinghouse; and (2) relates to the past, present, or future physical or mental health or condition of an individual; the provision of health care to an individual; or the past, present, or future payment for the provision of health care to an individual."[53] HIPAA also applies when PHI is transmitted or maintained by a covered entity. The rule also discusses individually identifiable health information, including demographic data such as name, Social Security number, date of birth, and other identifiers that "identify the individual or for which there is a reasonable basis to believe can be used to identify the individual."[53]

Disclosure of Protected Health Information PHI should be shared with the clear understanding that only the minimum amount of information required to accomplish the purpose of the disclosure will be released. These "minimum" necessary standards do not apply to information that is given to patients themselves, used for treatment, or required by law.[54] Covered entities should have procedures in place, including limitations on access to electronic medical records, to ensure that users are able to obtain only that information necessary to their job or business purpose.

HIPAA allows covered entities to use PHI, without authorization, for purposes of treatment, payment, and operations. Treatment is the provision, management, and coordination of health care and related services, including consultations and referrals.[55] The payment exclusion allows a healthcare provider to use PHI to obtain payment or be reimbursed for the care provided to an individual.[55] Operations include a number of activities, including, but not limited to, quality improvement, employee evaluation and credentialing, auditing programs, and business activity such as planning, development, management, and administration.[55] An exception to this rule is that psychotherapy notes often require written consent for their use except for treatment, certain legal matters, and the protection of the public from a serious threat.[56]

There are 12 national priorities, as shown in **Table 303-3**,[57,58] in addition to treatment, payment, and operations usage, for which covered entities are allowed to disclose PHI without authorization. These disclosures are permitted by the law and have specific conditions or limitations to balance the privacy of the individual and the public interest for the information.[57]

Under the privacy rule, the risk of every possible incidental use or disclosure of PHI does not have to be eliminated.[57] Provided the incidental disclosure or use occurs as the unintentional result of a legitimate use or disclosure of PHI, the entity has in place reasonable safeguards (as defined in the rule), and has applied the minimum necessary standard, there is likely to be no violation of the rule.[59]

TABLE 303-3 The 12 National Priorities for Which Protected Health Information May Be Disclosed or Used without Written Authorization

1. As required by law (statute, regulation, or court order)
2. For public health reporting (e.g., vital statistics, disease, adverse event reporting)
3. For reporting abuse, neglect, or domestic violence
4. For health oversight activities (e.g., inspections, audits)
5. For judicial and administrative proceedings
6. For law enforcement purposes (e.g., criminal investigations) under certain circumstances
7. For disclosures about deceased persons to medical examiners, coroners, and funeral directors
8. For organ, eye, and tissue donation purposes
9. For some types of research (e.g., in cases where an institutional review board has waived the authorization requirement)
10. To avert a serious threat to the health or safety of the public
11. For specialized government functions, such as military missions or correctional activities
12. For workers' compensation claims

Patient Rights to Protected Health Information The HIPAA regulations also require that a notice of privacy practices be given to all patients, informing them of their rights regarding their health information.[60] Patients are asked to sign these documents and receive a copy of the notice.

These rights to PHI include access to records in the patient's preferred format, request for amendments, request for additional restrictions, notice of PHI use, and an accounting of disclosures made from their PHI.[61-64] In general, most of these functions will be handled by a hospital's medical records department, but requests to amend records must be addressed by the provider promptly (60 days). If the request is denied, the patient has the right to place a written statement in the medical record disagreeing with the denial.[61]

Law Enforcement Rights to Protected Health Information HIPAA allows the limited release of PHI for certain law enforcement purposes. Release is permitted to respond to a judicially issued warrant, subpoena, court order, or grand jury subpoena. Release is allowed to assist law enforcement in identifying or locating a suspect, fugitive, material witness, or missing person by releasing only the following information: "name and address, date and place of birth, Social Security number, ABO blood type and Rh factor, type of injury, date and time of treatment, date and time of death, if applicable, and a description of distinguishing physical characteristics, including height, weight, gender, race, hair and eye color, presence or absence of facial hair (beard or moustache), scars, and tattoos."[65] Providers may notify authorities of a person's death if a possible criminal activity was the cause of the death. PHI may be released in response to law enforcement requests for information about a victim or suspected victim of crime, with the patient's consent. When a patient, who may be a victim of a crime, is unable to consent, the provider may release information to law enforcement if they believe the release is in the patient's best interests and that the information is not intended to be used against the patient by law enforcement.[53]

Impact of Protected Health Information on Emergency Physicians HIPAA allows for open discussions with primary providers, consultants, and other persons involved in the care of an individual. Primary providers are allowed to discuss a patient, without first obtaining the patient's consent, if the patient is under their care in the ED. Providers are able to release information under the national priorities and as required under state law. If family or friends call and ask about a patient by name, "directory" information may be released unless the patient has requested they not be listed in the directory. Providers are cautioned about releasing additional information over the phone unless

TABLE 303-4 Health Insurance Portability and Accountability Act (HIPAA) Do's and Don'ts

HIPAA Do's

1. Talk openly with patient's primary physician.
2. Discuss protected health information with consultants and other members of the patient's healthcare team.
3. Use protected health information for reimbursement and operational issues.
4. Release records to the patient or an authorized representative.*
5. Discuss patient protected health information with family or friends if the patient is in an emergency situation, unable to consent, and the information would be beneficial to the patient.

HIPPA Don'ts

1. Discuss patients or protected health information in public or unsecured areas.
2. Leave computers with access to protected health information logged on and unattended.
3. Discuss protected health information in front of others without permission.
4. Speak loudly when discussing protected health information, particularly in public areas.
5. Look at records for which you have no legitimate purpose as a provider.

*May require the patient to sign an authorization form.

they can reasonably confirm the identity of the caller and, if possible, have the patient's permission to release additional health information.

Do not access records for which you are not the treating provider, unless such information is needed for operations, for law enforcement, or for another legitimate reason. Document the reason for access to any chart where you are not the treating provider. Failure to comply with these regulations can lead to significant monetary and even criminal penalties for providers. See **Table 303-4** for some HIPAA do's and don'ts.

Need to Report Protected Health Information **Privacy and confidentiality are not absolute rights.** Ethicists, courts, and legislators have agreed that in some situations, the rights of the individual are overridden by the needs of the public. In many cases, this takes the form of permitted or mandatory reporting of certain diseases, pathogens, forms of abuse, and other medical conditions or situations. Providers should balance confidentiality, patient autonomy, the public good, and legal mandates with possible sanctions for noncompliance and medical-legal risk when deciding when to report a given condition.

Abuse All states require the reporting of suspected child abuse or neglect and generally give providers legal protection as long as reports are made in good faith.[43] Most states have similar reporting requirements for elder abuse. Some of these laws only pertain to those elderly patients who are incapacitated or in care facilities, whereas other states include all persons above a certain age.[66] Mandatory reporting laws for domestic partner violence have been passed in a few states. In some domestic violence cases, reporting may be required based on state laws that mandate reporting of injury during the commission of a crime or injuries from deadly weapons.[67,68] Key to the reporting of all types of abuse is the willingness of the provider to consider and discuss potential abuse cases with patients.[67,69]

Injury by Deadly Weapon or due to a Criminal Act Most states mandate the reporting of injuries from deadly weapons, including stab and gunshot wounds.[67] A number of states also require reporting of injuries that occur as a result of a criminal act but do not require reporting of so-called "victimless" crimes such as drug abuse.[43]

Driving Impairment Many patients have medical conditions that may cause care providers, family, and the public to question their ability to safely operate motor vehicles. In some states, providers are required to report drivers with epilepsy to the department of motor vehicles. Patients with a variety of other medical conditions, such as dementia, vision impairment, Parkinson's disease, and other degenerative conditions, as well as patients on certain medications, may be unable to safely operate a vehicle.[70] A majority of states provide physicians with immunity when reporting impaired drivers. In other states, immunity is not provided, and providers could be found liable for damages resulting from reporting or nonreporting.[67] Many providers have concerns about reporting these patients, and the American Academy of Neurology supports optional reporting of medically impaired or potentially impaired drivers.[70] A study of California emergency physicians found very low reporting rates in compliance with a state law requiring physicians to report all patients with lapses of consciousness.[71] In addition, some states require that providers report drivers who are in accidents while intoxicated.[67]

Infectious Disease Reporting The U.S. federal government requires the reporting of contagious diseases for surveillance purposes.[41] The annual lists of diseases and conditions under national surveillance are available on the Centers for Disease Control and Prevention website.[72] Pathogens on this list commonly encountered by emergency providers may include *Chlamydia trachomatis*, gonorrhea, viral hepatitis, human immunodeficiency virus, Lyme disease, pertussis, and resistant *Streptococcus pneumoniae*. Other pathogens, such as methicillin-resistant *Staphylococcus aureus*, may be reportable to other databases or to state health departments. The diseases under surveillance change as new pathogens are discovered and priorities change; other diseases are deleted from the list as they lose relevance.

Reporting of Medical Errors A number of states and organizations have enacted a combination of mandatory and voluntary reporting systems in an attempt to improve healthcare processes and reduce patient morbidity and mortality due to hospital errors and adverse events.[73] Providers should comply with these systems as required by law.

Reporting of Breaches and Penalties under HIPAA Under HIPAA, any disclosure, access, or use of PHI in a manner not permitted under the law is assumed to be a breach.[74] The covered entity must demonstrate that there is a low probability that the PHI has been compromised based on a risk assessment or face penalties. If a breach is found, notification may be required to the party whose information was compromised, the secretary of the Department of Health and Human Services, and in the case of large breaches the public at large.[75-77] Penalties for violation of HIPAA range from $100 per violation if the covered entity was unaware of the violation and should not reasonably have been aware to $1.5 million per violation if the breach was considered due to willful neglect and not adequately addressed in the required time frame.[75] Federal law also provides for criminal penalties of up to 10 years in jail and $250,000 in fines for HIPAA violations.[78] Providers are strongly encouraged to discuss with their attorney or hospital privacy officer or legal counsel any potential HIPAA violation immediately upon learning of a potential breach to minimize the risk of penalties against providers and organizations.

EMERGENCY MEDICAL TREATMENT AND ACTIVE LABOR ACT

Congress enacted EMTALA in 1985 in response to situations where hospitals refused care to uninsured patients.

EMTALA OBLIGATIONS

EMTALA imposes numerous obligations on hospitals operating EDs. These include the provision of a "medical screening exam," performed by "qualified medical personnel," to look for an "emergency medical condition" (EMC) for all patients who "come to the ED" seeking care for a medical condition. If an EMC is found, the patient must be stabilized (as defined under EMTALA) within the capability of the hospital or transferred, in a specified manner, if necessary, to complete stabilization. Each element will be considered in turn.

"Comes to the ED" Under EMTALA a "dedicated emergency department" is "any department or facility of the hospital, regardless of whether it is located on or off the main hospital campus that": (1) is licensed by the state as an emergency room or ED; (2) is held out to the public as providing unscheduled care for EMCs on an urgent basis; or (3) provides one-third of its outpatient visits for the treatment of EMCs on an urgent, unscheduled basis.[79] Many hospital-owned urgent care centers may meet this definition.

Hospitals must provide a screening examination to any patient who comes to the "dedicated ED" (hereafter "ED") and requests, or has a request made by another, for evaluation or treatment of a medical condition. If a prudent layperson observer would believe the person needed evaluation or treatment for a medical condition, the hospital's obligation under EMTALA is triggered.[79] Note that the language says for a "medical condition," not an "emergency medical condition." Other hospital locations, such as labor and delivery, psychiatric intake areas, and urgent care areas, which meet the above definition, are subject to EMTALA obligations as well.[80] An infant born alive is considered an individual under the law, and therefore, the same EMTALA obligations apply, including when the infant was born in the ED.[31]

Emergency Medical Condition An EMC is a "medical condition manifesting itself by acute symptoms of sufficient severity (including severe pain, psychiatric disturbances and/or symptoms of substance abuse) such that the absence of immediate medical attention could reasonably be expected to result in: 1) Placing the health of the individual (or, with respect to a pregnant woman, the health of the woman or her unborn child) in serious jeopardy; 2) Serious impairment to bodily functions; or 3) Serious dysfunction of any bodily organ or part; or with respect to a pregnant woman who is having contractions: 1) That there is inadequate time to effect a safe transfer to another hospital before delivery; or 2) That transfer may pose a threat to the health or safety of the woman or the unborn child."[79] For pregnant women with contractions, an EMC exists if there is insufficient time to transfer the patient before delivery or the transfer may pose a risk to mother or child.[79] Ultimately, this is a medical decision. If it is determined that no EMCs exists, then EMTALA no longer applies to that patient. It is good practice to note the time that this decision was made. The courts have generally ruled that the physician must be aware an EMC exists before he or she is liable under EMTALA. It is important to understand that for an EMC to be present the patient must have a condition such that the lack of immediate medical attention could result in the consequences outlined above. The rule does not suggest that any particular symptom, including severe pain, is in and of itself an EMC, only that the presence of such symptoms mandates a screening, as described below, to determine if the patient has an EMC.[81]

Medical Screening Examination A medical screening examination is the process required to reach, with reasonable clinical confidence and based on the patient's presenting signs and symptoms, the point at which it can be determined whether an EMC does or does not exist.[31] This may involve a simple process, such as a brief history and physical examination, or a complex process involving ancillary studies, consultants, and procedures.[31]

The screening must be the same for every patient presenting with similar symptoms or complaints to be EMTALA compliant. The courts have generally held that so long as screening examinations are performed in a consistent manner across all patients and in accordance with a hospital's own policies, the EMTALA screening obligation has been met.[80] This is true even in cases of misdiagnosis. The courts have also held that misdiagnosis and the adequacy of screening are issues of negligence and should be addressed under state malpractice statutes. **Nurse triage does not meet the hospital obligation to provide a medical screening examination.**[80]

EMTALA dictates that a hospital may not delay the screening examination and stabilizing treatment to inquire about method of payment or insurance status.[82] Hospitals may follow reasonable registration procedures, including inquiring about insurance, provided that it does not delay the medical screening examination or discourage patients from remaining for evaluation.[82] Requests for copayments or down payments should be deferred until after the screening examination and any indicated stabilization to avoid the appearance that the request for payment could have deterred a patient from continuing to seek care. Similarly, advance beneficiary notices and managed care organization authorizations should be deferred.[80]

Providers are allowed to contact a patient's personal physician for advice regarding the patient's history, treatment, and evaluation (but not to obtain prior authorization) as long as this does not delay the medical screening examination.[83]

Qualified Medical Personnel The statute states that "The examination must be conducted by an individual(s) who is determined qualified by hospital bylaws or rules and regulations."[84] These individuals must be formally recognized by the hospital governing body as qualified to perform this type of examination.[31] Although the regulations do not specify what type of provider (e.g., registered nurse, medical doctor, physician's assistant) should perform the medical screening examination, the qualifications of the provider may be retrospectively reviewed and found inadequate.[80] The regulations specifically allow a certified nurse midwife to certify false labor.[79]

Stabilized The concept of stabilization under EMTALA is not what most clinicians would expect. To have a duty to stabilize, the treating providers must be aware of the presence of an EMC. Under EMTALA, stabilize means to provide "treatment as necessary to assure, within reasonable medical probability, that no material deterioration of the condition is likely to result from or occur during the transfer of an individual from a facility or that . . . the woman has delivered the child and placenta."[79] **Stabilization does not require that the underlying medical condition be resolved.** For example, a patient with difficulty breathing and a history of asthma may be stable once provided with medication and oxygen, despite the fact that the underlying condition of asthma is still present.[85]

The decision regarding whether or not the patient is stable rests with the physician actually treating the patient.[86,87] However, this decision is subjective and may be reviewed with medical hindsight. In an investigation, the burden of proof for stability rests with the transferring hospital.

After stabilization, EMTALA no longer applies, and patients may be discharged or admitted for further care. Once a patient is admitted to inpatient status in good faith, not just for the purposes of avoiding EMTALA obligations, the admitting hospital's EMTALA duty is considered complete.[88]

Transfers in accordance with local protocols, such as a trauma system protocol, will generally meet the stabilization requirement, but the transferring hospital must stabilize within its means first.[31] If a hospital is unable to stabilize the patient, then transfer to a higher level of care is appropriate, and all efforts made to stabilize by the transferring hospital should be documented in the patient chart.[31]

The U.S. Supreme Court has ruled that the hospital or physician does not need to have an improper motive for a transfer to be successfully sued for failure to stabilize under EMTALA.

Below are the definitions for two specific situations (discharges and psychiatric patients) as written in the State Operations Manual used by EMTALA investigators.

Stable for Discharge "Discharge home with follow-up instructions. An individual is considered stable and ready for discharge when, within reasonable clinical confidence, it is determined that the individual has reached the point where his/her continued care, including diagnostic work-up and/or treatment, could be reasonably performed as an outpatient or later as an inpatient, provided the individual is given a plan for appropriate follow-up care as part of the discharge instructions. The EMC that caused the individual to present to the dedicated ED must be resolved, but the underlying medical condition may persist. Hospitals are expected within reason to assist/provide discharged individuals the necessary information to secure the necessary follow-up care to prevent relapse or worsening of the medical condition upon release from the hospital."[85]

Therefore, the availability of follow-up and content of discharge instructions may be reviewed should a complaint trigger an investigation. One area where this is problematic is follow-up for uninsured patients. An emergency physician may be liable for a violation, for not requiring an on-call specialist to come in, if a patient is referred for needed follow-up care, such as fracture reduction, and is subsequently refused care—if the emergency physician was aware, or should have been aware, that the follow-up was unlikely to occur. Should there be any question about the patient's ability to obtain the needed follow-up care, the specialist should be asked to come to the ED to see the patient and provide the needed care.[86]

All discharge instructions should educate patients to return to the ED if they have any problem accessing follow-up care as planned.

Psychiatric Patients "Psychiatric patients are considered stable when they are protected and prevented from injuring or harming him/herself or others. The administration of chemical or physical restraints for purposes of transferring an individual from one facility to another may stabilize a psychiatric patient for a period of time and remove the immediate EMC, but the underlying medical condition may persist, and if not treated for longevity the patient may experience exacerbation of the EMC. Therefore, practitioners should use great care when determining if the medical condition is in fact stable after administering chemical or physical restraints."[85] Psychiatric patients present one of the greatest challenges under EMTALA due to the difficulty of determining stability and the lack of available psychiatric resources in most communities.

Transfers Under EMTALA, transfer is "the movement (including discharge) of an individual outside a hospital's facilities at the direction of any person" representing the hospital, regardless of that person's employment status with the hospital.[79]

Hospitals are expected to appropriately transfer patients if they do not possess either the "capability" or "capacity" to care for the patient. Capability would include the availability of technology, specialists with the needed skills to care for a patient, and equipment or supplies required by the patient's condition. Capacity looks at numbers and availability of qualified staff, beds, and equipment and what the hospital "customarily does to accommodate patients in excess of its occupancy limits."[79] Therefore, if a hospital routinely opens extra beds to accommodate patients, they must do so if necessary to avoid the transfer of a patient for whom they could otherwise provide care.

Hospitals may not transfer a patient who has not been stabilized unless an appropriate transfer is performed and either (1) the patient requests the transfer and the request is documented in writing, including the patient's awareness of the risks and benefits of the transfer; or (2) a physician documents that the medical benefits of transfer to a hospital with greater resources reasonably outweigh the increased risk to the patient, pregnant woman, or unborn child.[89] An "appropriate transfer" is defined in the EMTALA regulations. The following four elements are required for an appropriate transfer.[89]

1. The transferring hospital stabilized the patient and, when applicable, the unborn child to the best of its ability, minimizing the risks of the transfer to the patient or, in the case of a woman in labor, her unborn child.
2. The receiving (accepting) hospital has the capability and capacity to care for the patient and agrees to accept the individual and provide appropriate medical treatment.
3. The transferring facility sends all pertinent medical records, including test and study results, treatment provided, and the written consent for the transfer. Information not available at the time of transfer must be sent as soon as possible. If the transfer is necessary due to the failure of an on-call physician to appear, that physician's name and address must be provided to the accepting hospital.
4. The transfer must be performed through qualified personnel and transportation as determined by the transferring physician. The accepting facility may not condition its acceptance on the use of a specific transport service or method.[87,90]

If a hospital attempts to transfer a patient to meet its EMTALA obligation and the patient, or person acting on the patient's behalf, refuses the transfer, then the hospital's EMTALA obligation is considered met. The hospital is expected to attempt to obtain written informed refusal, including a discussion of the risks and benefits of the refusal of transfer and describe both the facts of the transfer that was proposed and the stated reasons for refusal.[91]

Hospitals may not penalize a provider who refuses to authorize the transfer of a patient with an unstabilized EMC or take negative action against any employee who reports a violation of EMTALA.[89]

Duties of Receiving Hospitals A hospital with specialized capabilities or facilities such as (but not limited to) burn units, trauma units, or regional referral centers may not refuse to accept a transfer from a referring hospital anywhere in the United States when the patient in question requires the specialized capabilities *and* the receiving hospital has the capacity to treat the patient.[92] The failure of centers with specialized capabilities to appropriately accept patients requiring their services has been colorfully referred to as "reverse dumping." This rule applies even if the receiving hospital does not have its own dedicated ED.[92]

Due to the risk of a citation or lawsuit should a hospital with specialized or higher level services fail to accept a transfer as required by the law, some authors suggest that all transfers be accepted by hospitals with specialized conditions without inquiry into the patient's insurance status.[86] Should the accepting hospital find that the transfer was not appropriate or improperly motivated, it is both their duty and remedy to report the transferring hospital for a potential violation of EMTALA.[86,93] Delays in accepting a patient in transfer who has an unstabilized EMC to receive or confirm financial information may be considered an EMTALA violation by the receiving hospital.[94]

Failure to report an EMTALA violation is itself a violation.

On-Call Responsibilities Hospitals are required to maintain an on-call list of physicians "who are on the hospital's medical staff or who have privileges at the hospital, or who are on the staff or have privileges at another hospital participating in a formal community call plan in accordance with the resources available to the hospital."[95] The call list must specifically name an individual physician with accurate contact information, not solely the name of a group or specialty.[96] The stipulation that the hospital provide these services "in accordance with the resources available to the hospital" leaves considerable leeway for hospitals to decide what services to offer. Physicians who are formally on call must assist when requested to determine if an EMC exists, to help stabilize patients, and to accept appropriate transfers. They must do this in a reasonable amount of time.[31] Although regulations allow for physicians to be on call at multiple hospitals and to perform elective surgery while on call, a clear plan must exist to provide EMTALA care in these situations.[97] It is the responsibility of the emergency physician to determine if the on-call provider needs to appear in person to see a patient. In general, EMTALA does not allow patients to be sent to private physician offices for examination or stabilization, except possibly in cases where the office is part of the hospital-owned facility and on campus with the hospital. One exception may be that of ophthalmologists, who often have specialized equipment not available in many EDs. Hospitals that allow physicians to selectively take call only for their own established patients who present to the ED must ensure the availability of adequate on-call services to all ED patients requiring similar care.[96] If the on-call doctor will not come after substantial efforts from the emergency provider, then the patient should be transferred to receive necessary care. The emergency provider must inform the accepting hospital that is why the patient is being sent and provide them with the on-call doctor's name and address (failure to do so is an EMTALA violation).

The widespread adoption of communications technology has made consults by a variety of electronic methods increasingly common. There is no restriction to the use of any means of communication with consultants.[96]

Table 303-5 outlines some EMTALA do's and don'ts.

ENFORCEMENT OF EMTALA

The U.S. Department of Health and Human Services is responsible for enforcing EMTALA at the federal level. A complaint is required to initiate an investigation of a hospital for an EMTALA violation. The complaint may come from a patient, hospital, hospital employee, or anyone who thinks care has been denied someone inappropriately. Hospitals may not penalize employees who report violations.[89] Punishments under EMTALA can be severe and may include a hospital's exclusion from participating in Medicare and Medicaid in addition to substantial fines. Providers found to violate EMTALA can also be fined and/or excluded from federal programs, making them nearly unemployable.[98]

Physicians, particularly on-call physicians, are relatively unaware of their obligations under EMTALA,[99] and hospitals should educate their staff regarding EMTALA.[88] An EMTALA violation does not imply medical malpractice.

Situations Where EMTALA Does Not Apply or Ceases to Apply Once a patient is admitted, in good faith, as an inpatient to the hospital for further care, EMTALA ceases to apply. However, EMTALA still applies to patients in the ED and patients on observation status such as patients in an ED chest pain unit, an observation area of labor and delivery, or in observation status within the main hospital even if they are on

TABLE 303-5 EMTALA Do's and Don'ts

EMTALA Do's
1. Treat all patients in the same way.
2. Provide a medical screening examination appropriate to the patient's complaints.
3. Appropriately transfer patients you cannot stabilize.
4. Accept transfers who require specialized services your hospital offers, as long as the specialized services have the capacity for care.
5. Involve on-call specialists when needed to diagnose or stabilize an EMC.
6. Educate ED, hospital staff, and faculty on the EMTALA rules.
7. See patients quickly and efficiently.
8. Document the completion of the MSE and if an EMC was identified or not during the visit.
EMTALA Don'ts
1. Substitute triage for an MSE.
2. Discourage or coerce patients away from receiving their screening exams and stabilization.
3. Allow yourself to be convinced that a specialist does not need to come to the ED.
4. Fail to stabilize within your capabilities.
5. Delay the MSE for preauthorization or registration.
6. Fail to follow your own rules, policies, and procedures.

Abbreviations: EMC = emergency medical condition; EMTALA = Emergency Medical Treatment and Active Labor Act; MSE = medical screening exam.

a unit that also contains patients on inpatient status.[80,87,100] Although Centers for Medicare and Medicaid Services regulations do identify that under the above conditions EMTALA does not apply to inpatients, the subject is not settled law as far as the courts are concerned, so careful documentation of why patients were admitted (to validate the good faith clause) and what status they were in the hospital on (to validate that they were an inpatient) is very important.[100] Inpatients who subsequently develop an EMC are not covered by EMTALA, even if they are physically moved back to the ED; however, they are covered by the Medicare Conditions of Participation. EMTALA does not apply to outpatients who have already begun a scheduled appointment. EMTALA may not apply during a declared national emergency or pursuant to a state emergency or pandemic preparedness plan following the issuance of a waiver under law.[101]

Ambulance "Parking" Prolonged delays in moving patients from EMS care to hospital care, referred to as "parking," is not acceptable and may be considered a violation.[90] This does not mean that every ambulance patient must instantly be taken from the care of EMS, particularly in instances where the hospital may lack capacity or capability to immediately care for the patient.[90] The hospital has an EMTALA obligation to the patient once on hospital property.

Patient-Initiated Transfers Any transfer not for medical reasons is considered a patient-requested transfer. The chart should reflect the patient's reason for wanting the transfer. The transfer must still be an "appropriate transfer."

Use of the ED for Nonemergency Services If a request is made by, or for, a patient presenting for treatment of a medical condition but the "nature of the request makes it clear that the medical condition is not of an emergency nature, the hospital is required only to perform such screening as would be appropriate for anyone presenting in a similar manner to determine" if an EMC exists.[102]

Withdrawal of Request for Screening Patients who fail to start or complete the screening and treatment process fall into one of three categories: patients who arrive at the ED and then fail to even begin their medical screening examination (often classified as left without being seen or left before examination); patients who leave or "elope" without informing staff at any point during the evaluation[103]; and patients who refuse recommended treatment or admission and leave "against medical advice."

In each scenario, the hospital should make a clear, well-documented effort to find a missing patient by overhead paging and a search of the department. The medical record should contain a description of the services offered (examination and treatment) that were refused. The hospital should take all reasonable steps to procure the individual's written refusal on a document that also outlines the risks and benefits of examination and treatment. These issues are very important under EMTALA, as regulations state "that hospitals should be very concerned about patients leaving without being screened. Since every patient who presents seeking emergency services is entitled to a screening examination, a hospital could violate the patient antidumping statute if it routinely keeps patients waiting so long that they leave without being seen, particularly if the hospital does not attempt to determine and document why individual patients are leaving, and reiterate to them that the hospital is prepared to provide medical screening if they stay."

Triage Down Downgrading a patient's triage level from the level required under hospital protocol risks an EMTALA citation and could form the basis for a civil lawsuit.[103,104]

State Law Some states have passed laws that impose additional duties or requirements on emergency physicians and hospitals. Such laws should be followed unless they directly conflict with the federal EMTALA rule, in which case the federal statute takes precedence.

Requests for Testing In some cases, patients may present to the ED for testing, such as x-rays or blood work, under the order of their personal physician. Because these patients are not requesting examination or treatment of a medical condition, EMTALA does not apply. Should the hospital choose to provide the patient with the testing services, these patients should be differentiated from standard ED patients. Separate paperwork defining consent, that a medical screening examination was not requested (signed by the patient), and interactions with the ordering physician should be recorded. Patients who independently present for testing, such as pregnancy testing, should receive a medical screening examination before testing, and if they refuse the screening examination, they should be referred elsewhere for the requested testing.

A common scenario is the patient brought in by law enforcement for alcohol or drug screening. In these cases, if it appears that the patient should be screened (prudent layperson) or the patient or police request an examination, then the screening examination should be done.

Screen Away Programs Such programs aim to comply with the letter of the EMTALA law by performing medical screening examinations and then either sending away those patients found not to have an EMC or requesting payment before treatment. The ethical implications of these programs are beyond the scope of this chapter. Physicians and hospitals should consider the legal risk and ethical and moral implications of such programs, particularly in those cases where alternative sources of care are not provided.[105]

Private Patients in the ED In some EDs, it is common for staff physicians to send their patients to the ED, with plans to meet the patient in the ED. Although this is acceptable, these patients should go through the standard triage process, and if any concern exists about the presence of an EMC, patients should be evaluated in the standard manner by the emergency physician present and stabilized while waiting for the private physician.

"The Guarantee" Some hospitals have begun programs in which they promise a patient will be triaged or seen by a doctor within a specific amount of time. These guarantees are problematic from an EMTALA point of view, as the hospital will likely be held to these times during an investigation.

Pain and EMTALA An epidemic of prescription drug abuse in the United States has led to substantial risk for patients and growing difficulties for providers.[106] Legislation both enacted and pending in many states attempts to address this problem, often placing emergency physicians in a difficult position.[106] While EMTALA indicates that pain may be a symptom suggestive of an EMC, it only requires that the patient with pain receive a medical screening exam consistent with the patient's presenting complaints. Once a patient has been identified as not having an EMC, providers can make reasoned clinical determinations about the appropriateness of opioids and other medications. The Centers for Medicare and Medicaid Services has clarified that the posting of signage that, even when intended as education, discusses restrictions on ED prescribing or use of opioids may discourage patients from receiving their medical screening exam and therefore would be in violation of EMTALA.[107] Providers and staff should also not discuss with patients the results of state pharmacy database queries prior to the completion of the medical screening exam to prevent the patient from feeling coerced not to complete their exam.[107] The best course in dealing with patients with painful complaints is to provide a medical screening exam each and every time they present to the ED, and once an EMC is determined not to exist, to treat the patient as clinically appropriate based on the clinical scenario, risk for pharmaceutical abuse, and applicable state law.[106]

RISK MANAGEMENT

The ED presents a unique setting in health care where numerous factors interact to create the potential for error.[108,109] These errors can create adverse outcomes for patients and increased medical-legal risks for ED providers. Risk management is the process of identifying and mitigating factors that may be a source of errors. This section will focus on important sources of error in the ED and suggestions for the individual provider to mitigate risk within the confines of their existing care setting.

Studies looking at data from malpractice lawsuits have consistently found that certain presenting complaints and disease processes are associated with poor outcomes leading to legal action. These are summarized in **Table 303-6.**[108-111]

The error types most commonly reported in emergency medicine include diagnostic error or delay, treatment error or delay, improper performance of procedure or treatment, misinterpretation of tests, failure to supervise or monitor a case, and a failure or delay to consult or refer.[108,110] Of these, diagnostic error, which includes failure to diagnose, delay in diagnosis, and wrong diagnosis, is consistently the most frequent and costly, in terms of malpractice claims paid, both in emergency medicine and across all specialties.[108,109,112] Diagnostic error can be defined as a diagnosis that is "missed, wrong, or delayed."[113] These errors lead to permanent injury or death in almost half of filed malpractice cases related to diagnostic error.[109]

One study evaluated the sources of these diagnostic errors in the ED.[111] The study found that cognitive errors encompassing errors in judgment, knowledge, and vigilance or memory contributed to 96% of claims with identified errors. Communication errors, particularly as they relate to patient handoffs, were involved in 35% of diagnostic errors. System errors, including issues with supervision, workload, and fatigue, were noted in 37% of cases; these errors were more prevalent where students or residents were involved. Patient-related factors were involved in an additional 34% of cases. Of note, two-thirds of the errors involved cases in which more than one provider participated in the patient's care, further suggesting the importance of communication-related factors.

TABLE 303-6 Complaints and Diagnoses Associated with High Risk of Diagnostic Error
Chest pain/missed acute myocardial infarction (AMI)*
Wounds (retained foreign body, nerve or tendon damage, poor healing)
Fractures (vertebral, forearm, leg)
Symptom involving the abdomen and pelvis (including appendicitis and abdominal aneurysm)
Pediatric fever
Meningitis
CNS bleed
Stroke
Embolism
Trauma related
Spinal cord injuries
Ectopic pregnancy

*Missed AMI is the most frequently alleged missed diagnosis, is the diagnosis most associated with death, and had an average payout of $245,000 to $600,000.

REDUCING RISK

Improving patient safety and reducing risk in emergency medicine requires a broad focus involving multiple disciplines and addressing numerous issues including, but not limited to, medication administration, electronic health records, ED staffing, flow, and culture, and available equipment and resources.[108,109] Although these systemic changes are often beyond the ability of the individual physician to influence, there are a number of steps each physician can take to reduce the risk of error and of being named in a malpractice suit. Providers can address both interpersonal and clinical issues that may reduce risk.

Some actions that providers can take to establish a good patient–provider relationship are noted in **Table 303-7.**[114] This relationship is key to facilitating good communications and reducing risk. Introductions are simple and important. Tell the patient your name and your place on the healthcare team (e.g., attending or supervising doctor, resident physician, student). Engage the family in addition to the patient, when appropriate and permitted by the patient. Ensure that the patient and family or caretaker understand the diagnosis and discharge instructions, particularly those related to follow-up, treatment, and when to return to the ED. The physician should, whenever possible, personally review the discharge instructions with patients and provide the opportunity for patients and caregivers to ask questions prior to discharge to ensure comprehension.

Providers can also work to change other practice behaviors that may perpetuate or lead to error and risk. Patient handoffs are a significant area of risk for patients and providers. Avoiding limited or rushed patient handoffs and bedside transfers of care, when possible, may reduce the risk associated with shift change and multiple providers on the care team. Providers may fail to consider all the diagnostic possibilities in a transferred or signed-out patient because they receive the patient with a preexisting plan and diagnosis. It is a good practice for providers to meet each patient signed out to them and to evaluate them at least once before discharge.[115] Errors around procedures were the second highest category of error in one ED study.[108] Provide adequate supervision of residents and students performing procedures, provide comprehensive informed consent for every procedure when possible, and follow established best practices and guidelines when present or available for a given procedure to reduce this risk. Avoid criticizing the care provided by other providers, and never make guarantees about patient outcomes.

SPECIFIC HIGH-RISK DIAGNOSES AND TREATMENTS

Certain diagnoses, covering a wide variety of systems and mechanisms, present a high risk to emergency providers, as noted in Table 303-6. Providers should be aware of these diagnoses and their atypical presentations and consider the possibility of a high-risk problem in every patient. Avoid placing a diagnosis on a patient without sufficient clinical certainty. When a diagnosis is uncertain, describe the patient's assessment with symptoms.

The optimal treatment of certain diseases is unclear. Numerous situations exist in which the standard of care is not well defined. Providers should have careful and well-documented discussions with patients and families about what treatments are or are not being given, and why. Although the management of risk and errors in emergency medicine is highly complex, each physician should take it upon himself or herself to do what they can to reduce risk in their own practice and behavior.

TABLE 303-7 Provider Interpersonal Behaviors That Can Reduce Risk
Introduce yourself to the patient and family.
Dress neatly and professionally.
Address patients respectfully.
Sit down at the bedside.
Discuss with patients their expectations of care.
Speak in clear, simple language, avoiding medical terms.
Provide emotional support and show empathy.
Meet each signed-out patient.
Personally provide discharge instructions and answer questions prior to patient departure.

EMERGENCY PHYSICIANS AND DEATH CERTIFICATES

The registration of death is a state function governed by the laws and regulations of the state in which the death occurs. The death certificate is the permanent record of the fact of the death. Information from the death certificate is used as the source for many health statistics, to help determine funding for research, and to help settle the estate of the deceased, and in some states, it is required to get a burial permit.[116] To ensure consistency of the data reported to the National Vital Statistics System, a standard death certificate was created, and all state certificates conform closely to the standard.

The patient's personal (attending) physician usually fills out the death certificate. This physician likely knows the patient better than other healthcare providers and is in the most favorable position to certify the cause of death.[117] In cases in which there is no primary physician and the patient dies in the ED, the emergency physician may be called on to certify the death. Despite the fact that many death certificates contain errors in the assessment of cause of death, a search of the literature has not revealed any reports of physician liability for death certificate errors.[118] In many ED cases, the death will require referral to the coroner or medical examiner's office to certify the death. Cases requiring referral vary by state but may include the situations listed in **Table 303-8**.

The physician who completes the certificate is required to fill out the document in a timely fashion, often within 24 to 72 hours, using black ink and legible writing. In addition to documenting the time and date of death, the physician should indicate an opinion as to the immediate and underlying causes of the death. The immediate cause of death is the final entity causing death. The underlying cause of death is the original condition or diagnosis from which the chain of events leading to death originated. The chain of events should be listed on the certificate from most recent to the final, underlying cause.[118] The manner of death (e.g., natural, accident, homicide) and other significant but not directly linked conditions should be listed separately. In cases in which the disease processes involved are unclear, in some states physicians may qualify their opinions by listing them as "probable."

Terminal events such as cardiac or respiratory arrest should not be listed as the proximate cause of death because they do not indicate the disease process that caused death.

NEWBORNS LEFT AT THE ED

All U.S. states, the District of Columbia, and Puerto Rico have enacted laws allowing a mother and, in some states, either a custodial parent or an agent of the parent to leave a newborn infant at a "safe haven" in an attempt to reduce the numbers of infanticides and abandonments of children in unsafe places.[119] These laws vary with respect to who may leave the infant, how long after birth the child may be left, whom the child may be entrusted to, and the amount of legal protection and anonymity due the person leaving the child.[119] In most states, a healthcare provider or emergency services provider is authorized to accept the child.[119] Providers should be aware of the laws in their state, and every ED should have a policy to deal with this situation.

DUTY TO THIRD PARTIES

The *Tarasoff* ruling set the precedent that a physician owes a duty to a foreseeable third party when the physician is aware of a reasonable risk to that individual. Over the years, courts have extended that duty to include an obligation to warn or protect others against a variety of dangers, including communicable diseases, impaired drivers, employment physicals, and medication or treatment reactions.[120] Physicians have varying obligations and protections under state laws for reporting patients and warning potential victims or authorities when third parties may be at risk.[121] Good patient education, including medication side effects, driving and work restrictions, and strict compliance with state reporting laws, is a good start to minimize this risk.

TABLE 303-8 Cases That May Require Referral to the Medical Examiner/Coroner
Traumatic death
Death due to natural disaster
Individuals in police custody or jail inmates
Death under suspicion of homicide or suicide
Suspicion of poisoning
Sudden, unexplained death not clearly related to preexisting disease

TELEPHONE ADVICE

Calls for telephone advice should be routed to an established "advice line" operated by the hospital, an insurer, or other entity. By dispensing telephone medical advice, a physician may inadvertently enter into a binding physician–patient relationship.[122] ED staff should be taught a standard response to unsolicited phone calls from the general public: they should state that they are not allowed to give advice over the phone and should encourage the patient to come to the ED for evaluation and treatment.[123]

EXTENSION OF CARE OUTSIDE OF THE ED ENCOUNTER

Emergency providers can be exposed to liability extending beyond the ED. Two common sources of this risk are the writing of inpatient orders and responding to emergencies elsewhere in the hospital.[124] Emergency physician orders that cover any part of the inpatient stay are risky because there is a lack of clarity about when the transfer of care to the inpatient provider takes place. The American College of Emergency Physicians recommends that the emergency physician not be compelled to write any orders extending outside of the ED and that medical staff policies provide for timely orders for and evaluation of admitted patients by the inpatient medical staff.[125]

In some EDs, the emergency physician is expected to address a variety of medical issues that may arise on the inpatient floors.[124] Hospitals are responsible for the treatment of inpatients and should not rely on the ED physician to care for inpatients. In cases in which no other option is available, inpatients could be brought to the ED for evaluation and treatment.[126]

NEGLIGENCE STANDARDS

Physicians are generally expected to exercise reasonable care and practice within the accepted standard of care. A failure to do so is considered negligence and is the standard used in most medical malpractice lawsuits. Efforts to protect the healthcare safety net provided by EDs and specialists treating ED patients have led some states to enact a more rigorous standard of negligence for care provided in the ED. This standard is often referred to as "gross negligence." Gross negligence is more serious than negligence and has various definitions across jurisdictions that include "conduct so reckless as to demonstrate a substantial lack of concern for whether an injury results" and a "failure to exercise slight care or diligence."[127,128] The term *reckless* is sometimes used to describe a standard of negligence and generally seems to be equivalent to gross negligence.[127] A third standard, "willful or wanton" misconduct, although not universally seen as separate from the "gross negligence" standard, is often found in "Good Samaritan" laws.[127,129] "Willful or wanton" misconduct suggests behavior "where someone knew that an injury was likely to result from an action and, despite this knowledge, acted with a conscious disregard for the safety of another person."[127] The "willful and wanton" standard requires the provider to know that what they were doing was almost certain to lead to injury.[127]

ROLE AND RESPONSIBILITY OF EXPERT WITNESSES IN EMERGENCY MEDICINE

In a malpractice lawsuit, the plaintiff must prove that the physician has violated the standard of care and was therefore negligent. In most jurisdictions, expert witnesses are brought into court to state their "expert" opinion of the care given and if it violated the standard of care.[129]

The rules about who can provide expert witness testimony vary widely, with some jurisdictions requiring that the expert be of the same specialty as the defendant and others requiring only that the expert be a licensed physician without regard to specialty.[130] The quality of some expert testimony has become a concern of specialty societies, and some societies have begun to call for action against or attempt to sanction members providing misleading or inaccurate testimony.[131,132] The American College of Emergency Physicians has released guidelines for its members when acting as expert witnesses including the belief that expert testimony constitutes the practice of medicine.[133] These guidelines include the expectations that: (1) "the expert witness should review the medical facts in a thorough, fair, and objective manner and should not exclude any relevant information to create a view favoring either the plaintiff or the defendant"; (2) "the expert witness should not provide expert medical testimony that is false, misleading, or without medical foundation"; (3) the expert "be in the active clinical practice of emergency medicine for three years immediately preceding the date of the event giving rise to the case"; (4) the expert is willing to allow their testimony to be submitted to peer review; and (5) "misconduct as an expert, including the provision of false, fraudulent, or misleading testimony, may expose the physician to disciplinary action."[133,134] Emergency physicians acting as expert witnesses should be aware of these guidelines and strive to provide testimony that is a credit to themselves, the legal process, and the specialty of emergency medicine.

OTHER LEGAL ISSUES OF CONCERN

Other areas of ED practice with legal implications are listed in **Table 303-9**. The legal risk varies from state to state, and clearly written guidelines, an understanding of local laws, and an honest approach that avoids any appearance of conflict of interest can minimize risk.

TABLE 303-9 Other Legal Issues of Concern to Emergency Providers
Peer review
Business arrangements (antikickback Stark laws)
Credentialing
Recommendation writing
Emergency situations arising outside of the hospital
Compliance
Medical malpractice
Translation services for patients

DISCLAIMER

This chapter does not address state-specific issues or replace the advice of the hospital attorney in a given situation. The information provided in this chapter is not intended to be legal advice. Laws and regulations are always changing, and this chapter does not replace a timely consultation with an attorney specialized in healthcare issues.

REFERENCES

The complete reference list is available online at www.TintinalliEM.com.

Index

Page numbers followed by an *f* indicate figure; page numbers followed by a *t* indicate tables. **Bold** indicates the start of the main discussion.

O

V

W